BMA LIBRARY
WITHDRAWN
FROM LIBRARY
BRITISH MEDICAL ASSOCIATION

BRITISH MEDICAL ASSOCIATION

1003510

Shackelford's

SURGERY *of the* ALIMENTARY TRACT

SECTION
EDITORS

Volume
1

Volume
2

Steven R. DeMeester, MD, FACS

Division of Foregut and Minimally Invasive Surgery
The Oregon Clinic
Portland, Oregon

Section I Esophagus and Hernia

David W. McFadden, MD, MBA, FACS

Chairman, Department of Surgery
University of Connecticut
Surgeon-in-Chief
University of Connecticut Health
Farmington, Connecticut

Section II Stomach and Small Intestine

Jeffrey B. Matthews, MD, FACS

Dallas B. Phemister Professor and Chairman of Surgery
The University of Chicago
Chicago, Illinois

Section III Pancreas, Biliary Tract, Liver, and Spleen

James W. Fleshman, MD, FACS

Seeger Professor and Chairman of Surgery
Baylor University Medical Center
Professor of Surgery
Texas A&M Health Science Center
Dallas, Texas

Section IV Colon, Rectum, and Anus

EIGHTH EDITION

Shackelford's

SURGERY *of the* ALIMENTARY TRACT

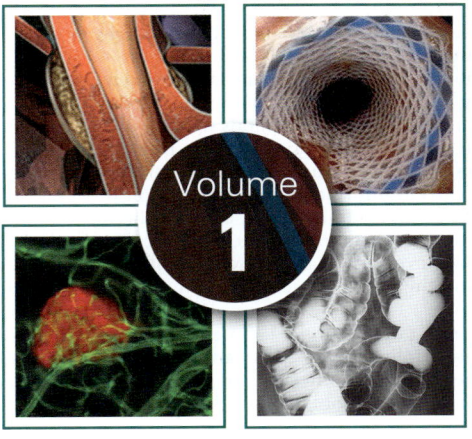

Volume **1**

Charles J. Yeo, MD, FACS

Samuel D. Gross Professor and Chair

Department of Surgery

Sidney Kimmel Medical College at
Thomas Jefferson University

Philadelphia, Pennsylvania

ELSEVIER

ELSEVIER

1600 John F. Kennedy Blvd.
Ste 1800
Philadelphia, PA 19103-2899

SHACKELFORD'S SURGERY OF THE ALIMENTARY
TRACT, EIGHTH EDITION

ISBN: 978-0-323-40232-3
Volume 1 part number: 9996118169
Volume 2 part number: 9996118223

Copyright © 2019 by Elsevier, Inc. All rights reserved.

No part of this publication may be reproduced or transmitted in any form or by any means, electronic or mechanical, including photocopying, recording, or any information storage and retrieval system, without permission in writing from the publisher. Details on how to seek permission, further information about the Publisher's permissions policies and our arrangements with organizations such as the Copyright Clearance Center and the Copyright Licensing Agency, can be found at our website: www.elsevier.com/permissions.

This book and the individual contributions contained in it are protected under copyright by the Publisher (other than as may be noted herein).

Notices

Knowledge and best practice in this field are constantly changing. As new research and experience broaden our understanding, changes in research methods, professional practices, or medical treatment may become necessary.

Practitioners and researchers must always rely on their own experience and knowledge in evaluating and using any information, methods, compounds, or experiments described herein. In using such information or methods they should be mindful of their own safety and the safety of others, including parties for whom they have a professional responsibility.

With respect to any drug or pharmaceutical products identified, readers are advised to check the most current information provided (i) on procedures featured or (ii) by the manufacturer of each product to be administered, to verify the recommended dose or formula, the method and duration of administration, and contraindications. It is the responsibility of practitioners, relying on their own experience and knowledge of their patients, to make diagnoses, to determine dosages and the best treatment for each individual patient, and to take all appropriate safety precautions.

To the fullest extent of the law, neither the Publisher nor the authors, contributors, or editors, assume any liability for any injury and/or damage to persons or property as a matter of products liability, negligence or otherwise, or from any use or operation of any methods, products, instructions, or ideas contained in the material herein.

Previous editions copyrighted 2013, 2007, 2002, 1996, 1991, 1986, 1983, 1982, 1981, 1978, 1955.
Mayo Foundation retains copyright to their original artwork.

Library of Congress Cataloging-in-Publication Data

Names: Yeo, Charles J., editor.
Title: Shackelford's surgery of the alimentary tract / [edited by] Charles J. Yeo.
Other titles: Surgery of the alimentary tract
Description: Eighth edition. | Philadelphia, PA : Elsevier, [2019] | Includes bibliographical references and index.
Identifiers: LCCN 2017042680 | ISBN 9780323402323 (hardcover : alk. paper)
Subjects: | MESH: Digestive System Surgical Procedures–methods | Digestive System Diseases–surgery
Classification: LCC RD540 | NLM WI 900 | DDC 617.4/3–dc23 LC record available at https://lccn.loc.gov/2017042680

Executive Content Strategist: Russell Gabbedy
Content Development Specialist: Mary Hegeler
Publishing Services Manager: Patricia Tannian
Senior Project Manager: Amanda Mincher
Design Direction: Patrick Ferguson

Printed in China

Last digit is the print number: 9 8 7 6 5 4 3 2 1

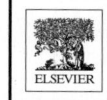

Working together
to grow libraries in
developing countries

www.elsevier.com • www.bookaid.org

To my wife, Theresa, and my children, William and Scott; to my many mentors (some now deceased, many still alive) who have contributed to the science of surgery and to my education; to the many colleagues and friends whose contributions have made this eighth edition possible; and to those young alimentary tract surgeons and other health care professionals who will learn from these pages, move the field forward, and continue to improve our understanding of alimentary tract diseases.

CHARLES J. YEO

To my father, Tom DeMeester, whose passion for understanding the pathophysiology of esophageal and foregut disorders and applying this knowledge to better the lives of patients has been and remains an inspiration for me; to my many mentors who have helped me learn the craft of surgery and encouraged me to constantly strive for perfection; to my colleagues who give up many hours of their evenings, weekends, and vacations to contribute to abstracts, papers, and book chapters; to my fellows and residents who diligently train to be the next generation of expert surgeons; and to my family and friends who support me and graciously accept my long hours away at work caring for people in need of help.

STEVEN R. DeMEESTER

I would like to dedicate this book to all the past residents and fellows with whom I have worked and to thank them for making education such a wonderful part of my life; I hope this will help us to remember the times we've spent together taking care of complex patients and will encourage you to continue to pass on your knowledge to those whom you mentor.

JAMES W. FLESHMAN

To Dr. William Silen and my late grandfather, Dr. Benjamin M. Banks, for their wisdom; to the surgical residents and students, for their thirst for knowledge; and to my wife, Joan, and our boys, Jonathan, David, and Adam, for their love and support.

JEFFREY B. MATTHEWS

To my wife, Nancy, and my children, William, Hunter, and Nora; and to all of my mentors, colleagues, and patients who challenge and inspire me every day.

DAVID W. McFADDEN

Contributors

Abbas E. Abbas, MD, MS, FACS
Professor and Chief, Division of Thoracic Surgery, Department of Thoracic Medicine and Surgery; Director, Thoracic and Foregut Surgery, Temple University School of Medicine, Philadelphia, Pennsylvania

David B. Adams, MD
Professor of Surgery, Medical University of South Carolina, Charleston, South Carolina

Piyush Aggarwal, MBBS
Fellow, Division of Colorectal Surgery, Mayo Clinic, Phoenix, Arizona

Bestoun H. Ahmed, MD, FRCS, FACS, FASMBS
Associate Professor of Surgery, University of Pittsburgh School of Medicine, Pittsburgh, Pennsylvania

Craig Albanese, MD, MBA
Division of Pediatric Surgery, Department of Surgery, Stanford University School of Medicine, Stanford, California

Matthew R. Albert, MD, FACS, FASCRS
Program Director, Florida Hospital Colorectal Fellowship, Department of Colon and Rectal Surgery, Center for Colon and Rectal Surgery, Florida Hospital, Orlando, Florida

Abubaker Ali, MD
Assistant Professor of Surgery, Wayne State University, Detroit, Michigan

Evan Alicuben, MD
General Surgery Resident, Keck School of Medicine of the University of Southern California, Los Angeles, California

Marco E. Allaix, MD, PhD
Department of Surgical Sciences, University of Torino, Torino, Italy

Ashley Altman, MD
Department of Radiology, The University of Chicago Medicine, Chicago, Illinois

Hisami Ando, MD
President, Aichi Prefectural Colony; Emeritus Professor, Department of Pediatric Surgery, Nagoya University Graduate School of Medicine, Nagoya-city, Aichi, Japan

Ciro Andolfi, MD
Department of Surgery, The University of Chicago Pritzker School of Medicine, Chicago, Illinois

Alagappan Annamalai, MD
Surgery, Cedars-Sinai Medical Center, Los Angeles, California

Elliot A. Asare, MD, MS
Chief Resident, General Surgery, Department of Surgery, Medical College of Wisconsin, Milwaukee, Wisconsin

Emanuele Asti, MD, FACS
Assistant Professor, General and Emergency Surgery, IRCCS Policlinico San Donato, University of Milano, Milan, Italy

Hugh G. Auchincloss, MD, MPH
Cardiothoracic Fellow, Massachusetts General Hospital, Boston, Massachusetts

Benjamin Babic, MD
Department of Surgery, Agaplesion Markus Hospital, Frankfurt, Germany

Talia B. Baker, MD
Associate Professor of Surgery, Transplantation Institute, The University of Chicago Medicine, Chicago, Illinois

Chad G. Ball, MD, MSC, FRCSC, FACS
Associate Professor of Surgery, University of Calgary, Foothills Medical Center, Calgary, Alberta, Canada

Arianna Barbetta, MD
Research Fellow, General Surgery Department, Thoracic Surgery Service, Memorial Sloan Kettering Cancer Center, New York, New York

John M. Barlow, MD
Assistant Professor, Department of Radiology, Mayo Clinic College of Medicine, Rochester, Minnesota

Justin Barr, MD, PhD
Department of Surgery, Duke University Medical Center, Durham, North Carolina

Juan Camilo Barreto, MD
Assistant Professor of Surgery, Division of Surgical Oncology, University of Arkansas for Medical Sciences, Little Rock, Arkansas

Linda Barry, MD, FACS
Associate Professor of Surgery, University of Connecticut School of Medicine; Chief Operating Officer, Connecticut Institute for Clinical and Translational Science, Farmington, Connecticut

Eliza W. Beal, MD
Department of Surgery, The Ohio State University Wexner Medical Center, Columbus, Ohio

Kristin Wilson Beard, MD
Baylor Scott and White Medical Center, Round Rock, Texas

David E. Beck, MD, FACS, FASCRS
Professor and Chair, Department of Colon and Rectal Surgery, Ochsner Clinic Foundation, New Orleans, Louisiana; Professor of Surgery, Ochsner Clinical School, University of Queensland, Brisbane, Queensland, Australia

Kevin E. Behrns, MD
Dean, School of Medicine, VP for Medical Affairs, St. Louis University, St. Louis, Missouri

Oliver C. Bellevue, MD
General Surgery Resident, Department of Surgery, Swedish Medical Center, Seattle, Washington

Omar E. Bellorin-Marin, MD
Chief Resident, General Surgery, NewYork-Presbyterian/Queens, Flushing, New York

Jacques Bergman, MD, PhD
Professor of Gastrointestinal Endoscopy, Department of Gastroenterology and Hepatology, Academic Medical Center, Amsterdam, The Netherlands

James Berry, MD
Department of Surgery, University of Connecticut Health Center, Farmington, Connecticut

Marc G.H. Besselink, MD, MSc, PhD
Department of Surgery, Academic Medical Center, Amsterdam, The Netherlands

Adil E. Bharucha, MBBS, MD
Professor of Medicine, Division of Gastroenterology and Hepatology, Mayo Clinic, Rochester, Minnesota

Anton J. Bilchik, MD, PhD
Professor of Surgery, Chief of Medicine, Chief of Gastrointestinal Research, Gastrointestinal Oncology, John Wayne Cancer Institute at Providence Saint John's Health Center, Santa Monica, California

Nikolai A. Bildzukewicz, MD, FACS
Assistant Professor of Clinical Surgery, Division of Upper GI and General Surgery, Associate Program Director, General Surgery Residency and Advanced GI/MIS Fellowship, Keck School of Medicine of the University of Southern California, Los Angeles, California

Jason Bingham, MD
Department of General Surgery, Madigan Army Medical Center, Tacoma, Washington

Elisa Birnbaum, MD
Professor of Surgery, Section of Colon and Rectal Surgery, Washington University School of Medicine, St. Louis, Missouri

Sylvester M. Black, MD, PhD
Assistant Professor of Surgery, Division of Transplant, The Ohio State University Wexner Medical Center, Columbus, Ohio

Shanda H. Blackmon, MD, MPH
Associate Professor of Surgery, Division of Thoracic Surgery, Mayo Clinic, Rochester, Minnesota

Joshua I.S. Bleier, MD
Associate Professor of Surgery, University of Pennsylvania, Philadelphia, Pennsylvania

Adam S. Bodzin, MD
Assistant Professor, Department of Surgery, Section of Transplantation, The University of Chicago, Chicago, Illinois

C. Richard Boland, MD
Chief, Division of Gastroenterology, Internal Medicine, Baylor Scott and White, La Jolla, California

John Bolton, MD
Chairman Emeritus, Department of Surgery, Ochsner Health Systems, New Orleans, Louisiana

Nathan Bolton, MD
Resident, General Surgery, Ochsner Medical Center, New Orleans, Louisiana

Luigi Bonavina, MD, PhD
Professor and Chief of General Surgery, Department of Biomedical Sciences for Health, IRCCS Policlinico San Donato, University of Milano, Milan, Italy

Morgan Bonds, MD
Surgical Resident, University of Oklahoma Health Science Center, Oklahoma City, Oklahoma

Stefan A.W. Bouwense, MD, PhD
Department of Surgery, Radboud University Medical Center, Nijmegen, The Netherlands

Joshua A. Boys, MD
Thoracic Surgery Research Fellow, Department of Surgery, University of Southern California, Los Angeles, California

Raquel Bravo-Infante, MD
Gastrointestinal Surgery Department, Hospital Clinic of Barcelona, Barcelona, Spain

Ross M. Bremner, MD, PhD
Executive Director, Norton Thoracic Institute, St. Joseph's Hospital and Medical Center, Phoenix, Arizona

Bruce M. Brenner, MD
Associate Professor of Surgery, University of Connecticut, Farmington, Connecticut

Shaun R. Brown, DO, FACS
Clinical Fellow, Department of Colon and Rectal Surgery, Ochsner Medical Center, New Orleans, Louisiana

Mark P. Callery, MD
Professor of Surgery, Harvard Medical School; Chief, Division of General Surgery, Beth Israel Deaconess Medical Center, Boston, Massachusetts

John L. Cameron, MD
Alfred Blalock Distinguished Service Professor of Surgery, Professor of Surgery, The Johns Hopkins Hospital, Baltimore, Maryland

Michael Camilleri, MD
Atherton and Winifred W. Bean Professor, Professor of Medicine, Pharmacology, and Physiology, Consultant, Division of Gastroenterology and Hepatology, Department of Medicine, Mayo Clinic, Rochester, Minnesota

Jacob Campbell, DO, MPH
Department of Surgery, University of Connecticut Health Center, Farmington, Connecticut

Riaz Cassim, MD, FACS, FASCRS
Associate Professor, Department of Surgery, West Virginia University, Morgantown, West Virginia; Chief of Surgery, Louis A. Johnson VA Medical Center, Clarksburg, West Virginia

Manuel Castillo-Angeles, MD, MPH
Research Fellow, Department of Surgery, Beth Israel Deaconess Medical Center, Boston, Massachusetts

Christy Cauley, MD, MPH
Resident, Department of Surgery, Massachusetts General Hospital, Boston, Massachusetts

Keith M. Cavaness, DO, FACS
Surgery, Baylor Scott and White Health, Dallas, Texas

Robert J. Cerfolio, MD, MBA, FACS, FACCP
Professor of Surgery, Chief of Clinical Division Thoracic Surgery, Director of the Lung Cancer Service Line, New York University; Senior Advisor, Robotic Committee, New York, New York

Bradley J. Champagne, MD, FACS, FASCRS
Chairman of Surgery, Fairview Hospital; Director of Services, DDSI West Region; Professor of Surgery, Cleveland Clinic Lerner School of Medicine; Medical Director, Fairview Ambulatory Surgery Center, Cleveland, Ohio

Parakrama Chandrasoma, MD, MRCP
Chief, Surgical and Anatomic Pathology, Los Angeles County + University of Southern California Medical Center; Emeritus Professor of Pathology, Keck School of Medicine of the University of Southern California, Los Angeles, California

Alex L. Chang, MD
Department of General Surgery, University of Cincinnati, Cincinnati, Ohio

Christopher G. Chapman, MD
Assistant Professor of Medicine, Director, Bariatric and Metabolic Endoscopy, Center for Endoscopic Research and Therapeutics, The University of Chicago Medicine and Biological Sciences, Chicago, Illinois

William C. Chapman, MD, FACS
Surgery, Washington University, St. Louis, Missouri

Susannah Cheek, MD
Clinical Instructor in Surgery, University of Pittsburgh, Pittsburgh, Pennsylvania

Harvey S. Chen, MD
Department of Surgery, Mayo Clinic, Rochester, Minnesota

Clifford S. Cho, MD
Department of Surgery, University of Michigan, Ann Arbor, Michigan

Eric T. Choi, MD
Chief, Vascular and Endovascular Surgery, Professor of Surgery, Professor, Center for Metabolic Disease Research, Temple University Lewis Katz School of Medicine, Philadelphia, Pennsylvania

Eugene A. Choi, MD
Associate Professor of Surgery, Baylor College of Medicine, Houston, Texas

Karen A. Chojnacki, MD, FACS
Associate Professor of Surgery, Thomas Jefferson University, Philadelphia, Pennsylvania

Michael A. Choti, MD, MBA
Professor, Department of Surgery, University of Texas Southwestern Medical Center, Dallas, Texas

Ian Christie
Research Assistant, Department of Cardiothoracic Surgery, University of Pittsburgh, Pittsburgh, Pennsylvania

Heidi Chua, MD
Consultant, Department of Colon and Rectal Surgery, Mayo Clinic, Rochester, Minnesota

James M. Church, MBChB, MMedSci, FRACS
Staff Surgeon, Colorectal Surgery, Digestive Disease and Surgery Institute, Cleveland Clinic, Cleveland, Ohio

Jessica L. Cioffi, MD
Assistant Professor of Surgery, University of Florida, Gainesville, Florida

Susannah Clark, MS, MPAS
Boston, Massachusetts

Pierre-Alain Clavien, MD, PhD
Professor and Chairman, Department of Surgery, Division of Visceral and Transplant Surgery, University Hospital Zurich, Zurich, Switzerland

Adam Cloud, MD
Assistant Professor of Surgery, University of Connecticut, Farmington, Connecticut

Paul D. Colavita, MD
Gastrointestinal and Minimally Invasive Surgery, Carolinas Medical Center, Charlotte, North Carolina

Steven D. Colquhoun, MD
Professor of Surgery, Chief, Section of Hepatobiliary Surgery, Director of Liver Transplantation, Department of Surgery, University of California, Davis, Davis, California

William Conway, MD
Surgical Oncology, Ochsner Medical Center, New Orleans, Louisiana

Jonathan Cools-Lartigue, MD, PhD
Assistant Professor of Surgery, McGill University, Montreal, Quebec, Canada

Willy Coosemans, MD, PhD
Professor in Surgery, Clinical Head, Department of Thoracic Surgery, University Hospital Leuven, Leuven, Belgium

Edward E. Cornwell III, MD, FACS, FCCM, FWACS
The LaSalle D. Leffal Jr., Professor and Chairman of Surgery, Howard University Hospital, Washington, D.C.

Mario Costantini, MD
Department of Surgical, Oncological, and Gastroenterological Sciences, University and Azienda Ospedaliera of Padua, Padua, Italy

Yvonne Coyle, MD
Medical Director, Oncology Outpatient Services at the Baylor T. Boone Pickens Cancer Hospital; Texas Oncology and the Baylor Charles A. Sammons Cancer Center at the Baylor University Medical Center; Clinical Associate Professor, Texas A&M Health Science Center, College of Medicine, Dallas, Texas

Daniel A. Craig, MD
Assistant Professor of Radiology, Mayo Clinic, Rochester, Minnesota

Kristopher P. Croome, MD, MS
Assistant Professor of Transplant Surgery, Mayo Clinic, Jacksonville, Florida

Joseph J. Cullen, MD
Professor of Surgery, University of Iowa College of Medicine; Chief Surgical Services, Iowa City VA Medical Center, Iowa City, Iowa

Anthony P. D'Andrea, MD, MPH
Department of Surgery, Division of Colon and Rectal Surgery, Icahn School of Medicine at Mount Sinai, New York, New York

Themistocles Dassopoulos, MD
Adjunct Professor of Medicine, Texas A&M University; Director, Baylor Scott and White Center for Inflammatory Bowel Diseases, Dallas, Texas

Marta L. Davila, MD
Professor, Department of Gastroenterology, Hepatology, and Nutrition, The University of Texas MD Anderson Cancer Center, Houston, Texas

Raquel E. Davila, MD
Associate Professor, Department of Gastroenterology, Hepatology, and Nutrition, The University of Texas MD Anderson Cancer Center, Houston, Texas

Steven R. DeMeester, MD, FACS
Division of Foregut and Minimally Invasive Surgery, The Oregon Clinic, Portland, Oregon

Tom R. DeMeester, MD
Professor and Chairman Emeritus, Department of Surgery, University of Southern California, Los Angeles, California

Daniel T. Dempsey, MD, MBA
Professor of Surgery, University of Pennsylvania; Assistant Director, Perioperative Services, Hospital of the University of Pennsylvania, Philadelphia, Pennsylvania

Gregory dePrisco, MD
Diagnostic Radiologist, Baylor University Medical Center, Dallas, Texas

Lieven Depypere, MD
Joint Clinical Head, Department of Thoracic Surgery, University Hospital Leuven, Leuven, Belgium

David W. Dietz, MD, FACS, FASCRS
Chief, Division of Colorectal Surgery, Vice Chair, Clinical Operations and Quality, Vice President, System Surgery Quality and Experience, University Hospitals, Cleveland, Ohio

Mary E. Dillhoff, MD, MS
Assistant Professor of Surgery, The Ohio State University College of Medicine, Columbus, Ohio

Joseph DiNorcia, MD
Assistant Professor of Surgery, David Geffen School of Medicine, University of California, Los Angeles, Los Angeles, California

Stephen M. Doane, MD
Advanced Gastrointestinal Surgery Fellow, Department of Surgery, Thomas Jefferson University Hospital, Philadelphia, Pennsylvania

Epameinondas Dogeas, MD
Resident, Department of Surgery, University of Texas Southwestern Medical Center, Dallas, Texas

Eric J. Dozois, MD, FACS, FASCRS
Colon and Rectal Surgery, Mayo Clinic, Rochester, Minnesota

Kristoffel Dumon, MD
Associate Professor of Surgery, Hospital of the University of Pennsylvania, Philadelphia, Pennsylvania

Stephen P. Dunn, MD
Chairman, Department of Surgery, Nemours/Alfred I. Dupont Hospital for Children, Wilmington, Delaware; Professor of Surgery, Sidney Kimmel Medical College, Thomas Jefferson University, Philadelphia, Pennsylvania

Christy M. Dunst, MD
Co-Program Director, Advanced GI-Foregut Fellowship, Cancer Center, Providence Portland Medical Center; Foregut Surgeon, Gastrointestinal and Minimally Invasive Surgery, The Oregon Clinic, Portland, Oregon

John N. Dussel, MD
Fellow in Vascular Surgery, University of Connecticut, Farmington, Connecticut

Matthew Dyer, BA
Case Western Reserve University School of Medicine, Cleveland, Ohio

Jonathan Efron, MD
Associate Professor of Surgery and Urology, Johns Hopkins University, Baltimore, Maryland

Yousef El-Gohary, MD
Department of General Surgery, Stony Brook University School of Medicine, New York, New York

Mustapha El Lakis, MD
Thoraco-Esophageal Postdoctoral Research Fellow, General, Vascular, and Thoracic Surgery, Virginia Mason Medical Center, Seattle, Washington

E. Christopher Ellison, MD
Robert M. Zollinger and College of Medicine Distinguished Professor of Surgery, The Ohio State University College of Medicine, Columbus, Ohio

James Ellsmere, MD, MSc, FRCSC
Division of General Surgery, Dalhousie University, Halifax, Nova Scotia, Canada

Rahila Essani, MD, FACS
Department of Surgery, Baylor Scott and White Healthcare, Texas A&M University College of Medicine, Temple, Texas

Douglas B. Evans, MD
Professor and Chair of Surgery, Medical College of Wisconsin, Milwaukee, Wisconsin

Sandy H. Fang, MD
Assistant Professor, Department of Surgery, Johns Hopkins Medical Institutions, Baltimore, Maryland

Geoffrey Fasen, MD, MS
Clinical Instructor in General Surgery, University of Virginia, Charlottesville, Virginia

Hiran C. Fernando, MBBS, FRCS, FRCSEd
Department of Surgery, Inova Fairfax Medical Campus, Falls Church, Virginia

Lorenzo Ferri, MD, PhD
Professor of Surgery, McGill University, Montreal, Quebec, Canada

Alessandro Fichera, MD, FACS, FASCRS
Professor and Section Chief, Gastrointestinal Surgery, University of Washington Medical Center, Seattle, Washington

Christine Finck, MD
Chief, Division of Pediatric Surgery, Donald Hight Endowed Chair, Surgery, Connecticut Children's Medical Center, Hartford, Connecticut; Associate Professor of Pediatrics and Surgery, University of Connecticut Health Center, Farmington, Connecticut

Oliver M. Fisher, MD
Gastroesophageal Cancer Program, St. Vincent's Centre for Applied Medical Research, Department of Surgery, University of Notre Dame School of Medicine, Sydney, Australia

James W. Fleshman, MD, FACS
Seeger Professor and Chairman of Surgery, Baylor University Medical Center; Professor of Surgery, Texas A&M Health Science Center, Dallas, Texas

Yuman Fong, MD
Chairman, Department of Surgery, City of Hope National Medical Center, Duarte, California

Michael L. Foreman, MS, MD
Chief, Division of Trauma, Critical Care, and Acute Care Surgery, Department of Surgery, Baylor University Medical Center; Professor of Surgery, Texas A&M Health Science Center, College of Medicine, Dallas, Texas

Todd D. Francone, MD, MPH, FACS, FASCRS
Chief, Division of Colon and Rectal Surgery, Newton-Wellesley Hospital; Director, Robotic Surgery, Newton-Wellesley Hospital; Associate Chair, Department of Surgery, Newton-Wellesley Hospital; Staff Surgeon, Massachusetts General Hospital; Assistant Professor of Surgery, Tufts Medical School, Boston, Massachusetts

Edward R. Franko, MD, FACS
Assistant Professor of Surgery, Texas A&M University College of Medicine, Dallas, Texas

Daniel French, MD, MASc, FRCSC
Assistant Professor, Division of Thoracic Surgery, Dalhousie University, Halifax, Nova Scotia, Canada

Hans Friedrich Fuchs, MD
Department of Surgery, University Hospital Cologne, Cologne, Germany

Karl Hermann Fuchs, MD
Professor, Department of Surgery, Agaplesion Markus Hospital, Frankfurt, Germany

Brian Funaki, MD
Professor of Radiology, The University of Chicago Pritzker School of Medicine; Section Chief, Division of Vascular and Interventional Radiology, The University of Chicago Medicine, Chicago, Illinois

Geoffrey A. Funk, MD, FACS
Trauma and General Surgery, Surgical Critical Care, Assistant Professor of Surgery, Texas A&M University College of Medicine, Dallas, Texas

Joseph Fusco, MD
Children's Hospital of Pittsburgh, University of Pittsburgh, Pittsburgh, Pennsylvania

Shrawan G. Gaitonde, MD
Fellow, Surgical Oncology, John Wayne Cancer Institute at Providence Saint John's Health Center, Santa Monica, California

Julio Garcia-Aguilar, MD, PhD
Chief, Colorectal Service, Department of Surgery, Benno C. Schmidt Chair in Surgical Oncology, Memorial Sloan Kettering Cancer Center; Professor of Surgery, Weill Cornell Medical College, New York, New York

Susan Gearhart, MD
Associate Professor of Surgery, Johns Hopkins Medical Institutions, Baltimore, Maryland

David A. Geller, MD, FACS
Richard L. Simmons Professor of Surgery, Chief, Division of Hepatobiliary and Pancreatic Surgery, University of Pittsburgh, Pittsburgh, Pennsylvania

Comeron Ghobadi, MD
Department of Radiology, The University of Chicago Medicine, Chicago, Illinois

Sebastien Gilbert, MD
Associate Professor of Surgery, University of Ottawa; Chief, Division of Thoracic Surgery, Department of Surgery, Clinician Investigator, The Ottawa Hospital Research Institute, The Ottawa Hospital, Ottawa, Ontario, Canada

David Giles, MD
Associate Clinical Professor of Surgery, University of Connecticut School of Medicine, Farmington, Connecticut

Erin Gillaspie, MD
Assistant Professor, Department of Thoracic Surgery, Vanderbilt University Medical Center, Nashville, Tennessee

Micah Girotti, MD
Division of Vascular Surgery, Northwestern University Feinberg School of Medicine, Chicago, Illinois

George K. Gittes, MD
Professor of Surgery, Surgeon-in-Chief, Children's Hospital of Pittsburgh, University of Pittsburgh School of Medicine, Pittsburgh, Pennsylvania

Michael D. Goodman, MD
Assistant Professor of Surgery, University of Cincinnati, Cincinnati, Ohio

Hein G. Gooszen, MD, PhD
Professor, Department of Operating Room/Evidence Based Surgery, Radboud University Medical Center, Nijmegen, The Netherlands

Gregory J. Gores, MD
Executive Dean for Research, Professor of Medicine, Division of Gastroenterology and Hepatology, Mayo Clinic, Rochester, Minnesota

James F. Griffin, MD
Surgical Resident, Department of Surgery, The Johns Hopkins Hospital, Baltimore, Maryland

S. Michael Griffin, OBE, MD, FRCSEd
Professor, Consultant Oesophagogastric Surgeon, Northern Oesophagogastric Cancer Unit, Royal Victoria Infirmary, Newcastle-upon-Tyne, United Kingdom

Leander Grimm Jr., MD, FACS, FASCRS
Assistant Professor of Surgery, Division of Colon and Rectal Surgery, University of South Alabama, Mobile, Alabama

L.F. Grochola, MD, PhD
Department of Visceral and Transplant Surgery, University Hospital Zurich, Zurich, Switzerland

Fahim Habib, MD, MPH, FACS
Esophageal and Lung Institute, Allegheny Health Network, Pittsburgh, Pennsylvania

John B. Hanks, MD
C. Bruce Morton Professor and Chief, Division of General Surgery, Department of Surgery, University of Virginia Health System, Charlottesville, Virginia

James E. Harris Jr., MD
Assistant Professor of Surgery, The Johns Hopkins Hospital, Baltimore, Maryland

Matthew G. Hartwig, MD
Associate Professor of Surgery, Division of Thoracic and Cardiovascular Surgery, Department of Surgery, Duke University Hospital, Durham, North Carolina

Imran Hassan, MD, FACS
Clinical Associate Professor of Surgery, Carver College of Medicine, University of Iowa Health Care, Iowa City, Iowa

Traci L. Hedrick, MD, MS
Associate Professor of Surgery, University of Virginia Health System, Charlottesville, Virginia

Terry C. Hicks, MD, FACS, FASCRS
Colorectal Surgeon, Department of Colon and Rectal Surgery, Ochsner Medical Center, New Orleans, Louisiana

Richard Hodin, MD
Department of Surgery, Massachusetts General Hospital, Boston, Massachusetts

Wayne L. Hofstetter, MD
Professor of Surgery and Deputy Chair, Department of Thoracic and Cardiovascular Surgery, The University of Texas MD Anderson Cancer Center, Houston, Texas

Melissa Hogg, MD, MS
Assistant Professor of Surgery, Division of Surgical Oncology, University of Pittsburgh Medical Center, Pittsburgh, Pennsylvania

Yue-Yung Hu, MD, MPH
Pediatric Surgery Fellow, Connecticut Children's Medical Center, Hartford, Connecticut

Eric S. Hungness, MD
S. David Stulberg, MD Research Professor, Associate Professor in Gastrointestinal and Endocrine Surgery and Medical Education, Northwestern University Feinberg School of Medicine; Attending Surgeon, Northwestern Memorial Hospital, Chicago, Illinois

Steven R. Hunt, MD
Associate Professor of Surgery, Division of General Surgery, Section of Colon and Rectal Surgery, Washington University School of Medicine, St. Louis, Missouri

Khumara Huseynova, MD
Assistant Professor of Vascular and Endovascular Surgery, West Virginia University, Morgantown, West Virginia

Neil H. Hyman, MD
Chief, Section of Colon and Rectal Surgery, Co-Director, Digestive Disease Center, Department of Surgery, The University of Chicago Medicine, Chicago, Illinois

David A. Iannitti, MD
Chief, Division of Hepatobiliary and Pancreatic Surgery, Department of Surgery, Carolinas HealthCare System, Charlotte, North Carolina

Jeffrey Indes, MD
Associate Professor of Surgery, Section of Vascular Surgery, University of Connecticut, Farmington, Connecticut

Megan Jenkins, MD
Department of Surgery, New York University Langone Medical Center, New York, New York

Todd Jensen, MSc
Research Associate, University of Connecticut, Farmington, Connecticut

Paul M. Jeziorczak, MD
Senior Fellow, Division of Pediatric Surgery, St. Louis Children's Hospital, St. Louis, Missouri

Danial Jilani, MD
Department of Radiology, The University of Chicago Medicine, Chicago, Illinois

Marta Jiménez-Toscano, MD, PhD
Gastrointestinal Surgery Department, Hospital Clinic of Barcelona, Barcelona, Spain

Blair A. Jobe, MD, FACS
Director, Esophageal and Lung Institute, Allegheny Health Network; Clinical Professor of Surgery, Temple University School of Medicine, Pittsburgh, Pennsylvania

Lily E. Johnston, MD, MPH
Resident, Department of Surgery, University of Virginia Health System, Charlottesville, Virginia

Peter J. Kahrilas, MD
Gilbert H. Marquardt Professor of Medicine, Northwestern University Feinberg School of Medicine, Chicago, Illinois

Matthew F. Kalady, MD
Professor of Surgery, Colorectal Surgery, Co-Director, Comprehensive Colorectal Cancer Program, Digestive Disease and Surgery Institute, Cleveland Clinic, Cleveland, Ohio

Noor Kassira, MD
Assistant Professor of Surgery, Division of Pediatric Surgery, University of South Florida, Morsani College of Medicine, Tampa, Florida

Namir Katkhouda, MD, FACS
Professor of Surgery, Division of Upper Gastrointestinal and General Surgery, Keck School of Medicine of the University of Southern California, Los Angeles, California

Philip O. Katz, MD, FACG
Director of Motility Laboratories, Jay Monahan Center for Gastrointestinal Health, Weill Cornell Medicine, New York, New York

Deborah S. Keller, MS, MD
Department of Surgery, Baylor University Medical Center, Dallas, Texas

Matthew P. Kelley, MD
General Surgery Resident, Johns Hopkins Medical Institutions, Baltimore, Maryland

Gregory D. Kennedy, MD, PhD
Professor of Surgery, University of Alabama Birmingham, Birmingham, Alabama

Tara Sotsky Kent, MD, MS
Assistant Professor of Surgery, Harvard Medical School, Beth Israel Deaconess Medical Center, Boston, Massachusetts

Leila Kia, MD
Department of Medicine, Northwestern University Feinberg School of Medicine, Chicago, Illinois

Melina R. Kibbe, MD
Chair, Department of Surgery, The University of North Carolina at Chapel Hill, Chapel Hill, North Carolina

John Kim, DO, MPH, FACS
Clinical Assistant Professor of Surgery, Clerkship Director, Surgery, University of Illinois College of Medicine, Champaign-Urbana, Illinois; Attending Surgeon, Acute Care Surgery and Trauma, Carle Foundation Hospital, Urbana, Illinois

Alice King, MD
Junior Fellow, Division of Pediatric Surgery, St. Louis Children's Hospital, St. Louis, Missouri

Ravi P. Kiran, MBBS, MS, FRCS (Eng), FRCS (Glas), FACS, MSc EBM (Oxford)
Kenneth A. Forde Professor of Surgery in Epidemiology, Division Chief and Program Director, Director, Center for Innovation and Outcomes Research, Division of Colorectal Surgery, NewYork-Presbyterian Hospital/Columbia University Medical Center, New York, New York

Orlando C. Kirton, MD, FACS, MCCM, FCCP, MBA
Surgeon-in-Chief, Chairman of Surgery, Abington-Jefferson Health; Professor of Surgery, Sidney Kimmel Medical College of Thomas Jefferson University, Abington, Pennsylvania

Andrew Klein, MD, MBA, FACS
Professor and Vice Chairman, Department of Surgery, Director, Comprehensive Transplant Center, Cedars-Sinai Medical Center, Los Angeles, California

Eric N. Klein, MD
Acute Care Surgeon, North Shore University Hospital, Manhasset, New York

Geoffrey P. Kohn, MBBS(Hons), MSurg, FRACS, FACS
Senior Lecturer, Department of Surgery, Monash University, Melbourne, Australia; Upper Gastrointestinal Surgeon, Melbourne Upper Gastrointestinal Surgical Group, Melbourne, Victoria, Australia

Robert Caleb Kovell, MD
Assistant Professor of Clinical Urology in Surgery, Department of Urology Surgery, Perelman School of Medicine, University of Pennsylvania, Philadelphia, Pennsylvania

Robert Kozol, MD
General Surgery, JFK Medical Center, Atlantis, Florida

Antonio M. Lacy, MD, PhD
Chief, Gastrointestinal Surgery, Hospital Clinic of Barcelona, Barcelona, Spain

Daniela P. Ladner, MD, MPH, FACS
Associate Professor of Transplant Surgery, Division of Organ Transplantation, Feinberg School of Medicine, Northwestern University; Director, Northwestern University Transplant Outcomes Research Collaborative, Northwestern University, Chicago, Illinois

S.M. Lagarde, MD, PhD
Department of Surgery, Erasmus MC–University Medical Center Rotterdam, Rotterdam, The Netherlands

Carrie A. Laituri, MD
Assistant Professor of Surgery, Division of Pediatric Surgery, University of South Florida, Morsani College of Medicine, Tampa, Florida

Alessandra Landmann, MD
Resident Physician, Department of Surgery, University of Oklahoma, Oklahoma City, Oklahoma

Janet T. Lee, MD, MS
Clinical Assistant Professor of Surgery, University of Minnesota, St. Paul, Minnesota

Lawrence L. Lee, MD, PhD, FRCSC
Department of Colon and Rectal Surgery, Center for Colon & Rectal Surgery, Florida Hospital, Orlando, Florida

Jennifer A. Leinicke, MD, MPHS
Department of Surgery, Washington University School of Medicine, St. Louis, Missouri

Toni Lerut, MD, PhD
Emeritus Professor of Surgery, Clinical Head, Department of Thoracic Surgery, University Hospital Leuven, Leuven, Belgium

David M. Levi, MD
Transplant Surgeon, Carolinas Medical Center, Charlotte, North Carolina

Chao Li, MD, MSc, FRCSC
Division of General Surgery, Dalhousie University, Halifax, Nova Scotia, Canada

Yu Liang, MD
Department of Surgery, University of Connecticut Health Center, Farmington, Connecticut

Andrew H. Lichliter, MD
Diagnostic Radiology Resident, Baylor University Medical Center, Dallas, Texas

Warren E. Lichliter, MD
Chief, Colon and Rectal Surgery, Baylor Scott and White Health, Dallas, Texas

Amy L. Lightner, MD
Senior Associate Consultant, Department of Colon and Rectal Surgery, Mayo Clinic, Rochester, Minnesota

Deacon J. Lile, MD
Department of General Surgery, Temple University Hospital, Philadelphia, Pennsylvania

Keith D. Lillemoe, MD, FACS
W. Gerald Austen Professor of Surgery, Harvard Medical School; Surgeon-in-Chief, The Massachusetts General Hospital, Boston, Massachusetts;

Jules Lin, MD, FACS
Associate Professor, Mark B. Orringer Professor, Section of Thoracic Surgery, University of Michigan, Ann Arbor, Michigan

Shu S. Lin, MD, PhD
Associate Professor of Surgery, Pathology, and Immunology, Duke University Medical Center, Durham, North Carolina

John C. Lipham, MD, FACS
Chief, Division of Upper Gastrointestinal and General Surgery, Associate Professor of Surgery, Keck School of Medicine of the University of Southern California, Los Angeles, California

Virginia R. Litle, MD
Professor of Surgery, Division of Thoracic Surgery, Boston University, Boston, Massachusetts

Nayna A. Lodhia, MD
Resident, Department of Internal Medicine, The University of Chicago Medicine, Chicago, Illinois

Walter E. Longo, MD, MBA
Colon and Rectal Surgery, Yale University School of Medicine, New Haven, Connecticut

Reginald V.N. Lord, MBBS, MD, FRACS
Director, Gastroesophageal Cancer Program, St. Vincent's Centre for Applied Medical Research; Professor and Head of Surgery, University of Notre Dame School of Medicine, Sydney, Australia

Brian E. Louie, MD, MPH, MHA
Director, Thoracic Research and Education, Division of Thoracic Surgery, Swedish Cancer Institute and Medical Center, Seattle, Washington

Donald E. Low, MD, FACS, FRCS(C)
Head of Thoracic Surgery and Thoracic Oncology, General, Vascular, and Thoracic Surgery, Virginia Mason Medical Center, Seattle, Washington

Val J. Lowe, MD
Professor of Radiology/Nuclear Medicine, Mayo Clinic, Rochester, Minnesota

Jessica G.Y. Luc, MD
Faculty of Medicine and Dentistry, University of Alberta, Alberta, Canada

James D. Luketich, MD
Henry T. Bahnson Professor and Chairman, Department of Cardiothoracic Surgery, Chief, Division of Thoracic and Foregut Surgery, University of Pittsburgh School of Medicine, Pittsburgh, Pennsylvania

Yanling Ma, MD
Pathologist, Department of Surgical Pathology, Los Angeles County + University of Southern California Medical Center; Associate Professor of Pathology, Keck School of Medicine of the University of Southern California, Los Angeles, Los Angeles, California

Robert L. MacCarty, MD
Professor of Diagnostic Radiology, Emeritus, Mayo Clinic College of Medicine, Rochester, Minnesota

Blair MacDonald, MD, FRCPC
Associate Professor of Medical Imaging, University of Ottawa; Clinical Investigator, The Ottawa Hospital Research Institute; Gastrointestinal Radiologist, The Ottawa Hospital, Ottawa, Ontario, Canada

Robert D. Madoff, MD
Professor of Surgery, University of Minnesota, Minneapolis, Minnesota

Deepa Magge, MD
Fellow in Surgical Oncology, Division of Surgical Oncology, University of Pittsburgh Medical Center, Pittsburgh, Pennsylvania

Anurag Maheshwari, MD
Clinical Assistant Professor of Medicine, Division of Gastroenterology and Hepatology, University of Maryland School of Medicine; Consultant Transplant Hepatologist, Institute for Digestive Health and Liver Diseases, Mercy Medical Center, Baltimore, Maryland

Najjia N. Mahmoud, MD
Professor of Surgery, Division of Colon and Rectal Surgery, University of Pennsylvania, Philadelphia, Pennsylvania

David A. Mahvi, MD
Brigham and Women's Hospital, Boston, Massachusetts

David M. Mahvi, MD
Professor of Surgery, Northwestern University School of Medicine, Chicago, Illinois

Grace Z. Mak, MD
Associate Professor, Section of Pediatric Surgery, Department of Surgery, The University of Chicago Medicine and Biological Sciences, Chicago, Illinois

Sara A. Mansfield, MD, MS
Clinical Housestaff, Department of Surgery, The Ohio State University Wexner Medical Center, Columbus, Ohio

Maricarmen Manzano, MD
Division of Gastroenterology, National Cancer Institute of Mexico, Mexico City, Mexico

David J. Maron, MD, MBA
Vice Chair, Department of Colorectal Surgery, Director, Colorectal Surgery Residency Program, Cleveland Clinic Florida, Weston, Florida

Melvy S. Mathew, MD
Assistant Professor of Radiology, The University of Chicago Pritzker School of Medicine; Division of Body Imaging, The University of Chicago Medicine, Chicago, Illinois

Kellie L. Mathis, MD
Surgery, Mayo Clinic, Rochester, Minnesota

Jeffrey B. Matthews, MD, FACS
Dallas B. Phemister Professor and Chairman of Surgery, The University of Chicago, Chicago, Illinois

David W. McFadden, MD, MBA, FACS
Chairman, Department of Surgery, University of Connecticut; Surgeon-in-Chief, University of Connecticut Health, Farmington, Connecticut

Amit Merchea, MD, FACS, FASCRS
Assistant Professor of Surgery, Colon and Rectal Surgery, Mayo Clinic, Jacksonville, Florida

Evangelos Messaris, MD, PhD
Associate Professor of Surgery, Pennsylvania State University, College of Medicine, Hershey, Pennsylvania

Daniel L. Miller, MD
Clinical Professor of Surgery, Medical College of Georgia, Augusta University, Augusta, Georgia; Chief, General Thoracic Surgery, Program Director, General Surgery Residency Program, Kennestone Regional Medical Center, WellStar Health System/Mayo Clinic Care Network, Marietta, Georgia

Heidi J. Miller, MD, MPH
Assistant Professor of Surgery, University of New Mexico, Sandoval Regional Medical Center, Albuquerque, New Mexico

J. Michael Millis, MD, MBA
Professor of Surgery, Transplant Surgery, The University of Chicago, Chicago, Illinois

Sumeet K. Mittal, MD, FACS, MBA
Surgical Director, Esophageal and Foregut Program, Norton Thoracic Institute, St. Joseph's Hospital and Medical Center, Phoenix, Arizona

Daniela Molena, MD
Surgical Director, Esophageal Cancer Surgery Program, General Surgery Department, Thoracic Surgery Service, Memorial Sloan Kettering Cancer Center, New York, New York

Stephanie C. Montgomery, MD, FACS
Director of Surgery Education, Saint Francis Hospital and Medical Center; Assistant Professor, University of Connecticut School of Medicine, Hartford, Connecticut

Ryan Moore, MD
Department of General Surgery, Temple University Hospital, Philadelphia, Pennsylvania

Katherine A. Morgan, MD, FACS
Professor of Surgery, Chief, Division of Gastrointestinal and Laparoscopic Surgery, Medical University of South Carolina, Charleston, South Carolina

Melinda M. Mortenson, MD
Department of Surgery, Permanente Medical Group, Sacramento, California

Michael W. Mulholland, MD, PhD
Department of Surgery, University of Michigan, Ann Arbor, Michigan

Michael S. Mulvihill, MD
Resident Surgeon, Department of Surgery, Duke University, Durham, North Carolina

Matthew Mutch, MD
Chief, Section of Colon and Rectal Surgery, Associate Professor of Surgery, Washington University, St. Louis, Missouri

Philippe Robert Nafteux, MD, PhD
Assistant Professor in Surgery, Clinical Head, Department of Thoracic Surgery, University Hospital Leuven, Leuven, Belgium

Arun Nagaraju, MD
Department of Radiology, The University of Chicago Medicine, Chicago, Illinois

David M. Nagorney, MD, FACS
Professor of Surgery, Mayo Clinic, Rochester, Minnesota

Hari Nathan, MD, PhD
Department of Surgery, University of Michigan, Ann Arbor, Michigan

Karen R. Natoli, MD
Department of Surgery, Community Hospital, Indianapolis, Indiana

Rakesh Navuluri, MD
Department of Radiology, The University of Chicago Medicine, Chicago, Illinois

Nicholas N. Nissen, MD
Director, Liver Transplant and Hepatopancreatobiliary Surgery, Cedars-Sinai Medical Center, Los Angeles, California

Tamar B. Nobel, MD
Department of Surgery, Mount Sinai Hospital, New York, New York

B.J. Noordman, MD
Department of Surgery, Erasmus MC–University Medical Center Rotterdam, Rotterdam, The Netherlands

Jeffrey A. Norton, MD
Professor of Surgery, Stanford University School of Medicine, Stanford, California

Yuri W. Novitsky, MD
Director, Cleveland Comprehensive Hernia Center, University Hospitals Cleveland Medical Center; Professor of Surgery, Case Western Reserve School of Medicine, Cleveland, Ohio

Michael S. Nussbaum, MD, FACS
Professor and Chair, Department of Surgery, Virginia Tech Carilion School of Medicine, Roanoke, Virginia

Scott L. Nyberg, MD, PhD
Professor of Biomedical Engineering and Surgery, Department of Transplantation Surgery, Mayo Clinic, Rochester, Minnesota

Brant K. Oelschlager, MD
Byers Endowed Professor of Esophageal Research, Chief, Division of General Surgery, University of Washington Medical Center; Vice Chair, Department of Surgery, University of Washington, Seattle, Washington

Daniel S. Oh, MD
Assistant Professor of Surgery, Thoracic Surgery, University of Southern California, Los Angeles, California

Ana Otero-Piñeiro, MD
Gastrointestinal Surgery Department, Hospital Clinic of Barcelona, Barcelona, Spain

Aytekin Oto, MD
Professor of Radiology, The University of Chicago Pritzker School of Medicine; Section Chief, Division of Body Imaging, The University of Chicago Medicine, Chicago, Illinois

H. Leon Pachter, MD
Chairman, Department of Surgery, New York University Langone Medical Center, New York, New York

Charles N. Paidas, MD, MBA
Professor of Surgery and Pediatrics, Chief, Pediatric Surgery, Vice Dean for Graduate Medical Education, University of South Florida, Morsani College of Medicine, Tampa, Florida

Francesco Palazzo, MD
Associate Professor of Surgery, Thomas Jefferson University, Philadelphia, Pennsylvania

Alessandro Paniccia, MD
General Surgery Resident, University of Colorado School of Medicine, Aurora, Colorado

Harry T. Papaconstantinou, MD, FACS, FACRS
Department of Surgery, Baylor Scott and White Healthcare, Texas A&M University College of Medicine, Temple, Texas

Theodore N. Pappas, MD, FACS
Distinguished Professor of Surgical Innovation, Chief of Advanced Oncologic and Gastrointestinal Surgery, Duke University School of Medicine, Durham, North Carolina

Emmanouil P. Pappou, MD, PhD
Assistant Professor of Colorectal Surgery, Columbia University Medical Center, New York, New York

Manish Parikh, MD
Associate Professor of Surgery, New York University Langone Medical Center/Bellevue Hospital, New York, New York

Jennifer L. Paruch, MD, MS
Lahey Hospital and Medical Center, Burlington, Massachusetts

Asish D. Patel, MD
Chief Resident, Department of Surgery, University of Nebraska Medical Center, Omaha, Nebraska

Mikin Patel, MD
Department of Radiology, The University of Chicago Medicine, Chicago, Illinois

Marco G. Patti, MD
Center for Esophageal Diseases and Swallowing, University of North Carolina at Chapel Hill, Chapel Hill, North Carolina

Emily Carter Paulson, MD, MSCE
Assistant Professor of Surgery, University of Pennsylvania; Assistant Professor of Surgery, Corporal Michael Crescenz VA Medical Center, Philadelphia, Pennsylvania

Timothy M. Pawlik, MD, MPH, PhD
Professor of Surgery and Oncology, The Urban Meyer III and Shelley Meyer Chair for Cancer Research, Ohio State University; Chair, Department of Surgery, Wexner Medical Center, Columbus, Ohio; Division of Surgical Oncology, Department of Surgery, The Johns Hopkins School of Medicine, Baltimore, Maryland

Isaac Payne, DO
Surgical Resident, University of South Alabama, Mobile, Alabama

John H. Pemberton, MD
Professor of Surgery, College of Medicine, Consultant, Department of Colon and Rectal Surgery, Mayo Clinic, Rochester, Minnesota

Michael Pendola, MD
Staff Colorectal Surgeon, Department of Surgery, Baylor University Medical Center, Dallas, Texas

Alexander Perez, MD, FACS
Chief of Pancreatic Surgery, Duke University Medical Center, Durham, North Carolina; Associate Professor of Surgery, Duke University School of Medicine, Durham, North Carolina

Luise I.M. Pernar, MD
Assistant Professor of Surgery, Boston University School of Medicine; Minimally Invasive and Weight Loss Surgery, Boston Medical Center, Boston, Massachusetts

Walter R. Peters Jr., MD, MBA
Chief, Division of Colon and Rectal Surgery, Baylor University Medical Center, Dallas, Texas

Henrik Petrowsky, MD
Professor of Surgery, Vice Chairman, Department of Visceral and Transplant Surgery, University Hospital Zurich, Zurich, Switzerland

Christian G. Peyre, MD
Division of Thoracic and Foregut Surgery, Department of Surgery, University of Rochester School of Medicine and Dentistry, Rochester, New York

Alexander W. Phillips, MA, FRCSEd, FFSTEd
Consultant Oesophagogastric Surgeon, Northern Oesophagogastric Cancer Unit, Royal Victoria Infirmary, Newcastle-upon-Tyne, United Kingdom

Lashmikumar Pillai, MD
Associate Professor of Vascular and Endovascular Surgery, West Virginia University Medical Center, Morgantown, West Virginia

Joseph M. Plummer, MBBS, DM
Department of Surgery, Radiology, and Intensive Care, University of the West Indies, Mona, Jamaica

David T. Pointer Jr., MD
Surgery, Tulane University School of Medicine, New Orleans, Louisiana

Katherine E. Poruk, MD
Surgical Resident, Department of Surgery, The Johns Hopkins Hospital, Baltimore, Maryland

Mitchell C. Posner, MD, FACS
Thomas D. Jones Professor of Surgery and Vice-Chairman, Chief, Section of General Surgery and Surgical Oncology, Physician-in-Chief, The University of Chicago Medicine Comprehensive Cancer Center, The University of Chicago Medicine, Chicago, Illinois

Russell Postier, MD
Chairman, Department of Surgery, University of Oklahoma, Oklahoma City, Oklahoma

Vivek N. Prachand, MD
Associate Professor, Director of Minimally Invasive Surgery, Chief Quality Officer, Executive Medical Director, Procedural Quality and Safety, Section of General Surgery, Department of Surgery, The University of Chicago Medicine and Biological Sciences, Chicago, Illinois

Timothy A. Pritts, MD, PhD
Professor of Surgery, University of Cincinnati, Cincinnati, Ohio

Gregory Quatrino, MD
Surgical Resident, University of South Alabama, Mobile, Alabama

Sagar Ranka, MD
Resident, Department of Internal Medicine, John H. Stroger Hospital of Cook County, Chicago, Illinois

David W. Rattner, MD
Chief, Division of General and Gastrointestinal Surgery, Massachusetts General Hospital; Professor of Surgery, Harvard Medical School, Boston, Massachusetts

Kevin M. Reavis, MD
Division of Gastrointestinal and Minimally Invasive Surgery, The Oregon Clinic, Portland, Oregon

Vikram B. Reddy, MD, PhD
Colon and Rectal Surgery, Yale University School of Medicine, New Haven, Connecticut

Feza H. Remzi, MD, FACS, FTSS (Hon)
Director, Inflammatory Bowel Disease Center, New York University Langone Medical Center; Professor of Surgery, New York University School of Medicine, New York, New York

Rocco Ricciardi, MD, MPH
Chief, Section of Colon and Rectal Surgery, Massachusetts General Hospital, Boston, Massachusetts

Thomas W. Rice, MD
Professor of Surgery, Cleveland Clinic Lerner College of Medicine; Emeritus Staff, Department of Thoracic Cardiovascular Surgery, Cleveland Clinic, Cleveland, Ohio

Aaron Richman, MD
Department of Surgery, Boston Medical Center, Boston, Massachusetts

Paul Rider, MD, FACS, FASCRS
Associate Professor of Surgery, Division of Colon and Rectal Surgery, University of South Alabama, Mobile, Alabama

John Paul Roberts, MD, FACS
Professor and Chief, Division of Transplant Surgery, University of California, San Francisco, San Francisco, California

Patricia L. Roberts, MD
Chair, Department of Surgery, Senior Staff Surgeon, Division of Colon and Rectal Surgery, Lahey Hospital and Medical Center, Burlington, Massachusetts; Professor of Surgery, Tufts University School of Medicine, Boston, Massachusetts

Kevin K. Roggin, MD
Professor of Surgery and Cancer Research, Program Director, General Surgery Residency Program, Associate Program Director, Surgical Oncology Fellowship, The University of Chicago Medicine, Chicago, Illinois

Garrett Richard Roll, MD, FACS
Assistant Professor of Surgery, Department of Surgery, Division of Transplant, University of California, San Francisco, San Francisco, California

Kais Rona, MD
Chief Resident in General Surgery, Keck School of Medicine of the University of Southern California, Los Angeles, California

Charles B. Rosen, MD
Chair, Division of Transplantation Surgery, Mayo Clinic, Rochester, Minnesota

Samuel Wade Ross, MD, MPH
Chief Resident, Department of Surgery, Carolinas Medical Center, Charlotte, North Carolina

J. Scott Roth, MD
Professor of Surgery, Chief, Gastrointestinal Surgery, Department of Surgery, University of Kentucky, Lexington, Kentucky

Amy P. Rushing, MD, FACS
Assistant Professor, Division of Trauma, Critical Care, and Burn, The Ohio State University Wexner Medical Center, Columbus, Ohio

Bashar Safar, MBBS
Assistant Professor of Surgery, Johns Hopkins Medicine, Baltimore, Maryland

Pierre F. Saldinger, MD
Chairman, Surgery, NewYork-Presbyterian/Queens, Flushing, New York

Kamran Samakar, MD, MA
Assistant Professor of Surgery, Division of Upper Gastrointestinal and General Surgery, Keck School of Medicine of the University of Southern California, Los Angeles, California

Kulmeet K. Sandhu, MD, FACS, MS
Assistant Professor of Clinical Surgery, Division of Upper Gastrointestinal and General Surgery, Keck School of Medicine of the University of Southern California, Los Angeles, California

Lara W. Schaheen, MD
Cardiothoracic Surgery Resident, Department of Cardiothoracic Surgery, University of Pittsburgh, Pittsburgh, Philadelphia

Bruce Schirmer, MD
Stephen H. Watts Professor of Surgery, University of Virginia Health System, Charlottesville, Virginia

Andrew Schneider, MD
General Surgery Resident, The University of Chicago Medicine, Chicago, Illinois

Richard D. Schulick, MD, MBA
Professor and Chair, Department of Surgery, University of Colorado School of Medicine, Aurora, Colorado

Ben Schwab, MD, DC
General Surgery Resident, Northwestern University Feinberg School of Medicine, Chicago, Illinois

Stephanie Scurci, MD
Resident, University of Miami Miller School of Medicine, Palm Beach Regional Campus, Palm Beach, Florida

Anthony Senagore, MD, MS, MBA
Professor, Chief of Gastrointestinal Surgery, Surgery, University of Texas–Medical Branch, Galveston, Texas

Adil A. Shah, MD
Resident, Department of Surgery, Howard University Hospital and College of Medicine, Washington, D.C.

Shimul A. Shah, MD
Director, Liver Transplantation and Hepatobiliary Surgery, Associate Professor of Surgery, University of Cincinnati, Cincinnati, Ohio

Brian Shames, MD
Chief, Division of General Surgery, General Surgery Residency Program Director, University of Connecticut Health Center, Farmington, Connecticut

Skandan Shanmugan, MD
Assistant Professor of Surgery, Division of Colon and Rectal Surgery, University of Pennsylvania, Perelman School of Medicine, Philadelphia, Pennsylvania

David S. Shapiro, MD, FACS, FCCM
Chairman, Department of Surgery, Saint Francis Hospital and Medical Center–Trinity Health New England, Hartford, Connecticut; Assistant Professor of Surgery, University of Connecticut School of Medicine, Farmington, Connecticut

Matthew Silviera, MD
Washington University, St. Louis, Missouri

Douglas P. Slakey, MD, MPH, FACS
Professor, Surgery, Tulane University, New Orleans, Louisiana

Joshua Sloan, DO
Division of Gastroenterology, Einstein Healthcare Network, Philadelphia, Pennsylvania

Nathan Smallwood, MD
Division of Colon and Rectal Surgery, Baylor University Medical Center, Dallas, Texas

Shane P. Smith, MD
General Surgery Resident, Department of Surgery, Swedish Medical Center, Seattle, Washington

B. Mark Smithers, MBBS, FRACS, FRCSEng, FRCSEd
Professor of Surgery, University of Queensland; Director, Upper Gastrointestinal and Soft Tissue Unit, Princess Alexandra Hospital, Brisbane, Queensland, Australia

Rory L. Smoot, MD, FACS
Assistant Professor, Mayo Clinic, Rochester, Minnesota

Kevin C. Soares, MD
Resident, General Surgery, Department of Surgery, Johns Hopkins Medical Institutions, Baltimore, Maryland

Edy Soffer, MD
Professor of Clinical Medicine, Director, GI Motility Program, Keck School of Medicine of the University of Southern California, Los Angeles, California

Julia Solomina, MD
Department of Surgery, The University of Chicago, Chicago, Illinois

Nathaniel J. Soper, MD
Loyal and Edith Davis Professor of Surgery, Northwestern University Feinberg School of Medicine; Chair, Department of Surgery, Northwestern Memorial Hospital, Chicago, Illinois

Stuart Jon Spechler, MD
Chief, Division of Gastroenterology, Co-Director, Center for Esophageal Research, Baylor University Medical Center at Dallas; Co-Director, Center for Esophageal Research, Baylor Scott and White Research Institute, Dallas, Texas

Praveen Sridhar, MD
Department of Surgery, Boston Medical Center, Boston, Massachusetts

Scott R. Steele, MD, FACS, FASCRS
Chairman, Department of Colorectal Surgery, Cleveland Clinic; Professor of Surgery, Case Western Reserve University School of Medicine, Cleveland, Ohio

Joel M. Sternbach, MD, MBA
Bechily-Hodes Fellow in Esophagology, Department of Surgery, Northwestern University Feinberg School of Medicine, Chicago, Illinois

Christina E. Stevenson, MD
Assistant Professor of Surgery, Department of Surgery and Neag Comprehensive Cancer Center, University of Connecticut, Farmington, Connecticut

Scott A. Strong, MD
James R. Hines Professor of Surgery, Northwestern University Feinberg School of Medicine, Chicago, Illinois

Iswanto Sucandy, MD
Clinical Instructor, Department of Surgery, University of Pittsburgh School of Medicine, Pittsburgh, Pennsylvania

Magesh Sundaram, MD, MBA, FACS
Senior Associate Medical Director, Carle Cancer Center, Carle Foundation Hospital, Urbana, Illinois

Sudhir Sundaresan, MD, FRCSC, FACS
Surgeon-in-Chief, The Ottawa Hospital; Wilbert J. Keon Professor and Chairman, Department of Surgery, University of Ottawa, Ottawa, Ontario, Canada

Lee L. Swanstrom, MD
The Institute of Image-Guided Surgery of Strasbourg, University of Strasbourg, Strasbourg, Alsace, France; Director, Division of Gastrointestinal and Minimally Invasive Surgery, The Oregon Clinic, Portland, Oregon

Patricia Sylla, MD
Associate Professor of Surgery, Division of Colorectal Surgery, Icahn School of Medicine at Mount Sinai Hospital, New York, New York

Tadahiro Takada, MD, FACS, FRCSEd
Emeritus Professor, Department of Surgery, Teikyo University School of Medicine, Tokyo, Japan

Ethan Talbot, MD
Resident, General Surgery, Bassett Medical Center, Cooperstown, New York

Vernissia Tam, MD
Resident in General Surgery, University of Pittsburgh Medical Center, Pittsburgh, Pennsylvania

Eric P. Tamm, MD
Professor, Diagnostic Imaging, The University of Texas MD Anderson Cancer Center, Houston, Texas

Talar Tatarian, MD
Department of Surgery, Jefferson Gastroesophageal Center, Sidney Kimmel Medical College at Jefferson University, Philadelphia, Pennsylvania

Ali Tavakkoli, MD, FACS, FRCS
Associate Professor of Surgery, Director, Minimally Invasive and Weight Loss Surgery Fellowship, Co-director, Center for Weight Management and Metabolic Surgery, Brigham and Women's Hospital, Harvard Medical School, Boston, Massachusetts

Helen S. Te, MD
Associate Professor of Medicine, Department of Medicine, Center for Liver Diseases, The University of Chicago Medicine, Chicago, Illinois

Ezra N. Teitelbaum, MD, MEd
Foregut Surgery Fellow, Providence Portland Medical Center, Portland, Oregon

Charles A. Ternent, MD, FACS
Section of Colon and Rectal Surgery, Creighton University School of Medicine, University of Nebraska College of Medicine, Omaha, Nebraska

Jon S. Thompson, MD
Professor of Surgery, University of Nebraska Medical Center, Omaha, Nebraska

Iain Thomson, MBBS, FRACS
Senior Lecturer, University of Queensland; Upper Gastrointestinal and Soft Tissue Unit, Princess Alexandra Hospital, Brisbane, Queensland, Australia

Alan G. Thorson, MD, FACS
Clinical Professor of Surgery, Creighton University School of Medicine, University of Nebraska College of Medicine, Omaha, Nebraska

Chad M. Thorson, MD, MSPH
Pediatric Surgery Fellow, Stanford University, Palo Alto, California

Crystal F. Totten, MD
Department of Surgery, University of Kentucky College of Medicine, Lexington, Kentucky

Mark J. Truty, MD, MsC, FACS
Assistant Professor, Mayo Clinic, Rochester, Minnesota

Susan Tsai, MD, MHS
Associate Professor of Surgical Oncology, Department of Surgery, Medical College of Wisconsin, Milwaukee, Wisconsin

Jennifer Tseng, MD
Surgical Oncology Fellow, The University of Chicago, Chicago, Illinois

Tom Tullius, MD
Department of Radiology, The University of Chicago Medicine, Chicago, Illinois

Andreas G. Tzakis, MD, PhD
Director, Transplant Center, Cleveland Clinic Florida, Weston, Florida

J.J.B. van Lanschot, MD, PhD
Professor, Department of Surgery, Erasmus MC–University Medical Center Rotterdam, Rotterdam, The Netherlands

Hjalmar C. van Santvoort, MD, PhD
Department of Surgery, St. Antonius Hospital, Nieuwegein, The Netherlands

Hans Van Veer, MD
Joint Clinical Head, Department of Thoracic Surgery, University Hospital Leuven, Leuven, Belgium

Jorge A. Vega Jr., MD
Department of Surgery, University of South Florida Morsani College of Medicine, Tampa, Florida

Vic Velanovich, MD
Professor, Department of Surgery, University of South Florida Morsani College of Medicine, Tampa, Florida

Sarah A. Vogler, MD, MBA
Clinical Assistant Professor of Surgery, University of Minnesota, Minneapolis, Minnesota

Huamin Wang, MD, PhD
Professor of Pathology, The University of Texas MD Anderson Cancer Center, Houston, Texas

Mark A. Ward, MD
Minimally Invasive Surgery Fellow, Gastrointestinal and Minimally Invasive Surgery, The Oregon Clinic, Portland, Oregon

Brad W. Warner, MD
Division of Pediatric Surgery, St. Louis Children's Hospital, St. Louis, Missouri

Susanne G. Warner, MD
Assistant Professor of Surgery, City of Hope National Medical Center, Duarte, California

Thomas J. Watson, MD, FACS
Professor of Surgery, Georgetown University School of Medicine; Regional Chief of Surgery, MedStar Washington, Washington, D.C.

Irving Waxman, MD
Sara and Harold Lincoln Thompson Professor of Medicine, Director of the Center for Endoscopic Research and Therapeutics, The University of Chicago Medicine and Biological Sciences, Chicago, Illinois

Carissa Webster-Lake, MD
University of Connecticut, Farmington, Connecticut

Benjamin Wei, MD
Assistant Professor, Division of Cardiothoracic Surgery, University of Alabama-Birmingham Medical Center, Birmingham, Alabama

Martin R. Weiser, MD
Stuart H.Q. Quan Chair in Colorectal Surgery, Department of Surgery, Memorial Sloan Kettering Cancer Center; Professor of Surgery, Weill Cornell Medical College, New York, New York

Dennis Wells, MD
Resident in Thoracic Surgery, Department of Surgery, University of Cincinnati College of Medicine, Cincinnati, Ohio

Katerina Wells, MD, MPH
Director of Colorectal Research, Baylor University Medical Center; Adjunct Assistant Professor, Texas A&M Health Science Center, Dallas, Texas

Mark Lane Welton, MD, MHCM
Chief Medical Officer, Fairview Health Services, Minneapolis, Minnesota

Yuxiang Wen, MD
General Surgery, Cleveland Clinic Florida, Weston, Florida

Mark R. Wendling, MD
Acting Instructor and Senior Fellow, Advanced Minimally Invasive Surgery, CVES, Division of General Surgery, University of Washington, Seattle, Washington

Hadley K.H. Wesson, MD
Assistant Professor of Surgery, The Johns Hopkins Hospital, Baltimore, Maryland

Steven D. Wexner, MD, PhD(Hon)
Director, Digestive Disease Center, Chair, Department of Colorectal Surgery, Cleveland Clinic Florida, Weston, Florida

Rebekah R. White, MD
Associate Professor of Surgery, University of California, San Diego, La Jolla, California

Charles B. Whitlow, MD, FACS, FASCRS
Chairman, Department of Colon and Rectal Surgery, Ochsner Clinic Foundation, New Orleans, Louisiana

B.P.L. Wijnhoven, MD, PhD
Department of Surgery, The Erasmus University Medical Center, Rotterdam, The Netherlands

Justin Wilkes, MD
Department of Surgery, Maine Medical Center, Portland, Maine; Research Fellow, Department of Surgery, University of Iowa, Iowa City, Iowa

Rickesha L. Wilson, MD
General Surgical Resident, Department of Surgery, University of Connecticut, Farmington, Connecticut

Piotr Witkowski, MD, PhD
Associate Professor of Surgery, Department of Surgery, The University of Chicago, Chicago, Illinois

Christopher L. Wolfgang, MD, PhD
Chief, Hepatobiliary and Pancreatic Surgery, Professor of Surgery, Pathology, and Oncology, The Johns Hopkins Hospital, Baltimore, Maryland

Stephanie G. Worrell, MD
Surgery, Keck School of Medicine of the University of Southern California, Los Angeles, California

Jian Yang, MD
Department of Liver Transplantation Center, West China Hospital of Sichuan University, Chengdu, Sichuan Province, China

Charles J. Yeo, MD, FACS
Samuel D. Gross Professor and Chair, Department of Surgery, Sidney Kimmel Medical College at Thomas Jefferson University, Philadelphia, Pennsylvania

Ching Yeung, MD
Thoracic Surgery Fellow, University of Ottawa, The Ottawa Hospital–General Campus, Ottawa, Canada

Evan E. Yung, MD
Fellow in Surgical Pathology, Los Angeles County + University of Southern California Medical Center, Los Angeles, California

Syed Nabeel Zafar, MD MPH
Chief Resident, Department of Surgery, Howard University Hospital, Washington, D.C.

Giovanni Zaninotto, MD
Professor, Department of Surgery and Cancer, Imperial College, London, United Kingdom

Herbert Zeh III, MD
Professor of Surgery, Division of Surgical Oncology, University of Pittsburgh Medical Center, Pittsburgh, Pennsylvania

Joerg Zehetner, MD, MMM, FACS
Adjunct Associate Professor of Surgery, Klinik Beau-Site Hirslanden, Berne, Switzerland

Michael E. Zenilman, MD
Professor of Surgery, Weill Cornell Medicine; Chair, Department of Surgery, NewYork-Presbyterian Brooklyn Methodist Hospital, Brooklyn, New York

Pamela Zimmerman, MD
Associate Professor of Vascular and Endovascular Surgery, West Virginia University, Morgantown, West Virginia

Gregory Zuccaro Jr., MD
Department of Gastroenterology and Hepatology, Cleveland Clinic, Cleveland, Ohio

Preface

The time has come to release the eighth edition of the classic textbook *Shackelford's Surgery of the Alimentary Tract*. This publication has served as an important resource for surgeons, internists, gastroenterologists, residents, medical students, and other medical professionals over the past 61 years. I hope that you will find the eighth edition brimming with new information, beautifully illustrated, up to date, and educationally fulfilling.

BRIEF HISTORY

The first edition of *Surgery of the Alimentary Tract* was written solely by Dr. Richard T. Shackelford, a Baltimore surgeon, and was published in 1955. Following the success of the first edition, the book's publisher, W.B. Saunders Company, urged Dr. Shackelford to produce a second edition. Considerable time passed. A second edition was released, as separate five-volume tomes, between 1978 and 1986, with Dr. Shackelford enlisting the assistance of Dr. George D. Zuidema, the Chairman of the Department of Surgery at Johns Hopkins, as co-editor. It was the second edition that served as my "bible" for alimentary tract diseases during my surgical residency and early faculty appointment.

The third edition, edited by Dr. Zuidema, was published as a five-volume set in 1991 and proved to be a major tour de force. The field of alimentary tract surgery had advanced, new research findings were included in the edition, and emerging techniques were illustrated. For the third edition, Dr. Zuidema enlisted the help of a guest editor for each of the five volumes.

The fourth edition, again headed by Dr. Zuidema, was published in 1996 and remained encyclopedic in scope, breadth, and depth of coverage. The textbook had become a classic reference source for surgeons, internists, gastroenterologists, and other health care professionals involved in the care of patients with alimentary tract diseases.

The fifth edition was published in 2002. At that time, Dr. Zuidema asked me to join him as a co-editor. The fifth edition remained a five-volume set, and it was filled with new operative techniques, advances in molecular biology, and noninvasive therapies. It marked progress in the co-management of patients by open surgical, laparoscopic surgical, and endoscopic techniques.

In 2007, the sixth edition of *Shackelford's Surgery of the Alimentary Tract* was published. The look of the sixth edition was changed. The book went from five volumes to two volumes with the deletion of outdated material, and it included a four-color production scheme, emphasized new procedures, and focused on advances in technology. In 2012, the seventh edition was published.

THE EIGHTH EDITION

The eighth edition maintains the exterior changes and look of the sixth and seventh editions. However, the eighth edition has been carefully planned by me and the four expert section editors to represent the current state of alimentary tract surgery as practiced throughout the world. This edition has been completed with an enormous amount of assistance from my four colleagues, who have served as editors for the four major sections of the book. These section editors have worked tirelessly, planning, organizing, and developing this massive textbook. They have incorporated numerous changes in surgical practice, operative techniques, and noninvasive therapies within the text. Although each area does retain sections on anatomy and physiology, the numerous advances in genomics, proteomics, laparoscopic techniques, and robotics are included. The eighth edition includes the contributions of two new and two retained section editors from the seventh edition, providing both innovation and stability.

Section I, Esophagus and Hernia, is now edited by Dr. Steven R. DeMeester, a Professor of Surgery at the University of Southern California, in Los Angeles. Dr. DeMeester is a nationally and internationally known expert who brings his detailed knowledge of the esophagus and esophageal diseases to the textbook. Dr. DeMeester is the son of Dr. Tom DeMeester, a legendary individual who has made numerous contributions to the field. Steve has enlisted new authors for his chapters and has put together a spectacular section on esophageal diseases, including pathology and ambulatory diagnostics, extensive sections on gastroesophageal reflux disease, esophageal motility disorders, and esophageal neoplasia.

Dr. David W. McFadden remains as the editor for Section II, Stomach and Small Intestine. Dr. McFadden works at the University of Connecticut in Farmington, Connecticut, serving as the Professor and Chairman of the Department of Surgery and the Surgeon in Chief of their health system. Dr. McFadden is an expert in alimentary tract diseases, surgical research, and education. He served for many years as the co-editor-in-chief of the *Journal of Surgical Research*, and he has served as the president of the Society for Surgery of the Alimentary Tract. He has done a superb job of enlisting many new chapter authors so as to present an updated section regarding the luminal structures of the upper gastrointestinal system. Dr. McFadden's section is an outstanding contribution to this area.

For Section III, Pancreas, Biliary Tract, Liver, and Spleen, we have retained our section editor, Dr. Jeffrey B. Matthews, the Dallas B. Phemister Professor and Chairman of the Department of Surgery at the University of Chicago, in Chicago, Illinois. Dr. Matthews' surgical career has focused on diseases of the nonluminal structures of the alimentary tract, and he has done a superb job in enlisting new contributors and reorganizing this section. Dr. Matthews' credentials include serving as the editor-in-chief of the *Journal of Gastrointestinal Surgery*, and he is also a recent past president of the Society for Surgery of the Alimentary Tract. This section serves as an outstanding contribution to the field.

Finally, Section IV, Colon, Rectum, and Anus, has been designed and reorganized by Dr. James W. Fleshman, the Seeger Professor and Chairman of the Department of Surgery at Baylor University Medical Center. Dr. Fleshman is an internationally known figure in his field, and his section has been totally reorganized. Included are various new developments in the field, updates on pelvic floor anatomy and physiology, new therapies for inflammatory bowel disease, increased emphasis on laparoscopic interventions, and new chapters dealing with the topics not previously presented.

ACKNOWLEDGMENTS

The eighth edition would have been impossible to complete without the expertise, dedication, and hard work of each of these four expert section editors. They have been helped immensely by their colleagues, staff, and all the chapter contributors. I would like to thank each of these section editors for their vision, dedication, expertise, and incredible hard work in bringing this project to fruition.

As is often the case with printed works of this size, hundreds of individuals have contributed chapters to this edition. In fact, hundreds of contributors are listed in the contributors section. We understand how difficult it is to produce superb chapters, and I wish to recognize these individuals and thank them for their dedication and commitment. Most of these contributors are nationally and internationally known leaders in their fields. I am deeply indebted to them for sharing their knowledge and enthusiasm about their topic, culminating in an outstanding overall product.

I would also like to thank the publishing team at Elsevier, who again have been instrumental in making this edition a reality. My thanks go out to Michael Houston, Mary Hegeler, Amanda Mincher, and many others who have been involved in overseeing this project. This edition represents an enormous amount of new work, and thousands of hours have been spent on its production. These professionals have made it a labor of love to work on this project.

Finally, I must thank individuals who have helped me during this new edition process over the past three years. Here in my office at Thomas Jefferson University, accolades go out to Claire Reinke, Dominique Vicchairelli, and Laura Mateer who have been outstanding assistants in bringing this work to fruition.

Charles J. Yeo, MD

Contents

SECTION **II**

Stomach and Small Intestine

SECTION IV

Colon, Rectum, and Anus

PART ONE

Anatomy, Physiology, and Diagnosis of Colorectal and Anal Diseases

PART TWO

Benign Colon, Rectal, and Anal Conditions

PART FIVE

Techniques and Pearls

Esophagus and Hernia

Anatomy and Physiology of the Esophagus

Esophageal Sphincters in Health and Disease

Karl Hermann Fuchs | Benjamin Babic | Hans Friedrich Fuchs

The esophagus is a muscular tube connecting the mouth with the stomach. The main function of the esophagus is transport of fluids and food to ensure regular nutrition of the body. At the proximal and distal end of the tube, special boundaries are necessary to fulfill complex functional tasks such as swallowing, belching, and vomiting and allowing breathing and coughing, while preventing substantial reflux of gastric contents into the esophagus. The proximal part of the esophagus and its upper esophageal sphincter (UES) comprise mainly striated musculature.[1] In the esophageal corpus, a few centimeters below the UES, the structure switches through a zone of mixed striated-smooth muscle to the distal esophagus including the lower esophageal sphincter (LES) with complete smooth muscle structures. The complex function of the two sphincters is regulated and influenced by nerval innervations, pressure systems, hormonal and chemical influences, and external and possible psychological factors.

UPPER ESOPHAGEAL SPHINCTER IN HEALTH

SWALLOWING PROCESS

The UES is involved in the swallowing process. This process is complex and requires a number of important features to temporarily change the pathway of breathing air between the mouth, nose, pharynx, and the trachea into the channel for passing liquid and food farther into the esophagus.

The main anatomic structures of the upper boundary of the esophagus are the cricopharyngeal muscle connected to the cricoid cartilage. Because there is no circular symmetric muscle structure, but instead a ventral cartilage with lateral and dorsal muscular parts, the resulting pressure profile of the UES is not symmetric. It is important to note that the anatomic relations functionally change during swallowing. The UES moves upward approximately 1 cm because of the laryngeal upward swing. The innervation of the UES is mainly achieved by the vagus nerve and, to a lesser extent, by cranial nerves IX and XII.[1]

Swallowing is a complex process and the UES is involved in the pharyngeal phase, which occurs later in the swallowing process. Depending on the respective author,

swallowing can be described in three to six different phases.[2-6] Three main phases are often differentiated: the oral, pharyngeal, and esophageal phase.

In the oral phase, the tongue and the surrounding structures of the pharynx, the soft and hard palate, and the closed glossopalatal area form a bolus (Fig. 1.1). This process is started by will of the individual. The first step of bolus formation is performed by the soft palate and the posterior aspect of the tongue. The second component of the oral phase is the upward movement of the soft palate toward the hard palate, closing the nasopharynx, and the upward swing of the hyoid bone more ventrally.

When the tongue creates more pressure on the bolus toward the soft and hard palates, the bolus is propelled through the glossopalatal opening and enters the pharyngeal area, thus representing the transition to the pharyngeal phase (Fig. 1.2). The sequences of the pharyngeal phase happen involuntarily. In health, the most important part of the process is the well-coordinated closure of the airway during the passage of the bolus. The nasopharyngeal area is closed by the soft palate and the posterior pharyngeal wall. The muscles of the floor of the mouth pull the hyoid bone, and subsequently the larynx and cricoid, anteriorly and upward, thus allowing the epiglottis to flip downward and close off the airways.

The constrictor pharyngeal muscle contracts, and the UES is opened by approximately 1 second of relaxation. The bolus leaves the pharyngeal area, moves through the hypopharynx, and into the esophagus. The esophageal phase begins as the bolus enters the proximal esophagus through the opened cricopharyngeal sphincter (Fig. 1.3). The peristaltic contractions take over propulsion of the bolus and assist gravity in transporting the bolus through the esophageal corpus. Finally, all structures return to their resting positions, and the airway is opened again as the UES closes.

ASSESSMENT OF THE UPPER ESOPHAGEAL SPHINCTER

The UES comprises cricoid cartilage at the ventral border and cricopharyngeal muscle toward its lateral and posterior borders.[1] This structure creates the asymmetric pressure

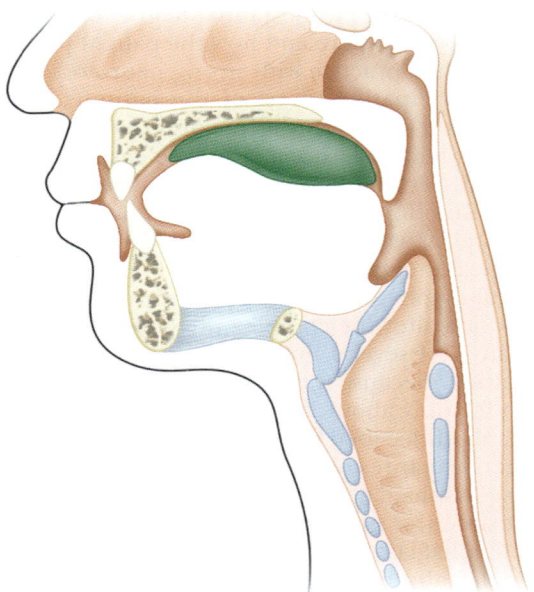

FIGURE 1.1 The swallowing process: The tongue has formed a bolus between the ventral part of the tongue and its posterior part against the soft palate.

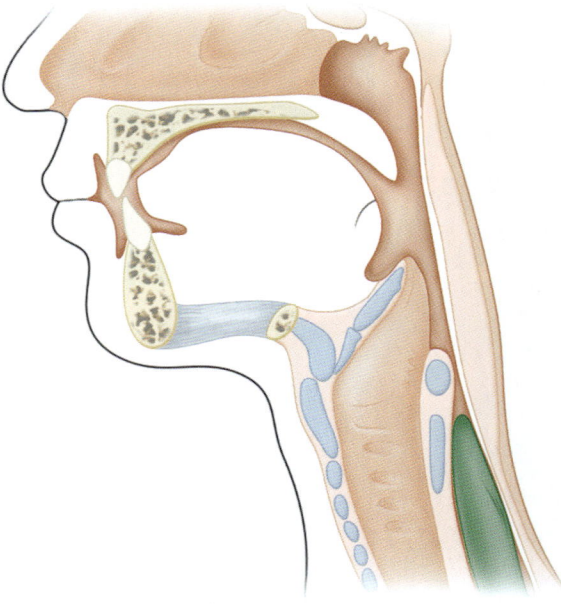

FIGURE 1.3 The swallowing process: The upper esophageal sphincter is fully relaxed for a short time in which the bolus passes into the proximal esophagus, where it is pushed farther by gravity and esophageal peristalsis. The larynx and epiglottis then resume their resting positions.

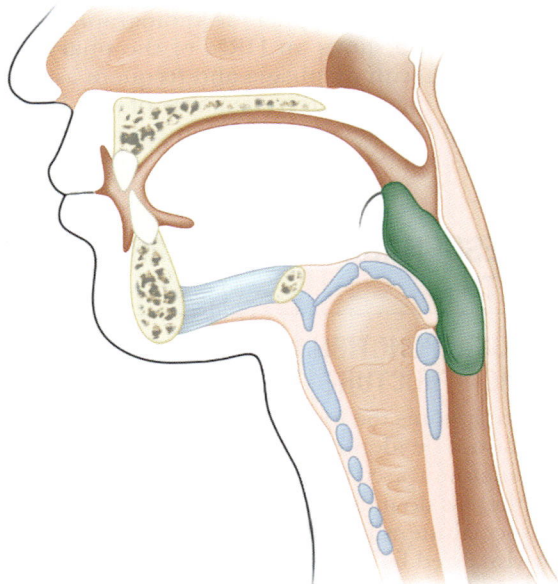

FIGURE 1.2 The swallowing process: The soft palate is lifted upward toward the hard palate, thus closing off the nasopharynx. The tongue pushes the bolus backward into the pharynx. The hyoid bone and the larynx are pulled upward, thus causing the epiglottis to flip down and close off the trachea. The upper esophageal sphincter relaxes to prepare the passage of the bolus.

profile of the sphincter. Functional assessment of the UES is usually performed by radiographic studies or manometric techniques.[2-5] Routine radiographic investigations by barium swallow provide insight into the swallowing process and demonstrate pathologic anatomic alterations such as a Zenker diverticulum. However, a subtle functional failure of the regular swallowing process—for example, as a result of a discrete neurologic defect causing cervical dysphagia—might be missed. High-speed photography using a specialized kinematographic analysis may be necessary to describe dysfunctions in detail.[4] Video documentation allows for repetitive visualization and analysis of the findings.

Clinical assessment of symptoms is necessary to clearly determine the underlying functional problem and the impact of the disorder on the patient's quality of life. Endoscopy is important in detecting or excluding malignant disease and obstruction.

Pharyngoesophageal manometric studies can demonstrate the physiologic swallowing function through the UES and possibly its pathologic changes.[5,7-10] The UES is asymmetric and changes its pressure profile in milliseconds during swallowing. Consequently, traditional perfusion manometry with a few recorded openings and manometry probes with only a few solid-state pressure transducers cannot demonstrate subtle pressure increases or relaxations or coordination features along the vertical axis. Manometry systems with multiple recording sites along the probe and circumferentially on the probe are necessary to record sufficient data to fully describe the complex process of

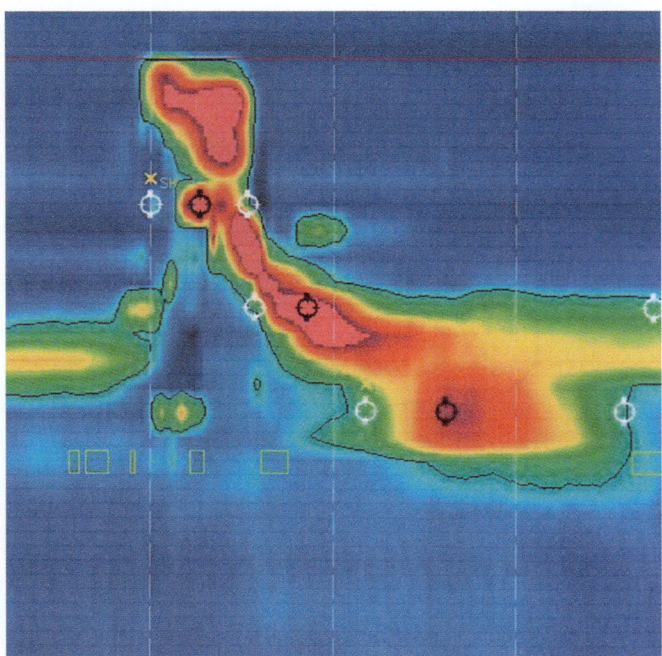

FIGURE 1.4 High-resolution manometry of the pharynx and upper esophageal sphincter (UES) in a healthy individual. The contraction of the soft palate, subsequent pharyngeal contraction, and relaxation of the UES is demonstrated. In addition, the pressurization proximal to the original level of the UES can be noticed, reflecting the upward movement of the larynx and the UES during the closure of the airways.

swallowing, not to mention the possible pathologic changes that occur in a functional disorder.

Manometry allows assessment of the pressure changes during swallowing, the relaxation of the UES, and the subsequent contractions of the esophagus. Because the UES is asymmetric, the actual opening of the UES is sometimes not accurately detected.[8]

More recently, high-resolution manometry (HRM) techniques have provided better insight into the process of swallowing, pressure changes at the UES, and their association with esophageal pressurization.[10] In HRM, the swallowing process at the UES can be followed quite accurately (Fig. 1.4). Pharyngeal contractions and UES relaxation are monitored, and their coordination can be appreciated along the timeline. HRM allows for investigations in different circumstances.

CHANGES OF THE UPPER ESOPHAGEAL SPHINCTER IN DISEASE

There are many disorders that can cause cervical or oropharyngeal dysphagia, including myogenic, neurogenic, iatrogenic, mechanical, and psychogenic disorders, as well as idiopathic dysfunctions of the UES, the esophageal corpus, and the LES with associated gastroesophageal reflux disease (GERD), and other esophageal and gastric disorders or obstructions that influence sensation and swallowing at the UES.[6,8,9]

The composition of a patient population with cervical dysphagia depends to a substantial degree on individual circumstances and where and how the patient population is evaluated. In a practice with strong neurologic and/or geriatric participation, most of the patients will have neurogenic and possibly myogenic disorders. In a practice with more esophageal, surgical, and/or gastroenterologic background, cervical dysphagia is often related to idiopathic dysfunctions of the UES, LES, and esophageal corpus as well as associated motor disorders and problems after surgical therapy or radiotherapy.

Cervical dysphagia is often caused by neurogenic disorders, which alter the complex physiologic process and coordination of several muscles and structures involved in swallowing. Because the UES opens in the physiologic situation for only about 1 second to let the bolus pass, it can be easily understood that slight failures of coordination with other structures or insufficient opening of the UES can cause dysphagia.

There are three groups of possible reasons for oropharyngeal dysphagia: anatomic reasons, neurologic reasons, or muscular abnormalities.[6] Possible anatomic sources include a local tumor, an enlarged thyroid, an abscess, a Zenker diverticulum, or scarring as a result of accidents, surgery, or irradiation. Neurologic causes are cerebral infarction, poliomyelitis, neuronal disease, Parkinson disease, multiple sclerosis, and other cerebral diseases and disorders. Muscular disorders include polymyositis, muscular dystrophy, and myasthenia gravis. Usually, precise coordination and/or muscular strength are lost, causing cervical dysphagia.

Functional testing is useful to determine the cause of the dysphagia and should include radiographic studies and HRM. Fig. 1.5 shows an HRM of the pharynx and UES in a patient with dysphagia and frequent aspiration resulting from incomplete relaxation of the UES and hypertensive pharyngeal contraction associated with a neurologic disorder.

LOWER ESOPHAGEAL SPHINCTER IN HEALTH

PHYSIOLOGIC FUNCTION AND ANATOMIC STRUCTURE

The LES represents the lower boundary of the esophageal tube. It cannot be identified from inside the abdomen as a visible anatomic area at the lower end of the esophagus because there is no muscular thickening of the esophageal wall or special identifiable muscular structure. It can be roughly visualized by endoscopy and radiographic studies, but it can be best demonstrated and assessed quantitatively with esophageal manometry.

The major function of the LES is closure of the gastric reservoir to prevent reflux of gastric contents back into the esophagus. This is important because gastric juice can be toxic for the esophageal mucosa.[11] However, the LES cannot exclusively function as a one-way valve just for ingested liquid and food to pass into the stomach, because it must also allow for selective retrograde passage of gas, usually ingested air, from the stomach. In healthy

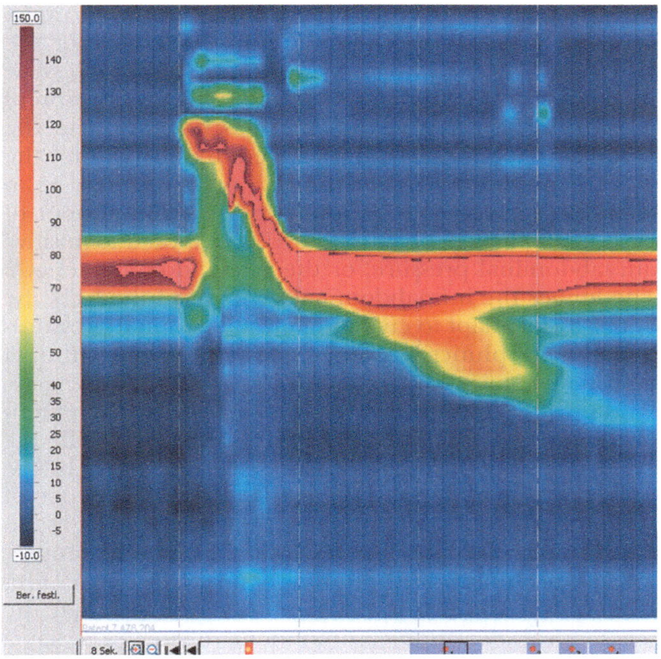

FIGURE 1.5 High-resolution manometry of the pharynx and upper esophageal sphincter in a patient with dysphagia, based on insufficient relaxation of the upper esophageal sphincter and hypertensive contractions because of a neurologic disorder.

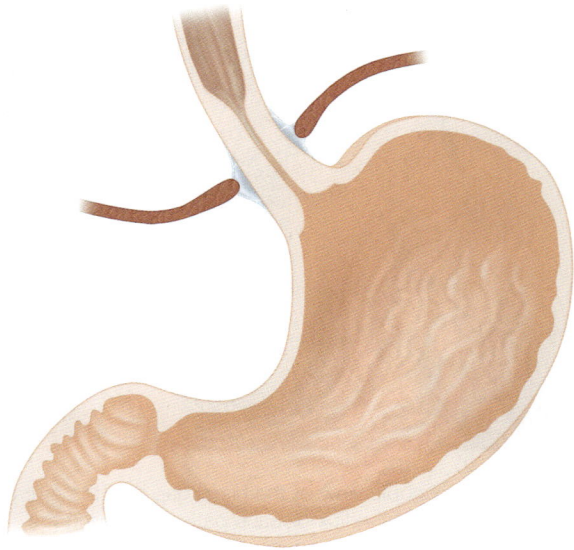

FIGURE 1.6 Schematic demonstration of the lower esophageal sphincter and the gastroesophageal junction showing the lower esophageal sphincter, the stomach, the diaphragm, and the phrenoesophageal membrane.

individuals, mechanisms prevent an overload of air in the stomach and small bowel with subsequent substantial discomfort for the individual. Excessive intragastric air can be vented through the LES back into the esophagus and outside transorally.

In several diseases, particularly those with partial or total obstruction of a normal gastric emptying or small bowel paralysis, vomiting can be an important mechanism to solve the problem. Thus, the physiologic LES must allow for this retrograde emptying of the stomach.

The anatomic structure of the LES was best studied by Liebermann-Meffert.[1] A detailed analysis of fiber specimens shows, in the distal esophagus and proximal stomach, several different bundles of muscle fibers that create this high-pressure zone. Although in the esophageal corpus there is a distinct two-layer formation of longitudinal and circular muscles, at the gastroesophageal junction, one can find so-called semicircular muscular claps toward the lesser curvature. On the left side of the cardia at the angle of His, gastric sling fibers create the lower end of the LES, forming the left part of the high-pressure zone. These structural elements create a certain thickening at the LES with an asymmetric structural and functional high-pressure zone. Vagal branches regulate the neurologic function of the LES.

The second important anatomic structure that is responsible for the lower boundary of the esophagus is the diaphragm and its crura, the diaphragmatic arch at the hiatal opening, and the phrenoesophageal membrane, fixing the distal esophagus in its position within the hiatal opening (Fig. 1.6). Inspiration creates a negative pressure in the thoracic environment and an increased positive pressure environment in the abdominal cavity. Additional body activity of a person will further increase intraabdominal pressure. The phrenoesophageal membrane and the esophagus itself, filling the hiatal gap, are under constant pressure changes because of the positive intraabdominal pressure environment and the negative thoracic pressure environment during respiration.

In healthy individuals, the phrenoesophageal membrane is not just a circular ligament, because the hiatal opening or gap is not a circular structure. Depending on the size of the individual, this transition zone of the distal esophagus through the hiatal opening has a length of 1 to 3 cm. The main body of the crura develop their muscle structure from a caudal posterior position toward the ventral and more cranial position to unify at the hiatal arch, thus surrounding the LES in an almost circular fashion, usually with an open posterior part on the aorta. The posterior part of the opening is represented by the aorta, on which the crura are also fixed partially or sometimes completely. The latter carries a certain risk because clinical observations have shown that quite often in young reflux patients, the left crus is shorter than the right one, and its insertion is weakened by spreading out on the anterior aspect of the aorta, which limits its stable fixation point posteriorly (Fig. 1.7).

In healthy individuals, the structures at the hiatal gap have to keep the cardia in its position over decades despite a constant tendency to wear out secondary to respiratory movements, coughing, and pressure increases from the abdominal and the thoracic environments, while still allowing for some flexibility such as movements of the esophagus during swallowing.[11] Given this situation, it is not surprising that over decades, the system becomes insufficient in some people. The tissue in some people

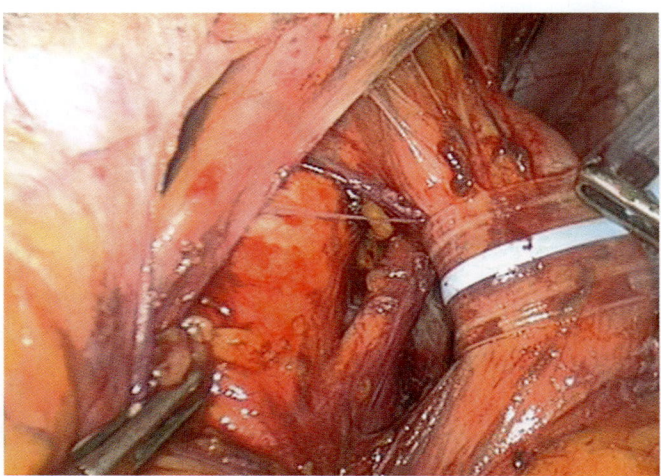

FIGURE 1.7 Laparoscopic view of the hiatal gap and the crura in a young gastroesophageal reflux disease patient, showing the shortage of the left crus, causing insufficient fixation of the lower esophageal sphincter by the phrenoesophageal membrane.

weakens and structures elongate, finally resulting in sliding of structures within the hiatal opening and into the chest, thus creating a sliding hiatal hernia.

FUNCTIONAL CHARACTERISTICS OF THE LOWER ESOPHAGEAL SPHINCTER AND THE ANTIREFLUX BARRIER

The major functional finding at the distal esophagus is a high-pressure zone. Over decades, traditional esophageal manometry was performed by perfusion catheters with multiple radially oriented recording openings. Over the past 40 years there have emerged two major concepts regarding the quantitative manometric description of the antireflux barrier. One is a more mechanical description by the surgical DeMeester school.[11-13] The second was developed mainly by gastroenterologists Dent and Dodds, and invokes a more dynamic concept involving transient lower esophageal sphincter relaxations (tLESR).[14,15]

Following the DeMeester school, the LES can be characterized by three manometrically assessed components: the overall length of the high-pressure zone, the sphincter pressure, and the sphincter position, expressed by the intraabdominal length of the high-pressure zone.[11,12] The quantitative assessment of the sphincter was based on the rather limited measurements provided by traditional perfusion manometry. The perfusion catheter usually consisted of five radially oriented side holes, through which water was perfused and pressure changes were recorded initially on paper and later on computer software. Considering the complex movements and subtle pressure changes as well as positional changes of LES during breathing and swallowing, the harvest of data using the early water-perfused systems was very limited.

In healthy individuals, the high-pressure zone in the distal esophagus can be measured from the thoracic part of the distal esophagus through the hiatal opening to the intraabdominal part of the esophagus and the proximal stomach. In the normal physiologic condition, this high-pressure zone is 3 to 5 cm long and has a mean pressure of 14 mm Hg depending on the size of the individual.[11,12] The LES must create an effective pressure (resistance) over a certain length to fulfill its function of preventing substantial reflux of gastric juice into the esophagus. It should be emphasized that the shorter the overall length, the higher the LES pressure must be to maintain its barrier function. A critical component of overall length is the length of the LES exposed to positive intraabdominal pressure, or the intraabdominal length. The longer the intraabdominal segment of the LES, the better it can adapt to changing intraabdominal pressures to maintain sphincter competence and prevent reflux of gastric juice into the esophagus.

Many publications have shown that the measurement of these three characteristics of the LES is clinically relevant.[13,16-18] As GERD severity worsens, as assessed by the presence of symptoms, esophagitis, and the presence of complications such as stricture or Barrett esophagus, an increasing number of deficiencies in overall length, intraabdominal length, and pressure can be demonstrated.[16,18] Therefore, it can be clearly stated that the mechanical measurable components of the LES play a major role in the function of the antireflux barrier and these criteria can be used for decision making and assessment of disease severity.

The gastroenterologists Dent and Dodds described the concept of tLESR as a significant mechanism of gastroesophageal reflux in normal individuals and in patients with GERD.[14,15] These tLESRs are identified by manometric sleeve technology systems as further developed by Dent, which allow for pressure measurement over the complete length of the high-pressure zone. It must be emphasized that these relaxations of the high-pressure zone occurred without previous swallowing and without pharyngeal contractions. They also showed that these relaxations are coordinated with crural diaphragmatic relaxations.[19] Based on these findings, tLESR became accepted in gastroenterology as the major mechanism of gastroesophageal reflux.

However, there is controversy regarding this phenomenon because studies in healthy subjects and patients showed that tLESRs were most severe in the postprandial phase. This may indicate that LES relaxations could be associated with gastric filling and/or gastric distention.[14] Further controversies around the concept of the tLESR arose when manometric studies showed that postprandial distention of the stomach caused sphincter shortening. Radiographic studies supported this finding. Fig. 1.8 demonstrates the enlargement of the gastric fundus by overfilling of the fundus, which is a common phenomenon in Western societies as a result of overeating. Excessive filling of the gastric fundus will pull the distal part of the high-pressure zone apart because of fundic accommodation, thus shortening the LES even in healthy persons. As mentioned previously, the shorter the overall length of the high-pressure zone, the higher the pressure must be for the LES to remain competent. If the stomach is filled by food and/or ingested air, sphincter shortening can occur. With progressive shortening and loss if intraabdominal sphincter length, the LES pressure becomes unable to maintain competency, and once the intragastric pressure reaches the LES residual pressure, the LES gives

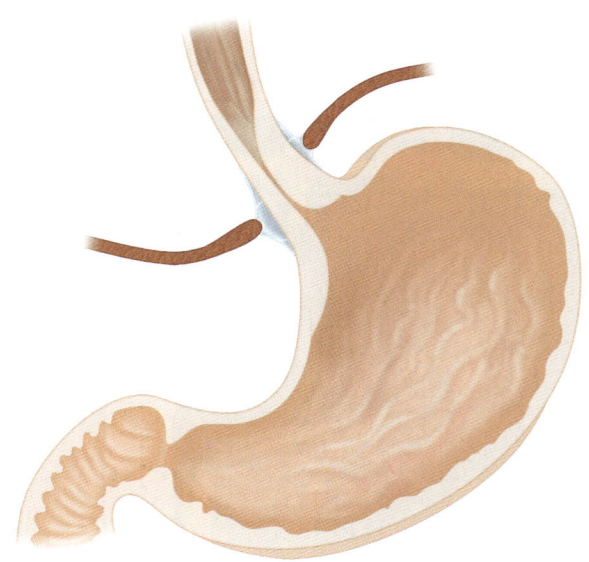

FIGURE 1.8 Schematic demonstration of the stepwise shortening of the lower esophageal sphincter and weakening of the phrenoesophageal membrane by enlargement of the fundus, for example, because of overeating.

way and will manometrically appear as tLESRs because the LES pressure drops to zero during opening of the sphincter. Thus, critics of the tLESR concept argue that tLESRs may in fact represent transient LES shortenings resulting from gastric distention.[19,20] This would explain why tLESRs increase in the postprandial phase and why, in patients with advanced reflux disease and a destroyed LES, there is not a substantial increase in tLESRs as one would otherwise expect if the tLESRs were the cause of the reflux.[20]

With the advent of HRM, the number of pressure-detecting recording sites has increased tremendously.[21-23] Current HRM technology has 36 recording site levels that are 1 cm apart on the probe, with circumferential recording at each level. This technology allows for an integral assessment of pressure changes of the complete esophageal corpus, the proximal and distal high-pressure zones, as well as pressure changes of the surrounding structures such as the diaphragm and its respiratory-dependent changes. This new technology has clinical advantages because it allows for the assessment of complex pressure profiles in the physiologic situation as well as in pathologic circumstances. Fig. 1.9 demonstrates an LES area with a pressure profile of the complete antireflux barrier, that is, the LES and the diaphragmatic pressure influences are combined in the gastroesophageal junction high-pressure zone.

LOWER ESOPHAGEAL SPHINCTER IN DISEASE

The most frequent form of failure of the LES is weakening or incompetence leading to increased gastroesophageal reflux.[12,13,16-18] This phenomenon is usually accompanied by structural changes of the hiatal architecture and the cardia. The weakening of the sphincter and the weakening of the phrenoesophageal ligament with changing position of the sphincter within the diaphragm can result in a total loss of antireflux barrier function.

Other disorders of the LES are isolated hypertension of the LES causing increased resistance during swallowing and therefore dysphagia, or a failure of relaxation during swallowing. A well-described disease entity is achalasia. One major element of achalasia is the nonrelaxing LES, often in combination with hypertensive muscular tone of the high-pressure zone and loss of peristaltic abilities of the esophageal corpus.

LOWER ESOPHAGEAL SPHINCTER IN GASTROESOPHAGEAL REFLUX DISEASE

In patients with GERD, the high-pressure zone and the other structural components of the antireflux barrier such as the phrenoesophageal membrane can weaken over time. Very often, a sequence of changes occurs over many years, leading to progressively worsening gastroesophageal reflux. There is a high prevalence of GERD in Western industrial societies. One can speculate that the initial problem is overeating, which enlarges the fundus and effaces the intraabdominal portion of the LES. This exposes the effaced portion of the LES to the acid pocket in the stomach after a meal, with subsequent injury to the distal portion of the LES. Over time the damage gradually leads to loss of the intraabdominal length of the LES, and progressively more effacement until the sphincter completely loses competence and frank GERD develops. In addition, increased intraabdominal pressure because of intraabdominal fat leads to weakening of the supporting structures of the esophagus within the hiatal opening. Combined with tissue weakening as a result of age, the initially strong phrenoesophageal membrane becomes a loose fatty hernia sac, which facilitates a temporary sliding of the LES in the chest. Later, the LES will move to a permanent position in the lower mediastinum (Fig. 1.10).

Many publications have shown the loss of LES competence in GERD and the relationships among disease severity, the presence of its complications, and the increasing incidence of LES incompetence in these patients.[11-18] Patients with advanced GERD typically have a hiatal hernia and an incompetent LES on manometry. Using HRM, the LES and the pressure influences from the diaphragm are displayed. In someone without a hiatal hernia, these pressures are superimposed to form one gastroesophageal junction pressure (see Fig. 1.9). When a hiatal hernia is present, the LES and the hiatal structure separate and the separate pressure influences of the LES and the diaphragm become evident (Fig. 1.11). This allows for the description of a hiatal hernia in the HRM pressure profile.

These findings can be important for therapeutic decision making regarding further medical treatment or a laparoscopic antireflux procedure.[24,25] The manometric finding of a loss of mechanical sphincter function has a prognostic component. Kuster showed that patients with GERD and an incompetent sphincter on manometry have a higher probability of having GERD problems after 10

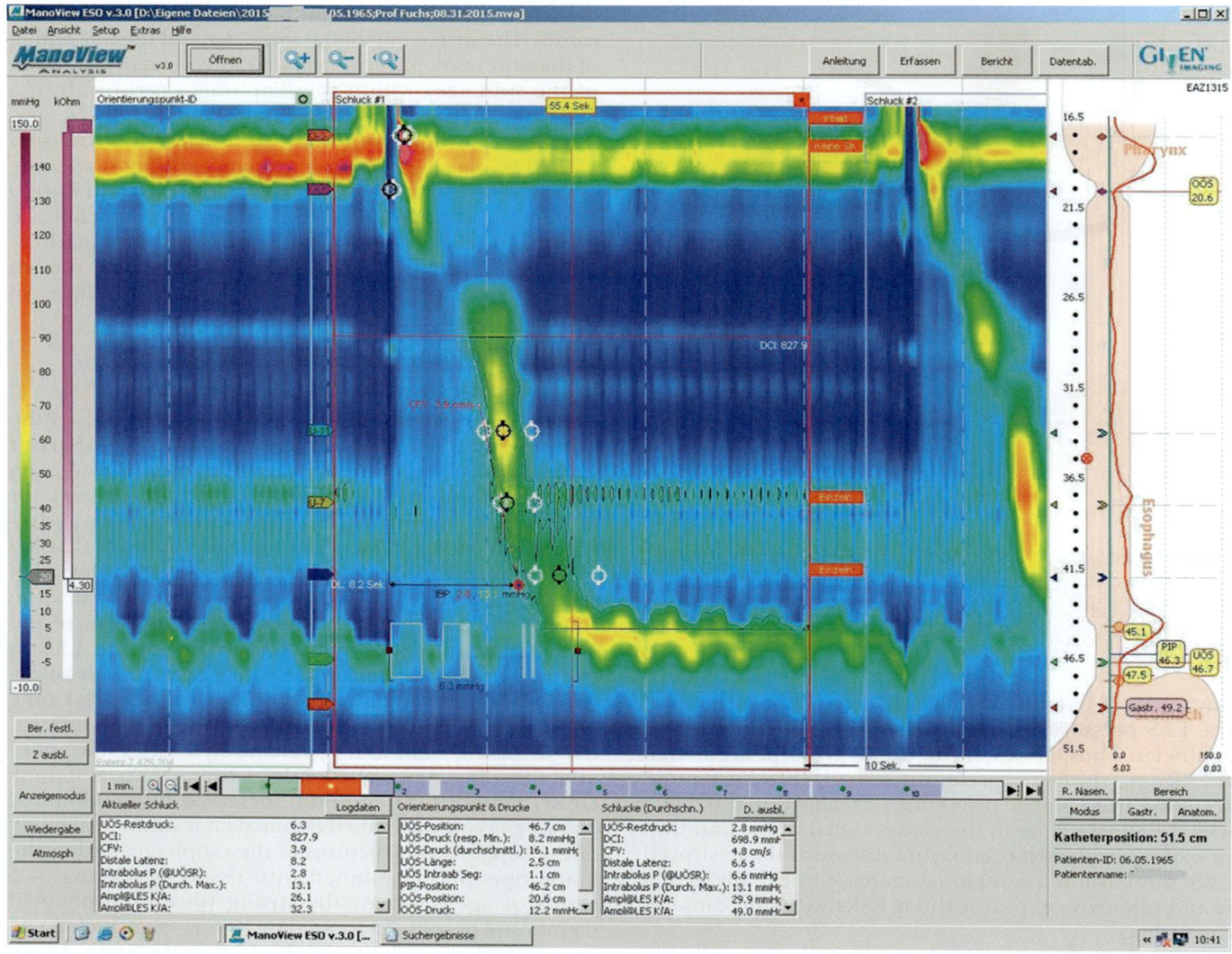

FIGURE 1.9 High-resolution manometry of the esophagus: demonstration of the esophageal body and lower esophageal sphincter in a healthy individual, showing swallowing and relaxation of the lower esophageal sphincter.

years, which could be an argument for earlier surgical therapy.[26]

LOWER ESOPHAGEAL SPHINCTER FUNCTION IN PATIENTS WITH ACHALASIA AND OTHER ESOPHAGEAL MOTILITY DISORDERS

Dysphagia related to solids and liquids is the most common complaint in patients with esophageal motility disorders. Some patients also experience chest pain. Although most of the esophageal motility disorders are rather nonspecific changes of peristaltic contractions, achalasia is the best-defined and probably best-described esophageal motility disorder.

One major sign of achalasia is a failure of the LES to relax during swallowing. This leads to obstruction of the bolus transport. In addition to relaxation failure, the esophageal body loses its ability to develop a normal peristalsis leading to a total failure of transport.[22,27,28] Retrosternal pain or burning can occur in achalasia as a

result of simultaneous and/or spastic contractions and/or retention esophagitis, caused by long-standing remainders of food in the esophageal body because of obstruction. Interestingly, the resting pressure of the nonrelaxing LES can vary in achalasia from physiologic values up to massive hypertension. An unfavorable relationship between persisting pressure in the LES and the absence of esophageal peristalsis is important when considering obstruction. As a result, only gravity and/or a rise in intraluminal hydrostatic pressure because of the food and fluid column can overcome the persistent pressure in the LES.

The diagnostic work-up for patients with achalasia and all other esophageal motility disorders should consist of a combination of investigations to describe the alterations at the LES.[21,27,28] Endoscopy should be done to rule out any malignant disease, scarring, or a peptic stricture. An upper gastrointestinal (GI) radiographic study performed as a timed barium swallow can demonstrate and quantify the degree of esophageal outflow obstruction at the LES. HRM will confirm the diagnosis and can be used to subclassify the type of achalasia, which has implications for treatment.[21,22,29] The working group in Chicago has published the Chicago classification based on the difference in esophageal motility in patients with achalasia.[22] Currently, achalasia patients can be subdivided in Chicago type I (hypomotile esophageal body), Chicago type II (simultaneous tonic contraction after swallowing), and Chicago type III (massive, simultaneous, high-pressure contractions of the distal esophagus). All types show a loss of normal LES relaxations.

HYPERTENSIVE LOWER ESOPHAGEAL SPHINCTER

Another disorder of the LES, which has been called *hypertensive LES*, can be documented in some patients with dysphagia and retrosternal pain.[30,31] In these patients, the LES pressure is elevated and there may be impaired opening, but there is preserved esophageal body peristalsis, which separates this entity from achalasia. Treatment is aimed at lowering the LES pressure with onabotulinumtoxinA (Botox), pneumatic dilation, or myotomy of the sphincter laparoscopically or using a peroral technique.

CONCLUSION

The esophageal tube is responsible for the transport of food from the mouth to the stomach, and to keep gastric

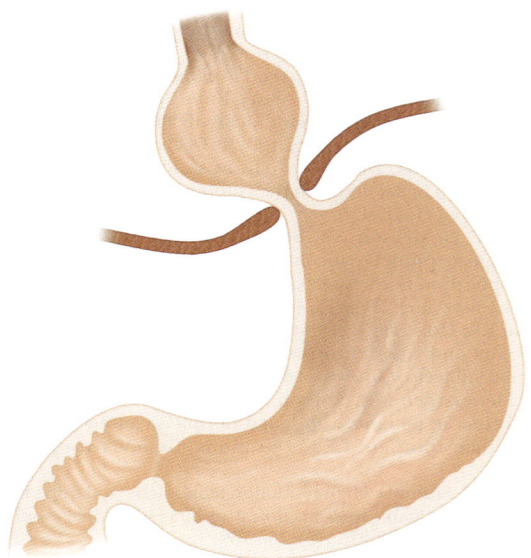

FIGURE 1.10 Schematic demonstration of the gastroesophageal junction and the alterations as a result of a hiatal hernia. The phrenoesophageal membrane has deteriorated from a firm ligament into a floppy and fatty hernia sac.

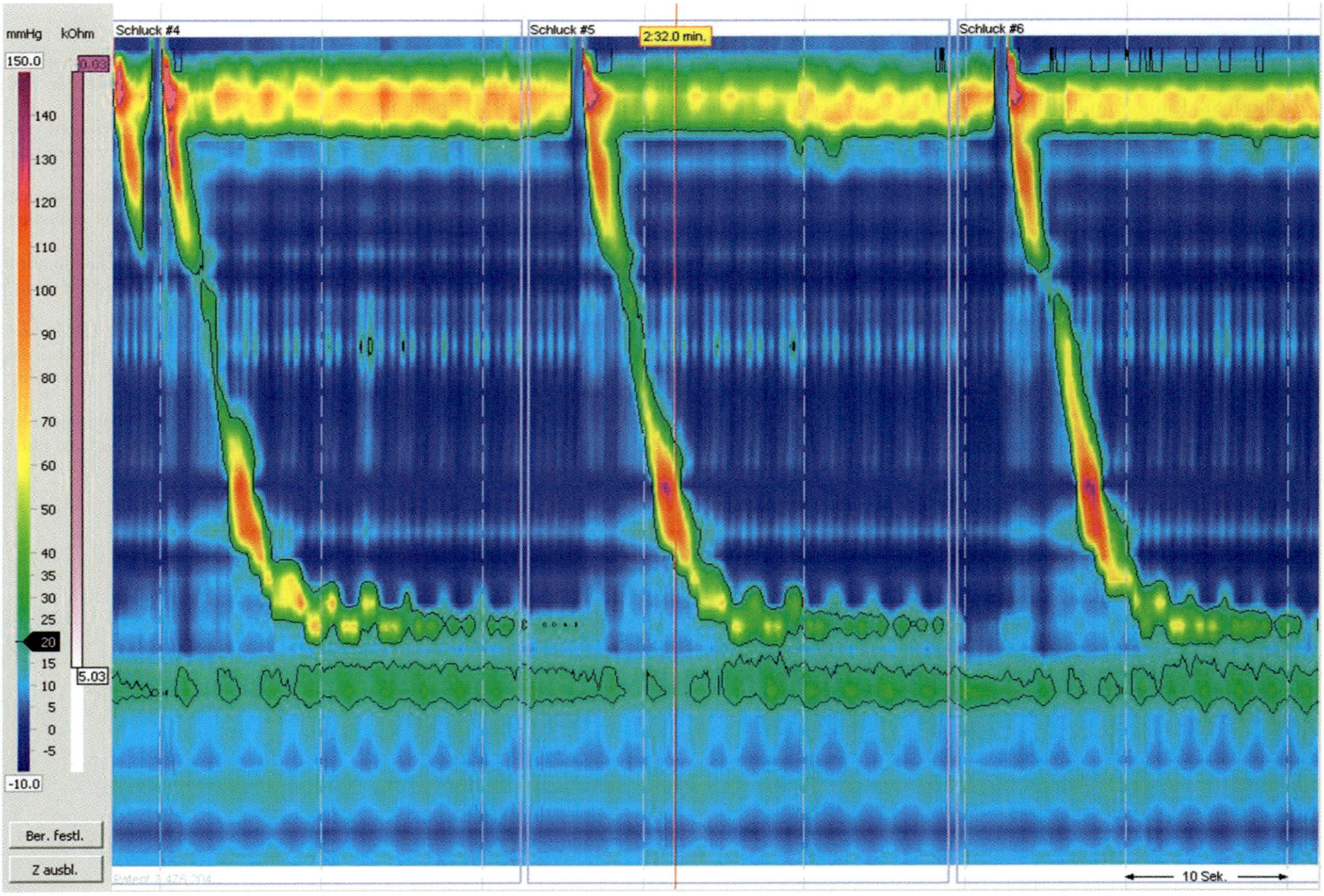

FIGURE 1.11 High-resolution manometry in a patient with gastroesophageal reflux disease and hiatal hernia. The weak lower esophageal sphincter can be noted as well as the separation of the remaining pressure level of the lower esophageal sphincter and the diaphragmatic structures.

contents in the stomach once they reach it. This simple requirement involves complex interactions involving pharyngeal muscles, the diaphragm, the UES and LES, and coordinated peristalsis in the esophageal body. These complex physiologic mechanisms allow for a number of critical points where malfunction can create symptoms.

REFERENCES

1. Liebermann-Meffert D, Duranceau A. Anatomy and embryology of the esophagus. In: Orringer MB, Zuidema GD, eds. *Shackelford's Surgery of the Alimentary Tract, Vol 1, The Esophagus.* 4th ed. Philadephia: Saunders; 1996:3-38.
2. Dodds WJ, Hogan WJ, Lyndon SB. Quantification of pharyngeal motor function in human subjects. *J Appl Physiol.* 1975;39:960.
3. Donner MW, Bosma JF, Robertson DL. Neuromuscular disorders of the pharynx. *Gastrointest Radiol.* 1985;10:196.
4. Hannig C, Wuttge-Hannig A. Status of high-frequency roentgen cinematography in the diagnosis of the pharynx and esophagus. *Rontgenpraxis.* 1987;40(10):358-377.
5. Kahrilas PJ, Dodds WJ, Dent J, Logemann JA, Shaker R. Upper esophageal sphincter function during deglutition. *Gastroenterology.* 1988;95(1):52-62.
6. Duranceau A. Disorders of the pharyngoesophageal junction. In: Yeo CJ, ed. *Shackelford's Surgery of the Alimentary Tract.* Vol. 1. 6th ed. Philadelphia: Saunders; 2007:374-390.
7. Castell JA, Dalton CB, Castell DO. Pharyngeal and upper esophageal sphincter manometry in humans. *Am J Physiol.* 1990;21:G73.
8. Cook IJ, Gabb M, Panagopoulos V, et al. Pharyngeal (Zenker's) diverticulum is a disorder of upper esophageal sphincter opening. *Gastroenterology.* 1992;103(4):1229-1235.
9. Goyal RK, Martin SB, Shapiro J, Spechler SJ. The role of cricopharyngeus muscle in pharyngoesophageal disorders. *Dysphagia.* 1993;8(3):252-258.
10. Ghosh SK, Pandolfino JE, Zhang Q, Jarosz A, Kahrilas PJ. Deglutitive upper esophageal sphincter relaxation: a study of 75 volunteer subjects using solid-state high-resolution manometry. *Am J Physiol Gastrointest Liver Physiol.* 2006;291(3):G525-G531.
11. DeMeester TR. Definition, detection and pathophysiology of gastroesophageal reflux disease. In: DeMeester TR, Matthews HR, eds. *International Trends in General Thoracic Surgery, Vol 3, Benign Esophageal Disease.* St. Louis: Mosby; 1987:99-127.
12. Zaninotto G, DeMeester TR, Schwizer W, Johansson KE, Cheng SC. The lower esophageal sphincter in health and disease. *Am J Surg.* 1988;155(1):104-111.
13. Fuchs KH, Freys SM, Heimbucher J, Fein M, Thiede A. Pathophysiologic spectrum in patients with gastroesophageal reflux disease in a surgical GI function laboratory. *Dis Esophagus.* 1995;8:211-217.
14. Dent J, Holloway RH, Toouli J, Dodds WJ. Mechanisms of lower oesophageal sphincter incompetence in patients with symptomatic gastro-oesophageal reflux. *Gut.* 1988;29:1020-1028.
15. Mittal RK, Holloway RH, Penagini R, Blackshaw A, Dent J. Transient lower esophageal sphincter relaxations. *Gastroenterology.* 1995;109:601-610.
16. Stein HJ, Barlow AP, DeMeester TR, Hinder RA. Complications of gastroesophageal reflux disease. Role of the lower esophageal sphincter, esophageal acid and acid/alkaline exposure, and duodenogastric reflux. *Ann Surg.* 1992;216(1):35-43.
17. Fein M, Ritter M, DeMeester TR, et al. Role of lower esophageal sphincter and hiatal hernia in the pathogenesis of GERD. *J Gastrointest Surg.* 1999;3(4):405-410.
18. Lord RV, DeMeester SR, Peters JH, et al. Hiatal hernia, lower esophageal sphincter incompetence, and effectiveness of Nissen fundoplication in the spectrum of gastroesophageal reflux disease. *J Gastrointest Surg.* 2009;13(4):602-610.
19. Mittal RK, Holloway R, Dent J. Effect of atropine on the frequency of reflux and transient lower esophageal sphincter relaxation in normal subjects. *Gastroenterology.* 1995;109(5):1547-1554.
20. Van Herwaarden MA, Samson M, Smout AJP. Excess gastroesophageal reflux in patients with hiatal hernia is caused by mechanisms other than transient LES relaxations. *Gastroenterology.* 2000;119:1439.
21. Kahrilas PJ, Sifrim D. High-resolution manometry and impedance-pH/manometry: valuable tools in clinical and investigational esophagology. *Gastroenterology.* 2008;135(3):756-769.
22. Pandolfino JE, Kwiatek MA, Nealis T, Bulsiewicz W, Post J, Kahrilas PJ. Achalasia: a new clinically relevant classification by high-resolution manometry. *Gastroenterology.* 2008;135(5):1526-1533.
23. Kahrilas PJ. Esophageal motor disorders in terms of high-resolution esophageal pressure topography: what has changed? *Am J Gastroenterol.* 2010;105(5):981-987.
24. Stefanidis D, Hope WW, Kohn GP, et al. Guidelines for surgical treatment of GERD. *Surg Endosc.* 2010;24(11):2647-2669.
25. Fuchs KH, Babic B, Breithaupt W, et al. EAES recommendations for the management of gastroesophageal reflux disease. *Surg Endosc.* 2014;28(6):1753-1773.
26. Kuster E, Ros E, Toledo-Pimentel V, et al. Predictive factors of the long term outcome in gastro-oesophageal reflux disease: six year follow up of 107 patients. *Gut.* 1994;35(1):8-14.
27. Zaninotto G, Costantini M, Rizetto C, et al. Four hundred laparoscopic myotomies for esopahegal achalasia—a single center experience. *Ann Surg.* 2008;248:986-993.
28. Campos GM, Vittinghoff E, Rabel C, et al. Endoscopic and surgical treatments of achalasia: a system review and meta-analysis. *Ann Surg.* 2009;249:45-57.
29. Kahrilas PJ, Bredenoord AJ, Fox M, et al. The Chicago Classification of esophageal motility disorders, v3.0. *Neurogastroenterol Motil.* 2015;27:160-174.
30. Gockel I, Lord RV, Bremner CG, Crookes PF, Hamrah P, DeMeester TR. The hypertensive lower esophageal sphincter: a motility disorder with manometric features of outflow obstruction. *J Gastrointest Surg.* 2003;7(5):692-700.
31. Tamhankar AP, Almogy G, Arain MA, et al. Surgical management of hypertensive lower esophageal sphincter with dysphagia or chest pain. *J Gastrointest Surg.* 2003;7(8):990-996.

Esophageal Body in Health and Disease

Marco E. Allaix | Marco G. Patti

High-resolution manometry (HRM) is a well-established diagnostic tool that evaluates esophageal motility. It dynamically measures intraluminal pressure changes in the esophagus by using closely spaced pressure sensors. Data are acquired, displayed, and interpreted by esophageal pressure topography plots.[1]

The Chicago Classification aims to define esophageal motility disorders according to HRM findings. This classification was first proposed in 2008[2] and then updated in 2011[3] and in 2014.[4,5] The latest version, the Chicago Classification, version 3.0,[4,5] evaluates new parameters when compared with the previous versions, including esophagogastric junction (EGJ) morphology and contractility at rest, "fragmented" contractions, and ineffective esophageal motility (IEM). This classification categorizes (1) disorders of the EGJ outflow, such as achalasia and EGJ outflow obstruction, (2) major peristalsis disorders such as absent contractility, distal esophageal spasm and hyper contractile esophagus, and (3) minor disorders characterized by impaired bolus transit.

The aim of this chapter is to review the esophageal function in the healthy esophagus and in the most frequent esophageal motility disorders.

ESOPHAGEAL BODY IN HEALTH

The evaluation of esophageal motility by HRM is based on the assessment of ten 5-mL water swallows performed in supine position (Fig. 2.1). During each swallow the following features are evaluated:
- EGJ relaxation
- esophageal contractile activity
- esophageal pressurization
  The pressure topographic measurements used are
- *integrated relaxation pressure (IRP)*
- *distal contractile integral (DCI)*
- *contractile deceleration point (CDP)*
- *distal latency (DL)*

EVALUATION OF THE ESOPHAGOGASTRIC JUNCTION MORPHOLOGY AND DEGLUTITIVE ESOPHAGEAL CONTRACTION

During swallowing, the pressure detected at the level of the EGJ is defined by lower esophageal sphincter (LES) pressure, contraction of crural diaphragm (CD), and intrabolus pressure as the swallowed bolus passes through the EGJ.[6] IRP, defined as the mean pressure for the 4 seconds of maximal deglutitive relaxation in the 10-second window starting with deglutitive upper esophageal sphincter (UES) relaxation, is the best metric to differentiate between normal and impaired EGJ relaxation.[7] IRP is influenced not only by LES relaxation but also by CD contraction and intrabolus pressure. In addition, normal values depend on the HRM device used: the upper limit value in normal subjects varies between the transducer used, ranging from 15 mm Hg in the Sierra design transducers to 28 mm Hg in the Unisensor design transducers in the supine position.[5]

The EGJ can be classified into three subtypes based on the axial relationship between the LES and CD[8]:
- *Type I*: LES and CD are completely overlapped.
- *Type II*: LES and CD are separated, with the separation between the pressure peaks being 2 cm or less.
- *Type III*: the separation between LES and CD is greater than 2 cm.
  - *Type IIIa*: the pressure inversion point remains at the level of CD.
  - *Type IIIb*: the pressure inversion point is localized at the level of LES.

When food passes through the UES, a contraction is initiated in the upper esophagus, which progresses distally toward the stomach (Fig. 2.2). The wave initiated by swallowing is referred as primary peristalsis. It travels at a speed of 3 to 4 cm/s and reaches amplitudes of 60 to 140 mm Hg in the distal esophagus. Local stimulation by distention at any point in the body of the esophagus will elicit a peristaltic wave from the point of stimulus. This is called secondary peristalsis and aids esophageal emptying when the primary wave has failed to clear the lumen of ingested food, or when gastric contents reflux from the stomach. Tertiary waves are considered abnormal, but they are frequently seen in elderly people who have no symptoms of esophageal disease.

Postdeglutitive esophageal contraction is evaluated by using the following metrics:
- *CDP* represents the inflection point in the contractile front propagation velocity in the distal esophagus.[9–11]
- *DL* represents the interval between UES relaxation and the CDP. It is considered an important metric indicating the integrity of the inhibitory pathway in the distal esophagus. A value less than 4.5 seconds defines a premature contraction, indicative of spasm.[12]
- *DCI* describes the vigor of the distal esophageal contraction.[13] It is measured as the "volume" of the esophageal contraction spanning from the transition zone to the EGJ. The DCI is the product of the integral of the amplitude exceeding 20 mm Hg, the duration, and the length of the contractile segment between the transition zone and the EGJ. Cutoff values defining different diagnostic categories depend on the type of HRM hardware and software used. DCI in normal subjects ranges between 450 and 8000 mm Hg-s-cm. Hypercontractility is defined by a DCI greater than 8000 mm Hg-s-cm. A DCI ranging between 100 and 450 mm Hg-s-cm defines weak peristalsis, whereas a DCI lower than 100 mm Hg-s-cm identifies failed peristalsis. Both failed and weak contractions are considered ineffective.[4,5,14–16]

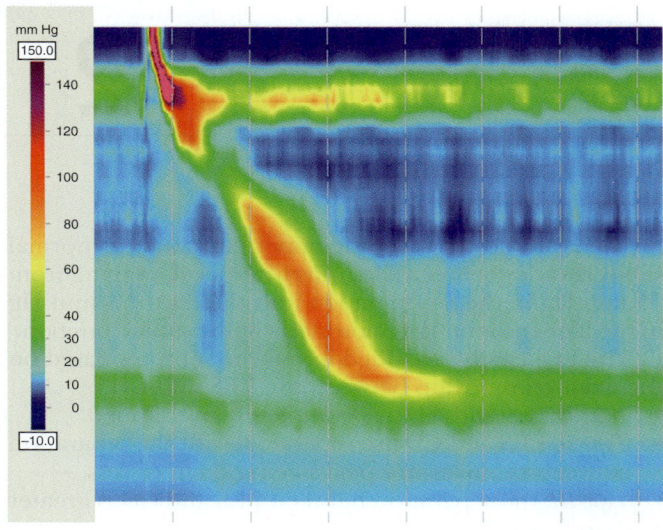

FIGURE 2.1 Normal peristalsis.

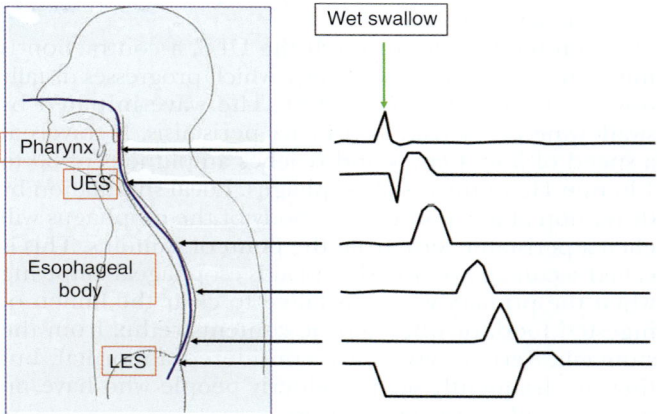

FIGURE 2.2 Physiology of swallowing. *UES,* Upper esophageal sphincter.

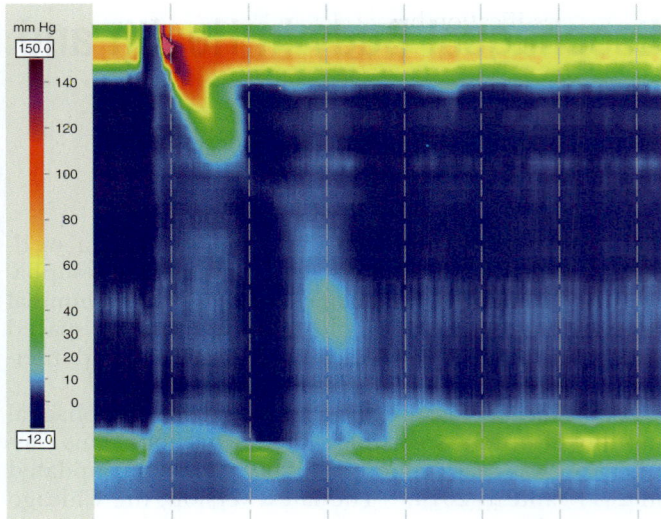

FIGURE 2.3 Achalasia type I.

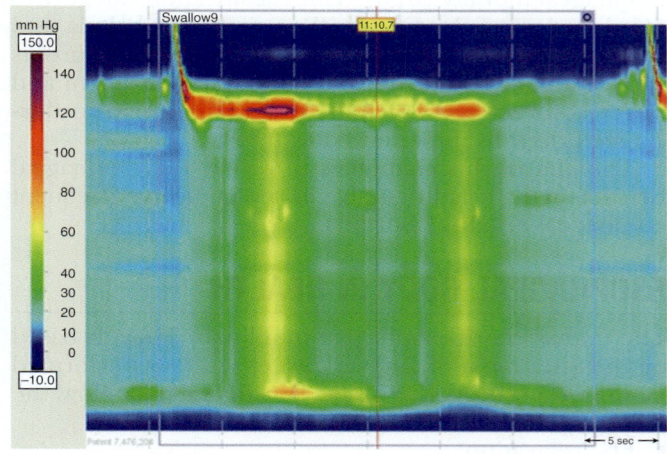

FIGURE 2.4 Achalasia type II.

Contraction integrity, contraction pattern, and intrabolus pressure pattern characterize each swallow.[6] Contraction integrity is defined based on the integrity of the 20-mm Hg isobaric contour. Small (2 to 5 cm in length) interruptions, or breaks, in the 20-mm Hg isobaric contour between the UES and EGJ are considered normal, whereas large (>5 cm in length) breaks define weak contractions. The associated intrabolus pressure pattern is assessed using the 30-mm Hg isobaric contour. Intrabolus pressure is qualified as panesophageal pressurization if it spans from UES to EGJ and as compartmentalized pressurization if it is restricted to the segment between the deglutitive contractile front and the EGJ.[4,5]

ESOPHAGEAL BODY IN DISEASE

ACHALASIA AND ESOPHAGOGASTRIC JUNCTION OUTFLOW OBSTRUCTION

EGJ outflow obstruction is defined by a median IRP greater than 15 mm Hg.[3] Disorders of EGJ outflow obstruction

are subdivided based on the patterns of contractions and pressurization in the esophageal body into
- achalasia subtypes
- EGJ outflow obstruction.[4,5]

Although EGJ outflow obstruction is defined by the presence of high median IRP in association with normal or weak peristalsis, the presence of impaired EGJ relaxation in the absence of peristalsis defines achalasia. Achalasia is further subdivided in three subtypes[4,5,17]:

- *Type I achalasia (classic)*: It is characterized by 100% failed contractions (DCI <100 mm Hg-s-cm) and no esophageal pressurization (Fig. 2.3);
- *Type II achalasia (with esophageal compression)*: It is defined as 100% failed contraction and panesophageal pressurization for at least 20% of swallows (Fig. 2.4);
- *Type III achalasia (spastic)*: It is defined as the presence of preserved fragments of distal peristalsis or premature contractions (DCI >450 mm Hg-s-cm) for at least 20% of the swallows.

This classification has a relevant clinical impact because there is evidence that the preoperative manometric pattern predicts the outcome of pneumatic balloon dilatation[18] and surgical treatment for esophageal achalasia.[19] For instance, Pratap et al.[18] found in 45 patients treated with pneumatic dilatation that type II achalasia had a better response to the endoscopic treatment (18/20, 90.0%) than did type I (14/22, 63.3%) and type III (1/3, 33.3%).

Salvador et al.[19] evaluated 246 consecutive achalasia patients who underwent surgery as their first treatment. Treatment failure was defined as a postoperative symptom score greater than the 10th percentile of the preoperative score. Treatment failure rates differed significantly in the three groups: I = 14.6% (14/96), II = 4.7% (6/127), and III = 30.4% (7/23; P = .0007). At univariate analysis, the manometric pattern, a low LES resting pressure, and a high chest pain score were the factors predicting treatment failure. At multivariate analysis, the manometric pattern and a LES resting pressure less than 30 mm Hg predicted a negative outcome.

Recently, partial recovery of peristalsis was observed in association with reduction or normalization of the EGJ relaxation pressure in some achalasia type III patients after pneumatic dilatation or Heller myotomy.[20] Roman et al.[20] have speculated that esophageal pressurization might have hidden some instances of peristalsis in the pretreatment HRM. Further studies are needed to better understand if the return of peristalsis is predictive of improved outcomes in these patients.

MAJOR MOTILITY DISORDERS

They include aperistalsis, distal esophageal spasm, and hypercontractile (jackhammer) esophagus. Patients with these motility disorders complain of dysphagia, chest pain and gastroesophageal reflux disease (GERD)-like symptoms.[4,5]

Aperistalsis

Aperistalsis is characterized by the presence of normal IRP in association with 100% failed contractions (DCI <100 mm Hg-s-cm). Aperistalsis can be detected in patients with severe GERD and in collagen vascular diseases, such as scleroderma.[4,5]

Distal Esophageal Spasm

Distal esophageal spasm is defined by normal EGJ relaxation (normal IRP) and 20% or more swallows with premature contractions (DCI greater than 450 mm Hg-s-cm and DL lower than 4.5 s) (Fig. 2.5).[4,5,10]

Hypercontractile (Jackhammer) Esophagus

Hypercontractile esophagus (nicknamed jackhammer esophagus) is a disorder that might occur as a primary esophageal motility disorder or be present in the context of other esophageal diseases, including GERD, EGJ outflow obstruction, and eosinophilic esophagitis. Hypercontractile esophagus is defined by the presence repetitive contractions in at least 20% of swallows with a DCI greater than 8000 mm Hg-s-cm.[4,5,14]

Minor Motility Disorders

They include IEM and fragmented peristalsis.

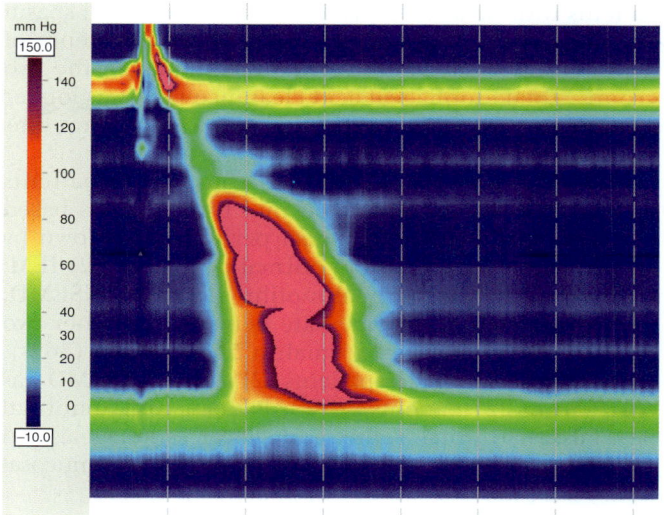

FIGURE 2.5 Distal esophageal spasm.

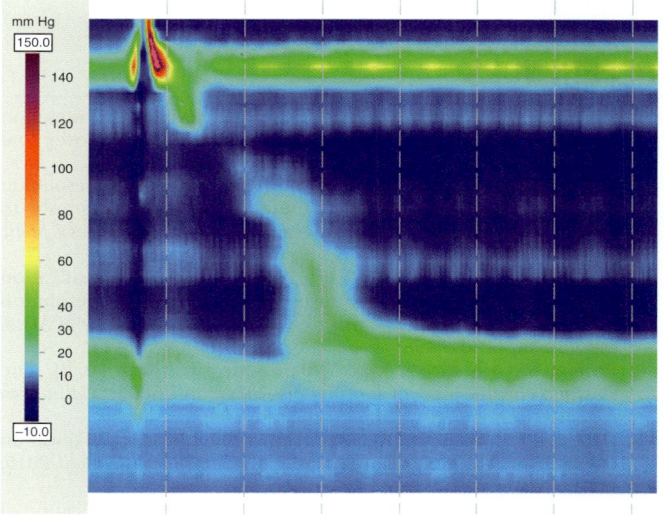

FIGURE 2.6 Ineffective esophageal motility.

Ineffective Esophageal Motility

By conventional manometry, IEM is defined by distal esophageal amplitude less than 30 mm Hg or simultaneous waves in more than 50% of wet swallows.[21] By HRM, IEM is defined as the presence of more than 50% of ineffective swallows (DCI <450 mm Hg-s-cm) (Fig. 2.6).[4,5]

IEM is frequently observed in patients with GERD, particularly those with erosive esophagitis and extraesophageal symptoms of GERD. For instance, Fouad et al.[22] reviewed 98 consecutive patients with respiratory symptoms and abnormal reflux shown by pH-metry. This group of patients was compared with 66 patients with heartburn with no extraesophageal manifestations. IEM was found to be the most common motility disorder in both groups of GERD patients. It was detected more frequently in patients with chronic cough (41%) (P = .003) or asthma (53%) (P = .01) and in patients with laryngitis (31%) than in patients with heartburn (19%). Distal esophageal spasm and nutcracker esophagus were rarely seen. Incidence of hypertensive or hypotensive LES was similar in the two groups. Total esophageal acid clearance time was longer in patients with GERD-associated respiratory symptoms than in patients with heartburn.

Diener et al.[23] evaluated 1006 consecutive patients with GERD, who were divided into three groups based on the character of esophageal peristalsis as shown by esophageal manometry: (1) normal peristalsis; (2) IEM; (3) nonspecific esophageal motility disorder (NSEMD; motor dysfunction intermediate between the other two groups). Peristalsis was normal in 563 patients (56%), IEM was detected in 216 patients (21%), and NSEMD was observed in 227 patients (23%). Patients with abnormal peristalsis had worse reflux and slower esophageal acid clearance. Heartburn, respiratory symptoms, and mucosal injury were all more severe in patients with IEM.

Fragmented Peristalsis

This motility disorder is defined as the presence of fragmented contractions in more than 50% of swallows without meeting the IEM criteria.[4,5]

REFERENCES

1. Soudagar AS, Sayuk GS, Gyawali CP. Learners favour high resolution oesophageal manometry with better diagnostic accuracy over conventional line tracings. *Gut.* 2012;61(6):798-803.
2. Pandolfino JE, Fox MR, Bredenoord AJ, Kahrilas PJ. High-resolution manometry in clinical practice: utilizing pressure topography to classify oesophageal motility abnormalities. *Neurogastroenterol Motil.* 2009;21:796-806.
3. Bredenoord AJ, Fox M, Kahrilas PJ, et al. Chicago classification criteria of esophageal motility disorders defined in high resolution esophageal pressure topography (EPT). *Neurogastroenterol Motil.* 2012;24(suppl 1):57-65.
4. Roman S, Gyawali CP, Xiao Y, Pandolfino JE, Kahrilas PJ. The Chicago classification of motility disorders: an update. *Gastrointest Endosc Clin N Am.* 2014;24:545-561.
5. Kahrilas PJ, Bredeboord AJ, Fox M, et al. The Chicago Classification of esophageal motility disorders, v3.0. *Neurogastroneterol Motil.* 2015; 27:160-174.
6. Kahrilas PJ, Roman S, Pandolfino JE. The Chicago Classification of esophageal motility disorders. In: Fisichella PM, Soper NJ, Pellegrini CA, Patti MG, eds. *Surgical Management of Benign Esophageal Disorders. The "Chicago Approach".* London: Springer-Verlag; 2014:25-38.
7. Ghosh SK, Pandolfino JE, Rice J, Clarke JO, Kwiatek M, Kahrilas PJ. Impaired deglutitive EGJ relaxation in clinical esophageal manometry: a quantitative analysis of 400 patients and 75 controls. *Am J Physiol.* 2007;293:G878-G885.
8. Pandolfino JE, Kim H, Ghosh SK, Clarke JO, Zhang Q, Kahrilas PJ. High-resolution manometry of the EGJ: an analysis of crural diaphragm function in GERD. *Am J Gastroenterol.* 2007;102:1056-1063.
9. Pandolfino JE, Leslie E, Luger D, Mitchell B, Kwiatek MA, Kahrilas PJ. The contractile deceleration point: an important physiologic landmark on oesophageal pressure topography. *Neurogastroenterol Motil.* 2010;22:395-400.
10. Pandolfino JE, Roman S, Carlson D, et al. Distal esophageal spasm in high-resolution esophageal pressure topography: defining clinical phenotypes. *Gastroenterology.* 2011;141:469-475.
11. Lin Z, Pandolfino JE, Xiao Y, et al. Localizing the contractile deceleration point (CDP) in patients with abnormal esophageal pressure topography. *Neurogastroenterol Motil.* 2012;24:972-975.
12. Roman S, Lin Z, Pandolfino JE, Kahrilas PJ. Distal contraction latency: a measure of propagation velocity optimized for esophageal pressure topography studies. *Am J Gastroenterol.* 2011;106:443-451.
13. Ghosh SK, Pandolfino JE, Zhang Q, Jarosz A, Shah N, Kahrilas PJ. Quantifying esophageal peristalsis with high-resolution manometry: a study of 75 asymptomatic volunteers. *Am J Physiol.* 2006;290(5):G988-G997.
14. Roman S, Pandolfino JE, Chen J, Boris L, Luger D, Kahrilas PJ. Phenotypes and clinical context of hypercontractility in high resolution pressure topography (EPT). *Am J Gastroenterol.* 2012;107:37-45.
15. Xiao Y, Kahrilas PJ, Kwasny MJ, et al. High-resolution manometry correlates of ineffective esophageal motility. *Am J Gastroenterol.* 2012;107(11):1647-1654.
16. Xiao Y, Kahrilas PJ, Nicodème F, Lin Z, Roman S, Pandolfino JE. Lack of correlation between HRM metrics and symptoms during the manometric protocol. *Am J Gastroenterol.* 2014;109:521-526.
17. Pandolfino JE, Kwiatek MA, Nealis T, Bulsiewicz W, Post J, Kahrilas PJ. Achalasia: a new clinically relevant classification by high-resolution manometry. *Gastroenterology.* 2008;135:1526-1533.
18. Pratap N, Kalapala R, Darisetty S, et al. Achalasia cardia subtyping by high-resolution manometry predicts the therapeutic outcome of pneumatic balloon dilatation. *J Neurogastroenterol Motil.* 2011;17:48-53.
19. Salvador R, Costantini M, Zaninotto G, et al. The preoperative manometric pattern predicts the outcome of surgical treatment for esophageal achalasia. *J Gastrointest Surg.* 2010;14:1635-1645.
20. Roman S, Kahrilas PJ, Mion F, et al. Partial recovery of peristalsis after myotomy for achalasia; more the rule than the exception. *JAMA Surg.* 2013;148:157-164.
21. Blonski W, Vela M, Safder A, Hila A, Castell DO. Revised criterion for diagnosis of ineffective esophageal motility is associated with more frequent dysphagia and greater bolus transit abnormalities. *Am J Gastroenterol.* 2008;103:699-704.
22. Fouad YM, Katz PO, Hatlebakk JG, Castell DO. Ineffective esophageal motility: the most common motility abnormality in patients with GERD-associated respiratory symptoms. *Am J Gastroenterol.* 1999;94: 1464-1467.
23. Diener U, Patti MG, Molena D, Fisichella PM, Way LW. Esophageal dysmotility and gastroesophageal reflux disease. *J Gastrointest Surg.* 2001;5:260-265.

Esophageal Mucosa in Health and Disease

Parakrama Chandrasoma | Yanling Ma | Evan E. Yung

Pathology has no clinical value at the present time in the diagnosis and management of gastroesophageal reflux disease (GERD) before the occurrence of visible columnar lined esophagus (vCLE). Its only value is in the diagnosis of intestinal metaplasia, increasing dysplasia and adenocarcinoma in the patient with Barrett esophagus.

We will only consider GERD in this chapter. We will explore the pathophysiology of GERD through its entire progression from the normal state to severe GERD. This will lead to the proposal of a new pathologic test for lower esophageal sphincter (LES) damage that is based on mucosal changes defined by histology. The new ability to measure LES damage has the potential to open the door to a new method of diagnosis and management of GERD that has the potential to eradicate GERD-induced esophageal adenocarcinoma.

The evidence base in support of the new test is solid, albeit small. Its acceptance requires the removal of two long-held and powerful dogmas that presently preclude acceptance of the new method. One is a histology dogma and the other an endoscopic dogma. The histologic dogma that must be discarded is that cardiac epithelium normally lines the proximal stomach and is present at the normal gastroesophageal junction (GEJ). The endoscopic dogma that must be discarded is that the GEJ is accurately defined by the proximal limit of the rugal folds and/or the end of the tubular esophagus. The evidence shows clearly that these are both false even as they continue to be accepted.

What is being proposed is revolutionary.

PRESENT STATUS OF GASTROESOPHAGEAL REFLUX DISEASE

GERD is regarded as a chronic progressive disease. When defined by the presence of symptoms that reach a point where they are considered troublesome,[1] 20% to 40% of the population has GERD. Approximately 70% of these patients are well controlled throughout life with proton pump inhibitors (PPIs). Their disease does not seem to be progressive, although some dose escalation may be needed for control.

From this perspective, progression of GERD is limited to the approximately 30% of GERD patients in whom PPI therapy fails to control symptoms (Fig. 3.1). There is no ability or attempt to prevent the progression of 30% of GERD patients into the stage of refractory GERD defined by treatment failure. Patients who fail to be controlled with PPIs live a life whose quality is compromised to varying degrees by their symptoms. It is only when they reach this stage defined by failure of PPIs to control symptoms, or when they develop alarm symptoms such as dysphagia, that endoscopy is indicated.[2]

From the different perspective of endoscopy, GERD progresses from no visible endoscopic change to erosive esophagitis of increasing severity (Los Angeles [LA] grade A to D), to vCLE, Barrett esophagus (defined as vCLE with intestinal metaplasia in the United States), and through increasing dysplasia, to adenocarcinoma.

Biopsy is currently not recommended by most societies in patients who do not have an endoscopic abnormality at the GEJ.[2] Biopsy of the endoscopically normal squamous epithelium may show histologic changes of reflux, but these are not sufficiently sensitive or specific to have practical value. Biopsy of the "normal" squamocolumnar junction (SCJ) is not recommended, although it is known that a small but significant number of patients will have intestinal metaplasia if biopsies are taken, particularly if the SCJ is slightly irregular.[3]

Endoscopy in the patient who has failed PPI therapy changes management only in the patient with Barrett esophagus, who enters an endoscopic surveillance program aimed at detecting early neoplastic changes (see Fig. 3.1). In patients without Barrett esophagus, endoscopy provides little if any useful information that impacts symptom control with PPIs. Often symptoms are diminished in patients with Barrett esophagus, and the efficacy of medical therapy to prevent Barrett's progression remains unproven. Progression to dysplasia and adenocarcinoma in all patients cannot be effectively prevented.[4]

Symptoms of GERD and endoscopic findings are often not concordant. A person without symptoms of GERD can have long segment Barrett esophagus or present with an advanced GERD-induced adenocarcinoma. Conversely, a patient with symptoms of GERD can be endoscopically normal (nonerosive reflux disease [NERD]). Treatment of GERD with PPIs can heal erosive esophagitis without completely resolving GERD symptoms.[2] Patients with NERD are more resistant to symptom control with PPIs than those with erosive esophagitis.[2]

GERD is generally diagnosed when typical reflux symptoms such as heartburn and regurgitation are present. Objective testing with ambulatory pH monitoring can confirm the diagnosis, but is infrequently done when patients first present with symptoms. Instead, most patients receive empiric acid suppressive treatment with the sole objective of symptom control. A positive empiric test of PPI therapy is commonly used to confirm the symptom-based diagnosis of GERD.[2]

There is no symptom complex or test at present that can accurately predict which GERD patient under empiric treatment will progress to failure of PPI therapy in the future. Failure is recognized only when maximum PPI therapy fails to control symptoms. There is no symptom complex or endoscopic finding short of Barrett esophagus that can predict with sufficient accuracy to warrant surveillance endoscopy that a GERD patient will develop

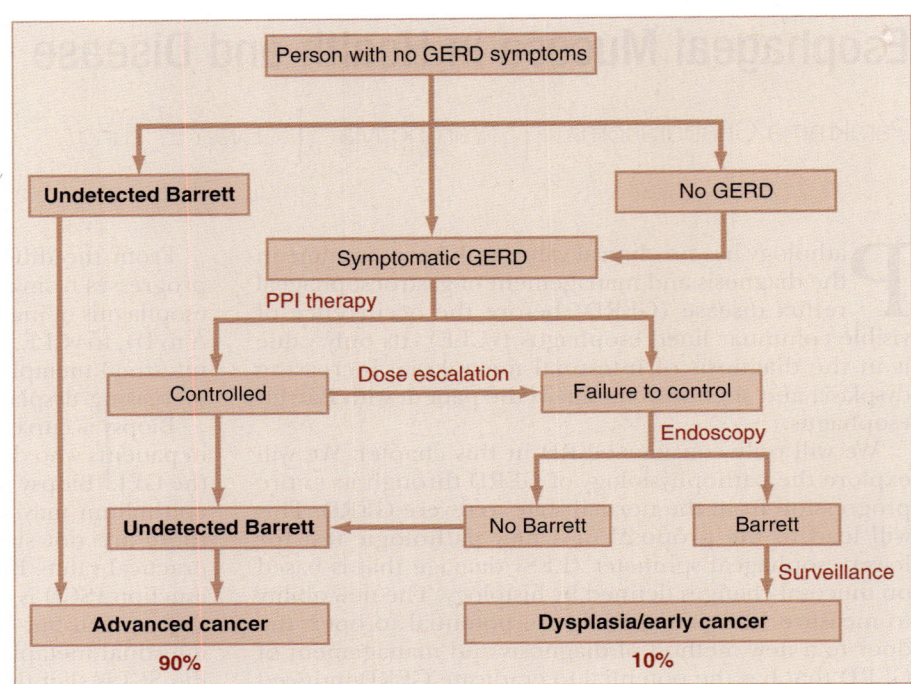

FIGURE 3.1 The failure of the present treatment algorithm of gastroesophageal reflux disease *(GERD)* to prevent mortality from esophageal adenocarcinoma. Endoscopy is limited to patients who fail medical therapy and surveillance is limited to those patients who have Barrett esophagus at endoscopy. Ninety percent of adenocarcinomas occur in asymptomatic people, patients well controlled by proton pump inhibitor *(PPI)* therapy, and people who do not have Barrett esophagus at endoscopy. Only 10% are found in early stages of cancer and can be treated effectively with a mortality of less than 30%, compared with 90% for advanced cancer.

adenocarcinoma in the future. Screening for Barrett esophagus is not recommended.[3]

This treatment algorithm therefore precludes any method that can prevent the progression of GERD to its severe end points of treatment failure and adenocarcinoma. When the end point of severe GERD is compromised quality of life, antireflux surgery offers the only hope of control. However, surgery has its own problems and is performed relatively rarely. Many patients who opt to not have surgery continue to live a life that is disrupted by fear of eating, sleep deprivation, and loss of productivity at work.[5]

When the end point is advanced adenocarcinoma, hope exists for very few patients and too commonly for a very short period of time (see Fig. 3.1). Only 10% of patients developing adenocarcinoma have ever had a diagnosis of Barrett esophagus. If carefully followed with surveillance endoscopy, these patients can be detected with early-stage cancer that is amenable to endoscopic therapy, which is often curative and obviates the need for esophagectomy, chemotherapy, and radiation. Unfortunately, most patients have a dismal outcome, with a 5-year survival of around 15%.

This is a sad commentary of our present management of GERD. We have abandoned the hallowed principles of early diagnosis and prevention in favor of an illogical and unrealized hope that PPIs will cure the disease. We simply permit the development severe GERD and then struggle with few good answers to prevent the inevitable impaired quality of life and progression to adenocarcinoma in a highly significant minority of patients with GERD.

There is no attempt to control progression of GERD. There is no attempt to prevent adenocarcinoma or its premalignant state, Barrett esophagus. There is no attempt to prevent the state of misery associated with GERD that becomes refractory to PPI therapy.

A revolution is essential if there is to be any control of the ever-increasing incidence of adenocarcinoma.[6] This is the first attempt at such a revolution.

PROGRESSION OF GASTROESOPHAGEAL REFLUX DISEASE WITH EMPIRIC PROTON PUMP INHIBITOR THERAPY

The best available scientific prospective study of long-term outcomes associated with treating symptomatic GERD with acid suppressive medical therapy is the Pro-GERD study.[7] A total of 6215 patients older than 18 years old with the primary symptom of heartburn were enrolled into this prospective multicenter open cohort study in Europe. The study was largely conducted under the auspices of Astra-Zeneca, makers of esomeprazole, which makes any result that suggests a negative effect of PPI therapy highly credible.

All patients underwent an index endoscopy done in selected centers by endoscopists who received special training. Endoscopic findings were recorded and the patients given 4 to 8 weeks of PPI therapy with assessment of symptom control and repeat endoscopy to assess healing. They were then sent back to their primary care physicians for continuation of empiric acid suppressive treatment at their discretion. Treatment used during follow-up and symptom control was monitored by questionnaires, and 2721 of this cohort of patients reported to the study centers for repeat endoscopic assessment at 5 years.

At the initial endoscopy, the distribution of endoscopic changes of these 2721 patients was as follows: nonerosive disease, 1224; erosive disease LA A/B, 1044; erosive disease LA C/D, 213; and 240 (8.8%) patients with vCLE. (Note: vCLE was reported as "Barrett oesophagus, endoscopic" and "Barrett oesophagus with histologic confirmation," the latter with intestinal metaplasia.) The patients with vCLE at the initial endoscopy were not included in this study.

Reversal and prevention of progression of erosive esophagitis at 5 years was impressive. Of the 1041 patients with nonerosive disease at baseline, 784 remained nonerosive, 248 progressed to LA A/B, and 9 to LA C/D erosive disease. Of the 918 patients with LA A/B erosive disease at baseline, 578 had reversed to nonerosive disease, 331 remained LA A/B, and 9 had progressed to LA C/D erosive disease. Of the 188 patients with LA C/D erosive disease at baseline, 94 now had nonerosive disease, 78 had LA A/B, and 16 stayed at LA C/D erosive disease. Over a period of 5 years, the number of patients with severe erosive esophagitis had decreased from 188 to 34. Regular intake of PPI reduced the likelihood of progression compared with on-demand PPI or other therapy. The severity of symptoms at baseline was not a predictor of progression to severe erosive esophagitis. It could reasonably be concluded that PPI therapy was highly effective in healing erosive esophagitis.

In contrast, 241 (9.7%) patients who did not have vCLE initially had developed this at 5 years. These patients who progressed included 72 of 1224 (5.9%) who originally had NERD, 127 of 1044 (12.1%) with LA grade A/B, and 42 of 213 (19.7%) with LA grade C/D erosive esophagitis. The factors significantly associated with progression to vCLE at 5 years were (1) female gender, which had a negative association ($P = .041$); (2) alcohol intake ($P = .033$); (3) erosive esophagitis compared with NERD ($P < .001$); and (4) regular PPI use ($P = .019$).

These data show that empiric PPI therapy titrated to control symptoms in the primary care setting heals erosive esophagitis effectively but simultaneously results in an endoscopic progression to vCLE with and without intestinal metaplasia. Whether PPI therapy causes this conversion is unproven. However, the study data prove that nearly 10% of the GERD population under empiric acid reducing treatment will progress from not having vCLE to vCLE within 5 years.

When one considers that 20% to 40% of the population have symptomatic GERD, 10% translates to an absolute number that easily explains why GERD-induced adenocarcinoma has increased sevenfold in the past 4 decades.[6]

VALUE OF PATHOLOGY IN THE DIAGNOSIS OF GASTROESOPHAGEAL REFLUX DISEASE

Pathologic criteria for diagnosis of GERD are presently limited to changes in the squamous epithelium of the esophagus that result from exposure to gastric contents. Reflux esophagitis is characterized by intercellular edema (dilated intercellular spaces), basal cell hyperplasia, papillary elongation, and infiltration by eosinophils and neutrophils. These changes do not have the necessary sensitivity or specificity for the diagnosis of GERD. As such, histologic examination of biopsies has no practical value in the diagnosis of GERD.

Pathologic criteria do not exist at present for assessment of the LES. In this chapter, we will develop a new set of pathologic criteria that can define the presence and extent of damage to the abdominal segment of the LES (a-LES).

We will also explore how this simple histologic test for a-LES damage can transform the future management of GERD.

A PROPOSED NEW OBJECTIVE IN THE MANAGEMENT OF GASTROESOPHAGEAL REFLUX DISEASE

The present treatment algorithm for GERD (see Fig. 3.1) can be described as totally reactive. There is no defined objective aimed at detecting or preventing any cellular change that may be a harbinger of adenocarcinoma. We simply wait for symptoms that are "troublesome" to begin empiric PPI therapy[1]; then wait for failure of PPI therapy to perform endoscopy[2]; and then wait for the occurrence of high-grade dysplasia and adenocarcinoma. The only proactive event in this algorithm that improves outcomes is Barrett esophagus surveillance, but current recommendations for surveillance intervals often render this effort a failure too.

Even worse, most physicians convince themselves that PPI therapy is a wonderful method of treating GERD that brings comfort to millions of GERD sufferers. This is true. However, we hide and ignore the greatest increase of a specific cancer type in the history of medicine that has concurrently occurred while patients are being treated with increasingly effective acid reducing drugs.[6]

In this chapter, we will attempt to change the present outcomes of GERD with a new approach based on the development of a new understanding of GERD based on the pathogenesis of progression of a-LES damage.

It is well known that GERD is the result of LES damage. As such, focus on LES damage attacks the problem at its root. The primary objective of the new approach is to turn the curve of increasing incidence of adenocarcinoma downward all the way to zero. A secondary objective is to prevent failure of medical therapy.

DEFINING A CRITERION OF IRREVERSIBILITY: VISIBLE COLUMNAR LINED ESOPHAGUS

The first step in preventing adenocarcinoma is to recognize the point of irreversibility that signals the inability to prevent progression to adenocarcinoma. In GERD, at this point in time, that point of irreversibility is the occurrence of vCLE. In the United Kingdom, vCLE defines Barrett esophagus.[8] In the United States and Europe, intestinal metaplasia is required for the diagnosis of Barrett esophagus.

Medical treatment does not reverse vCLE or prevent its progression to intestinal metaplasia, increasing dysplasia, and adenocarcinoma. Present medical treatment of GERD therefore commits 10% of all patients to irreversibility every 5 years.[7]

The advantage with defining irreversibility in GERD by the presence of vCLE is that there is no evidence that any patient who does not have vCLE progresses to adenocarcinoma. If we prevent vCLE, we will prevent adenocarcinoma.

It can be reasonably argued that the person who is endoscopically normal with intestinal metaplasia at the normal SCJ is at risk for adenocarcinoma of the "gastric cardia." However, present management guidelines recommend that such patients with GERD should not undergo biopsies because the risk of cancer in patients who have intestinal metaplasia is unknown.[2] The argument, therefore, has no practical merit at this time. It may change in the future if an increased cancer risk is defined in this group. If and when that happens, preventing intestinal metaplasia at the SCJ in the endoscopically normal person will become necessary.

The detection of vCLE requires endoscopy. The present management guidelines delay endoscopy to the point of treatment failure. At this point a significant number of patients will already have vCLE. If endoscopy is performed proactively without waiting for treatment failure, as was done in the Pro-GERD study, 240 of 2721 (8.8%) patients would already have vCLE.[7] In addition, the following endoscopic findings were predictive of progression to vCLE in the next 5 years: (1) presence of erosive esophagitis with risk increasing to 19.7% in patients with severe erosive esophagitis[7]; and (2) presence of intestinal metaplasia in a biopsy taken from the SCJ of an endoscopically normal patient, with such patients having a 25% risk of progression to vCLE within 5 years.[9] The patients in the Pro-GERD study had well-established GERD, often with severe symptoms and a long duration.[7] It is probable that endoscopy performed at the onset of GERD would have a lower prevalence of vCLE.

In the Pro-GERD study, the nonendoscopic findings that were significantly associated with progression to vCLE in GERD patients under medical therapy were male gender, alcohol use, and regular PPI use.

None of the nonendoscopic criteria that are predictive for development of vCLE within 5 years listed previously are indications for endoscopy in the GERD patient. The indication remains the occurrence of treatment failure. The main reason for this is the lack of any desire to prevent vCLE in the minds of the medical community. To them, vCLE is simply another inevitable event in the course of GERD that occurs in a minority of GERD patients. The fact that it is a cellular change whose end point is a lethal malignancy is ignored.

This is a nihilistic attitude that permits conversion of the patient without risk to one whose progression to adenocarcinoma becomes inevitable. The only excuse for this attitude is that cancer is rare in GERD patients. With the sevenfold increase in the incidence of GERD-induced adenocarcinoma over the past 4 decades,[6] this excuse has become increasingly lame and unacceptable.

If the presence of vCLE is recognized as the point of irreversibility in GERD, there can be a new objective of management of the GERD patient: *the prevention of progression to vCLE.*

This would then provide an incentive and demand for earlier endoscopy before failure with empiric treatment with PPI in the patient with GERD. Early endoscopy presently has the ability only to recognize the presence of vCLE and predict its occurrence within the next 5 years by the presence of severe erosive esophagitis (19.7%) and intestinal metaplasia at the normal SCJ (25%). Successful repair of the damaged LES in the patient with a high risk of vCLE in 5 years has a high probability of preventing vCLE.

These reasons for early endoscopy are presently not justified because of the cost associated with increasing the number of endoscopies. However, it emphasizes the fact that any push to prevent adenocarcinoma must change the indications for endoscopy to an earlier stage in the progression of GERD. This will only happen if a new and more accurate method of predicting progression of GERD to vCLE becomes available. The new histologic measure of LES damage that we propose can be that test.

CAUSE OF VISIBLE COLUMNAR LINED ESOPHAGUS

To be effective in preventing vCLE, we must identify its cause. It is certain that vCLE is the result of exposure of the esophagus above the endoscopic GEJ to gastric contents as a result of reflux. As such, it is also certain that if reflux can be prevented, vCLE will not occur.

There is strong evidence that the risk of vCLE increases with increasing severity of reflux (demonstrated by objective evidence of acid exposure by a pH test), increasing duration of reflux, male gender, regular PPI therapy, and possibly alcoholism and smoking. Nason et al.[10] showed that the prevalence of Barrett esophagus was higher in patients whose symptoms were controlled with PPI therapy. They suggested that the present practice of waiting for treatment failure was irrational if the objective for endoscopy was the detection of Barrett esophagus.

The most dominant factors in the etiology of vCLE are the severity and duration of reflux. Patients with Barrett esophagus are known to have a higher prevalence of an abnormal pH test than any other category of GERD. There is no specifically defined level of abnormality in the pH test or a specific number of years of reflux that correlates with the occurrence of vCLE. If the objective is preventing vCLE, success will demand intervention at the earliest practical time after the onset of reflux. For prevention of vCLE to be certain, intervention must occur before any significant reflux occurs into the thoracic esophagus.

From a practical standpoint, it is necessary to identify criteria that separate very low and high risk of impending and future vCLE by some defined severity and/or duration of reflux. This is not possible by presently available tests. We will propose that the new test of LES damage provides accurate criteria for predicting future vCLE.

It is certain that the severity of reflux into the thoracic esophagus correlates with the frequency of LES failure, which in turn correlates with the severity of LES damage. In relation to our objective of preventing vCLE, this recognition establishes a new more practical objective: *prevention of reflux into the thoracic esophagus that is severe enough to cause vCLE.*

LOWER ESOPHAGEAL SPHINCTER

One of the great obstacles to the study of GERD is the absence of a pathologic method of assessing the LES by pathology at autopsy and resection specimens. Careful study of the region has identified complicated arrangement of the muscle fibers that may represent the LES,[11] but these cannot be translated into routine pathology practice. The LES can only be defined and measured by manometry (Fig. 3.2).

The LES acts as a beautifully designed barrier that prevents reflux of gastric contents into the esophagus.[12,13] The LES pressure is normally greater than 15 mm Hg, exceeding the baseline luminal pressure in the esophagus (normally around −5 mm Hg) proximally, and the baseline luminal pressure in the stomach (normally around +5 mm Hg) distally. The LES therefore acts as a valve that effectively prevents reflux along the natural pressure gradient that exists from the stomach into the esophagus (Figs. 3.3 and 3.4).

DEFINING THE NORMAL AND DEFECTIVE LOWER ESOPHAGEAL SPHINCTER BY MANOMETRY

The functional state of the LES can be defined manometrically by three separate components[12,13]: its mean pressure, its total length, and the length of its abdominal segment. Manometric studies of asymptomatic subjects indicate that the LES pressure is greater than 15 mm Hg, the total LES length is 40 to 50 mm, and the length of the abdominal segment (a-LES) is 30 to 35 mm.

The criteria that define a defective LES that correlates with the presence of sufficient reflux into the esophagus to produce clinical GERD are[13] (1) a decrease in the mean LES pressure to less than 6 mm Hg, (2) a decrease in total LES length to less than 20 mm, and (3) a decrease in a-LES length to less than 10 mm. At these levels of LES damage, sphincter failure occurs so frequently that it results in an abnormal pH test and significant exposure of the squamous epithelium in the body of the esophagus

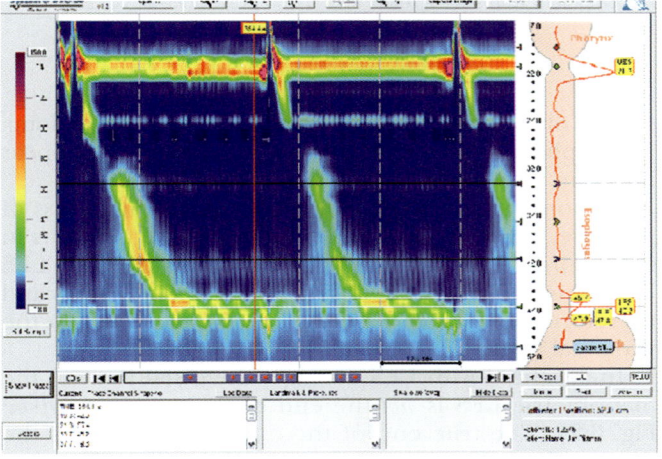

FIGURE 3.2 High-resolution manometry showing the esophageal pressure tracing during three swallows. The lower esophageal sphincter is the high-pressure zone defined by an increase of 2 mm from baseline esophageal pressure at the proximal end and from baseline gastric pressure at the distal end. The lower esophageal sphincter relaxes during the swallow and regains its resting pressure between swallows.

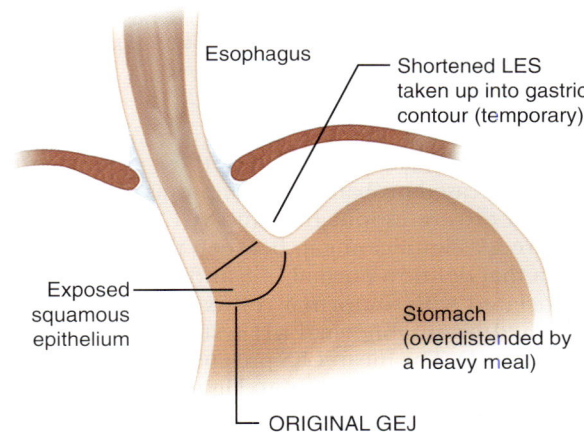

FIGURE 3.4 Mechanism of exposure of the squamous epithelium of the distal esophagus to acid. When the stomach overdistends with a heavy meal, the lower esophageal sphincter shortens, the distal lower esophageal sphincter becomes effaced (i.e., moves down into the contour of the gastric fundus), and the squamous epithelium becomes exposed to gastric contents of the full stomach. There is, at the top of the food column, an acid pocket that meets the descending squamous epithelium. *GEJ*, Gastroesophageal junction.

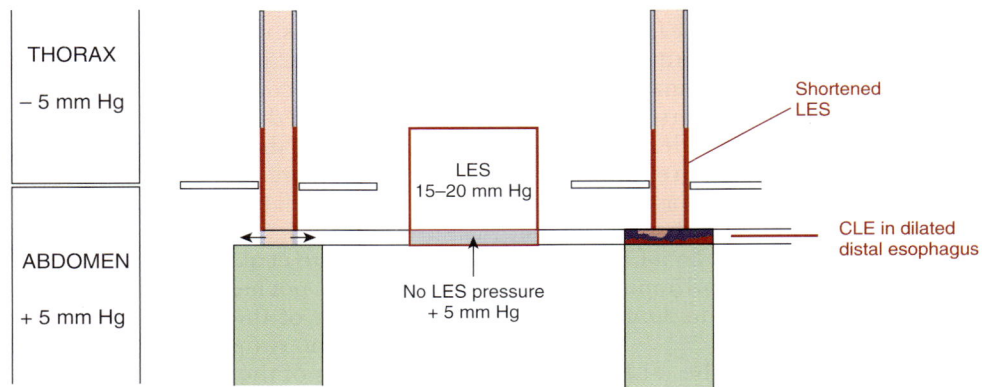

FIGURE 3.3 Effect of loss of pressure in the abdominal segment of the lower esophageal sphincter *(LES)*. The normal resting pressure of the abdominal LES overcomes the positive intraluminal pressure in the abdominal esophagus and maintains the tubal shape of the esophagus. When the LES pressure is lost, the intraluminal pressure causes this part of the distal esophagus to dilate. *CLE,* Columnar lined esophagus.

TABLE 3.1 Length of Abdominal Segment of Lower Esophageal Sphincter (a-LES) Damage (Measured by the New Test), Length of the Residual Functional a-LES, and Their Correlation With Lower Esophageal Sphincter Failure and Severity of Reflux*

a-LES Damage	Residual a-LES Length	Postprandial a-LES Length	Probability of LES Failure	Severity of Reflux (% time pH < 4)
Zero	35 mm	25 mm	Zero	Zero
>0–<5 mm	30–35 mm	20–25 mm	Zero	Zero
5–<10 mm	25–30 mm	15–20 mm	Zero	Zero
10–<15 mm	20–25 mm	10–15 mm	Postprandial—rare	>zero–4.5%
15–<20 mm	15–20 mm	5–10 mm	Postprandial—frequent	>zero–4.5%
20–25 mm	10–15 mm	0–5 mm	Postprandial—very frequent	>4.5%
25–30 mm	5–10 mm	Zero	Incessant	>>4.5%
30–35 mm	Zero–5 mm	Zero	Incessant	>>>4.5%

*We assume that the patient has an initial a-LES length of 35 mm, that a heavy meal causes 10 mm of dynamic shortening of the a-LES in the postprandial phase, and that LES failure occurs at an a-LES length of less than 10 mm.
GERD, Gastroesophageal reflux disease; *LES,* lower esophageal sphincter. *Green areas,* The LES is competent with damage that is within its reserve capacity. *Orange areas,* Clinical GERD from onset of symptoms to point of transition from postprandial reflux to incessant reflux and an increasing prevalence of visible columnar-lined esophagus (vCLE). *Red areas,* The LES is incompetent with severe reflux and a high prevalence of vCLE.

to reflux.[13] LES damage defined by these criteria correlate with an increased probability of symptoms of GERD, severe grades of erosive esophagitis, and vCLE.

There is a significant gap between the previously listed criteria that define a normal LES and a defective LES that is associated with abnormal reflux into the esophagus, as defined by an abnormal pH test and the presence of clinical GERD. The mean LES pressure must decrease from a normal of greater than 15 mm Hg to less than 6 mm Hg; the total LES length must decrease from a normal of 40 to 50 mm to less than 20 mm; and the a-LES length must decrease from 30 to 35 mm to less than 10 mm before it becomes a criterion of LES failure.

At least part of this gap between a normal and defective LES represents the reserve capacity of the LES. As LES damage increases, its reserve capacity is progressively reduced. However, as long as it is not exhausted, the LES maintains its competence (green zone in Table 3.1).

This early LES damage cannot be recognized by any present criterion for the diagnosis of GERD: the patient has no symptoms, no endoscopic abnormality, no manometric criteria of a defective LES, and no abnormal pH test. This state where the LES is damaged within its reserve functional capacity can be called the *phase of compensated LES damage.* We will show that histologic examination with new criteria can define and measure this early LES damage.

Before the onset of LES damage, all persons have an initial a-LES length that is equal to the length of the abdominal esophagus. Zaninotto et al.[13] reported that the manometric length of the a-LES in 49 asymptomatic volunteers had the following distribution (I have taken the liberty of removing one outlier that had an a-LES length of >50 mm): less than 10 mm in 1; 10 to 15 mm in 6; 15 to 20 mm in 10; 20 to 25 mm in 17; 25 to 30 mm in 11; and 30 to 35 mm in 5 persons.

The manometric measurement of the a-LES at any given point in a person's life after the LES has developed completely can be expressed by the following formula:

$$\text{Initial a-LES length} = \text{manometric a-LES length} + \text{LES damage}$$

This only assumes that the anatomic part of the abdominal esophagus that contains the a-LES does not disappear into thin air when LES pressure is lost.

Manometrically, LES damage is equivalent to loss of pressure. When this occurs at the distal end, it results in shortening of the manometric a-LES. The damaged LES is distal to the end of the residual LES at manometry and therefore identical in its pressure characteristics to the proximal stomach.

In a patient with LES damage, the distal limit of the manometric LES is *not* the end of the esophagus (see Fig. 3.2). The true end of the esophagus includes the damaged a-LES. Any manometric interpretation that makes the assumption that the esophagus ends at the distal end of the manometric LES is potentially wrong by as much as 35 mm (the entire initial a-LES length). For example, if the distal limit of the manometric LES is above the diaphragmatic pressure impression, this is not necessarily a hiatal hernia because the true end of the esophagus cannot be defined by manometry.

At present, the previous formula that defines the LES cannot be applied because two elements, LES damage and the initial LES length, are unknown. As a result, manometry has no practical value in the diagnosis of GERD. However, it illustrates the critically important and misunderstood concept that the manometric definition of the distal end of the a-LES is not the end of the esophagus. The true end of the esophagus must include the damaged a-LES that is present distal to the manometric end of the LES in virtually all people This cannot be measured at present.

In Zaninotto et al.[13], therefore, the measured manometric a-LES does not necessarily represent individual variation of the length of the normal a-LES, simply because the subjects had no symptoms of GERD. It could be the result of shortening of the a-LES by progressive a-LES damage. The data in the study can be explained by assuming that the initial a-LES length was 35 mm (the highest length) in all patients, and the distribution represents different degrees of a-LES damage. For example, an asymptomatic person with a measured manometric a-LES length of

22 mm (the median a-LES length in the study) could have an initial length of 35 mm with 13 mm of a-LES damage (see Table 3.1). That person is asymptomatic because the LES, though damaged, is still sufficiently competent to prevent reflux.

The distribution of acid exposure in these volunteers in Zaninotto et al.[13] showed a pH less than 4 for a mean of 1.57%, a median of 1.1%, and a range of 0% to 6% of the 24-hour period. This shows that these asymptomatic persons had evidence of mild reflux with 5% reaching the pH test definition for abnormal reflux. This was objective evidence of LES failure, despite the fact that they did not have symptoms.

The data in Zaninotto et al.[13] raise the intriguing but obvious probability that the LES has a reserve capacity. It can shorten significantly from its initial length while remaining competent—that is, there is a phase of compensated LES damage where patients have LES damage within its reserve capacity without significant LES failure and reflux into the thoracic esophagus. A person without significant reflux into the thoracic esophagus will be at zero risk for developing vCLE.

Based on this understanding, we can divide the severity of LES damage into (1) compensated, (i.e., LES damage is such that it does not produce LES failure, where the pH test is zero; green zone in Table 3.1); (2) LES damage that causes infrequent LES failure and mild reflux (i.e., pH test is greater than zero but pH test normal; <4.5% of time pH < 4 or DeMeester score < 14), noting that vCLE is extremely unlikely in such patients (orange zone in Table 3.1); and (3) severe LES damage with LES failure sufficient to produce an abnormal pH test and a high prevalence of vCLE (red zone in Table 3.1).

This further refines our objective into an LES-based objective to prevent vCLE: *prevention of a-LES damage beyond the point where reflux is sufficiently severe to cause vCLE*. In Table 3.1, this corresponds to preventing a-LES damage from reaching 25 mm. When there is a measure of a-LES damage, there is a range of zero to 25 mm of LES damage that is available for intervention to prevent progression of LES damage. Prevention of vCLE becomes theoretically very feasible in this method.

This new objective clearly shows the futility of present management of GERD. The presently accepted criteria that define GERD (troublesome symptoms, erosive esophagitis, an abnormal pH test, and a defective LES on manometry where the a-LES is <10 mm) are the very things that must be prevented if we hope to prevent esophageal adenocarcinoma.

RESULT OF ABDOMINAL LOWER ESOPHAGEAL SPHINCTER DAMAGE: THE DILATED DISTAL ESOPHAGUS

A largely unappreciated normal function of the a-LES is to maintain the tubular shape of the abdominal esophagus. The high resting pressure of the a-LES continually opposes the dilatory tendency of the positive (around +5 mm Hg) intraluminal pressure of the abdominal esophagus.

When the a-LES is damaged, the protection provided by the tonic contraction of the LES is lost. The dilatory positive intraluminal pressure will be accentuated during meals when the stomach distends and the intragastric pressure increases. The distal abdominal esophagus that has lost LES pressure will therefore dilate to form the dilated distal esophagus (see Fig. 3.3).[14]

With LES damage, the tubular abdominal esophagus shortens, the damaged esophagus dilates[15] and takes up the gastric contour and becomes part of the reservoir, and the angle of His becomes more obtuse.[16] Mucosal rugal folds, which are a feature of all reservoir organs, develop in this dilated distal esophagus that results from loss of abdominal LES function (as discussed later).

The dilated distal esophagus has a variable length that is equal to the amount of shortening of the a-LES due to damage. The equation that defines the a-LES now resolves as follows:

Initial length of a-LES = length of residual a-LES
    (= tubular abdominal esophagus)
    + length of LES damage (= dilated distal esophagus)

The end of the tubular esophagus, which has been used by pathologists to define the GEJ since Hayward in 1961[17], is proximal to the true GEJ by the length of the dilated distal esophagus.

This "gastricization" of the abdominal esophagus that has lost LES tone occurs at a manometric, endoscopic, and gross anatomic level. This has led to confusion that has created error in this region from the beginning of time and continues to the present.[18]

We will show that it is only the correct interpretation of the histology of this region that can resolve this error.

MECHANISM OF ABDOMINAL LOWER ESOPHAGEAL SPHINCTER DAMAGE

LES damage is the result of pressure exerted from below, as a result of a heavy meal that causes gastric overdistention. Ayazi et al.[19] and Robertson et al.[20] showed elegantly that gastric overdistention causes "effacement" of the distal part of the LES, resulting in a temporary decrease in LES length. The squamous epithelium lining the effaced LES is exposed to gastric juice because the pH transition point has moved proximally (see Fig. 3.4).

The phenomenon of effacement of the distal end of the LES can be demonstrated at endoscopy. In a person with normal endoscopy, the SCJ is the GEJ. In retroflex view, when the stomach is insufflated with air, the SCJ moves downward and becomes visible. When the same thing happens during a heavy meal, the squamous epithelium is in the stomach, below the pH transition point.

There is a pocket of strong acid at the height of the food column during a meal.[21] Repeated and frequent exposure of the squamous epithelium to this acid pocket during gastric overdistention during heavy meals results first in reversible injury to the distal esophageal squamous epithelium, followed by permanent columnar metaplasia of the squamous epithelium.

If LES damage occurs because of pressure from below, it must follow that LES damage begins at its distal end and progresses upward. Loss of length therefore begins in the distal a-LES. Robertson et al.[20] showed that early LES shortening produced by a heavy meal in asymptomatic volunteers was entirely in the abdominal segment and did not affect the thoracic LES.

TABLE 3.2 Changes With Age of the Functional Residual Length of the Abdominal Lower Esophageal Sphincter*

Rate of LES Damage	At 25 Years	At 35 Years	At 45 Years	At 55 Years	At 65 Years	At 75 Years
1 mm/decade	34 mm	33 mm	32 mm	31 mm	30 mm	29 mm
2 mm/decade	33 mm	31 mm	29 mm	27 mm	25 mm	23 mm
3 mm/decade	32 mm	29 mm	26 mm	23 mm	20 mm	17 mm
4 mm/decade	31 mm	27 mm	23 mm	19 mm	15 mm	11 mm
5 mm/decade	30 mm	25 mm	20 mm	15 mm	10 mm	5 mm
6 mm/decade	29 mm	23 mm	17 mm	11 mm	5 mm	0 mm
7 mm/decade	28 mm	21 mm	14 mm	7 mm	0 mm	0 mm
8 mm/decade	27 mm	19 mm	11 mm	3 mm	0 mm	0 mm
9 mm/decade	26 mm	17 mm	8 mm	0 mm	0 mm	0 mm
10 mm/decade	25 mm	15 mm	5 mm	0 mm	0 mm	0 mm

*Assuming that the original length at maturity is 35 mm, that lower esophageal sphincter (LES) damage begins at age 15 years, and that LES damage has a linear progression over the long term. Note: The abdominal LES lengths in *green* represent lengths at which the LES is likely to be competent. The lengths in *orange* represent an LES that is susceptible to failure with gastric distention (i.e., at risk of postprandial reflux). The lengths in *red* represent an LES that is below the length at which LES failure occurs at rest.

LES damage can therefore be considered to be basically the result of an eating disorder. Viewed in this light, each person can be regarded as having a unique relationship between his/her eating habit, the response of the LES to this overeating, and the damage caused to the esophageal squamous epithelium by exposure to gastric juice.

At one extreme, the patient's LES is not damaged by the effect of his/her eating habit on the LES. This patient never has LES failure and reflux, the pH test is zero, and this person never gets GERD. At the other extreme, the patient's LES is damaged early in life by an excessive eating habit and/or an LES susceptible to damage and progresses rapidly to LES incompetence and severe reflux into the thoracic esophagus at a relatively young age. This damage includes erosive esophagitis and becomes irreversible when vCLE occurs.

Between these two extremes is the entire clinicopathologic spectrum of GERD. Progression of GERD can therefore be defined by the rate of progression of LES damage resulting from a person's eating habit (Table 3.2).

RELATIONSHIP BETWEEN ABDOMINAL LOWER ESOPHAGEAL SPHINCTER LENGTH AND LOWER ESOPHAGEAL SPHINCTER FAILURE

LES damage is a progressive phenomenon. When looked at from the perspective of LES damage, progression is inexorable from the onset of LES damage to the end point defined as the end of life, or some intervention that stops the progression, such as an antireflux procedure.

PPI therapy has no positive impact on the rate of progression of LES damage. By removing the pain associated with reflux and allowing the patient to eat excessively, PPIs may actually prevent the body's natural defense against progression of LES damage.

In general, the greater the LES damage, the greater is the severity of reflux. Kahrilas et al.[22] beautifully demonstrated the close relationship between decreasing LES length and LES failure. They measured baseline total LES length in three groups with increasing severity of GERD: patients who had no symptoms of GERD ("normal"), patients with GERD without a hiatal hernia, and patients with GERD who had a hiatal hernia.

The baseline LES length in the fasting state was progressively less in normal persons compared to nonhernia GERD with hernia GERD. This correlated with an increase in baseline reflux as measured by a pH electrode placed 5 cm above the upper border of the LES.

In this study, Kahrilas et al.[22] infused air into the stomach at 15 mL/min, causing progressive gastric distention. This caused an additional shortening of the LES of 5 to 7 mm from baseline in all three groups as distention increased. The additional temporary shortening of the LES was similar in the three groups, suggesting that gastric overdistention caused LES exposure to gastric contents in a linear manner. During the temporary shortening of the LES with gastric distention, the number of reflux episodes and total acid exposure in the esophagus increased significantly and most prominently in the hernia-GERD group. This showed that a damaged LES with a shorter baseline length was more susceptible to failure when exposed to gastric distention.

This study confirms that a-LES length is a critical determinant of the severity of reflux (objectively measured in a pH test). It also shows that significant reflux can occur during the postprandial phase in asymptomatic persons.

HISTOLOGIC MEASUREMENT OF ABDOMINAL LOWER ESOPHAGEAL SPHINCTER DAMAGE

The objective of preventing vCLE is not possible at the present time, because there is no test that has the ability to predict with sufficient accuracy those patients at high risk of progressing to vCLE. The use of symptom severity has no value; some patients with vCLE are asymptomatic. The control of symptoms with PPIs has a negative correlation with prevalence of vCLE.[10] There is no defined value in the pH test or manometry that can predict impending or future vCLE. The presence of severe erosive esophagitis and intestinal metaplasia in a biopsy of the SCJ in the endoscopically normal GERD patient has a 20% to 25% known progression to vCLE within 5 years, but this has not led to a recommendation to intervene in some way to prevent vCLE.

We propose a new method of achieving the ability to predict high risk of impending and future vCLE. This is the measurement of the dilated distal esophagus by histology. We will show that the length of the dilated distal esophagus is equal to the length of metaplastic columnar epithelium that is found *distal* to the endoscopic GEJ.[14] In turn, this is equal to the shortening by damage of the a-LES.

This provides, for the first time, a method of measuring a-LES damage, the cause of GERD. This is of such fundamental value to the understanding of GERD that it has the potential to transform the management of GERD.

At the present time, two false dogmas prevent the application of this new method of diagnostic testing: (1) the false dogma that cardiac epithelium is a normal proximal gastric epithelium, and (2) that the proximal limit of rugal folds and/or the distal limit of the tubular esophagus define the GEJ. The result of these two false dogmas is that the entire pathology of LES damage is mistaken as "normal proximal stomach." The failure of understanding at such a fundamental level explains the present chaos in the diagnosis and management of GERD with its disastrous patient outcomes of refractory GERD and adenocarcinoma.

DEFINITION OF NORMAL HISTOLOGY OF THE ESOPHAGUS AND STOMACH

It is remarkable that GERD, a disease that results from damage to esophageal epithelium by gastric acid, has no histopathologic criteria that have practical value in present diagnosis. Before we accept the fact that histology does not play a role in the diagnosis of early GERD, it is important to ask the right questions: *Is there any possibility that we are overlooking some histologic change that is diagnostic of GERD? Are we looking in the right places? Is there any possibility of error in our definitions? Could we be calling the distal esophagus damaged by GERD the proximal stomach? Is it possible that we are so wrong?* The simple answer to all these questions is a vehement "yes."

To begin to answer these questions and explore histologic criteria for defining early GERD, it is important to first define the epithelial types seen in the esophagus and stomach.[23] There are only three basic epithelial types that occur from the proximal end of the esophagus to the pyloric antrum.[23,24] These are (1) stratified squamous epithelium, which is limited to the esophagus in the human and is *always* present; (2) gastric oxyntic mucosa, which is limited to the proximal stomach and not found in the esophagus, and is *always* present (Fig. 3.5); and (3) metaplastic columnar epithelia, which are *always* derived from chronic exposure of esophageal squamous epithelium to gastric juice and are *not always* present. When present, however, metaplastic columnar epithelia are *always* interposed between the distal limit of esophageal squamous epithelium and the proximal limit of gastric oxyntic epithelium (Fig. 3.6).

Metaplastic columnar epithelium is cardiac epithelium. Cardiac epithelium *never* occurs normally in the proximal stomach. It consists of three histologic variants (Fig. 3.7): (1) pure cardiac epithelium composed of only mucous

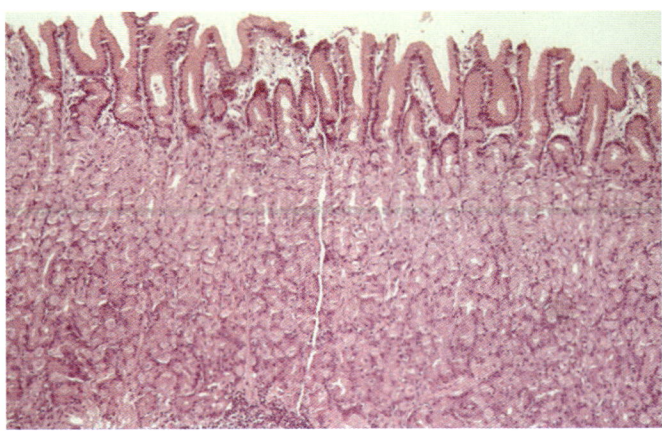

FIGURE 3.5 Normal gastric oxyntic epithelium. This shows a surface layer and short foveolar pit composed of mucous cells and a long, straight tubular gland that contains parietal and chief cells. No mucous cells are seen below the foveolar pit. Hematoxylin and eosin stain.

cells; (2) cardiac epithelium with parietal cells admixed with mucous cells in the glands (oxyntocardiac epithelium); and (3) cardiac epithelium with goblet cells, which define intestinal metaplasia. The prevalence of these three columnar epithelial types is variable. Intestinal epithelium is the least common and oxyntocardiac epithelium the most prevalent.

The four columnar epithelial types (i.e., three metaplastic and gastric oxyntic epithelium) can be precisely defined by simple histologic criteria based on the presence or absence of mucous cells, parietal cells, and goblet cells (Table 3.3). The definition of the epithelial type is applied to every unit of the epithelium, which is defined as a single foveolar-gland complex. Multiple epithelial types can therefore be present in a small area (see Fig. 3.7).

The diagnosis of these four epithelial types has high precision with minimal requirement for training and experience. It is easy. More important than training is a belief in the pathologist that differentiating between these epithelial types has value. Careful study of routine sections stained by hematoxylin and eosin is adequate for accurate diagnosis.

The extent of cardiac epithelium (with and without parietal and/or goblet cells) distal to the endoscopic GEJ (proximal limit of rugal folds and/or end of tubular esophagus) defines the length of the dilated distal esophagus and is therefore a measure of a-LES damage. This can be measured with a high level of accuracy with an appropriate tissue sample.

DEFINITION OF THE GASTROESOPHAGEAL JUNCTION

From an anatomic standpoint, it is very important to have a precise and accurate definition of the GEJ. The most widely used definition of the GEJ is the proximal limit of rugal folds.[2,25] This is a reasonably precise endoscopic landmark and can usually be seen in gross specimens. However, there is absolutely no evidence that it accurately represents the GEJ. The basis of the definition is the opinion of experts.[2,26] For an opinion-based definition

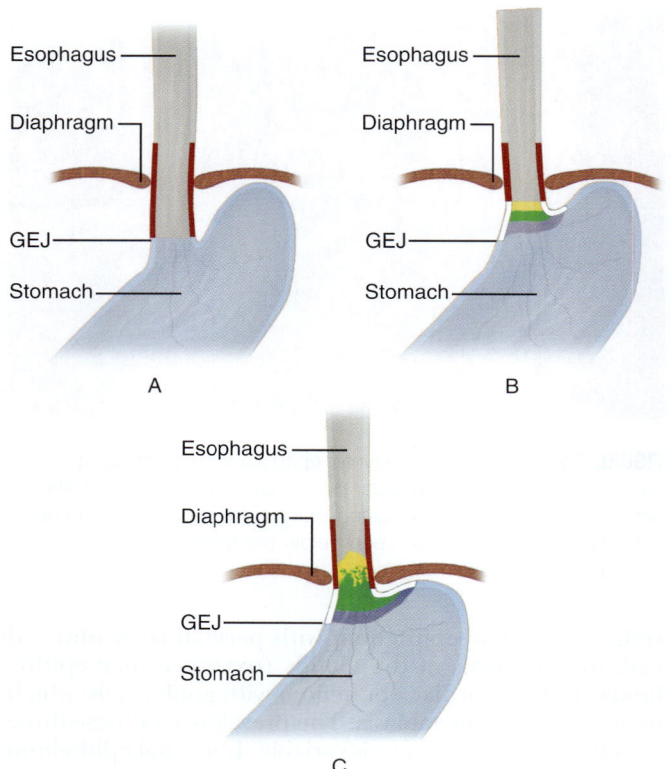

FIGURE 3.6 Progression of the gap between the squamocolumnar junction and gastric oxyntic epithelium with increasing severity of gastroesophageal reflux disease. (A) Normal state with no gap; the squamous epithelium *(gray)* transitions directly to gastric oxyntic epithelium *(blue)*; note rugal folds *(lines)*. (B) Metaplastic columnar epithelium limited to the dilated distal esophagus. This is depicted with intestinal metaplasia *(yellow)*, cardiac epithelium *(green)*, and oxyntocardiac epithelium *(purple)*. Note that these epithelia have replaced squamous epithelium. The proximal limit of gastric oxyntic epithelium has not moved. The area of columnar metaplasia of squamous epithelium is dilated and has developed rugal folds. This is the dilated distal esophagus resulting from abdominal lower esophageal sphincter (LES) damage. This is presently mistaken for proximal stomach (gastric cardia), because it is distal to the end of the tubular esophagus and the proximal limit of rugal folds. (C) Final phase of progression where LES damage has led to sufficient reflux into the esophageal body to cause visible columnar-lined esophagus (vCLE). (*Note:* The damaged LES is shown as a *white wall* that has replaced the *red wall* where the LES is intact.) *GEJ*, Gastroesophageal junction.

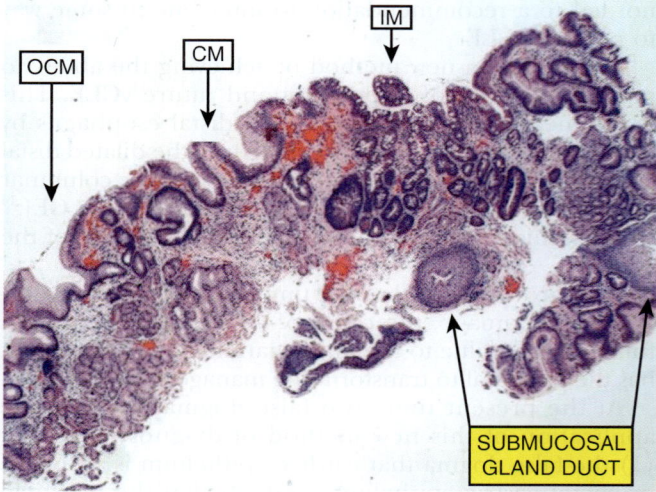

FIGURE 3.7 The histologic composition of the dilated distal esophagus, showing the three metaplastic columnar epithelial types. Intestinal metaplasia with goblet cells *(IM)* is proximal, cardiac epithelium *(CM)* is in the middle, and oxyntocardiac epithelium with parietal cells *(CCM)* is distal (on the *left*). Note the presence of submucosal gland ducts. Ducts of submucosal glands are specific for the esophagus; their presence proves that the location of this tissue is esophageal.

TABLE 3.3 Histologic Criteria for Diagnosis of Four Columnar Epithelial Types Encountered in the Esophagus and Proximal Stomach*

	Mucous Cells in Glands†	Parietal Cells	Goblet Cells
Gastric oxyntic epithelium	−	+	−‡
Cardiac epithelium	+	−	−
Oxyntocardiac epithelium	+	+	−
Intestinal epithelium	+	−	+

*Gastric oxyntic epithelium lined the entire proximal stomach. Cardiac, oxyntocardiac, and intestinal epithelia are, when present, interposed between the squamous epithelium and gastric oxyntic epithelium (i.e., form the squamo-oxyntic gap). *Note:* There is no epithelium defined in this scheme that has both parietal and goblet cells in one foveolar-gland complex. This is an extremely rare finding; when found, goblet cells take precedence and the epithelium is designated as intestinal.

†Mucous cells are present at the surface and foveolar pit in all epithelial types; it is the presence of mucous cells in glands below the foveolar pit that are relevant to the definitions.

‡Gastric oxyntic epithelium with atrophic gastritis can have goblet cells. This is intestinal metaplasia in gastric oxyntic epithelium, which is different than cardiac (metaplastic esophageal) epithelium with intestinal metaplasia.

for which evidence is lacking, this definition of the GEJ has incredible universal acceptance.

Chandrasoma et al.[27] have shown conclusively that this endoscopic definition of the GEJ is incorrect (Fig. 3.8A and B). They showed that the area distal to the endoscopic GEJ lined by cardiac epithelium (with and without parietal and/or goblet cells) was the esophagus, by virtue that submucosal glands that are specific to the esophagus were present in and concordant with the length of the dilated distal esophagus (Fig. 3.9).

The correct definition of the true GEJ is the proximal limit of gastric oxyntic epithelium. This never changes its position. In the person with LES damage, whether symptoms or GERD are present or not, the true GEJ is separated from the endoscopic GEJ by cardiac epithelium (with and without parietal and/or goblet cells; see Fig. 3.6).

The present use of the endoscopic GEJ results in an error that is equal to the length of the dilated distal esophagus. Ironically, the greater the amount of LES damage (i.e., the more severe the GERD), the greater the error. This error is made at endoscopy, manometry, and

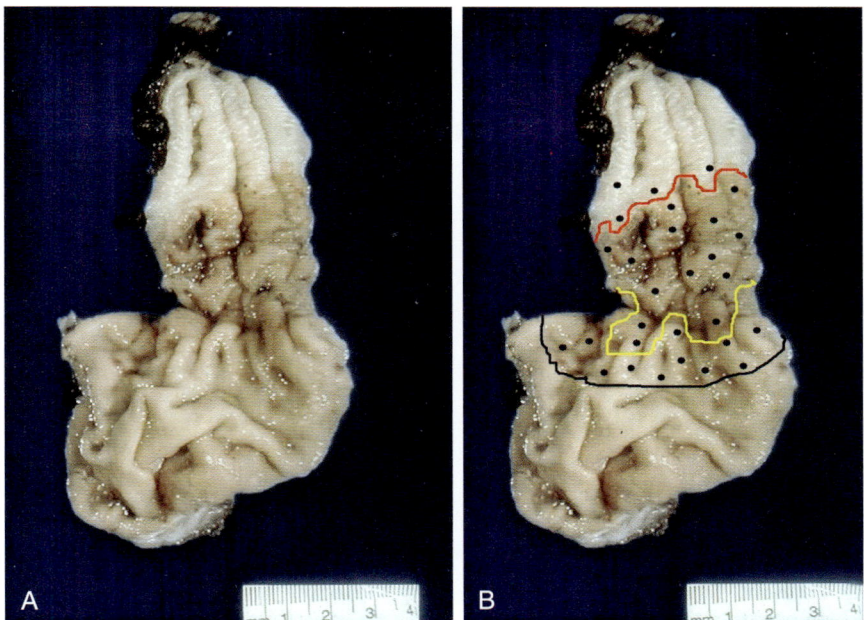

FIGURE 3.8 Present incorrect and correct interpretation of an esophagectomy specimen. (A) This specimen shows a tubular esophagus lined by 5.5 cm of visible columnar-lined esophagus *(vCLE)* above the proximal limit of rugal folds. There is an ulcerated adenocarcinoma immediately distal to the squamocolumnar junction. The area distal to the end of the tubular esophagus is lined by rugal folds. This area will be interpreted as proximal stomach by present criteria for defining the gastroesophageal junction (GEJ) at endoscopy and gross dissection. (B) Histologic findings show that 20.5 mm of the area distal to the end of the tubular esophagus and containing rugal folds is lined by cardiac epithelium with intestinal metaplasia proximally and oxyntocardiac epithelium distally. The *red line* is the squamocolumnar junction; the *yellow line* is the distal limit of intestinal metaplasia; the *black line* is the proximal limit of gastric oxyntic epithelium, which is the true GEJ. The dilated distal esophagus between the end of the tubular esophagus and the true GEJ contains submucosal glands *(black dots)*, whose extent is concordant with the length of cardiac epithelium (with parietal and goblet cells). This is proof of the dilated distal esophagus.

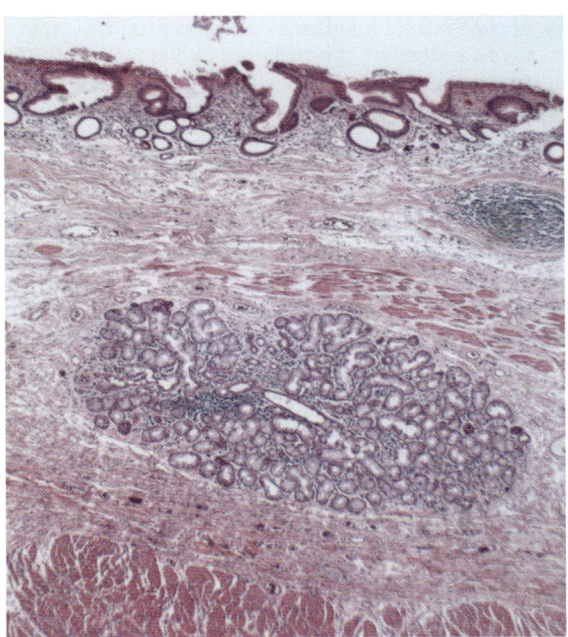

FIGURE 3.9 Full-thickness section of dilated distal esophagus showing cardiac epithelium with an underlying submucosal gland.

gross pathology. It is also made at histology by pathologists who believe that cardiac epithelium is part of the normal stomach. Only pathologists who understand that cardiac epithelium is always an abnormal metaplastic esophageal epithelium have the key to the truth.

MEASUREMENT OF THE LENGTH OF THE DILATED DISTAL ESOPHAGUS

The dilated distal esophagus can be precisely measured by examining the mucosa distal to the endoscopic GEJ. This can be done at autopsy and in resected specimens by taking a vertical section with its proximal end at the SCJ (in a person without vCLE), extending distally till the proximal limit of gastric oxyntic epithelium is reached (30 mm beyond the SCJ to ensure that gastric oxyntic epithelium is reached).[27,28] When vCLE is present, the dilated distal esophagus is measured from the endoscopic GEJ (end of tubular esophagus or proximal limit of rugal folds) to the proximal limit of gastric oxyntic epithelium (see Fig. 3.8).

The length of the dilated distal esophagus can be assessed at endoscopy by measured biopsies taken at 5 mm intervals from the SCJ, extending distally to a point 30 mm distal to the SCJ (Fig. 3.10). It is unlikely that this labor-intensive, endoscopist-dependent, and cumbersome multilevel biopsy protocol will be acceptable or accurate. The inability to orient each biopsy will result in an error in the measurement of at least 1 to 2 mm. Ideally, a new

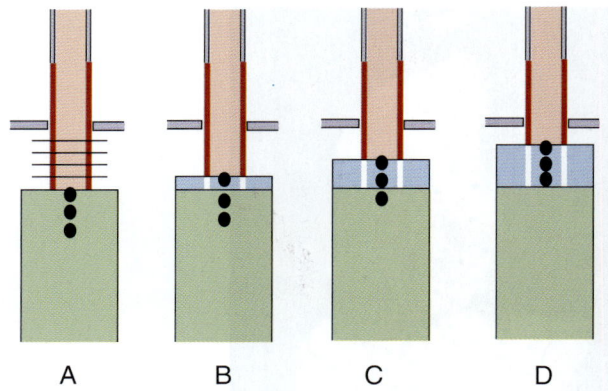

FIGURE 3.10 Multilevel biopsy protocol for measuring the length of cardiac epithelium in the dilated distal esophagus *(blue)* between the distal limit of squamous epithelium *(pink)* and the proximal limit of gastric oxyntic epithelium *(green)*. Three biopsies *(black circles)* are taken at 5 mm intervals. (A) Normal state with no cardiac epithelium. (B) Cardiac epithelium present in the zero to 5 mm biopsy. (C) Cardiac epithelium present in the zero to 10 mm biopsies. (D) Cardiac epithelium present in all three biopsies up to 15 mm distal to the squamocolumnar junction.

biopsy instrument should be developed that can obtain a single, intact 25 mm vertical biopsy of the mucosa. This will provide a measurement that has a level of accuracy within a micrometer, identical to a vertical section taken from a resection specimen.

VARIATION IN THE LENGTH OF THE DILATED DISTAL ESOPHAGUS

The reported length of the dilated distal esophagus varies in published reports from zero to 28 mm in patients without vCLE. Its theoretical length is the initial length of the a-LES, which is 35 mm. When the entire a-LES has been destroyed, the angle of His essentially disappears and hiatal hernia occurs.

Normally, in a person with a completely intact LES, there is no dilated distal esophagus. The entire abdominal esophagus is tubular, lined by squamous epithelium to its end (the GEJ) where it transitions to gastric oxyntic epithelium. There is no metaplastic columnar epithelium (i.e. cardiac epithelium). Chandrasoma et al.[24] and other groups[29] have illustrated an SCJ with a direct transition of squamous to gastric oxyntic epithelium without cardiac epithelium (Fig. 3.11A and B).

The abnormal state where the LES is damaged is defined by the presence of a dilated distal esophagus. The length of the dilated distal esophagus, as measured by histology, has a strong correlation with the cellular changes associated with GERD.

Chandrasoma et al.[24] reported a length of 0 to 8.05 mm in persons without symptoms of GERD at autopsy (Fig. 3.12). Kilgore et al.[30] in a study of 30 pediatric autopsies confirmed that cardiac epithelium measured a maximum of 4 mm.

Robertson et al.[20] in a study of asymptomatic volunteers reported that the length of cardiac epithelium was a median of 2.50 mm in persons with central obesity, significantly greater than the 1.75 mm in those without obesity. The patients with central obesity also had a shorter a-LES.

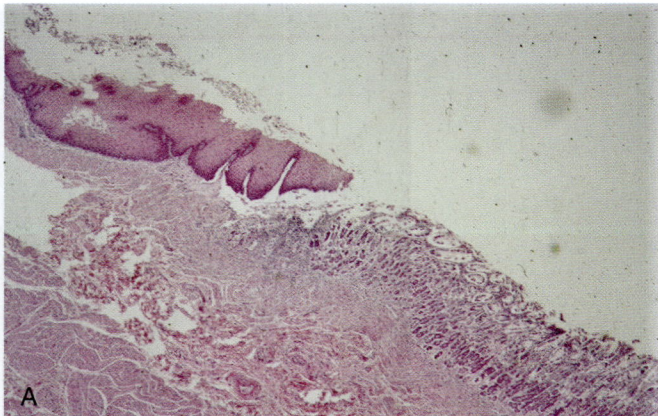

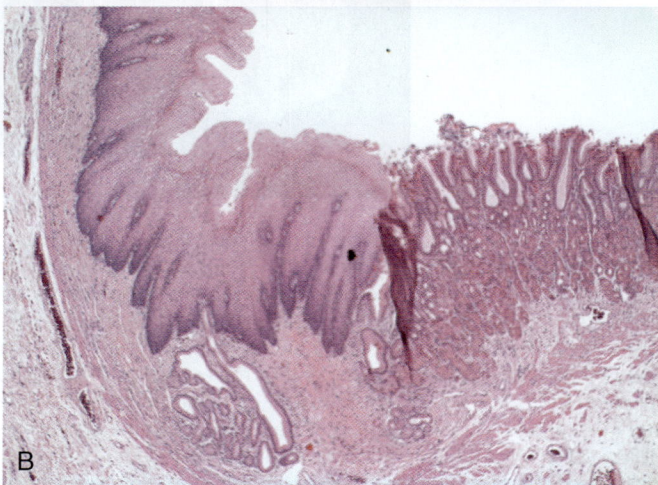

FIGURE 3.11 (A) A section across the squamocolumnar junction at autopsy showing direct transition of squamous epithelium to gastric oxyntic epithelium, characterized by the typical straight tubular glands containing only parietal and chief cells below the foveolar pit. (B) A zero squamo-oxyntic gap in a 77-year-old male undergoing esophagectomy for squamous carcinoma. Exactly at the end of the esophagus is a small mucous gland with a duct.

The dilated distal esophagus is longer in patients with GERD and correlates with the severity of GERD. In the only study with multilevel biopsies in a population of GERD patients, Ringhofer et al.[31] reported the findings at the endoscopic GEJ and on both sides of it at intervals of 0.5 cm. Cardiac epithelium (with and without parietal and/or goblet cells) was found in 100% at the GEJ, in 81% in the biopsy taken 5 mm distal to the GEJ, and in 28% in the biopsy taken 10 mm distal to the GEJ.

Chandrasoma et al.[27] reported the findings in 10 esophagectomy specimens that had a sharp transition from the tube to the sac at the exact location of well-defined proximal rugal folds. Eight patients had adenocarcinoma of the esophagus secondary to Barrett esophagus; in these patients, the dilated distal esophagus measured 10.3 to 20.5 mm (Fig. 3.13). In two patients who had squamous carcinoma without vCLE, the dilated distal esophagus measured 3.1 and 4.3 mm (see Fig. 3.13). Sarbia et al.[28] in a similar study of esophagectomy specimens in 36 patients with squamous carcinoma showed that cardiac epithelium (with and without parietal and/or goblet cells) was present distal to the end of the tubular esophagus to a length that varied from a minimum of 4 mm (median) to a maximum length of 11 mm (median). In eight patients (25%), cardiac and/or oxyntocardiac epithelium was situated over submucosal glands.

The true GEJ cannot be seen at endoscopy because the dilated distal esophagus and proximal stomach both have rugal folds. With standard endoscopy, it is not possible to differentiate cardiac and gastric oxyntic epithelium. It is possible that newer endoscopic modalities, such as confocal microscopy and optical coherence tomography, can do this. At present, though, only histologic examination is capable of identifying the true GEJ.

NEW PATHOLOGIC TEST OF LOWER ESOPHAGEAL SPHINCTER DAMAGE

We have proposed a new test that can accurately measure the presence and severity of a-LES damage in any person, whether or not there are symptoms of GERD. LES damage is equal to the measured length of the dilated distal esophagus. This is the length of cardiac epithelium (with and without parietal and/or goblet cells) between the SCJ and the proximal limit of gastric oxyntic epithelium in persons without a visible CLE at endoscopy.

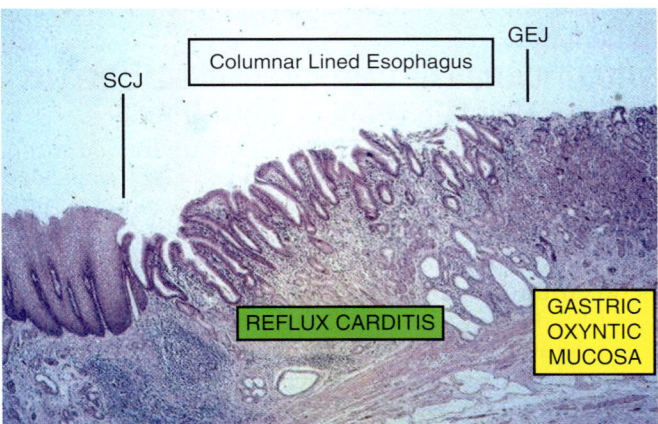

FIGURE 3.12 The histologic gap composed of cardiac and oxyntocardiac epithelia between the distal end of the squamous epithelium and proximal limit of gastric oxyntic epithelium (2 mm long in this section). This is the histologic definition of the dilated distal esophagus. This patient has 2 mm of abdominal lower esophageal sphincter damage. *GEJ,* Gastroesophageal junction; *SCJ,* squamocolumnar junction.

With a suitable specimen, this can be measured with an accuracy within 1 μm. The measurement is made on a standard histologic slide with a standard microscope that has an ocular micrometer. These are available in every pathology laboratory the world over. The test is inexpensive.

CLASSIFICATION OF GASTROESOPHAGEAL REFLUX DISEASE BY THE RESULTS OF THE NEW TEST

The ability to measure a-LES damage opens a new dimension in the diagnosis and management of GERD. The entire spectrum of the disease from the normal state to the most severe disease can be understood by the extent of damage to the 35 mm of the a-LES (see Table 3.1). Correlations between severity of a-LES damage and frequency of LES failure, severity of reflux, and severity of cellular changes in the esophagus are likely to be more accurate than with any other measure.

Theoretically, we can divide GERD into four stages based on the amount of a-LES damage. To do this, we will make the following assumptions: (1) the initial length of the a-LES is 35 mm; (2) LES failure correlates with a functional a-LES length of less than 10 mm; (3) a-LES damage has a linear progression with a variable rate in any person; and (4) dynamic shortening of the a-LES with a meal has a maximum of 10 mm.

Four stages of GERD emerge in this new method:

1. **Normal**. There is no LES damage. The residual a-LES length is 35 mm. Defined by the absence of a dilated distal esophagus. This is rare in adults. However, I have encountered a 67-year-old male without cardiac epithelium in an esophagectomy done for squamous carcinoma (Fig. 3.11).

2. **The phase of compensated a-LES damage**. There is a-LES damage less than 15 mm defined by a dilated distal esophagus of less than 15 mm. Residual a-LES length is greater than 20 mm. This is the finding in 70% of the population at large who do not have symptoms of GERD. Their LES is competent at all times, and there is no significant reflux on a pH test (zero to well below normal).

3. **Mild GERD**. There is a-LES damage of 15 to 25 mm, defined by a dilated distal esophagus of 15 to 25 mm. Residual a-LES length is 10 to 20 mm. This is the finding in 70% of patients with GERD. Their symptoms are controlled with PPIs, and there is a low prevalence of vCLE. Their LES tends to fail during the postprandial period when dynamic shortening decreases the a-LES length to less than 10 mm. At the low end of this range, the patients are at the onset of disease with infrequent postprandial reflux. At the high end, they are at the cusp of severe GERD. Somewhere in the higher end of this

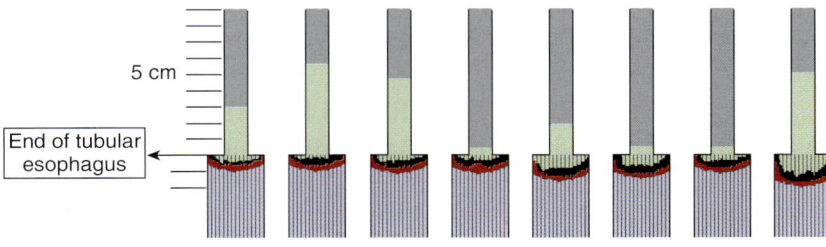

5 cm

End of tubular esophagus

FIGURE 3.13 Esophagectomy specimens in eight patients with adenocarcinoma arising in Barrett esophagus. The dilated distal esophagus measures 10.3 to 20.5 mm and is associated with visible columnar-lined esophagus (vCLE) in the tubular esophagus. *Green,* intestinal metaplasia; *Black,* cardiac epithelium; *Red,* oxyntocardiac epithelium; *Lilac,* gastric oxyntic epithelium; black vertical lines indicate rugal folds.

range, they may develop vCLE. They have significant reflux with a high normal or abnormal pH test.

4. **Severe GERD**. There is a-LES damage of greater than 25 mm. The residual a-LES in the fasting state is below the threshold at which LES failure occurs. Reflux is severe and unrelated to meals. There is a high prevalence of refractory GERD and vCLE.

EVIDENCE BASE SUPPORTING THE NEW DIAGNOSTIC METHOD

We have presented the data that show strong support that the length of the dilated distal esophagus, measured by the length of cardiac epithelium (with and without parietal and/or goblet cells) between the endoscopic GEJ and proximal limit of gastric oxyntic epithelium, accurately represents LES damage. We have shown that the length of a-LES damage can be measured accurately within 1 μm in autopsy and resected specimens.

Unfortunately, there is almost no data relating to the measured a-LES damage in either asymptomatic people or patients with GERD. This is the result of the erroneous beliefs that cardiac epithelium lines the normal proximal stomach and the GEJ is defined by the proximal limit of rugal folds. These false dogmas have resulted in a general recommendation by all gastroenterology societies that biopsies should not be taken in the person who is endoscopically normal, which has inhibited data being accumulated.[2,8] As a result, there has never been a systematic study of the dilated distal esophagus.

We have made several assumptions in using the new test to classify patients into four stages based on a-LES damage. These assumptions are based on a careful examination of the best available evidence. However, the evidence base is scanty. There is an opportunity to study the dilated distal esophagus at every upper endoscopy. Our hope is that knowledge of this new diagnostic test will stimulate esophagologists to produce data that will refine the criteria for defining these various stages of GERD.

PREDICTION OF PROGRESSION OF LOWER ESOPHAGEAL SPHINCTER DAMAGE

LES damage is irreversible. There is evidence that a-LES damage progresses in an inexorably relentless manner. Progression is not impacted in any way by medical therapy. The cause of LES damage is an eating disorder that can be described as LES-unfriendly. Once this eating habit is established, the rate of progression of a-LES damage is likely to be linear over the long term.

The new test of a-LES damage provides a unique ability to predict the status of the a-LES in the future if it is assumed that progression of LES damage is linear over the long term. Theoretically, if a-LES damage is measured on two occasions separated by a significant interval, a simple straight-line slope can be drawn that extrapolates the extent of damage back into the past and forward into the future.

The prediction is also possible with one measurement with the assumption that a-LES damage begins at an early age, say 15 years old, when a person's adult eating habit is established. There are now two points that permit the slope of future a-LES damage to be drawn.

The ability to predict future a-LES damage permits the identification of persons who are at risk of progressing to severe GERD defined by vCLE in the future long before the point at which the person is in danger. This permits intervention to slow the progression of LES damage. If a successful intervention can be developed, progression to severe GERD and vCLE can be prevented. *The objective of preventing vCLE is achieved. Adenocarcinoma will not occur without vCLE.*

POTENTIAL VALUE OF THE NEW TEST IN THE MANAGEMENT OF GASTROESOPHAGEAL REFLUX DISEASE

The new test has obvious value in the management of GERD.

EXCLUSION OF GASTROESOPHAGEAL REFLUX DISEASE AS A CAUSE OF SYMPTOMS

At the present time, there is no diagnostic test that can accurately determine whether symptoms that could possibly be caused by GERD are actually caused by GERD. Diagnosis commonly depends on an empiric PPI test that is known to have a significant false-positive rate.[2] The consequence of a false-positive empiric PPI test is that many people are unnecessarily placed on long-term PPI therapy who do not have GERD. The new test provides a definitive answer: *If the measured a-LES damage is less than 15 mm (or a number based on new data), the symptoms are not caused by GERD.*

STRATIFICATION OF GASTROESOPHAGEAL REFLUX DISEASE TREATMENT ACCORDING TO RISK

At the present time, all GERD patients are treated with a one-size-fits-all regimen of acid reducing drugs as needed to control symptoms. The ability of the new test to identify the minority of people who are at risk to progress to vCLE allows a concentrated attack on this group. The interval between the test and the predicted time of occurrence of a-LES damage sufficient to cause vCLE is likely to be many decades. This allows time to watch the patient, repeat testing to verify findings, try a test of dietary control, and intervene to prevent progression of LES damage before vCLE develops.

WHAT NEEDS TO HAPPEN FOR THE NEW TEST TO WORK

Like any new scientific test, there is much research, development, and testing that needs to be done to bring the test to fruition. We can conceive some of these at this time. However, when the test is recognized as being valuable, novel developments yet not conceived are likely to emerge.

NEED TO REMOVE ERRORS IN INTERPRETATION

The evidence base that cardiac epithelium is always a metaplastic esophageal epithelium is powerful. The present dogma that cardiac epithelium is the normal lining of the proximal stomach must be eliminated.

The evidence that the true GEJ is the proximal limit of gastric oxyntic epithelium and cannot be seen at endoscopy is powerful. The opinion-based definitions that are universally used to define the GEJ at endoscopy and gross dissection (proximal limit or rugal folds and end of the tubular esophagus) must be eliminated.

NEED FOR A NEW BIOPSY DEVICE

Accurate measurement of the dilated distal esophagus is not possible with present biopsy forceps. A critical length of between 15 and 25 mm of a-LES damage differentiates mild GERD at its onset to severe GERD. Accuracy is vital. With present biopsy forceps, multiple level biopsies distal to the endoscopic GEJ need to be performed. These are likely to be extremely difficult and time consuming, and therefore fraught with error. A simple new biopsy device that can remove a piece of mucosa measuring 25 mm long, 2 mm wide, and 1 mm deep should be easy to produce. This will provide a mucosal biopsy sample that is equivalent to a section taken from a resected specimen that we know can produce a measurement of the dilated distal esophagus that is accurate to within 1 μm.

NEED FOR DATA ON ASYMPTOMATIC PERSONS AND GASTROESOPHAGEAL REFLUX DISEASE PATIENTS

A large database is the essential requirement for defining criteria for length of a-LES damage that is associated with vCLE. This is the critical value, because preventing vCLE is the objective and basis of preventing adenocarcinoma. We have used the best available evidence at this time to suggest that greater than 25 mm of a-LES damage is the earliest point at which vCLE occurs. This may be optimistic; it is possible that this number is closer to 20 mm. The important thing is that examination of a sufficient number of people *will* provide that number.

NONENDOSCOPIC MEASUREMENT OF A-LOWER ESOPHAGEAL SPHINCTER DAMAGE

At present, all biopsy methods are designed for use with an endoscope. The need for endoscopy to perform the new test will seriously limit its usage. Endoscopy will have low value in the assessment of GERD if the new test becomes a stand-alone diagnostic test. In that event, it will be important to develop nonendoscopic methods of inserting the biopsy device to the appropriate location and orientation to allow the required biopsy to be taken. If such a method can be developed that is safe, quick, and inexpensive, with the ability to be done in the doctor's office without the need for sedation, the scope of the test can be expanded dramatically to the general population, allowing screening and early diagnosis.

NEW EFFECTIVE METHOD FOR PREVENTING PROGRESSION OF A-LOWER ESOPHAGEAL SPHINCTER DAMAGE

Many procedures are presently available to repair or augment a defective LES. Some are done by endoscopy and others require laparoscopic surgery. These all have less than perfect and variable effectiveness with significant complications.

The new need is simpler. The objective is not to repair or augment a defective LES; it is to prevent progression of a damaged LES with significant residual function that is predicted to progress to severe damage in the future. This is a far easier surgical problem. It is very likely that many of the techniques that currently have low success rates in augmenting a defective LES will have more success in preventing progression of damage in a partially damaged LES.

CONCLUSION

We envision the management of GERD in the future to be very different with the availability of the new test. At its ultimate end point of development, a biopsy device will be used in a doctor's office as a screening test in the population at around age 30 to 35 years, unless symptoms appear earlier. The test will be simple, inexpensive, and relatively painless. It will identify those at risk in the future, with a timeline that shows the exact status of the a-LES at specific times in the life of the patient. We can equate it to a Pap smear for cancer of the uterine cervix.

The patient will have choices depending on the results of the test:

1. The test predicts that a-LES damage will remain within the reserve capacity, indicating that there will be no GERD. The person can be confident that esophageal adenocarcinoma will not occur. No treatment will ever be necessary. The senior author (PC) has had this assessment. He knows that at age 56 years, he had 4 mm of a-LES damage, measured in an endoscopic biopsy of the normal SCJ. Biopsies greater than 5 mm, greater than 10 mm, greater than 15 mm, and greater than 20 mm distal to the SCJ consisted of normal gastric oxyntic epithelium. By the algorithm that predicts linear progression, he is predicted to have 8 mm of a-LES damage at age 97 years. He will always stay in the green zone of Table 3.1 with LES damage that is within its reserve capacity. He will never develop GERD, Barrett esophagus, or esophageal adenocarcinoma. No one else in the world has that certainty.

2. The test predicts the occurrence of LES damage that is likely to cause mild GERD during the expected life span that can be easily controlled with acid reducing therapy without progression to severe GERD, vCLE, or cancer. This person can opt to let GERD arise and be treated with PPIs for the entire lifetime or undergo the procedure to protect the LES and prevent GERD.

3. The test predicts future severe LES damage with a high risk of refractory GERD, vCLE, and adenocarcinoma. These persons can develop a long-term treatment protocol with repeat testing, dietary control to slow progression of a-LES damage, and timely intervention with a simple procedure well before the predicted time of LES damage sufficient to cause severe GERD and vCLE.

In all scenarios, knowledge of future a-LES damage allows for stratification of treatment according to the risk of future cellular complications of GERD.

We can only guess whether this vision of a world without GERD and esophageal adenocarcinoma will come true. What is important is that this new method provides us with the possibility that there may be a way to this goal. It will change the perspective toward a belief that GERD, Barrett esophagus, and esophageal adenocarcinoma are preventable. This is better than the present nihilistic attitude, where we do nothing and simply hope that our patients will not progress to severe GERD that is refractory to therapy or, worse, be complicated by adenocarcinoma.

REFERENCES

1. Vakil N, van Zanten SV, Kahrilas P, Dent J, Jones B, The Global Consensus Group. The Montreal definition and classification of gastroesophageal reflux disease: a global evidence-based consensus. *Am J Gastroenterol.* 2006;101:1900-1920.
2. Kahrilas PJ, Shaheen NJ, Vaezi MF. American Gastroenterological Association medical position statement on the management of gastroesophageal reflux disease. *Gastroenterology.* 2008;135:1383-1391.
3. Chandrasoma PT, Der R, Ma Y, Peters J, DeMeester T. Histologic classification of patients based on mapping biopsies of the gastroesophageal junction. *Am J Surg Pathol.* 2003;27:929-936.
4. Spechler SJ, Sharma P, Souza RF, Inadomi JM, Shaheen NJ. American Gastroenterological Association medical position statement on the management of Barrett's esophagus. *Gastroenterology.* 2011;140:1084-1091.
5. Toghanian S, Wahlqvist P, Johnson DA, Bolge SC, Liljas B. The burden of disrupting gastro-esophageal disease: a database study in US and European cohorts. *Clin Drug Investig.* 2010;30:167-178.
6. Pohl H, Sirovich B, Welch HG. Esophageal adenocarcinoma incidence: are we reaching the peak? *Cancer Epidemiol Biomarkers Prev.* 2010;19:1468-1470.
7. Malfertheiner P, Nocon M, Vieth M, et al. Evolution of gastro-oesophageal reflux disease over 5 years under routine medical care—the ProGERD study. *Aliment Pharmacol Ther.* 2012;35:154-164.
8. Fitzgerald RC, di Pietro M, Ragunath K, et al. British Society of Gastroenterology guidelines on the diagnosis and management of Barrett's oesophagus. *Gut.* 2014;63:7-42.
9. Leodolter A, Nocon M, Vieth M, et al. Progression of specialized intestinal metaplasia at the cardia to macroscopically evident Barrett's esophagus: an entity of concern in the Pro-GERD study. *Scand J Gastroenterol.* 2012;47:1429-1435.
10. Nason KS, Wichienkuer PP, Awais O, et al. Gastroesophageal reflux disease symptom severity, proton pump inhibitor use, and esophageal carcinogenesis. *Arch Surg.* 2011;146:851-858.
11. Stein HJ, Liebermann-Meffert D, DeMeester TR, Siewert JR. Three-dimensional pressure image and muscular structure of the human lower esophageal sphincter. *Surgery.* 1995;117:692-698.
12. Bonavina L, Evander A, DeMeester TR, et al. Length of the distal esophageal sphincter and competency of the cardia. *Am J Surg.* 1986;151:25-34.
13. Zaninotto G, DeMeester TR, Schwizer W, Johansson KE, Cheng SC. The lower esophageal sphincter in health and disease. *Am J Surg.* 1988;155:104-111.
14. Chandrasoma P, Wijetunge S, Ma Y, DeMeester S, Hagen J, DeMeester T. The dilated distal esophagus: a new entity that is the pathologic basis of early gastroesophageal reflux disease. *Am J Surg Pathol.* 2011;35:1873-1881.
15. Korn O, Csendes A, Burdiles P, Braghetto I, Stein HJ. Anatomic dilatation of the cardia and competence of the lower esophageal sphincter: a clinical and experimental study. *J Gastrointest Surg.* 2000;4:398-406.
16. Curcic J, Roy S, Tech M, et al. Abnormal structure and function of the esophagogastric junction and proximal stomach in gastroesophageal reflux disease. *Am J Gastroenterol.* 2014;109:658-666.
17. Hayward J. The lower end of the oesophagus. *Thorax.* 1961;16:36-41.
18. Chandrasoma PT. Histologic definition of gastro-esophageal reflux disease. *Curr Opin Gastroenterol.* 2013;29:460-467.
19. Ayazi S, Tamhankar A, DeMeester SR, et al. The impact of gastric distension on the lower esophageal sphincter and its exposure to acid gastric juice. *Ann Surg.* 2010;252:57-62.
20. Robertson EV, Derakhshan MH, Wirz AA, et al. Central obesity in asymptomatic volunteers is associated with increased intrasphincteric acid reflux and lengthening of the cardiac mucosa. *Gastroenterology.* 2013;145:730-739.
21. Clarke AT, Wirz AA, Manning JJ, Ballantyne SA, Alcorn DJ, McColl KE. Severe reflux disease is associated with an enlarged unbuffered proximal gastric acid pocket. *Gut.* 2008;57:292-297.
22. Kahrilas PJ, Shi G, Manka M, Joehl RJ. Increased frequency of transient lower esophageal sphincter relaxation induced by gastric distension in reflux patients with hiatal hernia. *Gastroenterology.* 2000;118:688-695.
23. Chandrasoma P. Controversies of the cardiac mucosa and Barrett's esophagus. *Histopathology.* 2005;46:361-373.
24. Chandrasoma PT, Der R, Ma Y, Dalton P, Taira M. Histology of the gastroesophageal junction: an autopsy study. *Am J Surg Pathol.* 2000;24:402-409.
25. McClave SA, Boyce HW Jr, Gottfried MR. Early diagnosis of columnar lined esophagus: a new endoscopic diagnostic criterion. *Gastrointest Endosc.* 1987;33:413-416.
26. Sharma P, McQuaid K, Dent J, et al. A critical review of the diagnosis and management of Barrett's esophagus: the AGA Chicago Workshop. *Gastroenterology.* 2004;127:310-330.
27. Chandrasoma P, Makarewicz K, Wickramasinghe K, Ma YL, DeMeester TR. A proposal for a new validated histologic definition of the gastroesophageal junction. *Hum Pathol.* 2006;37:40-47.
28. Sarbia M, Donner A, Gabbert HE. Histopathology of the gastroesophageal junction. A study on 36 operation specimens. *Am J Surg Pathol.* 2002;26:1207-1212.
29. Park YS, Park HJ, Kang GH, Kim CJ, Chi JG. Histology of gastroesophageal junction in fetal and pediatric autopsy. *Arch Pathol Lab Med.* 2003;127:451-455.
30. Kilgore SP, Ormsby AH, Gramlich TL, et al. The gastric cardia: fact or fiction? *Am J Gastroenterol.* 2000;95:921-924.
31. Ringhofer C, Lenglinger J, Izay B, et al. Histopathology of the endoscopic esophagogastric junction in patients with gastroesophageal reflux disease. *Wien Klin Wochenschr.* 2008;120:350-359.

Relevant Anatomic Relations of the Esophagus

Jules Lin

The primary purpose of the esophagus is to transport food from the mouth to the stomach, and the esophagus has no digestive or absorptive function. The esophagus is a muscular tube that starts at the inferior border of the cricoid cartilage in the neck and traverses the chest, ending as it enters the stomach in the upper abdomen. Esophageal surgeons need to be familiar with the anatomy and clinical importance of the relationship of the esophagus to surrounding structures in all three areas of the body.

The esophagus is anchored superiorly to the cricoid cartilage and inferiorly to the diaphragm. Its length from the cricoid cartilage at C6 to the gastric orifice at T11 ranges from 22 to 28 cm (Fig. 4.1).[1] The length of the esophagus varies with the height of the patient. The esophageal bed lies in the posterior mediastinum along the ventral surface of the vertebra. This is the shortest distance for reconstruction after esophagectomy and measures approximately 30 cm. When the orthotopic route is not available due to previous surgery, the retrosternal (32 cm) or subcutaneous (34 cm) routes are alternatives.[2,3]

On endoscopy, the upper esophageal sphincter is approximately 15 cm from the incisors, the carina at 25 cm, and the lower esophageal sphincter at 38 to 40 cm in men and 36 to 38 cm in women. When planning the surgical approach to the esophagus, it is useful to consider the location of the tumor relative to the carina at 25 cm in deciding whether to perform a left or a right thoracotomy to avoid the aortic arch, which blocks access to the upper thoracic esophagus on the left.

While the cervical esophagus is flattened by surrounding structures, the thoracic esophagus is more round due to negative intrathoracic pressure. Once the esophagus enters the abdomen, it becomes more flattened again as a result of positive intraabdominal pressure. The overall diameter of the esophagus is approximately 2.5 cm.[1] There are three anatomic narrowings of the esophagus (Fig. 4.2). The narrowest part of the gastrointestinal tract is at the cricopharyngeal constriction at the upper esophageal sphincter, where the esophagus is 1.5 cm in diameter. In the superior mediastinum, the aortic arch, left atrium, and left mainstem bronchus compress the left anterolateral aspect of the esophagus around 22 cm from the incisors. The third area of narrowing is at the lower esophageal sphincter. These areas are important since swallowed foreign bodies often lodge in these areas.

The esophageal wall is composed of four layers, including an inner squamous mucosal layer, submucosa, muscularis propria, and adventitia. The mucosal layer consists of the squamous epithelium, lamina propria, and muscularis mucosa, while the muscularis propria consists of an inner circular and outer longitudinal layer of muscle (Fig. 4.3). The longitudinal layer originates from the cricoid cartilage as two muscle bundles that converge 3 cm distal to the cricopharyngeus muscle, leaving a V-shaped weakened area posteriorly covered only with circular muscle fibers, known as Laimer triangle (Fig. 4.4). The cricopharyngeal muscle and up to 2 cm of the cervical esophagus are composed mostly of striated muscle.[4,5] There is a gradual transition from striated muscle, which is only present in the upper 40% of the esophagus, to smooth muscle (Fig. 4.5). As a result, most dysmotility disorders, which involve smooth muscle, predominantly affect the distal two-thirds of the esophagus.

CERVICAL ESOPHAGUS

The cervical esophagus shifts to the left at the base of the neck, so the best approach to the cervical esophagus is a left neck incision (e.g., during the cervical anastomosis for a transhiatal esophagectomy or resection of a Zenker diverticulum). The cervical esophagus is 5 cm in length and extends from the cricoid cartilage at the C6 vertebra to the suprasternal notch anteriorly and the T1-T2 interspace posteriorly. The esophagus is surrounded by loose fibroareolar tissue, and unlike the remainder of the gastrointestinal tract, there is no serosal lining or mesentery.

The pretracheal fascia anteriorly, prevertebral fascia posteriorly, and carotid sheaths laterally create two cervical compartments, the paraesophageal space anteriorly, and the retroesophageal space posteriorly. The pretracheal fascia extends to the pericardium, while the prevertebral fascia extends to the diaphragm, connecting compartments in the neck and chest, allowing infections from tonsillar or dental abscesses to spread quickly into the mediastinum. A descending infection can rapidly lead to potentially fatal necrotizing mediastinitis, emphasizing the importance of early surgical drainage. Iatrogenic perforations most commonly occur above the narrowing of the cricopharyngeal muscle, resulting in a posterior pharyngeal perforation (see Fig. 4.4).[6]

The arterial blood supply for the cervical esophagus originates from the right and left superior and inferior thyroid arteries (Fig. 4.6). There are also smaller branches from the common carotid and subclavian arteries. Venous drainage is through the inferior thyroid vein. The middle thyroid vein crosses from the internal jugular vein to the thyroid gland, and often is divided to improve exposure of the cervical esophagus. Innervation of the cervical esophagus is from the recurrent laryngeal nerves and the sympathetic chains.

UPPER ESOPHAGEAL SPHINCTER

The posterior pharynx consists of three bilateral constrictor muscles originating from the base of the skull, the

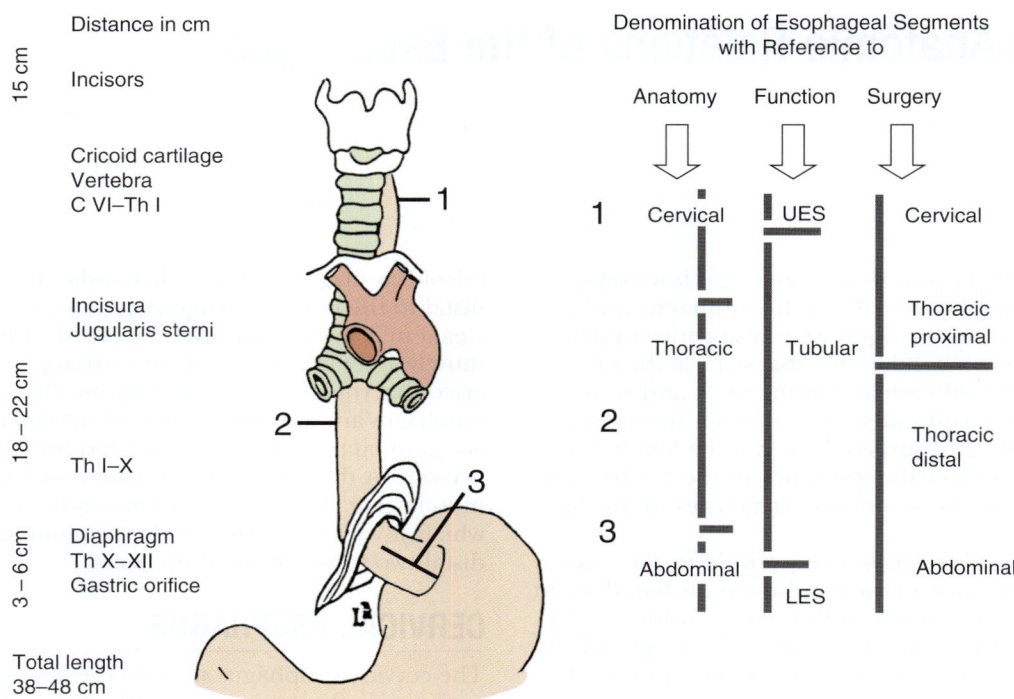

Distance in cm

15 cm

Incisors

Cricoid cartilage
Vertebra
C VI–Th I

Incisura
Jugularis sterni

18 – 22 cm

Th I–X

3 – 6 cm

Diaphragm
Th X–XII
Gastric orifice

Total length
38–48 cm

Denomination of Esophageal Segments
with Reference to

	Anatomy	Function	Surgery
1	Cervical	UES	Cervical
2	Thoracic	Tubular	Thoracic proximal
			Thoracic distal
3	Abdominal	LES	Abdominal

FIGURE 4.1 Division of the esophagus into cervical, thoracic, and abdominal segments *(Anatomy)*. The approximate length of each segment is shown with its relationship to the cervical *(C)* and thoracic *(Th)* vertebrae. The esophagus can also be subdivided according to functions of the upper or lower esophageal sphincters *(Function)* or based on cranial or caudal lymphatic drainage *(Surgery)*. *LES*, Lower esophageal sphincter; *UES*, upper esophageal sphincter.

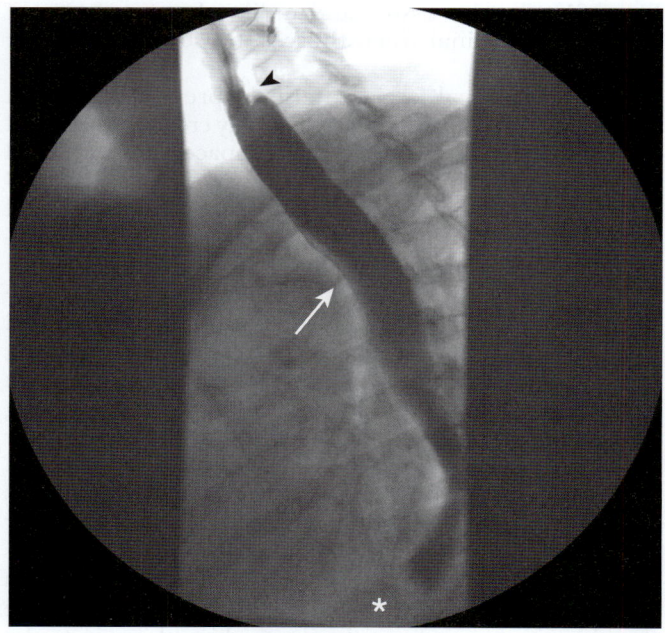

FIGURE 4.2 Barium esophagram demonstrating the normal anatomic narrowings of the esophagus, including the cricopharyngeal muscle at the upper esophageal sphincter *(arrowhead)*, the aortic impression *(arrow)*, and the lower esophageal sphincter *(asterisk)*.

Microhistological cross section of esophagus

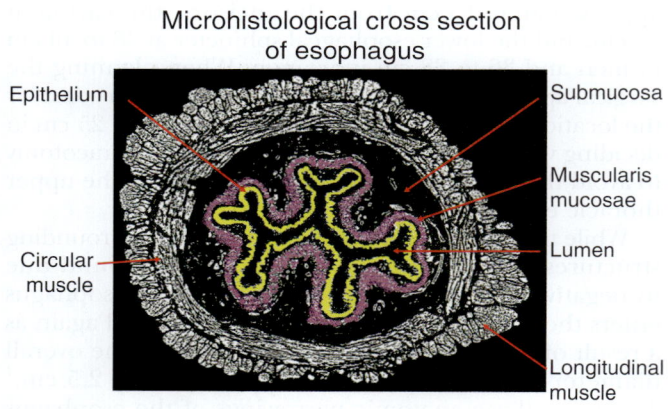

Epithelium

Circular muscle

Submucosa

Muscularis mucosae

Lumen

Longitudinal muscle

FIGURE 4.3 Histologic cross section showing the layers of the esophageal wall, including the epithelium (mucosa), submucosa, and the circular and longitudinal muscle layers.

hyoid bone, and the thyroid and cricoid cartilages. These constrictor muscles converge in the midline posteriorly to form a median raphe. The cricopharyngeus forms a continuous band of muscle originating from the cricoid cartilage without a raphe and blends with the oblique fibers of the inferior pharyngeal constrictor and the circular muscles of the esophagus. Between the inferior constrictor muscle and the cricopharyngeal muscle is a relatively weak area known as Killian triangle (see Fig. 4.4). A pulsion pharyngoesophageal, or Zenker, diverticulum can form in Killian triangle, due to hypertrophy of the

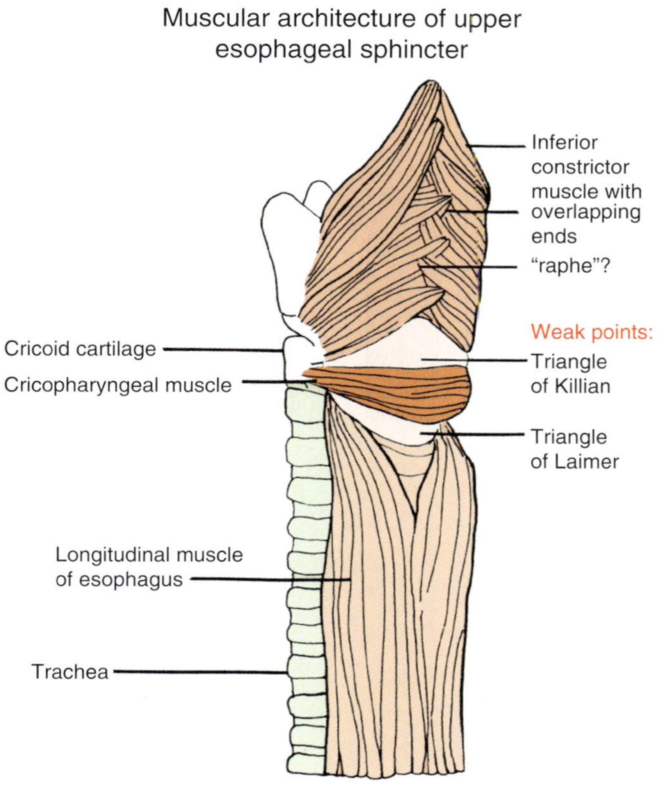

Muscular architecture of upper esophageal sphincter

FIGURE 4.4 Drawing of the structures of the pharyngoesophageal junction seen posteriorly. A Zenker diverticulum can develop at a relatively weak area (Killian triangle) proximal to the cricopharyngeal muscle in the setting of underlying esophageal dysmotility.

cricopharyngeus muscle or underlying dysmotility. There is a 2- to 4-cm high-pressure zone between the pharynx and the cervical esophagus, corresponding to the semicircular cricopharyngeal muscle.[7,8] The upper esophageal sphincter is composed of the cricoid cartilage, the hyoid bone, and the cricopharyngeal and inferior pharyngeal constrictor muscles. The cricopharyngeus muscle includes a mixture of fast- and slow-twitch striated muscle fibers, allowing a basal tone but also permitting rapid changes for swallowing. The upper esophageal sphincter relaxes as intrapharyngeal pressure increases during swallowing, allowing the food bolus to enter the cervical esophagus.

TRACHEA AND SPINE

The esophagus is closely related to the membranous trachea, and care must be taken during dissection of the cervical esophagus to avoid injury to the trachea (Fig. 4.7). A tracheoesophageal fistula can also result from direct invasion, radiation of tumors in this area, or dilation of proximal radiation-associated or anastomotic strictures. Laterally, the esophagus is adjacent to the common carotid arteries and the thyroid gland.

The cervical esophagus is directly anterior to the vertebra. A cervical esophageal perforation or anastomotic leak can lead to a spinal abscess and should be drained by opening the neck to help prevent this complication. Anterior spinal procedures can also result in inadvertent esophageal injury. In addition, esophageal surgeons should be aware of previous anterior cervical spinal operations that could lead to adhesions to the esophagus and potential infection of spinal hardware.

RECURRENT LARYNGEAL NERVES

The recurrent laryngeal nerves originate from the vagus nerves (Fig. 4.8). The right nerve recurs posteriorly around the right subclavian artery, while the left nerve recurs around the aortic arch. Both recurrent nerves ascend in the tracheoesophageal groove, although the left nerve comes closer to the esophagus, since the cervical esophagus deviates to the left and the right nerve recurs around the subclavian more laterally. A nonrecurrent nerve occurs rarely on the right. Toniato et al. report an incidence of 0.1% (31/6000) of patients on the right, with none on the left.[9] The recurrent laryngeal nerves also innervate the cricopharyngeal muscle and the cervical esophagus. Care must be taken to protect the left recurrent laryngeal nerve when dissecting out the cervical esophagus during a transhiatal esophagectomy or Zenker diverticulectomy. The fat in the tracheoesophageal groove containing the nerve should be sharply dissected from the wall of the esophagus, and care should be taken to gently retract the trachea medially with a finger to expose the esophagus, avoiding the use of any metal retractors on the nerve. With experience and these precautions, the incidence of recurrent laryngeal injury should be approximately 1%.[10] Injury to the recurrent laryngeal nerve not only results in hoarseness but also affects the mobility of the cervical esophagus and function of the cricopharyngeal muscle, with impaired swallowing and an increased risk of aspiration. Injury to both recurrent nerves can result in bilateral vocal cord paralysis, with airway obstruction and the need for a tracheostomy.

THORACIC ESOPHAGUS

The thoracic esophagus is 20 cm in length and extends from the thoracic inlet to the diaphragmatic hiatus (see Fig. 4.1). The esophagus passes through the middle mediastinum and shifts to the right at the level of the seventh thoracic vertebra, so the best approach to the mid-esophagus is through a right thoracotomy or thoracoscopy, for example, during an Ivor-Lewis or minimally invasive three-hole esophagectomy. However, the esophagus angulates to the left after passing through the diaphragmatic crura, and along with the location of the liver on the right, the best approach to the distal thoracic esophagus is from the left for a transthoracic hiatal hernia repair or resection of an epiphrenic diverticulum, even when the hernia or diverticulum extend into the right chest.

The arterial blood supply originates from the bronchial arteries, and the majority of patients have one right-sided branch and one to two left-sided branches. There are usually two esophageal branches from the descending aorta between the sixth and ninth thoracic vertebrae. There is a vast network of collateral vessels within the wall of the esophagus, allowing the esophagus to receive blood supply from larger vessels perfusing other organs such as the thyroid, trachea, and stomach (Fig. 4.9).[11,12] Because of this rich intramural network of small vessels, the

Types of muscles in the esophagus

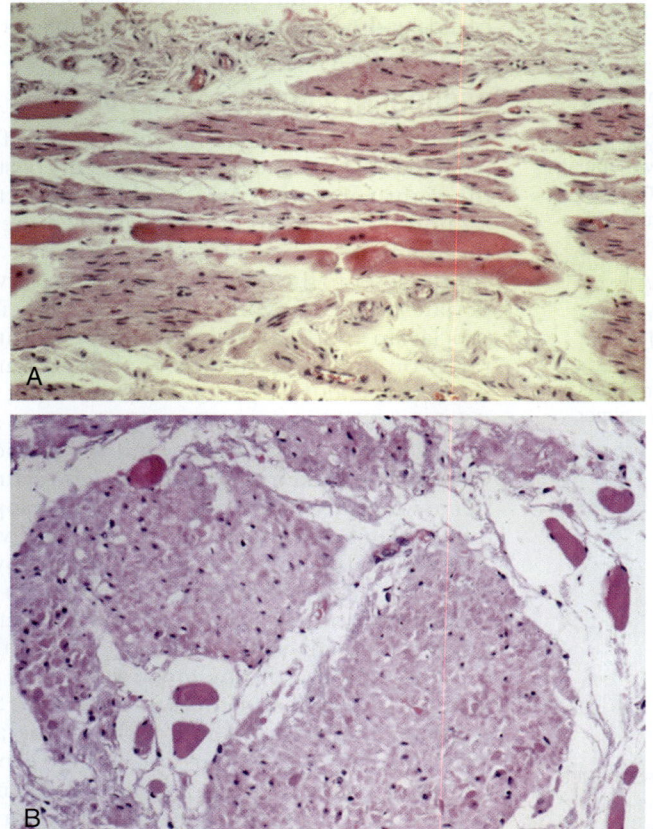

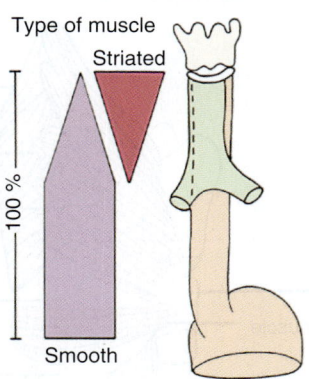

FIGURE 4.5 Transverse (A) and longitudinal (B) histologic sections of the esophageal muscle 4 cm superior to the tracheal bifurcation, showing the transition between striated and smooth muscle. There are individual striated muscle fibers among the smooth muscle fibers. The diagram illustrates the gradual transition from striated to smooth muscle in the proximal to distal esophagus. (Specimen and photo courtesy D. Liebermann-Meffert, Geissdorfer, and Winter, Munich.)

esophagus can be completely mobilized from the stomach to the aortic arch, yet continue to be well perfused.[11-13] However, care should be taken if the inferior thyroid artery has been ligated during a previous thyroidectomy. The arterial vessels supplying the esophagus branch into small, fine vessels at a distance from the esophageal wall, and bleeding can be controlled by packing the mediastinum, allowing for blunt dissection during a transhiatal esophagectomy.[14] Venous drainage is through the azygos vein, with some drainage through the hemiazygos and bronchial veins.

The thoracic esophagus is bordered by the mediastinal pleura on either side. The esophagus is surrounded by loose fibroareolar tissue. This loose investing tissue, with no dense fibrous attachments in the chest, allows the esophagus to be bluntly dissected during a transhiatal esophagectomy. During transhiatal or laparoscopic dissection of the esophagus, it is important to recognize entry into either pleural space. A chest tube is placed for drainage of blood during an esophagectomy, and a tension pneumothorax must be recognized during laparoscopy. In the upper thorax, the trachea is anterior, the azygos is on the right (Fig. 4.10), and the left subclavian artery and

aortic arch are to the left of the esophagus (Fig. 4.11). The descending aorta turns posteriorly and continues to the left of the esophagus until T8, where the esophagus moves anterior to the aorta.

In the lower thorax, the pericardium and left atrium lie anterior to the esophagus (Fig. 4.12). Invasion of the heart or the aorta in locally advanced esophageal cancer is unresectable and can be evaluated on a chest computed tomography with contrast or endoscopic ultrasound. Direct invasion of the aorta can also lead to an aortoesophageal fistula. Hematemesis in a patient with esophageal cancer can represent sentinel bleeding from an aortoesophageal fistula, which must be recognized early to prevent fatal exsanguinating hemorrhage. However, if the tumor just abuts these structures, often there is no invasion at intraoperative exploration. Posteriorly, the esophagus is adjacent to the spine from the thoracic inlet to T8, where the esophagus moves anteriorly to enter the esophageal hiatus. The left lateral distal esophagus is covered only with mediastinal pleura. As a result of the relative weakness in this area, spontaneous Boerhaave perforation occurs most commonly along the left lateral aspect of the distal esophagus.

Reconstruction of macrovascular blood supply to esophagus

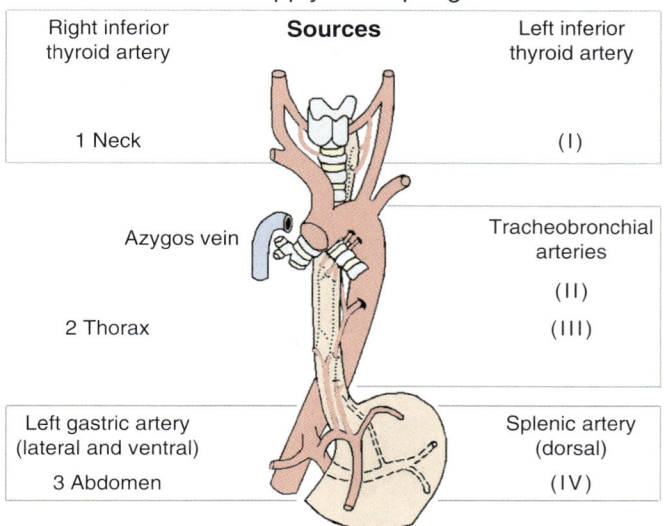

	Sources	
Right inferior thyroid artery		Left inferior thyroid artery
1 Neck		(I)
Azygos vein		Tracheobronchial arteries (II) (III)
2 Thorax		
Left gastric artery (lateral and ventral)		Splenic artery (dorsal)
3 Abdomen		(IV)

FIGURE 4.6 The esophagus receives blood from larger vessels, perfusing other organs such as the thyroid, trachea, and stomach through a rich network of collateral vessels within the wall of the esophagus *(dotted lines)*.

Esophagogastric innervation

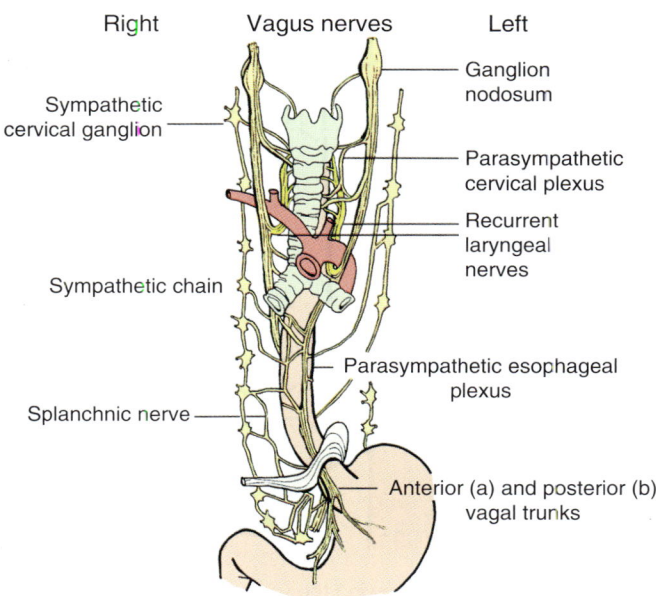

Right   Vagus nerves   Left

Sympathetic cervical ganglion

Sympathetic chain

Splanchnic nerve

Ganglion nodosum

Parasympathetic cervical plexus

Recurrent laryngeal nerves

Parasympathetic esophageal plexus

Anterior (a) and posterior (b) vagal trunks

FIGURE 4.8 Esophageal sympathetic and parasympathetic innervation (vagal nerves) are shown. The right and left recurrent laryngeal nerves arise from the vagus nerves and recur around the right subclavian artery and the aorta, respectively, and travel in the tracheoesophageal groove where they are at risk of injury during dissection of the cervical esophagus. The anterior and posterior vagal trunks pass through the hiatus and must be identified during a Nissen fundoplication or hiatal hernia repair. (From Liebermann-Meffert D, Walbrun B, Hiebert CA, Siewert JR. Recurrent and superior laryngeal nerves: a new look with implications for the esophageal surgeon. *Ann Thorac Surg.* 1999;67:217.)

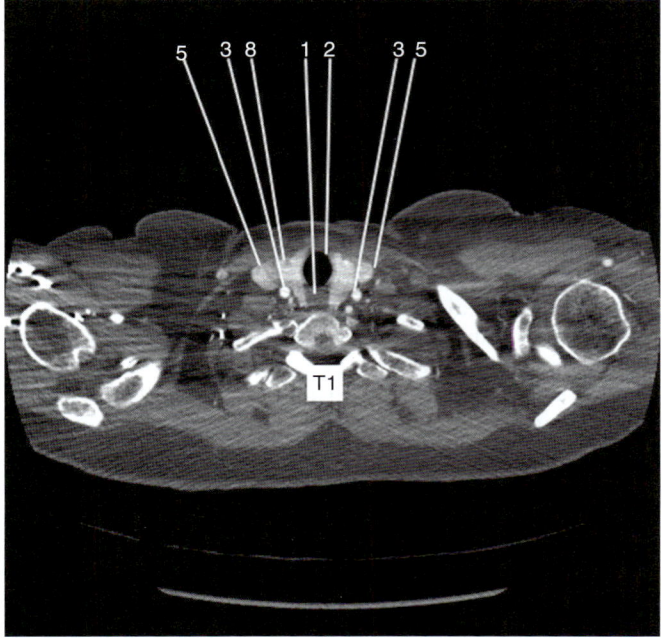

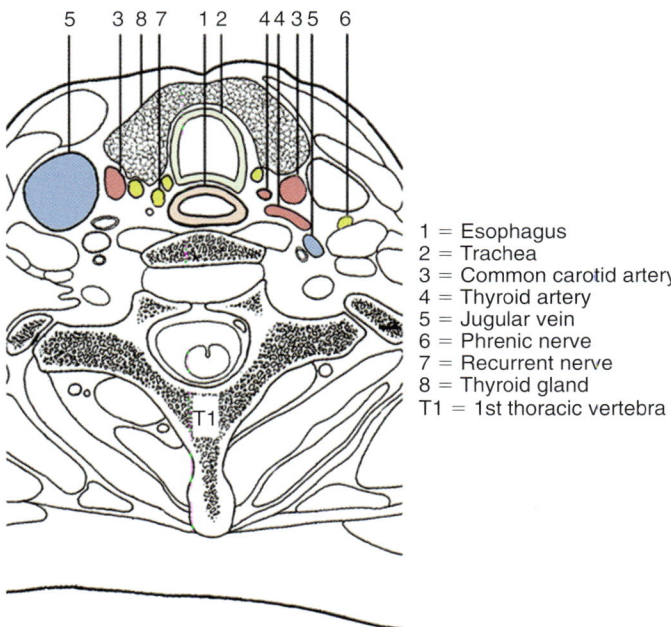

1 = Esophagus
2 = Trachea
3 = Common carotid artery
4 = Thyroid artery
5 = Jugular vein
6 = Phrenic nerve
7 = Recurrent nerve
8 = Thyroid gland
T1 = 1st thoracic vertebra

FIGURE 4.7 Topographic anatomy of the cervical esophagus at the level of the thyroid gland with a corresponding computed tomography image. (Modified from Koritké H, Sick J. *Atlas of Sectional Human Anatomy.* 2nd ed. Baltimore: Urban & Schwarzenberg; 1988.)

Cast of esophageal blood supply

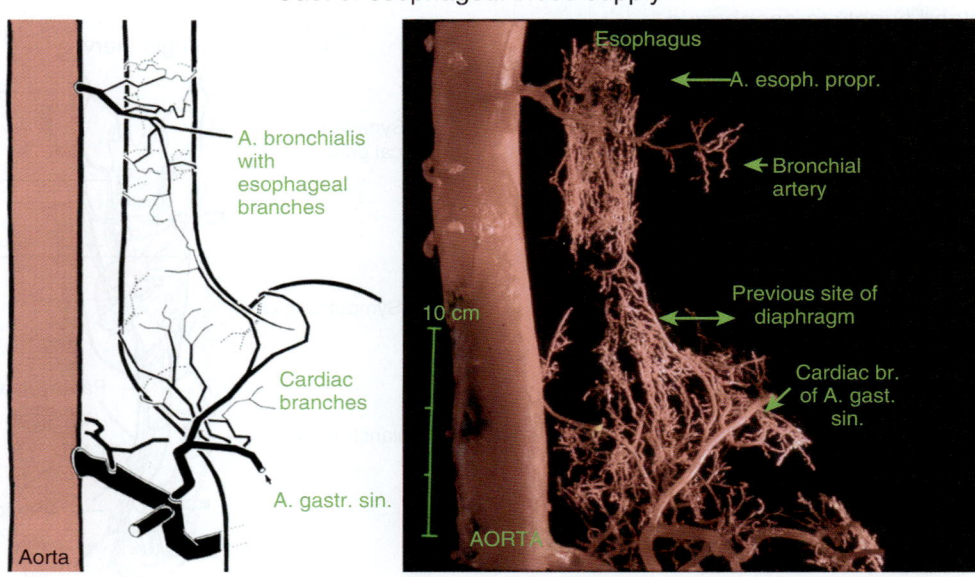

FIGURE 4.9 Arterial cast showing the vascular supply to the middle and lower esophagus. There is a rich intramural network of small vessels, allowing the mobilized esophagus to remain well perfused, even after extensive mobilization. (Photo courtesy D. Liebermann-Meffert, Munich.)

The azygos vein

From lateral =
Right thoracic approach

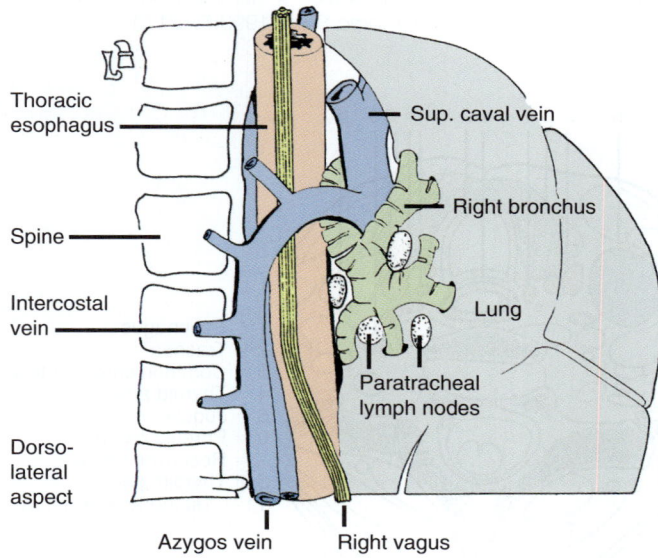

FIGURE 4.10 From a right thoracotomy approach, the azygos is to the right of the esophagus and can be divided to improve exposure of the esophagus. (Diagram courtesy D. Liebermann-Meffert, Munich.)

VAGUS NERVES

The recurrent laryngeal nerves recur around the subclavian artery on the right and the aortic arch on the left (see Fig. 4.8). The nerves may be injured when dissecting the esophagus or lymph nodes in these areas, resulting in hoarseness, difficulty swallowing, and possible aspiration. Care should be taken to avoid the use of cautery in these areas.

The vagus nerves provide parasympathetic innervation to the esophageal musculature. Branches from the vagus nerves and the sympathetic chain enter the wall of the esophagus and form a myenteric (Auerbach) plexus between the longitudinal and circular muscle layers, which control contraction of the esophageal musculature. The submucosal (Meissner) plexus regulates contraction of the muscularis mucosae and secretions. Achalasia results from degeneration of the ganglion in Auerbach plexus, leading to aperistalsis of the esophagus with impaired relaxation of the lower esophageal sphincter.

At the tracheal bifurcation, the right and left vagus nerves form pulmonary and esophageal plexuses. Along the distal esophagus, the anterior fibers from the left vagus coalesce into the anterior vagus, and the posterior fibers from the right vagus form the posterior vagal trunk, although both vagal trunks can contain nerve fibers originating from the left or right vagal nerves. The vagal trunks pass through the esophageal hiatus, along with the esophagus.

TRACHEA

The esophagus is closely related to the membranous trachea anteriorly. Care must be taken during dissection of the esophagus, especially with energy devices, to avoid injury to the membranous trachea, which if not recognized,

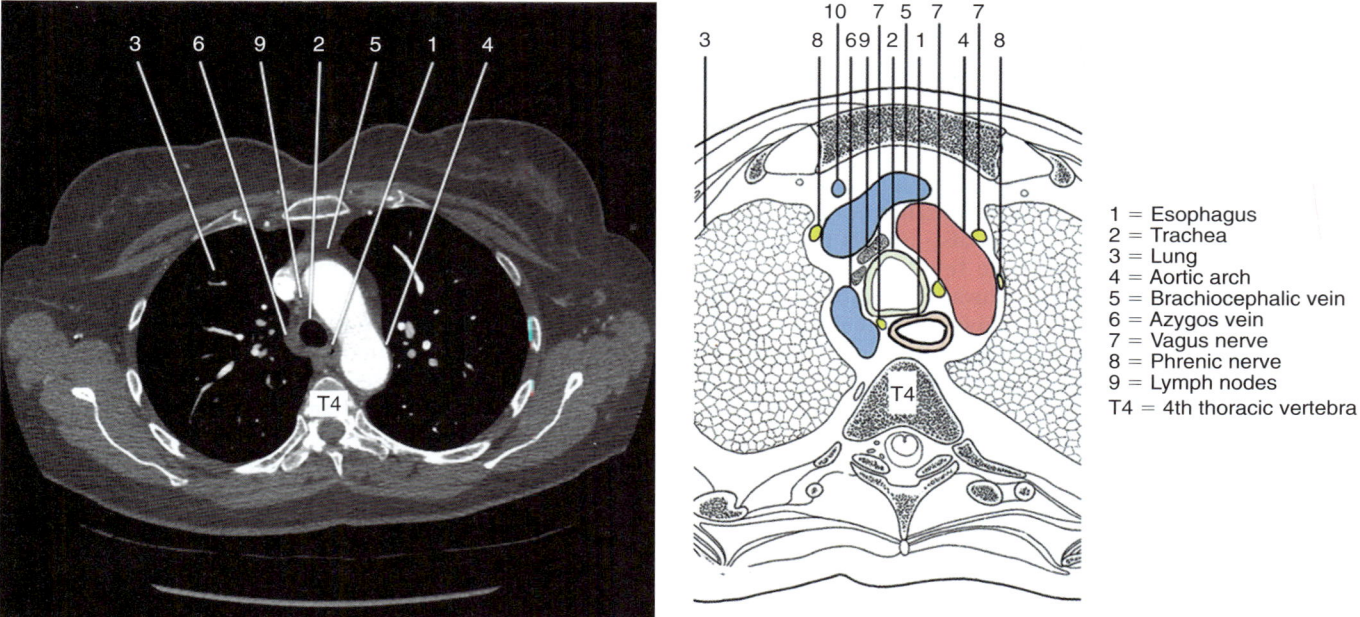

FIGURE 4.11 Topographic anatomy of the upper thoracic esophagus at the level of the aortic arch, along with a corresponding computed tomography image. (Modified from Koritké H, Sick J. *Atlas of Sectional Human Anatomy*. 2nd ed. Baltimore: Urban & Schwarzenberg; 1988.)

1 = Esophagus
2 = Trachea
3 = Lung
4 = Aortic arch
5 = Brachiocephalic vein
6 = Azygos vein
7 = Vagus nerve
8 = Phrenic nerve
9 = Lymph nodes
T4 = 4th thoracic vertebra

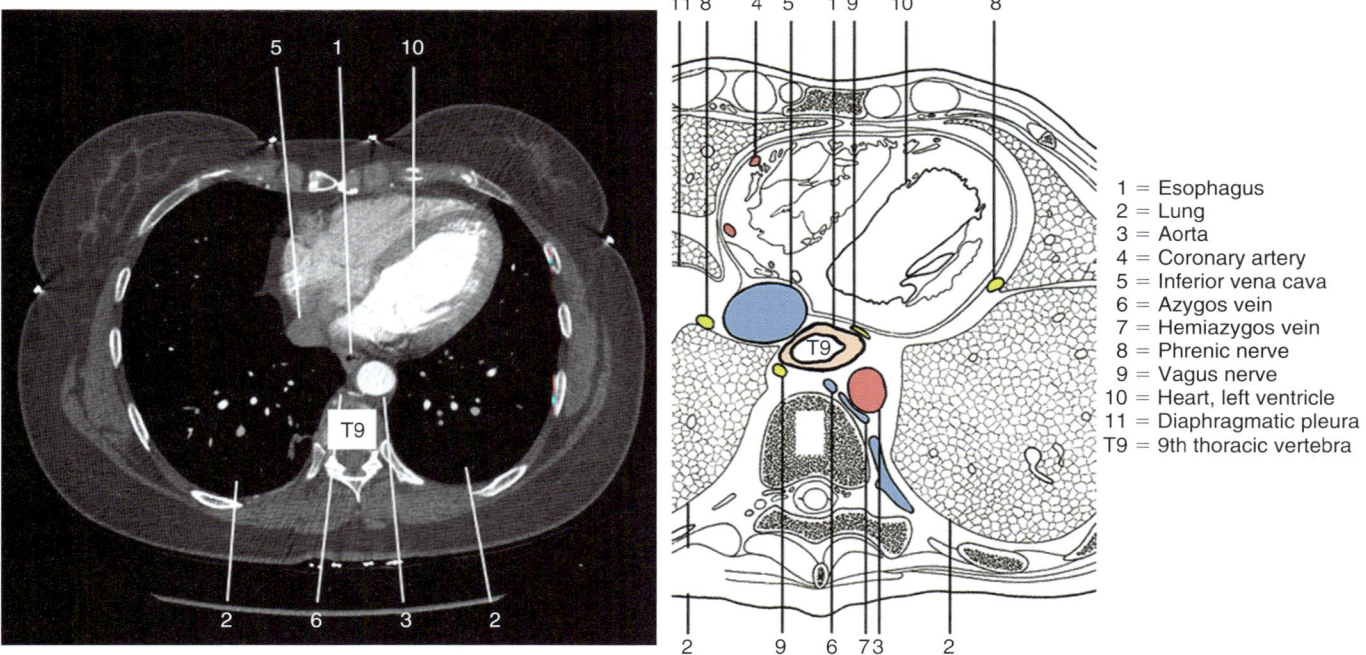

FIGURE 4.12 Topographic anatomy of the lower thoracic esophagus at the level of the left atrium, along with a corresponding computed tomography image. (Modified from Koritké H, Sick J. *Atlas of Sectional Human Anatomy*. 2nd ed. Baltimore: Urban & Schwarzenberg; 1988.)

1 = Esophagus
2 = Lung
3 = Aorta
4 = Coronary artery
5 = Inferior vena cava
6 = Azygos vein
7 = Hemiazygos vein
8 = Phrenic nerve
9 = Vagus nerve
10 = Heart, left ventricle
11 = Diaphragmatic pleura
T9 = 9th thoracic vertebra

can lead to a delayed tracheoesophageal fistula. The carina is located at 25 cm from the incisors, and patients with esophageal tumors proximal to this point may require a bronchoscopy to evaluate for any tracheal invasion. Below the carina, the esophagus is in contact initially with the left mainstem bronchus, and tumor invasion can result in a bronchoesophageal fistula.

AZYGOS VEIN

The azygos vein is adjacent and to the right of the upper thoracic esophagus (see Fig. 4.10). It can become involved via direct invasion by midesophageal tumors. Care must be taken during dissection during a transhiatal esophagectomy not to avulse the azygos vein. The vein is often divided during an Ivor-Lewis esophagectomy to improve exposure of the upper thoracic esophagus.

LYMPHATIC DRAINAGE AND THORACIC DUCT

Understanding esophageal lymphatic drainage is important in tumor staging and treatment planning. A rich submucosal lymphatic network transports lymph to subadventitial lymphatics. The vast network of lymphatics not only drains fluid, debris, and bacteria, but also allows the spread of tumor cells. While there are few lymphatics in the superficial mucosa, once tumors invade the submucosa, the submucosal lymphatic plexus allows tumor cells to spread widely (Fig. 4.13). Sakata first noted that the esophageal lymphatic drainage was longitudinal and intramural.[15] Lehnert believed that these longitudinal lymphatic channels within the submucosa allow lymph to flow most easily up and down the esophagus, which is consistent with the longitudinal spread of esophageal cancer sometimes far away from the primary tumor.[16]

While lymph from the esophagus above the tracheal bifurcation drains superiorly to paratracheal, subcarinal, and paraesophageal lymph nodes, lymph below the carina drains inferiorly toward the lower mediastinal, celiac, and left gastric lymph nodes (Fig. 4.14).[16] However, the direction of lymphatic flow may change when the lymphatics become blocked by tumor, and the pattern of metastatic spread may not follow normal lymphatic drainage, allowing the cephalad spread of distal tumors. Collecting lymphatic ducts also originate intermittently from the submucosal network. These collecting ducts connect directly to the thoracic duct in 40% of patients.[17]

The importance of the submucosal lymphatic network in nodal metastases is highlighted by the association of the depth of tumor invasion (T stage) with the incidence of nodal disease.[18,19] T1a tumors localized to the mucosa with limited lymphatics have a low incidence of nodal spread of 2.6%, while T1b tumors crossing the muscularis mucosa into the submucosa have a 22.2% incidence.[20] Nodal involvement increases to 43.2% in T2, 77.2% in T3, and 66.7% in T4 esophageal tumors.

The main lymphatic vessel is the thoracic duct, which begins in the abdomen as the cisterna chyli at T12 and passes through the aortic hiatus along with the aorta and the azygos and hemiazygos veins. The duct lies on the anterior surface of the vertebra and is posterior to the esophagus between the azygos on the right and the descending aorta on the left. To perform a mass ligation for a chylothorax, the tissue between the azygos vein and aorta is ligated just above the diaphragm. In greater than 50% of patients, the duct turns behind the left mainstem

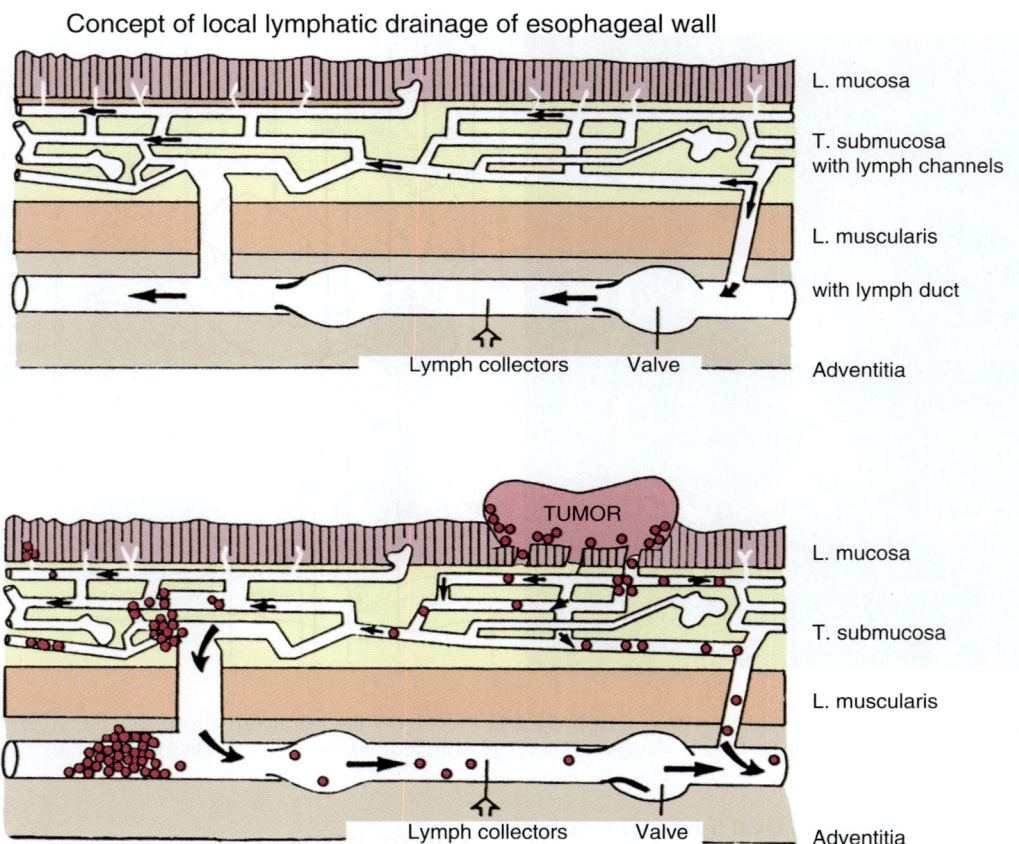

Concept of local lymphatic drainage of esophageal wall

L. mucosa

T. submucosa with lymph channels

L. muscularis

with lymph duct

Lymph collectors   Valve   Adventitia

TUMOR

L. mucosa

T. submucosa

L. muscularis

Lymph collectors   Valve   Adventitia

FIGURE 4.13 The diagram illustrates the extensive submucosal lymphatics that allow tumor cells to travel longitudinally a distance away from the primary tumor. When lymphatics become blocked, tumor cells can travel retrograde, demonstrating how cells from a distal esophageal tumor can be found in the proximal esophagus. *L*, Lamina; *T*, tunica. (From Liebermann-Meffert D, Duranceau A, Stein HJ. Anatomy and embryology. In: Orringer MB, Heitmiller R, eds. *The Esophagus*. Vol 1. In: Zuidema GD, Yeo CJ, series eds. *Shackelford's Surgery of the Alimentary Tract*. 5th ed. Philadelphia: Saunders; 2002:3.)

Concept of lymphatic drainage

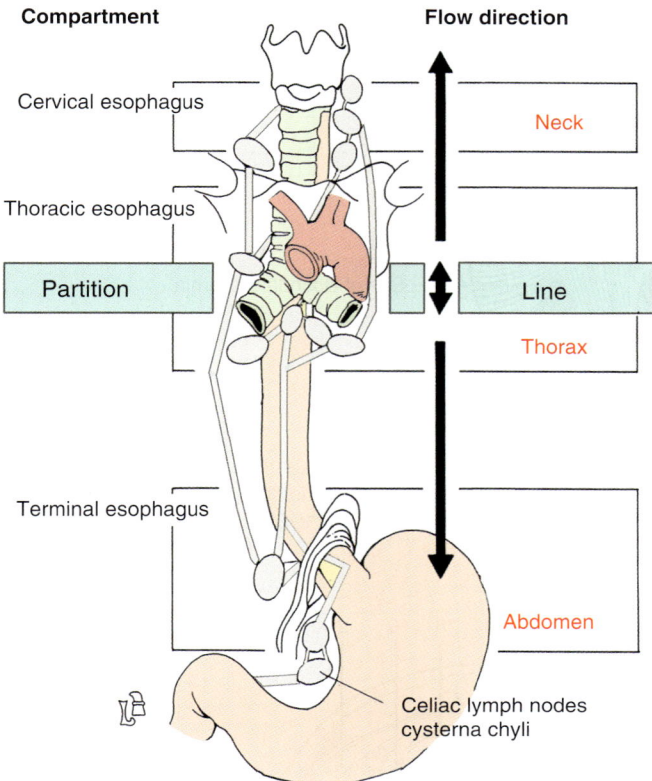

FIGURE 4.14 Lymph from the esophagus above the tracheal bifurcation *(partition line)* drains mostly toward the neck, while lymph below the tracheal bifurcation drains toward the lower mediastinum and the celiac axis. Lymph at the tracheal bifurcation can flow in either direction. When lymphatics become blocked, tumor cells can travel in the opposite direction. (From Liebermann-Meffert D, Duranceau A, Stein HJ. Anatomy and embryology. In: Orringer MB, Heitmiller R, eds. *The Esophagus.* Vol 1. In: Zuidema GD, Yeo CJ, series eds. *Shackelford's Surgery of the Alimentary Tract.* 5th ed. Philadelphia: Saunders; 2002:3.)

bronchus, at the level of the fifth and sixth thoracic vertebrae, to eventually empty into the junction of the left subclavian and jugular veins.[21] There are also a number of possible anatomic variations.[22] The thoracic duct is adjacent to the thoracic esophagus and is damaged in 1% to 2% of esophagectomies, resulting in a chylothorax.[10,14] If there is suspicion for a thoracic duct injury postoperatively, with high pink, clear chest tube output, which becomes milky once fat is added to the patient's diet, the thoracic duct should either be surgically ligated or embolized by interventional radiology to prevent complications associated with the loss of the protein and leukocyte-rich lymph.

The thoracic esophagus is in contact with lymph nodes from several stations, allowing endoscopic ultrasound imaging and fine-needle aspiration of stations 2 (upper paratracheal), 3P (posterior mediastinal), 4 (lower paratracheal), 7 (subcarinal), 8 (paraesophageal), and 9 (inferior pulmonary ligament) lymph nodes in the staging of lung

and esophageal cancer.[23,24] The proximity of the esophagus to the left atrium also allows optimal transesophageal echocardiographic imaging of the mitral valve.

ABDOMINAL ESOPHAGUS

The abdominal esophagus and proximal stomach are approached through a laparotomy or laparoscopy. Normally, the abdominal esophagus is 3 to 6 cm in length.[1] The abdominal esophagus angulates to the left after passing through the diaphragmatic hiatus, and care must be taken to carefully guide an esophageal bougie during a Nissen fundoplication or a rigid esophagoscope through this area to avoid perforation (see Fig. 4.1). The distal esophagus is the second most common site of perforation after the pharynx, just proximal to the cricopharyngeus. The esophagus ends as it enters the cardia along the lesser curvature of the stomach. The abdominal esophagus receives blood supply from small arteries derived from the left gastric artery and the inferior phrenic artery (see Fig. 4.6). Venous drainage is through the left gastric vein. Intraesophageal veins are located in a subepithelial plexus located in the lamina propria. In the distal esophagus, this venous plexus connects with the portal system, leading to esophageal varices with elevated portal pressures.[25] Regional lymph nodes in the abdomen include stations 15 (diaphragmatic), 16 (paracardial), 17 (left gastric), 18 (common hepatic), 19 (splenic), and 20 (celiac).[26]

The esophagus passes through the esophageal hiatus at the level of the 10th thoracic vertebra (Fig. 4.15). Distal esophageal tumors can directly invade the crura, which can be resected en bloc with the esophageal tumor. The crura originate from the anterior aspect of the first three to four lumbar vertebrae. As the esophagus passes through the hiatus, the left lobe of the liver lies anteriorly, and the triangular ligament can be divided to help expose the hiatus (Fig. 4.16). The aorta is posterior to the esophagus and passes through its own hiatus in the diaphragm. The aortic hiatus is bordered by the median arcuate ligament anteriorly, which is used to anchor sutures in performing a Hill repair for gastroesophageal reflux.[27,28] The inferior vena cava lies lateral and inferior to the right crus.

VAGUS NERVES

The anterior and posterior vagal nerves run along the distal esophagus through the esophageal hiatus (see Fig. 4.8). The anterior nerve is usually located adjacent to the esophageal wall, while the posterior nerve can be farther away. The anterior nerve should be carefully identified after the phrenoesophageal membrane is opened and preserved during a Heller myotomy, continuing the myotomy underneath the nerve when necessary. Both nerves should be identified during a Nissen fundoplication, especially with a hiatal hernia repair where the nerves can become involved in the hernia sac and inadvertently divided. If the nerves are injured, approximately 15% of patients will develop delayed gastric emptying.[29]

DIAPHRAGM

The left and right edges of the esophageal hiatus most commonly originate from the deep and superficial layers of the right crus, while the left crus forms one edge of

Diaphragm and location of hernia

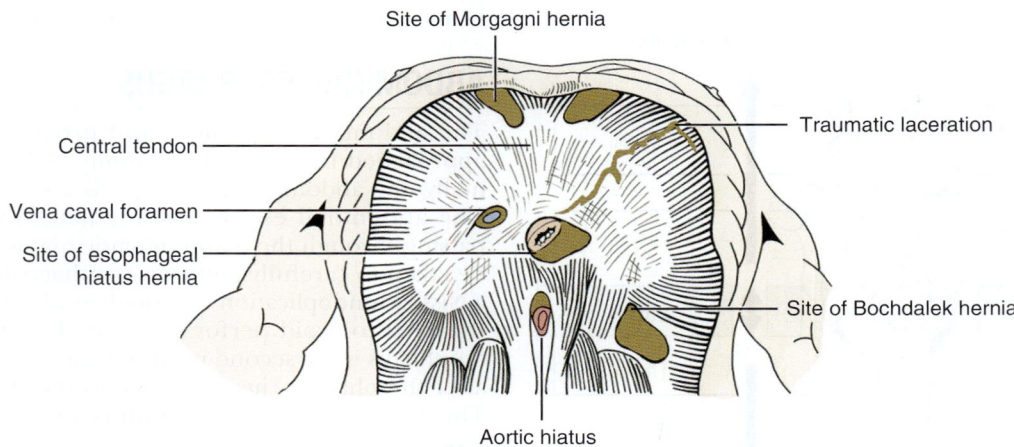

FIGURE 4.15 The esophagus passes through the diaphragm at the esophageal hiatus, while the aorta passes through its own hiatus posteriorly. The inferior vena cava is lateral to the right crus. The location of various diaphragmatic hernias is shown. (Diagram courtesy D. Liebermann-Meffert. In: *Shackelford's Surgery of the Alimentary Tract.* 3rd ed. Philadelphia: Saunders; 1991.)

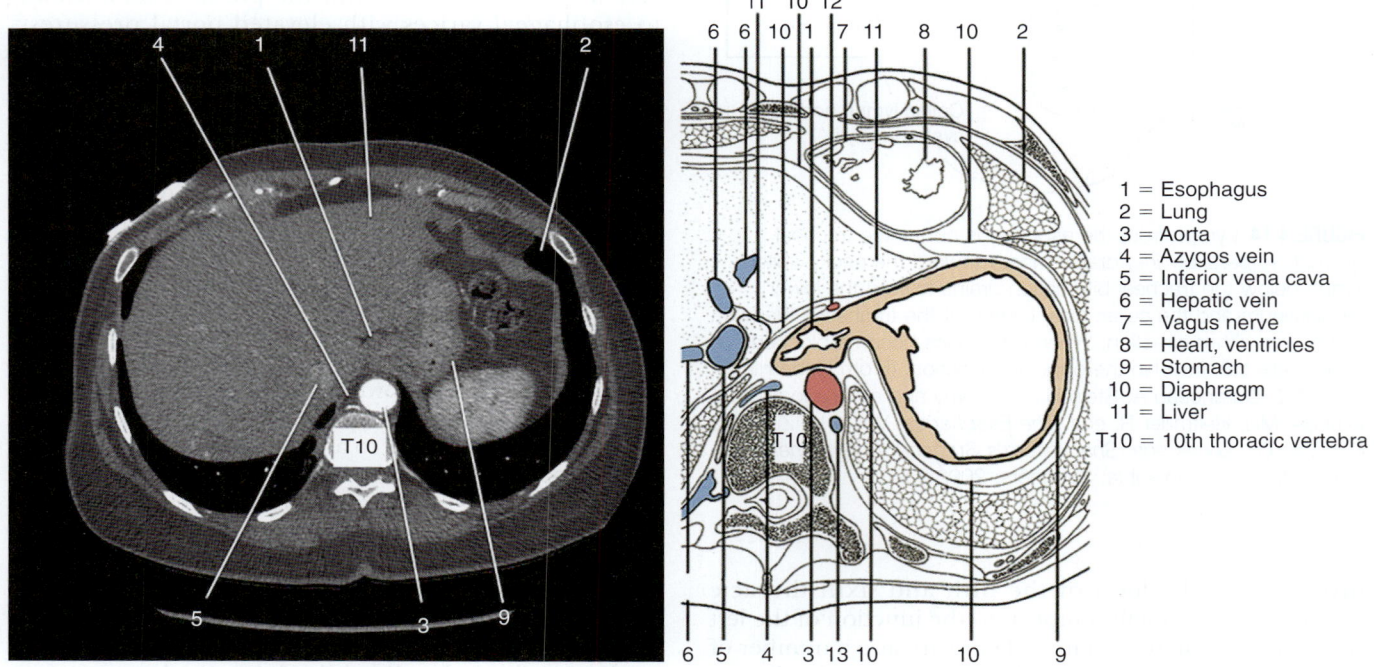

1 = Esophagus
2 = Lung
3 = Aorta
4 = Azygos vein
5 = Inferior vena cava
6 = Hepatic vein
7 = Vagus nerve
8 = Heart, ventricles
9 = Stomach
10 = Diaphragm
11 = Liver
T10 = 10th thoracic vertebra

FIGURE 4.16 Topographic anatomy of the abdominal esophagus along with a corresponding computed tomography image. (Modified from Koritké H, Sick J. *Atlas of Sectional Human Anatomy.* 2nd ed. Baltimore: Urban & Schwarzenberg; 1988.)

the aortic hiatus. The phrenoesophageal membrane, also known as Laimer or Allison membrane, arises from the subdiaphragmatic fascia and attaches the esophagus to the diaphragm (Fig. 4.17). The phrenoesophageal membrane is composed of two sheaths. One sheath passes superior from the diaphragm for 2 to 4 cm along the distal esophagus, and its fibers insert into the submucosa of the esophagus.[4,30] The other sheath extends inferiorly across the cardia and blends into the gastric serosa, muscle, dorsal mesentery, and the gastrohepatic ligament. The

phrenoesophageal membrane allows the esophagus to move dynamically relative to the diaphragm.

Abnormalities in the phrenoesophageal membrane may lead to hiatal hernia formation. The elastic fibers of the phrenoesophageal membrane are replaced by inelastic fibers with aging.[30] Eliska et al. believe that abnormal anchorage of the phrenoesophageal membrane, along with increasing adipose tissue between the membrane and the cardia, may lead to the development of a hiatal hernia.[30] Mittal reported that the phrenoesophageal membrane and its esophageal attachments may also contribute to the function of the lower esophageal sphincter, although hiatal hernia experiments in cats found no effect on lower esophageal sphincter function with complete disruption of the phrenoesophageal membrane and positioning the cardia in the chest.[31,32]

Attachment fibers of PEM

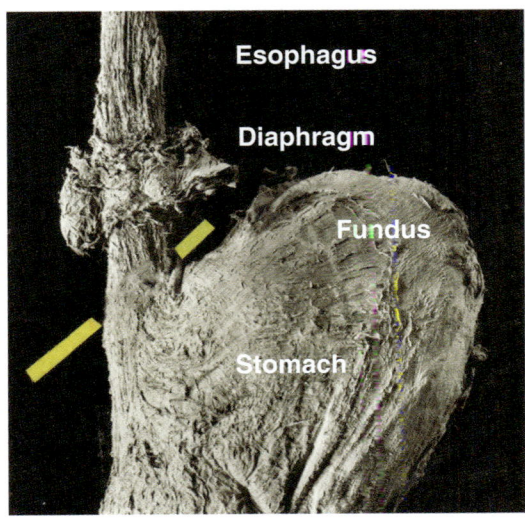

FIGURE 4.17 The fibers attaching the phrenoesophageal membrane (PEM) to the muscle wall of the terminal esophagus are shown, along with its relationship to the gastroesophageal junction. (Courtesy Dr. Owen Korn, Munich and Santiago di Chile.)

GASTROESOPHAGEAL JUNCTION

The location of the gastroesophageal junction remains controversial and can vary depending on the criteria used, which can be based on histologic, endoscopic, or surgical findings. Histologically, the gastroesophageal junction has been defined as the point where there are no longer any submucosal esophageal glands or the proximal extent of the gastric oxyntic glands. Endoscopically, the junction has been defined as the squamocolumnar junction, or Z-line, and the proximal extent of the gastric mucosal folds. Surgically, the gastroesophageal junction has been identified as the peritoneal reflection on the stomach and the junction of the tubular esophagus and the stomach. It is important to remove the gastric fat pad to accurately identify the gastroesophageal junction during a Nissen fundoplication or a Heller myotomy.

LOWER ESOPHAGEAL SPHINCTER

Approximately 3 cm proximal to the gastroesophageal junction, the circular muscle layer increases in thickness.[4,33] Although there is no palpable circular sphincter at the gastroesophageal junction, the circular fibers become short muscular clasps along the lesser curvature (Figs. 4.18 and 4.19). Along the greater curvature and the angle of His, the circular fibers become oblique gastric sling fibers. This muscular arrangement extends 3 to 4 cm above the gastroesophageal junction and 1 to 2 cm onto the stomach, forming a high-pressure zone allowing the lower esophageal sphincter to be identified on manometry.[7,34,35] The muscle is thicker along the greater curvature, and three-dimensional manometry findings have shown that the pressure measurements are also asymmetric, which is thought to contribute to the antireflux mechanism of the lower esophageal sphincter (Fig. 4.20).[33] The angle of His between the lower esophagus and the gastric fundus and the attachment of the phrenoesophageal membrane

Architecture of esophagogastric musculature

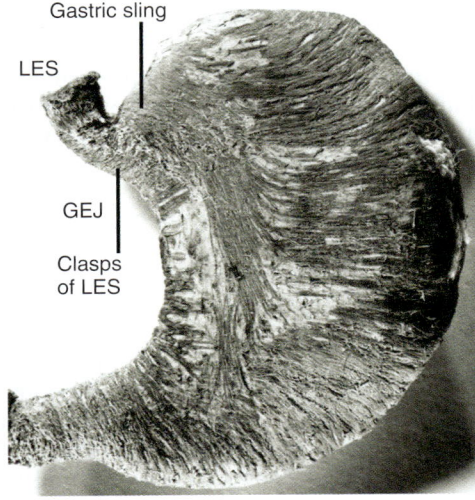

FIGURE 4.18 The dry muscle fiber specimen shows the muscle orientation at the gastroesophageal junction (GEJ) with the outer, longitudinal muscle (left) and the inner, circular fibers (right). Along the lesser curvature, the circular fibers become short muscular clasps, while the circular fibers become oblique gastric sling fibers along the gastric curve at the angle of His, forming a functional and anatomic lower esophageal sphincter (LES). (Specimens from the collection of D. Liebermann-Meffert.)

Closure Mechanisms
Pharynx, Esophagus, Stomach

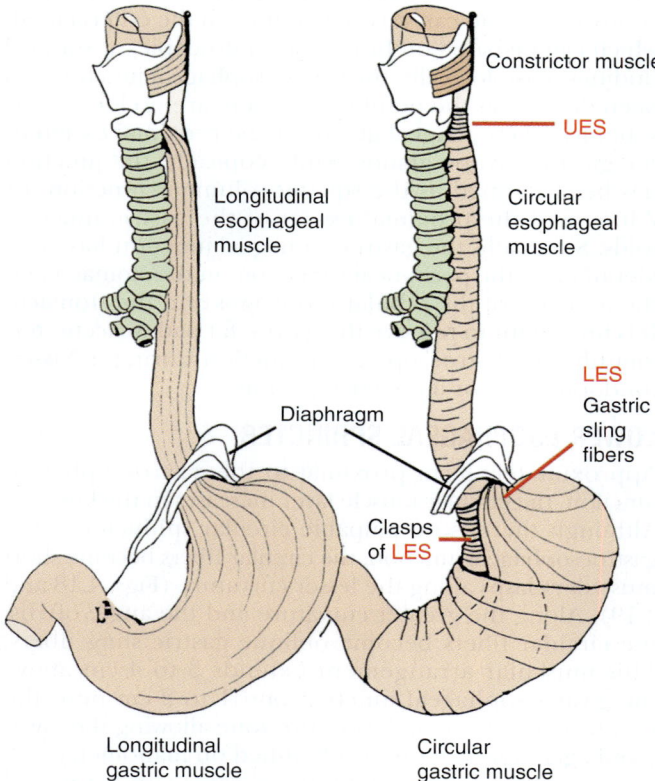

FIGURE 4.19 The outer, longitudinal *(left)* and inner, circular *(right)* muscle layers are shown. The upper *(UES)* and lower *(LES)* esophageal sphincters are composed of inner circular fibers. (Diagram courtesy D. Liebermann-Meffert, Munich.)

Correlation of muscular structures *(left)* and manometric pressure measurement *(right)*

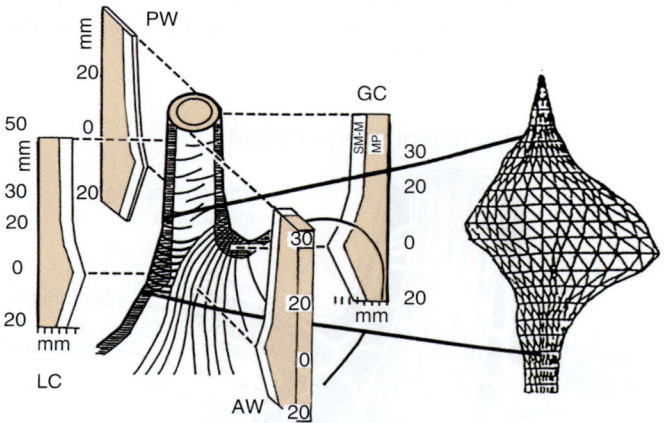

FIGURE 4.20 The illustration shows the correlation between the mean *(n* = 15) radial muscle thickness at the posterior gastric wall *(PW)*, greater curvature *(GC)*, anterior gastric wall *(AW)*, and lesser curvature *(LC)* *(left)* and a three-dimensional manometric pressure image *(right)* at the gastroesophageal junction. There is asymmetry of the radial and axial muscular thickness and manometric pressure profiles. (From Liebermann-Meffert D, Allgöwer M, Schmid P, Blum AL. Muscular equivalent of the lower esophageal sphincter. *Gastroenterology.* 1979;76:31; and Stein HJ, Liebermann-Meffert D, DeMeester TR, Siewert JR. Three-dimensional pressure image and muscular structure of the human lower esophageal sphincter. *Surgery.* 1995;117:692.)

to the diaphragmatic hiatus are also felt to contribute to the antireflux mechanism at the gastroesophageal junction. The lower esophageal sphincter provides a barrier to gastroesophageal reflux and relaxes 3 seconds after swallowing is initiated allowing the food bolus to enter the stomach.[36,37] Some have suggested that an esophagomyotomy for achalasia should be performed between the short clasp fibers and the oblique gastric sling fibers to maintain the strength of the sling mechanism.[38–40]

CONCLUSION

The esophagus is a muscular tube that starts at the cricoid cartilage in the neck and traverses the chest before ending in the stomach in the upper abdomen. The primary purpose of the esophagus is to transport food from the mouth to the stomach. While the esophagus seems like a simple organ at first glance, esophageal surgeons must be familiar with the complex anatomy and function of the upper and lower esophageal sphincters, the extensive lymphatic and vascular submucosal networks, and the clinical importance of the relationship of the esophagus to surrounding structures in all three areas of the body for effective surgical planning and the prevention of potential complications.

REFERENCES

1. Liebermann-Meffert D. Anatomy, embryology, and histology. In: Pearson FG, Cooper JD, Delauriers J, et al., eds. *Esophageal Surgery.* Philadelphia: WB Saunders; 2000.
2. Goldsmith HS, Akiyama H. A comparative study of Japanese and American gastric dimensions. *Ann Surg.* 1979;190:690-693.
3. Ngan SY, Wong J. Lengths of different routes for esophageal replacement. *J Thorac Cardiovasc Surg.* 1986;91:790-792.
4. Liebermann-Meffert D, Duranceau A, Stein HJ. Anatomy and embryology. In: Orringer MB, Heitmiller R, eds. *The Esophagus.* Vol. 1. 5th ed. Philadelphia: Saunders; 2002.
5. Liebermann-Meffert D, Geissdörfer K. Is the transition of striated into smooth muscle precisely known? In: Giuli R, McCallum RW, Skinner DB, eds. *Primary Motility Disorders of the Esophagus: 450 Questions—450 Answers.* Paris: Libbey Eurotext; 1991.
6. Savary M, Miller G. *The Esophagus: Handbook and Atlas of Endoscopy.* Solothurn, Switzerland: Gassman; 1978.
7. Winans CS. The pharyngoesophageal closure mechanism: a manometric study. *Gastroenterology.* 1972;63:768-777.
8. Lerche W. *The Esophagus and Pharynx in Action.* Springfield, IL: Charles C Thomas; 1950.
9. Toniato A, Rubello D, Merante Boschin I. Nonrecurrent and ipsilateral recurrent inferior laryngeal nerves. *Minerva Chir.* 2012;67:286-287.
10. Orringer MB, Marshall B, Chang AC, et al. Two thousand transhiatal esophagectomies: changing trends, lessons learned. *Ann Surg.* 2007;246:363-372; discussion 72-74.
11. Liebermann-Meffert D, Siewert JR. Arterial anatomy of the esophagus: a review of literature with brief comments on clinical aspects. *Gullet.* 1992;2:3.
12. Liebermann-Meffert DM, Meier R, Siewert JR. Vascular anatomy of the gastric tube used for esophageal reconstruction. *Ann Thorac Surg.* 1992;54:1110-1115.
13. Liebermann-Meffert DM, Luescher U, Neff U, Rüedi TP, Allgöwer M. Esophagectomy without thoracotomy: is there a risk of

intramediastinal bleeding? A study on blood supply of the esophagus. *Ann Surg.* 1987;206:184-192.

14. Orringer MB, Orringer JS. Esophagectomy without thoracotomy: a dangerous operation? *J Thorac Cardiovasc Surg.* 1983;85:72-80.

15. Sakata K. Ueber die Lymphgefasse des Oesophagus und uber seine regionaren Lymphdrusen mit Berucksichtigung der Verbrietung des Carcinoms. *Mitt Grenzgeb Med.* 1903;11:629-656.

16. Akiyama H. Surgery for carcinoma of the esophagus. *Curr Probl Surg.* 1980;17:53-120.

17. Murakami G, Sato I, Shimada K, Dong C, Kato Y, Imazeki T. Direct lymphatic drainage from the esophagus into the thoracic duct. *Surg Radiol Anat.* 1994;16:399-407.

18. Matsubara T, Ueda M, Abe T, Akimori T, Kokudo N, Takahashi T. Unique distribution patterns of metastatic lymph nodes in patients with superficial carcinoma of the thoracic oesophagus. *Br J Surg.* 1999;86:669-673.

19. Nigro JJ, DeMeester SR, Hagen JA, et al. Node status in transmural esophageal adenocarcinoma and outcome after en bloc esophagectomy. *J Thorac Cardiovasc Surg.* 1999;117:960-968.

20. Rice TW, Zuccaro G Jr, Adelstein DJ, Rybicki LA, Blackstone EH, Goldblum JR. Esophageal carcinoma: depth of tumor invasion is predictive of regional lymph node status. *Ann Thorac Surg.* 1998;65:787-792.

21. Wirth W, Frommhold H. Thoracic duct and its variations. Lymphography studies. *Fortschr Geb Rontgenstr Nuklearmed.* 1970;112:450-459.

22. Netter FH. *The Ciba Collection of Medical Illustrations. Digestive System. Part 1: Upper Digestive Tract.* Vol. 3. New York: Ciba Pharmaceutical Embassy; 1971.

23. Fritscher-Ravens A, Sriram PV, Bobrowski C, et al. Mediastinal lymphadenopathy in patients with or without previous malignancy: EUS-FNA-based differential cytodiagnosis in 153 patients. *Am J Gastroenterol.* 2000;95:2278-2284.

24. Hyer JD, Silvestri G. Diagnosis and staging of lung cancer. *Clin Chest Med.* 2000;21:95-106, viii-ix.

25. Vianna A, Hayes PC, Moscoso G, et al. Normal venous circulation of the gastroesophageal junction. A route to understanding varices. *Gastroenterology.* 1987;93:876-889.

26. Casson AG, Rusch VW, Ginsberg RJ, Zankowicz N, Finley RJ. Lymph node mapping of esophageal cancer. *Ann Thorac Surg.* 1994;58:1569-1570.

27. Aye RW, Rehse D, Blitz M, Kraemer SJ, Hill LD. The Hill antireflux repair at 5 institutions over 25 years. *Am J Surg.* 2011;201:599-604.

28. Lindner HH, Kemprud E. A clinicoanatomical study of the arcuate ligament of the diaphragm. *Arch Surg.* 1971;103:600-605.

29. Swanson EW, Swanson SJ, Swanson RS. Endoscopic pyloric balloon dilatation obviates the need for pyloroplasty at esophagectomy. *Surg Endosc.* 2012;26:2023-2028.

30. Eliska O. Phreno-oesophageal membrane and its role in the development of hiatal hernia. *Acta Anat (Basel).* 1973;86:137-150.

31. Mittal RK. Current concepts of the antireflux barrier. *Gastroenterol Clin North Am.* 1990;19:501-516.

32. Liebermann-Meffert D, Heberer M. Allgöwer M. The muscular counterpart of the lower esophageal sphincter. In: DeMeester TR, Skinner DB, eds. *Esophageal Disorders: Pathology and Therapy.* New York: Raven Press; 1985.

33. Liebermann-Meffert D, Allgower M, Schmid P, Blum AL. Muscular equivalent of the lower esophageal sphincter. *Gastroenterology.* 1979;76:31-38.

34. Code CF, Fyke FE Jr, Schlegel JF. The gastroesophageal sphincter in healthy human beings. *Gastroenterologia.* 1956;86:135-150.

35. Winans CS. Manometric asymmetry of the lower-esophageal high-pressure zone. *Am J Dig Dis.* 1977;22:348-354.

36. Friedland GW, Melcher DH, Berridge FR, Gresham GA. Debatable points in the anatomy of the lower oesophagus. *Thorax.* 1966;21:487-498.

37. Pope CE 2nd. The esophagus: 1967 to 1969. I. *Gastroenterology.* 1970;59:460-476.

38. Bombeck CT, Nyhus LM, Donahue PE. How far should the myotomy extend on the stomach? In: Giuli R, McCallum RW, Skinner DB, eds. *Primary Motility Disorders of the Esophagus.* Paris: Libbey Eurotext; 1991:455.

39. Korn O, Stein HJ, Richter TH, Liebermann-Meffert D. Gastroesophageal sphincter: a model. *Dis Esophagus.* 1997;10:105-109.

40. Preiksaitis HG, Tremblay L, Diamant NE. Regional differences in the in vitro behaviour of muscle fibers from the human lower esophageal sphincter. *J Gastrointest Motility.* 1991;3:195.

Esophageal Symptoms and Selection of Diagnostic Tests

Ross M. Bremner | Sumeet K. Mittal

A surgeon evaluating a patient prior to a possible esophageal operation must spend enough time in conversation with that patient to ensure a clear understanding of their symptoms. Such dialogue not only illuminates potential causes of those symptoms, but more importantly, it indicates whether a given surgical procedure may resolve them. The spectrum of symptoms in esophageal disease is wide, ranging from common typical symptoms (e.g., heartburn, regurgitation, and dysphagia) to atypical symptoms (e.g., cough, voice changes, chest pain, and globus sensation). Esophageal symptoms are often vague in nature, which should prompt further questioning of the patient. Surgeons should be familiar with the concept of "functional heartburn" so that surgery is not performed for patients who would not benefit from surgical intervention.

The tests used to evaluate symptoms should be selected in accordance with the suspected underlying pathology. Functional testing is critical when a functional operation is planned, and in the present era of justified cost containment, exhaustive testing is not always necessary. Nonetheless, shortcuts should be avoided, as most functional testing is additive in the assessment of a patient's pathology and generally carries meaning. An operation performed for the incorrect indication can be disastrous, particularly because the esophagus is a relatively unforgiving organ. The most common cause of failure after antireflux surgery is poor patient selection[1]; therefore, thoughtful analysis of presenting symptoms and a complete work-up to identify the cause of these symptoms are necessary before the surgeon advises a surgical procedure for a functional disorder. Surgeons whose patients experience dysphagia should be aware of the possibility of malignancy, as dysphagia is the most common presenting symptom associated with esophageal cancer.

ORIGIN OF ESOPHAGEAL SENSATION

Sensory nerve fibers in the esophagus are present in both the muscle and mucosa, and are carried in the vagus nerve and in the spinal nerves. The vagus nerve afferents have been described as tension-sensitive fibers with low thresholds for response. They are thought to contribute to physiologic reflexes. The spinal afferents likely provide a nociceptor function and convey noxious intensity of various stimuli. Stimuli that excite these afferents include distention and exposure to acid. The afferent nerves have been classified as muscle-tension-sensitive, mucosal mechano/chemosensitive, and tension/mucosal receptors; however, most afferent fibers respond to both mechanical and chemical stimuli.[2,3] Acid excites primary sensory neurons in the esophagus by activating two proton-gated channels: transient receptor potential vanilloid-1 (TRPV1) and acid-sensing ion channels. The latter is thought to mediate heartburn in nonerosive reflux disease (NERD).[4] The activation of the TRPV1 channel by acid can initiate neurogenic inflammation and the release of proinflammatory substances from the surrounding cellular matrix, with a resulting increase in noxious stimuli. Visceral hypersensitivity in patients with NERD appears to involve neurogenic inflammation, with an increase in both release of substance P and expression of neurokinin 1 receptor, which in turn activates TRPV1 and protease-activated receptor 2.[4]

A number of tests have historically been used to understand esophageal symptomatology, including acid infusion (i.e., the Bernstein test) and balloon distention. These proved to be useful for understanding the stimulus-symptom axis of the esophagus, but they are seldom used in today's clinical practice. The sensory neurons from the heart and the esophagus converge on the dorsal horns of the spinal cord, which likely explains the overlap of pain from either organ and often prompts suspicion of myocardial infarction in patients with severe esophageal spastic syndromes. A gender difference in esophageal symptom perception has also been described, with males having both lower tolerance to acid perfusion and greater sensitivity to balloon distention after acid sensitization.[5] Hyperalgesia (i.e., the heightened perception of painful stimuli) appears to occur over a greater anatomic region in females.[5]

Sensory hypersensitivity includes both hyperalgesia and allodynia (i.e., the perception of pain from nonpainful stimuli) and can be caused by exposure to acid, among other things. *Functional heartburn* is a term used to describe a symptom of retrosternal burning that occurs without objective evidence of abnormal exposure of the esophagus to gastric juice. Early studies[6] that characterized symptom perception in patients after balloon distension showed highly variable patient responses. Stimulus localization was poor, and perception of the distention as pain, nausea, or heartburn was also quite variable. These findings underscore the need for complete testing in patients presenting with various esophageal symptoms, especially when surgery is considered as a treatment option.

SYMPTOMS

Gastroesophageal reflux disease (GERD) is an extremely common condition that causes most esophageal symptoms. GERD symptoms may be classified as typical or atypical. Typical symptoms of GERD include heartburn and regurgitation (some authors include dysphagia); atypical symptoms include noncardiac chest pain, chronic cough and asthma, hoarseness and dental caries, nausea and vomiting, and globus sensation. A global consensus group defined GERD as troublesome symptoms or complications that result from reflux of gastric contents into the esophagus.[7] GERD has been further classified into cases with endoscopically visible injury and cases without, the latter now commonly referred to as NERD. Patients with NERD may make up as much as 70% of patients who experience reflux symptoms.[8] Erosive disease and esophageal stricture may be related to the concentration of the acid that is refluxed, as well as overall duration of exposure.[9]

TYPICAL SYMPTOMS OF GASTROESOPHAGEAL REFLUX DISEASE

Heartburn

The most common esophageal symptom of GERD is heartburn, usually resulting from reflux of acidic gastric juice into the esophagus. Acid irritates the esophageal mucosa, stimulating nociceptors and causing heartburn. The relationship between acid exposure and heartburn is quite complex, as evidenced by the variable response to acid suppression therapy (especially in patients with NERD). Up to 60% of the Western population experience heartburn at least once every year, and 20% to 30% have weekly symptoms.[10,11] Heartburn is usually described as retrosternal burning that ascends from the epigastrium toward the throat. The classic billboard advertisements for proton pump inhibitors (PPIs) that feature a patient with a grimace and a balled-up hand held to the chest are an apt representation of the sensation.

Many patients describe aggravation of their heartburn brought about by eating spicy or fatty meals, drinking citrus juices, or consuming chocolate, alcohol, or coffee. It is frequently associated with regurgitation, which is exacerbated by postural changes. Heartburn is usually relieved by antacids or antisecretory medications, and the availability of over-the-counter PPIs and oft-prescribed antisecretory medications have led to widespread use of

BOX 5.1 **Nighttime Heartburn Is an Underappreciated Clinical Problem**

50 million Americans have nighttime heartburn at least once per week

45% of heartburn sufferers report that current remedies do not relieve all the symptoms they experience

63% report that it affects their ability to sleep and affects their work the next day

72% are taking prescription medications

80% had nocturnal symptoms; 65% both day and night

TABLE 5.1 Normal Values of Six Components of the 24-Hour Record for 50 Healthy Volunteers

	Mean	95th Percentile
Total time pH <4 (%)	1.51	4.45
Upright time pH <4 (%)	2.34	8.42
Supine time pH <4 (%)	0.63	3.45
Number of episodes	19.00	46.90
Number of episodes ≥5 min	0.84	3.45
Longest episode	6.74	19.80

these remedies. Not infrequently, physicians may find that their patient is completely dependent on these medications, and withdrawal of PPIs results in the rapid return of heartburn. It is therefore important to ask the patient about their use of these medications and what symptoms they experience when the medication is withheld. Nocturnal heartburn appears to be an especially serious symptom, as noted by a Gallup poll conducted by the American Gastroenterologic Society (Box 5.1).[12]

The most appropriate objective measurement of refluxed gastric acid as a cause of the patient's symptoms is a 24-hour pH test. This test has been well studied and documented by Johnson and DeMeester, and their composite score helps distinguish normal acid exposure from abnormal levels, as described in Table 5.1.[13]

Functional Heartburn

The term *functional heartburn*, which is a concept developed further over the past decade, refers to the manifestation of heartburn in a patient with no objective evidence that relates the symptom to abnormal esophageal exposure of refluxed gastric juice. Similarly, functional chest pain is presumed to be of esophageal origin but has a negative work-up on routine testing. Galmiche and colleagues[14] have defined the criteria for the diagnosis of functional heartburn. Diagnosing this condition requires a negative impedance study to exclude patients experiencing symptoms with either weak-acid or alkaline reflux. A recent study of pH impedance testing showed that 30% of PPI-refractory patients experience functional heartburn.[15] These patients may have altered visceral hypersensitivity, as their condition frequently overlaps with other functional abnormalities and various psychiatric disorders. In patients with functional heartburn, antireflux surgery outcomes are often poor,[16] which drives home the importance of pH testing before antireflux surgery is considered. Treatment for functional heartburn usually includes antidepressants, which are thought to have a neuromodulatory role in hypersensitivity disorders. However, scant data prove their efficacy.

The functional heartburn category of patients again reaffirms the sometimes-vague presentation of esophageal pathologies, and certainly adds weight to the argument that GERD must be objectively diagnosed with pH or pH impedance testing before surgery is considered.

Regurgitation

Regurgitation is the effortless return of gastric juice or recently ingested food or liquid into the back of the throat or mouth, and it is often exacerbated by postural changes. This symptom is most frequently accompanied by heartburn, but it may occur in isolation in patients with adequate acid-suppression therapy (i.e., with PPIs). Regurgitation occurring at night is especially significant, as it may result in silent aspiration and lung damage. Delayed gastric emptying may exacerbate regurgitation.

Dysphagia

Dysphagia may be either oropharyngeal or esophageal in origin. Oropharyngeal dysphagia may result from mechanical, obstructive, functional, or neurologic causes. Esophageal dysphagia usually results from a mechanical obstruction, or from poor bolus transport (i.e., hypomotility or uncoordinated, spastic contractions). Patients can frequently identify the general area in which dysphagia is occurring, but this is not always reliable. The symptom of dysphagia is often referred to as an *alarm symptom*, as it is usually the primary presenting symptom of esophageal cancer. It is a common symptom, however, and can accompany GERD with or without stricture and a number of other benign disorders. Symptom duration and rapidity of symptom progression often offer clues regarding the pathology. Rapid progression of dysphagia that inhibits swallowing solids first and ultimately impedes swallowing of liquids over a period of weeks or months forebodes a malignant process, whereas a slow progression over years suggests an underlying motility disorder such as achalasia. Patients often initially compensate for solid-food dysphagia by avoiding dense solid foods (e.g., steak, chicken breast), chewing food very well, or eating only very soft food.

If dysphagia is accompanied by a prominent history of heartburn, the surgeon should consider peptic stricture, but patients with achalasia sometimes experience heartburn, and reflux disease is the culprit behind the development of most esophageal carcinomas. Generally speaking, dysphagia should prompt a structural investigation such as endoscopy or dedicated barium esophagram. The former is more invasive but allows for biopsy of any abnormalities, whereas the latter provides evidence of narrowing from stricture or malignancy and offers some information on the propulsive capability of the esophagus. Potential causes of esophageal dysphagia are listed in Box 5.2.

The least invasive study in the work-up of patients with dysphagia is the barium esophagram. When done correctly, this test should identify spastic motor disorders, diverticula, achalasia, and strictures (benign or malignant).

BOX 5.2 Potential Causes of Dysphagia

Cancer
Congenital webs
Congenital aberrant subclavian artery (i.e., dysphagia lusoria)
Schatzki ring
Benign stricture
- Peptic
- Eosinophilic esophagitis
- Pill-induced or caustic-induced
Motility abnormalities
- Achalasia
- Diffuse esophageal spasm
- Hypertensive lower esophageal sphincter
- Muscular A-ring
- Hypomotility of the esophagus
Diverticula
- Zenker diverticulum
- Mid-esophageal traction diverticulum
- Pulsion diverticulum associated with spastic motor disorders

---

Barium studies performed with liquids and foods of various consistencies or with a large barium tablet, as described later, provide additional information. Endoscopy is both diagnostic and therapeutic, as it can facilitate biopsy and provide an opportunity to dilate a Schatzki ring or stricture. More subtle motility abnormalities often require manometry for diagnosis, and this test is necessary before surgery for a manometric disorder is considered.

ATYPICAL SYMPTOMS OF GASTROESOPHAGEAL REFLUX DISEASE

Noncardiac Chest Pain

One of the more difficult GERD symptoms to diagnose and treat is noncardiac chest pain. It is frequently of esophageal origin, and although it may be on the spectrum of GERD or of a motility disorder, surgeons should approach this symptom with caution. A convergence of sensory neurons from both the heart and the esophagus exists on the dorsal horns of the spinal cord, so myocardial infarction is often suspected in patients with severe esophageal spastic syndromes. Unfortunately, the fear of missing a myocardial infarction results in significant expense in examining patients presenting with chest pain. It is thought that as many as 150,000 of the 500,000 coronary angiograms performed annually in the United States are performed for functional disorders.[17,18] Manometry is generally required to confirm suspicion of a motor disorder, but it is not always diagnostic, as many of these motor disorders are episodic in nature. Twenty-four-hour manometry (often combined with 24-hour pH monitoring) has been useful in diagnosing these patients, but is not widely available and is rarely used in clinical practice. pH testing has been found to be predictive of a therapeutic response to omeprazole in patients with severe reflux and noncardiac chest pain.[19]

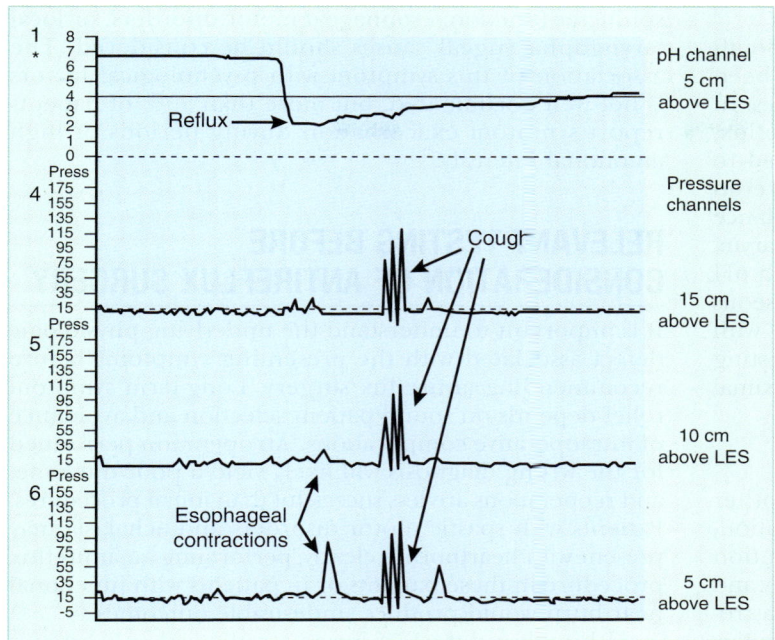

A

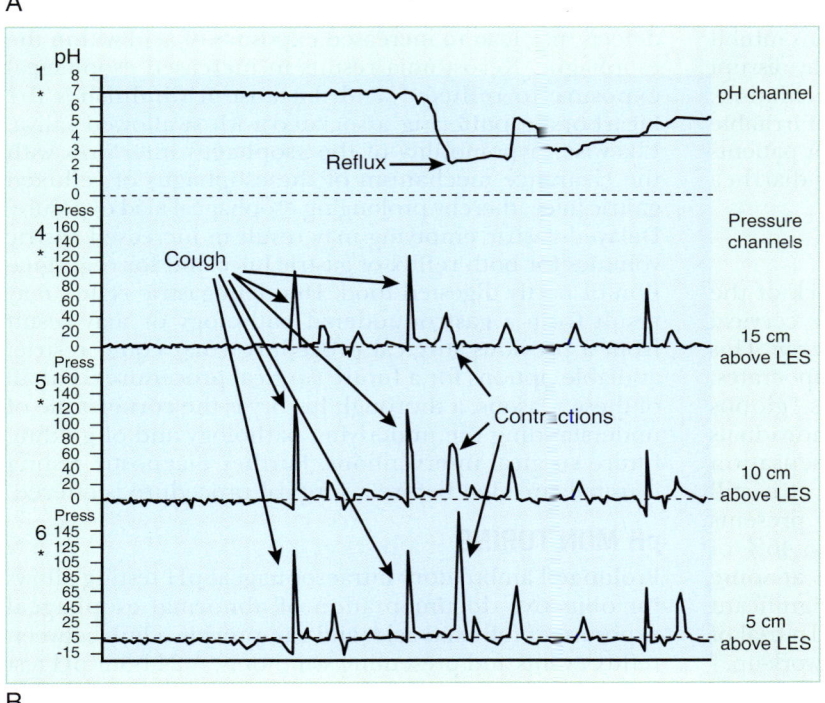

B

FIGURE 5.1 Cause-and-effect relationship between cough and esophageal acid exposure. (A) Coughing precipitated by a reflux episode may be the result of occult aspiration of refluxed gastric juice or a reflex brought on by esophageal acidification. (B) Conversely, increased intraabdominal pressure, as occurs with coughing, may overcome antireflux mechanisms and result in a gastroesophageal reflux episode. *LES,* Lower esophageal sphincter.

Chronic Cough and Asthma

Reflux as a cause of chronic cough is a challenge to diagnose. Silent aspiration is presumed to inflame and irritate the airway. Alexander and colleagues[20] observed an increased prevalence of GERD symptoms and increased esophageal exposure to acid in asthmatic patients. Schnatz and Castell[21] also noted a high proportion (~8%) of positive pH tests in patients with chronic cough or asthma. Increased esophageal exposure to gastric juice in these patients is probably both the cause and the effect: Severe coughing with wheezing increases intraabdominal pressure, driving gastric juice into the relatively negative-pressure environment of the chest, and esophageal acidification can result in a reflexive bronchospastic response (Fig. 5.1). Furthermore, as discussed later, chronic aspiration contributes to ongoing cough and to progressive parenchymal fibrosis. Evidence of pharyngeal reflux on pH testing helps identify patients with respiratory symptoms who may benefit from an antireflux operation.[22]

Hoarseness and Dental Caries

Reflux of gastric juice to the laryngeal aditus or the mouth is called laryngopharyngeal reflux (LPR), and has been associated with laryngeal symptoms and dental caries. In the work-up of patients thought to have significant reflux, catheters with two or more probes have been used to assess reflux into the more proximal esophagus or even the pharynx.[23,24] Furthermore, the addition of impedance catheter monitoring has shown that reflux into the pharynx is more frequent than previously thought, even with pH monitoring. Kawamura et al.[25] have shown that gaseous reflux with weak acidity is more common in patients with reflux-related laryngeal lesions. Again, objective testing with pH or pH impedance is needed to diagnose proximal reflux as a possible cause of LPR.

Nausea and Vomiting

Although nausea and vomiting may accompany other foregut symptoms such as heartburn and regurgitation, they should alert the surgeon to proceed with caution when considering an antireflux procedure. Early satiety and bloating may indicate delayed gastric emptying or gastroparesis, especially in diabetic patients. Severe preoperative nausea and vomiting should be relative contraindications to antireflux surgery, as most antireflux operations inhibit the ability to vomit, and postoperative heaving may disrupt the fundoplication or result in recurrent herniation. Similarly, patients with concomitant symptoms of irritable bowel syndrome, postcholecystectomy patients, or patients with other prominent bowel symptoms such as diarrhea should be treated conservatively, if possible.

Globus Sensation

The sensation of a lump or fullness in the back of the throat, or of having a foreign sensation in the cervical esophageal region, has been termed *globus sensation*. This symptom was recognized 2500 years ago by Hippocrates, and in the 19th century it was referred to as "globus hystericus" due to its frequent appearance in individuals with psychological disorders. Although the sensation is generally associated with benign disorders, it is still extremely irritating to most patients. It usually presents in the fifth and sixth decades of life, and up to 46% of healthy individuals experience this sensation at some point in their lives.[26,27] Globus sensation has a significant association with GERD, and some have suggested a trial of high-dose PPIs for 3 to 6 months prior to further work-up.[28] It may require a more prolonged and intensive trial of PPIs than is required for typical heartburn.[29]

Objective pH testing may reveal abnormal esophageal acid exposure in many patients with globus sensation, but some have suggested that pH impedance studies are more sensitive, as some patients are found to have symptoms associated with weak acid reflux.[30–32] Patients who respond to PPIs only partially or not at all should not expect good outcomes after antireflux surgery, and antireflux surgery should not be considered as treatment for globus sensation alone. If the disorder is associated with other symptoms, such as dysphagia or weight loss, immediate work-up should be carried out to rule out a malignant cause. The origin of the globus sensation is poorly understood, but if it is persistent, local causes such as abnormal upper esophageal sphincter function, esophageal motor disorders, or local laryngopharyngeal causes should be considered. The association of this symptom with psychological factors is not well documented, but more than 90% of patients report symptom exacerbation during periods of high emotional intensity.[33]

RELEVANT TESTING BEFORE CONSIDERATION OF ANTIREFLUX SURGERY

It is important to understand the underlying physiologic defect associated with the presenting symptoms before recommending antireflux surgery. Long-term symptom relief depends on sound patient selection and avoidance of intraoperative complications. An operation performed for the wrong diagnosis will likely yield a poor outcome, and reoperations are less successful than initial procedures. Patients with spastic motor disorders and achalasia may present with heartburn[34]; clearly, performing an antireflux procedure in these patients or in patients with functional heartburn would produce undesirable outcomes.

Although a defective lower esophageal sphincter is the most common underlying pathology of GERD, other defects may lead to increased exposure of acid within the esophagus. Xerostomia results in increased esophageal exposure to refluxed acid, because it diminishes the bicarbonate buffering associated with swallowed saliva. Likewise, hypomotility of the esophagus interferes with the clearance mechanism of the esophagus of refluxed gastric juice, thereby prolonging esophageal acid exposure. Delayed gastric emptying may result in increased gastric volumes for both reflux of gastric juice and for regurgitation of partly digested food. Duodenogastric reflux may result from a gastroduodenal pathology or may result from a previous surgical procedure (that could restrict available options for a future surgical procedure). For all of these reasons, a thorough history is the cornerstone of understanding the underlying pathology and of guiding future surgical interventions. Further diagnostic testing is usually needed before a surgical procedure is offered.

pH MONITORING

Prolonged ambulatory intraesophageal pH testing allows for objective documentation of abnormal esophageal exposure to refluxed acid, and can provide a link between reflux events and presenting symptoms. A 24-hour pH test is the most accurate means of confirming suspected GERD and provides details on the extent of the esophageal acid exposure (see Table 5.1). A pH test may be performed with either a 24-hour transnasal probe or a small capsule (Bravo capsule, Medtronic, Dublin, Ireland) that is affixed to the esophageal mucosa and transmits pH data via a radiotelemetry device (Figs. 5.2 to 5.4). Both catheter- and capsule-based technology have been shown to be valid and reproducible,[35,36] although the capsule allows for prolonged recordings (up to 48 or 72 hours). This may add additional diagnostic information and can provide a greater database for correlation of symptoms. The catheter system, on the other hand, allows for a proximal and a distal pH sensor, which may aid in identifying patients with LPR and increase understanding of the effect of reflux on chronic cough.

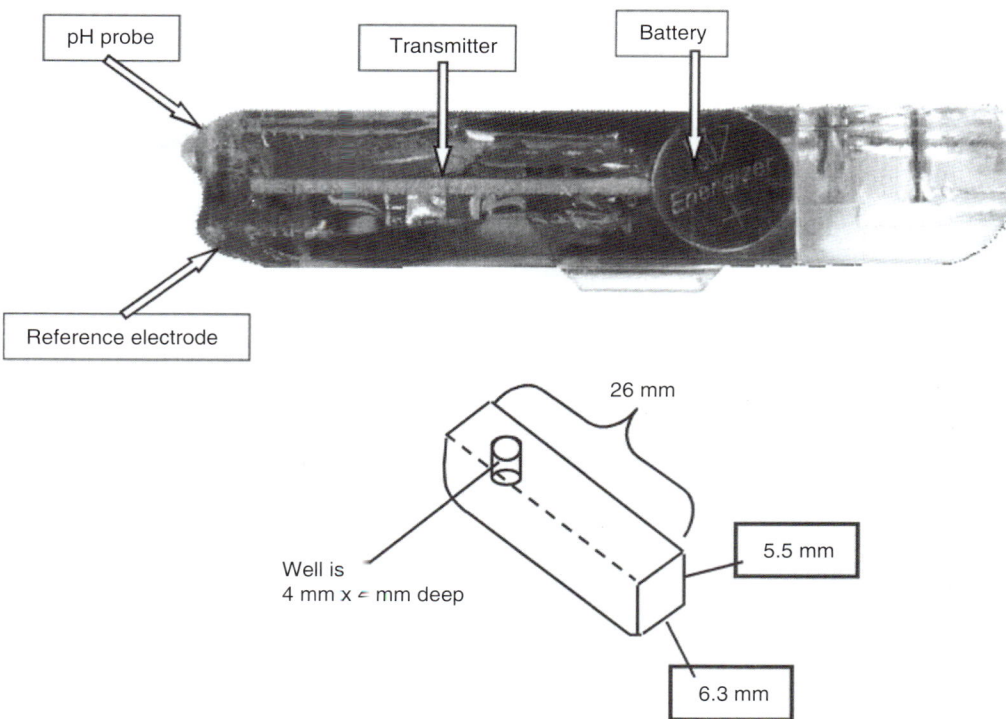

FIGURE 5.2 Dimensions and electronics of the Bravo pH capsule (Medtronic, Dublin, Ireland). The capsule is oblong (6.3 × 5.5 × 26 mm). A well (diameter, 4 mm; depth, 4 mm) is located on the superior-lateral aspect of the probe. The well is connected to a custom-made vacuum unit capable of generating 600 mm Hg vacuum pressure to the well via the delivery system. An antimony pH electrode and reference electrode are located on the distal tip of the capsule, and an internal battery and transmitter are contained within the capsule.

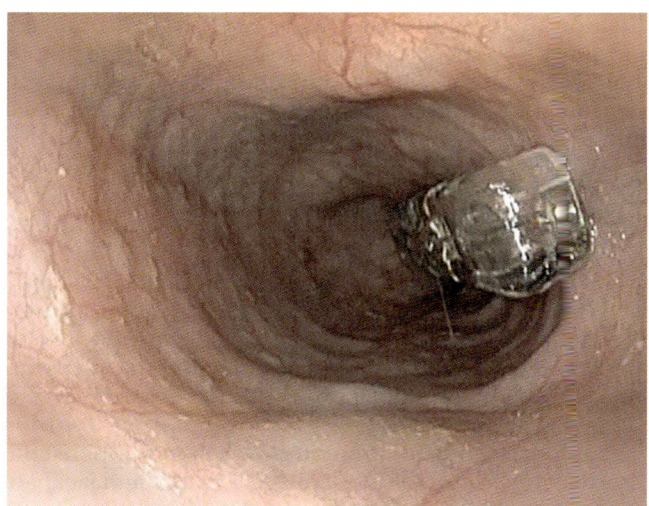

FIGURE 5.3 Endoscopic view of the Bravo pH capsule (Medtronic, Dublin, Ireland) properly deployed in the esophagus. *(Used with permission from Norton Thoracic Institute, Phoenix, Arizona.)*

A 24-hour pH study also facilitates characterization of the reflux—for example, whether it occurs predominantly in the postprandial period, the duration of reflux episodes (thereby providing an indication of esophageal insensitivity or poor clearance), and the time of day during which it usually occurs.

Before antireflux surgery can be safely considered, it is important to document abnormal esophageal exposure to gastric juice. The pH catheter and Bravo capsule can provide objective evidence of acid exposure, but patients must cease taking PPI medications for at least 1 week before the test is performed. Many patients cannot tolerate cessation of their PPIs, and some may "cheat" during the absence period, which may explain a negative test in an otherwise symptomatic patient. Histamine-2 (H_2) blockers can be used up to 48 hours before the test; thereafter, only over-the-counter antacids are appropriate up until the time of the study. Understanding a patient's symptoms without PPIs is important, as severe heartburn after withholding PPIs is in itself a reasonably reliable diagnostic test. As a corollary, if a patient's symptoms are not significantly changed when PPIs are withheld, the surgeon should exercise caution when considering surgical treatment—functional heartburn may be the more accurate diagnosis.

A pH test may not be necessary in a patient with an obviously defective lower esophageal sphincter (as seen on manometry) or with obvious esophagitis (as seen on endoscopy). However, mild esophagitis has poor interobserver agreement,[37] and esophagitis may result from pill injury or infection. In patients experiencing both reflux and regurgitation, endoscopic ulcerative esophagitis is 97% specific for GERD.[38] A pH test may be unnecessary if the patient has a very large paraesophageal hernia and the surgery is primarily directed at this defect, especially

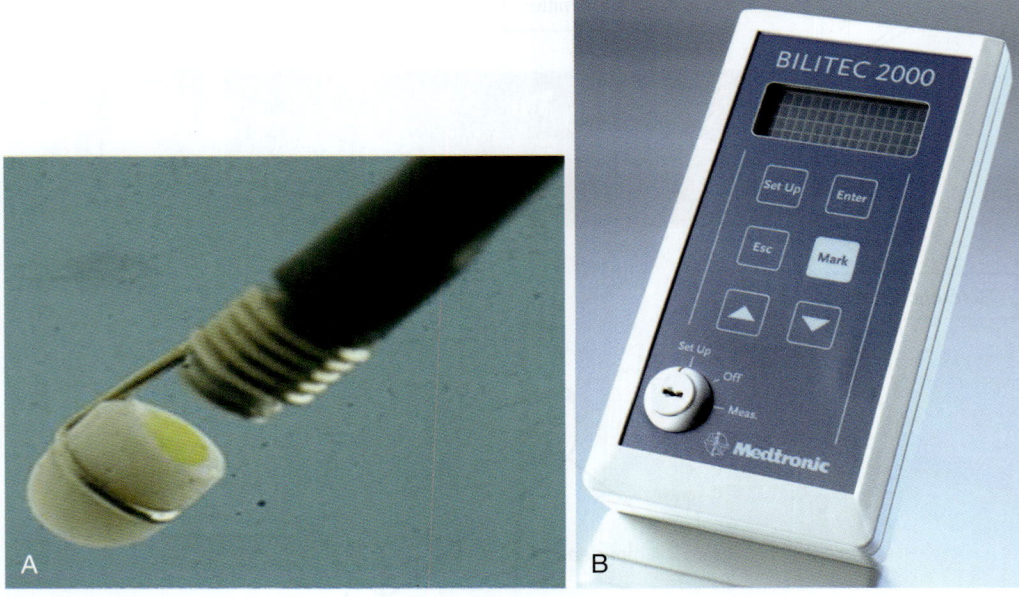

FIGURE 5.4 Bilitec probe (A) and electronic data logger (B) for 24-hour esophageal bilirubin monitoring.

since an antireflux procedure usually accompanies repair of the paraesophageal hernia, regardless of whether the patient experienced heartburn preoperatively.

Antireflux surgery performed in patients with normal 24-hour pH tests is associated with significantly worse outcomes than when it is performed in patients with abnormal tests; therefore, routine pH testing is recommended prior to antireflux surgery.[16] As a corollary, 24-hour pH testing or pH impedance testing is very useful in selecting those patients with functional heartburn or with visceral hyperesthesia for whom surgery may prove ineffective.

IMPEDANCE TESTING

Multichannel intraluminal impedance testing relies on the change in resistance to an electrical current when a bolus, liquid, or gas passes between the metallic rings on a catheter. When the esophagus is empty, the electrical current is conducted by the ions on the mucosa. Liquids with more ions increase conductivity and decrease resistance, which can be measured and recorded in much the same way acid is measured in 24-hour monitoring scenarios. By measuring impedance at many sites along a catheter, the direction of the bolus's movement can be determined. In this way, a swallow of a liquid will be antegrade, whereas a reflux episode will be retrograde.

The benefit of this type of testing is that the fluid bolus (i.e., refluxate) can be measured regardless of its acidity. By combining pH testing with impedance testing, all types of reflux can be measured. This allows practitioners to determine acid episodes, weak acid episodes, and nonacid episodes, and to correlate symptoms to each type.[39] Although most patients undergoing antireflux surgery will have a positive acid pH test, a subgroup of patients with weakly acid or nonacid reflux who may benefit from surgery has been described.[39] Impedance testing may also have value in identifying the cause of chronic cough in patients with normal pH studies. Impedance studies are relatively new; therefore, they are still being evaluated in the surgical arena. The test has the potential to add substantially more information, although the testing does require a transnasal catheter for 24 hours.

MANOMETRY

Manometry provides information on the tone and coordination of the upper and lower esophageal sphincters and on the propulsive function of the esophageal body. It allows for identification of motility disorders and also provides information that may preclude some surgical approaches.

Most historical, water-perfused manometry systems have been replaced with high-resolution manometry that uses sensitive, solid-state pressure transducers. The data that can be collected with this test have allowed for more precise evaluation of esophageal motility disorders, and a new classification system (i.e., the Chicago Classification System) has been proposed to capture this new level of precision. This classification system uses the pressure tomography plots from high-resolution manometry to categorize various disorders by prioritizing (1) disorders of esophagogastric junction outflow, (2) major peristaltic disorders (i.e., aperistalsis, esophageal spasm, and jackhammer or nutcracker esophagus), and (3) minor peristaltic disorders (i.e., those that impede bolus transport; namely, ineffective esophageal motility and fragmented peristalsis). Already this system has facilitated clarification of subtypes I, II, and III for achalasia, and implications of therapy and potential surgical outcomes for each subtype have been delineated.[40,41]

The success of the Nissen fundoplication in patients with hypomotility of the esophageal body has been the subject of much debate. Some have shown that motility of the esophageal body may improve slightly in some patients after fundoplication.[42–47] Although it is likely true that mildly depressed contraction amplitudes do not significantly impact postoperative dysphagia in expert hands,[48–50] severely depressed contractions and the so-called aperistaltic esophagus (as seen in connective tissue disorders) will likely result in poor esophageal clearance after a 360° fundoplication. Manometric evaluation of the esophagus is the only objective way to provide a clear evaluation of the esophageal pressure profiles that guide a surgeon performing functional surgery. Data are emerging on the benefits of the Chicago Classification System in predicting outcomes after surgery depending on various motility abnormalities.[41] High-resolution manometry may identify abnormalities that contraindicate surgery; others may help a surgeon counsel patients and manage expectations of surgical outcomes.

Spastic motor disorders (e.g., diffuse esophageal spasm or achalasia) may present with heartburn-like discomfort.[51] In a large retrospective study of 1081 patients referred for antireflux surgery, 1 in 14 were found to have abnormalities on high-resolution manometry that were considered absolute or relative contraindications for antireflux surgery.[51] The researchers further noted that almost 25% of patients would have undergone antireflux surgery without clear evidence of GERD, had pH monitoring and manometry not been performed during work-up. Of all 1081 patients, 2.5% were found to have abnormalities on the achalasia spectrum. An antireflux operation in this context would obviously have a poor outcome that would likely require a second, corrective operation. In patients for whom manometry is impossible (e.g., the patient refuses or the catheter cannot be passed through the nose), a partial fundoplication should be performed to minimize the risk of postoperative dysphagia. In this situation, a well-performed barium study may provide some insight on peristaltic function.

IMPEDANCE MANOMETRY

The recent addition of impedance to esophageal manometry may provide further information on esophageal clearance in real time, but the role this technology plays in surgical planning is presently unclear. This modality may help evaluate the propulsive efficiency of the esophagus for different bolus consistencies and for different body positions.[52] This method may be useful for evaluation of esophageal function both before and after fundoplication in the future.

BARIUM ESOPHAGRAM

Continuous digital or video barium esophagram can identify structural abnormalities and can provide functional information about the esophagus. If the patient is unable to tolerate a manometric study, the barium esophagram can offer insight into the peristaltic activity of the esophagus, especially if the test is done with both solids and liquids. A barium esophagram can also help identify the nature and position of a hiatal hernia. Interestingly, the standard barium esophagram performed in many institutions today has changed little over the 30 years it has been in use.[53] Effervescent crystals are still used to provide information on mucosal relief, and prone oblique views are still used, even when achalasia is suspected. Some specialized centers have modified the barium study to better understand

functional esophageal disorders, as is well described later in this book.

Perhaps the most important aspect of performing the barium esophagram is effective communication between the surgeon and the radiologist with regard to the patient's symptoms and suspected diagnoses. The study can be modified to concentrate on mucosal relief (for patients with ulcerative esophagitis, infections, or early tumors), propulsive action (recumbent swallows with different barium consistencies), emptying of the esophagus in the upright position in patients with achalasia,[54,55] or evaluation of strictures. Certain provocative maneuvers, such as leg raising or a Valsalva maneuver while the patient is supine, can elicit free reflux, which—although not a sensitive test—is usually quite specific for GERD.[56] The radiologist should have some understanding of the concepts of deglutitive inhibition (i.e., rapid swallowing followed only by a terminal peristaltic wave), and the refractory period of the esophagus, as swallows closer together than 20 seconds may have poorer quality propulsive function. Overall, the barium study—when performed correctly—is a wonderful screening tool in patients with esophageal symptoms.

ENDOSCOPY

Endoscopy is considered a critical preoperative study before recommending antireflux surgery and provides necessary biopsy material in patients with Barrett esophagus, suspected malignancy, or eosinophilic esophagitis. Endoscopy can identify esophagitis, strictures, hiatal hernia, the presence of Barrett esophagus, or malignancy, and provide a qualitative look at the function of the lower esophageal sphincter. This analysis has been well described by Hill.[57]

Endoscopy facilitates categorization of esophagitis; the most commonly used scale is the Los Angeles classification system (Table 5.2).[58] Endoscopy also allows diagnosis of Barrett esophagus via biopsy, as the presence of high-grade dysplasia or intramucosal carcinoma in a segment of the esophagus with Barrett esophagus may alter the surgeon's approach. In that situation, further studies may be indicated, and ablation or resection may be the

TABLE 5.2 The Los Angeles Classification of Esophagitis

Grade A	One (or more) mucosal break no longer than 5 mm that does not extend between the tops of two mucosal folds
Grade B	One (or more) mucosal break more than 5 mm long that does not extend between the tops of two mucosal folds
Grade C	One (or more) mucosal break that is continuous between the tops of two or more mucosal folds, but which involves less than 75% of the circumference
Grade D	One (or more) mucosal break that involves at least 75% of the esophageal circumference

Reprinted from Sami SS, Ragunath K. The Los Angeles classification of gastroesophageal reflux disease. *Video J Encyclopedia GI Endoscopy.* 2013;1:103–104. Used with permission under Creative Commons license CC BY-NC-ND 4.0.

first course of action. The length of a Barrett segment, the size of a hiatal hernia, the presence of esophagitis or stricture, and the ease of eructation in the retroflexed position on insufflation should all be noted. Patients with Barrett esophagus should undergo biopsies at four quadrants every one to two centimeters, and should be placed on a surveillance program regardless of whether they undergo fundoplication.

GASTRIC EMPTYING STUDIES

For patients with prominent symptoms of nausea, vomiting, postprandial fullness, or bloating, an evaluation of gastric emptying should be considered. A bezoar visible after an overnight fast is usually a good indication of delayed gastric emptying, but the best objective study is a scintigraphic radionucleotide study using both solids and liquids.[59] Unfortunately, the methods and normal values vary significantly between centers, and the results are not always reliable.[60,61] A recent consensus report suggested using a standardized meal of radiolabeled low-fat egg whites with imaging up to 4 hours after the meal.[59] A Nissen fundoplication may improve gastric emptying,[62] but a significantly delayed gastric emptying study should alert the surgeon to the need for other procedures, such as pyloric injection of botulinum toxin type A, pyloroplasty, or a Roux-en-Y procedure.

RELEVANT PREOPERATIVE TESTING FOR SPECIFIC INDICATIONS

PREOPERATIVE TESTING FOR BARRETT ESOPHAGUS

Barrett esophagus can only be diagnosed on endoscopy with confirmation of intestinal metaplasia on biopsy. The finding of goblet cells intermingled in a columnar lining of the tubular esophagus is pathognomonic of Barrett esophagus. The disease is considered to be a metaplastic response to severe GERD,[63] and its clinical significance is the premalignant potential of the unstable epithelium. The definition has changed slightly over the years, but biopsy is required for confirmation.

The finding of Barrett esophagus has significance outside its potential for malignancy, as patients with Barrett esophagus often have associated esophageal hypomotility and generally have severely abnormal esophageal exposure to both refluxed acid and duodenal contents. Patients with Barrett esophagus may also have a shorter-than-normal esophagus, which may have implications for a planned surgical procedure.

PREOPERATIVE TESTING FOR GIANT HERNIAS OR LARGE PARAESOPHAGEAL HERNIAS

The aging population, coupled with the ubiquitous use of PPIs for heartburn control (often of decades' duration), has led to an epidemic of large paraesophageal hernias or the so-called intrathoracic stomach. Presumably, heartburn has been adequately controlled in these patients, but the hernia has progressively enlarged to the point that the hernia itself is responsible for the presenting symptoms. These symptoms may include chest discomfort, postprandial fullness or discomfort, dyspnea, dysphagia, or anemia. Dysphagia may be related to the

accordion-like shortening of the esophagus, with the external pressure of the paraesophageal stomach pressing on the esophagus itself, or from a coexisting motility disorder. Chest discomfort and bloating may be related to distention of the intrathoracic stomach and the slow emptying of this compartment. Dyspnea as a symptom is poorly understood, but is usually improved after surgical intervention. Not infrequently, patients with giant hernias or large paraesophageal hernias describe only a remote history of heartburn, but it is either no longer an issue or is easily controlled with PPIs.

Large hernias occasionally present acutely with torsion, which usually mandates immediate surgical intervention (although decompression and de-torsion with endoscopy has been described). Severe abdominal and chest pain is usually attributed to ischemia of the herniated stomach, and patients with these presenting symptoms often progress rapidly to being critically ill with hemodynamic instability.

For the most part, patients' symptoms progress slowly, and an outpatient work-up can be performed. This work-up should include barium studies, endoscopy, and manometry. pH studies are likely unnecessary, as the indication for surgery is the large hernia itself, and the surgical repair of the hernia is usually accompanied by some sort of fundoplication. Barium studies will show the size and position of the hernia, and if performed with a 13-mm barium tablet, will reveal any delay during passage through the esophagus. Endoscopy will identify Barrett esophagus, dysplasia, and Cameron ulcers in the stomach. Manometry will identify any marked motility abnormalities—which is especially important, as the incidence of spastic motor disorders increases in the older population.

PREOPERATIVE TESTING FOR MYOTOMY FOR ACHALASIA OR DIVERTICULA

The diagnosis of spastic motor disorders and achalasia depends on a well-performed manometric study, and manometry is critical before surgery is considered for these disorders. Barium studies usually show areas of corkscrewing or the tapered bird-beak appearance of the distal esophagus associated with achalasia. Endoscopy is recommended to rule out pseudoachalasia, in which the motility disorder of the esophagus is secondary to an infiltrating process (usually adenocarcinoma) at the gastroesophageal junction.[64,65] Chagas disease may give a similar picture.[66]

Barium esophagram and a manometric study can indicate how far the myotomy should extend, especially in patients with a diverticulum that is situated more than a few centimeters above the gastroesophageal junction. Manometry can also help counsel patients with different variants of achalasia regarding expected outcomes.[40,41]

PREOPERATIVE TESTING FOR END-STAGE LUNG DISEASE AND TRANSPLANTATION

The effect of GERD in patients with end-stage lung disease and in patients who have undergone lung transplantation has historically been underestimated. A high proportion of patients with end-stage lung disease have pathologic GERD, and it has been suggested that silent aspiration contributes to pulmonary injury in many of these patients.

Similarly, the chronic cough associated with many end-stage lung diseases is thought to promote reflux, as it increases intraabdominal and transsphincteric pressure (see Fig. 5.1). Recently, GERD has also been implicated as a significant adverse contributor to the development of bronchiolitis obliterans syndrome after lung transplantation.[67,68] Davis and colleagues[67] have shown that 73% of patients who have undergone lung transplantation have GERD (diagnosed by pH monitoring). This may be due to the significant number of patients with unrecognized GERD before transplantation, to vagal damage at the time of surgery, or to the reflux-promoting side effects of postoperative immunosuppressive medications. Nonetheless, Davis et al.[67] have shown that fundoplication in lung transplant recipients with GERD is associated with significantly improved lung function, particularly if the fundoplication is performed before bronchiolitis obliterans syndrome reaches advanced stages. Others have suggested that performing a fundoplication more than 6 months after lung transplantation is associated with worse long-term allograft function.[69,70] Many patients with progressive deterioration in lung function and the diagnosis of pulmonary fibrosis referred for transplantation have experienced stabilization of their pulmonary disease after fundoplication, again emphasizing the negative effects that GERD and silent aspiration have on pulmonary function.

It is now the standard of care to have a solid understanding of a patient's reflux history before considering lung transplantation, and in many centers all patients considered for lung transplantation undergo manometry, videoesophagraphy, and 24-hour pH testing to assess for GERD. Patients with severe reflux and a nonprohibitive surgical risk will undergo fundoplication before transplantation. Antireflux surgery in the early posttransplant period is considered for patients who cannot undergo surgery before transplantation, or who develop GERD after transplantation.

pH monitoring has provided tremendous insight into the significance of GERD in this complex group of patients, and continues to provide important information that directs therapy. A mere symptom assessment is completely inadequate when evaluating patients slated to undergo lung transplantation, and pH or pH impedance testing is required to identify patients who may be at risk of aspiration as a result of GERD. Soresi and colleagues[71] found almost 60% of lung transplantation patients suffered from postoperative GERD. Similarly, Tamhankar et al.[72] showed that PPIs only affect the pH of the refluxate—not the occurrence or frequency of the reflux episodes. As such, it may be prudent to have all transplant patients undergo multichannel pH impedance testing posttransplantation, especially as patients with abnormal proximal esophageal reflux are more likely to be readmitted to the hospital. This group of patients should be treated aggressively (i.e., early antireflux surgery) to protect the implanted allograft, especially in the face of immunosuppression.[69]

The problematic effects of reflux in the patients who have undergone lung transplantation are complex. Clearly, aspiration occurs more frequently than previously thought, as bile salts and pepsin have been found in bronchoalveolar lavage fluid, and thorough testing pre- and posttransplant

are indicated. pH impedance studies are diagnostic, but manometry is also important, as abnormalities in peristalsis or function of the lower esophageal sphincter may occur in up to 66% of patients[73] and may contribute to poor esophageal clearance of refluxed fluid. Endoscopy is important, as Barrett esophagus may be more prevalent in the lung transplant population.[74] Early antireflux surgery should be considered in patients with GERD; if the patient can tolerate such a procedure, this is optimal, because the patient can recover when they are not taking steroids or other immunosuppressive medications, as they will be posttransplant. If antireflux surgery cannot be performed before transplantation, it should be considered soon after transplant to protect the transplanted organ. By the time the organ shows evidence of decline (i.e., decreased forced expiratory volume in 1 second [FEV_1]), it may be too late to prevent the progression of organ dysfunction.

PREOPERATIVE TESTING FOR REOPERATION AFTER FAILURE OF PREVIOUS ANTIREFLUX SURGERY

A very detailed patient history is critical when evaluating a patient who has undergone an antireflux procedure that has presumably failed. It is useful to review any preoperative studies carried out before the initial operation, if the results of those studies are available. An attempt should be made to prioritize the patient's symptoms to understand the nature of the failure (Box 5.3). When considering a reoperation, it is crucial to perform all necessary testing to optimize the outcome, because the second and third procedures are usually less successful than the initial procedure, especially if dysphagia is a prominent symptom.[75–77]

Manometry is particularly important because it provides the surgeon with useful information about the motor function of the esophagus, as it may differ from its status before the first operation. A gastric emptying study is also important, particularly if bloating and early satiety are prominent symptoms. Operative options include takedown of the previous wrap, redo fundoplication, possible pyloroplasty, and gastric diversion such as Roux-en-Y esophagoenterostomy or gastroenterostomy, all of which are discussed in greater detail later in this book.

BOX 5.3 Questions to Ask Your Patient Prior to Redo Surgery

What were your symptoms before your first operation?
What tests did you undergo before your first operation?
Did you have a hiatal hernia or a paraesophageal hernia? If so, did your surgeon use mesh to repair the hernia?
How long were you in the hospital?
Did you have any side effects of the operation?
Did your symptoms improve or resolve after your first operation?
What are your main symptoms currently?
When did these start? Are they progressively getting worse?
Did anything precipitate the onset of these symptoms?
Were any of these present prior to your initial operation?
Please describe any symptoms of dysphagia, heartburn, regurgitation, bloating, nausea, or early satiety in detail.

PREOPERATIVE TESTING FOR ESOPHAGEAL CANCER

The presenting symptom for esophageal cancer is, invariably, some degree of dysphagia. Depending on the severity of the dysphagia, the patient may also have experienced some degree of weight loss. Unfortunately, dysphagia usually has an insidious beginning and patients often adapt, sometimes for months, as the symptoms progress before scheduling an appointment with a physician—which can be particularly troubling, as dysphagia usually occurs late in the course of esophageal cancer. It only occurs when more than 60% of the circumference of the esophagus is involved, or when the lumen is decreased to a diameter of less than 12 mm. Other symptoms, such as chest pain or hematemesis, are less common and are usually accompanied by dysphagia. If the tumor invades the tracheobronchial tree, symptoms such as cough, stridor, hemoptysis, and pneumonia may be present. Distant metastases may produce symptoms of bone pain, neurologic symptoms, or jaundice. Dysphagia has been called an "alarm symptom" for this reason, and while there are many benign causes (e.g., GERD, motility disorders, and esophageal stricture), the physician should take this symptom seriously.

The work-up of a patient with suspected cancer involves obtaining a tissue biopsy and diagnosis, and performing staging procedures to plan treatment. A barium study may show narrowing or an apple-core-like stricture in the esophagus, but an endoscopy will facilitate biopsy and (together with an endoscopic ultrasound) can provide information on the extent of the cancer and possible lymph node involvement. Positron emission tomography and computed tomography are considered critical in identifying the stage of the disease.

CONCLUSION

Complete physiologic testing and a thorough understanding of a patient's symptoms are necessary before surgery can be recommended for patients with functional esophageal disorders. Surgeons should understand the value of the various modalities of esophageal testing (e.g., pH impedance testing and manometry studies), as the information gleaned from these tests can direct therapeutic intervention. Symptoms alone should not direct a surgical procedure. Patients who experience dysphagia should be taken seriously and should undergo a complete work-up, as dysphagia is the most common presenting symptom of esophageal cancer.

SUGGESTED READINGS

Bremner RM, Bremner CG, DeMeester TR. Gastroesophageal reflux: the use of pH monitoring. *Curr Probl Surg.* 1995;32(6):429-558.

Goyal R, Shaker R. *GI Motility Online;* 2016. http://www.nature.com/gimo/index.html.

Kahrilas PJ, Bredenoord AJ, Fox M, et al. The Chicago Classification of esophageal motility disorders, v3.0. *Neurogastroenterol Motil.* 2015;27(2):160-174.

Khajanchee YS, Hong D, Hansen PD, Swanstrom LL. Outcomes of antireflux surgery in patients with normal preoperative 24-hour pH test results. *Am J Surg.* 2004;187(5):599-603.

Yoshida N, Kuroda M, Suzuki T, et al. Role of nociceptors/neuropeptides in the pathogenesis of visceral hypersensitivity of nonerosive reflux disease. *Dig Dis Sci.* 2013;58(8):2237-2243.

REFERENCES

1. Campos GM, Peters JH, DeMeester TR, et al. Multivariate analysis of factors predicting outcome after laparoscopic Nissen fundoplication. *J Gastrointest Surg.* 1999;3(3):292-300.
2. Drewes AM, Schipper KP, Dimcevski G, et al. Multimodal assessment of pain in the esophagus: a new experimental model. *Am J Physiol Gastrointest Liver Physiol.* 2002;283(1):G95-G103.
3. Drewes AM, Schipper KP, Dimcevski G, et al. Multi-modal induction and assessment of allodynia and hyperalgesia in the human oesophagus. *Eur J Pain.* 2003;7(6):539-549.
4. Bulsiewicz WJ, Shaheen NJ, Hansen MB, Pruitt A, Orlando RC. Effect of amiloride on experimental acid-induced heartburn in non-erosive reflux disease. *Dig Dis Sci.* 2013;58(7):1955-1959.
5. Reddy H, Arendt-Nielsen L, Staahl C, et al. Gender differences in pain and biomechanical responses after acid sensitization of the human esophagus. *Dig Dis Sci.* 2005;50(11):2050-2058.
6. Polland WS, Bloomfield AL. Experimental referred pain from the gastrointestinal tract. Part I. The esophagus. *J Clin Invest.* 1931;10(3):435-452.
7. Vakil N, van Zanten SV, Kahrilas P, Dent J, Jones R. The Montreal definition and classification of gastroesophageal reflux disease: a global evidence-based consensus. *Am J Gastroenterol.* 2006;101(8):1900-1920; quiz 1943.
8. Fass R, Tougas G. Functional heartburn: the stimulus, the pain, and the brain. *Gut.* 2002;51(6):885-892.
9. Bremner RM, Crookes PF, DeMeester TR, Peters JH, Stein HJ. Concentration of refluxed acid and esophageal mucosal injury. *Am J Surg.* 1992;164(5):522-526; discussion 526–527.
10. Amos JA. Acid Reflux (GERD) Statistics and Facts; 2012. http://www.healthline.com/health/gerd/statistics#2.
11. Zhao Y, Encinosa W. Gastroesophageal Reflux Disease (GERD) Hospitalizations in 1998 and 2005; 2008. http://www.hcup-us.ahrq.gov/reports/statbriefs/sb44.jsp.
12. Shaker R, Castell DO, Schoenfeld PS, Spechler SJ. Nighttime heartburn is an under-appreciated clinical problem that impacts sleep and daytime function: the results of a Gallup survey conducted on behalf of the American Gastroenterological Association. *Am J Gastroenterol.* 2003;98(7):1487-1493.
13. Johnson LF, DeMeester TR. Development of the 24-hour intraesophageal pH monitoring composite scoring system. *J Clin Gastroenterol.* 1986;8(suppl 1):52-58.
14. Galmiche JP, Clouse RE, Balint A, et al. Functional esophageal disorders. *Gastroenterology.* 2006;130(5):1459-1465.
15. Herregods TV, Troelstra M, Weijenborg PW, Bredenoord AJ, Smout AJ. Patients with refractory reflux symptoms often do not have GERD. *Neurogastroenterol Motil.* 2015;27(9):1267-1273.
16. Khajanchee YS, Hong D, Hansen PD, Swanstrom LL. Outcomes of antireflux surgery in patients with normal preoperative 24-hour pH test results. *Am J Surg.* 2004;187(5):599-603.
17. Clouse RE, Richter JE, Heading RC, Janssens J, Wilson J. Functional esophageal disorders. In: Drossman DA, ed. *The Functional Gastrointestinal Disorders.* 2nd ed. McLean, VA: Degnon Associates; 2000:147-298.
18. Richter JE. Chest pain and gastroesophageal reflux disease. *J Clin Gastroenterol.* 2000;30(3 suppl):S39-S41.
19. Fass R, Fennerty MB, Johnson C, Camargo L, Sampliner RE. Correlation of ambulatory 24-hour esophageal pH monitoring results with symptom improvement in patients with noncardiac chest pain due to gastroesophageal reflux disease. *J Clin Gastroenterol.* 1999;28(1):36-39.
20. Alexander JA, Hunt LW, Patel AM. Prevalence, pathophysiology, and treatment of patients with asthma and gastroesophageal reflux disease. *Mayo Clin Proc.* 2000;75(10):1055-1063.
21. Schnatz PF, Castell JA, Castell DO. Pulmonary symptoms associated with gastroesophageal reflux: use of ambulatory pH monitoring to diagnose and to direct therapy. *Am J Gastroenterol.* 1996;91(9):1715-1718.
22. Oelschlager BK, Eubanks TR, Oleynikov D, Pope C, Pellegrini CA. Symptomatic and physiologic outcomes after operative treatment for extraesophageal reflux. *Surg Endosc.* 2002;16(7):1032-1036.
23. Hanson DG, Conley D, Jiang J, Kahrilas P. Role of esophageal pH recording in management of chronic laryngitis: an overview. *Ann Otol Rhinol Laryngol Suppl.* 2000;184:4-9.
24. Harrell S, Evans B, Goudy S, et al. Design and implementation of an ambulatory pH monitoring protocol in patients with suspected laryngopharyngeal reflux. *Laryngoscope.* 2005;115(1):89-92.

25. Kawamura O, Aslam M, Rittmann T, Hofmann C, Shaker R. Physical and pH properties of gastroesophagopharyngeal refluxate: a 24-hour simultaneous ambulatory impedance and pH monitoring study. *Am J Gastroenterol.* 2004;99(6):1000-1010.

26. Drossman DA, Li Z, Andruzzi E, et al. U.S. householder survey of functional gastrointestinal disorders. Prevalence, sociodemography, and health impact. *Dig Dis Sci.* 1993;38(9):1569-1580.

27. Moloy PJ, Charter R. The globus symptom. Incidence, therapeutic response, and age and sex relationships. *Arch Otolaryngol.* 1982;108(11):740-744.

28. Lee BE, Kim GH. Globus pharyngeus: a review of its etiology, diagnosis and treatment. *World J Gastroenterol.* 2012;18(20):2462-2471.

29. Remacle M. The diagnosis and management of globus: a perspective from Belgium. *Curr Opin Otolaryngol Head Neck Surg.* 2008;16(6):511-515.

30. Bajbouj M, Becker V, Neuber M, Schmid RM, Meining A. Combined pH-metry/impedance monitoring increases the diagnostic yield in patients with atypical gastroesophageal reflux symptoms. *Digestion.* 2007;76(3-4):223-228.

31. Lee BE, Kim GH, Ryu DY, et al. Combined dual channel impedance/pH-metry in patients with suspected laryngopharyngeal reflux. *J Neurogastroenterol Motil.* 2010;16(2):157-165.

32. Malhotra A, Freston JW, Aziz K. Use of pH-impedance testing to evaluate patients with suspected extraesophageal manifestations of gastroesophageal reflux disease. *J Clin Gastroenterol.* 2008;42(3):271-278.

33. Harris MB, Deary IJ, Wilson JA. Life events and difficulties in relation to the onset of globus pharyngis. *J Psychosom Res.* 1996;40(6):603-615.

34. Crookes PF, Corkill S, DeMeester TR. Gastroesophageal reflux in achalasia. When is reflux really reflux? *Dig Dis Sci.* 1997;42(7):1354-1361.

35. Ayazi S, Lipham JC, Portale G, et al. Bravo catheter-free pH monitoring: normal values, concordance, optimal diagnostic thresholds, and accuracy. *Clin Gastroenterol Hepatol.* 2009;7(1):60-67.

36. Johnson LF, DeMeester TR. Twenty-four-hour pH monitoring of the distal esophagus. A quantitative measure of gastroesophageal reflux. *Am J Gastroenterol.* 1974;62(4):325-332.

37. Bytzer P, Havelund T, Hansen JM. Interobserver variation in the endoscopic diagnosis of reflux esophagitis. *Scand J Gastroenterol.* 1993;28(2):119-125.

38. Tefera L, Fein M, Ritter MP, et al. Can the combination of symptoms and endoscopy confirm the presence of gastroesophageal reflux disease? *Am Surg.* 1997;63(10):933-936.

39. Hila A, Agrawal A, Castell DO. Combined multichannel intraluminal impedance and pH esophageal testing compared to pH alone for diagnosing both acid and weakly acidic gastroesophageal reflux. *Clin Gastroenterol Hepatol.* 2007;5(2):172-177.

40. Pandolfino JE, Fox MR, Bredenoord AJ, Kahrilas PJ. High-resolution manometry in clinical practice: utilizing pressure topography to classify oesophageal motility abnormalities. *Neurogastroenterol Motil.* 2009;21(8):796-806.

41. Pandolfino JE, Kwiatek MA, Nealis T, Bulsiewicz W, Post J, Kahrilas PJ. Achalasia: a new clinically relevant classification by high-resolution manometry. *Gastroenterology.* 2008;135(5):1526-1533.

42. Fibbe C, Layer P, Keller J, Strate U, Emmermann A, Zornig C. Esophageal motility in reflux disease before and after fundoplication: a prospective, randomized, clinical, and manometric study. *Gastroenterology.* 2001;121(1):5-14.

43. Herbella FA, Tedesco P, Nipomnick I, Fisichella PM, Patti MG. Effect of partial and total laparoscopic fundoplication on esophageal body motility. *Surg Endosc.* 2007;21(2):285-288.

44. Lund RJ, Wetcher GJ, Raiser F, et al. Laparoscopic Toupet fundoplication for gastroesophageal reflux disease with poor esophageal body motility. *J Gastrointest Surg.* 1997;1(4):301-308; discussion 308.

45. Pizza F, Rossetti G, Del Genio G, Maffettone V, Brusciano L, Del Genio A. Influence of esophageal motility on the outcome of laparoscopic total fundoplication. *Dis Esophagus.* 2008;21(1):78-85.

46. Rydberg L, Ruth M, Abrahamsson H, Lundell L. Tailoring antireflux surgery: a randomized clinical trial. *World J Surg.* 1999;23(6):612-618.

47. Tsereteli Z, Sporn E, Astudillo JA, Miedema B, Eubanks WS, Thaler K. Laparoscopic Nissen fundoplication is a good option in patients with abnormal esophageal motility. *Surg Endosc.* 2009;23(10):2292-2295.

48. Booth M, Stratford J, Dehn TC. Preoperative esophageal body motility does not influence the outcome of laparoscopic Nissen fundoplication for gastroesophageal reflux disease. *Dis Esophagus.* 2002;15(1):57-60.

49. Patti MG, Perretta S, Fisichella PM, et al. Laparoscopic antireflux surgery: preoperative lower esophageal sphincter pressure does not affect outcome. *Surg Endosc.* 2003;17(3):386-389.

50. Zornig C, Strate U, Fibbe C, Emmermann A, Layer P. Nissen vs Toupet laparoscopic fundoplication. *Surg Endosc.* 2002;16(5):758-766.

51. Chan WW, Haroian LR, Gyawali CP. Value of preoperative esophageal function studies before laparoscopic antireflux surgery. *Surg Endosc.* 2011;25(9):2943-2949.

52. Gao F, Gao Y, Hobson AR, Huang WN, Shang ZM. Normal esophageal high-resolution manometry and impedance values in the supine and sitting positions in the population of Northern China. *Dis Esophagus.* 2016;29(3):267-272.

53. Levine MS, Rubesin SE, Herlinger H, Laufer I. Double-contrast upper gastrointestinal examination: technique and interpretation. *Radiology.* 1988;168(3):593-602.

54. Kostic S, Andersson M, Hellstrom M, Lonroth H, Lundell L. Timed barium esophagogram in the assessment of patients with achalasia: reproducibility and observer variation. *Dis Esophagus.* 2005;18(2):96-103.

55. Vaezi MF, Baker ME, Achkar E, Richter JE. Timed barium oesophagram: better predictor of long term success after pneumatic dilation in achalasia than symptom assessment. *Gut.* 2002;50(6):765-770.

56. Christiansen T, Funch-Jensen P, Jacobsen NO, Thommesen P. Radiologic quantitation of gastro-oesophageal reflux. Correlation between height of food stimulated gastro-oesophageal reflux and level of histologic changes in reflux oesophagitis. *Acta Radiol.* 1987;28(6):731-734.

57. Hill LD, Kozarek RA, Kraemer SJ, et al. The gastroesophageal flap valve: in vitro and in vivo observations. *Gastrointest Endosc.* 1996;44(5):541-547.

58. Lundell LR, Dent J, Bennett JR, et al. Endoscopic assessment of oesophagitis: clinical and functional correlates and further validation of the Los Angeles classification. *Gut.* 1999;45(2):172-180.

59. Abell TL, Camilleri M, Donohoe K, et al. Consensus recommendations for gastric emptying scintigraphy: a joint report of the American Neurogastroenterology and Motility Society and the Society of Nuclear Medicine. *Am J Gastroenterol.* 2008;103(3):753-763.

60. Guo JP, Maurer AH, Fisher RS, Parkman HP. Extending gastric emptying scintigraphy from two to four hours detects more patients with gastroparesis. *Dig Dis Sci.* 2001;46(1):24-29.

61. Ziessman HA, Bonta DV, Goetze S, Ravich WJ. Experience with a simplified, standardized 4-hour gastric-emptying protocol. *J Nucl Med.* 2007;48(4):568-572.

62. Hinder RA, Stein HJ, Bremner CG, DeMeester TR. Relationship of a satisfactory outcome to normalization of delayed gastric emptying after Nissen fundoplication. *Ann Surg.* 1989;210(4):458-464; discussion 464–455.

63. Bremner CG, Lynch VP, Ellis FH Jr. Barrett's esophagus: congenital or acquired? An experimental study of esophageal mucosal regeneration in the dog. *Surgery.* 1970;68(1):209-216.

64. Rosenzweig S, Traube M. The diagnosis and misdiagnosis of achalasia. A study of 25 consecutive patients. *J Clin Gastroenterol.* 1989;11(2):147-153.

65. Tucker HJ, Snape WJ Jr, Cohen S. Achalasia secondary to carcinoma: manometric and clinical features. *Ann Intern Med.* 1978;89(3):315-318.

66. de Oliveira RB, Rezende Filho J, Dantas RO, Iazigi N. The spectrum of esophageal motor disorders in Chagas' disease. *Am J Gastroenterol.* 1995;90(7):1119-1124.

67. Davis RD Jr, Lau CL, Eubanks S, et al. Improved lung allograft function after fundoplication in patients with gastroesophageal reflux disease undergoing lung transplantation. *J Thorac Cardiovasc Surg.* 2003;125(3):533-542.

68. Verleden GM, Dupont LJ, Van Raemdonck DE. Is it bronchiolitis obliterans syndrome or is it chronic rejection: a reappraisal? *Eur Respir J.* 2005;25(2):221-224.

69. Lo WK, Goldberg HJ, Burakoff R, Feldman N, Chan WW. Increased proximal acid reflux is associated with early readmission following lung transplantation. *Neurogastroenterol Motil.* 2016;28(2):251-259.

70. Lo WK, Goldberg HJ, Wee J, Fisichella PM, Chan WW. Both pre-transplant and early post-transplant antireflux surgery prevent development of early allograft injury after lung transplantation. *J Gastrointest Surg.* 2016;20(1):111-118; discussion 118.

71. Soresi S, Zeriouh M, Sabashnikov A, et al. GORD symptoms in lung transplantation: how efficient is the reflux symptom index questionnaire compared to the esophageal impedance test? *Clin Transplant.* 2016;30(1):44-51.

72. Tamhankar AP, Peters JH, Portale G, et al. Omeprazole does not reduce gastroesophageal reflux: new insights using multichannel intraluminal impedance technology. *J Gastrointest Surg.* 2004;8(7):890-897; discussion 897–898.

73. Basseri B, Conklin JL, Pimentel M, et al. Esophageal motor dysfunction and gastroesophageal reflux are prevalent in lung transplant candidates. *Ann Thorac Surg.* 2010;90(5):1630-1636.

74. Davis CS, Shankaran V, Kovacs EJ, et al. Gastroesophageal reflux disease after lung transplantation: pathophysiology and implications for treatment. *Surgery.* 2010;148(4):737-744; discussion 744–735.

75. Khajanchee YS, O'Rourke R, Cassera MA, Gatta P, Hansen PD, Swanstrom LL. Laparoscopic reintervention for failed antireflux surgery: subjective and objective outcomes in 176 consecutive patients. *Arch Surg.* 2007;142(8):785-901; discussion 791–782.

76. Papasavas PK, Yeaney WW, Landreneau RJ, et al. Reoperative laparoscopic fundoplication for the treatment of failed fundoplication. *J Thorac Cardiovasc Surg.* 2004;128(4):509-516.

77. Wee JO. Redo laparoscopic repair of benign esophageal disease. *J Thorac Cardiovasc Surg.* 2012;144(3):S71-S73.

Radiology of the Esophagus: Barium, Computed Tomography Scan, Positron Emission Tomography Scan, Magnetic Resonance Imaging

John M. Barlow | Daniel A. Craig | Val J. Lowe | Robert L. MacCarty

Radiologic evaluation of esophageal diseases can be performed by fluoroscopic barium examination (esophagram), computed tomography (CT) scan, positron emission tomography (PET) scan, fused CT and PET images (PET/CT), and magnetic resonance imaging (MRI). These five imaging modalities constitute the radiologic options currently available for esophageal evaluation. Which test is best for the diagnosis of esophageal disease? It depends. The choice of esophageal imaging modality depends on the goal of esophageal imaging. Indeed, the choice of esophageal testing, in general, depends on the goal of the testing. When the diagnostic questions are esophageal obstruction, characterization of hiatal hernia, esophageal perforation, or achalasia, the esophagram is the best test to perform. When the diagnostic questions are gastroesophageal reflux disease (GERD), other esophagitis, mass, or motility disorder other than achalasia, the esophagram can be useful, although it is not the best test available for these entities. When the diagnostic question is the staging of esophageal tumors, esophagram is not indicated because it demonstrates the luminal margin of the esophagus only. Tumor staging questions are best answered by cross-sectional imaging modalities.

The barium esophagram remains a test of definite utility in the 21st century, along with cross-sectional imaging (CT, MRI, and PET), endoscopy, endoscopic ultrasound (EUS), high-resolution manometry, pH monitoring, and multichannel intraluminal impedance. In fact, all of these tests are complementary for the diagnosis of esophageal diseases.

In our practice over the last decade, the volume of radiographic contrast studies of the stomach, small bowel, and colon has continued to decline; however, the volume of esophagrams has increased each year. This increasing utilization of a nearly 100-year-old test by gastroenterologists and other referring physicians and surgeons indicates its continuing relevance for the evaluation of dysphagia. The utility of the esophagram is increased further when, in the appropriate clinical context of dysphagia, it is paired with a fluoroscopic video swallow. Between them, these two examinations can demonstrate the structure and function of the oropharynx, hypopharynx, cervical esophagus, and thoracic esophagus. Their relatively low cost and almost universal availability make them a logical starting point for the evaluation of dysphagia.

This chapter begins by describing the essential technical elements, normal findings, and common artifacts of the esophagram. Then, the utility of the esophagram is discussed in the settings of GERD, esophageal motility disorders, esophageal neoplasms, and the postoperative esophagus. The discussion of esophageal neoplasms includes a discussion of the role of cross-sectional imaging, especially PET/CT, for tumor staging. Subsequently, miscellaneous conditions such as hiatal hernias, esophageal rings and webs, less common types of esophageal strictures, caustic injury, and esophageal perforation, diverticula, and varices are discussed and illustrated.

ESOPHAGRAM

An understanding of the imaging techniques of the esophagram helps the referring physician evaluate the quality of images, the completeness of the study, and the validity of the conclusions reached by the radiologist. The essential techniques of the esophagram are not complex. The performance of the radiologist performing esophagrams improves when referring physicians and surgeons provide follow-up regarding the accuracy of his or her diagnoses. Indeed, a team approach to the care of esophageal diseases not only benefits the patient; it also benefits the physicians caring for the patient. They learn from each other.

A complete esophagram is a multiphasic examination performed in upright and recumbent positions with variable consistencies of barium resulting in air-contrast, single-contrast, and mucosal relief images.[1] Unfortunately, radiologists typically refer to this complete esophagram as an *air-contrast esophagram*; nevertheless, they know that single-contrast, recumbent images are necessary, in addition to air-contrast images, to consider an esophagram complete. The images obtained during air-contrast, single-contrast, and mucosal relief phases of the examination are complementary.

The air-contrast technique is performed in the upright position, typically with the patient in the left posterior oblique position with respect to the vertical fluoroscopy table. This technique allows for detailed evaluation of the esophageal mucosa. Maximum gaseous distention of the esophagus is achieved when the patient ingests an effervescent agent that releases carbon dioxide when mixed with water. Immediately after the esophagus is distended by gas, the patient drinks high-density barium as quickly as possible in the upright position. Uniform distribution of this thick barium on the luminal surfaces of the gas-distended esophagus allows demonstration of the entire mucosa of the esophagus. Normally, the esophageal mucosa is featureless on these air-contrast images. Occasionally,

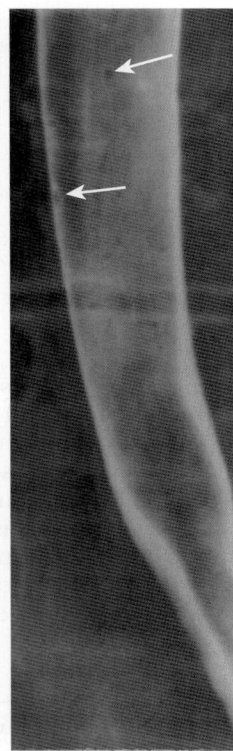

FIGURE 6.1 Normal air-contrast esophagram. The mucosa is featureless, except for the occasional tiny filling defect caused by undissolved effervescent crystals *(arrows)*.

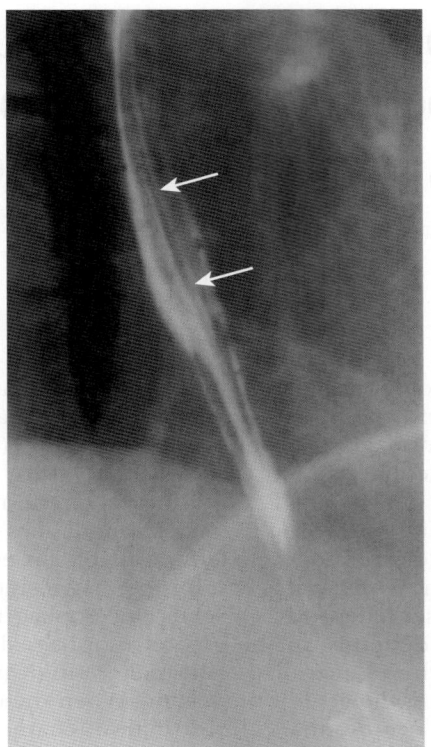

FIGURE 6.2 Normal mucosal relief esophagram. The longitudinal mucosal folds *(arrows)* appear smooth and continuous. They measure less than 3 mm in thickness.

tiny filling defects, representing undissolved effervescent crystals, are present on the mucosal surface (Fig. 6.1). These artifactual filling defects usually change position on sequential upright images.

Because the esophagus remains distended by gas for only a short time in the upright position, the radiologist needs to obtain air-contrast images quickly. As the esophageal lumen collapses, residual barium is trapped between redundant longitudinal mucosal folds of the esophagus, resulting in a mucosal relief image of the esophagus. These longitudinal folds should appear as smooth and linear structures less than 3 mm thick on mucosal relief images (Fig. 6.2). Mild thickening and irregularity of the distal longitudinal folds may be a subtle sign of reflux esophagitis.

Before tilting the table into the horizontal position, the radiologist should determine the need for upright evaluation of swallowing and the cervical esophagus. Anatomically, the two main sites of abnormalities resulting in dysphagia are the oropharynx and the esophagus. When patients report food sticking, and point to the neck or thoracic inlet as the level of obstruction, their symptoms may result from oropharyngeal dysphagia or esophageal dysphagia. However, when patients report food sticking, and point to the substernal region as the level of obstruction, their symptoms typically result from an esophageal dysphagia. Therefore, referring physicians and surgeons, as well as radiologists, should ask the patient two questions: (1) Does food stick? (2) Where does it stick?

When the patient indicates that food sticks at the level of the neck or thoracic inlet, the oropharynx and cervical esophagus should be evaluated in the upright position. For example, the radiologist puts the patient in the upright lateral position and observes a swallow fluoroscopically. Structural causes of oropharyngeal dysphagia such as cricopharyngeal bar, cervical esophageal stricture, or cervical esophageal web are readily identified in the lateral position. When a neuromuscular cause of dysphagia is suggested by this single upright view, it is best evaluated by a speech pathologist trained in the evaluation of dysphagia. The speech pathologist interviews and examines the patient before performing a video swallow study with multiple consistencies of barium. In fact, we often perform the video swallow, in consultation with speech pathologist, and the esophagram during a single patient visit to the fluoroscopy suite. This patient convenience is facilitated by our referring physicians and surgeons, who are aware of the variable etiology of so-called high dysphagia (when the patient indicates that food sticks at the level of neck or thoracic inlet). Consequently, they can order both the video swallow study and the esophagram initially, or they can give us permission to evaluate the esophagus as necessary based on the result of the video swallow. A motion-recording device that captures 30 frames per second is very helpful for the evaluation of swallowing. This type of continuous recording captures the dynamic events of swallowing far better than rapid sequential radiographic images captured at 4 to 8 frames per second.

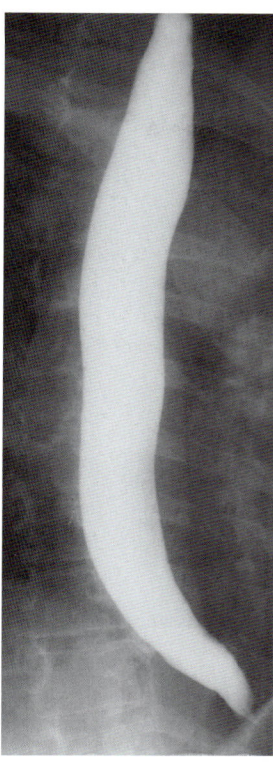

FIGURE 6.3 Normal single-contrast esophagram in prone position. The luminal margins are smooth.

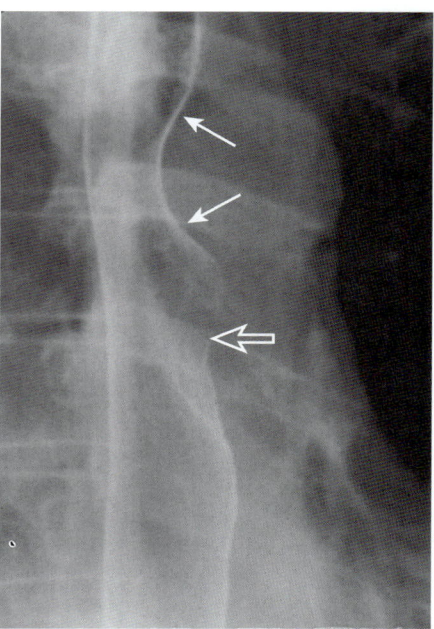

FIGURE 6.4 Upright, left posterior oblique air-contrast view demonstrating normal extrinsic impressions on the esophagus from the aortic arch *(closed arrows)* and left main bronchus *(open arrow)*.

The single-contrast phase of esophagram is performed in the prone, right anterior, oblique position with respect to the horizontal fluoroscopy table. Patients drink as rapidly as possible in this position to produce maximal esophageal distention. Fixed segments of subtle esophageal narrowing become apparent only during maximal esophageal distention. If the patient cannot drink barium rapidly enough to sufficiently distend the lumen, areas of segmental narrowing are likely to go undetected.[2]

When fully distended, the margins of the esophagus should be smooth on these single-contrast images (Fig. 6.3). Normal extrinsic impressions occur at the level of the transverse aorta and the left main stem bronchus (Fig. 6.4). Extrinsic impressions occurring elsewhere should be viewed with suspicion.

Esophageal motility should be tested by single swallows of barium with patient in the prone, right anterior, oblique position. In this position, gravity does not contribute to esophageal emptying. To prevent esophageal peristaltic inhibition, patients are asked not to swallow between swallows. In addition, the time between swallows should be at least 20 seconds. The primary peristaltic wave initiated by swallowing should propagate through the entire esophagus and result in bolus passage into the stomach. The trailing edge of the peristaltic wave resembles an inverted V, as sequential muscular contractions obliterate the esophageal lumen from proximal to distal. Frequently, a small amount of barium remains in the middle third of the esophagus after passage of the primary peristaltic wave. This small residual volume of barium should not be interpreted as abnormal motility since this esophageal

segment is normally the zone of lowest normal contractile amplitude. Completion of the peristaltic contraction is accompanied by relaxation of the lower esophageal sphincter (LES) as the bolus passes into the stomach.

In normal patients, 95% of swallows are accompanied by normal esophageal peristalsis.[3] The incidence of failed and low-amplitude peristaltic contractions probably increases with age.[4] This increased incidence with age may represent normal aging or subclinical disease. Therefore, abnormal peristaltic function, especially nonpropulsive (tertiary) contractions, should be interpreted with caution in older individuals.

As the esophagram comes to an end, we return the fluoroscopy table and the patient to the upright position. When patients complain of difficulty swallowing pills, or we are suspicious of an esophageal stricture based on prone, single-contrast images, we ask them if they are willing to swallow a 12.5-mm barium tablet with 60 mL of water in the upright position. In normal subjects, the tablet should pass into the stomach within 60 seconds.[5] One-half or one-third of a marshmallow, swallowed with thin barium in upright position, may hang up at areas of narrowing not otherwise visible during routine examination.[6,7] Single bites of other foods, such as bread, may also be used to assess the functional severity of a stricture. None of these items should be administered by the radiologist to a patient at risk of aspiration. In addition, patients have the right to refuse to swallow a tablet or other food bolus. Many patients, especially those with oropharyngeal causes of dysphagia, are frightened of choking on the pill or food bolus.

With the patient in the upright position again, the radiologist has one more chance to evaluate swallowing

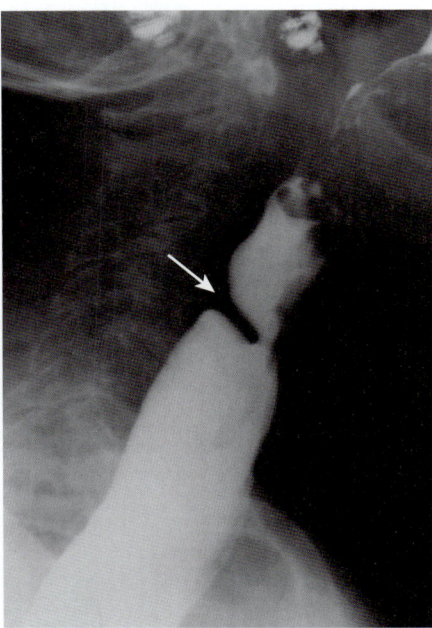

FIGURE 6.5 Cricopharyngeal bar. A smooth posterior impression at the pharyngoesophageal junction *(arrow)* caused by failure of cricopharyngeus muscle to relax.

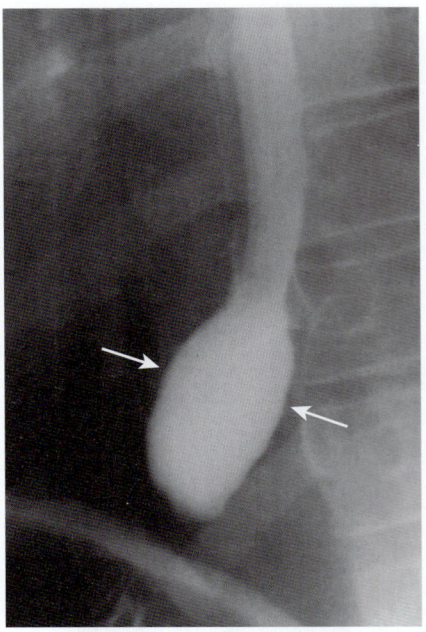

FIGURE 6.6 Esophageal ampulla (vestibule). The caliber of the normal esophagus increases slightly just superior to the level of the gastroesophageal junction *(arrows)*.

in the cervical esophagus in the lateral position. This evaluation is especially relevant in patients who report food sticking in region of neck or thoracic inlet. The likelihood of an oropharyngeal cause of dysphagia in these patients is more likely than it is in those patients who report food sticking in the substernal region. This upright lateral view may suggest neuromuscular causes of dysphagia, best evaluated by speech pathologists. The abnormality revealed most commonly by these lateral images is a cricopharyngeal bar at the pharyngoesophageal junction. This failure of the cricopharyngeus muscle to relax occasionally accompanies more distal disease and may contribute to the dysphagia symptoms (Fig. 6.5).[8] Cervical esophageal webs, rings, and strictures can also be demonstrated by this lateral view.

A brief examination of the stomach contributes to the evaluation of patients complaining of dysphagia. Neoplasms of the gastric cardia can present with dysphagia, and may be overlooked if the stomach is not evaluated.[9] In patients with GERD, gastric dysfunction may be an important contributory factor, so evidence of delayed gastric emptying should be noted.

The normal esophageal ampulla (vestibule) is sometimes confused with a hiatal hernia. It appears as a smoothly marginated, mildly dilated segment of the esophagus just superior to the esophageal hiatus (Fig. 6.6). Unlike a hiatal hernia, the ampulla does not contain gastric folds and will demonstrate typical esophageal peristalsis. The transient appearance of fine, evenly spaced, transverse folds is called "feline esophagus" (Fig. 6.7). This condition has been reported to be more frequent in patients with GERD,[10] but is also demonstrated in asymptomatic patients. It is thought to result from contraction of the longitudinal muscle layer of the esophagus, usually in response to gastroesophageal reflux (GER).

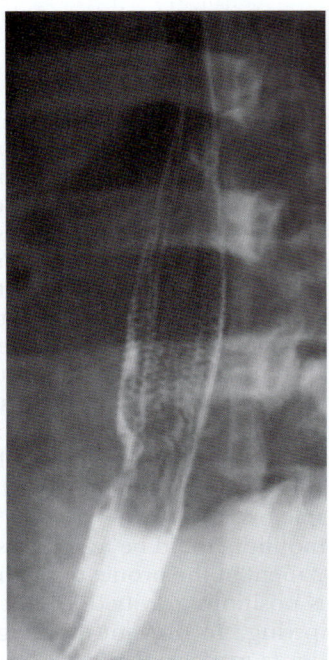

FIGURE 6.7 Feline esophagus. Closely spaced, transient, transverse mucosal folds, presumed secondary to longitudinal muscle contractions, typically occur immediately after an episode of gastroesophageal reflux.

GASTROESOPHAGEAL REFLUX DISEASE

One of the earliest reports of abnormal reflux of gastric contents into the esophagus was based on observations made during GI contrast studies.[11] Today the esophagram remains useful in evaluating GERD patients especially those considering surgical intervention.

The cause of GERD is multifactorial. The most common etiologic factor is abnormality of the LES leading to loss of the normal antireflux barrier. Contributory factors include the volume and composition of the gastric refluxate, altered esophageal mucosal resistance, and the effectiveness of esophageal clearance. Although other tests are more accurate in quantifying these etiologic factors, the esophagram may provide clues that point to the need for further evaluation. For example, the demonstration of a hiatal hernia by esophagram suggests alteration of the normal antireflux barrier that can be confirmed with LES manometry. Radiographic signs of abnormal esophageal motility suggest poor esophageal clearance of any refluxed material that can be evaluated with esophageal manometry.

UTILITY OF ESOPHAGRAM IN GASTROESOPHAGEAL REFLUX DISEASE

Exclusion of Motility Disorder

The classic symptoms of GERD—namely, heartburn and regurgitation—are nonspecific and may accompany a variety of esophageal diseases, including motility disorders. About 10% of patients with motility disorders present with symptoms suggestive of GERD—namely, heartburn and regurgitation. Furthermore, dysphagia and chest pain, more typical symptoms of motility disorders, may be absent in these patients. Symptoms of heartburn are even more common in achalasia, occurring in 40% of patients. In patients with classic achalasia, the esophagram is usually characteristic, confirming the diagnosis. In patients complaining of heartburn, the correct diagnosis of achalasia prevents a potential catastrophe resulting from inappropriate antireflux surgery.

Detection of Gastroesophageal Reflux

Ambulatory pH monitoring is the gold standard for the diagnosis of GER. A pH of 4 or less during greater than 5% of the 24-hour monitoring period constitutes a positive test.[12] A few studies have correlated pH results with radiographic detection of GER. One study[13] demonstrated relatively good correlation, showing a radiographic sensitivity of 70% and specificity of 74%, with both spontaneous reflux and the water siphon test. A subsequent study[14] failed to confirm this correlation and concluded that barium radiography lacks sufficient sensitivity and specificity to be used as a screening procedure for GERD. In general, the response to trials of proton pump inhibitors in patients with typical symptoms of heartburn and regurgitation are more predictive of pH test results than the presence of radiologically detectable GER.

Small volumes of barium transiently refluxing into the distal esophagus are probably not significant. However, repeated episodes of reflux into the upper esophagus, particularly in the presence of a large hiatal hernia, are often predictive of a high pH score.

Detect Evidence of Esophageal Injury

Esophageal injury is manifested by acute inflammation, scarring, stricture, Barrett metaplasia, and alterations in esophageal motility. Radiographic detection of acute

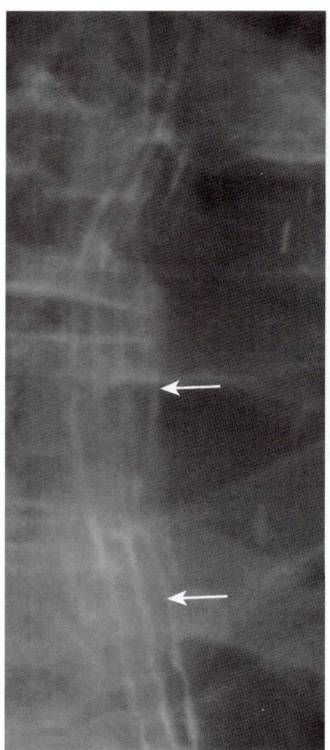

FIGURE 6.8 Acute reflux esophagitis. Mucosal relief view demonstrates irregular thickening of the longitudinal folds of the esophagus *(arrows)*.

esophagitis depends on the severity of the disease. Mild to moderate degrees of inflammation are frequently not demonstrated radiographically.[16] Signs of acute esophagitis include thickening and irregularity of the distal esophageal folds, best demonstrated by mucosal relief images (Fig. 6.8). Less frequently, mucosal nodularity and erosions are visible on air-contrast images.

Esophageal scars and strictures secondary to GERD are generally visible radiographically. The appearance of these scars and strictures can be typical enough to exclude malignancy.[17] Reflux strictures usually occur at the gastroesophageal junction (GEJ); they may be smoothly tapered or irregular (Fig. 6.9). When compared with a mucosal ring (Schatzki ring), strictures are generally more eccentric and thicker. When an otherwise typical-appearing reflux stricture occurs well above the GEJ, it suggests the possibility of Barrett metaplasia between the GEJ and the stricture (Fig. 6.10).

Single-contrast evaluation of the esophagus in the prone position is superior to endoscopy for detecting areas of segmental esophageal narrowing, especially larger-diameter strictures and those that taper gradually.[2,18] These strictures may only be demonstrated when the esophagus is maximally dilated by rapidly ingested barium. They may not be appreciated endoscopically, particularly with smaller-diameter endoscopes. Many esophageal strictures and rings may be missed if the esophagus is examined only in the upright position.

Initial reports suggested high sensitivity of air-contrast esophagrams for the detection of columnar epithelium

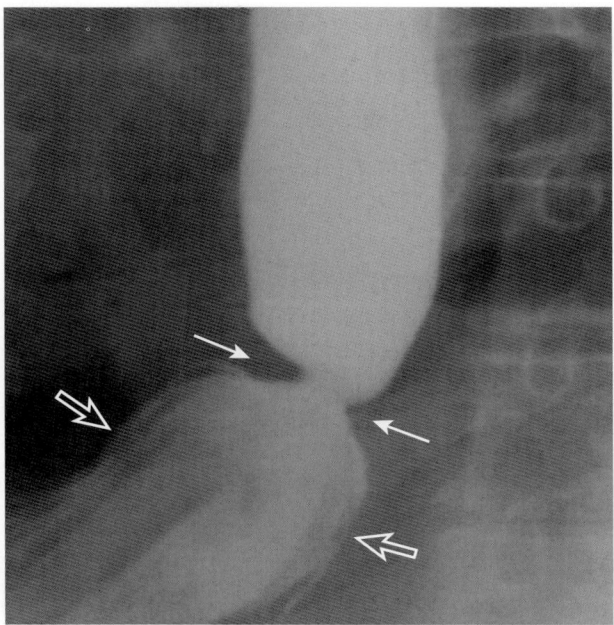

FIGURE 6.9 Esophageal stricture secondary to gastroesophageal reflux disease. Asymmetric narrowing *(closed arrows)* is evident at the gastroesophageal junction above a hiatal hernia *(open arrows)*. This stricture is thicker, more asymmetric, and slightly more irregular than the Schatzki ring demonstrated in Fig. 6.36.

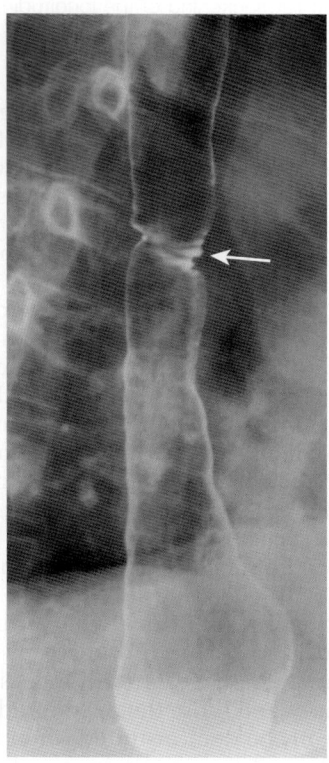

FIGURE 6.10 Midesophageal scarring secondary to gastroesophageal reflux disease. Transverse scars *(arrow)* are typical for a benign stricture caused by gastroesophageal reflux disease. However, the location of this stricture, many centimeters proximal to the gastroesophageal junction, suggests the presence of Barrett metaplasia between gastroesophageal junction and this stricture.

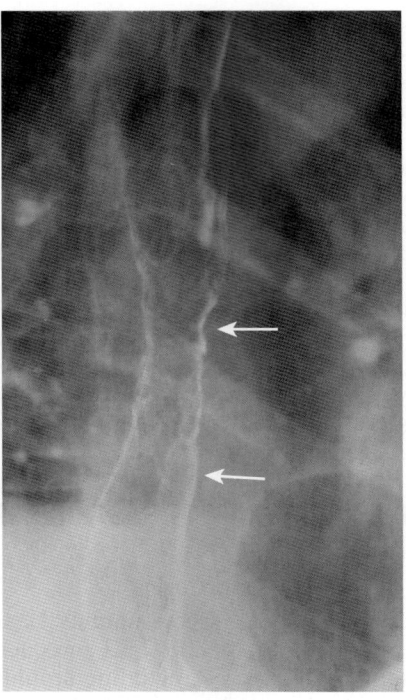

FIGURE 6.11 Barrett esophagus. Mild narrowing and a reticular mucosal pattern are apparent in the midesophagus on this upright, air-contrast image (between *arrows*).

in Barrett esophagus.[19] The findings were described as a reticular mucosal pattern (Fig. 6.11). However, other investigators found this radiographic feature to be present in only 23% of cases.[20] The findings of hiatal hernia, GER, and esophageal stricture are better clues to the presence of Barrett metaplasia than the reticular mucosal pattern described initially.[21,22] In addition, a midesophageal stricture suggests Barrett metaplasia between the stricture and the GEJ (see Fig. 6.10).

Evaluation of Esophageal Clearance

Abnormal motility causing poor clearance of refluxed material promotes esophageal damage by prolonging exposure of the mucosa to the noxious effects of the refluxate. Studies have shown relatively good correlation between the results of synchronous manometry and fluoroscopic observation of the barium bolus progressing through the esophagus, suggesting that barium examination may provide accurate estimates of esophageal motility.[15] Therefore evidence of poor esophageal motility radiographically may help identify patients who will be resistant to conventional-dose proton pump inhibitor therapy. This information is also helpful in selection of the appropriate surgical approach and type of antireflux repair.

Preoperative Planning

The presence of a large hiatal hernia (>5 cm) or evidence of a shortened esophagus can influence the type of surgical repair and operative approach during surgery for GERD. In fact, failure to recognize these conditions may lead to surgical failure as a result of an inappropriate surgical approach or type of repair. The size of a hiatal hernia

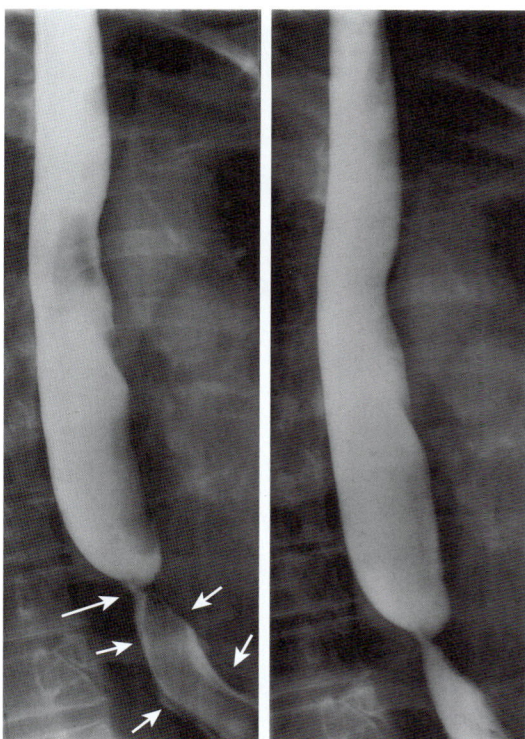

FIGURE 6.12 Scleroderma with esophageal shortening. A tight stricture at the gastroesophageal junction *(large arrow)* causes proximal dilatation on these prone single-contrast images. Notice that the herniated portion of the stomach demonstrates tapered shoulders and elongation *(small arrows)*, suggesting that t has been "pulled" into the chest by the shortened esophagus

is best estimated during a barium study. Hernia size is determined by measuring the distance from the GEJ to the esophageal hiatus during maximum filling of the hernia in the prone position. Hernia size can be underestimated by endoscopy, perhaps because of partial reductior of the hernia during passage of the endoscope.

Esophageal shortening is the result of longitudinal scarring, often caused by severe GERD. In such cases, inadequate surgical dissection during laparoscopic fundoplication may leave the repair under tension and lead to early surgical failure. Clues to the diagnosis of esophageal shortening include esophageal scarring, stricture, and the size and shape of the hiatal hernia. A hiatal hernia with tapered, rather than bulging, shoulders suggests shortening (Fig. 6.12).

ESOPHAGEAL MOTILITY DISORDERS

Conditions associated with abnormal esophageal motor function are classified as motility disorders. Established manometric criteria exist for all of the motility disorders.[23] The diagnosis of a motility disorder is based on a combination of manometric and clinical findings. Esophagram may suggest dysmotility and help referring physicians and surgeons select patients who would benefit from further evaluation by manometry.

The efficacy of the esophagram for detection of esophageal dysmotility is dependent on the type of motility disorder. Although the examination is very sensitive for the detection of achalasia (95%), it is less sensitive for diffuse esophageal spasm (DES; 71%) and nonspecific esophageal motility disorder (NEMD; 46%).[24] In a group of patients with dysphagia, the overall sensitivity of esophagram for the detection of a motility disorder was 56%. The sensitivity increased to 89% when patients with nutcracker esophagus and NEMD were excluded.[25]

Symptoms of dysmotility are nonspecific and include dysphagia, regurgitation, chest pain, and heartburn. Dysphagia to both liquids and solids is more common in motility disorders. When present, regurgitation is usually described as bland rather than acidic, as a result of its origin from the esophagus rather than the stomach. Chest pain varies from intermittent and sharp to constant and pressure-like. It may mimic pain of cardiac origin. The presence of dysphagia increased the likelihood of an esophageal, rather than cardiac, cause of chest pain. Heartburn is a common complaint, especially in patients with achalasia. The nonspecificity of the symptoms of motility disorders, especially their overlap with symptoms of GERD, makes additional diagnostic studies necessary to clarify the nature of the disease.

PRIMARY MOTILITY DISORDERS

Motility disorders are classified as either primary or secondary. This distinction is based on whether the esophagus is primarily involved or whether the esophageal involvement is part of a systemic process.

Achalasia is characterized manometrically by absent peristalsis in the distal two-thirds of the esophagus and abnormally high LES resting pressure. In classic achalasia, the esophagus is markedly dilated. As the patient drinks in the upright position, the barium column is usually distorted by retained food and fluid within the dilated lumen. Nevertheless, the lower end of the barium column is typically tapered to a point, resembling a bird's beak (Fig. 6.13). A barium-fluid level results when barium, which is denser than water, accumulates inferior to the retained secretions in the esophagus. The height of this barium-fluid level is usually characteristic for each patient—the more severe the obstruction, the higher the level. With severe achalasia, the esophagus becomes redundant and the distal esophagus assumes a sigmoid configuration (Fig. 6.14). The configuration contributes another cause of poor esophageal emptying to the absent peristalsis and LES relaxation failure of less severe achalasia.

Vigorous achalasia is a variant of classic achalasia in which prominent tertiary contractions of the distal two-thirds of the esophagus accompany the esophageal dilatation and tapered narrowing of the GEJ (Fig. 6.15) of classic achalasia.

Pseudoachalasia results from mural infiltration by malignancies at the GEJ. The esophageal findings mimic classic achalasia. In many cases, no intraluminal mass is demonstrated by esophagram or by endoscopy. In these cases, the diagnosis is often suspected because of the older age of the patient and the rapid onset of dysphagia. One paper suggests that the length of the "bird's beak" is greater in patients with pseudoachalasia than in those with classic

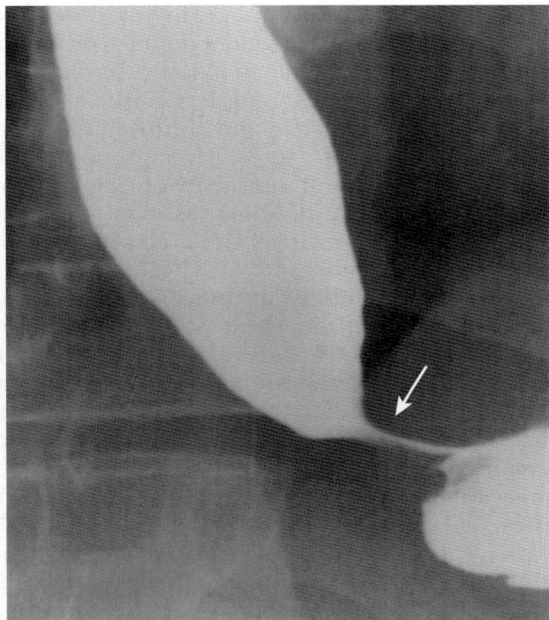

FIGURE 6.13 Classic achalasia. Prone single-contrast image demonstrates markedly dilated and atonic esophagus with tapered narrowing, "bird's beak" deformity *(arrow)*, at the gastroesophageal junction.

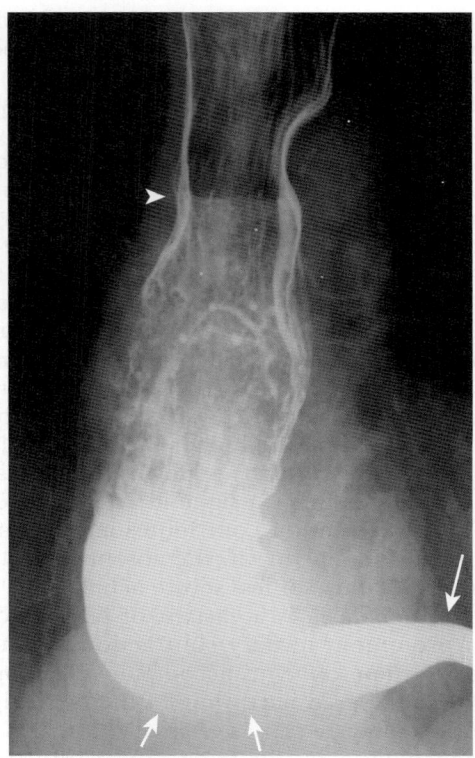

FIGURE 6.14 "Sigmoid" esophagus on upright, air-contrast, frontal image. Severe achalasia has resulted in an elongated, tortuous esophagus. The level of the distal esophagus *(large arrow)* is inferior to the level of the gastroesophageal junction *(small arrows)* contributing to even worse esophageal drainage than occurs with less-severe achalasia. Note the retained debris and air-fluid level *(arrowhead)* near the aortic arch.

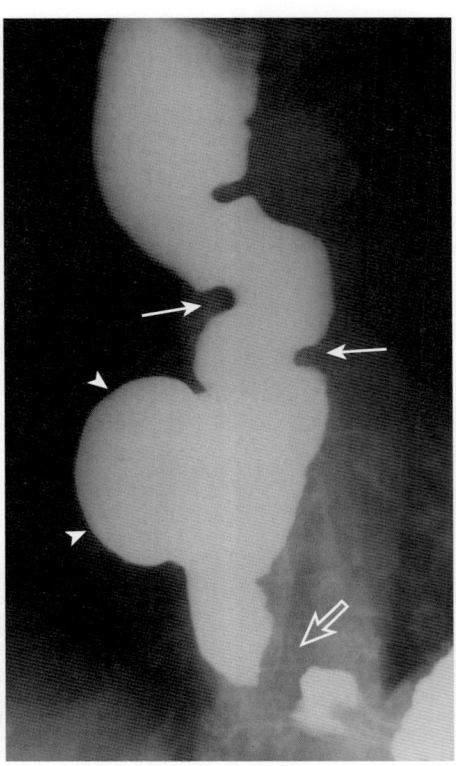

FIGURE 6.15 Vigorous achalasia suggested by a dilated esophagus with prominent tertiary contractions *(arrows)* and a narrow gastroesophageal junction *(open arrow)* above a tiny hiatal hernia. A large pulsion diverticulum *(arrowheads)* of the distal esophagus is also demonstrated.

achalasia.[26] When pseudoachalasia is suspected, CT of the chest and abdomen with intravenous contrast material sometimes demonstrates the infiltrative intramural mass.

DES is a disorder of unknown cause characterized by intermittently abnormal motility associated with symptoms of chest pain and dysphagia. The dysphagia is variably present and does not necessarily accompany the chest pain. Manometrically, simultaneous contractions occur in greater than 10% of wet swallows. Radiographic features reflect the manometric findings; peristalsis is intermittently replaced by tertiary contractions, producing a "corkscrew" appearance of the esophagus (Fig. 6.16). Normal peristalsis is usually present in the proximal esophagus. One report has suggested that delayed esophageal emptying, secondary to abnormalities of the LES, may be a more common esophagraphic finding in DES than a corkscrew appearance of the esophagus.[27]

Radiographic sensitivity in the diagnosis of DES is low in comparison to its sensitivity in the diagnosis of achalasia. Tertiary contractions are common in both normal patients and those with motility disorders, and should not be interpreted as indicative of DES unless confirmed by manometry. Thickening of the distal esophageal wall by thoracic CT scans has been reported in 21% of patients with DES.[28] The thickness of the esophageal wall by CT in normal subjects should not exceed 5.5 mm.[29] Therefore DES should be considered in the differential diagnosis

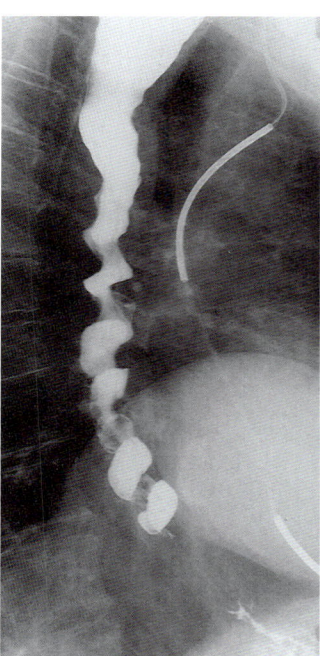

FIGURE 6.16 Diffuse esophageal spasm. Multiple tertiary contractions produce a "corkscrew" appearance of the esophagus.

of concentric distal esophageal wall thickening by CT, along with infectious, inflammatory, and neoplastic causes.

NEMD is a "waste basket" category used that includes motility disorders that do not meet established manometric criteria for other motility disorders. Manometric abnormalities include failed peristalsis, low-amplitude contractions, prolonged duration of peristalsis, simultaneous contractions, tertiary contractions, and incomplete relaxation of the LES. Symptoms are nonspecific and include chest pain and dysphagia. Radiographic findings are frequently normal. When present, radiographic findings are nonspecific, and include ineffective peristalsis and tertiary contractions causing stasis of esophageal barium.

Recently, a subgroup of patients with NEMD defined manometric criteria demonstrating hypocontraction of the distal esophagus. GERD is common in these patients. However, radiographic findings in these patients are nonspecific, and are similar to those of other patients with NEMD.[30]

SECONDARY MOTILITY DISORDERS

Secondary motility disorders are systemic disorders that secondarily affect the esophagus. With few exceptions, the radiographic appearance is nonspecific. Of the collagen vascular diseases, scleroderma most often involves the esophagus. The pathologic changes of scleroderma result in hypomotility of the distal esophagus and a hypotensive LES. The combination of these two motor abnormalities sets the stage for severe GERD, secondary to recumbent GER and poor acid clearance.

The radiographic changes of scleroderma include poor distal esophageal peristalsis, stasis, and esophageal injury secondary to GERD. Eventually, the severe GERD caused by esophageal scleroderma results in distal esophageal scarring, an esophageal shortening resulting in proximal dilatation, distal stricture, and hiatal hernia with tapered, rather than shouldered, margins (see Fig. 6.12). When esophageal scleroderma reaches this advanced stage, it can be difficult to distinguish from achalasia because of the similar radiographic findings of poor esophageal peristalsis, distal stenosis, and proximal dilatation.

Chagas disease is caused by the tropical protozoan *Trypanosoma cruzi*. It is endemic to South and Central America. Cardiac muscle and smooth muscle of the gastrointestinal tract are commonly involved. The radiographic appearance of esophageal Chagas disease is identical to classic achalasia.

ESOPHAGEAL NEOPLASMS

Patients with malignant esophageal neoplasms usually present with dysphagia. Conversely, benign esophageal tumors tend to be incidental radiographic or endoscopic findings. However, when these tumors are symptomatic, excision is usually curative. CT can occasionally suggest the diagnosis of esophageal neoplasm, but it is more useful in staging esophageal malignancies, along with more specific modalities such as PET and EUS.

CARCINOMA

The symptoms causing patients with esophageal malignancy to seek medical care are typically dysphagia of recent onset (1 to 4 months) and weight loss. The prognosis for symptomatic patients is dismal. Historically, more than 95% of esophageal cancers have been squamous cell carcinomas. However, in recent decades, the incidence of esophageal adenocarcinoma has increased dramatically.[31] Radiographically, these two types of carcinoma are indistinguishable. However, adenocarcinoma predominantly occurs in the distal esophagus within regions of the Barrett esophagus. Squamous cell carcinoma, by comparison, tends to occur in the upper two-thirds of the esophagus. Other primary malignancies of the esophagus, such as sarcomas, gastrointestinal stromal tumors (GISTs), melanoma, and lymphoma, are rare.

Radiologic Appearance

The esophagram can contribute to the initial diagnosis of esophageal cancer. It can characterize the size, location, and morphology of the mass. It can demonstrate complications that make the cancer unresectable, such as a fistula to the tracheobronchial tree. It can also demonstrate coexisting esophageal disorders, such as benign strictures, hiatal hernias, motility disorders, and rare synchronous second tumors.

Early resectable esophageal carcinomas can be suggested on air-contrast images of the esophagus performed with careful technique. Early disease has a variety of subtle radiographic appearances, including fixed mucosal irregularity, irregular strictures, polypoid filling defects, or plaque-like filling defects (Fig. 6.17). When radiographic findings of a smooth benign-appearing stricture are demonstrated, they can reliably be considered benign.[17] However, endoscopy may still be useful to search for signs of acute esophagitis or Barrett esophagus. When radiographically equivocal or malignant-appearing strictures are demonstrated,

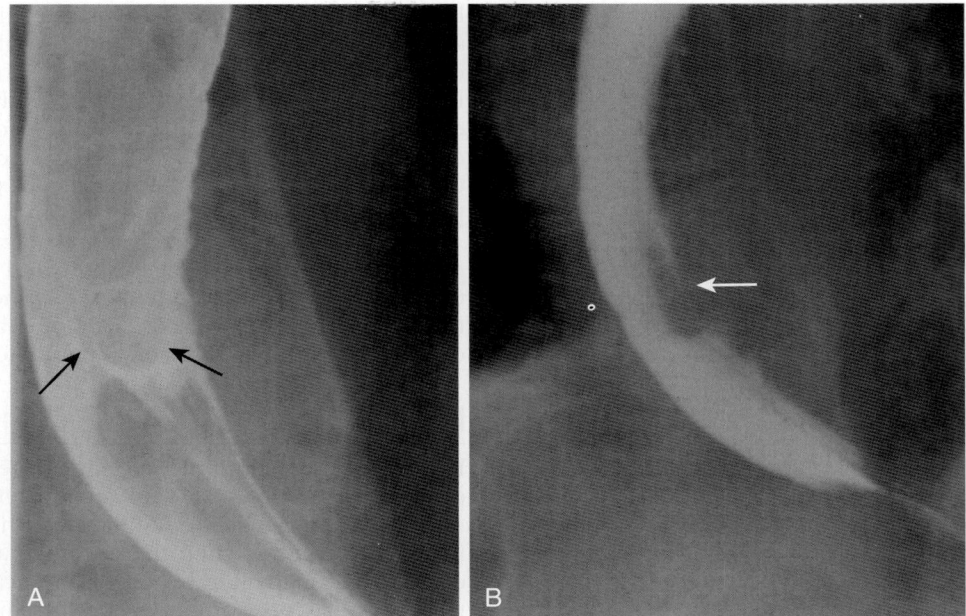

FIGURE 6.17 Adenocarcinoma arising from a region of Barrett esophagus in a 71-year-old man. (A) An air-contrast image in the left posterior oblique projection shows barium outlining subtle areas of mucosal irregularity *(arrows)* of this subtle, round 1-cm cancer demonstrated en face. (B) A single-contrast, prone image shows a plaque-like lesion *(arrow)* in profile along the left side of the distal esophagus.

endoscopy is required for definitive diagnosis. It has been said that esophagram is highly accurate for the detection of esophageal neoplasm, but this has been found to be true only in symptomatic (and therefore high-risk) patients.[9] Early, curable esophageal malignancy is best found by endoscopy in high-risk patients (such as those with known Barrett esophagus).

More advanced esophageal cancer can readily be detected with a single-contrast or air-contrast barium technique. Advanced esophageal cancer is usually manifested as a focal ulcerated or fungating mass extending into the lumen causing irregular, eccentric luminal narrowing (Fig. 6.18). The luminal caliber is often narrowed by 50% to 75%, frequently with at least two-thirds of the circumference involved.[32] By esophagram, the transition from normal esophagus to carcinoma is usually abrupt, not tapered. Aspiration can occur as a result of partial esophageal obstruction, particularly in high esophageal lesions (Fig. 6.19). A carcinoma near the GEJ can cause high-grade obstruction with dilation of the proximal esophagus, retention of barium, and significant luminal narrowing at the GEJ. This appearance has been referred to as *secondary achalasia*, because of an appearance and functional behavior similar to true achalasia (Fig. 6.20).

The esophagram can detect some complications of high-stage disease, such as the formation of a fistula to the tracheobronchial tree (Fig. 6.21). The ability of the esophagram to give a "global" view of the esophagus, even in the presence of tight strictures, makes it useful in detecting coexistent esophageal disorders, including benign strictures, hiatal hernia, motility disorders, and rare synchronous neoplasms (Fig. 6.22).

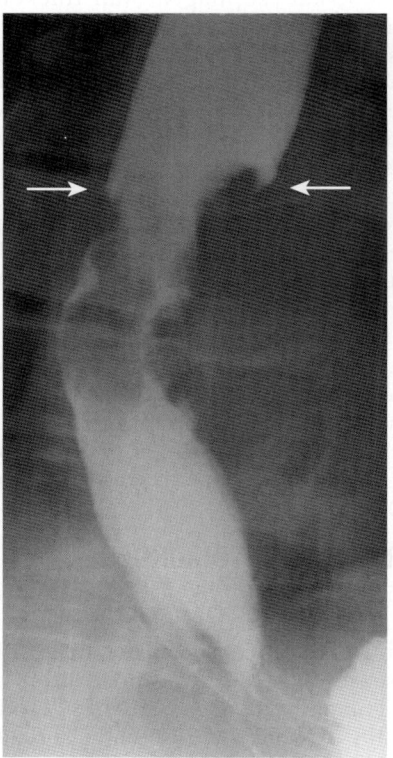

FIGURE 6.18 Adenocarcinoma of the lower esophagus in a 54-year-old man. Single-contrast esophagram shows asymmetric circumferential luminal narrowing, mucosal ulceration, and abrupt transition zone, or shoulders *(arrows)*, at the proximal margin of the mass.

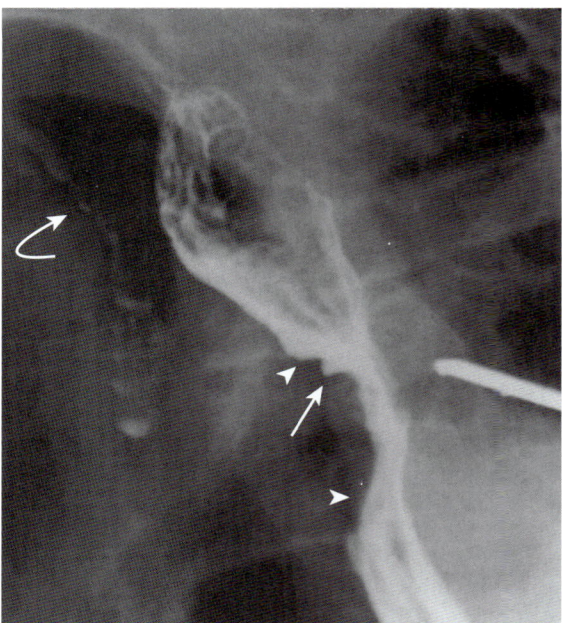

FIGURE 6.19 Adenocarcinoma in the upper thoracic esophagus in an 83-year-old man. This is a broad-based, eccentric mucosal mass *(arrowheads)* with ulceration *(arrow)*. Note the aspirated barium in the trachea *(curved arrow)* related to the dysphagia caused by the stricture resulting from this mass.

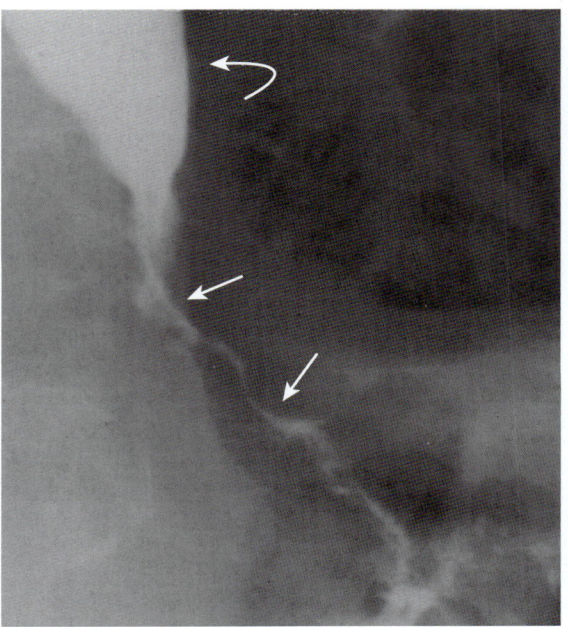

FIGURE 6.20 A 77-year-old man with grade 4 adenocarcinoma within Barrett esophagus located at the esophagogastric junction causing the appearance of secondary achalasia. Note the retained barium in the dilated esophagus *(curved arrow)* above the fixed, narrowed esophagogastric junction from this nearly obstructive carcinoma *(arrows)*.

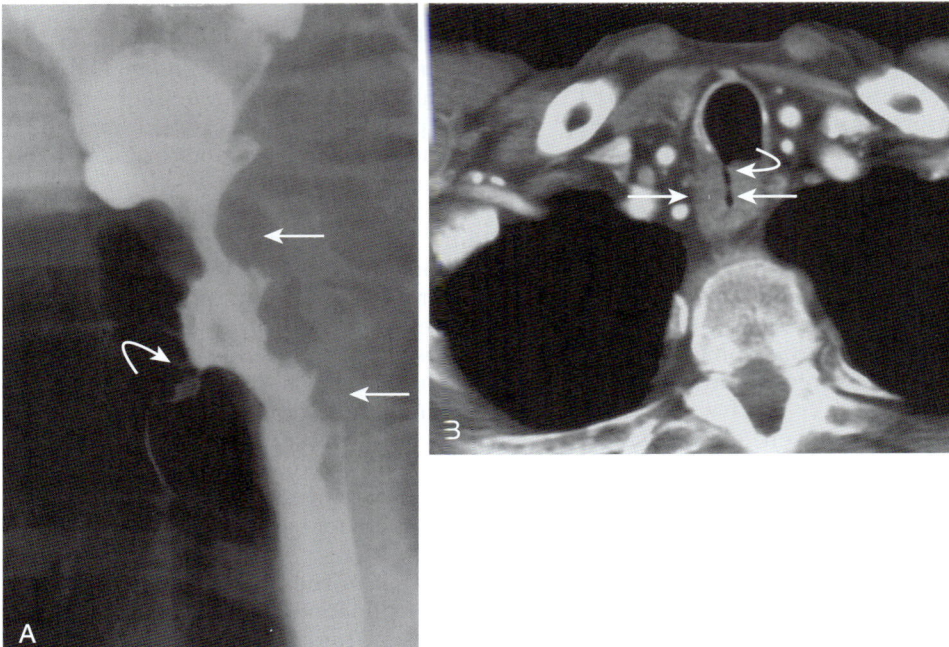

FIGURE 6.21 Squamous cell carcinoma of the upper thoracic esophagus in a 60-year-old man. (A) Upright esophagram image demonstrates irregular luminal narrowing secondary to ulcerated mass *(arrows)* and a tracheoesophageal fistula *(curved arrow)*. (B) Axial computed tomography image with intravenous contrast material confirms the tracheoesophageal fistula *(curved arrow)* traversing the malignant esophageal mass *(arrows)*.

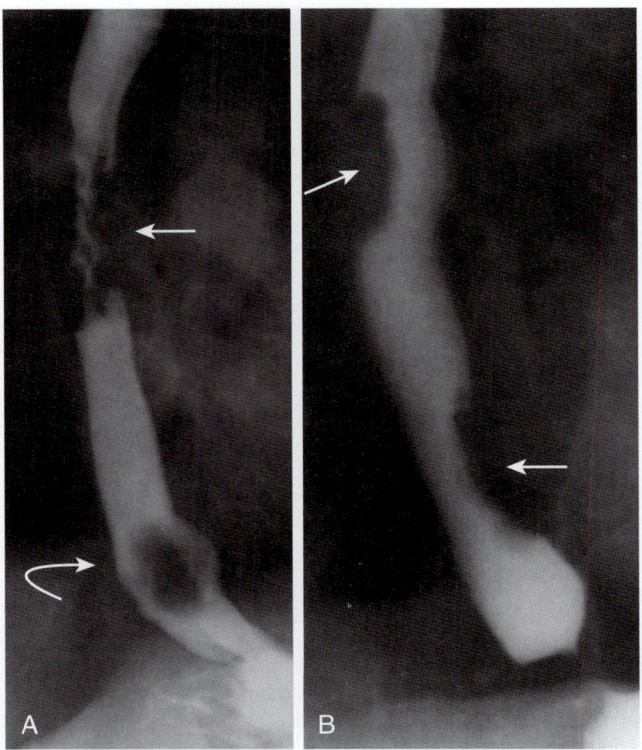

FIGURE 6.22 Synchronous squamous cell carcinomas in two separate patients. (A) Ulcerated infiltrating mass *(arrow)* in the midesophagus and an unusual polypoid intraluminal mass *(curved arrow)* in the lower esophagus. (B) Broad-based sessile polypoid masses *(arrows)* arising eccentrically from opposite sides of the mid and lower esophagus.

Staging

The depth of invasion of esophageal cancer within the wall of the esophagus determines whether a tumor is T1 (limited to the lamina propria or submucosa), T2 (invading the muscularis propria), or T3 (invading the adventitia). Whereas lesions that are T2 or lower have a 5-year survival rate of 40%, T3 (or higher) lesions have a 5-year survival rate of 4%.[33] In addition, involvement beyond the mucosa is associated with nodal disease in 50% of patients.[33] The presence of direct invasion of adjacent structures (T4) or the presence of distant metastases (M1) portends a poor prognosis. Unfortunately, many esophageal cancers are unresectable at the time of initial evaluation, thus precluding curative therapy.

A multimodality imaging approach, often including esophagram, CT, endoscopy, EUS, and PET, is usually necessary to determine if an esophageal cancer is resectable. CT and PET/CT cannot determine the depth of invasion, and are not useful for evaluating low-stage disease. However, they are useful in detecting the presence of metastatic disease, confirming high-stage disease.

Esophagram. Barium esophagram plays little role in the staging of recently diagnosed esophageal cancer, unless it happens to show the unusual finding of direct invasion of the tracheobronchial tree (see Fig. 6.21), thereby confirming a T4 lesion. If a newly diagnosed esophageal cancer is thought to be possibly early stage (see Fig. 6.17),

EUS is useful to determine the depth of invasion within the esophageal wall.

Computed Tomography. CT can detect primary changes of esophageal cancer and suggest its diagnosis, but it is inferior to esophagram and endoscopy in this role. CT can demonstrate asymmetric esophageal wall thickening, particularly when it is severe or when esophageal contrast has been used (Fig. 6.23). However, the confident detection of esophageal wall thickening near the GEJ (where many adenocarcinomas develop in the setting of Barrett esophagus) is difficult because of the oblique course of the esophagus through the diaphragmatic hiatus. This obliquity can simulate mural thickening.

CT can confirm high-stage, often unresectable disease. CT can demonstrate direct invasion of adjacent structures (see Fig. 6.21) and worrisome adenopathy (greater than 1 cm in diameter) in mediastinal and subdiaphragmatic locations (see Fig. 6.23). In the setting of known esophageal cancer, most lymph nodes detected by CT with a short-axis diameter greater than 1 cm will represent metastatic adenopathy. Unfortunately, lymph nodes that are less than a centimeter can also be metastatic. These subcentimeter lymph nodes can sometimes be confirmed as metastatic when PET/CT fusion scans show abnormally increased metabolism in these smaller nodes. When PET/CT is not available, these small nodes may remain indeterminate in the staging process.

Distant metastases are often well demonstrated by CT. Percutaneous biopsy guidance by CT is common. MRI has most of the same advantages and disadvantages as CT. The most common problem of MRI is motion artifact; in addition, it is more expensive and less available than CT. Currently, MRI has no routine role in esophageal cancer staging.

Positron Emission Tomography

Staging of Esophageal Cancer. The usefulness of PET is in evaluating biopsy-proven, high-grade malignancies of the esophagus. There is no documented role for PET in differentiating benign tumors, or inflammatory conditions, from malignancy.

PET staging of proven esophageal cancer can provide additive information in several respects. One potential PET contribution is detection of metastatic disease in lymph nodes smaller than the standard CT criteria for nodal enlargement. In addition, for enlarged lymph nodes without metastasis, PET can improve specificity by excluding any nodes that may be enlarged because of inflammation alone. Nevertheless, PET can be falsely negative for metastases when the nodal disease is below the detection threshold of PET, such as nodal micrometastases, and falsely positive for metastases when inflamed lymph nodes that do not harbor malignancy demonstrate elevated uptake by PET.

Variation in the ability of PET to detect lymph node metastases depends a great deal on two things: (1) the proximity of nodal regions to the primary tumor, with nodal metastases adjacent to a metabolically active tumor being more difficult to detect, and (2) the demographic characteristics of the patient groups assessed by PET. In one study of esophageal cancer patients, PET demonstrated sensitivity for local nodal metastases of 76% (22/29) versus

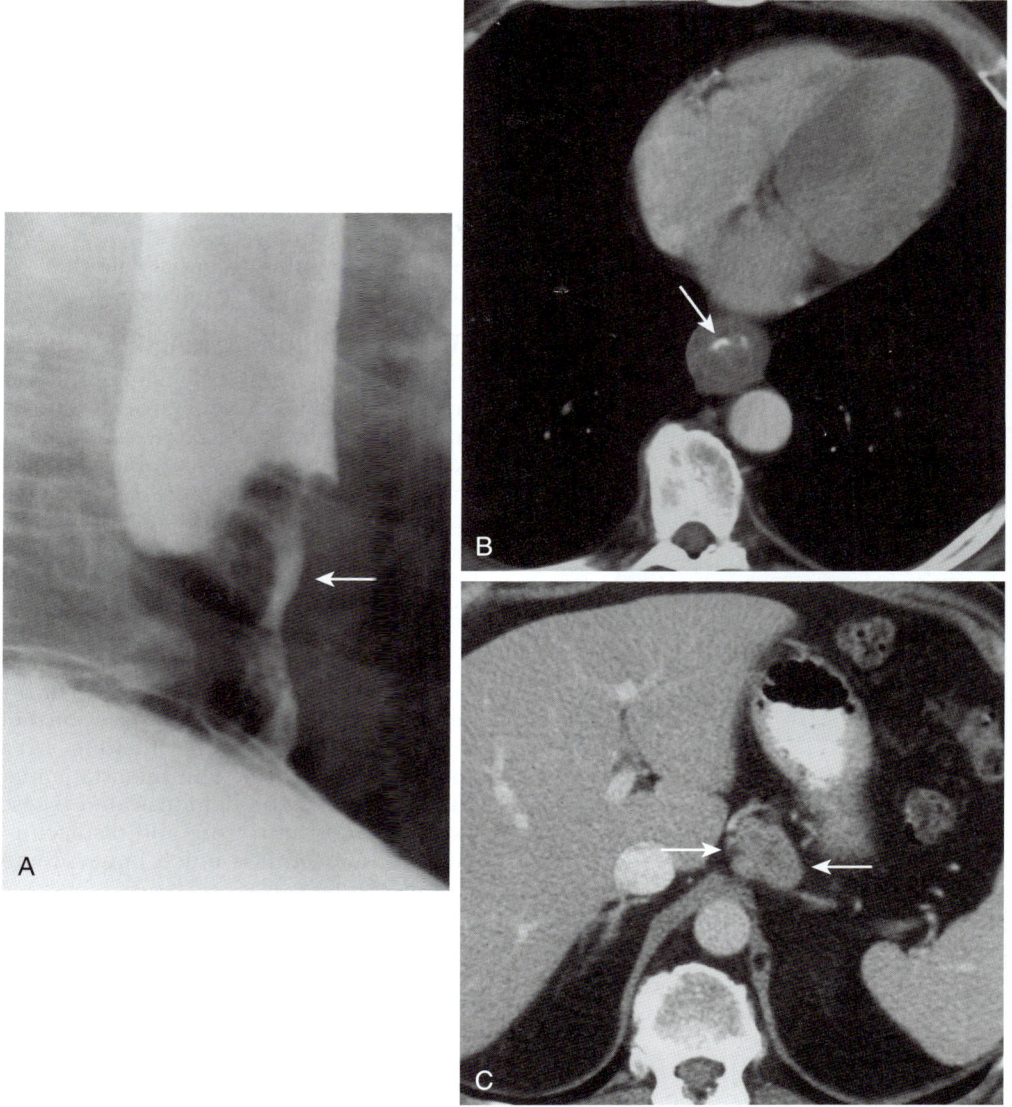

FIGURE 6.23 Adenocarcinoma of the distal esophagus with an area of Barrett esophagus in a 65-year-old man. (A) A single-contrast esophagram shows an abruptly marginated (shouldered), ulcerated mass causing asymmetric, nearly occlusive, luminal narrowing *(arrow)*. (B) An axial computed tomography image with intravenous contrast material shows asymmetric esophageal wall thickening, confirmed by the presence of oral contrast *(arrow)* in the eccentrically narrowed lumen. (C) An axial computed tomography image with intravenous contrast material demonstrates celiac lymphadenopathy *(arrows)*. Fine-needle aspiration of these nodes, with endoscopic ultrasound guidance, confirmed metastatic adenocarcinoma.

45% (13/29) for CT.[34] However, the PET sensitivity for detection of nodal metastasis has also been reported to be as low as 33% for local nodal disease in other studies.[35–37] In our experience, local nodal staging has been roughly equivalent between EUS, CT, and PET when all referred patients are included. However, in about 10% of cases one imaging method does identify disease not demonstrated by the other.

Identifying distant metastatic disease has some important caveats for PET. Relative to distant nodal disease, identification of M1a disease can be difficult without the use of CT fusion imaging to provide anatomic guidance on location of the celiac axis. For M1b disease, CT fusion with PET may

not be as important but can help in locating metastases (e.g., in bone versus soft tissue). These issues make the use of PET with CT fusion of significant importance when performing PET imaging for esophageal cancer.

PET can improve the staging of distant metastases. In one study of seven patients who did not undergo surgery, PET detected distant metastases that were not identified by CT in five cases, and another patient had an unsuspected concomitant primary lung tumor discovered by PET alone. In another study of 35 patients with potentially resectable esophageal cancer by CT, PET identified distant metastatic disease in 20%. The accuracy of PET in determining distant metastatic disease in this group was 91%.[38] Other

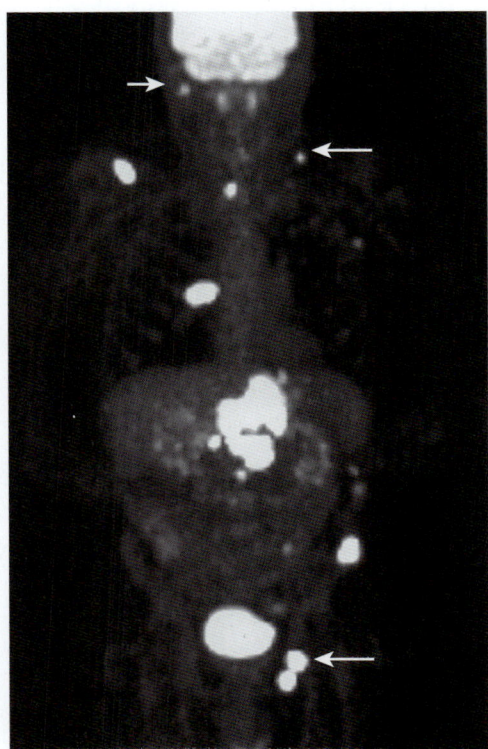

FIGURE 6.24 Coronal image from positron emission tomography scan in a patient with esophageal cancer. Endoscopic ultrasound had previously demonstrated the tumor and suspicious peritumoral lymphadenopathy. Computed tomography had previously demonstrated the tumor and suspicious gastrohepatic lymphadenopathy. Positron emission tomography showed multiple distant metastases not demonstrated previously, some of which—right neck, left supraclavicular, and left inguinal (arrows)—would be easily accessible for biopsy.

investigators have reported similar findings. Fig. 6.24 illustrates the case of a patient with esophageal cancer in whom widespread distant metastases identified by PET had been underestimated by other imaging modalities.

Detection and Staging of Recurrent Esophageal Cancer.
Attempts to improve the survival of patients with esophageal cancer are leading to new treatment regimens. The use of PET to select successful treatment regimens, early in the course of therapy, holds the promise of more rapid discovery of treatment regimens that improve survival. Research has shown that PET is able to detect therapeutic tumor response as early as 14 days into therapy. In a group of 40 patients with locally advanced adenocarcinoma of the GEJ, Weber et al. showed that reduction of tumor fluorodeoxyglucose (FDG) metabolism after 14 days of therapy was significantly different between responding and nonresponding tumors. Optimal differentiation was achieved by a cutoff value of 35% reduction of initial FDG uptake. Applying this cutoff value as a criterion for a metabolic response after 14 days predicted clinical response with a sensitivity of 93% (14 of 15 patients) and specificity of 95% (21 of 22). Furthermore, patients without a metabolic response at 14 days demonstrated a

significantly shorter time to progression or recurrence ($P = .01$) and shorter time of overall survival ($P = .04$).[39]

In patients suspected of recurrence, PET imaging has been shown to be more sensitive than evaluation by CT and EUS for the detection and staging of recurrent esophageal cancer.[40] However, the survival benefit of the higher sensitivity of PET for recurrent cancer is uncertain, since there is little benefit to additional therapy after esophageal cancer recurrence. No data are yet available regarding the potential role that PET could play in esophageal cancer surveillance.

OTHER ESOPHAGEAL MALIGNANCIES

Leiomyosarcoma and malignant esophageal GIST are rare. An esophageal GIST, while rare, is 3 times more common than an esophageal leiomyosarcoma.[41] Lymphoma is exceedingly rare as a primary esophageal lesion. Melanoma accounts for 0.1% to 0.2% of all primary esophageal malignancies. These unusual primary esophageal malignancies are usually diagnosed in symptomatic patients by endoscopic biopsy. Their imaging characteristics are generally nonspecific.

Metastases to the esophagus are most commonly from stomach, lung, or breast cancer. Esophageal metastases can result from direct invasion, lymphatic spread, or hematogenous spread. Metastases of the periesophageal lymph nodes can occur with lung, breast, head/neck, and pancreas cancer. This metastatic mediastinal lymphadenopathy may be demonstrated by esophagram as an extrinsic mass narrowing and displacing the esophageal lumen; however, it is much better demonstrated by CT (Fig. 6.25).

Benign Esophageal Neoplasms

Benign neoplasms of the esophagus are rare, with the exception of leiomyoma, which is the most common esophageal neoplasm. Most benign esophageal tumors are asymptomatic and found incidentally. Symptoms, when they occur, are usually those of obstruction. Some of these lesions can be confidently diagnosed on the basis of their CT characteristics. The remainder can be diagnosed by EUS or endoscopy with biopsy. Treatment of these rare benign lesions is based on the presence and severity of symptoms.

Intraluminal masses usually arise from the esophageal mucosa. By esophagram, a well-circumscribed intraluminal mass often expands the lumen and causes a filling defect by displacing surrounding barium (Fig. 6.26). These lesions need to be differentiated from retained food above an esophageal stricture.

Intramural lesions arise within the wall of the esophagus and generally are covered by normal, intact mucosa. An intramural lesion appears as a smooth convex impression on the esophagus that causes focal narrowing of the lumen. These lesions form a right angle or slightly obtuse angle with the normal esophageal wall as they protrude into the lumen. EUS with biopsy is useful for diagnosing these lesions. Fibrovascular polyps are intramural masses that manifest themselves as intraluminal masses (see Fig. 6.26). Typically they arise from the upper esophagus where they are tethered by a relatively long, narrow pedicle. They can be quite mobile within the esophagus.

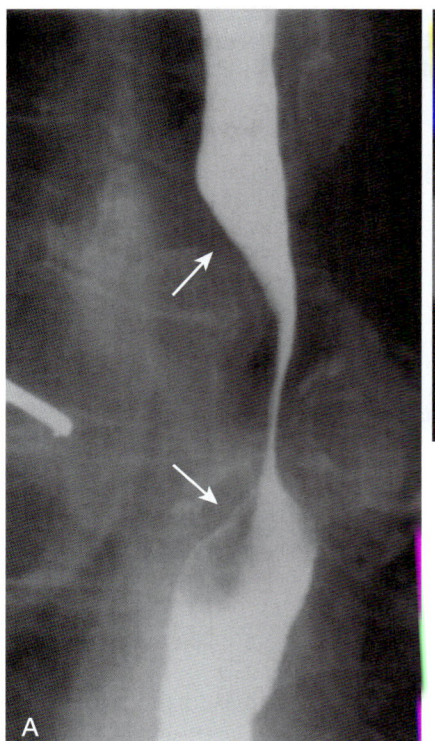
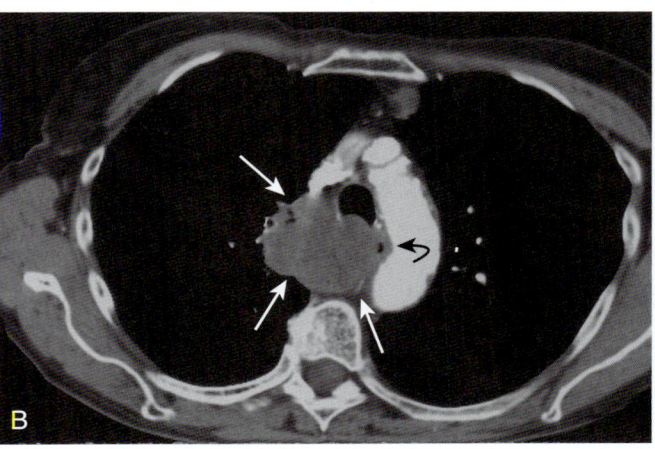

FIGURE 6.25 Adenocarcinoma of the right lung in a 78-year-old woman. (A) An esophagram shows a long extrinsic impression on the right side of the midesophagus *(arrows)*. (B) Axial computed tomography image with intravenous contrast material demonstrates bulky, metastatic, mediastinal lymphadenopathy *(arrows)*, displacing the esophagus *(curved arrow)* to the left and compressing it against the aorta, is the cause of the esophagram finding.

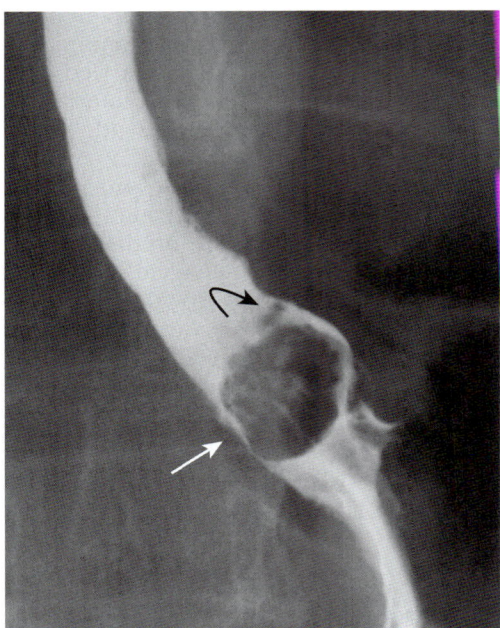

FIGURE 6.26 A 45-year-old woman with a pedunculated fibrovascular polyp demonstrated as an intraluminal filling defect *(arrow)* expanding the distal esophagus. At fluoroscopy, the mass demonstrated several centimeters of movement within the esophagus, made possible by a thin stalk *(curved arrow)* attaching the mass to the esophageal wall.

Extrinsic lesions arise outside of the wall of the esophagus. By esophagram, an extrinsic mass appears as a smooth, convex impression narrowing the esophageal lumen. These extrinsic masses cause a shallower, longer, more obtuse impression on the esophageal lumen than intrinsic masses that cause a more abrupt transition between the normal and narrow lumen.

Leiomyomas (Fig. 6.27) are the most common benign esophageal neoplasm. They are often asymptomatic, discovered incidentally, and can be multiple. Leiomyoma is the classic example of an intramural lesion with smooth contour that causes focal narrowing. Despite being the most common esophageal neoplasm, leiomyomas often go undetected in imaging studies because of their frequent lack of symptoms, intact overlying mucosa, and often subtle impression on the esophageal lumen. EUS demonstrates a benign-appearing mass, usually arising from the muscularis mucosae, and biopsy is not generally necessary for small, asymptomatic incidental lesions.

The main exophytic mass arising from the esophagus is a duplication cyst. Pathologically, it is a congenital lesion and not a true neoplasm. By esophagram, a duplication cyst mimics an extrinsic mass. On CT, an esophageal duplication cyst appears as a well-circumscribed, benign-appearing, thin-walled cystic structure. Mediastinal neoplasms or adenopathy (see Fig. 6.25) can also cause extrinsic narrowing of the esophageal lumen; chest CT is the best modality to demonstrate these mediastinal abnormalities.

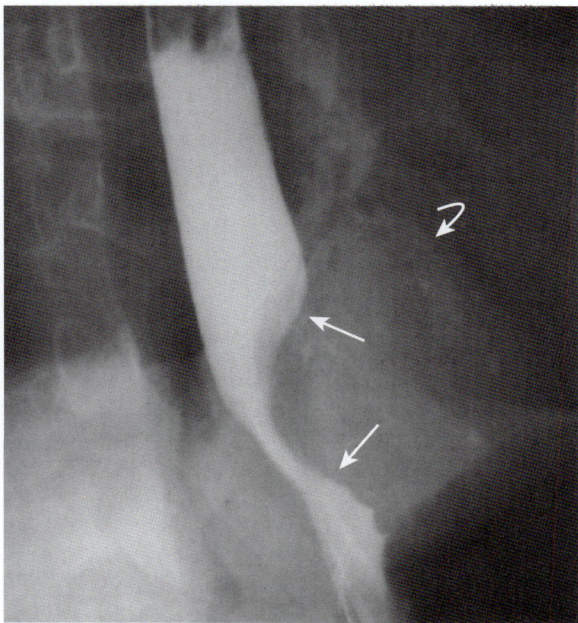

TABLE 6.1 Barium Versus Water-Soluble Contrast Material for Postoperative Esophagrams

	Barium	Water-Soluble Contrast Material
Advantages	Increased density shows leaks missed by water-soluble contrast material	Leak into the mediastinum does not cause mediastinitis
	Aspiration does not cause pulmonary edema	Reabsorption of leaked contrast from the mediastinum makes future esophagrams easier to interpret
Disadvantages	Risk of mediastinitis with leak into mediastinum	Aspiration can cause pulmonary edema
	Leaked barium remaining in the mediastinum may suggest new leak on future esophagrams	Leaks can be missed because of decreased density of water-soluble contrast material

FIGURE 6.27 Asymptomatic 52-year-old woman with an abnormal chest radiograph (not shown). A barium esophagram shows mass effect on the left side of lower esophagus causing a smooth, obtuse impression on the esophageal lumen *(arrows)*. This intramural mass was shown by biopsy to be a large benign leiomyoma with a prominent exophytic component *(curved arrow)*.

POSTOPERATIVE ESOPHAGUS

TECHNIQUES OF POSTOPERATIVE ESOPHAGEAL IMAGING

Radiologic evaluation of the postoperative esophagus demonstrates the postoperative anatomy, effectiveness of surgical intervention, and complications.[42] During the early postoperative period (<4 weeks), the most common complications after esophageal surgery include leak, obstruction, and stasis. During the late postoperative period (>4 weeks), the most common complications include GER, stricture, and recurrent carcinoma.[42]

IMAGING MODALITIES

Chest radiography plays an important role in the early postoperative period, especially after esophagectomy, because of the high incidence of respiratory complications in these patients, particularly those who have undergone thoracotomy.[43] Complications such as pneumothorax, pleural effusion, and pneumonia are the most frequent causes of morbidity shortly after esophagectomy.[44] Chest radiographs can also provide indirect evidence of esophageal leak. Findings such as pneumomediastinum, mediastinal widening, or a rapidly growing pleural effusion suggest esophageal leaks. However, chest radiographic findings are relatively insensitive in the diagnosis of leaks. A normal chest radiograph in a clinical setting suspicious for postoperative leak should not discourage further investigation of the esophagus.[42]

Esophagraphy is the major imaging modality for evaluation of a postoperative esophagus. This fluoroscopic examination is performed as the patient drinks contrast material to opacify the esophageal lumen. Radiographs obtained during (spot images) and after (overhead images) fluoroscopy tell only part of the story. The radiologist who observed the dynamic fluoroscopic images may report findings that are not included or poorly demonstrated on the radiographic images.

In the early postoperative period, esophagrams are often limited to examination in the recumbent position. Decreased ability to swallow and poor patient mobility add to the difficulty of performing the examination. These early postoperative esophagrams are carried out, at least initially, with water-soluble contrast material in case of leaks. Later in the postoperative period, esophagrams are typically performed with upright, air-contrast images obtained with high-density barium and prone, single-contrast images with low-density barium.[42]

CT is not a primary imaging modality in the early postoperative period after esophageal surgery. However, as a secondary modality, CT provides important additional information after the discovery of a postoperative esophageal leak by esophagram. Chest CT demonstrates the severity and extent of mediastinal inflammation associated with the leak and the size and location of any mediastinal fluid collection or abscess. CT can guide the placement of drains into these collections by surgeons or interventional radiologists.[45]

ENTERIC CONTRAST MATERIALS

Two types of enteric (oral) contrast material are used during postoperative esophagrams: barium and water soluble. Each of these contrast materials has advantages and disadvantages (Table 6.1). The type of contrast material employed by the radiologist is at least partially dependent on the time since surgery. Water-soluble contrast material is used, at least initially, for early postoperative esophagrams (<4 weeks), and barium is used later in the postoperative period (>4 weeks).

Leaks can occur after any esophageal surgery, but they are most common after esophagectomy. The development of pain and fever after esophagectomy warrants emergency esophagraphy[43] performed initially with water-soluble contrast material. If this initial esophagram is negative, the examination should be immediately repeated with thick barium. As a result of the greater radiographic density of barium, small leaks may be diagnosed only with barium.

In a retrospective study of 24 esophagectomy patients with postoperative leaks, 16 (67%) of these leaks were demonstrated only with the use of high-density 250% weight per volume [w/v]) barium.[46] The benefit of demonstrating a leak often outweighs the risk for mediastinitis secondary to mediastinal barium.[47] Nevertheless, each patient presents unique challenges. Therefore, these difficult cases require close communication between radiologist and referring surgeon.

The risk for pulmonary edema after the aspiration of water-soluble contrast material depends on the volume and osmolarity of the material aspirated. Aspiration of high-osmolar water-soluble contrast material, such as diatrizoate meglumine or diatrizoate sodium, is more likely to cause pulmonary edema than aspiration of a similar amount of low-osmolar water-soluble contrast material, such as iohexol. Therefore the use of low-osmolar water-soluble contrast material should be considered in postoperative patients at risk for aspiration whose evaluation requires the use of water-soluble contrast material.[47]

SPECIFIC POSTOPERATIVE FINDINGS

Cricopharyngeal Myotomy

Cricopharyngeal myotomy is typically combined with Zenker diverticulectomy or diverticulopexy. Postoperative esophagrams in successfully treated patients show resolution of the prominent cricopharyngeus muscle and nonfilling of the diverticulum (Fig. 6.28). Mild mucosal

irregularity and mild protrusion of the pharyngoesophageal segment posteriorly are not worrisome findings.[48]

Because the major complication of cricopharyngeal myotomy is leak, the postoperative esophagram should be performed initially with water-soluble contrast material. This contrast material needs to be administered cautiously, because transient postoperative pharyngeal dysfunction predisposes these patients to aspiration (low-osmolar water-soluble contrast material can be considered for these examinations). If the water-soluble contrast study is negative, reexamination with high-density barium should be performed. Leaks often appear as blind-ending tracts extending from the esophagus posteriorly into the prevertebral space.[48]

Cardiomyotomy

After cardiomyotomy, the esophagram usually demonstrates prompt esophageal emptying and a widely patent GEJ.[42] Eccentric ballooning of the esophageal mucosa through the myotomy defect is a common finding (Fig. 6.29) and occurs in 50% of patients after cardiomyotomy.[49] Frequently, an antireflux procedure (usually partial fundoplication) is performed in conjunction with the cardiomyotomy, and radiographic evidence of this procedure may also be demonstrated on the postoperative esophagram.

An early complication of cardiomyotomy is leak. Radiographic evaluation for leak should begin with water-soluble esophagram. If this study is negative, it should be followed by barium esophagram to more confidently exclude a perforation. Late complications include dysphagia secondary to inadequate myotomy or tight fundoplication.

Antireflux Procedures

The esophagram after antireflux procedures demonstrates reduction of esophageal hiatal hernia, restoration of an intraabdominal esophageal segment, and gastric fundal wrap. Common antireflux surgeries include the Nissen,

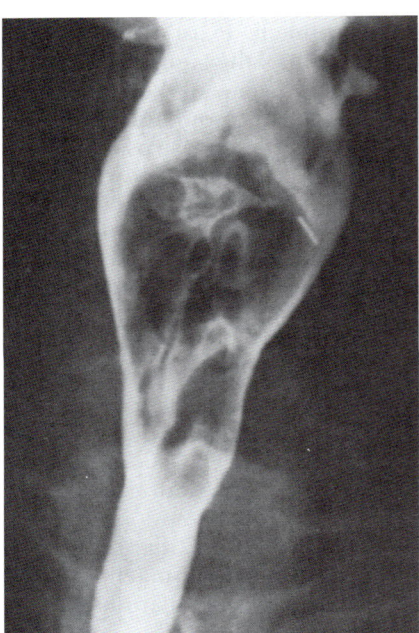
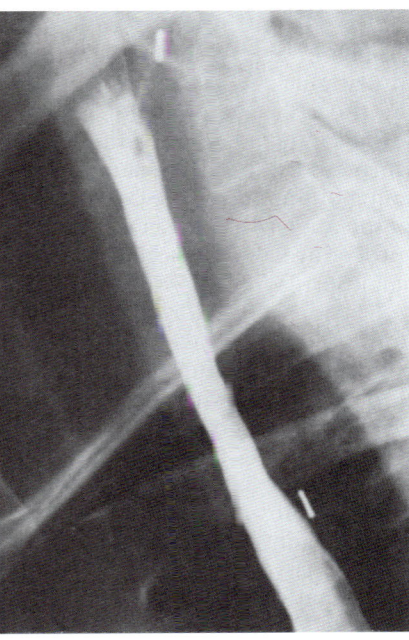

FIGURE 6.28 Cricopharyngeal myotomy. Frontal and lateral views from a barium esophagram, performed several months after surgery, demonstrate the myotomy extending superiorly and inferiorly to the level of the cricopharyngeus muscle (the surgical clips mark the superior and inferior limits of the myotomy). A cricopharyngeal bar is not evident.

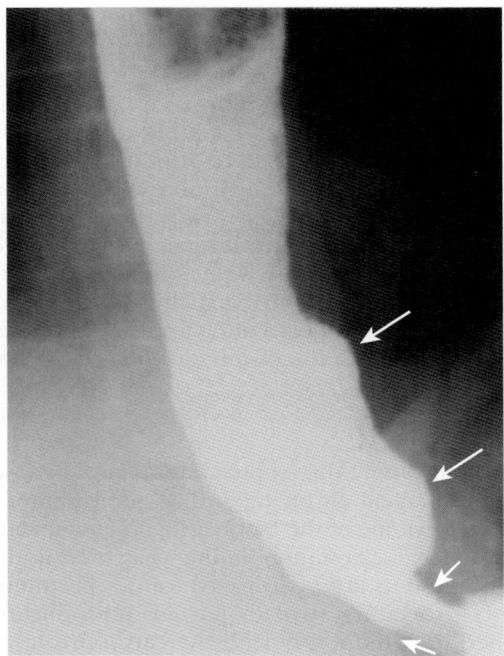

FIGURE 6.29 Cardiomyotomy (Heller myotomy). An upright, frontal view from a postoperative barium esophagram, performed several months after surgery, demonstrates protrusion of the distal esophageal mucosa through the myotomy defect *(arrows)*. Decreased caliber of the esophagus distal to the myotomy deformity *(small arrows)* should result from partial anterior fundoplication.

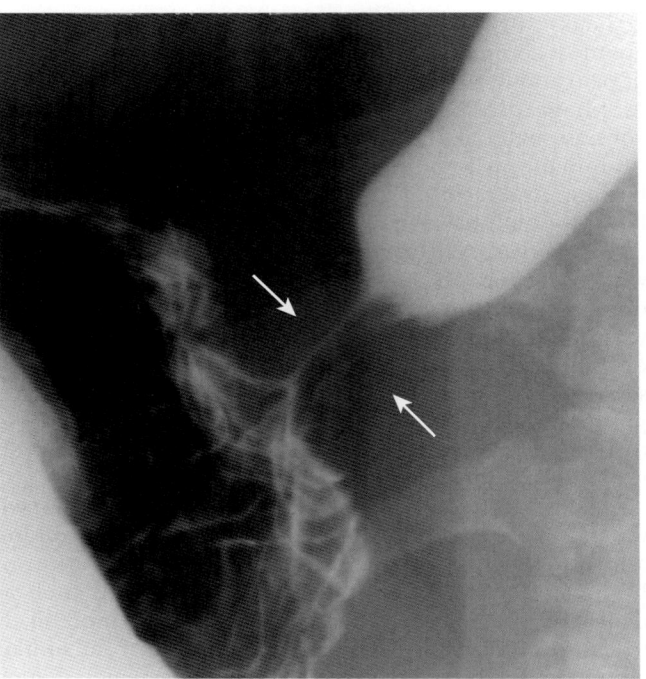

FIGURE 6.30 Nissen fundoplication. Prone, oblique, single-contrast view of the gastroesophageal junction from a barium esophagram performed 6 weeks after laparoscopic Nissen fundoplication. A smooth, symmetric, fundal pseudomass results from the 360-degree fundal wrap around the intraabdominal esophagus *(arrows)*. The esophagus passes through the center of this pseudomass.

Belsey Mark IV, and Hill procedures.[42] The Nissen procedure results in a 360-degree wrap of the gastric fundus around the esophagus. Radiographically, the Nissen wrap creates a smooth, symmetric, fundal soft-tissue pseudomass. The esophagus passes through the center of this pseudomass (Fig. 6.30). The Belsey Mark IV procedure uses a 240-degree fundal wrap with suturing of the esophagus to the gastric fundus to recreate an acute angle (of His) at the GEJ. By esophagram, this procedure results in a smaller soft tissue pseudomass in the fundus and angulation of the intraabdominal esophagus. During the Hill procedure, the GEJ is sutured to the median arcuate ligament posteriorly. No fundoplication is performed. By esophagraphy, this procedure results in lengthening of the intraabdominal esophagus and exaggeration of the angle of His. Regardless of the specific antireflux procedure, the esophagram should not demonstrate a hiatal hernia or evidence of reflux esophagitis.[42]

The most common early complication of fundoplication demonstrated by esophagram is obstruction of the distal esophagus secondary to edema of the fundal wrap. This process usually resolves in a matter of weeks. Late complications include (1) esophageal obstruction caused by a tight fundal wrap or tight esophageal hiatus, (2) recurrent hiatal hernia and GER caused by disruption of fundoplication sutures (fundal pseudomass no longer visible), and (3) recurrent hiatal hernia (fundal pseudomass remains visible) caused by dehiscence of diaphragmatic sutures.[42]

Esophageal Resection

The radiographic appearance after esophagectomy depends on the bowel segment used as an esophageal substitute. Stomach, colon, and jejunum are used as esophageal substitutes, with gastric substitution being the most common. Gastric substitution requires resection of the esophagus and cardia, mobilization of the stomach, and anastomosis of the esophagus to the stomach. Pyloromyotomy, or pyloroplasty, and partial resection of the gastric fundus may also be performed to facilitate drainage of the denervated stomach.[42] A normal postoperative esophagram should demonstrate patency of the esophagogastrostomy (Fig. 6.31), patency of the stomach as it passes through the esophageal hiatus, and patency of the pylorus.

Leak is the most feared early postoperative complication of esophagectomy and esophagogastrostomy. The leak may occur at the esophagogastric anastomosis, at the pyloroplasty or pyloromyotomy, or along the gastric staple line resulting from partial gastric resection.[42] Pain and fever after esophagectomy warrant emergency esophagram[47] with water-soluble contrast material and, if necessary, barium. High-density barium has been reported to be more effective in demonstrating leaks.[46]

Early postoperative obstruction may result from edema at the esophagogastrostomy or pyloroplasty/pyloromyotomy sites. Obstruction may also result from diaphragmatic compression of the distal part of the stomach or from gastric volvulus.[42] Gastric atony causes similar obstructive symptoms.

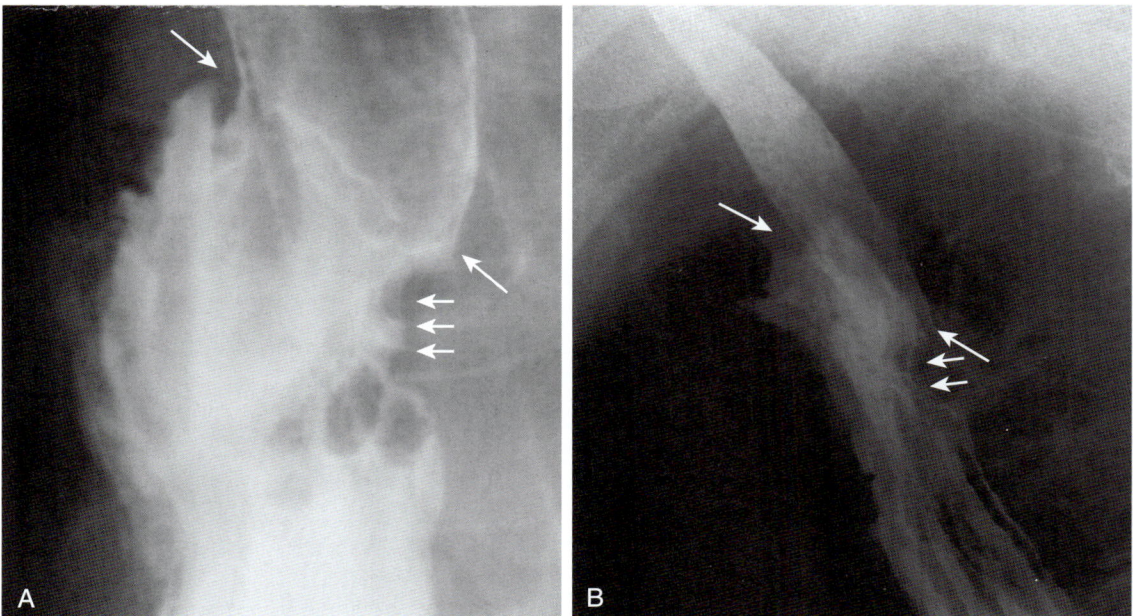

FIGURE 6.31 Esophagogastrostomy. Upright, frontal (magnified) (A) and lateral air-contrast images (B) from a barium esophagram performed 1 month after esophagectomy for T1N0 adenocarcinoma demonstrate an esophagogastric anastomosis (*large arrows* in both images). A possible ulcerated mass along the left posterior margin of the gastrostomy, just distal to the anastomosis (*small arrows* in both images), should represent a benign postoperative finding since the patient had no evidence of recurrent disease 10 months after this esophagram.

Late complications after esophagectomy and esophagogastrostomy include GER, stricture, and tumor recurrence. GER can cause reflux esophagitis, stricture (above the esophagogastric anastomosis), Barrett esophagus, and eventually adenocarcinoma.[42] Postesophagectomy patients with dysphagia should be initially evaluated by esophagram. Anastomotic strictures, typically resulting from chronic reflux esophagitis, are usually well demonstrated (Fig. 6.32). Reflux esophagitis and Barrett esophagus are best evaluated with endoscopy. CT and PET are best for detection of recurrent tumor and are discussed in another section of this chapter.

MISCELLANEOUS CONDITIONS

HIATAL HERNIAS

Although the correlation between GER and sliding hiatal hernias is far from perfect, such hernias are thought to predispose to GER.[50] Hiatal hernias can be classified into several types, depending on their esophagraphic appearance. By far, the most common type is a sliding hiatal hernia, characterized by superior migration, often transient, of the GEJ into the chest (Fig. 6.33).

The second major type of hiatal hernia (Fig. 6.34) is a paraesophageal hernia, in which the GEJ remains near the esophageal hiatus, and all or part of the stomach herniates through the esophageal hiatus to lie adjacent to the esophagus (paraesophageal). Such hernias are important to recognize because they are more likely than sliding hernias to be associated with symptomatic gas entrapment, obstruction, incarceration, and strangulation. These complications are more common with large

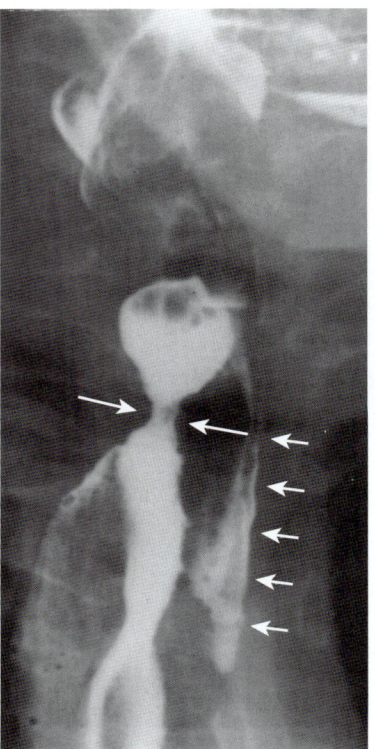

FIGURE 6.32 Stricture of esophagogastrostomy. An upright, frontal air-contrast view from a barium esophagram was performed 6 weeks after esophagectomy for T2N0 adenocarcinoma of the esophagus. A partially obstructing anastomotic stricture (*large arrows*) secondary to chronic reflux esophagitis is causing aspiration of barium into the trachea (*small arrows*).

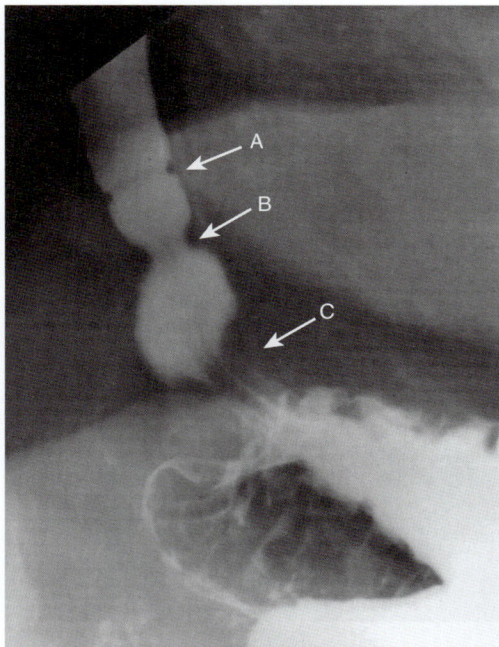

FIGURE 6.33 Single-contrast barium esophagram demonstrates a small sliding hiatal hernia. *Arrows* indicate an esophageal mucosal ring (A), muscular ring (B), and extrinsic diaphragmatic impression at the esophageal hiatus (C).

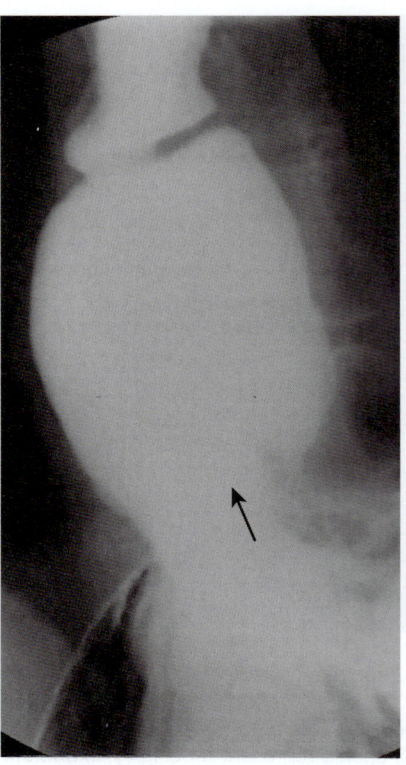

FIGURE 6.35 Abrupt shoulders superiorly and bulging margins bilaterally, typical of a sliding hiatal hernia, are well demonstrated by this image obtained while this hernia was well distended by refluxing barium *(arrow)*.

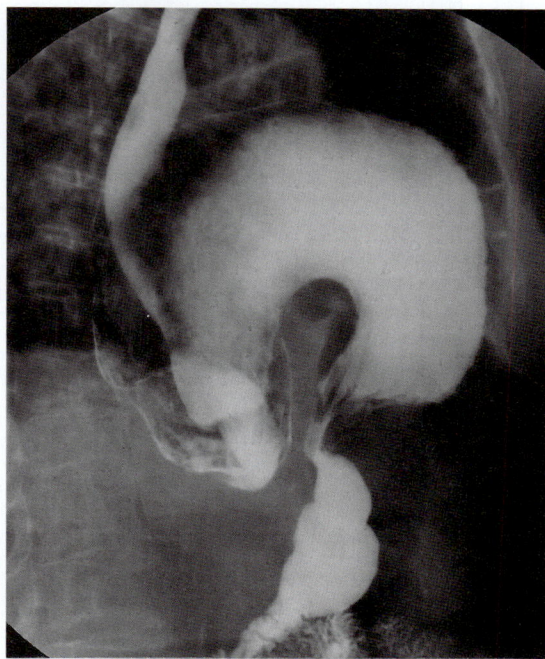

FIGURE 6.34 Upside-down, intrathoracic stomach. Double-contrast upper gastrointestinal examination shows a large paraesophageal hiatal hernia. The greater curvature of the stomach has rotated 180 degrees, with respect to the long axis of the stomach, to become superior to the lesser curve (upside-down, intrathoracic stomach). The gastroesophageal junction has remained within the esophageal hiatus of the diaphragm.

paraesophageal hernias, in which the greater curvature of the stomach rotates 180 degrees, with respect to the long axis of the stomach, to lie superior to the lesser curvature (upside-down, intrathoracic stomach). Elective surgical repair can be performed to prevent these severe complications of large paraesophageal hernias.[51,52]

When the GEJ is located above the esophageal hiatus and a portion of the stomach is located adjacent to the herniated esophagus, a combined or mixed hiatal hernia, consisting of sliding and paraesophageal components, is present. These hernias behave similar to sliding hiatal hernias, until the paraesophageal component becomes dominant. When superior rotation of the greater curvature is observed, they should be considered paraesophageal hernias.

A short-esophagus type of hiatal hernia results from esophageal shortening (see Fig. 6.12) caused by longitudinal scarring secondary to chronic GERD. The tapered shoulders and elongation of the herniated stomach in short-esophagus hiatal hernia contrast with the abrupt shoulders and bulging margins of the gastric component of a sliding hiatal hernia (Fig. 6.35).

ESOPHAGEAL RINGS AND WEBS

A mucosal ring is a short (2 to 3 mm in thickness), diaphragm-like, circumferential indentation commonly observed at the junction of esophageal squamous epithelium above and columnar gastric epithelium below. These rings are visible only when they are located above

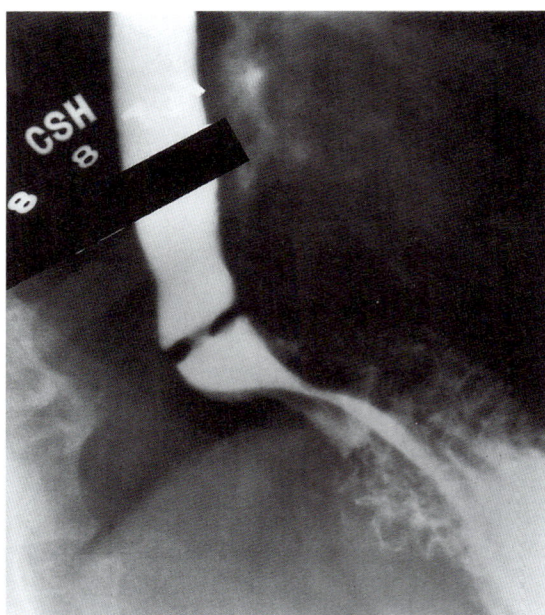

FIGURE 6.36 Single-contrast barium esophagram in a patient with dysphagia. A Schatzki ring (a short, stenotic, diaphragm-like indentation of the esophageal wall circumferentially) is demonstrated at the gastroesophageal junction. The diameter of the ring measures less than 1 cm.

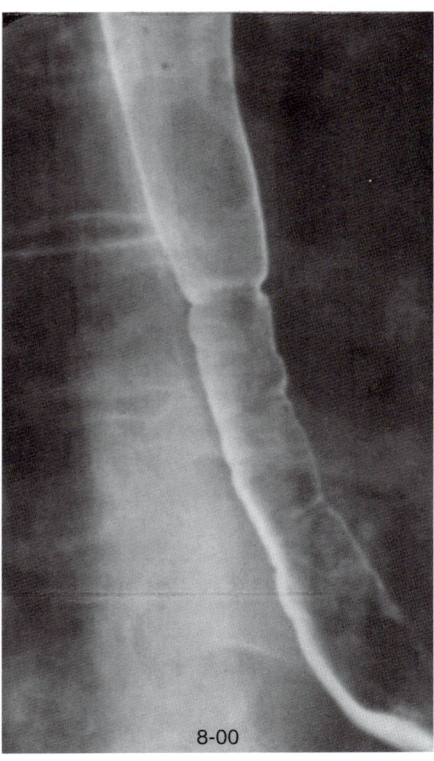

FIGURE 6.37 Double-contrast barium esophagram in a 45-year-old woman with medically refractory gastroesophageal reflux disease. Note mild diffuse narrowing and scarring of the lower esophagus indicative of chronic reflux esophagitis. The most superior scar is thin and circumferential, mimicking a Schatzki ring. However, it is located well above the gastroesophageal junction.

the esophageal hiatus and when the herniated esophagus and stomach are well distended (see Fig. 6.35). In fact, they are a useful sign to confirm the presence of a hiatal hernia. Most mucosal rings have a luminal diameter of at least 2 cm and are asymptomatic. When the diameter is less than 20 mm, the mucosal ring may cause dysphagia. In Schatzki's original article,[53] all patients with ring diameters less than 14 mm were symptomatic. Although many radiologists use the terms "mucosal ring" and "Schatzki ring" interchangeably, the term "Schatzki ring" should be reserved for stenotic mucosal rings measuring less than 14 mm in diameter (Fig. 6.36). These are the rings associated with dysphagia and the risk of food impaction.

Schatzki rings are idiopathic and not thought to be causally related to reflux esophagitis. Occasionally, a ring-like stricture secondary to chronic GERD may resemble a Schatzki ring. These strictures can usually be distinguished from Schatzki rings by their more superior location relative to the GEJ, and their association with additional findings of chronic reflux esophagitis (Fig. 6.37).

The classic esophageal web occurs in the cervical esophagus, just below the cricopharyngeal muscle (Fig. 6.38). Unlike esophageal rings, cervical esophageal webs are not usually circumferential; rather, they are U-shaped and indent the anterior and lateral walls but spare the posterior wall. Most cervical esophageal webs measure 1 to 2 mm in thickness, do not narrow the esophageal lumen significantly, and are asymptomatic. The common observation of cervical esophageal webs as incidental findings in asymptomatic, otherwise healthy individuals calls into question the classic association of cervical esophageal webs with iron deficiency, splenomegaly, and an underlying

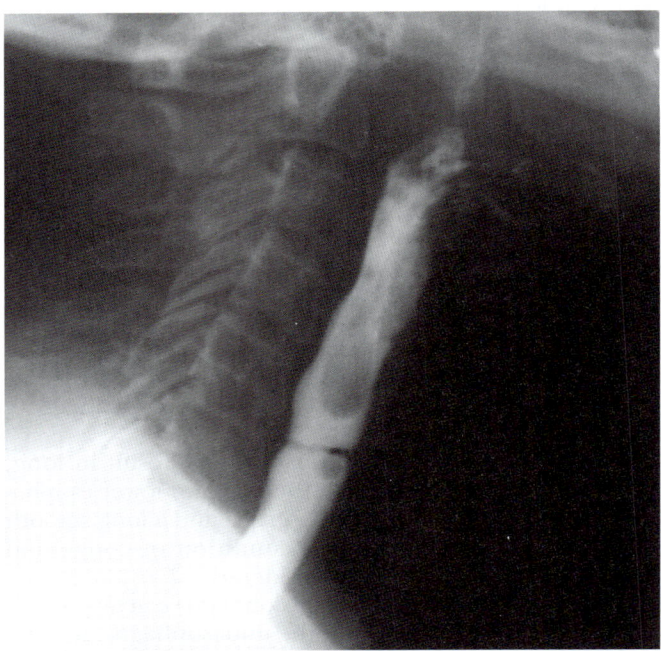

FIGURE 6.38 Lateral, single-contrast, upright view of hypopharynx and cervical esophagus demonstrates a nonobstructive, cervical esophageal web, resulting from 1 mm thick indentation of the cervical esophageal lumen, most prominent anteriorly.

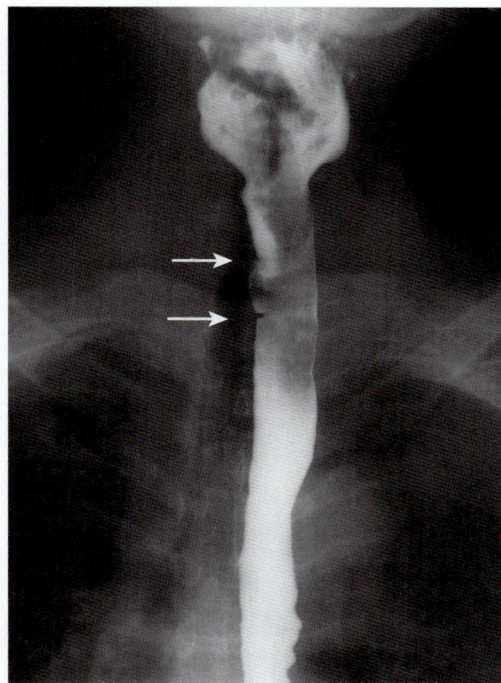

FIGURE 6.39 Single-contrast esophagram (frontal view) shows ectopic gastric mucosa. Two indentations of the right lateral aspect of the cervical esophageal lumen *(arrows)* result from a patch of ectopic gastric mucosa confirmed by endoscopic biopsy.

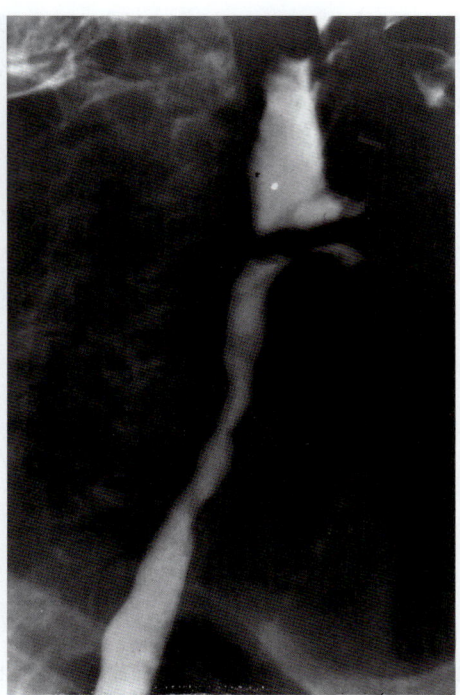

FIGURE 6.40 Single-contrast esophagram, left oblique view, from an 86-year-old man with cicatricial pemphigoid causing a lengthy stricture of moderate severity of the hypopharynx and cervical esophagus.

predisposition to hypopharyngeal and esophageal cancer (Plummer-Vinson or Paterson-Kelly syndrome).[54,55] Cervical esophageal webs should be differentiated from ectopic gastric mucosa, which produces two indentations laterally (Fig. 6.39). Ectopic gastric mucosa has a classic appearance and location and is asymptomatic.

LESS COMMON TYPES OF STRICTURES

The blistering skin diseases cicatricial pemphigoid and epidermolysis bullosa occasionally involve the esophagus.[56,57] Webs and strictures of various length are typical findings (Fig. 6.40), usually more common in the upper part of the esophagus. The associated skin lesions are the key to diagnosis of the esophageal lesions. The rare skin disorder lichen planus may also involve the esophagus. These strictures may be demonstrated in any portion of the esophagus and are typically long and mildly irregular (Fig. 6.41); they may be difficult to detect without adequate luminal distention.

Prolonged nasogastric intubation may result in long, smoothly tapered strictures in the mid and lower esophagus. In patients with lifelong dysphagia and a long smooth esophageal stricture, the rare condition of congenital esophageal stenosis can be considered.[58,59]

Smooth strictures of the midesophagus can also result from radiation therapy, when the midesophagus must be included in the radiation field. Extrinsic compression of the esophagus by mediastinal lymphadenopathy can mimic an intrinsic esophageal stricture (Fig. 6.42).

Eosinophilic esophagitis is another cause of esophageal stricture that may be a component of the more

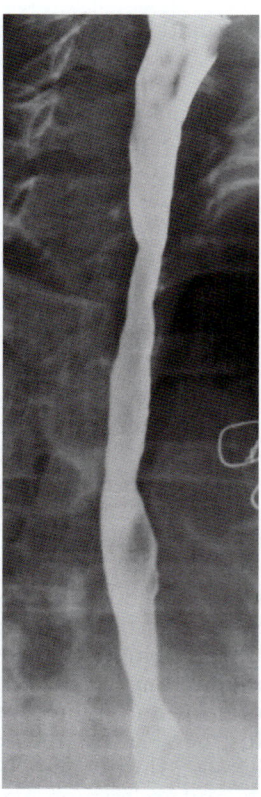

FIGURE 6.41 Single-contrast esophagram in a 73-year-old woman with known oral lichen planus and a mild-moderate, smooth stricture of the midesophagus, about 10 cm in length. Endoscopic biopsies were consistent with esophageal involvement by lichen planus.

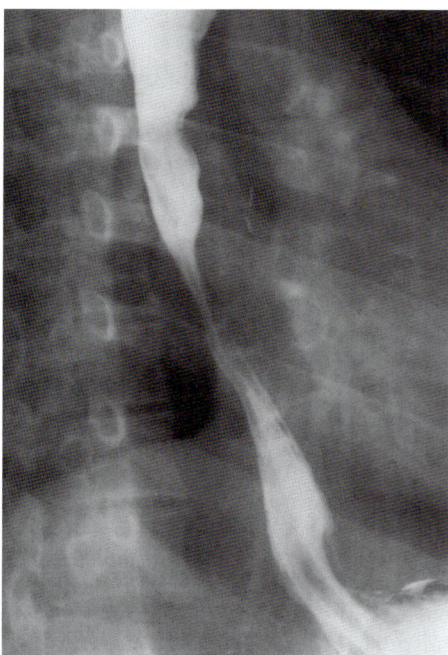

FIGURE 6.42 Single-contrast esophagram in a 26-year-old man with mediastinal histoplasmosis. Extrinsic compression of the midesophagus by mediastinal lymphadenopathy mimics an intrinsic esophageal stricture.

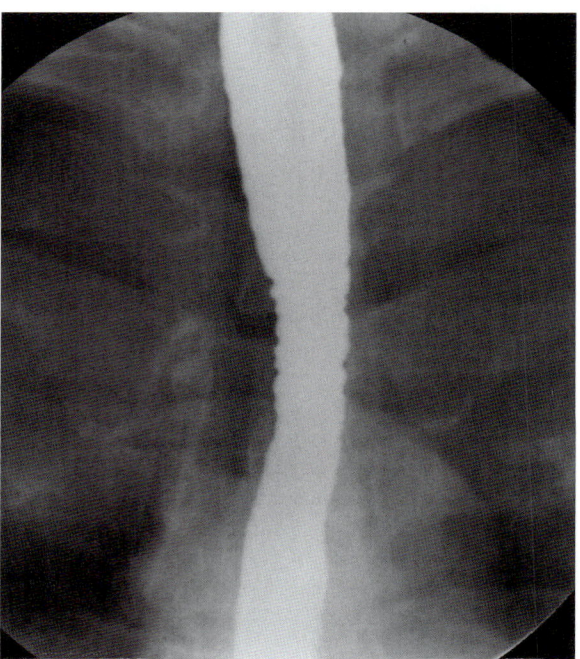

FIGURE 6.43 Single-contrast esophagram in a 38-year-old man with a long history of dysphagia and multiple food impactions. A midesophageal stricture with corrugated margins results from biopsy-proven eosinophilic esophagitis.

general condition of eosinophilic gastroenteritis, but it is increasingly being recognized as a disorder confined to the esophagus.[60] Strictures usually involve the upper or midportion of the esophagus. Some eosinophilic esophagitis strictures have a "corrugated" appearance (Fig. 6.43), while others result from diffuse and uniform narrowing of the esophagus (Fig. 6.44).[61]

Patients with Crohn disease may rarely have esophageal involvement. Manifestations of esophageal Crohn disease are variable and include ulceration, fold thickening, stricture, and obstruction (Figs. 6.45 and 6.46). Involvement by Crohn disease elsewhere in gut is almost always present, so the diagnosis has usually been established when esophageal lesions are discovered.

CAUSTIC INJURY

Caustic esophagitis usually results from ingestion of a liquid solution of concentrated lye. The severity of esophageal injury depends on the volume and concentration of the caustic agent and the duration of mucosal contact.[62] Mild injuries may be confined to the mucosa and heal without sequelae. Severe injuries may result in esophageal perforation, mediastinitis, and death. Patients who survive severe injury are typically left with long, irregular strictures of the midesophagus. The entire esophagus may be affected, with marked narrowing of the lumen producing a threadlike appearance.[63]

Less severe injury to the esophagus may result from the ingestion of other household products, including ammonium chloride. Also, a variety of medications,[64] such as tetracycline, doxycycline, potassium chloride, quinidine, nonsteroidal antiinflammatory drugs, and alendronate sodium (Fosamax) can cause esophageal strictures.

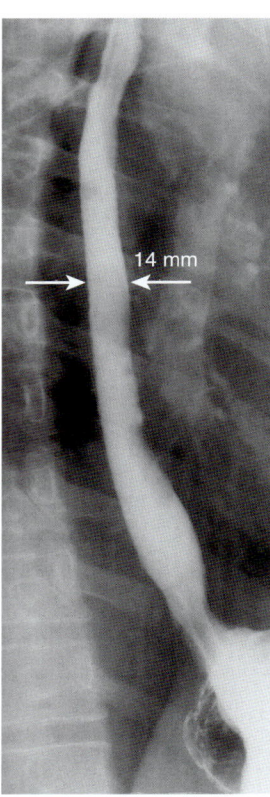

14 mm

FIGURE 6.44 Single-contrast, recumbent image demonstrating smooth, diffuse narrowing of the midesophagus, with maximum diameter of 14 mm (arrows), also results from biopsy-proven eosinophilic esophagitis.

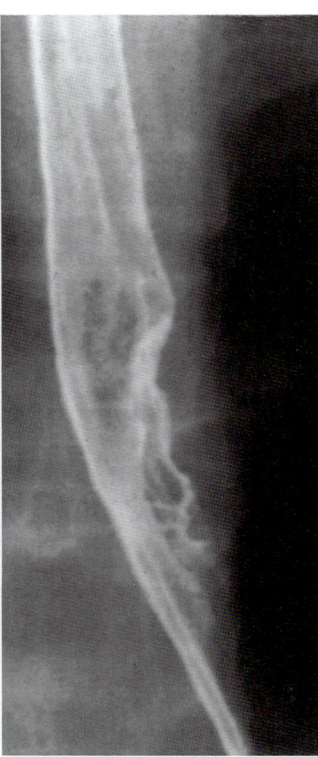

FIGURE 6.45 Double-contrast esophagram, in left posterior oblique projection, in a 25-year-old man. Irregularity and ulceration of the lower esophagus are nonspecific. These findings could result from an esophageal mass such as an adenocarcinoma. However, in this young male, they resulted from esophageal Crohn disease.

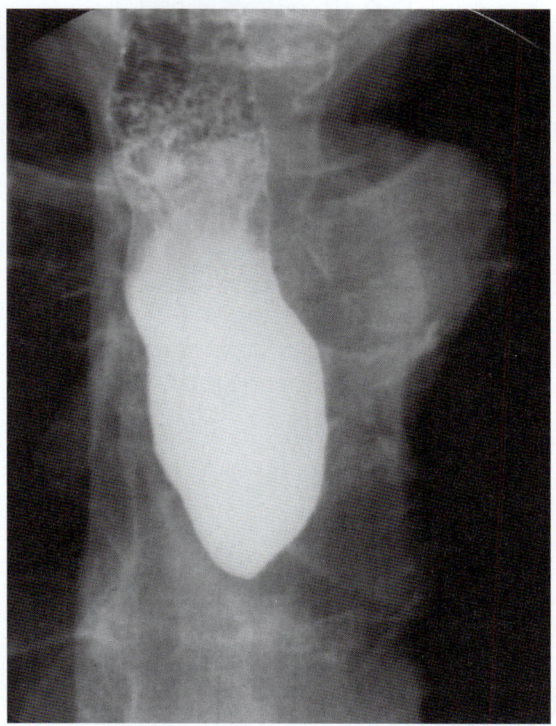

FIGURE 6.46 Upright image from single-contrast esophagram in a 78-year-old woman with Crohn disease and a midesophageal stricture causing complete obstruction.

ESOPHAGEAL PERFORATION

Esophageal perforation may result from blunt or penetrating chest trauma, foreign body ingestion, instrumentation, or caustic ingestion. Spontaneous esophageal perforation (Boerhaave syndrome) results from a sudden increase in intraluminal pressure, usually from extreme vomiting or retching, classically occurring after alcoholic binge drinking.

Regardless of the cause, esophageal perforations are potentially life threatening and require immediate attention. Localized perforations, especially of the cervical esophagus, may be managed nonoperatively, but perforations of the thoracic esophagus almost always require surgical intervention.[65]

Plain film findings of esophageal rupture include retropharyngeal gas, cervical subcutaneous emphysema, widening of the mediastinum, pneumomediastinum, pleural effusion, and hydropneumothorax (more commonly on the left; Fig. 6.47A). Because plain films are relatively insensitive and nonspecific, contrast esophagrams should be used early in the investigation of clinically suspected esophageal perforations (see Fig. 6.47B). Water-soluble contrast agents, swallowed or injected through a nasogastric tube, are the agents of first choice. For patients at risk for aspiration (or fistula to the airway), low-osmolar agents are less likely to cause pulmonary edema, if aspirated, than high-osmolar agents.

When water-soluble agents leak into the mediastinum, they are rapidly absorbed and do not incite an inflammatory response, conferring a margin of safety over barium contrast agents, which are nonabsorbable and may incite foreign body granuloma formation.[66,67] Nevertheless, a negative esophagram with water-soluble contrast should be immediately followed by a barium esophagram, which because of its higher density, has been reported to increase the sensitivity for detecting esophageal leaks by 15% to 25%.[68,69] The low risk for mediastinal complications from barium extravasation is more than offset by the benefits of earlier diagnosis.

Chest CT is more sensitive in detecting pneumomediastinum than plain films are, and is useful after a negative contrast esophagram in high-risk patients or when contrast esophagrams are difficult to perform in seriously ill patients. With modern scanners, chest CT can be combined with contrast esophagraphy to expedite the diagnosis of esophageal rupture.[70]

DIVERTICULA

Esophageal diverticula vary greatly in size, shape, location, cause, and significance. Even incidentally discovered diverticula are important to document, because they may predispose the patient to injury during instrumentation.[71]

Traditionally, esophageal diverticula are classified as either traction diverticula, occurring primarily in the midesophagus, or pulsion diverticula, occurring primarily in the upper or lower esophagus. In reality, many midesophageal diverticula are pulsion type,[72] caused by increased intraluminal pressure resulting in "ballooning" of mucosal and submucosal layers through localized weak areas of the esophageal wall. True traction diverticula are recognized by elongation, or "tenting," of the diverticulum

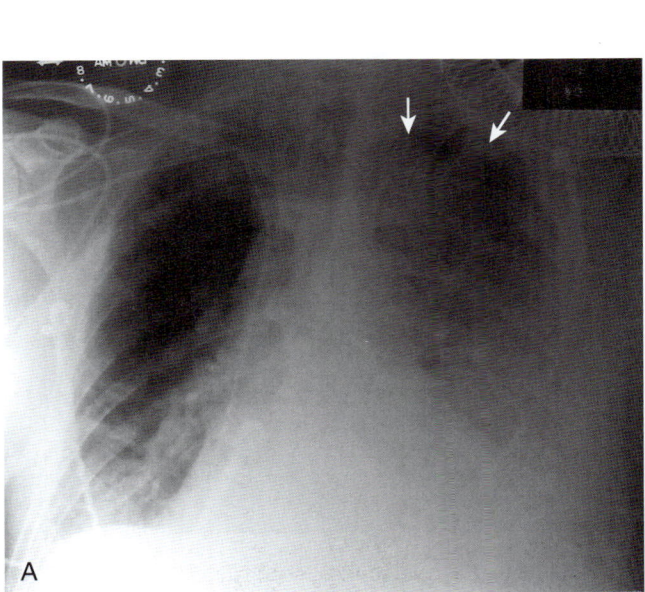

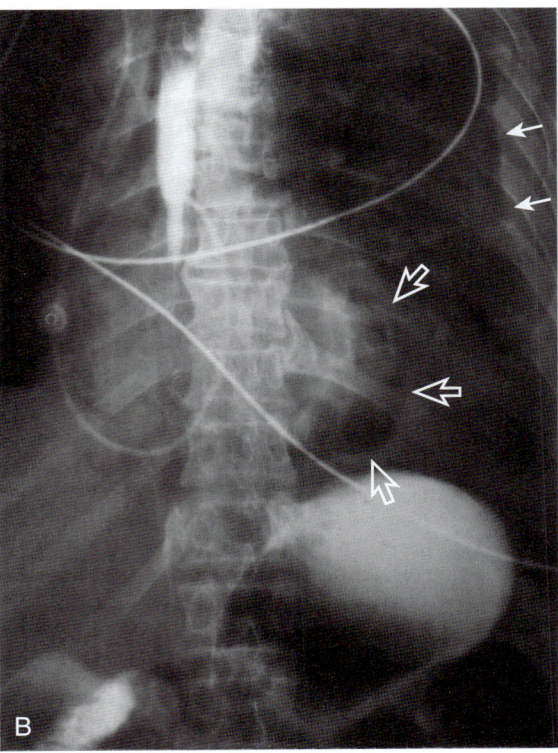

FIGURE 6.47 (A) Anteroposterior portable chest radiograph in a patient with Boerhaave syndrome and left apical pneumothorax *(arrows)*. Diffusely increased density of the left hemothorax results from a pleural effusion. (B) Supine image from water-soluble contrast upper gastrointestinal examination shows a left pleural effusion *(closed arrows)*. A retrocardiac, mediastinal collection of gas and leaked contrast material *(open arrows)* indicates esophageal rupture.

(Fig. 6.48), typically the result of fibrosis in adjacent lymph nodes involved by granulomatous inflammation.

Pulsion diverticula of the mid- and lower esophagus are often associated with an underlying esophageal motility disorder, especially those characterized by strong, non-peristaltic tertiary contractions. These pulsion diverticula are often multiple. In this clinical setting, the motility disorder is more likely to be the cause of symptoms than the diverticula. When large, especially when located near the diaphragm (epiphrenic), pulsion diverticula may retain food and liquids and become symptomatic (Fig. 6.49).[73]

A Zenker diverticulum is pulsion diverticulum occurring at the junction of the hypopharynx and cervical esophagus.[74] It results from posterior herniation of hypopharyngeal mucosa and submucosa through a triangular region of mural thinning between the oblique fibers of the thyropharyngeus muscle superiorly and the transverse fibers of the cricopharyngeus muscle inferiorly known as Killian dehiscence. Larger Zenker diverticula typically retain food and are associated with regurgitation, aspiration, hoarseness, and halitosis. They occur in association with a prominent cricopharyngeus muscle, which is the cause of dysphagia (Fig. 6.50).

VARICES

Although less sensitive than endoscopy, barium esophagram may demonstrate esophageal varices as undulating, serpentine, and sometimes nodular filling defects, often transient. They are more commonly demonstrated in the lower esophagus as the result of portal venous hypertension

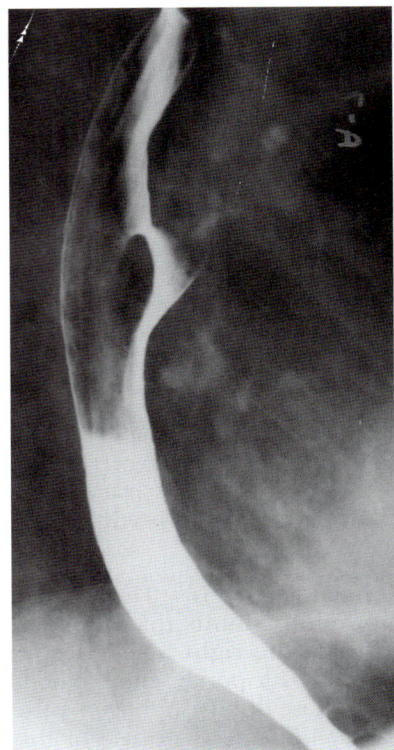

FIGURE 6.48 Double-contrast esophagram demonstrating a midesophageal traction diverticulum. Note the elongated, or "tented," appearance of the diverticulum.

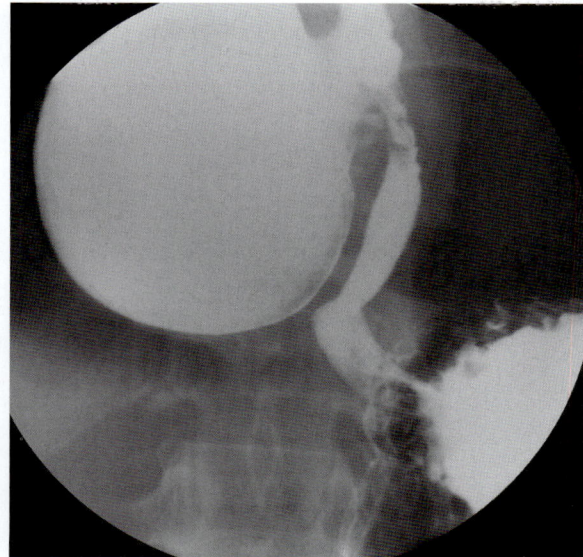

FIGURE 6.49 Double-contrast esophagram in a 62-year-old man with dysphagia and regurgitation. A large epiphrenic diverticulum bulges to the right. Barium preferentially filled the diverticulum rather than the distal esophagus. Subsequently, barium in the diverticulum refluxed into the more proximal esophagus.

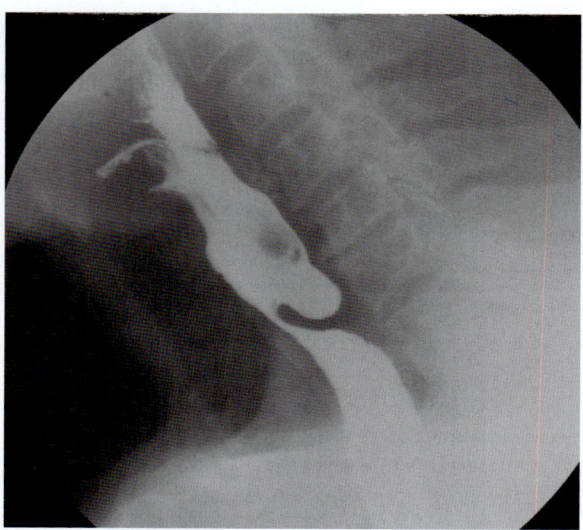

FIGURE 6.50 Lateral, upright, single-contrast image of hypopharynx and cervical esophagus shows a Zenker diverticulum immediately superior to prominent cricopharyngeus muscle causing extrinsic compression of the pharyngoesophageal lumen.

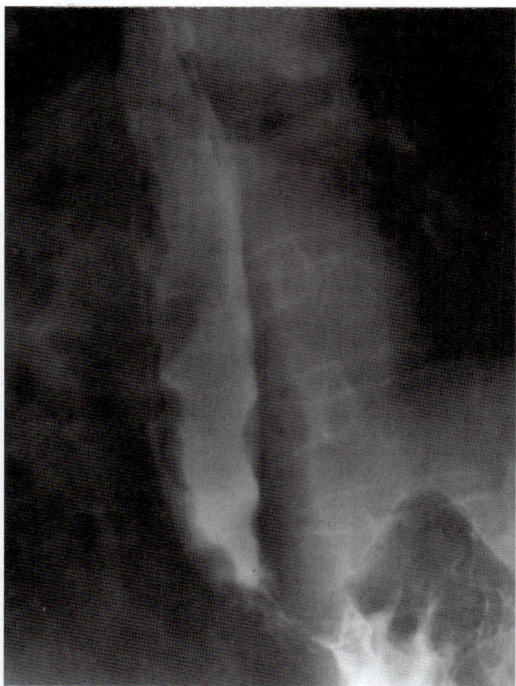

FIGURE 6.51 Single-contrast esophagram revealing moderate uphill varices. Serpentine filling defects are present in the lower esophagus.

obstruction of the superior vena cava. These varices are often referred to as *downhill varices* (Fig. 6.52) because of the direction of blood flow inside them (see Fig. 6.52).

SUMMARY

This chapter has described the essential technical elements of the esophagram and its normal structural and functional findings, as well as common artifacts and normal variants; the efficiency of the esophagram for the investigation of structural and functional causes of dysphagia (in conjunction with a video swallow study when an oropharyngeal cause of dysphagia is suspected); the appropriateness of the esophagram for evaluating the postoperative esophagus; the detection of benign and malignant esophageal neoplasms; and the role of cross-sectional imaging, especially PET/CT, for staging of esophageal cancer. Specific esophagraphic findings such as hiatal hernias, esophageal rings and webs, less common types of esophageal strictures, caustic injury, and esophageal perforation, diverticula, and varices have also been described and illustrated.

The barium esophagram remains a valuable test in the 21st century. The esophagram is complementary to CT, PET, MRI, endoscopy, EUS, high-resolution manometry, pH monitoring, and multichannel intraluminal impedance. These complementary esophageal examinations are especially beneficial to patients with esophageal disease when the radiologists and other physicians and surgeons ordering and performing them collaborate. This team approach to the diagnosis and management of esophageal diseases also increases the understanding of these diseases by all collaborating physicians.

secondary to hepatic cirrhosis. These varices represent portosystemic venous shunts that allow portal venous blood to return to the right heart, despite increased resistance to intrahepatic portal venous blood flow secondary to cirrhosis. These distal esophageal varices are often referred to as *uphill varices* because of the inferior to superior direction of blood flow inside them (Fig. 6.51). Rarely, varices may be demonstrated in the upper part of the esophagus; these varices represent venous shunts between the superior and inferior vena cava secondary to

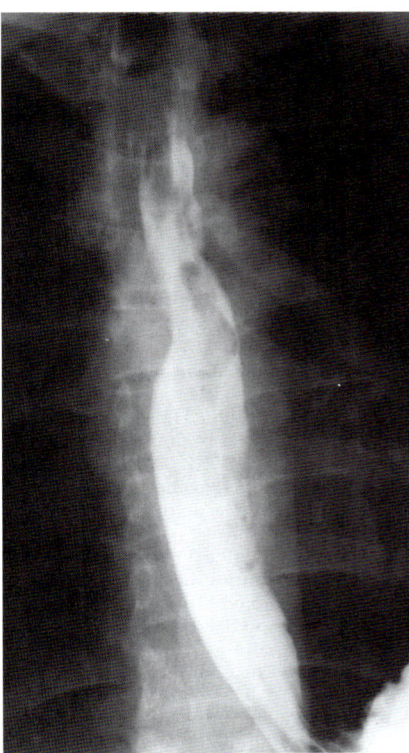

FIGURE 6.52 Single-contrast esophagram demonstrating small downhill varices in a 26-year-old man with mediastinal histoplasmosis and superior vena caval obstruction. Serpentine filling defects are present in the upper esophagus.

REFERENCES

1. Gelfand DW. The multiphasic upper gastrointestinal examination. *Radiol Clin North Am.* 1994;32:1067.
2. Ott DJ, Chen YM, Wu WC, Gelfand DW, Munitz HA. Radiographic and endoscopic sensitivity in detecting lower esophageal mucosal ring. *AJR Am J Roentgenol.* 1986;147:261.
3. Richter JE, Wu WC, Johns DN, et al. Esophageal manometry in 95 healthy adult volunteers. Variability of pressures with age and frequency of "abnormal" contractions. *Dig Dis Sci.* 1987;32:583.
4. Khan TA, Shragge BW, Crispin JS, Lind JF. Esophageal motility in the elderly. *Am J Dig Dis.* 1977;22:1049.
5. Gallo SH, McClave SA, Makk LJ, Looney SW. Standardization of clinical criteria required for use of the 12.5 millimeter barium tablet in evaluating esophageal luminal patency. *Gastrointest Endosc.* 1996;44:181.
6. Ott DJ, Kelley TF, Chen MY, Gelfand DW. Evaluation of the esophagus with a marshmallow bolus: clarifying the cause of dysphagia. *Gastrointest Radiol.* 1991;16:1.
7. Ott DJ, Kelley TF, Chen MY, Gelfand DW, Wu WC. Use of a marshmallow bolus for evaluating lower esophageal mucosal rings. *Am J Gastroenterol.* 1991;86:817.
8. Ekberg O, Lindgren S. Gastroesophageal reflux and pharyngeal function. *Acta Radiol.* 1986;27:421.
9. Levine MS, Chu P, Furth PP, Rubesin SE, Laufer I, Herlinger H. Carcinoma of the esophagus and esophagogastric junction: sensitivity of radiographic diagnosis. *AJR Am J Roentgenol.* 1997;168:1423.
10. Samadi F, Levine M, Rubesin S, Katzka DA, Laufer I. Feline esophagus and gastroesophageal reflux. *AJR Am J Roentgenol.* 2010;194:972.
11. Robins S, Jankelson IR. Cardioesophageal relaxation. *JAMA.* 1926;87:1961.
12. DeMeester T, Johnson LF. The evaluation of objective measurements of gastroesophageal reflux and their contribution to patient management. *Surg Clin North Am.* 1976;56:39.
13. Thompson JK, Koehler RE, Richter JE. Detection of gastroesophageal reflux: value of barium studies compared with 24-hr pH monitoring. *AJR Am J Roentgenol.* 1994;162:621.
14. Johnston BT, Troshnisky MB, Castell JA, Castell DO. Comparison of barium radiology with esophageal pH monitoring in the diagnosis of gastroesophageal reflux disease. *Am J Gastroenterol.* 1996;91:1181.
15. Hewson EG, Ott DJ, Dalton CB, Chen YM, Wu WC, Richter JE. Manometry and radiology. Complementary studies in the assessment of esophageal motility disorders. *Gastroenterology.* 1990;98:626.
16. Ott DJ, Gelfand DW, Wu WC. Reflux esophagitis: radiographic and endoscopic correlation. *Radiology.* 1979;130:583.
17. Gupta S, Levine MS, Rubesin SE, Katzka DA, Laufer I. Usefulness of barium studies for differentiating benign and malignant strictures of the esophagus. *AJR Am J Roentgenol.* 2003;180:737.
18. Ott DJ, Chen YM, Wu WC, Gelfand DW. Endoscopic sensitivity in the detection of esophageal strictures. *J Clin Gastroenterol.* 1985;7:121.
19. Glick SN, Teplick SK, Amenta PS. The radiologic diagnosis of Barrett esophagus: importance of mucosal surface abnormalities on air-contrast barium studies. *AJR Am J Roentgenol.* 1991;157:951.
20. Chen M, Frederick MG. Barrett esophagus and adenocarcinoma. *Radiol Clin North Am.* 1994;32:1167.
21. Glick SN. Barium studies in patients with Barrett's esophagus: importance of focal areas of esophageal deformity. *AJR Am J Roentgenol.* 1994;163:65.
22. Yamamoto AJ, Levine MS, Katzka DA, Furth EE, Rubesin SE, Laufer I. Short-segment Barrett's esophagus: findings on double-contrast esophagography in 20 patients. *AJR Am J Roentgenol.* 2001;176:1173.
23. Spechler SJ, Castell DO. Classification of esophageal motility abnormalities. *Gut.* 2001;49:145.
24. Ott DJ. Motility disorders of the esophagus. *Radiol Clin North Am.* 1994;32:1117.
25. Ott DJ, Richter JE, Chen YM, Wu WC, Gelfand DW, Castell DO. Esophageal radiography and manometry: correlation in 172 patients with dysphagia. *AJR Am J Roentgenol.* 1987;149:307.
26. Woodfield CA, Levine CA, Rubesin SE, Langlotz CP, Laufer I. Diagnosis of primary versus secondary achalasia: reassessment of clinical and radiographic criteria. *AJR Am J Roentgenol.* 2000;175:727.
27. Prabhakar A, Levine MS, Rubesin S, Laufer I, Katzka D. Relationship between diffuse esophageal spasm and lower esophageal sphincter dysfunction on barium studies and manometry in 14 patients. *AJR Am J Roentgenol.* 2004;183:409.
28. Goldberg MF, Levine MS, Torigan DA. Diffuse esophageal spasm: CT findings in seven patients. *AJR Am J Roentgenol.* 2008;191:758.
29. Xia F, Mao J, Ding J, Yang H. Observation of normal appearance and wall thickness of esophagus on CT images. *Eur J Radiol.* 2009;72:406.
30. Shakespear JS, Blom D, Huprich JE, Peters JH. Correlation of radiographic and manometric findings in patients with ineffective esophageal motility. *Surg Endosc.* 2004;18:459.
31. Blot WJ, Devesa SS, Kneller RW, Fraumeni JF Jr. Rising incidence of adenocarcinoma of the esophagus and gastric cardia. *JAMA.* 1991;265:1287.
32. Gore RM. Esophageal cancer: clinical and pathologic features. *Radiol Clin North Am.* 1997;35:243.
33. Iyer RB, Silverman PM, Tamm EP, Dunnington JS, DuBrow RA. Diagnosis, staging, and follow-up of esophageal cancer. *AJR Am J Roentgenol.* 2003;181:785.
34. Flanagan FL, Dehdashti F, Siegel BA, et al. Staging of esophageal cancer with ^{18}F-fluorodeoxyglucose positron emission tomography. *AJR Am J Roentgenol.* 1997;168:417.
35. Flamen P, Lerut A, Van Cutsem E, et al. Utility of positron emission tomography for the staging of patients with potentially operable esophageal carcinoma. *J Clin Oncol.* 2000;18:3202.
36. Rasanen JV, Sihvo EI, Knuuti MJ, et al. Prospective analysis of accuracy of positron emission tomography, computed tomography, and endoscopic ultrasonography in staging of adenocarcinoma of the esophagus and the esophagogastric junction. *Ann Surg Oncol.* 2003;10:954.
37. Rice TW. Clinical staging of esophageal carcinoma. CT, EUS, and PET. *Chest Surg Clin N Am.* 2000;10:471.
38. Luketich JD, Schauer PR, Meltzer CC, et al. Role of positron emission tomography in staging esophageal cancer. *Ann Thorac Surg.* 1997;64:765.
39. Weber WA, Ott K, Becker K, et al. Prediction of response to preoperative chemotherapy in adenocarcinomas of the esophagogastric junction by metabolic imaging. *J Clin Oncol.* 2001;19:3058.

40. Flamen P, Lerut A, Van Cutsem E, et al. The utility of positron emission tomography for the diagnosis and staging of recurrent esophageal cancer. *J Thorac Cardiovasc Surg.* 2000;120:1085.

41. Miettinen M, Sarlomo-Rikala M, Sobin LH, Lasota J. Esophageal stromal tumors: a clinicopathologic, immunohistochemical, and molecular genetic study of 17 cases and comparison with esophageal leiomyomas and leiomyosarcomas. *Am J Surg Pathol.* 2000;24:211.

42. Rubesin S, Williams N. Postoperative esophagus. In: Gore RM, Levine MS, eds. *Textbook of Gastrointestinal Radiology.* 2nd ed. Philadelphia: WB Saunders; 2000:495.

43. Orringer M. Complications of esophageal surgery. In: Orringer M, Heitmiller R, eds. *Shackelford's Surgery of the Alimentary Tract.* 5th ed. Philadelphia: WB Saunders; 2002:443.

44. Kim SH, Lee KS, Shim YM, Kim K, Yang PS, Kim TS. Esophageal resection: indications, techniques, and radiologic assessment. *Radiographics.* 2001;21:1119; discussion 1138.

45. Maher M, Lucey BC, Boland G, Gervais DA, Mueller PR. The role of interventional radiology in the treatment of mediastinal fluid collections caused by esophageal anastomotic leaks. *AJR Am J Roentgenol.* 2002;178:649.

46. Swanson JO, Levine MS, Redfern RO, et al. Usefulness of high-density barium for detection of leaks after esophagogastrectomy, total gastrectomy, and total laryngectomy. *AJR Am J Roentgenol.* 2003;181:415.

47. Levine MS. *Miscellaneous Abnormalities of the Esophagus.* Philadelphia: WB Saunders; 2000:465.

48. Sydow BD, Levine MS, Rubesin SE, Laufer I. Radiographic findings and complications after surgical or endoscopic repair of Zenker's diverticulum in 16 patients. *AJR Am J Roentgenol.* 2001;177:1067.

49. Rubesin SE, Kennedy M, Levine MS, Rosato EF, Laufer I. Distal esophageal ballooning following Heller myotomy. *Radiology.* 1988;167:345.

50. Ott DJ, Gelfand DW, Chen YM, Wu WC, Munitz HA. Predictive relationship of hiatal hernia to reflux esophagitis. *Gastrointest Radiol.* 1985;10:317.

51. Hill LD. Incarcerated paraesophageal hernia: a surgical emergency. *Am J Surg.* 1973;126:286.

52. Dunn DB, Quick G. Incarcerated paraesophageal hernia. *Am J Emerg Med.* 1990;8:36.

53. Schatzki RGJ. Dysphagia due to diaphragm-like localized narrowing in the lower esophagus (lower esophageal ring). *Radiology.* 1953;70:911.

54. Waldenström J, Kjeulberg SR. The roentgenological diagnosis of sideropenic dysphagia (Plummer-Vinson's syndrome). *Acta Radiol.* 1939;20:618.

55. Chisholm M. The association between webs, iron and postcricoid carcinoma. *Postgrad Med J.* 1974;50:215.

56. Mauro MA, Parker LA, Hartley WS, Renner JB, Mauro PM. Epidermolysis bullosa: radiographic findings in 16 cases. *AJR Am J Roentgenol.* 1987;149:925.

57. Naylor MF, MacCarty RL, Rogers RS 3rd. Barium studies in esophageal cicatricial pemphigoid. *Abdom Imaging.* 1995;20:97.

58. Dominiquez R, Zarabi M, Oh KS, Bender TM, Girdany BR. Congenital esophageal stenosis. *Clin Radiol.* 1985;36:263.

59. Pokieser P, Schima W, Schober E, et al. Congenital esophageal stenosis in a 21-year-old man: clinical and radiographic findings. *AJR Am J Roentgenol.* 1998;170:147.

60. Croese J, Fairley SK, Masson JW, et al. Clinical and endoscopic features of eosinophilic esophagitis in adults. *Gastrointest Endosc.* 2003;58:516.

61. Vasilopoulos S, Murphy P, Auerbach A, et al. The small-caliber esophagus: an unappreciated cause of dysphagia for solids in patients with eosinophilic esophagitis. *Gastrointest Endosc.* 2002;55:99.

62. Goldman LP, Weigert JM. Corrosive substance ingestion: a review. *Am J Gastroenterol.* 1984;79:85.

63. Franken EA. Caustic damage of the gastrointestinal tract: Roentgen features. *AJR Am J Roentgenol.* 1973;118:77.

64. Bova JG, Dutton NE, Goldstein HM, Hoberman LJ. Medication-induced esophagitis: diagnosis by double-contrast esophagography. *AJR Am J Roentgenol.* 1987;148:731.

65. Port JL, Kent MS, Korst RJ, Bacchetta M, Altorki NK. Thoracic esophageal perforations: a decade of experience. *Ann Thorac Surg.* 2003;75:1071.

66. James AE, Montali RJ, Chaffee V, Strecker EP, Vessal K. Barium or Gastrografin: which contrast media for diagnosis of esophageal tears? *Gastroenterology.* 1975;68:1103.

67. Vessal K, Montali RJ, Larson SM, Chaffee V, James AE Jr. Evaluation of barium and Gastrografin as contrast media for the diagnosis of esophageal ruptures or complications. *AJR Am J Roentgenol.* 1975;123:307.

68. Buecker A, Wein BB, Neuerburg JM, Guenther RW. Esophageal perforation: comparison of use of aqueous and barium-containing contrast media. *Radiology.* 1997;202:683.

69. Foley MJ, Ghahremani GG, Rogers LF. Reappraisal of contrast media used to detect upper gastrointestinal perforations. *Radiology.* 1982;144:213.

70. Fadoo F, Ruiz DE, Dawn SK, Webb WR, Gotway MB. Helical CT esophagography for the evaluation of suspected esophageal perforation or rupture. *AJR Am J Roentgenol.* 2004;182:1177.

71. Nutter KM, Ball OG. Esophageal diverticula: current classification and important complications. *J Miss State Med Assoc.* 2004;45:131.

72. Schima W, Schober E, Stacher G, et al. Association of mid esophageal diverticula with esophageal motor disorders: videofluoroscopy and manometry. *Acta Radiol.* 1997;38:108.

73. Fasano NC, Levine MS, Rubesin SE, Redfern RO, Laufer I. Epiphrenic diverticulum: clinical and radiographic findings in 27 patients. *Dysphagia.* 2003;18:9.

74. Perrott JW. Anatomical aspects of hypopharyngeal diverticula. *Aust N Z J Surg.* 1962;31:307.

Endoscopic Evaluation of the Esophagus and Endoscopic Ultrasonography of the Esophagus

Daniel S. Oh | Stuart Jon Spechler | Jacques Bergman |

Thomas W. Rice | Gregory Zuccaro Jr.

The endoscopist who examines the esophagus evaluates a muscular tube whose primary function is to convey swallowed material from the mouth to the stomach. The esophagus is approximately 25 cm in length measured from its origin in the neck just below the cricoid cartilage (C6 level, approximately 15 cm from the incisor teeth as measured by the endoscopist) to its termination in the abdomen at the gastric cardia (T10 to T11 level, approximately 40 cm from the incisor teeth).[1] Proximally, the upper esophageal sphincter (UES) separates the pharynx from the esophagus. The UES extends approximately 3 cm in length and comprises three skeletal muscle groups including the distal portion of the inferior pharyngeal constrictor, the cricopharyngeus, and the circular muscle of the proximal esophagus.[2] Introduction of the endoscope into the UES often causes gagging, and the muscles relax only briefly during a swallow. Consequently, the endoscope typically is passed quickly through the UES, and endoscopic visualization of its mucosal lining often is limited.

The esophagus passes from the chest into the abdomen through the diaphragmatic hiatus, a canal-shaped opening in the right crus of the diaphragm. Approximately 2 cm of the distal esophagus normally lie within the abdomen.[3] The lower esophageal sphincter (LES) comprises both the skeletal muscle of the crural diaphragm (external LES muscle) and the circular smooth muscle of the distal esophagus itself (internal LES muscle), although endoscopists often refer to only the latter when describing the LES. Unlike the UES, endoscopic examination of the LES region generally is not limited either by sustained sphincter muscle contraction or by patient discomfort.

The esophageal lumen is collapsed at rest and must be distended with air during endoscopy so that the stratified squamous epithelial lining can be visualized well. When so distended, the squamous epithelium appears pale, glossy, and relatively featureless. In the proximal esophagus, within a few centimeters of the UES, it is common to find patches of columnar epithelium that have a reddish color and velvetlike texture similar to the epithelium of the stomach (Fig. 7.1).[4] These so-called inlet patches are believed to be congenital rests of heterotopic gastric epithelium. They are often overlooked during routine endoscopic examinations, but, if sought specifically, they can be found in up to 11% of patients who have endoscopic examinations. Inlet patches usually are of no clinical importance, but they can produce acid and, in rare cases, can cause peptic ulcerations in the proximal esophagus. In addition, they occasionally contain intestinal metaplasia,

and rare instances of adenocarcinoma have been described developing from an inlet patch.

Within the chest at about the T4 level, the esophagus is indented on its left side by the aortic arch. This pulsating indentation can be noted during endoscopic examination at a distance of approximately 23 cm from the incisor teeth (Fig. 7.2).[5] Just below the arch at approximately 25 cm, the left main bronchus causes a subtle indentation on the left anterior aspect of the esophagus (see Fig. 7.2). Below the bronchus, the esophagus abuts the left atrium. The heart normally causes no prominent indentation of the esophageal lumen, but atrial pulsations often can be visualized at a level approximately 30 cm from the incisor teeth.

ENDOSCOPIC EVALUATION OF THE GASTROESOPHAGEAL JUNCTION

The gastroesophageal junction (GEJ) is the level at which the esophagus ends and the stomach begins. Unfortunately, there are no universally accepted landmarks that clearly delimit the distal esophagus and the proximal stomach, and the GEJ has been defined differently by anatomists, radiologists, physiologists, and endoscopists.[6] Landmarks suggested by anatomists, such as the peritoneal reflection or the character of the muscle bundles in the esophageal wall, are not useful for endoscopists. Radiologists refer to the region of the GEJ as the vestibule, and they seldom attempt to localize the precise point at which the esophagus joins the stomach.[7] Physiologists have used the distal border of the LES (determined manometrically) to define the GEJ,[8] but it is not feasible to identify this border precisely by endoscopic techniques. Indeed, one study has shown that manometric and endoscopic localizations of the LES often differ by several centimeters.[9] This has implications for placement of a wireless pH capsule endoscopically based on the GEJ versus based on manometry because the location and consequently the findings may differ based on technique (see later).

When considering any proposed landmark for the GEJ, it is important to appreciate that there is no clear-cut "gold standard" for the structure and, consequently, all of the suggested landmarks can be considered arbitrary. For most disorders of the esophagus and stomach that are diagnosed endoscopically, furthermore, it is not important that the GEJ be identified with great precision. For some disorders, most notably Barrett esophagus, for which the endoscopist must determine the extent of esophageal

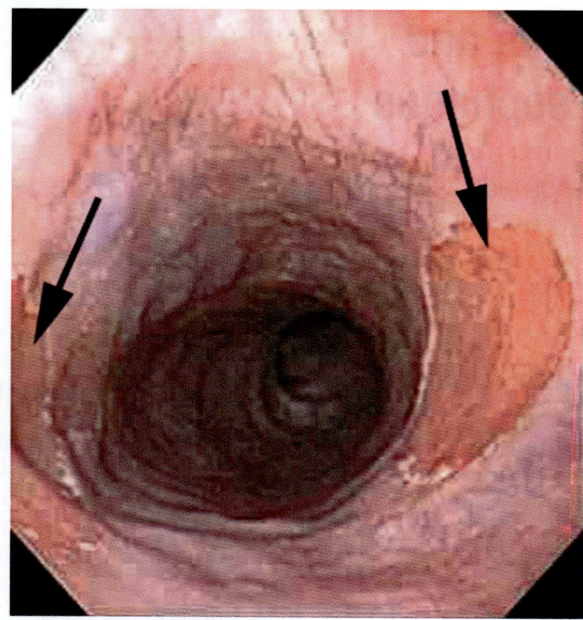

FIGURE 7.1 Endoscopic photograph of the proximal esophagus, just distal to the upper esophageal sphincter, showing two inlet patches *(arrows)*, which are rests of heterotopic gastric epithelium.

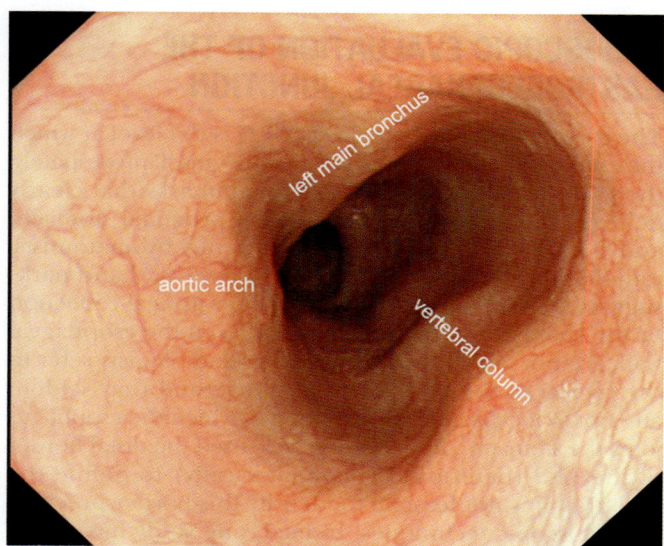

FIGURE 7.2 Endoscopic photograph of the proximal esophagus showing the normal indentations caused by the aortic arch, the left main bronchus, and the vertebral column.

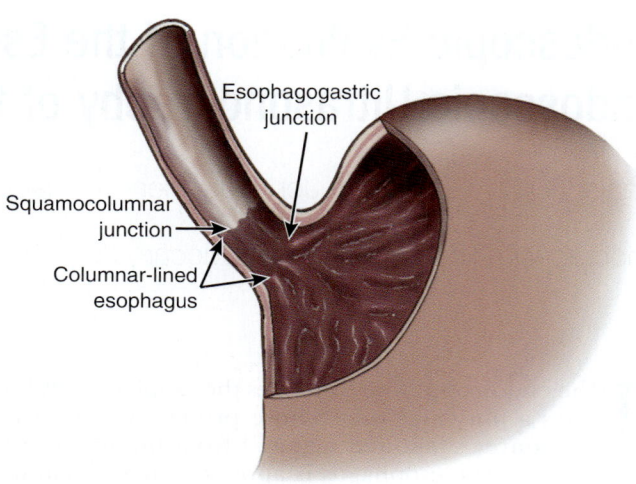

FIGURE 7.3 Endoscopic landmarks. The squamocolumnar junction (or Z-line) is the visible line formed by the juxtaposition of squamous and columnar epithelia. The gastroesophageal junction (GEJ) is the imaginary line at which the esophagus ends and the stomach begins. The most proximal extent of the gastric folds has been proposed as a marker for the GEJ. When the squamocolumnar junction is located proximal to the GEJ, there is a columnar-lined segment of esophagus. (Reprinted with permission from Spechler SJ. The role of gastric carditis in metaplasia and neoplasia at the gastroesophageal junction. *Gastroenterology.* 1999;117:218.)

columnar lining, precise localization of the GEJ can be critical for establishing the diagnosis.

Suggested endoscopic criteria for the GEJ include: (1) the level at which the tubular esophagus flares to become the sack-like stomach,[10] (2) the proximal margin of the gastric rugal folds when the esophagus and stomach are partially distended,[11] and (3) the distal end of the esophageal palisade vessels.[12,13] Although these landmarks may be recognized readily in still photographs of the junction region, the distal esophagus in vivo is a dynamic structure whose appearance changes from moment to moment. The location of the point of flare changes with respiratory and peristaltic activity. The proximal gastric folds can prolapse transiently up into the esophagus. The appearance of the junction region also varies with the degree of distention of the esophagus and stomach, and the palisade vessels can be difficult to identify using conventional endoscopes.

The proximal extent of the gastric folds is the landmark for the GEJ used frequently by Western endoscopists (Figs. 7.3 to 7.5).[14] This landmark was proposed by McClave et al. in 1987 based on their endoscopic observations in only four subjects who were identified as normal controls because they had "no clinical evidence of esophageal disease."[11] The junction between squamous and columnar epithelia (the SCJ) was located within 2 cm of the gastric folds in all of those four subjects, and so the authors concluded that the diagnosis of columnar-lined esophagus should be considered only when the SCJ is located more than 2 cm above the GEJ (i.e., the proximal level of the gastric folds). This study can be criticized both for the small number of control subjects and for the lack of documentation that the four controls were indeed normal. Esophageal pH monitoring studies were not performed, and so it is not clear that the control subjects had normal esophageal acid exposure. Biopsy specimens of the columnar-lined esophagus were not taken, and so short-segment Barrett esophagus was not excluded (see later). Furthermore, three of the four control subjects had hiatus hernias and one had reflux esophagitis. It seems surprising that a proposed landmark based on such questionable data has been so widely accepted by endoscopists.

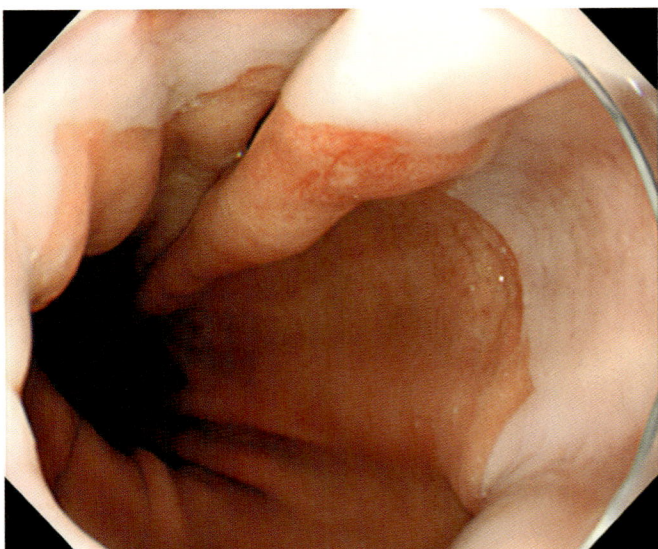

FIGURE 7.4 Endoscopic photograph of the gastroesophageal junction region in a patient who has a hiatal hernia. The squamocolumnar junction is located above some of the gastric folds (i.e., there is a columnar-lined segment of esophagus), whereas for others the squamocolumnar junction seems to coincide with the proximal extent of the folds.

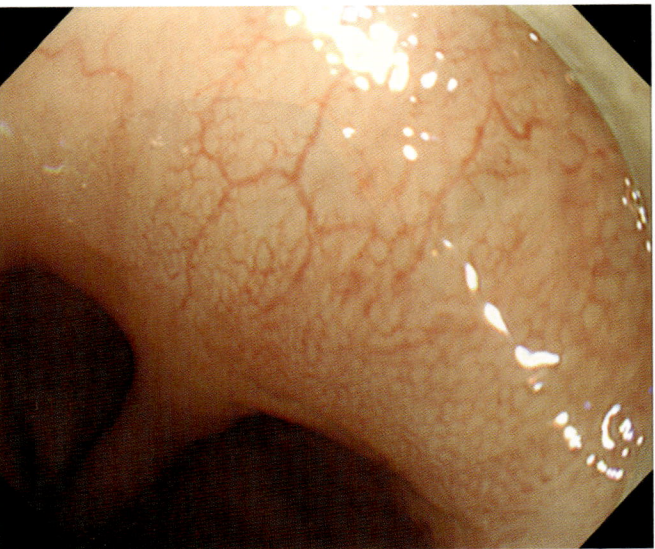

FIGURE 7.6 Palisade vessels in the distal esophagus are fine, longitudinal veins in the lamina propria. The distal end of the palisade vessels has been proposed as an endoscopic landmark for the gastroesophageal junction.

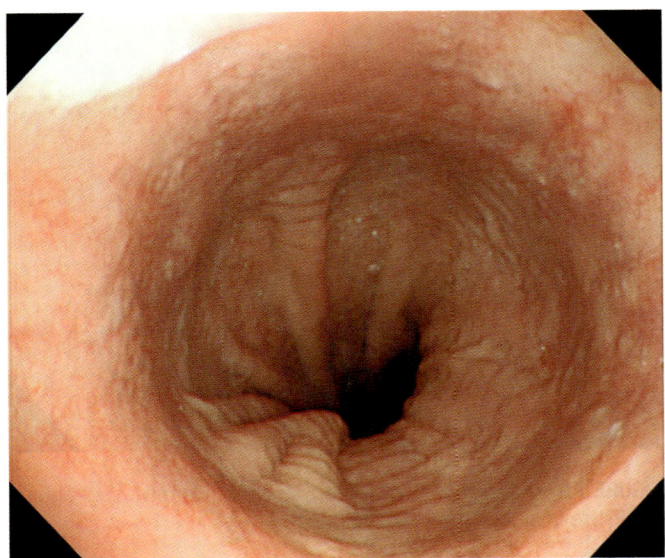

FIGURE 7.5 Endoscopic photograph of the gastroesophageal junction region in a patient with long-segment Barrett esophagus. Columnar epithelium extends above the tops of the gastric folds to involve the distal esophagus in a circumferential fashion.

A number of Asian investigators use the end of the esophageal palisade vessels as their landmark for the GEJ (Fig. 7.6).[13] Elegant anatomic studies of the GEJ have revealed four distinct zones of venous drainage, including a gastric zone, a palisade zone, a perforating zone, and a truncal zone.[15] The palisade zone comprises a group of fine, longitudinal veins located largely within the lamina propria of the distal esophagus. The palisade

vessels pierce the muscularis mucosae distally to join the submucosal vessels of the gastric zone and proximally to join the submucosal vessels of the perforating zone. The palisade vessels can be difficult to visualize by conventional endoscopy, especially if there is inflammation in the distal esophagus. The appearance of these vessels can be enhanced by narrow band imaging endoscopy, which uses primarily blue light that penetrates only the superficial layers of the mucosa (where the palisade vessels are found) and that is absorbed by the hemoglobin within the vessels. Furthermore, even in autopsy studies in which blood vessels of the GEJ region are injected with resins that provide exquisite detail of the venous structures, it is difficult to identify precisely the termination of the palisade vessels.[15] Finally, it is not clear conceptually why the distal end of the palisade vessels should be considered the precise end of the esophagus.

Few studies have addressed specifically the problem of endoscopic localization of the GEJ and, even in those that have done so, the accuracy of the criteria used cannot be assessed meaningfully in the absence of a gold standard. It is not clear which is the best diagnostic criterion for the GEJ, and the reproducibility of the various criteria have not been established. If one cannot determine with certainty where the esophagus ends and the stomach begins, then any assessment of the extent of esophagus lined by columnar epithelium will be inherently imprecise. This unresolved problem continues to confound clinicians and investigators who deal with Barrett esophagus.

CONVENTIONAL ENDOSCOPIC DIAGNOSIS OF BARRETT ESOPHAGUS

Barrett esophagus is the condition in which metaplastic columnar epithelium that predisposes to cancer

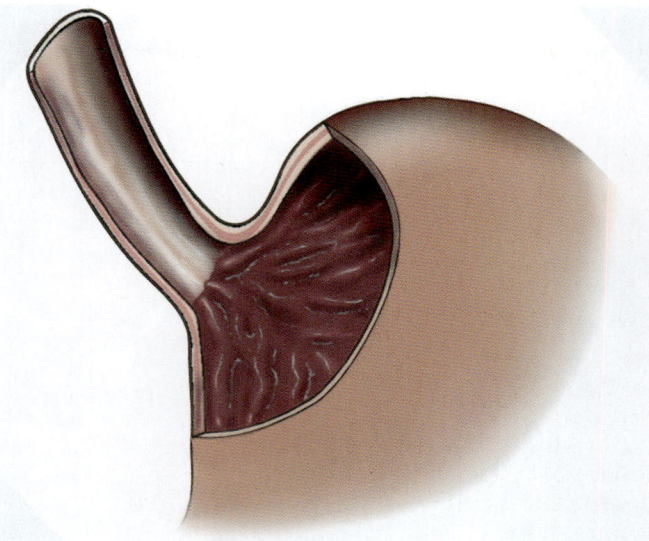

FIGURE 7.7 In this drawing, the gastroesophageal junction and the Z-line coincide, and there is no columnar-lined segment of esophagus. (Reprinted with permission from Spechler SJ. The role of gastric carditis in metaplasia and neoplasia at the gastroesophageal junction. *Gastroenterology*. 1999;117:218.)

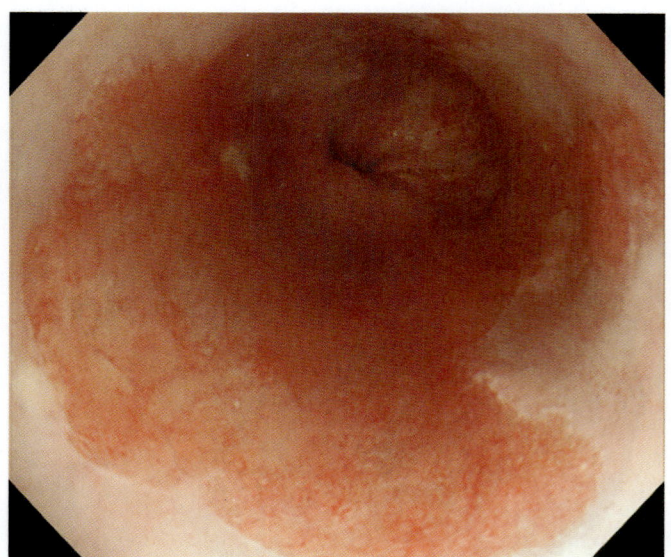

FIGURE 7.8 In this patient with long-segment Barrett esophagus, the Z-line is relatively smooth.

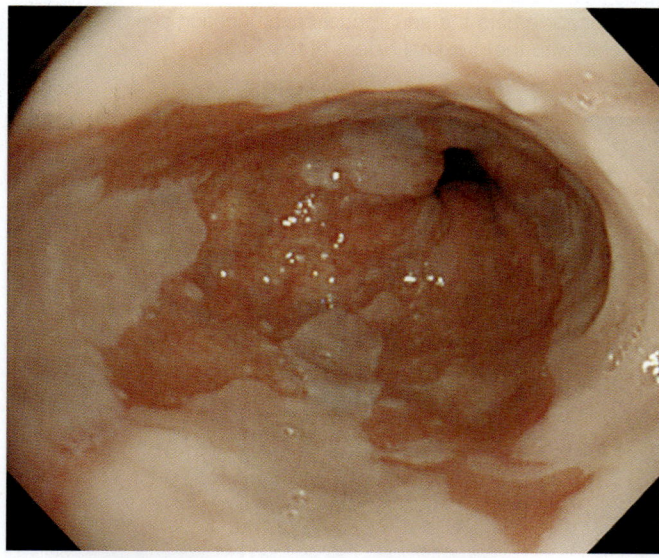

FIGURE 7.9 In this patient with short-segment Barrett esophagus, the Z-line is jagged and eccentric.

development replaces the stratified squamous epithelium that normally lines the distal esophagus.[16] Endoscopic examination is required to establish a diagnosis of Barrett esophagus, and the endoscopic impression must be confirmed by histologic evaluation of biopsy specimens from the columnar-lined esophagus. Specifically, the endoscopist must ensure that the following two criteria are fulfilled[14]: (1) columnar epithelium lines the distal esophagus and (2) biopsy specimens of the columnar-lined esophagus show specialized intestinal metaplasia. To document that columnar epithelium lines the esophagus, the endoscopist must identify both the SCJ and GEJ (see Fig. 7.3). Columnar epithelium has a reddish color and coarse texture on endoscopic examination, whereas squamous epithelium has a pale, glossy appearance. Narrow band imaging is invaluable for assessing this. The juxtaposition of these epithelia at the SCJ forms a visible line called the Z-line. When the SCJ and GEJ coincide (Fig. 7.7), then the entire esophagus is lined by squamous epithelium. When the SCJ is located proximal to the GEJ (see Fig. 7.3), then there is a columnar-lined segment of esophagus. If the endoscopist takes biopsy specimens from that columnar-lined segment and histologic evaluation shows specialized intestinal metaplasia, then the patient has Barrett esophagus (in the United States definition of Barrett).

Several classification systems for Barrett esophagus have been proposed based on the extent of columnar-lined esophagus and on the appearance of the Z-line. Perhaps the most widely used system classifies patients as having either "long segment" or "short segment" Barrett esophagus.[17] Patients have long-segment Barrett esophagus when the distance between the GEJ and the most proximal extent of the Z-line is 3 cm or more, and they have short-segment Barrett esophagus when that distance is less than 3 cm. The cutoff value of 3 cm is arbitrary, and this classification

has no clear implications regarding the pathogenesis of the condition or the clinical management of affected patients. Furthermore, there can be substantial variation in the appearance of the Z-line among patients with Barrett esophagus (Figs. 7.8 to 7.10), and the short-long classification provides no specific information about that appearance.

In 2000 Wallner et al. proposed the ZAP (*Z*-line *AP*pearance) classification for evaluating the SCJ. The ZAP classification has four categories as follows[18]: Grade 0—the Z-line is sharp and circular; grade I—the Z-line is irregular and there are tonguelike protrusions and/or islands of columnar epithelium; grade II—there is a distinct, obvious tongue of columnar epithelium less than

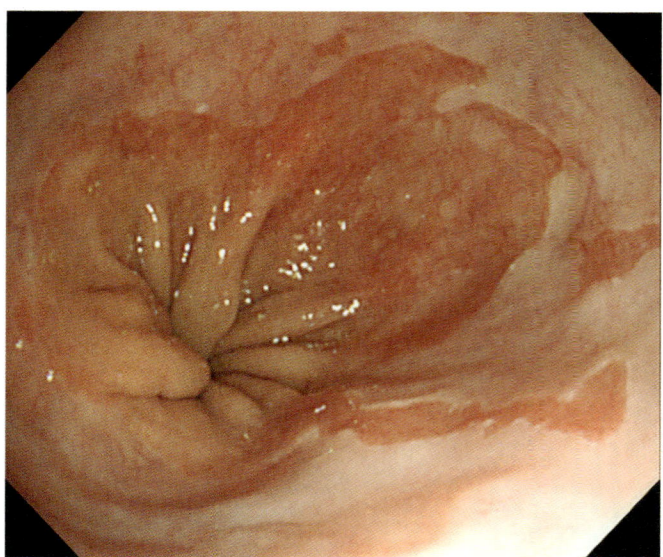

FIGURE 7.10 In this patient with short-segment Barrett esophagus, the Z-line extends approximately 2 cm above the gastroesophageal junction (the tops of the gastric folds) on the right, but there is virtually no columnar-lined esophagus on the left.

3 cm in length; grade III—there are distinct tongues of columnar epithelium greater than 3 cm in length, or there is a cephalad displacement of the Z-line greater than 3 cm. The likelihood of finding intestinal metaplasia (and hence having Barrett esophagus) was shown to increase significantly with increasing ZAP grades, and the classification was found to have excellent reproducibility among endoscopists.[19] However, the clinical utility of the ZAP classification has not been established, and the system has not been used widely in clinical practice.

Recently, a new system has been proposed for grading Barrett esophagus called the Prague C and M criteria.[20] This system describes both the extent of circumferential metaplasia (C, measured from the GEJ to the most proximal extent of circumferential esophageal metaplasia) and the extent of the longest tongue of esophageal metaplasia (M, measured from the GEJ to the most proximal extent of esophageal metaplasia). For example, a patient classified as C2M5 has columnar metaplasia involving the distal 2 cm of the esophagus in a circumferential fashion with a tongue of metaplasia that extends 5 cm above the GEJ. One study has demonstrated excellent interobserver agreement among endoscopists using the Prague C and M criteria when columnar epithelium extends at least 1 cm above the GEJ, but poor agreement for shorter segments of esophageal columnar lining.[20] The clinical utility of this system has not been established. Some have argued that the term *Barrett esophagus* itself is artificial and that the condition has been defined variably by investigators who have imposed arbitrary criteria that fit their personal perspectives.[21] In 1996 Spechler and Goyal proposed a simple classification system as follows: Whenever columnar epithelium is seen in the esophagus, regardless of extent, the condition is called "columnar-lined esophagus." In these cases, biopsy specimens can be obtained from the esophageal columnar lining to seek specialized intestinal

metaplasia. The condition then can be classified as either "columnar-lined esophagus with specialized intestinal metaplasia" or "columnar-lined esophagus without specialized intestinal metaplasia." Despite the simplicity and conceptual appeal of this system, the term *Barrett esophagus* has become so firmly entrenched among clinicians that it is unlikely to be abandoned.

SPECIALIZED ENDOSCOPIC TECHNIQUES FOR BARRETT ESOPHAGUS

A variety of specialized endoscopic techniques are available for the evaluation of Barrett esophagus including chromoendoscopy, magnification endoscopy, narrow band imaging, endosonography, optical coherence tomography, and spectroscopy using reflectance, absorption, light-scattering, fluorescence, and Raman detection methods.[22–27] These techniques have been used to enhance the identification of both intestinal metaplasia in the esophagus and neoplasia in Barrett esophagus. Only chromoendoscopy, magnification endoscopy, and narrow band imaging will be discussed in this chapter.

In chromoendoscopy the esophageal mucosa is painted with dyes that either stain the cells that absorb them or that accumulate in mucosal crevices to enhance the architectural features of the epithelium. When potassium iodide is absorbed by squamous epithelial cells, it binds to their glycogen and stains them brown. The application of this dye can help to delineate the SCJ. For individuals who are at high risk for squamous cell cancers of the esophagus (e.g., patients who have had cancers of the head and neck, individuals living in high-incidence areas for squamous cell carcinoma such as northern China), potassium iodide staining also has been used to identify areas of early neoplasia in the squamous epithelium. Methylene blue dye is absorbed by intestinal-type cells, and this dye can be applied to identify areas of intestinal metaplasia in a columnar-lined esophagus. In addition, areas of dysplasia and early cancer in the specialized intestinal metaplasia of Barrett esophagus can be identified by their failure to absorb methylene blue. One report has shown that methylene blue application may cause DNA damage in Barrett esophagus, and so the use of this dye conceivably could be dangerous.[28] Indigo carmine is a chromoendoscopy dye that is not absorbed and is used to enhance architectural features. Cresyl violet dye stains the columnar cells that absorb it purple, and the dye also accumulates in crevices to enhance architectural features. Acetic acid, although not a dye, is often sprayed on the mucosa before chromoendoscopy as a mucolytic agent. Acetic acid application also causes the columnar epithelium to swell, and this effect may enhance the evaluation of architectural features.

In magnification endoscopy an optical zoom device is used to magnify the mucosa up to 150-fold. Magnification endoscopy can also be combined with chromoendoscopy. Investigators using this technique have identified a variety of "pit-patterns" that might be typical of the intestinal metaplasia of Barrett esophagus (Figs. 7.11 and 7.12).[29–31] Magnification endoscopy also can be combined with narrow band imaging (Fig. 7.13).

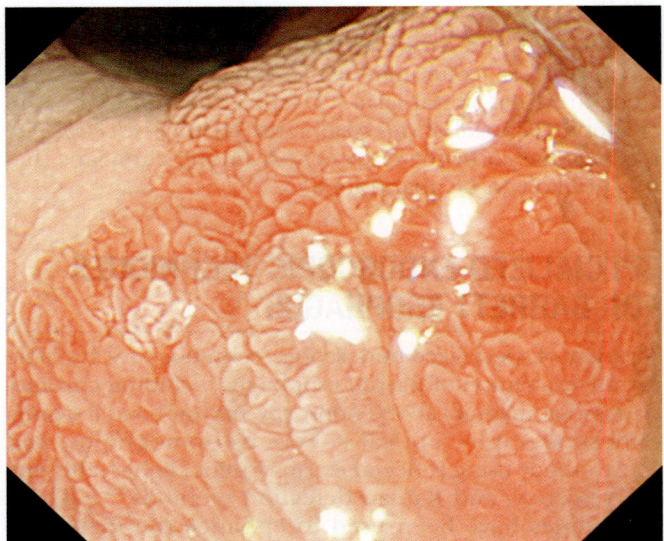

FIGURE 7.11 Magnification endoscopy of mucosa sprayed with acetic acid showing the pit pattern of columnar epithelium at the squamocolumnar junction. The relatively featureless squamous epithelium is seen adjacent to the columnar epithelium in the upper left corner of the slide.

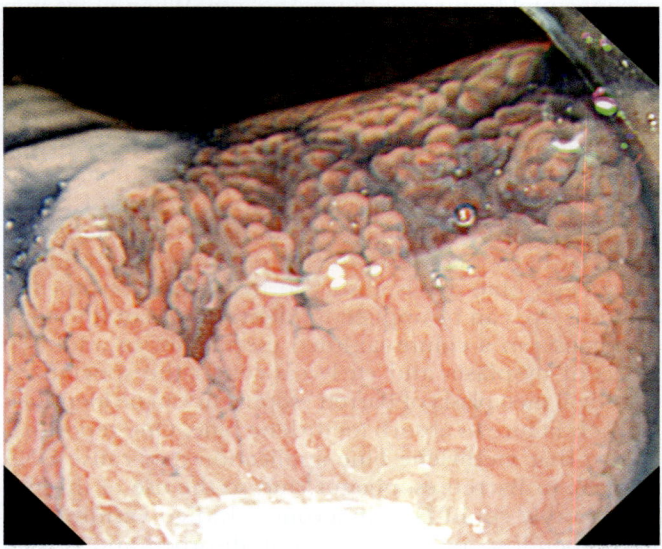

FIGURE 7.12 Magnification endoscopy of the region shown in Fig. 7.11 after application of indigo carmine dye.

ENDOSCOPIC DIAGNOSIS OF REFLUX ESOPHAGITIS

Gastroesophageal reflux disease (GERD) has been defined as the condition that develops when the reflux of stomach contents causes troublesome symptoms and/or complications.[32] Heartburn is the most common symptom of GERD, and tissue injury results when esophageal epithelial cells succumb to the damaging effects of the refluxed acid and pepsin. When these caustic agents cause macroscopic injury to the esophageal epithelium, the endoscopist can

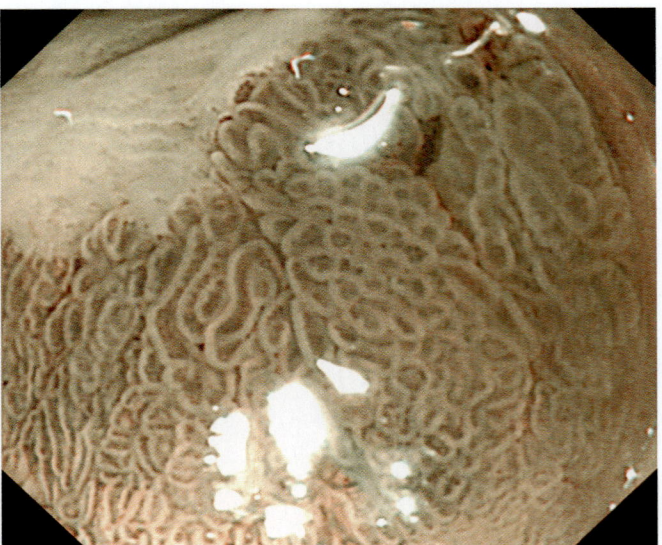

FIGURE 7.13 Magnification endoscopy of the region shown in Fig. 7.11 combined with narrow band imaging.

make a diagnosis of reflux esophagitis. However, more than 50% of patients who have typical GERD symptoms have normal endoscopic examinations.[33,34] Thus it appears that GERD usually does not cause visible damage to the esophageal mucosa in most patients.

Mild changes of GERD that may be visible to the endoscopist include mucosal erythema, edema, hypervascularity, friability, and blurring of the SCJ. However, identification of those changes is a subjective skill, and agreement among endoscopists regarding the presence of such minimal signs of reflux esophagitis can be very poor.[35,36] More severe GERD can result in esophageal erosions and ulcerations. Histologically, erosions are defined as superficial necrotic defects that do not penetrate the muscularis mucosae, whereas ulcerations are deeper defects that extend through the muscularis mucosae into the submucosa.[37] Endoscopically, these peptic esophageal lesions are identified on the basis of their gross features, and clinicians seldom have histologic confirmation that the lesions they call "esophageal ulcers" in fact have breached the muscularis mucosae. Thus the distinction between an esophageal ulceration and an erosion usually is based on a subjective assessment of the depth of the necrotic lesion. One modern system for grading the severity of reflux esophagitis, the Los Angeles classification, avoids the problem of distinguishing erosions from ulcerations by referring to both as "mucosal breaks."[38]

More than 30 systems for the classification of reflux esophagitis have been proposed over the past few decades.[38] The endoscopic criteria for three of the most widely used systems are listed in Table 7.1.[36,38,39] All of the proposed systems have limitations, and no one system has been shown to be clearly superior to another for establishing the diagnosis of GERD or for predicting the response to treatment. Arguably the best validated and most widely used system now is the Los Angeles classification that was proposed at the World Congress of Gastroenterology meeting in Los Angeles in 1994.[38] In this system a

TABLE 7.1 Classification Systems for Reflux Esophagitis

THE SAVARY-MILLER CLASSIFICATION

Grade 0	Normal mucosa
Grade I	Discrete areas of erythema
Grade II	Noncircumferential erosions
Grade III	Circumferential erosions
Grade IV	Gastroesophageal reflux disease complications (ulcers, strictures, Barrett esophagus)

THE MUSE (*M*ETAPLASIA, *U*LCERATION, *S*TRICTURE, *E*ROSION) CLASSIFICATION

	Metaplasia	Ulceration	Stricture	Erosion
Grade 0	M0 absent	U0 absent	S0 absent	E0 absent
Grade 1	M1 one	U1 one	S1 > 9 mm	E1 one
Grade 2	M2 circumferential	U2 ≥ 2	S2 ≤ 9 mm	E2 circumferential

THE LOS ANGELES CLASSIFICATION

Grade A	≥1 mucosal break <5 mm long that does not extend between the tops of 2 mucosal folds
Grade B	≥1 mucosal break >5 mm long that does not extend between the tops of 2 mucosal folds
Grade C	≥1 mucosal break that extends between the tops of ≥2 mucosal folds involving <75% of the esophageal circumference
Grade D	≥1 mucosal break that involves ≥75% of the esophageal circumference

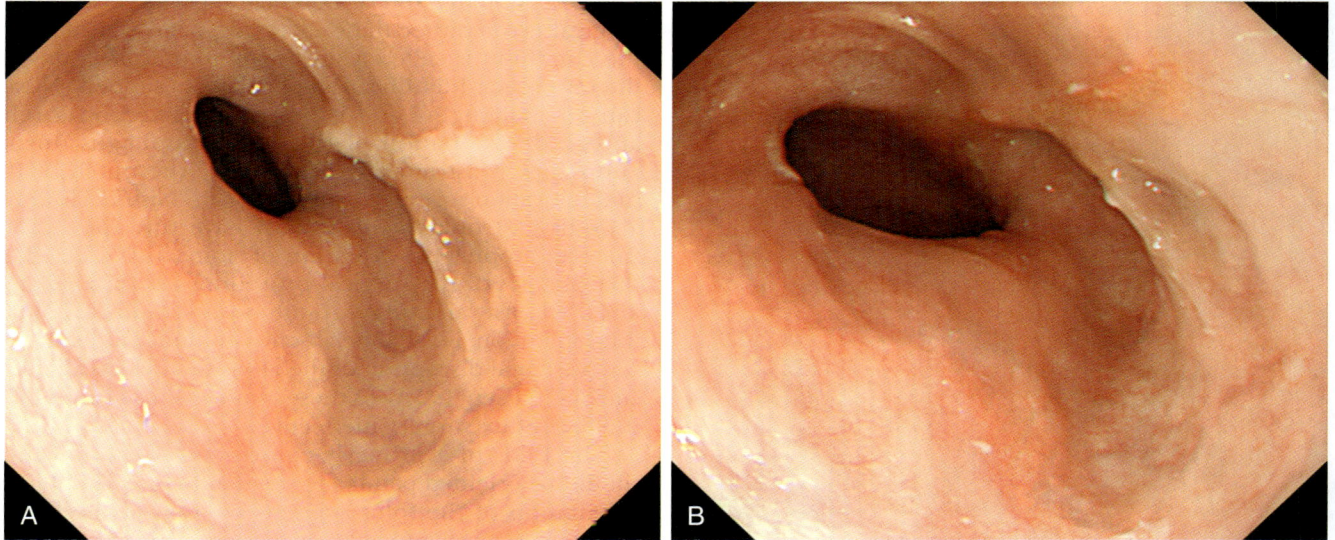

FIGURE 7.14 (A) Endoscopic photograph of Los Angeles grade B esophagitis. There is a mucosal break defined as "an area of slough or erythema with a discrete line of demarcation from the adjacent, more normal-looking mucosa." Notice the whitish exudates covering the mucosal break, which is greater than 5 mm in length. In addition, there is scarring of the distal esophagus, indicated by the fibrous strands that run perpendicular to the mucosal break at the 12- and 5-o'clock positions. (B) Same area as shown in (A) after the whitish exudates have been washed off. The mucosal break is still visible but less prominent.

mucosal break is defined as "an area of slough or erythema with a discrete line of demarcation from the adjacent, more normal-looking mucosa" (Fig. 7.14). Esophagitis is graded on a scale of A to D depending on the length and circumferential extent of the mucosal breaks (Figs. 7.14 and 7.15). Los Angeles grades C and D represent severe reflux esophagitis. Originally, grade D esophagitis was defined as a mucosal break that involved the entire circumference of the esophagus, but this was modified in 1999 to the criterion shown in Table 7.1 because it can be difficult to ascertain that a mucosal break is completely circumferential.[36]

ENDOSCOPIC EVALUATION OF PATIENTS WHO HAVE HAD ANTIREFLUX SURGERY

The two most commonly used fundoplication procedures (Nissen and Toupet) create characteristic folds in the proximal stomach that are best appreciated with the endoscope in the retroflexed position.[40] The folds of the fundoplication should be located just below the diaphragm (Fig. 7.16). If the folds are seen above the diaphragm, it is an indication that the fundoplication has herniated into the chest, which usually results from

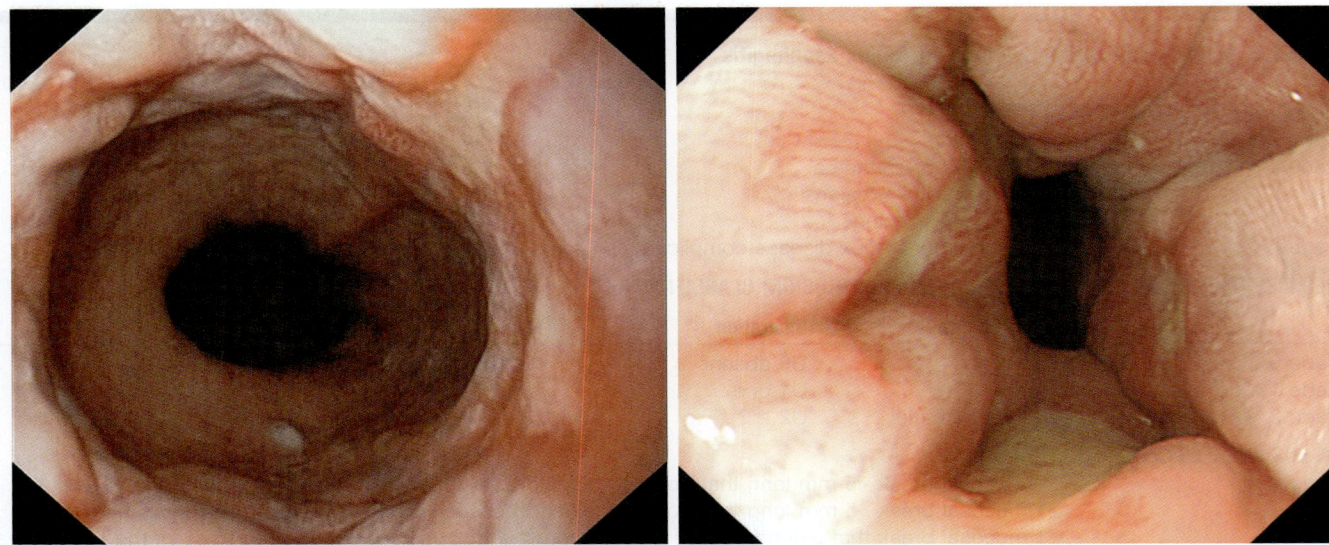

FIGURE 7.15 Two examples of Los Angeles grade C esophagitis.

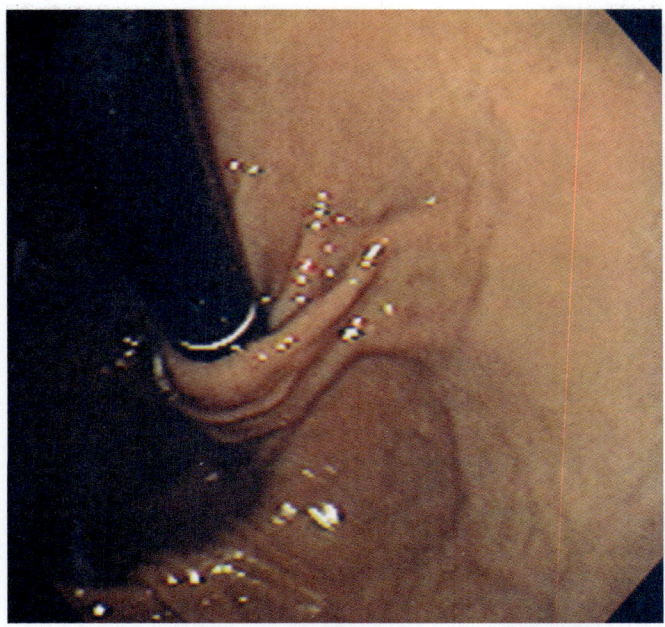

FIGURE 7.16 Endoscopic photograph of an anatomically correct Nissen fundoplication, retroflexed view. The fundoplication folds' span is located below the diaphragm, and the folds run parallel to the white distance line on the endoscope. (Reprinted with permission from Spechler SJ. The management of patients who have "failed" antireflux surgery. *Am J Gastroenterol.* 2004;99:552.)

disruption of the crural repair. If there is a pouch of stomach proximal to the folds of the fundoplication, the condition is called a "slipped" fundoplication (e.g., a "slipped Nissen"). A slipped fundoplication can occur in two ways: (1) the fundoplication is fashioned in the correct location but a portion of the stomach later herniates ("slips") through the fundoplication, or (2) the surgeon mistakes the proximal stomach for the distal esophagus and inadvertently fashions the fundoplication around the stomach. Although the latter situation represents an initial surgical error rather than a later slippage (herniation), the condition is called a slipped fundoplication despite the misnomer. Identification of a low or "slipped" Nissen can be challenging and is best appreciated on careful antegrade evaluation of the distal esophagus during endoscopy. Gastric rugal folds above the pinch of the fundoplication suggest a low or "slipped" Nissen. However, a Collis gastroplasty will usually have this appearance since an esophageal extension of stomach is created, so the specifics of the surgical procedure are important to know when evaluating patients with symptoms after a fundoplication. Finally, the absence of fundoplication folds suggests total disruption of the antireflux procedure (the "missin' Nissen"). Any of these abnormalities can render the antireflux surgery ineffective.

The folds of a properly constructed fundoplication should be oriented parallel to the diaphragm. An oblique orientation of the folds suggests twisting of the fundoplication or improper construction of the wrap using the body rather than the fundus of the stomach (Fig. 7.17).[40] Either of these conditions can cause postoperative gastroesophageal reflux, dysphagia, or both. The folds should measure approximately 1 to 2 cm in span. A wider span indicates a too-generous fundoplication that can cause dysphagia. A paraesophageal hernia also can cause dysphagia by pressing on the distal esophagus (Fig. 7.18). The herniated portion of the stomach in these cases often originates from the fundoplication itself and may result from attempts to construct a "floppy" wrap.

ESOPHAGEAL CANCER

Esophageal cancers that are recognizable by conventional endoscopy appear as masses that protrude into the lumen of the esophagus. The masses are often nodular, irregular, and ulcerated, and the tumors may have a different color and texture than the surrounding normal mucosa. Squamous cell and adenocarcinomas of the esophagus cannot

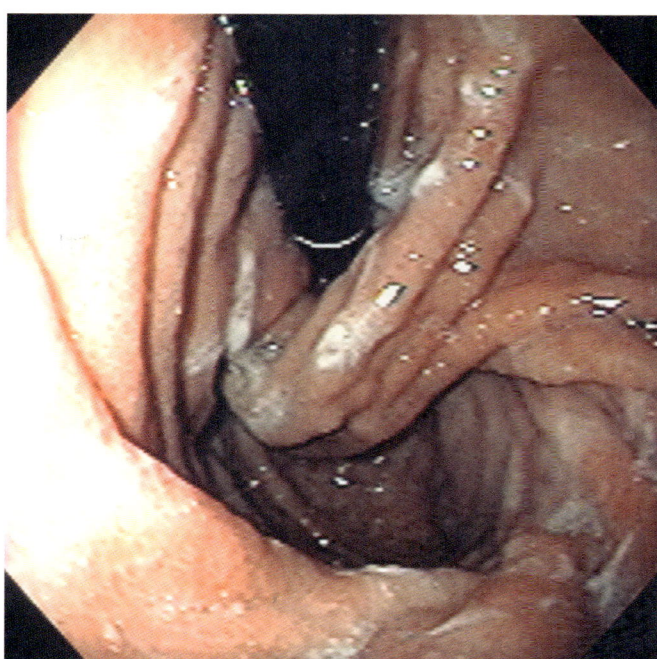

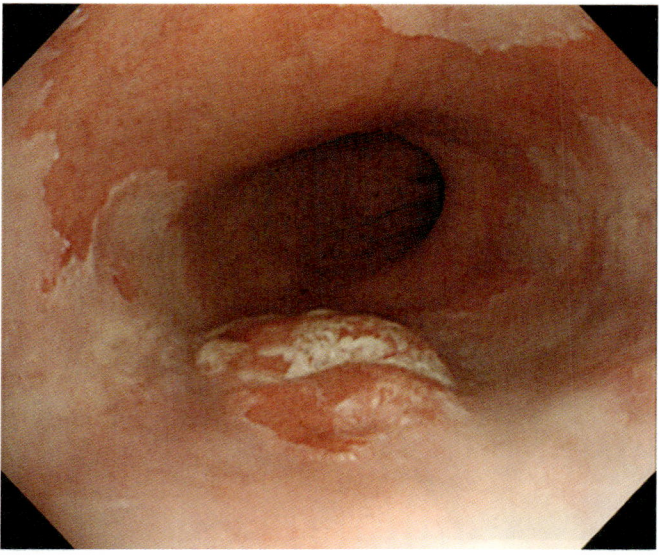

FIGURE 7.19 Early cancer in Barrett esophagus. Note the background of flat Barrett epithelium with the nodular mass in the foreground.

FIGURE 7.17 Endoscopic photograph of a slipped Nissen fundoplication, retroflexed view. The fundoplication folds are oriented obliquely to the white distance line on the endoscope, and there is a pouch of stomach proximal to the folds. (Reproduced with permission from Spechler SJ. The management of patients who have "failed" antireflux surgery. *Am J Gastroenterol.* 2004;99:552.)

be differentiated on the basis of endoscopic appearance, but the location of the tumor and its associated features may provide important clues regarding the histology. Tumors that involve the proximal and middle esophagus and that are separated from the stomach by a segment of squamous epithelium are very likely to be squamous cell carcinomas. Tumors of the distal esophagus can be either squamous cell carcinomas or adenocarcinomas. If there is associated Barrett esophagus, the tumor is likely to be an adenocarcinoma (Figs. 7.19 and 7.20). However, adenocarcinomas that cause symptoms often have grown so large that they have obliterated any evidence of the Barrett esophagus that spawned them. It can be especially difficult to determine the origin of an adenocarcinoma that straddles the GEJ (Fig. 7.21). Such tumors can arise either from Barrett esophagus or from the proximal stomach. If no Barrett esophagus is apparent, investigators have relied on the location of the tumor epicenter to classify the tumor as esophageal or "cardiac."

EOSINOPHILIC ESOPHAGITIS

Eosinophilic esophagitis (EoE) is a modern esophageal disorder that has become recognized widely only within the past decade.[41,42] EoE appears to be a manifestation of food allergy in which eosinophils infiltrate the esophageal epithelium, causing symptoms and tissue damage mediated by cytokines released from the eosinophils and surrounding tissues. The disorder commonly is diagnosed in men in the fourth and fifth decades of life who describe a long history of dysphagia for solid foods, often with hospital visits for food impactions. Heartburn is also a common complaint, and it can sometimes be difficult to distinguish EoE from GERD. Patients frequently have a personal and family history of allergic disorders such as asthma, atopic dermatitis, eczema, hay fever, and food allergies. Children with EoE may have symptoms of abdominal

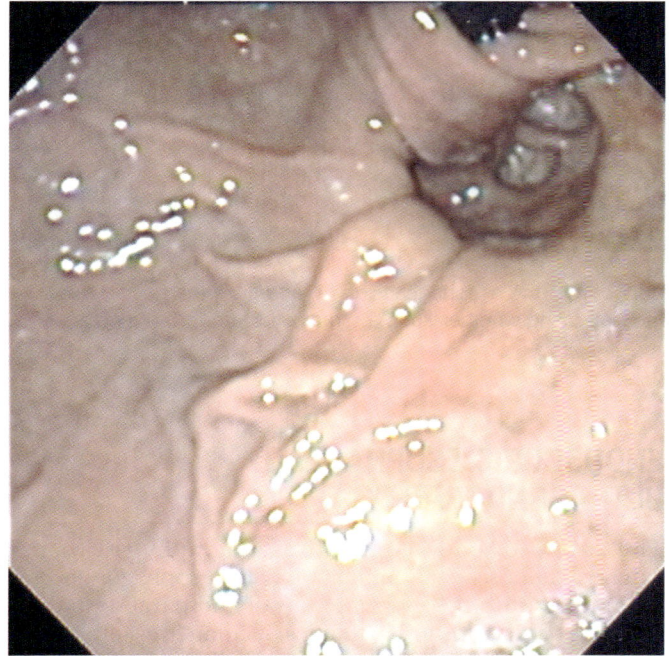

FIGURE 7.18 Endoscopic photograph of a paraesophageal hernia, retroflexed view. The herniated pouch of stomach is located next to the fundoplication folds. (Reproduced with permission from Spechler SJ. The management of patients who have "failed" antireflux surgery. *Am J Gastroenterol.* 2004;99:552.)

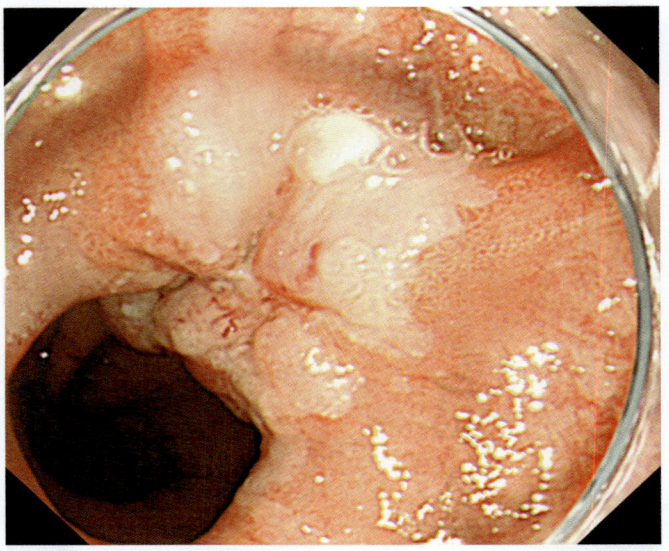

FIGURE 7.20 Ulcerated cancer of the distal esophagus.

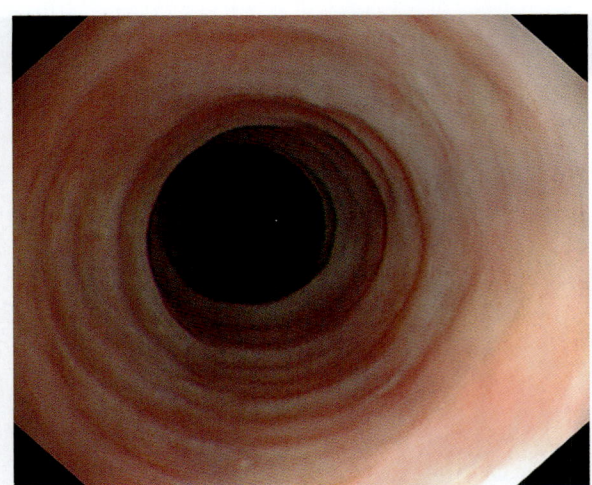

FIGURE 7.22 Ringed esophagus in a patient with eosinophilic esophagitis.

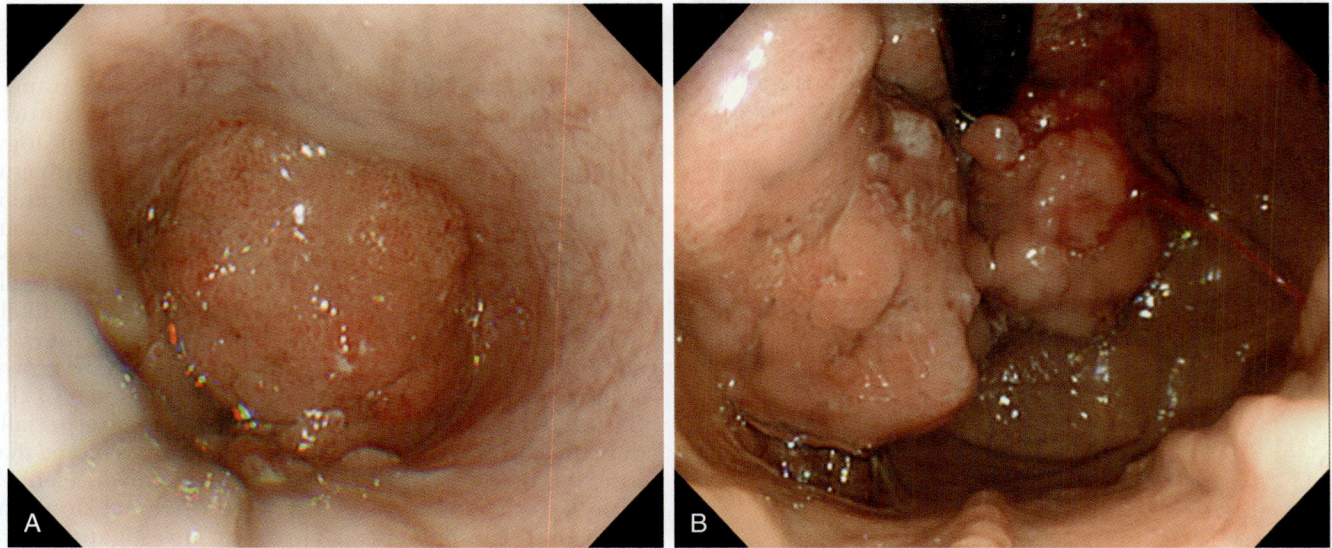

FIGURE 7.21 Adenocarcinoma of the gastroesophageal junction photographed from the esophageal side (A) and from the gastric side (B). If there is no Barrett epithelium seen in the esophagus, it is not possible to determine whether such a tumor originated from the distal esophagus or from the gastric cardia.

pain, heartburn, vomiting, feeding disorders, and failure to thrive.

Multiple esophageal rings are common endoscopic findings in patients with EoE (Fig. 7.22). When pronounced, the rings may give the esophagus a trachea-like appearance. Other common esophageal endoscopic abnormalities include vertical furrows (Fig. 7.23), strictures, "white specks" (which are 1- to 3-mm-diameter eosinophilic exudates), and small-caliber esophagus. In up to 25% of cases the esophagus appears normal endoscopically. Esophageal biopsy is needed to establish the diagnosis. The esophageal mucosa is unusually fragile in EoE, and esophageal dilations often are complicated by extensive mucosal tears that can be quite painful.

ENDOSCOPIC ESOPHAGEAL ULTRASONOGRAPHY

The advent of endoscopic ultrasonography (EUS) has extended endoscopic examination of the esophagus beyond the mucosa into the esophageal wall and paraesophageal tissues. The diagnostic capabilities of cutaneous ultrasound have been expanded by endoscopic placement of ultrasound transducers adjacent to the gastrointestinal mucosa. These transducers, operating at relatively high frequencies, provide detailed examination of the esophageal wall and surrounding tissues. EUS is the most significant advance in the diagnosis of esophageal disease since the introduction

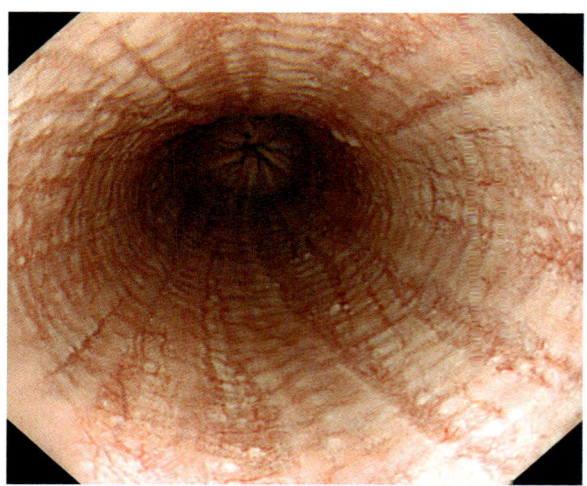

FIGURE 7.23 Vertical furrows in the esophagus of a patient with eosinophilic esophagitis.

of flexible fiberoptic endoscopy. These intracorporeal examinations have proved beneficial in the diagnosis and treatment of both benign and malignant diseases of the esophagus and adjacent structures.

FUNDAMENTALS OF ULTRASONOGRAPHY

Sound is produced by vibration of a source within a medium. Vibration produces waves, cyclic compression, and rarefaction (expansion) of molecules in the medium, thus transmitting the sound wave through the medium. The number of cycles (compression and rarefaction) of a sound wave occurring in 1 second is the frequency and is measured in hertz (Hz). The frequency of sound waves audible to the human ear is between 20 and 20,000 Hz. Sound waves with frequencies higher than 20,000 Hz are ultrasound waves. Frequencies used in medical ultrasound imaging range from 1 to 20 million Hz (1 to 20 MHz).

Ultrasound waves may be produced by electrical excitation of a piezoelectric crystal. The application of voltage across a crystal causes it to deform. Alternating electrical energy vibrates the crystal and produces sound waves. Conversely, if a sound wave deforms a crystal, electrical energy is produced. It is this ability to convert electrical energy into sound energy and, conversely, to convert sound energy into electrical energy that allows these crystals to function as both transmitters and receivers (i.e., as *transducers*). These transducers are responsive to a limited range of frequencies; hence more than one transducer may be required for an ultrasound examination.

The speed of a sound wave within a medium (tissue) is defined by the following relationship: $V = (K/p)^{1/2}$, where V is the velocity of the sound wave, K is the bulk modulus of the tissue (a measure of stiffness), and p is the density of the tissue.

The resistance to passage of a sound wave through tissue is called the acoustic impedance (Z), which is defined by the following relationship: $Z = pV = (pK)^{1/2}$.

Sound waves travel best through dense or elastic tissue. Absorption of some of the energy of an ultrasound wave occurs as the wave passes through tissue. The amount of absorption is determined by tissue characteristics and the frequency of the sound wave. Higher-frequency waves have greater absorption.

Interactions occurring as a sound wave encounters different tissues are critical to the diagnostic capabilities of ultrasound. As a sound wave passes from one tissue to the next, a portion of the wave is transmitted and a portion is reflected. The reflected wave is received by the transducer, thereby providing the diagnostic information of ultrasound. The difference in acoustic impedance between the two tissues and the angle at which the sound wave enters the new medium (angle of incidence) determine the portion of the wave that is reflected and the portion that is transmitted. In tissue with similar acoustic impedance, most of the wave is transmitted. Soft tissue has excellent transmission qualities; the density and velocity vary only by 12% to 14% among different soft tissues. Because acoustic impedance is the product of velocity and density, the product of these small changes results in a 22% difference in acoustic impedance between fat and muscle.[43] Useless, bright echo images are obtained when an ultrasound wave encounters air or bone. Air is very compressible and of low density, whereas bone, although dense, has low compressibility and high reflectivity. These properties account for the poor transmission of ultrasound waves from tissue to air or tissue to bone. The amount of reflected sound is also related to the angle of incidence: as the angle of incidence increases, less sound is reflected. In addition, sound waves are bent as they travel from one tissue to the next. This process is termed *refraction*.

Absorption, reflection, and refraction are major sources of energy loss. Some ultrasound wave energy is also lost by scattering (diffusion), which occurs when a sound wave encounters heterogeneous tissue. Tiny particles within tissue (such as fat in muscle), smaller than the ultrasound wavelength, scatter the ultrasound wave. As a sound wave passes through tissue, a portion of its energy is lost; this is called *attenuation*. Attenuation increases as more tissues are encountered and as the wave travels farther from the source. If the returning ultrasound wave is not processed, the same tissue would be imaged differently, depending on its distance from the transducer. The intensity of the returning waves must be amplified (gain) to ensure that distant waves are correctly represented. Attenuation increases as ultrasound frequency increases.

Resolution is the ability to discriminate among different tissues with ultrasound waves. Depth or axial resolution is the ability to differentiate between two tissues along the path of the ultrasound wave. Lateral resolution is the ability to distinguish between adjacent tissues. Transducer characteristics and focus determine resolution. Higher frequencies allow better resolution but decreased tissue penetration.

Pulse-echo technique is used in EUS. Ultrasound waves are emitted for a brief period, followed by a subsequent listening period during which the reflected waves are received. The returning ultrasound waves are displayed such that the brightness is proportional to the amplitude of the returning ultrasound waves. This is known as *B-mode ultrasonography*. Because the amplitude is presented in a range from white to gray to black, the display is also termed *grayscale ultrasound*. Individual scans are shown at a rate at which the eye cannot detect single images (12/ second). This fast-frame display is called *real-time ultrasound* and allows the ultrasonographer to study tissue temporally as well as spatially.

INSTRUMENTS AND TECHNIQUES

Because EUS does not provide adequate endoscopic inspection of the upper gastrointestinal tract, every ultrasound study should be preceded by a standard flexible endoscopic upper gastrointestinal examination. This provides precise location and mucosal definition (including biopsy) of the esophageal lesion and guides the ultrasound examiner. The ultrasound endoscope is generally passed blindly through the oropharynx and hypopharynx. Care must be taken because the distal tip containing the transducer is rigid. For complete examination, the endoscope must be passed beyond the esophagus into the stomach.

In the past, the radial mechanical ultrasound endoscope (Fig. 7.24) was the principal instrument used for EUS. The ultrasound transducer is housed in the tip of the endoscope. It produces up to a 360-degree sector scan perpendicular to the transducer tip. Because the transducer is adjacent to tissues to be examined, higher frequencies than those used in extracorporeal ultrasound can be used. In the newest models, a range of transducer frequencies, from 5 to 20 MHz, are available. These transducers allow adequate visualization of anatomic structures to a depth of 3 to 12 cm. An acceptable acoustic interface between the transducer and the tissue being examined must be obtained to ensure good-quality ultrasound images. This is most commonly accomplished by covering the tip of the endoscope with a latex balloon, which can be filled with water to provide an excellent acoustic interface (see Fig. 7.24). A less commonly used technique is rapid insufflation of the esophageal lumen with water. This provides an excellent, but transient acoustic interface without the tissue compression that may occur with the latex balloon. Current echoendoscopes also provide a video endoscopic image, albeit with a somewhat limited view in a forward oblique direction. The control section contains the deflection controls and air/water and suction valves, similar to those on a standard endoscope (see Fig. 7.24). A water inflation/ deflation system for the balloon is incorporated into the air/water and suction valve mechanisms. A direct-current motor and drive mechanism that rotates the ultrasound transducer are housed in the control section. Current ultrasound endoscopes are totally immersible in liquids.

A radial mechanical blind probe (Fig. 7.25) is available for the evaluation of esophageal strictures. This echoendoscope provides images similar to those of larger-diameter radial mechanical echoendoscopes, but it has no endoscopic optical capabilities and is less than 8 mm in diameter. More commonly used in current practice are higher-frequency miniprobes passed through the operating channel of standard endoscopes (Fig. 7.26); these miniprobes provide radial images from 12 to 30 MHz.

These three instruments are used in conjunction with an image processor (Fig. 7.27). The image processor allows for adjustment of gain, contrast, and sensitivity time control to regulate the strength of the returning echo at different depths. Onscreen calibration and labeling can be done with the image processor. The image may be displayed on a video monitor or stored digitally or on videotape. The image processor has been refined and

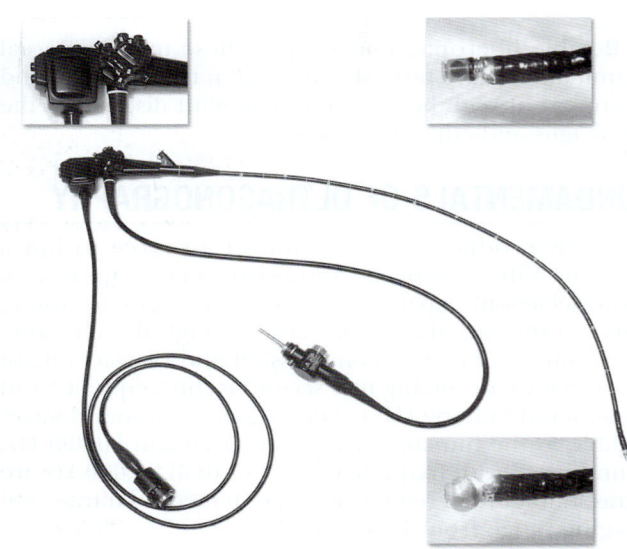

FIGURE 7.24 The Olympus GF-UM130 ultrasound endoscope. *Upper left inset*, The control section contains the deflection controls and air/water and suction valves similar to those on a standard endoscope. *Upper right inset*, The ultrasound transducer is housed in the tip of the endoscope. The forward oblique viewing endoscope and suction channel are proximal to the ultrasound transducer. *Lower right inset*, The distal tip of the ultrasound endoscope with the water-inflated contact balloon, which covers the ultrasound transducer.

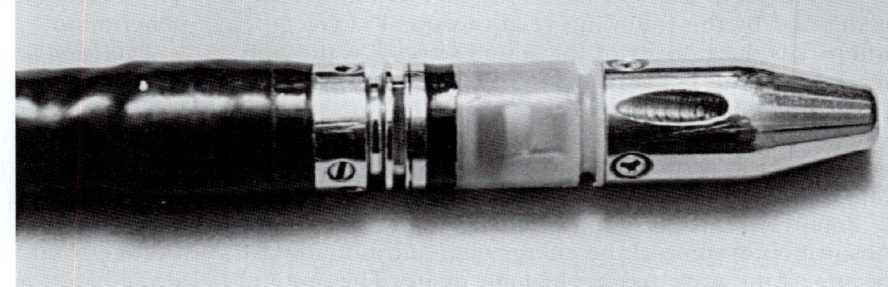

FIGURE 7.25 Radial mechanical blind probe. The tip is tapered to allow passage through tight strictures. The radial ultrasound transducer is positioned behind the tapered tip.

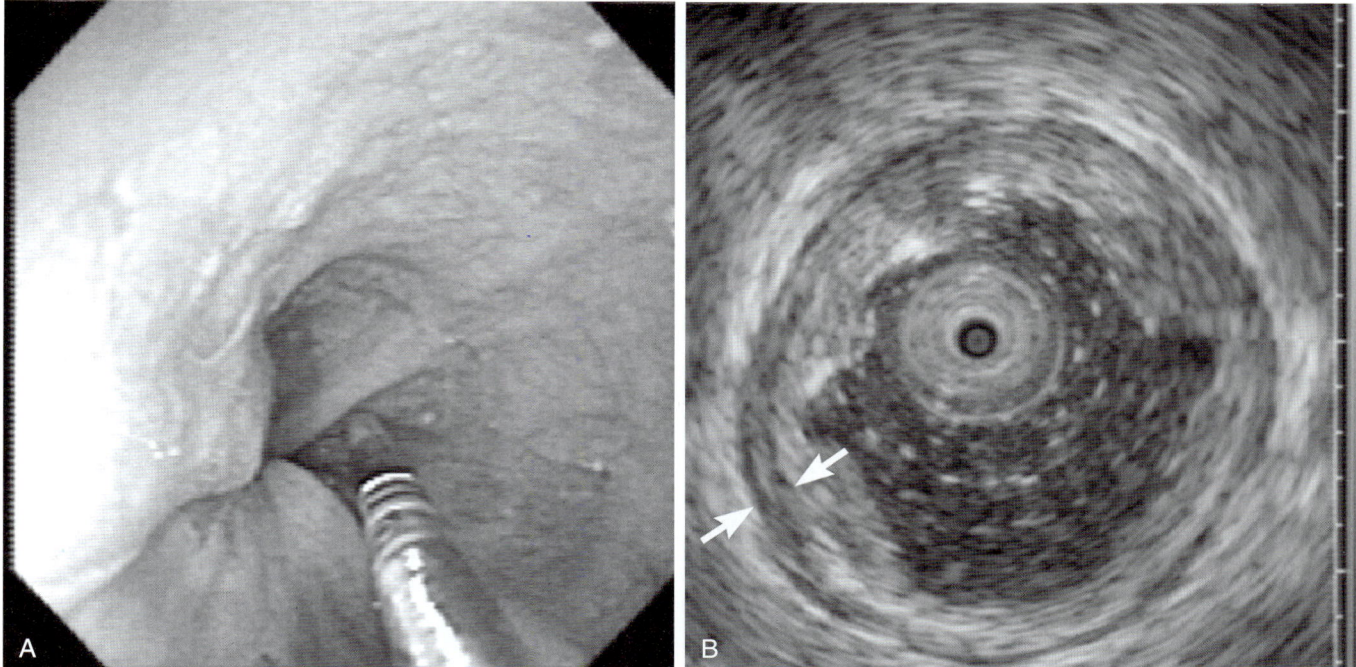

FIGURE 7.26 (A) High-frequency (12 to 30 MHz) miniprobe passed through the operating channel of a standard endoscope. (B) Miniprobe ultrasound image of a normal esophagus. The probe is not centered in the nondistended esophageal lumen. The mucosa and submucosa are the inner hyperechoic layer. The muscularis propria *(arrows)* is the inner hypoechoic layer.

miniaturized with successive generations of endoscopic ultrasound equipment.

Newer electronic endoscopes are now more commonly used. The electronic radial echoendoscope provides an enhanced image as a result of use of tissue harmonic echo and can provide color and power Doppler (Fig. 7.28). The curvilinear electronic echoendoscope (Fig. 7.29) also has video endoscopic capability and can produce up to a 180-degree oblique forward field. It allows a range of scanning frequencies from 5 to 10 MHz with a depth of penetration of 4 cm or greater. This echoendoscope provides color and power Doppler examination and direct visualization of cytology needles passed into and beyond the esophageal wall.

Radial and curvilinear echoendoscopes have increased the accuracy of EUS. For diagnostic purposes, the radial scanner is preferable because it allows a 360-degree view and is known as the "workhorse" of EUS. Because the radial scanner does not allow safe directed passage of a needle into the esophageal wall or adjacent tissue if a tissue sample is required for cytologic evaluation, the electronic curvilinear echoendoscope is used. It is possible to perform both diagnosis and fine-needle aspiration (FNA) with the electronic linear echoendoscope alone, but the limitation in viewing field requires significant torque on the insertion tube to image the esophageal wall and adjacent tissues for a 360-degree view. However comparable results for staging examinations have been reported with the electronic curvilinear echoendoscope.[44] Both systems must be available for adequate EUS evaluation. Electronic radial and linear echoendoscopic examinations can be accomplished using one image processor (Fig. 7.30).

ESOPHAGEAL WALL AND ULTRASOUND ANATOMY

The esophageal wall is composed of three distinct layers: mucosa, submucosa, and muscularis propria (Fig. 7.31). The mucosa has three elements: epithelium, lamina propria, and muscularis mucosae. The innermost layer is stratified, nonkeratinizing squamous epithelium. It is separated and isolated from the remainder of the esophageal wall by a basement membrane. Immediately beneath is the lamina propria. This loose matrix of collagen and elastic fibers forms a superficial undulating layer; invaginations into the epithelium produce epithelial papillae. Lymphatic channels in the lamina propria are an anatomic feature unique to the esophagus. The muscularis mucosae surrounds the lamina propria. This smooth muscle layer pleats the two inner layers of the mucosa into folds that disappear with distention of the lumen.

The submucosa is composed of connective tissues that contain a rich network of blood vessels and lymphatics. The dense submucosal lymphatic plexus facilitates early dissemination of esophageal malignancies. Submucosal glands of mixed type are characteristic of the esophagus.

The muscularis propria is the muscular sleeve that provides the propulsive force necessary for swallowing. There are two layers of muscle: an inner circular layer and an outer longitudinal layer. The upper cervical esophagus is composed entirely of striated muscle. There is a gradual transition from striated to smooth muscle within muscle bundles until the esophagus is entirely smooth muscle at the upper and midthird junction. Lymphatic channels

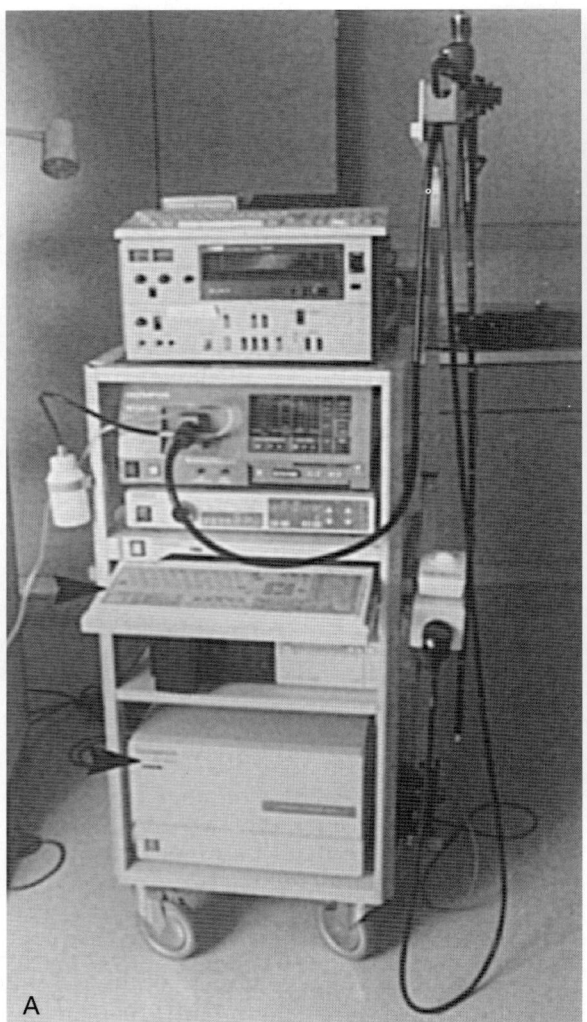
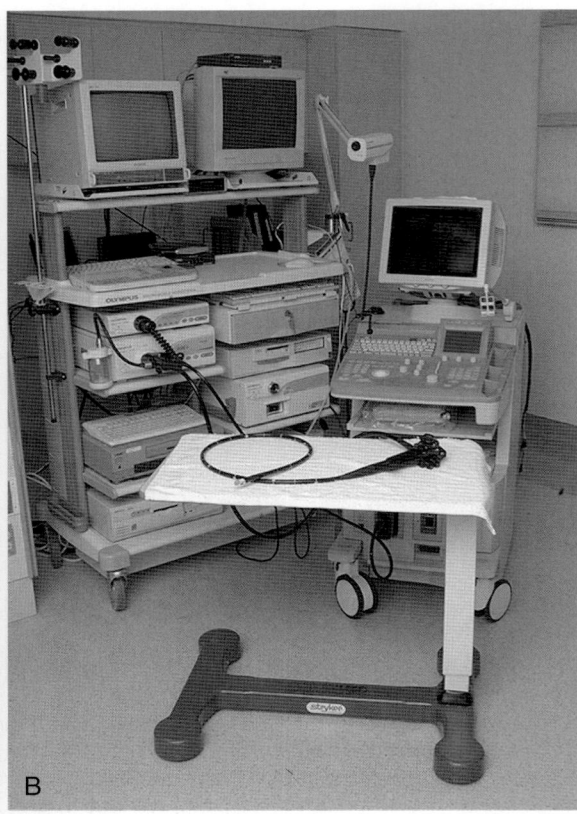

FIGURE 7.27 (A) The Olympus EU-M20 image processor *(lower arrowhead)* is rack-mounted in a standard cart, which includes the other essential endoscopic equipment. The keyboard *(upper arrowhead)* can be used to measure and mark ultrasound findings. (B) The complete system includes the light source rack, image processor, and ultrasound endoscope.

pierce the muscularis propria and drain into regional lymphatics or directly into the thoracic duct.

The esophagus has no investing adventitia. The paraesophageal tissue is composed of fibrofatty tissue that lies directly against the outer fibers of the muscularis propria.

The normal esophagus is usually viewed as five discrete layers by EUS (Fig. 7.32). These layers are seen as alternating hyperechoic (white) and hypoechoic (black) rings. Studies demonstrate that the five layers seen by EUS correspond to the balloon-mucosa interface, the mucosa deep to this interface, the submucosa and the acoustic interface between the submucosa and muscularis propria, the muscularis propria minus the acoustic interface between the submucosa and the muscularis propria, and the periesophageal tissue.[45,46] For clinical purposes, these layers represent the superficial mucosa, deep mucosa, submucosa, muscularis propria, and periesophageal tissue. In the upper part of the esophagus, with overdistention of the examining balloon or if the transducer is too close to the esophageal wall, only three layers of the esophageal

wall may be apparent because the superficial mucosa, deep mucosa, and submucosa compose one hyperechoic layer. The thickness of each ultrasound layer is about equal and does not represent the thickness of the tissue layer but, instead, the time that it takes the ultrasound wave to traverse this layer.

ESOPHAGEAL CARCINOMA

Staging of cancer of the esophagus and esophagogastric junction (EGJ) has been extensively changed and improved in the seventh edition of the American Joint Committee on Cancer/International Union Against Cancer (AJCC/UICC) Cancer Staging Manual (Box 7.1).[47] Changes address problems of empiric stage grouping and lack of harmonization with stomach cancer. This was accomplished by assembling worldwide data and using modern machine learning techniques for data-driven staging.[48-51] Improvements include new definitions of Tis, T4, regional lymph node, N classification, and M classification, and addition

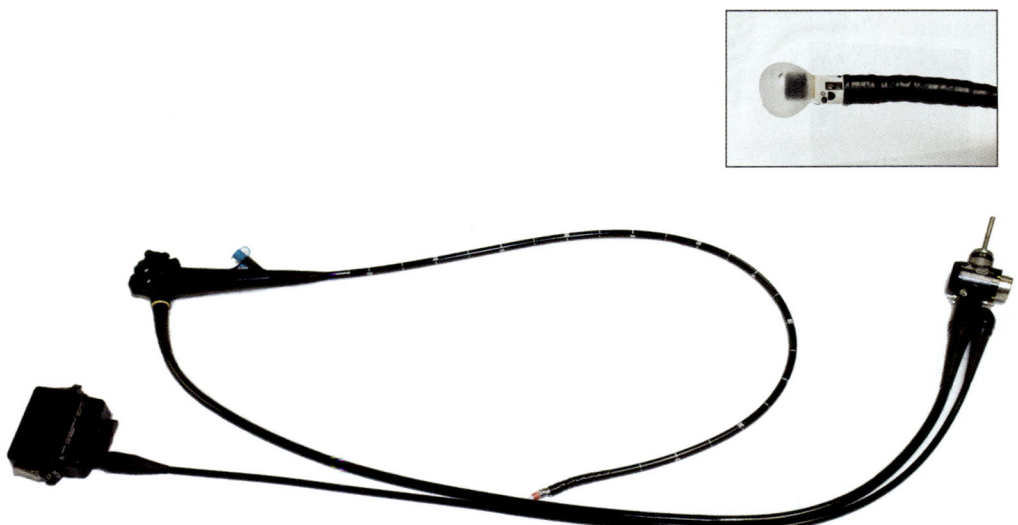

FIGURE 7.28 The Olympus GF-UE160 electronic radial echoendoscope. The electronic radial echoendoscope provides an enhanced image as a result of use of tissue harmonic echo and can provide color and power Doppler, not available in mechanical radial design. *Inset,* The tip of the Olympus GF-UE160 electronic radial echoendoscope with water-filled balloon. This tip is easier to maneuver endoscopically compared with prior models.

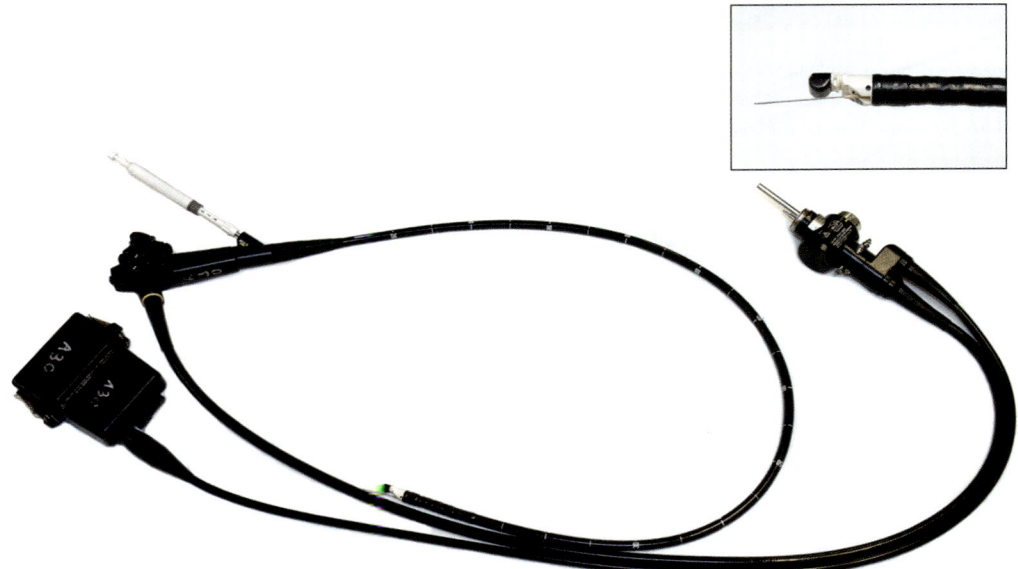

FIGURE 7.29 The Olympus GF-UC140P convex scanning linear echoendoscope. This endoscope has a high-resolution CCD (charge-coupled device) chip that provides outstanding optics and four imaging frequencies (5 to 10 MHz). It is shown with the Olympus EZ Shot aspiration needle. *Inset,* The tip of the Olympus GF-UC140P echoendoscope. Like the electronic radial echoendoscope, insertion and maneuverability are improved compared to previous iterations.

of the nonanatomic cancer characteristics: histopathologic cell type, histologic grade, and tumor location. Stage groupings were constructed by adherence to principles of staging, including monotonic decreasing survival with increasing stage group, distinct survival between groups, and homogeneous survival within groups.

Depth of tumor invasion classifies the primary tumor (T). Tis tumors are intraepithelial malignancies confined to the epithelium without invasion of the basement membrane and are now termed *high-grade dysplasia.* Tis

includes all noninvasive neoplastic epithelium that was previously called carcinoma in situ. T1 tumors breach the basement membrane to invade the lamina propria, muscularis mucosae, or the submucosa but do not invade beyond the submucosa. T1 tumors may be subclassified into T1a, tumors that invade only the mucosa, and T1b, tumors that invade the submucosa.[52] T2 tumors invade into but not beyond the muscularis propria. T3 tumors invade beyond the esophageal wall into the periesophageal tissue but do not invade adjacent structures. T4 tumors

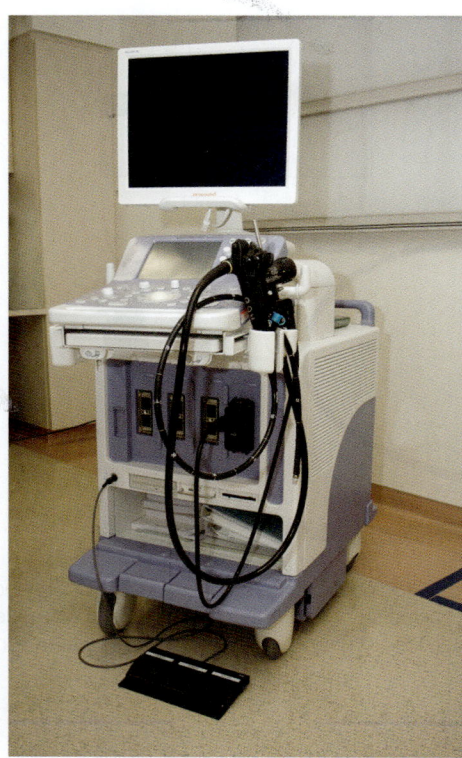

FIGURE 7.30 The Aloka ProSound ALPHA10 System. This unit supports both electronic radial and linear echoendoscopes, eliminating the need for two separate processors for esophageal ultrasonography.

directly invade structures in the vicinity of the esophagus. T4 has been subclassified as T4a and T4b; T4a tumors are resectable cancers invading adjacent structures, such as pleura, pericardium, or diaphragm. T4b tumors are unresectable cancers invading other adjacent structures, such as aorta, vertebral body, or trachea.

A regional lymph node has been redefined to include any paraesophageal lymph node extending from cervical nodes to celiac nodes. Data analyses support convenient coarse groupings of number of cancer-positive nodes (7 to 9). Regional lymph node (N) classification comprises N0 (no cancer-positive nodes), N1 (1 or 2), N2 (3 to 6), and N3 (7 or more). N classifications for cancers of the esophagus and EGJ are identical to stomach cancer N classifications.

The subclassifications M1a and M1b have been eliminated, as has MX. Distant metastases are simply designated M0, no distant metastasis, and M1, distant metastasis.

Three nonanatomic cancer characteristics— histopathologic cell type, histologic grade, and tumor location—are necessary for staging. Because AJCC seventh edition staging of cancer of the esophagus and EGJ is based on cancers arising from the epithelium, histopathologic cell type is either adenocarcinoma or squamous cell carcinoma. Because the data indicate that squamous cell carcinoma has a poorer prognosis than adenocarcinoma, a tumor of mixed histopathologic type is staged as squamous cell carcinoma. Nonmucosal cancers arising in the wall are classified according to their cell of origin.

The nonanatomic cancer characteristic histologic grade is categorized as G1, well differentiated; G2, moderately

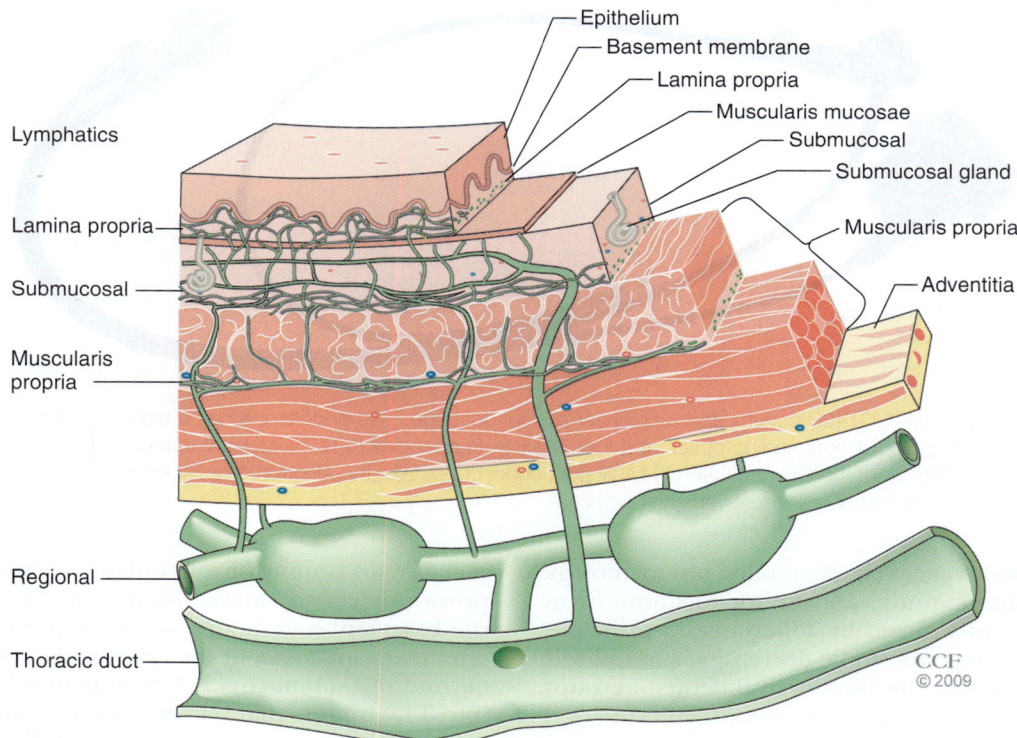

FIGURE 7.31 The esophageal wall is composed of mucosa, submucosa, and muscularis propria. The mucosa is composed of epithelium, lamina propria, and muscularis mucosae.

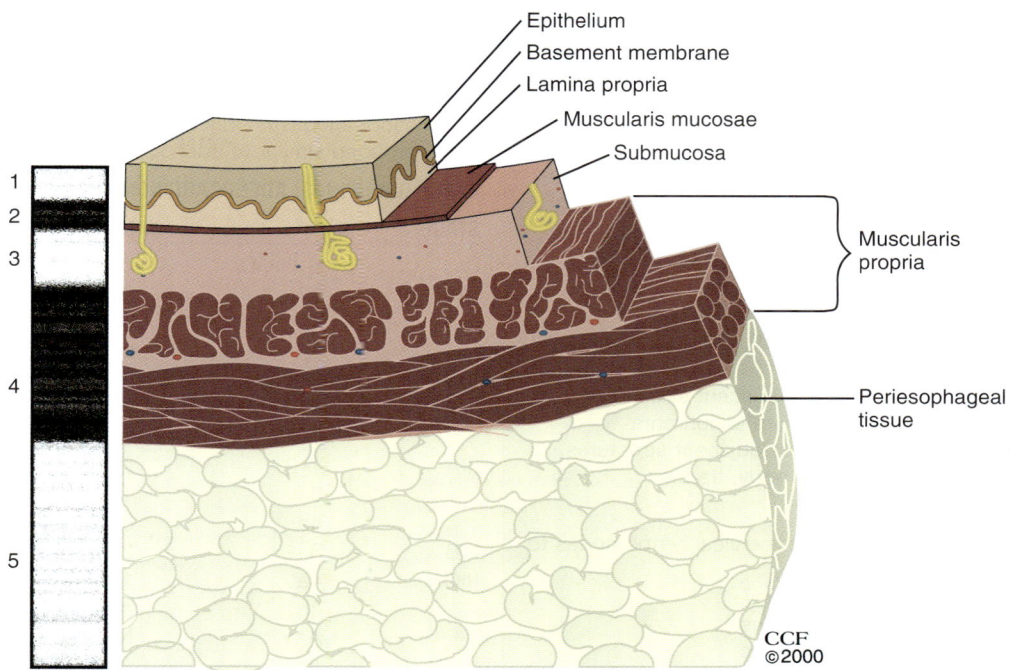

FIGURE 7.32 The esophageal wall is visualized as five alternating layers of differing echogenicity by esophageal ultrasound. The first layer, which is hyperechoic *(white),* represents the superficial mucosa (epithelium and lamina propria). The second layer, which is hypoechoic *(black),* represents the deep mucosa (muscularis mucosae). The third layer, which is hyperechoic *(white),* represents the submucosa. The fourth layer, which is hypoechoic *(black),* represents the muscularis propria. The fifth layer, which is hyperechoic *(white)* is the periesophageal tissue.

differentiated; G3, poorly differentiated; or G4, undifferentiated. Because the data indicate that squamous cell carcinoma has a poorer prognosis than adenocarcinoma, G4, undifferentiated cancers, are staged similar to G3 squamous cell carcinoma.

Tumor location is defined by position of the upper end of the cancer in the esophagus (Fig. 7.33). It is best expressed as distance from incisors to proximal edge of the tumor, and conventionally by its location within broad regions of the esophagus. Typical esophagoscopy measurements of cervical esophageal cancer measured from the incisors are from 15 to less than 20 cm. If esophagoscopy is not available, location can be assessed by computed tomography (CT). If thickening of the esophageal wall begins above the sternal notch, location is cervical. Typical esophagoscopy measurements of upper thoracic esophageal cancer from the incisors is from 20 to less than 25 cm. CT location of an upper thoracic cancer is esophageal wall thickening that begins between the sternal notch and azygos vein. Typical esophagoscopy measurements of middle thoracic esophageal cancer from the incisors is from 25 to less than 30 cm. CT location is wall thickening that begins between the azygos vein and inferior pulmonary vein. Typical esophagoscopy measurements of lower thoracic esophageal cancer from the incisors are from 30 to 40 cm (see Fig. 7.33). CT location is wall thickening that begins below the inferior pulmonary vein. The abdominal esophagus is included in the lower thoracic esophagus. Cancers whose epicenter is in the lower thoracic esophagus, EGJ, or within the proximal 5 cm of the stomach (cardia) that extend into the EGJ

or esophagus (Siewert III) are staged as adenocarcinoma of the esophagus. All other cancers with an epicenter in the stomach greater than 5 cm distal to the EGJ, or those within 5 cm of the EGJ but not extending into it or the esophagus, are stage grouped using the gastric (non-EGJ) cancer staging system.[47]

TNM descriptors are grouped into stages to assemble subgroups with similar behavior and prognosis (see Box 7.1). Stages 0 and IV are by definition (not data driven) TisN0M0 and Tany Nany M1, respectively. The difference in survival between adenocarcinoma and squamous cell carcinoma was best managed by separate stage groupings for stages I and II. For T1N0M0 and T2N0M0 adenocarcinoma, subgrouping is by histologic grade, G1 and G2 (not G3) versus G3. For T1N0M0 squamous cell carcinoma, subgrouping is by histologic grade: G1 versus all other G. For T2N0M0 and T3N0M0 squamous cell carcinoma, stage grouping is by histologic grade and location. The four combinations range from G1 lower thoracic squamous cell carcinoma (stage IB), which has the best survival, to G2–G4 upper and middle thoracic squamous cell carcinomas (stage IIB), which have the worst. G2–G4 lower thoracic squamous cell carcinomas and G1 upper and middle thoracic squamous cell carcinomas are grouped together (stage IIA) with intermediate survival.

Stages 0, III, and IV adenocarcinoma and squamous cell carcinoma are stage grouped identically. Adenosquamous carcinomas are staged as squamous cell carcinoma.

EUS may be used at different periods in the course of esophageal carcinoma. The principal times are at the initial staging examination (cStage) and after induction or

BOX 7.1 American Joint Committee on Cancer Staging of Cancer of the Esophagus and Esophagogastric Junction

T: PRIMARY TUMOR

TX Tumor cannot be assessed
T0 No evidence of tumor
Tis High-grade dysplasia
T1 Tumor invades the lamina propria, muscularis mucosae, or submucosa. It does not breach the submucosa
T2 Tumor invades into but not beyond the muscularis propria
T3 Tumor invades the paraesophageal tissue but does not invade adjacent structures
T4 T4a Resectable tumor invades adjacent structures, such as pleura, pericardium, diaphragm
   T4b Unresectable tumor invades adjacent structures, such as aorta, vertebral body, trachea

N: REGIONAL LYMPH NODES

Any periesophageal lymph node from cervical lymph nodes to celiac node
N0 No regional lymph node metastases
N1 1 to 2 positive regional lymph nodes
N2 3 to 6 positive regional lymph nodes
N3 7 or more positive regional lymph nodes

M: DISTANT METASTASIS

M0 No distant metastases
M1 Distant metastases

NONANATOMIC CANCER CHARACTERISTICS

Histopathologic cell type
   Adenocarcinoma
   Squamous cell carcinoma
Histologic grade
   G1 Well differentiated
   G2 Moderately differentiated
   G3 Poorly differentiated
   G4 Undifferentiated
Tumor location
   Upper thoracic   20–25 cm from incisors
   Middle thoracic   >25–30 cm from incisors
   Lower thoracic   >30–40 cm from incisors
   Esophagogastric junction   Includes cancers whose epicenter is in the distal thoracic esophagus, esophagogastric junction, or within the proximal 5 cm of the stomach (cardia) that extend into the

esophagogastric junction or esophagus and are stage grouped similar to adenocarcinoma of the esophagus

STAGE GROUPINGS: ADENOCARCINOMA

STAGE	T	N	M	G
0	is (HGD)	0	0	1
IA	1	0	0	1–2
IB	1	0	0	3
	2	0	0	1–2
IIA	2	0	0	3
IIB	3	0	0	Any
	1–2	1	0	Any
IIIA	1–2	2	0	Any
	3	1	0	Any
	4a	0	0	Any
IIIB	3	2	0	Any
IIIC	4a	1–2	0	Any
	4b	Any	0	Any
	Any	N3	0	Any
IV	Any	Any	1	Any

STAGE GROUPINGS: SQUAMOUS CELL CARCINOMA

STAGE	T	N	M	G	LOCATION
0	is (HGD)	0	0	1	Any
IA	1	0	0	1	Any
IB	1	0	0	2–3	Any
	2–3	0	0	1	Lower
IIA	2–3	0	0	1	Upper, middle
	2–3	0	0	2–3	Lower
IIB	2–3	0	0	2–3	Upper, middle
	1–2	1	0	Any	Any
IIIA	1–2	2	0	Any	Any
	3	1	0	Any	Any
	4a	0	0	Any	Any
IIIB	3	2	0	Any	Any
IIIC	4a	1–2	0	Any	Any
	4b	Any	0	Any	Any
	Any	N3	0	Any	Any
IV	Any	Any	1	Any	Any

HGD, High-grade dysplasia.

definitive chemotherapy/chemoradiotherapy (ycStage). It may also be used to diagnose and stage cancer recurrence (rStage), also referred to as retreatment stage.

CLINICAL STAGE (cTNM)

DETERMINATION OF COMPUTED TOMOGRAPHY CLASSIFICATION

Detailed images of the esophageal wall by EUS make it the most accurate modality available for clinical determination of the depth of tumor invasion (T) before treatment (Figs. 7.34 to 7.37).[53–58] The same definition of the esophageal wall is not offered by CT. A thickened esophageal wall, the principal CT finding in esophageal carcinoma, is not specific for esophageal carcinoma and lacks the definition required to distinguish T1, T2, and T3 tumors.[59] In differentiation of T3 from T4 tumors, EUS is superior to CT. Evaluation of the fat planes is used to define local invasion at CT examination. The obliteration or lack of fat planes is not sensitive in predicting local invasion, but preservation of these planes is specific for the absence of T4 disease.[60–67] When compared with CT, EUS provides a more sensitive and reliable determination of vascular involvement.[68]

Experience with both examination technique and ultrasound interpretation is critical to accurately determine the clinical depth of tumor invasion. Seventy-five to 100 examinations are required before competence is obtained.[69,70] A center that does a high volume of EUS

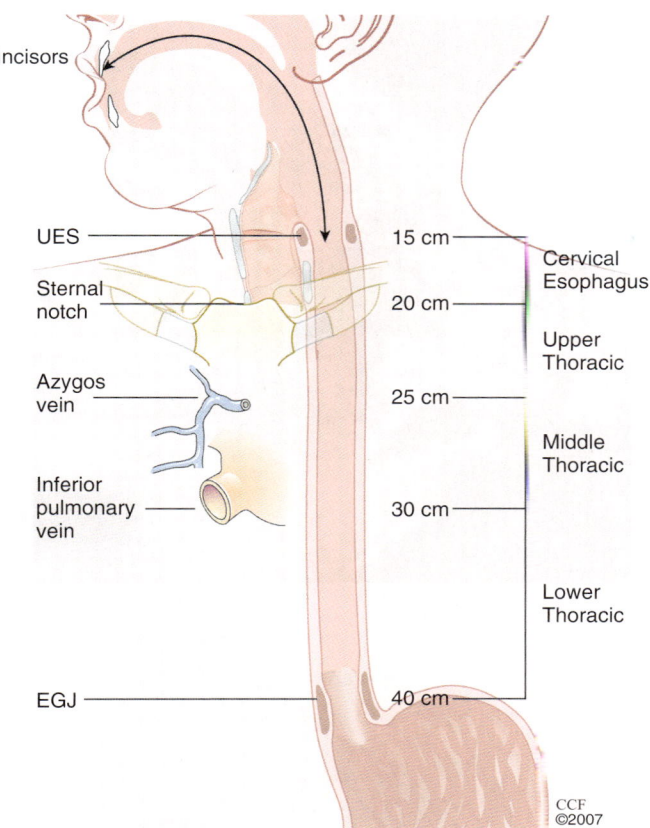

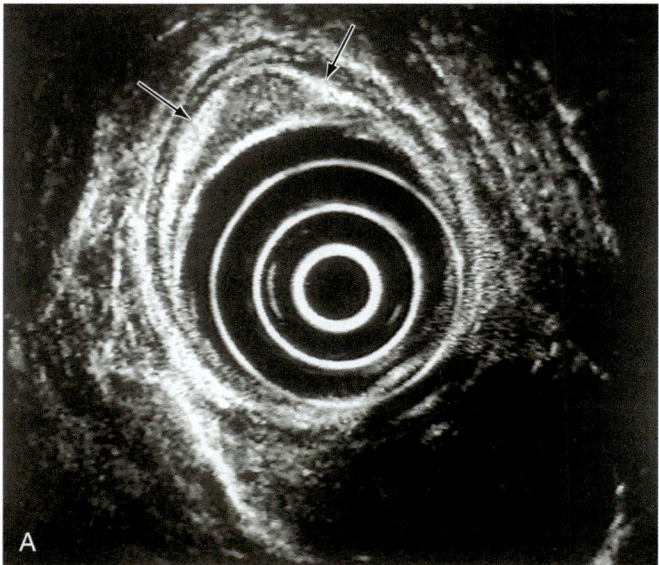

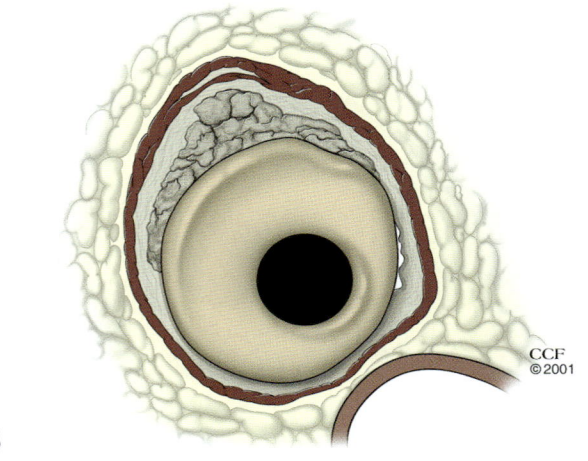

FIGURE 7.33 Cancer location. *Cervical esophagus,* bounded superiorly by the cricopharyngeus and inferiorly by the sternal notch, is typically 15 to 20 cm from the incisors at esophagoscopy. *Upper thoracic esophagus,* bounded superiorly by the sternal notch and inferiorly by the azygos arch, is typically less than 20 to 25 cm from the incisors at esophagoscopy. *Middle thoracic esophagus,* bounded superiorly by the azygos arch and inferiorly by the inferior pulmonary vein, is typically less than 25 to 30 cm from the incisors at esophagoscopy. *Lower thoracic esophagus,* bounded superiorly by the inferior pulmonary vein and inferiorly by the lower esophageal sphincter, is typically less than 30 to 40 cm from the incisors at esophagoscopy; it includes cancers whose epicenter is within the proximal 5 cm of the stomach that extend into the esophagogastric junction or lower thoracic esophagus. *EGJ,* Esophagogastric junction; *UES,* upper esophageal sphincter.

FIGURE 7.34 (A) A T1 tumor as seen on esophageal ultrasound. The hypoechoic *(black)* tumor invades the hyperechoic *(white)* third ultrasound layer (submucosa) but does not breach the boundary between the third and fourth layers *(arrows).* (B) A T1 tumor invades but does not breach the submucosa.

examinations is more likely to perform a better examination than a low-volume center.[71]

A review of 21 series reported an 84% accuracy of EUS for T classification.[72] Accuracy is not constant and varies with the T classification. In this meta-analysis, accuracy for T1 carcinomas was 83.5%, with 16.5% of tumors overstaged; accuracy for T2 was 73%, with 10% understaged and 17% overstaged; accuracy for T3 was 89%, with 5% understaged and 6% overstaged; and accuracy for T4 was 89%, with 11% understaged.[72] This review reported variation in accuracy with T classification: 75% to 82% for T1, 64% to 85% for T2, 89% to 94% for T3, and 88% to 100% for T4. A meta-analysis of 27 articles demonstrated EUS to be highly effective in the differentiation of T1 and T2 from T3 and T4 cancers.[73] A recent meta-analysis

found that EUS better staged advanced (T4) than early (T1) cancers.[74]

The greatest inaccuracy is reported for T2 tumors.[75–78] EUS anatomy, in part, accounts for this problem. The muscularis propria is vital in defining T1, T2, and T3 tumors. For clinical assessment the fourth ultrasound layer is interpreted as the muscularis propria. However, this layer does not include the interface between the submucosa and muscularis propria; it is contained in the third ultrasound layer. Thus the border necessary to completely differentiate T1 from T2 tumors is contained in the third ultrasound layer. As two boundaries must be assessed for determination of T2 and errors might occur at each, the inaccuracy is potentially twice that of T1 and T4 tumors.

Because invasion beyond the esophageal wall is important in determining therapy, some investigators have examined the accuracy of EUS in determining T

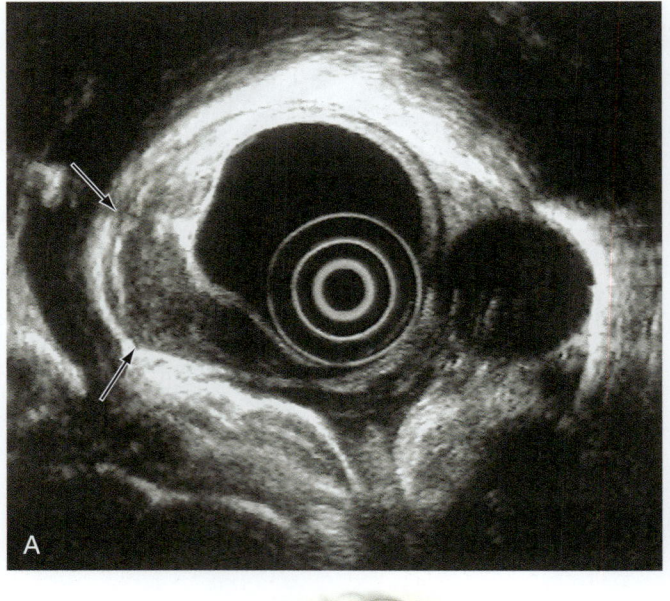

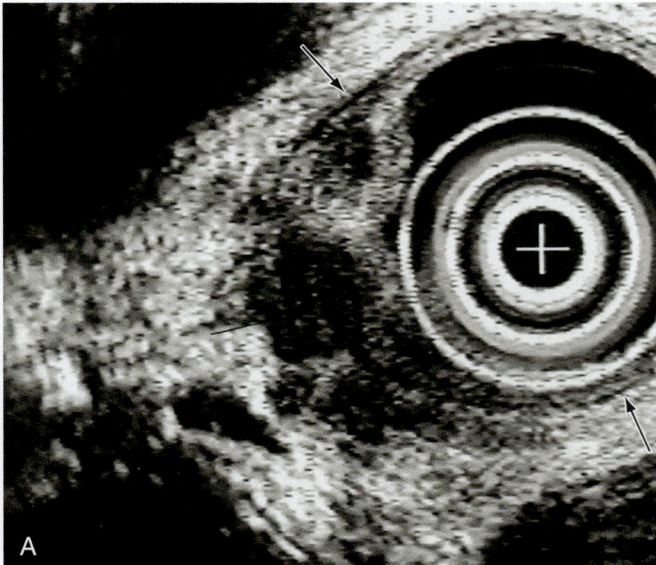

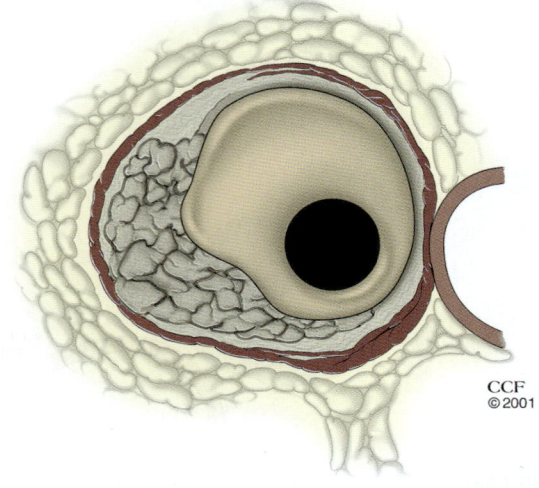

FIGURE 7.35 (A) A T2 tumor as seen on esophageal ultrasound. The hypoechoic *(black)* tumor invades the hypoechoic *(black)* fourth ultrasound layer but does not breach the boundary between the fourth and fifth layers *(arrows)*. (B) A T2 tumor invades but does not breach the muscularis propria.

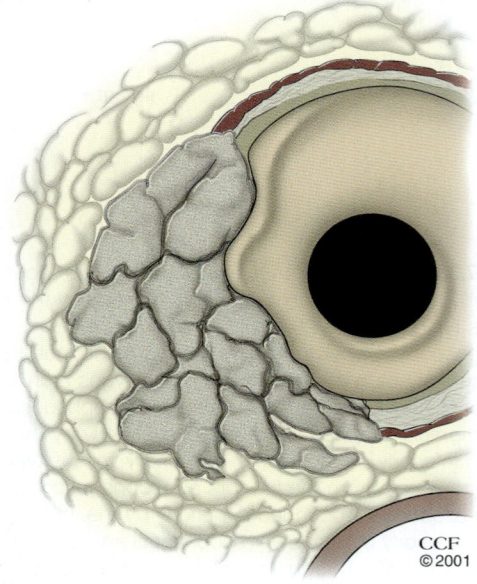

FIGURE 7.36 (A) A T3 tumor as seen on esophageal ultrasound. The hypoechoic *(black)* tumor breaches the boundary between the fourth and fifth ultrasound layers *(arrows)* and invades the hyperechoic *(white)* fifth ultrasound layer (periesophageal tissue). (B) A T3 tumor invades the periesophageal tissue but does not involve adjacent structures.

classification dichotomously. When compared with T classification determined pathologically, EUS was 87% accurate, 82% sensitive, 91% specific, 89% positively predictive, and 86% negatively predictive of tumors confined to the esophageal wall (<T2) or invading beyond the esophageal wall (>T2).[79] A systematic review of 13 studies also confirmed that EUS was highly effective in differentiating T1/T2 from T3/T4 tumors.[80] Although EUS can determine the extent of invasion of the periesophageal tissue (cT3), this distinction has not been clinically useful because the extent of periesophageal invasion is not associated with either cancer mortality or recurrence.[81]

EUS interpretation is not done in the absence of clinical information; patient history and preceding esophagoscopy and imaging are usually available. This fact was illustrated by Meining et al., who reported that a blinded review of EUS studies was significantly less accurate than a retrospective review of EUS reports, 53% versus 73%, respectively.[82] When interpreters were unblinded and given endoscopy tapes, accuracy improved to 62%. Tumor length and luminal obstruction are known at the time of EUS and are predictive of the T classification.[83] In this report, tumor length greater than 5 cm had a sensitivity of 89% and specificity of 92% for diagnosing T3 tumors. Thirteen patients with luminal obstruction had at least T3 tumors. EUS-determined tumor volume based on EUS-defined tumor length was reported to be a significant prognosticator in esophageal cancer.[84]

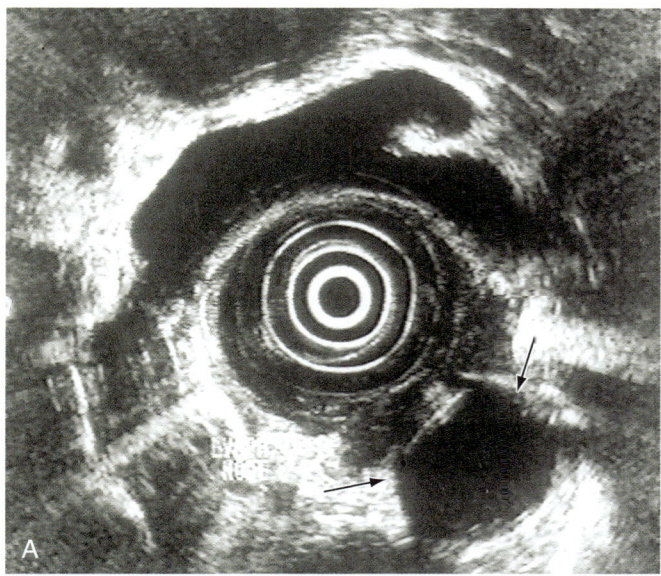

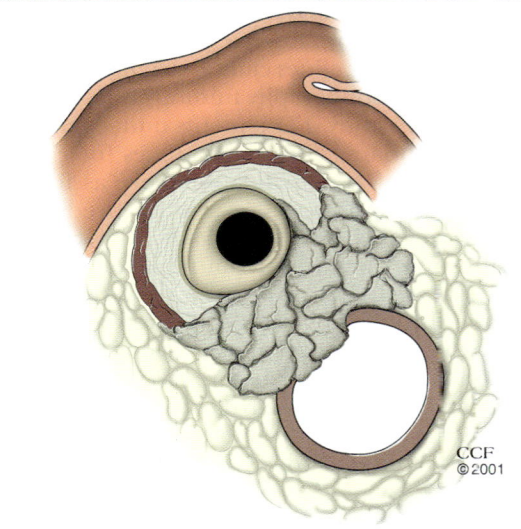

CCF
©2001

B

FIGURE 7.37 (A) A T4 tumor as seen on esophageal ultrasound. The hypoechoic *(black)* tumor invades the aorta. The tumor breaches the boundary between periesophageal tissue and the aorta *(arrows)*. (B) A T4 tumor invades the aorta.

Esophageal obstruction caused by a malignant high-grade stricture prohibits staging in 3% to 63% of examinations.[58,85–87] Two studies have reported that EUS may be less reliable in nontraversable esophageal cancers.[57,88] Failure to pass an ultrasound probe beyond a malignant stricture is an accurate predictor of advanced stage. More than 90% of these patients have stage III or IV disease.[89] These discordant findings may be reconciled when viewed in the context of a study by Hordijk et al.[86] that assessed the severity of malignant strictures. In this study the accuracy of T classification was 87% for nontraversable strictures, 46% for tight strictures that were difficult to pass, and 92% for easily traversable strictures. Options in the case of nontraversable strictures include limited examination of the proximal tumor margin, dilation and subsequent EUS examination, and the use of miniprobes. Limited examination of the tumor above the stricture has variable accuracy but may be useful in staging if T3 or N1 disease is seen. Dilation of malignant strictures followed by EUS examination may be associated with an increased incidence of perforation.[89] However, it allows a complete examination in 42% to 97% of patients with high-grade strictures[87,90–92] and is not associated with perforation if careful stepwise dilation is performed. Careful dilation followed by EUS allowed Wallace et al.[92] to detect advanced disease in 19% of patients, mostly because of the detection of celiac lymph node metastases. This problem may be overcome by the use of miniature ultrasound catheter probes (see Fig. 7.26). Passed through the biopsy channel of the endoscope and advanced through the stricture, these probes accurately determined T classification in 85% to 90% of patients.[93–96] Because most of these data are uncontrolled, it is not clear whether the additional effort and cost provide staging benefits. These 20-MHz probes have limited depth of penetration, which may prevent full ultrasound assessment. Because most nontraversable tumors are at least T3, it is crucial to evaluate the outer boundary of the tumor and adjacent structures and regional lymph nodes, which may be outside the range of the miniprobe. As a rule of thumb, if the tumor stricture is not allowing passage of the EUS scope, the most practical option is to abort the procedure and manage the patient as at least cT3N1 and treat with neoadjuvant therapy prior to esophagectomy.[97]

Because conventional EUS does not image the mucosa well, EUS has not proven useful to stage patients suspected of having high-grade dysplasia or intramucosal cancer and has been abandoned in favor of endoscopic resection and pathologic staging in most centers. However, in instances of larger superficial tumors or those with lymphovascular invasion that have a higher risk of lymph node metastases, EUS may provide some value.[98–101] The duplicate muscularis mucosae seen in the majority of patients with Barrett esophagus may result in the overstaging of intramucosal cancer (T1a) as submucosal (T1b) cancers.[102] Although high-resolution EUS better assesses the mucosa than conventional EUS, it is of limited value in superficial esophageal cancer.[103–106]

DETERMINATION OF N CLASSIFICATIONS

In addition to size, EUS evaluates nodal shape, border, and internal echo characteristics in lymph node assessment (Fig. 7.38). Large (>1 cm in long axis), round, hypoechoic, nonhomogeneous, sharply bordered lymph nodes are more likely to be malignant; small, oval or angular, hyperechoic, homogeneous lymph nodes with indistinct borders are more likely to be benign.[107] In a retrospective review of 100 EUS examinations, determination of N was 89% sensitive, 75% specific, and 84% accurate.[107] Positive predictive value of EUS for N+ disease was 86%; negative predictive value was 79%. A patient was 24 times more likely to have N+ cancer if EUS detected regional lymph nodes. The single most sensitive predictor in detecting N+ cancer was a hypoechoic internal echo pattern, followed by a sharp border, a round shape, and size greater than 1 cm. When all four factors are present, the accuracy of N1 detection is 80% to 100%.[107,108] Unfortunately, all four features are present in only 25% of N+ lymph nodes.[108] The ability to use EUS to diagnose nodal metastases varies with the

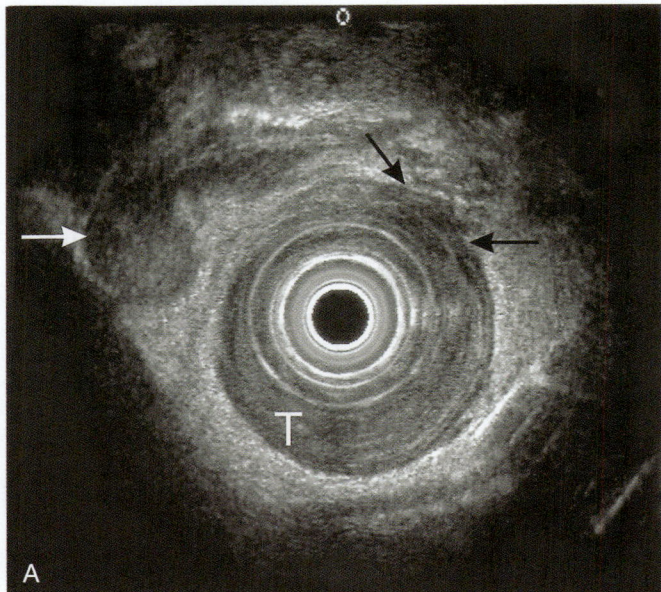

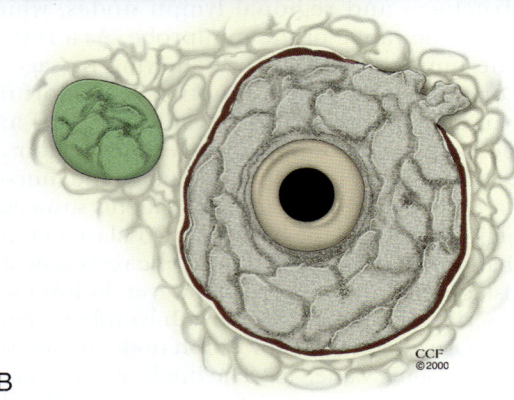

FIGURE 7.38 T3N1 esophageal carcinoma. (A) A T3 tumor *(T)* obliterates the ultrasound anatomy at this level. At the 1 o'clock position *(black arrows),* the tumor breaks through the fourth ultrasound layer and invades the fifth. An N1 regional lymph node *(white arrow),* close to the primary tumor, is large (2.2 cm in diameter), round, hypoechoic, and sharply demarcated. (B) A T3N1 tumor breaches the muscularis propria to invade periesophageal tissue and metastasizes to a single regional lymph node.

location. It is better in the assessment of celiac lymph nodes (accuracy, 95%; sensitivity, 83%; specificity, 98%; positive predictive value, 91%; negative predictive value, 97%) than in mediastinal lymph nodes (accuracy, 73%; sensitivity, 79%; specificity, 63%; positive predictive value, 79%; and negative predictive value, 63%).[109]

A meta-analysis of 21 series reported EUS as being 77% accurate for N, 69% for N0, and 89% for N+.[72] Endoscopic ultrasound–guided fine-needle aspiration (EUS-FNA) further refines clinical staging by adding tissue sampling to endosonography findings. In a multicenter study, 171 patients had EUS-FNA of 192 lymph nodes.[110] EUS-FNA for determination of lymph node status was 92% sensitive, 93% specific, 100% positively predictive, and 86% negatively predictive. Combined EUS and EUS-FNA assessment of celiac lymph nodes was 72% sensitive, 97%

specific, 95% positively predictive, and 82% negatively predictive.[111] FNA confirmed positive EUS celiac lymph nodes in 88% of patients. More recent experience of this group reported 98% accuracy of EUS-FNA detection of malignant celiac lymph nodes.[112]

Subclassification of N+ requires determination of number of regional lymph nodes containing metastases (positive nodes). EUS can accurately determine number of positive regional lymph nodes, and this clinical assessment is predictive of survival.[113–115]

There are associations between the primary tumor and N classification. Close proximity of the regional node to the primary tumor is a predictor of N+ cancer. Comparison of the echo characteristic of the tumor and regional lymph nodes is useful for EUS lymph node evaluation. The relationship of T classification to N+ must be considered during EUS examinations. The incidence of N+ cancer increases with deeper tumor invasion: For a patient with poorly differentiated adenocarcinoma, the probability of N1 is 17% for T1 tumors, 55% for T2, 83% for T3, and 88% for T4.[116] For T3 and T4 cancers, an EUS assessment of N0 does not ensure absence of N+ disease.

EUS-FNA further refines clinical staging by adding tissue sampling to endosonography findings (Fig. 7.39).[111,117–122] In a multicenter study, 171 patients underwent EUS-FNA of 192 lymph nodes.[122] Referent values for EUS-FNA in determination of N classification were as follows: sensitivity, 92%; specificity, 93%; positive predictive value, 100%; and negative predictive value, 86%. Accuracy of N classification increased from 69% for EUS alone to 92% for EUS-FNA. Two to three passes of the needle were made through each node. There was one nonfatal complication: an esophageal perforation during dilation of an esophageal stricture before EUS-FNA. Subsequent studies from Vazquez-Sequeiros et al. confirm and extend these findings.[120,121] In the most recent report the first prospective, blinded study, EUS-FNA was more accurate than EUS (87% vs. 74%, respectively) as determined by histopathologic review of surgical specimens.[121] When compared with CT, EUS-FNA changed the tumor stage in 38% of patients. Complications are extremely rare.[123] Unfortunately, some lymph nodes cannot be aspirated because of proximity to the primary tumor. Only nodes in which the needle path avoids the primary tumor are appropriate for EUS-FNA because false-positive results might otherwise be obtained.

The combination of EUS and EUS-FNA of celiac lymph nodes, deemed positive by EUS, had a sensitivity of 77%, specificity of 85%, positive predictive value of 89%, and negative predictive value of 71%.[124] EUS-FNA confirmed a positive celiac node in 94% of patients and was 98% accurate. EUS detection of nodal metastases makes EUS-FNA the least costly pathologic staging strategy in patients with non-M1 esophageal cancer.[125]

For preoperative EUS examinations, N classification best predicts patient survival.[126] It is a superior predictor of patient survival than EUS determination of T classification. The use of EUS-FNA is associated with improved recurrence-free and overall survival.[127] Therefore careful EUS N classification with aggressive EUS-FNA lymph node sampling is mandatory and critical to treatment planning and prognostication.

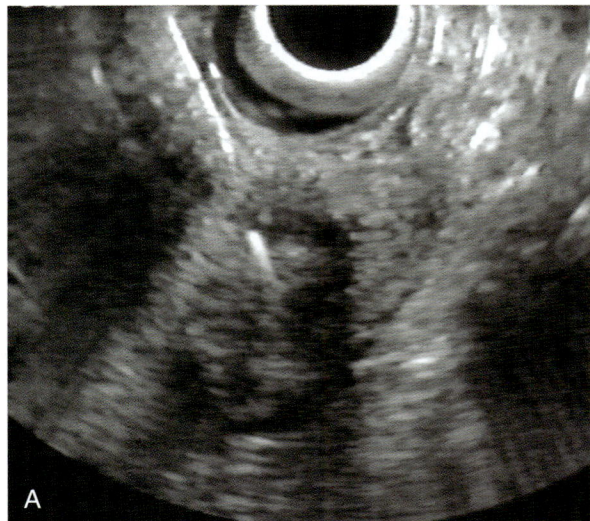

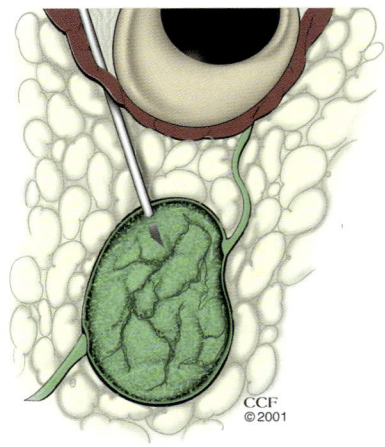

FIGURE 7.39 Esophageal ultrasound–guided fine-needle aspiration of an N1 regional lymph node. (A) Ultrasound image with a needle passed through the esophageal wall and into the N1 node. (B) An N1 regional lymph node undergoing fine-needle aspiration under curvilinear electronic endoscopic examination.

DETERMINATION OF M CLASSIFICATION

EUS has limited value in screening for distant metastases (M1). The distant organ must be in direct contact with the upper gastrointestinal tract for EUS to be useful. The left lateral segment of the liver[128] and retroperitoneum are two such sites (Fig. 7.40). EUS is capable of detecting low-volume ascites not apparent on CT. This finding is associated with unresectable cancer in one-half of patients with low-volume ascites, and in the remaining patients with low-volume ascites, only half were able to undergo R0 resections.[129]

POSTTHERAPY STAGE (ycTNM)

After induction therapy, a subset of patients with esophageal cancer will be disease free. Because significant morbidity is associated with surgery for esophageal cancer, the ability to detect patients who have no residual cancer (ycT0N0M0)

after induction therapy is theoretically desirable. However, ycT0N0M0 does not ensure ypT0N0M0 or freedom from cancer recurrence. Esophageal ultrasonography has been used in multiple clinical series for this purpose. Early series indicated that EUS was very accurate in determining T classification after chemotherapy. However, in these series the presurgical therapy was largely ineffective in causing pathologic downstaging; therefore EUS was accurate by merely indicating that no significant change had occurred.[130-133] In two series in which radiation therapy was provided along with chemotherapy, the accuracy of determination of T classification was again high (72% to 78%), but the prevalence of pathologic T0 disease was low or not reported.[134,135] Accuracy of T classification can therefore be attributed primarily to a lack of tumor response to chemoradiotherapy.

Later series incorporated more aggressive regimens of chemoradiotherapy, with higher rates of significant downstaging of tumor and pathologic T0N0M0 cancer. In these series, up to 31% of patients had pathologic T0N0M0 stage grouping after chemoradiotherapy.[134] EUS was poor in accurately determining T classification, with reported rates of 27% to 47%.[136-139] The most common mistake made in determining T classification was overstaging because EUS is unable to distinguish tumor from inflammation and fibrosis produced by chemoradiotherapy. Similar difficulties in this differentiation also have been reported with EUS staging of rectal cancer.[140]

EUS accuracy for N classification after chemoradiotherapy has been reported in only four clinical series. The reported accuracy ranged from 49% to 71%.[135,137-139] The accuracy of N classification in patients who undergo chemoradiotherapy is lower than in patients not treated with chemoradiotherapy. Primary reasons for this inaccuracy are alterations in the ultrasound appearance of nodes after chemoradiotherapy such that established EUS criteria do not apply and there is residual foci of cancer within the nodes that are too small for detection by any modality other than pathologic analysis.

Change in maximal cross-sectional area before and after chemoradiotherapy appears to be a more useful means of assessing the response of esophageal cancer to preoperative therapy.[136,141] Chak et al. defined a response as a 50% or greater reduction in tumor area. Improved survival was reported in responders and responder subgroups who had surgery after chemoradiotherapy, adenocarcinoma, and T3N1M0 cancer before treatment.[141] Identification of persistent tumor in lymph nodes by EUS-FNA has been used to modify the treatment of patients receiving preoperative chemoradiotherapy.[142]

Despite these shortcomings, in a systematic review of the literature EUS and CT have similar overall diagnostic accuracy for assessment of response to neoadjuvant therapy in patients with esophageal cancer.[143] However, in most centers positron emission tomography (PET)-CT is the preferred staging study after neoadjuvant therapy to exclude metastatic disease, with limited use of repeat EUS.

RECURRENCE STAGE (rTNM)

EUS has been useful in the diagnosis and restaging of patients with anastomotic recurrence that is not endoscopically visible.[144,145]

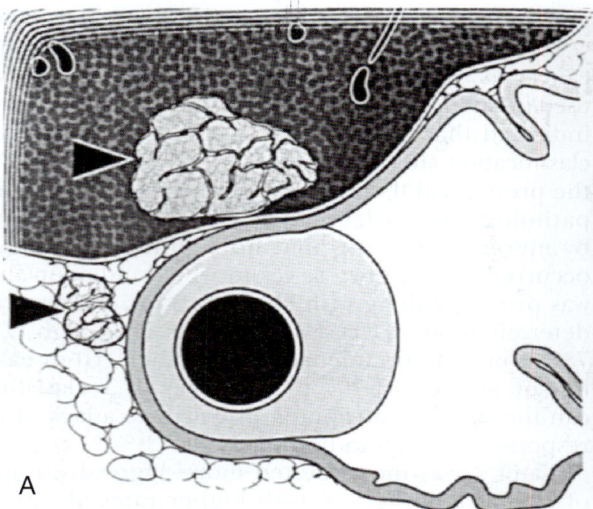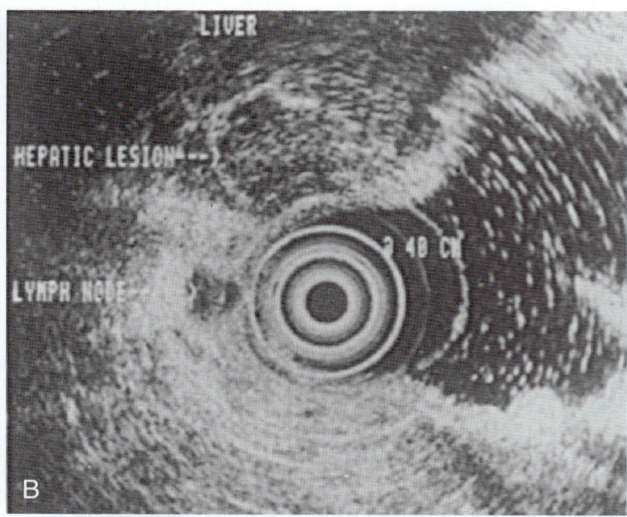

FIGURE 7.40 (A) Hepatic metastasis *(upper arrowhead)* in the left lateral segment of the liver. A perigastric lymph node metastasis is shown *(lower arrowhead)*. The esophageal ultrasound probe is seen in the gastric cardia. (B) Hepatic metastasis *(upper arrow)* as seen from the gastric cardia by esophageal ultrasound. The metastasis was imaged only by esophageal ultrasound. A perigastric lymph node metastasis is shown *(lower arrow)*. (From Rice TW, Boyce GA, Sivak MV, et al. Esophageal carcinoma: esophageal ultrasound assessment of preoperative chemotherapy. *Ann Thorac Surg.* 1992;53:972.)

TABLE 7.2 Endoscopic Ultrasonographic Classification of Benign Esophageal Tumors

EUS Layer	Esophageal Tumor
First/second (mucosa/deep mucosa)	Fibrovascular polyp
	Granular cell tumor
	Retention cyst
	Leiomyoma*
Third (submucosa)	Lipoma
	Fibroma
	Neurofibroma
	Granular cell tumor
Fourth (muscularis propria)	Leiomyoma*
	Cysts
Fifth	Cysts

*Leiomyomas may arise from the second or fourth ultrasound layer.

BENIGN ESOPHAGEAL DISEASES

BENIGN ESOPHAGEAL TUMORS

Detailed EUS examination of the esophageal wall has improved the diagnosis of benign esophageal tumors. EUS identification of intramural masses relies on both the layer from which the tumor arises (Table 7.2) and the ultrasound characteristics of the tumor. Homogeneous lesions that are anechoic, of intermediate echogenicity, or hyperechoic are almost exclusively benign.[146] A heterogeneous echo pattern may be seen in benign tumors, but this endosonographic finding, particularly in lesions greater than 3 to 4 cm in largest diameter, may be indicative of malignancy.

TUMORS OF THE MUCOSA

Fibrovascular polyps are collections of fibrous, vascular, and adipose tissue lined by normal squamous epithelium.

Microscopically, fibrovascular polyps are expansions of the lamina propria.[147] These polyps usually arise in the cervical esophagus, extend into the esophageal lumen, and may reach into the stomach. Most patients eventually complain of dysphagia or respiratory symptoms, or both. Spectacular manifestations include regurgitation into the hypopharynx and mouth with subsequent aspiration and, occasionally, sudden death by asphyxiation. Barium esophagography and CT best detect these lesions. Because fibrovascular polyps fill the esophageal lumen and have a composition similar to the mucosa, definition by esophagoscopy or EUS may be difficult or impossible.[148] EUS-guided FNA and cytologic examination may be diagnostic if benign fibrofatty elements are demonstrated originating from the mucosa/submucosa.[149]

Granular cell tumors are the third most common benign esophageal tumor, and the esophagus is the most common gastrointestinal site of these tumors. Most are located in the distal end of the esophagus. Their origin is neural from the Schwann cell. Most patients with granular cell tumors are asymptomatic and rarely require surgery. At endoscopy, these lesions are yellow, firm nodules. Endoscopic biopsy is diagnostic in only 50% of patients.[150] EUS evaluation typically demonstrates a tumor less than 2 cm in diameter that has an intermediate or hypoechoic, mildly inhomogeneous solid pattern with smooth borders and rising from the inner two EUS layers.[150,151] Less than 5% of granular cell tumors originate from the submucosa. Malignant variants are rare and distinguished by size (>4 cm), nuclear pleomorphism, and mitotic activity.[152] Atypical EUS findings may predict the rare malignant granular cell tumors.

TUMORS OF THE SUBMUCOSA

Esophageal stromal tumors are rare and include lipomas, fibromas, and hemangiomas. Lipomas are indirectly detected at esophagoscopy as a bulging of the overlying esophageal mucosa. They have a pale yellow appearance and soft texture when probed with an esophagoscope. Endoscopic biopsy usually produces normal overlying squamous epithelium because these samplings rarely penetrate the submucosa. EUS demonstrates a hyperechoic homogeneous lesion that originates in and is confined to the submucosal layer. Generally asymptomatic and most often found incidentally, lipomas require no EUS follow-up. Fibromas and neurofibromas are very uncommon. At endoscopy, they are firm "to the touch." These lesions are less hyperechoic than lipomas. Symptomatic submucosal tumors are uncommon, and the symptoms may be unrelated. These tumors are typically incidental findings of a "shotgun" investigation of atypical symptoms such as chest pain and cough. EUS is critical in diagnosis and thus in avoiding excision.

Hemangiomas may present with dysphagia and bleeding. Most hemangiomas are in the lower part of the esophagus and may be mistaken for esophageal varices. EUS examination reveals a hypoechoic mass with sharp margins arising from the second or third EUS layer.[153,154]

TUMORS OF THE MUSCULARIS PROPRIA

Leiomyomas are benign smooth muscle tumors of the muscularis propria. Symptomatic tumors arising from the muscularis mucosae are rare, with the majority arising from the inner circular muscle layer in the distal and midthoracic esophagus.[155] EUS examinations reveal that the majority of esophageal leiomyomas are greater than 1 cm in diameter and are most frequently found in the muscularis mucosae.[156] Leiomyomas are the most common benign esophageal tumors and account for more than 70% of all benign tumors. There is no gender preponderance, and they typically occur in patients 20 to 50 years old (i.e., patients who are significantly younger than patients with esophageal carcinoma). Although frequently asymptomatic and discovered incidentally, leiomyomas can cause dysphagia, pain, or bleeding. Distal esophageal leiomyomas are often associated with symptoms of GERD. Barium esophagography demonstrates smooth filling defects; esophagoscopy reveals a normal overlying mucosa. EUS displays a hypoechoic, sharply bordered tumor arising in the fourth ultrasound layer (Fig. 7.41). The diagnosis of small leiomyomas (<1 cm in diameter) may be enhanced with the use of miniature ultrasound probes.[156] Atypical EUS findings are a tumor larger than 4 cm, irregular margins, mixed internal echo characteristics, and associated regional lymphadenopathy. Endoscopic biopsies do not reach the muscularis propria. EUS-FNA is unlikely to provide the cellular architectural characteristics necessary to differentiate leiomyomas from leiomyosarcomas, which are exceedingly rare.[157] Malignant transformation of benign leiomyomas has been infrequently reported. Surgical resection, by minimally invasive or endoscopic techniques if possible, is indicated for symptomatic leiomyomas. In asymptomatic tumors with typical EUS features, expectant therapy plus EUS observation is indicated.

Esophageal gastrointestinal stromal tumors are exceedingly rare tumors arising from the cells of Cajal in the muscularis propria. They may be differentiated from more common leiomyomas by EUS-FNA.[158,159]

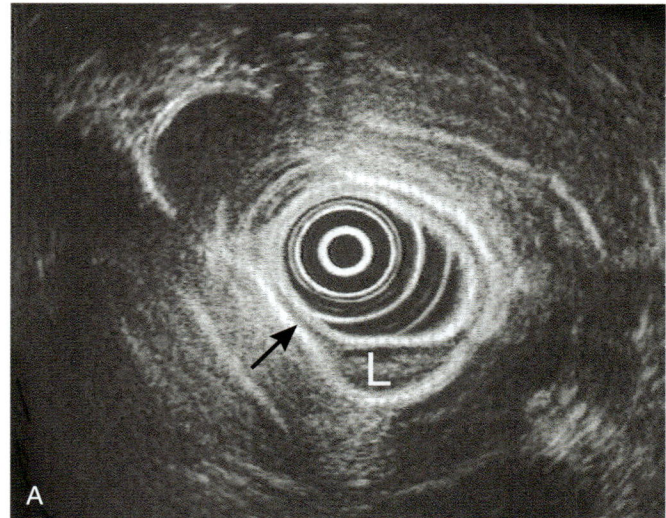

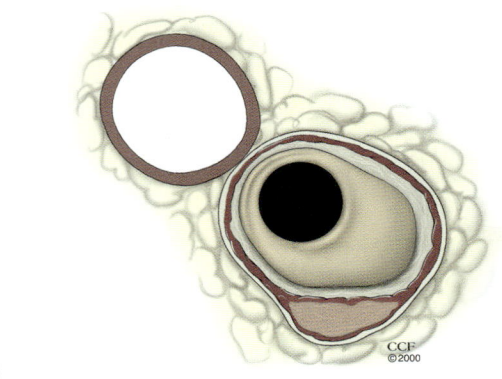

FIGURE 7.41 Esophageal leiomyoma. (A) Endoscopic ultrasonography (EUS) of this most common benign tumor demonstrates a hypoechoic, homogeneous, well-demarcated tumor with no associated lymphadenopathy. EUS balloon overdistention blends the first three ultrasound layers into one hyperechoic layer. The tumor arises from and is confined to the fourth ultrasound layer *(arrow)*. (B) A benign leiomyoma arises from and is confined to the muscularis propria.

MISCELLANEOUS ESOPHAGEAL DISEASES

ESOPHAGEAL CYSTS

Esophageal cysts, the second most common benign esophageal tumors, account for 20% of these lesions. The minority are acquired epithelial cysts arising in the lamina propria. Submucosal glandular inflammation is the suspected cause. The majority of esophageal cysts are congenital foregut cysts. They are lined with squamous, respiratory, or columnar epithelium and may contain smooth muscle, cartilage, or fat. Esophageal duplication is a subtype of foregut cyst; it is lined with squamous epithelium, and its submucosal and muscularis elements interdigitate with the muscularis propria of the esophagus. EUS can clearly define the intramural or extraesophageal nature of these tumors and further determine their anechoic, cystic nature (Fig. 7.42).[160–163] Transesophageal EUS drainage of a foregut

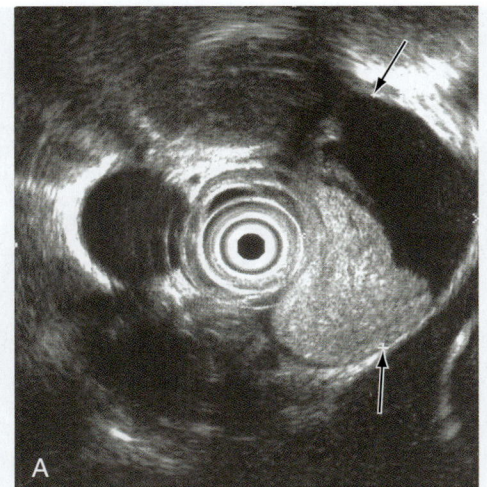

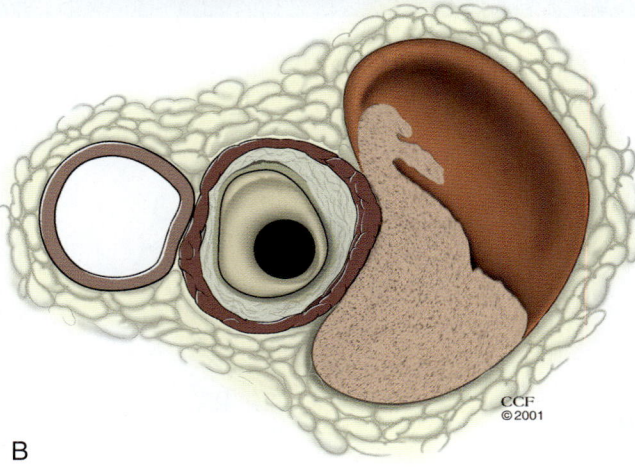

FIGURE 7.42 Foregut cyst. (A) Esophageal ultrasonography demonstrates a mass *(arrows)* adjacent to the trachea and esophagus. The cyst has two components, one hyperechoic *(white),* representing proteinaceous material, and one hypoechoic *(black),* representing fluid. (B) A foregut cyst in close proximity to the esophagus and trachea.

cyst has been reported, but drainage of the cyst without destruction of its lining may result in recurrence.[164]

ESOPHAGEAL VARICES

Esophageal varices have the typical appearance of blood vessels at EUS. Appearing as tubular, round, or serpiginous echo-free structures, they may be visualized within the submucosa or in tissues adjacent to the esophagus (Fig. 7.43). These EUS patterns change after sclerosis.[165] Intravariceal sclerosis fills the varix with echogenic material representing thrombus. Paravariceal injection leads to obliteration of the varix with hypoechoic extravariceal thickening. EUS in combination with color-flow Doppler may be useful in the hemodynamic assessment of the portal venous system and treatment effects upon hepatic blood flow.[166]

ACHALASIA

EUS findings in achalasia are controversial. Some authors report thickened esophageal wall in most patients examined.[167,168] However, this excessive thickening may be artifactual. In a dilated and convoluted esophagus, the ultrasound transducer may orient at an angle oblique to the esophageal wall and give a false appearance of wall thickening.[169] The main role of EUS in achalasia is to exclude other mural abnormalities.[170–172]

PARAESOPHAGEAL DISEASES

EUS has been used to examine the mediastinal lymph nodes in patients with bronchogenic carcinoma.[140–142,173–175] In this setting, EUS has a reported positive predictive value of 77%, a negative predictive value of 93%, and an overall accuracy of 92% when using criteria similar to regional lymph node evaluation in esophageal carcinoma.[141,174] Anatomic constraints limit its usefulness for evaluation of lymph nodes in proximity to the airway. EUS-FNA provides cytologic differentiation between benign and malignant lymphadenopathy[143,176] and has successfully diagnosed solid lesions of the mediastinum and lung.[118,144–146,177–179]

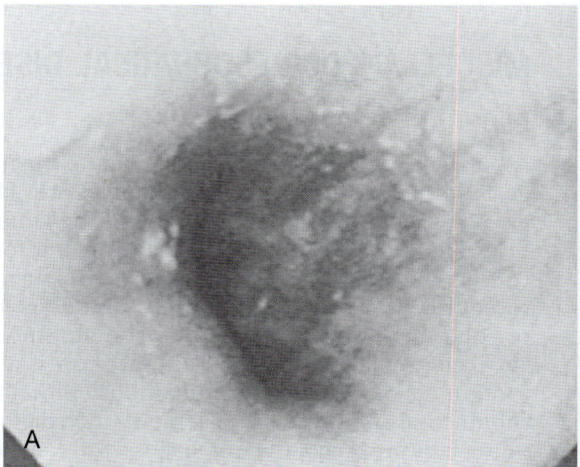

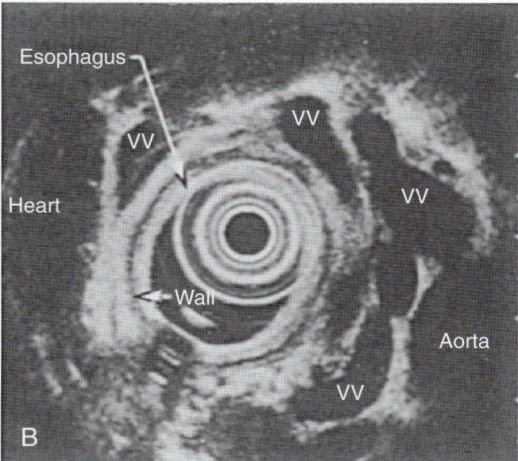

FIGURE 7.43 Paraesophageal varices. (A) At endoscopy, small varices are not visible. (B) On esophageal ultrasound, the varices *(VV)* are prominent anechoic, tubular, and rounded structures outside the esophageal wall.

CONCLUSION

EUS and EUS-FNA are essential in determining the clinical stage and directing treatment of esophageal cancer. The diagnosis of benign esophageal tumors requires EUS examination, which determines both the layer of origin in the esophageal wall and the ultrasound characteristics of the tumor. Because many of these tumors are asymptomatic, EUS affords simple follow-up and avoids unnecessary excision. EUS is a useful adjuvant for the diagnosis and treatment of paraesophageal disease.

REFERENCES

1. Netter FH. Anatomy of the esophagus. In: Oppenheimer E, ed. *The CIBA Collection of Medical Illustrations.* Vol 3. Digestive System. Part I. Upper Digestive Tract. New York: CIBA Pharmaceutical Company; 1959:34.
2. Goyal RK, Martin SB, Shapiro J, Spechler SJ. The role of cricopharyngeal muscle in pharyngoesophageal disorders. *Dysphagia.* 1993;8:252.
3. Mittal RK, Balaban DH. The esophagogastric junction. *N Engl J Med.* 1997;336:924.
4. Weickert U, Wolf A, Schröder C, Autschbach F, Vollmer H. Frequency, histopathological findings, and clinical significance of cervical heterotopic gastric mucosa (gastric inlet patch): a prospective study in 300 patients. *Dis Esophagus.* 2011;24:63.
5. Johnson LF, Moses FM. Endoscopic evaluation of esophageal disease. In: Castell DO, Johnson LF, eds. *Esophageal Function in Health and Disease.* New York: Elsevier Science Publishing Co., Inc.; 1983:237.
6. Goyal RK, Bauer J, Spiro HM. The nature and location of the lower esophageal ring. *N Engl J Med.* 1971;284:1175.
7. Ott DJ. Radiology of the oropharynx and esophagus. In: Castell DO, ed. *The Esophagus.* Boston: Little, Brown and Company; 1995:41.
8. Paull A, Trier JS, Dalton MD, Camp RC, Loeb P, Goyal RK. The histologic spectrum of Barrett's esophagus. *N Engl J Med.* 1976;295:476.
9. Kim SL, Waring PJ, Spechler SJ, et al.; the Department of Veterans Affairs Gastroesophageal Reflux Study Group. Diagnostic inconsistencies in Barrett's esophagus. *Gastroenterology.* 1994;107:945.
10. Bozymski EM. Barrett's esophagus: endoscopic characteristics. In: Spechler SJ, Goyal RK, eds. *Barrett's Esophagus: Pathophysiology, Diagnosis, and Management.* New York: Elsevier Science Publishing Co., Inc.; 1985:113.
11. McClave SA, Boyce HW Jr, Gottfried MR. Early diagnosis of columnar-lined esophagus: a new endoscopic criterion. *Gastrointest Endosc.* 1987;33:413.
12. De Carvalho CA. Sur l'angio-architecture veineuse de la zone de transition esophago-gastrique et son interprétation fonctionnelle. *Acta Anat.* 1966;64:125.
13. Choi DW, Oh SN, Baek SJ, et al. Endoscopically observed lower esophageal capillary patterns. *Korean J Intern Med.* 2002;17:245.
14. Spechler SJ. The role of gastric carditis in metaplasia and neoplasia at the gastroesophageal junction. *Gastroenterology.* 1999;117:218.
15. Vianna A, Hayes PC, Moscoso G, et al. Normal venous circulation of the gastroesophageal junction. A route to understanding varices. *Gastroenterology.* 1987;93:876.
16. Spechler SJ, Fitzgerald RC, Prasad GA, Wang KK. History, molecular mechanisms, and endoscopic treatment of Barrett's esophagus. *Gastroenterology.* 2010;138:854.
17. Sharma P, Morales TG, Sampliner RE. Short segment Barrett's esophagus. The need for standardization of the definition and of endoscopic criteria. *Am J Gastroenterol.* 1998;93:1033.
18. Wallner B, Sylvan A, Stenling R, Janunger KG. The esophageal Z-line appearance correlates to the prevalence of intestinal metaplasia. *Scand J Gastroenterol.* 2000;35:17.
19. Wallner B, Sylvan A, Janunger KG. Endoscopic assessment of the "Z-line" (squamocolumnar junction) appearance: reproducibility of the ZAP classification among endoscopists. *Gastrointest Endosc.* 2002;55:65.
20. Sharma P, Dent J, Armstrong D, et al. The development and validation of an endoscopic grading system for Barrett's esophagus: the Prague C & M criteria. *Gastroenterology.* 2006;131:1392.
21. Spechler SJ, Goyal RK. The columnar lined esophagus, intestinal metaplasia, and Norman Barrett. *Gastroenterology.* 1996;110:614.
22. Canto MIF, Setrakian S, Willis J, et al. Methylene blue-directed biopsies improve detection of intestinal metaplasia and dysplasia in Barrett's esophagus. *Gastrointest Endosc.* 2000;51:560.
23. Scotiniotis IA, Kochman ML, Lewis JD, Furth EE, Rosato EF, Ginsberg GG. Accuracy of EUS in the evaluation of Barrett's esophagus and high-grade dysplasia or intramucosal carcinoma. *Gastrointest Endosc.* 2001;54:689.
24. Kobayashi K, Izatt JA, Kulkarni MD, Willis J, Sivak MV Jr. High-resolution cross-sectional imaging of the gastrointestinal tract using optical coherence tomography: preliminary results. *Gastrointest Endosc.* 1998;47:515.
25. Georgakoudi I, Jacobson BC, Van Dam J, et al. Fluorescence, reflectance, and light-scattering spectroscopy for evaluating dysplasia in patients with Barrett's esophagus. *Gastroenterology.* 2001;120:1620.
26. Kendall C, Stone N, Shepherd N, et al. Raman spectroscopy, a potential tool for the objective identification and classification of neoplasia in Barrett's oesophagus. *J Pathol.* 2003;200:602.
27. Bergman JJ, Tytgat GN. New developments in the endoscopic surveillance of Barrett's oesophagus. *Gut.* 2005;54:i38.
28. Olliver JR, Wild CP, Sahay P, Dexter S, Hardie LJ. Chromoendoscopy with methylene blue and associated DNA damage in Barrett's oesophagus. *Lancet.* 2003;362:373.
29. Amano Y, Kushiyama Y, Ishihara S, et al. Crystal violet chromoendoscopy with mucosal pit pattern diagnosis is useful for surveillance of short-segment Barrett's esophagus. *Am J Gastroenterol.* 2005;100:21.
30. Toyoda H, Rubio C, Befrits R, Hamamoto N, Adachi Y, Jaramillo E. Detection of intestinal metaplasia in distal esophagus and esophagogastric junction by enhanced-magnification endoscopy. *Gastrointest Endosc.* 2004;59:15.
31. Endo T, Awakawa T, Takahashi H, et al. Classification of Barrett's epithelium by magnifying endoscopy. *Gastrointest Endosc.* 2002;55:641.
32. Vakil N, van Zanten SV, Kahrilas P, et al.; Global Consensus Group. The Montreal definition and classification of gastroesophageal reflux disease: a global evidence-based consensus. *Am J Gastroenterol.* 2006;101:1900.
33. Armstrong D. Endoscopic evaluation of gastro-esophageal reflux disease. *Yale J Biol Med.* 1999;72:93.
34. Richter JE, Peura D, Benjamin SB, Joelsson B, Whipple J. Efficacy of omeprazole for the treatment of symptomatic acid reflux disease without esophagitis. *Arch Intern Med.* 2000;160:1810.
35. Bytzer P, Havelund T, Hansen JM. Interobserver variation in the endoscopic diagnosis of reflux esophagitis. *Scand J Gastroenterol.* 1993;28:119.
36. Lundell LR, Dent J, Bennett JR, et al. Endoscopic assessment of oesophagitis: clinical and functional correlates and further validation of the Los Angeles classification. *Gut.* 1999;45:172.
37. Grossman MI, ed. *Peptic Ulcer: A Guide for the Practicing Physician.* Chicago: Year Book Medical Publishers, Inc.; 1981.
38. Armstrong D, Bennett JR, Blum AL, et al. The endoscopic assessment of esophagitis: a progress report on observer agreement. *Gastroenterology.* 1996;111:85.
39. Savary M, Miller G. *The Esophagus. Handbook and Atlas of Endoscopy.* Solothurn, Switzerland: Verlag Gassman; 1978.
40. Spechler SJ. The management of patients who have "failed" antireflux surgery. *Am J Gastroenterol.* 2004;99:552.
41. Furuta GT, Liacouras CA, Collins MH, et al.; First International Gastrointestinal Eosinophil Research Symposium (FIGERS) Subcommittees. Eosinophilic esophagitis in children and adults: a systematic review and consensus recommendations for diagnosis and treatment. *Gastroenterology.* 2007;133:1342.
42. Rothenberg ME. Biology and treatment of eosinophilic esophagitis. *Gastroenterology.* 2009;137:1238.
43. Kimmey MB, Martin RW. Fundamentals of endosonography. *Gastrointest Endosc Clin N Am.* 1992;2:557.
44. Vilmann P, Khattar S, Hancke S. Endoscopic ultrasound examination of the upper gastrointestinal tract using a curved-array transducer. A preliminary report. *Surg Endosc.* 1991;5:79.
45. Bolondi L, Casanova P, Santi V, Caletti G, Barbara L, Labò G. The sonographic appearance of the normal gastric wall: an in vitro study. *Ultrasound Med Biol.* 1986;12:991.
46. Kimmey MB, Martin RW, Haggitt RC, Wang KY, Franklin DW, Silverstein FE. Histologic correlates of gastrointestinal ultrasound images. *Gastroenterology.* 1989;96:433.

47. Edge SB, Byrd DR, Compton CC, Fritz AG, Greene F, Trotti A. *AJCC Cancer Staging Manual.* 7th ed. New York: Springer; 2009.

48. Rice TW, Rusch VW, Apperson-Hansen C, et al. Worldwide esophageal cancer collaboration. *Dis Esophagus.* 2009;22:1.

49. Ishwaran H, Blackstone EH, Apperson-Hansen C, Rice TW. A novel approach to cancer staging: application to esophageal cancer. *Biostatistics.* 2009;10:603.

50. Rice TW, Rusch VW, Ishwaran H, et al. Cancer of the esophagus and esophagogastric junction: data-driven staging for the 7th edition of the AJCC cancer staging manual. *Cancer.* 2010;16:3763.

51. Rice TW, Blackstone EH, Rusch VW. A cancer staging primer: esophagus and esophagogastric junction. *J Thorac Cardiovasc Surg.* 2010;139:527.

52. Rice TW, Blackstone EH, Rybicki LA, et al. Refining esophageal cancer staging. *J Thorac Cardiovasc Surg.* 2003;125:1103.

53. Botet JF, Lightdale CJ, Zauber AG, Gerdes H, Urmacher C, Brennan MF. Preoperative staging of esophageal cancer: comparison of endoscopic US and dynamic CT. *Radiology.* 1991;181:419.

54. Date H, Miyashita M, Sasajima K, et al. Assessment of adventitial involvement of esophageal carcinoma by endoscopic ultrasonography. *Surg Endosc.* 1990;4:195.

55. Heintz A, Hohne U, Schweden F, Junginger T. Preoperative detection of intrathoracic tumor spread of esophageal cancer: endosonography versus computed tomography. *Surg Endosc.* 1991;5:75.

56. Tio TL, Cohen P, Coene PP, Udding J, den Hartog Jager FC, Tytgat GN. Endosonography and computed tomography of esophageal carcinoma. Preoperative classification compared to the new (1987) TNM system. *Gastroenterology.* 1989;96:1478.

57. Vilgrain V, Mompoint D, Palazzo L, et al. Staging of esophageal carcinoma: comparison of results with endoscopic sonography and CT. *AJR Am J Roentgenol.* 1990;155:277.

58. Ziegler K, Sanft C, Zeitz M, et al. Evaluation of endosonography in TN staging of oesophageal cancer. *Gut.* 1991;32:16.

59. Reinig JW, Stanley JH, Schabel SI. CT evaluation of thickened esophageal walls. *AJR Am J Roentgenol.* 1983;140:931.

60. Consigliere D, Chua CL, Hui F, Yu CS, Low CH. Computed tomography for oesophageal carcinoma: its value to the surgeon. *J R Coll Surg Edinb.* 1992;37:113.

61. Duignan JP, McEntee GP, O'Connell DJ, Bouchier-Hayes DJ, O'Malley E. The role of CT in the management of carcinoma of the oesophagus and cardia. *Ann R Coll Surg Engl.* 1987;69:286.

62. Kasbarian M, Fuentes P, Brichon PY. *Usefulness of Computed Tomography in Assessing the Extension of Carcinoma of the Esophagus and Gastroesophageal Junction.* Berlin: Springer-Verlag; 1988.

63. Kirk SJ, Moorehead RJ, McIlrath E, Gibbons JP, Spence RA. Does preoperative computed tomography scanning aid assessment of oesophageal carcinoma? *Postgrad Med J.* 1990;66:191.

64. Markland CG, Manhire A, Davies P, Beggs D, Morgan WE, Salama FD. The role of computed tomography in assessing the operability of oesophageal carcinoma. *Eur J Cardiothorac Surg.* 1989;3:33.

65. Rice TW, Boyce GA, Sivak MV. Esophageal ultrasound and the preoperative staging of carcinoma of the esophagus. *J Thorac Cardiovasc Surg.* 1991;101:536, [discussion 543–544].

66. Ruol A, Rossi M, Ruffatto A. *Reevaluation of Computed Tomography in Preoperative Staging of Esophageal and Cardial Cancers: A Prospective Study.* New York: Springer-Verlag; 1987.

67. Sondenaa K, Skaane P, Nygaard K, Skjennald A. Value of computed tomography in preoperative evaluation of resectability and staging in oesophageal carcinoma. *Eur J Surg.* 1992;158:537.

68. Ginsberg GG, Al-Kawas EH, Nguyen CC. Endoscopic ultrasound evaluation of vascular involvement in esophageal cancer: a comparison with computed tomography [abstract]. *Gastrointest Endosc.* 1993;39:A276.

69. Fockens P, Van den Brande JH, van Dullemen HM, van Lanschot JJ, Tytgat GN. Endosonographic T-staging of esophageal carcinoma: a learning curve. *Gastrointest Endosc.* 1996;44:58.

70. Schlick T, Heintz A, Junginger T. The examiner's learning effect and its influence on the quality of endoscopic ultrasonography in carcinoma of the esophagus and gastric cardia. *Surg Endosc.* 1999;13:894.

71. van Vliet EP, Eijkemans MJ, Poley JW, Steyerberg EW, Kuipers EJ, Siersema PD. Staging of esophageal carcinoma in low-volume EUS center compared with reported results from high-volume centers. *Gastrointest Endosc.* 2006;63:938.

72. Rosch T. Endosonographic staging of esophageal cancer: a review of literature results. *Gastrointest Endosc Clin N Am.* 1995;5:537.

73. Kelly S, Harris SM, Berry E, et al. A systematic review of the staging performance of endoscopic ultrasound in gastroesophageal carcinoma. *Gut.* 2001;49:534.

74. Puli SR, Reddy JB, Bechtold ML, Antillon D, Ibdah JA, Antillon MR. Staging accuracy of esophageal cancer by endoscopic ultrasound: a meta-analysis and systematic review. *World J Surg.* 2008;14:1479.

75. Rice TW, Blackstone EH, Adelstein DJ, et al. Role of clinically determined depth of tumor invasion in the treatment of esophageal carcinoma. *J Thorac Cardiovasc Surg.* 2003;125:1091.

76. Heidemann J, Schilling MK, Schmassmann A, Maurer CA, Büchler MW. Accuracy of endoscopic ultrasonography in preoperative staging of esophageal carcinoma. *Dig Surg.* 2000;17:219.

77. Rice TW, Mason DP, Murthy SC, et al. T2N0M0 esophageal cancer. *J Thorac Cardiovasc Surg.* 2007;133:317.

78. Pech O, Günter E, Dusemund F, Origer J, Lorenz D, Ell C. Accuracy of endoscopic ultrasound in preoperative staging of esophageal cancer: results from a referral center for early esophageal cancer. *Endoscopy.* 2010;42:456.

79. Rice TW, Blackstone EH, Adelstein DJ, et al. Role of clinically determined depth of tumor invasion in the treatment of esophageal carcinoma. *J Thorac Cardiovasc Surg.* 2003;125:1091.

80. Kelly S, Harris KM, Berry E, et al. A systematic review of the staging performance of endoscopic ultrasound in gastro-oesophageal carcinoma. *Gut.* 2001;49:534.

81. Yusuf TE, Harewood GC, Clain JE, Levy MJ, Topazian MD, Rajan E. Clinical implications of the extent of invasion of T3 esophageal cancer by endoscopic ultrasound. *J Gastroenterol Hepatol.* 2005;20:1880.

82. Meining A, Dittler HJ, Wolf A, et al. You get what you expect? A critical appraisal of imaging methodology in endosonographic cancer staging. *Gut.* 2002;50:599.

83. Bhutani MS, Barde CJ, Markert RJ, Gopalswamy N. Length of esophageal cancer and degree of luminal stenosis during upper endoscopy predict T stage by endoscopic ultrasound. *Endoscopy.* 2002;34:461.

84. Twine CP, Roberts SA, Lewis WG, et al. Prognostic significance of endoluminal ultrasound-defined disease length and tumor volume (EDTV) for patients with the diagnosis of esophageal cancer. *Surg Endosc.* 2010;24:870.

85. Dancygier H, Classen M. Endoscopic ultrasonography in esophageal diseases. *Gastrointest Endosc.* 1989;35:220.

86. Hordijk ML, Zander H, van Blankenstein M, Tilanus HW. Influence of tumor stenosis on the accuracy of endosonography in preoperative T staging of esophageal cancer. *Endoscopy.* 1993;25:171.

87. Morgan MA, Twine CP, Lewis WG, et al. Prognostic significance of failure to cross esophageal tumors by endoluminal ultrasound. *Dis Esophagus.* 2008;21:508.

88. Catalano MF, Van Dam J, Sivak JMV. Malignant esophageal strictures: staging accuracy of endoscopic ultrasonography. *Gastrointest Endosc.* 1995;41:535.

89. Van Dam J, Rice TW, Catalano MF, Kirby T, Sivak MV Jr. High-grade malignant stricture is predictive of esophageal tumor stage: risks of endosonographic evaluation. *Cancer.* 1993;71:2910.

90. Kallemanis GE, Gupta PK, al-Kawas FH, et al. Endoscopic ultrasound for staging esophageal cancer, with and without dilation, is clinically important and safe. *Gastrointest Endosc.* 1995;41:540.

91. Pfau PR, Ginsberg GG, Lew RJ, Faigel DO, Smith DB, Kochman ML. Esophageal dilation for endosonographic evaluation of malignant esophageal strictures is safe and effective. *Am J Gastroenterol.* 2000;95:2813.

92. Wallace MB, Hawes RH, Sahai AV, Van Velse A, Hoffman BJ. Dilation of malignant esophageal stenosis to allow EUS guided fine-needle aspiration: safety and effect on patient management. *Gastrointest Endosc.* 2000;51:309.

93. Binmoeller KF, Seifert H, Seitz U, Izbicki JR, Kida M, Soehendra N. Ultrasonic esophagoprobe for TNM staging of highly stenosing esophageal carcinoma. *Gastrointest Endosc.* 1995;41:547.

94. Hunerbein M, Ghadimi BM, Haensch W, Schlag PM. Transendoscopic ultrasound of esophageal and gastric cancer using miniaturized ultrasound catheter probes. *Gastrointest Endosc.* 1998;48:371.

95. McLoughlin RF, Cooperberg PL, Mathieson JR, Stordy SN, Halparin LS. High resolution endoluminal ultrasonography in the staging of esophageal carcinoma. *J Ultrasound Med.* 1995;14:725.

96. Menzel J, Hoepffner N, Nottberg H, Schulz C, Senninger N, Domschke W. Preoperative staging of esophageal carcinoma: miniprobe sonography versus conventional endoscopic ultrasound

in a prospective histopathologically verified study. *Endoscopy.* 1999;31:291.

97. Worrell SG, Oh DS, Greene CL, Demeester SR, Hagen JA. Endoscopic ultrasound staging of stenotic esophageal cancers may be unnecessary to determine the need for neoadjuvant therapy. *J Gastrointest Surg.* 2014;18:318-320.

98. Buskens CJ, Westerterp M, Lagarde SM, Bergman JJ, ten Kate FJ, van Lanschot JJ. Prediction of appropriateness of local endoscopic treatment for high-grade dysplasia and early adenocarcinoma by EUS and histopathologic features. *Gastrointest Endosc.* 2004;60:703.

99. Scotiniotis IA, Kochman ML, Lewis JD, Furth EE, Rosato EF, Ginsberg GG. Accuracy of EUS in the evaluation of Barrett's esophagus and high-grade dysplasia or intramucosal carcinoma. *Gastrointest Endosc.* 2001;54:689.

100. Pech O, May A, Günter E, Gossner L, Ell C. The impact of endoscopic ultrasound and computed tomography on TNM stage of early cancer in Barrett's esophagus. *Am J Gastroenterol.* 2006;101:2223.

101. Rampado S, Bocus P, Battaglia G, Ruol A, Portale G, Ancona E. Endoscopic ultrasound: accuracy in staging superficial carcinomas of the esophagus. *Ann Thorac Surg.* 2008;85:251.

102. Mandal RV, Forcione DG, Brugge WR, Nishioka NS, Mino-Kenudson M, Lauwers GY. Effect of tumor characteristics and duplication of the muscularis mucosae on the endoscopic staging of superficial Barrett esophagus-related neoplasia. *Am J Surg Pathol.* 2009;33:620.

103. May A, Gunter E, Roth F, et al. Accuracy of staging in early oesophageal cancer using high resolution endoscopy and high resolution endosonography: a comparative, prospective, and blinded trial. *Gut.* 2004;53:634.

104. Murata Y, Napoleon B, Odegaard S. High-frequency endoscopic ultrasonography in the evaluation of superficial esophageal cancer. *Endoscopy.* 2003;35:429, [discussion 436].

105. Waxman I, Raju GS, Critchlow J, Antonioli DA, Spechler SJ. High-frequency probe ultrasonography has limited accuracy for detecting invasive adenocarcinoma in patients with Barrett's esophagus and high-grade dysplasia or intramucosal carcinoma: a case series. *Am J Gastroenterol.* 2006;101:1773.

106. Thomas T, Gilbert D, Kaye PV, Penman I, Aithal GP, Ragunath K. High-resolution endoscopy and endoscopic ultrasound for evaluation of early neoplasia in Barrett's esophagus. *Surg Endosc.* 2010;24:1110.

107. Catalano MF, Sivak MV Jr, Rice T, Gragg LA, Van Dam J. Endosonographic features predictive of lymph node metastasis. *Gastrointest Endosc.* 1994;40:442.

108. Bhutani MS, Hawes RH, Hoffman BJ. A comparison of the accuracy of echo features during endoscopic ultrasound (EUS) and EUS-guided fine-needle aspiration for diagnosis of malignant lymph node invasion. *Gastrointest Endosc.* 1997;45:474.

109. Catalano MF, Alcocer E, Chak A, et al. Evaluation of metastatic celiac axis lymph nodes in patients with esophageal carcinoma: accuracy of EUS. *Gastrointest Endosc.* 1999;50:352.

110. Wiersema MJ, Vilmann P, Giovannini M, Chang KJ, Wiersema LM. Endosonography-guided fine-needle aspiration biopsy: diagnostic accuracy and complication assessment. *Gastroenterology.* 1997;112:1087.

111. Reed CE, Mishra G, Sahai AV, Hoffman BJ, Hawes RH. Esophageal cancer staging: improved accuracy by endoscopic ultrasound of celiac lymph nodes. *Ann Thorac Surg.* 1999;67:319.

112. Eloubeidi MA, Wallace MB, Reed CE, et al. The utility of EUS and EUS-guided fine needle aspiration in detecting celiac lymph node metastasis in patients with esophageal cancer: a single-center experience. *Gastrointest Endosc.* 2001;54:714.

113. Natsugoe S, Yoshinaka H, Shimada M, et al. Number of lymph node metastases determined by presurgical ultrasound and endoscopic ultrasound is related to prognosis in patients with esophageal carcinoma. *Ann Surg.* 2001;234:613.

114. Chen J, Xu R, Hunt GC, Krinsky ML, Savides TJ. Influence of the number of malignant regional lymph nodes detected by endoscopic ultrasonography on survival stratification in esophageal adenocarcinoma. *Clin Gastroenterol Hepatol.* 2006;4:573.

115. Twine CP, Roberts SA, Rawlinson CE, et al. Prognostic significance of the endoscopic ultrasound defined lymph node metastasis count in esophageal cancer. *Dis Esophagus.* 2010;23:652.

116. Rice TW, Zuccaro G Jr, Adelstein DJ, Rybicki LA, Blackstone EH, Goldblum JR. Esophageal carcinoma: depth of tumor invasion is predictive of regional lymph node status. *Ann Thorac Surg.* 1998;65:787.

117. Wiersema MJ, Hawes RH, Tao LC, et al. Endoscopic ultrasonography as an adjunct to fine needle aspiration cytology of the upper and lower gastrointestinal tract. *Gastrointest Endosc.* 1992;38:35.

118. Wiersema MJ, Kochman ML, Chak A, Cramer HM, Kesler KA. Real-time endoscopic ultrasound-guided fine-needle aspiration of a mediastinal lymph node. *Gastrointest Endosc.* 1993;39:429.

119. Mortensen MB, Pless T, Durup J, Ainsworth AP, Plagborg GJ, Hovendal C. Clinical impact of endoscopic ultrasound-guided fine needle aspiration biopsy in patients with upper gastrointestinal tract malignancies. A prospective study. *Endoscopy.* 2001;33:478.

120. Vazquez-Sequeiros E, Norton ID, Clain JE, et al. Impact of EUS-guided fine-needle aspiration on lymph node staging in patients with esophageal carcinoma. *Gastrointest Endosc.* 2001;53:751.

121. Vazquez-Sequeiros E, Wiersema MJ, Clain JE, et al. Impact of lymph node staging on therapy of esophageal carcinoma. *Gastroenterology.* 2003;125:1626.

122. Wiersema MJ, Vilmann P, Giovannini M, Chang KJ, Wiersema LM. Endosonography-guided fine-needle aspiration biopsy: diagnostic accuracy and complication assessment. *Gastroenterology.* 1997;112:1087.

123. O'Toole D, Palazzo L, Arotcarena R, et al. Assessment of complications of EUS-guided fine-needle aspiration. *Gastrointest Endosc.* 2001;53:470.

124. Eloubeidi MA, Wallace MB, Reed CE, et al. The utility of EUS and EUS-guided fine needle aspiration in detecting celiac lymph node metastasis in patients with esophageal cancer: a single-center experience. *Gastrointest Endosc.* 2001;54:714.

125. Harewood GC, Wiersema MJ. A cost analysis of endoscopic ultrasound in the evaluation of esophageal cancer. *Am J Gastroenterol.* 2002;97:452.

126. Pfau PR, Ginsberg GG, Lew RJ, Brensinger CM, Kochman ML. EUS predictors of long-term survival in esophageal carcinoma. *Gastrointest Endosc.* 2001;53:463.

127. Harewood GC, Kumar KS. Assessment of clinical impact of endoscopic ultrasound on esophageal cancer. *J Gastroenterol Hepatol.* 2004;19:433.

128. McGrath K, Brody D, Luketich J, Khalid A. Detection of unsuspected left hepatic lobe metastases during EUS staging of cancer of the esophagus and cardia. *Am J Gastroenterol.* 2006;101:1742.

129. Sultan J, Robinson S, Hayes N, Griffin SM, Richardson DL, Preston SR. Endoscopic ultrasonography-detected low-volume ascites as a predictor of inoperability for oesophagogastric cancer. *Br J Surg.* 2008;95:1127.

130. Adelstein DJ, Rice TW, Boyce GA, et al. Adenocarcinoma of the esophagus and gastroesophageal junction. Clinical and pathologic assessment of response to induction chemotherapy. *Am J Clin Oncol.* 1994;17:14.

131. Hordijk ML, Kok TC, Wilson JH, Mulder AH. Assessment of response of esophageal carcinoma to induction chemotherapy. *Endoscopy.* 1993;25:592.

132. Roubein LD, DuBrow R, David C, et al. Endoscopic ultrasonography in the quantitative assessment of response to chemotherapy in patients with adenocarcinoma of the esophagus and esophagogastric junction. *Endoscopy.* 1993;25:587.

133. Dittler HJ, Fink U, Siewert GR. Response to chemotherapy in esophageal cancer. *Endoscopy.* 1994;26:769.

134. Giovannini M, Seitz JF, Thomas P, et al. Endoscopic ultrasonography for assessment of the response to combined radiation therapy and chemotherapy in patients with esophageal cancer. *Endoscopy.* 1997;29:4.

135. Zuccaro G Jr, Rice TW, Goldblum J, et al. Endoscopic ultrasound cannot determine suitability for esophagectomy after aggressive chemoradiotherapy for esophageal cancer. *Am J Gastroenterol.* 1999;94:906.

136. Isenberg G, Chak A, Canto MI, et al. Endoscopic ultrasound in restaging of esophageal cancer after neoadjuvant chemoradiation. *Gastrointest Endosc.* 1998;48:158.

137. Laterza E, de Manzoni G, Guglielmi A, Rodella L, Tedesco P, Cordiano C. Endoscopic ultrasonography in the staging of esophageal carcinoma after preoperative radiotherapy and chemotherapy. *Ann Thorac Surg.* 1999;67:1466.

138. Kalha I, Kaw M, Fukami N, et al. The accuracy of endoscopic ultrasound for restaging esophageal carcinoma after chemoradiation therapy. *Cancer.* 2004;101:940.

139. Beseth BD, Bedford R, Isacoff WH, Holmes EC, Cameron RB. Endoscopic ultrasound does not accurately assess pathologic stage

of esophageal cancer after neoadjuvant chemoradiotherapy. *Am Surg.* 2000;66:827.

140. Fleshman JW, Myerson RJ, Fry RD, Kodner IJ. Accuracy of transrectal ultrasound in predicting pathologic stage of rectal cancer before and after preoperative radiation therapy. *Dis Colon Rectum.* 1992;35:823.

141. Chak A, Canto MI, Cooper GS, et al. Endosonographic assessment of multimodality therapy predicts survival of esophageal carcinoma patients. *Cancer.* 2000;88:1788.

142. Agarwal B, Swisher S, Ajani J, et al. Endoscopic ultrasound after preoperative chemoradiation can help identify patients who benefit maximally after surgical esophageal resection. *Am J Gastroenterol.* 2004;99:1258.

143. Ngamruengphong S, Sharma VK, Nguyen B, Das A. Assessment of response to neoadjuvant therapy in esophageal cancer: an updated systematic review of diagnostic accuracy of endoscopic ultrasonography and fluorodeoxyglucose positron emission tomography. *Dis Esophagus.* 2010;3:216.

144. Catalano MF, Sivak MV Jr, Rice TW, Van Dam J. Postoperative screening for anastomotic recurrence of esophageal carcinoma by endoscopic ultrasonography. *Gastrointest Endosc.* 1995;42:540.

145. Lightdale CJ, Botet JF, Kelsen DP, Turnbull AD, Brennan MF. Diagnosis of recurrent upper gastrointestinal cancer at the surgical anastomosis by endoscopic ultrasound. *Gastrointest Endosc.* 1989;35:407.

146. Kawamoto K, Yamada Y, Utsunomiya T, et al. Gastrointestinal submucosal tumors: evaluation with endoscopic US. *Radiology.* 1997;205:733.

147. Lewin KJ, Appelman HD. Mesenchymal tumors and tumor-like proliferations of the esophagus. In: Rosai J, Sobin LH, eds. *Tumors of the Esophagus and Stomach.* Washington, DC: Armed Forces Institute of Pathology; 1996:145 Atlas of Tumor Pathology; 3rd series, fascicle 18.

148. Schuhmacher C, Becker K, Dittler HJ, Höfler H, Siewert JR, Stein HJ. Fibrovascular esophageal polyp as a diagnostic challenge. *Dis Esophagus.* 2000;13:324.

149. Devereaux BM, LeBlanc JK, Kesler K, Burttet LM, Kruel CD, da Rosa AP. Giant fibrovascular polyp of the esophagus. *Endoscopy.* 2003;35:970.

150. Palazzo L, Landi B, Cellier C, et al. Endosonographic features of esophageal granular cell tumors. *Endoscopy.* 1997;29:850.

151. Love MH, Glaser M, Edmunds SE, Mendelson RM. Granular cell tumour of the oesophagus: endoscopic ultrasound appearances. *Australas Radiol.* 1999;43:253.

152. Goldblum JR, Rice TW, Zuccaro G, Richter JE. Granular cell tumors of the esophagus: a clinical and pathologic study of 13 cases. *Ann Thorac Surg.* 1996;62:860.

153. Araki K, Ohno S, Egashira A, et al. Esophageal hemangioma: a case report and review of the literature. *Hepatogastroenterology.* 1999;46:3148.

154. Maluf-Filho F, Sakai P, Amico EC, Pinotti HW. Giant cavernous hemangioma of the esophagus: endoscopic and echo-endoscopic appearance. *Endoscopy.* 1999;31:S32.

155. Takada N, Higashino M, Osugi H, Tokuhara T, Kinoshita H. Utility of endoscopic ultrasonography in assessing the indications for endoscopic surgery of submucosal esophageal tumors. *Surg Endosc.* 1999;13:228.

156. Xu GM, Niu YL, Zou XP, Jin ZD, Li ZS. The diagnostic value of transendoscopic miniature ultrasonic probe for esophageal diseases. *Endoscopy.* 1998;30(suppl 1):A28.

157. Stelow EB, Jones DR, Shami VM. Esophageal leiomyosarcoma diagnosed by endoscopic ultrasound guided fine-needle aspiration. *Diagn Cytopathol.* 2007;35:167.

158. Gouveia AM, Pimenta AP, Lopes JM, et al. Esophageal GIST: therapeutic implications of an uncommon presentation of a rare tumor. *Dis Esophagus.* 2005;18:7.

159. Blum MG, Bilimoria KY, Wayne JD, de Hoyos AL, Talamonti MS, Adley B. Surgical considerations for the management and resection of esophageal gastrointestinal stromal tumors. *Ann Thorac Surg.* 2007;84:1717.

160. Bhutani MS, Hoffman BJ, Reed C. Endosonographic diagnosis of an esophageal duplication cyst. *Endoscopy.* 1996;28:396.

161. Faigel DO, Burke A, Ginsberg GG, Stotland BR, Kadish SL, Kochman ML. The role of endoscopic ultrasound in the evaluation and management of foregut duplications. *Gastrointest Endosc.* 1997;45:99.

162. Lim LL, Ho KY, Goh PM. Preoperative diagnosis of a paraesophageal bronchogenic cyst using endosonography. *Ann Thorac Surg.* 2002;73:633.

163. Massari M, De Simone M, Cioffi U, Gabrielli F, Boccasanta P, Bonavina L. Endoscopic ultrasonography in the evaluation of leiomyoma and extramucosal cysts of the esophagus. *Hepatogastroenterology.* 1998;45:938.

164. Van Dam J, Rice TW, Sivak MV Jr. Endoscopic ultrasonography and endoscopically guided needle aspiration for the diagnosis of upper gastrointestinal tract foregut cysts. *Am J Gastroenterol.* 1992;87:762.

165. Yasuda K, Cho E, Nakajima M, Kawai K. Diagnosis of submucosal lesions of the upper gastrointestinal tract by endoscopic ultrasonography. *Gastrointest Endosc.* 1990;36(suppl 2):S17.

166. El-Saadany M, Jalil S, Irisawa A, Shibukawa G, Ohira H, Bhutani MS. EUS for portal hypertension: a comprehensive and critical aapprasal of clinical and experimental indications. *Endoscopy.* 2008;40:690.

167. Bergami GL, Fruhwirth R, Di Mario M, Fasanelli S. Contribution of ultrasonography in the diagnosis of achalasia. *J Pediatr Gastroenterol Nutr.* 1992;14:92.

168. Deviere J, Dunham F, Rickaert F, Bourgeois N, Cremer M. Endoscopic ultrasonography in achalasia. *Gastroenterology.* 1989;96:1210.

169. Falk GW, Van Dam J, Sivak MV. Endoscopic ultrasonography (EUS) in achalasia. *Gastrointest Endosc.* 1991;37:241.

170. Barthet M, Mambrini P, Audibert P, et al. Relationships between endosonographic appearance and clinical or manometric features in patients with achalasia. *Eur J Gastroenterol Hepatol.* 1998;10:559.

171. Ponsot P, Chaussade S, Palazzo L, et al. Endoscopic ultrasonography in achalasia. *Gastroenterology.* 1990;98:253.

172. Ziegler K, Sanft C, Friedrich M, Gregor M, Riecken EO. Endosonographic appearance of the esophagus in achalasia. *Endoscopy.* 1990;22:1.

173. Kobayashi H, Danabara T, Sugama Y, Saito T, Kitamura S, Kira S. Observation of lymph nodes and great vessels in the mediastinum by endoscopic ultrasonography. *Jpn J Med.* 1987;26:353.

174. Kondo D, Imaizumi M, Abe T, Naruke T, Suemasu K. Endoscopic ultrasound examination for mediastinal lymph node metastases of lung cancer. *Chest.* 1990;98:586.

175. Potepan P, Meroni E, Spagnoli I, et al. Non–small-cell lung cancer: detection of mediastinal lymph node metastases by endoscopic ultrasound and CT. *Eur Radiol.* 1996;6:19.

176. Mishra G, Sahai AV, Penman ID, et al. Endoscopic ultrasonography with fine-needle aspiration: an accurate and simple diagnostic modality for sarcoidosis. *Endoscopy.* 1999;31:377.

177. Fritscher-Ravens A, Petrasch S, Reinacher-Schick A, Graeven U, König M, Schmiegel W. Diagnostic value of endoscopic ultrasonography-guided fine-needle aspiration cytology of mediastinal masses in patients with intrapulmonary lesions and nondiagnostic bronchoscopy. *Respiration.* 1999;66:150.

178. Hunerbein M, Ghadimi BM, Haensch W, Schlag PM. Transesophageal biopsy of mediastinal and pulmonary tumors by means of endoscopic ultrasound guidance. *J Thorac Cardiovasc Surg.* 1998;116:554.

179. Pedersen BH, Vilmann P, Folke K, et al. Endoscopic ultrasonography and real-time guided fine-needle aspiration biopsy of solid lesions of the mediastinum suspected of malignancy. *Chest.* 1996;110:539.

High-Resolution Esophageal Manometry: Techniques and Use in the Diagnosis of Esophageal Motility Disorders and for Surgical Decision Making

Ezra N. Teitelbaum | Christy M. Dunst

Esophageal motility disorders may be implicated as an explanation for dysphagia and noncardiac chest pain after exclusion of esophageal structural lesions by endoscopy, with the caveat that eosinophilic esophagitis has been ruled out with histology. Gastroesophageal reflux disease (GERD) must also be carefully considered, and most patients will be given a course of proton pump inhibitor therapy or evaluated with a 24- or 48-hour pH monitoring study to exclude that possibility even in the absence of endoscopic lesions. The best-defined esophageal motor disorder is achalasia; however, other motility disorders such as distal esophageal spasm (DES), hypercontractile (or jackhammer) esophagus, absent peristalsis, and ineffective esophageal motility (IEM) have also been reported to be associated with dysphagia and/or chest pain.[1]

Esophageal manometry is the clinical test that defines the contractile characteristics of the esophagus to identify and classify motility disorders. Manometric evaluation of the tubular esophagus assesses the integrity, rate of progression, and morphology of the contractile complex (amplitude, duration, repetitive contractions). Classification strategies grounded in conventional manometry have characterized esophageal motor patterns with three to eight pressure sensors spaced 3 to 5 cm apart, using pressure displayed along a time axis. However, with recent advances in pressure transduction hardware, computer processing, and analysis software, conventional manometry has been rapidly supplanted by high-resolution manometry (HRM) and esophageal pressure topography (EPT) analysis as the methodology of choice. HRM and EPT were initially described experimentally by Clouse in the 1990s[2] and have now become widely available for clinical practice through his initiatives with industry partners. Using EPT, pressure data are presented as a seamless dynamic not only in time but also along the length of the esophagus. A key advantage is in the ability to assess pressure profiles along the vertical (length) axis of the esophagus (spatial-pressure variation plots) improving both the accuracy and detail of the study compared with the conventional techniques that it replaces.

In addition to its use as a tool to diagnose esophageal motility disorders, HRM plays an important role in the evaluation of esophageal function in patients before and after foregut operations, particularly laparoscopic antireflux surgery. Long-term functional complications such as dysphagia and gas bloat syndrome are concerning sequelae that occur in some patients after laparoscopic fundoplication. To identify patients who may be at risk for developing postoperative dysphagia, it is recommended that patients undergo routine preoperative HRM. HRM can diagnose previously unrecognized major disorders of esophageal motility, such as achalasia, and identify patients with partially impaired esophageal body function, or IEM. How to approach patients with IEM who are undergoing fundoplication is an area of considerable controversy. Some surgeons preferred a strategy of "tailored" fundoplication in which a partial wrap is constructed in such patients, whereas others do not feel this is necessary and perform a complete, or Nissen, fundoplication regardless of preoperative HRM results. This chapter will focus on describing esophageal motor disorders using HRM and EPT interpretation and will illustrate how these techniques are used in the management of esophageal motility disorders. In addition, it will discuss the use of HRM in the perioperative evaluation of patients undergoing foregut operations, with a focus on antireflux surgery.

TECHNIQUES OF ESOPHAGEAL MANOMETRY

The utility of esophageal manometry in clinical practice resides in two domains: (1) to accurately define esophageal motor function and (2) to delineate a treatment plan based on motor abnormalities.

TECHNICAL ASPECTS

Esophageal manometry is a test in which intraluminal pressure sensors, either water perfused or solid state, are positioned axially within the esophagus to quantify the contractile characteristics of the esophagus and segregate it into functional regions. The probe/catheter is inserted transnasally and connected to a recording unit (via a hydraulic pump in case of perfused pressure sensors). Whereas conventional technique used probes with 3 to 8 pressure sensors spaced 3 to 5 cm apart, HRM typically uses 36 solid-state pressure sensors spaced at 1-cm intervals. The concept of HRM is to use a sufficient number of pressure sensors within the esophagus such that intraluminal pressure can be monitored as a continuum along the entire length of the esophagus, much as time is viewed as a continuum in line tracings of conventional manometry. Fig. 8.1 superimposes representative conventional and HRM recordings with the HRM displayed in EPT format. The most common currently available HRM catheters consist of 36 pressure sensors spaced 1 cm apart. These devices provide sufficient recording length (35 cm) for the recording to span from the hypopharynx to the stomach (with several intragastric sensors) without need for probe repositioning during the course of a study. HRM

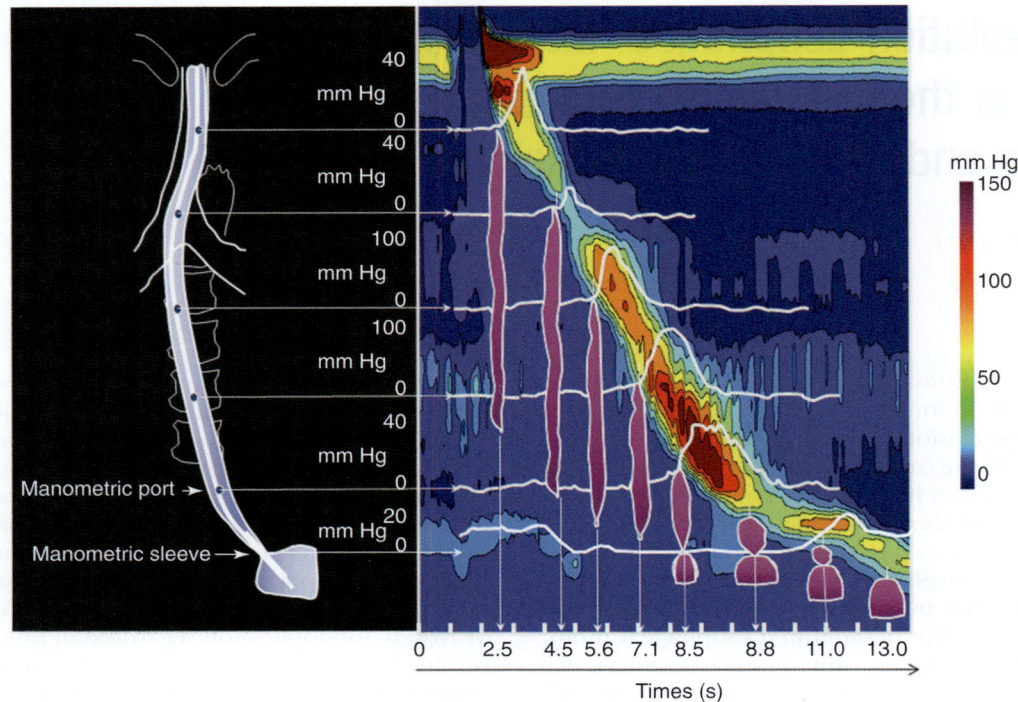

FIGURE 8.1 Depiction of normal esophageal motility by fluoroscopy *(pink tracings)*, conventional manometry *(white line tracings),* and high-resolution manometry with esophageal pressure topography (EPT). The positions of pressure sensors in the esophagus for the conventional manometry are indicated in the anatomic drawing *on the left* with a sleeve device across the esophagogastric junction (EGJ). *On the right* the conventional manometry tracings, bolus distribution, and EPT are overlaid to illustrate how they correspond with each other. The peristaltic wave strips the bolus from the esophagus, with the pressure upstroke (conventional) or isobaric contour (EPT) demarcating the bolus/no bolus interface. Note the tremendously enhanced detail provided by EPT, especially in the area of the EGJ.

offers several theoretical advantages over conventional manometry: (1) the technique lends itself to standardized objective metrics of interpretation, (2) it is easier to perform studies of uniform high quality, (3) movement artifact attributable to a relative change in the position of a sensor and contractile zone (especially sphincters) is minimized, and (4) the process of interpretation is more intuitive and more easily learned by trainees naïve to either conventional or high-resolution manometric formats.[3]

MANOMETRIC PROTOCOL

Esophageal manometry is usually performed in the supine position. This position allows the testing of peristaltic function without the effect of gravity on bolus transit and esophageal contractile pressures are augmented when supine. Historically, using perfused pressure sensors, the supine position was mandatory to have all the sensors at the same height as the external pressure transducers, thereby avoiding pressure offsets secondary to hydrostatic pressure. With solid-state transducers, this is no longer an issue and studies can be performed in the upright position, which some argue to be more physiologic. However, all currently available normative data have been established in the supine position.

A typical manometry protocol consists of a 30-second basal period without swallowing followed by 10 test 5-mL water swallows. Test swallows are separated by at least 20 seconds to reestablish basal activity and avoid having deglutitive inhibition from the prior swallow modulating

the subsequent swallow. The manometric diagnosis is based on the analysis of the 10 5-mL test swallows. Increased water volume (10, 20 mL) can be given to stress peristalsis, and multiple rapid swallows may be used to assess deglutitive inhibition,[4] but these challenges have not yet been sufficiently standardized to serve as diagnostic criteria. However, multiple rapid swallows are a simple method for assessing the integrity of deglutitive inhibition, defects of which are thought to be responsible for some motility disorders. Finally, the consistency of the bolus can be varied using viscous solutions or solids such as marshmallow or bread. However, again, these challenges have not yet been sufficiently standardized to serve as diagnostic criteria.

ESOPHAGEAL PRESSURE TOPOGRAPHY

When HRM is coupled with sophisticated algorithms to display the manometric data as pressure topography plots, esophageal contractility is visualized with isobaric conditions among sensors indicated by isocoloric regions on the pressure topography plots. In EPT plots (or Clouse plots) the y-axis represents the axial length of the esophageal body, with the pharynx and upper esophageal sphincter (UES) at the top of the graph and the esophagogastric junction (EGJ) and proximal stomach at the bottom. The x-axis represents time, so that peristaltic pressure waves can be seen propagating to the right during swallows. Pressure is represented as color, with "hot" colors (red, orange) representing higher pressures and "cool" colors (green, blue) depicting lower pressures.

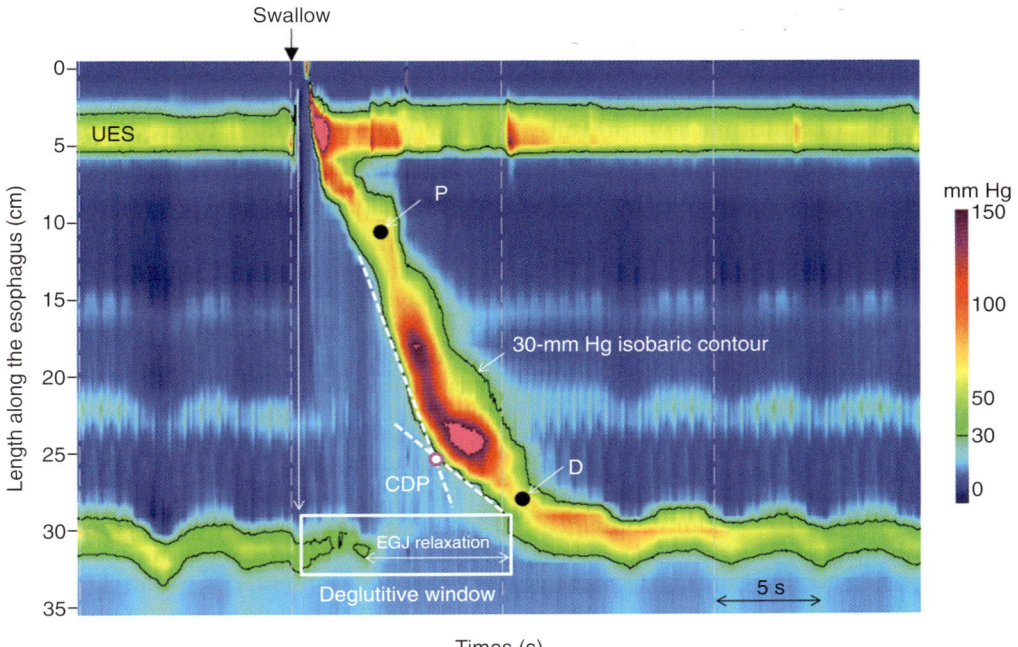

FIGURE 8.2 A normal swallow in an esophageal pressure topography plot. Before and after the swallow, two high-pressure zones are visualized: the upper esophageal sphincter *(UES)* and the esophagogastric junction *(EGJ)*. The highlighted *black line* is the 30-mm Hg isobaric contour circumscribing areas on the plot with intraluminal pressure greater than 30 mm Hg. The peristaltic esophageal contraction is characterized by two troughs, one proximal *(P)* and one distal *(D)*. The contractile deceleration point *(CDP)* represents the inflexion point in the contractile front propagation. It is localized by fitting two tangential lines to the initial and terminal portions of the 30-mm Hg isobaric contours and noting intersection of the lines *(white dot)*. The EGJ relaxation window, extending for 10 seconds after UES relaxation, is the area in which deglutitive EGJ relaxation is assessed.

Fig. 8.2 depicts a normal swallow in a high-resolution EPT plot encompassing both sphincters and the intervening esophagus; the relative timing of sphincter relaxation and segmental contraction as well as the position of the transition zone are all readily demonstrated. The swallowing sequence is described as follows. The UES relaxation induced by swallowing is followed by a peristaltic contraction in the esophageal body that is dependent on the regional gradient of inhibitory neurons within the myenteric plexus. The peristaltic esophageal contraction is preceded by a period of latency or quiescence in the esophageal body and contractile activity is not generated until the period of inhibition or latency is supplanted by excitatory activity at that particular location. Swallow-induced EGJ relaxation also begins just after UES relaxation and ends when the propagated esophageal contraction reaches the EGJ. The peristaltic contraction is characterized by two major pressure troughs, one proximal and one distal (see P and D in Fig. 8.2). A middle pressure trough is sometimes evident, but this is variable among individuals. Another notable feature of peristalsis is an inflexion point in propagation velocity as the contraction nears the EGJ. This inflexion point, termed the contractile deceleration point (CDP), demarcates the initial segment of the esophageal contraction dominated by esophageal peristalsis from the later portion of the contraction during which ampullary emptying transpires. The CDP can be localized objectively by fitting tangential lines to the initial

and terminal portions of the 30-mm Hg isobaric contour and noting intersection of the lines as illustrated in Fig. 8.2.

ALGORITHM OF ANALYSIS USING PRESSURE TOPOGRAPHY PARAMETERS

The algorithm for classifying esophageal motor disorders using EPT is based on a systematic analysis that begins by separating the plot into two functional domains: the EGJ and esophageal body. This system for analysis was developed after the advent of HRM and relies on the use of computer calculations to measuring metrics specific to EPT. The resulting algorithm for HRM measurement and subsequent classification and diagnosis of esophageal contractility disorders has been termed the Chicago Classification.[5] Drawing on an initial experience using the system, the Chicago Classification has subsequently been updated by international working groups to the current version 3.0 (v3.0).[6] The remainder of the chapter will be based on this current iteration.

Chicago Classification analysis begins with an assessment of EGJ function because abnormal EGJ pressure morphology or impaired deglutitive EGJ relaxation can profoundly affect peristalsis and pressure topography within the esophageal body. EGJ abnormalities are also of important clinical significance because bolus transport depends on the balance among resistance through the EGJ, intrabolus pressure (IBP), and esophageal closure pressure behind the bolus.[7] Consequently, the first step in analyzing esophageal motility should focus on the EGJ. Consistent with this, a stepwise analysis algorithm first characterizes EGJ pressure morphology (presence of hiatus hernia) and the adequacy of deglutitive EGJ relaxation. The implications of abnormal EGJ pressure morphology on clinical classification have yet to be fully defined, but physiologic data support the concept that there is a strong interaction between EGJ structure and esophageal function, as well as competence of the EGJ valve mechanism in preventing gastroesophageal reflux (GER).[7] The consequences of impaired deglutitive EGJ relaxation are more obvious, leading to increased distal esophageal (or panesophageal) IBP. Hence, although EGJ pressure morphology will likely be incorporated into future diagnostic categories, the first branch point in the current scheme is of normal or impaired EGJ relaxation because this consistently affects esophageal function.

After defining EGJ anatomy and deglutitive relaxation, the next step in analysis is focused on the esophageal peristalsis. The topography pattern of individual swallows are each classified according to the Chicago Classification parameters shown in Table 8.1. Earlier versions of the Chicago Classification focused on the integrity of peristalsis (i.e., whether breaks in the peristaltic waves

occurred). However, subsequent studies demonstrated that significant breaks in peristalsis frequently occur in healthy individuals, especially at the transition zone in the proximal esophagus between striated and smooth muscle, and that these breaks are not a reliable measure for defining clinically relevant diagnostic categories.[8] As a result, the Chicago Classification v3.0 focuses on assessing the effectiveness of individual swallows based on contractile vigor, or the summed pressure front of the peristaltic wave of each swallow, irrespective of breaks in the wave pattern. This is done by measuring the distal contractile integral (DCI), which can be conceptualized as the volume of the pressure topography graph in the peristaltic wave distal to the transition zone. Swallows are classified as failed, weak, normal, or hypercontractile, based on DCI. This method of analysis both simplifies the classification of swallows and makes it a more clinically relevant assessment of bolus clearance. Swallows are then further characterized by distal latency (DL) and peristaltic breaks to identify instances of premature contraction (i.e., spasm) or fragmented peristalsis (currently defined as a minor disorder of esophageal motility of unclear clinical significance).

In addition to the contractile pattern, each swallow is examined for an abnormal esophageal pressurization with the contractile activity. This is a unique feature of EPT as these patterns are much more evident in pressure topography compared with the conventional line-tracing format. After all test swallows are characterized, the study results are summarized using the classification algorithm, as presented in Fig. 8.3 and Table 8.2.

Esophagogastric Junction Morphology

Both the lower esophageal sphincter (LES) and the surrounding crural diaphragm (CD) contribute to measured intraluminal EGJ pressure. The CD component is most evident during inspiration but probably also contributes a minor component to EGJ pressure during expiration. Thus there are two major confounding variables in describing EGJ intraluminal pressure: phase of the respiratory cycle and the relative positions of the LES and the CD. No consensus was ever achieved with conventional manometry on how to deal with either of these variables. Indeed, there was generally little recognition of the EGJ as a complex sphincter, instead simply referring to it as the LES on manometry studies. With HRM, the sphincteric contributions of the CD and LES become somewhat obvious and the relative localization of the LES and CD elements defines EGJ morphologic subtypes (Fig. 8.4). The magnitude of CD augmentation of EGJ pressure during normal respiration is readily quantified. A retrospective analysis of the relationship between these attributes of EGJ pressure topography and GERD found that GERD patients had significantly greater CD-LES separation (i.e., hiatal hernia) compared with either controls or non-GERD patients.[9] GERD patients also had significantly less inspiratory CD augmentation compared with controls or non-GERD patients. Furthermore, in a logistic regression model, only inspiratory augmentation was found to have a significant independent association with GERD, suggesting that CD impairment was the mediator of both the hiatus hernia and LES hypotension effects.

TABLE 8.1 Esophageal Pressure Topography Scoring of Individual Swallows

CONTRACTION VIGOR

Failed	DCI <100 mm Hg-s-cm
Weak	DCI >100 mm Hg-s-cm, but <450 mm Hg-s-cm
Ineffective	Failed or weak
Normal	DCI ≥450 mm Hg-s-cm, but <8000 mm Hg-s-cm
Hypercontractile	DCI ≥8000 mm Hg-s-cm

CONTRACTION PATTERN

Premature	DL <4.5 s
Fragmented	Large break (>5 cm length) in the 20 mm Hg isobaric contour with DCI >450 mm Hg-s-cm
Normal contraction	Not achieving any of the above diagnostic criteria

INTRABOLUS PRESSURE PATTERN (30-mm Hg ISOBARIC CONTOUR)

Panesophageal pressurization	Uniform pressurization extending from the UES to the EGJ
Compartmentalized esophageal pressurization	Pressurization extending from the contractile front to the EGJ
EGJ pressurization	Pressurization restricted to zone between the LES and CD with LES-CD separation (i.e., presence of a hiatal hernia)
Normal pressurization	No bolus pressurization >30 mm Hg

CD, Crural diaphragm; *DCI*, distal contractile integral; *DL*, distal latency; *EGJ*, esophagogastric junction; *LES*, lower esophageal sphincter; *UES*, upper esophageal sphincter.
From Kahrilas PJ, Bredenoord AJ, Fox M, et al. The Chicago Classification of esophageal motility disorders, v3.0. *Neurogastroenterol Motil.* 2015;27:160–174.

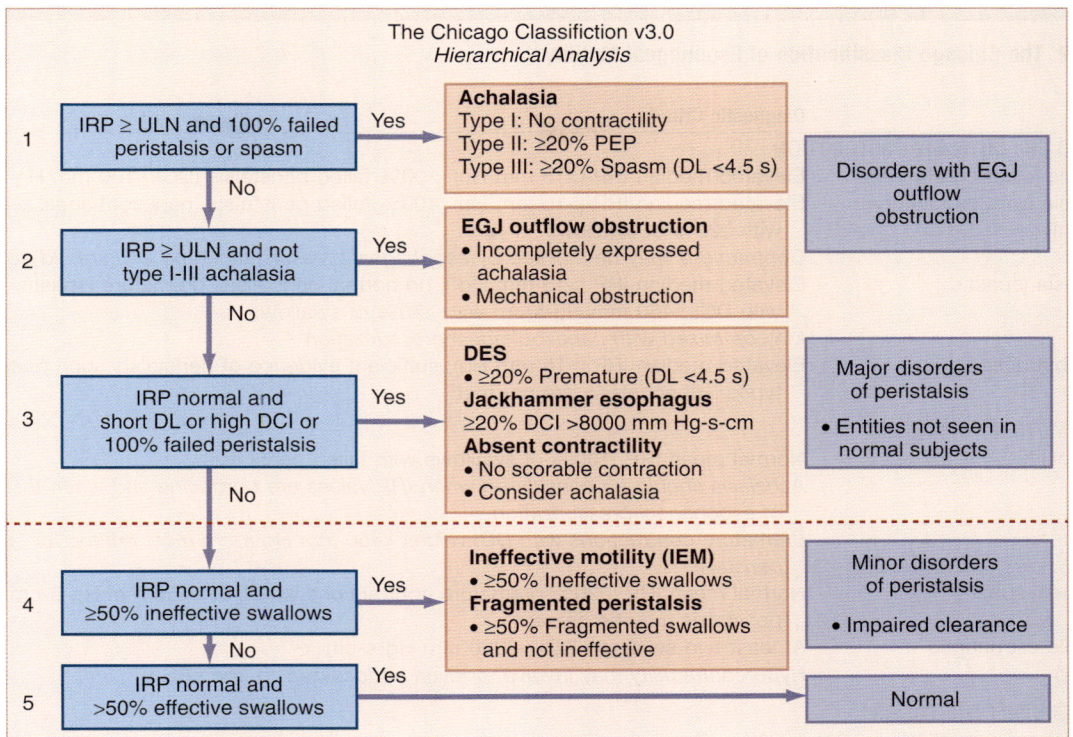

FIGURE 8.3 Algorithm for analysis of esophageal pressure topography studies according to the Chicago Classification v3.0. Note that motility disorders should be considered as a cause of dysphagia and/or chest pain only after first evaluating for structural disorders, eosinophilic esophagitis, and, where appropriate, cardiac disease. The first branch point is to identify patients meeting criteria for achalasia (elevated integrated relaxation pressure *[IRP]* and absent peristalsis), which is then subclassified. If IRP is normal, then other peristaltic abnormalities such as spasm and hypercontractility are identified if present. Major disorders of peristalsis are shown above the dotted line, with minor disorders and normal peristalsis below it. *DCI,* Distal contractile integral; *DES,* distal esophageal spasm; *DL,* distal latency; *EGJ,* esophagogastric junction; *PEP,* panesophageal pressurization; *ULN,* upper limit of normal.

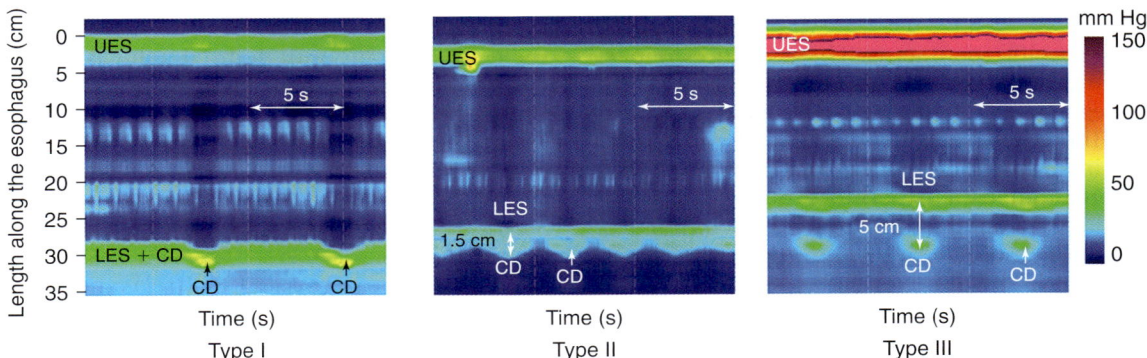

FIGURE 8.4 Esophagogastric junction (EGJ) morphology characterized in esophageal pressure topography. The two main EGJ components are lower esophageal sphincter *(LES)* and crural diaphragm *(CD),* which cannot be independently quantified when superimposed, classified as type I EGJ. With a type II EGJ, the LES and CD are separated by 1 to 2 cm, and in a type III the LES and CD are separated by more than 2 cm. A type III EGJ is the manometric criterion for hiatal hernia. *UES,* Upper esophageal sphincter.

Finally, dynamic HRM studies during reflux monitoring revealed that this is not a static situation. Rather, GERD patients oscillated between types I and II EGJ conformations. Reflux events preferentially occurred during the periods of type II conformation characterized by a small separation of the two high-pressure areas.[10] Paradoxically, in contrast to the findings related to the CD and EGJ morphology, it is less clear that any measure of basal EGJ pressure has much significance.

Esophagogastric Junction Relaxation

Incomplete deglutitive EGJ relaxation is an essential feature in the diagnosis of achalasia, and achalasia is not only the best-defined esophageal motor disorder but also the one

TABLE 8.2 The Chicago Classification of Esophageal Motility

	Diagnostic Criteria
ACHALASIA AND EGJ OUTFLOW OBSTRUCTION	
Type I achalasia (classic achalasia)	Elevated median IRP (>15 mm Hg), 100% failed peristalsis (DCI <100 mm Hg-s-cm)
Type II achalasia (with esophageal compression)	Elevated median IRP (>15 mm Hg), 100% failed peristalsis, panesophageal pressurization with ≥20% of swallows
	Contractions may be masked by esophageal pressurization and DCI should not be calculated
Type III achalasia (spastic achalasia)	Elevated median IRP (>15 mm Hg*), no normal peristalsis, premature (spastic) contractions with DCI >450 mm Hg-s-cm with ≥20% of swallows
	May be mixed with panesophageal pressurization
EGJ outflow obstruction	Elevated median IRP (>15 mm Hg), sufficient evidence of peristalsis such that the criteria for types I–III achalasia are not met[†]
OTHER MAJOR MOTILITY DISORDERS	
Absent contractility	Normal mean IRP, 100% of swallows with failed peristalsis
	Achalasia should be considered when IRP values are borderline and when there is evidence of esophageal pressurization
	Premature contractions with DCI values <450 mm Hg-s-cm meet criteria for failed peristalsis
Distal esophageal spasm	Normal mean IRP, ≥20% premature contractions with DCI >450 mm Hg-s-cm. Some normal peristalsis may be present.
Hypercontractile esophagus (jackhammer)	At least two swallows DCI >8000 mm Hg-s-cm
	Hypercontractility may involve, or even be localized to, the LES
MINOR DISORDERS OF PERISTALSIS	
Ineffective esophageal motility (IEM)	≥50% ineffective swallows
	Ineffective swallows may be failed or weak (DCI <450 mm Hg-s-cm)
	Multiple repetitive swallow assessment may be helpful in determining peristaltic reserve
Fragmented peristalsis	≥50% fragmented contractions with DCI >450 mm Hg-s-cm
Normal esophageal motility	Not fulfilling any of the above classifications

*Cutoff values dependent on the manometric hardware; these are the cutoffs for the Sierra device.
[†]Potential etiologies: early achalasia, mechanical obstruction, esophageal wall stiffness, or manifestations of hiatal hernia.
DCI, Distal contractile integral; *DL*, distal latency; *EGJ*, esophagogastric junction; *IRP*, integrated relaxation pressure; *LES*, lower esophageal sphincter.
From Kahrilas PJ, Bredenoord AJ, Fox M, et al. The Chicago Classification of esophageal motility disorders, v3.0. *Neurogastroenterol Motil.* 2015;27: 160–174.

with the most specific treatments. These features impart important clinical relevance on the accurate detection of incomplete deglutitive EGJ relaxation. Despite this cardinal significance, there has never been a unified convention for defining incomplete deglutitive EGJ relaxation with conventional manometry. Furthermore, numerous potential confounding factors exist, including CD contraction during respiration, esophageal shortening, hiatal hernia, IBP through the EGJ, sphincter radial asymmetry, and movement of the recording sensor relative to the EGJ. With HRM, the ease and reliability of measurement of EGJ relaxation is greatly improved. Pressure topography plotting facilitates accurate localization of the EGJ and the deglutitive relaxation window, as illustrated in Fig. 8.2. An exploratory study comparing criteria for detecting impaired deglutitive EGJ relaxation within that relaxation window in a large group of patients and control subjects concluded that the optimal measure for quantifying deglutitive relaxation was the integrated relaxation pressure (IRP), with normal being defined as less than 15 mm Hg. The IRP is amenable to automated calculation, and conceptually it is the lowest average pressure for 4 seconds (either contiguous or noncontiguous) within the 10-second relaxation window (Fig. 8.5). This single measure of deglutitive EGJ relaxation exhibited 98% sensitivity and 96% specificity

for distinguishing well-defined achalasia patients from control subjects and patients with other diagnoses.[11] It should be noted that the measurement of IRP is variable depending on the manometry probe and analysis software that is being used. The Chicago Classification v3.0 set the cutoff for normal at less than 15 mm Hg for the Sierra design catheters and less than 28 mm Hg for the Unisensor design. A model-specific cutoff value should be used when categorizing EGJ relaxation.

Contraction Vigor

The vigor of the distal esophageal contraction between the major pressure nodes P and D is quantified using the DCI. Conceptually the DCI corresponds to the volume of the distal contraction in dimensions of time, length, and amplitude between the proximal and the distal troughs using the 20-mm Hg isobaric contour at the base and expressed as (mm Hg-s-cm) (Fig. 8.6B). It is calculated by multiplying the mean pressure of the contraction (less 20 mm Hg), duration of the contraction, and the length of the esophageal segment between the proximal and distal troughs. Based on this value, swallows are classified as failed (DCI < 100 mm Hg-s-cm), weak (DCI > 100, but < 450 mm Hg-s-cm), normal (DCI from 450 to 8000 mm Hg-s-cm) or hypercontractile (DCI >

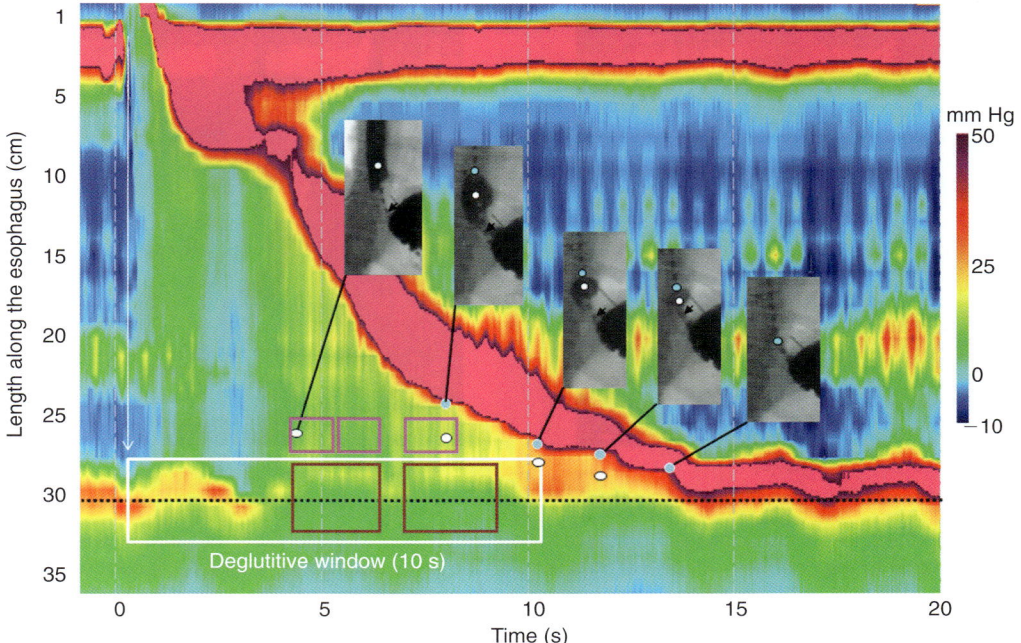

FIGURE 8.5 Concomitant esophageal pressure topography (EPT) and fluoroscopy during esophageal emptying illustrating the transition from peristaltic transport to ampullary emptying. The fluoroscopic images in the windows are synchronized with the EPT plot. The *white* and *blue dots* indicate areas of intrabolus pressure and the onset of luminal closure, respectively. The second image (at about time 8 seconds) is near the contractile deceleration point, evident both by the transition of the fluoroscopic image to ampullary conformation and slowing of the luminal closure front. The *colored rectangles* within the deglutitive relaxation window indicate the time fragments used to compute the integrated relaxation pressure, whereas the *pink rectangles* above the esophagogastric junction show the times used to compute intrabolus pressure.

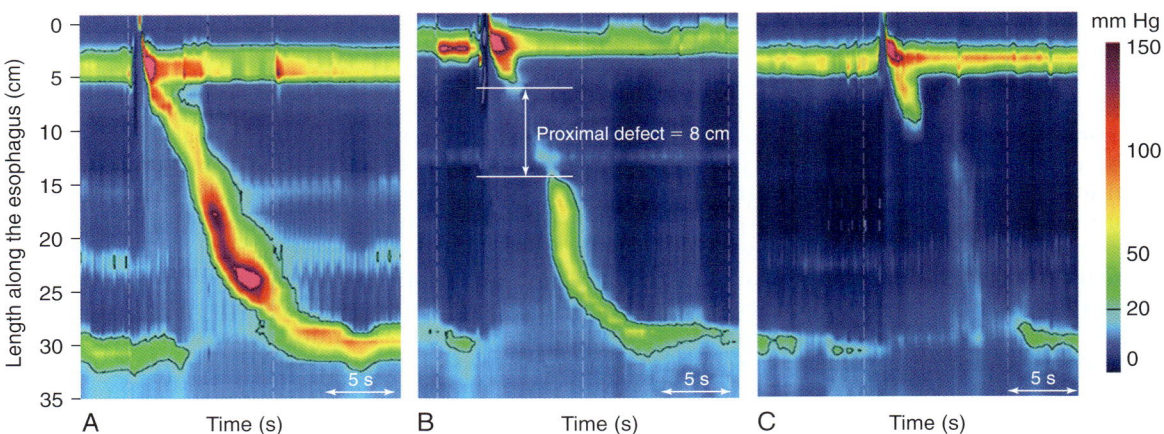

FIGURE 8.6 Varying degrees of peristaltic integrity. In each panel, the *black line* represents the 20-mm Hg isobaric contour. The swallow in (A) is intact (no disruption in the 20 mm Hg isobaric contour). (B) A swallow with a large break in the 20 mm Hg isobaric contour. (C) A failed swallow (absence of 20 mm Hg integrity in the distal two-thirds of the esophagus resulting in a DCI <100 mm Hg-s-cm).

8000 mm Hg-s-cm). Failed and weak swallows are together classified as "ineffective" swallows.

Distal Contractile Latency

The esophageal deglutitive response is initiated with the oropharyngeal swallow. However, the subsequent peristaltic contraction in the distal esophagus is preceded by a period of quiescence. Behar and Biancani introduced the concept of latency to quantify this period of quiescence and suggested that patients with spasm had a substantial reduction in contractile latency.[12] Distal contractile latency, measured from the onset of the swallow to the onset of the contraction, was shorter in patients with simultaneous contractions than in those with normal peristaltic velocity. In EPT terms, distal contractile latency (DL) is defined as the duration of the interval between UES relaxation and

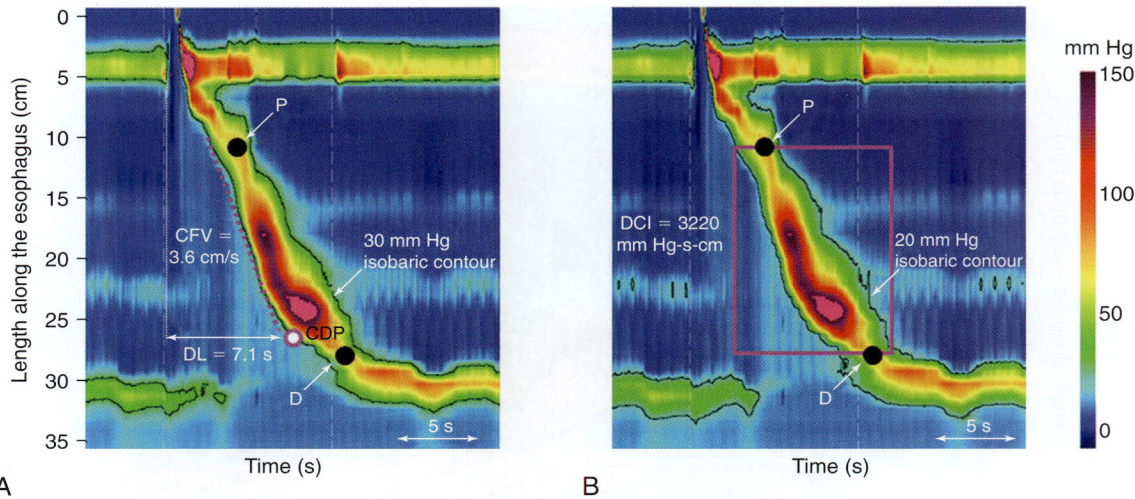

FIGURE 8.7 Metrics used in the analysis of esophageal pressure topography. The distal latency is measured from the onset of the UES relaxation *(dashed vertical line)* to the contractile deceleration point (A). The distal contractile integral (DCI) corresponds to the entire volume (amplitude × time × duration) of the distal contraction spanning from the proximal to the distal troughs *(pink box)* above 20 mm Hg (B). The DCI is calculated by multiplying the average pressure × the duration × the length of the contractile segment contained in the *pink box. CFV,* Contractile front velocity; *D,* distal; *DCI,* distal contractile integral; *DL,* distal latency; *P,* proximal.

the CDP (see Fig. 8.6A). A DL shorter than 4.5 seconds is defined as a premature, or spastic, contraction. This classification system has replaced the use of contractile front velocity (CFV) as a marker of esophageal spasm in Chicago Classification v3.0.

Contraction Pattern

Although the measurement in breaks in the peristaltic wave (as measured by continuity of the 20 mm Hg isobaric pressure contour) is no longer used as the primary method for assessing peristaltic efficacy, contractile pattern still serves as a secondary metric in the Chicago Classification v3.0. Small breaks in peristalsis (<3 cm) are of limited clinical significance; however, breaks of greater than 5 cm are more common in patients with dysphagia than in healthy controls (14% vs. 4%).[13] Thus swallows with such large breaks (>5 cm) are classified as having a "fragmented" pattern (Fig. 8.7). These swallows must have normal DL (>4.5 seconds) and DCI (≥450 mm Hg-s-cm) or else they would be primarily classified as premature or ineffective.

Esophageal Pressurization

Esophageal pressurization patterns during swallowing and measure of IBP are evaluated because they provide an indirect assessment of the adequacy of EGJ relaxation and bolus transit. The occurrence of pressurization in the esophageal body to greater than 30 mm Hg is qualified as panesophageal or compartmentalized, depending on whether it spans from the EGJ to the UES (panesophageal) or from a partially preserved peristaltic contraction to the EGJ (compartmentalized). The EPT metric for IBP during swallowing is measured 1 cm above the proximal border of the EGJ and quantifies the greatest mean pressure for 3 contiguous or noncontiguous seconds during the deglutitive window (see Fig. 8.5).

ESOPHAGEAL MOTOR DISORDERS

ACHALASIA

Apart from improving the sensitivity of manometry in the detection of achalasia, EPT has also defined a clinically relevant subclassification of achalasia.[14] Type I achalasia occurs in the setting of esophageal dilation with an absence pressurization within the esophagus (Fig. 8.8A). Type II achalasia is defined by esophageal compression characterized by panesophageal pressurization (see Fig. 8.8B). The last, type III, is a less common pattern of spastic achalasia in which there is a spastic contraction within the distal esophageal segment (see Fig. 8.8C). Although not definitely proven, it is thought that type II likely represents an earlier presentation of the disease and that these patients, if left untreated, will evolve into type I as the esophagus dilates and loses any contractile ability. Type III likely represents a separate disease entity. These subtypes play an important role in prognostication for treatment outcomes. In the European Achalasia Trial, which randomized patients to either endoscopic pneumatic dilation or laparoscopic Heller myotomy with partial fundoplication, patients with type II achalasia had the highest rates of symptom resolution following either treatment modality (96%), followed by those with type II (81%) and type III (66%).[15]

Because the underlying neuropathology of achalasia cannot be corrected, treatment is directed at compensating for the poor esophageal emptying by reducing outflow resistance through the EGJ to a level that is less than the pressure within the esophageal body. In practical terms, this amounts to reducing LES pressure so that gravity promotes esophageal emptying. LES pressure can be reduced by pharmacologic therapy, forceful dilation, or surgical myotomy. Pharmacologic treatments, on the whole, are not very effective, making them more appropriate as

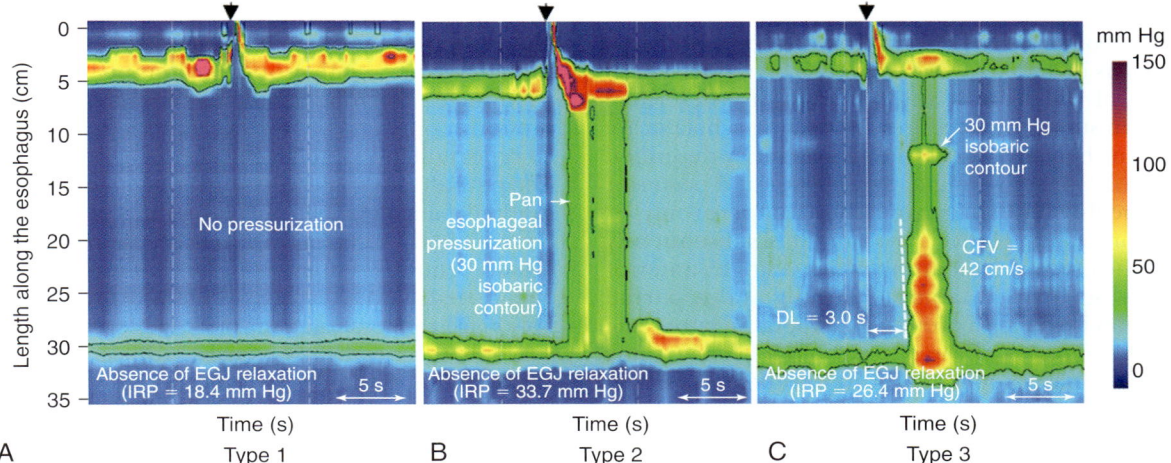

FIGURE 8.8 Achalasia subtypes. All three subtypes are characterized by impaired esophagogastric junction *(EGJ)* relaxation (integrated relaxation pressure *[IRP]* >15 mm Hg) and absent peristalsis. In type 1 (A), there is negligible pressurization in the esophageal body, evident by the absence of any area circumscribed by the 30-mm Hg isobaric contour *(black line)*. In type 2 (B), panesophageal pressurization occurs evident by the banding pattern of the 30-mm Hg isobaric contour spanning from the upper esophageal sphincter to the EGJ. This represents elevated intrabolus pressure and is associated with contraction of the longitudinal muscle on the muscularis propria. Type 3 achalasia (C) is characterized by spastic contractions (short distal latency *[DL]*) in the esophageal body.

temporizing maneuvers than as definitive therapies. The definitive treatments of achalasia are disruption of the LES either surgically (laparoscopic Heller myotomy or peroral endoscopic myotomy [POEM]) or with endoscopic pneumatic dilation.

Pharmacologic Therapy

Smooth muscle relaxants such as nitrates (isosorbide dinitrate) or sildenafil and calcium channel blockers (diltiazem, nifedipine, verapamil) have been proposed as pharmacologic treatment of achalasia. They are administered immediately before eating, and they can relieve dysphagia in achalasia by reducing the LES pressure. However, placebo-controlled crossover trials have found only minimal benefit.[16] Side effects also limit the use of these drugs (headache, hypotension for nitrates; flushing, dizziness, headache, peripheral edema, and orthostasis for nifedipine).

Botulinum Toxin Injection

Because LES tone is partially mediated via a cholinergic pathway, blockade of acetylcholine release from excitatory motor neurons should partially eliminate the neurogenic component of LES pressure, thereby decreasing LES pressure. Botulinum toxin (Botox) irreversibly inhibits the release of acetylcholine from presynaptic cholinergic terminals. However, because this effect is eventually reversed by the growth of new axons, botulinum toxin is not long-lasting therapy. The initial landmark study of botulinum toxin in achalasia reported that intrasphincteric injection of 80 units of botulinum toxin decreased LES pressure by 33% and improved dysphagia in 66% of patients for a 6-month period.[17] Although some efficacy is noted in a majority of achalasia patients, the effects are temporary. Success rates drop from 80% to 90% after 1 month to 53% to 54% after 1 year. Although there are data to suggest that repeat treatments can be effective,

no data exist on botulinum toxin as a long-term treatment strategy for achalasia. Studies comparing botulinum toxin injection with pneumatic dilation suggest that the expense of repeated injection outweighs the potential economic benefits of added safety, unless the patient's life expectancy is minimal. Thus this option is mainly reserved for elderly or frail individuals who are poor risks for definitive treatments.

Pneumatic Dilation

Therapeutic dilation for achalasia requires distention of the LES to a diameter of at least 30 mm to effect a lasting reduction of LES pressure, presumably by partially disrupting the circular muscle of the sphincter. Dilation with an endoscope, standard bougies (up to 60 French), or with through-the-scope balloon dilators (up to 2 cm) provides very temporary benefit at best, and these are not considered to be definitive treatments. Only dilators specifically designed to treat achalasia are able to achieve adequate sphincter disruption for lasting effectiveness. The basic element of an achalasia dilator is a long, noncompliant, cylindrical balloon that can be positioned fluoroscopically (Rigiflex dilator) or endoscopically (Witzel dilator) across the LES and then inflated to a characteristic diameter in a controlled fashion using a hand-held manometer. Failure of response with a 30-mm dilator can be retreated with greater-diameter balloons, sequentially progressing to 35 to 40 mm diameters if needed.

The reported success rates for pneumatic dilation vary from 70% to 90%.[18] The need for further dilations is determined by the persistence of symptoms approximately 4 weeks after treatment. In this case, a larger-diameter balloon (35 mm, sometimes 40 mm) may be used. The major complication of pneumatic dilation is esophageal perforation; however, mortality is very rare. The reported incidence of esophageal perforation from pneumatic dilation ranges between 0.4% and 5%.[18]

Laparoscopic Heller Myotomy

Although a more detailed description of surgical therapy for achalasia is included elsewhere in this textbook, a brief description of the surgery and outcomes are described here. Modern surgical procedures for treating achalasia are variations on the esophagomyotomy originally described by Heller in 1913, consisting of an anterior and posterior myotomy performed through either a laparotomy or a thoracotomy. The Heller myotomy has subsequently evolved to the current standard in which a single, anterior myotomy is performed laparoscopically and a partial fundoplication is added to prevent postoperative iatrogenic GER. Published series of the efficacy of Heller myotomy in treating achalasia report good to excellent results in around 90% of patients, with persistent dysphagia troubling fewer than 10% of patients.[19]

Peroral Endoscopic Myotomy

POEM is a novel operation for the treatment of achalasia and other esophageal dysmotility disorders. First described by Haru Inoue in Japan in 2008,[20] POEM is performed completely endoscopically using a standard flexible gastroscope. A small (approximately 1 to 2 cm) incision is made in the mucosa of the distal esophagus, and then a submucosal tunnel in the wall of the esophagus is created, extending caudally from this point across the EGJ and onto the stomach. A controlled myotomy across the EGJ high-pressure zone is then performed using an endoscopic electrocautery knife, and the entry mucosotomy is closed with clips.

Although POEM has yet to be compared with either endoscopic dilation or laparoscopic Heller myotomy in a randomized trial, initial reports from single-center series have shown excellent outcomes out to 2 year postoperatively. Hungness et al. reported a treatment success rate of 92% at a mean of 2.4 years, which is comparable to prior studies of Heller myotomy that used similar outcome measures.[21,22] Bhayani et al. compared outcomes between POEM and laparoscopic Heller myotomy performed in a nonrandomized fashion and found similar efficacy at 6 months postoperatively, as well as similar rates of postoperative GER (39% for POEM and 32% for laparoscopic Heller myotomy).[23] One potential advantage of POEM over laparoscopic Heller is the ability to perform a long myotomy that extends further cephalad than is possible via a laparoscopic approach. This could benefit patients with type III achalasia or jackhammer esophagus in which the pathologically hypercontractile segment extends to the transition zone in the proximal esophagus. A multicenter nonrandomized comparison found better outcomes after POEM than laparoscopic Heller in patients with type III achalasia, but due to the relative rarity of such patients, this result will need to be verified in future studies.[24]

Treatment Failure

Persistent dysphagia after treatment for achalasia can be due to a number of causes and should be evaluated with a combination of endoscopy, esophageal manometry, and contrast esophagram. Endoscopy may detect reflux esophagitis, peptic stricture, candidiasis, hiatal hernia, or other anatomic deformities. Manometry may be useful to quantify residual EGJ pressure, with IRP values exceeding 15 mm Hg arguing for further therapy targeting the EGJ. Fluoroscopy is useful both to identify anatomic problems, as well as to evaluate esophageal emptying.[25]

In the case of a patient who failed therapy and was not previously operated on, further treatment could potentially be repeat dilation, Heller myotomy, or POEM. In patients who have already undergone myotomy, manometric demonstration of an inadequate myotomy or functional esophageal obstruction from the antireflux component of the surgery usually requires reoperation, but pneumatic dilation can be pursued as an alternative. POEM provides an attractive option for reoperation after prior Heller myotomy because it avoids the need for extensive adhesiolysis, reopening of the hiatus, and takedown of the prior fundoplication. In extremely advanced or refractory cases of achalasia, esophageal resection may be the only surgical option.

ESOPHAGEAL SPASM

The pathophysiology of DES involves an impairment of inhibitory mechanisms, leading to both premature and rapidly propagated or simultaneous contractions in the distal esophagus. Experimental inhibition of nitric oxide in control subjects induces simultaneous esophageal contraction, and hence the mechanism appears to be related to a reduction in the DL of the contraction. In contrast, the administration of nitric oxide donors prolongs the DL in patients with DES and decreases the contraction amplitude.[26]

The manometric definition of DES is based on the presence of rapidly propagated contraction associated with short DL in a context of normal EGJ relaxation (Fig. 8.9A). The incidence of this disorder is extremely low, and it has almost certainly been overdiagnosed using conventional manometry.[27] Even using EPT, overdiagnosis occurs when one uses a rapid CFV without considering impaired latency or abnormalities of hypercontractility. This is one of the weaknesses of prior versions of the Chicago Classification that has been improved upon in v3.0, which uses DL less than 4.5 seconds as the sole criteria for spasm (see Fig. 8.9B).

Pharmacologic Treatment

As with achalasia, nitrates and calcium channel blockers have been proposed to treat esophageal spastic motility disorders. However, these treatments have limited demonstrated efficacy in treating chest pain that is thought to be related to spasm. Sildenafil represents a new option to treat spastic motility disorders. It reduces pressure amplitude and propagation velocity in controls and in patients with motility disorders. Preliminary data suggest it to be effective on relieving esophageal symptoms and in improving manometric findings in patients with spastic motility disorders.[28]

Finally, low-dose antidepressants can improve a patient's reaction to pain without objectively improving motility function. A trial using the anxiolytic trazodone (serotonin uptake inhibitor) suggested that reassurance and control of anxiety are important therapeutic goals.[29]

Endoscopic Treatment

Although the rationale for dilation is unclear, some success has been reported in treating spastic disorders

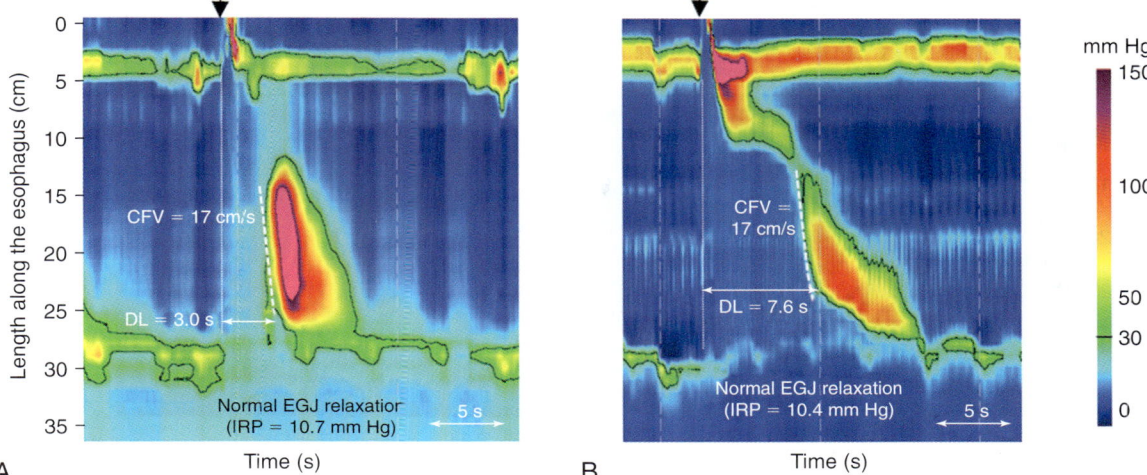

FIGURE 8.9 Examples of spasm and rapidly propagated peristalsis. In the context of normal esophagogastric junction *(EGJ)* relaxation, a rapidly propagated contraction with short latency (distal latency *[DL]* < 4.5 seconds) defines esophageal spasm (A). However, this example of a rapidly propagated contraction occurring with normal DL was encountered in an asymptomatic control (B). *CFV,* Contractile front velocity; *IRP,* integrated relaxation pressure.

with dilation. However, an important caveat is that it is completely uncertain as to whether or not patients who benefited by pneumatic dilation would not be more properly categorized as spastic achalasia or achalasia with esophageal compression, emphasizing the need for accurate manometric classification.

Botulinum toxin injection is a pathophysiologically attractive approach to treating patients with spastic disorders. Therapeutic trials suggest it can reduce chest pain.[30] The technique has not been standardized in this application with some reports injecting botulinum toxin only at the level of the EGJ and others also injecting the distal esophagus. No trial has yet compared botulinum toxin injection with other treatments.

Surgical Treatment

Long myotomy extending from the LES proximally onto the esophageal body has been used to treat patients with spastic disorders. The extent of the myotomy may be guided by manometric findings. In an uncontrolled study, surgical treatment seemed more effective than the medical treatment.[31] Due to its ability to create an extended proximal myotomy, POEM also offers a potentially superior surgical option for the treatment of DES. Only a handful of small case series have reported results after POEM performed for DES and other spastic esophageal motility disorders, so far showing excellent outcomes with a meta-analysis reporting symptomatic success in 88% of patients.[32]

JACKHAMMER ESOPHAGUS

Vigorous esophageal contractions with normal propagation have been reported in association with chest pain.[33] The pathophysiology of hypertensive peristalsis is unclear but is believed to be related to either excessive excitation, reactive compensation for increased EGJ obstruction, or myocyte hypertrophy.[34]

The conventional manometric definition of hypertensive peristalsis used the term *nutcracker esophagus* and peak peristaltic amplitude greater than 180 mm Hg between 3 and 8 cm above the LES.[35] Subsequently, the defining peristaltic amplitude has been debated, and more recent work suggests that this should be increased to 260 mm Hg, a value more likely to be associated with chest pain and dysphagia.[33]

The introduction of HRM and EPT has allowed further stratification of hypertensive peristalsis to account for both excessive amplitude and abnormal morphology of the peristaltic contraction. The summary metric for contractile vigor in the entire distal segment is the DCI with a value of 5000 mm Hg-s-cm being the 95th percentile of normal. DCI values greater than 5000 mm Hg-s-cm but less than 8000 mm Hg-s-cm are found in individuals with hypertensive peristalsis akin to nutcracker esophagus in conventional terms. However, because values in this range are also encountered in normal individuals, they have now been classified as normal in the Chicago Classification v3.0. In contrast, DCI values greater than 8000 mm Hg-s-cm are almost universally associated with chest pain and dysphagia, and these patients appear to have a more exaggerated pattern of hypercontractility that is repetitive and more akin to a jackhammer than a nutcracker (Fig. 8.10). The current version of the Chicago Classification refers to this condition as jackhammer esophagus to fit better with the contractile morphology. Having said that, the clinical relevance of these conditions is still unclear. Nonetheless, it seems likely that focusing future trials on patients with a DCI greater than 8000 mm Hg-s-cm rather than a lower threshold is more likely to identify a homogeneous population potentially amenable to specific pharmacologic treatment.

Pharmacologic Treatment

The same therapeutic options used for DES have also been advocated for patients with hypertensive peristalsis. Smooth muscle relaxants, such as calcium channel blockers and nitrates, have been used for these disorders because

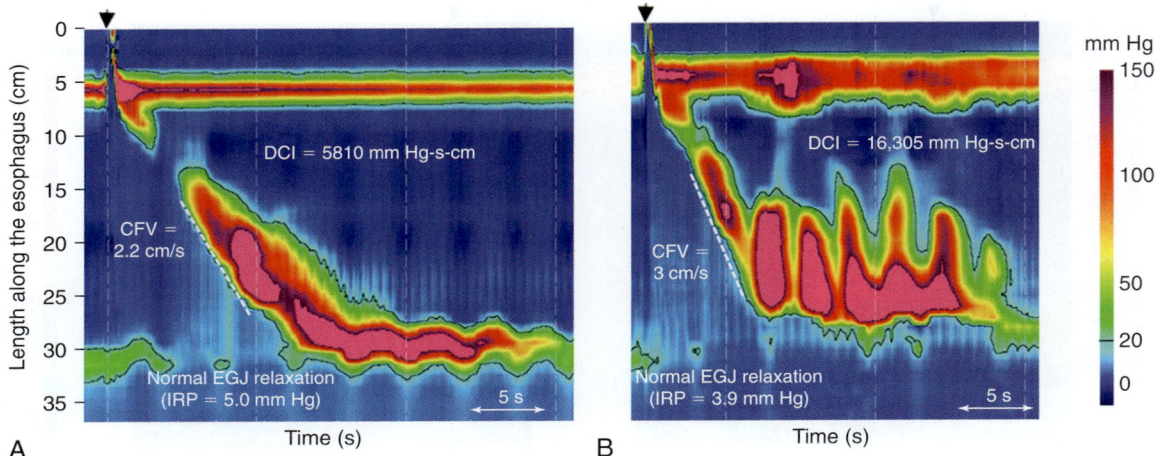

FIGURE 8.10 Hypercontractile (jackhammer) esophagus. Hypercontractile swallows are defined by a distal contractile integral *(DCI)* greater than 8000 mm Hg-s-cm (A). This example is associated with a hypercontractile lower esophageal sphincter but normal esophagogastric junction *(EGJ)* relaxation. (B) An extremely abnormal contraction in a jackhammer esophagus patient with repetitive prolonged contractions evoking the action of the jackhammer. *CFV,* Contractile front velocity; *IRP,* integrated relaxation pressure.

they reduce peristaltic amplitude even though neither has been shown to relieve chest pain or dysphagia in clinical trials. Alternatively, sildenafil is appealing because of its profound effect of reducing contraction amplitude and potentially reducing the occurrence of repetitive contractions.[36] Again, there are no supportive clinical trial data yet. Finally, botulinum toxin injection in the esophageal muscle with or without endoscopic ultrasound guidance may be an option for patients with refractory symptoms.

Because of the potential overlap of hypertensive peristalsis with GERD and the observation that many of these patients have coexistent psychologic distress, therapy focused on modulating acid secretion, visceral sensitivity, and stress has been attempted. Proton pump inhibitors have been proposed to treat hypertensive peristalsis based on the hypothesis that GERD can induce chest pain and hypertensive peristalsis.[37] Similarly, treatment with low-dose tricyclic antidepressants may reduce contractions via the anticholinergic effect and may alter visceral sensitivity. Akin to DES, POEM has been proposed as an ideal surgical option for treatment of patients with jackhammer esophagus who are refractory to medical therapy. With POEM, the myotomy can be extended proximally to encompass the entire hypercontractile segment of the smooth muscle esophagus, from the transition zone through the EGJ. Again, due to the scarcity of the condition, reports of POEM performed for jackhammer esophagus are just beginning to appear and further data regarding its efficacy are needed.[32]

ROLE OF MANOMETRY IN ANTIREFLUX SURGERY

HRM is an important component of the physiologic evaluation of patients prior to antireflux surgery and is now recommended by many as a routine preoperative test, although this has not be universally accepted as standard of care.[38,39] HRM serves several roles in the preoperative evaluation of such patients: first, it confirms conclusively that the patient does not have a previously undiagnosed major disorder of esophageal motility, such as achalasia. This is important because a significant number of patients with achalasia will have chest pain that they describe as "heartburn" and are initially misdiagnosed with GERD. Conversely, a number of patients with true GERD will complain of dysphagia as a result of esophageal hypersensitivity and partially impaired motility resulting from prolonged reflux. Second, some surgeons choose to "tailor" their fundoplication (i.e., decide to perform either a partial or complete fundoplication) based on the results of preoperative HRM, in conjunction with the patient's symptoms. Lastly, having a preoperative HRM serves as an important baseline if a patient develops troublesome symptoms postoperatively, such as dysphagia. Being able to compare preoperative and postoperative HRM studies is invaluable in determining whether such patients' symptoms are due to elevated EGJ pressure or impaired esophageal peristalsis as a result of the fundoplication.

FUNDOPLICATION TAILORING

Long-term functional problems, including dysphagia, gas bloat, diarrhea, and increased flatulence, are feared complications of antireflux surgery. Some surgeons use a tailored approach in which they perform a partial fundoplication (either anterior or posterior) in patients determined to be at high risk of postoperative dysphagia, as shown in Fig. 8.11. Several studies have shown partial fundoplication to result in lower rates of dysphagia as compared with Nissen[40]; therefore if at-risk patients could be identified by preoperative HRM and other factors, they could potentially benefit from such a modification. However, the precise means for identifying such patients and the role of HRM measurements in this algorithm remain matters of considerable controversy.

The presence of preoperative dysphagia is an important risk factor for worsening, or persistence, of dysphagia after fundoplication.[41] In addition, patients with IEM

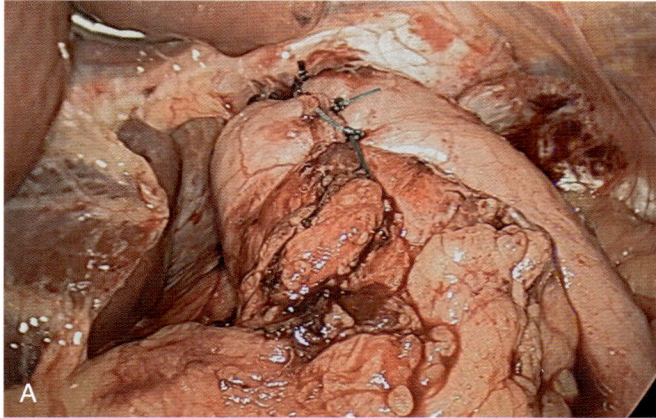

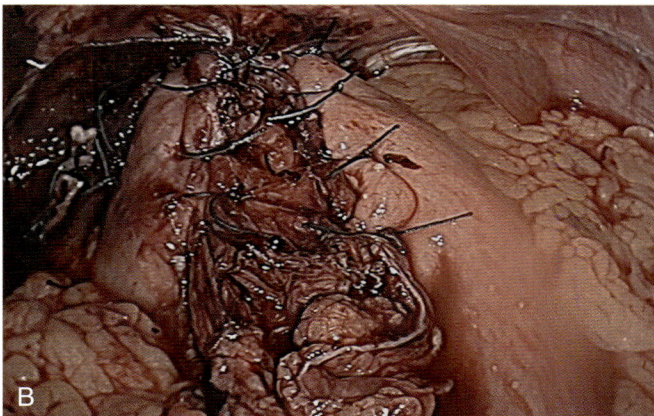

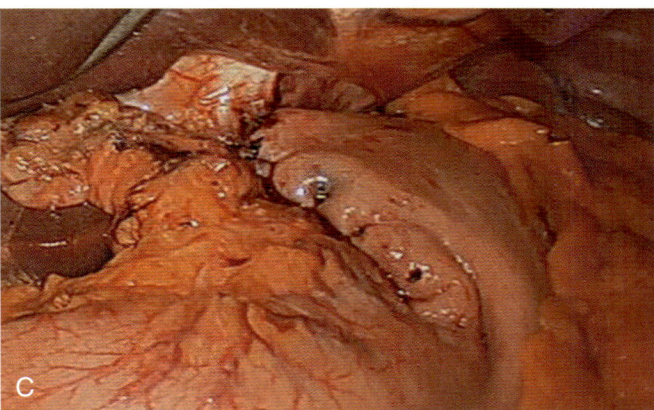

FIGURE 8.11 Examples of complete and partial fundoplications performed during laparoscopic antireflux surgery. A Nissen (A) is a complete 360-degree fundoplication that provides the most effective and durable antireflux barrier but may result in increased rates of postoperative dysphagia. Some surgeons choose to tailor their fundoplications based on manometry results and other patient factors by performing a partial wrap, either a posterior Toupet fundoplication (B) or an anterior Dor fundoplication (C).

on HRM are more likely to have dysphagia at baseline.[42] Therefore it would seem that preoperative IEM would be a significant risk factor for dysphagia after fundoplication and that such patients would be better served with a partial wrap. However, most randomized trials comparing partial and complete fundoplication have failed to show

that patients with IEM have improved outcomes and less dysphagia with a partial fundoplication.[43,44] In addition, it does not appear that patients with IEM are at higher risk for development of new-onset dysphagia after Nissen fundoplication than patients with normal esophageal motility preoperatively.[45] Further complicating this issue is the fact that the majority of these studies evaluated motility using conventional, rather than high-resolution, manometry. They also uniformly used older metrics for evaluating peristaltic function, such as contraction amplitude and fragmented peristalsis, rather than DCI.

Taken together, the available evidence suggests that HRM is an important tool in the evaluation of patients prior to antireflux surgery. However, no standardized algorithm can reliably predict which patients will experience postoperative dysphagia or would have improved outcomes with a partial, rather than complete, fundoplication. Based on the best available evidence, our recommendation would be that patients with absent or severely impaired peristalsis on preoperative HRM or those with preoperative dysphagia *and* IEM should undergo a partial fundoplication. In other patients, a Nissen can safely be performed.

CONCLUSION

Esophageal motility disorders are diagnosed and classified using esophageal manometry, with HRM now being the gold standard. The Chicago Classification is an evolving classification scheme based on the consensus of an international working group that periodically meets for updates and clarifications, with v3.0 serving as the most current edition.[6] The major recognized disorders are the three subtypes of achalasia, EGJ outflow obstruction, DES, jackhammer esophagus, absent contractility, with IEM and fragmented peristalsis now categorized as minor motility disorders. HRM serves an important role, not only in the diagnosis of these disorders, but also in prognostication and guiding the most appropriate treatment option. In addition, HRM forms an important component in the preoperative evaluation of patients undergoing laparoscopic antireflux surgery and can help to guide the choice of fundoplication in a patient-specific manner. For these reasons, it is important that surgeons have a firm understanding of the principles of HRM diagnosis and its application in surgical decision making.

ACKNOWLEDGMENTS

The authors thank and acknowledge Sabine Roman, MD, Peter J. Kahrilas, MD, and John E. Pandolfino, MD, for their contributions to the prior edition of this chapter.

REFERENCES

1. Pandolfino JE, Kahrilas PJ, American Gastroenterological Association. American Gastroenterological Association medical position statement: clinical use of esophageal manometry. *Gastroenterology.* 2005;128:207-208.
2. Clouse RE, Staiano A, Alrakawi A. Development of a topographic analysis system for manometric studies in the gastrointestinal tract. *Gastrointest Endosc.* 1998;48:395-401.
3. Grubel C, Hiscock R, Hebbard G. Value of spatiotemporal representation of manometric data. *Clin Gastroenterol Hepatol.* 2008;6:525-530.

4. Fornari F, Bravi I, Penagini R, Tack J, Sifrim D. Multiple rapid swallowing: a complementary test during standard oesophageal manometry. *Neurogastroenterol Motil.* 2009;21:718-e41.

5. Pandolfino JE, Fox MR, Bredenoord AJ, Kahrilas PJ. High-resolution manometry in clinical practice: utilizing pressure topography to classify oesophageal motility abnormalities. *Neurogastroenterol Motil.* 2009;21:796-806.

6. Kahrilas PJ, Bredenoord AJ, Fox M, et al. The Chicago Classification of esophageal motility disorders, v3.0. *Neurogastroenterol Motil.* 2015;27:160-174.

7. Mittal RK, Fisher M, McCallum RW, Rochester DF, Dent J, Sluss J. Human lower esophageal sphincter pressure response to increased intra-abdominal pressure. *Am J Physiol.* 1990;258:G624-G630.

8. Kumar N, Porter RF, Chanin JM, Gyawali CP. Analysis of intersegmental trough and proximal latency of smooth muscle contraction using high-resolution esophageal manometry. *J Clin Gastroenterol.* 2012;46:375-381.

9. Pandolfino JE, Kim H, Ghosh SK, Clarke JO, Zhang Q, Kahrilas PJ. High-resolution manometry of the EGJ: an analysis of crural diaphragm function in GERD. *Am J Gastroenterol.* 2007;102:1056-1063.

10. Bredenoord AJ, Weusten BL, Timmer R, Smout AJ. Intermittent spatial separation of diaphragm and lower esophageal sphincter favors acidic and weakly acidic reflux. *Gastroenterology.* 2006;130:334-340.

11. Ghosh SK, Pandolfino JE, Rice J, Clarke JO, Kwiatek M, Kahrilas PJ. Impaired deglutitive EGJ relaxation in clinical esophageal manometry: a quantitative analysis of 400 patients and 75 controls. *Am J Physiol Gastrointest Liver Physiol.* 2007;293:G878-G885.

12. Behar J, Biancani P. Pathogenesis of simultaneous esophageal contractions in patients with motility disorders. *Gastroenterology.* 1993;105:111-118.

13. Roman S, Lin Z, Kwiatek MA, Pandolfino JE, Kahrilas PJ. Weak peristalsis in esophageal pressure topography: classification and association with dysphagia. *Am J Gastroenterol.* 2011;106:349-356.

14. Pandolfino JE, Kwiatek MA, Nealis T, Bulsiewicz W, Post J, Kahrilas PJ. Achalasia: a new clinically relevant classification by high-resolution manometry. *Gastroenterology.* 2008;135:1526-1533.

15. Rohof WO, Salvador R, Annese V, et al. Outcomes of treatment for achalasia depend on manometric subtype. *Gastroenterology.* 2013;144:718-725; quiz e13–e14.

16. Traube M, Hongo M, Magyar L, McCallum RW. Effects of nifedipine in achalasia and in patients with high-amplitude peristaltic esophageal contractions. *JAMA.* 1984;252:1733-1736.

17. Pasricha PJ, Ravich WJ, Hendrix TR, Sostre S, Jones B, Kalloo AN. Intrasphincteric botulinum toxin for the treatment of achalasia. *N Engl J Med.* 1995;332:774-778.

18. Boeckxstaens GE. Achalasia. *Best Pract Res Clin Gastroenterol.* 2007;21:595-608.

19. Schoenberg MB, Marx S, Kersten JF, et al. Laparoscopic Heller myotomy versus endoscopic balloon dilatation for the treatment of achalasia: a network meta-analysis. *Ann Surg.* 2013;258:943-952.

20. Inoue H, Minami H, Kobayashi Y, et al. Peroral endoscopic myotomy (POEM) for esophageal achalasia. *Endoscopy.* 2010;42:265-271.

21. Hungness ES, Sternbach JM, Teitelbaum EN, Kahrilas PJ, Pandolfino JE, Soper NJ. Per-oral endoscopic myotomy (POEM) after the learning curve: durable long-term results with a low complication rate. *Ann Surg.* 2016;264:508-517.

22. Boeckxstaens GE, Annese V, des Varannes SB, et al. Pneumatic dilation versus laparoscopic Heller's myotomy for idiopathic achalasia. *N Engl J Med.* 2011;364:1807-1816.

23. Bhayani NH, Kurian AA, Dunst CM, Sharata AM, Rieder E, Swanstrom LL. A comparative study on comprehensive, objective outcomes of laparoscopic Heller myotomy with per-oral endoscopic myotomy (POEM) for achalasia. *Ann Surg.* 2014;259:1098-1103.

24. Kumbhari V, Tieu AH, Onimaru M, et al. Peroral endoscopic myotomy (POEM) vs laparoscopic Heller myotomy (LHM) for the treatment of Type III achalasia in 75 patients: a multicenter comparative study. *Endosc Int Open.* 2015;3:E195-E201.

25. Vaezi MF, Baker ME, Achkar E, Richter JE. Timed barium oesophagram: better predictor of long term success after pneumatic dilation in achalasia than symptom assessment. *Gut.* 2002;50:765-770.

26. Grubel C, Borovicka J, Schwizer W, Fox M, Hebbard G. Diffuse esophageal spasm. *Am J Gastroenterol.* 2008;103:450-457.

27. Pandolfino JE, Ghosh SK, Rice J, Clarke JO, Kwiatek MA, Kahrilas PJ. Classifying esophageal motility by pressure topography characteristics: a study of 400 patients and 75 controls. *Am J Gastroenterol.* 2008;103:27-37.

28. Eherer AJ, Schwetz I, Hammer HF, et al. Effect of sildenafil on oesophageal motor function in healthy subjects and patients with oesophageal motor disorders. *Gut.* 2002;50:758-764.

29. Clouse RE, Lustman PJ, Eckert TC, Ferney DM, Griffith LS. Low-dose trazodone for symptomatic patients with esophageal contraction abnormalities. A double-blind, placebo-controlled trial. *Gastroenterology.* 1987;92:1027-1036.

30. Storr M, Allescher HD, Rosch T, Born P, Weigert N, Classen M. Treatment of symptomatic diffuse esophageal spasm by endoscopic injections of botulinum toxin: a prospective study with long-term follow-up. *Gastrointest Endosc.* 2001;54:754-759.

31. Patti MG, Pellegrini CA, Arcerito M, Tong J, Mulvihill SJ, Way LW. Comparison of medical and minimally invasive surgical therapy for primary esophageal motility disorders. *Arch Surg.* 1995;130:609-615, discussion 615–616.

32. Khan MA, Kumbhari V, Ngamruengphong S, et al. Is POEM the answer for management of spastic esophageal disorders? A systematic review and meta-analysis. *Dig Dis Sci.* 2017;62:35-44.

33. Agrawal A, Hila A, Tutuian R, Mainie I, Castell DO. Clinical relevance of the nutcracker esophagus: suggested revision of criteria for diagnosis. *J Clin Gastroenterol.* 2006;40:504-509.

34. Dogan I, Puckett JL, Padda BS, Mittal RK. Prevalence of increased esophageal muscle thickness in patients with esophageal symptoms. *Am J Gastroenterol.* 2007;102:137-145.

35. Spechler SJ, Castell DO. Classification of oesophageal motility abnormalities. *Gut.* 2001;49:145-151.

36. Fox M, Sweis R, Wong T, Anggiansah A. Sildenafil relieves symptoms and normalizes motility in patients with oesophageal spasm: a report of two cases. *Neurogastroenterol Motil.* 2007;19:798-803.

37. Pehlivanov N, Liu J, Mittal RK. Sustained esophageal contraction: a motor correlate of heartburn symptom. *Am J Physiol Gastrointest Liver Physiol.* 2001;281:G743-G751.

38. Stefanidis D, Hope WW, Kohn GP, et al. Guidelines for surgical treatment of gastroesophageal reflux disease. *Surg Endosc.* 2010;24:2647-2669.

39. Kahrilas PJ, Shaheen NJ, Vaezi MF, et al. American Gastroenterological Association medical position statement on the management of gastroesophageal reflux disease. *Gastroenterology.* 2008;135:1383-1391, 1391.e1–e5.

40. Varin O, Velstra B, De Sutter S, Ceelen W. Total vs partial fundoplication in the treatment of gastroesophageal reflux disease: a meta-analysis. *Arch Surg.* 2009;144:273-278.

41. Tsuboi K, Lee TH, Legner A, Yano F, Dworak T, Mittal SK. Identification of risk factors for postoperative dysphagia after primary anti-reflux surgery. *Surg Endosc.* 2011;25:923-929.

42. Xiao Y, Kahrilas PJ, Kwasny MJ, et al. High-resolution manometry correlates of ineffective esophageal motility. *Am J Gastroenterol.* 2012;107:1647-1654.

43. Fibbe C, Layer P, Keller J, Strate U, Emmermann A, Zornig C. Esophageal motility in reflux disease before and after fundoplication: a prospective, randomized, clinical, and manometric study. *Gastroenterology.* 2001;121:5-14.

44. Chrysos E, Tsiaoussis J, Zoras OJ, et al. Laparoscopic surgery for gastroesophageal reflux disease patients with impaired esophageal peristalsis: total or partial fundoplication? *J Am Coll Surg.* 2003;197:8-15.

45. Biertho L, Sebajang H, Anvari M. Effects of laparoscopic Nissen fundoplication on esophageal motility: long-term results. *Surg Endosc.* 2006;20:619-623.

pH and Impedance Evaluation of the Esophagus

Geoffrey P. Kohn

Gastroesophageal reflux disease (GERD) is a very common global disorder that poses a significant public health burden. GERD affects approximately 20% of the population of the Western world[1-5] and has been ranked as the fourth most prevalent gastrointestinal disease and the most expensive disease of the alimentary tract.[6]

There can be no standard diagnostic criteria for the definition of GERD because the threshold distinction between physiologic reflux and reflux disease is arbitrary.[7] A consensus panel of experts, the so-called Montreal consensus, has defined GERD as "a condition which develops when the reflux of stomach contents causes troublesome symptoms and/or complications."[8]

GERD patients report "typical" symptoms of heartburn and regurgitation. The regurgitation is often acidic in nature, leading to the sour taste of water brash. "Atypical" or so-called extraesophageal symptoms include chest pain and respiratory symptoms, including cough, wheeze, and dysphonia. Extraesophageal manifestations of reflux disease may result from direct action of the primary refluxate or may be due to reflex neurologic arcs.

It is problematic to define a disease based on symptoms, especially when symptoms are not specific to the disease. Therapy directed at GERD will be ineffective if the etiology of the symptoms is from a nonreflux condition. Therefore objective assessment of GERD is often required, with ambulatory pH evaluation the most widely used technique.

HISTORY OF ESOPHAGEAL pH MONITORING

The first attempt to objectively detect gastroesophageal reflux (GER) was accomplished by Reichman in 1884.[9,10] He lowered gelatin-coated sponges into the esophagus of patients with heartburn and showed that they contained acid when retrieved. Several decades later Aylwin found acid and pepsin in esophageal juice retrieved with a tube from a patient with esophagitis.[11] Bernstein and Baker recognized the relationship between the presence of acid in the esophagus and symptoms of heartburn and regurgitation.[12] They developed the acid infusion test, which is based on reproducing esophageal symptoms by the instillation of 0.1 N hydrochloric acid in the esophagus. The first in situ measurement of acid reflux in the esophagus was achieved by Tuttle and Grossman in 1958[13] using pH-metry equipment previously described for studies of gastric acidity. Although this approach greatly improved the detection of acid reflux, it was limited by its failure to differentiate normal subjects from abnormal subjects. Prolonged esophageal pH measurements were first described by Spencer in 1969.[14] This technique soon became the standard method to quantify GER. Initially, the recording machines were not portable, forcing patients to

remain attached to large equipment, making the procedure an inpatient system. In 1974 Johnson and DeMeester performed landmark studies in controls and GERD patients, establishing the technique and normal values for 24-hour ambulatory pH monitoring, and subsequently ambulatory pH monitoring has been widely applied in both clinical and research settings.[15]

INDICATIONS FOR pH TESTING

For patients with the typical symptoms of reflux, lifestyle changes of weight loss, avoidance of refluxogenic foods, and avoidance of the full recumbent position, particularly in the postprandial period, relieve symptoms. For others a therapeutic trial of acid suppressant medications, such as proton pump inhibitors (PPIs) and histamine H_2 channel antagonists, will suffice, after excluding alternative pathologies. However, it is prudent to objectively document GER before considering invasive procedures such as antireflux surgery. Objective endoscopic evidence of GERD includes "mucosal breaks" of esophagitis in the distal esophagus, Barrett metaplasia, and the reflux-related complication of peptic esophageal stricture. In the absence of endoscopic evidence of reflux, objective evidence can be obtained by 24-hour ambulatory esophageal pH monitoring.[16] The presence of an abnormal 24-hour pH score has been shown to be the strongest predictor of a good outcome after antireflux surgery.[17] In addition, pH monitoring is useful in the evaluation of patients with persisting reflux symptoms despite medical or surgical therapy.[10]

ELECTROCHEMICAL PROPERTIES OF pH ELECTRODES

Esophageal pH monitoring techniques are designed to measure the intraluminal hydrogen ion concentration.[10] The negative logarithm of the hydrogen ion concentration defines the pH value (pH = +log $1/[H^+]$). The hydrogen activity can be detected by a number of different electrodes with different characteristics depending on the electrode material. The electrical potential difference, generated by a concentration gradient of hydrogen ions between two electrodes, can be extrapolated to give a pH value. Esophageal pH systems consist of glass, antimony, or ion-sensitive field effect transistor (ISFET) pH sensors and a reference electrode.[18] The reference electrode is either external, placed on the patients' skin, or built into the catheter. A disadvantage of using external cutaneous reference electrodes is the risk of disturbed skin contact during the pH recording, which can lead to artifactual pH values. External electrodes are also associated with a risk of erroneous results as a consequence of influence of the mucosal potential difference. Based on these observations, pH catheters with an internal reference electrode are considered superior[19] and are much more common in modern clinical practice. Glass electrodes measure the electrical potential difference across a thin glass membrane. The monocrystalline antimony electrode is a metal/metal oxide electrode that measures the corrosion potential at the hydrogen ion and antimony interface.[20] The ISFET is a modification of the normal field effect transistor and combines in one device the sensing surface and a signal amplifier.[21] Laboratory studies suggest that the more expensive glass electrodes are superior to monocrystal-line antimony electrodes because they respond much quicker to changes in pH and have less drift and a better linear response.[22] However, in a clinical setting, the less expensive antimony electrodes provide similar results and better patient comfort as compared with the larger glass electrodes.[23,24] There is some evidence that ISFET electrodes produce the most accurate in vivo measurements of acid exposure, but they are not in widespread use.[18]

Calibration of the pH electrodes is performed in all pH systems prior to each study, using reference buffer solutions, usually either nitrate or phthalate based. The pH value of the calibration solution varies among manufacturers, but most systems calibrate the pH sensor at room temperature to an acidic pH (range, 1.0 to 4.0) and a more neutral pH (range, 6.0 to 7.0). When the patient returns after completion of the test, the calibration should be repeated to rule out electrode failure and to allow correction for slow pH drift.

CATHETER-BASED pH MONITORING

The conventional catheter-based pH monitoring system principally consists of a flexible catheter, usually made from polyurethane, with one or more pH sensors and a data recorder. The catheter is passed through the nose, along the posterior wall of the pharynx, and is placed with the pH sensor in the distal esophagus 5 cm above the manometrically determined upper border of the lower esophageal sphincter (LES). It is connected to a data recorder that is carried by the patient during the study. The system samples pH data every 1 to 10 seconds, depending on the manufacturer of the catheter system. Ambulatory catheter-based pH monitoring is generally performed over a 24-hour period because a complete circadian cycle allows for determining the effect of physical activity and body positions on esophageal acid exposure, as well as allowing for an increased detection of symptoms for the calculation of symptom associations.[25]

In general, esophageal pH monitoring is carried out while the patient is off acid-suppressant medication. Patients are normally instructed to discontinue the use of PPIs at least 7 days prior, histamine H$_2$-antagonists 5 days prior, and simple antacids 24 hours prior to the investigation. Only when the aim of the study is to measure the esophageal acid exposure that persists during treatment should acid suppressants be continued.

During the study, patients are instructed to keep a diary and to record symptoms, mealtimes, and times for supine and upright postures. Patients are often asked to avoid foods with a pH below 4, such as coffee, tea, citrus, tomato products, wine, and carbonated beverages, although the intake of these products has a rather short-lived effect on esophageal pH. Meal periods can be excluded from the analysis to avoid potential artifacts produced by acidic meal ingestion, and this may improve the clinical reliability of the test.[26] The activity and the diet of the patients during the study should ideally be identical to that of the control population from which the normative values for esophageal acid exposure were developed. Some centers encourage the patients to eat their usual meals and may include one meal likely to precipitate their symptoms, the so-called refluxogenic or challenge meal, which often is a burger, fries, and shake at a fast-food restaurant. This challenge meal is useful because the process of esophageal pH monitoring has been shown to reduce reflux-provoking activities and patients tend to be more sedentary.[27] In part this is related to social embarrassment and discomfort related to having the catheter coming out of the nose. When patients change their routines during pH testing, the degree of esophageal acid reflux may theoretically be underestimated, which could potentially decrease the sensitivity of the pH test. Therefore patients should be strongly encouraged to return to work and to engage in all normal daily activities. The catheter itself does not induce reflux.[28] The test is not tolerated by all patients, and adverse symptoms may lead to interference with daily activities and eating and interruption of normal sleep,[29] possibly leading to underestimation of reflux related to physical activity and meals and hampering the evaluation of nocturnal reflux.[10]

WIRELESS pH MONITORING

Some of the limitations of the catheter-based technique have been avoided with the introduction of the catheter-free, wireless pH system (Bravo, Medtronic, Minnesota). In addition to improved patient comfort[29] and less effect on reflux-provoking activities, the capsule-based pH system has the advantages of fixed placement of the pH electrode, minimizing the risk of slipping into the stomach and allowing for prolonged recordings. The longer duration of pH monitoring has been suggested to increase the sensitivity of reflux monitoring in identifying patients with gastroesophageal reflux.[30] Contraindications for the use of the Bravo capsule are hemorrhagic diathesis, esophageal varices, severe esophagitis, patients with a pacemaker or a defibrillator, and pregnancy. The delivery system for the pH capsule is most commonly passed transorally after completion of an upper endoscopy and measurements of the distance between the incisors to the base of the squamocolumnar junction (SCJ). Some centers recommend that application should be performed under direct endoscopic vision and not blindly after the endoscopy.[31] The pH capsule can also be placed transnasally based on prior manometric localization of the LES.[32] The capsule should be positioned 6 cm above the gastroesophageal junction (GEJ) identified endoscopically or 5 cm above the manometrically determined LES.

The pH system consists of a capsule attached to the end of a catheter delivery system and a telemetry receiver (Fig. 9.1). The capsule ($6 \times 5.5 \times 25$ mm^3) has an antimony pH electrode and a reference electrode located on the distal

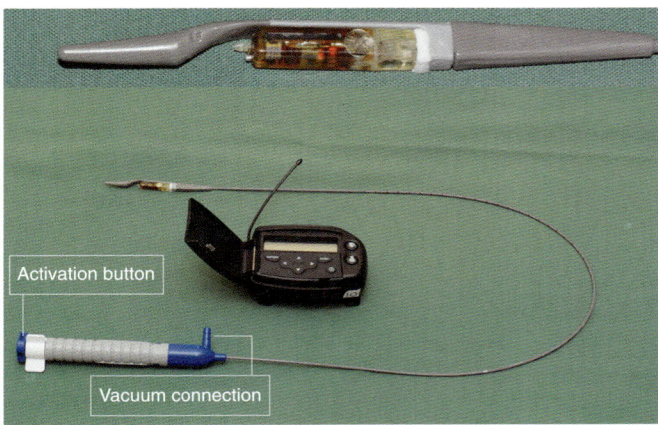

FIGURE 9.1 The Bravo wireless pH monitoring system.

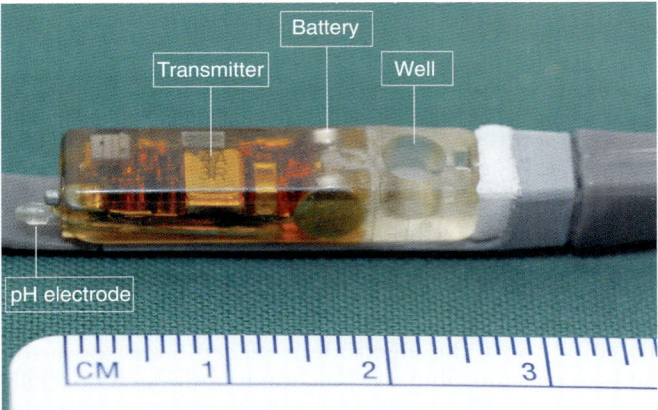

FIGURE 9.2 The Bravo capsule.

tip and contains an internal battery and a transmitter, all encapsulated in epoxy (Fig. 9.2). The capsule has a well that fills with mucosa when suction is applied, and the device is deployed by firing a pin through the mucosa in the well. This attaches the capsule at the desired position in the esophagus. The delivery system is removed, leaving only the capsule in place in the esophagus. The capsule simultaneously measures and transmits pH data using radiotelemetry to a portable receiver worn by the patient. The receiver has two recording channels, allowing placement of up to two capsules simultaneously. The patient is instructed to remain within 6 ft (2 m) of the recorder during the study period to ensure effective telemetry signal strength. The capsule is designed to detach in 3 to 7 days and then pass through the gastrointestinal tract. There are reports of the probe remaining attached for longer periods usually without consequence[30] but sometimes requiring endoscopic removal.[30]

The data sampling rate at 6-second intervals of the wireless pH system is often slower than the 1- to 10-second intervals used by the catheter-based pH systems. Prior studies show that faster sampling frequencies up to 1 Hz (i.e., 1 per second) lead to detection of a greater total number of reflux events as events with shorter durations are able to be recorded, but the greater sampling frequency does not change the overall value for esophageal acid exposure.[33]

Wireless esophageal pH monitoring is associated with fewer adverse symptoms and less interference with normal daily activities and is preferred by patients,[34] although there are limitations associated with the wireless technique. The wireless pH capsule is associated with thoracic discomfort in 10% to 65% of the patients. The severity of chest symptoms ranges from a mild foreign body sensation to severe chest pain, although the latter is uncommon. In rare cases the pain is so severe that endoscopic removal of the capsule is necessary.[35–37]

Limitations of the capsule-based pH system also include technical problems, such as premature detachment of the capsule or interruption of the radiotelemetry signal. Detachment of the pH capsule is suggested by an abrupt pH drop as the sensor dislocates into the stomach with an increasing pH reaching greater than 7 as gastric motility propels the pH capsule into the duodenum. Interruption of the pH signal can potentially be attributable to interference with other wireless systems using the same 433-MHz band or, more commonly, by the receiver being beyond the range of the signal emanating from the radio-transmitting capsule. The interruption of the recording of pH data normally constitutes only a small fraction of the total monitored time.[31] In general, the technical limitations of early capsule detachment and interruption of the radiotelemetry signal do not significantly affect the interpretation of the recorded pH data. However, in a small proportion of patients with unsuccessful recordings, pH monitoring has to be repeated as a consequence of these technical problems.

DURATION OF pH MONITORING

The standard duration of recording for catheter-based esophageal pH testing is 24 hours and for the wireless pH system is 48 hours, although approximately 10% of wireless probes detach prior to the completion of this period.[30,38] The reported proportion of successful wireless pH recordings of at least 36 hours range from 89% to 96%.[30,31,36,39,40]

Recording of pH data from the wireless capsule is commonly carried out over a period of 48 hours but may be extended to even longer periods of time. The extended recording capabilities of the wireless pH system as compared with the conventional catheter-based technique appear to increase the sensitivity of the test. Studies have demonstrated that by increasing the pH recording time from 24 to 48 hours, the yield of the procedure increased in capturing more abnormal pH tests or symptom-associated reflux events.[35]

The 48-hour data can be interpreted using an average of the 2 days, or alternatively using only the 24-hour period with the greatest acid exposure, termed "worst day analysis." Using this approach a pH test is considered abnormal if either or both days of the test show increased esophageal acid exposure, with patients with both days abnormal having in general more severe reflux disease. A significant increase in the sensitivity of the pH testing is seen, together with a small decrease in specificity, when

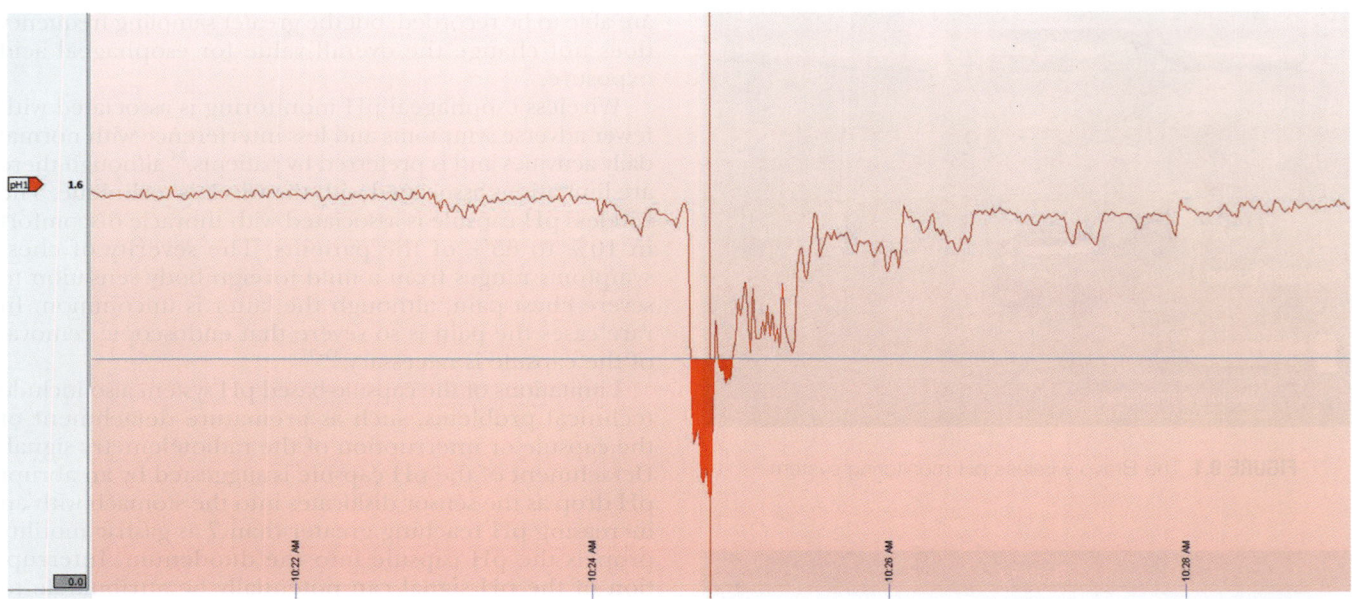

FIGURE 9.3 A gastroesophageal reflux event shown by an abrupt decline in intraesophageal pH.

using the worst day data as compared with either 24-hour data or averaged 48-hour data.[25]

Shorter recording periods have also been investigated with the catheter-based study so as to improve patient comfort and tolerance. Sensitivity of a 3-hour catheter-based study has been reported to have 88% of the sensitivity and 98% of the specificity in reflux detection of a 24-hour catheter-based study.[41] However, studies that contain less than 16 hours of data are generally considered to be inadequate.

pH ELECTRODE PLACEMENT

Consistent positioning of the pH electrode is vital for obtaining reliable esophageal pH data and for comparison with normal values. Studies performed using catheters with multiple pH sensors for simultaneous pH recording at different levels in the esophagus have shown, as would be expected, greater acid exposure in the distal esophagus compared with more proximally.[42,43] Consequently, esophageal acid detection will be significantly reduced when the distance from the LES to the recording level increases, and therefore accurate pH probe placement is essential for a reliable diagnosis of GERD. Typically, the pH electrode should be placed close enough to the stomach to sample the region of esophageal mucosa most affected by GER, without displacing into the stomach during the course of the study. During swallowing, the GEJ migrates approximately 2 to 4 cm,[44,45] and so positioning of the pH probe must consider this. By convention, the catheter-based pH electrode is placed 5 cm above the manometrically defined upper border of the LES.[46] This position should avoid inadvertent dislocation of the electrode into the stomach during breathing, movements induced by changes in body position, or swallow-induced esophageal shortening. Thus to determine this location, esophageal manometry must be performed prior to the pH

study. Placement on the basis of the pH profile recorded on withdrawal of the electrode from the stomach has been found to be inferior to placement based on manometric LES localization.[47]

In wireless esophageal pH monitoring the pH sensor is most commonly placed according to endoscopic landmarks. By convention, the electrode is placed 6 cm above the GEJ (or squamocolumnar junction if positioned normally at the GEJ). This position has been derived from the findings of concurrent manometry and fluoroscopy studies that show the upper border of the LES high-pressure zone typically extends 1 to 1.5 cm above the SCJ.[48] Positioning the pH electrode 6 cm above the SCJ therefore approximates the standard 5 cm above the upper border of the manometrically defined LES electrode position of the catheter-based technique. Transnasal placement of the pH capsule requires prior manometry and provides the most accurate placement of the capsule.[32] If placed transnasally using measurements obtained via endoscopy or transoral manometry, a conversion factor of 4 cm is typically applied,[49] approximating the distance between the nares and oropharynx. However, there is significant patient variability in this number and this technique is not recommended.

INTERPRETATION OF ESOPHAGEAL pH STUDIES

Due to swallowed saliva and esophageal bicarbonate secretion, esophageal pH is normally maintained between pH 5 and pH 7. Gastric acid secretion generates a highly acidic environment within the stomach, with a pH of 1 to 2 and rarely more than 3. During esophageal pH monitoring (Fig. 9.3), GER events are detected as abrupt declines in intraesophageal pH. Episodes in which pH falls below 4 are counted as reflux events. The choice of the cutoff of pH 4 is

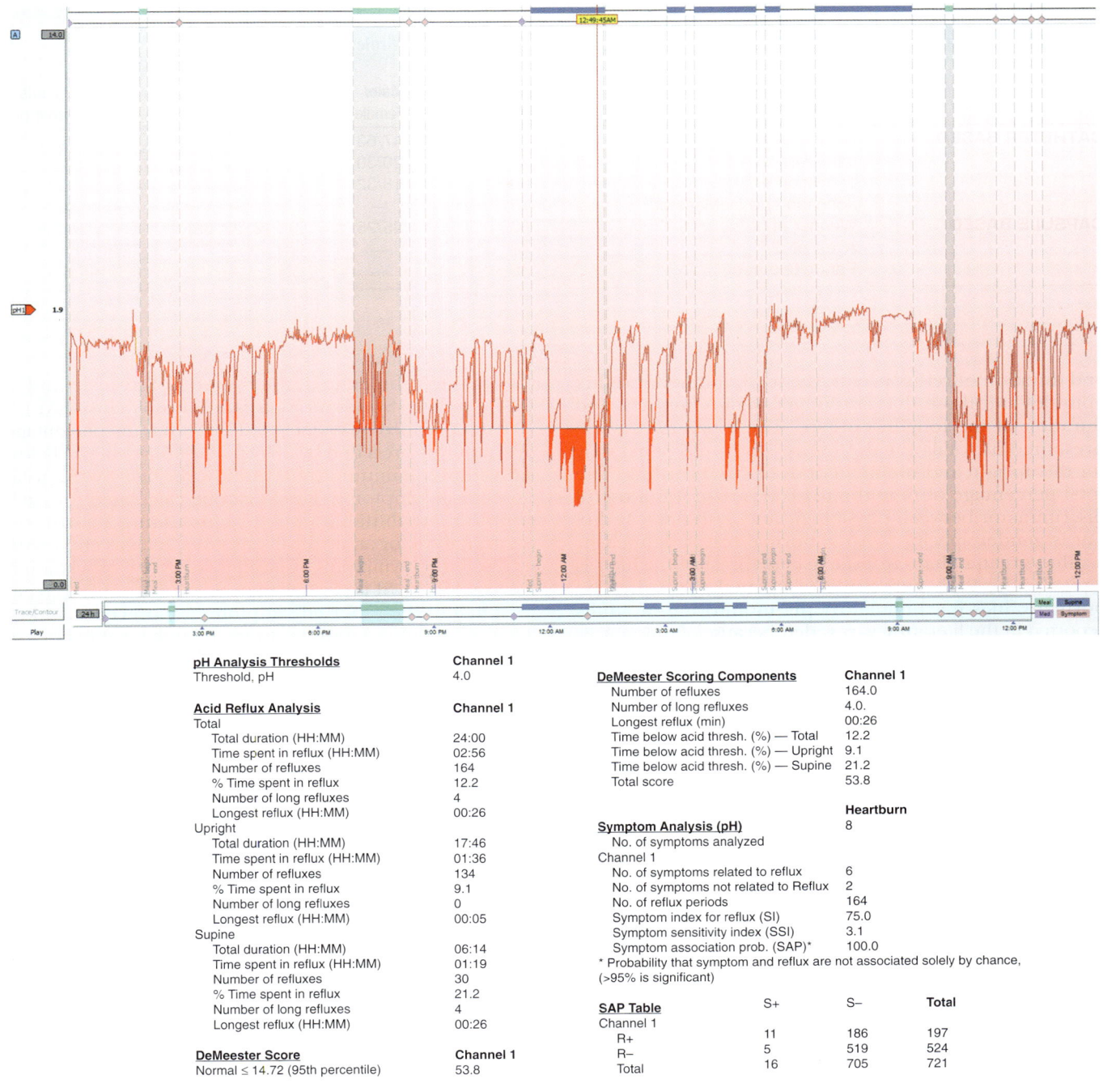

pH Analysis Thresholds	Channel 1
Threshold, pH	4.0

Acid Reflux Analysis	Channel 1
Total	
Total duration (HH:MM)	24:00
Time spent in reflux (HH:MM)	02:56
Number of refluxes	164
% Time spent in reflux	12.2
Number of long refluxes	4
Longest reflux (HH:MM)	00:26
Upright	
Total duration (HH:MM)	17:46
Time spent in reflux (HH:MM)	01:36
Number of refluxes	134
% Time spent in reflux	9.1
Number of long refluxes	0
Longest reflux (HH:MM)	00:05
Supine	
Total duration (HH:MM)	06:14
Time spent in reflux (HH:MM)	01:19
Number of refluxes	30
% Time spent in reflux	21.2
Number of long refluxes	4
Longest reflux (HH:MM)	00:26

DeMeester Score	Channel 1
Normal ≤ 14.72 (95th percentile)	53.8

DeMeester Scoring Components	Channel 1
Number of refluxes	164.0
Number of long refluxes	4.0.
Longest reflux (min)	00:26
Time below acid thresh. (%) — Total	12.2
Time below acid thresh. (%) — Upright	9.1
Time below acid thresh. (%) — Supine	21.2
Total score	53.8

Symptom Analysis (pH)	Heartburn
No. of symptoms analyzed	8
Channel 1	
No. of symptoms related to reflux	6
No. of symptoms not related to Reflux	2
No. of reflux periods	164
Symptom index for reflux (SI)	75.0
Symptom sensitivity index (SSI)	3.1
Symptom association prob. (SAP)*	100.0

* Probability that symptom and reflux are not associated solely by chance, (>95% is significant)

SAP Table	S+	S–	Total
Channel 1			
R+	11	186	197
R–	5	519	524
Total	16	705	721

FIGURE 9.4 Example of an automated 24-hour ambulatory single-channel pH study report.

supported by the observation that patients with symptomatic reflux usually report heartburn at an intraesophageal pH below this threshold.[50] When the pH recording is complete, the software generates a report that includes a graphical pH tracing, reflux parameters, and symptom-reflux correlations (Fig. 9.4). In the analysis of esophageal pH tracings the pattern of acid reflux can provide important information. Physiologic acid reflux seen in healthy subjects typically occurs in the upright position after a meal and is rapidly cleared from the esophagus. In patients with early reflux disease the number of reflux events increases, but the

pattern typically remains as upright, postprandial reflux. With increasing severity of GERD the reflux may become bipositional, with increased acid exposure in both the upright and supine postures.[51–53] Often both the duration and number of acid reflux episodes increase, resulting in prolonged esophageal acid exposure times. Isolated supine reflux is rare and can reflect stasis or pooling of refluxed gastric juice in the esophagus, leading to very prolonged reflux episodes.

Several discrete parameters are routinely calculated by the software of the pH system, including the frequency of

TABLE 9.1 Reports on Normal Values for 24-Hour Catheter-Based and 48-Hour Wireless pH Monitoring

	Author	Number of Subjects	Male/ Female	Median Age (Range)	Upper Limit of Normal (%)
CATHETER BASED	Richter et al.[54]	110	47/63	30 (20–84)	5.8
	Jamieson et al.[55]	50	20/30	—	4.5
	Johnsson et al.[56]	50	18/32	38 (30–77)	3.4
	Johnson and DeMeester[15]	15	—	—	4.2
CAPSULE BASED	Wenner et al.[31]	50	25/25	42 (22–65)	4.34
	Ayazi et al.[32]	48	—	—	4.8
	Pandolfino et al.[30]	36	—	—	5.4

and duration of reflux events, the total number of reflux episodes and those that last longer than 5 minutes, and duration of the longest episode. These parameters are presented as totals for the entire study and separately for the upright and supine periods of the recording. The total percentage of time the pH is less than 4 is a useful discriminator between physiologic and pathologic reflux but is gender specific.[46] An abnormal test is defined by a value greater than an established threshold, which is typically the 95th percentile of normal controls. The normal values for ambulatory pH monitoring in adults reported in the literature vary widely because of differences in the selection and the age and gender distribution of the control population. Table 9.1 shows reports on normal data for catheter-based and capsule-based pH monitoring.[10]

A more precise method of presenting esophageal acid exposure data is calculation of a composite score, originally proposed by Johnson and DeMeester.[15] The DeMeester Score includes six parameters: (1) total percent time pH less than 4.0; (2) percent time pH less than 4.0 in the upright period; (3) percent time pH less than 4.0 in the recumbent period; (4) the total number of reflux episodes; (5) the total number of reflux episodes longer than 5 minutes; and (6) the duration of the longest reflux episode. The score is automatically calculated and reported in most commercially available pH software. Unlike total time pH less than 4, the score is gender independent. The most referenced value for an abnormal DeMeester composite score is a value larger than 14.7.[15] The DeMeester composite score was also calculated based on normals for use with the Bravo pH system and are slightly different than the catheter normals (day 1 = 14, day 2 = 14, combined = 16). Regardless of whether the composite score or individual acid exposure time is used, a detailed evaluation of the pH tracing is of fundamental importance to recognize and exclude artifacts and to assess symptom association.

SYMPTOMS ASSOCIATION

Reflux symptoms such as heartburn and regurgitation are very common, but because these symptoms are not very specific for GERD, it can be useful to determine if there is a temporal relationship between symptoms and reflux events. The relationship between symptoms and reflux episodes can be expressed numerically using symptom association analysis.[57] The most frequently used indices are the Symptom Index (SI), the Symptom Sensitivity Index (SSI), and the Symptom Association Probability (SAP).[10]

First described by Wiener et al.[58] the SI is the percentage of symptoms preceded by a drop in esophageal pH below 4.0 within a 5-minute time window divided by the total number of symptoms. The SI can be calculated for each symptom attributable to reflux, including heartburn, regurgitation, or an atypical symptom, such as chest pain or respiratory symptoms. A positive symptom association is declared if the SI is greater than or equal to 50% (i.e., at least half of the reported symptoms are preceded within a 5-minute time window by an intraesophageal pH below 4.0).[59] Over the years the definition and use of the SI have been challenged. Based on a sensitivity analysis in patients with chest pain, it has been proposed to use a shorter, 2-minute time window after the onset of a reflux episode in which a symptom has to occur for it to be considered associated with reflux.[60] The SI does not take into account the total number of reflux events, and there currently is insufficient evidence to use SI as a reliable determination of the presence or absence of reflux disease.

The SSI is defined as the percentage of symptoms associated with reflux events.[58,61] The SI does not consider the total number of reflux episodes, and the SSI does not include the total number of symptom events. As a consequence, the probability that the SI becomes positive increases with an increasingly high number of reflux episodes and SSI is more likely to be positive when the number of symptom episodes is high. An SSI greater than 10% is usually considered positive and suggests an association between symptom and reflux.

The SAP is a statistical method to determine the relationship between symptoms and reflux episodes. The SAP is calculated by dividing the entire study's pH data into consecutive 2-minute segments. For each of these segments, it is determined whether reflux occurred in the segment, allowing for calculation of the total number of 2-minute segments with and without reflux. Subsequently, it is determined whether or not a reflux episode occurred in the 2-minute period before each symptom. A 2 × 2 contingency table is constructed in which the number of 2-minute segments with and without symptoms and with and without reflux are tabulated. Using the Fisher exact test, a P value is calculated, and the SAP index is calculated as $(1 - P) \times 100\%$.[62] The cutoff value for a positive test is often defined as SAP greater than or equal to to 95%. However, even a statistically significant relationship between reflux events and symptoms does not necessarily imply causality. The yield of the SI and SAP is greater when performed off rather than on acid-suppressant therapy.[25]

pH TESTING ON VERSUS OFF ACID SUPPRESSIVE MEDICATION

For patients complaining of reflux symptoms, current clinical practice guidelines recommend empirical trials of PPIs instead of pH testing.[63] The favorable side effect profile of PPIs has encouraged this initial step, although the sensitivity and specificity of this approach are only 78% and 54%, respectively.[64] If symptoms persist, then esophageal pH testing is performed. Studies suggest that a more cost-effective approach is to study all patients with pH testing as an initial approach because many patients are put on PPI medication for nonreflux symptoms and stay on the medications for years inappropriately. If patients are started on PPIs for reflux symptoms without confirmation of the disease and present with persistent symptoms, objective testing is necessary. At this point an important decision has to be made whether to perform testing on or off medications. Esophageal pH testing without acid-suppressant medication is more accurate, and there are established normal values. A test showing normal distal esophageal acid exposure is very helpful in suggesting that the symptoms are not caused by reflux.

A positive pH test while off acid-suppressant therapy confirms the diagnosis of reflux disease but may not explain why the patient is still having symptoms while taking PPIs. If the symptoms are regurgitation, it can be reliably assumed that these symptoms are reflux related because it is well established that reflux continues on PPI therapy; only the nature of the refluxed material is changed from acid to weak or nonacid. These persistent regurgitation symptoms are well addressed with antireflux procedures, including transoral incisionless fundoplication, the LINX device, or a fundoplication. In contrast, if the symptoms on PPI are persistent heartburn, testing on therapy may allow assessment of the efficacy of PPI therapy, with continued acid reflux, suggesting that additional medication or a change in medication may be effective to improve symptomatic control of the GERD. In these patients the use of dual pH electrodes to monitor both distal esophageal and gastric pH are sometimes recommended (Fig. 9.5).[25] Although intragastric pH measurement can help to determine the efficacy of acid-suppressive medications or suggest poor patient compliance, its clinical relevance is unclear because

there is a paucity of data showing a correlation between intragastric pH and GER.[65,66] Alternatively, combining intraluminal impedance with pH testing can provide additional information on the nature of refluxed material while on medications, but these studies are limited by the lack of clearly defined normal values for the impedance portion of the test, unreliable automated reading of the study, and poor interobserver agreement particularly for proximal reflux events.

LIMITATIONS OF ESOPHAGEAL pH MONITORING

Ambulatory esophageal pH monitoring is not without some limitations. The sensitivity and specificity of catheter-based pH monitoring have traditionally been reported to be in the range of 87% to 96% and 97% to 100%, respectively.[55,56] As there is a relationship between the severity of the disease and the discriminatory power of the test,[67] the published data on sensitivity and specificity reflect the severity of reflux disease in the populations tested, and patients with mild reflux may be missed.[10] In studies of patients with typical reflux symptoms and esophagitis, a sensitivity of 76% to 78% and a specificity of 93% to 95% were reported for the capsule-based technique for esophageal pH monitoring.[30,67] In contrast, other studies suggest increased sensitivity with capsule pH monitoring based on the longer duration of monitoring, up to 96 hours.

In patients with typical symptoms and endoscopy-proven Los Angeles Classification of Gastroesophageal Reflux Disease (LA) grade C or D esophagitis or Barrett esophagus, the diagnosis of GERD is confirmed and additional investigation with esophageal pH monitoring is unnecessary.[16] However, with lesser degrees of esophagitis and in patients without endoscopic evidence of GERD, who constitute up to two-thirds of all patients with typical reflux symptoms, objective GERD testing is recommended.[68] A negative pH test in most cases excluded the presence of significant reflux disease. However, because normal values are based on the 95th percentile, there by definition are 5% false-negative studies. In addition, patients with typical reflux symptoms and no esophagitis (so-called NERD or nonerosive reflux disease patients) are likely a heterogeneous group with different etiologies for their symptoms, including esophageal motor events, reflux of nonacid contents, acid hypersensitivity, functional heartburn, or emotional or psychologic abnormalities that cannot be reliably detected using pH testing alone.[69,70]

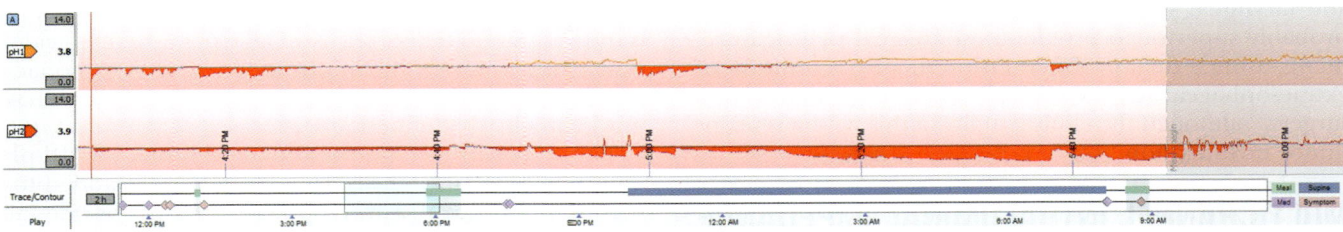

FIGURE 9.5 Double-channel pH study with sensors in the stomach ("pH2") and 5 cm above the upper border of the lower esophageal sphincter ("pH1"), showing intragastric acidification.

Perhaps one of the most important roles of pH testing is in the diagnosis of a patient considering antireflux surgery. Particularly with typical heartburn and regurgitation symptoms of reflux, a good patient outcome from antireflux surgery can be predicted by an abnormal preoperative pH study, and unsatisfactory outcomes are much more likely if surgery is performed after a normal pH study. Atypical esophageal symptoms, such as cough, globus sensation, dysphonia, throat pain, and respiratory symptoms, are often multifactorial, but if due to GERD, they may arise from proximal extension of the refluxate. The diagnosis of reflux in these patients can be challenging, and abnormal proximal acid exposure can occur in some patients despite normal distal esophageal acid exposure related to proximal jetting of refluxed gastric juice and the lower thresholds for abnormal acid exposure in the proximal esophagus. Dual probe monitoring with a distal and a proximal probe can be useful in these patients. In addition, new technologies for proximal esophageal pH assessment using a pharyngeal pH probe (Restech pH, California) and multichannel intraluminal impedance (MII) studies may be of use.

PROXIMAL ESOPHAGEAL pH ASSESSMENT

The association between reflux of acidic gastric contents into the larynx and laryngeal symptoms was initially proposed in 1968.[71] There are multiple potential causes for these respiratory and laryngeal symptoms, and establishing reflux as part of or the major cause based on symptoms alone is unreliable.[72,73] Distal esophageal acid measurement can confirm increased esophageal acid exposure in patients with extraesophageal symptoms, but that does not confirm that the symptoms are caused by reflux.[74] Proximal esophageal pH abnormalities have been identified in patients with normal distal esophageal acid exposure,[75] and standardization of placement of the proximal esophageal pH probe has been proposed using the upper esophageal sphincter as the anatomic landmark.[76] Normative values (95th percentile) for upper esophageal acid exposure have been defined (24 episodes and 0.9 for % time pH < 4).[73] These values are lower than those in the distal esophagus.

Probes for the measurement of pH require liquid to be presented to the sensor for accurate measurement. For example, drying of the pH sensor when the pH sensor is placed in the hypopharynx or proximal esophagus can cause artifacts in the pH recording. Certain sensors, such as the Dx-pH probe (Restech, California) are specifically designed not to dry out in the pharynx and also allow for measurement of aerosolized pH. This probe is designed to help to diagnose reflux as the cause of respiratory and laryngeal symptoms. Pharyngeal pH monitoring is probably superior to proximal esophageal pH measurements using a dual probe when predicting resolution of extraesophageal atypical GERD symptoms after antireflux surgery,[77] although the clinical utility of this system remains under investigation.[78,79]

MULTICHANNEL INTRALUMINAL IMPEDANCE

First described by Silny[80] in 1991 MII is a relatively new technique for evaluating esophageal bolus transit during swallowing, without the use of radiation and for monitoring GER independent of its pH.

The presence and movement of an intraesophageal bolus is detected on MII based on measuring differences in electrical conductivity affected by the presence of various materials within the esophagus.[81] An MII catheter requires an alternating current source connected to a series of metal rings located along segments of the esophageal lumen. An isolator separates the rings so that the electrical circuit is closed by the electrical charges (i.e., ions) surrounding the catheter. The impedance within a given segment is then determined by measuring the electrical resistance as a substance passes through the current established by the rings. Once placed in the esophagus, the ions of the esophageal mucosa close the circuit and the system measures a relatively stable resistance of approximately 2000 to 3000 ohms.

Liquid boluses conduct better than the empty esophagus, leading to a rapid decline in intraluminal impedance when the bolus enters the impedance measuring segment.[81] Impedance returns to baseline once the bolus has exited the segment. Multiple impedance measuring segments mounted on the same catheter allow determination of the direction of bolus movement based on the timing of changes in impedance at individual levels. Proximal to distal (antegrade) progression of impedance changes is indicative of swallowing (Fig. 9.6), whereas a distal to proximal (retrograde) progression indicates a reflux episode (Fig. 9.7).[82]

When combined with pH, MII can evaluate the presence of a reflux event and its pH, thereby allowing the detection and differentiation of both acid and nonacid reflux (see Fig. 9.6).

COMBINED MULTICHANNEL INTRALUMINAL IMPEDANCE AND pH

Esophageal pH monitoring quantifies the amount of distal esophageal acid exposure but requires the refluxed gastric juice to have a pH of less than 4 to be considered a reflux event. Reflux with a pH greater than 4 in a patient off medications may be related to gastric achlorhydria or to excessive bile in the gastric juice. Different approaches (e.g., bilirubin monitoring and scintigraphy) have been proposed to evaluate these patients. Adding impedance assessment to pH measurements is a new method to evaluate the function of the antireflux barrier.[83]

Because impedance can detect the presence of refluxate in the esophagus independent of its composition and can be mounted on a regular pH catheter, MII has several advantages in monitoring gastroesophageal reflux. MII-pH is the best test to detect reflux of all types, whether acid or nonacid.[83] However, the implications of weak or nonacid reflux events and normal thresholds for these events have not been clearly defined.

For monitoring of gastroesophageal reflux via MII-pH, multiple impedance-measuring segments are added to a regular pH probe. Gastroesophageal reflux episodes are detected by retrograde declines in intraluminal impedance produced by increased conductivity of the liquid reflux, and data from the esophageal pH sensor are used to

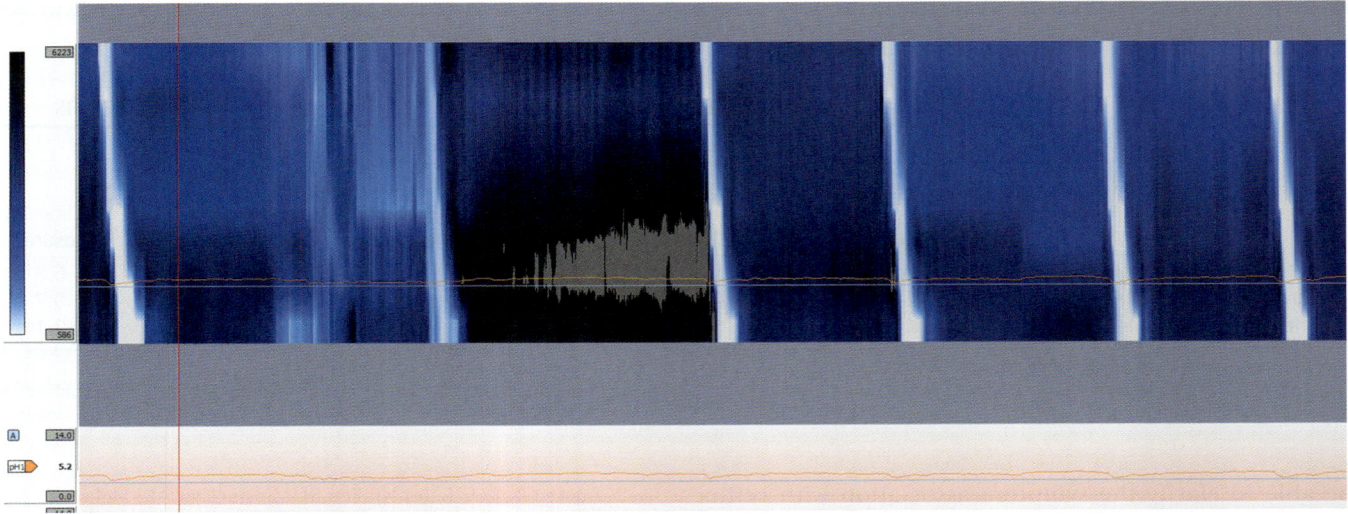

FIGURE 9.6 Impedance trace of antegrade bolus movement—normal swallows.

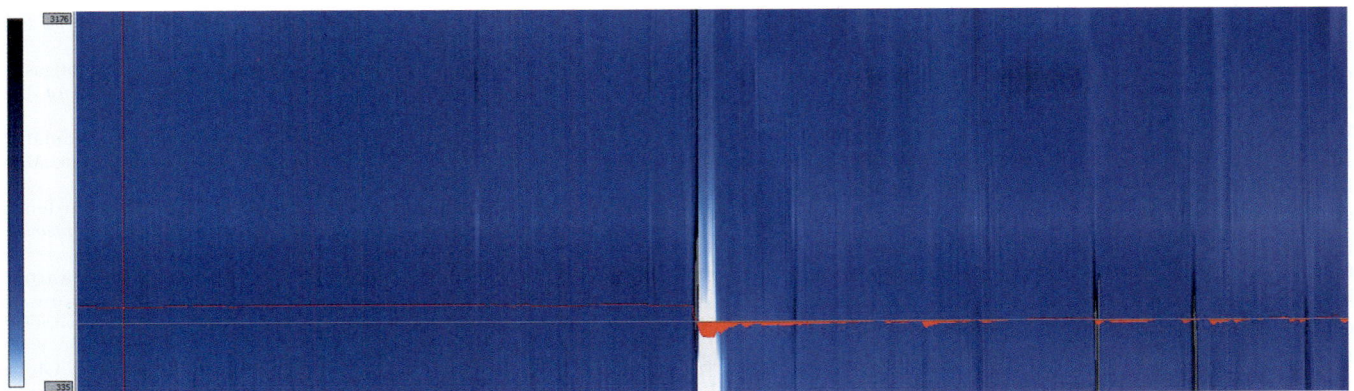

FIGURE 9.7 An impedance trace of retrograde bolus movement—an acidic reflux event.

categorize the reflux as acid or nonacid. The refluxate is considered acidic if the pH drops from greater than to less than 4, weakly acidic if the pH is between 4 and 7, and nonacidic if the intraesophageal pH during an MII-detected reflux episode remains greater than 7.[83]

In addition to the chemical properties of the gastroesophageal refluxate, MII has the ability to determine its physical state; MII can differentiate between liquid only, gas only, and mixed gas-liquid reflux episodes based on changes in intraluminal impedance. Gas or air has very poor electrical conductivity and, when present between impedance-measuring rings, will produce a rise in impedance to greater than 7000 ohms; in contrast, liquid, which has better electrical conductivity, will produce a decline in impedance.[81]

Nonacid reflux (i.e., a reflux episode with a pH greater than 4) is relatively infrequent in subjects not taking acid-suppressive therapy; it occurs primarily in the postprandial periods[84] and rarely at night.[85] However, in subjects taking acid-suppressive therapy, the medications typically change the composition of the gastroesophageal refluxate without affecting the total number of reflux episodes.[86,87] Normal values for the number of acid and nonacid reflux events on and off acid-suppressive therapy[85] have been published

(Table 9.2), as have various population-specific norms.[88–90] However, of all reflux parameters the number of reflux events has the most variability in normals and appears to be affected by body mass index (BMI) and other factors. This problem limits the utility of MII for the reliable diagnosis of GERD, unless the pH component confirms increased esophageal acid exposure.

Esophageal mucosal healing rates of up to 90% have been documented in patients taking potent acid–suppressive therapy,[91] and therefore nonacid reflux is presumed less likely to cause esophageal lesions. Nonacid reflux does appear to have a role in causing persistent symptoms in patients taking acid-suppressive therapy, particularly regurgitation symptoms. There are both direct evidence of postprandial symptoms being associated with nonacid reflux[86] and indirect data from a large PPI trial indicating that 35% to 40% of patients receiving acid-suppressive therapy continue to have symptoms.[91]

Quantifying the type and proximal extent of reflux may be of interest in patients with extraesophageal atypical symptoms. Furthermore, gas-containing reflux episodes may participate in proximal extension of reflux and extraesophageal symptoms.[92,93] Combined MII-pH monitoring of patients with refractory symptoms has been shown to

TABLE 9.2 24-Hour pH/Impedance Normal Values

| | IMPEDANCE PARAMETERS | | | | | pH PARAMETERS | |
| | All Reflux Episodes | | Frequency of Reflux Types | | | | | |
	Total	Duration (s)	Acid (pH < 4)	Weakly Acidic (4 ≤ pH ≤ 7)	Nonacid pH > 7	% Time Bolus Exposure (by Impedance)	pH Only Reflux Events*	% Time Acid Exposure
Total (95th percentile)	73	44	55	26	1	1.4	3	6.3
Upright (95th percentile)	67	43	52	24	1	2.1	3	9.7
Supine (95th percentile)	7	51	5	4	0	0.7	1	2.1

*Reflux events (pH only): a pH fall from greater than to less than 4 without concomitant liquid reflux by impedance.
From Shay S, Tutuian R, Sifrim D, et al. Twenty-four hour ambulatory simultaneous impedance and pH monitoring: a multicenter report of normal values from 60 healthy volunteers. *Am J Gastroenterol.* 2004;99(6):1037–1043.

be able to clarify the symptom association with reflux events and has revealed that about 50% of patients with persistent symptoms on therapy do not have a temporal correlation between their symptoms and any type of reflux, whereas 40% have temporal association between their symptoms and nonacid reflux.[94–96] A poor symptom correlation may suggest that reflux is not the cause for a patient's symptoms. There may be a subset of patients with normal pH studies on medications but abnormal MII tests that will have good short-term outcomes after fundoplicaiton,[97] but these patients have to be approached cautiously because the outcomes with surgery are less predictable. It is advised that these patients have pH testing off medications to confirm the diagnosis of GERD before offering an antireflux procedure given the absence of clearly defined normal values for impendence-detected number of reflux events. Nonetheless, MII-pH monitoring is being increasingly used in the assessment of patients with atypical symptoms of GERD.[98–100] With studies showing a postfundoplication improvement in extraesophageal symptoms after diagnosis based on pH-only criteria of 15% to 95%,[101] comparison with outcomes of reflux diagnosed by impedance or pH-impedance will be challenging due to the wide range of the results, and these studies are currently lacking.

CONCLUSION

Ambulatory pH monitoring has become widely available and well-established normal thresholds allow confirmation of the presence of increased esophageal acid exposure in patients with GERD symptoms to allow selection of an appropriate therapy. New techniques to add further information on pharyngeal reflux and to assess weak and nonacid reflux events can be useful in some patients. A complete understanding of the strengths and weaknesses of all these studies is beneficial to ensure cost-effective and appropriate evaluation and therapy for patients with both typical and atypical reflux symptoms.

REFERENCES

1. Fedorak RN, Veldhuyzen van Zanten S, Bridges R. Canadian Digestive Health Foundation Public Impact Series: gastroesophageal reflux disease in Canada: incidence, prevalence, and direct and indirect economic impact. *Can J Gastroenterol.* 2010;24(7):431-434.
2. Locke GR 3rd, Talley NJ, Fett SL, Zinsmeister AR, Melton LJ 3rd. Prevalence and clinical spectrum of gastroesophageal reflux: a population-based study in Olmsted County, Minnesota. *Gastroenterology.* 1997;112(5):1448-1456.
3. Mohammed I, Cherkas LF, Riley SA, Spector TD, Trudgill NJ. Genetic influences in gastro-oesophageal reflux disease: a twin study. *Gut.* 2003;52(8):1085-1089.
4. Isolauri J, Laippala P. Prevalence of symptoms suggestive of gastro-oesophageal reflux disease in an adult population. *Ann Med.* 1995;27(1):67-70.
5. Knox SA, Harrison CM, Britt HC, Henderson JV. Estimating prevalence of common chronic morbidities in Australia. *Med J Aust.* 2008;189(2):66-70.
6. Sandler RS, Everhart JE, Donowitz M, et al. The burden of selected digestive diseases in the United States. *Gastroenterology.* 2002;122(5):1500-1511.
7. Kahrilas PJ, Shaheen NJ, Vaezi MF, et al. American Gastroenterological Association Medical Position Statement on the management of gastroesophageal reflux disease. *Gastroenterology.* 2008;135(4):1383-1391, 1391.e1–e5.
8. Vakil N, van Zanten SV, Kahrilas P, Dent J, Jones R, Global Consensus Group. The Montreal definition and classification of gastroesophageal reflux disease: a global evidence-based consensus. *Am J Gastroenterol.* 2006;101(8):1900-1920; quiz 1943.
9. Babey A. Observations on the nature of heartburn. *Am J Dig Dis.* 1937;4:600.
10. Öberg S. Esophageal pH monitoring. In: Yeo CJ, ed. *Shackelford's Surgery of the Alimentary Tract.* 7th ed. Philadelphia: Saunders; 2013:147-153.
11. Aylwin JA. The physiological basis of reflux oesophagitis in sliding hiatal diaphragmatic hernia. *Thorax.* 1953;8(1):38-45.
12. Bernstein LM, Baker LA. A clinical test for esophagitis. *Gastroenterology.* 1958;34(5):760-781.
13. Tuttle SG, Grossman MI. Detection of gastro-esophageal reflux by simultaneous measurement of intraluminal pressure and pH. *Proc Soc Exp Biol Med.* 1958;98(2):225-227.
14. Spencer J. Prolonged pH recording in the study of gastro-oesophageal reflux. *Br J Surg.* 1969;56(12):912-914.
15. Johnson LF, DeMeester TR. Twenty-four-hour pH monitoring of the distal esophagus. A quantitative measure of gastroesophageal reflux. *Am J Gastroenterol.* 1974;62(4):325-332.
16. Stefanidis D, Hope WW, Kohn GP, et al. Guidelines for surgical treatment of gastroesophageal reflux disease. *Surg Endosc.* 2010;24(11):2647-2669.
17. Campos GM, Peters JH, DeMeester TR, et al. Multivariate analysis of factors predicting outcome after laparoscopic Nissen fundoplication. *J Gastrointest Surg.* 1999;3(3):292-300.
18. Hemmink GJ, Weusten BL, Oors J, Bredenoord AJ, Timmer R, Smout AJ. Ambulatory oesophageal pH monitoring: a comparison between antimony, ISFET, and glass pH electrodes. *Eur J Gastroenterol Hepatol.* 2010;22(5):572-577.
19. Opekun AR, Graham DY. Antimony electrodes for in vivo pH monitoring. *Dig Dis Sci.* 1991;36(8):1180-1181.
20. Emde C. Electrochemical aspects of pH electrodes. *Dig Dis.* 1990;8(suppl 1):18-22.

21. Duroux P, Emde C, Bauerfeind P, et al. The ion sensitive field effect transistor (ISFET) pH electrode: a new sensor for long term ambulatory pH monitoring. *Gut.* 1991;32(3):240-245.

22. McLauchlan G, Rawlings JM, Lucas ML, McCloy RF, Crean GP, McColl KE. Electrodes for 24 hours pH monitoring—a comparative study. *Gut.* 1987;28(8):935-939.

23. Ward BW, Wu WC, Richter JE, Lui KW, Castell DO. Ambulatory 24-hour esophageal pH monitoring. Technology searching for a clinical application. *J Clin Gastroenterol.* 1986;8(suppl 1):59-67.

24. Pandolfino JE, Ghosh S, Zhang Q, Heath M, Bombeck T, Kahrilas PJ. Slimline vs. glass pH electrodes: what degree of accuracy should we expect? *Aliment Pharmacol Ther.* 2006;23(2):331-340.

25. Hirano I, Richter JE; Practice Parameters Committee of the American College of Gastroenterology. ACG practice guidelines: esophageal reflux testing. *Am J Gastroenterol.* 2007;102(3):668-685.

26. Ter RB, Johnston BT, Castell DO. Exclusion of the meal period improves the clinical reliability of esophageal pH monitoring. *J Clin Gastroenterol.* 1997;25(1):314-316.

27. Fass R, Hell R, Sampliner RE, et al. Effect of ambulatory 24-hour esophageal pH monitoring on reflux-provoking activities. *Dig Dis Sci.* 1999;44(11):2263-2269.

28. Decktor DL, Krawet SH, Rodriguez SL, Robinson M, Castell DO. Dual site ambulatory pH monitoring: a probe across the lower esophageal sphincter does not induce gastroesophageal reflux. *Am J Gastroenterol.* 1996;91(6):1162-1166.

29. Wong WM, Bautista J, Dekel R, et al. Feasibility and tolerability of transnasal/per-oral placement of the wireless pH capsule vs. traditional 24-h oesophageal pH monitoring—a randomized trial. *Aliment Pharmacol Ther.* 2005;21(2):155-163.

30. Pandolfino JE, Richter JE, Ours T, Guardino JM, Chapman J, Kahrilas PJ. Ambulatory esophageal pH monitoring using a wireless system. *Am J Gastroenterol.* 2003;98(4):740-749.

31. Wenner J, Johnsson F, Johansson J, Oberg S. Wireless oesophageal pH monitoring: feasibility, safety and normal values in healthy subjects. *Scand J Gastroenterol.* 2005;40(7):768-774.

32. Ayazi S, Lipham JC, Portale G, et al. Bravo catheter-free pH monitoring: normal values, concordance, optimal diagnostic thresholds, and accuracy. *Clin Gastroenterol Hepatol.* 2009;7(1):60-67.

33. Emde C, Garner A, Blum AL. Technical aspects of intraluminal pH-metry in man: current status and recommendations. *Gut.* 1987;28(9):1177-1188.

34. Wenner J, Johnsson F, Johansson J, Oberg S. Wireless esophageal pH monitoring is better tolerated than the catheter-based technique: results from a randomized cross-over trial. *Am J Gastroenterol.* 2007;102(2):239-245.

35. Prakash C, Clouse RE. Value of extended recording time with wireless pH monitoring in evaluating gastroesophageal reflux disease. *Clin Gastroenterol Hepatol.* 2005;3(4):329-334.

36. Ahlawat SK, Novak DJ, Williams DC, Maher KA, Barton F, Benjamin SB. Day-to-day variability in acid reflux patterns using the BRAVO pH monitoring system. *J Clin Gastroenterol.* 2006;40(1):20-24.

37. Bhat YM, McGrath KM, Bielefeldt K. Wireless esophageal pH monitoring: new technique means new questions. *J Clin Gastroenterol.* 2006;40(2):116-121.

38. Hirano I, Zhang Q, Pandolfino JE, Kahrilas PJ. Four-day Bravo pH capsule monitoring with and without proton pump inhibitor therapy. *Clin Gastroenterol Hepatol.* 2005;3(11):1083-1088.

39. Lee YC, Wang HP, Chiu HM, et al. Patients with functional heartburn are more likely to report retrosternal discomfort during wireless pH monitoring. *Gastrointest Endosc.* 2005;62(6):834-841.

40. Remes-Troche JM, Ibarra-Palomino J, Carmona-Sanchez RI, Valdovinos MA. Performance, tolerability, and symptoms related to prolonged pH monitoring using the Bravo system in Mexico. *Am J Gastroenterol.* 2005;100(11):2382-2386.

41. Arora AS, Murray JA. Streamlining 24-hour pH study for GERD: use of a 3-hour postprandial test. *Dig Dis Sci.* 2003;48(1):10-15.

42. Anggiansah A, Sumboonnanonda K, Wang J, Linsell J, Hale P, Owen WJ. Significantly reduced acid detection at 10 centimeters compared to 5 centimeters above lower esophageal sphincter in patients with acid reflux. *Am J Gastroenterol.* 1993;88(6):842-846.

43. Wenner J, Johnsson F, Johansson J, Oberg S. Acid reflux immediately above the squamocolumnar junction and in the distal esophagus: simultaneous pH monitoring using the wireless capsule pH system. *Am J Gastroenterol.* 2006;101(8):1734-1741.

44. Lee YY, Whiting JG, Robertson EV, et al. Kinetics of transient hiatus hernia during transient lower esophageal sphincter relaxations and swallows in healthy subjects. *Neurogastroenterol Motil.* 2012;24(11):990-e539.

45. Edmundowicz SA, Clouse RE. Shortening of the esophagus in response to swallowing. *Am J Physiol.* 1991;260(3 Pt 1):G512-G516.

46. Kahrilas PJ, Quigley EM. Clinical esophageal pH recording: a technical review for practice guideline development. *Gastroenterology.* 1996;110(6):1982-1996.

47. Mattox HE 3rd, Richter JE, Sinclair JW, Price JE, Case LD. Gastroesophageal pH step-up inaccurately locates proximal border of lower esophageal sphincter. *Dig Dis Sci.* 1992;37(8):1185-1191.

48. Kahrilas PJ, Lin S, Chen J, Manka M. The effect of hiatus hernia on gastro-oesophageal junction pressure. *Gut.* 1999;44(4):476-482.

49. Lacy BE, O'Shana T, Hynes M, et al. Safety and tolerability of transoral Bravo capsule placement after transnasal manometry using a validated conversion factor. *Am J Gastroenterol.* 2007;102(1):24-32.

50. Tuttle SG, Rufin F, Bettarello A. The physiology of heartburn. *Ann Intern Med.* 1961;55:292-300.

51. Ouatu-Lascar R, Lin OS, Fitzgerald RC, Triadafilopoulos G. Upright versus supine reflux in gastroesophageal reflux disease. *J Gastroenterol Hepatol.* 2001;16(11):1184-1190.

52. Campos GM, Peters JH, DeMeester TR, Oberg S, Crookes PF, Mason RJ. The pattern of esophageal acid exposure in gastroesophageal reflux disease influences the severity of the disease. *Arch Surg.* 1999;134(8):882-887; discussion 887–888.

53. Saraswat VA, Dhiman RK, Mishra A, Naik SR. Correlation of 24-hr esophageal pH patterns with clinical features and endoscopy in gastroesophageal reflux disease. *Dig Dis Sci.* 1994;39(1):199-205.

54. Richter JE, Bradley LA, DeMeester TR, Wu WC. Normal 24-hr ambulatory esophageal pH values. Influence of study center, pH electrode, age, and gender. *Dig Dis Sci.* 1992;37(6):849-856.

55. Jamieson JR, Stein HJ, DeMeester TR, et al. Ambulatory 24-h esophageal pH monitoring: normal values, optimal thresholds, specificity, sensitivity, and reproducibility. *Am J Gastroenterol.* 1992;87(9):1102-1111.

56. Johnsson F, Joelsson B, Isberg PE. Ambulatory 24 hour intraesophageal pH-monitoring in the diagnosis of gastroesophageal reflux disease. *Gut.* 1987;28(9):1145-1150.

57. Bredenoord AJ, Weusten BL, Smout AJ. Symptom association analysis in ambulatory gastro-oesophageal reflux monitoring. *Gut.* 2005;54(12):1810-1817.

58. Wiener GJ, Richter JE, Copper JB, Wu WC, Castell DO. The symptom index: a clinically important parameter of ambulatory 24-hour esophageal pH monitoring. *Am J Gastroenterol.* 1988;83(4):358-361.

59. Tutuian R, Castell DO. Gastroesophageal reflux monitoring: pH and impedance. *GI Motility online.* Published May 16, 2006.

60. Lam HG, Breumelhof R, Roelofs JM, Van Berge Henegouwen GP, Smout AJ. What is the optimal time window in symptom analysis of 24-hour esophageal pressure and pH data? *Dig Dis Sci.* 1994;39(2):402-409.

61. Breumelhof R, Smout AJ. The symptom sensitivity index: a valuable additional parameter in 24-hour esophageal pH recording. *Am J Gastroenterol.* 1991;86(2):160-164.

62. Weusten BL, Roelofs JM, Akkermans LM, Van Berge-Henegouwen GP, Smout AJ. The symptom-association probability: an improved method for symptom analysis of 24-hour esophageal pH data. *Gastroenterology.* 1994;107(6):1741-1745.

63. Katz PO, Gerson LB, Vela MF. Guidelines for the diagnosis and management of gastroesophageal reflux disease. *Am J Gastroenterol.* 2013;108(3):308-328; quiz 329.

64. Numans ME, Lau J, de Wit NJ, Bonis PA. Short-term treatment with proton-pump inhibitors as a test for gastroesophageal reflux disease: a meta-analysis of diagnostic test characteristics. *Ann Intern Med.* 2004;140(7):518-527.

65. Fackler WK, Ours TM, Vaezi MF, Richter JE. Long-term effect of H2RA therapy on nocturnal gastric acid breakthrough. *Gastroenterology.* 2002;122(3):625-632.

66. Bell NJ, Burget D, Howden CW, Wilkinson J, Hunt RH. Appropriate acid suppression for the management of gastro-oesophageal reflux disease. *Digestion.* 1992;51(suppl 1):59-67.

67. Wenner J, Johansson J, Johnsson F, Oberg S. Optimal thresholds and discriminatory power of 48-h wireless esophageal pH monitoring in the diagnosis of GERD. *Am J Gastroenterol.* 2007;102(9):1862-1869.

68. Venables TL, Newland RD, Patel AC, Hole J, Wilcock C, Turbitt ML. Omeprazole 10 milligrams once daily, omeprazole 20 milligrams once daily, or ranitidine 150 milligrams twice daily, evaluated as

initial therapy for the relief of symptoms of gastro-oesophageal reflux disease in general practice. *Scand J Gastroenterol.* 1997;32(10):965-973.

69. Bredenoord AJ, Weusten BL, Curvers WL, Timmer R, Smout AJ. Determinants of perception of heartburn and regurgitation. *Gut.* 2006;55(3):313-318.

70. Tack J, Fass R. Review article: approaches to endoscopic-negative reflux disease: part of the GERD spectrum or a unique acid-related disorder? *Aliment Pharmacol Ther.* 2004;19(suppl 1):28-34.

71. Cherry J, Margulies SI. Contact ulcer of the larynx. *Laryngoscope.* 1968;78(11):1937-1940.

72. Mahieu HF. Review article: the laryngological manifestations of reflux disease: why the scepticism? *Aliment Pharmacol Ther.* 2007;26(suppl 2):17-24.

73. Ayazi S, Hagen JA, Zehetner J, et al. Proximal esophageal pH monitoring: improved definition of normal values and determination of a composite pH score. *J Am Coll Surg.* 2010;210(3):345-350.

74. Vaezi MF, Hicks DM, Abelson TI, Richter JE. Laryngeal signs and symptoms and gastroesophageal reflux disease (GERD): a critical assessment of cause and effect association. *Clin Gastroenterol Hepatol.* 2003;1(5):333-344.

75. Schnatz PF, Castell JA, Castell DO. Pulmonary symptoms associated with gastroesophageal reflux: use of ambulatory pH monitoring to diagnose and to direct therapy. *Am J Gastroenterol.* 1996;91(9):1715-1718.

76. McCollough M, Jabbar A, Cacchione R, Allen JW, Harrell S, Wo JM. Proximal sensor data from routine dual-sensor esophageal pH monitoring is often inaccurate. *Dig Dis Sci.* 2004;49(10):1607-1611.

77. Worrell SG, DeMeester SR, Greene CL, Oh DS, Hagen JA. Pharyngeal pH monitoring better predicts a successful outcome for extraesophageal reflux symptoms after antireflux surgery. *Surg Endosc.* 2013;27(11):4113-4118.

78. Ummarino D, Vandermeulen L, Roosens B, Urbain D, Hauser B, Vandenplas Y. Gastroesophageal reflux evaluation in patients affected by chronic cough: Restech versus multichannel intraluminal impedance/pH metry. *Laryngoscope.* 2013;123(4):980-984.

79. Patel DA, Harb AH, Vaezi MF. Oropharyngeal reflux monitoring and atypical gastroesophageal reflux disease. *Curr Gastroenterol Rep.* 2016;18(3):12.

80. Silny J. Intraluminal multiple electric impedance procedure for measurement of gastrointestinal motility. *Neurogastroenterol Motil.* 1991;3(3):151-162.

81. Tutuian R, Castell DO. Multichannel intraluminal impedance. In: Yeo CJ, ed. *Shackelford's Surgery of the Alimentary Tract.* 7th ed. Philadelphia: Saunders; 2013:154-161.

82. Mainie I, Tutuian R, Agrawal A, Adams D, Castell DO. Combined multichannel intraluminal impedance-pH monitoring to select patients with persistent gastro-oesophageal reflux for laparoscopic Nissen fundoplication. *Br J Surg.* 2006;93(12):1483-1487.

83. Sifrim D, Castell D, Dent J, Kahrilas PJ. Gastro-oesophageal reflux monitoring: review and consensus report on detection and definitions of acid, non-acid, and gas reflux. *Gut.* 2004;53(7):1024-1031.

84. Wildi SM, Tutuian R, Castell DO. The influence of rapid food intake on postprandial reflux: studies in healthy volunteers. *Am J Gastroenterol.* 2004;99(9):1645-1651.

85. Shay S, Tutuian R, Sifrim D, et al. Twenty-four hour ambulatory simultaneous impedance and pH monitoring: a multicenter report of normal values from 60 healthy volunteers. *Am J Gastroenterol.* 2004;99(6):1037-1043.

86. Vela MF, Camacho-Lobato L, Srinivasan R, Tutuian R, Katz PO, Castell DO. Simultaneous intraesophageal impedance and pH measurement of acid and nonacid gastroesophageal reflux: effect of omeprazole. *Gastroenterology.* 2001;120(7):1599-1606.

87. Tamhankar AP, Peters JH, Portale G, et al. Omeprazole does not reduce gastroesophageal reflux: new insights using multichannel intraluminal impedance technology. *J Gastrointest Surg.* 2004;8(7):890-897; discussion 897–898.

88. Ndebia EJ, Sammon AM, Umapathy E, Iputo JE. Normal values of 24-hour ambulatory esophageal impedance-pH monitoring in a rural South African cohort of healthy participants. *Dis Esophagus.* 2016;29(4):385-391.

89. Xiao YL, Lin JK, Cheung TK, et al. Normal values of 24-hour combined esophageal multichannel intraluminal impedance and pH monitoring in the Chinese population. *Digestion.* 2009;79(2):109-114.

90. Zerbib F, des Varannes SB, Roman S, et al. Normal values and day-to-day variability of 24-h ambulatory oesophageal impedance-pH monitoring in a Belgian-French cohort of healthy subjects. *Aliment Pharmacol Ther.* 2005;22(10):1011-1021.

91. Castell DO, Kahrilas PJ, Richter JE, et al. Esomeprazole (40 mg) compared with lansoprazole (30 mg) in the treatment of erosive esophagitis. *Am J Gastroenterol.* 2002;97(3):575-583.

92. Kawamura O, Aslam M, Rittmann T, Hofmann C, Shaker R. Physical and pH properties of gastroesophagopharyngeal refluxate: a 24-hour simultaneous ambulatory impedance and pH monitoring study. *Am J Gastroenterol.* 2004;99(6):1000-1010.

93. Ribolsi M, Savarino E, De Bortoli N, et al. Reflux pattern and role of impedance-pH variables in predicting PPI response in patients with suspected GERD-related chronic cough. *Aliment Pharmacol Ther.* 2014;40(8):966-973.

94. Mainie I, Tutuian R, Shay S, et al. Acid and non-acid reflux in patients with persistent symptoms despite acid suppressive therapy: a multicentre study using combined ambulatory impedance-pH monitoring. *Gut.* 2006;55(10):1398-1402.

95. Triadafilopoulos G. A closure without a closure: impedance pH monitoring expanding the indications for antireflux surgery. *Gastroenterology.* 2010;138(1):390-392; discussion 392.

96. Zerbib F, Roman S, Ropert A, et al. Esophageal pH-impedance monitoring and symptom analysis in GERD: a study in patients off and on therapy. *Am J Gastroenterol.* 2006;101(9):1956-1963.

97. del Genio G, Tolone S, del Genio F, et al. Prospective assessment of patient selection for antireflux surgery by combined multichannel intraluminal impedance pH monitoring. *J Gastrointest Surg.* 2008;12(9):1491-1496.

98. Malhotra A, Freston JW, Aziz K. Use of pH-impedance testing to evaluate patients with suspected extraesophageal manifestations of gastroesophageal reflux disease. *J Clin Gastroenterol.* 2008;42(3):271-278.

99. Bajbouj M, Becker V, Neuber M, Schmid RM, Meining A. Combined pH-metry/impedance monitoring increases the diagnostic yield in patients with atypical gastroesophageal reflux symptoms. *Digestion.* 2007;76(3-4):223-228.

100. Forootan M, Ardeshiri M, Etemadi N, Maghsoodi N, Poorsaadati S. Findings of impedance pH-monitoring in patients with atypical gastroesophageal reflux symptoms. *Gastroenterol Hepatol Bed Bench.* 2013;6(suppl 1):S117-S121.

101. Iqbal M, Batch AJ, Spychal RT, Cooper BT. Outcome of surgical fundoplication for extraesophageal (atypical) manifestations of gastroesophageal reflux disease in adults: a systematic review. *J Laparoendosc Adv Surg Tech A.* 2008;18(6):789-796.

Novel Diagnostic Technologies: Mucosal Impedance, Optical Coherence Tomography, Endomicroscopy

Fahim Habib | Blair A. Jobe

Endoscopy remains the fundamental diagnostic technique for the evaluation of a wide spectrum of esophageal disease. Its cardinal purposes are to perform a comprehensive visual assessment of the esophagus, and to obtain tissue for histologic evaluation. The current standard for endoscopic evaluation, white-light endoscopy (WLE), suffers from several limitations. Key among these is its inability to identify subtle mucosal abnormalities and to detect pathology beneath the surface of mucosa, thereby resulting in a failure to establish the diagnosis or an inability to make the diagnosis at an early stage when therapy is more likely to be potentially curative. This is especially important in the surveillance of Barrett esophagus, a rising problem in Western countries due to the significant increase in incidence of gastroesophageal reflux disease (GERD). Several advanced imaging options have been developed to overcome the limitations of conventional WLE. These include high-definition WLE, magnification endoscopy,[1] chemical chromoendoscopy,[2-5] and electronic chromoendoscopy including narrow band imaging.[6,7] These advanced imaging techniques have been shown to significantly increase the detection of dysplasia in Barrett esophagus, and reduce the number of biopsies needed to adequately screen patients.[8] In spite of these advances, our ability to accurately detect the presence of dysplasia and early carcinoma remains at best suboptimal, and the need for the development of novel diagnostic technologies remains critical. Among the novel diagnostic technologies under development, those with current clinical applicability include mucosal impedance, optical coherence tomography, and endomicroscopy. In addition, several other novel technologies are in the process of development but have yet to gain clinical utility. These include optical coherence tomography angiography (OCTA), capsule volumetric laser endomicroscopy (VLE), and Raman spectroscopy, among others.

MUCOSAL IMPEDANCE

Impedance is a measure of resistance to flow of current. Impedance of the esophageal mucosa can be measured by placing a specialized multichannel catheter with a series of conducting rings into the lumen of the esophagus. When there is movement of intraluminal material between these conducting rings, changes in impedance occur, and can be recorded in terms of amplitude of impedance change over time. Presence of intraluminal liquids as a result of oral intake or reflux results in a drop in impedance from the baseline, while gas due to burping or swallowing of air results in a rise in impedance above the baseline. The directionality of change in impedance allows us to

determine if the flow is anterograde or retrograde. When there is no measurable movement of liquid or gas through the esophagus, the catheter is in direct contact with the esophageal mucosa. The mucosal impedance measured under such conditions is termed the esophageal baseline impedance value. This baseline impedance correlates with transepithelial resistance (TER), which is reflective of the structural integrity of the esophageal mucosa. The TER is significantly influenced by the structural integrity of the intercellular junction complex,[9,10] a critical element in the maintenance of epithelial barrier function. These tight junctions function to seal off paracellular pathways, form paracellular ion channels, and act as transporters.[11] In the presence of reflux, both acid and nonacid, structural alterations in the mucosa occur, critical among which is the appearance of dilated intercellular spaces (DISs) with resultant impairment in esophageal mucosal integrity[12] and a decrease in TER, and as a consequence, a lowered baseline impedance value.[13]

Currently, preliminary studies demonstrate a potential for using measures of baseline mucosal impedance in the clinical evaluation of patients with GERD, assessing adequacy of acid suppression therapy in patients with Barrett esophagus, and in the diagnosis and response to treatment with fluticasone for eosinophilic esophagitis.

Baseline impedance can be measured using a specialized multichannel intraluminal impedance/pH catheter (ComfortTec, Sandhill Scientific, Inc, Highlands Ranch, Colorado). The length of the catheter selected for use is based on the height of the patient; each catheter has specialized circumferential electrodes located at 3, 5, 7, 9, 15, and 17 cm from the tip. The pH probe is placed 5 cm above the upper margin of the manometrically defined lower esophageal sphincter (LES). Impedance and pH signals are collected at a sampling rate resolution of 50 Hz. Data recorded over a 24-hour period are analyzed using a dedicated software program (BioView analysis; Sandhill Scientific, Inc, Highlands Ranch, Colorado). Distal baseline impedance is calculated using data obtained from the sensor at 3 cm, while proximal baseline impedance is calculated from data obtained at the sensor 17 cm above the LES. Measurements are made during four different periods of time over the 24 hours of recording. The first interval is the time between breakfast and lunch, the second interval is between lunch and dinner, the third interval is between dinner and going to sleep, and the fourth interval is during sleep. During each of these four time intervals, three different time periods are selected, each of 1-minute duration, where a constantly stable impedance tracing is noted without alterations due to swallowing or reflux events. Impedance during each

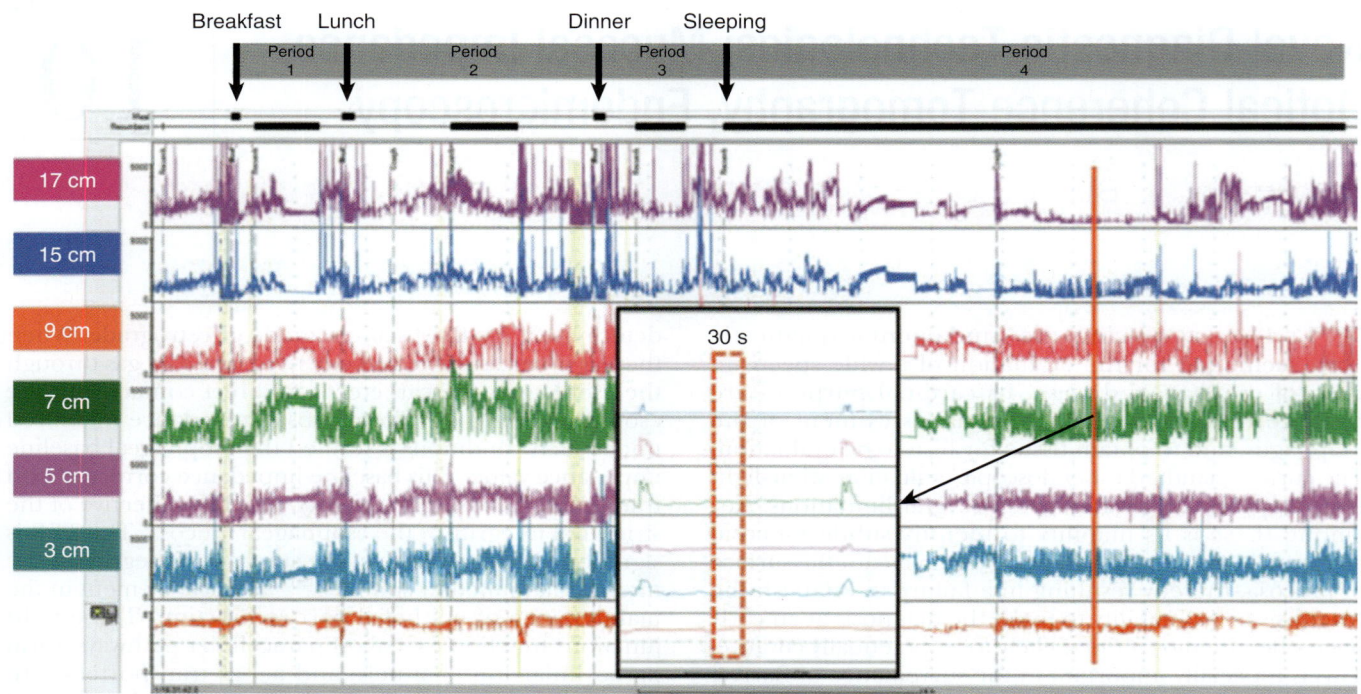

FIGURE 10.1 Protocol for measuring baseline impedance. The 24-hour impedance recording is divided into four periods: two periods between meals, one period before sleep, and one period during sleep. During each of these periods, three different 1-minute measurements are made at times when the impedance is at a stable level. The average of these three measurements is calculated. The final baseline impedance is calculated by averaging the average impedance of these four periods. (From Min YW. Impaired esophageal mucosal integrity may play a causative role in patients with nongastroesophageal reflux disease-related noncardiac chest pain. *Medicine [Baltimore].* 2015;94:1–6.)

of these intervals is calculated by averaging the three impedance readings obtained, and then overall baseline impedance at a particular site is calculated by averaging the measurements made at the four time intervals (Fig. 10.1).

Farré and colleagues placed impedance catheters in rabbits, and after obtaining baseline values, perfused a control solution with a pH of 7.2. During perfusion of the liquid solution, impedance dropped dramatically, and on cessation of perfusion the impedance recovered immediately. In contrast, when perfusion was performed using saline with a pH of 1.5 and 1.0, impedance values persistently remained lower at $39.1 \pm 7.0\%$ and $63.9 \pm 6.5\%$ $(P < .05)$ respectively. The in vivo basal impedance correlated positively with the TER obtained in vitro $(r = 0.72; P = .0021)$. Histologic evaluation of the mucosa demonstrated induction of the DIS even though the tissue showed no gross evidence of erosions. Similarly, in healthy volunteers, infusion with saline of pH 2.0 and 1.0 resulted in the baseline impedance remaining lower at $21.9 \pm 6.5\%$ and $52.7 \pm 5.0\%$ $(P < .0001)$ respectively.[14]

Kessing et al. studied esophageal baseline impedance levels in patients with GERD both on and off therapy, and in normal controls. They found a negative correlation between esophageal acid exposure time and distal baseline impedance, suggesting that acid reflux lowers baseline impedance levels. Further, use of proton pump inhibitors resulted in increases in baseline impedance, suggesting the role of acid exposure in altering mucosal integrity in lowering baseline impedance.[15] In addition to

median baseline impedance values being lower at 2 cm above the squamocolumnar junction in patients with GERD as compared to those without GERD, baseline impedance is decreased even further at sites of erosive esophagitis compared to those without erosion. Further, a graded increase in baseline impedance along the axis of the esophagus from distal to proximal is seen in patients with GERD. A similar gradient is not seen in individuals without reflux.[16]

Wright et al. performed a prospective observational study to determine if mucosal impedance values could help determine if patients with Barrett esophagus were compliant with their acid suppression regimen. All patients had histologically confirmed intestinal metaplasia. Measurements of mucosal impedance were made using a customized single-channel mucosal impedance catheter with unique sensors that was passed through the working channel of a standard endoscope. Mucosal impedance was measured at the site of Barrett epithelium as well as 2, 5, and 10 cm above the squamocolumnar junction. Mucosal impedance values in patients with Barrett esophagus who were not compliant with their acid suppression therapy were lower and similar to the values in patients with GERD. In contrast, mucosal impedance values in patients who were compliant with the acid suppression therapy were higher and similar to values found in patients without GERD (Fig. 10.2).[17]

In addition, a number of small studies have investigated the role of changes in baseline impedance of the

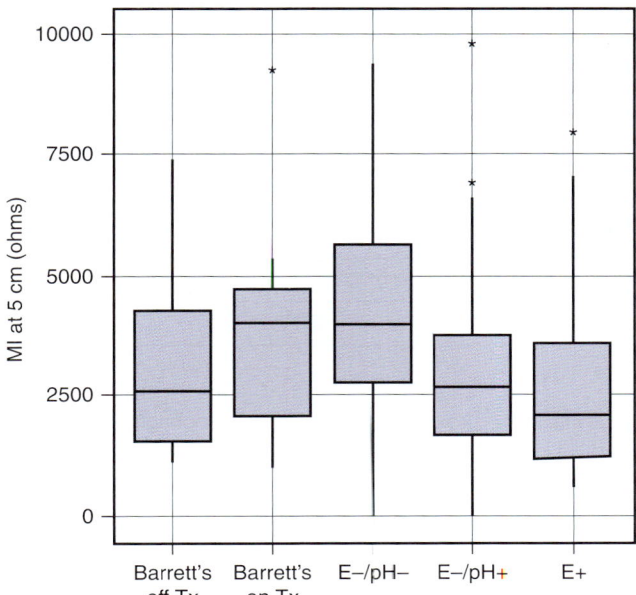

FIGURE 10.2 Basal mucosal impedance values 5 cm above the squamocolumnar junction of the esophagus: (1) Barrett esophagus off therapy, (2) Barrett esophagus on therapy, (3) nonerosive mucosa with normal pH, (4) nonerosive mucosa with abnormal pH, and (5) erosive esophagitis. (From Wright MR, Higginbotham T, Slaughter JC, Ates F, Yuksel ES, Vaezi M. Sa1260 mucosal impedance in Barrett's esophagus: can it assess compliance with medication? *Gastroenterology*. 2016;150[Suppl 1, April]:S260.)

esophageal mucosa in the diagnosis and management of a variety of esophageal pathology. These studies can at best be considered exploratory and further validation is needed before they can be applied clinically. Fukahori et al. evaluated the role of baseline impedance measurements as a parameter to assess the condition of the esophageal mucosa, with the ultimate aim being to replace the need for endoscopic examinations in patients where the procedure would be challenging, in this case neurologically impaired children. In the study, a cutoff value of 1500 ohms represented the baseline impedance that suggested the presence of reflux esophagitis.[18] Other investigators have noted a linear correlation between lower baseline impedance values and acid hypersensitivity, suggesting that lower mucosal baseline impedance is a surrogate marker for impaired mucosal integrity, with an increased sensitivity to acid exposure.[19] Studies on the role of mucosal impedance to diagnose functional heartburn have shown mixed results. Weijenborg et al. evaluated 12 patients with nonerosive reflux disease (NERD) and 9 patients with functional heartburn. Subjects underwent an acid perfusion test, assessment of mucosal integrity by measurement of tissue impedance, and upper endoscopy with biopsy. Obtained specimens were analyzed in Ussing chambers for transepithelial electrical resistance and transepithelial permeability. No difference in baseline impedance, transepithelial resistance, or permeability was found between the two groups, concluding thereby that alterations in baseline impedance were not helpful in

distinguishing patients with NERD from those with functional heartburn.[20] Kandulski et al. performed a prospective study in which 52 patients (19 with NERD, 16 with erosive reflux disease, and 17 with functional heartburn) were studied using endoscopy and multichannel intraluminal impedance studies after discontinuation of proton pump inhibitor therapy. Baseline impedance was assessed at 3, 5, 7, 9, 15, and 17 cm proximal to the LES. Biopsies were also taken 3 cm above the gastroesophageal junction and histologic assessment was performed to semiquantitatively assess the presence of dilated intercellular spaces. They found that baseline impedance was significantly lower in both forms of reflux disease when compared to that of functional heartburn. When a cutoff value of less than 2100 ohms was used, baseline impedance had 78% sensitivity and 71% specificity with positive and negative predictive values of 75% in distinguishing patients with reflux disease versus those with functional heartburn.[21] Although promising, the studies need further validation and more defined establishment of cutoff points, and they are not yet ready for clinical use.

EOSINOPHILIC ESOPHAGITIS

Over the last decade, much progress has been made in understanding the eosinophilic esophagitis, a chronic inflammatory disorder of the esophagus. Eosinophilic esophagitis is believed to be primarily mediated by penetration of the esophageal epithelium by food antigens, which induces a T-helper type 2 cell allergy and results in eosinophil predominant inflammation, decreased barrier function of the esophagus, and dilation in the cellular spaces. Clinically it is characterized by symptoms of esophageal dysfunction, presenting predominantly as feeding difficulties in children, and dysphagia or food impaction in adults. Diagnosis is established when one or more biopsy specimens obtained from the proximal and distal esophagus demonstrate eosinophilic predominant inflammation, with more than 15 eosinophils per high-power field (HPF), representing the minimum threshold value.[22] However, using histologic criteria alone may result in diagnostic error. In up to one-third of patients who did not meet the criteria for eosinophilic esophagitis (<15 eosinophils per HPF) on initial biopsy, subsequent biopsy at repeat endoscopy demonstrated more than 15 eosinophils per HPF, fulfilling the criteria for diagnosis.[23] Further, a proportion of patients with GERD may meet the criteria for eosinophilic esophagitis with 15 or more eosinophils per HPF[23,24] in the absence of eosinophilic esophagitis. Hence, there is great interest in diagnostic modalities that may help establish/support the diagnosis and monitor response to treatment. Because the cardinal pathophysiologic feature of eosinophilic esophagitis is impaired mucosal integrity with DIS and decreased barrier function, measurements of alterations in mucosal impedance have attracted significant attention.

Katzka and colleagues measured mucosal impedance in 10 patients with active eosinophilic esophagitis (>15 eosinophils per HPF), 10 patients with inactive eosinophilic esophagitis (<15 eosinophilic per HPF) following treatment of histologically confirmed eosinophilic esophagitis, and in 10 controls without esophageal symptoms. Mucosal impedance was significantly lower in patients with active

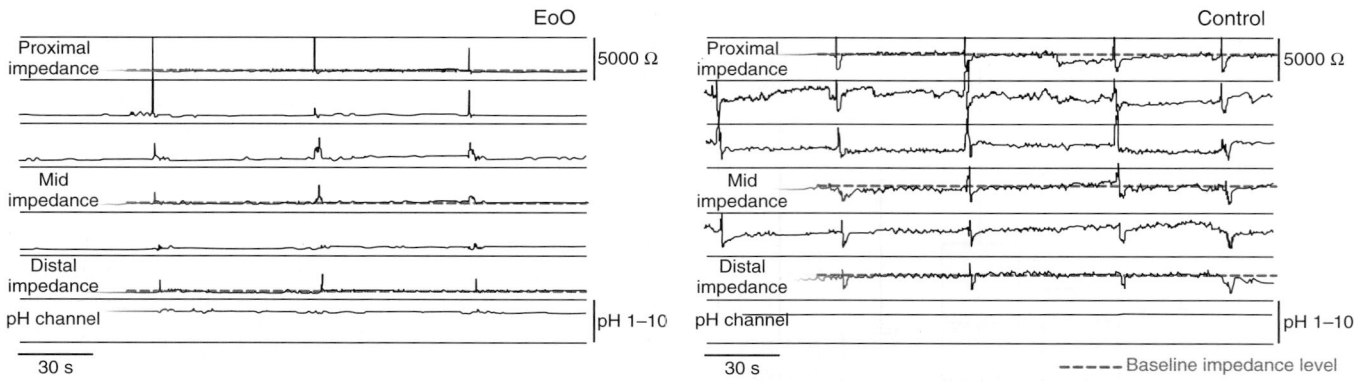

FIGURE 10.3 pH impedance showing significantly lower baseline impedance levels in the proximal, mid, and distal esophagus in patients with eosinophilic esophagitis as compared with normal controls. (From Van Rhijn BD, Kessing BF, Smout AJ, Bredenoord AJ. Oesophageal baseline impedance values are decreased in patients with eosinophilic oesophagitis. *United Eur Gastroenterol J.* 2013;1:242–248.)

eosinophilic esophagitis (1909 Ohms) than subjects with inactive disease (4349 Ohms) or in controls (5530 Ohms). There was a significant inverse correlation between mucosal impedance and the number of eosinophils per HPF on histology ($RS = -0.584$). When a mucosal impedance cutoff value of 2300 Ohms was used to define active eosinophilic esophagitis, test characteristics demonstrated 90% sensitivity and 91% specificity.[25] The low baseline impedance levels are apparent over the entire esophagus including the proximal, mid, and distal portions (Fig. 10.3). Serial changes in baseline impedance can also be used to determine response to therapy. Van Rhijn and colleagues in a prospective study of 15 patients with eosinophilic esophagitis, assessed esophageal mucosal barrier integrity before and after the 8-week course of swallowed fluticasone propionate (500 µg twice daily [BID]). Substantial increases in esophageal mucosal integrity were noted following treatment with increase in mucosal impedance and transepithelial electrical resistance, and decrease in transit epithelial molecular flux.[26]

The role of acid suppression therapy with proton pump inhibitors in patients with the eosinophilic esophagitis is unclear. Although some patients clearly benefit from being placed on acid suppression therapy, others do not. Studies of mucosal impedance suggest that eosinophilic esophagitis may not represent a single disease entity but rather represent a heterogeneous group of disorders. One such subgroup has been termed proton pump inhibitor responsive eosinophilia (PPI-REE). Although parameters of mucosal integrity (electrical tissue impedance, transepithelial electrical resistance, transit epithelial molecule flux) are reduced at baseline in both classic eosinophilic esophagitis and PPI-REE, treatment with high-dose acid suppression therapy using proton pump inhibitors partially restores mucosal integrity in patients with PPI-REE.[27] Measurement of mucosal impedance before and after an 8-week course of acid suppression using proton pump inhibitors may therefore help identify the subset of patients who may benefit from continued treatment, and allow the discontinuation of these medications in patients who do not show any improvement in mucosal impedance, thereby reducing the exposure to

the potential toxicities resulting from the long-term use of proton pump inhibitors.

OPTICAL COHERENCE TOMOGRAPHY

OCT represents a clinically useful "red flag technology" that allows for the evaluation of large mucosal surface areas at high resolution,[28] based on the principles of echo time delay and back scattering of light. Using a rotating optical laser probe that passes through the working channel of the endoscope and contacts the esophageal mucosa, near-infrared light is transmitted onto the surface of the esophagus and the light reflectivity of esophageal tissue is measured. This allows generation of real-time images that permit detection of mucosal surface changes, and changes in glandular architecture on a microscopic scale with an axial resolution of 10 µm. Although this degree of resolution is 10 times that of high-frequency endoscopic ultrasound, there is less depth of penetration. Changes in architecture facilitate identification of targets suspicious for intestinal metaplasia, which can subsequently be subjected to targeted biopsy.[29,30]

VLE is a second-generation frequency domain optical coherence tomography imaging technique that is currently available for clinical use in the United States (NinePoint Medical Inc., Bedford, Massachusetts). An integrated imaging system consisting of a console, monitor, and a near-infrared-light optical probe centered within a transparent balloon is used to deliver a 1350-nm wavelength laser that emanates from the probe in a helical manner with automated pullback. The system allows fast real-time imaging with a 6-cm length of esophagus being scanned in approximately 90 seconds and provides wide-field, cross-sectional imaging of the surface and subsurface of the esophagus with an axial resolution of up to 7 µm and down to a depth of 3 mm (Fig. 10.4).

Prior to performing VLE, a diagnostic endoscopy is performed with WLE using a high-definition diagnostic endoscope (HQ 190, Olympus, Tokyo, Japan) to identify the location of the gastroesophageal junction, and evaluate the esophagus for conditions that would preclude safe passage and inflation of the optical probe; these include

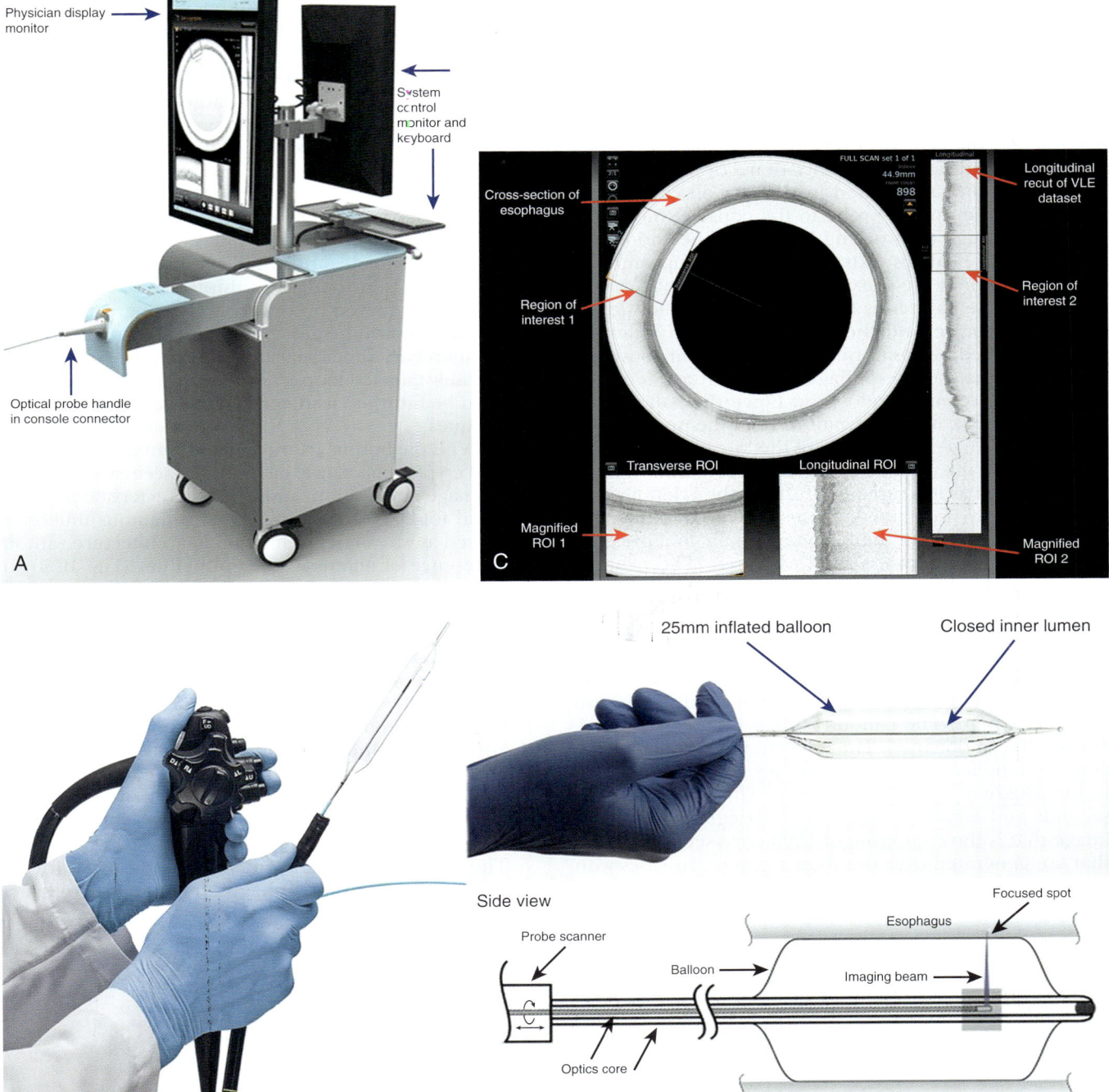

FIGURE 10.4 The Nvision volumetric laser endomicroscopy (VLE) system. (A) Imaging system console. (B) Optical probe with centering balloon. (C) The Nvision VLE display shows a complete circumferential cross-sectional view of the esophagus, with longitudinal recuts of the 3-dimensional VLE dataset displayed alongside, and magnified regions of interest in the circumferential and longitudinal views shown in separate insets. (From Wolfson HC. Safety and feasibility of volumetric laser endomicroscopy in patients with Barrett's esophagus [with videos]. *Gastrointest Endosc.* 2015;82:631–640.)

the presence of mass lesions or severe strictures. Caution should be exercised in patients with a tortuous esophagus, and in those with suspected eosinophilic esophagitis. The extent of the Barrett segment is recorded using the Prague criteria.[31] During endoscopy the appropriate size of the optical probe to be used can also be determined. Although the standard length of the optical probe is 6 cm, it is available in diameters of 14 mm, 17 mm, and 20 mm. In our experience, in the absence of major pathology the 20 mm balloon can be used in virtually all cases. After connecting the optical probe to the console, the probe is passed through the working channel of the endoscope until the entire balloon extrudes from the scope and the opaque marker at the proximal end of the probe can be visualized. The balloon is then positioned to lie with its distal tip 1 cm beyond the gastroesophageal junction. This is achieved by positioning the scope 7 cm above the location of the gastroesophageal junction as identified during the screening endoscopy. Once the balloon has been positioned, it is important to hold the probe firmly between the fingers at the level of the bite block, and as it emerges from the working channel, to prevent movement of the balloon as it is inflated. If the probe is left lax, the balloon tends to drop into the stomach. The custom syringe is then used to inflate the balloon with air to a pressure of 10 psi. A scout scan is then obtained. The primary purpose of the scout scan is to ensure that the obtained scan includes the gastric cardia, the gastroesophageal junction, and the distal portion of the esophagus. It is also used to confirm that the balloon is optimally centered. If the balloon has migrated, it can be deflated, repositioned, reinflated, and a repeat scout scan obtained to confirm ideal placement. The balloon is then inflated to 15 psi, and a full scan obtained. The full scan is generated by the automatic helical pullback of the probe from the distal to the proximal end of the balloon. This occurs over 90 seconds and creates a real-time 360-degree volumetric image that is the composite of 1200 cross-sectional scans that are generated over the 6-cm segment. In cases with a dilated esophagus, a higher inflation pressure of up to

20 psi may be necessary to center the balloon. On completion of the scan, the balloon is deflated, and the location of the registration line as described according to the face of the clock is noted. This then allows orientation of the cross-sectional imaging on the monitor with its location in the esophagus allowing for targeted biopsies. When the segment of interest is greater than 6 cm, multiple scans may be performed. Here it is critical to identify a unique anatomic characteristic that is visualized on both scans and to overlap them accurately such that the resultant scan represents a seamless continuum. In the absence of such a unique anatomic characteristic, cautery marks may be made, and will be visible on the scan and can then be used to align multiple scans. Localization of lesions is achieved by a process of triangulation based on the location of the gastroesophageal junction and the registration line. Superficial abnormalities can be subjected to precisely targeted biopsies, while submucosal abnormalities can be biopsied using endoscopic mucosal resection techniques.

On VLE the normal gastric mucosa demonstrates vertical pit and crypt architecture, has high surface reactivity, shows poor image penetration, and thick characteristic presence of rugal folds. Normal esophageal squamous mucosa is visualized as was a layered horizontal architecture without the presence of glands in the epithelium (Fig. 10.5). In contrast, esophageal mucosa with intestinal metaplasia shows a loss of layered architecture and the presence of glands in the epithelium (Fig. 10.6).

In the most recent version of the VLE, which has only just become available, a 1470-nm wavelength laser is used. A hand control attached to the endoscope allows the operator to navigate the optical probe in real time through the esophagus. On identification of areas of interest, the laser can be fired, creating a cautery mark on the surface of the esophagus. Subsequent WLE allows the endoscopist to identify the marked area and facilitate the performance of VLE-directed biopsies (Fig. 10.7).[32,33]

The most common current clinical indications for the use of VLE are Barrett esophagus, including surveillance

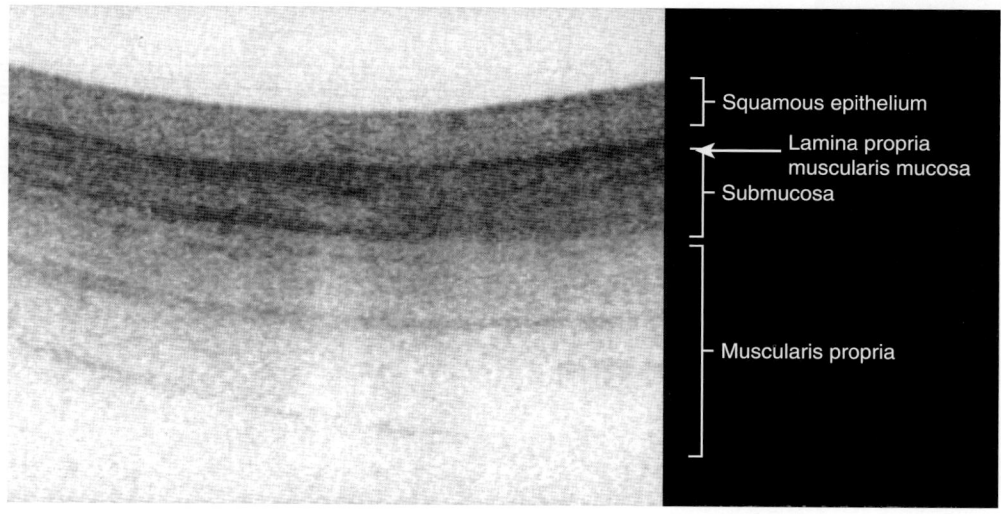

FIGURE 10.5 Histologic correlates of the layers of normal esophageal wall obtained by volumetric laser endomicroscopy. (From Lightdale CJ. Optical coherence tomography in Barrett's esophagus. *Gastrointest Endosc Clin N Am.* 2013;23:549–563.)

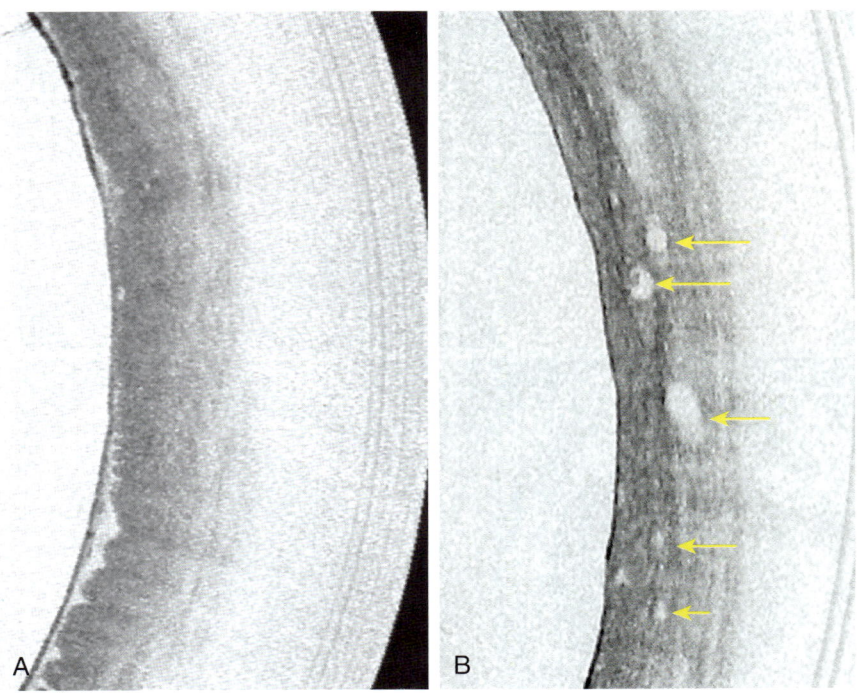

FIGURE 10.6 Volumetric laser endomicroscopy features of intestinal metaplasia. (A) Loss of layered architecture. (B) Glands seen in the epithelium. (From Trindale AJ. Volumetric laser endomicroscopy can target neoplasia not detected by conventional endoscopic measures in long segment Barrett's esophagus. *Endosc Int Open.* 2016;04[E3]:18–322.)

of high-risk, treatment-naive Barrett esophagus, and for postablation surveillance to detect recurrence or persistence.[34,35] VLE is also used to guide peroral endoscopic myotomy (POEM) for the treatment of achalasia.

SURVEILLANCE OF TREATMENT-NAIVE BARRETT ESOPHAGUS

The generated image allows differentiation between normal and abnormal tissue in the stomach and in the esophagus.[36] On VLE, normal gastric cardia demonstrates vertical pit and crypt architecture, high surface reflectivity, poor image penetration, and presence of rugal folds. Normal esophageal squamous mucosa demonstrates a layered horizontal architecture without the presence of glands in the epithelium. Loss of layered architecture and presence of glands in the epithelium are suggestive of intestinal metaplasia.[37] Presence of dysplasia is assessed on the basis of two features of the obtained image: signal intensity and glandular architecture. Signal intensity is assessed by comparing the surface signal intensity with the signal intensity in the subsurface tissue. Normally, surface intensity should be less than subsurface intensity. Partial effacement is present when this surface intensity is equivalent to that of subsurface tissue. Full effacement is present when the surface intensity is greater than that of the subsurface tissue. Glandular architecture is assessed by determining the presence or absence of glands, with or without atypia. Using these two features, Leggett et al. developed an OCT scoring index (OCT-SI) (Fig. 10.8). A score of 2 or higher is associated with 83% sensitivity and 75% specificity for dysplasia. They also used these characteristics to develop a VLE diagnostic algorithm based on ex vivo VLE assessment of specimens obtained by endoscopic mucosal resection. First, a comparative assessment of surface intensity versus the intensity of subsurface tissue is performed. Presence of full effacement

as characterized by surface intensity that is greater than the intensity of the subsurface tissue denotes a high suspicion for dysplasia. Then, in cases where effacement is partial, presence of atypical glands is assessed with the detection of more than five atypical glands, raising suspicion for the presence of dysplasia. Using this algorithm Legget et al. obtained a sensitivity of 86% and a specificity of 88% for the detection of dysplasia.[38]

Swager et al. recently presented results of her study investigating the feasibility of a computer algorithm for detection of early Barrett neoplasia using VLE. A total of 60 VLE images were used in the study, of which 30 were dysplastic and 30 nondysplastic. Decision making by the computer-based algorithm relied on features associated with dysplasia including (1) a higher optical frequency domain imaging (OFDI) surface signal than subsurface signal in tissue and (2) a lack of layering. The algorithm had a sensitivity of 93%, specificity of 70%, and accuracy of 82%. The area under the curve (AUC) on the receiver operating characteristic (ROC) curve was 0.91, which compares favorably with a recently developed clinical prediction model that had an AUC of 0.81.[39,40] In the latter model, Swager et al. found three independent predictors for neoplasia in Barrett esophagus: (1) lack of layering (6 points); (2) higher surface than subsurface signal (6 points for a surface signal that was equivalent to the subsurface tissue, and 8 points for a higher surface signal when compared to subsurface tissue); and (3) presence of irregular, dilated glands/ducts (5 points) (Fig. 10.9). The ROC curve in the validation phase showed an AUC of 0.81 (95% confidence interval [CI], 0.71 to 0.90). Using a cutoff value of more than 8 points, sensitivity of 83% and specificity of 71% were obtained. As with several studies involving VLE, histologic analysis was performed on ex vivo specimens. The applicability of these findings in vivo has yet to be determined.

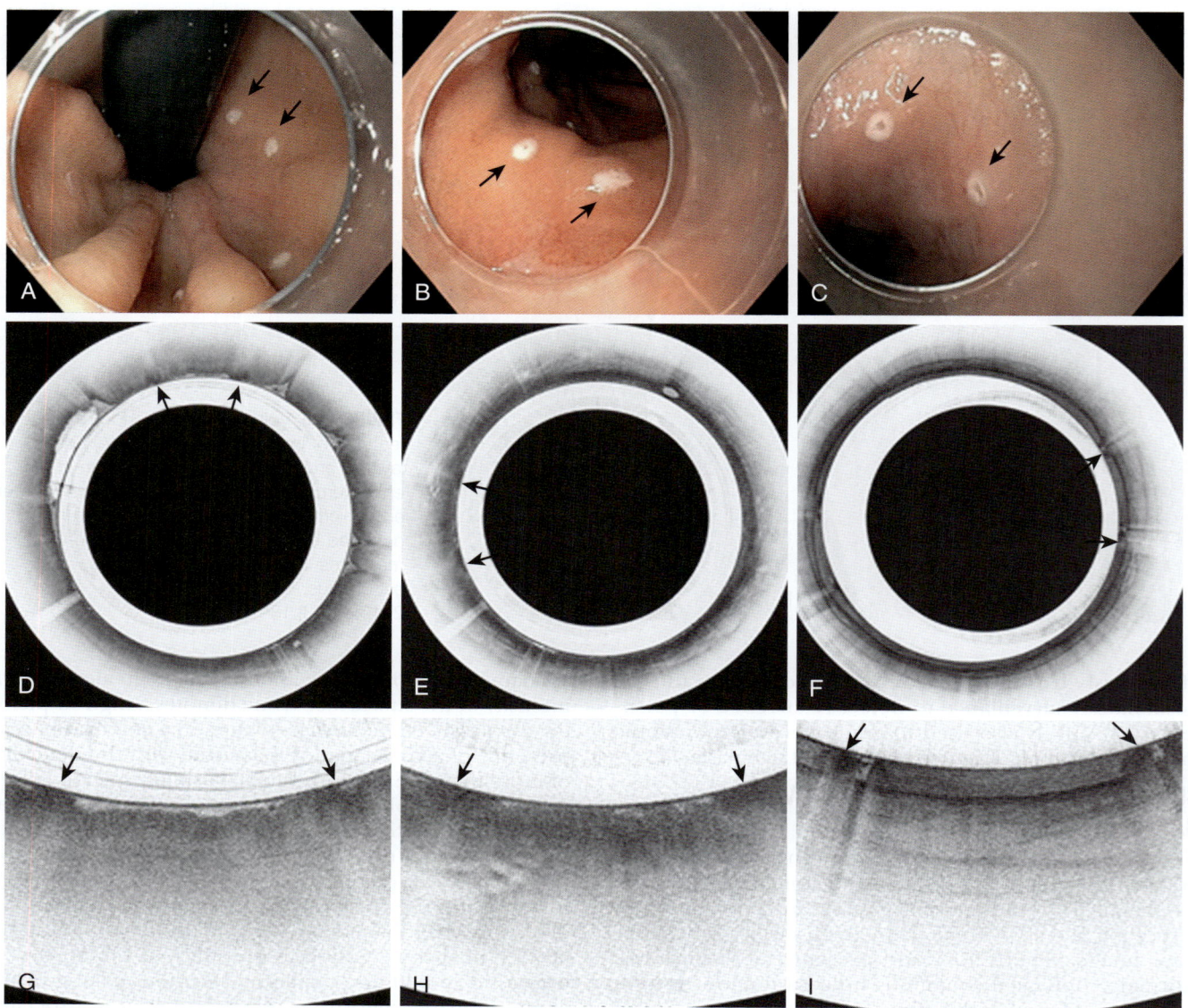

FIGURE 10.7 Visibility of laser marks *(arrows)* in gastric (A, D, G), nondysplastic (B, E, H), and squamous mucosa (C, F, I) on white-light endoscopy, circumferential volumetric laser endomicroscopy (VLE), and zoom-in views on VLE. (From Swager A, de Groof AJ, Meijer SL, Weusten BL, Curvers WL, Bergman JJ. Feasibility of laser marking in Barrett's esophagus with volumetric laser endomicroscopy: first-in-man pilot study. *Gastrointest Endosc*. pii:S0016-5107[17]30074-3.)

The ability to mark the area of interest during performance of VLE with subsequent targeted biopsy of the marked regions has potential to further improve the accuracy of image-guided biopsy for Barrett esophagus. Suter et al. first explored this in a pilot feasibility study involving 22 patients.[41] Burn marks using lasers of different wavelengths were made on either side of the VLE-detected abnormality. The optimal marking parameter was found to be 2 seconds at 410 mW, with separation of the two marks by 6 mm. All marks made were visible at endoscopy. There were no adverse events related to VLE or laser marking. Accuracy for corrected VLE postmarking images was 100% when compared to histologic interpretations. This approach has been further refined, and the newest version of the VLE imaging system incorporates a laser marking system. This

allows direct in vivo marking of suspicious areas as they are identified during real-time VLE. One of two marking options may be used. In the offset marking mode, two laser marks are placed automatically in the horizontal position 6 mm apart. In the point marking mode, a single laser mark is placed. The marking laser is activated and controlled by the operator with a handheld control that is attached to the endoscope. In a recent pilot feasibility study, the protocol for laser marking was developed in a primary learning phase. Subsequently the visibility on follow-up endoscopy of random laser markings made in squamous, Barrett, and gastric tissue was assessed; positional accuracy was tested; and finally, the most suspicious area for neoplasia as identified by VLE was targeted. The location of laser marks made could be identified on VLE in 100%

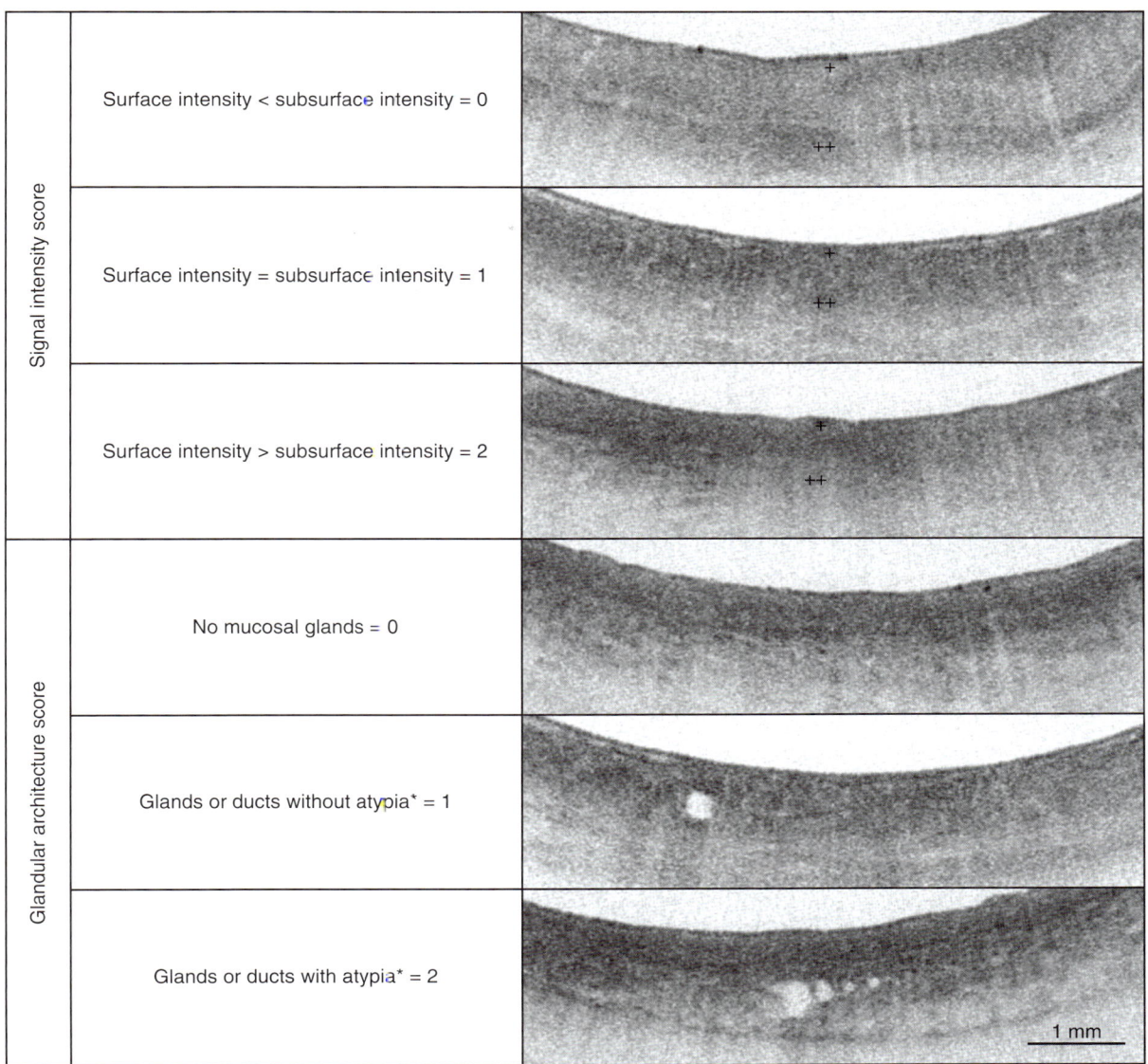

FIGURE 10.8 OCT Scoring Index (OCT-SI). A score of ≥2 has a sensitivity of 83% and specificity of 75% for detecting dysplasia. (From Leggett CL, Gorospe EC, Chan DK, et al. Comparative diagnostic performance of volumetric laser endomicroscopy and confocal laser endomicroscopy in the detection of dysplasia associated with Barrett's esophagus. *Gastrointest Endosc.* 2016;83:880–888.e2.)

of cases and on WLE in 97%. Areas found to be suspicious on VLE were successfully targeted by the laser marks in all cases.[33]

POSTABLATION SURVEILLANCE OF BARRETT ESOPHAGUS

When endoscopic ablation of Barrett esophagus is performed, residual metaplastic glands can remain under the layer of neosquamous epithelium that forms. In addition, buried glands may be present at the junction of Barrett epithelium and squamous epithelium. The incidence of buried glands is higher following photodynamic therapy (14.2%) than when radiofrequency ablation is employed as the treatment modality (0.9%).[42] However, these reported incidences may underestimate the true incidence of buried glands because biopsy specimens may not contain sufficient subepithelial tissue to make the diagnosis. This low incidence of buried Barrett glands following radiofrequency ablation was further confirmed by Swager and colleagues. Although VLE identified subsquamous granular structures following radiofrequency ablation of Barrett esophagus, the overwhelming majority of identified subsquamous glands were determined to be normal histologic structures such as dilated glands and blood vessels. Buried glands were identified in only 1 of 17 post-radiofrequency ablation patients. The development of high-grade dysplasia and adenocarcinoma in these varied subsquamous metaplastic tissues has been reported.[43,44] Characteristic VLE findings include increased signal intensity and atypical appearing glands with dilated ducts under a layer of squamous epithelium.

Trindade et al.[45] recently began to address the issue of reproducibility of the interpretation of VLE images. Eight high-frequency VLE users (who have read more than 50

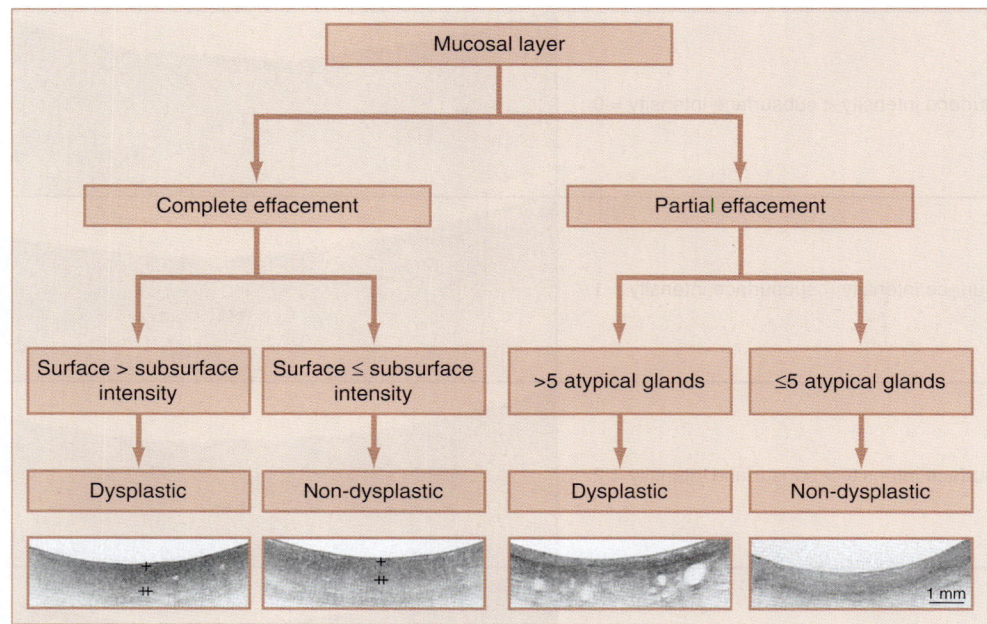

FIGURE 10.9 The volumetric laser endomicroscopy diagnostic algorithm index has a sensitivity of 86% and a specificity of 88% in detecting dysplasia. (From Leggett CL, Gorospe EC, Chan DK, et al. Comparative diagnostic performance of volumetric laser endomicroscopy and confocal laser endomicroscopy in the detection of dysplasia associated with Barrett's esophagus. *Gastrointest Endosc*. 2016;83:880–888.e2.)

VLE examinations) from academic tertiary care centers in the United States evaluated 120 identified images classifying them as gastric cardia, esophageal squamous mucosa, nonneoplastic Barrett esophagus (nondysplastic Barrett esophagus and low-grade dysplasia), and neoplastic Barrett esophagus. They were also instructed to distinguish nonneoplastic Barrett esophagus from neoplastic Barrett esophagus using the OCT-SI. An OCT-SI score of 2 or greater was used as the criteria of neoplastic disease. The overall agreement among users was excellent (kappa equals 0.81; 95% CI, 0.79 to 0.83). Agreement was near perfect for esophageal squamous and gastric cardia (kappa equals 0.95 and 0.86, respectively [95% CI, 0.92 to 0.98 and 0.83 to 0.89]). Agreement was strong for distinguishing nonneoplastic Barrett esophagus and neoplastic Barrett esophagus (Kappa = 0.66 [95% CI, 0.63 to 0.69] and Kappa = 0.79 [95% CI, 0.75 to 0.82], respectively). Overall median accuracy for identifying the correct tissue type was 96% (95% CI, 94% to 99%). These findings suggest that with increasing experience and application of uniform criteria, targeted biopsies can be made a clinical reality. However, one must take into account that these images were analyzed offline. Interpretation of images in real time as the study is in progress may not be as easily learned. Hence, at the present time, random biopsies obtained using the Seattle protocol should still remain the gold standard. Targeted biopsies as guided by abnormalities noted on VLE must be taken in addition.

VLE has only recently been adopted into clinical practice and largely at institutions specializing in the management of Barrett esophagus. Cost effectiveness data are therefore not available at this time. It does, however, seem plausible that replacement of extensive protocol biopsies such as those employed by the Seattle protocol with targeted biopsies and a reduction in the need for multiple subsequent endoscopic procedures has the potential to result in an overall cost saving in the long term.

VOLUMETRIC LASER ENDOMICROSCOPY IN ACHALASIA

Desai and colleagues recently described a novel application of optical coherence tomography. They incorporated VLE into the algorithm for assessing the esophagus and planning approach prior to POEM in the treatment of achalasia. VLE images were analyzed for regional differences in thickness of circular muscle, and for the presence of large vessels at the location of intended incision. Based on these features, a decision to perform an anterior POEM or a posterior POEM was made. Results were compared in patients who underwent the procedure prior to introduction of VLE for preoperative assessment with those who underwent the procedure after this new diagnostic modality was adopted into clinical practice. Less bleeding (8% vs. 43%; $P = .0001$) and a shorter procedural time (85.8 vs. 121.7 minutes; $P = .000097$) were noted when the use of VLE was introduced.[46] An additional use of optical coherence tomography is to assess the adequacy of myotomy after performance of a POEM procedure. A full scan of the esophagus can be performed, and demonstrates a break in the muscular layers at the site where the POEM was performed on (Fig. 10.10). This technique can therefore potentially be used to evaluate recurrence of symptoms following endoscopic myotomy.[47]

ENDOSCOPIC OPTICAL COHERENCE TOMOGRAPHY

Normal   Post-POEM procedure

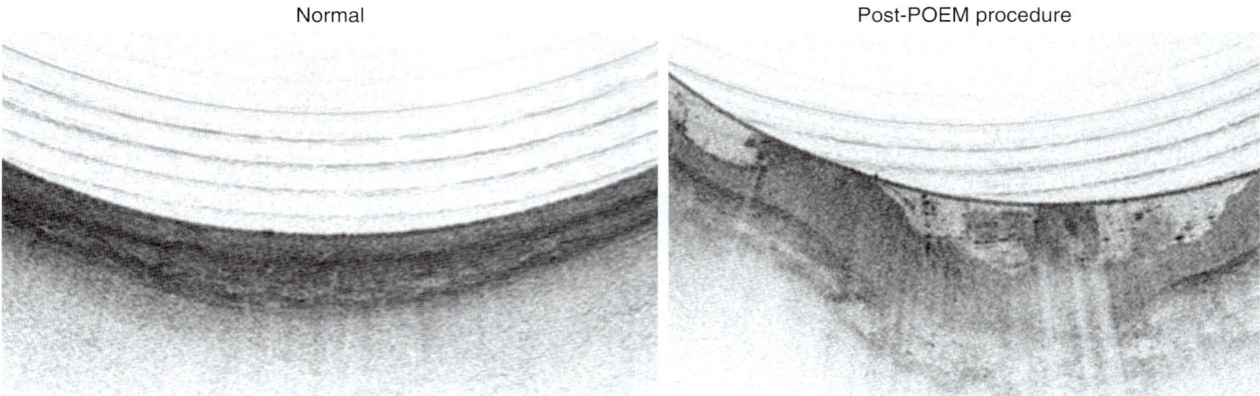

FIGURE 10.10 Use of optical coherence tomography to evaluate success of myotomy following peroral endoscopic myotomy (POEM). (From Parra V, Kedia P, Minami H, Sharaiha RZ, Kahaleh M. Endoscopic optical coherence tomography as a tool to evaluate successful myotomy after a peroral endoscopic myotomy. *Gastroint Endosc.* 2015;81;1251.)

CONFOCAL LASER ENDOMICROSCOPY

Confocal laser endomicroscopy (CLE) is an optical imaging modality that allows for real-time in vivo histologic evaluation of the esophageal mucosa during endoscopy. CLE can currently be performed using one of two available systems. With eCLE, imaging is performed using a special endoscope that incorporates the confocal laser endomicroscope (Pentax Medical, Montvale, New Jersey), whereas with pCLE, a probe is inserted through the working channel of the standard endoscope (Cellvizio Mauna Kea Technologies, Paris, France). Following the administration of intravenous fluorescein, an argon blue laser light with a wavelength of 488 nm is used to illuminate and then to detect fluorescent light reflected from the mucosa. It can achieve subcellular resolution up to 250 mcm in depth with 500 to 1000× magnification.[48] A standardized system to distinguish between nondysplastic Barrett, high-grade dysplasia, and adenocarcinoma has been developed by consensus and is termed the Miami classification.[49] These have since been validated in randomized controlled trials and are now widely accepted. Nondysplastic Barrett esophageal mucosa has a uniform villiform architecture and columnar epithelial cells with dark goblet cells, demonstrates minimal intracellular fluorescence, and has an organized cellular architecture. In contrast, dysplastic Barrett esophagus demonstrates intense intracellular fluorescence, heterogeneous cellular sizes, and disorganized cellular architecture with irregularly shaped crypts and dilated capillary vessels. In esophageal adenocarcinoma, there is complete loss of crypt and villiform architecture with irregular and dilated capillaries (Fig. 10.11). Kiesslich and colleagues were the first to demonstrate the value of CLE. In a study of 63 patients, CLE demonstrated a sensitivity of 98.1% and the specificity of 94.1%. The ability to detect associated neoplasia had a sensitivity of 92.9% and specificity of 98.4%.[50] Multiple studies since then have validated the utility of CLE. Dunbar et al. in a crossover study of 39 patient demonstrated a higher diagnostic yield for high-grade dysplasia or carcinoma when compared with conventional WLE with random biopsies (33.7% vs. 17.2%; *P* = .01).[51] Pohl et al. in a prospective study evaluated 296 lesions in 38 patients. They found that CLE had a high negative predictive value (98.8%) for high-grade dysplasia and adenocarcinoma. Sensitivity, however, was low at 75%.[52] Bajbouj et al. in contrast found a low positive predictive value (46%) and sensitivity (18%).[53] Sharma et al. demonstrated pCLE to be superior to high-definition WLE in the detection of neoplastic tissue in Barrett esophagus.[54] In a more recent study, Canto et al. using CLE with targeted biopsies, tripled the diagnostic yield for neoplasia when compared with random biopsies at the time of WLE (22% vs. 6%; *P* = .002). In a comparative study of pCLE versus VLE, 27 patients underwent 50 endoscopic mucosal resections (EMRs) while enrolled in a surveillance program for Barrett esophagus. The 34 neoplastic (high-grade dysplasia, intramucosal adenocarcinoma) and 16 nonneoplastic (low-grade dysplasia, nondysplastic) specimens were imaged using pCLE and VLE. The sensitivity, specificity, and diagnostic accuracy of pCLE for this study was 76% (95% CI, 59 to 88), 79% (95% CI, 53 to 92), and 77% (95% CI, 72 to 82), respectively. Gupta and colleagues performed a meta-analysis that compared the diagnostic accuracy of targeted biopsies guided by CLE with four-quadrant random biopsies in detecting the presence of high-grade dysplasia/adenocarcinoma. Due to the finding of relatively low sensitivity and negative predictive value, these authors felt that CLE-targeted biopsies should not replace the current standard biopsy protocols at the present time.[55]

Although the technology appears promising, there are several limitations that preclude clinical use in its present format. Key among these is the limited imaging depth and limited field of view, which would make evaluation of large extents of mucosal surfaces tedious and time consuming. Also, much of the available data come from academic centers treating high-risk subtype populations. The generalizability of these results to the community setting, where a large proportion of these patients are probably treated, is uncertain. Further, there is a need for special training in image interpretation. There is also

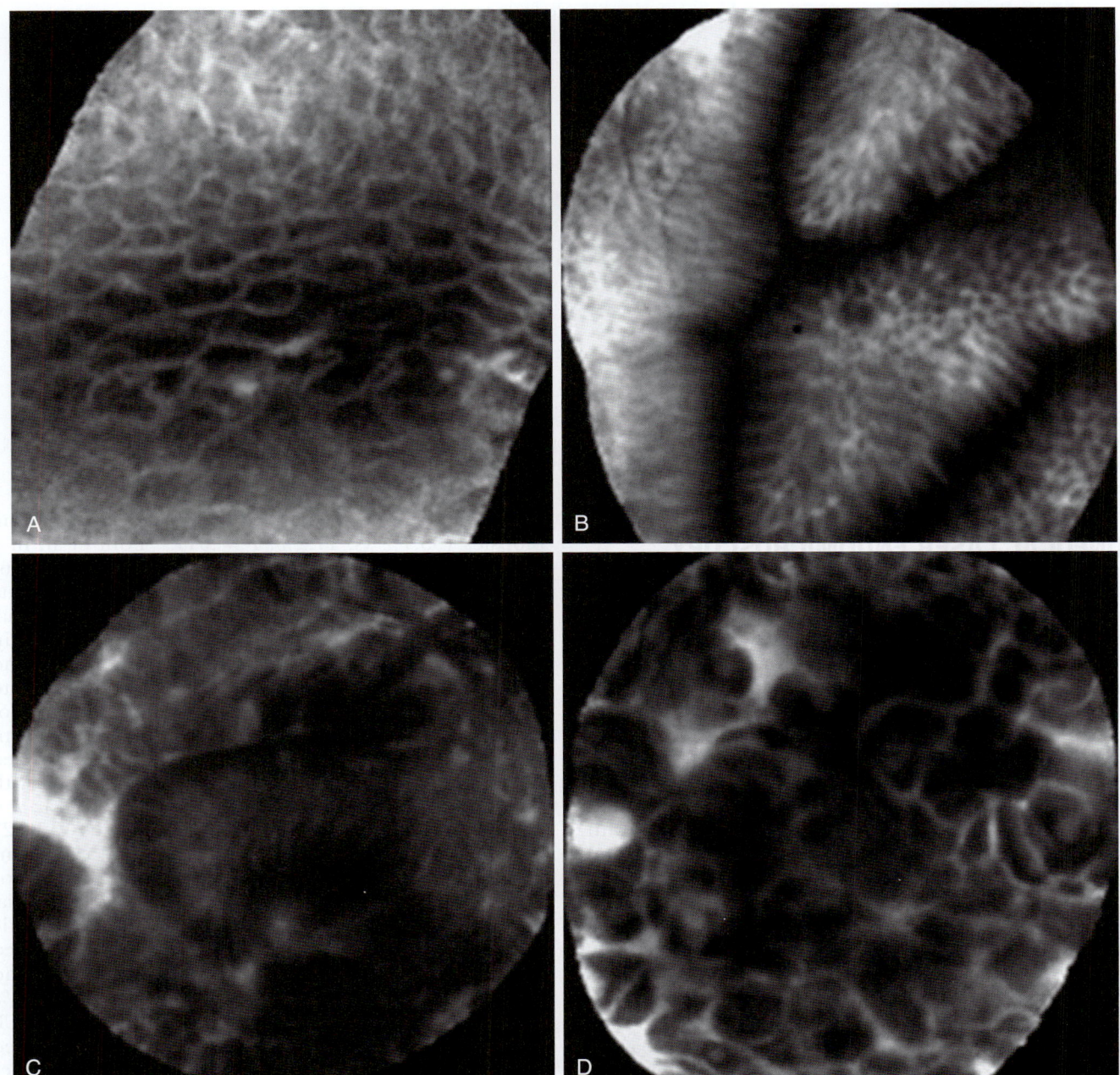

FIGURE 10.11 Confocal microscopy Miami criteria. (A) Normal squamous epithelium: Flat cells without crypts or villi. (B) Barrett without dysplasia: Uniform villiform architecture, columnar cells interspersed with dark goblet cells. (C) High-grade dysplasia: Villiform structure preserved, dark irregular thickened epithelial borders, dilated irregular vessels. (D) Adenocarcinoma: Villiform structure absent or significantly disorganized, multiple dark columnar cells with dilated irregular vessels. (From Shahid MW, Wallace MB. Endoscopic imaging for the detection of esophageal dysplasia and carcinoma. *Gastrointest Endosc Clin N Am*. 2010;20:17; with permission.)

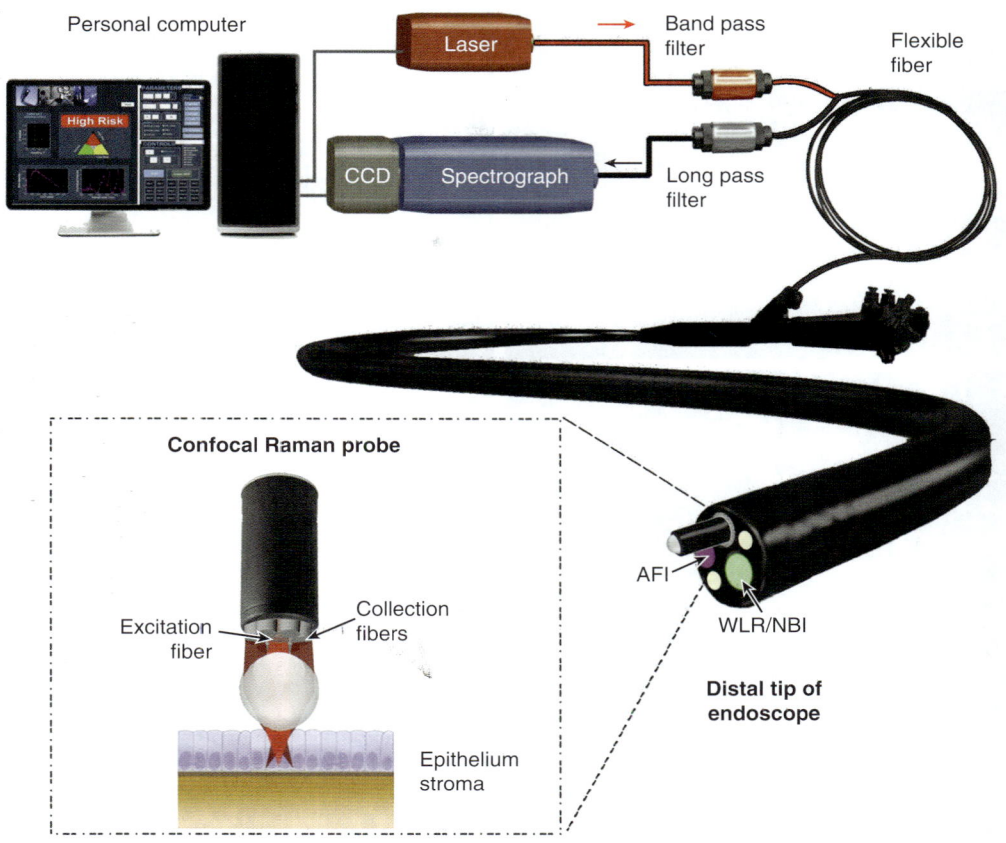

FIGURE 10.12 The rapid fiberoptic confocal Raman spectroscopy system. *AFI,* Autofluorescence imaging; *CCD,* charge-coupled device; *WLR/NBI,* white light reflectance/narrow band imaging. (From Bergholt MA, Zheng W, Ho KY, et al. Fiberoptic confocal Raman spectroscopy for real-time in vivo diagnosis of Barrett's esophagus. *Gastroenterology.* 2014;146:27–32.)

the necessity for intravenous administration of fluorescent contrast agents, which may temporarily cause the skin and urine to become yellow to orange for up to 24 hours.

OTHER EMERGING TECHNOLOGIES

Capsule VLE imaging: Liang and colleagues have developed an ultra-high-speed OCT tethered capsule that is capable of obtaining a large field of view, imaging the subsurface, and obtaining cross-sectional volumetric imaging of the esophagus. This capsule, which is 30 mm long and 12 mm in diameter, has a micro motor that scans at 300 frames per second. The capsule is attached to a semirigid tether and is introduced into the esophagus of sedated patients, with a pull-push technique to volumetrically map the esophagus. In its current form the technology suffers from an inability to image the full circumference of the esophagus. Regions of noncontact appear dark. The need for manual pull–push, movements due to respiration, cardiac motion, and peristalsis also produce image distortion. Further refinements in the technology are necessary to overcome these limitations.[56]

Raman spectroscopy is based on the principle of inelastic scattering of light with frequency shifts that correspond to the molecular composition of the tissue being evaluated, providing histopathologic assessments at the biomolecular level.[57] Early studies on ex vivo esophageal tissue demonstrated a sensitivity of 86% and a specificity of 88% in the detection of high-grade dysplasia and adenocarcinoma. The technique was also able to identify the presence of intestinal metaplasia and grade the degree of dysplasia.[58] Recently, a novel endoscopic confocal Raman probe was developed that allows rapid acquisition of data from large tissue areas (Fig. 10.12). The utility of this probe is currently under evaluation.[59]

Endoscopic optical coherence angiography is being developed to overcome limitations inherent to current OCT modalities including limited frame rate, narrow field of view, sensitivity to motion artifact, and limitation of analysis to surface vascular patterns. Using a micro motor catheter, circumferential cross-sectional scans in a helical pattern are performed at 400 frames per second with images from an area greater than 100 mm² being acquired in about 8 seconds (Fig. 10.13). Detection of the intensity correlation generated by moving erythrocytes allows further visualization of the microvasculature without the need for administration of exogenous contrast agents.[60]

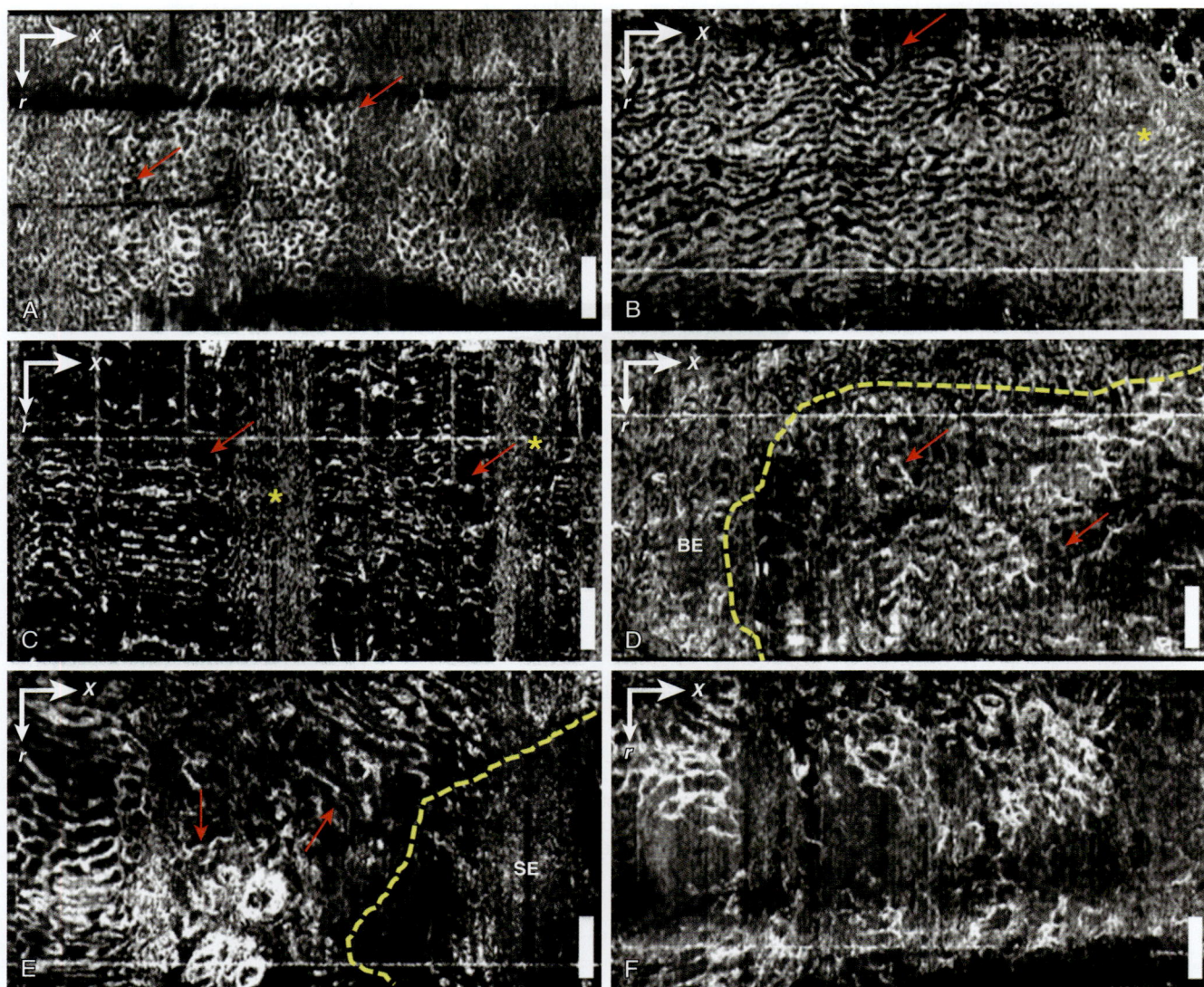

FIGURE 10.13 En face optical coherence tomography angiography. (A–C) Nondysplastic Barrett esophagus: Regular honeycomb microvascular pattern *(arrows)*, may be compressed or streaked in the longitudinal direction due to motion artifact *(stars)*. (D–E) High-grade dysplasia. The *dashed line* delineates the boundary between abnormal microvasculature and neighboring nondysplastic regions. (F) Low-grade dysplasia: Abnormal vessel branching with crowding, a corkscrew appearance, and heterogeneous vessel size *(arrows)*. (From Lee HC, Ahsen OO, Liang K, et al. Endoscopic optical coherence tomography angiography microvascular features associated with dysplasia in Barrett's esophagus. *Gastrointest Endosc.* 2017;pii:S0016-5107[17]30078-0.)

REFERENCES

1. Inoue H, Kaga M, Ikeda H, et al. Magnification endoscopy in esophageal squamous cell carcinoma: a review of the intrapapillary capillary loop classification. *Ann Gastroenterol.* 2015;28(1):41-48.
2. Chedgy FJ, Subramaniam S, Kandiah K, Thayalasekaran S, Bhandari P. Acetic acid chromoendoscopy: improving neoplasia detection in Barrett's esophagus. *World J Gastroenterol.* 2016;22(25):5753-5760.
3. Trivedi PJ, Braden B. Indications, stains and techniques in chromoendoscopy. *QJM.* 2013;106(2):117-131.
4. Coletta M, Sami SS, Nachiappan A, Fraquelli M, Casazza G, Ragunath K. Acetic acid chromoendoscopy for the diagnosis of early neoplasia and specialized intestinal metaplasia in Barrett's esophagus: a meta-analysis. *Gastrointest Endosc.* 2016;83(1):57-67.
5. Canto MI. Acetic-acid chromoendoscopy for Barrett's esophagus: the "pros". *Gastrointest Endosc.* 2006;64(1):13-16.
6. Singh R, Jayanna M, Wong J, et al. Narrow-band imaging and white-light endoscopy with optical magnification in the diagnosis of dysplasia in Barrett's esophagus: results of the Asia-Pacific Barrett's Consortium. *Endosc Int Open.* 2015;3(1):E14-E18.
7. Goda K, Tajiri H, Ikegami M, Urashima M, Nakayoshi T, Kaise M. Usefulness of magnifying endoscopy with narrow band imaging for the detection of specialized intestinal metaplasia in columnar-lined esophagus and Barrett's adenocarcinoma. *Gastrointest Endosc.* 2007;65(1):36-46.
8. Qumseya BJ, Wang H, Badie N, et al. Advanced imaging technologies increase detection of dysplasia and neoplasia in patients with Barrett's esophagus: a meta-analysis and systematic review. *Clin Gastroenterol Hepatol.* 2013;11(12):1562-1570.
9. Tobey NA, Hosseini SS, Argote CM, Dobrucali AM, Awayda MS, Orlando RC. Dilated intercellular spaces and shunt permeability in nonerosive acid-damaged esophageal epithelium. *Am J Gastroenterol.* 2004;99(1):13-22.
10. Farré R, De Vos R, Geboes K, et al. Critical role of stress in increased oesophageal mucosa permeability and dilated intercellular spaces. *Gut.* 2007;56(9):1191-1197.

11. Colegio OR, Van Itallie CM, McCrea HJ, Rahner C, Anderson JM. Claudins create charge-selective channels in the paracellular pathway between epithelial cells. *Am J Physiol Cell Physiol.* 2002;283(1):C142-C147.

12. Orlando LA, Orlando RC. Dilated intercellular spaces as a marker of GERD. *Curr Gastroenterol Rep.* 2009;11(3):190-194.

13. van Malenstein H, Farré R, Sifrim D. Esophageal dilated intercellular spaces (DIS) and nonerosive reflux disease. *Am J Gastroenterol.* 2008;103(4):1021-1028.

14. Farré R, Blondeau K, Clement D, et al. Evaluation of oesophageal mucosa integrity by the intraluminal impedance technique. *Gut.* 2011;60(7):885-892.

15. Kessing BF, Bredenoord AJ, Weijenborg PW, Hemmink GJ, Loots CM, Smout AJ. Esophageal acid exposure decreases intraluminal baseline impedance level. *Am J Gastroenterol.* 2011;106(12):2093-2097.

16. Yuksel ES, Higginbotham T, Slaughter JC, et al. Use of direct, endoscopic-guided measurements of mucosal impedance in diagnosis of gastroesophageal reflux disease. *Clin Gastroenterol Hepatol.* 2012;10(10):1110-1116.

17. Wright MR, Higginbotham T, Slaughter JC, Ates F, Yuksel ES, Vaezi M. Sa1260 mucosal impedance in Barrett's esophagus: can it assess compliance with medication? *Gastroenterology.* 2016;150(Suppl 1, April):S260.

18. Fukahori S, Yagi M, Ishii S, et al. A baseline impedance analysis in neurologically impaired children: a potent parameter for estimating the condition of the esophageal mucosa. *Neurogastroenterol Motil.* 2017;29(6):doi:10.1111/nmo.13012.

19. Lottrup C, Krarup AL, Gregersen H, Ejstrud P, Drewes AM. Patients with Barrett's esophagus are hypersensitive to acid but hyposensitive to other stimuli compared with healthy controls. *Neurogastroenterol Motil.* 2017;29(4):doi:10.1111/nmo.12992.

20. Weijenborg PW, Smout AJ, Bredenoord AJ. Esophageal acid sensitivity and mucosal integrity in patients with functional heartburn. *Neurogastroenterol Motil.* 2016;28(11):1649-1654.

21. Kandulski A, Weigt J, Caro C, Jechorek D, Wex T, Malfertheiner P. Esophageal intraluminal baseline impedance differentiates gastroesophageal reflux disease from functional heartburn. *Clin Gastroenterol Hepatol.* 2015;13(6):1075-1081.

22. Liacouras CA, Furuta GT, Hirano I, et al. Eosinophilic esophagitis: updated consensus recommendations for children and adults. *J Allergy Clin Immunol.* 2011;128(1):3-20.

23. Ravi K, Katzka DA, Smyrk TC, et al. Prevalence of esophageal eosinophils in patients with Barrett's esophagus. *Am J Gastroenterol.* 2011;106(5):851-857.

24. Mueller S, Neureiter D, Aigner T, Stolte M. Comparison of histological parameters for the diagnosis of eosinophilic oesophagitis versus gastro-oesophageal reflux disease on oesophageal biopsy material. *Histopathology.* 2008;53(6):676-684.

25. Katzka DA, Ravi K, Geno DM, et al. Endoscopic mucosal impedance measurements correlate with eosinophilia and dilation of intercellular spaces in patients with eosinophilic esophagitis. *Clin Gastroenterol Hepatol.* 2015;13(7):1242-1248.

26. van Rhijn BD, Verheij J, van den Bergh Weerman MA, et al. Histological response to fluticasone propionate in patients with eosinophilic esophagitis is associated with improved functional esophageal mucosal integrity. *Am J Gastroenterol.* 2015;110(9):1289-1297.

27. van Rhijn BD, Weijenborg PW, Verheij J, et al. Proton pump inhibitors partially restore mucosal integrity in patients with proton pump inhibitor-responsive esophageal eosinophilia but not eosinophilic esophagitis. *Clin Gastroenterol Hepatol.* 2014;12(11):1815-1823.

28. Anandasabapathy S. Advanced imaging in Barrett's esophagus: are we ready to relinquish the random? *Clin Gastroenterol Hepatol.* 2013;11(12):1571-1572.

29. Brand S, Poneros JM, Bouma BE, Tearney GJ, Compton CC, Nishioka NS. Optical coherence tomography in the gastrointestinal tract. *Endoscopy.* 2000;32(10):796-803.

30. Sivak MV Jr, Kobayashi K, Izatt JA, et al. High-resolution endoscopic imaging of the GI tract using optical coherence tomography. *Gastrointest Endosc.* 2000;51(4 Pt 1):474-479.

31. Sharma P, Dent J, Armstrong D, et al. The development and validation of an endoscopic grading system for Barrett's esophagus: the Prague C NM criteria. *Gastroenterology.* 2006;131(5):1392-1399.

32. Suter MJ, Gora MJ, Lauwers GY, et al. Esophageal-guided biopsy with volumetric laser endomicroscopy and laser cautery marking: a pilot clinical study. *Gastrointest Endosc.* 2014;79(6):886-896.

33. Swager A, de Groof AJ, Meijer SL, Weusten BL, Curvers WL, Bergman JJ. Feasibility of laser marking in Barrett's esophagus with volumetric laser endomicroscopy: first-in-man pilot study. *Gastrointest Endosc.* 2017;pii: S0016-5107(17)30074-3.

34. Leggett CL, Gorospe E, Owens VL, Anderson M, Lutzke L, Wang KK. Volumetric laser endomicroscopy detects subsquamous Barrett's adenocarcinoma. *Am J Gastroenterol.* 2014;109(2):298-299.

35. Swager AF, Tearney GJ, Leggett CL, et al. Identification of volumetric laser endomicroscopy features predictive for early neoplasia in Barrett's esophagus using high-quality histological correlation. *Gastrointest Endosc.* 2016;pii: S0016-5107(16)30581-8.

36. Sauk J, Coron E, Kava L, et al. Interobserver agreement for the detection of Barrett's esophagus with optical frequency domain imaging. *Dig Dis Sci.* 2013;58(8):2261-2265.

37. Evans JA, Bouma BE, Bressner J, et al. Identifying intestinal metaplasia at the squamocolumnar junction using optical coherence tomography. *Gastrointest Endosc.* 2007;65(1):50-56.

38. Leggett CL, Gorospe EC, Chan DK, et al. Comparative diagnostic performance of volumetric laser endomicroscopy and confocal laser endomicroscopy in the detection of dysplasia associated with Barrett's esophagus. *Gastrointest Endosc.* 2016;83(5):880-888.

39. Swager A, van der Sommen F, Klomp SR, et al. Computer-aided detection of early Barrett's neoplasia using volumetric laser endomicroscopy. *Gastrointest Endosc.* 2017;pii:S0016-5107(17)30191-8.

40. Deleted in review.

41. Deleted in review.

42. Gray NA, Odze RD, Spechler SJ. Buried metaplasia after endoscopic ablation of Barrett's esophagus: a systematic review. *Am J Gastroenterol.* 2011;106(11):1899-1908.

43. Titi M, Overhiser A, Ulusarac O, et al. Development of subsquamous high-grade dysplasia and adenocarcinoma after successful radiofrequency ablation of Barrett's esophagus. *Gastroenterology.* 2012;143(3):564-566.e1.

44. Deleted in review.

45. Trindade AJ, Inamdar S, Smith MS, et al. Volumetric laser endomicroscopy in Barrett's esophagus: interobserver agreement for interpretation of Barrett's esophagus and associated neoplasia among high-frequency users. *Gastrointest Endosc.* 2016;pii:S0016-5107(16)30807-0.

46. Desai AP, Tyberg A, Kedia P, et al. Optical coherence tomography (OCT) prior to peroral endoscopic myotomy (POEM) reduces procedural time and bleeding: a multicenter international collaborative study. *Surg Endosc.* 2016;30(11):5126-5133.

47. Parra V, Kedia P, Minami H, Sharaiha RZ, Kahaleh M. Endoscopic optical coherence tomography as a tool to evaluate successful myotomy after a peroral endoscopic myotomy. *Gastrointest Endosc.* 2015;81(5):1251.

48. De Palma GD. Confocal laser endomicroscopy in the "in vivo" histological diagnosis of the gastrointestinal tract. *World J Gastroenterol.* 2009;15(46):5770-5775.

49. Wallace M, Lauwers GY, Chen Y, et al. Miami classification for probe-based confocal laser endomicroscopy. *Endoscopy.* 2011;43(10): 882-891.

50. Kiesslich R, Gossner L, Goetz M, et al. In vivo histology of Barrett's esophagus and associated neoplasia by confocal laser endomicroscopy. *Clin Gastroenterol Hepatol.* 2006;4(8):979-987.

51. Dunbar KB, Okolo P 3rd, Montgomery E, Canto MI. Confocal laser endomicroscopy in Barrett's esophagus and endoscopically inapparent Barrett's neoplasia: a prospective, randomized, double-blind, controlled, crossover trial. *Gastrointest Endosc.* 2009;70(4):645-654.

52. Pohl H, Rösch T, Vieth M, et al. Miniprobe confocal laser microscopy for the detection of invisible neoplasia in patients with Barrett's oesophagus. *Gut.* 2008;57(12):1648-1653.

53. Bajbouj M, Vieth M, Rösch T, et al. Probe-based confocal laser endomicroscopy compared with standard four-quadrant biopsy for evaluation of neoplasia in Barrett's esophagus. *Endoscopy.* 2010;42(6):435-440.

54. Sharma P, Meining AR, Coron E, et al. Real-time increased detection of neoplastic tissue in Barrett's esophagus with probe-based confocal laser endomicroscopy: final results of an international multicenter, prospective, randomized, controlled trial. *Gastrointest Endosc.* 2011;74(3):465-472.

55. Gupta A, Attar BM, Koduru P, Murali AR, Go BT, Agarwal R. Utility of confocal laser endomicroscopy in identifying high-grade dysplasia and adenocarcinoma in Barrett's esophagus: a systematic review and meta-analysis. *Eur J Gastroenterol Hepatol.* 2014;26(4):369-377.

56. Liang K, Ahsen OO, Lee HC, et al. Volumetric mapping of Barrett's esophagus and dysplasia with en face optical coherence tomography tethered capsule. *Am J Gastroenterol.* 2016;111(11):1664-1666.

57. Shim MG, Song LM, Marcon NE, Wilson BC. In vivo near-infrared Raman spectroscopy: demonstration of feasibility during clinical gastrointestinal endoscopy. *Photochem Photobiol.* 2000;72(1):146-150.

58. Almond LM, Hutchings J, Lloyd G, et al. Endoscopic Raman spectroscopy enables objective diagnosis of dysplasia in Barrett's esophagus. *Gastrointest Endosc.* 2014;79(1):37-45.

59. Bergholt MS, Zheng W, Ho KY, et al. Fiberoptic confocal Raman spectroscopy for real-time in vivo diagnosis of dysplasia in Barrett's esophagus. *Gastroenterology.* 2014;146(1):27-32.

60. Tsai TH, Ahsen OO, Lee HC, et al. Endoscopic optical coherence angiography enables 3-dimensional visualization of subsurface microvasculature. *Gastroenterology.* 2014;147(6):1219-1221.

PART THREE

Esophageal Motility Disorders and Diverticula

Cricopharyngeal Dysfunction and Zenker Diverticulum

Giovanni Zaninotto | Mario Costantini

Disorders at the cricopharyngeal level lead to *oro-pharyngeal dysphagia*, or *transfer dysphagia*. With this term, we usually refer to the difficulty in making the food progress from the oropharynx to the esophagus, through the upper esophageal sphincter (UES), mostly but not exclusively constituted by the cricopharyngeal muscle. With this term, we differentiate it from esophageal dysphagia, which we define as difficulty in the progression of the bolus from the esophagus to the stomach after the bolus itself has been correctly transferred from the oropharynx to the esophagus.

Dysphagia has been recognized by the World Health Organization (WHO) as a medical disability associated with increased morbidity, mortality, and cost of care.[1] The real incidence is poorly understood, but it is continuously increasing, probably related to the longer overall survival of the general population, the development of degenerative and neurologic disease, treatment of other conditions and, probably, from a better understanding and assessment of this symptom. In the nonhospitalized elderly population, the prevalence of oropharyngeal dysphagia is 11% to 16%, whereas it may rise to 55% in hospitalized patients or nursing home residents.[2] Dysphagia is reportedly present in greater than 70% of patients after a stroke and remains severe in 15% of patients with early swallowing problems.[3] Moreover, dysphagia is now recognized as a symptom of concern in conditions such as acquired brain injury and cervical spine surgery. The treatment of head and neck cancer with chemoradiation or surgery has more pronounced adverse effects on swallowing function than on other functions such as breathing. Dysphagia may complicate an inflammatory myopathy in about half the cases and may represent the presenting symptom in different neuromuscular diseases, for example, inclusion body myositis. Finally, dysphagia is present in up to 57% of patients with established dementia.[5] The various causes of oropharyngeal dysphagia are listed in Box 11.1.

ASSESSMENT OF OROPHARYNGEAL DYSPHAGIA

CLINICAL EVALUATION

Symptom assessment of a patient with dysphagia is essential for a correct diagnosis. In the case of oropharyngeal dysphagia, the patient clearly describes his/her difficulty in transferring food from the mouth to the pharynx and the esophagus and to initiate the involuntary (esophageal) phase of swallowing. The patient is usually very accurate in describing the accumulation of food in the mouth, an inability to control the bolus in the oral cavity, the aspiration of food before, during, or after the swallowing act, and the location where the bolus has gotten stuck. Often patients with esophageal dysphagia also locate the level of food arrest at the cervical region, making the perceived location of food arrest inaccurate for determining the etiology of the process. Associated symptoms of oropharyngeal dysphagia include nasal regurgitation and cough related to the inadequacy of protective mechanisms, and dysarthria or nasal speech related to weakness of the palate. A gurgle sound may suggest a Zenker diverticulum (ZD; see later). Other symptoms, when present, may be useful for the final diagnosis, such as a speech disorder or other signs of impairment of cranial nerves. Often dysphagia is only part of the symptom complex of the patient, and the diagnosis of a neuromuscular disorder is well evident; however, sometimes dysphagia is the first symptom that causes the patient to be seen by a doctor, and only the subsequent physical and neurologic examination may reveal the underlying disease. Finally, weight loss may be the only sign of a swallowing disorder, since patients may avoid eating because of the difficulties they experience.

ENDOSCOPIC EVALUATION

Since dysphagia is an ominous sign, endoscopy is mandatory to rule out any anatomic abnormality or organic

BOX 11.1 Oropharyngeal Dysphagia: Causes and Classification

Anatomic
- Inflammation (abscesses, pharyngitis)
- Neoplasms
- Webs (Plummer-Vinson or Patterson-Kelly syndrome)
- Extrinsic causes (head and neck surgery and radiation, thyroid masses, lymphoadenopathy, other)

Neurologic
1. Central nervous system
   - Cerebrovascular accidents (Pseudobulbar palsy)
   - Amyotrophic lateral sclerosis
   - Parkinson disease
   - Multiple sclerosis
   - Wilson disease
   - Neoplasms
2. Peripheral nervous system
   - Bulbar poliomyelitis
   - Peripheral neuropathies (tetanus, botulism, alcoholic and diabetic neuropathy)
   - Iatrogenic
   - Neoplasms
3. Neuromuscular junction
   - Myasthenia gravis

Muscular
- Polymyositis and dermatomyositis
- Oculopharyngeal dystrophy
- Myotonic dystrophy (Steinert syndrome)
- Metabolic myopathies (myxedema, thyrotoxicosis)

Psychogenic

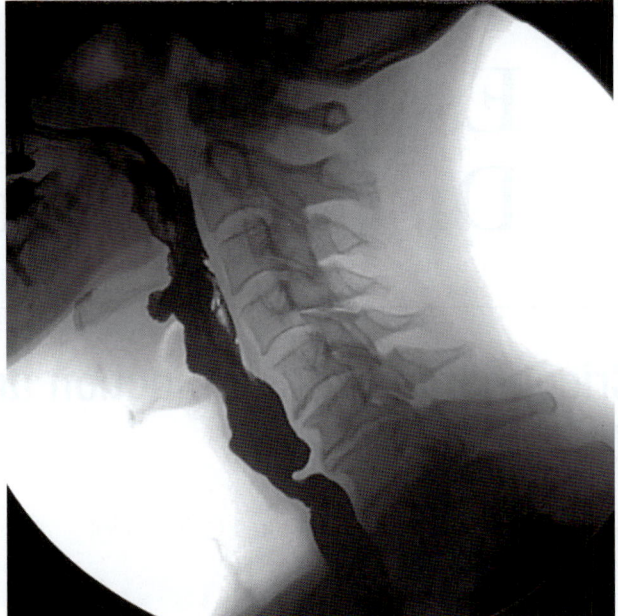

FIGURE 11.1 Radiologic appearance of a cricopharyngeal bar. This is to be considered the radiologic counterpart of a restricted sphincter opening and increased resistance to bolus flow across the sphincter, despite normal upper esophageal sphincter resting tone and "normal" manometric upper esophageal sphincter relaxation.

disease, especially cancer. It must be performed with the maximum care, avoiding undue efforts to penetrate the cervical esophagus if resistance or abnormalities are encountered, since iatrogenic perforation may occur, especially if a ZD is present. Careful examination of the entire esophageal body and cardia must be performed to rule out other gastroesophageal diseases, namely reflux, that may affect the swallowing capabilities of the patient. Rarely, rigid endoscopy under general anesthesia may be required. Laryngoscopy usually completes the endoscopic evaluation of the patient with oropharyngeal dysphagia. This can be also part of a functional evaluation of the swallowing act (see subsequent text).

RADIOLOGIC STUDIES

The definitive diagnosis and the exact quantification of the swallowing disorder are possible only through a careful examination. Conventional studies (barium swallow) are usually inadequate because of the rapidity of events during these initial phases of swallowing. They may reveal, however, possible anatomic abnormalities, such as strictures, webs, diverticula, or the so-called cricopharyngeal bar (Fig. 11.1). Videofluoroscopic evaluation of swallowing, with digital high-frequency recording, is the test of choice, since it allows recording of the rapid movements of mouth, pharynx, palate, epiglottis, larynx, and cervical esophagus during the act of swallowing a liquid or solid contrast bolus, typically using varied volume and consistency, and can identify the presence and mechanism of dysfunction. The

patient should be studied in both the anterior-posterior (AP) and lateral positions. Possible swallowing dysfunction can be categorized into four groups: (1) motility disorders, (2) stasis in the pharyngeal recesses, (3) pharyngeal stasis, and (4) incoordination (aspiration or laryngeal penetration).[4] The motility disorders may be represented by a delayed beginning of the swallowing itself; repetitive attempts may be observed with the tongue moving backward for several times before an effective swallow begins. A "lazy," or a completely disorganized, motor activity can be seen, which is often followed by stasis or aspiration. Pharyngeal stasis without a distal organic obstruction is another radiologic sign of a motility pharyngeal disorder. Finally, incoordination with penetration of the bolus into the larynx and aspiration is one of the most common alterations seen in a patient with pharyngoesophageal dysphagia. In a high percentage of patients, these alterations may be variously combined.

Videofluoroscopy has limitations, however, such as the need for radiation, the necessity to move the patient to the radiologic suite, and the mainly qualitative nature of information obtained. Numerical measures such as the timing of opening or closing of the glossopharyngeal junction, laryngeal vestibule, and UES are not routinely collected in clinical practice, presumably because they are considered too time-consuming and cumbersome. Some scoring systems have been proposed, however, and the Penetration-Aspiration Scale is the most used and validated scoring system to assess the presence and severity of aspiration and penetration related to swallowing.[5]

FIBEROPTIC ENDOSCOPIC EVALUATION OF SWALLOWING

The fiberoptic endoscopic evaluation of swallowing (FEES) using a flexible laryngoscope has been also introduced.[6] It allows evaluating pharyngeal and laryngeal structures before, during, and after deglutition, and is generally well-tolerated, easily repeatable, and can be performed at the bedside of the patient. During the test, the endoscope is introduced transnasally and advanced to enable visualization of the mucosal surface and movement of the tongue base, pharynx and larynx, as well as the bolus transit and airway protection. The patient is asked to swallow a variety of foods and liquids with a coloring contrast (blue dye). During the normal swallow, however, a blind period of approximately 0.5 second occurs when the epiglottis tilts backward and the pharynx squeezes, preventing the complete visualization of the actual passage of the bolus. The presence of secretion, residual colorized food in the pharynx, or its penetration or aspiration in the airway provides useful qualitative information on the deglutitive capacity of the patient and allows the calculation of a Penetration-Aspiration Scale, in a similar way as the videofluorography.[7] The main limitation of FEES is that it does not allow a direct evaluation of the swallow physiology but only relies on indirect and subjective interpretation of findings such as residual food and/or penetration.

MANOMETRY

Conventional, water-perfused manometry can evaluate the entire esophagus, in addition to the pharyngoesophageal region to rule out any esophageal motor disorders and to verify the function and competency of both the UES and the lower esophageal sphincter (LES). The evaluation of the pharyngoesophageal tract quantifies the strength and the coordination of the pharyngeal contractions, the completeness of the UES relaxation, and its coordination with the pharyngeal wave. The test can be very useful, provided some aspects are kept in consideration. First, during deglutition there is a 2-cm orad movement of the whole laryngopharyngoesophageal block; therefore if using a single recording point placed in the UES, this may be found to record the events in the cervical esophagus during swallowing. To avoid this problem, a sleeve sensor recording over a 6-cm length has been introduced and used in some important studies,[8] but its use may be cumbersome in the routine practice. Furthermore, the radial asymmetry of the sphincter requires multiple recording sites on different directions, or a circumferential pressure sensing microtransducer. A second and more relevant problem is given by the rapidity of the pressure events. In the normal state, pharyngeal contractions may reach 600 mm Hg with a duration of 0.5 to 1.0 second: perfused systems may therefore underestimate the real amplitude and coordination of these contractions. Modern catheters, based on solid-state microtransducers, allow for a better and more reliable recording of these rapid events.

Because of all these caveats, the real frequency and type of pharyngoesophageal alterations are highly underestimated and unknown. Other manometric parameters have been introduced to better evaluate these patients. Cook et al.[9] focused on the intrabolus pressure that is increased

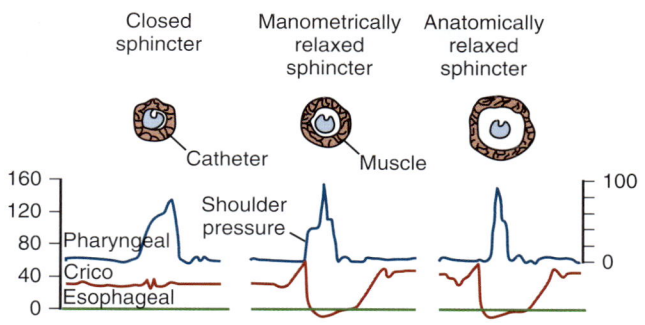

FIGURE 11.2 The intrabolus pressure (or "shoulder" pressure) in the hypopharynx, in a manometrically relaxed but incomplete anatomically relaxed upper esophageal sphincter *(middle)*. This finding indicates increased pharyngeal pressure because of increased resistance to the passage of a bolus through the pharyngoesophageal segment secondary to muscle pathology. (From DeMeester TR, Costantini M. Function tests. In: Patterson GA, Cooper JD, Deslaurier J, Lerut AEMR, Luketich JD, Rice TW, eds. *Pearson's Thoracic & Esophageal Surgery*. 3rd ed. Philadelphia: Churchill Livingstone; 2008:117–147, Fig. 9.13.)

in patients with pharyngoesophageal dysfunction and in those with a ZD, as a counterpart of a reduced compliance of the pharyngoesophageal segment and the UES that, in combined manometric and radiologic studies, may be shown to be manometrically but not anatomically relaxed (Fig. 11.2).[10]

The advent of the *high-resolution manometry* (HRM) in the past decade has greatly enhanced the possibility of further investigating the muscular function of the pharynx and UES during swallowing.[11] HRM measures contractile activity using a transnasal catheter with closely spaced pressure sensors along the entire length of pharynx, the UES segment, and the esophagus as well. HRM has improved the use of manometry in performing pharyngoesophageal function studies, but further work on its clinical implementation is needed. The possibility of combining this technique with videofluoroscopy has allowed for a more complete understanding of bolus transport because of the pharyngoesophageal motor patterns (Fig. 11.3).[3]

FUNCTIONAL LUMEN IMAGING PROBE

On the basis of impedance planimetry, the functional lumen imaging probe (FLIP) has been developed to test distensibility of a lumen.[12] A balloon is placed at the distal end of a FLIP and distended by filling it with a conductive solution. The FLIP provides multiple estimated diameter or cross-sectional area measures of the lumen and uses these to recreate a dynamic image of sphincter geometry. FLIP was originally designed to evaluate esophagogastric junction compliance in gastroesophageal reflux disease (GERD) and achalasia.[13] The role of FLIP in the evaluation of UES function has been also recently explored (Fig. 11.4). Quantitative UES distensibility data, UES diameter, relaxation time, and intraballoon pressure were measured in healthy adults and in patients after laryngectomy.[14] This new method has the potential to demonstrate in a new way the actual opening of the UES and could complement the information provided by swallow studies.

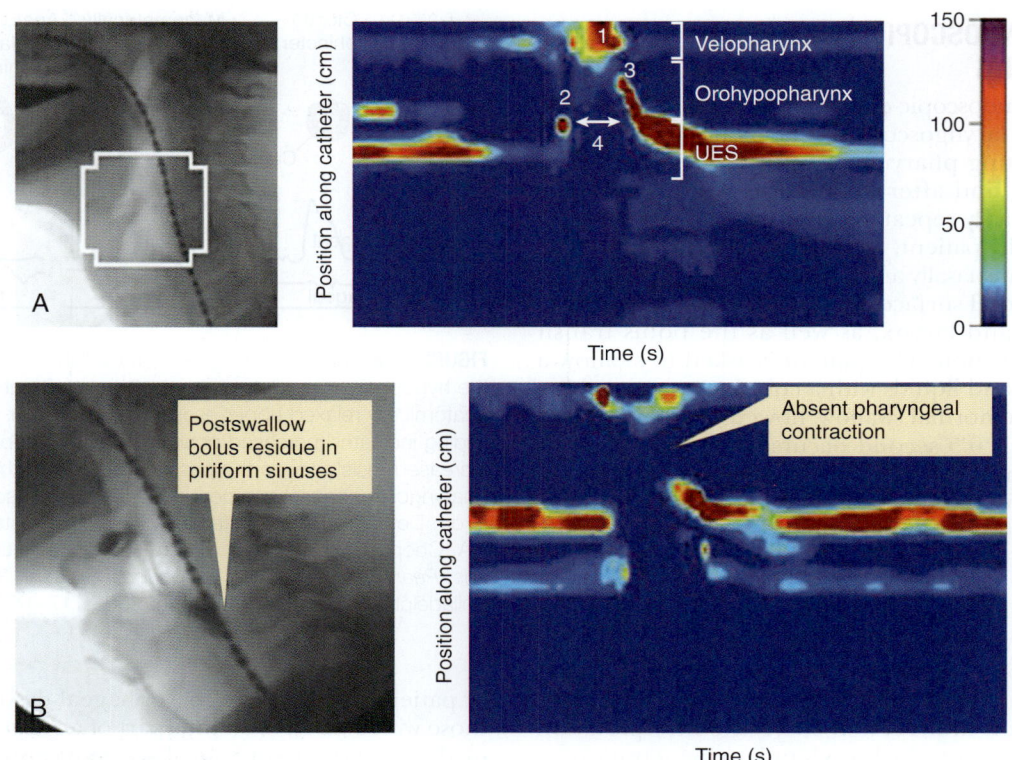

FIGURE 11.3 Lateral videofluoroscopic view and high-resolution manometry color plot of a liquid (10 mL water) swallow. The color panel indicates the corresponding pressure values along the pharyngoesophageal segment. (A) An individual with a normal swallow. During normal deglutition, three manometric regions can be identified along the pharyngoesophageal segment: the soft palate (velopharynx), the tongue base (oropharynx and hypopharynx), and the upper esophageal sphincter (UES) *(left)*. On the high-resolution manometry color plot *(right)*, the velopharyngeal closure *(1)*, elevation of the larynx *(2)*, initiation of the pharyngeal stripping wave *(3)*, and relaxation of the UES *(4)* can be directly visualized. (B) A patient with an oropharyngeal swallowing disorder. Videofluoroscopy shows residue in the piriform sinuses and inadequate opening of the UES. Manometrically, the swallow is characterized by pharyngeal paresis (absent pharyngeal peristalsis) and normal UES relaxation. The observed residue in the hypopharynx could be due to ineffective pharyngeal function or due to inadequate UES relaxation. (From Rommel M, Hamdy S. Oropharyngeal dysphagia: manifestations and diagnosis. *Nat Rev Gastroenterol Hepatol*. 2016;13:49–59, Fig. 2.)

TREATMENT

For patients with oropharyngeal dysphagia and/or cricopharyngeal dysfunction, treatment generally begins with behavioral intervention. The most important is modifications in texture, viscosity, consistency, composition, and bolus size of the prescribed food. Also, the posture and position of the body and head are important factors. The patient therefore must be cognitively alert, oriented, and responsive before food is given, and this unfortunately excludes a significant proportion of patients with neurogenic dysphagia. A variety of maneuvers and techniques are used to ensure feeding safety, including supraglottic swallow, supersupraglottic swallow, the Mendelsohn maneuver (to promote pharyngeal and laryngeal elevation), neck flexion, neck extension, head turning, and tongue-base retraction.[15] Behavioral interventions also include exercise programs to improve the range of motion of the structures involved in swallowing, such as the oral tongue, hyoid and larynx, and strengthening exercises to improve tongue and lip movement. Once therapy is initiated, these compensatory techniques can be varied as progress occurs, but some persons will always require

these strategies and risk-reduction diets to ensure that they minimize the risk of aspiration during a meal.[15,16]

Interventional procedures can be divided into those adapted to promote alimentation, those designed to protect the airway, and those specifically directed at alleviating the swallowing difficulty. Patients who are at high risk for aspiration and cannot meet their nutritional needs through oral feedings will need supplementary (or total) alternative nutrition. If these needs are short term, peripheral intravenous alimentation or nasogastric tube feeding may suffice. Because this is rarely the case and considering the shortcomings of nasogastric tubes for chronic feedings (discomfort, risk of aspiration), alternative methods such as a percutaneous endoscopic gastrostomy (PEG) should be considered. This can be performed with the patient under local anesthesia and minimal sedation with little discomfort.[17] If reflux or aspiration is suspected, a slow infusion rate of the formula or the conversion to a feeding jejunostomy is recommended. A gastrostomy may also be safely performed radiologically, avoiding the need for endoscopy.[18]

In patients unable to adequately clear their secretions from the tracheobronchial tree and aspiration of saliva

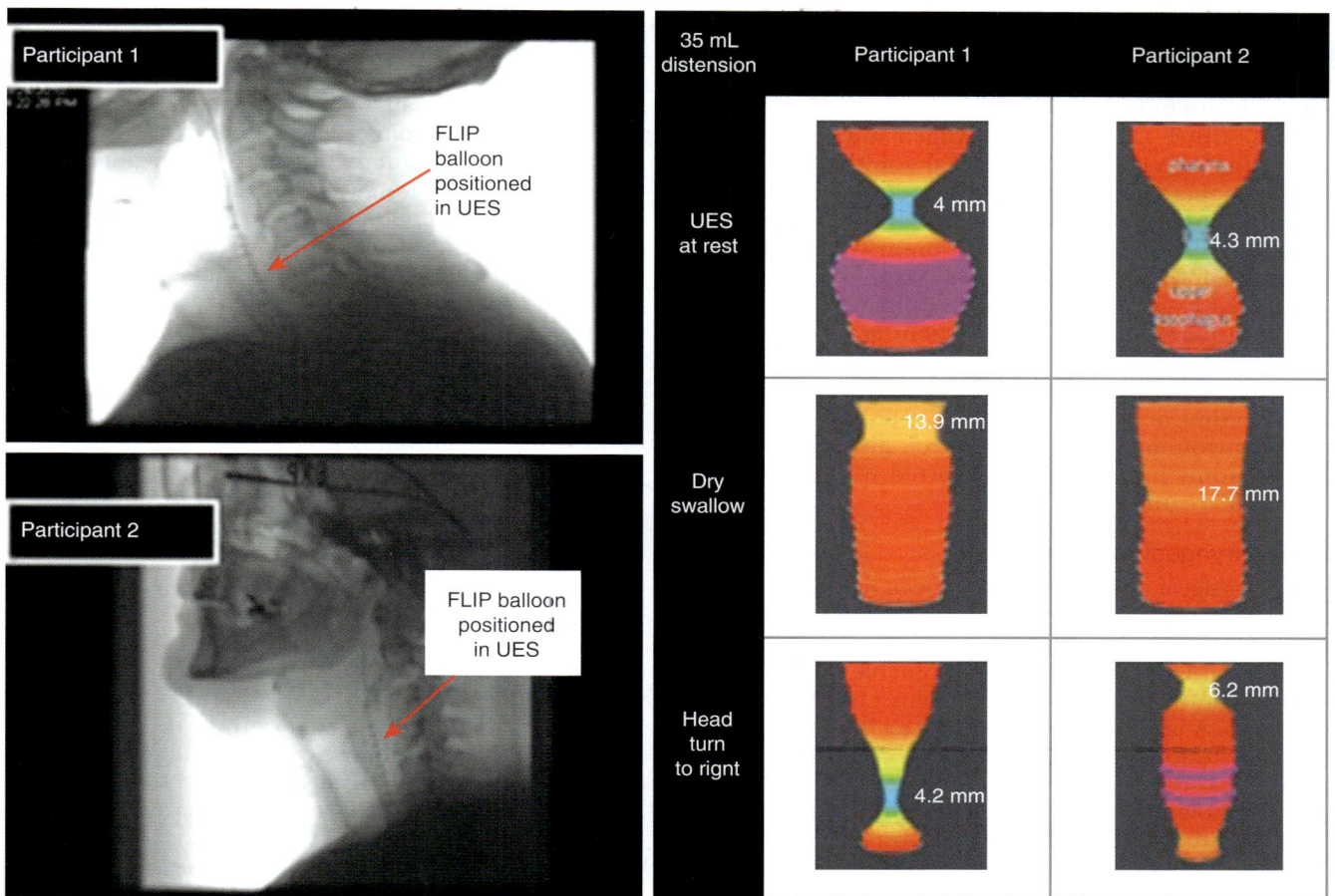

FIGURE 11.4 Still images from fluoroscopic studies of the functional lumen imaging probe (FLIP) in position in the upper esophageal sphincter (UES) of two healthy volunteers *(left)*. The volunteer turns the head in the bottom image. The FLIP can clearly be identified by the electrode arrays. The *right panel* shows FLIP studies on these participants indicating the profiles at rest, with estimated minimum diameters identified; the minimum diameter during dry swallows, clearly indicative of opening; and finally, profiles for both with minimum diameters during right head turns, indicating a shift in either the probe or the narrow region. (From Lottrup C, Reggersene H, Liao D, et al. Functional lumen imaging of the gastrointestinal tract. *J Gastroenterol*. 2015;50:1005–1016, Fig. 4.)

or gastric-refluxed material, a tracheostomy with a cuffed tube is probably one of the most common procedures used in such circumstances. This procedure can be performed with the patient under local anesthesia; it is reversible and allows vocalization to be maintained if the cuff can be deflated at times. Sometimes, however, more radical and irreversible procedures may be used, such as injection of Teflon or other substances to medialize vocal cords, laryngoplasty, subcricoid cricoidectomy, epiglottic sewdown, or the narrow-field laryngectomy.[16]

Interventional procedures specifically aimed to treat dysphagia are directed toward the UES region. The current operative management of UES dysfunction is quite variable, and there are little data to support the relative superiority in outcomes of one intervention over another.[19]

Endoscopic Dilations

Endoscopic dilations (with bougies or balloons) have been sometimes used, especially if an obvious organic or functional cause (e.g., strictures or webs) is detectable. Dilations have the advantages of being simple, relatively safe, and typically performed under conscious sedation.

The short-term outcome is similar to other more invasive procedures (e.g., cricopharyngeal myotomy) but requires repetition in about 50% of cases, and further treatment with surgical myotomy is eventually indicated in a consistent percentage of patients.[19,20]

Injection of Botulinum Toxin

Injection of botulinum toxin (BoT) in the cricopharyngeal muscle (transcutaneously with electromyography [EMG] guidance or endoscopically) has gained some popularity after its introduction in 1994.[21] BoT inhibits the tonic contraction of muscles by inhibiting the release of acetylcholine across the neuromuscular junction; therefore it will primarily benefit patients with hypertonicity of the UES and a retained ability to complete pharyngeal bolus formation. Furthermore, it has distinct appeal in patients who are not ideal candidates for surgery. A recent review has been performed.[22] Only two of the analyzed studies, however, reported on more than 20 patients, with the majority of articles being either case reports or limited series of less than 10 patients. The causes of CD in these published series encompassed numerous diagnoses, including neurologic diseases, multiple sclerosis, diabetic neuropathy, radiation treatment, and cerebrovascular accidents. The dosages and administration techniques of BoT were also quite variable. The techniques for administration of BoT to the cricopharyngeal muscle included endoscopic injection under general anesthesia or mask ventilation, percutaneous injection with or without EMG guidance, and injection via flexible endoscopy. In general, the majority of patients reported improved swallowing function: approximately 75% in the combined analysis. Complications were infrequent and included transient vocal fold paresis, temporary worsening of dysphagia, neck cellulitis, and aspiration pneumonia. There were no reported deaths directly related to the procedure. BoT injection may also be used as a test to determine whether myotomy would be effective, although success with myotomy has also been reported in patients who failed BoT treatment.[23]

Cricopharyngeal Myotomy

Cricopharyngeal myotomy has long been used for treating patients with cricopharyngeal dysfunction of neurologic or myogenic origin, with the aim to remove the obstructive effect of the UES below a pharynx unable to initiate an effective contraction to push the bolus into the cervical esophagus. A brief description of the technique adopted in our institution follows.[24] Under general anesthesia, the patient is positioned supine on the operating table with a small pillow under the shoulders and with the head hyperextended and slightly turned on the right side. An incision is performed along the anterior border of the left sternocleidomastoid muscle (Fig. 11.5A). After dividing the subcutaneous tissue and the platysma, the pharynx and esophagus are exposed by retracting the sternocleidomastoid muscle and vessels (carotid artery and jugular vein) laterally and the laryngothyroid block medially (see Fig. 11.5B). Exposure of the region is facilitated by dividing the omohyoid muscle and the middle thyroid vein (see Fig. 11.5C). Dividing the inferior thyroid artery helps in further exposing and preventing the risk of damaging the recurrent laryngeal nerve. This approach is the same as described later for the cricopharyngeal myotomy associated to the treatment of a ZD. The transverse fibers of the cricopharyngeal muscle are identified and the myotomy is performed from its upper border and the lower pharyngeal wall to the cervical esophagus, over a length of at least 5 cm, using the scalpel and scissors (see Fig. 11.5D). When the myotomy is complete, the mucosa bulges free through the muscle edges (see Fig. 11.5E). A drain is left for 24 hours to avoid hematomas in the neck region, and after a hydrosoluble contrast study, the patient is allowed to start a liquid and soft diet. Complications of the procedure may be the development of hematomas of the cervical region that can jeopardize the airway patency and require immediate surgical revision and perforations of the esophageal mucosa that can be repaired during the operation (a muscle flap from the sternocleidomastoid muscle may be used to buttress the repairing suture) or conservatively treated (with nil per os [NPO; nothing by mouth] and parenteral support) if discovered with the contrast control study. These surgical complications in patients with neurologic or myogenic

dysphagia are rare; other more severe and potentially lethal complications such as aspiration and pneumonia are related to the underlying pathology and the severity of the swallowing impairment.[25] The challenge in this category is to identify which patients will benefit from cricopharyngeal myotomy. Intact voluntary oral-phase of deglutition with good control of the tongue, good control of the laryngeal aditus with normal phonation, and absence of dysarthria are reliable prognostic factors for a successful outcome.[26] Poor coordination in the swallowing mechanism may still result after surgery in persistent silent aspiration and the potential for pulmonary infection. Cumulative analysis of published data (mostly uncontrolled case series) showed an overall favorable response rate of 63% with an average mortality of 1.8%.[15] Other reviews report a success rate of 78%, with a morbidity of 7%.[19] At present, there are no clear and accepted indications for cricopharyngeal myotomy in oropharyngeal dysphagia of neurologic or myogenic origin, and final clinical decisions need to be made on a case-by-case basis.

ZENKER DIVERTICULUM

Pharyngoesophageal diverticula are protrusions of pharyngeal mucosa through a weak zone in the posterior wall of the pharynx that are limited inferiorly by the upper border of the cricopharyngeal muscle and laterally by the oblique fibers of the thyropharyngeal muscle, the so-called Killian triangle. These diverticula are named after the German pathologist, Frederick Albert von Zenker who published a review of 27 patients with this disease.[27] Though not the first to describe this condition, Zenker is credited for realizing that the pathogenesis of the diverticula lay in an increased intrapharyngeal pressure, thus causing a "pulsion" diverticulum.

PHYSIOLOGY AND PATHOPHYSIOLOGY OF ZENKER DIVERTICULUM

After recognition of the central role of the UES in causing the diverticulum, different theories have been suggested during the years. An increased resting pressure of the UES, a lack of complete relaxation (achalasia), or premature or discoordinated UES relaxation with the incoming pharyngeal contraction have all been proposed.[28] The development of modern manometric techniques has shown, however, that the UES resting pressure is similar and even decreased in these patients compared with controls, that the UES appears to properly relax on manometry during deglutition and, finally, that pharyngosphincteral incoordination was an inconsistent finding. The demonstration of the real role of the UES in the pathogenesis of the diverticulum was finally demonstrated in the early 1990s by means of elegant concurrent manometric and videofluorographic studies, and it was confirmed by histologic examinations. Cook et al.[29] using a sleeve catheter for manometry and simultaneous video-radiographic recordings, demonstrated a significantly reduced radiologic sphincter opening despite a manometrically "complete" relaxation due to the loss of contact between the sphincter walls and recording catheter. Furthermore, in these patients, they found a greater "intrabolus" pressure, demonstrating therefore that the pathophysiologic abnormality is indeed a diminished

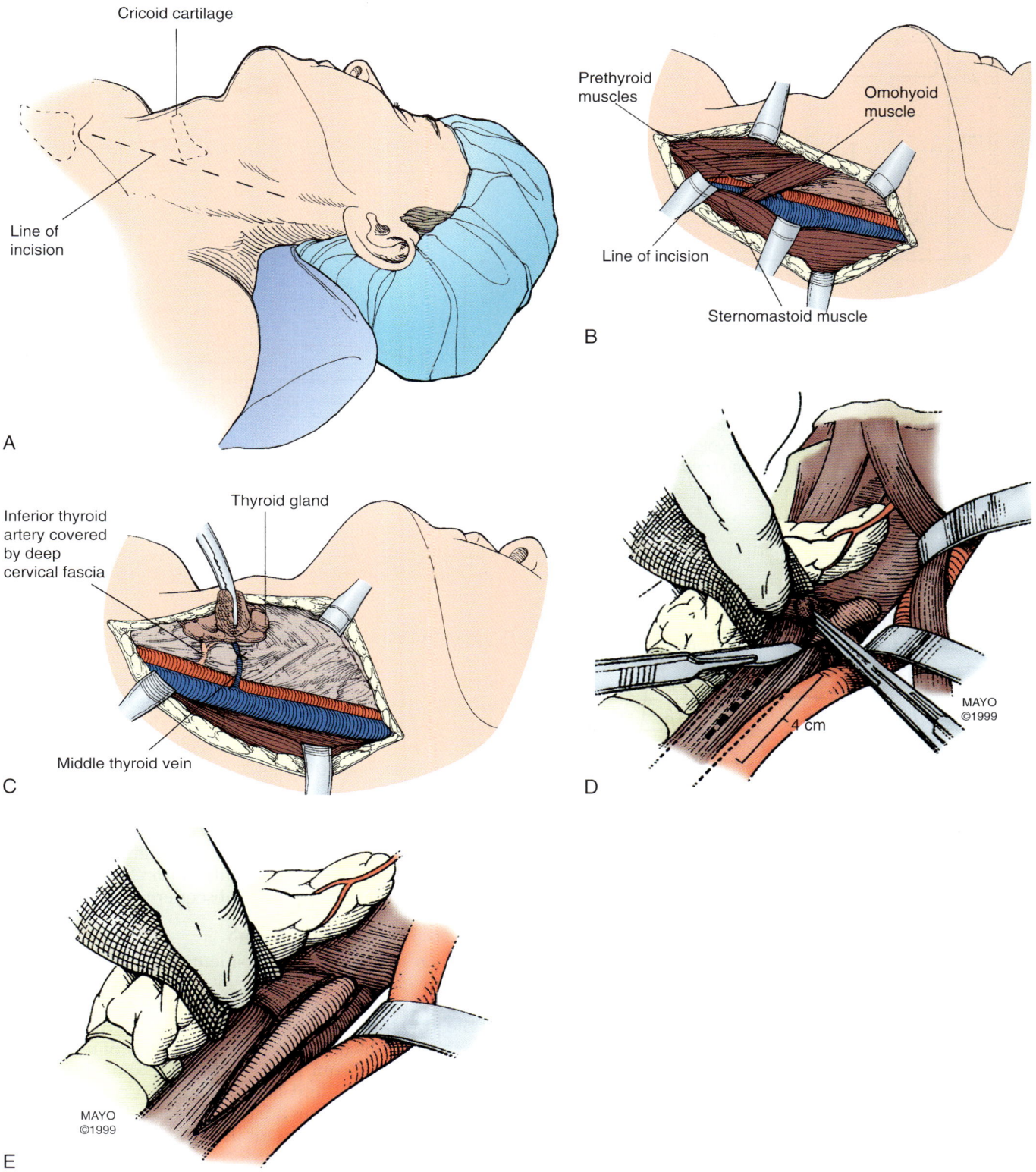

FIGURE 11.5 Surgical technique for the myotomy of the upper esophageal sphincter (cricomyotomy). (A) The patient is positioned supine on the operating table with a small pillow under the shoulders and with the head hyperextended and slightly turned on the right side; the incision is performed along the anterior border of the left sternocleidomastoid muscle. (B) The exposure of the pharyngoesophageal tract is facilitated by dividing the omohyoid muscle. (C) The middle thyroid vein and the inferior thyroid artery are also divided. (D) The transverse fibers of the cricopharyngeal muscle are identified and the myotomy is performed from its upper border and the lower pharyngeal wall to the cervical esophagus over a length of at least 4 cm using the scalpel and scissors. (E) When the myotomy is complete, the mucosa bulges free through the muscle edges. ([D and E] Copyright Mayo Clinic, 1999.)

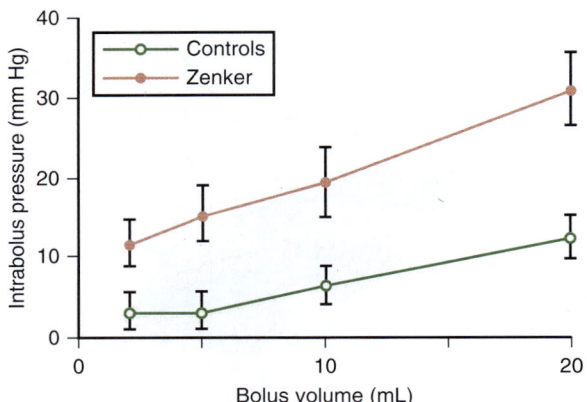

FIGURE 11.6 Relationship of swallow volume to intrabolus pressure in patients who have lost compliance of the cricopharyngeal and cervical esophageal muscle. Higher pressure for increased swallowed volume indicates that patients have sufficient pharyngeal muscle power to create an intrabolus pressure, and improvement of the compliance with a myotomy of the cricopharyngeal and cervical esophageal muscle should result in clinical improvement.

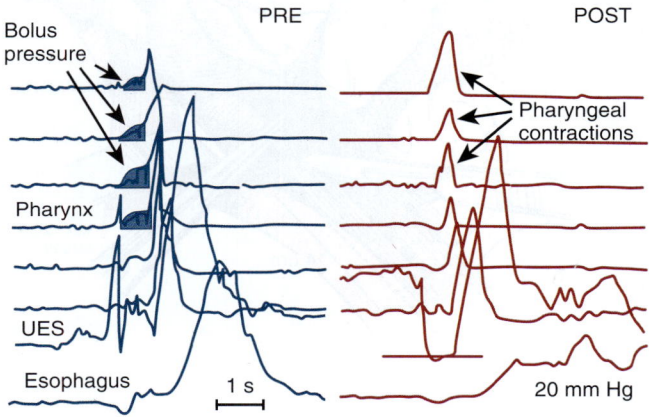

FIGURE 11.7 Pharyngoesophageal manometric tracing in a patient with Zenker diverticulum before and after diverticulectomy and myotomy. A nonrelaxing upper esophageal sphincter and a prominent bolus pressure are evident in the preoperative recording. Myotomy increased the compliance of the pharyngoesophageal segment, with complete disappearance of the "shoulder" of the bolus pressure in the pharyngeal contractions. *UES,* Upper esophageal sphincter.

UES opening with increased intrapharyngeal pressure that probably accounts for the development of the diverticulum (Fig. 11.6). They postulated that degenerative changes cause a lack of elasticity of the sphincter muscle preventing it from relaxing completely, and introduced the concept of reduced compliance of the pharyngoesophageal segment that can be seen manometrically by the appearance of a "shoulder" before the onset of the pharyngeal contraction, representing a higher pressure regimen in the pharynx (Fig. 11.7).

This theory has been subsequently endorsed by several histologic and contractility studies on biopsy specimens

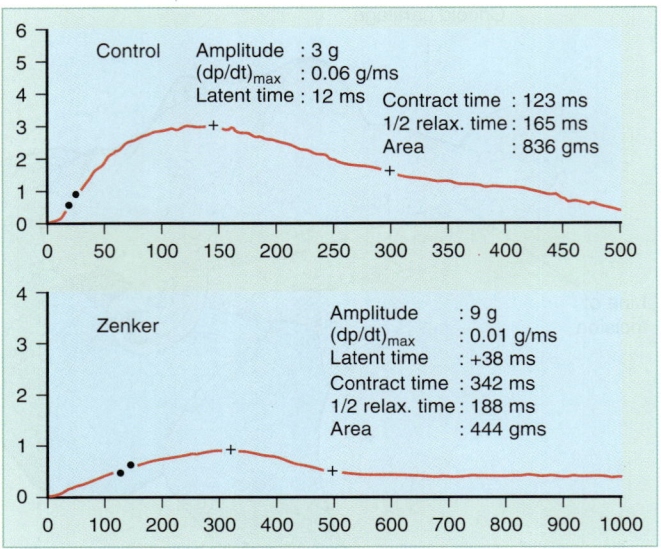

FIGURE 11.8 Contractility pattern of the cricopharyngeal muscle in a control specimen and Zenker diverticulum.

taken from patients with ZD and controls. Lerut et al.[30] showed a slower and weaker contraction curve with a lower amplitude, a longer time to peak twitch, and a much longer half relaxation time in muscle fibers of ZD patients (Fig. 11.8). They also found histologic, electron microscopic, and immunohistochemical alterations, prompting them to suggest the hypothesis that both neurogenic and myogenic abnormalities are the underlying cause for dysfunction of the UES in these patients. Further studies[31,32] confirmed these findings, by showing a significantly higher collagen content, higher isodesmosine/desmosine and collagen/ elastin ratios in the cricopharyngeal muscle and the cervical esophagus muscularis propria in patients compared with controls (Fig. 11.9). These findings also highlighted the role of the proximal muscle fibers of the cervical esophagus in the pathogenesis of the diverticulum, supporting the need to also divide these fibers for 2 to 3 cm when performing a myotomy (see subsequent text).

SYMPTOMS AND DIAGNOSIS

The main symptom in these patients is dysphagia, present in nearly all the cases. One can distinguish this *intrinsic* dysphagia from the extrinsic one, caused by the distention of the pouch by accumulated food that can further compress the esophageal lumen. Regurgitation of undigested food particles (from previous meals), abnormal noise during swallowing, and halitosis are also common. The most frequent symptoms are listed in Table 11.1. Dysphagia may lead to weight loss, and penetration and inhalation of food particles into the airway can cause coughing and recurrent pulmonary infections. This is particularly relevant since the majority of patients are elderly and often frail. Other symptoms related to the upper gastrointestinal tract are often present. In particular, a high frequency of reflux symptoms and esophagitis has been reported, with pH-proven GERD in as high as 44% of patients.[33] GERD has long been postulated as a chronic irritative element in causing damage to the cricopharyngeal muscle that

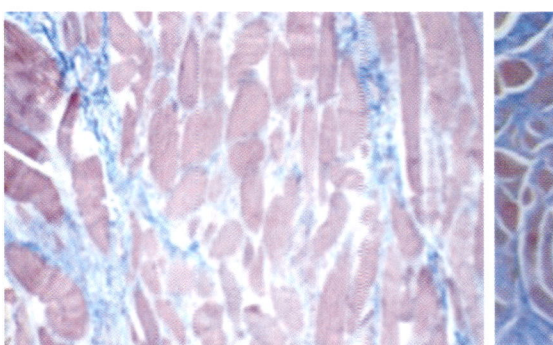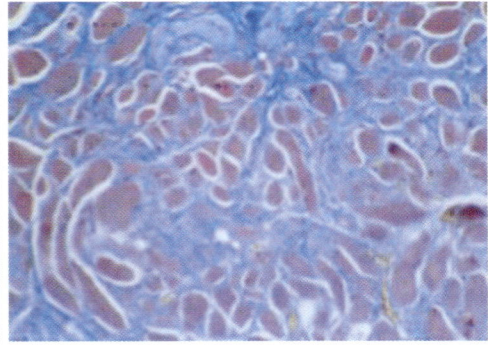

FIGURE 11.9 Histologic examination of a cricopharyngeal muscle specimen of a control subject *(left)* and of a patient with Zenker diverticula *(right)*. A marked decrease in the amount of muscle fibers is well evident in the patient. Therefore the muscle:connective ratio is lower in patients than in controls. (From Zaninotto G, Costantini M, Boccù C, et al. Functional and morphological study of the cricopharyngeal muscle in patients with Zenker's diverticulum. *Br J Surg*. 1996;83:1263–1267.)

TABLE 11.1 Zenker Diverticulum: Clinical Presentation and Symptoms

Mean Age	68 years (38–92)
>70 years	50%
>80 years	20%
SYMPTOMS	
Mean duration	37.4 months
Dysphagia	80%
Regurgitation	58%
Choking	20%
Coughing	18%
Globus sensation	21%
Weight loss	23%
Others	14%
ASSOCIATED PATHOLOGY	
Pulmonary infections	37%
Upper GI tract pathology	60%
Documented GERD	44%
Other comorbidity	52%

GERD, Gastroesophageal reflux disease; *GI*, gastrointestinal.
Modified from Lerut T, Coosemans W, Decaluwé H, et al. Pathophysiology and treatment of Zenker diverticulum. In: Yeo CJ, et al., eds. *Shackelford's Surgery of the Alimentary Tract*. 7th ed. Philadelphia: Saunders; 2013:336–348.

predisposes to the development of a ZD. GERD should be properly investigated in these patients, especially given the theoretic but unproven risk that a subsequent myotomy, by eliminating the barrier between pharynx and esophagus, may favor esophagopharyngeal and laryngeal reflux.

The diagnosis of a Zenker is radiologic in most patients. A barium or Gastrografin swallow will readily show the posteriorly located pouch in the neck. Penetration or aspiration in the airway may be also seen. In the lateral projection, the diverticulum can be adequately measured, especially as far as the distance from the septum to the bottom of the pouch is concerned, since this measure may guide the choice of the treatment (Fig. 11.10).[34] Radiologic evaluation should precede any endoscopic examination in a patient with dysphagia and suspected ZD, given the risk of iatrogenic perforation. Endoscopy may be useful in further evaluating the dimensions of the pouch and its neck and in assessing the morphology of the septum between the esophageal lumen and the diverticulum. It may reveal inflammation of the diverticular mucosa due to stasis, and even a possible, albeit anecdotal, neoplastic degeneration.

In dedicated centers, HRM combined with fluorography is the most useful tool to investigate the complex pharyngoesophageal swallowing events,[3] but dedicated pharyngoesophageal manometry, outside a research program, is not necessary for the routine diagnosis of ZD. However, it may reveal coexisting esophageal motility abnormalities and, combined with pH monitoring, detect any underlying GERD.

THERAPY

The standard surgical treatment for ZD consisted of myotomy of the UES and resection or suspension (pexy) of the pouch, or even myotomy alone for small diverticula.[35] Alternative endoscopic procedures that divided the septum between the diverticulum and the esophageal wall using a cautery or laser[36,37] were also described, but they gained little popularity because of the high risk of severe complications. The situation changed in 1993, when Collard proposed simultaneously dividing and suturing the diverticular and esophageal wall using a laparoscopic stapler introduced through a special endoscope (the Weerda diverticuloscope).[38] This procedure rapidly gained popularity and is now considered in many centers the treatment of choice for ZD. In 1995, Ishioka in Brazil[39] and Mulder in the Netherlands[40] reported their initial results using a flexible endoscope for cutting the diverticular septum. Most recently, per oral endoscopic myotomy techniques, similar to those used at the LES for achalasia, have been applied for the treatment of ZD. A description of therapeutic options for ZD is given as follows.

Cricopharyngeal Myotomy With or Without Diverticulectomy

The initial steps of the operation were described earlier (see Fig. 11.5A–C). After exposing the pharyngoesophageal region, the diverticulum is identified and isolated from the surrounding tissues by blunt dissection, until its neck is clearly identified on the posterior pharyngeal wall. The

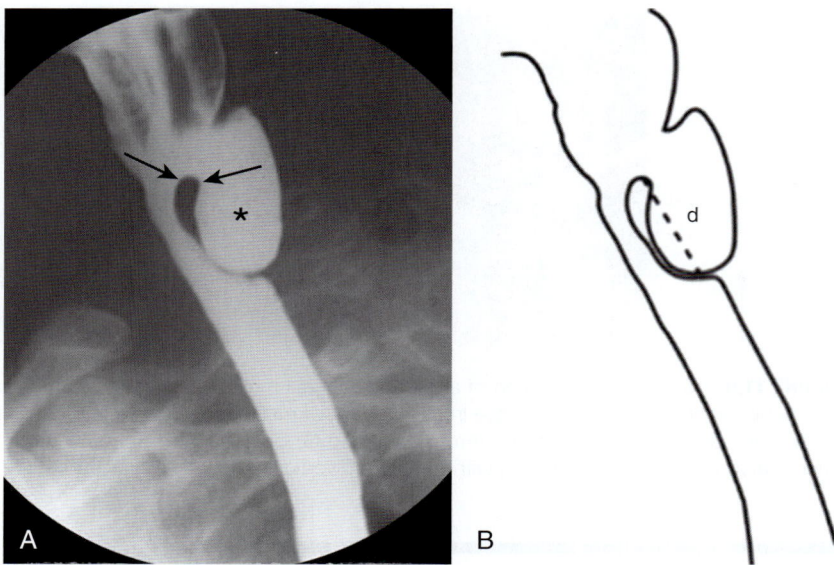

FIGURE 11.10 (A) Steep oblique view on preoperative barium study in a patient with dysphagia shows a 3.2-cm diverticulum *(asterisk)* above prominent cricopharyngeal muscle *(arrows)*. Note the well-distended pouch and esophagus and the profile of the septum. (B) Drawing shows Zenker diverticula depth measurement, defined by the distance *(d)* from the top of the septum to the bottom of the pouch. (From Pomerri F, Costantini M, Dal Bosco C, et al. Comparison of preoperative and surgical measurements of Zenker's diverticulum. *Surg Endosc.* 2012;26:2010–2015.)

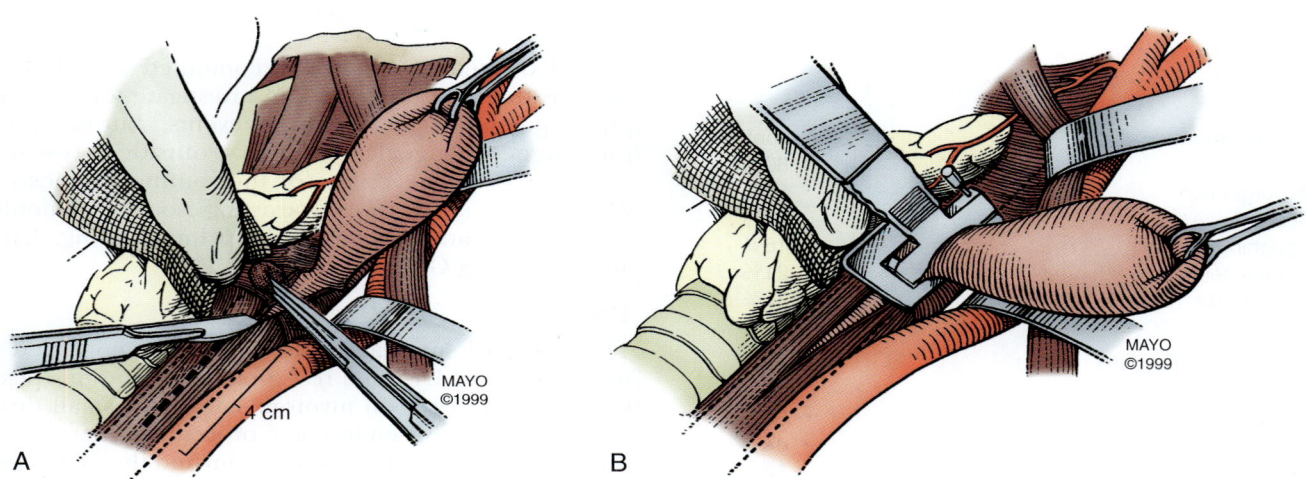

FIGURE 11.11 Treatment of a Zenker diverticulum. (A) After the myotomy is completed, the diverticulum bulges free through the muscle edges. (B) The diverticulum is then transected with a linear stapler if it is 2 cm or more in size. Smaller diverticula (1 cm or less) can be safely left in place, since the simple myotomy is sufficient to relieve patients' symptoms. Diverticula nearing 2 cm in size can be inverted below the pharyngeal muscles and sutured to the muscle layer, thus performing a sort of intramural suspension. (Copyright Mayo Clinic, 1999.)

transverse fibers of the cricopharyngeal muscle are easy to see below the neck of the diverticulum. The myotomy is performed from this level to the cervical esophagus over a length of at least 5 cm, using the scalpel and scissors (Fig. 11.11A). When the myotomy is complete, the mucosa bulges free through the muscle edges. If the diverticulum is 3 cm or more in size, it is transected with a linear stapler (see Fig. 11.11B). Smaller diverticula are best upended and sutured to the prevertebral fascia or the pharyngeal muscles to avoid the potential for leakage from the staple or suture line when resecting the pouch.[33] Very small (<1 cm) pouches can be safely left in place, since the myotomy alone suffices to reduce the pouch and alleviate the symptoms.

Endoscopic Stapling Diverticulostomy

Patients with diverticula larger than 2 cm can be considered for an endoscopic stapled technique. Smaller diverticula lead to an incomplete division of the dysfunctional cricopharyngeal muscle and diverticulum or symptom recurrence. Under general anesthesia with orotracheal intubation, the patient is placed supine on the operating table with a small pillow under the upper torso and the head hyperextended. The surgeon sits behind the patient's head. A Weerda diverticuloscope is inserted in the hypopharynx, positioning its anterior blade in the esophageal lumen and the posterior blade in the diverticulum. A 5-mm diameter telescope is passed through the scope. After visualization of the septum between the

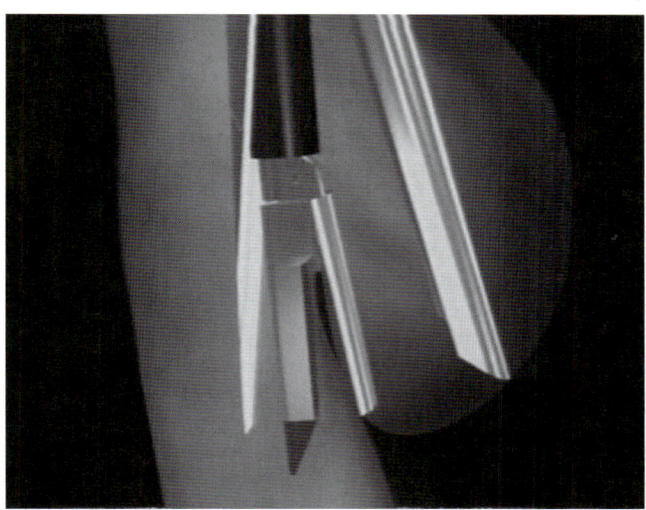

FIGURE 11.12 Schematic representation of the transoral stapling diverticulostomy. The diverticuloscope is inserted through the mouth, positioning its anterior blade in the esophageal lumen and the posterior blade in the diverticulum. With a modified surgical endostapler, the septum between the diverticulum and the esophageal lumen is divided and the diverticuloesophagostomy is performed. (From Costantini M, Zaninotto G, Rizzetto C, Narne S, Ancona E. Esophageal diverticula. *Best Pract Res Clin Gastroenterol.* 2004;18:3–17, Fig. 2.)

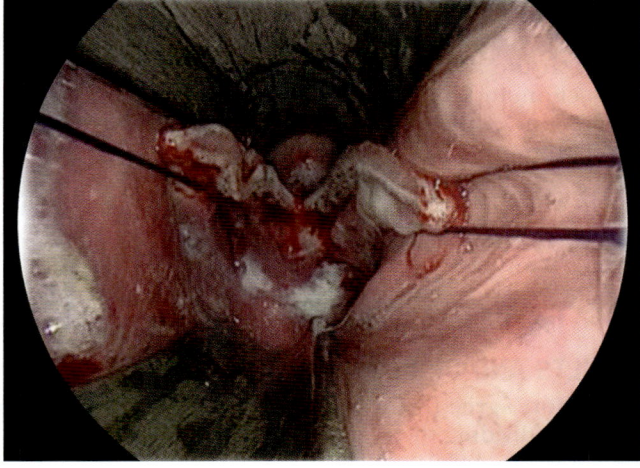

FIGURE 11.13 Endoscopic vision through the Weerda diverticuloscope. Two traction sutures applied on the septum between the diverticulum *(bottom)* and the esophagus *(top)* with a laparoscopic endostitching device can help to engage the septum between the stapler jaws and allow a more complete septal division.

esophagus and the diverticulum, the diverticuloscope is fixed with the help of a chest support. The length of the diverticulum is accurately measured with a graduated rod. A disposable, modified surgical endostapler is then inserted through the Weerda scope to divide the septum between the diverticulum and the esophageal lumen and to perform the diverticuloesophagostomy. The device has been modified by shortening its anvil, thus enabling complete tissue stapling and sectioning down to the very bottom of the diverticulum. The anvil is placed in the lumen of the diverticulum and the cartridge in the esophageal lumen. Stapling sutures the posterior esophageal wall to the anterior wall of the diverticulum over a length of about 30 mm and the tissue coming between three rows of staples on each side is transected (Fig. 11.12). With this technique, a second stapling step is typically required, depending on the actual size of the diverticulum. Two traction sutures applied at the apex of the septum with a laparoscopic endostitching device can help to engage the septum between the stapler jaws and allow a more complete septal division (Fig. 11.13). Electrocoagulation with endosurgical scissors may be used to complete the dissection of the septum at the distal end on the stapled line. The suture lines are then checked for hemostasis, and the scope is removed. The procedure takes about 20 minutes to complete with the major complication being inability to adequately extend the neck and damage to the teeth, tongue, jaw, or pharynx during attempts at insertion of the diverticuloscope.[38,41]

The harmonic scalpel (Ultracision, Ethicon) operating through the diverticuloscope has been used to divide the septum as an alternative to stapling.[42,43] This device can simultaneously cut and coagulate tissue with minimal thermal spreading and optimal hemostasis, and its small caliber allows for easy maneuverability through the scope. Also, the CO_2 laser, first introduced in 1981 by van Overbeek,[44] may represent another alternative to stapling. This is a very precise technique, but widespread adoption has been limited, since it is strictly operator-dependent and carries an intrinsic risk for perforation and mediastinitis.

Fiberoptic Endoscopic Treatment

A flexible endoscope avoids the issues with inability to place the diverticuloscope and several endoscopic techniques have been used to divide the septum between the esophageal lumen and the diverticulum. These can be valuable in elderly patients at high risk for general anesthesia or with contraindications for the previously described techniques (e.g., the inability to open their mouth wide, or diverticula <2 cm in size). Patients are under conscious sedation with propofol or intubated with general anesthesia. The procedure is usually performed in the endoscopy unit. It is generally possible to obtain a good view of the septum. In addition, a nasogastric tube is useful to optimize the exposure, and it helps to protect the anterior esophageal wall. A variety of different endoscopic accessories (capo, hood, overtube) can be used to improve the septum exposure and protect the esophagus and the pouch from thermal injury. The new soft diverticuloscope (Zenker overtube, Cook Endoscopy) is a transparent soft-rubber overtube that has two distal flaps that protect the esophagus anteriorly and the diverticulum posteriorly. The overtube is passed over the endoscope and advanced under direct vision to properly display the septum to be cut.[45] The incision is made starting from the rim between the esophageal orifice and the opening of the diverticulum. Different cutting devices can be used (e.g., needle-knife, monopolar forceps, hook-knife, argon plasma coagulator).[46] A clip-assisted technique has been introduced by some authors to reduce the risk of perforation and mediastinitis.[47] With this technique (clip and cut), prior to dissection, two endoclips are placed on either side of the septum. A metal endoclip may also be placed at the apex of the incision to prevent tearing of the section and microperforation.[45]

The aim of the procedure is to completely obliterate the septum, thus achieving a wide opening between the diverticulum and the esophagus (diverticulostomy). Only one session is usually needed for small diverticula (≤2 cm), whereas repeated sessions may become necessary if they are larger. At any one session, a 1.5- to 2.0-cm incision is performed, and it is repeated in 1-weeks' time. A nasogastric tube is usually placed for nutritional purposes for 2 days.

RESULTS AND DISCUSSION

All authors agree that a fundamental step in therapy for ZD lies in dividing the cricopharyngeus muscle fibers (i.e., the UES). As obvious as it may seem today, this notion is a recent acquisition that is based empirically on the finding of much lower complication (i.e., leakage) and recurrence rates when myotomy is added to the diverticulectomy.[35] As said, definitive support for this belief came from studies[29] which demonstrated that the muscle pathology of the UES with inflammation and fibrosis restricts the opening of the UES, leading to a higher pressure of the bolus arriving in the hypopharynx and ultimately to the formation of a pulsion diverticulum. Surgical cricopharyngeal myotomy, alone in the case of small (<2 cm) diverticula, or combined with either diverticulectomy or diverticulum suspension (diverticulopexy) ensures symptom relief in nearly all treated patients (Table 11.2; Fig. 11.14). The related morbidity may involve some local hematomas and recurrent nerve palsy in addition to leakages, which occur in about 2% of cases.[35] It should be emphasized, however, that the mortality rate of this procedure in frail, elderly patients, is far from negligible, mostly due to cardiopulmonary complications.

The risks of complications and even death cannot be completely overcome even with endoscopic techniques, but they are likely lower than with open surgery. Thus far, there have been no prospective trials comparing the different endoscopic treatment options with surgery. Information comes from retrospective series or prospectively recorded case series, using one or more of these techniques. Moreover, given the rarity of the disease and its prevalence in elderly patients, often with severe comorbidities, it is unlike that randomized studies can be performed in the near future.

We reviewed our experience a few years ago, reporting on 51 patients treated with endoscopic stapling diverticulostomy, and 77 patients were treated with surgical myotomy.[41] After the operation, there was a statistically significant improvement in the symptom score in both groups. In the endoscopic group, however, 11 patients (21.5%) still complained of severe dysphagia and were considered as procedure failures, requiring further endoscopic treatment (8 cases) or surgical myotomy (3 cases). On the other hand, only 4 patients (5.2%) of the surgical group had recurrent dysphagia ($P < .05$), successfully treated with pneumatic dilation in 3 (1 patient refused further treatment). A posterior pouch was still evident (Fig. 11.15) in all patients treated endoscopically and studied with postoperative barium swallow; however, most of the patients were asymptomatic. By further dividing the two groups of patients following the size of the diverticulum (≤3 cm and >3 cm), we found that 64% and 92% of asymptomatic patients were in the endoscopic group compared with 94.5% and 96%, respectively, in the surgical group. Therefore patients with a greater than 3-cm diverticulum may have the same probability of a good outcome with the endostapling procedure as the patients undergoing open surgery. Patients with smaller diverticula (≤3 cm) should be offered the open surgical approach or a flexible endoscopic approach whereby the entire cricopharyngeal muscle is divided using peroral myotomy techniques that continue the myotomy distal to the extent of the diverticulum.

Similar results are reported by the Brussels group,[48] which first proposed endoscopic stapling for ZD (Table 11.3). They retrospectively compared their experience

TABLE 11.2 Outcome of Open Surgical Treatment for Zenker Diverticulum

Author, Year	Time Period	Method	N	Complications (%)	Mortality (%)	RESULTS (%) Good	RESULTS (%) Partial	Recurrence (%)
Payne, 1992	1944–78	D, DM, M	888	7.9	2	82	11	3.6
		D	184	21	1.5	94		4.9
		DM	121	10				4.9
GEEMO, 1995 (n = 390)	1960–82	PM	55	12.7				1.8
		M	26	0				NA
		P	4	0				7.6
Bonafede, 1997	1976–93	M, DM, PM	87	24	3.5	78	13	NA
Zbaren, 1999	1987–97	D, DM	66	15	1.5	77	11	6
Feussner, 1999	1982–98	PM, DM	140	4.2	1	>90		0.8
Leporrier, 2001	1988–98	DM, PM	40	17.5	0	92	8	0
Jougon, 2003	1987–2000	DM	73	4	0	99	1	0
Colombo, 2003	1985–95	D, DM	79	15	0	76	19	2.5
Lerut, 2008	1975–2003	PM, M, DM	289	8.5	0	94.2	3.8	0.03
Total			2119	10.5	1.4			3.5

D, Diverticulectomy; *GEEMO*, Group Européen d'Etude des Maladies de l'Oesophage; *M*, myotomy; *NA*, not announced; *P*, diverticulopexy.
Modified from Lerut T, Coosemans W, Decaluwé H, et al. Pathophysiology and treatment of Zenker diverticulum. In: Yeo CJ, et al., eds. *Shackelford's Surgery of the Alimentary Tract*. 7th ed. Philadelphia: Saunders; 2013:336–348.

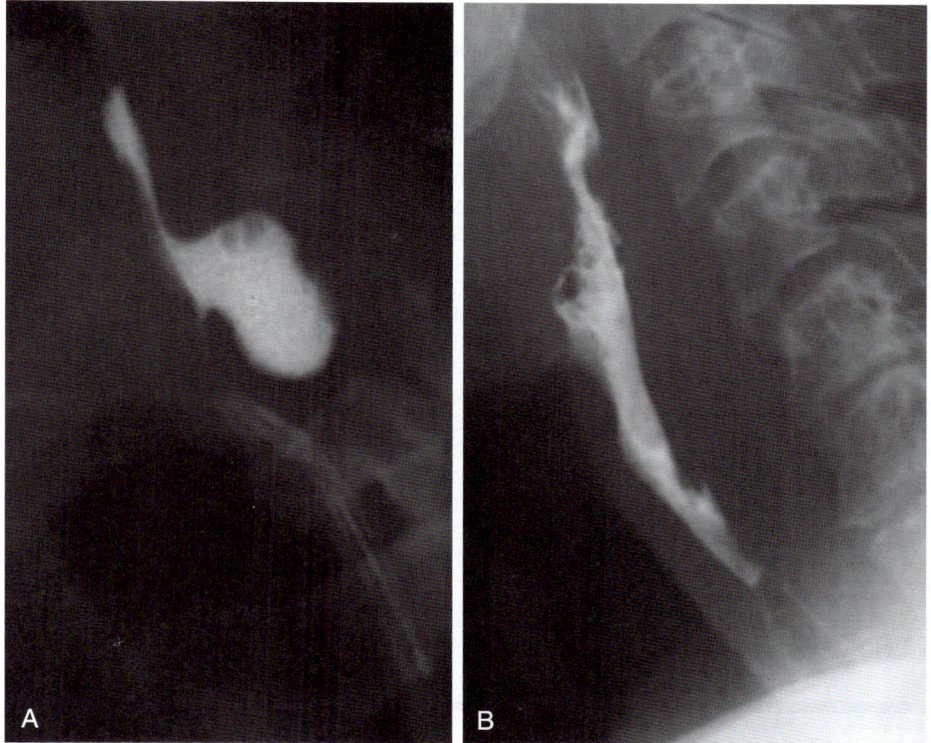

FIGURE 11.14 (A) Radiologic image of a pharyngoesophageal (Zenker) diverticulum. (B) The same patient, after myotomy of the upper esophageal sphincter and diverticulectomy. (From Costantini M, Zaninotto G, Rizzetto C, Narne S, Ancona E. Esophageal diverticula. *Best Pract Res Clin Gastroenterol*. 2004;18:3–17, Fig. 1.)

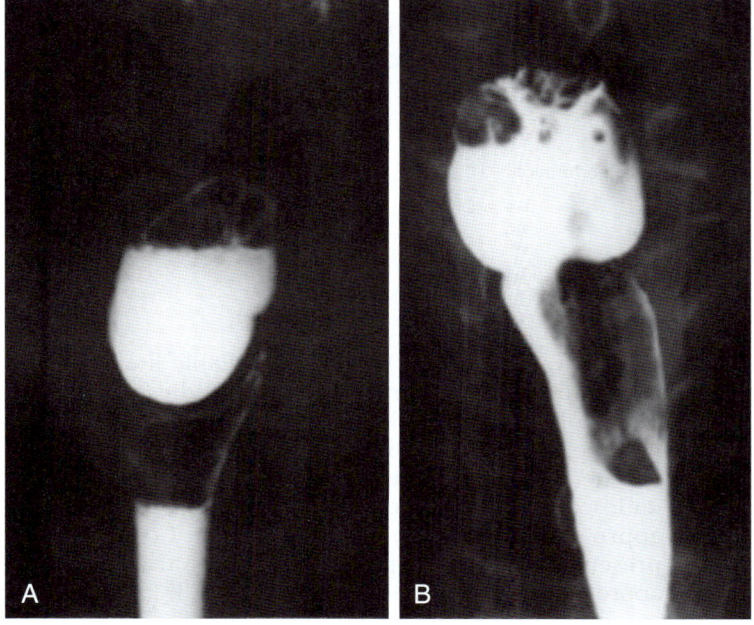

FIGURE 11.15 (A) Radiologic image of a pharyngoesophageal (Zenker) diverticulum. (B) The same patient, after endoscopic stapling diverticulostomy. A posterior pouch is still visible, representing the diverticulum widely anastomosed to the esophageal lumen. ([B] From Costantini M, Zaninotto G, Rizzetto C, Narne S, Ancona E. Esophageal diverticula. *Best Pract Res Clin Gastroenterol*. 2004;18:3–17, Fig. 3.)

with endoscopic treatment against traditional myotomy. Patients treated endoscopically had shorter hospital stays and fasting periods after the operation; they also had fewer complications (though two cervical abscesses and mediastinitis were recorded). Symptom outcome was less favorable than with open surgery, however, because only 75% of patients treated endoscopically were symptom free

at the follow-up (compared with 97% of the patients who had open surgery). Furthermore, only 57% of patients with a diverticulum less than 3 cm were satisfied with the treatment, whereas this was true of 98% of patients treated with open surgery ($P < .05$). Also, Bonavina et al.[49] in their series of 100 patients treated with endostapler reported a success rate of 88.4% in patients with greater than 3 cm

TABLE 11.3 Outcome of Transoral Rigid Procedures With Stapler for Zenker Diverticulum

Author	Year	Time Period	N	Complications (%)	Mortality (%)	RESULTS (%) Good	Partial	Recurrence (%)
Peracchia	1998	1992–96	95	0	0	92.2	7.8	5.4
Van Eeden	1999	1996–97	18	5.9	0	53	35	NA
Cook	2000	1995–99	74	5	0	71	24	8.7
Luscher	2000	1997–98	23	4.3	0	76	14	4.3
Philippsen	2000	1996–99	14	0	0	57	21	NA
Sood	2000	1992–99	44	4.5	1	70	24	9
Jaramillo	2001	1996–99	32	3.7	0	80		7.4
Stoeckli	2002	1997–2000	30	27	0	96		NA
Counter	2002	1993–97	31	9.7	0	50	44	22
Raut	2002	1994–98	25	8	0	48		32
Chang	2003	1995–2001	150	12.7	0	73.3	22	11.8
Chiari	2003	1997–2001	39	10	0	71	20	10.9
Wasserzug	2010	1997–2001	55	4	0	90		10
Bonavina	2015	2001–13	100	2	0	84	5.4	24
Total			730	7.8	0.02	48–92		10.9

NA, Not announced.
Modified from Lerut T, Coosemans W, Decaluwé H, et al. Pathophysiology and treatment of Zenker diverticulum. In: Yeo CJ, et al., eds. *Shackelford's Surgery of the Alimentary Tract*. 7th ed. Philadelphia: Saunders; 2013:336–348.

TABLE 11.4 Retrospective Studies Comparing Surgical Myotomy and Endoscopic Treatment for Zenker Diverticula

Author	SURGICAL MYOTOMY No. Patients	Complications	Good Results (%)	ENDOSCOPIC TREATMENT No. Patients	Complications	Good Results (%)	P*
Gutshow, 2002	67	6[†]	97	86	3[‡]	75	< .05
Rizzetto, 2008	77	10[§]	94.8	51	3[‖]	88.5	< .05
Seth, 2014	31	2[¶]	93	24	7[**]	67	.015
Shahawy, 2014	31	8[††]	100	36	20[‡‡]	61	< .01

*P significances relate to percent of good results with the two technique.
[†]5 leakages; 1 death for myocardial infarction.
[‡]2 cervical abscesses and mediastinitis; 1 dental injury.
[§]2 leakages, 4 hematomas, 1 pericarditis, 2 recurrent palsy (1 transient), 1 mucosal perforation.
[‖]1 mucosal perforation (conversion to open), 1 mucosal tearing, 1 bleeding.
[¶]2 sore throat.
[**]2 sore throat, 2 tongue numbness, 1 perioral burn.
[††]1 perforation, 3 aspiration, 4 other.
[‡‡]3 perforations, 5 aspiration, 1 esophageal stenosis, 11 other.

diverticula, as compared with 54.9% in those with smaller, less than 3 cm diverticula (*P* < .05).

Two recent papers reported the outcome of endoscopic and surgical treatment in Zenker patients.[50,51] Even with all the drawbacks of being retrospective analyses, all these papers agree in reporting a significantly better outcome with traditional surgery (Table 11.4). Furthermore, Lerut reports on a prospective randomized study comparing endoscopic stapling and open surgery that was initiated but terminated after 20 cases (9 surgical, 11 endoscopic) because of a higher number of complications and modest results in the endoscopic group.[33]

No differences in the failure and complications rate were observed when diverticulostomy was performed with a rigid endoscope, and the septum was transected with cautery or CO_2 laser, although two deaths were reported (Table 11.5), or with a flexible endoscope compared with the transoral stapled technique (Table 11.6).

Finally, a systematic review on available literature (28 comparative studies and 43 cohort studies), analyzing results of surgical and the various endoscopic techniques, has been recently published.[52]

The rate of failure was significantly higher with endoscopic techniques compared with external surgical approaches (18.4% vs. 4.2%; *P* < .001). Complications presented a different pattern with the various surgical approaches, since mediastinitis (1.2% vs. 0.3%; *P* < .01) and emphysema (3.0% vs. 0.1%; *P* < .01) occurred significantly more often with endoscopic treatment, compared with fistula (3.7% vs. 1.2%; *P* < .01), recurrent nerve palsy (3.4% vs. 0.3%; *P* < .001), and hematoma (2.2% vs. 0.6%; *P* < .01) with transcervical treatment. Surgery-related deaths were infrequent in both groups (0.9% for the open approach vs. 0.4% for endoscopic techniques). Overall postoperative complications tended to occur more frequently after transcervical approach (7% vs. 11%).

TABLE 11.5 Outcome of Transoral Rigid Procedures With Cautery or Laser for Zenker Diverticulum

Author	Year	Time Period	Method	N	Complications (%)	Mortality (%)	RESULTS (%) Good	RESULTS (%) Partial	Recurrence (%)
Van Overbeek	1994	1964–92	Cautery/CO₂L	545	6.7	1	90.6	8.6	NA
Ishioka	1995	1982–92	Cautery	42	4.8	0	92.9	7.1	7.1
Von Doersten	1997	1985–94	Cautery	40	25	0	92.5		0
Hashiba	1999	>1978	Cautery	47	14.9	0	96		4.3
Lippert	1999	1984–96	CO₂L	60	10	0	73	21	10
Nyrop	2000	1989–99	CO₂L	61	13.3	0	70	22	13
Mattinger	2002	1974–98	CO₂L	52	13.5	1	84.6		15.4
Krespi	2002	1989–2001	CO₂L	83	4.8	0	85.5	11	7.5
Total				930	8.7	0.02	70–96		7.2

CO_2L, Carbon dioxide laser; *NA*, not announced.
Data from Lerut T, Coosemans W, Decaluwé H, et al. Pathophysiology and treatment of Zenker diverticulum. In: Yeo CJ, et al., eds. *Shackelford's Surgery of the Alimentary Tract*. 7th ed. Philadelphia: Saunders; 2013:336–348.

TABLE 11.6 Outcome of Transoral Flexible Procedures for Zenker Diverticulum

Author	Year	N	Emphysema, Microperforation (%)	Bleeding (%)	Resolution of Symptoms (%)	Recurrence (%)
Ishioka	1995	42	2	2.4	92.8	7.1
Sakai	2001	10	—	—	100	—
Hashiba	1999	47	13	2.1	96	NA
Rubinstein	2007	41	3	—	95	17
Vogelsang	2007	31	23	3.3	84	35
Costamagna	2007	28	18	14	43	29
Christiaens	2007	21	4.8	—	100	10
Case	2010	22	27	23	82	18
Al Kadi	2010	18	6	17	77.7	11
Repici	2010	32	3	3	97	12.5
Total		292	10	5.5	43–100	16.7

NA, Not announced.
Modified from Lerut T, Coosemans W, Decaluwé H, et al. Pathophysiology and treatment of Zenker diverticulum. In: Yeo CJ, et al., eds. *Shackelford's Surgery of the Alimentary Tract*. 7th ed. Philadelphia: Saunders; 2013:336–348.

It is difficult to draw final conclusions from these studies. Endoscopic treatment is very attractive because it is less invasive and has a lower complication rate, although, when compared with surgery, it is sometimes less effective in relieving dysphagia completely. Endoscopic stapling also has other drawbacks, mainly related to the size of the diverticulum: in the case of a small diverticulum (≤2 cm), the stapler anvil is too long to be properly accommodated inside the pouch, and the cricopharyngeal fibers cannot be transected completely. In this sense, diverticulostomy with the laser or cautery may be more effective. On the other hand, very large diverticula (>5 cm) plunging into the mediastinum carry the risk of vascular lesions if they are transected blindly. Myotomy of the UES is probably more effectively achieved with open surgery, when the muscle fibers are cut under direct vision and the edges of the myotomy are further separated by blunt dissection, leaving the submucosa widely exposed. Furthermore, the inferior pharyngeal constrictor muscle layers of the proximal cervical esophagus may be easily divided. The major drawback of open surgery is the related morbidity, which is higher than with endoscopy mainly due to leakage from the suture line. Although this does not normally require further surgery and heals spontaneously (with nasogastric suction, NPO, and antibiotic therapy), it is nonetheless a potentially severe complication in patients with concurrent respiratory or heart disease.

CONCLUSION

ZD can be effectively treated with either endoscopic diverticulostomy or open surgery. Both approaches have advantages and disadvantages. An individual approach to ZD should therefore be recommended: High-risk patients with medium-size diverticula are probably better served by diverticulostomy; open surgery should be recommended for small (<2 cm) or giant ZD or in patients with a low surgical risk. New peroral flexible endoscopic techniques offer promise for patients with any size diverticulum but will probably be best for small to medium (0 to 5) cm diverticula.

REFERENCES

1. World Health Organization. *International Classification of Functioning, Disability and Health (ICF)*. Geneva: WHO; 2001.
2. Roden DF, Altman KW. Causes of dysphagia among different age groups: a systematic review of the literature. *Otolaryngol Clin North Am*. 2013;46:965-987.
3. Rommel M, Hamdy S. Oropharyngeal dysphagia: manifestations and diagnosis. *Nat Rev Gastroenterol Hepatol*. 2016;13:49-59.
4. Briani C, Marcon M, Ermani M, et al. Radiological evidence of sub-clinical dysphagia in motor neuron disease. *J Neurol*. 1998;245:211-216.
5. Rosenbek JC, Robbins JA, Roecker EB, Coyle JL, Wood JL. A penetration-aspiration scale. *Dysphagia*. 1996;11:93-98.
6. Langmore SE, Schatz K, Olson N. Fiberoptic endoscopic examination of swallowing safety: a new procedure. *Dysphagia*. 1988;2:216-219.
7. Butler SG, Markley L, Sanders B, Stuart A. Reliability of the penetration aspiration scale with flexible endoscopic evaluation of swallowing. *Ann Otol Rhinol Laryngol*. 2015;124:480-483.
8. Kahrilas PJ, Dent J, Dodds WJ, Hogan WJ, Arndorfer RC. A method for continuous monitoring of upper esophageal sphincter pressure. *Dig Dis Sci*. 1987;32:121-128.
9. Cook IJ, Dodds WJ, Dantas RO, et al. Opening mechanisms of the human upper esophageal sphincter. *Am J Physiol*. 1989;257:G748-G759.
10. DeMeester TR, Costantini M. Function tests. In: Patterson GA, Cooper JD, Deslaurier J, Lerut AEMR, Luketich JD, Rice TW, eds. *Pearson's Thoracic & Esophageal Surgery*. 3rd ed. Philadelphia: Churchill Livingstone Elsevier; 2008:117-147.
11. Ghosh SK, Pandolfino JE, Zhang O, Jarosz A, Kahrilas PJ. Deglutitive upper esophageal sphincter relaxation: a study of 75 volunteer subjects using solid-state high-resolution manometry. *Am J Physiol Gastrointest Liver Physiol*. 2006;291:G525-G531.
12. McMahon BP, Frøkjaer JB, Kunwald P, et al. The functional lumen imaging probe (FLIP) for evaluation of the esophagogastric junction. *Am J Physiol Gastrointest Liver Physiol*. 2007;292:G377-G384.
13. Lottrup C, Reggersene H, Liao D, et al. Functional lumen imaging of the gastrointestinal tract. *J Gastroenterol*. 2015;50:1005-1016.
14. Regan J, Walshe M, Timon C, McMahon BP. Endoflip® evaluation of pharyngo-oesophageal segment tone and swallowing in a clinical population: a total laryngectomy case series. *Clin Otolaryngol*. 2015;40:121-129.
15. Cook IJ, Kahrilas PJ. AGA technical review on management of oropharyngeal dysphagia. *Gastroenterology*. 1999;116:455-478.
16. Broniatowski M, Sonies BC, Rubin JS, et al. Current evaluation and treatment of patients with swallowing disorders. *Otolaryngol Head Neck Surg*. 1999;120:464-473.
17. Gauderer MWL, Ponsky JL, Izant RJ Jr. Gastrostomy without laparotomy: a percutaneous endoscopic technique. *J Pediatr Surg*. 1980;15:872-875.
18. Sacks BA, Glotzer DJ. Percutaneous reestablishment of feeding gastrostomies. *Surgery*. 1979;85:575-576.
19. Kocdor P, Siegel ER, Tulumay-Ugur O. Cricopharyngeal dysfunction: a systematic review comparing outcomes of dilation, Botulinum toxin injection, and myotomy. *Laryngoscope*. 2016;126:135-141.
20. Marston AP, Maldonado FJ, Ravi K, Kasperbauer JL, Ekbom DC. Treatment of oropharyngeal dysphagia secondary to idiopathic cricopharyngeal bar: surgical cricopharyngeal muscle myotomy versus dilation. *Am J Otolaryngol*. 2016;37(6):507-512.
21. Schneider I, Thumfart WF, Pototschnig C, Eckel HE. Treatment of dysfunction of the cricopharyngeal muscle with botulinum A toxin: introduction of a new, noninvasive method. *Ann Otol Rhinol Laryngol*. 1994;103:31-35.
22. Kelly EA, Koszewski IJ, Jaradeh SS, et al. Botulinum toxin injection for the treatment of upper esophageal sphincter dysfunction. *Ann Otol Rhinol Laryngol*. 2013;122:100-108.
23. Zaninotto G, Marchese Ragona R, Briani C, et al. The role of botulinum toxin injection and upper esophageal sphincter myotomy in treating oropharyngeal dysphagia. *J Gastrointest Surg*. 2004;8:997-1006.
24. Ancona E, Frasson P, Peracchia A. La myotomie du sphincter oesophagien supérieur dans les dyskinésies pharyngo-oesophagiennes. *Ann Chir*. 1979;33:467-473.
25. Brigand C, Ferraro P, Martin J, Duranceau A. Risk factors in patients undergoing cricopharyngeal myotomy. *Br J Surg*. 2007;94:978-983.
26. Duranceau A, Ferraro P. Pharyngeal and cricopharyngeal disorders. In: Patterson GA, Cooper JD, Deslaurier J, Lerut AEMR, Luketich JD, Rice TW, eds. *Pearson's Thoracic & Esophageal Surgery*. 3rd ed. Philadelphia: Churchill Livingstone Elsevier; 2008:677-701.
27. Zenker FA, von Ziemssen H. Krankheiten des oesophagus. In: von Ziemsen H, ed. *Handbuch der Speciellen Pathologie und Therapie*. Vol 7, Suppl. Leipzig: FC Vogel; 1877.
28. Costantini M, Zaninotto G, Rizzetto C, Narne S, Ancona E. Esophageal diverticula. *Best Pract Res Clin Gastroenterol*. 2004;18:3-17.
29. Cook IJ, Gabb M, Panagopoulos V. Zenker's diverticulum is a disorder of upper esophageal sphincter opening. *Gastroenterology*. 1993;103:1229-1235.
30. Lerut T, van Raemdonck D, Guelinckx P, et al. Zenker's diverticulum: is a myotomy of the cricopharyngeus useful? How long should it be? *Hepatogastroenterology*. 1992;39:127.
31. Zaninotto G, Costantini M, Boccù C, et al. Functional and morphological study of the cricopharyngeal muscle in patients with Zenker's diverticulum. *Br J Surg*. 1996;83:1263-1267.
32. Venturi M, Bonavina L, Colombo L, et al. Biochemical markers in upper esophageal sphincter compliance in patients with Zenker's diverticulum. *J Surg Res*. 1997;70:46.
33. Lerut T, Coosemans W, Decaluwé H, et al. Pathophysiology and treatment of Zenker diverticulum. In: Yeo CJ, et al., eds. *Shackelford's Surgery of the Alimentary Tract*. 7th ed. Philadelphia: Saunders; 2013:336-348.
34. Pomerri F, Costantini M, Dal Bosco C, et al. Comparison of preoperative and surgical measurements of Zenker's diverticulum. *Surg Endosc*. 2012;26:2010-2015.
35. Payne WS. The treatment of pharyngoesophageal diverticulum: the simple and the complex. *Hepatogastroenterol*. 1992;39:109-114.
36. Dohlman G, Mattson O. The endoscopic operation for hypopharyngeal diverticula. *Arch Otolaryngol*. 1960;71:744-752.
37. Knegt PP, de Jong PC, van der Schans EJ. Endoscopic treatment of the hypopharyngeal diverticulum with CO_2 laser. *Endoscopy*. 1985;17:205-206.
38. Collard JM, Otte IB, Kestens PJ. Endoscopic stapling technique of esophagodiverticulostomy for Zenker's diverticulum. *Ann Thorac Surg*. 1993;56:573-576.
39. Ishioka S, Sakai P, Maluf FF, Melo JM. Endoscopic incision of Zenker's diverticula. *Endoscopy*. 1995;27:433-437.
40. Mulder CJJ, Robijn RJ, Thies JE. Flexible endoscopic treatment of Zenker's diverticulum: a new approach. *Endoscopy*. 1995;27:438-442.
41. Rizzetto C, Zaninotto G, Costantini M, et al. Zenker's diverticula: feasibility of a tailored approach based on diverticulum size. *J Gastrointest Surg*. 2008;12:2057-2065.
42. Fama AF, Moore EJ, Kasperbauer JL. Harmonic scalpel in the treatment of Zenker's diverticulum. *Laryngoscope*. 2009;119:1265-1269.
43. Sharp DB, Newman JR, Magnuson JS. Endoscopic management of Zenker's diverticulum: stapler assisted versus Harmonic Ace. *Laryngoscope*. 2009;119:1906-1912.
44. van Overbeek J, Hoeksema PE, Edens ET. Microendoscopic surgery of the hypopharyngeal diverticulum using electrocoagulation or carbon dioxide laser. *Ann Otol Rhinol Laryngol*. 1984;93:34-36.
45. Costamagna G, Iacopini F, Tringali A, et al. Flexible endoscopic Zenker's diverticulotomy: cap-assisted technique vs. diverticuloscope-assisted technique. *Endoscopy*. 2007;39:146-152.
46. Aiolfi A, Scolari F, Saino G, Bonavina L. Current status of minimally invasive endoscopic management for Zenker diverticulum. *World J Gastrointest Endosc*. 2015;7:87-93.
47. Tang SJ, Jazrawi SF, Chen E, Tang L, Myers LL. Flexible endoscopic clip-assisted Zenker's diverticulotomy: the first case series (with videos). *Laryngoscope*. 2008;118:1199-1205.
48. Gutschow CA, Hamoir M, Rombaux P, et al. Management of pharyngoesophageal (Zenker's) diverticulum: which technique? *Ann Thorac Surg*. 2002;74:1677-1683.
49. Bonavina L, Aiolfi A, Scolari F, Bonma D, Lovece A, Asti E. Long-term out come and quality of life after transoral stapling for Zenker diverticulum. *World J Gastroenterol*. 2015;21:1167-1172.
50. Seth R, Rajasekaran K, Lee WT, et al. Patient reported outcomes in endoscopic and open transcervical treatment for Zenker's diverticulum. *Laryngoscope*. 2014;124:119-125.
51. Shahawy S, Janisiewicz AM, Annino D, Shapiro J. A comparative study of outcomes for endoscopic diverticulotomy versus external diverticulectomy. *Otolaryngol Head Neck Surg*. 2014;151:646-651.
52. Verdonck J, Morton RP. Systematic review on treatment of Zenker's diverticulum. *Eur Arch Otorhinolaringol*. 2015;272:3095-3107.

Surgical Management of Mid- and Distal Esophageal Diverticula

Brian E. Louie | Shane P. Smith | Oliver C. Bellevue

Diverticular diseases of the esophagus consist of variations of outpouchings of one or more layers of the gut wall that are epithelial lined. These outpouchings can be found along the entire length of the esophagus. They are described by their location along the esophagus: pharyngoesophageal, mid-esophagus, and epiphrenic. Often these diverticula are asymptomatic, but when they are symptomatic, they create a significant constellation of symptoms that reduce the patient's quality of life and may lead to life-threatening complications such as aspiration pneumonia. Because these occur often in the elderly or patients with comorbidities, careful surgical evaluation needs to be completed before treatment is rendered to ensure a good outcome. This chapter focuses on the presentation and treatment of mid- and distal esophageal diverticula.

DISTAL ESOPHAGEAL (EPIPHRENIC) DIVERTICULUM

An epiphrenic diverticulum is an outpouching of mucosa and submucosa through the muscularis propria layer of the esophagus that was first described by Mondiere.[1] It is generally accepted that this is a pulsion diverticulum most often found in the distal 10 cm of the esophagus.[2] These are considered false diverticula, because not all layers of the esophagus are involved in the outpouching, though in practical terms, the muscle layer can often be delineated overlying the diverticulum in a very thin layer.[3] The incidence of this diverticulum is unknown but occurs one third as frequently as a pharyngoesophageal diverticulum.[4]

The majority of epiphrenic diverticula are in middle-aged or elderly patients, but reported age ranges include patients in the teenage years[5] and mid-20s.[6] There is no gender predilection, with most recent series showing that it affects both men and women relatively equally.[6–9] The majority of patients will present with a single diverticulum, but up to 15% of patients can have two diverticula, with more than two diverticula (Fig. 12.1) occurring with decreasing frequency.[10–12] The diverticulum arises from the right side of the esophagus in approximately 70% of patients (Fig. 12.2), is usually within 5 cm of the gastroesophageal junction, and measures between 4 and 7 cm in maximal dimension (Fig. 12.3).[7,11–13]

PATHOPHYSIOLOGY

Despite advances in manometric evaluation, the pathogenesis of an epiphrenic diverticulum has not been fully elucidated. It is generally accepted that this type of diverticulum is almost always secondary to an underlying esophageal motility disorder.[2,6,7] Named motility disorders associated with these diverticula include achalasia, diffuse esophageal spasm, nutcracker esophagus, and hypertensive lower esophageal sphincter (LES), with the most common being achalasia followed by diffuse esophageal spasm.[2,14,15] One theory suggests that the presence of dysmotility causes an uncoordinated contraction between the distal esophagus and lower esophageal sphincter leading to increased intraluminal pressure and subsequent herniation through a weakened area of the esophagus.[16] Another study identified that esophageal diverticulum is associated with areas of low peristaltic pressure amplitude, bizarre peristaltic wave forms, and hypertensive peristaltic pressures.[17] Other reported etiologies such as a distal stricture, prior fundoplication, and hiatal hernia all act to create the same outflow pressure dynamics as a motility disorder.

SYMPTOMS AND DIAGNOSIS

Epiphrenic diverticula present either asymptomatically when they are incidentally identified on a radiographic study or with symptoms due to the underlying motility disorder and associated outpouching.[10,11,18] Symptomatic patients most commonly present with dysphagia (90%), regurgitation of undigested food (80%), and repetitive episodes of aspiration (30%).[11] However, there is a range of symptomatic patients, some who have minimal or only intermittent symptoms of dysphagia, and others who have incapacitating and at times life-threatening symptoms particularly from regurgitation of undigested food that is often precipitated by position and is most often at night.[11] Chest pain, pyrosis/heartburn, and weight loss are also commonly reported.

It is often difficult to determine whether the symptoms originate with the diverticulum itself or the underlying motility disorder. In one study comparing symptoms in different size diverticula in patients with and without a motility disorder, increasing diverticula size, particularly those 5 cm or greater, was more likely to produce symptoms irrespective of the presence of a motility disorder.[12] This suggests that symptoms are more likely derived from the motility disorder early in the disease process. However, with disease progression and increasing anatomic distortion, the diverticulum begins to drive symptoms.

The diagnosis of an epiphrenic diverticulum is initially confirmed by barium esophagram in which one or more diverticula are identified. However, for patients being considered for surgical treatment, the barium esophagram is only the start of a comprehensive evaluation. All patients should undergo a thorough history and physical examination to document comorbidities and guarantee surgical fitness. This is followed by three main studies:

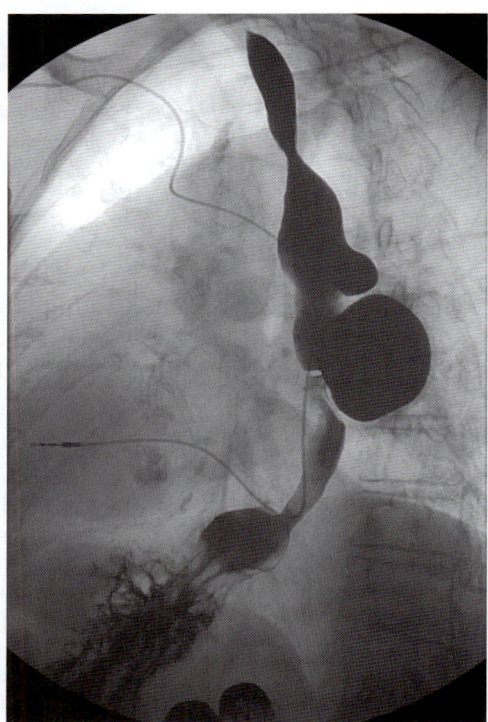

FIGURE 12.1 Barium swallow demonstrating two esophageal diverticula.

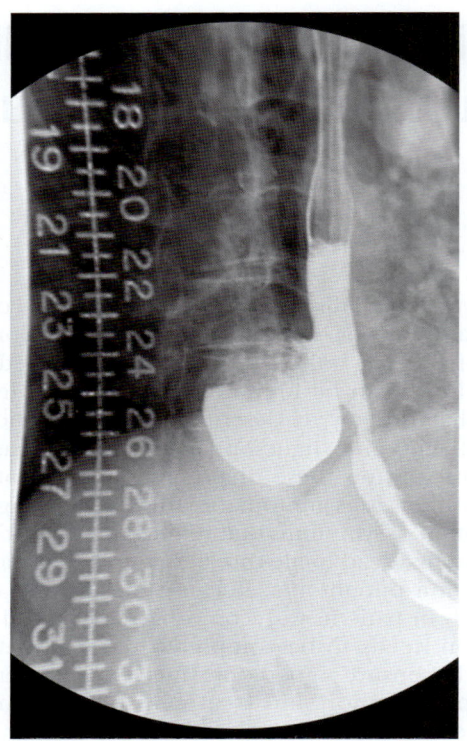

FIGURE 12.3 Barium swallow estimating the size of the diverticulum.

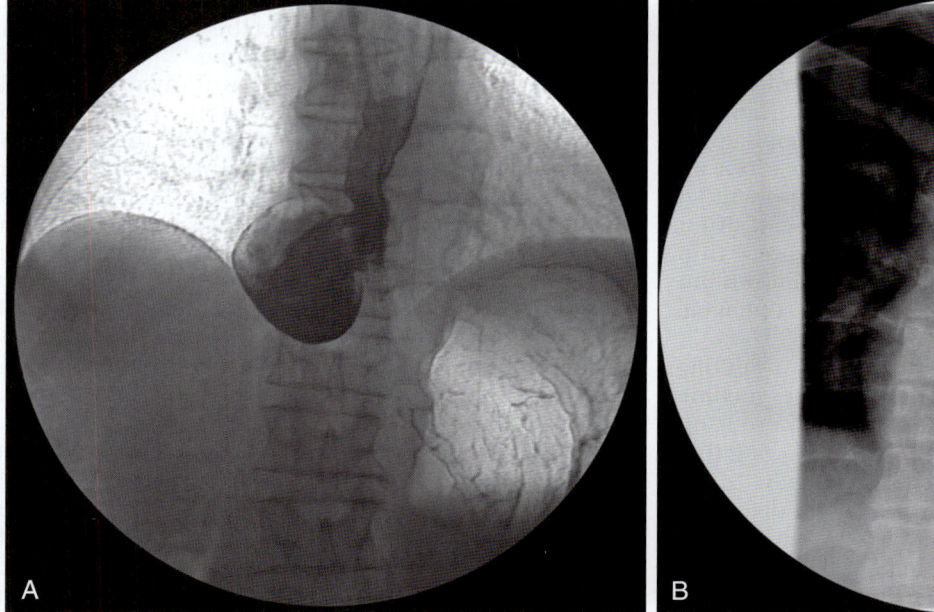

FIGURE 12.2 (A) Barium swallow demonstrating a right-side diverticulum. (B) Barium swallow demonstrating a left-side diverticulum.

Barium swallow
- Allows measurement of length and size of diverticulum
- Orients diverticulum (right/left)
- Identifies other pathology such as hiatal hernia, stricture
- Provides information about esophageal motility

Esophagogastroduodenoscopy (EGD)
- Defines anatomy of diverticulum, including precise location relative to the gastroesophageal junction (GEJ) (Fig. 12.4)
- Assesses for concomitant pathology such as ulceration or malignancy

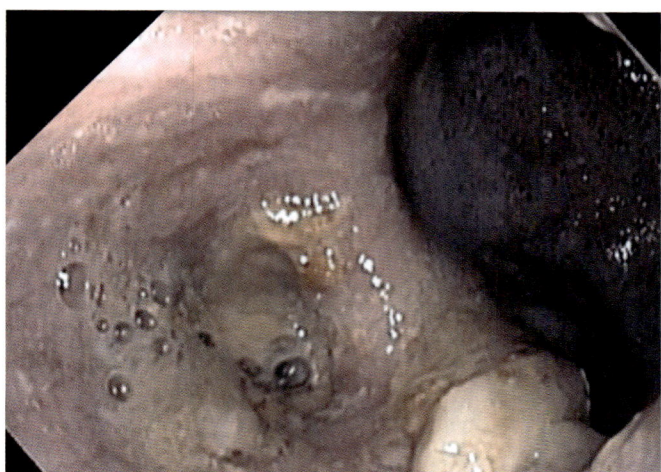

FIGURE 12.4 Esophagogastroduodenoscopy showing a wide-mouth diverticulum with the small esophageal opening just above the gastroesophageal junction.

- Used to treat bleeding, place manometry catheter, feeding tube

High-resolution manometry
- Defines underlying motility disorder
- May need to be placed endoscopically or under fluoroscopy
- Potentially guides length of myotomy

In addition to the primary studies, there are several additional studies that may provide additional information preoperatively and during long-term follow-up. A timed barium swallow has been used to manage patients treated for achalasia.[19,20] This standardized test when performed prior to surgery and then during follow-up provides a simple and objective method of esophageal emptying, since symptoms are unreliable in this setting. A computed tomography scan of the chest can be helpful in determining the true proximal extent of the diverticulum. When the superior edge of the diverticulum is beyond the inferior pulmonary veins, it may be very difficult to access laparoscopically and suggests the need for the addition of a thoracoscopic procedure to completely resect the diverticulum.[8] Lastly, patients with suspected symptoms of gastroesophageal reflux disease (GERD) may undergo pH testing as necessary.

TREATMENT

The decision to offer treatment to a patient with an epiphrenic diverticulum is based on the patient's symptoms and severity of those symptoms. Patients who are asymptomatic or minimally symptomatic may forgo any treatment, but whether they require ongoing follow-up is controversial. Two long-term follow-up studies from the Mayo Clinic provide conflicting data. Debas et al. in 1980 detailed the outcomes of 37 patients undergoing nonoperative treatment. In this group of patients, seven remained without symptoms and were followed, two underwent surgery elsewhere, and six were treated with esophageal dilation with resolution of symptoms. In the remaining 22, 15 had no details, but 4 of the remaining 7 experienced an aspiration event with one

death, 2 patients became malnourished, and 1 patient developed an esophageal carcinoma.[10] This suggests that continued follow-up is necessary because of the development of worsening symptoms. Comparatively, Benacci et al. in 1993 documented outcomes of 71 patients without symptoms or minimal symptoms. Of 47 patients who were asymptomatic, 27 were lost to follow-up, and 20 patients were followed for a median of 4 years (range 1–17) and remained stable. Of 24 patients with mild symptoms, 9 were lost to follow-up, and 15 were followed a median of 11 years (range 1–25 years) with either EGD or barium swallow with stable minimal symptoms.[11] Although many patients remained stable, the outcomes of many were lost in follow-up. Because the symptoms that develop can be devastating, it seems reasonable to follow these patients to ensure that progressive symptoms do not develop given the rarity of this disease and the unpredictable development of symptoms.

The indication for surgical treatment is symptoms attributable to the diverticulum or motility disorder. Surgical evaluation is mandatory if a patient developed incapacitating symptoms or respiratory compromise from aspiration of the esophageal contents. Regardless of the surgical approach, there are a number of surgical principles that have been articulated surrounding the treatment of these diverticula. These key steps include:
- Delineation of the entire diverticulum at the mucosal level
- Definition of the "neck" of the diverticulum
- Resection of the diverticulum
- Closure of the overlying muscle with or without buttress
- Distal myotomy with or without partial fundoplication

SURGICAL APPROACHES AND RESULTS

At present, there are a variety of approaches used to surgically treat an epiphrenic diverticulum including transthoracic, video-assisted thoracic surgery (VATS), laparoscopic, combined VATS-laparoscopic, and reports of endoscopic approaches have recently emerged.

TRANSTHORACIC APPROACH

Traditionally, an epiphrenic diverticulum is approached via a seventh or eighth interspace left thoracotomy though both thoracic cavities have been used (Fig. 12.5).[21] Most often the diverticulum resides on the right side of the esophagus; consequently, the entire distal esophagus is mobilized through the left chest including the diaphragmatic hiatus to allow access to the diverticulum. Once the diverticulum is identified, the overlying muscle is split along the length of the diverticulum taking care to avoid the vagus nerve. The mucosa can be grasped carefully and the muscle dissected away to expose the superior and inferior margins of the diverticulum along with the "neck" or "waist." Most surgeons will place either a bougie or an endoscope into the esophagus at this point in preparation for division of the diverticulum with an endoscopic stapler. After division of the diverticulum, the adjacent muscle and pleura are approximated with interrupted silk sutures. A buttress of pleura or an intercostal muscle can also be added to cover the suture line.

The esophagogastric myotomy is begun on the contralateral side of the esophagus at the location of the inferior

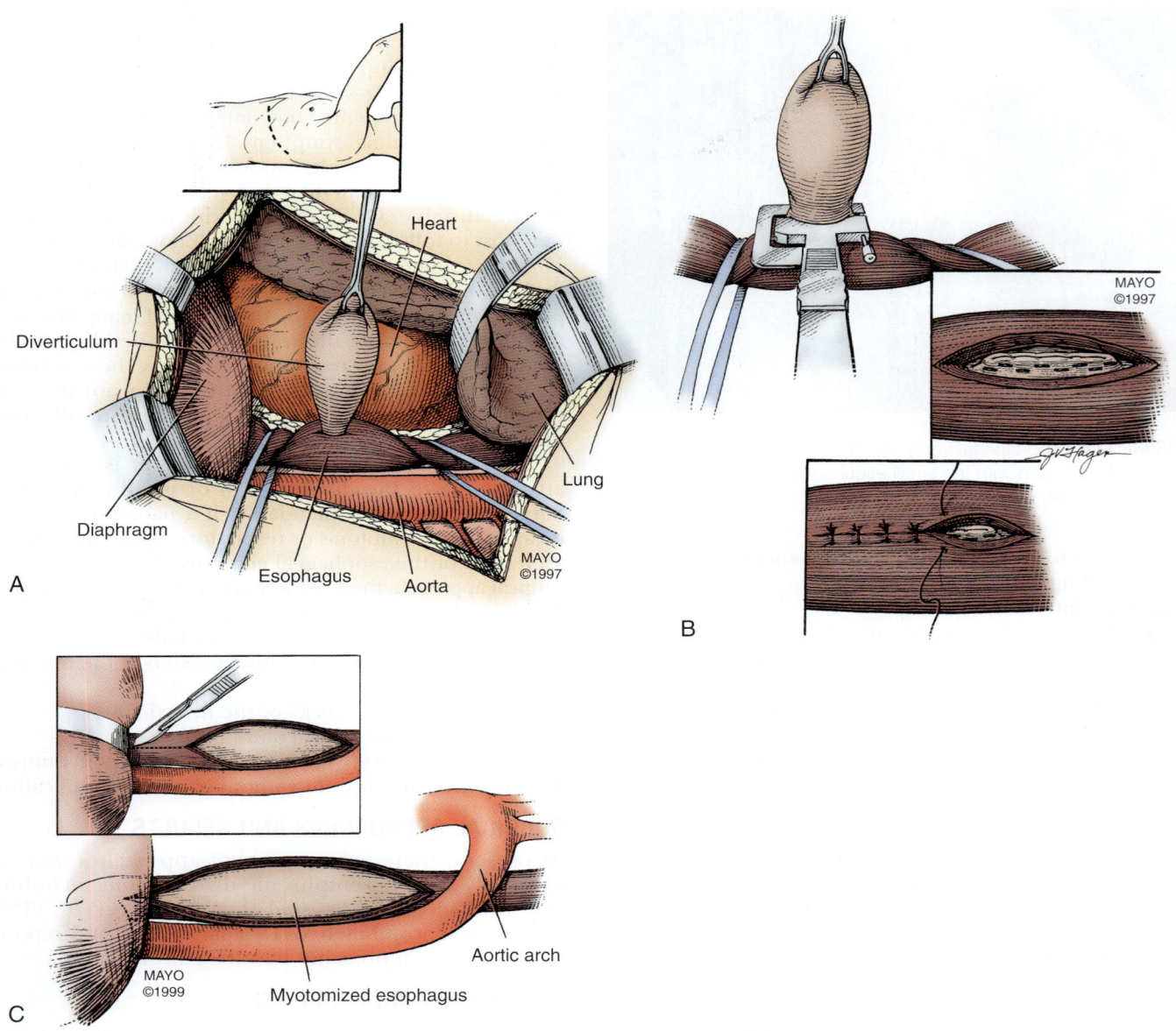

FIGURE 12.5 Surgical management of an epiphrenic esophageal diverticulum. A left posterolateral thoracotomy incision is shown in the *inset.* Exposure of the diverticulum is obtained when the chest is entered through the bed of the eighth rib. Note that the esophagus has been delivered from its mediastinal bed, tape has been passed around the esophagus, and the esophagus has been rotated to bring the diverticulum into view. The neck of the diverticulum has been dissected to identify the defect in the esophageal muscular wall (A). A TA stapling device is used to transect and close the diverticulum followed by closure of the esophageal musculature over a mucosal suture line (B). The site of the diverticular incision has been rotated back to the right and is not visible. A long esophagomyotomy extending from the esophagogastric junction to the aortic arch has been performed. The musculature of the esophagus has been freed from approximately 50% of the circumference of the esophageal mucosal tube to allow the mucosa to bulge through the muscular incision (C). (Copyright Mayo Clinic, 1999.)

aspect of diverticulectomy and extended onto the stomach for 2 cm. Some surgeons will also extend the myotomy proximally for a centimeter or two, whereas other surgeons will extend the myotomy up to the aortic arch as shown in Fig. 12.5. However, the value of this proximal extension is unclear, since the high-pressure zone is distal to the diverticulum. Many surgeons favor the addition of a partial antireflux repair to provide an element of reflux control,[22] and in this circumstance, most opt to create a Belsey Mark IV fundoplication.[23]

VIDEO-ASSISTED THORACIC APPROACH ± LAPAROSCOPIC MYOTOMY/FUNDOPLICATION

After placement of a double-lumen endotracheal tube, the patient is placed in the left lateral decubitus position with the bed flexed at the top of the iliac crest. A total of four ports are placed (seventh intercostal space [ICS] posterior axillary line for surgeon's left hand, stapler, ninth ICS in the line of the scapular tip for the camera, fourth ICS posterior axillary line for retraction and suctioning, and seventh ICS just inferior and posterior to the scapular tip for the surgeon's right hand) (Fig. 12.6). The diverticulum is identified and the muscular layers of the esophageal wall split to identify the mucosa at the inferior and superior aspect of the diverticulum. Once the neck of the diverticulum (Fig. 12.7A) is exposed and dissected free, the stapler is then applied over the neck of the diverticulum with either a bougie or upper endoscope in situ and resected with an endoscopic stapler (Fig. 12.7B). The muscular layers are closed with interrupted sutures and occasionally reinforced with pleura. A 24-French chest tube and/or a 24-French drain is placed adjacent to the esophagus prior to closure.

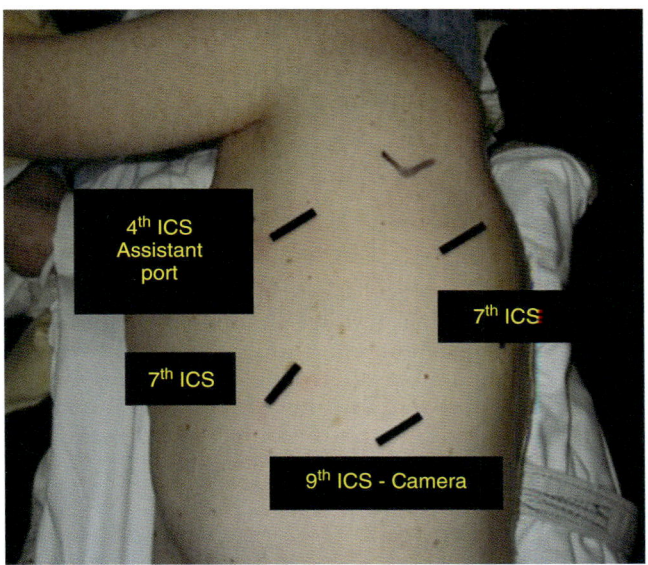

FIGURE 12.6 Example of video-assisted thoracic surgery ports.

The challenge in using a VATS-only approach is performing a distal esophageal myotomy. Since the majority of diverticula are found in the right chest and access to the proximal stomach is limited from this approach, several options have been proposed. First, it has been suggested to perform pneumatic dilation of the lower esophageal sphincter prior to diverticulectomy in patients with a documented motility disorder.[24] It is likely this will need to be repeated to achieve a similar result to surgical myotomy based on a recent trial.[25] Second, the patient can be repositioned supine or low lithotomy and a laparoscopic myotomy with or without partial fundoplication can be performed. To ensure the proper extent of the myotomy, the distal end of the diverticulum is marked with a clip on the anterior surface of the esophageal wall at the completion of the VATS portion. The clip can then be identified at laparoscopy and the esophagomyotomy performed from the clip on the left side of the esophagus onto the gastric cardia.[8] Lastly, if the diverticulum is left sided, the myotomy can be performed similar to the approach described by Pellegrini et al. though the relief of dysphagia and ability to create a fundoplication favors adding a laparoscopic myotomy.[26,27]

LAPAROSCOPIC APPROACH

A laparoscopic transhiatal approach is becoming increasingly common.[6,9,16,28–30] Most surgeons position the patient as they would for a modified Heller-Dor or Nissen fundoplication procedure. We favor the patient in low lithotomy with placement of five laparoscopic ports.[31] The initial exposure is to dissect and mobilize the entire esophageal hiatus for maximal exposure. The vagal nerves are identified as dissection is performed cranially up the esophagus until the distal aspect of the diverticulum is identified. Once identified, the dissection proceeds anterior and posterior along the diverticulum until circumferential dissection is complete. The distally identified vagus nerves are then traced toward the diverticulum; on occasion it is necessary to separate a nerve from the diverticulum. The neck of the diverticulum is then identified by separating any remaining muscle fibers and then dissecting down

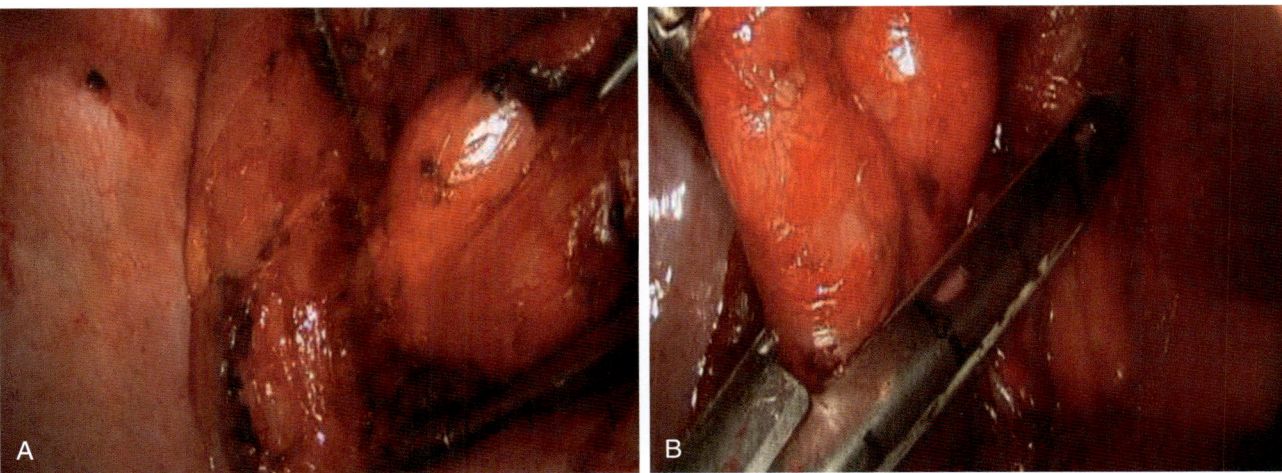

FIGURE 12.7 (A) Operative video-assisted thoracic surgery (VATS) photo showing the diverticulum and the narrow aspect of the neck or waist. (B) Operative VATS photo showing application of the stapler in line with the esophagus at the level of the neck of the diverticulum.

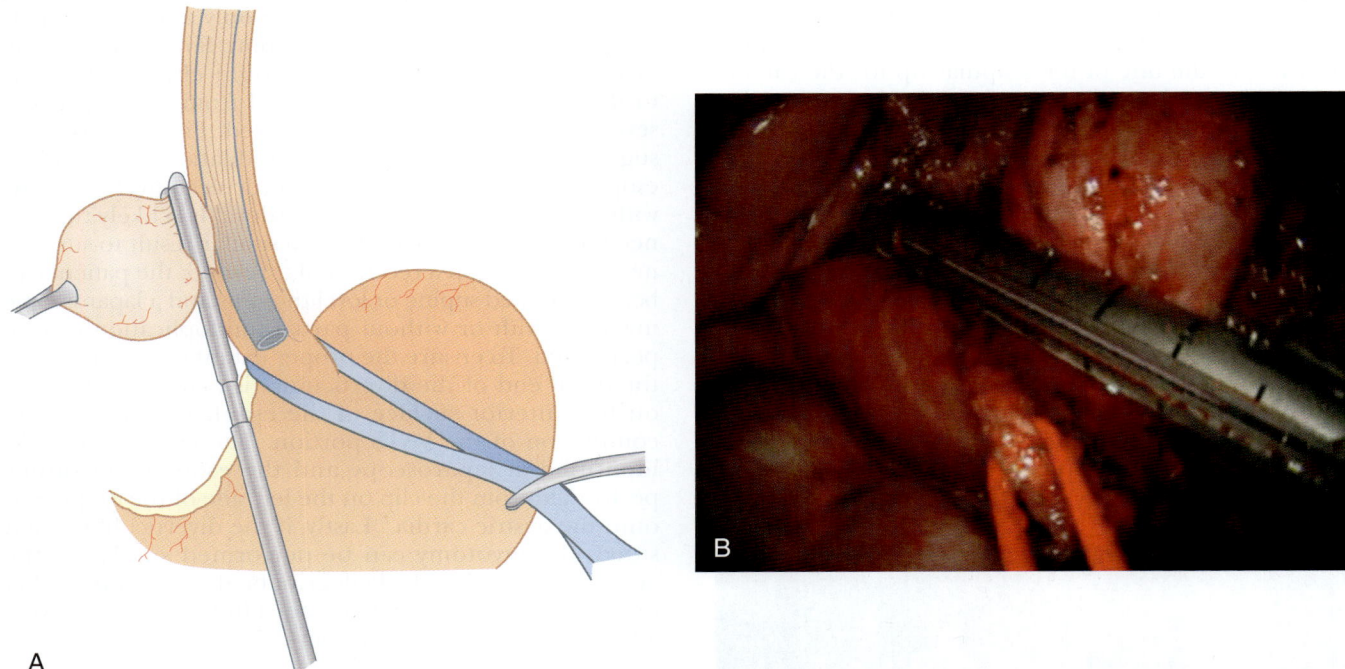

FIGURE 12.8 (A) Stapled resection of an epiphrenic diverticulum through a laparoscopic approach. (B) Operative laparoscopic photo of stapler across the neck of the diverticulum. Orange vessel loop around the vagus nerve.

to expose the mucosa. Similar to the open and VATS approaches, the neck of the diverticulum is exposed, and an endoscopic stapler is applied over the neck of the diverticulum with either a bougie or upper endoscope in situ (Fig. 12.8). The staple line is then imbricated using sutures.

The esophageal myotomy is performed along the left anterior wall of the esophagus just to the left of midline. The myotomy is extended inferiorly from at least the inferior aspect of the diverticulum through the lower esophageal sphincter and extended 2 cm onto the proximal stomach. The hiatus is then reapproximated posteriorly, and either a Toupet fundoplication is created posteriorly or a Dor fundoplication is created anteriorly (Fig. 12.9).

ENDOSCOPIC APPROACH

With the advent of endoscopic surgical techniques such as endoscopic tunneling and endoscopic myotomy,[32,33] it is possible to imagine that an epiphrenic diverticulum may be approached in this fashion. Two recent abstracts report on the use of these techniques to treat an epiphrenic diverticulum.[34,35] In both cases, a submucosal tunnel is created to facilitate a distal esophageal myotomy using the same technique used to perform per oral endoscopic myotomy for achalasia. However, treatment of the diverticulum differs. In one case, the diverticulum is inverted into the lumen, and an endoscopic snare placed around the neck of the diverticulum. The mucosa eventually sloughs and the defect is healed over time. In the second case, a channel is created between the diverticulum and the gastric body by means of a transdiverticulum-to-gastric puncture and subsequent dilation of the channel and placement of an endoscopic stent. The authors cautioned

about the development of gastroesophageal reflux. At the present time, an endoscopic approach should be considered experimental and while the distal myotomy can be performed successfully, endoscopic management of the diverticulum requires further thought and innovation to minimize the risk of gastroesophageal reflux and the potential stricture from mucosal sloughing.

CURRENT CONTROVERSIES IN SURGICAL APPROACH

Surgeons caring for patients with an epiphrenic diverticulum and who wish to approach these minimally invasively should be sufficiently skilled in both laparoscopy and thoracoscopy, because even though the diverticulum is commonly just above the gastroesophageal junction, it can be located anywhere in the distal esophagus with the cephalad edge located above the inferior pulmonary veins. During laparoscopic hiatal hernia repair, access to the level of the inferior pulmonary veins can consistently be achieved but rarely above this point. In the patient with a normal hiatus access, visualization into the mediastinum can be limited. It is likely then that diverticula that are greater than 5 cm from the GEJ will be inadequately addressed with a transhiatal dissection, with a higher propensity for incomplete resection or a staple line leak at the superior-most aspect of the diverticulectomy. This is supported by a recent report by Allaix et al.[36] in which 13 patients with achalasia and epiphrenic diverticulum underwent attempted resection. The diverticulum was excised in six patients but left in situ in seven patients. In four of the seven patients, the diverticulum was left in place because it was too far from the GEJ and could not be safely dissected laparoscopically. Postoperatively,

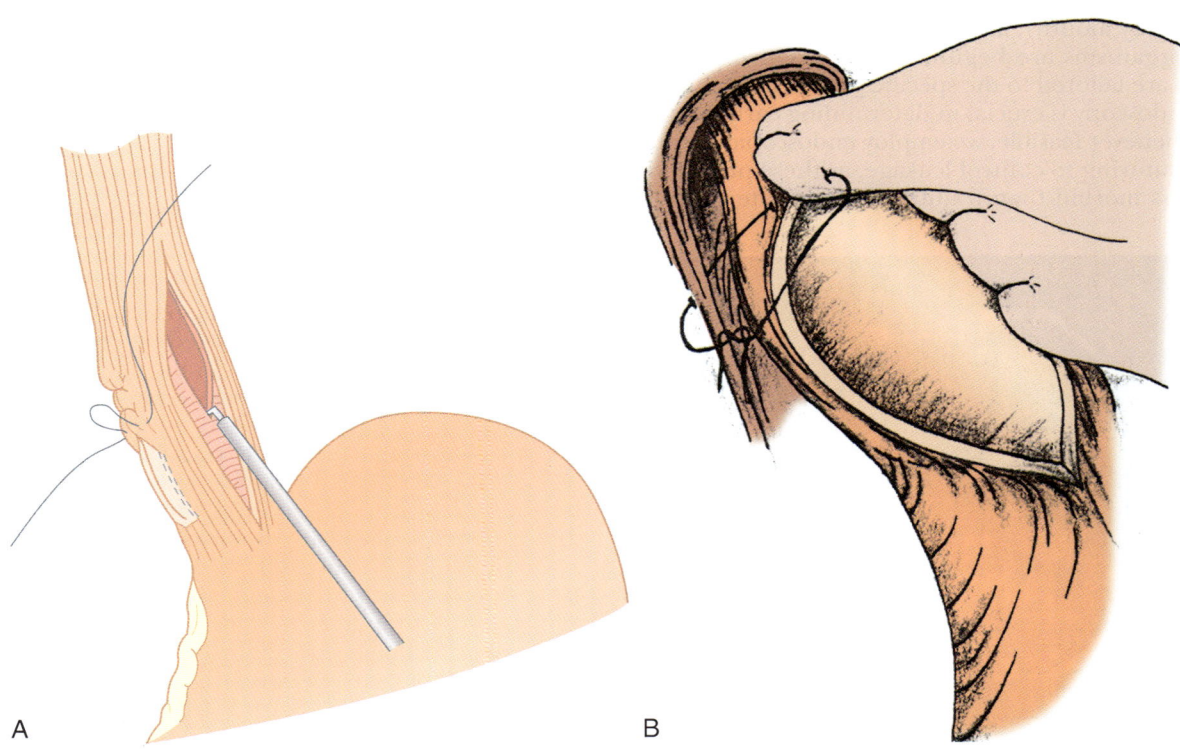

A   B

FIGURE 12.9 (A) Heller myotomy performed on the opposite esophageal wall of the stapled line and extending for approximately 2 cm on the gastric side. (B) A Dor fundoplication is constructed by suturing the anterior fundic wall to the edges of the myotomy.

patient symptoms were controlled as measured by the Eckardt score, but with only 2 years of follow-up. This contrasts with other reports recommending the addition of a VATS in these high diverticula.[8,30]

Regardless of symptoms, it is unclear what the impact is of leaving the diverticulum in situ with its long-term potential for bleeding, impaction, and stasis with regurgitation. Until further data are reported, it is advisable except in extenuating circumstances or a small diverticulum that disappears after myotomy to resect the diverticulum. In patients with high diverticula, a combined VATS and laparoscopic approach may be a more suitable and efficacious option. One strategy is to assess the location of the diverticulum based on the location of the upper border of the diverticulum in relation to the endoscopically identified GEJ. For diverticula less than 5 cm above the GEJ, a laparoscopic transhiatal approach is likely to be successful, whereas for those greater than 5 cm above the GEJ or above the inferior pulmonary vein, a combined thoracoscopic-laparoscopic minimally invasive approach is likely necessary.[8]

The need for an esophagomyotomy is accepted by most esophageal surgeons based on the fact that most diverticula are associated with an underlying motility disorder, and theoretically, a distal obstruction or high pressure zone potentially increases the risk for staple line dehiscence and subsequent leakage.[13,21] However, selective use of a myotomy in patients without a motility disorder has been proposed based on a small series of patients.[37] The rationale for abstaining from a myotomy is that patients with a normal LES will resolve their symptoms after diverticulectomy alone; myotomy creates the potential for GERD, which requires a fundoplication and/or the need for proton pump inhibitor medication, and leaks occur regardless of the presence of a myotomy. There has been no clear resolution about the use of a myotomy, but the majority of cases reported in the literature include a myotomy, and it is suggested to include a myotomy as part of treatment until additional data supporting its exclusion is provided.

COMPLICATIONS

Regardless of the surgical approach, the operative risks remain significant in a patient population that is often malnourished, elderly, has significant comorbidities, and potentially long-standing pulmonary soilage from aspiration. A wide variety of postoperative complications have been reported but complications specific to this operation include staple line leak, incomplete myotomy, vagal nerve injury (manifested by delayed gastric emptying), and pleural effusion. Broader complications that are more commonly associated with open resection have also been reported and include intraoperative hemorrhage, pulmonary complications (acute respiratory distress syndrome, pneumonia), and cardiac events (atrial fibrillation, infarction).

The most significant complication is a staple line leak (Fig. 12.10). These are best avoided by careful and meticulous dissection, reapproximation of the esophageal muscle, and complete myotomy.[9] When a staple line leaks occurs, treatment is individualized for the patient and the extent of leak. Patients are made nil per os (NPO, or nothing by mouth), antibiotics to cover gram-negative enteric organisms are begun, and alternative forms of nutrition are tailored to the specific patient and situation. Upper endoscopy is crucial in determining early management. Whenever feasible, we employ endoscopic stenting, clips, or suturing to control leakage, as these procedures are far less morbid than traditional open interventions.

One recent alternative is to consider placement of an endoluminal wound vac sponge to manage the staple line disruption.[38] However, if less invasive endoscopic measures prove unsuccessful in mitigating leakage, return to the operating room is always available for wide drainage, control of contamination, and diversion (when necessary).

OUTCOMES OF DIVERTICULECTOMY AND MYOTOMY

The surgical treatment results for epiphrenic diverticula in series reporting at least 10 cases are tabulated in Tables 12.1 and 12.2. Regardless of the approach, transthoracic or minimally invasive, the reported outcomes show good to excellent relief of symptoms in the majority of patients. The operative mortality rate has decreased with transition to a minimally invasive approach, but the rates of morbidity remain significant, likely reflecting the underlying age and comorbidities that are carried by patients with this disease. Lastly, the postoperative leak rate remains the Achilles heel of any operation on the esophageal mucosa though it appears the prompt treatment has been able to successfully manage the leak without mortality or compromise of long-term outcomes.

At present, epiphrenic diverticula remain a rare disease with most surgeons reporting on 20 to 30 cases over decades of care. Over the last two decades, there has been a slow but steady transition away from a transthoracic approach to the use of minimally invasive techniques that maintain the surgical principles outlined for the treatment of epiphrenic diverticula. The cumulative experience to date suggests that a laparoscopic approach is quickly

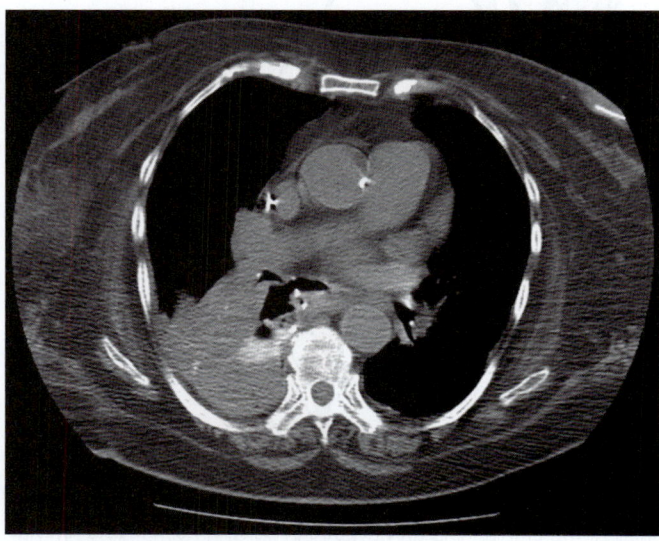

FIGURE 12.10 Computed tomography scan demonstrating a staple line leak with a large abscess cavity in the right chest.

TABLE 12.1 Outcomes of Transthoracic Epiphrenic Diverticulum Surgery

Author	Years	N	Approach	Operation	Mortality (%)	Morbidity (%)	Leak	Outcomes
Allen et al.[21]	1944–53	24	RT	D	4	25		10/24 persistent symptoms
	1954–63	17	LT	D/M	6	18		15/27 good to excellent relief of symptoms
Streitz et al.[37]	1960–90	18	LT	D (8) D/M (10)	0	33	6	Median follow-up = 7 years • 13/18 good to excellent relief of symptoms • Neurogenic
Fékéte et al.[43]	1969–89	27	RT/LT Lap	D (10) D/M/F (10) M/F (4)	11	19	7	
Altorki et al.[44]	1970–90	17	LT	D/M/F (14)	6			Median follow-up = 7 years • 13/17 symptom free • 1/17 poor result
Benacci et al.[11]	1975–91	33	LT	D (7) D/M (22) M (1) Resection (3)	9.1	33	18	Median follow-up = 7 years • 67% good to excellent outcomes • 33% poor to fair outcomes
Castrucci et al.[45]	1983–95	27	LT	D (5) D/M (5) D/M/F (17)	7	11	4	Mean follow-up = 47 months • 92% satisfied • Visick I and II
Nehra et al.[13]	1987–96	21	LT	D/M/F	5		5	Median follow-up = 24 months • 88% good to excellent outcomes
Varghese et al.[7]	1976–2005	35	LT	D/M/F (33)	2.8	9	6	Median follow-up = 33 months • 76% excellent resolution of symptoms • 21 mild dysphagia
D'Journo et al.[46]	1977–2008	23	LT	D/M/F	0	9		Median follow-up = 61 months • Significant symptom improvement

D, Diverticulectomy; *F,* fundoplication; *Lap,* Laparoscopic transhiatal; *LT,* left thoracotomy; *M,* myotomy; *RT,* right thoracotomy.

TABLE 12.2 Outcomes of Minimally Invasive Epiphrenic Diverticulum Surgery

Author	Years	N	Approach	Operation	Mortality (%)	Morbidity (%)	Leak (%)	Outcomes
Rosati et al.[47] Fumagalli et al.[48]	1994–2012	30	Lap	D/M/F	0	6	3.3	Median follow-up = 52 months • Excellent results • 3/19 mild symptoms
Klaus et al.[49]	1996–2000	10	Lap	D/M (6) D (4)	0	20	10	Median follow-up 26 months • Symptom score significantly improved
Fernando et al.[29] Macke et al.[6]	1997–2012	57	V (33) Lap (18) Lap/V (6)	D (6) D/M (27) D/M/F (20) D/F (3)	2	30	11	Mean follow-up = 21 months • Dysphagia improved • GERD-HRQL = 5
Del Genio et al.[50]	1994–2002	13	Lap	D/M/F	8	30	23	Median follow-up = 58 months • 100% good to excellent outcome
Soares et al.[30]	1997–2008	23	Lap (19) Lap/V (4)	D/M/F (16)	4.3	26	0	Median follow-up = 45 months • 85% Good to excellent
Zaninotto et al.[51]	1993–2010	24	Lap (17) Lap/RT (7)	D/M/F (14) D/F (3)	0	35	16.6	Median follow-up = 96 months • 71% successful treatment
Melman et al.[15]	1999–2006	13	Lap	D/M	0	15	8	Median follow-up = 13 months • 15% with persistent dysphagia • 8% with GERD
Palanivelu et al.[52]	—	12	Lap (8) V (4)	D (7) D/M (1) D/M/F (2) D/F (2)	0		8	Median follow-up = 24 months • 1 patient with GERD
Allaix et al.[36]	2009–13	13	Lap	M/F (7) D/M/F (6)	0		17	Mean follow-up = 21 and 11 months • Eckardt score = 0
Achim et al.[8]	2004–15	17	Lap (9) Lap/V (5) V (3)	D/M/F (14) D (3)	6	23.5	18	Median follow-up 10 months • Eckhardt score = 0 • GERD-HRQL = 1

D, Diverticulectomy; *F,* fundoplication; *GERD-HRQL,* Gastroesophageal Reflux Disease Health-Related Quality-of-Life score; *Lap,* Laparoscopic transhiatal; *M,* myotomy; *RT,* right thoracotomy; *V,* right video-assisted thoracic surgery (VATS).

becoming the approach of choice with the addition of VATS for diverticula placed higher in the mediastinum.

MIDDLE ESOPHAGEAL DIVERTICULUM

Mid-esophageal diverticula are true diverticula that involve all layers of the esophagus (mucosa, submucosa, and muscularis) and are found in the middle one-third of the esophagus within 4 to 5 cm of the tracheal carina. They are traditionally thought of as traction diverticula that occur due to mediastinal inflammation pulling on the esophageal wall to create the diverticulum in the middle third of the esophagus.[29] These adhesions are most often caused by a granulomatous inflammatory reaction in subcarinal lymph nodes or by scar tissue.[39] The granulomatous diseases typically associated with these adhesions include sarcoidosis, histoplasmosis, and tuberculosis (Fig. 12.11). In addition, etiologies include a congenital component related to an incomplete tracheal-esophageal fistula or foregut duplication. In addition to the traction etiology, there is most likely a pulsion component, as motility disorders are present in over 80% of patients who present with this type of diverticulum.[40]

SYMPTOMS AND DIAGNOSIS

Mid-esophageal diverticula are typically asymptomatic usually due to their wide-mouth opening and dependent

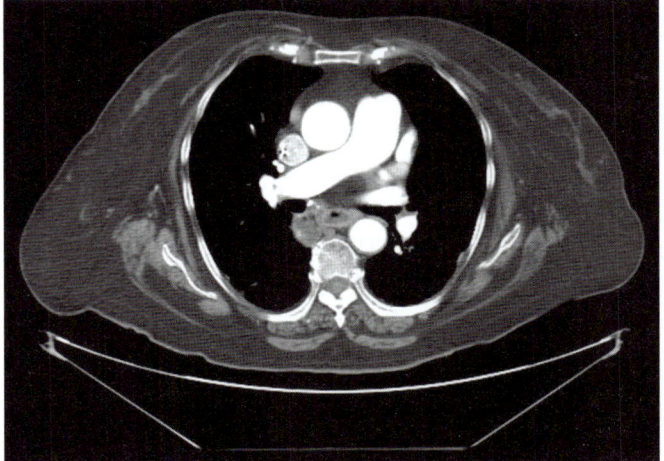

FIGURE 12.11 Computed tomography of the chest with a mid-esophageal diverticulum adjacent to a calcified station 7 mediastinal lymph node.

drainage. They are therefore often diagnosed on esophageal imaging in the work-up of another condition. When symptomatic, most patients present with intermittent dysphagia and some with occasional retrosternal pain, heartburn, and/or acid reflux.[14] Patients will also present due to complications of the traction diverticula. Ongoing

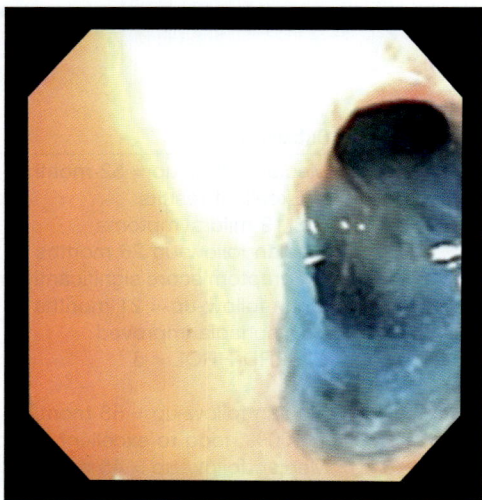

FIGURE 12.12 Bronchoscopy photo of methylene blue in the right upper lobe that was injected from the esophageal side of a diverticulum.

inflammation in the region can lead to the development of a fistula between the diverticulum and the airway[41] and bleeding secondary to erosion into a bronchial artery, small esophageal vessel, or even major vessel.[42] Bleeding is also caused by the friable granulation tissue found at the tip of the diverticulum.

The diagnostic approach to the mid-esophageal diverticulum involves the same investigations that were used for an epiphrenic diverticulum. However, the initial test that identifies the diverticulum is more likely to be a computed tomography scan of the chest during evaluation for mediastinal adenopathy or for chronic cough due to a small fistula. A contrast radiographic study should be included in the evaluation. In the absence of obvious mediastinal pathology being the causative agent, high-resolution manometry should be undertaken given that many of these patients will have an underlying disorder that may impact surgical decision making. During endoscopic evaluation, the option of bronchoscopy should be available, particularly if there is a suspicion for a fistula. This can often be difficult to ascertain, and an injection of dilute methylene blue into the esophagus may be visualized in the proximal airways (Fig. 12.12).

TREATMENT

The indications for surgical treatment are related to the presence of symptoms from the diverticulum. This is best approached with a right thoracotomy through the fifth intercostal space given the ease of access to the carina, mediastinal nodes, and esophagus. The surgeon should expect extreme scarring and distorted anatomy due to the ongoing inflammation. The first step will be to separate the esophagus and diverticulum from the adjoining mediastinal nodes. Once this is accomplished, any fistulous tract should be divided and controlled. The diverticulum should be isolated, and the mucosa should be evaluated and repaired or resected depending on the degree of damage. The overlying muscle layers should be reapproximated over top with an interposition graft usually

of intercostal muscle placed between the repair and the inflamed tissue to prevent recurrence. If an underlying motility disorder has been identified, a distal myotomy should be considered.

Expected outcomes from surgical management of a mid-esophageal diverticulum should approximate those of a distal diverticulum. Specific series addressing these outcomes are limited only to case reports or to a handful of cases included in a larger series of distal esophageal diverticula.

SUMMARY

Mid- and distal esophageal diverticula are uncommon diseases that often present without symptoms. However, some patients will have incapacitating or life-threatening symptoms from either the diverticulum, the underlying motility disorder, or both. After identification by barium swallow, careful evaluation of the patient followed by upper endoscopy, high-resolution manometry, and the occasional CT scan of the chest will provide the key information to decide upon surgical treatment. Similar to many esophageal procedures, treatment of these diverticula has moved toward minimally invasive surgery to perform the diverticulectomy, distal esophageal myotomy, and in most instances a partial fundoplication. Diverticula near the inferior pulmonary vein may be better addressed with a combined VATS and laparoscopy. For most patients, this results in relief of the presenting symptoms and a low rate of mortality but a not insignificant rate of morbidity. The staple line leak remains the key complication surgeons hope to avoid.

REFERENCES

1. Mondiere J. Notes sur quelques maladies de l'oesophage. *Arch Gen Med.* 1833;3:28-65.
2. Soares R, Herbella FA, Prachand VN, Ferguson MK, Patti MG. Epiphrenic diverticulum of the esophagus. From pathophysiology to treatment. *J Gastrointest Surg.* 2010;14(12):2009-2015.
3. Bruggeman LL, Seaman WB. Epiphrenic diverticula. An analysis of 80 cases. *Am J Roentgenol Rad Ther Nucl Med.* 1973;119(2):266-276.
4. Postlethwait RW. Diverticula of the esophagus. In: Postlethwait RW, ed. *Surgery of the Esophagus.* 2nd ed. Norwalk, CT: Appleton-Century-Crofts; 1986:129.
5. Vinson PP. Diverticula of the thoracic portion of the esophagus. *Arch Otolaryngol Head Neck Surg.* 1934;19:508-513.
6. Macke RA, Luketich JD, Pennathur A, et al. Thoracic esophageal diverticula: a 15-year experience of minimally invasive surgical management. *Ann Thorac Surg.* 2015;100(5):1795-1802.
7. Varghese TK, Marshall B, Chang AC, Pickens A, Lau CL, Orringer MB. Surgical treatment of epiphrenic diverticula: a 30-year experience. *Ann Thorac Surg.* 2007;84(6):1801-1809.
8. Achim V, Aye RW, Farivar AS, Vallières E, Louie BE. A combined thoracoscopic and laparoscopic approach for high epiphrenic diverticula and the importance of complete myotomy. *Surg Endosc.* 2017;31(2):788-794.
9. Bowman TA, Sadowitz BD, Ross SB, Boland A, Luberice K, Rosemurgy AS. Heller myotomy with esophageal diverticulectomy: an operation in need of improvement. *Surg Endosc.* 2016;30(8):3279-3288.
10. Debas HT, Payne WS, Cameron AJ, Carlson HC. Physiopathology of lower esophageal diverticulum and its implications for treatment. *Surg Gynecol Obstet.* 1980;151(5):593-600.
11. Benacci JC, Deschamps C, Trastek VF, Allen MS, Daly RC, Pairolero PC. Epiphrenic diverticulum: results of surgical treatment. *Ann Thorac Surg.* 1993;55(5):1109-1114.

12. Fasano NC, Levine MS, Rubesin SE, Redfern RO, Laufer I. Epiphrenic diverticulum: clinical and radiographic findings in 27 patients. *Dysphagia.* 2003;18(1):9-15.

13. Nehra D, Lord R V, DeMeester TR, et al. Physiologic basis for the treatment of epiphrenic diverticulum. *Ann Surg.* 2002;235(3):346-354.

14. Nascimento F, Lemme E, Costa M. Esophageal diverticula: pathogenesis, clinical aspects, and natural history. *Dysphagia.* 2006;198-205.

15. Melman L, Quinlan J, Robertson B, et al. Esophageal manometric characteristics and outcomes for laparoscopic esophageal diverticulectomy, myotomy, and partial fundoplication for epiphrenic diverticula. *Surg Endosc Other Interv Tech.* 2009;23(6):1337-1341.

16. Fisichella PM, Jalilvand A, Dobrowolsky A. Achalasia and epiphrenic diverticulum. *World J Surg.* 2015;39(7):1614-1649.

17. Dodds WJ, Stef JJ, Hogan WJ, Hoke SE, Stewart ET, Arndorfer RC. Radial distribution of esophageal peristaltic pressure in normal subjects and patients with esophageal diverticulum. *Gastroenterology.* 1975;69:584-590.

18. Orringer MB. Epiphrenic diverticula: fact and fable. *Ann Thorac Surg.* 1993;55(5):1067-1068.

19. Kostic SV, Rice TW, Baker ME, et al. Timed barium esophagogram: a simple physiologic assessment for achalasia. *J Thorac Cardiovasc Surg.* 2000;120(5):935-943.

20. Oezcelik A, Hagen JA, Halls JM, et al. An improved method of assessing esophageal emptying using the timed barium study following surgical myotomy for achalasia. *J Gastrointest Surg.* 2009;13(1):14-18.

21. Allen TH, Claggett OT. Changing concepts in the surgical treatment of pulsion diverticula of the lower esophagus. *J Thorac Cardiovasc Surg.* 1965;50(4):455-462.

22. Richards WO, Torquati A, Holzman MD, et al. Heller myotomy versus Heller myotomy with Dor fundoplication for achalasia: a prospective randomized double-blind clinical trial. *Ann Surg.* 2004;240(3):405-412.

23. Little AG, Soriano A, Ferguson MK, Winans CS, Skinner DB. Surgical treatment of achalasia: results with esophagomyotomy and Belsey repair. *Ann Thorac Surg.* 1988;45(5):489-494.

24. Peracchia A, Bonavina L, Rosati R. Thoracoscopic resection of epiphrenic esophageal diverticula. In: Peters JH, DeMeester T, eds. *Minimally Invasive Surgery of the Foregut.* St. Louis: Quality Medical Publishing; 1995:110.

25. Boeckxstaens GE, Annese V, des Varannes SB, et al. Pneumatic dilation versus laparoscopic Heller's myotomy for idiopathic achalasia. *N Engl J Med.* 2011;364(19):1807-1816.

26. Pellegrini C, Wetter L, Patti M, et al. Thoracoscopic esophagomyotomy. Initial experience with a new approach for the treatment of achalasia. *Ann Surg.* 1992;216(3):291-296.

27. Stewart KC, Finley RJ, Clifton JC, Graham AJ, Storseth C, Inculet R. Thoracoscopic versus laparoscopic modified Heller myotomy for achalasia: efficacy and safety in 87 patients. *J Am Coll Surg.* 1999;189(2):164-170.

28. Rosati R, Fumagalli U, Bona S, Bonavina L, Peracchia A. Diverticulectomy, myotomy, and fundoplication through laparoscopy: a new option to treat epiphrenic esophageal diverticula? *Ann Surg.* 1998;227(2):174-178.

29. Fernando HC, Luketich JD, Samphire J, et al. Minimally invasive operation for esophageal diverticula. *Ann Thorac Surg.* 2005;80(6):2076-2080.

30. Soares RV, Montenovo M, Pellegrini CA, Oelschlager BK. Laparoscopy as the initial approach for epiphrenic diverticulum. *Surg Endosc Other Interv Tech.* 2011;25(12):3740-3746.

31. Bellevue OC, Louie BE. Laparoscopic diverticulectomy and myotomy. In: Wee J, Linden PA, eds. *Thoracic and Esophageal Surgery.* Scientific American; In press.

32. Pasricha PJ, Hawari R, Ahmed I, et al. Submucosal endoscopic esophageal myotomy: a novel experimental approach for the treatment of achalasia. *Endoscopy.* 2007;39(9):761-764.

33. Inoue H. Peroral endoscopic myotomy (POEM) for esophageal achalasia. *Endoscopy.* 2010;42:265-271.

34. Khashab MA. Thoughts on starting a peroral endoscopic myotomy program. *Gastrointest Endosc.* 2013;77(1):109-110.

35. Liu B-R, Song J, Fan Q. 899 endoscopic esophageal epiphrenic diverticulum inversion by using the submucosal tunneling technique. *Gastrointest Endosc.* 2015;81(5):AB180.

36. Allaix ME, BorraezSegura BA, Herbella FA, Fisichella PM, Patti MG. Is resection of an esophageal epiphrenic diverticulum always necessary in the setting of achalasia? *World J Surg.* 2015;39(1):203-207.

37. Streitz JM, Glick ME, Ellis H Jr. Selective use of myotomy for treatment of epiphrenic diverticula. *Arch Surg.* 1992;127:585-588.

38. Smallwood N, Fleshman J, Leeds S, Burdick J. The use of endoluminal vacuum (E-Vac) therapy in the management of upper gastrointestinal leaks and perforations. *Surg Endosc.* 2016;30(6):2473-2480.

39. Dukes RJ, Strimlan CV, Dines DE, Payne WS, MacCarty RL. Esophageal involvement with mediastinal granuloma. *JAMA.* 1976;236(20):2313-2315.

40. Kaye MD. Oesophageal motor dysfunction in patients with diverticula of the mid-thoracic oesophagus. *Thorax.* 1974;29(6):666-672.

41. Wychulis AR, Ellis FH, Andersen HA. Acquired nonmalignant esophagotracheobronchial fistula. Report of 36 cases. *JAMA.* 1966;196(2):117-122.

42. Jonasson OM, Gunn LC. Midesophageal diverticulum with hemorrhage. *Arch Surg.* 1965;90:713-715.

43. Fékéte F, Vonns C. Surgical management of esophageal thoracic diverticula. *Hepatogastroenterology.* 1992;39(2):97-99.

44. Altorki NK, Sunagawa M, Skinner DB. Thoracic esophageal diverticula. Why is operation necessary? *J Thorac Cardiovasc Surg.* 1993;105(2):260-264.

45. Castrucci G, Porziella V, Granone PL, Picciocchi A. Tailored surgery for esophageal body diverticula. *Eur J Cardiothorac Surg.* 1998;14(4):380-387.

46. D'Journo XB, Ferraro P, Martin J, Chen LQ, Duranceau A. Lower oesophageal sphincter dysfunction is part of the functional abnormality in epiphrenic diverticulum. *Br J Surg.* 2009;96(8):892-900.

47. Rosati R, Fumagalli U, Elmore U, De Pascale S, Massaron S, Peracchia A. Long-term results of minimally invasive surgery for symptomatic epiphrenic diverticulum. *Am J Surg.* 2011;201(1):132-135.

48. Fumagalli Romario U, Ceolin M, Porta M, Rosati R. Laparoscopic repair of epiphrenic diverticulum. *Semin Thorac Cardiovasc Surg.* 2012;24(3):213-217.

49. Klaus A, Hinder RA, Swain J, Achem SR. Management of epiphrenic diverticula. *J Gastrointest Surg.* 2003;7(7):906-911.

50. Del Genio A, Rossetti G, Maffetton V, et al. Laparoscopic approach in the treatment of epiphrenic diverticula: long-term results. *Surg Endosc.* 2004;18(5):741-745.

51. Zaninotto G, Parise P, Salvador R, et al. Laparoscopic repair of epiphrenic diverticulum. *Semin Thorac Cardiovasc Surg.* 2012;24(3):218-222.

52. Palanivelu C, Rangarajan M, Maheshkumaar GS, Senthilkumar R. Minimally invasive surgery combined with peroperative endoscopy for symptomatic middle and lower esophageal diverticula: a single institute's experience. *Surg Laparosc Endosc Percutan Tech.* 2008;18(2):133-138.

Epidemiology, Diagnosis, and Medical Management of Achalasia

Edy Soffer

Achalasia is a rare esophageal disorder presenting primarily with dysphagia, characterized by well-defined esophageal motor abnormalities. This chapter addresses the epidemiology, pathophysiology, and diagnosis of achalasia, as well as the medical therapeutic options for this disorder.

EPIDEMIOLOGY

Epidemiologic data originate mostly from Western populations and vary among studies. The incidence rate ranges from a low of 0.03/100,000 per year to 1.63/100,000 per year, with the majority of rates clustering between 0.5 and 1.2/100,000 per year, with prevalence rates of approximately 10/100,000.[1,2] Hospitalizations for achalasia increase in frequency with age, with a peak incidence in those older than 65 years, reaching a high of 37/100,000 in patients older than 85 years.[3] The incidence of achalasia is comparable among males and females, and it can affect adults of all age groups.[1,4] A genetic etiology is documented in a fraction of patients with achalasia. The triple-A syndrome (Allgrove disease) is a rare condition presenting with achalasia, alacrima, adrenocorticotropic hormone (ACTH)–resistant adrenal insufficiency, and neurologic disturbances.[5–7] A few familial cases have been described.[8,9] Polymorphisms in the nitric oxide synthase gene have been investigated, but data are conflicting. No difference in polymorphisms was found between patients with achalasia and controls; however, a recent report described two siblings with infant-onset achalasia that were homozygous for a premature stop codon in the gene encoding nitric oxide synthase.[10,11] Idiopathic achalasia was also found to be associated with class II human leukocyte antigens (HLAs).[12]

DIAGNOSIS

Progressive dysphagia to both solids and liquids is the most common presenting symptom (90%), followed by regurgitation of undigested food (76% to 91%), respiratory complications (nocturnal cough [30%] and aspiration [8%]), chest pain (25% to 64%), heartburn (18% to 52%), and weight loss (35% to 91%).[13,14] However, symptoms are nonspecific, and the diagnosis is commonly delayed by a number of years after the onset of symptoms. Patients often accommodate to their dysphagia by changing their eating habits, avoiding solid food such as meat and bread, and drinking liquids with their meals. Unless specifically asked, they may not provide these clues to their condition. Heartburn, caused by fermentation of retained food in the esophagus, and regurgitation can lead to an incorrect

diagnosis of gastroesophageal reflux disease. In fact, in a series of 145 untreated patients with achalasia, 65% were taking acid-suppressing medications at the time of referral.[13]

Once the diagnosis of achalasia is suspected, anatomic evaluation is required to exclude other conditions that can mimic achalasia. Endoscopy is particularly useful for diagnosing mechanical obstruction or pseudoachalasia, a rare entity caused by tumors involving the gastroesophageal junction.[15] Occasionally tumors may infiltrate the tissue beneath the mucosa, and in such cases imaging studies such as endoscopic ultrasound or computed tomography scan are required for diagnosis. Endoscopic findings in the more advanced stage of achalasia include a dilated esophagus containing retained saliva or food residue, stasis changes in the mucosa, and occasionally the presence of candidiasis. However, early on endoscopic findings may be unremarkable. The puckered appearing gastroesophageal junction presents with mild resistance when attempting to intubate the stomach. The feeling of a stronger resistance should raise suspicion for pseudoachalasia, and the need for further evaluation. Careful inspection of the gastroesophageal junction (GEJ) and cardia, including a retroflex view, should help exclude infiltrating lesions.

RADIOLOGY

Typical findings on barium esophagram in advanced disease are a dilated esophagus with food and contrast retention, lack of peristaltic stripping waves, and a narrowed GEJ (the so-called *bird beak*). The type III variant can present radiographically with a corkscrew appearance, the result of spastic contractions. Comparable to endoscopy, radiologic findings in early disease may be nonspecific. Radiology is helpful in assessing esophageal emptying using the time barium esophagram (TBE). This simple technique involves drinking a large bolus of barium in an upright position and obtaining a radiograph after 1 and 5 minutes and assessing the height of the barium column in the esophagus (Fig. 13.1).[16] This measure proved useful in predicting symptomatic response to therapy, whether by balloon dilatation or by myotomy. Lack of adequate reduction in the height of the barium column after therapy was associated with higher risk of treatment failure during follow-up, and should prompt careful follow-up or reintervention in such patients.[17,18]

MANOMETRY

The diagnosis of achalasia is contingent upon the presence of impaired lower esophageal sphincter (LES) relaxation and apersiatalsis, in the absence of obstructive lesions involving the gastroesophageal junction.[19] While endoscopy

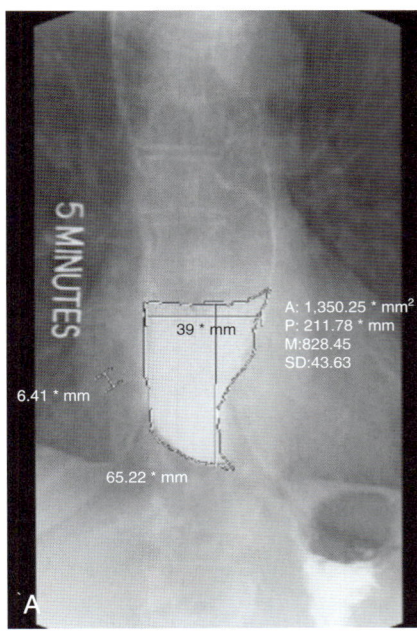
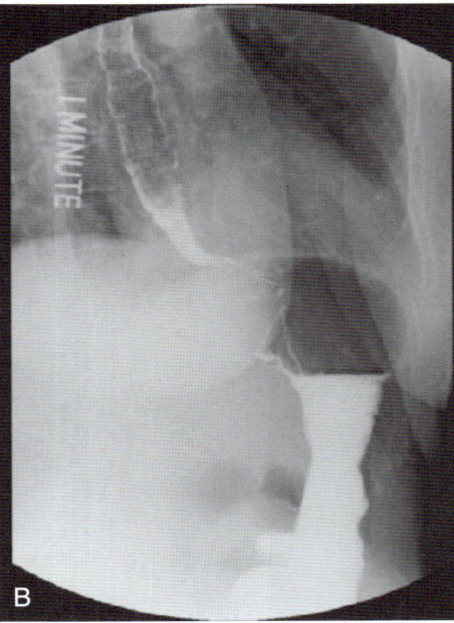

FIGURE 13.1 Time barium esophagram in achalasia. (A) Appearance at 5 minutes after swallow, with retention of contrast in a dilated esophagus. (B) Near complete clearance at 1 minute in a nondilated esophagus, following successful myotomy.

and imaging studies are complementary tests to the diagnosis, and can be highly suggestive in classic achalasia, they are frequently not sensitive enough, and manometry is required for proper diagnosis. Traditional esophageal manometry was performed with water-perfused or strain gauge systems, usually with sensors spaced a few centimeters apart, with a line mode display. The last decade saw the replacement of the traditional system by high-resolution manometry (HRM) systems. Originally conceived by Clouse, the system includes catheters that incorporate multiple sensors, spaced 1 cm apart, allowing recording from the upper esophageal sphincter to the stomach, and software that provides esophageal pressure topography (EPT) display, with an added presentation in color mode.[20] HRM simplifies the recording process and facilitates the identification of pressure events and pattern recognition. In the case of achalasia, it has tightened diagnostic criteria by the introduction of new metrics, and in particular the development of the integrated relaxation pressure (IRP) for better assessment of esophagogastric junction (EGJ) relaxation.[21] Esophageal pressure topography has allowed for the classification of achalasia into three variants on the basis of the contractile pattern of the esophageal body.[22] In type I achalasia (classic achalasia), no contractile activity is detected and no significant pressurization is within the esophageal body. In type II achalasia, swallowing water results in panesophageal pressurization, while type III achalasia (spastic/vigorous achalasia) is associated with premature contractions (characterized by short distal latency; Fig. 13.2). Most recently, a new recording method, the functional lumen imaging probe (FLIP), has detected esophageal contractile activity in achalasia not seen with the standard thin intraluminal manometric catheters.[23] The pathophysiologic and prognostic implications of these patterns require further study. A number of publications have highlighted the clinical prognostic value of these variants in predicting response to medical or surgical therapy, whereby patients with type II variant have the best response, those with type III have the poorest response but tend to do better with myotomy as compared to pneumatic dilation, and type I patients present with intermediate response that worsens with increasing dilatation of the esophagus.[22,24]

Another entity, recently detected by HRM, EGJ outflow obstruction, is characterized by impaired EGJ relaxation in the presence of preserved peristaltic contractions (see Fig. 13.2).[25] In some patients it is secondary to obstructive etiologies such as paraesophageal hernia, Schatzki ring, benign, or malignant tumors involving the EGJ, while in others, no obvious abnormality is found. Imaging studies are required to distinguish the secondary from the primary group. Some of the patients with primary GEJ outlet obstruction may go on to develop achalasia.[25,26] Various treatment modalities for symptomatic patients have been reported, including balloon dilation, botulinum toxin A (Botox) injection, and Heller myotomy, with varying degrees of success. In some patients spontaneous resolution has been documented.[25,27,28]

MEDICAL MANAGEMENT

Treatment modalities for achalasia, whether surgical, endoscopic, or medical, are aimed at reducing the resistance to esophageal emptying by reducing LES tone, since meaningful peristaltic activity cannot be restored by any intervention. The purpose of all treatment modalities is to relieve symptoms and prevent complications such as weight loss, aspiration pneumonia, and further dilation of the esophagus. Nonsurgical treatments consist primarily of pharmacologic therapy and pneumatic balloon dilation (PD).

PHARMACOLOGIC THERAPY

This approach uses smooth muscle relaxants to reduce LES tone. Nitrates and calcium channel blockers are the most commonly used. A review of randomized trials concluded

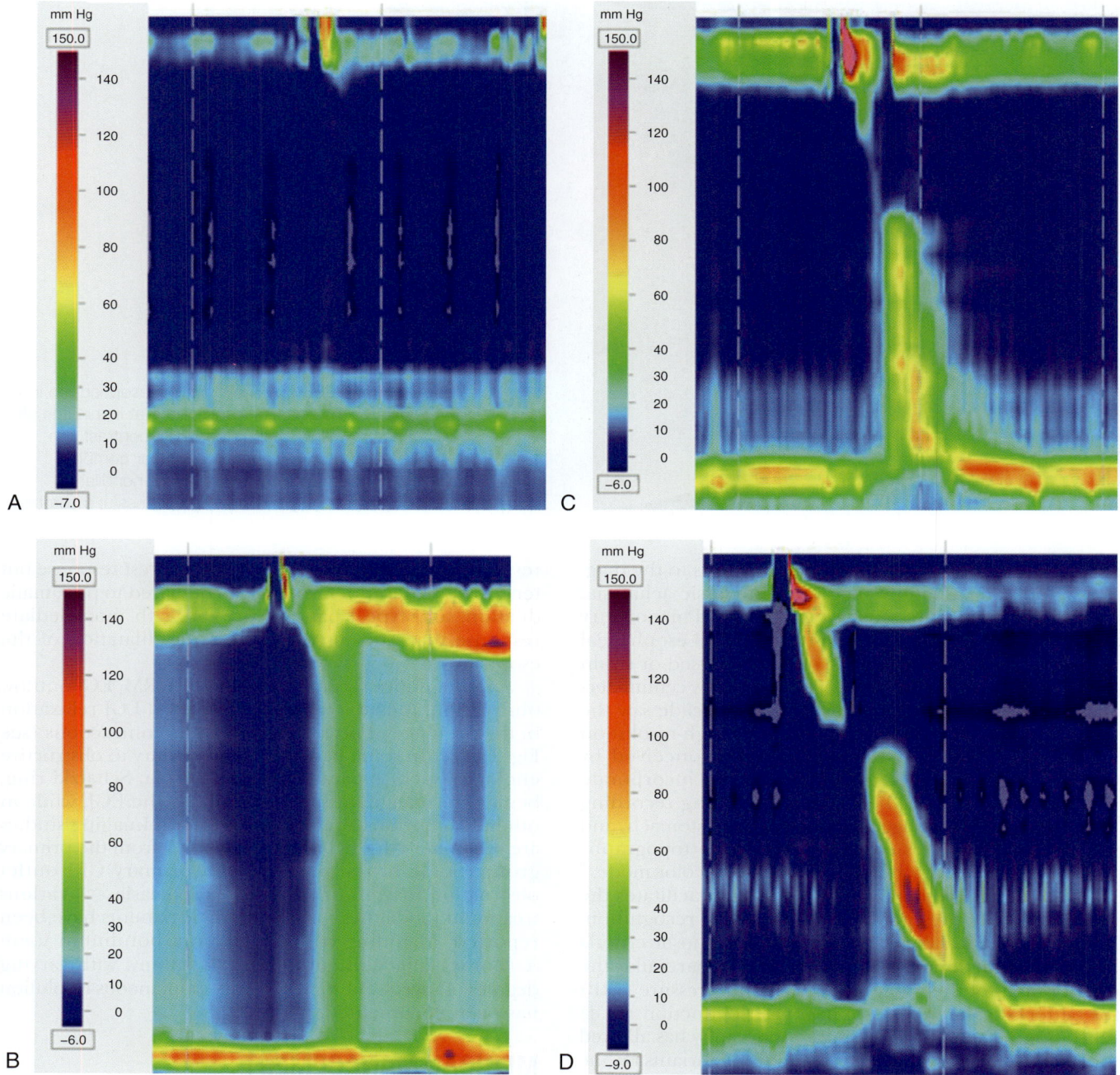

FIGURE 13.2 Subtypes of achalasia as they appear on high-resolution manometry. (A) Type I achalasia is characterized by absent peristalsis. (B) Type II achalasia is characterized by panesophageal pressurization, the result of pressure buildup within a closed cavity. (C) Type III achalasia is characterized by contractile activity with short latency (spastic) following a swallow. (D) Esophagogastric junction outflow obstruction in a patient with dysphagia. Incomplete swallow-induced lower esophageal sphincter relaxation (high integrated relaxation pressure) with normal contractile sequence.

that there was not enough evidence to determine the therapeutic efficacy of nitrates in achalasia.[29] When used, they should be delivered in sublingual form, such as isosorbide dinitrate 5 mg, taken 10 to 15 minutes before meals. Nifedipne, a calcium channel blocker, is also taken sublingually, at a dose of 10 to 30 mg) 30 to 45 minutes before meals.[30,31,32] Limited symptomatic response and side effects such as hypotension, dizziness, and headaches limit

the use of these agents. Hence these agents are useful in patients in whom more definitive interventions are deemed too risky, or when patients desire a low-risk therapy.

BOTULINUM TOXIN

This agent has been more thoroughly studied, and is more widely used. Botulinum toxin A is a neurotoxin that inhibits the release of acetylcholine from the nerve terminal, thus

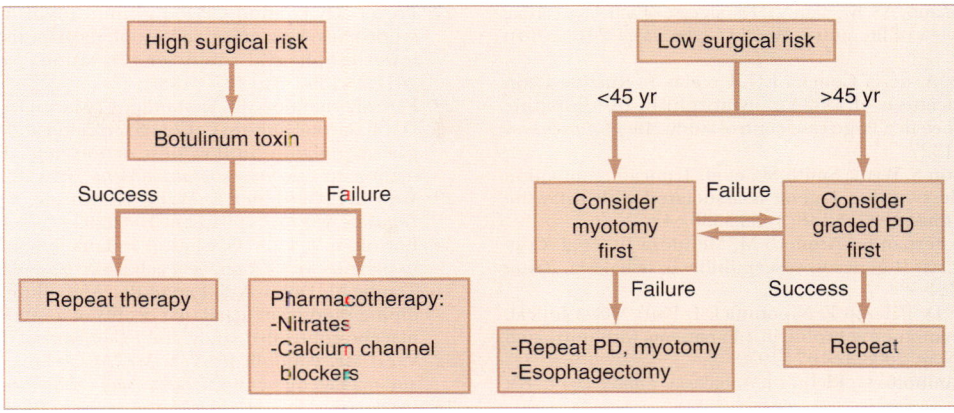

FIGURE 13.3 Suggested approach to the patient with dysphagia. *PD,* Pneumatic balloon dilation. (Modified with permission from Richter JE. Esophageal motility disorder achalasia. *Curr Opin Otolaryngol Head Neck Surg.* 2013;21:535–542.)

blocking the neurogenic but not the myogenic component of LES tone. It is injected into the LES endoscopically by a sclerotherapy needle, at a total dose of 100 U, usually divided in four aliquots, injected to the four quadrants of the LES, just above the squamocolumnar junction. Prospective randomized controlled trials compared its therapeutic efficacy with pneumatic dilation and with surgical intervention.[33,34] While the response rate early on is quite high and comparable to more invasive interventions, relapse is observed in approximately 50% of patients by 1 year, and repeat injections are required. Given the simplicity and good safety profile of this intervention, it is an attractive option in patients who are unsuitable for more risky interventions.

BALLOON DILATION

The main medical intervention for achalasia is PD. It is currently done with a standard noncompliant balloon (with a Rigiflex dilator by Boston Scientific) and comes in three sizes (30, 35, and 40 mm diameters). It is positioned across the LES, commonly under fluoroscopic control and with the aid of a guidewire, and is inflated with air to forcefully stretch the LES muscle. The balloon is kept inflated for about 15 to 60 seconds, while straightening of the balloon waist at the level of the LES is observed. Following dilation, patients are evaluated by a Gastrografin study followed by a barium esophagram to exclude esophageal perforation.[32] Graded dilation, starting with the smallest diameter, is the recommended approach, with symptomatic and radiographic assessment within 4 to 6 weeks after treatment, and repeat dilation with a larger size balloon in case of failed response. Clinical response following PD as the initial therapy for achalasia varies depending on the balloon size and number of dilations. A success rate of 28% versus 44% was achieved at 6 years with single versus serial dilation, respectively.[35] A number of variables have been associated with a favorable response to PD, including older age (>45 years), female gender, LES pressure of less than 10 mm Hg following PD, narrow esophagus prior to PD, and type II pattern on HRM, and may influence the selection of medical versus surgical treatment approach.[22,36,37] Balloon dilation can also be performed after failed Heller myotomy, though response

is suboptimal in patients with adequate reduction in LES pressure.[38] Chest pain is common after PD, but the feared complication is perforation. Previous data suggested rates of 0% to 16%, but a recent systematic review reported a rate of about 1%, comparable to the rate of unrecognized perforation during Heller myotomy.[39,40] Fig. 13.3 outlines a suggested algorithm for the treatment of patients with achalasia.

ESOPHAGEAL STENTS

Initial experience in a small number of patients demonstrated limited success but substantial morbidity.[41,42] Recently the use of temporary, self-expanding, fully covered metal stents or partially covered metal stents was reported.[43,44] Diameter varied between 20 and 30 mm, and stents were removed after 6 or 30 days, respectively. Follow-up of up to 36 months showed good remission rates with low morbidity related to stent migration in a few patients. This treatment modality may be attractive in high-risk patients, but further data are needed for better assessment of its role in the therapeutic approach to achalasia.

REFERENCES

1. O'Neill OM, Johnston BT, Coleman HG. Achalasia: a review of clinical diagnosis, epidemiology, treatment and outcomes. *World J Gastroenterol.* 2013;19(35):5806-5812.
2. Kim E, Lee H, Jung HK, Lee KJ. Achalasia in Korea: an epidemiologic study using a national healthcare database. *J Korean Med Sci.* 2014; 29(4):576-580.
3. Sonnenberg A. Hospitalization for achalasia in the United States 1997–2006. *Dig Dis Sci.* 2009;54:1680.
4. Podas T, Eaden J, Mayberry M, Mayberry J. Achalasia: a critical review of epidemiological studies. *Am J Gastroenterol.* 1998;93:2345-2347.
5. Allgrove J, Claden GS, Grant DB, Macaulay JC. Familial glucocorticoid deficiency with achalasia of the cardia and deficient tear production. *Lancet.* 1978;1:1284-1286.
6. Stuckey BG, Mastaglia FL, Reed WD, Pullan PT. Glucocorticoid insufficiency, achalasia, alacrima with autonomic motor neuropathy. *Ann Intern Med.* 1987;106(1):61-63.
7. Handschg K, Sperling S, Yoon SJ, Hennig S, Clark AJ, Huebner A. Triple A syndrome is caused by mutations in AAAS, a new WD-repeat protein gene. *Hum Mol Genet.* 2001;10:283-290.
8. Gordillo-González G, Guatibonza YP, Zarante I, Roa P, Jacome LA, Hani A. Achalasia familiar: report of a family with an autosomal dominant pattern of inherence. *Dis Esophagus.* 2011;24(1):E1-E4.

9. Evsyutina YV, Trukhmanov AS, Ivashkin VT. Family case of achalasia cardia: case report and review of literature. *World J Gastroenterol.* 2014;20(4): 1114-1118.

10. Vigo AG, Martínez A, de la Concha EG, Urcelay E, Ruiz de León A. Suggested association of OS2A polymorphism in idiopathic achalasia: no evidence in a large case-control study. *Am J Gastroenterol.* 2009;104(5):1326-1327.

11. Shteyer E, Edvardson S, Wynia-Smith SL, et al. Truncating mutation in the nitric oxide synthase 1 gene is associated with infantile achalasia. *Gastroenterology.* 2015;148(3):533-536.e4.

12. De la Concha EG, Fernandez-Arquero M, Mendoza JL, et al. Contribution of HLA class II genes to susceptibility in achalasia. *Tissue Antigens.* 1998;52:381-384.

13. Fisichella PM, Raz D, Palazzo F, Niponmick I, Patti MG. Clinical, radiological, and manometric profile in 145 patients with untreated achalasia. *World J Surg.* 2008;32:1974-1979.

14. Boeckxstaens G, Zaninotto G, Richter J. Achalasia. *Lancet.* 2014;383: 83-93.

15. Kahrilas PJ, Kishk SM, Helm JF, Dodds WJ, Harig JM, Hogan WJ. A comparison of pseudoachalasia and achalasia. *Am J Med.* 1987;82:439-446.

16. De Oliveira JM, Birgisson S, Doinoff C, et al. Timed barium swallow: a simple technique for evaluating esophageal emptying in patients with achalasia. *AJR Am J Roentgenol.* 1997;169:473-479.

17. Vaezi MF, Baker ME, Achkar E, Richter JE. Timed barium oesophagram: better predictor of long term success after pneumatic dilation in achalasia than symptom assessment. *Gut.* 2002;50:765-770.

18. Andersson M, Lundell L, Kostic S, et al. Evaluation of the response to treatment in patients with idiopathic achalasia by the timed barium esophagogram: results from a randomized clinical trial. *Dis Esophagus.* 2009;22:264-273.

19. Pandolfino JE, Kahrilas PJ. American Gastroenterological Association medical position statement: clinical use of esophageal manometry. *Gastroenterology.* 2005;128:207-208.

20. Clouse RE, Staiano A. Topography of the esophageal peristaltic pressure wave. *Am J Physiol.* 1991;261(4 Pt 1):G677-G684.

21. Ghosh SK, Pandolfino JE, Rice J, Clarke JO, Kwiatek M, Kahrilas P. Impaired deglutitive EGJ relaxation in clinical esophageal manometry: a quantitative analysis of 400 patients and 75 controls. *Am J Physiol Gastrointest Liver Physiol.* 2007;293:G878-G885.

22. Pandolfino JE, Kwiatek MA, Nealis T, Bulsiewicz W, Post J, Kahrilas PJ. Achalasia: a new clinically relevant classification by high-resolution manometry. *Gastroenterology.* 2008;135:1526-1533.

23. Carlson D, Zhiyue L, Kahrilas P, et al. The functional lumen imaging probe detects esophageal contractility not observed with manometry in patients with achalasia. *Gastroenterology.* 2015;149:1742-1751.

24. Rohof WO, Salvador R, Annese V, et al. Outcomes of treatment of achalasia depend on manometric subtype. *Gastroenterology.* 2013;144: 718-725.

25. Scherer JR, Kwiatek MA, Soper NJ, Pandolfino JE, Kahrilas PJ. Functional esophagogastric junction obstruction with intact peristalsis: a heterogeneous syndrome sometimes akin to achalasia. *J Gastrointest Surg.* 2009;13:2219-2225.

26. Van Hoeij FB, Smout AJ, Bredenoord AJ. Characterization of idiopathic esophagogastric junction outflow obstruction. *Neurogastroenterol Motil.* 2015;27:1310-1316.

27. Porter RF, Gyawali CP. Botulinum toxin injection in dysphagia syndromes with preserved esophageal peristalsis and incomplete lower esophageal sphincter relaxation. *Neurogastroenterol Motil.* 2011;23:139-144, e127–e138.

28. Pérez-Fernández MT, Santander C, Marinero A, Burgos-Santamaría D, Chavarría-Herbozo C. Characterization and follow up of esophagogastric junction outflow obstruction detected by high resolution manometry. *Neurogastroenterol Motil.* 2016;28:116-126.

29. Wen ZH, Gardener E, Wang YP. Nitrates for achalasia. *Cochrane Database Syst Rev.* 2004;(1):CD002299.

30. Bortolotti M, Labo G. Clinical and manometric effects of nifedipine in patients with esophageal achalasia. *Gastroenterology.* 1981;80:39-44.

31. Traube M, Dubovik S, Lange RC, McCallum RW. The role of nifedipine therapy in achalasia: results of a randomized, double-blind, placebo-controlled study. *Am J Gastroenterol.* 1989;84:1259-1262.

32. Vaezi MF, Pandolfi JE, Vela MF. ACG clinical guideline: diagnosis and management of achalasia. *Am J Gastroenterol.* 2013;108:1238-1249.

33. Leyden JE, Moss AC, MacMathuna P. Endoscopic pneumatic dilation versus botulinum toxin injection in the management of primary achalasia. *Cochrane Database Syst Rev.* 2006;(4):CD005046.

34. Campos GM, Vittinghoff E, Rabl C, et al. Endoscopic and surgical treatments for achalasia: a systematic review and meta-analysis. *Ann Surg.* 2009;249:45-57.

35. Vela MF, Richter JE, Khandwala F, et al. The long-term efficacy of pneumatic dilatation and Heller myotomy for the treatment of achalasia. *Clin Gastroenterol Hepatol.* 2006;4:580-587.

36. Farhoomand K, Connor JT, Richter JE, Achkar E, Vaezi MF. Predictors of outcome of pneumatic dilation in achalasia. *Clin Gastroenterol Hepatol.* 2004;2:389-394.

37. Pratap N, Kalapala R, Darisetty S, et al. Achalasia cardia subtyping by high resolution manometry predicts the therapeutic outcome of pneumatic balloon dilatation. *J Neurogastroenterol Motil.* 2011;17:48-53.

38. Guardino JM, Vela MF, Connor JT, Richter JE. Pneumatic dilation for the treatment of achalasia in untreated patients and patients with failed Heller myotomy. *J Clin Gastroenterol.* 2004;38:855-860.

39. Katzka DA, Castell DO. Review article: an analysis of the efficacy, perforation rates and methods used in pneumatic dilation for achalasia. *Aliment Pharmacol Ther.* 2011;34:832-839.

40. Lynch KL, Pandolfino JE, Howden CW, Kahrilas PJ. Major complications of pneumatic dilation and Heller myotomy for achalasia: single-center experience and systematic review of the literature. *Am J Gastroenterol.* 2012;107(12):1817-1825.

41. Mukherjee S, Kaplan DS, Parasher G, Sipple MS. Expandable metal stents in achalasia—is there a role? *Am J Gastroenterol.* 2000;95: 2185-2188.

42. De Palma GD, Lovino P, Masone S, Persico M, Persico G. Self-expanding metal stents for endoscopic treatment of esophageal achalasia unresponsive to conventional treatments: long-term results in eight patients. *Endoscopy.* 2001;33:1027-1030.

43. Zeng Y, Dai YM, Wan XJ. Clinical remission following endoscopic placement of retrievable, fully covered metal stents in patients with esophageal achalasia. *Dis Esophagus.* 2014;27:103-108.

44. Coppola F, Gaia S, Rolle E, Recchia S. Temporary endoscopic metallic stent for idiopathic esophageal achalasia. *Surg Innov.* 2014;21:11-14.

Endoscopic and Surgical Therapies for Achalasia

Paul D. Colavita | Lee L. Swanstrom

With an estimated annual incidence of 1 in 100,000 and prevalence of 10 in 100,000,[1,2] achalasia is a rare, primary motility disorder of the esophagus, defined by absence of normal peristalsis and failure of swallow-induced relaxation of the lower esophageal sphincter (LES). The first described treatment for "cardiospasm" in the 1600s was self-dilatation with oral passage of a whale rib-bone with an attached sponge.[3] In 1937 Lendrum proposed the pathologic mechanism of failed LES relaxation, leading to the new name of achalasia.[4] The etiology of achalasia remains unclear, but autoimmune, viral, and neurodegenerative factors have been implicated in the development of impaired LES relaxation through loss of ganglion cells in Auerbach myenteric plexus, leading to loss of neurotransmitters, such as vasoactive intestinal peptide and nitric oxide.[5–7] As the underlying mechanism for achalasia development remains unknown, current treatment options rely on disruption of the LES to relieve outflow obstruction.

Patients typically present with progressive dysphagia, volume regurgitation, and sometimes noncardiac chest pain.

PREOPERATIVE WORK-UP

An upper gastrointestinal series or esophagram is the usual initial test to evaluate dysphagia, although some clinicians include endoscopy as an initial assessment. An esophagram will often demonstrate a "bird's beak" tapering of the distal esophagus, with progressive dilatation and tortuosity of the esophagus demonstrated in later stages of the disease. The definitive diagnosis requires confirmation by manometry, preferably high-resolution manometry (HRM). Endoscopy is important to rule out pseudoachalasia from an obstruction, such as cancer, and endoscopic ultrasound can be considered when suspicion for malignancy causing obstruction is high. Endoscopy frequently appears normal in early stages of the disease, as dilation of the esophageal body may not have occurred, but esophagitis from stasis and/or yeast esophagitis may be present. Later stages of disease may demonstrate dilatation of the esophageal body with tortuosity or sigmoidization. A timed barium swallow (TBS)[8] provides objective data on esophageal emptying and is commonly used before and as follow-up after treatment for achalasia. TBS involves ingestion of 200 mL of oral contrast, with radiographs taken at baseline and then 1, 2, and 5 minutes after ingestion. The height and width of the barium column at each time period are recorded.

ACHALASIA MANOMETRIC SUBTYPES

With the advent of HRM, three manometric subtypes of achalasia have been described as part of the Chicago Classification.[9] All three require incomplete or failed relaxation of the LES defined by integrated relaxation pressure (IRP) thresholds. Type I is consistent with the classical consideration of achalasia: incomplete or failed relaxation of the LES with no esophageal body contractility. Type II requires absence of normal peristalsis with at least 20% of swallows having panesophageal pressurization. Type III consists of absent normal peristalsis with secondary and tertiary spastic distal esophageal contractions in at least 20% of swallows.[10] The response of these subtypes to various treatments will be discussed in the sections that follow.

TREATMENT OPTIONS

Surgical myotomy was initially described by Heller[11] in 1913, and was performed as a thoracotomy with two separate 8 cm myotomies, separated by 180 degrees. The technique has undergone several modifications and now involves a single anterior myotomy with addition of a partial fundoplication to reduce the incidence of iatrogenic reflux. Pneumatic dilatation became a common treatment in the 1970s and 1980s. In the early 1990s, laparoscopic and thoracoscopic approaches to the Heller myotomy were described.[12,13] Peroral endoscopic myotomy (POEM) was developed in the first decade of this century, but has roots in the 1980s. Ortega[14] described an endoscopic myotomy in 1980, consisting of division of the mucosa and muscle of the LES with two short full thickness incisions. Despite satisfactory outcomes, the technique was not adopted, due to concern for esophageal perforation. POEM was first described by Pasricha[15,16] in 2007 as a "submucosal endoscopic esophageal myotomy" in a porcine model. Inoue presented the first human experience in 2008 with four patients and coined the term "POEM." He published a series on 17 patients 2 years later.[17]

LAPAROSCOPIC HELLER MYOTOMY WITH PARTIAL FUNDOPLICATION

By the mid- to late-1990s, laparoscopic Heller myotomy had become the primary treatment for achalasia.[3] The authors' practice is to keep patients on a clear liquid diet for 24 hours before surgery. The procedure requires general anesthesia and is most commonly performed in a split leg position. The procedure is performed with both arms on arm boards. As with all procedures involving the hiatus, steep reverse Trendelenburg positioning is utilized, so patients should be well secured to the operating room table. The authors' preferred positioning involves foot boards at the base of the flat padded and abducted leg boards with sequential compression devices for deep venous thrombosis prophylaxis in place. The legs are covered with a warming device and blankets, and the legs are secured to the leg boards with tape above and below the knee.

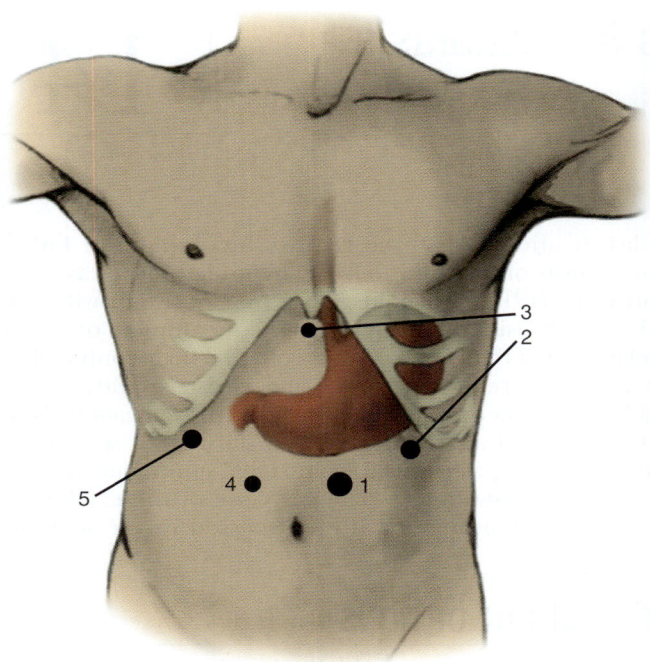

FIGURE 14.1 Position of the trocars: *1*, Camera (11 mm); *2*, surgeon's right hand (5 mm); *3*, surgeon's left hand (5 mm); *4*, assistant port for retraction (5 mm); *5*, liver retractor (5 mm).

The operating surgeon stands on the patient's left side, with the assistant standing between the legs (Fig. 14.1).

Standard laparoscopic equipment is required. Atraumatic graspers are necessary for handling the involved tissues, needle drivers for suturing, and a liver retractor to provide adequate visualization of the hiatus. The harmonic scalpel is useful for dissection, but other devices can also be used. Myotomy can be performed with a hook (with or without cautery), laparoscopic scissors (with or without cautery), or the harmonic scalpel. Five laparoscopic ports are necessary, and they can all be 5 mm trocars. Typically, we use a single 11-mm port to allow the use of a larger 45-degree laparoscope. Finally, an upper endoscope should be available for intraoperative evaluation of the anatomy before and after myotomy, as well as perform endoscopic leak test. A bougie can be used during myotomy to better spread the muscle fibers.

Technique

There are four steps to a laparoscopic Heller myotomy: port placement and exposure, dissection of the stomach and hiatus, myotomy, and fundoplication.

Port Placement and Exposure. The setup is identical to that of a laparoscopic fundoplication. A Veress needle is used to establish pneumoperitoneum followed by camera port placement at the same site, to the left of midline and roughly between the umbilicus and the xiphoid. Other ports are placed as illustrated (see Fig. 14.1).

Dissection of the Stomach and Hiatus. The amount of dissection depends on the planned fundoplication for the procedure. Most commonly, we perform a partial posterior fundoplication, as described by Toupet.[18] Further discussion of fundoplication choice is detailed

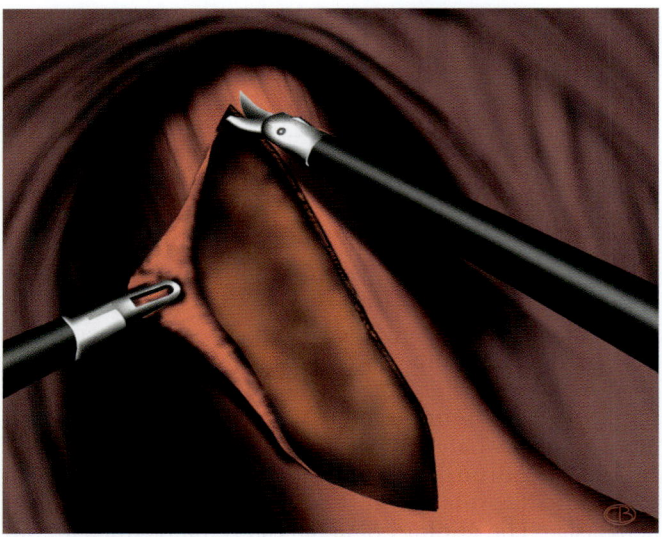

FIGURE 14.2 The intraoperative use of a bougie allows tension on the circular fibers to facilitate myotomy.

in subsequent text. To prepare for myotomy and posterior partial fundoplication, the stomach must be mobilized and the hiatus completely dissected. The assistant retracts the gastroesophageal fat pad inferiorly to reduce any hiatal hernia, and the surgeon then divides the gastrohepatic ligament to expose the right crus. The mediastinum is then entered anteriorly, and the esophagus is mobilized circumferentially. The short gastric arteries are divided. To expose the esophagus for myotomy, the gastroesophageal fat pad is removed, taking care to protect the left vagus nerve.

Myotomy. A bougie is inserted transorally. The myotomy is initiated with the hook cautery, 2 cm above the gastroesophageal junction (GEJ). The myotomy should be performed with a low power setting to avoid transmission to the esophageal mucosa. The longitudinal and circular fibers are dissected off the mucosa and are divided. A fine grasper, such as the Maryland forceps, can be used to elevate the muscle on either side of the myotomy to allow passage of the hook cautery, laparoscopic scissors, or harmonic scalpel into the submucosal plane (Fig. 14.2). Blunt dissection can be used to separate the muscle from the submucosa, which allows for elevation of the muscle away from the submucosa for continued proximal myotomy. The myotomy should be 4 to 5 cm onto the esophagus; bleeding muscle edges can be controlled with delicate cautery or compression. Extending the myotomy above the diaphragm should be avoided, as this can result in a diverticulum in the future. After completing the esophageal myotomy, the distal gastric myotomy is performed for a length of 2 to 3 cm with the energy device. After completing the myotomy, the muscle edges are mobilized laterally to each side to better expose the submucosa. Any remaining circular muscle fibers are divided. The bougie is removed, and an endoscope can be used to evaluate the myotomy and perform an air leak test.

Fundoplication. To prevent postoperative gastroesophageal reflux disease (GERD), a fundoplication should be

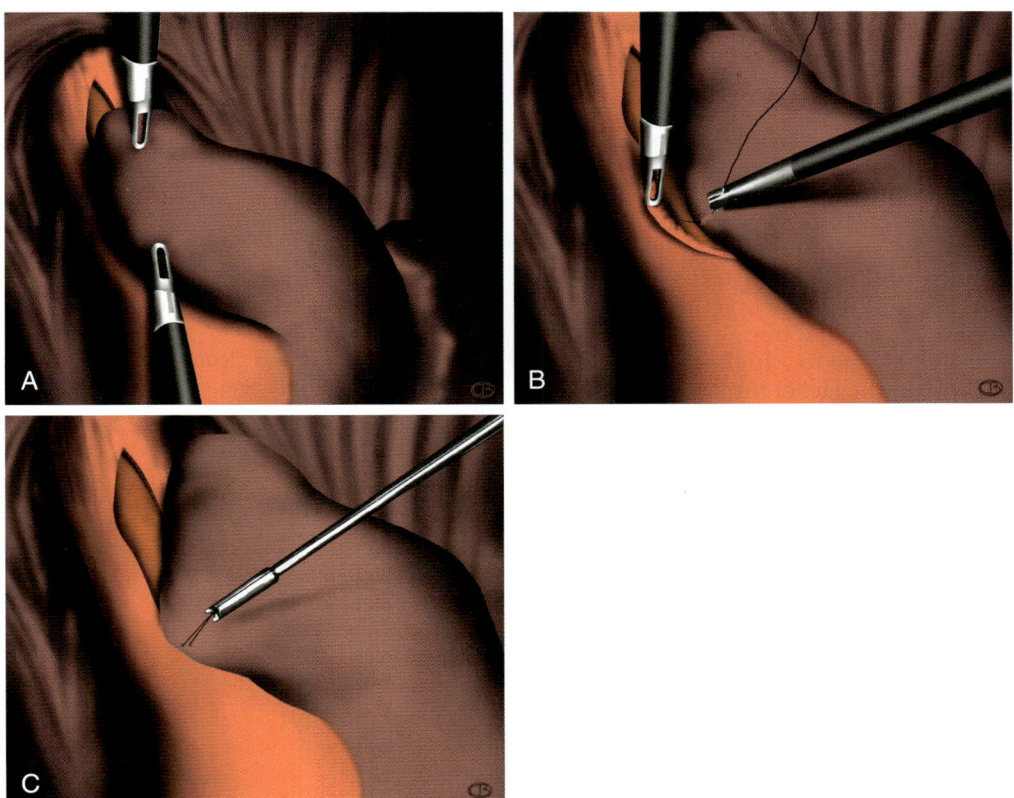

FIGURE 14.3 (A to C) A partial anterior fundoplication using the gastric fundus is added to the myotomy. The most proximal stitches also include the corresponding diaphragmatic pillar.

added. Given the aperistaltic nature of the esophageal body, a partial fundoplication is typically performed. A posterior partial fundoplication involves loose posterior crural closure and fastening the left and right wrap to the corresponding crura. Finally, the right and left sides of the wrap are secured to the esophageal myotomy edges with three interrupted nonabsorbable sutures.

An anterior partial fundoplication (Dor)[19] is used if there is no hiatal hernia and adequate intraabdominal esophageal length for myotomy. This requires minimal mobilization of the fundus and minimizes mediastinal dissection. The fundus is folded over the myotomy and secured to each arch of the hiatus and to each side of the myotomy with three permanent sutures (Fig. 14.3).

Postoperative Care

Before initiating oral intake, the authors' standard practice is to obtain a water-soluble contrast esophagram on postoperative day 1 to exclude perforation and obstruction, followed by 14 days of a pureed diet, and then a regular diet. A routine postoperative visit is planned for 3 to 4 weeks postoperatively with endoscopy, TBS, and pH testing planned for 6 months to evaluate for GERD. Due to the increased risk of squamous cell carcinoma, screening endoscopies are recommended every 5 years.

Complications

The most common complication of an esophageal myotomy is mucosal perforation. These are infrequent and are usually detected at the time of occurrence. These can be repaired laparoscopically with fine interrupted absorbable sutures. Rates of perforation during primary laparoscopic Heller myotomies range from 2.9% to 6.0% in large series, with increased rates of perforation after prior endoscopic treatments,[20–26] and can be as high as 31.2% in redo Heller myotomies.[20]

The outcome after repair of intraoperative mucosal injury is similar to patients who undergo uncomplicated laparoscopic Heller myotomies.[24]

Results

Early results for laparoscopic Heller myotomy demonstrate good improvement in dysphagia, generally greater than 90% with symptom improvement and with 80% to 96%[21,27–30] reporting no dysphagia in the first year after surgery. Dysphagia rates appear to increase with time, with only 63.4% to 88%[21,22,27] free from dysphagia in follow-up beyond 1 year. Studies demonstrate similar improvement with regurgitation with 93.1% to 95%,[27,28] reporting no regurgitation in the early postoperative period, and 79.1%[27] free from symptoms in long-term follow-up. Dilation after recurrent symptoms has been demonstrated to provide durable dysphagia relief in up to 75% of patients with recurrent dysphagia.[22]

Objective GERD identified with pH testing was found in 6% to 41.7%, with variance based on type of fundoplication performed and more reflux noted after Dor fundoplication.[22,31–34] Postoperative reflux has been noted in up to

100% of patients who undergo laparoscopic myotomy without fundoplication.[35]

PERORAL ENDOSCOPIC MYOTOMY

There are no current absolute contraindications to POEM, except inability to tolerate general anesthesia. No longer are patients with end stage "sigmoid" achalasia or those with prior interventions felt to be relative contraindications; patients have successfully undergone POEM after dilatation, Botulinum toxin (Botox) treatment, prior POEM, and even open and laparoscopic myotomy. The authors do consider a large hiatal hernia to be a relative contraindication to POEM due to a higher risk of GERD postprocedurally. Laparoscopic Heller myotomy with hernia repair and partial posterior fundoplication is preferred in these patients.

Similar to Heller myotomy candidates, the authors' practice is to place patients on a clear liquid diet for 24 hours prior to the procedure. Because of risk of yeast esophagitis, 5 days of preoperative nystatin swish and swallow are given prophylactically, as well as a single dose of first-generation cephalosporin within 30 minutes of mucosotomy. A single dose of dexamethasone (10 mg) is given intravenously in the preoperative holding area to minimize mucosal edema at the site of the mucosotomy and to facilitate closure. The procedure requires endotracheal intubation and general anesthesia, and most commonly occurs in the operating room to allow for close monitoring and potential intervention if complications occur.

Technique

There are five steps to POEM: endoscopic measurements, saline lift/mucosotomy, submucosal tunneling, circular myotomy, and mucosotomy closure. Reported operative times are 90 to 120 minutes. The learning curve has been estimated to be approximately 20 procedures,[36] with 30 procedures suggested before attempting POEM after failed Heller myotomy.[37] Basic equipment for the procedure is listed in Table 14.1.

Endoscopic Measurements. A short overtube is placed at the beginning of the case, with the exception of long endoscopic myotomies for spastic disorders or achalasia type 3. In addition to reducing the risk of oropharyngeal trauma, the overtube provides added stability to the endoscope and results in less tension at the mucosotomy, yielding less tearing and a smaller mucosotomy to close at the end of the procedure. Anatomic landmarks are measured in reference to the overtube. The length of the myotomy can be determined using intraoperative impedance planimetry using EndoFlip (Crospon, Galway, Ireland).

For achalasia types 1 and 2, a short myotomy is generally performed; the start of the myotomy is planned for 3 cm proximal to the high-pressure zone. For achalasia type 3, a longer myotomy is performed, based on impedance planimetry and preoperative HRM, to include the entire spastic segment in the planned myotomy.

Saline Lift and Mucosotomy. The site for the mucosal incision should be 3 to 4 cm proximal to the determined start of the myotomy. The authors prefer the anterior lesser curve position (2-o'clock position) for the myotomy, although the posterior position (6-o'clock) is possible as well. The saline lift is performed by injecting a dilute

TABLE 14.1 Peroral Endoscopic Myotomy Equipment

BASIC EQUIPMENT	MUCOSOTOMY/TUNNEL
Video tower	Generator/ground pad
Endoscope	(mucostomy: 60 cut)
CO_2 regulation unit with low flow tubing	(Tunnel: 60 spray tunnel; myotomy: 40 spray)
Flushing pump	Active cord
Large pitcher for lifting solution	Injection needle
10-cc controlled syringes for hydrodissection	Endoscopic knife
Alcohol swabs for lens cleaning	Sphincterotomy balloon
Toothbrushes for cleaning knives	Dissecting caps—soft, hard, or angled
Wire bucket for temporary wire storage	Hemostatic graspers
MEASUREMENT	**CLOSURE**
Data sheet	Clip—large and small
Overtube	Suture—overstitch—requires dual-channel scope
LIFTING SOLUTION	
1 mL Indigo Carmine diluted in 500 mL NS	
±epinephrine 1:1000 1 mg/mL	

methylene blue saline solution, with or without epinephrine ("lifting solution"), into the submucosal space through a 23-gauge endoscopic injection needle. A 1.5 cm mucosotomy is then performed using a hook or triangle-tip (TT) cautery device with cutting current.

Submucosal Tunnel. The endoscope, which is fitted with a vented, taper, or angled dissection cap, is inserted through the mucosotomy and into the submucosal plane. Insertion can be aided with the use of a 15-mm biliary extraction balloon to elevate the edges of the mucosa. Hydrostatic dissection can also be performed through the extraction balloon by instilling lifting solution. After initial hydrostatic dissection, the esophageal mucosa and submucosa are separated from the underlying circular muscle fibers using spray cautery (Fig. 14.4). Hydrostatic dissection is repeated every few centimeters. Large bridging vessels are occasionally encountered and can be controlled with a coag grasper and soft cautery. Difficult bleeding can be controlled with direct pressure by advancing the dissecting cap and holding the endoscope in place. The distal extent of the dissection can be identified by encountering the tattoo placed previously or by visualizing the transition from orderly esophageal vessels to the submucosal palisades characteristic of the gastric plane. Finally, a retroflexed view can confirm mucosal blanching caused by the tunnel extending across the GEJ.

During creating of the submucosal tunnel, care must be taken to avoid mucosal injury from cautery or shear injury from bowing of the endoscope; most inadvertent mucosotomies are small and can be repaired with an endoscopic clip from the lumen of the esophagus at the end of the procedure. Maintaining the same operative position and ensuring the circular fibers are parallel to the end of the cap will prevent spiraling of the tunnel.

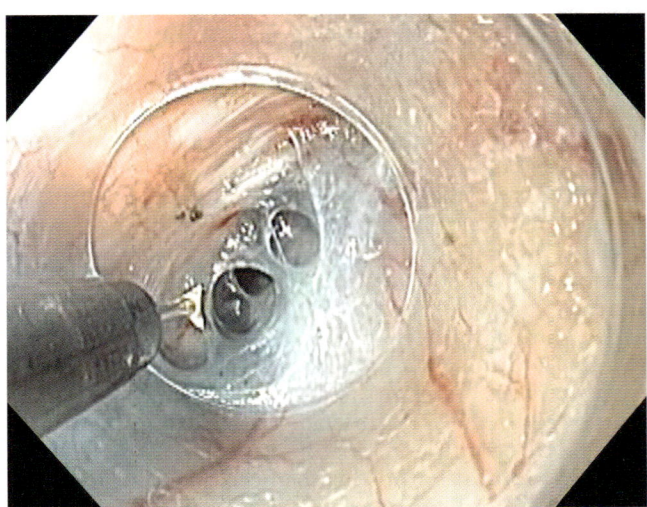

FIGURE 14.4 Hydrostatic dissection during peroral endoscopic myotomy.

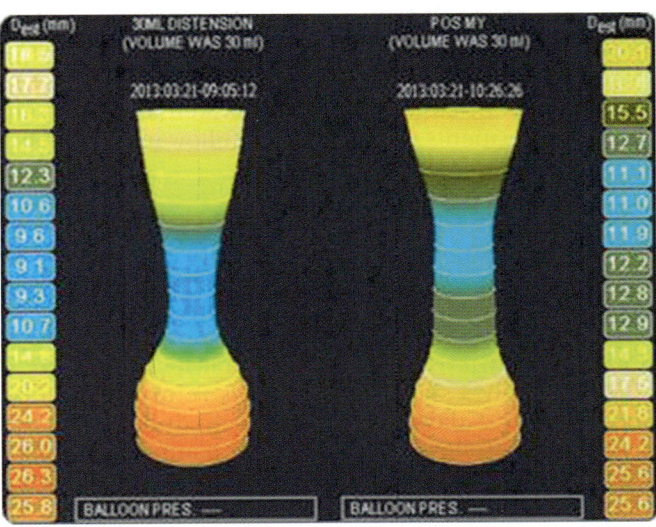

FIGURE 14.6 Impedance planimetry using EndoFlip (Crospon, Galway, Ireland).

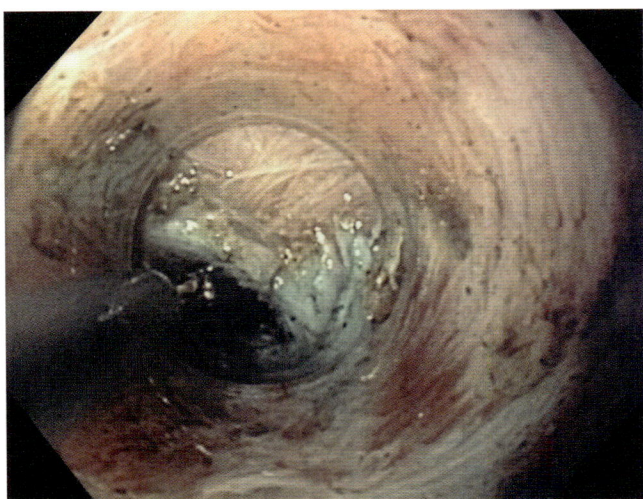

FIGURE 14.5 Division of circular fibers and exposure of longitudinal fibers during peroral endoscopic myotomy.

Circular Myotomy. The myotomy begins 2 to 3 cm distal to the most distal extent of the mucosotomy and proceeds antegrade to allow the dissecting cap to place tension on the muscle fibers. The myotomy consists of division of the circular muscle fibers using an Endocut current using a triangle tip or hook cautery. Once the circular fibers are divided, the longitudinal muscle fibers are easily visible (Fig. 14.5). The longitudinal fibers are very thin and splitting often occurs under the pressure of the dissecting cap, which will reveal mediastinal structures beyond the intact esophageal adventitia. This "mediastinal exposure" is common and does not indicate a full-thickness perforation.

The plane between the longitudinal and circular muscle fibers is followed distally with continued myotomy. The myotomy plane often becomes tight at the GEJ due to the thickened musculature, the curve from the esophagus

to the stomach, and the impression of the diaphragm. Progressive lifting and dissection will always eventually permit passage of the endoscope into the gastric submucosal plane. Forcing the dissecting cap through this area can cause endoscopic bowing and further mucosotomy tearing. The myotomy should be continued well onto the gastric wall, as confirmed by the previously placed tattoo and/or confirmation by retroflexion. We also repeat the impedance planimetry to ensure an increase in the cross-sectional area and, more importantly, an improvement in the compliance of the LES (Fig. 14.6).

Mucosotomy Closure. Once adequate dissection has occurred, the mucosotomy is then closed using endoscopic clips or endoscopic sutures. Any mucosal burns or perforations should be first clipped, and then the mucosotomy is closed from distal to proximal.

Other Considerations

Extended proximal myotomy should be considered for noncardiac chest pain and for type 3 achalasia, which can be extended from a few centimeters from the cricopharyngeus to the gastric cardia. POEM has been shown to be both safe and effective for these extended indications. Due to concerns for submucosal fibrosis from dilations or injections, previous treatments were initially felt to be contraindications to POEM. As experience has increased, POEM has been successfully completed with no increases in procedure length or perioperative complication rates after prior intervention.[38] POEM has also been reported after prior laparoscopic myotomy; it is technically difficult but safe and effective with published efficacy of 91.7% to 100%.[39–41] In the setting of failed Heller myotomy, some recommend creation of the submucosal tunnel in the posterior aspect of the esophagus[42] or the lateral wall.[43]

End-stage achalasia or "sigmoid" esophagus is more difficult technically to treat and has somewhat poorer clinical results. As with dilation or Heller myotomy, many end-stage patients will have continued functional deterioration, and up to 5% will require esophagectomy.[44] End-stage achalasia was felt to be a contraindication for POEM in the past, but successful therapy has been described in small subsets of larger studies,[17,41] as well as one recent study of 32 patients with long-term follow-up and a 96% success rate.[45]

Postprocedure Care

Before initiating oral intake, we obtain a water-soluble contrast esophagram on postoperative day 1, followed by 7 days of a pureed diet, and then a regular diet. The pureed diet is required so that the endoscopic clips are not dislodged too early. The hospital length of stay is approximately 1 day,[31] and patients return to regular activity after 4 days.[41] The same schedule for Heller myotomies is followed: office visit is planned for 3 to 4 weeks postoperatively with endoscopy, TBS, and pH testing planned for 6 months to evaluate for GERD. Due to the increased risk of squamous cell carcinoma, screening endoscopies are recommended every 5 years.

Results

Dysphagia relief after POEM has been demonstrated to be greater than 90% in short-term and long-term follow-up, with complete dysphagia relief occurring more commonly for achalasia than nonachalasia patients.[41,42,46–49] The Eckardt Clinical Score is used to evaluate subjective achalasia symptoms and postoperative results. It is a validated tool that allows for symptom grading in severity and frequency of dysphagia, chest pain, regurgitation, and degree of weight loss.[50] Scores of 3 or less are used to define successful symptom relief. Eckardt scores range from 5.5 to 8.8 before POEM to 0 to 1.4 after POEM.[41,43,46,49,51–53] There are objective improvements after POEM as well. TBS can be used to measure improvements in esophageal emptying; it has been shown to correlate with subjective improvements in swallowing in POEM patients.[51,52] HRM has also been used to demonstrate appropriate decreases in LES resting and residual pressures after POEM.[31,54] POEM has also been performed after failed POEM,[55] with 85% of patients having improvement in Eckardt scores to a threshold below 3.

Complications

Inadvertent mucosal injuries, such as burns and small perforations, can occur in up to 25% of cases during the learning curve, but can almost always be treated with simple endoscopic treatment such as clips or sutures, and rarely stents, Endoloops, or fibrin sealant. Full-thickness perforations are very rare but can cause serious harm to patients if not recognized and repaired at the time of the procedure. Mucosotomy dehiscence and postoperative bleeding are also rare and can almost always be controlled endoscopically.[41,49,56]

Pneumoperitoneum, pneumomediastinum, and pneumothorax are not felt to be complications, but rather side effects of the procedure. As long as carbon dioxide is used for the procedure, these rarely require intervention due to reabsorption. If necessary due to symptoms, sterile needle decompression, without indwelling drain placement, can be performed in the peritoneal cavity or the anterior chest during or after the procedure.[41,56]

Gastroesophageal Reflux Disease

Although POEM does not allow for a fundoplication at the time of myotomy, the intact phrenoesophageal ligaments and preservation of the longitudinal esophageal muscle fibers are believed to reduce the incidence of GERD after POEM. Approximately 10% to 40% of patients will demonstrate symptoms of reflux after POEM,[31,41,49,57] which is similar to rates after the Heller myotomy described previously. Objective testing demonstrates higher rates of acid exposure after POEM,[58,59] though many of these patients are asymptomatic.

Up to 50% of patients with post-POEM reflux can be asymptomatic,[41] and up to 44% of patients with symptoms of reflux have normal acid exposure[52]; the authors therefore recommend postoperative pH testing in all patients to identify those with increased acid exposure after POEM, and consideration of antacid medication or even selective fundoplication in this subset.

Peroral Endoscopic Myotomy Compared to Heller Myotomy

POEM has compared favorably with laparoscopic Heller myotomy with fundoplication.[53,60] The cost-effectiveness of the two procedures is also similar.[61] Three studies have demonstrated POEM to have improved outcomes. These included shorter operative times, lower blood loss, shorter hospital stay, better short-term Eckardt scores, similar intermediate Eckardt scores, similar reflux, and lower dysphagia rates,[31,51] as well as less postoperative pain.[62] Randomized controlled trials are underway to further compare the two procedures.

CONCLUSION

Achalasia is a devastating disease with no cure. Treatment, laparoscopic or endoscopic, aims at disrupting the esophageal outflow obstruction. POEM is a new technique that compares favorably with the standard laparoscopic myotomy with fundoplication. Long-term results and comparative studies are still in progress, but sufficient evidence currently exists to validate the technique as a primary treatment alternative.

REFERENCES

1. Sadowski DC, Ackah F, Jiang B, Svenson LW. Achalasia: incidence, prevalence and survival. A population-based study. *Neurogastroenterol Motil*. 2010;22(9):e256-e261.
2. Enestvedt BK, Williams JL, Sonnenberg A. Epidemiology and practice patterns of achalasia in a large multi-centre database. *Aliment Pharmacol Ther*. 2011;33(11):1209-1214.
3. Spiess AE, Kahrilas PJ. Treating achalasia: from whalebone to laparoscope. *JAMA*. 1998;280(7):638-642.
4. Lendrum FC. Anatomic features of the cardiac orifice of the stomach: with special reference to cardiospasm. *Arch Intern Med*. 1937;59(3):474-511.
5. Vaezi MF, Pandolfino JE, Vela MF. ACG clinical guideline: diagnosis and management of achalasia. *Am J Gastroenterol*. 2013;108(8):1238-1249; quiz 1250.
6. Gockel I, Bohl JR, Doostkam S, Eckardt VF, Junginger T. Spectrum of histopathologic findings in patients with achalasia reflects different etiologies. *J Gastroenterol Hepatol*. 2006;21(4):727-733.
7. Boeckxstaens GE. Novel mechanism for impaired nitrergic relaxation in achalasia. *Gut*. 2006;55(3):304-305.

8. de Oliveira JM, Birgisson S, Doinoff C, et al. Timed barium swallow: a simple technique for evaluating esophageal emptying in patients with achalasia. *AJR Am J Roentgenol.* 1997;169(2):473-479.

9. Bredenoord AJ, Fox M, Kahrilas PJ, et al. Chicago classification criteria of esophageal motility disorders defined in high resolution esophageal pressure topography. *Neurogastroenterol Motil.* 2012;24(suppl 1): 57-65.

10. Kahrilas PJ, Bredenoord AJ, Fox M, et al. The Chicago Classification of esophageal motility disorders, v3.0. *Neurogastroenterol Motil.* 2015;27(2):160-174.

11. Heller E. Extramuköse Cardiaplastik beim chronischen Cardiospasmus mit Dilatation des Oesophagus. *Mitt Grenzgeb Med Chir.* 1913;27:141-149.

12. Shimi S, Nathanson LK, Cuschieri A. Laparoscopic cardiomyotomy for achalasia. *J R Coll Surg Edinb.* 1991;36(3):152-154.

13. Pellegrini C, Wetter LA, Patti M, et al. Thoracoscopic esophagomyotomy. Initial experience with a new approach for the treatment of achalasia. *Ann Surg.* 1992;216(3):291-296; discussion 296–299.

14. Ortega JA, Madureri V, Perez L. Endoscopic myotomy in the treatment of achalasia. *Gastrointest Endosc.* 1980;26(1):8-10.

15. Pasricha PJ, Hawari R, Ahmed I, et al. Submucosal endoscopic esophageal myotomy: a novel experimental approach for the treatment of achalasia. *Endoscopy.* 2007;39(9):761-764.

16. Rajan E, Gostout CJ, Feitoza AB, et al. Widespread EMR: a new technique for removal of large areas of mucosa. *Gastrointest Endosc.* 2004;60(4):623-627.

17. Inoue H, Minami H, Kobayashi Y, et al. Peroral endoscopic myotomy (POEM) for esophageal achalasia. *Endoscopy.* 2010;42(4):265-271.

18. Toupet A. [Technic of esophago-gastroplasty with phrenogastropexy used in radical treatment of hiatal hernias as a supplement to Heller's operation in cardiospasms]. *Mem Acad Chir (Paris).* 1963;89:384-389.

19. Dor J, Humbert P, Paoli JM, Miorclerc M, Aubert J. [Treatment of reflux by the so-called modified Heller-Nissen technic]. *Presse Med.* 1967;75(50):2563-2565.

20. Zhang LP, Chang R, Matthews BD, et al. Incidence, mechanisms, and outcomes of esophageal and gastric perforation during laparoscopic foregut surgery: a retrospective review of 1,223 foregut cases. *Surg Endosc.* 2014;28(1):85-90.

21. Patti MG, Pellegrini CA, Horgan S, et al. Minimally invasive surgery for achalasia: an 8-year experience with 168 patients. *Ann Surg.* 1999;230(4):587-593; discussion 593–584.

22. Zaninotto G, Costantini M, Rizzetto C, et al. Four hundred laparoscopic myotomies for esophageal achalasia: a single centre experience. *Ann Surg.* 2008;248(6):986-993.

23. Rosemurgy A, Villadolid D, Thometz D, et al. Laparoscopic Heller myotomy provides durable relief from achalasia and salvages failures after botox or dilation. *Ann Surg.* 2005;241(5):725-733; discussion 733–725.

24. Salvador R, Spadotto L, Capovilla G, et al. Mucosal perforation during laparoscopic Heller myotomy has no influence on final treatment outcome. *J Gastrointest Surg.* 2016;20(12):1923-1930.

25. Patti MG, Molena D, Fisichella PM, et al. Laparoscopic Heller myotomy and Dor fundoplication for achalasia: analysis of successes and failures. *Arch Surg.* 2001;136(8):870-877.

26. Torquati A, Richards WO, Holzman MD, Sharp KW. Laparoscopic myotomy for achalasia: predictors of successful outcome after 200 cases. *Ann Surg.* 2006;243(5):587-591; discussion 591–583.

27. Finley CJ, Kondra J, Clifton J, Yee J, Finley R. Factors associated with postoperative symptoms after laparoscopic Heller myotomy. *Ann Thorac Surg.* 2010;89(2):392-396.

28. Hunter JG, Trus TL, Branum GD, Waring JP. Laparoscopic Heller myotomy and fundoplication for achalasia. *Ann Surg.* 1997;225(6):655-664; discussion 664–655.

29. Rosati R, Fumagalli U, Bonavina L, et al. Laparoscopic approach to esophageal achalasia. *Am J Surg.* 1995;169(4):424-427.

30. Frantzides CT, Moore RE, Carlson MA, et al. Minimally invasive surgery for achalasia: a 10-year experience. *J Gastrointest Surg.* 2004;8(1):18-23.

31. Bhayani NH, Kurian AA, Dunst CM, Sharata AM, Rieder E, Swanstrom LL. A comparative study on comprehensive, objective outcomes of laparoscopic Heller myotomy with per-oral endoscopic myotomy (POEM) for achalasia. *Ann Surg.* 2014;259(6):1098-1103.

32. Rawlings A, Soper NJ, Oelschlager B, et al. Laparoscopic Dor versus Toupet fundoplication following Heller myotomy for achalasia: results of a multicenter, prospective, randomized-controlled trial. *Surg Endosc.* 2012;26(1):18-26.

33. Khajanchee YS, Kanneganti S, Leatherwood AE, Hansen PD, Swanstrom LL. Laparoscopic Heller myotomy with Toupet fundoplication: outcomes predictors in 121 consecutive patients. *Arch Surg.* 2005;140(9):827-833; discussion 833–824.

34. Richards WO, Torquati A, Holzman MD, et al. Heller myotomy versus Heller myotomy with Dor fundoplication for achalasia: a prospective randomized double-blind clinical trial. *Ann Surg.* 2004;240(3):405-412; discussion 412–405.

35. Falkenback D, Johansson J, Oberg S, et al. Heller's esophagomyotomy with or without a 360 degrees floppy Nissen fundoplication for achalasia. Long-term results from a prospective randomized study. *Dis Esophagus.* 2003;16(4):284-290.

36. Kurian AA, Dunst CM, Sharata A, Bhayani NH, Reavis KM, Swanstrom LL. Peroral endoscopic esophageal myotomy: defining the learning curve. *Gastrointest Endosc.* 2013;77(5):719-725.

37. Dunst CM, Kurian AA, Swanstrom LL. Endoscopic myotomy for achalasia. *Adv Surg.* 2014;48:27-41.

38. Sharata A, Kurian AA, Dunst CM, Bhayani NH, Reavis KM, Swanstrom LL. Peroral endoscopic myotomy (POEM) is safe and effective in the setting of prior endoscopic intervention. *J Gastrointest Surg.* 2013;17(7): 1188-1192.

39. Onimaru M, Inoue H, Ikeda H, et al. Peroral endoscopic myotomy is a viable option for failed surgical esophagocardiomyotomy instead of redo surgical Heller myotomy: a single center prospective study. *J Am Coll Surg.* 2013;217(4):598-605.

40. Zhou PH, Li QL, Yao LQ, et al. Peroral endoscopic remyotomy for failed Heller myotomy: a prospective single-center study. *Endoscopy.* 2013;45(3):161-166.

41. Sharata AM, Dunst CM, Pescarus R, et al. Peroral endoscopic myotomy (POEM) for esophageal primary motility disorders: analysis of 100 consecutive patients. *J Gastrointest Surg.* 2015;19(1):161-170; discussion 170.

42. Ren Z, Zhong Y, Zhou P, et al. Perioperative management and treatment for complications during and after peroral endoscopic myotomy (POEM) for esophageal achalasia (EA) (data from 119 cases). *Surg Endosc.* 2012;26(11):3267-3272.

43. Chiu PW, Wu JC, Teoh AY, et al. Peroral endoscopic myotomy for treatment of achalasia: from bench to bedside (with video). *Gastrointest Endosc.* 2013;77(1):29-38.

44. Duranceau A, Liberman M, Martin J, Ferraro P. End-stage achalasia. *Dis Esophagus.* 2012;25(4):319-330.

45. Hu JW, Li QL, Zhou PH, et al. Peroral endoscopic myotomy for advanced achalasia with sigmoid-shaped esophagus: long-term outcomes from a prospective, single-center study. *Surg Endosc.* 2015;29(9): 2841-2850.

46. von Renteln D, Inoue H, Minami H, et al. Peroral endoscopic myotomy for the treatment of achalasia: a prospective single center study. *Am J Gastroenterol.* 2012;107(3):411-417.

47. Zhou P-H, Yao L, Zhang Y-Q, et al. Peroral endoscopic myotomy (POEM) for esophageal achalasia: 205 cases report. *Gastrointest Endosc.* 2012;75(4):AB132-AB133.

48. Stavropoulos SN, Brathwaite CE, Iqbal S, et al. P.O.E.M. (peroral endoscopic myotomy), a U.S. gastroenterologist perspective: initial 2 year experience. *Gastrointest Endosc.* 2012;75(4):AB149.

49. Hungness ES, Sternbach JM, Teitelbaum EN, Kahrilas PJ, Pandolfino JE, Soper NJ. Per-oral endoscopic myotomy (POEM) after the learning curve: durable long-term results with a low complication rate. *Ann Surg.* 2016;264(3):508-517.

50. Gockel I, Junginger T. The value of scoring achalasia: a comparison of current systems and the impact on treatment—the surgeon's viewpoint. *Am Surg.* 2007;73(4):327-331.

51. Hungness ES, Teitelbaum EN, Santos BF, et al. Comparison of perioperative outcomes between peroral esophageal myotomy (POEM) and laparoscopic Heller myotomy. *J Gastrointest Surg.* 2013;17(2):228-235.

52. Swanstrom LL, Kurian A, Dunst CM, Sharata A, Bhayani N, Rieder E. Long-term outcomes of an endoscopic myotomy for achalasia: the POEM procedure. *Ann Surg.* 2012;256(4):659-667.

53. Schneider AM, Louie BE, Warren HF, Farivar AS, Schembre DB, Aye RW. A matched comparison of per oral endoscopic myotomy to laparoscopic Heller myotomy in the treatment of achalasia. *J Gastrointest Surg.* 2016;20(11):1789-1796.

54. Familiari P, Gigante G, Marchese M, et al. EndoFLIP system for the intraoperative evaluation of peroral endoscopic myotomy. *United European Gastroenterol J.* 2014;2(2):77-83.

55. Tyberg A, Seewald S, Sharaiha RZ, et al. A multicenter international registry of redo per-oral endoscopic myotomy (POEM) after failed POEM. *Gastrointest Endosc.* 2017;85(6): 1208-1211.

56. Bechara R, Ikeda H, Inoue H. Peroral endoscopic myotomy: an evolving treatment for achalasia. *Nat Rev Gastroenterol Hepatol.* 2015;12(7):410-426.

57. Talukdar R, Inoue H, Reddy DN. Efficacy of peroral endoscopic myotomy (POEM) in the treatment of achalasia: a systematic review and meta-analysis. *Surg Endosc.* 2015;29(11):3030-3046.

58. Familiari P, Gigante G, Marchese M, et al. Peroral endoscopic myotomy for esophageal achalasia: outcomes of the first 100 patients with short-term follow-up. *Ann Surg.* 2016;263(1):82-87.

59. Stavropoulos SN, Modayil R, Friedel D. Per oral endoscopic myotomy for the treatment of achalasia. *Curr Opin Gastroenterol.* 2015;31(5): 430-440.

60. Zhang Y, Wang H, Chen X, et al. Per-oral endoscopic myotomy versus laparoscopic Heller myotomy for achalasia: a meta-analysis of nonrandomized comparative studies. *Medicine (Baltimore).* 2016;95(6): e2736.

61. Miller HJ, Neupane R, Fayezizadeh M, Majumder A, Marks JM. POEM is a cost-effective procedure: cost-utility analysis of endoscopic and surgical treatment options in the management of achalasia. *Surg Endosc.* 2017;31(4):1636-1642.

62. Docimo S Jr, Mathew A, Shope AJ, Winder JS, Haluck RS, Pauli EM. Reduced postoperative pain scores and narcotic use favor per-oral endoscopic myotomy over laparoscopic Heller myotomy. *Surg Endosc.* 2017;31(2):795-800.

PART FOUR

Gastroesophageal Reflux Disease

Gastroesophageal Reflux Disease: Definition and Scope of the Problem in the United States of America and Worldwide

Joshua Sloan | Philip O. Katz

Gastroesophageal reflux disease (GERD) is among the most common diseases seen by both primary care and gastrointestinal (GI) specialists worldwide. Its prevalence is increasing, with reflux symptoms ranging from 10% to 30% of the population of Western countries.[1-3] Compared to the numbers reported in North America, the prevalence of weekly GERD symptoms is slightly lower in Europe (8.8% to 25.9%) and substantially lower in Asia (approximately 10%).[1,2] Overall, the incidence of GERD remains somewhere around 5 per 1000 person years.[1,2] In this chapter we review the disease as it affects patients in the United States and around the world; discuss complications including its relation to strictures, Barrett esophagus, and esophageal adenocarcinoma; and address GERD's effect on patient quality of life.

DEFINITION

GERD is a condition that is defined as troublesome symptoms or complications that result from the reflux of gastric contents into the esophagus or beyond into the oral cavity or lung.[4,5] Troublesome is defined by consensus as mild symptoms that occur at least 2 times per week or moderate to severe symptoms at least once per week.[4] The pathogenesis is multifactorial. Overall, GERD is a disorder caused by abnormal function of the lower esophageal sphincter (LES). The most frequent abnormality is an increase in so-called transient lower esophageal sphincter relaxations (TLESR), a normal physiologic occurrence of sphincter opening without an antecedent swallow that results in reflux of gastric contents into the esophagus.[6,7] Basal LES pressure may be low, and transient increases in intraabdominal pressure and a hiatal hernia contribute to LES dysfunction and reflux. Traditional thinking is that acidic gastric contents cause symptoms and/or injury via direct contact with mucosa resulting in inflammation. The role of bile acids in producing symptoms and reflux

injury is controversial. In combination with acid there is likely synergy causing esophagitis. A recent study suggests that reflux injury may be a result of an inflammatory reaction.[8] Reflux is cleared by secondary peristalsis and neutralization by salivary bicarbonate. Failure of either of these clearance mechanisms may contribute to injury. In some cases, gastric emptying delay may contribute to GERD by increasing gastric volume and precipitating TLESRs. Other factors such as central obesity can increase intraabdominal pressure and result in GERD.[9,10]

Symptoms of GERD can be divided into typical, atypical, and extraesophageal (Fig. 15.1).[4,5] The most common typical symptoms of GERD are heartburn and regurgitation. Many consider dysphagia and chest pain as typical symptoms as well.[4,5] Atypical symptoms include dyspepsia, epigastric pain, nausea, bloating, and belching.[5] The most common extraesophageal symptoms include chronic cough, asthma, and throat symptoms including chronic voice disturbance and laryngitis.[4,5,11] The latter may be associated with typical symptoms or sometimes may be the presenting symptom of the disease. Direct aspiration of gastric contents are believed to be the most common cause of these extraesophageal symptoms, although rarely they may result from distal esophageal acid exposure alone via a reflex event.

SCOPE

GERD is a common disease affecting millions of people worldwide. The prevalence is up to 30% in Western countries and 10% in Asia (Table 15.1 and Fig. 15.2).[2] These data are based on a number of epidemiologic studies that have been performed and reviewed in the literature (see Table 15.1 and Fig. 15.2).[1,2]

In the United States, the prevalence ranges from 18.1% to 27.8%.[2] A study published in 2007 explored the prevalence of irritable bowel syndrome (IBS) and

GERD.[12] The researchers sent a questionnaire to 4194 people with 2273 returning the questionnaire.[12] The study found the overall prevalence of GERD to be 18.1% in a group representative of the United States Caucasian population.[2,12] The upper range of GERD prevalence in the United States of 27.8% was established in a cross-sectional survey asking questions pertaining to weekly heartburn or regurgitation symptoms.[1,2,12,13]

Studies have been performed in the United States to evaluate if the prevalence of GERD changes based on race. A 2004 cross-sectional survey studied the prevalence of GERD in African American and Caucasian Veterans Affairs (VA) employees.[13] The study included a survey followed by endoscopy. No statistically significant difference in GERD prevalence was found between the two groups (27% and 23% with heartburn, and 16% and 15% for regurgitation in African Americans and Caucasians, respectively). However, there were higher rates of esophagitis in Caucasians compared with African Americans.[13] The prevalence of GERD in Hispanics in the United States is thought to be similar to non-Hispanic whites.[14] A survey-based study performed in Philadelphia found that Hispanics had higher monthly heartburn than other racial groups with a prevalence of 50%.[15,16] Asians surveyed in the same study were found to have a 20% prevalence of monthly heartburn.[15,16]

In South America, the prevalence of weekly symptoms of heartburn or regurgitation was approximately 23% in a study published in 2005.[2,17] This study highlighted the prevalence of GERD only in an Argentinian population.[2,17] More recently, a Brazilian study echoed findings similar to the 2004 study.[17,18] In that study, monthly GERD symptoms were found to be approximately 22.7%.[18]

Based on eight studies in two separate epidemiologic reviews, the prevalence of GERD in Europe ranges from 8.8% to 25.9%.[2,19–26] This represents an increased prevalence from the previously presented data of 9.8% to 18%.[1] Two studies were large surveys sent via mail to Swedish populations, which established the increased prevalence.[25,26]

The prevalence of GERD in East Asian populations has increased from 2.5%–4.8% to 3.5%–7.8%.[1,2] In the epidemiologic review published in 2005, the prevalence was based on three studies conducted in mainland China

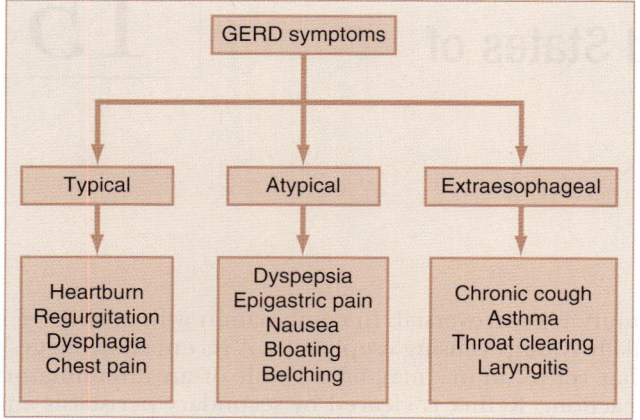

FIGURE 15.1 Gastroesophageal reflux disease (GERD) symptoms.

TABLE 15.1 Prevalence of Gastroesophageal Reflux Disease Worldwide

	Unites States	South America	Europe	East Asia	Middle East
Prevalence	18.1%–27.8%	22.7%–23.0%	8.8%–25.9%	3.5%–8.5%	8.7%–45.4%

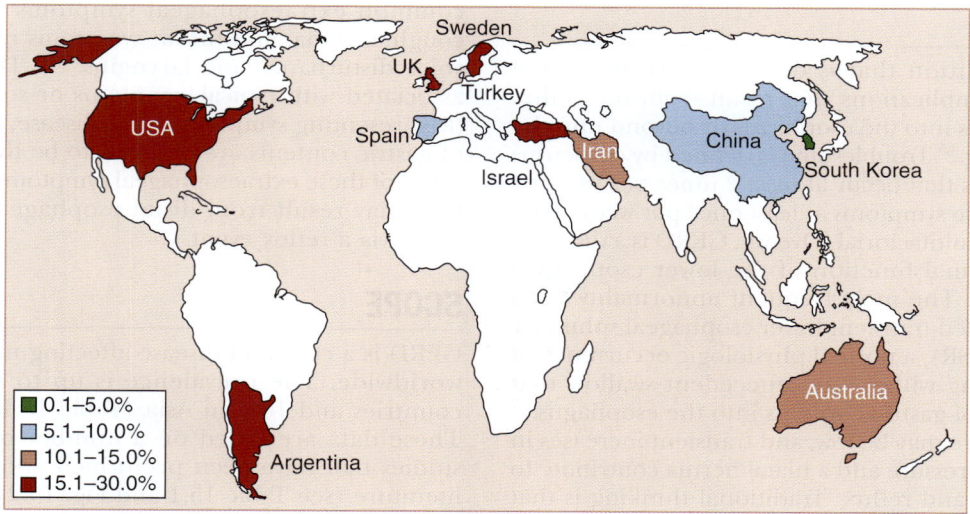

FIGURE 15.2 Worldwide epidemiology of gastroesophageal reflux disease. (From El-Serag HB, Sweet S, Winchester CC, Dent J. Update on the epidemiology of gastro-oesophageal reflux disease: a systematic review. *Gut.* 2014;63[6]:878.)

and Hong Kong.[27-29] Two of the studies were telephone surveys completed by 3858 individuals; the third was a survey of 5000 people and was conducted with the assistance of physicians and medical students.[27-29] More recently, the three studies included in the review by El-Serag were conducted in South Korea and China.[2] Between the three studies, 20,833 people were surveyed leading to the findings of 3.5% to 7.8% prevalence of GERD.[30-32] An additional review performed in Korea between 2005 and 2010 found that the prevalence in eastern Asia may range from 5.2% to 8.5%.[33]

Middle Eastern populations also have a significant prevalence of GERD ranging from 8.7% to 33.1%.[2,34-40] When evaluating the data there was one study in Turkey, one in Israel, and five studies in Iran. The Turkish study evaluated 630 patients and the prevalence of GERD symptoms, heartburn or regurgitation, ranged from 10% to 15.6%.[34] The study performed in Israel evaluated 981 patients and found a prevalence of 9.3%.[35] Finally, the Iranian studies of GERD showed a prevalence of 8.7% to 21.2% with the exception of one study evaluating nomads in Iran.[2,36-40] Similar to the Israeli study, this particular study evaluated only a subgroup of the population and may falsely increase the prevalence in the general population.[40] A more recent study suggests that the prevalence of GERD may range from 14% to 34% in Iran.[41] If we include a study published in 2014, which surveyed a Saudi Arabian population, the overall prevalence range in the Middle East ranges from 8.7% to 45.4%.[42]

The current body of data does not show a difference in prevalence of GERD in aging patients.[2,5,43,44] Available data do, however, suggest that esophageal sensitivity to acid decreases with age, thus predisposing those older than 55 to 65 years to an increase in higher grades of esophagitis than younger patients.[44,45] There does not appear to be a large difference in GERD symptoms between men and women. However, some studies suggest women tend to present with nonerosive disease, whereas men tend to have more esophagitis and Barrett esophagus.[2,43]

GERD is also prevalent in pregnancy and ranges from 30% to 80% at some point during the course of pregnancy.[46,47] A 2012 study evaluated prevalence throughout the course of pregnancy and found a prevalence of 26.1%, 36.1%, and 51.2% in trimesters one through three.[46] A separate study found that the incidence of GERD is approximately 25% in each trimester of pregnancy.[47] Little information is available on the end organ effects, if any, of GERD in pregnancy, though clinical experience suggests they are minimal. Although some feel that GERD in pregnancy is a risk for long-term disease, the data supporting this are lacking. GERD symptoms commonly resolve with delivery, but may start again at a later date in some patients.

Two longitudinal studies are worth reviewing in some detail. The first was a representative random sample of the normal population of two communities in northern Sweden.[25] Subjects were surveyed and a large number (*n* = 1000) underwent endoscopy. GERD symptoms increased with age, the lowest being the 20- to 34-year-old group and peaking in the 50- to 65-year-old and older groups. One thousand participants underwent esophagogastro-duodenoscopy (EGD); the prevalence rates for monthly,

weekly, and daily GERD symptoms were 40%, 20%, and 6%, respectively, with no statistical differences between females and males.[25] EGD showed normal endoscopic findings, esophagitis, and hiatal hernia in 77%, 15.5%, and 23.9% of subjects, respectively. Of the group with monthly GERD symptoms, 35%, 63%, and 53% had normal endoscopy, esophagitis, and hiatal hernia, respectively. When compared to females, men had more esophagitis (odds ratio: 2.83), especially in the younger age groups (32%). Compared to asymptomatic individuals, those with GERD symptoms, esophagitis, or both reported an increased prevalence of medical treatment—that is, antacids, proton pump inhibitors (PPIs) or any medication—0% to 3% in normal patients versus 8% to 33% in persons with GERD symptoms.[25]

The ProGERD study assessed symptoms and endoscopic findings in a cohort of GERD patients from Germany, Switzerland, and Austria with the intent to examine the natural history of the disease. A total of 3894 patients with GERD symptoms participated in a longitudinal study undergoing EGD at baseline and at 2-year follow-up.[48] After a baseline EGD, all patients received treatment with esomeprazole. Thereafter, further medical treatment was given at the discretion of the physician. After 2 years, 25% of those with non-erosive reflux disease (NERD) were noted to have grade A or B esophagitis, whereas 6% had grade C or D esophagitis. In patients with baseline grade A and B esophagitis, 1.6% progressed to grade C and D, and 61% with baseline A and B esophagitis regressed to NERD (no esophagitis; normal endoscopy) at 2 years. Among those with grade C and D esophagitis, 42% regressed to A and B esophagitis, and 50% of those with grade C and D regressed to NERD. The study tells us that although the endoscopic findings of GERD are not static, the vast majority of patients with esophagitis heal and those with NERD remain stable. A second study from Germany reproduced the trend of the above ProGERD study in a smaller group of GERD patients.[49] Overall GERD symptom prevalence remains stable over time.

Multiple logistic regression analyses show male gender, increased body mass index, regular alcohol consumption, history of GERD longer than 1 year, and smoking were risks for erosive esophagitis. A positive *Helicobacter pylori* status was associated with a lower risk.[50]

The ProGERD study also examined the history of GERD medication over a 4-year period.[51] PPIs were used in 79%, 84%, 85%, and 87% of patients after 1, 2, 3, and 4 years, respectively. Continuous PPI administration was needed in 53%, 49%, 56%, and 56% of patients after 1, 2, 3, and 4 years. On-demand PPI therapy was administered in 26%, 35%, 29%, and 29% of patients after 1, 2, 3, and 4 years, respectively. The need for continuous PPI treatment increased with advanced grades of esophagitis. After 1, 2, 3, and 4 years, 61%, 56%, 60%, and 60% of those with severe esophagitis at baseline, respectively, remained on continuous PPI treatment.[51]

The next analysis of the ProGERD study examined the effect of GERD on the quality of life of the patients over a 5-year period.[52] Over the 5-year period, medical treatment improved the categories emotional distress, sleep disturbances, eating problems, and vitality by 60%

to 69%. In 54% of patients, physical/social function remained unchanged, whereas it improved in 42%. In all dimensions, clinically relevant worsening was observed in less than 6% of patients. Impairment of the quality of life could largely be attributed to advanced disease with a high symptom load and the perception of nighttime reflux with sleep disturbances. These patients need more than medical treatment and should be offered surgical management of GERD.[52]

In addition to typical symptoms, GERD can impair the quality of life because of the generation of so-called extraesophageal or atypical symptoms (chest pain, cough, laryngeal symptoms, asthma). Jaspersen et al. examined the frequency of extraesophageal GERD symptoms in persons who participated in the ProGERD study (48% NERD, 52% GERD).[53] Extraesophageal symptoms were present in 34.9% and 30.5% of GERD and NERD patients, respectively, and included chest pain (14.5%), cough (13%), laryngeal complaints (10.4%), and asthma (4.8%). Except for asthma, all atypical symptoms were more prevalent in GERD. After 5 years, the prevalence of the symptoms remained unchanged, except for asthma, which increased from 4.5% to 7.8%. The resolution of the extraesophageal symptoms was independent of erosive disease, typical symptoms, disease duration, and PPI medication.[53] Risk factors for the presence and persistence of symptoms included female gender, increased age, more severe esophagitis (types C and D), GERD history longer than 1 year, and smoking.[54] The important epidemiologic data indicate that compared to typical symptoms, extraesophageal GERD symptoms may originate from a different or multifactorial pathogenesis, do not correlate with endoscopic findings, and do not reliably respond to medical treatment.

COMPLICATIONS

Complications associated with GERD include strictures, Barrett esophagus, and adenocarcinoma. In addition, significant decreases in quality of life and economic impact are associated with this disease.

STRICTURES

Since the era of PPIs, the incidence of peptic strictures has decreased.[55] Data from the mid-1980s, pre-PPI use, suggest a prevalence of esophageal stricture of approximately 0.07% to 0.12%.[55,56] Strictures develop from repeated acid exposure resulting in fibrosis and subsequent narrowing of the esophageal lumen.[55,57] With adequate acid suppression, namely by PPIs, stricture formation can be reduced.[55,58] However, even today with a wide array of PPIs in the armamentarium, stricture formation has an incidence of 1.1 per 10,000 person-years and 11.1 per 100 person-years of stricture recurrence.[55]

BARRETT ESOPHAGUS

Barrett esophagus is defined as a change from the normal squamous cell esophageal mucosa to columnar mucosa with intestinal metaplasia and is a premalignant condition (Fig. 15.3).[59,60] Intestinal metaplasia can subsequently degenerate further to dysplasia—both low and high grade—and adenocarcinoma. GERD patients have a 10% to 15% risk

of developing Barrett esophagus.[59,61–63] The prevalence of Barrett esophagus in the US general population without GERD symptoms may be as high as 5.6%.[60,63,64] In a study performed in Sweden, out of 3000 study participants, 1.6% had Barrett esophagus.[65] Out of their study population, 2.3% with reflux symptoms were found to have Barrett esophagus.[65] Having erosive esophagitis increases the likelihood of Barrett esophagus. Additional risk factors for the development of Barrett esophagus are male gender, Caucasian, central obesity, and the duration of GERD symptoms.[59,66–71] Several studies have evaluated the incidence of progression of nondysplastic Barrett esophagus to esophageal adenocarcinoma and have shown the rate to be anywhere from 0.33% to 0.63% annual risk.[72,73] A separate meta-analysis evaluated 41 studies and found an annual incidence of esophageal adenocarcinoma progressing from low-grade dysplasia of 0.54%, and an annual risk of high-grade dysplasia of 1.73%.[74] Finally, the annual incidence of developing esophageal adenocarcinoma from high-grade dysplasia ranges from 7% to 19%.[75,76] The 7% annual risk is based on a meta-analysis of four studies that included 236 patients.[75] The 19% annual risk is based on a study that randomized 127 patients into a high-grade dysplasia surveillance arm and an ablation arm. The surveillance arm was found to have the 19% annual incidence of esophageal adenocarcinoma.[76] In patients with Barrett esophagus, the use of PPIs resulted in a significant decrease in high-grade dysplasia and esophageal adenocarcinoma.[59,77]

QUALITY OF LIFE

In addition to the physical complications described earlier, GERD patients have a decrease in their quality of life as a result of their disease. A 1998 study evaluated 533 adults using the Medical Outcomes Study Short Form (SF-36) and found GERD patients had worse health-related quality of life than the general population. This study also found that the greatest impact was in areas pertaining to pain, social function, and mental health.[78] A subsequent study used the SF-36 questionnaire to evaluate the effects of nocturnal GERD symptoms compared to the general population and found subjects with nocturnal symptoms, again, had a worse quality of life.[79] Kulig et al. evaluated quality of life in GERD patients using the Reflux Disease Questionnaire (RDQ), Quality of Life in Reflux and Dyspepsia (QOLRAD), and SF-36. Their study further supported the claims that quality of life is negatively impacted with GERD, and additionally, treatment with a PPI helped to improve quality of life by controlling symptoms.[80] A meta-analysis of 19 studies showed that GERD led to a decrease in health-related quality of life, a decrease in physical and mental health, and resulted in increased missed days from work.[81] An additional meta-analysis of 9 studies further corroborated the previous findings that mental and physical health are impacted by GERD symptoms.[82]

ECONOMIC BURDEN

Not only does GERD affect quality of life, it also results in large economic consequences. This is partly a result of lost wages from missed days at work and lost productivity due to the decreases in quality of life. Suzuki

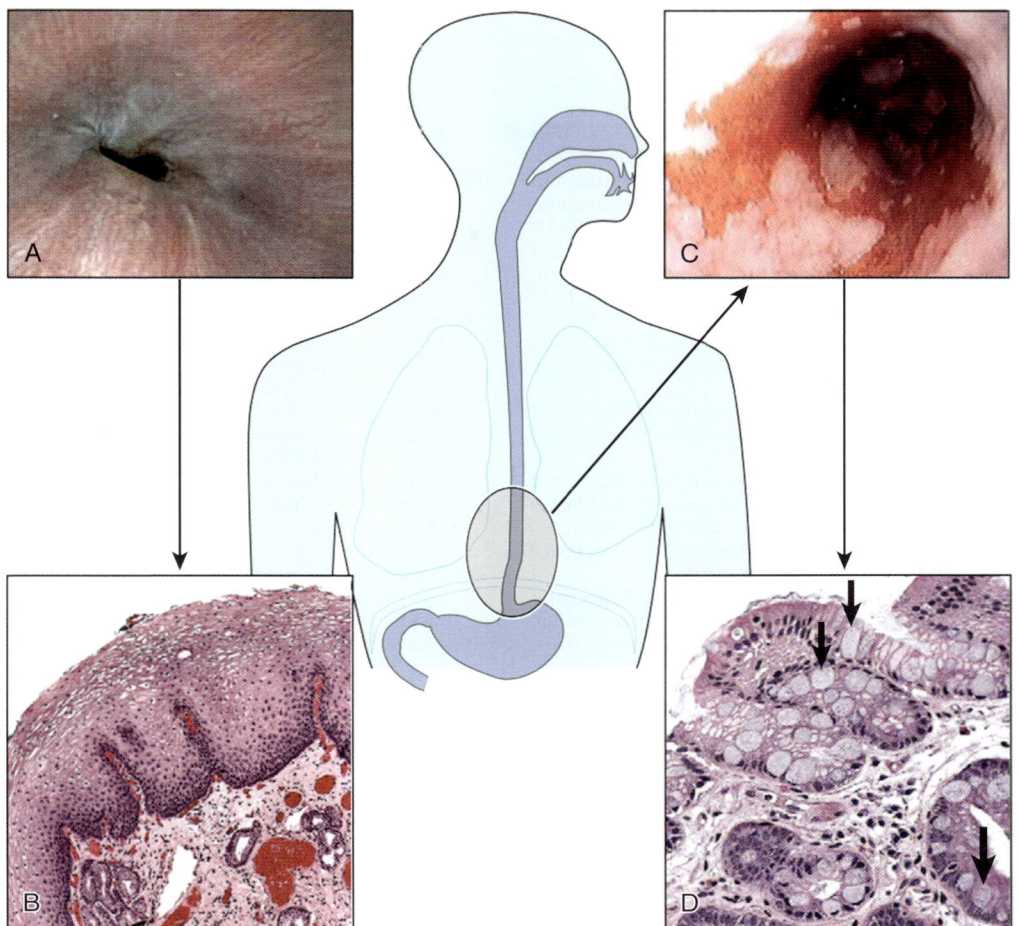

FIGURE 15.3 (A) Normal-appearing squamocolumnar junction seen on upper endoscopy. (B) Normal-appearing histology of esophageal squamous mucosa. (C) Barrett esophagus extending proximal from the gastroesophageal junction. (D) Intestinal metaplasia with *arrows* pointing to goblet cells. (From Shaheen NJ, Richter JE. Barrett's oesophagus. *Lancet.* 2009;373:851, Figure 1.)

et al. found that in Japanese workers with GERD there was a decrease in work productivity of about 0.7 hour per week resulting in a reduction in work productivity of 26.9%.[83] The severity of symptoms correlated with worse productivity at work and increased hours of absenteeism.[81]

In addition to the economic impact from lost productivity, the cost of GERD from direct and indirect medical costs is more than $12.1 billion per year and $515 million per year, respectively.[84] The number of visits to physician offices is in the millions and to emergency departments for GERD is in the hundreds of thousands.[85,86]

CONCLUSION

GERD is a prevalent disease across the world. It has a higher prevalence in the United States and other Western countries compared to locations such as East Asia.[2] GERD can be managed by a number of modalities, both medical and surgical, to help mitigate some of the effects of GERD ranging from strictures, Barrett esophagus, and esophageal adenocarcinoma to its impacts on quality of life, lost work productivity, and overall cost.

ACKNOWLEDGMENTS

This is an update of a previous chapter written by Martin Riegler, Sebastian Schoppmann, and Johannes Zacherl.

REFERENCES

1. Dent J, El-Serag HB, Wallander MA, Johansson S. Epidemiology of gastro-oesophageal reflux disease: a systematic review. *Gut.* 2005;54:710-717.
2. El-Serag HB, Sweet S, Winchester CC, Dent J. Update on the epidemiology of gastro-oesophageal reflux disease: a systematic review. *Gut.* 2014;63:871-880.
3. Ness-Jensen E, Hveem K, El-Serag H, Lagergren J. Lifestyle intervention in gastroesophageal reflux disease. *Clin Gastroenterol Hepatol.* 2016;14:175-182.e1-3.
4. Vakil N, van Zanten SV, Kahrilas P, Dent J, Jones R, Global Consensus Group. The Montreal definition and classification of gastroesophageal reflux disease: a global evidence-based consensus. *Am J Gastroenterol.* 2006;101:1900-1920.
5. Katz PO, Gerson LB, Vela MF. Guidelines for the diagnosis and management of gastroesophageal reflux disease. *Am J Gastroenterol.* 2013;108:303-328; quiz 329.
6. Hershcovici T, Mashimo H, Fass R. The lower esophageal sphincter. *Neurogastroenterol Motil.* 2011;23:819-830.
7. Mittal RK, Balaban DH. The esophagogastric junction. *N Engl J Med.* 1997;336:924-932.

8. Dunbar KB, Agoston AT, Odze RD, et al. Association of acute gastroesophageal reflux disease with esophageal histologic changes. *JAMA*. 2016;315:2104-2112.

9. Corley DA, Kubo A, Zhao W. Abdominal obesity, ethnicity and gastro-oesophageal reflux symptoms. *Gut*. 2007;56:756-762.

10. El-Serag HB, Ergun GA, Pandolfino J, Fitzgerald S, Tran T, Kramer JR. Obesity increases oesophageal acid exposure. *Gut*. 2007;56:749-755.

11. Irwin RS, Curley FJ, French CL. Chronic cough. The spectrum and frequency of causes, key components of the diagnostic evaluation, and outcome of specific therapy. *Am Rev Respir Dis*. 1990;141:640-647.

12. Jung HK, Halder S, McNally M, et al. Overlap of gastro-oesophageal reflux disease and irritable bowel syndrome: prevalence and risk factors in the general population. *Aliment Pharmacol Ther*. 2007;26:453-461.

13. El-Serag HB, Petersen NJ, Carter J, et al. Gastroesophageal reflux among different racial groups in the United States. *Gastroenterology*. 2004;126:1692-1699.

14. Sharma P, Wani S, Romero Y, Johnson D, Hamilton F. Racial and geographic issues in gastroesophageal reflux disease. *Am J Gastroenterol*. 2008;103:2669-2680.

15. Yuen E, Romney M, Toner RW, et al. Prevalence, knowledge and care patterns for gastro-oesophageal reflux disease in United States minority populations. *Aliment Pharmacol Ther*. 2010;32:645-654.

16. Friedenberg FK. GERD in minority populations. *Gastroenterol Hepatol (N Y)*. 2011;7:411-413.

17. Chiocca JC, Olmos JA, Salis GB, et al. Prevalence, clinical spectrum and atypical symptoms of gastro-oesophageal reflux in Argentina: a nationwide population-based study. *Aliment Pharmacol Ther*. 2005;22:331-342.

18. do Rosario Dias de Oliveira Latorre M, Medeiros da Silva A, Chinzon D, Eisig JN, Dias-Bastos TR. Epidemiology of upper gastrointestinal symptoms in Brazil (EpiGastro): a population-based study according to sex and age group. *World J Gastroenterol*. 2014;20:17388-17398.

19. Thompson WG, Heaton KW. Heartburn and globus in apparently healthy people. *Can Med Assoc J*. 1982;126:46-48.

20. Isolauri J, Laippala P. Prevalence of symptoms suggestive of gastro-oesophageal reflux disease in an adult population. *Ann Med*. 1995;27:67-70.

21. Valle C, Broglia F, Pistorio A, Tinelli C, Perego M. Prevalence and impact of symptoms suggestive of gastroesophageal reflux disease. *Dig Dis Sci*. 1999;44:1848-1852.

22. Terry P, Lagergren J, Wolk A, Nyrén O. Reflux-inducing dietary factors and risk of adenocarcinoma of the esophagus and gastric cardia. *Nutr Cancer*. 2000;38:186-191.

23. Mohammed I, Cherkas LF, Riley SA, Spector TD, Trudgill NJ. Genetic influences in gastro-oesophageal reflux disease: a twin study. *Gut*. 2003;52:1085-1089.

24. Diaz-Rubio M, Moreno-Elola-Olaso C, Rey E, Locke GR 3rd, Rodriguez-Artalejo F. Symptoms of gastro-oesophageal reflux: prevalence, severity, duration and associated factors in a Spanish population. *Aliment Pharmacol Ther*. 2004;19:95-105.

25. Ronkainen J, Aro P, Storskrubb T, et al. High prevalence of gastro-esophageal reflux symptoms and esophagitis with or without symptoms in the general adult Swedish population: a Kalixanda study report. *Scand J Gastroenterol*. 2005;40:275-285.

26. Lofdahl HE, Lane A, Lu Y, et al. Increased population prevalence of reflux and obesity in the United Kingdom compared with Sweden: a potential explanation for the difference in incidence of esophageal adenocarcinoma. *Eur J Gastroenterol Hepatol*. 2011;23:128-132.

27. Pan G, Xu G, Ke M, et al. Epidemiological study of symptomatic gastroesophageal reflux disease in China: Beijing and Shanghai. *Chin J Dig Dis*. 2000;1:2-8.

28. Hu WH, Wong WM, Lam CL, et al. Anxiety but not depression determines health care-seeking behaviour in Chinese patients with dyspepsia and irritable bowel syndrome: a population-based study. *Aliment Pharmacol Ther*. 2002;16:2081-2088.

29. Wong WM, Lai KC, Lam KF, et al. Prevalence, clinical spectrum and health care utilization of gastro-oesophageal reflux disease in a Chinese population: a population-based study. *Aliment Pharmacol Ther*. 2003;18:595-604.

30. Chen M, Xiong L, Chen H, Xu A, He L, Hu P. Prevalence, risk factors and impact of gastroesophageal reflux disease symptoms: a population-based study in South China. *Scand J Gastroenterol*. 2005;40:759-767.

31. He J, Ma X, Zhao Y, et al. A population-based survey of the epidemiology of symptom-defined gastroesophageal reflux disease: the systematic investigation of gastrointestinal diseases in China. *BMC Gastroenterol*. 2010;10:94.

32. Cho YS, Choi MG, Jeong JJ, et al. Prevalence and clinical spectrum of gastroesophageal reflux: a population-based study in Asan-si, Korea. *Am J Gastroenterol*. 2005;100:747-753.

33. Jung HK. Epidemiology of gastroesophageal reflux disease in Asia: a systematic review. *J Neurogastroenterol Motil*. 2011;17:14-27.

34. Kitapcioglu G, Mandiracioglu A, Caymaz Bor C, Bor S. Overlap of symptoms of dyspepsia and gastroesophageal reflux in the community. *Turk J Gastroenterol*. 2007;18:14-19.

35. Sperber AD, Halpern Z, Shvartzman P, et al. Prevalence of GERD symptoms in a representative Israeli adult population. *J Clin Gastroenterol*. 2007;41:457-461.

36. Solhpour A, Pourhoseingholi MA, Soltani F, et al. Gastro-esophageal reflux symptoms and body mass index: no relation among the Iranian population. *Indian J Gastroenterol*. 2008;27:153-155.

37. Nouraie M, Radmard AR, Zaer-Rezaii H, Razjouyan H, Nasseri-Moghaddam S, Malekzadeh R. Hygiene could affect GERD prevalence independently: a population-based study in Tehran. *Am J Gastroenterol*. 2007;102:1353-1360.

38. Nouraie M, Razjouyan H, Assady M, Malekzadeh R, Nasseri-Moghaddam S. Epidemiology of gastroesophageal reflux symptoms in Tehran, Iran: a population-based telephone survey. *Arch Iran Med*. 2007;10:289-294.

39. Nasseri-Moghaddam S, Mofid A, Ghotbi MH, et al. Epidemiological study of gastro-oesophageal reflux disease: reflux in spouse as a risk factor. *Aliment Pharmacol Ther*. 2008;28:144-153.

40. Mostaghni A, Mehrabani D, Khademolhosseini F, et al. Prevalence and risk factors of gastroesophageal reflux disease in Qashqai migrating nomads, southern Iran. *World J Gastroenterol*. 2009;15:961-965.

41. Delavari A, Moradi G, Elahi E, Moradi-Lakeh M. Gastroesophageal reflux disease burden in Iran. *Arch Iran Med*. 2015;18:85-88.

42. Almadi MA, Almousa MA, Althwainy AF, et al. Prevalence of symptoms of gastroesophageal reflux in a cohort of Saudi Arabians: a study of 1265 subjects. *Saudi J Gastroenterol*. 2014;20:248-254.

43. Locke GR 3rd, Talley NJ, Fett SL, Zinsmeister AR, Melton LJ 3rd. Prevalence and clinical spectrum of gastroesophageal reflux: a population-based study in Olmsted County, Minnesota. *Gastroenterology*. 1997;112:1448-1456.

44. Becher A, Dent J. Systematic review: ageing and gastro-oesophageal reflux disease symptoms, oesophageal function and reflux oesophagitis. *Aliment Pharmacol Ther*. 2011;33:442-454.

45. Johnson DA, Fennerty MB. Heartburn severity underestimates erosive esophagitis severity in elderly patients with gastroesophageal reflux disease. *Gastroenterology*. 2004;126:660-664.

46. Malfertheiner SF, Malfertheiner MV, Kropf S, Costa SD, Malfertheiner P. A prospective longitudinal cohort study: evolution of GERD symptoms during the course of pregnancy. *BMC Gastroenterol*. 2012;12:131.

47. Rey E, Rodriguez-Artalejo F, Herraiz MA, et al. Gastroesophageal reflux symptoms during and after pregnancy: a longitudinal study. *Am J Gastroenterol*. 2007;102:2395-2400.

48. Labenz J, Nocon M, Lind T, et al. Prospective follow-up data from the ProGERD study suggest that GERD is not a categorial disease. *Am J Gastroenterol*. 2006;101:2457-2462.

49. Bajbouj M, Reichenberger J, Neu B, et al. A prospective multicenter clinical and endoscopic follow-up study of patients with gastroesophageal reflux disease. *Z Gastroenterol*. 2005;43:1303-1307.

50. Labenz J, Jaspersen D, Kulig M, et al. Risk factors for erosive esophagitis: a multivariate analysis based on the ProGERD study initiative. *Am J Gastroenterol*. 2004;99:1652-1656.

51. Nocon M, Labenz J, Jaspersen D, et al. Long-term treatment of patients with gastro-oesophageal reflux disease in routine care—results from the ProGERD study. *Aliment Pharmacol Ther*. 2007;25:715-722.

52. Nocon M, Labenz J, Jaspersen D, et al. Health-related quality of life in patients with gastro-oesophageal reflux disease under routine care: 5-year follow-up results of the ProGERD study. *Aliment Pharmacol Ther*. 2009;29:662-668.

53. Jaspersen D, Nocon M, Labenz J, et al. Clinical course of laryngo-respiratory symptoms in gastro-oesophageal reflux disease during routine care—a 5-year follow-up. *Aliment Pharmacol Ther*. 2009;29:1172-1178.

54. Jaspersen D, Kulig M, Labenz J, et al. Prevalence of extra-oesophageal manifestations in gastro-oesophageal reflux disease: an analysis

based on the ProGERD Study. *Aliment Pharmacol Ther.* 2003;17:1515-1520.

55. Ruigomez A, Garcia Rodriguez LA, Wallander MA, Johansson S, Eklund S. Esophageal stricture: incidence, treatment patterns, and recurrence rate. *Am J Gastroenterol.* 2006;101:2685-2692.

56. Fennerty MB. The continuum of GERD complications. *Cleve Clin J Med.* 2003;70(suppl 5):S33-S50.

57. Spechler SJ. Clinical manifestations and esophageal complications of GERD. *Am J Med Sci.* 2003;326:279-284.

58. Marks RD, Richter JE, Rizzo J, et al. Omeprazole versus H2-receptor antagonists in treating patients with peptic stricture and esophagitis. *Gastroenterology.* 1994;106:907-915.

59. Shaheen NJ, Falk GW, Iyer PG, Gerson LB, American College of Gastroenterology. ACG Clinical guideline: diagnosis and management of Barrett's esophagus. *Am J Gastroenterol.* 2016;111:30-50.

60. Shaheen NJ, Richter JE. Barrett's oesophagus. *Lancet.* 2009;373: 850-861.

61. Halland M, Katzka D, Iyer PG. Recent developments in pathogenesis, diagnosis and therapy of Barrett's esophagus. *World J Gastroenterol.* 2015;21:6479-6490.

62. Dent J. Barrett's esophagus: a historical perspective, an update on core practicalities and predictions on future evolutions of management. *J Gastroenterol Hepatol.* 2011;26(suppl 1):11-30.

63. Sharma P. Clinical practice. Barrett's esophagus. *N Engl J Med.* 2009;361:2548-2556.

64. Rex DK, Cummings OW, Shaw M, et al. Screening for Barrett's esophagus in colonoscopy patients with and without heartburn. *Gastroenterology.* 2003;125:1670-1677.

65. Ronkainen J, Aro P, Storskrubb T, et al. Prevalence of Barrett's esophagus in the general population: an endoscopic study. *Gastroenterology.* 2005;129:1825-1831.

66. Rubenstein JH, Mattek N, Eisen G. Age- and sex-specific yield of Barrett's esophagus by endoscopy indication. *Gastrointest Endosc.* 2010;71:21-27.

67. Kubo A, Cook MB, Shaheen NJ, et al. Sex-specific associations between body mass index, waist circumference and the risk of Barrett's oesophagus: a pooled analysis from the international BEACON consortium. *Gut.* 2013;62:1684-1691.

68. Singh S, Sharma AN, Murad MH, et al. Central adiposity is associated with increased risk of esophageal inflammation, metaplasia, and adenocarcinoma: a systematic review and meta-analysis. *Clin Gastroenterol Hepatol.* 2013;11:1399-1412, e7.

69. Cook MB, Wild CP, Forman D. A systematic review and meta-analysis of the sex ratio for Barrett's esophagus, erosive reflux disease, and nonerosive reflux disease. *Am J Epidemiol.* 2005;162:1050-1061.

70. Lieberman DA, Oehlke M, Helfand M. Risk factors for Barrett's esophagus in community-based practice. GORGE consortium. Gastroenterolgy Outcomes Research Group in Endoscopy. *Am J Gastroenterol.* 1997;92:1293-1297.

71. Thrift AP, Kramer JR, Qureshi Z, Richardson PA, El-Serag HB. Age at onset of GERD symptoms predicts risk of Barrett's esophagus. *Am J Gastroenterol.* 2013;108:915-922.

72. Desai TK, Krishnan K, Samala N, et al. The incidence of oesophageal adenocarcinoma in non-dysplastic Barrett's oesophagus: a meta-analysis. *Gut.* 2012;61:970-976.

73. Sikkema M, de Jonge PJ, Steyerberg EW, Kuipers EJ. Risk of esophageal adenocarcinoma and mortality in patients with Barrett's esophagus: a systematic review and meta-analysis. *Clin Gastroenterol Hepatol.* 2010;8:235-244; quiz e.32.

74. Singh S, Manickam P, Amin AV, et al. Incidence of esophageal adenocarcinoma in Barrett's esophagus with low-grade dysplasia: a systematic review and meta-analysis. *Gastrointest Endosc.* 2014;79:897-909. e4; quiz 983.e1, 983.e3.

75. Rastogi A, Puli S, El-Serag HB, Bansal A, Wani S, Sharma P. Incidence of esophageal adenocarcinoma in patients with Barrett's esophagus and high-grade dysplasia: a meta-analysis. *Gastrointest Endosc.* 2008;67:394-398.

76. Shaheen NJ, Sharma P, Overholt BF, et al. Radiofrequency ablation in Barrett's esophagus with dysplasia. *N Engl J Med.* 2009;360:2277-2288.

77. Singh S, Garg SK, Singh PP, Iyer PG, El-Serag HB. Acid-suppressive medications and risk of oesophageal adenocarcinoma in patients with Barrett's oesophagus: a systematic review and meta-analysis. *Gut.* 2014;63:1229-1237.

78. Revicki DA, Wood M, Maton PN, Sorensen S. The impact of gastroesophageal reflux disease on health-related quality of life. *Am J Med.* 1998;104:252-258.

79. Farup C, Kleinman L, Sloan S, et al. The impact of nocturnal symptoms associated with gastroesophageal reflux disease on health-related quality of life. *Arch Intern Med.* 2001;161:45-52.

80. Kulig M, Leodolter A, Vieth M, et al. Quality of life in relation to symptoms in patients with gastro-oesophageal reflux disease—an analysis based on the ProGERD initiative. *Aliment Pharmacol Ther.* 2003;18:767-776.

81. Tack J, Becher A, Mulligan C, Johnson DA. Systematic review: the burden of disruptive gastro-oesophageal reflux disease on health-related quality of life. *Aliment Pharmacol Ther.* 2012;35:1257-1266.

82. Becher A, El-Serag H. Systematic review: the association between symptomatic response to proton pump inhibitors and health-related quality of life in patients with gastro-oesophageal reflux disease. *Aliment Pharmacol Ther.* 2011;34:618-627.

83. Suzuki H, Matsuzaki J, Masaoka T, Inadomi JM. Greater loss of productivity among Japanese workers with gastro-esophageal reflux disease (GERD) symptoms that persist vs resolve on medical therapy. *Neurogastroenterol Motil.* 2014;26:764-771.

84. Menees SB, Guentner A, Chey SW, Saad R, Chey WD. How do US gastroenterologists use over-the-counter and prescription medications in patients with gastroesophageal reflux and chronic constipation? *Am J Gastroenterol.* 2015;110:1516-1525.

85. Peery AF, Crockett SD, Barritt AS, et al. Burden of gastrointestinal, liver, and pancreatic diseases in the United States. *Gastroenterology.* 2015;149:1731-1741.e3.

86. Peery AF, Dellon ES, Lund J, et al. Burden of gastrointestinal disease in the United States: 2012 update. *Gastroenterology.* 2012;143:1179-1187, e1-3.

Etiology and Natural History of Gastroesophageal Reflux Disease and Predictors of Progressive Disease

Tom R. DeMeester

Gastroesophageal reflux disease (GERD) is the most common foregut disease in the world and accounts for approximately 75% of all esophageal pathology.[1] The majority of affected patients have mild disease and are successfully managed with lifestyle modification and acid suppression medication.[2] Fortunately, progression to erosive disease occurs in only 13% of patients over 5 years.[3] Unfortunately, progression to Barrett esophagus (BE), the premalignant lesion for adenocarcinoma of the esophagus, occurs in 10% of patients over 5 years.[3] This has led to concerns that proton pump inhibitor (PPI) therapy does not directly address the underlying cause of the disease. It is estimated that more than 113 million PPI prescriptions are filled globally each year.[4] A 10% progression to BE every 5 years is therefore an enormous problem.

GERD is currently defined as a condition that develops when the reflux of stomach contents into the esophagus causes troublesome symptoms such as heartburn and/or regurgitation.[5] This symptomatic definition is not a precise guide to the presence of disease because there is not always a clear correlation between reflux symptoms and objective evidence of the disease, such as esophagitis or increased esophageal acid exposure on 24-hour esophageal pH monitoring. Further, patients may have typical reflux symptoms in the absence of endoscopic esophagitis or have endoscopic esophagitis in the absence of typical reflux symptoms.[6] In both situations a 24-hour esophageal pH monitoring study is necessary to confirm the presence of disease.

In practice, it is common for primary care physicians to treat patients with GERD symptoms on their initial visit with a trial of PPIs. If symptoms are relieved, they accept that the diagnosis of GERD is confirmed despite studies showing that the "PPI trial" has a low accuracy for identifying the patient with GERD.[7,8] In the absence of a complete response to a trial of PPIs, it is recommended that the dose of PPIs be doubled.[9] If this does not lead to symptom resolution, a 24-hour esophageal pH monitoring study should be performed off medication to measure the esophageal acid exposure and confirm the diagnosis of GERD. If the study is positive, it is recommended that the PPI dose be further increased or an alternative PPI prescribed.[9] This approach has popularized the concept that patients with persistent symptoms while on PPI therapy are undermedicated. As a consequence, the possibility of progressive disease occurring under PPI therapy is rarely considered. A more prudent conclusion is that whether or not the patient's symptoms come under control with the escalation of the PPI dose, the possibility of progressive disease remains and must be assessed.

PROGRESSION OF GASTROESOPHAGEAL REFLUX DISEASE UNDER THERAPY

Two scenarios have been proposed regarding the natural history of GERD. The first is that GERD is a categorical disorder, and the patient can be categorized as having either nonerosive reflux disease (NERD) or erosive reflux disease (ERD) and patients remain in their diagnosed category.[10] The second is that GERD is a spectrum disorder with NERD at one end of the spectrum and BE and esophageal adenocarcinoma at the other end, with the ability of the disease to progress through the spectrum over time.[11] Current clinical evidence appears to support the spectrum concept in that there are several studies showing progression of patients from their initial category to a more advanced category.[12]

One of the largest studies of GERD progression was the ProGERD study involving 2721 patients from Germany, Switzerland, and Austria.[13] Patients were categorized endoscopically as having NERD or ERD based on the Los Angeles (LA) classification. Patients with BE were excluded. The study consisted of an initial endoscopy to categorize the patients, followed by 4 to 8 weeks of PPI therapy, followed by maintenance therapy provided by the patients' primary care physician. A follow-up endoscopy was performed at 2 and 5 years. Progression to BE, confirmed by endoscopy and biopsy during the 5 years of therapy, was observed in 5.9% of patients with NERD, 12.1% of patients with ERD (LA grade A/B), and 19.7% of patients with severe ERD (LA grade C/D). Patients with severe ERD on initial endoscopy had the highest incidence of progression to BE. Overall, 10% of patients progressed to BE during the 5-year follow-up period. This study clearly showed that disease progression occurred in a proportion of patients while receiving PPI therapy and established that, although regular and consistent PPI therapy can improve symptoms and heal erosive esophagitis, it does not stop progression to BE.

The second study consisted of a group of 33 patients who were referred to a gastrointestinal clinic in Milan, Italy with the diagnosis of NERD.[14] Patients were endoscopically normal but had an abnormal 24-hour esophageal pH monitoring study at baseline. The patients were observed for 10 years. During the first 5 years of follow-up, 18 patients had a repeat endoscopy and 17 (94.4%) had esophagitis. When active PPI therapy was discontinued after 10 years of follow-up, symptoms relapsed in 96.6% of the available patients (28/29). This study showed that GERD of all severities requires long-term medical therapy. It further showed the progressive capability of NERD and that the absence of endoscopic esophagitis at presentation is not a positive prognostic factor.

A third study of 40 Swedish patients with GERD, confirmed by an abnormal esophageal acid exposure on 24-hour pH monitoring, showed that when progression occurred during PPI treatment, it was associated with the development of manometric abnormalities of the lower esophageal sphincter (LES).[15] Patients in the study underwent endoscopy, esophageal manometry, and 24-hour esophageal pH monitoring at the beginning and end of a 21-year follow-up period. At baseline, 24 patients had NERD and 16 ERD. None had endoscopic or histologic evidence of BE. Of the 24 patients with NERD, a baseline 14 progressed to ERD and 10 (41.7%) to BE. Of the 16 patients with ERD at baseline, 8 developed BE (50%). Overall, 18 of 40 (45%) progressed to BE over the 21-year follow-up period. Progression was associated with a significantly shorter LES mean intraabdominal length ($P = .01$) and a significantly greater esophageal acid exposure on pH monitoring ($P = .004$) compared with patients who did not progress. Furthermore, the study population showed a trend toward increased use of PPIs over the 21-year follow-up period, and an increase in the number of patients who developed erosive esophagitis. These results indicate that patients with a long duration of GERD are more likely to progress despite PPI treatment, likely due to deterioration of the LES during the course of therapy.

The previous study was the first to introduce the concept that the progression of GERD while on PPI therapy was likely due to progressive LES damage during therapy. In practice the byword became, the greater the LES damage, the less effective the PPI therapy. This concept was examined prospectively in a study of GERD patients with different degrees of LES and esophageal body functionality prior to therapy.[16] A damaged LES was defined as a pressure less than 8 mm Hg and/or a LES abdominal length less than 1.2 cm. More than 20% ineffective peristaltic contractions were used to indicate a compromised esophageal body. PPI failure, shown by the recurrence of symptoms or esophagitis, occurred in 7.7% (2/26) of patients with a normal LES and normal esophageal body, 38.1% (24/63) of patients with a damaged LES and normal esophageal body, and 79.5% (31/39) of patients with a damaged LES and a compromised esophageal body. These results strongly indicated that PPI therapy was less effective in patients with a damaged LES than in those with a normal LES and that a compromised esophageal body added to their ineffectiveness.

In an effort to understand further the effects of mechanical factors in the progression of GERD under PPI therapy, we studied the existence of mechanical abnormalities in the spectrum of GERD. This included factors such as anatomic distortion of the hiatal anatomy by a hiatal hernia, abnormalities of the LES, and the effects of LES incompetency on esophageal exposure to acid and bile.[17] Fifty symptomatic consecutive patients were identified for each of the four stages of GERD from the preoperative records of those who had a laparoscopic Nissen fundoplication performed by us. The stages were (1) NERD, (2) mild ERD, defined as "healable esophagitis" with PPI therapy, (3) severe ERD, defined as "difficult to heal esophagitis" that persisted despite PPI therapy, and (4) BE. Exclusion criteria were normal preoperative esophageal acid exposure on pH monitoring, esophageal pH monitoring performed elsewhere, previous antireflux surgery, and a named esophageal motility disorder or a low contraction amplitude in distal half of the esophagus. Patients who could not be contacted for study approval were also excluded. All patients' records contained a detailed preoperative clinical questionnaire, and all underwent a preoperative upper gastrointestinal endoscopy, esophageal manometry, and distal esophageal pH monitoring. Patients who had received PPI therapy prior to their initial endoscopy were excluded from the NERD group. BE was diagnosed by the presence of microscopic intestinal metaplasia on biopsy of an endoscopic visible columnar-lined esophagus of any length. The final studied population consisted of 39 patients with NERD, 42 with mild ERD (i.e., healable esophagitis), 35 with severe ERD (i.e., difficult to heal esophagitis), and 44 with BE.

The significant anatomic and physiologic differences between the patient groups are shown in Fig. 16.1. The differences between the patient groups "healable esophagitis" and the "difficult to heal esophagitis" was the status of their LES. Preoperative mechanical factors (i.e., altered hiatal anatomy, LES resting pressure, and LES lengths) were significantly more impaired in patients with "difficult to heal esophagitis" and BE compared with those with "healable esophagitis" and NERD. Esophageal acid and bile exposure also was worse in the more severe GERD stages with the most severe in patients with BE. The composite pH score, which includes all the acid reflux measures in a weighted calculation of reflux severity, discriminated most clearly between the different GERD stages. These findings support the importance of LES length and resting pressure in the etiology and severity of GERD. The findings also link the extent and severity of endoscopic mucosal injury with the extent and severity of mechanical abnormalities at the gastroesophageal barrier. Furthermore, they suggest that progression of GERD in a patient on PPI therapy commonly requires a concomitant reduction in LES length and pressure and altered hiatal anatomy. These findings are similar to other studies of regression analysis which show that the status of the LES and size of the hiatal hernia are dominant determinants of esophagitis and its severity.[18,19]

Taken together, the above studies show most importantly the following: (1) the treatment of GERD with PPIs does not prevent progression of disease, (2) the stages of GERD severity correlate well to the altered mechanical features of the gastroesophageal reflux barrier, (3) damage to the LES is associated with altered hiatal anatomy, increased esophageal exposure to refluxed acid and bile, and (4) PPI therapy does not protect against continuing LES damage. These findings encourage the concept that to stop the progression of GERD requires (1) early recognition

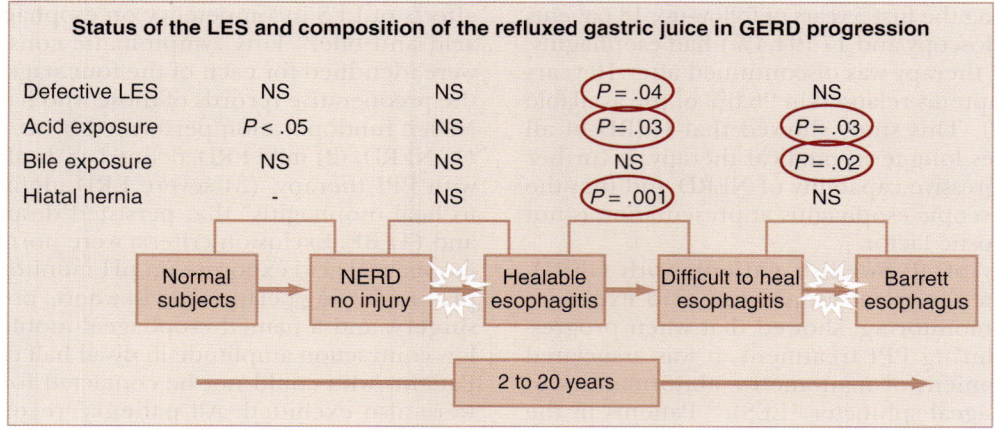

FIGURE 16.1 Status of the lower esophageal sphincter *(LES)*, esophageal acid exposure, esophageal bile exposure, and the anatomic distortion of the hiatal anatomy by a hiatal hernia in the spectrum of gastroesophageal reflux disease *(GERD)* categories: nonerosive reflux disease *(NERD)*, "healable esophagitis," "difficult to heal esophagitis," and Barrett esophagus *(BE)*. Significant anatomic and physiologic differences existed between the categories of healable esophagitis and difficult to heal esophagitis. BE differs from difficult to heal esophagitis only by the degree of esophageal acid and bile exposure. High bile exposure was unique to BE. *NS,* No significance. (From Lord RV, DeMeester SR, Peters JH, et al. Hiatal hernia, lower esophageal sphincter incompetence, and effectiveness of Nissen fundoplication in the spectrum of gastroesophageal reflux disease. *J Gastrointest Surg.* 2009;13:602–610.)

of the symptoms and signs of progressive disease, (2) manometric assessment of the LES, (3) measurements of esophageal acid exposure, (4) endoscopic examination of the esophagus, and, if indicated, (5) early surgical intervention to correct the LES abnormalities. To do so requires an understanding of the pathophysiology and the histopathology of GERD.

PATHOPHYSIOLOGY OF GASTROESOPHAGEAL REFLUX DISEASE

There are two fundamental determinants of GERD: the status of the LES and the composition of the gastric juice refluxed into the esophagus. Of the two, the status of the LES is the primary determinant. The LES is a measurable force located in the distal end of the esophagus where it straddles the diaphragm. Anatomically its boundaries are unmarked and its exact location can only be determined by using a pressure-sensitive catheter. The LES normally remains closed with two exceptions: during a swallow, when an induced reflex relaxation of the force occurs to allow a bolus of food to enter the stomach, or during a belch, when the force is disrupted to allow gas to be vented from a distended stomach. The common denominator for virtually all episodes of gastroesophageal reflux is the disappearance of the force. When this occurs, resistance to the flow of gastric juice from an environment of higher pressure—the stomach—to an environment of lower pressure—the esophagus—is lost. In early disease the loss of the force is a transient event. In advanced disease, the loss or deficiency of the force is permanent.

Dr. Charles Code discovered the force (i.e., the "high pressure zone," as he referred to it) in 1956.[20] The importance of its discovery in regard to GERD was nullified by Dr. Campbell McLaurin from Scotland. After a fairly extensive study, McLaurin concluded that the "high pressure zone"

was not of primary importance in the prevention of reflux because there was no direct relationship between its pressure and the existence of reflux.[21] This, along with other similar reports, shelved the LES as a curiosity.

The introduction of 24-hour esophageal pH monitoring resurfaced an interest to further investigate the LES as a barrier to reflux. The renewed interest resulted in studies of normal subjects and symptomatic GERD patients with esophageal manometry and 24-hour esophageal pH monitoring.[22] The results of these studies indicated there were three characteristics of the force, or LES, that worked together to provide a barrier to challenges of increased intragastric and intraabdominal pressure (Fig. 16.2A). One of these characteristics was the position of the LES. A portion of the LES length is normally exposed to the positive intraabdominal pressure environment and is commonly referred to as the abdominal length of the LES.[23] During periods of increased intraabdominal pressure, the resistance of the LES could easily be overcome if the challenge of intraabdominal pressure was unable to be applied equally to the abdominal esophagus (i.e., synonymous with abdominal length of LES) and stomach.[24–26] In situations in which the length of the abdominal esophagus has become permanently inadequate, the abdominal esophagus cannot collapse in response to challenges of intraabdominal pressure. This is called permanent failure of the LES (Fig. 16.2B), and with the encouragement from the negative intrathoracic pressure, results in persistent reflux of gastric juice into the esophagus with minimal abdominal pressure challenges.

The remaining two characteristics of the LES, overall length of the LES and the LES pressure, also provide a barrier to reflux. Both function together and depend on each other to provide resistance to flow of gastric juice from the stomach into the esophagus unrelated to intraabdominal pressure challenges. Critical to this function is the relationship between the LES overall length

LES pressure profile

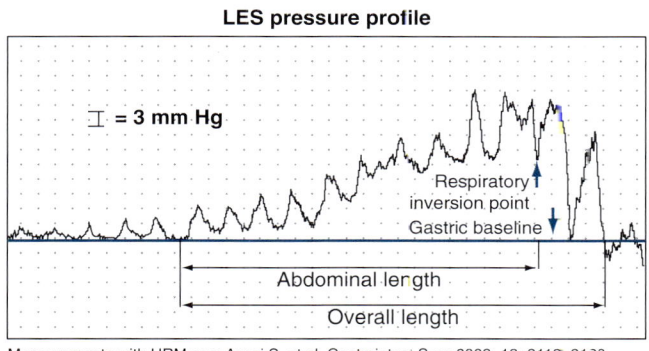

$\mathbb{I}$ = 3 mm Hg

Respiratory inversion point
Gastric baseline

Abdominal length

Overall length

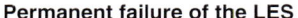

Measurements with HRM see: Ayazi S, et al. Gastrointes: Surg 2009; 13: 2113–2120

A

Permanent failure of the LES

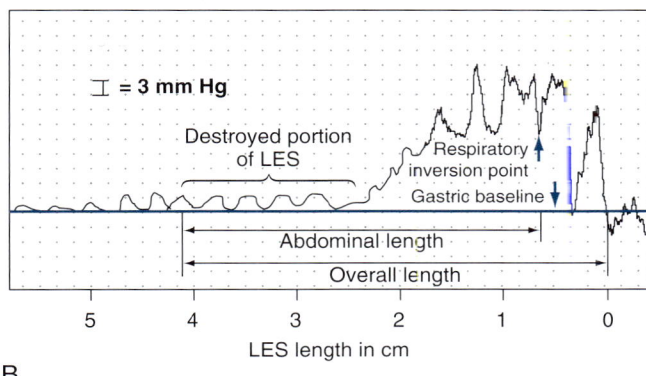

$\mathbb{I}$ = 3 mm Hg

Destroyed portion of LES

Respiratory inversion point
Gastric baseline

Abdominal length

Overall length

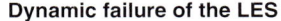

LES length in cm

B

Dynamic failure of the LES

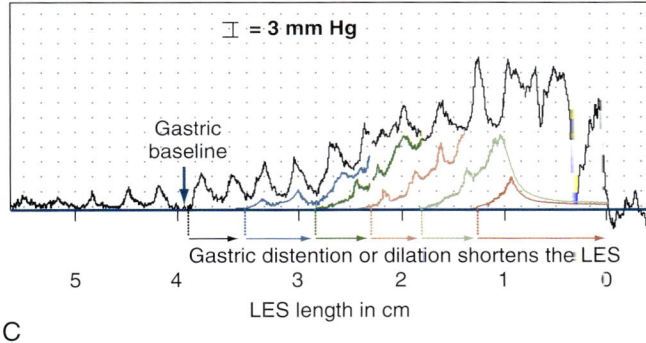

$\mathbb{I}$ = 3 mm Hg

Gastric baseline

Gastric distention or dilation shortens the LES

LES length in cm

C

FIGURE 16.2 (A) The pressure profile of the lower esophageal sphincter *(LES)* in normal subjects. Note the long intraabdominal length identified by the positive respiratory excursions. The abdominal length ends at the respiratory inversion point where the respiratory excursions change from positive excursions with breathing to negative excursion with breathing. A short intrathoracic portion of the LES is identified by the negative respiratory excursions. Adequate overall length, abdominal length, and pressure are necessary for the LES to function as a barrier to reflux. (B) An illustration of permanent failure of the LES. This is due to the permanent loss of abdominal LES length. This compromises the ability of the LES to prevent reflux caused by intraabdominal pressure challenges. (C) An illustration of dynamic failure of the LES. The overall and abdominal length of the LES shortens with gastric distention and returns back to its original length when the distention is relieved by a burp. As the LES shortens due to distention or nonpressurized gastric dilation, it reaches a point where the ratio of length to pressure is insufficient to keep the LES closed, allowing gastroesophageal reflux to occur. When the stomach is decompressed or gastric dilation recedes, the length of the LES returns to normal and competency is reestablished.

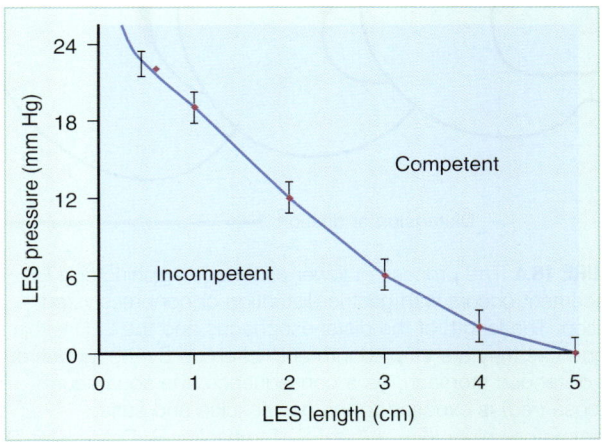

FIGURE 16.3 The relationship between lower esophageal sphincter *(LES)* pressure and overall length to its competency. Excessive eating results in gastric distention and dilation, which can shorten the length of the LES to the point where its existing pressure is ineffective in keeping the circumferential wall of the LES approximated. When this occurs, the walls of the LES separate, competency of the LES is lost, and reflux occurs.

and the LES pressure.[27] The shorter the overall length, the higher the pressure must be for the LES to maintain competency against challenges of intragastric pressure above intraabdominal pressure (Fig. 16.3). Consequently, a normal LES pressure can be nullified by a short overall LES length, and a normal overall LES length can be nullified by a low LES pressure. The fundamental principle is that the overall length of the LES, similar to the LES abdominal length, is important to the function of the LES as a barrier.[28–30] Shortening of the overall length of the LES occurs naturally with gastric filling because the distal end of the LES is "taken up" by the expanding fundus. This is similar to the shortening of the neck of a balloon as it is inflated. During the process the distal portion of the neck of the balloon becomes part of the expanded body of the balloon. The process is called effacement and also occurs with gastric distention (Fig. 16.4). With

voluminous gastric distention, the overall length of the LES shortens to a point at which the existing LES pressure is unable to maintain its closure and belching and/or reflux occurs. As a consequence the patient's gastric distention is relieved, effacement of the LES retreats, LES regains its overall length, and competency of the LES is restored. This is called dynamic failure of the LES because it is reversible after the distention is relieved (see Fig. 16.2C). If the length of the LES becomes permanently short (see Fig. 16.2B), then further shortening caused by normal amounts of gastric distention with meals will readily result in postprandial reflux and gastroesophageal reflux becomes an ever-constant clinical problem.[31]

If esophageal manometry, done at rest, in the recumbent position, and after an overnight fast shows the LES to have an abnormally low pressure, a short overall length, or a minimal length exposed to the abdominal pressure environment, it is called a permanent failure of the LES, and unhampered reflux of the gastric contents into the esophagus occurs (see Fig. 16.2B). The existence of a permanently failed LES is identified by one or more inadequate components: an average pressure of 6 mm Hg or less, an average overall length of 2 cm or less, or an average abdominal length of 1 cm or less. Compared with normal subjects, these values are less than the 2.5 percentile for each parameter.[28] Fig. 16.5 is a schema of the LES components showing their median normal values with the fifth and 95th percentile values and their point

of failure. The latter is the value for a specific component at which esophageal acid exposure becomes abnormal independent from the values of the other components.

The refocus on the LES also led to the realization that almost half of the patients with confirmed GERD by 24-hour esophageal pH monitoring have a normal LES on a motility study performed at rest, in the recumbent position, and after an overnight fast.[28] The proposed etiology of reflux in such patients was described by Dr. Jerry Dodds in 1982.[32] He observed transient relaxations of a normal LES that were unrelated to a swallow but were stimulated by gastric distention or nonpressurized gastric dilation.[33] The term he used to describe these events was "transient LES relaxations" (tLESRs).

There are two proposed explanations for the occurrence of tLSERs. The first is, tLESRs are due to a neuromediated reflex initiated by pressurized gastric distention or nonpressurized dilation from gastric adaptive relaxation induced by a meal.[34] It was hypothesized that these conditions stimulate stretch receptors in the gastric fundus, which in turn stimulate vagal afferent nerve fibers that relay the input from the receptors to the medulla. Medullary nuclei then orchestrate the efferent limb of the reflex via the vagal and phrenic nerves to elicit a tLESR, crural diaphragm inhibition, and distal esophageal shortening.[35] This explanation suggests that the basic etiology of GERD is a neuromuscular abnormality.

The second proposal is, tLESRs are due to transient shortening of the LES length due to it being taken up into the stomach during episodes of pressurized gastric distention or nonpressurized dilation from gastric adaptive relaxation.[36] Normally, in the fasting state and resting recumbent position, the median overall length of the LES is 3.6 cm.[28] With gastric distention or dilation, the length of the LES shortens as the effaced portion is taken up by the expanding fundus. When gastric distention or dilation is excessive, the length of the LES shortens to its point of failure of 2 cm or less. At this length the corresponding pressure of the LES can no longer maintain closure, the LES opens, and gastroesophageal reflux occurs.[27,30,37] This occurs predominately during the postprandial period[31] and is called "dynamic failure of the LES" in that when the gastric distention or dilation is relieved the LES returns to its normal initial length.

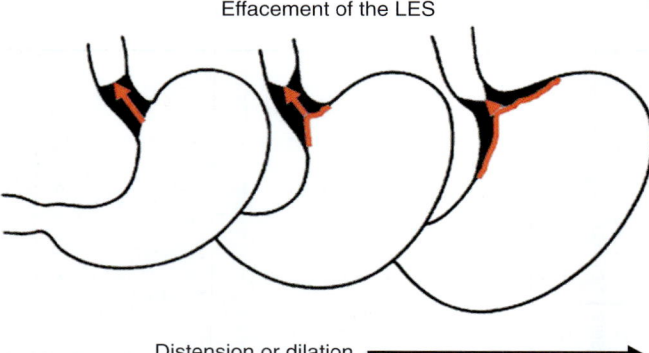

Effacement of the LES

Distension or dilation ⟶

FIGURE 16.4 The process of lower esophageal sphincter *(LES)* effacement occurs with gastric distention or nonpressurized dilation. The length of the distal esophagus and the LES within it shorten as they are effaced into and taken up by the fundus of the distended stomach. As a consequence, the squamous mucosa *(red)* is exposed to the gastric juice and suffers inflammatory injury. (From Ayazi S, Tamhankar R, DeMeester TR, et al. The impact of gastric distension on the lower esophageal sphincter and its exposure to acid gastric juice. *Ann Surg.* 2010;252:52-62.)

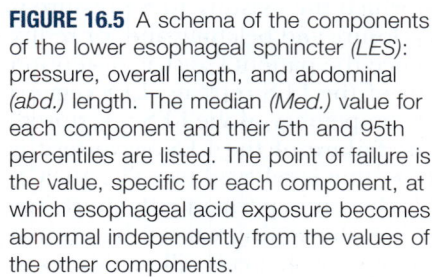

FIGURE 16.5 A schema of the components of the lower esophageal sphincter *(LES)*: pressure, overall length, and abdominal *(abd.)* length. The median *(Med.)* value for each component and their 5th and 95th percentiles are listed. The point of failure is the value, specific for each component, at which esophageal acid exposure becomes abnormal independently from the values of the other components.

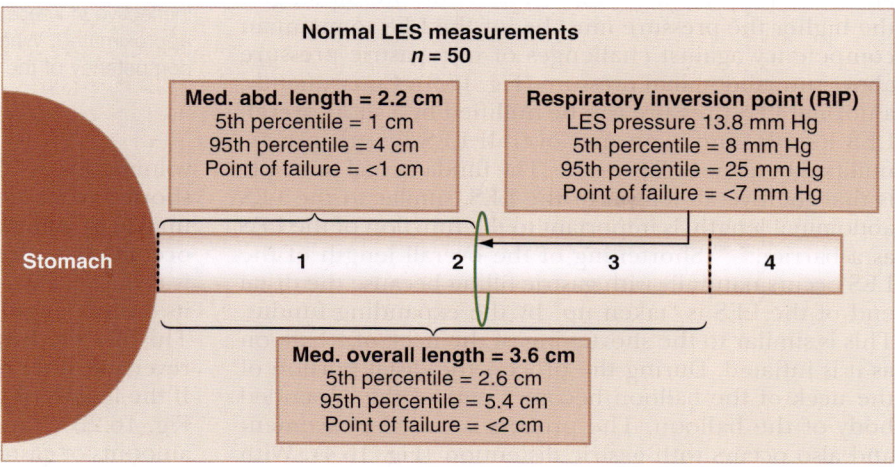

Normal LES measurements
n = 50

Med. abd. length = 2.2 cm
5th percentile = 1 cm
95th percentile = 4 cm
Point of failure = <1 cm

Respiratory inversion point (RIP)
LES pressure 13.8 mm Hg
5th percentile = 8 mm Hg
95th percentile = 25 mm Hg
Point of failure = <7 mm Hg

Stomach

1   2   3   4

Med. overall length = 3.6 cm
5th percentile = 2.6 cm
95th percentile = 5.4 cm
Point of failure = <2 cm

Understanding the concept of effacement is crucial to comprehending the pathophysiology of GERD. Not all effacement events result in the reflux of gastric juice through an open LES into the esophagus. During most effacement events, only the distal end of the LES with its squamous epithelial covering is taken up by the fundus and exposed to gastric juice while the proximal squamous epithelium remains protected.[36] Inflammation and ulceration does occur in the portion of the squamous epithelium exposed to gastric juice.[36] If the inflammation continues due to repetitive episodes of effacements, it can result in permanent damage with reduction of the abdominal length of the LES to 1 cm or less, limiting its ability to respond to intraabdominal pressure challenges and allowing unhampered reflux into the esophagus. Similarly, persistent inflammation can result in permanent damage with reduction of the overall length of the LES to 2 cm or less, limiting its ability to resist intragastric distention or nonpressurized gastric dilation. In both situations a "transient failure of the LES" has advanced to a "permanent failure of the LES" due to the permanent loss of a crucial amount of LES's abdominal and/or overall length secondary to inflammatory injury. The last component of the LES to go is pressure. The loss in pressure is due to injury of the complete underlying muscle by inflammatory by-products from the overlying inflamed squamous epithelium. "Permanent failure of the LES" is identified when one or more of the following LES abnormalities are seen on a resting motility study performed in the fasted patient: an abdominal length of 1 cm or less, an overall length of 2 cm or less, and a resting pressure of 6 mm Hg or less.[28] When all three components are abnormal, the LES is completely destroyed and will require reconstruction.[37] Fig. 16.6 shows that the damage to the LES parallels the severity of esophageal mucosal injury and corroborates a link between damage to the LES and mucosal injury.[38] The data in Fig. 16.7 further support this suggestion by showing the higher the esophageal acid exposure, the more extensive the damage to the LES as assessed by the number of failed LES components per patient. In summary, the greater the mucosal injury, the greater is the LES injury, resulting in greater esophageal acid exposure and the necessity for a higher dose of acid suppression therapy to control symptoms and heal epithelial and LES damage. The question is, does PPI therapy prevent progressive damage to the LES or does progressive damage occur to the LES despite PPI therapy?

The only guidance we have to answer this question is the study of Falkenback et al.[15] discussed previously, on the course of GERD in 40 patients treated with PPIs and followed for 20 years. Over the period of observation the studied population showed more use of PPI therapy ($P = .007$), and an increasing prevalence of esophagitis ($P = .001$) and BE ($P = .002$). While on PPI therapy, those who progressed differed from those who did not progress by a 1-cm shortening of their LES abdominal length ($P < .01$) and an increase of 11% in the time the esophageal pH was less than 4 during the supine period ($P < .004$). This supports the concept that progressive disease, despite increases in PPI dose, is associated with manometric abnormalities of the LES that develop during the course of PPI treatment. The logical inference is that preventing LES effacement due to gastric distention may be an effective means of preventing damage to the LES and the progression of GERD from early to advanced disease.

The second fundamental determinant of GERD is the composition of the gastric juice refluxed into the esophagus. Increased esophageal exposure to gastric juice can cause injury to the esophageal and/or respiratory epithelium, along with the loss of esophageal and lung function. Injury is manifested on endoscopy by linear or interlacing ulceration and repair by stricture and/

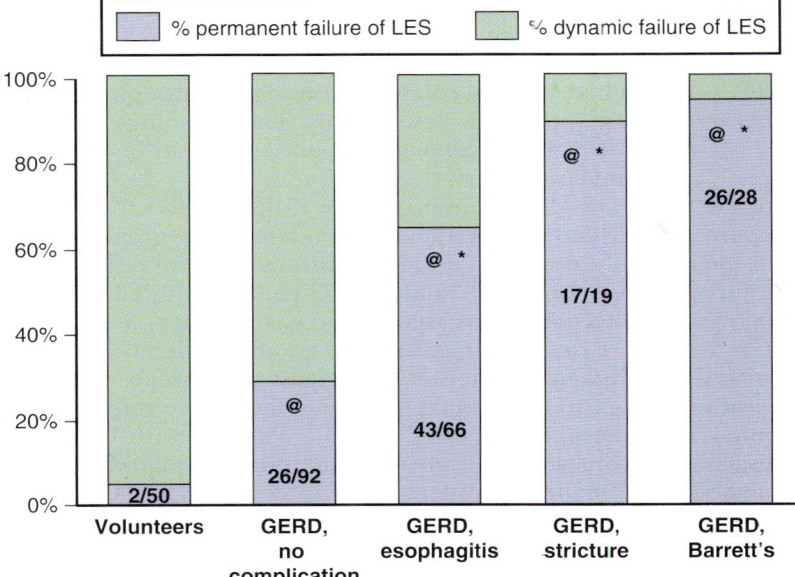

FIGURE 16.6 The relationship between various degrees of mucosal injury and the prevalence of a permanently failed lower esophageal sphincter *(LES)*. The majority of the patients with mucosal injury have a permanently failed LES. No injury vs. injury of any type *P* < .01. *GERD*, Gastroesophageal reflux disease. (From Stein HJ, Barlow AP, DeMeester TR, Hinder RA. Complications of gastroesophageal reflux disease: role of lower esophageal sphincter, esophageal acid and acid/alkaline exposure, and duodenogastric reflux. *Ann Surg*. 1992;216:35–43.)

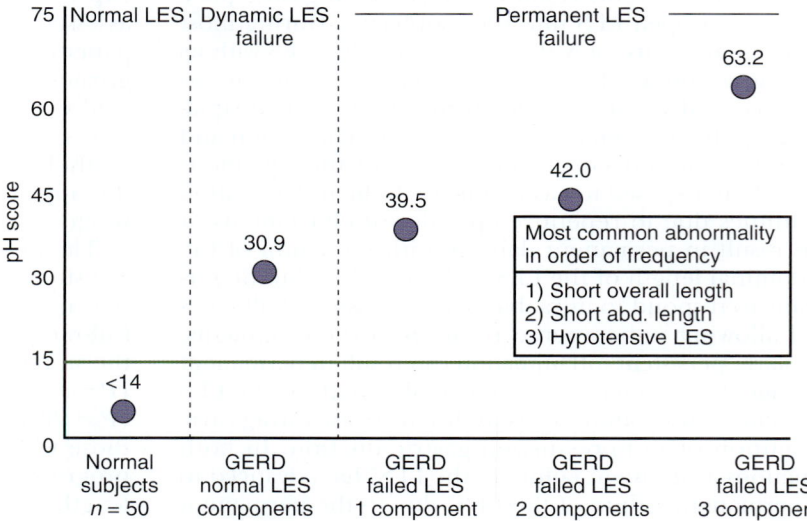

The extent of LES injury and acid exposure
918 GERD patients with abnormal 24-h pH score

FIGURE 16.7 The relationship between extent of lower esophageal sphincter *(LES)* damage and esophageal acid exposure. The more extensive the damage to the LES, assessed by the number of failed components per patient, the higher the esophageal acid exposure. *abd.,* Abdominal; *GERD,* gastroesophageal reflux disease.

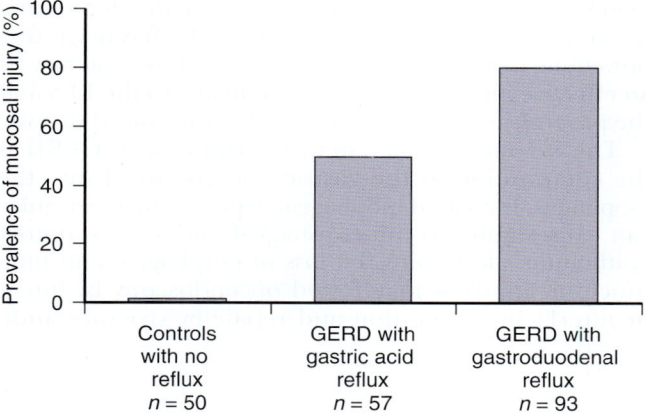

FIGURE 16.8 The relationship between the composition of the gastric juice refluxed and the prevalence of mucosal injury. Injury is highest when the refluxed gastric juice is a mixture of gastric acid and duodenal bile. *GERD,* Gastroesophageal reflux disease.

or metaplasia of the squamous epithelium to cardiac epithelium. The prevalence and severity of injury are not only related to a failure of the LES but also to the composition of the refluxed gastric juice. Mucosal injury is the highest when the refluxed gastric juice is a mixture of gastric acid and duodenal bile (Fig. 16.8).

The emphasis on acid suppression therapy has resulted in the misconception that GERD is associated only with esophageal exposure to gastric acid, while other components of refluxed gastric juice have been ignored. This has led to the hypothesis that an improvement in the potency of acid suppression therapy will reduce the incidence of epithelial damage and progressive disease. Indeed, clinical experience with potent acid suppression therapy has shown a marked reduction in acid-related complications such as esophagitis and strictures. Paradoxically, the incidence of

BE and esophageal adenocarcinoma has increased. This implies that abnormal acid exposure in the distal esophagus is only part of the problem in GERD and other components of the refluxed gastric juice are important. Acid alone in physiologic concentrations is not very damaging, but in high concentrations the incidence of epithelial damage is substantial. Similarly, the reflux of duodenal juice alone does little damage but when combined with gastric acid becomes particularly noxious (Fig. 16.8).[39,40]

Continuous esophageal aspiration studies with analysis of nonpooled samples have confirmed the presence of bile acid at toxic concentrations in the esophagus of patients with GERD compared with normal subjects (Fig. 16.9).[41] Patients with erosive esophagitis showed a 10-fold increase in bile acid concentration compared with those who had no injury while esophageal acid exposure was similar in both groups. Patients with strictures or BE had more esophageal acid exposure than the other groups but had bile acid concentrations significantly greater than those with erosive esophagitis. These findings reinforce the concept of an acid and bile synergism in the cause of mucosal injury.

The development of the Bilitec probe to monitor bilirubin as a marker for duodenal juice greatly simplified the study of duodenogastroesophageal reflux.[42] In a large population study of 273 patients with GERD, 30% reflux only increased acidic gastric juice, 56% reflux increased acidic gastric juice and duodenal juice and 14% had sufficient duodenogastric reflux to neutralize all gastric acid so that only duodenal juice refluxed into the esophagus (Fig. 16.10).[43] Patients with increased esophageal exposure to a mixture of acid and bile had the highest prevalence of endoscopic ($P < .0007$ vs. all groups) and histologic epithelial injury (data not shown) and the highest degree of functional loss for LES pressure, overall length and abdominal length ($P < .002$ to .0004) (Fig. 16.11). The common association of functional loss with mucosal injury, and the unlikelihood of functional loss in the absence of mucosal injury, suggest that the loss is due to the consequences of inflammatory injury.

The effect of duodenogastric reflux is the elevation of the pH of gastric juice. The height of the elevation depends on the baseline level of gastric pH, which varies depending on whether the patient is taking acid suppression therapy. Elevating the pH of gastric juice has four known effects. Frist, when the pH exceeds 4, heartburn and regurgitation diminish.[44] Second, when the pH enters the 3 to 5 range, it stimulates phenotypic differentiation of the cardiac mucosa toward intestinalization, with proliferation of the mucosal glandular cells.[45] Third, when the pH reaches 4.5, bacteria normally present in the mouth begin to grow in the stomach, and bile acids can be deconjugated to release the more noxious free bile acid.[46,47] Fourth, when the pH enters the 3 to 6 range, bile acids become soluble, and a portion dissociates into their ionized salt and free H[+] while the remainder persists as a lipophilic, nonionized acid. As the pH approximates 7, more than 90% of bile acid becomes soluble and completely ionized. Acidification of bile to a pH below 2 results in an irreversible bile-acid precipitation. Consequently, under normal physiologic conditions, bile acids in the stomach precipitate and have minimal effect in an acid gastric environment. On the other hand, in a more alkaline gastric environment, which occurs with excessive duodenogastric reflux or acid suppression therapy, bile acids remain in solution and are only partially dissociated. When nondissociated, nonpolar bile-acid molecules reflux into the esophagus, they can enter the mucosal cells. Once in the cell, where the pH is 7, they become completely dissociated into polar ions and are trapped intracellularly in concentrations of up to 7 times the luminal concentrations.[48] In the cell, bile acid salts can at low concentrations impair mitochondrial function[49]; at high concentrations they become cytotoxic[50] and function as co-mutagens[51] or likely direct mutagens.[52]

If soluble bile acids are to remain innocuous in a patient with chronic reflux managed by acid suppression therapy, they must remain completely ionized. This requires that a gastric pH of 6 to 7 be maintained 24 hours a day, 7 days a week, while the patient is on acid suppression therapy. This is not only impractical but probably impossible without very high doses of medication. Insufficient medication allows the pH to drift down to 4 to 5 and causes cellular mucosal damage while the patient remains relatively asymptomatic (Fig. 16.12).[53,54]

Throughout the 1950s and 1960s, complications of BE were mainly acid related (i.e., inflammation, ulceration, and stricture formation). There were only a few reports of adenocarcinoma of the esophagus, and most authors believed that when adenocarcinoma did occur at the GEJ, it was a gastric cancer that had crept up into the esophagus. Since the 1970s, when potent acid suppression therapy became available, the acid complications associated with BE became less common and the malignant complication more common. In the 1990s, convincing evidence emerged of an explosion in the incidence of BE and adenocarcinoma of the esophagus that has yet to be explained. Several studies were initiated to determine whether bile acids, now solubilized in gastric juice owing to the widespread use of acid suppression therapy, were responsible. If evidence continues to emerge showing that soluble bile salts contribute to the development of malignancy, then early surgical interventions to restore a competent LES and allow an acid gastric environment

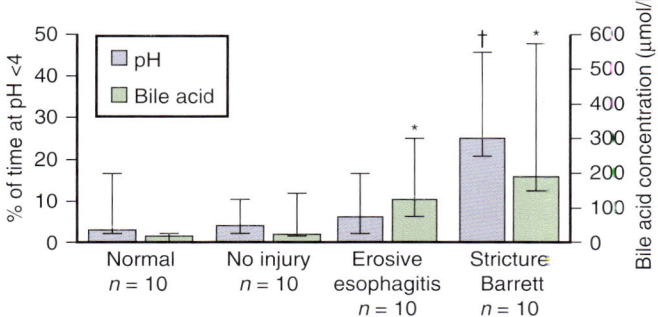

FIGURE 16.9 Comparison of esophageal exposure to bile acid concentration, measured by continuous aspiration and acid, measured by the percentage of time the pH is < 4 in normal subjects and patients with mucosal injury of varied severity. Values are shown in *bars* for medians and *whiskers* for interquartile range. *P < .05 vs. normal or no injury. †P < .05 vs. normal, no injury or erosive esophagitis.

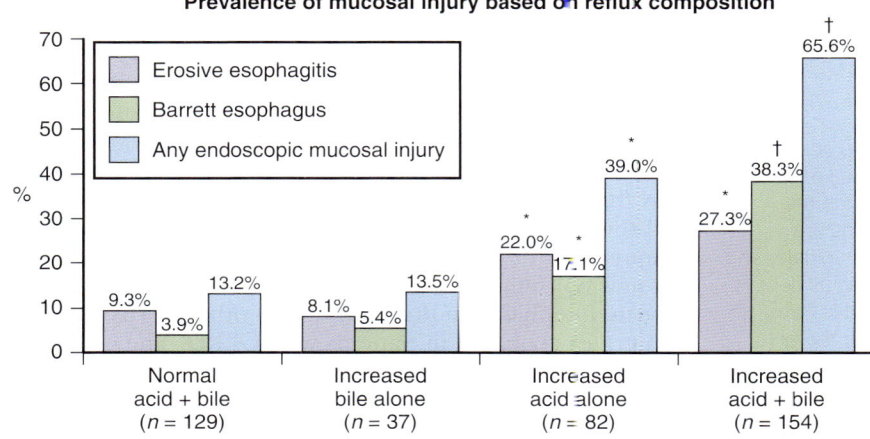

FIGURE 16.10 The prevalence of erosive esophagitis and Barrett esophagus in patients with normal esophageal exposure to acid and bile, increased exposure to bile alone, increased exposure to acid alone, and increased exposure to acid and bile. . Patients with exposure to increased acid and bile had the highest prevalence of endoscopic and histologic epithelial injury. *P ≤ .006 vs. normal acid and bile exposure. †P ≤ .0007 vs. other groups.

COMPOSITION OF GASTRIC JUICE AND ITS EFFECT ON ESOPHAGEAL FUNCTION

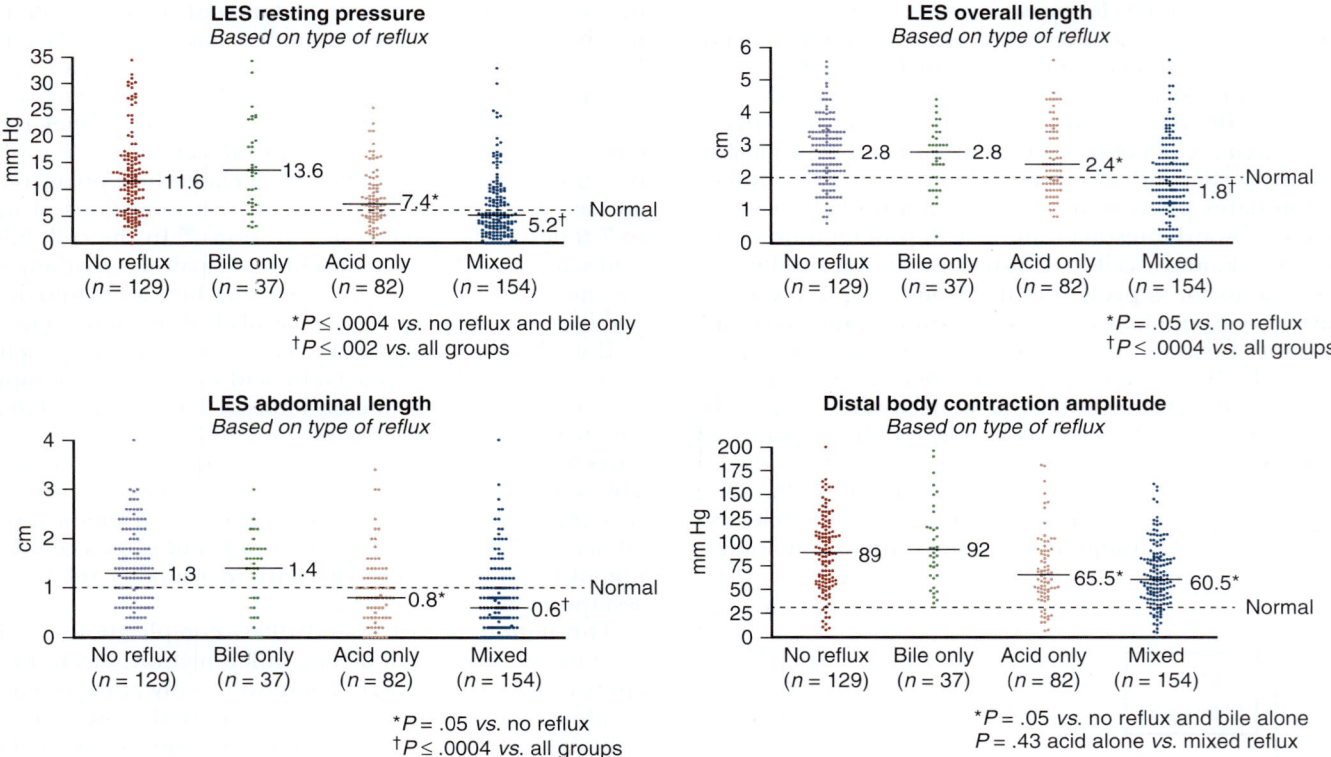

FIGURE 16.11 Lower esophageal sphincter (LES) pressure, overall length, abdominal length, and contraction amplitude of the distal esophagus in patients with normal esophageal exposure to acid and bile, increased exposure to bile alone, to acid alone, or both acid and bile on 24-hour pH and bile monitoring. An increased exposure to acid and bile was associated with the greatest reduction in LES pressure, overall length, and abdominal length. Increased bile exposure alone had no effect.

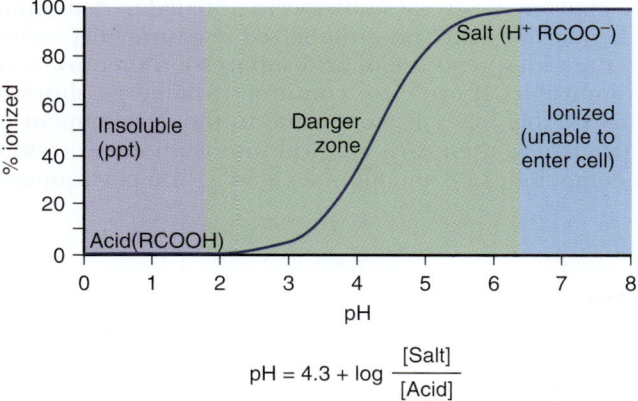

$$pH = 4.3 + \log \frac{[Salt]}{[Acid]}$$

FIGURE 16.12 A representative ionization curve for bile acids. At pH 2 or below, bile acids are in their associated form (i.e., un-ionized [RCOOH]). In this form and pH the bile acids are insoluble and precipitate. At pH 6 or greater, bile acids are completely dissociated (i.e., ionized = [H⁺ + RCOO⁻]), soluble, and nontoxic to the cells. Between these extremes, bile acids can exist in their associated form and remain soluble. In this form, they can enter the cell with detrimental effects; hence the pH range between 2 and 6.5 is called the danger zone.

to return by the discontinuation of PPI therapy should be encouraged.

HISTOPATHOLOGY OF GASTROESOPHAGEAL REFLUX DISEASE

There has been a mystery regarding the pathologic changes within the region of the gastroesophageal junction (GEJ) associated with GERD. This was due to the absence of dependable anatomic, endoscopic, or histologic landmarks regarding the position of the LES and the fact the LES cannot be recognized either during endoscopy, at surgery, or on gross examination of surgical specimens. To deepen the mystery, physiologic and pathologic studies have introduced the concept that GERD begins at the squamocolumnar junction (SCJ). In the absence of squamoepithelial injury, the position of the SCJ and GEJ are concordant. As squamoepithelial injury occurs, metaplastic cardiac epithelium forms, and a new SCJ emerges, separated from the GEJ, and lying further cephalad in the LES.[54a,54b] In other words, the SCJ migrates cephalad in patients with GERD. The extent of the cephalad migration correlates with the severity of disease. BE represents the extreme of this migration.[55] As a consequence of these ill-defined and moving landmarks, the pathology of the gastroesophageal junctional zone has been an enigma for many years. The early literature regarded BE as a congenital disorder, and not until 1959 had sufficient clinical evidence accumulated to suggest that it was an acquired abnormality caused by GERD. The acquired etiology was confirmed experimentally in the landmark report of Bremner et al. in 1970.[56]

Hayward in 1961 brought attention to the gastroesophageal and squamocolumnar junctional zone by stating that the lower 1 to 2 cm of the esophagus is normally lined by a mucus-secreting columnar epithelium that has the ability to resist acid-peptic digestion.[57] He argued that this epithelium prevents squamous epithelial digestion by providing a buffer between it and the acid-pepsin producing oxyntic mucosa of the fundus. Although Hayward's description placed this columnar mucosa in the lower esophagus, it has over time, without any logical or scientific basis, come to be regarded as the cardiac zone of the stomach and was termed cardiac mucosa. Hayward's thoughts persisted until 1976, when it was recognized that three different types of glandular epithelium could line the lower esophagus in patients with BE[58]: oxyntocardiac mucosa containing chief and parietal cells; cardiac mucosa containing mucous cells and no chief and parietal cells; and intestinalized cardiac mucosa with a villiform surface, mucous glands, alcian blue–staining goblet cells, and no parietal or chief cells. When present, the intestinalized cardiac mucosa is always most proximal and the oxyntocardiac mucosa most distal, with cardiac mucosa interposed between them.

In 1997 Chandrasoma[59,60] reviewed the histology of the GEJ in a large number of autopsied patients whose medical records did not mention GERD. He found that in the vast majority of children and adults under age 20, the squamous epithelium transitioned directly with the oxyntic epithelium of the gastric fundus. On the other hand, cardiac mucosa appeared in specimens from patients older than age 20, but its length was almost always less than 1 cm. Even in these older patients, there were a considerable number of individuals where the squamous epithelium transitioned directly to oxyntic mucosa in the fundus of the stomach without intervening cardiac mucosa.

Several authors have evaluated this finding further.[61,62] Oberg et al.[61] obtained endoscopic biopsies from above, at, and below the GEJ identified by the proximal extent of the rugal folds in 334 consecutive patients with symptoms of foregut disease and no prior history of gastric or esophageal surgery or endoscopic evidence of visible BE. In 88 of the 334 patients (26%), multiple biopsies revealed no cardiac mucosa. The absence of cardiac mucosa was strongly associated with the absence of the hallmarks of GERD (Table 16.1). Spechler's group[62] performed a similar study by obtaining multiple biopsies of the SCJ from patients with an endoscopically normal-appearing GEJ and also showed that cardiac mucosa was present in only a minority of patients. Based on these investigations, the traditional view that the anatomic gastric cardia is lined by cardiac mucosa may not be correct. Rather, cardiac mucosa may be a metaplastic mucosa that occurs as a sequel to reflux-induced squamous mucosal injury and is an early sign of GERD.

The current interpretation of these findings is that in the normal state, the squamous epithelial lining of the

TABLE 16.1 Hallmarks of Gastroesophageal Reflux Disease in Patients With and Without Cardiac Mucosa on Biopsies of the Gastroesophageal Junction

	FINDINGS ON MULTIPLE BIOPSIES OF THE CARDIA		
	No Cardiac Epithelium (n = 88)	Cardiac Epithelium (n = 246)	P Value
% Time pH <4	1.1 ± 4.6	6.0 ± 7.4	<0.01
% Hiatal hernia	25.0	55.1	<0.01
LES pressure (mm Hg)	13.2 ± 12.8	8.0 ± 8.0	<0.01
LES abdominal length (mm)	1.6 ± 1.1	1.0 ± 1.2	<0.01
LES overall length (mm)	3.0 ± 1.2	2.2 ± 1.6	<0.01
% Permanently failed LES	27.2	62.3	<0.01
% Esophagitis	11.2	33.2	<0.01
No. of patients with micro IM on biopsy of the SCJ	0%	29 (11.7%)	

Values are median ± interquartile range.
IM, Intestinal metaplasia; *LES,* lower esophageal sphincter; *SCJ,* squamous columnar junction.
From Oberg S, Peters JH, DeMeester TR, et al. Inflammation and specialized intestinal metaplasia of cardiac mucosa is a manifestation of gastroesophageal reflux disease. *Ann Surg.* 1997;226:522-532.

esophagus and LES changes abruptly to oxyntic mucosa of the gastric fundus without a "gastric cardia" mucosa. It is hypothesized that because oxyntic mucosa of the fundus of the stomach is not affected by gastric juice, cardiac mucosa must come from exposure of the esophageal squamous mucosa to gastric juice. This process likely represents a change in the direction of differentiation of the germinal cells of the squamous epithelium toward metaplastic cardiac epithelium.[63,64] Exposure of squamous mucosa to gastric juice is most likely to occur postprandial, when the stomach is distended and the squamous-lined distal esophagus is effaced into and taken up by the expanding fundus (see Fig. 16.4). Exposure of the effaced squamous epithelium to acidic gastric juice results in inflammatory damage and the formation of squamous epithelial islands separated by newly formed metaplastic cardiac epithelium. The underlying esophageal muscle is damaged in the process, and a portion of the abdominal length of the LES is destroyed, splayed out by intragastric pressure, and takes on the appearance of the stomach (Fig. 16.13). When the acid exposure is limited and in physiologic concentration, the newly formed metaplastic cardiac mucosa can undergo oxyntic transformation forming oxyntic-cardiac mucosa. This is a stable, glandular mucosa that is similar to the oxyntic mucosa of the stomach in that it contains both parietal and mucous cells and is more resistant to damage by refluxed gastric acid.

In nearly all circumstances, metaplastic cardiac mucosa, when present, shows inflammatory and reactive changes referred to as carditis.[61] This inflamed metaplastic cardiac mucosa is the only mucosal type that progresses to intestinal metaplasia.[59] When this occurs, the metaplastic cardiac mucous cells develop acid rather than neutral mucin and take on a positive stain with alcian blue. Subsequently, well-formed goblet cells appear. Once intestinalized, the metaplastic cardia mucosa seems to have an increased

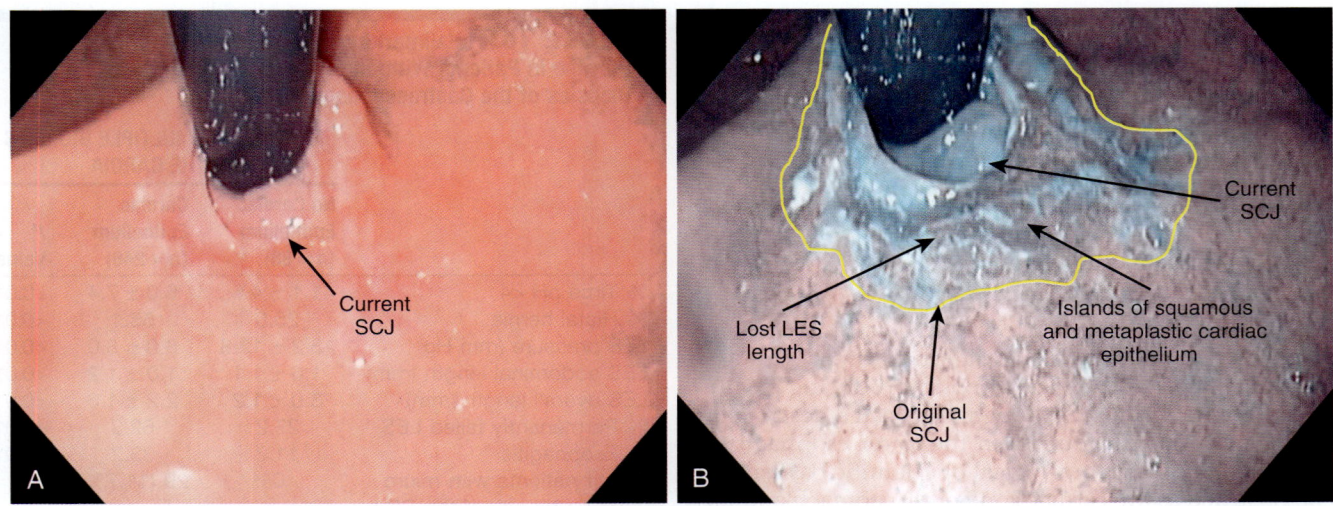

Normal light imaging   Narrow band imaging

FIGURE 16.13 Retroflex endoscopic images of the squamocolumnar junction *(SCJ)* and lower esophageal sphincter *(LES)* damage. (A) A normal white light image and displays a slightly irregular circular SCJ with normal squamous epithelium extending up the esophagus. The gastric mucosa below the SCJ appears normal with some erythematous streaking. (B) A narrow band image and shows the irregular circular SCJ and multiple islands of squamous epithelium separated by newly formed metaplastic cardiac epithelium. The original position of the SCJ is marked by a *yellow line*. The current irregular SCJ maintains its circular form while the splayed out original SCJ and the destroyed distal portion of the esophagus take on the appearance of the stomach. This is due to the loss of a portion of the LES muscle due to inflammatory injury. As a consequence, a portion of the LES's abdominal length has been destroyed and its ability to function as a barrier compromised.

ability to withstand damage by refluxed gastric juice, because biopsy shows little or no inflammation. The development of intestinal metaplasia within metaplastic cardiac mucosa is considered a detrimental change because this mucosa can progress to dysplasia and adenocarcinoma.[64] In contrast, intestinal metaplasia does not occur within metaplastic cardiac mucosa that has undergone oxyntic mucosal transformation (i.e., oxyntocardiac epithelium) as a result of exposure to gastric juice. Oxyntic transformation of metaplastic cardiac mucosa protects against the development of intestinal metaplasia and is a beneficial change.[59]

In the 1980s it became evident that the malignant transformation of BE occurred in the intestinalized cardiac mucosa.[65,66] After this association was recognized, the term BE was applied only to an esophagus lined by intestinalized cardiac mucosa. The length of the intestinalized cardiac mucosa could be as short as a few millimeters.[67] In other words, a patient is considered to have BE if any amount of cardia mucosa in the lower esophagus has histologic evidence of goblet cells (i.e., the sign of intestinalization). The length of the intestinalized mucosa is measured as limited to the GEJ, limited to the lower 3 cm of the esophagus, or involving less than 3 cm of the esophagus.

The observation that some patients have cardiac mucosa without intestinalization suggests that intestinalization requires a specific condition or stimulus. In other words, the development of the mucosal change typical of BE is a stepwise process. In the first step, metaplastic cardiac mucosa forms from the squamous epithelium. This is initiated by an inflammatory response to acid exposure

of the squamous mucosa covering the effaced portion of the LES.[61] Under proper luminal conditions and stimuli, intestinalization of the metaplastic cardiac mucosa follows.[68] This process may take a period of time. Indeed, in children younger than age 5 years who acquire a metaplastic cardiac mucosa–lined esophagus, intestinal metaplasia is rare.[69] Goblet cells begin to appear only later. Clinical studies have shown a time lag of 5 to 7 years after the onset of reflux symptoms for intestinalized cardiac mucosa to appear in adults.[70]

Oberg et al.[71] have shown that the prevalence of intestinalized metaplastic cardiac mucosa is related to the status of the LES and the severity of esophageal acid exposure. In 251 patients, who had a normal-appearing SCJ and GEJ on endoscopy, biopsy of the SCJ had microscopic cardiac mucosa of which 14% showed intestinal metaplasia. These patients had more LES damage and esophageal acid exposure. With time and further deterioration of the LES, metaplastic cardiac mucosa is endoscopically visible in the esophageal body for a distance greater than 3 cm, and 97% had intestinal metaplasia on biopsy. These patients had the most LES damage and esophageal acid exposure. At each step, the patients exhibit more profound hallmarks of GERD, including decreasing length and pressure of the LES, increasing esophageal acid exposure, and eventual loss of esophageal contraction amplitude (Table 16.2). The LES damage results from inflammatory changes in the muscularis propria secondary to increased esophageal acid exposure.[72] The same process causes the loss of esophageal body contractility classically seen in patients with long segments of BE. It is rare that the length of BE exceeds more than 8 to 9 cm up the esophagus from

TABLE 16.2 Functional Characteristics of Gastroesophageal Reflux Disease in Patients With Varied Lengths of Cardiac-Type Mucosa With Intestinal Metaplasia

	INTESTINAL METAPLASIA LIMITED TO:		
	Microscopic—Biopsy of SCJ GE Junction*	Visible on Endoscopy Distal 3 cm of Esophagus[†]	Visible on Endoscopy Esophageal Body
SPHINCTER			
Abdominal length (cm)	1.0	0.9	0.4[‡]
Overall length (cm)	2.2	2.1	1.8[§]
Resting pressure (mm Hg)	7.2	6.4	3.8[‡]
Permanently defective (%)	53	66	94[‡]
ESOPHAGEAL ACID EXPOSURE			
% Time pH <4.0	5.8	8.4[‡]	16.5[‡]
Increased exposure (%)	65	86[§]	93[§]
No. of reflux episodes	53	81[§]	197[‡]
ESOPHAGEAL BODY			
Distal amplitude (mm Hg)	79	61[§]	51[§]
No. of reflux episodes >5 min	2	5[§]	7[‡]
Duration of longest episodes (min)	10	18[§]	28[‡]

*Cardiac-type mucosa with intestinal metaplasia not seen on endoscopy but discovered on biopsies taken just below the squamocolumnar junction in an endoscopically normal-appearing gastroesophageal junction.
[†]Cardiac-type mucosa with intestinal metaplasia within the vicinity of the high-pressure zone.
[‡]$P < .05$ vs. all other groups.
[§]$P < .05$ vs. intestinal metaplasia limited to gastroesophageal junction.
GE, Gastroesophageal; SCJ, squamocolumnar junction.
From Oberg S, DeMeester TR, Peters JH, et al. The extent of Barrett's esophagus depends on the status of the lower esophageal sphincter and the degree of esophageal acid exposure. *J Thorac Cardiovasc Surg*. 1999;117:572-580.

the GEJ. This is due to the normal gradient between the positive pressure environment in the stomach and the negative pressure environment in the thoracic esophagus. When the LES completely deteriorates, gastric juice flows to the point of lowest esophageal pressure, which is in the mid-thoracic esophagus. Under these conditions, intestinalized metaplastic cardiac mucosa could appear within the lower half of the esophageal body without any apparent subsequent change in length over time. At any time during the process, specific luminal conditions or stimuli, such as exposure to a specific pH range in the presence of a specific solubilized bile acid, intestinalization of metaplastic cardiac mucosa can occur and set the stage for malignant degeneration. Studies have suggested that intestinalization of the metaplastic cardiac mucosa is initiated by exposure to a pH 3 to 5 resulting from the interaction of the reflux gastric juice, duodenal juice, and saliva at the squamocolumnar interface. Exposure to this pH range has been shown to encourage the phenotypic expression of intestinalization by metaplastic cardiac epithelial cells.[45,61]

The most controversial issue in the pathology of early BE is whether intestinalized cardiac epithelium found below the SCJ is due to *Helicobactor pylori*. Extensive studies have shown that the presence of inflamed cardiac mucosa at the SCJ was inversely related to *H. pylori* infection and strongly associated with increased esophageal acid exposure. Further, there was no association between the presence of intestinal metaplasia and *H. pylori*. In addition, the incidence of *H. pylori* in patients with esophageal adenocarcinoma was not different from the prevalence of *H. pylori* in patients with benign esophageal disease. Based

on these studies, *H. pylori* has no role in the pathogenesis of GERD or its complications.[73]

PREVENTION OF PROGRESSIVE DISEASE

Physicians have developed some concerns after 35 years of experience with more than 20 million GERD patients taking prescribed PPIs. Despite the introduction and use of new powerful acid suppression drugs over this time period, the incidence of GERD continues to increase by 30% every 10 years, and 30% to 40% of the patients have only partial relief of their symptoms. Every year between 2% and 3.5% of the 20 million patients receiving PPI therapy develop BE. Of those who develop BE, 0.5% to 1% will progress to esophageal adenocarcinoma.[74] Less than 1% of patients with a partial response and/or disease progression on PPI therapy seek surgical therapy. These concerns have given rise to the thought that the time has come for a change in the treatment strategy of GERD. Current treatment focuses on only one of the two determinants of the disease, the composition of the gastric juice, whereas the other determinant, failure of the LES, is ignored.

Taken together, the studies on histopathology have introduced the concept that GERD begins at the SCJ. In the absence of disease the SCJ and the GEJ are concordant. As LES damage occurs and progresses, the SCJ separates from the GEJ and moves up the esophagus. This results in a squamooxyntic gap between the oxyntic gastric mucosa in the proximal stomach and the remaining squamous esophageal mucosa within the LES (Fig. 16.14).[75] The gap is filled with metaplastic cardiac mucosa, making the

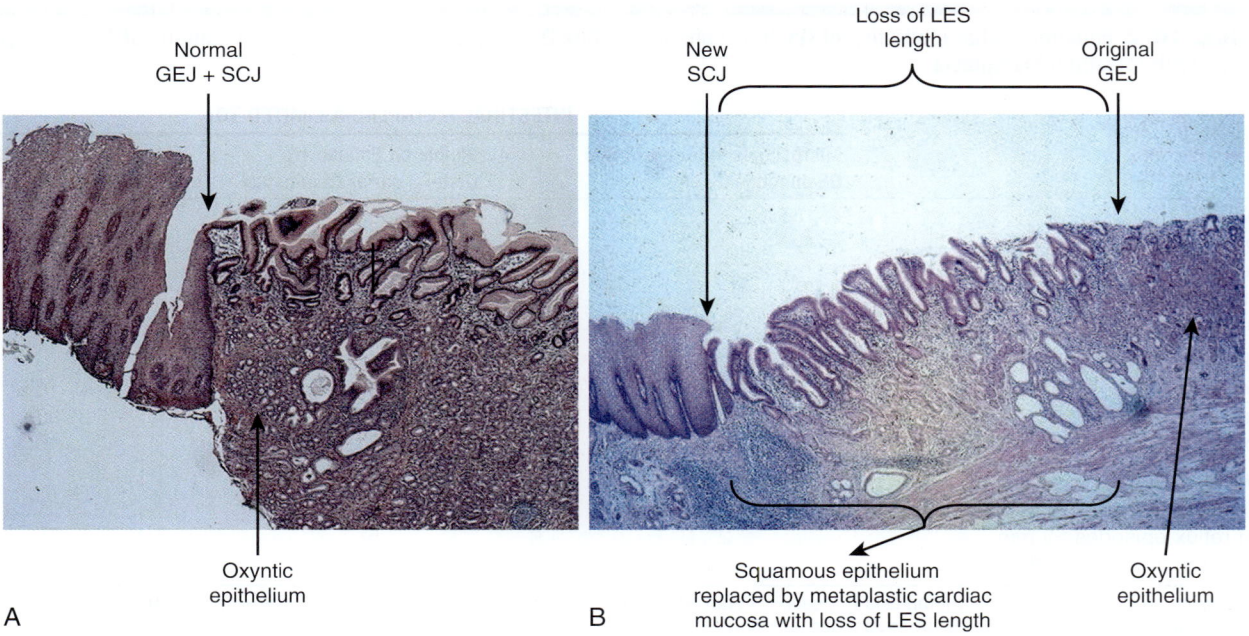

FIGURE 16.14 The squamooxyntic gap. (A) A photomicrograph of the normal squamocolumnar junction *(SCJ)* with squamous epithelium directly apposed to oxyntic gastric epithelium (i.e., normal gastric epithelium). In normal subjects, a biopsy of the SCJ shows a 0- to 2-mm gap between the two epithelia. (B) A photomicrograph of a patient with gastroesophageal reflux disease *(GERD)* showing a squamooxyntic gap between the oxyntic gastric mucosa in the proximal stomach and the remaining squamous esophageal mucosa within the lower esophageal sphincter *(LES)*. The gap is filled with metaplastic cardiac mucosa, which can become intestinalized and give rise to visible Barrett esophagus in 2 to 5 years. The submucosa and muscularis propria show inflammatory damage resulting in the loss of LES length. *GEJ,* Gastroesophageal junction.

determination between esophagus and stomach difficult because the gap appears like stomach but is actually esophagus. The prevalence of intestinal metaplasia of the metaplastic cardiac mucosa is directly proportional to the length of the squamooxyntic gap. In a study of 1655 patients with GERD, intestinal metaplasia was observed in 24% of patients with a gap shorter than 1 cm, 86% of patients with a gap of 1 to 5 cm, and 100% with a gap longer than 5 cm. It has been proposed that the squamooxyntic gap could be used as a cellular criterion to diagnose GERD. In other words, if you have microscopic metaplastic cardiac mucosa on biopsies of the SCJ margin of the gap you have GERD, the length of the gap provides an assessment of the severity of GERD, and intestinalized metaplastic cardiac mucosa within the gap is an early indicator of disease progression and risk of esophageal adenocarcinoma. This allows the diagnosis of GERD at a very early stage when the disease is intrasphincteric and prior to becoming transsphincteric and involving the esophageal body.

These initial histologic changes are subtle, and a patient with early GERD is likely to have a normal endoscopy. Consequently, clinical symptoms and endoscopy alone are not sufficient to confidently evaluate a patient with early disease. This requires a manometric assessment of the LES, a measurement of esophageal acid exposure, and biopsies of and just below the SCJ. Most important in the management of such patients is to prevent the development of visible BE, for this is the premalignant lesion of adenocarcinoma of the esophagus and is extremely

difficult to reverse after it has become large enough to be visible on endoscopy. The best opportunity to reverse the process is when intestinal metaplasia of cardiac mucosa is microscopic and not visible on endoscopy.

The primary method of identifying early disease in symptomatic patients is to obtain multiple biopsies of the SCJ. If one or more biopsies show microscopic intestinalized cardiac mucosa, the patient has early GERD and is at risk for visible BE. The treatment consists of stopping the reflux of gastric juice into the esophagus by repairing the LES and reestablishing gastric acidity by the discontinuation of PPI therapy. This should be done as early as possible in patients who have an incomplete response to PPI therapy, normal endoscopy, no visible BE, increased esophageal acid exposure on 24-hour esophageal pH monitoring, and a biopsy of the SCJ that shows microscopic intestinalized metaplastic cardiac mucosa. The earlier these patients undergo surgical correction of a defective LES, the more likely is the success in controlling symptoms and preventing progressive disease.

The grounds for this proposal are based on GERD progression in 171 such patients investigated in the ProGERD study.[76] These patients had microscopic nonvisible intestinal metaplasia on biopsy of the SCJ prior to any therapy. After the 4 to 8 weeks of initial PPI therapy, 128 of the patients had a follow-up endoscopy and biopsy of the SCJ. All had persistent microscopic intestinal metaplasia. These patients continued to receive PPI therapy and underwent endoscopy and biopsy after 2 and 5 years of follow-up. Endoscopic visible BE was seen in 25.8% (33/128) of the

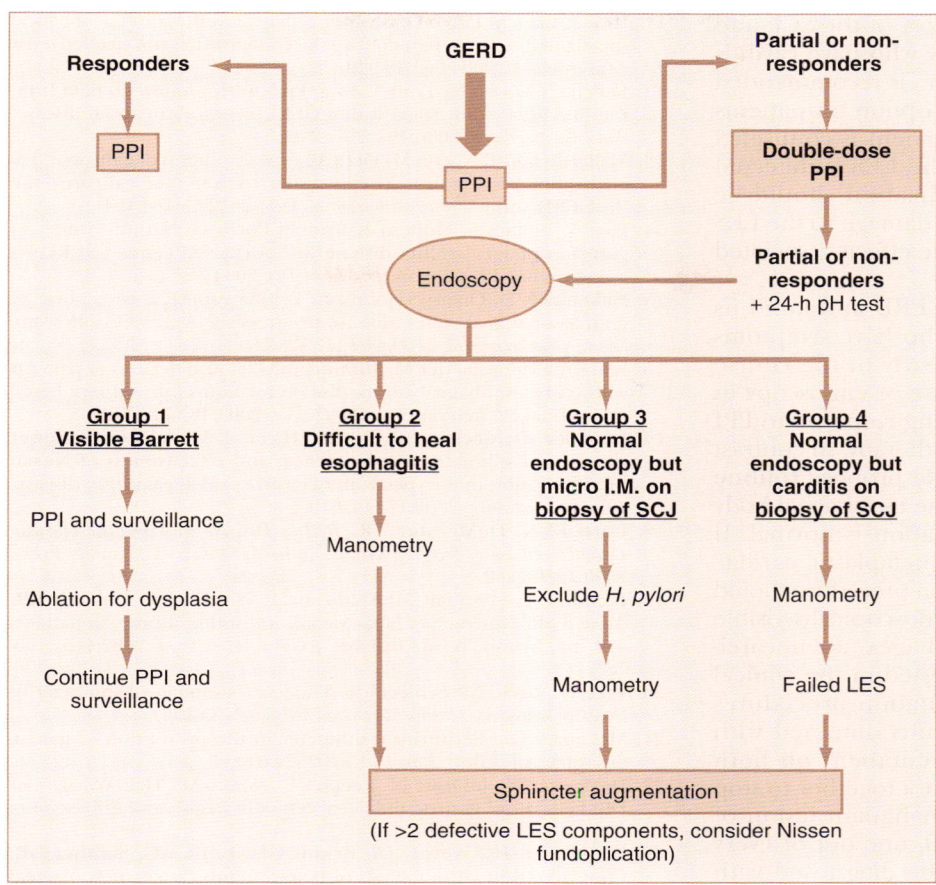

FIGURE 16.15 Proposed treatment algorithm for the early recognition and treatment of patients at risk for disease progression. See text for explanation. *GERD*, Gastroesophageal reflux disease; *I.M.*, intestinal metaplasia; *LES*, lower esophageal sphincter; *PPI*, proton pump inhibitor; *SCJ*, squamocolumnar junction.

patients. The conclusion of the study was that a biopsy of the SCJ showing microscopic intestinal metaplasia in a patient who is otherwise endoscopically normal is a strong indication of a high risk of progression to visible BE.

The problem with medical management of early GERD is that the available medications have not shown the ability to prevent the development of BE or induce regression of microscopic intestinal metaplasia that develops at the SCJ and is a precursor of visible BE. In contrast, a competent Nissen fundoplication has been shown to prevent BE if performed before endoscopically visible BE develops.[77,78] Furthermore, a competent Nissen fundoplication can induce complete regression of microscopic intestinal metaplasia at the SCJ and avoid the subsequent development of visible BE.[79] Despite these proven benefits of the fundoplication procedure, its side effects (i.e., dysphagia, postprandial bloating, and the inability to burp or vomit) have significantly limited its use early in the course of GERD.

Over the past decade, minimally invasive outpatient LES augmentation procedures have been developed. Examples include the implantation of a collar of magnetic beads around the inferior border of the LES to prevent its effacement into the stomach,[80] neuromodulation of the LES through electrical stimulation to increase LES resting pressure,[81] and incisionless partial fundoplication performed using a flexible endoscope introduced into the stomach through the mouth.[82] Clinical studies have shown the efficacy of LES augmentation in eliminating reflux symptoms and healing esophagitis in GERD patients suffering from an incomplete response to PPI therapy.[83,84] These procedures avoid the side effects associated with Nissen fundoplication, are reversible if required, and are appropriate for early surgical treatment of patients with progressive disease and the risk of BE, the premalignant lesion of esophageal adenocarcinoma.

A proposed treatment algorithm that features early use of LES augmentation procedures to prevent GERD progression is shown in Fig. 16.15. The algorithm emphasizes the use of early endoscopy with biopsy of the SCJ, manometry of the LES, and esophageal pH monitoring to assess patients with the likelihood of progression. The patients are initially identified by one or several of the following complaints or observations: (1) partial symptomatic response to PPI therapy, (2) deterioration of PPI effectiveness over time, (3) rigid dependency on daily PPI therapy, (4) esophagitis that is difficult to heal with PPI therapy, (5) increasing esophageal exposure to acid over time, (6) loss of LES overall and/or abdominal length on esophageal motility study, and (7) a normal endoscopy but microscopic intestinalized cardiac mucosa on biopsy of the SCJ. The early use of endoscopy in patients who are confirmed nonresponders stratifies the patients into four groups: (1) patients with visible BE; (2) patients with difficult to heal esophagitis; (3) patients with a normal endoscopy but have microscopic intestinalization of metaplastic cardiac mucosa on biopsy of the SCJ; and (4) patients with a normal endoscopy who have carditis on biopsy of the SCJ. LES augmentation is recommended for patients in groups 2 and 3 and an option for patients in group 4. In the latter group the patient is counseled toward augmentation if damage to the LES is detected on manometry. The Nissen fundoplication should be considered for patients with extensive damage to the LES after a thorough discussion on the side effects associated with the procedure.[85]

To improve our management of GERD and avoid its complication require that patients who have symptoms of progressive disease be identified early in the course of their disease. This requires early use of endoscopy in patients with a partial or a deteriorating response to PPI therapy, or a rigid dependency on PPI therapy. In contrast to current management guidelines, we propose routine biopsy of the SCJ in such patients if the esophageal body component of the endoscopic evaluation is normal. If microscopic intestinal metaplasia of metaplastic cardiac mucosa is identified, a LES augmentation procedure should be done to prevent progression to endoscopically visible BE, the premalignant lesion of esophageal adenocarcinoma. This approach must be first tested in the clinical setting to confirm that LES augmentation procedures can reproduce the encouraging results obtained with the Nissen fundoplication.[79] It is incumbent on both gastroenterologists and surgeons to work together to stop the rising incidence of BE, the premalignant lesion of esophageal adenocarcinoma. By 2030, one out of every 100 European men is projected to be diagnosed with esophageal adenocarcinoma before the age of 75 years.[86] The principle of the solution to this developing crisis is, Where there is no BE, there is no cancer.

REFERENCES

1. DeMeester TR, Stein HJ. Surgical treatment of gastroesophageal reflux disease. In: Castell DO, ed. *The Esophagus*. Boston: Little, Brown; 1992:579-626.
2. Tutuian R, Castell DO. Management of gastroesophageal reflux disease. *Am J Med Sci*. 2003;326(5):309-318.
3. Ronkainen J, Talley NJ, Storskrubb T, et al. Erosive esophagitis is a risk factor for Barrett's esophagus: a community-based endoscopic follow-up study. *Am J Gastroenterol*. 2011;106:1946-1952.
4. Shah NH, LePendu P, Bauer-Mehren A, et al. Proton pump inhibitor usage and the risk of myocardial infarction in the general population. *PLoS One*. 2015;10:e0124653.
5. Vakil N, van Zanten SV, Kahrilas P, Dent J, Jones R. Globale Konsensusgruppe. The Montreal definition and classification of gastroesophageal reflux disease: a global evidence-based consensus. *Am J Gastroenterol*. 2006;101:1900-1920.
6. Ronkainen J, Aro P, Stoeskrubb T, et al. High prevalence of gastroesophageal reflux symptoms and esophagitis with or without symptoms in the general adult Swedish population: a Kalixanda study report. *Scand J Gastroenterol*. 2005;40:275-285.
7. Bytzer P, Jones R, Vakil N, et al. Limited ability of the proton-pump inhibitor test to identify patients with gastroesophageal reflux disease. *Clin Gastroenterol Hepatol*. 2012;10:1360-1366.
8. Vakil N. Review article: how valuable are proton-pump-inhibitors in establishing a diagnosis of gastroesophageal reflux disease? *Aliment Pharmacol Ther*. 2006;22(suppl 1):64-69.
9. Katz PO, Gerson LB, Vela MF. Guidelines for the diagnosis and management of gastroesophageal reflux disease. *Am J Gastroenterol*. 2013;108:308-328.
10. Agrawal A, Castell DO. GERD is chronic but not progressive. *J Clin Gastroenterol*. 2006;40:374-375.
11. Pace F, Bianchi Porro G. Gastroesophageal reflux disease: a typical spectrum disease (a new conceptual framework is not needed). *Am J Gastroenterol*. 2004;99:946-949.
12. Labenz J, Nocon M, Lind T, et al. Prospective follow-up data from the ProGERD study suggest that GERD is not a categorial disease. *Am J Gastroenterol*. 2006;101:2457-2462.
13. Malfertheiner P, Nocon M, Vieth M, et al. Evolution of gastroesophageal reflux disease over 5 years under routine medical care—the ProGERD study. *Aliment Pharmacol Ther*. 2012;35:154-164.
14. Pace F, Bollani S, Molteni P, Bianchi Porro G. Natural history of gastroesophageal reflux disease without oesophagitis (NERD)—a reappraisal 10 years on. *Dig Liver Dis*. 2004;36:111-115.
15. Falkenback D, Oberg S, Johnsson F, Johansson J. Is the course of gastroesophageal reflux disease progressive? A 21-year follow-up. *Scand J Gastroenterol*. 2009;44:1277-1287.
16. Klaus A, Gadenstaetter M, Muhlmann G, et al. Selection of patients with gastroesophageal reflux disease for antireflux surgery based on esophageal manometry. *Dig Dis Sci*. 2003;48:1719-1722.
17. Lord RV, DeMeester SR, Peters JH, et al. Hiatal hernia, lower esophageal sphincter incompetence, and effectiveness of Nissen fundoplication in the spectrum of gastroesophageal reflux disease. *J Gastrointest Surg*. 2009;13:602-610.
18. Lord RVN, DeMeester TR. *Reflux Disease and Hiatal Hernia. Oxford Textbook of Surgery*. Vol. 2. Oxford: Oxford University Press; 2000:1239-1262.
19. Bammer T, Freeman M, Shahrian A, Hinder RA, DeVault KR, Achem SR. Outcome of laparoscopic antireflux surgery in patients with nonerosive reflux disease. *J Gastrointest Surg*. 2002;6(5):730-737.
20. Fyke FE, Code CF, Schlegel JF. The gastroesophageal sphincter in healthy humans. *Gastroenterologia*. 1956;86:135-150.
21. McLaurin C. The intrinsic sphincter in the prevention of gastroesophageal reflux. *Lancet*. 1963;282:801-805.
22. DeMeester TR, Johnson LF, Joseph GJ, Toscano MS, Hall AW, Skinner DB. Patterns of gastroesophageal reflux in health and disease. *Ann Surg*. 1976;184:459-470.
23. DeMeester TR, Wernly JA, Bryant GH, Little AG, Skinner DB. Clinical and in vitro analysis of determinants of gastroesophageal competence. *Am J Surg*. 1979;137:39-46.
24. Johnson LF, Lin YC, Hong SK. Gastroesophageal dynamics during immersion in water to the neck. *J Appl Physiol*. 1975;38:449-454.
25. Pellegrini CA, DeMeester TR, Skinner DB. Response of the distal esophageal sphincter to respiratory and positional maneuvers in humans. *Surg Forum*. 1976;27:380-382.
26. O'Sullivan GC, DeMeester TR, Joelsson BE, et al. The interaction of the lower esophageal sphincter pressure and length of sphincter in the abdomen as determinants of gastroesophageal competence. *Am J Surg*. 1982;143:40-47.
27. Bonavina L, Evander A, DeMeester TR, et al. Length of the distal esophageal sphincter and competency of the cardia. *Am J Surg*. 1986;151:25-34.
28. Zaninotto G, DeMeester TR, Schwizer W, Johansson KE, Cheng SC. The lower esophageal sphincter in health and disease. *Am J Surg*. 1988;155:104-111.
29. Pettersson GB, Bombeck CT, Nyhus LM. The lower esophageal sphincter: mechanism of opening and closure. *Surgery*. 1980;88:307-314.
30. Bonavina L, DeMeester TR, Evander A. Role of the overall length of the distal esophageal sphincter in the antireflux mechanism. In: Siewert JR, Holscher AH, eds. *Diseases of the Esophagus*. New York: Springer-Verlag; 1987:1031-1036.
31. Mason RJ, Oberg S, Bremner CG, et al. Postprandial gastroesophageal reflux in normal volunteers and symptomatic patients. *J Gastrointest Surg*. 1998;2:342-349.
32. Dodds WJ, Dent J, Hogan WJ, et al. Mechanics of gastroesophageal reflux in patients with reflux esophagitis. *N Engl J Med*. 1982;307:1549-1552.
33. Holloway RH, Hong M, Berger K, McCallum RW. Gastric distension: a mechanism for postprandial gastroesophageal reflux. *Gastroenterology*. 1985;89:779-784.
34. Jahnberg T, Martinson J, Hulten L, Fasth S. Dynamic gastric response to expansion before and after vagotomy. *Scand J Gastroenterol*. 1975;10:593-598.
35. Scheffer RC, Akkermans LM, Bais JE, Roelofs JMM, Smout AJPM, Gooszen HG. Elicitation of transient lower esophageal sphincter

relaxation in response to gastric distension and meal ingestion. *Neurogastroenterol Motil.* 2002;14:647-655.

36. Ayazi S, Tamhankar R, DeMeester TR, et al. The impact of gastric distension on the lower esophageal sphincter and its exposure to acid gastric juice. *Ann Surg.* 2010;252:52-62.

37. Mason RJ, Lund RJ, DeMeester TR, et al. Nissen fundoplication prevents shortening of the sphincter during gastric distension. *Arch Surg.* 1997;132:719-726.

38. Stein HJ, Barlow AP, DeMeester TR, Hinder RA. Complications of gastroesophageal reflux disease: role of lower esophageal sphincter, esophageal acid and acid/alkaline exposure, and duodenogastric reflux. *Ann Surg.* 1992;216:35-43.

39. Kauer WKH, Peters JH, DeMeester TR, Ireland AP, Bremner CG, Hagen JA. Mixed reflux of gastric and duodenal juice is more harmful to the esophagus than gastric juice alone: the need for surgical therapy re-emphasized. *Ann Surg.* 1995;222:525-533.

40. Stein HJ, Kauer WKH, Feussner H, Siewert JR. Bile reflux in benign and malignant Barrett's esophagus: effect of medical acid suppression and Nissen fundoplication. *J Gastrointest Surg.* 1998;2:333-341.

41. Nehra D, Howell P, Pye JK, Beynon J. Assessment of combined bile and acid pH profiles using an automated sampling device in gastro-oesophageal reflux disease. *Br J Surg.* 1998;85:134-139.

42. Kauer WKH, Burdiles P, Ireland AP, et al. Does duodenal juice reflux into the esophagus of patients with complicated GERD? Evaluation of a fiberoptic sensor for bilirubin. *Am J Surg.* 1995;169:98-104.

43. Oh DS, Hagen JA, Fein M, et al. The impact of reflux composition on mucosal injury and esophageal function. *J Gastrointest Surg.* 2006;10:787-797.

44. Marshall REK, Anggiansah A, Owen WA, Owen WJ. The relationship between acid and bile reflux and symptoms in gastro-oesophageal reflux disease. *Gut.* 1997;40:182-197.

45. Fitzgerald RC, Omary MB, Triadafilopoulos G. Dynamic effects of acid on Barrett's esophagus. *J Clin Invest.* 1996;98:2120-2128.

46. Karmeli Y, Stalnikowitz R, Eliakim R, Rahav G. Conventional dose of omerprazole alters gastric flora. *Dig Dis Sci.* 1995;401:2070-2073.

47. Domeliof L, Reddy BS, Weisburger H. Microflora and deconjugation of bile acids in alkaline reflux after partial gastrectomy. *Am J Surg.* 1980;140:291-295.

48. Schweitzer EJ, Bass BL, Batzri S, Harmon JW. Bile acid accumulation by rabbit esophageal mucosa. *Dig Dis Sci.* 1986;31:1105-1113.

49. Spirey JR, Bronk SF, Gores GJ. Glycochenodeoxycholate-induced hepatocellular injury in rat hepatocytes: role of ATP depletion and cytosolic free calcium. *J Clin Invest.* 1993;92:17-24.

50. Latta RK, Fiander H, Ross NW, Simpson C, Schneider H. Toxicity of bile acids to colon cancer cell lines. *Cancer Lett.* 1993;70:167-173.

51. Silverman SJ, Andrews HW. Bile acids: co-mutagenic activity in the salmonella-mammalian-microsome mutagenicity test. *J Natl Cancer Inst.* 1977;59:1557-1559.

52. Busby WF, Shuker DEG, Charnley G, Newberne PM, Tannenbaum SR, Wogan GN. Carcinogenicity in rats of the nitrosated bile acids conjugates N-nitroso-glycocholic acid and N-nitrosotaurocholic acid. *Cancer Res.* 1985;45:1367-1371.

53. Moersch RN, Ellis FH. Pathologic change occurring in severe reflux esophagitis. *Surg Gyn Obstet.* 1959;108:476-484.

54. Peghini PL, Katz PO, Bracy NA, Castell DO. Nocturnal recovery of gastric acid secretion with twice-daily dosing of proton pump inhibitors. *Am J Gastroenterol.* 1998;93:763-767.

54a. Chandrasoma P, Wijetunge S, Ma Y, et al. Histologic classification of patients based on mapping biopsies of the gastroesophageal junction. *Am J Surg Pathol.* 2003;27:929-936.

54b. Chandrasoma P, Wijetunge S, Ma Y, et al. The dilated distal esophagus: a new entity that is the pathological bases of early gastroesophageal reflux disease. *Am J Surg Pathol.* 2011;35:1873-1881.

55. Csendes A, Maluenda F, Braghetto I, Csendes P, Henriquez A, Quesada MS. Location of the lower esophageal sphincter and the squamous columnar mucosal junction in 109 healthy controls and 778 patients with different degrees of endoscopic esophagitis. *Gut.* 1993;94:21-27.

56. Bremner CJ, Lynch V, Ellis HF. Barrett's esophagus: congenital or acquired? An experimental study of esophageal mucosal regeneration in dog. *Surgery.* 1970;68:209-217.

57. Hayward J. The lower end of the esophagus. *Thorax.* 1961;16:36-41.

58. Paull A, Trier JS, Dalton MD, Camp RC, Loeb P, Goyal RK. The histologic spectrum of Barrett's esophagus. *N Engl J Med.* 1976;295:476-480.

59. Chandrasoma PT, Der R, Ma Y, et al. Histology of the gastroesophageal junction: an autopsy study. *Am J Surg Pathol.* 2000;24:402-409.

60. Chandrasoma P. Pathophysiology of Barrett's esophagus. *Semin Thorac Cardiovasc Surg.* 1997;9:270-278.

61. Oberg S, Peters JH, DeMeester TR, et al. Inflammation and specialized intestinal metaplasia of cardiac mucosa is a manifestation of gastroesophageal reflux disease. *Ann Surg.* 1997;226:522-532.

62. Jain R, Aquino D, Harford WV, Lee E, Spechler SJ. Cardiac epithelium is found infrequently in the gastric cardia. *Gastroenterology.* 1998;114:A160.

63. Lindahl H, Rintala R, Sariola H. Chronic esophagitis and gastric metaplasia are frequent late complications of esophageal atresia. *J Pediatr Surg.* 1993;28:1178-1180.

64. Gillen P, Byrne P, West AB, West AB, Hennessy TP. Experimental columnar metaplasia in the canine esophagus. *Br J Surg.* 1988;75:113-115.

65. Skinner DB, Bruno CW, Riddell R, Schmidt H, Iascone C, DeMeester TR. Barrett's esophagus: comparison of benign and malignant cases. *Ann Surg.* 1983;198:554-566.

66. Reid BJ, Weinstein WM. Barrett's esophagus and adenocarcinoma. *Annu Rev Med.* 1987;38:477-492.

67. Weinstein WM, Ippoliti AF. Editorial: the diagnosis of Barrett's esophagus; goblets, goblets, goblets. *Gastrointest Endosc.* 1996;44:91-95.

68. Qualman SJ, Murray RD, McClung J, Lucas J. Intestinal metaplasia is age related in Barrett's esophagus. *Arch Pathol Lab Med.* 1889;114:1236-1240.

69. Lieberman DA, Oehlke M, Helfand M. Risk factors for Barrett's esophagus in community-based practice. GORGE consortium. Gastroenterology Outcome Research Group in Endoscopy. *Gastroenterology.* 1997;921:1203-1297.

70. Qualman ST, Murray RD, McClung J, et al. Intestinal metaplasia is age related in Barrett's esophagus. *Arch Pathol Lab Med.* 1990;114:1236-1240.

71. Oberg S, Peters JH, DeMeester TR, et al. The extent of Barrett's esophagus depends on the status of the lower esophageal sphincter and the degree of esophageal acid exposure. *J Thorac Cardiovasc Surg.* 1999;117:572-580.

72. Iascone C, DeMeester TR, Little AG, Skinner DB. Barrett's esophagus: functional assessment, proposed pathogenesis and surgical therapy. *Arch Surg.* 1983;118:543-549.

73. Oberg S, Peters JH, Nigro JJ, et al. *Helicobacter pylori* is not associated with the manifestation of gastroesophageal reflux disease. *Arch Surg.* 1999;134:722-726.

74. Lagergren J, Lagergren P. Recent developments in esophageal adenocarcinoma. *CA Cancer J Clin.* 2013;63:232-248.

75. Chandrasoma P, Wijetunge S, DeMeester SR, et al. The histologic squamo-oxyntic gap: an accurate and reproducible diagnostic marker of gastroesophageal reflux disease. *Am J Surg Pathol.* 2010;34:1574-1581.

76. Leodolter A, Nocon M, Vieth M, et al. Progression of specialized intestinal metaplasia at the cardia to macroscopically evident Barrett's esophagus: an entity of concern in the ProGERD study. *Scand J Gastroenterol.* 2012;47:1429-1435.

77. Welscher GJ, Gadenstaetter M, Klingler PJ, et al. Efficacy of medical therapy and antireflux surgery to prevent Barrett's metaplasia in patients with gastroesophageal reflux disease. *Ann Surg.* 2001;234:627-632.

78. Gutschow CA, Schroder W, Prengel K, et al. Impact of antireflux surgery on Barrett's esophagus. *Langenbecks Arch Surg.* 2002;387:138-145.

79. DeMeester SR, Campos GM, DeMeester TR, et al. The impact of an antireflux procedure on intestinal metaplasia of the cardia. *Ann Surg.* 1998;228:547-556.

80. Ganz RA, Peters JH, Horgan S, et al. Esophageal sphincter device for gastroesophageal reflux disease. *N Engl J Med.* 2013;368:719-727.

81. Rodriguez L, Rodriguez PA, Gomez B, Netto MG, Crowell MD, Soffer E. Electronic stimulation therapy of the lower esophageal sphincter is successful in treating GERD: long-term 3-year results. *Surg Endosc.* 2016;30:2666-2672.

82. Trad KS, Barnes WE, Simoni G, et al. Transoral incisionless fundoplication effective in eliminating GERD symptoms in partial responders to

proton pump inhibitor therapy at 6 months: the TEMPO randomized clinical trial. *Surg Innov.* 2015;22:26-40.

83. Bonavina L, Saino G, Lipham JC, Demeester TR. LINX reflux management system in chronic gastroesophageal reflux: a novel effective technology for restoring the natural barrier to reflux. *Therap Adv Gastroenterol.* 2013;6:261-268.

84. Ganz RA, Edmundowicz SA, Taiganides PA, et al. Long-term outcomes of patients receiving a magnetic sphincter augmentation device for gastroesophageal reflux. *Clin Gastroenterol Hepatol.* 2016;14:671-677.

85. Warren HF, Louie BE, Farivar A, Wilshire C, Aye RW. Manometric changes to the lower esophageal sphincter after magnetic sphincter augmentation in patients with chronic gastroesophageal reflux disease. *Ann Surg.* 2017;266:99-104.

86. Arnold M, Laversanne M, Brown LM, Devesa SS, Bray F. Predicting the future burden of esophageal cancer by histological subtype: international trends in incidence up to 2030. *Am J Gastroenterol.* 2017;112: 1247-1255.

Respiratory Complications of Gastroesophageal Reflux Disease

Michael S. Mulvihill | Shu S. Lin | Matthew G. Hartwig

Gastroesophageal reflux (GER) refers to the reflux of stomach contents into the esophagus. GER can occur physiologically, particularly in the postprandial state.[1] When reflux is of small volume for limited durations and limited to the distal esophagus, this retrograde flow of stomach contents is generally of minor medical importance. In this chapter, the repercussions of reflux of gastric contents into the airway will be reviewed. In the acute setting, the reflux of large volumes of gastric contents proximally into the airway can present a life-threatening aspiration event, sometimes known as Mendelson syndrome.[2] However, for the purpose of this chapter, a focus will be maintained on the long-term sequelae of small volume reflux proximal to the esophagus.

Although the stomach benefits from the secretion of protective mucus, the lining of the esophagus lacks these protective features, and as such the mucosa of the esophagus may become irritated or damaged by the regurgitation of stomach contents. Gastroesophageal reflux disease (GERD) describes the presence of excessive reflux of acid or nonacid stomach contents, with unwanted resultant manifestations. A host of factors may contribute to the change from physiologic to pathologic state.[1,3] In particular, lifestyle factors (use of alcohol, use of cigarettes, obesity), medications (calcium channel blockade, theophyllines), diet (fatty food, fried foods, chocolate, caffeine, acidic foods, spicy foods), eating habits (large meals shortly before sleep), and other medical conditions (hiatus hernia, pregnancy, rapid weight gain) are known to contribute to GERD. A broad range of the most common symptoms associated with GERD include the traditional gastrointestinal manifestations. However, extraesophageal symptoms such as cough, hoarseness, sore throat, frequent throat clearing, asthma, bronchitis, and other laryngeal and pulmonary manifestations have been noted, and increasing attention is being paid to the extraesophageal sequelae of GERD. The high prevalence of extraesophageal manifestations of GERD in patients with respiratory illness highlights the importance of the consideration of gastrointestinal causes in the approach to the patient with respiratory illness. In this chapter, respiratory complications associated with GERD will be reviewed.

Patients with respiratory manifestations of GERD often do not report the more typical reflux symptoms, with estimates of 75% of patients with GER-related cough exhibiting otherwise "silent" reflux.[4] Because of this, clinicians need to maintain a high level of suspicion in patients with respiratory complaints that may be the only manifestation of their underlying GERD. Descriptive studies to assess the prevalence of respiratory complications of GERD have primarily focused on asthma and cough, the most common extraesophageal manifestations of GERD. Available evidence suggests that GERD is identified in approximately 30% to 80% of patients previously diagnosed with asthma.[5] In a longitudinal study, development of asthma occurred at a higher rate in patients with longer duration of GERD symptoms. Conversely, the prevalence of asthma in GERD patients is reported at approximately 4.6%.[5] Assessment of the prevalence of GERD-related cough is influenced heavily by the patient population, diagnostic testing modalities used, and the decision to attribute cough to a single or multiple etiologies. As such, estimates of the prevalence of GERD-related cough have ranged from 10% to 40% in the literature.[4]

In the following sections, the relationship between GER and respiratory disease will be reviewed. A growing body of evidence supports the finding that, although GER may not be uniquely causative of respiratory pathology, it is frequently a contributing factor. Treatment of GERD in the patient with respiratory illness, then, should be tailored to the individual patient based on his or her symptoms and the degree to which GER is thought to contribute to the respiratory pathology at hand.

ROLE OF GASTROESOPHAGEAL REFLUX DISEASE IN CHRONIC COUGH

The American College of Chest Physicians defines chronic cough as one lasting greater than 8 weeks in a nonsmoking, immunocompetent patient who takes no cough-inducing drugs (such as angiotensin-converting enzyme inhibitors) and has a normal chest radiograph.[6] Causative factors of chronic cough represent a vast array of clinical entities. Asthma, postnasal drip, and GER represent the most common etiologies of chronic cough. The epidemiologic link between GER and chronic cough was established in 1981 and subsequently verified across a range of patient cohorts.[7] Despite a clear association in the literature, estimates of prevalence have varied widely from 0% to 73%, driven by differences in populations, methodologies, and clinical awareness related to range of specialists (pulmonary medicine, gastroenterology, otolaryngology, general surgery) that evaluate these patients in the clinic setting.

As a theme that will appear in discussion of the interplay between GER and other respiratory disease states, GER contributes to the development and sequelae of chronic cough by way of a variety of mechanisms. The primary mechanisms for consideration are microaspiration, the esophagobronchial reflex, and an increased sensitivity of the cough reflex.

Microaspiration refers to the presence of gastric contents in the airway as evidenced by detection in bronchoalveolar lavage (BAL) fluid. At bronchoscopy, evidence for aspiration includes subglottic stenosis, hemorrhagic tracheobronchitis, and erythema of the subsegmental bronchi. Plain radiographs and axial imaging may also reveal parenchymal changes consistent with acute or chronic aspiration. Irritation of the lower respiratory tract by aspiration represents the most direct link between GER and cough.

Chronic cough may also be triggered indirectly through activation of an esophagobronchial reflex, a means by which cough may be stimulated by GER in the absence of bronchoscopic or radiographic evidence of aspiration. Mechanistically, esophageal innervation by sensory-type fibers that express acid-sensitive channel TRPV-1 and the subsequent convergence of these sensory afferents with vagal afferent neurons provides a means by which refluxate in the distal esophagus may stimulate a vagal reflex. Ing et al. provide evidence of this mechanism in humans by showing that instillation of acid into the distal esophagus of patients with both GERD and cough increased the frequency, duration, and intensity of cough compared with instillation of normal saline.[8] Such a response was subsequently attenuated by pretreatment with lidocaine. Further studies in humans suggest that repetitive exposure can lead to hypersensitivity and a lowering of the cough threshold.[9,10] Dynamic changes in the cough threshold may cause cough to become relatively stimulus agnostic, such that nonreflux stimuli precipitate symptoms previously associated with GER.

The approach to the patient with chronic cough attributed to GER may be guided by both national guidelines and systematic review of the available evidence. The American College of Chest Physicians recommends empiric acid suppression in patients thought to experience reflux-induced cough.[6] A Cochrane systematic review identified 13 randomized controlled trials examining GERD therapy for the treatment of cough in adults without primary lung disease.[11] Analysis of H$_2$-receptor antagonist, motility agents, and conservative treatment was not possible in the meta-analysis. The remaining nine trials compared proton pump inhibitor (PPI) with placebo. Although there was no difference in the rate of total resolution of cough, patients receiving PPI therapy were more likely to note improvement in cough scores. Thus, even though the primary outcome was not met, there appears to be a benefit to acid suppression in appropriately selected patients. Nonetheless, the long-term consequences of respiratory complications were not addressed in any of these studies.

To date, controlled studies of the efficacy of fundoplication or other surgical interventions for patients with cough and GER are lacking. In single-center studies, surgical intervention consistently demonstrates efficacy in key metrics. In particular, fundoplication is effective in reducing the number of reflux events by esophageal pH monitoring and produces symptomatic improvement. Traditionally, patients with extraesophageal GER symptoms such as cough have been found to benefit from fundoplication at a rate lower than those with typical GER symptoms, with estimates of approximately 60% of patients with

cough subsequently reporting improvements in cough scores, and freedom from PPI therapy.[12] This is most likely due to our inability to better confirm the direct causal effect of GERD on chronic cough in all patients.

LARYNGOPHARYNGEAL REFLUX

The earliest reports of acid-driven injury to the larynx (manifest by laryngeal ulcerations and granulomas) were noted by Cherry in 1968.[13] Pellegrini was among the first in 1979 to note that acid-containing reflux of gastric contents may then be a causative factor in this laryngeal pathology.[14] Although at the time the potential for a surgical cure of extraesophageal symptoms of reflux was noted to be achievable by way of an antireflux procedure, laryngitis was not formally recognized as an extraesophageal manifestation of GER until 2006 by the Montreal Definition and Classification System. Data regarding the prevalence of laryngopharyngeal reflux (LPR) are relatively limited, in part stemming from controversy in the professional organizations with respect to the appropriate diagnostic criteria for LPR. In particular, controversy exists with respect to the extent to which symptoms related to LPR should be attributed to reflux in the absence of traditional heartburn symptoms.

A high index of suspicion should be maintained for LPR in the patient with hoarseness, cough, globus, and throat clearing. A minority of patients (35%) found to have LPR report heartburn symptoms. Scoring systems such as the Reflux Symptom Index (RSI) or Hull Airway Reflux Questionnaire (HARQ) may be of utility in the screening of these patients for LPR and associated extraesophageal manifestations of GERD as a cause of symptoms. Patients who are subsequently evaluated by direct laryngoscopy following history and physical exam are assessed for posterior laryngeal edema, true vocal fold edema, and pseudosulcus. Although these findings may be sensitive for the diagnosis of LPR, they often are not specific because they are common findings in the general population and are not strictly linked to exposure of the larynx to gastric contents.

Detection of reflux into the pharynx requires diagnostic strategies that differ from the detection of reflux in the distal esophagus, on account of the neutralization of refluxate as it ascends the esophagus into the more alkaline environment of the pharynx. As such, pharyngeal pH monitoring is of low sensitivity in the diagnosis of LPR. Currently, pH/impedance monitoring offers a superior strategy for diagnosis, with a significant benefit of detection of both acid and nonacid reflux. pH/impedance monitoring may also identify the proximal extent of reflux. Reflux into the laryngopharynx is very rare in healthy patients, such that any evidence of reflux so far proximal from the gastroesophageal junction may be considered abnormal and thereby warrant treatment. The use of a dual-probe (or bifurcated) impedance pH catheter permits detection of both impedance and pH changes across the upper esophageal sphincter, thereby permitting detection of pharyngeal reflux. More novel techniques aim to detect the pH of aerosolized reflux, which reveal the finding that patients with chronic cough may reflux both liquid and gaseous stomach contents. Patients with predominantly cough-related symptoms may benefit from techniques that make use of physiologic changes associated with cough (such as pressure changes above and below the diaphragm) to demonstrate a temporal link between cough and reflux.

Mechanistically, as with exposure of other nonstomach structures to acid, the larynx has relatively little protection against both acid and enzymatic activity. The thinner epithelium and lack of peristalsis to wash away acid contribute to injury seen with relatively brief and short-duration exposures in animal models. In addition to the consequences of direct exposure to acid and other gastric contents, laryngeal injury may also manifest as an indirect consequence of exposure of the esophagus to refluxate. In the indirect model, irritation of the esophagus can generate vagally mediated reflexes such as cough and bronchoconstriction that can contribute to chronic laryngeal injury.

Successful treatment of LPR again requires adequacy of diagnosis. In the patient with modifiable risk factors, behavior modification such as minimization of tobacco and alcohol consumption is recommended. Those patients with LPR and evidence of esophageal symptoms of GERD should be treated with acid suppression. The role of acid suppression in patients with suspected or confirmed LPR but without evidence of esophageal manifestations of GERD is controversial, and success of therapy likely depends on the extent to which acid is a contributing factor in the symptoms associated with LPR. The American Gastroenterological Association recommends against PPI and H_2-receptor blockade for the treatment of suspected LPR in the absence of a concomitant GERD syndrome.[15] In contrast, the American Academy of Otolaryngology-Head and Neck Surgery recommends twice-daily PPI for no less than 6 months for patients with LPR.[16] Data regarding the use of acid suppression in the absence of esophageal manifestations are weak and are limited by a lack of standardized diagnostic criteria. Trials have also been limited by the possibility of placebo effect, such that, in small studies, for example, patients with no measurable pH response to PPI report symptom improvement.[17,18] Uncontrolled trials of surgery have shown some promise in patients with medication-refractory LPR, but a controlled trial of antireflux surgery in patients who failed aggressive acid suppression did not improve laryngeal symptoms despite showing successful control of reflux by way of pH studies.

ROLE OF GASTROESOPHAGEAL REFLUX DISEASE IN ASTHMA AND CHRONIC OBSTRUCTIVE PULMONARY DISEASE

Chronic obstructive pulmonary disease (COPD) and asthma are distinct clinical entities with unique risk factors, pathophysiology, and prognosis. However, they may exhibit overlapping clinical presentations. GER represents a comorbidity experienced by many patients with each disorder. Most broadly, abnormal GER may contribute to worsening asthma symptoms and has been associated with an increased risk of COPD exacerbation. Although results have been inconsistent, treatment of symptomatic GER leads to improvements in patient-related outcomes in both asthma and COPD. The prevalence and pathophysiology of GER in each entity are reviewed.

Asthma is common in the United States, with approximately 24 million Americans carrying the diagnosis. Of these patients with asthma, an estimated 30% to 90% of patients have GER.[5] Systematic review by Havemann revealed that 59.2% of asthmatics had evidence of GERD, whereas the prevalence in controls was 38.1%. Similarly, abnormal esophageal pH, esophagitis, and hiatal hernia are all more prevalent in patients with asthma.[19] GER is also a risk factor for asthma-related hospitalizations in older adults.[20]

The prevalence of GER in patients with COPD is more poorly understood. A retrospective study from the Veterans Health Administration found that of 101,366 veterans those with erosive esophagitis and esophageal stricture had higher rates of chronic bronchitis, asthma, and COPD. A smaller study demonstrated that pathologic GER was identified in 62% of patients with severe COPD. Notably, episodes of esophageal acid exposure were temporally linked to oxygen desaturations in this patient population. There is also evidence that GER contributes to detrimental outcomes in patients with COPD. The 2010 results of the ECLIPSE study (Evaluation of COPD Longitudinally to Identify Predictive Surrogate Endpoints) prospectively assessed 2138 patients with stages II–IV COPD to identify factors associated with increased frequency of COPD exacerbation. In this cohort, GER was independently associated with an increased risk of COPD exacerbation.[21]

Multiple mechanisms likely contribute to the interaction between esophageal pathology and injury to the respiratory system. A shared embryonic origin from the foregut of the respiratory and gastrointestinal systems contributes to the interplay between asthma, COPD, and GER.

Shared vagal innervation and resultant converging visceral sensory neural input contributes to pulmonary symptoms at the time of stimulation of esophageal receptors by stimuli such as acid exposure. Nonadrenergic neurons in the esophageal myenteric plexus communicate with the trachea. In animal models, instillation of acid in the esophagus subsequently results in the release of tachykinin-like substances in the airways and subsequent bronchoconstriction. This finding can be terminated by vagotomy, suggesting that vagal innervation is required for this interaction. This finding may contribute to the finding of increased airway reactivity common to this patient population. A single bolus of acid can result in rapid distribution through the lung and generate a wide range of histopathologic changes, including neutrophil sequestration, epithelial damage, pulmonary edema, and pulmonary hemorrhage.

Chronic aspiration results in inflammation, an altered immune response, and worsening of asthma symptoms. In animal studies, instillation of acid increases total lung resistance and leads to an aspiration pneumonia that is characterized by neutrophilic and lymphocytic peribronchiolar infiltrates, goblet cell hyperplasia, and thickening of the smooth muscle layer. Barbas et al. demonstrated that chronic aspiration of murine gastric fluid produced an injury pattern characterized by hyperplasia and neutrophil infiltration of the bronchioles that differs from the response seen in acute aspiration. This chronic aspiration model subsequently results in a shift to a Th2 inflammatory response.[22]

Although overlapping mechanisms may contribute to the relationship between COPD and GER, additional mechanisms are worthy of consideration. Reduction of lower esophageal sphincter (LES) tone may be due to multiple factors but regardless can contribute to the reflux of gastric contents. In particular, anatomic changes related to COPD, such as the flattening of the diaphragm, can result in a decrease in resting LES tone.[23] In addition, oral theophylline, although used less frequently in contemporary management of COPD, may reduce LES tone.

Evidence supports the treatment of symptomatic GER in the setting of asthma. Adequate studies in the management of GER in the patient with COPD are presently lacking. To date, three large randomized controlled trials represent the best evidence that high-dose PPI therapy improves symptoms of asthma. In the first trial, 207 patients with moderate to severe asthma and reflux symptoms experienced improvements in Asthma Quality of Life Questionnaire scores and decreased asthma exacerbations with lansoprazole therapy compared with controls, although neither the primary outcome (improvement in asthma symptoms) nor the secondary outcomes (peak expiratory flow [PEF] and forced expiratory volume [FEV]$_1$) were met.[24] A second trial randomized 961 patients with moderate to severe asthma and symptoms of GER to esomeprazole, finding that the treatment arm enjoyed small but significant improvements in PEF, FEV$_1$, and Asthma Quality of Life Questionnaire scores.[25] A third trial of patients with moderate to severe asthma and both nocturnal respiratory symptoms and GER found that esomeprazole improved PEF.[26]

Although a significant fraction (24% to 62% in the available literature) of patients with asthma may have clinically silent GER, the evidence does not support PPI therapy for patients with silent GER and asthma. Available trial data indicate that the addition of PPI for patients with poorly controlled asthma and minimal to no symptoms of reflux does not improve episodes of poor asthma control nor does it improve PEF.

A Cochrane systematic review synthesizes these findings with 12 randomized controlled trials of medical interventions (including histamine antagonists, PPIs, and lifestyle modification) of GER in patients with asthma. The review concludes that treatment of GER does provide a benefit with respect to management of asthma. No consistent improvement in secondary outcomes such as lung function, airway responsiveness, or asthma symptoms was identified.[11]

The role for antireflux surgery in patients with asthma and GER is poorly defined and without high-level evidence. Surgical therapy is associated with improved asthma symptom control, but improvements in pulmonary function have not been demonstrated in the asthmatic population. A meta-analysis of 24 studies estimates that antireflux surgery may improve asthma symptoms, suggesting that appropriately selected patients may find benefit to surgical therapy.[12] To date, the literature has not identified improvements in pulmonary function associated with antireflux surgery in this patient population.

Patients with asthma and extraesophageal reflux symptoms (and without warning signs such as dysphagia or weight loss) may be considered for an empiric trial of PPI. Those with improvements in asthma symptomatology or improvements in pulmonary function testing may warrant chronic therapy. Further diagnostic testing is warranted in those patients who do not experience improvement in symptoms after empiric therapy. Appropriately selected patients for whom goals of symptom relief and avoidance of long-term medication are prioritized may be suitable candidates for surgical antireflux procedures. At this time, management strategies for the patient with COPD and symptomatic GER are not widely generalizable and should be considered on a case-by-case basis.

ROLE OF GASTROESOPHAGEAL REFLUX DISEASE IN BRONCHIECTASIS

Patients with bronchiectasis (both due to cystic fibrosis [CF] and non-CF bronchiectasis) experience GER at a rate higher than the general population. Symptomatic GER may occur at a rate higher in the CF population than the general population, with reports ranging from 30% to 40% of CF patients reporting symptoms of GERD, and up to 90% of patients may have evidence of silent GER by esophageal monitoring in patients with severe disease. Patients with bronchiectasis may frequently have a clinical presentation that is atypical with respect to GER symptoms, thereby requiring a higher index of suspicion in the approach to the patient with bronchiectasis and possible GER.

There exist increasing data to suggest that increased GER (with or without aspiration) may lead to functional lung impairment in CF. Data from the European Epidemiologic Registry of Cystic Fibrosis demonstrate that patients with CF with GER have lower pulmonary function than those without GER.[27] Aspiration of gastric contents also appears to be associated in a dose-dependent fashion with an increase in the extent of airway inflammation in these patients.

The mechanisms for GER in the patient with CF or non-CF bronchiectasis appear similar to the broader patient population, namely relaxation of the LES, but additional mechanisms may contribute. In particular, the increased intraabdominal pressure due to chronic cough, wheezing, and lung hyperinflation—all common in the patient with bronchiectasis—may contribute to the development of GER. In addition, delayed gastric emptying and a decreased basal tone of the LES may be contributing factors. Delayed gastric emptying is seen in approximately 30% of GER patients and may be higher in patients with both CF and GER.[28] Approximately 30% of patients with CF appear to experience delayed gastric transit. Although increased gastric retention may lead to a higher (more proximal) extent of reflux, a formal causal relationship is yet to be defined. Manometric studies of CF patients reveal a rate of decreased basal LES tone in approximately 60% of patients.[29]

The sequelae of GER in patients with bronchiectasis manifest by mechanisms similar to the broader population.

In particular, microaspiration, reflex bronchospasm, and increased airway inflammation all contribute to pulmonary injury. As mentioned previously, GER may result in functional lung impairment in this patient population.

Optimal treatment strategies in this patient population are poorly defined. To date, there exist no randomized trial data on which to base consensus. Observational studies note an improvement in pulmonary function in patients with CF after initiation of PPI therapy for symptomatic GERD. However, acid suppression has been demonstrated to increase a rate of bacterial overgrowth in stomach contents, leading to altered respiratory flora when nonacid but bacterial-laden stomach contents are refluxed. Antireflux procedures should be considered in patients with GER refractory to medical management and in patients with complications of GER, such as erosive esophagitis, stricture, or failure to thrive. Surgical management of reflux in the pediatric CF patient population has been shown in observational studies to decrease the rate of pulmonary function decline.[30,31] Outcomes with respect to GER symptoms have been mixed following surgical intervention.

ROLE OF GASTROESOPHAGEAL REFLUX DISEASE IN INTERSTITIAL LUNG DISEASE

The interstitial lung diseases (ILDs) represent a heterogeneous group of progressive acute and chronic parenchymal lung diseases characterized by diffuse infiltrates and progressive fibrosis. The progressive nature of ILD can lead to worsening lung function and respiratory insufficiency.

In a manner similar to bronchiectasis, there is an increasing recognition of the interplay between GER and ILD, such as idiopathic pulmonary fibrosis (IPF), scleroderma, and other connective tissue disease (CTD). Although definitive proof that GER and subsequent microaspiration are the proximal cause of ILD, precipitate exacerbation, or promote disease progression is lacking, there exists a body of evidence that suggests a role for GER and microaspiration in each of these disease states.

Development of IPF is associated with a range of exposures, viral infections, and inherited genetic factors. It is characterized by a histopathologic pattern of usual interstitial pneumonia (UIP) on lung biopsy. Classic findings include areas of distorted parenchymal architecture interspersed with fibrotic lesions characterized by temporal heterogeneity. Beginning in the 1970s, studies of prevalence have estimated that in excess of 50% of patients with evidence of pulmonary fibrosis had evidence of GER.[32,33] Typical symptoms of GER are poor predictors of GER in patients with IPF.[34]

Although a high fraction of IPF patients have evidence of GER and although animal models of reflux described previously can result in chronic inflammatory changes to the lung tissue, no causal relationship between GER and the development of IPF has been established in humans. A small body of evidence suggests that a role exists for acid suppression therapy in the IPF patient population.[35,36] Three case series of IPF patients report stabilization of

oxygen requirements and improved long-term survival in patients treated with PPI followed by fundoplication if required to adequately suppress acid.[37,38]

GER is likewise common in patients with other connective tissue disorders, such as scleroderma. In particular, GER (as well as impaired esophageal motility and esophageal dilatation) is highly prevalent in those patients with CTD and evidence of pulmonary fibrosis. Although further mechanistic studies are again warranted, these data do suggest a possibility that patients with CTD exhibit a disordered response to microaspiration and reflux that ultimately places them at higher risk for pulmonary fibrosis. The patients with CTD and esophageal dysmotility, then, are subsequently most likely to suffer the pulmonary consequences of CTD. Randomized data to guide treatment for patients with scleroderma or other CTD and GER are lacking. Consideration of acid suppression therapy, whether by lifestyle modification, medical management, or surgical intervention, should be determined on a case-by-case basis.

ROLE OF GASTROESOPHAGEAL REFLUX DISEASE IN PATIENTS UNDER CONSIDERATION FOR LUNG TRANSPLANTATION

Special attention is warranted in the consideration of the patient with GER who has undergone or who is under evaluation for lung transplantation. Indeed, many of the disease states discussed in this chapter (COPD, CF, IPF) may progress to respiratory insufficiency and end-stage lung failure. GER is very common in both the pretransplant candidate and the posttransplant recipient, with estimates in the range of 50% of patients who receive an allograft having evidence of reflux before transplant and upward of 75% after lung transplantation.[39,40] For these patients, strategies for management are extremely limited and lung transplantation is the gold standard therapy.

The lung is relatively unique among solid-organ allografts because of its continuous exposure to the outside environment. As such, immunosuppressive strategies and the subsequent consequences of immunomodulation must be tailored to this need for the allograft to respond to antigen exposure. Exposure to gastric contents—both acid and nonacid containing—represent a critical source of environmental exposure in lung transplantation. Survival following lung transplantation is limited by the development of chronic lung allograft dysfunction (CLAD) that manifests clinically by a progressive decline in FEV_1 from peak posttransplant values. GERD has been recognized as an important risk factor for the development of CLAD posttransplant. Patients with GERD before transplant have also been identified as being at risk for premature graft dysfunction. In addition, patients with GERD before transplant are at risk for increasing severity of reflux posttransplant. As such, in retrospective clinical data, patients with GERD are at increased risk of negative outcomes after lung transplantation.[39]

In animal models, chronic aspiration of gastric fluid led to increased rates of acute rejection and fibrosis after orthotopic lung transplantation.[41–45] In addition, instillation of nonacid gastric contents in similar models can produce equivalent aspiration injury, in part due to higher rates of bacterial overgrowth that might otherwise be suppressed by low gastric pH.[46]

Taken together, multiple lines of evidence implicate GERD as a contributing factor to diminished pulmonary function posttransplant.[47] On account of the critical observation that exposure to nonacid gastric contents can contribute to lung allograft failure in animal models, there exists minimal role for medical therapy by way of acid suppression in the treatment of reflux after lung transplantation. Use of routine PPI posttransplantation has not abrogated the relationship between abnormal esophageal acid contact times and diminished FEV_1. Not surprisingly, then, PPI alone does not prevent aspiration of gastric contents and, as such, is inadequate therapy to minimize the risk of development of bronchiolitis obliterans in allograft recipients with evidence of reflux. Single-center data suggest that surgical intervention by way of fundoplication preserves 1-year and peak pulmonary allograft function.[48,49] Aggressive work-up and management, with consideration of early surgical intervention by way of fundoplication posttransplant, are warranted in patients evaluated for lung transplantation.

REFERENCES

1. Dodds WJ, Dent J, Hogan WJ, et al. Mechanisms of gastroesophageal reflux in patients with reflux esophagitis. *N Engl J Med.* 1982;307(25): 1547-1552. doi:10.1056/NEJM198212163072503.
2. Mendelson CL. The aspiration of stomach contents into the lungs during obstetric anesthesia. *Anesthesiology.* 1946;7(6):694-695.
3. Canning BJ, Mazzone SB. Reflex mechanisms in gastroesophageal reflux disease and asthma. *Am J Med.* 2003;115(3 suppl 1):45-48. doi:http://dx.doi.org/10.1016/S0002-9343(03)00192-X.
4. Irwin RS. Chronic cough due to gastroesophageal reflux disease: ACCP evidence-based clinical practice guidelines. *Chest.* 2006;129 (1 suppl):80S-94S. doi:10.1378/chest.129.1_suppl.80S.
5. Havemann BD, Henderson CA, El-Serag HB. The association between gastro-oesophageal reflux disease and asthma: a systematic review. *Gut.* 2007;56(12):1654-1664. doi:10.1136/gut.2007.122465.
6. Gibson P, Wang G, McGarvey L, et al. Treatment of unexplained chronic cough: CHEST Guideline and Expert Panel Report. *Chest.* 2016;149(1):27-44. doi:http://dx.doi.org/10.1378/chest.15-1496.
7. Christopher KL, Wood RP, Eckert RC, Blager FB, Raney RA, Souhrada JF. Vocal-cord dysfunction presenting as asthma. *N Engl J Med.* 1983;308(26):1566-1570. doi:10.1056/NEJM198306303082605.
8. Ing AJ, Ngu MC, Breslin AB. Pathogenesis of chronic persistent cough associated with gastroesophageal reflux. *Am J Respir Crit Care Med.* 1994;149(1):160-167. doi:10.1164/ajrccm.149.1.8111576; PubMed PMID: 8111576.
9. Javorkova N, Varechova S, Pecova R, et al. Acidification of the oesophagus acutely increases the cough sensitivity in patients with gastro-oesophageal reflux and chronic cough. *Neurogastroenterol Motil.* 2008;20(2):119-124. doi:10.1111/j.1365-2982.2007.01020.x; PubMed PMID: 17999650.
10. Benini L, Ferrari M, Sembenini C, et al. Cough threshold in reflux oesophagitis: influence of acid and of laryngeal and oesophageal damage. *Gut.* 2000;46(6):762-767. PubMed PMID: 10807885; PMCID: PMC1756455.
11. Gibson PG, Henry R, Coughlan JJL. Gastro-oesophageal reflux treatment for asthma in adults and children. *Cochrane Database Syst Rev.* 2003;(2):CD001496. doi:10.1002/14651858.CD001496; PubMed PMID: CD001496.
12. Garg SK, Gurusamy KS. Laparoscopic fundoplication surgery versus medical management for gastro-oesophageal reflux disease (GORD) in adults. *Cochrane Database Syst Rev.* 2015;(11):CD003243. doi:10.1002/14651858.CD003243.pub3; PubMed PMID: CD003243.
13. Cherry J, Margulies SI. Contact ulcer of the larynx. *Laryngoscope.* 1968;78(11):1937-1940. doi:10.1288/00005537-196811000-00007; PubMed PMID: 5722896.
14. Pellegrini CA, DeMeester TR, Johnson LF, Skinner DB. Gastro-esophageal reflux and pulmonary aspiration: incidence, functional abnormality, and results of surgical therapy. *Surgery.* 1979;86(1):110-119. PubMed PMID: 36677.
15. Kahrilas PJ, Shaheen NJ, Vaezi MF, American Gastroenterological Association Institute. Clinical Practice and Quality Management Committee. American Gastroenterological Association Institute technical review on the management of gastroesophageal reflux disease. *Gastroenterology.* 2008;135(4):1392-1413, 413 e1-5. doi:10.1053/j.gastro.2008.08.044; PubMed PMID: 18801365.
16. Koufman JA, Aviv JE, Casiano RR, Shaw GY. Laryngopharyngeal reflux: position statement of the Committee on Speech, Voice, and Swallowing Disorders of the American Academy of Otolaryngology-Head and Neck Surgery. *Otolaryngol Head Neck Surg.* 2002;127(1):32-35. PubMed PMID: 12161727.
17. Reichel O, Keller J, Rasp G, Hagedorn H, Berghaus A. Efficacy of once-daily esomeprazole treatment in patients with laryngopharyngeal reflux evaluated by 24-hour pH monitoring. *Otolaryngol Head Neck Surg.* 2007;136(2):205-210. doi:10.1016/j.otohns.2006.10.011; PubMed PMID: 17275540.
18. Reichel O, Dressel H, Wiederanders K, Issing WJ. Double-blind, placebo-controlled trial with esomeprazole for symptoms and signs associated with laryngopharyngeal reflux. *Otolaryngol Head Neck Surg.* 2008;139(3):414-420. doi:10.1016/j.otohns.2008.06.003; PubMed PMID: 18722223.
19. Field SK, Underwood M, Brant R, Cowie RL. Prevalence of gastro-esophageal reflux symptoms in asthma. *Chest.* 1996;109(2):316-322. PubMed PMID: 8620699.
20. Diette GB, Krishnan JA, Dominici F, et al. Asthma in older patients: factors associated with hospitalization. *Arch Intern Med.* 2002;162(10):1123-1132. doi:10.1001/archinte.162.10.1123.
21. Hurst JR, Vestbo J, Anzueto A, et al. Susceptibility to exacerbation in chronic obstructive pulmonary disease. *N Engl J Med.* 2010;363(12):1128-1138. doi:10.1056/NEJMoa0909883; PubMed PMID: 20843247.
22. Barbas AS, Downing TE, Balsara KR, et al. Chronic aspiration shifts the immune response from Th1 to Th2 in a murine model of asthma. *Eur J Clin Invest.* 2008;38(8):596-602. doi:10.1111/j.1365-2362.2008.01976.x.
23. Roussos C, Macklem PT. The respiratory muscles. *N Engl J Med.* 1982;307(13):786-797. doi:10.1056/NEJM198209233071304.
24. Littner MR, Leung FW, Ballard ED 2nd, Huang B, Samra NK, Lansoprazole Asthma Study Group. Effects of 24 weeks of lansoprazole therapy on asthma symptoms, exacerbations, quality of life, and pulmonary function in adult asthmatic patients with acid reflux symptoms. *Chest.* 2005;128(3):1128-1135. doi:10.1378/chest.128.3.1128; PubMed PMID: 16162697.
25. American Lung Association Asthma Clinical Research Centers, Mastronarde JG, Anthonisen NR, et al. Efficacy of esomeprazole for treatment of poorly controlled asthma. *N Engl J Med.* 2009;360(15):1487-1499. doi:10.1056/NEJMoa0806290; PubMed PMID: 19357404; PMCID: PMC2974569.
26. Kiljander TO, Harding SM, Field SK, et al. Effects of esomeprazole 40 mg twice daily on asthma: a randomized placebo-controlled trial. *Am J Respir Crit Care Med.* 2006;173(10):1091-1097. doi:10.1164/rccm.200507-1167OC; PubMed PMID: 16357331.
27. Navarro J, Rainisio M, Harms HK, et al. Factors associated with poor pulmonary function: cross-sectional analysis of data from the ERCF. *Eur Respir J.* 2001;18(2):298-305.
28. Pauwels A, Blondeau K, Dupont LJ, Sifrim D. Mechanisms of increased gastroesophageal reflux in patients with cystic fibrosis. *Am J Gastroenterol.* 2012;107(9):1346-1353. doi:10.1038/ajg.2012.213; PubMed PMID: 22777342.
29. Sabati AA, Kempainen RR, Milla CE, et al. Characteristics of gas-troesophageal reflux in adults with cystic fibrosis. *J Cyst Fibros.* 2010;9(5):365-370. doi:10.1016/j.jcf.2010.06.004; PubMed PMID: 20674518.
30. Fathi H, Moon T, Donaldson J, Jackson W, Sedman P, Morice AH. Cough in adult cystic fibrosis: diagnosis and response to fundoplication. *Cough.* 2009;5(1):1-6. doi:10.1186/1745-9974-5-1.
31. Boesch RP, Acton JD. Outcomes of fundoplication in children with cystic fibrosis. *J Pediatr Surg.* 2007;42(8):1341-1344. doi:http://dx.doi.org/10.1016/j.jpedsurg.2007.03.030.

32. Sweet MP, Patti MG, Leard LE, et al. Gastroesophageal reflux in patients with idiopathic pulmonary fibrosis referred for lung transplantation. *J Thorac Cardiovasc Surg*. 2007;133(4) 1078-1084. doi:10.1016/j.jtcvs.2006.09.085; PubMed PMID: 17382656.

33. Raghu G, Freudenberger TD, Yang S, et al. High prevalence of abnormal acid gastro-oesophageal reflux in idiopathic pulmonary fibrosis. *Eur Respir J*. 2006;27(1):136-142. doi:10.1183/09051936.06.00037005; PubMed PMID: 16387946.

34. Sweet MP, Herbella FA, Leard L, et al. The prevalence of distal and proximal gastroesophageal reflux in patients awaiting lung transplantation. *Ann Surg*. 2006;244(4):491-497. doi:10.1097/01.sla.0000237757.49687.03; PubMed PMID: 16998357; PMCID: PMC1856564.

35. Lee JS, Collard HR, Anstrom KJ, et al. Anti-acid treatment and disease progression in idiopathic pulmonary fibrosis: an analysis of data from three randomised controlled trials. *Lancet Respir Med*. 2013;1(5):369-376. doi:http://dx.doi.org/10.1016/S2213-2600(13)70105-X.

36. Lee JS, Ryu JH, Elicker BM, et al. Gastroesophageal reflux therapy is associated with longer survival in patients with idiopathic pulmonary fibrosis. *Am J Respir Crit Care Med*. 2011;184(12): 1390-1394. doi:10.1164/rccm.201101-0138OC.

37. Linden PA, Gilbert RJ, Yeap BY, et al. Laparoscopic fundoplication in patients with end-stage lung disease awaiting transplantation. *J Thorac Cardiovasc Surg*. 2006;131(2):438-446. doi:10 1016/j.jtcvs.2005.10.014; PubMed PMID: 16434276.

38. Hoppo T, Jarido V, Pennathur A, et al. Antireflux surgery preserves lung function in patients with gastroesophageal reflux disease and end-stage lung disease before and after lung transplantation. *Arch Surg*. 2011;146(9):1041-1047. doi:10.1001/archsurg.2011.216.

39. Cantu E 3rd, Appel JZ 3rd, Hartwig MG, et al. Maxwell Chamberlain memorial paper. Early fundoplication prevents chronic allograft dysfunction in patients with gastroesophageal reflux disease. *Ann Thorac Surg*. 2004;78(4):1142-1151; discussion 1151. doi:10.1016/j.athoracsur.2004.04.044; PubMed PMID: 15464462.

40. Hartwig MG, Appel JZ, Davis RD. Antireflux surgery in the setting of lung transplantation: strategies for treating gastroesophageal reflux disease in a high-risk population. *Thorac Surg Clin*. 2005;15(3):417-427. PubMed PMID: 16104132.

41. Li B, Hartwig MG, Appel JZ, et al. Chronic aspiration of gastric fluid induces the development of obliterative bronchiolitis in rat lung transplants. *Am J Transplant*. 2008;8(8):1614-1621. doi:10.1111/j.1600-6143.2008.02298.x; PubMed PMID: 18557728.

42. Hartwig MG, Appel JZ, Li B, et al. Chronic aspiration of gastric fluid accelerates pulmonary allograft dysfunction in a rat model of lung transplantation. *J Thorac Cardiovasc Surg*. 2006;131(1):209-217. doi:10.1016/j.jtcvs.2005.06.054; PubMed PMID: 16399314.

43. Chang JC, Leung JH, Tang T, et al. In the face of chronic aspiration, prolonged ischemic time exacerbates obliterative bronchiolitis in rat pulmonary allografts. *Am J Transplant*. 2012;12(11):2930-2937. doi:10.1111/j.1600-6143.2012.04215.x; PubMed PMID: 22882880; PMCID: PMC4332511.

44. Meers CM, De Wever W, Verbeken E, et al. A porcine model of acute lung injury by instillation of gastric fluid. *J Surg Res*. 2011;166(2):e195-e204. doi:10.1016/j.jss.2010.10.015; PubMed PMID: 21109258.

45. Meltzer AJ, Weiss MJ, Veillette GR, et al. Repetitive gastric aspiration leads to augmented indirect allorecognition after lung transplantation in miniature swine. *Transplantation*. 2008;86(12):1824-1849. doi:10.1097/TP.0b013e318190afe6; PubMed PMID: 19104429; PMCID: PMC2717556.

46. Tang T, Chang JC, Xie A, Davis RD, Parker W, Lin SS. Aspiration of gastric fluid in pulmonary allografts: effect of pH. *J Surg Res*. 2013;181(1):e31-e38. doi:10.1016/j.jss.2012.06.036; PubMed PMID: 22765998.

47. Atkins BZ, Petersen RP, Daneshmand MA, Turek JW, Lin SS, Davis RD Jr. Impact of oropharyngeal dysphagia on long-term outcomes of lung transplantation. *Ann Thorac Surg*. 2010;90(5):1622-1628. doi:10.1016/j.athoracsur.2010.06.089; PubMed PMID: 20971276.

48. Hartwig MG, Anderson DJ, Onaitis MW, et al. Fundoplication after lung transplantation prevents the allograft dysfunction associated with reflux. *Ann Thorac Surg*. 2011;92(2):462-468. doi:10.1016/j.athoracsur.2011.04.035; [discussion 8-9], PubMed PMID: 21801907; PMCID: PMC3617490.

49. Davis RD Jr, Lau CL, Eubanks S, et al. Improved lung allograft function after fundoplication in patients with gastroesophageal reflux disease undergoing lung transplantation. *J Thorac Cardiovasc Surg*. 2003;125(3):533-542. doi:10.1067/mtc.2003.166; PubMed PMID: 12658195.

Acid-Suppression Therapy for Gastroesophageal Reflux Disease and the Therapeutic Gap

Leila Kia | Peter J. Kahrilas

Over the past 40 years, there has been a remarkable evolution in our understanding of the pathophysiology, clinical manifestations, and treatment strategies underlying gastroesophageal reflux disease (GERD). Initially synonymous with esophagitis and presence of hiatal hernias, we now understand that reflux disease is a much more complicated and often nuanced diagnosis to make, wherein a myriad of potential nonspecific symptoms and absence of suitable biomarkers can make the diagnosis challenging.[1] In the absence of overt GERD manifestations (i.e., erosive esophagitis, Barrett metaplasia, adenocarcinoma) and in light of imperfect pH testing and symptom correlation, we find that a diagnosis of *potential GERD* has become a catchall for a constellation of gastrointestinal and supraesophageal symptoms. As such, proton pump inhibitor (PPI) therapy has become first line not only for symptoms attributable to reflux disease but also for numerous other complaints potentially associated with reflux disease. This has resulted in substantial overuse of PPIs. Complicating matters further, multiple epidemiologic studies and subsequent follow-up articles in the lay media have raised concerns over possible adverse events associated with long-term PPI use.[2,3] Hence, patients and clinicians alike are becoming wary of continued PPI use and are keen on investigating nonpharmacologic alternatives to GERD management. Furthermore, the concept of *refractory GERD,* which has traditionally referred to persistence of mucosal disease in spite of PPI therapy, has now evolved to define failure of symptomatic response for *potential* GERD symptoms, highlighting the need for alternative therapeutic approaches. Thus, as we find ourselves witnessing the indiscriminate use of PPIs, we also notice newly heightened concern for their long-term safety and the need for different therapies to bridge this therapeutic gap. The aim of this chapter is to review the pathophysiology of GERD and the indications and limitations of acid-suppressive therapy and to highlight other treatment modalities aimed at refractory symptoms and nonpharmacologic approaches.

PATHOPHYSIOLOGIC MECHANISMS UNDERLYING GASTROESOPHAGEAL REFLUX DISEASE

A discussion of therapeutic options for management of GERD requires an understanding of the underlying pathophysiology of reflux disease so that relevant therapeutic targets can be identified. Defined as "a condition which develops when the reflux of stomach contents causes troublesome symptoms and/or complications," GERD is multifactorial.[4] Anatomic impairment of antireflux defenses, poor clearance of refluxate, compromised mucosal defense mechanisms, slow gastric emptying, underlying motility disturbances, and altered neural sensitivity pathways can all play a role in the generation of troublesome symptoms.[5] Precisely how reflux evolves from a physiologic phenomenon to causing bothersome symptoms and mucosal disease is complex and variable among individuals. At its crux, the presence of a normal esophagogastric junction (EGJ) with a coordinated lower esophageal sphincter (LES) and crural diaphragm (CD) maintains a mechanical barrier, which is indispensable to preservation of normal physiologic function. As such, reflux occurs exclusively during transient lower esophageal sphincter relaxations (TLESRs), is largely restricted to gas, and refluxed fluid is confined to the distal esophagus and rapidly cleared.[6] If there is a disruption to any of the components of the mechanical barrier, normal function may be altered. The presence of a mechanically impaired EGJ, either due to an overt hiatal hernia or disruption of the LES-CD complex, results in an increase in non-TLESR reflux events, poor gas/liquid discrimination during gastric venting, and increased volume and extent of the refluxate leading to regurgitation. Coupled with hypersensitivity, this results in troublesome symptoms. Furthermore, other external factors such as obesity, diet, pregnancy, age, esophageal neuromuscular dysfunction, and trauma can instigate and/or exacerbate these mechanisms.

It is important to note that despite gastric acid secretion being the primary target for pharmacologic therapy, abnormal gastric acid secretion is not a mechanism for pathogenesis of GERD, except in rare cases of true acid hypersecretion as seen with some neuroendocrine tumors. In fact, the level of acid secretion in patients with GERD is similar to that of asymptomatic controls.[7] This highlights one of the main limitations of treatment with PPIs, largely that it does not address the root causes of GERD or the hypersensitivity pathways closely tied to bothersome symptoms.

MANAGEMENT OF GASTROESOPHAGEAL REFLUX DISEASE WITH ACID-SUPPRESSION THERAPY

In spite of limitations associated with acid-suppression therapy, their advent has revolutionized GERD treatment. In patients with mild symptoms, on-demand rapid-acting (and short-acting) antacids can be used with or without histamine-2 (H_2)-receptor antagonists to achieve adequate symptom response. However, in patients with moderate to severe symptoms or with evidence of mucosal damage, PPIs have become first-line therapy and can be titrated up to twice-a-day dosing for those with an insufficient response to daily dosing. PPIs are so effective in treating esophagitis that definitions of GERD early in the PPI era proposed the inclusion of response (or failure of response) to PPI therapy.[8] Moreover, mucosal manifestations of GERD (except for Barrett metaplasia) can be held in remission with sustained PPI therapy. The problem of refractory mucosal disease has essentially vanished and in its place has emerged the notion of refractory symptoms and syndromes potentially attributable to GERD. By the time a patient is referred to a gastroenterologist for refractory GERD, they have likely been on twice-daily PPI for some time and tried on-demand adjunctive antacid or H₂-receptor antagonist therapy. It has become the physician's task to determine whether these are, in fact, refractory patients, or whether there is an alternative diagnosis, such as dyspepsia, functional heartburn, irritable bowel, eosinophilic esophagitis, or a motility disorder as the cause of inadequate response to PPI therapy.

PPI treatment success for potential GERD syndromes is variable, and the best chance for success is in treating those with erosive esophagitis. Typical GERD symptoms (heartburn, regurgitation, and chest pain) also respond relatively well, particularly in patients with esophagitis or with abnormal pH testing off PPI therapy.[9] Atypical symptoms and those with normal pH testing are less likely to respond to PPI therapy and warrant evaluation for other causes before being labeled as PPI nonresponders.[10] There are rare instances of true *PPI failures*, as defined by persistence of abnormal acid exposure on adequate PPI therapy. In these cases, compliance must be questioned, and optimization of dosage and frequency of PPI therapy can be attempted. In rare cases, reduced bioavailability, rapid metabolism, and PPI resistance can be implicated as a cause for nonresponse, and it is reasonable to switch to a different PPI when such situations are suspected. However, for the majority of patients, the most likely reasons for PPI nonresponse are the absence of GERD as an etiology of their symptoms or persistence of regurgitation and/or hypersensitivity (i.e., not inadequate acid suppression). In partial responders, it appears that increased proximal reflux and hypersensitivity account for the lack of full response.[11] For these reasons, pH testing, either in the form of combined intraluminal pH-impedance monitoring or the radiocapsule technique (Bravo), is a first and crucial step in the evaluation of patients with refractory symptoms, along with exclusion of a symptomatic hiatal hernia. There is continued debate regarding the optimal approach to testing (i.e., on or off therapy and the use of impedance versus pH testing alone), but generally, the chance of establishing a correlation between reflux symptoms and events is greatest when a patient is studied off acid-suppression therapy.[12] Impedance testing can add useful information, particularly when regurgitation is the predominant symptom and nonacid reflux (i.e., adequately acid-suppressed on PPI) is thought to drive the main symptomatology.[13] Thus adequate phenotyping of the PPI nonresponder is critical in identifying appropriate targets for therapy beyond PPIs.

ALTERNATIVE PHARMACOLOGIC AND LIFESTYLE INTERVENTIONS FOR GASTROESOPHAGEAL REFLUX DISEASE

It is common to recommend dietary and lifestyle modifications for patients with symptomatic regurgitation and heartburn, particularly in those with persistent regurgitation on PPI therapy or those with mild symptoms. These alterations can minimize symptoms, but they do little to change the underlying mechanism leading to symptom generation. A more useful recommendation is that of weight loss, particularly in patients with central obesity. From a mechanistic standpoint, obesity promotes GERD by increasing intraabdominal pressure, thereby promoting reflux and the development of a hiatal hernia, and metabolically active visceral fat may also promote Barrett metaplasia via proinflammatory mechanisms.[14,15] Multiple studies have shown that reductions in body mass index (BMI) and central obesity result in improved GERD symptom control.[16,17] As such, the importance of weight loss should be highlighted to patients seeking optimization of their GERD management.

Beyond lifestyle modifications and acid-suppression therapy, other medical interventions are available, but their use is limited by side effects and/or minimal efficacy. As adjunctive therapy to PPIs, alginates have been found to have modest benefit in reducing the number of acid reflux episodes and the severity and frequency of heartburn, regurgitation, and nighttime symptoms by creating a pH-neutral raft at the site of the postprandial acid pocket.[18,19] However, alginate formulations differ between the United States and the world at large, and it is unclear if similar benefit can be achieved from the American preparation, which contains lower concentrations of alginate and higher concentrations of antacid. Prokinetics (e.g., metoclopramide, domperidone, and cisapride), which promote gastric emptying, increase LES pressure, and enhance esophageal clearance, have also been studied as adjunctive therapies, particularly in patients with predominant regurgitation.[20] However, their use has been limited by marginal efficacy and prohibitive safety concerns, including potentially fatal cardiac arrhythmias and irreversible neurologic side effects (tardive dyskinesia).[21] Baclofen, a γ-aminobutyric acid type B (GABA_B) receptor agonist, has been used to modulate TLESRs, which are, in part, regulated by GABA. Multiple studies have shown that modulating this pathway can lead to improved GERD symptoms and reduction in reflux events, acid exposure, and TLESR rate when compared with placebo.[22-26] Despite improvement in reflux events and symptoms, use of baclofen is limited by neurologic disturbances, including dizziness, fatigue, and drowsiness. Interestingly, when used at bedtime, the side effect profile is less problematic and may actually aid in reducing nighttime symptoms by improving sleep efficiency.[27] Thus it is reasonable to add baclofen as adjunctive therapy in patients with persistent nighttime symptoms on PPI therapy. Other novel GABA receptor agonists, including lesogaberan and arbaclofen, showed promising results in initial clinical trials, but subsequent phase IIb randomized control studies failed to show sufficient benefit when compared with placebo to warrant further development.[28,29]

An additional approach to management of refractory GERD symptoms, particularly in patients with predominant hypersensitivity, is to use neuromodulators to target pain-processing pathways and reduce symptom perception. Attempts to target esophageal acid-sensing targets mediated by transient receptor potential cation channel subfamily vanilloid member 1 (TRPV1) receptors, which are activated by acid, capsaicin, and heat and have been implicated in esophageal symptom perception, have not been successful thus far.[30] However, the use of psychotropic agents (particularly low-dose antidepressants), which modulate symptom perception by targeting pain pathways, has yielded encouraging results. There is evidence for both tricyclic antidepressants (TCAs) and selective serotonin reuptake inhibitors (SSRIs) in modulating these pathways and improving symptoms (and/or quality of life),[31,32] and these should be considered in patients with a hypersensitivity phenotype.[33–35] However, note that recent randomized control trials of TCAs have failed to show significant improvements compared with placebo, whereas studies evaluating SSRIs have yielded positive results, suggesting that the latter may be a preferred initial treatment choice.[36–38]

NONPHARMACOLOGIC TREATMENTS FOR GASTROESOPHAGEAL REFLUX DISEASE: BRIDGING THE THERAPEUTIC GAP?

Lifestyle and pharmacologic interventions, including use of PPIs, have been effective in improving symptoms in a majority of patients with GERD. However, none of these interventions addresses the associated underlying anatomic defects that are implicated in the pathogenesis of GERD. Surgical treatment, by way of a fundoplication, is the only intervention that targets competency of the EGJ, eliminates hiatus hernia, and creates a barrier for prevention of reflux. As such, laparoscopic fundoplication has been shown to effectively reduce episodes of all types of reflux, including acid and nonacid.[39] It is most effective in patients who have a favorable response to PPI therapy prior to surgery, good compliance with acid-suppressive medications, typical symptoms, and objective evidence of acid reflux (esophagitis, or abnormal pH testing).[40,41] Interestingly, 5-year results of the LOTUS trial, a randomized controlled trial comparing laparoscopic Nissen fundoplication to esomeprazole, showed no difference in esophagitis or heartburn control between treatments.[42] However, regurgitation was better controlled by fundoplication and adverse events, such as flatulence, dysphagia, and an inability to belch, were also more common in the surgical group. Hence, for patients with adequate symptom control on PPI therapy, continuation of PPI has fewer side effects, lower morbidity, and similar efficacy compared with surgery and should be recommended. Patients with persistent regurgitation as their main symptom, with at least partial response to PPI therapy (and proven abnormal pH testing), are the group most likely to benefit from antireflux surgery.

There has been considerable interest in developing alternative, minimally invasive, nonpharmacologic interventions for GERD other than fundoplication. To be successful, these interventions have to be conceptually valid, have a valid physiologic proof of concept, demonstrate symptom reduction, demonstrate pH control, have excellent safety profiles, and be reimbursable. However, these have proven to be difficult hurdles and the development of such novel therapeutics has been challenging. A number of devices and procedures have been developed over the years, but the majority have been ineffective or lacked durability. Currently there are three main types of interventions that are in use or in active stages of development: (1) radiofrequency ablation therapy (Stretta, Mederi Therapeutics, Greenwich, Connecticut), (2) transoral incisionless fundoplication (TIF; Esophyx, Endogastric Solutions, San Mateo, California); and Medigus Ultrasonic Surgical Endostapler (MUSE) (Medigus, Israel), and (3) magnetic sphincter augmentation device (Linx, Torax Medical, United Kingdom). A brief review of these interventions follows.

RADIOFREQUENCY ABLATION THERAPY: STRETTA

The Stretta procedure was designed to deliver radiofrequency energy to the EGJ via an endoscopically placed catheter, with the goal of mechanically altering the EGJ and/or modulating neural pathways using thermal energy. This process was proposed to promote tissue necrosis, local inflammation, and collagen deposition, thereby "tightening" the LES. Although an interesting concept, this effect has not been demonstrated to occur. Alternatively radiofrequency neurolysis may alter sensitivity and reduce TLESRs because this is a neuronally mediated reflex.[43–45] Randomized sham-controlled trials evaluating the efficacy of Stretta failed to show a reduction in acid exposure when compared with a sham procedure, and a recent meta-analysis evaluating three sham-controlled trials and one trial comparing Stretta with PPI therapy failed to show any benefit in reduction of PPI use or quality of life.[46,47] However, there has been a resurgence of interest after studies reported comparable symptom outcomes with fundoplication.[48–51] However, many of the studies were limited in their design and selection criteria, and most did not include long-term follow-up data.[52] Expert opinion and reviews of the current data have yielded conflicting results, with some proposing favorable outcomes, whereas others pointing out flaws in methodology and suggesting the technology to be ineffective.[53] At this time, the verdict is still out on Stretta, and high-quality studies are needed to determine its viability as a treatment option.

TRANSORAL INCISIONLESS FUNDOPLICATION: ESOPHYX AND MEDIGUS ULTRASONIC SURGICAL ENDOSTAPLER

TIF was envisioned as a less invasive alternative to laparoscopic fundoplication for restoring competency of the EGJ, by way of an endoluminal approach. The EsophyX device allows for the creation of a 210- to 300-degree fundoplication at the level of the EGJ by using full-thickness fasteners to create a valve. An initial randomized control trial comparing EsophyX to standard Nissen fundoplication reported similar benefit between the two therapies with a reduced length of stay in the TIF group.[54] More recently, the RESPECT trial, a randomized control trial evaluating 129 patients with troublesome regurgitation, showed significant improvement in problematic regurgitation in the TIF/placebo group compared with the sham/PPI group (67% vs. 45%) with few adverse events.[55] The main limitations of the TIF technique have been questions regarding durability and the inability to address the problem of hiatus hernia, making it unclear whether or not it is a viable alternative for patients seeking to avoid surgical fundoplication. As such, the ideal target population has yet to be elucidated.

The MUSE device, which also creates an incisionless fundoplication, differs from EsophyX in that it uses ultrasound guidance and a disposable endoscopic stapling device to place sets of transmural surgical staples to secure the fundoplication, which may address the issue of durability. Treatment data for the MUSE device are very preliminary but have shown promising results, with reductions in need for PPI and improvements in quality of life that have been sustained at 5-year follow-up.[56-58] Recently the company has suspended clinical use of the device.

MAGNETIC SPHINCTER AUGMENTATION DEVICE: LINX

Linx has emerged as a frontrunner in the realm of novel therapeutic modalities for minimally invasive antireflux treatments. The magnetic sphincter augmentation device is sized for each patient and surgically positioned around the LES with the intent of generating a barrier for reflux, while preserving bolus passage and the ability to belch.[59] Repair of a hiatal hernia can also be done at the time of the procedure. An initial pivotal study showed improvement in acid exposure (19.9% to 3.3%), symptoms, and PPI use in 100 patients undergoing the procedure but was limited by lack of a control group. The same group published 5-year follow-up data on 84 of these patients and found sustained response to treatment. They noted that at 5 years, only 15.3% of patients were on PPIs (compared with 100% prior), 1.2% reported moderate to severe regurgitation (vs. 57% prior), and all patients retained the ability to belch. No device erosions, migrations, or malfunctions were reported by this group, although a case report of perforation due to device erosion has been described in the literature and a case of dysphagia due to erosion into the esophagus has been reported to the US Food and Drug Administration.[60,61] Note that dysphagia was noted to be 6% after the procedure compared with 5% prior to intervention.[62] Overall the data for Linx have been promising, but further studies are needed. If further studies validate these findings, Linx may emerge as a viable alternative therapeutic option for patients with reflux disease dissatisfied with medical therapy, particularly in the phenotype of patients with persistent regurgitation as a predominant symptom.

CONCLUSION

There has been considerable advancement in our understanding, phenotyping, and management of GERD over the past two decades.

We have learned that the pathogenesis is complex and that treatment modalities that target one disease facet may fail to address the spectrum of potential phenotypes. We have also learned that there are a large number of patients with *potential* GERD symptoms, whose underlying symptoms are likely due to an alternative diagnosis, and warrant accurate phenotyping prior to being categorized as refractory GERD. Furthermore, we have witnessed a change in patients' perception of safety and long-term viability for pharmacologic therapy, particularly with PPIs, which has invigorated investigations into alternative lifestyle and surgical/endoluminal treatments. At the present time, the crux of adequate GERD management rests on a number of principles: (1) establishing an accurate diagnosis, (2) adequately phenotyping patients to determine the best targets for treatments, (3) educating patients on weight loss and the pros and cons of long-term PPI use, and (4) investigating other treatment options such as surgical and endoluminal therapies for patients with incomplete symptom control on medical therapy and those who are PPI intolerant or choose not to take these medications long term. We are still working to bridge the "therapeutic gap" in management of GERD, but new promising therapies may change the landscape of GERD management if they prove successful and safe.

ACKNOWLEDGMENTS

Supported by R01 DK56033 (PJK) from the Public Health Service. Peter J. Kahrilas is a consultant for Ironwood Pharmaceuticals.

REFERENCES

1. Kia L, Pandolfino JE, Kahrilas PJ. Biomarkers of reflux disease. *Clin Gastroenterol Hepatol*. 2016;14(6):790-797.
2. Kia L, Kahrilas PJ. Therapy: risks associated with chronic PPI use—signal or noise? *Nat Rev Gastroenterol Hepatol*. 2016;13(5):253-254.
3. Forgacs I, Loganayagam A. Overprescribing proton pump inhibitors. *BMJ*. 2008;336(7634):2-3.
4. Vakil N, van Zanten SV, Kahrilas P, Dent J, Jones R, Global Consensus Group. The Montreal definition and classification of gastroesophageal reflux disease: a global evidence-based consensus. *Am J Gastroenterol*. 2006;101(8):1900-1920; quiz 43.
5. Woodland P, Sifrim D. The refluxate: the impact of its magnitude, composition and distribution. *Best Pract Res Clin Gastroenterol*. 2010;24(6):861-871.
6. Boeckxstaens G, El-Serag HB, Smout AJ, Kahrilas PJ. Symptomatic reflux disease: the present, the past and the future. *Gut*. 2014;63(7):1185-1193.
7. Hirschowitz BI. A critical analysis, with appropriate controls, of gastric acid and pepsin secretion in clinical esophagitis. *Gastroenterology*. 1991;101(5):1149-1158.
8. Numans ME, Lau J, de Wit NJ, Bonis PA. Short-term treatment with proton-pump inhibitors as a test for gastroesophageal reflux disease: a meta-analysis of diagnostic test characteristics. *Ann Intern Med*. 2004;140(7):518-527.
9. Kahrilas PJ, Boeckxstaens G. Failure of reflux inhibitors in clinical trials: bad drugs or wrong patients? *Gut*. 2012;61(10):1501-1509.
10. Roman S, Keefer L, Imam H, et al. Majority of symptoms in esophageal reflux PPI non-responders are not related to reflux. *Neurogastroenterol Motil*. 2015;27(11):1667-1674.
11. Rohof WO, Bennink RJ, de Jonge H, Boeckxstaens GE. Increased proximal reflux in a hypersensitive esophagus might explain symptoms resistant to proton pump inhibitors in patients with gastroesophageal reflux disease. *Clin Gastroenterol Hepatol*. 2014;12(10):1647-1655.
12. Hemmink GJ, Bredenoord AJ, Weusten BL, Monkelbaan JF, Timmer R, Smout AJ. Esophageal pH-impedance monitoring in patients with therapy-resistant reflux symptoms: 'on' or 'off' proton pump inhibitor? *Am J Gastroenterol*. 2008;103(10):2446-2453.
13. Mainie I, Tutuian R, Shay S, et al. Acid and non-acid reflux in patients with persistent symptoms despite acid suppressive therapy:

a multicentre study using combined ambulatory impedance-pH monitoring. *Gut.* 2006;55(10):1398-1402.

14. El-Serag H. Role of obesity in GORD-related disorders. *Gut.* 2008;57(3):281-284.
15. El-Serag HB, Hashmi A, Garcia J, et al. Visceral abdominal obesity measured by CT scan is associated with an increased risk of Barrett's oesophagus: a case-control study. *Gut.* 2014;63(2):220-229.
16. Jacobson BC, Somers SC, Fuchs CS, Kelly CP, Camargo CA Jr. Body-mass index and symptoms of gastroesophageal reflux in women. *N Engl J Med.* 2006;354(22):2340-2348.
17. Singh M, Lee J, Gupta N, et al. Weight loss can lead to resolution of gastroesophageal reflux disease symptoms: a prospective intervention trial. *Obesity (Silver Spring).* 2013;21(2):284-290.
18. Rohof WO, Bennink RJ, Smout AJ, Thomas E, Boeckxstaens GE. An alginate-antacid formulation localizes to the acid pocket to reduce acid reflux in patients with gastroesophageal reflux disease. *Clin Gastroenterol Hepatol.* 2013;11(12):1585-1591; quiz e90.
19. Reimer C, Lodrup AB, Smith G, Wilkinson J, Bytzer P. Randomised clinical trial: alginate (Gaviscon Advance) vs. placebo as add-on therapy in reflux patients with inadequate response to a once daily proton pump inhibitor. *Aliment Pharmacol Ther.* 2016;Feb 22 [Epub ahead of print].
20. Tack J. Prokinetics and fundic relaxants in upper functional GI disorders. *Curr Opin Pharmacol.* 2008;8(6):690-696.
21. Scarpellini E, Ang D, Pauwels A, De Santis A, Vanuytsel T, Tack J. Management of refractory typical GERD symptoms. *Nat Rev Gastroenterol Hepatol.* 2016;13(5):281-294.
22. Lidums I, Lehmann A, Checklin H, Dent J, Holloway RH. Control of transient lower esophageal sphincter relaxations and reflux by the GABA(B) agonist baclofen in normal subjects. *Gastroenterology.* 2000;118(1):7-13.
23. Zhang Q, Lehmann A, Rigda R, Dent J, Holloway RH. Control of transient lower oesophageal sphincter relaxations and reflux by the GABA(B) agonist baclofen in patients with gastro-oesophageal reflux disease. *Gut.* 2002;50(1):19-24.
24. Vela MF, Tutuian R, Katz PO, Castell DO. Baclofen decreases acid and non-acid post-prandial gastro-oesophageal reflux measured by combined multichannel intraluminal impedance and pH. *Aliment Pharmacol Ther.* 2003;17(2):243-251.
25. Ciccaglione AF, Marzio L. Effect of acute and chronic administration of the GABA B agonist baclofen on 24 hour pH metry and symptoms in control subjects and in patients with gastro-oesophageal reflux disease. *Gut.* 2003;52(4):464-470.
26. Koek GH, Sifrim D, Lerut T, Janssens J, Tack J. Effect of the GABA(B) agonist baclofen in patients with symptoms and duodeno-gastro-oesophageal reflux refractory to proton pump inhibitors. *Gut.* 2003;52(10):1397-1402.
27. Lehmann A, Antonsson M, Holmberg AA, et al. (R)-(3-Amino-2-fluoropropyl) phosphinic acid (AZD3355), a novel GABAB receptor agonist, inhibits transient lower esophageal sphincter relaxation through a peripheral mode of action. *J Pharmacol Exp Ther.* 2009;331(2):504-512.
28. Shaheen NJ, Denison H, Bjorck K, Karlsson M, Silberg DG. Efficacy and safety of lesogaberan in gastro-oesophageal reflux disease: a randomised controlled trial. *Gut.* 2013;62(9):1248-1255.
29. Vakil NB, Huff FJ, Bian A, Jones DS, Stamler D. Arbaclofen placarbil in GERD: a randomized, double-blind, placebo-controlled study. *Am J Gastroenterol.* 2011;106(8):1427-1438.
30. Krarup AL, Ny L, Gunnarsson J, et al. Randomized clinical trial: inhibition of the TRPV1 system in patients with nonerosive gastro-esophageal reflux disease and a partial response to PPI treatment is not associated with analgesia to esophageal experimental pain. *Scand J Gastroenterol.* 2013;48(3):274-284.
31. Limsrivilai J, Charatcharoenwitthaya P, Pausawasdi N, Leelakusolvong S. Imipramine for treatment of esophageal hypersensitivity and functional heartburn: a randomized placebo-controlled trial. *Am J Gastroenterol.* 2016;111(2):217-224.
32. Keefer L, Kahrilas PJ. Editorial: low-dose tricyclics for esophageal hypersensitivity: is it all placebo effect? *Am J Gastroenterol.* 2016;111(2):225-227.
33. Broekaert D, Fischler B, Sifrim D, Janssens J, Tack J. Influence of citalopram, a selective serotonin reuptake inhibitor, on oesophageal hypersensitivity: a double-blind, placebo-controlled study. *Aliment Pharmacol Ther.* 2006;23(3):365-370.
34. Viazis N, Keyoglou A, Kanellopoulos AK, et al. Selective serotonin reuptake inhibitors for the treatment of hypersensitive esophagus:

a randomized, double-blind, placebo-controlled study. *Am J Gastroenterol.* 2012;107(11):1662-1667.
35. Peghini PL, Katz PO, Castell DO. Imipramine decreases oesophageal pain perception in human male volunteers. *Gut.* 1998;42(6):807-813.
36. Hershcovici T, Wendel CS, Fass R. Symptom indexes in refractory gastroesophageal reflux disease: overrated or misunderstood? *Clin Gastroenterol Hepatol.* 2011;9(10):816-817.
37. Forcelini CM, Tomiozzo JC Jr, Farre R, et al. Effect of nortriptyline on brain responses to painful esophageal acid infusion in patients with non-erosive reflux disease. *Neurogastroenterol Motil.* 2014;26(2):187-195.
38. Ostovaneh MR, Saeidi B, Hajifathalian K, et al. Comparing omeprazole with fluoxetine for treatment of patients with heartburn and normal endoscopy who failed once daily proton pump inhibitors: double-blind placebo-controlled trial. *Neurogastroenterol Motil.* 2014;26(5):670-678.
39. Bredenoord AJ, Draaisma WA, Weusten BL, Gooszen HG, Smout AJ. Mechanisms of acid, weakly acidic and gas reflux after anti-reflux surgery. *Gut.* 2008;57(2):161-166.
40. Campos GM, Peters JH, DeMeester TR, et al. Multivariate analysis of factors predicting outcome after laparoscopic Nissen fundoplication. *J Gastrointest Surg.* 1999;3(3):292-300.
41. Hayden J, Jamieson G. Optimization of outcome after laparoscopic antireflux surgery. *ANZ J Surg.* 2006;76(4):258-263.
42. Galmiche JP, Hatlebakk J, Attwood S, et al. Laparoscopic antireflux surgery vs esomeprazole treatment for chronic GERD: the LOTUS randomized clinical trial. *JAMA.* 2011;305(19):1969-1977.
43. Kim MS, Holloway RH, Dent J, Utley DS. Radiofrequency energy delivery to the gastric cardia inhibits triggering of transient lower esophageal sphincter relaxation and gastroesophageal reflux in dogs. *Gastrointest Endosc.* 2003;57(1):17-22.
44. Triadafilopoulos G. Stretta: an effective, minimally invasive treatment for gastroesophageal reflux disease. *Am J Med.* 2003;115(suppl 3A):192S-200S.
45. Kahrilas PJ. Radiofrequency therapy of the lower esophageal sphincter for treatment of GERD. *Gastrointest Endosc.* 2003;57(6):723-731.
46. Arts J, Bisschops R, Blondeau K, et al. A double-blind sham-controlled study of the effect of radiofrequency energy on symptoms and distensibility of the gastro-esophageal junction in GERD. *Am J Gastroenterol.* 2012;107(2):222-230.
47. Lipka S, Kumar A, Richter JE. No evidence for efficacy of radiofrequency ablation for treatment of gastroesophageal reflux disease: a systematic review and meta-analysis. *Clin Gastroenterol Hepatol.* 2015;13(6):1058-1067.e1.
48. Coron E, Sebille V, Cadiot G, et al. Clinical trial: radiofrequency energy delivery in proton pump inhibitor-dependent gastro-oesophageal reflux disease patients. *Aliment Pharmacol Ther.* 2008;28(9):1147-1158.
49. Liang WT, Wu JN, Wang F, et al. Five-year follow-up of a prospective study comparing laparoscopic Nissen fundoplication with Stretta radiofrequency for gastroesophageal reflux disease. *Minerva Chir.* 2014;69(4):217-223.
50. Liang WT, Yan C, Wang ZG, et al. Early and midterm outcome after laparoscopic fundoplication and a minimally invasive endoscopic procedure in patients with gastroesophageal reflux disease: a prospective observational study. *J Laparoendosc Adv Surg Tech A.* 2015;25(8):657-661.
51. Yan C, Liang WT, Wang ZG, et al. Comparison of Stretta procedure and Toupet fundoplication for gastroesophageal reflux disease-related extra-esophageal symptoms. *World J Gastroenterol.* 2015;21(45):12882-12887.
52. Das B, Reddy M, Khan OA. Is the Stretta procedure as effective as the best medical and surgical treatments for gastro-oesophageal reflux disease? A best evidence topic. *Int J Surg.* 2016;30:19-24.
53. Hopkins J, Switzer NJ, Karmali S. Update on novel endoscopic therapies to treat gastroesophageal reflux disease: a review. *World J Gastrointest Endosc.* 2015;7(11):1039-1044.
54. Svoboda P, Kantorova I, Kozumplik L, et al. Our experience with transoral incisionless plication of gastroesophageal reflux disease: NOTES procedure. *Hepatogastroenterology.* 2011;58(109):1208-1213.
55. Hunter JG, Kahrilas PJ, Bell RC, et al. Efficacy of transoral fundoplication vs omeprazole for treatment of regurgitation in a randomized controlled trial. *Gastroenterology.* 2015;148(2):324-333.e5.
56. Kim HJ, Kwon CI, Kessler WR, et al. Long-term follow-up results of endoscopic treatment of gastroesophageal reflux disease with the MUSE endoscopic stapling device. *Surg Endosc.* 2016;30(8):3402-3408.

57. Zacherl J, Roy-Shapira A, Bonavina L, et al. Endoscopic anterior fundoplication with the Medigus Ultrasonic Surgical Endostapler (MUSE) for gastroesophageal reflux disease: 6-month results from a multi-center prospective trial. *Surg Endosc.* 2015;29(1):220-229.

58. Roy-Shapira A, Bapaye A, Date S, Pujari R, Dorwat S. Trans-oral anterior fundoplication: 5-year follow-up of pilot study. *Surg Endosc.* 2015;29(12):3717-3721.

59. Ganz RA, Peters JH, Horgan S. Esophageal sphincter device for gastroesophageal reflux disease. *N Engl J Med.* 2013;368(21):2039-2040.

60. Bauer M, Meining A, Kranzfelder M, et al. Endoluminal perforation of a magnetic antireflux device. *Surg Endosc.* 2015;29(12):3806-3810.

61. US Food and Drug Administration. MAUDE adverse event report: Torax Medica, Inc. Linx Reflux management system anti-reflux implant;2016. Available at https://www.accessdata.fda.gov/scripts/cdrh/cfdocs/cfmaude/detail.cfm?mdrfoi__id=4208665.

62. Ganz RA, Edmundowicz SA, Taiganides PA, et al. Long-term outcomes of patients receiving a magnetic sphincter augmentation device for gastroesophageal reflux. *Clin Gastroenterol Hepatol.* 2016;14(5):671-677.

Fundoplication for Gastroesophageal Reflux Disease

Joel M. Sternbach | Nathaniel J. Soper

Gastroesophageal reflux disease (GERD) is the most common disorder of the esophagus and gastroesophageal junction. While transient reflux of stomach contents into the esophagus occurs physiologically, according to the Montreal Classification,[1] the criteria for GERD are met when reflux causes troublesome symptoms and/or complications. With 60% of American adults reporting intermittent heartburn symptoms, GERD is a serious health concern in the Western world. For the 20% of Americans who describe weekly reflux symptoms, GERD increases the risk for esophageal stricture, Barrett esophagus, and esophageal cancer, while significantly affecting health-related quality of life and work productivity.[1–5]

The modern era of GERD therapy has brought advances in diagnosis and treatment, and, subsequently, a better understanding of the pathophysiology of GERD. The single most important factor in the development of GERD is an incompetent lower esophageal sphincter.[6] Progressive dilation plus deterioration of the gastroesophageal flap-valve mechanism results in loss of the anatomic antireflux barrier and allows for acid and bile reflux. The goal of antireflux surgery is to reestablish the competency of the lower esophageal sphincter while preserving the patient's normal swallowing capacity.[7]

Acid suppression therapies in the form of histamine H_2 receptor antagonists and proton pump inhibitors (PPIs) have brought both symptomatic relief and effective resolution of esophageal inflammation. While these approaches may ameliorate some of the long-term sequelae of GERD, medical therapy must be continued indefinitely and does not address nonacid reflux. Antireflux surgery provides an anatomic and physiologic cure with durable symptomatic relief and prevention of the adverse consequences of ongoing esophageal exposure to caustic refluxate.

The current gold standard for the operative treatment of GERD is the laparoscopic Nissen fundoplication. This well-established procedure has proved to be both durable and safe over a period of more than 25 years. Following the introduction of the laparoscopic approach in 1991 by Dallemagne and Geagea, the number of Nissen fundoplications performed annually increased threefold. While efficacy of medical therapy and concerns regarding potential complications of fundoplication have led to a recent decline in the number of operations performed annually in the United States, the pendulum may be swinging back with increasing concerns over the sequelae of chronic acid suppression.[8,9]

Since Rudolf Nissen's original fundoplication in 1937, performed to protect a gastroesophageal anastomosis, the Nissen fundoplication has undergone many modifications. The principles of modern Nissen fundoplication are designed to most closely replicate the normal physiology of the gastroesophageal flap valve,[10] including secure crural closure and the creation of a short, 360-degree "floppy" wrap around 2 to 3 cm of intraabdominal esophagus. This chapter discusses the indications and technical aspects of laparoscopic and open fundoplication for the treatment of GERD.

CLINICAL FEATURES

As with all operations, proper patient selection is essential for a successful outcome. A thorough history and physical examination, as well as appropriate laboratory tests, should be completed to establish a diagnosis of GERD and eliminate other potential causes of symptoms. Patients should be queried regarding classic GERD symptoms including heartburn, regurgitation, and dysphagia. The frequency and timing of reflux symptoms, the relationship to meals, symptom exacerbation in the supine or upright position, and difficulty swallowing should be noted. The response and the duration of medical therapy are also recorded, as this information has prognostic significance following fundoplication.

In addition, patients may have atypical symptoms such as chronic cough, asthma, pulmonary disease, odynophagia, hoarseness, and chest pain. These patients should undergo cardiac evaluation, including a chest radiograph, electrocardiogram, and, if indicated, pulmonary function tests, in addition to the standard diagnostic evaluation for gastroesophageal reflux. Patients with atypical symptoms and those who fail to respond to medical therapy may show less improvement in symptoms after Nissen fundoplication than those with typical GERD symptoms.[11] Box 19.1 includes a list of classic and atypical GERD symptoms.

PREOPERATIVE EVALUATION

The preoperative evaluation of patients with GERD should be thorough. At a minimum, patients should undergo esophagogastroduodenoscopy (EGD). Performance of an esophageal motility study (EMS) is currently a preoperative standard to detect esophageal motility disorders that may lead to troublesome postoperative dysphagia. Although it has been dogma that patients with ineffective esophageal motility (IEM) (mean distal peristaltic amplitude <30 mm Hg or >20% loss of peristalsis) should undergo a partial fundoplication to prevent postoperative dysphagia, recent studies demonstrate that postoperative dysphagia after Nissen fundoplication is no greater with IEM than with normal esophageal motility.[12] We routinely perform a preoperative EMS because it also allows documentation of a motility "baseline" for comparison should postoperative dysphagia develop. In addition, it has been reported that up to a third of patients with achalasia report symptoms of heartburn and EMS can help rule out this disease.[13]

BOX 19.1 Signs and Symptoms of Gastroesophageal Reflux Disease

Typical
  Heartburn
  Regurgitation
  Water brash
  Chest pain
  Dysphagia
Atypical
  Cough
  Dental erosions
  Hoarseness
  Asthma

BOX 19.2 Primary Indications for Antireflux Surgery

Patients with esophageal and/or extraesophageal GERD symptoms that are responsive but not completely eliminated by PPIs
Patients with heartburn eliminated by PPIs but continued volume reflux (regurgitation)
Patients with well-documented reflux events preceding symptoms such as chest pain, cough, or wheezing
Patients with GERD complications such as peptic stricture, Barrett esophagus, or vocal cord injury while taking PPIs twice a day
Patients with well-documented GERD who desire to stop chronic PPI use despite excellent symptom control (e.g., side effects, lifestyle, expense)

GERD, Gastroesophageal reflux disease; *PPI,* proton pump inhibitors.

Twenty-four hour ambulatory pH monitoring is essential for the evaluation of patients with nonerosive reflux disease, extraesophageal, or atypical symptoms, and those who do not respond to PPI therapy. Patients with typical reflux symptoms and erosive esophagitis (or Barrett esophagus and peptic stricture) do not routinely need a pH study to prove the diagnosis of reflux preoperatively. In a multivariate analysis of factors predicting a good response to antireflux surgery, the best outcomes (98% good to excellent results) occurred in patients who had symptom relief with PPIs, typical GERD symptoms, and a positive 24-hour pH study.[14]

Other new diagnostic modalities that have become increasingly important in the diagnosis and understanding of GERD physiology are the BRAVO pH probe and multichannel intraluminal impedance (MII). The wireless (noncatheter based) BRAVO probe monitors distal esophageal pH and transmits the data to a small external recorder worn on the belt for a duration of 48 to 96 hours. It has the advantage of being more comfortable than standard 24-hour pH probes. In addition, data suggest that 48-hour BRAVO monitoring may have greater sensitivity for GERD than does standard 24-hour monitoring.[15] MII has also gained significant popularity for detecting both acid and nonacid GERD. MII measures electrical resistance (impedance) between a series of electrodes on a catheter placed across the gastroesophageal junction and up the esophagus. Air within the esophageal lumen causes an increase in impedance, whereas the presence of liquid refluxate within the esophageal lumen causes a decrease in impedance. By determining the temporal sequence of impedance events, one can establish the directional flow of gas and liquid within the esophagus (i.e., distal flow: swallow; proximal flow: reflux event or belch). By coupling this technology with data from a standard pH probe, one can correlate both acid and nonacid refluxate with patient symptomatology. Standardization of reference ranges for normal patients and in patients with reflux, and improvement of the software used for data interpretation, have moved this technology from a research tool to clinical practice.[16] However, the role of this technology in determining which patients will best respond to surgery is still being studied. Those with significant symptoms and concomitant reflux events (acid or nonacid) while taking acid-suppression therapy may be the ideal patients for surgical therapy.[17]

Impedance planimetry has emerged as a novel physiologic assessment tool and been applied to evaluating the esophagogastric junction (EGJ) in a variety of pathologic conditions, including the diagnosis of GERD.[18] Available commercially as the EndoFLIP device (EndoFLIP model EF-325N, Crospon Ltd., Galway, Ireland), the functional lumen imaging probe (FLIP) is a catheter-based system that provides a geometric evaluation of luminal structures by measuring 16 adjacent cross-sectional areas while simultaneously recording intraballoon pressure using a solid-state pressure transducer. When placed across the EGJ, dividing the minimum cross-sectional area by the intraballoon pressure allows a calculation of the distensibility index (DI) of the EGJ. Kwiatek and colleagues compared FLIP measurements of the EGJ DI in GERD patients and asymptomatic controls and found GERD patients to have a 2 to 3 times more distensible EGJ.[18]

INDICATIONS FOR SURGERY

Although several innovative methods for treating GERD have achieved modest popularity over the past 5 years, the indications for antireflux surgery have changed little, and a fundoplication remains the "gold standard" to which all other procedures should be compared. Box 19.2 lists the primary indications for antireflux surgery.

There is rarely an indication for antireflux surgery in patients with uncomplicated GERD who are satisfied with medical therapy (single- or double-dose PPI), unless there are concerns or side effects related to the use of these medications. Such patients are usually maintained on medical therapy as long as their symptoms are well controlled and are advised to pursue lifestyle modifications and most importantly weight loss to mitigate the physiologic challenges to EGJ competence. In contrast, antireflux surgery should be seriously considered in patients with severe GERD whose symptoms are not controlled by medical therapy, patients who would prefer to avoid lifelong acid-suppression therapy, and those with complicated GERD (Barrett esophagus, refractory esophagitis, stricture). In the latter group of patients, surgery may not be necessary if repeat EGD reveals healing of the esophagus or a 24-hour pH probe while taking medications confirms the absence of acid reflux. However, because elimination of excessive reflux is difficult to achieve in those patients with complications of GERD, a marker of disease severity, consideration should be given to antireflux surgery. Preoperative endoscopic or medical treatment of esophageal stricture or peptic ulcer disease must be accomplished before surgery. In a patient with esophageal stricture, preoperative dilation to at least 16 mm (48 French) is advisable to minimize the chance that the customary postoperative dysphagia (a result of edema and early postoperative esophageal dysmotility) will be compounded by a tight stricture. If preoperative dilation to 16 mm is successful—several sessions are sometimes necessary—it is usually possible to extend the dilation intraoperatively to 18 or 20 mm, the standard-size dilators used by surgeons for calibrating the fundoplication. Laparoscopic antireflux surgery has also been increasingly used in the treatment of GERD following lung transplantation, as acid suppression alone has been shown to be inadequate in preventing allograft injury secondary to aspiration of nonacid refluxate.[19]

In certain subgroups of patients with severe GERD, fundoplication may not be the optimal antireflux surgery. Medically complicated, morbidly obese (body mass index >35 kg/m^2) patients with significant GERD may be better served by undergoing Roux-en-Y gastric bypass as these patients have high failure rates following Nissen fundoplication.[20] Patients with Barrett esophagus and high-grade dysplasia or adenocarcinoma should be treated by mucosal ablation or esophageal resection. Severe strictures that are not responsive to dilation therapy should also be treated by esophageal resection. Patients with low-grade dysplasia should be treated with high-dose PPIs for 3 months, after which they should undergo repeat biopsy. Fundoplication may be considered in such patients if subsequent pathology shows no progression to high-grade dysplasia or carcinoma. Finally, GERD patients with previous gastric surgery should be approached cautiously. GERD in patients after gastric bypass, partial or sleeve gastrectomy, and vertical banded gastroplasty cannot be treated by fundoplication because the fundus has been anatomically disrupted by the prior surgery.

Once a decision is made to perform a surgical antireflux procedure on a patient with GERD, the next step is to decide which type of fundoplication to perform. Recent data support the concept that Nissen fundoplication is an effective therapy for GERD and is not associated with significant long-term dysphagia, even in patients with IEM.[21] These data, combined with data suggesting that partial fundoplication is associated with high long-term failure rates,[22] have led to a significant decrease in the application of partial fundoplication in patients with GERD, regardless of esophageal peristaltic function. Currently, partial fundoplication is reserved for patients with a "named" esophageal motility disorder, such as achalasia or scleroderma, those with both IEM and significant dysphagia, and those patients undergoing revision of a prior 360-degree fundoplication for refractory dysphagia. Despite the recent trend toward complete (Nissen) fundoplication in most patients, contrasting data suggest that long-term satisfactory results may be achieved with partial fundoplication.[23] Consequently, the debate regarding the role of partial fundoplication in the treatment of GERD persists, although the majority of experienced American surgeons prefer to perform complete fundoplication in most patients.

OPEN VERSUS LAPAROSCOPIC NISSEN FUNDOPLICATION

Laparoscopic Nissen fundoplication was first reported by Dallemagne et al. in 1991.[24] Since then, several large clinical series of Nissen fundoplication have been reported, including longitudinal studies with long-term follow-up that demonstrate the results of both open and laparoscopic fundoplication to be equivalent.[25–28] Several randomized clinical trials published in the past decade reached the same conclusion.[25,29–31] The laparoscopic approach is associated with shorter hospital stays, less postoperative pain, fewer wound-related complications, and earlier return to work. Despite these advantages, selection of the open versus the laparoscopic approach should depend on surgeon experience and the patient's previous surgical history. The intraoperative steps of surgical repair are relatively similar in both approaches. Laparoscopic Nissen fundoplication, however, requires that the surgeon possess advanced laparoscopic skills.

The approach to reoperative Nissen fundoplication should be individualized with the goal being long-term success of the procedure, since at the end of the day that is what will restore quality of life, independent of the approach. Most first-time redo procedures can be done laparoscopically, and several large series have demonstrated equivalent results with laparoscopic and open reoperation.[32] Laparoscopic reoperation after open surgery, although feasible, may be tedious because the intraabdominal adhesions associated with open surgery may be formidable. It is important when planning a reoperation to consider why the prior procedure failed and address the cause of failure. An unrecognized short esophagus is one such potential cause, and a Collis gastroplasty may be an important addition during the reoperation in some patients. In the multiply reoperative foregut, consideration should be given to an alternative approach, such as an open thoracic or thoracoscopic approach or resection of the stomach or esophagus.

PRINCIPLES OF NISSEN FUNDOPLICATION

Basic surgical principles guide the successful performance of Nissen fundoplication, regardless of the approach (laparoscopic or open). Box 19.3 lists the fundamental principles of Nissen fundoplication.

LAPAROSCOPIC NISSEN FUNDOPLICATION
Position and Port Placement

Pneumatic sequential compression devices are applied to the calves, and 5000 units of subcutaneous heparin may be administered before the induction of general anesthesia, with placement of a Foley catheter, if indicated. The patient is placed in a split-leg position with both arms tucked and secured to the operating table. A vacuum beanbag mattress can aid in supporting the arms and perineum to prevent patient migration during repositioning of the operating table. The surgeon stands between the patient's legs with the primary monitor over the patient's head. The first assistant stands to the patient's right, and the scrub technician stands to the patient's left. The first step involves safe entry into the abdomen, which is achieved in most patients by inserting a Veress needle at the umbilicus and establishing pneumoperitoneum. In patients with a history of prior abdominal surgery, either an open cut-down approach or alternative Veress location can be used.

A five-port (one or two 10-mm ports and three or four 5-mm ports) technique is used (Fig. 19.1). Additional ports may be placed as necessary. A camera port, to accommodate a 5-mm or 10-mm laparoscope, is placed just superior and to the left of the umbilicus, approximately 12 cm below the xiphoid and approximately 2 to 3 cm to the left of midline. A 30- or 45-degree laparoscope is placed through this port. The laparoscopic camera may be managed by the first assistant, a dedicated camera operator, or with a robotic camera holder. A thorough abdominal exploration with the laparoscope is routinely performed before initiating dissection. All secondary ports are placed under direct vision. After positioning the patient in steep reverse Trendelenburg, allowing the omentum and abdominal organs to fall away from the diaphragm, a second port (10 mm) is placed approximately 10 cm from the xiphoid process along the left costal margin for the surgeon's right hand. The 10-mm port accommodates an SH or V-20 size needle to allow for intracorporeal suturing. The third port, for liver retraction, is a 5-mm port placed on the right costal margin 12 to 15 cm from the xiphoid (depending on the size of the liver). A 5-mm articulating liver retractor is placed through the right lateral port under laparoscopic visualization, and the left lateral lobe of the liver is retracted anteriorly and superiorly to expose the hiatus (Fig. 19.2). The right crus and caudate lobe of the liver should be clearly visible through the gastrohepatic ligament or pars flaccida if the liver retraction is adequate. Alternatively, the liver

---

BOX 19.3 Primary Principles of Nissen Fundoplication

Careful positioning to protect patient and surgeon from neuromuscular injury

Safe entry into the abdomen

Circumferential hiatal dissection near the crura, limiting manipulation and avoiding injury to the esophagus

Circumferential dissection of the esophagus under direct vision, with preservation of the vagus nerves

Adequate mobilization of the esophagus (or Collis gastroplasty) to attain 2–3 cm of intraabdominal esophagus without inferior traction

Complete mobilization of the gastric fundus including division of the short gastric vessels and any posterior attachments to the pancreas

Closure of hiatal defect by reapproximation of the diaphragmatic crura.

Creation of a short (2 cm), "floppy" (tension-free) fundoplication around the distal esophagus only and anchored to the esophagus

---

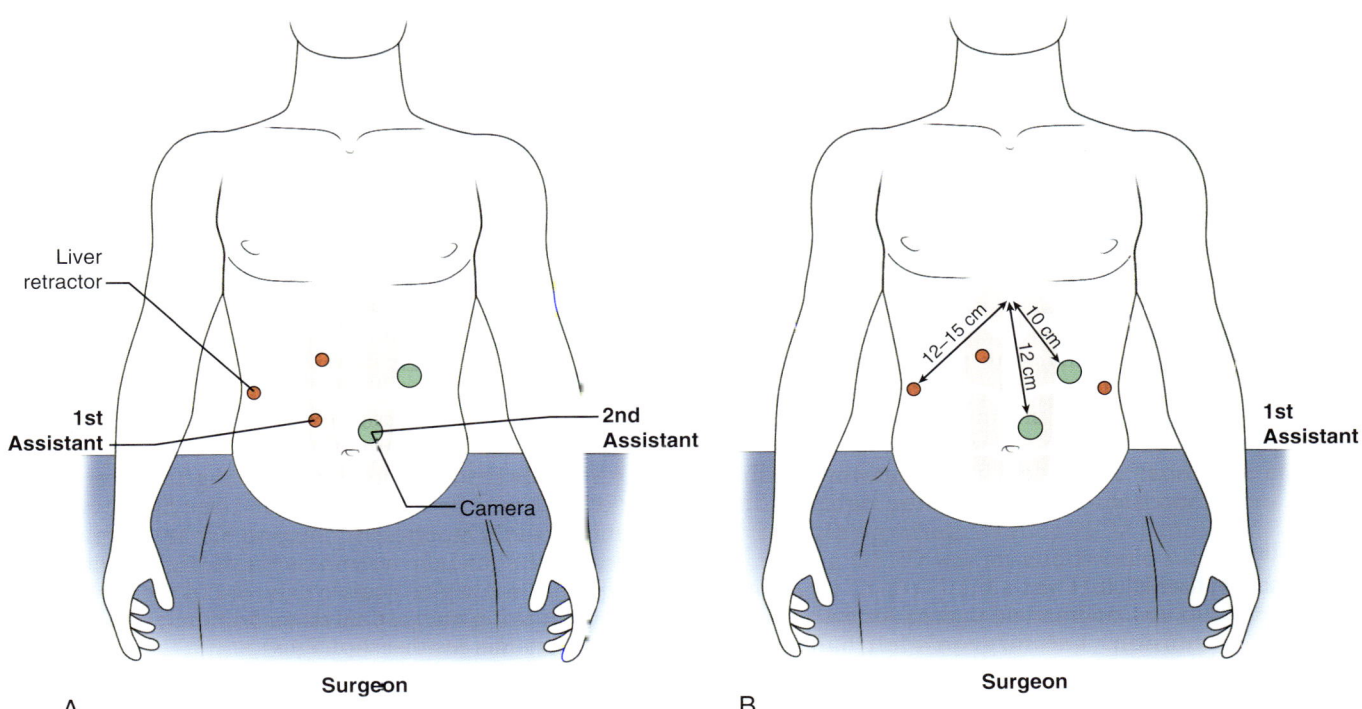

FIGURE 19.1 (A) Arrangement of laparoscopic ports during a standard Nissen fundoplication and (B) alternative port site positioning, with the first assistant to the left of the patient, for cases in which a dedicated camera driver is unavailable. *Small circles* represent 5-mm radially dilating trocars and *large circles* denote 11- to 12-mm trocars.

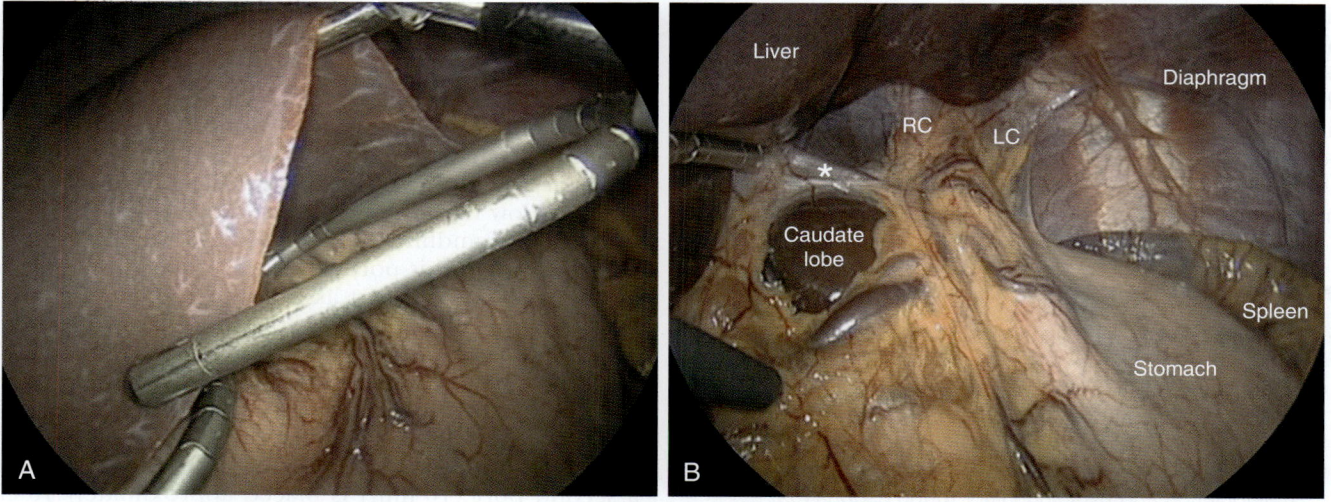

FIGURE 19.2 (A) The liver is reflected anteriorly to expose the esophageal hiatus using a snake-type retractor through the most lateral port on the patient's right side. (B) The liver retractor is secured in place to provide exposure of the gastrohepatic ligament, esophagus, and hiatus. The caudate lobe of the liver is visible through the thin tissue of the pars flaccida. *Hepatic branch of the anterior vagus nerve running along a replaced left hepatic artery. *LC,* Left crus; *RC,* right crus.

can be retracted with a Nathanson retractor placed just inferior and to the right of the xiphoid process. The liver retractor is stabilized with an endoscopic instrument holder attached to the operating table. The fourth port (5 mm), for the assistant, is generally placed midway between the liver retractor and the camera port. Finally, based on the location of the inferior edge of the liver after securing the retractor, a 5-mm port is placed to the right of midline, at the level of the 10-mm dissecting port, so that instruments in the surgeon's left hand triangulate the hiatus without hitting the falciform ligament or left lobe of the liver.

In the absence of a dedicated camera holder, the assistant can stand on the left side of the patient and control the laparoscope with the left hand. Should this be necessary, the fourth port is moved from the right upper quadrant to a location along the left costal margin, at least 5 cm below the 10 mm port used for the surgeon's right hand.

Exposure

An atraumatic grasper is used by the assistant to provide retraction of the stomach. The phrenoesophageal fat pad along the lesser curvature just below the EGJ is used for inferior retraction to minimize the risk of gastric or esophageal injury. The operating surgeon uses an atraumatic grasper in the left hand and an ultrasonic scalpel or advanced energy device in the right hand.

Dissection

Exposure of the Hiatus. The assistant retracts the stomach inferolaterally to the patient's left, putting the gastrohepatic ligament on tension. The surgeon's left hand grasps just above the pars flaccida, which is opened using the ultrasonic scalpel (Fig. 19.3). An aberrant left hepatic artery may be present in the pars flaccida in up to 13% of patients and often requires division as the dissection of the gastrohepatic ligament is carried superiorly toward the base of the right crus of the diaphragm. Preservation

of prominent vessels, as well as the hepatic branch of the anterior vagus nerve (Fig. 19.2B), can be attempted, but clinically significant liver ischemia has not been reported in cases where division is necessary. Dissection of the lesser curve is extended superiorly, up to the EGJ, to reveal the caudate lobe below and expose the hiatus and the right crus of the diaphragm. The peritoneum just medial to the right crus is incised and the esophagus carefully dissected away from its border (Fig. 19.4). The posterior vagus nerve is identified and preserved as the posterior mediastinal tissue is bluntly swept medially. Using the open jaws of the atraumatic grasper to provide anterolateral retraction on the right crus of the diaphragm, the dissection is continued clockwise up to the phrenoesophageal membrane. The thin anterior leaf of the phrenoesophageal membrane is divided along the apex of the hiatus (see Fig. 19.3) and dissection is continued across the top of the crural arch until the left crus is exposed. The anterior vagus nerve runs along the esophagus in this region and should be identified and preserved. The dissection is then carried down the border of the left crus until the angle of His and the gastric fundus limit further inferior dissection. Circumferential hiatal dissection is initiated bluntly and extended into the mediastinum by introducing the closed tip of round-nosed atraumatic graspers between the right crus and the esophagus and opening them vertically (12-o'clock and 6-o'clock positions) (see Fig. 19.4). The open jaws of the grasper are then used to retract the right crus laterally, while the instrument in the right hand gently sweeps the esophagus medially. The use of thermal devices is limited during mediastinal dissection to minimize injury to the vagus nerves or esophagus.

Complete Mobilization of the Gastric Fundus. Dissection of the fundus of the stomach is begun by identifying the point on the greater curvature approximately a third of the distance from the angle of His to the antrum. A convenient landmark for this point is the inferior pole of the spleen, roughly 10 to 15 cm inferior to the angle

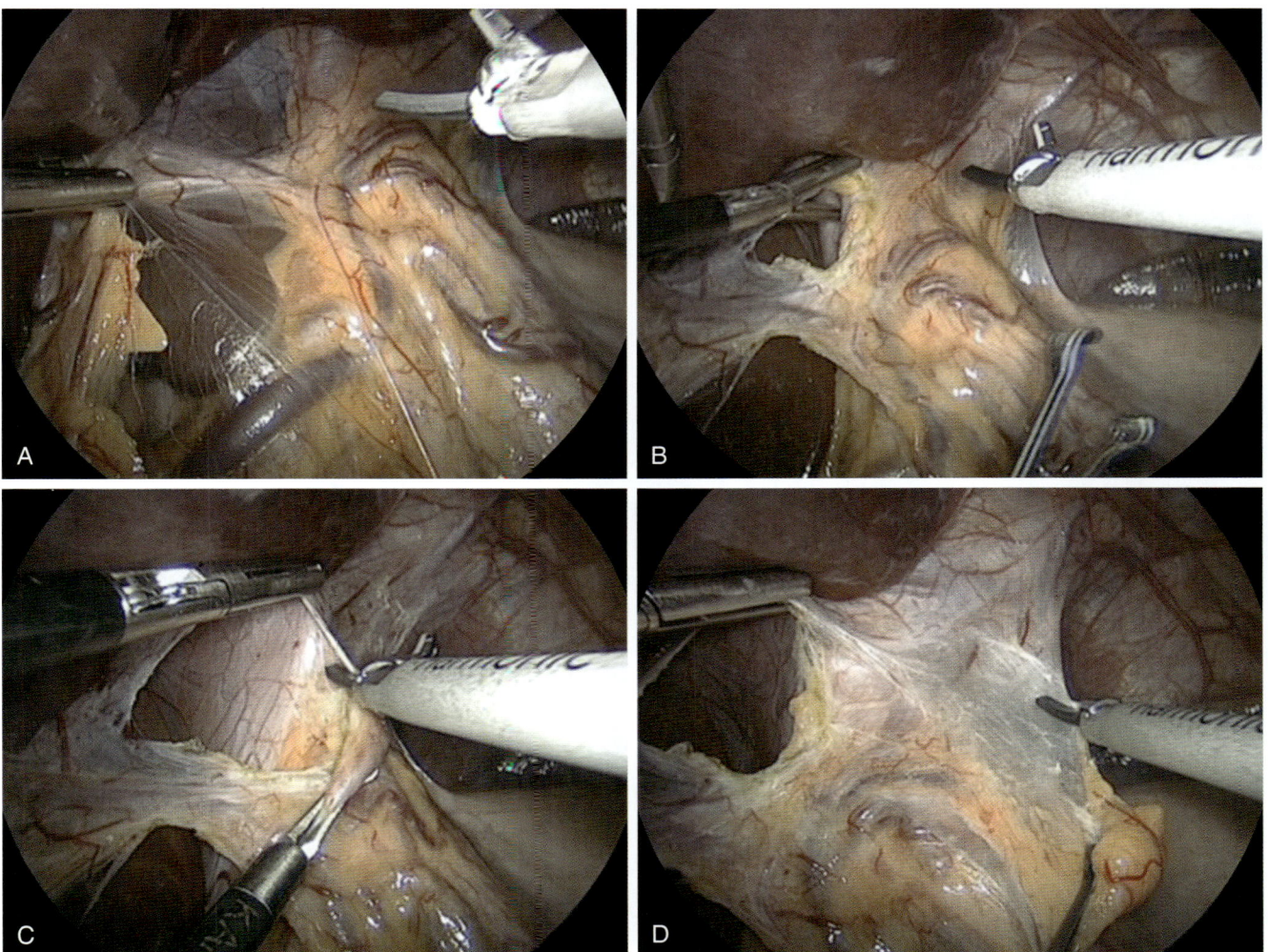

FIGURE 19.3 (A) Opening of the pars flaccida with the ultrasonic scalpel to begin dissection of the gastrohepatic ligament. (B) Dissection of the lesser curve (extending superiorly) exposes the right crus of the diaphragm. (C) Division of the phrenoesophageal ligament is continued along the apex of the hiatus, with (D) the assistant providing retraction by grasping the fat pad overlying the gastroesophageal junction, elevating the tissue away from the underlying esophagus.

of His. The lateral border of the fundus is grasped and retracted anteriorly and to the right, while the gastrocolic omentum is grasped and retracted ventrally and to the left. The lesser sac is entered approximately 5 to 10 mm away from the greater curve of the stomach, using the ultrasonic scalpel (Fig. 19.5). Injury to the greater curvature of the stomach can be avoided by rocking the surgeon's left hand up and down to visualize the posterior and anterior surface of the short gastric vessels as they are divided. Any visible thermal injury to the stomach may warrant placement of an imbricating suture. The short gastric vessels are divided individually with the ultrasonic scalpel until the superior pole of the spleen is reached. As one proceeds superiorly, three strategies may help dissection in this area:

1. Expose the superior pole of the spleen with "triangular retraction." The three corners of retraction in the axial plane are the spleen tip, the surgeon's left-hand instrument retracting anteromedially on the anterior wall of the fundus, and the first assistant retracting posteromedially on the posterior wall of the stomach.

2. If the greater omentum obscures the superior pole of the spleen, it should be retracted inferiorly. This may be accomplished by increasing the degree of reverse Trendelenburg, introducing an additional port and grasper in the left flank or placing a broad-based, figure-of-eight "reefing" suture in the greater omentum and retracting the omentum through the left lateral port with the two long ends of this suture.

3. Layer the dissection of the vascular structures at the superior pole of the spleen, starting with the visceral peritoneal reflection, then the short gastric vessels, and then the retroperitoneal gastrophrenic tissues. Dividing the pancreaticogastric peritoneal fold and the posterior gastric artery is necessary to fully mobilize the fundus and reach the base of the left crus posteriorly.

Mediastinal and Posterior Esophagus. After fully mobilizing the fundus, the base of the left crus is reached. If the earlier dissection reached the base of the right crus, the plane behind the esophagus is complete. Passing a Babcock grasper from right to left through the retroesophageal window and grasping the apex of the fundus near the

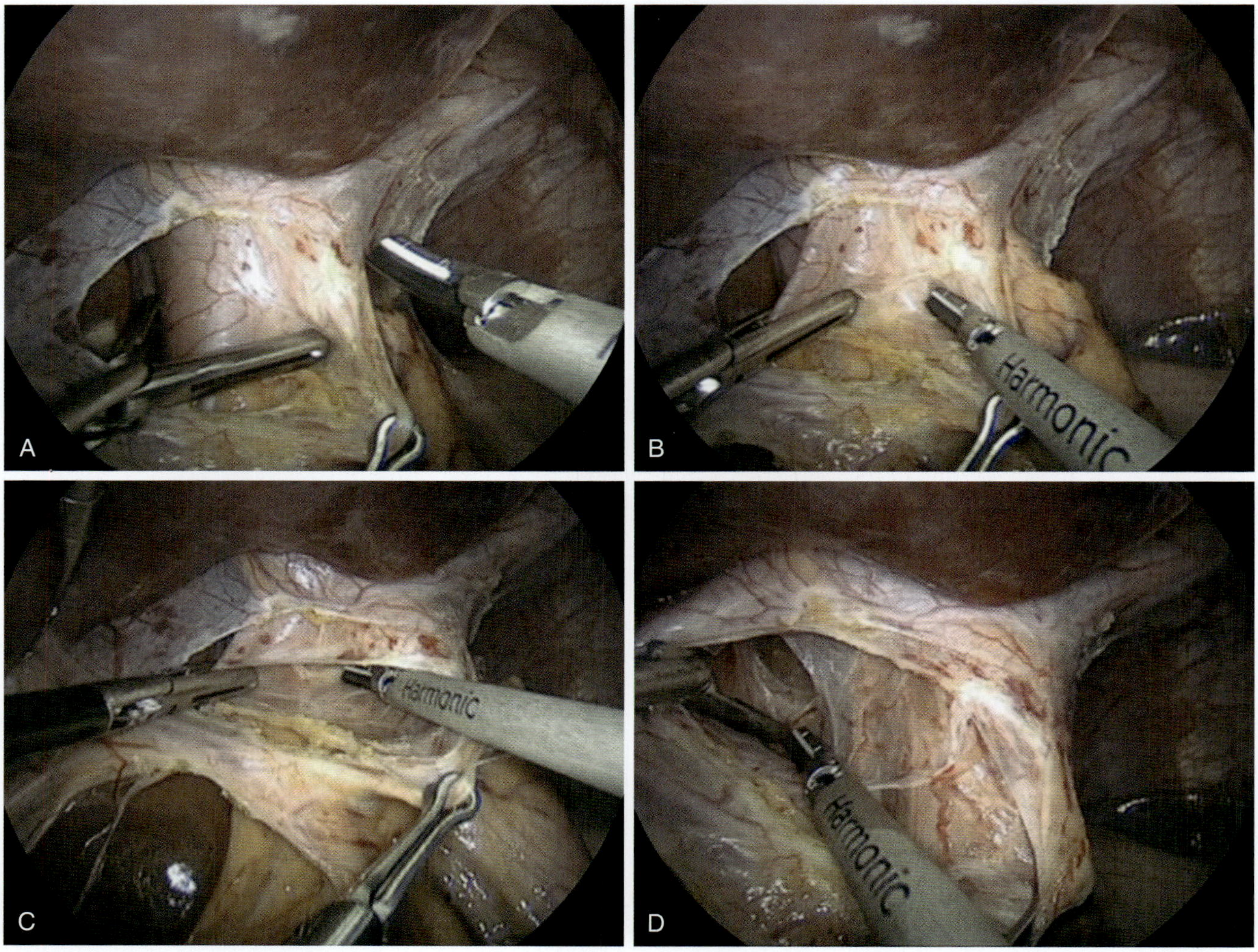

FIGURE 19.4 Initiation of the mediastinal dissection. (A) The right crus is grasped and (B) retracted laterally, while the right-handed instrument is used to bluntly dissect the esophageal tissue medially. (C) As the dissection is carried higher into the mediastinum, the assistant provides caudal retraction and (D) the left-handed instrument, with jaws opened, is moved inside the hiatus and provides countertraction.

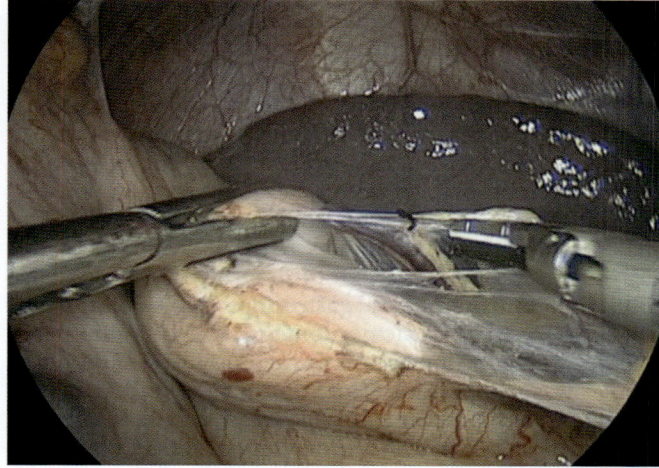

FIGURE 19.5 Mobilization of the gastric fundus is initiated by dividing the short gastric vessels along the greater curvature of the stomach.

divided short gastric vessels allows the fundus to be pulled through the window, to the right side of the esophagus (Fig. 19.6). Alternatively, a 4-inch-long, $\frac{1}{4}$ inch-wide Penrose drain is passed around the esophagus and secured with an Endoloop. The first assistant places a toothed locking grasper on the secured Penrose drain and retracts inferiorly and to the patient's left. The esophagus is freed circumferentially within the mediastinum by blunt dissection. Prior dissection of the posterior vagus away from the esophagus exposes the nerve to injury during posterior mediastinal dissection; this is why the dissection aims to maintain the posterior vagus alongside the posterior esophageal wall. Although most of the mediastinal dissection can be done bluntly, an occasional aortoesophageal artery is encountered (usually high on the left) and should be controlled with the ultrasonic scalpel. The proximal extent of the mediastinal dissection depends on the length of available intraabdominal esophagus. In the presence of Barrett esophagus, severe inflammation, stricture, giant hiatal hernia, or previous surgery, the esophagus may be foreshortened, necessitating further mediastinal dissection, an esophageal lengthening procedure (i.e., Collis gastroplasty), or both (see Acquired Short Esophagus, later).

To best assess intraabdominal esophageal length, the fundus or Penrose drain is released and the distance from the gastroesophageal junction to the crural closure is measured. At least 2.5 cm of esophagus must be within the abdomen and under no tension. If the maximal mediastinal dissection does not adequately reduce more than 2.5 cm of intraabdominal esophagus, a Collis gastroplasty should be performed. The gastric fundus is then passed posteriorly from the patient's left to right with atraumatic graspers to assess for adequate mobilization. The "shoeshine maneuver" involves sliding the fundus back and forth behind the esophagus to confirm good

position and confirm the absence of redundant tissue posteriorly (Fig. 19.7). Grasping a point too low on the greater curvature may predispose to the latter error. The fundoplication should not retract when the graspers are released; the presence of such a "spring sign" suggests excessive rotational tension and mandates reassessment of the completeness of the dissection.

Reconstruction

Crural Closure. The crura are closed from the right of the esophagus with interrupted nonabsorbable 0-Ethibond sutures placed 8 to 10 mm apart, 5 to 10 mm back from the crural edge. The peritoneal covering of the crura should be incorporated into the repair, and the sutures should be "staggered" in the anterior–posterior plane on the crura to avoid splitting the crural musculature along the length of the repair. The completed crural closure should be calibrated such that the crura just touch the walls of the empty esophagus (Fig. 19.8). To prevent reherniation, a variety of techniques have been used to reduce tension at the crural closure including buttressing with 1-cm² Teflon felt patches, felt strips, or a piece of absorbable or nonabsorbable mesh. More recently, diaphragmatic relaxing incisions have allowed for significant reduction in tension at the crural closure while avoiding the risk of erosion associated with foreign material surrounding the esophagus.[33,34]

Fundoplication. A 56- or 60-French esophageal dilator is passed transorally into the stomach by the anesthesiologist under direct laparoscopic vision by the surgeon. Good communication and slow advancement of the dilator are essential to minimize the risk of perforation at the EGJ. The dilator should pass without resistance. If resistance is encountered, the dilator is removed and a smaller dilator is passed. An indication that esophageal injury may have occurred is the appearance of blood on the dilator when it is removed. The size of the dilator is then increased until resistance is noted.

After dilator placement, the central stitch of the fundoplication is placed 1.5 cm proximal to the EGJ with

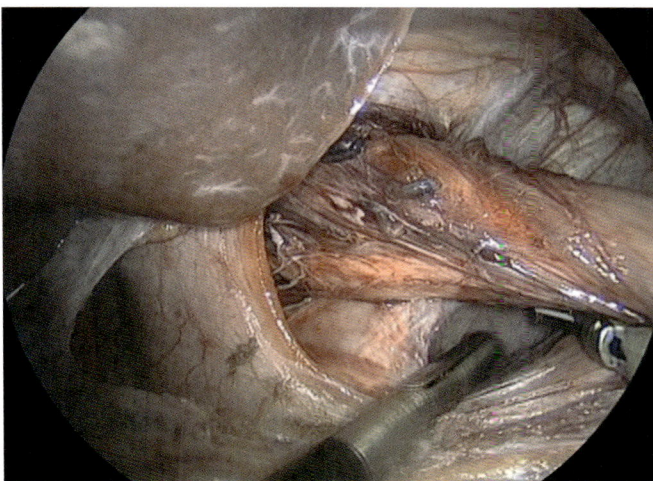

FIGURE 19.6 Following completion of circumferential hiatal dissection, an atraumatic instrument is used to grasp the apex of the gastric fundus and pass the tissue through the retroesophageal window from left to right.

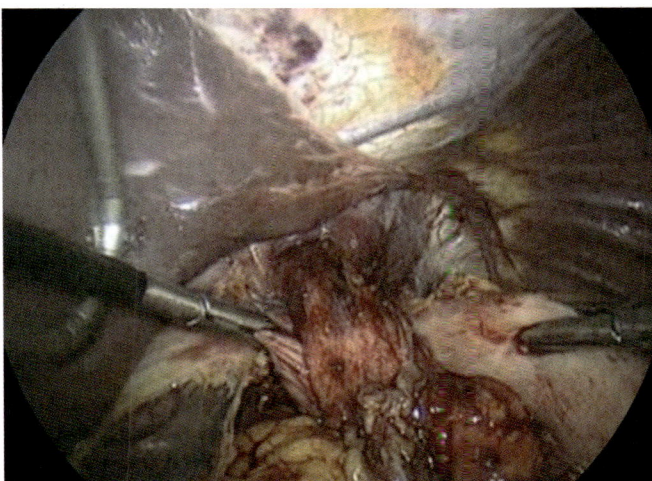 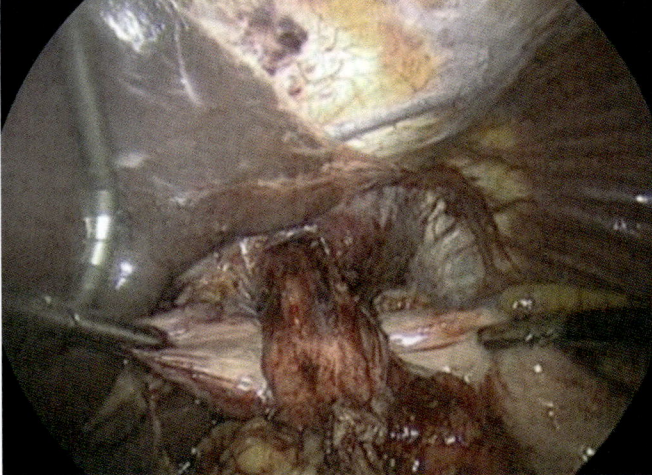

FIGURE 19.7 The "shoeshine maneuver," one-to-one movement of the fundus through the retroesophageal window, is performed to ensure that the fundoplication is in good position without tension or excess tissue posterior to the esophagus.

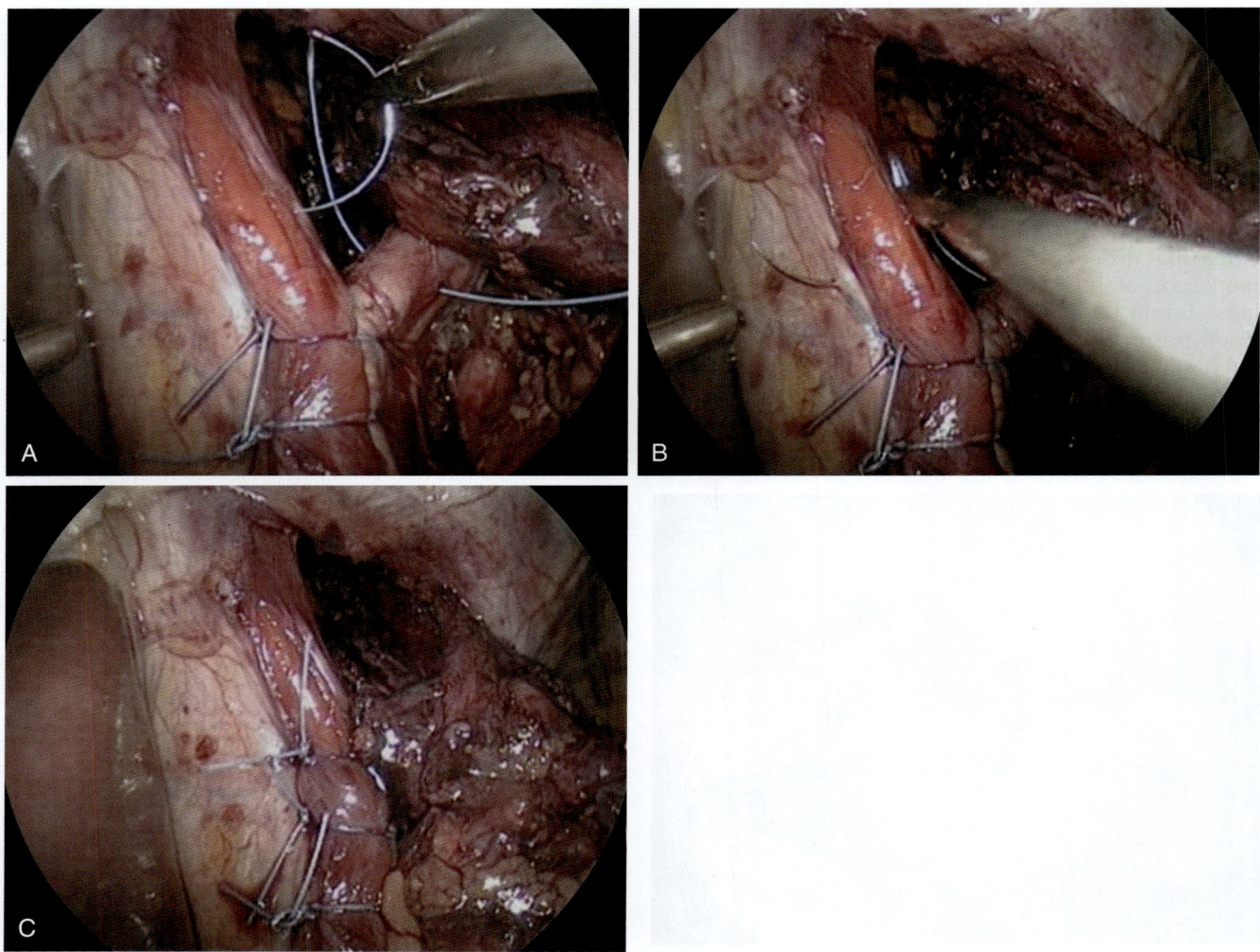

FIGURE 19.8 (A) Crural closure with nonabsorbable suture starting posteriorly and working anteriorly. (B) Each bite should incorporate endoabdominal fascia along with the musculature of the left and right crus. (C) Sutures are placed to close the hiatus such that it abuts the esophageal wall without impinging it or causing anterior angulation.

simple interrupted 2-0 nonabsorbable suture; seromuscular bites are taken through each side of the fundoplication, without incorporating the esophagus as the first stitch can be under increased tension as the wrap is being constructed. Additional sutures are placed 1 cm above and below the initial suture, including partial-thickness bites of the esophageal wall, to create a 2-cm-long fundoplication that is secured to the esophagus just above the level of the EGJ (Fig. 19.9). The tightness of the fundoplication is tested after placing each suture by gently sliding a blunt-ended gasper between the esophagus and the wrap. The grasper should easily slide along the esophagus, and lateral retraction of the wrap should visualize the diaphragm between the wrap and the esophagus. Knots may be tied extracorporeally, but intracorporeal knotting decreases tissue trauma and optimizes knot tension and position. Some authors advocate infradiaphragmatic fixation of the fundoplication to the crura to prevent reherniation, but there is no evidence that this decreases failure rates if adequate, tension-free intraabdominal esophageal length

is attained, either through mediastinal dissection or via an esophageal lengthening procedure.

OPEN NISSEN FUNDOPLICATION

The principal steps in performing an open Nissen fundoplication are similar to the laparoscopic approach. Open Nissen fundoplication is indicated if surgeons do not have adequate laparoscopic experience, patients have dense adhesions because of previous upper gastrointestinal operations, or a complication occurs that requires laparotomy to address. Despite the improved tactile feedback with an open approach, visual exposure of the hiatus may be less easily achieved than with a laparoscopic approach. Because the techniques involved in open and laparoscopic fundoplication are similar, the following sections address only significant differences.

Exploration and Exposure

An upper midline incision with the use of a self-retaining retractor allows adequate exposure. A liver retractor placed

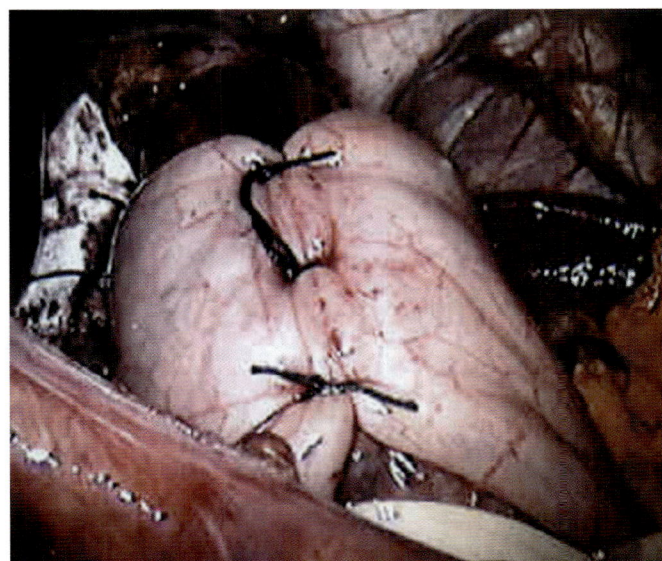

FIGURE 19.9 The completed Nissen fundoplication with three nonabsorbable sutures 1 cm apart.

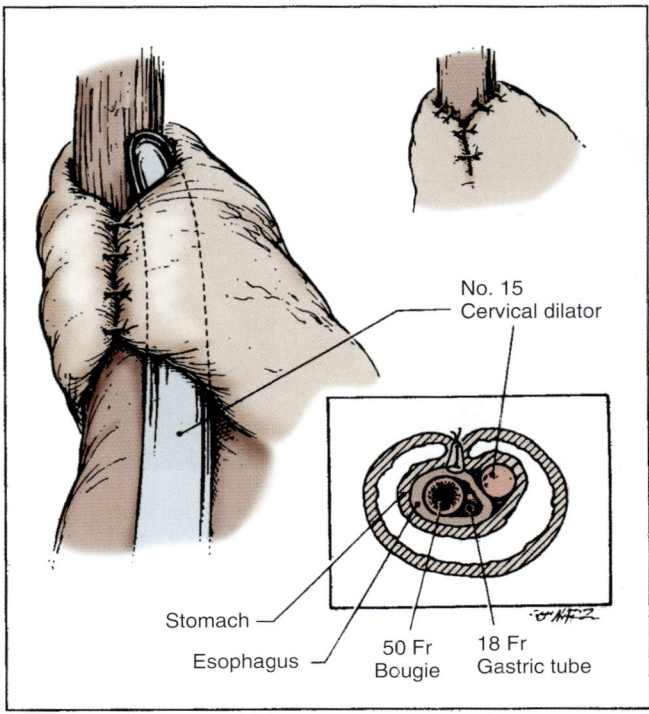

FIGURE 19.10 The original description of a "floppy" Nissen fundoplication by Donahue and Bombeck et al. in 1977. *Fr,* French. (From Donahue PE, Larson GM, Stewardson RH, Bombeck CT. Floppy Nissen fundoplication. *Rev Surg.* 1977;34:223.)

close to the most posterior part of the left lateral lobe of the liver permits improved visualization. Optimal exposure is obtained when the diaphragm is seen to run vertically from the upper end of the incision directly posteriorly to the hiatus. In patients with large left lateral lobe of the liver, mobilization of the left lateral liver by dividing the left coronal ligament may be necessary to achieve adequate exposure.

Lesser Curve. The thin gastrohepatic ligaments are incised, extended superiorly, and carried over the anterior surface of the esophagus as described earlier. Similarly, an aberrant left hepatic artery and hepatic branch of the vagus are protected if encountered in the pars flaccida. The anterior vagus is likewise identified and protected.

Crus. By retracting the lesser curve inferolaterally and to the right, the left crus is exposed. The right crus is dissected bluntly with the left fingers to create a retroesophageal space. A Penrose drain is passed around the lower part of the esophagus, excluding the posterior vagus nerve, and used as a retractor to provide better visualization of the retroesophageal space.

Mediastinal and Posterior Esophagus. With retraction on the Penrose drain, the esophagus can be dissected circumferentially. Similarly, the mediastinal dissection can be carried superiorly.

Fundus and Greater Curve. The loose attachments between the fundus and the left diaphragm are taken down. The short gastric vessels are sequentially divided with clamps and suture or ligated with the ultrasonic shears, as described earlier (see Fig. 19.5).

Repair and Fundoplication. Crural repair and fundoplication are performed as described earlier. A "floppy" Nissen fundoplication requires that the fundic wrap admit the surgeon's index finger between the wrap and the esophagus with the dilator in place (Fig. 19.10). Factors that influence the tightness of the wrap are the degree of mobilization of the fundus, the size of the esophageal dilator, and the sutures placed to create the fundoplication.

ACQUIRED SHORT ESOPHAGUS

The presence of a short esophagus increases the difficulty of laparoscopic Nissen fundoplication. Up to 20% of surgical failures with Nissen fundoplication may be the result of not recognizing a short esophagus. A short esophagus is discovered more frequently in patients with esophageal stricture, Barrett esophagus, and type III paraesophageal hernia. Esophageal foreshortening is thought to occur as a result of recurrent transmural inflammation from acid peptic injury and subsequent fibrosis of the mediastinal esophagus. Given its pathogenesis, it is not surprising that esophageal stricture is often associated with esophageal foreshortening. Large hiatal hernias may also be associated with a short esophagus as a result of chronic cephalad displacement of the gastroesophageal junction. Preoperative results of barium swallow and EGD may provide an indication of a short esophagus, but no combination of preoperative clinical variables reliably predicts the presence of a short esophagus, and the diagnosis of this entity continues to be made definitively at the time of operation, where it is defined as failure to achieve 2.5 cm of intraabdominal esophagus after maximal mediastinal dissection techniques.

Collis gastroplasty achieves esophageal lengthening by using the gastric cardia to create a neoesophagus.

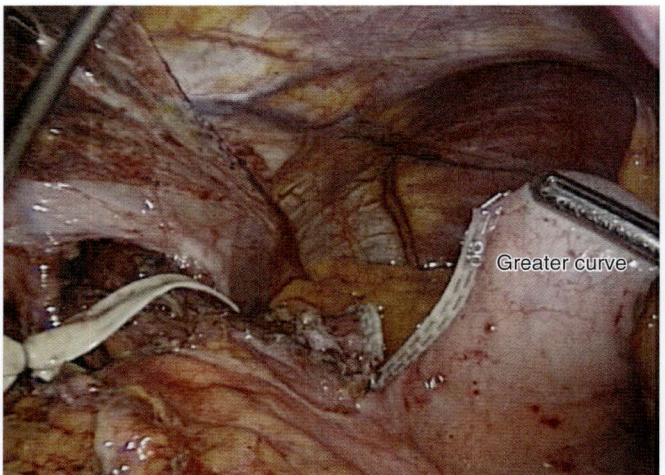

FIGURE 19.11 Laparoscopic stapling of the fundus from the greater curve toward the lesser curve to initiate a wedge fundectomy.

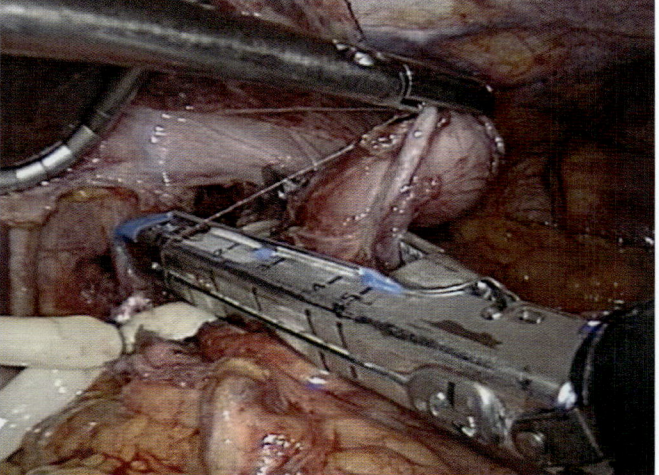

FIGURE 19.12 Lengthening of the esophagus by laparoscopic stapling parallel to the esophagus (with a dilator in place) in the cranial direction.

In open surgery, this can be performed easily by applying a linear stapler on the left side and parallel to the esophagus with a 56- or 60-French dilator in place. When a minimally invasive approach is used, the complexity of the procedure is increased. It can be accomplished either by a combined thoracoscopic–laparoscopic approach or by a totally laparoscopic approach.[35,36]

With the esophageal dilator in place, a thoracoscope is inserted through the third intercostal space in the anterior axillary line and passed through the chest until it meets the mediastinal pleura. This is visualized with a laparoscope in place in the abdomen. The thoracoscope is then removed, and a linear stapler is inserted through the same port until it meets the mediastinal pleura at the crura as seen with the laparoscope. Dissection from the abdomen allows for passage of the stapler into the abdomen, which is then applied to the stomach alongside the esophageal bougie at the gastroesophageal junction at the angle of His. Application of this stapler divides the upper part of the stomach from the angle of His distally along the esophageal dilator, thus creating a neoesophagus very similar to that performed with an open Collis gastroplasty.

The totally laparoscopic approach to a short esophagus currently used by most surgeons involves the use of a linear stapler inserted through the left subcostal port to perform a stapled wedge fundectomy.[37] An esophageal dilator (40 to 50 French) is placed to calibrate the width of the gastric tube. A marking suture is placed 3 cm inferior to the angle of His adjacent to the dilator. The linear stapler is fired horizontally from the greater curve toward the marking suture with the esophageal dilator in place (Fig. 19.11). Two firings of the laparoscopic linear stapler, using 45 mm, tissue thickness loads, are usually required to reach the marking suture. The gastroplasty is completed by firing a staple line parallel to the dilator in the cranial direction to the angle of His, thereby creating a tubular neoesophagus based on the proximal lesser curve (Fig. 19.12). This technique usually removes only a small triangular piece of stomach, and the adjacent remaining fundus can be used as the leading edge of

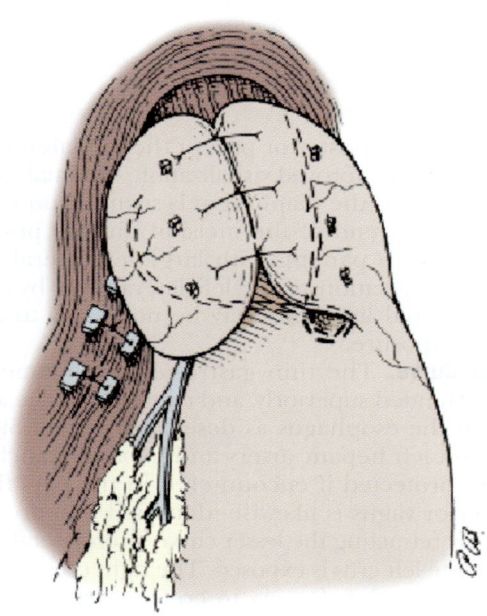

FIGURE 19.13 Final appearance of the fundoplication with the gastric portion of the staple line placed against the neoesophagus.

the fundoplication. After performing the fundectomy, an intraoperative endoscopy with a bubble test is performed to check for a leak at the staple line.

Elements of importance in fashioning the fundoplication include placing the initial suture of the fundoplication on the esophagus, immediately above the gastroesophageal junction, to ensure that acid-secreting (gastric) mucosa does not reside above the fundoplication. A second element, which ensures safety and avoids wrap deformation, is to place the gastric portion of the staple line against the neoesophagus such that the tip of the gastric staple line sits adjacent to the middle suture of the fundoplication on the right side of the esophagus (Fig. 19.13). Before initiating a liquid diet, a water-soluble contrast study can be performed to ensure the absence of a leak.

POSTOPERATIVE CARE

A nasogastric tube is unnecessary after laparoscopic Nissen fundoplication. However, liberal use of scheduled, and as needed, antiemetic medications is used to prevent retching that could disrupt the wrap in the immediate postoperative period. Patients are monitored on the general surgery floor and start clear liquids once they are awake and alert on the evening of surgery. The diet can be advanced to soft foods the following day. Patients are usually discharged home on the first postoperative day. Although outpatient laparoscopic Nissen fundoplication has been performed, patient satisfaction is low, and management of pain and nausea may be difficult without parenteral access. Patients are advised to consume a mechanical (dental) soft diet for the first 2 to 4 weeks, especially avoiding bread, meat, and raw vegetables. After the first 24 hours, postoperative pain can usually be managed with liquid oral analgesia. We encourage 1-month follow-up after discharge. No routine imaging or physiologic studies are obtained at the first postoperative visit, but a barium swallow serves as an excellent screening test to evaluate postoperative dysphagia or reflux-like symptoms. In brief, if the fundoplication is intact and if a 12.5-mm barium tablet passes without difficulty, it is extremely unlikely that the symptoms are related to a technical deficiency of the repair.

SPECIFIC INTRAOPERATIVE AND POSTOPERATIVE COMPLICATIONS

Intraoperative complications include esophageal perforation, splenic injury, bleeding, and missed visceral injury. Although these complications occur in less than 2% of all series,[38] the consequences can be grave.[39] Esophageal and gastric perforations occur in approximately 1% of cases and should be repaired primarily and buttressed with the fundoplication, if technically feasible. When an esophageal repair has been performed, progression to a solid diet is typically delayed by 5 to 7 days.

Injury to the mediastinal pleura during the intrathoracic dissection can lead to capnothorax (5% to 15%), which is usually well tolerated, but may cause immediate or delayed hemodynamic or respiratory consequences. When a pleural tear is detected, the first step is to make the hole larger (to avoid a tension capnothorax created by a one-way valve phenomenon). If increased airway pressure or decreased blood pressure develops, the pneumoperitoneum pressure is decreased and the positive-pressure ventilation setting increased. A chest tube is almost never necessary. At the end of the case, suction is applied to the mediastinum, as the pneumoperitoneum is released, and the patient is administered several vital capacity breaths. A chest radiograph is unnecessary unless the patient has specific cardiopulmonary issues requiring this diagnostic test.

Splenic injury can take the form of infarction or bleeding. Superior pole infarction can occur with ligation of the short gastric arteries. Occasionally, some of these vessels enter the spleen directly without passing through the hilum and are end arteries to the upper pole. No further intervention is required if the tip of the spleen is infarcted.

Rarely do patients have additional pain or fever under these conditions. Splenic bleeding, however, may require conversion to laparotomy and urgent splenectomy (0.5% to 1%). Incidental electrocautery burns to hollow viscera from arcing or incomplete insulation of the instruments can result in delayed perforation and peritonitis. Thorough inspection of the laparoscopic instruments, meticulous dissection, and gentle retraction can help prevent injury. An abdominal survey before closure can help identify any signs of bleeding.

Late complications can usually be attributed to the underlying disease process or technical issues with the fundoplication or hernia repair. Even though Nissen fundoplication has greater than a 90% success rate in eliminating reflux symptoms, over time, new or recurrent foregut symptoms will develop in 2% to 17% of patients. Although some dysphagia, gas bloat, and mild residual esophagitis are not uncommon in the early postoperative period, these symptoms generally resolve by 3 to 6 months. Severe or persistent symptoms may indicate failure. Large series have reported 2% to 6% of patients undergoing antireflux surgery will eventually require a reoperation.[34,39] Reported causes of failure vary significantly between studies, but a slipped or misplaced fundoplication and dehiscence are each responsible in approximately 15% to 30% of cases, transthoracic herniation occurs in 10% to 60%, and tight fundoplication, missed motility disorders, and paraesophageal hernias account for other causes of antireflux surgery failure.

SHORT-TERM RESULTS

The overall short-term results in appropriately selected patients are excellent.[25,39] Minor self-limited symptoms may occur in the early postoperative period in some patients. Up to 20% of patients will experience transient dysphagia, which is usually caused by postoperative edema secondary to surgical manipulation of the gastroesophageal junction. These symptoms typically improve without intervention within 6 weeks. EGD or barium swallow is indicated if symptoms persist. Dilation may provide relief of persistent dysphagia, but reoperation may be necessary in patients who are not responsive to dilation. The failure rate of Nissen fundoplication is approximately 1% per year for the first 10 years.[30,40] Bloating is common in GERD patients, and the severity is generally not significantly different before or after surgery, but may cause troublesome symptoms.[30] Other common symptoms after Nissen fundoplication are early satiety, nausea, and diarrhea. These symptoms are likely to improve with time and tend to respond to nonoperative therapy. Bilateral vagus nerve injury may result in gastroparesis.

LONG-TERM RESULTS

Studies of Nissen fundoplication with 10 or greater years of follow-up demonstrate excellent procedure satisfaction, durable symptom relief, improved quality of life, and high rates of cessation of acid-suppression therapy.[41,42] In a randomized control trial comparing open to laparoscopic Nissen fundoplication, patient procedure satisfaction was 72.7% and 78.5% at 10-year follow-up, respectively. The same study reported relief of GERD symptoms in 92.4% and 90.7% of patients after 10 years for laparoscopic and open Nissen fundoplications, respectively. Acid-suppression therapy was used in 20% of the patients at 10 years, but 65% of these patients did not have objective evidence of reflux based on 24-hour pH-impedance studies.[41] Eleven-year follow-up of laparoscopic Nissen fundoplication revealed that 92.5% of patients were satisfied with the results of their surgery, 90% had durable improvement of their symptoms, 70% of patients were off acid-suppression therapy, and the revisional surgery rate was 8.3%.[42] Surgical failure is most often attributable to (1) complete disruption of the wrap, (2) a slipped Nissen fundoplication (in which part of the stomach lies above and part lies below the fundoplication), or (3) herniation of an intact wrap through the hiatus into the chest.[32,43] Surgical failures may require reoperation.[27,39] Patients should be cautioned that the results of reoperation for GERD are never as favorable as the results after a primary operation and that residual atypical symptoms may persist. Laparoscopic reoperative fundoplication is technically feasible by experienced surgeons.

CONCLUSION

Antireflux surgery is an excellent treatment option for patients with symptoms of GERD that are inadequately treated with medication, for patients who desire to avoid lifelong medical therapy, or for patients with significant complications from acid reflux. The effect of antireflux surgery on progression of Barrett esophagus is not fully understood, and patients with Barrett esophagus who undergo antireflux surgery still require routine endoscopic surveillance. The introduction of a laparoscopic approach to fundoplication should not alter the operative indications. Finally, to ensure successful surgical outcomes, an understanding of disease pathophysiology, preoperative diagnostic evaluation, appropriate patient selection, and complete familiarity with the various types of antireflux procedures available are essential.

The introduction of endoscopic therapies for reflux control has provided new options for the patient with GERD. However, the effectiveness and durability of these endoscopic therapies have yet to approximate the outcomes of surgical fundoplication. Regardless of these advances, surgical therapy for GERD will continue to play an important role in patients with complicated disease, such as those with large hiatal hernias or a shortened esophagus.

REFERENCES

1. Shaker R, Castell DO, Schoenfeld PS, Spechler SJ. Nighttime heartburn is an under-appreciated clinical problem that impacts sleep and daytime function: the results of a Gallup survey conducted on behalf of the American Gastroenterological Association. *Am J Gastroenterol.* 2003;98:1487.
2. Wu AH, Tseng CC, Bernstein L. Hiatal hernia, reflux symptoms, body size, and risk of esophageal and gastric adenocarcinoma. *Cancer.* 2003;98:940.
3. Srinivasan R, Tutuian R, Schoenfeld P, et al. Profile of GERD in the adult population of a northeast urban community. *J Clin Gastroenterol.* 2004;38:651.
4. Vakil N, van Zanten SV, Kahrilas P, Dent J, Jones R, Global Consensus Group. The Montreal definition and classification of gastroesophageal reflux disease: a global evidence-based consensus. *Am J Gastroenterol.* 2006;101:1900.
5. Friedenburg FK, Hanlon A, Vanar V, et al. Trends in gastroesophageal reflux disease as measured by the National Ambulatory Medical Care Survey. *Dig Dis Sci.* 2010;55:1911.
6. Zaninotto G, DeMeester TR, Schwizer W, Johansson KE, Cheng SC. The lower esophageal sphincter in health and disease. *Am J Surg.* 1988;155:104.
7. Stein HJ, Crookes PF, DeMeester TR. Three-dimensional manometric imaging of the lower esophageal sphincter. *Surg Annu.* 1995;27:199.
8. Finlayson SR, Laycock WS, Birkmeyer JD. National trends in utilization and outcomes of antireflux surgery. *Surg Endosc.* 2003;17:864.
9. Fuchs KH, DeMeester TR, Albertucci M. Specificity and sensitivity of objective diagnosis of gastroesophageal reflux disease. *Surgery.* 1987;102:575.
10. Hunter JG, Trus TL, Branum GD, Waring JP, Wood WC. A physiologic approach to laparoscopic fundoplication for gastroesophageal reflux disease. *Ann Surg.* 1996;223:673; discussion 685.
11. Farrell TM, Richardson WS, Trus TL, Smith CD, Hunter JG. Response of atypical symptoms of gastro-oesophageal reflux to antireflux surgery. *Br J Surg.* 2001;88:1649.
12. Rydberg L, Ruth M, Abrahamsson H, et al. Tailoring antireflux surgery: a randomized clinical trial. *World J Surg.* 1999;23:612.
13. Spechler SJ, Souza RF, Rosenberg SJ, Ruben RA, Goyal RK. Heartburn in patients with achalasia. *Gut.* 1995;37:305.
14. Campos GM, Peters JH, DeMeester TR, et al. Multivariate analysis of factors predicting outcome after laparoscopic Nissen fundoplication. *J Gastrointest Surg.* 1999;3:292.
15. Tseng D, Rizvi AZ, Fennerty MB, et al. Forty-eight-hour pH monitoring increases sensitivity in detecting abnormal esophageal acid exposure. *J Gastrointest Surg.* 2005;9:1043; discussion 1051.
16. Shay S, Tutuian R, Sifrim D, et al. Twenty-four hour ambulatory simultaneous impedance and pH monitoring: a multicenter report of normal values from 60 healthy volunteers. *Am J Gastroenterol.* 2004;99:1037.
17. Castell DO, Vela M. Combined multichannel intraluminal impedance and pH-metry: an evolving technique to measure type and proximal extent of gastroesophageal reflux. *Am J Med.* 2001;111(suppl 8A):157S.
18. Kwiatek MA, Pandolfino JE, Hirano I, Kahrilas PJ. Esophagogastric junction distensibility assessed with an endoscopic functional luminal imaging probe (EndoFLIP). *Gastrointest Endosc.* 2010;72:272.
19. Robertson AG, Krishnan A, Ward C, et al. Anti-reflux surgery in lung transplant recipients: outcomes and effects on quality of life. *Eur Respir J.* 2012;39:691.
20. Morgenthal CB, Lin E, Shane MD, Hunter JG, Smith CD. Who will fail laparoscopic Nissen fundoplication? Preoperative prediction of long-term outcomes. *Surg Endosc.* 2007;21:1978.
21. Pizza F, Rossetti G, Del Genio G, Maffettone V, Brusciano L, Del Genio A. Influence of esophageal motility on the outcome of laparoscopic total fundoplication. *Dis Esophagus.* 2008;21:78.
22. Horvath KD, Jobe BA, Herron DM, Swanstrom LL. Laparoscopic Toupet fundoplication is an inadequate procedure for patients with severe reflux disease. *J Gastrointest Surg.* 1999;3:583.
23. Watson DI, Jamieson GG, Lally C, et al. Multicenter, prospective, double-blind, randomized trial of laparoscopic Nissen vs anterior 90 degrees partial fundoplication. *Arch Surg.* 2004;139:1160.
24. Dallemagne B, Weerts JM, Jehaes C, Markiewicz S, Lombard R. Laparoscopic Nissen fundoplication: preliminary report. *Surg Laparosc Endosc.* 1991;1:138.
25. Ackroyd R, Watson DI, Majeed AW, Troy G, Treacy PJ, Stoddard CJ. Randomized clinical trial of laparoscopic versus open fundoplication for gastro-oesophageal reflux disease. *Br J Surg.* 2004;91:975.
26. Terry M, Smith CD, Branum GD, Galloway K, Waring JP, Hunter JG. Outcomes of laparoscopic fundoplication for gastroesophageal reflux disease and paraesophageal hernia. *Surg Endosc.* 2001;15:691.
27. Granderath FA, Kamolz T, Schweiger UM, et al. Long-term results of laparoscopic antireflux surgery. *Surg Endosc.* 2002;16:753.
28. Viljakka MT, Luostarinen ME, Isolauri JO. Complications of open and laparoscopic antireflux surgery: 32-year audit at a teaching hospital. *J Am Coll Surg.* 1997;185:446.
29. Lundell L, Dalenback J, Hattlebakk J, et al. Outcome of open antireflux surgery as assessed in a Nordic multicentre prospective clinical trial. Nordic GORD-Study Group. *Eur J Surg.* 1998;164:751. Erratum in *Eur J Surg* 165:1104, 1999.

30. Laine S, Rantala A, Gullichsen R, Ovaska J. Laparoscopic vs conventional Nissen fundoplication. A prospective randomized study. *Surg Endosc.* 1997;11:441.

31. Heikkinen TJ, Haukipuro K, Bringman S, Ramel S, Sorasto A, Hulkko A. Comparison of laparoscopic and open Nissen fundoplication 2 years after operation. A prospective randomized trial. *Surg Endosc.* 2000;14:1019.

32. Hunter JG, Smith CD, Branum GD, et al. Laparoscopic fundoplication failures: patterns of failure and response to fundoplication revision. *Ann Surg.* 1999;230:595; discussion 604.

33. Crespin OM, Yates RB, Martin AV, Pellegrini CA, Oelschlager BK. The use of crural relaxing incisions with biologic mesh reinforcement during laparoscopic repair of complex hiatal hernias. *Surg Endosc.* 2016;30:2179. doi:10.1007/s00464-015-4522-1.

34. Alicuben ET, Worrell SG, DeMeester SR. Impact of crural relaxing incisions, Collis gastroplasty, and non-cross-linked human dermal mesh crural reinforcement on early hiatal hernia recurrence rates. *J Am Coll Surg.* 2014;219:988. doi 10.1016/j.jamcollsurg.2014.07.937.

35. Swanstrom LL, Marcus DR, Galloway GQ. Laparoscopic Collis gastroplasty is the treatment of choice for the shortened esophagus. *Am J Surg.* 1996;171:477.

36. Johnson AB, Oddsdottir M, Hunter JG. Laparoscopic Collis gastroplasty and Nissen fundoplication. A new technique for the management of esophageal foreshortening. *Surg Endosc.* 1998;12:1055.

37. Terry ML, Vernon A, Hunter JG. Stapled-wedge Collis gastroplasty for the shortened esophagus. *Am J Surg.* 2004;188:195.

38. Watson DI, Jamieson GG. Antireflux surgery in the laparoscopic era. *Br J Surg.* 1998;85:1173.

39. Watson DI, Jamieson GG, Game PA, Williams RS, Devitt PG. Laparoscopic reoperation following failed antireflux surgery. *Br J Surg.* 1999;86:98.

40. Power C, Maguire D, McAnena O. Factors contributing to failure of laparoscopic Nissen fundoplication and the predictive value of preoperative assessment. *Am J Surg.* 2004;187:457.

41. Broeders JA, Jong R, Draaisma W, Bredenoord AJ, Smout AJ, Gooszen HG. Ten-year outcome of laparoscopic and conventional Nissen fundoplication. *Ann Surg.* 2009;250:698.

42. Morgenthal CB, Shane MD, Stival A, et al. The durability of laparoscopic Nissen fundoplication: 11-year outcomes. *J Gastrointest Surg.* 2007;11:693.

43. Hinder RA, Klingler PJ, Perdikis G, Smith SL. Management of the failed antireflux operation. *Surg Clin North Am.* 1997;77:1083.

Magnetic Sphincter Augmentation for Gastroesophageal Reflux Disease

Luigi Bonavina | Emanuele Asti

The continuous search for the ideal antireflux procedure reflects a widely held perception among surgeons, gastroenterologists, and patients that therapy for gastroesophageal reflux disease (GERD) remains unsatisfactory. About 30% to 40% of patients are resistant or only partial responders to proton pump inhibitor (PPI) therapy,[1,2] and even high-dose escalation may be inadequate to maintain individuals in a symptom-free state with a mechanically defective lower esophageal sphincter (LES). Additionally, there are growing concerns over the long-term effects of chronic acid suppression. Many patients suffer from persistent nonacid reflux and nocturnal acid breakthrough, and may progress to serious complications of the disease, such as volume regurgitation with pulmonary aspiration and Barrett metaplasia, the leading risk factor for esophageal adenocarcinoma.[3] A large European open cohort multicenter study showed that about 10% of patients under routine medical care progressed to Barrett esophagus in 5 years of follow-up.[4] Recent literature also indicates that chronic acid suppression with PPIs can reduce the absorption of vitamin B_{12} and magnesium, the effectiveness of medications such as clopidogrel, and increase the risk of *Clostridium difficile* infection.[5] Other consequences of prolonged PPI therapy include hypergastrinemia, enterochromaffin-like cell hyperplasia, and parietal cell hypertrophy, leading to rebound acid hypersecretion.[6] Finally, there is some evidence suggesting that chronic acid suppression may be associated with an increased incidence of gastric cancer.[7]

The laparoscopic Nissen fundoplication is the current surgical gold standard for the treatment of GERD. It is a safe, effective, and durable antireflux procedure when performed in specialized centers. A multicenter European trial comparing medical therapy with total or partial fundoplication performed in selected centers by expert surgeons showed that 92% of medical patients and 85% of surgical patients remained in remission at 5 years of follow-up.[8] However, despite remarkably low morbidity and mortality rates, the operation is underused due to the perception of long-term side effects and fear of failure, which impacts referral patterns.[9] Also, wide variability in clinical outcomes related to interindividual surgical expertise and/or technical modifications[10] have limited the adoption of this procedure especially in patients with early GERD. Patients undergoing a Nissen fundoplication are especially at risk for potential side effects of the procedure such as bloating, the inability to belch and vomit, and the occurrence of persistent dysphagia that may occasionally require revisional surgery.[11] These are the main reasons why gastroenterologists tend to limit their referrals for fundoplication only to patients with long-lasting severe disease and large hiatal hernias. A downward trend in the use of surgical fundoplication has been noted in the United States over the past decade.[12–14] The decline in surgical volume has been attributed to the perceived risk of fundoplication failure, to the availability of over-the-counter PPI and endoscopic therapies, and to the rise of bariatric surgery.

The limitations of both PPI therapy and fundoplication have left many patients and clinicians in the equivocal position of tolerating a lifetime drug dependence with incomplete symptom relief, or undertaking the risk of a surgical procedure that alters gastric anatomy, may have considerable side effects, and may deteriorate over time. The Linx Reflux Management System (Torax Medical, St. Paul, Minnesota) is a US Food and Drug Administration–approved device designed to provide a permanent solution to GERD by augmenting the LES barrier with a standardized laparoscopic procedure.

MAGNETIC SPHINCTER AUGMENTATION

The Linx is a simple mechanical device designed to augment the physiologic barrier to reflux by magnetic force. The device consists of a series of biocompatible titanium beads with magnetic cores hermetically sealed inside. The beads are interlinked with independent titanium wires to form a flexible and expandable ring. At rest, each bead is in contact with adjacent beads. The beads can move independent of the adjacent beads, creating a dynamic implant that does not compress the esophagus and does not limit its range of motion upon swallowing, belching, and vomiting (Fig. 20.1). For reflux to occur, the intragastric pressure must overcome the resistance to opening of both the patient's native LES pressure and the magnetic bonds of the device. The Linx is manufactured in different sizes and is capable of nearly doubling its diameter when all beads are separated. The magnetic attraction force to be counteracted to allow bead separation is independent of the number of beads contained in the device. The Linx device, while augmenting the LES, allows for expansion to accommodate a swallowed bolus or the escape of elevated gastric pressure associated with belching or vomiting. Once healing is complete after the implant, the device is encapsulated in fibrous tissue but is not incorporated in the esophageal wall[15]; this makes it possible to remove the device without damage to the esophagus. The Linx has recently received magnetic resonance imaging (MRI) approval for scanning in systems up to 1.5 Tesla.

SURGICAL TECHNIQUE

Compared to the current surgical standard of a fundoplication, the Linx procedure requires less dissection and fewer

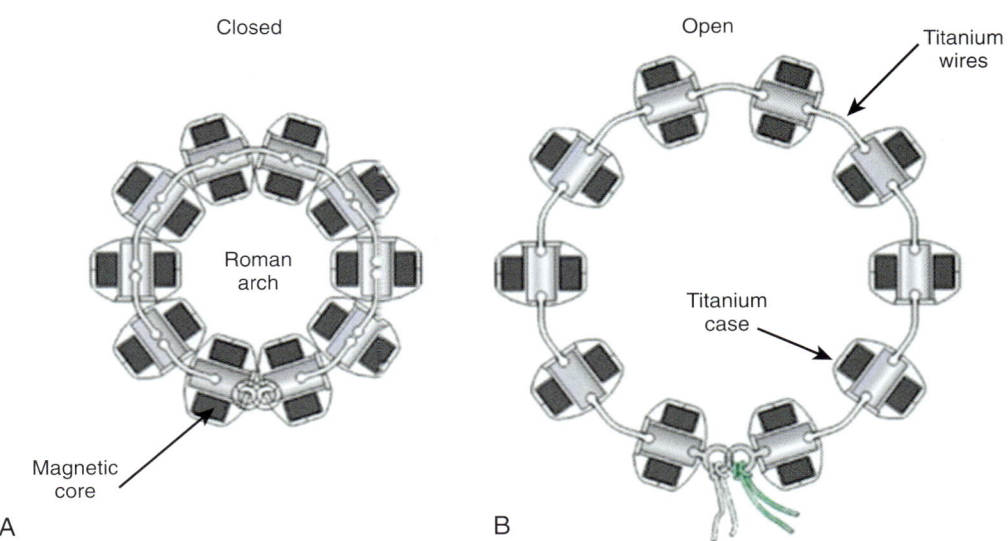

Closed

Open

Titanium wires

Roman arch

Titanium case

Magnetic core

A

B

FIGURE 20.1 An engineering schematic of the magnetic sphincter augmentation device. The device consists of an expansible bracelet of magnetic beads designed to be placed surgically around the exterior surface of the distal end of the lower esophageal sphincter (LES). Each bead is composed of a titanium case containing a magnetic core of small disk-shaped magnets. The beads are connected by titanium wires of specific lengths that limit the distance any two individual beads can move apart. When the device is closed (A), the magnetic force is sufficient to prevent effacement and opening of the LES yet is weak enough to allow the device to open (B) with the esophageal peristalsis. When the device is closed, the Roman arch construction prevents compression of the esophageal tissues. (From DeMeester, TR. New approaches to gastroesophageal reflux disease [LINX]. In: Cameron JL, et al, eds. *Current Surgical Therapy*. 12th ed. Philadelphia: Elsevier; 2017:19-24.)

steps. The device is implanted with a standard laparoscopic approach under general anesthesia. Ideally the dissection should be minimal with preservation of the phrenoesophageal ligament. The steps of the procedure are illustrated in Fig. 20.2. The first step is division of the peritoneum on the anterior surface of the gastroesophageal junction below the insertion of the inferior leaf of the phrenoesophageal ligament and above the junction of the hepatic branch to the anterior vagus nerve. The lateral surface of the left crus is freed from the posterior fundic wall without dividing any short gastric vessels. The gastrohepatic ligament is opened above and below the hepatic branch to facilitate the preparation of the retroesophageal window. Gentle dissection from the right side is made toward the left crus just above the crural decussation to identify the posterior vagus nerve. A tunnel is then created between the vagus and the posterior esophageal wall, and a Penrose drain is passed in a left-to-right direction. The circumference of the esophagus is measured to determine the proper size of the Linx device to be implanted. The sizing tool is a laparoscopic instrument with a soft, circular curved tip actuated by coaxial tubes through a handset. The handset contains a numerical indicator that corresponds to the size range of the Linx device. The sizing tool is placed around the esophagus in the dissected space between the esophageal wall and the posterior vagus nerve bundle. Once the appropriate Linx device has been selected, it is introduced through the posterior tunnel. The opposing ends are then brought to the anterior surface of the esophagus and connected together by engaging the two clasps. The decision to proceed with a posterior crural repair depends on the size of the hernia that is found

intraoperatively. Operative time is generally less than 1 hour. Patients are discharged the same day of surgery or on the first postoperative day and are counseled to gradually return to a normal diet and to discontinue use of acid suppression medication.

SUMMARY OF CLINICAL EXPERIENCE

Since the first human implantation in 2007, all reported studies investigating the long-term clinical outcomes of the Linx device have confirmed a high rate of symptom relief, discontinuation of PPI therapy, objective reduction of esophageal acid exposure, and improved quality of life. Two prospective, single-arm, multicenter, controlled clinical studies have been conducted to evaluate the Linx System. The feasibility study included 44 patients implanted with the Linx at four study centers in the United States and in Europe between February 2007 and October 2008; the short-term, mid-term, 4-year, and final results of this study have been previously published.[16–19] In the feasibility study, patients served as their own control to assess the effect of treatment on esophageal acid exposure, symptoms, and use of PPI. The primary criteria for inclusion in the feasibility trial were patients between ages 18 and 85 years, typical reflux symptoms at least partially responsive to PPI therapy, abnormal esophageal acid exposure, and normal contractile amplitude and wave form in the esophageal body. The primary criteria for exclusion from the trial were a history of dysphagia, previous upper abdominal surgery, previous endoluminal antireflux procedures, sliding hiatal hernia greater than 3 cm, esophagitis greater than grade A, and/or the presence of histologically documented Barrett

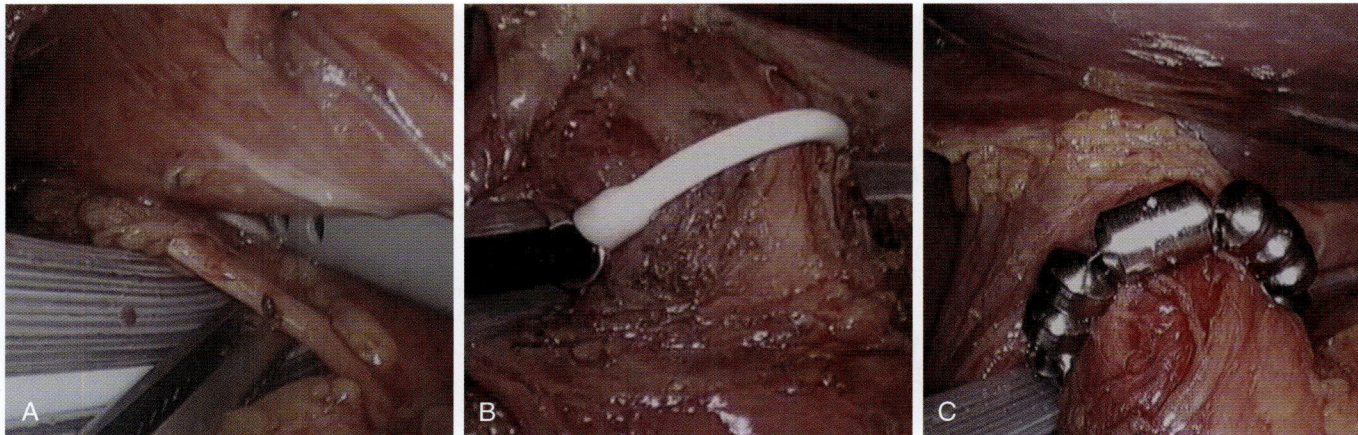

FIGURE 20.2 Surgical steps of the Linx procedure. (A) Establish the area for device placement by preservation of the phrenoesophageal ligament. A tunnel behind the esophageal wall is made after identification of the posterior vagus nerve. (B) The esophagus is measured using a special sizing tool. (C) The Linx device is locked in front of the esophagus after alignment and engagement of the two clasps.

esophagus. Patients with abnormal manometric findings (distal esophageal contraction amplitude of less than 35 mm Hg on wet swallows or less than 70% propulsive peristaltic sequences) were also excluded. Preoperative evaluation consisted of a symptom questionnaire and the Gastroesophageal Reflux Disease–Health Related Quality of Life (GERD-HRQL) questionnaire, upper gastrointestinal endoscopy, barium swallow, standard esophageal manometry, and 24- to 48-hour esophageal pH monitoring. All Linx devices were successfully implanted via a standard laparoscopic approach. The median operative time was 40 (19 to 104) minutes. No intraoperative complications occurred. Patients were instructed to resume a regular diet after a chest film and radiologic assessment of the esophageal transit were performed. All patients except one were discharged within 48 hours. Thirty-three patients (75%) were followed at 5 years. The mean total GERD-HRQL score off PPIs decreased from 25.7 at baseline to 2.9 at year 5 ($P < .001$), and 94% (31/33) patients had a greater than 50% reduction in the total score compared to baseline; 91% of patients reported being satisfied with their current condition. Esophageal pH testing was completed in 20 patients at 5 years: 85% of patients achieved normal esophageal acid exposure or had at least a 50% reduction from baseline. Normalization of esophageal pH was achieved in 70% of patients. Complete cessation of PPIs or a reduction of 50% or more of the daily dose at 5 years was achieved by 88% and 94% of patients, respectively.

Forty-three percent of patients complained of mild dysphagia during the postoperative period; in all individuals the symptom resolved by 90 days without treatment. Three patients were explanted: one because of persistent dysphagia, one because of the need to undergo MRI, and the last one who elected to have a Nissen fundoplication for persisting GERD symptoms. All removals were safely performed by a laparoscopic procedure.

Similar rigorous inclusion criteria and perioperative subjective and objective evaluations were used in the larger second study involving 100 patients at 14 centers in the United States.[20] Significant improvements were seen in GERD-related quality of life, regurgitation, and esophageal acid exposure. Use of PPIs dropped to 13% at 3 years and patient satisfaction with reflux control increased to 94% after implantation. Importantly, these positive results were stable and showed no degradation over the study time period. Although 14% of patients reported some bloating after implantation, no patients rated this symptom as severe. Patients retained their ability to belch and vomit. Dysphagia proved to be quite common, present to some extent in 68% of patients but decreasing to 4% by 3 years. Five percent of patients rated the dysphagia as severe and the device was removed in three of them with complete resolution.

Two single-center studies have further validated the efficacy of the Linx procedure. In Milan, Italy, 100 consecutive patients underwent Linx implantation between 2007 and 2012. The median implant duration was 3 years, ranging from 378 days to 6 years. There was a significant reduction of acid exposure time and improvement of GERD-HRQL score; freedom from daily dependence on PPIs was achieved in 85% of the patients.[21] Another study from the United States, including 66 patients with an average follow-up of 5.8 months, showed similar satisfactory results.[22]

Three recent case-control studies found comparable control of reflux symptoms after surgical fundoplication or Linx implant up to 1-year follow-up. However, the fundoplication group showed a higher rate of patients who were unable to belch and vomit, along with more severe gas-bloat symptoms.[23–26]

Concerns regarding the safety of this operation, especially the fear of erosions, stem from past adverse experience with the Angelchik device and, more recently, with the gastric banding device. A recent analysis of the safety profile of the first 1000 worldwide implants in 82 hospitals showed 1.3% hospital readmission rate, 5.6% need of postoperative endoscopic dilations, and 3.4% reoperation rate.[27] All reoperations were performed on a nonemergent basis for device removal. Among the 36 patients who had the device removed, the most common symptoms were dysphagia and recurrence of reflux symptoms. In addition, 7% of patients enrolled in the US multicenter single-arm trial had the device removed due to persistent dysphagia in four, vomiting in one, chest pain in one, and reflux in one.[28] A recent study focused on reoperations for Linx removal and reported the long-term results of one-stage laparoscopic removal and fundoplication.[29] Eleven (6.7%) out of 164 patients who underwent a laparoscopic Linx implant with a median follow-up of 48 months were explanted at a later date. The main presenting symptom requiring device removal was recurrence of heartburn or regurgitation in 46%, dysphagia in 37%, and chest pain in 18%. In two patients (1.2%) full-thickness erosion of the esophageal wall with partial endoluminal penetration of the device occurred. Although the course of this complication appeared to be benign and easy to treat, it is possible that the long-term erosion rate of the Linx device will be higher than has been reported so far. The median implant duration was 20 months, with 82% of the patients being explanted between 12 and 24 months after the implant. Device removal was most commonly combined with partial fundoplication. There were no conversions to laparotomy and the postoperative course was uneventful in all patients. At the latest follow-up after reoperation (12 to 58 months), the GERD-HRQL score was within normal limits in all patients.

CONCLUSION

The Linx procedure was developed as a less disruptive and more standardized surgical option for patients who have early evidence of progressive GERD. The Linx addresses the limitations of existing medical, endoscopic, and surgical therapies, and provides a more physiologic solution to GERD with a favorable side-effect profile. The results of clinical trials have shown that augmentation of the gastroesophageal junction barrier using the Linx procedure is highly effective in decreasing esophageal acid exposure, reducing typical GERD symptoms, reducing daily PPI dependence, and improving patients' quality of life. Safety issues such as device erosions or migrations have been rare and not associated with mortality. The device can be easily removed if necessary, thereby preserving the option of fundoplication or other therapies in the future.

The Linx device is mainly intended for use in patients with unsatisfactory response to medical therapy and in those with early, uncomplicated GERD who would not usually be considered ideal candidates for fundoplication.[30,31] The potential limitations of this innovative procedure are the untested efficacy in the presence of a large hiatal hernia and Barrett esophagus, the current contraindication to undergo scanning in MRI systems greater than 1.5 Tesla, and the potential long-term consequences of a permanent foreign body implant. Future randomized trials comparing Linx and fundoplication are needed to definitely test the effectiveness of the procedure and, possibly, to establish the disease level at which lower sphincter augmentation may prove superior to reconstruction.

REFERENCES

1. Toghanian S, Johnson DA, Stalhammar NO, Zerbib F. Burden of gastro-oesophageal reflux disease in patients with persistent and intense symptoms despite proton pump inhibitor therapy: a post-hoc analysis of the 2007 national health and wellness survey. *Clin Drug Investig.* 2011;31:703-715.
2. Kahrilas PJ, Howden CW, Hughes N. Response of regurgitation to proton pump inhibitor therapy in clinical trials of gastroesophageal reflux disease. *Am J Gastroenterol.* 2011;106:1419-1425.
3. Lord R, DeMeester S, Peters J, et al. Hiatal hernia, lower esophageal sphincter incompetence, and effectiveness of Nissen fundoplication in the spectrum of gastroesophageal reflux disease. *J Gastrointest Surg.* 2009;13:602-610.
4. Malfertheiner P, Nocon M, Vieth M, et al. Evolution of gastro-oesophageal reflux disease over 5 years under routine medical care—the ProGERD study. *Aliment Pharmacol Ther.* 2012;35:154-164.
5. Heidelbaugh JJ, Kim AH, Chang R, Walker PC. Overutilization of proton-pump inhibitors: what the clinician needs to know. *Ther Adv Gastroenterol.* 2012;5(4):219-232.
6. McColl K, Gillen D. Evidence that proton-pump inhibitor therapy induces the symptoms it is used to treat. *Gastroenterology.* 2009;137:20-22.
7. Poulsen AH, Christensen S, McLaughlin JK, et al. Proton pump inhibitors and risk of gastric cancer: a population-based cohort study. *Br J Cancer.* 2009;100:1503-1507.
8. Galmiche JP, Hatlebakk J, Attwood S, et al. Laparoscopic antireflux surgery vs esomeprazole treatment for chronic GERD: the LOTUS randomized clinical trial. *JAMA.* 2011;305(19):1969-1977.
9. Niebisch S, Fleming FJ, Galey KM, et al. Perioperative risk of laparoscopic fundoplication: safer than previously reported—analysis of the American College of Surgeons National Surgical Quality Improvement Program 2005 to 2009. *J Am Coll Surg.* 2012;215: 61-69.
10. Richter JE, Dempsey DT. Laparoscopic antireflux surgery: key to success in the community setting. *Am J Gastroenterol.* 2008;103:289-291.
11. Khajanchee YS, O'Rourke R, Cassera MA, Gatta P, Hansen PD, Swanström LL. Laparoscopic reintervention for failed antireflux surgery: subjective and objective outcomes in 176 consecutive patients. *Arch Surg.* 2007;142:785-791.
12. Finks JF, Wei Y, Birkmeyer JD. The rise and fall of antireflux surgery in the United States. *Surg Endosc.* 2006;20:1698-1701.
13. Colavita PD, Belyansky I, Walters AL, et al. Nationwide inpatient sample: have antireflux procedures undergone regionalization? *J Gastrointest Surg.* 2013;17:6-13.
14. Khan F, Maradey-Romero C, Ganocy S, Frazier R, Fass R. Utilisation of surgical fundoplication for patients with gastro-oesophageal reflux disease in the USA has declined rapidly between 2009 and 2013. *Aliment Pharmacol Ther.* 2016;43:1124-1131.
15. Ganz R, Gostout C, Grudem J, Swanson W, Berg T, DeMeester TR. Use of a magnetic sphincter for the treatment of GERD: a feasibility study. *Gastrointest Endosc.* 2008;67:287-294.
16. Bonavina L, Saino G, Bona D, et al. Magnetic augmentation of the lower esophageal sphincter: results of a feasibility clinical trial. *J Gastrointest Surg.* 2008;12:2133-2140.
17. Bonavina L, DeMeester TR, Fockens P, et al. Laparoscopic sphincter augmentation device eliminates reflux symptoms and normalizes esophageal acid exposure. *Ann Surg.* 2010;252:857-862.
18. Lipham JC, DeMeester TR, Ganz RA, et al. The Linx reflux management system: confirmed safety and efficacy now at 4 years. *Surg Endosc.* 2012;26:2944-2949.
19. Saino G, Bonavina L, Lipham J, Dunn D, Ganz RA. Magnetic sphincter augmentation for gastroesophageal reflux at 5 years: final results of a pilot study show long-term acid reduction and symptom improvement. *J Laparoendosc Adv Surg Tech.* 2015;25:787-792.
20. Ganz RA, Peters JH, Horgan S, et al. Esophageal sphincter device for gastroesophageal reflux disease. *N Engl J Med.* 2013;368:719-727.
21. Bonavina L, Saino G, Bona D, Sironi A, Lazzari V. One hundred consecutive patients treated with magnetic sphincter augmentation for gastroesophageal reflux disease: 6 years of clinical experience from a single center. *J Am Coll Surg.* 2013;217:577-585.
22. Smith CD, Devault KR, Buchanan M. Introduction of mechanical sphincter augmentation for gastroesophageal reflux disease into practice: early clinical outcomes and keys to successful adoption. *J Am Coll Surg.* 2014;218:776-781.
23. Louie BE, Farivar AS, Schultz D, Brennan C, Vallières E, Aye RW. Short-term outcomes using magnetic sphincter augmentation versus Nissen fundoplication for medically resistant gastroesophageal reflux disease. *Ann Thorac Surg.* 2014;98:498-504.
24. Riegler M, Schoppman SF, Bonavina L, Ashton D, Horbach T, Kemen M. Magnetic sphincter augmentation and fundoplication

for GERD in clinical practice: one-year results of a multicenter, prospective observational study. *Surg Endosc.* 2015;29:1123-1129.

25. Reynolds J, Zehetner J, Wu P, Shah S, Bildzukewicz N, Lipham JC. Laparoscopic magnetic sphincter augmentation vs laparoscopic Nissen fundoplication; a matched-pair analysis of 100 patients. *Ann Surg.* 2015;221:123-128.

26. Asti E, Bonitta G, Lovece A, Lazzari V, Bonavina L. Longitudinal comparison of quality of life in patients undergoing laparoscopic Toupet fundoplication versus magnetic sphincter augmentation: observational cohort study with propensity score analysis. *Medicine (Baltimore).* 2016;95(30):e4366.

27. Lipham JC, Taiganides PA, Louie BE, Ganz RA, DeMeester TR. Safety analysis of first 1000 patients treated with magnetic sphincter augmentation for gastroesophageal reflux disease. *Dis Esophagus.* 2015;28:305-311.

28. Ganz RA, Edmundowicz SA, Taiganides PA, et al. Long-term outcomes of patients receiving a magnetic sphincter augmentation device for gastroesophageal reflux. *Clin Gastroenterol Hepatol.* 2016;14:671-677.

29. Asti E, Siboni S, Lazzari V, Bonitta G, Sironi A, Bonavina L. Removal of the magnetic sphincter device. Surgical technique and results of a single-center cohort study. *Ann Surg.* 2016;doi:10.1097/SLA.0000000000001785.

30. Worrel SG, Greene CL, DeMeester TR. The state of surgical treatment of gastroesophageal reflux disease after five decades. *J Am Coll Surg.* 2014;219:819-830.

31. Bonavina L, Attwood S. Laparoscopic alternatives to fundoplication for gastroesophageal reflux: the role of magnetic augmentation and electrical stimulation of the lower esophageal sphincter. *Dis Esophagus.* 2015;29(8):996-1001. doi:10.1111/dote.12425.

Endoscopic Management of Gastroesophageal Reflux Disease

Aaron Richman | Praveen Sridhar | Hiran C. Fernando

Gastroesophageal reflux disease (GERD) is defined by the reflux of gastric fluid into the esophagus causing troublesome symptoms and/or complications, such as mucosal inflammation and metaplasia.[1] Functional disturbances of the lower esophageal sphincter (LES), along with anatomic abnormalities of the esophagogastric junction (EGJ) such as hiatal hernia, allow the reflux of gastric fluid up into the esophagus. Treatment of GERD is focused on providing relief of symptoms and reducing reflux-related mucosal injury. The choice of treatment modality is based on symptom severity, the degree of esophageal injury, the presence and severity of hiatal hernia, and the degree of esophageal dysmotility.

The mainstay of therapy is medical with gastric acid suppression through the use of proton pump inhibitors (PPIs). PPIs are recommended as first-line therapy based on their rapid impact on symptoms and efficient control of esophageal inflammation. PPIs have a well-known safety profile that allows for long-term use. Such additional measures as weight loss, head-of-bed elevation, and elimination of food triggers are also used but are less effective. Because none of the medical therapies address the incompetent LES, their efficacy is somewhat limited.[2,3]

Surgical therapy is the preferred treatment in patients with recalcitrant symptoms, especially those with esophagitis, Barrett esophagus, or extraesophageal pathology. Surgical repair includes two fundamental principles: restoration of the gastroesophageal flap valve (Fig. 21.1) with reinforcement of the LES and placement of the EGJ below the diaphragm. Laparoscopic fundoplication with correction of the hiatal hernia, if indicated, is the gold standard, with well-established efficacy. Postoperative dysphagia and gas-bloat syndrome continue to be troublesome side effects for surgical fundoplication despite modifications to the original procedure.[4] Over the past 10 to 15 years a number of endoscopic approaches have been developed to treat GERD and will be described in this review.

INDICATIONS FOR ENDOSCOPIC THERAPY OF GASTROESOPHAGEAL REFLUX DISEASE

Endoscopic antireflux (EAR) procedures aim to reinforce the mechanical antireflux barrier, thereby reducing symptoms and preventing pathologic progression of esophagitis. Indications for EAR intervention are similar to those for surgical intervention, namely relapsing or recalcitrant symptoms despite adequate medical therapy, PPI intolerance, desire to stop chronic drug therapy, and progressive esophagitis. In addition, there are patients who want to avoid surgical fundoplication and the associated side effects, such as dysphagia, bloating, or meteorism, and who will seek an EAR approach. Endoscopic therapy also provides a less invasive option for patients who are not good candidates for laparoscopic interventions due to previous laparotomies, or are not candidates for open repair due to medical comorbidities. In addition, there may be situations when patients with recurrent reflux after an operative fundoplication may find benefit from EAR therapy.

Due to the limitations of endoscopic manipulation, patients with hiatal hernias larger than 2 cm and GERD are not candidates for endoscopic therapy and are best managed with a standard laparoscopic repair. Patients with moderate to severe mucosal inflammation (Los Angeles endoscopic classification grade C and D), as well as patients with Barrett esophagitis, have been excluded from most studies evaluating EAR therapies. Although these characteristics are not an absolute contraindication to an EAR approach, the efficacy for these patients is not yet known.

TECHNIQUES

The primary endoscopic therapies for GERD can be classified into three major categories: (1) endoscopic suturing or plication (full or partial thickness), (2) thermal remodeling and neurolysis of the LES zone by radiofrequency energy delivery, and (3) bulking or reinforcement of the LES zone by injection of inert material. These methods, along with a recently described technique using endoscopic mucosal resection (EMR), will be examined next.

ENDOSCOPIC PLICATION

Endoscopic suturing techniques were first described in the 1980s when Swain and colleagues developed a miniature sewing machine that attached to the end of a standard upper gastrointestinal endoscope.[5] The first US Food and Drug Administration (FDA)-approved method for treating GERD was an endoscopic suturing method introduced by Bard (Murray Hill, New Jersey) under the name EndoCinch. This method was the commercial version of the miniature sewing machine as developed by Swain and Mills in London. This technique involved a partial-thickness plication on the gastric side of the EGJ.[6] Clinical outcomes with the EndoCinch have generally been marginal.[7] As a result, the EndoCinch, like many endoscopic therapies, has been withdrawn from clinical use.

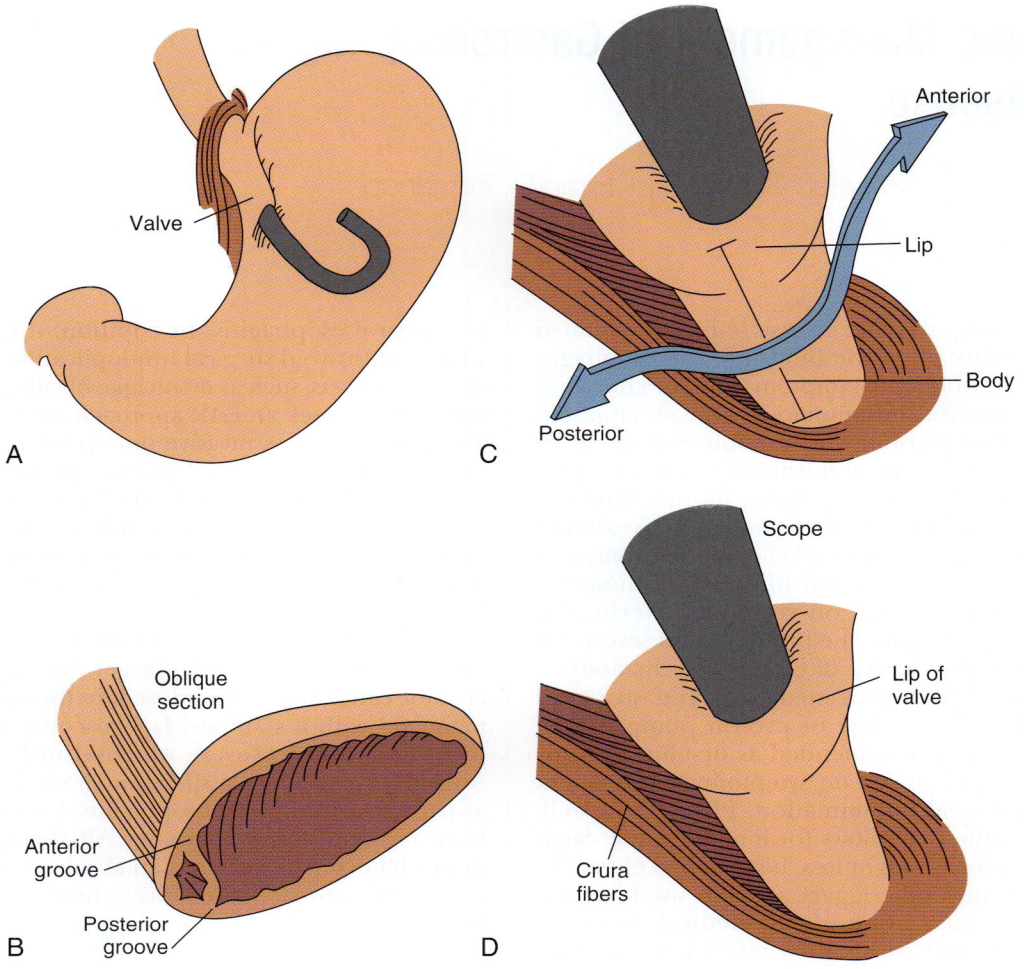

FIGURE 21.1 Endoscopic appraisal of the gastroesophageal flap valve. (Redrawn from Jobe BA, Kahrilas PJ, Vernon AH, et al. Endoscopic appraisal of the gastroesophageal valve after antireflux surgery. *Am J Gastroenterol.* 2004;99:233.).

Currently there are two endoscopic plication systems that are FDA approved for patients with reflux. These are the Medigus Ultrasonic Endostapling system (MUSE; Medigus, Omer, Israel) and the EsophyX device (Endo-gastric Solutions, Redmond, Washington). Each is described later.

Medigus Ultrasonic Endostapling System (MUSE) Method

The MUSE system uses an endostapler (titanium 4.8-mm staples), ultrasonic range finder, insufflation pump, suction-irrigation, and an endoscopic console (Fig. 21.2). Compared with the EsophyX device, the MUSE is a single operator system with the fundoplication completed in the supine position. The stapler is inserted transorally through a rigid overtube, advanced under direct vision into the stomach, and retroflexed once the stapler is 5 cm past the EGJ to view the gastric fundus and the EGJ. An anchoring staple is placed between the fundus and the esophagus at the left lateral position, with subsequent stapling at 60 to 180 degrees along the circumference of the EGJ.[8]

There are limited long-term data examining the effectiveness of the MUSE system. Zacherl et al. examined 69 patients prospectively from six centers who underwent transoral fundoplication with the MUSE system using GERD Health-Related Quality of Life (HRQL) question-naires, PPI dose reduction, and pH monitoring as their objective measures of outcome, with the most notable exclusion criteria being patients who had hiatal hernias larger than or equal to 3 cm. A reduction of at least 50% in GERD-HRQL scores was achieved in 73% of patients at 6-month follow-up. In addition, 65% of patients were no longer using PPIs, and 85% of patients were able to halve their dose. Esophageal pH studies showed a signifi-cant post-procedure reduction in the number of episodes of reflux, as well as a reduction in the total time of pH less than 4.[9] Kim et al. then updated results in this same cohort of patients at 4 years. Thirty-seven of the initial cohort of patients were followed for a total of 4 years. At follow-up, 69% of patients remained off daily PPIs and mean HRQL scores remained significantly reduced. No patients required repeat procedures or conversion to laparoscopic fundoplication.[10] Similar findings were

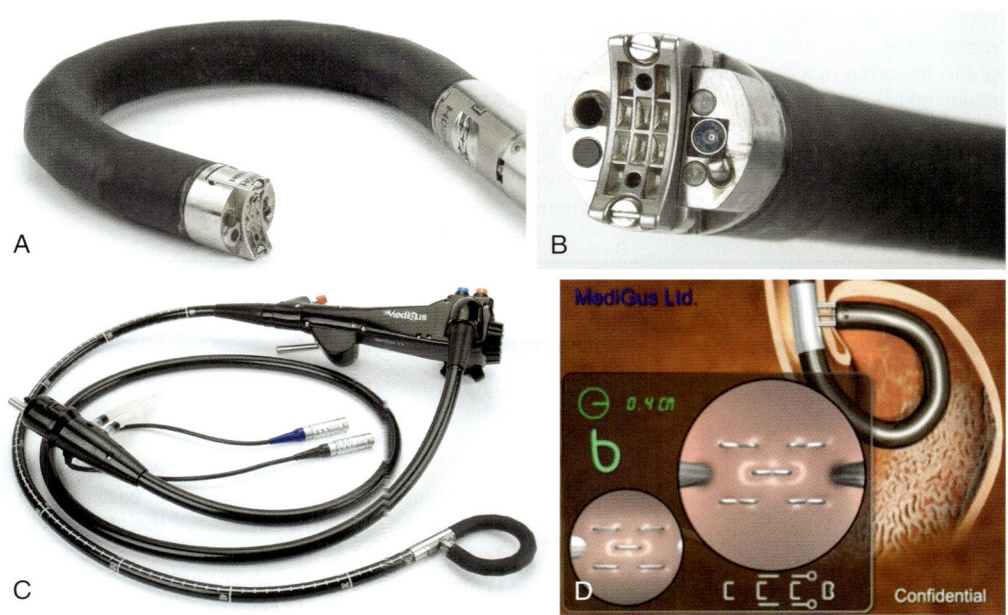

FIGURE 21.2 The Medigus SRS device. (A to C) This procedure is done by using an adapted endoscope that has two stapler components; the anvil is located at the tip and the cartridge is located at the shaft. Their accurate alignment is guided by ultrasonic sights. (D) The endoscope is inserted transorally, and the top of the fundus is caught by the anvil located at the tip of the device and brought against the shaft, which contains the stapler cartridge that is fired with standard 4.8-mm staples. The device is then partially withdrawn, rotated 120 degrees, and the procedure is repeated. (From http://www.medigus.com/AboutGerd/GERD.aspx.)

described by Roy-Shapira et al. in a small cohort of patients followed out to 5 years.[11] The most significant complications encountered were empyema and pneumothorax in one patient and bleeding requiring transfusion from an endoscopically unidentified source in one patient.[9,10]

EsophyX Transoral Incisionless Fundoplication

Clinical experience has been greater with the EsophyX system, and currently this is the most widely used endoscopic approach in the United States. Reports with follow-up as long as 6 years are now available for the EsophyX technique.[12] The device is composed of a handle, a chassis containing a channel for passage of the endoscope, a tissue invaginator, a tissue mold, a screw, and stylets through which fasteners can be deployed. Patients are positioned in left lateral decubitus position, and completion of the procedure requires two operators—one to operate the endoscope and one to handle the instrument. After insertion of the instrument, the stomach is insufflated and the instrument retroflexed. The tissue mold creates apposition between the stomach and the EsophyX device within the esophageal lumen, and polypropylene fasteners are deployed as the greater curve is rotated within the tissue mold and around the EGJ to create a new valve with a circumference of greater than 240 degrees (Fig. 21.3A).[8,13,14]

Although there have been a small number of studies examining the long-term safety and effectiveness of fundoplication using the MUSE, there have been considerably more data regarding the use of the EsophyX device. There have been several prospective studies that have examined long-term outcomes after transoral fundoplication with the EsophyX device up to 6 years postoperatively.[12] Most recently, Witteman et al. prospectively compared

transoral incisionless fundoplication (TIF) with maximal medical therapy in a randomized controlled trial, using GERD-HRQL as well as postoperative pH studies as end points. Patients treated with TIF experienced significantly improved quality-of-life (QoL) scores despite showing a lack of improvement in esophageal acid exposure.[15] Most studies demonstrated effectiveness and safety of TIF at 6-, 12-, and 24-month follow-up because 61% to 93% of patients in these studies were able to discontinue these medications (follow-up endoscopic findings seen in Fig. 21.3B). Furthermore, symptom response was shown in 86% of patients followed up to 6 years in one study.[12,16–19] Notably, factors that negatively impacted outcomes in patients undergoing TIF were hiatal hernias larger than 2 cm and preoperative Hill esophageal valve grade of III or IV.[12]

Our group previously reported on our early experience with the EsophyX procedure in 46 patients.[20] One patient was readmitted with an aspiration pneumonia, and three patients had minor complications. Mean GERD-HRQL scores improved significantly (23 vs. 7), and 4 (8.6%) patients had no improvement in symptoms. More recently we have looked at longer follow-up (mean 24 months) in 41 patients (unpublished data—currently submitted). Among these 41 patients, 63% had either stopped or reduced their PPI dose (Table 21.1).

RADIOFREQUENCY ABLATION

The Stretta system was one of the first endoscopic approaches introduced into clinical practice and is still currently available. It is believed that radiofrequency ablation induces a thickened scar and that augments the LES. This is based on animal data demonstrating that the

FIGURE 21.3 The EsophyX device. (A) The EsophyX device is inserted into the gastric cavity and positioned into the cardia. A retractor is applied to the gastroesophageal flap valve. A flexible endoscope serves for viewing the procedure (1). The gastroesophageal flap valve is retracted and brought to the arms of the device (2). The device is closed and the H-shape fasteners are deployed (3 and 4). The device is retracted (5). Final antireflux valve configuration after finishing the procedure, showing enlargement of the gastroesophageal flap valve (6). (B) Endoscopic view of the cardia; the *top photos* show pre-EsophyX procedure; the *bottom photos* show 12 months after treatment. ([A] Redrawn from Cadière GB, Buset M, Muls V, et al. Antireflux transoral incisionless fundoplication using EsophyX: 12-month results of a prospective multicenter study. *World J Surg.* 2008;32:1676; [B] from Cadière GB, Rajan A, Germay O, et al. Endoluminal fundoplication by a transoral device for the treatment of GERD: a feasibility study. *Surg Endosc.* 2008;22:333.)

TABLE 21.1 Current Data Regarding the Efficacy and Durability of Transoral Incisionless Fundoplication (TIF)

Author	Year	Study Type	N	Follow-Up (months)	Preoperative GERD-HRQL	Last Recorded Postoperative GERD-HRQL	Percentage Reduction of Postoperative PPI Use at Last Follow-Up	Percentage Postoperative Normalization of pH
Cadière et al.	2008	Prospective	84	12	24 (median)	7 (median)	68%	37%
Cadière et al.	2009	Prospective	19	24	17 (median)	7 (median)	—	—
Testoni et al.	2010	Prospective	20	6	45 (mean)	16 (mean)	78%	—
Velanovich et al.	2010	Retrospective	24	7 (mean)	25 (median)	5 (median)	79%	—
Repici et al.	2010	Prospective	20	12	40 (median)	7 (median)	47%	—
Demyttanaere et al.	2010	Retrospective	26	10 (mean)	22 (mean)	10 (mean)	55%	—
Hoppo et al.	2010	Retrospective	19	11 (mean)	—	—	42%	—
Barnes et al.	2011	Retrospective	124	7 (median)	28 (median)	2 (median)	93%	—
Bell et al	2011	Retrospective	37	6 (median)	16 (median)	4 (median)	82%	61%
Ihde et al.	2011	Retrospective	48	6 (median)	29 (median)	3 (median)	76%	—
Trad et al.	2012	Retrospective	34	14 (median)	26 (median)	4 (median)	82%	—
Testoni et al.	2012	Retrospective	35	27 (mean)	22 (mean)	18 (mean)	69.2%	—
Petersen et al.	2012	Retrospective	23	7 (median)	—	—	42%	26%
Bell et al.	2012	Prospective	100	6	26 (median)	4 (median)	89%	54%
Muls et al.	2013	Prospective	86	36	25 (median)	6 (median)	61%	82%*
Trad et al.[†]	2014	Prospective	63	6	19 (median)	2 (median)	95%	54%
Testoni et al.	2015	Prospective	50	53 (mean)	20 (mean)	17 (mean)[‡]	86%[‡]	—

*11 of the initially enrolled 86 patients underwent pH testing at 3-year follow-up, 9 of whom had normalization.
[†]Trad et al. recently (2016) published updated results at 30 months of follow-up for patients undergoing TIF in this initial TEMPO trial showing GERD Health-Related Quality of Life (HRQL) scores improving to 5 (median) and 70% of patients completely off PPIs.
[‡]GERD-HRQL scores completed at 36-month follow-up: at 6-year follow-up; 12 of 14 patients had stopped or halved proton pump inhibition (PPI) use.[12,13,16–19,21–31]

fibrosis from chemical sclerosants reduces compliance and relaxation of the gastroesophageal junction and reduces reflux.[32,33]

The Stretta system is an endoscopic instrument that uses radiofrequency ablation to treat GERD. Originally introduced in 2000, the device and its protocols have been refined over the years to improve its efficacy and safety.[34] The device is composed of a flexible balloon basket assembly with four electrode needle sheaths introduced orally that delivers radiofrequency energy to the muscular layer of the EGJ. The device and electrodes are positioned in the distal esophagus, the needles are deployed into the circular muscle layer, and radiofrequency energy is delivered (Fig. 21.4). The delivery of heat is controlled using thermocouples at the base and tip of each needle with a target temperature of 85°C. The mucosa is protected from thermal injury by maintaining its temperature less than 50°C using concurrent irrigation.[35] Serial applications are repeated every 0.5 cm such that an area approximately 2 cm above and below the squamocolumnar junction receives treatment.[36] Treatment can be repeated if there is not substantial improvement in symptoms.

The therapeutic effect appears to occur via two primary mechanisms. Anatomically, the heating causes collagen contraction, yielding a mechanical alteration of the EGJ and a tightening of the LES. There is an associated increase in smooth muscle fiber size with larger fibers and more smooth muscle cells per bundle. This effect can be seen immediately after the procedure, and the collagen deposition continues up to 12 months as wound healing ensues. Physiologically, there is ablation of aberrant esophageal nerve pathways leading to an increase in both LES pressure and gastric yield pressure, as well as a decrease in transient LES relaxation.[37–39] In addition, an improvement in gastroparesis associated with GERD has been noted after ablation. It is not clear what the mechanism of this effect is, but likely it is related to vagal neurolysis.[40]

Multiple studies, including a multicenter sham-controlled randomized trial, have demonstrated the Stretta

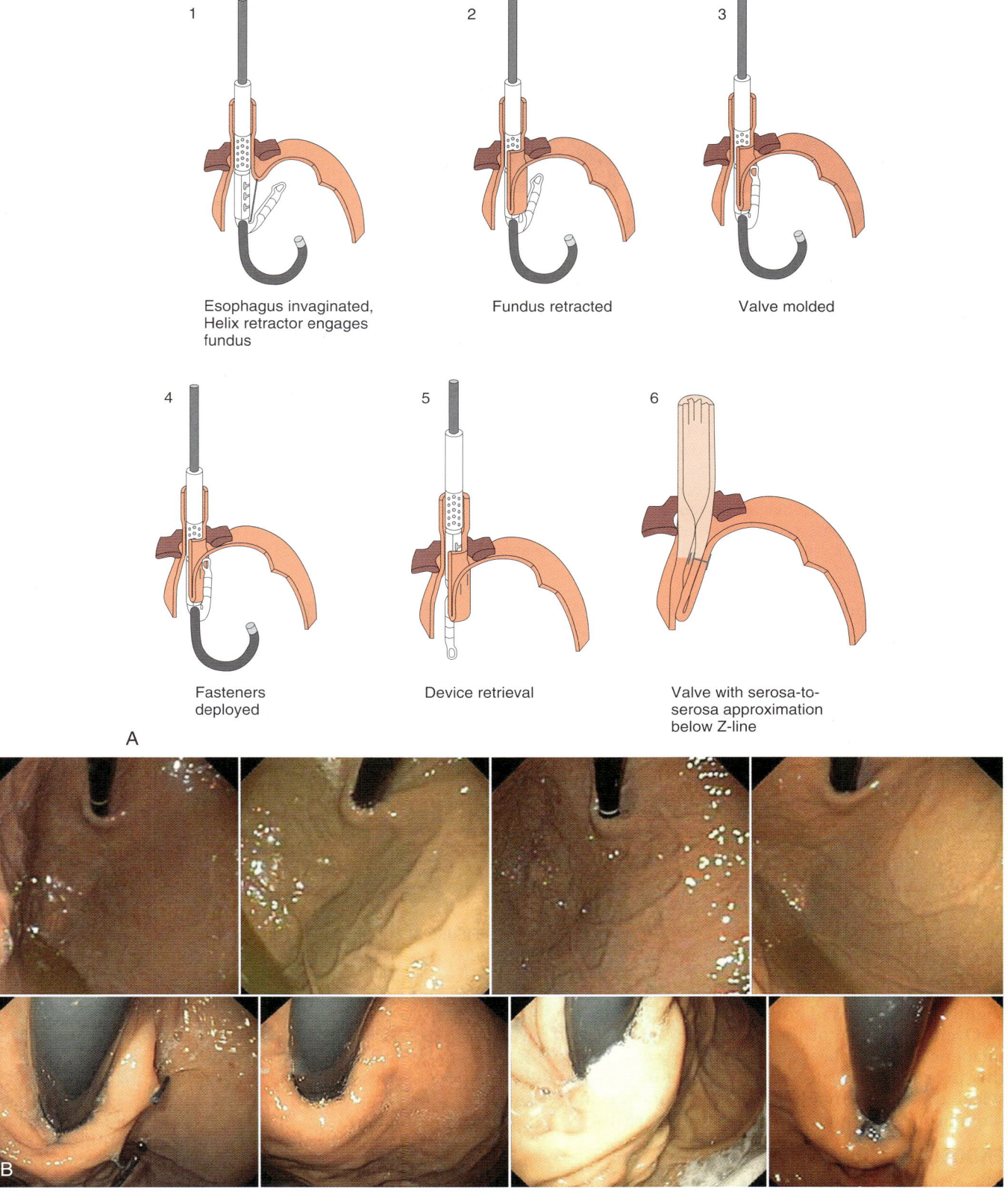

1 Esophagus invaginated, Helix retractor engages fundus

2 Fundus retracted

3 Valve molded

4 Fasteners deployed

5 Device retrieval

6 Valve with serosa-to-serosa approximation below Z-line

A

B

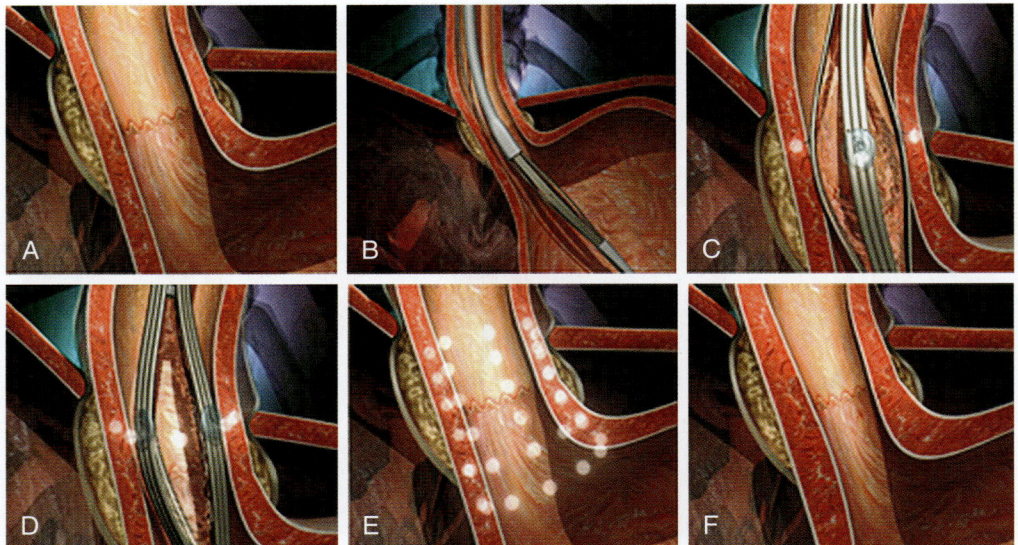

FIGURE 21.4 The Stretta procedure. (A) The gastroesophageal junction is inspected and measured. (B) The radiofrequency catheter is introduced over the guidewire. (C) The balloon is inflated proximal to the squamocolumnar junction, and the electrode needles are used for delivering radiofrequency energy for more than 90 seconds for a desired tissue temperature of 85°C. (D) The needles are then withdrawn, the balloon is deflated, the scope is rotated 45 degrees, and the procedure is repeated. (E) These steps should be serially repeated every 0.5 cm such that an area covering 2 cm above and 1.5 cm below the squamocolumnar junction receives treatment. (F) Postprocedure changes such as enlargement of the muscular layer at the esophagogastric junction area can be expected. (From Hogan WJ. Endoscopic therapy for gastroesophageal reflux disease. *Curr Gastroenterol Rep.* 2003;5:206.)

system is a safe and effective treatment for GERD. Adverse events associated with radiofrequency ablation are mostly transient and mild. The most common include bleeding, mucosal injury, chest pain, fever, dysphagia, and effusion.[35] When evaluated at 6 to 12 months, the procedure significantly improved heartburn symptoms and GERD-specific QoL and decreased the need for PPI therapy.[34,41–44] Preexisting Barrett metaplasia regressed in a set of patients evaluated with endoscopic biopsy.[45] Despite a number of smaller studies showing excellent results with greater than 70% of patients remaining off PPIs and continued high QoL scores out to 10 years, the long-term durability of the intervention remains somewhat controversial.[44–47] Two independently performed meta-analyses found conflicting results for symptomatic relief, reduction of acid exposure, and QoL scores beyond 48 months from therapy.[43,48] When Stretta is compared head to head with surgical treatments, fundoplication demonstrated improved symptomatic relief, elimination of PPI use, and overall satisfaction, albeit with slightly higher rates of adverse events.[49–51]

Overall the ease of the procedure, efficacy, and low incidence of complication or adverse events have made this procedure an attractive option for appropriately selected patients. In addition, it does not preclude subsequent surgical intervention for refractory disease.

ENDOSCOPIC BULKING TECHNIQUES

The principle of these techniques is to create a mechanical barrier in the EGJ and augment the LES so as to prevent gastroesophageal reflux. Three products have been used: (1) biopolymer augmentation (Enteryx), (2) polymethylmethacrylate (PMMA) implantation, and (3) expandable hydrogel prosthesis (Gatekeeper Reflux

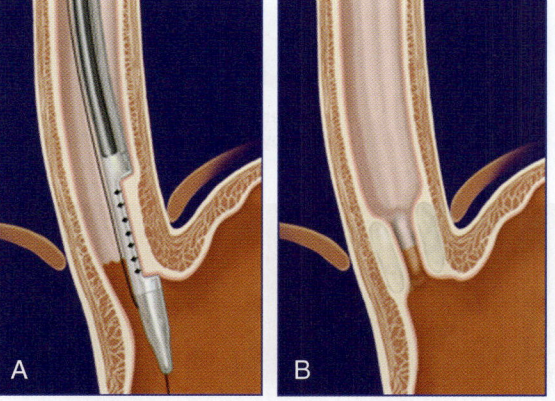

FIGURE 21.5 The Gatekeeper procedure. (A) Insertion of the delivering system positioned at the esophagogastric junction. (B) Bulking effect seen at esophagogastric junction after the device being deployed and fully expanded. (Modified from Fockens P, Cohen L, Edmundowicz SA, et al. Prospective randomized controlled trial of an injectable esophageal prosthesis versus a sham procedure for endoscopic treatment of gastroesophageal reflux disease. *Surg Endosc.* 2010;24:1387.)

Repair System) (Fig. 21.5). Enteryx was the first product to be approved by the FDA (Fig. 21.6). Although each showed initially promising results, all have subsequently been taken off the market due to poor durability and significant complications.[52,53]

ANTIREFLUX MUCOSECTOMY

Antireflux mucosectomy (ARMS) is a new EAR approach currently being investigated in Japan. Based on their

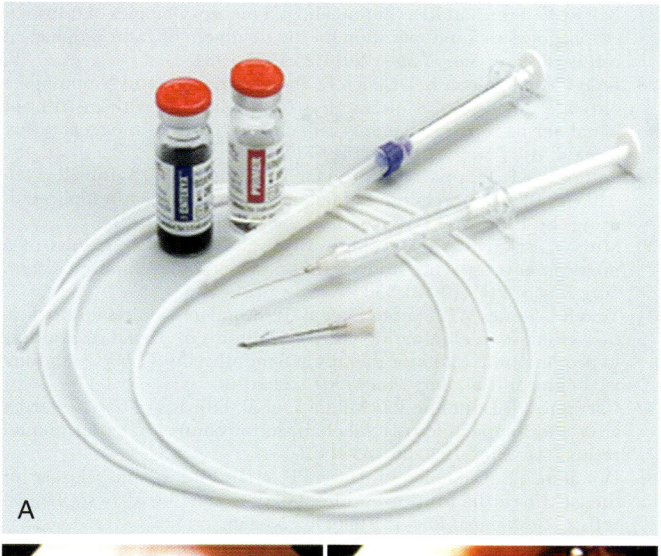

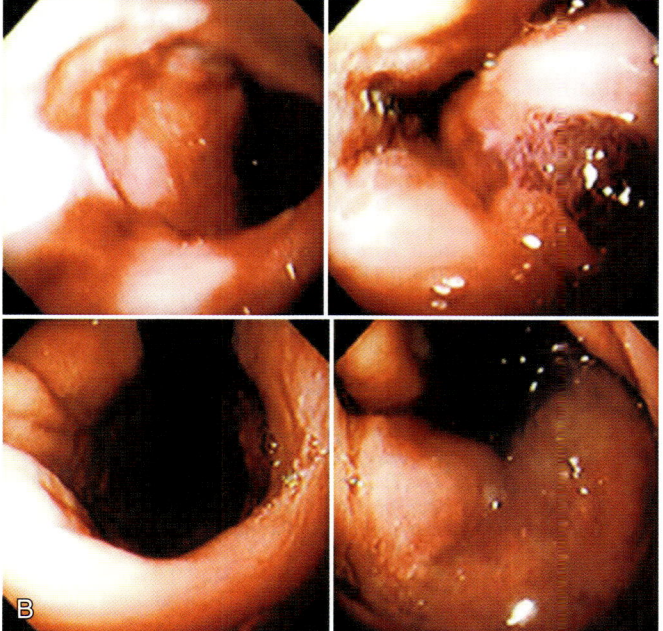

FIGURE 21.6 EnteryX procedure. (A) Flasks containing injectable solution of 8% ethylene vinyl alcohol copolymer and dimethyl sulfoxide and dedicated endoscopic needles for injection. (B) Bulking effect at the esophagogastric junction after intramuscular injection. (From Hogan WJ. Endoscopic therapy for gastroesophageal reflux disease. *Curr Gastroenterol Rep.* 2003; 5:206.)

experiences with EMR and endoscopic submucosal dissection (ESD) for management of Barrett esophagitis, Inoue et al. performed a pilot study to evaluate the use of this technique for management of GERD. Their previous studies had demonstrated improved reflux symptoms thought to be related to the stricture formation along the resected segment. Currently ARMS is performed using EMR and ESD of at least 3-cm length (1 cm in the esophagus and 2 cm in the stomach), with the length of mucosal resection at the cardia measured in retroflexion from the gastric side. To preserve the sharp mucosal valve at the cardia, a hemicircumferential, crescentic resection is performed along the lesser curve of the stomach.[54,55]

Although small, the studies evaluating ARMS have demonstrated encouraging results. GERD symptoms improved significantly. The DeMeester scores for heartburn and regurgitation decreased from 2.7 to 0.3 and from 2.5 to 0.3, respectively. Evaluations of esophageal pH showed that the fraction of time at pH less than 4 improved from 29.1% to 3.1%. Follow-up endoscopy performed at 2 months demonstrated well-healed mucosa with improved appearance of the flap valve. Balloon dilation was required to manage stenosis in two cases in which total circumferential resection was performed. All patients were off of PPIs at the completion of the trial.[54–56]

These early, uncontrolled data from experienced endoscopists show promising results. However, larger controlled trials with longer-term follow-up will be needed to validate the procedure's efficacy and safety, particularly if this approach is adopted by other physicians.

CONCLUSION

Over the past decade, EAR therapies have emerged as an alternative therapy for patients suffering from GERD. Initially there was great interest in these approaches; however, several of the techniques introduced earlier into practice have been abandoned either because of poor efficacy or adverse outcomes. A few approaches, such as the EsophyX, are still being used in several centers, and the introduction of new techniques, such as ARMS, suggests that physicians and patients have continued interest in an incisionless approach to treat GERD. Although there are only a few large studies, the data for these techniques show promise. The currently available techniques appear safe, with an acceptable and manageable side effect profile. Refinements in technology and technique for radiofrequency ablation and endoscopic plication appear to have improved their efficacy. With more experience, further improvements with EAR instrumentation and technique may also be expected. The long-term durability of EAR remains a challenge, and well-controlled studies will need to be performed to ensure that insurance providers are willing to pay for EAR as a routine therapy. Although use of these techniques remains confined mostly to research protocols and specialized centers, the large number of patients with GERD who fail to see complete resolution with current medical therapies but who are willing to pursue or are not candidates for surgical therapy will drive continued adoption and research.

REFERENCES

1. Vakil N, van Zanten SV, Kahrilas P, Dent J, Jones R. The Montreal definition and classification of gastroesophageal reflux disease: a global evidence-based consensus. *Am J Gastroenterol.* 2006;101:1900-1920; quiz 1943.
2. Katz PO, Gerson LB, Vela MF. Guidelines for the diagnosis and management of gastroesophageal reflux disease. *Am J Gastroenterol.* 2013;108:308-328.
3. Kahrilas PJ, Shaheen NJ, Vaezi MF. American Gastroenterological Association Institute technical review on the management of gastroesophageal reflux disease. *Gastroenterology.* 2008;135:1392-1413.
4. Zaninotto G, Attwood SEA. Surgical management of refractory gastro-oesophageal reflux. *Br J Surg.* 2010;97:139-140.

5. Paul SC, Mills TN. An endoscopic sewing machine. *Gastrointest Endosc.* 1986;32:36-38.

6. Swain CP, Brown GJ, Mills TN. An endoscopic stapling device: the development of a new flexible endoscopically controlled device for placing multiple transmural staples in gastrointestinal tissue. *Gastrointest Endosc.* 1989;35:338-339.

7. Filipi CJ, Lehman GA, Rothstein RI, et al. Transoral, flexible endoscopic suturing for treatment of GERD: a multicenter trial. *Gastrointest Endosc.* 2001;53:416-422.

8. Testoni PA, Mazzoleni G, Testoni SGG. Transoral incisionless fundoplication for gastro-esophageal reflux disease: techniques and outcomes. *World J Gastrointest Pharmacol Ther.* 2016;7:179-189.

9. Zacherl J, Roy-Shapira A, Bonavina L, et al. Endoscopic anterior fundoplication with the Medigus Ultrasonic Surgical Endostapler (MUSE™) for gastroesophageal reflux disease: 6-month results from a multi-center prospective trial. *Surg Endosc.* 2015;29:220-229.

10. Kim HJ, Kwon CI, Kessler WR, et al. Long-term follow-up results of endoscopic treatment of gastroesophageal reflux disease with the MUSE™ endoscopic stapling device. *Surg Endosc.* 2015;doi:10.1007/s00464-015-4622-y.

11. Roy-Shapira A, Bapaye A, Date S, Pujari R, Dorwat S. Trans-oral anterior fundoplication: 5-year follow-up of pilot study. *Surg Endosc.* 2015;29:3717-3721.

12. Testoni PA, Testoni S, Mazzoleni G, Vailati C, Passaretti S. Long-term efficacy of transoral incisionless fundoplication with EsophyX (Tif 2.0) and factors affecting outcomes in GERD patients followed for up to 6 years: a prospective single-center study. *Surg Endosc.* 2015;29:2770-2780.

13. Testoni PA, Vailati C, Testoni S, Corsetti M. Transoral incisionless fundoplication (TIF 2.0) with EsophyX for gastroesophageal reflux disease: long-term results and findings affecting outcome. *Surg Endosc.* 2012;26:1425-1435.

14. Cadière GB, Rajan A, Rqibate M, et al. Endoluminal fundoplication (ELF)—evolution of EsophyX, a new surgical device for transoral surgery. *Minim Invasive Ther Allied Technol.* 2006;15:348-355.

15. Witteman BPL, Conchillo JM, Rinsma NF, et al. Randomized controlled trial of transoral incisionless fundoplication vs. proton pump inhibitors for treatment of gastroesophageal reflux disease. *Am J Gastroenterol.* 2015;110:531-542.

16. Bell RCW, Mavrelis PG, Barnes WE, et al. A prospective multicenter registry of patients with chronic gastroesophageal reflux disease receiving transoral incisionless fundoplication. *J Am Coll Surg.* 2012;215:794-809.

17. Trad KS, Turgeon DG, Deljkich E. Long-term outcomes after transoral incisionless fundoplication in patients with GERD and LPR symptoms. *Surg Endosc.* 2012;26:650-660.

18. Cadière GB, Buset M, Muls V, et al. Antireflux transoral incisionless fundoplication using EsophyX: 12-month results of a prospective multicenter study. *World J Surg.* 2008;32:1676-1688.

19. Repici A, Fumagalli U, Malesci A, Barbera R, Gambaro C, Rosati R. Endoluminal fundoplication (ELF) for GERD using EsophyX: a 12-month follow-up in a single-center experience. *J Gastrointest Surg.* 2010;14:1-6.

20. Narsule CK, Burch MA, Ebright MI, et al. Endoscopic fundoplication for the treatment of gastroesophageal reflux disease: initial experience. *J Thorac Cardiovasc Surg.* 2012;143:228-234.

21. Cadière GB, Van Sante N, Graves JE, Gawlicka AK, Rajan A. Two-year results of a feasibility study on antireflux transoral incisionless fundoplication using EsophyX. *Surg Endosc.* 2009;23:957-964.

22. Testoni PA, Corsetti M, Di Pietro S, et al. Effect of transoral incisionless fundoplication on symptoms, PPI use, and pH-impedance refluxes of GERD patients. *World J Surg.* 2010;34:750-757.

23. Velanovich V. Endoscopic, endoluminal fundoplication for gastroesophageal reflux disease: initial experience and lessons learned. *Surgery.* 2010;148:646-653.

24. Demyttenaere SV, Bergman S, Pham T, et al. Transoral incisionless fundoplication for gastroesophageal reflux disease in an unselected patient population. *Surg Endosc.* 2010;24:854-858.

25. Hoppo T, Immanuel A, Schuchert M, et al. Transoral incisionless fundoplication 2.0 procedure using EsophyX™ for gastroesophageal reflux disease. *J Gastrointest Surg.* 2010;14:1895-1901.

26. Barnes WE, Hoddinott KM, Mundy S, Williams M. Transoral incisionless fundoplication offers high patient satisfaction and relief of therapy-resistant typical and atypical symptoms of GERD in community practice. *Surg Innov.* 2011;18:119-129.

27. Bell RCW, Freeman KD. Clinical and pH-metric outcomes of transoral esophagogastric fundoplication for the treatment of gastroesophageal reflux disease. *Surg Endosc.* 2011;25:1975-1984.

28. Ihde GM, Besancon K, Deljkich E. Short-term safety and symptomatic outcomes of transoral incisionless fundoplication with or without hiatal hernia repair in patients with chronic gastroesophageal reflux disease. *Am J Surg.* 2011;202:740-747.

29. Petersen RP, Filippa L, Wassenaar EB, Martin AV, Tatum R, Oelschlager BK. Comprehensive evaluation of endoscopic fundoplication using the EsophyX™ device. *Surg Endosc.* 2012;26:1021-1027.

30. Muls V, Eckardt AJ, Marchese M, et al. Three-year results of a multicenter prospective study of transoral incisionless fundoplication. *Surg Innov.* 2013;20:321-330.

31. Trad KS, Barnes WE, Simoni G, et al. Transoral incisionless fundoplication effective in eliminating GERD symptoms in partial responders to proton pump inhibitor therapy at 6 months: the TEMPO randomized clinical trial. *Surg Innov.* 2015;22:26-40.

32. Carvalho PJ, Donahue PE, Miidla I, et al. Fibrosis of gastric cardia after endoscopic sclerosis. Mechanism for control of experimental reflux? *Am Surg.* 1990;56:163-166.

33. Donahue PE, Carvalho PJ, Davis PE, et al. Endoscopic sclerosis of the gastric cardia for prevention of experimental gastroesophageal reflux. *Gastrointest Endosc.* 1990;36:253-256.

34. Aziz AMA, El-Khayat HR, Sadek A, et al. A prospective randomized trial of sham, single-dose Stretta, and double-dose Stretta for the treatment of gastroesophageal reflux disease. *Surg Endosc.* 2010;24:818-825.

35. Yeh RW, Triadafilopoulos G. Endoscopic antireflux therapy: the Stretta procedure. *Thorac Surg Clin.* 2005;15:395-403.

36. Go MR, Dundon JM, Karlowicz DJ, Domingo CB, Muscarella P, Melvin WS, et al. Delivery of radiofrequency energy to the lower esophageal sphincter improves symptoms of gastroesophageal reflux. *Surgery.* 2004;136:786-794.

37. DiBaise JK, Brand RE, Quigley EMM. Endoluminal delivery of radiofrequency energy to the gastroesophageal junction in uncomplicated GERD: efficacy and potential mechanism of action. *Am J Gastroenterol.* 2002;97:833-842.

38. Tam WCE. Delivery of radiofrequency energy to the lower oesophageal sphincter and gastric cardia inhibits transient lower oesophageal sphincter relaxations and gastro-oesophageal reflux in patients with reflux disease. *Gut.* 2003;52:479-485.

39. Utley DS, Kim M, Vierra MA, Triadafilopoulos G. Augmentation of lower esophageal sphincter pressure and gastric yield pressure after radiofrequency energy delivery to the gastroesophageal junction: a porcine model. *Gastrointest Endosc.* 2000;52:81-86.

40. Noar MD, Noar E. Gastroparesis associated with gastroesophageal reflux disease and corresponding reflux symptoms may be corrected by radiofrequency ablation of the cardia and esophagogastric junction. *Surg Endosc.* 2008;22:2440-2444.

41. Corley DA, Katz P, Wo JM, et al. Improvement of gastroesophageal reflux symptoms after radiofrequency energy: a randomized, sham-controlled trial. *Gastroenterology.* 2003;125:668-676.

42. Wolfsen HC, Richards WO. The Stretta procedure for the treatment of GERD: a registry of 558 patients. *J Laparoendosc Adv Surg Tech A.* 2002;12:395-402.

43. Perry KA, Banerjee A, Melvin WS. Radiofrequency energy delivery to the lower esophageal sphincter reduces esophageal acid exposure and improves GERD symptoms. *Surg Laparosc Endosc Percutan Tech.* 2012;22:283-288.

44. Dughera L, Rotondano G, De Cento M, Cassolino P, Cisar F. Durability of Stretta radiofrequency treatment for GERD: results of an 8-year follow-up. *Gastroenterol Res Pract.* 2014;2014:531907.

45. Noar M, Squires P, Noar E, Lee M. Long-term maintenance effect of radiofrequency energy delivery for refractory GERD: a decade later. *Surg Endosc.* 2014;28:2323-2333.

46. Dughera L, Navino M, Cassolino P, et al. Long-term results of radiofrequency energy delivery for the treatment of GERD: results of a prospective 48-month study. *Diagn Ther Endosc.* 2011;2011:507157.

47. Reymunde A, Santiago N. Long-term results of radiofrequency energy delivery for the treatment of GERD: sustained improvements in symptoms, quality of life, and drug use at 4-year follow-up. *Gastrointest Endosc.* 2007;65:361-366.

48. Lipka S, Kumar A, Richter JE. No evidence for efficacy of radiofrequency ablation for treatment of gastroesophageal reflux disease: a systematic review and meta-analysis. *Clin Gastroenterol Hepatol.* 2015;13:1058-1067.e1.

49. Liang WT, Yan C, Wang ZG, et al. Early and midterm outcome after laparoscopic fundoplication and a minimally invasive endoscopic procedure in patients with gastroesophageal reflux disease: a prospective observational study. *J Laparoendosc Adv Surg Tech A*. 2015;25:657-661.

50. Liang WT, Wang ZG, Wang F, et al. Long-term outcomes of patients with refractory gastroesophageal reflux disease following a minimally invasive endoscopic procedure: a prospective observational study. *BMC Gastroenterol*. 2014;14:178.

51. Yan C, Liang WT, Wang ZG, et al. Comparison of Stretta procedure and Toupet fundoplication for gastroesophageal reflux disease-related extra-esophageal symptoms. *World J Gastroenterol*. 2015;21:12882-12887.

52. Fockens P, Cohen L, Edmundowicz SA, et al. Prospective randomized controlled trial of an injectable esophageal prosthesis versus a sham procedure for endoscopic treatment of gastroesophageal reflux disease. *Surg Endosc*. 2010;24:1387-1397.

53. Wong RF, Davis TV, Peterson KA. Complications involving the mediastinum after injection of Enteryx for GERD. *Gastrointest Endosc*. 2003;61:753-756.

54. Ota K, Takeuchi T, Harada S, et al. A novel endoscopic submucosal dissection technique for proton pump inhibitor-refractory gastroesophageal reflux disease. *Scand J Gastroenterol*. 2014;49(12):1409-1413.

55. Inoue H, Ito H, Ikeda H, et al. Anti-reflux mucosectomy for gastroesophageal reflux disease in the absence of hiatus hernia: a pilot study. *Ann Gastroenterol*. 2014;27(4):346-351.

56. Bechara R, Inoue H. Recent advancement of therapeutic endoscopy in the esophageal benign diseases. *World J Gastrointest Endosc*. 2015;7:481-495.

Options to Address Delayed Gastric Emptying in Gastroesophageal Reflux Disease

John C. Lipham | Kulmeet K. Sandhu

Gastroparesis is described as delayed gastric emptying (DGE) without evidence of mechanical outlet obstruction. Common symptoms of gastroparesis include chronic nausea, emesis, abdominal pain, early satiety, and bloating. Abdominal pain can be significant and is associated with narcotic dependence in some patients. The true prevalence of this potentially debilitating disease is unknown, but it has been estimated to affect up to 4% of the population.[1] Some affected with this disorder have mild symptoms that can be medically controlled. Others have a chronic debilitating issue that is refractory to conservative management with antiemetic and prokinetic medications. Causes of DGE are varied and include diabetes, gastric surgery, central nervous system disorders, and metabolic and systemic disorders. Approximately one third of cases are idiopathic.[1-3]

DIAGNOSIS OF DELAYED GASTRIC EMPTYING

Gastroparesis is diagnosed based on the presence of typical signs and symptoms combined with objective tests to verify DGE and the absence of mechanical obstruction. Upper gastrointestinal endoscopy can be performed to exclude luminal obstruction and can also be used to note retained food products despite fasting status.[1]

DGE is most often evaluated using scintigraphy, which is performed with a meal labeled with radioactive markers.[1,2,4] Liquids and solids can both be marked with tracers and then followed for rate of emptying using gamma cameras. The stomach can be segmented so that emptying of the proximal and distal stomach can be assessed separately. Some recommend that the study should be performed for at least 4 hours, as shorter test times underrepresent patients with gastroparesis.[2] It should be noted that results of gastric emptying scintigraphy can have significant variability; this is partly dependent on how the food and tracer are prepared.[4] A standardized protocol should therefore be followed to decrease variability of results. Of note, the degree of DGE, usually measured as the gastric retention percentage or the half emptying time, does not correlate well with the severity of symptoms of gastroparesis.[1]

Another technique used to measure DGE is the stable isotope breath test. [13]C is a stable isotope that is used as a substrate, combined with food, and ingested. The substrate is absorbed in the small bowel and then oxidized to $^{13}CO_2$ and exhaled. The ratio of the substrate to its oxidized counterpart is used to determine gastric emptying.[2,4]

Several other techniques are being used to investigate gastric emptying. Magnetic resonance imaging (MRI), which is noninvasive, can evaluate motility in addition to emptying. Ultrasonography, another noninvasive technique, has also been used to evaluate patients for DGE but is dependent on the presence of a skilled technician.

Antroduodenal manometry can be used to evaluate gastric, pyloric, and duodenal motor activity and assess motor dysfunction. This includes antral hypomotility, migrating motor complex (MMC) activity, and focal dysfunction. This procedure is performed with a perfusion manometry system or a solid-state catheter to measure intraluminal pressure of gastric and duodenal wall contractions. Antroduodenal manometry findings can be abnormal in multiple disorders including DGE and gastroesophageal reflux disease (GERD).[2,4]

DELAYED GASTRIC EMPTYING IN GASTROESOPHAGEAL REFLUX DISEASE

Gastric emptying is a complex process involving multiple mechanisms and incorporates transport, storage, and digestion. The proximal stomach, or fundus, gradually dilates with receptive relaxation and stores food boluses. In the fundus, relaxation is followed by low-amplitude contractions to transport the food bolus to the distal stomach. The gastric antrum then assists in grinding food and maneuvering it toward the pylorus. The pylorus must then relax to allow for transit of the bolus into the duodenum. The gastric pacemaker, located in the body along the greater curvature, produces approximately three cycles per minute and is responsible for this movement from the body and antrum into the duodenum.[4,5] This rate of emptying is affected by the meal composition, with liquids passing more quickly than solids.[2] All of these elements involved in gastric emptying are potential sites of therapeutic intervention for the treatment of gastroparesis.

GERD is a failure of the antireflux barrier and is contributed to by a defective lower esophageal sphincter (LES) with reduced pressure, transient LES relaxations (TLESRs), impaired esophageal peristalsis, and possibly DGE.[6,7] Surgical intervention is warranted for GERD when patients with objective reflux fail medical management, prefer surgical treatment to a lifelong medication requirement, suffer from complications of GERD, or have extraesophageal symptoms.[7] Preoperative evaluation in reflux patients can include esophagogastroduodenoscopy (EGD), esophageal pH monitoring, esophageal manometry, and video esophagram or barium swallow.

It is possible that DGE affects the occurrence of gastroesophageal reflux and has an influence on the refluxate composition. In theory it makes sense that DGE may lead to larger quantities of food in the stomach available to be refluxed. This gastric distention may also cause increased episodes of reflux by generating TLESRs.[6,8-10] Yet the relationship between the rate of gastric emptying and GERD has been studied in multiple articles without a consensus on the exact nature or significance of their association.

Maddern et al. assessed solid and liquid gastric emptying simultaneously in 72 patients with symptomatic GERD. Of these, 44% were found to have delayed solid emptying and 37% delayed liquid emptying. There was no significant correlation noted between gastric emptying and the resting LES pressure. Symptoms of regurgitation and epigastric fullness also did not correlate with gastric emptying.[9] Cunningham et al. also demonstrated DGE of solids in 46% of patients with GERD.[10] The authors noted that this may indicate that the role of delayed emptying in GERD was related to gastric distention leading to alteration of gastric wall tension in the region of the LES, thereby increasing reflux events.[9,10]

Whereas the aforementioned studies noted DGE in a significant percentage of patients with GERD, Schwizer et al. found DGE with similar frequency in GERD patients versus controls. In this study, DGE was associated with a decreased incidence of esophagitis, suggesting that retained food had a buffering effect on the acidity of the stomach. This study concluded that DGE was not a major contributing factor to GERD.[11]

The previous studies demonstrate that it is unclear whether there is a significant link between abnormal gastric emptying and increased gastroesophageal reflux. Yet it has been speculated that gastric distention can contribute to reflux episodes by triggering TLESRs. This theory suggests that although total gastric emptying may be similar in patients with GERD and controls, the difference may lie in the time taken to empty different sections of the stomach. The gastric fundus and antrum have different functions in gastric emptying, and dysfunctional motor activity at either of these sites could have a role in the production of reflux episodes. Herculano et al. compared gastric emptying and food retention in the proximal stomach in these two groups using scintigraphy. This study found that total gastric emptying was similar in GERD patients and controls but patients had decreased proximal retention of a liquid meal with an increased number of reflux episodes. This indicated a negative correlation between proximal gastric retention and reflux episodes.[12] These results are in contrast to the results of Stacher et al., who, using scintigraphy, evaluated total and proximal stomach emptying of a semisolid meal in patients with symptoms of DGE and GERD. Their data showed that delayed proximal gastric emptying was associated with increased reflux episodes.[13]

Attention has also been given to the evaluation of the distal stomach and to assessing its role in GERD. Barbieri et al. used dynamic antral scintigraphy to monitor postprandial antral contractions and their relationship to GERD and DGE. They found that the amplitude of the contractions was linked to gastric emptying time but negatively correlated with reflux episodes.[14] These findings of increased amplitude of antral contractions in the setting of DGE contrast with results that show a similar pattern of distal antral contractions in these two groups.[15]

Carmagnola et al. took a different approach in attempting to determine whether DGE plays a role in the number of reflux episodes in GERD. They evaluated gastric emptying with ultrasonography and esophageal pH monitoring after patient use of cisapride, a prokinetic medication, and compared these results with placebo. Forty percent of their GERD patients were noted to have DGE. Cisapride was seen to increase gastric emptying and decrease the number of reflux episodes and esophageal acid exposure. However, no correlation was seen between changes in gastric emptying and the medication-induced changes in reflux variables.[16]

As these previous reports found discordant results, Gourcerol et al. used combined esophageal pH-impedance measurements to evaluate whether the occurrence of gastroesophageal reflux correlated with gastric emptying rate. Esophageal impedance monitoring was used to help identify the type of reflux (less acidic or nonacidic). Gastric emptying was assessed using the ^{13}C-octanoic acid breath test. This study found that delay in gastric emptying increased daily liquid and mixed reflux events without affecting esophageal acid exposure. This may be attributed to acid buffering due to gastric food retention and the production of nonacidic or weakly acidic refluxate or reflux of larger volume. Compared with normal gastric emptying, DGE patients had symptomatic reflux with higher proximal extension and a longer bolus clearance time.[6] These patients with DGE and higher proximal extension may be more symptomatic despite a similar number of reflux episodes.[8]

All of these studies indicate that gastric function may affect GERD pathogenesis, but an unequivocal connection between DGE and the degree of reflux symptoms has not been confirmed. In fact, as evidenced by a few of the noted articles, some studies have failed to demonstrate an association between GERD and DGE. This may be because many of these studies differ in inclusion criteria, have small sample sizes, and vary in the ingested meal that is studied. Even when studies show a significant association between GERD and DGE, it remains to be considered whether this has an effect on clinical symptoms or esophageal acid exposure. As noted earlier, it has been described that medication-induced acceleration of gastric emptying does not correlate with decreased acid exposure at the esophagus or other reflux variables.[16] At this time it appears that the studies on gastric motility and emptying in regard to GERD have variable and contradictory results.[17] DGE may play a larger role in less acidic or nonacidic reflux events because of buffering effects and may not be a major determinant of the number of reflux episodes.[6,8]

TREATMENT OPTIONS

There is no universally accepted treatment option for patients with DGE in the setting of GERD. Multiple medical therapies and surgical procedures are available for both of these disorders, but the number of options for treatment is indicative of the complex nature of this combination of disorders. Treatment may oftentimes be geared toward the predominating symptoms.

MEDICAL MANAGEMENT

Prokinetic medications augment gastrointestinal tract contractility and stimulate forward flow and gastric emptying. Dopamine receptor antagonists are often used as treatment for gastroparesis because they have antiemetic and prokinetic effects. Metoclopramide has been shown to be effective for short-term treatment of gastroparesis, but long-term maintenance of symptoms has not been well described. Prolonged use can also cause tardive dyskinesia, and these symptoms sometimes do not improve even after medication use is discontinued. Domperidone, a peripheral dopamine receptor antagonist, does not cross the blood-brain barrier and therefore has decreased risk of central nervous system side effects. The macrolide antibiotic and motilin receptor agonist erythromycin has also been used to treat gastroparesis, but it may cause the development of tachyphylaxis.[1,2,18]

Prokinetics have been shown to stimulate gastric emptying and decrease gastroparesis symptoms, but do they have an effect on GERD? Manzotti et al. performed a review of randomized control trials (RCTs) to evaluate the value of prokinetic medication for the treatment of gastroesophageal reflux esophagitis. Prokinetic drugs may ameliorate symptoms in patients with GERD by improving gastric emptying and increasing LES pressure. Eighteen studies were included in this review, and an increase was noted in the probability of symptom and endoscopic improvement.[19] Of note, many of the RCTs used cisapride, a 5-hydroxytryptamine type 4 (5-HT$_4$) receptor agonist, as the prokinetic medication. Cisapride has since been removed from the market in the United States due to adverse effects associated with cardiac dysrhythmias. Metoclopramide, a dopamine D$_2$ receptor antagonist, has both prokinetic and antiemetic effects and is often used for the treatment of gastroparesis.[2] Metoclopramide has also been shown to be significantly more effective than placebo in the treatment of GERD by significantly improving gastric emptying and LES pressure.[20]

ENDOSCOPIC BOTULINUM TOXIN INJECTION

An imbalance of acetylcholine and nitric oxide (NO) neurotransmitters may contribute to pylorospasm, with resultant nausea and vomiting in gastroparesis.[5] Botulinum toxin inhibits cholinergic neuromuscular transmission and may ameliorate the symptoms of DGE. If symptomatic improvement is noted, the treatment may be repeated at several-month intervals.

Mirbagheri et al. studied the effect of endoscopic pyloric botulinum toxin injection in patients with GERD associated with DGE.[21] Their methodology involved dilution of 200 units of botulinum toxin A into 4 mL of saline. A 25-gauge needle was then used to inject 50 units into each of the four quadrants of the pyloric sphincter. Of the 11 patients studied, 8 showed response with improvement of reflux or gastroparesis symptoms. The period of symptom relief was brief, with a mean duration of a little over 10 weeks. The authors concluded that although this method of treatment is not a permanent solution, it may act as a marker to predict which patients are most likely to respond to surgical intervention.

RADIOFREQUENCY ABLATION

Since 2000, GERD has been managed using a noninvasive radiofrequency treatment. This option has been used in patients whose symptoms are uncontrolled with medication but who do not wish to undergo surgical intervention. The Stretta procedure involves endoluminal delivery of low-level radiofrequency waves to the gastroesophageal junction. This therapy leads to inflammation, with collagen accumulation and thickening of the LES muscle. Noar and Noar studied 31 patients with GERD and DGE who underwent the Stretta procedure with ablation of the gastroesophageal junction and cardia.[22] Of these 31 patients, 73% had normalization of gastric emptying at 6 months postprocedure. Both responders and nonresponders had significant improvements in GERD–Health Related Quality of Life (GERD-HRQL) scores, but symptoms of dyspepsia were significantly improved only in the responder group. The mechanism of action for this effect is unclear. It may partly be due to a stronger esophagogastric barrier in the setting of radiofrequency-induced modification of the gastric pacemaker, leading to decreased numbers of TLESRs.

GASTRIC ELECTRICAL STIMULATION

As noted earlier in this chapter, the intrinsic gastric pacemaker produces antral stimulation at three cycles per minute. Gastric electrical stimulation (GES) delivers high-frequency, low-energy electrical stimulation to the gastric smooth muscle cells using surgically implanted electrodes. GES is used to treat intractable nausea and vomiting due to diabetic or idiopathic gastroparesis. The mechanism for this improvement of symptoms is unclear, and emptying studies after stimulator placement may show minimal change in gastric emptying despite symptom improvement.[1,2] This device can be placed laparoscopically or with an open procedure (Table 22.1). Risks of gastric stimulator placement include erosion of the leads into the gastric lumen with resultant infection, lead dislodgement, intestinal obstruction due to the intraabdominal portions of the wires, and infection at the stimulator site.[5] Stimulator placement has been shown to improve quality of life, reduce hospital visits, improve glycemic control in diabetic patients, and reduce the need for parenteral and enteral nutritional supplementation. Stimulation is

---

TABLE 22.1 Gastric Electrical Stimulator Implantation

1. A small upper midline incision is made in the epigastric area.
   - If laparoscopy is used, a 10-mm camera trocar is placed above the umbilicus and two working trocars are placed below the right and left subcostal margins.
2. The electrodes are placed 10 cm proximal to the pylorus approximately 1 cm apart along the greater curvature.
3. A subcutaneous pocket is created for the GES device using the same midline incision but away from the fascial incision on top of the anterior fascia.
4. The electrodes are connected to the GES device and the fascia and subcutaneous pocket are closed.

GES, Gastric electrical stimulator.

TABLE 22.2 Laparoscopic Subtotal Gastrectomy

1. Patient is placed in low lithotomy with the surgeon between the patient's legs.
2. A 12-mm camera port is placed above and to the left of the umbilicus. Two 12-mm working ports are placed at the bilateral subcostal margins in the midclavicular line. A Nathanson liver retractor is placed in the subxiphoid position. A 12-mm port in the left anterior axillary line is placed as an assistant port.
3. The gastrohepatic ligament is divided and the lesser sac entered. The proximal extent of the dissection is the lesser curvature where the left gastric vessels enter the stomach.
4. The distal extent of dissection is the pylorus and here the right gastric vessels are ligated and divided.
5. The right gastroepiploic vessels are identified and ligated and posterior adhesions from the stomach are divided.
6. Distal resection is performed using a laparoscopic linear cutting stapler at the duodenal bulb just distal to the pylorus.
7. The proximal resection is performed at the previously chosen site from the lesser curvature to the greater curvature using the laparoscopic linear cutting stapler.
8. After division of the proximal jejunum approximately 20 cm from the ligament of Treitz, the alimentary limb is brought up to the gastric pouch and a stapled end-to-side anastomosis is performed.
9. The camera port site is enlarged, a wound protector is placed, and the gastrectomy specimen is removed.
10. This incision is then used to perform a stapled side-to-side jejunojejunostomy between the biliary limb and the distal jejunum. The alimentary limb is measured approximately 50–60 cm to prevent bile reflux.

more effective if the predominant symptoms are nausea and vomiting; it is less effective if a patient's primary complaints are pain, fullness, and early satiety.[1]

Long-term outcomes and symptom evaluation has been performed by Lin et al.[23] They reviewed 55 patients who had placement of the gastric electrical stimulator and were followed up beyond 3 years. Six patients had device removal for infection, small bowel volvulus around the wires, or conversion to total gastrectomy for refractory symptoms. For the 37 patients who completed 3 years of stimulation, the average total symptom score decreased by 62.5%. These patients also had decreased requirements for nutritional support and significant improvements in HbA$_{1c}$ levels if they were diabetic.

Zehetner et al. compared outcomes in patients treated with the gastric electrical stimulator versus laparoscopic subtotal or total gastrectomy for gastroparesis (Table 22.2).[24] In this study, 72 patients were treated with GES and there was a 26% (19 patients) failure rate. Thirty-day morbidity and mortality rates were similar. Sixty-three percent of the GES group reported improvement in symptoms, compared with 87% in the primary gastrectomy group. Thirteen patients who failed GES eventually underwent subtotal gastrectomy, and all of these patients reported symptomatic improvement. This study concluded that GES is an effective treatment for gastroparesis that does not respond to medical therapy, and it can be converted to laparoscopic subtotal gastrectomy for continuing symptoms.

The previous studies indicate that GES is an effective treatment strategy for gastroparesis. Whether it may be of benefit in GERD has yet to be definitively determined. GES in a dog model has shown resultant increased LES pressure.[25] This augmentation of the sphincter may decrease TLESRs and suggests a potential role for the treatment of GERD symptoms. Reflux was also studied in 65 patients who underwent implantation of a gastric stimulator for weight loss. Twenty-seven of these patients had signs of GERD on endoscopy and almost all of these patients reported symptom improvement after GES. They also noted increased LES tone in 40% and length in 95%.[26]

In one case report, gastric stimulator placement was performed in conjunction with a laparoscopic Nissen fundoplication in a bilateral lung transplant patient with severe GERD and DGE. These procedures were performed to decrease the risk of aspiration pneumonitis and possible lung transplant rejection. The patient noted improvement of her reflux and DGE symptoms with decreased medication requirements and weight gain.[27] This novel approach to DGE in GERD requires further study.

PYLOROMYOTOMY AND PYLOROPLASTY

DGE associated with reflux in the pediatric population is often treated with a gastric emptying procedure such as pyloromyotomy or pyloroplasty. Okuyama et al. compared 54 pediatric patients who underwent fundoplication in addition to either pyloromyotomy or pyloroplasty for DGE and GERD. Of note, approximately 80% of these patients had an associated neurologic disorder. Postoperative gastric emptying was significantly improved in both groups. No significant difference was noted between postoperative emptying in the pyloromyotomy and pyloroplasty groups.[28] This suggests that both of these gastric drainage procedures improve gastric emptying when performed together with fundoplication for reflux.

Studies in adult patients have also shown the benefit of addition of a gastric drainage procedure to fundoplication. Masqusi et al. offered pyloroplasty with fundoplication to GERD patients with bloating symptoms and abnormal gastric emptying scintigraphy. Thirty-five patients underwent this combined procedure, and postoperatively, 80% reported significant symptomatic improvement, and gastric emptying improved by greater than 50%.[29]

Although fundoplication may improve gastric emptying, associated impaired gastric motility may result in an increased number of postoperative symptoms. Farrell et al. reviewed 25 patients with GERD and DGE.[30] These patients underwent laparoscopic Nissen fundoplication and 12 underwent concurrent pyloroplasty. One patient who underwent pyloroplasty had a gastric emptying half-time of 100 to 150 minutes, and the remaining 11 had emptying times greater than 150 minutes. Symptom scores at 1-year after fundoplication showed improvement in heartburn and regurgitation in both DGE and normal emptying groups. The investigators noted that bloating remained the same in both groups. Of the DGE patients, 8 (32%) had postoperative gastric emptying studies performed. All of these showed normalization of emptying half-times, with a 38% increase in emptying in the fundoplication-only group and a 70% improvement in the fundoplication with pyloroplasty group. Pyloroplasty decreases outflow

TABLE 22.3 Laparoscopic Heineke–Mikulicz Pyloroplasty

1. A camera port is placed above and to the left of the umbilicus. Two 5-mm ports are placed at the bilateral subcostal margins in the midclavicular line. A 5-mm port is placed above and to the right of the umbilicus. A liver retractor is placed in the subxiphoid position.
2. The pylorus is mobilized from superior and inferior attachments to decrease suture line tension.
3. A Kocher maneuver is performed, if needed, to improve visualization and decrease tension with incision of the peritoneum at the lateral aspect.
4. Two stay sutures are placed at the superior and inferior aspects of the pylorus.
5. A 5-cm full-thickness antroduodenal transverse incision is performed.
6. Traction is applied at the stay sutures and the incision is closed in a single layer transversely using absorbable suture in either a running or interrupted fashion.

Data From Hibbard M, Dunst C, Swanstrom L. Laparoscopic and endoscopic pyloroplasty for gastroparesis results in sustained symptom improvement. *J Gastrointest Surg.* 2011;15(9):1513.

resistance and facilitates gastric emptying and should be considered as an addition to fundoplication in patients with moderate to severe DGE.

Hibbard et al. explored the use of laparoscopic and endoscopic pyloroplasty for the treatment of gastroparesis.[31] They had 28 patients undergo either laparoscopic Heineke-Mikulicz pyloroplasty or laparoscopically assisted flexible transoral circular stapled pyloroplasty (Table 22.3). Significant symptom improvement was noted for nausea, vomiting, GERD symptoms, bloating, and abdominal pain. There was normalization in gastric emptying studies in 71% of patients, and prokinetic medication usage was also significantly reduced. Three patients eventually underwent gastric stimulator placement for unrelenting symptoms. This study reinforces the idea that minimally invasive gastric drainage procedures can be performed safely with good effect on gastroparesis symptoms. It also demonstrates that these procedures do not preclude the use of other treatment strategies in the setting of refractory symptoms.

GASTRIC FUNDOPLICATION

In the previous section it was illustrated that the addition of a gastric drainage procedure to fundoplication may improve GERD and DGE symptoms. Gastric fundoplication alone has also been evaluated in the setting of DGE and GERD (Table 22.4). The postprandial proximal stomach accommodates ingested food by relaxation. In DGE, prolongation of this step in the proximal stomach may contribute to increased reflux episodes.[8] Nissen fundoplication has a significant success rate in the control of gastroesophageal reflux symptoms by augmenting LES pressure and possibly reducing the number of TLESRs. Vu et al. used gastric barostat, gastric emptying studies, and measurement of vagus nerve integrity to study post–Nissen fundoplication patients.[32] Their results demonstrated that postprandial gastric relaxation correlated with gastric emptying of solids. In postprandial post-Nissen patients, gastric relaxation was significantly reduced and emptying of solids was significantly increased.

TABLE 22.4 Laparoscopic Nissen Fundoplication

1. The patient is placed in low lithotomy with the surgeon between the patient's legs.
2. A 12-mm camera port is placed above and to the left of the umbilicus. A 12-mm working port is placed at the left subcostal margin and a 5-mm port at the right subcostal margin in the midclavicular line. A Nathanson liver retractor is placed in the subxiphoid position. A 5-mm port in the left anterior axillary line is placed as an assistant port.
3. Circumferential dissection of the esophagus is performed with identification of the vagus nerves. A Penrose drain placed around the esophagus can aid in the production of an adequately sized retroesophageal window and crural closure.
4. The gastric fundus is mobilized with division of the short gastric vessels.
5. An esophageal bougie (50–60 French) is placed prior to passage of the fundus posterior to the esophagus.
6. The fundus is sutured to itself using three interrupted sutures to produce an approximately 2-cm loose, floppy wrap.

Bais et al. also noted post-Nissen enhancement of gastric emptying of solids.[33] Thirty-six patients were studied, of which 10 had preoperative DGE. Postoperatively, in the delayed emptying group, three patients had normalization of their gastric emptying, five had acceleration of emptying, and two were not affected. They noted that preoperative intragastric distribution differences seen on gastric emptying studies between patients with and without DGE were eliminated by Nissen fundoplication. Interestingly, this study noted that, based on symptom scores, this postoperative improvement of gastric emptying may not correct symptoms of delayed emptying and that fundoplication can bring about symptoms such as nausea and early satiety. This may be due in part to accelerated intragastric distribution.

It has been indicated that preoperative upright reflux is associated with worse outcomes after antireflux surgery, so Wayman et al. attempted to assess the interaction between preoperative DGE and reflux patterns and their effect on outcomes after laparoscopic fundoplication.[34] Thirty-one percent of the evaluated patients had DGE, and no association was found between the pattern of reflux and DGE. This study also did not show an influence of preoperative DGE or reflux pattern on surgical outcomes after fundoplication.

Despite multiple studies indicating improved gastric emptying after Nissen fundoplication, up to 12% to 15% of patients have persistent reflux symptoms and 19% to 25% suffer from postoperative gas-related symptoms.[35,36] As we have seen, it is unclear whether this is affected by the pattern of reflux. These symptoms may possibly be associated with weakly acidic reflux or combined (acidic and weakly acidic) reflux. Rebecchi et al. looked at the effect of DGE in patients after total laparoscopic fundoplication with combined or weakly acidic reflux.[35] This was a prospective study with a 5-year follow-up. Of the 172 GERD patients analyzed, 24.4% had mild to moderate DGE preoperatively. There was a significant reduction of acidic and liquid reflux occurrences in both DGE and normal gastric emptying patients, but significant improvement in weakly acidic reflux and mixed gas and liquid reflux was noted in only patients with normal emptying. In normal emptying patients, esophageal manometry showed a significant increase in gastroesophageal pressure at 1 and 5 years. In DGE patients, the gastroesophageal pressure significantly increased at 1 year but deteriorated at 5 years, with a return to baseline in 66.7%. These findings translated into clinical findings. Postoperative symptom scores were significantly improved in the normal emptying group, and less than 10% of these patients required proton pump inhibitor (PPI) therapy at 60 months. This was in contrast with the DGE patients, who did not have any meaningful improvement in symptoms, and over 90% were on medical therapy with PPIs and prokinetics at 5 years without adequate control of their symptoms. These results indicate that symptoms and reflux are not well controlled in DGE patients who undergo laparoscopic total fundoplication alone.

PARTIAL AND TOTAL GASTRECTOMY

Subtotal or total gastrectomy is performed for refractory gastroparesis, but its true effectiveness is unclear.[3] It has been shown that laparoscopic subtotal gastrectomy can be considered as a primary surgical treatment for gastroparesis since it is associated with significant symptomatic improvement with acceptable morbidity and mortality.[24] Gastrectomy has also been evaluated in the treatment of recurrent reflux disease after fundoplication. Twelve patients underwent gastrectomy (near-total, proximal, or total) and 25 had refundoplication for unsuccessful fundoplication with mean follow-up over 3 years.[37] Both groups showed improvement in symptom severity scores, but gastrectomy had a higher resolution of the primary symptom (89% vs. 50%). There was a higher morbidity and mortality rate in the gastrectomy patients, but four of the patients in the refundoplication group required an additional surgical procedure. This suggests that gastrectomy is an option for recurrent reflux in certain patients, especially those who have had numerous failures in the past.

Clark et al. reviewed nine patients who underwent gastrectomy (total, near-total, proximal) for postfundoplication debilitating gastric dysfunction.[38] Patients may have symptoms due to undiagnosed DGE prior to the fundoplication or because of vagal nerve dysfunction postoperatively. Three patients had postoperative complications. Seven of the patients continued to have symptoms despite gastrectomy, and three continued to require enteral nutrition via feeding tube. These findings show that although gastrectomy has been shown to improve gastroparesis and recurrent reflux separately, its effect on gastric dysfunction after fundoplication is associated with suboptimal results.

BARIATRIC SURGERY FOR GASTROESOPHAGEAL REFLUX DISEASE AND DELAYED GASTRIC EMPTYING

Bariatric surgery has become more prevalent over time. The influence of bariatric procedures on both gastroparesis and gastroesophageal reflux is now being considered. It is well known that obesity is related to GERD, with overweight patients having up to 3 times the incidence of reflux symptoms.[39,40] Fundoplication for GERD in the obese does not have any effect on the other comorbidities suffered by this population and has been found to have variable results.[39,40] Roux-en-Y gastric bypass (RYGB) has been shown to improve reflux symptoms. A study of 58 patients with preoperative GERD and morbid obesity who underwent laparoscopic RYGB demonstrated that symptoms improved or resolved in the majority of patients.[41]

RYGB can also improve symptoms of gastroparesis. Seven patients with a mean body mass index (BMI) of 39.5 kg/m² and gastroparesis underwent laparoscopic RYGB. Mean follow-up at 315 days showed that BMI was reduced by a mean of 9.1 units. Patients were also found to have significant improvement in their symptom scores with a resultant decrease in prokinetic and antiemetic medications.[42] These studies indicate that RYGB is a feasible option for patients with DGE and GERD.

Another bariatric procedure that has widespread use and may also have some effect on gastric emptying is the sleeve gastrectomy (SG). An Australian study evaluated four patients with laparoscopic SG with simultaneous fundoplication for DGE and GERD.[43] Postoperatively, all of these patients were able to stop PPI usage. Gastric emptying improved 67% and GERD-HRQL scores bettered in all patients, suggesting this technique should be studied further for possible broader applicability.

CONCLUSION

The pathophysiology of DGE may include decreased motility, compromised gastric tone, impaired antroduodenal coordination, and pyloric hypercontractility.[1-3] There is no cure, and symptom control is the mainstay of therapy. This disorder becomes even more difficult to manage once it is associated with GERD. Medical management with prokinetics has shown variable results, and the options have become more limited with removal of certain medications with significant side effects from the market. Endoscopic pyloric botulinum toxin A injection can give short-term respite from symptoms of both GERD and DGE but is not a viable permanent solution.[21] Radiofrequency ablation of the gastroesophageal junction and gastric cardia for reflux has been shown to improve gastric emptying and symptoms. The patient population in this study was limited; hence further study is warranted.[22] GES has been shown to have a significant effect on gastroparesis symptoms, and there is a suggestion that it may also contribute to the improvement of reflux symptoms. GES also has been used in conjunction with gastric fundoplication in a case report but further evaluation of this technique is required.[27] Fundoplication alone has shown conflicting results in terms of efficacy. As noted, one prospective study to 5 years showed that DGE patients had poor symptom control after fundoplication.[35] The addition of gastric drainage procedures such as pyloroplasty has been shown to improve symptoms in patients with GERD and DGE.[30] Gastric resection, from SG to total gastrectomy, is the most invasive procedure for the treatment of DGE in the setting of GERD, but it does not always result in symptom improvement and is often used as the last resort. However, with the growth of minimally invasive techniques, the morbidity of these procedures has become more reasonable.[24] Also, surgeons now have newer therapies in their armamentarium, many of which can be used in conjunction, to help battle this problematic issue. Laparoscopic magnetic sphincter augmentation, for example, has been shown to have similar reflux symptom control as Nissen fundoplication but with a lower frequency of severe gas-bloat; it has been recommended for patients with mild to moderate GERD.[44] It is conceivable that this technology could be used in combination with gastric drainage procedures to also improve DGE symptoms.

REFERENCES

1. Abell T, Bernstein R, Cutts T, et al. Treatment of gastroparesis: a multidisciplinary clinical review. *Neurogastroenterol Motil.* 2006;18(4):263.
2. Haans J, Masclee A. Review article: the diagnosis and management of gastroparesis. *Aliment Pharmacol Ther.* 2007;26(2):37.
3. Jones M, Maganti K. A systematic review of surgical therapy for gastroparesis. *Am J Gastroenterol.* 2003;98(10):2122.
4. Fuchs K-H. Tests of gastric function and their use in the evaluation of esophageal disease. In: Yeo CJ, Matthews JB, McFadden DW, et al., eds. *Shackelford's Surgery of the Alimentary Tract.* 7th ed. Philadelphia: Saunders; 2013:162-173 [Chapter 12].
5. Meilahn J. Motility disorders of the stomach and small intestine. In: Yeo CJ, Matthews JB, McFadden DW, et al., eds. *Shackelford's Surgery of the Alimentary Tract.* 7th ed. Philadelphia: Saunders; 2013:781-790 [Chapter 63].
6. Gourcerol G, Benanni Y, Boueyre E, Leroi AM, Ducrotte P. Influence of gastric emptying on gastro-esophageal reflux: a combined pH-impedance study. *Neurogastroenterol Motil.* 2013;25(10):800.
7. Stefanidis D, Hope W, Kohn G, et al. Guidelines for surgical treatment of gastroesophageal reflux disease. *Surg Endosc.* 2010;24(11):2647.
8. Emerenziani S, Sifrim D. Gastroesophageal reflux and gastric emptying, revisited. *Curr Gastroenterol Rep.* 2005;7(3):190.
9. Maddern G, Chatterton B, Collins P, Horowitz M, Shearman DJ, Jamieson GG. Solid and liquid gastric emptying in patients with gastro-oesophageal reflux. *Br J Surg.* 1985;72(5):344.
10. Cunningham K, Horowitz M, Riddell P, et al. Relations among autonomic nerve dysfunction, oesophageal motility, and gastric emptying in gastro-oesophageal reflux disease. *Gut.* 1991;32(12):1436.
11. Schwizer W, Hinder R, DeMeester T. Does delayed gastric emptying contribute to gastroesophageal reflux disease? *Am J Surg.* 1989;157(1):74.
12. Herculano J, Troncon L, Aprile L, et al. Diminished retention of food in the proximal stomach correlates with increased acidic reflux in patients with gastroesophageal reflux disease and dyspeptic symptoms. *Dig Dis Sci.* 2004;49(5):750.
13. Stacher G, Lenglinger J, Bergmann H, et al. Gastric emptying: a contributory factor in gastro-oesophageal reflux activity? *Gut.* 2000;47(5):661.
14. Barbieri C, Troncon L, Herculano J, et al. Postprandial gastric antral contractions in patients with gastro-oesophageal reflux disease: a scintigraphic study. *Neurogastroenterol Motil.* 2008;20(5):471.
15. King P, Pryde A, Heading R. Transpyloric fluid movement and antroduodenal motility in patients with gastro-oesophageal reflux. *Gut.* 1987;28(5):545.
16. Carmagnola S, Fraquelli M, Cantù P, Conte D, Penagini R. Relationship between acceleration of gastric emptying and oesophageal acid exposure in patients with endoscopy-negative gastro-oesophageal reflux disease. *Scand J Gastroenterol.* 2006;41(7):767.
17. Penagini R, Bravi I. The role of delayed gastric emptying and impaired oesophageal body motility. *Best Pract Res Clin Gastroenterol.* 2010;24(6):831.
18. Stapleton J, Wo J. Current treatment of nausea and vomiting associated with gastroparesis: antiemetics, prokinetics, tricyclics. *Gastrointest Endosc Clin N Am.* 2009;19(1):57.
19. Manzotti M, Catalano H, Serrano F, Di Stilio G, Koch MF, Guyatt G. Prokinetic drug utility in the treatment of gastroesophageal reflux esophagitis: a systematic review of randomized controlled trials. *Open Med.* 2007;1(3):e171.
20. McCallum R, Fink S, Winnan G, Avella J, Callachan C. Metoclopramide in gastroesophageal reflux disease: rationale for its use and results of a double-blind trial. *Am J Gastroenterol.* 1984;79(3):165.
21. Mirbagheri S, Sadeghi A, Amouie M, et al. Pyloric injection of botulinum toxin for the treatment of refractory GERD accompanied with gastroparesis: a preliminary report. *Dig Dis Sci.* 2008;53(10):2621.
22. Noar MD, Noar E. Gastroparesis associated with gastroesophageal reflux disease and corresponding reflux symptoms may be corrected by radiofrequency ablation of the cardia and esophagogastric junction. *Surg Endosc.* 2008;22(11):2440.
23. Lin Z, Sarosiek I, Forster J, McCallum RW. Symptom responses, long-term outcomes and adverse events beyond 3 years of high-frequency gastric electrical stimulation for gastroparesis. *Neurogastroenterol Motil.* 2006;18(1):18.
24. Zehetner J, Ravari F, Ayazi S, et al. Minimally invasive surgical approach for the treatment of gastroparesis. *Surg Endosc.* 2013;27(1):61.
25. Xing J, Felsher J, Soffer E. Gastric electrical stimulation significantly increases canine lower esophageal sphincter pressure. *Dig Dis Sci.* 2005;50(8):1481.
26. Cigaina V. Long-term follow-up of gastric stimulation for obesity: the Mestre 8-year experience. *Obes Surg.* 2004;14(suppl 1):S14.
27. Filichia LA, Baz M, Cendan JC. Simultaneous fundoplication and gastric stimulation in a lung transplant recipient with gastroparesis and reflux. *JSLS.* 2008;12(3):303.
28. Okuyama H, Urao M, Starr G, et al. A comparison of the efficacy of pyloromyotomy and pyloroplasty in patients with gastroesophageal reflux and delayed gastric emptying. *J Pediatr Surg.* 1997;32(2):316.
29. Masqusi S, Velanovich V. Pyloroplasty with fundoplication in the treatment of combined gastroesophageal reflux disease and bloating. *World J Surg.* 2007;31(2):332.
30. Farrell T, Richardson W, Halkar R, et al. Nissen fundoplication improves gastric motility in patients with delayed gastric emptying. *Surg Endosc.* 2001;15(3):271.
31. Hibbard M, Dunst C, Swanström L. Laparoscopic and endoscopic pyloroplasty for gastroparesis results in sustained symptom improvement. *J Gastrointest Surg.* 2011;15(9):1513.
32. Vu M, Straathof J, Schaar P, et al. Motor and sensory function of the proximal stomach in reflux disease and after laparoscopic Nissen fundoplication. *Am J Gastroenterol.* 1999;94(6):1481.
33. Bais J, Samsom M, Boudesteijn E, van Rijk PP, Akkermans LM, Gooszen HG. Impact of delayed gastric emptying on the outcome of antireflux surgery. *Ann Surg.* 2001;234(2):139.
34. Wayman J, Meyers J, Jamieson G. Preoperative gastric emptying and patterns of reflux as predictors of outcome after laparoscopic fundoplication. *Br J Surg.* 2007;94(5):592.
35. Rebecchi F, Allaix M, Giaccone C, Morino M. Gastric emptying as a prognostic factor for long-term results of total laparoscopic fundoplication for weakly acidic or mixed reflux. *Ann Surg.* 2013;258(5):831.
36. Broeders J, Mauritz F, Ahmed Ali U, et al. Systematic review and meta-analysis of laparoscopic Nissen (posterior total) versus Toupet (posterior partial) fundoplication for gastro-oesophageal reflux disease. *Br J Surg.* 2010;97(9):1318.
37. Williams V, Watson T, Gellersen O, et al. Gastrectomy as a remedial operation for failed fundoplication. *J Gastrointest Surg.* 2007;11(1):29.
38. Clark C, Sarr M, Arora A, Nichols FC, Reid-Lombardo KM. Does gastric resection have a role in the management of severe postfundoplication gastric dysfunction. *World J Surg.* 2011;35(9):2045.
39. Nadaleto B, Herbella F, Patti M. Gastroesophageal reflux disease in the obese: pathophysiology and treatment. *Surgery.* 2016;159(2):475.
40. Khan A, Kim A, Sanossian C, Francois F. Impact of obesity treatment on gastroesophageal reflux disease. *World J Gastroenterol.* 2016;22(4):1627.
41. Schauer P, Ikramuddin S, Gourash W, Ramanathan R, Luketich J. Outcomes after laparoscopic Roux-en-Y gastric bypass for morbid obesity. *Ann Surg.* 2000;232(4):515.
42. Papasavas P, Ng J, Stone A, Ajayi OA, Muddasani KP, Tishler DS. Gastric bypass surgery as treatment of recalcitrant gastroparesis. *Surg Obes Relat Dis.* 2014;10(5):795.
43. Le Page P, Martin D. Laparoscopic partial sleeve gastrectomy with fundoplication for gastroesophageal reflux and delayed gastric emptying. *World J Surg.* 2015;39(6):1460.
44. Reynolds J, Zehetner J, Wu P, Shah S, Bildzukewicz N, Lipham JC. Laparoscopic magnetic sphincter augmentation vs laparoscopic Nissen fundoplication: a matched-pair analysis of 100 patients. *J Am Coll Surg.* 2015;221(1):123.

Management of Failed Fundoplications, End-Stage Gastroesophageal Reflux Disease, and Scleroderma

Hugh G. Auchincloss | David W. Rattner

Patients with recurrent, persistent, or new symptoms after antireflux surgery can be a challenging problem for the foregut surgeon. Determining who will benefit from reoperation and what operation to perform requires that the surgeon be able to interpret a host of preoperative studies and be familiar with the common methods of failure associated with antireflux procedures. When reoperation is contemplated, the anticipated functional outcome must be balanced against both the efficacy of resuming medical therapy and the morbidity of a second, third, or fourth procedure. The relative modesty of these functional outcomes requires that patients' expectations be managed carefully. However, an experienced surgeon may reasonably offer many of these patients improvement in alimentary function and quality of life.

Patients nowadays rarely present with end-stage gastroesophageal reflux disease (GERD) in the absence of prior failed antireflux surgery due to the near ubiquitous use of proton pump inhibitors (PPIs). However, the occasional patient will present with complications related to chronic GERD, including profound esophageal dysmotility or long-segment Barrett esophagus with strictures, that preclude standard antireflux procedures. Such cases require thoughtful management by a surgeon and/or multidisciplinary team that includes expertise in performing complex foregut reconstruction. Patients with scleroderma—otherwise known as systemic sclerosis (SSc)—and esophageal involvement represent a particularly challenging subset of patients. Surgery in these patients should be approached with caution given the increased risk associated with intervention and the diminished prospects for functional improvement. However, well-selected patients with SSc can benefit from surgery to relieve regurgitation, heartburn, and occasionally dysphagia.

OUTCOMES AFTER FUNDOPLICATION

Laparoscopic Nissen fundoplication was introduced in 1991[1] and has become the standard approach to the surgical management of GERD. Variations on the 360-degree fundoplication—including the Hill repair, 180-degree anterior Dor fundoplication, and the 270-degree posterior Toupet fundoplication—are also commonly performed. Transthoracic fundoplication (e.g., the Belsey Mark IV fundoplication) has become increasingly uncommon as a primary antireflux procedure. Several large series have examined long-term outcomes following laparoscopic antireflux surgery. Although enthusiasts claim that 90% of patients experience durable symptom relief and improvement in quality of life,[2,3] nonsurgical series generally report that 20% to 50% of patients undergoing

antireflux operations require ongoing medical therapy.[4] Many patients who resume PPIs have nonreflux-related causes for their symptoms[5]; it is therefore more accurate to state that between 75% and 80% of patients undergoing primary antireflux surgery will have no further pathologic acid reflux, as documented by pH probe testing, for the remainder of their life span. Many patients who experience mild recurrent heartburn can be managed medically, but between 3% and 6% will ultimately require reoperation.[6,7] Interestingly, failures do not always occur in the early postoperative period but rather increase in incidence over time; the occasional patient will experience early improvement but ultimately experience failure of fundoplication a decade or more later.[2]

In patients presenting for reoperation after failed antireflux surgery the most common complaint is recurrent heartburn or regurgitation. These symptoms are present in 60% of patients with failed fundoplications. Dysphagia as a dominant symptom is present in 30% of patients. Other complaints include hiatal hernia, gas bloat, and atypical symptoms such as chest or abdominal pain.[8–10] Often a combination of symptoms is present, making it difficult to distinguish anatomic and functional reasons for failure.

WHY DO FUNDOPLICATIONS FAIL?

It is important for the foregut surgeon to understand how and why fundoplications fail. In addition to guiding the surgeon away from similar failures in their own practice, this understanding allows the surgeon to put the signs and symptoms of the "failed" patient into context. An educated assessment about the need and strategy for further operations follows. Generally speaking, fundoplications fail because of patient factors that existed prior to surgery, technical problems that lead to compromise of the operation, or early postoperative coughing or retching.

When failure is attributed to patient factors, it can be reasonably said that the preoperative assessment of the patient was inadequate, data gathered during that assessment were misinterpreted, or that poor judgment was used in developing a surgical strategy. Alternatively, the patient may experience progression of a condition that was present but insignificant prior to surgery, such as deterioration in esophageal peristalsis. The ideal patient for antireflux surgery is a nonobese individual with relatively preserved esophageal peristalsis, documented abnormal pH testing with good symptom correlation, typical symptoms of GERD, and symptoms that are at least partially responsive to PPIs.[11] Patients with concomitant esophageal motility disorder (such as achalasia or diffuse esophageal spasm), those in whom obesity contributes to reflux, and those with nonacid reflux or atypical symptoms including laryngospasm, chest pain, and recurrent aspiration have demonstrably inferior outcomes following fundoplication. Similarly, those with overlooked anatomic or functional abnormalities, such as esophageal strictures, fistula, or delayed gastric emptying, are unlikely to have their symptoms relieved by fundoplication alone. Advanced age, female gender, and the presence of a large hiatal hernia have also been noted as potential risk factors for failure.[12]

Technical failures of fundoplication have been well described and may compromise the early technical success of the operation or the durability of the repair. A typical fundoplication involves restoring the gastroesophageal junction and several centimeters of esophagus to an intraabdominal position, construction of a tension-free, "floppy" fundoplication wrap composed of the gastric fundus around a short segment of the intraabdominal esophagus, and securing the wrap and closure of the diaphragmatic crura with permanent suture. Variation exists with regard to the type of fundoplication performed, the need for division of the short gastric arteries, and the use of bioprosthetic mesh to reinforce the closure of the hiatus. Studies by Awais,[6] Dallemagne,[7] Khajanchee,[10] Furnée[13] found that migration of fundoplication wrap was the most common anatomic defect encountered at the time of reoperation, occurring in approximately two-thirds of patients (Table 23.1). Several types of wrap migration can occur, including transhiatal herniation of an intact wrap into the mediastinum or herniation of the proximal stomach through the wrap into a supra- or infradiaphragmatic position (i.e., the "slipped" Nissen). Other technical problems encountered at reoperation include a crural closure or wrap that is too tight or too long, a malpositioned or twisted wrap, or complete disruption of the wrap. An important cause of dysfunction after antireflux surgery stems from a failure to recognize or address a shortened esophagus. The importance of thorough mediastinal dissection with restoration of intraabdominal esophagus to the success of antireflux surgery cannot be overstated. Inability to create sufficient intraabdominal esophagus despite this dissection should be addressed with a Collis gastroplasty. Omission of these steps results in a wrap that is improperly situated and is subject to tensile forces that make it prone to transhiatal herniation. Lastly,

injury to the vagus nerves probably contributes to some patients' symptoms postfundoplication, particularly if these symptoms can be attributed to poor gastric emptying, diarrhea, or perhaps gas bloat syndrome.

The most dangerous cause of early failure is herniation of the wrap in the immediate postoperative period. This creates an iatrogenic incarcerated hiatal hernia with potential compromise of regional blood flow. An episode of violent coughing or retching with increase in intraabdominal pressure may precede such event. Without prompt intervention, the patient is at risk for necrosis of the stomach leading to significant morbidity or death. If a portion of the stomach becomes infarcted, the reconstruction options are limited by the patient's physiologic condition and the availability of a viable conduit to restore alimentary continuity. A staged repair is sometimes necessary in this circumstance.

APPROACH TO THE PATIENT WITH A FAILED FUNDOPLICATION

Many patients with recurrent or new symptoms after antireflux surgery are reluctant to seek the advice of a surgeon because of the perception that surgery has contributed to their situation or has little to offer by way of palliation. Such patients may only present after years of marginally beneficial medical and minimally invasive therapy. Symptoms and secondary sequelae of failed fundoplication may therefore be quite advanced. Evaluation of all patients begins with a careful attempt to understand the circumstances of the prior operation. When available, the patient's preoperative studies and operative report should be reviewed to look for clues as to the nature of the failure. Attention should be paid to similarities and differences between the patient's previous GERD symptoms and their current symptom complex. For example, dysphagia that was present prior to the first operation and remains speaks to a different etiology of failure than dysphagia that developed only after the fundoplication.

Even in a patient with a history and symptoms that strongly suggest a specific reason for failure of fundoplication, it is necessary to obtain objective data prior to proceeding with reoperation. It is recognized that symptoms and objective findings in primary and secondary GERD are imperfectly correlated; however, the information gained from such studies—which include upper gastrointestinal contrast imaging, high-resolution manometry, pH testing, multichannel intraluminal impendance testing, and endoscopy—guides surgical decision making and provides a baseline against which the outcome of reoperation may be measured.

CONTRAST IMAGING

Contrast imaging—traditionally a dynamic barium swallowing study—is essential for all patients with symptoms after fundoplication. A well-situated, intact fundoplication appears as a filling defect of the gastric fundus that is smooth in contour and located mostly anteriorly. The distal esophagus is narrowed slightly as it transverses this defect.[15] A barium swallow in a patient with recurrent

TABLE 23.1 Causes of Fundoplication Failure

Type of Failure	Incidence	Symptoms
Hiatal hernia	40%–65%	Reflux, dysphagia, asymptomatic
Slipped wrap	4%–16%	Reflux, dysphagia, early satiety, postprandial pain
Loose or disrupted wrap	3%–23%	Reflux
Tight or twisted wrap	1%–10%	Dysphagia
Underlying esophageal dysmotility	1%–2%	Dysphagia

Data from references 6–8, 10, 14.

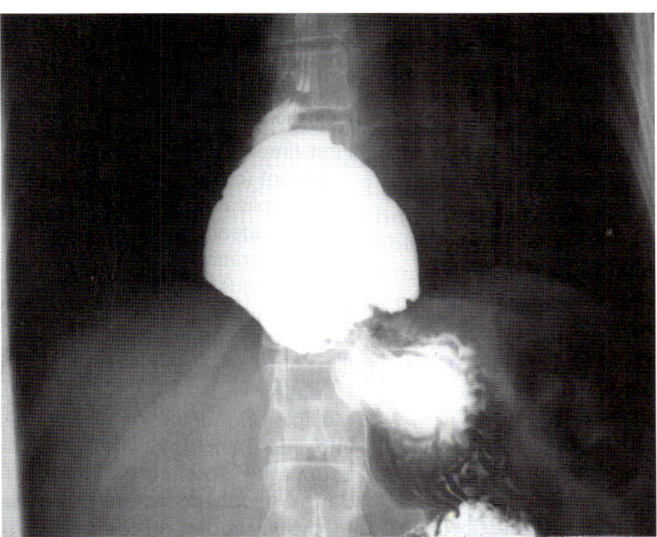

FIGURE 23.1 A barium swallow demonstrating a migrated or "slipped" fundoplication.

symptoms may demonstrate reflux or delayed passage of liquid or tablet-form contrast, suggesting that the wrap is too tight, too long, herniated, or disrupted (Fig. 23.1). Secondary findings of GERD may be present, including strictures and ulcerations. Lastly, dynamic video swallowing studies may provide clues about abnormal esophageal or gastric motility.

MANOMETRY

The primary role of esophageal manometry prior to initial or revision antireflux surgery is to exclude an alternative diagnosis of esophageal dysmotility, namely achalasia.[16] Manometry should be performed in all patients in whom revision surgery is contemplated because the presence of esophageal dysmotility may alter surgical planning considerably. In general, esophageal motility is never completely normal in the presence of GERD with or without a prior fundoplication. However severe dysmotility should be recognized as a relative contraindication to revision fundoplication. While several studies have shown that manometric findings are not predictive of postoperative dysphagia, it is important to understand the contribution, if any, that impaired peristalsis plays in symptom generation.

ESOPHAGEAL pH TESTING

Esophageal pH testing may be done with a transnasal catheter–based pH monitor or an implantable probe. For patients with confirmed erosive esophagitis on endoscopy and typical symptoms of GERD, pH testing is probably unnecessary.[16] However, abnormal esophageal acid exposure has been shown to be an important predictor of a successful outcome after fundoplication.[1] Postfundoplication the presence of reflux-like symptoms and findings of esophagitis on endoscopy must be viewed critically. Establishing the presence of abnormal esophageal acid exposure clarifies that recurrent reflux is at least part of the patient's problem. Given the complexity of both the

evaluation and treatment of patients with failed fundoplications, it is a good principle to obtain all potentially relevant data prior to reoperation. Should patients have persistent complaints postoperatively, comparison with preoperative objective data can be helpful. However, patients whose sole postfundoplication complaint is dysphagia and who have a clear-cut anatomic cause, such as a slipped fundoplication identified on barium swallow, do not need preoperative manometry.

MULTICHANNEL INTRALUMINAL IMPEDANCE TESTING

Multichannel intraluminal impedance (MII) testing is a valuable addition to the work-up of the patient with symptoms after fundoplication. MII documents both acid and nonacid reflux, as well as bolus transit in the esophagus. Coupled with manometry, it can establish the presence of ineffective peristalsis. MII is indicated for patients in whom symptoms strongly suggest reflux or dysmotility but objective findings on pH studies or manometry are discordant.

ENDOSCOPY

Direct examination of the esophageal mucosa is necessary to establish the degree of esophagitis and ulceration, confirm the presence or absence of a stricture, and exclude a diagnosis of Barrett esophagus or carcinoma. The presence of erosive esophagitis may also be sufficient to establish a diagnosis of recurrent GERD without the need for pH monitoring. However, a normal endoscopic examination in a patient with severe symptoms of reflux does not preclude the need for reoperation in the presence of other findings.

OTHER STUDIES

Delayed gastric emptying may confound a diagnosis of failed fundoplication and change reoperative strategy. Patients whose predominant symptoms include regurgitation, abdominal pain, or bloating should undergo nuclear gastric emptying studies. In complex revision operations in which esophagectomy with colon interposition is considered, mesenteric angiography is an important part of the preoperative evaluation. Debate about this routine practice exists in the literature, but we believe there is value in establishing the continuity of the marginal artery and the presence of a late-branching middle colic artery when contemplating using the colon as an esophageal substitute.[17] Angiography is unnecessary when small bowel reconstruction is planned. Computed tomography scans have no prescribed role in the evaluation of primary or recurrent GERD. The main value of axial imaging is to exclude other causes of abdominal pain.

CHOICE OF OPERATION

The threshold to perform reoperative surgery should be somewhat higher than for primary operations. Many patients whose original fundoplication has loosened and complain primarily of heartburn can be effectively managed with PPIs and avoid the risks associated with reoperative surgery. Some of these patients may ultimately opt to have a redo fundoplication because they felt better with

Of the many techniques for performing esophageal resection—thoracoabdominal, Ivor Lewis, McKeown, transhiatal, minimally invasive—none is clearly superior in patients with benign disease, and most surgeons opt for the technique with which they are most familiar and easiest for the patient to tolerate. Chang[31] and Shen[32] both reported large series of esophagectomy after antireflux surgery and found no difference in approach. Luketich[33] reported on outcomes after minimally invasive esophagectomy and noted no difference in the 111 out of 1011 patients who had undergone prior gastric or esophageal surgery. It seems that the optimal approach should be tailored to both the patient's disease and the surgeon's expertise. For example, a left thoracoabdominal approach provides excellent exposure to the stomach and gastroesophageal junction and is particularly useful in obese patients who have undergone multiple hiatal repairs. A final note should be made of vagal-sparing esophagectomy, a technique that can be combined with either a gastric or alternative conduit and has been shown to result in a decreased incidence of postoperative dumping syndrome and conduit dysfunction.[34] Unfortunately, in patients with multiple prior antireflux procedures, this technique is seldom possible due to extensive scarring of the hiatus, nor is preservation of the vagus nerves necessarily desirable.

The choice of conduit to replace the esophagus is controversial. A gastric conduit is the preferred reconstruction option following resection of the esophagus for cancer. This factors in the relative ease and safety of constructing a gastric conduit and the modest life expectancy of many patients with esophageal malignancy. In contrast, for patients with benign disease the outcome measure of interest is functional performance over a presumably normal life span. This has led some surgeons to suggest that, although the body of the stomach is frequently usable as a conduit despite multiple prior surgeries,[31,32] a short- or long-segment colon or jejunum interposition graft may provide superior quality of life. The theoretical advantages of a colon or jejunum interposition are that it allows the junction of the stomach and the neoesophagus to remain in the abdomen and preserves the reservoir function of the stomach. If the stomach is absent, a Roux limb can be used to complete the distal colonic anastomosis. Colonic mucosa in particular appears to be reasonably resistant to changes associated with acid exposure. The blood supply to the colon and jejunum is also robust and the incidence of anastomotic leaks—thought to be a consequence of ischemia—is probably less than with a gastric conduit. The disadvantages of colon or jejunum interposition are apparent. The operation is more technically challenging and requires at least three enteric anastomoses. The colon is not always available as a conduit due to intrinsic pathology. The jejunum usually does not reach to the neck for a long-segment esophageal replacement without the addition of a microvascular anastomosis.[35] Despite these technical challenges, some centers have found that patient satisfaction after colon interposition for benign disease is above 90%,[36] and others have reported equivalent or superior outcomes when colon or jejunum interposition is compared with a gastric conduit.[37,38] When a colon or jejunum interposition is constructed and anastomosed to the stomach, a pyloromyotomy should be performed because of the high incidence of gastric emptying dysfunction.

APPROACH TO THE PATIENT WITH END-STAGE GASTROESOPHAGEAL REFLUX DISEASE

It is rare to see a patient present with severe complications of reflux disease in the absence of prior antireflux surgery. These complications include intractable esophagitis, dysmotility, ulceration or fistula, or undilatable stricture. In some cases these complications are mild or moderate and may be expected to improve or resolve after fundoplication as a primary antireflux surgery. However, beyond this, more extensive resection and reconstruction is usually required. Options include Roux-en-Y gastric bypass, esophagojejunostomy, or esophageal replacement as discussed previously.

APPROACH TO THE PATIENT WITH SCLERODERMA

SSc affecting the esophagus is a particularly challenging problem that leads to significant morbidity in patients suffering from this progressive disease. SSc is a rare disorder with 10 new cases per million people each year. Women are 4 times more likely than men to be affected. Symptoms typically begin in the third or fourth decade of life. Gastrointestinal manifestations are the third most common presenting symptom (behind Raynaud disease and cutaneous findings) and are seen in 90% of patients. Nearly half of patients with SSc will have symptomatic esophageal involvement,[39,40] primarily manifested as dysphagia or GERD symptoms due to severely impaired esophageal peristalsis.

SSc is characterized by atrophy of the smooth muscle found in the distal two-thirds of the esophagus and replacement with fibrosis. This transforms the esophagus from propulsive muscular tube into a static, inflexible structure. Characteristic manometry findings include absent or diminished peristalsis of the esophageal body and weakening of the lower esophageal sphincter. The esophagus frequently becomes shortened due to fibrosis, resulting in a hiatal hernia. Patients experience often debilitating GERD with or without dysphagia. Symptoms are exacerbated by autonomic nerve dysfunction, gastroparesis and other gastrointestinal dysmotility, and the frequent coexistence of sicca syndrome (characterized by absent or ineffective saliva production). Endoscopy frequently finds *Candida* esophagitis (not a feature of typical GERD), which is thought to be related to immunosuppressive drugs and stasis within the distal esophagus. Strictures have been documented in between 15% and 30% of patients. It is unknown if Barrett esophagus and esophageal carcinoma are more common in patients with SSc, but this is presumed to be the case.[39]

The treatment of esophageal dysfunction in patients with SSc is typically medical. PPIs and other acid-suppressing medications are used along with lifestyle modification to reduce GERD symptoms. Dysphagia is more difficult to manage. Promotility agents, laxatives, and antibiotics to reduce bacterial overgrowth have been used with variable efficacy. Systemic treatment of SSc may delay progression of the disease but does not reverse the end-organ dysfunction.[41,42]

Surgery should be avoided in most patients with SSc because of the poor prospects for functional improvement and risk of impaired wound healing. Patients with severe symptoms refractory to medical therapy and those with complications of GERD including undilatable stricture, recurrent aspiration from regurgitation, or esophageal erosion may benefit from carefully planned surgery. Options include partial fundoplication, gastric resection with Roux-en-Y reconstruction, and esophageal replacement. Few series have looked at the outcome of antireflux surgery in patients with SSc, and results have been variable.

FUNDOPLICATION

Laparoscopic fundoplication is the most common operation performed in patients with SSc because it is most familiar to the majority of foregut surgeons and it avoids the morbidity of a gastrointestinal anastomosis. However, it has significant drawbacks that limit its utility. Chief among these limitations is high incidence of refractory postoperative dysphagia in the setting of poor underlying esophageal motility. This problem is particularly pronounced in patients with gastric or diffuse intestinal dysmotility. Also important is the difficulty in achieving an adequate length of intraabdominal esophagus in the setting of severe fibrosis, which may be impossible. Surgeons taking on these cases need to be able to perform esophageal lengthening procedures, such as a Collis gastroplasty, when indicated. This in turn creates an aperistatic segment of neoesophagus that contributes to postoperative dysphagia. Orringer[43] and Poirier[44] found that 17 out of 20 and 10 of 14 patients, respectively, had resolution of reflux symptoms over a short period of follow-up after open Collis-Nissen fundoplication. The rates of postoperative dysphagia were 39% and 69%, respectively. Objective improvement based on pH monitoring, esophageal manometry, and endoscopy to assess for esophagitis was marginal. Although fundoplication is a potential option for some patients with SSc, we would limit its use to those with relatively preserved esophageal length and peristalsis. Partial fundoplication is favored over complete fundoplication for the reasons stated previously.

GASTRECTOMY WITH ROUX-EN-Y RECONSTRUCTION

Roux-en-Y reconstruction of the foregut offers several advantages over fundoplication in patients with SSc. The reflux barrier is achieved by the addition of Roux limb of sufficient length rather than by restoring the function of the lower esophageal sphincter resulting in a decreased chance of postoperative dysphagia. Resecting the stomach is beneficial in patients in whom gastroparesis contributes to reflux disease. Lastly, a Roux limb can be made to reach to the distal or even mid-esophagus and can therefore be used as a reconstructive option in the presence of severe distal esophageal stricture or erosion requiring partial resection. Drawbacks include increased technical complexity and the addition of two anastomoses.

However, in experienced hands the operation can be performed laparoscopically with low morbidity. Patients with SSc suffering from both esophageal and small bowel dysmotility—particularly those with small bowel bacterial overgrowth—are at theoretical risk for worsening dysphagia and esophagitis after Roux-en-Y reconstruction.

Kent and colleagues[45] at the University of Pittsburgh have advocated for Roux-en-Y gastric bypass or esophagojejunostomy as the operation of choice in patients with SSc. This is based on a series demonstrating improvement in reflux symptoms, dysphagia, and overall quality of life at 21 months in patients undergoing Roux-en-Y reconstruction as opposed to fundoplication. The incidence of bloating and diarrhea were also decreased but not significantly. Though small in size, this study establishes credible support for the hypothesized benefits of Roux-en-Y reconstruction over standard fundoplication in patients with SSc.

ESOPHAGEAL REPLACEMENT

Esophageal replacement is a morbid procedure in patients with SSc and should be reserved for those patients with long-segment undilatable strictures, intractable esophageal ulcerations, or esophageal carcinoma. In 1988 Mansour et al.[46] recommended that esophagectomy with colon interposition be the primary operation for SSc; however, this thinking does not reflect current advances in medical therapy or laparoscopic surgical techniques. As recently as 2007 Kent[45] found that of five patients undergoing esophagectomy for SSc, one died and three of the remaining four suffered serious morbidity. In rare cases in which esophagectomy is necessary there is no consensus as to which approach is best. However, a colon interposition may provide a superior reflux barrier and alleviate some of the problems associated with gastric conduit dysfunction in patients with preexisting autonomic dysfunction.

CONCLUSION

Surgical management of patients with failed fundoplications, end-stage GERD, and scleroderma requires a great deal of judgment and technical skill. Care must be individualized based on many of the factors discussed in this chapter. For primary reoperations in nonobese patients, a redo fundoplication is usually the best option. However, patients who have had two or more prior fundoplications and those who are morbidly obese may be better served by gastric resection or bypass with Roux-en-Y reconstruction. In patients with extensive scarring, complications from prior mesh placement, or end-stage damage to the distal esophagus, resection of the fundus and distal esophagus may be necessary. In these situations the surgeon must have experience with a variety of options to restore continuity of the alimentary tract.

REFERENCES

1. Dallemagne B, Weerts JM, Jehaes C, Markiewicz S, Lombard R. Laparoscopic Nissen fundoplication: preliminary report. *Surg Laparosc Endosc.* 1991;1(3):138-143.
2. Broeders JA, Rijnhart-de Jong HG, Draaisma WA, Bredenoord AJ, Smout AJ, Gooszen HG. Ten-year outcome of laparoscopic and conventional Nissen fundoplication: randomized clinical trial. *Ann Surg.* 2009;250(5):698-706.

3. Morgenthal CB, Shane MD, Stival A, et al. The durability of laparoscopic Nissen fundoplication: 11-year outcomes. *J Gastrointest Surg.* 2007;11(6):693-700.

4. Spechler SJ, Lee E, Ahnen D, et al. Long-term outcome of medical and surgical therapies for gastroesophageal reflux disease: follow-up of a randomized controlled trial. *JAMA.* 2001;285(18):2331-2338.

5. Wijnhoven BP, Lally CJ, Kelly JJ, Myers JC, Watson DI. Use of antireflux medication after antireflux surgery. *J Gastrointest Surg.* 2008;12(3):510-517.

6. Awais O, Luketich JD, Schuchert MJ, et al. Reoperative antireflux surgery for failed fundoplication: an analysis of outcomes in 275 patients. *Ann Thorac Surg.* 2011;92(3):1083-1089; discussion 1089-1090.

7. Dallemagne B, Arenas Sanchez M, Francart D, et al. Long-term results after laparoscopic reoperation for failed antireflux procedures. *Br J Surg.* 2011;98(11):1581-1587.

8. van Beek DB, Auyang ED, Soper NJ. A comprehensive review of laparoscopic redo fundoplication. *Surg Endosc.* 2011;25(3):706-712.

9. Kim M, Navarro F, Eruchalu CN, Augenstein VA, Heniford BT, Stefanidis D. Minimally invasive Roux-en-Y gastric bypass for fundoplication failure offers excellent gastroesophageal reflux control. *Am Surg.* 2014;80(7):696-703.

10. Khajanchee YS, O'Rourke R, Cassera MA, Gatta P, Hansen PD, Swanström LL. Laparoscopic reintervention for failed antireflux surgery: subjective and objective outcomes in 176 consecutive patients. *Arch Surg.* 2007;142(8):785-901; discussion 791-793.

11. Campos GM, Peters JH, DeMeester TR, et al. Multivariate analysis of factors predicting outcome after laparoscopic Nissen fundoplication. *J Gastrointest Surg.* 1999;3(3):292-300.

12. Grover BT, Kothari SN. Reoperative antireflux surgery. *Surg Clin North Am.* 2015;95(3):629-640.

13. Furnée EJ, Draaisma WA, Broeders IA, Smout AJ, Gooszen HG. Surgical reintervention after antireflux surgery for gastroesophageal reflux disease: a prospective cohort study in 130 patients. *Arch Surg.* 2008;143(3):267-274; discussion 274.

14. Furnée EJ, Draaisma WA, Broeders IA, Gooszen HG. Surgical reintervention after failed antireflux surgery: a systematic review of the literature. *J Gastrointest Surg.* 2009;13(8):1539-1549.

15. Carbo AI, Kim RH, Gates T, D'Agostino HR. Imaging findings of successful and failed fundoplication. *Radiographics.* 2014;34(7):1873-1884.

16. Jobe BA, Richter JE, Hoppo T, et al. Preoperative diagnostic workup before antireflux surgery: an evidence and experience-based consensus of the Esophageal Diagnostic Advisory Panel. *J Am Coll Surg.* 2013;217(4):586-597.

17. Wain JC, Wright CD, Kuo EY, et al. Long-segment colon interposition for acquired esophageal disease. *Ann Thorac Surg.* 1999;67(2):313-317; discussion 317-318.

18. Wilshire CL, Louie BE, Shultz D, Jutric Z, Farivar AS, Aye RW. Clinical outcomes of reoperation for failed antireflux operations. *Ann Thorac Surg.* 2016;101(4):1290-1296.

19. Pennathur A, Awais O, Luketich JD. Minimally invasive redo antireflux surgery: lessons learned. *Ann Thorac Surg.* 2010;89(6):S2174-S2179.

20. Symons NR, Purkayastha S, Dillemans B, et al. Laparoscopic revision of failed antireflux surgery: a systematic review. *Am J Surg.* 2011;202(3):336-343.

21. Furnée EJ, Draaisma WA, Broeders IA, Smout AJ, Vlek AL, Gooszen HG. Predictors of symptomatic and objective outcomes after surgical reintervention for failed antireflux surgery. *Br J Surg.* 2008;95(11):1369-1374.

22. Oelschlager BK, Pellegrini CA, Hunter JG, et al. Biologic prosthesis to prevent recurrence after laparoscopic paraesophageal hernia repair: long-term follow-up from a multicenter, prospective, randomized trial. *J Am Coll Surg.* 2011;213(4):461-468.

23. Awais O, Luketich JD, Tam J, et al. Roux-en-Y near esophagojejunostomy for intractable gastroesophageal reflux after antireflux surgery. *Ann Thorac Surg.* 2008;85(6):1954-1959; discussion 1959-1961.

24. Awais O, Luketich JD, Reddy N, et al. Roux-en-Y near esophagojejunostomy for failed antireflux operations: outcomes in more than 100 patients. *Ann Thorac Surg.* 2014;98(6):1905-1911; discussion 1911-1913.

25. Makris KI, Panwar A, Willer BL, et al. The role of short-limb Roux-en-Y reconstruction for failed antireflux surgery: a single-center 5-year experience. *Surg Endosc.* 2012;26(5):1279-1286.

26. Mittal SK, Légner A, Tsuboi K, Juhasz A, Bathla L, Lee TH. Roux-en-Y reconstruction is superior to redo fundoplication in a subset of patients with failed antireflux surgery. *Surg Endosc.* 2013;27(3):927-935.

27. Stefanidis D, Navarro F, Augenstein VA, Gersin KS, Heniford BT. Laparoscopic fundoplication takedown with conversion to Roux-en-Y gastric bypass leads to excellent reflux control and quality of life after fundoplication failure. *Surg Endosc.* 2012;26(12):3521-3527.

28. Williams VA, Watson TJ, Gellersen O, et al. Gastrectomy as a remedial operation for failed fundoplication. *J Gastrointest Surg.* 2007;11(1):29-35.

29. Kellogg TA, Andrade R, Maddaus M, Slusarek B, Buchwald H, Ikramuddin S. Anatomic findings and outcomes after antireflux procedures in morbidly obese patients undergoing laparoscopic conversion to Roux-en-Y gastric bypass. *Surg Obes Relat Dis.* 2007;3(1):52-57; discussion 58-59.

30. Gadenstatter M, Hagen JA, DeMeester TR, et al. Esophagectomy for unsuccessful antireflux operations. *J Thorac Cardiovasc Surg.* 1998;115(2):296-300, 302; discussion 300-301.

31. Chang AC, Lee JS, Sawicki KT, Pickens A, Orringer MB. Outcomes after esophagectomy in patients with prior antireflux or hiatal hernia surgery. *Ann Thorac Surg.* 2010;89(4):1015-1021; discussion 1022-1023.

32. Shen KR, Harrison-Phipps KM, Cassivi SD, et al. Esophagectomy after anti-reflux surgery. *J Thorac Cardiovasc Surg.* 2010;139(4):969-975.

33. Luketich JD, Pennathur A, Awais O, et al. Outcomes after minimally invasive esophagectomy: review of over 1000 patients. *Ann Surg.* 2012;256(1):95-103.

34. Banki F, Mason RJ, DeMeester SR, et al. Vagal-sparing esophagectomy: a more physiologic alternative. *Ann Surg.* 2002;236(3):324-335; discussion 335-336.

35. Gaur P, Blackmon SH. Jejunal graft conduits after esophagectomy. *J Thorac Dis.* 2014;6(suppl 3):S333-S340.

36. Watson TJ, DeMeester TR, Kauer WK, Peters JH, Hagen JA. Esophageal replacement for end-stage benign esophageal disease. *J Thorac Cardiovasc Surg.* 1998;115(6):1241-1247; discussion 1247-1249.

37. Young MM, Deschamps C, Allen MS, et al. Esophageal reconstruction for benign disease: self-assessment of functional outcome and quality of life. *Ann Thorac Surg.* 2000;70(6):1799-1802.

38. Stephens EH, Gaur P, Hotze KO, Correa AM, Kim MP, Blackmon SH. Super-charged pedicled jejunal interposition performance compares favorably with a gastric conduit after esophagectomy. *Ann Thorac Surg.* 2015;100(2):407-413.

39. Ebert EC. Esophageal disease in scleroderma. *J Clin Gastroenterol.* 2006;40(9):769-775.

40. Arif T, Masood Q, Singh J, Hassan I. Assessment of esophageal involvement in systemic sclerosis and morphea (localized scleroderma) by clinical, endoscopic, manometric and pH metric features: a prospective comparative hospital based study. *BMC Gastroenterol.* 2015;15:24.

41. Nagaraja V, McMahan ZH, Getzug T, Khanna D. Management of gastrointestinal involvement in scleroderma. *Curr Treatm Opt Rheumatol.* 2015;1(1):82-105.

42. Carlson DA, Hinchcliff M, Pandolfino JE. Advances in the evaluation and management of esophageal disease of systemic sclerosis. *Curr Rheumatol Rep.* 2015;17(1):475.

43. Orringer MB, Orringer JS, Dabich L, Zarafonetis CJ. Combined Collis gastroplasty—fundoplication operations for scleroderma reflux esophagitis. *Surgery.* 1981;90(4):624-630.

44. Poirier NC, Taillefer R, Topart P, Duranceau A. Antireflux operations in patients with scleroderma. *Ann Thorac Surg.* 1994;58(1):66-72; discussion 72-73.

45. Kent MS, Luketich JD, Irshad K. Comparison of surgical approaches to recalcitrant gastroesophageal reflux disease in the patient with scleroderma. *Ann Thorac Surg.* 2007;84(5):1710-1715; discussion 1715-1716.

46. Mansour KA, Malone CE. Surgery for scleroderma of the esophagus: a 12-year experience. *Ann Thorac Surg.* 1988;46(5):513-514.

Esophageal Complications of Bariatric Procedures

Joerg Zehetner

Over the last three decades bariatric surgery moved from open to laparoscopic procedures, with all the benefits of minimally invasive surgery. All existing restrictive bariatric procedures may affect the esophagus over time, with the possibility of mild or sometimes severe complications.

Depending on the procedure performed, the esophagus can be affected minimally or severely. The gold standard of bariatric surgery is still the laparoscopic Roux en-Y gastric bypass. Despite the rise of the gastric sleeve, the gastric bypass is still one of the most favored bariatric procedures, and because of its low side-effect profile, with low mortality and morbidity, many bariatric surgeons consider it the preferred treatment option. Although the gastric bypass has little or no effect on the esophagus—it is even described as a protective procedure regarding problems with reflux and acid exposure—other restrictive procedures have a high potential for leading to esophageal complications.

COMPLICATIONS

ESOPHAGEAL DILATION

With the overuse of the adjustable gastric band in the late 1990s up to the year 2012, as well as uncontrolled overfilling of the gastric band, esophageal dilation can be found at different degrees of severity. Gastric bands should be surveyed and the patient seen once or twice a year by a physician. Bands were often overfilled to achieve rapid weight loss. Nausea and vomiting in combination with the outlet obstruction of the esophagus may lead to reversible and sometimes irreversible dilation of the esophagus. Esophageal dilation can be reversed if the band filling is reduced early in the process. Large esophageal dilation allows the patient to eat into the esophagus (as a neo-stomach), therefore making the gastric banding of no use for controlling weight, and removal or conversion to a gastric bypass or gastric sleeve are the next necessary steps.

MOTILITY DISORDERS

The adjustable gastric band can cause difficulties for the esophagus if the restriction is too high and therefore causing an outflow obstruction. While it will initially cause esophageal dilation and tertiary contractions, it can lead to aperistalsis called pseudoachalasia.

In cases of a severe motility disorder the gastric band has to be emptied to give the esophagus a chance to recover. If the overfilled band is left in place with the patient vomiting frequently, progressive esophageal dilation may lead to worsened motility and potentially permanent damage.

After emptying the band completely for 2 months another attempt via increasing the restriction—filling the band again—can be made. If the motility disorders are

recurrent and not reversible, the band should be removed and conversion to a laparoscopic gastric bypass or gastric sleeve recommended.

PSEUDOACHALASIA

The full picture of severe outflow obstruction caused by a narrow gastric band can lead to a type of aperistalsis called *pseudoachalasia*. Early on, it can be a reversible process, as described with the motility disorders, and immediate emptying of the band is warranted. This complication is rare after gastric sleeve or gastric bypass unless a severe stenosis at the incisura of the stomach or at the anastomosis is present.

REFLUX ESOPHAGITIS

Although the laparoscopic gastric bypass is a known antireflux procedure, since with a small pouch only a very small amount of acid can reflux into the esophagus, other procedures—including gastric banding, gastric sleeve, and duodenal switch—are known for the associated increased postoperative incidence of reflux esophagitis. If a patient after gastric bypass develops reflux esophagitis, there should be a high suspicion for a gastrogastric fistula. Diagnosis can be made with a contrast-swallow study of the esophagus, a computed tomography (CT) scan with oral contrast, or an endoscopy. Even negative endoscopic or contrast studies cannot rule out fistulas. Indirect signs on CT could be air in the remnant stomach or increased acid exposure on pH studies. Treatment for reflux esophagitis is aimed at the cause and may include excision of the fistula, pouch revision with narrowing of the pouch, or, if the alimentary limb is too short, lengthening the alimentary limb to 100 cm.

In general, reflux esophagitis in bariatric patients is treated with high-dose proton pump inhibitors (PPIs) for 4 weeks followed by a repeat upper endoscopy. In patients with reflux esophagitis after gastric banding, the initial treatment is opening the band—by emptying about half of the amount of fluid in the band—to provide better emptying of the esophagus. Most of the time a tight band creates an outflow obstruction, which might still allow reflux but can potentially reduce clearance, especially in patients where the band is high on the stomach and close to the gastroesophageal (GE) junction.

The gastric sleeve procedure is associated with the highest incidence of postoperative reflux and reflux esophagitis. Although different publications report controversial results, it is known that the gastric sleeve facilitates reflux, especially in patients with a hiatal hernia or a known weak distal esophageal sphincter and where no concurrent hiatal hernia repair is performed. It is also known that patients with prior reflux esophagitis and chronic gastroesophageal reflux disease (GERD) symptoms are poor candidates for the gastric sleeve procedure because of the higher associated incidence of postoperative GERD. Studies have shown that the gastric sleeve—especially when performed with too narrow an angle of His—can lead to dysfunction of the lower esophageal sphincter, as shown by its increased distensibility on planimetry.

An evaluation for GERD symptoms is recommended before sleeve gastrectomy. In patients with GERD symptoms, an upper endoscopy to rule out reflux esophagitis is mandatory. A contrast-swallow study should be performed to evaluate for esophageal motility disorders. In patients with reflux esophagitis and/or poor esophageal motility, a laparoscopic gastric bypass is the preferred procedure.

In patients with reflux esophagitis after a gastric sleeve procedure, the initial treatment is high-dose PPIs for 4 weeks or, if reflux is recurrent, PPIs as long-term treatment. In patient with persistent symptoms of GERD or persistent reflux esophagitis despite medical therapy or side effects from long-term PPI treatment and if insufficient weight loss was achieved with the gastric sleeve, conversion to a gastric bypass should be implemented.

In patients with sufficient weight loss and more than 1 year after gastric sleeve surgery, several surgical options are available. In those with good esophageal motility, the LINX reflux management system (Torax Medical, Inc., Shoreview, Minnesota) can be implanted. This laparoscopic procedure should be combined with a hiatal hernia repair in patients with hiatal hernias. Another option is the endoscopic Stretta procedure (Mederi Therapeutics, Inc., Norwalk, Connecticut), which is a radiofrequency application into the distal esophageal sphincter. Another option is the ENDOSTIM stimulator implantation (EndoStim, Inc., Dallas, Texas), whereby two electrodes are placed close to the lower esophageal sphincter to improve sphincter tone. There are currently no evidence-based data at the level of randomized studies; most of the recommendations are based on expert opinion.

ULCERS AND STENOSIS

Severe acid exposure of the distal esophagus can lead to ulcers and strictures, especially in patients with poor esophageal motility and hence poor clearance of the esophagus. In patients with severe reflux esophagitis and ulcers, biopsies should be taken on upper endoscopy to rule out malignancy. If the biopsies are negative, repeat studies with biopsies should be performed, as well as an endoscopic ultrasound of the distal esophagus and a CT scan of the chest and abdomen to rule out

underlying malignancy and esophageal cancer. In patients with strictures or stenosis, esophageal dilation with endoscopic balloon dilation is the first option. Recurrent strictures can be treated with a combination of high-dose PPIs, balloon or Savary dilation, and/or steroid injections.

Patients with persistent ulcers or stenosis after gastric sleeve or banding should be converted to a laparoscopic Roux-en-Y gastric bypass.

ESOPHAGEAL PERFORATION

Esophageal perforation is very rare after bariatric surgery and reported only in patients with severe vomiting after gastric banding. Treatment is similar to that for primary esophageal perforation, with immediate surgery and primary closure if diagnosed within 24 hours and drainage and stenting if diagnosed after 24 hours. If the perforation is in the distal esophagus under a migrated gastric band, laparoscopic gastric band removal and fundoplication over the perforated area as well as drainage would be the recommended salvage procedure.

SUMMARY

The frequency of esophageal complications after bariatric surgery depends on the type of procedure performed:

Gastric banding: The main complications are motility disorder, pseudoachalasia, esophageal dilations, and reflux esophagitis.
Gastric sleeve: The main complications are reflux esophagitis, possible ulcers, and strictures.
Gastric bypass: This is still the gold standard for bariatric patients with symptomatic GERD.

SUGGESTED READINGS

Naef M, Mouton WG, Naef U, van der Weg B, Maddern GJ, Wagner HE. Esophageal dysmotility disorders after laparoscopic gastric banding—an underestimated complication. *Ann Surg.* 2011;253(2):285-290. doi:10.1097/SLA.0b013e318206843e.

Reynolds JL, Zehetner J, Shiraga S, Lipham JC, Katkhouda N. Intraoperative assessment of the effects of laparoscopic sleeve gastrectomy on the distensibility of the lower esophageal sphincter using impedance planimetry. *Surg Endosc.* 2016; Apr 12 [Epub ahead of print].

Zehetner J, Holzinger F, Triaca H, Klaiber CH. A 6-year experience with the Swedish adjustable gastric band Prospective long-term audit of laparoscopic gastric banding. *Surg Endosc.* 2005;19(1):21-28.

Paraesophageal Hernia: Etiology, Presentation, and Indications for Repair

Jorge A. Vega Jr. | Vic Velanovich

Paraesophageal hernias are the results of defects in the diaphragmatic hiatus. Widening of the hiatus between the left and right diaphragmatic crura provides the pathway for upward displacement of abdominal contents into the mediastinum. Paraesophageal hernias are an increasingly common type of hiatal hernia. They can be associated with life-threatening complications such as gastric volvulus leading to necrosis or perforation of the stomach. Due to these potential complications, it was thought that all paraesophageal hernias should be repaired upon diagnosis. Recent evidence, however, has suggested that a nonsurgical approach is reasonably safe in asymptomatic patients. Symptoms can be subtle and include chest pain or pressure after meals, dysphagia for solids, dyspnea on exertion out of proportion to general health, early satiety, and the need to eat very small meals to avoid feeling uncomfortable. In addition, anemia is a common condition in patients with a paraesophageal hernia and typically resolves with correction of the hernia. Surgical intervention is recommended for patients who are exhibiting symptoms or signs associated with a paraesophageal hernia. The general etiology, presentation, and indications for repair of paraesophageal hernias are reviewed here.

ETIOLOGY

Hiatal hernias occur when portions of the stomach or other abdominal contents herniate superiorly into the mediastinum through a defect in the esophageal hiatus. Hiatal hernias have been associated with gastroesophageal reflux disease (GERD), and the prevalence and size of the hiatal hernia has been described to correlate with the severity of reflux.[1] The presence of a hiatal hernia has also been identified in nearly 40% of obese patients.[2] Some of the causes of hiatal hernias have been attributed to age, stress, and degenerative processes on the diaphragm.[3] Most cases of hiatal hernia are acquired rather than congenital, although familial clustering has been reported.[4]

CLASSIFICATION

Four types of hiatal hernias have traditionally been described. Type I hiatal hernia is a migration of the gastroesophageal (GE) junction into the posterior mediastinum, which is usually the result of deterioration of the phrenoesophageal ligament.[5] The forces exerted during swallowing and the negative intrathoracic pressure combined with the positive intraabdominal pressure contribute to the stretching of the phrenoesophageal ligament. Different types of collagen, particularly types I and III, have been found to be reduced in the phrenoesophageal ligament of patients with GERD and hiatal hernia.[6] Type I hiatal hernia is also known as the "sliding" hiatal hernia (Fig. 25.1). Sliding hiatal hernias can be large, but importantly, the GE junction remains above the herniated stomach.

Types II, III, and IV hiatal hernias are the paraesophageal hernias, where the stomach and esophagus are juxtaposed. A paraesophageal hernia is a true hernia with a hernia sac. The key feature that defines a paraesophageal hernia is that the fundus of the stomach is located above the GE junction, which can either be in a normal intraabdominal location or also herniated into the chest. The location of the fundus relative to the GE junction defines a sliding versus a paraesophageal hernia. Type II, or "rolling" hiatal hernias, occur when the gastric fundus herniates anterior to the esophagus, with a normally positioned intraabdominal GE junction. Type II is also referred to as a "true" paraesophageal hernia. Congenital defects in the esophageal hiatus can lead to paraesophageal hernias.[7] Type III hiatal hernias are a combination of types I and II, in which both the GE junction and a portion of the stomach—usually the gastric fundus—herniate into the mediastinum. Type IV hiatal hernias contain stomach and other abdominal organs such as small bowel, colon, pancreas, or spleen in the mediastinum. The term *giant paraesophageal hernia* refers to large hiatal hernias where at least 50% of the stomach is in the mediastinum or the hernia measures at least 6 cm on endoscopy.[8]

PREVALENCE

The actual prevalence of paraesophageal hernias is not known. The most common hiatal hernia is type I, which accounts for up to 95% of all hiatal hernias.[9] Paraesophageal hernias may account for up to 14% of all hiatal hernias, and the majority of paraesophageal hernias are

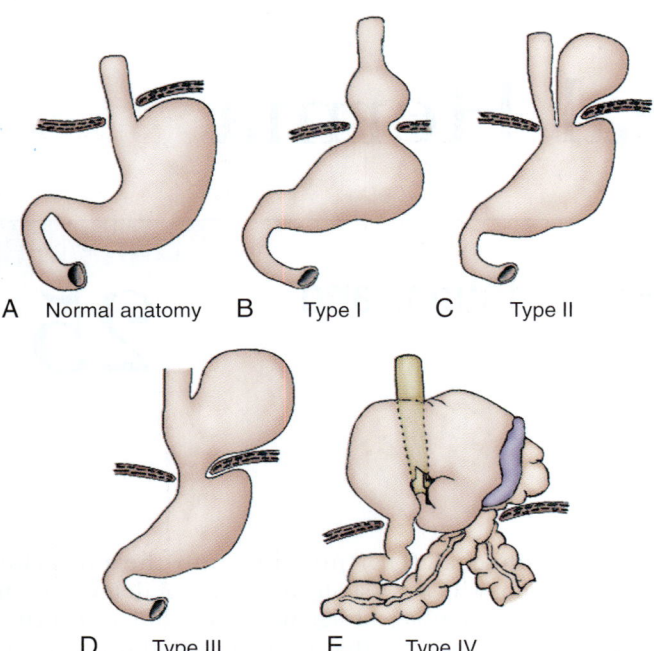

A   Normal anatomy   B   Type I   C   Type II

D   Type III   E   Type IV

FIGURE 25.1 Types of hiatus hernia. (A) Normal anatomy. (B) Type I, or sliding, hiatal hernia. (C) Type II or "true" paraesophageal hernia. (D) Type III or "mixed" paraesophageal hernia. (E) Type IV paraesophageal hernia, containing other intraabdominal organs. (Modified from Duranceau A, Jamieson GG. Hiatal hernia and gastroesophageal reflux. In: Sabiston DC Jr, ed. *Textbook of Surgery and the Biological Basis of Modern Surgical Practice.* 15th ed. Philadelphia: Saunders; 1997:775.)

TABLE 25.1 Paraesophageal Hernias: Preoperative Symptoms and Findings

Typical heartburn	47%
Dysphagia	35%
Epigastric pain	26%
Vomiting	23%
Anemia	21%
Barrett epithelium	13%
Aspiration	7%

Caveat: Many paraesophageal hernias are asymptomatic.
From Pierre AF, Luketich JD, Fernando HC, et al. Results of laparoscopic repair of giant paraesophageal hernias: 200 consecutive patients. *Ann Thorac Surg.* 2002;74:1909.

of the type III variety.[10] The incidence of paraesophageal hernias increases with age. Paraesophageal hernias tend to develop on the left anterior aspect of the esophageal hiatus. Women are more likely to develop paraesophageal hernias compared to men, and kyphosis is a risk factor.

PRESENTATION

Symptoms in patients with a paraesophageal hernia may be completely absent, minor and overlooked (Table 25.1), or quite debilitating and interfere with quality of life. Symptomatic patients commonly have typical GERD symptoms including heartburn, regurgitation, and water brash. However, some patients can present with obstructive symptoms, such as dysphagia, anemia secondary to chronic gastric blood loss, and respiratory complaints, such as dyspnea, asthma, chronic obstructive pulmonary disease, and aspiration pneumonia. Other symptoms associated with paraesophageal hernia include lower chest pain or discomfort, bloating, gassiness, and early satiety. Other patients develop these symptoms after undergoing upper gastrointestinal operations. For example, the incidence of symptomatic hiatal hernia after esophagectomy ranges between 1.0% and 4.5%.[11] Many patients have endoscopic evidence of gastritis and Cameron ulcers. It has been postulated these gastric ulcers can result from gastric torsion and poor gastric emptying. Because many of these symptoms are vague or can be attributed to other causes, their relationship to paraesophageal hernia is commonly missed. Therefore, it is not unusual for patients to be suffering from these symptoms for many years.

INCARCERATION AND STRANGULATION

Overall, the risk of incarceration and strangulation in patients with paraesophageal hernia is rare. It is even more rare that incarceration and strangulation would be the first symptoms manifested by a paraesophageal hernia. Many patients with gastric incarceration secondary to paraesophageal hernias present with epigastric pain or anterior chest pain.[12] Gastric incarceration can lead to obstruction, ischemia and strangulation, anemia, perforation, and even death. A gastric volvulus can occur when the stomach turns on its long axis, called organoaxial, or when it turns on its short axis, called mesenteroaxial. The classic symptoms for a gastric volvulus include chest pain, retching with the inability to vomit, and inability to pass a nasogastric tube. These findings make up Borchardt triad.[13] These symptoms, however, are not always present. Acute gastric volvulus is a surgical emergency. The presentation of gastric incarceration or strangulation, however, is often misdiagnosed initially.

COMPRESSION OF THE ESOPHAGUS OR STOMACH

Paraesophageal hernias can cause symptoms because of mechanical forces from the displaced stomach. When gastric volvulus occurs, there is compression of the stomach and GE junction, leading to symptoms such as chest pain or epigastric pain, and retching without emesis. As the stomach distends, the esophagus can be compressed, and this can result in dysphagia or chest pain. Many patients with heartburn report that their acid reflux symptoms went away about the same time they began to notice symptoms attributed to mechanical obstruction or compression such as retching or chest pain.[3] Compression and herniation of the stomach can cause compression of the stomach against other organs and structures. Aortogastric fistula secondary to a foreign body in the stomach has been described as a result of a herniated stomach into the mediastinum.[14]

ANEMIA

An important sign of paraesophageal hernia is chronic anemia. About one third of patients with paraesophageal hernias can develop anemia secondary to bleeding. Bleeding can be caused by ischemia or by ulcers within the herniated stomach. Cameron lesions are single or multiple gastric erosions or ulcerations that can be seen at the diaphragmatic hiatus, and they can be the source of bleeding in patients with hiatal hernias.[15] The most common location of these ulcerations is on the lesser curve of the stomach, at the level of the diaphragmatic hiatus. In those patients with hiatal hernias, Cameron lesions are visualized in up to 4.7%.[15] Haurani et al. reported that patients with paraesophageal hernia and anemia were greater than seven times more likely to have evidence of linear ulcerations or erosions in gastric mucosa compared with patients who had paraesophageal hernias without evidence of bleeding.[16] They also demonstrated that anemia secondary to these lesions resolved in the majority of patients undergoing surgical repair of their paraesophageal hernias.

RESPIRATORY SYMPTOMS

Patients with paraesophageal hernias can also develop dyspnea and cough. These patients report a progression of their symptoms throughout the day. GE reflux is an infrequent complication of type II hiatal hernia and may present in the form of respiratory complaints.[17] Evaluation of paraesophageal hernia should be started in patients with a history of reflux who present with unexplained dyspnea or new-onset bronchospasm. There have been multiple reports that pulmonary symptoms attributed to paraesophageal hernias improve after operative repair. The size of hiatal hernia inversely correlates with total lung capacity and vital capacity, and improvements in lung volumes have been reported after surgical repair.[18]

DIAGNOSTIC APPROACH

Evaluation of paraesophageal hernias begins with a history and physical examination. Many patients with paraesophageal hernias are asymptomatic. Physical examination can

appear benign in the majority of cases. Sometimes, however, chest examination can reveal decreased breath sounds on the affected side, or the presence of bowel sounds within the chest. Many patients undergo evaluation for chest pain that eventually leads to upper gastrointestinal evaluation, and the diagnosis of a paraesophageal hernia. Radiographic or endoscopic evaluation for other reasons may reveal the presence of a paraesophageal hernia in an asymptomatic patient.

RADIOGRAPHIC STUDIES

Chest radiographs are obtained many times as part of the work-up of chest pain. An upright radiograph of the chest may be diagnostic for paraesophageal hernia, revealing the pathognomic retrocardiac air-fluid level.[19] Lateral radiographs usually demonstrate retrocardiac opacities or air-fluid levels (Fig. 25.2). A radiograph demonstrating coiling of a nasogastric tube in the thorax can be used to help demonstrate the presence of an intrathoracic stomach. Computed tomography (CT) scans can be useful in demonstrating anatomic details in a patient with a hiatal hernia, but they are not typically used as part of the work-up for a hiatal hernia. CT scan is useful to differentiate between other types of hernias of the diaphragm such as Morgagni hernia or traumatic hernias.

CONTRAST ESOPHAGOGRAPHY

Barium esophagram can be useful in the diagnosis of paraesophageal hernias and often gives the most accurate information regarding the hernia's anatomy and location. An esophagram can help differentiate between type II and type III hiatal hernias (Fig. 25.3). An esophagram can also help provide functional information regarding esophageal peristalsis and reflux. Diagnostic accuracy of hiatal hernias can be improved using the right anterior

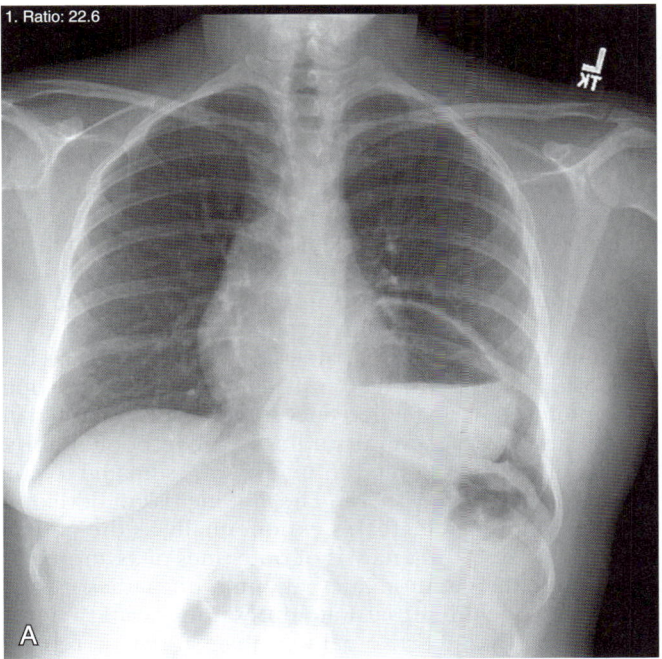
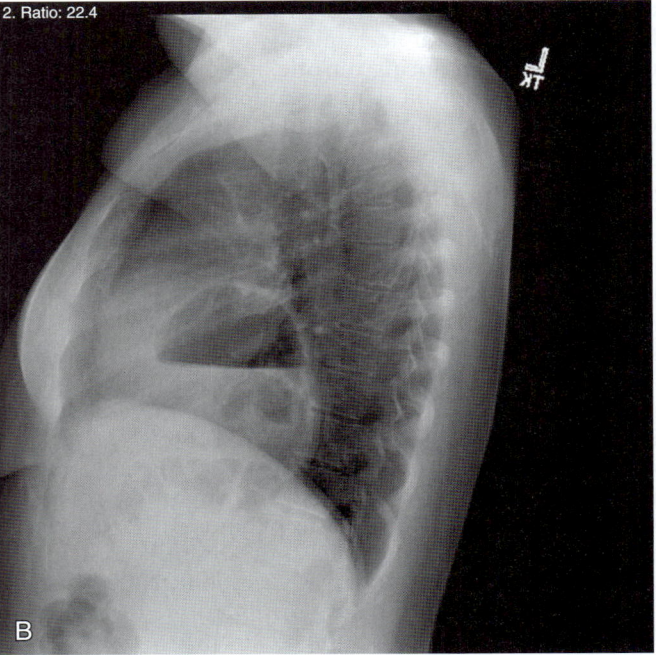

FIGURE 25.2 Chest radiographs. Posteroanterior (A) and lateral (B) views of a patient with a paraesophageal hernia. Notice the large air-fluid level behind the cardiac silhouette because of the intrathoracic stomach.

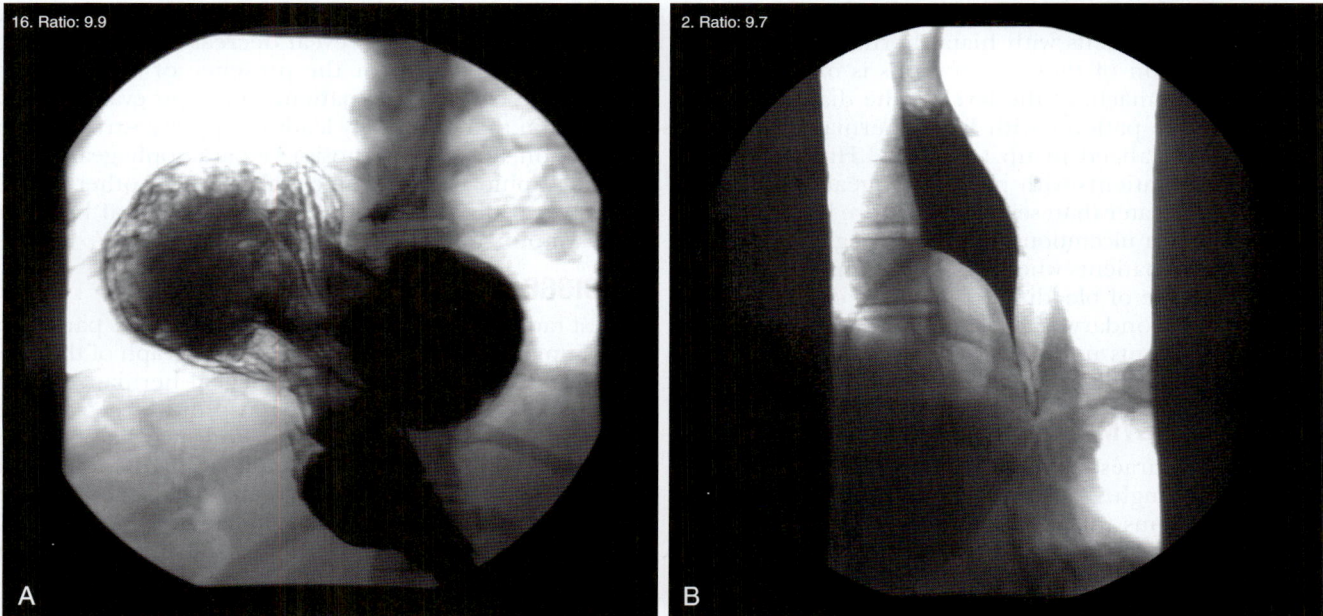

FIGURE 25.3 Barium swallow of a patient with a paraesophageal hernia (same patient as in Fig. 25.2). (A) The majority of the stomach is in an intrathoracic position. (B) Esophageal narrowing is seen because of compression from the intrathoracic portion of the stomach.

oblique esophagram technique in patients undergoing bariatric surgery.[20]

UPPER ENDOSCOPY

Esophagogastroduodenoscopy (EGD) can be used to assess the presence of esophageal or gastric pathology, such as ulceration and mucosal ischemia. EGD allows for evaluation of the GE junction and the size of the hernia. Retroflexion during EGD allows for better visualization of these areas. For example, noticing a second orifice next to the GE junction during retroflexion can help diagnose a type II hiatal hernia. Upper endoscopy also helps to screen for Barrett esophagus and malignancy, which can alter management for the hiatal hernia.

ESOPHAGEAL MANOMETRY AND pH MONITORING

Manometry studies and pH monitoring are not routinely used when evaluating patients with paraesophageal hiatal hernias. These tests may be difficult to perform, since intubation of the lower esophageal sphincter may be difficult to achieve due to anatomic distortion from the large hernia. Manometry is therefore rarely used to plan fundoplication as an adjunct procedure in these patients, since the anatomy is distorted and peristalsis may not be accurately depicted with this study. Instead, many surgeons rely on the functional information provided by the esophagram. However, in patients with dysphagia for whom a mechanical cause is not present, esophageal manometry is useful to identify weak esophageal peristalsis and plan the appropriate fundoplication. In patients with a symptomatic paraesophageal hernia, pH testing is not necessary since, unlike sliding hiatal hernias, the indication for repair is the presence of symptoms, and repair should include a fundoplication in these patients.

INDICATIONS FOR REPAIR

The approach to manage patients with paraesophageal hernias can be challenging, especially since many patients are older and have associated comorbidities. In the past, operative repair was implemented for all paraesophageal hernias once diagnosed. Symptomatic and asymptomatic patients underwent surgical repair due to fear that incarceration and strangulation would lead to life-threatening complications. In the 1960s, Skinner and Belsey followed 21 patients without surgery, and 6 of these patients (29%) died of causes related to the paraesophageal hernia.[21] This led to the preference of elective surgery, with the lower mortality rate of 1% compared with emergency surgery.[21] In the 1970s, Hill reported that the incidence of incarceration developed in up to 30% of patients with paraesophageal hernias.[22] There are reports suggesting that paraesophageal hernias should be repaired in good-risk surgical patients.[23–25] Additionally, there are also reports that laparoscopic repair of large hiatal hernias can be effective and durable.[26]

The true incidence of paraesophageal hernias has been reported to be less than 30%. The probability of developing symptoms requiring emergency surgery has been estimated from analyses of several studies.[27–31] The pooled annual probability of developing symptoms was estimated to range between 0.69% and 1.93%. The lifetime risk of developing acute symptoms decreases exponentially as the patient's age increases.[32] An analysis of outcomes of asymptomatic or minimally symptomatic patients with paraesophageal hernias concluded that watchful waiting would be more beneficial than elective paraesophageal hernia repair in over 80% of patients.[32] A detailed assessment of symptoms and a thorough discussion regarding risks versus benefits should drive the decision for operative repair.

An analysis of 1005 patients with paraesophageal hernia examined the morbidity and mortality in octogenarians after nonelective repair. A six- to sevenfold increase in mortality was associated with nonelective repair compared with elective repair.[33] This same analysis revealed that nonelective repairs were associated with a 50% longer length of stay versus elective repair and were found to be the predictor of inpatient mortality in patients over the age of 80. It is important to distinguish between asymptomatic patients and those patients with symptoms attributed to their paraesophageal hernia. Patients who have symptoms of acute incarceration or strangulation should undergo prompt surgical repair. Patients with obstructive symptoms, bleeding, or respiratory symptoms attributed to their paraesophageal hernia should also undergo surgical repair. Surgical management of the elderly patient with a paraesophageal hernia should be individualized. A study of 354 patients who underwent paraesophageal hernia repair revealed that mortality was highest in patients over the age of 75.[34] This study also revealed that morbidity was higher in patients with an American Society of Anesthesiologists class 3 or 4 and in patients with a type IV hiatal hernia.

Another topic of discussion in paraesophageal hernia repair is the need for an antireflux procedure. Most patients develop symptoms of GERD after paraesophageal hernia repair, and unless there is a contraindication, these patients would benefit from a fundoplication procedure in addition to their hiatal hernia repair. Adding a fundoplication to the paraesophageal hernia repair can help prevent GERD symptoms in these patients, which can result from the extensive dissection required during the procedure.[35]

Surgical management of paraesophageal hernias should be offered to symptomatic patients, but it should be individualized, especially in the elderly patient with high surgical risk.

REFERENCES

1. Maish MS, DeMeester SR. Paraesophageal hernia. In: Cameron JL, ed. *Current Surgical Therapy*. 8th ed. Philadelphia: Mosby; 2004:38.
2. Che F, Nguyen B, Cohen A, Nguyen NT. Prevalence of hiatal hernia in the morbidly obese. *Surg Obes Relat Dis*. 2013;9(6):920-924.
3. Kissane NC, Rattner DW. Paraesophageal and other complex diaphragmatic hernias. In: Yeo CJ, ed. *Shackelford's Surgery of the Alimentary Tract*. 7th ed. Philadelphia: Saunders; 2012:494.
4. Baglaj SM, Noblett HR. Paraesophageal hernia in children: familial occurrence and review of the literature. *Ped Surg Int*. 1999;15:85-87.
5. Hashemi M, Sillin LF, Peters JH. Current concepts in the management of paraesophageal hiatal hernia. *J Clin Gastroenterol*. 1999;29:8-13.
6. Von Diemen V, Trindade EN, Trindade ME. Hiatal hernia and gastroesophageal reflux: study of collagen in the phrenoesophageal ligament. *Surg Endosc*. 2016;30(11):5091-5098.
7. Kleitsch WP. Embryology of congenital diaphragmatic hernia. I. Esophageal hiatus hernia. *Arch Surg*. 1958;76:868.
8. Melvin WS, Perry KA. Paraesophageal hernia-open repair. In: Fischer JE, ed. *Fischer's Mastery of Surgery*. 6th ed. Philadelphia: Lippincott Williams & Wilkins; 2012:760.
9. Hyun JJ, Bak YT. Clinical significance of hiatal hernia. *Gut Liver*. 2011;5(3):267-277.
10. Postlewaite RW. *Surgery of the Esophagus*. 2nd ed. Norwalk, CT: Appleton Century-Crofts; 1986.
11. Oor JE, Wiezeer MJ, Hazebroek EJ. Hiatal hernia after open versus minimally invasive esophagectomy: a systematic review and meta-analysis. *Ann Surg Oncol*. 2016;23(8):2690-2698.
12. Chang CC, Tseng CL, Chang YC. A surgical emergency due to an incarcerated paraesophageal hernia. *Am J Emerg Med*. 2009;27:134.
13. Ghosh RK, Fatima K, Ravakhah K, et al. Gastric volvulus: an easily missed diagnosis of chest pain in the emergency room. *BMJ Case Rep*. 2016;2016:pii: bcr2015213888. doi:10.1136/bcr-2015-213888;
14. Kabayashi F, Saiki M, Nakamura Y, et al. Aortogastric fistula caused by a foreign body in a hiatal hernia. *Ann Thorac Surg*. 2016;101:1976-1978.
15. Gray DM, Kushnir V, Kalra G, et al. Cameron lesions in patients with hiatal hernias: prevalence, presentation, and treatment outcome. *Dis Esophagus*. 2015;28:448-452.
16. Haurani C, Carlin AM, Hammoud ZT, Velanovich V. Prevalence and resolution of anemia with paraesophageal hernia repair. *J Gastrointest Surg*. 2012;6:1817-1820.
17. Greub G, Liaudet L, Wiesel P, Bettschart V, Schaller MD. Respiratory complications of gastroesophageal reflux associated with para-esophageal hiatal hernia. *J Clin Gastroenterol*. 2003;37:129.
18. Naoum C, Kritharides L, Ing A, Falk GL, Yiannikas J. Changes in lung volumes and gas trapping in patients with large hiatal hernia. *Clin Respir J*. 2015;11(2):139-150. doi:10.1111/crj.12314.
19. Kahrilas PJ, Kim HC, Pandolfino JE. Approaches to the diagnosis and grading of hiatal hernia. *Best Pract Res Clin Gastroenterol*. 2008;22:601-616.
20. Heacock L, Parikh M, Jain R, Balthazar E, Hindman N. Improving the diagnostic accuracy of hiatal hernia in patients undergoing bariatric surgery. *Obes Surg*. 2012;22:1730-1733.
21. Skinner DB, Belsey RH. Surgical management of esophageal reflux and hiatus hernia. Long-term results with 1,030 patients. *J Thorac Cardiovasc Surg*. 1967;53:33.
22. Hill LD. Incarcerated paraesophageal hernia. A surgical emergency. *Am J Surg*. 1973;126:286-291.
23. Oddsdottir M, Franco AL, Laycock WS, et al. Laparoscopic repair of paraesophageal hernia. New access, old technique. *Surg Endosc*. 1995;9:164-168.
24. Hawasli A, Zonca S. Laparoscopic repair of paraesophageal hiatal hernia. *Am Surg*. 1998;64:703-710.
25. Wiechmann RJ, Ferguson MK, Naunheim KS, et al. Laparoscopic management of giant paraesophageal herniation. *Ann Thorac Surg*. 2001;71:1080-1087.
26. Asti E, Lovece A, Bonavina L, et al. Laparoscopic management of large hiatus hernia: five-year cohort study and comparison of mesh-augmented versus standard crura repair. *Surg Endosc*. 2016;30(12):5404-5409.
27. Allen MS, Trastek VF, Deschamps C, et al. Intrathoracic stomach. Presentation and results of operation. *J Thorac Cardiovasc Surg*. 1993;105:253-259.
28. Pitcher DE, Curet MJ, Martin DT, Vogt DM, Mason J, Zucker KA. Successful laparoscopic repair of paraesophageal hernia. *Arch Surg*. 1995;130:590-596.
29. Gantert WA, Patti MG, Arcerito M, et al. Laparoscopic repair of paraesophageal hiatal hernias. *J Am Coll Surg*. 1998;186:428-433.
30. Hallissey MT, Ratliff DA, Temple JG. Paraoesophageal hiatus hernia: surgery for all ages. *Ann R Coll Surg Engl*. 1992;74:23-25.
31. Carlson MA, Condon RE, Ludwig KA, Schulte WJ. Management of intrathoracic stomach with polypropylene mesh prosthesis reinforced transabdominal hiatus hernia repair. *J Am Coll Surg*. 1998;187:227-230.
32. Stylopoulos N, Gazeelle GS, Rattner DW. Paraesophageal hernias: operation or observation? *Ann Surg*. 2002;236:492-501.
33. Poulose BK, Gosen C, Marks JM, et al. Inpatient mortality analysis of paraesophageal hernia repair in octogenarians. *J Gastrointest Surg*. 2008;122:1888.
34. Larusson JH, Zingg U, Hahnloser D, Delport K, Seifert B, Oertli D. Predictive factors for morbidity and mortality in patients undergoing laparoscopic paraesophageal hernia repair: age, ASA score and operation type influence morbidity. *World J Surg*. 2009;33:980.
35. Casabella F, Sinanan M, Horgan S, Pellegrini CA. Systematic use of gastric fundoplication in laparoscopic repair of paraesophageal hernias. *Am J Surg*. 1996;171:485.

Laparoscopic Paraesophageal Hernia Repair: Technique, Outcomes, and Management of Complications

Lara W. Schaheen | Ian Christie | James D. Luketich

PATHOPHYSIOLOGY, INCIDENCE, AND CLINICAL PRESENTATION

In normal esophageal anatomy the gastroesophageal junction (GEJ) is located below the hiatal orifice. It is held in place by both the phrenoesophageal ligaments and an aggregate of posterior attachments between the GEJ and cardia of the stomach. The phrenoesophageal ligament is formed from the fascia transversalis on the abdominal aspect of the diaphragm and the endothoracic fascia on the thoracic aspect of the diaphragm. Both leaves then insert on the muscular wall of the esophagus.[1] During normal swallowing-initiated peristalsis, the elastic properties of the phrenoesophageal ligament allow the esophagus to shorten, resulting in slight movement of the GEJ cephalad. Physiologic stressors, such as gastroesophageal reflux, obesity, chronic cough, and normal changes in tissue architecture associated with aging may result in the attenuation and weakening of the ligament, with widening of the hiatal aperture and herniation of the stomach into the chest and the paraesophageal space.

Hiatal hernias are generally classified into four types (Fig. 26.1). Type I is often referred to as a sliding hiatal hernia, with the GEJ frequently moving in and out of the chest. Paraesophageal hernia (PEH) occurs when part or all of the stomach translocates from the abdomen through the esophageal hiatus and into the posterior mediastinum. When the GEJ remains in the normal intraabdominal position, the PEH is a "true" PEH because the fundus of the stomach herniates through an anterolateral weakening of the phrenoesophageal ligament and lies next to the esophagus in the mediastinum. This type of PEH is known as a type II PEH, which is quite uncommon. In the more common type III PEH, the GEJ has also migrated cephalad, likely as a result of some genetic predisposition to this type of hernia and often preceded by long-standing gastroesophageal reflux. It is hypothesized that ongoing reflux leads to fibrotic changes to the esophagus wall, leading to a foreshortening of the esophageal longitudinal muscles and, subsequently, the esophagus itself.

One of the world's most renowned experts on this topic, Dr. Griffith Pearson, measured the length of the esophagus, from the upper esophageal sphincter to the lower esophageal sphincter, in a group of patients with type III PEH and found this to be on average approximately 5 cm shorter than the same measurement in patients without a PEH.[2] Over time, this scarring pulls the GEJ into the posterior mediastinum, along with the proximal stomach, stretching and lengthening the phrenoesophageal ligament and widening the crural aperture. Eventually, the GEJ becomes fixed within the posterior mediastinum with varying degrees of gastric herniation and is known as a type III PEH. Patients with large type III PEH are usually symptomatic and may present with symptoms suggestive of obstruction, including chest pain, early satiety, postprandial bloating, or dysphagia. Anemia, cough, aspiration, and shortness of breath are also common symptoms of the PEH that are often attributed to other causes. When other abdominal organs follow the stomach into the chest, such as omentum, colon, spleen, and/or portions of the pancreas, the hernia is referred to as type IV PEH.

PEHs comprise approximately 5% to 10% of all hiatal hernias, and in addition to their common symptomatology listed previously, they can in extreme situations lead to gastric volvulus with resultant gastric and/or esophageal necrosis, sepsis, and death. Despite frequent symptoms and the potential for significant morbidity associated with acute presentation, there is significant debate regarding the need for and timing of operative intervention, as well as the approach to operation. Part of the reluctance to send patients for elective surgery is the significant morbidity that was associated with historical open operations, which frequently included a thoracotomy and/or thoracoabdominal incisions. Currently, many experienced centers can perform repair of PEH minimally invasively but are still criticized by significant recurrence rates and side effects that may occur.[3] However, a combination of significant minimally invasive esophageal surgery experience and a thorough understanding of the anatomy, pathophysiology, and historical management of PEH may help to provide surgeons with the necessary tools to manage this difficult disease process and provide patients with durable outcomes.[4,5]

INDICATIONS/CONTRAINDICATIONS

Over the past decade, the laparoscopic approach for PEH repair has become a standard approach in many centers, enabling PEH to be repaired with less pain, faster recovery, and reduced morbidity. However, it has become clear that only a few centers have published successful outcomes with minimally invasive approaches that have recurrence rates that are reasonably comparable to the best open series.[2] Optimal outcomes with durable results are much more likely to occur when performed by experienced surgeons with significant open and minimally invasive esophageal surgery experience.[6–8]

When evaluating a patient with a PEH for possible surgery, the physician should be familiar with the full

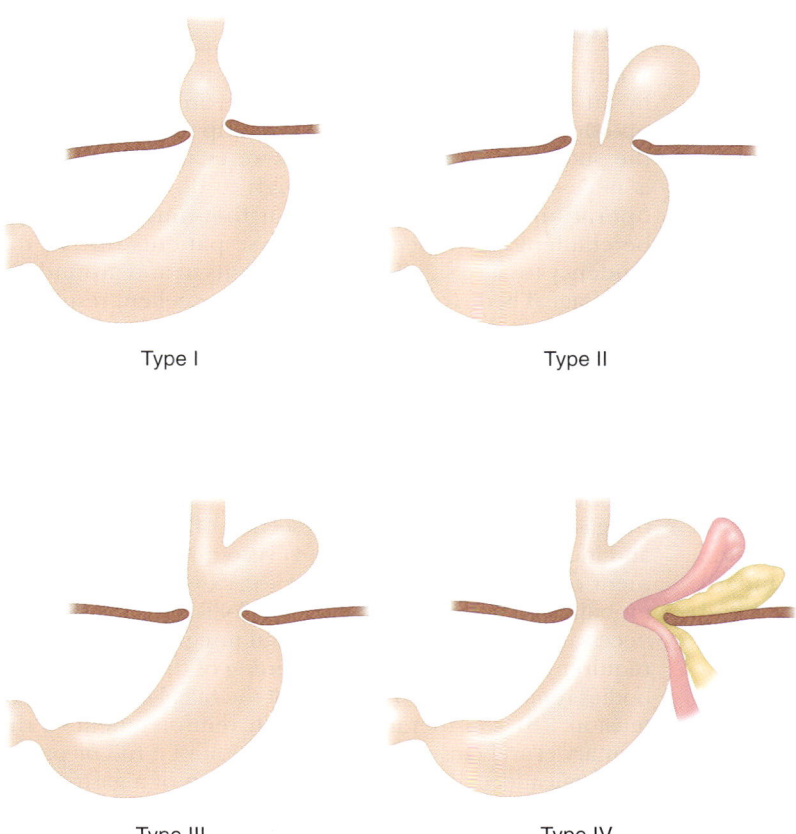

Type I   Type II

Type III   Type IV

FIGURE 26.1 Types of hiatal hernia (types I to IV) are depicted. (From Sun R. *Imaging for Surgical Disease.* Philadelphia: Lippincott Williams & Wilkins; 2014.)

spectrum of associated symptoms because less than 5% of patients are truly asymptomatic when questioned thoroughly.[4] Repair is generally recommended for all symptomatic patients. The management of a truly asymptomatic hernia remains a topic of debate. The incidence of a truly asymptomatic PEH is uncommon, and often patients billed as asymptomatic frequently co suffer from significant symptoms such as shortness of breath that may not be attributed to the hernia. Often these symptoms have occurred insidiously and patients have learned to live with these troublesome limitations and symptoms. In the previous era of primarily open repair, some studies estimated that the risk of life-threatening complications from a PEH was greater than 25% within a relatively short-term follow-up.[9] More recently, it has been recognized that life-threatening events are much less common and some authors have created risk-benefit algorithms to support the notion that life-threatening events are lower than the risk of undergoing repair.[10,11] However, when analyzing the findings of these studies, it is important to make note of the definition of minimally symptomatic or asymptomatic used; in the paper by Stylopoulos, minimal symptoms were defined as "heartburn that did not affect patient quality of life." In our experience, the vast majority of patients with radiographic findings of large PEH will have obstructive symptoms, including dysphagia, postprandial bloating, and chest pain and may not suffer from actual heartburn. On occasion, elderly patients in our clinics may deny difficulty swallowing but, when questioned further, will report significant and unintentional weight loss over

the previous 5 to 10 years and substantial changes to their diet to avoid hard and sometimes even soft solids.

When these hernias progress to requiring semiurgent, nonelective repair in our series, as well as by other surgeons, they are associated with a significantly increased risk of perioperative morbidity and mortality. In our series of 662 patients who underwent laparoscopic repair of a giant PEH, patients admitted electively for laparoscopic repair had a postoperative mortality rate of 0.5% compared with 7.5% for patients who underwent urgent repair.[12] This can be markedly higher when patients present with gastric necrosis, massive hemorrhage, or severe aspiration pneumonia, albeit the incidence of these more life-threatening situations is less common. Thus, when evaluating patients who may be minimally symptomatic, it is important to keep these data in mind. The risk of perioperative mortality and/or morbidity with elective and nonelective operation can be estimated to some degree by the size of the PEH, the patient's functional status, the presence of comorbid conditions, and the patient's symptom complex. In patients with age-adjusted Charleston Comorbidity Index scores of 5 or less, perioperative morbidity and mortality with elective laparoscopic repair is low and increases dramatically when performed urgently. Furthermore, patients with very large PEH were much more likely to have obstructive symptoms and to present urgently when compared with patients with smaller (<75% gastric herniation) PEH.[13] Urgent presentations often occur in patients in whom the presence of the PEH was known much earlier. As such, we recommend elective surgical repair for most patients who have minimal symptoms and very large PEH because of the higher risk of mortality or complications after emergency surgery.

Relative contraindications to laparoscopic PEH repair include conditions that might preclude or increase the risk of all laparoscopic surgery, such as portal hypertension, significant hematologic clotting disorders, and contraindications to surgery in general, such as inadequate cardiovascular function or the inability to tolerate general anesthesia. All of these relative contraindications must be weighed against the complications of an incarcerated, necrotic stomach or the morbidity of an urgent repair for acute problems. Age itself should not be considered a complication because most of these patients are elderly and will be even less likely to tolerate urgent or emergent surgery but typically do very well with elective laparoscopic repair.

PREOPERATIVE ASSESSMENT

PEH can be visualized with a variety of radiographic studies. We consider the barium esophagram as the gold standard for evaluating PEH because it is inexpensive, low risk, and provides an accurate assessment of the degree of gastric herniation and the anatomic relationship between the stomach, GEJ, and diaphragmatic hiatus. When combined with video imaging, the barium esophagram provides useful information on reflux and esophageal motility. In less experienced hands, endoscopic evaluation can be difficult due to changes in the anatomic orientation of the esophagus, stomach, and diaphragm. In cases of a large volvulized PEH navigating the endoscope through the GEJ, stomach, and pylorus can be challenging. Computed tomography (CT) scans can provide complementary data and are often useful in identifying type IV hernias and evaluating coexisting pathology. However, we do not routinely require a CT scan prior to surgery. Additional studies, such as 24-hour pH monitoring and manometry, are used selectively in patients with smaller PEH (~30% to 50%). Although these functional tests are important when evaluating patients with smaller hernias, they provide less reliable information in patients with larger PEH. Furthermore, in contrast to sliding hiatal hernias, objective evidence of reflux disease is not necessary prior to repair of a symptomatic PEH.

Manometric assessment of the lower esophageal sphincter in large PEH is frequently difficult and at times inaccurate due to proximal displacement of the GEJ, tortuosity, and inability to position the catheter into the distal stomach. However, obtaining a simple manometric analysis of the body of the esophagus can be quite helpful in assessing the esophageal peristaltic wave and contractions to help determine the type of fundoplication as part of PEH repair. Preoperative or intraoperative endoscopy is always performed by the operating surgeon to evaluate gastric and esophageal viability and to identify associated abnormalities, such as Barrett esophagus, strictures, diverticula, esophageal malignancy, and the location of the GEJ. It is critical for the surgeons to perform their own endoscopy, if not prior to surgery, then at a minimum, the day of surgery, and not rely on the findings on endoscopy reported by others, because important features can be missed or underestimated when unaccustomed to endoscopic evaluation of a PEH.

SURGICAL TECHNIQUE

When performed in esophageal centers of excellence, by an experienced esophageal surgeon, the short-term outcomes of laparoscopic repair compare favorably with the outcomes of open repair.[8,9] However, not every surgeon is necessarily experienced enough to do these complex operations independently. Even first-time repairs can be challenging, especially in obese patients due to the tendency to have significant fat deposits in and around the esophageal bed. To obtain consistently excellent results, we recommend that less-experienced surgeons be proctored by senior esophageal surgeons early in their career.

To optimize repair durability and to ensure long-term symptom resolution, PEH repair requires strict attention to several key elements: (1) complete reduction of the hernia sac and contents; (2) careful preservation of the anterior and posterior vagus nerves; (3) mobilization of the gastroesophageal fat pad, resection of excess hernia sac, and identification of the GEJ; (4) recognition and management of a shortened esophagus; (5) extensive mediastinal mobilization and performance of a Collis gastroplasty when necessary; (6) preservation of crural integrity with absolute requirement that the peritoneal lining of the crural muscle bodies remain intact; (7) closure of the hiatal defect without tension; (8) consideration of mesh reinforcement of the primary crural closure; and (9) addition of a full or partial fundoplication, or in select cases addition of a gastropexy.

In the operating room, general endotracheal anesthesia is induced and flexible endoscopy performed by the surgeon if not done preoperatively. Care is taken to minimize air insufflation during the endoscopic evaluation; one should be particularly attentive if endoscopy is being taught at this stage because it is easy to overinsufflate, which can cause significant technical challenges with regard to laparoscopic visualization. The esophagus is inspected, and the stomach is decompressed as much as possible at the end of the endoscopic exam. The patient is then positioned for laparoscopy. Our preferred approach for positioning of the patient is supine with the surgeon on the patient's right side and the assistant on the left, although many prefer the split leg position with the surgeon between the patient's legs. A subhepatic liver retractor is used, so the patient is placed to the far right of the operating room table to allow proper positioning of the retractor. A foam-padded foot stop is placed on the operating table to facilitate reverse Trendelenburg positioning. The patient's arms are rotated away from the patient, secured to an arm board at no more than a 45-degree angle from the bed in an effort to minimize the risk of stretch injury to the brachial plexus.

Proper port placement is one of the important early steps in the successful execution of the operation. Due to the extensive mediastinal dissection required to reduce the hernia sac and fully mobilize the esophagus, placement of the ports in the upper aspect of the abdominal wall is critical. To accomplish this, we identify the midline from the xiphoid to the umbilicus and use a skin marker to divide the distance into thirds (Fig. 26.2). In the majority of patients, five ports are used. Using the open cutdown technique, a 10-mm Hassan port is placed in the right paramedian line approximately one-third of the way from the xiphoid to the umbilicus, taking care to avoid

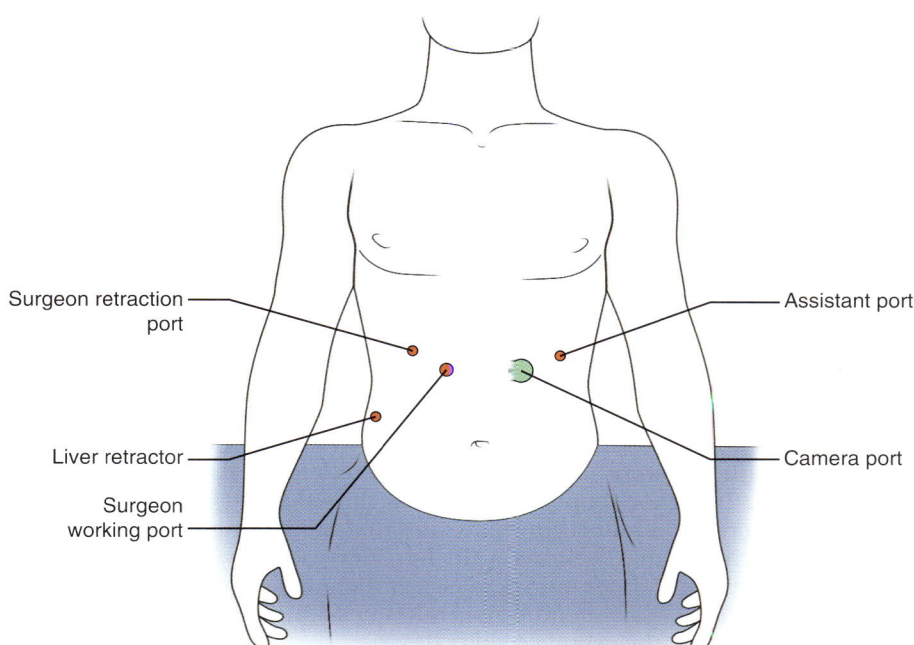

Surgeon retraction port

Liver retractor

Surgeon working port

Assistant port

Camera port

FIGURE 26.2 Surgeon, port placement, and instrument positions are shown. The ports are positioned one-third of the distance from the xiphoid to the umbilicus.

dissection into the falciform ligament. In patients with a large protuberant abdomen, dividing the distance from the xiphoid to umbilicus can be misleading; therefore the initial right paramedian port should be placed approximately 2 to 3 inches from the xiphoid process. Insufflation pressures are set at between 12 and 15 mm Hg, with attention paid to the patient's hemodynamic state. In patients with poor cardiopulmonary risk, insufflation pressure in the 8- to 10-mm Hg range can be used with reasonable visualization if blood pressure problems occur. The remainder of the ports are then placed under direct vision. The assistant's ports are positioned to the left of the midline. The assistant's left hand holds the camera through a 10-mm port in the left paramedian line slightly lower than the position of the initial Hassan port at the right paramedian line. Two 5-mm ports are then placed after full insufflation and just below the costal margins bilaterally. In general, we like to maintain a hand's breath (9 to 10 cm) between working ports to avoid "scissoring" of instruments. Liver retraction can be accomplished through a 5-mm port in the far right lateral subcostal position.

REDUCING THE HERNIA SAC

Following port placement and liver retraction, the operating room table is placed in steep reverse Trendelenburg to facilitate visualization of the hiatus and aid in reducing the herniated abdominal contents. It is important to remember that the combination of the patient's dehydrated preoperative fasting state and shift in intravascular volume to the lower extremities upon steep Trendelenburg positioning can lead to a precipitous fall in blood pressure. Thus gradual patient repositioning and initiation of abdominal insufflation will allow time for the anesthesiologist to volume load the patient with intravenous fluids and allow the patient to respond more favorably to these changes.

Reduction of herniated contents, such as omentum and bowel, is performed upon initial assessment of the hiatus. Excessive traction or pulling on the stomach should be avoided because this causes unnecessary trauma. To accomplish sac reduction, the surgeon and assistant grasp the hernia sac just inside the hiatus at or near the 12 o'clock position and attempt an atraumatic eversion. By everting this sac, we attempt to enter the layers of the elongated and attenuated phrenoesophageal ligament. By careful dissection, the surgeon can then use hemostatic energy devices such as the harmonic scalpel (Ethicon, Cincinnati, Ohio) to open and identify the foamy, areolar type plane, reminiscent of working in the retroperitoneum or perinephric fat. The appearance of this foamy layer is quite characteristic and critical to the technical success and ease of the operation. Once this plane is identified, it is important to try to stay within this plane as it is extended up into the mediastinum. While working within this plane, one can visualize the esophagus, the anterior vagus, the aorta, and the pleura bilaterally. It is important to note that failure to identify this areolar plane can significantly increase the difficulty of the entire operation. Even though these areolar attachments are only minimally vascularized, we use energy here and minimize blunt dissection to keep the mediastinum meticulously dry and hemostatic. Extensive, circumferential mobilization of the esophagus is performed high into the mediastinum, laterally to the pleura and into the posterior mediastinum, and periaortic area. The dissection can be carried as high as the inferior pulmonary veins and beyond if needed.

Next, we exit the mediastinum and examine the right crus and divide the gastrohepatic ligament. Occasionally, a significantly sized accessory hepatic artery may be encountered, which can be spared with some extra technical work. However, in most cases, even if sizeable, a temporary clip can be placed and liver perfusion reassessed in 15 to 20 minutes; if in the judgment of the surgeon, this vessel should be spared, it can be but with some technical challenges. In most cases it can be divided with no significant sequela.

During dissection of the hernia sac, the pleural reflection should be identified. During the early steps of the operation, we try to avoid entering the pleura. Entering the pleura early can lead to a "billowing" of the planes, blood pressure instability, and increased CO_2 absorption. Prior to crural approximation, we intentionally enter the left pleural space with a small 5 mm port and pigtail to reduce tension on the diaphragm induced by the pneumoperitoneum and facilitate crural reapproximation. An added benefit of entering the pleural space is that it allows drainage of any hematoma that otherwise might occur in the mediastinum after reduction of the hernia contents.

After the sac has been reduced from the mediastinum, and the areolar dissection complete, the stomach generally has completely returned tension free, to its normal subdiaphragmatic location. At all times during the procedure, care is taken to avoid injury to the peritoneal lining covering the crura so to preserve the integrity and allow for successful primary closure. We have found that, if after complete mobilization of the hernia and sac, if crural tension is still present, inducing or augmenting an existing left-sided pneumothorax (as described earlier) may yield a more prominent "floppy diaphragm sign," allowing for a tension-free primary repair. Clear communication with the anesthesiologist is important when inducing or augmenting the pneumothorax to allow him or her to monitor and correct any hemodynamic instability. If crural integrity has been compromised or there is still tension preventing primary repair, one should consider the addition of a right- or left-sided crural-relaxing incision and mesh reinforcement. In our experience, this occurs less than 5% of the time.

ESTABLISHING ADEQUATE INTRAABDOMINAL ESOPHAGEAL LENGTH

The next step in the PEH repair is to assess and reestablish adequate intraabdominal esophageal length. If this is not achieved, the esophagus and stomach continue to exert axial forces on the crural closure and a recurrence is more likely to result.

To accurately assess the location of the true GEJ, the gastric fat pad is mobilized off of the stomach and distal esophagus to allow for clear visualization of the junction of the longitudinal muscle fibers of the esophagus and the serosa of the stomach along with the angle of His. The fat pad dissection is then continued around the GEJ to create a posterior window between the esophagus and posterior vagus nerve through which to perform the fundoplication. Constant visualization of the anterior and posterior vagus nerves is important to avoid injury to these structures. If there is significant esophageal shortening, which is common with type III PEH, additional attempts at high mediastinal esophageal mobilization should be made. In the event that 2 cm of tension-free intraabdominal esophagus cannot be established, a Collis gastroplasty should be performed if the plan is to proceed with a fundoplication. We have found over the years, that with more experience and better esophageal mobilization, the need for a Collis gastroplasty has been reduced and when it is needed, the length of the Collis gastroplasty can be kept to a smaller distance.

REPAIRING THE DIAPHRAGMATIC DEFECT

A key element to durable repair of PEH is a tension-free closure of the hiatal defect. There has been debate regarding primary closure versus the routine use of mesh to reinforce the hiatal repair. Two prospective randomized trials have compared primary closure with mesh-reinforced repair, with short-term outcomes initially favoring a reduction in recurrent herniation in the mesh-reinforced group.[3,14] However, in the study of biologic mesh repair, early failure rates at 6 months were suboptimal in both groups, 9% in the mesh group, and 24% in the nonmesh group, leaving significant room for improvement in both arms. In a subsequent analysis at a median follow-up of 58 months, 59% of patients who received a primary hiatal repair and 54% who received a mesh-buttressed repair were noted to have a recurrence.[15] Although the need for reoperation was less than this, no one can be happy about recurrence rates that high. Longer-term outcomes may well see a further increase in symptoms requiring reoperation, and clearly the outcomes of this trial showed no benefit to the routine use of mesh reinforcement for the crural repair.

In our center, we have found that in the vast majority of patients, we can achieve primary crural repair if the principles of complete esophageal and sac mobilization and preservation of crural integrity are followed. The crura are approximated with two or three interrupted nonabsorbable sutures placed posteriorly with the esophagus lying in a neutral, tension-free position within the hiatus. If any tension is present, we make sure the crura are mobilized by using a number of routine steps. For example, freeing up the spleen from the edge of the left crus can relieve some of the tension in this location. Normally, the spleen lives in the left upper quadrant and is not adherent to the left crus. However, after years of gastric migration into the chest, the short gastrics and residual posterior hernia sac can "drag" the spleen toward the crus and actually leads to scarification at the left crural edge. This can generally be easily mobilized with little risk to the spleen if care is taken. Next, if tension remains, we consider adding a controlled tension pneumothorax (as previously described) to the left side. This creates a very favorable "floppy diaphragm" and, in almost all cases, allows a tension-free approximation of the crus both posteriorly and anteriorly. It is not uncommon to have to reintroduce carbon dioxide into the left hemithorax every few minutes to maintain this floppiness, thus we often place a 5-mm port above the left costal margin. Alternatively, simply opening the left pleura in the mediastinum accomplishes this purpose. Care is taken to avoid an artificial angulation or "speed-bump" deformity of the esophagus as it passes through the hiatus from excessive posterior crural closure. However, because many of these patients are kyphotic, and posterior crural closure actually adds intraabdominal length to the esophagus, some surgeons will add additional posterior sutures. After placing the sutures posteriorly, the hiatus is reevaluated. If the hiatal space continues to be patulous (i.e., more than a centimeter of space between the crura and esophagus with introduction of a grasper through the opening), additional interrupted horizontal sutures are placed either posteriorly or anteriorly on the upper aspect of the crura.

In some patients, there is a favorable angle for a lateral suture into the left crus at approximately "3 o'clock." At the completion of the closure, a grasper should be easily introduced through the hiatus, with a small visible space surrounding the esophagus circumferentially. This is very much an experience and judgment decision: you want the space to be minimal because, if too patulous, you risk herniation of the wrap and/or other abdominal contents, and too tight can produce dysphagia.

REESTABLISHING THE ANTIREFLUX BARRIER

Gastroesophageal reflux is present in only approximately 50% of patients at the time of PEH repair, but a number of experts have published results showing the majority of patients with GPEH have a history of GERD. In addition, the reduction of the mediastinal sac and dissection of the esophagus disrupts the phrenoesophageal ligament further and potentially the integrity of the lower esophageal antireflux barrier contributing to post-op GERD symptoms if a wrap is omitted. There are some recent trials of PEH repair comparing groups with and without an antireflux fundoplication after the other steps of the hernia repair are complete, and the data have shown that a higher percent of patients undergoing surgical PEH correction have postoperative reflux, if a fundoplication is not performed.[11,15,16] Surgeon preference and preoperative esophageal manometry may help to determine the type of fundoplication to be performed: a circumferential "floppy" fundoplication (two-stitch Nissen over a 54 or 56 bougie)[17] or a partial fundoplication[18,19] are the two most commonly reported. In the past, we routinely performed the circumferential "floppy" Nissen fundoplication but more recently have moved onto a partial fundoplication or "near" Nissen to minimize side effects such as dysphagia, gas bloat, and flatulence in our generally elderly PEH population.

We have noted that certain patients, particularly elderly, frail patients with an upside-down stomach and essentially 100% intrathoracic location, have primarily obstructive symptoms and minimal heartburn. In this group, we are evaluating repair without a fundoplication and are putting these data together in an attempt to better clarify who might be predicted to do well without a wrap. In this very specific population, a gastropexy can be considered following careful adherence to the principles of PEH repair, including careful and complete sac dissection, complete stomach mobilization, vagal preservation, and careful crural closure. Some surgeons have described gastropexy as a single point of fixation using suture or the placement of a gastrostomy tube. We begin the gastropexy near the angle of His to the left crus and then follow the cardia and fundus along the diaphragm, just above the spleen, essentially in a line very near to where the short gastrics used to live. We place multiple interrupted horizontal mattress sutures (2 to 0 ethibond). Gastropexy sutures are placed on a diaphragmatic fold just a few millimeters above the spleen, approximately 2 cm apart over a distance of 10 to 14 cm. By more or less duplicating what used to be the line of the short gastrics, we are attempting to recreate normal anatomy of the intraabdominal stomach, not just a "pexy." We realize that until we have analyzed and published our outcomes in this series of patients, the addition of a fundoplication should be used in most patients.

At the completion of the operation a nasogastric tube can be placed by the anesthesiologist or surgeon under direct laparoscopic visualization. It is critical that the surgeon and anesthesiologist approach this placement with care because the obstruction created by the wrap and the closure can easily cause resistance to passage of a nasogastric (NG) tube and potential for esophageal perforation or at a minimum, suboptimal placement. Although we believe this tube can be removed early on postoperative day 1, we believe it is essential to enter the recovery room with an NG tube and an empty stomach to avoid postoperative retching, vomiting, or hiccupping.

MESH USE AT THE HIATUS

The use of mesh at the hiatus remains controversial. Early trials with permanent synthetic mesh suggested a reduction in hernia recurrence rates, but for most esophageal surgeons the potential complications associated with synthetic mesh, including erosion and difficult reoperations, outweigh the potential benefit. Two randomized trials using biologic absorbable mesh have failed to show a benefit for the use of this type of mesh. However, it is important to recognize that neither trial aggressively assessed or treated tension. The fundamentals of hernia surgery dictate that tension is the enemy of any hernia repair, and it is logical that this tenet holds true at the hiatus as well. Consequently, future studies need to focus on adequately addressing tension in the form of relaxing incisions for crural tension or adding an intentional pneumothorax to create a "floppy diaphragm" to relieve tension during crural repair. In addition, the role of Collis gastroplasty for axial esophageal tension should be further evaluated in controlled trials, and further evaluation of the role of nonpermanent and permanent mesh reinforcement of the crural closure.

COMPLICATIONS AND OUTCOMES

In our center, routine postoperative care includes a barium esophagram on postoperative day 1 to establish a new anatomic baseline and rule out perforation or leak prior to initiating oral intake. In addition, given the results of a number of reports of high recurrence rates, the onus is on the surgical team to document their surgical results immediately postoperatively and then to follow this group of patients and establish your own recurrence rates. Patients are discharged on liquid narcotic pain medication for 1 to 3 days and early are converted to oral liquid Tylenol. Patients are advised to refrain from heavy lifting long term and limit lifting to 15 to 20 pounds. In addition, we educate the patient on the avoidance of constipation and to watch for and treat early symptoms of gas bloat, using dietary manipulation and simethicone as needed. Patients follow up in clinic in 2 weeks with a chest x-ray and then annually with a barium esophagram to monitor for radiographic recurrence. If any abnormal or concerning symptoms are present at any time point, the first step is an interview with the patient and to review carefully a barium esophagram, with direct comparison with the one taken the first postoperative day. This close attention to detail facilitates early recognition of relevant symptoms, including dysphagia, and appropriate interventions to assist with patient comfort and satisfaction with quality of life. It is important for the surgeon to remain engaged in this process because the patient's primary care physicians and even their gastroenterologists may fail to recognize correctible problems that are related to the PEH repair. Routine dietary changes should include avoiding gassy foods and slowing down the eating process to avoid excess gas swallowing, following what we call the "25 chew" rule (i.e., chewing each bite of food 25 times). We also recommend four to five small meals per day and avoiding large feast-type meals.

In the early postoperative period, major postoperative complications include pneumonia, congestive heart failure, and pulmonary embolisms can occur in a small subset of patients. Postoperative mortality in the setting of elective repair should be less than 1% but is higher in patients older than 80 years and in patients requiring urgent repair.[11,13] In a review of outcomes from more than 650 patients who underwent laparoscopic giant paraesophageal hiatal hernia repairs, Luketich and colleagues reported major adverse outcomes including pneumonia (4%), pulmonary embolism (3.4%), congestive heart failure (2.6%), need for reintubation (2.6%), and postoperative leak (2.5%).[12] Laparoscopic repair by experienced laparoscopic esophageal surgeons is associated with a significant decrease in postoperative morbidity as compared with most series of open repair (~25% of patient's experience complications after laparoscopic repair as compared with ~60% after open repair), although there are no randomized comparative studies that have been performed.[7] The outcomes from the University of Pittsburgh revealed short postoperative hospitalizations (2 to 3 days) and low 30-day mortality when PEH repair is performed electively. Importantly, 90% of patients reported good to excellent scores on evaluation of their symptomatic outcomes, with only 3.4% requiring re-repair for symptom recurrence at long-term (7 years) follow-up.[10,12] We acknowledge that another 10% or so have small hiatal hernia recurrences, of which the majority will be manageable without surgery. However, we are not accepting these "small recurrences" as ideal, and we are continuing to evaluate our surgical results and hope to achieve "Pearson-like outcomes" of a less than 2% reoperation rate at long-term follow-up.[2]

SUMMARY

There are several key elements to laparoscopic repair of PEH: (1) complete reduction of the hernia sac and contents; (2) careful preservation of the anterior and posterior vagus nerves; (3) mobilization of the gastroesophageal fat pad and identification of the GEJ; (4) recognition and management of a shortened esophagus (extensive mediastinal mobilization and performance of a Collis gastroplasty when necessary); (5) preservation of crural integrity and closure of the hiatal defect without tension with liberal use of an induced pneumothorax to yield a "floppy" diaphragm during repair; selective use of mesh reinforcement only if other measures fail; and (6) performance of an antireflux procedure or perhaps in select patients a gastropexy. Laparoscopic repair of PEH can provide excellent patient satisfaction and symptom resolution when performed by surgeons with extensive experience in minimally invasive and open esophageal surgery. In this setting, we have shown that the outcomes, both short and long term, and the reoperation rates with a minimally invasive approach can be comparable with the best open series.[2,12]

REFERENCES

1. Kwok H, Marriz Y, Al-Ali S, Windsor JA. Phrenoesophageal ligament re-visited. *Clin Anat*. 1999;12:164-170.
2. Maziak DE, Todd TR, Pearson FG. Massive hiatus hernia: evaluation and surgical management. *J Thorac Cardiovasc Surg*. 1998;115(1):53-60, discussion 61–62.
3. Oelschlager BK, Pellegrini CA, Hunter J, et al. Biologic prosthesis reduces recurrence after laparoscopic paraesophageal hernia repair: a multicenter, prospective, randomized trial. *Ann Surg*. 2006;244:481-490.
4. Luketich JD, Raja S, Fernando HC, et al. Laparoscopic repair of giant paraesophageal hernia: 100 consecutive cases. *Ann Surg*. 2000;232(4):608-618.
5. Luketich JD, Maddaus MA. Laparoscopic Collis gastroplasty. In: Pearson FG, Patterson GA, eds. *Pearson's Thoracic and Esophageal Surgery*. 3rd ed. Philadelphia: Churchill Livingstone/Elsevier; 2008:326-336.
6. Mattar SG, Bowers SP, Galloway KD, Hunter JG, Smith CD. Long-term outcome of laparoscopic repair of paraesophageal hernia. *Surg Endosc*. 2002;16(5):745-749. [Epub 2002 Feb 8].
7. Karmali S, McFadden S, Mitchell P, et al. Primary laparoscopic and open repair of paraesophageal hernias: a comparison of short-term outcomes. *Dis Esophagus*. 2008;21(1):63-68.
8. Nason KS, Luketich JD, Qureshi I, et al. Laparoscopic repair of giant paraesophageal hernia results in long-term patient satisfaction and a durable repair. *J Gastrointest Surg*. 2008;12(12):2066-2075, discussion 2075–2077.
9. Skinner DB, Belsey RH. Surgical management of esophageal reflux and hiatus hernia: long-term results with 1,030 patients. *J Thorac Cardiovasc Surg*. 1967;53:33-54.
10. Allen MS, Trastek VF, Deschamps C, Pairolero PC. Intrathoracic stomach. Presentation and results of operation. *J Thorac Cardiovasc Surg*. 1993;105(2):253-258, discussion 258–259.
11. Stylopoulos N, Gazelle GS, Rattner DW. Paraesophageal hernias: operation or observation? *Ann Surg*. 2002;236(4):492-500, discussion 500–501.
12. Luketich JD, Nason KS, Christie NA, et al. Outcomes after a decade of laparoscopic giant paraesophageal hernia repair. *J Thorac Cardiovasc Surg*. 2010;139(2):395-404.
13. Ballian N, Luketich JD, Levy RM, et al. A clinical prediction rule for perioperative mortality and major morbidity after laparoscopic giant paraesophageal hernia repair. *J Thorac Cardiovasc Surg*. 2013;145(3):721-729.
14. Frantzides CT, Madan AK, Carlson MA, Stavropoulos GP. A prospective, randomized trial of laparoscopic polytetrafluoroethylene (PTFE) patch repair vs simple cruroplasty for large hiatal hernia. *Arch Surg*. 2002;137:649-652.
15. Oelschlager BK, Petersen RP, Brunt LM, et al. Laparoscopic paraesophageal hernia repair: defining long-term clinical and anatomic outcomes. *J Gastrointest Surg*. 2012;16(3):453-459.
16. Fuller CB, Hagen JA, DeMeester TR, Peters JH, Ritter M, Bremmer CG. The role of fundoplication in the treatment of type II paraesophageal hernia. *J Thorac Cardiovasc Surg*. 1996;111:655-661.
17. Davis RE, Awad ZT, Filipi CJ. Technical factors in the creation of a "floppy" Nissen fundoplication. *Am J Surg*. 2004;187(6):724-727.
18. O'Reilly MJ, Mullins SG, Saye WB, et al. Laparoscopic posterior partial fundoplication: analysis of 100 consecutive cases. *J Laparoendosc Surg*. 1996;6(3):141-150.
19. el-Sherif AE, Adusumilli PS, Pettiford BL, et al. Laparoscopic clam shell partial fundoplication achieves effective reflux control with reduced postoperative dysphagia and gas bloating. *Ann Thorac Surg*. 2007;84(5):1704-1709.

Open Paraesophageal Hernia Repair

Daniel L. Miller

Hiatal hernia (HH) was first recognized more than 400 years ago. In 1610 Ambrose Paré described a patient with the stomach herniating through the esophageal hiatus.[1] Bowditch was the first to report repair of an HH in 1853, and Akerlund first reported paraesophageal herniation in 1926.[2,3] In 1945 Harrington described the first series of patients who underwent HH repair.[4] In 1951 Allison was the first to attribute the symptoms of gastroesophageal reflux disease (GERD) and acid ingestion to an HH and also described an anatomic repair.[5] In 1968 Hill and Tobias were the first to clearly understand the anatomy (gastroesophageal junction [GEJ] and stomach) and clinical implications of paraesophageal hernias (PEHs).[6]

HHs were first classified into three types by the Swedish radiologist, Ake Akerlund.[2] The current classification scheme defines four types of hiatal or PEHs. The four types are classified based on the location of the GEJ and the fundus of the stomach in relationship to the diagrammatic crura (hiatus). Type I (sliding) hernia is when the GEJ migrates into the chest only, type II (true) is when the GEJ remains in the abdomen and the fundus of the stomach herniates into the chest, type III (mixed) is the combination of type I and II with herniation of both the GEJ and fundus into the chest, and type IV (complex) is when other abdominal viscera (colon [Fig. 27.1], small bowel, spleen, pancreas, or omentum) migrate into the chest with the GEJ and/or stomach. Type I, or sliding hernias, are the most common type and account for approximately 95% of all HHs, with the remaining three types (PEHs) making up the remaining 5% of HHs; 90% of the PEHs are the type III mixed PEHs (Fig. 27.2), and the rarest (<5%) are the type II true PEHs.

An HH is characterized by enlargement of the opening between the diaphragmatic crura, which allows the stomach and other abdominal viscera to elevate into the chest. The cause of enlargement of the hiatus is related to increased intraabdominal pressure creating a transdiaphragmatic pressure gradient between the thoracic and abdominal cavities at the GEJ. This pressure gradient results in weakness of the phrenoesophageal membrane and widening of the esophageal hiatus. Conditions that cause an increase in intraabdominal pressure include obesity, pregnancy, chronic constipation, chronic obstructive pulmonary disease (COPD) with chronic coughing, and strenuous jobs with significant amount of lifting. Aging is also a significant risk factor for development of PEH. PEH mainly affects older adults, with the median age of presentation between 65 and 75 years of age.[7] The US population, older than 65 years of age, increased from 13% to 17% between 2000 and 2015 and is predicted to increase to 24% by 2060.[8] With this increase in the elderly population and the rise of obesity within the United States, the incidence of patients with PEH that will require surgical care will increase significantly over time, so timing of surgical correction and what approach and repair is paramount to decrease operative morbidity and mortality and to improve short- and long-term outcomes.

INDICATION FOR SURGICAL REPAIR

Surgical repair is indicated in patients with symptomatic or complications of PEHs, the timing of which depends upon the acuity of presentation and significance of symptoms. Emergency repair is required in patients with acute gastric volvulus (Fig. 27.3), uncontrolled gastrointestinal bleeding, obstruction, strangulation, perforation, or irreversible respiratory comprise secondary to the PEH. As expected a patient with a PEH that presents as an emergency and requires surgical correction is associated with higher mortality rates.[9] Elective repair is recommended in patients with PEH who experience chronic symptoms that are increasing in frequency and severity, such as GERD refractory to medical therapy, dysphagia, early satiety, postprandial chest or abdominal pain, postprandial shortness of breath, aspiration, chronic anemia (Cameron erosions), or vomiting. Surgical repair of these patients electively is associated with improved symptoms and better quality of life (QoL).[10] Prophylactic PEH repair (PEHR) in asymptomatic patients is controversial. There is no consensus, but traditionally most surgeons feel that the very old or debilitated patients should not undergo surgery, whereas younger and healthier patients with life expectancy of 5 to 10 years should consider surgery to prevent both risk of acute gastric volvulus, especially if greater than 50% of stomach in the chest, and potentially progressive symptoms. In a recent study, the mortality rate from elective repair was estimated to be 1.4%, while the probability of developing acute symptoms that would necessitate emergency surgery was 1.1%. Allen and colleagues followed 23 patients with large PEHs who refused surgery and preferred medical management, for a median of 78 months (range, 12 to 268 months).[11] In four patients, progressive symptoms developed, and one patient died from aspiration. They concluded that patients with an intrathoracic upside-down stomach who have obstructive symptoms at initial presentation should undergo repair and that elective operation is safe and effective. However, gastric strangulation is extremely rare. The lifetime risk of developing acute symptoms requiring emergency surgery decreases exponentially with age older than 65 years.

PREOPERATIVE EVALUATION

Detailed history, physical exam, and endoscopic and radiographic evaluation are warranted in patients with

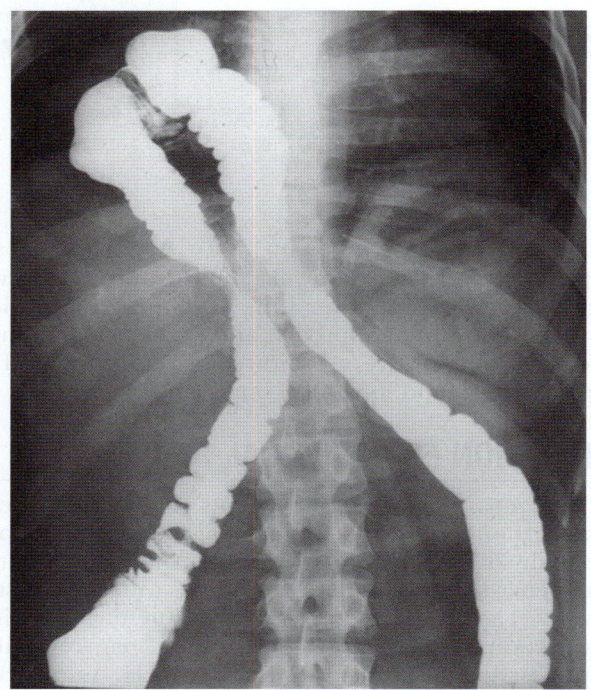

FIGURE 27.1 Type IV complex paraesophageal hernia (PEH) (colon). Barium enema of a patient with type IV PEH showing transverse colon that has passed through dilated hiatus into the hernia sac within the left chest.

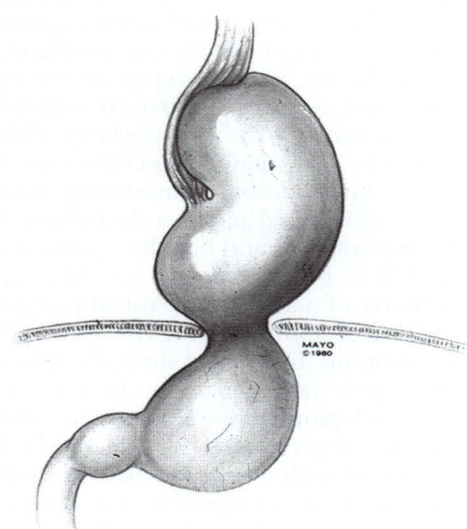

FIGURE 27.2 Large type III paraesophageal hernia (PEH). Schematic of a type III PEH demonstrating both the gastroesophageal junction and fundus of stomach above the normal positioned diaphragmatic hiatus. (Used with permission of Mayo Foundation for Medical Education and Research. All rights are reserved.)

PEHs to maximize the best surgical treatment, approach, and type of procedure for symptomatic and asymptomatic PEH patients. Current symptoms, previous medical therapies, comorbidities, and operative reports are recorded. All patients undergo upper endoscopy, barium swallow/

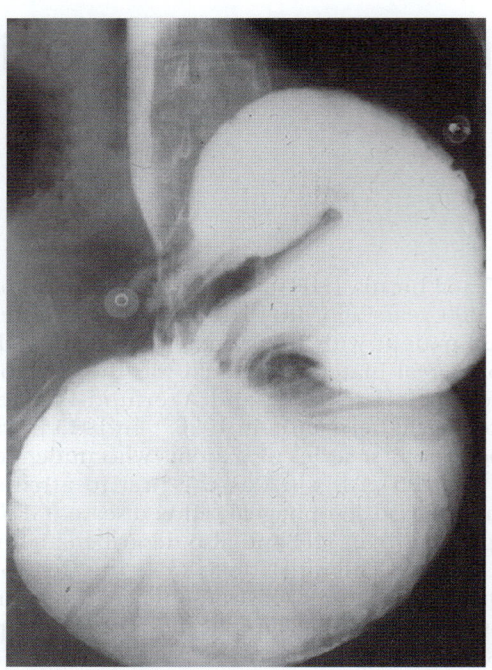

FIGURE 27.3 Large paraesophageal hernia (PEH) with gastric volvulus. Upper gastrointestinal series radiograph of a patient with large type III PEH with an organoaxial gastric volvulus.

upper gastrointestinal (UGI) series, computed tomography (CT) scan of chest and upper abdomen, and review of pathology biopsies if performed. Upper endoscopy is performed prior to surgery in an elective situation or at the time of emergency surgery to evaluate the hernia, including retroflexion maneuver, and to rule out possible esophageal or gastric pathology. In addition, a gastric volvulus can be determined, as well as mucosal ischemia or perforation related to strangulation. Oral contrast studies provide important information of gastric anatomy but most importantly length of the esophagus. Esophageal manometry and pH analysis are not required because they are unreliable and difficult to perform. Review of previous operative reports is paramount for success if you are performing a redo procedure. Attention should focus on type of crura repair, if mesh was used and how it was anchored, type of fundoplication, if the hernia sac was removed, if a gastroplasty or esophageal lengthening procedure was performed, and if an abdominal incisional hernia was repaired and if mesh was used for the repair.

OPERATIVE APPROACHES

PEHs can be repaired transabdominally or transthoracically. Transabdominal repairs can be performed open or laparoscopically. In most practices currently in the United States, laparoscopic PEHR is preferred for most patients in both elective and emergency situations. The first report of laparoscopic HH repair was published by Cuschieri and colleagues in 1992.[12] Even in the earliest of series, laparoscopic PEHR was associated with less morbidity compared with the open repair. The enthusiasm of laparoscopic community was dampened in 2000 when

Hashemi and colleagues demonstrate a 42% recurrence rate for the laparoscopic approach as opposed to 15% for the open approach.[13] Open transabdominal approach is used in patients who have had a limited number of upper abdominal procedures in the past, and reserve the transthoracic approach for patients who have failed previous transabdominal procedures, a history of abdominal wall mesh, history of abdominal abscess, infection, and contamination, and significant elevated body mass index (BMI) (>40). The three operative approaches have not been compared with one another in randomized trials, and the optimal operative approach for PEHR remains controversial and varies most depending on surgeon training and experience.[14]

In an analysis of approximately 40,000 patients from 1999 through 2008 from the Nationwide Inpatient Sample (NIS) database, 74%, 17%, and 9% were performed open transabdominally, transthoracically, and laparoscopically, respectively.[15] Currently, laparoscopic PEHR has surpassed open transabdominal repair as the most commonly performed procedure for PEHs. In the NIS study, transthoracic approach was associated with the longest hospital stay (7.8 days), the greatest need for mechanical ventilation (5.6%), and the greatest risk of having pulmonary embolism.[15] Laparoscopic approach was associated with the shortest hospital stay (4.5 days) and the lowest risk of requiring mechanical ventilation (2.3%). In a second study using the NIS database, published in 2017, 63,800 patients were analyzed from 2000 through 2013 to assess the effect of minimally invasive PEH surgery (MIS PEH) on patient outcomes.[16] Abdominal approach was used in 94.2% of patients (67.1% laparoscopically and 32.9% open) and 5.8% via the thoracic approach (24.5% thoracoscopically and 75.5% open). Patients undergoing MIS PEH experienced shorter hospital stay and decreased overall cost. Long-term outcome data are not known in these NIS studies. Other uncontrolled studies suggest that morbidity and mortality rates appear lower for laparoscopic PEHR compared with the other approaches. Although the risk of radiographic recurrence is higher with laparoscopic approach, reoperation rates are similar.

TRANSABDOMINAL REPAIR

An open or laparoscopic PEHR involves the same sequence of steps and principles of repair. An open transabdominal incision is usually performed via an upper abdominal incision from the xiphoid to just above the umbilicus. At times to facilitate further hiatal exposure the upper portion of the incision is extended to the left of the xiphoid. An upper hand retractor is preferred, which is connected to the bed bilaterally and is used instead of circumferential incisional retractor to allow elevation of the foregut for maximal exposure of the hiatal anatomy. Sequence of open surgical steps will now be described in detail.

Dissection of Hiatus

To prevent reherniation after PEHR, complete dissection and removal of the hernia sac from the mediastinum is mandatory. This dissection should be performed meticulously to avoid injury to mediastinal pleural, pericardium, aorta, and vagal nerves. If a pneumothorax occurs, it is not a hemodynamic issue during an open approach and

a chest tube is placed laterally above the diaphragm at completion of the repair prior to closure. The peritoneal covering of the crus on the abdominal side is preserved when dividing the gastrohepatic omentum from the right crus of the diaphragm to improve stability of the hiatus tightening. A Penrose drain is used and placed around the esophagus at the GEJ to elevate the esophagus and stomach to improve dissection of the posterior hiatus. Short gastric vessels are divided with an energy device (bipolar) to allow complete mobilization of the stomach into a normal configuration and for facilitation of the planned fundoplication.

Esophageal Mobilization

Distal mobilization of the esophagus and GEJ into the abdomen with sufficient length (4 to 5 cm) of intra-abdominal esophagus is essential for a tension-free PEHR and reduction of recurrence. Energy-assisted intrathoracic dissection is warranted to prevent injury to associated anatomic structures and more importantly to minimize the injury to the vagus nerves. This dissection is usually carried up to the level of the aortic arch to allow for a tension-free esophagus. If adequate intraabdominal esophagus cannot be achieved, a lengthening procedure is required; a true shortened esophagus is rare, usually less than 5% of patients. Chronicity of the PEH may lead to a higher incidence of a shortened esophagus. Lengthening of the esophagus is performed by a Collis gastroplasty.[17] The Collis procedure creates a gastric tube by vertically stapling the proximal stomach from the angle of His, parallel to a large bougie, 48 to 51 French, positioned along the lesser curvature of the stomach (Fig. 27.4). The neoesophagus is an elongated gastric tube, thus creating an extension of the esophagus that allows for the new esophagogastric junction to be greater than 4 cm in the abdomen. The Collis procedure was originally performed via a left thoracotomy, but more recently it has been performed transabdominally via open approach or laparoscopically.[18] The open or laparoscopic technique is called a wedge Collis gastroplasty because a wedge of fundus is resected to allow for vertical placement of the endoscopic stapler parallel to the lesser curvature, thus creating an elongated intraabdominal esophagus (Fig. 27.5).

Closure of Hiatus

After complete mobilization of the esophagus, the crura of the diaphragm are closed posteriorly to the esophagus. The closure of the hiatal defect is one of the most crucial steps in repair of a PEH. The repair must be tension free. The repair can be performed primarily, with a patch only, or a combination of primary repair and patch reinforcement. Primary closure is usually performed with nonabsorbable sutures, usually 3 to 5, depending on the size of hiatal defect, in an interrupted fashion; some surgeons prefer pledgeted horizontal mattress sutures because the cura have no fascial layer. If the crural fibers are disrupted during the dissection or the primary repair is under tension, the crural closure can be reinforced with biologic mesh, such as porcine dermal matrix or bovine pericardium. In addition, new bioresorbable materials are being evaluated and may prove useful at the hiatus to help

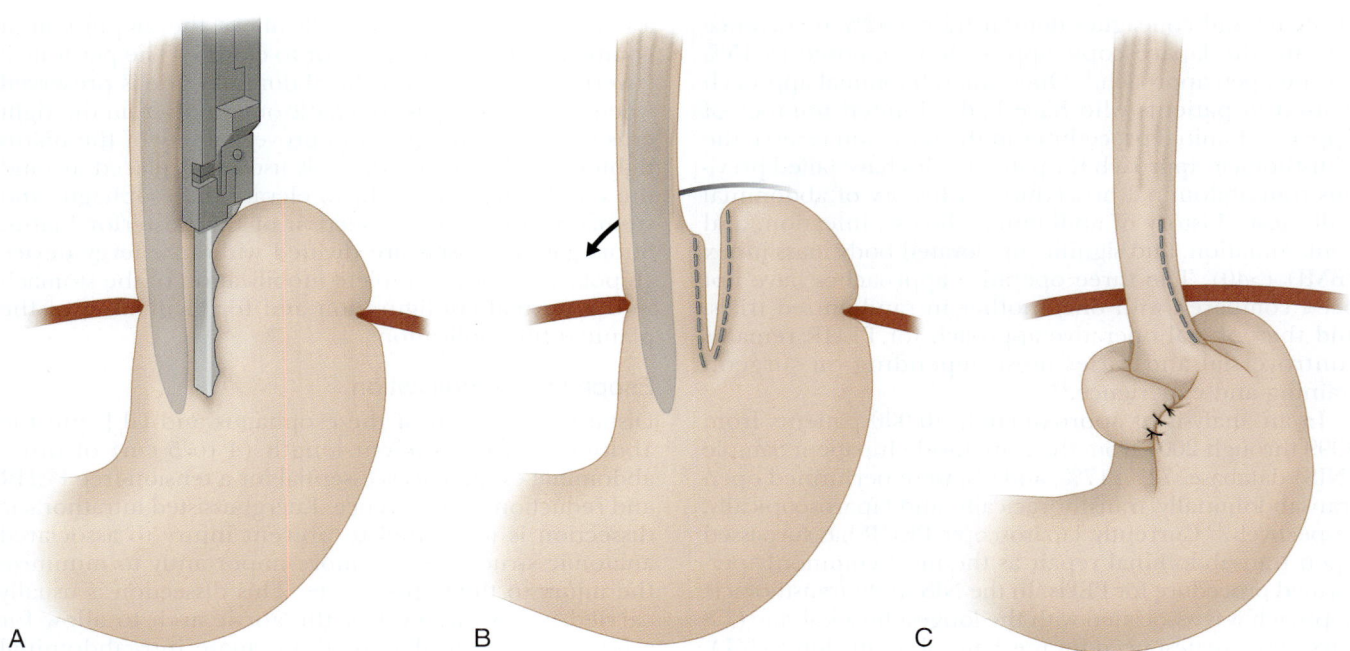

A   B   C

FIGURE 27.4 Sequence of surgical maneuvers for creation of Collis-Nissen gastroplasty for a shortened esophagus. (A) Placement of 60-mm linear staple parallel to an esophageal bougie (51 French) along the lesser curvature of the stomach. (B) Successful firing of the linear stapler with creation of the neoesophagus. The fundus of the stomach is being wrapped around the neoesophagus posteriorly. (C) Completion of the Nissen fundoplication below the diaphragm with primary closure of hiatus.

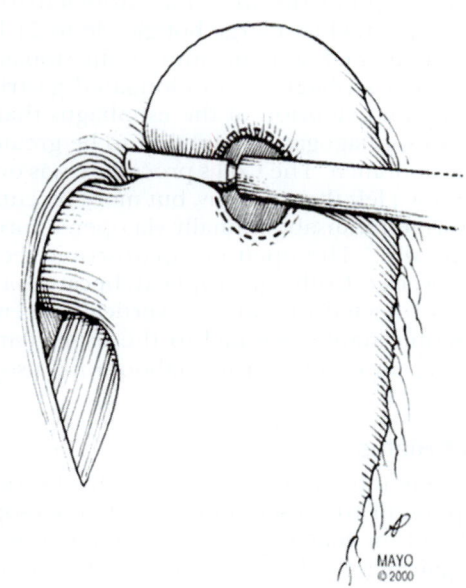

FIGURE 27.5 Laparoscopic gastroplasty. Drawing of a laparoscopic gastroplasty technique during an open transabdominal procedure for shortened esophagus. An end-to-end anastomosis stapler has been fired with creation of an opening in the fundus of stomach for placement of a linear stapler to complete the wedge gastroplasty. (Used with permission of Mayo Foundation for Medical Education and Research. All rights are reserved.)

reduce hernia recurrence. Synthetic permanent material such as polytetrafluoroethylene (PTFE) or polypropylene (Prolene) mesh is contraindicated for reinforcement or primary repair of hiatal defect because of serious and even life-threatening complications, including esophageal erosion with ulceration and perforation as well as abscess formation.

Reinforcement of a hiatal closure at the time of PEHR has been shown to reduce recurrence and reoperations.[19] In a 2016 meta-analysis of four randomized trials including 406 patients, compared with suture closure, mesh reinforcement of the hiatal closure reduced reoperations 2% versus 9% and recurrences 16% versus 27%, but not the complication rate of 10% for both, respectively.[20] Only the reoperation rate was statistically significant. In our practice, we selectively use mesh reinforcement during PEHR. When we reinforce, we usually use bovine pericardium in older patients, especially women greater than 80 years of age, steroid-dependent patients, reoperations, and significant COPD patients. The complication rate related to mesh reinforcement is related to the type of mesh and the configuration used. Biologic and bioresorbable mesh complications are usually only dysphagia as compared with erosion, perforation, stenosis, fibrosis, and the need for complex reoperations because of synthetic nonabsorbable mesh (Fig. 27.6).[21]

Fundoplication

We perform a fundoplication on all patients who undergo a PEHR. We usually perform a total 360-degree (Nissen) fundoplication with an open transabdominal PEHR, except in patients with severe preoperative dysphagia, for whom

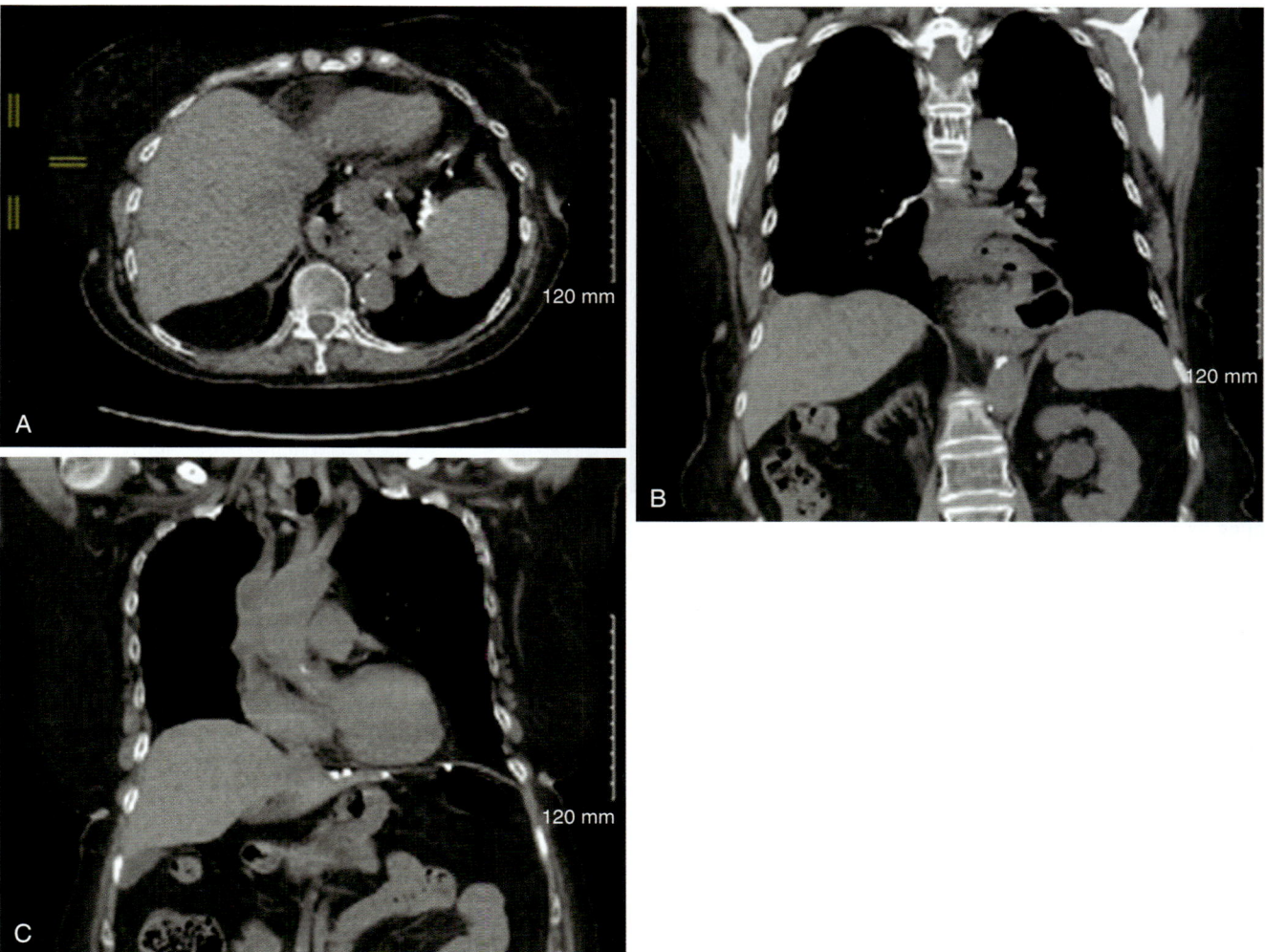

FIGURE 27.6 Recurrent type III paraesophageal hernia (PEH)—status post-mesh reinforcement. Recurrent type III PEH after mesh reinforcement. (A) Axial computed tomography (CT) scan tomogram of patient showing a recurrent PEH after undergoing laparoscopic PEH repair (PEHR) with synthetic mesh reinforcement. (B) Coronal CT scan tomogram of patient showing a recurrent PEH after undergoing laparoscopic PEHR with synthetic mesh reinforcement. (C) Coronal CT scan tomogram of patient showing metal surgical screws used to secure mesh during hiatus reinforcement.

we perform an anterior partial (Dor) fundoplication to minimize possible worsening dysphagia postoperatively. By adding a fundoplication you will reduce the incidence of postoperative GERD symptoms by restoring competency to the lower esophageal sphincter (LES). We routinely secure the fundoplication, partial or full, to the anterior portion of the hiatus to complete the closure of the defect and hopefully reduce the possibility of recurrence. The total fundoplication usually measures 2.0 to 2.5 cm in width to help prevent postoperative gas bloat syndrome and is anchored to the esophagogastric junction after removal of the esophageal fat pad to prevent slippage of the fundoplication.

In a randomized study, 40 patients who underwent either a cardiophrenicopexy (suture the cardia of the stomach to the diaphragm) or total fundoplication at the time of PEHR were analyzed. Patients who underwent fundoplication had significantly fewer postoperative GERD symptoms at 3 and 12 months and significantly lower rates of postoperative esophagitis, 17% versus 53%.[22] Other postoperative complications such as dysphagia and gas bloating did not differ between the two groups.

Postoperative Management

Patients are admitted to our surgical floor after PEHR. Intraoperative orogastric tubes are removed at the completion of the PEHR in the operating room (OR). Patients are given antiemetics for the first 24 hours postoperatively to reduce the risk of postoperative nausea and vomiting, which can disrupt the PEHR and cause early recurrence.[23] We have the patient ambulate the night of surgery, as well as start chewing gum 3 times a day for 20-minute intervals. We do not routinely perform a barium swallow the morning after surgery. We allow the patients to start sips of clear liquids 24 hours after surgery. The patient's chest and abdomen with respect to reherniation and gastric motility

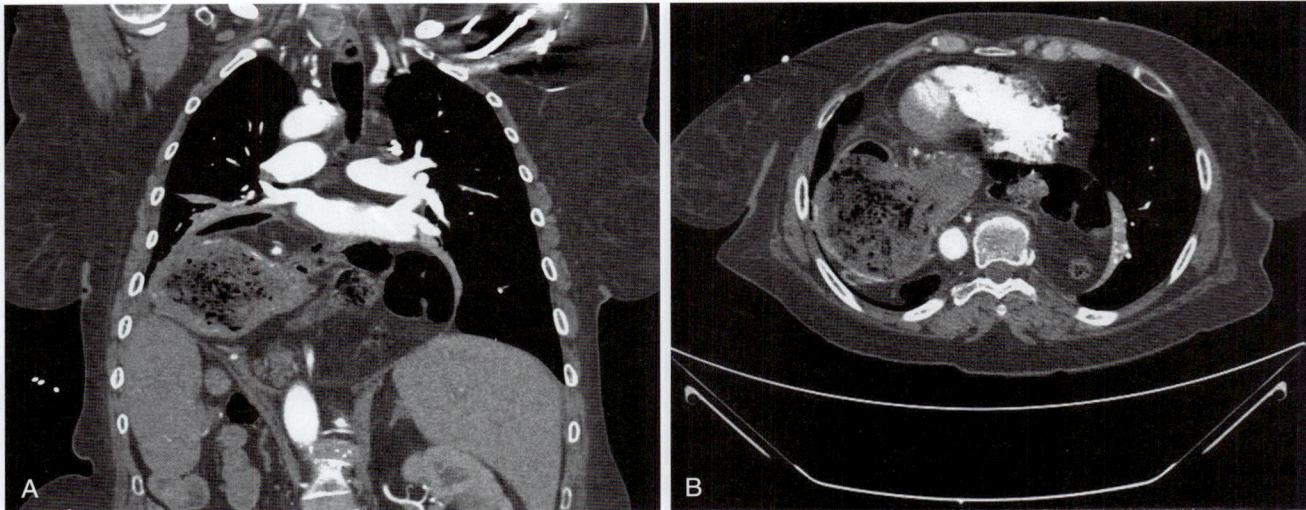

FIGURE 27.7 Type IV paraesophageal hernia (PEH) in patient with situs inversus. Large type IV PEH containing stomach, colon, and small bowel in patient with situs inversus. (A) Coronal computed tomography (CT) scan tomogram of patient showing a large type IV PEH containing stomach, colon, and small bowel in patient with situs inversus. (B) Axial CT scan tomogram of patient showing a large type IV PEH containing stomach, colon, and small bowel in patient with situs inversus.

is assessed by daily chest x-rays (CXRs). Postoperative pain management after an open transabdominal PEHR is controlled by intraoperative field blocks with 20 mL of bupivacaine liposome (Exparel; Pacira Pharmaceuticals, Inc., Parsippany, New Jersey) diluted to a total of 300 mL with injectable normal saline. Patients are discharged from the hospital usually 3 to 5 days after surgery once bowel function returns and the patient is tolerating a low-residue diet.

TRANSTHORACIC REPAIR

Transthoracic PEHR was the mainstay approach for all PEHs. Proponents now advocate that a transthoracic PEH should be performed instead of a transabdominal repair in patients who are obese, have a true shortened esophagus, have associated esophageal dysmotility disorders, have a complex type IV PEH, have failed at least two transabdominal repairs, or have had a midline abdominal incisional hernia repair with mesh. Thoracic surgeons argue that an open transthoracic PEHR is more durable compared with transabdominal repair because it permits more accurate intraoperative assessment of esophageal length, greater ease of performing an esophageal lengthening procedure (true Collis), greater ease of closing the hiatus without tension, and a better exposure in obese patients.[24] We generally proceed with a transthoracic repair in patients who are extremely obese (BMI >40), failed multiple transabdominal repairs (open and laparoscopically), with a complex type IV PEH with or without gastric volvulus, and in patients with situs inversus (Fig. 27.7). If we are evaluating an obese patient who has a large PEH, we refer the patient to bariatric surgery to determine if it would be best to have a combined PEHR and specific bariatric procedure (depending on the patient's BMI) to correct both conditions so that the patient can have the best outcome possible.

Transthoracic Approach

The patient is placed in a right lateral decubitus position after an oral gastric tube is placed. Single-lung aesthesia is facilitated by a double-lumen endotracheal tube; a left anteriolateral thoracotomy is usually performed through the bed of the unresected eighth rib.

Esophageal Mobilization

Adhesions between the PEH and the lung, chest wall, and diaphragm are lysed. The mediastinum pleura is opened at the level of the inferior pulmonary vein and the esophagus and both vagus nerves are encircled with a Penrose drain. The esophagus is mobilized distally to the hiatus. The phrenoesophageal membrane is opened at its apex in the chest and the stomach exposed. The entire hernia sac is dissected free from the hiatus and stomach and removed, making sure not to injure the vagus nerves. The stomach is examined for areas of ischemia if performed emergently and resected if present. Correct anatomic configuration of the stomach is confirmed, and the stomach is reduced. The esophagus is accessed for possible shortening. If it is present, a traditional Collis gastroplasty is performed, usually over a 51-French bougie with a usual staple length of 45 mm. The lengthening procedure reduces the tension on the native esophagus to prevent recurrence of the PEH.

Fundoplication

When an open transthoracic approach is used, the fundoplication that is included with the PEHR is a near-total (240 degrees) fundoplication—Belsey Mark IV repair.[25] This repair is a six-suture fundoplication of three sutures per two rows evenly positioned over the 240 degrees of the anterior stomach to cover 4 cm of intraabdominal esophagus (Fig. 27.8). The final row of nonabsorbable

Belsey Mark IV Procedure

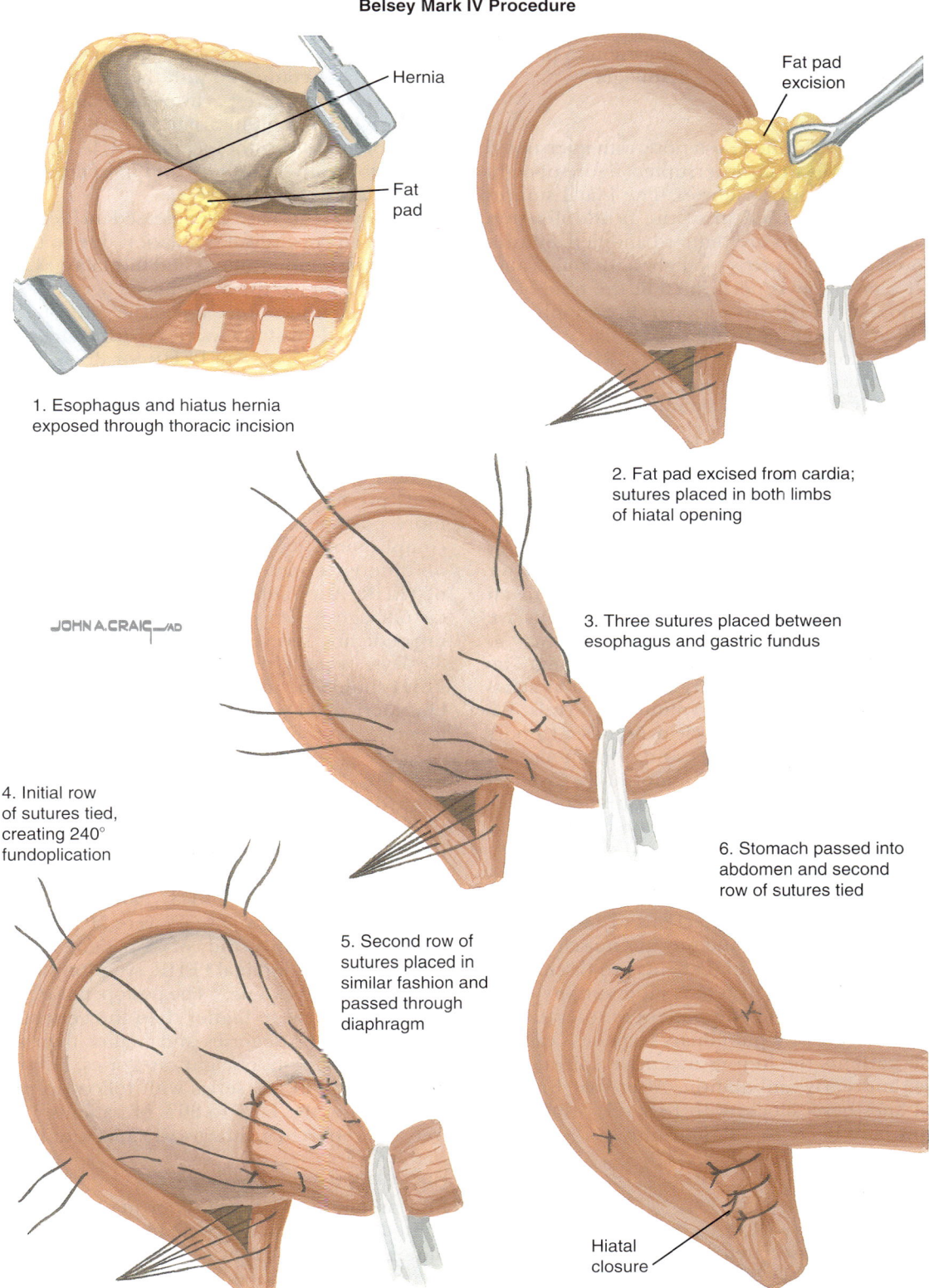

1. Esophagus and hiatus hernia exposed through thoracic incision

2. Fat pad excised from cardia; sutures placed in both limbs of hiatal opening

3. Three sutures placed between esophagus and gastric fundus

4. Initial row of sutures tied, creating 240° fundoplication

5. Second row of sutures placed in similar fashion and passed through diaphragm

6. Stomach passed into abdomen and second row of sutures tied

Hernia

Fat pad

Fat pad excision

JOHN A. CRAIG — AD

Hiatal closure

FIGURE 27.8 Belsey Mark IV repair. (Netter illustration used with permission of Elsevier, Inc. All rights reserved.)

sutures is secured below the diaphragm and tied to the anterior portion of the hiatus. The Belsey repair is an excellent long-term functional fundoplication to prevent GERD symptoms, recurrence, and dysphagia.[26]

Hiatus Repair

The hiatal closure is performed posteriorly with interrupted nonabsorbable sutures in an interrupted figure-of-eight configuration, usually 4 to 5 sutures. The hiatal sutures are placed first but not tied until the fundoplication transdiaphragmatic sutures are reduced and tied. Sutures can be removed if the closure is too tight and could cause dysphagia. If a myotomy is performed at the time of an open transthoracic PEHR for preoperative esophageal dysmotly, then the center sutures from each row are eliminated with continued excellent GERD symptom prevention. Reinforcement material is not needed in an open transthoracic repair, which significantly reduces the intraoperative cost. The chest is drained with a single 28-French chest tube that can cross the midline and drain the right chest if the pleura was entered during dissection of the hernia sac.

Postoperative Management

Patients are again admitted to our surgical floor after PEHR. Intraoperative oral gastric tubes are removed at the completion of the PEHR in the OR. Patients are given antiemetics for the first 24 hours postoperatively to reduce the risk of postoperative nausea and vomiting. The patient ambulates the night of surgery, as well as starts chewing gum 3 times a day for 20-minute intervals. We allow the patients to start sips of clear liquids 24 hours after surgery. The patient's chest and abdomen with respect to reherniation and gastric motility is assessed by daily CXRs. We do not use epidural catheters in our open transthoracic PEHR patients because of issues with medication-induced hypotension in the elderly and Foley-related issues in elderly men. Postoperative pain management after an open transthoracic PEHR is controlled by intraoperative parasympathetic injections (T2 to T11), as well as full-thickness latissimus and serratus muscle blocks with 300 mL of diluted Exparel. Patients are discharged from the hospital usually 4 to 6 days after surgery once bowel function returns and the patient is tolerating a low-residue diet. Aggressive pulmonary hygiene is carried out in these patients, including incentive spirometry, flutter valve, and early ambulation. After switching to the regional anesthesia blocks with Exparel, respiratory complications have decreased significantly.

PATIENT OUTCOMES

Morbidity and Mortality

Laparoscopic PEHR is associated with low overall morbidity (<3%) and mortality (<2.0%).[7,27] The mortality and morbidity rates are higher in patients who are 70 years of age or older, who underwent an emergent procedure, and those patients with multiple comorbid conditions. As expected, open transabdominal and transthoracic PEHR are associated with higher morbidity and mortality rates, but not as high as expected. In a retrospective study of 1005 patients who underwent an open transabdominal PEHR

and were older than 80 years of age, operative mortality was 8.2%.[28] Emergent repair, which was performed in 43% of those patients, was associated with a much higher mortality rate compared with the elective repair patients, 15.7% versus 2.4%, respectively, and was the only predictor of mortality in a multivariate analysis. In the two largest series of open transthoracic PEHR, 94 and 240 patients, the postoperative morbidity and mortality rates were 1.7% and 2.1%, respectively.[29,30]

Older patients have an increased incidence of PEH and can be denied surgical evaluation due to the perception of increased complications and mortality. El Lakis and colleagues examined the influence of age and comorbidities on early complications and other short-term outcomes of PEHR.[31] The study was a retrospective review of 524 patients who underwent PEHR for PEHs with more than 50% of stomach involved and were stratified by age (<70, 70 to 79, ≥80 years of age) to determine outcomes. Patients 80 years of age or older had higher American Society of Anesthesiologists (ASA) class, more comorbidities, larger PEHs, and higher incidence of type IV PEHs and acute presentation. Patients 80 years of age or older had more postoperative complications but not more major complications; hospital stay was 1 day longer. There was no difference in recurrence of their PEH based on age of PEHR. After adjustment for comorbidities and other factors, age 80 years or older was not a significant factor in predicting severe complications, readmissions within 30 days, or early recurrence. Older patients with giant PEHs should be given the opportunity to be evaluated by experienced surgeons for PEHR. Advanced age is no longer a contraindication for PEHR.

Efficacy

Regardless of approach, PEHRs have been shown to significantly alleviate preoperative symptoms related to the PEH. A prospective study of 111 patients found laparoscopic PEHR to be associated with improved symptoms and better QoL at 1 and 3 years after surgery.[32] The overall QoL scores at 3 years were 50% higher than the baseline scores. In a study of 72 patients who underwent an open transabdominal PEHR, symptoms were improved compared with baseline.[14] The postoperative Short Form-36 (SF-36) scores were higher than the general population in six of eight categories and higher than age-matched population in eight of eight categories. In two large open transthoracic PEHR series with follow-up ranging from 42 to 92 months, 80% to 86% of patients were symptom free and reported satisfactory results with the surgery.[29,30]

Recurrence

Interpretation of studies reporting recurrence rates are limited by different outcome measures used. The rate of radiographic recurrence is higher than that of clinical recurrence. Most patients with a radiographic recurrence after PEHR are asymptomatic, whereas patients with clinical recurrence can usually have symptoms controlled with medication. Only a small percentage of patients will require re-PEHR for complications or intractable symptoms. Laparoscopic PEHRs have a higher radiologic recurrence rate than the two open approaches, but most of these recurrences are clinically silent and do not require reoperation. A meta-analysis of 13 retrospective studies of laparoscopic PEHR reported a clinical recurrence rate of 10.2% (range, 3% to 33%) and radiographic recurrence rate of 25%.[33] The reported rates of clinical recurrence after an open transabdominal PEHR vary from 0% to 44%.[14,33,34] The majority of recurrences were sliding hernias less than 2 cm in size. In the two largest open transthoracic repair series of 94 and 240 patients who underwent transthoracic PEHR, only 1.7% and 2.1% developed clinical recurrence that required reoperation, respectively.[29,30]

Reoperation

Reoperation for a symptomatic PEH presents a technical challenge, especially if synthetic mesh was used at the time of the original PEH operation. If the initial approach for a redo PEHR is laparoscopic, there should be a low threshold at the time of reoperation to convert to an open procedure, especially in the presence of perforation, ischemia, significant blood loss, or undissectable adhesions. In complex reoperative cases, such as multiple failed transabdominal repairs, a transthoracic approach can provide a surgeon-friendly virgin chest with undissected planes for a successful PEHR. However, the dissection along the left lateral segment of the liver and fully mobilizing the fundus can be tedious and require a concomitant diaphragmatic incision to allow adequate exposure. A retrospective population-based analysis was performed using the NIS for the period 2000–2013 of adults undergoing PEHR to determine if perioperative results were impacted by surgical volume.[16] Hospital surgical volume was categorized as small (<6 operations/year), intermediate (6 to 20 operations/year), and high (>20 operations/year). A total of 63,812 patients were included. Over the time period, the rate of procedures across high-volume centers increased from 65.8% to 94.4%. The rate of open PEHR was significantly different among the groups (small volume—61.6%, intermediate volume—58.2%, and high volume—32.6%). Patients undergoing PEHR at high-volume centers had fewer postoperative complications and shorter hospital stay. This solidifies further that initial PEHRs and reoperative PEHRs should be performed by highly experienced surgeons at high-volume centers.

CONCLUSION

Indication for PEHR has changed over the past 20 years. Traditional indications for PEHR are medically refractory GERD, dysphagia, regurgitation, and obstructive symptoms, as well as complications such as chronic anemia and recurrent aspiration pneumonia, but more recently shortness of breath and dyspnea on exertion, as well as decreased cardiac function should be addressed. Advanced age is not a contraindication for PEHR. Even though laparoscopic approach has become the standard approach for elective and emergent PEHR, an open transabdominal or transthoracic approach should also be in a surgeon's surgical armamentarium to offer patients with complex type IV PEHs, who have failed multiple laparoscopic PEHR, who had prior mesh use, and with significant obesity. Open procedures have similar associated morbidity and mortality as laparoscopic PEHR. Conversion to an open approach,

transabdominal for general surgeons or transthoracic for thoracic surgeons is warranted to improve outcomes in patients with a complex or recurrent PEHs. Elective PEHR is preferred.

REFERENCES

1. Ohler WR, Rivto M. Diaphragmatic (hiatus) hernia—a clinical study. *N Engl J Med.* 1943;229:191-196.
2. Bowditch HI. *A Treatise on Diaphragmatic Hernia.* Buffalo: Jewett Thomas; 1853.
3. Akerlund A, Onnell H, Key E. Hernia diaphragmatica hiatus oesophagei vom anastomischen und roentgenologischen gesichtspunkt. *Acta Radiol.* 1926;6:3-22.
4. Harrington SW. The surgical treatment of the more common types of diaphragmatic hernia: esophageal hiatus, traumatic, pleuroperitoneal hiatus, congenital absence and foramen of Morgagni: report of 404 cases. *Ann Surg.* 1945;122:546-568.
5. Allison PR. Reflux esophagitis, sliding hiatal hernia and anatomy of repair. *Surg Gynecol Obstet.* 1951;92:419-431.
6. Hill LD, Tobias JA. Paraesophageal hernia. *Arch Surg.* 1968;96:735-744.
7. Luketich JD, Nason KS, Christie NA, et al. Outcomes after a decade of laparoscopic giant paraesophageal hernia repair. *J Thorac Cardiovasc Surg.* 2010;139:395-406.
8. Colby SI, Ortman JM. *Projections of the Size and Composition of the US Population: 2014 to 2060, Current Population Reports, P25—1143.* Washington, DC: US Census Bureau; 2015.
9. Zaman JA, Lidor AO. The optimal approach to symptomatic paraesophageal hernia repair: important technical considerations. *Curr Gastroenterol Rep.* 2016;18:1-8.
10. Lebenthal A, Waterford SA, Fisichelia PM. Treatment and controversies in paraesophageal hernia repair. *Front Surg.* 2015;2:1-6.
11. Allen MS, Trastek VF, Deschamps C, Pairolero PC. Intrathoracic stomach: presentation and results of operation. *J Thorac Cardiovasc Surg.* 1993;105:253-259.
12. Cuschieri A, Shimi S, Nathanson LK. Laparoscopic reduction, crural repair and fundoplication of large hiatal hernia. *Am J Surg.* 1992;163:425-430.
13. Hashemi M, Peters JH, DeMeester TR, et al. Laparoscopic repair of large type III hiatal hernia: objective followup reveals high recurrence rate. *J Am Coll Surg.* 2000;190:553-561.
14. Low DE, Unger T. Open repair of paraesophageal hernia: reassessment of subjective and objective outcomes. *Ann Thorac Surg.* 2005;80:287-294.
15. Paul S, Nasar A, Port JL, et al. Comparative analysis of diaphragmatic hernia outcomes using the nationwide inpatient sample database. *Arch Surg.* 2012;147:607-620.
16. Schlottmann F, Strassle PD, Allaix ME, Patti MG. Paraesophageal hernia repair in the USA: trends of utilization stratified by surgical volume and consequent impact on perioperative outcomes. *J Gastrointest Surg.* 2017;21:1199-1205.
17. Collis JL. An operation for hiatal hernia with short esophagus. *Thorax.* 1957;12:181-186.
18. Mattioli S, Lugaresi M, Ruffato A, et al. Collis-Nissen gastroplasty for short oesophagus. *Multimed Man Cardiothorac Surg.* 2015 Nov 18;2015.
19. Frantzides CT, Madan AK, Carlson MA, Stavropoulos GP. A prospective, randomized trial of laparoscopic polytetrafluoroethylene (PTFE) patch repair vs simple cruroplasty for large hiatal hernia. *Arch Surg.* 2002;137:649-657.
20. Memon MA, Memon B, Yunus RM, Khan S. Suture cruroplasty versus prosthetic hiatal herniorrhaphy for large hiatal hernia: a meta-analysis and systematic review of randomized controlled trials. *Ann Surg.* 2016;263:258-266.
21. Stadhuber RJ, Sherif AE, Mittal SK, et al. Mesh complications after prosthetic reinforcement of hiatal closure: a 28-case series. *Surg Endosc.* 2009;23:1219-1226.
22. Muller-Stich BP, Achtstatter V, Diener MK, et al. Repair of paraesophageal hiatal hernia—is a fundoplication needed? A randomized controlled pilot trial. *J Am Coll Surg.* 2015;221:602-610.
23. Puri V, Kakarlapudi GV, Awad ZT. Filipi CJ. Hiatal hernia recurrence: 2004. *Hernia.* 2004;8:311-317.
24. Itano H, Okamoto S, Kodama K, Horita N. Transthoracic Collis-Nissen repair of massive type IV paraesophageal hernia. *Gen Thorac Cardiovasc Surg.* 2008;56:446-450.

25. Belsey R. Mark IV repair of hiatal hernia by the transthoracic approach. *World J Surg.* 1977;1:475-481.

26. Allen MS. Open repair of hiatus hernia: thoracic approach. *Chest Surg Clin N Am.* 1998;8:431-440.

27. Larusson HJ, Zingg U, Hahnloser D, et al. Predictive factors for morbidity and mortality in patients undergoing laparoscopic para-esophageal hernia repair: age, ASA score and operation type influence morbidity. *World J Surg.* 2009;33:980-985.

28. Poulose BK, Gosen C, Marks JM, et al. Inpatient mortality analysis of paraesophageal hernia repair in octogenarians. *J Gastrointest Surg.* 2008;12:1888-1892.

29. Patel HJ, Tan BB, Ye J, et al. A 25-year experience with open primary transthoracic repair of paraesophageal hernia repair. *J Thorac Cardiovasc Surg.* 2004;127:843-849.

30. Mazaiak DE, Todd TR, Pearson FG. Massive hiatus hernia; evaluation and surgical management. *J Thorac Cardiovasc Surg.* 1998;115:53-62.

31. El Lakis MA, Kaplan SJ, Hubka M, Mohiuddin K, Low DE. The importance of age on short-term outcomes associated with repair of giant paraesophageal hernias. *Ann Thorac Surg.* 2017;103:1700-1709.

32. Lidor AO, Steele KE, Stem M, et al. Long-term quality of life and risk factors for recurrence after laparoscopic repair of paraesophageal hernia. *JAMA Surg.* 2015;150:424-431.

33. Carlson MA, Condon RE, Ludwig KA, Schulte WJ. Management of intrathoracic stomach with polypropylene mesh prosthesis reinforced transabdominal hiatus repair. *J Am Coll Surg.* 1998;187:227-230.

34. Ferri LE, Feldman LS, Stanbridge D, et al. Should laparoscopic paraesophageal hernia repair be abandoned in favor of the open approach? *Surg Endosc.* 2005;19:4-8.

Diaphragmatic Relaxing Incisions for Crural Tension During Hiatal Hernia Repair

Marc A. Ward | Steven R. DeMeester

Laparoscopic repair of a large hiatal hernia with a widened hiatus is challenging and objective hernia recurrence rates are high. In a recent randomized trial, the recurrence rate exceeded 50% at 5 years after laparoscopic paraesophageal hernia.[1] Tension on the repair of any hernia contributes to an increased risk for recurrence. This was first recognized for inguinal hernias and led to the incorporation of relaxing incisions and tension-free repairs. Subsequently component separation has been adopted to release tension during ventral hernia repair.[2-4] Logically this concept can be extended to the hiatus for patients with large crural defects where achieving primary approximation of the crural pillars would be difficult or impossible without significant tension. Similar to the tension-free inguinal hernia repair, bridging the crural defect with mesh has been considered. However, bridging with synthetic mesh has been associated with mesh erosion into the esophagus and is ill-advised (Fig. 28.1).[5] Bridging with a biologic mesh is only a temporary solution since the bridged biologic or absorbable material will go away, setting the stage for hernia recurrence. Park et al. proposed using the mobilized falciform ligament to bridge the hiatal defect, but the long-term efficacy of this approach is unknown.[6] In our opinion a better alternative is a relaxing incision in either the right or left diaphragm, and occasionally in both.

The concept of a relaxing incision is to create a defect adjacent to the area of interest that is less critical (muscle or fascia) to allow the principal tissues to come together. In the case of the hiatus, relaxing incisions are ideal since there is available diaphragm on either side. In addition, there is little (if any) downside to making a relaxing incision in the diaphragm. Because there is a pressure differential between the thorax (negative pressure) and the abdomen (positive pressure), all relaxing incisions must be closed. Even small diaphragmatic defects can lead to herniation of abdominal contents into the chest.[7] We routinely close these defects with polytetrafluoroethylene (PTFE), since there is a large experience with this mesh for chest wall and diaphragm reconstruction. Unlike other types of synthetic mesh, the lung does not typically fuse to PTFE mesh, so future thoracic surgical procedures, if needed, will not be made more complex. While there is concern about the use of PTFE mesh in a clean-contaminated case, six of our patients in our published series had a concomitant wedge fundectomy Collis gastroplasty, and no patient developed an infection of the PTFE mesh used in the reconstruction.[8] Unlike ventral hernia repairs with mesh, the use of simple interrupted sutures to sew the PTFE mesh to the edges of the defect with no overlap works well on the diaphragm. This is likely possible because as the mesh contracts, the diaphragm has enough give to accommodate without tearing the stitches out. In fact, the large amount of shrinkage that occurs with PTFE mesh may be beneficial in restoring a more natural contour to the diaphragm over time after a relaxing incision. Absorbable or biologic mesh should be avoided, since it will not permanently repair the defect.

Both right- and left-sided relaxing incisions are relatively straightforward laparoscopic procedures, provided that important landmarks are recognized. In our study, none of our patients suffered complications or paralyzed diaphragms related to the relaxing incisions.[8] Furthermore, it is important to recognize that a wide communication between the abdomen and thorax during a laparoscopic procedure with 15 mm Hg carbon dioxide capnoperitoneum is well tolerated. Small pleural holes can lead to a ball-valve effect and tension pneumothorax, but large openings are not associated with such problems. In fact, large openings of the pleura are standard when we repair large hiatal defects, even without a relaxing incision. This allows the mediastinal space to drain into the right, left, or both pleural cavities once the hernia has been repaired. After the pleura is opened or a relaxing incision has been created, I do not routinely leave drains in the mediastinum or chest unless a lung injury with air leak was created or suspected during the dissection.

IMPORTANT INITIAL MANEUVERS

The first step to allow crural movement and approximation is to ensure that the posterior sac has been well dissected off of the left crus. When the sac remains attached to the left crus, it can restrict movement and reapproximation of the crura. The second step is to create a left pneumothorax. This will equilibrate the capnoperitoneum on both sides of the diaphragm, allowing the left diaphragm to become floppy and facilitating its movement toward the right crus. Just this maneuver alone is enough to reduce measured tension during crural approximation by 35.8%, as shown in an elegant study by Bradley and colleagues, where a tensometer was used intraoperatively to evaluate the effect of tension-reducing techniques.[9] If there is still excessive tension when trying to approximate the crura despite these maneuvers, a relaxing incision is the next recommended step.

TECHNIQUE FOR RIGHT-SIDED RELAXING INCISION

The right-sided relaxing incision is straightforward and adds only 15 to 30 minutes to the overall procedure. It is the preferred release, but the right crus must be at least a

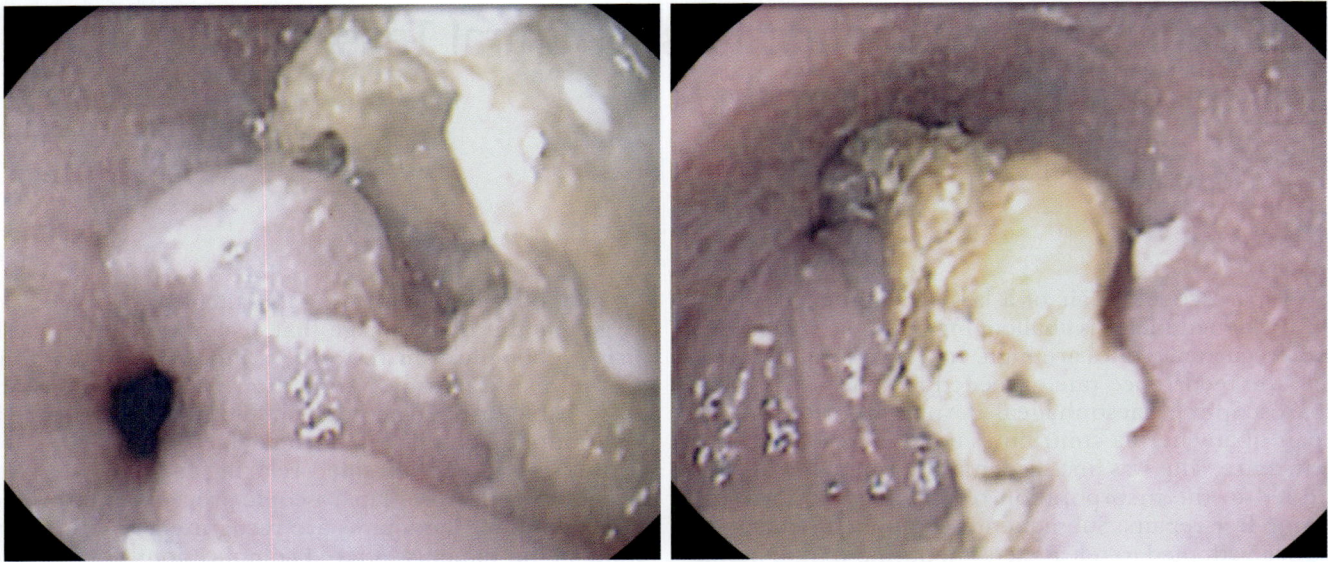

FIGURE 28.1 The use of synthetic mesh near the diaphragmatic hiatus can result in erosion of the mesh into the esophagus, as seen in this figure.

centimeter wide to have enough tissue to reconstruct the hiatus following this maneuver. Rarely, but particularly in reoperations, the right crus may be so thin and scarred that there is insufficient room between the edge of the crus and the inferior vena cava to do a right-sided relaxing incision. In these patients, or in the rare patient where a right-sided relaxing incision is insufficient to allow tension-free crural closure, a left-sided relaxing incision is necessary. It is important that the relaxing incision be made anterior to the apex of the hiatus, not posteriorly at the base. Vital structures, such as the aorta and thoracic duct, are near the base, and any incision in the diaphragm should stay above this area. Also, in the vast majority of cases, the base of the hiatus will come together with one or two stitches.

A right relaxing incision is performed by opening the right crus parallel to the inferior vena cava, saving a 3-mm cuff of tissue along the cava to allow a patch to be sewn into place. The right-sided relaxing incision entails a full-thickness incision through the right crus into the right pleural space. It is started in the midportion of the right crus and ends below the anterior crural vein (Fig. 28.2). The diaphragm in this area is quite tendinous, so ultrasonic energy or a hook cautery work well to make the incision on the right side. Typically, the incision only needs to go anteriorly to the level of the crural vein, but if that is insufficient, the crural vein can be ligated and the incision carried further anterior and medially to allow additional release. It is surprising how well this release will allow the right crus to move medially, and in the process leave a gaping defect in the right diaphragm (Fig. 28.3A). The only structure of significance to avoid injuring with the right-sided relaxing incision is the intrathoracic vena cava, but this should be anterior and lateral to the incision, if made as described previously. If not used routinely, pledgeted sutures are recommended after a right relaxing incision to minimize the risk that the crural closure sutures pull through the residual right crural pillar. Once the hiatus

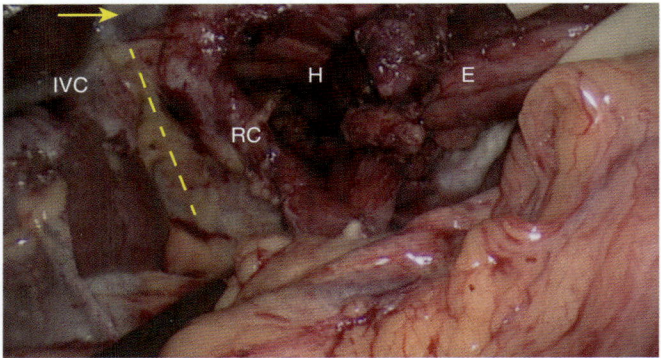

FIGURE 28.2 Site for right relaxing incision is indicated by the *dashed line*. *Arrow* indicates the anterior crural vein. *E,* Esophagus; *H,* hiatus; *IVC,* inferior vena cava; *RC,* right crus.

is reconstructed, the defect created by the relaxing incision is repaired with a permanent mesh. My preference is 1 mm PTFE sewn in with interrupted 3-0 monofilament sutures (see Fig. 28.3B). I then prefer to reinforce the primary crural closure with absorbable biologic or biosynthetic mesh (see Fig. 28.3C). The absorbable mesh is secured to the diaphragm using absorbable tacks.

TECHNIQUE FOR LEFT-SIDED RELAXING INCISION

The left-sided relaxing incision is not difficult, but requires more time to repair the defect since a larger incision is required than the right. Unlike the radial incision paralleling the crus on the right side, the left-sided incision should be made laterally following the seventh rib. The phrenic nerve is protected on the right side by the vena cava, but a radial incision on the left side puts the phrenic nerve at risk, which could lead to paralysis of

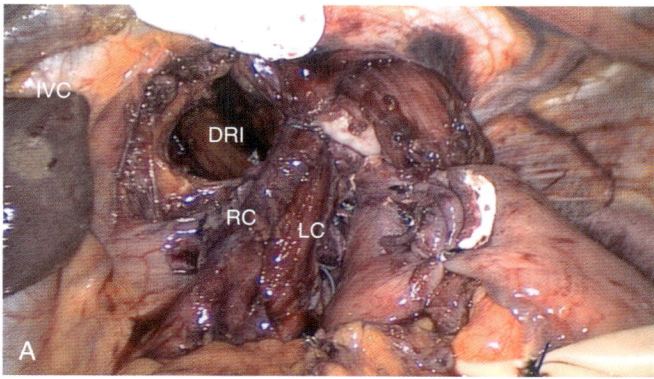

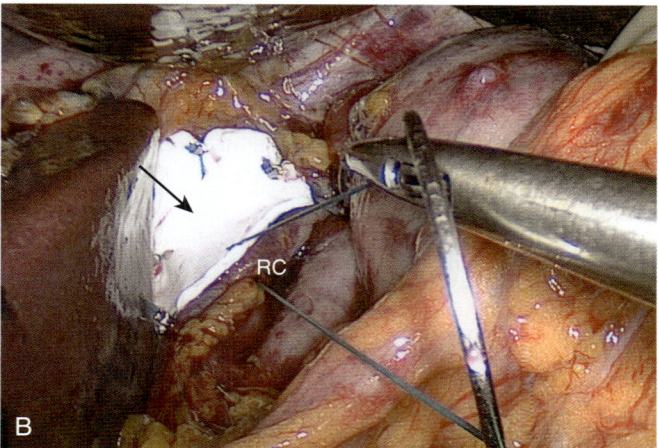

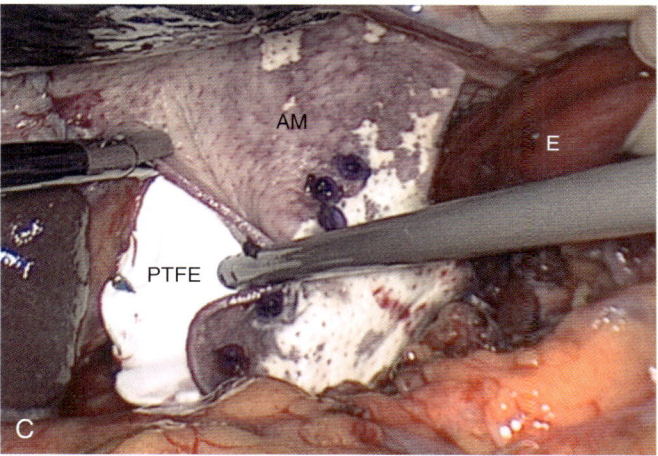

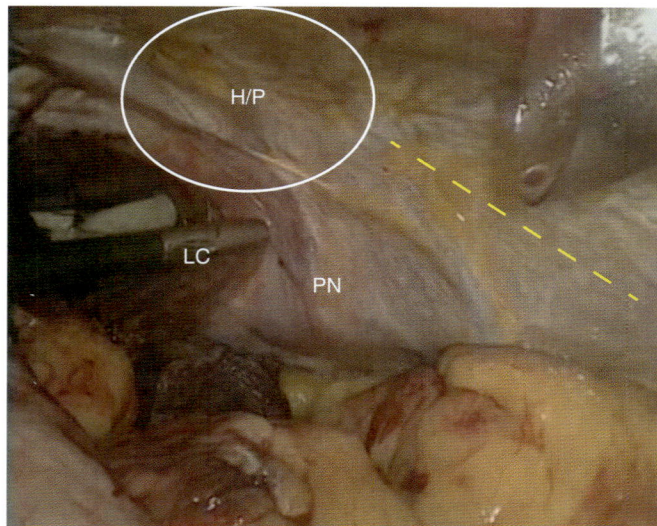

FIGURE 28.4 *Dashed line* indicates site for left diaphragmatic relaxing incision. The incision needs to be done radially to avoid injury to structures including the heart/pericardium *(H/P)* as well as the phrenic nerve *(PN)*. *LC,* Left crus.

FIGURE 28.3 (A) After a right relaxing incision the hiatus closed nicely with minimal tension. (B) The defect is being closed with 1 mm PTFE mesh, indicated with *arrow*. *RC* indicates the location of the right crus in relation to the mesh. (C) The primary crural closure is reinforced with an absorbable biologic mesh that also covers the PTFE patch. *AM,* Absorbable mesh; *DRI,* diaphragmatic relaxing incision; *E,* esophagus; *IVC,* inferior vena cava; *LC,* left crus; *PTFE,* nonabsorbable PTFE patch *RC,* right crus.

the left hemidiaphragm. The only other structure of significance with a left-sided relaxing incision is the heart, which should be anterior and medial to the site of the incision (Fig. 28.4). Prior to starting the left relaxing incision, it is important to create a left capnothorax by

opening the left pleura, if not done already. This takes the left diaphragm off tension, making it easier to begin the relaxing incision. As previously discussed, this may obviate the need for a relaxing incision in some cases. Further, this allows the diaphragm to be pulled away from the heart, which minimizes the risk of injury.

The incision is started lateral to the heart approximately 1 to 2 cm below the seventh rib. The 1 to 2 cm of diaphragm attached to the rib is necessary to allow subsequent closure of the defect. The incision is full thickness, extending into the left pleural space. Typically this incision needs to be carried laterally toward the spleen to allow sufficient release. For this incision, I prefer ultrasonic energy to minimize diaphragm twitching and bleeding, given that the left diaphragm is more muscular than tendinous. Once sufficient release has been achieved to allow tension-free closure of the hiatus, the diaphragmatic defect can be reconstructed. On occasion the left diaphragm slides medially without creating a wide defect, and the relaxing incision can be closed primarily with interrupted figure-of-eight permanent sutures. Often though a patch is necessary, and here we prefer 2 mm PTFE sewn in with interrupted 0-Ethibond or similar suture (see Figs. 28.4 and 28.5). Like right-sided diaphragmatic closures, we reinforce the tension-free hiatal repair with an absorbable biologic or biosynthetic mesh to complete the hiatal reconstruction (see Fig. 28.3C).

OUTCOMES WITH CRURAL RELAXING INCISIONS

The use of crural relaxing incisions, when necessary, has eliminated the need for a bridged crural repair. In our initial series of 15 patients published in 2013, the hiatal reconstruction was completed laparoscopically in all patients with primary crural closure. No drains were

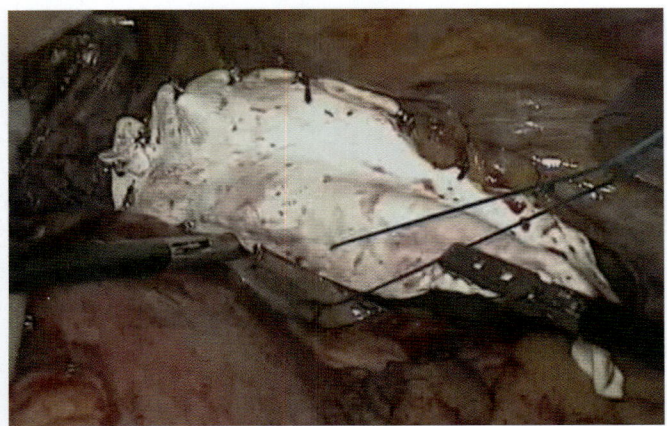

FIGURE 28.5 A left relaxing incision is being closed with 2 mm PTFE mesh.

left in the pleural space or mediastinum, and no patient developed a pleural effusion prior to discharge. On follow-up chest x-ray, three patients had developed a pleural effusion and two patients required pigtail drainage. An asymptomatic mild elevation of the left hemidiaphragm was seen in one patient. At short-term follow-up, no patient had required reoperation, and no patient developed a diaphragmatic hernia through the repaired relaxing incision or evidence of PTFE mesh infection. Objective follow-up in 11 of the 15 patients showed that the repair was intact in all but one patient who had an asymptomatic, trivial (<2 cm) recurrent hernia at 4.5 months.[8]

CONCLUSION

A crural relaxing incision will allow crural repair with reduced tension in patients with a wide hiatus. Since tension is the enemy of any hernia repair, it is likely that the use of a crural relaxing incision when necessary will lead to reduced hernia recurrence rates and better patient outcomes after hiatal hernia repair. The techniques for a right- and left-sided relaxing incision are straightforward and should be in the armamentarium of surgeons who take on the repair of paraesophageal or large sliding hiatal hernias.

DISCLOSURES

Dr. DeMeester is a consultant for Gore and Davol/Bard, and has received a research grant from Davol/Bard.

REFERENCES

1. Oelschlager B, Pellegrini C, Hunter J, et al. Biologic prosthesis to prevent recurrence after laparoscopic paraesophageal hernia repair: long-term follow-up from a multicenter, prospective, randomized trial. *J Am Coll Surg.* 2011;213:461-468.
2. Read RC. The contributions of Usher and others to the elimination of tension from groin herniorrhapy, 2004. *Hernia.* 2004;9:208-211.
3. Read RC. Herniology: past, present and future. *Hernia.* 2009;13:577-580.
4. Halvorson EG. On the origins of components separation. *Plast Reconstr Surg.* 2009;124:1545.
5. Stadlhuber R, Sherif A, Mittal S, et al. Mesh complications after prosthetic reinforcement of hiatal closure: a 28-case series. *Surg Endosc.* 2009;23:1219-1226.
6. Park A, Hoogerboord C, Sutton E. Use of the falciform ligament flap for closure of the esophageal hiatus in giant paraesophageal hernia. *J Gastrointest Surg.* 2012;16(7):1417-1421.
7. Crespin OM, Yates RB, Martin AV, Pellegrini CA, Oelschlager BK. The use of crural relaxing incisions with biologic mesh reinforcement during laparoscopic repair of complex hiatal hernias. *Surg Endosc.* 2016;30(6):2179-2185.
8. Greene CL, DeMeester SR, Zehetner J, Worrell SG, Oh DS, Hagen JA. Diaphragmatic relaxing incisions during laparoscopic paraesophageal hernia repair. *Surg Endosc.* 2013;27(12):4532-4538.
9. Bradley DD, Louie BE, Farivar AS, Wilshire CL, Baik PU, Aye RW. Assessment and reduction of diaphragmatic tension during hiatal hernia repair. *Surg Endosc.* 2015;29(4):796-804.

Collis Gastroplasty for a Foreshortened Esophagus

Stephanie G. Worrell | Joshua A. Boys | Steven R. DeMeester

Normally, several centimeters of the distal esophagus and the gastroesophageal junction (GEJ) lie below the hiatus within the abdomen. When the GEJ, the fundus of the stomach, or both migrate into the chest above the hiatus, a hiatal hernia is present. Intrinsic to the repair of a hiatal hernia is the need to bring the GEJ, stomach, and distal esophagus back into the abdomen. However, since 1950 it has been known that in some patients this can be challenging, particularly those with severe gastroesophageal reflux disease (GERD) or a large hiatal hernia. In these patients esophageal shortening can lead to loss of intraabdominal esophageal length and put tension on the repair of a hiatal hernia. Dr. John. Leigh Collis described a technique in 1957 to address acquired esophageal shortening.[1] His technique, now referred to as a Collis gastroplasty, creates an extension to the esophagus from the high lesser curvature of the stomach. His gastroplasty was done as a transthoracic procedure. Subsequently, several techniques have been described to create a similar gastroplasty using a laparoscopic approach. However, more than 50 years after Dr. Collis described his procedure for lengthening the esophagus there is still controversy about the existence and prevalence of a foreshortened esophagus. Furthermore, the laparoscopic management of a short esophagus is challenging, and as a result there is a tendency by many surgeons to ignore esophageal length and proceed with a standard repair. Importantly, tension is the enemy of any hernia repair, and long-term successful outcomes with hiatal hernia repairs, as for all other abdominal hernias, require addressing tension when encountered.

IDENTIFYING THE SHORT ESOPHAGUS

Patients at risk for acquired esophageal shortening include those with advanced GERD with esophagitis, stricture, long-segment Barrett esophagus, a history of sarcoidosis, caustic ingestion, or scleroderma and those with a large sliding or paraesophageal hernia (PEH).[2,3] In some reports patients with a PEH have the highest frequency of a short esophagus.[4] The presence of a foreshortened esophagus in patients with severe GERD is understandable because exposure to refluxed gastric juice causes mucosal injury and can lead to transmural inflammation, fibrosis, and collagen contraction. An esophageal stricture is strongly associated with a shortened esophagus and the need for a gastroplasty. The presence of both a large hiatal hernia (>5 cm) and an esophageal stricture further increases the risk of a shortened esophagus.[2] In addition, a history of a previous failed antireflux procedure with recurrent hiatal hernia should raise suspicion that the length of the esophagus is short. The etiology of esophageal shortening in patients with a PEH is unclear but may be related to loss of elasticity in the longitudinal esophageal muscle related to chronic loss of intraabdominal fixation of the GEJ. Although any of these histories should increase the suspicion that a patient may have a short esophagus, none are definitive. Objective studies in patients with GERD or PEH are useful to define the size, type, and reducibility of any hiatal hernia, presence of a stricture or erosive esophagitis, esophageal function, and the presence and severity of increased esophageal exposure to refluxed gastric juice. A foreshortened esophagus can effectively be ruled out when a hiatal hernia fully reduces on barium esophagram, but in any nonreducing hiatal hernia a short esophagus may be present. Therefore, although objective studies can rule out a short esophagus, none can accurately identify its presence. Instead, a foreshortened esophagus can be confirmed only by the intraoperative inability to reduce the GEJ below the hiatus by 2 to 3 cm after mediastinal esophageal mobilization and posterior crural closure.

MANAGEMENT OF THE SHORT ESOPHAGUS

Failure to obtain an adequate length of intraabdominal esophagus during hiatal hernia repair has been proposed as a leading cause for reherniation and breakdown of the repair.[3] Mediastinal mobilization and posterior crural closure, particularly in a kyphotic patient, are routinely used to add esophageal length. To accomplish a fundoplication without tension there should be 2 to 3 cm of intraabdominal esophagus below the hiatal closure. The amount of intraabdominal esophagus during laparoscopic surgery is deceptive because the pneumoperitoneum artificially elevates the diaphragm and gives the appearance of more esophageal length than what is actually present. With deflation of the pneumoperitoneum, the diaphragm descends and some of the apparent esophageal length is lost. If standard methods for esophageal mobilization are insufficient to provide 2 to 3 cm of abdominal esophagus, esophageal lengthening is recommended.

There are several methods to accomplish a Collis gastroplasty during a laparoscopic procedure, including advancing a linear stapler through a port in the thorax and using a circular stapler to make a hole in the stomach and then completing the gastroplasty with a linear stapler.[5,6] Our preferred approach was described by Terry and colleagues and is the wedge fundectomy Collis gastroplasty (WFCG) technique.[7] The WFCG was created with a 52-French bougie in place using a 45-mm Endo GIA blue load stapler. The goal was to excise as small a wedge of fundus as possible. Given the limitations of articulating Endo GIA staplers, we found that to excise only a small portion of the fundus it was necessary to create a starfish-shaped piece of the proximal fundus by successively cutting through the inferior staple line with each successive staple load until a mark approximately 3 cm below the angle of His was reached. The staple line was not reinforced but was buried by the fundoplication. A partial Toupet or complete Nissen fundoplication was added to the WFCG in all patients. Importantly the fundoplication was kept as high on the gastroplasty as possible, preferably at the top near the GEJ. The importance of this is the fact that the gastroplasty is made from stomach, and acid production by the gastroplasty above the fundoplication can lead to erosive esophagitis in some patients, particularly if there are several centimeters of gastroplasty above the fundoplication. It is also important to recognize that the gastroplasty tube is aperistaltic. Therefore bolus transport through the gastroplasty relies on the motility of the distal esophagus above the gastroplasty. Consequently, we are more liberal with the use of a partial fundoplication in patients who have a WFCG added for a shortened esophagus.

OUTCOME WITH A COLLIS GASTROPLASTY

Before the introduction of laparoscopic surgery, most antireflux procedures were performed in patients with severe GERD, often with impaired esophageal body function. A Collis gastroplasty in these patients frequently led to protracted postoperative dysphagia. In a series reported from our center in 1998 a transthoracic Collis gastroplasty in the presence of preoperative dysphagia was significantly associated with a poor postoperative outcome. Many of these patients had strictures and severe reflux disease.[8] The availability of potent acid-suppressing medications has led to a reduction in the acid-related complications of reflux disease including strictures. Furthermore, the number of patients presenting for elective repair of a PEH in the era of laparoscopic surgery is increasing. In these patients a Collis gastroplasty seems to be better tolerated. In contrast to our earlier series, a recent evaluation of our laparoscopic Collis gastroplasties showed that severe reflux disease was less common.[9] The Collis gastroplasty was done in 72% of patients, either for a PEH or during reoperation for a failed fundoplication. Dysphagia was a common preoperative symptom; however, it resolved in the majority (71%) postoperatively. Importantly, new-onset dysphagia occurred in only two patients (5.5%) and resolved after one endoscopic dilatation in both patients. Dysphagia that was present preoperatively and persisted was typically mild and did not significantly impact the patient's diet or lifestyle. The relief of dysphagia in most patients was likely related to repair of the large hiatal hernia and healing of esophagitis. However, we also attributed the low rate of new-onset dysphagia to our "tailored approach" for a fundoplication, using a Toupet rather than a Nissen in patients with manometric evidence of ineffective esophageal motility.

A second potential issue with a Collis gastroplasty is acid production by the neoesophagus above the fundoplication. In our recent series we found that the prevalence of esophagitis after laparoscopic Collis gastroplasty was much lower (11%) than reported by others. It is not clear why our prevalence was much less than the 36% rate reported by Jobe et al., but it may in part be related to our efforts to keep the fundoplication as high on the

neoesophagus as possible without inducing excessive tension on the repair.[5] It is also possible that the degree of shortening in our patients was less than that in the series by Jobe et al., because in patients with a very short esophagus, the Collis gastroplasty can extend above the hiatus. In that circumstance it is not possible to position the fundoplication at the top of the gastroplasty. Importantly, esophagitis in these patients is often asymptomatic. Consequently, we recommend that at least one postoperative endoscopy be done after a Collis gastroplasty to evaluate for esophagitis. If esophagitis is found in the setting of an intact fundoplication, treatment with a proton pump inhibitor is recommended to prevent stricture formation or other complications related to ongoing mucosal injury.

A transthoracic Collis gastroplasty has been associated with complications not typically seen with standard antireflux surgery, including staple line leaks, abscesses, and fistulas.[10] We are always careful to ensure adequate perfusion of the Collis segment and would avoid a Collis gastroplasty if there was any compromise of the lesser curve blood supply due to interruption of the left gastric artery. In our series of laparoscopic WFCGs we did not have any of these complications. We routinely cover the Collis staple line with the fundoplication to minimize the risk of a leak or fistula. Furthermore, the wedge fundectomy technique may lead to a wider and more robust portion of fundus that lessens the tension that was sometimes present with a fundoplication after a traditional transthoracic Collis gastroplasty.

The key issue of course with a Collis gastroplasty is whether it reduces hernia recurrence rates. We recently reviewed our experience in 83 patients who had primary laparoscopic PEH repair (manuscript submitted for publication). In 46 patients (55%), we identified a short esophagus, and these patients were given a WFCG. The remainder had a fundoplication alone. At a median follow-up of 9 months there was objective evidence of a 2-cm or greater recurrent hernia in two (5.4%) of the fundoplication-alone group compared with one (2.2%) in the WFCG group (P = .583). Two of the three recurrent hernias were small (2 to 3 cm). The single large recurrent hernia developed in a patient who had a fundoplication alone and required reoperation for recurrent symptoms. Based on these data, one could conclude that a Collis gastroplasty does not alter the frequency of hernia recurrence. However, an alternative conclusion is that without a Collis gastroplasty, patients with a short esophagus would have had a higher recurrence rate. If true, then the finding of a similar recurrent hernia rate in patients deemed to have a short esophagus who had a WFCG compared with those with no esophageal shortening would suggest that addressing a short esophagus is warranted and improves outcomes.

The expected objective hernia recurrence rate after laparoscopic PEH repair is known. The randomized trial by Oelschlager and colleagues reported a greater than 50% hernia recurrence rate, and the use of biologic mesh did not reduce the rate at 5-year follow-up.[11] Recognizing this high failure rate, which we also reported in 2000, we have modified our approach.[12] It is likely that the high recurrence rate is related to the inherent weakness of the crural tissue and to unaddressed tension on the repair. Tension on the repair of any hernia is a harbinger for failure. Consequently, we now address lateral tension on the crural closure with a diaphragm-relaxing incision and axial tension from a short esophagus with WFCG. Furthermore, we routinely reinforce the primary crural closure with biologic or absorbable mesh. Using this approach we have excellent short-term outcomes with a very low objective hernia recurrence rate.[13]

CONCLUSION

Patients found to have a short esophagus during laparoscopic hiatal hernia repair are likely at increased risk for breakdown of the repair and a recurrent hiatal hernia. The first steps to gain esophageal length are mediastinal esophageal mobilization and posterior crural closure. If these steps are inadequate a Collis gastroplasty should be added. The wedge fundectomy technique allows esophageal lengthening laparoscopically and is associated with a low rate of complications. Clear-cut evidence that a laparoscopic Collis gastroplasty reduces hernia recurrence rates is lacking; however, tension on the repair of any hernia is associated with an increased failure rate. Consequently, a Collis gastroplasty in the setting of a foreshortened esophagus is likely to prove beneficial in the long term and should be part of the armamentarium of modern laparoscopic esophageal surgeons.

REFERENCES

1. Collis JL. An operation for haitus hernia with short esophagus. *J Thorac Surg.* 1957;34:768-778.
2. Gastal OL, Hagen JA, Peters JH, et al. Short esophagus: analysis of predictors and clinical implications. *Arch Surg.* 1999;134(6):633-636, discussion 637-638.
3. Horvath KD, Swanstrom LL, Jobe BA. The short esophagus: pathophysiology, incidence, presentation, and treatment in the era of laparoscopic antireflux surgery. *Ann Surg.* 2000;232(5):630-640.
4. Herbella FAM, Del Grande JC, Colleoni R. Short esophagus: literature incidence. *Dis Esophagus.* 2002;15(2):125-131.
5. Jobe BA, Horvath KD, Swanstrom LL. Postoperative function following laparoscopic Collis gastroplasty for shortened esophagus. *Arch Surg.* 1998;133(8):867-874.
6. Luketich JD, Grondin SC, Pearson FG. Minimally invasive approaches to acquired shortening of the esophagus: laparoscopic Collis-Nissen gastroplasty. *Semin Thorac Cardiovasc Surg.* 2000;12(3):173-178.
7. Terry ML, Vernon A, Hunter JG. Stapled-wedge Collis gastroplasty for the shortened esophagus. *Am J Surg.* 2004;188(2):195-199.
8. Ritter MP, Peters JH, DeMeester TR, et al. Treatment of advanced gastroesophageal reflux disease with Collis gastroplasty and Belsey partial fundoplication. *Arch Surg.* 1998;133(5):523-528, discussion 528-529.
9. Zehetner J, DeMeester SR, Ayazi S, Kilday P, Alicuben ET, DeMeester TR. Laparoscopic wedge fundectomy for Collis gastroplasty creation in patients with a foreshortened esophagus. *Ann Surg.* 2014;260: 1030-1033.
10. Patel HJ, Tan BB, Yee J, Orringer MB, Iannettoni MD. A 25-year experience with open primary transthoracic repair of paraesophageal hiatal hernia. *J Thorac Cardiovasc Surg.* 2004;127(3):843-849.
11. Oelschlager BK, Petersen RP, Brunt LM, et al. Laparoscopic paraesophageal hernia repair: defining long-term clinical and anatomic outcomes. *J Gastrointest Surg.* 2012;16(3):453-459.
12. Hashemi M, Peters JH, DeMeester TR, et al. Laparoscopic repair of large type III hiatal hernia: objective followup reveals high recurrence rate. *J Am Coll Surg.* 2000;190(5):553-560, discussion 560-561.
13. Alicuben E, Worrell SG, DeMeester SR. Impact of crural relaxing incisions, Collis gastroplasty and non-cross-linked human dermal mesh crural reinforcement on early hiatal hernia recurrence rates. *J Am Coll Surg.* 2014;219(5):988-992.

Mesh at the Hiatus

Sumeet K. Mittal | Ross M. Bremner

Crural repair and reduction of hiatal hernia (HH) are paramount to the success of an antireflux surgery. Case series from the early laparoscopic era (i.e., the 1990s) reported an unacceptably high recurrence rate of HHs. In addition, some patients were found to be naturally predisposed to hernia formation, and recurring hernias were thought to be due in part to inherent defects in healing. Simultaneously, the routine use of synthetic mesh in inguinal and ventral hernia repair was gaining widespread acceptance and was found to be both safe and effective.

These findings set the stage for some practitioners to advocate for the use of mesh at the hiatus. Soon thereafter, several case series described experience with various types of synthetic mesh materials and configurations of mesh at the hiatus, and these studies were strengthened by significantly lower recurrence rates in their series. However, these early reports were followed by isolated case reports describing complications related to mesh use, including catastrophic cases that required esophagogastric resections.[1] These disastrous complications were thought to result from the synthetic nature of the mesh materials being used, so bioprosthetic materials were suggested as attractive alternatives to synthetic mesh. A randomized prospective trial described outcomes in patients with and without use of biologic mesh and found a significant decline in recurrence at 6 months' follow-up when mesh reinforcement was used.[2] A large series of 28 patients undergoing reoperation with either synthetic or biologic mesh at the hiatus was published that demonstrated that both types of mesh were associated with significant mesh-related complications.[3] Since then, others have reported that reoperation after the use of mesh is significantly more challenging than reoperation in patients in whom mesh was not used and that the patients with mesh are at greater risk of needing an esophagogastric resection.[4,5]

Perhaps the benchmark for HH repair, with or without mesh, is the sizable open transthoracic series by Maziak et al.[6] They achieved a mean follow-up of 94 months in 90 of 94 patients in their cohort who underwent surgical repair of a large paraesophageal hernia (PEH) over a 36-year period. They reported excellent results in 72 of 90 patients (80%), with anatomic recurrence in only two patients, both of whom underwent reoperation. Table 30.1 summarizes the findings of studies on open PEH repair with objective follow-up.

Since the publication of these early laparoscopic reports, advancements in minimally invasive surgery (e.g., improved visualization, better instrumentation, and greater experience) have helped surgeons achieve more extensive mediastinal dissection, better crus closure, and use of Collis gastroplasty. All of these are associated with improved outcomes with primary crus repair of the hiatus, even for larger HHs. The goal of this chapter is to briefly review the advantages and disadvantages of using mesh at the hiatus.

HIATAL HERNIA: RECURRENCE AND OUTCOMES

RECURRENCE RATES WITH PRIMARY CLOSURE IN THE EARLY LAPAROSCOPIC ERA

A 2004 review described a high recurrence rate of eight HH case series published up to that point.[8] The studies that were evaluated incorporated systematic radiographic follow-up for laparoscopic PEH repair, and objective follow-up was available for 277 of 460 patients. The mean overall reported recurrence rate was 27% (range, 7% to 43%). In 2000 Hashemi et al.[9] reported their experience with 54 patients who underwent surgery for repair of large PEH at the University of Southern California, a large and well-respected esophageal center. In the subset of patients who underwent laparoscopic repair of large PEH ($n = 27$), objective follow-up was available for 21 patients (78%). These authors found HH recurrence in 9 of 21 patients (43%), with 8 of 21 patients (38%) also reporting recurrent symptoms.[9] This report led to widespread uncertainty about the safety and efficacy of laparoscopy for PEH repair. However, the authors' high rate of recurrent symptoms is unusual because most patients who undergo laparoscopic PEH repair report good to excellent symptom control, which may not correlate with radiographic recurrence.[2,9]

RECURRENCE RATES WITH PRIMARY CLOSURE IN THE MODERN LAPAROSCOPIC ERA

Andujar et al.[10] reported their systematic radiographic follow-up for 166 patients who underwent laparoscopic repair of large PEH. At a mean follow-up of 15 months, they stated a recurrence rate of 25% (5% PEH and 20% sliding HH). Nine years later, Gibson et al.[11] described the outcomes of their single-center experience of HH repair in 100 consecutive patients. They reported a very low recurrence rate of 9 of 100 patients, 7 of whom had only a small (<2 cm) recurrent HH. The same group later reported medium-term follow-up, describing a total recurrence rate of 25% at mean follow-up of 24 months (5% PEH and 20% small HH).[12] They also reported excellent continued gastroesophageal reflux disease–related quality-of-life scores.

Nason et al.[13] reported their long-term follow-up of 187 patients who underwent laparoscopic repair of a giant PEH from 1997 to 2003. Over their median follow-up of 77 months, they found a radiographic recurrence rate of 15%. Mittal et al.[14] later reported 5-year follow-up findings in their 73 patients who underwent surgical intervention for intrathoracic stomach. They reported 5%, 11%, and 17% radiographic failure rates at 1, 3, and 5 years, respectively, after surgery. Table 30.2 summarizes outcomes after laparoscopic PEH repair.

RECURRENCE RATES WITH MESH-REINFORCED CRUS CLOSURE

An early review of the literature summarized outcomes of 432 patients in 22 studies who underwent mesh-reinforced HH repair.[8] Recurrence rates ranged from 0% to 24%, but most of the studies in this review reported zero recurrences.

Different mesh configurations and materials were used in different series. A recent 1-year contrast study described follow-up after laparoscopic PEH repair and reported a 27% recurrence of HH larger than 2 cm after biologic mesh reinforcement of HH.[21] Lee et al.[22] reported an even higher recurrence rate of 40% at 5-year follow-up with routine use of AlloDerm (LifeCell Corporation, Branchburg, New Jersey) for all cruroplasty (not just PEH). Table 30.3 summarizes recurrence rates and other follow-up data from studies reporting mesh-reinforced closure.

MESH CONFIGURATIONS AND MATERIALS

Early on, synthetic meshes (e.g., polypropylene and polytetrafluoroethylene) were used for hiatus reinforcement as a direct extension of use in ventral and inguinal hernias. Multiple configurations of varying mesh sizes and shapes were described and are too simply numerous to list individually. The mesh was generally placed either as a bridge to cover a gap in the crural defect (either anterior or posterior) or as an overlay over the primary crus closure. Some practitioners advocated circumferential placement of mesh with a keyhole-shaped opening to accommodate the esophagus.[28] Others advised creation of relaxing incisions in the diaphragm to allow for primary crus closure and recommended using mesh to bridge the created defect.[29] Fig. 30.1 shows the various mesh placement configurations described previously.

TABLE 30.1 Open Hiatal Hernia Repair

Author, Year	Study Design	Findings
Maziak et al., 1998[6]	94 patients with massive incarcerated PEH.	Mean follow-up: 94 months. 93% of patients had good or excellent outcome; only 2% had symptomatic recurrence.
Low and Unger, 2005[7]	72 patients with large PEH.	Mean follow-up: 29.8 months. 13% of patients had recurrent hernia. No patient required revision surgery.

PEH, Paraesophageal hernia.

TABLE 30.2 Laparoscopic Hiatal Hernia Repair

Author, Year	Study Design	Findings
Hashemi et al., 2000[9]	54 patients: 13 open surgery, 14 thoracotomy, 27 laparoscopic HH repair.	Symptomatic outcomes: excellent/good in 76% laparoscopic; 88% in open. Recurrence in 12 patients, symptomatic in 5/12. (Laparoscopic 42% recurrence, open 15% recurrence).
Mattar et al., 2002[15]	136 patients: Laparoscopic PEH repair.	Mean follow-up: 40 months. Significant improvement of all symptoms. Three patients had symptomatic recurrence.
Targarona et al., 2004[8]	Review of eight case series. Objective follow-up for 277 of 460 patients.	Mean overall recurrence rate: 27% (range, 7%–43%).
Ferri et al., 2005[16]	60 patients: 25 open surgery, 35 laparoscopic HH repair.	Recurrence rate: 44% open, 23% laparoscopic.
Rathore et al., 2007[17]	Meta-analysis of 13 retrospective reviews. 965 patients.	Overall recurrence rate for laparoscopic PEH repair: 10.2%. True recurrence rate with video barium esophagram 25.5%. No associated learning curve. Hiatoplasty and esophageal lengthening had significant protective influence.
White et al., 2008[18]	10-year follow-up for 52 patients with laparoscopic PEH repair.	Significant improvement in symptoms at 10 years compared with preoperative symptoms. Ten recurrences (2 within 1 postoperative year).
Luketich et al., 2010[19]	662 patients with laparoscopic giant PEH repair.	Mesh and Collis use decreased over time with stable morbidity rates. QOL scores were excellent or good in 90%; radiologic recurrence in 16%. Symptomatic recurrence in none. Reoperation in 3%.
Mittal et al., 2011[14]	73 patients with ITS, 7 transthoracic, 64 laparoscopic, 1 open, 1 laparoscopic-to-open conversion. Mesh used in 14%.	Objective failure at 1, 3, and 5 years was 5%, 11%, and 17%, respectively. Subjective outcome was similar at each follow-up period. Subjective satisfaction remained high throughout follow-up.
Le Page et al., 2015[20]	455 patients with attempted laparoscopic repair of giant HH.	Mean follow-up: 42 months. Laparoscopy in 95% (mesh in 6%). Overall recurrence: 35.6%; follow-up at over 10 years: 50%. Recurrence in 14.8%; revision surgery in 4.8%.

HH, Hiatal hernia; *ITS*, intrathoracic stomach; *PEH*, paraesophageal hernia; *QOL*, quality of life.

TABLE 30.3 Mesh-Reinforced Hiatal Hernia Repair

Author, Year	Study Design	Findings
Carlson et al., 1998[1]	44 large PEH and ITS. Posterior cruroplasty and onlay Prolene mesh.	Mean follow-up: 52 months. No clinical recurrence.
Lee et al., 2008[22]	52 patients, cruroplasty with AlloDerm.	Early recurrence: 4%. 5-year follow-up of 47%.
Frantzides et al., 2010[23]	5486 HH repairs: 77% laparoscopic, 23% open.	Most common mesh types: biomaterial (28%), polytetrafluoroethylene (25%), and polypropylene (21%). Suture anchorage in 56%. Failure rate: 3%, stricture rate: 0.2%, erosion rate: 0.3%. Biomaterial tended to be associated with failure; nonabsorbable mesh tended to be associated with stricture and erosion.
Alicuben et al., 2014[24]	114 patients (72% laparoscopic) with crural closure and Bio-A mesh reinforcement. Crural relaxing incision in 4%, Collis in 39%.	Recurrence in 0.9%.
Lidor et al., 2015[21]	111 patients. Type III PEH with biologic mesh buttressed over primary cruroplasty.	Mean follow-up: 43.5 months. Significant relief of symptoms and improved QOL. Recurrence in 27%. Four patients required reoperation (1 of whom had symptomatic recurrence).
Ward et al., 2015[25]	54 patients: all laparoscopic: 37 patients had Flex HD and 17 patients had AlloDerm mesh.	Median follow-up: 33 months. Recurrence in 15% (18% with AlloDerm; 14% with Flex HD).
Chang and Thackeray, 2016[26]	172 patients: laparoscopic HH repair with biologic mesh.	Mean follow-up: 14.5 months. Significant decline in GERD health-related QOL. Recurrence in eight patients. Reoperation required in one. One perioperative death.
Priego et al., 2017[27]	93 patients: CruraSoft mesh.	Median follow-up: 76 months. Recurrence in 8 patients (9%). Reoperation in three patients (3%).

HH, Hiatal hernia; *ITS*, intrathoracic stomach; *PEH*, paraesophageal hernia; *QOL*, quality of life.

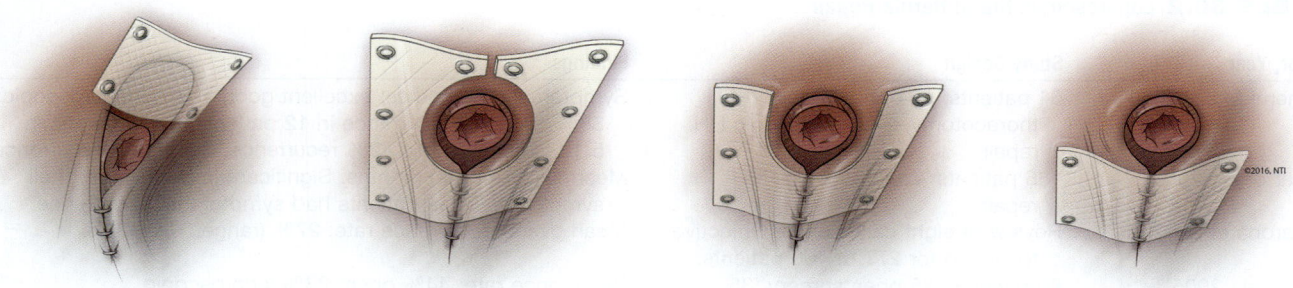

FIGURE 30.1 Various mesh placement configurations for repair of a hiatal hernia. (Used with permission from Norton Thoracic Institute, Phoenix, Arizona.)

Due to the safety concerns described earlier, biologic mesh was the preferred material for reinforcement. Many types of available biologic mesh have been reported and recommended for use, including porcine submucosa (Surgisis, Cook Medical, Bloomington, Indiana), bovine pericardium (Varitas, Baxter International, Deerfield, Illinois), human acellular dermis (AlloDerm, LifeCell Corporation, Branchburg, New Jersey), and porcine dermal collagen (Permacol, Medtronic, Dublin, Ireland). More recently, synthetic bioabsorbable meshes have gained acceptance; the most widely used of these is Bio-A (Gore Medical, Flagstaff, Arizona), which comes as a prefashioned rectangular mesh that can be tailored for posterior hiatal reinforcement. In the present era, the use of nonabsorbable mesh has been all but abandoned, as has circumferential mesh placement.

MESH-RELATED COMPLICATIONS

Reports of mesh-related complications were initially isolated in the literature, but they raised safety concerns nonetheless. A series of 28 patients from several different institutions included 17 patients with mesh erosions and 1 case of mesh extraction via the esophagus.[3] A significant number of patients in these series required esophagogastric resection. Parker et al.[5] subsequently reported a series of 78 patients from a single institution who required reoperation for antireflux surgery. They compared 10 patients who had prior mesh at the hiatus with the 68 patients who did not and concluded that the incidence of HH recurrence did not differ between the groups, which suggested that mesh does not provide complete protection from recurrence. However, they also reported a significantly higher need (30%) for esophagogastric resection in patients who had prior mesh at the hiatus. The authors cautioned against the liberal use of mesh, advising surgeons to weigh the higher recurrence rate with no mesh against the need for esophagogastric resection associated with mesh in the event that reoperation was needed.

Nandipati et al.[4] reported the largest single-center experience with reoperation for patients in whom mesh had previously been used at the hiatus. Their series of 26 patients included three mesh erosions, and they found that 70% of patients had recurrent HH, indicating that mesh does not eliminate the risk of developing a recurrent HH. They also reported that 8 of 26 patients (31%) required esophagogastric resection as a corrective procedure and there was high associated perioperative morbidity, although no postoperative mortalities was reported.

Priego et al.[27] recently described long-term follow-up of 93 patients who had mesh placed at the hiatus at the time of primary surgery. They reported 4.3% 30-day mortality, including 1% mesh-specific mortality. In addition, reoperation was required in five patients (5.4%) at

a mean follow-up of 76 months, including three patients (3.2%) who required removal of the mesh. The overall rate of recurrent HH was 9% in this series during the same follow-up.

MESH VERSUS NO MESH

COMPARATIVE STUDIES

Ten prospective and retrospective comparative studies have been carried out that examine primary crus suture closure versus synthetic mesh reinforcement. Tam et al.[30] summarized these as part of a systematic review, but the review was hindered by differences in surgical technique, mesh type, duration of follow-up, variation in diagnostic tests, and definition of recurrence. The overall recurrence rate of primary suture closure was 63 of 312 (20%); with mesh reinforcement, that rate was 32 of 293 (11%) (9 of 10 studies included adequate data). The rate of reoperation in the same cohort for primary suture closure patients was 16 of 200 (8%) and 14 of 214 (6.5%) for patients who received mesh reinforcement (6 of 10 studies included adequate data). Of all reported complications in the entire cohort, six were mesh-related. Two of these required esophageal resection.[30] Table 30.4 summarizes outcomes in comparative, nonrandomized studies.

TABLE 30.4 Mesh Versus No Mesh

Author, Year	Study Design	Findings
COMPARATIVE STUDIES		
Schmidt et al., 2014[31]	Retrospective review of 38 patients with biologic mesh versus 32 patients with suture cruroplasty only.	At 1-year objective follow-up: Recurrence 0% in mesh group versus 16% in suture cruroplasty group.
Asti et al., 2016[32]	84 patients with laparoscopic HH repair; 41 with mesh and 43 without.	Median follow-up: 24 months. 12 endoscopic recurrences (4 mesh, 8 nonmesh). Recurrence symptomatic in three patients, no revision surgery. Earlier recurrence in nonmesh group.
RANDOMIZED CONTROLLED TRIALS		
Frantzides et al., 2002[28]	72 patients: 36 with PTFE mesh repair; 36 with primary closure.	22% recurrence in primary repair group; no recurrence in mesh repair group.
Granderath et al., 2005[33]	100 laparoscopic Nissen fundoplication patients: 50 with primary suture closure alone; 50 with onlay Prolene mesh reinforcement.	Comparable 3-month and 1-year functional outcomes. Higher postoperative dysphagia in mesh group. Intrathoracic wrap migration in 26% of primary closure versus 8% in mesh group ($P < .001$).
Oelschlager et al., 2011[34]	108 patients with laparoscopic HH repair: 57 with primary repair alone; 51 with primary repair buttressed with biologic prosthesis, SIS ($n = 51$). Long-term follow-up in 72 patients.	Median follow-up: 58 months. Radiographic recurrence (≥ 20 mm) was 14% at 6 months and 57% at 58 months. At the time of follow-up, significant improvement in all symptoms in both groups. 14 (54%) in the SIS group developed recurrent hernia >2 cm; 20 (59%) recurrent HH in the primary repair group. No significant difference in relevant symptoms or QOL. No strictures, erosions, dysphagia, or other complications related to mesh.
Watson et al., 2015[35] Koetje et al., 2015[36]	126 patients with laparoscopic HH repair: 43 with primary sutures, 41 with absorbable mesh, 42 with nonabsorbable mesh.	No difference in QOL or outcome. Recurrence: 23.1% after suture repair, 30.8% after absorbable mesh, 12.8% after nonabsorbable mesh. Similar clinical outcomes. Overall outcomes after suture repair were similar to those after mesh repair.

HH, Hiatal hernia; *PTFE*, polytetrafluoroethylene; *QOL*, quality of life; *SIS*, small intestinal submucosa.

RANDOMIZED CONTROLLED TRIALS

To date, four randomized controlled trials (RCTs) have compared primary crus closure and mesh-reinforced crus closure. The first trial, carried out by Frantzides et al. in 2002,[28] reported mean objective follow-up of 36 months. They showed a definitive decline in recurrent HH with the use of mesh—from 22% recurrence with primary crus closure to 0% with mesh reinforcement (polytetrafluoroethylene circular mesh). In 2005 Granderath et al.[33] reported outcomes in a larger RCT of 100 patients in whom Prolene mesh (Ethicon, Somerville, New Jersey) was used for posterior crus reinforcement. At 12-month follow-up, Granderath et al.[33] found significantly less intrathoracic wrap migration in patients with mesh versus patients with primary crus closure (8% vs. 26%, respectively). In 2011 Oelschlager et al.[34] reported 5-year follow-up of a multicenter RCT of patients who received a U-shaped biologic prosthesis and patients who did not. They defined hernia recurrence as a herniation of 2 cm or more on contrast study and found that the rate of recurrence was alarmingly high, with 59% recurrence in the primary suture repair group and 54% in the prosthesis group. They therefore concluded that biologic mesh does not protect patients against recurrent HH, but that it may decrease the need for reoperation. Most recently, Watson et al.[35] reported 12-month follow-up of a three-armed RCT that evaluated primary crus closure, nonabsorbable mesh reinforcement, and absorbable mesh reinforcement. They found no significant difference in recurrence among the groups (primary closure: 23%, absorbable mesh: 31%, nonabsorbable mesh: 13%). They will report long-term follow-up as it becomes available. Table 30.4 summarizes the outcomes of these RCTs.

In 2016 Memon et al.[37] performed a meta-analysis of the four previously mentioned RCTs. They concluded that prosthetic hiatal herniorrhaphy and suture cruroplasty produce comparable results, and routine use of mesh cannot be endorsed. Table 30.5 summarizes the main meta-analyses and systematic reviews comparing primary suture repair with mesh-reinforced HH repair.

CONCLUSION

Most studies report a short-term higher recurrence rate of HH when it has been repaired without mesh. Only one study has produced long-term data on the use of bioabsorbable mesh, and that study reports equally alarmingly high rates of recurrent HH, both with and without the use of a biologic prosthesis. All prospective series, comparative studies, and RCTs report significant improvement in quality-of-life parameters, both with and without mesh reinforcement—a finding not necessarily associated with endoscopic or radiographic recurrence. Other initial comparative and randomized studies have not reported long-term follow-up, and this paucity of long-term data from large centers that experienced initial success with synthetic mesh is troubling. The long-term outcomes regarding recurrence rate and mesh-related complications would greatly help resolve the controversy.

Until further studies are available, the only conclusion that can be drawn at present is that, although mesh reinforcement at the hiatus seems to lessen the likelihood of short-term radiographic recurrence, no evidence shows that this is still the case at longer-term follow-up. In addition, reoperation when mesh has been used previously (regardless of mesh composition) is in the least case tedious—and in the worst case, hazardous—commonly leading to the need for esophagogastric resection. The routine use of mesh cannot be justified at present, and its use should be restricted to individual cases based on the treating surgeon's discretion based on intraoperative findings.

TABLE 30.5 Meta-Analyses and Systematic Reviews

Author, Year	Study Design	Findings
Antoniou et al., 2015[38]	Review of five case series; laparoscopic repair of HH; suture repair versus biologic mesh.	Suture versus biologic mesh: Short-term recurrence: 16.6% versus 3.5%; long-term recurrence: 51.3% versus 42.4%; short-term benefit for biologic mesh, but no confirmed long-term benefit by the same.
Huddy et al., 2016[39]	Review of nine case series; synthetic versus biologic mesh versus suture repair.	No significant difference in complications. Overall recurrence rate significantly less with mesh compared with suture repair (synthetic mesh < biologic mesh < suture repair). 20% mesh erosions.
Memon et al., 2016[37]	Review of 406 patients in 4 RCTs. 186 primary suture repair, 220 prosthetic mesh repair.	Prosthetic hiatal herniorrhaphy and suture cruroplasty produced comparable results for repair of large HH in terms of recurrence, wrap migration, and complication rates. Reoperation rate was lower in prosthetic mesh repair patients.
Tam et al., 2016[30]	Systematic review and meta-analysis of 13 studies; 10 had adequate data.	Recurrence rate in primary suture group: 20%; mesh reinforcement group: 11%. Reoperation in primary suture group: 8%; mesh reinforcement group: 6.5%.

HH, Hiatal hernia; *RCT,* randomized controlled trial.

REFERENCES

1. Carlson MA, Condon RE, Ludwig KA, Schulte WJ. Management of intrathoracic stomach with polypropylene mesh prosthesis reinforced transabdominal hiatus hernia repair. *J Am Coll Surg.* 1998;187(3):227-230.
2. Oelschlager BK, Pellegrini CA, Hunter J, et al. Biologic prosthesis reduces recurrence after laparoscopic paraesophageal hernia repair: a multicenter, prospective, randomized trial. *Ann Surg.* 2006;244(4):481-490.

3. Stadlhuber RJ, Sherif AE, Mittal SK, et al. Mesh complications after prosthetic reinforcement of hiatal closure: a 28-case series. *Surg Endosc.* 2009;23(6):1219-1226.
4. Nandipati K, Bye M, Yamamoto SR, Pallati P, Lee T, Mittal SK. Reoperative intervention in patients with mesh at the hiatus is associated with high incidence of esophageal resection—a single-center experience. *J Gastrointest Surg.* 2013;17(12):2039-2044.
5. Parker M, Bowers SP, Bray JM, et al. Hiatal mesh is associated with major resection at revisional operation. *Surg Endosc.* 2010;24(12):3095-3101.
6. Maziak DE, Todd TR, Pearson FG. Massive hiatus hernia: evaluation and surgical management. *J Thorac Cardiovasc Surg.* 1998;115(1):53-60; discussion 61–62.
7. Low DE, Unger T. Open repair of paraesophageal hernia: reassessment of subjective and objective outcomes. *Ann Thorac Surg.* 2005;80(1):287-294.
8. Targarona EM, Bendahan G, Balague C, Garriga J, Trias M. Mesh in the hiatus: a controversial issue. *Arch Surg.* 2004;139(12):1286-1296; discussion 1296.
9. Hashemi M, Peters JH, DeMeester TR, et al. Laparoscopic repair of large type III hiatal hernia: objective followup reveals high recurrence rate. *J Am Coll Surg.* 2000;190(5):553-560; discussion 560–561.
10. Andujar JJ, Papasavas PK, Birdas T, et al. Laparoscopic repair of large paraesophageal hernia is associated with a low incidence of recurrence and reoperation. *Surg Endosc.* 2004;18(3):444-447.
11. Gibson SC, Wong SC, Dixon AC, Falk GL. Laparoscopic repair of giant hiatus hernia: prosthesis is not required for successful outcome. *Surg Endosc.* 2013;27(2):618-623.
12. Furtado RV, Vivian SJ, van der Wall H, Falk GL. Medium-term durability of giant hiatus hernia repair without mesh. *Ann R Coll Surg Engl.* 2016;98(7):450-455.
13. Nason KS, Luketich JD, Qureshi I, et al. Laparoscopic repair of giant paraesophageal hernia results in long-term patient satisfaction and a durable repair. *J Gastrointest Surg.* 2008;12(12):2066-2075; discussion 2075-2077.
14. Mittal SK, Bikhchandani J, Gurney O, Yano F, Lee T. Outcomes after repair of the intrathoracic stomach: objective follow-up of up to 5 years. *Surg Endosc.* 2011;25(2):556-566.
15. Mattar SG, Bowers SP, Galloway KD, Hunter JG, Smith CD. Long-term outcome of laparoscopic repair of paraesophageal hernia. *Surg Endosc.* 2002;16(5):745-749.
16. Ferri LE, Feldman LS, Stanbridge D, Mayrand S, Stein L, Fried GM. Should laparoscopic paraesophageal hernia repair be abandoned in favor of the open approach? *Surg Endosc.* 2005;19(1):4-8.
17. Rathore MA, Andrabi SI, Bhatti MI, Najfi SM, McMurray A. Meta-analysis of recurrence after laparoscopic repair of paraesophageal hernia. *JSLS.* 2007;11(4):456-460.
18. White BC, Jeansonne LO, Morgenthal CB, et al. Do recurrences after paraesophageal hernia repair matter?: ten-year follow-up after laparoscopic repair. *Surg Endosc.* 2008;22(4):1107-1111.
19. Luketich JD, Nason KS, Christie NA, et al. Outcomes after a decade of laparoscopic giant paraesophageal hernia repair. *J Thorac Cardiovasc Surg.* 2010;139(2):395-404, 404.e1.
20. Le Page PA, Furtado R, Hayward M, et al. Durability of giant hiatus hernia repair in 455 patients over 20 years. *Ann R Coll Surg Engl.* 2015;97(3):188-193.
21. Lidor AO, Steele KE, Stem M, Fleming RM, Schweitzer MA, Marohn MR. Long-term quality of life and risk factors for recurrence after laparoscopic repair of paraesophageal hernia. *JAMA Surg.* 2015;150(5):424-431.
22. Lee YK, James E, Bochkarev V, Vitamvas M, Oleynikov D. Long-term outcome of cruroplasty reinforcement with human acellular dermal matrix in large paraesophageal hiatal hernia. *J Gastrointest Surg.* 2008;12(5):811-815.
23. Frantzides CT, Carlson MA, Loizides S, et al. Hiatal hernia repair with mesh: a survey of SAGES members. *Surg Endosc.* 2010;24(5):1017-1024.
24. Alicuben ET, Worrell SG, DeMeester SR. Resorbable biosynthetic mesh for crural reinforcement during hiatal hernia repair. *Am Surg.* 2014;80(10):1030-1033.
25. Ward KC, Costello KP, Baalman S, et al. Effect of acellular human dermis buttress on laparoscopic hiatal hernia repair. *Surg Endosc.* 2015;29(8):2291-2297.
26. Chang CG, Thackeray L. Laparoscopic hiatal hernia repair in 221 patients: outcomes and experience. *JSLS.* 2016;20(1).
27. Priego P, Perez de Oteyza J, Galindo J, et al. Long-term results and complications related to Crurasoft® mesh repair for paraesophageal hiatal hernias. *Hernia.* 2017;21:291-298.
28. Frantzides CT, Madan AK, Carlson MA, Stavropoulos GP. A prospective, randomized trial of laparoscopic polytetrafluoroethylene (PTFE) patch repair vs simple cruroplasty for large hiatal hernia. *Arch Surg.* 2002;137(6):649-652.
29. DeMeester SR. Laparoscopic paraesophageal hernia repair: critical steps and adjunct techniques to minimize recurrence. *Surg Laparosc Endosc Percutan Tech.* 2013;23(5):429-435.
30. Tam V, Winger DG, Nason KS. A systematic review and meta-analysis of mesh vs suture cruroplasty in laparoscopic large hiatal hernia repair. *Am J Surg.* 2016;211(1):226-238.
31. Schmidt E, Shaligram A, Reynoso JF, Kothari V, Oleynikov D. Hiatal hernia repair with biologic mesh reinforcement reduces recurrence rate in small hiatal hernias. *Dis Esophagus.* 2014;27(1):13-17.
32. Asti E, Lovece A, Bonavina L, et al. Laparoscopic management of large hiatus hernia: five-year cohort study and comparison of mesh-augmented versus standard crura repair. *Surg Endosc.* 2016;30(12):5404-5409.
33. Granderath FA, Schweiger UM, Kamolz T, Asche KU, Pointner R. Laparoscopic Nissen fundoplication with prosthetic hiatal closure reduces postoperative intrathoracic wrap herniation: preliminary results of a prospective randomized functional and clinical study. *Arch Surg.* 2005;140(1):40-48.
34. Oelschlager BK, Pellegrini CA, Hunter JG, et al. Biologic prosthesis to prevent recurrence after laparoscopic paraesophageal hernia repair: long-term follow-up from a multicenter, prospective, randomized trial. *J Am Coll Surg.* 2011;213(4):461-468.
35. Watson DI, Thompson SK, Devitt PG, et al. Laparoscopic repair of very large hiatus hernia with sutures versus absorbable mesh versus nonabsorbable mesh: a randomized controlled trial. *Ann Surg.* 2015;261(2):282-289.
36. Koetje JH, Irvine T, Thompson SK, et al. Quality of life following repair of large hiatal hernia is improved but not influenced by use of mesh: results from a randomized controlled trial. *World J Surg.* 2015;39(6):1465-1473.
37. Memon MA, Memon B, Yunus RM, Khan S. Suture cruroplasty versus prosthetic hiatal herniorrhaphy for large hiatal hernia: a meta-analysis and systematic review of randomized controlled trials. *Ann Surg.* 2016;263(2):258-266.
38. Antoniou SA, Muller-Stich BP, Antoniou GA, et al. Laparoscopic augmentation of the diaphragmatic hiatus with biologic mesh versus suture repair: a systematic review and meta-analysis. *Langenbecks Arch Surg.* 2015;400(5):577-583.
39. Huddy JR, Markar SR, Ni MZ, et al. Laparoscopic repair of hiatus hernia: does mesh type influence outcome? A meta-analysis and European survey study. *Surg Endosc.* 2016;30(12):5209-5221.

PART SIX

Barrett Esophagus

Controversies in the Definition of Barrett Esophagus

Thomas J. Watson

Esophageal adenocarcinoma (EAC) is a highly lethal disease associated with a survival of less than 20% at 5 years.[1] The American Cancer Society estimates that 16,940 new esophageal cancer cases will be diagnosed in the United States in 2017, the majority from EAC, with 15,690 cancer-related deaths.[2] The incidence of EAC has been climbing for more than 40 years at a rate greater than any other malignancy and with a greater than sevenfold increase in the United States between 1975 and 2006.[3] The poor prognosis relates to the common presentation of patients with advanced malignancy at the time symptoms manifest, as well as the lack of effective systemic therapies. Early diagnosis and curative treatment of locoregional disease are essential for improving overall survival, factors emphasizing the importance of appropriate screening and follow-up of at-risk populations prior to symptom development.

Barrett esophagus (BE) is the only known precursor to EAC and is a strong risk factor, imparting a 30-fold to 125-fold increased risk over that of the general population.[4] Ample evidence supports the value of BE surveillance in detecting EAC at an earlier stage, requiring less aggressive treatment and with a better prognosis, than tumors first presenting at the time symptoms arise.[5,6] The development of BE is due to metaplasia of the esophageal lining from squamous to columnar epithelium resulting from the effects of refluxed gastric contents, including acid, bile, and pancreatic enzymes, in susceptible individuals. Depending on how it is defined and the diligence with which it is detected, BE is found in approximately 10% to 15% of patients with symptomatic gastroesophageal reflux disease (GERD) undergoing endoscopic biopsies.[7] The pathogenesis of EAC places BE as the important link between GERD, the most common malady affecting the foregut, and EAC, the cancer most rapidly increasing in incidence in Western societies.[8]

Despite being common and playing a key role in EAC development, BE has been shrouded in controversy since it was first described 50 years ago.[9] Even today, debate continues over the correct definition relative to the location and type of columnar metaplasia required to establish the diagnosis. The debate is by no means esoteric, given

that it is centered on the question of which subtypes of metaplastic epithelium arising in the esophagus or esophagogastric junction (EGJ) are at risk for neoplastic progression. The definition of BE is best determined by its malignant potential because what patients carrying the diagnosis ultimately want to know is whether they are at risk of developing esophageal cancer.

CURRENT DEFINITIONS OF BARRETT ESOPHAGUS

The definition of BE according to the current American Gastroenterological Association (AGA) medical position statement on the management of BE is "the condition in which any extent of metaplastic columnar epithelium that predisposes to cancer development replaces the stratified squamous epithelium that normally lines the distal esophagus."[10] The manuscript goes on to state, "Intestinal metaplasia is required for the diagnosis of Barrett's esophagus because intestinal metaplasia is the only type of esophageal columnar epithelium that clearly predisposes to malignancy."[10] Therefore the diagnosis of BE requires a combination of endoscopic and histologic findings, in that the columnar metaplasia must involve the tubular esophagus on endoscopy and must contain goblet cells, which define the presence of intestinal metaplasia (IM), on biopsy specimens.

Agreement does not exist worldwide on the requirement for goblet cells to diagnose BE.[11] The British Society of Gastroenterology mandates only histologic proof of columnar mucosa on biopsies taken from the tubular esophagus; goblet cells do not need to be documented.[12] In Japan the presence of any endoscopically detectable columnar lining of the distal esophagus is adequate to prove the diagnosis of BE; biopsy confirmation is not mandated.[13] The main controversies underlying these differing definitions are the potential for development of EAC in the setting of a columnar-lined esophagus (CLE) with or without the presence of goblet cells, as well as in IM developing distal to the tubular esophagus, so-called cardia intestinal metaplasia (CIM).[14]

HISTORICAL PERSPECTIVE

Fundamental to the definition of BE is the definition of the esophagus. In 1950 Norman Barrett (Fig. 31.1) determined the distal boundary of the esophagus to be the squamocolumnar junction (SCJ), believing that an organ should be defined by its mucosa.[15] Because of this

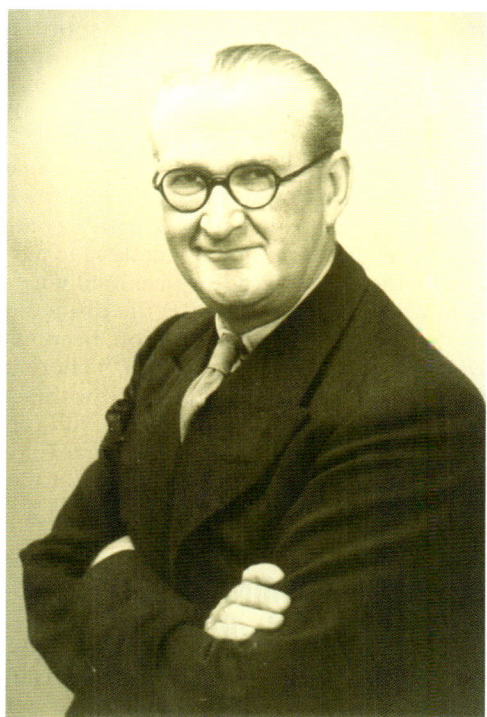

FIGURE 31.1 Norman Barrett. (Courtesy Julia Gough.)

interpretation, a columnar-lined tubular structure subjacent to the esophagus was not recognized as CLE but rather was thought to represent an intrathoracic tubular stomach caused by a congenitally foreshortened esophagus (Fig. 31.2A). An irony is that Barrett initially misdiagnosed the condition later bearing his name!

In 1953, based on the recognition that columnar-lined intrathoracic tubular structures as described by Barrett lacked a peritoneal lining (characteristic of the stomach) and contained esophageal submucosal glands, Allison and Johnstone concluded that the tubular structures were of esophageal, as opposed to gastric, origin.[16] Barrett later agreed with Allison and Johnstone, and introduced the term *columnar-lined esophagus* in 1957 (see Fig. 31.2B).[17] Over the next 6 decades, the definition of BE evolved as the genesis of CLE, and its relationship to EAC, became better understood. In the early 1980s Haggitt and Dean first recognized the association between CLE with IM and the risk of developing EAC.[18] Since then, documentation of the presence of IM has been necessary to establish the diagnosis of BE in the United States and most of the world.

With the introduction and popularization of the flexible fiberoptic upper endoscope came the need for a reliable method to identify the gastroesophageal junction (GEJ) from within the esophageal lumen. External landmarks, such as the location of the peritoneal reflection, and the presence of esophageal glands are not discernible at the time of endoscopy. The first endoscopic definition of the GEJ was proposed by Hayward in 1961 and determined the stomach to start where the esophageal tube flared into a gastric pouch.[19] In this publication, Hayward also described what he believed to be the normal histology spanning the GEJ. Specifically, he stated that the lower 1 to 2 cm of the esophagus could be lined by columnar epithelium and that this "cardiac (or junctional) mucosa" extended 3 cm onto the stomach (Fig. 31.3).

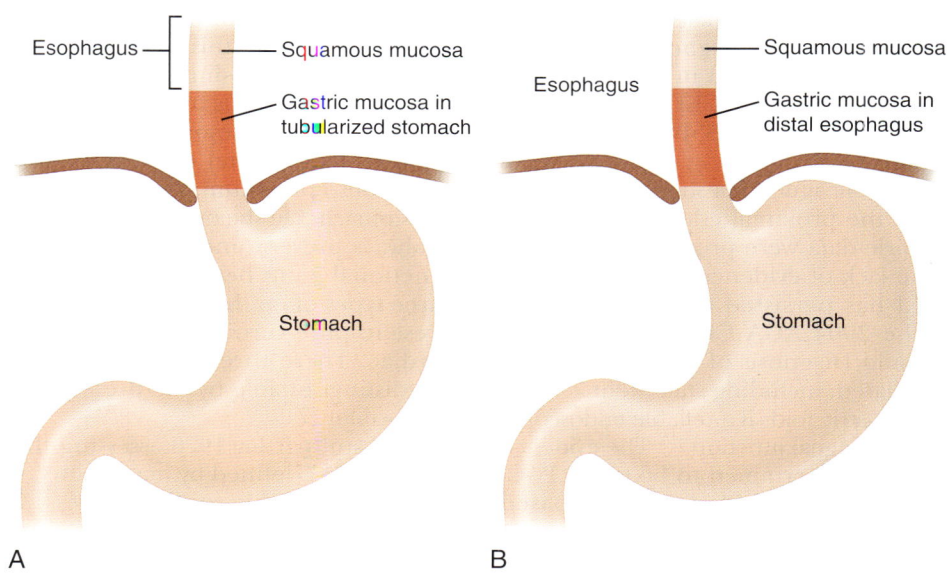

A   B

FIGURE 31.2 (A) Barrett's original conception (1950) of the etiology of a columnar-lined tubular structure in the chest subjacent to the esophagus, what he believed to be an intrathoracic stomach. (B) Allison and Johnstone's interpretation (1953) of the etiology of a columnar-lined tubular structure in the chest, later termed by Barrett (1957) to be *columnar-lined esophagus*.

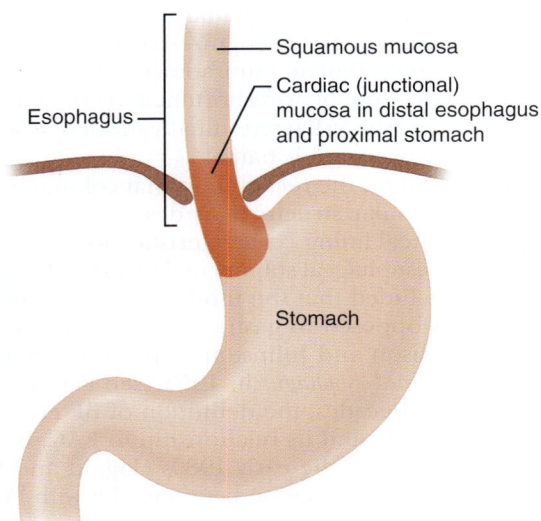

Esophagus —

— Squamous mucosa

— Cardiac (junctional) mucosa in distal esophagus and proximal stomach

Stomach

FIGURE 31.3 Hayward's description (1961) of cardiac mucosa spanning the gastroesophageal junction.

Despite the lack of strong evidence supporting his conclusions, Hayward's observation that a 5-cm segment of cardiac epithelium normally lined the distal 2 cm of the esophagus and proximal 3 cm of the stomach was accepted as fact for the next 30 years. He hypothesized that this "junctional" epithelium served to buffer the esophageal squamous lining from the noxious effects of gastric acid. The theory was based, at least in part, on the premise that the juxtaposition of gastric oxyntic mucosa directly with squamous esophageal mucosa was not teleologically sound due to the potential for inducing erosive reflux esophagitis; a buffer zone was thought necessary. The dogma that the distal 2 cm of the esophagus could be lined by cardiac epithelium led to the dictum that at least 3 cm of CLE had to be present to establish the diagnosis of BE.[20] To this day, the 3-cm cutoff has persisted in distinguishing long-segment BE (LSBE), defined as CLE 3 cm or more in length, from short-segment BE (SSBE), defined as CLE less than 3 cm.

In 1987 McClave and colleagues first suggested that the GEJ was delineated by the proximal edge of the gastric rugal folds.[21] No empiric data were provided to support the claim. Despite the lack of evidence, this endoscopic landmark of the GEJ has persisted and is commonly used currently. At the 2004 AGA Chicago Workshop on the Management and Diagnosis of BE, a number of statements were formulated, including statement 7: "The proximal margin of the gastric folds is a reliable endoscopic marker for the gastroesophageal junction."[22] The evidence behind this statement was determined to be grade IV-C, or from the "opinions of respected authorities based on clinical experience, descriptive studies, or reports of expert committees" and with "poor evidence to support the statement." Furthermore, the manuscript stated, "The group universally favored using the proximal margin of the gastric folds to identify the GEJ but recognized that there are scant data that validate it."

Given the lack of a universally accepted endoscopic criterion for the location of the GEJ, the most recent position of the AGA (in 2011) was, "A majority of published studies on Barrett's esophagus conducted over the past 20 years have used the proximal extent of the gastric folds as the landmark for the GEJ. In the absence of compelling data for the use of alternative markers, we advocate the continued use of this landmark."[10] Thus in the United States the definition of the GEJ continues out of tradition and convenience rather than out of scientific proof of the validity of the proximal rugal folds as an appropriate landmark. To the contrary, the GEJ is defined in Japan by the distal limit of palisade vessels visualized in the lower esophagus.[13]

Countering the validity of the rugal folds as an accurate determinant of the GEJ is the theory that, as the lining of the esophagus is damaged by reflux of gastric contents, the squamous epithelium undergoes metaplasia to a columnar cell type with the SCJ migrating proximally as a result. In addition, with progressive GERD the distal esophagus dilates and loses its tubular configuration, becomes part of the gastric sac, and develops rugal folds.[23] Therefore what had once been tubular esophagus lined with squamous epithelium becomes gastric in appearance with rugal folds. The use of the proximal limit of the rugal folds as the criterion for determining the GEJ in this model would shift it inappropriately cephalad.

HISTOLOGIC DETERMINATION OF THE GASTROESOPHAGEAL JUNCTION

Given the importance of the location of the GEJ in determining the presence of BE, alternative definitions of the junction have been sought. Due to the inability to rely on external landmarks at the time of endoscopy, and the lack of data confirming the validity of the proximal extent of the gastric rugal folds as an appropriate marker, histologic assessment has been proposed as the definitive manner to denote this junction.

Critical to assessing histologic abnormalities in the region of the GEJ is an understanding of the epithelia residing within the esophagus and stomach in health and disease. The normal esophagus is lined with stratified squamous epithelium; this epithelium is never found in the stomach. On the other hand, gastric oxyntic epithelium is always present and confined to the stomach. In the junctional zone between the esophagus and stomach, three types of epithelium may be found and are variably present: pure cardiac, oxyntocardiac, and intestinalized cardiac. These three subtypes of columnar epithelium are distinguishable by the presence of mucous, parietal, and goblet cells.[24]

In a study from 1976 assessing the histology of CLE, with the GEJ defined by manometry, Paull et al. detected these three variable epithelial types.[25] Cardiac ("junctional type") epithelium (Fig. 31.4), comprised exclusively of mucus-secreting cells, and oxyntocardiac ("gastric fundic type") epithelium (Fig. 31.5), comprised of mucus-secreting cells as well as some parietal and chief cells, were found in all patients; intestinalized cardiac ("specialized type") epithelium (Fig. 31.6), containing mucus-secreting cells

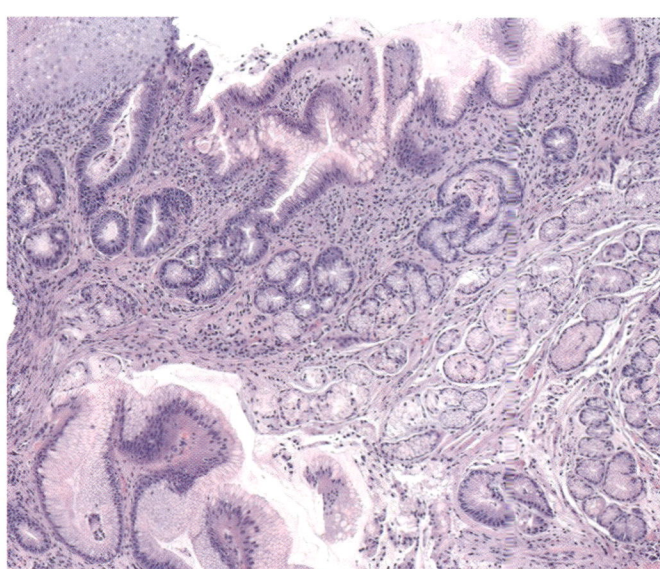

FIGURE 31.4 Cardiac (junctional) epithelium with mucous cells. *(Photomicrographs courtesy Wei Xu, MD.)*

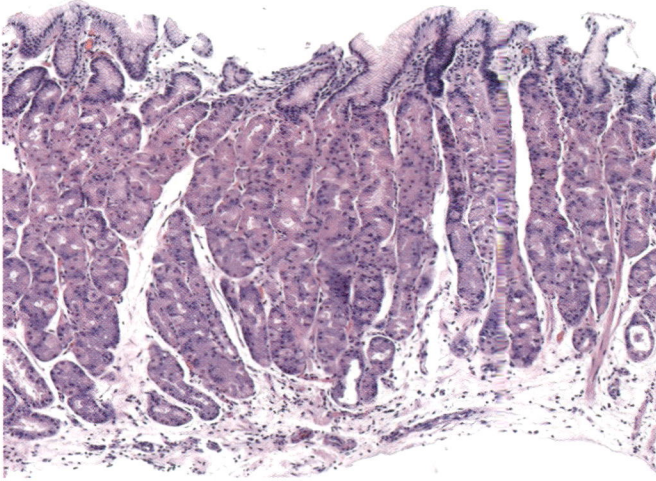

FIGURE 31.5 Oxyntocardiac (fundic) epithelium with mucous, parietal, and chief cells. *(Photomicrographs courtesy Wei Xu, MD.)*

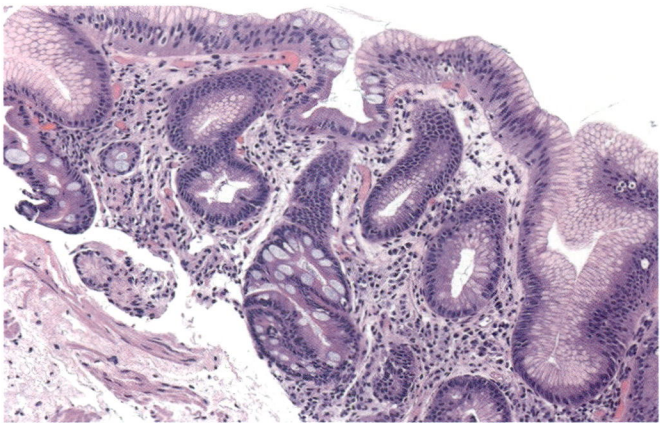

FIGURE 31.6 Intestinal (specialized) epithelium with mucous and goblet cells. *(Photomicrographs courtesy Wei Xu, MD.)*

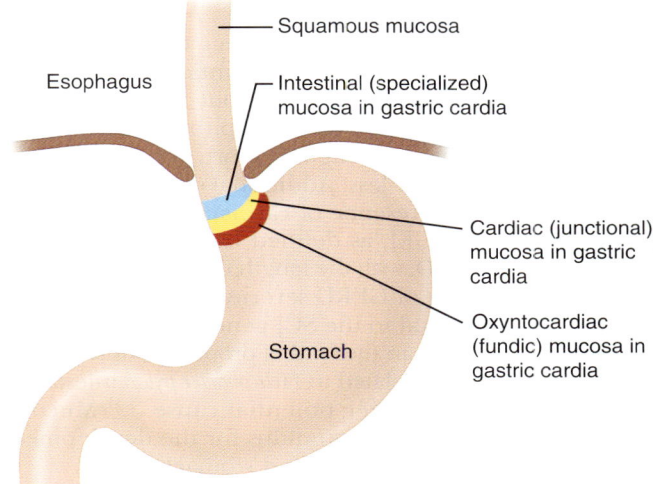

FIGURE 31.7 The squamo-oxyntic gap.

and prominent goblet cells, was found in some. Of note, these three cell types have been detected without visible CLE in the region just distal to the GEJ, as defined by the proximal extent of the gastric rugal folds.[26]

When present, these epithelia always reside between the squamous lining of the esophagus and gastric oxyntic mucosa, creating what Chandrasoma and colleagues have termed a *squamo-oxyntic gap* (Fig. 31.7).[26] Of note, when only one epithelium is present, such as is found only in short gaps generally less than 5 mm, it is oxyntocardiac.[27] In longer gaps, cardiac and oxyntocardiac mucosa may both be present, with cardiac in a more proximal location. When all three epithelial types are present intestinalized cardiac epithelium is proximal, cardiac epithelium is in the middle, and oxyntocardiac epithelium is distal, although admixing may occur. Thus the distribution of

types of columnar epithelium within CLE is not random, with IM residing at the most proximal region of CLE and extending downward while nonintestinalized columnar epithelia occupy a more distal position.[25–27] In patients with CLE the squamo-oxyntic gap traverses the GEJ as defined by the rugal folds, whereas in patients who have a normal-appearing GEJ on endoscopy, the gap is entirely subjacent to the tubular esophagus.

An extensive body of literature has emerged from the University of Southern California disproving the dogma that 5 cm of cardiac mucosa normally reside within the distal esophagus and proximal stomach. The competing theory proposed by Chandrasoma and co-authors from that institution is that cardiac mucosa is not present at the normal GEJ but rather represents metaplastic esophageal epithelium resulting from pathologic exposure to refluxed gastric juice.[27]

The proof of their theory comes in several forms. An assessment of biopsies taken just distal to the normal-appearing GEJ, using a retroflexed endoscope, found cardiac epithelium usually less than 5 cm in length and occasionally absent.[14] Patients with cardiac and oxyntocardiac epithelium were more likely to have an abnormal 24-hour ambulatory esophageal pH study and a mechanically defective lower esophageal sphincter on manometry, both suggesting the presence of GERD, than patients lacking those epithelial types.

An autopsy study reported in 2000 assessed the histology of the GEJ in adult subjects who had no evidence of GERD throughout their lives.[28] Cardiac epithelium was absent in more than half of specimens, and the length of cardiac and oxyntocardiac epithelia ranged from 0.4 to 8.05 mm, with a squamo-oxyntic gap of less than 5 mm in the majority. Half of subjects were found to have a direct transition from squamous to gastric oxyntic mucosa in at least part of the circumference of the SCJ. These findings were validated by a later independent study.[29] An additional autopsy study in children found cardiac epithelium in all subjects, but limited to a length between 1 and 4 mm, with a median of 1.8 mm, far less than the 50-mm length previously thought to be normal.[30]

Based on these findings, a direct transition from esophageal squamous mucosa to oxyntic gastric mucosa does exist in some individuals, without a buffer zone of cardiac epithelium. When cardiac epithelium is present in normal individuals, its length is short, generally limited to a few millimeters or less. Additional studies have demonstrated that the presence of cardiac epithelium distal to the endoscopic GEJ, as defined by the rugal folds, is associated with GERD, with the length of the segment being a sensitive indicator of GERD severity.[31,32] Finally, cardiac mucosa residing distal to the SCJ generally demonstrates chronic inflammation in the lamina propria, consistent with GERD, and likely not related to *Helicobacter pylori* infestation of the stomach, the other potential cause.[33,34] Mucosal inflammation is the major stimulus for the development of IM, both in the esophagus and stomach.

If the premise is accepted that cardiac epithelium at the GEJ is pathologic, related to GERD-induced metaplasia of the esophageal mucosa rather than a normal lining of the proximal stomach, an accurate histologic determination of the GEJ becomes possible. In this model the GEJ is defined by the proximal border of gastric oxyntic mucosa as assessed on biopsies. In a normal subject the GEJ is located where esophageal squamous mucosa transitions to gastric oxyntic mucosa. In patients with GERD the GEJ is located where metaplastic columnar epithelium residing within the squamocolumnar gap transitions to gastric oxyntic mucosa. Because this latter transition is not discernible at the time of endoscopy, the true GEJ in such circumstances can only be determined by extensive, meticulous, and accurately recorded biopsies.

IMPLICATIONS OF THE LOCATION OF THE GASTROESOPHAGEAL JUNCTION

DEFINITION OF THE CARDIA

The location of the GEJ has several implications relative to the diagnosis, classification, and management of metaplasia or neoplasia arising in the distal esophagus or proximal stomach. The term *gastric cardia* has been used to denote the region of the stomach just distal to the GEJ, although its boundaries are poorly defined and its definition is controversial. The theory that metaplastic cardiac epithelium has a derivation similar to metaplastic esophageal epithelium means that the cardia has its origins in the esophagus, not the stomach, contrary to common terminology and conceptualization. Cancers of the cardia, according to this theory, are best classified as esophageal not gastric,[35] consistent with the most recent staging of the American Joint Committee on Cancer, seventh edition.[36] Remarkable in this theory is the premise that, in a complete reversal of the original contention of Norman Barrett that the tubularized CLE he observed was stomach, what has been called proximal stomach (the "gastric cardia") lined by metaplastic columnar epithelium is, in fact, esophagus.

Several types of evidence support the esophageal origin of cardia adenocarcinoma. Cancers arising in the cardia are associated with symptomatic GERD, albeit to a lesser extent than EAC.[8] The increasing incidence of cardia adenocarcinoma has paralleled the rise in EAC over the past four decades, although it has deviated from the trend in incidence of cancer arising in the distal stomach.[37] In addition, the vast majority of cases of both EAC and cardia adenocarcinoma occur in association with IM.[38,39] The presence of dysplastic epithelium arising in cardiac (junctional) or fundic mucosa is uncommon in the absence of coexisting IM.[22]

SCREENING AND SURVEILLANCE BIOPSY PROTOCOLS FOR BARRETT ESOPHAGUS

Given that IM arising in columnar epithelium below the proximal limit of the gastric folds (i.e., CIM) has the same pathogenesis as IM arising from the tubular esophagus (i.e., BE), both sites of IM would be expected to have the same neoplastic potential. As IM is a GERD-related phenomenon, it represents a continuum of disease starting at the most distal esophagus, where reflux is most severe, and progressing cephalad; CIM and BE are not distinct clinical entities. The differentiation of CIM from SSBE can be quite difficult and arbitrary, given that the conventional boundary is the top of the gastric rugal folds, a landmark that can be indiscrete. If the pathogenesis and risk of malignant progression is the same for the two entities, then distinguishing them is not necessary.

Although studies have shown an increased risk of EAC with longer segments of IM, a length threshold relative to risk has not been established.[40–44] In a prospective study, Sikkema et al. found that for every additional centimeter in BE length the risk of developing high-grade dysplasia (HGD) or EAC increased by 11% over 4 years.[45] The preponderance of evidence, as well as common sense, suggests that the rate of development of EAC increases with a larger at-risk surface area of metaplastic epithelium; arbitrary cutoffs between CIM, SSBE, and LSBE relative to that risk do not seem justified.

Some authors have argued that CIM and SSBE are, in fact, distinct clinical entities with differing etiologies and risks of neoplastic progression.[46] As evidence, proponents of this belief cite differing cytokeratin 7 and 20 immunoreactivity between CIM and BE noted in one study, a finding that has not been verified in subsequent reports.[47–49] The preponderance of literature would suggest that there are no other immunohistochemical biomarkers either specific for mucin or intestinalization (such as CDX2, DAS-1, Hep Par 1, Villin, or MUC2) that can differentiate metaplasia occurring in the tubular esophagus from the cardia.[49–51] In addition, IM arising in the proximal stomach possesses immunohistochemical features similar to BE and not to IM arising in the distal stomach.[52]

The conceptualization of a continuum of metaplasia arising within the esophagus, rather than the discrete entities of CIM, SSBE, and LSBE, has implications regarding the need to biopsy both above and below the top of the rugal folds at the time of endoscopy for BE. Most studies of BE screening, surveillance, and progression have assessed biopsies taken from the tubular esophagus alone, not the gastric cardia. As a result, the cancer risk in patients with CIM is poorly defined.[53–56]

In the AGA Chicago Workshop Recommendations on the Diagnosis and Management of BE from 2004, statement 9 is: "The normal appearing and normally located squamocolumnar junction should not be biopsied."[22] The subsequent AGA medical position statement on the management of BE from 2011 is quiet on the matter.[10] In addition, the AGA recommendations from 2004 are to perform systematic biopsies of both SSBE and LSBE, the consensus opinion being that they are not distinct clinical entities.[22] Given the continuum of IM length, the omission of biopsies from the proximal columnar mucosa just distal to the upper limit of the gastric rugal folds does not appear justified, despite the dearth of data delineating neoplastic risk of IM at this location. Although the risk of progression is likely lower than for longer segments of IM based on surface area considerations alone, a discrete recommendation differing from that for SSBE does not seem appropriate.

RISK OF NEOPLASTIC PROGRESSION IN SUBTYPES OF ESOPHAGEAL COLUMNAR METAPLASIA

LIMITATIONS OF USING GOBLET CELLS TO DETERMINE THE PRESENCE OF INTESTINAL METAPLASIA

Most cases of adenocarcinoma of the esophagus or GEJ arise in a background of IM as defined by the presence of goblet cells, which normally reside in the intestines.[6,38,54–56] Therefore detecting goblet cells in screening or surveillance biopsies for BE is critical for determining the risk of subsequent neoplastic progression and the need for follow-up. The dictum "no goblets—no Barrett's" has arisen to underscore their fundamental importance.[57] That being said, the highly differentiated goblet cell is unlikely the precursor to EAC because cancers typically arise from more poorly differentiated cell lines. The goblet cell merely serves as a marker for the malignant potential of the surrounding metaplastic epithelium.

A number of factors can affect the detection of goblet cells, including:

1. Differentiation of goblet cells from pseudogoblet cells;

2. Sampling error, which depends upon the thoroughness of biopsies, the length of CLE, and goblet cell density; and

3. Goblet cell dynamics.

Pseudogoblet cells are mucin-containing columnar cells that are difficult to differentiate from true goblet cells. In contrast to goblet cells, which typically form as single cells in a random distribution, pseudogoblet cells tend to occur in rows within the superficial epithelium. Pseudogoblet cells also lack the triangular nucleus characteristic of true goblet cells.[58]

The number of goblet cells may be small in patients with CIM or SSBE. Chandrasoma et al. found IM in 56% of patients with a 1-cm length of CLE, progressing to 100% with a CLE length greater than 5 cm.[59] The likelihood of detecting goblet cells has been shown to correlate directly with the number of biopsies performed at endoscopy as well as the length of CLE.[26,60] Harrison and co-authors found a progressive increase in the detection of IM with a higher number of biopsies, reaching 100% when more than 16 biopsies were taken.[61] In addition, goblet cell density has been shown in some studies to vary with the position along the length of CLE, being highest near the SCJ and lower in the more distal portions.[24,62] However, other reports have shown a more random distribution.[59,63]

Current guidelines recommend four quadrant biopsies every 1 to 2 cm along CLE, with special attention given to regions of mucosal nodularity or irregularity.[10,64,65] If an adequate number of biopsies is not taken along the entire length of CLE, and if the biopsies are not appropriately dispersed with particular attention paid to the region of the SCJ, the presence of goblet cells may be missed. Finally, goblet cells may vary over time, with therapy, and with progression of disease.[60,66] Repeat endoscopy with biopsies may be necessary to establish the diagnosis of IM.[60,66] Each of these factors contributes to the unreliability of using the identification of goblet cells as the pathognomonic criterion for the presence of IM.

STEPS IN THE DEVELOPMENT OF INTESTINAL METAPLASIA

Chronic esophageal inflammation and ulceration resulting from the reflux of gastric contents, including both acid and bile, drive metaplasia within the esophageal lining. The conversion of esophageal squamous epithelium to IM is thought to be a stepwise process. Inflamed esophageal squamous epithelium is first replaced by a multilayer, transitional epithelium followed by a single-layer, nonintestinal columnar epithelium; a specialized intestinal-type metaplastic epithelium is the final step.[67] According to this model, the previously described phenotypes of columnar metaplasia, including cardiac, oxyntocardiac, and intestinal types, represent points along a continuum rather than distinct entities. The first step in intestinalization appears to be mediated by upregulation of the Sonic hedgehog (SHH)–bone morphogenetic protein 4 (BMP-4) signaling path, leading to phosphorylation of SMAD proteins (pSMAD), and is modulated by a number of antagonists and downstream factors. SHH-BMP-4/pSMAD signaling is responsible for the induction of genes responsible for the nonintestinal type of metaplasia. The next step is the induction of genes responsible for intestinalization and is mediated by the interaction of pSMAD with CDX2, an intestine-specific homeobox gene critical to intestinal epithelial functions. In the final stages of intestinal differentiation, Wnt and Notch signaling also are key.[67]

Metaplastic columnar epithelium can reveal biochemical or molecular evidence of intestinal differentiation prior to the development of goblet cells. Studies have shown that metaplastic columnar mucosa without goblet cells may express proteins or transcription factors specific to intestinalization, such as CDX2, DAS-1, and Villin, or intestine-specific mucopolysaccharides, such as MUC2, early in the process of differentiation, although may be expressed further once goblet cells appear.[48,49,68–70] Metaplastic esophageal columnar epithelium not containing goblet cells on histology may still be "biologically intestinalized,"[58] with studies finding similar DNA content and chromosomal abnormalities to epithelium containing goblet cells.[71,72] Thus goblet cell formation likely represents the end of a chain of genetic and signaling events ultimately culminating in histologic intestinalization of metaplastic cardiac epithelium.

RISK OF NEOPLASTIC PROGRESSION IN COLUMNAR-LINED ESOPHAGUS WITH OR WITHOUT GOBLET CELLS

Given the genetic and molecular abnormalities identifiable in nongoblet esophageal metaplasia, questions exist as to whether such an epithelium is at risk for progression to EAC and whether the risk is similar to progression of IM in the presence of goblet cells.

A study of 141 patients who underwent endoscopic resection (ER) of small (<2 cm diameter) EAC found that 71% had cardiac or fundic epithelium, not IM, adjacent to the cancer.[73] In addition, IM was not observed in any areas of the ER specimens in 57% of cases. Of note, areas of CLE outside of the ER specimens were not biopsied in this study, so the true incidence of IM in their patient population is not known.

Two large retrospective studies from the United Kingdom found the rates of development of dysplasia or EAC to be similar in patients with IM compared with those with CLE without IM.[74,75] Gatenby et al. analyzed 3568 biopsies of nondysplastic CLE from 1751 patients with and without IM and found no difference in the rate of development of dysplasia or EAC between the two groups.[74] The mean length of CLE in the two cohorts was 5.75 cm and 4.93 cm, respectively. Because the mean number of biopsies was only 2.04 per patient and the biopsies were randomly distributed with no targeting of the SCJ, a strong argument can be made that IM was missed in many patients due to sampling error. This argument is bolstered by the authors' findings that the rate of IM detection increased with the number of biopsies taken (a 24% increase noted for each additional biopsy), and the fact that 90.8% of the patients initially not found to have IM developed it on subsequent biopsies over the course of the next 10 years. Sampling error likely was a major factor negating their conclusion that cancer risk was not affected by the presence or absence of IM.

Kelty et al. analyzed 712 patients with CLE with or without IM over a mean follow-up of 12 years and found

no difference in the rate of progression to EAC (4.5% and 3.6%, respectively). However, the same questions can be raised about their findings relative to errors in sampling for the presence of goblet cells.[75]

Other studies have contradicted the claim that adenocarcinomas of the esophagus and EGJ can arise from nongoblet columnar metaplasia. A large population-based analysis of 8522 patients with CLE with or without IM was undertaken by Bhat et al. using the Northern Ireland BE Registry.[76] At a mean follow-up of 7 years, the risk of cancer progression was 0.07% per year in patients without IM compared with 0.38% per year in patients with IM at initial biopsy ($P < .001$). In a study of 214 patients by Chandrasoma et al. using a rigorous biopsy protocol of CLE and the GEJ, dysplasia or EAC developed only in patients with proven IM; the risk of malignant progression was thought either nonexistent or extremely low for patients without goblet cells.[61] Similarly, Westerhoff et al. found EAC or dysplasia to arise only in patients with documented goblet cells.[77] Elimination of the requirement for identification of goblet cells would have increased the diagnosis of BE by 147% in their study population without identifying any additional patients who subsequently developed dysplasia or neoplasia. Finally, in a study of 45 patients with BE, biopsies of IM revealed a higher frequency of cancer-associated mutations than those obtained from nongoblet metaplastic mucosa.[78]

At present, whether nongoblet cell metaplasia of the esophagus is a premalignant condition remains controversial. What is known is that if the definition of BE were expanded to include all patients with CLE without documented IM, the number of patients in need of surveillance would escalate greatly, adding significant cost without proof of increasing cancer detection and saving lives. More data clearly are necessary regarding the natural history of non-goblet esophageal metaplasia, including the cancer risk in both long and short segments, other risk factors for malignant progression, potential lives saved with surveillance, and the cost-effectiveness of various management strategies, before recommendations can be made to change current practice.

CONCLUSION

The definition of BE has evolved over the past 60 years since CLE was first recognized as an understanding of its pathogenesis has emerged. At the core of the definition of BE is the malignant potential of metaplastic esophageal columnar epithelium, whether or not it contains goblet cells and whether or not it is located in the tubular esophagus. The risk of developing esophageal cancer is, after all, what concerns patients diagnosed with BE, their families, and their care providers and determines the need for surveillance.

In the United States and most of the world the presence of IM must be documented to establish the diagnosis of BE, given the malignant potential of metaplastic columnar epithelium containing goblet cells. Although the presence of IM is not a requirement for the diagnosis of BE in Great Britain and Japan, a paucity of data exists delineating the malignant risk associated with nongoblet columnar epithelium. The available literature in support of the precancerous nature of CLE not demonstrating IM must be interpreted with caution in light of the potential for significant sampling error, leading to an underappreciation of the presence of goblet cells in patients assessed in those studies.

Although metaplasia found within what has been termed the *gastric cardia* has not received as much attention as IM arising in the tubular esophagus, an extensive body of investigation into the histology of the GEJ supports an esophageal origin to the metaplastic mucosa arising just beyond the proximal limit of the gastric folds. Because CIM shares a common pathogenesis with BE, both entities should be handled as a spectrum of metaplastic changes spanning the GEJ and extending proximally into the esophagus. Only with further study of cohorts of patients undergoing an aggressive biopsy protocol, including adequate sampling of the mucosa just beyond the SCJ, will the significance of IM in the "gastricized" esophagus be clarified.

Until the malignant potential of nongoblet IM arising in CLE is clarified with additional longitudinal studies on adequate numbers of patients undergoing a thorough biopsy protocol, the diagnosis of BE is best reserved for cases of documented IM. Expanding the definition of BE to include all types of columnar metaplasia would greatly increase the pool of patients in need of long-term surveillance, with an associated increase in costs and without proven benefit. The impact of the diagnosis of BE on the individual, both in terms of the psychologic costs of a precancerous diagnosis and the monetary costs of serial endoscopic assessments, is not trivial. In addition, a diagnosis of BE can escalate the price of life insurance, with a reported increase of 118% for an otherwise healthy, nonsmoking male.[79]

Much remains to be learned about BE, including ways to improve the diagnosis, stratify risk, and predict the response to therapy. Molecular profiling has been studied, particularly in nongoblet CLE, although it needs to be validated for cancer risk independent of the presence of IM. The current position of the AGA is that molecular biomarkers should not be used for risk stratification.[10] Similarly, serum biomarkers have been studied, although the available data do not support their utility at present.[80]

For now, the presence of IM, as determined by the histologic confirmation of goblet cells, remains the key to establishing the diagnosis of BE. Until additional data dictate otherwise, those of us providing care to the patient with BE should not be ready to "throw down the goblet"!

REFERENCES

1. Pohl H, Sirovich B, Welch HG. Esophageal adenocarcinoma incidence: are we reaching the peak? *Cancer Epidemiol Biomarkers Prev.* 2010;19(6):1468-1470.
2. https://www.cancer.org/cancer/esophagus-cancer/about/key-statistics.html. Accessed 5 December 2017.
3. Pera M, Manterola C, Vidal O, Grande L. Epidemiology of esophageal adenocarcinoma. *J Surg Oncol.* 2005;92:151-159
4. Cameron AJ, Ott BJ, Payne WS. The incidence of adenocarcinoma in columnar-lined (Barrett's) esophagus. *N Engl J Med.* 1985;313(14):857-859.
5. Corley DA, Levin TR, Habel LA, Weiss NS, Buffler PA. Surveillance and survival in Barrett's adenocarcinomas: a population-based study. *Gastroenterology.* 2002;122:633-640.
6. Peters JH, Clark GWB, Ireland AP, Chandrasoma P, Smyrk TC, DeMeester TR. Outcome of adenocarcinoma arising in Barrett's esophagus in endoscopically surveyed and nonsurveyed patients. *J Thorac Cardiovasc Surg.* 1994;108:813-821.
7. Dent J, El-Serag HB, Wallander ME, Johansson S. Epidemiology of gastro-oesophageal reflux disease: a systematic review. *Gut.* 2005;54(5):710-717.
8. Lagergren J, Bergstrom R, Lindgren A, Nyren O. Symptomatic gastroesophageal reflux as a risk factor for esophageal adenocarcinoma. *N Engl J Med.* 1999;340(11):825-831.
9. Barrett NR. The lower esophagus lined by columnar epithelium. *Surgery.* 1957;41:881-894.
10. Spechler SJ, Sharma P, Souza RF, Inadomi JM, Shaheen NJ. American Gastroenterological Association medical position statement on the management of Barrett's esophagus. *Gastroenterology.* 2011;140:1084-1091.
11. Riddell RH, Odze RD. Definition of Barrett's esophagus: time for a rethink—is intestinal metaplasia dead? *Am J Gastroenterol.* 2009;104:2588-2594.
12. Fitzgerald RC, di Pietro M, Raganuth K, et al. British Society of Gastroenterology guidelines on the diagnosis and management of Barrett's oesophagus. *Gut.* 2014;63:7-42.
13. Ogiya K, Kawano T, Ito E, et al. Lower esophageal palisade vessels and the definition of Barrett's esophagus. *Dis Esophagus.* 2008;21:645-649.
14. Oberg S, Peters JH, DeMeester TR, et al. Inflammation and specialized intestinal metaplasia of cardiac mucosa is a manifestation of gastroesophageal reflux disease. *Ann Surg.* 1997;226:522-532.
15. Barrett NR. Chronic peptic ulcer of the oesophagus and 'oesophagitis'. *Br J Surg.* 1950;38:175-182.
16. Allison PR, Johnstone AS. The oesophagus lined with gastric mucous membrane. *Thorax.* 1953;8:87-101.
17. Barrett NR. The lower esophagus lined by columnar epithelium. *Surgery.* 1957;41:881-894.
18. Haggitt RC, Dean PJ. Adenocarcinoma in Barrett's epithelium. In: Spechler SJ, Goyal RK, eds. *Barrett's Esophagus: Pathophysiology, Diagnosis and Management.* New York: Elsevier Science Publishing; 1985:153-166.
19. Hayward J. The lower end of the oesophagus. *Thorax.* 1961;16:36-41.
20. Bremner CG, Hamilton DG, DeMeester TR, et al. Barrett's esophagus: controversial aspects. In: DeMeester TR, Skinner DB, eds. *Esophageal Disorders: Pathophysiology and Therapy.* New York: Raven Press; 1985:233.
21. McClave SA, Boyce HW Jr, Gottfried MR. Early diagnosis of columnar lined esophagus: a new endoscopic diagnostic criterion. *Gastrointest Endosc.* 1987;33:413-416.
22. Sharma P, McQuaid K, Dent J, et al. A critical review of the diagnosis and management of Barrett's esophagus: the AGA Chicago Workshop. *Gastroenterology.* 2004;127:310-330.
23. Ayazi S, Tamhankar A, DeMeester SA, et al. The impact of gastric distention on the lower esophageal sphincter and its exposure to acid gastric juice. *Ann Surg.* 2010;252:57-62.
24. Chandrasoma PT, Makarewicz K, Wickramasinghe K, Ma YL, DeMeester TR. A proposal for a new validated histologic definition of the gastroesophageal junction. *Hum Pathol.* 2006;37:40-47.
25. Paull A, Trier JS, Dalton MD, Camp RC, Loeb P, Goyal RK. The histologic spectrum of Barrett's esophagus. *N Engl J Med.* 1976;295:476-480.
26. Chandrasoma PT, Wijetunge S, DeMeester SR, Hagen JA, DeMeester TR. The histologic squamo-oxyntic gap: an accurate and reproducible marker of gastroesophageal reflux disease. *Am J Surg Pathol.* 2010;34:1574-1581.
27. Chandrasoma PT, Der R, Ma Y, Peters J, DeMeester TR. Histologic classification of patients based on mapping biopsies of the gastroesophageal junction. *Am J Surg Pathol.* 2003;27:929-936.
28. Chandrasoma PT, Der R, Ma Y, Dalton P, Taira M. Histology of the gastroesophageal junction: an autopsy study. *Am J Surg Pathol.* 2000;24:402-409.
29. Sarbia M, Donner A, Gabbert HE. Histopathology of the gastroesophageal junction. A study on 36 operation specimens. *Am J Surg Pathol.* 2002;26:1207-1212.
30. Park YS, Park HJ, Kang GH, Kim CJ, Chi JG. Histology of gastroesophageal junction in fetal and pediatric autopsy. *Arch Pathol Lab Med.* 2003;127:451-455.
31. Kilgore SP, Ormsby AH, Gramlich TL, et al. The gastric cardia: fact or fiction? *Am J Gastroenterol.* 2000;95:921-924.
32. Glickman JN, Fox V, Antonioli DA, Wang HH, Odze RD. Morphology of the cardia and significance of carditis in pediatric patients. *Am J Surg Pathol.* 2002;26:1032-1039.

33. Der R, Tsao-Wei DD, DeMeester TR, et al. Carditis: a manifestation of gastroesophageal reflux disease. *Am J Surg Pathol.* 2001;25:245-252.

34. Spechler SJ, Wang HH, Chen YY, Zeroogian JM, Antonioli DA, Goyal RK. GERD vs. *H. pylori* infections as potential causes of inflammation in the gastric cardia. *Gastroenterology.* 1997;112:A297.

35. Chandrasoma PT, Makarewicz K, Wickramasinghe K, Ma YL, DeMeester TR. Adenoarcinomas of the distal esophagus and "gastric cardia" are predominantly esophageal adenocarcinomas. *Am J Surg Pathol.* 2007;31:569-575.

36. Stephen B Edge, American Joint Committee on Cancer. *AJCC Cancer Staging Manual.* 7th ed. New York: Springer; 2010:103-115.

37. Devesa SS, Blot WJ, Fraumeni JF. Changing patterns in the incidence of esophageal and gastric carcinoma in the United States. *Cancer.* 1998;83:2049-2053.

38. Haggitt RC, Tryzelaar J, Ellis FH, Colcher H. Adenocarcinoma complicating columnar epithelium-lined (Barrett's) esophagus. *Am J Clin Pathol.* 1978;70:1-5.

39. Smith RRL, Hamilton SR, Boitnott JK, Rogers EL. The spectrum of carcinoma arising in Barrett's esophagus. *Am J Surg Pathol.* 1984;8:563-573.

40. Rudolph RE, Vaughan TL, Storer BE, et al. Effect of segment length on risk for neoplastic progression in patients with Barrett's esophagus. *Ann Intern Med.* 2000;132:612-620.

41. Weston AP, Badr AS, Hassanein RS. Prospective multivariate analysis of clinical, endoscopic, and histologic factors predictive of the development of Barrett's multifocal high-grade dysplasia or adenocarcinoma. *Am J Gastroenterol.* 1999;94:3413-3419.

42. Menke-Pluymers MB, Hop WC, Dees J, van Blankenstein M, Tilanus HW. Risk factors for the development of an adenocarcinoma in columnar-lined (Barrett) esophagus. The Rotterdam Esophageal Tumor Study Group. *Cancer.* 1993;72:1155-1158.

43. Wani S, Falk G, Hall M, et al. Patients with nondysplastic Barrett's esophagus have low risks for developing dysplasia or esophageal adenocarcinoma. *Clin Gastroenterol.* 2011;9:2207.

44. Desai TK, Krishnan K, Samala N, et al. The incidence of esophageal adenocarcinoma in non-dysplastic Barrett's esophagus: a meta-analysis. *Gut.* 2012;61:970-976.

45. Sikkema M, Looman CW, Steyergerg EW, et al. Predictors for neoplastic progression in patients with Barrett's esophagus: a prospective cohort study. *Am J Gastroenterol.* 2011;106:1231-1238.

46. Sharma P, Weston AP, Morales T, Topalovski M, Mayo MS, Sampliner RE. Relative risk of dysplasia for patients with intestinal metaplasia in the distal oesophagus and in the gastric cardia. *Gut.* 2000;46:9-13.

47. Glickman JN, Wang H, Das KM, et al. Phenotype of Barrett's esophagus and intestinal metaplasia of the distal esophagus and gastroesophageal junction. An immunohistochemical study of cytokeratins 7 and 20, DAS-1 and 45M1. *Am J Surg Pathol.* 2001;25:87-94.

48. Mohammed IA, Streutker CJ, Riddell RH. Utilization of cytokeratins 7 and 20 does not differentiate between Barrett's esophagus and gastric cardiac intestinal metaplasia. *Mod Pathol.* 2002;15:611-616.

49. DeMeester SR, Wickramasinghe KS, Lord RV, et al. Cytokeratin and DAS-1 immunostaining reveal similarities among cardiac mucosa, CIM and Barrett's esophagus. *Am J Gastroenterol.* 2002;97:2514-2523.

50. Phillips RW, Frierson HF Jr, Moskaluk CA. Cdx2 as a marker of epithelial intestinal differentiation in the esophagus. *Am J Surg Pathol.* 2003;27:1442-1447.

51. Chu PG, Jiang Z, Weiss LM. Hepatocyte antigen as a marker of intestinal metaplasia. *Am J Surg Pathol.* 2003;27:952-959.

52. White NM, Gabril M, Ejeckam G, et al. Barrett's esophagus and cardiac intestinal metaplasia: two conditions within the same spectrum. *Can J Gastroenterol.* 2008;22:369-375.

53. Spechler SJ, Zeroogian JM, Antonioli DA, Wang HH, Goyal RK. Prevalence of metaplasia at the gastro-oesophageal junction. *Lancet.* 1994;344:1533-1536.

54. Hirota WK, Loughney TM, Lazas DJ, Maydonovitch CL, Rholl V, Wong RKH. Specialized intestinal metaplasia, dysplasia and cancer of the esophagus and esophagogastric junction: prevalence and clinical data. *Gastroenterology.* 1999;116:277-285.

55. Ruol A, Parenti A, Zaninotto G, et al. Intestinal metaplasia is the probable common precursor of adenocarcinoma in Barrett esophagus and adenocarcinoma of the gastric cardia. *Cancer.* 2000;88:2520-2528.

56. Cameron AJ, Souto EO, Smyrk TC. Small adenocarcinomas of the esophagogastric junction: association with intestinal metaplasia and dysplasia. *Am J Gastroenterol.* 2002;97:1375-1380.

57. Batts KP. Barrett's esophagus—more steps forward. *Hum Pathol.* 2001;32:357-359.

58. Naini BV, Chak A, Ali MA, Odze RD. Barrett's oesophagus diagnostic criteria: endoscopy and histology. *Best Pract Res Clin Gastroenterol.* 2015;29:77-96.

59. Chandrasoma P, Wijetunge S, DeMeester S, Ma Y, et al. Columnar-lined esophagus without intestinal metaplasia has no proven risk of adenocarcinoma. *Am J Surg Pathol.* 2012;36:1-7.

60. Oberg S, Johansson J, Wenner J, et al. Endoscopic surveillance of columnar lined esophagus: frequency of intestinal metaplasia detection and impact of antireflux surgery. *Ann Surg.* 2001;234:619-626.

61. Harrison R, Perry I, Haddadin W, et al. Detection of intestinal metaplasia in Barrett's esophagus: an observational comparator study suggests the need for a minimum of eight biopsies. *Am J Gastroenterol.* 2007;102:1154-1161.

62. Chandrasoma PT, Der R, Dalton P, et al. Distribution and significance of epithelial types in columnar-lined esophagus. *Am J Surg Pathol.* 2001;25:1188-1193.

63. Thompson JJ, Zinsser KR, Enterline HT. Barrett's metaplasia and adenocarcinoma of the esophagus and gastroesophageal junction. *Hum Pathol.* 1983;14:42-61.

64. Wang KK, Sampliner RE. Updated guidelines 2008 for the diagnosis, surveillance and therapy of Barrett's esophagus. *Am J Gastroenterol.* 2008;103:788-797.

65. ASGE Standards of Practice Committee, Evans JA, Early DS, Fukami N, et al. The role of endoscopy in Barrett's esophagus and other premalignant conditions of the esophagus. *Gastrointest Endosc.* 2012;76:788-797.

66. Jones TF, Sharma P, Daaboul B, et al. Yield of intestinal metaplasia in patients with suspected short-segment Barrett's esophagus (SSBE) on repeat endoscopy. *Dig Dis Sci.* 2002;47:2108-2111.

67. Krishnadath KK, Wang KK. Molecular pathogenesis of Barrett esophagus. *Gastroenterol Clin North Am.* 2015;44:233-247.

68. Hahn HP, Blount PL, Ayub K, et al. Intestinal differentiation in metaplastic, nongoblet columnar epithelium in the esophagus. *Am J Surg Pathol.* 2009;33:1006-1015.

69. Groisman GM, Amar M, Meir A. Expression of the intestinal marker Cdx2 in the columnar-lined esophagus with and without intestinal (Barrett's) metaplasia. *Mod Pathol.* 2004;17:1282-1288.

70. Chaves P, Cruz C, Dias Pereira A, et al. Gastric and intestinal differentiation in Barrett's metaplasia and associated adenocarcinoma. *Dis Esophagus.* 2005;18(6):383-387.

71. Liu W, Hahn H, Odze RD, Goyal RK. Metaplastic esophageal columnar epithelium without goblet cells shows DNA content abnormalities similar to goblet-containing epithelium. *Am J Gastroenterol.* 2009;104:816-824.

72. Chaves P, Crespo M, Ribeiro C, et al. Chromosomal analysis of Barrett's cells: demonstration of instability and detection of the metaplastic lineage involved. *Mod Pathol.* 2007;20:788-796.

73. Takubo K, Aida J, Naomoto Y, et al. Cardiac rather than intestinal-type background in endoscopic resection specimens of minute Barrett adenocarcinoma. *Hum Pathol.* 2009;40:65-74.

74. Gatenby PA, Ramus JR, Caygill CP, Shepherd NA, Watson A. Relevance of the detection of intestinal metaplasia in non-dysplastic columnar-lined oesophagus. *Scand J Gastroenterol.* 2008;43:524-530.

75. Kelty CJ, Gough MD, Van Wyk Q, Stephenson TJ, Ackroyd R. Barrett's oesophagus: intestinal metaplasia is not essential for cancer risk. *Scand J Gastroenterol.* 2007;42:1271-1274.

76. Bhat S, Coleman HG, Yousef F, et al. Risk of malignant progression in Barrett's esophagus patients: results from a large population-based study. *J Natl Cancer Inst.* 2011;103(13):1049-1057. (Erratum: *J Natl Cancer Inst.* 2013;105(8):581.)

77. Westerhoff M, Hovan L, Lee C, Hart J. Effects of dropping the requirement for goblet cells from the diagnosis of Barrett's esophagus. *Clin Gastroenterol Hepatol.* 2012;10:1232-1236.

78. Bandla S, Peters JH, Ruff D, et al. Comparison of cancer-associated genetic abnormalities in columnar-lined esophagus tissues with and without goblet cells. *Ann Surg.* 2014;260:72-80.

79. Shaheen NJ, Dulai GS, Ascher B, et al. Effect of a new diagnosis of Barrett's esophagus on insurance status. *Am J Gastroenterol.* 2005;100:577-580.

80. Bansal A, Fitzgerald RC. Biomarkers in Barrett's esophagus: role in diagnosis, risk stratification, and prediction of response to therapy. *Gastroenterol Clin North Am.* 2015;44:373-390.

Epidemiology of Barrett Esophagus and Risk Factors for Progression

Oliver M. Fisher | Reginald V.N. Lord

PREVALENCE AND INCIDENCE OF BARRETT ESOPHAGUS

Barrett esophagus (BE) is the disease in which the normal squamous lining of the distal esophagus is replaced by a metaplastic columnar cell epithelium (termed intestinal metaplasia [IM]) in response to chronic severe gastroesophageal reflux disease (GERD). Its clinical importance is as the precursor lesion and major risk factor for esophageal adenocarcinoma (EAC). The epidemiology of EAC has been investigated thoroughly because of this cancer's high lethality and recent extraordinary increase in incidence rates. Less extensive and less consistent data are available for the epidemiology of BE, which is a difficult disease to study in populations, because the majority of individuals with BE are undiagnosed as they have not undergone upper gastrointestinal endoscopy. Access to endoscopy is influenced by demographic and other factors such as the availability of public health care. BE epidemiology studies may thus suffer from population selection bias; for example, the possibility that diagnosed BE cases have a different profile to undiagnosed cases or other confounding factors.

Considering these difficulties, it is not surprising that, as shown in Table 32.1, the reported estimates of BE prevalence vary widely. Studies designed to reduce the risk of bias include an autopsy study[1] and a study that screened for BE in colonoscopy patients with and without heartburn[2]; and the estimated prevalence of BE in patients without reflux symptoms in these studies is 0.4% to 6%. A widely cited estimate of BE prevalence is from an endoscopic screening study of 1000 unselected residents who underwent upper gastrointestinal endoscopy in two communities in northern Sweden.[3] Endoscopic findings of possible BE were present in 10.3% of individuals, with BE (IM) confirmed by histopathology in 1.6% of cases. Thus a standard estimate is that Barrett disease affects approximately 1% to 2% of Western populations.

Some data indicate that BE affects white non-Hispanic Westerners more than Asian or Hispanic people,[4,5] but a recent meta-analysis including 51 studies with over greater than 450,000 patients from Asia suggests that the histologically proven pooled-prevalence of BE is 1.3% (95% confidence interval [CI], 0.7 to 2.2%; 28 studies, and 298,850 subjects) and thus comparable to Western estimates.[6] Allowing for the limitations of pooled analyses, such as varying study time periods, BE definitions, and study populations (the meta-analysis only included one population-based study with 1029 participants), this suggests that BE is not uncommon in Asian (particularly Eastern Asian) countries.

Although puzzlingly much lower than the incidence rate increase for EAC, studies from several countries have reported an increase in the incidence of BE.[7–11] This seems to be a true increase as only some of this rise in incidence can be attributed to increased use of endoscopy.[7,8]

RISK FACTORS FOR BARRETT ESOPHAGUS

FACTORS ASSOCIATED WITH INCREASED RISK OF BARRETT ESOPHAGUS

Sex and Age

Most epidemiologic data show a 2:1 male preponderance among diagnosed cases of BE.[5,12] BE patients are also typically slightly older than non-BE GERD patients at between 50 and 65 years at the time of diagnosis.[5,13,14] BE is rare in pediatric populations, being confirmed by histologic presence of IM in approximately 0.12% of patients less than 20 years of age referred for upper endoscopy for any indication.[15] There are no reports of IM containing BE in a child under the age of 5 years,[16] and within children/adolescent study cohorts, the risk of BE is increased after the age of 12 years,[15] supporting a timeline of some years for BE development.

Gastroesophageal Reflux

Chronic GERD is the main cause of BE,[17] with the risk and length of Barrett disease correlating with the amount and duration of reflux exposure in the distal esophagus.[18–20] The exact mechanism by which GERD triggers Barrett formation remains elusive, but some have postulated that the refluxate causes an erosive episode during which there is a denuding of the normal squamous epithelium, allowing it to be subsequently repopulated by columnar cells. Where these cells are derived from remains a matter of ongoing scientific debate.[21,22]

Clinical studies have confirmed that severe GERD is present in patients with BE and that these patients have more esophageal dysmotility and lower distal esophageal sphincter pressures compared with patients with erosive or nonerosive esophagitis.[18,23,24] Equally, other studies have shown that BE patients have long exposure to gastric content with very low pH levels (pH < 2.0 to 3.0)[25] and a high frequency of hiatal hernia (76% in BE vs. 36% in GERD patients).[23,24,26,27] In addition to gastric acid, duodenal juices in the refluxate are thought to be important contributors to the formation and propagation of BE.[28] The combined exposure of esophageal cells to bile acids and low pH results in DNA damage and oxidative stress,[29] which in turn propagates BE formation and progression. Similarly, in vitro treatment of esophageal

TABLE 32.1 Summary of Studies Estimating the Prevalence of Barrett Esophagus in Different Populations

Author	Year	N	Study Design	Study Population	Ethnicity	BE Prevalence Estimate	BE Prevalence in GERD Patients	BE Prevalence in Non-GERD Patients	Potential Source of Bias	Comments
Winters et al.	1987	97	Prospective, observational study	Patients with ≥1×/week symptoms of GERD	—	12.40%	12.40%	—	Selection bias	BE specialized epithelium was histologically confirmed in 50% of the patients determined as having BE. Columnar gastric and junctional epithelium was also regarded as "BE" if it was confirmed to be in the tubular esophagus and/or ≥5 cm proximal of the gastroesophageal junction.
Mann et al.	1989	180	Prospective, cohort study	GERD patients with or without reflux esophagitis	"Vast majority Caucasian"	11.00%	11.00%	—	Selection bias	—
Cameron et al.	1990	959	Prospective, observational study including autopsy data	Population-based study + prospective search of Mayo Clinic autopsy material	—	0.34%	—	—	—	While retrospective in nature, this paper is regarded as one of the first articles to suggest that most Barrett esophagus patients are unrecognized.
Clark et al.[228]	1997	241	Prospective, observational study	GERD patients undergoing upper endoscopy	—	29.00%	29.00%	—	Selection bias	Biased population as patients have GERD symptoms and 68% of study population males.
Voutilainen et al.[229]	2000	1128	Prospective, observational study	Patients referred for upper endoscopy from primary care setting with GERD/dyspepsia and other upper-GI symptoms warranting endoscopic investigation	—	1.00%	4.40%	—	Selection bias	BE prevalence estimate is only applicable to patients presenting with upper GI symptoms.
Gerson et al.[230]	2002	110	Prospective, observational study	"Asymptomatic" individuals presenting for screening sigmoidoscopy	73% Caucasian, 14% African American, 10% Hispanic, 4% Pacific Islander/Asian	25.00%	—	—	Selection bias	Only 53% of participants had no GERD symptoms; biased population as 92% males with mean age of >60 years.

Author	Year	N	Study type	Population	Race				Bias	Comments
Rex et al.	2003	961	Prospective, observational study	Patients undergoing colonoscopy	78% Caucasian, 20.3% black, 1.6% Latin-American/Asian	6.80%	8.30%	5.60%	Selection bias	Biased population as presenting for colonoscopy, 78% white and predominantly male (~60%).
Malfertheiner et al.	2005	6215	Prospective, observational study	Patients undergoing upper endoscopy for GERD symptoms	—	8.39%	8.39%		Selection bias	In patients who had erosive reflux disease prevalence of Barrett was up to 14%, whereas in patients with NERD BE prevalence was 2.3%. This study population is also biased toward GERD patients.
Ronkainen et al.	2005	1000	Prospective, multicenter cohort study	Random population sample invited to participate in screening upper endoscopy	—	1.60%	2.30%	1.20%	—	Regarded as a robust assessment of the true prevalence of BE in a general population. Problems exist with regard to generalizability as only two northern Swedish communities were studied.
Westhoff et al.	2005	378	Prospective, cohort study	GERD patients presenting for first-time upper endoscopy	86% white	13.20%	13.20%	—	Selection bias	86% white and 95% male, with median age of 56 years, all of whom had GERD.
Veldhuyzen van Zanten et al.[231]	2006	1040	Prospective, cohort study	Dyspepsia patients recruited from primary care setting	95% Caucasian, 2% black, 1% Asian, 1% Aboriginal/Metis	2.40%	2.40%	—	Selection bias	Analyses patients who were promptly referred for endoscopy from a primary care setting; selection bias exists for true BE population prevalence estimates, as these are "symptomatic" patients.

Continued

TABLE 32.1 Summary of Studies Estimating the Prevalence of Barrett Esophagus in Different Populations—cont'd

Author	Year	N	Study Design	Study Population	Ethnicity	BE Prevalence Estimate	BE Prevalence in GERD Patients	BE Prevalence in Non-GERD Patients	Potential Source of Bias	Comments
Corley et al.	2008	4205	Observational study	Evaluation of BE diagnosis among all patients with a membership in an integrated health services delivery organization (Kaiser Permanente, Northern California; n ~3.3 million)	Study population included Caucasians, African Americans, Asians and Hispanics. Specific percentages are not provided, but it is noted that the endoscopy volume/rate did not vary between demographic groups	0.13%	—	—	Potential diagnostic bias as incidence of a new diagnosis of BE increased over time	This study documents that, in a fairly unbiased population, the frequency of a diagnosis of BE is rare. It also demonstrates a linear increase in the diagnosed prevalence of disease. It also finds that white non-Hispanic males aged 61 to 70 have the highest risk of BE. Note: Prevalence defined as number of active members with a new diagnosis of BE divided by number of person-years in the membership for the respective year.
Abrams et al.	2008	2100	Retrospective, cross-sectional study	Patients undergoing upper endoscopy for any indication	37.7% Caucasian, 11.8% African American, 22.2% Hispanic, 28.3% unknown	4.40%	—	—	Selection bias	Main indications for endoscopy were GERD symptoms (23.5%), nonreflux dyspepsia (34.7%), and overt/occult GI bleeding (and/or anemia; 16.5%). Consequently, this is a highly preselected cohort of patients. Main focus of the study was to study racial disparities in BE incidence rates, limited by that over 1/4 of the study population had an "unknown" ethnicity.

Author	Year	N	Study type	Method	Race				Limitations/bias	Comments
Zagari et al.	2008	1033	Prospective cohort study	Population sample invited to participate in completion of reflux questionnaire and screening upper endoscopy	—	1.30%	1.50%	1.00%	—	This study was performed similarly to the Scandinavian study and provides a fairly robust estimate of the true prevalence of BE in the Italian population. Also shows that frequent reflux symptoms are a risk factor for BE, but almost half (46.2%) of patients with BE report no reflux symptoms whatsoever.
Fan et al.	2009	4457	Retrospective study	Racial distribution in GERD group was 68% Caucasian, 19% African American, 11% Hispanic, 2% other. In the non-GERD group 65% Caucasian, 21% African American, 11% Hispanic and 3% other.	1.72%	4.39%	1.56%	Selection bias	Selection bias as all patients had to be referred for endoscopy; thus not generalizable to the general population.	
Hayeck et al.[232]	2010	—	Computer simulation	Computer simulation model with SEER data verification	—	5.57%	—	—	Computer modeling aligned to available (published) data	A computer-modeling study that aimed to estimate the population prevalence of BE by adjusting the model inputs based on published data and aligning results to EAC incidence rates in the SEER data.
Shiota et al.	2015	453,147	Meta-analysis of observational studies	Various: Inclusion criteria (and subgroup analyses) were performed according to whether population sampling was population-based, from health checkups, screening, or for symptomatic patients	Asian as categorized according to International Agency for Research on Cancer: Eastern, South Eastern, South Central and Western Asia	1.30%	1.40%	0.70%	Included studies own selection biases, methodologic limitations inherent to meta-analyses	This meta-analysis mainly included studies from Eastern Asian countries (38/51), and therefore the prevalence estimates cannot be generalized to the rest of Asia. Indicates that BE may be more frequent in Asian countries than originally estimated.

BE, Barrett esophagus; *EAC*, esophageal adenocarcinoma; *GERD*, gastroesophageal reflux disease; *GI*, gastrointestinal; *SEER*, Surveillance, Epidemiology and End Results Reporting database.

cells with both bile and acid leads to the expression of intestinal and/or columnar cell markers.[30–32]

While GERD can affect up to 20% of Western populations,[33] only 5% to 10% of patients with GERD develop BE.[34–39] A higher frequency (e.g., ≥weekly) of GERD symptoms is associated with a greatly (10 times) increased risk of BE in population control studies.[40,41] A weaker association between symptoms and BE is found in endoscopy studies of patients with typical symptoms of GERD.[13,40,42] It thus remains unclear if BE patients have considerably more frequent or only slightly more frequent symptoms of reflux compared with non-BE GERD patients.[3,38] Frequency and number of years of reflux symptoms (i.e., chronicity of reflux) are better predictors of BE.[43,44] Patients with BE may report that their GERD symptoms have improved in recent years, which is postulated to be related to BE development and perhaps reduced esophageal sensitivity.

Obesity

There is a strong reproducible association between obesity and the risk for EAC, indicating that patients with a body mass index (BMI) $\geq$ 30 kg/m^2 bear a 2 to 3 times higher risk of developing this malignancy,[45–49] but the associations with BE have been less consistent. A recent meta-analysis[50] concluded that there was no significant association with BMI and BE when comparing BE and GERD patients. However, when using the pooled estimates from three studies comparing BE patients with general population controls, a significant association between BMI and risk for BE could be determined (pooled odds ratio [OR], 1.02 per kg/m^2; 95% confidence interval [CI], 1.01 to 1.04; I^2 = 0%). Other data from population-based studies suggest that there is no more than a 50% increase in risk for BE with BMIs 30 kg/m^2 or greater.[40,42,45,51–53]

Central visceral adiposity may be a more important risk factor for BE formation than BMI itself.[51,52,54] A case-control study found that visceral adipose tissue was 1.5 times higher in patients with BE compared with controls[54] and population-based studies have identified a significant association between BE and either increasing waist circumference[51] or waist-to-hip ratio.[52] Interestingly, when controlling for waist-to-hip ratio, the association between BMI and BE has been shown to be almost completely attenuated, suggesting that the obesity effect is mediated through visceral adiposity.[52]

A mechanistic explanation for the relationship with central adiposity includes the unproven postulates that increased abdominal visceral fat elevates intraabdominal pressure[55] or intragastric pressure.[56] More likely is that the pressure gradient across the antireflux barrier is increased, resulting in hiatus hernia and GERD, and the metabolic and endocrine activity of visceral adipose tissue in those with central obesity (who interestingly are more likely to be male)[9,57–59] may also be important. Central obesity alters expression levels of obesity-related and proinflammatory cytokines such as leptin, adiponectin, tumor necrosis factor (TNF)-alpha, interleukin (IL)-6, and insulin-like growth factor.[60–63]

As leptin is upregulated in obesity and increases proliferation of EAC cells in vitro,[64] the association between serum leptin levels and BE has been examined.[9,59,65] Two studies found an increased risk of BE if leptin levels were elevated, but the association was stronger in men in one study[9] and stronger in women in the other study.[59] Another study did not show an association with leptin, but it did show a significant inverse association of elevated adiponectin levels and BE risk compared with colon screening controls (adjusted OR, 0.42; 95% CI, 0.22 to 0.80).[65] Thus while recent studies on the interaction of central obesity and EAC have elucidated the molecular pathways by which adipocytokines contribute to EAC formation and propagation, more data from larger studies are required to further clarify the role for leptin and other obesity-related cytokines in BE development.

Smoking and Alcohol Consumption

Most, but not all, population-based studies have documented an approximately twofold increase in risk of BE in patients who have ever smoked.[40–42,66,67] Contrary to some earlier findings,[68] recent data suggest that a greater number of pack-years smoked may be associated with a greater risk of BE,[67] but this effect may plateau at approximately 20 pack-years.[69] Furthermore, a recent population-based study showed that smoking and GERD may exert a synergistic effect on disease development and progression.[49] There are no convincing data supporting an increased risk of BE due to alcohol consumption. On the contrary, an inverse association of wine consumption and risk of BE has been reported[70,71] and a pooled analysis of Barrett cases compared with controls found a moderate reduction of risk with consumption of wine (OR, 0.71; 95% CI, 0.60 to 1.00), although without a dose-response relationship.[72]

Family History and Genetic Predisposition

There is most probably a heritable or familial aspect for BE and EAC development in some cases.[73,74] This is supported by the following observations: concordance of cases in both mono- and dizygous twins,[75–77] increased disease risk in patients with a positive family history,[78–81] and the identification through genome-wide association studies (GWAS) of single-nucleotide polymorphisms (SNPs) in genes that render individuals susceptible to the development of BE and EAC.[82–84] SNPs affecting at least seven genes (MHC locus, FOXF1, CRCT1, BARX1, FOXP1, TBX5, and GDF7), some of which are involved in esophageal development and inflammatory response processes, are thought to be significantly associated with the risk of BE and EAC development.[82–84]

The prevalence estimates of familial Barrett cases vary, with one series reporting confirmed family cases of BE in 6% of subjects,[79] whereas another study found a familial prevalence rate of up to 24%.[80] The aforementioned twin studies have suggested a heritability of up to 30% to 40%.[75–77] One study estimated 35% (standard error [SE], 6%) of overall BE risk variance to be explained by common germline genetic variants,[85] whereas another recent report provided a more conservative estimate of 9.99% (SE, 1.2%).[84] Similarly, another recent study estimated 7% (95% CI, 3% to 11%) of phenotypic variance for GERD to be explained by inheritable SNPs.[86] More importantly, however, this study also showed that there is approximately 77% (SE, 24%) genetic correlation between GERD and

BE and approximately 88% (SE, 25%) between GERD and EAC, thus providing first evidence for a polygenic basis for GERD and supporting a polygenic overlap for GERD with both BE and EAC.[86] Taken together, these data also suggest that much of the genetic basis for EAC may lie in the development of BE, rather than in the progression of BE to EAC. It is thus important to assess a complete family history for patients with BE or EAC.

FACTORS ASSOCIATED WITH DECREASED RISK OF BARRETT ESOPHAGUS

Patient Height

A study including 999 cases of EAC, 2061 cases of BE, and 2168 population controls found that height is inversely associated with the risk of BE (OR, 0.69; 95% CI, 0.62 to 0.77 for every 10-cm increase in height) and EAC (OR, 0.70; 95% CI, 0.62 to 0.79 for each 10 cm increase in height). This effect was irrespective of gender and the estimates were similar across all strata of age, patient education levels, BMI, weight, and whether or not the patients had GERD symptoms or if they smoked.[87]

Helicobacter pylori Infection

The historic decline of *Helicobacter pylori* infection prevalence in developed countries is temporally aligned with an increased incidence in GERD complications such as BE and EAC. One explanation for this has been that *H. pylori* infections reduce intragastric acidity through the generation of ammonia or by causing severe corpus gastritis with concomitant destruction of gastric parietal cells, thus reducing acid production and protecting against GERD complications.[88] While infection with *H. pylori* (particularly CagA+ strains) has consistently been shown to reduce risks of EAC,[89] the evidence for this effect has been less consistently shown for BE.[90] A first meta-analysis of 12 case-control studies published in 2009 showed that overall there was no significant difference in *H. pylori* infection rates between BE and controls (42.9% vs. 43.9%; OR, 0.74; 95% CI, 0.40 to 1.37), although in a subgroup analysis comparing BE patients with endoscopically normal controls, *H. pylori* infection was significantly less frequent in BE patients (23.1% vs. 42.7%; OR, 0.50; 95% CI, 0.27 to 0.93). An explanation for these discrepancies may be that many of the included studies provided heterogeneous effect estimates, as they were prone to selection and information biases. A later meta-analysis[91] included only four high-quality studies,[2,3,92,93] finding an overall protective effect of *H. pylori* infection on BE risk compared with population-based controls (OR, 0.46; 95% CI, 0.35 to 0.60). Importantly, two of these studies[92,93] also showed that this risk was reduced even when controlling for reflux symptoms, hence suggesting that the protective effect of *H. pylori* infection cannot be explained simply by reduced gastric acid production. The exact mechanism by which *H. pylori* infection exerts a protective mechanism on BE formation thus remains uncertain.

Nonsteroidal Antiinflammatory Drugs and Statins

There is compelling evidence that nonsteroidal antiinflammatory drugs (NSAIDs), including aspirin, may prevent a variety of cancers, particularly of the esophagus, stomach, colon, and rectum.[94,95] Combined observational data suggest a reduction of 44% to 58% in esophageal cancer mortality rates in aspirin users.[95] NSAIDs, including aspirin, inhibit the enzymes cyclooxygenase (COX) 1 and 2. Elevated COX-2 expression, as found in BE and EAC[96–99] can be induced by inflammation, growth factors, mitogens, and other cytokines. COX-2 inhibition can restore apoptosis[100,101] and inhibit cell growth and proliferation[101,102] and neoangiogenesis.[103] The potential for COX-2 inhibition through aspirin or other NSAID administration to prevent BE progression is supported by cohort and case-control studies,[104] but further evidence is needed, and the risk/benefit ratio is unclear.[105] Whether this should be routine therapy in patients with BE will hopefully become evident with the results of a large (5000 patients) randomized-controlled aspirin and proton pump inhibitor (PPI) trial in the United Kingdom (The Aspirin Esomeprazole Chemoprevention Trial, AspECT; UKCRN ID 1339, anticipated trial end date October 2018).[106,107]

Patients who take statin medications for treatment of hypercholesterolemia or as preventive therapy for coronary heart disease may have a reduced risk of developing both BE and EAC.[108–110] A meta-analysis suggests that statin use is significantly associated with a reduced risk of BE compared with controls with a pooled OR of 0.63 (95% CI, 0.51 to 0.77; 1090 Barrett cases vs. 2085 controls).[109] A preventive role against BE progression is suggested by a recent nested case-control study with more than 1000 US veterans, which found that BE patients who develop EAC are less likely to have used statins compared with BE patients who never develop cancer (40.2% vs. 54.0%; $P < .01$).[111] With further data, the routine use of NSAIDs or statins for chemoprevention in Barrett disease may be recommended.[112]

Acid Suppressive Medical Therapy and Antireflux Surgery

The main treatment options for GERD are medical acid suppression therapy and antireflux surgery by fundoplication. Whether medical or surgical therapies protect patients with GERD against the development of BE or against BE progression to EAC remains highly contentious.[113] A Cochrane review that pooled data from two randomized controlled trials (RCTs) failed to show any major protective effect of PPI therapy on BE progression,[114] and it is thus reasonable to state that PPIs are indicated for symptom relief but that they are not BE chemopreventive agents.[112]

With regard to antireflux surgery, a thorough prospective trial from Sweden in particular[115] and other surgical series suggest that fundoplication promotes BE regression and prevents dysplasia formation.[116–118] Two RCTs comparing surgery versus medical therapy concluded that both provided good symptom control, but slightly better outcomes were observed in the surgical group.[119,120] Four meta-analyses have examined whether medical therapy or surgery is better at preventing BE development and/or progression to EAC.[113,121–123] Two of these studies found no protective effect of antireflux surgery for the development of EAC compared with medical therapy,[121,122] and a third study concluded that because of an observed high postoperative tumor progression rate, antireflux surgery does not prevent EAC formation in BE patients.[123] These three meta-analyses had methodologic limitations, as each type of therapy was pooled into one group irrespective of whether the original studies were comparative. Thus the most recent meta-analysis, published in 2016 by Maret-Ouda,[113] aimed to have more rigorous inclusion criteria by only including comparative studies that contained both treatment arms. This systematic review included 10 studies comparing the risk of EAC after antireflux surgery with nonoperated GERD patients, 7 studies including patients with BE and 2 studies comparing the EAC risk following surgery to the background population. The study found that the risk of EAC was not significantly reduced in operated patients compared with medically treated GERD patients irrespective of if they had BE or not. However, if the studies were restricted to those performed after 2000, then a significant reduction in pooled incidence rate ratios (IRR) could be found in surgically treated BE patients compared with medically treated patients (IRR, 0.26; 95% CI, 0.09 to 0.79). The authors also found that the risk for EAC does not revert to that of the background population for surgically treated patients (IRR, 10.78; 95% CI, 8.48 to 13.71), indicating that patients undergoing antireflux surgery need ongoing endoscopic surveillance. In summary, there is a discrepancy between single-center surgery studies finding BE regression after fundoplication, whereas this is not shown by multicenter and population data studies that have so far failed to show that this occurs more frequently than expected by chance alone.

Nutrition

High intakes of fruits, vegetables, fibers, and even meat may be inversely associated with the risk of developing BE, whereas high intake of trans-fats may be linked to an increased risk of BE.[124] Another study in the same cohort found dietary antioxidants, vitamin C, beta-carotene, and vitamin E are also associated with a reduced risk of BE, but the use of antioxidant supplements did not influence BE risk.[125] A recent population-based study from Ireland suggests that high dietary intake of magnesium significantly reduces the risk of reflux esophagitis and BE (adjusted OR, 0.31; 95% CI, 0.11 to 0.87 and adjusted OR, 0.29; 95% CI, 0.12 to 0.71, respectively) and that this effect is most prominent in the setting of a low calcium:magnesium intake ratio.[126]

RISK FACTORS FOR THE NEOPLASTIC PROGRESSION OF BARRETT ESOPHAGUS

OVERALL RISK OF NEOPLASTIC BARRETT PROGRESSION

Estimates of the risk of cancer development in patients with BE range from approximately 0% to 3% per patient-year.[127,128] The reasons for higher risk estimates have been discussed widely[127–129] and include factors such as publication bias and not accounting for the presence of baseline dysplasia, which is an intermediate stage of EAC development.[129] Many of the observational studies included in earlier meta-analyses of BE progression risk were from the 1980s, which is prior to the widespread

recognition of short-segment BE (SSBE, BE < 3 cm in length) as true Barrett disease,[130] including only patients with long-segment BE (LSBE) is likely to increase EAC risk estimates.[129,131]

A widely used estimate of the annual incidence of EAC in patients with BE was approximately 0.5%, or 1 in 200 patients per year,[128,132] although it has been noted that even this low frequency of EAC may not be observed in clinical practice.[133] Both Wani et al.[134] and Sikkema et al.[135] also estimated an annual incidence of EAC of approximately 0.6% in pooled analyses but included some patients with a baseline diagnosis of low-grade dysplasia (LGD). When patients with early incident EACs and a baseline diagnosis of high-grade dysplasia (HGD) were excluded, as in the study by Yousef et al.,[136] an annual EAC incidence rate of 0.41% was estimated. Subsequently, another meta-analysis by Desai et al. aimed to determine the risk of BE progression in patients with a baseline diagnosis of nondysplastic BE (NDBE).[129] This study combined data from 57 studies with 11,434 histologically confirmed cases of NDBE and a total of 58,547 patient-years of follow-up. With a total of 186 incident cases of EAC during follow-up, a pooled incidence rate of 0.33% (95% CI, 0.28 to 0.38%) was estimated. This estimate remained the same when only the highest quality studies were included in a post hoc sensitivity analysis (0.33%; 95% CI, 0.26 to 0.40%). This risk of EAC dropped further in a subgroup analysis of 16 studies focusing on patients with nondysplastic SSBE (967 patients and 4456 patient-years of follow-up), in whom an annual EAC incidence rate of 0.19% (95% CI, 0.08 to 0.34%) was estimated. Importantly, this study also found that patients with NDBE were more than 10 times more likely to die of another cause than to develop EAC.

Four large-scale population-based studies that include more than 30,000 study subjects have been published, essentially confirming this low incidence rate with annual cancer risks ranging from 0.12% to 0.43% in patients with BE.[137–140] Thus as illustrated in Fig. 32.1, there has been a continuous downward trend in estimates of EAC incidence rates in patients with BE over recent decades; it is currently considered that the risk of developing EAC in nondysplastic BE is *low* at approximately 1 case per 300 to 500 patients per year and that BE patients' risk of mortality is increased due to other causes.

As a result of these newer data, the effectiveness of routine surveillance endoscopy among patients with histologically confirmed non- and never dysplastic BE is increasingly being questioned,[141–144] particularly in light of other data showing the inadequacies of current surveillance protocols: up to 60% of incidence EAC cases are diagnosed within 1 year of the diagnosis of BE, indicating that they are probably missed at index endoscopy.[138] Current clinical practice (the Seattle protocol) includes four-quadrant biopsies every 1 to 2 cm.[145] But even such rigorous biopsy strategies typically sample less than 5% of the Barrett epithelium, thus rendering sampling error unavoidable.[146] Furthermore, up to 90% of endoscopists do not adhere to this laborious surveillance protocol.[147] These factors demonstrate the importance of identifying patients at higher risk of BE progression through determining clinical and molecular risk factors of progression, as discussed in the subsequent section.

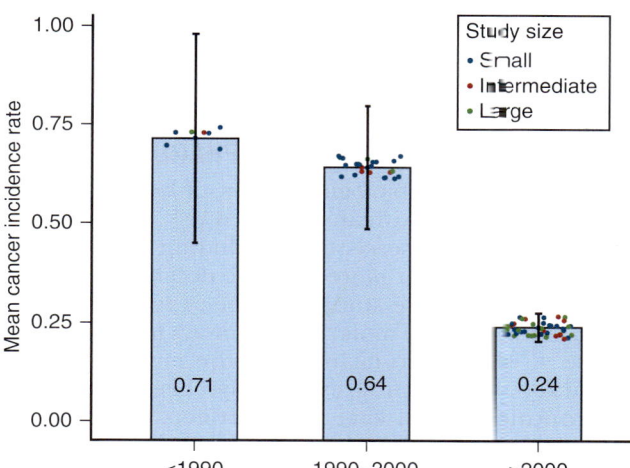

FIGURE 32.1 Changes in estimates of the annual risk of esophageal adenocarcinoma formation in patients with Barrett esophagus over time. Study sizes have been classfed as small *(blue)*, intermediate *(red)*, or large *(green)* depending on the number of patient follow-up years. Small studies had less than 500, intermediate 500 to 1000, and large greater than 1000 patient-years of follow-up. The figure shows how with increasing study cohort size/follow-up the annual cancer incidence rate has decreased.

CLINICAL RISK FACTORS FOR THE PROGRESSION OF BARRETT ESOPHAGUS

Age and Sex

Men are at increased risk of developing EAC compared with women.[148] A recent international registry analysis including over 100,000 cases of EAC showed that only 22.3% of cases occurred in women, and male-to-female ratios of up 6 : 1 were reported.[149] However, there is some paucity of data regarding the association of male sex and the risk of BE progression to cancer. One of the most recent population-based studies indicates that men with BE are 2 to 4 times more likely to develop EAC compared with females.[137,150]

The risk of EAC increases with age,[149] typically peaking around the sixth to seventh decade of life.[46,137] The duration of patients' diagnosis of BE is also a risk factor for malignant progression, with patients having BE for 10 or more years displaying a greater than 2 times higher risk of HGD/EAC development compared with those with a diagnosis less than 10 years.[151] Consequently, while screening strategies have not been formally adopted, it is widely accepted that (Caucasian) men over the age of 50 years with BE are at increased risk of developing EAC.[112,145,152,153]

Obesity and Smoking

EAC is a cancer with one of the strongest associations with obesity,[154,155] whether measured as increased BMI or abdominal obesity.[155,156] Whether increased BMI also translates to a higher risk of malignant progression in patients with BE is not clear, but some data suggest that, particularly in males, increased waist-to-hip ratio and waist circumference may confer a higher risk of BE progression.[157]

Tobacco use is a risk factor for EAC.[49] The risk is increased for both current (OR 2.3; 95% CI, 1.5 to 3.5) and former smokers (OR 1.5; 95% CI, 1.1 to 2.1) and the risk of EAC increases with cumulative exposure.[49] Smoking has also been found to increase the risk of progression to HGD and EAC in patients with BE (hazard ratio [HR], 2.03; 95% CI, 1.2 to 3.17).[158] Importantly, this risk of progression persists across all strata of smoking intensity, and current smokers display the highest risk of malignant BE progression.[158] Alcohol consumption, on the other hand, has not consistently shown an association with increased risk of EAC and/or BE progression.[47,49,71]

Recurrent Gastroesophageal Reflux Disease

Large-scale population-based studies suggest that approximately 40% of EAC cases arise in patients with frequently *recurring* symptoms of GERD, noticed as heartburn and/or regurgitation of gastric acid/content at least once a week.[159–161] The EAC risk also increases with longer symptom duration: patients with 20 years or longer of reflux symptoms have an almost 3 times higher risk of EAC compared with those with less than 10 years' duration.[162] Moreover, patients who have reflux symptoms have an approximately 6 times higher risk of EAC compared with those without symptoms.[161] The clinical relevance of this association, especially for EAC screening, is limited by the lack of typical GERD symptoms in many patients with EAC, the prevalence of GERD symptoms in the community (~20% of the population report at least weekly symptoms of GERD),[163] and the low annual incidence rates for EAC of 2.7 per 100,000 in the general population and 6.0 per 100,000 in white males.[164] It is nevertheless clear that severe, long-standing and frequent GERD are associated with an increased risk of EAC. Consequently, and despite uncertainty with regard to effectiveness, current management guidelines recommend BE patients with severe and uncontrolled symptoms of reflux require acid suppressive therapy to help prevent progression.[112,152,153]

Barrett Segment Length

The risk of neoplastic progression increases with the length of Barrett epithelium.[129,131,151] This was elegantly demonstrated in the study from Germany by Pohl et al.[131] in which the annual cancer progression rates of patients with long-segment (≥3 cm), short-segment (≥1 to <3 cm), and ultra-short segment (<1 cm) BE were 0.22%, 0.03%, and 0.01%, respectively. These data imply that to detect one case of EAC, 450 patients with LSBE would require annual surveillance endoscopy, whereas in SSBE and ultra-short BE, the corresponding number of patients increases to 3440 and 12,364, respectively. As a result of these differences in cancer incidence rates, recent guidelines suggest that patients with greater than 3 cm of Barrett segment length and no dysplasia should undergo screening endoscopy with quadrantic biopsies every 2 to 3 years, whereas in patients with SSBE, the screening interval can be extended to every 3 to 5 years.[153] If a nodule, ulcer, or stricture is present, however, there is a high risk of malignancy irrespective of Barrett segment length and reassessment without delay is needed.[165]

Dysplasia

The accumulation of genetic and epigenetic alterations in Barrett mucosa produces phenotypic changes seen histologically as dysplasia. These changes are cytologic, for example nuclear shape and size, and tissue architectural, such as cell polarization and glandular crowding. Dysplasia is graded according to the severity of these changes into LGD, HGD, and indefinite for dysplasia (IND). The presence and grade of dysplasia is used as the main predictor of risk of BE progression to EAC, as dysplastic BE has a higher risk of progression than NDBE. Estimates of this increased risk vary considerably, however, because of the subjective nature of histologic interpretation resulting in substantial interobserver and even intraobserver variation. For example, a consensus study with a panel of expert BE pathologists found majority agreement on diagnosis could be reached in only 27 of 42 cases of LGD and 27 of 52 cases of HGD.[166] Other studies report similar findings with kappa-values of 0.18 to 0.35,[166–169] indicating only moderate agreement at best. When an expert panel of pathologists at a tertiary referral center used rigorously standardized dysplasia criteria to reassess histologic specimens of patients with an initial diagnosis of LGD, only approximately 25% of cases could effectively be confirmed.[170] As a result of this diagnostic unreliability, estimates of cancer progression risk in LGD range from 0.5% to 13.4% per year.[134,137,138,171,172]

Some studies have used a consensus diagnosis by multiple pathologists in an attempt to overcome this problem. In these studies, the incidence of HGD or EAC is substantially higher in patients in whom LGD is diagnosed through consensus compared with patients in whom the initial diagnosis of LGD is subsequently downstaged to NDBE by a panel of experts in a tertiary referral center.[170,173] The risk of HGD or EAC development is as high as approximately 13% per patient-year in the LGD cases, compared with approximately 0.5% in those with disease downstaged to NDBE.[170,173,174] These data have therefore supported the notion that aggressive eradication of BE with "true" LGD through ablation therapy is warranted.[174] These findings are controversial because HGD/EAC incidence is so much higher than generally observed, leading to concerns that some of the LGD cases may be HGD cases. In practice, access to expert consensus panels is presently limited.

Data on the accuracy of diagnosing HGD and the risk of progression from HGD to EAC are less controversial. The few reports of significant interobserver variability between pathologists are mainly related to the separation of HGD from early invasive EAC.[175] The risk of malignant transformation of HGD is regularly reported to be approximately 6% to 7% per year,[134,176] although substantially higher rates of progression have also been noted.[177] The high rate of progression warrants the eradication of HGD, as discussed elsewhere.[165]

In summary, despite some existing controversies, dysplasia remains the basis for clinical decision making. As discussed earlier, the risk of EAC development is higher in patients with LGD compared with those with NDBE and highest for patients with HGD.[112,134,145,152,153] Dysplasia confirmed by two gastrointestinal pathologists is currently the best available biomarker for the assessment of risk of BE progression,[112,153] but due to the variation in pathology interpretation, sampling error, lack of endoscopic examination, cost of endoscopy and pathology, and other factors, this situation needs to be improved.

MOLECULAR RISK FACTORS FOR THE PROGRESSION OF BARRETT ESOPHAGUS

The identification of biologic markers, or biomarkers, that identify cases of BE with an increased risk of progression to more advanced disease stages including EAC has been a focus of research for more than two decades. The major achievement of these studies has been to increase our understanding of the molecular pathways involved in this disease,[178] whereas so far none of the many promising biomarkers for BE progression have been introduced into routine clinical care. This reflects most studies' methodologic limitations such as the use of cross-sectional convenience samples from heterogeneous patient cohorts, lack of power, insufficient follow-up periods, a lack of reproducibility[21,169] or external validation, and a lack of RCT data.[179] Many studies have used the same BE segment with the risk of field effects.[180–182]

The molecular pathogenesis of Barrett progression involves a series of complex pathways leading to increased genetic and epigenetic instability within singular or multiple Barrett cell clones.[178] Whether these changes occur through a linear progression model or branched evolution remains a matter of debate,[183] but recent data suggest that many EACs evolve from BE through a direct path in which the tumor suppressor gene TP53 (often simply called p53) is mutated, as found in most EAC,[184] and these cells undergo genome doubling events followed by oncogene amplification.[185] Equally, recent genome sequencing data suggest that neoplasia formation can be accelerated through increasing overall genetic mutation rates and even more rapidly through catastrophic, so-called chromothriptic, chromosomal events, which may occur during a single or just a few cell divisions.[186,187] Evidence for the latter being a frequent occurrence in EAC has emerged.[188] EAC has one of the highest pan-genomic mutational burdens of all human solid cancers,[189,190] and even NDBE displays a mutation frequency that is comparable to and sometimes even higher than many invasive malignancies, indicating that these genomic processes are likely to be relevant to BE development and to the risk of progression.[185]

Flow cytometry, comparative genomic hybridization, and other studies have shown that increasing cellular aneuploidy (an abnormal increase or decrease in the number of chromosomes within a cell) is more frequent in dysplastic BE and EAC.[191–194] Likewise, large chromosomal arm losses resulting in the loss of a gene copy (loss-of-heterozygosity, LOH),[195–197] and severe cell-cycle changes are more frequent in advanced disease stages.[198–201] Changes in clonal evolutionary dynamics within the Barrett segment are also thought to predispose to EAC formation.[183] Clonal expansion, potentially driven by CDKN2A mutation and methylation, 9p and 17p LOH, and direct TP53 gene mutations, show promise as molecular predictors for BE progression.[202] Moreover, the size of Barrett clones with 17p LOH or severe DNA content abnormalities (such as tetraploidy or aneuploidy) also increases the risk of EAC formation, potentially through the expansion of genetically unstable clones.[203,204] These aspects are further supported by studies showing that increased clonal diversity as measured by the number of unique clones, Shannon diversity index, and genetic divergence of clones, increases the risk of EAC even when DNA content abnormalities and 17p LOH are taken into account.[205] A recent study on clonal diversity in Barrett suggests that there is strong clonal selection in NDBE disease over time, implying that the malignant potential of these lesions may be largely predetermined.[206]

Finally, a variety of complex molecular regulatory pathways have been suggested to be disrupted during the development of EAC,[178] as evidenced by altered transcriptomic,[207–213] methylomic[214–218] and proteomic profiles.[219–222] These types of studies are helping elucidate the alterations in regulatory pathways, including disturbances in critical cycle and proliferation processes,[223] that are involved in BE progression. Whole-transcriptome RNA-sequencing has shown that aside from protein coding genes interacting in complex gene regulatory networks, a plethora of noncoding genomic elements such as long noncoding RNAs, and repeat elements are also differentially expressed in EAC compared with less advanced BE stages.[213]

While encouraging new data for biomarker panels exist,[207,217,224,225] these biomarkers have not progressed past stages 2 or 3 of the National Institutes of Health (NIH)/National Cancer Institute (NCI) Early Detection Research Network (EDRN; https://edrn.nci.nih.gov/) clinical biomarker development stages,[226] indicating that they are largely preclinical, lacking both external and prospective validation.[169,179] The largest body of evidence concerns the potential clinical utility of p53 immunohistochemistry to assess protein expression (as reviewed in reference 112). Numerous studies have proposed that the addition of p53 immunohistochemistry may improve the diagnosis of dysplasia and improve patient stratification, as either overexpression or loss of p53 protein expression seems to be an accurate predictor of the risk of BE progression.[112,227] The British Society for Gastroenterology is the first professional society to recommend the clinical use of p53 immunostaining to help guide management of patients with BE.[112]

More objective means of disease evaluation through biomarkers remains the most viable approach to overcome current management limitations as well as biases. This will ultimately lead to those patients who are assessed as being at low risk of progression based on their molecular and clinical disease characteristics being spared laborious and unnecessary surveillance, while those at highest risk of cancer development can be guided toward more aggressive eradication treatments. This will reduce the individual and societal burden of EAC.

REFERENCES

1. Cameron AJ, Zinsmeister AR, Ballard DJ, Carney JA. Prevalence of columnar-lined (Barrett's) esophagus. Comparison of population-based clinical and autopsy findings. *Gastroenterology.* 1990;99(4):918-922.
2. Rex DK, Cummings OW, Shaw M, et al. Screening for Barrett's esophagus in colonoscopy patients with and without heartburn. *Gastroenterology.* 2003;125(6):1670-1677.
3. Ronkainen J, Aro P, Storskrubb T, et al. Prevalence of Barrett's esophagus in the general population: an endoscopic study. *Gastroenterology.* 2005;129(6):1825-1831.
4. Abrams JA, Fields S, Lightdale CJ, Neugut AI. Racial and ethnic disparities in the prevalence of Barrett's esophagus among patients who undergo upper endoscopy. *Clin Gastroenterol Hepatol.* 2008;6(1):30-34.
5. Corley DA, Kubo A, Levin TR, et al. Race, ethnicity, sex and temporal differences in Barrett's oesophagus diagnosis: a large community-based study, 1994–2006. *Gut.* 2009;58(2):182-188.
6. Shiota S, Singh S, Anshasi A, El-Serag HB. Prevalence of Barrett's esophagus in Asian countries: a systematic review and meta-analysis. *Clin Gastroenterol Hepatol.* 2015;13(11):1907-1918.
7. Prach AT, MacDonald TA, Hopwood DA, Johnston DA. Increasing incidence of Barrett's oesophagus: education, enthusiasm, or epidemiology? *Lancet.* 1997;350(9082):933.
8. Conio M, Cameron AJ, Romero Y, et al. Secular trends in the epidemiology and outcome of Barrett's oesophagus in Olmsted County, Minnesota. *Gut.* 2001;48(3):304-309.
9. Kendall BJ, Macdonald GA, Hayward NK, et al. Leptin and the risk of Barrett's oesophagus. *Gut.* 2008;57(4):448-454.
10. van Soest EM, Dieleman JP, Siersema PD, Sturkenboom MCJM, Kuipers EJ. Increasing incidence of Barrett's oesophagus in the general population. *Gut.* 2005;54(8):1062-1066.
11. Coleman HG, Bhat S, Murray LJ, McManus D, Gavin AT, Johnston BT. Increasing incidence of Barrett's oesophagus: a population-based study. *Eur J Epidemiol.* 2011;26(9):739-745.
12. Cook MB, Wild CP, Forman D. A systematic review and meta-analysis of the sex ratio for Barrett's esophagus, erosive reflux disease, and nonerosive reflux disease. *Am J Epidemiol.* 2005;162(11):1050-1061.
13. Edelstein ZR, Bronner MP, Rosen SN, Vaughan TL. Risk factors for Barrett's esophagus among patients with gastroesophageal reflux disease: a community clinic-based case–control study. *Am J Gastroenterol.* 2009;104(4):834-842.
14. Eloubeidi MA, Provenzale D. Clinical and demographic predictors of Barrett's esophagus among patients with gastroesophageal reflux disease: a multivariable analysis in veterans. *J Clin Gastroenterol.* 2001;33(4):306-309.
15. El-Serag HB, Gilger MA, Shub MD, Richardson P, Bancroft J. The prevalence of suspected Barrett's esophagus in children and adolescents: a multicenter endoscopic study. *Gastrointest Endosc.* 2006;64(5):671-675.
16. Sherman PM, Hassall E, Fagundes-Neto U, et al. A global, evidence-based consensus on the definition of gastroesophageal reflux disease in the pediatric population. *Am J Gastroenterol.* 2009;104(5):1278-1295.
17. Falk GW. Barrett's esophagus. *Gastroenterology.* 2002;122(6):1569-1591.
18. Iascone C, Demeester TR, Little AG, Skinner DB. Barrett's esophagus. Functional assessment, proposed pathogenesis, and surgical therapy. *Arch Surg.* 1983;118(5):543-549.
19. Taylor JB, Rubenstein JH. Meta-analyses of the effect of symptoms of gastroesophageal reflux on the risk of Barrett's esophagus. *Am J Gastroenterol.* 2010;105(8):1729-1730; quiz 1738.
20. Fass R, Hell RW, Garewal HS, et al. Correlation of oesophageal acid exposure with Barrett's oesophagus length. *Gut.* 2001;48(3):310-313.
21. Phillips WA, Lord RV, Nancarrow DJ, et al. Barrett's esophagus. *J Gastroenterol Hepatol.* 2011;26:639-648.
22. Souza RF, Krishnan K, Spechler SJ. Acid, bile, and CDX: the ABCs of making Barrett's metaplasia. *Am J Physiol Gastrointest Liver Physiol.* 2008;295(2):G211-G218.
23. Öberg S, DeMeester TR, Peters JH, et al. The extent of Barrett's esophagus depends on the status of the lower esophageal sphincter and the degree of esophageal acid exposure. *J Thorac Cardiovasc Surg.* 1999;117(3):572-580.
24. Lord RVN, DeMeester SR, Peters JH, et al. Hiatal hernia, lower esophageal sphincter incompetence, and effectiveness of Nissen fundoplication in the spectrum of gastroesophageal reflux disease. *J Gastrointest Surg.* 2008;13(4):602-610.
25. Stein HJ, Hoeft S, Demeester TR. Functional foregut abnormalities in Barrett's esophagus. *J Thorac Cardiovasc Surg.* 1993;105(1):107-111.
26. Avidan B, Sonnenberg A, Schnell TG, Sontag SJ. Hiatal hernia and acid reflux frequency predict presence and length of Barrett's esophagus. *Dig Dis Sci.* 2002;47(2):256-264.
27. Cameron AJ. Barrett's esophagus: prevalence and size of hiatal hernia. *Am J Gastroenterol.* 1999;94(8):2054-2059.
28. Vaezi MF, Richter JE. Role of acid and duodenogastroesophageal reflux in gastroesophageal reflux disease. *Gastroenterology.* 1996;111(5):1192-1199.
29. Dvorak K, Payne CM, Chavarria M, et al. Bile acids in combination with low pH induce oxidative stress and oxidative DNA damage:

relevance to the pathogenesis of Barrett's oesophagus. *Gut.* 2007;56(6):763-771.

30. Marchetti M, Caliot E, Pringault E. Chronic acid exposure leads to activation of the cdx2 intestinal homeobox gene in a long-term culture of mouse esophageal keratinocytes. *J Cell Sci.* 2003;116(8):1429-1436.

31. Bajpai M, Liu J, Geng X, Souza RF, Amenta PS, Das KM. Repeated exposure to acid and bile selectively induces colonic phenotype expression in a heterogeneous Barrett's epithelial cell line. *Lab Invest.* 2008;88(6):643-651.

32. Fitzgerald RC, Omary MB, Triadafilopoulos G. Dynamic effects of acid on Barrett's esophagus. An ex vivo proliferation and differentiation model. *J Clin Invest.* 1996;98(9):2120.

33. Locke GR, Talley NJ, Fett SL, Zinsmeister AR, Melton LJ. Prevalence and clinical spectrum of gastroesophageal reflux: a population-based study in Olmsted County, Minnesota. *Gastroenterology.* 1997;112(5):1448-1456.

34. Winters C, Spurling TJ, Chobanian SJ, et al. Barrett's esophagus. A prevalent, occult complication of gastroesophageal reflux disease. *Gastroenterology.* 1987;92(1):118-124.

35. Mann NS, Tsai MF, Nair PK. Barrett's esophagus in patients with symptomatic reflux esophagitis. *Am J Gastroenterol.* 1989;84(12):1494-1496.

36. Malfertheiner P, Lind T, Willich S, et al. Prognostic influence of Barrett's oesophagus and *Helicobacter pylori* infection on healing of erosive gastro-oesophageal reflux disease (GORD) and symptom resolution in non-erosive GORD: report from the ProGORD study. *Gut.* 2005;54(6):746-751.

37. Westhoff B, Brotze S, Weston A, et al. The frequency of Barrett's esophagus in high-risk patients with chronic GERD. *Gastrointest Endosc.* 2005;61(2):226-231.

38. Zagari RM, Fuccio L, Wallander M-A, et al. Gastro-oesophageal reflux symptoms, oesophagitis and Barrett's oesophagus in the general population: the Loiano-Monghidoro study. *Gut.* 2008;57(10):1354-1359.

39. Fan X, Snyder N. Prevalence of Barrett's esophagus in patients with or without GERD symptoms: role of race, age, and gender. *Dig Dis Sci.* 2009;54(3):572-577.

40. Johansson J, Hakansson H-O, Mellblom L, et al. Risk factors for Barrett's oesophagus: a population-based approach. *Scand J Gastroenterol.* 2007;42(2):148-156.

41. Anderson LA, Watson RGP, Murphy SJ, et al. Risk factors for Barrett's oesophagus and oesophageal adenocarcinoma: results from the FINBAR study. *World J Gastroenterol.* 2007;13(10):1585-1594.

42. Smith KJ, O'Brien SM, Green AC, Webb PM, Whiteman DC. Current and past smoking significantly increase risk for Barrett's esophagus. *Clin Gastroenterol Hepatol.* 2009;7(8):840-848.

43. Conio M, Filiberti R, Blanchi S, et al. Risk factors for Barrett's esophagus: a case-control study. *Int J Cancer.* 2002;97(2):225-229.

44. Eisen GM, Sandler RS, Murray S, Gottfried M. The relationship between gastroesophageal reflux disease and its complications with Barrett's esophagus. *Am J Gastroenterol.* 1997;92(1):27-31.

45. Wild CP, Hardie LJ. Reflux, Barrett's oesophagus and adenocarcinoma: burning questions. *Nat Rev Cancer.* 2003;3(9):676-684.

46. Brown LM, Devesa SS, Chow W-H. Incidence of adenocarcinoma of the esophagus among white Americans by sex, stage, and age. *J Natl Cancer Inst.* 2008;100(16):1184-1187.

47. Vaughan TL, Davis S, Kristal A, Thomas DB. Obesity, alcohol, and tobacco as risk factors for cancers of the esophagus and gastric cardia: adenocarcinoma versus squamous cell carcinoma. *Cancer Epidemiol Biomarkers Prev.* 1995;4(2):85-92.

48. Lagergren J, Bergström R, Nyren O. Association between body mass and adenocarcinoma of the esophagus and gastric cardia. *Ann Intern Med.* 1999;130(11):883-890.

49. Whiteman DC, Sadeghi S, Pandeya N, et al. Combined effects of obesity, acid reflux and smoking on the risk of adenocarcinomas of the oesophagus. *Gut.* 2008;57(2):173-180.

50. Cook MB, Greenwood DC, Hardie LJ, Wild CP, Forman D. A systematic review and meta-analysis of the risk of increasing adiposity on Barrett's esophagus. *Am J Gastroenterol.* 2008;103(2):292-300.

51. Corley DA, Kubo A, Levin TR, et al. Abdominal obesity and body mass index as risk factors for Barrett's esophagus. *Gastroenterology.* 2007;133(1):34-41.

52. Edelstein ZR, Farrow DC, Bronner MP, Rosen SN, Vaughan TL. Central adiposity and risk of Barrett's esophagus. *Gastroenterology.* 2007;133(2):403-411.

53. Jacobson BC, Chan AT, Giovannucci EL, Fuchs CS. Body mass index and Barrett's oesophagus in women. *Gut.* 2009;58(11):1460-1466.

54. El-Serag HB, Kvapil P, Hacken-Bitar J, Kramer JR. Abdominal obesity and the risk of Barrett's esophagus. *Am J Gastroenterol.* 2005;100(10):2151-2156.

55. Wilson LJ, Ma W, Hirschowitz BI. Association of obesity with hiatal hernia and esophagitis. *Am J Gastroenterol.* 1999;94(10):2840-2844.

56. Berstad A, Weberg R, Larsen IF, Hoel B, Hauer-Jensen M. Relationship of hiatus hernia to reflux oesophagitis: a prospective study of coincidence, using endoscopy. *Scand J Gastroenterol.* 2009;21(1):55-58.

57. Donohoe CL, Doyle SL, McGarrigle S, et al. Role of the insulin-like growth factor 1 axis and visceral adiposity in oesophageal adenocarcinoma. *Br J Surg.* 2012;99(3):387-396.

58. Howard JM, Pidgeon GP, Reynolds JV. Leptin and gastro-intestinal malignancies. *Obes Rev.* 2010;11(12):863-874.

59. Thompson OM, Beresford SAA, Kirk EA, Bronner MP, Vaughan TL. Serum leptin and adiponectin levels and risk of Barrett's esophagus and intestinal metaplasia of the gastroesophageal junction. *Obesity (Silver Spring).* 2010;18(11):2204-2211.

60. Housa D, Housová J, Vernerová Z, Haluzík M. Adipocytokines and cancer. *Physiol Res.* 2006;55(3):233-244.

61. Kelesidis I, Kelesidis T, Mantzoros CS. Adiponectin and cancer: a systematic review. *Br J Cancer.* 2006;94(9):1221-1225.

62. Garofalo C, Surmacz E. Leptin and cancer. *J Cell Physiol.* 2006;207(1):12-22.

63. Doyle SL, Donohoe CL, Finn SP, et al. IGF-1 and its receptor in esophageal cancer: association with adenocarcinoma and visceral obesity. *Am J Gastroenterol.* 2011;107(2):196-204.

64. Ogunwobi O, Mutungi G, Beales ILP. Leptin stimulates proliferation and inhibits apoptosis in Barrett's esophageal adenocarcinoma cells by cyclooxygenase-2-dependent, prostaglandin-E2-mediated transactivation of the epidermal growth factor receptor and c-Jun NH 2-terminal kinase activation. *Endocrinology.* 2006;147(9):4505-4516.

65. Greer KB, Falk GW, Bednarchik B, Li L, Chak A. Associations of serum adiponectin and leptin with Barrett's esophagus. *Clin Gastroenterol Hepatol.* 2015;13(13):2265-2272.

66. Kubo A, Levin TR, Block G, et al. Cigarette smoking and the risk of Barrett's esophagus. *Cancer Causes Control.* 2008;20(3):303-311.

67. Andrici J, Cox MR, Eslick GD. Cigarette smoking and the risk of Barrett's esophagus: a systematic review and meta-analysis. *J Gastroenterol Hepatol.* 2013;28(8):1258-1273.

68. Phillips WA, Lord RV, Nancarrow DJ, Watson DI, Whiteman DC. Barrett's esophagus. *J Gastroenterol Hepatol.* 2011;26(4):639-648.

69. Cook MB, Shaheen NJ, Anderson LA, et al. Cigarette smoking increases risk of Barrett's esophagus: an analysis of the Barrett's and esophageal adenocarcinoma consortium. *Gastroenterology.* 2012;142(4):744-753.

70. Kubo A, Levin TR, Block G, et al. Alcohol types and sociodemographic characteristics as risk factors for Barrett's esophagus. *Gastroenterology.* 2009;136(3):806-815.

71. Anderson LA, Cantwell MM, Watson RGP, et al. The association between alcohol and reflux esophagitis, Barrett's esophagus, and esophageal adenocarcinoma. *Gastroenterology.* 2009;136(3):799-805.

72. Thrift AP, Cook MB, Vaughan TL, et al. Alcohol and the risk of Barrett's esophagus: a pooled analysis from the International BEACON Consortium. *Am J Gastroenterol.* 2014;109(10):1586-1594.

73. di Pietro M, Fitzgerald RC. Barrett's oesophagus: an ideal model to study cancer genetics. *Hum Genet.* 2009;126(2):233-246.

74. Sun X, Elston R, Barnholtz-Sloan J, et al. A segregation analysis of Barrett's esophagus and associated adenocarcinomas. *Cancer Epidemiol Biomarkers Prev.* 2010;19(3):666-674.

75. Cameron AJ, Lagergren J, Henriksson C, Nyren O, Locke GR III, Pedersen NL. Gastroesophageal reflux disease in monozygotic and dizygotic twins. *Gastroenterology.* 2002;122(1):55-59.

76. Mohammed I, Cherkas LF, Riley SA, Spector TT, Trudgill NJ. Genetic influences in gastro-oesophageal reflux disease: a twin study. *Gut.* 2003;52(8):1085-1089.

77. Lembo A, Zaman M, Jones M, Talley NJ. Influence of genetics on irritable bowel syndrome, gastro-oesophageal reflux and dyspepsia: a twin study. *Aliment Pharmacol Ther.* 2007;25(11):1343-1350.

78. Groves C, Jankowski J, Barker F, Holdstock G. A family history of Barrett's oesophagus: another risk factor? *Scand J Gastroenterol.* 2005;40(9):1127-1128.

79. Chak A, Ochs-Balcom H, Falk G, et al. Familiality in Barrett's esophagus, adenocarcinoma of the esophagus, and adenocarcinoma

174. Phoa KN, van Vilsteren FG, Weusten BL, et al. Radiofrequency ablation vs endoscopic surveillance for patients with Barrett esophagus and low-grade dysplasia: a randomized clinical trial. *JAMA.* 2014;311(12):1209-1217.

175. Downs-Kelly E, Mendelin JE, Bennett AE, et al. Poor interobserver agreement in the distinction of high-grade dysplasia and adenocarcinoma in pretreatment Barrett's esophagus biopsies. *Am J Gastroenterol.* 2008;103(9):2333-2340.

176. Rastogi A, Puli S, El-Serag HB, Bansal A, Wani S, Sharma P. Incidence of esophageal adenocarcinoma in patients with Barrett's esophagus and high-grade dysplasia: a meta-analysis. *Gastrointest Endosc.* 2008;67(3):394-398.

177. Shaheen NJ, Sharma P, Overholt BF, et al. Radiofrequency ablation in Barrett's esophagus with dysplasia. *N Engl J Med.* 2009;360(22):2277-2288.

178. Clemons NJ, Phillips WA, Lord RV. Signaling pathways in the molecular pathogenesis of adenocarcinomas of the esophagus and gastroesophageal junction. *Cancer Biol Ther.* 2013;14(9):782-795.

179. Ong CA, Lao-Sirieix P, Fitzgerald RC. Biomarkers in Barrett's esophagus and esophageal adenocarcinoma: predictors of progression and prognosis. *World J Gastroenterol.* 2010;16(45):5669-5681.

180. Brabender J, Marjoram P, Salonga D, et al. A multigene expression panel for the molecular diagnosis of Barrett's esophagus and Barrett's adenocarcinoma of the esophagus. *Oncogene.* 2004;23(27):4780-4788.

181. Brabender J, Marjoram P, Lord RVN, et al. The molecular signature of normal squamous esophageal epithelium identifies the presence of a field effect and can discriminate between patients with Barrett's esophagus and patients with Barrett's-associated adenocarcinoma. *Cancer Epidemiol Biomarkers Prev.* 2005;14(9):2113-2117.

182. Lord RVN, Salonga D, Danenberg KD, et al. Telomerase reverse transcriptase expression is increased early in the Barrett's metaplasia, dysplasia, adenocarcinoma sequence. *J Gastrointest Surg.* 2000;4(2):135-142.

183. Reid BJ, Paulson TG, Li X. Genetic insights in Barrett's esophagus and esophageal adenocarcinoma. *Gastroenterology.* 2015;149(5):1142-1143.

184. Fisher OM, Lord SJ, Falkenback D, Clemons NJ, Eslick GD, Lord RV. The prognostic value of TP53 mutations in oesophageal adenocarcinoma: a systematic review and meta-analysis. *Gut.* 2017;66(3):399-410.

185. Stachler MD, Taylor-Weiner A, Peng S, et al. Paired exome analysis of Barrett's esophagus and adenocarcinoma. *Nat Genet.* 2015;47(9):1047-1055.

186. Carter SL, Cibulskis K, Helman E, et al. Absolute quantification of somatic DNA alterations in human cancer. *Nat Biotechnol.* 2012;30(5):413-421.

187. Stephens PJ, Greenman CD, Fu B, et al. Massive genomic rearrangement acquired in a single catastrophic event during cancer development. *Cell.* 2011;144(1):27-40.

188. Nones K, Waddell N, Wayte N, et al. Genomic catastrophies frequently arise in esophageal adenocarcinoma and drive tumorigenesis. *Nat Commun.* 2014;5:5224.

189. Dulak AM, Stojanov P, Peng S, et al. Exome and whole-genome sequencing of esophageal adenocarcinoma identifies recurrent driver events and mutational complexity. *Nat Genet.* 2013;45(5):478-486.

190. Weaver JM, Ross-Innes CS, Shannon N, et al. Ordering of mutations in preinvasive disease stages of esophageal carcinogenesis. *Nat Genet.* 2014;46(8):837-843.

191. Reid BJ, Li X, Galipeau PC, Vaughan TL. Barrett's oesophagus and oesophageal adenocarcinoma: time for a new synthesis. *Nat Rev Cancer.* 2010;10(2):87-101.

192. Wijnhoven BPL, Tilanus HW, Dinjens WNM. Molecular biology of Barrett's adenocarcinoma. *Ann Surg.* 2001;233(3):322-337.

193. Jenkins GJS, Doak SH, Parry JM, D'Souza FR, Griffiths AP, Baxter JN. Genetic pathways involved in the progression of Barrett's metaplasia to adenocarcinoma. *Br J Surg.* 2002;89(7):824-837.

194. Galipeau PC, Li X, Blount PL, et al. NSAIDs modulate CDKN2A, TP53, and DNA content risk for progression to esophageal adenocarcinoma. *PLoS Med.* 2007;4(2):e67.

195. Nancarrow DJ, Handoko HY, Smithers BM, et al. Genome-wide copy number analysis in esophageal adenocarcinoma using high-density single-nucleotide polymorphism arrays. *Cancer Res.* 2008;68(11):4163-4172.

196. Lai LA, Paulson TG, Li X, et al. Increasing genomic instability during premalignant neoplastic progression revealed through high resolution array-CGH. *Genes Chromosomes Cancer.* 2007;46(6):532-542.

197. Li X, Galipeau PC, Sanchez CA, et al. Single nucleotide polymorphism-based genome-wide chromosome copy change, loss of heterozygosity, and aneuploidy in Barrett's esophagus neoplastic progression. *Cancer Prev Res (Phila).* 2008;1(6):413-423.

198. Ouatu Lascar R, Fitzgerald RC, Triadafilopoulos G. Differentiation and proliferation in Barrett's esophagus and the effects of acid suppression. *Gastroenterology.* 1999;117(2):327-335.

199. Sirieix PS, O'Donovan M, Brown J, Save V, Coleman N, Fitzgerald RC. Surface expression of minichromosome maintenance proteins provides a novel method for detecting patients at risk for developing adenocarcinoma in Barrett's esophagus. *Clin Cancer Res.* 2003;9(7):2560-2566.

200. Murray L, Sedo A, Scott M, et al. TP53 and progression from Barrett's metaplasia to oesophageal adenocarcinoma in a UK population cohort. *Gut.* 2006;55(10):1390-1397.

201. Bani-Hani K, Martin IG, Hardie LJ, et al. Prospective study of Cyclin D1 overexpression in Barrett's esophagus: association with increased risk of adenocarcinoma. *J Natl Cancer Inst.* 2000;92(16):1316-1321.

202. Maley CC, Galipeau PC, Li X, Sanchez CA, Paulson TG, Reid BJ. Selectively advantageous mutations and hitchhikers in neoplasms. *Cancer Res.* 2004;64(10):3414-3427.

203. Barrett MT, Sanchez CA, Prevo LJ, et al. Evolution of neoplastic cell lineages in Barrett oesophagus. *Nat Genet.* 1999;22(1):106-109.

204. Maley CC, Galipeau PC, Li X, et al. The combination of genetic instability and clonal expansion predicts progression to esophageal adenocarcinoma. *Cancer Res.* 2004;64(20):7629-7633.

205. Maley CC, Galipeau PC, Finley JC, et al. Genetic clonal diversity predicts progression to esophageal adenocarcinoma. *Nat Genet.* 2006;38(4):468-473.

206. Timmer MR, Martinez P, Lau L, et al. 139 Longitudinal single cell clonal analysis reveals evolutionary stasis and re-determined malignant potential in non-dysplastic Barrett's esophagus. *Gastroenterology.* 2016;150(4):S34.

207. Varghese S, Newton R, Ross-Innes CS, et al. Analysis of dysplasia in patients with Barrett's esophagus based on expression pattern of 90 genes. *Gastroenterology.* 2015;149(6):1511-1518.

208. van Baal JWPM, Milana F, Rygiel AM, et al. A comparative analysis by SAGE of gene expression profiles of esophageal adenocarcinoma and esophageal squamous cell carcinoma. *Cell Oncol.* 2008;30(1):63-75.

209. van Baal JWPM, Milano F, Rygiel AM, et al. A comparative analysis by SAGE of gene expression profiles of Barrett's esophagus, normal squamous esophagus, and gastric cardia. *Gastroenterology.* 2005;129(4):1274-1281.

210. Helm J, Enkemann SA, Coppola D, Barthel JS, Kelley ST, Yeatman TJ. Dedifferentiation precedes invasion in the progression from Barrett's metaplasia to esophageal adenocarcinoma. *Clin Cancer Res.* 2005;11(7):2478-2485.

211. Barrett MT, Yeung KY, Ruzzo WL, et al. Transcriptional analyses of Barrett's metaplasia and normal upper GI mucosae. *Neoplasia.* 2002;4(2):121-128.

212. Nancarrow DJ, Clouston AD, Smithers BM, et al. Whole genome expression array profiling highlights differences in mucosal defense genes in Barrett's esophagus and esophageal adenocarcinoma. *PLoS One.* 2011;6(7):e22513.

213. Fisher OM, Maag JL, Levert-Mignon A, et al. Tu1135 whole transcriptome sequencing reveals previously unrecognized alterations in Barrett's esophagus and esophageal adenocarcinoma. *Gastroenterology.* 2016;150(4):S854-S865, e1; quiz e16-e17.

214. Krause L, Nones K, Loffler KA, et al. Identification of the CIMP-like subtype and aberrant methylation of members of the chromosomal segregation and spindle assembly pathways in esophageal adenocarcinoma. *Carcinogenesis.* 2016;37(4):356-365.

215. Smith E, De Young NJ, Pavey SJ, et al. Similarity of aberrant DNA methylation in Barrett's esophagus and esophageal adenocarcinoma. *Mol Cancer.* 2008;7(1):1.

216. Wang JS, Guo M, Montgomery EA, et al. DNA promoter hypermethylation of p16 and APC predicts neoplastic progression in Barrett's esophagus. *Am J Gastroenterol.* 2009;104(9):2153-2160.

217. Jin Z, Cheng Y, Gu W, et al. A multicenter, double-blinded validation study of methylation biomarkers for progression prediction in Barrett's esophagus. *Cancer Res.* 2009;69(10):4112-4115.

218. Rakyan VK, Down TA, Thorne NP, et al. An integrated resource for genome-wide identification and analysis of human tissue-specific differentially methylated regions (tDMRs). *Genome Res.* 2008;18(9):1518-1529.

219. Shah AK, Lê Cao K-A, Choi E, et al. Glyco-centric lectin magnetic bead array (LeMBA)—proteomics dataset of human serum samples from healthy, Barrett's esophagus and esophageal adenocarcinoma individuals. *Data Brief.* 2016;7:1058-1062.

220. Kraly JR, Jones MR, Gomez DG, et al. Reproducible two-dimensional capillary electrophoresis analysis of Barrett's esophagus tissues. *Anal Chem.* 2006;78(17):5977-5986.

221. Peng D, Sheta EA, Powell SM, et al. Alterations in Barrett's -related adenocarcinomas: a proteomic approach. *Int J Cancer.* 2007;122(6): 1303-1310.

222. Zhao J, Chang AC, Li C, et al. Comparative proteomics analysis of Barrett metaplasia and esophageal adenocarcinoma using two-dimensional liquid mass mapping. *Mol Cell Proteomics.* 2007;6(6): 987-999.

223. Chao DL, Sanchez CA, Galipeau PC, et al. Cell proliferation, cell cycle abnormalities, and cancer outcome in patients with Barrett's esophagus: a long-term prospective study. *Clin Cancer Res.* 2008;14(21):6988-6995.

224. Bird Lieberman EL, Dunn JM, Coleman HG, et al. Population-based study reveals new risk-stratification biomarker panel for Barrett's esophagus. *Gastroenterology.* 2012;143(4):927-935, e3.

225. Critchley-Thorne RJ, Duits LC, Prichard JW, et al. A tissue systems pathology assay for high-risk Barrett's esophagus. *Cancer Epidemiol Biomarkers Prev.* 2016;25(6):958-968.

226. Pepe MS, Etzioni R, Feng Z, et al. Phases of biomarker development for early detection of cancer. *J Natl Cancer Inst.* 2001;93(14): 1054-1061.

227. Kastelein F, Biermann K, Steyerberg EW, et al. Aberrant p53 protein expression is associated with an increased risk of neoplastic progression in patients with Barrett's oesophagus. *Gut.* 2013;62(12):1676-1683.

228. Clark GW, et al. Short-segment Barrett's esophagus: a prevalent complication of gastroesophageal reflux disease with malignant potential. *J Gastrointest Surg.* 1997;1:113-122.

229. Voutilainen M, et al. Gastroesophageal reflux disease: prevalence, clinical, endoscopic and histopathological findings in 1,128 consecutive patients referred for endoscopy due to dyspeptic and reflux symptoms. *Digestion.* 2000;61:6-13.

230. Gerson LB, et al. Prevalence of Barrett's esophagus in asymptomatic individuals. *Gastroenterology.* 2002;123:461-467.

231. Veldhuyzen van Zanten SJ, et al. The prevalence of Barrett's oesophagus in a cohort of 1040 Canadian primary care patients with uninvestigated dyspepsia undergoing prompt endoscopy. *Aliment Pharmacol Ther.* 2006;23:595-599.

232. Hayeck TJ, et al. The prevalence of Barrett's esophagus in the US: estimates from a simulation model confirmed by SEER data. *Dis Esophagus.* 2010;23:451-457.

Medical and Surgical Therapy for Gastroesophageal Reflux Disease and Barrett Esophagus

Mark R. Wendling | Brant K. Oelschlager

The British surgeon Norman Barrett is famously credited for his early description of the lower esophagus lined by columnar epithelium. However, he himself did not claim to be the first to describe the condition that would later bear his name. His original article in 1950 details numerous previous reports that likely represented this pathology.[1] Throughout Barrett's impressive career, he proposed many theories that later proved to be correct, but in this instance, he concluded that the columnar epithelium he observed was gastric tissue in the setting of a congenitally short esophagus.[2] It was not until 3 years later when Allison and Johnstone published their own findings that this was corrected.[3] They demonstrated not only that the columnar-lined viscus was indeed the esophagus, but they also proposed that the ulcer associated with this condition should be referred to as "Barrett's ulcer."

If the initial description was difficult to come by, then it may have been foreshadowing of things to come. The controversies regarding the definition of Barrett esophagus and the epidemiologic descriptions of the disease are so extensive that they have been granted their own chapters in this edition. In contrast, something that has been correctly postulated from the beginning is that Barrett esophagus is a reaction of the esophageal mucosa to chronic injury from refluxate. The tools available in the physician's armamentarium for the treatment of Barrett esophagus are diverse. These include medication for prophylaxis and treatment, antireflux operations, ablation therapies, and surgical resection in select cases. The indications for each continue to evolve with time. The holy grail of treatment remains prevention of progression along the pathway from metaplasia to neoplasia, and whether the natural history of Barrett esophagus can be altered remains a topic of debate. Current goals of therapy are directed at relief of associated reflux symptoms and healing of esophagitis to prevent complications of nondysplastic Barrett esophagus and removal or obliteration of the tissue when it progresses on the continuum toward cancer.

CLINICAL FEATURES OF BARRETT ESOPHAGUS

The mucosa of the esophagus consists of stratified squamous epithelium. Barrett esophagus is the metaplastic replacement of this squamous epithelium with intestinal columnar epithelium, which predisposes to the development of adenocarcinoma. Barrett esophagus has been described across all demographics, but in the Western world, where it is the most prominent, the highest incidence is in middle-aged white males. It is diagnosed by recognition of columnar mucosa on endoscopy and confirmed histologically from tissue obtained from biopsy during the upper endoscopy. The mean age at time of diagnosis is in the 6th decade of life[4] and demonstrates a male-to-female predominance of approximately 2:1.[5] Obesity is a risk factor for gastroesophageal reflux disease (GERD) due to its effects on the body's normal antireflux mechanisms and is consequently a likely risk factor for Barrett esophagus. Body mass index (BMI) exists as the most common quantifier of obesity; however, many have suggested that an increased abdominal circumference or waist-to-hip ratio may carry more significance, as it is a better measure of abdominal adiposity.[6,7] Other independent risk factors that have been suggested include smoking[8] and presence of a hiatal hernia.[9] Conversely, the presence of *Helicobacter pylori* has demonstrated an inverse association with risk of Barrett esophagus for reasons that are not entirely clear.[10] The majority of available data suggest that the prevalence of Barrett esophagus is significantly lower in African Americans compared with non-Hispanic whites by several times.[11–13] Although it is not entirely understood whether this imbalance exists due to differences in risk factor profiles or genetic susceptibility, a genetic predisposition seems likely. Variances at specific genetic loci have been implicated in increasing the genetic susceptibility to developing Barrett esophagus.[14] Also, the vast majority of patients are diagnosed on their first endoscopy.[15] This suggests that reflux acts as a trigger in the right genetic environment for the development of Barrett esophagus.

Barrett esophagus has been categorized by its extent either as long (>3 cm) or short (<3 cm) segments. A third, more controversial, description is intestinal metaplasia at the gastroesophageal junction. This likely represents either very short segment Barrett or intestinal metaplasia of the gastric cardia, and the malignant potential is less clear. Short-segment Barrett represents the large majority of cases, while long segments likely represent more severe reflux both in terms of acid exposure and its proximal extent.[16] There has been theoretical concerns that long-segment disease may be associated with a higher incidence of both dysplasia and adenocarcinoma due to disease burdens on the cellular level, and there is some retrospective data to support this.[17,18] However, the available evidence has not been sufficient to justify incorporating length consistently across current surveillance guidelines. Instead, the presence and degree of dysplasia has provided the marker of risk and has driven the clinical management. Histologically

Barrett esophagus is classified as nondysplastic, indefinite for dysplasia, low-grade dysplasia (LGD), or high-grade dysplasia (HGD). A specimen indefinite for dysplasia is often a result of active inflammation, which precludes accurate histologic classification. This is an interim diagnosis only, which requires close follow-up for definitive characterization of the histologic pattern. Acid suppression therapy should be maximized and repeat biopsies obtained after a brief period to allow healing. Regardless of the classification, there remains a subjective element to histologic grading, which has been demonstrated by relatively low interobserver agreement within specimens, particularly for LGD. Consequently, a second opinion from an expert gastrointestinal pathologist is recommended to confirm a diagnosis of LGD or HGD.

SURVEILLANCE

The development of esophageal adenocarcinoma represents the most feared complication of Barrett esophagus, with mortality increasing with the stage at diagnosis. The goal of early detection forms the rationale of surveillance. This efficacy of surveillance has been questioned recently, but poor efficacy is likely related to an excessively long interval between surveillance endoscopies and an inadequate number of biopsies to adequately evaluate the Barrett segment.[19,20] Surveillance for nondysplastic Barrett esophagus should include the use of high-definition endoscopy with systematic four-quadrant biopsies every 2 cm with separate endoscopic mucosal resection (EMR) of mucosal abnormalities at an interval of 1 to 2 years. If there is a history of LGD, biopsies should be obtained every 1 cm with an interval of 6 to 12 months, although increasingly patients with dysplasia are undergoing ablation rather than continued surveillance. There is evidence that surveillance results in the detection of esophageal adenocarcinoma at an earlier stage. For instance, in a retrospective review of 224 patients, Grant et al.[21] found that those who underwent surveillance had significantly lower stage tumors at the time of diagnosis. One would then expect this to translate to a benefit in mortality but concern exists that this may represent lead-time bias instead of a true survival benefit. Disputing this is data from multiple centers showing that with endoscopic resection of early adenocarcinoma patients are cured of their disease and have survival similar to the general population. Corley et al.[22] did not demonstrate an association between surveillance and a decreased risk of death in a case-control study of 70 patients with esophageal adenocarcinoma diagnosed greater than 6 months after Barrett esophagus, although these results have been criticized for high overall mortality rates, not using endoluminal therapy in early disease and not differentiating between adequate surveillance and any surveillance.[23] In contrast, shortly thereafter, Verbeek et al.[24] demonstrated decreased esophageal adenocarcinoma mortality at 2 and 5 years for those adhering to a surveillance program (hazard ratio [HR], 0.79) (Fig. 33.1). Logically, if early-stage cancer is curative in most patients, it makes sense that surveillance at an appropriate interval that allows detection of progression to HGD or early adenocarcinoma will be beneficial.

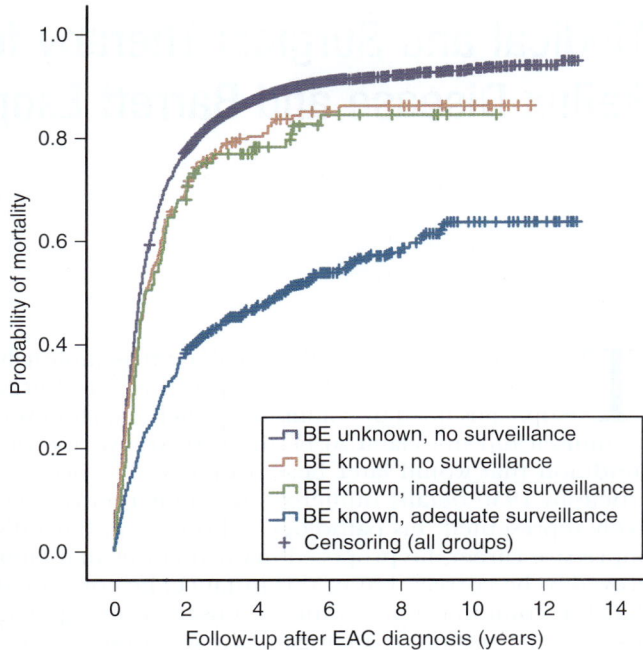

FIGURE 33.1 Mortality related to a prior Barrett esophagus (BE) diagnosis and surveillance participation. Kaplan–Meier survival analysis (+log-rank test) for mortality in esophageal adenocarcinoma (EAC) patients, with and without a prior BE diagnosis, with or without participating in an (adequate) surveillance program. BE unknown vs. BE known, no surveillance: $P = .006$; BE unknown vs. inadequate surveillance: $P = .007$, BE unknown vs. adequate surveillance: $P < .001$; adequate vs. inadequate surveillance: $P < .001$. Adequate surveillance vs. BE known, no surveillance: $P < .001$. (From Verbeek RE, Leenders M, Ten Kate FJ, et al. Surveillance of Barrett's esophagus and mortality from esophageal adenocarcinoma: a population-based cohort study. *Am J Gastroenterol.* 2014;109:1215–1222.)

TREATMENT OF NONDYSPLASTIC BARRETT ESOPHAGUS

MEDICAL TREATMENT

See Box 33.1.

Chemoprophylaxis

In recent years, there has been much attention paid to the subject of chemoprophylaxis against the development of esophageal adenocarcinoma. Statins originally were shown to have some efficacy in in vitro cell lines. This is thought to be secondary to induction of apoptosis and cyclooxygenase (COX)-2 inhibition.[25,26] There have since been several observational studies published investigating the translational significance of these findings. Although these studies have had conflicting results, they are also heterogeneous and likely underpowered. The largest case-control study to investigate the effect of statins in the setting of Barrett esophagus (311 cases, 856 controls) found approximately 35% lower odds of developing esophageal adenocarcinoma in those on statin therapy.[27] Two meta-analyses have attempted addressing the role of statins,

---

BOX 33.1 Management of Barrett Esophagus or Early Carcinoma

NONDYSPLASTIC BARRETT
Repeat EGD with surveillance biopsies in 1–2 years

INDEFINITE FOR DYSPLASIA
Maximize acid suppression therapy (High dose PPI plus a nocturnal H_2 blocker)
   Repeat EGD with surveillance biopsies after a period for healing (weeks to months)

LOW-GRADE DYSPLASIA
Aggressive reflux control with recommendation for antireflux surgery in appropriate candidates and second opinion from expert GI pathologist
   Repeat EGD with surveillance biopsies in 6 months
   Regression on two consecutive exams → De-escalate to nondysplastic Barrett
   Persistent or high-risk features → Ablative therapy to reduce progression risk

HIGH-GRADE DYSPLASIA OR INTRAMUCOSAL ADENOCARCINOMA
Second opinion from expert GI pathologist
Endoscopic resection of visible lesions
Ablation of Barrett mucosa
   Consider esophagectomy in patients with ultra-long (8 cm or more Barrett), when multifocal disease present, or in patients with difficult to control or severe GERD especially in the setting of poor esophageal motility and large hiatal hernia

EGD, Esophagogastroduodenoscopy; *GERD,* gastroesophageal reflux disease; *GI,* gastrointestinal; *PPI,* proton pump inhibitor.

---

and both have reported inverse associations of similar magnitude between statin use and adenocarcinoma.[28,29]

Nonsteroidal antiinflammatory drugs (NSAIDs) including aspirin are the other class of medication that has received the majority of attention regarding chemoprophylaxis in the setting of Barrett esophagus. Again, this is due to the implication of cyclooxygenases in the oncogenic transformation of Barrett esophagus to esophageal adenocarcinoma.[30] This has been supported in both in vitro Barrett cell lines and in animal models. However, a multicenter randomized placebo-controlled trial of celecoxib in patients with either LGD or HGD did not find that 200 mg twice daily prevented progression of Barrett dysplasia to adenocarcinoma over a 48-week study period.[31] Aspirin in conjunction with proton pump inhibitors (PPIs) has been found to decrease prostaglandin E_2 levels in patients with either nondysplastic Barrett or LGD. The Aspirin Esomeprazole Chemoprevention Trial (AspECT) is currently ongoing with an estimated study completion in 2017. This may help explain on the issue. Both NSAIDs and statins have shown promise and require further investigation, but there is inadequate evidence currently to support a recommendation for use of any medication for chemoprophylaxis alone.

Acid Suppression

There are no randomized controlled trials that demonstrate that PPI usage prevents progression along the pathway of metaplasia to carcinoma. The introduction and widespread use of PPIs has, in fact, coincided with a continued increase in the incidence of esophageal adenocarcinoma. That being said, a theoretical benefit for removing the inciting insult would appear logically sound and is supported by multiple cohort studies.[32–34] PPIs are the most effective pharmacologic inhibitors of gastric acid secretion available and are first-line therapy solutions for patients with Barrett esophagus. They are highly effective at obtaining symptomatic relief, but obtaining objective normalization of acid exposure has proven more difficult. In 48 patients with Barrett esophagus, pathologic esophageal acid exposure was demonstrated in 50% on PPI therapy doses that resulted in symptomatic control.[35] More recently and favorably, rabeprazole 20 mg twice daily can achieve normal acid exposure in 26 of 29 patients. This was improved further with an increased dose of 40 mg twice daily.[36] These data demonstrate that, although our goal is often symptom control, this does not equate to acid control (much less other potential pathogens such as bile and pepsin). The discordance between the two may be due to decreased sensitivity of Barrett esophagus to acid, but this is yet to be proven. Spechler et al.[37] attempted to define why objective control remains difficult. They compared gastric and esophageal acidity in 31 patients with Barrett esophagus on varied doses of esomeprazole. Between 16% and 23% of subjects continued to have a time pH < 4.0 greater than 5% depending on the PPI dose. This was in the setting of a gastric % time pH >4 more than 80%. This suggests that it is not gastric resistance to acid suppression but rather decreased anatomic antireflux mechanisms that are responsible for continued acid exposure.

SURGICAL TREATMENT

The primary goal of surgical therapy in patients with Barrett esophagus, like in GERD patients without Barrett, is the relief of GERD-related symptoms that are not adequately controlled with medical therapy. The presence of Barrett esophagus itself is not an indication for surgery. However, Barrett esophagus does represent GERD on the severe end of the spectrum (Table 33.1), and as previously stated, obtaining acid control in these patients has proven difficult. Furthermore, patients with Barrett commonly have a weak lower esophageal sphincter and a hiatal hernia and often suffer from regurgitation symptoms even if heartburn is controlled with acid suppression medications. Patients with Barrett esophagus have been found to have an earlier onset of symptoms[38] and more frequent complications of reflux such as esophagitis and strictures, and although absence of symptoms is not uncommon in Barrett esophagus patients, they have been found to have more severe symptoms versus age- and gender-matched controls.[39] There is also a question of bile acids in the role of Barrett esophagus development and progression.[40] Bile acids have been shown to be important in the development of Barrett esophagus in animal models,[41] and several studies have suggested a synergistic nature of gastric and duodenal reflux in mucosal injury.[42,43] Patients with Barrett esophagus are more likely to have mixed reflux of both gastric and duodenal contents than GERD patients without Barrett.[40,44] It is not clear if this is causative or just another marker of severe reflux barrier impairment. The role of duodenal contents has been controversial for some time, and we

TABLE 33.1 Clinical Features of Patients With Barrett Esophagus and Gastroesophageal Reflux Disease and Esophagogastroduodenoscopy Controls

	Barrett (n = 79)	GERD Controls (n = 94)	EGD Controls (n = 84)
Duration of symptoms (year)*	16.4	11.8	13
Mean age at onset*	35.3	43.7	42.7
Esophagitis[†]	51 (65%)	33 (35%)	24 (29%)
Esophageal ulcer[†]	17 (22%)	7 (7%)	6 (7%)
Esophageal stricture[†]	21 (27%)	7 (7%)	5 (6%)
Hiatal hernia[†]	60 (76%)	41 (44%)	31 (37%)
Severe GERD[‡]	67 (85%)	55 (59%)	53 (63%)

EGD, Esophagogastroduodenoscopy; *GERD*, gastroesophageal reflux disease.

*$P < .05$ for the Barrett esophagus group versus either control group (Kruskal-Wallis test).

[†]Odds ratios for esophagitis, esophageal ulcer, esophageal stricture, and hiatal hernia greater than 3 cm for the Barrett esophagus group versus either control group.

[‡]Severe GERD was defined as heartburn so painful that it awoke the patient or prevented sleeping.

EGD, Esophagogastroduodenoscopy; *GERD*, gastroesophageal reflux disease.

Modified from Eisen GM, Sandler RS, Murray S, Gottfried M. The relationship between gastroesophageal reflux disease and its complications with Barrett's esophagus. *Am J Gastroenterol.* 1997;92:27.

TABLE 33.2 Comparison of Pre- and Postoperative Symptoms in 106 Patients With Barrett Esophagus Who Underwent Laparoscopic Antireflux Surgery

Symptom	Preoperative Incidence: n (%)	Resolution: n (%)	Improvement: n (%)	No Improvement: n (%)
Heartburn	98 (92%)	69 (70%)	25 (26%)	4 (4%)
Regurgitation	69 (65%)	52 (75%)	6 (9%)	11 (16%)
Dysphagia	33 (31%)	21 (64%)	6 (18%)	6 (18%)
Cough	31 (29%)	22 (71%)	2 (6%)	7 (23%)
Chest pain	30 (28%)	20 (67%)	6 (20%)	4 (13%)
Hoarseness	25 (24%)	21 (84%)	1 (4%)	3 (12%)

From Oelschlager BK, Barreca M, Chang L, Oleynikov D, Pellegrini CA. Clinical and pathologic response of Barrett's esophagus to laparoscopic antireflux surgery. *Ann Surg.* 2003;238:458–464.

are currently without a satisfying answer. Nevertheless, return of a competent mechanical antireflux barrier that prevents all types of reflux would have advantages over medical therapy by addressing both the acid and nonacid components. It is important to remember, however, that the anatomic findings that correlate with severe GERD and Barrett esophagus such as a large hiatal hernia, decreased motility, stricture, and a shortened esophagus also make obtaining a successful surgical result more challenging. One must identify these factors prior to an operation. Furthermore, evidence indicates that patients with Barrett and a failed fundoplication are at increased risk for disease progression. Thus it is imperative to select patients with Barrett esophagus carefully for antireflux surgery and perform the surgery well to minimize the potential for breakdown of the repair.

Subjective and Objective Outcomes

In general, patients with Barrett esophagus have good symptomatic and functional outcomes after antireflux surgery (Table 33.2 and Fig. 33.2), although it has been suggested that results are inferior to those with uncomplicated GERD. The LOTUS trial,[45] published in 2011, represents the first multicenter, randomized trial comparing laparoscopic antireflux surgery with PPIs. Importantly, only patients with good symptomatic control on PPIs were eligible for the study. Both therapies were found to be effective at 5 years. A subset analysis of patients with Barrett esophagus from this study was published by Attwood[46] and has provided insight into the subject. Sixty patients were randomized to either standardized laparoscopic antireflux surgery or dose-adjusted esomeprazole. Again, both treatment modalities were found to be effective, with only four treatment failures between the groups (1 surgery, 3 PPI,

not significant). There was no difference found in the level of symptom control at 3-year follow-up. Also, there was no difference found when comparing symptomatic outcomes or dysphagia rates between those with Barrett esophagus and those without. Objectively, pH monitoring performed at 6 months post treatment demonstrated significantly lower percent acid exposure times for those randomized to surgical therapy compared with PPIs (13.2% to 0.4% and 7.4% to 4.9%, respectively; $P = .002$).

Hofstetter et al.[47] also demonstrated excellent results in 97 patients with Barrett esophagus who underwent antireflux surgery. At median 5-year follow-up, 79% of patients had complete resolution of all reflux symptoms with a 97% patient satisfaction rate reported. The vast majority of pH studies normalized as well (81%). This is consistent with a randomized prospective trial comparing medical therapy with fundoplication prior to the popularization of the laparoscopic approach. Fifty-eight patients with Barrett esophagus were randomized to the surgical arm with median 5-year follow-up. Satisfactory symptomatic outcomes were achieved in 91% of patients. The total % time of pH < 4 decreased from 19.0% preoperatively to just 0.6% postoperatively with positive studies found in 15% of patients. Bilitec monitoring to detect duodenogastric reflux was also used with 92% of these studies being normal in the surgical arm versus just 25% in those receiving medical therapy.[48]

We have examined the outcomes of those with Barrett esophagus who received laparoscopic antireflux surgery in our own experience. We demonstrated 86% of patients reported improvement in symptoms of heartburn and regurgitation and 10/10 median patient satisfactions at 8-year follow-up. Also, we demonstrated a mean decrease in DeMeester score from 54 to 9.[49] We have also demonstrated that approximately three-quarters of our patients have normal objective pH data following antireflux surgery.[50] This likely underrepresents the success as it is relatively difficult to convince the asymptomatic patient to undergo objective testing compared with those who are experiencing recurrent gastroesophageal reflux. It seems obvious that nothing inherent to the metaplastic epithelium itself would result in inferior results to surgical attempts of reflux control. Most likely, the relationship between Barrett esophagus and surgery represents somewhat of a catch-22

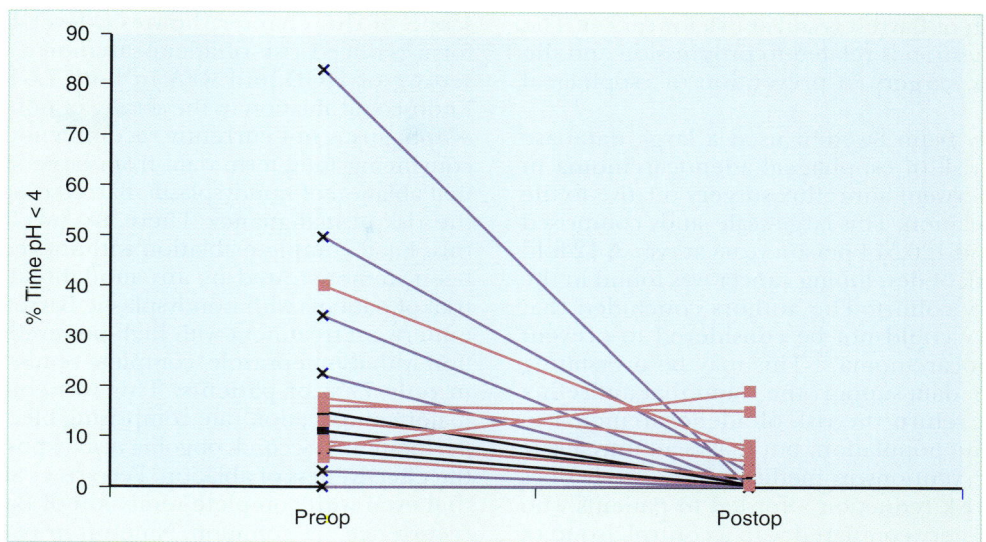

FIGURE 33.2 Twenty-four-hour distal esophageal pH results before and after Nissen fundoplication in 21 patients with Barrett esophagus studied preoperatively and postoperatively. *Postop,* Postoperative; *Preop,* preoperative. (From Hofstetter WA, Peters JH, DeMeester TR, et al. Long term outcome of antireflux surgery in patients with Barrett's esophagus. *Ann Surg.* 2001;234:532.)

where the same anatomic factors that lead to severe gastroesophageal reflux, Barrett esophagus, and need for surgical intervention also result in more clinically challenging patients and technically challenging operations, making the pursuit of quality outcomes more difficult.

Impact of Antireflux Surgery on the Metaplasia-Dysplasia-Neoplasia Continuum

Since GERD is an essential component to the development of Barrett, it is reasonable to assume that effective treatment of GERD would have a positive effect on the natural history of the disease. Although heavily debated, some also hold the belief that once Barrett metaplasia has occurred, its natural history cannot be altered. Theoretically, on the continuum from metaplasia to neoplasia, there must be a point of no return at which the development of esophageal adenocarcinoma is inevitable. The uncertain point of this biologic Rubicon coupled with the relatively low incidence of the disease makes determining the effect of surgical therapy on the prevention of esophageal adenocarcinoma extremely difficult and thus far elusive.

In 1980 Brand et al.[51] first described regression in 4 of 10 patients with Barrett esophagus. Since then, there has been an abundance of surgical literature from observational studies demonstrating varying rates of regression after antireflux surgery. In a cohort study of 91 symptomatic patients with Barrett esophagus, Gurski et al.[52] demonstrated a regression rate of 36.4% after antireflux surgery. This was compared with a regression rate of 7.1% for 14 patients receiving medical therapy. In the surgical group, the regression was composed of 17 patients with LGD who reverted to nondysplastic Barrett and 11 patients with Barrett who regressed to nonmetaplastic epithelium. Eight patients progressed (five and three to LGD and HGD, respectively). Zaninotto et al.[53] compared a cohort of 45 postsurgical patients with 44 with medical management. There was a statistically significant increase in the rate of

regression for those who underwent antireflux surgery compared with the medically managed group (40 vs. 16%; $P = .04$). Both these investigations demonstrated significantly higher rates of regression in those with short-segment compared with long-segment disease.

The other factor that seems to play a role in the rate of regression is, perhaps unsurprisingly, actual success in reconstructing a competent gastric cardia. A cohort of 75 patients with median follow-up of 8.9 years demonstrated a rate of regression of 31%. The rate of progression in this population was 8%. Patients with progression were much more likely to have a failed fundoplication based on endoscopic evaluation than those who did not progress (67% vs. 16%; $P = .0129$).[54] In our own experience, we described a 55% regression rate in 90 consecutive patients at median 40-month follow-up. Of those who underwent functional testing, 89% were found to have normalized pH studies.[50]

Rates of regression have not been universally reproducible. Randomized prospective data by Parrilla et al.[48] did not find complete regression in any of the 101 patients receiving either medical or surgical therapy despite high rates of acid normalization on functional studies. There was significantly less de novo dysplasia found in the surgical group (2% vs. 20%). There are several possible explanations for the wide variability in findings between studies. It has been proposed that incorporation of metaplastic epithelium in a fundoplication makes identification and biopsy more difficult in short-segment disease resulting in frequent sampling error, although most endoscopists dismiss any increased difficulty with biopsies after a fundoplication.

The likelihood of regression has been shown repeatedly to be related to both disease length and acid normalization. However, the clinical relevance of regression is unknown, as it is possible that Barrett esophagus that is susceptible to regression may never have progressed at all, and any length of Barrett is still at risk for cancer. The more pressing question is related to progression and the role of antireflux surgery in prevention of esophageal adenocarcinoma.

A flawed study from Sweden used a large database to compare the risk of esophageal adenocarcinoma in patients who underwent antireflux surgery relative to the background population. This large-scale study comprised 14,102 patients and 120,514 person-years at risk. A 12-fold increase in the risk of developing cancer was found in the antireflux surgery cohort. The authors concluded that antireflux surgery could not be considered to prevent esophageal adenocarcinoma.[55] This may be overstating the evidence. The data support the claim that antireflux surgery does not return the risk of adenocarcinoma to that of the baseline population, but that is an unrealistic bar for most interventions in medicine. The study does not address the risk reduction afforded to patients who had antireflux surgery compared with a control group of patients with reflux disease treated with acid suppression medications. In a follow-up analysis of this study population, Lofdahl et al.[56] identified 55 cases where patients developed esophageal adenocarcinoma more than 5 years after antireflux surgery. They were compared with 240 controls matched to age, sex, and calendar year of antireflux surgery. They found that those who developed esophageal adenocarcinoma were 3 times more likely to have recurrent pathologic reflux after their operation than the control population. This led the authors to conclude that perhaps recurrent GERD was responsible for the lack of protective effect of antireflux surgery. This is supported by randomized prospective data that found no difference in progression to carcinoma between medically and surgically treated patients (5% vs. 3%) at 5 years' follow-up. In the latter group, all progression was associated with clinical and objective recurrence of GERD.[48] Logically, if recurrent GERD and a failed fundoplication is a risk factor for disease progression, a functioning fundoplication must reduce or stabilize the risk.

TREATMENT OF DYSPLASIA AND EARLY CANCER

ENDOSCOPIC THERAPY FOR DYSPLASTIC BARRETT ESOPHAGUS

The efficacy of medical and surgical therapy for Barrett esophagus as it relates to progression to carcinoma continues to be described and debated. In the meantime, several endoscopic ablative modalities proved beneficial to alter the natural history of Barrett esophagus. In theory, if the metaplastic cells could be eradicated completely in a safe and reliable manner, the risk of progression could be completely removed. This would negate the need for further surveillance and make many current issues of no consequence. There are several methods of eradication of Barrett esophagus including radiofrequency ablation (RFA), photodynamic therapy (PDT), cryoablation, argon plasma coagulation (APC), and EMR (Fig. 33.3), each with their own advantages and proponents. The differentiation between ablative therapies is beyond the

scope of this chapter; however, level 1 evidence exists for a reduced risk of adenocarcinoma with PDT in the setting of HGD and RFA in both LGD and HGD.[57–59] Endoscopic ablation in the setting of nondysplastic Barrett esophagus is not currently recommended, as there is no convincing long-term data from large studies to suggest that ablation of nondysplastic Barrett esophagus decreases the risk of malignancy. There are two likely reasons for this. First, complete ablation without recurrence has not been demonstrated by any modality. In a multicenter trial of patients with nondysplastic Barrett esophagus who underwent treatment with high-powered APC in conjunction with esomeprazole, complete remission was obtained in only 77% of patients. This was coupled with 9.8% major complication rate comprising bleeding, stenosis, or perforation.[60] Second, ongoing acid exposure may sabotage the effectiveness of ablation. Ferraris et al.[61] demonstrated that even with complete remission of Barrett esophagus, recurrence was common. Ninety-four patients underwent endoscopic ablation with APC and had reflux control with either medical or surgical therapy. At a mean follow-up of 36 months, recurrence of intestinal metaplasia was identified in 18% of patients. The risk of recurrence was found to be significantly lower in those who underwent surgical fundoplication (OR, 0.30). In addition to concerns about incomplete ablation, ongoing acid exposure, and recurrence of intestinal metaplasia, there is concern regarding buried Barrett glands under the neosquamous epithelium. The risk of these glands is unknown; however, they may also confer an ongoing risk of progression to cancer.[62]

Low-Grade Dysplasia

LGD in the setting of Barrett esophagus represents a diagnostic entity where the ideal treatment is largely unknown. Large variance has been shown in the interobserver reliability of the diagnosis. This has led to wide-ranging results in the literature for treatment and outcome. Certainly, inflammation from ongoing reflux can lead to histologic changes that mimic dysplasia, and these resolve with control of reflux, particularly with antireflux surgery. However, true dysplasia likely does not regress.

The historically believed rate of progression of Barrett esophagus to adenocarcinoma of 1% per year has more recently thought to be an overestimation. In fact, recently, a cohort of patients with LGD was followed for over 950 patient-years. The rate of progression to HGD was found to be 1.6% per year, and progression to esophageal adenocarcinoma was 0.44% per year.[63] In terms of merely making the diagnosis, a Dutch study of 293 patients where Barrett esophagus was designated with LGD found that when reviewed by an expert panel, only 27% of the initial diagnoses were confirmed. The remainder of the cases were downstaged to either nondysplastic Barrett or indefinite for dysplasia. Interestingly, the rate of progression was 9.1% per year in the confirmed group and only 0.6% per year for those with downstaged nondysplastic Barrett esophagus.[64] Importantly, this 0.6% rate is still higher than many reports for true nondysplastic Barrett esophagus, suggesting that even if not confirmed by a second pathologist, a patient found to have LGD is someone who needs to be watched closely.

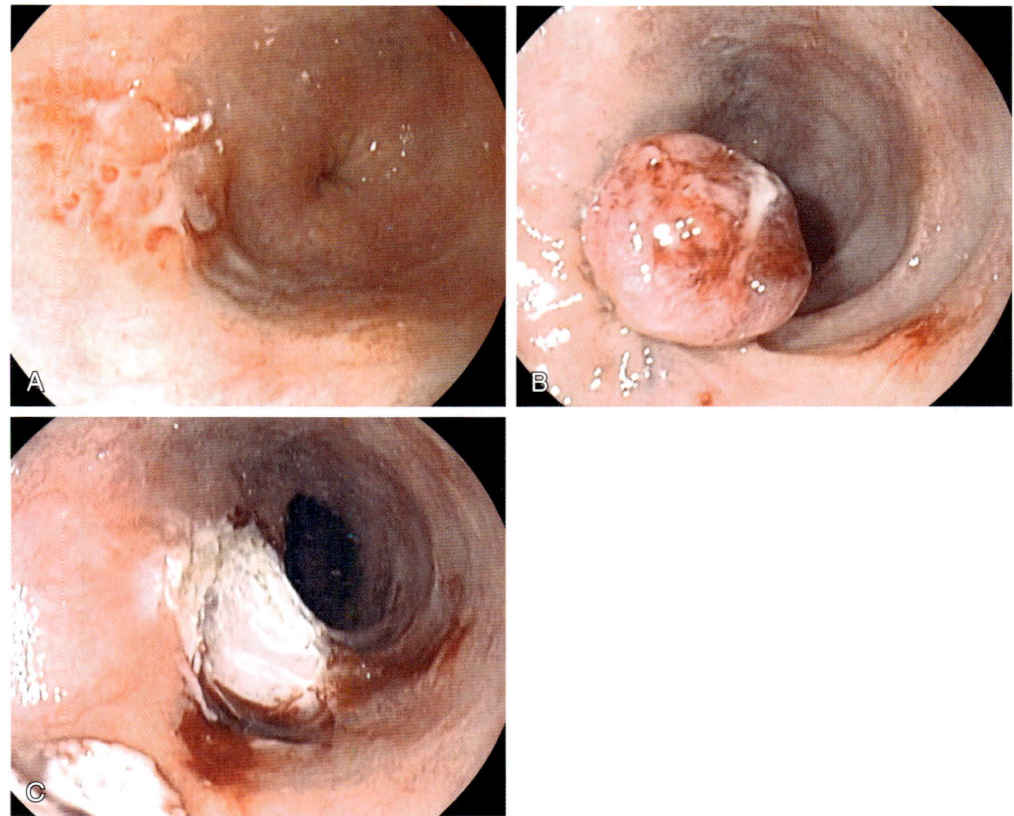

FIGURE 33.3 Endoscopic photographs of a mucosal resection. (A) Biopsy shows 1-cm lesion at 9 o'clock position, which is high-grade dysplasia and intramucosal adenocarcinoma. (B) Pseudopolyp after endoscopic cap/band application. (C) Completed resection. The lesion was completely excised.

Since there is risk associated with ablative therapy and the risk of progression seems variable within the patient population of LGD, emphasis has been placed on identifying those who are at increased risk within this population. There is some consensus that a patient with Barrett esophagus and LGD on a single biopsy should undergo continued surveillance in the absence of high-risk features such as mucosal irregularity, multifocal, or long-segment disease. The timing of the second endoscopy has been recommended at a wide interval from 8 weeks to 12 months depending on the guidelines of several societies. LGD present on a second endoscopy is classified as persistent dysplasia. A recent multicenter, randomize trial found that the number of endoscopies with LGD was an independent predictor of progression in their multi-variate analysis.[58] When LGD is not found on subsequent examination, this is characterized as regressive disease. It is recognized that this may represent true regression, sampling error, or interobserver variability in the histologic examination. The significant effect that this determination has on treatment decisions makes the need for evaluation by two expert pathologists of paramount importance. A large retrospective cohort of the Netherlands' nationwide registry found that the risk of progression to HGD or esophageal adenocarcinoma was higher for those who had a diagnosis of LGD confirmed by expert patholo-gist compared with those where the diagnosis was not

confirmed.[64] Conflicting these data is evidence from a large Norwegian study showing a significant increase in the rate of progression of LGD compared with nondysplastic Barrett even when unconfirmed by a second pathologist. In the setting of persistent, multifocal, or long-segment disease, a detailed discussion regarding the risks of abla-tion (bleeding, stricture, perforation, continued need for surveillance, progression despite ablation) should be weighed against potentially decreasing the risk of progression to carcinoma. These risks were demonstrated by Phoa et al.[58] with 136 patients randomized at a 1:1 ratio to either ablative therapy or continued surveillance for 3 years. Ablation reduced the risk of progression to HGD or adenocarcinoma by 25.0% and the risk of progression to adenocarcinoma by 7.4%. Complete eradication occurred in 92.6% for dysplasia among patients in the ablation group and 88.2% for intestinal metaplasia. In addition, 19.1% of patients receiving ablation experienced adverse events related to their treatment, with eight patients developing an esophageal stricture. This study was terminated early due to the superiority of ablation in reducing risk of adenocarcinoma. The available evidence suggests that at a diagnosis of LGD, patients should undergo aggressive management of their reflux disease, ideally with antireflux surgery given multiple studies showing regression of LGD postfundoplication. Repeat endoscopy and biopsies are recommended at 3 to 6 months, and if dysplasia persists, ablation with a low-risk modality such as RFA is recommended to reduce the risk of progression to HGD or adenocarcinoma in suitable candidates.

High-Grade Dysplasia and Intramucosal Adenocarcinoma

Although esophagectomy was once the standard of care for those diagnosed with HGD or early carcinoma, EMR has recently gained favor, as it has been shown to be safe, effective, and less invasive than traditional resection.[65] EMR allows for better, more definitive histologic examination of the specimen for diagnosis or staging and is curative in nearly all patients with disease limited to the mucosa. Patients with Barrett esophagus and either HGD or superficial esophageal adenocarcinoma should undergo an in-depth evaluation prior to treatment with endoscopic therapies. Again, the histopathology evaluation by two independent pathologists with expertise in this area is emphasized to decrease the rate of false-positive results and subsequent risk of unnecessary therapy. A thorough endoscopic evaluation at centers with high proficiency should be undertaken, using high-resolution endoscopes and a meticulous systematic approach to biopsy and EMR of concerning areas. High-resolution modalities such as narrow band imaging (NBI) have shown promise for identifying mucosal abnormalities. However, the vascular and mucosal patterns seen with NBI have currently not been standardized or validated, making utilization outside of high-volume centers limited. If referral to a high-volume center is not possible, we recommend using the Seattle protocol[66] in which four-quadrant biopsies are taken at 1-cm increments, beginning at the proximal gastric folds to the most proximal extent of intestinal metaplasia. It is imperative that all mucosal abnormalities receive separate targeted biopsies, as they are especially high risk of harboring pathology of interest. The authors of this system concluded that 50% of cancers detected using this approach would have been missed by standard protocol techniques.

For patients with nonnodular Barrett esophagus and HGD, ablative therapy is preferable to both intense surveillance and surgery due to the risk of progression and favorable morbidity profile.[65] Pradad et al.[67] performed a retrospective review of treatment of HGD in 129 patients who received treatment with a combination of EMR and PDT. This was compared with 70 patients who underwent esophagectomy. Mean follow-up was 5 years. None of the patients in either cohort died of esophageal cancer, although one patient did die because of a postoperative complication. In a multicenter, sham-controlled trial of 127 patients by Shaheen et al.,[57] complete eradication was obtained in 81% of patients with HGD. The rate of progression to esophageal adenocarcinoma was decreased from 19% to 2.4% ($P = .04$). No perforations or deaths were associated with the treatment.

In instances of mucosal irregularity due to nodularity, ulceration, or irregular mucosal contour, EMR can be both diagnostic and therapeutic. The pathologic findings from the EMR specimen should guide the next steps in therapy. If EMR is used in the setting of nondysplastic Barrett esophagus for mucosal irregularities and no dysplasia is found after complete resection, then surveillance may continue without change. Mucosal irregularities that demonstrate either LGD or HGD on EMR should undergo ablation of the remainder of the intestinal metaplasia. An intramucosal (T1a) lesion may be treated with endoscopic ablative therapy to the surrounding Barrett, as the risk of lymph node metastasis is low. The presence of poorly differentiated histology, lymphovascular invasion, or invasion into the submucosa (T1b) should prompt discussion of further treatment plan in the setting of a multidisciplinary oncology group, considering the patient's functional status, specific risk tolerances, and goals of care. In most circumstances, submucosal (T1b) invasion represents a significant risk for lymph node metastases and is an indication for esophagectomy and lymph node dissection.

Endoscopic techniques have demonstrated safety and efficacy in the treatment of early esophageal adenocarcinoma. Pech et al.[65] evaluated a cohort of 114 patients treated with either transthoracic esophagectomy or EMR in conjunction with APC for T1 lesions. The major complication rate was found to be 32% in the surgery group, and 0% in the endoscopic group. There was one mortality in the surgery group, which was not tumor related, and none in the endoscopic group at approximately 4 years' follow-up. The recurrence rate after endoscopic therapy was 6.6%, of which all were managed endoscopically. EMR of the known lesion is not adequate therapy as up to one-third of patients with complete resection develop metachronous lesions in the residual Barrett mucosa. Ablation or resection of the remainder of the intestinal metaplasia is needed to decrease this risk.

Complete resection of T1b lesions is possible with EMR or endoscopic submucosal dissection (ESD). The major factor limiting this as a curative therapy is that the risk of lymph node metastasis becomes significant as the tumor invades into the submucosa.[68] Sepesi et al.[69] demonstrated lymph node metastasis in 21% to 50% of patients depending on the level of submucosa involved (sm1-3) in 29 patients. Increasing rates of lymph node involvement have not been dependably shown based on the depth of the submucosa involved, and neither positron emission tomography nor endoscopic ultrasound has proven sensitive enough in these situations to warrant routine use. The first and most critical step in staging is endoscopic resection of the lesion with pathologic evaluation of the depth of invasion and risk factors for node metastases including size greater than 2 cm, poor differentiation, and lymphovascular invasion. There is some evidence that low-risk submucosal lesions may be treated endoscopically, particularly in patients at increased risk for esophagectomy.

RESECTION FOR DYSPLASTIC BARRETT ESOPHAGUS

As mentioned earlier, until recently, esophagectomy was the standard of care for the treatment of Barrett esophagus with HGD. Reported rates of esophageal adenocarcinoma found in the final pathology around 40% made any other approach prohibitively risky in the surgical candidate.[70] Two major changes have occurred that have shifted the use of formal resection to a second-line treatment. First, endoscopic therapy has emerged with a favorable risk and efficacy profile as detailed earlier. Second, the rate of esophageal adenocarcinoma seems be below previous estimations (as biopsy protocols and EMR make understaging less likely). Recent studies have demonstrated values between 6% and 13%.[71-73] However, this does not mean that there is no longer a role for surgical resection in the treatment of dysplastic Barrett or intramucosal adenocarcinoma. Although the rate of occult invasive esophageal cancer is much lower than 40%, it is not 0%, and factors such as multifocal or nodular disease have been associated with increased risk[73,74]; treatment with esophagectomy in this group was recently found to have increased utility and cost effectiveness compared with EMR-RFA.[75] Patients who have a relatively low operative risk estimation based on a lack of comorbid conditions in the setting of high-risk tumor features should be carefully counseled regarding the treatment options and potential outcomes.

Finally, esophagectomy should be considered in those who fail endoscopic therapy. A multicenter sham-controlled trial found that after four sessions (12 months' follow-up), HGD persisted in 19% of patients.[57] With continued treatment this number was decreased to 7% at 2 years.[76] The study protocol excluded those with nodular Barrett or disease segments greater than 8 cm, which likely improved their results. Pech et al. reported a failure rate of 3.7% of endoscopic therapy in a population of patients with HGD[65] and 1000 consecutive patients with T1a lesions.[77] The definition of failed endoscopic therapy remains largely subjective, although failure to make progress in eradication of disease is commonly used. Hunt et al.[78] studied 15 patients who underwent esophagectomy after endoscopic therapy. They found that those with invasive esophageal cancer on final pathology underwent more procedures to attempt eradication on average (6.5 vs. 3). Following esophagectomy at specialized high-volume centers, the 5-year survival rates approach 90%.[79]

CONCLUSION

Much has been learned in the 66 years since Norman Barrett's early description of the condition that bears his name. There have been several paradigm shifts in the way that we think about and treat the disease. This trend is sure to continue and our current practices will someday be historic, as interventions become increasingly efficacious and less invasive. As for now, treatment of Barrett esophagus remains steeped in controversy, complex, and highly challenging across its spectrum and highlights the importance of a multispecialty and modality approach to these patients.

REFERENCES

1. Barrett NR. Chronic peptic ulcer of the esophagus and "oesophagitis". *Br J Surg*. 1950;38:175-182.
2. Lord RV. Norman Barrett, "doyen of esophageal surgery". *Ann Surg*. 1999;229:428-439.
3. Allison PR, Johnstone AS. The oesophagus lined with gastric mucous membrane. *Thorax*. 1953;8:87-101.
4. Spechler SJ. Barrett's esophagus. *Semin Gastrointest Dis*. 1996;7:51-60.
5. Cook MB, Wild CP, Forman D. A systematic review and meta-analysis of the sex ratio for Barrett's esophagus, erosive reflux disease, and nonerosive reflux disease. *Am J Epidemiol*. 2005;162:1050-1061.
6. Corley DA, Kubo A, Levin TR, et al. Abdominal obesity and body mass index as risk factors for Barrett's esophagus. *Gastroenterology*. 2007;133:34-41, quiz 311.
7. Kramer JR, Fischbach LA, Richardson P, et al. Waist-to-hip ratio, but not body mass index, is associated with an increased risk of Barrett's esophagus in white men. *Clin Gastroenterol Hepatol*. 2013;11:373-381, e1.
8. Rubenstein JH, Morgenstern H, Appelman H, et al. Prediction of Barrett's esophagus among men. *Am J Gastroenterol*. 2013;108:353-362.
9. Andrici J, Tio M, Cox MR, Eslick GD. Hiatal hernia and the risk of Barrett's esophagus. *J Gastroenterol Hepatol*. 2013;28:415-431.
10. Fischbach LA, Graham DY, Kramer JR, et al. Association between *Helicobacter pylori* and Barrett's esophagus: a case-control study. *Am J Gastroenterol*. 2014;109:357-368.
11. Wang A, Mattek NC, Holub JL, Lieberman DA, Eisen GM. Prevalence of complicated gastroesophageal reflux disease and Barrett's esophagus among racial groups in a multi-center consortium. *Dig Dis Sci*. 2009;54:964-971.
12. Corley DA, Kubo A, Levin TR, et al. Race, ethnicity, sex and temporal differences in Barrett's oesophagus diagnosis: a large community-based study, 1994–2006. *Gut*. 2009;58:182-188.
13. Nguyen TH, Thrift AP, Ramsey D, et al. Risk factors for Barrett's esophagus compared between African Americans and non-Hispanic Whites. *Am J Gastroenterol*. 2014;109:1870-1880.
14. Su Z, Gay LJ, Strange A, et al. Common variants at the MHC locus and at chromosome 16q24.1 predispose to Barrett's esophagus. *Nat Genet*. 2012;44:1131-1136.
15. Rodriguez S, Mattek N, Lieberman D, Fennerty B, Eisen G. Barrett's esophagus on repeat endoscopy: should we look more than once? *Am J Gastroenterol*. 2008;103:1892-1897.
16. Loughney T, Maydonovitch CL, Wong RK. Esophageal manometry and ambulatory 24-hour pH monitoring in patients with short and long segment Barrett's esophagus. *Am J Gastroenterol*. 1998;93:916-919.
17. Rudolph RE, Vaughan TL, Storer BE, et al. Effect of segment length on risk for neoplastic progression in patients with Barrett's esophagus. *Ann Intern Med*. 2000;132:612-620.
18. Hirota WK, Loughney TM, Lazas DJ, Maydonovitch CL, Rholl V, Wong RK. Specialized intestinal metaplasia, dysplasia, and cancer of the esophagus and esophagogastric junction: prevalence and clinical data. *Gastroenterology*. 1999;116:277-285.
19. Shaheen NJ, Falk GW, Iyer PG, Gerson LB. ACG clinical guideline: diagnosis and management of Barrett's esophagus. *Am J Gastroenterol*. 2016;111:30-50.
20. Fitzgerald RC, di Pietro M, Ragunath K, et al. British Society of Gastroenterology guidelines on the diagnosis and management of Barrett's oesophagus. *Gut*. 2014;63:7-42.
21. Grant KS, DeMeester SR, Kreger V, et al. Effect of Barrett's esophagus surveillance on esophageal preservation, tumor stage, and survival with esophageal adenocarcinoma. *J Thorac Cardiovasc Surg*. 2013;146:31-37.
22. Corley DA, Mehtani K, Quesenberry C, Zhao W, de Boer J, Weiss NS. Impact of endoscopic surveillance on mortality from Barrett's esophagus-associated esophageal adenocarcinomas. *Gastroenterology*. 2013;145:312-319.e1.
23. Demeester SR, Demeester TR. Ineffective surveillance does not improve survival in patients with Barrett's who progress to adenocarcinoma. *Gastroenterology*. 2014;146:588.
24. Verbeek RE, Leenders M, Ten Kate FJ, et al. Surveillance of Barrett's esophagus and mortality from esophageal adenocarcinoma: a population-based cohort study. *Am J Gastroenterol*. 2014;109:1215-1222.
25. Konturek PC, Burnat G, Hahn EG. Inhibition of Barret's adenocarcinoma cell growth by simvastatin: involvement of COX-2 and apoptosis-related proteins. *J Physiol Pharmacol*. 2007;58(suppl 3):141-148.
26. Ogunwobi OO, Beales IL. Statins inhibit proliferation and induce apoptosis in Barrett's esophageal adenocarcinoma cells. *Am J Gastroenterol*. 2008;103:825-837.
27. Nguyen T, Duan Z, Naik AD, Kramer JR, El-Serag HB. Statin use reduces risk of esophageal adenocarcinoma in US veterans with Barrett's esophagus: a nested case-control study. *Gastroenterology*. 2015;149:1392-1398.
28. Singh S, Singh AG, Singh PP, Murad MH, Iyer PG. Statins are associated with reduced risk of esophageal cancer, particularly in patients with Barrett's esophagus: a systematic review and meta-analysis. *Clin Gastroenterol Hepatol*. 2013;11:620-629.

29. Beales IL, Hensley A, Loke Y. Reduced esophageal cancer incidence in statin users, particularly with cyclo-oxygenase inhibition. *World J Gastrointest Pharmacol Ther.* 2013;4:69-79.

30. Buttar NS, Wang KK, Anderson MA, et al. The effect of selective cyclooxygenase-2 inhibition in Barrett's esophagus epithelium: an in vitro study. *J Natl Cancer Inst.* 2002;94:422-429.

31. Heath EI, Canto MI, Piantadosi S, et al. Secondary chemoprevention of Barrett's esophagus with celecoxib: results of a randomized trial. *J Natl Cancer Inst.* 2007;99:545-557.

32. Kastelein F, Spaander MC, Steyerberg EW, et al. Proton pump inhibitors reduce the risk of neoplastic progression in patients with Barrett's esophagus. *Clin Gastroenterol Hepatol.* 2013;11:382-388.

33. El-Serag HB, Aguirre TV, Davis S, Kuebeler M, Bhattacharyya A, Sampliner RE. Proton pump inhibitors are associated with reduced incidence of dysplasia in Barrett's esophagus. *Am J Gastroenterol.* 2004;99:1877-1883.

34. Nguyen DM, El-Serag HB, Henderson L, Stein D, Bhattacharyya A, Sampliner RE. Medication usage and the risk of neoplasia in patients with Barrett's esophagus. *Clin Gastroenterol Hepatol.* 2009;7:1299-1304.

35. Gerson LB, Boparai V, Ullah N, Triadafilopoulos G. Oesophageal and gastric pH profiles in patients with gastro-oesophageal reflux disease and Barrett's oesophagus treated with proton pump inhibitors. *Aliment Pharmacol Ther.* 2004;20:637-643.

36. Yachimski P, Maqbool S, Bhat YM, Richter JE, Falk GW, Vaezi MF. Control of acid and duodenogastroesophageal reflux (DGER) in patients with Barrett's esophagus. *Am J Gastroenterol.* 2015;110:1143-1148.

37. Spechler SJ, Sharma P, Traxler B, Levine D, Falk GW. Gastric and esophageal pH in patients with Barrett's esophagus treated with three esomeprazole dosages: a randomized, double-blind, crossover trial. *Am J Gastroenterol.* 2006;101:1964-1971.

38. Thrift AP, Kramer JR, Qureshi Z, Richardson PA, El-Serag HB. Age at onset of GERD symptoms predicts risk of Barrett's esophagus. *Am J Gastroenterol.* 2013;108:915-922.

39. Eisen GM, Sandler RS, Murray S, Gottfried M. The relationship between gastroesophageal reflux disease and its complications with Barrett's esophagus. *Am J Gastroenterol.* 1997;92:27-31.

40. Kauer WK, Peters JH, DeMeester TR, Ireland AP, Bremner CG, Hagen JA. Mixed reflux of gastric and duodenal juices is more harmful to the esophagus than gastric juice alone. The need for surgical therapy re-emphasized. *Ann Surg.* 1995;222:525-531, discussion 31-33.

41. Sun D, Wang X, Gai Z, Song X, Jia X, Tian H. Bile acids but not acidic acids induce Barrett's esophagus. *Int J Clin Exp Pathol.* 2015;8:1384-1392.

42. Vaezi MF, Richter JE. Synergism of acid and duodenogastroesophageal reflux in complicated Barrett's esophagus. *Surgery.* 1995;117:699-704.

43. Fein M, Ireland AP, Ritter MP, et al. Duodenogastric reflux potentiates the injurious effects of gastroesophageal reflux. *J Gastrointest Surg.* 1997;1:27-32, discussion 33.

44. Stein HJ, Feussner H, Kauer W, DeMeester TR, Siewert JR. Alkaline gastroesophageal reflux: assessment by ambulatory esophageal aspiration and pH monitoring. *Am J Surg.* 1994;167:163-168.

45. Galmiche JP, Hatlebakk J, Attwood S, et al. Laparoscopic antireflux surgery vs esomeprazole treatment for chronic GERD: the LOTUS randomized clinical trial. *JAMA.* 2011;305:1969-1977.

46. Attwood SE, Lundell L, Hatlebakk JG, et al. Medical or surgical management of GERD patients with Barrett's esophagus: the LOTUS trial 3-year experience. *J Gastrointest Surg.* 2008;12:1646-1654, [discussion 54-55].

47. Hofstetter WL, Peters JH, DeMeester TR, et al. Long-term outcome of antireflux surgery in patients with Barrett's esophagus. *Ann Surg.* 2001;234:532-538, discussion 538-539.

48. Parrilla P, Martinez de Haro LF, Ortiz A, et al. Long-term results of a randomized prospective study comparing medical and surgical treatment of Barrett's esophagus. *Ann Surg.* 2003;237:291-298.

49. Morrow E, Bushyhead D, Wassenaar E, et al. The impact of laparoscopic anti-reflux surgery in patients with Barrett's esophagus. *Surg Endosc.* 2014;28:3279-3284.

50. Oelschlager BK, Barreca M, Chang L, Oleynikov D, Pellegrini CA. Clinical and pathologic response of Barrett's esophagus to laparoscopic antireflux surgery. *Ann Surg.* 2003;238:458-464, discussion 464-466.

51. Brand DL, Ylvisaker JT, Gelfand M, Pope CE 2nd. Regression of columnar esophageal (Barrett's) epithelium after anti-reflux surgery. *N Engl J Med.* 1980;302:844-848.

52. Gurski RR, Peters JH, Hagen JA, et al. Barrett's esophagus can and does regress after antireflux surgery: a study of prevalence and predictive features. *J Am Coll Surg.* 2003;196:706-712, discussion 712-713.

53. Zaninotto G, Parente P, Salvador R, et al. Long-term follow-up of Barrett's epithelium: medical versus antireflux surgical therapy. *J Gastrointest Surg.* 2012;16:7-14, discussion 14-15.

54. Zehetner J, DeMeester SR, Ayazi S, et al. Long-term follow-up after anti-reflux surgery in patients with Barrett's esophagus. *J Gastrointest Surg.* 2010;14:1483-1491.

55. Lagergren J, Ye W, Lagergren P, Lu Y. The risk of esophageal adenocarcinoma after antireflux surgery. *Gastroenterology.* 2010;138:1297-1301.

56. Lofdahl HE, Lu Y, Lagergren P, Lagergren J. Risk factors for esophageal adenocarcinoma after antireflux surgery. *Ann Surg.* 2013;257:579-582.

57. Shaheen NJ, Sharma P, Overholt BF, et al. Radiofrequency ablation in Barrett's esophagus with dysplasia. *N Engl J Med.* 2009;360:2277-2288.

58. Phoa KN, van Vilsteren FG, Weusten BL, et al. Radiofrequency ablation vs endoscopic surveillance for patients with Barrett esophagus and low-grade dysplasia: a randomized clinical trial. *JAMA.* 2014;311:1209-1217.

59. Overholt BF, Lightdale CJ, Wang KK, et al. Photodynamic therapy with porfimer sodium for ablation of high-grade dysplasia in Barrett's esophagus: international, partially blinded, randomized phase III trial. *Gastrointest Endosc.* 2005;62:488-498.

60. Manner H, May A, Miehlke S, et al. Ablation of nonneoplastic Barrett's mucosa using argon plasma coagulation with concomitant esomeprazole therapy (APBANEX): a prospective multicenter evaluation. *Am J Gastroenterol.* 2006;101:1762-1769.

61. Ferraris R, Fracchia M, Foti M, et al. Barrett's oesophagus: long-term follow-up after complete ablation with argon plasma coagulation and the factors that determine its recurrence. *Aliment Pharmacol Ther.* 2007;25:835-840.

62. Gray NA, Odze RD, Spechler SJ. Buried metaplasia after endoscopic ablation of Barrett's esophagus: a systematic review. *Am J Gastroenterol.* 2011;106:1899-1908, quiz 1909.

63. Wani S, Falk GW, Post J, et al. Risk factors for progression of low-grade dysplasia in patients with Barrett's esophagus. *Gastroenterology.* 2011;141:1179-1186, 1186.e1.

64. Duits LC, Phoa KN, Curvers WL, et al. Barrett's oesophagus patients with low-grade dysplasia can be accurately risk-stratified after histological review by an expert pathology panel. *Gut.* 2015;64:700-706.

65. Pech O, Bollschweiler E, Manner H, Leers J, Ell C, Holscher AH. Comparison between endoscopic and surgical resection of mucosal esophageal adenocarcinoma in Barrett's esophagus at two high-volume centers. *Ann Surg.* 2011;254:67-72.

66. Reid BJ, Blount PL, Feng Z, Levine DS. Optimizing endoscopic biopsy detection of early cancers in Barrett's high-grade dysplasia. *Am J Gastroenterol.* 2000;95:3089-3096.

67. Prasad GA, Wang KK, Buttar NS, et al. Long-term survival following endoscopic and surgical treatment of high-grade dysplasia in Barrett's esophagus. *Gastroenterology.* 2007;132:1226-1233.

68. Badreddine RJ, Prasad GA, Lewis JT, et al. Depth of submucosal invasion does not predict lymph node metastasis and survival of patients with esophageal carcinoma. *Clin Gastroenterol Hepatol.* 2010;8:248-253.

69. Sepesi B, Watson TJ, Zhou D, et al. Are endoscopic therapies appropriate for superficial submucosal esophageal adenocarcinoma? An analysis of esophagectomy specimens. *J Am Coll Surg.* 2010;210:418-427.

70. Edwards MJ, Gable DR, Lentsch AB, Richardson JD. The rationale for esophagectomy as the optimal therapy for Barrett's esophagus with high-grade dysplasia. *Ann Surg.* 1996;223:585-589, discussion 589-591.

71. Nasr JY, Schoen RE. Prevalence of adenocarcinoma at esophagectomy for Barrett's esophagus with high grade dysplasia. *J Gastrointest Oncol.* 2011;2:34-38.

72. Wang VS, Hornick JL, Sepulveda JA, Mauer R, Poneros JM. Low prevalence of submucosal invasive carcinoma at esophagectomy for high-grade dysplasia or intramucosal adenocarcinoma in Barrett's esophagus: a 20-year experience. *Gastrointest Endosc.* 2009;69:777-783.

73. Konda VJ, Ross AS, Ferguson MK, et al. Is the risk of concomitant invasive esophageal cancer in high-grade dysplasia in Barrett's esophagus overestimated? *Clin Gastroenterol Hepatol.* 2008;6:159-164.

74. Buttar NS, Wang KK, Sebo TJ, et al. Extent of high-grade dysplasia in Barrett's esophagus correlates with risk of adenocarcinoma. *Gastroenterology.* 2001;120:1630-1639.

75. Hu Y, Puri V, Shami VM, Stukenborg GJ, Kozower BD. Comparative effectiveness of esophagectomy versus endoscopic treatment for esophageal high-grade dysplasia. *Ann Surg.* 2016;263:719-726.

76. Shaheen NJ, Overholt BF, Sampliner RE, et al. Durability of radiofrequency ablation in Barrett's esophagus with dysplasia. *Gastroenterology.* 2011;141:460-468.

77. Pech O, May A, Manner H, et al. Long-term efficacy and safety of endoscopic resection for patients with mucosal adenocarcinoma of the esophagus. *Gastroenterology.* 2014;146:652-660.e1.

78. Hunt BM, Louie BE, Dunst CM, et al. Esophagectomy for failed endoscopic therapy in patients with high-grade dysplasia or intramucosal carcinoma. *Dis Esophagus.* 2014;27:362-367.

79. Peters JH, Clark GW, Ireland AP, Chandrasoma P, Smyrk TC, DeMeester TR. Outcome of adenocarcinoma arising in Barrett's esophagus in endoscopically surveyed and nonsurveyed patients. *J Thorac Cardiovasc Surg.* 1994;108:813-821, discussion 21-22.

Ablation for Patients With Barrett or Dysplasia

B. Mark Smithers | Iain Thomson

Compared with the general population, patients with Barrett esophagus (BE) have a higher risk of developing esophageal adenocarcinoma (EAC) with the risk increasing in those patients who develop dysplasia—low-grade dysplasia (LGD) or high-grade dysplasia (HGD).[1] In the past, patients with HGD or proven intramucosal adenocarcinoma (IMC) will have been considered for an esophagectomy, if they were medically suitable. This major procedure clearly removes the pathology, as well as the whole Barrett segment, but at a cost of morbidity and mortality. Now the evidence supports the use of endoscopic therapies with endoscopic resection of localized lesions such as early mucosal adenocarcinoma or segments of HGD, aiming to completely remove the neoplastic segment. However, the residual untreated BE is left in situ with a significant risk of recurrent neoplasia, being reported in up to one-third of patients.[2,3] This has led to a focus on therapies aimed at eradicating this high-risk mucosa allowing regrowth of squamous epithelium. With the incidence of BE and adenocarcinoma increasing in Western countries along with improved outcomes and greater experience of Barrett mucosal ablation, there has been a trend to expand ablation to patients who have not had HGD or IMC but may have LGD or even consider ablation in patient with nondysplastic BE (NDBE). Thus for every patient the role and value of these treatments must be weighed against the impact of the treatment on the individual from a cancer prevention perspective, the impact on quality of life both after treatment and in the long term, and the cost implications to the community.

The optimal ablative therapy would completely eliminate the mucosa to the submucosa, in a single session, with very few side effects, and offer the patient a lifetime guarantee of no recurrence following complete squamous re-epithelialization of the treated segment.[4] We are not there yet. The ablation techniques that have been used include endoscopic resection of a focal lesion or of the complete BE segment and mucosal ablation techniques such as radiofrequency ablation (RFA), photodynamic therapy (PDT), argon plasma coagulation (APC), laser therapy, and cryotherapy. Presently the most commonly applied techniques are endoscopic resection of a focal abnormality with RFA of the residual dysplastic or non-dysplastic Barrett esophagus (NDBE). The indications for Barrett ablation, along with the techniques and their outcomes, will be described in this chapter.

WHICH PATIENTS WITH BARRETT SHOULD HAVE ABLATION?

For a clinician to consider performing a significant intervention on a patient, one must be secure the diagnosis is

BE and when dysplastic changes are reported, that this is a true reflection of a potential neoplastic process. Chapter 31 has addressed the issues related to the definition of Barrett intestinal metaplasia that, when present, will lead to endoscopic surveillance. If there is a diagnosis of dysplasia at endoscopy, the management implications change for the patient and the clinician. However, pathologic consensus of the histologic diagnosis can be a problem, and the dysplastic changes may not be present on subsequent biopsies, particularly LGD. The diagnosis of HGD, confirmed by a second pathologist with gastrointestinal (GI) expertise, carries a clear risk for progression to adenocarcinoma such that all these patients should be considered for definitive treatment of the neoplastic lesion as well as ablation of the whole BE segment. The alternative is an esophagectomy.[5-7] The presence of visible lesions (nodules or ulceration) in a segment of HGD carries significant implications. If nodules are present, there is a 2.6 times potential for progression to EAC,[8] and if ulceration is present, the risk of the presence of EAC in a high-grade dysplastic segment has been reported to be 80%, compared with 52% if there was no ulceration.[9] Endoscopic resection of these abnormalities, if possible, offers better pathologic staging and complete resection and should be performed before attempts at BE ablation. Patients with a diagnosis of IMC that has been endoscopically completely removed will need ablation of the residual BE segment.

Patients with confirmed LGD in BE will require more regular endoscopic surveillance, and there is evidence to support considering this group for complete BE ablation. However, the diagnosis of LGD needs to be secure. There has been a meta-analysis of the outcomes from endoscopic therapies for LGD, which assessed 37 studies comprising 521 patients. The multiple techniques of ablation used provided complete eradication (CE) of dysplasia in 88.9% and intestinal metaplasia (IM) in 67.8%, with a pooled incidence of progression to cancer of 3.9 (95% CI, 1.27 to 9.1) per 1000 patient-years. The authors concluded that there was likely to be histologic overdiagnosis of LGD. RFA was the most safe and effective option in this group, but ablation did not eliminate the risk of progression to HGD or EAC.[10]

The potential for "overdiagnosis" of LGD and the consequences have been highlighted by a number of studies. In a group of patients diagnosed with LGD by community pathologists, where subsequent review by expert GI pathologists occurred, the diagnosis was downgraded in 85% of patients to NDBE or indefinite dysplasia.[11] In the "downgraded group" the risk of progression to HGD or EAC was 0.49% per patient per year, compared with the group confirmed to have LGD where the progression was 13.4%.[11] In a Dutch study, the percentage of diagnoses downgraded from LGD to indeterminate or NDBE was

73%, where expert pathologists reviewed the histology of 293 referred patients. At a median follow-up of 39 months, 21 of the 75 (27%) confirmed LGD patients progressed to HGD/EAC. The rate of progression was measured at 9.1% per patient-year compared with the pathologically reviewed NDBE group who had a rate of progression of 0.6 per patient-year.[12]

The multicenter European SURF trial randomized 136 patients with LGD to receive RFA ablation to the BE or surveillance, with both groups receiving proton pump inhibitor (PPI) therapy. There was CE of the dysplasia in 93% of the RFA group and 28% of the controls and CE of the IM in 88% of the RFA group compared with zero in the controls. At 3-year follow-up, the rate of progression to HGD was 1.5% after RFA compared with 26.5% in the surveillance group, and the rate of progression to EAC was 1.5% compared with 8.8%, respectively. They reported a neoplasia progression rate of 8% per year.[13] The rate of progression of LGD confirmed by an expert pathologist was further assessed in a cohort study of 170 patients, with 45 undergoing RFA ablation and 125 surveillance with median follow-up of more than 2 years. The rate of progression to HGD or EAC in the RFA group was 0.77% compared with 6.6% in the surveillance group. The measured risk of progression after RFA had a hazard ratio of 0.08 (95% CI, 0.01 to 0.61). In the surveillance group, following a multivariate analysis, independent factors associated with the risk of progression were nodularity in the BE and multifocal dysplasia.[14]

For LGD to be considered *confirmed*, guidelines recommend a second pathologist with GI expertise review the biopsies, and for a second endoscopy and biopsy after 6 months to reassess the BE and confirm the continued presence of the LGD.[15–18] In this group of patients with confirmed LGD, the data for a higher risk for progression to HGD and IMC are clear.[13] Using this definition for LGD, guidelines in the United States recommend endoscopic ablation to be appropriate for patients with confirmed LGD.[18] In the UK the published guidelines in 2014[15] were updated in 2016 when reviewed evidence supported the role of RFA to ablate confirmed LGD.[19] The factors that have been associated with higher rates of progression of LGD to HGD/EAC include male gender, NDBE present for more than 10 years, length of BE (>3 cm), persistent esophagitis, multifocal dysplasia, and the presence of nodules in the BE mucosa.[5,20] In a consensus statement from the BOBCAT group, it was agreed that there was "moderate quality evidence" to support the ablation of the high-risk LGD group. The criteria for considering ablating this group were consensus of the diagnosis by two expert pathologists, persistence of the LGD over time, multifocal dysplasia, and longer BE segments.[17]

ISSUES RELATING TO NONDYSPLASTIC BARRETT ESOPHAGUS AND ABLATION

With the improvement in the outcomes of the techniques for ablative therapy, the pendulum has swung to consider the role of this therapy for patients with NDBE. Reasons stated include anxiety to the potential for malignant progression that may not be identified from the random sampling, performed at the surveillance endoscopy. The patient perspective was highlighted in a study assessing patient preference in the management of NDBE where the options, hypothetically, were put for either chemoprevention with aspirin and 3 to 5 yearly surveillance endoscopies or endoscopic ablation. The patients preferred ablation.[21]

For ablation to be a realistic option in asymptomatic patients with NDBE, the treatment must be safe, be effective, have durable long-term results, and be cost effective. The safest, most effective treatment is RFA. In a cohort study of patients with NDBE who had RFA and regular follow-up with treatment of residual or recurrent IM, the complete regression rate was 70% at 1 year[22] and 92% at 5 years.[23] This group of patients required multiple endoscopies and the need for more intense surveillance than recommended for nontreated NDBE. The impact of this approach on the patients' longevity and quality of life along with the cost effectiveness is yet to be clearly defined.

With respect to cost effectiveness of BE ablation, in 2004, a study examined the management of HGD comparing endoscopic surveillance, endoablation (using PDT), and esophagectomy. Endoablation with PDT was shown to be the most effective strategy.[24] A recent literature review concluded that endoscopic therapy for dysplastic BE, using PDT or RFA, was cost effective compared with esophagectomy.[25] One single-institution cohort study reported the cost of PDT to be 5 times that of RFA.[26] Using a Markov model, assessing patients with HGD, RFA with continued surveillance is more cost effective than endoscopic surveillance and esophagectomy when a cancer develops.[27]

For patients with LGD, if confirmed by two pathologists and the diagnosis remains stable on repeated endoscopies when assessing quality-adjusted life years (QALYs), RFA is more cost effective than continued regular surveillance and performing the RFA when HGD develops.[27] Although the American Society of Gastroenterology (ASGE) has recommended ablation is an "option" for NDBE,[16] the evidence suggests this is not cost effective, due to the low rate of progression to adenocarcinoma in this group of patients.[25,27]

At this time, for NDBE there is no evidence that supports the routine use of ablative therapies. In the future, for ablation to be considered, there will need to be a number of factors better defined. They may include selection of patients with longer life expectancy than average BE patients; identifying patients with higher risk for progression than the average patient without dysplasia, most likely through a panel of biomarkers; identifying which patients will do well with RFA and which group has a higher risk of failing; and finally creating a situation whereby minimal surveillance is required, as well as a reduced need to "touch up" the ablated segments.[28]

ABLATIVE TECHNIQUES: METHODS, OUTCOMES, AND COMPLICATIONS

The aims of ablation are to eliminate all the intestinal metaplasia/dysplasia and provide a uniform depth of treatment to allow squamous reepithelialization with minimal residual IM. Assessment of the outcomes of these procedures relates to the efficacy of the eradication of the dysplastic and NDBE, as well as the durability with respect to the long-term eradication of the at-risk mucosa,[26] along with the rate of adverse effects from the procedure.

ENDOSCOPIC RESECTION

ER techniques include endoscopic mucosal resection (EMR) of a focal lesion typically combined with other ablation techniques, complete EMR or serial radical endoscopic resection (SRER) aiming to remove the whole segment in a piecemeal stepwise fashion, or more rarely endoscopic submucosal dissection (ESD), which resects en bloc the mucosa and submucosa to the muscularis propria aiming to remove en bloc a lesion or Barrett segment.

ENDOSCOPIC MUCOSAL RESECTION

Not only potentially therapeutic, by completely removing a neoplastic lesion, EMR also provides a specimen large enough to offer the pathologist a better assessment with the potential to alter the histologic diagnosis in nearly 50% of patients. EMR is typically aimed at removal of lesions less than 1.5 cm; otherwise the lesion may need piecemeal resection. The larger specimens offered to the pathologist may reduce the variation of interpretation that can occur when small sample biopsies are assessed among multiple pathologists. The larger specimen offers better T staging of an early adenocarcinoma.[29,30] As previously outlined, targeted EMR should be performed if there are identified visible abnormalities. Once an invasive cancer is excluded or IMC is completely resected endoscopically or HGD confirmed, patients will need the residual BE segment eradicated.

Endoscopic Mucosal Resection Technique

Single or multiple applications may be required depending upon the area of abnormal mucosa. The ER cap ("suck and cut") technique with oblique caps (12.8/14.8/18 mm diameter) allows piecemeal resection after a submucosal injection of a mixture containing a variable combination of the agents (NaCl, adrenaline 1:20,000, methylene blue, and hydroxymethyl cellulose). The lesion is sucked into cap and then cut with a preloaded snare. Multiband mucosectomy (MBM; "band and snare") uses a modified variceal band ligator (six bands) with a transparent cap and a channel that allows passage of a 7-French hexagonal snare. This technique allows the suction of mucosa to form a pseudopolyp, the base of which is "ligated" with a band. The polyp is resected with the snare, with up to six resections being possible. It can be performed with or without submucosal injection. The ER cap was compared with the MBM techniques and was found to be faster and less expensive, but it delivered smaller specimens although there was no difference in depth or complications. A simple band and snare technique, with or without submucosal injection, can also be performed.

STEPWISE RADICAL ENDOSCOPIC RESECTION

In this procedure, following a targeted resection of the abnormal neoplastic focus, multiple resections are then performed to remove the rest of the BE segment in a piecemeal fashion. The aim is to attempt 50% to 70% of

TABLE 34.1 Outcomes Following Stepwise Radical Endoscopic Resection for Barrett Esophagus

Outcomes	% of Patients
EFFICACY	
Complete eradication of dysplasia	95% (95% CI, 87%–99%)
Complete eradication of IM	89% (95% CI, 79%–95%)
DURABILITY	
2 years complete eradication of dysplasia	85%–100%
Complete eradication of IM	75%–100%
3–5 years complete eradication of IM	68%–95%
COMPLICATIONS	
Stricture	26%–88%
Perforation	2%–3%
Bleeding	2%–3%
Buried Barrett	3%–11%

IM, Intestinal metaplasia.

circumference resection at the first session. The technique usually requires two to three ER sessions per patient.[31,32]

In patients with HGD or IMC, SRER has been reported to provide CE of the neoplastic pathology in 81% to 100% and IM in 71% to 100%.[33–36] In a randomized controlled trial (RCT) of SRER compared with focal EMR and RFA, CE of BE was reported following SRER in 100%, compared with 96% who had EMR and RFA.[37] A systematic review assessing complete EMR (SRER) reported the efficacy to eradicate dysplastic BE to be 95% (95% CI, 87% to 99%) and IM 89% (95% CI, 79% to 95%). At a median follow-up time of 23 months, the durability was 85% to 100% for dysplastic BE and 75% to 100% for IM. In this study the upper limit of the length of BE was 5 cm.[38]

Although the incidence is low, the rate of bleeding and perforation (2% to 3%) is higher in patients having SRER than the other ablative techniques, with the majority managed endoscopically. In the RCT, the stricture rate in the SRER group was 88% compared with 14% in the EMR/RFA group.[37] The outcomes are summarized in Table 34.1.

ENDOSCOPIC SUBMUCOSAL DISSECTION

ESD has been widely used in Asia, notably for early neoplasia of the stomach, esophagus, and colorectum. The advantage is the ability to remove larger lesions en bloc in the plane between the submucosa and the muscularis propria. The lesion is outlined with a normal margin using cautery and is elevated using a submucosal fluid injection. An Endoknife is used to cut and coagulate the mucosa and submucosa, with Endograspers used for localized bleeding. A meta-analysis of ESD compared with EMR for removal of neoplastic lesions in the stomach, colorectum, and esophagus (three esophageal studies) confirmed ESD provided better rates of en bloc removal and curative resections with less local recurrence, but the procedure was more time-consuming, with higher rates of bleeding and perforation.[39] The largest series of patients who had ESD was reported from a unit where the procedure was selected to be performed in 75 patients from more than

TABLE 34.2 Summary Outcomes from Endoscopic Submucosal Dissection for Barrett Esophagus

Outcomes	% of Patients
EFFICACY	
Complete eradication of dysplasia	97%–100%
Complete eradication of IM	60%
DURABILITY	
2 years complete eradication of dysplasia	92%
2 years complete eradication of IM	75%
COMPLICATIONS	
Stricture	60%
Perforation	4%
Bleeding	3%
Buried Barrett	NS

IM, Intestinal metaplasia; *NS*, not stated.

300 patients being considered for endoscopic resection. The selection criteria were visible lesion, multiple lesions, and lesions larger than 15 mm or poorly lifting with submucosal injection.[40] En bloc resection of the relevant lesion occurred in 90%. Residual IM required further treatment (median 2) in 62%, using EMR, ESD, APC, or RFA. At a median of 20 months, the CE rate of neoplasia was 92% and IM 73%. There were two patients who had a delayed hemorrhage and three with perforation, all treated endoscopically. The stricture rate was 60% with regular dilations required; for some patients this was long term.[40] A study of 30 patients reported IMC and HGD complete resection rates of 97%, with en bloc removal of the abnormal lesion in 90%. The R0 rate was 39% due to lateral margin involvement with dysplasia.

ESD is more time-consuming, has more serious complications, and requires an extra level of expertise. There is no clear evidence for improved rates of CE of dysplasia or IM or reduced rate of progression to EAC, compared with SRER or focal EMR followed by BE ablation notably using RFA. It would seem that selective use of ESD in specialist units will remain the standard unless there are RCTs showing a benefit over EMR in the future. The outcomes are summarized in Table 34.2.

MUCOSAL ABLATION

The most frequently used mucosal ablation technique is RFA, because this procedure produces a more predictable degree of mucosal eradication and has a low side-effect profile.

RADIOFREQUENCY ABLATION

Ablation occurs through the transfer of heat using radiofrequency energy applied to the mucosa of the esophagus. The energy is delivered with an RFA delivery HALO device (BARRX Medical, Sunnydale, California) 10 to 12 J/cm², 40 W/cm². The devices used to transfer the energy are a HALO 360, 10 cm balloon used for circumferential energy transfer, or HALO 90 and 60 devices to allow treatment of Barrett islands. The energy delivered causes water vaporization, protein coagulation, and tissue necrosis. The HALO 360 involves a sizing balloon that generates pressure volume data and determines the esophageal

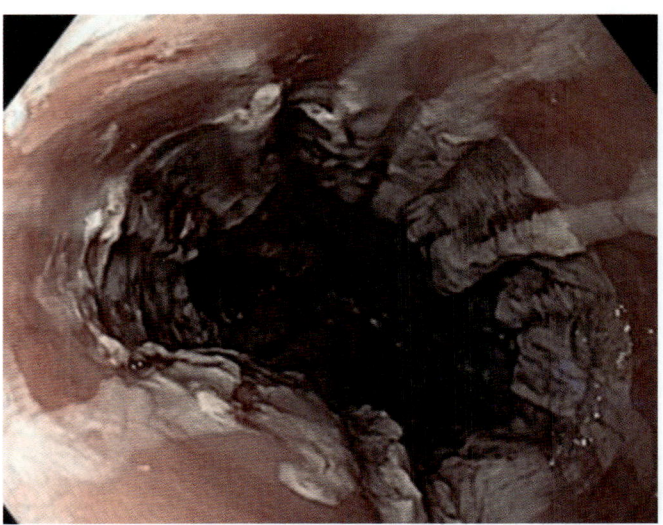

FIGURE 34.1 Appearance post radiofrequency ablation.

diameter to allow selection of the correct size ablation balloon catheter.[42] The ablation catheter is positioned, and then there is a double application of the energy applied (Fig. 34.1). RFA offers the most reliable destruction of the mucosa to the level of the submucosa. The efficacy of this technique at the time of the first application is reduced if there is a large hiatus hernia, longer segments of BE, esophagitis, and a narrow esophagus.[42]

The pivotal AIM trial was an RCT, which compared RFA with a sham endoscopy, with both groups receiving high-dose PPI therapy, and with recruitment on a 2:1 ratio, respectively. The 127 patients were stratified for the grade of dysplasia and the length of IM, and had intensive postprocedural surveillance. In the patients with HGD, at 12 months, on an intention-to-treat (ITT) analysis, following a mean of 3.5 treatments per patient, there was CE of the dysplasia in 81% compared with 19% in the controls. The segment of intestinal metaplasia was eradicated in 74% in the RFA group, compared with zero in the control group. In this high-risk population, one patient (2%) in the RFA group progressed to EAC and four (19%) in the sham group.[6] This trial also recruited patients with LGD. At 12 months, in the RFA group CE of the dysplasia occurred in 91% of the patients compared with 23% in the control patients. The number needed to treat (NNT) to avoid one persistent dysplasia was 1.5 patients.[6] At 3 years, the RFA group had CE of all dysplasia in 94% of patients and IM in 91%.[43]

Patients may require a number of treatments to achieve complete BE ablation. A study in the United States reported CE after one treatment in 29%, two treatments 35%, and for the rest it took up to 10 treatments. CE was achieved more quickly in younger patients and those with short-segment BE. This group reported a recurrence rate of IM of 20% at 1 year and 33% at 2 years. Others have also reported up to 55% of patients will require repeat ablations after the first 12 months to achieve ablation levels above 90%.[43]

Larger cohort studies have confirmed the efficacy of RFA. Most of these studies included patients with neoplastic lesions endoscopically removed with subsequent RFA

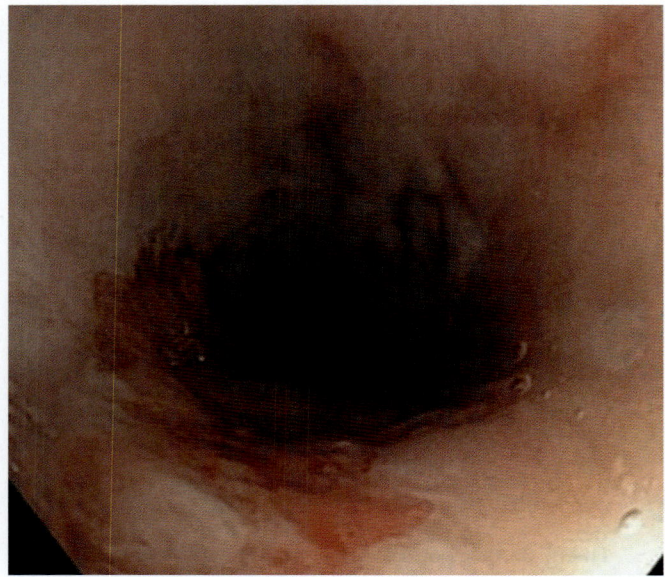

FIGURE 34.2 Post radiofrequency ablation recurrent intestinal metaplasia.

ablation. A US study with 244 patients (94%—dysplasia/IMC) reported CE of dysplasia in 87% and IM in 80%.[44] From the UK, the RFA registry reported results from 335 patients (HGD 72%, IMC 24%, LGD 4%) who had endoscopic resection of visible lesions and then RFA. At 12 months, the CE rate for HGD was 86%, dysplasia 81%, and IM 62%. Invasive carcinoma occurred in 3%. There was progression of neoplasia in 5% at 19 months' follow-up.[45] A multicenter European study with 132 patients (IMC 59%, HGD 23%, LGD 5%) reported CE of dysplasia in 91% and IM in 88%.[46]

Predictors of a poor response to RFA include active reflux esophagitis, EMR scar regeneration with new BE mucosa, esophageal lumen narrowing pre-RFA, and the number of years of neoplasia pretreatment.[47] Recurrence after RFA (Fig. 34.2) has been reported to present in three distinct patterns, including endoscopic invisible IM underneath the neosquamous epithelium (buried glands), visible recurrence in the tubular esophagus, and intestinal metaplasia typically seen at the gastroesophageal junction.[48] Usually the recurrence histologic grade is no worse than the pretreatment grade.[49]

The durability of RFA to treat IM was demonstrated from the longitudinal study (AIM II), which followed patients who had RFA to a segment of NDBE (2 to 6 cm). In the first year, RFA was repeated at 4 months if IM was present. At 1 year the CE rate was 70%, following further treatments the rate was 98% at 2.5 years, and when assessed at 5 years the rate was 92% with further ablation performed in those with residual IM. No patient had dysplasia or buried Barrett. The probability of CE of IM at 4 years was calculated to be 0.91 (95% CI, 0.77 to 0.97). Those who failed to convert to CE were treated with other modalities.[22,23]

The length of the BE may impact on the ability to clear the dysplasia and IM. When the ablation rates for a BE 4 to 8 cm were compared with the rates for segments greater than 8 cm, at follow-up of 45 and 34 months, respectively, equivalent dysplasia eradication rates of 88% and 90% and IM eradication rates of 82% and 77% were reported. The IM recurrence rate in the 4 to 8 cm group was 16% compared with 23% for the longer segments.[50] The 3-year IM CE rates were 82% and 65%, respectively. It was estimated that the potential for successful eradication of IM decreased by 13% for each extra 1 cm of BE.[51] A similar figure of 15% was reported when the effect of the length of BE and RFA efficacy was assessed from data in the UK registry.[45]

The potential for recurrence of dysplasia and IM after RFA is clear. At 5 years the CE rate of dysplasia and IM has been reported to be 90%.[46] The UK registry reported 4% of patients with recurrent dysplasia requiring further RFA, two of these patients 4 years post CE. A study from the United States with follow-up beyond 8 years reports the presence of IM in 33% of their cohort. Dysplastic histology was diagnosed in 22% of this group.[51] Using the US RFA registry to assess the risk of recurrence of IM, the 1634 patients confirmed to have histologic CE following treatment for IM (nondysplastic or indeterminate; 48%), LGD (20%), HGD (25%), or carcinoma (7%) were assessed for rate of recurrence of IM. With an average follow-up of 2.4 years, 20% developed recurrent IM (NDBE, 86%), 6% having upgraded histology. The progression to malignancy was 1.2%. The annual rate of recurrence was 9%. Using multivariate analysis, recurrence was more likely if patients were older, had longer lengths of BE, or were non-Caucasian.[52]

Lower long-term recurrence rates have been reported from other national studies. The UK registry reported a 9% recurrence rate and a study from the Netherlands reported 6% recurrence.[46] The US study included biopsies at the esophagogastric junction (EGJ) and cardia, with 28% of patients with IM at EGJ developing dysplasia by 3 years (75% of this group being HGD). However, the Netherlands study had IM at EGJ in 35% of patients but none developed dysplasia with a 61-month follow-up. The reason for the differences is not clear. Many reports of the recurrence or persistence of IM do not state the site. If the biopsies are from the cardia, the implication is unclear. The presence of intestinal metaplasia at the cardia is reported in 25% in a normal population.[53] In the Netherlands study, there were no neoplastic events in the cardia in their patients; however, the US study reported dysplastic progression. The relevance of these findings is to be defined in longer term studies where surveillance biopsies have included the cardia routinely.[49] It is clear that continued careful surveillance is necessary after patients have had RFA ablation and that the surveillance biopsies should include the cardia.

A systematic review and meta-analysis of studies, between 2008 and 2012, assessing RFA efficacy (18 studies, 3802 patients) and durability (6 studies, 540 patients) to ablate BE, with or without dysplasia, reported CE of dysplasia in 91% (95% CI, 87% to 95%), IM 78% (95% CI, 70% to 86%), with IM recurrence of 13% (95% CI, 9% to18%). Using the data to estimate the rate of progression to EAC related to the histology being ablated, the authors report the risk for NDBE to be 0.09%; LGD, 0.2%; HGD, 0.4%; and IMC 0.9%. These rates are less than the reported

TABLE 34.3 Outcomes from Radiofrequency Ablation With and Without Focal Endoscopic Mucosal Resection

Outcomes	EMR + RFA	RFA
EFFICACY		
Complete eradication of dysplasia	91% (95% CI, 87%–95%)	74%
Complete eradication of IM	78% (95% CI, 70–86)	80%–90%
DURABILITY		
4 years complete eradication of IM	91% (95% CI, 77%–97%)	
5 years complete eradication of IM		92%
COMPLICATIONS		
Stricture	4%–12%	4%
Buried Barrett	0	0.9%

EMR, Endoscopic mucosal resection; *IM,* intestinal metaplasia; *RFA,* radiofrequency ablation.

annual risk for untreated NDBE (0.12% to 0.6%)[1,5] and LGD/HGD (1.7/6.6%).[54]

It has been advocated that the gold standard is to concentrate the care of the patients in high-volume centers with the RFA performed in an environment of multidisciplinary expertise that includes well-trained endoscopists who have experience with the procedure and other endoscopic therapies and who will be involved in the follow-up, recognizing residual or recurrent lesions, expert GI pathology, and surgical backup.[4,55]

A systematic review comparing SRER with RFA (usually with focal EMR) assessed 22 studies (SRER 10, RFA 8, RCT 2). At 23 months, the eradication rate for dysplasia from SRER was 85% to 100% and at 21 months for RFA 79% to 100%. For IM, the rates were for SRER 75% to 100% and RFA 54% to 100%. Further treatments for persistent or recurrent disease was required more often following EMR (50%) compared with RFA (11%).[38] There were fewer short-term complications in the EMR with RFA group with no perforations, and one patient with bleeding. The stricture rate was 38% for SRER and 4% for RFA. Buried Barrett was found in 3% of the SRER group and none of the RFA group.

Stricture formation is the most common complication following RFA, with the incidence reported to be between 7% and 12%.[6,13,38] The predictors for a higher stricture rate were the use of nonsteroidal antiinflammatory drugs (NSAIDs), previous antireflux surgery, and a history of esophagitis.[6] Less common complications include upper GI hemorrhage, dysphagia, and transient retrosternal chest pain.[13] The outcomes for RFA and focal EMR with RFA are summarized in Table 34.3.

PHOTODYNAMIC THERAPY

Photochemical ablation using PDT uses a photosensitizer that accumulates in the Barrett mucosa and is activated by light energy applied during endoscopy. There is good tissue penetration and thus a good depth of necrosis. PDT is intensive, expensive, requires specialized equipment, and has a large side-effect profile, so the procedure has been confined to specialized units.[26,56] The photosensitizing drugs used are activated by light at specific wavelengths, resulting in a photodynamic reaction causing direct cytotoxicity, inflammation, and necrosis. The drugs used include porfimer sodium (PS), aminolevulinic acid (ALA), or meta-tetrahydroxyphenyl chlorine (mTHPC). ALA has less photosensitivity due to its shorter half-life and has a lower stricture rate due to a more limited absorption of light. The patients receive the photosensitizing agent prior to the endoscopy treatment; PS (2 mg/kg) is given intravenously 72 hours prior, whereas ALA (30 to 60 mg/kg) can be given orally on the day of procedure. The lasers deliver light, at a specific wavelength, via optical fibers contained within a specifically designed balloon or bare cylinder. The majority of PDT data are from red light at 630 to 635 nm, with some series using green light at 514 nm. Technical considerations include the application of even light dosimetry with diffusing fibers/perspex dilators and balloon devices, as well as ensuring the esophageal folds are flattened.[57]

PDT is a targeted therapy that will specifically treat the Barrett segment, allowing replacement by neosquamous epithelium in 50% to 80% of patients.[58,59] The majority of the reported data on the role of PDT ablation of BE relates to the eradication of HGD rather than the whole BE segment. There is long-term evidence in an RCT for a significant reduction in HGD and in the progression to EAC patients treated with PDT, compared with patients who were observed and treated with a PPI. Following PDT the probability of maintaining complete ablation of the HGD was 48%, compared with 4% in the surveillance group.[60] This has been confirmed in systematic reviews.[61,62] The risk of recurrence of the HGD is up to 8% of patients. The risk is higher if the BE is longer than 8 cm and if multiple treatments were required to eliminate the IM.[60] It has been recommended that PDT may be worthy of consideration as an effective salvage procedure in patients with HGD resistant to other endoscopic therapies,[61] although other less technically difficult procedures are likely to be preferred to PDT. With respect to eradication of the complete BE segment, at 12 months, one group had a 50% incidence of macroscopic neosquamous epithelium, with the other patients having various degrees of reduction in the area of the IM.[63] An RCT comparing PS and ALA as sensitizers for PDT demonstrated CE of HGD in 40% versus 47%, a stricture rate of 33% versus 9%, and a difference in photosensitivity of 43% versus 6%, respectively.[56]

The outcomes from PDT have been compared with RFA in a single center over two time periods as the investigators moved from PDT to RFA in their patient cohort. In the PDT group, 33 patients with HGD had up to three treatments and at 1 year had a CE rate of 54.5%. The RFA group of 53 patients (LGD 47, HGD 6) had a CE rate of 89% (P = .001). The stricture rate was 28% in the PDT group, and it cost 5 times more than the RFA treatment per patient.[26]

The complication profile of PDT includes strictures, photosensitivity, pleural effusions, hypotension, and transient liver function test abnormalities. Stricture rates as high as 36% have been reported.[64] Strictures occurred less with ALA PDT, and with the use of newer, longer balloons, which may allow for less overlapping of the treated area.[57]

TABLE 34.4 Outcomes from Photodynamic Therapy for Barrett Esophagus

Outcomes	% of Patients
EFFICACY	
Complete eradication of dysplasia	50%–80%
Complete eradication of IM	13%–52%
DURABILITY	
5 years complete eradication of dysplasia	48%
COMPLICATIONS	
Stricture	9%–36%
Photosensitivity	6%–43%
Buried Barrett	14%–20%

IM, Intestinal metaplasia.

TABLE 34.5 Outcomes from Argon Plasma Coagulation for Barrett Esophagus

Outcomes	% of Patients
EFFICACY	
Complete eradication of dysplasia	67%
Complete eradication of IM	38%–99%
DURABILITY	
1 year complete eradication of IM	84%
8 years complete eradication of IM	66%
16 years complete eradication of IM	50%
COMPLICATIONS	
Stricture	9%–11%
Buried Barrett	21%–24%

IM, Intestinal metaplasia.

The rate of buried Barrett glands varies but can be as high as 48%.[42,56] The outcomes are summarized in Table 34.4.

ARGON PLASMA COAGULATION

APC is a no contact technique using the delivery of ionized argon gas to cause tissue coagulation. Superficial mucosal necrosis occurs to a variable depth due to the increased resistance in coagulated tissue. Newer devices have multiple power settings that can influence depth of ablation. The energy settings reported vary from 40 to 90 W, with gas flow of 1.8 to 2 L/min.[65] Complete eradication of BE has been reported to occur between 38% and 99%, with a recurrence rate of 3% to 16%.[64–68]

Assessing the long-term results from APC, in 32 patients (NDBE 28, LGD 5), one group achieved CE after multiple treatments (1 to 5 applications). One month after CE, at endoscopy the status of the IM was complete in 25 (78%), partial, 4 (13%), and no change, 3 (9%). At 16 years, 16 patients (50%) had sustained eradication, 11 (35%) partial, and 6% were lost to follow-up. Carcinoma occurred in three patients (9%), two from buried Barrett glands, and one from a residual IM segment.[69] No patient died from carcinoma. This study used outdated APC techniques, and acid suppression was prescribed for 1 year and then subsequently for symptom control only.

In two RCTs examining APC ablation for eradication of predominately nondysplastic Barrett, APC was compared with surveillance, where the difference in the trials was the type of long-term acid control. One study used continuous PPI and the other a fundoplication. The recruitment criteria were the same. The combined results in 129 patients were reported with short- (12 months), medium- (42 to 75 months), and long-term (>84 months) outcomes. Greater than 95% eradication of the IM was possible in 97% after multiple treatments. The CE rate was 84% at 12 months, 67% medium term, and in the long term 66%. The presence of dysplasia, LGD, and HGD each occurred in a single patient. In the surveillance group, the BE length regressed from an average of 4.2 to 2.7 cm (mainly in the fundoplication group), with HGD and LGD developing in 3 (9%) and 6 (19%), respectively.[70]

The role of APC following EMR for IMC or HGD was compared with focal EMR and a PPI with no ablation in an RCT.[3] "Complete ablation" was considered to be greater than 90% eradication of the residual BE segment

and took an average of four sessions (range 2 to 7). In the 33 patients who had BE ablation at a follow-up time of 23 months, 1 patient (3%) in the ablation group had recurrence of the neoplasia. In the 30 patients undergoing surveillance, at follow-up time 25 months, 11 patients (37%) had recurrent neoplasia ($P = .005$). All neoplastic recurrences were treated with endoscopic resection. The study was ceased early in 2010 when the results from RFA trials became apparent, and the standard became the ablation of all patients who had had neoplastic segments resected.[3]

APC ablation has been compared with PDT in a number of studies. A small RCT assessed ablation in patients with NDBE. At 12 months, APC, following a median of three treatments, achieved CE of IM in 97% compared with PDT, where the rate was 50%, after a median of five treatments.[63] With regard to dysplastic BE, an RCT with 13 patients in each arm compared PDT with APC ablation. At 12 months the CE rate for APC was 67% and for PDT 77%. In the APC group, 4 of 13 (30%) were excluded from the 12-month follow-up.[66] Finally, a study comparing single and fractionated PDT with APC in 40 BE patients (LGD 20%, NDBE 80%) reported CE of IM in 86% for PDT, compared with 67% following APC. However, any residual BE in both groups were allowed APC treatment; there was one death 72 hours post PDT from a presumed arrhythmia.[71]

Stricture formation has been reported to occur in 9% to 11%.[3,70] In one study, one patient had bleeding and one a localized perforation treated conservatively.[3] The incidence of buried Barrett has been reported to be up to 24% patients.[62] In the RCT, the incidence of buried Barrett was similar in both groups: PDT, 24%, and APC, 21%.[63] The outcomes are summarized in Table 34.5.

CRYOTHERAPY ABLATION

Cryotherapy (CRYO) destroys tissue with cycles of rapid freezing and slow thawing. It is a no-contact therapy using liquid nitrogen (N_2) or carbon dioxide (CO_2). The mechanism of action causes an immediate effect, with failure of cellular metabolism due to intracellular and extracellular ice. The cell damage leads to vascular stasis and ischemic necrosis. The console system contains the tank and equipment for regulation of flows and pressure

TABLE 34.6 Outcomes from Cryotherapy Ablation for Barrett Esophagus

Outcomes	% of Patients
EFFICACY	
Complete eradication of dysplasia	87%–100%
Complete eradication of IM	53%–84%
DURABILITY	
Two year complete eradication of HGD	100%
Two year complete eradication of IM	84%
COMPLICATIONS	
Stricture	3%–9%
Perforation	<1%
Chest pain	2%
Buried Barrett	3%

HGD, High-grade dysplasia; *IM*, intestinal metaplasia.

(22 pounds/inch^2, 151.7 psi).[65] A spray catheter is used for application with multiple areas (three to five) able to be treated at once. The liquidized gas is applied until white frost appears, and then allowed to thaw after a period of at least 45 seconds. The dosing has varied from three cycles of 20 seconds to four cycles of 10 seconds and recently two cycles of 20 seconds.[65] The system includes the insertion of a passive and active orogastric decompression tube, which is placed in the stomach, prior to treatment, to allow decompression of the evaporated cryogen. A 20-second application of liquid nitrogen will produce 6 to 7 L of gas at room temperatures.[65] There may be technical difficulties with frosting of the lens and applying the treatment around the decompression tube.[65]

In a cohort of 60 patients who had CRYO for HGD, at 10 months' mean follow-up, CE of the HGD occurred in 97% and IM in 57%.[72] A study of 32 patients treated with liquid nitrogen CE reported, at 2 years, a number of "touch-ups" during surveillance, the CE rate for HGD was 100%, and from IM 84%. The recurrence rate of HGD during that time was 18% and for IM 41%, with 34% at the neosquamo-columnar junction.[73] There are no RCTs assessing the efficacy of CRYO compared with the other ablative techniques. Typically multiple treatments are required to achieve ablation of the BE segment when higher recurrence of the segment is greater than 3 cm.[74] This procedure may be beneficial in patients with irregular or scarred areas due to the noncontact technique for ablation.

There has been concern with respect to perforation rates because of the gaseous distention,[74] and this was reported in a single study.[75] The stricture rate has been reported to be 3%[72] and 9%[74] in separate studies. The outcomes are summarized in Table 34.6.

SUBSQUAMOUS BARRETT GLANDS (BURIED BARRETT)

The issue of BE under the neosquamous epithelium occurring after ablative therapies is a concern, given reports of malignancy developing in this epithelium. It is apparent that the BE may be subsquamous at the squamo-columnar

junction in a typical Barrett segment. This was found to be the case in 98% of patients who had the Barrett/squamous junction resected as part of an EMR for focal neoplasia The average subsquamous length was 3.3 mm (0.2 to 9.6 mm), and it was present as "finger-like" projections.[76] The relevance of this with respect to the risk of buried Barrett following ablation is not clear.

The incidence of malignancy in these residual buried glands is not clear. One series of patients who had APC ablation with a long-term follow-up reported two cases in 35 patients treated. In the authors' assessment of the literature, they amassed 35 cases that occurred after PDT, APC, and RFA.[69] It has been proposed that the neoplastic BE may be more resistant to the ablative therapies and are more likely to remain as residual segments or as buried cells.[77,78] However, there has also been the suggestion that there is a biologic change in the DNA of these residual segments, which may relate to a lower neoplastic potential.[77,79] Buried glands may regress in some patients after ablation. One study of patients who had APC ablation reported a decreased incidence at later time points on surveillance biopsies.[80]

The reported incidence of buried Barrett is lowest following RFA, with a review of 18 studies containing 1004 patients and follow-up of 8 weeks to 5 years reporting an incidence of 0.9%. In 22 reports of PDT ablation, containing 953 patients, the incidence was 14%,[81] although rates as high as 20% have been reported.[26,63,69,71] Buried metaplasia can also be seen in patients who have not had any ablative therapy, with theories that this is a result of extensive biopsy sampling and subsequent healing.[81,82] This has been documented in 20% to 25% of patients.[56]

The incidence of this entity may be higher than seen from surveillance biopsies. Three-dimensional optical coherence tomography (3D-OCT) performed at endoscopy will image the mucosa to a depth of 1 to 2 mm so that the tissue morphology under the squamous epithelium can be assessed. This technology will assess 30 to 60 times the area compared with biopsies. In a small study, the presence of buried Barrett was 63% (10 of 16 patients) that had complete ablation following RFA of a short BE segment. The majority of these deposits were within 5 mm of the neosquamo-columnar junction. There are no data on the natural history of these findings,[83] which is relevant given the very low incidence of buried Barrett from biopsies in the post-RFA ablation studies.

SUMMARY OF ABLATIVE THERAPIES

When assessing the efficacy, the incidence of sustained eradication, ease of application, consistency of outcomes, and safety profile, RFA is the superior method for eradication of BE segments. For visible lesions, the combination of focal EMR and RFA is the gold standard. SRER removes the whole segment but has been restricted to shorter BE segments, has a similar incidence of persistent or recurrent IM compared with RFA, and although relatively safe, there is a high stricture rate. For BE, the role of ESD is not clear. It may be relevant to a group of highly selected patients and should be performed in specialist units. PDT has disappointing results with respect to long-term CE rates, requires specific expertise, and has a high complication profile that includes a high rate of stricture formation and photosensitivity. APC is relatively easy to apply, but durability of the CE rate is disappointing, with recurrence of the IM occurring in long-term studies. The results from APC can be dependent upon the operator, as well as factors such as the energy settings, APC mode, and the distance of the catheter from the mucosa and time of energy transmission. For longer segments of Barrett the procedure can be very time-consuming. The complication profile is not high, but strictures do occur. The data from CRYO studies have not suggested equivalent efficacy or durability when compared with RFA, and the numbers relate to small cohort studies. CRYO or APC may be reasonable alternative therapies if a patient had recurrence following previous RFA ablative therapy.

ROLE OF ACID CONTROL BEFORE AND AFTER ABLATION TREATMENT

Following the mucosal injury, most studies recommend a minimum medical therapy of a double-dose PPI following ablation. Once the injury has healed, patients are maintained with a normal dose of PPI. One of the lower rates of recurrence of IM (6%) following RFA has been reported from a study in the Netherlands where patients received high-dose PPI (twice daily esomeprazole 40 mg), ranitidine (300 mg at night), and sucralfate (5 mL [200 mg/mL] 4 times a day for 2 weeks) and then a normal dose of maintenance PPI.[46] The role of maintenance therapy is not clear. In the general population there is a paucity of data to support routine use of regular acid suppression in a patient with BE. PPI therapy is typically prescribed for symptom control of gastroesophageal reflux disease (GERD). A systematic review of cohort studies reported that the use of PPIs in patients with NDBE produced a decreased risk of progression to neoplastic BE compared with no acid suppression.[84] There is evidence that incomplete control of GERD may be associated with increased recurrence rates of IM following successful ablation,[85,86] although there is no evidence for the degree of control and the relationship to the rate of recurrence. The presence of uncontrolled acid reflux before RFA ablation predisposes patients to a higher rate of incomplete response after RFA.[87] Thus at this time, despite the level of evidence not being high, patients should have their GERD controlled with a PPI prior to ablative therapy, and it is recommended that patients are maintained on a regular PPI following ablation therapy.

The role of antireflux surgery in the form of a fundoplication to control GERD long term has been assessed through analysis of data in the US RFA registry. There was no difference in the CE of dysplastic epithelium or intestinal metaplasia among 301 patients who had a fundoplication, compared with those who had not had antireflux surgery.[88] Another group assessed the role of APC and acid control compared with surveillance and acid control. They performed two RCTs where the difference in each trial was the form of long-term acid control, one trial with regular PPI and the other group having antireflux surgery. The group who had antireflux surgery (a fundoplication) had a rate of at least 95% IM ablation at 1 year of 87% and at 7 years 74%, compared with the medically treated patients who had an IM ablation rate of 79% at 1 year and 54% at 7 years. The numbers in the trial were small and the difference between methods of acid control was not significant. There was also no difference in the rate of dysplasia in each group.[70] Presently antireflux surgery is not considered to be an antineoplastic measure in patients with BE, so that the indications for surgery in patients who have had BE ablation is the same as for a population of patients with GERD who have not had the procedure.[18]

SURVEILLANCE

It will typically take a number of episodes of treatments to achieve CE or near CE of the BE segment, no matter which ablative technique is being used. There are varying rates of recurrence of dysplasia and IM with the different ablative techniques, with RFA ablation achieving the more durable results. One study reported a 9% per year rate of recurrence of IM post apparent complete BE eradication by RFA ablation. Often further treatment episodes will be required after the first year.[43] The mean time to IM recurrence in patients with NDBE has been reported to be around 2 years.[52] A study of 166 patients, assessing the long-term control following treatment of neoplastic BE with multiple modalities including endoscopic resection, PDT, and RFA, or a combination of these treatments, reported CE of the neoplastic BE in 95% and IM 83%. At follow-up of 33 months (range 18 to 58 months), the recurrent IM rate was 35% and dysplasia 9%. Retreatment achieved remission in 90%.[89] It is clear that for patients treated with Barrett neoplasia, long-term careful surveillance will be necessary.[26]

Presently the data used to inform the surveillance periods following BE ablation is based on cohort studies with the longer term follow-up details, and recommendations have been reported in recent guideline documents.[18,45,46] For patients who have had HGD and/or IMC resected with subsequent BE ablation, it is recommended they should have 3-monthly reviews in the first year, 6-monthly reviews in the second year, and then annually. For patients who have had ablation for LGD, it is recommended they have 6-monthly reviews in the first year and then annually. The tubular esophagus and the gastroesophageal junction should be assessed visually, and four-quadrant biopsies at 1 cm levels over the previous IM segment and the cardia should be taken. Recurrent metaplasia/dysplasia should be treated according to the histology of the lesion.[18]

Whether the surveillance periods can be extended will remain a source of research with assessment of longer-term data. The AIM II trial assessed the durability of RFA in patients with NDBE, 2 to 6 cm in length, at 5 years posttreatment, in 50 out of the 70 patients recruited. The CE rate was 92%, and those who had focal IM had this successfully eradicated with focal RFA. In this group of patients there were no patients with dysplasia or buried Barrett.[23] It may be that once dysplasia is cleared, the times between surveillance endoscopies can be extended.

ROLE OF BIOMARKERS

There is a need to develop and validate biomarkers that will inform the management of patients with BE. The information achieved may define the mucosa, which has a higher risk of neoplastic transformation, confirm the diagnosis of LGD, or predict risk of progression of LGD to HGD/IMC. In an overview of molecular markers in BE, it was reported that testing for p53 immunohistochemistry could be a useful adjunct to risk stratify and clarify dysplasia, notably LGD. It is becoming clear that it is likely that panels of biomarkers that assess genomic instability and other specific abnormalities will be used to risk stratify patients with NDBE.[90] Using a panel of biomarkers of genomic instability in patients with NDBE has been shown to increase the prediction of the development of carcinoma from 10% if the abnormalities did not exist to 79% at 10 years if three of the abnormalities were present.[91] Indeed when the role of RFA ablation for NDBE is assessed, where the therapy is selected on the basis of risk stratification using a panel of biomarkers obtained by biopsy of the BE, ablation in this subgroup becomes cost effective.[92]

In a cost-effective analysis, in patients with NDBE the four modes of therapy used in the Markov model were stratify selection to ablation based upon high rates of genomic instability being present, no treatment, typical endoscopic guidelines for surveillance, and RFA ablation for all cases. The selection of ablation only in the group who had high rates of genomic instability had the best value for QALYs. At this time guidelines in managing patients with BE do not recommend the use of biomarkers in managing BE.[18] It is likely that this technology will improve, and with validation in clinical studies, these assessments may become reality in clinical practice.

CONCLUSION

Endoscopic therapy for patients at high risk of developing an invasive carcinoma in their BE is now a treatment standard. It has been stated that for ablation to be preferable to surveillance, there should be a decreased risk of the important endpoints such as cancer, or worse cancer death; the decrease in risk should be durable without the need for repeated treatments, and the treatment should be relatively easy to administer, without excessive cost or treatment risk.[93] The combination of endoscopic resection of visible or known pathology in combination with RFA ablation of the residual BE fulfils the criteria to allow this to be considered a standard of therapy for IMC and HGD in BE, as it does reduce the risk of invasive adenocarcinoma.

For patients with intermediate or low risk of malignant transformation, the decision between continued surveillance only or ablation with surveillance is complicated by the lack of comparative studies with the important endpoints of esophagectomy or cancer death. The presence of persistent dysplasia is a surrogate marker.[93] The evidence does support selecting patients considered high risk with LGD to undergo ablation with RFA but not patients with NDBE.

REFERENCES

1. Hvid-Jensen F, Pedersen L, Drewes AM, Sorensen HT, Funch-Jensen P. Incidence of adenocarcinoma among patients with Barrett's esophagus. *N Engl J Med.* 2011;365(15):1375-1383.
2. Pechz O, Behrens A, May A, et al. Long-term results and risk factor analysis for recurrence after curative endoscopic therapy in 349 patients with high-grade intraepithelial neoplasia and mucosal adenocarcinoma in Barrett's oesophagus. *Gut.* 2008;57(9):1200-1206.
3. Manner H, Rabenstein T, Pech O, et al. Ablation of residual Barrett's epithelium after endoscopic resection: a randomized long-term follow-up study of argon plasma coagulation vs. surveillance (APE study). *Endoscopy.* 2014;46(1):6-12.
4. Pouw RE, Bergman JJGHM. Radiofrequency ablation for Barrett's esophagus, for whom and by whom? *Clin Gastroenterol Hepatol.* 2013;11(10):1256-1258.
5. Sikkema M, Looman CWN, Steyerberg EW, et al. Predictors for neoplastic progression in patients with Barrett's esophagus: a prospective cohort study. *Am J Gastroenterol.* 2011;106(7):1231-1238.
6. Shaheen NJ, Sharma P, Overholt BF, et al. Radiofrequency ablation in Barrett's esophagus with dysplasia. *N Engl J Med.* 2009;360(22):2277-2288.
7. Rastogi A, Puli S, El-Serag HB, Bansal A, Wani S, Sharma P. Incidence of esophageal adenocarcinoma in patients with Barrett's esophagus and high-grade dysplasia: a meta-analysis. *Gastrointest Endosc.* 2008;67(3):394-398.
8. Buttar NS, Wang KK, Sebo TJ, et al. Extent of high-grade dysplasia in Barrett's esophagus correlates with risk of adenocarcinoma. *Gastroenterology.* 2001;120(7):1630-1639.
9. Montgomery E, Bronner MP, Greenson JK, et al. Are ulcers a marker for invasive carcinoma in Barrett's esophagus? Data from a diagnostic variability study with clinical follow-up. *Am J Gastroenterol.* 2002;97(1):27-31.
10. Almond LM, Hodson J, Barr H. Meta-analysis of endoscopic therapy for low-grade dysplasia in Barrett's oesophagus. *Br J Surg.* 2014;101(10):1187-1195.
11. Curvers WL, ten Kate FJ, Krishnadath KK, et al. Low-grade dysplasia in Barrett's esophagus: overdiagnosed and underestimated. *Am J Gastroenterol.* 2010;105(7):1523-1530.
12. Duits LC, Phoa KN, Curvers WL, et al. Barrett's oesophagus patients with low-grade dysplasia can be accurately risk-stratified after histological review by an expert pathology panel. *Gut.* 2015;64(5):700-706.
13. Phoa KN, van Vilsteren FGI, Weusten BLAM, et al. Radiofrequency ablation vs endoscopic surveillance for patients with Barrett esophagus and low-grade dysplasia a randomized clinical trial. *JAMA.* 2014;311(12):1209-1217.
14. Small AJ, Araujo JL, Leggett CL, et al. Radiofrequency ablation is associated with decreased neoplastic progression in patients with Barrett's esophagus and confirmed low-grade dysplasia. *Gastroenterology.* 2015;149(3):567-576.
15. Fitzgerald RC, di Pietro M, Ragunath K, et al. British Society of Gastroenterology guidelines on the diagnosis and management of Barrett's oesophagus. *Gut.* 2014;63(1):7-42.
16. Evans JA, Early DS, Fukami N, et al. The role of endoscopy in Barrett's esophagus and other premalignant conditions of the esophagus. *Gastrointest Endosc.* 2012;76(6):1087-1094.
17. Bennett C, Moayyedi P, Corley DA, et al. BOB CAT: a large-scale review and Delphi consensus for management of Barrett's esophagus with no dysplasia, indefinite for, or low-grade dysplasia. *Am J Gastroenterol.* 2015;110(5):662-682.
18. Shaheen NJ, Falk GW, Iyer PG, Gerson LB. ACG clinical guideline: diagnosis and management of Barrett's esophagus. *Am J Gastroenterol.* 2016;111(1):30-50.
19. Endoscopic radiofrequency ablation for Barrett's oesophagus with low-grade dysplasia or no dysplasia. 2014; https://www.nice.org.uk/guidance/IPG496/chapter/1-Recommendations. Accessed June 2016.
20. Thota PN, Lee HJ, Goldblum JR, et al. Risk stratification of patients with Barrett's esophagus and low-grade dysplasia or indefinite for dysplasia. *Clin Gastroenterol Hepatol.* 2015;13(3):459-465.
21. Yachimski P, Wani S, Givens T, et al. Preference of endoscopic ablation over medical prevention of esophageal adenocarcinoma by patients with Barrett's esophagus. *Clin Gastroenterol Hepatol.* 2015;13(1):84-90.

22. Sharma VK, Wang KK, Overholt BF, et al. Balloon-based, circumferential, endoscopic radiofrequency ablation of Barrett's esophagus: 1-year follow-up of 100 patients. *Gastrointest Endosc*. 2007;65(2):185-195.

23. Fleischer DE, Overholt BF, Sharma VK, et al. Endoscopic radiofrequency ablation for Barrett's esophagus: 5-year outcomes from a prospective multicenter trial. *Endoscopy*. 2010;42(10):781-789.

24. Shaheen NJ, Inadomi JM, Overholt BF, Sharma P. What is the best management strategy for high grade dysplasia in Barrett's oesophagus? A cost effectiveness analysis. *Gut*. 2004;53(12):1736-1744.

25. Gerson LB. Cost-analyses studies in Barrett's esophagus: what is their utility? *Gastroenterol Clin N Am*. 2015;44(2):425-438.

26. Ertan A, Zaheer I, Correa AM, Thosani N, Blackmon SH. Photodynamic therapy vs radiofrequency ablation for Barrett's dysplasia: efficacy, safety and cost-comparison. *World J Gastroenterol*. 2013;19(41):7106-7113.

27. Hur C, Choi SE, Rubenstein JH, et al. The cost-effectiveness of radiofrequency ablation for Barrett's esophagus. *Gastroenterology*. 2012;142(5):S73.

28. Bergman JJGHM, Corley DA. Barrett's esophagus: who should receive ablation and how can we get the best results? *Gastroenterology*. 2012;143(3):524-526.

29. Peters FR, Brakenhoff KPM, Curvers WL, et al. Histologic evaluation of resection specimens obtained at 293 endoscopic resections in Barrett's esophagus. *Gastrointest Endosc*. 2008;67(4):604-609.

30. Mino-Kenudson M, Hull MJ, Brown I, et al. EMR for Barrett's esophagus-related superficial neoplasms offers better diagnostic reproducibility than mucosal biopsy. *Gastrointest Endosc*. 2007;66(4):660-666.

31. May A, Gossner L, Behrens A, et al. A prospective randomized trial of two different endoscopic resection techniques for early stage cancer of the esophagus. *Gastrointest Endosc*. 2003;58(2):167-175.

32. Peters FR, Kara MA, Curvers WL, et al. Multiband mucosectomy for endoscopic resection of Barrett's esophagus: feasibility study with matched historical controls. *Eur J Gastroenterol Hepatol*. 2007;19(4):311-315.

33. Pouw RE, Seewald S, Gondrie JJ, et al. Stepwise radical endoscopic resection for eradication of Barrett's oesophagus with early neoplasia in a cohort of 169 patients. *Gut*. 2010;59(9):1169-1177.

34. Lopes CV, Hela M, Pesenti C, et al. Circumferential endoscopic resection of Barrett's esophagus with high-grade dysplasia or early adenocarcinoma. *Surg Endosc*. 2007;21(5):820-824.

35. Larghi A, Lightdale CJ, Ross AS, et al. Long-term follow-up of complete Barrett's eradication endoscopic mucosal resection (CBE-EMR) for the treatment of high grade dysplasia and intramucosal carcinoma. *Endoscopy*. 2007;39(12):1086-1091.

36. Peters FP, Kara MA, Rosmolen WD, et al. Stepwise radical endoscopic resection is effective for complete removal of Barrett's esophagus with early neoplasia: a prospective study. *Am J Gastroenterol*. 2006;101(7):1449-1457.

37. van Vilsteren FGI, Pouw RE, Seewald S, et al. Stepwise radical endoscopic resection versus radiofrequency ablation for Barrett's oesophagus with high-grade dysplasia or early cancer: a multicentre randomised trial. *Gut*. 2011;60(6):765-773.

38. Chadwick G, Groene O, Markar SR, Hoare J, Cromwell D, Hanna GB. Systematic review comparing radiofrequency ablation and complete endoscopic resection in treating dysplastic Barrett's esophagus: a critical assessment of histologic outcomes and adverse events. *Gastrointest Endosc*. 2014;79(5):718-731.

39. Cao Y, Liao C, Tan A, Gao Y, Mo Z, Gao F. Meta-analysis of endoscopic submucosal dissection versus endoscopic mucosal resection for tumors of the gastrointestinal tract. *Endoscopy*. 2009;41(9):751-757.

40. Chevaux JB, Piessevaux H, Jouret-Mourin A, Yeung R, Danse E, Deprez PH. Clinical outcome in patients treated with endoscopic submucosal dissection for superficial Barrett's neoplasia. *Endoscopy*. 2015;47(2):103-112.

41. Neuhaus H, Terheggen G, Rutz EM, Vieth M, Schumacher B. Endoscopic submucosal dissection plus radiofrequency ablation of neoplastic Barrett's esophagus. *Endoscopy*. 2012;44(12):1105-1113.

42. Subramanian CR, Triadafilopoulos G. Endoscopic treatments for dysplastic Barrett's esophagus: resection, ablation, what else? *World J Surg*. 2015;39(3):597-605.

43. Shaheen NJ, Overholt BF, Sampliner RE, et al. Durability of radiofrequency ablation in Barrett's esophagus with dysplasia. *Gastroenterology*. 2011;141(2):460-468.

44. Bulsiewicz WJ, Kim HP, Dellon ES, et al. Safety and efficacy of endoscopic mucosal therapy with radiofrequency ablation for patients with neoplastic Barrett's esophagus. *Clin Gastroenterol Hepatol*. 2013;11(6):636-642.

45. Haidry RJ, Dunn JM, Butt MA, et al. Radiofrequency ablation and endoscopic mucosal resection for dysplastic Barrett's esophagus and early esophageal adenocarcinoma: outcomes of the UK National Halo RFA Registry. *Gastroenterology*. 2013;145(1):87-95.

46. Phoa KN, Pouw RE, Van Vilsteren FGI, et al. Remission of Barrett's esophagus with early neoplasia 5 years after radiofrequency ablation with endoscopic resection: a Netherlands cohort study. *Gastroenterology*. 2013;145(1):96-104.

47. van Vilsteren FGI, Herrero LA, Pouw RE, et al. Predictive factors for initial treatment response after circumferential radiofrequency ablation for Barrett's esophagus with early neoplasia: a prospective multicenter study. *Endoscopy*. 2013;45(7):516-525.

48. Korst RJ, Santana JS, Rutledge JR, et al. Patterns of recurrence and persistent intestinal metaplasia after successful radiofrequency ablation of Barrett's esophagus. *J Thorac Cardiovasc Surg*. 2013;145:1529-1534.

49. Orman ES, Kim HP, Bulsiewicz WJ, et al. Intestinal metaplasia recurs infrequently in patients successfully treated for Barrett's esophagus with radiofrequency ablation. *Am J Gastroenterol*. 2013;108(2):187-195.

50. Dulai PS, Pohl H, Levenick JM, Gordon SR, MacKenzie TA, Rothstein RI. Radiofrequency ablation for long- and ultralong-segment Barrett's esophagus: a comparative long-term follow-up study. *Gastrointest Endosc*. 2013;77(4):534-541.

51. Gupta M, Iyer PG, Lutzke L, et al. Recurrence of esophageal intestinal metaplasia after endoscopic mucosal resection and radiofrequency ablation of Barrett's esophagus: results from a US multicenter consortium. *Gastroenterology*. 2013;145(1):79-86.

52. Pasricha S, Bulsiewicz WJ, Hathorn KE, et al. Durability and predictors of successful radiofrequency ablation for Barrett's esophagus. *Clin Gastroenterol Hepatol*. 2014;12(11):1840-1847.

53. Morales TG, Camargo E, Bhattacharyya A, Sampliner RE. Long-term follow-up of intestinal metaplasia of the gastric cardia. *Am J Gastroenterol*. 2000;95(7):1677-1680.

54. Wani S, Puli SR, Shaheen NJ, et al. Esophageal adenocarcinoma in Barrett's esophagus after endoscopic ablative therapy: a meta-analysis and systematic review. *Am J Gastroenterol*. 2009;104(2):502-513.

55. Haidry R, Lovat L, Sharma P. Radiofrequency ablation for Barrett's dysplasia: past, present and the future? *Curr Gastroenterol Rep*. 2015;17(3):13.

56. Dunn JM, Mackenzie GD, Banks MR, et al. A randomised controlled trial of ALA vs. Photofrin photodynamic therapy for high-grade dysplasia arising in Barrett's oesophagus. *Lasers Med Sci*. 2013;28(3):707-715.

57. Kelty CJ, Marcus SL, Ackroyd R. Photodynamic therapy for Barrett's esophagus: a review. *Dis Esophagus*. 2002;15(2):137-144.

58. Zoepf T, Alsenbesy M, Jakobs R, Apel D, Rosenbaum A, Riemann JF. Photodynamic therapy (PDT) versus argon plasma coagulation (APC) for ablative therapy of Barrett's esophagus. *Gastrointest Endosc*. 2003;57(5):Ab139.

59. Ackroyd R, Brown NJ, Davis MF, et al. Photodynamic therapy for dysplastic Barrett's oesophagus: a prospective, double blind, randomised, placebo controlled trial. *Gut*. 2000;47(5):612-617.

60. Overholt BF, Wang KK, Burdick JS, et al. Five-year efficacy and safety of photodynamic therapy with photofrin in Barrett's high-grade dysplasia. *Gastrointest Endosc*. 2007;66(3):460-468.

61. Gray J, Fullarton GM. Long term efficacy of photodynamic therapy (PDT) as an ablative therapy of high grade dysplasia in Barrett's oesophagus. *Photodiagn Photodyn*. 2013;10(4):561-565.

62. Fayter D, Corbett M, Heirs M, Fox D, Eastwood A. A systematic review of photodynamic therapy in the treatment of pre-cancerous skin conditions, Barrett's oesophagus and cancers of the biliary tract, brain, head and neck, lung, oesophagus and skin. *Health Technol Asses*. 2010;14(37):1-7.

63. Kelty CJ, Ackroyd R, Brown NJ, Stephenson TJ, Stoddard CJ, Reed MWR. Endoscopic ablation of Barrett's oesophagus: a randomized-controlled trial of photodynamic therapy vs. argon plasma coagulation. *Aliment Pharm Therap*. 2004;20(11-12):1289-1296.

64. Attwood SE, Lewis CJ, Caplin S, Hemming K, Armstrong G. Argon beam plasma coagulation as therapy for high-grade dysplasia in Barrett's esophagus. *Clin Gastroenterol Hepatol*. 2003;1(4):258-263.

65. Dumot JA, Greenwald BD. Argon plasma coagulation, bipolar cautery, and cryotherapy: ABC's of ablative techniques. *Endoscopy*. 2008;40(12):1026-1032.

66. Ragunath K, Krasner N, Raman VS, Haqqani MT, Phillips CJ, Cheung I. Endoscopic ablation of dysplastic Barrett's oesophagus comparing

argon plasma coagulation and photodynamic therapy: a randomized prospective trial assessing efficacy and cost-effectiveness. *Scand J Gastroenterol.* 2005;40(7):750-758.

67. Pereira-Lima JC, Busnello JV, Saul C, et al. High power setting argon plasma coagulation for the eradication of Barrett's esophagus. *Am J Gastroenterol.* 2000;95(7):1661-1668.

68. Madisch A, Miehlke S, Bayerdoerffer E, et al. Long-term follow-up after complete ablation of Barrett's esophagus with argon plasma coagulation. *World J Gastroenterol.* 2005;11(8):1182-1186.

69. Milashka M, Calomme A, Van Laethem JL, et al. Sixteen-year follow-up of Barrett's esophagus, endoscopically treated with argon plasma coagulation. *United Eur Gastroenterol.* 2014;2(5):367-373.

70. Sie C, Bright T, Schoeman M, et al. Argon plasma coagulation ablation versus endoscopic surveillance of Barrett's esophagus: late outcomes from two randomized trials. *Endoscopy.* 2013;45(11):859-865.

71. Hage M, Siersema PD, van Dekken H, et al. 5-am nolevulinic acid photodynamic therapy versus argon plasma coagulation for ablation of Barrett's oesophagus: a randomised trial. *Gut.* 2004;53(6):785-790.

72. Shaheen NJ, Greenwald BD, Peery AF, et al. Safety and efficacy of endoscopic spray cryotherapy for Barrett's esophagus with high-grade dysplasia. *Gastrointest Endosc.* 2010;71(4):680-685.

73. Gosain S, Mercer K, Twaddell WS, Uradomo L, Greenwald BD. Liquid nitrogen spray cryotherapy in Barrett's esophagus with high-grade dysplasia: long-term results. *Gastrointest Endosc.* 2013;78(2):260-265.

74. Pasricha PJ, Hill S, Wadwa KS, et al. Endoscopic cryotherapy: experimental results and first clinical use. *Gastrointest Endosc.* 1999;49(5):627-631.

75. Greenwald BD, Dumot JA, Horwhat JD, Lightdale CJ, Abrams JA. Safety, tolerability, and efficacy of endoscopic low-pressure liquid nitrogen spray cryotherapy in the esophagus. *Dis Esophagus.* 2010;23(1):13-19.

76. Anders M, Lucks Y, El-Masry MA, et al. Subsquamous extension of intestinal metaplasia is detected in 98% of cases of neoplastic Barrett's esophagus. *Clin Gastroenterol Hepatol.* 2014;12(3):405-410.

77. Chennat J, Ross AS, Konda VJA, et al. Advanced pathology under squamous epithelium on initial EMR specimens in patients with Barrett's esophagus and high-grade dysplasia or intramucosal carcinoma: implications for surveillance and endotherapy management. *Gastrointest Endosc.* 2009;70(3):417-421.

78. Prasad GA, Wang KK, Halling KC, et al. Utility of biomarkers in prediction of response to ablative therapy in Barrett's esophagus. *Gastroenterology.* 2008;135(2):370-379.

79. Hornick JL, Mino-Kenudson M, Lauwers GY, Liu WT, Goyal R, Odze RD. Buried Barrett's epithelium following photodynamic therapy shows reduced crypt proliferation and absence of DNA content abnormalities. *Am J Gastroenterol.* 2008;103(1):38-47.

80. Ackroyd R, Tam W, Schoeman M, Devitt PG, Watson DI. Prospective randomized controlled trial of argon plasma coagulation ablation vs. endoscopic surveillance of patients with Barrett's esophagus after antireflux surgery. *Gastrointest Endosc.* 2004;59(1):1-7.

81. Gray NA, Odze RD, Spechler SJ. Buried metaplasia after endoscopic ablation of Barrett's esophagus: a systematic review. *Am J Gastroenterol.* 2011;106(11):1899-1908.

82. Bronner MP, Overholt BF, Taylor SL, et al. Squamous overgrowth is not a safety concern for photodynamic therapy for Barrett's esophagus with high-grade dysplasia. *Gastroenterology.* 2009;136(1):56-64.

83. Zhou C, Tsai TH, Lee HC, et al. Characterization of buried glands before and after radiofrequency ablation by using 3-dimensional optical coherence tomography (with videos). *Gastrointest Endosc.* 2012;76(1):32-40.

84. Singh S, Garg SK, Singh PP, Iyer PG, El-Serag HB. Acid-suppressive medications and risk of oesophageal adenocarcinoma in patients with Barrett's oesophagus: a systematic review and meta-analysis. *Gut.* 2014;63(8):1229-1237.

85. Kahaleh M, Van Laethem JL, Nagy N, Cremer M, Deviere J. Long-term follow-up and factors predictive of recurrence in Barrett's esophagus treated by argon plasma coagulation and acid suppression. *Endoscopy.* 2002;34(12):950-955.

86. Ferraris R, Fracchia M, Foti M, et al. Barrett's oesophagus: long-term follow-up after complete ablation with argon plasma coagulation and the factors that determine its recurrence. *Aliment Pharm Therap.* 2007;25(7):835-840.

87. Krishnan K, Pandolfino JE, Kahrilas PJ, Keefer L, Boris L, Komanduri S. Increased risk for persistent intestinal metaplasia in patients with Barrett's esophagus and uncontrolled reflux exposure before radiofrequency ablation. *Gastroenterology.* 2012;143(3):576-581.

88. Shaheen NJ, Kim HP, Bulsiewicz WJ, et al. Prior fundoplication does not improve safety or efficacy outcomes of radiofrequency ablation: results from the US RFA Registry. *J Gastrointest Surg.* 2013;17(1):21-28.

89. Guarner-Argente C, Buoncristiano T, Furth EE, Falk GW, Ginsberg GG. Long-term outcomes of patients with Barrett's esophagus and high-grade dysplasia or early cancer treated with endoluminal therapies with intention to complete eradication. *Gastrointest Endosc.* 2013;77(2):190-199.

90. Zeki S, Fitzgerald RC. The use of molecular markers in predicting dysplasia and guiding treatment. *Best Pract Res Clin Gastroenterol.* 2015;29(1):113-124.

91. Galipeau PC, Li XH, Blount PL, et al. NSAIDs modulate CDKN2A, TP53, and DNA content risk for progression to esophageal adenocarcinoma. *PLoS Med.* 2007;4(2):342-354.

92. Das A, Singh V, Fleischer DE, Sharma VK. A comparison of endoscopic treatment and surgery in early esophageal cancer: an analysis of Surveillance, Epidemiology and End Results data. *Am J Gastroenterol.* 2008;103(6):1340-1345.

93. Corley DA, Mehtani K, Quesenberry C, Zhao W, de Boer J, Weiss NS. Impact of endoscopic surveillance on mortality from Barrett's esophagus-associated esophageal adenocarcinomas. *Gastroenterology.* 2013;145(2):312-319, e311.

PART SEVEN
Esophageal Cancer

Epidemiology, Risk Factors, and Clinical Manifestations of Esophageal Cancer

Talar Tatarian | Francesco Palazzo

Esophageal cancer accounts for 1% of new cancer diagnoses in the United States annually and 2.6% of cancer-related deaths.[1] An estimated 0.5% of men and women will be diagnosed with esophageal cancer at some point during their lifetime. The two most common subtypes of primary esophageal cancer include adenocarcinoma (EAC) and squamous cell carcinoma (SCC). These differ tremendously in their natural history, epidemiologic pattern, and risk factors. SCC arises from the native squamous epithelium of the esophagus. Chronic inflammation due to environmental exposures causes progression to dysplasia and eventually malignant change.[2] EAC typically arises in areas of the esophagus where the squamous epithelium is replaced by columnar-lined metaplastic epithelium (Barrett esophagus), usually due to the presence of gastroesophageal reflux.[3]

This chapter reviews the epidemiologic pattern, risk factors, and clinical manifestations of esophageal cancer and its histologic subtypes.

EPIDEMIOLOGY

INCIDENCE

In 2016, an estimated 16,910 people will be diagnosed with esophageal cancer in the United States alone.[4] Worldwide, over 450,000 people are diagnosed annually. Over the past few decades, there has been a major shift in the incidence of esophageal cancer worldwide with trends differing by histologic subtype.[5,6]

In the United States, the overall incidence of esophageal cancer has been falling an average of 1.4% per year over the past decade (Fig. 35.1). The most recent Surveillance Epidemiology, and End Results (SEER) data estimate 4.3 new cases annually per 100,000 men and women. Across all races, EAC is the most common histologic subtype in the United States and Europe. Since the 1970s, the incidence of EAC has increased at a rate greater than any other malignancy in the United States.[7] The absolute incidence of EAC has increased from 0.4 case per 100,000 in 1975 to 2.58 cases per 100,000 in 2009.[8] During this same period, the incidence of SCC has steadily decreased.[7,9,10]

Worldwide, the incidence of esophageal cancer varies by more than 21-fold, with SCC being the predominant subtype.[6] The highest-risk area, referred to as the *esophageal cancer belt,* extends from the Middle East to northeast China, where the incidence of SCC is more than 100 cases per 100,000 people annually.[5,6,11,12] High rates of esophageal SCC are also seen in Southern and Eastern Africa, whereas the lowest rates are found in Western Africa.[6]

MORTALITY AND PROGNOSIS OF PATIENTS WITH ESOPHAGEAL CANCER

Esophageal cancer is the 11th leading cause of cancer-related death in the United States.[1] It accounted for an estimated 15,690 deaths in 2016.[4] Over the past decade, the death rate due to esophageal cancer has been declining an average of 0.8% per year (see Fig. 35.1). Across all races, the death rate is approximately 5 times higher in men than women. The overall relative 5-year survival rate has increased from 4% in the 1970s to 18.7% currently.[1]

Improved prognosis is seen in patients with localized disease. With complete surgical resection, the relative 5-year survival rate is approximately 90% for pTis tumors, 75% for pT1, 45% for pT2, 30% for pT3, and 10% to 15% for pT4 disease.[13] Unfortunately, more than 30% of patients have metastatic disease at the time of presentation, with a relative 5-year survival of 4.5% (Table 35.1).[1,4]

AGE, SEX, AND RACE DISTRIBUTION

Esophageal cancer is more common with increased age. The majority of new cases are diagnosed in people aged 65 to 74 years with a median age at diagnosis of 67.[1] Overall, it has a male preponderance (7:1) with a high of 11:1 in those aged 50 to 54 and a low of 4:1 in those aged 75 to 79. This predilection for males is seen irrespective of race/ethnicity.[14]

Across races, substantial differences are seen in the incidence of esophageal cancer and the distribution of the histologic subtypes. The age-adjusted incidence rate of esophageal cancer is highest in white and black men (7.9 and 7.2 per 100,000 people, respectively) and lowest in men of Asian/Pacific Islander descent (3.4 per 100,000). Over the past three decades, the incidence of

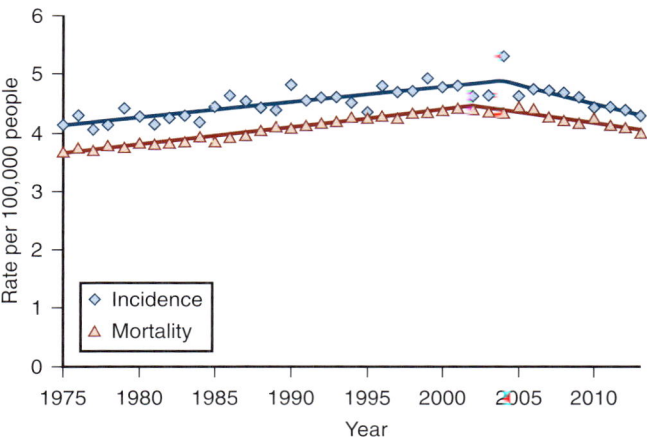

FIGURE 35.1 Trend in incidence and mortality from esophageal cancer (1975–2013, all ages, all races, both sexes). (Data from Howlader N, Noone AA, Krapcho M, et al. SEER Cancer Statistics Review, 1975–2013. http://seer.cancer.gov/csr/1975_2013/.)

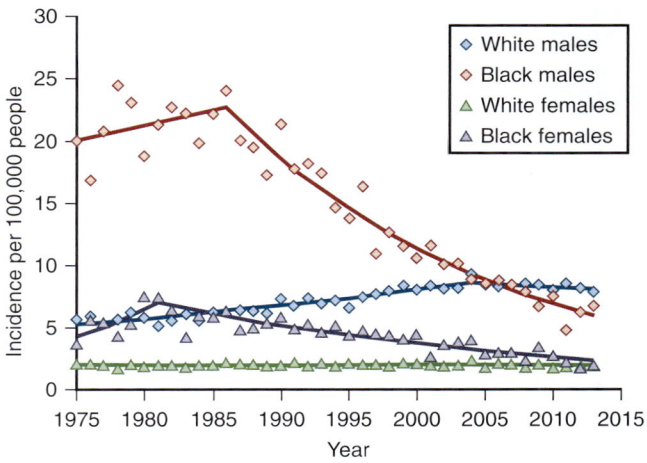

FIGURE 35.2 Trend in age-adjusted incidence rate of esophageal cancer by race and sex (1975–2013). (Data from Howlader N, Noone AA, Krapcho M, et al. SEER Cancer Statistics Review, 1975–2013. http://seer.cancer.gov/csr/1975_2013/.)

TABLE 35.1 Stage Distribution at Diagnosis and Respective 5-Year Relative Survival

Stage at Diagnosis	Stage Distribution (%)	5-year Relative Survival (%)
Localized (confined to primary site)	20	41.3
Regional (spread to regional lymph nodes)	31	22.8
Distant (cancer has metastasized)	38	4.5
Unknown (unstaged)	11	12.4

Data based on SEER 18, 2006–2012, both sexes, all races.
Data from Howlader N, Noone AA, Krapcho M, et al. SEER Cancer Statistics Review, 1975–2013. <http://seer.cancer.gov/csr/1975_2013/>.

esophageal cancer has steadily decreased in black men and women, whereas it has increased in white men (Fig. 35.2). The overall incidence has been relatively stable in white women. Histologically, the rate of SCC is fourfold greater in black versus white men, whereas EAC is fivefold greater in white versus black men.[15] The SEER data from 2009–2013 demonstrated that SCC accounted for 78.7% of esophageal cancer in blacks and 68.5% of Asian/Pacific Islanders, compared with only 25.4% in whites. The opposite was true for EAC, which was the primary histologic subtype in 69.1% of whites, 61.3% of American Indians/Alaskan Natives, and 57.4% of Hispanics, but only 16.6% of blacks.[1]

ANATOMIC DISTRIBUTION OF ESOPHAGEAL CANCER

Cancer of the cervical esophagus is rare. SCC is evenly distributed within the middle and lower thoracic esophagus, whereas 75% of all EAC is located in the distal esophagus.[16]

Tumors of the esophagogastric junction (EGJ) represent an entity that has historically been difficult to classify. EGJ tumors are defined as those located between the distal 5 cm of the esophagus and the proximal 5 cm of the gastric cardia. Siewert and Stein subclassified these tumors into three types based on their location with relation to the Z line: type I (esophageal), type II (cardiac), and type III (subcardiac).[17] The 7th edition of the American Joint Commission on Cancer (AJCC) Cancer Staging Manual grouped EGJ tumors with esophageal cancer for purposes of staging and treatment.[18]

RISK FACTORS FOR ESOPHAGEAL CANCER

There are several risk factors that are associated with the development of EAC and SCC. The risk factors and their effects are summarized in Table 35.2.

TOBACCO/ALCOHOL

Tobacco use and alcohol consumption have been identified as strong independent risk factors that also act synergistically in the development of esophageal cancer, particularly SCC.[19] In the United States, tobacco and alcohol use account for 90% of esophageal SCC cases.[6] The risk of esophageal cancer is dependent on the duration of tobacco use, with current smokers having a three- to sevenfold increase in the risk of SCC and a twofold increase in the risk of EAC.[20,21] Studies have shown that consuming more than three alcoholic beverages per day increases the risk of SCC.[22–24] An association has not been shown with alcohol use and EAC.[24]

ACHALASIA

Achalasia has been associated with an increased risk of esophageal SCC, presumably due to chronic mucosal irritation caused by nitrosamines released from bacteria in stagnant food debris.[25] The incidence rate of malignancy in these patients varies significantly throughout the literature, with a 10- to 50-fold increase in relative risk compared with the general population.[26–28] Leeuwenburgh et al. found an incidence of 0.34% per year of follow-up with

TABLE 35.2 Risk Factors for the Development of Esophageal Adenocarcinoma and Squamous Cell Carcinoma (Presented in Alphabetical Order)

	Esophageal Adenocarcinoma	Esophageal Squamous Cell Carcinoma
Achalasia	↑	↑
Age	↑	↑
Alcohol	0	↑
Fruit and vegetable intake	↓	↓
GERD/Barrett esophagus	↑	0
H. pylori infection	↓	?
Low socioeconomic status	↓	↑
Lower sphincter-relaxing medication	↑	0
Male sex	↑	↑
NSAIDs	↓	↓
Obesity	↑	↓
Proton pump inhibitors	↑	0
Tobacco	↑	↑
White race	↑	↓

↓, Negative association; ↑, positive association; 0, no association; ?, unknown association; *GERD*, gastroesophageal reflux disease; *NSAIDs*, nonsteroidal antiinflammatory drugs.

malignancy developing an average of 24 years after the onset of achalasia symptoms.[29] An association with EAC has also been reported but is less well established.[26,30]

DIET AND NUTRITION

High intake of fruits and vegetables has been shown to be protective against esophageal cancer.[31–33] The majority of data is from case-control or cohort studies evaluating the risk of SCC in high-risk populations. In high-risk areas, such as countries within the esophageal cancer belt, poor nutritional status, low intake of fruits and vegetables, and drinking hot beverages are suggested to be partially responsible.[34–37]

Deficiencies in vitamin A, vitamin E, selenium, and zinc are also believed to contribute to the development of SCC.[38] The Seattle Barrett Esophagus Research Program demonstrated an association between daily use of multivitamins, vitamin C, and vitamin E, and a reduced risk of EAC.[39] In contrast, epidemiologic studies suggest a possible link between carbohydrate intake and esophageal cancer, as the rise in carbohydrate intake in the United States has correlated with the rise in EAC and decline in SCC.[40]

NONSTEROIDAL ANTIINFLAMMATORY DRUGS

Overexpression of the enzyme cyclooxygenase-2 (COX-2) has been implicated in the development of Barrett esophagus and esophageal cancer.[41] COX-2 contributes to tumorigenesis by several mechanisms, including inhibition of apoptosis and increase in angiogenesis, cellular adhesion, and invasion.[42] Epidemiologic studies have shown that long-term use of nonsteroidal antiinflammatory drugs (NSAIDs) and aspirin (ASA) are associated with a decreased risk of esophageal cancer.[43,44] Liao et al. performed a pooled analysis of six population-based studies within the Barrett's and Esophageal Adenocarcinoma Consortium (BEACON).[43] They found a protective association between NSAID or ASA use and EAC compared with nonusers,

with odds ratios (ORs) of 0.68 (95% CI, 0.56 to 0.83) and 0.77 (95% CI, 0.69 to 0.97), respectively. Specifically, with NSAIDs, the risk reduction was increased with more frequent (at least daily) or long-term (≥10 years) use. It is presumed that by inhibiting COX, these drugs act early in the inflammation-metaplasia-cancer sequence to prevent the development or esophageal cancer or its precursor.[45]

RISK FACTORS SPECIFIC TO ESOPHAGEAL ADENOCARCINOMA

OBESITY

The rising incidence of EAC has coincided with the obesity epidemic in the United States. As such, several studies have identified a correlation between obesity and the risk of esophageal cancer.[46–49] A recent meta-analysis by Turati et al. demonstrated that both men and women with a body mass index (BMI) greater than 30 kg/m^2 have a threefold increase in risk (relative risk [RR] = 2.73), and an RR of 1.11 for every 5 kg/m^2 increase in BMI.[50] Corley et al. found abdominal diameter specifically to correlate with an increased risk of EAC (BMI-adjusted OR, 4.78; 95% CI, 1.14 to 20.11) but not SCC (OR, 0.78; 95% CI, 0.32 to 1.92).[47] Similarly, a recent study by Steffen et al. concluded that abdominal obesity (measured by waist circumference) as opposed to general obesity (reflected by BMI) contributed to a considerable risk for EAC.[48]

The mechanism through which obesity contributes to esophageal cancer risk is not fully understood. It has been suggested that the increased incidence of gastroesophageal reflux disease (GERD) and low-grade systemic inflammation associated with adipose tissue all contribute to progression along the inflammation-metaplasia-cancer sequence.[51]

GASTROESOPHAGEAL REFLUX DISEASE

GERD is a highly prevalent disorder worldwide, with prevalence estimates considerably higher in Western populations (18% to 28%) compared with East Asia (2% to 8%).[52] Several studies have investigated the role of GERD in the development of EAC. Lagergren et al. were among the first to evaluate this association in a case-control study comparing 189 patients with EAC and 820 control subjects.[53] They demonstrated an exposure-dependent increase in risk. Compared with asymptomatic patients, those with recurrent symptoms of reflux had an OR of 7.7 (95% CI, 4.3 to 11.5) of developing EAC, while those with long-lasting and severe symptoms had an OR of 43.5 (95% CI, 11.3 to 103.5). It has been reported that up to two-thirds of patients undergoing esophagectomy for EAC have preoperative GERD symptoms.[54] Even still, despite the high prevalence of GERD, the absolute risk of esophageal cancer in a given patient with reflux is low.[55] Therefore the American Gastroenterological Association does not recommend routine endoscopic surveillance in the setting of chronic GERD without troublesome symptoms such as dysphagia.[56]

BARRETT ESOPHAGUS

More so than GERD, Barrett esophagus is the most important risk factor in the development of EAC. In patients without dysplasia, the annual risk of esophageal cancer is 0.25%, compared with 6% for those with high-grade dysplasia.[57] Risk factors for progression to cancer include chronic GERD, presence of hiatal hernia, advanced age, male sex, white race, tobacco use, and obesity. The risk of cancer also increases as the segment length of Barrett increases, with long-segment Barrett (≥ 3 cm) having a transition rate of 0.22% per year compared with 0.01% in ultra-short segment Barrett (<1 cm).[58]

PROTON PUMP INHIBITORS

The increased incidence of EAC has correlated with the increased use of proton pump inhibitors (PPIs) since their discovery in the 1980s. Studies have shown that up to half of patients with EAC report PPI use.[4] While PPIs decrease the acidity of the refluxate into the esophagus, they do not eliminate reflux. In fact, studies have shown that reflux of bile salts also contributes to the development of Barrett esophagus.[59,60]

LOWER-SPHINCTER RELAXING MEDICATIONS

Medications that lower the resting pressure of the lower esophageal sphincter (LES) are thought to increase the risk of esophageal cancer by promoting increased gastroesophageal reflux. A case-control study by Lagergren et al. found a positive association between past use of sphincter-relaxing medications (nitroglycerin, anticholinergics, β-adrenergic agonists, aminophyllines, and benzodiazepines) and the risk of EAC.[61] They also demonstrated a higher prevalence of reflux symptoms among users of LES-relaxing agents. After adjusting for reflux symptoms, the positive association almost disappeared suggesting that promotion of reflux is the link between the use of sphincter-relaxing drugs and EAC. Ranka et al. demonstrated a similar positive association with cancer risk and the use of bronchodilators, theophylline, and calcium channel blockers.[62]

HELICOBACTER PYLORI

Helicobacter pylori infection is linked to several gastrointestinal malignancies including gastric cancer.[63] Conversely, studies have shown that colonization of the stomach with *H. pylori*, particularly cytotoxin-associated gene A (CagA)-positive strains, may protect against the development of EAC.[64] A recent meta-analysis also demonstrated a negative association with SCC in East Asian populations but no effect in Western populations.[65] It is hypothesized that *H. pylori* induces gastric atrophy and decreased acid production, hence decreasing acid reflux into the distal esophagus.[66] Another suggested mechanism is through decreased gastric secretion of the hormone ghrelin, which subsequently decreases appetite, leading to lower rates of obesity, a known risk factor for EAC.[67]

WHY IS THE EPIDEMIOLOGY CHANGING?

Several theories have been proposed to explain the changing epidemiology of esophageal cancer worldwide. The rise in EAC has been the most dramatic change. Some have raised the question of whether the rise in the incidence of EAC is actually a result of reclassification of related cancers or improved diagnosis due to better-quality endoscopy. Pohl and Welch used the SEER database to assess these hypotheses.[7] They noted a shift in the anatomic distribution of esophageal cancer with an increased incidence only in the distal third of the esophagus where EAC is usually found. This would argue that reclassification of SCC does not account for the increased incidence of EAC. Similarly, it cannot be explained by reclassification of tumors of the gastric cardia because the incidence of tumors below the gastroesophageal junction has also increased over the past three decades. Finally, they noted that over the past 30 years, the mortality from EAC has increased over sevenfold with only a minor change in the proportion of patients diagnosed with localized disease, excluding improved diagnosis as a cause for the rise in incidence. Because of these data, they concluded that the increased incidence of EAC represented a true increase in disease burden.

The increase in esophageal cancer may be explained by changes in the prevalence of its known risk factors. The most notable change has been in the increased prevalence of obesity, especially in the United States. As reviewed earlier in this chapter, several studies have identified obesity and central adiposity as risk factors for EAC, possibly due to hormonal effects or due to the increased prevalence of GERD among obese individuals. Over the past three decades, the increased incidence of EAC has been greatest in the Netherlands, United States, and Spain, in decreasing order. However, Kroep et al. identified that the prevalence of obesity has not followed the same trend, signifying that there must be other key drivers in the rise of EAC incidence.[68] Parallels have also been noted with the rising prevalence of GERD, PPI use, and *H. pylori* eradication, particularly in the Western world.

CLINICAL MANIFESTATIONS

The symptoms of esophageal cancer vary by stage. Early-stage tumors are typically asymptomatic, which is why over 50% of patients present with regionally advanced or metastatic disease.[4] The most common presenting symptoms include dysphagia (74%), weight loss (57%), and odynophagia (17%).[69,70] Other symptoms such as cough, dyspnea, hoarseness, and pain (abdominal, back, retrosternal) may indicate more extensive disease.[71] In patients with EAC, up to two-thirds of patients have a history of reflux symptoms.[54]

For early-stage disease, the physical examination is usually unremarkable. Patients with metastatic disease may have hepatomegaly, pleural effusion, or lymphadenopathy, particularly in the left supraclavicular fossa (Virchow node).[71]

Routine endoscopic screening of the general population is generally not recommended, as the incidence of esophageal cancer is low. The American College of Gastroenterology 2016 guidelines recommend endoscopic screening for Barrett esophagus in men with chronic or frequent symptomatic GERD with two or more risk factors for EAC (i.e., age >50, Caucasian race, central obesity, current or past tobacco use, family history of Barrett or esophageal cancer in a first-degree relative).[72] In women, they recommend considering screening on a case-by-case basis as determined by the presence of multiple risk factors listed above. In patients with Barrett esophagus, surveillance is recommended every 3 to 5 years in the absence of dysplasia, with more frequent intervals and/or therapy in the setting of dysplasia.

REFERENCES

1. Howlader N, Noone AA, Krapcho M, et al. SEER Cancer Statistics Review, 1975–2013. http://seer.cancer.gov/csr/1975_2013/.
2. Dawsey SM, Lewin KJ, Wang GQ, et al. Squamous esophageal histology and subsequent risk of squamous cell carcinoma of the esophagus. A prospective follow-up study from Linxian, China. *Cancer.* 1994;74:1686-1692.
3. Conteduca V, Sansonno D, Ingravallo G, et al. Barrett's esophagus and esophageal cancer: an overview. *Int J Oncol.* 2012;41:414-424.
4. Siegel RL, Miller KD, Jemal A. Cancer statistics, 2016. *CA Cancer J Clin.* 2016;66:7-30.
5. Pennathur A, Gibson MK, Jobe BA, et al. Oesophageal carcinoma. *Lancet.* 2013;381:400-412.
6. Torre LA, Bray F, Siegel RL, et al. Global cancer statistics, 2012. *CA Cancer J Clin.* 2015;65:87-108.
7. Pohl H, Welch HG. The role of overdiagnosis and reclassification in the marked increase of esophageal adenocarcinoma incidence. *J Natl Cancer Inst.* 2005;97:142-146.
8. Hur C, Miller M, Kong CY, et al. Trends in esophageal adenocarcinoma incidence and mortality. *Cancer.* 2013;119:1149-1158.
9. Trivers KF, Sabatino SA, Stewart SL. Trends in esophageal cancer incidence by histology, United States, 1998–2003. *Int J Cancer.* 2008;123: 1422-1428.
10. Giri S, Pathak R, Aryal MR, et al. Incidence trend of esophageal squamous cell carcinoma: an analysis of Surveillance Epidemiology, and End Results (SEER) database. *Cancer Causes Control.* 2015;26:159-161.
11. Torre LA, Siegel RL, Ward EM, et al. Global cancer incidence and mortality rates and trends—an update. *Cancer Epidemiol Biomarkers Prev.* 2016;25:16-27.
12. Kamangar F, Dores GM, Anderson WF. Patterns of cancer incidence, mortality, and prevalence across five continents: defining priorities to reduce cancer disparities in different geographic regions of the world. *J Clin Oncol.* 2006;24:2137-2150.
13. Rice TW, Rusch VW, Apperson-Hansen C, et al. Worldwide esophageal cancer collaboration. *Dis Esophagus.* 2009;22:1-8.
14. Mathieu LN, Kanarek NF, Tsai HL, et al. Age and sex differences in the incidence of esophageal adenocarcinoma: results from the Surveillance, Epidemiology, and End Results (SEER) Registry (1973–2008). *Dis Esophagus.* 2014;27:757-763.
15. Cook MB, Chow WH, Devesa SS. Oesophageal cancer incidence in the United States by race, sex, and histologic type, 1977–2005. *Br J Cancer.* 2009;101:855-859.
16. Zhang Y. Epidemiology of esophageal cancer. *World J Gastroenterol.* 2013; 19:5598-5606.
17. Siewert JR, Stein HJ. Classification of adenocarcinoma of the oesophagogastric junction. *Br J Surg.* 1998;85:1457-1459.
18. Rice TW, Blackstone EH, Rusch VW. 7th edition of the AJCC cancer staging manual: esophagus and esophagogastric junction. *Ann Surg Oncol.* 2010;17:1721-1724.
19. Prabhu A, Obi KO, Rubenstein JH. The synergistic effects of alcohol and tobacco consumption on the risk of esophageal squamous cell carcinoma: a meta-analysis. *Am J Gastroenterol.* 2014;109:822-827.
20. Pandeya N, Williams GM, Sadhegi S, et al. Associations of duration, intensity, and quantity of smoking with adenocarcinoma and squamous cell carcinoma of the esophagus. *Am J Epidemiol.* 2008;168:105-114.
21. Kamangar F, Chow WH, Abnet CC, et al. Environmental causes of esophageal cancer. *Gastroenterol Clin North Am.* 2009;38:27-57, vii.
22. Corrao G, Bagnardi V, Zambon A, et al. A meta-analysis of alcohol consumption and the risk of 15 diseases. *Prev Med.* 2004;38:613-619.
23. Bagnardi V, Blangiardo M, La Vecchia C, et al. A meta-analysis of alcohol drinking and cancer risk. *Br J Cancer.* 2001;85:1700-1705.
24. Freedman ND, Abnet CC, Leitzmann MF, et al. A prospective study of tobacco, alcohol, and the risk of esophageal and gastric cancer subtypes. *Am J Epidemiol.* 2007;165:1424-1433.
25. Eckardt AJ, Eckardt VF. Current clinical approach to achalasia. *World J Gastroenterol.* 2009;15:3969-3975.
26. Zendehdel K, Nyren O, Edberg A, et al. Risk of esophageal adenocarcinoma in achalasia patients, a retrospective cohort study in Sweden. *Am J Gastroenterol.* 2011;106:57-61.
27. Sandler RS, Nyren O, Ekbom A, et al. The risk of esophageal cancer in patients with achalasia. A population-based study. *JAMA.* 1995;274: 1359-1362.
28. Dunaway PM, Wong RK. Risk and surveillance intervals for squamous cell carcinoma in achalasia. *Gastrointest Endosc Clin N Am.* 2001;11:425-434, ix.
29. Leeuwenburgh I, Scholten P, Alderliesten J, et al. Long-term esophageal cancer risk in patients with primary achalasia: a prospective study. *Am J Gastroenterol.* 2010;105:2144-2149.
30. Brucher BL, Stein HJ, Bartels H, et al. Achalasia and esophageal cancer: incidence, prevalence, and prognosis. *World J Surg.* 2001;25: 745-749.
31. Riboli E, Norat T. Epidemiologic evidence of the protective effect of fruit and vegetables on cancer risk. *Am J Clin Nutr.* 2003;78:559S-569S.
32. Freedman ND, Park Y, Subar AF, et al. Fruit and vegetable intake and esophageal cancer in a large prospective cohort study. *Int J Cancer.* 2007;121:2753-2760.
33. Yamaji T, Inoue M, Sasazuki S, et al. Fruit and vegetable consumption and squamous cell carcinoma of the esophagus in Japan: the JPHC study. *Int J Cancer.* 2008;123:1935-1940.
34. Jemal A, Center MM, DeSantis C, et al. Global patterns of cancer incidence and mortality rates and trends. *Cancer Epidemiol Biomarkers Prev.* 2010;19:1893-1907.
35. Tran GD, Sun XD, Abnet CC, et al. Prospective study of risk factors for esophageal and gastric cancers in the Linxian general population trial cohort in China. *Int J Cancer.* 2005;113:456-463.
36. Islami F, Kamangar F, Nasrollahzadeh D, et al. Oesophageal cancer in Golestan Province, a high-incidence area in northern Iran—a review. *Eur J Cancer.* 2009;45:3156-3165.
37. Islami F, Boffetta P, Ren JS, et al. High-temperature beverages and foods and esophageal cancer risk—a systematic review. *Int J Cancer.* 2009;125:491-524.
38. Lukanich JM. Section 1. Epidemiological review. *Semin Thorac Cardiovasc Surg.* 2003;15:158-166.
39. Dong LM, Kristal AR, Peters U, et al. Dietary supplement use and risk of neoplastic progression in esophageal adenocarcinoma: a prospective study. *Nutr Cancer.* 2008;60:39-48.
40. Thompson CL, Khiani V, Chak A, et al. Carbohydrate consumption and esophageal cancer: an ecological assessment. *Am J Gastroenterol.* 2008;103:555-561.
41. Zimmermann KC, Sarbia M, Weber AA, et al. Cyclooxygenase-2 expression in human esophageal carcinoma. *Cancer Res.* 1999;59:198-204.
42. Trifan OC, Hla T. Cyclooxygenase-2 modulates cellular growth and promotes tumorigenesis. *J Cell Mol Med.* 2003;7:207-222.
43. Liao LM, Vaughan TL, Corley DA, et al. Nonsteroidal antiinflammatory drug use reduces risk of adenocarcinomas of the esophagus and esophagogastric junction in a pooled analysis. *Gastroenterology.* 2012;142:442-452. e445, quiz e422–443.
44. Vaughan TL, Dong LM, Blount PL, et al. Non-steroidal antiinflammatory drugs and risk of neoplastic progression in Barrett's oesophagus: a prospective study. *Lancet Oncol.* 2005;6:945-952.
45. Anderson LA, Johnston BT, Watson RG, et al. Nonsteroidal antiinflammatory drugs and the esophageal inflammation-metaplasia-adenocarcinoma sequence. *Cancer Res.* 2006;66:4975-4982.
46. Calle EE, Rodriguez C, Walker-Thurmond K, et al. Overweight, obesity, and mortality from cancer in a prospectively studied cohort of U.S. adults. *N Engl J Med.* 2003;348:1625-1638.
47. Corley DA, Kubo A, Zhao W. Abdominal obesity and the risk of esophageal and gastric cardia carcinomas. *Cancer Epidemiol Biomarkers Prev.* 2008;17:352-358.
48. Steffen A, Huerta JM, Weiderpass E, et al. General and abdominal obesity and risk of esophageal and gastric adenocarcinoma in the European Prospective Investigation into Cancer and Nutrition. *Int J Cancer.* 2015;137:646-657.
49. Thrift AP, Shaheen NJ, Gammon MD, et al. Obesity and risk of esophageal adenocarcinoma and Barrett's esophagus: a Mendelian randomization study. *J Natl Cancer Inst.* 2014;106.
50. Turati F, Tramacere I, La Vecchia C, et al. A meta-analysis of body mass index and esophageal and gastric cardia adenocarcinoma. *Ann Oncol.* 2013;24:609-617.
51. Long E, Beales IL. The role of obesity in oesophageal cancer development. *Therap Adv Gastroenterol.* 2014;7:247-268.
52. El-Serag HB, Sweet S, Winchester CC, et al. Update on the epidemiology of gastro-oesophageal reflux disease: a systematic review. *Gut.* 2014;63:871-880.

53. Lagergren J, Bergstrom R, Lindgren A, et al. Symptomatic gastro-esophageal reflux as a risk factor for esophageal adenocarcinoma. *N Engl J Med.* 1999;340:825-831.

54. Lada MJ, Nieman DR, Han M, et al. Gastroesophageal reflux disease, proton-pump inhibitor use and Barrett's esophagus in esophageal adenocarcinoma: trends revisited. *Surgery.* 2013;154:856-864, discussion 864–856.

55. Shaheen N, Ransohoff DF. Gastroesophageal reflux, Barrett esophagus, and esophageal cancer: scientific review. *JAMA.* 2002;287:1972-1981.

56. Kahrilas PJ, Shaheen NJ, Vaezi MF, et al. American Gastroenterological Association medical position statement on the management of gastroesophageal reflux disease. *Gastroenterology.* 2008;135:1383-1391. 1391 e1381–1385.

57. Spechler SJ. Barrett esophagus and risk of esophageal cancer: a clinical review. *JAMA.* 2013;310:627-636.

58. Pohl H, Pech O, Arash H, et al. Length of Barrett's oesophagus and cancer risk: implications from a large sample of patients with early oesophageal adenocarcinoma. *Gut.* 2016;65:196-201.

59. Nasr AO, Dillon MF, Conlon S, et al. Acid suppression increases rates of Barrett's esophagus and esophageal injury in the presence of duodenal reflux. *Surgery.* 2012;151:382-390.

60. Alsalahi O, Dobrian AD. Proton pump inhibitors: the culprit for Barrett's esophagus? *Front Oncol.* 2014;4:373.

61. Lagergren J, Bergstrom R, Adami HO, et al. Association between medications that relax the lower esophageal sphincter and risk for esophageal adenocarcinoma. *Ann Intern Med.* 2000 133:165-175.

62. Ranka S, Gee JM, Johnson IT, et al. Non-steroidal anti-inflammatory drugs, lower oesophageal sphincter-relaxing drugs and oesophageal cancer. A case-control study. *Digestion.* 2006;74:109- 15.

63. Parsonnet J, Friedman GD, Vandersteen DP, et al. *Helicobacter pylori* infection and the risk of gastric carcinoma. *N Engl J Med.* 1991;325: 1127-1131.

64. Islami F, Kamangar F. *Helicobacter pylori* and esophageal cancer risk: a meta-analysis. *Cancer Prev Res (Phila).* 2008;1:329-338.

65. Xie FJ, Zhang YP, Zheng QQ, et al. *Helicobacter pylori* infection and esophageal cancer risk: an updated meta-analysis. *World J Gastroenterol.* 2013;19:6098-6107.

66. Chow WH, Blaser MJ, Blot WJ, et al. An inverse relation between cagA+ strains of *Helicobacter pylori* infection and risk of esophageal and gastric cardia adenocarcinoma. *Cancer Res.* 1998;58:588-590.

67. Whiteman DC, Sadeghi S, Pandeya N, et al. Combined effects of obesity, acid reflux and smoking on the risk of adenocarcinomas of the oesophagus. *Gut.* 2008;57:173-180.

68. Kroep S, Lansdorp-Vogelaar I, Rubenstein JH, et al. Comparing trends in esophageal adenocarcinoma incidence and lifestyle factors between the United States, Spain, and the Netherlands. *Am J Gastroenterol.* 2014;109:336-343, quiz 335, 344.

69. Daly JM, Fry WA, Little AG, et al. Esophageal cancer: results of an American College of Surgeons Patient Care Evaluation Study. *J Am Coll Surg.* 2000;190:562-572, discussion 572–563.

70. Fein R, Kelsen DP, Geller N, et al. Adenocarcinoma of the esophagus and gastroesophageal junction. Prognostic factors and results of therapy. *Cancer.* 1985;56:2512-2518.

71. Enzinger PC, Mayer RJ. Esophageal cancer. *N Engl J Med.* 2003;349: 2241-2252.

72. Shaheen NJ, Falk GW, Iyer PG, et al. ACG clinical guideline: diagnosis and management of Barrett's esophagus. *Am J Gastroenterol.* 2016;111: 30-50.

Esophageal Cancer Diagnosis and Staging

Mustapha El Lakis | Donald E. Low

EPIDEMIOLOGY

The incidence of esophageal cancer has increased in recent decades, with an estimated 17,990 new cases in the United States in 2013.[1] Histologically, in the United States esophageal adenocarcinoma is the fastest-growing subtype, surpassing the incidence of esophageal squamous cell carcinoma (SCC), in contrast to worldwide incidence where SCC still predominates.[2,3] There is a marked variation in histologic incidence of esophageal cancer with respect to race, sex, geographic area, and economical status. SCC is three times more frequent in blacks as compared with whites.[4] In the United States, the age-adjusted incidence among whites is up to 5 per 100,000 versus 12.5 per 100,000[5] in France versus more than 100 per 100,000 in some parts of China.[6] In most countries the male-to-female ratio is 6 to 1.[7] Genetic predisposition has also been clearly established; however, other risk factors, such as smoking and alcohol, have been strongly associated with SCC, and gastroesophageal reflux disease (GERD) has been associated with Barrett esophagus and adenocarcinoma.

Esophageal cancer remains one of the deadliest cancers with an overall 5-year survival rate estimated to be less than 18%.[8] Esophagectomy has historically been the gold standard for regional invasive cancers; however, less invasive therapy such as endoscopic mucosal resection (EMR) has become an accepted alternative treatment for intramucosal carcinoma.[9] Moreover, multimodality therapy (neoadjuvant chemotherapy, or chemoradiotherapy followed by esophagectomy) has shown increased survival benefits when compared with surgery alone in locally advanced cases.[10] Therefore, accurate staging is essential for a stage-directed treatment approach, for prognostication, for quality control in clinical trials, and for proper communication among health care workers as well as patients.

Both invasive and noninvasive staging techniques are employed. Although new technologies have upgraded staging accuracy, the best overall approach remains controversial. This chapter describes the current staging classifications and methods for esophageal cancer and highlights some of the difficulties and controversies.

ANATOMY

The esophagus is approximately 20 to 30 cm in length and is located in the posterior mediastinum. It extends from the hypopharynx, posterior to the trachea and the heart, to the stomach, passing through the esophageal hiatus. Through its descent, three critical anatomic points of narrowing are identified: the cricopharyngeus muscle, the bronchoaortic constriction, and the esophagogastric junction, which are also the most common sites of iatrogenic

and mechanical perforation. The esophagus, a muscular tube, is composed of three general layers as follows: mucosa (stratified squamous epithelium), submucosa, and muscularis propria. The tissue immediately attached to the esophagus is called the adventitia.

The esophagus is divided into three anatomic areas comprising cervical, upper and middle thoracic, and lower thoracic/esophagogastric junction (Fig. 36.1). The esophagus also can be divided into thirds with 50% of adenocarcinoma occurring in the lower third.[11] The location of the tumor is an important prognostic element and has been included in the tumor, node, metastasis (TNM) seventh edition staging system of the SCC. Tumors in the middle or upper esophagus are considered higher stage compared with the lower one-third of the esophagus.

1. The cervical esophagus extends from the esophageal orifice (lower border of the cricoid cartilage) to the sternal notch (or thoracic inlet). Typical endoscopic measurements for the cervical esophagus from the incisors are from 15 to less than 20 cm.
2. The upper thoracic esophagus extends from the sternal notch to the azygos vein arch. Typically, this is located from 20 to less than 25 cm from the incisors. The middle thoracic esophagus is bordered superiorly by the lower border of the azygos vein and inferiorly by the inferior pulmonary vein. Typical endoscopic measurements from the incisors are from 25 to less than 30 cm.
3. The lower thoracic esophagus extends from below the inferior pulmonary vein to the gastroesophageal junction (GEJ). Typical measurements from the incisors are from 30 to 40 cm.

Lymph node involvement and the number of lymph node metastases are important prognostic factors. The esophagus has a complex pattern of a dense and rich interconnected network of lymphatic vessels deep within submucosa that communicate freely longitudinally and transversally with the lymphatics of the muscular layers; thus, the pattern of lymph node metastases is very complex. Lymphatic channels in the submucosa facilitate the longitudinal spread of neoplastic cells along the esophageal wall. They can drain to cervical, tracheobronchial, mediastinal nodes, and gastric and celiac nodes.

Many patients will present late in the disease process with unresectable tumors or distant metastasis. The most common metastatic sites are retroperitoneal or celiac lymph nodes, liver, lungs, and adrenals.[12] Metastatic disease can also manifest as malignant pleural effusion, ascites, and bone pain of the affected site in bone metastasis or as hypercalcemia secondary to paraneoplastic syndrome. Adenocarcinomas most frequently metastasize to intraabdominal sites, while metastases from SCCs more commonly spread to intrathoracic or cervical locations.

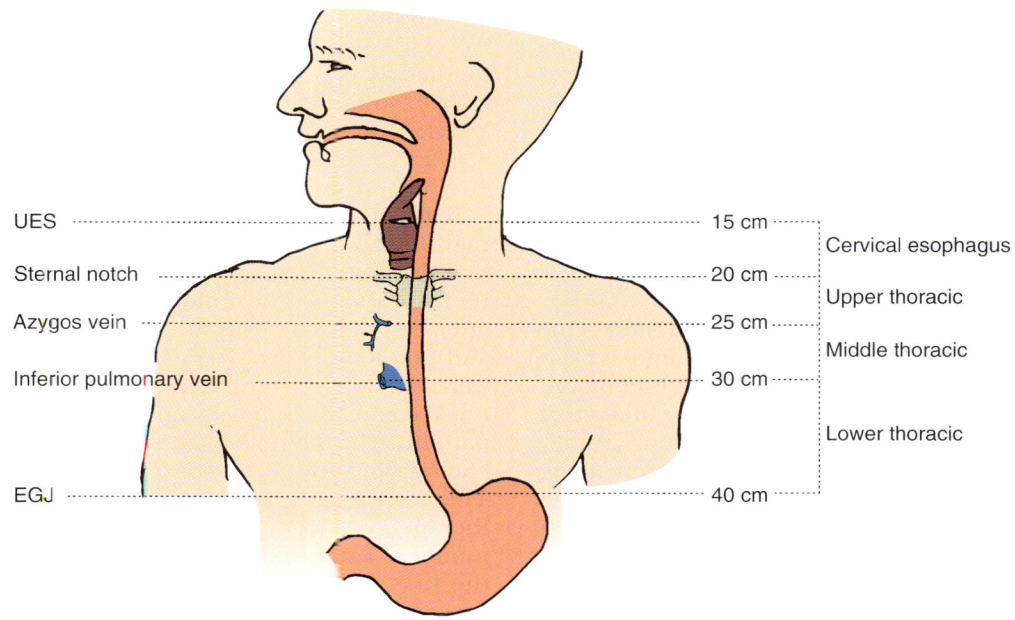

UES ·········· 15 cm ········
Cervical esophagus

Sternal notch ·········· 20 cm ········
Upper thoracic

Azygos vein ·········· 25 cm ········
Middle thoracic

Inferior pulmonary vein ·········· 30 cm ········

Lower thoracic

EGJ ·········· 40 cm ········

FIGURE 36.1 Description of the anatomic landmarks of the esophagus. *EGJ*, Esophagogastric junction; *UES*, upper esophageal sphincter.

NOMENCLATURE

Different-stage nomenclatures are used to define the state of the disease at specific phases in the care of the cancer patients. These include pretreatment stage or *clinical stage,* and postsurgical or *pathologic stage.* In addition, stage is further classified according to neoadjuvant therapy or at the time of recurrence.

The clinical stage or pretreatment stage is the extent of disease defined by diagnostic studies such as physical examination, imaging tests, endoscopic examination, biopsies of the primary tumor, and surgical exploration without resection of the affected areas. The nomenclature for clinical staging is cT, cN, and cM.

The pathologic stage is defined by the same diagnostic studies used for clinical staging supplemented by findings from surgical resection and histologic examination of the surgically removed tissues. This pathologic extent of disease is expressed as pT, pN, and pM.

The posttherapy stage documents the extent of the disease after neoadjuvant therapy or when systemic therapy or radiation is the only treatment. The posttherapy stage may be recorded as clinical or pathologic, depending on the source of posttreatment information. The nomenclature is recorded by adding the prefix "yc" or "yp" such as: ycT, ycN, ycM, ypT, ypN, and ypM.

Restaging is used to determine the extent of the disease following the completion of neoadjuvant therapy, and if a cancer recurs after treatment. This is done to determine if additional treatment is warranted or appropriate.

In addition to the TNM components, residual tumor and surgical margins are two important elements that may have a prognostic implication on the cancer patients after surgery. Residual tumor is denoted by the symbol "R";

it reflects the effect of therapy and the completeness of surgical resection, and is a strong predictor of prognosis. Although not formally integrated into TNM staging, "R" status is an important component of the pathologic record within the cancer registry.

The "R" categories for the primary tumor site are as follows:
- R0 no residual tumor
- R1 microscopic residual tumor
- R2 macroscopic residual tumor
- RX presence of residual tumor cannot be assessed

It should be noted that the "R1" designation varies between countries. In the United States, which uses the American College of Pathology designation of R1, it is "tumors at the surgical margin." In the United Kingdom, the definition of the Royal College of Pathology is used, which designates R1 as a "tumor within 1 mm of the surgical margin."

HISTOLOGIC TYPE

Esophageal cancers are histologically classified as SCC or adenocarcinoma.[13] Adenocarcinoma is a malignant epithelial tumor with glandular differentiation arising predominantly from Barrett esophagus mucosa in the lower third of the esophagus. Occasionally they originate from heterotopic gastric mucosa in the upper esophagus, or from mucosal and submucosal glands. SCC is a malignant epithelial tumor with squamous cell differentiation, microscopically characterized by keratinocyte-like cells with intercellular bridges and/or keratinization. SCC and adenocarcinoma are assumed to have different biologic behaviors, which might influence treatment choices. SCC seems to be more sensitive to chemotherapy, chemoradiation, and radiotherapy than adenocarcinoma, but the long-term outcome of therapy appears to be similar. Adenocarcinoma may be associated with a better long-term prognosis after resection than SCC.[14] Another histologic subtype that has been reported is the *primary mixed adenosquamous carcinoma*. It is a rare kind of malignancy characterized by mixed glandular and squamous differentiation as well as a propensity for aggressive clinical behavior.[15]

HISTOLOGIC GRADE

The tumor grade reflects the histologic aggressiveness of the cancer. It can be an indicator of how quickly a tumor is likely to grow and spread. Cancers that are "well-differentiated" tend to grow and spread at a slower rate than tumors that are "undifferentiated" or "poorly differentiated." Tumor grade is defined by numbers: 1, 2, 3, or 4 or by X depending on the amount of abnormality, shown as[16]:

- GX: Grade cannot be assessed (undetermined grade)
- G1: Well differentiated (low grade)
- G2: Moderately differentiated (intermediate grade)
- G3: Poorly differentiated (high grade)
- G4: Undifferentiated (high grade)

TUMOR, NODE, METASTASIS CLASSIFICATION AND UPDATES IN THE SEVENTH EDITION

The TNM staging system for all solid tumors was devised by Pierre Denoix between 1943 and 1952. Currently, it is maintained and developed by the American Joint Committee on Cancer (AJCC) and the Union for International Cancer Control (UICC). The TNM staging system is updated every 6 to 8 years to include advances in our understanding of cancer prognostication. The TNM system classifies and groups cancers primarily by the extent of local tumor invasion into the esophageal wall and advanced invasion into adjacent structures (T), the status of regional draining lymph nodes (N), and the presence or absence of distant metastases (M). The T stage is assessed by evaluation of the depth of invasion into the four distinct layers involving the esophageal wall and adventitia according to the following nomenclature:

- TX: Primary tumor cannot be assessed
- T0: No evidence of primary tumor
- Tis: High-grade dysplasia
- T1: Tumor invading mucosal lamina propria, muscularis mucosae, or submucosa
  - T1a: Tumor invading into the lamina propria or muscularis mucosae
  - T1b: Tumor invading submucosa
- T2: Tumor invading muscularis propria
- T3: Tumor invading adventitia
- T4: Tumor invading adjacent structures
  - T4a: Resectable tumor invading pleura, pericardium, or diaphragm
  - T4b: Unresectable tumor invading other adjacent structures, such as aorta, vertebral body, or trachea.

T stage is important in the prognostication and is crucial to determining suitability for surgical resection and establishing a treatment plan.

The nodal classification (N) is one of the most controversial aspects in TNM staging. Different N stages are defined as:

- N0: No positive node
- N1: 1 to 2 nodes
- N2: 3 to 6 nodes
- N3: 7 or more nodes

There is no consensus on the ideal number of nodes that must be resected for optimal staging. Data suggest that the number of lymph nodes recovered—rather than their location—is an independent predictor of survival after esophagectomy. In the Surveillance, Epidemiology, and End Results (SEER) database, when 12 lymph nodes were examined, significant reduction in mortality was noted compared with no lymph node evaluation. Moreover, patients who had 30 or more lymph nodes examined had significantly lower mortality than any other groups.[17] This may be secondary to enhanced N staging, or to a therapeutic effect of lymphadenectomy. In addition, the number of involved lymph nodes can be used to predict the likelihood of systemic disease.[18] There is general agreement that a two-field lymph node dissection should be done in an invasive cancer. For lymph node mapping, a lymph node map that extends the nomenclature and numbering system used for the staging of non–small cell lung cancer can be used (Fig. 36.2).

Distant metastasis is simply designated as:

- M0: no distant metastases
- M1: distant metastases.

UPDATES IN THE SEVENTH EDITION

The seventh edition of TNM staging is the most updated version published in 2010. This update involved the analysis of data on 4627 patients treated with esophagectomy without induction or adjuvant therapy.[19] Changes as compared with the AJCC sixth edition are reviewed in Table 36.1.

Two major revisions were made for the T stage: Tis, or high-grade dysplasia, now includes all noninvasive neoplastic epithelium, which was previously termed carcinoma-in-situ. T1–T3 stages remained the same as in the sixth edition. T4 lesions have been subcategorized into T4a, resectable cancers infiltrating the pleura, pericardium, or diaphragm; and T4b, unresectable cancers infiltrating structures, such as the aorta, vertebral body, or tracheabronchi and carotid vessels.

In the seventh TNM edition, major modifications were observed for the N stage. The sixth edition defined regional nodes (N1) as those in the periesophageal, mediastinal, and perigastric areas, but cervical and celiac nodes were regarded as "distant" metastases and designated M1a and M1b. Stage M1b included visceral organ metastases.

In the seventh edition, a regional node was redefined to include any paraesophageal node extending from the thoracic inlet to celiac axis. The subclassifications of M1a and M1b have been eliminated, as has MX. In addition, the seventh edition accounted for the nodal burden by classifying the number of involved lymph nodes into categories: N1, 1 to 2; N2, 3 to 6; N3, 7 or more.

The seventh edition also noted the following changes: a different staging system for adenocarcinoma and SCC (Table 36.2); the precise definition of the three types of GEJ tumors based on location, including all three exclusively

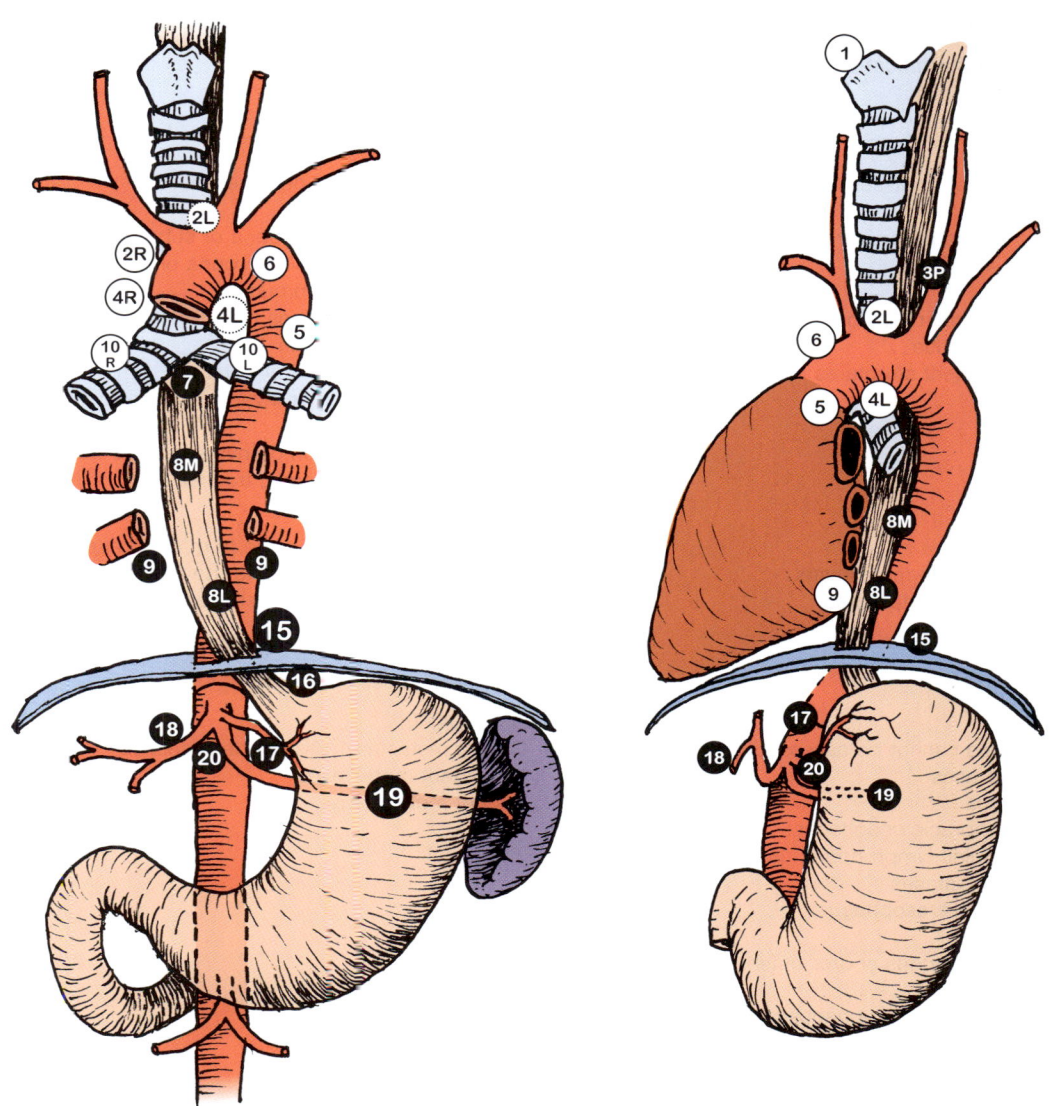

FIGURE 36.2 Lymph node stations suggested by the American Joint Committee on Cancer manual. *1*, Supraclavicular; *2R*, right upper paratracheal nodes; *2L*, left upper paratracheal nodes; *3P*, posterior mediastinal nodes; *4R*, right lower paratracheal nodes; *4L*, left lower paratracheal nodes; *5*, aortopulmonary nodes; *6*, anterior mediastinal nodes; *7*, subcarinal nodes; *8M*, middle paraesophageal nodes; *8L*, lower paraesophageal nodes; *9*, pulmonary ligament nodes; *10R*, right tracheobronchial nodes; *10L*, left tracheobronchial nodes; *15*, diaphragmatic nodes; *16*, paracardial nodes; *17*, left gastric nodes; *18*, common hepatic nodes; *19*, splenic nodes; *20*, celiac nodes.

in the esophageal staging system; and lastly, the inclusion of tumor grade as part of the system.

STAGE GROUPINGS

SCC and adenocarcinomas are grouped differently (see Table 36.2). For lower-staged squamous cell cancers (stage 0 to IIB), tumor grade and location come into play to assign the stage grouping. G1 lower thoracic squamous cell (stage IB) has the best prognosis, G2 to G4 upper- and middle-third cancers (stage IIB) have the worst survival, and G2 to G4 lower thoracic SCC and G1 upper- and middle-third cancers (stage IIA) have intermediate survival. For adenocarcinomas, only tumor differentiation influences the stage grouping from stage 0 to IIA. Stage 0, III, and IV squamous cell and adenocarcinomas are identically stage grouped.

ANATOMIC LOCATION AND ESOPHAGOGASTRIC JUNCTION TUMORS

The classification of adenocarcinoma of the esophagogastric junction (EGJ) was originally described by Siewert et al. They divided it into three types according to the anatomic location of the epicenter or the location of the tumor mass. When the epicenter, or more than two-thirds of the mass, is located more than 1 cm above the anatomic EGJ, the tumor is considered in the distal esophagus as type I. When the epicenter or tumor is located within 1 cm proximal and 2 cm distal to the anatomic EGJ, it is classified as type II. When the epicenter or more than two-thirds of the mass is located more than 2 cm below the anatomic EGJ, the tumor is classified as type III. In 2000, the classification was

TABLE 36.1 TNM Classification Changes

AJCC Sixth Edition	AJCC Seventh Edition
T CLASSIFICATION*	**T CLASSIFICATION**
Tx: Primary tumor cannot be assessed	Tx: Primary tumor cannot be assessed
Tis: Carcinoma in situ	Tis: High-grade dysplasia[†]
T1: Tumor invades lamina propria or submucosa	T1: Tumor invades lamina propria or submucosa
	T1a: Tumor invades lamina propria or muscularis mucosae
	T1b: Tumor invades submucosa
T2: Tumor invades muscularis propria	T2: Tumor invades muscularis propria
T3: Tumor invades adventitia	T3: Tumor invades adventitia
T4: Tumor invades adjacent structures	T4: Tumor invades adjacent structures[‡]
	T4a for resectable tumor invading pleura, pericardium, or diaphragm
	T4b for unresectable tumor invading other adjacent structures such as aorta, vertebral body, trachea, etc.
N CLASSIFICATION	**N CLASSIFICATION[†,‡]**
	Any periesophageal lymph node from cervical nodes to celiac nodes
N0: No regional lymph node metastases	Nx: Regional lymph nodes cannot be assessed
N1: Regional lymph node metastases	N0: No regional lymph node metastases
	N1: 1–2 involved nodes
	N2: 3–6 nodes
	N3: 7 or more nodes
M CLASSIFICATION	**M CLASSIFICATION[‡]**
Mx: Distant metastases cannot be assessed	Mx: Distant metastases cannot be assessed
M0: No distant metastases	M0: No distant metastases
M1: Distant metastases	M1: Distant metastases
Tumors of the lower thoracic esophagus:	
M1a: Metastases in celiac lymph nodes	
M1b: Other distant metastases	
Tumors of the midthoracic esophagus:	
M1a: Not applicable	
M1b: Nonregional lymph nodes and/or other distant metastases	
Tumors of the upper thoracic esophagus:	
M1a: Metastases in cervical nodes	
M1b: Other distant metastases	

*Maximal dimension of the tumor should be recorded.
[†]Redefined.
[‡]Subclassified.
AJCC, American Joint Committee on Cancer.

modified. For Siewert type I or adenocarcinoma of the distal esophagus, the epicenter of the tumor is identified within 1 to 5 cm above the anatomic EGJ. For Siewert type II or true carcinoma of the cardia, the epicenter is identified within 1 cm above and 2 cm below the EGJ. For Siewert type III or cardial carcinoma, the epicenter is identified between 2 and 5 cm below the EGJ, infiltrating the EGJ and the distal esophagus from below (Fig. 36.3).

In the revised AJCC seventh edition staging system, tumors whose midpoint are in the lower thoracic esophagus, EGJ, or within the proximal 5 cm of the stomach that extends into the EGJ or esophagus (Siewert types I and II) are classified as adenocarcinoma of the esophagus for the purpose of staging. All other cancers with a midpoint in the stomach lying more than 5 cm distal to the EGJ, or those within 5 cm of the EGJ, but not extending into the EGJ or esophagus (Siewert type III), are staged using the gastric cancer staging system.

DIAGNOSTIC TOOLS

TUMOR DETECTION

Esophageal cancers are usually discovered upon investigation of upper gastrointestinal (UGI) symptoms, such as dysphagia and weight loss, or on follow-up for Barrett esophagus via surveillance upper flexible endoscopy and biopsy.[20]

UPPER GASTROINTESTINAL CONTRAST STUDIES

Traditionally, before endoscopy and as a "road map," barium swallow was performed when patients presented with dysphagia. Barium swallow can clearly identify a polypoid tumor, strictures with mucosal irregularity, and "apple core" constrictions (Fig. 36.4). Additional diagnostic information, such as location of the tumor, the axis of the esophagus at the level of the tumor, and the presence of other pathology (such as a hiatal

TABLE 36.2 American Joint Committee on Cancer Seventh Edition Stage Groupings

Stage	ADENOCARCINOMA T	N	M	Grade	SQUAMOUS CELL CARCINOMA T	N	M	Grade	Location*
0	is	0	0	1	is	0	0	1	Any
IA	1	0	0	1–2	1	0	0	1	Any
IB	1	0	0	3	1	0	0	2–3	Any
	2	0	0	1–2	2–3	0	0	1	Lower
IIA	2	0	0	3	2–3	0	0	1	Upper, middle
					2–3	0	0	2–3	lower
IIB	3	0	0	Any	2–3	0	0	2–3	Upper, middle
	1–2	1	0	Any	1–2	1	0	Any	Any
IIIA	1–2	2	0	Any	1–2	2	0	Any	Any
	3	1	0	Any	3	1	0	Any	Any
	4a	0	0	Any	4a	0	0	Any	Any
IIIB	3	2	0	Any	3	2	0	Any	Any
IIIC	4a	1–2	0	Any	4a	1–2	0	Any	Any
	4b	Any	0	Any	4b	Any	0	Any	Any
	Any	3	0	Any	Any	3	0	Any	Any
IV	Any	Any	1	Any	Any	Any	1	Any	Any

*Location of the primary cancer site is defined by the position of the upper (proximal) edge of the tumor in the esophagus.

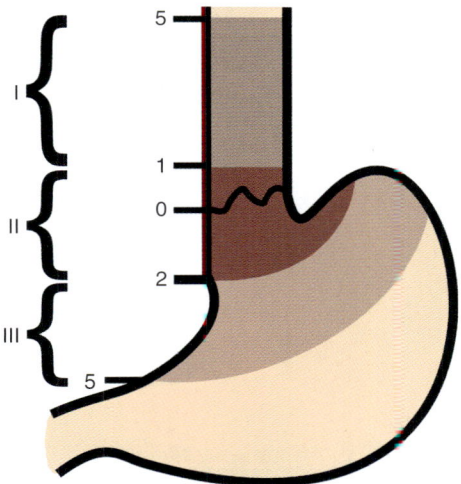

FIGURE 36.3 Siewert and Stein classification of adenocarcinomas around the gastroesophageal junction. *Type I*, Esophageal; *type II*, cardiac; *type III*, subcardiac.

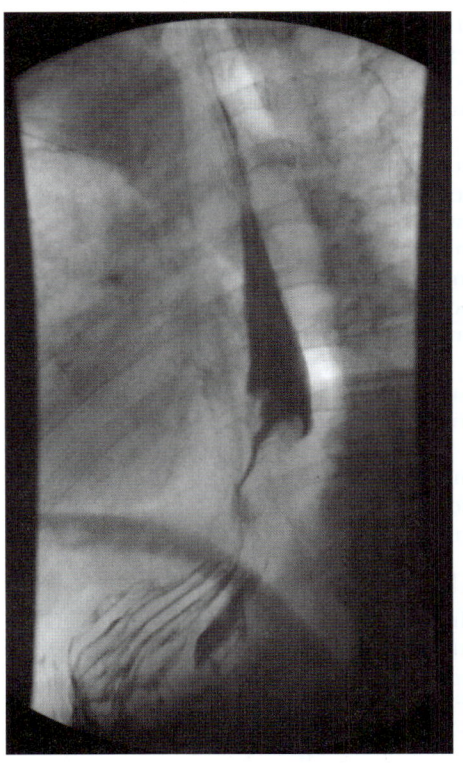

FIGURE 36.4 Barium contrast study showing distal thoracic apple core lesion.

hernia or diverticulum) are also provided by barium swallow. Double-contrast barium studies have been found to be a useful technique in the absence or delayed availability of endoscopy, although the positive predictive value (PPV) is 42%.[21] With the routine availability of endoscopy, UGI barium studies are not a routine component of initial assessment due to decreased accuracy and the inability to biopsy suspicious lesions. UGI studies should be considered when patients present with dysphagia and weight loss, and when endoscopy is not readily available. In situations where stricture precludes a complete endoscopic evaluation, barium studies may help to demarcate the distal extent of the tumor.

UPPER ENDOSCOPY AND BIOPSY

Flexible upper endoscopy is the standard initial diagnostic modality for evaluating the esophagus in patients with dysphagia and weight loss when cancer is part of the differential diagnosis. Endoscopy provides valuable and necessary details of the esophageal lumen morphology and can identify other abnormal lesions. Endoscopic reports should include visual description of any gross lesion characteristics, such as tumor morphology, the distance measured from the incisors, the length of the lesion, the percentage of circumferential involvement, and the position in relation to the GEJ (length of extension into cardia if present), in addition to a description of any skip lesions. The presence, location, and length of Barrett esophagus should also be noted.

Lesions seen endoscopically within the columnar-lined portion of the esophagus are at high risk to be cancerous. Therefore, in addition to visual details, tissues for histologic evaluation are obtained. Several biopsies should be performed that will increase the diagnostic accuracy of the study. The diagnostic yield approaches 100% when six or more samples are obtained using a standard endoscopic biopsy protocol.[22,23] Biopsy of necrotic or fibrotic areas will decrease diagnostic accuracy. Brush cytology also can be used in cases of tight malignant strictures where conventional biopsies may be difficult to obtain.[24] In these cases, to maximize the yield, brushings should be obtained before biopsy.[25] In situations where standard biopsy or brushings do not yield a diagnosis in cases with high suspicion, endoscopic ultrasonography (EUS) should be considered.[26] Suspicious lesions other than the index lesions should also be biopsied as submucosal spread or skip lesions within the esophagus are not uncommon.[27]

Once the histologic diagnosis of cancer has been established, subsequent studies are warranted in patients who might be considered surgical candidates for an accurate staging, which will guide the treatment plan.[28] Transmural tumors have a higher possibility of lymph node or systemic involvement; therefore, they will relatively benefit from multimodality therapy compared with very early lesions that may be amenable to surgery alone or curative endoscopic therapy.

Staging usually begins with a computed tomography (CT) scan or positron emission tomography (PET) scan to evaluate the presence of metastatic disease (see later). If distant metastases are excluded, a more detailed evaluation of locoregional disease extent (T and N stage) should be obtained.

FDG-PET/CT SCANS

2-[^{18}F]-fluoro-2-deoxyglucose-PET/CT (FDG-PET/CT) is now routinely used in the staging of esophageal cancer. By highlighting the metabolically active tissue via the use of a glucose analogue (FDG), which remains trapped in cancer cells during metabolism, PET scans can detect primary tumors as well as provide a functional assessment of metabolically active lymph nodes or metastatic sites (Fig. 36.5). By determining the degree of metabolic activity via standardized uptake value, PET may also be able to distinguish between inflammatory and malignant lymph node involvement. PET scanners have been integrated with CT scanners, which enabled direct comparison of metabolic information with anatomic location. Combined PET/CT has many advantages over PET scan alone, and it significantly improves the diagnostic accuracy.[29]

Histologically, SCCs were found to highly accumulate FDG at the primary tumor site in contrast to

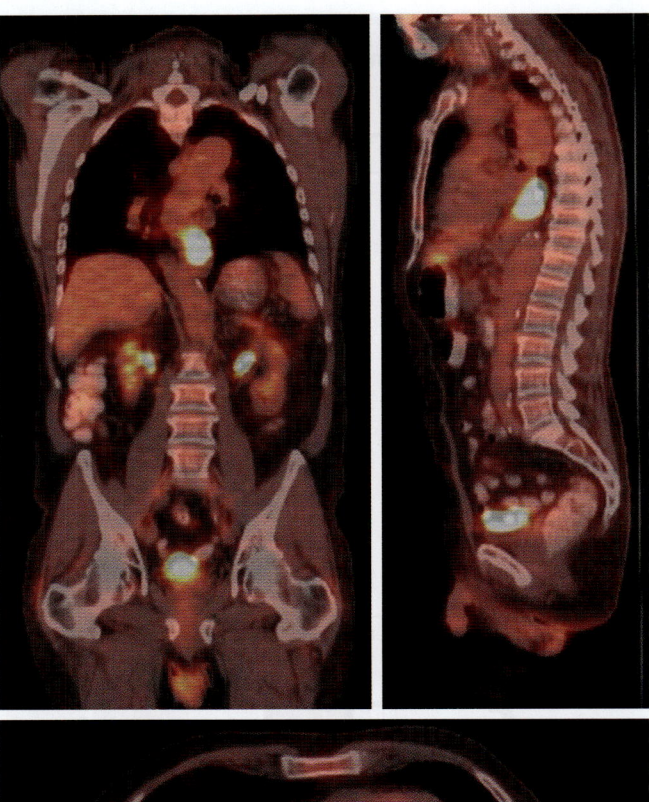
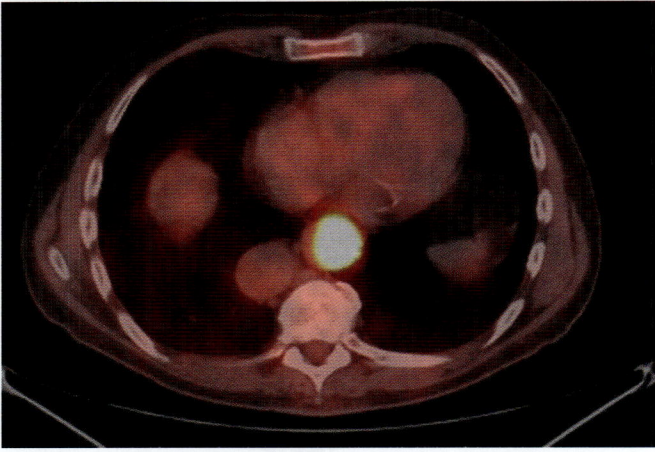

FIGURE 36.5 PET-avid lesion in the distal esophagus on coronal, cross-sectional, and sagittal view positron emission tomography–computed tomography (PET/CT) images.

adenocarcinomas, which demonstrate more limited FDG accumulation. FDG avidity in adenocarcinoma was found to be related to tumor growth type, differentiation degree, and mucus content. Nonavid tumors were often poorly differentiated, showing a diffuse, nonintestinal growth type and mucus-containing tumor type.[30]

Sensitivity and specificity of the study in the assessment of the TNM stage might be affected by different factors. In the detection of a primary tumor, the sensitivity ranges between 78% and 95%, with most false-negative tests occurring in patients with small tumors (T1 and T2).[31] PET does not provide enough definition of the esophageal wall and thus has no value in T staging. In addition, PET has a poor spatial resolution, which renders it insufficient to separate the primary tumor from juxtatumoral lymph nodes secondary to the interference from the primary tumor. The sensitivity of PET is poor in the identification of lymph node involvement ranging from 38% to 82%. This is especially true for nodes in the middle and lower mediastinum, where most primary tumors are found. In one study, the sensitivity of PET for detecting cervical, upper thoracic, and abdominal nodes was 78%, 82%, and 60%, respectively, but it was only 38% and 0%, respectively, for the mid- and lower mediastinum.[31] PET scan specificity is much better than its sensitivity for the N staging with a high pooled specificity ranging from 76% to 95% as compared with 77% to 89% in CT scans.[32,33]

The main utility of PET scanning is in its ability to identify the presence of distant metastasis as compared with contrast CT alone. A study recently demonstrated a change in the plan of management from curative into palliative in 47% of cases seen to be negative on CT, but were positive for distant metastasis on PET.[34] In addition, Luketich et al. reported 69% sensitivity, 93.4% specificity, and 84% accuracy in detecting metastases with PET compared with 46.1% sensitivity, 73.8% specificity, and 63% accuracy with CT.[35] A meta-analysis of 12 publications on the use of PET in esophageal cancer showed that the pooled sensitivity and specificity for the detection of locoregional metastases were 0.51 and 0.84, respectively. The PPV and negative predictive value (NPV) were 0.60 and 0.46, respectively. For distant metastases the pooled sensitivity and specificity were 0.67 and 0.97, respectively. The corresponding PPV and NPV were 0.92 and 0.83. When two studies that had particularly low sensitivities for the detection of distant metastases were excluded (probably because they included more early tumors), the pooled sensitivity improved to 0.72 and the specificity to 0.95.[36] This study highlights that the accuracy of PET in detecting locoregional nodes is only moderate. EUS fine-needle aspiration (FNA) is more accurate in this regard. However, PET is clearly more accurate for identifying distant nodal and visceral metastases.

The diagnostic utility of PET in early-stage disease (Tis, T1) may be low because the incidence of lymph node metastases increases with the increasing T stage. Cost studies to support PET in early-stage disease are unlikely. PET should routinely be performed in patients in whom standard staging methods (CT and EUS) demonstrate regional invasive cancer with no distant metastatic disease as it has been shown to be an independent predictor of overall survival in patients with nonmetastatic esophageal cancer. PET/CT improves the detection of metastatic disease and, thus, can often result in a change of the management strategy.[37] Overall management strategies were reported to be changed because of PET findings in 3% to 20% of patients in a recent meta-analysis.[36]

CT SCAN AND MAGNETIC RESONANCE IMAGING

CT is typically performed as the first radiologic test in the staging evaluation of an endoscopically diagnosed esophageal cancer. An esophageal wall thickness of greater than 5 mm on a CT scan is generally regarded as abnormal and warrants further investigation. A CT scan can display the lesion and surrounding structures, regional organ invasion, and lymph node metastasis (Fig. 36.6). Its role is particularly important to exclude T4 disease with a

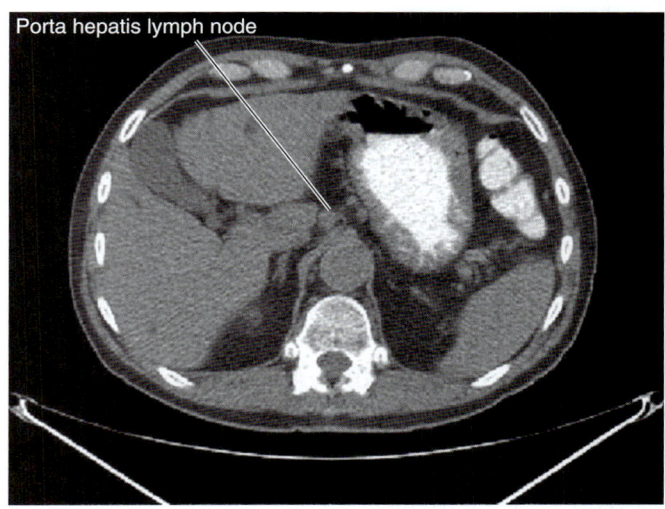
Porta hepatis lymph node

FIGURE 36.6 Enlarged porta hepatis lymph node on cross-sectional computed tomography scan.

sensitivity and specificity of 25% and 94%, respectively.[38] A CT performed with intravenous and oral contrast provides anatomic details that are critical before considering surgical treatment. Obliteration of the fat plane between the esophagus and the aorta, trachea and bronchi, and the pericardium is suggestive of invasion, but the paucity of fat often makes this assessment unreliable. Thickening or indentation of the normally flat membranous trachea and left main bronchus also is suggestive of invasion, but it should always be confirmed by bronchoscopic examination. When the area of contact between the esophagus and the aorta extends beyond 90 degrees of the circumference, an 80% accuracy of infiltration is reported. However, a CT scan cannot reliably distinguish the various T stages; T1 and T2 lesions generally show an esophageal wall thickness between 5 and 15 mm, and T3 lesions have a thickness greater than 15 mm, but this is far from accurate.

The sensitivity of detecting mediastinal and abdominal nodal involvement is suboptimal with CT because size alone is used as a diagnostic criterion. Intrathoracic and abdominal nodes greater than 1 cm are considered enlarged, and supraclavicular nodes with a short axis greater than 0.5 cm and retrocrural nodes greater than 0.6 cm are pathologic.[39] However, normal-sized lymph nodes may contain metastatic deposits, and enlargement of lymph nodes may be due to reactive and inflammatory processes. Sensitivity and specificity of detecting lymph node involvement is 50% and 83%, respectively.[32]

The main value of CT lies in its ability to detect distant systemic disease, such as hepatic, adrenal, and lung metastases. With adenocarcinoma of the GEJ and gastric cardia, peritoneal metastases are more likely than with squamous cell cancer of the tubular esophagus. CT scanning is inferior to laparoscopy in detecting peritoneal metastases. Solitary lung metastases are rare in patients with esophageal carcinoma and, thus, when seen on CT, are more likely to be primary lung cancer or benign nodules and additional assessment including PET is required.

Magnetic resonance imaging (MRI) presents the advantage of direct multiplanar imaging capabilities, which may be of particular use in assessing tracheobronchial, aortic, and pericardial invasion. Conventional MRI correctly assessed the T stage in 60% of patients[40] versus 81% when using high-resolution T2-weighted MRI.[41] A study performed using high-resolution T2-weighted MRI with faster sequences and cardiorespiratory motion gating in combination with diffusion-weighted imaging demonstrated detection rates of 33% for T1, 58% for T2, 96% for T3, and 100% for T4 carcinomas.[42] Experience with MRI has shown limitations similar to those of CT, especially with respect to the low detection rate of mediastinal lymph nodes.[43]

ENDOSCOPIC ULTRASOUND AND ENDOSCOPIC ULTRASONOGRAPHY/FINE-NEEDLE ASPIRATION

Several modalities have been used to assess the depth of invasion of cancer into the tubular esophagus. Dedicated EUS operating at frequencies of 7.5 and 12 MHz are able to identify the wall as a five-layered structure (Fig. 36.7) with relatively accurate sensitivities ranging from 81% to 92%[44] and provide information on the presence of abnormal or enlarged lymph nodes. However, low-frequency endoscopes cannot visualize the muscularis mucosae. Therefore authorities consider the deeper the tumor, the higher the sensitivity of EUS.[45,46] There are conflicting data on the ability to accurately discriminate invasion of the mucosa and submucosa (i.e., the T1a versus T1b stages). A comparative prospective blinded trial concluded that neither standard probes nor newer high-resolution 20-MHz probes are able to accurately distinguish intramucosal from submucosal tumor invasion.[47] In contrast, Thosani et al. demonstrated a sensitivity and a specificity for T1a tumors of 85% and 87%, respectively, and 86% for both sensitivity and specificity for T1b tumors.[48] The accuracy of EUS in determining T4 stage was found to be 86%.[49]

Overstaging may occur as peritumoral edematous changes may be mistaken for a tumor; on the other hand, understaging can result when tumor penetration is below the resolution of sonography.[50] Other technical obstacles might preclude complete EUS examination, such as stenotic esophageal tumors. To negotiate the stenotic esophagus, maneuvers such as dilatation of the lumen can be selectively considered, or different instruments, such as small-caliber ultrasound catheter or a wire-guided echoendoscope without fiberoptics, might be used. However, there are currently no comparative studies to determine their accuracy. In view of these conflicting results, the only method that is currently capable of accurately determining the depth of invasion of a small visible lesion is EMR (see later).[51]

EUS improves the accuracy of N staging by identifying suspicious nodal characteristics and by providing cytologic confirmation of nodal metastatic disease aspirated by FNA biopsy. Optimal criteria for identifying malignant lymph nodes based upon EUS criteria and for helping to select patients for whom EUS/FNA is required continue to evolve. The modified EUS criteria (four standard criteria plus EUS-identified celiac lymph nodes, >5 lymph nodes, or EUS T3/4 tumor) were more accurate than standard criteria (hypoechoic, smooth border, round, or width >5 to 10 mm) at identifying malignant lymph nodes.[52] Compared with the gold standard final pathologic evaluation of esophageal resected specimen along with dissected lymph nodes, sensitivity, specificity, and accuracy of EUS/FNA for locoregional lymph nodes are all over 85%[53,54]; in particular, sensitivity is highest for cervical and upper thoracic paraesophageal, infracarinal, left paratracheal, and recurrent laryngeal nodes. A prospective study comparing the performance characteristics of CT, EUS, and EUS/FNA for preoperative lymph node staging of esophageal carcinoma in 125 patients demonstrated that EUS/FNA was more sensitive than CT (83% vs. 29%) and more accurate than CT (87% vs. 51%) or EUS (87% vs. 74%) for nodal staging.[55]

EUS accuracy is operator-dependent and interobserver reliability was found to be influenced by experience and tumor stage.[56] Agreement among experienced endosonographers for both T and N stage was good, except for T2 tumors in which agreement was poor. There is a tendency to overstage T2 cancers by expert endosonographers in 8% to 14% of cases due to peritumoral inflammation.[57]

However, FNA nodal aspiration should be considered in all cases of celiac, porta hepatis, cervical, and upper thoracic adenopathy. It should only be performed when nodes are accessible and when the primary tumor is not in the pathway of the aspiration needle.

ENDOSCOPIC RESECTION

Any malignant, visible lesion cannot be assumed to be limited to the mucosa; in fact, very small cancers may penetrate into the submucosa. EMR is a technique by which the mucosa, and in most patients part or all of the submucosa, are resected down to the muscularis propria for definitive histologic diagnosis. It was first described in 1992 by Dr. Inoue from Japan.[58] Different techniques have been described, but the more popular method involves the use of a cap that fits over the end of a standard endoscope. The aim is to excise the specimen in one piece; however, piecemeal excision remains acceptable, but raises the potential for incomplete resection and makes pathologic evaluation of the resection margins more complex. This technique has evolved and revolutionized the staging and treatment of superficial

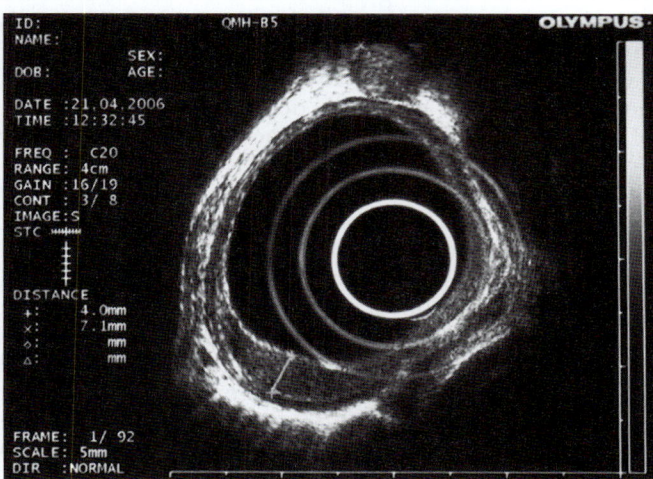

FIGURE 36.7 Esophageal wall layers identified by endoscopic ultrasound.

esophageal adenocarcinoma—particularly the 20% of all esophageal adenocarcinoma in the United States presenting at early stage (T1) with disease confined to the mucosa or submucosa.[59] It permits accurate assessment of depth of infiltration, presence of lymphovascular invasion, and degree of differentiation, thus providing a relevant estimation of the risk for local lymph node metastasis. However, histopathologic interpretation of esophageal reflux (ER) specimens may not be straightforward. There is a high rate of discordance (up to 48%) between pathologists' assessment for the depth of tumor invasion in ER specimens, particularly for lesions called T1b.[60]

The appropriate treatment modality is best selected in a multidisciplinary fashion with EMR providing the most accurate staging. Several studies have demonstrated that ER is safe and effective for complete resection with excellent comparable long-term disease control, lower rate of complications but higher rate of recurrence when compared with surgery for high-grade dysplasia and intramucosal adenocarcinoma (T1aN0). In these lesions the risk of lymph node involvement or hematogenous dissemination is estimated to be less than 2%,[61] justifying a nonsurgical approach.[62,63] For lesions penetrating into the submucosa, more definitive treatment, such as esophagectomy with lymphadenectomy, is advocated.

BRONCHOSCOPY AND ENDOBRONCHIAL ULTRASOUND

Flexible bronchoscopy is performed to assess tumor invasion into the tracheobronchial tree and to evaluate mediastinal lymph nodes, especially in situations where the presence of an obstructing esophageal tumor prevents the progression of an echoendoscope to perform EUS or when the tumor is located in the mid- and upper portions of the esophagus.

Signs of involvement include a widened carina, external compression, tumor infiltration, and fistulization. The last two signs contraindicate resection.[64] The gross macroscopic bronchoscopic appearance may not be accurate; in fact, a bulge of the posterior tracheobronchial wall or minimal mucosal changes (erythema, edema) do not confirm neoplastic invasion of the wall, and biopsy plus brush cytology is recommended. In one study involving patients with supracarinal cancer, endoluminal tumor mass, protrusion of the posterior tracheal wall, and signs of mucosal invasion were visible in 5.9%, 28.6%, and 4.1% of bronchoscopic examinations, respectively. However, in only 8.6% of 220 bronchoscopic examinations, cancer invasion was proved by biopsy or cytology. Bronchoscopy excluded 18.1% of otherwise potentially operable patients from surgery because of airway invasion, with an overall accuracy of 93.3%.[65]

Endobronchial ultrasound has been investigated as a staging tool. The diagnosis of tracheobronchial invasion was based on an interruption in the most external hyperechoic layer of the tracheobronchus (corresponding to its adventitia). In one study of 26 patients determined to be invasion-free by bronchoscopic ultrasound, only 2 had invasion. This compares with 7 of 22 patients who were found to have invasion not suggested by CT alone. In another study evaluating esophageal or thyroid cancer patients with suspicion of tracheobronchial invasion, the

sensitivity and specificity of tracheal involvement were 92% and 83%, respectively, compared with 59% and 56%, and 75% and 73% in CT and MRI, respectively.[66] In addition, other recent studies have demonstrated that endobronchial ultrasound (EBUS) has a greater accuracy in evaluating tracheobronchial invasion by esophageal neoplasia when compared with conventional bronchoscopy, CT, and EUS.[67]

A study by Liberman et al. highlighted the utility of EBUS combined with EUS in sampling peritumoral esophageal lymph nodes as EUS/FNA run a high risk of false-positive cytopathology secondary to contamination of the sample by piercing the primary tumor. Adding EBUS to EUS for staging esophageal cancer in this study added valuable information for patients with upper and mid-esophageal tumors owing to the inability to assess local lymph node invasion in the peritracheal area and subcarinal region. A total of 12% of patients were upstaged with the addition of EBUS to EUS in this study, and that has an important impact on patient prognostication and treatment planning. However, this technique has not yet seen wide application.[68]

LAPAROSCOPY AND THORACOSCOPY

To improve preoperative staging, diagnostic laparoscopy or thoracoscopy is selectively performed. Small-volume intraperitoneal metastases can be difficult to diagnose noninvasively by either CT or PET scans. Laparoscopic or thoracoscopic assessment can help in identifying occult intraperitoneal or intrathoracic distant metastases as well as sampling regional lymph nodes in some situations, such as in cancers at the GEJ or in the distal esophagus.[69,70] This approach might limit aggressive treatment to patients with locally advanced or metastatic disease.

Laparoscopic staging includes visual inspection of the peritoneal cavity and surface of the liver, as well as the potential for laparoscopic ultrasound examination of the liver, collection of peritoneal fluid for cytologic examination, and biopsy of suspicious lesions.

In a study of 53 patients who underwent preoperative evaluation including minimally invasive staging, a change in the stage originally assigned by CT scan and EUS occurred in 32.1% of patients with adenocarcinoma of the esophagus.[71] The multiinstitutional study from the Cancer and Leukemia Group B (CALGB 9380) reported on combined thoracoscopic and laparoscopic staging in 113 patients; the strategy was feasible in 73% of patients. Thoracoscopy and laparoscopy identified nodes or metastatic disease missed by CT in 50% of patients, by MRI in 40%, and by EUS in 30%. Although no deaths or major complications occurred, it did involve general anesthesia, one-lung anesthesia, a median operating time of 210 minutes, and a hospital stay of 3 days.[72]

Currently diagnostic thoracoscopic assessment is not used except in highly selective cases where other staging studies suggest metastatic disease. Many consider diagnostic laparoscopy in patients with adenocarcinoma with extensive gastric involvement, or in patients with suspicious CT and PET findings.

EUS/FNA is an effective approach for sampling mediastinal nodes. However, laparoscopy has its role, especially for adenocarcinoma of the lower esophagus or GEJ tumors since the chance of metastases in the abdomen is considerably greater compared with SCC of the esophagus. Laparoscopy can be of use in diagnosing abdominal metastases, such as peritoneal secondaries or identifying unsuspected cirrhosis, which is a relative contraindication to surgical resection. Its value is minimal for more proximally located tumors.[73] Following CT and EUS, laparoscopy may upstage nodal status in 0% to 21% of patients and downstage it in 4% to 19%. Together with other findings, change in management can occur in up to 20% of patients.[74] Even though thoracoscopy and laparoscopy can identify some additional patients with advanced disease, the application of these approaches should involve our highly selected patients.[75]

The increased accuracy of PET/CT may decrease the application of other invasive staging methods, especially with regard to distant disease. It does seem that with better PET, CT, and EUS, staging laparoscopy is less indicated. Laparoscopic assessment is indicated in cases where liver metastases or peritoneal metastases are suspected and confirmation is required.

Proper staging of esophageal cancer patients is critical in view of the wide available variation in treatment approaches. Fig. 36.8 highlights all steps for the work-up of patients with esophageal cancer. Following the completion of staging and physiologic assessment, patients should be considered for presentation at a multidisciplinary tumor board whenever it is feasible.

THERAPY MONITORING

Neoadjuvant chemoradiotherapy followed by surgery has demonstrated a favorable long-term outcome compared with surgery alone.[76] However, in a proportion of patients, the objective anticipated response will be insufficient, or the disease will progress in spite of neoadjuvant therapy. These findings can result in changing the management strategy as chemoradiotherapy side effects could lead to increased perioperative morbidity. In addition, prolonged but ineffective preoperative treatment will inevitably delay appropriate surgical therapy. In addition, the ability to identify nonresponders will increase the ability to tailor therapy.

Conventional imaging techniques for monitoring nonsurgical therapy, such as CT and EUS, are based on morphologic imaging. General restrictions of these methods include difficulty in distinguishing a viable tumor from necrotic or fibrotic tissue and delay between cell kill and tumor shrinkage.[77] Nevertheless, CT scanning is still widely applied for this purpose, partly because of its wide availability. In a study involving the use of CT scans, CT after chemoradiotherapy accurately staged the T classification in only 42%; it overstaged 36% of patients, and understaged 20%. CT had a sensitivity of 65%, a specificity of 33%, a PPV of 58%, and an NPV of 41% in evaluating the pathologic tumor response.[78]

EUS is typically not recommended for response assessment because of its limited accuracy and poor reproducibility. Moreover, EUS is invasive and not always feasible, especially in case of postradiation esophagitis or severe stricturing.[79] A study assessing the prognostic value of endoscopic biopsy and EUS demonstrated an accuracy of approximately 50% when correlated with the percentage of residual viable cells in the surgical specimen and survival.[80]

A potentially more accurate diagnostic modality that has the potential to predict tumor response early in the course of neoadjuvant treatment is FDG-PET scanning, which has been shown to be moderately sensitive in esophageal cancer. The evaluation of FDG-PET for early monitoring of nonsurgical therapy response is described in several small studies and in one large phase II trial, with promising results.[80–84]

The MUNICON study recruited 110 patients who underwent neoadjuvant chemotherapy, of whom 54 had metabolic response after 2 weeks of induction therapy. Nonresponders underwent immediate surgery while responders had surgery after a full course of treatment. Survival in nonresponders (median, 26 months) was inferior to responders, but did not appear to be worse than a historical cohort who received chemotherapy and surgery, despite incomplete chemotherapy.[85] This study suggests the potential feasibility of a PET-guided treatment algorithm.

In a study on patients who were assessed before and after chemoradiation, Brücher et al. demonstrated a sensitivity in detecting a response of 100%, with a corresponding specificity of 55%. The PPV and NPV were 72% and 100%, respectively.[81] Flamen et al. also demonstrated the value of PET for evaluation of response. Serial PET had a predictive accuracy of 78% for a major response, with a sensitivity of 71% and a specificity of 82%.[82]

False negatives (overestimation of response) is due to residual micrometastatic cancer foci falling below the detection threshold. False positives (underestimation of response) usually occur at the primary tumor site where inflammatory reactions may increase FDG uptake. FDG-PET scanning cannot demonstrate a complete pathologic response to neoadjuvant chemoradiation, although clinical trials examining this issue are ongoing.

SURVEILLANCE STRATEGY

Surveillance, following either surgical or medical management of esophageal cancer, is typically done to implement salvage therapy in cases of locoregional failure. However, the number of salvageable cases after recurrences is small. Sudo et al. demonstrated that only 2% of 518 esophageal adenocarcinoma patients who underwent trimodality therapy were salvageable when they recurred at a median of 29.3 months of follow-up, which raised the question of the benefit of the surveillance/salvage strategies.[86]

Following nonsurgical management, it is difficult to evaluate the lesion as distinguishing between fibrosis, inflammation, and true histologic response is not easy. The posttreatment surveillance strategy suggested by the consensus-based guidelines from the National Comprehensive Cancer Network include the following steps:

- History and physical examination every 3 to 6 months for 1 to 3 years, then every 6 months for years 4 and 5, then annually
- Complete blood count and chemistry profile, as clinically indicated

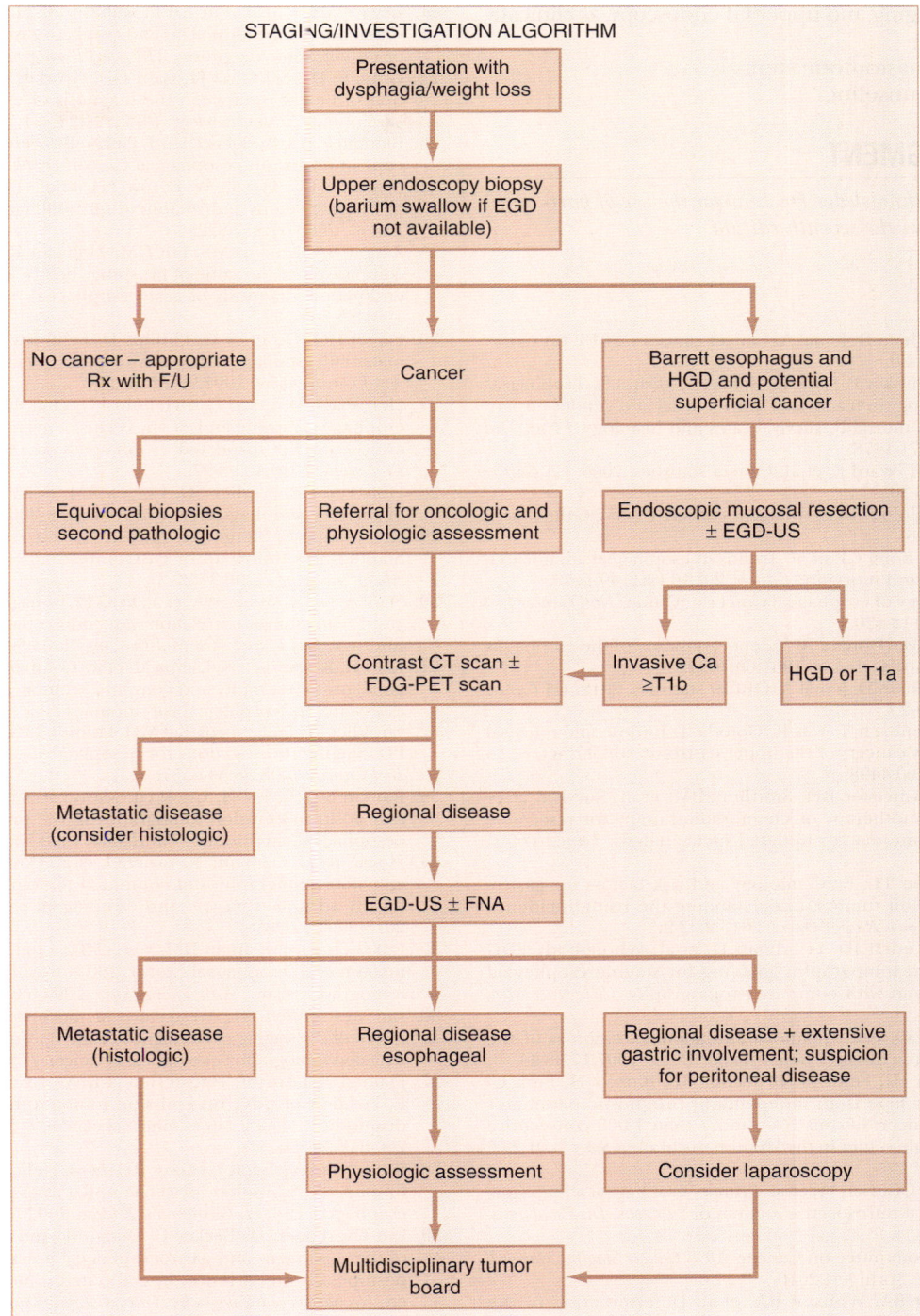

FIGURE 36.8 Scheme of stepwise approach in diagnosing suspected cancer in the esophagus. *Ca,* Cancer; *CT,* computed tomography; *EGD,* esophagogastroduodenoscopy; *FDG,* 2-[^{18}F]-fluoro-2-deoxyglucose; *FNA,* fine-needle aspiration; *F/U,* follow-up; *HGD,* high-grade dysplasia; *PET,* positron emission tomography; *Rx,* treatment; *US,* ultrasound.

- Radiologic imaging and upper GI endoscopy, as clinically indicated
- Dilation for anastomotic stenosis
- Nutritional counseling.

ACKNOWLEDGMENT

We would like to acknowledge Dr. Law for the use of parts of his chapter published in the seventh edition.

REFERENCES

1. Siegel R, Naishadham D, Jemal A. Cancer statistics, 2013. *CA Cancer J Clin.* 2013;63:11-30.
2. Baquet CR, Commiskey P, Mack K, Meltzer S, Mishra SI. Esophageal cancer epidemiology in blacks and whites: racial and gender disparities in incidence, mortality, survival rates and histology. *J Natl Med Assoc.* 2005;97:1471-1478.
3. Jemal A, Murray T, Ward E, et al. Cancer statistics, 2005. *CA Cancer J Clin.* 2005;55:10-30.
4. Zhang Y. Epidemiology of esophageal cancer. *World J Gastroenterol.* 2013;19:5598-5606.
5. Hur C, Miller M, Kong CY, et al. Trends in esophageal adenocarcinoma incidence and mortality. *Cancer.* 2013;119:1149-1158.
6. Li JY. Epidemiology of esophageal cancer in China. *Natl Cancer Inst Monogr.* 1982;62:113-120.
7. MacDonald WC, MacDonald JB. Adenocarcinoma of the esophagus and/or gastric cardia. *Cancer.* 1987;60:1094.
8. Siegel R, Naishadham D, Jemal A. Cancer statistics, 2012. *CA Cancer J Clin.* 2012;62:10-29.
9. Soetikno R, Kaltenbach T, Yeh R, Gotoda T. Endoscopic mucosal resection for early cancers of the upper gastrointestinal tract. *J Clin Oncol.* 2005;23:4490-4498.
10. Sjoquist KM, Burmeister BH, Smithers BM, et al. Survival after neoadjuvant chemotherapy or chemoradiotherapy for resectable oesophageal carcinoma: an updated meta-analysis. *Lancet Oncol.* 2011;12:681.
11. Buas MF, Vaughan TL. Epidemiology and risk factors for gastroesophageal junction tumors: understanding the rising incidence of this disease. *Semin Radiat Oncol.* 2013;23:3-9.
12. Meltzer CC, Luketich JD, Friedman D, et al. Whole-body FDG positron emission tomographic imaging for staging esophageal cancer: comparison with computed tomography. *Clin Nucl Med.* 2000;25:882.
13. Siewert JR, Katja O. Are squamous and adenocarcinomas of the esophagus the same disease? *Semin Radiat Oncol.* 2007;17:38-44.
14. Siewert JR, Stein HJ, Feith M, Bruecher BL, Bartels H, Fink U. Histologic tumor type is an independent prognostic parameter in esophageal cancer: lessons from more than 1,000 consecutive resections at a single center in the Western world. *Ann Surg.* 2001;234:360-367.
15. Zhang HD, Chen CG, Gao YY, et al. Primary esophageal adenosquamous carcinoma: a retrospective analysis of 24 cases. *Dis Esophagus.* 2014;27:783-789.
16. American Joint Committee on Cancer. *AJCC Cancer Staging Manual.* 7th ed. New York: Springer; 2010.
17. Groth SS, Virnig BA, Whitson BA, et al. Determination of the minimum number of lymph nodes to examine to maximize survival in patients with esophageal carcinoma: data from the Surveillance, Epidemiology and End Results database. *J Thorac Cardiovasc Surg.* 2010;139:612-620.
18. Peyre CG, Hagen JA, DeMeester SR, et al. Predicting systemic disease in patients with esophageal cancer after esophagectomy: a multinational study on the significance of the number of involved lymph nodes. *Ann Surg.* 2008;248:979-985.
19. Rice TW, Rusch VW, Ishwaran H, Blackstone EH; Worldwide Esophageal Cancer Collaboration. Cancer of the esophagus and esophagogastric junction: data-driven staging for the seventh edition of the American Joint Committee on Cancer/International Union Against Cancer Cancer Staging Manuals. *Cancer.* 2010;116:3763-3773.
20. Enzinger PC, Mayer RJ. Esophageal cancer. *N Engl J Med.* 2003;349:2241-2252.
21. Levine MS, Chu P, Furth EE, Rubesin SE, Laufer I, Herlinger H. Carcinoma of the esophagus and esophagogastric junction: sensitivity of radiographic diagnosis. *AJR Am J Roentgenol.* 1997;168:1423.
22. Graham DY, Schwartz JT, Cain GD, Gyorkey F. Prospective evaluation of biopsy number in the diagnosis of esophageal and gastric carcinoma. *Gastroenterology.* 1982;82:228-231.
23. Bloomfeld RS, Bridgers DI 3rd, Pineau BC. Sensitivity of upper endoscopy in diagnosing esophageal cancer. *Dysphagia.* 2005;20:278-282.
24. Jacobson BC, Hirota W, Baron TH, et al. The role of endoscopy in the assessment and treatment of esophageal cancer. *Gastrointest Endosc.* 2003;57:817-822.
25. Zargar SA, Khurro MS, Jan GM, Mahajan R, Shah P. Prospective comparison of the value of brushings before and after biopsy in the endoscopic diagnosis of gastroesophageal malignancy. *Acta Cytol.* 1991;35:549-552.
26. Faigel DO, Deveney C, Phillips D, Fennerty MB. Biopsy negative malignant esophageal stricture: diagnosis by endoscopic ultrasound. *Am J Gastroenterol.* 1998;93:2257-2260.
27. Heresbach D, Leray E, d'Halluin PN, et al. Diagnostic accuracy of esophageal capsule endoscopy versus conventional upper digestive endoscopy for suspected esophageal squamous cell carcinoma. *Endoscopy.* 2010;42:93-97.
28. Hofstetter W, Swisher SG, Correa AM, et al. Treatment outcomes of resected esophageal cancer. *Ann Surg.* 2002;236:376-385.
29. Rosenbaum S, Stergar H, Antoch G, Veit P, Bockisch A, Kühl H. Staging and follow-up of gastrointestinal tumors with PET/CT. *Abdom Imaging.* 2006;31:25-35.
30. Stahl A, Ott K, Weber WA, et al. FDG PET imaging of locally advanced gastric carcinomas: correlation with endoscopic and histopathological findings. *Eur J Nucl Med Mol Imaging.* 2003;30:288-295.
31. Kato H, Kuwano H, Nakajima M, et al. Comparison between positron emission tomography and computed tomography in the use of the assessment of esophageal carcinoma. *Cancer.* 2002;94:921.
32. van Vliet EP, Heijenbrok-Kal MH, Hunink MG, Kuipers EJ, Siersema PD. Staging investigations for oesophageal cancer: a meta-analysis. *Br J Cancer.* 2008;98:547-557.
33. Rankin SC, Taylor H, Cook GJ, Mason R. Computed tomography and positron emission tomography in the pre-operative staging of oesophageal carcinoma. *Clin Radiol.* 1998;53:659-665.
34. Hocazade C, Özdemir N, Yazici O, et al. Concordance of positron emission tomography and computed tomography in patients with locally advanced gastric and esophageal cancer. *Ann Nucl Med.* 2015;29:621-626.
35. Luketich JD, Friedman DM, Weigel TL, et al. Evaluation of distant metastases in esophageal cancer: 100 consecutive positron emission tomography scans. *Ann Thorac Surg.* 1999;68:1133.
36. van Westreenen HL, Westerterp M, Bossuyt PM, et al. Systematic review of the staging performance of 18F-fluorodeoxyglucose positron emission tomography in esophageal cancer. *J Clin Oncol.* 2004;22:3805.
37. Flamen P, Lerut T, Haustermans K, Van Cutsem E, Mortelmans L. Position of positron emission tomography and other imaging diagnostic modalities in esophageal cancer. *Q J Nucl Med Mol Imaging.* 2004;48:96-108.
38. Romagnuolo J, Scott J, Hawes RH, et al. Helical CT versus EUS with fine needle aspiration for celiac nodal assessment in patients with esophageal cancer. *Gastrointest Endosc.* 2002;55:648.
39. van Overhagen H, Becker C. Diagnosis and staging of carcinoma of the esophagus and gastroesophageal junction, and detection of postoperative recurrence, by computed tomography. In: Myers M, ed. *Neoplasms of the Digestive Tract: Imaging, Staging and Management.* Philadelphia: Lippincott-Raven; 1998:31.
40. Wu LF, Wang BZ, Feng JL, et al. Preoperative TN staging of esophageal cancer: comparison of miniprobe ultrasonography, spiral CT and MRI. *World J Gastroenterol.* 2003;9:219-224.
41. Riddell AM, Allum WH, Thompson JN, Wotherspoon AC, Richardson C, Brown G. The appearances of oesophageal carcinoma demonstrated on high-resolution, T2-weighted MRI, with histopathological correlation. *Eur Radiol.* 2007;17:391-399.
42. Sakurada A, Takahara T, Kwee TC, et al. Diagnostic performance of diffusion-weighted magnetic resonance imaging in esophageal cancer. *Eur Radiol.* 2009;19:1461-1469.
43. Lehr L, Rupp N, Siewert JR. Assessment of resectability of esophageal cancer by computed tomography and magnetic resonance imaging. *Surgery.* 1998;103:344.
44. Hasegawa N, Niwa Y, Arisawa T, Hase S, Goto H, Hayakawa T. Preoperative staging of superficial esophageal carcinoma: comparison

of an ultrasound probe and standard endoscopic ultrasonography. *Gastrointest Endosc.* 1996;44:388.

45. Puli SR, Reddy JB, Bechtold ML, Antillon D, Ibdah JA, Antillon MR. Staging accuracy of esophageal cancer by endoscopic ultrasound: a meta-analysis and systematic review. *World J Gastroenterol.* 2008;14:1479-1490.

46. Young PE, Gentry AB, Acosta RD, Greenwald BD, Riddle M. Endoscopic ultrasound does not accurately stage early adenocarcinoma or high-grade dysplasia of the esophagus. *Clin Gastroenterol Hepatol.* 2010;8:1037.

47. May A, Gunter E, Roth F, et al. Accuracy of staging in early esophageal cancer using high resolution endoscopy and high resolution endosonography: a comparative, prospective, and blinded trial. *Gut.* 2004;53:624-640.

48. Thosani N, Singh H, Kapadia A, et al. Diagnostic accuracy of EUS in differentiating mucosal versus submucosal invasion of superficial esophageal cancers: a systematic review and meta-analysis. *Gastrointest Endosc.* 2012;75:242.

49. Rösch T. Endosonographic staging of esophageal cancer: a review of literature results. *Gastrointest Endosc Clin N Am.* 1995;5(3):537.

50. Saunders HS, Wolfman NT, Ott DJ. Esophageal cancer radiologic staging. *Radiol Clin North Am.* 1997;35:281-294.

51. Pouw RE, Heldoorn N, Alvarez Herrero L, et al. Do we still need EUS in the workup of patients with early esophageal neoplasia? A retrospective analysis of 131 cases. *Gastrointest Endosc.* 2011;73:662.

52. Vazquez-Sequeiros E, Levy MJ, Clain JE, et al. Routine vs. selective EUS-guided FNA approach for preoperative nodal staging of esophageal carcinoma. *Gastrointest Endosc.* 2006;63:204-211.

53. Eloubeidi MA, Wallace MB, Reed CE, et al. The utility of EUS and EUS-guided fine needle aspiration in detecting celiac lymph node metastasis in patients with esophageal cancer: a single-center experience. *Gastrointest Endosc.* 2001;54:714.

54. Giovannini M, Seitz JF, Monges G, Perrier H, Rabbia I. Fine-needle aspiration cytology guided by endoscopic ultrasonography: results in 141 patients. *Endoscopy.* 1995;27:171.

55. Vazquez-Sequeiros E, Wiersema MJ, Clain JE, et al. Impact of lymph node staging on therapy of esophageal carcinoma. *Gastroenterology.* 2003;125:1626.

56. Fockens P, Van den Brande JH, van Dullemen HM, van Lanschot JJ, Tytgat GN. Endosonographic T-staging of esophageal carcinoma: a learning curve. *Gastrointest Endosc.* 1996;44:58.

57. Souquet JC, Napoleon B, Pujol B, Valette PJ, Cholet R, Lambert R. Endosonography-guided treatment of esophageal carcinoma. *Endoscopy.* 1992;1:324.

58. Inoue H, Takeshita K, Hori H, Muraoka Y, Yoneshima H, Endo M. Endoscopic mucosal resection with a cap-fitted panendoscope for esophagus, stomach, and colon mucosal lesions. *Gastrointest Endosc.* 1993;39:58-62.

59. Das A, Singh V, Fleischer DE, Sharma VK. A comparison of endoscopic treatment and surgery in early esophageal cancer an analysis of Surveillance, Epidemiology and End Results data. *Am J Gastroenterol.* 2008;103:1340-1345.

60. Worrell SG, Boys JA, Chandrasoma P, et al. Inter-observer variability in the interpretation of endoscopic mucosal resection specimens of esophageal adenocarcinoma: interpretation of ER specimens. *J Gastrointest Surg.* 2016;20:140-145.

61. Manner H, Pech O, Heldmann Y, et al. Efficacy, safety, and long-term results of endoscopic treatment for early stage adenocarcinoma of the esophagus with low-risk sm1 invasion. *Clin Gastroenterol Hepatol.* 2013;11:630-635.

62. Fernando HC, Luketich JD, Buenaventura PO, Perry Y, Christie NA. Outcomes of minimally invasive esophagectomy (MIE) for high-grade dysplasia of the esophagus. *Eur J Cardiothorac Surg.* 2002;22:1.

63. Schmidt HM, Mohiuddin K, Bodnar AM, et al. Multidisciplinary treatment of T1a adenocarcinoma in Barrett's esophagus: contemporary comparison of endoscopic and surgical treatment in physiologically fit patients. *Surg Endosc.* 2016;30:3391-3401.

64. Cheung HC, Siu KF, Wong J. A comparison of flexible and rigid endoscopy in evaluating esophageal cancer patients for surgery. *World J Surg.* 1988;12:117.

65. Riedel M, Stein HJ, Mounyam L, Lembeck R, Siewert JR. Extensive sampling improves preoperative bronchoscopic assessment of airway

invasion by supracarinal esophageal cancer: a prospective study in 166 patients. *Chest.* 2001;119:1652.

66. Nishimura Y, Osugi H, Inoue K, Takada N, Takamura M, Kinosita H. Bronchoscopic ultrasonography in the diagnosis of tracheobronchial invasion of esophageal cancer. *J Ultrasound Med.* 2002;21:49-58.

67. Wakamatsu T, Tsushima K, Yasuo M, et al. Usefulness of preoperative endobronchial ultrasound for airway invasion around the trachea: esophageal cancer and thyroid cancer. *Respiration.* 2006;73:651-657.

68. Liberman M, Hanna N, Duranceau A, Thiffault V, Ferraro P. Endobronchial ultrasonography added to endoscopic ultrasonography improves staging in esophageal cancer. *Ann Thorac Surg.* 2013;96:232.

69. Kaushik N, Khalid A, Brody D, Luketich J, McGrath K. Endoscopic ultrasound compared with laparoscopy for staging esophageal cancer. *Ann Thorac Surg.* 2007;83:2000.

70. Bryan RT, Cruickshank NR, Needham SJ, et al. Fielding laparoscopic peritoneal lavage in staging gastric and oesophageal cancer. *Eur J Surg Oncol.* 2001;27:291.

71. Luketich JD, Meehan M, Nguyen NT, et al. Minimally invasive surgical staging for esophageal cancer. *Surg Endosc.* 2000;14:700.

72. Krasna MJ, Reed CE, Nedzwiecki D, et al. CALGB 9380: a prospective trial of the feasibility of thoracoscopy/laparoscopy in staging esophageal cancer. *Ann Thorac Surg.* 2001;71:1073.

73. Stein HJ, Kraemer SJ, Feussner H, Fink U, Siewert JR. Clinical value of diagnostic laparoscopy with laparoscopic ultrasound in patients with cancer of the esophagus or cardia. *J Gastrointest Surg.* 1997;1:167.

74. Yoon HH, Lowe VJ, Cassivi SD, Romero Y. The role of FDG-PET and staging laparoscopy in the management of patients with cancer of the esophagus or gastroesophageal junction. *Gastroenterol Clin North Am.* 2009;38:105.

75. Wallace MB, Nietert PJ, Earle C, et al. An analysis of multiple staging management strategies for carcinoma of the esophagus: computed tomography, endoscopic ultrasound, positron emission tomography, and thoracoscopy/laparoscopy. *Ann Thorac Surg.* 2002;74:1026.

76. Gebski V, Burmeister B, Smithers BM, et al. Survival benefits from neoadjuvant chemoradiotherapy or chemotherapy in oesophageal carcinoma: a meta-analysis. *Lancet Oncol.* 2007;8:226-234.

77. Westerterp M, van Westreenen HL, Reitsma JB, et al. Esophageal cancer: CT, endoscopic US, and FDG PET for assessment of response to neoadjuvant therapy—systematic review. *Radiology.* 2005;236:841-851.

78. Jones DR, Parker LAJ, Detterbeck FC, Egan TM. Inadequacy of computed tomography in assessing patients with esophageal carcinoma after induction chemoradiotherapy. *Cancer.* 1999;85:1026.

79. Sloof GW. Response monitoring of neoadjuvant therapy using CT, EUS, and FDG-PET. *Best Pract Res Clin Gastroenterol.* 2006;20:941-957.

80. Schneider PM, Metzger R, Schaefer H, et al. Response evaluation by endoscopy, rebiopsy, and endoscopic ultrasound does not accurately predict histopathologic regression after neoadjuvant chemoradiation for esophageal cancer. *Ann Surg.* 2008;248:902.

81. Brücher BL, Weber W, Bauer M, et al. Neoadjuvant therapy of esophageal squamous cell carcinoma: response evaluation by positron emission tomography. *Ann Surg.* 2001;233:300.

82. Flamen P, Van Cutsem E, Lerut A, et al. Positron emission tomography for assessment of the response to induction radiochemotherapy in locally advanced oesophageal cancer. *Ann Oncol.* 2002;13:361.

83. Wieder HA, Brucher BL, Zimmermann F, et al. Time course of tumor metabolic activity during chemoradiotherapy of esophageal squamous cell carcinoma and response to treatment. *J Clin Oncol.* 2004; 22:900-908.

84. Cerfolio RJ, Bryant AS, Ohja B, Bartolucci AA, Eloubeidi MA. The accuracy of endoscopic ultrasonography with fine-needle aspiration, integrated positron emission tomography with computed tomography, and computed tomography in restaging patients with esophageal cancer after neoadjuvant chemoradiotherapy. *J Thorac Cardiovasc Surg.* 2005;129:1232-1241.

85. Lordick F, Ott K, Krause BJ, et al. PET to assess early metabolic response and to guide treatment of adenocarcinoma of the oesophagogastric junction: the MUNICON phase II trial. *Lancet Oncol.* 2007; 8:797-805.

86. Sudo K, Taketa T, Correa AM, et al. Locoregional failure rate after preoperative chemoradiation of esophageal adenocarcinoma and the outcomes of salvage strategies. *J Clin Oncol.* 2013;31:4306-4310.

Endoscopic Management of High-Grade Dysplasia and Superficial Esophageal Carcinoma

Wayne L. Hofstetter | Raquel E. Davila | Marta L. Davila

The detection and treatment of high-grade dysplasia and early esophageal cancer overlap to the point that they are a continuum. In some situations they can be difficult to separate and exist simultaneously. Because existing studies often combine the descriptions of the two, for the purposes of this chapter we will consider both as superficial neoplasia.

Esophagectomy, long considered the only curative option for esophageal cancer, is no longer standard therapy for high-grade dysplasia (HGD) and early esophageal cancer limited to the mucosa. Recognition of disease biology in combination with bridging technologic gaps have brought about a change in the treatment paradigm that is both disruptive to previous therapies and represents a clear advance in therapy. Organ-sparing procedures including endoscopic resection (ER) in combination with various forms of ablation have been shown to be the preferable option for the treatment of early esophageal neoplasia in the vast majority of cases.[1–4]

In the United States the incidence of esophageal adenocarcinoma (EAC) has been increasing, whereas squamous cell cancers of the esophagus are decreasing.[5] In fact, the rise in incidence of EAC is inconsistent with most other cancers, which are either stable or declining. The reasons for this are not completely clear, but what is known is that this is an insidious disease. Symptoms occur late in the disease process, leaving most cases of EAC diagnosed at an advanced stage, a point where the disease is lethal in the majority of patients. Therefore an early diagnosis constitutes our best hope of impacting survival. Emphasis on public awareness regarding the risk factors for EAC has perhaps stimulated a trend toward esophageal surveillance, despite a lack of clarity within the gastroenterology society guidelines. People with long-standing reflux who are not realizing benefits from medical therapy or those who are simply undergoing routine colon screening and describe a long history of reflux to their gastroenterologists are often undergoing screening. This informal screening method has been one of the only mechanisms for us to routinely observe and treat early stage esophageal disease.

SCREENING AND SURVEILLANCE

Screening for squamous cell carcinoma (SCC) of the esophagus should be considered for patient populations with known risk factors, such as tobacco and alcohol use, Plummer-Vinson syndrome, tylosis palmaris et plantaris, history of head and neck cancer, caustic injury, and achalasia. Increased body mass index (BMI), hiatal hernia, and gastroesophageal reflux disease (GERD) are all considered to be contributors to the formation of intestinal metaplasia (Barrett esophagus [BE]), a precursor lesion to EAC.[3–6] On the other hand, many patients presenting with a new diagnosis of EAC do not have BE and have never had symptoms of reflux. Perhaps that is because "silent" reflux is present in this subgroup of patients or there are other variables driving the progression to neoplasia that are not fully understood. We have a little better understanding about disease progression when BE is present. Through an accumulation of incompletely understood genetic alterations, disease can progress from nondysplastic intestinal metaplasia to low-grade dysplasia (LGD), HGD, and invasive EAC.[7] However, an orderly progression through the metaplasia-dysplasia-cancer sequence may not be recognized or even present in every patient with a Barrett-associated cancer. It is possible that episodic observation of the esophagus misses those events in real time, if they have occurred. Another explanation may be that the disease has the ability to skip intermediate stages of progression once a critical genetic mutation or mutational load is reached. Nonetheless, screening endoscopies are one of the most important elements in discovering early, curable disease that can be treated without removal of the esophagus. Unfortunately, it is the rare patient with early disease who manifests observable symptoms that would set into motion the need for an endoscopy. It is far more common that symptoms are the harbinger of locally advanced or advanced disease. Therefore devising a cost-effective screening strategy that will detect early disease is challenging. Given the low yield of endoscopy/cancer diagnoses, current recommendations by expert consensus panels indicate that there is a lack of sufficient evidence to support routine screening for Barrett-related disease. According to the American Gastroenterological Association report "well-established risk factors for Barrett's esophagus include advanced age, male sex, white ethnicity, GERD, hiatal hernia, elevated body mass index, and a predominantly intraabdominal distribution of body fat. [However], despite the considerable published data available on risk factors for Barrett's esophagus, few attempts have been made to apply this information systematically in the design of guidelines on who to screen for the condition."[1] The vexing issue is that we are unable to focus screening efforts upon a sufficiently high-risk population to justify the expense.

Notwithstanding the lack of concrete guidelines, most experts would recommend that any patient who has had long-standing reflux, has a family history of esophageal neoplasia, continues to be symptomatic with GERD despite therapy, or has unexplained anemia should consider endoscopic screening of the esophagus. Likewise, longitudinal studies have shown that initial presentation with erosive esophagitis (Los Angeles [LA] Classification of GERD grade C/D) and regular proton pump inhibitor (PPI) use were independently associated with progression

TABLE 37.1 Guidelines for Patients With Barrett Esophagus With and Without Dysplasia

Diagnosis	Recommendations
Nondysplastic BE	EGD every 3–5 years
	Four-quadrant biopsies every 2 cm
	Focused biopsy on areas of abnormality
Low-grade dysplasia	Confirm results with expert pathologist
	Follow-up EGD with biopsies in 6 months
	Consider endoscopic resection and/or ablation
	Surveillance after therapy is necessary
High-grade dysplasia	Confirm results with expert pathologist
	Refer for endoscopic resection and/or ablation
	Consider esophagectomy in refractory cases
	Surveillance after endoscopic therapy is necessary

BE, Barrett esophagus; *EGD,* esophagogastroduodenoscopy.

to BE, warranting screening in these populations.[8] After BE has been discovered, endoscopic efforts convert from screening to surveillance, the purpose of which is to detect the presence of esophageal lesions that are at high risk of progressing to EAC. Although the benefit of surveillance has also not been conclusively proved, several studies have shown that patients who contracted EAC while under surveillance presented at a lower stage of disease and had improved survival when compared with those not undergoing surveillance.[9,10] In fact, surveillance guidelines have been developed under the assumption that the practice will reduce deaths.

Surveillance guidelines vary according to the degree of dysplasia detected in the esophageal biopsies (Table 37.1). Mucosal irregularities identified on endoscopy need particular attention and should be biopsied with multiple bites taken to increase accuracy. An expert pathologist should confirm the detection of dysplasia or cancer.[11]

Although older literature advocated for surveillance, patients with confirmed HGD should now be referred for treatment.[11–14] As discussed in the introduction, bridging a technology gap that enables efficient and safe therapy has changed the recommendations for treatment of HGD. Without intervention, the progression risk from *flat* HGD to EAC is high, ranging from 6% to 19% per year. Patients with visible lesions, such as a nodular esophagus, have a much higher risk of progression (40% to 70%).[13] There is also a risk of concomitant adenocarcinoma in patients diagnosed with HGD. Historical data have given us somewhat of a perspective on this risk. In one study, patients who underwent esophagectomy for HGD actually harbored invasive cancer in approximately 50% of the resected specimens.[13] But to be equitable, other more recent studies using better endoscopy techniques and superior equipment suggest that the rate of undiagnosed cancer may be as low 11% in patients without visible lesions.[15]

Surveillance as a treatment strategy for HGD should be reserved for those who are unable or unwilling to undergo therapy. In these cases endoscopy should be scheduled every 3 months, with random four-quadrant biopsies every 1 cm with focused biopsies on any mucosal irregularity.

ENDOSCOPIC DIAGNOSIS AND STAGING

A detailed inspection of the Barrett segment with high-definition white light endoscopy with or without magnification is essential for the detection of mucosal abnormalities, nodularity, and cancer. Studies reveal that the longer the time spent inspecting the Barrett segment, the higher the likelihood of detecting suspicious lesions. In a study of 112 patients undergoing surveillance, the authors reported that endoscopists who averaged greater than 1 minute of inspection time per centimeter of Barrett detected more suspicious lesions than those who spent less time.[16]

Topographic detection of suspicious lesions is probably also aided by various techniques for mucosal enhancement. A number of visual aids such as chromoendoscopy, narrow band imaging (NBI; Olympus, Center Valley, Pennsylvania), autofluorescence imaging, confocal laser endomicroscopy, and volumetric laser endomicroscopy have become available for detailed visualization and characterization of mucosal and cellular architecture. Although the literature has not clearly defined the benefit of these advanced imaging techniques, we advocate using mucosal enhancements that are either electronic or vital staining as a routine practice to facilitate the detection of HGD and early neoplasia. These modalities can be very helpful in targeting biopsies.[17]

Upper endoscopy with ultrasound plays an important role in the diagnosis and staging of esophageal cancer. In cases of intermediate to locally advanced EAC, endoscopic ultrasound (EUS) is the principal method used to estimate the depth and regional nodal status of the disease. In contrast, EUS maintains a limited role for the evaluation of patients with HGD and early EAC. The accuracy of EUS staging in these disease categories is modest at best.[18] In a study describing the accuracy of endoscopy compared with EUS, the sensitivity of EUS staging for mucosal tumors was 90%, whereas for submucosal tumors it was 46%, which was not significantly different from the sensitivity of high-resolution endoscopy in experienced hands.[19] A systematic review compared EUS with endoscopic mucosal resection (EMR) or surgical pathology for early (T1-T2) tumors. In that study EUS predicted the depth of the target lesion with 67% accuracy (12 studies, $n = 132$). Because some patients had multiple lesions, analysis on an individual patient basis reduced the accuracy to only 56%.[20] Given the available data, most experts would not recommend EUS in patients with a flat Barrett segment and HGD detected by biopsy. There are several factors that may contribute to the suboptimal accuracy of EUS in early EAC, including wall thickening due to chronic inflammation, presence of a duplicated muscularis mucosa often seen around the junction, anatomic changes at the level of the gastroesophageal junction (GEJ)/cardia, and endoscopist's experience.[20] Despite these drawbacks, we continue to advocate for EUS in select cases in which there is a possibility of detecting malignant lymphadenopathy. Fine-needle aspiration (FNA) is especially important to verify the presence of disease in any suspicious lymph nodes. In a study of 25 patients undergoing EUS evaluation (13 with intramucosal adenocarcinoma), 7 patients were found to have suspicious lymphadenopathy. FNA confirmed malignancy in five of these seven patients. EUS identified five patients (20%) who were unsuitable candidates for endoscopic therapy.[21] Studies like this one highlight the importance of a careful, individual approach to patients with early esophageal cancer.

EMR is the preferred diagnostic and therapeutic tool for patients with nodular Barrett or early adenocarcinoma. EMR is capable of removing small- to moderate-sized mucosal and superficial submucosal lesions. It is superior to EUS for the assessment of depth of invasion by the simple fact that depth is determined by histologic examination under the microscope. In practice, studies that compared EMR with esophagogastroduodenoscopy [EGD]-EUS report that the pathologic assessment was changed by EMR in 30% to 48% of cases.[22,23] A prospective study of 75 patients with biopsy-proven HGD or early cancer reports that the pathology from an EMR changed the tumor grading or staging in 48% of patients (downgrading in 28% and upgrading in 20%).[22] Another study of 293 EMR procedures performed on focal lesions indicated that 30% of patients changed therapy as a result of ER compared with clinical assessment.[23] These are very significant findings; imagine redirecting the recommended therapy of an individual patient from combined multimodality therapy consisting of chemoradiation followed by esophagectomy to an organ-sparing, curative EMR.

In summary, optimal evaluation is fundamental to the management of dysplastic and early-stage mucosal and selected submucosal lesions. ER is an important diagnostic and potentially therapeutic tool for patients with early neoplastic disease.

ENDOSCOPIC TREATMENT OF HIGH-GRADE DYSPLASIA/INTRAMUCOSAL CANCER

ABLATION

- Endoscopic therapy currently consists of methods that either ablate (destroy) or resect tissue.
- Advantages of ablation therapies include ability to apply over large surface areas.
- Repeat applications are possible and typically required to eradicate long segments of metaplasia/dysplasia.
- Ablation therapies do not provide a pathologic specimen and are not as effective in treating elevated or ulcerated lesions.
- Ablative therapies include photodynamic therapy, thermal laser, argon plasma coagulation (APC), multipolar electrocoagulation, radiofrequency ablation (RFA), and cryoablation. This chapter will focus on describing RFA and cryoablation, given the evidence of effectiveness, ease of application, and low risk of adverse effects.

RADIOFREQUENCY ABLATION

RFA destroys tissue through a heat-energy system applied to the esophageal mucosa. Mucosal ablation is performed under endoscopic guidance followed by immediate débridement of the ablated area (Fig. 37.1). The ablation treatment is then immediately repeated in the same area, so that there is full treatment of the Barrett segment all within one endoscopy session. The depth of ablation is typically between 500 and 1000 μm, depending on the

intrinsic properties of the esophagus and the energy setting used for the RFA. This will typically ablate through the epithelium and into the lamina propria layer of the esophageal mucosa. Multiple endoscopic treatments may be required to attain complete eradication of dysplasia (CE-D) and/or metaplasia, with the goal being total resolution of metaplasia. Treatments are usually performed every 2 to 3 months until therapeutic goals are met, after which surveillance is continued.

Several studies have demonstrated the efficacy, safety, and durability of RFA to treat dysplastic Barrett.[14,24-26] In the AIM trial, a randomized multicenter study, 127 patients with dysplastic BE were assigned to receive either RFA or sham procedure.[14] Eighty-four patients were randomized to the RFA treatment group (42 patients with HGD and 42 with LGD). After an average of 3.5 treatments per patient, CE-D occurred in 81% of HGD patients assigned to the ablation group as compared with 19% of those assigned to the control group ($P < .001$). Overall, 77.4% of patients in the RFA group had complete eradication of intestinal metaplasia (CE-IM) compared with 2.3% of those in the control group ($P < .001$). Progression from HGD to cancer occurred in 4 of 21 patients in the control group and in 1 of 42 patients in the RFA treated group ($P = .045$). Longer follow-up at 2 years indicated that among subjects with initial HGD, there was CE-D in 93% and CE-IM in 89%. At 3 years, CE-D was reported in 98% of patients and CE-IM in 91%. The annual rate of progression to EAC among those treated with RFA was 0.55% per patient per year.[24]

The safety profile of RFA has also been described. The most common complications reported include: chest pain lasting less than 1 week, strictures requiring dilation (6% to 8%), and gastrointestinal hemorrhage (1%).[14,27] Although operator experience has been shown to impact the success of RFA and the number of sessions needed to achieve CE-IM, it does not appear to impact the risk of complications including stricture formation, gastrointestinal hemorrhage, perforation, or hospitalization.

Several factors have been identified as predictors of a poor response after RFA. In a large, multicenter study of 278 patients, poor initial response was defined less than 50% regression of the BE 3 months after circumferential balloon-based RFA. Thirty-six patients (13%) were deemed to have a poor initial response. Predictive factors for a poor response included the presence of active reflux esophagitis, regeneration of Barrett at the ER scar, relative esophageal narrowing prior to RFA, and number of years with dysplastic changes before RFA.[28]

Following RFA, endoscopic surveillance is indicated to monitor for recurrence, which can occur with an incidence at 1 year ranging from 5% to 25%.[29,30] Currently, there are no consensus recommendations regarding surveillance interval in postablation patients. Some experts recommend surveillance endoscopy every 3 months for the first year, every 6 months for the second year, and then annually.[30,31]

CRYOTHERAPY

Cryotherapy is an ablative technique that causes tissue destruction by application of liquid nitrogen or carbon dioxide gas (Fig. 37.2). Small areas can be treated (2 to 3 cm) while covering approximately one-third or one-half

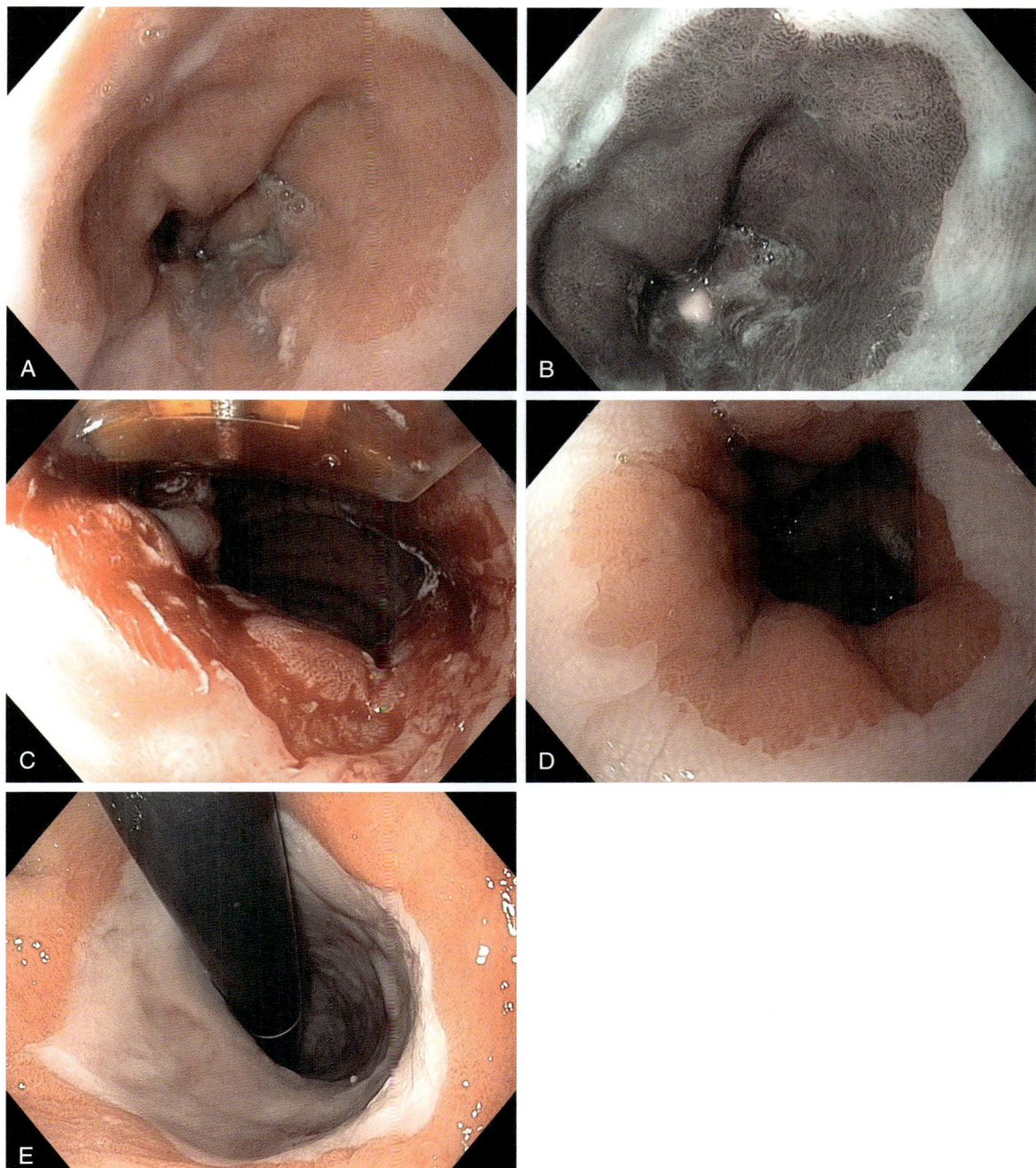

FIGURE 37.1 (A) Long-segment circumferential Barrett esophagus with dysplasia/intramucosal cancer. (B) Endoscopic view with narrow band imaging (Olympus). (C) Treatment with the HALO 90 (Medtronic) device. (D) Endoscopic appearance postradiofrequency ablation treatment, new Z-line. (E) Retroflex view of neosquamous lining.

of the luminal circumference with each application. Multiple areas can be treated in one endoscopic session. On average, three to four endoscopies are needed to completely ablate a long segment of disease, and the procedures can be performed approximately every 6 to 8 weeks.[31,32]

There are no randomized controlled studies assessing the efficacy of cryotherapy in the treatment of dysplastic BE. In a multicenter retrospective study of liquid nitrogen in patients with BE-HGD, 97% of patients had CE of HGD and

87% had CE of all dysplasia.[33] The most common adverse events reported included strictures in 3% that responded to endoscopic dilation, and chest pain in 2%, managed on an outpatient basis. With regard to cryoablation for early cancer, a multicenter retrospective study of liquid nitrogen for esophageal cancer was published in 2010. CE of cT1a tumors occurred in 18 of 24 (75%) patients. For cT1b (submucosal) tumors, CE was seen in four of six patients (60%) with a mean follow-up of 11.8 months.[33] Caveats must be made that these cancers were clinically

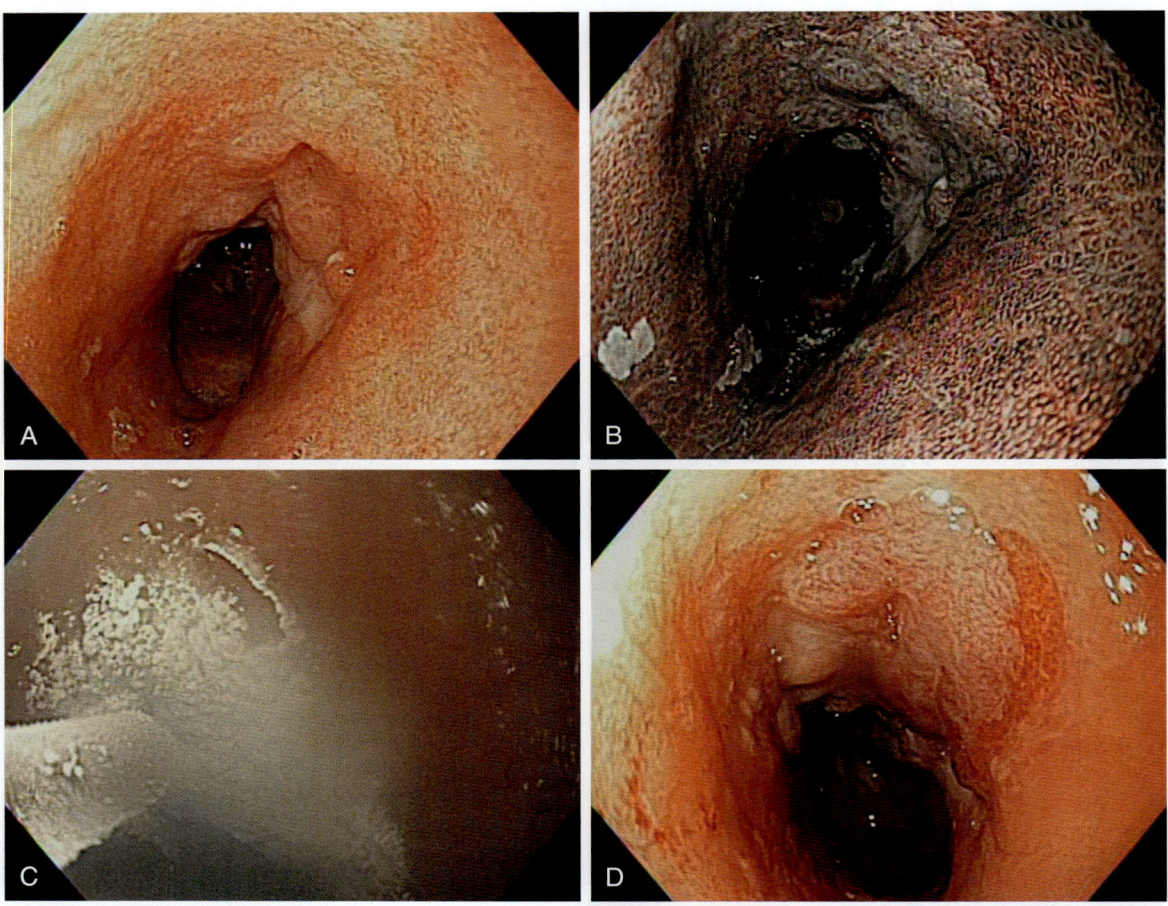

FIGURE 37.2 (A and B) Endoscopic appearance of nodular dysplastic Barrett esophagus with intramucosal cancer. (C) Cryotherapy application. (D) Appearance immediately after cryotherapy.

staged with the inherent deficiencies of EUS staging, and because ablation was chosen over ER no tissue was provided to pathology for analysis. Overall, it seems that cryotherapy has a bit better pain profile and may be more durable in applications where the mucosa is not flat. As example, a single-center retrospective cohort study of 121 patients with Barrett with dysplasia or intramucosal cancer, 16 patients who failed RFA[14] or had recurrent dysplasia[2] underwent cryotherapy as salvage. After cryotherapy, 75% of patients had CE-D and 31% had CE-IM.[34]

ENDOSCOPIC RESECTION

ER is currently the leading therapy for nodular BE and suspected early esophageal tumors.[35–43] This procedure originally gained acceptance as a treatment for polyps and early-staged cancers within the colon. It later translated into treatment for esophageal squamous cell carcinoma within Asian medical centers. Now it is used throughout the world after groups in Germany, the Netherlands, and North America have shown that this modality is a preferable treatment option over surgery for HGD and early EAC.[37–40] In patients diagnosed with HGD, the main goal of ER is to resect visible lesions within the esophagus. Solitary nodules, areas of nodularity, and superficial ulcers are all high-risk areas for concurrent, unrecognized carcinoma or progression to invasive disease. Areas of flat HGD

are often adequately managed by endoscopic ablation therapies alone, but there are times when a strategy of resection may be more definitive, cheaper, and effective. Short segments of flat HGD are amenable to complete ER with a low risk of complication.[44] This is especially true when the area is not circumferential (circumferential resections will cause serious stricture issues).[45]

Invasive lesions amenable to EMR must be superficial (T1) and small enough to be completely resected endoscopically. Patients with the lowest risk for regional or systemic disease will have lesions that are less than 2 cm in maximal dimension. Well-differentiated mucosal adenocarcinomas are associated with very low rates of lymph node metastases (<3%) and can be managed with endoscopic therapies, whereas tumors invading the submucosa may have a substantial risk of lymph node metastases (in excess of 20%) and should be referred for esophagectomy.[46]

Step by step ER (Fig. 37.3):

1. *Procedure setup and setting.* Patients are advised to remain nothing by mouth (NPO) overnight and preferably stay on a liquid diet the evening before. Performing this procedure with food in the stomach is inconvenient and perhaps incurs a bit more risk. The appropriate setting is in a monitored suite with full anesthesia capability. We perform the procedure with monitored sedation in

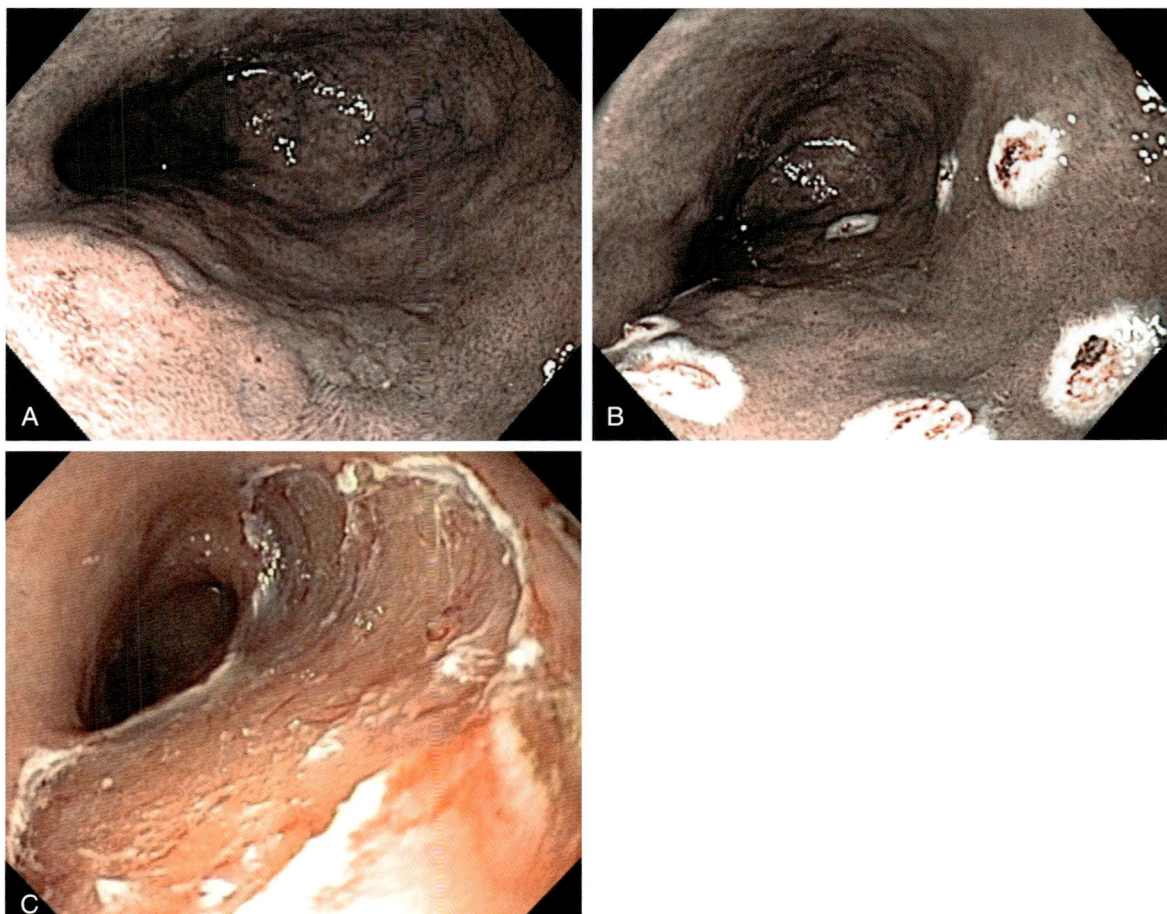

FIGURE 37.3 (A) Endoscopic appearance of an early adenocarcinoma. (B) Cautery marks the margins of resection. (C) Immediate postresection appearance.

most cases, but it is not absolutely imperative that the patient is under a general anesthetic. Avoiding cough, hiccoughs, and excess patient movement does help at the most critical point of the case when the tissue is acquired into a cap or band.

2. *Identification of the lesion.* High-definition equipment is mandatory. The endoscopy equipment is critical to the outcome of therapy. Techniques that improve topographic visualization are encouraged because early lesions around the GEJ/cardia can be easily overlooked. Endoscopists must be experienced at detecting early esophageal/gastroesophageal pathology.

3. *Outline the area of resection.* The area to be removed should be marked prior to introducing a cap for therapy. We are frequently surprised at how an obvious lesion becomes difficult to see once a scope with a cap partially obstructs our view in the esophagus. Chromoendoscopy of some sort can facilitate marking the lesion with adequate margins. The endoscopist may also choose to place marks (cautery, ink, or clips) on the tissue to be resected that will orient the tissue margins for the clinician and pathologist. This is probably only relevant in situations in which there is a single resection because piecemeal resections render peripheral margins interpretable in most situations.

4. *Choose a method of resection.* Multiple methods of EMR or endoscopic submucosal dissection (ESD) are currently used. EMR with a cap and snare technique or mucosal banding followed by a cauterized snare will resect into the submucosal layer of the esophagus, and the procedure is facile after a relatively short learning curve. Smaller lesions and selected lesions that are up to 2 cm can be removed entirely en bloc with suction cap techniques. Larger lesions resected with an EMR-cap typically require a "piecemeal" approach in which the lesion is removed by multiple applications of the cap and snare to include overlapping areas, ultimately resulting in a complete resection. In cases where a lesion is tough to lift or is a little larger, we will often use a larger oblique cap as these are capable of handling larger tissue areas. Another alternative is ESD. This more aggressive approach has the potential to achieve an en bloc resection for larger or deeper lesions; however, ESD skills are more difficult to master and there are more frequent reports of complications, such as perforation or bleeding. For this reason it is performed only in selected centers where specialized training has been performed and there is adequate system support to increase the acuity of care.

Retrieve all of the tissue samples and grossly examine the specimen to confirm complete capture and adequate margins. Take more tissue around the margins with additional ER if necessary to achieve a complete resection. Pinning the tissue to cork will help the pathologist to orient the deepest margin; omitting this step allows the tissue to invert its shape into a little mushroom button that may lead to misinterpretation of the deep margin.

5. *Postresection management.* Patients are discharged home on the same day unless there are comorbidities or complications that direct otherwise. We typically allow full liquid diet on the first day, then liberalize the diet when symptoms allow, starting on a soft diet for the first few days after the procedure. Patients and caregivers need to be educated on expected outcomes and potential signs of complications. Expected short-term outcomes will include mild to moderate chest discomfort and odynophagia for a few days after resection so we may provide a prescription compound that includes an ionic binder to help heal the iatrogenic ulcer and a local anesthetic to alleviate symptoms. Narcotics are not usually required; in our experience, GEJ ER is more easily tolerated than a high to mid-esophageal lesion. Mild to moderate dysphagia can be a frequent complaint associated with healing but most often subsides after 6 to 8 weeks. Most patients are already on an acid reduction medication, so we recommend continuing with a high-dose PPI for at least 2 weeks after the ER, then resuming the previous dose that the patient was taking. If not on a PPI previously, we will typically keep a patient on them at least until the next endoscopic evaluation. Patients with lower EAC with or without Barrett are typically maintained on PPIs indefinitely, but the evidence for this practice after eradication of IM is lacking.

Complications specific to EMR include perforation, an event that is seen in less than 0.1% of cases using most cap techniques. This is in contrast to reports of perforation upward of 40% for aggressive ESD procedures. Fortunately almost all perforations associated with ER can be managed nonoperatively. Bleeding risk is approximately 2% for EMR.[47] Stricture may occur, and this depends on previous pathology in the individual patient and the extent of circumferential resection. Removing more than 50% circumference significantly increases the risk of stricture.[48] Complete circumferential resections can be performed, but we typically like to stage procedures that will require circumferential resections into several episodes. Single-session circumferential resection is associated with healing to high-grade stenosis; therefore stenting at the time of resection should be considered.[45,48]

6. *Individualizing therapy based on interpretation of pathology.* Lesions that are treated successfully with EMR are most often limited to the mucosa. Submucosal invasion increases the risk of lymph node invasion and/or cancer related events of recurrence or death. Lymphovascular invasion (LVI) is the most important prognostic determinant of outcome for resected early-stage cancer.[38] In current surgical literature the risk of nodal involvement has been estimated to increase from 2% to 3% for a T1a lesion without LVI to 60%+ for T1b lesions with LVI.[38,40] Size of tumor and differentiation are other factors that have been shown to be independent prognostic variables in some studies, in which lesions less than 2 cm and well to moderately differentiated are less likely to harbor concurrent adenopathy.[38,40]

According to some reports it is possible to identify patients with early submucosal disease at low risk for nodal disease that may be adequately treated by ER alone.[49] Given that there is still some question about interobserver variability regarding submucosal invasion and the presence of LVI even among expert pathologists, selecting appropriate patients who can avoid resection should be done only at centers of excellence and in the presence of a multidisciplinary group.

7. *Follow-up.* It has been our practice to perform endoscopy every 2 to 3 months while in the process of ablating residual metaplasia/dysplasia, followed by increasing intervals between procedures depending on individual findings. The need for cross-sectional imaging is debated in small T1a lesions given the low risk of regional or distant metastasis, and it is not at all indicated for patients with dysplasia only. Patients at higher risk for regional and distant disease such as those with deeper, or larger lesions, or those patients with LVI who have opted for endoscopic treatment alone based on risk for esophageal resection should undergo imaging every 4 to 6 months and consider EUS to screen for regional disease.

ENDOSCOPIC RESECTION, MUCOSAL ABLATION, OR BOTH?

After initial endoscopic therapy directed at nodular areas, any remaining areas of metaplasia/dysplasia should undergo ablation with the goal of total eradication. Past reports indicated that untreated segments increased the risk of metachronous lesions to as high as 30%.[43,44] Combining EMR with ablation to eradicate residual intestinal metaplasia is both safe and efficacious. Pouw et al. reported their experience with 23 patients who underwent EMR for visible lesions; 16 patients had early cancer and 7 patients had BE-HGD. In this study, RFA was performed at least 6 weeks after the EMR. CE-neoplasia was achieved in 100% of patients (median follow-up 22 months) and CE-IM in 88% of patients.[42]

Another retrospective study reported on the treatment of 65 patients with EMR and RFA for nodular disease and an additional 104 patients treated with RFA alone for flat segments of Barrett disease. There were no significant differences in eradication of dysplasia and intramucosal carcinoma between the two groups. The complication rates were also similar, including strictures that occurred in 4.6% of the EMR-before-RFA patient group and in 7.7% of patients in the RFA only group.[43] This study suggests that similar results may be achieved when ER is reserved for dysplasia-associated lesions that are visible while RFA alone may suffice for flat pathology.

Of course there is the possibility that one could resect the entire area of pathology in the esophagus using ER techniques. This may be favorable in situations in which there is limited, noncircumferential disease. In contrast, combined EMR with ablation may be the preferred approach over stepwise radical ER for the treatment of Barrett associated with early cancer. In a Dutch multicenter study, patients with a BE segment less than or equal to 5 cm containing HGD/early cancer were randomized to stepwise radical endoscopic resection (SRER) or ER followed by RFA. Although both groups achieved excellent (>90%) and comparable rates of CE-neoplasia and CE-IM, those in the SRER group developed a significantly higher number of strictures requiring endoscopic dilation (88% in the SRER group compared with 14% in the EMR-RFA group; $P < .001$).[42]

Endoscopic treatment compares favorably with esophagectomy as well. A retrospective comparison of endoscopic therapy performed in 40 patients (22 with HGD and 18 with intramucosal cancer [IMC]) with esophagectomy in 61 patients (13 with HGD and 48 with IMC) reported that there was no difference in survival between the two groups (94% at 3 years). However, compared with esophagectomy, endoscopic therapy was associated with significantly lower morbidity (39% vs. 0%; $P < .0001$).[46] One should note that endoscopic therapy was not finite in this study, consisting of 102 ERs and 79 ablations in 40 patients. Nonetheless, cost comparisons still seem to favor endoscopic treatment over esophageal resection in most situations.[50]

In summary, EMR followed by ablation is an effective treatment modality for early cancer arising in the setting of BE. However, these techniques are best performed at high-volume referral centers by experienced endoscopists. The outcomes may not apply to general practices.

CONCLUSION

Endoscopic therapies have been shown to be effective and safe in the treatment of patients with BE-HGD and early esophageal cancer while preserving the esophagus. Attempts at total eradication of all dysplasia/metaplasia followed by close surveillance is recommended after endoscopic therapy because of the risk of recurrence. Given the complexities in the evaluation and management of these patients, they are best managed by a multidisciplinary team in a tertiary referral center with expertise in esophageal diseases.

REFERENCES

1. Spechler SJ, Sharma P, Souza RF, et al. American Gastroenterological Association Medical Position Statement on the management of Barrett's esophagus. *Gastroenterology.* 2011;140:1084-1091.
2. Sampliner RE. Practice guidelines on the diagnosis, surveillance and therapy of Barrett's esophagus. *Am J Gastroenterol.* 1998;93:1028-1031.
3. Jung KW, Talley NJ, Romero Y, et al. Epidemiology and natural history of intestinal metaplasia of the gastroesophageal junction and Barrett's esophagus: a population-based study. *Am J Gastroenterol.* 2011;106:1447-1455.
4. Hvid-Jensen F, Pedersen L, Drewes AM, Sørensen HT, Funch-Jensen P. Incidence of adenocarcinoma among patients with Barrett's esophagus. *N Engl J Med.* 2011;365:1375-1383.
5. Hur C, Miller M, Kong CY, et al. Trends in esophageal adenocarcinoma incidence and mortality. *Cancer.* 2013;119(6):1149-1158.
6. Yates M, Cheong E, Luben R, et al. Body mass index, smoking, and alcohol and risks of Barrett's esophagus and esophageal adenocarcinoma: a UK prospective cohort study. *Dig Dis Sci.* 2014;59(7):1552-1559.
7. Goldblum JR. Barrett's esophagus and Barrett's-related dysplasia. *Mod Pathol.* 2003;16:316-324.
8. Malfertheiner P, Nocon M, Vieth M, et al. Evolution of gastro-oesophageal reflux disease over 5 years under routine medical care—the ProGERD study. *Aliment Pharmacol Ther.* 2012;35(1):154-164.
9. Corley DA, Levin HR, Habel LA, Weiss NS, Buffler PA. Surveillance and survival in Barrett's adenocarcinoma: a population based study. *Gastroenterology.* 2002;122:633-640.
10. Fountoulakis A, Zafirellis K, Donlan K, et al. Effect of surveillance of Barrett's oesophagus on clinical outcome of oesophageal cancer. *Br J Surg.* 2004;91:997-1003.
11. Fernando HC, Murthy SC, Hofstetter W, et al. The Society of Thoracic Surgeons practice guideline series: guidelines for the management of Barrett's esophagus with high-grade dysplasia. *Ann Thorac Surg.* 2009;87:1993-2002.
12. Phoa KN, van Vilsteren FG, Weusten BL, et al. Radiofrequency ablation vs endoscopic surveillance for patients with Barrett esophagus and low-grade dysplasia: a randomized clinical trial. *JAMA.* 2014;311(12):1209-1217.
13. Rastogi A, Puli S, El-Serag HB, Bansal A, Wani S, Sharma P. Incidence of esophageal adenocarcinoma in patients with Barrett's esophagus and high-grade dysplasia: a meta-analysis. *Gastrointest Endosc.* 2008;67:394-398.
14. Shaheen NJ, Sharma P, Overholt BF, et al. Radiofrequency ablation in Barrett's esophagus with dysplasia. *N Engl J Med.* 2009;360:2277-2288.
15. Konda VJ, Ross AS, Ferguson MK, et al. Is the risk of concomitant invasive esophageal cancer in high-grade dysplasia in Barrett's esophagus overestimated? *Clin Gastroenterol Hepatol.* 2008;6:159-164.
16. Gupta N, Gaddam S, Wani SB, Bansal A, Rastogi A, Sharma P. Longer inspection time is associated with increase detection of high-grade dysplasia and esophageal adenocarcinoma in Barrett's esophagus. *Gastrointest Endosc.* 2012;76:531-538.
17. Panossian AM, Raimondo M, Wolfsen HC. State of the art in the endoscopic imaging and ablation of Barrett's esophagus. *Dig Liver Dis.* 2011;43:365-373.
18. Thosani N, Singh H, Kapadia A, et al. Diagnostic accuracy of EUS in differentiating mucosal versus submucosal invasion of superficial esophageal cancers: a systematic review and meta-analysis. *Gastrointest Endosc.* 2012;75(2):242-253.
19. May A, Günter E, Roth F, et al. Accuracy of staging in early oesophageal cancer using high resolution endoscopy and high resolution endosonography: a comparative, prospective, and blinded trial. *Gut.* 2004;53:634-640.
20. Young PE, Gentry AB, Acosta RD, Greenwald BD, Riddle M. Endoscopic ultrasound does not accurately stage early adenocarcinoma or high-grade dysplasia of the esophagus. *Clin Gastroenterol Hepatol.* 2010;8:1037-1041.
21. Shami VM, Villaverde A, Stearns L, et al. Clinical impact of conventional endosonography and endoscopic ultrasound-guided fine needle aspiration in the assessment of patients with Barrett's esophagus and high-grade dysplasia or intramucosal carcinoma who have been referred for endoscopic ablation therapy. *Endoscopy.* 2006;38:157-161.
22. Moss A, Bourke MJ, Hourigan LF, et al. Endoscopic resection for Barrett's high-grade dysplasia and early esophageal adenocarcinoma: an essential staging procedure with long-term therapeutic benefit. *Am J Gastroenterol.* 2010;105:1276-1283.
23. Peters FP, Brakenhoff KP, Curvers WL, et al. Histologic evaluation of resection specimens obtained at 293 endoscopic resections in Barrett's esophagus. *Gastrointest Endosc.* 2008;67:604-609.
24. Shaheen NJ, Overholt BF, Sampliner RE, et al. Durability of radiofrequency ablation in Barrett's esophagus with dysplasia. *Gastroenterology.* 2011;141:460-468.
25. Ganz RA, Overholt BF, Sharma VK, et al. Circumferential ablation of Barrett's esophagus that contains high-grade dysplasia: a U.S. multicenter registry. *Gastrointest Endosc.* 2008;68:35-40.
26. Fleischer DE, Overholt BF, Sharma VK, et al. Endoscopic radiofrequency ablation for Barrett's esophagus: 5-year outcomes from a prospective multicenter trial. *Endoscopy.* 2010;42:781-789.
27. Bulsiewicz WJ, Kim HP, Dellon ES, et al. Safety and efficacy of endoscopic mucosal therapy with radiofrequency ablation for patients with neoplastic Barrett's esophagus. *Clin Gastroenterol Hepatol.* 2013;11(6):636-642.
28. Van Vilsteren FG, Alvarez Herrero L, Pouw RE, et al. Predictive factors for initial treatment response after circumferential radiofrequency

ablation for Barrett's esophagus with early neoplasia: a prospective multicenter study. *Endoscopy.* 2013;45:516-525.

29. Orman ES, Kim HP, Bulsiewicz WJ, et al. Intestinal metaplasia recurs infrequently in patients successfully treated for Barrett's esophagus with radiofrequency ablation. *Am J Gastroenterol.* 2013;108(2):187-195, [quiz 196].

30. Titi M, Overhiser A, Ulusarac O, et al. Development of subsquamous high-grade dysplasia and adenocarcinoma after successful radiofrequency ablation of Barrett's esophagus. *Gastroenterology.* 2012;143: 564-566.

31. Greenwald BD, Dumot JA. Cryotherapy for Barrett's esophagus and esophageal cancer. *Curr Opin Gastroenterol.* 2011;27:363-367.

32. Shaheen NJ, Greenwald BD, Peery AF, et al. Safety and efficacy of endoscopic spray cryotherapy for Barrett's esophagus with high-grade dysplasia. *Gastrointest Endosc.* 2010;71:680-685.

33. Greenwald BD, Dumot JA, Abrams JA, et al. Endoscopic spray cryotherapy for esophageal cancer: safety and efficacy. *Gastrointest Endosc.* 2010;71:686-693.

34. Sengupta N, Ketwaroo GA, Bak DM, et al. Salvage cryotherapy after failed radiofrequency ablation for Barrett's esophagus-related dysplasia is safe and effective. *Gastrointest Endosc.* 2015;82:443-448.

35. Pech O, Bollschweiler E, Manner H, Leers J, Ell C, Holscher AH. Comparison between endoscopic and surgical resection of mucosal esophageal adenocarcinoma in Barrett's esophagus at two high-volume centers. *Ann Surg.* 2011;254(1):67-72.

36. Pech O, Behrens A, May A, et al. Long-term results and risk factor analysis for recurrence after curative endoscopic therapy in 349 patients with high-grade intraepithelial neoplasia and mucosal adenocarcinoma in Barrett's oesophagus. *Gut.* 2008;57(9):1200-1206.

37. Manner H, Pech O, Heldmann Y, et al. Efficacy, safety, and long-term results of endoscopic treatment for early-stage adenocarcinoma of the esophagus with low-risk sm1 invasion. *Clin Gastroenterol Hepatol.* 2013;11(6):630-635. [quiz e45].

38. Lee L, Ronellenfitsch U, Hofstetter WL, et al. Predicting lymph node metastases in early esophageal adenocarcinoma using a simple scoring system. *J Am Coll Surg.* 2013;217(2):191-199.

39. Pouw RE, van Vilsteren FG, Peters FP, et al. Randomized trial on endoscopic resection-cap versus multiband mucosectomy for piecemeal endoscopic resection of early Barrett's neoplasia. *Gastrointest Endosc.* 2011;74(1):35-43.

40. Alvarez Herrero L, Pouw RE, van Vilsteren FG, et al. Risk of lymph node metastasis associated with deeper invasion by early adenocarcinoma of the esophagus and cardia: study based on endoscopic resection specimens. *Endoscopy.* 2010;42(12):1030-1036.

41. May A, Gossner L, Pech O. Local endoscopic therapy for intraepithelial high-grade neoplasia and early adenocarcinoma in Barrett's esophagus: acute-phase and intermediate results of a new treatment approach. *Eur J Gastroenterol Hepatol.* 2002;14:1085-1091.

42. Pouw RE, Wirths K, Eisendrath P, et al. Efficacy of radiofrequency ablation combined with endoscopic resection for Barrett's esophagus with early neoplasia. *Clin Gastroenterol Hepatol.* 2010;8:23-29.

43. Kim HP, Bulsiewicz WJ, Cotton CC, et al. Focal endoscopic mucosal resection before radiofrequency ablation is equally effective and safe compared with radiofrequency ablation alone for the eradication of Barrett's esophagus with advanced neoplasia. *Gastrointest Endosc.* 2012;76:733-739.

44. Van Vilsteren FG, Pouw RE, Seewald S, et al. Stepwise radical endoscopic resection versus radiofrequency ablation for Barrett's oesophagus with high-grade dysplasia or early cancer: a multicenter randomized trial. *Gut.* 2011;60:765-773.

45. Conio M, Fisher DA, Blanchi S, Ruggeri C, Filiberti R, Siersema PD. One-step circumferential endoscopic mucosal cap resection of Barrett's esophagus with early neoplasia. *Clin Res Hepatol Gastroenterol.* 2014;38(1):81-91.

46. Zehetner J, DeMeester SR, Hagen JA, et al. Endoscopic resection and ablation versus esophagectomy for high-grade dysplasia and intramucosal adenocarcinoma. *J Thorac Cardiovasc Surg.* 2011;141:39-47.

47. Pech O, May A, Manner H, et al. Long-term efficacy and safety of endoscopic resection for patients with mucosal adenocarcinoma of the esophagus. *Gastroenterology.* 2014;146(3):652-660.

48. Hanaoka N, Ishihara R, Uedo N, et al. Refractory strictures despite steroid injection after esophageal endoscopic resection. *Endosc Int Open.* 2016;4(3):E354-E359.

49. Manner H, May A, Pech O, et al. Early Barrett's carcinoma with "low-risk" submucosal invasion: long-term results of endoscopic resection with a curative intent. *Am J Gastroenterol.* 2008;103(10):2589-2597.

50. Pohl H, Sonnenberg A, Strobel S, Eckardt A, Rösch T. Endoscopic versus surgical therapy for early cancer in Barrett's esophagus: a decision analysis. *Gastrointest Endosc.* 2009;70(4):623-631.

Multimodality Therapy in the Management of Locally Advanced Esophageal Cancer

Jonathan Cools-Lartigue | Lorenzo Ferri

Esophageal cancer (EC) remains a devastating malignancy with a low rate of cure. Results in patients with early-stage disease (stage I to II) remain more promising, with long-term survival rates between 60% and 90%.[1-4] Unfortunately the majority of patients present with locally advanced or advanced disease.[1-5] This is associated with high rates of systemic recurrence and has demonstrated poor outcomes when treated with surgery alone. Thus while surgery continues to play a central role in curative intent therapy for EC, a significant number of patients present with a burden of disease precluding upfront surgery.[1] Accordingly, the modern approach to the majority of patients with locally advanced disease is the implementation of multimodality treatment strategies.[1]

Complementary therapeutic modalities include chemotherapy and radiation therapy, which have demonstrated efficacy with respect to improved local and distant control.[1] However, considerable variability in the application of multimodality regimens is observed in the literature to date.[1] This includes the application of neoadjuvant or adjuvant chemotherapy alone or in conjunction with radiation therapy, as well as the exact drug regimens and radiation doses employed.[1] Furthermore, considerable variability in the surgical approach to esophagectomy is evident in the literature. In keeping with these observations, controversy regarding the optimal regimen persists. What remains clear is that a meticulous approach to this vulnerable patient population with respect to staging, surgical technique, and adjuvant local and systemic therapies is necessary to provide the best possible outcome.[1] Herein, the literature providing the rationale for modern multimodality approaches is reviewed, and the advantages and disadvantages of each are laid out.

PERIOPERATIVE CHEMOTHERAPY VERSUS SURGERY ALONE

The addition of chemotherapy to the management of esophageal cancer has the potential to confer several important benefits. First, the majority of esophageal cancer patients will ultimately die of metastatic disease, thus supporting the implementation of systemic therapy.[1-4] This propensity for systemic spread is manifest by the observation that even in patients with seemingly localized disease successfully managed operatively, death from metastasis is a common occurrence.[5] From a practical standpoint, the questions regarding the timing of chemotherapy (pre-, post-, or perioperative) as well as the optimum regimen are evident. With respect to the former, a number of

theoretic advantages have been put forward favoring both approaches.

Given the observation that a majority of patients present with locally advanced disease, preoperative chemotherapy could serve to downstage seemingly unresectable lesions, rendering them amenable to complete oncologic (R0) resection. Furthermore, in the preoperative setting, optimal drug delivery may be achieved given an intact blood supply. Finally, the administration of chemotherapy in the preoperative setting provides a unique opportunity to observe the clinical efficacy of the drug regimen in question. Assessment of tumor response has important prognostic significance and by identifying patients who do not respond, alternate treatment strategies can be selected in lieu of an initial ineffective and morbid approach.[6] Proponents for the postoperative approach highlight the possibility of overtreatment based on inaccurate staging. Pathologic analysis of surgical specimens provides ultimate staging and can thus direct treatment to patients with risk factors for recurrence who stand to benefit the most.[7,8] Finally, controversy does exist regarding the optimum chemotherapeutic regimen. The majority of randomized controlled trials (RCTs) to date have employed doublet platinum–based therapy, but triplet regimens have been employed and may demonstrate improved efficacy with regard to tumor regression and survival.

Based on these postulates, a number of important questions can be formulated. *First, does perioperative chemotherapy improve survival in patients with esophageal cancer and, if so, does this depend on tumor histology? Second, if so, is chemotherapy more effective when administered in the preoperative or postoperative setting? Third, do triplet regimens confer an advantage over doublets?*

DOES PERIOPERATIVE CHEMOTHERAPY IMPROVE SURVIVAL IN PATIENTS WITH ESOPHAGEAL CANCER AND, IF SO, DOES THIS DEPEND ON HISTOLOGY?

Table 38.1 lists high-quality randomized studies comparing survival outcomes in patients receiving perioperative chemotherapy compared with curative intent surgery alone.[7-19] A number of early studies failed to demonstrate a clear survival advantage in patients receiving preoperative chemotherapy compared with curative intent surgery alone. However, despite these overarching findings, important information regarding the utility of chemotherapy in the management of EC can be inferred. For example, in the negative studies conducted by Roth et al., Schlag, Law et al., Ancona et al., and Kelsen et al., subgroup

TABLE 38.1 Randomized Trials Comparing Neoadjuvant Chemotherapy to Surgery Alone

Study	Year	N	Histology	Regimen	R0	Survival	P
Schlag et al.	1992	69	SCC	Cisplatin, 5FU 3 cycles preop. Restaged after first cycle. If response, 2 additional; if no response, surgery.	44% vs. 42%	Median 8 mo vs. 9 mo	NS
Law et al.	1997	147	SCC	Cisplatin, 5FU 2 preop cycles	67% vs. 24%	Median 16.8 mo vs. 13 mo 2 yr 44% vs. 21%	NS
Ando et al.	1997	205	SCC	Cisplatin, vindesine 2 cycles postop	NA	5 yr 45% vs. 48%	NS
Roth et al.	1998	36	SCC	Cisplatin, vinblastine, bleomycin 3 cycles preop, 3 cycles postop	NA	3 yr 25% vs. 5% Median 10 mo vs. 10 mo	NS
Ancona et al.	2001	96	SCC	Cisplatin, 5FU, 2 cycles preop, +1 additional if response	79% vs. 74%	Median 25 mo vs. 24 mo 5 yr 44% vs. 22%	NS
MRC/OE2	Sep-02	802	SCC/EAC	Cisplatin, 5FU, 2 cycles preop	60% vs. 54%	Median 16.8 mo vs. 13.3 mo 2 yr 43% vs. 34%	0.004
Ando et al.	2003	242	SCC	Cisplatin, 5FU, 2 cycles postop	100% (enrollment criteria)	5 yr 45% vs. 55%	0.037
Cunningham et al. (MAGIC)	2006	503	EAC	Epirubicin, cisplatin, 5FU, 3 cycles preop and postop	79.3% vs. 70.3%	5 yr 36% vs. 29%	0.009
Kelsen et al.	2007	440	SCC/EAC	Cisplatin, 5FU, 3 cycles preop	63% vs. 59%	5 yr 19.4% vs. 21%	NS
Boonstra et al.	2011	169	SCC	Etoposide, cisplatin, up to 4 preop cycles	71% vs. 57%	1 yr 64% vs. 52% 5 yr 26% vs. 17%	0.003
Ychou et al.	2011	224	GEJ AC	Cisplatin, 5FU, 3 cycles preop, 3 cycles postop	87% vs. 73%	5 yr 38% vs. 24%	0.02
Ando et al.	2012	330	SCC	Cisplatin, 5FU, 2 cycles preop OR postop	96% vs. 91%	5 yr 55% vs. 43%	0.04

GEJ AC, Gastroesophageal junction adenocarcinoma; *EAC,* esophageal adenocarcinoma; *5FU,* 5-fluorouracil; *NA,* not available; *NS,* not significant; *SCC,* squamous cell carcinoma.

analysis demonstrates improved survival outcomes in patients who demonstrate a response to the preoperative regimen.[10,11,13,14,19]

Roth et al. demonstrated improved survival in squamous cell carcinoma (SCC) patients who demonstrated a major (47%) or complete (5%) response to vinblastine-, cisplatin-, and bleomycin-based chemotherapy (median survival, 20 months vs. 6 months; P = .008). Patients who responded to preoperative therapy also fared better than patients who received surgery alone.[13] Schlag similarly demonstrated significant increases in survival for patients with SCC who demonstrated a response (minor 12%, major 32%, complete 6%) to 3 cycles of cisplatin and 5-fluorouracil (5FU)-based chemotherapy.[14] Schlag et al. randomized SCC patients to receive 2 cycles of cisplatin and 5FU-based chemotherapy in the preoperative setting or to curative intent surgery alone. The authors demonstrated reduced recurrence rates, predominantly as a result of improved locoregional control in patients who received chemotherapy compared with surgery alone. This finding likely relates to higher R0 resection rates in chemotherapy-treated patients (67% vs. 35%; P = .003). This did not translate into an overall survival (OS) advantage (median and 2-year survival in chemotherapy vs. surgery alone, 16.8 months vs. 13 months, and 44% vs. 31%, respectively; P = .17).[14] However, in patients who demonstrated a response, as

in the previous studies, median and 2-year survival times were improved (chemotherapy vs. surgery, 42.2 months vs. 13.8 months; P = .008 and 59% vs. 33%, respectively). Ancona et al. similarly randomized patients with SCC to two cycles of preoperative cisplatin and 5FU or curative intent surgery alone.[19] Combined complete and major response rates of resected tumors in the neoadjuvant arm were 40%, with a complete response rate of 12.8%. No difference in median survival was noted on an intention to treat basis (24 and 25 months for surgery alone vs. neoadjuvant chemotherapy, respectively).[19] In the 40% of patients who demonstrated a major response to chemotherapy, a significant improvement with respect to median (53 months) and 3-year (74%) and 5-year (60%) survival was observed compared with patients undergoing surgery alone (28 months, 46%, 26%; P = .01) and nonresponders to chemotherapy (19 months, 38%, 19%; P < .05). In keeping with this theme, the survival benefit was most pronounced in the 12.8% of patients who demonstrated a complete response, leading the authors to conclude that pathologic response is a significant determinant of long-term outcome in addition to R0 resection.[19]

Kelsen et al. randomized patients with both SCC and esophageal adenocarcinoma (EAC) in roughly equal proportions to three cycles of preoperative cisplatin and 5FU or curative intent surgery alone.[10] Complete response rate in patients receiving chemotherapy was 2.5%, with a major objective response observed in 19%.[10] In keeping with previous studies, survival was only improved in patients who demonstrated a major response (response vs. no response, hazard ratio [HR], 2.83; 95% confidence interval [CI], 1.84 to 4.35; $P < .001$).[10]

Collectively, these data suggest that effective chemotherapy, as measured by an objective regression response, is protective and confers a significant survival advantage, in addition to R0 resection in patients with both SCC and EAC compared with surgery alone. Furthermore, effective chemotherapy may improve R0 resection rates and thus contribute to improved survival through improved locoregional control.

More recent studies, including the MRC/OE2, Boonstra, Ychou, and Cunningham (MAGIC) trials, were positive on an intent to treat basis, supporting the use of neoadjuvant chemotherapy over surgery alone in patients with locally advanced esophageal cancer.[9,12,15,17,18] In these studies, histologies were commonly mixed. Therapeutic regimens included cisplatin and 5FU-based doublets, with the exception of the Cunningham (MAGIC) trial, which administered triplet therapy encompassing an anthracycline in addition to cisplatin and 5FU. All studies administered chemotherapy in the preoperative and postoperative periods, with the exception of the MRC study, where chemotherapy was administered in the preoperative setting only.

In the MRC study and its subsequent follow-up (OE2), preoperative cisplatin and 5FU was associated with a significant reduction in primary tumor size and regional lymph node positivity, compared with specimens from untreated patients.[12,18] This was associated with improved R0 resection rates in patients subject to neoadjuvant chemotherapy (60% vs. 54%, $P < .001$). Similarly, OS was improved in patients subject to neoadjuvant treatment (median and 2-year survival, neoadjuvant chemotherapy followed by surgery versus surgery alone: 16.8 months vs. 13.3 months and 43% vs. 34%, respectively; HR, 0.79; 95% CI, 0.67 to 0.93; $P = .004$).[12,18] In long-term follow-up (OE2), patients subject to chemotherapy demonstrated reduced T and N stage compared with patients receiving surgery alone following pathologic analysis. Overall 5-year survival was 23% in neoadjuvant group versus 17.1% in patients randomized to surgery alone ($P < .001$).[12,18]

Boonstra et al. conducted a clinical trial comparing perioperative chemotherapy using a regimen of cisplatin and etoposide in patients with SCC.[17] Following chemotherapy, a partial response rate of 40% and complete response rate of 7% were observed. No difference in R0 resection (71% vs. 57%) rate or lymph node positivity between the two treatment arms was noted; however, significantly more patients in the surgery alone arm demonstrated unresectable tumors or underwent an R2 resection.[17] Accordingly, a significant survival advantage in patients receiving chemotherapy was noted (median, 2- and 5-year survival CS vs. surgery alone, 16 months vs. 12 months, 42% vs. 30%, and 26% vs. 17%, respectively; $P = .03$).[17]

The trials by Ychou and Cunningham et al. included patients with adenocarcinoma of the esophagus and stomach.[9,15] Ychou et al. randomized patients, of whom 75% harbored lower esophageal or gastroesophageal (GE) junction tumors to receive perioperative cisplatin

and 5FU versus surgery alone.[15] Patients randomized to preoperative therapy demonstrated improved outcome with respect to R0 resection rate (87% vs. 74%; $P = .04$) and OS (5-year survival chemotherapy vs. surgery alone 38% vs. 24%; $P < .05$).[15] In the study by Cunningham et al., patients with gastric and lower esophageal/GE junction tumors (25%) were randomized to receive perioperative chemotherapy with 5FU, cisplatin, and epirubicin. In patients receiving perioperative therapy, an improvement in R0 (CS vs. surgery alone, 79.3% vs. 70.3%; $P = .03$) resection rate and a tendency for smaller tumors and less advanced nodal disease was noted.[9] In keeping with these findings, improved OS was noted in the chemotherapy arm compared with surgery alone (HR, 0.75; 95% CI, 0.6 to 0.93; $P = .009$; 5-year survival, 36.3% vs. 23%).[9]

Collectively, the data demonstrate that when given in the perioperative setting, chemotherapy can effectively reduce tumor burden, facilitate curative resection, and impart a significant survival benefit in patients with locally advanced SCC or EAC. With respect to whether efficacy differs according to tumor histology, overall the data suggest that chemotherapy provides a benefit in both SCC and EAC. The MRC/OE2 study specifically assessed treatment effects according to histology and found no evidence of a difference in the two, with a significant reduction in both T and N stage overall.[12,18] Furthermore, the benefits of chemotherapy with respect to survival did not differ according to histology, with absolute 5-year survival rates in chemotherapy versus surgery alone of 22.6% versus 17.6% in EAC patients and 25.5% versus 17% in SCC patients, respectively.[12,18] Thus effective chemotherapy may be considered in esophageal cancer patients in addition to surgery, regardless of histology.

DO TRIPLET REGIMENS CONFER AN ADVANTAGE OVER DOUBLETS?

The studies mentioned thus far have predominantly employed chemotherapy regimens composed of a doublet.[7,8,10–12,14–19] These are typically composed of a platinum agent and 5FU. The rationale for this regimen stems from the observation of significant response rates in conjunction with a good toxicity profile. The MAGIC trial suggests that treatment with a chemotherapy triplet via the addition of an anthracycline to the cisplatin and 5FU doublet is also highly effective.[9] Proponents of triplet therapy highlight the potential to improve response rates with acceptable toxicity.[5,20–26] A recent meta-analysis examined 21 randomized studies comparing a doublet to triplet regimen in patients with distal esophageal, esophagogastric, and gastric adenocarcinoma.[20] Overall, outcomes in 3475 patients were assessed. The authors demonstrated improved OS (HR, 0.9; 95% CI, 0.83 to 0.97) and progression-free survival (PFS) (HR, 0.8; 95% CI, 0.69 to 0.93), favoring taxane-based triplet therapies. Fluoropyrimidine-based triplets were associated with an objective response rate (ORR) compared with doublets alone (RR, 1.25; 95% CI, 1.09 to 1.44). This benefit, however, was associated with increased incidence of grade 3 to 4 thrombocytopenia, infection, and mucositis by a factor of approximately 2.[20]

With respect to SCC, doublet therapies composed of cisplatin and 5FU have demonstrated effectiveness, as demonstrated by the studies noted previously.[7,8,10-12,14-19] Similarly, triplet therapies comprising an additional taxane have also demonstrated efficacy.[20-26] However, to date no extensive randomized data exist specifically comparing doublet to triplet regimens in patients with squamous histology.

Recently there has been much interest in taxane-based triplets in the neoadjuvant setting, with excellent oncologic results from phase II studies employing docetaxel in both major histologic subtypes.[20-26] We have previously shown excellent tolerance and response (pathologic complete response [pCR] of 10%) in a phase II trial in patients with locally advanced (cT3 and/or N1) adenocarcinoma of the esophagus, GE junction, and stomach using a regimen of docetaxel, cisplatin, and 5FU (DCF).[21] Long-term results demonstrated an impressive 5-year survival of over 55%, despite a high burden of residual disease (median positive pathologic lymph nodes = 5).[5] These results have been replicated in several German series, including a recent study employing a docetaxel-based regimen, but replacing cisplatin with oxaliplatin (FLOT: 5-Flourouracil, Leucovorin, Oxaliplatin, and Taxotere [Docetaxel]) for esophagogastric adenocarcinoma with impressive pathologic response rates—20% pCR and another 20%, with near pCR (<10% residual tumor).[23] Another German study employing a similar regimen demonstrated a pCR rate of 15% and a median OS of just over 4 years.[24] These strong data set the foundation for a large German multicenter phase three trial investigating FLOT versus the regimen established by the MAGIC trial (ClinicalTrials.gov identifier, NCT01216644), ECF (epirubicin, cisplatin, and 5-fluorouracil regimen) in patients with locally advanced esophagogastric adenocarcinoma. This study has completed accrual. Several Japanese studies have supported the use of taxane-based triplets, most notably docetaxel, in esophageal SCC.[22,25,26] Indeed, impressive results from these studies have led to inclusion of DCF as one of three arms in the ongoing large Japanese multiinstitutional NExT (JCOG1109) trial investigating neoadjuvant chemotherapy (cisplatin/5FU or docetaxel/cisplatin/5FU) versus cisplatin/5FU with concurrent radiotherapy.[27] This study is well underway, with preliminary results due in 2017.

IS CHEMOTHERAPY MORE EFFECTIVE WHEN ADMINISTERED IN THE PRE- OR POSTOPERATIVE SETTING?

Current data are conflicted regarding the use of postoperative chemotherapy alone in the adjuvant setting only.[7,8] The 1997 study by Ando et al. randomized patients with esophageal SCC to receive either curative intent surgery alone or adjuvant chemotherapy with cisplatin and vindesine, delivered in two cycles.[8] Patients predominantly harbored locally advanced disease; however, in this study the exact rate of curative R0 resection was not clearly indicated. No survival benefit was observed with the addition of postoperative chemotherapy, although the efficacy of the regimen and uncertainty regarding the extent of resection diminish the generalizability of the study.[8]

In 2003, Ando and colleagues published a Japanese Clinical Oncology Group multiinstitutional phase III trial investigating postoperative cisplatin and 5FU in patients with SCC versus surgery alone. In patients who were ultimately found to harbor node positive disease, adjuvant chemotherapy was associated with a significant improvement in 5-year disease-free survival (DFS) compared with surgery alone (52% vs. 38%; P = .041). Conversely, there was a nonsignificant trend toward worse DFS outcomes in node negative patients receiving adjuvant chemotherapy compared with surgery alone (70% vs. 76%; P = .433).[7]

These seemingly contradictory results led to a follow-up study comparing the same regimen given either pre- or postoperatively. In this study, the authors directly compared preoperative versus postoperative chemotherapy in 330 patients with locally advanced esophageal SCC. Patients received two cycles of cisplatin and 5FU, either preceding or following curative intent surgery.[16] OS was significantly improved in patients who received preoperative compared with postoperative therapy, with 5-year survival of 55% versus 43% (P = .04).[16] Overall response rates to chemotherapy were 38%, which translated into fewer preoperative-treated patients being found to harbor T4 or N+ tumors. Furthermore, significantly more patients who received neoadjuvant chemotherapy underwent curative (R0) resection (96% vs. 91%; P = .04). Patients in the adjuvant arm experienced increased toxicity and reduced completion (75% vs. 85%; P = .04) of therapy compared with patients in the neoadjuvant arm. Overall, the results of the studies to date support the use of preoperative chemotherapy with respect to compliance, assessment of tumor response, and survival.[16]

NEOADJUVANT CHEMORADIATION VERSUS SURGERY ALONE

The studies looking at chemotherapy administration in the perioperative setting demonstrated that patients with a marked tumor response to therapy experienced improved survival outcomes.[10,16,17,19] This benefit was observed when tumor response was noted both within the primary tumor and regional lymph nodes.[10,16,17,19] In an attempt to improve local response and R0 resection rates, the addition of radiation to chemotherapy in the preoperative setting has been attempted and extensively studied. A useful framework for assessing the added benefit of chemoradiation to surgery alone is to look at its efficacy with respect to local/regional control and any additional control of systemic recurrence. Furthermore, the toxicity of various treatment regimens needs to be determined. Stated otherwise, *does neoadjuvant chemoradiation improve local/regional control compared with surgery alone in patients with esophageal SCC and EAC? Does it provide improved systemic control compared with surgery alone? Can any benefits be achieved with acceptable toxicity?* Along these lines, the bulk of evidence to date has helped establish neoadjuvant chemoradiation as a standard of care in the management of EC. Randomized trials comparing chemoradiation (CRT) to surgery alone are outlined in Table 38.2.[28-40]

Until the publication of the CROSS trial in 2008, the bulk of the studies examining neoadjuvant CRT failed to demonstrate a significant survival benefit over surgery alone with the exception of the Walsh and Tepper trials.

TABLE 38.2 Randomized Trials Comparing Chemoradiotherapy to Surgery Alone

Study	Year	Patients	Histology	Regimen	Response Rate	R0	Survival	P
Nygaard et al.	1992	186 (88 XRT)	SCC	1. Sx alone 2. 2 cycles cisplatin, bleomycin preop 3. 35 Gy preop 4. Chemo + XRT	NA	1. 37% 2. 44% 3. 40% 4. 55%	3 yr 1. 19%, 2. 3%, 3. 21%, 4. 17% 1+2. 6% 3+4. 19%	Any XRT vs. no XRT P = .009
Le Prise et al.	1994	104	SCC	Sequential 5FU, cisplatin + 20 Gy	pCR 10.3%	NA	Median 10 mo in both groups	NS
Walsh et al.	1996	113	EAC	Concurrent 5FU, cisplatin + 40 Gy	pCR 25% 42% N+ vs. 82% Sx alone	NA	Median (ITT) 16 mo vs. 11 mo Median (pp) 32 mo vs. 11 mo 3 yr (pp) 37% vs. 7%	P = .01 P = .06
Bosset et al.	1997	282	SCC	Sequential cisplatin + 18.5 Gy	pCR 26% 25% N+ vs. 57% Sx alone	81% vs. 69%	Median survival 18.6% overall	NS
Urba et al.	2001	100	SCC/ EAC	Concurrent cisplatin, 5FU, vinblastine + 45 Gy	pCR 28% pCR SCC 38% pCR EAC 24%	96% vs. 90%	Median 19.9 mo vs. 17.6 mo 3 yr 30% vs. 16%	NS
Burmeister et al.	2002	257	SCC/ EAC	Concurrent cisplatin, 5FU + 35 Gy	pCR 16% pCR SCC 27% pCR EAC 9%	80% vs. 59%	Median 22.2 mo vs. 19.3 mo	NS
Tepper et al.	2008	56	SCC/ EAC	Cisplatin, 5FU + 50.4 Gy	pCR 40%	NA	Median 4.48 yr vs. 1.79 yr 5 yr 39% vs. 16%	P = .002
Van Hagen/ Shapiro et al. (CROSS)	2008/15	368	SCC/ EAC	Concurrent paclitaxel, carboplatin + 41.4 Gy	pCR 29% pCR SCC 49% pCR EAC 23%	92% vs. 69%	Median 49.4 mo vs. 24 mo 5 yr 47% vs. 34%	P = .003
Cao et al.	2009	473	SCC	1. Cisplatin, 5FU, mitomycin + Sx 2. 40 Gy + Sx 3. 1 + 40 Gy 4. Sx alone	1. 1.7% 2. 15.2% 3. 22.3%	1. 86.6% 2. 95.7% 3. 98.3% 4. 73.3%	3 yr 1. 57.1% 2. 69.5% 3. 73.3% 4. 53.4%	Any XRT vs. no XRT P < .05
Lv et al.	2010	238	SCC	Preop cisplatin, paclitaxel + 40 Gy vs. postop cisplatin, paclitaxel + 40 Gy vs. Sx alone	NA	1. 97.4% 2. 78% 3. 80%	Median preop 53 mo vs. postop 48 mo vs. 36 mo Sx 5 yr preop 43.5% vs. postop 42.3% vs. Sx 34%	P = .004 vs. Sx alone
Bass et al.	2014	211	SCC/ EAC	5FU, cisplatin + 40 Gy	pCR SCC 31% pCR AC 25% 29% N+ vs. 64% Sx alone	NA	Median 63.8 mo vs. 23.41 mo	P < .001
Mariette et al.	2014	195	SCC/ EAC	5FU, cisplatin + 45 Gy	pCR 33.3%	CRT 93.8% vs. Sx 92.1%	5 yr CRT 41.1% vs. Sx 33.8%	NS

CRT, Chemoradiotherapy; *EAC,* esophageal adenocarcinoma; *5FU,* 5-fluorouracil; *ITT,* intention to treat; *N+,* node positive; *NA,* not available; *NS,* not significant; *pCR,* pathologic complete response; *SCC,* squamous cell carcinoma; *Sx,* surgery; *XRT,* radiation therapy.

However, while grossly negative, the additional trials listed provide important information concerning the effectiveness of various neoadjuvant CRT regimens with respect to both local and distant control.

DOES NEOADJUVANT CHEMORADIATION IMPROVE LOCAL/REGIONAL CONTROL COMPARED WITH SURGERY ALONE IN PATIENTS WITH ESOPHAGEAL SCC AND EAC? DOES IT PROVIDE IMPROVED SYSTEMIC CONTROL COMPARED WITH SURGERY ALONE?

With respect to local control, the evidence to date suggests that neoadjuvant CRT is beneficial.[28,31–33,35–37,39,40] In particular, the benefit is greater in SCC compared with adenocarcinoma. For example, the Nygaard study, conducted exclusively in patients with SCC, demonstrated a trend toward improved R0 resection rates with neoadjuvant CRT.[28] This translated into improved survival compared with patients who received no radiation at all.[28] In the Le Prise study, also exclusively conducted in SCC patients, a significant downstaging effect can be inferred based on the finding of significantly more T3 and T4 tumors in the non-CRT group.[29] However, no difference in R0 resection and a very low pCR rate were observed, which may have contributed to the negative nature of the study overall. Similarly, a relatively low dose of chemotherapy and radiation (20 Gy) were used.[29] The Walsh study, which was a positive study in patients with adenocarcinoma, demonstrated a pCR rate of 25% and a significant downstaging effect, with 42% of patients treated with CRT found to harbor positive lymph nodes at the time of surgery, compared with 82% of patients in the surgery alone arm ($P < .001$).[30] The Bosset study, again a negative study in patients with SCC, demonstrated a 26% pCR and significantly fewer lymph node metastases at the time of surgery (25% vs. 57%) in patients who received CRT compared with surgery alone.[31] The authors also demonstrated a significant increase in R0 resection rate following neoadjuvant CRT (81% vs. 69%).[31]

The study by Urba et al. yielded similarly results and was a powerful indicator of improved local/regional control in patients treated with neoadjuvant CRT.[32] Furthermore, it suggested differential efficacy in patients harboring SCC versus adenocarcinoma, with the former deriving a greater benefit.[32] Patients with mixed histology were enrolled. pCR rates differed between SCC and adenocarcinoma patients, with the latter exhibiting a 25% response rate consistent with previous studies. SCC patients exhibited an improved response at 38%. R0 resection rate was improved in the CRT group (96% vs. 90%), although surgical quality was excellent in both arms. Overall no survival benefit was observed as a result of CRT. However, in patients who exhibited a pCR, a survival benefit could be appreciated (median, 1-, 3-year survival pCR vs. no pCR 49.7 months, 86%, 64% vs. 12 months, 52%, 19% respectively; $P = .01$). Importantly this benefit appeared to be driven by improved local control with no difference in systemic recurrence rates between the two groups.[32] The trial by Burmeister et al. also showed improved R0 resection rates in patients randomized to neoadjuvant CRT compared with surgery alone (80% vs. 59%), although R0 resection rates overall were low, particularly in patients receiving surgery alone.[33] As in previous studies, pCR was higher in SCC at 27% versus 9% in EAC patients, which was lower than response rates observed in contemporary studies. No appreciable difference in survival was noted between groups.[33]

The CROSS trial is the largest positive trial performed to date comparing neoadjuvant CRT to surgery alone and has established a standard therapy for both esophageal SCC and adenocarcinoma in much of the West.[35,36] The authors employed a slightly different chemotherapeutic approach composed of a weekly regimen of relatively low-dose taxane and carboplatin in conjunction with concurrent radiation at a dose of 41.4 Gy. With respect to local control, in the adenocarcinoma arm a pCR rate of 25% was again noted compared with 49% in patients with SCC.[35,36] In keeping with previous studies, R0 resection was achieved in a greater proportion of patients receiving neoadjuvant CRT compared with surgery alone (92% vs. 69%).[35,36] In addition, significantly more patients undergoing surgery alone were found to harbor metastatic lymph nodes compared with patients receiving neoadjuvant CRT (75% vs. 31%), despite comparable preoperative clinical staging.[35,36] Finally, on long-term follow-up, a significant reduction in locoregional recurrence was noted in patients with either adenocarcinoma or SCC following neoadjuvant CRT compared with surgery alone (22% vs. 38%; HR, 0.45; 95% CI, 0.3 to 0.66; $P < .001$), thus supporting the locoregional benefit of neoadjuvant CRT.[35,36]

Bass and colleagues demonstrated analogous findings in 211 esophageal cancer (SCC and EAC) patients with respect to pCR and improved locoregional control following neoadjuvant CRT.[38] For patients with EAC pCR rates were lower than for patients with SCC, again at 25% versus 31%.[38] Downstaging of mediastinal disease following neoadjuvant CRT was inferred based on a 64% rate of lymph node positivity in patients treated with surgery alone versus 29% in patients undergoing neoadjuvant CRT. Again, this effect was more pronounced in SCC patients, with 85% being node negative following CRT versus 58% in adenocarcinoma patients.[38]

The two final studies performed to date by Lv et al. and Cao et al. included patients with SCC exclusively and similarly showed comparable results with respect to oncologic resection, with improved R0 resection rates in patients following neoadjuvant CRT, along with an elevated pCR (22.3%), albeit lower than what was observed in the CROSS trial.[39,40] The preoperative regimen was 5FU and cisplatin-based, which may account for this disparity.

Taken together, the bulk of evidence to date demonstrates improved local control following neoadjuvant CRT compared with surgery alone, as evidenced by a significant clinical and pathologic response rate, a significant reduction in lymph node disease burden within the mediastinum, and consequently, an improved R0 resection rate. However, this benefit is more pronounced in patients with SCC compared with EAC. Another interesting finding is that for chemoradiotherapy (CRT) in EAC, the pCR rate hovers around a consistent 20% to 25% irrespective of the chemotherapy regimen and amount of radiotherapy. However, in patients who do respond to neoadjuvant therapy, this improved local control translates into improved survival.

DOES NEOADJUVANT CHEMORADIATION PROVIDE IMPROVED SYSTEMIC CONTROL COMPARED WITH SURGERY ALONE?

Since the bulk of mortality related to esophageal cancer is related to systemic disease, any curative intent therapy should ideally minimize the incidence of systemic recurrence. Of the studies that indicate an OS advantage in patients treated with neoadjuvant chemoradiation, a few specifically mention control of systemic recurrence. The trial by Bosset et al., although a negative trial, assessed both local and systemic control and determined that the benefit using their CRT regimen was only effective with respect to local control, with no difference in systemic recurrence rates between both treatment arms.[31] Indeed, Urba et al. arrived at the same conclusion, with an approximate 60% overall systemic recurrence rate in both treatment arms as site of first recurrence.[32] Similarly, in the study by Cao et al., although neoadjuvant CRT improved R0 resection rate and reduced the incidence of mediastinal lymph node positivity, no improvement in 5-year survival was noted in these patients compared with surgery alone.[39] Thus, in this particular study, improved local control, as evidenced by improved 1- and 3-year survival, did not translate into increased rates of cure.[39] Finally, although the trial by Walsh et al. did demonstrate a survival advantage at 3 years in patients randomized to multimodal therapy compared with surgery alone, some of the findings are problematic.[30] For example, the authors demonstrate 3-year survival in CRT-treated patients of 32% to 36%. In patients subject to surgery alone, 3-year survival was only 6% to 7%.[30] Furthermore, no data were provided regarding R0 resection rate in either treatment arm. Collectively, these observations cast doubt regarding the surgical quality achieved in the study, as evidenced by an unacceptable 3-year survival in patients treated with surgery alone.[1,28,32] Contemporary studies demonstrate survival rates ranging from 15% to 30% over similar time periods.[1,28,32] Given that patients in the surgery alone group fared so poorly, the conclusion that multimodal therapy translated to improved survival in that particular study must be interpreted with caution.

The CROSS trial was one of the few studies to clearly demonstrate improved systemic control in patients treated with neoadjuvant CRT.[35,36] However, the benefit depended on histology and was only significant in patients with SCC (HR for death of 0.75 [0.56 to 1.01] on multivariate analysis at 5 years).[35,36] There was a trend toward improved survival in EAC patients, but this was not as pronounced and did not achieve statistical significance on multivariate analysis (0.75 [0.57 to 1.01]).[35,36] For the entire cohort of patients, however, the HR for distant recurrence was 0.63 (0.46 to 0.87).[35,36] Similarly, Bass et al. demonstrated a durable improvement in survival for both EAC and SCC patients following neoadjuvant CRT, with follow-up times of more than 200 months.[38] This suggests at least some element of systemic control, which is thought to be due to the systemic effects of the chemotherapy administered with radiation.

In keeping with the observation that neoadjuvant CRT is more effective in patients with esophageal SCC, the results of the study by Lv et al. demonstrate improved survival in patients receiving neoadjuvant CRT, compared with patients undergoing radical resection alone.[40] The survival benefit was noted for up to 10 years, indicating a higher rate of cure (24.5% neoadjuvant CRT vs. 12.5% surgery alone; $P = .04$).[40] Furthermore, significantly more patients in the surgery alone arm died as a result of systemic recurrence than patients receiving neoadjuvant CRT (38% vs. 25%; $P = .011$).[40] A similar finding was noted by Burmeister et al., in which 5-year PFS rates were significantly improved following CRT, compared with surgery alone at 5 years in patients with squamous histology, but not in patients with adenocarcinoma.[33] Collectively these data suggest that neoadjuvant CRT provides a survival benefit as a result of the control of systemic disease, particularly in patients with squamous histology. This effect may be observed in some patients with adenocarcinoma, albeit with a markedly attenuated response.

CAN THE BENEFITS OF NEOADJUVANT CHEMORADIATION BE ACHIEVED WITH ACCEPTABLE TOXICITY?

One of the main criticisms regarding the use of multimodality therapy with the incorporation of radiation is an increase in treatment-related morbidity and mortality. To date, the data regarding the magnitude of this effect on OS are conflicting. Bosset et al. did show reduced cancer-related mortality in patients receiving neoadjuvant CRT, compared with those receiving surgery alone.[31] However, the survival benefit related to improved disease control was offset by a significant increase in treatment-related mortality. In patients receiving combined modality therapy, treatment-related mortality was 12%, compared with 4% for patients subject to surgery alone. The authors attributed this in part to the high dose of radiation administered per fraction, and this speaks to the overall toxicity of their regimen.[31] Similarly, treatment-related deaths were higher in patients who received neoadjuvant CRT than in those who received surgery alone in the study by Lv et al. (3.8% vs. 0%).[40] The remaining studies outlined in Table 38.2 failed to demonstrate any association between CRT and adverse events.

The benefit of CRT in patients with earlier stage (I, II) disease is less clear. The RCT by Mariette et al. compared neoadjuvant chemoradiation in patients with stage I and II esophageal cancer followed by surgery to surgery alone with respect to overall and DFS.[41] A total of 195 patients with both SCC and EAC were randomly assigned to preoperative radiation therapy with 5FU and cisplatin with concurrent 45 Gy of radiation or surgery alone. All patients who underwent surgery were subject to a transthoracic approach with two-field lymphadenectomy. R0 resection rate was comparable between the two groups and did not differ significantly at 92.9% (CRT) and 92.1% surgery (Sx). pCR rate was 33% in the CRT group, and significant downstaging of the primary tumor and associated lymph node positivity was noted at final pathology in CRT-treated patients, compared with surgery alone. This was associated with improved locoregional control, with CRT patients demonstrating a local failure rate of 28.6%, compared with 44.3% of patients treated with surgery alone ($P = .02$).[41] However, no difference was observed with respect to distant recurrence (22.5% vs. 28.9%; P = .31) or OS (median OS 31.8 months).[41] Furthermore, in-hospital mortality was significantly higher in patients randomized to CRT (11.1% vs. 3.4%; P = .049).[41] Taken together, the data demonstrate an oncologic benefit for neoadjuvant CRT in patients with locally advanced EC (T3 and/or N+ stage III and above), which is not maintained in patients with earlier stage disease, owing to increased treatment-related complications.

CHEMOTHERAPY VERSUS CHEMORADIATION BEFORE SURGERY

In patients with locally advanced esophageal cancer, the omission of perioperative therapy represents substandard care by modern standards.[1] However, both chemotherapy and chemoradiation therapy have demonstrated efficacy in the neoadjuvant setting, and the superiority of one strategy over another has not been clearly demonstrated.[1] Advantages for both modalities have been put forward—namely improved R0 resection rates and locoregional control in regimens employing radiation, compared with a focus on systemic control in regimens employing chemotherapy alone. Several oncologic surrogate metrics are frequently employed when comparing studies, most notably pCR and complete resection (R0) rate. However, it must be stressed that irrespective of these two pathologic results, the ultimate goal of treatment for patients with esophageal cancer is improving long-term outcomes, measured by OS and DFS. With this in mind, we can look at the available modalities of treatment for esophageal cancer in two broad terms—systemic therapy (chemotherapy and targeted agents) versus local therapy (radiotherapy and surgery). Theoretically, the goal of these two approaches is different; systemic therapies should address distant disease with its effectiveness measured by OS and the rate of distant metastatic failure, and local therapies should address the primary tumor and regional lymph node disease, the effectiveness of which is measured by the metrics of complete resection (R0) and local-regional recurrence.

THE CASE FOR NEOADJUVANT CHEMORADIATION

In early studies looking at the perioperative use of chemotherapy or radiation therapy, patients who demonstrate a pathologic response to therapy and in particular a complete response tend to derive the greatest survival benefit. To date, the highest rates of pCR have been achieved with CRT regimens.[31,35,37,40] From the standpoint of locoregional control, CRT is associated with improved R0 resection rates and significant mediastinal lymph node sterilization, which adds to the local benefit provided by surgery.[31,35,37,40] Furthermore, a benefit with respect to distant control has been observed with CRT.[13,30,31,34,35,37,40] This has been attributed to the systemic effect of chemotherapy on any micrometastatic disease present, as well as on the improved rates of lymph node clearance.[13,30,31,34,35,37,40]

THE CASE FOR NEOADJUVANT CHEMOTHERAPY

Administration of chemotherapy in the preoperative setting provides a number of advantages. First, response to the regimen can be observed prior to surgery, providing a marker of the efficacy of the regimen and an opportunity to modify treatment in the face of failure of a given regimen. Second, effective regimens aimed at controlling systemic disease seem logical, given that the bulk of mortality in EC patients stems from distant, rather than local, disease. Third, omitting radiation therapy prior to surgery may minimize treatment-related morbidity and allow it to be reserved for recurrent disease.[41] Finally, the results of radiation therapy in EAC, the predominant histology in the West, are somewhat disappointing, hovering consistently in the vicinity of 25% regardless of the CRT regimen in question.[30,31,35–37]

In addition to the potential benefits of chemotherapy, no study to date has specifically mandated en bloc esophagectomy and involved field lymphadenectomy in surgical patients. This may contribute to the improved local control observed in patients receiving CRT. Such a scenario has been observed in patients with gastric cancer, as demonstrated by the Macdonald study, wherein rates of D2 dissection were low, necessitating additional local therapy in the form of radiation for adequate disease control.[42] Results from several single-institution series in which en bloc esophagectomy was routinely performed reveal a local-regional recurrence rate of 5% to 10%,[21,43,44] significantly lower than the consistent 25% to 30% rate seen with a standard esophagectomy.[11,35,36,45,46] Furthermore, in a randomized trial of transhiatal versus transthoracic esophagectomy (with modified en bloc), local recurrence and DFS were significantly improved in the transthoracic study arm.[47] Thus it is possible that adequate local control can be achieved in at least a subset of patients with locally advanced disease with high-quality surgery, as represented by an en bloc esophagectomy, potentially obviating the need for additional local therapy in the form of radiotherapy. Accordingly, it is possible that in patients in whom an en bloc esophagectomy is performed, the only additional therapy required is systemic treatment, given the low rate of local-regional recurrence in these patients.

The literature directly comparing neoadjuvant CRT and chemotherapy are limited. Nonetheless, several randomized trials on this topic have been performed and are demonstrated in Table 38.3. The published studies to date suffer from low accrual and the fact that en bloc esophagectomy was not part of the treatment plan. Regardless, no trial to date has demonstrated a clearly superior modality, and both represent currently acceptable standards.[48–50]

Stahl et al. randomized patients with distal one-third and esophagogastric junction (EGJ) adenocarcinoma to receive preoperative chemotherapy with cisplatin and 5FU, or preoperative concurrent CRT with the same regimen in addition to 30 Gy of radiation.[48] In total, 126 patients were enrolled, with 64 patients randomized to chemotherapy and surgery and 62 randomized to CRT, with the trial being terminated early due to poor accrual. Patients receiving CRT demonstrated improved pCR (15.6% vs. 3%; P = .03) and a node-negative surgical specimen (36.7% vs. 64.4%; P = .01). R0 resection rates were comparable in the two groups (69.5% chemotherapy [CT] and 72% CRT). In-hospital mortality was increased in patients receiving neoadjuvant CRT compared with CT at 10.2% vs. 3.8%, but this difference did not reach statistical significance, likely due to low power (P = .26).

TABLE 38.3 Randomized Trials Comparing Neoadjuvant Chemotherapy to Neoadjuvant Chemoradiotherapy

Study	Year	N	Regimen	Response Rate	R0	Survival	P	Histology
Stahl et al.	2009	119	Chemo: 2 cycles cisplatin, 5FU	Chemo: pCR 2%	69.5% vs. 72%	Median 21.1 mo vs. 33.2 mo	NS closed early due to poor accrual	GEJ/EAC
			CRT: 2 cycles cisplatin, 5FU + cisplatin, 5FU, etoposide – 30 Gy (concurrent)	CRT: pCR 15.6%*		3 yr 27.7% vs. 47.4%		
				Chemo: ypN0 36.7% CRT: ypN0 64.4%*				
Burmeister et al.	2011	75	Chemo: 2 cycles cisplatin, 5FU	Chemo: pCR 0% CRT: pCR 13%*	80.5% vs. 84.6%*	Median 26 mo vs. 32 mo	NS	EAC
			CRT: 2 cycles cisplatin, 5FU + 35 Gy			5 yr 36% vs. 45%		
Klevebro et al.	2016	181	Chemo: 3 cycles cisplatin, 5FU	Chemo: pCR 9%	74% vs. 87%*	3 yr 47% vs. 49%	NS	SCC/EAC
			CRT: 3 cycles cisplatin, 5FU + 40 Gy	CRT: pCR 28%*				
Nakamura et al. (JCOG1109)	2013	501 (target)	Arm A: 2 cycles preop cisplatin 5FU	NA	NA	NA	NA	NA
			Arm B: 3 cycles preop docetaxel, cisplatin, 5FU					
			Arm C: 2 cycles preop cisplatin, 5FU + 30 Gy					
Keegan et al. (NeoAEGIS)	2014	366 (target)	MAGIC vs. CROSS	NA	NA	NA	NA	NA
Leong et al. (TOPGEAR)	2015	752 (target)	Chemo: 3 cycles epirubicin, cisplatin, and 5FU 3 cycles preop and 3 cycles postop	NA	NA	NA	NA	NA
			CRT: 2 cycles ECF preop + 45 Gy + 3 cycles ECF postop					

*CRT vs. CT achieved statistical significance.

CRT, Chemoradiotherapy; *EAC*, esophageal adenocarcinoma; *ECF*, epirubicin, cisplatin, and fluorouracil regimen; *5FU*, 5-fluorouracil; *GEJ*, gastroesophageal junction; *NA*, not available; *NS*, not significant; *pCR*, pathologic complete response; *SCC*, squamous cell carcinoma; *XRT*, radiation therapy.

Median and 3-year survival were improved in the CRT arm (see Table 38.3), but this did not reach significance. Subgroup analysis revealed that OS was improved in patients who underwent R0 resection and had negative lymph nodes following surgery, irrespective of which group they were randomized to.[48] However, because the rate of pathologically negative nodes was higher in the CRT group, the authors posit that CRT could provide a significant survival advantage in addition to R0 resection, as evidenced by the trend toward improved survival.

The study by Burmeister was similar in that patients with esophageal or EGJ adenocarcinoma were randomized to undergo neoadjuvant chemotherapy alone or concurrent chemoradiation.[49] Patients received a 5FU/cisplatin-based regimen either alone or in conjunction with 35 Gy of radiation. Overall, 75 patients were randomized, with 36 receiving chemotherapy and 39 receiving CRT prior to surgery. As in the study by Stahl, the study was terminated early due to poor accrual. R0 resection rate was comparable, at 80.5% and 84.6% in patients receiving chemotherapy or CRT, respectively. The pCR rate was 13% in patients who received CRT versus 0% in those who received chemotherapy alone. This difference was not associated with reduced locoregional, distant recurrence, or survival benefit.[49]

The most recent study from Sweden by Klevebro et al. randomized 181 patients to neoadjuvant chemotherapy (nCT), comprising three cycles of cisplatin and 5FU or neoadjuvant chemoradiation (nCRT) therapy with concomitant 40 Gy.[50] Surgery included a two-field lymphadenectomy in all cases. A total of 91 and 90 patients were allocated to each arm, respectively. The study predominantly included patients with EAC; however, nearly one-third had squamous histology. As in the prior two studies, pCR was increased in patients receiving nCRT compared with nCT (28% vs. 9%, P = .002). Similarly, pCR was associated with negative regional nodes on final pathology in 90% of patients. Accordingly, 35% of nCT treated patients were found to be node negative, compared with 65% of nCRT patients, despite a 63% rate of node positivity on initial staging in both groups. However, this did not translate into a survival benefit on an intention-to-treat or per protocol analysis. Subgroup analysis revealed improved outcomes following nCRT in patients with SCC that did not reach statistical significance compared with nCT. No trend was observed in adenocarcinoma patients. Furthermore, a trend toward increased severe postoperative complications was appreciated.[50]

Several criticisms with respect to each of these trials can be put forward. First, all were relatively underpowered to detect a clear difference in treatments. Second, none of the regimens employed in either treatment arm (nCT or nCRT) reflect those employed in the landmark studies to date for each modality.[9,35] Proponents of chemotherapy alone highlight the positive results in GEJ adenocarcinoma patients following the MAGIC trial, which employed triplet therapy with epirubicin, cisplatin, and 5FU in the pre- and postoperative setting, as well as the promising results of regimens incorporating docetaxel (DCF or FLOT).[9,35] Similarly, the CROSS trial employed carboplatin, paclitaxel, and concurrent 41.4 Gy.[9,35] No randomized trial to date has directly compared these regimens. Finally, none of these studies have required en bloc esophagectomy with involved field lymphadenectomy in their treatment protocols, which may explain the findings noted in the Stahl study, wherein node negativity correlated with improved survival, despite an equal R0 resection rate with both treatment modalities. However, there are retrospective data on this topic that attempt to address the influence of en bloc esophagectomy on the choice of neoadjuvant therapy. Spicer and colleagues combined data on locally advanced (cT3N+) EAC patients from three centers, all performing routine en bloc esophagectomy, two of which prefer neoadjuvant chemotherapy (cisplatin and 5FU [CF] or DCF) and one CRT.[51] No difference in any of the pathologic surrogates of oncologic efficacy (R0 or lymph node retrieval) differed, although CRT was associated with an increased pCR rate, as would be expected. With more than 100 patients in each study group, there was no difference in either DFS or OS between patients who received chemotherapy or CRT.[51]

Several ongoing trials will help resolve this ongoing question. The Japanese JCOG1109 (NExT trial) is a three-arm phase III trial comparing neoadjuvant chemotherapy with radiation therapy in patients with locally advanced esophageal SCC undergoing en bloc esophagectomy—the only trial to do so.[27] The chemotherapy regimens include preoperative docetaxel/cisplatin/5FU and cisplatin/5FU versus preoperative cisplatin/5FU-based CRT. Similarly, the ongoing Irish ICORG 10 to 14 trial (Neo-AEGIS) will directly compare the treatment outcomes in patients with locally advanced esophageal adenocarcinoma using

a modified MAGIC protocol versus CRT, according to the CROSS protocol. An Australian trial (TOP-GEAR) is randomizing patients with esophageal and gastric adenocarcinoma to chemotherapy (ECF), then surgery versus ECF, followed by CRT then surgery, with a series of adjuvant cycles of ECF. The latest trial to investigate this topic is a German initiative (ESOPEC) randomizing EAC patients to the docetaxel-based FLOT or CROSS (taxol/carboplatin with concurrent radiotherapy) regimens in the neoadjuvant setting. Results from these trials are expected over the next 5 years and hope to provide some clarity to this topic.

DEFINITIVE CHEMORADIATION

An examination of the data following combined CRT for esophageal cancer reveals that a significant number of patients experience a pCR as well as mediastinal downstaging and nodal clearance. This finding begs the question as to whether patients who demonstrate a complete response require surgery at all. Instead, should it be reserved for patients who fail to respond adequately? A number of studies have addressed this question specifically and are outlined in Table 38.4.[52–57] Overall, the main drawback is a prohibitive rate of local failure, even in seemingly complete responders in the range of 40% to 60%.[52–57] Thus the current standard in many centers is to reserve definitive chemoradiation for poor surgical candidates, a strategy that is best suited for SCC histology, given the poorer response rate of adenocarcinoma to radiotherapy.

The initial study demonstrating a survival benefit for combined CF-based CRT in EC patients was conducted by Herskovic et al.[52,53] The authors randomized patients with predominantly squamous histology to undergo CRT with 50 Gy, compared with radiation alone with 64 Gy. The authors showed improved outcomes with CRT versus radiation alone with respect to local and distant recurrence, as well as a significant survival advantage (5 year 26% vs. 0% radiation alone). Despite a high local failure rate approaching 50%, the 5-year survival observed was in line with standard surgery–based treatment at that time, thus suggesting a role for definitive chemoradiation.[52,53] In an attempt to improve upon these results, Minsky et al., performed a similarly structured trial, this time randomizing patients to receive combined CF-based CRT with either 50.4 or 64.8 Gy of concurrent radiation.[54] Squamous histology was present in 95% of included patients, and as in the previous study, there was a high local failure rate regardless of radiation dose in the vicinity of 50% to 60%. Survival rates, however, were similarly comparable.[54]

Given the relatively favorable survival outcomes noted in these studies and the observation that adequate local control is achieved in nearly half the patients subject to definitive chemoradiation without exposure to the morbidity associated with esophagectomy, a prospective comparison between chemoradiation with and without surgery was undertaken by Stahl et al.[55] Induction chemotherapy with cisplatin, etoposide, and 5FU in three cycles was followed by concurrent etoposide, cisplatin, and 65 Gy in the CRT alone group. In the surgery arm, this regimen was given with 40 Gy of radiation, followed by transthoracic esophagectomy. Following surgery, pCR and

TABLE 38.4 Randomized Trials of Definitive Chemoradiotherapy Alone

Study	Year	Patients	Regimen	Histology	Local Failure (CRT vs. XRT)	pCR	R0	Survival (CRT vs. XRT)
Herskovic/ Cooper et al. (RTOG 85-01)	1992	129	5FU, cisplatin +50 Gy vs. 64 Gy	SCC/EAC	PD 27%, LR 16% vs. PD 40%, LR 24%	NA	NA	Median 12.5 mo vs. 8.9 mo 5 yr 26% vs. 0%*
Minsky et al. (RTOG 94-05/ INT 0123)	2002	236	5FU, cisplatin + 50.4 Gy vs. 5FU, cisplatin + 64.8 Gy	SCC/EAC	50% vs. 55%	NA	NA	Median 13 mo vs. 18.1 mo 2 yr 31% vs. 40%
Stahl et al.	2005	172	Induction 5FU, cisplatin, etoposide + concurrent cisplatin, etoposide + 65 Gy vs. 5FU, cisplatin, etoposide + concurrent cisplatin, etoposide + 40 Gy + Sx	SCC	2 yr 59% vs. 36%*	35%	82%	Median 14.9 mo vs. 16.4 mo 3 yr 24.4% vs. 31.3%
Bedenne et al.	2007	259	Induction 5FU, cisplatin + 45 Gy Concurrent 5FU, cisplatin + 15–20 Gy vs. induction + Sx	SCC/EAC	43% vs. 33.6%*	23%	75%	Median 19.3 mo vs. 17.7 mo 2 yr 39.8% vs. 33.6%
Conroy et al. (PRODIGE5/ ACCORD17)	2014	267	FOLFOX + 50 Gy vs. 5FU, cisplatin + 50 Gy	SCC/EAC	PD 45% vs. 46%	NA	NA	Median 20.2 mo vs. 17.5 mo 3 yr 19.9% vs. 26.9%

*Denotes statistical significance.

CRT, Chemoradiotherapy; *EAC,* esophageal adenocarcinoma; *FOLFOX,* folinic acid, *5FU,* and oxaliplatin; *5FU,* 5-fluorouracil; *LR,* local recurrence; *pCR,* pathologic complete response; *PD,* persistent disease; *SCC,* squamous cell carcinoma; *Sx,* surgery; *XRT,* radiation therapy.

node negativity was appreciated in 35% of patients with nodal sterilization alone in an additional 33%. Survival analysis revealed a significant reduction in cancer-related mortality in patients who underwent surgery. However, this was associated with a greater incidence of treatment-related death. In-hospital mortality was 12.8% in patients who received surgery, versus 3.5% in patients who did not (P = .03). Survival at 2 and 3 years was equivalent in both groups (39.9%, 95% CI, 29.4 to 50.4, CRT + Sx; 35.4%, 95% CI, 25.2 to 45.6, and 31.3% vs. 24.4%). In keeping with the data presented thus far, local control was improved in patients subject to surgery. Freedom from progression in CRT alone was 40.7% versus 64.3% in CRT + Sx (P ≥ .003). Multivariate analysis revealed that the most important prognostic factor, however, was tumor response to therapy. Those patients in whom a response was noted demonstrated survival approaching 50% at 5 years, irrespective of treatment arm. In nonresponders, however, R0 resection improved survival, increasing survival from 17.9% at 3 years to 32%.[55]

Additional high-quality evidence supports these findings.[56] Bedenne et al. randomized patients to surgery or definitive chemoradiation therapy following induction therapy with a CF-based regimen. Patients who demonstrated a response were subsequently randomized to surgery or additional chemoradiation, for a total dose of 45 to 66 Gy. Patients who did not respond proceeded to surgery. Patients predominantly harbored SCC (90%). R0 resection was achieved in 75% of patients, and pCR was noted in 23% of surgical specimens. Treatment-related

mortality was 1% in the nonsurgical arm and 9% in the surgical arm (P = .002). No difference in survival was appreciated between treatment groups, with median and 2-year survival between the CRT and surgical arms of 19.3 months versus 17.7 months and 39.8% versus 33.6%, respectively. Although there was no difference in the frequency of metastasis between the two groups, local failures were more common in patients randomized to CRT alone (HR no surgery vs. surgery, 1.63; 95% CI, 1.04 to 2.55; P = .03). Collectively these data indicate that chemoradiation provides comparable survival outcomes to multimodality therapy in appropriately selected patients. Although surgery is associated with improved local control, it comes at the cost of increased treatment-associated mortality.[56]

Taken together, these results suggest that in patients with locally advanced SCC, definitive CRT and CRT + surgery offer equivalent survival results, with a reduction in treatment-associated morbidity and mortality compared with the addition of surgery. Although local control was improved in patients subject to surgery, subgroup analysis suggests that surgery is rescuing patients who do not demonstrate an adequate response to CRT, thus providing local control because of CRT failure. This is evidenced by the survival rates observed in patients who responded to treatment versus those who did not.

Given the collective results thus far, the majority of centers employ definitive CRT for patients who are unfit for surgery, and numerous studies are underway in search of the optimal regimen.

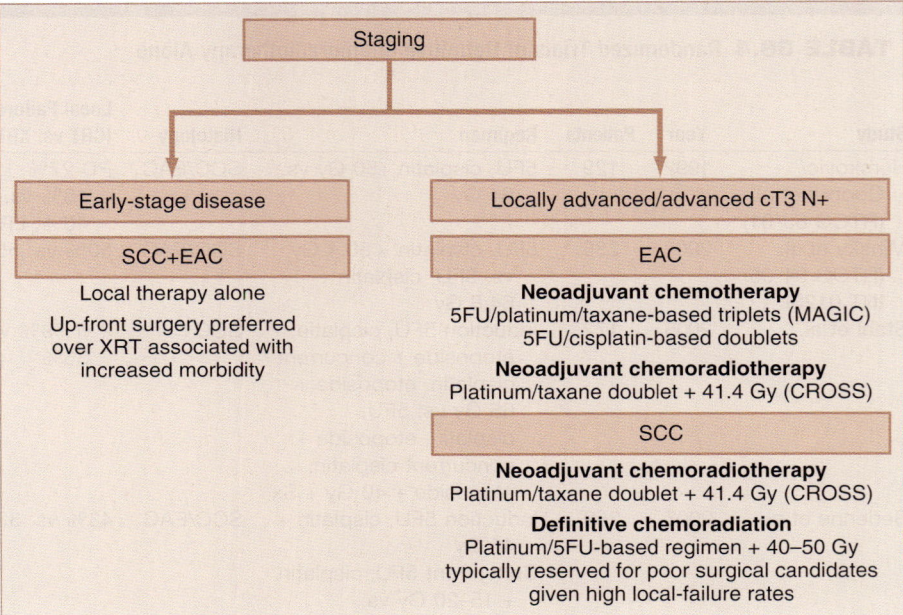

FIGURE 38.1 Conceptual framework outlining the neoadjuvant treatment of locally advanced esophageal carcinoma. *EAC*, Esophageal adenocarcinoma; *SCC*, squamous cell carcinoma; *XRT*, radiation therapy.

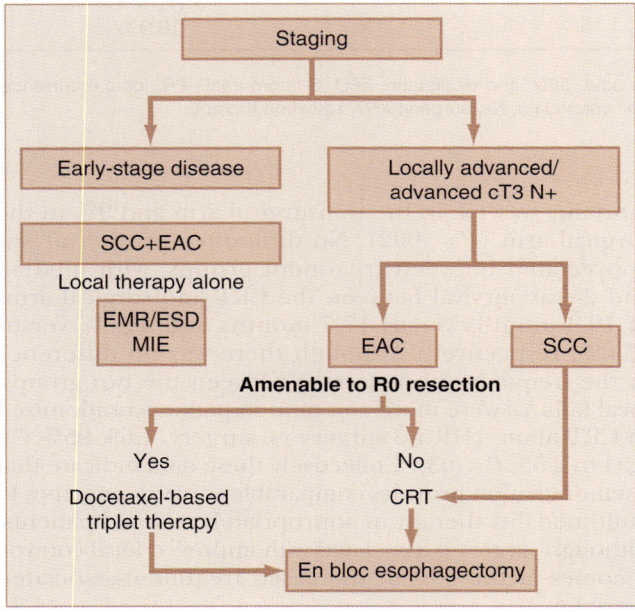

FIGURE 38.2 Local institutional approach to the management of patients presenting with locally advanced esophageal carcinoma. *CRT*, Chemoradiotherapy; *EAC*, esophageal adenocarcinoma; *EMR*, endoscopic mucosal resection; *ESD*, endoscopic submucosal dissection; *MIE*, minimally invasive esophagectomy; *SCC*, squamous cell carcinoma.

CONCLUSION

The management of locally advanced esophageal cancer remains complex and necessitates a multimodality approach to achieve favorable survival outcomes. Fig. 38.1 represents a summary of the data outlined in the current chapter,

and our institutional evidence-based preference is outlined in Fig. 38.2.

Given the evidence to date, several generalizations regarding the optimal management of patients with locally advanced esophageal cancer can be drawn. With respect to local control, excellent surgery remains paramount, as evidenced by improved outcomes associated with R0 resection. En bloc esophagectomy has been shown to provide excellent results, and its impact with respect to survival in large randomized trials is currently under elucidation in the NeXT, TOP GEAR, and Neo AEGIS trials. The inability to achieve R0 resection in a significant proportion of patients mandates additional local therapy. For patients with SCC, neoadjuvant CRT provides excellent results and represents standard therapy. That being said, excellent results with neoadjuvant chemotherapy alone have been reported, and this remains an acceptable standard in appropriate situations where R0 resection is possible.

With respect to patients with EAC, the benefit of neoadjuvant CRT is less pronounced but remains an acceptable standard. Excellent results have been reported with docetaxel-based triplets, which appears to be borne out in contemporary meta-analysis. Accordingly, neoadjuvant chemotherapy alone remains an acceptable standard in this patient population.

Because the majority of patients die of systemic recurrence, effective systemic therapy remains critical, with future improvements in patient outcome likely to be dictated by the efficacy of their chemotherapy/targeted therapy regimen. This underscores the rationale for treatment regimens that employ neoadjuvant chemotherapy alone, thus affording the opportunity to assess treatment response over clinically meaningful time frames, in addition to facilitating complete oncologic resection while avoiding the potential toxicity of added radiation.

With these concepts in mind, a reasonable approach to patients with SCC is the implementation of a neoadjuvant

CRT regimen, as opposed to neoadjuvant CT alone for appropriately selected patients with EAC. In both groups, surgery is aimed at achieving an R0 resection, which is effectively achieved with en bloc esophagectomy. Thus the optimal treatment of esophageal cancer necessitates a multidisciplinary approach tailored to the individual patient, taking into account their tumor location, histology, and performance status. In this manner, the selection of a regimen most likely to improve their survival and limit their treatment-related morbidity becomes increasingly possible. The spectrum of available regimens is likely to increase in the future, and a number of randomized studies are underway that may answer some of the ongoing questions in the treatment of this devastating disease.

REFERENCES

1. Cools-Lartigue J, Spicer J, Ferri LE. Current status of management of malignant disease: current management of esophageal cancer. *J Gastrointest Surg*. 2015;19:964-972.
2. Amin RN, Parikh SJ, Gangireddy VG, Kanneganti P, Talla S, Daram S. Early esophageal cancer specific survival is unaffected by anatomical location of tumor: a population-based study. *Can J Gastroenterol Hepatol*. 2016;2016:613-640.
3. Tapias LF, Mathisen DJ, Wright CD, et al. Outcome with open and minimally invasive Ivor Lewis esophagectomy after neoadjuvant therapy. *Ann Thorac Surg*. 2016;101:1097-1103.
4. Defoe SG, Pennathur A, Flickinger JC, et al. Retrospective review of patients with locally advanced esophageal cancer treated at the University of Pittsburgh. *Am J Clin Oncol*. 2011;34:587-592.
5. Sudarshan M, Alcindor T, Ades S, et al. Survival and recurrence patterns after neoadjuvant docetaxel, cisplatin, and 5-fluorouracil (DCF) for locally advanced esophagogastric adenocarcinoma. *Ann Surg Oncol*. 2015;22:324-330.
6. Ku GY, Kriplani A, Janjigian YY, et al. Change in chemotherapy during concurrent radiation followed by surgery after a suboptimal positron emission tomography response to induction chemotherapy improves outcomes for locally advanced esophageal adenocarcinoma. *Cancer*. 2016;122:2083-2090.
7. Ando N, Iizuka T, Ide H, et al. Surgery plus chemotherapy compared with surgery alone for localized squamous cell carcinoma of the thoracic esophagus: a Japan Clinical Oncology Group Study—JCOG9204. *J Clin Oncol*. 2003;21:4592-4596.
8. Ando N, Iizuka T, Kakegawa T, et al. A randomized trial of surgery with and without chemotherapy for localized squamous carcinoma of the thoracic esophagus: the Japan Clinical Oncology Group Study. *J Thorac Cardiovasc Surg*. 1997;114:205-209.
9. Cunningham D, Allum WH, Stenning SP, et al. Perioperative chemotherapy versus surgery alone for resectable gastroesophageal cancer. *N Engl J Med*. 2006;355:11-20.
10. Kelsen DP, Winter KA, Gunderson LL, et al. Long-term results of RTOG trial 8911 (USA Intergroup 113): a random assignment trial comparison of chemotherapy followed by surgery compared with surgery alone for esophageal cancer. *J Clin Oncol*. 2007;25:3719-3725.
11. Law S, Fok M, Chow S, Chu KM, Wong J. Preoperative chemotherapy versus surgical therapy alone for squamous cell carcinoma of the esophagus: a prospective randomized trial. *J Thorac Cardiovasc Surg*. 1997;114:210-217.
12. Medical Research Council Esophageal Cancer Working Group. Surgical resection with or without preoperative chemotherapy in esophageal cancer: a randomised controlled trial. *Lancet*. 2002;359:1727-1733.
13. Roth JA, Pass HI, Flanagan MM, Graeber GM, Rosenberg JC, Steinberg S. Randomized clinical trial of preoperative and postoperative adjuvant chemotherapy with cisplatin, vindesine, and bleomycin for carcinoma of the esophagus. *J Thorac Cardiovasc Surg*. 1988;96:242-248.
14. Schlag PM. Randomized trial of preoperative chemotherapy for squamous cell cancer of the esophagus. The Chirurgische Arbeitsgemeinschaft Fuer Onkologie der Deutschen Gesellschaft Fuer Chirurgie Study Group. *Arch Surg*. 1992;127:1446-1450.
15. Ychou M, Boige V, Pignon JP, et al. Perioperative chemotherapy compared with surgery alone for resectable gastroesophageal adenocarcinoma: an FNCLCC and FFCD multicenter phase III trial. *J Clin Oncol*. 2011;29:1715-1721.
16. Ando N, Kato H, Igaki H, et al. A randomized trial comparing postoperative adjuvant chemotherapy with cisplatin and 5-fluorouracil versus preoperative chemotherapy for localized advanced squamous cell carcinoma of the thoracic esophagus (JCOG9907). *Ann Surg Oncol*. 2012;19:68-74.
17. Boonstra JJ, Kok TC, Wijnhoven BP, et al. Chemotherapy followed by surgery versus surgery alone in patients with resectable esophageal squamous cell carcinoma: long-term results of a randomized controlled trial. *BMC Cancer*. 2011;11:181.
18. Allum WH, Stenning SP, Bancewicz J, Clark PI, Langley RE. Long-term results of a randomized trial of surgery with or without preoperative chemotherapy in esophageal cancer. *J Clin Oncol*. 2009;27:5062-5067.
19. Ancona E, Ruol A, Santi S, et al. Only pathologic complete response to neoadjuvant chemotherapy improves significantly the long term survival of patients with resectable esophageal squamous cell carcinoma: final report of a randomized, controlled trial of preoperative chemotherapy versus surgery alone. *Cancer*. 2001;91:2165-2174.
20. Mohammad NH, ter Veer E, Ngai L, Mali R, van Oijen MGH, van Laarhoven HWM. Optimal first-line chemotherapeutic treatment in patients with locally advanced or metastatic esophagogastric carcinoma: triplet versus doublet chemotherapy: a systematic literature review and meta-analysis. *Cancer Metastasis Rev*. 2015;34:429-441.
21. Ferri LE, Ades S, Alcindor T, et al. Perioperative docetaxel, cisplatin, and 5-fluorouracil (DCF) for locally advanced esophageal and gastric adenocarcinoma: a multicenter phase II trial. *Ann Oncol*. 2012;23:1512-1517.
22. Watanabe M, Nagai Y, Kinoshita K, et al. Induction chemotherapy with docetaxel/cisplatin/5-fluorouracil for patients with node-positive esophageal cancer. *Digestion*. 2011;83:146-152.
23. Schulz C, Kullmann F, Kunzmann V, et al. NeoFLOT: multicenter phase II study of perioperative chemotherapy in resectable adenocarcinoma of the gastroesophageal junction or gastric adenocarcinoma—very good response predominantly in patients with intestinal type tumors. *Int J Cancer*. 2015;137:678-685.
24. Lorenzen S, Thuss-Patience P, Al-Batran SE, et al. Impact of pathologic complete response on disease-free survival in patients with esophagogastric adenocarcinoma receiving preoperative docetaxel-based chemotherapy. *Ann Oncol*. 2013;24:2068-2073.
25. Hara H, Tahara M, Daiko H, et al. Phase II feasibility study of preoperative chemotherapy with docetaxel, cisplatin, and fluorouracil for esophageal squamous cell carcinoma. *Cancer Sci*. 2013;104:1455-1460.
26. Watanabe M, Baba Y, Yoshida N, et al. Outcomes of preoperative chemotherapy with docetaxel, cisplatin, and 5-fluorouracil followed by esophagectomy in patients with resectable node-positive esophageal cancer. *Ann Surg Oncol*. 2014;21:2838-2844.
27. Nakamura K, Kato K, Igaki H, et al. Three-arm phase III trial comparing cisplatin plus 5-FU (CF) versus docetaxel, cisplatin plus 5-FU (DCF) versus radiotherapy with CF (CF-RT) as preoperative therapy for locally advanced esophageal cancer (JCOG1109, NExT study). *Jpn J Clin Oncol*. 2013;43:752-755.
28. Nygaard K, Hagen S, Hansen HS, et al. Pre-operative radiotherapy prolongs survival in operable esophageal carcinoma: a randomized, multicenter study of pre-operative radiotherapy and chemotherapy. The second Scandinavian trial in esophageal cancer. *World J Surg*. 1992;16:1104-1109, discussion 1110.
29. Le Prise E, Etienne PL, Meunier B, et al. A randomized study of chemotherapy, radiation therapy, and surgery versus surgery for localized squamous cell carcinoma of the esophagus. *Cancer*. 1994;73:1779-1784.
30. Walsh TN, Noonan N, Hollywood D, Kelly A, Keeling N, Hennessy TP. A comparison of multimodal therapy and surgery for esophageal adenocarcinoma. *N Engl J Med*. 1996;335:462-467.
31. Bosset JF, Gignoux M, Triboulet JP, et al. Chemoradiotherapy followed by surgery compared with surgery alone in squamous-cell cancer of the esophagus. *N Engl J Med*. 1997;337:161-167.
32. Urba SG, Orringer MB, Turrisi A, Iannettoni M, Forastiere A, Strawderman M. Randomized trial of preoperative chemoradiation versus surgery alone in patients with locoregional esophageal carcinoma. *J Clin Oncol*. 2001;19:305-313.
33. Burmeister BH, Smithers BM, Gebski V, et al. Surgery alone versus chemoradiotherapy followed by surgery for resectable cancer of the esophagus: a randomised controlled phase III trial. *Lancet Oncol*. 2005;6:659-668.

34. Tepper J, Krasna MJ, Niedzwiecki D, et al. Phase III trial of trimodality therapy with cisplatin, fluorouracil, radiotherapy, and surgery compared with surgery alone for esophageal cancer: CALGB 9781. *J Clin Oncol.* 2008;26:1086-1092.
35. van Heijl M, van Lanschot JJ, Koppert LB, et al. Neoadjuvant chemoradiation followed by surgery versus surgery alone for patients with adenocarcinoma or squamous cell carcinoma of the esophagus (CROSS). *BMC Surg.* 2008;8:21.
36. Shapiro J, van Lanschot JJ, Hulshof MC, et al. Neoadjuvant chemoradiotherapy plus surgery versus surgery alone for esophageal or junctional cancer (CROSS): long-term results of a randomised controlled trial. *Lancet Oncol.* 2015;16:1090-1098.
37. van Hagen P, Hulshof MC, van Lanschot JJ, et al. Preoperative chemoradiotherapy for esophageal or junctional cancer. *N Engl J Med.* 2012;366:2074-2084.
38. Bass GA, Furlong H, O'Sullivan KE, Hennessy TP, Walsh TN. Chemoradiotherapy, with adjuvant surgery for local control, confers a durable survival advantage in adenocarcinoma and squamous cell carcinoma of the esophagus. *Eur J Cancer.* 2014;50:1065-1075.
39. Cao XF, He XT, Ji L, Xiao J, Lv J. Effects of neoadjuvant radiochemotherapy on pathological staging and prognosis for locally advanced esophageal squamous cell carcinoma. *Dis Esophagus.* 2009;22:477-481.
40. Lv J, Cao XF, Zhu B, Ji L, Tao L, Wang DD. Long-term efficacy of perioperative chemoradiotherapy on esophageal squamous cell carcinoma. *World J Gastroenterol.* 2010;16:1649-1654.
41. Mariette C, Dahan L, Mornex F, et al. Surgery alone versus chemoradiotherapy followed by surgery for stage I and II esophageal cancer: final analysis of randomized controlled phase III trial FFCD 9901. *J Clin Oncol.* 2014;32:2416-2422.
42. Macdonald JS, Smalley SR, Benedetti J, et al. Chemoradiotherapy after surgery compared with surgery alone for adenocarcinoma of the stomach or gastroesophageal junction. *N Engl J Med.* 2001;345:725-730.
43. Altorki N, Skinner D. Should en bloc esophagectomy be the standard of care for esophageal carcinoma? *Ann Surg.* 2001;234:581-587.
44. Hagen JA, DeMeester SR, Peters JH, Chandrasoma P, DeMeester TR. Curative resection for esophageal adenocarcinoma: analysis of 100 en bloc esophagectomies. *Ann Surg.* 2001;234:520-530, discussion 530–521.
45. Dresner SM, Griffin SM. Pattern of recurrence following radical oesophagectomy with two-field lymphadenectomy. *Br J Surg.* 2000;87:1426-1433.
46. Hulscher JB, van Sandick JW, Tijssen JG, Obertop H, van Lanschot JJ. The recurrence pattern of esophageal carcinoma after transhiatal resection. *J Am Coll Surg.* 2000;191:143-148.
47. Omloo JM, Lagarde SM, Hulscher JB, et al. Extended transthoracic resection compared with limited transhiatal resection for adenocarcinoma of the mid/distal esophagus: five-year survival of a randomized clinical trial. *Ann Surg.* 2007;246:992-1000, discussion 1000–1001.
48. Stahl M, Walz MK, Stuschke M, et al. Phase III comparison of preoperative chemotherapy compared with chemoradiotherapy in patients with locally advanced adenocarcinoma of the esophagogastric junction. *J Clin Oncol.* 2009;27:851-856.
49. Burmeister BH, Thomas JM, Burmeister EA, et al. Is concurrent radiation therapy required in patients receiving preoperative chemotherapy for adenocarcinoma of the esophagus? A randomised phase II trial. *Eur J Cancer.* 2011;47:354-360.
50. Klevebro F, Alexandersson von Dobeln G, Wang N, et al. A randomized clinical trial of neoadjuvant chemotherapy versus neoadjuvant chemoradiotherapy for cancer of the esophagus or gastro-esophageal junction. *Ann Oncol.* 2016;27:660-667.
51. Spicer JD, Stiles BM, Sudarshan M, et al. Preoperative chemoradiation therapy versus chemotherapy in patients undergoing modified en bloc esophagectomy for locally advanced esophageal adenocarcinoma: is radiotherapy beneficial? *Ann Thorac Surg.* 2016;101:1262-1269, discussion 1269–1270.
52. Herskovic A, Martz K, al-Sarraf M, et al. Combined chemotherapy and radiotherapy compared with radiotherapy alone in patients with cancer of the esophagus. *N Engl J Med.* 1992;326:1593-1598.
53. Cooper JS, Guo MD, Herskovic A, et al. Chemoradiotherapy of locally advanced esophageal cancer: long-term follow-up of a prospective randomized trial (RTOG 85-01). Radiation Therapy Oncology Group. *JAMA.* 1999;281:1623-1627.
54. Minsky BD, Pajak TF, Ginsberg RJ, et al. INT 0123 (Radiation Therapy Oncology Group 94-05) phase III trial of combined-modality therapy for esophageal cancer: high-dose versus standard-dose radiation therapy. *J Clin Oncol.* 2002;20:1167-1174.
55. Stahl M, Stuschke M, Lehmann N, et al. Chemoradiation with and without surgery in patients with locally advanced squamous cell carcinoma of the esophagus. *J Clin Oncol.* 2005;23:2310-2317.
56. Bedenne L, Michel P, Bouche O, et al. Chemoradiation followed by surgery compared with chemoradiation alone in squamous cancer of the esophagus: FFCD 9102. *J Clin Oncol.* 2007;25:1160-1168.
57. Conroy T, Galais MP, Raoul JL, et al. Definitive chemoradiotherapy with FOLFOX versus fluorouracil and cisplatin in patients with esophageal cancer (PRODIGE5/ACCORD17): final results of a randomised, phase 2/3 trial. *Lancet Oncol.* 2014;15:305-314.

Surgical Approaches to Remove the Esophagus: Open

B.J. Noordman | S.M. Lagarde | B.P.L. Wijnhoven

J.J.B. van Lanschot

SURGICAL THERAPY

Surgical resection remains the cornerstone of therapy for patients with resectable cancer of the esophagus in the absence of systemic metastases. Surgery, most of the time combined with neoadjuvant therapy in current practice, offers the highest likelihood of cure for patients with locoregional disease. To obtain the best results, the management of esophageal cancer should be individualized and based on a combination of factors including the physiologic status of the patient, tumor type and location, and stage of disease. In this chapter, we describe the different open surgical approaches to remove the esophagus in patients with esophageal cancer. Although minimally invasive techniques (see Chapter 39B) are increasingly applied, the benefits of fully minimally invasive esophagectomy have not yet been proven unequivocally, and an open or hybrid esophagectomy remains the standard procedure to remove the esophagus in many leading high-volume centers worldwide.[1] At present, the only strong available evidence comes from preliminary results of the French randomized MIRO trial comparing hybrid transthoracic esophagectomy (TTE, laparoscopic gastric mobilization, and open thoracotomy) with fully open TTE. These results suggest that hybrid TTE significantly reduces postoperative complications compared with open TTE (odds ratio [OR] for postoperative morbidity, 0.31; 95% confidence interval [CI], 0.18 to 0.55; $P = .0001$; percentage of pulmonary complications: 17.7% vs. 30.1% vs. $P = .037$).[2] The open thoracic part of hybrid TTE is similar to that of fully open TTE (this chapter), whereas the laparoscopic (abdominal) part is described in detail in Chapter 39B.

PATIENT ASSESSMENT

Esophageal cancer is a disease that occurs predominantly in the sixth and seventh decades of life. Advanced age alone should not be considered a contraindication for esophageal resection. Although the risk of mortality is higher in patients older than 70 years of age, this increased risk is due to the higher frequency of medical comorbidities such as heart, liver, and kidney disease in the elderly population rather than age per se.[3] It is important to note that when operative mortality is excluded, long-term survival after resection in the elderly population is similar to that observed in younger patients.[4,5] As a result, octogenarians and nonagenarians can be considered candidates for potentially curative resection, but particular attention needs to be paid to the preoperative assessment of patients' general condition.

The strong etiologic ties between (squamous cell) cancer of the esophagus and alcohol and tobacco usage make it imperative that patients be carefully screened for the presence of cardiovascular, pulmonary, and hepatic dysfunction regardless of their age. It has been estimated that between 20% and 30% of patients with esophageal cancer will have evidence of cardiovascular disease if carefully screened.[6] This evaluation should at least consist of electrocardiography for all patients. The preoperative evaluation should also include pulmonary function testing. Patients with significant impairment in the forced expiratory volume at 1 second ($FEV_1 < 1$ L) and those with chronic obstructive pulmonary disease are at increased risk of respiratory complications following surgery.[7,8] Cirrhosis of the liver is not uncommon in patients with esophageal cancer, particularly those with squamous cell carcinoma. Well-compensated cirrhosis (Child classification A) alone is not a contraindication to resection of an otherwise curable esophageal cancer, but one should be careful when considering resection in the setting of more advanced stages of cirrhosis, especially in the presence of ascites. Furthermore, patients who are planned to undergo neoadjuvant chemo(radio)therapy should be screened for renal insufficiency.

EXTENT OF RESECTION FOR LOCOREGIONAL ESOPHAGEAL CANCER

For several decades, the optimal surgical strategy for the potentially curative treatment of patients with locoregional esophageal cancer has been under debate. Historically, the Ivor-Lewis procedure has been widely applied, including a thoracotomy with limited lymphadenectomy and thoracic anastomosis.[9] Ever since, two main surgical techniques have evolved. First, the extended en bloc TTE was developed. With extensive two-field lymphadenectomy (upper abdomen and posterior mediastinum), this technique attempts to increase locoregional tumor control by enhancing the radicality of the resection.[10–14] It is established that extensive lymphadenectomy provides the benefit of more accurate staging, but its beneficial effect on survival is still unclear.[15–18] Second, the limited transhiatal esophagectomy (THE) was introduced, which focused on minimization of postoperative morbidity and mortality by preventing a thoracotomy.

Lymphatic dissemination in esophageal cancer occurs early and is unpredictable.[19] Once the tumor

TABLE 39A.1 Relationship Between Tumor Depth (T-stage) and Lymph Node Status (N-stage) for Esophageal Adenocarcinoma

Tumor Depth	Prevalence of Node Metastases (%)*	Number of Involved Nodes (Median [IQR])†	Number With 1–4 Involved Nodes (%)‡	Number With >4 Involved Nodes (%)§
Intramucosal (T1A)	1/16 (6)	2 (n/a)	1/16 (6)	0/16 (0)
Submucosal (T1B)	5/16 (31)	1 (n/a)	4/16 (25)	1/16 (6)
Intramuscular (T2)	10/13 (77)	2 (1–4)	9/13 (69)	1/13 (8)
Transmural (T3)	47/55 (85)	5 (3–13.5)	22/55 (40)	25/55 (45)

*$\chi^2 = 42.0$, $P < .0001$ (chi-square test for trend).
†$\chi^2 = 11.02$, $P = .0116$ (Kruskal-Wallis; includes only patients with involved nodes).
‡$\chi^2 = 13.64$, $P = .0035$ (chi-square test for trend).
§$\chi^2 = 21.38$, $P < .0001$ (chi-square test for trend).
Modified from Hagen JA, DeMeester SR, Peters JH, Chandrasoma P, DeMeester TR. Curative resection for esophageal adenocarcinoma: analysis of 100 en bloc esophagectomies. *Ann Surg.* 2001;234:520-530.

has penetrated the submucosal layer, up to one-half of patients will have nodal metastases.[20] More than 80% of patients with invasion of the muscularis propria will have at least one involved lymph node.[21] In the presence of transmural invasion, nodal involvement will be present in more than 85%, and the median number of involved nodes and the proportion of patients with more than four involved nodes increases (Table 39A.1).[22] Extended lymphadenectomy as performed during TTE increases the chance of removal of all tumor-positive lymph nodes and theoretically improves regional tumor control and perhaps even long-term survival. However, high-quality clinical evidence on the optimal extent of lymphadenectomy is absent, especially in the present era of neoadjuvant treatment. Consequently, individual opinions and institutional preferences currently dominate the choice of surgical technique and extent of lymphadenectomy.

TECHNIQUE OF OPEN EN BLOC TRANSTHORACIC ESOPHAGECTOMY

En bloc TTE is performed through a right thoracotomy and a midline laparotomy. The proximal anastomosis is performed either through an extra incision made at the left side of the neck or in the chest (see "Anastomosis"). When a cervical anastomosis is performed, the procedure starts with a thoracotomy followed by the abdominal part of the operation, whereas in case of an intrathoracic anastomosis the laparotomy is performed prior to the thoracic phase.

The thoracic dissection includes removal of the azygos vein with its associated nodes, the thoracic duct, and the paratracheal, subcarinal, paraesophageal, and parahiatal nodes in continuity with the resected esophagus. Nodes in the aortopulmonary window are removed separately. The block of tissue removed is bounded laterally on each side by the excised mediastinal pleura, anteriorly by the pericardium and membranous part of the trachea, and posteriorly by the aorta and vertebral bodies.

During the thoracic phase the patient is placed in the left lateral decubitus position with a posterolateral thoracotomy performed entering the chest through the fifth or sixth intercostal space. The inferior pulmonary ligament is divided to the level of the inferior pulmonary vein. The pleura overlying the right main bronchus is divided, taking into account its membranous part. The

pleura lying on both sides of the azygos arch is incised, and the arch is ligated or closed with a stapling device and subsequently transected. The pleura cranial to the azygos arch is incised and saved to create a pedicled "flap" to cover the subsequent intrathoracic anastomosis. The right paratracheal nodes are removed in between the trachea, superior vena cava, and the azygos arch. The right vagal nerve and the bronchial artery are divided. The vagal nerve should not be divided with use of electrocautery to prevent injury to the right recurrent nerve. The pleura overlying the lateral aspect of the vertebral bodies is incised from the level of the azygos arch to the diaphragm, and the intercostal veins are divided between ligatures or clips where they enter the azygos vein. A dissection plane is then created following each intact intercostal artery to reach the adventitial plane of the aorta. Dissection continues across the anterior surface of the aorta until the left mediastinal pleura is reached. Direct branches of the thoracic aorta to the esophagus should be carefully ligated before dividing. One or two communicating veins to the hemiazygos need to be ligated as they pass behind the aorta. The mediastinal tissue posteriorly between the azygos vein and the aorta just above the diaphragm includes the thoracic duct, which should be identified and transected at this stage. A heavy nonresorbable ligature should be placed caudally to prevent the development of a chylothorax. The dissection can be ended at the level of both crura of the diaphragm.

The anterior portion of the dissection is performed along the previously incised inferior pulmonary ligament. Hereby, the posterior aspect of the pericardium is freed by blunt and sharp dissection. The pericardium should only be removed when the tumor is adherent. Once the left mediastinal pleura is reached, the plane can be connected with the previous dissection over the aorta. Sometimes the left pleura is incised. The thoracic esophagus is then encircled with a Penrose drain for traction. The anterior dissection is then continued cephalad along the pericardium until the subcarinal nodes are encountered. Careful dissection along the right main bronchus up to the carina and then distally along the left main bronchus allows for removal of the entire subcarinal node basin in continuity with the resected esophagus. At this point, the anterior dissection is also transitioned to the wall of the esophagus by dividing the left vagal nerve where it crosses the left main bronchus.

The esophagus is separated from the membranous part of the trachea. In case of an intrathoracic anastomosis, the esophagus is divided above the level of the azygos arch. In case of a cervical anastomosis, the dissection is continued toward the root of the neck. The lymph nodes in the aortopulmonary window can be dissected after identification of the left vagal nerve. The left vagal nerve is divided between ligatures at the level of the left main bronchus. The proximal side is carefully moved upward with use of the same ligature, thus preventing damage to the left recurrent nerve when dissecting the aortopulmonary window nodes. The proximal thoracic duct is also ligated and cut at the level of the fourth vertebral body where it crosses from right to left.

The abdominal portion of the operation begins with a midline laparotomy and inspection of the peritoneal cavity and liver. Normally, segments two and three of the liver are mobilized by incising the left triangular ligament with electrocautery. The flaccid part of the lesser omentum is identified and incised in the direction of the right crus. The right gastric artery is identified, and the lesser omentum is further mobilized. Then the gastrocolic omentum is divided, carefully preserving the gastroepiploic arcade. This dissection should begin distally at the level of the pylorus, continuing proximally to include division of the short gastric vessels. The short gastric vessels should be divided as close as possible to the spleen to preserve as many collateral vessels to the fundus as possible. In this fashion, an omental wrap around the future anastomosis can also be created.

All of the lymph node–bearing tissue overlying the proximal border of the hepatic artery and portal vein is removed. This dissection is continued proximally along the hepatic artery to its origin from the celiac axis. The retroperitoneal tissue above the pancreas overlying the right crus of the diaphragm is dissected medially and superiorly to remain attached to the esophagectomy specimen. Attention is then turned to the greater curvature of the stomach where the gastrocolic omentum is divided. The gastric fundus is rotated to the right to continue the dissection in the retroperitoneum, removing all of the node-bearing tissue above the splenic artery and overlying the left crus of the diaphragm. The musculature of the diaphragmatic hiatus is then incised (in case of a bulky tumor) to meet the incision made in the diaphragm during the thoracic dissection. Often the diaphragmatic vein needs to be ligated. Retracting the stomach anteriorly, ample exposure of the celiac axis can be achieved to allow for ligation of the coronary vein (=left gastric vein). After this, the upper abdominal lymph adenectomy around the celiac trunk can be completed. The left gastric artery is divided at its origin. A Kocher maneuver can be performed if needed to allow additional mobility of the stomach.

Reconstruction is preferably performed by creation of a gastric tube after resection of the gastric cardia. The gastric tube is created using a linear stapling device. The staple line should begin on the upper fundus at least 5 cm from the distal limit of the tumor and should continue to a point along the lesser curvature corresponding to the fourth or fifth branch of the right gastric artery in the case of a cervical anastomosis, where more length can be achieved by staying closer to the greater curve

(consequently a narrower tube). When an intrathoracic anastomosis is performed, more of the right gastric vessels can be preserved; consequently, a wider tube can be created. Finally, the staple line is oversewn.

Technique of Transhiatal Esophagectomy

The operation begins with an abdominal lymph node dissection and gastric mobilization (see "Technique of Open En Bloc Transthoracic Esophagectomy"). Next, the tendinous part of the esophageal hiatus is incised anteriorly or the muscular part is incised circumferentially after division of the diaphragmatic vein with ligatures. This ensures removal of any potentially involved parahiatal nodes, but it also enlarges the hiatal opening that facilitates the lower mediastinal dissection. Placement of appropriate retractors through the widened esophageal hiatus allows for en bloc dissection of all the fatty tissue and lymph nodes surrounding the lower thoracic esophagus under visual control as far as possible. Under normal circumstances, this can be done up to the level of the inferior pulmonary veins. To not damage the thoracic duct, care should be taken not to dissect at the right side of the thoracic aorta. Subsequently, the gastric tube is created and the cervical esophagus is exposed (see "Cervical Anastomosis"). The upper thoracic esophagus is delivered into the cervical wound and it is divided in the neck. A large-bore vein stripper is inserted through the cervical esophagus and brought to the gastric remnant. After a long tape is tied to the distal part of the transected esophagus, it is bluntly stripped from the neck toward the abdomen, while the adhesions between the esophagus and surrounding structures are manually freed via the widened hiatus. In the lower mediastinum, the vagal nerve trunks that are separated from the esophagus by this maneuver can be divided below the carina with use of scissors. The right lateral attachments are mobilized by a similar maneuver passing the right hand anterior to the esophagus and using the thumb and index finger to bluntly dissect the right lateral attachments. The tape tied follows the inverting esophagus from the neck to the abdomen. The esophagus is everted again and the resection specimen is sent for pathologic examination. The tape is now sutured onto the top of the gastric tube (which has been created at an earlier stage; see previous text). The gastric tube can be wrapped in a bowel bag or laparoscopic camera bag to facilitate atraumatic passage and can be brought up to the neck by pulling gently on the tape and pushing the gastric tube into the mediastinum. Care should be taken to avoid rotation of the gastric tube. A cervical anastomosis can subsequently be performed (see "Cervical Anastomosis").

RECONSTRUCTION

In the far majority of patients undergoing resection for esophageal cancer, reconstruction is performed using a gastric conduit, where only a single anastomosis is required.

The major disadvantages of using the stomach include the almost complete lack of peristaltic activity and the tendency for persistent reflux into the remaining cervical esophagus that is directly connected to the acid-secreting stomach. In long-term survivors, this ongoing reflux can result in the development of interstitial metaplasia (Barrett) in the cervical remnant.[23] The need to preserve length may also result in more limited margins, especially for large or very distal tumors that can result in local recurrence. As a result, when there is extensive involvement of the stomach and the esophagus, the use of an antiperistaltic or isoperistaltic left colon interposition is preferred. Also, in cases where creation of a (sufficiently oxygenated) gastric tube is technically not possible (e.g., history of gastric surgery or aberrant blood supply of the stomach), reconstruction is performed using a colonic interposition.

During TTE, the surgeon can choose between an anastomosis at the cervical level or in the chest. In contrast, a THE always requires an anastomosis in the neck. Despite the increased rate of recurrent laryngeal nerve damage, leakage, and possible stricture formation, some surgeons prefer a cervical anastomosis during TTE, because of a longer proximal tumor-free margin and a theoretically reduced morbidity in case of an anastomotic leak.[24,25] The latter is founded on the assumption that a leakage of a cervical anastomosis is more likely to be confined to the neck instead of leaking into the pleural cavity and mediastinum. However, a meta-analysis on this topic did not show differences in pulmonary complications (OR, 0.86; 95% CI, 0.13 to 5.59; $P = .87$) and tumor recurrence (OR, 2.01; 95% CI, 0.68 to 5.91; $P = .21$), which suggests that a cervical anastomosis after TTE does not decrease the risk of thoracic complications compared with an intrathoracic anastomosis.[26] Interestingly, two large retrospective studies showed that the risk of intrathoracic manifestations due to leakage of a cervical anastomosis is significantly less in patients after THE than in patients who underwent TTE. This is probably explained by the difference in mediastinal dissection and pleural resection. After THE, the bilaterally intact parietal pleura may confine infections, which prevents extension to the pleural cavity and mediastinum.[27,28] Notably, these studies were performed before the introduction of neoadjuvant therapy. Studies comparing cervical with intrathoracic anastomoses in patients who underwent neoadjuvant therapy are lacking. The CROSS trial comparing neoadjuvant chemoradiotherapy plus surgery with surgery alone, in which most anastomoses were performed at cervical level, showed no significant difference in leakage rate.[29] Nevertheless, preoperative radiotherapy likely affects anastomotic healing, especially if the fundus (i.e., the future tip of the gastric tube) was located within the radiation field. Theoretically, the gastric tube can be shorter in case of an intrathoracic anastomosis, with potentially improved oxygenation of the tip and thus enhanced anastomotic healing. On the contrary, radiation damage on the intrathoracic esophageal remnant might hamper intrathoracic anastomotic healing. This topic is currently subject of investigation in an ongoing Dutch randomized trial comparing cervical with intrathoracic anastomosis after neoadjuvant chemoradiotherapy (ICAN trial, Dutch Trial Registry number: NTR4333).

CERVICAL ANASTOMOSIS

When a cervical anastomosis is performed after TTE, dissection of the proximal part of the thoracic esophagus should be performed as far as possible into the base of the neck to facilitate the later dissection. Exposure of the cervical esophagus is accomplished through an oblique left neck incision placed along the anterior border of the sternocleidomastoid muscle. This incision should extend from the sternal notch to a point halfway to the ear lobe. The omohyoid, sternohyoid, and sternothyroid muscles are divided laterally, and the jugular vein and carotid sheath are lateralized. The middle thyroid vein and inferior thyroid artery are ligated. Dissection is then continued posteriorly to the esophagus, down to the dissection plane with the prevertebral fascia, into the thoracic inlet where the dissection plane performed during the thoracotomy is reached. A dissection plane is then created between the esophagus and the trachea. The esophagus is encircled with a Penrose drain and the upper thoracic esophagus is delivered into the neck. The esophagus is divided at the level of the thoracic inlet and the specimen is removed via the abdomen after tying a tape to the esophagus. The cervical remnant should not be too long, thus preventing that the anastomosis will ultimately retract into the upper chest with a possibly increased risk of intrathoracic manifestation in case of leakage.

With use of the tape, which is tied to top of the gastric tube, the gastric pull-up can be completed. The previously created gastric tube can be wrapped in a plastic bag to facilitate atraumatic passage to the neck. Care should be taken to avoid excessive tension on the stomach or its gastroepiploic arcade during this maneuver and to avoid twisting of the stomach. The anastomosis is performed between the remaining cervical esophagus and the gastric tube. We prefer to perform an end-to-end anastomosis with single-layer running suture. Several nonabsorbable sutures should be placed to normalize the size of the hiatus to prevent visceral herniation into the thorax. A nasogastric decompression tube is then carefully passed as well as a nasojejunal feeding tube. Alternatively, one can choose for a percutaneous jejunal feeding tube.

INTRATHORACIC ANASTOMOSIS

In the case of an intrathoracic anastomosis, the proximal part of the esophagus is divided just above the arch of the azygos vein. With care to prevent rotation, the cardia together with the gastric tube is delivered through the hiatus into the thoracic cavity, and the surgical specimen (i.e., esophagus and cardia) is removed. After placement of four to eight sutures around the esophagus (PDS 3.0), a purse-string Prolene 1.0 suture is placed, and after careful inflation of a 30-mL balloon of a catheter, the diameter of the circular stapler is estimated and the anvil is placed. Subsequently, the gastrotomy is made at the tip of the gastric tube, the circular stapling device is introduced, and an end-to-side anastomosis is created using a 25 mm or 29 mm circular stapling device. The gastrotomy is closed with a linear stapler and the linear staple line is oversewn. A nasogastric tube is passed into the distal stomach. After completion of the anastomosis, omental tissue is wrapped around the anastomosis (omentoplasty).

COLON INTERPOSITION

When a colon interposition is performed, the complete stomach is removed with the esophagectomy specimen by dividing the duodenum just distal from the pylorus. There are several alternatives to use the colon for interposition. Frequently the left colon is used in an isoperistaltic position. For this purpose, the ascending and descending colon are mobilized completely. The left segment of the colon to be interposed derives its arterial supply from the ascending branch of the left colic artery and usually corresponds to the segment extending from the midtransverse colon to the proximal descending colon. This segment is mobilized by dissecting the middle colic artery back to its origin from the superior mesenteric artery where it arises as a single trunk in most patients. After the middle colic artery and vein have temporarily been occluded to ensure adequate collateral flow through the marginal artery, these vessels are ligated and divided.

The apex of the arc portended by the vascular pedicle is then marked with a suture and the distance from this point to the neck is measured with an umbilical tape. This tape is used to measure proximally from the first marking stitch to determine the point of transection of the proximal colon. The divided colon is then passed through the bed of the resected esophagus wrapped in a bowel bag, and a single-layer monofilament running anastomosis is performed to the remaining cervical esophagus. Traction is gently applied to the colon from within the abdomen to eliminate redundancy, and the colon is secured to the left crus of the diaphragm with a nonabsorbable suture.

The colon is then divided with a linear stapler 5 to 10 cm below the point where it enters the abdomen. Care should be exercised not to leave too long of an intraabdominal segment of colon, as this will result in food retention. The mesentery should be divided immediately adjacent to the wall of the colon to avoid injury to the vascular pedicle. A single-layered anastomosis is then performed between the distally divided colon and the Roux-en-Y jejunal loop, and colon continuity is restored by a colocolostomy.

Alternatively, the left colon can be used in antiperistaltic position, which is based on a vascular pedicle of the middle colic artery and vein. In this way, the interposed segment can be longer by making use not only of the descending colon, but also (part of) the sigmoid colon.

Finally, the right colon can be used including the ileocecal valve in an isoperistaltic position and again based on the middle colic vessels. The advantage of this technique is that the ileocecal valve will act as an antireflux mechanism at the proximal anastomosis.

We routinely perform a catheter jejunostomy to provide early postoperative enteral feeding and to avoid the need for parenteral nutrition in the event of postoperative complications such as an anastomotic leak. The jejunostomy catheter is removed when the patient is able to maintain body weight by oral feedings, usually 3 to 4 weeks postoperatively.

COMPLICATIONS

Despite recent improvements in perioperative management, postoperative morbidity and mortality following esophagectomy for cancer remain significant. These are large, technically demanding operations that are often performed on patients with compromised cardiopulmonary function. Nutritional disturbances are also common because of the combined effects of the cancer itself and the obstructing mass in the esophagus.

Recent audits suggest a hospital mortality rate varying from 3.5% to 9% in the West.[30,31] Complication rates varying from 17% to 74% are reported in both open and minimally invasive esophagectomy series.[32,33] This wide range of complication rates can be explained by the variations in definitions of complications and the absence of standardization of time periods defining postoperative deaths.[34,35] Accurate comparison of outcomes between centers to improve the quality of care requires consistency in definitions and data collection. Therefore an international system for defining and recording postoperative complications associated with esophagectomy has been developed.[36]

Complications occurring in a randomized trial comparing open TTE with open THE for esophageal adenocarcinoma are summarized in Table 39A.2.[37] Pulmonary complications including pneumonia (defined as isolation of a pathogen from a sputum culture and an infiltrate on chest x-ray) and atelectasis (defined as lobar collapse on chest x-ray) are among the most common complications, occurring in 57% and 27% of patients who underwent TTE or THE, respectively. These complications can be minimized by early ambulation and careful attention to adequate pain control. Prevention of aspiration can

TABLE 39A.2 Postoperative Complications Occurring in 220 Primary Resections for Esophageal Adenocarcinoma in a Randomized Trial Comparing Transthoracic Esophagectomy and Transhiatal Esophagectomy

Complication	Transthoracic Esophagectomy (%)	Transhiatal Esophagectomy (%)	P Value
Pulmonary complications*	65 (57)	29 (27)	<.001
Cardiac complications	30 (26)	17 (16)	.10
Anastomotic leakage[†]	18 (16)	15 (14)	.85
Subclinical	8 (7)	9 (8)	
Clinical	10 (9)	6 (6)	
Vocal-cord paralysis[‡]	24 (21)	14 (13)	.15
Chylous leakage	11 (10)	2 (2)	.02
Wound infection	11 (10)	8 (8)	.53

*Pulmonary complications include pneumonia (indicated by isolation of a pathogen from a sputum culture and an infiltrate on chest x-ray) and atelectasis (indicated by lobar collapse on chest x-ray).
[†]The definition for subclinical anastomotic leakage was anastomotic leakage seen only on contrast radiography, and clinical anastomotic leakage was defined as anastomotic leakage resulting in a cervical salivary fistula (all patients had cervical anastomoses).
[‡]In most cases, vocal-cord paralysis was temporary.
Data from Hulscher JB, van Sandick JW, de Boer AG, et al. Extended transthoracic resection compared with limited transhiatal resection for adenocarcinoma of the esophagus. *N Engl J Med.* 2002;347 1662–1669.

be achieved by keeping the patient constantly in the semi-upright position and by meticulous attention to maintaining a functioning nasogastric tube. When necessary, a mini-tracheostomy can provide invaluable assistance in clearing retained secretions.

Cardiac complications occur in approximately 26% and 16% of TTE and THE patients, with the development of atrial fibrillation accounting for the majority of these complications. The shift of body fluids and the extensive mediastinal dissection that causes a systemic inflammatory response likely play a role in the pathogenesis. Although these are generally self-limiting, they do require cardiac monitoring and treatment, which can prolong the intensive care unit stay. Atrial fibrillation can also, for example, be caused by anastomotic dehiscence with secondary mediastinitis or by mechanical irritation by a chest tube. For these underlying causes, specific measures are needed.

Anastomotic complications occur in 10% to 30% of patients depending on the definition and the type of reconstruction performed.[38] Most of these leaks can be managed with local drainage and antibiotic administration if the vascular supply to the reconstruction is adequate. We recommend early endoscopy in any patient who is known or suspected to have a substantial leak to exclude potentially life-threatening conduit ischemia, which can be present in as many as 14% of patients with an anastomotic leak.[39]

RESULTS

Long-term survival following esophagectomy depends on several factors including age, gender, weight loss, histologic subtype, depth of tumor invasion, radicality of the resection, and the number of involved lymph nodes.[29,40,41] The impact of surgical approach on long-term survival remains the subject of debate.

In a retrospective analysis from nine high-volume centers on 2303 patients (60% adenocarcinoma [AC], 40% squamous cell carcinoma [SCC]) who underwent R0 resections, it was shown that a high total number of resected nodes is an independent prognostic factor of (favorable) survival after primary surgery. The optimal threshold for survival benefit was removal of 23 nodes, and the operation most likely to achieve this number was found to be an en bloc transthoracic resection.[42] These findings are arguments in favor of TTE over THE. In contrast, a nonrandomized study by two British high-volume centers showed similar long-term survival after THE and TTE for patients with SCC (12%) or AC (88%), while hospital stay was significantly shorter after THE.[43] This advantage in short-term recovery after THE over TTE without substantially jeopardizing oncologic outcome was confirmed in a recent meta-analysis of 52 studies that included 3389 TTE patients and 2516 THE patients (48% SCC, 52% AC). In addition to the significantly shorter hospital stay (4 days less in patients who underwent THE; 95% CI, 1 to 7; $P < .01$), THE was associated with shorter operation time (85 minutes shorter; 95% CI, 40 to 129; $P < .001$), less pulmonary complications (17.3% vs. 21.4%; OR, 1.37; 95% CI, 1.05 to 1.79; $P = .02$), and lower postoperative mortality (7.2% vs. 10.6%; OR, 1.48; 95% CI, 1.20 to 1.83; $P < .001$). On the other hand, anastomotic leaks and recurrent nerve palsies occurred

more frequently after THE than after TTE. Moreover, lymph node yield was higher after TTE (mean difference of eight nodes; 95% CI, 1 to 14; $P = .02$). The results of this meta-analysis should be interpreted with caution, because both randomized and nonrandomized studies were included. This probably introduced a selection bias in favor of the THE group, because patients with more advanced tumors probably have been treated preferentially via the chest.[44] On the other hand, more frail patients may have been offered a THE because of no need for a thoracotomy. Finally, the enhanced short-term recovery after THE could not be confirmed in a large (more than 17,000 patients), multicenter observational study that compared TTE with THE; no differences were found in morbidity and mortality. However, a preference for THE in patients with poor performance status probably resulted in selection bias in favor of patients who underwent TTE.[45]

Proponents of the transhiatal approach explain differences in survival by stage that have been consistently reported as being due to stage migration. This occurs when positive nodes in the extended part of the dissection increase pN stage in patients with a more favorable prognosis compared with patients with the same number of positive nodes after a limited dissection during THE. To address this issue, Altorki et al. have reported outcome following en bloc TTE and transhiatal resections performed in patients with T3N-positive (stage III) disease.[46] In this group of patients, the effect of stage migration was supposed to be limited, because all had locally advanced tumors with lymph node involvement. They reported 4-year survival of 35% after en bloc resection, which was significantly better than the 11% survival observed after THE. Ultimately, this debate can only be resolved by the completion of a large randomized controlled trial. To date, only one such large trial (HIVEX) has been reported by Hulscher et al.[37] This trial randomized 220 patients with AC of the mid-to-distal esophagus or the gastric cardia substantially involving the esophagus between THE and TTE. By avoiding a thoracotomy, artificial ventilation time (1 day after THE vs. 2 days after TTE; $P < .001$) and hospital stay (15 days after THE vs. 19 days after TTE; $P < .001$) were shorter, and pulmonary complications were reported less frequently (27% after THE vs. 57% after TTE; $P < .001$) after THE than after TTE. Nevertheless, in-hospital mortality was comparable between both groups (2% after THE and 4% after TTE; $P = .45$). Interestingly, the more extended TTE was not associated with a higher percentage of tumor-free resection margins (72% after THE vs. 71% after TTE), whereas the median number of resected lymph nodes was 2 times higher after TTE than after THE (median 31 vs. 16; $P < .001$). This high lymph node yield did not translate into a significantly better 5-year overall survival (34% after THE and 36% after TTE; $P = .71$).[47] However, in a subsequent subgroup analysis of patients with a truly esophageal (Siewert type 1) cancer, and more specifically in patients with a limited number (1–8) of positive lymph nodes, an improved long-term survival was found after TTE (23% after THE vs. 64% TTE; $P = .02$). Given the post hoc design of this analysis, the effect of stage migration on improved survival of TTE patients cannot be excluded, because more lymph nodes were resected after TTE. Furthermore, the relevance of these results is unclear for patients with SCC (only patients with AC were included). The conclusion of the HIVEX trial was that in patients with advanced, truly esophageal cancer (Siewert type 1), TTE is the preferred technique (especially in case of a limited number of positive nodes), while THE suffices in patients with a tumor located at the esophagogastric junction (EGJ) (Siewert type 2) and in patients with a poor performance status (especially in case of pulmonary comorbidities), without clinically suspected nodes at or above the carina.[47]

ROLE OF NEOADJUVANT THERAPY

Increasingly, the management of esophageal cancer has focused nowadays on multimodality therapy, with neoadjuvant chemotherapy or chemoradiotherapy being administered to nearly all patients with locally advanced disease in many centers. The concept of neoadjuvant therapy in esophageal cancer was spurred by a general disappointment in the results of primary resections, which resulted in survival of 35% or less at 5 years.[37]

Many studies have been performed to test the additional value of preoperative neoadjuvant therapy to surgical resection. A meta-analysis showed that both neoadjuvant chemotherapy and neoadjuvant chemoradiotherapy improve long-term survival.[48] Furthermore, this meta-analysis showed a (nonsignificant) benefit of neoadjuvant chemoradiotherapy (nCRT) over neoadjuvant chemotherapy (nCT) by comparison of the treatment arms of several trials (hazard ratio [HR] for overall mortality for nCRT vs. nCT, 0.88; 95% CI, 0.76 to 1.01; $P = .07$). Unfortunately, direct comparisons are limited, especially for patients with AC.

Since the publication of this meta-analysis, the multicenter randomized CROSS trial was completed, comparing nCRT plus surgery with surgery alone in patients with esophageal or junctional cancer (both SCC and AC).[29,49] The applied regimen (carboplatin and paclitaxel with 41.4 Gy concurrent radiotherapy) had low toxicity compared with earlier trials that mostly used cisplatin and fluorouracil. Median survival doubled from 24% in the surgery-alone group to 49% in the nCRT group (HR, 0.68; 95% CI, 0.53 to 0.88; $P = .003$), with a 5-year survival advantage of 14% (33% vs. 47%). The superior survival in the surgery-alone arm of the CROSS trial compared with that in earlier randomized trials, indicates that the survival benefit can be attributed to improved survival in the multimodality arm, and is not due to poor survival in the surgery-alone arm.[50,51] Based on these results, nCRT according to the CROSS regimen plus surgery is now considered standard of care in many countries.

The favorable results of the CROSS trial were not confirmed in a recently completed French randomized trial (Fédération Francophone de Cancérologie Digestive [FFCD] 9901 trial) comparing nCRT plus surgery with surgery alone in stage I and II esophageal cancer patients. The applied neoadjuvant regimen consisted of cisplatin and fluorouracil with 45 Gy concurrent radiotherapy. No differences in 3-year overall survival rate and radical resection rate were found between both treatment arms.[52]

Based on the FFCD 9901 trial, the standard use of nCRT for early-stage tumors can be debated. Possibly, surgery alone suffices in this subgroup of patients. This is supported by the high rate of radical resections (92%) in the surgery-alone arm of the French trial. However, the generalizability of the FFCD 9901 trial is questionable due to the low case volume of most participating centers, the high toxicity of the nCRT regimen with less sophisticated radiation techniques compared with the CROSS trial, and a remarkably high postoperative mortality rate (11.1%). Therefore we caution to conclude that patients with early-stage esophageal cancer should not undergo nCRT. We believe that in the absence of high-quality evidence on the specific effect of nCRT on early-stage tumors, the results from the CROSS trial (which also included stage II cancers) should be leading.[53]

The CROSS trial and the FFCD 9901 trial included both AC and SCC. Although nCRT also significantly improves survival in patients with AC, the maximum benefit of nCRT is observed in SCC, which is known to be more radiosensitive than AC.[29,49] Three small underpowered randomized trials comprising 119, 75, and 131 patients, respectively, with esophageal AC did not show significant differences in survival between nCRT followed by surgery and nCT followed by surgery. Nevertheless, higher rates of pCR, R0, and ypN0 were found in the nCRT groups, and two of these three trials showed a (nonsignificant) benefit in favor of nCRT.[54-57] The optimal neoadjuvant treatment for esophageal AC remains undetermined and is currently investigated in the randomized Neo-AEGIS (perioperative MAGIC chemotherapy vs. preoperative CROSS chemoradiotherapy, in adenocarcinoma of the esophagus and esophagogastric junction) trial, which is likely to be reported in 2021.[58]

nCRT has a significant downstaging effect on both the primary tumor and the regional lymph nodes. In the nCRT-arm of the CROSS trial, a substantial number of patients (29% overall, 49% SCC, 23% AC) did not have any vital tumor left in the resection specimen. This observation led to the imperative to reconsider the necessity of standard esophagectomy in all patients who undergo nCRT. Therefore the feasibility of an active surveillance strategy in patients with a clinically complete response (cCR) after nCRT is currently being explored. In this so-called SANO (Surgery As Needed in Oesophageal cancer patients) approach, surgical resection would be offered only to patients in whom residual disease is highly suspected or proven after nCRT. Before SANO can be tested in a prospective clinical trial, we aim to determine the accuracy of clinical detection of residual disease after nCRT in the present preSANO trial.[59] Furthermore, the French phase II/III randomized ESOSTRATE trial comparing standard surgery with surgery on demand in case of recurrence in patients with a cCR after nCRT is currently being initiated (ClinicalTrials.gov identifier: NCT02551458).[60]

As outlined previously, the randomized HIVEX trial comparing THE with TTE for subcarinal AC only included patients with primary surgery. In that trial, TTE did not improve the rate of tumor-free margins (72% after THE vs. 71% after TTE) but roughly doubled the number of resected nodes (median ± standard deviation = 16 ± 9 after THE vs. 31 ± 14 after TTE; $P < .001$). As discussed previously, a retrospective international study has shown that after primary surgery, the number of resected nodes is correlated with a favorable long-term survival.[42] However, it has been reported that chemoradiotherapy reduces lymph node yield from within the radiotherapy field.[61–63] Importantly, in the patients after primary surgery from the CROSS trial, the total number of resected nodes and the number of resected positive nodes were positively correlated. However, this positive association completely disappeared in patients who underwent nCRT. Furthermore, after surgery alone, the total number of removed nodes was positively correlated with overall survival (HR per 10 additionally resected nodes, 0.76; P = .007), which corresponds with the earlier retrospective international study.[42,64] Interestingly, this positive correlation between the number of resected nodes and survival was absent after nCRT (HR, 1.00; P = .98). The randomized design of the CROSS trial renders differences between both treatment groups unlikely as an explanation for the (disappearance of the) association in this post hoc analysis. These results question the necessity of maximization of surgical lymph node dissection after nCRT, both for prognostication and for therapeutic purposes.

The same phenomenon was identified in a large retrospective comparison of 307 patients who underwent nCRT according to CROSS plus surgery and 301 patients who underwent nCT according to MAGIC followed by surgery. In the nCRT group, the association between lymph node harvest and survival was absent. However, in the nCT group, extent of lymphadenectomy seemed to be positively correlated with progression-free survival. Again, these data question the necessity for maximization of surgical lymph node retrieval specifically after nCRT. However, extended lymphadenectomy seems of importance in patients who undergo nCT followed by surgery (or surgery alone).[65]

These indirect arguments need confirmation in a randomized trial comparing TTE with extended lymphadenectomy and THE with limited lymphadenectomy in patients with (Siewert type 1) esophageal cancer who undergo nCRT. We believe that such trial should focus on truly esophageal cancer, and not on junctional cancer, because it already has been shown that THE suffices in junctional cancer if the patients undergo primary surgery, let alone in patients with junctional cancer who have been treated with preoperative nCRT.

SALVAGE SURGERY

Definitive CRT (dCRT) is frequently applied in patients with SCC of the proximal part of the esophagus (i.e., above the carina) and in patients not fit for surgery. Although organ preservation is a considerable advantage in the nonoperative strategy of dCRT, this approach is associated with high rates (up to 51%) of recurrence or persistence of locoregional disease.[66] In these patients, salvage esophagectomy is an option after failed dCRT with curative intent. This selective surgery is more demanding than primary esophagectomy. Thanks to centralization of care with improvement in patient selection, in surgical technique and in perioperative management, perioperative morbidity and mortality nowadays have substantially decreased.[67] Furthermore, the increased application of

nCRT has familiarized surgeons with surgical resection in an irradiated surgical field.

Results of salvage surgery after failed dCRT were analyzed in a nonrandomized phase II trial.[68] Forty-three patients were treated with induction CT (5-fluorouracil [5-FU], cisplatin and paclitaxel) followed by CRT (5-FU and cisplatin with concurrent 50.4 Gy). CT scans of the chest and abdomen, positron emission tomography (PET, optional but encouraged), esophagogastroscopy with biopsies, and endoscopic ultrasound (EUS) were performed after completion of CRT and serially thereafter. Twenty patients underwent salvage esophagectomy because of residual or recurrent disease without signs of distant metastases. One-year overall survival was 71% (95% CI, 54% to 82%). Nevertheless, a subsequent phase III trial was not initiated, because the intended predefined minimal 1-year survival rate of 77.5% was not achieved. This predefined 1-year survival rate was deducted from the RTOG database, consisting mainly of SCC patients. The proportion of ACs in this trial was 73%. Moreover, three CRT-related deaths were reported. Theoretically, elimination or mitigation of induction CT from the regimen might have reduced treatment-related toxicity and increased the chance of achieving the target 1-year survival rate of 77.5%.[68]

Furthermore, a more recent retrospective propensity matched analysis compared patients undergoing salvage esophagectomy (n = 308) with patients who underwent neoadjuvant chemoradiotherapy followed by planned esophagectomy (n = 540). In-hospital mortality was comparable (but high) in both groups (8.4% vs. 9.3%). Differences in postoperative complications were found for anastomotic leak (17.2% vs. 10.7%; P = .007) and wound infection (18.5% vs. 12.3%; P = .026), which were both more frequent in patients who underwent salvage surgery. At 3-year follow-up, groups had comparable overall (43.3% vs. 40.1%; P = .542) and disease-free survival rates (39.2% vs. 32.8%; P = .232), suggesting that salvage surgery can offer acceptable short- and long-term results in a selected group of patients.[69]

SUMMARY

Changes in the diagnosis, evaluation, and pre- and postoperative treatment of cancer of the esophagus and esophagogastric junction have resulted in improved prognosis for patients with this uncommon, but deadly, disease. A tailored approach to the management of these patients can now result in an overall 5-year survival of about 50%, which is a dramatic improvement compared with the dismal results reported in the (recent) past. Nevertheless, the optimal surgical approach remains unclear. The widely applied use of multimodality treatment (especially nCRT) questions the necessity of maximization of surgical lymph node retrieval, and the introduction of MIE might further decrease postoperative morbidity with reduction of especially pulmonary complications. However, the lack of high-quality evidence on these topics has led to persistence of substantial differences in the treatment approach between individual institutions. These differences underline the ongoing need for well-designed clinical trials on specific topics in the field of esophageal cancer surgery.

ACKNOWLEDGMENT

This chapter is a revised version of Chapter 35, 'Surgical Treat-ment of Cancer of the Esophagus and Esophagogastric Junction,' of the seventh edition of this work, written by J. A. Hagen and K. Grant. Their important input is gratefully acknowledged.

REFERENCES

1. Thomas N. With minimally invasive esophagectomy, thoracic surgeons must avoid falling into the same trap again! *Semin Thorac Cardiovasc Surg.* 2015;27:216-217.
2. Mariette C, Meunier B, Pezet D, et al. Hybrid minimally invasive versus open oesophagectomy for patients with oesophageal cancer: a multicenter, open-label, randomized phase III controlled trial, the MIRO trial. *J Clin Oncol.* 2015;33.
3. Sugimachi K, Inokuchi K, Ueo H, Matsuura H, Matsuzaki K, Mori M. Surgical treatment for carcinoma of the esophagus in the elderly patient. *Surg Gynecol Obstet.* 1985;160:317-319.
4. Zehetner J, Lipham JC, Ayazi S, et al. Esophagectomy for cancer in octogenarians. *Dis Esophagus.* 2010;23:666-669.
5. van Nistelrooij AM, Andrinopoulou ER, van Lanschot JJ, Tilanus HW, Wijnhoven BP. Influence of young age on outcome after esophagectomy for cancer. *World J Surg.* 2012;36:2512-2621.
6. Konder H, Ponitz-Pohl E, Roher HD, Lennartz H. [Risk assessment and preliminary treatment in patients with esophageal cancer]. *Anasth Intensivther Notfallmed.* 1988;23:9-13.
7. Giuli R, Sancho-Garnier H. Diagnostic, therapeutic, and prognostic features of cancers of the esophagus: results of the international prospective study conducted by the OESO group (790 patients). *Surgery.* 1986;99:614-622.
8. Chan K, Wong J. Mortality after esophagectomy for carcinoma of the esophagus: an analysis of risk factors. *Dis Esophagus.* 1990;3:49-53.
9. Lewis I. The surgical treatment of carcinoma of the oesophagus; with special reference to a new operation for growths of the middle third. *Br J Surg.* 1946;34:18-31.
10. Chu KM, Law SY, Fok M, Wong J. A prospective randomized comparison of transhiatal and transthoracic resection for lower-third esophageal carcinoma. *Am J Surg.* 1997;174:320-324.
11. Goldminc M, Maddern G, Le Prise E, Meunier B, Campion JP, Launois B. Oesophagectomy by a transhiatal approach or thoracotomy: a prospective randomized trial. *Br J Surg.* 1993;80:367-370.
12. Hulscher JB, Tijssen JG, Obertop H, van Lanschot J. Transthoracic versus transhiatal resection for carcinoma of the esophagus: a meta-analysis. *Ann Thorac Surg.* 2001;72:306-313.
13. Jacobi CA, Zieren HU, Muller JM, Pichlmaier H. Surgical therapy of esophageal carcinoma: the influence of surgical approach and esophageal resection on cardiopulmonary function. *Eur J Cardiothorac Surg.* 1997;11:32-37.
14. Muller JM, Erasmi H, Stelzner M, Zieren U, Pichlmaier H. Surgical therapy of oesophageal carcinoma. *Br J Surg.* 1990;77:845-857.
15. Altorki N, Kent M, Ferrara C, Port J. Three-field lymph node dissection for squamous cell and adenocarcinoma of the esophagus. *Ann Surg.* 2002;236:177-183.
16. Jamieson GG, Lamb PJ, Thompson SK. The role of lymphadenectomy in esophageal cancer. *Ann Surg.* 2009;250:206-209.
17. Lerut T, Nafteux P, Moons J, et al. Three-field lymphadenectomy for carcinoma of the esophagus and gastroesophageal junction in 174 R0 resections: impact on staging, disease-free survival, and outcome: a plea for adaptation of TNM classification in upper-half esophageal carcinoma. *Ann Surg.* 2004;240:962-972, [discussion 972-974].
18. Tong D, Law S. Extended lymphadenectomy in esophageal cancer is crucial. *World J Surg.* 2013;37:1751-1756.
19. Raja S, Rice TW, Goldblum JR, et al. Esophageal submucosa: the watershed for esophageal cancer. *J Thorac Cardiovasc Surg.* 2011;142:1403-1411.e1.
20. Stein HJ, Feith M, Bruecher BL, Naehrig J, Sarbia M, Siewert JR. Early esophageal cancer: pattern of lymphatic spread and prognostic factors for long-term survival after surgical resection. *Ann Surg.* 2005;242:566-573, [discussion 573-575].
21. Nigro JJ, Hagen JA, DeMeester TR, et al. Prevalence and location of nodal metastases in distal esophageal adenocarcinoma confined to the wall: implications for therapy. *J Thorac Cardiovasc Surg.* 1999;117:16-23, [discussion 23-25].
22. Hagen JA, DeMeester SR, Peters JH, Chandrasoma P, DeMeester TR. Curative resection for esophageal adenocarcinoma: analysis of 100 en bloc esophagectomies. *Ann Surg.* 2001;234:520-530, [discussion 530-531].
23. Oberg S, Johansson J, Wenner J, Walther B. Metaplastic columnar mucosa in the cervical esophagus after esophagectomy. *Ann Surg.* 2002;235:338-345.
24. Markar SR, Arya S, Karthikesalingam A, Hanna GB. Technical factors that affect anastomotic integrity following esophagectomy: systematic review and meta-analysis. *Ann Surg Oncol.* 2013;20:4274-4281.
25. Chasseray VM, Kiroff GK, Buard JL, Launois B. Cervical or thoracic anastomosis for esophagectomy for carcinoma. *Surg Gynecol Obstet.* 1989;169:55-62.
26. Biere SS, Maas KW, Cuesta MA, van der Peet DL. Cervical or thoracic anastomosis after esophagectomy for cancer: a systematic review and meta-analysis. *Dig Surg.* 2011;28:29-35.
27. Korst RJ, Port JL, Lee PC, Altorki NK. Intrathoracic manifestations of cervical anastomotic leaks after transthoracic esophagectomy for carcinoma. *Ann Thorac Surg.* 2005;80:1185-1190.
28. van Heijl M, van Wijngaarden AK, Lagarde SM, Busch OR, van Lanschot JJ, van Berge Henegouwen MI. Intrathoracic manifestations of cervical anastomotic leaks after transhiatal and transthoracic oesophagectomy. *Br J Surg.* 2010;97:726-731.
29. van Hagen P, Hulshof MC, van Lanschot JJ, et al. Preoperative chemoradiotherapy for esophageal or junctional cancer. *N Engl J Med.* 2012;366:2074-2084.
30. Dutch Institute for Clinical Auditing. Annual report 2014.
31. Finks JF, Osborne NH, Birkmeyer JD. Trends in hospital volume and operative mortality for high-risk surgery. *N Engl J Med.* 2011;364:2128-2137.
32. Dunst CM, Swanstrom LL. Minimally invasive esophagectomy. *J Gastrointest Surg.* 2010;14(suppl 1):S108-S114.
33. Courrech Staal EF, Aleman BM, Boot H, van Velthuysen ML, van Tinteren H, van Sandick JW. Systematic review of the benefits and risks of neoadjuvant chemoradiation for oesophageal cancer. *Br J Surg.* 2010;97:1482-1496.
34. Blencowe NS, Strong S, McNair AG, et al. Reporting of short-term clinical outcomes after esophagectomy: a systematic review. *Ann Surg.* 2012;255:658-666.
35. Talsma AK, Lingsma HF, Steyerberg EW, Wijnhoven BP, Van Lanschot JJ. The 30-day versus in-hospital and 90-day mortality after esophagectomy as indicators for quality of care. *Ann Surg.* 2014;260:267-273.
36. Low DE, Alderson D, Cecconello I, et al. International Consensus on Standardization of Data Collection for Complications Associated with Esophagectomy: Esophagectomy Complications Consensus Group (ECCG). *Ann Surg.* 2015;262:286-294.
37. Hulscher JB, van Sandick JW, de Boer AG, et al. Extended transthoracic resection compared with limited transhiatal resection for adenocarcinoma of the esophagus. *N Engl J Med.* 2002;347:1662-1669.
38. Nederlof N, Tilanus HW, Tran TC, Hop WC, Wijnhoven BP, de Jonge J. End-to-end versus end-to-side esophagogastrostomy after esophageal cancer resection: a prospective randomized study. *Ann Surg.* 2011;254:226-233.
39. Portale G, Hagen JA, Peters JH, et al. Modern 5-year survival of resectable esophageal adenocarcinoma: single institution experience with 263 patients. *J Am Coll Surg.* 2006;202:588-596, [discussion 596-598].
40. Lagarde SM, ten Kate FJ, Reitsma JB, Busch OR, van Lanschot JJ. Prognostic factors in adenocarcinoma of the esophagus or gastroesophageal junction. *J Clin Oncol.* 2006;24:4347-4355.
41. Shapiro J, van Klaveren D, Lagarde SM, et al. Prediction of survival in patients with oesophageal or junctional cancer receiving neoadjuvant chemoradiotherapy and surgery. *Br J Surg.* 2016;103(8):1039-1047.
42. Peyre CG, Hagen JA, DeMeester SR, et al. The number of lymph nodes removed predicts survival in esophageal cancer: an international study on the impact of extent of surgical resection. *Ann Surg.* 2008;248:549-556.
43. Davies AR, Sandhu H, Pillai A, et al. Surgical resection strategy and the influence of radicality on outcomes in oesophageal cancer. *Br J Surg.* 2014;101:511-517.
44. Boshier PR, Anderson O, Hanna GB. Transthoracic versus transhiatal esophagectomy for the treatment of esophagogastric cancer: a meta-analysis. *Ann Surg.* 2011;254:894-906.

45. Connors RC, Reuben BC, Neumayer LA, Bull DA. Comparing outcomes after transthoracic and transhiatal esophagectomy: a 5-year prospective cohort of 17,395 patients. *J Am Coll Surg.* 2007;205: 735-740.

46. Altorki NK, Girardi L, Skinner DB. En bloc esophagectomy improves survival for stage III esophageal cancer. *J Thorac Cardiovasc Surg.* 1997;114:948-955, [discussion 955-956].

47. Omloo JM, Lagarde SM, Hulscher JB, et al. Extended transthoracic resection compared with limited transhiatal resection for adenocarcinoma of the mid/distal esophagus: five-year survival of a randomized clinical trial. *Ann Surg.* 2007;246:992-1000, [discussion 1000-1001].

48. Sjoquist KM, Burmeister BH, Smithers BM, et al. Survival after neoadjuvant chemotherapy or chemoradiotherapy for resectable oesophageal carcinoma: an updated meta-analysis. *Lancet Oncol.* 2011;12:681-692.

49. Shapiro J, van Lanschot JJ, Hulshof MC, et al. Neoadjuvant chemoradiotherapy plus surgery versus surgery alone for oesophageal or junctional cancer (CROSS): long-term results of a randomised controlled trial. *Lancet Oncol.* 2015;16:1090-1098.

50. Walsh TN, Noonan N, Hollywood D, Kelly A, Keeling N, Hennessy TP. A comparison of multimodal therapy and surgery for esophageal adenocarcinoma. *N Engl J Med.* 1996;335:462-467.

51. Tepper J, Krasna MJ, Niedzwiecki D, et al. Phase III trial of trimodality therapy with cisplatin, fluorouracil, radiotherapy, and surgery compared with surgery alone for esophageal cancer: CALGB 9781. *J Clin Oncol.* 2008;26:1086-1092.

52. Mariette C, Dahan L, Mornex F, et al. Surgery alone versus chemoradiotherapy followed by surgery for stage I and II esophageal cancer: final analysis of randomized controlled phase III trial FFCD 9901. *J Clin Oncol.* 2014;32:2416-2422.

53. Shapiro J, van Lanschot JJ, Hulshof MC, van der Gaast A. Effectiveness of neoadjuvant chemoradiotherapy for early-stage esophageal cancer (letter to the editor). *J Clin Oncol.* 2015;33:288-289.

54. Stahl M, Walz MK, Stuschke M, et al. Phase III comparison of preoperative chemotherapy compared with chemoradiotherapy in patients with locally advanced adenocarcinoma of the esophagogastric junction. *J Clin Oncol.* 2009;27:851-856.

55. Burmeister BH, Thomas JM, Burmeister EA, et al. Is concurrent radiation therapy required in patients receiving preoperative chemotherapy for adenocarcinoma of the oesophagus? A randomised phase II trial. *Eur J Cancer.* 2011;47:354-360.

56. Klevebro F, Alexandersson von Dobeln G, Wang N, et al. A randomized clinical trial of neoadjuvant chemotherapy versus neoadjuvant chemoradiotherapy for cancer of the oesophagus or gastro-oesophageal junction. *Ann Oncol.* 2016;27(4):660-667.

57. Stahl M, Riera-Knorrenschild J, Stuschke M, et al. Preoperative chemoradiotherapy and the long-term run in curative treatment of locally advanced oesophagogastric junction adenocarcinoma: update of the POET phase III study. *J Clin Oncol.* 2016;34(suppl; abstr 4031).

58. Keegan N, Keane F, Cuffe S. Neo-AEGIS: a randomized clinical trial of neoadjuvant and adjuvant chemotherapy (modified MAGIC regimen) versus neoadjuvant chemoradiation (CROSS protocol) in adenocarcinoma of the esophagus and esophagogastric junction. *J Clin Oncol.* 2014;32(suppl; abstr TPS4145).

59. Noordman BJ, Shapiro J, Spaander MC, et al. Accuracy of detecting residual disease after cross neoadjuvant chemoradiotherapy for esophageal cancer (preSANO Trial): rationale and protocol. *JMIR Res Protoc.* 2015;4:e79.

60. Putora PM, Bedenne L, Budach W, et al. Oesophageal cancer: exploring controversies overview of experts' opinions of Austria, Germany, France, Netherlands and Switzerland. *Radiat Oncol.* 2015;10:116.

61. Robb WB, Dahan L, Mornex F, et al. Impact of neoadjuvant chemoradiation on lymph node status in esophageal cancer: post hoc analysis of a randomized controlled trial. *Ann Surg.* 2015;261:902-908.

62. Taflampas P, Christodoulakis M, Gourtsoyianni S, Leventi K, Melissas J, Tsiftsis DD. The effect of preoperative chemoradiotherapy on lymph node harvest after total mesorectal excision for rectal cancer. *Dis Colon Rectum.* 2009;52:1470-1474.

63. Lykke J, Roikjaer O, Jess P. Danish Colorectal Cancer Group. Tumour stage and preoperative chemoradiotherapy influence the lymph node yield in stages I–III rectal cancer: results from a prospective nationwide cohort study. *Colorectal Dis.* 2014;16:O144-O149.

64. Talsma AK, Shapiro J, Looman CW, et al. Lymph node retrieval during esophagectomy with and without neoadjuvant chemoradiotherapy: prognostic and therapeutic impact on survival. *Ann Surg.* 2014;260:786-793.

65. Markar SR, Noordman BJ, Mackenzie H, et al. Multimodality treatment for esophageal adenocarcinoma: multi-center propensity-score matched study. *Ann Oncol.* 2017;28:519-527.

66. Cooper JS, Guo MD, Herskovic A, et al. Chemoradiotherapy of locally advanced esophageal cancer: long-term follow-up of a prospective randomized trial (RTOG 85-01). Radiation Therapy Oncology Group. *JAMA.* 1999;281:1623-1627.

67. Markar SR, Schmidt H, Kunz S, Bodnar A, Hubka M, Low DE. Evolution of standardized clinical pathways: refining multidisciplinary care and process to improve outcomes of the surgical treatment of esophageal cancer. *J Gastrointest Surg.* 2014;18:1238-1246.

68. Swisher SG, Winter KA, Komaki RU, et al. A Phase II study of a paclitaxel-based chemoradiation regimen with selective surgical salvage for resectable locoregionally advanced esophageal cancer: initial reporting of RTOG 0246. *Int J Radiat Oncol Biol Phys.* 2012;82:1967-1972.

69. Markar S, Gronnier C, Duhamel A, et al. Salvage surgery after chemoradiotherapy in the management of esophageal cancer: is it a viable therapeutic option? *J Clin Oncol.* 2015;33:3866-3873.

Surgical Approaches to Remove the Esophagus: Minimally Invasive

Arianna Barbetta | Daniela Molena

The first reports of minimally invasive esophagectomy (MIE) were published in the early 1990s by Cuschieri et al., who described a thoracoscopic esophageal mobilization in 1992,[1] and DePaula et al., who reported an MIE with a laparoscopic transhiatal approach in 1995.[2] The technique was popularized almost 10 years later at the University of Pittsburgh Medical Center by James Luketich, who initially adopted a modified McKeown approach with a thoracoscopic esophageal mobilization, followed by a laparoscopic preparation of the gastric conduit and its transposition to the neck for the final cervical anastomosis.[3] Since then many different techniques have been described to perform either a completely MIE or a hybrid combination of open, hand-assisted, and minimally invasive options.

This chapter reviews the current indications, techniques, limitations, and outcomes of minimally invasive surgery for the treatment of esophageal cancer.

INDICATIONS AND CONTRAINDICATION FOR MINIMALLY INVASIVE ESOPHAGECTOMY

Patients' selection for MIE is similar to the classic open esophagectomy. Accurate staging is warranted to tailor treatment to the extension of disease, and multimodality treatment is recommended for locally advanced cancers. Timing of esophagectomy after induction chemoradiation is important to allow patients' complete recovery yet avoiding disease progression and potential technical difficulties and late complications related to treatment. Surgery is therefore performed approximately 6 to 8 weeks after completion of induction therapy, similarly to the open esophagectomy.[4] There are no absolute contraindications to a minimally invasive approach, however, extensive abdominal or thoracic adhesions can make the approach difficult to perform, extension of the tumor in other structures or organs can be difficult to assess due to lack of tactile feedback and single lung ventilation is preferred—although not always necessary—to maximized exposure.

The most important prerequisites to perform an MIE are the institutional availability of advanced minimally invasive equipment and the surgeon's skill with minimally invasive procedures. This operation is, in fact, technically demanding, and a significant learning curve is necessary to limit complications. Improved surgical and oncologic outcomes are usually achieved after 35 to 40 cases.[5–8] A recent British general consensus reported that the appropriate learning curve to perform MIE is estimated to include between 20 and 50 cases.[9]

MINIMALLY INVASIVE IVOR LEWIS ESOPHAGECTOMY

In the Western world, the minimally invasive Ivor Lewis approach is the most commonly used because the adenocarcinoma of the lower esophagus is the most prevalent subtype in the United States and Europe. This approach is a particularly well-suited technique for this tumor, which often does not require a complete esophageal resection, and it is also our preferred option for this disease.[10,11]

The first description of a complete minimally invasive Ivor Lewis esophagectomy was reported in 1999 when Watson et al. performed a laparoscopic and thoracoscopic esophagectomy with an intrathoracic handsewn anastomosis.[12]

A summary of our technique is reported in subsequent text.

ABDOMINAL PHASE

The patient is positioned supine with a foot board to allow steep reverse Trendelenburg during the procedure. A double-lumen endotracheal tube is placed for lung isolation during the thoracoscopic phase. An esophagogastroduodenoscopy is performed to evaluate the proximal and distal extension of the tumor and the presence of Barrett esophagus and to evaluate the stomach, which will be used for reconstruction. As previously described,[11] we use five abdominal ports and the Nathanson liver retractor to expose the hiatus.

The abdominal cavity and the liver are carefully inspected to rule out any metastatic disease. We start our dissection in the lesser curvature of the stomach by opening the gastrohepatic ligament and exposing the branches of the celiac trunk. A complete lymph node dissection of the hepatic, the left gastric, and the splenic arteries is performed, and the nodes are sent separately to pathology for evaluation (Fig. 39B.1). The left gastric vein and artery are then divided with a vascular stapler. This allows exposure and nodal dissection at the base of the celiac artery and the diaphragmatic crus.

Mobilization of the greater curvature of the stomach includes complete division of the gastrocolic ligament just distal to the gastroepiploic arcade. Dissection is extended to the fundus by dividing the short gastric vessels and phrenoesophageal attachments and to the proximal duodenum by completely separating the colon from the gastric attachments. When the greater curvature is completely mobilized, the stomach is lifted to dissect the retroperitoneal attachments and mobilize the right gastroepiploic pedicle to its base. This maneuver is very

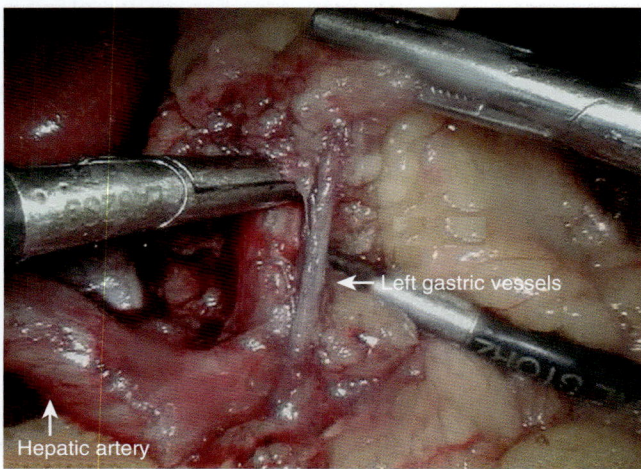

FIGURE 39B.1 A complete abdominal lymphadenectomy is performed around the celiac trunk vessels skeletonizing the hepatic, splenic, and left gastric arteries. The left gastric vessels identified in this figure are then divided at their base with an endoscopic stapler.

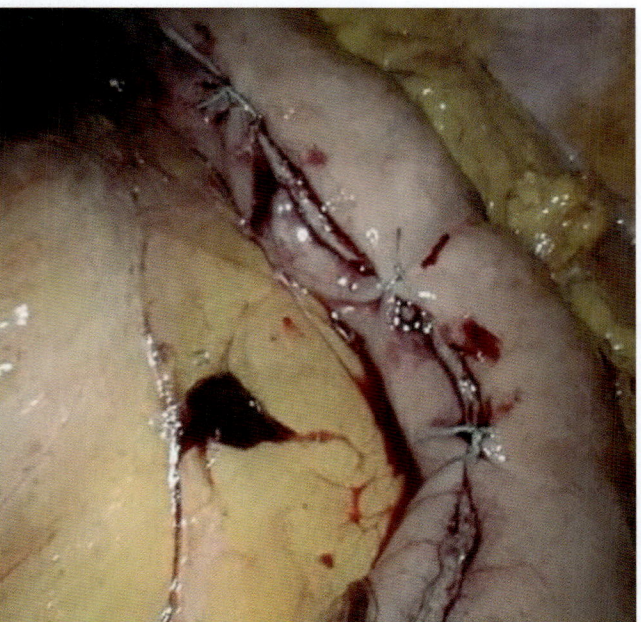

FIGURE 39B.2 The gastric conduit is completely mobilized and tubulized to ensure adequate length. Interrupted stitches are used to reinforce the staple line without shortening the conduit and help with gauging conduit length during the thoracic phase. The conduit is left undivided at the fundus to allow easy retrieval from the chest.

important to obtain transposition of the conduit within the chest without tension on the anastomosis. A Kocher maneuver is not routinely performed to avoid conduit redundancy, which may cause herniation of the gastric antrum and duodenum in the mediastinum. After the stomach is completely mobilized, a transhiatal dissection of the esophagus is performed, exposing and carefully removing the paracardial and lower paraesophageal nodes, which are harder to expose from the chest. A Penrose drain is used to encircle the distal esophagus for retraction, and it is left in the mediastinum to help the esophageal dissection during the thoracic phase.

Pyloric drainage can be achieved either with pyloromyotomy or with a pyloroplasty. Our preference is to use botulinum toxin (Botox) percutaneously injected into the pylorus in both the gastric and duodenal side. This technique has shown good results and is very quick to perform.[13]

A 5-cm-wide gastric tube is created by dividing the stomach with multiple firings of a linear stapler, starting below the incisura to allow complete unfurling of the stomach (Fig. 39B.2). Interrupted Lembert sutures can be used to reinforce the gastric staple line and as a way of measuring conduit length after the conduit has been transposed in the chest. To facilitate retrieval from the chest and avoid torsion, the gastric conduit is left undivided at the fundus. Several studies reported an increase risk of ischemia and leak with a too-narrow diameter (3 to 4 cm) of the gastric tube[14]; however, leaving the entire stomach can lead to severe regurgitation and offers limited length for chest transposition.[3] A 12-French feeding jejunostomy is inserted percutaneously with a Seldinger technique and is fixed to the abdominal wall with five transfascial sutures.

THORACIC PHASE

The patient is positioned in a left lateral decubitus, and the right lung is collapsed. A right video-assisted thoracoscopic surgery (VATS) approach with four trocars and CO_2 insufflation is used. Insufflation at 8 mm Hg is well tolerated and allows flattening of the diaphragm with easier exposure of the hiatus and stabilization of the mediastinum during dissection. An alternative choice in the thoracic phase is the prone positioning. Several authors favor this approach, which offers a good view of the operating field without collapse of the right lung and report shorter anesthesia time and better postoperative respiratory function than the standard left lateral decubitus.[15] We find that this prone approach requires training to identify anatomic structures and their relationship from an unusual perspective and also makes it harder to perform a stapled anastomosis because the space between the ribs gets tighter closer to the spine.

After dividing the pulmonary ligament to the level of the inferior pulmonary vein to allow the lung to fall anteriorly, the posterior mediastinal pleura is opened from the hiatus up to the level of the azygos vein. The azygos vein is divided with a vascular stapler to allow exposure of the entire esophagus. The Penrose drain left around the esophagus is retrieved and used to retract the esophagus and facilitate dissection. The esophagus and periesophageal soft tissues are dissected en bloc from the pericardium, aorta, airways, and contralateral pleura. Once freed up from its circumferential attachments, the esophagus is divided at the thoracic inlet with a stapler (Fig. 39B.3) and the proximal margin is sent for frozen-section pathologic evaluation to rule out cancer or Barrett mucosa. We then perform a complete infracarinal lymphadenectomy. For squamous cell histology or tumors located in the

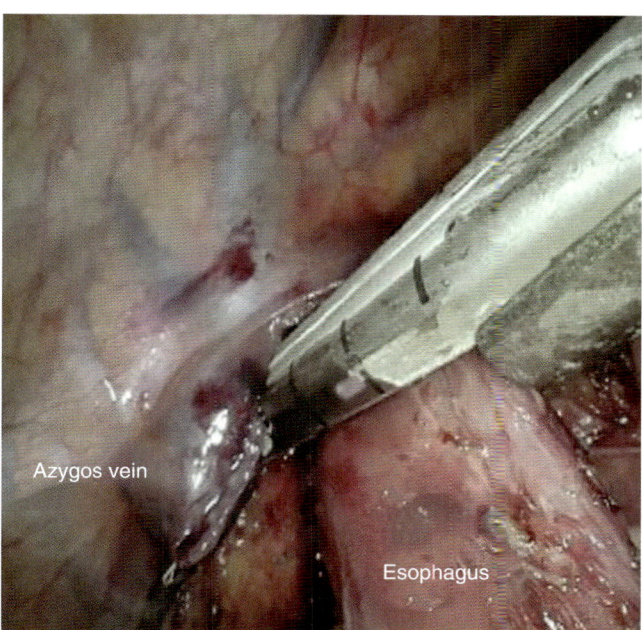

FIGURE 39B.3 The esophagus is completely mobilized to the thoracic inlet and divided with an endoscopic stapler. The esophageal stump is completely freed up from the trachea and the other mediastinal structures.

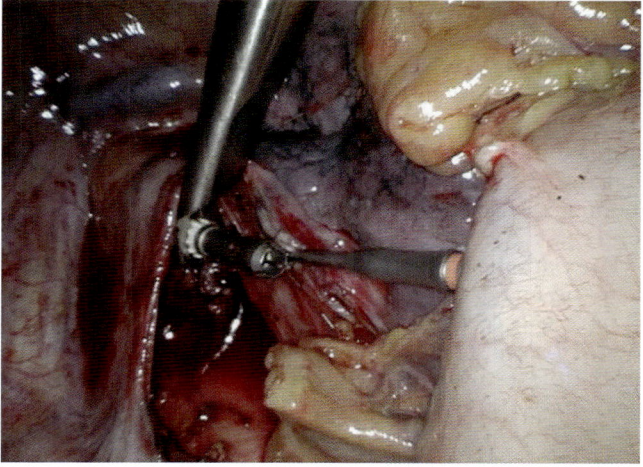

FIGURE 39B.4 The Orvil is engaged with a circular mechanical stapler to complete the anastomosis along the greater curvature of the gastric conduit.

midesophagus or higher, the lymphadenectomy is extended to the paratracheal nodal stations. A cervical anastomosis is also considered in these cases.

The gastric conduit is then pulled up into the chest and completely divided from the esophagus with a linear stapler. It is extremely important that the gastric tube has a proper orientation to avoid spiraling or twisting of the conduit. The inferomedial port site is extended up to approximately 3 cm and a wound protector is placed to allow the retrieval of the specimen and the introduction of a circular stapler in the chest. The specimen is removed into a bag through the wound protector and sent for pathologic analysis of the gastric margin. The operation is completed with an intrathoracic anastomosis (Fig. 39B.4).

Several different intrathoracic anastomoses have been performed with MIE; these include both handsewn and stapled techniques. Transthoracic circular, transoral circular, and side-to-side linear stapled are among the most common mechanical anastomoses.

Transoral circular stapler: This is our preferred approach. The Orvil is inserted through the patient's mouth into the esophageal stump. The orogastric tube connected with the anvil is passed through a small opening next to the staple line and removed through one of the trocars. After transposing the conduit into the posterior mediastinum, we use fluorescence imaging and indocyanine green to evaluate the microvascular perfusion to target our anastomoses. Correct assessment of the gastric conduit length is also necessary to avoid either an excessive tension on the anastomosis or twisting and folding of the distal stomach above the diaphragm and impairment in gastric emptying.[16]

The EEA (Covidien; Minneapolis, Minnesota) stapler is introduced through an opening made in the proximal gastric conduit. The conduit is pulled over the stapler to allow the piston to come out next to the greater curvature of the stomach in the area chosen for the anastomoses. The anvil and the stapler are engaged, and the stapler is fired to complete the anastomosis. We most often use the largest Orvil (25 mm), and due to the esophageal thickness we prefer using the green stapler (4.8-mm staples). Using a linear stapler, the excess gastric tip is resected, leaving at least 1 cm of tissue between this staple line and the anastomosis. To protect the anastomosis posteriorly and avoid fistulization into the airways in case of leakage, the greater fat pad is positioned between the conduit and the airways. Finally, to avoid abdominal organ herniation into the chest, the gastric conduit is bound to the right diaphragm by an interrupted suture.

Transthoracic end-to-side anastomosis using a circular stapler: With this technique, a 25- or 28-mm anvil is placed into the esophageal stump from the operating field, and the stump is tightly closed around the anvil with a purse string. The anastomosis is then completed in the same fashion as explained earlier.

Intrathoracic side-to-side anastomosis using a linear stapler: The proximal stump of the esophagus and the gastric conduit are aligned with the esophagus coming over the stomach. The esophageal stump can be left completely open or closed with a stapler. The stapler is introduced through a small gastrostomy placed next to the greater curve, approximately 5 or 6 cm away from the top of the gastric conduit. If the esophagus was divided with a stapler, a small esophagostomy is performed in the middle of the esophageal stump to introduce the stapler. The side-to-side anastomosis is then completed with an Endo GIA stapler. The common enterotomy can be closed with a linear stapler (a longer anastomosis is required in this case) or with interrupted stitches or running suture.

A stapled anastomosis is often preferred with the Ivor Lewis approach and has been shown to be associated with lower incidence of stricture (especially with the linear stapling).[17] The circular anastomosis is usually quicker to perform and does not require a long esophageal stump.[18] Although with distal esophageal cancer the proximal margin of resection is often not a problem to obtain, we prefer to place the anastomosis above the azygos vein so that there is not much redundant stomach within the abdomen, which can predispose to severe gastroesophageal reflux.

For patients with a proximal thoracic tumor located near the airways or with extensive Barrett esophagus or if there is a concern with obtaining a proximal margin free of tumor, a modified McKeown esophagectomy or three-hole esophagectomy with a cervical anastomosis may represent a better option.

MCKEOWN MINIMALLY INVASIVE ESOPHAGECTOMY

This approach is often the preferred approach when transitioning from open to minimally invasive techniques because the intrathoracic anastomosis is the most challenging portion of the Ivor Lewis approach. It is also a better choice for cervical and upper thoracic esophageal cancers, patients with a long-segment Barrett esophagus, and patients with multifocal disease.

A minimally invasive three-hole esophagectomy involves a thoracoscopic esophageal mobilization, followed by a laparoscopic creation of the gastric conduit and a cervical anastomosis. Mediastinal and abdominal lymphadenectomy are also performed with this technique. Analyzing patients with stage T1 and T2 esophageal squamous cell carcinoma, Ye et al. reported a similar lymph node dissection with MIE as with open surgery. The advantage of this approach is the improved proximal margin; the disadvantages are a higher rate of recurrent laryngeal nerve injury and anastomotic leak.[19]

TRANSHIATAL MINIMALLY INVASIVE ESOPHAGECTOMY

Transhiatal esophagectomy (THE) offers the advantage of resection—avoiding the morbidity associated with thoracotomy[20]; however, this technique is losing popularity because only an abdominal and limited periesophageal lymphadenectomy are possible with this approach. Moreover, a transthoracic approach should be preferred in cases of large tumors of the middle esophagus, tumors abutting the airway or mediastinal vasculature, and patients with suspected mediastinal fibrosis.[4,21] The operation involves an abdominal laparoscopic approach for the preparation of the gastric conduit and abdominal lymphadenectomy and a transhiatal dissection of the esophagus. The diaphragm is often enlarged to expose the mediastinum, and under direct vision, the surgeon proceeds with esophageal dissection within the posterior mediastinum, usually as high as the carina. The proximal esophagus is usually identified through a left cervical incision and divided with a stapler. The transected esophagus is then inverted and pulled into the abdominal cavity by retracting on a Penrose sutured

to the proximal end. After the specimen is retrieved from the abdomen, the gastric conduit is pulled up into the neck through the posterior mediastinum and anastomosed to the cervical esophagus. The anastomoses can be done with handsewn or stapled techniques (usually linear stapler).

The minimally invasive approach as compared with open THE offers a superior visualization of the mediastinum. The magnified visualization by the laparoscopic camera associated with a less "blind" dissection may account for decreased blood loss and transfusion rates.[22,23] Decreased rates of respiratory complication, a shorter hospital and intensive care unit stay, faster return of bowel function, and lower costs have also been reported.[23,24]

LAPAROSCOPIC HAND-ASSISTED ESOPHAGECTOMY

An alternative or intermediate approach to a complete minimally invasive technique is the use of hand-assisted laparoscopic surgery (HALS), where a hand access device (Lap Disc) is placed into a 7-cm midline incision and the surgeon can use laparoscopic instruments as well as the assistance of his or her hand. The advantage of the tactile sensation with the surgeon's hand facilitates gentle manipulation, blunt dissection, leading to a quicker operation. This approach was also associated with lower rate of complication and short recovery and may represent an adjunctive tool for training surgeons to minimally invasive surgery.[25]

ROBOTIC ESOPHAGECTOMY

Despite the progress achieved with laparoscopy and thoracoscopy, MIE has still several intrinsic limitations, including a two-dimensional view and a decreased freedom of movement that can cause some difficulties, especially during the thoracoscopic phase, due to the rigidity of the chest cavity. Robotic systems have been used to overcome some of these limitations offering three-dimensional views, wristlike range of motion, and innovative tools. Data suggest the robotic approach for esophageal resection to be safe and feasible and easier to use for some surgeons than the laparoscopic/thoracoscopic alternative; although definitive results regarding oncologic efficacy are limited, perioperative outcomes are similar to other techniques for MIE and open surgery.[26]

RESULTS

Potential outcome benefits have been reported with MIE when compared with open surgery.

SURGICAL OUTCOMES

As with other minimally invasive procedures, avoiding a thoracotomy and/or a laparotomy, MIE minimizes postoperative pain, allows for a faster recovery, decreases the risk of wound infection, cardiopulmonary complications, blood loss, and length of hospital stay. Several prospective and retrospective studies have shown that perioperative outcomes are positively affected by a minimally invasive approach.[27-32]

Pulmonary complication rate—in particular pneumonia and acute respiratory distress syndrome (ARDS)—has been shown to decrease with MIE.[30-34] There are several reasons why this may occur: smaller incisions and avoiding rib spreading significantly reduce postoperative pain, lung contusion is minimized as retraction of the right lung is no longer necessary, and occasionally single lung ventilation can be avoided by using a prone position.[3-] This option is particularly valuable in patients with severely impaired lung function because avoiding total lung collapse reduces arteriovenous shunts, preserving better oxygenation and decreasing the risk of pulmonary infection.[30] The immune system seems to also play an important role: improved leukocyte counts, interleukin (IL)-8 levels, and stress response were in fact observed in patients who underwent MIE.[36]

In a recent meta-analysis including 15,790 esophagectomies, MIE was associated with significantly higher operative time but significantly shorter hospital stay, mortality, and overall morbidity. Most of the morbidity advantage with MIE was attributable to pulmonary and cardiovascular complications, which were significantly lower for MIE, whereas gastrointestinal complications, anastomotic leak rate, and recurrent laryngeal nerve injury were similar in both groups.[37]

In contrast, a recent analysis of the Society of Thoracic Surgeons National Database showed equivalent rates of mortality and overall morbidity in both open and MIEs but significantly higher rates of empyema and reoperations in the MIE group.[38]

Only one randomized controlled study has published its results so far and showed significantly decreased respiratory complications, shorter length of hospital stay, and improved short-term quality of life with MIE.[30] One year follow-up of the TIME-trial showed a similar rate of late complications among the groups and improved 1-year quality of life for MIE patients.[28]

ONCOLOGIC AND SURVIVAL OUTCOMES

Several retrospective studies showed oncologic equivalence between MIE and open esophagectomy.[39,40] In some cases a higher lymph node harvest has been reported with MIE,[40,41] and this might be explained by a magnified visualization using the laparoscopic and thoracoscopic camera during lymphadenectomy.[42]

The adequacy of the resected margins is still a controversial topic, with no definitive results in the literature. Most of the studies showed that there are no differences in the ability to achieve a complete tumor resection (R0) between open esophagectomy and MIE.[41,43-45]

Survival outcomes are being investigated in several ongoing trials.[46,47] A recent 3-year follow-up of the TIME-trial[48] showed similar survival outcomes in patients who underwent MIE or open esophagectomy for cancer with a 36% disease-free 3-year survival in the open group versus 40% in the MIE group.[48]

In conclusion, MIE is feasible and safe. The operation is technically challenging but can offer reduced morbidity, faster recovery, improved short-term quality of life yet with similar oncologic results to the open approach.

REFERENCES

1. Cuschieri A, Shimi S, Banting S. Endoscopic oesophagectomy through a right thoracoscopic approach. *J R Coll Surg Edinb.* 1992;37:7-11.
2. DePaula AL, Hashiba K, Ferriera EAB, et al. Laparoscopic transhiatal esophagectomy with esophagogastroplasty. *Surg Laparosc Endosc.* 1995;5:1-5.
3. Luketich JD, Alvero-Rivera M, Christie NA, et al. Minimally invasive esophagectomy. *Ann Thorac Surg.* 2000;70:906-911.
4. Grimm JC, Valero V, Molena D. Surgical indications and optimization of patients for resectable esophageal malignancies. *J Thorac Dis.* 2014;6(3):249-257.
5. Dhamija A, Rosen JE, Dhamija A, et al. Learning curve to lymph node resection in minimally invasive esophagectomy for cancer. *Innovations.* 2014;9:286-291.
6. Guo W, Zou YB, Ma Z, et al. One surgeon's learning curve for video-assisted thoracoscopic esophagectomy for esophageal cancer with the patient in lateral position: how many cases are needed to reach competence? *Surg Endosc.* 2013;27:1346-1352.
7. Tapias LF, Morse CR. Minimally invasive Ivor Lewis esophagectomy: description of a learning curve. *J Am Coll Surg.* 2014;218(6):1130-1140.
8. Osugi H, Takemura M, Higashino M, et al. Learning curve of video-assisted thoracoscopic esophagectomy and extensive lymphadenectomy for squamous cell cancer of the thoracic esophagus and results. *Surg Endosc.* 2003;17(3):515-519.
9. Hardwick RH. *Association of Upper Gastrointestinal Surgeons, Association of Laparoscopic Surgeons. A Consensus View and Recommendations on the Development and Practice of Minimally Invasive Oesophagectomy.* London: AUGIS; 2008 http://www.augis.org/wp-content/uploads/2014/05/MIO_Consensus.pdf. Accessed April 2017.
10. Noble F, Kelly JJ, Bailey IS, et al. South Coast Cancer Collaboration Oesophago-Gastric. A prospective comparison of totally minimally invasive versus open Ivor Lewis esophagectomy. *Dis Esophagus.* 2013;26:263-271.
11. Mungo B, Lidor AO, Stem M, et al. Early experience and lessons learned in a new minimally invasive esophagectomy program. *Surg Endosc.* 2016;30:1692-1698.
12. Watson DI, Davies N, Jamieson GG. Totally endoscopic Ivor Lewis esophagectomy. *Surg Endosc.* 1999;13(3):293-297.
13. Martin JT, Federico JA, McKelvey AA, et al. Prevention of delayed gastric emptying after esophagectomy: a single center's experience with botulinum toxin. *Ann Thorac Surg.* 2009;87:1708-1713.
14. Berrisford RG, Wajed SA, Sanders D, et al. Short-term outcomes following total minimally invasive oesophagectomy. *Br J Surg.* 2008;95:602-610.
15. Palanivelu C, Prakash A, Senthilkumar R, et al. Minimally invasive esophagectomy: thoracoscopic mobilization of the esophagus and mediastinal lymphadenectomy in prone position: experience of 130 patients. *J Am Coll Surg.* 2006;203(1):7-16.
16. Tsai WS, Levy RM, Luketich JD. Technique of minimally invasive Ivor-Lewis esophagectomy. *Oper Tech Thorac Cardiovasc Surg.* 2009;14:176-192.
17. Blackmon SH, Correa AM, Wynn B, et al. Propensity-matched analysis of three techniques for intrathoracic esophagogastric anastomosis. *Ann Thorac Surg.* 2007;83:1805-1813.
18. Irino T, Tsai JA, Ericson J, et al. Thoracoscopic side-to-side esophagogastrostomy by use of linear stapler—a simplified technique facilitating a minimally invasive Ivor-Lewis operation. *Langenbecks Arch Surg.* 2016;401:315-322.
19. Ye B, Zhong C, Yang Y, et al. Lymph node dissection in esophageal carcinoma: minimally invasive esophagectomy vs open surgery. *World J Gastroenterol.* 2016;22(19):4750-4756.
20. Macha M, Whyte RI. The current role of transhiatal esophagectomy. *Chest Surg Clin N Am.* 2000;10:499-518.
21. Perry Y, Fernando HC. Three-field minimally invasive esophagectomy: current results technique. *J Thorac Cardiovasc Surg.* 2012;144:S63-S66.
22. Cash JC, Zehetner J, Hedayati B, et al. Outcomes following laparoscopic transhiatal esophagectomy for esophageal cancer. *Surg Endosc.* 2014;28:492-499. doi:10.1007/s00464-013-3230-y.
23. Ecker BL, Savulionyte GE, Datta J, et al. Laparoscopic transhiatal esophagectomy improves hospital outcomes and reduces cost: a single-institution analysis of laparoscopic-assisted and open techniques. *Surg Endosc.* 2016;30:2535-2542.

24. Bhayani NH, Gupta A, Dunst CM, et al. Esophagectomy with thoracic incisions carry increased pulmonary morbidity. *JAMA Surg.* 2013;148(8):733-738.

25. Suzuki Y, Urashima M, Ishibashi Y, et al. Hand-assisted laparoscopic and thoracoscopic surgery (HALTS) in radical esophagectomy with three-field lymphadenectomy for thoracic esophageal cancer. *Eur J Surg Oncol.* 2005;31:1166-1174.

26. Huang L, Onaitis M. Minimally invasive and robotic Ivor Lewis esophagectomy. *J Thorac Dis.* 2014;6(S3):S314-S321.

27. Tapias LF, Mathisen DJ, Wright CD, et al. Outcomes with open and minimally invasive Ivor Lewis esophagectomy after neoadjuvant therapy. *Ann Thorac Surg.* 2016;101(3):1097-1103.

28. Maas KW, Cuesta MA, van Berge Henegouwen MI, et al. Quality of life and late complication after minimally invasive compared to open esophagectomy: results of a randomized trial. *World J Surg.* 2015;39(8):1986-1993.

29. Luketich JD, Pennathur A, Franchetti Y, et al. Minimally invasive esophagectomy: results of a prospective phase II multicenter trial—the Eastern Cooperative Oncology Group (E2202) study. *Ann Surg.* 2015;261(4):702-707.

30. Biere SS, van Berge Henegouwen MI, Maas KW, et al. Minimally invasive versus open oesophagectomy for patients with oesophageal cancer: a multicenter, open-label, randomised controlled trial. *Lancet.* 2012;379:1887-1892.

31. Lv L, Hu W, Ren Y, et al. Minimally invasive esophagectomy versus open esophagectomy for esophageal cancer: a meta-analysis. *Onco Targets Ther.* 2016;9:6751-6762.

32. Gurusamy KS, Pallari E, Midya S, et al. Laparoscopic versus open transhiatal oesophagectomy for oesophageal cancer. *Cochrane Database Syst Rev.* 2016;(3):CD011390.

33. Wang H, Yaxing S, Mingxiang F, et al. Outcomes, quality of life, and survival after esophagectomy for squamous cell carcinoma: a propensity score-match comparison of operative approaches. *J Thorac Cardiovasc Surg.* 2015;149:1006-1015.

34. Luketich J, Alvero-Rivera M, Buenaventura PO, et al. Minimally invasive esophagectomy. Outcomes in 222 patients. *Ann Surg.* 2003;238:486-495.

35. Mao T, Fang W, Gu Z, et al. Comparison of perioperative outcomes between open and minimally invasive esophagectomy for esophageal cancer. *Thorac Cancer.* 2015;6:303-306.

36. Maas KW, Biere SS, Van Hoogstraten IM, et al. Immunological changes after minimally invasive or conventional esophageal resection for cancer. A randomized trial. *World J Surg.* 2014;38(1):131-137. doi:10.1007/s00268-013-2233-0.

37. Yibulayin W, Abulizi S, Lv H, et al. Minimally invasive oesophagectomy versus open esophagectomy for resectable esophageal cancer: a meta-analysis. *World J Surg Oncol.* 2016;14:304.

38. Sihag S, Kosinski S, Gaissert HA, et al. Minimally invasive versus open esophagectomy for esophageal cancer: a comparison of early surgical outcomes from the Society of Thoracic Surgeons national database. *Ann Thorac Surg.* 2016;101:1281-1289.

39. Dantoc MM, Cox MR, Eslick GD. Does minimally invasive esophagectomy (MIE) provide for comparable oncologic outcomes to open techniques? A systematic review. *J Gastrointest Surg.* 2012;16(3):486-494.

40. Dolan JP, Kaur T, Diggs BS, et al. Impact of comorbidity on outcomes and overall survival after open and minimally invasive esophagectomy for locally advanced esophageal cancer. *Surg Endosc.* 2013;27(11):4094-4103.

41. Palazzo F, Rosato E, Chaudhary A, et al. Minimally invasive esophagectomy provides significant advantage compared with open or hybrid esophagectomy for patient with cancer of the esophagus and gastroesophageal junction. *J Am Coll Surg.* 2015;4:672-679.

42. Shen Y, Zhang Y, Tan L, et al. Extensive mediastinal lymphadenectomy during minimally invasive esophagectomy: optimal results from a single center. *J Gastrointest Surg.* 2012;16:715-721.

43. Sihag S, Wright CD, Wain JC, et al. Comparison of perioperative outcomes following open versus minimally invasive Ivor Lewis oesophagectomy at a single, high-volume centre. *Eur J Cardiothorac Surg.* 2012;42:430-437.

44. Sudarshan M, Ferri L. A critical review of minimally invasive esophagectomy. *Surg Laparosc Endosc Percutan Tech.* 2012;22(4):310-318.

45. Sundaram A, Geronimo JC, Willer BL, et al. Survival and quality of life after minimally invasive esophagectomy: a single surgeon experience. *Surg Endosc.* 2012;26(1):168-176.

46. Briez N, Piessen G, Bonnetain F, et al. Open versus laparoscopically-assisted oesophagectomy for cancer: a multicenter randomized controlled phase III trial—the MIRO trial. *BMC Cancer.* 2011;11:310.

47. Avery KN, Metcalfe C, Berrisford R, et al. The feasibility of a randomized controlled trial of esophagectomy for esophageal cancer—the ROMIO (Randomized Oesophagectomy: Minimally Invasive or Open) study: protocol for a randomized control trial. *Trials.* 2014;15:2000.

48. Straatman J, van der Wielen N, Cuesta MA, et al. Minimally invasive versus open esophagectomy resection. Three-year follow-up of the previously reported randomized controlled trial: the TIME trial. *Ann Surg.* 2017;266(2):232-236.

Surgical Approaches to Remove the Esophagus: Vagal-Sparing

Steven R. DeMeester

To date, no therapy has been proven superior to esophagectomy for the cure of patients with early-stage esophageal cancer. The primary goal of surgery is complete (R0) resection of the tumor to maximize the opportunity for cure and minimize the incidence of local recurrence. However, with early-stage disease and a high likelihood of long-term survival, there is an increasing focus on postesophagectomy quality of life, especially since there are endoscopic alternatives for these early lesions. This has prompted us to scale back the extent of the resection and preserve the vagal nerves to try to provide the benefits of complete resection, while minimizing some of the morbidity associated with esophagectomy in appropriate candidates.

WHY A VAGAL-SPARING ESOPHAGECTOMY?

An esophagectomy is a major operation associated with significant perioperative and long-term physiologic alterations. During the procedure, the dissection, typically involving the mediastinum and the abdomen, leads to extensive third spacing and volume shifts in the perioperative period. These volume shifts frequently produce hemodynamic alterations and in some patients cardiopulmonary compromise. Later, the gastrointestinal alterations associated with esophagectomy and reconstruction often include dumping, diarrhea, early satiety, and gastroesophageal reflux symptoms. A laparoscopic vagal-sparing esophagectomy minimizes the dissection associated with an esophagectomy, since the esophagus is stripped out of the mediastinum without formal dissection. In addition, many of the gastrointestinal alterations associated with an esophagectomy are secondary to division of the vagus nerves, and vagal preservation minimizes dumping, diarrhea, and depending on the type of reconstruction early satiety and reflux symptoms compared with other types of esophagectomy and reconstruction.[1,2] Lastly, the technique for a vagal-sparing esophagectomy with gastric pull-up allows preservation of the left gastric arterial trunk and branches to the pylorus. This improves the perfusion of the proximal portion of the graft and may reduce anastomotic leaks and stenosis.

INDICATIONS FOR A VAGAL-SPARING ESOPHAGECTOMY

A vagal-sparing procedure should be considered in any patient with a benign process such as end-stage achalasia or gastroesophageal reflux disease, in patients with high-grade dysplasia in squamous mucosa or Barrett esophagus,

and in patients with esophageal cancer limited to the mucosa. Importantly, a vagal-sparing procedure is only applicable to patients with intramucosal tumors and no evidence of lymphadenopathy since preserving the vagus nerves precludes the ability to perform an adequate lymphadenectomy along the left gastric artery and in the periesophageal mediastinal tissues. Therefore a biopsy showing cancer in an area of nodularity or ulceration requires initial endoscopic resection to confirm that the tumor is limited to the mucosa.[3] Submucosal tumors have a significant risk for lymph node metastases and tumor invasion into this layer is a contraindication for a vagal-sparing approach. Relative contraindications to a vagal-sparing esophagectomy include the presence of an esophageal stricture, history of caustic injury to the esophagus, or prior antireflux or esophageal surgery (repair of perforation or congenital trachea-esophageal fistula) since in these circumstances mediastinal scaring may prohibit safe stripping of the esophagus or may lead to vagal disruption even if the stripping is accomplished safely. Further, diabetes or evidence of impaired gastric emptying should be considered a relative contraindication for a vagal-sparing procedure using a colon interposition to the intact stomach. Lastly, prior gastric surgery such as a pyloroplasty may preclude an advantage to preserving the vagal nerves, although even in this setting avoidance of postvagotomy diarrhea may be a sufficient reason to spare the vagus nerves, if possible.

SURGICAL APPROACH

A vagal-sparing esophagectomy with gastric pull-up has some similarities to a transhiatal operation, except the esophagus is stripped out of the mediastinum and no mediastinal or transhiatal dissection is done, and the left gastric arterial trunk is preserved, along with vagal innervation to the pylorus. The operation commences in the abdomen, and with a minimum of dissection, the hiatus is opened and the anterior and posterior vagal trunks are encircled with a vessel loop. The vagus nerves are retracted gently toward the patient's right, and the gastroesophageal fat pad is dissected, beginning on the left of the esophagus and stomach, such that it allows the anterior vagus nerve to be brought well over to the right of the esophagus. Failure to do this step will lead in most cases to inadvertent injury of the anterior vagus nerve during the subsequent steps of the procedure. Once the anterior vagus is safely over to the right of the esophagus, a highly selective vagotomy is performed starting just above the crow's foot near the antrum of the stomach. This is necessary if the stomach is to be used as the esophageal replacement, and is beneficial with a colon interposition to reduce gastric acidity and the potential for ulceration in the colon graft. The highly selective vagotomy precisely follows the lesser curve of the stomach up to the point where the distal esophagus is reached and the vagal nerve trunks are completely separated from the esophagus. This dissection is facilitated by sequential grasping of the stomach with Babcock clamps along the lesser curve, and by using an advanced energy source in this very vascular area. Avoidance of a hematoma or bleeding during this dissection is critical to prevent unintended injury to the distal vagal branches.

At this point, the gastroesophageal junction should be completely exposed and the lesser curve above the crow's foot skeletonized. If the stomach is to be used for esophageal replacement, then the greater curve is mobilized in the same fashion as for a standard gastric pull-up. However, if the colon is to be used then there is no need to mobilize the greater curve completely. Instead, the omentum is detached from the transverse colon and a window created near the left crus by dividing the most proximal one or two short gastric and posterior pancreaticogastric vessels. This creates a passage from the lesser sac to the hiatus for the colon graft. The colon is mobilized in standard fashion based on the ascending branch of the left colic artery whenever possible.[4] The necessary length of colon is marked out by measuring the distance from the tip of the left ear to the xiphoid anteriorly with an umbilical tape, and then marking a similar distance on the colon starting from the point where the left colic vessels tether the graft and going proximally. The colon can then be divided and placed in the pelvis for later use.

Next, attention is directed to the left neck. The esophagus is exposed, and after placing a Penrose drain around the esophagus to facilitate traction, blunt dissection is accomplished with a finger to free the upper mediastinal portion of the esophagus, a nasogastric tube is inserted, and the esophagus is irrigated with a dilute povidone-iodine (Betadine) solution to reduce mediastinal contamination during the subsequent stripping procedure. The nasogastric tube is then removed. Next, a gastrotomy is made near the gastroesophageal junction, or alternatively the cardia is divided with a stapler and a small portion of the staple line is opened to provide access to the esophageal lumen. A standard vein stripper is then passed retrograde up the esophagus and brought out the anterior wall of the cervical esophagus, as distally as possible. The esophagus is ligated distal to the exit site of the vein stripper in the neck using a heavy suture, and the cervical esophagus is divided at the site where the vein stripper comes out. The divided distal end of the esophagus is then suture ligated and tied securely. The use of several Endoloops can facilitate secure ligation of the esophagus around the vein stripper head. This is a critical step since, if the ligatures slip, the vein stripper will merely pull out, leaving the partially stripped esophagus somewhere in the mediastinum. After changing the vein stripper to the large head, the esophagus is inverted on itself by pulling the vein stripper from below. It is useful to leave a long umbilical tape tied to the distal end of the cervical esophagus to provide access to the tract in the posterior

mediastinum after the esophagus has been removed. The esophagus comes out inverted with the mucosa external to the muscular wall similar to taking off a sock inside-out. In general, bleeding is minimal, and very little force is required to pull the esophagus out. Resistance should raise concern, and excessive resistance should prompt conversion to a transhiatal procedure.

Importantly, in patients with high-grade dysplasia or intramucosal cancer, all layers of the esophagus are stripped out so as not to inadvertently leave any dysplastic mucosa or tumor behind. However, in patients with achalasia, only the mucosa need be stripped out. This is accomplished in a similar fashion, except a cervical esophageal myotomy is made and the mucosa alone is encircled with a heavy tie, leaving the remaining muscular wall of the esophagus intact. After carefully securing the mucosal tie around the vein stripper, the mucosa can be stripped out from below, leaving the muscular wall of the esophagus in place. This works nicely through a gastrotomy high on the anterior fundus of the stomach. The mucosa is stapled off just distal to the squamocolumnar junction, and the anterior gastrotomy is closed.

The next step is to dilate the mediastinal tract to prevent constriction of the graft. I sequentially dilate the tract using a 90 cc balloon Foley catheter progressively filled with saline and pulled up through the mediastinum. Typically two to three passes are made to ensure an adequate tract is created. This is particularly important in patients who have a normal-caliber esophagus at the time of stripping. The graft can then be brought up through the posterior mediastinal tract.

When a gastric pull-up is being used, the stomach is tubularized in standard fashion, leaving the crow's foot intact. The gastric tube is then pulled up through the posterior mediastinum and an esophagogastric anastomosis is constructed in standard fashion. The vascular supply of the gastric tube is typically excellent, since the left gastric artery has been preserved and only the branches to the skeletonized lesser curve region were divided. This usually leaves several branches intact to the antrum, and in combination with preserved right gastric and gastroepiploic arteries, this leads to excellent graft perfusion in most patients. After completing the cervical anastomosis, the graft is gently pulled into the abdomen to eliminate redundancy and sutured to the crura to prevent herniation of abdominal organs into the mediastinum. At this point, the operation is complete with the exception of passing a nasogastric tube and placing a feeding jejunostomy tube. Since the antral innervation has been preserved, no pyloroplasty should be performed.

When a gastric pull-up is planned, the vagal-sparing procedure is readily adapted to a fully laparoscopic approach. The gastric mobilization as well as the highly selective vagotomy are straightforward laparoscopic procedures. I have found that the use of a 4-cm incision in the midline with placement of a hand port facilitates stripping the esophagus out (via the hand port) and subsequent dilatation of the mediastinal tract. The graft is pulled up attached to a chest tube, and the cervical esophagogastric anastomosis is accomplished in standard fashion. Similar to an open procedure, the gastric tube should be sutured to the left crus to prevent torsion of the graft or herniation of abdominal organs into the posterior mediastinum.

When a colon graft is used with preservation of the intact, innervated stomach, there are several important technical considerations. First, only the cardia immediately below the gastroesophageal junction is excised, leaving the remaining stomach in place. A highly selective vagotomy is performed along the lesser curvature to reduce acid secretion and provide protection from the development of cologastric anastomotic ulcers. There is no need to do an extensive mobilization of the greater curvature. Instead, only the proximalmost one to two short gastric vessels, along with the posterior pancreaticoduodenal vessels, are divided, so that there is an approximately 10 cm window created near the left crus of the diaphragm. Importantly, the colon graft is passed up *posterior* to the stomach through this window, into the hiatus, and then up through the posterior mediastinum. In patients with achalasia, where only the mucosa was stripped out through an anterior gastrotomy, the entire muscular tube of the native esophagus remains intact, and a sufficient-sized hole must be cut into the residual muscular tube along the left lateral aspect near the hiatus to allow the colon graft to be pulled up inside. If all layers of the esophagus have been stripped out, as in patients with high-grade dysplasia or intramucosal cancer, then that issue does not exist since the muscular wall of the esophagus is gone and only the mediastinal tract is present at the hiatus. The esophago-colo anastomosis is done either with a stapled or hand-sewn technique in an end-to-end fashion. If the muscular tube of the esophagus has been preserved, it can be pulled up like a sheath to cover the anastomosis proximally. The colon is then pulled firmly down into the abdomen to eliminate any redundancy and sutured to the left crus of the diaphragm to prevent twisting of the graft or herniation of abdominal contents into the mediastinum. In particular, sutures should be placed between the colon graft and the posterior aspect of the hiatus near crural decussation since herniation can occur underneath the colon graft if these sutures are omitted.

The colon is divided approximately 10 to 15 cm distal to the hiatus, taking care not to injure the vascular arcade.

A stapled cologastric anastomosis is then done to the proximal posterior fundus, using a 75-mm GIA stapler, and a nasogastric tube is guided into the stomach. Next, the colocolostomy is accomplished in standard fashion, with care taken to avoid traction on the left colic vessels or the marginal artery supplying the graft. Typically this requires that the right colon be brought up into the left upper quadrant. Lastly, the mesenteric defects are closed and a feeding jejunostomy is placed.

CONCLUSION AND SUMMARY

A vagal-sparing esophagectomy is the ideal operation for high-grade dysplasia or cancer confined to the mucosa, and in patients with end-stage benign disease. It is nearly always a "one and done" therapy that eliminates the diseased mucosa and the need for further interventions, and offers reduced side effects and better functional outcome compared with other types of esophagectomy. A vagal-sparing procedure is only an option with patients at low risk for lymph node metastases, since no formal lymphadenectomy is performed. Therefore any nodules or lesions in a patient with Barrett or squamous cell cancer must first undergo endoscopic resection to confirm if they are malignant and to pathologically determine the depth of invasion. Long-term good outcome can be achieved using either the tubularized stomach with pyloric innervation maintained or a colon interposition to the intact, innervated stomach for esophageal replacement.

REFERENCES

1. Banki F, Mason RJ, DeMeester SR, et al. Vagal-sparing esophagectomy: a more physiologic alternative. *Ann Surg.* 2002;236(3):324-335; discussion 335–336.
2. Peyre CG, DeMeester SR, Rizzetto C, et al. Vagal-sparing esophagectomy: the ideal operation for intramucosal adenocarcinoma and Barrett's with high-grade dysplasia. *Ann Surg.* 2007;246:665-674.
3. Greene CL, Worrell SG, Attwood SE, et al. Emerging concepts for the endoscopic management of superficial esophageal adenocarcinoma. *J Gastrointest Surg.* 2016;20(4):851-860.
4. Maish MS, DeMeester SR. Indications and technique of colon and jejunal interpositions for esophageal disease. *Surg Clin North Am.* 2005;85(3):505-514.

Benjamin Wei | Robert J. Cerfolio

The use of minimally invasive esophagectomy (MIE) has increased over the past several years. The term *minimally invasive* can refer to performing either or both the thoracic and abdominal phases of the operation with either laparoscopic or robotic assistance. Transhiatal esophagectomy is another form of MIE that avoids a chest incision. Recent studies have demonstrated that MIE has benefits with decreases in blood loss, chest tube duration, length of stay, and respiratory complications versus open esophagectomy[1-4] and maybe even reduces cost.[5] Melvin et al. were the first to report robotic esophagectomy in 2002.[6] Since then, the use of robotic technology for either/both the abdominal and thoracic phases of the operation, whether a transhiatal, Ivor Lewis, or modified McKeown approach is taken, has become increasingly common.

INDICATIONS

Most candidates for esophagectomy are also candidates for attempted MIE and therefore also candidates for robotic esophagectomy. There are few specific contraindications for the use of robotic technology. The need to perform an en bloc resection of aorta or intrathoracic trachea or carina along with the esophagectomy, which has been safely applied to selected patients, would generally be considered a contraindication to robotic esophagectomy.[7,8] Prior thoracic or abdominal surgery can make a robotic approach more challenging due to the presence of adhesions, but lysis of adhesions can be performed to permit its use. Comorbidities or poor functional status that would otherwise make patients suboptimal candidates for esophagectomy generally would also apply to offering robotic esophagectomy, although robotic esophagectomy may permit surgeons to offer esophagectomy to somewhat older and sicker patients by decreasing the perioperative complication rate (especially respiratory complications).[9] However, caution in patient selection should be applied, as the physiologic effects of complications such as anastomotic leak and chylothorax remain significant regardless of whether they occur in a robotic or open esophagectomy.

Early-stage (T1a and early T1b) esophageal cancers can be managed with endoscopic mucosal resection (EMR). Generally, if a lesion is not amenable to EMR or is T1b or deeper on final pathologic analysis, esophagectomy may be considered. If EMR for early-stage esophageal cancer is performed in the context of Barrett esophagus, radiofrequency ablation (RFA) to promote regression of Barrett should also be considered. Patients with persistent high-grade dysplasia following attempted RFA are also candidates for esophagectomy. Benign indications for esophagectomy include end-stage achalasia or mega-esophagus, refractory stricture, intractable reflux resistant to surgical interventions, and multiple failed hiatal hernia operations.

EQUIPMENT

The Da Vinci Surgical System is currently the only US Food and Drug Administration (FDA)-approved robotic system for surgery. The surgeon sits at a console some distance from the patient, who is positioned on an operating table close to the robotic unit with its four robotic arms. The robotic arms incorporate remote center technology, in which a fixed point in space is defined, and about it the surgical arms move so as to minimize stress on the thoracic or abdominal wall during manipulations. The small proprietary Endowrist instruments attached to the arms are capable of a wide range of high-precision movements. These are controlled by the surgeon's hand movements via "master" instruments at the console. The "master" instruments sense the surgeon's hand movements and translate them electronically into scaled-down micromovements to manipulate the small surgical instruments. Hand tremor is filtered out by a 6-Hz motion filter. The surgeon observes the operating field through console binoculars. The image comes from a maneuverable high-definition stereoscopic camera (endoscope) attached to one of the robot arms. The console also has foot pedals that allow the surgeon to engage and disengage different instrument arms, reposition the console "master" controls without the instruments themselves moving, and activate electric cautery. A second optional console allows tandem surgery and training. Da Vinci currently offers both the Xi and Si systems. The Xi system is newer and features an overhead beam that permits rotation of the instrument arms, allowing for greater flexibility in terms of direction of approach of the robot to the patient. Compared with the Si, the Xi also has thinner instrument arms, longer instruments themselves, and the option to switch the camera to any arm/port.

PREOPERATIVE EVALUATION

A thorough history and physical should be performed, focusing on key points such as Barrett esophagus, gastroesophageal reflux disease, motility disorders such as achalasia, prior surgeries, functional status, and cardiac and respiratory comorbidities. Smoking cessation should be encouraged and alcohol use should be noted to screen for cirrhosis and warn of possible withdrawal issues in the perioperative period. Patients undergoing esophagectomy for neoplasm should receive a whole-body positron emission tomography (PET)-computed tomography (CT) scan to evaluate for possible metastatic disease, unless this is obvious from chest/abdominal CT scans alone. If fairly convincing combined radiologic and clinical evidence exists for metastatic disease (e.g., weight loss, widespread adenopathy or liver/lung nodules), biopsy confirmation of metastatic disease may not be necessary. However, single-site M1 disease should likely be confirmed with tissue diagnosis. Location of tumor, synchronous lesions, and presence/extent of Barrett esophagus should be noted on the preoperative endoscopy. Tumors extending into the proximal stomach may require a partial gastrectomy and different reconstructive approach; tumors in the mid-esophagus should generally be approached via a McKeown type operation rather than Ivor Lewis. An adequate margin may be difficult to achieve for tumors in the proximal one-third of the esophagus; these patients are better suited for definitive chemoradiation, although in some centers, laryngoesophagectomy may be an option. Some investigators have suggested that patients with preoperative dysphagia may not need an endoscopic ultrasound (EUS) given that 90% of them had T3 to T4 disease, a finding that has been corroborated by others.[10,11] However, although the presence of symptoms such as dysphagia is a very specific finding for the presence of a T3 or greater lesion, the absence of symptoms does not necessarily indicate that the patient does not have a T3 or greater lesion. Given that being T3 or deeper and/or the presence of N1 or greater disease dictates the performance of induction chemoradiation at our institution, we also consider EUS a critical part of the preoperative evaluation. Performance of induction chemoradiation for T2N0 lesions is variable. We prefer preoperative therapy since a significant percentage will have nodal disease, although there is a controversy regarding patients who are older than 75 years. Brain imaging is performed if the patient has neurologic symptoms or headaches that are concerning for intracranial metastases. Bronchoscopy is done if the patient has an esophageal cancer of the proximal or middle esophagus to rule out airway invasion. Patients who remain candidates for esophagectomy after the aforementioned testing generally also receive pulmonary function testing and stress testing. No specific diagnostic procedures are performed for robotic esophagectomy per se.

After the completion of induction chemoradiation, restaging PET-CT should be performed. Patients who develop progression of disease or metastases are offered palliative management strategies. Patients who have persistent disease or show a response (complete or partial resolution of fluorodeoxyglucose (FDG) avidity of the lesion on PET-CT scan) are scheduled for esophagectomy from 8 to 12 weeks after the conclusion of chemoradiation, once they have recovered reasonably well from the side effects of induction therapy. Data on the optimal interval between completion of chemoradiation and surgery are mixed. Kim et al. showed no difference in terms of perioperative risk, pathologic response, or overall survival between patients who were resected more than 8 weeks after chemoradiation versus those resected less than 8 weeks after.[12] Lee et al. demonstrated that prolonging the interval after chemoradiation for esophageal adenocarcinoma increased the pathologic complete response rate

to induction therapy; however, this did not translate to survival.[13] Chiu et al., though, found that delayed surgery (defined as >8 weeks after chemoradiation) was associated with decreased 5-year survival for patients with *squamous cell carcinoma* that demonstrated a complete clinical response.[14]

CHOICE OF OPERATION

The abdominal and/or thoracic phase of the esophagectomy can be performed with robotic assistance. Choice of type of esophagectomy (Ivor Lewis, McKeown, or transhiatal) can be surgeon-dependent, with some preferring a neck anastomosis due to the decreased incidence of mediastinal leaks, and others preferring a chest anastomosis due to the risk of recurrent laryngeal nerve injury. Location of the tumor may dictate this decision; for instance, a midthoracic tumor is best suited for resection of the entire intrathoracic esophagus with a neck anastomosis.

TECHNICAL DETAILS

ABDOMINAL PHASE

The operation starts in the abdomen for Ivor Lewis or transhiatal esophagectomies. Port placement is shown in Fig. 39D.1. The camera port is located 18 cm inferior from the xiphoid process and is generally placed first. A 30-degree down camera or a 0-degree lens is used. Inspection of the abdomen is performed for liver and peritoneal metastases prior to placing the other ports. A single left robotic arm and two right robotic arms are used. These ports should be placed no more than 2 to 3 cm superior to the camera port to avoid problems with the angle of the instruments when dividing the greater omentum off the greater curvature of the stomach toward the pylorus. The robotic arms should be around 9 cm apart from each other if an Si system is used (8 cm if an Xi system is used). If there is not enough room on the left side of the abdomen to place the ports straight across, the robotic arm closer to the camera can be staggered slightly in front of the other one. If using the Si system, the second right robotic arm can be a 5 mm and the other robotic arms 8 mm. Stapling of the conduit is performed via the assistant port. If using the Xi system and robotic stapling is desired, the left robotic arm should be a 12-mm port; the rest of the robotic ports are 8-mm ports. A 5-mm port for the liver retractor is placed as close to the costal margin and laterally as possible (just over the right colon). A 12-mm assistant port is placed in the patient's right lower quadrant and triangulated behind the left robotic arm port and camera port. Insufflation should be delivered via this port during the case.

The patient is placed in steep reverse Trendelenburg position and the liver retractor is positioned under the left lateral lobe of the liver to expose the esophageal hiatus. We use a Snowden Pencer articulating pretzel retractor (Becton Dickinson; Franklin Lakes, New Jersey) for this purpose. If using an Si system, the head of the bed is turned so that the robot can approach it from over the head. If using an Xi system, the bed does not have to be turned. The robot is carefully driven in, making sure that its arms do not collide with the patient's head and upper

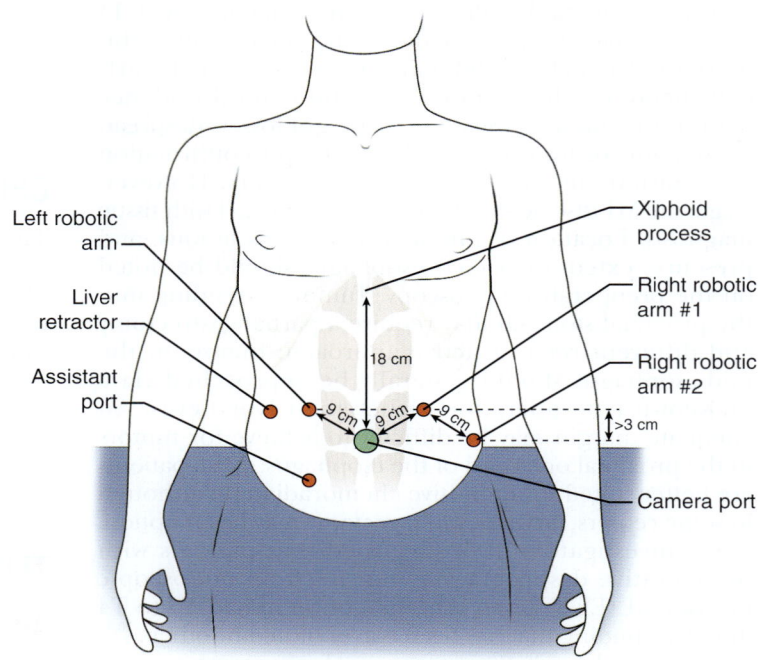

Left robotic arm

Liver retractor

Assistant port

Xiphoid process

Right robotic arm #1

Right robotic arm #2

Camera port

18 cm

9 cm 9 cm 9 cm

>3 cm

FIGURE 39D.1 Port placement for abdominal phase of robotic esophagectomy.

body. The robotic arms are docked to the ports, and the robotic phase begins.

We generally use the following instruments during the dissection: left robotic arm—Cadiere forceps; right robotic arm—Vessel Sealer; second right robotic arm—thoracic grasper (Si system), tip-up fenestrated grasper (Xi system). Division of the greater omentum from the greater curvature of the stomach starts by entering the lesser sac between the stomach and the left side of the transverse colon. Care is taken to identify the gastroepiploic vessels and assiduously avoid them. The greater omentum is divided from the patient's left toward the right until the pylorus is reached. The surgeon then switches direction and goes from the entry point into the lesser sac toward the spleen and fundus while paying extra attention to the short gastric vessels. During this process, the second robotic arm is used to hold the greater omentum/colon in one direction; the assistant can grasp the stomach and retract in the other direction. An omental flap should be preserved during this dissection to be wrapped around the anastomosis and protect the airway. Once the short gastric vessels are divided, the surgeon then works on the left side of the esophageal hiatus, working from the top of the hiatus down underneath the esophagus so that the area beneath the esophagus is as clear as possible to facilitate encircling the esophagogastric junction later. Attachments of the stomach to the retroperitoneum should also be divided at this point.

Next, the lesser sac is entered through the lesser omentum. An accessory or replaced left hepatic artery originating from the left gastric artery can be located in this area, as up to 12% of patients may have this variation.[15] Our practice is to test clamp any significant vessel in this location and perform a visual check for liver perfusion prior to dividing it. We have not had this occur, but if liver appears ischemic with the test clamp, the operation could be aborted, or the surgeon could attempt to divide the

left gastric artery above the replaced left hepatic artery. We then perform a circumferential dissection around the esophagus at the hiatus, carrying it into the mediastinum for a few centimeters but trying to avoid excessive trauma or widening of the hiatus or entering the left pleura, to avoid increasing the risk of paraconduit herniation. If a transhiatal esophagectomy is planned, however, this mediastinal dissection should be performed as high as possible. The use of the fenestrated bipolar forceps in the right hand can be helpful for atraumatically dissecting the underside of the esophagus. During this, the second right robotic arm is used to retract the esophagus up and to the patient's left (screen right). A 1-inch-thick or greater Penrose drain is placed around the esophagus and the ends are either tied or stapled together. The left gastric pedicle is identified and the surrounding fat is dissected off of the vein and artery. Depending on the patient, this vessel can be approached either from the lesser curvature side or from underneath the stomach as it is lifted (greater curvature side). Test clamp of the pedicle is then performed prior to division of the left gastric artery and vein with the stapler. The vessels may be stapled individually or together.

Next, botulinum toxin injection with 100 units in 4 mL of saline at the pylorus is performed. Alternatively, a gastric emptying procedure such as pyloromyotomy or pyloroplasty may be done at the discretion of the surgeon, although this increases the operative time without a significant improvement in results.[16] The pylorus should be able to reach the esophageal hiatus with little tension; if tension exists or it cannot reach, further mobilization of the pylorus from the greater omentum and a Kocher maneuver should be performed. Care should be taken to avoid injuring structures in the portal triad during mobilization. At this point, the surgeon needs to confirm that the nasogastric tube has been withdrawn to 20 cm or so. A starting point on the lesser curvature of the stomach is selected, and the perigastric fat going from the edge of the stomach to the opening in the lesser omentum is divided with the Vessel Sealer. The gastric conduit is created with a stapler (4 mm staple height, 45 to 60 mm length) using right robotic arm #2 (placed on the fundus) and the assistant (grasping or retracting the antrum) to stretch the stomach out. The specimen is not completely divided from the conduit so that the conduit may be pulled up into the chest or neck with the abdomen. A suture is placed at the distal part of the staple line near the pylorus so that the end of the staple line can be easily seen from the chest. If a neck anastomosis is being performed, part of the lesser curve of the specimen may be resected at this point to help facilitate its passage through the thoracic inlet. The Penrose drain and specimen are pushed up into the mediastinum.

Finally, a jejunostomy tube is placed. If the anatomy is suitable (e.g., exposure to the proximal jejunum is in front of the camera rather than directly below or behind it), this can be done robotically. In general, however, we have found it simpler and quicker to perform this laparoscopically after undocking the robot. Three 2-0 absorbable sutures are placed in the proximal jejunum in a triangulated fashion and the ends are exteriorized. The jejunostomy tube is placed with a Seldinger technique over a wire after dilating the tract and tying the sutures.

THORACIC PHASE

The single-lumen endotracheal tube may be exchanged for a double-lumen endotracheal tube during closure of the skin incisions to expedite transition to the thoracic phase. The patient is positioned in a nearly prone position. It is important to keep the right arm/shoulder low during positioning so it will not get in the way of the right robotic arm. Patient positioning and port placement are demonstrated in Fig. 39D.2. The right robotic arm port (8 mm; 12 mm if completely robotic linear stapling technique is desired) is placed in the axilla. A long trocar can be used to help avoid collisions with the patient. The camera port is placed about 9 cm (10 cm in Si system) from

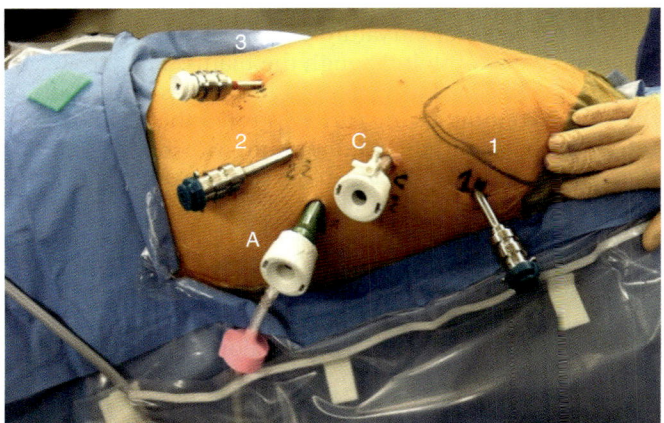

FIGURE 39D.2 Patient positioning and port placement for thoracic phase of robotic esophagectomy. *1*, Right robotic arm; *2*, left robotic arm; *3*, second left robotic arm; *A*, assistant port; *C*, camera port.

the right robotic arm port (8 mm in Xi system, 12 mm in Si system), which is in line with the anterior superior iliac spine. The left robotic arm port (12 mm in Xi system if completely robotic linear stapling of anastomosis is desired, 8 mm if not desired or in Si system) is placed 9 cm (10 cm in Si system) away from the camera port in line with the anterior iliac spine. The second left robotic arm port (8 mm in Xi system, 5 mm in Si system) is placed posterior to the midaxillary line just above the diaphragm. The assistant port (12 mm) is placed in a position triangulated behind the left robotic arm and camera port just above the diaphragm. We generally use the following instruments during the dissection: left robotic arm—Cadiere forceps, right robotic arm—thoracic dissector, second right robotic arm—thoracic grasper (Si system), and tip-up fenestrated grasper (Xi system). The lung is retracted anteriorly with the second left robotic arm, and the inferior pulmonary ligament is divided. Lymph nodes from stations 8 and 9 are resected. The esophagus is dissected off of the pericardium until the carina is exposed. Lymph nodes from station 7 are resected so that the right mainstem bronchus, carina, and left mainstem are clearly visible. Thermal injury to the airway is carefully avoided. The dissection is carried toward the azygos vein, which is then isolated and divided with a vascular load staple fired as posteriorly as possible. The dissection of the esophagus is then carried proximally and into the thoracic inlet, now staying closer to the esophagus to avoid a tracheal injury. If performing a cervical anastomosis, this dissection is carried as high as possible. Next, the esophagus is dissected off of the aorta posteriorly, taking care to avoid the thoracic duct, which runs especially close to the esophagus near the azygos vein. This is carried from the thoracic inlet toward the diaphragm until the dissection plane from the abdominal phase is reached and the Penrose drain is grasped. The Penrose drain can then be retracted with the second left robotic arm both anteriorly and laterally to help facilitate the remainder of the dissection. We try not to enter the left pleural space unless this needs to be resected for gross disease.

If a McKeown esophagectomy is to be performed, the Penrose is pushed up into the thoracic inlet to be retrieved through the neck. Much of the esophagus in the distal neck can be dissected via the chest with a right robotic approach; we believe that this is an added advantage of a robotic approach and may significantly decrease the incidence of recurrent laryngeal nerve injury. The chest tube is placed (additional tube placed in left pleural space if entered), insufflation gas turned off, ports removed, port sites are checked for bleeding, the lung reinflated, and incisions closed. Then the abdominal and cervical phases of the operation are begun.

If an Ivor Lewis esophagectomy is to be performed, the specimen and conduit are brought up into the thorax, mostly with the assistant using an atraumatic grasper such as empty ring forceps, making sure that the conduit is not twisted (staple line directed laterally). The previously placed suture at the distal staple line in the lesser curve should be visible and brought just into the chest above the hiatus. The esophagus is transected at the desired length with robotic shears and the proximal and distal margins are sent for pathologic examination. The specimen is divided from the gastric conduit with the stapler (4-mm staple height) and together with the Penrose removed. The gastric conduit is oriented so that the anastomosis will be located posteriorly. The conduit is tacked to pleura and/or transected vagus nerve to keep it in place during the anastomosis, which orients it and prevents tension. The anastomosis can be completely hand-sewn, completely stapled (linear or circular stapler), or a combination of the two (linear stapler "posterior" wall and hand-sewn "anterior" wall). The optimal approach to performing the anastomosis has not been described. We have performed all of these and will describe each technique:

Hand-Sewn Anastomosis

- The gastrotomy is made on the posterior wall of the conduit for an "end-to-side" anastomosis, at least 2 cm proximal to the tip of the conduit and away from the staple line.
- A row of 3-0 silk sutures is placed for the outer layer ("posterior").
- An inner layer of 3-0 absorbable sutures is placed for the inner layer ("posterior").
- The "anterior" wall for the anastomosis is closed with interrupted 3-0 absorbable sutures.
- An outer "anterior" layer of 3-0 silk sutures is placed.

Combination Stapled and Hand-Sewn Anastomosis

- After the gastrotomy is performed, the esophagus and conduit are lined up and a stapler is fired to create a 20 to 30 mm common wall for the "posterior" wall for the anastomosis. The stapler can be deployed either by the assistant or in the left robotic arm (Xi system).
- The "anterior" wall is closed in two layers as described earlier.

Completely Stapled Anastomosis (Linear Stapler)

- The "posterior" wall of the anastomosis is created as described previously.
- Five 3-0 silk interrupted sutures are placed and tied to approximate the muscle and mucosa of the "anterior" wall.
- These sutures are held up and the "anterior" wall of the anastomosis is created with the linear stapler. The stapler generally needs to be deployed in the location of the right robotic arm port (either robotically, in which case the surgeon needs to upsize to a 12-mm port, or after undocking that port and having the assistant place a stapler through it).

Completely Stapled Anastomosis (Circular Stapler)

- A purse string with 3-0 nonabsorbable monofilament suture is placed in the esophagus, making sure to incorporate the mucosal layer.
- The anvil is placed in the esophagus and the purse string is tied.
- An additional purse-string suture is placed if there is any gap around the anvil.
- A gastrotomy is created at the tip of the conduit. Retraction sutures can be placed to help.
- The stapler is positioned through the gastrotomy with the end directed toward the posterior aspect of the conduit. The tip of the stapler is extended, going through the wall of the conduit. Caution should be exercised to avoid

deployment of the tip of the stapler into the aorta. Multiple attempts at extending the tip through the conduit wall should also be avoided. The tip of the stapler is linked to the anvil, which can be facilitated with the use of the laparoscopic anvil grasper.
- The stapler is fired. The rims of tissue excised by the stapler should be examined; if they are not complete, the corresponding area of the anastomosis should be checked and closed with sutures.

The anastomosis should be inspected and any questionable areas should have sutures placed to close them. Endoscopy can be performed routinely if so desired and the integrity of the anastomosis checked by insufflating it while it is submerged under saline or water. The omental flap is wrapped around the anastomosis, protecting the airway from it, and sutured in place. The gastric conduit is secured to the diaphragm at the hiatus. A chest tube is placed and this phase of the operation concluded as described before.

CERVICAL PHASE

The cervical phase of the operation is similar to that performed during open operations. During the thoracic phase of a McKeown esophagectomy, we perform extensive periesophageal dissection into the thoracic inlet. We find it helpful to place a Penrose drain around the esophagus and either staple or tie the ends together and push the drain into the superior mediastinum so that the esophagus can be more easily encircled during the neck dissection. An incision anterior and parallel to the left sternocleidomastoid is made. The platysma is divided. The omohyoid muscle is encountered and divided. The carotid sheath containing the common carotid artery and the internal jugular vein is gently retracted laterally. The trachea is gently retracted medially, taking care to avoid the use of metal retractors that could injure the recurrent laryngeal nerve in the tracheoesophageal groove. The esophagus is followed inferiorly until the intrathoracic dissection plane is reached and the Penrose drain is identified. The Penrose is used to pull the esophagus into the incision. The specimen and conduit are pulled gently up through the chest. This can be done with the camera in the abdomen to make sure that the conduit does not twist during the process and to facilitate passage of the lesser curvature of the specimen or omental fat attached to conduit through the hiatus. The esophagus is then divided sharply, and the specimen is stapled off of the gastric conduit, taking care to prevent the conduit from retracting back into the mediastinum with a nontraumatic clamp. A gastrotomy is made in the conduit on the posterior wall, and a 3.5 to 4.5 mm tall stapler is fired to create the posterior wall of the anastomosis. Interrupted silk sutures are placed and tied anteriorly to approximate the mucosa and muscle, and a stapler is used to create the anterior wall of the anastomosis, making sure to incorporate mucosa of both the esophagus and stomach along the entire edge. If there is concern about the integrity of the anastomosis and enough redundancy exists, a buttressing layer over the staple line can be created by Lembert-type interrupted 3-0 silk sutures. We do not routinely test the anastomosis for leaks intraoperatively or leave a nasogastric tube. We do not typically leave a drain in place. The incision is then closed in layers with absorbable suture.

RESULTS

The results from series of robotic esophagectomy to date are shown in Table 39D.1 and compared with the largest nonrobotic MIE series currently in the literature.[30] Overall operative times of robotic esophagectomy have been comparable to nonrobotic MIE; a significant improvement in speed after the first 20 cases has been described.[18,29] Perioperative morbidity and postoperative parameters have also been similar to that reported from series of nonrobotic MIE. The single retrospective study comparing robotic esophagectomy with nonrobotic MIE showed similar operative times, estimated blood loss, resected lymph nodes, postoperative length of stay, and complications.[22] Direct comparisons of robotic esophagectomy with open esophagectomy have not been reported in the literature, but one randomized trial (ROBOT trial) is currently accruing patients to investigate differences in outcome between the techniques.[31] The robotic platform allows for real-time assessment of perfusion of the gastric conduit with the injection of indocyanine green (ICG) and near-infrared fluorescence imaging, which can help guide the surgeon to optimal area of transection of the specimen from the conduit and also for placement of the anastomosis. Investigators have described a 0% leak rate in 39 cases after instituting routine perfusion assessment using ICG to guide creation of the esophagotomy and performance of the anterior part of the anastomosis during the thoracic phase of Ivor Lewis esophagectomy, although it is possible that improvements in anastomotic technique also contributed to this remarkable result.[27] The use of ICG and near-infrared fluorescence imaging can also help with assessment of the vascular arcade during mobilization of the gastric conduit during the abdominal phase of the operation.[32] Some of the advantages of robotic esophagectomy over nonrobotic MIE may be difficult to quantify and relate to subjective experiences of the surgeon such as the three-dimensional nature of the

TABLE 39D.1 Results of Series of Robotic Esophagectomy

Name, Year	# Pts	Lymph Nodes Dissected	Operative Approach	Estimated Blood Loss (mL)	Operative Time (min)	Leak Rate	Overall Major Morbidity	Mortality
Cerfolio, 2016[17]	85	22	Ivor Lewis (lap/robot abd, robot chest)	35	361	4.3%	36.4%	3.5% 30-day 11% 90-day
Hernandez, 2013[18]	52	20	Ivor Lewis (robot abd/chest)	NR	442	3.8%	26.9%	0% ("hospital")
De la Fuente, 2013[19]	50	18.5	Ivor Lewis (robot abd/chest)	NR	445	4%	28%	0% ("hospital")
Sarkaria, 2013[20]	21	20	Ivor Lewis (n = 17 and McKeown n = 4), robot abd/chest	300	556	14% (grade II or greater)	24% (grade III or greater)	4.8% ("postoperative")
Dunn, 2013[21]	40	20	Transhiatal (robot mediastinal dissection)	100	311	25%	NR	2.5% 30-day
Weksler, 2012[22]	11	19	McKeown (robot abd/chest)	200	445	9.1%	36.4%	0% ("hospital")
Park, 2016[23]	114	44	McKeown (lap/robot abd, robot chest)	209	420	12.3% (grade II or greater)	NR	2.5% 90-day
Boone, 2009[24]	47	29	Ivor Lewis (lap abd, robot chest)	625	450	21%	NR	6.4% ("postoperative")
Kernstine, 2007[25]	14	18	Ivor Lewis (lap/robot abd, robot chest)	275	11.2 hours (total room time)	14%	29%	0% 30-day 1 patient (7.1%) died at 72 days
Galvani, 2008[26]	18	14	Transhiatal (robot abd)	54	267	33%	NR	0% 30-day
Hodari, 2015[27]	54	16	Ivor Lewis (lap abd, robot chest)	74.4	362	6.8%	NR	2% 30-day
Coker, 2014[28]	23	15	Transhiatal (robot abd)	100	231	9%	NR	4% 30-day
Harrison, 2015[29]	43	12	Transhiatal (28), McKeown (7), Ivor Lewis (5); robot abd	NR	309	23%	41.8%	4.7% ("postoperative")
Luketich, 2012[30]	1033	21	McKeown (n = 481), Ivor Lewis (n = 530) Lap abd/VATS chest	NR	NR	5% (requiring surgery)	NR	1.68% 30-day 2.8% 30-day or hospital

abd, Abdominal; *lap,* laparoscopic; *NR,* not recorded; *VATS,* video-assisted thoracoscopic surgery.

optics, improved dexterity, favorable ergonomics, and the ability to control the retraction and camera without an assistant.[33,34] Disadvantages of the robotic platform include cost, and complexity in terms of developing robotic skills, personnel issues, room layout, and robot docking, although these may be surmounted with a formal training paradigm.[35] Long-term oncologic outcomes specific to robotic esophagectomy are not yet well described, although it would be expected that they would be comparable to those for nonrobotic MIE.

CONCLUSION

Robotic esophagectomy can be done safely with comparable intraoperative parameters, morbidity, and outcomes to nonrobotic MIE, while offering certain more subjective advantages to the surgeon.

REFERENCES

1. Xie MR, Liu CQ, Guo MF, Mei XY, Sun XH, Xu MQ. Short-term outcomes of minimally invasive Ivor-Lewis esophagectomy for esophageal cancer. *Ann Thorac Surg.* 2014;97:1721-1727.
2. Biere SS, van Berge Henegouwen MI, Maas KW, et al. Minimally invasive versus open oesophagectomy for patients with oesophageal cancer: a multicenter, open-label, randomized controlled trial. *Lancet.* 2012;379:1887-1892.
3. Weksler B, Sharma P, Moudgill N, Chojnacki KA, Rosato EL. Robot-assisted minimally invasive esophagectomy is equivalent to thoracoscopic minimally invasive esophagectomy. *Dis Esophagus.* 2012;25:403-409.
4. Clark J, Sodergren MH, Purkayastha S, et al. The role of robotic assisted laparoscopy for oesophagogastric oncological resection; an appraisal of the literature. *Dis Esophagus.* 2011;24:240-250.
5. Lee S, Sudarshan M, Li C, et al. Cost-effectiveness of minimally invasive versus open esophagectomy for esophageal cancer. *Ann Surg Oncol.* 2013;20:3732-3739.
6. Melvin WS, Needleman BJ, Krause KR, et al. Computer-enhanced robotic telesurgery: initial experience in foregut surgery. *Surg Endosc.* 2002;16:1790-1792.
7. Cong Z, Diao Q, Yi J, et al. Esophagectomy combined with aortic segment replacement for esophageal cancer invading the aorta. *Ann Thorac Surg.* 2014;97:460-466.
8. Van Raemdonck D, Van Cutsem E, Menten J, et al. Induction therapy for clinical T4 oesophageal carcinoma; a plea for continued surgical exploration. *Eur J Cardiothorac Surg.* 1997;11:828-837.
9. Li J, Shen Y, Tan L, et al. Is minimally invasive esophagectomy beneficial to elderly patients with esophageal cancer? *Surg Endosc.* 2015;29:925-930.
10. Ripley RT, Sarkaria IS, Grosser R, et al. Pretreatment dysphagia in esophageal cancer patients may eliminate the need for staging by endoscopic ultrasonography. *Ann Thorac Surg.* 2016;101:226-230.
11. Fang TC, Oh YS, Szabo A, Khan A, Dua KS. Utility of dysphagia grade in predicting endoscopic ultrasound T-stage of non-metastatic esophageal cancer. *Dis Esophagus.* 2016;29(6):642-648.
12. Kim JY, Correa AM, Vaporciyan AA, et al. Does the timing of esophagectomy after chemoradiation affect outcome? *Ann Thorac Surg.* 2012;93:207-212.
13. Lee A, Wong AT, Schwartz D, Weiner JP, Osborn VW, Schreiber D. Is there a benefit to prolonging the interval between neoadjuvant chemoradiation and esophagectomy in esophageal cancer? *Ann Thorac Surg.* 2016;102(2):433-438.
14. Chiu C, Chao Y, Chang H, et al. Interval between neoadjuvant chemoradiotherapy and surgery for esophageal squamous cell carcinoma: does delayed surgery impact outcome? *Ann Surg Oncol.* 2013;20:4245-4251.
15. Hiatt JR, Gabbay J, Busuttil RW. Surgical anatomy of the hepatic arteries in 1000 cases. *Ann Surg.* 1994;220:50-52.
16. Cerfolio RJ, Bryant AS, Canon CL, Dhawan R, Eloubeidi MA. Is botulinum toxin injection of the pylorus during Ivor Lewis esophagogastrectomy the optimal drainage strategy? *J Thorac Cardiovasc Surg.* 2009;137:565-572.
17. Cerfolio RJ, Wei B, Hawn MT, Minnich DJ. Robotic esophagectomy for cancer: early results and lessons learned. *Semin Thorac Cardiovasc Surg.* 2016;28(1):160-169.
18. Hernandez JM, Dimou F, Weber J, et al. Defining the learning curve for robotic-assisted esophagogastrectomy. *J Gastrointest Surg.* 2013;17:1346-1351.
19. De la Fuente SG, Weber J, Hoffe SE, Shridhar R, Karl R, Meredith KL. Initial experience from a large referral center with robotic-assisted Ivor Lewis esophagogasrectomy for oncologic purposes. *Surg Enodsc.* 2013;27:3339-3347.
20. Sarkaria IS, Rizk NP, Finley DJ, et al. Combined thoracoscopic and laparoscopic robotic-assisted minimally invasive esophagectomy using a four-arm platform: experience, technique and cautions during early procedure development. *Eur J Cardiothorac Surg.* 2013;43:e107-e115.
21. Dunn DH, Johnson EM, Morphew JA, Dilworth HP, Krueger JL, Banerji N. Robot-assisted transhiatal esophagectomy: a 3-year single-center experience. *Dis Esophagus.* 2013;26:159-166.
22. Weksler B, Sharm P, Moudgill N, Chojnacki KA, Rosato EL. Robot-assisted minimally invasive esophagectomy is equivalent to thoracoscopic minimally invasive esophagectomy. *Dis Esophagus.* 2012;25:403-409.
23. Park SY, Kim DJ, Yu WS, Jung HS. Robot-assisted thoracoscopic esophagectomy with extensive mediastinal lymphadenectomy: experience with 114 consecutive patients with intrathoracic esophageal cancer. *Dis Esophagus.* 2016;29(4):326-332.
24. Boone J, Schipper ME, Moojen WA, Borel Rinkes IH, Cromheecke GJ, van Hillegersberg R. Robot-assisted thoracoscopic oesophagectomy for cancer. *Br J Surg.* 2009;96:878-886.
25. Kernstine KH, DeArmond DT, Shamoun DM, Campos JH. The first series of completely robotic esophagectomies with three-field lymphadenectomy: initial experience. *Surg Endosc.* 2007;21:2285-2292.
26. Galvani CA, Gorodner MV, Moser F, et al. Robotically assisted laparoscopic transhiatal esophagectomy. *Surg Endosc.* 2008;22(1):188-195.
27. Hodari A, Park KU, Lace B, Tsiouris A, Hammoud Z. Robot-assisted minimally invasive Ivor Lewis esophagectomy with real-time perfusion assessment. *Ann Thorac Surg.* 2015;100(3):947-952.
28. Coker AM, Barajas-Gamboa JS, Cheverie J, et al. Outcomes of robotic-assisted transhiatal esophagectomy for esophageal cancer after neoadjuvant chemoradiation. *J Laparoendoscopic Adv Surg Tech A.* 2014;24:89-94.
29. Harrison LE, Yiengpruksawan A, Patel J, Itskovich A, Lee B, Korst R. Robotic gastrectomy and esophagogastrectomy: a single center experience of 105 cases. *J Surg Oncol.* 2015;112:888-893.
30. Luketich JD, Pennathur A, Awais O, et al. Outcomes after minimally invasive esophagectomy: review of over 1000 patients. *Ann Surg.* 2012;256:95-103.
31. Van der Sluis PC, Ruurda JP, van der Horst S, et al. Robot-assisted minimally invasive thoraco-laparoscopic esophagectomy versus open transthoracic esophagectomy for resectable esophageal cancer, a randomized controlled trial (ROBOT trial). *Trials.* 2012;13:230.
32. Sarkaria IS, Bains MS, Finley DJ, et al. Intraoperative near-infrared fluorescence imaging as an adjunct to robotic-assisted minimally invasive esophagectomy. *Innovations (Phila).* 2014;9:391-393.
33. Wei B, D'Amico TA. Thoracoscopic versus robotic approaches: advantages and disadvantages. *Thorac Surg Clin.* 2014;24:177-188.
34. Ruurda JP, van der Sluis PC, van der Horst S, van Hillegersberg R. Robot-assisted minimally invasive esophagectomy for esophageal cancer: a systematic review. *J Surg Oncol.* 2015;112:257-265.
35. Cerfolio RJ, Bryant AS, Minnich DJ. Starting a robotic program in general thoracic surgery: why, how, and lessons learned. *Ann Thorac Surg.* 2011;91:1729-1737.

Extent of Lymphadenectomy for Esophageal Cancer

Alexander W. Phillips | S. Michael Griffin

The extent of lymphadenectomy as part of an esophagectomy for cancer remains a controversial issue. The aggressive nature of the disease often means that both local nodal and distant metastases exist at the time of presentation. As such, locally advanced disease in which potential cure is intended is frequently treated with neoadjuvant modalities. The debate on degree of lymphadenectomy hinges largely on the belief that a radical dissection provides improved locoregional control and thus improved survival. However, it is also worth noting that extended lymphadenectomy also provides improved staging, which can allow better patient counseling and may influence the use of adjuvant treatment as further studies are performed into its role.

LYMPHATIC DRAINAGE OF THE ESOPHAGUS AND PATTERNS OF SPREAD

Knowledge of the lymphatic drainage of the esophagus is a key component for having a rationale for lymphadenectomy. The esophagus traverses three body compartments, and lymph flow can occur in a wide pattern of spread. The embryologic origin of the esophagus is from the branchial arches and pharyngeal pouches from above, and the splanchnic mesoderm below. These join during early embryologic development but remain demarcated at the level of the tracheal bifurcation leading to bilateral lymphatic drainage (Fig. 40.1).

In early esophageal cancer the suggestion is that lymph node spread, when it occurs, follows these anatomic pathways, implying that the tumor location is key to determining which nodes are likely to be involved. Thus nodal involvement for tumors above the tracheal bifurcation is preferentially to those in the upper mediastinum and neck, whereas those below this point will metastasize toward the celiac axis. Tumors located at the bifurcation may metastasize in either direction. Skipping of lymph node stations in these early tumors is rare.[1]

Lymph node involvement appears to be more common with squamous cell carcinoma (SCC) compared with adenocarcinoma when the tumor has invaded into the muscularis mucosae (T1a-M3), approaching up to 12%,[2,3] compared with only 1.3% in adenocarcinoma.[-6]

There is also an extensive submucosal lymphatic network that allows longitudinal communication between the proximal and distal drainage systems. In tumors that are more advanced and have potentially led to a blockage of one of the primary pathways, this submucosal system allows eccentric lymph node involvement. This is an important consideration because most patients are diagnosed at a more advanced state and T3 disease is associated with an up to 85% chance of lymph node involvement.[7,8]

LYMPH NODE TIERS

Extent of lymph node dissection is commonly divided into three fields: the upper abdomen, the mediastinum, and the neck (Fig. 40.2). Three-field dissection therefore relates to removal of nodal tissue from each of these areas. A lack of clarity exists on the exact definition of a two-field lymph node resection. The lack of clarity is because of differences in prevalence of squamous cell cancer in Japan and the East and in those patients from Western countries where adenocarcinoma has become the prevalent cause.

Where SCC of the esophagus is the common pathology, a two-field dissection is usually described as removal of nodal tissue from the upper abdomen (around the celiac artery) and in the inferior and superior mediastinum and along both recurrent laryngeal nerves. To contrast this, in countries where adenocarcinoma has become the common variant, a two-field dissection is usually regarded as removal of tissue from the upper abdomen and inferior mediastinum. This usually extends only to the level of the carina and reflects the usual anatomic location of these tumors in the lower esophagus or at the esophagogastric junction.

Although some surgeons do not perform a formal lymphadenectomy irrespective of the surgical approach, the following describes what is commonly accepted to be the groups of nodes resected with each "field" of dissection.

ABDOMINAL LYMPH NODE DISSECTION

This is commonly regarded as the first "field" of lymphadenectomy and includes the following abdominal lymph node stations: the superior gastric group, celiac trunk nodes, and common hepatic nodes (see Fig. 40.1 and Table 40.1).

The superior gastric nodes include those that are paracardial, which are frequently involved and are related to the most superior branch of the left gastric artery, and so both left and right paracardial should be considered a single group. The lesser curve nodes are involved with tumor spread to the celiac trunk and are also considered part of the superior gastric group, as are the nodes found along the length of the left gastric artery.

The celiac trunk nodes include those around the celiac axis at the root of the left gastric artery, common hepatic artery, and splenic artery, and they should be removed en bloc with the primary lesion. Disease beyond this drainage point represents metastatic disease. Similarly, disease involvement beyond the hepatic nodes equates to metastatic disease.

The involvement of nodes in both paracardial regions and lesser curve are the most commonly involved with

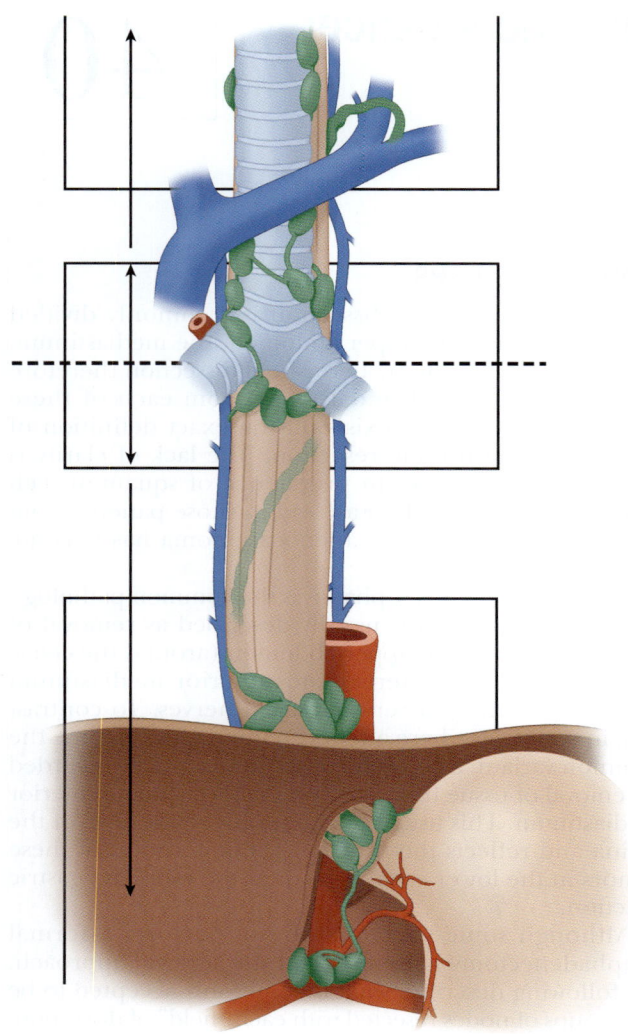

FIGURE 40.1 Direction of lymph flow from the esophagus. (From Stein HJ, Theisen J, Siewert J-R. Surgical resection for esophageal cancer: role of extended lymphadenectomy. In: Fielding JWL, Hallissey MT, eds. *Upper Gastrointestinal Surgery.* London: Springer; 2005:318.)

tumors of the lower esophagus. Nodes close to the left gastric artery and celiac trunk and hepatic artery are also commonly involved, which is consistent with the lymphatic drainage of the proximal stomach and lower esophagus.

Intramural spread distally and hence involvement of these abdominal nodes, for patients with lower esophageal cancers, is greater with adenocarcinoma (54%) compared with SCCs (10%), indicating the need for a wide resection margin in these patients.[9]

THORACIC LYMPH NODE DISSECTION

The second field of dissection commonly includes the mediastinal nodes, thoracic duct, nodes at both pulmonary hilar, paraesophageal nodes and those at the carina, both bronchi, and paratracheal nodes. These nodes are commonly involved with the tumor, as would be expected

given their close proximity, and should be taken as an en bloc resection with the esophagus.

Extended mediastinal dissection may be carried out, and this involves a lymphadenectomy including the nodes on the right side of the trachea. A "total mediastinal lymphadenectomy" involves the additional removal of nodes along the left recurrent laryngeal nerve and subaortic nodes.[10]

CERVICAL NODE DISSECTION

A three-field dissection involves removal of nodes from both the first two fields, as well as dissection in the neck to clear those nodes in the brachiocephalic, deep internal and external cervical nodes (see Table 40.1). This includes nodes by the left and right recurrent laryngeal nerve. With regard to those nodes that can be regarded as cervical, involvement of deep external nodes (found lateral to the internal jugular vein) and deep internal nodes (which approximate the recurrent laryngeal nerve) is more common than in the deep lateral nodes (the spinal accessory lymphatic chain) in thoracic carcinomas.

Of these groups, involvement of the deep internal and external nodes is more common than the lateral nodes.

SQUAMOUS CELL CANCERS VERSUS ADENOCARCINOMAS

The pattern of spread can to some extent be correlated with the histologic type of cancer found; however, the extensive lymphatic drainage system of the esophagus makes this difficult, particularly in more advanced cancers (Figs. 40.3 and 40.4). Squamous cell cancer, commonly found in the middle and proximal parts of the esophagus, rarely has nodal involvement when the tumor is confined to the mucosa (0% to 7%).[5,11–14] However, this increases dramatically with deeper invasion, and nodal involvement occurs in up to 50% of patients once the tumor has invaded the submucosa and in more than 73% in patients with transmural tumors.

The involvement of lymph nodes in adenocarcinomas also correlates with the depth of tumor invasion. For those tumors confined to the mucosa, the incidence mirrors that of squamous cell cancers at 0% to 7%. The low incidence of tumor involvement in these patients has led to the increased use of endoscopic resection for these cancers. Although lymph node involvement on penetration of the submucosa has been reported at between 15% and 50%, invasion through the muscularis propria is associated with up to 80% involvement.

A difference in pattern of spread between SCCs and adenocarcinomas of the lower esophagus and junction exists. Law et al. reviewed 108 patients undergoing esophagectomy with two-field lymphadenectomy for SCC. Two-thirds of recurrences were in the first year after surgery, and the majority of recurrences were extrathoracic. Of the extrathoracic recurrences, 28 were to distant organs, implying hematogenous spread, whereas 17 were to lymph nodes (12 cervical and 5 abdominal). There was an incidence of local recurrence of 25%.[15] This compares with a reported local recurrence rate of 9% for lower esophageal adenocarcinoma and 15% for junctional cancers.[16] Despite

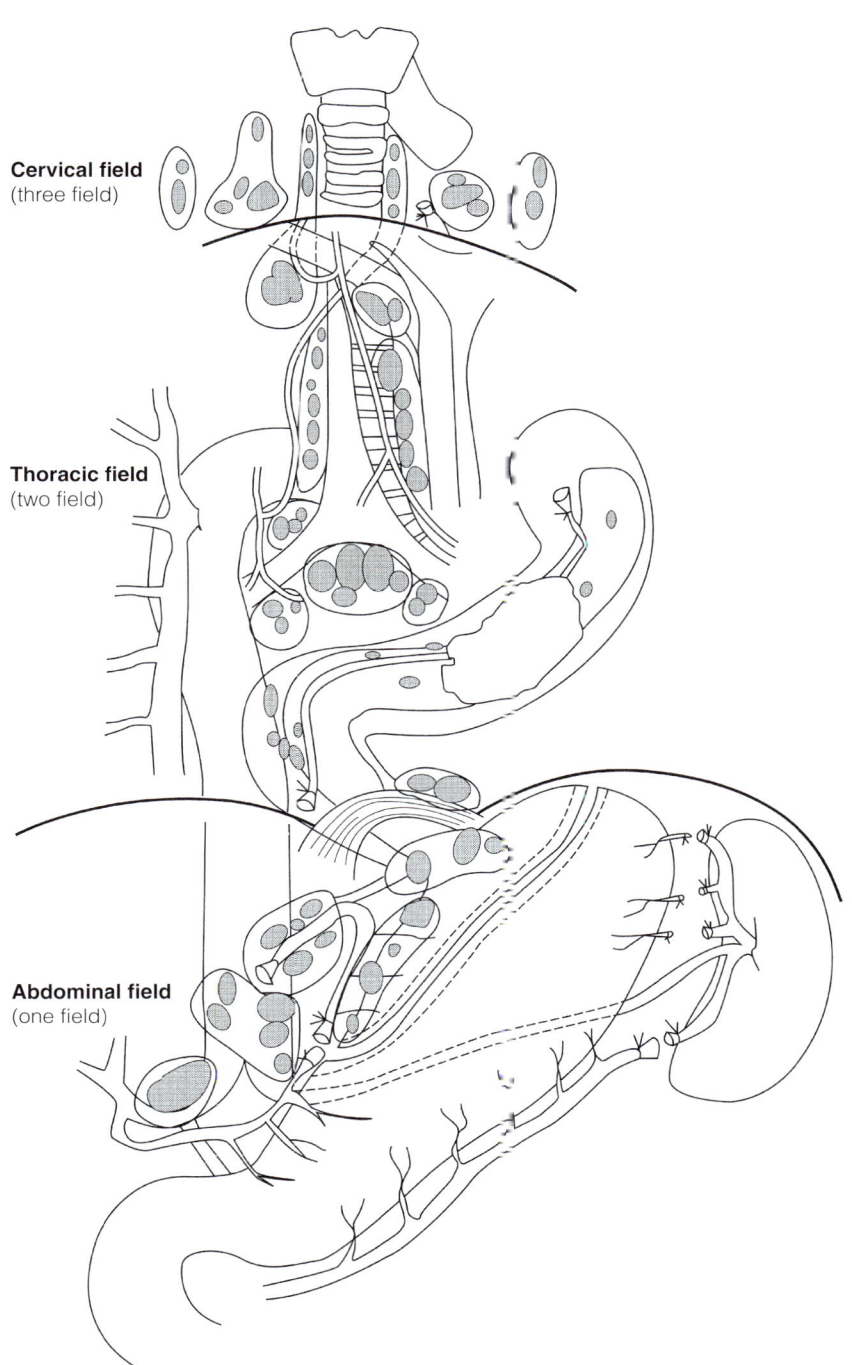

Cervical field
(three field)

Thoracic field
(two field)

Abdominal field
(one field)

FIGURE 40.2 Extent of resection and fields of lymph node dissection routinely carried out for cancer of the esophagus. (From Griffin SM, Raimes SA, Shenfine J, eds. *Oesophagogastric Surgery: A Companion to Specialist Surgical Practice.* 5th ed. Edinburgh: Saunders Ltd; 2013.)

these suggestions, the incidence of local recurrence for either subtype is between 25% and 50%, indicating that a meticulous lymphadenectomy may have a profound impact on providing locoregional control.

IMPLICATIONS OF LYMPHADENECTOMY

There is still a great deal of debate regarding the extent of lymphadenectomy that should be performed and whether a more radical resection confers any survival advantage. The argument for an extensive lymphadenectomy lies in a belief that it confers improved locoregional control, and hence cure rates, as well as improving the overall staging of the disease.[17]

It has been established that complete resection (R0) is an important indicator of prognosis and that those patients with microscopic (R1) or macroscopic (R2) residual disease have a significantly bleaker prognosis. Approximately 25% to 50% of patients may develop locoregional recurrence after a two-field lymphadenectomy. Anderegg et al. indicated that the location of nodal involvement is an independent predictor of survival in

TABLE 40.1   **Nodes According to Anatomic Region**

Cervical lymph nodes
  Deep lateral nodes
  Deep external nodes
  Deep internal nodes
Superior mediastinal lymph nodes
  Recurrent nerve lymphatic chain
  Paratracheal nodes
  Brachiocephalic artery nodes
  Infraaortic-arch nodes
Middle mediastinal lymph nodes
  Tracheal bifurcation nodes
  Pulmonary hilar nodes
  Paraesophageal nodes
Lower mediastinal lymph nodes
  Paraesophageal nodes
  Diaphragmatic nodes
Superior gastric lymph nodes
  Paracardial nodes
  Lesser curve nodes
  Left gastric artery nodes
Celiac trunk nodes
Common hepatic nodes

From Akiyama H. *Surgery for Cancer of the Esophagus.* Baltimore: Lippincott Williams & Wilkins; 1990.

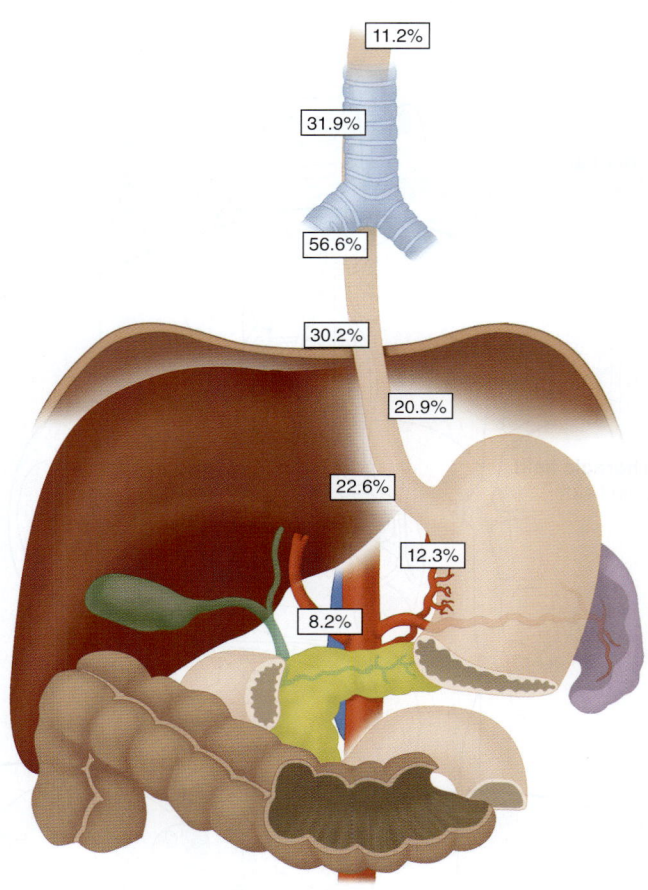

FIGURE 40.3 Distribution of lymph node metastases in squamous cell carcinoma from 100 patients. (From Stein HJ, Theisen J, Siewert J-R. Surgical resection for esophageal cancer: role of extended lymphadenectomy. In: Fielding JWL, Hallissey MT, eds. *Upper Gastrointestinal Surgery.* London: Springer; 2005:322.)

patients with adenocarcinoma of the distal esophagus and esophagogastric junction. In their series of 479 patients who underwent transthoracic esophagectomy and two-field lymphadenectomy, 253 patients had nodal metastases. Survival in those who had only locoregional lymph node involvement was 35 months compared with 16 months for those with nodes at the celiac trunk and 15 months for those with involvement in the proximal field.[18] In an earlier study, Hulscher demonstrated a trend toward greater survival at 5 years of patients undergoing transthoracic esophagectomy with extended en bloc lymphadenectomy when compared with a transhiatal approach in patients with lower esophageal and junctional adenocarcinomas.[19]

The risk of involvement of lymph nodes in early cancers has been previously established. Griffin et al. demonstrated that 12% of patients with adenocarcinoma invading the submucosa may have lymph node involvement, although none of the patients with tumor confined to the mucosa were lymph node positive.[20] Although this highlights that local endoscopic resection is not appropriate in patients with submucosal invasion, it also reiterates the importance of carrying out a meticulous lymphadenectomy even when the cancer is deemed as at an early stage.

A number of studies have attempted to determine the impact of the extent of lymphadenectomy by using the number of nodes retrieved as a surrogate for the extent of dissection. Van der Schaaf et al. reviewed the outcomes from a Swedish nationwide study of 1044 resections over a 23-year period, by comparing outcomes according to nodal yield quartiles.[21] They concluded that more extensive clearance did not equate to improved survival. Similarly Lagergren et al. looked at patients from a single center again using lymph node yield as a surrogate for extent of lymphadenectomy. Again, the results from this study did

not suggest that a higher yield of lymph nodes equated to better overall survival.[22] It is worth noting that in both these studies the lymph node yields were generally low with the upper border of the third quartile only 15 nodes in van der Schaaf's study, and 20 nodes in Lagergren's study. Both papers demonstrated that, as expected, a greater number of metastatic nodes is associated with decreased survival but also that a higher ratio of positive to negative nodes was associated with increased mortality.

Indeed the aspect of lymph node ratio has been evaluated a number of times. Several studies have demonstrated that lymph node ratio is a prognostic factor; however, this is often coupled with the caveat that if insufficient nodes are obtained, this ratio ceases to be useful as a prognostic tool due to the fact that there has been, in essence, incomplete sampling.

Chen et al. evaluated the impact of lymph node ratio for esophageal squamous cell cancers from more than 2000 patient in China and concluded that this was a better predictor of prognosis than using the "N" category. Their suggestion was to use an "Nr" ratios category of 0, 0% to 10%, 10% to 20%, and greater than 20% rather than N0-N3 with predicted survivals of 61%, 41%, 33%, and 23%, respectively.[23] Similar findings were made by Bhamidipati

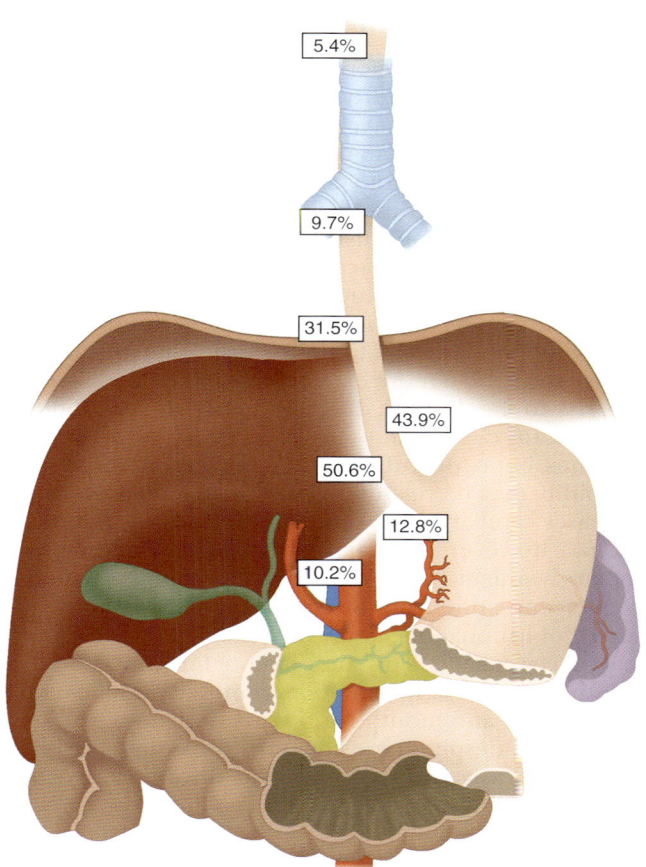

5.4%

9.7%

31.5%

43.9%

50.6%

12.8%

10.2%

FIGURE 40.4 Distribution of lymph node metastases in 100 patients with adenocarcinoma. (Modified from Stein HJ, Theisen J, Siewert J-R. Surgical resection for esophageal cancer: role of extended lymphadenectomy. In: Fielding JWL, Hallissey MT, eds. *Upper Gastrointestinal Surgery.* London: Springer; 2005:323.)

et al. in a cohort of US patients who predominantly had adenocarcinoma. They also concluded that lymph node ratio was an independent predictor of prognosis in their cohort of 347 patients undergoing surgery and was more useful than "N" category.[24]

The idea that an extensive lymphadenectomy leads to better locoregional control is founded in a belief that leaving positive lymph nodes behind equates to leaving disease behind. High lymph node yields do not necessarily equate to an extensive lymphadenectomy, and it is the location from which the nodes come that is of higher importance. Most recently Phillips et al. attempted to evaluate the impact of the extent of lymphadenectomy on outcomes from patients with adenocarcinoma undergoing transthoracic esophagectomy following neoadjuvant treatment. This study looked at the location of positive nodes after resection, and evaluated how many extra recurrences would have occurred had nodes in respective fields been left behind. This study suggested a 23% decrease in survival had no formal lymphadenectomy been carried out, but interestingly the impact of leaving abdominal nodes behind in this cohort of patients with lower esophageal and junctional adenocarcinomas was predicted as minimal.[25]

Another potential concern is the presence of micrometastases. It is difficult to determine what impact their occurrence has on potential recurrence, but their presence has been used to explain why node-negative patients develop recurrence. Micrometastases have been shown to be present in up to 50% of N0 patients.[26] Although some studies have found that immunohistochemically detected deposits are associated with poorer prognosis,[26,27] others have suggested they have no prognostic consequence.[28,29]

Current staging techniques do not allow easy identification of patients who are more likely to benefit from a more radical resection. There have been previous suggestions that an increased lymphadenectomy is more beneficial in patients with fewer than eight lymph node metastases,[30] and Rizk et al. determined that the optimum lymph node yield was dependent on the "T" category of disease, recommending 31 to 42 nodes in those with T3 disease or worse.[31] Patients who are considered for neoadjuvant treatment are likely to have more locally advanced disease, and this would suggest they will benefit from a more extensive lymphadenectomy.

Ideally it would be possible to tailor the lymphadenectomy according to disease stage. However, this is reliant on accurate assessment of which nodes are involved, and this currently remains difficult. Sentinel node techniques have been attempted, but the occurrence of skip metastases and unpredictability of nodal involvement makes this currently unreliable.[21]

Peyre et al. looked at whether systemic disease could be predicted by the number of lymph nodes involved.[32] Their review of 1053 patients with both adenocarcinoma and SCC, without neoadjuvant treatment, indicated that the probability of systemic disease exceeds 50% when more than three nodes are involved and approaches 100% when greater than eight nodes are involved.

A further study by the same group sought to evaluate the impact on the number of lymph nodes removed on outcomes in esophageal cancer. This study looked at 2303 esophageal cancer patients, again who did not receive neoadjuvant or adjuvant treatment. Their findings demonstrated that the number of nodes recovered was an independent predictor of survival after esophagectomy and suggested an optimum threshold of 23 nodes. Furthermore, they suggested that this optimum finding of 23 lymph nodes indicated that it was not only the number of nodes that affected survival but also their location.[33]

Omloo et al. found that an extended resection is beneficial in patients with fewer than eight lymph node metastases.[30] Thus, given the difficulty in identifying such patients, a complete two-field lymphadenectomy should be carried out in all patients where nodal involvement is a concern. Ideally, based on an individual's risk factors, it would be possible to tailor surgical approach[34] to try and optimize outcomes and minimize risks. The ability to tailor the lymphadenectomy so that metastatic nodes are removed, although technically possible, is fraught with a high false-negative rate.[35]

THREE-FIELD LYMPHADENECTOMY

Debate around the benefit of a three-field lymphadenectomy is long-standing. In Japan its practice has been widely used for many years, but in the West this approach is still performed relatively infrequently. This may be in part due to concerns regarding morbidity and mortality when including a cervical lymphadenectomy and also due to extrapolation of the already discussed argument that lymph node involvement equates to systemic disease and lymphadenectomy does not confer a survival advantage.

Lerut et al. looked at the long-term outcomes of three-field lymphadenectomy in a cohort of patients who received only unimodality treatment (prior to the integration of neoadjuvant treatment for locally advanced disease). Their findings are of interest, with a 0% survival for adenocarcinomas of the gastroesophageal junction and 12% survival for distal-third adenocarcinomas where cervical nodes were involved. This rose to 28% 5-year survival in middle-third squamous cell cancers. The implication was that cervical nodes should not necessarily be regarded as metastatic. There were other interesting findings from this study; 25% of patients had cervical lymph node involvement, and in three-quarters of these patients this had not been detected on the initial staging investigations. (It is worth noting that endoscopic ultrasound was used routinely as part of staging, but positron emission tomography was introduced only in the final year of this cohort.) A further interesting finding was that although the 5-year survival for distal-third adenocarcinomas with positive nodes was 12%, 4-year survival was 36%, perhaps indicating this surgery has a role in palliating disease.[8] There was no significant apparent increase in complications, and recurrent laryngeal nerve damage was low at 2.6%.

Although Lerut et al. evaluated a mixed cohort of adenocarcinomas and SCCs, Japanese studies involving patients with SCC indicate almost a third of patients will have cervical node involvement, explaining why three-field lymphadenectomy is widely used in Japan.

A number of surgeons have attempted to determine if anatomic location of the tumor should influence the need for cervical lymphadenectomy. Chen et al. reviewed 1715 patients with SCC and found that there was increased cervical node involvement the more proximal the tumor occurred, with 44% of proximal-third tumors having cervical node involvement, but strikingly 23% of lower-third tumors also had cervical node involvement.[36] This may indicate the importance of three-field lymphadenectomy for squamous cell cancers. Indeed, a number of systematic reviews, of predominantly squamous populations, have demonstrated superior survival with three-field lymphadenectomy.[37–39]

There is a paucity of data for three-field lymphadenectomy in patients with adenocarcinoma, particularly in the era of neoadjuvant treatments, and the poor overall survival demonstrated by Lerut indicates that routine cervical dissection may not be merited. Each patient with adenocarcinoma presenting with extensive mediastinal nodal disease should be considered for a three-field dissection. The decision will be dictated by extent of disease, likelihood of recurrence, and overall fitness. The protocol in our department is to consider each patient in the multidisciplinary setting and give the options to the patient and their family.

MORBIDITY OF LYMPHADENECTOMY

Extended lymphadenectomy has been associated by some with increased morbidity. Transhiatal esophagectomy has been shown to have fewer complications than a transthoracic esophagectomy with extended en bloc lymphadenectomy.[19] Respiratory problems are the main cause of major problems after esophagectomy, due to pneumonia and acute respiratory distress syndrome (ARDS). The extensive dissection places the tracheobronchial tree at risk of direct injury and may also occur in a delayed fashion if cautery has been used inadvertently in close proximity. Similarly risk to the recurrent laryngeal nerve is increased with a more extensive lymph node dissection, as is risk to the thoracic duct and hence the possibility of a significant chyle leak.

It has been postulated that increased respiratory morbidity may be related to one-lung ventilation, which increases capillary permeability and leads to pulmonary edema; however, mediastinal lymphadenectomy also impairs lymphatic flow, which can compound this edema.

A recent study from Sweden sought to establish the impact of lymphadenectomy on quality of life on esophageal cancer patients. This study did not find any association with the number of lymph nodes removed and the quality of life either at 6 months or 5 years post surgery.[40]

However, despite these concerns regarding morbidity, it is inconclusive that a significant difference exists in experienced hands.

SUMMARY

The American Joint Committee on Cancer revised the seventh edition of the TNM staging system for esophageal cancer in 2010. The revised system evaluated the N category by looking at the number of positive lymph nodes. This has continued on into the eighth edition of the TNM staging system, which has been published and should be used from 2018.[41] However, neither system specifies the number of nodes that constitutes an adequate yield to allow accurate staging, and it is well known that an inadequate yield may lead to understaging and thus stage migration.

It is felt by some that a comprehensive lymphadenectomy is associated with increased morbidity due to the increased surgical trauma. However, a number of studies have refuted this claim and found little difference in morbidity when a more extensive lymphadenectomy is carried out.

Although it is true that an extensive lymphadenectomy will lead to more accurate staging, advocates of a minimal dissection will point to the fact that there is little evidence for postoperative adjuvant treatment on long-term survival. However, such information may be valuable in counseling a patient regarding prognosis, and future studies may reveal that postoperative chemotherapy does confer a survival advantage.

Although there has been a variation in findings of the impact of lymphadenectomy, it would be intuitive to suppose that leaving positive nodes behind is likely to hasten recurrence. However, the effect of neoadjuvant treatments may in some patients sterilize any remaining disease. It is impossible to predict this impact and so we would unequivocally advocate an en bloc lymphadenectomy.

REFERENCES

1. Stein HJ, Feith M, Bruecher BLDM, Naehrig J, Sarbia M, Siewert JR. Early esophageal cancer: pattern of lymphatic spread and prognostic factors for long-term survival after surgical resection. *Ann Surg.* 2005;242(4):566-573, discussion 573–575.

2. Endo M, Yoshino K, Kawano T, Nagai K, Inoue H. Clinicopathologic analysis of lymph node metastasis in surgically resected superficial cancer of the thoracic esophagus. *Dis Esophagus Off J Int Soc Dis Esophagus.* 2000;13(2):125-129.

3. Kodama M, Kakegawa T. Treatment of superficial cancer of the esophagus: a summary of responses to a questionnaire on superficial cancer of the esophagus in Japan. *Surgery* 1998;123(4):432-439.

4. Alvarez Herrero L, Pouw R, van Vilsteren F, et al. Risk of lymph node metastasis associated with deeper invasion by early adenocarcinoma of the esophagus and cardia: study based on endoscopic resection specimens. *Endoscopy.* 2010;42(12):1030-1036.

5. Ancona E, Rampado S, Cassaro M, et al. Prediction of lymph node status in superficial esophageal carcinoma. *Ann Surg Oncol.* 2008;15(11):3278-3288.

6. Leers JM, DeMeester SR, Oezcelik A, et al. The prevalence of lymph node metastases in patients with T1 esophageal adenocarcinoma. *Ann Surg.* 2011;253(2):271-278.

7. Hagen JA, DeMeester SR, Peters JH, Chandrasoma P, DeMeester TR. Curative resection for esophageal adenocarcinoma: analysis of 100 en bloc esophagectomies. *Ann Surg.* 2001;234(4):520-530, discussion 530–531.

8. Lerut T, Nafteux P, Moons J, et al. Three-field lymphadenectomy for carcinoma of the esophagus and gastroesophageal junction in 174 R0 resections: impact on staging, disease-free survival, and outcome: a plea for adaptation of TNM classification in upper-half esophageal carcinoma. *Ann Surg.* 2004;240(6):962-972, discussion 972–974.

9. Akiyama H. *Surgery for Cancer of the Esophagus.* Baltimore: Lippincott Williams & Wilkins; 1990.

10. Fujita H, Sueyoshi S, Tanaka T, Shirouzu K. Three-field dissection for squamous cell carcinoma in the thoracic esophagus. *Ann Thorac Cardiovasc Surg.* 2002;8(6):328-335.

11. Takahashi H, Arimura Y, Masao H, et al. Endoscopic submucosal dissection is superior to conventional endoscopic resection as a curative treatment for early squamous cell carcinoma of the esophagus (with video). *Gastrointest Endosc.* 2010;72(2):255-264, 264.e1–2.

12. Araki K, Ohno S, Egashira A, Saeki H, Kawaguchi H, Sugimachi K. Pathologic features of superficial esophageal squamous cell carcinoma with lymph node and distal metastasis. *Cancer.* 2002;94(2):570-575.

13. Bollschweiler E, Baldus SE, Schröder W, et al. High rate of lymph-node metastasis in submucosal esophageal squamous-cell carcinomas and adenocarcinomas. *Endoscopy.* 2006;38(2):149-156.

14. Siewert JR, Stein HJ, Feith M, Bruecher BL, Bartels H, Fink U. Histologic tumor type is an independent prognostic parameter in esophageal cancer: lessons from more than 1,000 consecutive resections at a single center in the Western world. *Ann Surg.* 2001; 234(3):360-367, discussion 368–369.

15. Law SY, Fok M, Wong J. Pattern of recurrence after oesophageal resection for cancer: clinical implications. *Br J Surg.* 1996;83(1):107-111.

16. Wayman J, Bennett MK, Raimes SA, Griffin SM. The pattern of recurrence of adenocarcinoma of the oesophago-gastric junction. *Br J Cancer.* 2002;86(8):1223-1229.

17. Griffin SM, Raimes SA, Shenfine J, eds. *Oesophagogastric Surgery: A Companion to Specialist Surgical Practice.* 5th ed. Edinburgh: Saunders Ltd; 2013.

18. Anderegg MCJ, Lagarde SM, Jagadesham VP, et al. Prognostic significance of the location of lymph node metastases in patients with adenocarcinoma of the distal esophagus or gastroesophageal junction. *Ann Surg.* 2016;264(5):847-853.

19. Hulscher JBF, van Sandick JW, de Boer AGEM, et al. Extended transthoracic resection compared with limited transhiatal resection for adenocarcinoma of the esophagus. *N Engl J Med.* 2002;347(21):1662-1669.

20. Griffin SM, Burt AD, Jennings NA. Lymph node metastasis in early esophageal adenocarcinoma. *Ann Surg.* 2011;254(5):731-737.

21. van der Schaaf M, Johar A, Wijnhoven B, Lagergren P, Lagergren J. Extent of lymph node removal during esophageal cancer surgery and survival. *JNCI J Natl Cancer Inst.* 2015;107(5):djv043.

22. Lagergren J, Mattsson F, Zylstra J, et al. Extent of lymphadenectomy and prognosis after esophageal cancer surgery. *JAMA Surg.* 2016;151(1):32-39.

23. Chen J-W, Xie J-D, Ling Y-H, et al. The prognostic effect of perineural invasion in esophageal squamous cell carcinoma. *BMC Cancer.* 2014;14:313.

24. Bhamidipati CM, Stukenborg GJ, Thomas CJ, Lau CL, Kozower BD, Jones DR. Pathologic lymph node ratio is a predictor of survival in esophageal cancer. *Ann Thorac Surg.* 2012;94(5):1643-1651.

25. Phillips AW, Lagarde SM, Navidi M, Disep B, Griffin SM. Impact of extent of lymphadenectomy on survival, post neoadjuvant chemotherapy and transthoracic esophagectomy. *Ann Surg.* 2017;265(4):750-756.

26. Hosch S, Kraus J, Scheunemann P, et al. Malignant potential and cytogenetic characteristics of occult disseminated tumor cells in esophageal cancer. *Cancer Res.* 2000;60(24):6836-6840.

27. Izbicki JR, Hosch SB, Pichlmeier U, et al. Prognostic value of immunohistochemically identifiable tumor cells in lymph nodes of patients with completely resected esophageal cancer. *N Engl J Med.* 1997;337(17):1188-1194.

28. Glickman JN, Torres C, Wang HH, et al. The prognostic significance of lymph node micrometastasis in patients with esophageal carcinoma. *Cancer.* 1999;85(4):769-778.

29. Vazquez-Sequeiros E, Wang L, Burgart L, et al. Occult lymph node metastases as a predictor of tumor relapse in patients with node-negative esophageal carcinoma. *Gastroenterology.* 2002;122(7):1815-1821.

30. Omloo JMT, Lagarde SM, Hulscher JBF, et al. Extended transthoracic resection compared with limited transhiatal resection for adenocarcinoma of the mid/distal esophagus. *Ann Surg.* 2007;246(6):992-1001.

31. Rizk NP, Ishwaran H, Rice TW, et al. Optimum lymphadenectomy for esophageal cancer. *Ann Surg.* 2010;251(1):46-50.

32. Peyre CG, Hagen JA, DeMeester SR, et al. Predicting systemic disease in patients with esophageal cancer after esophagectomy. *Ann Surg.* 2008;248(6):979-985.

33. Peyre CG, Hagen JA, DeMeester SR, et al. The number of lymph nodes removed predicts survival in esophageal cancer: an international study on the impact of extent of surgical resection. *Ann Surg.* 2008;248(4):549-556.

34. de Bekker-Grob EW, Niers EJ, van Lanschot JJB, Steyerberg EW, Wijnhoven BPL. Patients' preferences for surgical management of esophageal cancer: a discrete choice experiment. *World J Surg.* 2015;39(10):2492-2499.

35. Grotenhuis BA, Wijnhoven BPL, van Marion R, et al. The sentinel node concept in adenocarcinomas of the distal esophagus and gastroesophageal junction. *J Thorac Cardiovasc Surg.* 2009;138(3):608-612.

36. Chen J, Wu S, Zheng X, et al. Cervical lymph node metastasis classified as regional nodal staging in thoracic esophageal squamous cell carcinoma after radical esophagectomy and three-field lymph node dissection. *BMC Surg.* 2014;14(1):110.

37. Ma G-W, Situ D-R, Ma Q-L, et al. Three-field vs two-field lymph node dissection for esophageal cancer: a meta-analysis. *World J Gastroenterol.* 2014;20(47):18022-18030.

38. Ye T, Sun Y, Zhang Y, Zhang Y, Chen H. Three-field or two-field resection for thoracic esophageal cancer: a meta-analysis. *Ann Thorac Surg.* 2013;96(6):1933-1941.

39. Shang Q-X, Chen L-Q, Hu W-P, Deng H-Y, Yuan Y, Cai J. Three-field lymph node dissection in treating the esophageal cancer. *J Thorac Dis.* 2016;8(10):E1136-E1149.

40. Schandl A, Johar A, Lagergren J, Lagergren P. Lymphadenectomy and health-related quality of life after oesophageal cancer surgery: a nationwide, population-based cohort study. *BMJ Open.* 2016;6(8):e012624.

41. Rice TW, Ishwaran H, Ferguson MK, Blackstone EH, Goldstraw P. Cancer of the esophagus and esophagogastric junction: an eighth edition staging primer. *J Thorac Oncol.* 2017;12(1):36-42.

Options for Esophageal Replacement

Lieven Depypere | Hans Van Veer | Philippe Robert Nafteux |

Willy Coosemans | Toni Lerut

MILESTONES IN SURGERY FOR ESOPHAGEAL CARCINOMA

1877—V. Czerny: first successful resection of the cervical esophagus for carcinoma[1]

1913—F. Torek: first successful transthoracic resection of the esophagus[2]

1913—W. Denk: cadaver and experimental animal studies on the transhiatal resection of the esophagus[3]

1933—T. Ohsawa: first report on transthoracic esophageal resection and esophagogastrostomy[4]

1933—G. Turner: first transhiatal resection[5]

1938—W. Adams and D. Phemister: first single stage transthoracic resection and reconstruction in the United States[6]

1946—I. Lewis: esophageal resection and esophagogastrostomy via a right thoracotomy and laparotomy[7]

1976—K. McKeown: description of a three-hole esophagectomy[8]

1978—M. Orringer: popularizes transhiatal esophagectomy in the Western hemisphere[9]

1992—A. Cushieri: first report on thoracoscopic esophagectomy[10]

2003—J. Luketich: popularizes total thoracoscopic and laparoscopic esophagectomy[11]

Milestones in esophageal reconstruction

1879—T. Billroth: attempt of reconstruction with skin[12]

1886—J. Mikulicz: Reconstruction of the cervical esophagus by skin flaps[13]

1905—C. Beck and A. Carrel: experimental animal study on tubulization of the greater curvature of the stomach[14]

1906—A. Carrel: successful transplantation of autologous small bowel into the neck of dogs[15]

1907—C. Roux: first use of a presternal jejunal loop combined with skin tube for benign esophageal stricture[16]

1911—H. Vuillet[17] and G. Kelling[18] separately introduced colon as a substitute: first attempt of two-stage resection followed by colonic interposition

The end of the 19th century was characterized by a true race to perform the first esophagectomy. Although Czerny[1] had already performed a successful partial resection of the cervical esophagus for a cancer as early as in 1877, further attempts to successfully resect an intrathoracic esophageal cancer had failed.

It is Franz Torek[2] who is to be credited on the first successful transthoracic (and transpleural) resection of the esophagus in 1913. Reconstruction was not attempted and the patient was fed using a rubber tube connecting the proximal esophagostomy with a gastrostomy; she lived for 13 years.

Further attempts made in the following years were mostly unsuccessful due to lack of technology to adequately ventilate the lungs. Only after the introduction of safe oro-tracheal intubation in the late 1920s by Rowbotham[19] and Magill[20] could surgeons undertake such a complex operation as a transthoracic esophagectomy more safely. Over the following decades pioneers, such as Denk,[3] Ohsawa,[4] Grey Turner,[5] Adam and Phemister,[6] Sweet,[21] Ivor Lewis,[7] McKeown,[8] Belsey,[22] and Orringer,[9] further developed and refined the surgical techniques as we use them today. However, postoperative mortality remained high well into the 1970s. Better insights in medical operability and better perioperative management hallmarked the 1980s and 1990s where operative mortality was brought down to below 5%,[23] and is now approximately 1% to 2% in many centers of experience.

Better selection in terms of oncologic operability through the introduction of the computed tomography scan, the positron emission tomography scan, and endoscopic ultrasound have resulted in a sharp decrease of futile exploratory thoracotomies. Better surgical techniques and the advent of induction therapy substantially increased the R0 resection rates in locally advanced (T3) carcinoma reaching greater than 90% today, in many published series.

Consequently, the resulting long-term survival has been constantly on the rise over the last decades, reaching an overall 5-year survival today between 35% and 45%.[24]

As a result of these improvements in oncologic outcome, increasing attention is now being paid to the functional outcome both short and long term. This is reflected by the high number of publications in recent years focusing on quality of life (QOL).[25]

Ideally the conduit substituting for the esophagus should mimic as closely as possible the function of a normal esophagus to preserve QOL. It should allow the undisturbed transport of the alimentary bolus from mouth to stomach, providing an adequate antireflux mechanism that protects the lungs from aspiration, but allowing the possibility to belch or vomit when necessary.

An equally important objective is to reduce mortality and morbidity inherent to major surgery, such as resection and reconstruction for cancer of the esophagus. In this respect, the choice of the type of conduit to restore continuity may play an important role. Indeed one can imagine that there is a potentially higher risk in postoperative morbidity, eventually mortality, when using a vascularized, so-called supercharged, long-segment, jejunal graft requiring five different anastomoses by two different teams, as compared to a gastric pull-up requiring only one anastomosis.

Furthermore, suboptimal nutritional, immunological, cardiopulmonary status, old age, or impaired performance status (e.g., due to severe arthrosis) may play a role in the choice of the substitute. In this context, the surgeon will preferably make use of a gastric pull-up with one single anastomosis versus a colon interposition requiring three anastomoses, which carries a higher potential for infectious complications.

Organ availability may play a role in the choice of the substitute; for example, previous total gastrectomy or partial or total colectomy, which will preclude the use of the stomach or the colon, respectively, as a substitute.

During surgery, the surgeon may encounter unforeseen situations, for example, former division of the right gastroepiploic artery as a consequence of a right colectomy with lymphadenectomy for colon cancer. Such a finding at the time of surgery will oblige the surgeon to switch to another conduit (e.g., the jejunum). Unforeseen metastatic intramural deposits higher up in the esophagus may require the surgeon to switch the level of the anastomosis from the chest to the neck.

Finally, a critical determinant is the surgeon's expertise, and that of the whole team involved in the pre- and postoperative management.

In other words, esophagectomy followed by reconstruction is one of the most complex and difficult operations on the alimentary tract, which requires an experienced surgical team familiar with all available conduits, and who are able to adapt to every situation in order to offer the patient the best possible type of reconstruction.

Historically, the first attempts for reconstruction were tried by Billroth[12] as early as 1879. Skin was the first material used for reconstruction,[13] but the stomach, colon, and jejunum—in order of their frequency of use—became the three classic substitutes over time. They are mostly used as a single pedicled transposition, but can be used as free vascularized grafts (in particular the jejunum) or occasionally as composite replacements.

Combining conduit choice with a multitude of different access routes, including the recent minimally invasive techniques, and different levels of anastomosis, it is clear that there are a myriad of options available when planning an esophagectomy and reconstruction for cancer. A tailored approach for each individual patient guided by an experienced surgeon is the key to success.

STOMACH

Today, gastroplasty is by far the most preferred conduit for replacing the esophagus in over 95% of cases. It is indeed the quickest and "simplest" organ surgery for reconstruction. It has a robust arterial and venous supply and submucosal plexus. After mobilization, the stomach will receive its blood supply from the right gastroepiploic artery with the venous blood drained via the right gastroepiploic vein (Fig. 41.1). There is only the need for a single anastomosis. As the stomach is a very flexible organ, it can easily reach the neck for a cervical or even hypopharyngeal anastomosis. Its main disadvantage is the potential of reflux and related aspiration problems.

Regarding the "robustness" of the blood supply, the surgeon must be aware of some anatomic variations

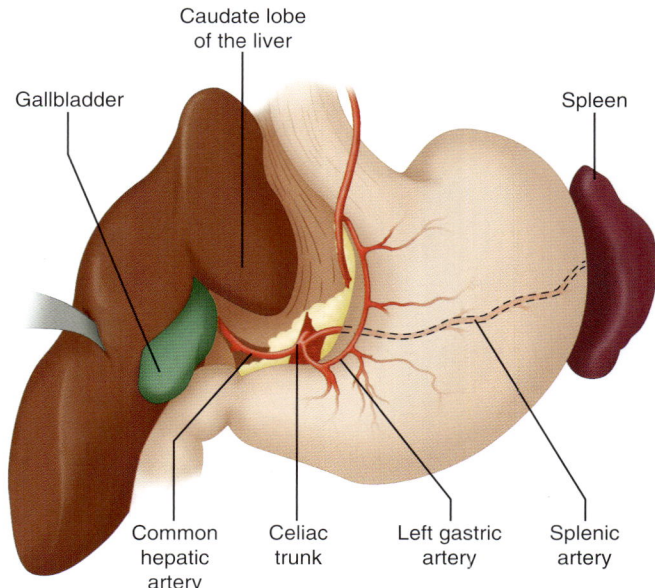

FIGURE 41.1 View on the upper abdominal compartment with vascularization of the stomach.

at the level of the gastroepiploic arcade. In some instances, the right gastroepiploic artery may end about half way up the greater curvature connecting to the left gastroepiploic artery only through delicate arterioles in the omentum, which need to be respected during mobilization (Fig. 41.2). Moreover, the pioneering work by Liebermann-Meffert et al.,[26] using corrosion casts on cadaver specimens, clearly shows that the submucosal plexus is thinning out near the top of the fundus, and that there is a watershed zone with a clear decrease of the intertwining connections between the submucosal microcirculation of the left side (lesser curvature) and the right side (greater curvature).

Studies have shown that after full mobilization of the greater curvature of the stomach and ligation of the left and right gastric artery, the oxygen tension at the top of the fundus decreases substantially, and, after transposing the conduit up to the neck, it falls to approximately 50%.[27,28] Efforts have been made to prevent this effect by preoperative conditioning of the vascular supply; that is, ligating or embolizing the left gastric artery a few days before the planned esophagectomy and reconstruction.[29–32] However, the results have been equivocal and one prospective, randomized trial failed to show any advantage. Therefore, it is of paramount importance not to traumatize the top end of the stomach in order to avoid anastomotic leak or eventually fundic necrosis.[30]

TECHNIQUE OF GASTROPLASTY WITH THE CREATION OF A GASTRIC TUBE

In general, most surgeons prefer to start with a laparotomy/laparoscopy in order to first inspect the abdominal cavity to exclude the presence of unforeseen metastasis before mobilization of the stomach. Alternatively, one may prefer to start with a thoracotomy/video-assisted thoracoscopic surgery (VATS) in order to assess resectability, particularly in the case of a questionable T3-4 tumor. Mobilization of the stomach is started by opening the gastrohepatic

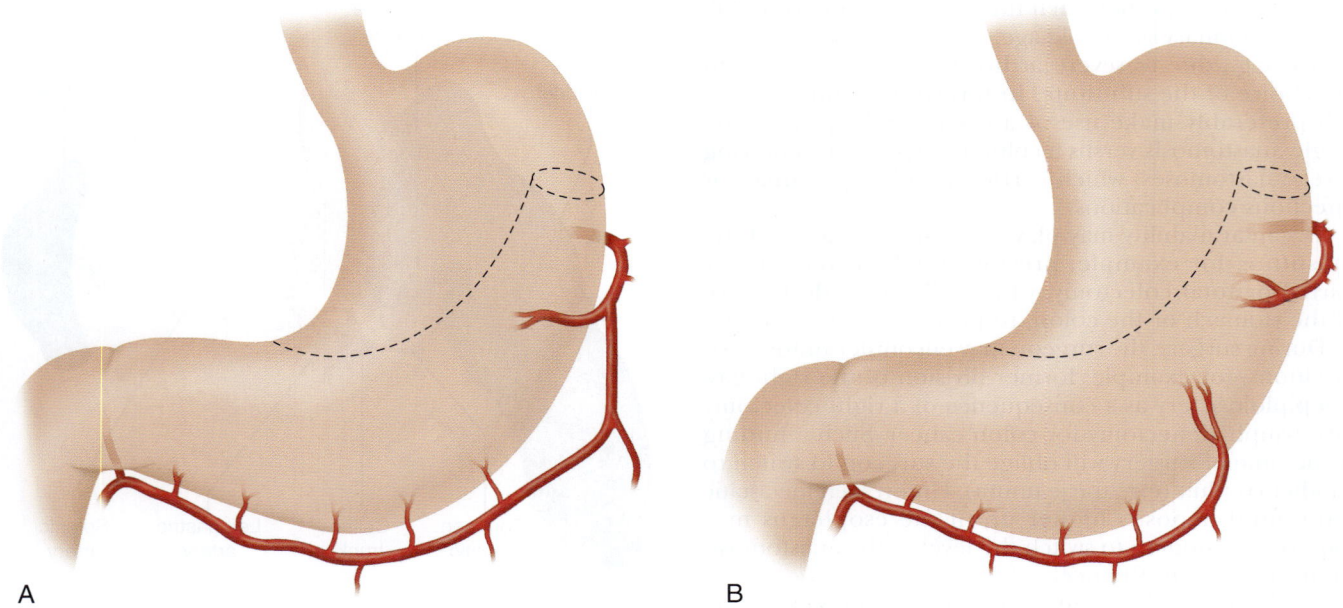

A

B

FIGURE 41.2 Favorable (A) and unfavorable (B) pattern of the right gastroepiploic arcade. (From Siewert R, Hölscher A. 3 Eingriffe beim Ösophaguskarzinom. Jejunuminterposition. In: Siewert, ed. *Breitner Chirurgische Operationslehre. Band IV: Ösophagus, Magen und Duodenum*. Vienna: Urban & Schwarzenberg; 1989:33. Fig. 3-36a,b.)

ligament so that the hiatus and the right pillar of the right crus come into view. In some patients, there will be a separate left hepatic artery present. If this artery is small, a couple of millimeters in diameter, it can be ligated without causing harm to the liver. A larger size left hepatic artery needs to be dissected carefully down to its origin, usually at the left gastric artery, and both need to be preserved in order to avoid major, possibly lethal, hepatic necrosis.

This is followed by the mobilization of the greater curvature by dividing, distally to the gastroepiploic vascular arcade, the omentum and its feeding vascular branches, as well as the attachments to the transverse colon in this area. Usually, the easier point to start the dissection of the greater curvature is about halfway up the greater curvature.

In some cases, due to previous episodes of pancreatitis for example, the retrogastric area will be obliterated making the dissection more difficult. The utmost care has to be taken not to damage the gastroepiploic vessels. Especially in laparoscopic mobilization, care should be taken never to grab the gastroepiploic vessels nor the greater curvature of the stomach with the laparoscopic forceps because of the earlier described very important but fragile microcirculation. In laparoscopic mobilization, it is very helpful to pull on the lesser curvature, as it will be stapled out afterward.

The dissection is further continued upward along the greater curvature and the gastroepiploic arcade is divided at the level of the inferior pole of the spleen at the point where the left gastroepiploic artery ends in the splenic artery.

In a number of patients, the right gastroepiploic artery interrupts somewhere midway or two-thirds of the way down on the greater curvature (Fig. 41.2). The connections with the left gastroepiploic artery or the short gastric vessels here come through the omental intertwining small vessels. At this level, it is important to stay away from the greater curvature and dissect more on the periphery of the omentum so these connections can be preserved. Coming at the level of the short gastric vessels connecting the spleen and the proximal greater curvature, it is again preferable to stay as close to the spleen as possible when dividing the vessels. Again this allows preservation of the small delicate connections within the submucosal plexus. Preserving as much as possible of the omentum at that level also allows it to be used to protect the anastomosis later on. Obviously, great care is taken not to damage the spleen. Today, with the help of ultrasonic devices, the risk of damage requiring eventually iatrogenic splenectomy has substantially decreased and, in fact, should no longer occur. Once the short gastric vessels are divided, the gastrodiaphragmatic area is dissected so that, after retraction of the fundus to the right, the left pillar of the right crus will come into view, allowing further dissection of the entire retrogastric area covering the hiatus.

The hiatus can now be opened by incising the phreno-esophageal ligament (if not already done from above during the thoracic portion of the case). In case of a gastroesophageal junction (GEJ) tumor, a rim of the diaphragmatic hiatus is excised and left in continuity with the esophagus in order to ensure a complete R0 resection. Now the inferior mediastinum becomes widely opened and accessible so the distal esophagus can be dissected out and a tape passed around it.

Next comes the ligation of the left gastric artery. This is done after the dissection of lymph nodes around the left gastric artery and the celiac axis extending over the common hepatic and the splenic artery.

Both the left gastric artery and accompanying vein are ligated and divided separately. The further dissection is continued toward the right toward the pylorus—first at the side of the greater curvature, again making sure not to damage the right gastroepiploic vessels, then on the lesser curvature where the right gastric artery is ligated and divided.

In order to obtain maximal mobility and length, it may be useful to perform a Kocher maneuver elevating the duodenum and the head of the pancreas anteriorly off the inferior vena cava. By doing so, the pylorus easily can be brought up to the level of the esophageal hiatus.

Most surgeons today prefer to create a rather narrow gastric tube with a width of about 4 cm (which is about on the watershed zone between the earlier described left and right microcirculation). To do so, the lesser curvature needs to be resected. This is also an essential oncologic act since the lymph nodes on the lesser curvature are known to be at risk for metastatic involvement—definitely in the lower half and in GEJ cancers.[33]

The creation of a gastric tube has been enormously facilitated by the introduction of the staplers. If the access route is a left thoracoabdominal one, the stapling starts from above, at the top of the fundus. A linear cutting stapler will be placed at the top end of the fundus about 5 cm laterally from the GEJ (Fig. 41.3). The staplers are then placed in a vertical direction. Several staplers will be necessary. The end result is a long gastric tube with a width of approximately 4 to 5 cm. If the access is through a laparoscopic approach, the stapling starts from the lesser curvature at the level of the crow's foot, about 4 cm proximal to the pylorus.

Many surgeons will oversew the staple line with separate or running sutures. This will help not only to protect against leakage but also (arguably) to prevent early postoperative dilatation of the tube (Fig. 41.4).[34] However, it can shorten the gastric tube and when performed laparoscopically, it is very time consuming.

The gastric tube is temporarily fixed to the divided lesser curvature with two stay sutures and the whole complex of esophagus, lesser curvature, and gastric tube will be pulled up via the cervical or thoracic incision and exteriorized. It is important to make sure that the tube is not twisted around its axis, with the staple line being on the medial side.

ANASTOMOSIS

After exteriorizing the whole complex, the anastomosis will be constructed.

In case of an Ivor Lewis approach, the anastomosis will be fashioned in the chest via a right thoracotomy or VATS. In a McKeown fashion, the anastomosis will be in the neck, preferably on the left side.

The anastomosis is the Achilles heel of the operation. Anastomotic leak once carried a high mortality. Fortunately, today, mortality has become very low but its relation to early and late morbidity is a source of concern and will be discussed in Chapter 43.

Because of these serious consequences, over time different techniques, either handsewn, mechanical, or combined, have been developed. This chapter will describe cervical handsewn and semimechanical anastomosis, and the intrathoracic stapled anastomosis.

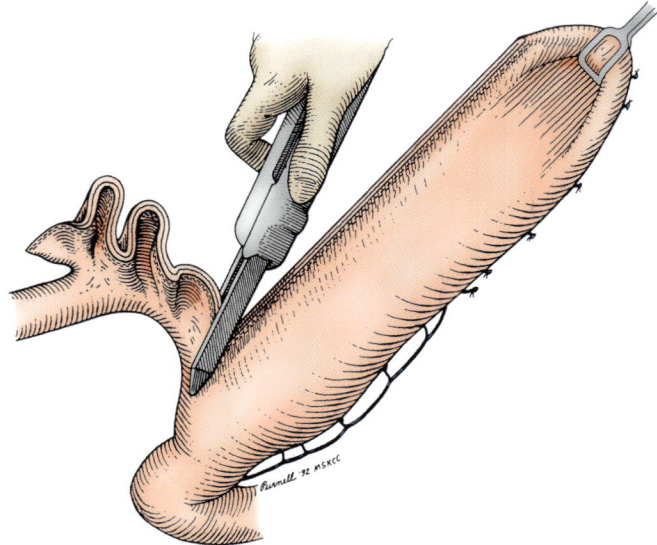

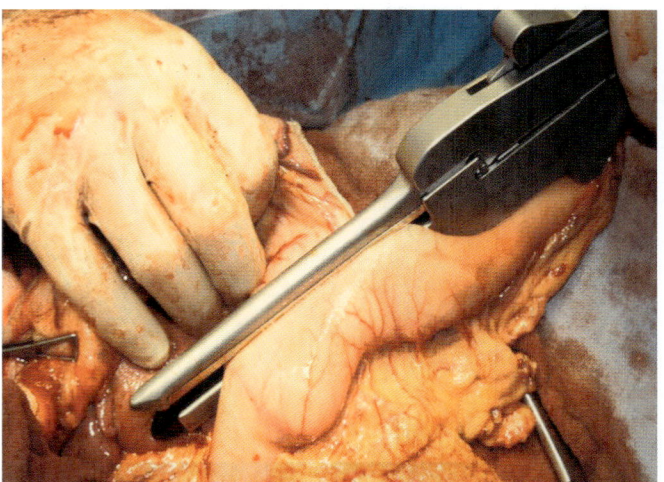

FIGURE 41.3 Resection of lesser curvature starting at the top of the fundus. ([A] Reprinted with permission from the Journal of the American College of Surgeons, formerly Surgery Gynecology & Obstetrics.)

Cervical Anastomosis

In the setting of a McKeown (three-hole) intervention, the patient is positioned and draped for laparotomy, or laparoscopy and cervicotomy, so that the surgical team can proceed simultaneously with the abdominal phase together with a left-sided cervicotomy. After the transection of the platysma and omohyoid muscles, the medial border of the sternocleidomastoid muscle is identified and retracted laterally. After division of the inferior thyroid artery, access to the cervical esophagus is achieved. There, the esophagus can be hooked with the surgeon's finger, exteriorizing the esophagus from the neck and chest. In the same movement, the gastric conduit is carefully brought up through the diaphragmatic hiatus into the posterior mediastinum and eventually into the neck. Attention should be paid during this maneuver to not injure the left recurrent laryngeal nerve.

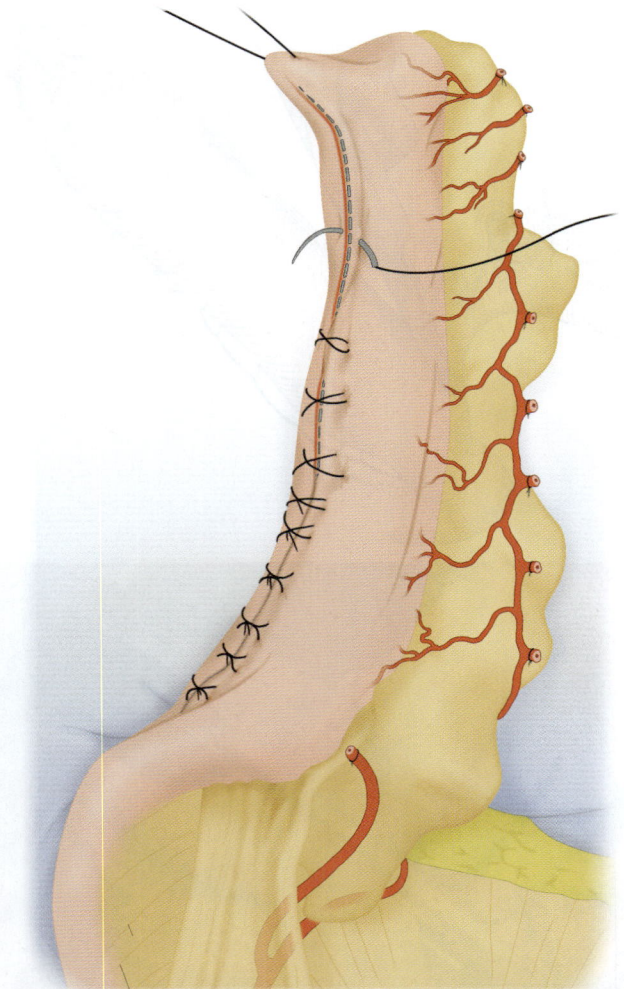

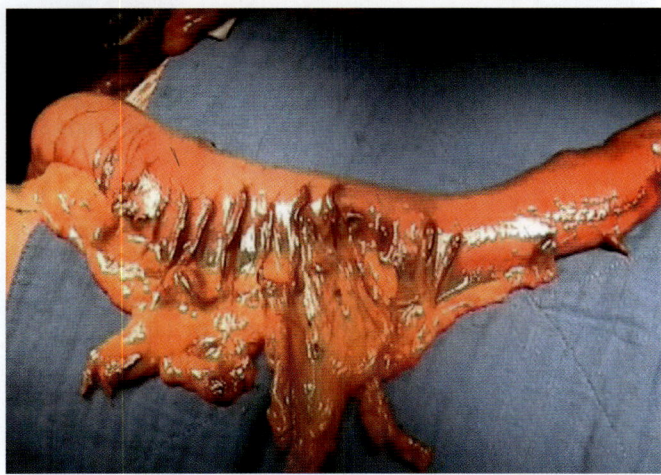

FIGURE 41.4 Oversewing the staple line and completed well-vascularized gastric tube.

To prevent damage to the vascular pedicle, the conduit should be carefully guided by one hand of the surgeon through the hiatus (or in the case of a laparoscopic procedure, by guiding the vascular pedicle through the hiatus without grasping it with the forceps when pulling up the conduit with the other hand). Care is taken not to axially twist the gastric tube at the cervical level.

At the thoracic inlet, there has to be sufficient width (about three fingers) to allow free passage into the cervical field without compression of the tube. Once the gastric tube is brought in the operative field in the neck, the temporary stay sutures are cut. The proximal esophagus is now lying side by side with the gastric conduit ready to construct an end (esophagus) to side (gastric tube) anastomosis. The place to incise the gastric tube is chosen well away from the lateral staple line. After reflecting the esophagus upward, the same is done on the esophageal wall.

Handsewn Anastomosis

On the outer sides of the esophagus and gastric tube, two sutures of nonresorbable monofilament 3-0 are placed between the muscularis of the esophagus and the seromuscular layer of the stomach. Separate sutures or continuous running suture will complete the posterior outer layer of the anastomosis. Care is taken to avoid any tension between the two conduits (Fig. 41.5).

Then with the electrocautery an incision of approximately 2 cm (maximum 3 cm) is made, widely opening the lumen of the stomach. This incision is made at a minimum distance of 1 cm away from the posterior outer layer.

The same maneuver is done on the esophageal wall comprising the whole width of the esophagus and again a minimum of 1 cm away from the outer layer. The slimy mucous content of the gastric tube and esophagus are carefully removed with suction and swabs, avoiding any spillage in the operative field, and both lumina are disinfected with a povidone-iodine (Betadine) swab.

Two 3-0 monofilament resorbable sutures are placed in each corner from the esophagus outside to inside, then to the stomach inside to outside, to start off the posterior inner layer. After tying the stitches, the inner layer is further completed out from one corner toward the opposite corner with a running suture similar to a vascular anastomosis. After finishing the posterior inner row, the nasogastric tube, partially withdrawn into the proximal esophagus, is advanced through the anastomosis well into the gastric tube.

At this point the residual anterior wall of the esophagus is transected so the anterior part of the anastomosis can start beginning from the opposite corner and running in a similar way back to the corner where the suturing initially started. Some surgeons will prefer to use separate sutures. One has to make sure to always incorporate both the mucosal and seromuscular layer into each stitch in such a way that the mucosal layer is "tucked away" underneath the seromuscular layer. This results in a smooth watertight anastomosis. Five to six mattress sutures taking muscularis on the esophageal side and seromuscularis on the gastric side complete the anterior outer layer. A mattress suture helps to have a better grip on the muscularis layer of the esophagus, which is rather fragile. For this reason, it is advisable not to tie the mattress sutures immediately one after the other, but rather to gently pull them up all together to equally spread out the traction over all sutures before tying them.

Mostly the length of the gastric tube and the chosen location of the anastomosis allow for the resection of a

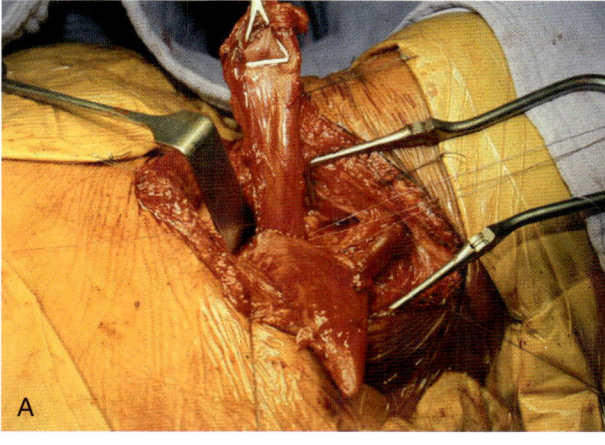

FIGURE 41.5 Handsewn anastomosis: (A) posterior mucosal layer; (B) posterior inner layer starting from corner to corner in a running fashion.

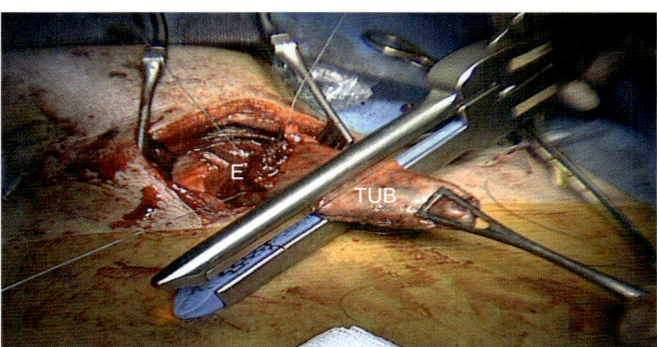

FIGURE 41.6 Trimming of the tip of the gastric tube by a linear stapler. *E*, Esophagus; *TUB*, gastric tube.

redundant proximal part. Otherwise, a blind sac would form, which can act as a pseudodiverticulum, possibly impairing the passage of food down the tube. This resection is done using a stapler, taking care that the line of transection is about 2 cm away from the anastomosis line to avoid ischemia with the risk of necrosis of the gastric wall in between (Fig. 41.6). The staple line is oversewn via a running nonabsorbable 3-0 monofilament suture. Usually, some omentum is available to wrap around the suture line as a protection against potential leaking. It is of paramount importance to avoid any traumatization of the tissues by clamps, forceps, or other instruments.

As the anastomosis is now finished, the esophagus-gastric tube complex is gently pushed back into the thoracic inlet and, after leaving behind a Redon-type drain, the cervicotomy is closed in layers.

Semimechanical Anastomosis

If the length of the conduit is sufficient (>5 cm overlap), a semimechanical Orringer or modified Collard end-to-side anastomosis is preferred (Fig. 41.7).[35] To avoid leakage, from traumatizing the tissues the tip of the gastric conduit will be resected with another linear stapler as described. It starts by placing five separate 3-0 nonresorbable stitches, in the form of a pentagon, between the muscular esophageal wall and the gastric serosal layer, with the tip being at

the deepest point. The gastric tube is incised at the base of the pentagon (see Fig. 41.7). Next, monofilament 3-0 resorbable sutures are placed in the corners outwards. Then, two monofilament 4-0 resorbable sutures are placed in the middle of the incision, bringing the base of the pentagon together and aligning the gastric and esophageal walls. In between these sutures, a 45-mm linear stapler is fired over a distance of ~35 mm (Fig. 41.8). This will create a V-shaped back wall, allowing a wider passage (Fig. 41.9). This technique prevents narrowing down during the cicatrization of the anastomosis, resulting in less dysphagia for semi-solid and solid food, thus limiting the need for repetitive anastomotic dilatations and improving the patient's QOL.[36,37] The base of the back wall, lateral to the stapler line, is completed with separate 4-0 monofilament sutures. Then, the nasogastric tube can be pushed through the anastomosis, down in the gastric conduit, to decompress the stomach after surgery. The front wall of the anastomosis is closed with a continuous two-layer suture with the earlier placed monofilament resorbable suture for the inner layer and the nonresorbable suture for the outer layer, as shown in Fig. 41.6. The tip of the gastric tube is resected by using a linear stapler as described. After careful hemostasis, a small Redon-type drain is placed in the neck to prevent the accumulation of blood, and the incision is closed. This semimechanical anastomosis results in improved dysphagia scores for solids and semi-solids, and significantly reduces the need for dilations, in particular repeat dilatations.[37]

Whether performing a handsewn or semimechanical anastomosis, before closing the cervicotomy, a minitracheostomy tube may be inserted through the cricothyroid ligament under tracheoscopic guidance from the anesthesiologist. A mini-tracheostomy facilitates the aspiration of secretions, which can be of particular assistance to patients who have insufficient strength to cough them up. Then, the platysma muscle is closed, followed by the skin suture.

Intrathoracic Stapled Anastomosis

In recent years, as a result of the increased interest in minimally invasive esophagectomy (MIE), there has

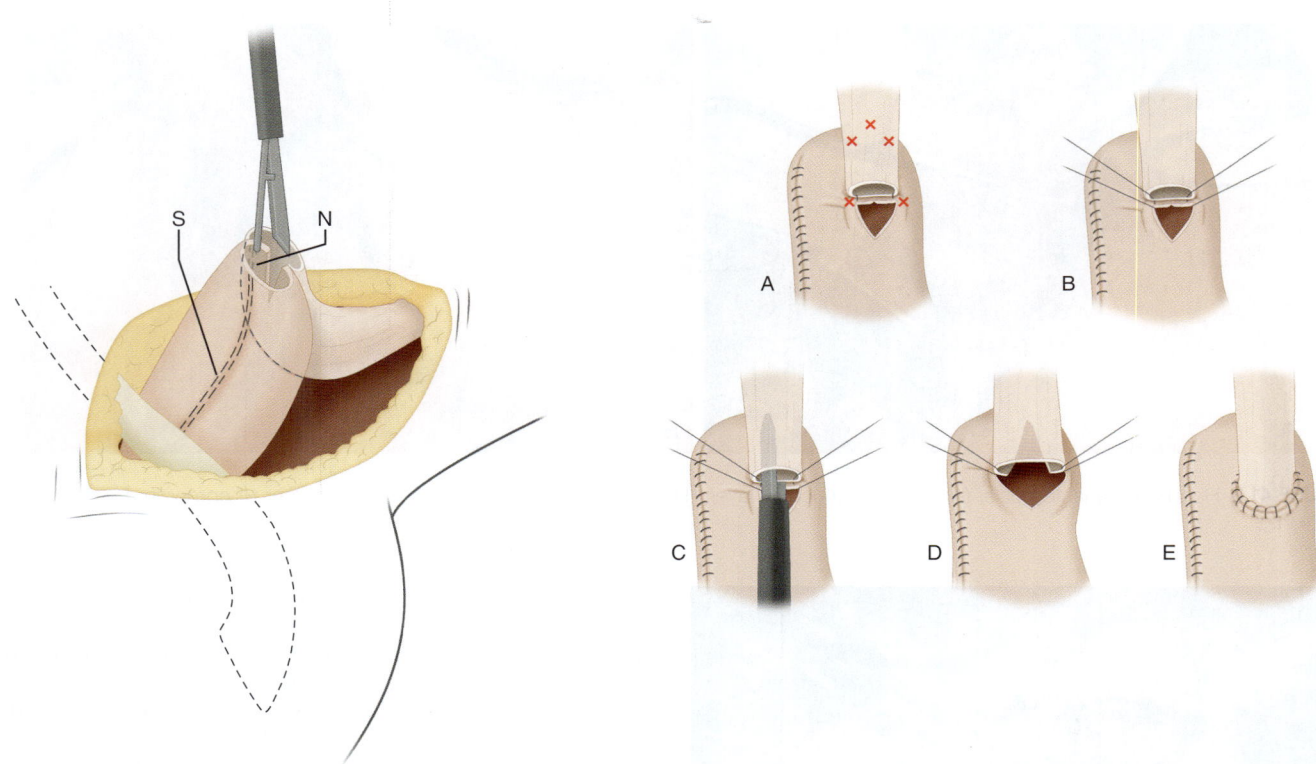

FIGURE 41.7 *(Left)* The modified Collard anastomosis: creation of an esophagogastrostomy on a gastric tube. *(Right)* (A) Serosal stitches in pentagonic form. (B) Placement of corner stitches. (C) Linear stapler insertion. (D) Status after firing the stapler resulting in a V-shaped posterior wall. (E) Manual running closure of the front wall. (*Left* from Collard JM, et al. Terminalized semimechanical side-to-side suture technique for cervical esophagogastrostomy. *Ann Thorac Surg.* 1998;65:814–817. *Right* from Ferguson M, ed. Esophagus. In: *Thoracic Surgery Atlas.* Philadelphia: Saunders; 2007:222.)

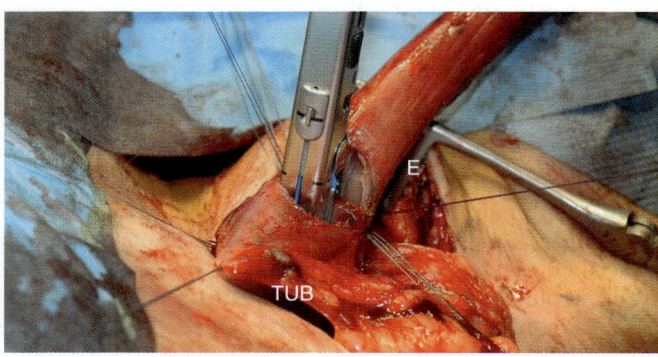

FIGURE 41.8 The stapler fired on the posterior walls of gastric tube and esophagus during the anastomosis to provide a wider passage. *E*, Esophagus; *TUB*, gastric tube.

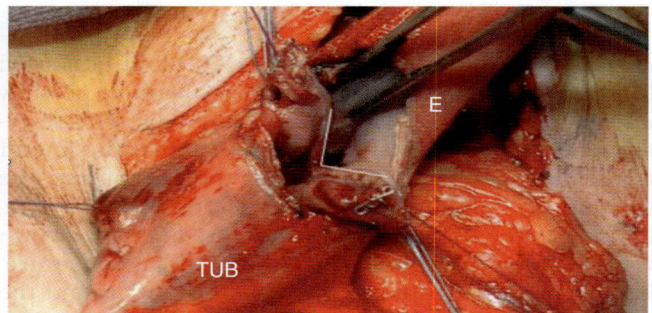

FIGURE 41.9 Demonstration of the V-shaped back wall of the esophagogastrostomy after firing of the linear stapler. *E*, Esophagus; *TUB*, gastric tube.

been a growing trend to perform the anastomosis in the chest. The advantage is that it saves time, but obviously an intrathoracic location of the anastomosis must be oncologically safe; that is, at least 5 cm proximal to the upper pole of the tumor.[38] Furthermore, the anastomosis should be located high in the apex of the right chest to reduce the risk of reflux and related aspiration.

There are two variations on how to proceed. The first option is not to fully complete the gastric tube during the abdominal phase and, after bringing up the mobilized stomach in the chest, to open the lesser curvature remnant to introduce the circular stapler and to resect the lesser curvature remnant after firing the stapler.

The second variant is to first complete the creation of the gastric tube and after bringing it up in the chest, to open the proximal part of the tube to introduce the circular stapler, resecting the top end of the tube after firing the stapler.

First, the anvil of the circular stapler, usually a 25-mm or 28-mm diameter is introduced in the esophagus. To do so, a purse string suture is applied around the cut end

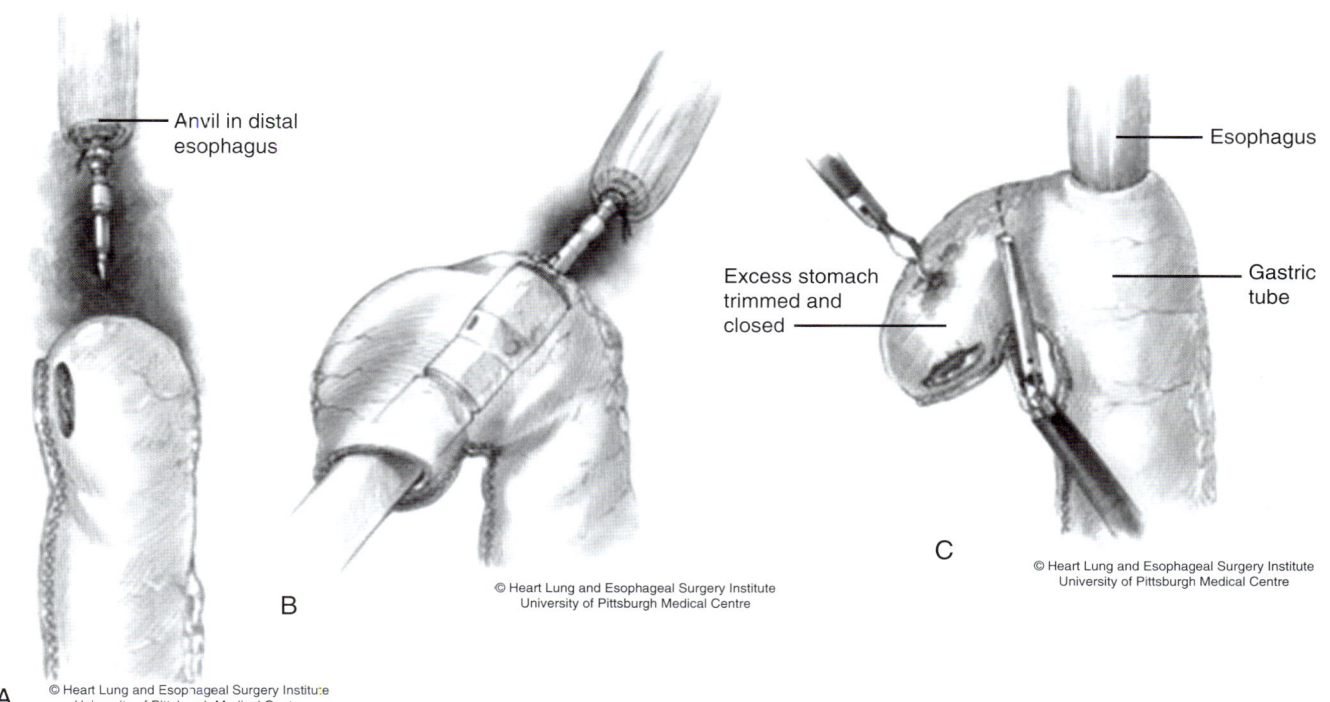

Anvil in distal esophagus

Excess stomach trimmed and closed

Esophagus

Gastric tube

© Heart Lung and Esophageal Surgery Institute
University of Pittsburgh Medical Centre

© Heart Lung and Esophageal Surgery Institute
University of Pittsburgh Medical Centre

© Heart Lung and Esophageal Surgery Institute
University of Pittsburgh Medical Centre

A

B

C

FIGURE 41.10 Intrathoracic EEA anastomosis during minimally invasive Ivor Lewis esophagectomy. (A) The EEA anvil is positioned in the proximal esophagus and secured with a purse-string suture. (B) A gastrotomy is made along the staple line near the tip of the gastric conduit, through which the EEA stapler is delivered. (C) After the anastomosis is completed, the tip of the gastric conduit is excised to complete the reconstruction. (From Schuchert MJ, Luketich JD, Landreneau RJ. Management of esophageal cancer. *Curr Probl Surg*. 2010;47:845–946.)

of the transected esophageal wall after making sure the frozen section is free of tumor. This purse string is inserted loosely using a monofilament nonabsorbable 3-0 suture (Fig. 41.10A). Second, the detached anvil is introduced. This can be somewhat tricky requiring the help of one or two Babcock-type clamps to exert counter traction. The purse string is now securely tied around the central rod of the anvil. Often after this maneuver, there may still be some tissue protruding that requires the placement of a second purse string.

In both variants, a gastrotomy is then performed to introduce the head of the circular stapler with the tip of the shaft fully retracted. The head is carefully positioned well away from the vertical staple line and ensures that the gastric conduit is not twisted. By turning the screw system of the gun, the central rod with pin is pushed through the gastric wall. Then the anvil and shaft are clicked together with the help of clamps (Fig. 41.10B). Further turning on the screw mechanism on the stapler device approximates the head and anvil tightly. The stapler is then firmly fired and removed and the two "doughnuts" are inspected for completeness. The esophageal doughnut is submitted for final pathologic examination of the margin. A nasogastric tube is passed through the anastomosis and the gastric remnant is resected using a linear stapler (Fig. 41.10C).

REVERSED GASTRIC TUBE

The principle of the reversed gastric tube was described by Beck and Carrel[14] as early as in 1905, and later by Jianu,[39] but it is mainly the Rumanian surgeon, Gavriliu,[40]

who popularized the technique in the 1980s. Claimed advantages are that it preserves part of the stomach and related gastric function and that it has the ability to reach the pharynx. In this respect, it also has been advocated for benign diseases. For malignant diseases it is rarely used nowadays.

The blood supply is based on the left gastroepiploic artery, which arises from the splenic artery and from the short gastric vessels, and requires a careful dissection in the hilum of the spleen. In essence, the liberation of the greater curvature is as described earlier. Typically, the right gastroepiploic artery is divided about 4 cm proximal to the pylorus (Fig. 41.11). The stomach is now divided starting at the greater curvature with a linear cutting stapler placed vertically, the subsequent staplers being placed in parallel with the greater curvature at a distance of approximately 3 to 4 cm away from the border and up to about two-thirds the length of the greater curvature. If a greater length is needed, a modification can be done by incorporating the pylorus into the tube (Fig. 41.12). The branches from the right gastroepiploic artery to the pylorus are preserved and the artery itself is divided close to its origin from the gastroduodenal artery. To make the conduit, the first stapler is placed at the lesser curvature at the level of the antrum and then further worked out in parallel with the greater curvature. The duodenum is transected with a linear cutting stapler just below the pylorus. Bringing up a Roux-en-Y jejunal limb to the distal stomach in order to avoid biliary reflux restores continuity with the duodenum.

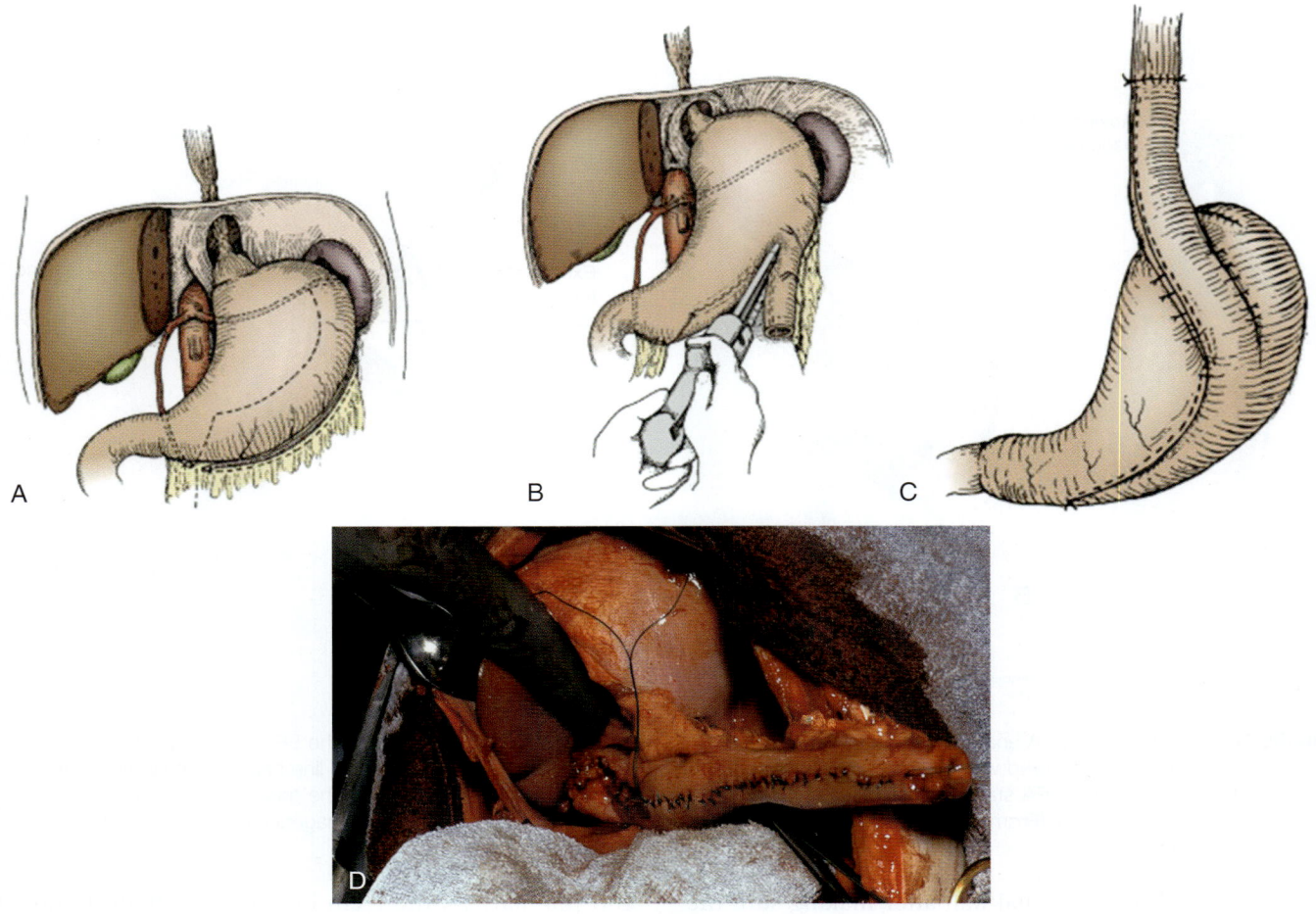

FIGURE 41.11 Graphic depiction of the technique to create a reversed gastric tube (Gavriliu) for esophageal replacement. (A) Inspection of the blood supply to the stomach and preservation of the gastroepiploic artery for creating the tube. (B) The use of a stapler to create the tube along the greater curvature of the stomach. (C) The completed reversed tube is brought up to the chest for the esophageal anastomosis. (D) Perioperative view. ([A, B, C] From Chandler NM, Colombani PM. *Ashcroft's Pediatric Surgery*. Philadelphia: Elsevier; 2014:351–364.)

NONREVERSED GASTRIC TUBE OR SPLIT STOMACH

An interesting variant is the split nonreversed gastric tube or split stomach (Fig. 41.13).[41]

Approximately 4 to 5 cm proximal to the pylorus, the shaft with a pin of a 28-mm circular stapler is pushed through both the anterior and posterior walls of the stomach. After clicking the anvil in the central rod the gun is fired, resulting in a 28-mm circular opening in the stomach. This opening suffices to introduce a linear cutting stapler cephalad. The end result is an isoperistaltic nonreversed gastric tube in connection with the antrum. The lesser curvature retains its continuity with the cardia and esophagus, the left gastric artery remaining intact and the gastric tube being pedicled on the right gastroepiploic artery, so only the left gastroepiploic artery and the short gastric vessels are taken down. This technique can be used in the rare case a bypass is needed for an unresectable cancer.

COMPLICATIONS

Gastroplasty is by far the most commonly used substitute after esophagectomy for cancer.

Over recent decades, due to the tremendous advances not only in surgical technique but also in peri- and postoperative management, the outcomes have substantially improved, both in terms of postoperative mortality and oncological outcome.

Nevertheless, this surgery still suffers from a high morbidity related to complications—reportedly 30% to 80% according to the literature. Pulmonary morbidity is responsible for two-thirds of the late non-cancer-related hospital mortality. In late follow-up, functional complications negatively influence QOL in about half of the patients, being persistently disabling in about 5% to 10% of them. Early complications, in particular leakage, necrosis, and stenosis, will be discussed in Chapter 43.

Reflux

Despite a significant reduction of acid output related to truncal vagotomy, persistence of acid secretion is the rule. Gutschow et al.[42] noted that, early on after esophagectomy and reconstruction with a denervated whole stomach, intraluminal acidity initially decreased in approximately two-thirds of the patients, but recovered its normal pH

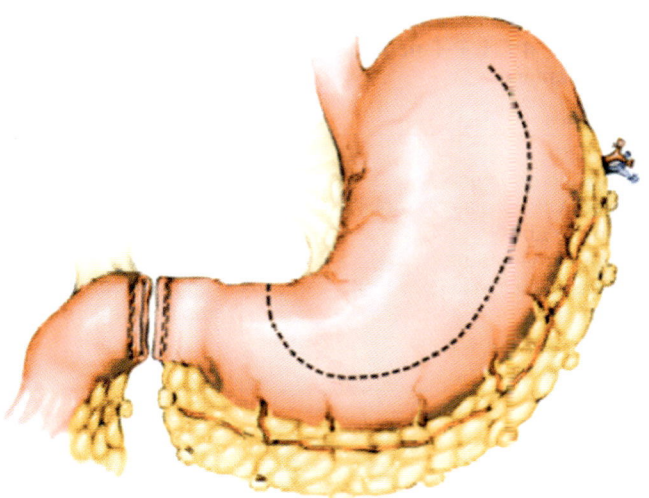

FIGURE 41.12 Extended reversed gastric tube. (Illustration reprinted with permission from Steichen FM, Wolsch RA, eds. *Mechanical Sutures in Operations on the Esophagus & Gastroesophageal Junction*. Woodbury, CT: Cine-Med; 2005.)

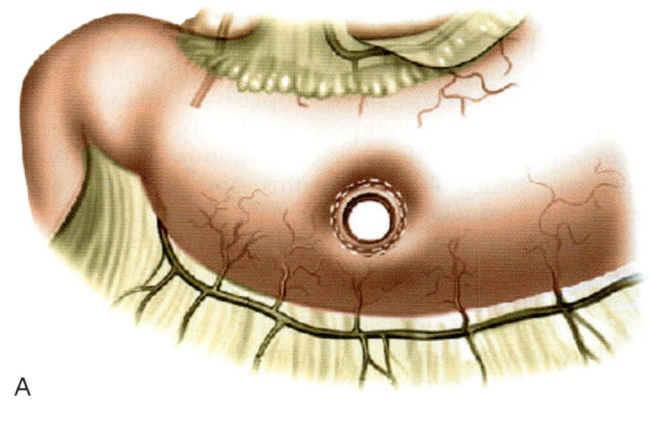

A

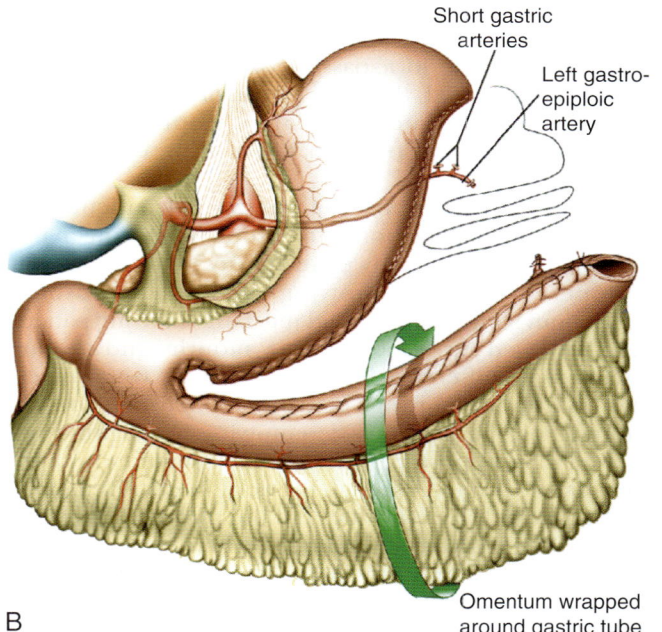

Short gastric arteries

Left gastro-epiploic artery

Omentum wrapped around gastric tube

B

FIGURE 41.13 (A) Preparation of the nonreversed gastric tube. The circular stapler creates the defect required for insertion of the linear stapler. (B) Omental wrap of the nonreversed gastric tube before cervical transposition. (From Fell SC, Ximenes-Netto M. Gastric tubes: reversed and nonreversed. In: Patterson G, et al. *Pearson's Thoracic and Esophageal Surgery*. 3rd ed. Philadelphia: Churchill Livingstone; 2008:656–662.)

profile over time. This is due to autonomous recovery of acid secretion from the parietal cells.

Consequently, a substantial number of patients will suffer from reflux symptoms after esophagectomy and gastroplasty. The main symptoms are heartburn, regurgitation, dysphagia, vomiting, and aspiration pneumonia. Shibuya et al.[43] reported that up to 58% of patients complained of reflux symptoms. On endoscopy, severe reflux esophagitis, grade C or D, was observed in 76% of the patients complaining of reflux symptoms. There was a significantly higher incidence of reflux esophagitis in patients with an intrathoracic anastomosis than in patients with a cervical anastomosis (89% vs. 56%; $F = .0039$).

De Leyn et al.[44] reported a 15% incidence of heartburn and regurgitation at 3 months, increasing to 21% after 1 year. There was a significant difference in the incidence of reflux symptoms, esophagitis, and anastomotic stenosis when comparing infraaortic intrathoracic anastomosis with cervical anastomosis. At 3 months, reflux symptoms were present in 5% of patients with a cervical anastomosis, and in 30% of patients with an intrathoracic anastomosis ($P = .097$). At 1 year, these figures were 4% and 50%, respectively ($P = .001$).

Esophagitis at 3 months was present in 6% after cervical anastomosis and 43% after intrathoracic anastomosis ($P = .02$). At 1 year, these figures were 8% and 53%, respectively ($P = .001$).

Anastomotic stenosis was present at 3 months in 12% after cervical anastomosis and 30% after intrathoracic anastomosis (6% and 17%, respectively [not significant], at 1 year). The latter figures suggest that, contrary to general opinion, cervical anastomosis does not necessarily result in a higher incidence of stenosis when compared with intrathoracic anastomosis. Gutschow et al.[42] reported that 38% of patients had reflux in the remnant esophagus at 3 years or more after esophagectomy. Fortunately, the introduction of potent antiacid medication (i.e., proton

pump inhibitors) has resulted in a major decrease of persistent disabling reflux-related problems.

Gastric Emptying–Related Symptoms: Pyloric Drainage, Yes or No?

Vagal denervation results in chronic dysmotility of the gastric remnant and an outlet dysfunction of the pylorus, which may cause delayed emptying. This may induce a wide spectrum of symptoms: early satiety, postprandial fullness, heartburn, high dysphagia, aspiration, and pneumonia. This spectrum of symptoms affects up to half of the patients and is truly disabling in approximately 5% to 10%.

The addition of a gastric drainage procedure, which can be a pyloroplasty, pyloromyotomy, digitoclasy, or botulinum toxin injection of the pylorus, has been advocated to remediate these undesired side effects. However, the need for such a drainage procedure has been criticized as being in fact harmful because of pyloroplasty-related technical complications (leaks), dumping, and biliary reflux. Several reports, including a number of randomized, controlled trials, have been published on this topic, but the results seem to be inconclusive.

Manjari et al.[45] compared the different types of pyloric drainage, which showed no difference in gastric emptying at 2 weeks for solid food. Huang et al.[46] randomly compared esophagectomy with or without a Heinecke-Mikulicz type of pyloroplasty in 35 patients. Gastric emptying was studied using a standard barium swallow. In both groups, there was a marked shortening of the postoperative first pyloric passage time when compared with preoperative findings. However, there was no difference between the two groups, either in the first pyloric passage or in the total emptying time. From this trial, the authors concluded that routine pyloroplasty is not necessary after esophageal cancer resection and reconstruction when using the stomach as a substitute.

Chattopadhyay et al.[47] randomized 24 patients who underwent esophagectomy for esophageal cancer into a pyloroplasty and a no pyloroplasty group. Pre- and postoperative gastric emptying was evaluated using a technetium 99m–labeled liquid meal. All surviving patients were followed up for between 6 months and 4 years. There was no difference in clinical outcome (i.e., fullness, regurgitation, vomiting, heartburn) between the two groups. Postoperative gastric emptying was significantly delayed in both postoperative groups compared with the preoperative results. Although the delay in gastric emptying was significantly less ($P = .001$) in the pyloroplasty group, it was still significantly prolonged when compared with preoperative values ($P = .001$). The authors concluded that postoperatively, patients may have symptoms as a result of this delayed emptying, but pyloroplasty fails to effectively prevent them, thus questioning the need for pyloroplasty.

Mannell et al.[48] compared clinical symptoms after randomizing 20 patients in the pyloroplasty and 20 patients in the no pyloroplasty group following esophagectomy for carcinoma and retrosternal gastric pull-up of the whole stomach with cervical esophagogastric anastomosis. In the pyloroplasty group, aspiration, food vomiting, and heartburn were absent. One patient complained of early satiety. In the no pyloroplasty group, aspiration occurred in four patients, with three fatal outcomes, food vomiting in one, early satiety in two, and heartburn in two. The results of this trial suggest that pyloroplasty should be performed on the retrosternal stomach in order to prevent the potentially lethal effects of gastric stasis.

The largest randomized study was performed by Fok et al.[49] with a meticulous analysis of eating abilities and gastric emptying function in the early postoperative period as well as during long-term follow-up. In this study, the whole stomach had been used for reconstruction in all patients. In the early postoperative period, the daily nasogastric aspirate was not significantly different. Subjective eating abilities at 2 weeks were as follows: for the pyloroplasty group the ability to consume a solid bolus

TABLE 41.1 Pyloric Drainage: Advantages and Disadvantages

Advantages	Disadvantages

Improved:
    Gastric emptying
    Recovery of gastric motility
    Eating ability
    Nutritional status
Decreased pulmonary
    aspiration
Decreased pyloric outlet
    obstruction
	Increased enterogastric-
	    esophageal biliary reflux
	Increased:
	    Esophagitis
	    Intestinal metaplasia in
	        esophageal remnant
	    Dumping syndrome (?)

was 65% and a full meal 73% (82% being asymptomatic); the results for the no pyloroplasty group were 41% ($P = .01$), 52% ($P = .001$), and 49% ($P = .01$), respectively. At 6 months, the differences between the two groups became smaller (for a solid bolus, 92% vs. 89%; for a full meal, 88% vs. 73%), but the percentage of asymptomatic patients in the pyloroplasty group remained significantly higher than that in the no pyloroplasty group (86% vs. 53%; $P = .01$). Gastric emptying was further assessed by studying the 50% emptying time of an indium 113–labeled semi-solid meal at 6 months. There was significantly slower emptying in the no pyloroplasty group compared with the pyloroplasty group (24.3 and 6.6 minutes, respectively; $P = .01$).

These studies seem to indicate a trend favoring pyloric drainage for both the early and late outcome of gastric emptying, food intake, and related nutritional status. Nevertheless, some patients, although asymptomatic, may have delayed gastric emptying, whereas others are symptomatic while having normal gastric emptying, indicating that there is a great variation in the individual pattern of gastric emptying, and thus reflecting individual differences in gastric tube activity (Table 41.1).

A meta-analysis by Urschel et al.[50] of all existing randomized, controlled trials showed a nonsignificant trend favoring drainage to improve emptying, nutritional status, and obstructive foregut symptoms, but favoring no drainage to prevent bile reflux-related complications.

Finally, a recent meta-analysis by Akkerman et al.[51] concluded that the results regarding the benefit of pyloric drainage procedures on gastric function remain contradictory, but do not support its routine use. More recently, the botulinum toxin (Botox) injection directly into the sphincter has been advocated as a promising method to prevent or relieve obstructive symptoms. Cerfolio et al.[52] compared pyloroplasty, pyloromyotomy, no drainage, and preoperative Botox injection into the pylorus. At day four, gastric delay as measured by a timed barium swallow was 96%, 93%, 96%, and 59%; $P = .001$. Hospital length of stay ($P = .015$) and operative times ($P = .037$) were shorter in the Botox group. Follow-up (mean, 40 months) showed symptoms of biliary reflux to be lowest in the Botox group ($P = .024$). They concluded that injection of the pylorus with Botox at the time of esophagogastrectomy is safe, and decreases operative time when compared with pyloroplasty or pyloromyotomy. In addition, it can improve early gastric emptying, decrease respiratory complications, shorten hospital stay, and reduce late bile reflux. In contrast, the study by Eldaif et al.[53] comparing Botox versus pyloroplasty and, -myotomy showed a significantly shorter operative time ($P \le .001$), but delayed emptying ($P = .08$), reflux ($P = .001$), the need for prokinetics and pyloric dilatation ($P < .001$) in the Botox group. The authors concluded that the intrapyloric botulinum injection should not be used as an alternative to standard drainage procedures.

It has been suggested that the individual variations in gastric tube activity may be related to different access routes. Finley et al.[54] studied the effect of different access routes, comparing right-sided, left-sided, and transhiatal esophagectomies. Esophagectomy carried out through a right-sided posterolateral thoracotomy with cervical esophagogastric anastomosis, had a significantly higher incidence of delayed gastric emptying (11%), pneumonia (26%), and hospital death (9%). The incidence of reflux for this access route was 20%. The left-sided thoracoabdominal approach was associated with 5% delayed emptying, 14% pneumonia, and 10% reflux. For transhiatal esophagectomy, these figures were 4%, 5%, and 14%, respectively.

Gastric Emptying–Related Symptoms: Gastric Tube Versus Whole Stomach?

Bemelman et al.[55] studied the impact of the size of the gastric substitute on delayed postoperative emptying. Delayed gastric emptying was seen in 38% of patients in whom the whole stomach was used; 14% of patients in whom substitution with distal two-thirds stomach was performed; and 3% of patients in whom a tubulized stomach was used. The addition of a pyloroplasty in each of the three groups did not affect the incidence of delayed gastric emptying. The authors suggest that the small gastric tube leads to a rapid increase of intraluminal gastric pressure when the stomach is filled, facilitating gastric emptying by the effect of the law of Laplace. Consequently, more gastric stasis occurs when the whole stomach is used for esophageal replacement. Similar results were reported by Barbera et al.[56]

Collard et al.,[57] on the other hand, found a better recovery of gastric motility, as reflected on manometric tracings, when using the whole stomach versus a gastric tube. The motility index progressively increased with time in both groups of patients, but motor recovery was better in whole-stomach patients than in those receiving a gastric tube. Even after 3 years, motor recovery remained significantly higher in whole-stomach patients. These differences might be explained by the fact that resection of the lesser curvature partly destroys both the organizer and effector command ganglia in the myenteric plexus. Long-term alimentary comfort was suggested to be significantly better with an interposed whole stomach than after gastric tube reconstruction.

The results of the studies by Bemelman et al. and Collard et al. are clearly in conflict, and further elucidation of strictly mechanical effects versus intrinsic functional effects is necessary. From a systematic literature review, Akkerman et al.[51] found a superiority of the gastric tube compared with the whole stomach in most of the studies. Pyloric drainage is not significantly associated with the risk of developing delayed gastric emptying after esophagectomy.

Treatment of Delayed Gastric Emptying and/or Gastric Outlet Obstruction

Irrespective of the size of the gastric conduit, the access route, or whether or not a pyloric drainage procedure has been performed, a number of patients may suffer from persistent delayed gastric emptying and/or gastric outlet obstruction. Balloon dilatation of the pylorus can be an effective procedure to solve this problem in some patients. Bemelman et al.[55] reported a successful outcome with balloon dilatation in 6 out of 18 patients. Swanson et al.[58] on the other hand reported that preoperative balloon dilatation of the pylorus 2 weeks before surgery in 25 patients obviated the need for pyloroplasty. (Only one patient needed another dilatation postoperatively.)

An alternative is to administer erythromycin. Erythromycin is a motilin agonist and has been demonstrated to improve gastric emptying in normal subjects and in patients with diabetic gastroparesis or postvagotomy gastroparesis. In a randomized, clinical trial, Burt et al.[59] showed that the percentage of gastric retention, as measured by a technetium 99m–labeled solid meal, at 90 minutes was 37% in patients receiving erythromycin versus 88% in patients receiving a placebo ($P < .001$). These studies were performed in the immediate postoperative period. Further studies are needed to investigate the impact of prolonged administration of erythromycin.

In patients with persistent symptoms of gastric outlet obstruction, balloon dilatation has become a valuable option. Lanuti et al.[60] reported a successful outcome in 36 out of 38 of the patients after pylorus dilatation for refractory gastric outlet symptoms. A total of 42% had no previous pyloric drainage procedure, while 52% did. Finally, in cases of persistent disabling symptoms despite such treatment, rescue pyloroplasty is a valuable last resort option as reported by Datta et al.[61] In this report, 9 out of 13 patients were successfully treated.

Intestinal Metaplasia and Gastric Drainage Procedures

The combination of biliary and acid reflux is commonly believed to play a central role in the pathogenesis of Barrett metaplasia in patients suffering from gastroesophageal reflux disease. The ablation of the lower esophageal sphincter mechanism at the time of esophagectomy and the vagotomy-induced pyloric dysfunction with possible related enterogastric biliary reflux, are of increasing concern in relation to the risk of developing Barrett metaplasia, especially in long-term survivors. As early as 1992, da Rocha et al.[62] reported that 8.3% of 48 patients developed Barrett metaplasia in the esophageal remnant in the long term, after subtotal esophagectomy. Franchimont et al.[63] found a 13.5% incidence of newly developed Barrett esophagus in the cervical stump after esophagectomy for cancer with a median time to diagnosis of 489 days (range 43 to 1172 days). Proton pump inhibition early after surgery did not appear to influence the development of Barrett esophagus.

In a series of 39 patients, Oberg et al.[64] noticed a 47% prevalence of metaplastic columnar mucosa within the cervical esophagus. Intestinal-type metaplasia was found in three patients, who all showed an abnormal exposure to both acid and bilirubin on 24-hour monitoring.

Other studies suggested that gastric drainage procedures favor enterogastric bile reflux.

Wang et al.[65] compared patients with and without pyloroplasty. Those with pyloroplasty were found to have a higher incidence of bile regurgitation (55.5% vs. 8.6%, respectively). Thirty-three of these patients underwent a technetium 99m–hydroxyiminodiacetic acid (HIDA) test showing a high incidence of enterogastric bile reflux (60%), whereas no enterogastric bile reflux could be demonstrated in patients who had not had a gastric drainage procedure.

Gutschow et al.[66] found a prevalence of esophagitis of 26.5% in patients who received a gastric drainage procedure versus 9.5% in patients who did not. In the group of patients receiving a gastric drainage procedure, 6.7% developed Barrett metaplasia. It is currently unknown whether these patients have the same risk of developing adenocarcinoma as is seen in the classic reflux-induced Barrett's population. But these data are suggesting that it is better not to perform any type of drainage procedure. In cases of persistent disabling symptoms, balloon dilatation appears to be a viable option.

Dumping and Diarrhea

After esophagectomy followed by gastroplasty, many patients complain of diarrhea and dumping (-like) symptoms, with a reported incidence of between 10% and 50%. McLarty et al.[67] suggested that symptoms are early postprandial abdominal and vasomotor symptoms resulting from osmotic fluid shifts and the release of vasoactive neurotransmitters, and late symptoms are secondary to reactive hypoglycemia. Diarrhea, abdominal cramps, nausea, dizziness, postprandial sweating, and hypotension are the main complaints. These dumping symptoms are thought to be provoked by the accelerated gastric emptying. Hölscher et al.[68] demonstrated a markedly accelerated emptying of semi-solid food in comparison to the stomach of a control group, but complete emptying of the intrathoracic stomach was very much delayed compared with transit through a normal esophagus. Banki et al.[69] compared the results of a vagal nerve sparing esophagectomy plus coloplasty versus a control group and a group of patients after standard esophagectomy with gastric pull-up. Patients with a vagal sparing esophagectomy had a complete absence of postoperative diarrhea and a low (7%) incidence of dumping. In the gastric pull-up group, the incidence of diarrhea was 50% and that of dumping 10%. Some authors argue that a gastric drainage procedure increases the incidence of dumping. In fact, 10% to 30% of patients undergoing pyloroplasty will develop dumping syndrome, 1% to 5% being refractory to conservative management.[70] Sinha et al.[71] compared the results of subtotal esophagectomy and cervical esophagogastrostomy with and without pyloroplasty. Evidence of dumping on a provocation test was noted in 18% of the pyloroplasty group but in none of the nonpyloroplasty group. An effective relief of dumping symptoms can be achieved with dietary modifications to minimize the ingestion of simple carbohydrates and to exclude fluid intake during the ingestion of the solid portion of a meal. More severely affected patients may respond to agents such as pectin and guar, which increase the viscosity of the intraluminal contents, or to drugs such as the α-glucosidase inhibitor acarbose, which decreases the rapid absorption of glucose, or native somatostatin or the somatostatin analogue octreotide, which alters gut transit and inhibits the release of vasoactive mediators into the bloodstream.[72]

Quality of Life After Surgery

Advances in proper selection, surgical techniques, including MIE, as well as the multimodality strategies, have resulted in significantly better outcomes for esophageal carcinoma patients over the last two decades. Currently, 5-year survival figures close to 50% are no longer an exception. However, significant morbidity as a consequence of postoperative complications can affect up to half of all patients who have surgery.[73] This morbidity can be related to a multitude of factors, but is mainly due to anastomotic complications (e.g., leak or stenosis), pulmonary complications as a direct consequence of the surgery itself (e.g., blood loss, length of surgery with prolonged intraoperative atelectasis), or as the consequence of reflux-related chronic aspiration, or due to undesired functional side effects as described earlier (e.g., gastric outlet obstruction). It takes up to 1 year for patients to recover their baseline health-related quality of life (HRQL), and this baseline level is never achieved if disease recurs within 2 years.[74] As a result, a paradigm shift is causing more focus on QOL.

Obviously, it is of paramount importance for surgeons to make relentless efforts to minimize complications through meticulous surgical techniques or by developing newer less traumatic techniques. In this respect, the advent of minimally invasive surgery seems to be promising, as shown in a randomized, controlled trial by Biere et al.[75] Several studies have shown that MIE has a beneficial effect on postoperative outcome and HRQL. A study by Nafteux et al.[76] compared the outcome between open esophagectomy (OE) and MIE for early cancer. The blood loss was less ($P = .01$) and the duration of operation longer ($P = .001$) in MIE. Hospital mortality ($P = .66$) and postoperative complications ($P = .34$) were comparable. However, respiratory complications ($P = .008$) and intensive care unit admission ($P = .02$) were higher in OE. Gastrointestinal complications ($P = .005$), that is, gastroparesis ($P = .004$) were more frequent in MIE. At 3 months, postoperative fatigue, pain (general), and gastrointestinal pain were less in MIE ($P = .09$, $P = .05$, and $P = .01$, respectively). In the following months, these differences faded out, and at 1 year there was no longer a difference. However, the values did stay below the preoperative baseline, indicating long-term persistence of the impact of the intervention on HRQL.

Reducing postoperative complications and related morbidity also translates into earlier discharge, which may have a beneficial effect on postoperative overall HRQL. This was clearly shown in another study by Nafteux et al.[77] Indeed, patients with early discharge (length of stay [LOS] <10 days) indicated, at 3 and 12 months postoperatively, significantly better HRQL scores in the functional scales (physical, emotional, social, and role functioning) and in the symptoms scales (fatigue, nausea, dyspnea, appetite loss, and dry mouth) when compared to those patients with LOS greater than 10 days. Return to the level of the reference population scores was achieved at 1 year in the LOS 10 days or less group for almost all the scales but not in the LOS greater than 10 days' group.

A well-known downside of MIE is its steep learning curve. It is generally accepted that a minimum of 25 MIEs is required to overcome the learning curve. This may be difficult to obtain given the fact that most centers are dealing with a rather limited number of annual esophagectomies. Therefore the experience of the surgeon and the entire team involved is of paramount importance to optimize not only the oncologic but also the functional outcome of esophagectomy. This is particularly true in an era where other nonsurgical approaches (endoluminal resections for early cancer, definitive radiochemotherapy for advanced squamous cell carcinoma) are increasingly challenging the outcomes of surgery as the cornerstone when aiming at therapy with curative options for esophageal cancer.

COLON

Vuillet[17] using the left colon on a cadaver, and Kelling[18] using transverse colon in a patient with esophageal cancer, in 1911 independently described the clinical principles for the use of the colon as an esophageal substitute. In the 1950s and 1960s, the use of the colon as a substitute was further popularized by Orsoni,[78] Reboud,[79] Waterston,[80] Belsey,[81] Lortat-Jacob,[82] and others.

The main advantage of using a colon is its versatility. The length is freely available for replacement of the entire esophagus up to the pharynx. The blood supply from the left colic artery is robust, and the presence of a marginal artery, the artery of Drummond, close to the colon, permits a linear interposition procedure without redundancy or mechanical kinking (Fig. 41.14A). If the stomach is retained, it offers the potential of reduced delayed gastric emptying and reduced reflux. However, it is a complex procedure requiring at least three anastomoses and thus longer operative time and higher rates of necrosis, morbidity, and mortality have been reported.

Its use is contraindicated in the presence of an aortic aneurysm or extensive atheromatosis disease involving the superior mesenteric artery, previous colon surgery, severe colonic inflammatory bowel disease (IBD), or tumors. Scattered diverticulosis may be a relative contraindication.

In the past, colonic interposition was preferred over gastric pull-up in young patients with early cancer and thus a long life expectancy. However, since early cancers (T1aN0M0) are now mostly treated by endoluminal resection, and due to the increasing experience with gastric pull-up and the related excellent-to-very-good functional results obtained, the colon nowadays is rarely used as the first option. A colon interposition is used as a second option substitute when the stomach cannot be used or when the stomach has to be resected for oncological reasons, such as adenocarcinoma involving the distal esophagus as well as the majority of the lesser curvature .

The blood supply from the colon comes from both the superior and the inferior mesenteric artery. Classically,

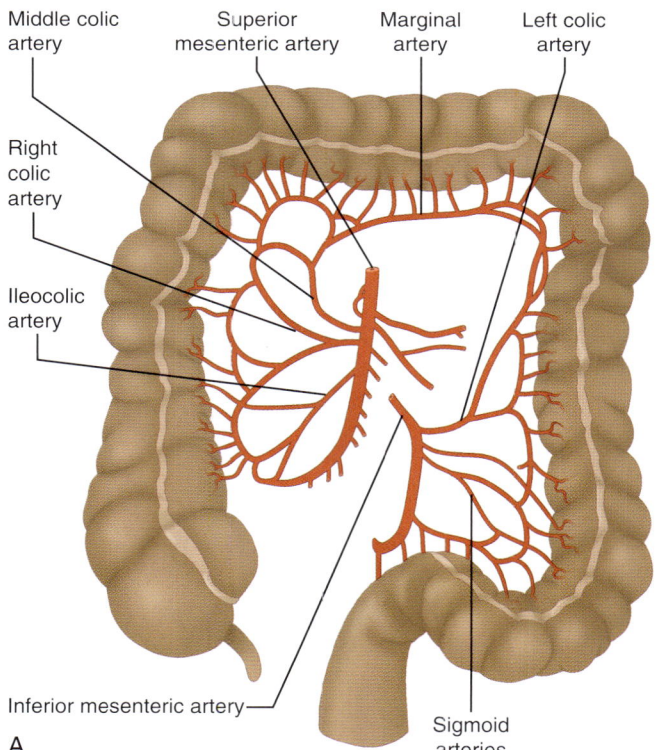
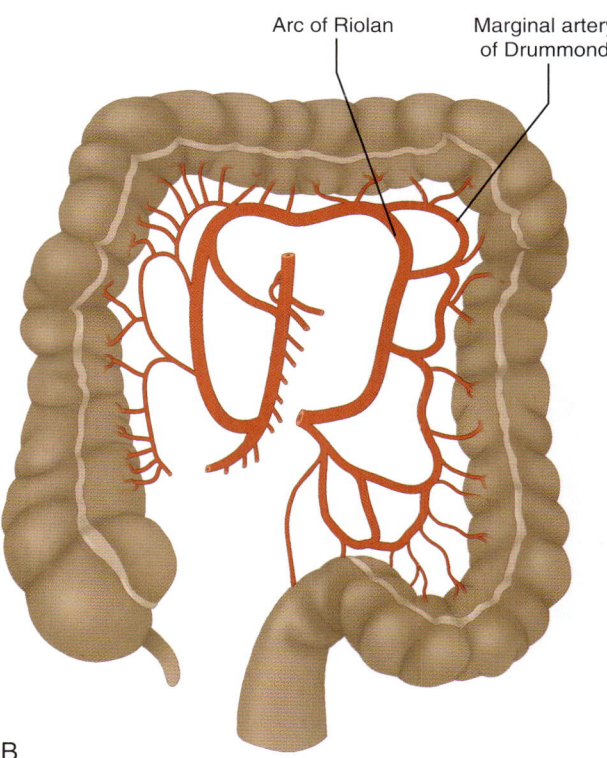

FIGURE 41.14 Vascularization of the colon. (A) Classic pattern. (B) Arc of Riolan. ([A] from Albright JB, Beaty J. *Colorectal Surgery*. Philadelphia: Elsevier; 2013:403–425. [B] from Gordon PH, Nivatvongs S, eds. *Principles and Practice of Surgery for the Colon, Rectum and Anus*. 2nd ed. St. Louis: Quality Medical Publishing; 1999:27.)

the middle, the right, and the ileocolic artery originate from the superior mesenteric artery, while the inferior mesenteric artery is the feeding artery for the left colic artery. All colonic arteries are interconnected by the marginal arcades (Drummond artery).

However, there are a number of variations that may compromise the use of the colon—in particular, a long-segment colon. The right colic artery can arise from the middle colic artery and in approximately 5% to 10% there are multiple right colic arteries with variable origins from middle, ileocolic, and superior mesenteric arteries. The marginal arcades are interrupted or interconnected by multiple small ramifications in about 10%, and sometimes are completely missing. A variation of the marginal artery of Drummond is the arc of Riolan, also known as the meandering mesenteric artery or central anastomotic mesenteric artery (Fig. 41.14B). It is an arterioarterial anastomosis between the superior and inferior mesenteric arteries proximal to the roots of the superior mesenteric artery, whereas the marginal of Drummond exists well distal to the roots of the mesenteric artery. The presence of an arc of Riolan usually precludes the use of a long-segment colon interposition. Among the many technical options, there are two main types of grafts traditionally used for esophageal reconstruction (Fig. 41.15). The *right* colon graft is created using the middle colic vessels as a pedicle; this usually involves dividing the right colic and ileocolic vessels. A segment from the terminal ileum to the ascending colon is interposed in an isoperistaltical fashion. A *left* colon graft is created based off the ascending branch of the left colic artery and the inferior mesenteric vein as a pedicle. The middle colic vessels are divided, preserving the communication between the right and left branches of these vessels. A segment from the transverse colon to the splenic flexure is used for interposition in an isoperistaltic fashion. In a long-segment interposition, the hepatic flexure is also included. This may require the division of a right colic artery.

Preoperative Management

Preoperative angiography of the colic vessels is typically of no value since the applicability of the colon as a substitute can only be decided at the time of surgery. It may be indicated in cases of previous abdominal surgery with potential involvement of the colonic vessels, or previous surgery on major abdominal vessels. A colonoscopy should be performed in elderly patients or patients with a history of colonic polyps. Prior to surgery, a mechanical bowel preparation such as polyethylene glycol is usually performed for all patients. Enemas are rarely required. However, the need for preoperative bowel preparation has been recently questioned.

In a retrospective series of 164 pediatric patients who underwent esophagocoloplasty, Leal et al.[83] showed that the incidence of cervical leakage was significantly decreased in patients without bowel preparation in comparison with the classical preparation group ($P = .03$). The addition of oral antibiotics may further reduce the risk of infection, but this is controversial. Just before the start of the surgery and for the subsequent 48 hours, broad spectrum antibiotics, including anaerobe covering, are administered intravenously (Table 41.2).

Technique of Left Colon Interposition

The preferred technique is a left colonic interposition. The arterial flow comes from the left vessels, and is interposed in an isoperistaltic way.[84] This technique allows for adequate length to make an anastomosis either in the thorax or in the neck with an excellent vascular supply if no compromising anatomic variations are present. The left colon is almost completely mobilized from its peritoneal attachments by incising the white line of Toldt down to where the inferior mesenteric artery is identified. The transverse colon is detached from the omentum and the splenic flexure is mobilized as well. On the right side, if a long-segment interposition is planned, the hepatic

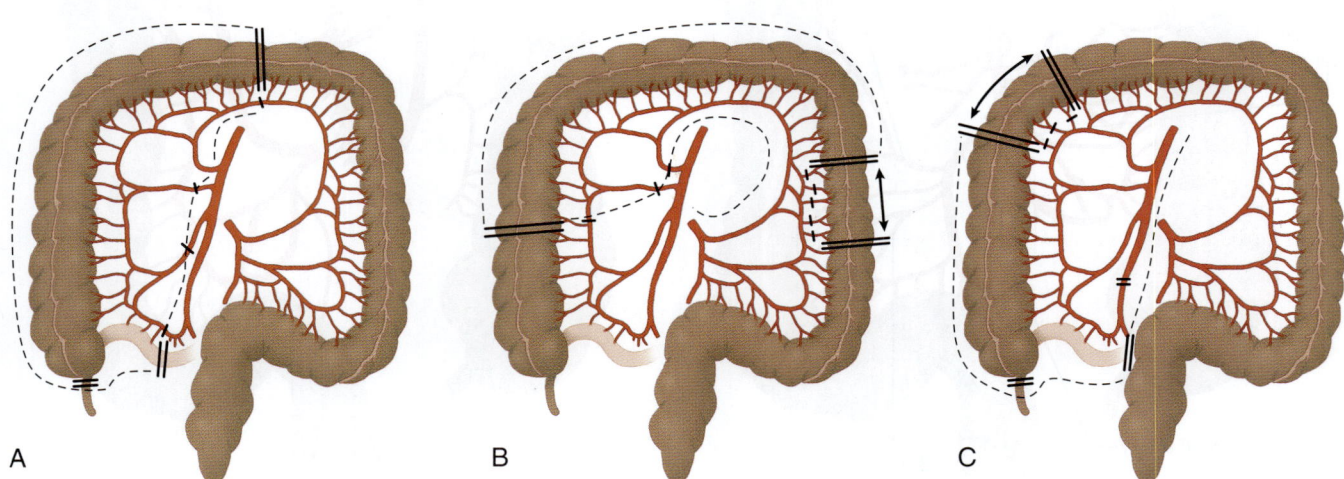

A   B   C

FIGURE 41.15 Modalities for colon interposition. (A) Right colon pedicled on middle colic artery. (B) Left colon pedicled on the ascending branch of left colic artery. (C) Ileocolic graft pedicled on the right colic artery. (From Watanabe M, Mine S, Nishida K, Kurogochi T, Okamura A, Imamura Y. Reconstruction after esophagectomy for esophageal cancer patients with a history of gastrectomy. *Gen Thorac and Cardiovasc Surg.* 2016;64:457–463.)

TABLE 41.2 Advantages and Disadvantages of Right and Left Colon Grafts

	Right Colon Graft	Left Colon Graft
Advantages	Bauhin valve prevents regurgitation	More reliable blood supply
	Reservoir-like capacity of the cecum	Adequate length for reconstruction
	Close match in the diameters of the esophagus and ileum	Smaller diameter
Disadvantages	High variation in blood vessels	Possible atherosclerosis of the inferior mesenteric artery
	Larger diameter, bulky cecum	
	More frequent regurgitation	

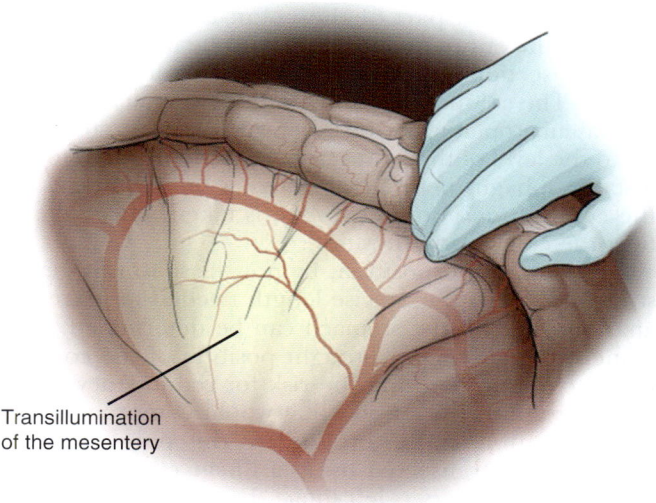

Transillumination of the mesentery

FIGURE 41.16 Transillumination. (From Popovici ZI. *Atlas of Advanced Operative Surgery*. Philadelphia: Elsevier; 2013:113–125.)

flexure, the right colon, and the cecum are mobilized by incising the peritoneal fold. Once the colon is fully mobilized, the arterial vascularization is identified. In a slim patient, the vessels can be easily seen in the mesentery of the colon. In obese patients, this may be more difficult as the mesenteric fat obscures the view. This can be solved using transillumination (Fig. 41.16). A thorough inspection of all the vessels is performed with special attention to the continuity of the marginal arteries and possible anatomic variations of the colic arteries. The ascending branch of the left colic artery is identified. Usually, this is a robust artery, and pulsations can easily be palpated. In a left colic transposition, this will be the artery on which the vascularization will be based. The middle colic and right colic artery are also visualized and vertical incisions are made in the mesenterium alongside these arteries. Then, a first assessment of the needed length of the conduit is made. With a white linen tape, the length from the neck to the origin of the ascending branch of the left colic artery is measured. The real length needed is now measured over the artery and marginal arteries—not by measuring the length of the colon (Fig. 41.17).

Atraumatic vascular clamps (e.g., bulldogs) are placed at the base of the middle colic artery; if more length is needed, they are also placed at the base of the right colic artery and on the marginal artery at the site of the proximal part of the colon selected for transection according to the measurement. The blood to the future conduit now comes only from the ascending branch of the left colic artery. Usually, pulsations are visible and palpable over the entire length of the isolated segment. This may require some time as the colon may have gone into spasm as a result of the dissection. The topical application of lidocaine or papaverine may relieve the spasm. If pulsations are not evident, removing the clamps and reapplying them after some 20 to 30 minutes may be needed to solve the problem. In the absence of visible/palpable pulsations, Doppler flow measurement may be used.

The middle colic artery can now be divided and ligated. To do so, both the artery and the vein are dissected out as close as possible to their origin. This is a most delicate maneuver and should be done using fine clamps. The

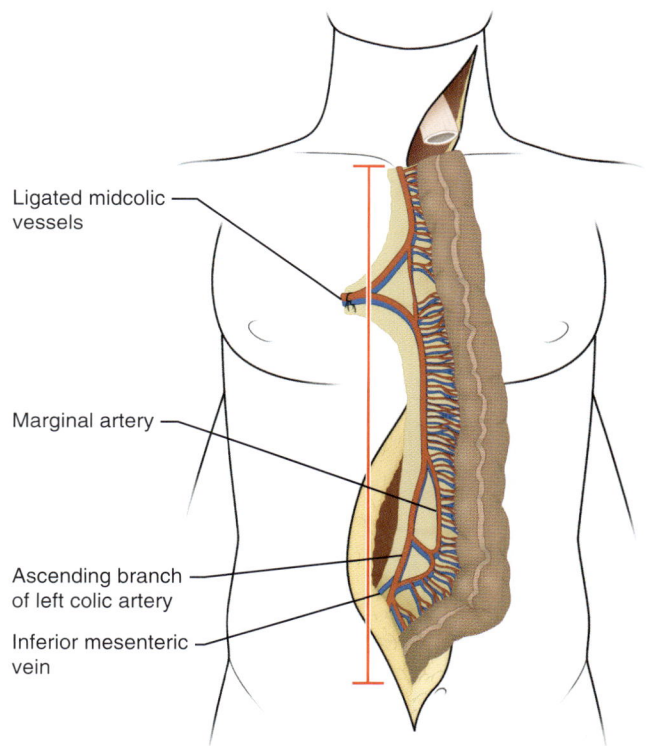

Ligated midcolic vessels

Marginal artery

Ascending branch of left colic artery

Inferior mesenteric vein

FIGURE 41.17 The measurement of the coloplasty is based on the length of vascular arcades rather than on the length of the colon itself. (From DeMeester TR. Esophageal replacement with colon interposition. *Oper Techn Cardiac Thorac Surg.* 1997;2:73–86.)

marginal artery at the point of proximal transection of the colon is clamped, but only at the side of the colon remaining in situ. After the transection of the marginal artery, the flow to the nonclamped side can be immediately evaluated.

The proximal part of the colon is now transected allowing the entire mobilized loop to be moved upward. The transection is performed by using a linear cutting stapler. The colon is passed behind the stomach through an avascular opening in the lesser gastrohepatic omentum up to the level of the hiatus, usually by attaching it to the distal esophagus before exteriorizing the esophagus via the cervical incision. Great care is taken not to axially twist the colonic interposition.

The colon interposition, by now in spasm, is gently stretched out so the precise length needed to make the anastomosis with the stomach can be determined. This maneuver guarantees a straight position of the conduit in the chest, minimizing the risk for redundancy whilst avoiding too much tension that would compromise the vascularization at the top end. At this point, the left colon will be transected using a linear cutting stapler. The marginal artery is left intact, but its small branches to the colon are dissected and divided over a distance of about 1 cm on both sides of the transection line each Figs. 41.18 and 41.19.

The first anastomosis is the cologastric anastomosis (Fig. 41.20). This is an end-to-side anastomosis. The linear staple line at the top end is removed and the colon is opened and carefully cleaned with an iso-Betadine swab. On the gastric side, the anastomosis is placed close to the greater curvature one-third of the length down from the fundus to the pylorus on the posterior side of the stomach. An 8- to 10-cm segment of the graft is retained underneath the diaphragm in the high pressure zone, creating an antireflux device similar to the principles governing a classic antireflux procedure (Fig. 41.21). After finishing the anastomosis, the fundus will fall as a flap valve over the intraabdominal part of the colon acting as the additional, second component of an effective antireflux barrier against reflux colitis. This is an essential feature of the procedure. The anastomosis is made with an inner layer of 3-0 absorbable and an outer layer of 3-0 nonabsorbable suture material, with both layers using a running suture.

The colocolic anastomosis is now fashioned between the right and left colon, which are easily brought together given the extensive mobilization. The opening in the mesenterium of colon can be closed to avoid herniation and possible strangulation of the small intestines, or can be left widely open.

The cervical anastomosis is fashioned in exactly the same way as described before when using the stomach. However, the preference is here to use handsewn anastomosis as

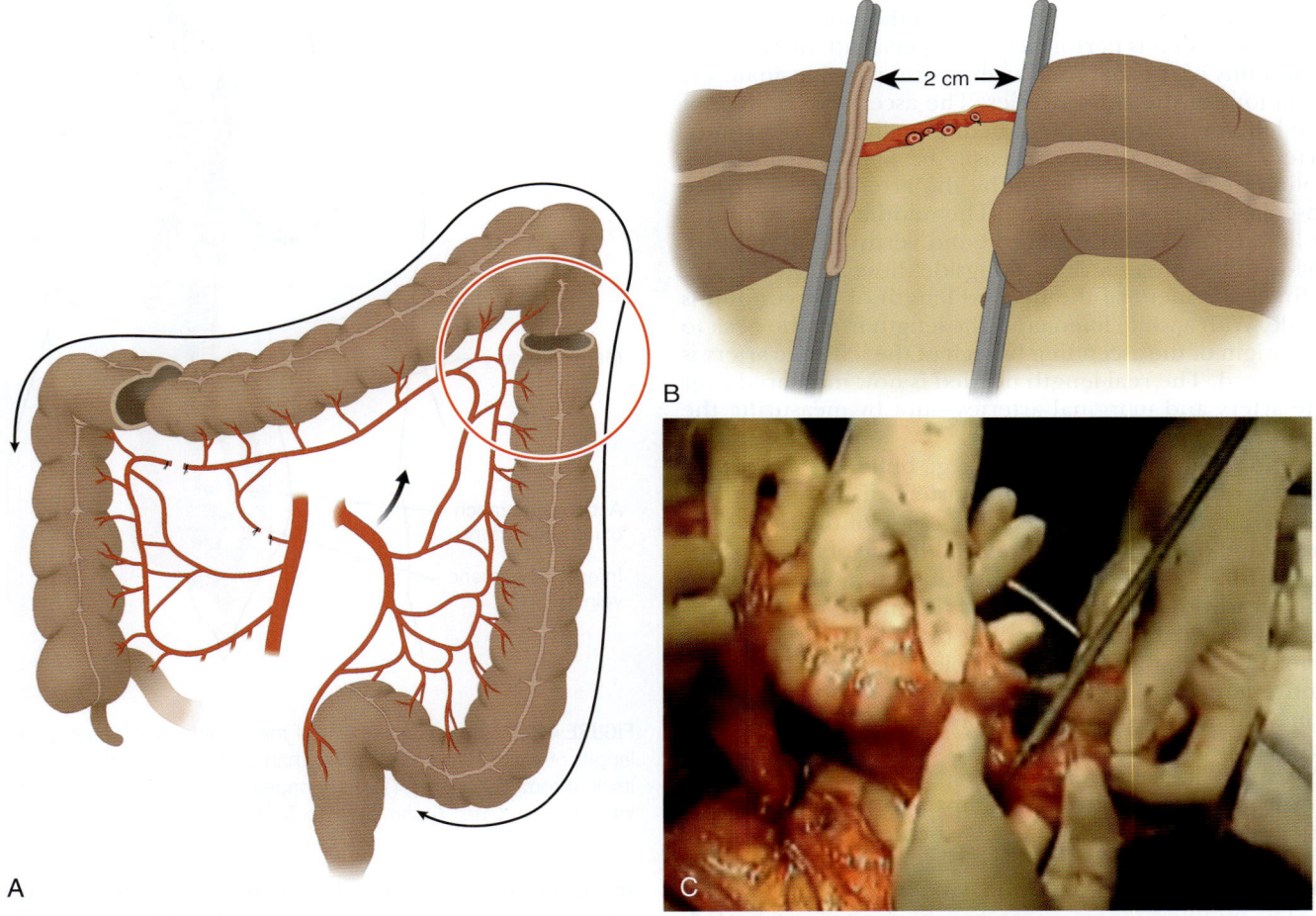

FIGURE 41.18 (A) Preparation of a left colon loop pedicled on the ascending branch of the left colic artery. (B) The distal marginal artery is not interrupted; the branches to the colon are divided. (C) Perioperative view. ([B] from DeMeester TR. Esophageal replacement with colon interposition. *Oper Techn Cardiac Thorac Surg.* 1997;2:73–86.)

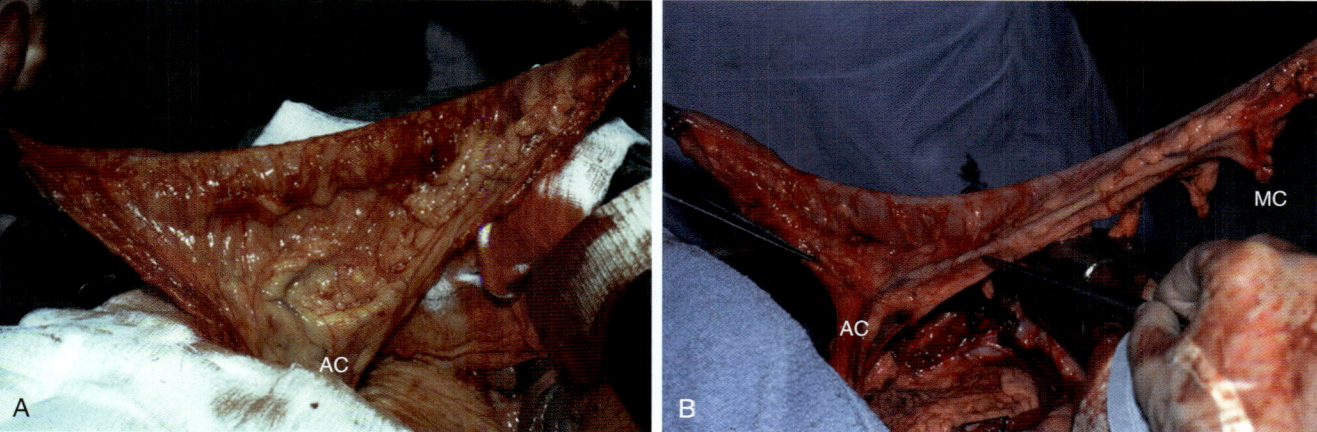

FIGURE 41.19 Perioperative view: (A) Short segment (B) Long sement. *AC,* Ascending branch of left colic artery; *MC,* ligated middle colic artery.

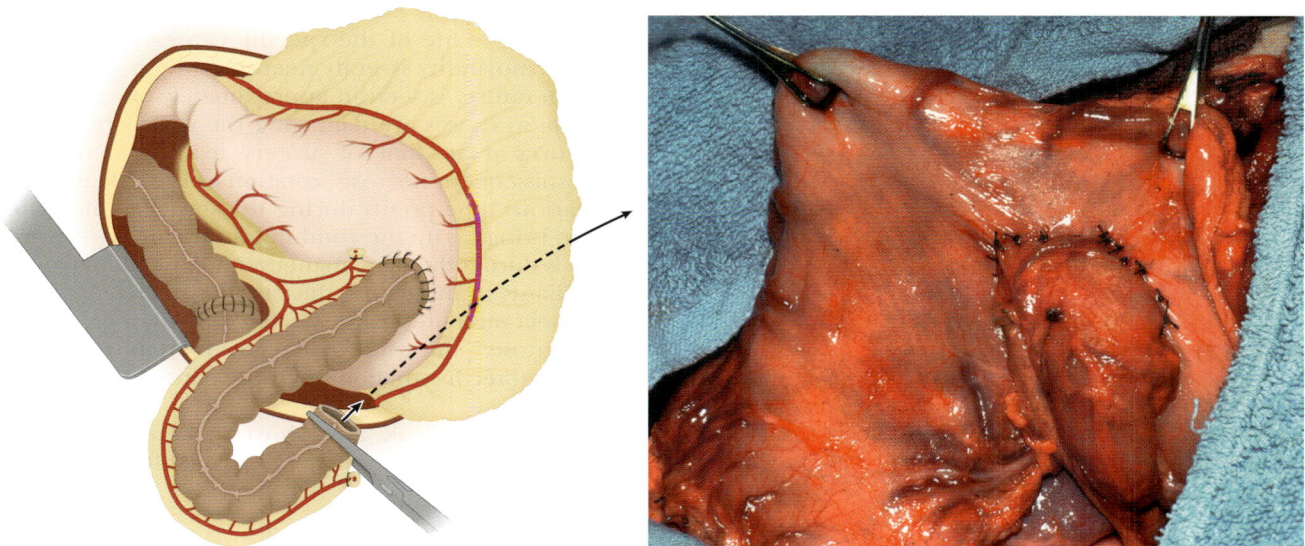

FIGURE 41.20 Cologastric anastomosis on the posterior wall of the stomach close to the greater curvature one-third of the length down from the top of the fundus to the pylorus. (Illustration based on *La Chirurgia dell'esofago*. Stipa – Belsey. Atlante: trattamento del carcinome dell'esofago e del cardias. Esofago-colo-gastroplastica. Piccin Editore Padova; 1980:463. Fig 14A.)

it allows for better adaptation for possible incongruence between cervical esophagus and the colon (Fig. 41.22). At the time of the cervical anastomosis, a nasogastric tube is pushed down through the anastomosis into the colon and through the cologastric anastomosis in order to decompress the stomach. A temporary placement of a gastrostomy may be useful as well.

Technique of Right Colon Interposition

The right colon is used as a first choice by some surgeons, or in case the vascularization of the left colon is compromised, such as after previous sigmoid resection.[85] The graft will be based on the middle colic artery. The principles of dissection and measuring the length needed are the same as for the left colon interposition. The right colic artery is identified and along this artery the mesenterium is incised. Test clamping is performed to assess sufficient

vascularization at the future top end of the marginal artery. In the scenario of a long segment, the cecum and last ileal loop may be needed as part of the interposition. In this situation, the right ileocolic artery also has to be divided. The further steps of the intervention are similar to those described for the left colon.

Variations

Most authors prefer isoperistaltic colon interposition assuming that the colon as substitute retains its capacity to episodically propel the solid bolus in an aboral direction. Therefore, placing the conduit in an antiperistaltic fashion is believed to increase the risk for aspiration.[84] However, in some situations where the surgeon, due to variations in the vascular anatomy, is forced to pedicle the conduit on the right colic artery, an antiperistaltic interposition of the conduit may be the only option.

Other variations are often related to technical, mostly vascular, difficulties discovered at the time of surgery. Occasionally the middle colic artery may split immediately after its origin from the superior mesenteric artery and without an overarching marginal artery in between the

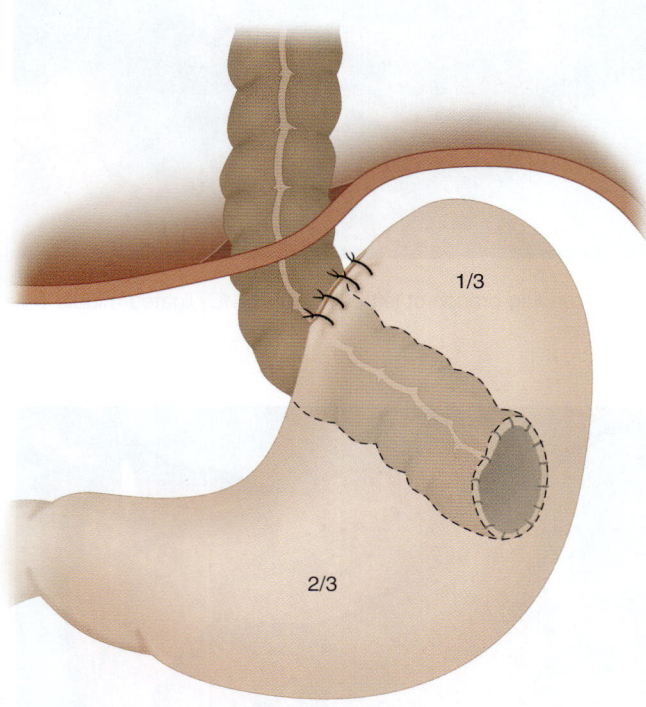

FIGURE 41.21 Fundus of the stomach falling as a flap valve over the intraabdominal part of the coloplasty. (Based on *La Chirurgia dell'esofago*. Stipa – Belsey. Atlante: trattamento del carcinome dell'esofago e del cardias. Esofago-colo-gastroplastica. Piccin Editore Padova; 1980:461. Fig 12.)

"V." In such a situation, the solution is to place a DeBakey vascular clamp on the mesenteric artery followed by the resection of the middle colic artery with a patch suturing the mesenteric artery and the patch with fine Prolene 6-0 (Fig. 41.23).

When impaired venous drainage is suspected, a "super-drainage" can be performed in order to avoid congestion of the transplant. The marginal vein is anastomosed to the anterior or exterior jugular vein, or the internal thoracic vein, using microsurgical techniques.[85,86] The so-called "supercharged colon interposition" consists of an arterial anastomosis to avoid ischemic necrosis of the graft, usually between the stump of the right or middle colic artery and the superior thyroid artery or internal mammary artery.[87]

Outcomes

Colon interposition is a very complex intervention, and the reported postoperative mortality after esophagectomy for cancer ranges between 10% and 20% being somewhat higher than the postoperative mortality after gastric pull-up.[88,89] One of the specific causes of mortality or severe morbidity is graft necrosis, which, according to the literature, is seen in approximately 5% of the cases. Common causes are damaging the vessels by clamps or ligatures at the time of surgery, leading to thrombosis and subsequent necrosis, rotation of the vascular pedicle at various time points during the surgery—in particular when bringing up the conduit into the neck—tearing off vessels during the same maneuver, too much narrowing of the hiatus strangulating the vascular pedicle, and failure to detect mesenteric atherosclerosis. When graft necrosis is diagnosed, the conduit needs to be removed, followed by staged reconstruction when the patient has completely recovered.

Anastomotic leaks after short-segment coloplasty with intrathoracic anastomosis are rare, but after long-segment

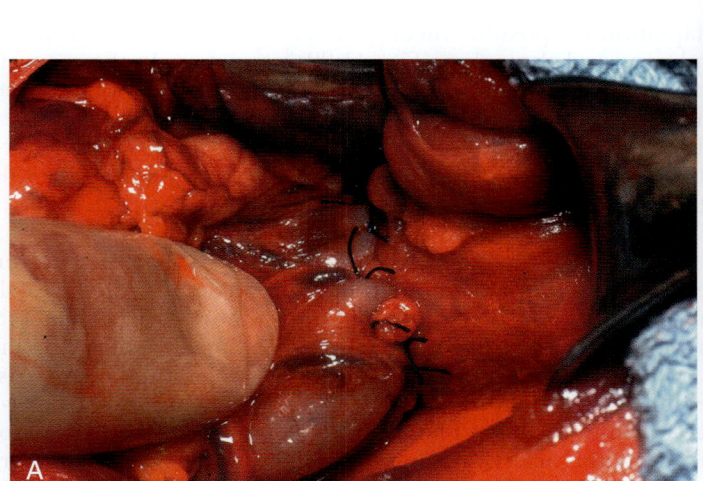
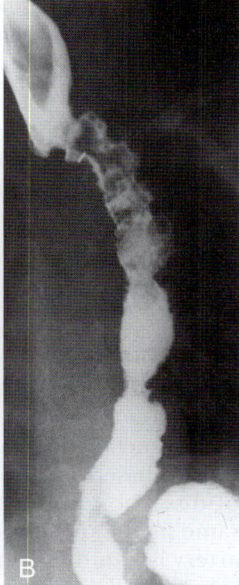

FIGURE 41.22 Termino lateral cervical anastomosis (A), and postoperative barium swallow 1 year postoperatively (B).

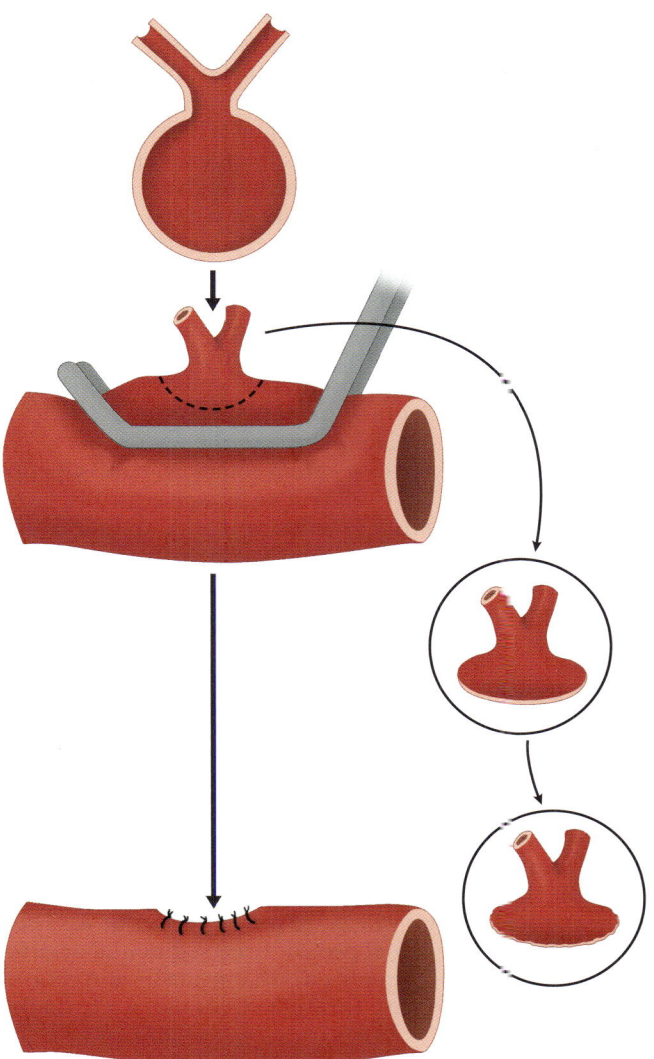

FIGURE 41.23 Middle colic artery with V split close to the superior mesenteric artery: resection with patch. (Based on DeMeester TR. Esophageal replacement with colon interposition. *Oper Techn Cardiac Thorac Surg.* 1997;2:73–86.)

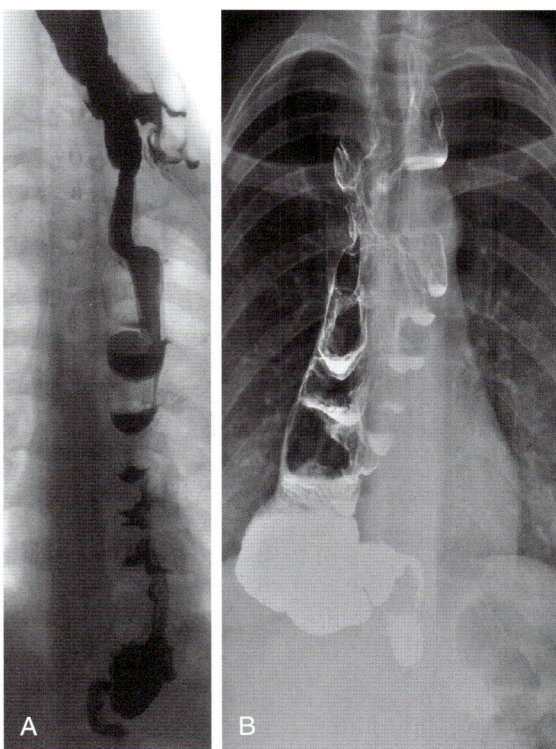

FIGURE 41.24 (A) Protruding colon at the cervical anastomosis level. (B) Redundancy of the colon interposition after retrosternal placement.

interposition with anastomosis in the neck, leaks are observed in about 10%. They usually can be treated conservatively and require rarely revisional surgery.[88,89] A particular problem at the cervical level of the coloplasty is bulging of its supraclavicular portion. Due to air swallowing during speech or while eating, the thin walled colon bulges out. Beside the unaesthetic aspect, the bulging may, in the long term, cause dysphagia so the patient has to manually push down the food bolus. This would eventually require revisional surgery by excising the protruded part (Fig. 41.24A). An important complication, in particular in later follow-up, is redundancy of the interposed colon (Fig. 41.24B). This is seen more after retrosternal interposition, when using right-sided access for the esophagectomy and, to a lesser extent, after left-sided or transhiatal esophagectomy. The redundancy will increase in size over time and eventually will result in a mechanical kinking. The symptoms are dysphagia and aspiration due to stasis

and regurgitation. The best treatment is prevention by a meticulous surgical technique and measurement of the length of the colon needed to replace the esophagus. It is believed that the posterior mediastinal route provides a better guarantee to prevent redundancy.

Jeyasingham et al.[90] reviewed a series of 69 long-segment coloplasties. Long-term follow-up ranged between 1 and 38 years. Seventeen patients (25%) developed redundancy, which was noticed at three levels: supraortic, supradiaphragmatic, and infradiaphragmatic. All patients were symptomatic, requiring revisional surgery in 15 cases to solve the problem. de Delva et al.[91] described their experience with revisional surgery for late complications. They treated 12 patients for redundancy, performing what they called a "box car" resection. This is a segmental resection of the redundant part, preserving the marginal artery followed by reanastomosis.

Another late complication is the occurrence of fibrosis at the top end of the graft. This is believed to be the result of a venous ischemia caused by congestion of the venous drainage. Such strictures are very difficult to dilate. de Delva et al.[91] described stricturoplasty, which is a longitudinal incision through the stricture that will be closed horizontally to solve the problem.

Reflux related colitis may occur. The best treatment is prevention using an appropriate surgical technique to minimize the risk of reflux as described earlier. Reflux-related colitis usually responds well to proton pump inhibitors. Occasionally, a reflux ulcer may cause a cologastric stenosis requiring surgical revision.

More problematic may be regurgitation and aspiration due to reflux and/or stasis in the conduit. If it does not respond to conservative therapy, revisional surgery may be required to remediate it. Within this context, some authors, especially when dealing with benign disorders in children or young adults, advocate to add a partial type of antireflux procedure,[92] claiming a significant improvement in reflux control without increasing stasis and dysphagia in late follow-up.

The occurrence of intrinsic pathology in the interposed segment, such as IBD or colon cancer in late follow-up has been described on an anecdotal basis, and is treated according to the related standards of care.

JEJUNOPLASTY (JEJUNAL INTERPOSITION)

César Roux is credited for having performed the first jejunoplasty in 1907 in a 12-year-old child suffering from a severe caustic injury. It was a presternal esophago-jejuno-gastrostomy. That patient died at the age of 53.[16]

Longmire[93] was the first to describe a long-segment jejunal interposition with microvascular augmentation. The complexity of the operation and a lack of appropriate microsurgical instrumentarium precluded widespread use in spite of these early reports, demonstrating the technical feasibility of the augmented blood supply to the long-segment pedicled jejunal interposition. The utility of a small bowel conduit for esophageal reconstruction was confirmed by Allison et al.[94] who, in 1957, reported that most patients had normal nutritive intake and work capacity at the 3-year follow-up. In 1945, Thompson[95] performed a presternal jejunoplasty as the first step to treat a mid-one-third squamous cell cancer, with the resection being performed as the second step.

Jejunal interposition is the third most commonly used modality for esophageal reconstruction. The reason for this is its rather segmental vascular configuration, making it more difficult to prepare a long segment compared to the stomach and colon, putting it at a higher risk for ischemia and necrosis.[96] Jejunum can be used as an interposition, a Roux-en-Y loop, or as a free vascular graft. It is most commonly used in esophageal cancer surgery to reconstruct continuity in patients who had previous gastrectomy or in patients in whom a total gastrectomy is needed for oncologic reasons, such as GEJ tumors extending into the stomach.

In general, a relatively short segment Roux-en-Y will suffice to allow an intrathoracic anastomosis at the level of the inferior pulmonary vein or somewhat higher up at the level of the aortic arch. The longer the segment needed, the more jejunal arteries that must be divided in order to obtain an adequate length.

The blood supply to the jejunum comes from the superior mesenteric artery (Fig. 41.25A). The branches are displayed in a segmental pattern. However, anatomic variations frequently occur causing technical difficulties when preparing a jejunal loop. In an unfavorable setting, there is a ladder-type distribution with the formation of secondary arches (Fig. 41.25B). In this setting, there is a tendency of the jejunum to retain its curved redundant appearance.

Technique of Roux-en-Y Jejunoplasty

The ligament of Treitz is identified and the vascularization is inspected. In a slim patient this will be quite easy, but in more obese patients with a fatty mesenterium a transillumination is necessary. The first jejunal artery is identified and preserved to guarantee adequate vascularization of the first 15 cm departing from the ligament of Treitz. Then the length that will be required has to be assessed after which the proximal two to three segmental arteries of this segment are visualized, with transillumination if needed. The arteries are carefully dissected out from the

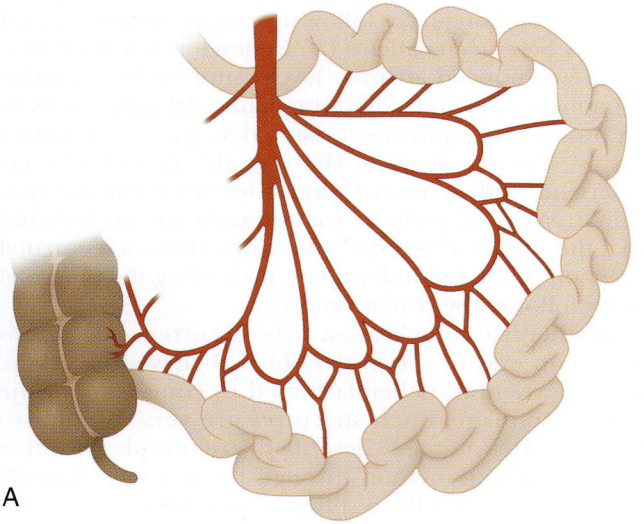
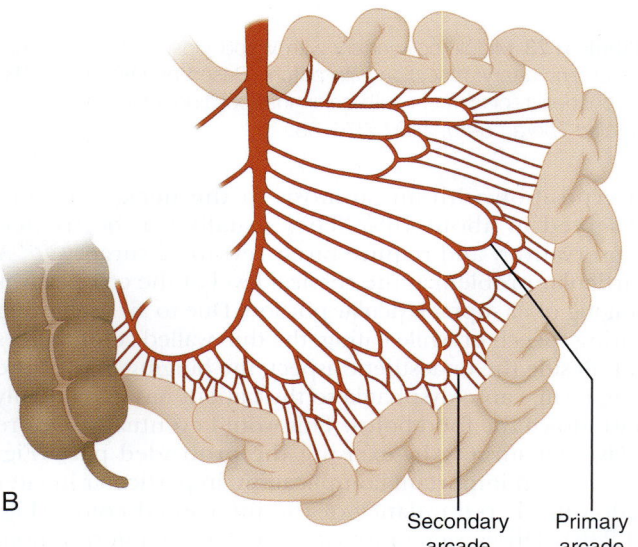

FIGURE 41.25 Segmental vascularization of the jejunum arising from the superior artery. (A) Favorable; (B) Unfavorable "ladder type" pattern. *PA,* Primary arcade; *SA,* secondary arcade. (Based on Siewert R, Hölscher A. 3 Eingriffe beim Ösophaguskarzinom. Jejunuminterposition. In: Siewert R, ed. *Breitner Chirurgische Operationslehre. Band IV: Ösophagus, Magen und Duodenum.* Urban & Schwarzenberg; 1989:47. Fig 3-60.)

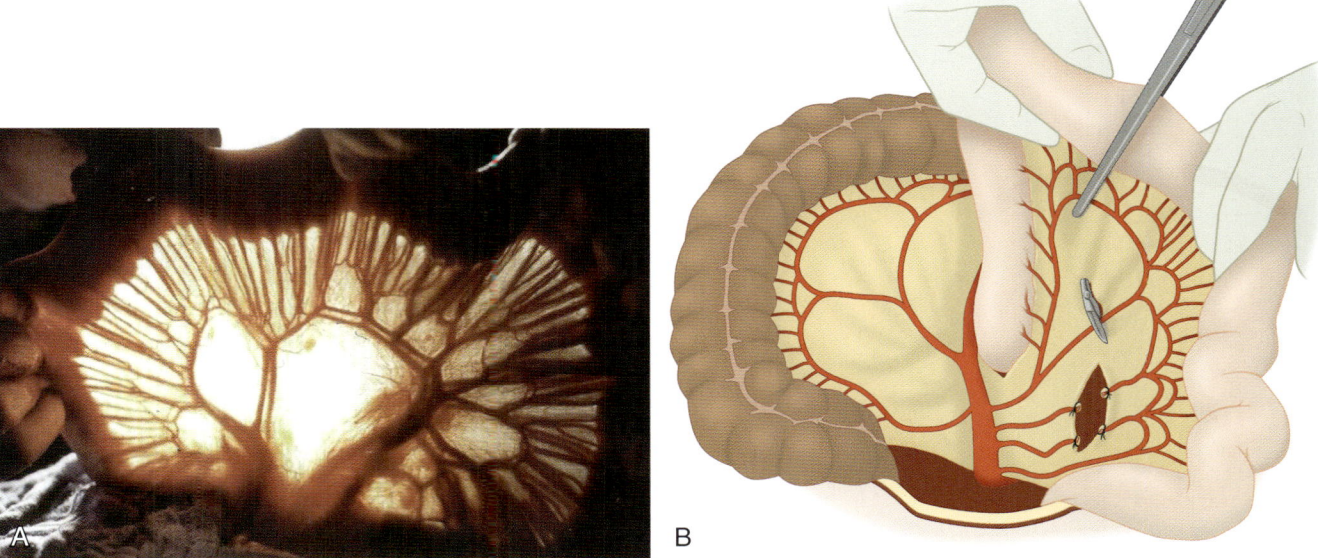

FIGURE 41.26 Preparation of a jejunal loop. (A) Transillumination. (B) Clamping the segmental arteries to be divided. ([A] from Maier A, Pinter H, Tomaselli F, et al. Retrosternal pedicled jejunum interposition: an alternative for reconstruction after total esophago-gastrectomy. *Eur J Cardiothorac Surg.* 2002;22:661–665; [B] from Siewert R, Hölscher A. 3 Eingriffe beim Ösophaguskarzinom. Jejunuminterposition. In: Siewert R, ed. *Breitner Chirurgische Operationslehre. Band IV: Ösophagus, Magen und Duodenum.* Urban & Schwarzenberg; 1989:48. Fig 3-62.)

mesenterium. With atraumatic bulldog vascular clamps, the adequacy of the vascularization is assessed (Fig. 41.26). The arteries and veins are now individually ligated and divided. With two or three arteries divided, sufficient length of the conduit is obtained to bring the conduit up to the level of the inferior pulmonary vein or even higher up to the level of the aortic arch. If a longer segment is needed, an additional artery can be divided, although the more arteries that are interrupted the higher the risk for ischemia at the top end of the conduit (Fig. 41.27A and B).

Some additional maneuvers can be done to increase the length. One is to divide and ligate one or two primary arcades—the vascular continuity being guaranteed through the secondary arcades close to the jejunum. This maneuver also can be used to avoid too much redundancy of the conduit resulting from the segmental aspect of the vascularization. After preparation of the loop, the jejunum is transected about 15 cm from the ligament of Treitz using a cutting linear stapler, and the jejunal loop is brought up into the chest through the mesentery of the transverse colon. For a short segment this is easy, but if the loop has to be longer this can be more difficult due to the fact that the jejunum has the tendency to retain its curved structure. This may cause problems in the later follow-up (e.g., stasis leading to distention, dysphagia, and regurgitation with aspiration). Segmental resection(s) of a redundant jejunum preserving the vascular integrity has been described.[97] In case of compromised vascularization at the top end of the jejunum, a supercharged arterial anastomosis on the internal mammary artery or inferior thyroid artery may rescue the situation (Fig. 41.27C).[98–100]

The esophago-jejunal anastomosis can be performed manually as described earlier with two layers of either interrupted or running suture, or by using a circular stapler.

For the latter, a 25 or 28 mm diameter device is used. The anvil is introduced in the transected esophagus and a purse string is placed around its central rod as described earlier (Fig. 41.28). After inspecting the completeness of the anastomosis, the jejunal stump is closed using a linear cutting stapler close to the circular anastomosis in order to prevent the formation of a pseudodiverticulum in the long run. The anastomosis can be performed in the same way via a VATS approach.

Another alternative to be used in an open setting is to perform a semimechanical anastomosis. Two stay sutures are placed between the top end of the jejunum and the esophagus approximately 4 cm cranial of its cut end. Then a small incision is made in the jejunum on its antimesenteric side. The two halves of a linear cutting device are introduced in the esophagus and jejunum, respectively, and fired. This will be the posterior, mechanical, wall of the anastomosis. The remaining open part of the esophageal circumference and the jejunal incision (i.e., the anterior wall) is closed with two layers of running sutures (Fig. 41.29).[101] This type of anastomosis of course requires at least 4 cm of esophagus available proximal from its cut end—the latter requiring another 5 cm proximal from the upper extent of the tumor.

The jejuno-jejunal end-to-side anastomosis finally concludes the reconstruction. The proximal 15 cm are anastomosed to the vertical limb of the jejunum at a distance of at least 70 cm from the top end in order to maximally prevent biliary reflux.

Technique of Jejunal Interposition

An alternative to the Roux-en-Y limb is the interposition of a jejunal loop known as the Merendino operation (Fig. 41.30).[102] This can be an option in the cases where the colon

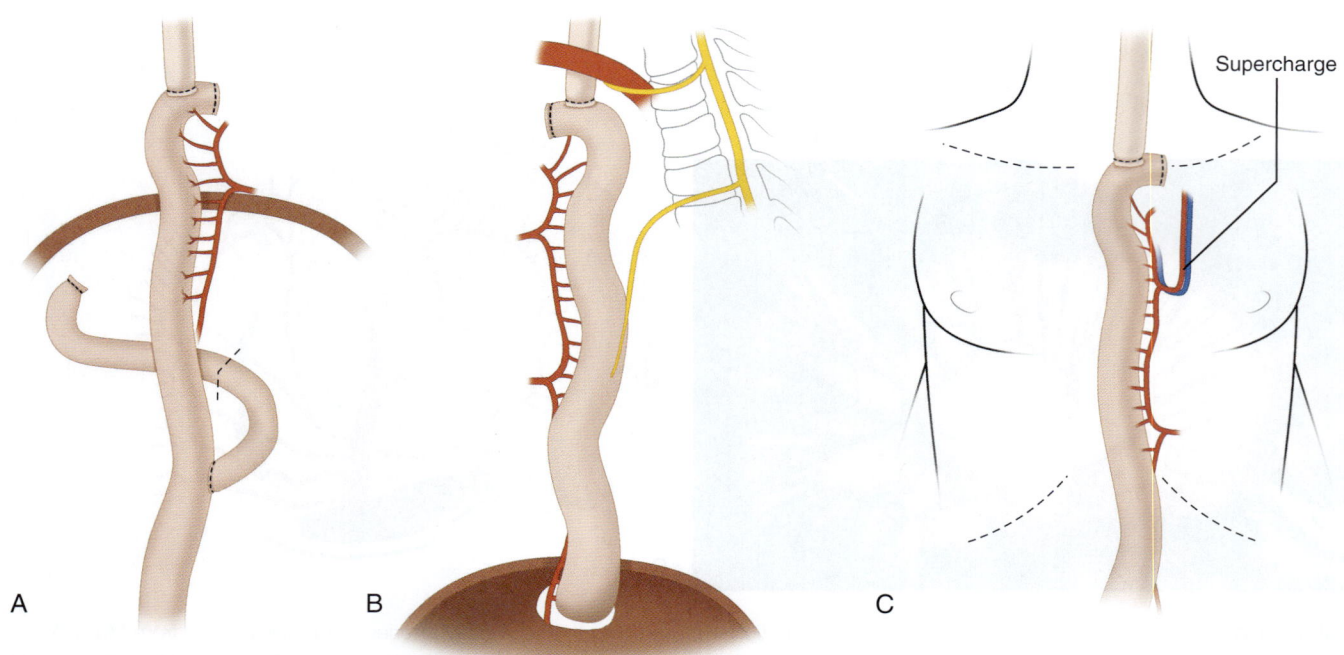

FIGURE 41.27 Esophageal reconstruction using a pedicled jejunum. (A) Roux-en-Y reconstruction anastomosis between the middle esophagus and pedicled jejunum. (B) Intrathoracic anastomosis with upper esophagus and elongated pedicled jejunum. (C) Cervical anastomosis using a supercharged jejunal pedicle. (From Watanabe M, Mine S, Nishida K, Kurogochi T, Okamura A, Imamura Y. Reconstruction after esophagectomy for esophageal cancer patients with a history of gastrectomy. *Gen Thorac Cardiovasc Surg.* 2016;64:457–463.)

is unavailable, and when preservation of the gastric reservoir function is preferred. Some authors have advocated it as the first choice in cases of high grade dysplasia (HGD) of early T1aN0M0.[103] However, as these conditions are now increasingly treated by endoscopic resections, this operation is rarely indicated in cancer surgery.

The principles of preparation of the conduit are exactly the same as described for the Roux-en-Y loop preparation, and the different anastomoses: esophago-jejunal, gastro-jejunal, and jejuno-jejunal are identical.

Functional Results

The results of jejunal Roux-en-Y and interposition are generally good. Postoperative mortality is around 3% to 5%, and the leak rate around 5% to 10%.[104] Dysphagia, regurgitation, diarrhea, and reflux-related heartburn are rare. However, some patients with Roux-en-Y reconstruction, even if adhering to a 70-cm distance from proximal to distal anastomosis, will suffer from persistent debilitating biliary reflux. This may be very difficult to treat and may eventually require revisional surgery replacing the anastomosis further down on the jejunum.

Given its technical difficulty, long-segment jejunoplasty is infrequently performed, but from the available data in literature the results seem to be similar to those obtained after short-segment jejunoplasty.[105,106] In a study by Ascioti et al.,[99] a long segment supercharged pedicled jejunoplasty was attempted in 26 patients. There was no postoperative mortality. Functional results were available in 95.4% (21/22) of the patients who survived at least 6 months after reconstruction. At the time of follow-up, 95% (20/21) of the patients were tolerating a regular diet, and 76.2% (16/21) did not require any supplemental alimentation. Ninety-five percent (20/21) of the patients were free from reflux symptoms, and 80.9% (17/21) had no dumping symptoms. Similar results are reported by Stephens et al.[107]

Free Vascular Grafts

The introduction and popularization of microsurgical technology in the 1970s boosted the interest in using free vascularized intestinal grafts, which, until then, had been performed only on an anecdotal basis, but were described by Alexis Carrel in dogs in 1906.[15] In theory, stomach based on the right gastroepiploic artery,[108] colon based on the middle colic artery, and jejunum based on the most robust segmental artery, can be used.

In practice, jejunum is the preferred option. It is claimed that jejunum, because of its preserved peristaltic mechanism, has the better functional outcome. Free vascularized bowel segments also can be used as onlay patches to cover localized large defects in the esophagus that cannot be closed primarily.[109] Free vascularized colon or jejunum grafts are mostly used in patients who need a laryngopharyngectomy for oncologic reasons, as a primary indication or as a rescue option.[110,111] The intervention is performed by two teams: a visceral surgery team and a plastic surgery team; the latter is specifically for the microvascular anastomoses.

The intervention starts in the abdomen with the preparation of the jejunal loop. A suitable segment of jejunum is

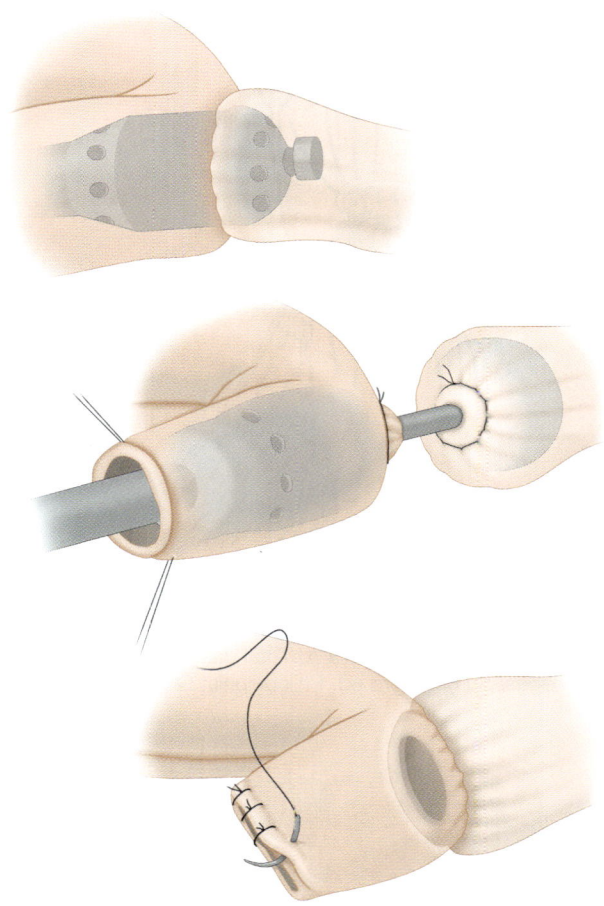

FIGURE 41.28 Stapled esophagojejunal anastomosis. (From Siewert R, Hölscher A. 3 Eingriffe beim Ösophaguskarzinom. Jejunuminterposition. In: Siewert R, ed. *Breitner Chirurgische Operationslehre. Band IV: Ösophagus, Magen und Duodenum.* Urban & Schwarzenberg; 1989:184. Figs. 9-112 & 9-113.)

chosen about 40 cm from the ligament of Treitz offering the better chance to obtain a segment of jejunum with an optimal length of both artery and vein to allow an easy anastomosis in the neck (Fig. 41.31). Equally important is to retrieve a segment of jejunum that has a sufficiently large diameter to match with the base of the pharynx. The jejunum is transected proximally and distally with a linear cutting stapler. Then the mesentery is divided on both sides of the feeding artery and draining vein. After removing the specimen, the blood vessels are flushed with a cold heparin-containing solution to prevent thrombosis after which they are occluded with small nontraumatic microsurgery bulldogs. The loop is brought up to the neck and the anastomosis between the pharynx and the jejunum is performed in two layers. This first anastomosis stabilizes the jejunum protecting against inadvertent movements/ displacements during and after the microsurgery. The loop is placed in an isoperistaltic fashion. Then the plastic surgery team comes in to perform the vascular microanastomosis, making the connection with the inferior thyroid artery and the external jugular vein with 10-0 monofilament suture material (Fig. 41.32). If the length of the vascular

pedicle is too short, vascular grafts are to be interposed (e.g., forearm radial artery and vein). While the plastic surgery team is working in the neck, the abdominal team creates the jejuno-jejunal anastomosis. After finishing the vascular anastomosis, the distal anastomosis between the jejunum and the esophagus is performed also as an end-to-end two-layer interrupted handsewn anastomosis. A nasogastric tube or, if the stomach is available, preferably a gastrostomy, is placed to improve gastric drainage. A piece of mesenterial fat can be exteriorized whilst closing the cervicotomy to monitor the viability of the loop in the first couple of days after surgery.

SKIN

Historically, skin tubes were among the first attempts to restore continuity,[13] but since the introduction of the technique of microvascular anastomosis, skin tubes are no longer used with the exception of myocutaneous flaps to cover large defects in the neck or radial forearm flaps to close defects in the esophageal wall or to bridge short gaps. Skin or myocutaneous flaps are other options, particularly in pharyngeal–cervical esophageal reconstructions. Bulky myocutaneous flaps from the pectoralis major or deltoideopectoral muscle are used if soft tissue is needed to cover cervical defects, especially after extensive neck dissection and/or radiation therapy. Forearm flaps are thinner and based on the radial artery and vein, and are used as free vascular grafts. They are most useful as an onlay patch for lateral pharyngeal defects and salivary fistulas. Also, they can be rolled into a tube to replace a short circumferential defect of pharynx and cervical esophagus as a last rescue when a bowel segment is not available, such as a frozen abdomen.[112,113]

Like free bowel transfers, these are highly specialized plastic and reconstructive techniques primarily used by head and neck tumor surgeons to restore the continuity of pharyngeal defects with associated loss of a short segment of cervical esophagus, or for repair of secondary leaks or salivary fistulas in a heavily irradiated neck.

NO REPLACEMENT

The idea of esophageal resection without replacement was originated by Theodor von Billroth.[12] In 1879, he resected an upper esophageal carcinoma together with the larynx and the thyroid gland. The wound was "encouraged to close" with the hope of reepithelialization of the neck channel. Bougies were passed to maintain the lumen. Unfortunately the patient died of mediastinitis when a bougie was passed through the mediastinum.

Very recently, the interventional endoscopy group from Marseille reported their experience with the so-called "rendezvous" technique for stenosis or partial necrosis of an interposition, where there is a mediastinal segment of more than 5 cm without reconstruction. In the described technique they use a scope from the pharynx down to the mediastinum and another one going up from the stomach, trying to reach each other. When necessary, a stent is placed, or several dilatations are performed, in order to create a tube of controlled fibrotic tissue to bridge the defect.[114,115]

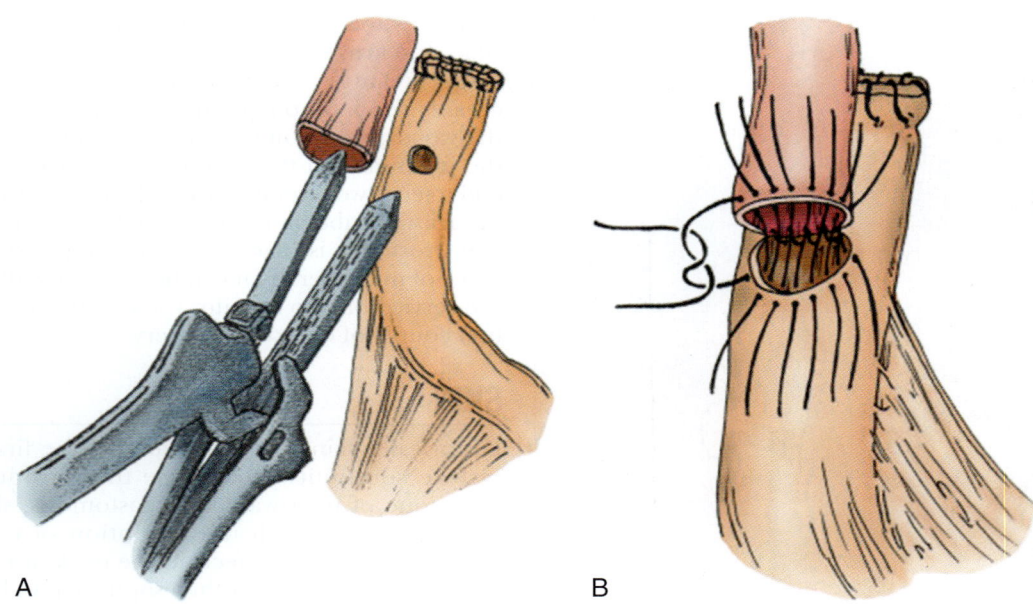

A   B

FIGURE 41.29 Semimechanical anastomosis. (A) The linear stapler introduced into a jejunal opening and into the severed esophageal stump creates the posterior wall. (B) The anterior wall is completed by manual suture. (From Peracchia A. Total gastrectomy and Roux-en-Y reconstruction. In: Patterson G, et al. *Pearson's Thoracic and Esophageal Surgery*. 3rd ed. Philadelphia: Churchill Livingstone; 2008:613-619.)

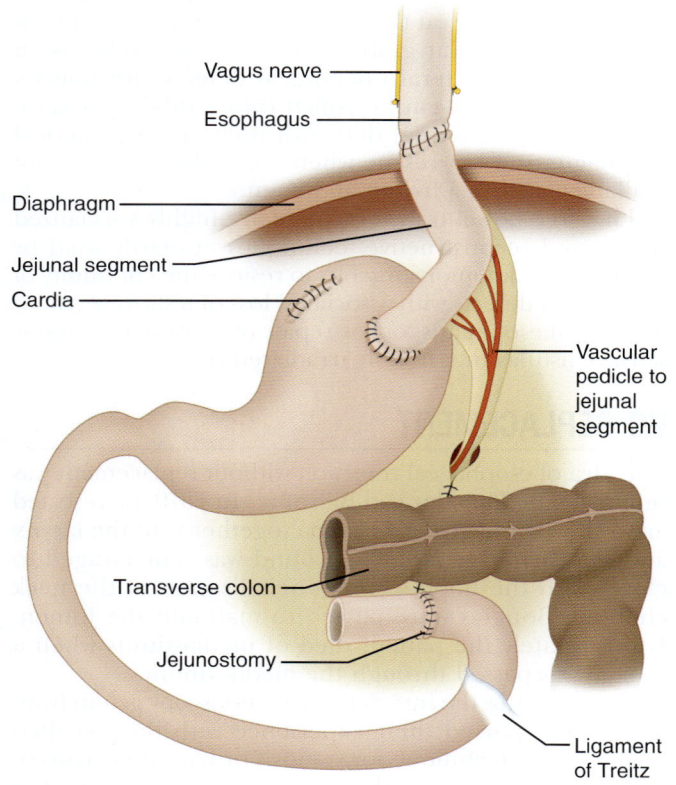

FIGURE 41.30 Merendino procedure: interposition of a jejunum loop. (From Merendino KA, Dillard DH. The concept of sphincter substitution by an interposed jejunal segment for anatomic and physiologic abnormalities at the esophagogastric junction. With special reference to reflux esophagitis, cardiospasm and esophageal varices. *Ann Surg.* 1955;September:488. Fig 1.)

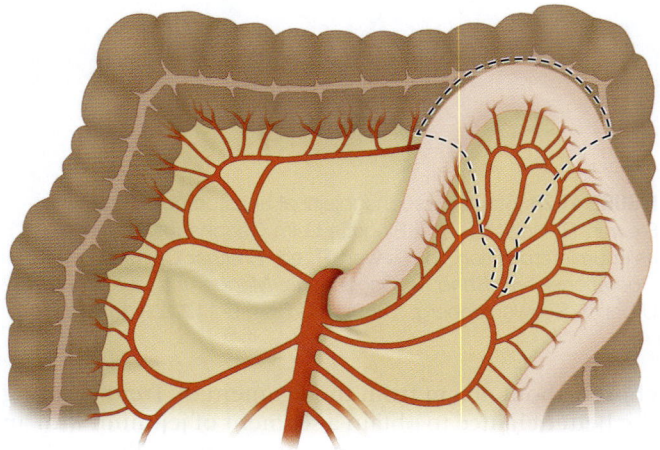

FIGURE 41.31 Free vascular graft preparation: the isolation of a suitable loop. (From Siewert R, Hölscher A. 3 Eingriffe beim Ösophaguskarzinom. Jejunuminterposition. In: Siewert R, ed. *Breitner Chirurgische Operationslehre. Band IV: Ösophagus, Magen und Duodenum.* Urban & Schwarzenberg; 1989:51. Fig 3-66.)

CONDUIT PLACEMENT

The route used to position the esophageal substitute is often determined by the extent of visceral resection, the location of the anastomosis, and the incisions and exposure required for the resection. The classic interventions for cancer of the esophagus are the left thoracoabdominal approach with intrathoracic anastomosis as popularized by Sweet, and with a cervical anastomosis as advocated by Belsey; right thoracotomy and laparotomy with intrathoracic anastomosis by Ivor Lewis; three-hole right thoracotomy, laparotomy, and cervicotomy by McKeown;

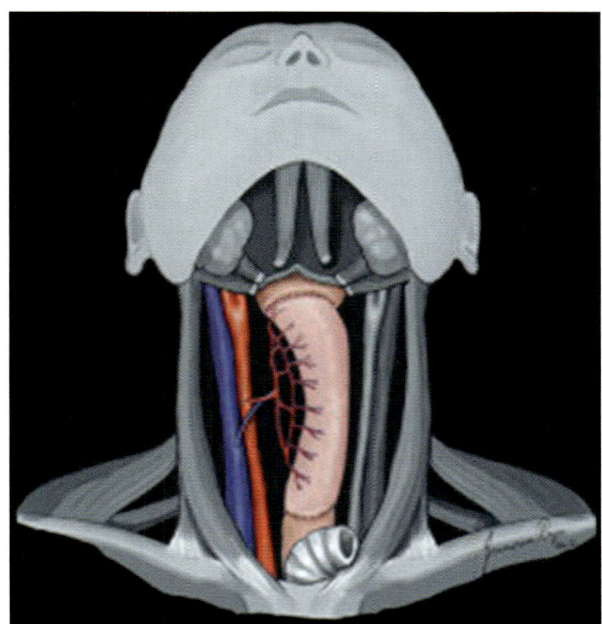

FIGURE 41.32 Free vascular jejunal graft after implantation. (From Lee HS, et al. Free jejunal graft for esophageal reconstruction using end-to-side vascular anastomosis and extended pharyngo-jejunostomy. *Ann Thorac Surg.* 2012;93:1850–1854.)

TABLE 41.3 Most Commonly Used Available Routes, Advantages and Disadvantages

Route	Advantages	Disadvantages
POSTERIOR MEDIASTINAL	Shortest route	Not available when mediastinum is scarred (e.g., previous surgery)
Transhiatal	No opening of the chest	Limitation of lymph node and lateral section plane clearance
Transthoracic: left or right sided, VATS	Direct visualization and lymph nodes allows more radical surgery	Displacement lung, atelectasis, more risk of pulmonary complications
SUBSTERNAL	Ease of dissection Useful when posterior mediastinum is unavailable	Long route Angulation at level of xiphoid and neck Previous cardiac surgery may block access
SUBCUTANEOUS	Ease of dissection Easy detection of graft failure, obstruction	Cosmetically disturbing

VATS, Video-assisted thoracoscopic surgery.

and transhiatal resection through laparotomy and with cervical anastomosis popularized by Orringer. More recently, MIE via laparoscopy and right-sided VATS has been introduced by Luketich, and is widely used today.

As to the route of replacement, four options are available (Fig. 41.33 and Table 41.3).

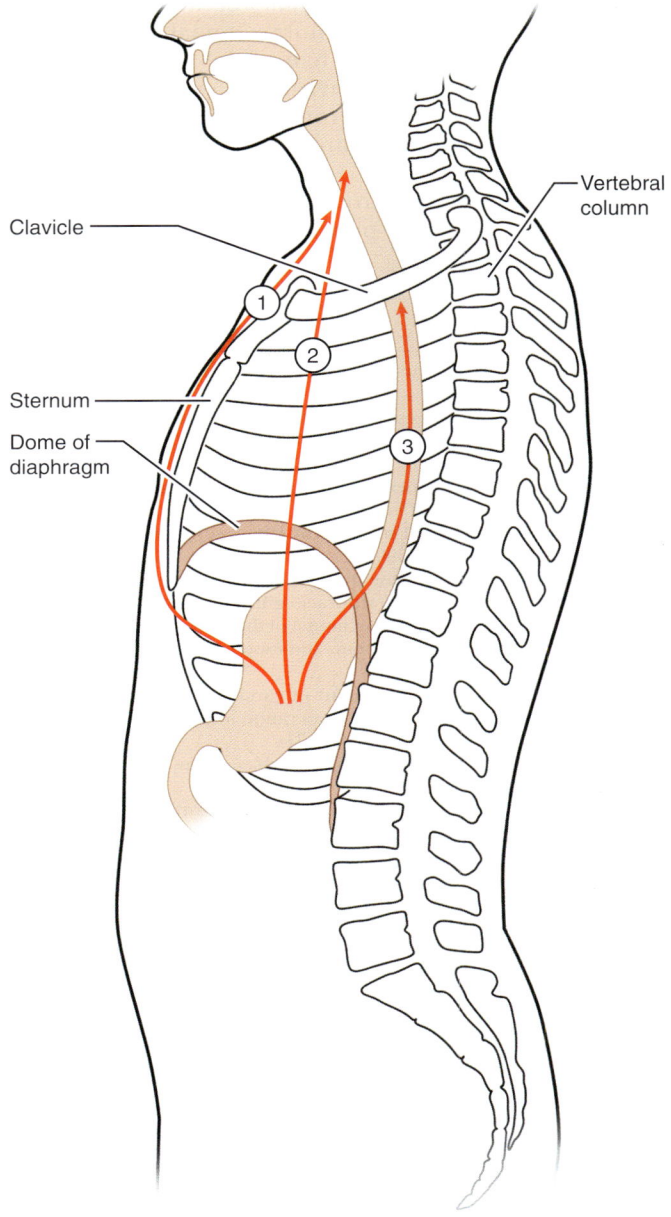

FIGURE 41.33 Options for the route of replacement.

The most commonly used route is the posterior mediastinal route through the bed of the native esophagus. It is the shortest route for reaching the neck, being 5 to 10 cm shorter than the substernal route.

The substernal route, usually without a sternal split, is most useful when the posterior mediastinal route is blocked by previous surgery. This is rarely the case in cancer surgery.

The substernal route is longer, and has two angulations, one from the xiphoid to the stomach and one at the cervical level from the substernal tunnel to the posterior part of the neck. This may cause dysphagia and a delay in the passage of the bolus. When using the colon as a substitute via the substernal route, it seems that there is a higher tendency toward redundancy because of the larger retrosternal space. Some authors systematically perform a resection of the overlying half of the manubrium and the attached head of the clavicle.

The lateral transpleural route, anterior to or behind the lung hilum, and the antethoracic route, are very rarely used.

Finally, a subcutaneous route is available in the extremely rare case that any of the previously mentioned routes are not available.

REFERENCES

1. Czerny V. Neue operationen: resection des oesophagus. *Zentr Chir.* 1877;4:433-434.
2. Torek F. The first successful case of resection of the thoracic portion of the esophagus for carcinoma. *Surg Gynecol Obstet.* 1913;16:614-617.
3. Denk W. Zur Radikaloperation des Oesophaguskarzinoms (vorläufige Mittelung). *Zentralbl Chir.* 1913;40:1065-1068.
4. Ohsawa T. Esophageal surgery (in Japanese). *Nippon Geka Gakkai Zasshi.* 1933;34:1318-1590.
5. Turner GG. Excision of the thoracic oesophagus for carcinoma with reconstruction of an extrathoracic gullet. *Lancet.* 1933;ii:315-316.
6. Adams W, Phemister DB. Carcinoma of the lower thoracic esophagus. Report of a successful resection and esophago-gastrostomy. *J Thorac Surg.* 1938;7:621-627.
7. Lewis I. The surgical treatment of carcinoma of the oesophagus with special reference to a new operation for growths of the middle third. *Br J Surg.* 1946;34(133):18-31.
8. McKeown KC. Total three-stage esophagectomy for cancer of the esophagus. *Br J Surg.* 1976;63(4):259-262.
9. Orringer MB. Esophagectomy without thoracotomy. *J Thorac Cardiovasc Surg.* 1978;76(5):643-654.
10. Cushieri A. Endoscopic oesophagectomy through a right thoracoscopic approach. *J R Coll Surg Edinb.* 1992;37(1):7-11.
11. Luketich JD, Alvelo-Rivera M, Buenaventura PO, et al. Minimally invasive esophagectomy: outcomes in 222 patients. *Ann Surg.* 2003;238(4):486-494.
12. Billroth CAT. Totalextirpation des Ganzenoesophagus vom Pharynx bis zum sternum: ein Totalextirpation des Ganzenlarynx mit des ganzen Schilddruse. *Verhandl Deut Ges Chir.* 1879;8:7-9.
13. von Mikulicz J. Ein fall von Resektion des Carcinomatosen Oesophagus mit plastischen Ersatz des exeidirten Stuckes. *Prag Med Wochenschr.* 1886;11:93-94.
14. Beck C, Carrel A. Demonstration of specimens illustrating a method of formation of a prethoracic esophagus. *Ill Med J.* 1905;7:463-464.
15. Carrel A. The surgery of blood vessels. *Bull Johns Hopkins.* 1907;190:18-27.
16. Roux CK. L'oesophago-jejuno gastromose: nouvelle operation pour retreeissement infranchissable de l'oesophage. *Sem Med.* 1907;27:37-40.
17. Vuillet H. De l'oesophagoplastie et des diverses modifications. *Semin Med.* 1911;31:529.
18. Kelling G. Oesophagoplastik mit hilfe des quercolon. *Zentralbl Chir.* 1911;38:1209-1212.
19. Rowbotham S. Laryngeal intubation in anaesthetics. *Br Med J.* 1923;1(3261):1090-1091.
20. Magill W. Endotracheal anesthesia. *Proc R Soc Med.* 1928;22(2):83-88.
21. Sweet RH. Carcinoma of the esophagus and cardiac end of the stomach: immediate and late results of treatment by resection of primary esophagogastric anastomosis. *JAMA.* 1947;135:485.
22. Belsey RH. Surgical exposure of the esophagus. In: Skinner DBJ, Belsey RH, eds. *Management of Esophageal Disorders.* Philadelphia: WB Saunders; 1988:192-201.
23. Jamieson GG, Mathew G, Ludemann R, et al. Postoperative mortality following oesophagectomy and problems in reporting its rate. *Br J Surg.* 2004;91(8):943-947.
24. Lerut T, Moons J, Coosemans W, et al. Multidisciplinary treatment of advanced cancer of the esophagus and gastroesophageal junction: a European center's approach. *Surg Oncol Clin N Am.* 2008;17:485-502.
25. Straatman J, Joosten PJ, Terwee CB, et al. Systematic review of patient-reported outcome measures in the surgical treatment of patients with esophageal cancer. *Dis Esophagus.* 2015 Oct 15; doi:10.1111/dote.12405; [Epub ahead of print].
26. Liebermann-Meffert DM, Meier R, Siewert JR. Vascular anatomy of the gastric tube used for esophageal reconstruction. *Ann Thorac Surg.* 1992;54:1110-1115.
27. Cooper GJ, Sherry KM, Thorpe JA. Changes in gastric tissue oxygenation during mobilisation for oesophageal replacement. *Eur J Cardiothorac Surg.* 1995;9(3):158-160.
28. Jacobi CA, Zieren HU, Müller JM, et al. Anastomotic tissue oxygen tension during esophagogastrostomy in patients with esophageal carcinoma. *Eur Surg Res.* 1996;28(1):26-31.
29. Bludau M, Hölscher AH, Vallböhmer D, et al. Ischemic conditioning of the gastric conduit prior to esophagectomy improves mucosal oxygen saturation. *Ann Thorac Surg.* 2010;90(4):1121-1126.
30. Farran L, Miro M, Alba E, et al. Preoperative gastric conditioning in cervical gastroplasty. *Dis Esophagus.* 2011;24(4):205-210.
31. Schröder W, Hölscher AH, Bludau M, et al. Ivor-Lewis esophagectomy with and without laparoscopic conditioning of the gastric conduit. *World J Surg.* 2010;34(4):738-743.
32. Veeramootoo D, Shore AC, Wajed SA. Randomized controlled trial of laparoscopic gastric ischemic conditioning prior to minimally invasive esophagectomy, the LOGIC trial. *Surg Endosc.* 2012;26(7):1822-1829.
33. Akiyama H, Tsurumaru M, Udagawa H, et al. Radical lymph node dissection for cancer of the thoracic esophagus. *Ann Surg.* 1994;220(3):364-372.
34. Silberhumer G, Györi G, Burghuber C, et al. The value of protecting the longitudinal staple line with invaginating sutures during esophageal reconstruction by gastric tube pull-up. *Dig Surg.* 2009;26(4):337-341.
35. Collard JM, Romagnoli R, Goncette L, et al. Terminalized semimechanical side-to-side suture technique for cervical esophagogastrostomy. *Ann Thorac Surg.* 1998;65(3):814-817.
36. Deng XF, Liu QX, Zhou D, et al. Hand-sewn vs linearly stapled esophagogastric anastomosis for esophageal cancer: a meta-analysis. *World J Gastroenterol.* 2015;21(15):4757-4764.
37. Nafteux P. The continuous quest for quality improvement after esophagectomy for cancer. thesis. Chapter 8: Impact of change in anastomotic type on complications and health-related quality of life after esophagectomy, gastric tubulation and cervical anastomosis for cancer: semimechanical and hand-sewn. 201;157-181Ed. Peeters, Leuven.
38. Barbour AP, Rizk NP, Gonen M, et al. Adenocarcinoma of the gastroesophageal junction: influence of esophageal resection margin and operative approach on outcome. *Ann Surg.* 2007;246(1):1-8.
39. Jianu A. Gastrostomie und Oesophagoplastik. *Dtsch Z Chir.* 1912;118:383.
40. Gavriliu D. Replacement of the esophagus by a reverse gastric tube. *Curr Probl Surg.* 1975;12(10):36-64.
41. Ximenes Netto M, Silva RO, Vieira LF, et al. The reversed gastric tube revisited: a useful replacement for benign disease. *South Am J Thorac Surg.* 1998;5:22.
42. Gutschow C, Collard JM, Romagnoli R, et al. Denervated stomach as an esophageal substitute recovers intraluminal acidity with time. *Ann Surg.* 2001;233:509-514.
43. Shibuya S, Fukudo S, Shineha R, et al. High incidence of reflux esophagitis observed by routine endoscopic examination after gastric pull-up esophagectomy. *World J Surg.* 2003;27:580-583.
44. De Leyn P, Coosemans W, Lerut T. Early and late functional results in patients with intrathoracic gastric replacement after oesophagectomy for carcinoma. *Eur J Cardiothorac Surg.* 1992;6:79-85.
45. Manjari R, Padhy AK, Chattopadhyay TK. Emptying of the intrathoracic stomach using three different pylorus drainage procedures: results of a comparative study. *Surg Today.* 1996;26(8):581-585.
46. Huang G, Zhang DC, Zhang DW. A comparative study of resection of carcinoma of the esophagus with and without pyloroplasty. In: Demeester T, Skinner D, eds. *Esophageal Disorders: Pathophysiology and Therapy.* New York: Raven Press; 1985:383-388.
47. Chattopadhyay T, Gupta S, Padhy A, et al. Is pyloroplasty necessary following intrathoracic transposition of stomach? Results of a prospective clinical study. *Aust N Z J Surg.* 1991;61:366-369.
48. Mannell A, McKnight A, Esser J. Role of pyloroplasty in the retrosternal stomach: result of prospective, randomized controlled trial. *Br J Surg.* 1990;77:57-59.
49. Fok M, Cheng S, Wong J. Pyloroplasty versus no drainage in gastric replacement of the esophagus. *Am J Surg.* 1991;162:447-452.

50. Urschel JD, Blewett CJ, Young JE, et al. Pyloric drainage (pyloroplasty) or no drainage in gastric reconstruction after esophagectomy: a meta-analysis of randomized controlled trials. *Dig Surg.* 2002;19:160-164.

51. Akkerman RD, Haverkamp L, van Hillegersberg R, et al. Surgical techniques to prevent delayed gastric emptying after esophagectomy with gastric interposition: a systematic review. *Ann Thorac Surg.* 2014;98(4):1512-1519.

52. Cerfolio RJ, Bryant AS, Canon CL, et al. Is botulinum toxin injection of the pylorus during Ivor Lewis [corrected] esophagogastrectomy the optimal drainage strategy? *J Thorac Cardiovasc Surg.* 2009;137(3):565-572.

53. Eldaif SM, Lee R, Adams KN, et al. Intrapyloric botulinum injection increases postoperative esophagectomy complications. *Ann Thorac Surg.* 2014;97(6):1959-1964.

54. Finley R, Lamy A, Clifton J, et al. Gastrointestinal function following esophagectomy for malignancy. *Am J Surg.* 1995;169:471-475.

55. Bemelman WA, Taat CW, Slors JFM, et al. Delayed postoperative emptying after esophageal resection is dependent on the size of the gastric substitute. *J Am Coll Surg.* 1995;180:461-464.

56. Barbera L, Kemen M, Wegener M, et al. Effect of site and width of stomach tube after esophageal resection on gastric emptying. *Zentralbl Chir.* 1994;119:240-244.

57. Collard JM, Tinton N, Malaise J, et al. Esophageal replacement: gastric tube or whole stomach? *Ann Thorac Surg.* 1995;60:261-266.

58. Swanson EW, Swanson SJ, Swanson RS. Endoscopic pyloric balloon dilatation obviates the need for pyloroplasty at esophagectomy. *Surg Endosc.* 2012;26(7):2023-2028.

59. Burt M, Scott A, Williard W, et al. Erythromycin stimulates gastric emptying after esophagectomy with gastric replacement: a randomized clinical trial. *J Thor Cardiovasc Surg.* 1996;11:649-654.

60. Lanuti M, DeDelva P, Morse CR, et al. Management of delayed gastric emptying after esophagectomy with endoscopic balloon dilatation of the pylorus. *Ann Thorac Surg.* 2011;91(4):1019-1024.

61. Datta J, Williams NN, Conway RG, et al. Rescue pyloroplasty for refractory delayed gastric emptying following esophagectomy. *Surgery.* 2014;156(2):290-297.

62. da Rocha JR, Cecconello I, Zilberstein B, et al. Barrett esophagus in the esophageal stump after subtotalesophagectomy with cervical esophagogastroplasty. *Rev Hosp Clin Fac Med Sao Paulo.* 1992;47:69-70.

63. Franchimont D, Covas A, Brasseur C, et al. Newly developed Barrett's esophagus after subtotalesophagectomy. *Endoscopy.* 2003;35:850-853.

64. Oberg S, Johansson J, Wenner J, et al. Metaplastic columnar mucosa in the cervical esophagus after esophagectomy. *Ann Surg.* 2002;235:338-345.

65. Wang L, Huang MH, Huang BS, et al. Gastric substitution for resectable carcinoma of the esophagus; an analysis of 368 cases. *Ann Thorac Surg.* 1992;53:289-294.

66. Gutschow C, Collard J, Romagnoli R, et al. Bile exposure of the denervated stomach as an esophageal substitute. *Ann Thorac Surg.* 2001;71:1786-1791.

67. McLarty AJ, Deschamps C, Trastek F, et al. Esophageal resection for cancer of the esophagus: long-term function and quality of life. *Ann Thorac Surg.* 1997;63:1568-1572.

68. Hölscher A, Voit H, Buttermann G, et al. Function of the intrathoracic stomach as esophageal replacement. *World J Surg.* 1988;12:835-844.

69. Banki F, Mason RJ, DeMeester SR, et al. Vagal-sparing esophagectomy: a more physiologic alternative. *Ann Surg.* 2002;236:324-335.

70. Humphrey C, Johnston D, Walker B, et al. Incidence of dumping after truncal and selective vagotomy with pyloroplasty and highly selective vagotomy without drainage procedure. *Br Med J.* 1972;3:785-788.

71. Sinha S, Padhy A, Chattopadhyay T. Dumping syndrome in the intra-thoracic stomach. *Trop Gastroenterol.* 1997;8:131-133.

72. Hasler W. Dumping syndrome. *Curr Treat Options Gastroenterol.* 2002;5:139-145.

73. Hulscher JB, van Sandick JW, de Boer AG, et al. Extended transthoracic resection comhapared with limited transhiatal resection for adenocarcinoma of the esophagus. *N Engl J Med.* 2002;347:1662-1669.

74. Lagergren P, Avery KN, Hughes R, et al. Health-related quality of life among patients cured by surgery for esophageal cancer. *Cancer.* 2007;110:686-693.

75. Biere SS, van Berge-Henegouwen MI, Maas KW, et al. Minimally invasive versus open oesophagectomy for patients with oesophageal cancer: a multicentre, open-label, randomised controlled trial. *Lancet.* 2012;379:1887-1892.

76. Nafteux P, Durnez J, Moons J, et al. Assessing the relationships between health-related quality of life and postoperative length of hospital stay after oesophagectomy for cancer of the oesophagus and the gastro-oesophageal junction. *Eur J Cardiothorac Surg.* 2013;44(3):525-533.

77. Nafteux P, Moons J, Coosemans W, et al. Minimally invasive oesophagectomy: a valuable alternative to open oesophagectomy for the treatment of early oesophageal and gastro-oesophageal junction carcinoma. *Eur J Cardiothorac Surg.* 2011;40(6):1455-1463.

78. Orsoni P, Lemaire M. Technique des oesophagoplasties par le colon transverse et descendant. *J Chir (Paris).* 1951;67:491-505.

79. Reboud E, Picaud R, Rouzaud R, et al. Left colon transplants in esophageal surgery. *Mem Acad Chir (Paris).* 1968;94(10):324-333.

80. Waterston D. Colonic replacement of esophagus. *Surg Clin North Am.* 1964;44:1441-1447.

81. Belsey R. Reconstruction of the esophagus with left colon. *J Thorac Cardiovasc Surg.* 1965;49:33-53.

82. Lortat-Jacob JL, Giuli R. Esophageal replacement. *Prog Surg.* 1973;12:77-95.

83. Leal AJ, Tannuri AC, Tannuri U. Mechanical bowel preparation for esophagocoloplasty in children: is it really necessary? *Dis Esophagus.* 2013;26(5):475-478.

84. Thomas PA, Gilardoni A, Trousse D, et al. Colon interposition for oesophageal replacement. *Multimed Man Cardiothorac Surg.* 2009;2009(603).

85. Hamai Y, Hihara J, Emi M, et al. Esophageal reconstruction using the terminal ileum and right colon in esophageal cancer surgery. *Surg Today.* 2012;42:342-350.

86. Saeki H, Morita M, Harada N, et al. Esophageal replacement by colon interposition with microvascular surgery for patients with thoracic esophageal cancer: the utility of superdrainage. *Dis Esophagus.* 2013;26:50-56.

87. Shirakawa Y, Naomoto Y, Noma K, et al. Colonic interposition and supercharge for esophageal reconstruction. *Langenbecks Arch Surg.* 2006;391:19-23.

88. Pompeo E, Nofroni I, Van Raemdonck D, et al. Esophagocoloplasty for congenital, benign and malignant diseases. Surgical and long-term functional results. *Eur J Cardiothorac Surg.* 1996;10(7):561-567.

89. Gust L, Ouattara M, Coosemans W, et al. European perspective in thoracic surgery-eso-coloplasty: when and how? *J Thorac Dis.* 2016;8(suppl 4):S387-S398.

90. Jeyasingham K, Lerut T, Belsey RH. Functional and mechanical sequelae of colon interposition for benign oesophageal disease. *Eur J Cardiothorac Surg.* 1999;15(3):327-331. [discussion 331–332].

91. de Delva PE, Morse CR, Austen WG Jr, et al. Surgical management of failed colon interposition. *Eur J Cardiothorac Surg.* 2008;34(2):432-437.

92. Vasseur Maurer S, Estremadoyro V, Reinberg O. Evaluation of an antireflux procedure for colonic interposition in pediatric esophageal replacements. *J Pediatr Surg.* 2011;46(3):594-600.

93. Longmire WP Jr, Ravitch MM. A new method for constructing an artificial esophagus. *Ann Surg.* 1946;123:819-835.

94. Allison PR, Wooler GH, Gunning AJ. Esophagojejunogastrostomy. *J Thorac Surg.* 1957;33:738-748.

95. Thompson VC. Oesophagectomy for carcinoma: restoration of function by an ante-thoracic jejunal graft. *Proc R Soc Med.* 1946;39:310.

96. Gaur P, Blackmon SH. Jejunal graft conduits after esophagectomy. *J Thorac Dis.* 2014;6(suppl 3):S333-S340.

97. Wright C, Cuschieri A. Jejunal interposition for benign esophageal disease. Technical considerations and long-term results. *Ann Surg.* 1987;205(1):54-60.

98. Watanabe W, Mine S, Nishida K, et al. Reconstruction after esophagectomy for esophageal cancer patients with a history of gastrectomy. *Gen Thorac Cardiovasc Surg.* 2016;64(8):457-463.

99. Ascioti AJ, Hofstetter WL, Miller MJ, et al. Long-segment, supercharged, pedicled jejunal flap for total esophageal reconstruction. *J Thorac Cardiovasc Surg.* 2005;130:1391-1398.

100. Blackmon SH, Correa AM, Skoracki R, et al. Supercharged pedicled jejunal interposition for esophageal replacement: a 10-year experience. *Ann Thorac Surg.* 2012;94:1104-1111. [discussion 1111-1113].

101. Peracchia A, Rosati R. Total gastrectomy and Roux-en-Y reconstruction. In: Patterson AG, Cooper JD, Deslauriers J, Lerut A, Luketich JD, Rice T, eds. *Pearson's Thoracic and Esophageal Surgery.* Philadelphia: Churchill Livingstone; 2008:613-619 [Chapter 57].

102. Merendino KA, Dillard DH. The concept of sphincter substitution by an interposed jejunal segment for anatomic and physiologic abnormalities at the esophagogastric junction; with special reference to reflux esophagitis, cardiospasm and esophageal varices. *Ann Surg.* 1955;142(3):486-506.

103. Stein H, Feith M, Siewert JR. Distal esophageal resection and jejunum interposition for early Barrett carcinoma. *Zentralbl Chir.* 2001;126(suppl 1):9-13. [German].

104. Blackmon SH, Correa AM, Skoracki R, et al. Supercharged pedicled jejunal interposition for esophageal replacement: a 10-year experience. *Ann Thorac Surg.* 2012;94(4):1104-1111.

105. Maier H, Pinter H, Tomaselli F, et al. Retrosternal pedicled jejunum interposition: an alternative for reconstruction after total esophagogastrectomy. *Eur J Cardiothorac Surg.* 2002;22(5):661-665.

106. Ring WS, Varco RL, L'Heureux PR, et al. Esophageal replacement with jejunum in children: an 18 to 33 year follow-up. *J Thorac Cardiovasc Surg.* 1982;83:918.

107. Stephens EH, Gaur P, Hotze KO, et al. Super-charged pedicled jejunal interposition performance compares favorably with a gastric conduit after esophagectomy. *Ann Thorac Surg.* 2015;100(2):407-413.

108. Yamagishi M, Ikeda N, Yonemoto T. An isoperistaltic gastric tube. New method of esophageal replacement. *Arch Surg.* 1970;100(6):689-692.

109. Jurkiewicz MJ, Paletta CEL. Free jejunal graft. In: *Current Therapy in Cardiothoracic Surgery.* Philadelphia: B.C. Decker; 1989:206.

110. Jurkiewicz MJ. Vascularized intestinal graft for reconstruction of the cervical esophagus and pharynx. *Plast Reconstr Surg.* 1965;36:509-517.

111. Hester TR, McConnel FM, Nahal F, et al. Reconstruction of cervical esophagus, hypopharynx and oral cavity using free jejunal transfer. *Am J Surg.* 1980;140(4):487-491.

112. Chen H, Tang Y. Microsurgical reconstruction of the esophagus. *Semin Surg Oncol.* 2000;19:235.

113. Nakatsuka T, Harii K, Asato H, et al. Comparative evaluation in pharyngo-oesophageal reconstruction: radial forearm flap compared with jejunal flap: a 10 year experience. *Scand J Plast Reconstr Surg Hand Surg.* 1997;32:307.

114. Gonzalez JM, Vanbiervliet G, Gasmi M, et al. Efficacy of the endoscopic rendez-vous technique for the reconstruction of complete esophageal disruptions. *Endoscopy.* 2016;48:179-183.

115. Perbtani Y, Suarez AL, Wagh MS. Emerging techniques and efficacy of endoscopic esophageal reconstruction and lumen restoration for complete esophageal obstruction. *Endosc Int Open.* 2016;4(2):E136-E142.

Palliative Therapy for Esophageal Cancer

Dennis Wells | Virginia R. Litle

The American Cancer Society estimates that 16,940 new cases of esophageal cancer will be diagnosed in 2016, and in the same year there will be 15,690 deaths from esophageal cancer.[1] Unfortunately, more than half of patients present with advanced disease with symptoms of dysphagia, weight loss, and less often bleeding.[2] Palliative interventions are needed to optimize quality of life by reducing hospital admissions for aspiration and bleeding, as well as allow them to enjoy eating. The goals for treating malignant dysphagia are ease of treatment and short hospital stay. For patients who may be candidates for palliative chemotherapy or chemoradiation therapy, the only palliative procedural intervention may be a need for a percutaneous gastrostomy tube for caloric supplementation.

Depending on the degree of dysphagia and the performance status of the patient, a significant number of patients may need endoscopic interventions to improve oral intake and nutritional status as the first step in their treatment algorithm. Patients who cannot swallow their saliva need an urgent endoscopic intervention to reduce their risk of aspiration, a potentially fatal event.

Most endoscopic therapies provide initial improvement in dysphagia but vary in their durability. After improvement in oral nutrition, performance may improve and other therapies may be tolerated. In this chapter, we review all the commonly used methods for endoscopic palliation of malignant dysphagia. In general, these methods deliver rapid relief and allow intake of a soft to regular diet with some modifications depending on the individual. Dilation and endoscopic stents are considered the mainstay of palliative options. As the durability of the relief of dysphagia is variable, a multimodality approach is often required. Laser therapy with thermal ablation and nonthermal photodynamic therapy have been options for many years; however, cryoablation has now joined the ranks. The palliative options for bleeding or obstructing esophageal cancer are summarized in Table 42.1. On the rare occasion, in a very good performance with incurable disease, esophagectomy may be indicated for palliation when other interventions fail. In our practice, advances in endoscopic palliative modalities have made this unusual.

ESOPHAGEAL DILATION

Malignant esophageal dysphagia can be relieved immediately to some degree with dilation with a bougie or a balloon dilator. If this is the only therapy, recurrent dysphagia will occur in almost all patients within 1 to 2 weeks. This temporary intervention may allow improvement of oral intake, particularly fluids, for a short period of time while other therapies, including chemotherapy and radiation, are initiated. Dilation is more commonly carried out in conjunction with other modalities such as stenting or ablation to provide longer relief for the patient. The Savary bougie dilators produce both radial and longitudinal forces to the esophagus (Fig. 42.1), whereas a balloon dilator produces only a radial force (Fig. 42.2). The balloon dilator is better for a longer stricture, such as a malignant stricture, and the bougie is better for the more focal anastomotic or postfundoplication stricture. The balloon dilation can be done under direct vision with a through-the-scope dilator or over a guidewire and with fluoroscopic guidance to confirm safe placement of the balloon across the tumor. When the esophageal lumen is very narrow, expandable metal stent placement without initial dilation may lead to stent infolding and an initial dilation may be indicated. Similarly, after expandable metal stent placement, careful balloon dilation may facilitate immediate expansion. However, overzealous dilation may lead to a less snug fit of the stent and early migration. Dilation is often used before and after ablative therapy including cryoablation or laser therapy to allow passage of the endoscope and laser fiber. Complications after esophageal dilation range from pain and fever to perforation. Although risk of perforation is uncommon in experienced hands, the endoscopist should have a low threshold for further diagnostic studies, such as an intraoperative esophagram with gastroview or postoperative barium esophagography, to rule this out, in particular in the patient with excessive pain or pneumomediastinum, pneumoperitoneum, or a pneumothorax after dilation. If there is no leak, the patient can be started on clear liquids for 24 hours, followed by a soft diet as tolerated. In some cases, if the perforation is minor and contrast agent shows no or minimal extravasation, with good drainage into the esophageal lumen, patients can be conservatively managed and treated with antibiotics and nothing by mouth for a short period of observation. In some cases, immediate deployment of a covered, expandable metal stent will seal more substantial leaks. It is imperative that an experienced thoracic surgeon evaluate these patients because, even in the era of covered expandable stents, surgical intervention may be indicated for perforations.

STENTS

With the advent of the self-expanding metal stent (SEMS), now more than 20 years ago, endoscopic palliation is now easier and associated with fewer complications than with the historical open traction and push-through techniques.[3] A SEMS can be placed via upper endoscopy with fluoroscopic guidance and does not require general anesthesia. The primary risks are aspiration at time of placement, so general anesthesia may reduce the risk of periprocedural aspiration. Communication with the anesthesiologist is paramount to optimize safety. Perforation is uncommon. One of the earlier reports on the SEMS involved placing a Wallstent, which was originally designed for vascular stenosis. In a small series the endoluminal tumor was partially obliterated with laser and then the SEMS was placed with safe and effective results.[4] Ell et al. also reported a small series of 20 patients with malignant obstruction treated with Gianturco-Z stents 20 years ago.[5] Of the 20 patients, 19 (95%) reported immediate relief in their dysphagia, and there were no technical problems. Fifty percent of the patients complained of chest or epigastric pain after the procedure. The migration rate was 5%.

TABLE 42.1 Palliative Options for Bleeding or Obstructing Esophageal Cancer

Modality	Bleeding	Obstruction	Weight Loss
Balloon dilation	N	Y	N
Self-expanding metal stent	N	Y	N
LASER			
Thermal laser (Nd:YAG)	Y	Y	N
Photodynamic therapy	Y	Y	N
Cryoablation	Y	Y	N
Radiation therapy	N	Y	N
Chemotherapy	N	Y	N
Percutaneous gastrostomy tube	N	N	Y

Nd:YAG, Neodymium:yttrium-aluminum-garnet.

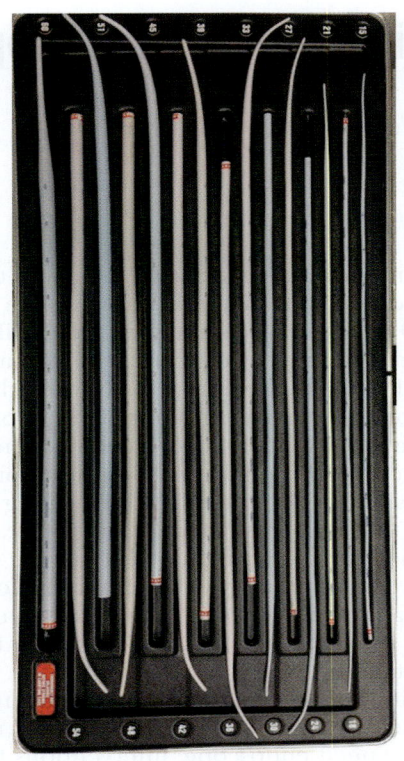

FIGURE 42.1 The Savary dilators (up to 60 French in size) are placed over a wire to dilate benign and malignant esophageal strictures with fluorosopic guidance.

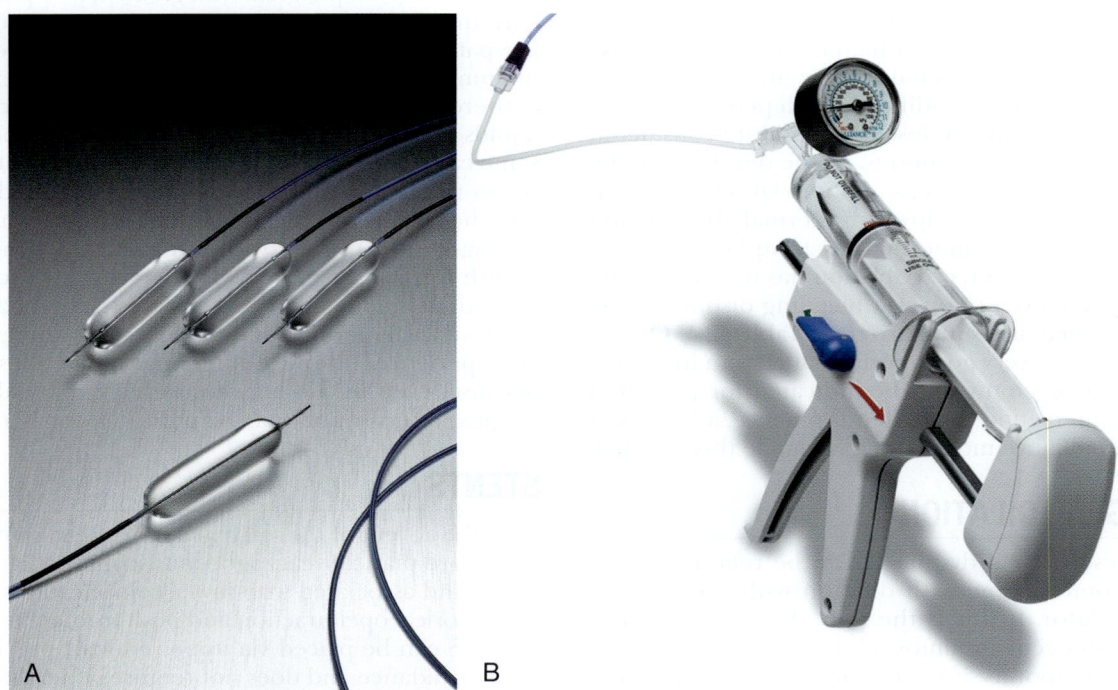

A   B

FIGURE 42.2 The balloon dilators (A) can be placed through the endoscope working channel and then inflated under direct vision or with fluoroscopic guidance with a handheld pump (B). (Images used with permission from Boston Scientific Corp.)

TABLE 42.2 Stent Options for Palliation of Malignant Dysphagia

Stent Type	Manufacturer	Covered	Stent Material	Release	Foreshortening
Ultraflex	Boston Scientific	Partially Fully	Nitinol	Proximal and distal	35%
Wallflex	Boston Scientific	Partially Fully	Cobalt based	Distal	35%
Evolution	Cook Medical	Partially Fully	Stainless steel	Distal	None
Alimaxx-ES	Merit Medical	Fully	Nitinol	Distal	None

Table 42.2 summarizes the more commonly used SEMS for malignant obstruction. There are several types of expandable metal stents, and all share many features but have minor design modifications, which may offer advantages of one over the other. The Evolution Controlled-Release Stent or Z-stent (Wilson Cook, Winston-Salem, North Carolina) is composed of stainless steel in either a mesh or zigzag design. It is released with a sheath and pusher rod mechanism, which is meant to optimize accurate placement. The Ultraflex and WallFlex SEMS (Boston Scientific, Watertown, Massachusetts) are knitted stents deployed with the removal of a string. After deployment, typical stent diameter ranges from 18 to 23 mm and stent length is 10 to 15 cm.[6]

The high radial force of SEMS may result in postoperative pain, which is usually mild and transient. In unusual cases it may persist and require removal. A SEMS is available covered or uncovered. The covered stents reduce tumor ingrowth except at the ends, which are uncovered to reduce stent migration. When tumor ingrowth of the stent occurs or overgrowth at the end of the stent occurs, additional stents can be applied, or neodymium:yttrium-aluminum-garnet (Nd:YAG) laser or photodynamic therapy (PDT) laser can be used to ablate the tumor. Thermal laser may be limited in these situations because the laser can damage the stent nitinol itself. Some of the newer designs of expandable metal stents (Alveolus) offer full-length coverage with options for more stable esophageal wall contact that may minimize migration yet allow full-length coverage.

Self-expanding plastic stents (SEPSs), including Polyflex (Boston Scientific), have more commonly been used to treat benign esophageal lesions because these stents are easier to retrieve given less tissue reaction in comparison to metal stents. Other benefits of plastic stents include lower cost, although they are prone to stent migration. Malignant esophageal disease and palliation has typically been addressed with SEMS. Conio et al. randomized patients to receive either the Polyflex or the Ultraflex stent and reported no difference in palliation of dysphagia but a significantly higher rate of complication, particularly stent migration,[7] in the SEPS group. In addition, a meta-analysis conducted by Yakoub et al. in London also reported metal stents performed superiorly to plastic stent for palliative management of malignant dysphagia.[8]

In our practice, we use a combination of endoscopic and fluoroscopic guidance to measure the length of esophageal obstruction before deploying the expandable metal stents.

After adequate seating in the esophagus, the intrinsic radial force of the most expandable metal stents leads to continued expansion to its maximal diameter, depending on the severity of the obstruction. Thus, if a stent appears patent but not open completely on initial placement, the clinician can repeat the endoscopy the next day or obtain a barium esophagram to see if the stent has expanded fully. Poor initial stent deployment, especially with significant infolding, may indicate an improper stent diameter or length. Immediate intervention, such as gentle dilation, or even stent removal may be necessary if an obvious failure is observed. Complications from stent placement can occur early and late. The early complications include aspiration pneumonia during the procedure, esophageal perforation, malpositioned stent, airway compression and compromise with mid to upper esophageal stents, persistent obstruction, and pain. Late complications include intractable reflux, stent obstruction, or migration. The risk of delayed perforation or erosion into adjacent structures is rare but has been described.[9] Delayed removal or repositioning of expandable esophageal stents is generally avoided but in experienced hands has been done. The obvious risk is esophageal trauma with the potential for esophageal perforation. In summary, expandable metal stents provide rapid improvement in malignant dysphagia, allowing patients a short or no hospital stay and improved quality of life. The need for repeat intervention is common in patients who live longer than a few months. In these cases a careful investigation of the causes for stent failure should be made to determine if additional dilation, stent placement, or laser therapy may be indicated to provide continued relief of obstruction.

Recent advancements in stents also include the development of drug-eluting stents,[10] radioactive stents,[11,12] as well as biodegradable stents.[13] The role of these types of stents for palliation of esophageal malignancy remains to be determined.

NEODYMIUM:YTTRIUM-ALUMINUM-GARNET LASER TREATMENT

Thermal laser therapy for esophageal cancer was initially described in 1982 and involved use of argon or Nd:YAG lasers. The Nd:YAG laser has since been proven to be more effective than the argon laser but suffers from some technical limitations and a perforation rate as high as 7% to 10%. PDT was approved by the US Food and Drug

Administration in 1996 for the treatment of malignant dysphagia and has a low perforation rate (1%) and is more durable than Nd:YAG laser ablation. Thermal laser remains a useful tool for ablating the unusual bleeding esophageal tumor acutely. The Nd:YAG laser uses a wavelength of 1064 nm. For both bleeding and obstructing esophageal lesions, 50 to 90 W is used with a pulse duration of 0.3 to 1.0 second. The greatest risk with thermal laser use is esophageal perforation, which can occur directly from the laser or with concurrent dilation. The laser treatment often begins with esophageal dilation either with a pneumatic balloon or Savary dilator with a guidewire and fluoroscopic guidance. The general concept is to work off the luminal surface of the tumor to minimize the risk of perforation. The tumor is then circumferentially ablated with the endoscopically placed Nd:YAG laser in a point-by-point method. Depending on the length of the endoluminal tumor, Nd:YAG can be more time consuming than PDT as the nonthermal laser diffuser probe allows administration of light over a greater surface area. Tumors with a significant component of extraluminal mass may fail laser therapy due to extrinsic compression and may be better palliated with an expandable metal stent. One study comparing thermal laser to esophageal stenting found similar relief in dysphagia and survival, but the dysphagia relief lasted significantly longer in the laser-treated group in whom the patients had significant gastric involvement.[14] The main complication of Nd:YAG laser therapy is esophageal perforation, which occurred in 7% of 118 patients in a randomized multicenter trial of patients undergoing PDT versus Nd:YAG therapy for palliation of esophageal cancer. Esophageal dilation had accompanied laser therapy in half of the perforation cases. Fever, nausea, and postoperative respiratory insufficiency are all potential perioperative morbidities of the laser treatment.[15] Fistulas and strictures occur as late complications in 10% of patients.[16] Thermal laser therapy may be valuable in cases where a stent cannot be placed easily, such as in the cervical esophagus where proximal airway compression or obstruction may result from the stent. Distal esophageal stents placed across the gastroesophageal junction can result in significant reflux, and laser therapy may minimize this problem. Stenting across the gastroesophageal junction (GEJ) may be reduced with an antireflux valve. However, in an early randomized study of 30 patients, the valve did not prevent gastroesophageal reflux.[17] More recently 38 patients were enrolled at nine centers to covered SEMS with antireflux valve or SEMS without a valve.[18] The conclusion was gastroesophageal reflux disease (GERD) was improved but there were more obstructions of the SEMS in the valve group.

PHOTODYNAMIC THERAPY

Photodynamic therapy is a nonthermal laser process using selective endoscopic delivery of light with a specific wavelength to activate a photosensitizing agent that results in tumor ablation and restores endoluminal patency. Currently PDT is primarily performed with porfimer sodium (Photofrin; Concordia Laboratories Inc., Oakville, Ontario), a hematoporphyrin derivative with a light activation wavelength of 630 nm. The depth of penetration and

tumor necrosis after PDT is limited to 5 mm. This provides a safety factor in minimizing risk of esophageal perforation but also can limit its effectiveness for large bulky tumors, especially when significant extrinsic compression is present. Full-thickness perforation can occur, but in the largest series to date, esophageal perforation occurred in only 5 of 215 patients (1.5%).[19] Balloon dilation was performed before PDT to allow passage of the endoscope through the obstructing tumor. It was unclear whether the mechanical dilation of the esophagus, the use of PDT, or a combination of the two factors contributed to this complication. In the same series of 215 patients, esophageal stricture after PDT occurred in only 1.5% of patients; however, in more contemporary series of PDT for palliation and treatment, the stricture rate approaches 20%.[20] This lower rate of stricture after PDT for palliation may be explained by the fact that less normal esophagus is exposed to the laser light when a bulky tumor is present. The combination of radiation therapy, chemotherapy, and PDT typically increases the risk of stricture formation. Whether a true PDT-induced stricture or tumor progression results in luminal narrowing is sometimes difficult to ascertain in the palliative setting. Ideal candidates for palliative PDT have locally advanced esophageal carcinoma with primarily endoluminal disease and minimal stricture or extrinsic compression. The overall advantages of PDT for treating locally advanced esophageal cancer include improvement in malignant dysphagia within days of treatment, minimal pain, and, in some cases of gastroesophageal junction tumors, less reflux; and in cases of high cervical esophageal obstruction, there is less concern over tracheal compression resulting from stent expansion of the cervical esophagus. The main disadvantages include the skin photosensitivity in patients with a limited life expectancy, the costs of specialized equipment and the photosensitizing agent, and limitations in efficacy when significant, bulky, extrinsic compression is present. The more common side effects are chest pain, nausea, odynophagia, and vomiting. Mediastinitis and tracheoesophageal fistulas are rare.[21]

CRYOTHERAPY

Cryotherapy can involve the use of nitrogen, a rapidly expanding gas, or carbon dioxide. The truFreeze (CSA Medical, Baltimore, Maryland) system has been available for several years, and despite the paucity of literature for palliative options, it has been reported for ablative purposes for more than 10,000 treatments.[22] TruFreeze involves spraying liquid nitrogen directly on the bulky tumor. A gastric decompression tube is required to reduce the risk of injury to the enteric viscera from the rapidly expanding nitrogen gas. If a decompression tube cannot be placed across a bulky endoluminal obstruction, then cryospray is not an initial palliative option. As the cryogen is released into the esophagus, a transmural freeze occurs. Cardiac arrhythmias may occur from the freeze affecting the heart. A preoperative cardiac assessment including a recent electrocardiogram is recommended in the preoperative setting. These risks and side effects should be discussed with the patient prior to surgery.

For the truFreeze cryotherapy technique, an orogastric decompression tube is placed, the cryospray catheter is

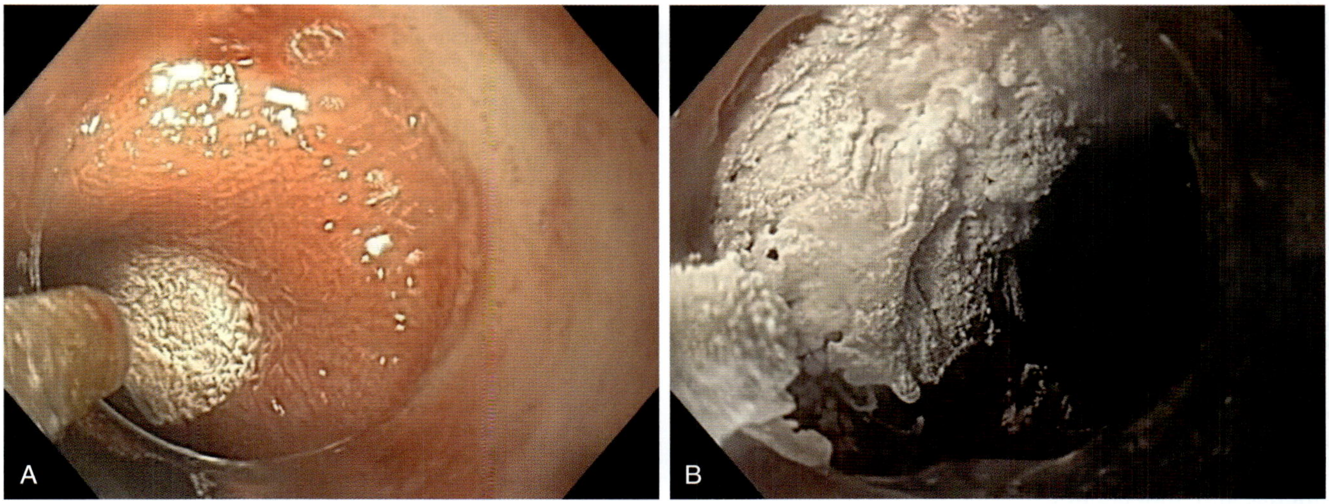

FIGURE 42.3 (A and B) TruFreeze liquid nitrogen is delivered through the endoscope to ablate the endoluminal tumor under direct vision.

primed, and the decompression tube is placed on continuous suction. Expose the upper abdomen and apply gentle pressure consistently throughout the procedure. Typically the clinician applies the cryospray (−196°C) under direct vision for 10 to 20 seconds and allows complete thawing of tissue in between freezes (~2 to 3 minutes) (Fig. 42.3). Three separate freezes are administered, then the catheter is defrosted with the decompression tube on suction still. Cryotherapy complications are uncommon but can include perforation, chest pain, and arrhythmias. The other technology is the carbon dioxide cryospray (Polar Wand; GI Supply, Camp Hill, Pennsylvania) and is also administered with a through-the-scope delivery system. The delivered temperature reaches −78°C. A decompression tube is not needed, but a suction channel is connected to spray catheter to allow a flow of CO_2 at 6 to 8 L/min. We await future reports of the palliative success with the Polar Wand.

BRACHYTHERAPY AND EXTERNAL BEAM RADIATION THERAPY

Endoluminal brachytherapy (BT) with high-dose rate radiation is another modality to locally ablate obstructing esophageal cancer. It has been used as a salvage therapy after external beam radiation therapy (EBRT), as well as resulting in greater than 50% relief in dysphagia.[23] The benefits are a good tumor response but with stricture rates of 38% with high-dose rate BT (3 weekly fractions of 500 cGy).[23] Patients typically return for several treatment fractions over 2 to 3 weeks to obtain the full treatment dose. In addition, BT requires specialized staff and expensive delivery equipment with limited availability. For each treatment the patient undergoes esophageal dilation and placement of the after loading catheter. Afterward they are transported to the BT delivery room, where the catheter is loaded and approximately 500 cGy is administered, which penetrates to a depth of 0.5 to 1 cm. Contraindications to the procedure include the presence of an esophageal fistula because this is a known potential complication of the procedure. Other complications include perforation

and stricture formation, the latter of which can be treated successfully with dilation. In a German retrospective study of 139 patients with incurable esophageal cancer treated with EBRT alone, EBRT with BT, or with BT alone, EBRT ± BT provided the longest dysphagia-free survival, at greater than 90% at 6 months.[24] Overall symptom relief occurred in 72% of patients for up to 5 months. Complications of the EBRT with BT in a series of 148 patients included fistula (5% of cases), stricture (27%), and bleeding (4%),[25] and the combination of EBRT with BT is not considered safe by all radiation oncologists.[26]

CHEMORADIATION THERAPY

Palliation of malignant dysphagia with radiation therapy alone requires 4 to 6 weeks for improvement in swallowing.[27] The addition of chemotherapy to a 3-week course of external beam radiation (35 to 40 Gy) results in significant improvement in malignant dysphagia, as demonstrated in a large study by Harvey et al.[28] Treatment regimens included a combination of 5-fluorouracil, cisplatin, and paclitaxel. Of 102 patients available for dysphagia scoring after treatment, 78% had an improvement in at least one grade of the dysphagia scoring system. The minor complication rate was low and included radiation pneumonitis and infections. There was a 6% treatment-related mortality rate. The median time to improvement was 6 weeks after the start of chemoradiation therapy. Part of the delay to clinical improvement is undoubtedly related to the significant incidence of esophagitis secondary to the treatment. Thus, although a tumor may be shrinking, esophagitis may contribute to the delay to satisfactory oral intake. In a phase III trial of palliative epirubicin, oxaliplatin, and capecitabine (EOX) versus docetaxel, cisplatin, 5-fluorouracil, and leucovorin (DCF) for esophageal and gastric adenocarcinomas, DCF provided a longer median survival by 2.4 months and with fewer side effects than EOX, with primary complications being nausea, pain, and thromboembolic events up to 13.8%.[29]

Chemotherapy alone as palliation is suboptimal because of the delay in relief. Clinicians reported in an observational study in the United Kingdom that only 53% of patients completed their course of palliative chemotherapy and only 9% of those older than 75 years completed it.[30] Patients who cannot tolerate chemoradiation therapy should be offered a palliative stent. Chemoradiation therapy can take longer than a month to see a benefit but may be a good choice for cervical esophageal lesions. For distal esophageal cancers, SEMS can produce significant reflux when placed across the gastroesophageal junction, and ablative therapies may be better endoscopic options.

COMMENTS

This chapter reviews the palliative approaches to the patient with dysphagia who has inoperable disease. The recent addition to the armamentarium is cryoablation. There is no single palliative therapy that works well for all patients, and, indeed, not all patients with mild degrees of dysphagia need palliation. It is critical that we recognize that the ability to restore oral nutrition is a valuable aspect of allowing the patient to regain an important component of his or her quality of life, which is far superior and more cost effective than feeding tubes or parenteral nutrition. In a retrospective cohort study of 736 patients in The Netherlands, investigators found an amalgam of approaches to palliate patients with inoperable esophageal cancer, with best supportive care begin the most common approach.[31] Ideally, the clinician dealing with esophageal cancer patients should be well versed in all endoscopic interventions and the palliative aspects and limitations of chemotherapy and radiation therapy; however, tools are available to allow patients to be comfortable and at home in their final days.

REFERENCES

1. Siegel RL, Miller KD, Jemal A. Cancer statistics, 2017. *CA Cancer J Clin.* 2017;67:7-30.
2. Homs MY, Kuipers EJ, Siersema PD. Palliative therapy. *J Surg Oncol.* 2005;92(3):246-256.
3. Cusumano A, Ruol A, Segalin A, et al. Push-through intubation: effective palliation in 409 patients with cancer of the esophagus and cardia. *Ann Thorac Surg.* 1992;53(6):1010-1014.
4. Knyrim K, Wagner HJ, Bethge N, Keymling M, Vakil N. A controlled trial of an expansile metal stent for palliation of esophageal obstruction due to inoperable cancer. *N Engl J Med.* 1993;329(18):1302-1307.
5. Ell C, May A, Hahn EG. Gianturco-Z stents in the palliative treatment of malignant esophageal obstruction and esophagotracheal fistulas. *Endoscopy.* 1995;27(7):495-500.
6. Hindy P, Hong J, Lam-Tsai Y, Gress F. A comprehensive review of esophageal stents. *Gastroenterol Hepatol (N Y).* 2012;8(8):526-534.
7. Conio M, Repici A, Battaglia G, et al. A randomized prospective comparison of self-expandable plastic stents and partially covered self-expandable metal stents in the palliation of malignant esophageal dysphagia. *Am J Gastroenterol.* 2007;102(12):2667-2677.
8. Yakoub D, Fahmy R, Athanasiou T, et al. Evidence-based choice of esophageal stent for the palliative management of malignant dysphagia. *World J Surg.* 2008;32(9):1996-2009.
9. Christie NA, Buenaventura PO, Fernando HC, et al. Results of expandable metal stents for malignant esophageal obstruction in 100 patients: short-term and long-term follow-up. *Ann Thorac Surg.* 2001;71(6):1797-1801, discussion 1801-1802.
10. Shaikh M, Choudhury NR, Knott R, Garg S. Engineering stent based delivery system for esophageal cancer using docetaxel. *Mol Pharm.* 2015;12(7):2305-2317.
11. Tian D, Wen H, Fu M. Comparative study of self-expanding metal stent and intraluminal radioactive stent for inoperable esophageal squamous cell carcinoma. *World J Surg Oncol.* 2016;14(1):18.
12. Liu N, Liu S, Xiang C, et al. Radioactive self-expanding stents give superior palliation in patients with unresectable cancer of the esophagus but should be used with caution if they have had prior radiotherapy. *Ann Thorac Surg.* 2014;98(2):521-526.
13. Krokidis M, Burke C, Spiliopoulos S, et al. The use of biodegradable stents in malignant oesophageal strictures for the treatment of dysphagia before neoadjuvant treatment or radical radiotherapy: a feasibility study. *Cardiovasc Intervent Radiol.* 2013;36(4):1047-1054.
14. Loizou LA, Grigg D, Atkinson M, Robertson C, Bown SG. A prospective comparison of laser therapy and intubation in endoscopic palliation for malignant dysphagia. *Gastroenterology.* 1991;100(5 Pt 1):1303-1310.
15. Lightdale CJ, Heier SK, Marcon NE, et al. Photodynamic therapy with porfimer sodium versus thermal ablation therapy with Nd:YAG laser for palliation of esophageal cancer: a multicenter randomized trial. *Gastrointest Endosc.* 1995;42(6):507-512.
16. Heier SK, Rothman KA, Heier LM, Rosenthal WS. Photodynamic therapy for obstructing esophageal cancer: light dosimetry and randomized comparison with Nd:YAG laser therapy. *Gastroenterology.* 1995;109(1):63-72.
17. Homs MY, Wahab PJ, Kuipers EJ, et al. Esophageal stents with antireflux valve for tumors of the distal esophagus and gastric cardia: a randomized trial. *Gastrointest Endosc.* 2004;60(5):695-702.
18. Coron E, David G, Lecleire S, et al. Antireflux versus conventional self-expanding metallic stents (SEMS) for distal esophageal cancer: results of a multicenter randomized trial. *Endosc Int Open.* 2016;4(6):E730-E736.
19. Litle VR, Luketich JD, Christie NA, et al. Photodynamic therapy as palliation for esophageal cancer: experience in 215 patients. *Ann Thorac Surg.* 2003;76(5):1687-1692, discussion 1692-1693.
20. Brantingham CR, Beekman BE, Te Groen DM. Peripheral venous incompetence and the urban terrain. The relationship of venous incompetence and flat surfaces, and a system for artificially varying the terrain. *J Am Podiatry Assoc.* 1967;57(12):547-554.
21. Yi E, Yang CK, Leem C, et al. Clinical outcome of photodynamic therapy in esophageal squamous cell carcinoma. *J Photochem Photobiol B.* 2014;141:20-25.
22. Sreenarasimhaiah J. Endoscopic applications of cryospray ablation therapy—from Barrett's esophagus and beyond. *World J Gastrointest Endosc.* 2016;8(16):546-552.
23. Grazziotin Reisner R, Reisner ML, Ferreira MA, et al. Measuring relief of dysphagia in locally advanced esophageal carcinoma patients submitted to high-dose-rate brachytherapy. *Brachytherapy.* 2015;14(1):84-90.
24. Welsch J, Kup PG, Nieder C, et al. Survival and symptom relief after palliative radiotherapy for esophageal cancer. *J Cancer.* 2016;7(2):125-130.
25. Laskar SG, Lewis S, Agarwal JP, Mishra S, Mehta S, Patil P. Combined brachytherapy and external beam radiation: an effective approach for palliation in esophageal cancer. *J Contemp Brachytherapy.* 2015;7(6):453-461.
26. Tai P, Yu E. Esophageal cancer management controversies: radiation oncology point of view. *World J Gastrointest Oncol.* 2014;6(8):263-274.
27. Siersema PD, Dees J, van Blankenstein M. Palliation of malignant dysphagia from oesophageal cancer. Rotterdam Oesophageal Tumor Study Group. *Scand J Gastroenterol Suppl.* 1998;225:75-84.
28. Harvey JA, Bessell JR, Beller E, et al. Chemoradiation therapy is effective for the palliative treatment of malignant dysphagia. *Dis Esophagus.* 2004;17(3):260-265.
29. Ochenduszko S, Puskulluoglu M, Konopka K, et al. Comparison of efficacy and safety of first-line palliative chemotherapy with EOX and mDCF regimens in patients with locally advanced inoperable or metastatic HER2-negative gastric or gastroesophageal junction adenocarcinoma: a randomized phase 3 trial. *Med Oncol.* 2015;32(10):242.
30. Groene O, Crosby T, Hardwick RH, Riley S, Greenaway K, Cromwell D. A population-based observational study on the factors associated with the completion of palliative chemotherapy among patients with oesophagogastric cancer. *BMJ Open.* 2015;5(3):e006724.
31. Opstelten JL, de Wijkerslooth LR, Leenders M, et al. Variation in palliative care of esophageal cancer in clinical practice: factors associated with treatment decisions. *Dis Esophagus.* 2017;30(2):1-7.

Anastomotic Complications After Esophagectomy: Frequency, Prevention, and Management

Tamar B. Nobel | Jessica G.Y. Luc | Daniela Molena

Since Dobromysslow described the first esophageal resection with successful anastomotic reconstruction in 1901, the outcomes of esophagectomy have significantly improved and this surgery is now the mainstay of treatment for esophageal cancer.[1] Data from the Society of Thoracic Surgeons (STS) National Database reported a major complication rate of 33.1% and mortality rate of 3.1%.[2] However, anastomotic complications continue to pose a technical challenge for surgeons and negatively impact patient postoperative recovery. Familiarity with such complications and the associated principles of management may better guide perioperative patient care and thus mitigate the long-term sequelae of such events. In this chapter, we discuss the etiology, diagnosis, and treatment of anastomotic complications after esophagectomy.

It is important to understand the techniques used for esophageal resection in order to better address diversions from the anticipated postoperative course. Currently, the most commonly used surgical approaches to esophagectomy include the Ivor Lewis esophagectomy (ILE); transhiatal esophagectomy (THE); McKeown, or tri-incisional esophagectomy (TIE); and thoracoabdominal esophagectomy (TAE). The procedure type dictates the anastomotic site; TAE and ILE use an intrathoracic anastomosis, whereas TIE and THE use a cervical anastomotic location. When reconstructing the esophagus, the stomach is most commonly used as a conduit. Alternatives include pedicled colonic or small bowel, and rarely, small bowel free graft. Finally, there are multiple methods for performing the anastomosis. The double layer handsewn technique was first described in 1942 by Churchill and Sweet and has since been modified; it now includes several variations including continuous versus interrupted suture, single- or double- layer sutures, and different suture types. More recent developments have led to increased use of mechanical stapling devices, which include both circular and linear techniques.[3,4] These differences in methodologic approaches may impact the likelihood and presentation of anastomotic complications following esophagectomy.

Leakage at the anastomotic site is the Achilles heel of every esophagectomy. It is associated with a threefold increased risk of postoperative death and up to 60% mortality. Furthermore, such events lead to increased length of hospital stay, delayed initiation of oral feeding, and increased risk of reoperation. Anastomotic leak may also influence oncologic outcome; in a multicenter study of 2994 postoperative patients with esophageal cancer, Markar et al. demonstrated a significant reduction in both overall and disease-free survival in patients with severe anastomotic leak (35.8 vs. 54.8 months, and 34 vs. 47.9 months, respectively) and 35% increased risk of recurrence.[5,6] These grave consequences make prevention, when possible, and early identification of leaks of utmost importance to minimize the impact of such events.

CLASSIFICATION AND INCIDENCE

The incidence of anastomotic leak after esophagectomy ranges from 0% to 35%.[7] Analyses of STS database results reported a 12% incidence of leaks requiring medical or surgical intervention.[2] Variability in the definition of anastomotic leak has led to wide discrepancies in reported rates. Bruce et al. determined that fewer than 40% of articles pertaining to anastomotic leak after esophagectomy included the criteria used to establish the diagnosis, and another systematic review noted definitions included in only 28.3% of studies with 22 different descriptions used.[7,8]

Possible explanations for differences in reported outcomes in the literature include variable diagnostic tools used to identify a leak, time frame used for evaluation (e.g., 30 vs. 90 day), and anastomotic location.[5] There have been multiple groups that have sought to reach a consensus on a definition for anastomotic leak. The International Multispecialty Anastomotic Leak Global Improvement Exchange group (IMAGINE) defined gastrointestinal postoperative anastomotic leak as "a defect of the integrity in a surgical join between two hollow viscera with communication between the intraluminal and extraluminal compartments."[9] In 2015 the Esophagectomy Complications Consensus Group (ECCG), a group of 21 high-volume esophageal surgeons from 14 countries, met to create a standardized system for defining and recording complications after esophagectomy (Table 43.1).[10]

Another commonly referenced classification system was proposed by Lerut et al. (Table 43.2).[11] In this definition, clinically occult leaks diagnosed on routine postoperative imaging comprise the most minor end of the spectrum while conduit necrosis is the most severe presentation. The type of leak has significant clinical implications, with grade I/II being relatively low risk and grade III and IV having mortality rates near 60% and 90%, respectively.[4]

RISK FACTORS

Failed anastomotic healing is affected by multiple inter-related factors. An understanding of these predictive variables is important in the preoperative setting because modifiable factors may be better optimized, and fixed

TABLE 43.1 Definitions

ANASTOMOTIC LEAK

Defined as: Full thickness GI defect involving esophagus, anastomosis, staple line, or conduit irrespective of presentation or method of identification

Type I: Local defect requiring no change in therapy or treated medically or with dietary modification

Type II: Localized defect requiring interventional but not surgical therapy, for example, interventional radiology drain, stent or bedside opening, and packing of incision

Type III: Localized defect requiring surgical therapy

CONDUIT NECROSIS

Type I: Conduit necrosis focal
- Identified endoscopically
- Treatment—additional monitoring or non-surgical therapy

Type II: Conduit necrosis focal
- Identified endoscopically and not associated with free anastomotic or conduit leak
- Treatment—surgical therapy not involving esophageal diversion

Type III: Conduit necrosis extensive
- Treatment—treated with conduit resection with diversion

CHYLE LEAK

Type I: Treatment – enteric dietary modifications
Type II: Treatment – total parenteral nutrition
Type III: Treatment – interventional or surgical therapy*
Severity Level
    < 1 liter output/day
    > 1 liter output/day

For example, a chyle leak initially producing 1200 ml/day and successfully treated by stopping enteric feeds and initiating TPN, Final Type IIB

VOCAL CORD INJURY/PALSY

Defined as: Vocal cord dysfunction post-resection. Confirmation and assessment should be by direct examination.

Type I: Transient injury requiring no therapy
    Dietary modification allowed

Type II: Injury requiring elective surgical procedure, for example, thyroplasty or medialization procedure

Type III: Injury requiring acute surgical intervention (due to aspiration or respiratory issues), for example, thyroplasty or medialization procedure

Severity Level
    Unilateral
    Bilateral

For example, a unilateral vocal cord injury requiring elective medialization procedure. Final Type IIA

*Does not include elective insertion of additional surgical or interventional chest drains.
GI, Gastrointestinal; TPN, total perenteral nutrition.
From Low DE, Alderson D, Cecconello I, et al. International consensus of standardization of data collection for complications associated with esophagectomy: esophagectomy Complications Consensus Group (ECCG). *Ann Surg* 2015;262:286-294.

TABLE 43.2 Lerut Classification of Anastomotic Leak

Leak (Grade)	Definitions	Treatment
Radiologic (I)	No clinical signs	No change in management
Clinical Minor (II)	Local inflammation (cervical wound)	Drain wound
	X-ray contained leak (thoracic anastomosis)	Delay oral intake
	Fever, leukocytosis	Antibiotics
Clinical Major (III)	Severe disruption on endoscopy	Change management: CT-guided drainage (reintervention)
	Sepsis	
Conduit Necrosis (IV)	Endoscopic confirmation	Reintervention

Lerut T, Coosemans W, Decker G, et al. Anastomotic complications after esophagectomy. *Dig Surg.* 2002;19:92-98.

characteristics may be used for risk stratification and patient selection in attempts to minimize poor outcomes.[12]

Esophagectomy is most often used to treat esophageal cancer and also has a role in management of motility disorders; therefore it is not surprising that patients undergoing esophagectomy often present with malnutrition. Poor nutritional status, commonly defined as hypoalbuminemia or weight loss, has previously been demonstrated to be associated with increased risk of anastomotic leak.[12,13] Analysis of the STS database found that heart failure, hypertension, renal insufficiency, and procedure type were predictive of anastomotic leak.[14] Use of neoadjuvant therapy has been associated with increased risk of leak in some series, although this appears to be dependent on radiation dose given. A review of 1939 patients demonstrated no increase in complications in patients who underwent preoperative neoadjuvant therapy.[5,15,16] The presence of diabetes mellitus or advanced patient age surprisingly does not seem to affect leak.[13]

The esophagus has several unique characteristics that make anastomosis after esophageal resection more technically challenging. Unlike the other organs of the gastrointestinal system, the esophagus does not have a serosal layer. This, in combination with the longitudinal orientation of the muscle fibers of the esophagus, contributes to increased fragility and decreased suture security.[4,13,17] Attempts to create additional protection using a free peritoneal patch did not impact the rate of leak but did increase the rate of stricture.[18] Furthermore, the esophagus is primarily located within the thorax, which may create a unique challenge for esophageal anastomoses when compared with other types of gastrointestinal leaks. The negative intrathoracic pressure may draw gastric fluid across anastomotic lines and result in leakage. Such leaks into the pleural space may affect the dynamics of intrathoracic pressure and result in respiratory and hemodynamic instability.[19]

The ability of an anastomosis to heal successfully is directly associated with maintenance of adequate tissue perfusion to the conduit. In the course of gastric mobilization and resection of the lesser curvature, the major vessels are ligated; this leaves approximately 60% of the gastric tube to be supplied by the right gastroepiploic vessels and the remaining proximal portion is supplied by small collateral vessels. As such, the anastomosis, which is usually made at the fundus, is within the most ischemic part. Caution must be exercised to minimize trauma to the collateral vessels during dissection. Tension on the anastomosis can lead to impaired blood supply and result in ischemia. Some authors have suggested that the utilization of the whole stomach as opposed to a gastric tube may better preserve blood supply by not disturbing collateral circulation. Arguments against use of the whole stomach claim that use of a gastric tube yields less gastric distention and decreased surface area for acid secretion, both of which can be detrimental to the anastomosis and also lead to poor quality of life. A narrow gastric conduit with longer length can better reach the cervical anastomosis site without tension but must be balanced against excessive narrowing leading to impaired blood supply.[11,12,19] Controversy remains as to whether other types of conduit, most commonly colonic, have a similar incidence of leak; however, colonic interposition does require three anastomoses as opposed to one when using a gastric conduit.[4]

Cervical anastomosis has been associated with a higher incidence of leakage than thoracic, with rates ranging from 2% to 26%.[20] This may possibly be explained by the longer distance required for blood supply to travel to the anastomosis site in the neck.[14] In comparison, thoracic anastomoses are associated with leak rates of 0% to 9.3%.[11,14,20] There was previously suggestion in the literature that thoracic leaks are associated with higher postoperative mortality, but more recent data do not support this finding when considering early (30-day) outcomes.[14,20,21] The higher leak rate associated with cervical anastomosis is more accepted because it is generally contained and thus associated with lower risk. Thoracic anastomotic breakdown is often associated with mediastinal soilage and may have a more severe clinical course.[19]

The type of anastomotic technique selected most often depends upon the surgeon's preference. Stapled anastomotic technique has been used for approximately 25 years and began to increase in popularity due to easier reconstruction, especially in areas where exposure and access are limited. Heitmiller et al. described an 0.8% leak rate after two-layer handsewn anastomosis.[3,22] Blackmon et al. published a propensity-matched analysis comparing outcomes between side-to-side stapled anastomosis, end-to-end circular stapled anastomosis, and handsewn, with no significant difference in leak rate noted.[23] Multiple randomized control trials have compared various techniques in attempt to identify the safest approach but have failed to identify a significant difference in leak rate.[24-26] Reconstruction can be performed either via an anterior retrosternal route or a posterior mediastinal route when performing a cervical anastomosis. Urschel et al. performed a meta-analysis that failed to demonstrate a significant difference in leak rate; however the posterior route is alleged to have the advantages of shorter distance to the anastomosis, resulting in decreased tension, avoidance of foregut angulation, less cardiopulmonary morbidity, soft tissue coverage of potentially devascularized airways, and preservation of the skeletal structures of the thoracic inlet. Anterior reconstruction is primarily justified due to the minimization of tumor recurrence by avoiding the posterior tumor bed.[27]

Laparoscopic surgery has become the standard approach to many gastrointestinal operations because it has been demonstrated to be safe with better postoperative results. Similarly, there has been increased utilization of minimally invasive approaches to esophagectomy. A 2016 Cochrane Review evaluating open versus laparoscopic THE observed fewer overall complications and decreased length of stay.[28] Biere et al. performed a randomized control trial comparing open versus minimally invasive transthoracic esophagectomy and demonstrated significant postoperative benefits, including decreased incidence of pulmonary infections, decreased length of stay, decreased operative blood loos, and improved quality of life at 6 weeks postoperatively and postoperative pain scores. In addition, no differences were demonstrated in number of lymph nodes harvested and rate of R0 resection.[29]

PREVENTION OF LEAK

Preoperative patient optimization with correction of malnutrition, optimization of medical conditions, and decreasing steroid use have been demonstrated to help decrease risk of leak.[5] Procedures performed at low-volume centers have been associated with increased risk of postoperative and long-term mortality, as well as increased risk of any (and severe) leaks, which highlights the importance of careful surgical technique in minimizing the incidence of leak. Intraoperatively, there have been attempts to better characterize perfusion to the anastomosis because there is no standardized therapy. Multiple approaches exist, including assessment of graft color, temperature, and checking Doppler signals. Doppler is limited to assessment of macrocirculation. Fluorescence imaging is a promising approach to assessment of the microcirculation and macrocirculation of the gastric conduit. Weaker perfusion, as assessed by intraoperative laser-assisted fluorescent dye angiography, has been demonstrated to be correlated to leak and may be a promising approach.[30]

Following stomach mobilization, a 50% drop in gastric fundus oxygen tension has been measured, and further study has described a direct correlation between intraoperative gastric fundus oximetry and resultant anastomotic success. Ischemic preconditioning has been described as an attempt to preoperatively redistribute gastric blood supply. Embolization of the left and right gastric and splenic arteries was performed 2 to 3 weeks before esophagectomy, thus leaving the stomach dependent on the right gastroepiploic artery. Results in animal models have demonstrated decreased anastomotic leak using these techniques, but similar results have not been demonstrated in humans. An additional technical consideration includes division of the interclavicular ligament to alleviate conduit venous obstruction.[4,5]

Postoperatively, gastric distention may contribute to anastomotic tension and inhibit venous drainage. Minimization of distention with use of nasogastric tube and promotility agents may help to alleviate this. Pyloromyotomy or pyloroplasty at time of original procedure may also reduce incidence of this complication. In addition, use of pharmacologic agents has been previously studied. Administration of prostaglandin E_1 within an hour of gastric tube creation has been shown to increase blood flow to the tissue but has failed to show a clinical benefit to date.[4]

DIAGNOSIS OF LEAK

Diagnosis of anastomotic leaks is dependent upon the size and location of the leak. In cases of conduit necrosis, patients often present within 48 to 72 hours with catastrophic sepsis. Clinical suspicion is necessary to correctly diagnose more subtle leaks. The most obvious signs include bilious output in surgical drains. Cervical leaks usually present within 5 to 10 days with associated fever, drainage, and wound erythema. Intrathoracic leaks may be less apparent. Unexplained low-grade fever, tachycardia, or leukocytosis should prompt suspicion.[4,5,13] A proposed risk assessment score found that C-reactive protein, white blood cell count, and albumin levels could be used to predict major complications with sensitivity of 89% and specificity of 63%.[31]

Many practices perform routine contrast esophagram studies postoperatively. Usually water-soluble contrast is used initially followed by barium. Grade I leaks are usually clinically silent and detected on such routine imaging. Computed tomography (CT) scan with oral contrast is more sensitive than contrast swallow study, and it is our preferred approach when suspicious for leak. Endoscopy is a useful adjunctive tool to confirm leak and guide potential intervention. Despite concern regarding an invasive procedure in the setting of a fresh anastomosis, systematic endoscopy following esophagectomy has been demonstrated to be safe.[5,13]

MANAGEMENT

General principles for management of anastomotic leak include intensive care treatment, maintenance of perfusion to the conduit through minimization of hypotension, optimization of respiratory function, broad-spectrum antibiotics, and nutrition, preferably enteral downstream from the site of leakage. Furthermore, collections near the site of the anastomosis should be drained.[5,32] In the absence of diffuse conduit necrosis, further treatment is dependent upon the location of leak and severity of clinical presentation.

Cervical leaks that are small and well contained may be managed conservatively with nothing by mouth. Antibiotics may often not be necessary in the absence of sepsis. Repeat contrast study or endoscopy may be performed to document healing. Larger, contained cervical leaks with associated wound erythema or fluctuance require drainage. This may often be accomplished by opening up the surgical wound. In cases in which a small defect is observed, direct suture closure or stenting may be performed to accelerate healing. Median time to closure is approximately 2 to 3 weeks. If patients fail to respond promptly to management with the above approaches, inadequate drainage or conduit necrosis should be considered and further investigation should be undertaken. Surgical management in the setting of uncontrolled sepsis includes débridement and assessment of the viability of the conduit, with possible resection in setting of necrosis. Subsequently, there is a high risk of stricture formation following cervical anastomotic leaks.[4,5,11]

The management of intrathoracic leaks depends upon the degree of sepsis. Patients with contained collections may be treated with percutaneous drainage. Patients with hemodynamic stability in the setting of sepsis should be taken to the operating room for washout and drainage. Conservative operative treatment, with débridement and refashioning of the anastomosis, has been described with 25% risk of recurrent leak.[5,11,33]

Recently, there has been increased interest in stenting as a mechanism of closure of anastomotic defects with possible adjunctive percutaneous drainage of associated fluid collections. In cases in which less than 30% of circumference of the anastomosis has broken down, stent placement may be appropriate. Covered self-expanding stents are preferred to facilitate future removal. Stent migration is a common problem, which may be minimized with the use of longer stents or with adjuncts, including clipping or suturing. Other risks associated include inadequate coverage resulting in persistent leak, plugging, and erosion into surrounding structures. Freeman et al. reported outcomes of 17 patients treated with stents after intrathoracic anastomotic leak and demonstrated 94% success in healing with 18% stent migration. The majority (82%) of patients were able to resume a diet 72 hours after stenting, and stents were removed at a mean of 17 days.[5,12,34] Endoluminal vacuum therapy has emerged as a new alternative approach to anastomotic leak after esophagectomy; the sponge is placed endoscopically into an intraluminal or intracavitary position and the vacuum then closes the esophageal defect and drains any associated collection via an intranasal route.[35]

CONDUIT NECROSIS

Incidence of gastric conduit ischemia ranges from 0.5% to 10.4%, which includes cases ranging from self-resolving, subclinical ischemia to frank necrosis.[36] The sequelae of conduit ischemia may be quite serious. Patients with ischemia may ultimately develop a stricture or, more concerning, an anastomotic leak requiring reoperation. Conduit necrosis is the most severe grade of anastomotic leak, as described previously. Mortality after conduit necrosis may exceed 90%, highlighting the importance of rapid identification and treatment of this problem, and when possible, prevention.[37]

Multiple risk factors for conduit necrosis have been identified, including improper technique in the creation or manipulation of the gastric tube, radiation, low perioperative cardiac output, postoperative hypotension, previous upper abdominal surgery, malnutrition, peptic ulcer disease, twisting of the stomach conduit as it passes into the mediastinum, and a tight hiatal opening. Radiation creates a fibrotic reaction that decreases the microvascular blood supply of the conduit. By using caution while mobilizing the conduit and taking caution in maintaining adequate patient perfusion in the perioperative period, these factors may be minimized.[36,38]

Patients with conduit necrosis most commonly present with severe sepsis within the first week postoperatively. They may initially have an unexplained tachycardia or leukocytosis with rapid clinical decompensation. The most important principle for management of such patients is to have a

TABLE 43.3 Endoscopic Grading of Anastomotic Ischemia

Grade	Findings
1	Dusky bluish-colored mucosa near anastomosis covered with metallic appearing mucus
2	Partial anastomotic disruption with equivocal viability or normal pink mucosa margins
3	Complete circumferential anastomotic breakdown with normal pink mucosa margins
4	Completely necrotic black mucosa throughout the conduit with intact anastomosis

From Oezcelik A, Banki F, Ayazi S, et al. Detection of gastric conduit ischemia or anastomotic breakdown after cervical esophagogastrostomy: the use of computed tomography scan versus early endoscopy. *Surg Endosc.* 2010;24:1948–1951.

high clinical suspicion. In patients with a questionable diagnosis, there are multiple diagnostic options available. Traditionally, an upper gastrointestinal contrast study may be used to identify presence of an anastomotic leak and may possibly demonstrate cobblestoning of the mucosa. CT with oral contrast may yield additional information regarding associated effusions, although a normal exam does not exclude the possibility of ischemia and fluid and air within the mediastinum may be normal in the postoperative state. Endoscopy should be the next diagnostic modality used.[37,38] Although there was historical concern regarding anastomotic disruption with this study, Page et al. demonstrated that endoscopy within 1 week of operation was safe and effective in detecting anastomotic leakage.[39]

A proposed endoscopic grading system identifies various degrees of ischemia with the goal of guiding management (Table 43.3).[40] In the setting of a small leak, nonoperative management with possible stenting will allow the patient to recover. Patients with a completely necrotic conduit are most often septic and brought to the operating room for emergent exploration. A video-assisted thorascopic investigation or thoracotomy in the case of an intrathoracic anastomosis or reopening of the neck incision must be performed to visualize the conduit. If this confirms necrosis, then the conduit must be resected and the patient should be diverted with an end esophagostomy, venting gastrostomy, and feeding jejunostomy. Care should be taken to maintain the longest possible length of remaining esophagus to facilitate future reconstruction; however, patients should be resuscitated and sepsis should resolve prior to any such attempts. Options for reconstruction include colonic interposition or jejunal transfer.[37,38]

ANASTOMOTIC STRICTURE

Anastomotic strictures often arise in the setting of previous anastomotic leak. Reported incidence of stricture after esophagectomy is 10% to 40%; however, as strictures are often diagnosed in the setting of patient-reported dysphagia, it is possible that the true incidence is much higher. Strictures that present early postoperatively are most often benign. Later presentation should raise suspicion for tumor recurrence.[4,5]

Anastomotic technique has been correlated with incidence of stricture and is associated with the resultant size of the anastomosis and wound retraction. Two-layer handsewn anastomoses have demonstrated higher rates of stricture than one layer. When comparing stapled versus handsewn anastomoses, circular end-to-end stapled anastomoses demonstrate higher rate of associated stricture; however, the semimechanical end-to-side anastomosis as described by Orringer creates a larger cross-sectional area and appears to have a lower stricture rate (48% of handsewn vs. 35% semimechanical).[4,41]

Early postoperative endoscopy has a high predictive value for subsequent stricture development. Anastomotic leak, more than one endoscopically visible stitch, and mucosal ulceration involving more than 50% of the anastomosis have been identified as factors correlated with stricture development.[42] Benign strictures can be well-managed using Savary or pneumatic endoscopic dilation, with 93% of patients experiencing initial relief of dysphagia symptoms.[43] Strictures that arise in the setting of severe anastomotic failure, secondary to ischemia, are more likely to be resistant to serial dilation. In addition to endoscopic dilation, it is important to administer proton-pump inhibitor treatment to prevent recurrence.[11]

CONDUIT AIRWAY FISTULA

The esophagogastric anastomosis lies close to the lung parenchyma and membranous airway, which increases the risk of possible fistulization between the airway and the conduit. Such events, although rare with reported incidence of 0.04% to 0.3%, may be life-threatening and must be rapidly identified.[38]

Multiple patient characteristics and perioperative complications may precipitate this event. A strong correlation has been made between neoadjuvant therapy and risk of fistula formation, likely due to secondary tissue injury and ischemia. Most often, conduit airway fistulas occur in the setting of anastomotic leak secondary to leakage of enteric contents resulting in tissue necrosis and erosion. Intraoperative tracheobronchial injury is a rare event with reported incidence of 1.8% during THE and 0.8% during transthoracic esophagectomy. It may serve as another potential source of airway conduit fistulization postoperatively due to the opening in the airway.[44] Additional etiologies may include ischemia due to extensive dissection around the trachea, stent erosion after management of leak, after endoscopic dilation of anastomotic stricture, or cuff-induced tracheal necrosis in the setting of prolonged endotracheal intubation.[38,45]

Patients may initially present with mild symptoms, such as cough with oral intake, or more serious symptoms, such as recurrent pneumonia. In the most extreme cases, patients may present with mediastinitis. A high index of suspicion will enable more prompt identification, which is of utmost importance as aspiration of gastric secretions into the lungs can lead to a severe pneumonitis and respiratory compromise. Oral contrast radiologic studies are usually the first diagnostic tool but may not visualize very small fistulas. Endoscopic evaluation is the preferred diagnostic modality to localize the fistula although mucosal folding within the conduit may obscure small openings. As such, bronchoscopic evaluation at same time as endoscopic assessment is the best way to characterize the size and location of the fistula.[12,38,45]

The management of fistulas should be based upon the size and site of the fistula in addition to the severity of the symptoms. In patients with benign clinical presentation, attempts at conservative treatment (nothing by mouth, antibiotics) may be considered; however, failure to heal within 4 to 6 weeks should prompt further intervention. Endoscopic approaches have been described including attempts at closure using fibrin glue, hemostatic clips, and mesh plugs.[38,45] Stent placement may be considered as a temporizing measure in severe cases to control contamination. Ultimately, a surgical repair may be required. The preferred approach is to repair the anastomosis and close the airway defect with interposition of vascularized soft tissue interposed between the suture lines to prevent recurrent fistulization. In severe cases in which the conduit must be excised, the preferred approach is with resection and esophagostomy with delayed reconstruction after the patient is clinically stabilized from sepsis. When performing reconstruction, colonic interposition in the substernal space can be used to avoid reoperation in the area of inflammation. In addition, jejunal interposition can be used.[12,38,45,46]

SUMMARY

Anastomotic complications after esophagectomy can be rapidly life-threatening. Awareness of the types of complications that can occur and their clinical presentations is critical for early recognition and diagnosis.

REFERENCES

1. Dobromysslow VD. Ein fall von transpleuraler osophagektomie ein brustabschitte. *Zentralbl Chir.* 1901;28:1.
2. The Society of Thoracic Surgeons General Thoracic Surgery Database Task Force. The Society of Thoracic Surgeons composite score for evaluating esophagectomy for esophageal cancer. *Ann Thorac Surg.* 2017;103:1661-1667.
3. Churchill ED, Sweet RH. Transthoracic resection of tumors of the stomach and esophagus. *Ann Surg.* 1942;115:897-920.
4. Cassivi SD. Leaks, strictures and necrosis: a review of anastomotic complications following esophagectomy. *Semin Thorac Cardiovasc Surg.* 2004;16:124-132.
5. Messager M, Warlaumont M, Renaud F, et al. Recent improvements in management of esophageal anastomotic leak after surgery for cancer. *Eur J Surg Oncol.* 2017;43:258-269.
6. Markar S, Gronnier C, Duhamel A, et al. The impact of severe anastomotic leak on long-term survival and cancer recurrence after surgical resection for esophageal malignancy. *Ann Surg.* 2015;262:972-980.
7. Blencowe NS, Strong S, McNair AGK, et al. Reporting of short-term clinical outcomes after esophagectomy: a systematic review. *Ann Surg.* 2012;255:658-666.
8. Bruce J, Krukowski ZH, Al-Khairy G, et al. Systematic review of the definition and measurement of anastomotic leak after gastrointestinal surgery. *Br J Surg.* 2001;88:1157-1168.
9. Chadi SA, Fingergut A, Berho M, et al. Emerging trends in the etiology, prevention and treatment of gastrointestinal anastomotic leakage. *J Gastrointest Surg.* 2016;20:2035-2051.
10. Low DE, Alderson D, Cecconello I, et al. International consensus of standardization of data collection for complications associated with esophagectomy: Esophagectomy Complications Consensus Group (ECCG). *Ann Surg.* 2015;262:286-294.
11. Lerut T, Coosemans W, Decker G, et al. Anastomotic complications after esophagectomy. *Dig Surg.* 2002;19:92-98.
12. Jones CE, Watson TJ. Anastomotic leakage following esophagectomy. *Thorac Surg Clin.* 2015;25:449-459.
13. Mitchell JD. Anastomotic leak after esophagectomy. *Thorac Surg Clin.* 2006;16:1-9.
14. Kassis ES, Kosinski AS, Ross P Jr, et al. Predictors of anastomotic leak after esophagectomy: an analysis of the Society of Thoracic Surgeons General Thoracic Database. *Ann Thorac Surg.* 2013;96:1919-1926.
15. Escofet X, Manjunath A, Twine C, et al. Prevalence and outcome of esophagogastric anastomotic leak after esophagectomy in a UK regional cancer network. *Dis Esophagus.* 2010;23:112-116.
16. Mungo B, Molena D, Stem M, et al. Does neoadjuvant therapy for esophageal cancer increase postoperative morbidity or mortality? *Dis Esophagus.* 2015;28:644-651.
17. Akiyama H. Esophageal anastomosis. *Arch Surg.* 1973;107:512-514.
18. Van Oosterom FJ, Van Lanschot JJ, Oosting J, et al. A free peritoneal patch does not affect the leakage rate but increases stricture formation of a cervical esophago-gastrostomy. *Dig Surg.* 1999;16:379-384.
19. Chen KN. Managing complications I: leaks, strictures, emptying, reflux, chylothorax. *J Thorac Dis.* 2014;6:S355-S363.
20. Biere SS, Maas KW, Cuesta MA, et al. Cervical or thoracic anastomosis after esophagectomy for cancer: a systematic review and meta-analysis. *Dig Surg.* 2011;28:29-35.
21. Chang AC, Ji H, Birkmeyer NJ, et al. Outcomes after transhiatal and transthoracic esophagectomy for cancer. *Ann Thorac Surg.* 2008;85:424-429.
22. Heitmiller RF, Fischer A, Liddicoat JR. Cervical esophagogastric anastomosis: results following esophagectomy for carcinoma. *Dis Esophagus.* 1999;12:264-269.
23. Blackmon SH, Correa AM, Wynn B, et al. Propensity-matched analysis of three techniques for intrathoracic esophagogastric anastomosis. *Ann Thorac Surg.* 2007;83:1805-1813.
24. Beitler AL, Urschel JD. Comparison of stapled and hand-sewn esophagogastric anastomoses. *Am J Surg.* 1998;175:337-340.
25. Law S, Fok M, Chu KM, et al. Comparison of hand-sewn and stapled esophagogastric anastomosis after esophageal resection for cancer: a prospective randomized controlled trial. *Ann Surg.* 1997;226:169-173.
26. Soluja SS, Ray S, Pal S, et al. Randomized trial comparing side-to-side stapled and hand-sewn esophagogastric anastomosis in neck. *J Gastrointest Surg.* 2012;16:1287-1295.
27. Urschel JD, Urschel DM, Miller JD, et al. A meta-analysis of randomized controlled trials of route of construction after esophagectomy for cancer. *Am J Surg.* 2001;182:470-475.
28. Gurusamy KS, Pallari E, Midya S, et al. Laparoscopic versus open transhiatal oesophagectomy for oesophageal cancer. *Cochrane Database Syst Rev.* 2016;(3):CD011390, doi:10.1002/14651858.CD011390.pub2.
29. Biere SS, van Berge Henegouwen MI, Maas KW, et al. Minimally invasive versus open oesophagectomy for patients with oesophageal cancer: a multicentre, open-label, randomised controlled trial. *Lancet.* 2012;379:1887-1892.
30. Zehetner K, DeMeester SR, Alicuben ET, et al. Intraoperative assessment of perfusion of the gastric graft and correlation with anastomotic leaks after esophagectomy. *Ann Surg.* 2015;262:74-78.
31. Noble F, Curtis N, Harris S, et al. Risk assessment using a novel score to predict anastomotic leak and major complications after oesophageal resection. *J Gastrointest Surg.* 2012;16:1083-1095.
32. Martin LW, Hofstetter W, Swisher SG, et al. Management of intrathoracic leaks following esophagectomy. *Adv Surg.* 2006;40:173-190.
33. Whooley BP, Law S, Alexandrou A, et al. Critical appraisal of the significance of intrathoracic anastomotic leakage after esophagectomy for cancer. *Am J Surg.* 2001;181:198-203.
34. Freeman RK, Vyverberg A, Ascioti AJ. Esophageal stent placement for the treatment of acute intrathoracic anastomotic leak after esophagectomy. *Ann Thorac Surg.* 2011;92:204-208.
35. Kuehn F, Loske G, Schiffmann L, et al. Endoscopic vacuum therapy for various defects of the upper gastrointestinal tract. *Surg Endosc.* 2017;doi:10.1007/s00464-016-5404-x; [Epub ahead of print].
36. Wormuth JK, Heitmiller RF. Esophageal conduit necrosis. *Thorac Surg Clin.* 2006;16:11-22.
37. Dickinson KJ, Blackmon SH. Management of conduit necrosis following esophagectomy. *Thorac Surg Clin.* 2015;25:461-470.
38. Meyerson SL, Mehta CK. Managing complications II: conduit failure and conduit airway fistulas. *J Thorac Dis.* 2014;6:S364-S371.
39. Page RD, Asmat A, McShane J, et al. Routine endoscopy to detect anastomotic leakage after esophagectomy. *Ann Thorac Surg.* 2013;95:292-298.
40. Oezcelik A, Banki F, Ayazi S, et al. Detection of gastric conduit ischemia or anastomotic breakdown after cervical esophagogastrostomy: the

use of computed tomography scan versus early endoscopy. *Surg Endosc.* 2010;24:1948-1951.

41. Orringer MB, Marshall B, Stirling MC. Transhiatal esophagectomy for benign and malignant disease. *J Thorac Cardiovasc Surg.* 1993;105:265-276.

42. Tretino P, Pompeo E, Nofroni I, et al. Predictive value of early postoperative esophagoscopy for occurrence of benign stenosis after cervical esophagogastrostomy. *Endoscopy.* 1997;29:840-844.

43. Briel JW, Tamhankar AP, Hagen JA, et al. Prevalence and risk factors for ischemia, leak and stricture of esophageal anastomosis: gastric pull-up versus colon interposition. *J Am Coll Surg.* 2004;198:536-541.

44. Hulscher JB, ter Hofstede E, Kloek J, et al. Injury to the major airways during subtotal esophagectomy: incidence, management and sequelae. *J Thorac Cardiovasc Surg.* 2000;120:1093-1096.

45. Buskens CJ, Hulscher JBF, Fockens P, et al. Benign trachea-neo-esophageal fistulas after subtotal esophagectomy. *Ann Thorac Surg.* 2001;72:221-224.

46. Boyd M, Rubio E. The utility of stenting in the treatment of airway gastric fistula after esophagectomy for esophageal cancer. *J Bronchology Interv Pulmonol.* 2012;19:232-236.

PART EIGHT

Miscellaneous Esophageal Conditions

Nonreflux Esophagitis

Deacon J. Lile | Ryan Moore | Abbas E. Abbas

The esophagus has been dubbed the organ of symptoms not signs. Inflammation of this dynamic conduit will elicit manifestations that can severely impact a patient's life. These symptoms are universal regardless of the cause of inflammation. They may include dysphagia, odynophagia, heartburn (pyrosis?), chest pain, nausea, vomiting, hematemesis, anorexia, and weight loss. So-called atypical respiratory symptoms may also occur, such as cough, bronchospasm, and aspiration. Due to the high prevalence of reflux disease, the vast majority of these patients who have very similar symptoms will be labeled as having gastroesophageal reflux disease (GERD) and will receive antireflux medication that will fail to resolve their symptoms.

Depending on the etiology, patients may experience septic symptoms in infectious cases or manifest stigmata of a systemic inflammatory disease, such as in autoimmune disorders.

As in any other inflammatory disorder, chronicity may cause a fibrotic reaction leading to benign strictures. Deep ulceration may occasionally cause severe bleeding or, more rarely, even perforation and mediastinitis. In addition, malignancy has been associated with long-standing esophagitis, especially with reflux when associated with intestinal metaplasia.

While you cannot directly examine the esophagus, a careful physical exam may elicit signs of a systemic disease or show manifestations of wider spread orogastrointestinal inflammation, such as oral thrush or rectal Crohn disease.

DIAGNOSIS

When presented with a patient who shows symptoms and signs of a possible esophagitis, the goal of the physician is to confirm the diagnosis, determine the cause (Table 44.1), prescribe a management plan, and follow up on this plan to ensure full remission. It is also important to treat complications of this disease as they arise.

As can be expected, careful endoscopic examination of the pharynx, esophagus, and stomach is an essential first step in diagnosing esophagitis and attempting to determine its etiology. An endoscopist must be prepared to take appropriate biopsies at the time of the procedure.

Radiologic studies may also help to shed light on the cause and to rule out complications, such as stricture formation or abnormal anatomy. The specific esophageal study is double-contrast barium swallow. This study should be avoided in patients with severe dysphagia who are at risk for aspiration. Otherwise it provides a "roadmap" prior to endoscopy. Other tests including chest computed tomography (CT), manometry, pH/impedance, and nuclear scintigraphy are obtained only on an individual basis to confirm a specific suspicion.

Laboratory tests can be helpful to rule out immunosuppression or systemic autoimmune disease.

MANAGEMENT

Of course, management of these patients will depend on the cause of the esophagitis. It may be necessary to initially treat the complications of this disease, such as severe bleeding, malnutrition, or esophageal perforation.

Esophagitis frequently causes clinical symptoms, including dysphagia, odynophagia, and regurgitation, which compel patients to seek evaluation and treatment. The most common cause of these symptoms is esophageal inflammation related to reflux; however, causes of nonreflux esophagitis are an increasingly important diagnostic consideration. Nonreflux esophagitis remains relatively rare in clinical practice, but its incidence has seen a dramatic increase over the last two decades. In particular, there has been a rapid expansion in the incidence and prevalence of eosinophilic esophagitis (EoE). Other causes include infectious esophagitis (fungal, viral, and tuberculous), medication-induced esophagitis, radiation esophagitis, and acute esophageal necrosis (AEN). When suspected, it is important to diagnose and treat esophagitis in a definitive fashion to avoid the uncommon but devastating outcomes of complicated esophagitis, including bleeding, malnutrition, stricture, perforation, and even cancer. This chapter outlines these causes and examines the clinical presentation, epidemiology, diagnostic work-up, and management of each distinct cause.

TABLE 44.1 Causes of Nonreflux Esophagitis

Eosinophilic esophagitis
Infectious esophagitis

- *Candida*
- Cytomegalovirus
- Herpes
- Tuberculosis

Radiation-induced esophagitis
Pill esophagitis
Acute esophageal necrosis

EOSINOPHILIC ESOPHAGITIS

EoE is a chronic inflammatory condition, characterized by symptomatic esophageal dysfunction with intraepithelial eosinophilic infiltration on pathologic examination.[1] The presence of esophageal eosinophilia was initially described in the presence of GERD.[2] Individual case reports of symptomatic eosinophilia in the absence of GERD began to emerge in the 1970s[3] and 1980s,[4,5] but it was not until 1993 that Attwood et al. described the current entity.[6] Over the last two decades, there has been tremendous growth in the observed incidence of this disease and a parallel growth in our understanding.[3]

CLINICAL PRESENTATION

EoE can present at any age, but the clinical presentation differs between adults and children.[2] In adults, the most common symptom of EoE is dysphagia, particularly to solid foods. In one series, dysphagia was the presenting complaint in 83% of patients.[7] The dysphagia is usually intermittent and rarely accompanied by odynophagia. In severe circumstances, persistent dysphagia and odynophagia can lead to malnutrition.[8] Other symptoms include heartburn (30% to 60% of patients) and noncardiac chest pain.[2] Of particular clinical importance is the frequency with which EoE causes food impaction requiring acute intervention (Fig. 44.1). In one series, food impaction was the presenting complaint in 42% of patients with EoE,[9] and more than half of adult patients with impaction may have esophageal eosinophilia.[10] When interviewing patients complaining of dysphagia, it is important to elicit a history of impaction events leading to retching or regurgitation, and EoE must be considered in all patients presenting with impaction.[2]

In children, the most common presenting complaints are heartburn and abdominal pain, with vomiting or decreased appetite.[11] One large series demonstrated that 38% of children with EoE report heartburn as their primary complaint upon presentation and 31% report abdominal pain or dyspepsia.[12] Other symptoms include growth failure and, rarely, hematemesis.[13] Infants and toddlers present with difficulty feeding, described by caregivers as "gagging" or "choking." In contrast to adults, dysphagia is uncommon in children until adolescence.[12]

EPIDEMIOLOGY

In children and adults, EoE is a chronic disease that does not resolve spontaneously and often recurs after

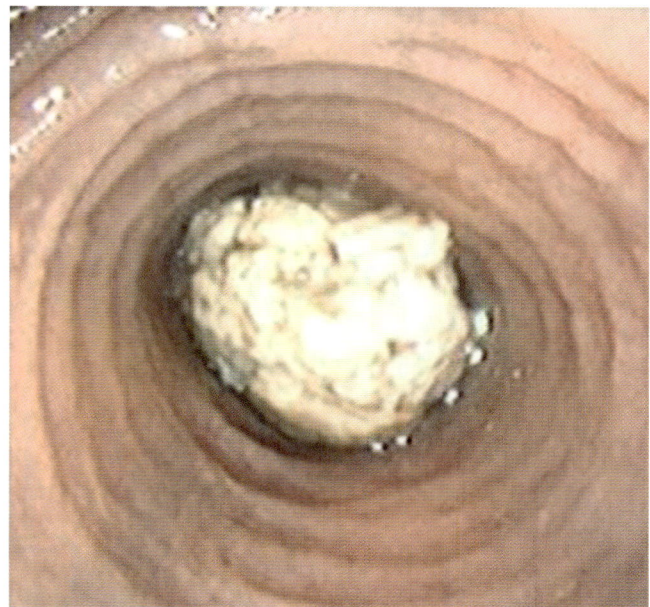

FIGURE 44.1 Food impaction in eosinophilic esophagitis with characteristic concentric rings. (From Gonsalves N, Policarpio-Nicolas M, Zhang Q, Rao MS, Hirano I. Histopathologic variability and endoscopic correlates in adults with eosinophilic esophagitis. *Gastrointest Endosc.* 2006;64:313–319.)

treatment cessation.[14] With years of persistent inflammation, the disease seems to progress toward a fibrostenotic phenotype; according to one large case series, the risk of fibrostenotic complications doubles with each decade.[15] The disease is more common in Caucasians and has a male predominance, which is consistently reported at 3 to 4:1 across all ages.[16,17] There is also a strong association with atopic diseases, including a correlation with environmental and food allergies.[18]

There is an increasingly large body of evidence showing that EoE is rapidly increasing in incidence and in prevalence, and that this increase cannot be explained simply by increased awareness. Current estimates indicate that the prevalence is likely between 40 and 90 cases per 100,000 persons in the United States.[16] This prevalence is consistent with other Western countries, namely Australia, Switzerland, Spain, and Canada.[14] In patients undergoing endoscopy for dysphagia, the prevalence of EoE is between 12% and 22%.[11,19]

In terms of incidence, multiple studies suggest that the incidence of EoE has been rapidly increasing since its discovery 20 years ago. In a case series from Hamilton County, Ohio, the incidence increased from 9 per 100,000 to 12.8 per 100,000 people over a 3-year period.[20] This finding is consistent with another report from Olmsted County, Minnesota, showing a dramatic increase in incidence over the 15-year period from 1990 until 2005.[21] A population-based, prospective study from the Swiss EoE study group provides more evidence for a marked increase in incidence. Like the Minnesota group, the Swiss study compares the observed incidence with the rate of upper endoscopy.[22] In both studies, the rise in EoE incidence in excess of increases in the upper endoscopy

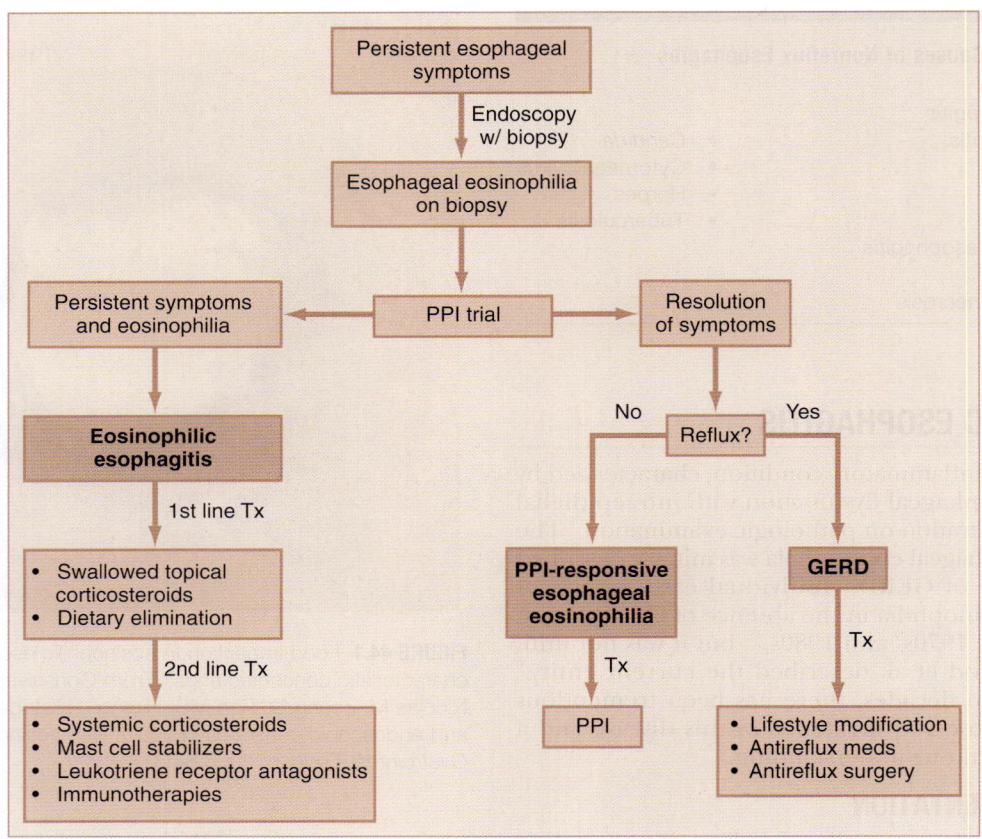

FIGURE 44.2 Diagnostic and therapeutic algorithm for eosinophilic esophagitis. *GERD*, Gastroesophageal reflux disease; *PPI*, proton pump inhibitor; *Tx*, therapy.

rate suggests that there is a real increase in disease rather than just an increase in awareness and detection.

The marked increase in incidence of EoE parallels increases in other allergic disease, including asthma, allergic rhinitis, atopic dermatitis, and various food allergies.[14] One potential explanation is the "hygiene hypothesis," which is a frequently cited and much-discussed theory initially based on epidemiologic studies. It points to the decreased infection burden in industrialized nations with an associated increase in atopic diseases and proposes a causative link. There are animal models that support the "hygiene hypothesis" for certain specific autoimmune diseases, but therapeutic approaches to allergic disease based on the reintroduction of specific infections have shown mixed results.[23] The "hygiene hypothesis" holds a plausible explanation for the rising incidence of EoE, but requires further study. Overall, the rapid rise of EoE is an area of much debate and research. Current thinking is that the increase is likely multifactorial, and hypotheses include a variety of immunologic-, environmental-, and microbiome-related topics.[14]

DIAGNOSTIC WORK-UP

According to the recently published guideline from the American College of Gastroenterology (ACG), EoE is defined as, "a clinicopathologic disorder diagnosed by clinicians taking into consideration both clinical and pathologic information without either of these parameters

interpreted in isolation."[24] Thus, the diagnostic criteria include a combination of clinical and pathologic findings; no single finding is pathognomonic (Fig. 44.2).

First, the patient must have symptoms of esophageal dysfunction. Second, pathologic examination of esophageal biopsy specimens must demonstrate eosinophil-predominant inflammation with a characteristic peak value of at least 15 eosinophils per high-power field (HPF); previous guidelines have used various thresholds for diagnosis, ranging from 15 to 30 eosinophils/HPF.[1] Third, secondary causes of esophageal eosinophilia should be excluded. Fourth, the mucosal eosinophilia is confined to the esophagus and persists after a proton pump inhibitor (PPI) trial. Patients who meet other criteria for EoE but have histologic and symptomatic resolution with PPI therapy may fall into the diagnostic criteria for a separate entity called PPI-responsive esophageal eosinophilia (REE), which is considered distinct from both EoE and GERD. Finally, a response to EoE-specific treatment, such as dietary elimination or topical corticosteroids, supports the diagnosis of EoE.[23]

To fulfill the ACG histologic criteria for diagnosis, an endoscopic evaluation with biopsy is required. Current recommendations call for two to four biopsy specimens from both the proximal and distal portions of the esophagus.[23] The physician performing the initial endoscopic evaluation should also obtain biopsies of the antrum and/or duodenum in patients with small intestine symptoms or endoscopic abnormalities to rule out other causes of esophageal eosinophilia, such as Crohn disease or rare infectious causes.[25] To evaluate for GERD in patients with esophageal eosinophilia, pH monitoring has historically been a useful diagnostic test.[24] However, a more recent cohort study of patients with esophageal eosinophilia showed a high incidence (71%) of pathologic reflux, and many patients without reflux had improvement in symptoms and pathologic response to PPI therapy. This group found that pH testing was not a useful predictor of patient response to PPI therapy.[26] Therefore, pH testing may be useful in select patients, but it is not required in the work-up of EoE.[24]

The ACG diagnostic criteria are devoid of radiographic or endoscopic findings; however, there are several characteristics of EoE that may be apparent and are increasingly important clinically. Endoscopic findings of EoE include the development of multiple concentric rings (see Fig. 44.1), "trachealization" or "feline esophagus," narrowing, linear furrows, white exudates, and edema.[1] These endoscopic findings may be present in 90% to 95% of cases.[2] Furthermore, the endoscopic appearance of EoE is under examination as a clinically relevant therapeutic outcome measure, and an endoscopic grading system to classify disease severity has been introduced.[23,24]

PATHOPHYSIOLOGY

The progression of chronic inflammation to fibrostenotic complications helps demonstrate the effect of prolonged eosinophilic infiltration on esophageal function.[15] Manometry studies in patients with biopsy-confirmed EoE show a potential association with nonspecific dysmotility, particularly of the lower esophagus, and lower esophageal sphincter dysfunction.[27,28] In severe cases, fibrostenotic pathology including ring and stricture formation, or narrowing, are a source of morbidity. These fibrostenotic complications are associated with increased symptom duration and underscores the importance of managing the characteristic inflammation of EoE.[13]

At a biochemical level, the pathogenesis of EoE is driven by myriad genetic, environmental, and immunologic factors.[2] Early descriptions of the disease observed an association with atopic conditions that has been supported by more recent work, earning the disease its early name, *esophageal asthma*.[1] Put succinctly, EoE appears to be a host response to environmental allergens. A T helper (Th)2-cell-mediated immune response involving interleukin (IL)-13,[29] and to a lesser extent IL-4 and IL-5,[30] stimulates the allergic response and recruits eosinophils into the esophagus.[13]

Analysis of RNA specimens of patients with biopsy-confirmed EoE demonstrates that IL-13-induced pathways are major drivers of inflammation. Under the influence of an IL-13-induced keratinocyte transcriptome that includes eotaxin-3 (a potent recruiter of eosinophils), the esophageal tissue experiences an influx of eosinophils, mast cells, and lymphocytes. Subsequent epithelial cell hyperplasia, elongation of papillae, and lamina propria remodeling correlate with the fibrostenotic changes observed grossly.[28] Histopathologic analysis of biopsy specimens taken from patients with EoE, and esophageal tissue from a mouse model of EoE, suggests that IL-5-mediated eosinophilia promotes esophageal tissue remodeling and is essential for the fibrostenotic changes observed in chronic EoE.[29] This work in the disease's biochemical pathogenesis suggests a role for targeted anti-IL-13 or anti-IL-5, which are currently under development.[28]

Outside of the observed association with other atopic conditions, there do not appear to be direct systemic consequences of the esophageal inflammation of EoE. There is some evidence of associated changes in serum laboratory values. To date, several studies in adults and children have demonstrated that approximately 40% to 50% of patients with EoE have an increased number of circulating eosinophils.[24] This systemic eosinophilia has led to research into potential biomarkers to gauge the response to treatment. Currently, there is insufficient evidence to support the routine monitoring of peripheral eosinophil count, total immunoglobulin E levels, or any other surrogate biomarker.[24]

ALLERGIC TRIGGERS

The environmental triggers that initiate the immunologic cascades outlined previously have also received a good deal of attention since the first descriptions of EoE in the 1990s. The success of dietary therapies targeting the identification and removal of dietary antigens suggests an essential role for food-borne allergens in the pathogenesis of EoE.[13] In contrast, there is much debate about the role of aeroallergens.

An early case report of a 21-year-old female with EoE showed symptomatic and histologic exacerbations during pollen season with remission during the winter months; in subsequent years, several other small case series suggested a potential role of aeroallergens.[31] More recently, work from a national US pathology database demonstrated clear geographic variability in the prevalence of EoE with a strong correlation between colder climates and increased disease prevalence in the United States.[32] Because climate is a major determinant of local flora, the authors of this study hypothesize that airborne antigens could trigger EoE in these climates. However, a recent meta-analysis found no seasonal variation in EoE incidence, which speaks against the importance of aeroallergens as triggers.[33] To date, there is no consensus on the causative role of aeroallergens in EoE and, outside the clear role of food-borne allergens, there remains much debate about the types of antigens that initiate the immunologic cascade of EoE.

MANAGEMENT

Medical management of EoE is challenging due to the disease's chronic nature and its propensity to relapse upon cessation of therapy. Therapeutic options are somewhat limited and can be broadly grouped into medical therapy and dietary elimination. There are a number of targeted immunotherapies currently under investigation, but at present the classes of medication available are corticosteroids, leukotriene inhibitors, mast cell stabilizers, and PPIs. Endoscopic dilation is an option for patients with strictures. (See Fig. 44.2.)

The challenge of effectively managing EoE is compounded by the lack of a consensus regarding therapeutic endpoints. The most recent ACG guidelines stipulate, "while complete resolution of symptoms and pathology is an ideal endpoint, acceptance of a range of reductions in symptoms and histology is a more realistic and practical goal of clinical practice."[24] The recommendation is graded as conditional, and the strength of evidence is graded as low. The guideline reflects a paucity of data regarding the degree of reduction in eosinophil density required to protect against esophageal injury, and treatment endpoints in the literature have shown considerable variation. Furthermore, symptom-based endpoints have proven difficult to quantify.[24] In spite of these difficulties, some medicines have proven to be effective in obtaining symptomatic relief and histologic improvement.

As part of the diagnostic work-up for EoE, other causes for esophageal eosinophilia must be excluded and a PPI trial must be initiated. Two clinical scenarios exist where patients with symptomatic esophageal eosinophilia will respond to PPI therapy: patients with reflux causing esophagitis with eosinophilia, and patients without reflux, who for somewhat unclear reasons have an eosinophilia that responds to PPI therapy.[24] The latter group falls under the diagnosis of PPI-REE. To exclude underlying reflux or PPI-REE and thus confirm the diagnosis of EoE, all patients who meet the diagnostic criteria should be given a 2-month course of PPI therapy.[2] The mechanism of PPI efficacy in PPI-REE remains unclear, but some in vitro evidence suggests that PPIs may have intrinsic eosinophil-reducing effects. This is due to direct inhibition of cytokine-stimulated increase in eotaxin-3 mRNA[34] and effect is independent of acid reduction effects.

The frequency with which esophageal eosinophilia responds to PPI therapy has led some authors to speculate on the role of acid-reducing procedures as a treatment of EoE, particularly in children. Early case reports of patients who underwent fundoplication for refractory reflux symptoms and were later found to have EoE showed no benefit. Theoretic concern over increasing the incidence of food impaction makes fundoplication potentially more risky, but there may be a role for "surgical" management of EoE. Some others posit that more research into the role of fundoplication is warranted.[35]

Once a PPI trial has confirmed the diagnosis of EoE, first-line therapy is swallowed topical steroids, either budesonide or fluticasone, for an initial 8-week trial.[24] Several randomized controlled trials in children showed significant symptomatic relief and histologic improvement with topical steroids, with the most robust responses to viscous formulations.[36,37]

In adults, multiple trials have demonstrated histologic remission with topical corticosteroid therapy.[2] A trial of swallowed aerosolized fluticasone against placebo in 42 patients showed a complete histologic response in 62% of patients compared with 0% in the placebo group.[38] Another randomized, double-blind, placebo-controlled trial examined the efficacy of a budesonide suspension in 36 patients over 14 years of age. This group found a significant reduction in eosinophils from 68.2 to 5.5/HPF in the treatment arm, compared with an insignificant reduction in the placebo group. Furthermore, patients had significantly improved dysphagia scores and many patients had resolution of endoscopic findings.[39]

In general, topical corticosteroids are well tolerated. There is no evidence of adrenal axis suppression after an 8- or 12-week course. The most common adverse effect is oral candidiasis, which may occur in up to 20% of patients.[2] Consensus guidelines state that the type and duration of steroid therapy depends upon the specific clinical circumstance. More research is required to guide optimum dosing, duration, and potential consequences of prolonged use.[25]

Systemic steroids are only recommended for cases refractory to topical steroids or where a rapid improvement in symptoms is needed.[24] There is one clinical trial that demonstrates the efficacy of oral steroids in children. In comparison to topical fluticasone, oral prednisone led to a more robust histologic resolution, but it was at the expense of an increased number of adverse events.[37] In general, the side-effect profile of systemic steroid therapy makes it a less desirable option.

There is little current evidence to support the use of other medical therapies for EoE. Some data suggest significant symptomatic improvement with the leukotriene receptor antagonist montelukast,[8] but there is no evidence that it induces a histologic response.[25] There is a theoretic role for the mast cell stabilizer cromolyn, but no evidence of therapeutic benefit in clinical practice.[24] Current research is ongoing to evaluate the highly selective anti-IL-5 antibodies (mepolizumab and reslizumab), and there also may be a role for a monoclonal antibody against IL-13, but there is not yet enough evidence to support the use of any biologic agent.[2]

DIETARY THERAPY

Dietary therapy consists of strategies to remove the food-borne allergens that trigger EoE.[3] There are three strategies currently accepted as effective treatment for EoE in both children and adults.[24] The first is conversion to elemental or amino-acid-based formula. This method completely eliminates all food allergens, but there are practical limitations in terms of cost and alterations in quality of life. The second is targeted elimination of foods guided by allergy testing. The third is empiric removal of the six most common triggers of EoE: soy, egg, milk, wheat, nuts, and seafood. Multiple retrospective studies and several meta-analyses have demonstrated the superiority of the elemental diet, although it is also the most labor intensive and disruptive.[2] Targeted elimination using results from specific allergy testing have proven to be generally ineffective, without evidence of widespread clinical or histologic remission.[13]

In the pediatric population, there is strong evidence for the effectiveness of dietary approaches. Some trials demonstrate efficacy in adults; however, in general, dietary therapy is less well studied in the adult population.[13] The treatment generally lasts for 4 to 6 weeks, with stepwise reintroduction of foods after achieving remission.[24] Patients who opt for elemental diets have the longest reintroduction process. Food groups are generally reintroduced one at a time to facilitate identification of individual triggers.[2]

Current recommendations call for clinical assessment and endoscopy with biopsy to monitor inflammatory response whenever foods are being withdrawn or reintroduced to the diet.[24] Clearly dietary elimination and allergen identification is incredibly time and labor intensive. It is also quite costly. A multidisciplinary approach involving the patient, important family members, the gastroenterologist, a nutritionist, and an allergist may be helpful.[24,25]

ENDOSCOPIC DILATION

In patients with severe fibrostenotic complications of EoE, including focal stricture and narrow-caliber esophagus, endoscopic dilation is an effective treatment. Current recommendations call for dilation in symptomatic patients with strictures that have persisted in spite of medical or dietary therapy, or in patients with "severely symptomatic esophageal stenosis."[24]

Esophageal dilation was one of the original therapies for symptomatic EoE, and dilation produces long-lasting symptom relief.[40] Dilation was initially associated with high complication rates; in particular, rates of perforation in some early series were as high as 8%.[13] A more recent meta-analysis from 2011 demonstrated symptomatic relief in 92% of patients for up to 1 to 2 years after dilation with a very low rate of true perforation (<0.1%).[41] It is important to note that the symptomatic improvement following dilation has no effect on the eosinophil-induced inflammation.[13]

Current guidelines advocate for small increases in esophageal diameter over multiple sessions, but do not make recommendations on dilation technique.[24] Regardless of the specific technique, whether wire-guided or non-wire-guided bougie or through-the-scope balloons, patients must be counseled on the expected postoperative pain associated with dilation[13] and the potential for complication.[25]

INFECTIOUS ESOPHAGITIS

Fungal, viral, bacterial, and parasitic causes of infectious esophagitis have all been described.[42] On the whole, infectious esophagitis is rare and tends to occur in patients with systemic or local immunosuppression.[8] Risk factors include steroid use, immunodeficiency syndromes, radiation or chemotherapy, malignancy, esophageal dysmotility, and antibiotic use.[43] The prognosis is generally tied to the severity of comorbid conditions.[8] Regardless of the causative agent, infectious esophagitis usually presents with acute onset of symptoms such as dysphagia or odynophagia.[42]

CANDIDA ESOPHAGITIS

Candida is by far the most common cause of fungal esophagitis, although there are reports of esophagitis due to cryptococcosis, histoplasmosis, blastomycosis, and aspergillosis.[42] Fungal esophagitis usually occurs in patients with impaired immunity, and most commonly in patients with hematologic malignancy, AIDS, or recent steroid use.[8] Although uncommon, *Candida*-induced esophagitis has been observed in immunocompetent individuals without associated risk factors.[44] The characteristic symptom of esophageal candidiasis is odynophagia.[42] There is a strong association with oropharyngeal candidiasis (thrush),[45] although the absence of thrush does not preclude a diagnosis of esophagitis.[46]

The diagnosis of *Candida* esophagitis can be confirmed with endoscopic evaluation, which shows mucosal plaque-like lesions (Fig. 44.3). The endoscopic findings range from white or yellow exudates less than 2 mm to

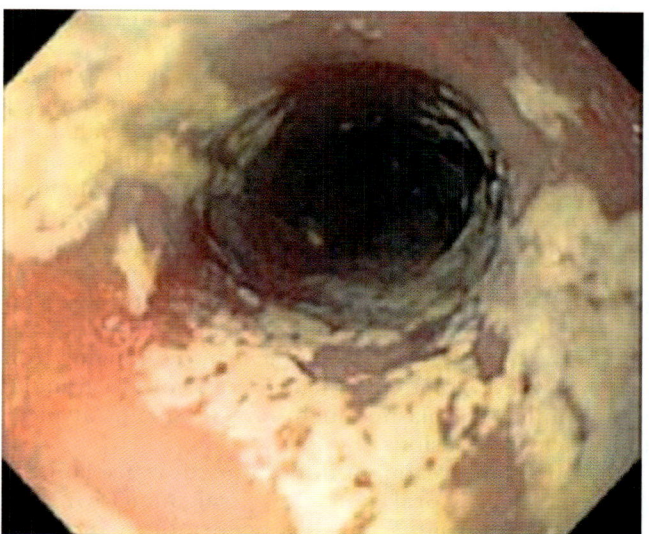

FIGURE 44.3 White exudates characteristic of *Candida* esophagitis. (From Rosolowski M, Kierzkiewicz M. Etiology, diagnosis and treatment of infectious esophagitis. *Prz Gastroenterol.* 2013;8:333–337.)

pseudomembranes causing esophageal stenosis. The findings can be graded on a scale of one to four.[8] Endoscopic evaluation has a sensitivity of 100% and a specificity of 83%.[8] Biopsy, which is not required for diagnosis, shows yeast and pseudohyphae invading mucosal cells.[42]

In patients with AIDS and acute-onset odynophagia, empiric systemic antifungal treatment without endoscopic evaluation is appropriate and symptoms should resolve in 3 to 5 days. If there is no timely resolution of symptoms, endoscopy with biopsy is needed due to the high incidence of viral coinfection.[42]

Candida esophagitis requires systemic antifungal therapy for 2 to 3 weeks. Intravenous antibiotics may be necessary if the disease is severe enough to limit intake by mouth. The current recommendation is for oral fluconazole with a loading dose of 400 mg followed by 200 to 400 mg daily. In refractory cases, other azoles may be used; echinocandins or amphotericin B are also acceptable alternatives. Amphotericin B is recommended for the treatment of esophageal candidiasis during pregnancy. In patients who have had recurrent infections, suppressive therapy with 100 to 200 mg of fluconazole 3 times per week is recommended.[47]

CYTOMEGALOVIRUS ESOPHAGITIS

With the advent of modern immunosuppression and the spread of the AIDS epidemic, cytomegalovirus (CMV) has emerged as a significant opportunistic pathogen. CMV is a DNA virus and has a seroprevalence in adults of 80% to 90% worldwide.[48] It may exist in isolation or with concomitant *Candida* esophagitis.[8] Disease can occur anywhere along the gastrointestinal (GI) tract, with colitis being the most common manifestation. CMV esophagitis usually occurs in patients with AIDS and a CD4 count below 50 cells/μL.[48] It has also been seen in patients on long-term immunosuppression after solid organ transplant, or patients on chemotherapy, and there are rare case reports in immunocompetent individuals.[49]

Immunosuppressed patients presenting with dysphagia or odynophagia who do not have resolution of symptoms with antifungal therapy warrant endoscopic evaluation. The presence of ulcerative esophagitis on endoscopy is 60% predictive of CMV esophagitis, but the gold standard remains endoscopic biopsy.[48] Endoscopic findings include segmental erosive changes or frank ulceration that can reach several centimeters in diameter.[48] Viral antigens or viral DNA can be detected using immunofluorescent antibodies or polymerase chain reaction. Histology can demonstrate a variety of cytopathic features, ranging from classic "owl eye" large intranuclear inclusions to granular, eosinophilic, cytoplasmic inclusions or small, "atypical" intranuclear inclusions.[1]

The first-line treatment in both organ transplant and AIDS patients is oral ganciclovir; valganciclovir is an acceptable alternative but has been more extensively studied in CMV retinitis.[50] For ganciclovir-resistant disease, other antiviral therapies include cidofovir and foscarnet. CMV immunoglobulin, in combination with antiviral medications or as a monotherapy, is not currently indicated due to heterogeneity among studies evaluating its use.[48]

HERPES ESOPHAGITIS

Herpes esophagitis, caused by the herpes simplex virus (HSV), is typically seen in immunocompromised patients. It usually occurs as an opportunistic infection secondary to viral reactivation in patients with underlying HIV infection, malignancy, immunosuppressive therapy, or severe illness.[51] It occurs less frequently than CMV esophagitis and the two viral infections may coexist.[8] There are case reports of HSV esophagitis in immunocompetent hosts, but these are exceedingly rare; in these patients the disease appears to be self-limited.[51] Within the last few years there have been several published reports of acute herpes esophagitis in immunocompetent patients with EoE; many of these cases were identified in the absence of steroid therapy. The coincidence of these two rare conditions raises the possibility of a causal relationship.

Patients generally present with symptoms of odynophagia, dysphagia, retrosternal chest pain, or fever, and there is often a recent history of upper respiratory infection or orolabial lesions.[1,51] On endoscopy, lesions are composed of small vesicles, 1 to 3 mm in diameter, which slough to leave well-circumscribed ulcers with discrete edges (Fig. 44.4).[8] The lesions are most commonly found in the mid- to lower esophagus.[51] Biopsies of herpes esophagitis is similar to herpesvirus infection at other sites; cytopathic effects include enlarged and multinucleated cells with marginated chromatin and nuclear molding. Intranuclear inclusions may be large, eosinophilic and glassy, or powdery and homogeneous. Optimal histologic diagnosis requires sampling of ulcer edges, because the virus infects squamous cells of intact epithelium.[1] Pharmacologic management is with antiviral medicines, and acyclovir is frequently used.[51]

TUBERCULOUS ESOPHAGITIS

Tuberculous esophagitis (TE) is rare, even in countries where tuberculosis is relatively common.[52] Reports of

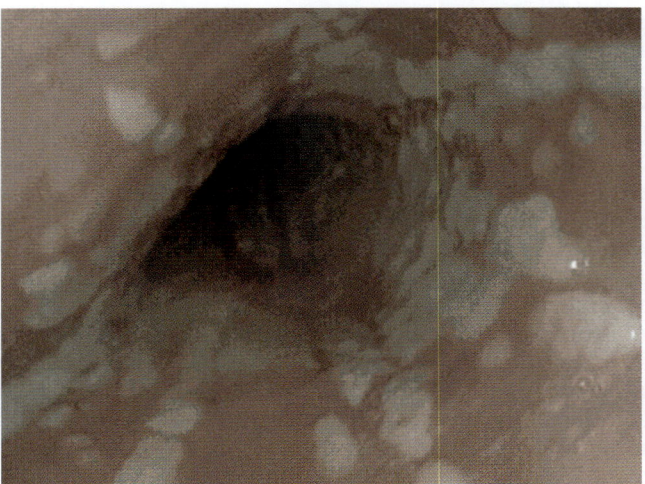

FIGURE 44.4 Herpetic ulcers in herpes simplex virus esophagitis. (From Gurvits GE, Shapsis A, Lau N, Gualtieri N, Robilotti JG. Acute esophageal necrosis: a rare syndrome. *J Gastroenterol.* 2007;42:29–38.)

individual cases suggest that the condition occurs most often in immunocompromised individuals.[1] TE can occur as a result of direct extension of tuberculosis from contiguous mediastinal structures. Symptoms of dysphagia or odynophagia may result, and ulceration or fistula formation may be evident on endoscopy. The diagnosis should be considered in patients with esophageal fistulas or sinus tracts on endoscopy; reports describe the development of bronchoesophageal and tracheoesophageal fistulas.[8] The differential diagnosis of esophageal fistulas must include Crohn disease and esophageal carcinoma; work-up should include bronchoscopy, endoscopy with biopsy, and CT scan. Histologic features may include caseating and noncaseating granulomas in combination with chronic inflammation and scarring. Acid-fast bacilli may be recognized on Ziehl–Neelsen staining.[1]

Most cases of fistulas require surgical resection with antituberculous treatment, although recent reports demonstrate that endoscopic intervention or nonoperative management may be effective in select patients.[53,54] One case series, albeit with just two patients, demonstrated efficacy of fistula resection with pedicled pleural flaps securing suture lines.[55] Another case series of six Chinese patients with dysphagia caused by TE demonstrated the efficacy of surgical management. In this series, five patients underwent video-assisted thoracoscopic surgery (VATS) with excision or enucleation and drainage of large mediastinal lymph nodes, and one patient with an esophagopleural fistula underwent thoracotomy with débridement and fistula repair coverage with a diaphragmatic muscle flap. These patients had uneventful postoperative courses, with relief from dysphagia at the time of discharge.[52]

DRUG-INDUCED ESOPHAGITIS

Drug-induced esophagitis, or "pill esophagitis," occurs when direct esophageal injury occurs as a result of an ingested medicine.[1] Since the original description in

1970, over 100 different medicines have been reported to cause drug-induced esophagitis.[56] The most commonly implicated medicines include bisphosphonates, nonsteroidal antiinflammatory drugs (NSAIDs), tetracyclines, vitamin C, and potassium chloride tablets.[8] Patients usually present with retrosternal pain or heartburn, less commonly odynophagia or dysphagia. The pathogenesis is linked to systemic and local actions of the ingested medicine, and the injury is most likely to occur at sites of anatomic or pathologic narrowing.[57]

On endoscopy, drug-induced esophagitis most commonly causes ulcers (82% of patients) with occasional bleeding (24% of patients); erosions are less common (18% of patients) and strictures are rare (3%).[58] Histologic features are generally nonspecific; they range from tiny, punctate erosions to large circumferential ulcers with granulation tissue and fibrinopurulent exudate.[1] Specific medicines tend to cause consistent patterns of injury; for example, the polarizable crystalline foreign material characteristic of alendronate causes a histiocytic giant-cell reaction.[1]

In the majority of cases, pill esophagitis is self-limiting and resolves without complications. The key to prompt resolution is correct and timely diagnosis with removal of the causative agent whenever possible.[57] Symptoms generally improve in 7 to 10 days. Rarely, cases may be complicated by significant bleeding, which may require endoscopic intervention and local epinephrine injection.[58] Endoscopic dilation may be required in cases of stricture formation; in rare circumstances these can take weeks to improve without dilation. Surgery is reserved for the management of complications that may develop during treatment.[57]

RADIATION ESOPHAGITIS

Radiation esophagitis is extremely common in patients who receive radiation therapy to the thorax, head, or neck region.[1] It occurs in adults and children.[59,60] Some authors refer to esophagitis as an "inevitable" result of radiotherapy and concurrent chemotherapy for thoracic cancer[61]; the associated dysphagia, odynophagia, and pain represent the major dose-limiting toxicity of treatment.[62] Given the frequency of symptomatic esophagitis in patients receiving therapeutic radiation, the National Cancer Institute has published a common terminology criterion for adverse events that grade dysphagia and esophagitis on a scale from 1 to 5.[63]

Radiotherapy causes congestion, edema, and erosion of the esophageal mucosa. This damage likely occurs due to obliterative endarteritis and microvascular damage that renders the esophageal mucosa ischemic, leading to fibrosis.[64] There appears to be a sensitization effect of chemotherapy. Symptoms of dysphagia, odynophagia, and substernal pain are extremely common; the incidence of esophagitis is as high as 40% in head/neck cancer patients, and the incidence of grade 1 to 2 acute esophagitis was 81% in patients undergoing concurrent radiation and chemotherapy for small-cell lung cancer (SCLC).

The management of radiation esophagitis depends upon the grade. Low-grade esophagitis (grade 1 to 2) may be managed with dietary modifications and local anesthetics; supportive care with calorie supplementation or intravenous hydration may be required if adequate intake by mouth becomes difficult. Grade 3 esophagitis generally requires inpatient management and some patients require enteric access with a gastrostomy tube to ensure adequate hydration and nutrition.

The risk of stricture formation correlates with the grade of esophagitis. In patients receiving treatment for SCLC, 24% of patients with grade 3 esophagitis developed an esophageal stricture compared with just 2% of patients with grade 1 or 2 disease.[62] In both adults and children, esophageal strictures are generally amenable to endoscopic dilation.[65]

Both anterograde and retrograde approaches have been shown to be safe and effective; regardless of the technique, patients usually require multiple dilations.[64] Dilation can be successful even in cases of complete stricture.[64] Surgical intervention is generally not required; cases of iatrogenic esophageal perforation following attempted dilation may be managed conservatively. The strongest predictor for failure of endoscopic dilation appears to be time to onset of esophageal stricture.[65]

ACUTE ESOPHAGEAL NECROSIS

AEN is a rare but potentially lethal disease; it likely represents a final common pathway for a number of conditions that can lead to severe esophageal injury.[66] The pathogenesis is believed to be multifactorial and an ischemic phenomenon is likely the major driver of the esophageal lesions. Hypoperfusion due to shock, atherosclerosis, thromboembolic disease, and cardiac arrhythmias have been implied in the development of AEN. Gastric outlet obstruction causing reflux and contributing to chemical esophageal injury may also play a role. There are known associations with alcoholism, cocaine abuse, malnutrition, malignancy, and general debilitation.[67]

Patients with AEN are generally quite ill, with myriad comorbid conditions. The most common presenting symptoms are hematemesis and/or melena (71% to 90% of cases).[66,67] On endoscopy, the disease is characterized by a circumferential black appearance, giving the condition its alternate name of "black esophagus" (Fig. 44.5). The mortality is high, but depends upon the comorbid conditions, and reports range from 15% to 36%.[66]

The treatment is generally supportive, and is directed at treating underlying medical conditions and maximizing tissue perfusion. This includes aggressive resuscitation, optimization of acid suppression, and treatment with antibiotics if sepsis is present. Surgical intervention is warranted in cases where AEN progresses to perforation, or in the presence of mediastinitis or a mediastinal abscess. If these conditions arise, surgery should be pursued expediently. Patients who survive are at risk for esophageal strictures, which may occur as early as 1 week after the initial diagnosis. These strictures may require serial endoscopy with dilation.[67] In our experience, the resulting strictures are frequently long segment, and endoscopic dilation is less likely to be effective. Surgical management is often necessary.

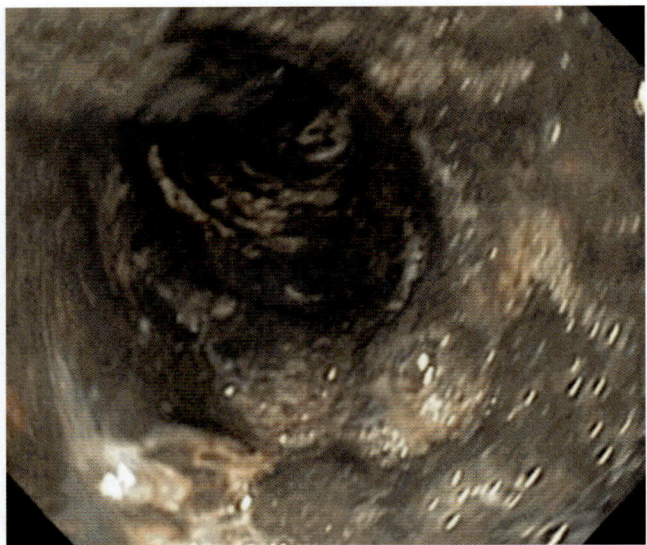

FIGURE 44.5 Characteristic "black esophagus" in acute esophageal necrosis. (From Shafa S, Sharma N, Keshishian J, Dellon ES. The black esophagus: a rare but deadly disease. *ACG Case Rep J.* 2016;3:88–91.)

REFERENCES

1. Almashat SJ, Duan L, Goldsmith JD. Non-reflux esophagitis: a review of inflammatory diseases of the esophagus exclusive of reflux esophagitis. *Semin Diagn Pathol.* 2014;31:89-99.
2. Kavitt RT, Hirano I, Vaezi MF. Diagnosis and treatment of eosinophilic esophagitis in adults. *Am J Med.* 2016;129:924-934. http://dx.doi.org/10.1016/j.amjmed.2016.04.024.
3. Attwood S, Furuta GT. Eosinophilic esophagitis: historical perspective on an evolving disease. *Gastroenterol Clin North Am.* 2015;43(2):185-199.
4. Picus D, Frank PH. Eosinophilic esophagitis. *AJR Am J Roentgenol.* 1981;136(5):1001-1003.
5. Feczko PJ, Halpert RD, Zonca M. Radiographic abnormalities in eosinophilic esophagitis. *Gastrointest Radiol.* 1985;10(4):321-324.
6. Attwood SEA, Smyrk TC, Demeester TR, Jones JB. Esophageal eosinophilia with dysphagia: a distinct clinicopathologic syndrome. *Dig Dis Sci.* 1993;38(1):106-119.
7. Potter JW, Saeian K, Staff D, et al. Eosinophilic esophagitis in adults: an emerging problem with unique esophageal features. *Gastrointest Endosc.* 2004;59(3):335-361.
8. Attwood SEA, Lamb CA. Eosinophilic oesophagitis and other non-reflux inflammatory conditions of the oesophagus: diagnostic imaging and management. *Best Pract Res Clin Gastroenterol.* 2008;22(4):639-660.
9. Remedios M, Campbell C, Jones DM, Kerlin P. Eosinophilic esophagitis in adults: clinical, endoscopic, histologic findings, and response to treatment with fluticasone propionate. *Gastrointest Endosc.* 2006;63:3-12.
10. Desai TK, Stecevic V, Chang CH, Goldstein NS, Badizadegan K, Furuta GT. Association of eosinophilic inflammation with esophageal food impaction in adults. *Gastrointest Endosc.* 2005;61:795-801.
11. Prasad GA, Talley NJ, Romero Y, et al. Prevalence and predictive factors of eosinophilic esophagitis in patients presenting with dysphagia: a prospective study. *Am J Gastroenterol.* 2007;102:2627-2632.
12. Kapel RC, Miller JK, Torres C, Aksoy S, Lash R, Katzka DA. Eosinophilic esophagitis: a prevalent disease in the United States that affects all age groups. *Gastroenterology.* 2008;134:1316-1321.
13. Dellon ES, Liacouras CA. Advances in clinical management of eosinophilic esophagitis. *Gastroenterology.* 2014;147(6):1238-1254.
14. Dellon ES. Epidemiology of eosinophilic esophagitis. *Gastroenterol Clin North Am.* 2014;43(2):201-218.
15. Dellon ES, Kim HP, Sperry SLW, Rybnicek DA, Woosley JT, Shaheen NJ. A phenotypic analysis shows eosinophilic esophagitis is a progressive fibrostenotic disease. *Gastrointest Endosc.* 2014;79(4):577-585.
16. Dellon ES, Jensen ET, Martin CF, Shaheen NJ, Kappelman MD. The prevalence of eosinophilic esophagitis in the United States. *Clin Gastroenterol Hepatol.* 2014;12(4):589-596.
17. Francios JP, Tam V, Liacouras CH, Spergel JM. A case-control study of sociodemographic and geographic characteristics of 335 children with eosinophilic esophagitis. *Clin Gastroenterol Hepatol.* 2009;7(4):415-419.
18. Roy-Ghanta S, Larosa DF, Katzka DA. Atopic characteristics of adult patients with eosinophilic esophagitis. *Clin Gastroenterol Hepatol.* 2008;6(5):531-535.
19. Ricker J, McNear S, Cassidy T, et al. Routine screening for eosinophilic esophagitis in patients presenting with dysphagia. *Therap Adv Gastroenterol.* 2011;4(1):27-35.
20. Noel RJ, Putnam PE, Rothenberg ME. Eosinophilic esophagitis. *N Engl J Med.* 2004;351(9):940-941.
21. Prasad GA, Alexander GA, Schleck CD, et al. Epidemiology of eosinophilic esophagitis over 3 decades in Olmsted County, Minnesota. *Clin Gastroenterol Hepatol.* 2009;7(10):1055-1061.
22. Hruz P, Straumann A, Bussmann C, et al. Escalating incidence of eosinophilic esophagitis: a 20-year prospective, population-based study in Olten County, Switzerland. *J Allergy Clin Immunol.* 2011;128(6):1349-1350.
23. Okada H, Kuhn C, Feillet H, Back JF. The 'Hygiene Hypothesis' for autoimmune and allergic disease: an update. *Clin Exp Immunol.* 2010;160:1-9.
24. Dellon ES, Gonsalves N, Hirano I, Furuta GT, Liacouras CA, Katzka DA. ACG clinical guideline: evidence based approach to the diagnosis and management of esophageal eosinophilia and eosinophilic esophagitis (EoE). *Am J Gastroenterol.* 2013;108:679-692.
25. Liacouras CA, Furuta GT, Hirano I, et al. Eosinophilic esophagitis: updated consensus recommendations for children and adults. *J Allergy Clin Immunol.* 2011;128(1):3-20.
26. Molina-Infante J, Ferrando-Lamana L, Ripoll C, et al. Esophageal eosinophilic infiltration responds to proton pump inhibition in most adults. *Clin Gastroenterol Hepatol.* 2011;9(2):110-117.
27. Lucendo AJ, Pascual-Turrion JM, Navarro M, et al. Endoscopic, bioptic, and manometric findings in eosinophilic esophagitis before and after steroid therapy: a case series. *Endoscopy.* 2007;39:765-771.
28. Lucendo AJ, Castillo P, Martin-Chavarri S, et al. Manometric findings in adult eosinophilic oesophagitis: a study of 12 cases. *Eur J Gastroenterol Hepatol.* 2007;19(5):417-424.
29. Blanchard C, Mingler MK, Vicario M, et al. IL-13 involvement in eosinophilic esophagitis: transcriptome analysis and reversibility with glucocorticoids. *J Allergy Clin Immunol.* 2007;120(6):1292-1300.
30. Mishra A, Wang M, Pemmaraju VR, et al. Esophageal remodeling develops as a consequence of tissue specific IL-5-induced eosinophilia. *Gastroenterology.* 2008;134(1):204-214.
31. Fogg MI, Ruchelli E, Spergel JM. Letters to the editor: pollen and eosinophilic esophagitis. *J Allergy Clin Immunol.* 2003;112(4):796-797.
32. Hurrell JM, Genta RM, Dellon ES. Prevalence of esophageal eosinophilia varies by climate zone in the United States. *Am J Gastroenterol.* 2012;107(5):698-706.
33. Lucendo AJ, Arias A, Redondo-Gonzalez O, Gonzalez-Cervera J. Seasonal distribution of initial diagnosis and clinical recrudescence of eosinophilic esophagitis: a systematic review and meta-analysis. *Allergy.* 2015;70:1640-1650.
34. Cheng E, Zhang X, Huo X, et al. Omeprazole blocks eotaxin-3 expression by oesophageal squamous cells from patients with eosinophilic oesophagitis and GORD. *Gut.* 2013;62:824-832.
35. Rea F, Caldara T, Tambucci R, et al. Eosinophilic esophagitis: is it also a surgical disease? *J Pediatr Surg.* 2013;48:304-308.
36. Aceves SS, Bastian JF, Newbury RO, Dohil R. Oral viscous budesonide: a potential new therapy for eosinophilic esophagitis in children. *Am J Gastroenterol.* 2007;102:2271-2279.
37. Schaefer ET, Fitzgerald JF, Molleston JP, et al. Comparison of oral prednisone and topical fluticasone in the treatment of eosinophilic esophagitis: a randomized trial in children. *Clin Gastroenterol Hepatol.* 2008;6(2):165-173.
38. Alexander JA, Jung KW, Arora AS, et al. Swallowed fluticasone improves histologic but not symptomatic response of adults with eosinophilic esophagitis. *Clin Gastroenterol Hepatol.* 2012;10(7):742-749.
39. Staumann A, Conus S, Degen L, et al. Budesonide is effective in adolescent and adult patients with active eosinophilic esophagitis. *Gastroenterology.* 2010;139:1526-1537.

40. Schoepfer AM, Gonsalves N, Bussmann C, et al. Esophageal dilation in eosinophilic esophagitis: effectiveness, safety, and impact on the underlying inflammation. *Am J Gastroenterol.* 2010;105:1062-1070.
41. Bohn ME, Richter JE. Review article: oesophageal dilation in adults with eosinophilic oesophagitis. *Aliment Pharmacol Ther.* 2011;33:748-757.
42. Rosolowski M, Kierzkiewicz M. Etiology, diagnosis and treatment of infectious esophagitis. *Prz Gastroenterol.* 2013;8(6):333-337.
43. Underwood JA, Williams JW, Keat RF. Clinical findings and risk factors for *Candida* esophagitis in outpatients. *Dis Esophagus.* 2006;16(2):66-69.
44. Mimidis K, Papadopoulos V, Margaritis V, et al. Predisposing factors and clinical symptoms in HIV-negative patients with *Candida* oesophagitis: are they always present? *Int J Clin Pract.* 2005;59(2):210-213.
45. Samonis G, Skordilis P, Maraki S, et al. Oropharyngeal candidiasis as a marker for esophageal candidiasis in patients with cancer. *Clin Infect Dis.* 1998;27(2):283-286.
46. Kanda N, Yasuba H, Takahashi T, et al. Prevalence of esophageal candidiasis among patients treated with inhaled fluticasone propionate. *Am J Gastroenterol.* 2003;98(10):2146-2148.
47. Pappas PG, Kauffman CA, Andes D, et al. Clinical practice guidelines for the management of candidiasis: 2009 update by the Infectious Diseases Society of America. *Clin Infect Dis.* 2009;48:503-535.
48. Baroco AL, Oldfield EC. Gastrointestinal cytomegalovirus disease in the immunocompromised patient. *Curr Gastroenterol Rep.* 2008;10:409-416.
49. Ozaki T, Yamashita H, Kaneko S, et al. Cytomegalovirus disease of the upper gastrointestinal tract in patients with rheumatic disease: a case series and literature review. *Clin Rheumatol.* 2013;32:1683-1690.
50. Martin D, Sierra-Madero J, Walmsley S, et al. A controlled trial of valganciclovir as induction therapy for cytomegalovirus retinitis. *N Engl J Med.* 2002;346:1119-1126.
51. Canalejo E, Duran FG, Cabello N, Martinez JG. Herpes esophagitis in healthy adults and adolescents: report of 3 cases and review of the literature. *Medicine (Baltimore).* 2010;89:204-210.
52. Ni B, Lu X, Gong Q, et al. Surgical outcome of esophageal tuberculosis secondary to mediastinal lymphadenitis in adults: experience from a single center in China. *J Thorac Dis.* 2013;5(4):498-505.
53. Manca S, Fois AG, Santoru L, et al. Unusual clinical presentation of thoracic tuberculosis: the need for a better knowledge of illness. *Am J Case Rep.* 2015;16:240-244.
54. Catano J, Cardeno J. Perforated tuberculosis lymphadenitis. *Am J Trop Med Hyg.* 2013;88(6):1009-1010.
55. Ramo OJ, Salo JA, Isolauri J, Luostarinen M, Mattila SP. Tuberculous fistula of the esophagus. *Ann Thorac Surg.* 1996;62:1030-1032.
56. Abid S, Mumtaz K, Jafri W, et al. Pill-induced esophageal injury: endoscopic features and clinical outcomes. *Endoscopy.* 2005;37(8):740-744.
57. Zografos GN, Georgiadou D, Thomas D, Kaltsas G, Digalakis M. Drug-induced esophagitis. *Dis Esophagus.* 2009;22:633-637.
58. Kim SH, Jeong JB, Kim JW, et al. Clinical and endoscopic characteristics of drug-induced esophagitis. *World J Gastroenterol.* 2014;20(31):10994-10999.
59. Lar DR, Foroutan HR, Su WT, Wolden SL, Boulad F, La Quaglia MP. The management of treatment-related esophageal complication in children and adolescents with cancer. *J Pediatr Surg.* 2006;41:495-499.
60. Werner-Wasik M. Treatment-related esophagitis. *Semin Oncol.* 2005;32(3):S60-S66.
61. Yu Y, Guan H, Done Y, Xing L, Li X. Advances in dosimetry and biological predictors of radiation-induced esophagitis. *Onco Targets Ther.* 2016;9:597-603.
62. Grant JD, Shirvani SM, Tang C, et al. Incidence and predictors of severe acute esophagitis and subsequent esophageal stricture in patients treated with accelerated hyperfractionated chemoradiation for limited-stage small cell lung cancer. *Pract Radiat Oncol.* 2015;5:e383-e391.
63. Cancer Therapy Evaluation Program, Common Terminology Criteria for Adverse Events, Version 3.0, DCTD, NCI, NIH, DHHS; 2003. http://ctep.cancer.gov. Accessed 9 August 2006.
64. Francis DO, Hall E, Dang JH, Vlacich GR, Netterville JL, Vaezi MF. Outcomes of serial dilation for high grade radiation-related esophageal strictures in head and neck cancer patients. *Laryngoscopy.* 2015;125(4):856-862.
65. Tuna Y, Kocak E, Dincer D, Koklu S. Factors affecting the success of endoscopic bougie dilation of radiation-induced esophageal stricture. *Dig Dis Sci.* 2012;57:424-428.
66. Shafa S, Sharma N, Keshishian J, Dellon ES. The black esophagus: a rare but deadly disease. *ACG Case Rep J.* 2016;3(2):88-91.
67. Gurvits GE, Shapsis A, Lau N, Gualtieri N, Robilotti JG. Acute esophageal necrosis: a rare syndrome. *J Gastroenterol.* 2007;42:29-38.

Esophageal Duplication Cyst

Ching Yeung | Blair MacDonald | Sebastien Gilbert

Esophageal duplication cyst is one of two types of foregut duplication cysts. The other type is the bronchogenic duplication cyst, and they are both classified together due to their common embryologic origin. Duplication cysts are a rare entity, with most literature consisting of case reports or small case series. It is estimated that foregut duplication cysts make up 20% of all gastrointestinal duplication cysts. Esophageal duplication cysts are the second most common benign posterior mediastinal lesion in children after bronchogenic cyst.[1] A review of almost 50,000 autopsies revealed an incidence of esophageal duplication cyst of 1 in 8200, with 60% occurring in the lower third esophagus, 17% in middle third, and 23% in upper third.[2] There is a male predominance in a ratio of 2:1, and duplication cyst has been associated with congenital abnormalities such as small intestinal duplication, esophageal atresia, and spinal abnormalities.[3]

PATHOPHYSIOLOGY

During the fifth to eighth week of fetal life, as the esophagus elongates, its epithelium grows and the cells obliterate the lumen of the esophagus. The esophagus produces secretions, which form into vacuoles. If the vacuoles persist because of failure of proper alignment and coalescence, duplication cysts may be formed. The cyst often occurs on the right because of the elongation of the viscera and dextrorotation of the stomach.[2] Esophageal duplication cysts are more commonly of the cystic form (80%), which has no communication with the lumen of the esophagus. The tubular form, which comprises 20% of esophageal duplication cysts, typically communicates with the esophageal lumen.[4] They vary in size, averaging 4.5 cm for the cystic form, and as large as 25 cm in tubular form.[2] Both esophageal duplication cyst and bronchogenic cyst are lined with ciliated epithelium because of their common embryologic origin. They differ histologically in that bronchogenic duplication cysts contain cartilage, whereas esophageal duplication cysts have two layers of smooth muscle.[5] Esophageal duplication cyst may also contain heterotopic gastric or pancreatic mucosa.[6]

Palmer's pathologic criteria are often used to define an esophageal duplication cyst. The criteria are (1) the lesion should be within or attached to esophageal wall, (2) there should be two layers of smooth muscle (inner circular and outer longitudinal), and (3) the cyst wall lining should contain ciliated epithelium or other cells found in embryologic tissue (squamous, columnar, cuboid, pseudostratified, ciliated).[7] However, there have been noteworthy exceptions in which intraabdominal duplication cysts did not meet the first criterion.[5]

CLINICAL PRESENTATION

The presentation of an esophageal duplication cyst depends on its size, location, and effect on surrounding structures. It is also related to the age of the patient. For instance, infants and children often present with respiratory distress, cough, or recurrent pneumonias.[8,9] Although the majority of adults are asymptomatic, presenting symptoms include progressive dysphagia to solids and liquids, epigastric or abdominal pain, and retrosternal chest discomfort.[8,10-13] Physical examination is often noncontributory. There are isolated reports of acute, severe abdominal pain in patients who present with cyst perforation or hemorrhage.[3,8]

There are also rare cases of patients presenting weight loss and lymphadenopathy due to malignancy arising from within the cyst.[14-16]

Malignant transformation within an esophageal duplication cyst is an extremely rare event, with only a handful of reported cases.[14-17] The age at presentation ranged widely from 18 to 60 years old, with no gender predominance and variable size from 3 to 10 cm. The clinical presentation of these malignancies varied from an incidental finding to dysphagia, fever, and pain.

The differential diagnosis for a submucosal esophageal lesion includes other nonepithelial tumors such as leiomyoma, gastrointestinal stromal tumor (GIST), sarcoma, lymphoma, lipoma, and other posterior mediastinal masses. For intraabdominal esophageal duplication cyst the differential diagnosis should include pancreatic pseudocyst, dermoid cyst, cystadenoma, and cystadenocarcinoma.[5]

INVESTIGATIONS

IMAGING STUDIES

Plain film chest radiographs have incidentally detected esophageal duplication cysts by showing an enlarged mediastinum or a retrocardiac mass.[7,18] Today, computed tomography (CT) scan is a more common detection modality. It usually reveals a smooth, well-defined hypodense lesion in the posterior mediastinum in close proximity to the esophagus.[7] Irregularity within the cyst wall may be associated with malignancy.[16] In the event of a rupture, the CT scan may show gas and debris within the area of the cyst, which can be confused with a paraesophageal hernia.[3] Magnetic resonance imaging (MRI) can be helpful to further delineate anatomic relationships and rule out other abnormalities, such as GIST or leiomyomas. Esophageal duplication cysts have high signal intensity on T2-weighted images due to the high proportion of water within the cyst contents.[5,19]

In rare cases, duplication cysts have been diagnosed using technetium 99m to detect ectopic gastric mucosa in the adult patient, or ultrasound in the prenatal (third trimester) period.[20] The use of prenatal ultrasound to detect esophageal duplication cyst has not been commonly reported, and other infants with esophageal duplication cysts have had normal prenatal ultrasounds.[21]

ENDOSCOPY

Esophagogastroduodenoscopy reveals a submucosal lesion. Depending on the size of the lesion, they can cause narrowing of the esophageal lumen as well as signs of extrinsic compression.[22] In cases of malignant transformation an associated esophageal stricture may be present.[15] Since the mid-1990s there has been increasing use of endoscopic ultrasound (EUS). EUS has been useful to determine if the lesion is intramural or extramural and cystic or solid.[4] On EUS, there is usually a three- to five-layer cyst wall with anechoic or hypoechoic, homogeneous internal contents. The lesion has regular margins and arises from the submucosal layer or extrinsic to the gut wall.[23] However, in a case series of 19 mediastinal cysts, the EUS findings were not as consistent.[24] EUS with a 12-MHz probe described the presence of both hypoechoic and anechoic cysts with and without the presence of cell wall layers on EUS. Three of the patients without a visible cystic wall on EUS underwent surgical resection that histologically confirmed the diagnosis of esophageal duplication cyst. The others without cell wall layers were managed conservatively and classified as nonspecific simple cysts. The role of EUS–fine-needle aspiration (FNA) is controversial because of the risk of infection. In the aforementioned case series, four patients developed infections following endoscopic drainage, one of which was life-threatening. FNA should be avoided when the lesion is clearly cystic in nature (i.e., anechoic). However, if the lesion is hypoechoic, FNA can be considered after appropriate prophylactic antibiotics have been administered.[4,24]

TREATMENT

ENDOSCOPIC

There has been recent interest in the endoscopic management of esophageal duplication cyst. Fine-needle aspiration under EUS guidance represents the least invasive treatment option for these patients. Although major surgery may be avoided, there should be a discussion about the potential for recurrence, and of the fact that this treatment modality cannot prevent potential complications, such as bleeding, ulceration, perforation, or malignant transformation, especially in young individuals.[18,22,25]

OPERATIVE

Surgical resection is often recommended because of the risks of ulceration, hemorrhage, perforation, and the small risk of malignant transformation associated with esophageal duplication cyst. As opposed to simple observation, surgery provides a definitive diagnosis and decreases the frequency of follow-up investigations. Complete surgical excision can be safely conducted via open or thoracoscopic approach.[7,10,12,13] The cystic lesion may need to be decompressed to facilitate dissection from the esophagus and surrounding structures and intercostal extirpation. The vagus nerves should be identified and preserved. The operation is similar to enucleation of a submucosal tumor of the esophagus. There can be significant adhesions to adjacent structures and, more importantly, to the underlying mucosa of the esophagus.

Patients should be informed of the risk and potential implications of esophageal injury as a result of cyst resection. This significant complication has been previously reported and is typically managed with immediate primary repair with or without soft tissue buttressing (e.g., intercostal muscle, pedicled pericardial fat pad–Brewer's patch, omentum, etc.). In some instances, successful management of a perforation at the time of resection has required esophagectomy.[5,26] If possible, the esophageal muscularis propria should be reapproximated to prevent the formation of a pseudodiverticulum, which may require further surgical correction.[7,13] Before reapproximation of the muscularis, the mucosal integrity at the repair site should always be assessed. This is preferably accomplished with the flexible esophagoscope, which allows for both direct mucosal examination and insufflation of the esophageal lumen to test for leakage while the posterior mediastinum is submerged under irrigation fluid.

Thoracoscopic resection may be associated with a shorter hospital stay.[7] Incomplete resection can lead to recurrence.[11] Resection of cysts near the gastroesophageal junction may result in incompetence of the lower esophageal sphincter and the development or exacerbation of gastroesophageal reflux symptoms. This can usually be managed medically.[13]

For the rare cases of malignant transformation, and locally advanced disease, patients should be treated on a case-by-case basis. In our review, patients with locally advanced disease received adjuvant chemotherapy and radiation.[16] If they were not considered surgical candidates because of morbidity of resection or distant metastasis, they received palliative chemoradiation.[14,15]

The management of this rare condition is best illustrated by an actual case from our institution. An 18-year-old female, who is otherwise healthy, presented to the emergency room with a 4-week history of progressively worsening cough associated with chest pain. She had a past medical history of asthma. A chest x-ray showed a posterior mediastinal mass (Fig. 45.1). The chest CT scan revealed an 8.5×4.5 cm homogeneous, well-circumscribed posterior mediastinal mass (Figs. 45.2 to 45.5). An esophagogastroduodenoscopy and EUS confirmed extrinsic compression of the esophagus from 30 to 36 cm from the level of the incisors. The mass was extrinsic to the wall of the esophagus on EUS. The patient underwent thoracoscopic enucleation of the esophageal duplication cyst (Fig. 45.6). The muscularis of the esophagus was repaired with a monofilament suture (Figs. 45.7 and 45.8). Intraoperative endoscopy confirmed the absence of any mucosal injury. The final pathology report was consistent with the preoperative diagnosis. Follow-up barium swallow at 1 and 6 years revealed a normal-appearing esophagus (Fig. 45.9). She has developed no postoperative complications at 6 years.

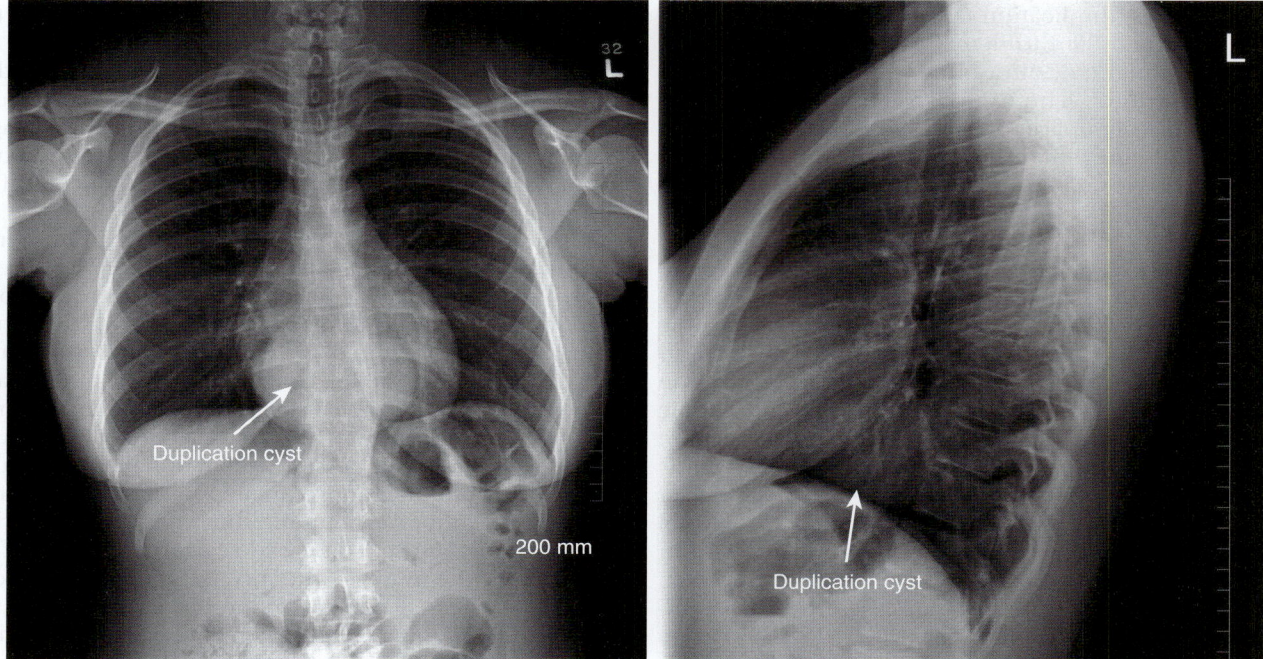

FIGURE 45.1 Frontal and lateral radiographic projections of the chest showing a large round retrocardiac mass with smooth interface with the adjacent lung. Differential includes esophageal solid mass and hiatal hernia. The normal position of the gastric fundus is below the diaphragm. The lack of air fluid level makes hiatal hernia less likely on the differential.

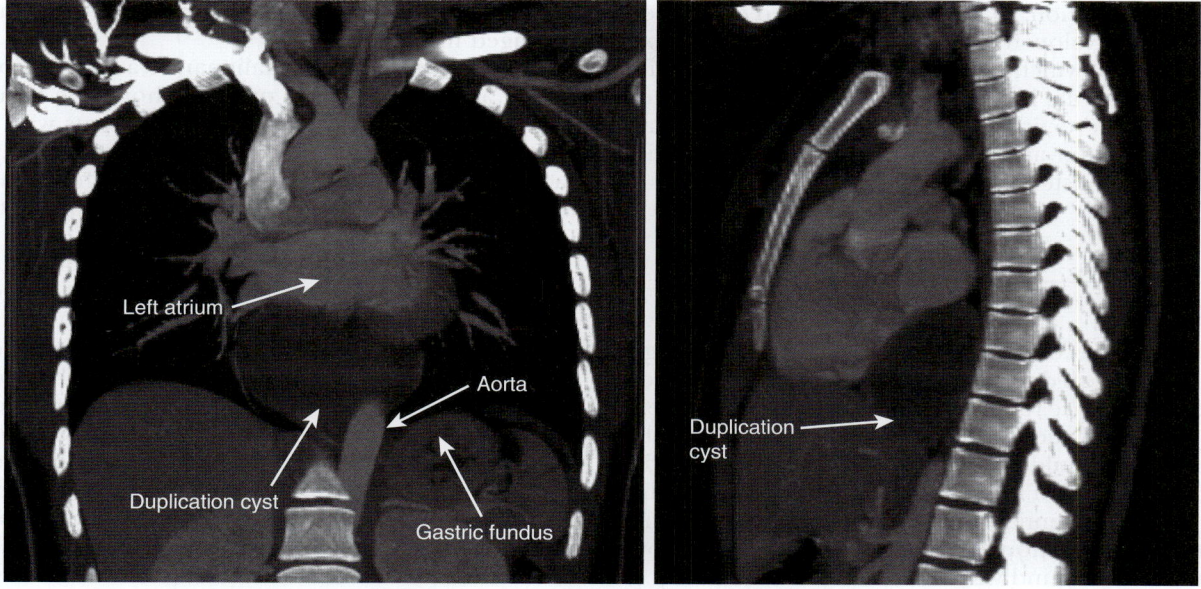

FIGURE 45.2 Maximum intensity projection (MIP) 12-mm slab images in coronal and sagittal plane showing the esophageal duplication cyst in relation to the posterior mediastinal structures (esophagus, left atrium, aorta, thoracic spine) and the diaphragm, and gastric fundus. Images obtained in the pulmonary circulatory vascular phase after injection of intravenous contrast on Toshiba Aquilion One (Toshiba Canada, Markham, ON, Canada) with axial volume acquisition at 0.625 mm and postprocessing reconstruction on Terarecon Aquarius Intuition software (Terarecon, Foster City, California).

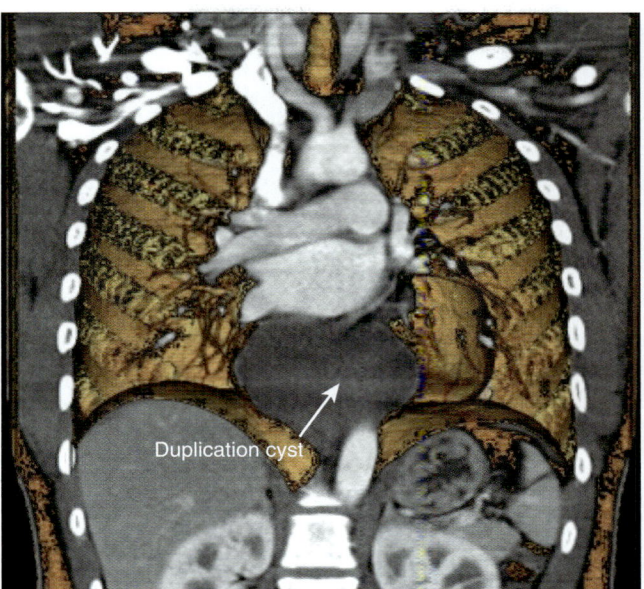
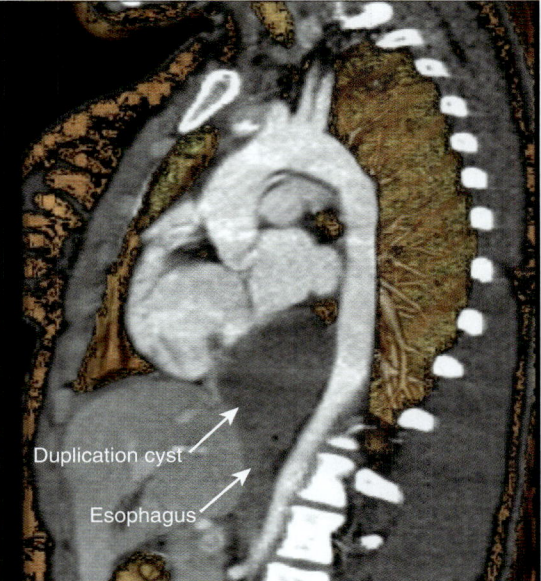

FIGURE 45.3 Volume-rendered computed tomography images with half volume coronal and oblique sagittal cut views showing the esophageal duplication cyst in relation to the posterior mediastinal structures (esophagus, left atrium, aorta, thoracic spine) and the diaphragm, and gastric fundus. Lower density structures (lungs, fat) projected as a color mask for emphasis. Images obtained in the pulmonary circulatory vascular phase after injection of intravenous contrast on Toshiba Aquilion One (Toshiba Canada, Markham, Ontario, Canada) with axial volume acquisition at 0.625 mm and postprocessing reconstruction on Terarecon Aquarius Intuition software (Terarecon, Foster City, California).

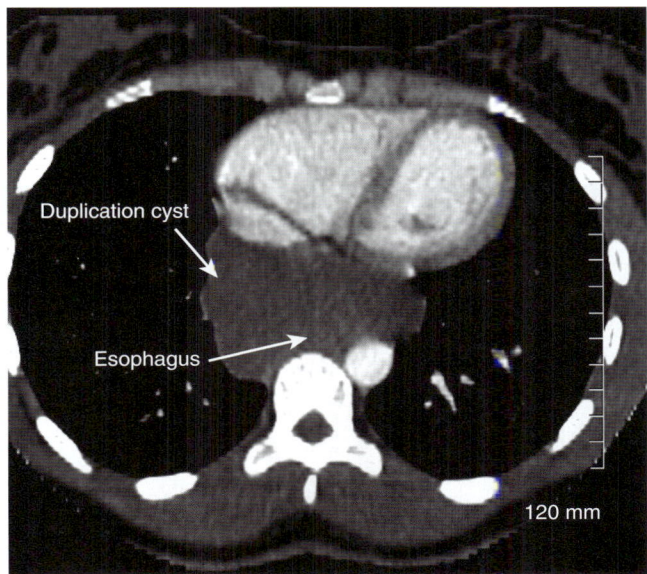

FIGURE 45.4 Axial 5-mm computed tomography image showing the esophageal duplication cyst in relation to the posterior mediastinal structures (esophagus, left atrium, aorta, thoracic spine). Images obtained in the pulmonary circulatory vascular phase after injection of intravenous contrast on Toshiba Aquilion One (Toshiba Canada, Markham, Ontario, Canada) with axial volume acquisition at 0.625 mm and postprocessing reconstruction on Terarecon Aquarius Intuition software (Terarecon, Foster City, California).

SUMMARY

Although surgical management is most commonly recommended, there is some controversy on how to manage asymptomatic patients. The very low incidence of the disease unfortunately precludes large group comparisons between conservative, endoscopic, and surgical treatment strategies. There will always be anecdotal reports of successful long-term observation or endoscopic fine-needle aspiration.[27] For the asymptomatic patient who is healthy enough to undergo surgery, age and size of the lesion should probably be taken into consideration in determining the optimal treatment approach. For instance, in an elderly patient with a small asymptomatic cyst, a period of observation with serial imaging to ensure stability may be a reasonable approach after detailed discussion of the potential complications related to esophageal duplication cysts.

Of all treatment options reviewed herein, we favor surgical excision because it is the best modality to obtain a definitive diagnosis and because it probably has the best likelihood of preventing long-term complications and recurrence. Esophageal duplication cyst is a relatively rare condition and, as a result, the scientific evidence to support our recommendation is and will likely remain limited. In that light, we acknowledge that it is appropriate to individualize management decisions on a case-by-case basis.

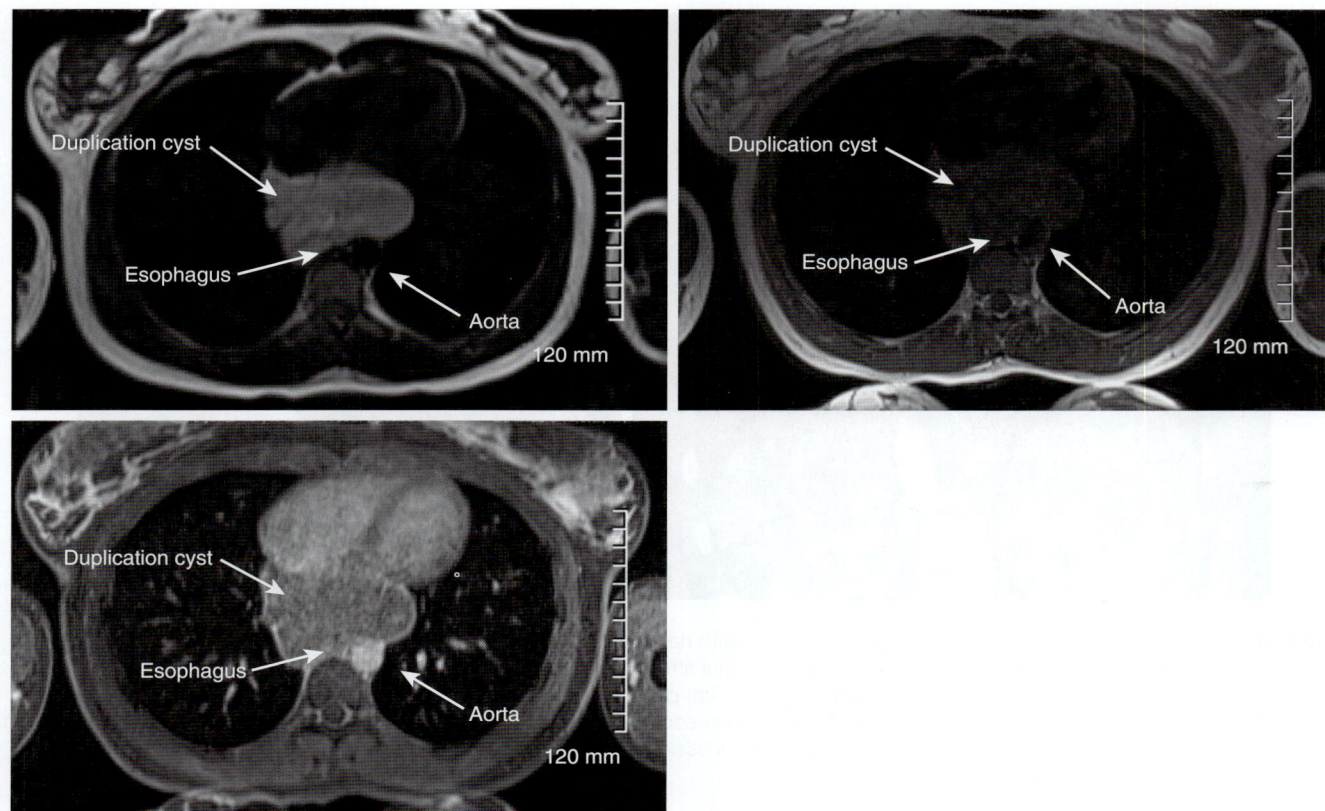

FIGURE 45.5 Axial T2 turbo spin echo (TSE) 5-mm, axial T1 TSE 5-mm, and axial T1 three-dimensional volumetric interpolated breath-hold examination fat-saturated (3D VIBE FS) postcontrast images showing the cyst in the same plane as the accompanying axial computed tomography scan. High signal intensity (SI) on T2 and low SI on T1 are consistent with water or near-water cystic contents. On postcontrast image there is a thin enhancing wall with no solid nodular components. Images obtained on a Siemens Symphony 1.5T magnet (Siemens Healthcare, Erlangen, Germany).

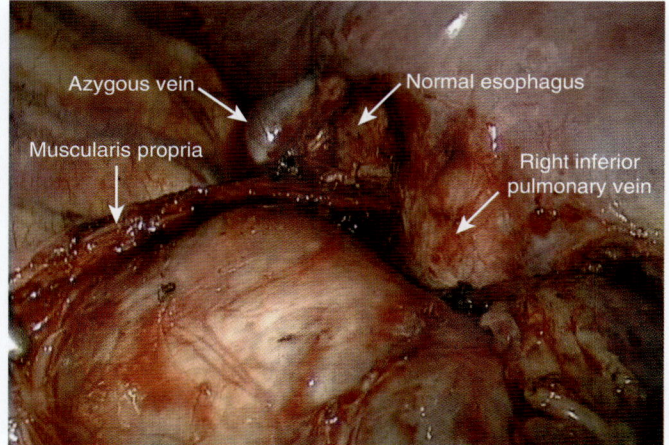

FIGURE 45.6 View from a right thoracoscopic approach. The mediastinal pleural and esophageal muscularis overlying the large duplication cyst have been incised to begin the enucleation.

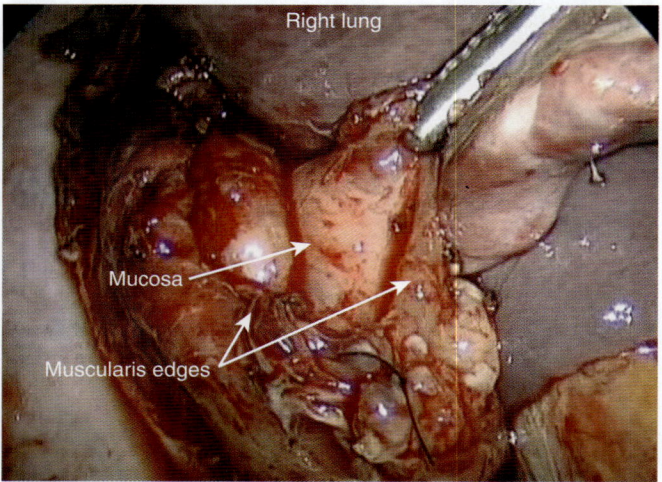

FIGURE 45.7 After the cyst has been removed, the muscularis propria is reapproximated over the loose esophageal mucosa.

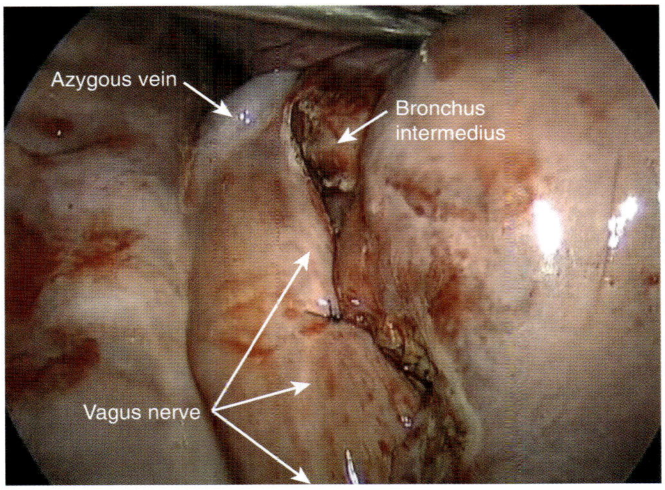

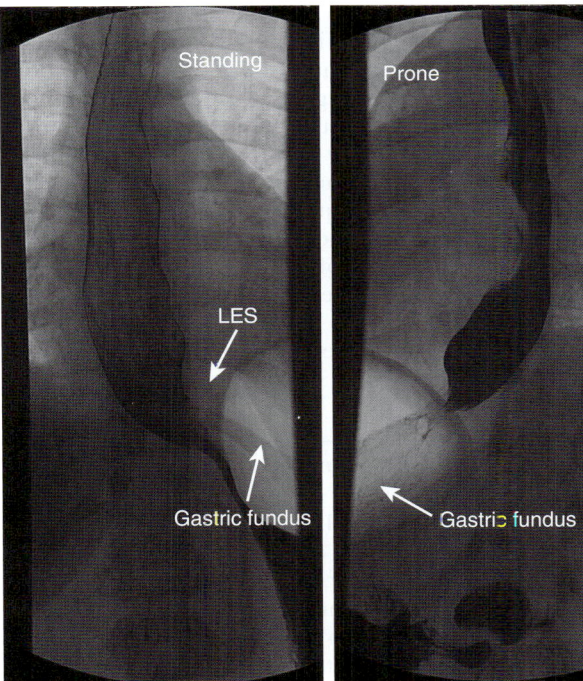

FIGURE 45.8 The mediastinal pleural is reapproximated over the enucleation. Care was taken to preserve both vagus nerves.

FIGURE 45.9 Postoperative standing double contrast upper gastrointestinal view with barium and gas crystals, and prone oblique view single barium contrast view of the lower esophagus, lower esophageal sphincter (LES), and gastric fundus, demonstrating normal mucosal, caliber, and LES relaxation during swallowing. No residual mass or deformity several weeks after surgery.

REFERENCES

1. Watanobe I, Ito Y, Akimoto E, et al. Laparoscopic resection of an intra-abdominal esophageal duplication cyst: a case report and literature review. *Case Rep Surg.* 2015;2015:940768.
2. Arbona JL, Fazzi JG, Mayoral J. Congenital esophageal cysts: case report and review of literature. *Am J Gastroenterol.* 1984;79(3):177-182.
3. Neo EL, Watson DI, Bessell JR. Acute ruptured esophageal duplication cyst. *Dis Esophagus.* 2004;17(1):109-111.
4. Faigel D, Burke A, Ginsberg G, Stotland BR, Kadish SL, Kochman ML. The role of endoscopic ultrasound in the evaluation and management of foregut duplications. *Gastrointest Endosc.* 1997;45(1):99-103.
5. Martin N, Kim J, Verma S, et al. Intra-abdominal esophageal duplication cysts: a review. *J Gastrointest Surg.* 2007;11:773-777.
6. Uppal P, Kaur J, Agarwala S, Gupta AK, Safaya R, Kabra SK. Communicating oesophageal duplication cyst with heterotopic pancreatic tissue—an unusual cause of recurrent pneumonia in an infant. *Acta Paediatr.* 2010;99:1432-1433.
7. Cioffi U, Bonavina L, De Simone M, et al. Presentation and surgical management of bronchogenic and esophageal duplication cysts in adults. *Chest.* 1998;113(6):1492-1496.
8. Lee HS, Jeon HJ, Song CW, et al. Esophageal duplication cyst complicated with intramural hematoma—case report. *J Korean Med Sci.* 1994;9(2):188-196.
9. Rangasami R, Chandrasekharan A, Archana L, Santhosh J. Case report: antenatal MRI diagnosis of esophageal duplication cyst. *Indian J Radiol Imaging.* 2009;19(1):75-77.
10. Achildi O, Grewal H. Congenital anomalies of the esophagus. *Otolaryngol Clin North Am.* 2007;40(1):219-244.
11. Al-Sadoon H, Wiseman N, Chernick V. Recurrent thoracic duplication cyst with associated mediastinal gas. *Can Respir J.* 1998;5(2):149-151.
12. Chaudhary V, Rana SS, Sharma V, et al. Esophageal duplication cyst in an adult masquerading as submucosal tumor. *Endosc Ultrasound.* 2013;2(3):165-167.
13. Herbella FA, Tedesco P, Muthusamy R, Patti MG. Thoracoscopic resection of esophageal duplication cysts. *Dis Esophagus.* 2006;19(2):132-134.
14. Lee MY, Jensen E, Kwak S, Larson RA. Metastatic adenocarcinoma arising in a congenital foregut cyst of the esophagus: a case report with review of the literature. *Am J Clin Oncol.* 1998;21(1):64-66.
15. McGregor D, Mills G, Boudet R. Intramural squamous cell carcinoma of the esophagus. *Cancer.* 1976;37:1556-1561.
16. Singh S, Lal P, Sikora SS, Datta NR. Squamous cell carcinoma arising from congenital duplication cyst of the esophagus in a young adult. *Dis Esophagus.* 2001;14:258-261.
17. Suzuki K, Koyama S, Yamada S, Kawabata Y. Adenocarcinoma arising in a mediastinal enteric cyst. *Intern Med.* 2007;46(11):781-784.
18. Kolomainen D, Hurley PR, Ebbs SR. Esophageal duplication cyst: case report and review of the literature. *Dis Esophagus.* 1998;11(1):62-65.
19. Rafal RB, Markisz JA. Magnetic resonance imaging of an esophageal duplication cyst. *Am J Gastroenterol.* 1991;86(12):1809-1811.
20. Jeung MY, Gasser B, Gangi A, et al. Imaging of cystic masses of the mediastinum. *Radiographics.* 2002;22 Spec:S79-S93.
21. Wootton-Gorges SL, Eckel GM, Poulos ND, Kappler S, Milstein JM. Duplication of the cervical esophagus: a case report and review of the literature. *Pediatr Radiol.* 2002;32(7):533-535.
22. Novellis P, Graffeo M, Sparano L, et al. Endoultrasonography (EUS) examination of the esophagus in the diagnosis of esophageal duplication: a case report and a review of a literature. *Eur Rev Med Pharmacol Sci.* 2015;19(16):3041-3045.
23. Liu R, Adler DG. Duplication cysts: diagnosis, management, and the role of endoscopic ultrasound. *Endosc Ultrasound.* 2014;3(3):152-160.
24. Wildi S, Hoda RS, Fickling W, et al. Diagnosis of benign cysts of the mediastinum: the role and risks of EUS and FNA. *Gastrointest Endosc.* 2003;58:362-368.
25. Will U, Meyer F, Bosseckert H. Successful endoscopic treatment of an esophageal duplication cyst. *Scand J Gastroenterol.* 2005;40(8):995-999.
26. Hirose S, Clifton MS, Bratton B, et al. Thoracoscopic resection of foregut duplication cysts. *J Laparoendosc Adv Surg Tech A.* 2006;16(5):526-529.
27. Versleijen MW, Drenth JP, Nagengast FM. A case of esophageal duplication cyst with a 13-year follow-up period. *Endoscopy.* 2005;37(9):870-872.

Submucosal Tumors of the Esophagus and Gastroesophageal Junction

Kristin Wilson Beard | Kevin M. Reavis

Submucosal tumors (SMTs) of the esophagus and gastroesophageal junction (GEJ) are a group of rare, benign lesions. This chapter will review the various types of esophageal and GEJ SMTs. We intend to focus on advancements in the imaging modalities, medical treatment, and surgical options for these tumors, including descriptions of evolving surgical techniques.

Our understanding of the prevalence of esophageal SMTs comes largely from autopsy studies from the mid-20th century, which identified an overall prevalence of about 0.5% for benign esophageal tumors and cysts.[1,2] Only 18% of all esophageal tumors were benign; the remaining 82% were malignant.[1] Benign esophageal and GEJ SMTs are found in people of all ages from infancy to elderly, with the majority presenting in the fourth through sixth decades, and with male predominance.

The development of symptoms related to esophageal SMTs is largely correlated to the size of the tumor. Presenting symptoms may include dysphagia and regurgitation due to intraluminal obstruction, pain, pulmonary symptoms due to extramural mass effect on the airways, or bleeding.[3] Physical examination is usually unrevealing unless the tumor is quite large; therefore, discovery of these tumors is often incidental. About 50% of esophageal SMTs are asymptomatic, and identified on endoscopy or imaging obtained for other reasons. A chest x-ray may show a mediastinal prominence in the case of a large tumor. Computed tomography (CT) of the chest can provide a clearer depiction of a small lesion, but findings may be subtle, suggesting esophageal wall thickening only. A contrast esophagram usually shows a smooth-walled indentation on the column of contrast.[2] The differential diagnosis for SMTs is broad, including benign solid tumor, cyst, vascular anomaly, or cancer. As advancements in imaging technology have developed, confidence in determining the benign nature of these lesions without tissue for diagnosis has grown. However, in some cases, multiple imaging modalities may still not definitively rule out malignancy. Standard endoscopic forceps biopsy or endoscopic ultrasound (EUS)-guided fine-needle aspiration (FNA) may be inadequate or indeterminate due to the submucosal location of the tumor, and whether biopsy is advisable. For large or symptomatic SMTs, surgical resection is generally recommended. However, surveillance versus surgical resection may be considered for small, asymptomatic tumors.

Due to the overall rare incidence of SMTs, evidence-based recommendations are mostly limited to findings from a few small series. The exception to this is leiomyoma, which is relatively frequent. Observation has been generally recommended for asymptomatic lesions less than 3 cm in diameter. However, concerns for patient compliance, the cost of repeat surveillance, the potential for delayed diagnosis of malignancy, and patient anxiety may lead physicians to recommend resection of small esophageal SMTs.[4]

Treatment options for esophageal SMTs have evolved in recent years. Targeted molecular therapy has greatly improved outcomes for gastrointestinal stromal tumors (GIST), and recommendations for optimizing medical therapy are evolving. Observation and surveillance of small and asymptomatic esophageal SMTs may be possible now with better diagnostic techniques in cases of well defined, small, asymptomatic, benign esophageal lesions with low potential for malignancy.[2] Historically, surgical resection was recommended for esophageal or GEJ SMTs, for both treatment and definitive diagnosis. Open laparotomy or thoracotomy for surgical enucleation or esophagectomy was recommended. Minimally invasive techniques including laparoscopy, video-assisted thoracoscopic surgery (VATS), and robotic surgical techniques have gained acceptance with improved outcomes in postoperative pain, pulmonary complications, and length of stay. More recently, purely endoscopic techniques for resection of select esophageal SMTs have been shown to be feasible and safe when performed by experienced endoscopists.

SURGERY

Surgical resection is the mainstay of treatment for leiomyoma. Indications for surgical resection include symptomatic lesions, inability to rule out malignancy or distinguish from GIST, atypical imaging findings, overlying mucosal erosion or dysplastic changes, regional lymphadenopathy, large tumors (size recommendation is variable), and tumor growth during surveillance.[5]

Traditionally SMTs, particularly leiomyomas, were resected by either enucleation via right or left thoracotomy, or laparotomy for GEJ tumors. With open access to the esophagus or GEJ, the surgeon can visualize and palpate the tumor to precisely localize it. The overlying pleura is incised, and the longitudinal and circular muscle split. The tumor is dissected from the surrounding muscle, submucosa, and enucleated from the underlying mucosa. Any mucosal injuries (incidence reported at 7% in open cases) are closed primarily, and the overlying muscle layers and pleura are generally closed (Fig. 46.1).[2,6] The safety and efficacy of the open approach has been well documented.[5,7,8] Mortality of thoracotomy with enucleation is less than 1.3%, and around 90% of patients were reported to be symptom free after 5 years.[5] Esophagectomy may be indicated for tumors greater than 8 cm or diffuse

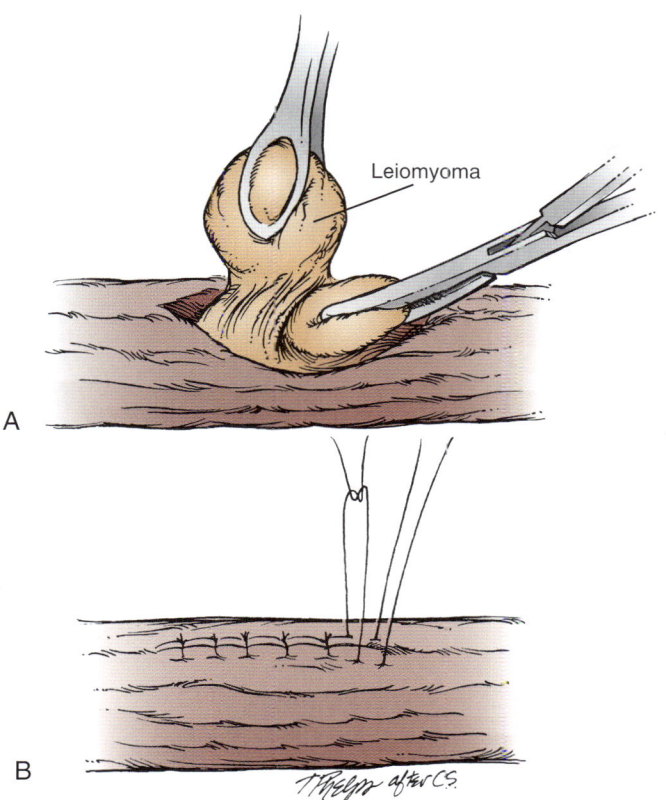

FIGURE 46.1 (A) The esophageal muscular fibers are split and the leiomyoma is bluntly extracted from the esophageal wall. (B) Once removed, the muscular defect is reapproximated.

leiomyomatosis. Esophagectomy historically has been required for about 5% to 10% of leiomyoma patients.[2,8,9]

Laparoscopic and video-assisted thoracoscopic resection is now widely accepted and found to be safe in case series.[10,11] Robotic minimally invasive surgery is also a safe and feasible option.[6,12] The length of stay for minimally invasive enucleation is about half that expected for open thoracic surgery.[8] Laparoscopic enucleation guided by intraoperative frozen section has been reported for tumors that displayed features concerning for GIST.[13] However, frozen section has been shown to be unreliable for differentiating GIST from leiomyoma, as immunohistochemistry is required to confirm the diagnosis.[14] The thoracoscopic approach may be required for more proximal lesions, and the esophagus is usually accessed through the right chest. Compared to thoracotomy, VATS reduces pulmonary complications, postoperative pain, and length of stay.[8,15] Intraoperative endoscopy is beneficial for the identification of small tumors and testing mucosal integrity after enucleation (Fig. 46.2).[15] A few cases of robotic enucleation for esophageal leiomyoma have been reported. Surgeons who have used this technique suggest that the benefits include improved dexterity, precision, and visibility, allowing minimized esophageal mobilization and avoidance of mucosal injury.[6] Up-front cost, the requirement of a bedside surgeon, and docking time are concerns that must be individually weighed against the potential benefits of this approach.[6,12]

Minimally invasive tumor localization can be improved with intraoperative endoscopy for specific localization of small lesions, and intraluminal balloons or bougies to help optimize the position of the lesion for surgical resection.[5,15,16] Laparoscopic transgastric or intragastric surgery has been reported for difficult-to-reach leiomyomas that are posteriorly located at the GEJ (Fig. 46.3).[17] With this technique, trocars are placed through the abdominal wall and then directly into the lumen of the stomach.

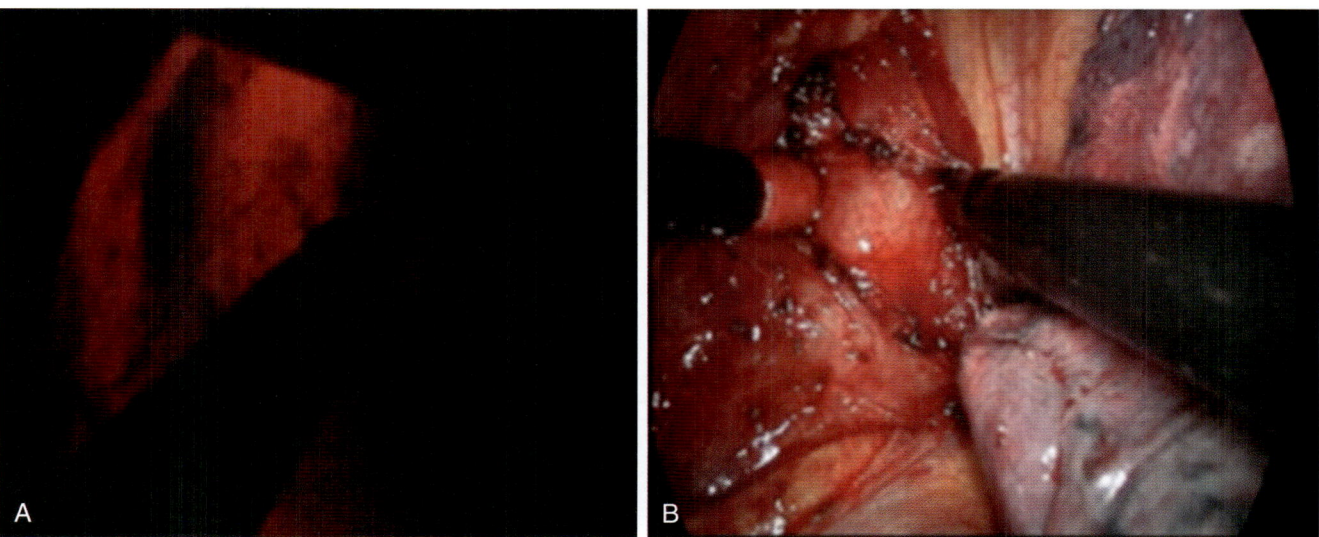

FIGURE 46.2 Tumor localization was performed under esophagoscopy, and myotomy was performed at the tumor level. (A) Tumor localization by transillumination. (B) Myotomy at the tumor level. (From Jeon HW, Choi MG, Lim CH, Park JK, Sung SW. Intraoperative esophagoscopy provides accuracy and safety in video-assisted thoracoscopic enucleation of benign esophageal submucosal tumors. *Dis Esophagus*. 2015;28:438.)

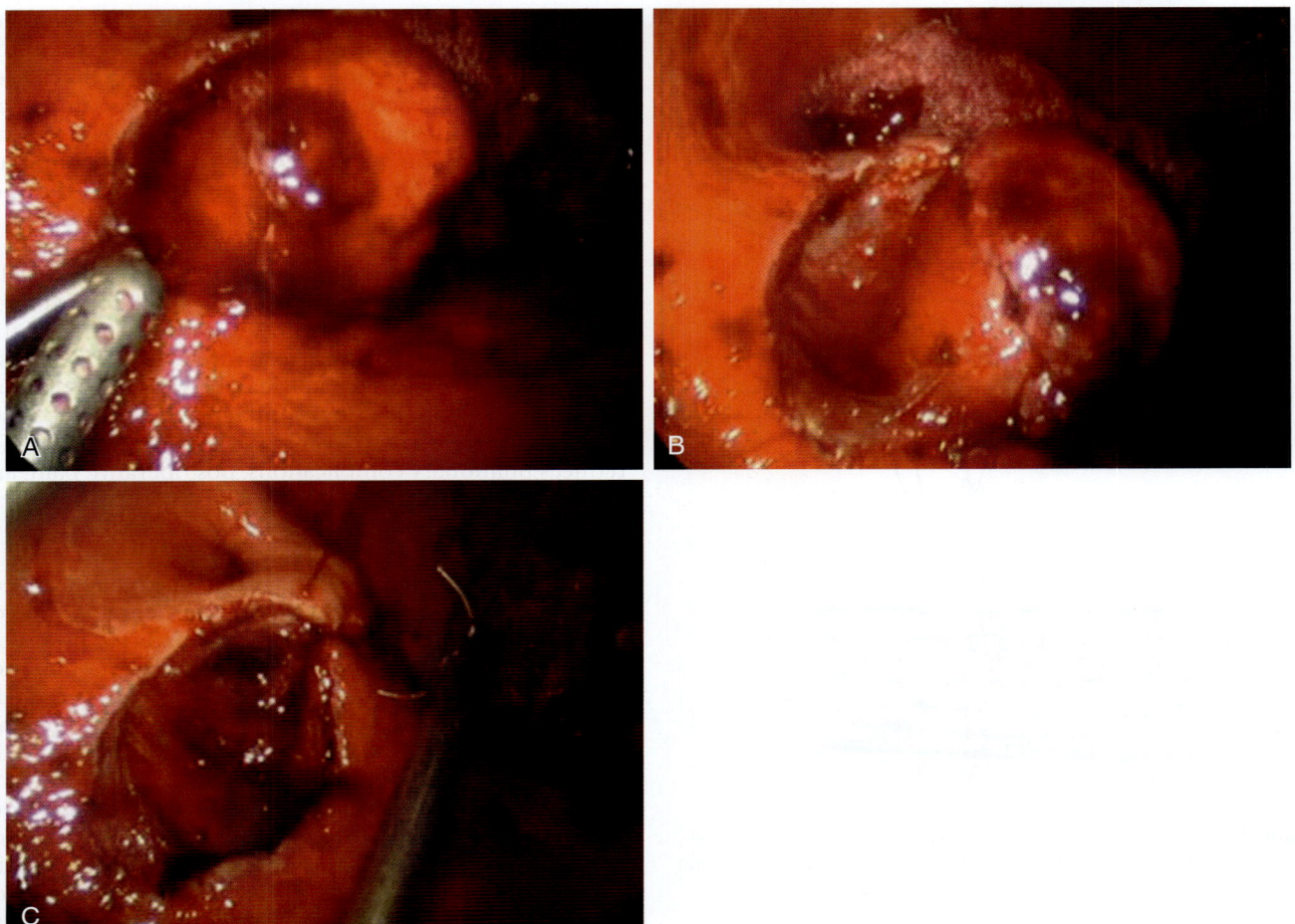

FIGURE 46.3 (A) Intraluminal submucosal lesion. (B) Partially enucleated lesion. (C) Intracorporeal closure of the mucosal and submucosal defect. (From Mino JS, Guerron AD, Monteiro R, et al. Long-term outcomes of combined endoscopic/laparoscopic intragastric enucleation of presumed gastric stromal tumors. *Surg Endosc.* 2016;30:1749.)

Capnogastrum is achieved with or without the aid of a coda balloon to occlude the gastric outlet. This approach may help to avoid excess resection and minimize the disruption of the angle of His at the GEJ, and has been successful for tumors as large as 7 cm.[18-20] Enucleation may be possible with combined endoscopic and laparoscopic instruments, but full-thickness resection is performed if enucleation with clear margins is not possible. The specimen can be removed via a specimen bag through a trocar site or transorally with the endoscope via a grasper or snare. The gastrotomy incisions are primarily closed with suture, but large defects from resection may be closed with an endoscopic stapler. If resection of a portion of the cardia is required and will leave a significant deformity of the GEJ, fundoplication should be considered to prevent postoperative reflux. The development of subsequent worsened or new onset gastroesophageal reflux disease (GERD) after resection of GEJ lesions or enucleation of midesophageal lesions has been reported.[8,16]

Endoscopic resection has been used more frequently in the last several years. Originally endoscopic resection techniques were used for the curative resection of well-differentiated squamous cell carcinoma of the esophagus.

Later, the technique was used for Barrett esophagus with high-grade dysplasia or intramucosal adenocarcinoma. The endoscopic submucosal dissection (ESD) technique is commonly used for tunneling in peroral endoscopic myotomy (POEM), a natural orifice transluminal endoscopic surgery (NOTES) procedure for the treatment of achalasia. Endoscopic resection has grown in popularity and indications have expanded as more surgeons and gastroenterologists gain experience with ESD and resection techniques. The particular approach depends upon the characteristics of the tumor and the experience of the endoscopist. A disadvantage of endoscopic resection is the learning curve, though it is reported to be relatively short for experienced endoscopists.[21]

ENDOSCOPIC MUCOSAL RESECTION

Endoscopic mucosal resection (EMR; Fig. 46.4) may be used for small, superficial tumors (<2 cm, superficial to submucosa). EMR separates the full thickness of mucosa from the underlying muscle layers. With this technique, a lifting solution is injected into the submucosal layer beneath the tumor to create a pseudopolyp, which can then be banded and snared to complete the resection.[22,23]

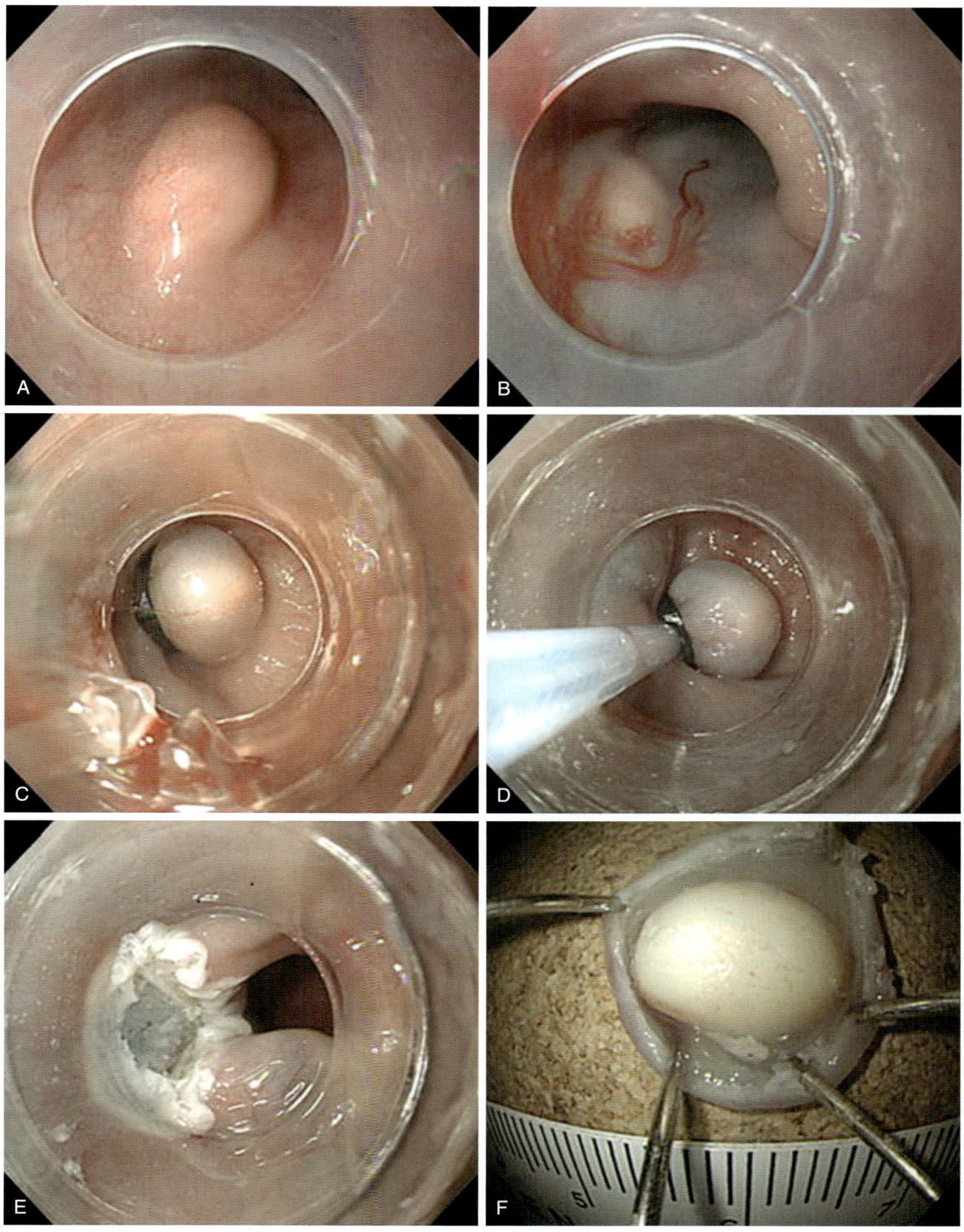

FIGURE 46.4 Endoscopic mucosal resection of a submucosal tumor (SMT) using a ligation device in the esophagus. (A) An SMT is observed in the lower esophagus. (B) Saline solution with a small amount of epinephrine and indigo carmine dye is injected beneath the lesion to elevate it. (C) The lesion is then aspirated into the ligation device, followed by deployment of the elastic band. (D) Snare resection is performed using a blended electrosurgical current. (E) The lesion is completely removed. (F) Inner surface of the resected specimen. (From Kahng DH, Kim GH, Park DY, et al. Endoscopic resection of granular cell tumors in the gastrointestinal tract: a single center experience. *Surg Endosc*. 2013;27:3230.)

ENDOSCOPIC MUCOSAL RESECTION TECHNIQUE

Endoscopy is performed with a high-definition single- or double-channel endoscope. A 23- or 25-gauge endoscopic needle is used to infiltrate the submucosa deep to the lesion with dilute indigo carmine or methylene blue solution, with or without epinephrine, to lift the lesion and expand and highlight the plane between it and the adjacent layers. To aid visualization in the limited working space of the esophagus, the injection is begun distal to the lesion and then sequential injections are placed proximally. The lesion should lift on the cushion of infiltrated submucosa in order to allow for en bloc resection. Failure to lift indicates a misplaced tip of the needle, most commonly too deep into the muscle, which can be adjusted by slowly withdrawing while gently injecting. If adjusting the needle fails to create an adequate lift, this suggests infiltration or scarring of the tumor into the deeper muscle layers. A simple cautery snare can be used for a well-lifted small lesion, but usually other techniques may be required to avoid piecemeal resection for an adherent tumor.

Cap-assisted EMR can be used with a single-channel endoscope with the cap in place. The targeted lesion then can be fully suctioned into the cap prior to snaring it. For more precise resection, a variceal band can be applied to ligate and position the lesion as a pseudopolyp so that the snare can be placed under direct vision. As an alternative to the cap-assisted technique, an endoscopic grasper can be used to lift the lesion for snaring, but this requires a dual-channel endoscope. The resection bed is then checked for bleeding or perforation. The specimen can be sucked into the cap and retrieved with the scope, or with grasping forceps or a retrieval net.

Endoscopic Submucosal Dissection

ESD (Fig. 46.5), though currently performed most frequently in Asia, endoscopists worldwide have begun to accept and use this technique. ESD is indicated for larger, deeper tumors. ESD variations include endoscopic submucosal tunneling or, in select cases, even full-thickness resection. ESD is indicated for tumors larger than 2 cm or involving layers deep into the mucosa, which cannot be captured en bloc by the limited dimensions of the EMR cap. Feasible size ranges from 2 to 8 cm depending on author, though greater than 5 cm usually requires piecemeal resection or at least dividing the lesion to allow extraction.[24,25] ESD involves a customized incision through the normal mucosa and dissection beneath and around the lesion through the submucosal plane. The dissection is performed with one of several varieties of endoscopic electrosurgical knives.

ENDOSCOPIC SUBMUCOSAL DISSECTION TECHNIQUE

The line of the planned incision is demarcated with cautery, marking every few millimeters along the circumference of the lesion as the intended margin of resection, a few millimeters away from the lesion to allow for shrinkage of the tissue while still preserving the pathologic margin (5 mm for malignant lesion to avoid a coagulation effect on the tumor). The margin of the specimen may be similarly marked for subsequent pathologic orientation. A dissecting cap is used to aid in retraction and visualization without the dissected tissues obscuring the lens of the scope. A lifting solution (2 mL indigo carmine/methylene blue, 1 mL epinephrine, 100 mL saline) is injected into the submucosal layer at the marked margin of resection, moving from a distal to a proximal direction, similar to the technique used for EMR. A small mucosal incision is created circumferentially with the electrosurgical knife into the submucosal layer. For a small lesion, a snare may now be used to complete the resection through the submucosal layer. For most lesions, the submucosal tissue is dissected directly, gradually separating and peeling the overlying lesion off of the muscular layers beneath. Once completely resected, the resection bed is inspected for bleeding or full-thickness violation of the muscular layers. Judicious use of cautery is used to achieve hemostasis, avoiding injury to the thin tissue. The specimen is then collected with a snare, grasping forceps, or retrieval nets, and extracted.

TUNNEL TECHNIQUE

For submucosal tunneling (Figs. 46.6 and 46.7), a lift is established similar to that described in the previous sections, except starting 2 to 3 cm proximal to the proximal edge of the lesion. A 1 to 2 cm mucosotomy is made and a submucosal tunnel created to approach the lesion—as described in the POEM technique first described by Inoue in humans.[26] Continue in this plane to lift the mucosa off the lesion; then it can be dissected off of and out of the muscularis. This may require full muscle thickness incision, exposing the mediastinal connective tissue, but the risk of infection or leak is minimized by careful preservation and clip closure of the mucosa. Once it is completely freed, the lesion is extracted with forceps or a snare. The tunneling technique has been recommended when feasible, with the potential benefit over standard ESD of being able to completely close the mucosal defect. This technique is suggested to have faster recovery and healing time over standard ESD.[24] In this case, even if the resection was full thickness through the circular and longitudinal muscle fibers, the closed mucosa should prevent leak or development of mediastinitis or peritonitis, similar to full-thickness POEM.

Intraoperative concerns including capnothorax, capnomediastinum, or capnoperitoneum are usually conservatively managed as the CO_2 (which should be used exclusively as opposed to air insufflation) is quick to absorb. Occasionally needle or Veress needle decompression or a percutaneous drain may be needed if the patient is symptomatic or if ventilator pressures become supraphysiologic.

Delayed perforation, leak, or fistula are dreaded postoperative concerns.[4,24] A follow-up swallow study can help rule out leak before feeding. A liquid diet is allowed for several days to allow healing before advancing to solid meals. Bleeding or persistence of a painful ulcer is of concern, particularly if the mucosal defect is not closed. Proton pump inhibitor (PPI) or mucosal protecting agents may be required for short-term use while ulcers heal, and follow-up endoscopy should be performed to ensure healing. Stricture formation may occur, particularly for large lesions requiring extensive resection. For any endoscopic resection technique, local recurrence due to inadequate resection is

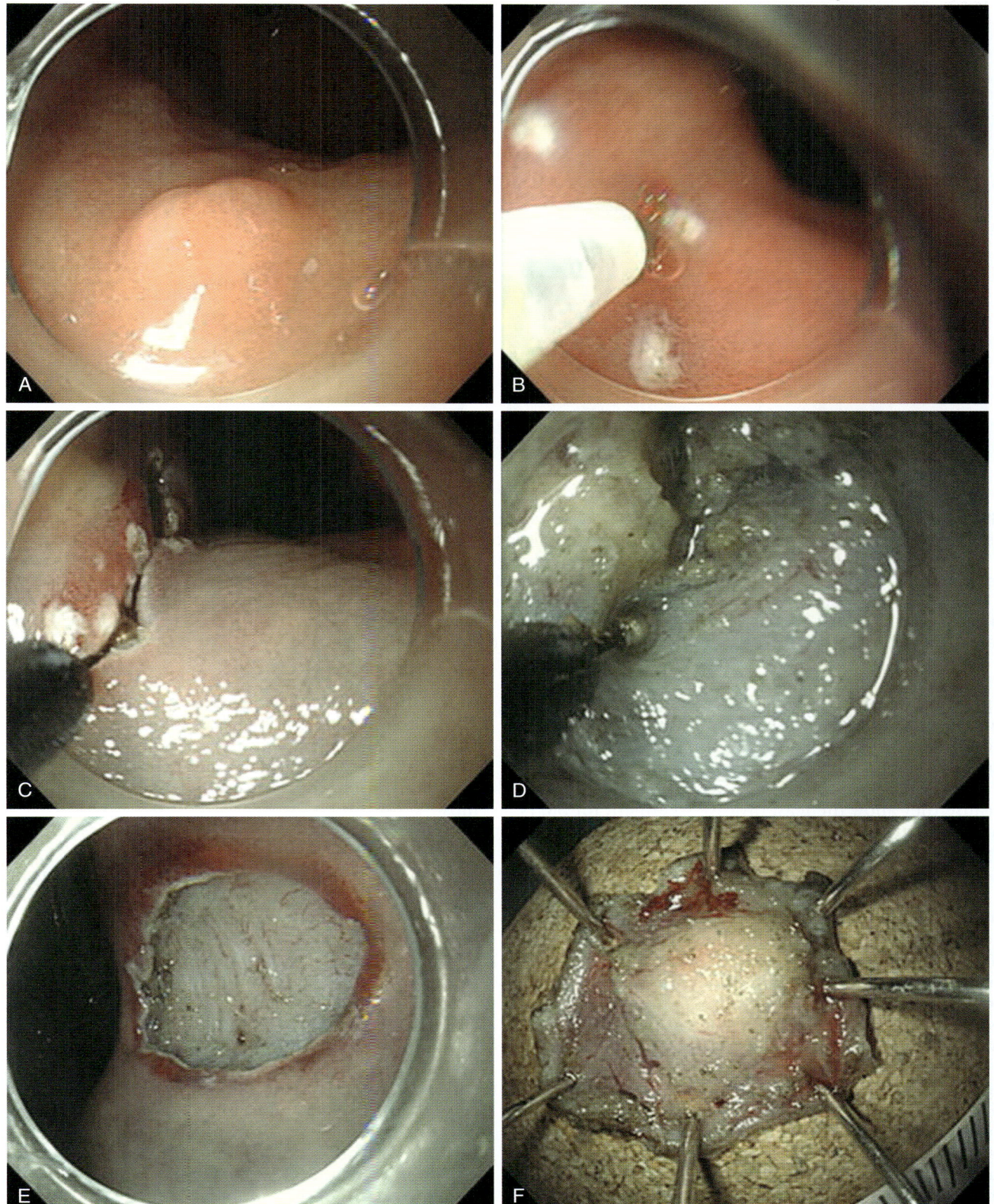

FIGURE 46.5 Endoscopic submucosal dissection of a submucosal tumor (SMT) in the stomach. (A) An SMT is observed in the upper body of the stomach. (B) Marking dots are made around the lesion and saline with epinephrine and indigo carmine is then injected into the submucosa beneath the lesion. (C) A complete circumferential incision is made using an insulated-tip (IT) knife. (D) Submucosal dissection is made using an IT knife. (E) The lesion is completely removed. (F) Inner surface of the resected specimen. (From Kahng DH, Kim GH, Park DY, et al. Endoscopic resection of granular cell tumors in the gastrointestinal tract: a single center experience. *Surg Endosc*. 2013;27:3230.)

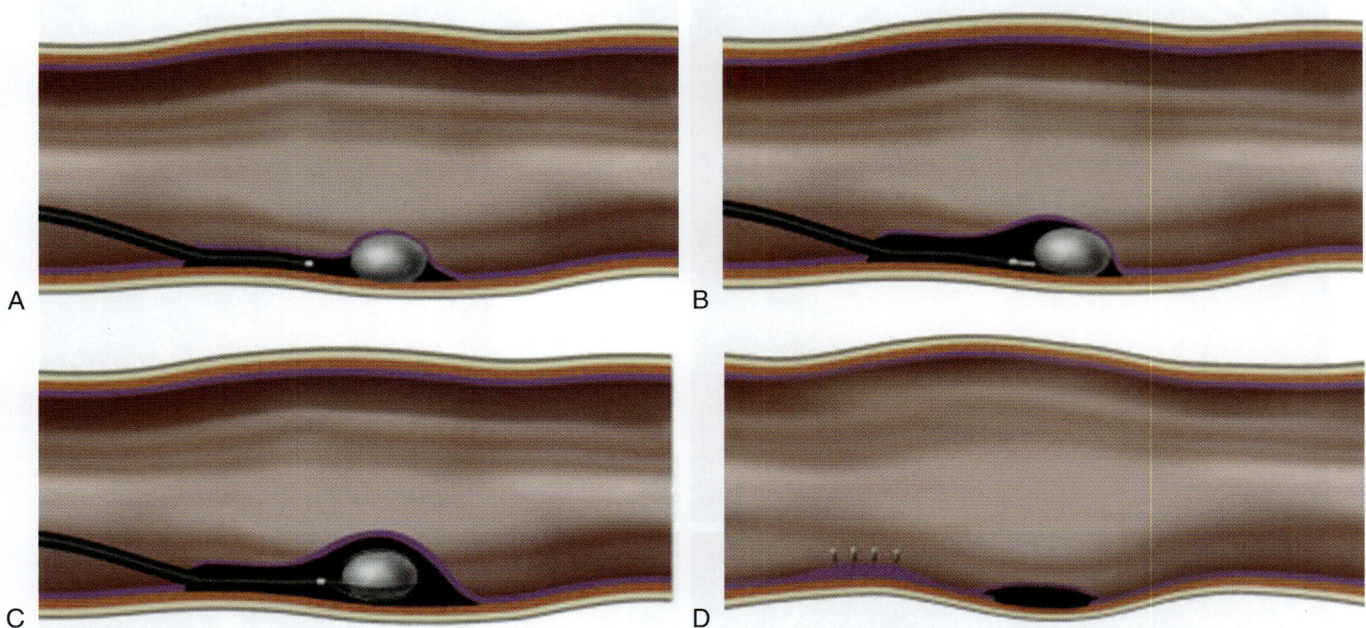

FIGURE 46.6 (A) Submucosal tunneling: a submucosal tunnel 5 cm above the tumor is created by endoscopic mucosectomy. Epinephrine or similar solution is injected into submucosa to separate the superficial mucosa from muscularis propria and create a submucosal cavity. (B) Tumor separation and resection: the submucosal tumor is separated from surrounding tissue and dissected from muscularis propria and mucosa. (C) Removal of the submucosal tumor: the submucosal tumor is totally extracted and carefully removed with an insulated-tip knife through the submucosal tunnel. (D) Closure of the mucosal entry orifice: after complete hemostasis in the submucosal tunnel, the mucosal entry orifice is tightly closed with hemostatic tips. (From Chen WS, Zheng XL, Jin L, Pan XJ, Ye MF. Novel diagnosis and treatment of esophageal granular cell tumor: report of 14 cases and review of the literature. *Ann Thorac Surg*. 2014;97:298.)

of primary concern. Follow-up interval endoscopy (in some protocols even before discharge) and EUS at 3 months and 12 months is generally recommended, though this may vary depending on tumor pathology.

Endoscopic resections appeal to patients and clinicians because they allow the least invasive treatment for SMTs. Outcomes are good, with few serious complications, improved postoperative pain, and length of stay compared to other surgical techniques. In the largest study to date of ESD for SMT by He et al, 224 cases were reviewed.[4] The SMTs were localized 41% esophageal and 6% cardia and were resected with en bloc ESD. These were mostly small tumors, mean diameter 13.6 mm, 39% originating from muscularis mucosae, 51% from muscularis propria, and 10% from submucosa. Submucosal tunnel endoscopic resection was performed for lesions greater than 2 cm, involving muscularis propria, or at the GEJ. The majority of tumors in the esophagus were leiomyomas, and the majority of those at the cardia were GIST. Of these patients 5% of attempts at ESD failed; 1.8% required conversion to surgery for bleeding or perforation. Overall, 6.25% of cases included perforation, and all but one were managed conservatively. There were no cases of mediastinitis or fistula, and no development of diverticulum at the resection site during the course of follow-up. Procedure time varied from 10 to 180 minutes with a mean of 47 minutes. Length of stay mean was 4.9 days, with a range of 1 to 31 days. There was a 1.3% incidence of incomplete resection. All of these cases of incomplete resection were identified on the first surveillance EUS postoperatively and were treated

successfully with repeat endoscopic resection. At the 12-month follow-up there were no instances of recurrence.[4] Declining morbidity and mortality have been observed over time with all surgical techniques.[2] SMTs overall have excellent prognosis; most require limited resection and most patients fully recover without persistent symptoms.

TUMORS BY TYPE: LEIOMYOMA

A leiomyoma is the most common benign esophageal or GEJ tumor of mesenchymal origin, sharing a common cell origin with GIST and schwannoma.[1,2] Sixty to seventy percent of benign esophageal tumors are leiomyomas. Twelve percent of all gastrointestinal leiomyomas originate in the esophagus.[27] Leiomyomas of the esophagus are rare, representing only 0.4% to 1% of all esophageal tumors; esophageal cancer is 50-fold more common.[2,13,28] The ratio of leiomyoma of the esophagus in men and women is 2:1. These tumors have been reported in both adults and children. Though rare in children younger than 12 years of age, 90% of cases in children have diffuse leiomyomatosis affecting extensive portions of the esophagus, and may be related to other syndromes.[2,29,30]

The most common location for leiomyomas is in the distal two-thirds of the esophagus. A large study reported the esophageal location as upper third in 8.5%, middle third in 38.2%, lower third in 46.5%, and at the GEJ in 6.8%.[31] Most commonly, leiomyomas originate in intramural layers of the esophagus, but variations may develop extraluminally, extending into the mediastinum, or intraluminally with polypoid features.[2] Leiomyomas

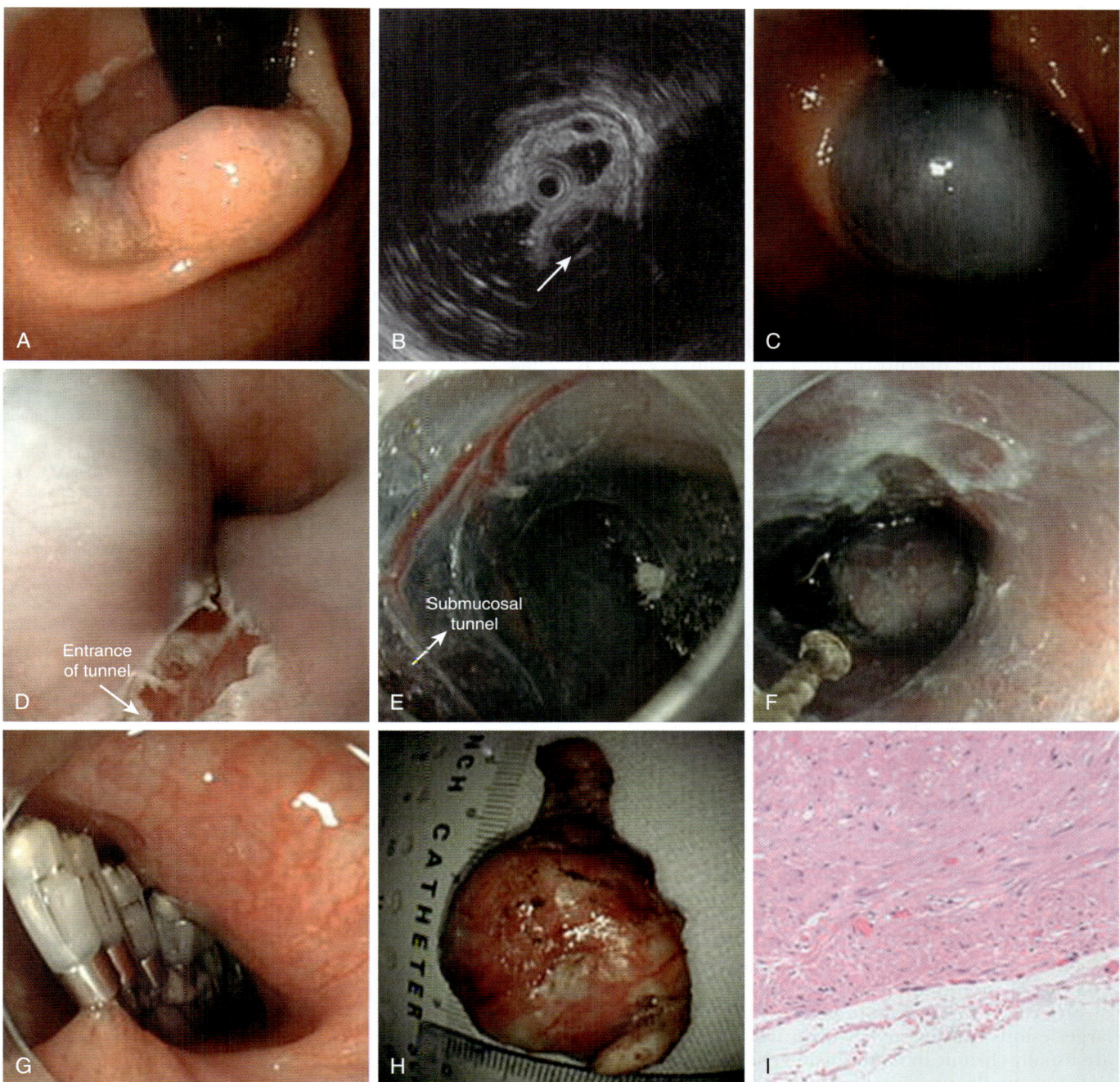

FIGURE 46.7 Submucosal tunnel endoscopic resection for a submucosal tumor (SMT) of the esophagogastric junction (EGJ). (A) SMT at the EGJ. (B) Endoscopic ultrasound (EUS) showing a lesion originating from the muscularis propria (MP) layer *(arrow)*. (C) Submucosal injection for marking tumor location preoperatively to prevent mistaking the target tissue in the tunnel cavity. (D) A 2-cm longitudinal mucosal incision was made approximately 5 cm proximal to the SMT *(arrow)*. (E) The submucosal tunnel is established *(arrow)*. (F) Separating the tumor from the MP layer using the hybrid knife. (G) The mucosal entry incision is sealed with several clips. (H) Irregularly-shaped, completely resected specimen (maximum diameter 30 mm). (I) Macroscopic findings of the resected specimen revealed a leiomyoma (H&E, ×20). (From Wang XY, Xu MD, Yao LQ, et al. Submucosal tunneling endoscopic resection for submucosal tumors of the esophagogastric junction originating from the muscularis propria layer: a feasibility study (with videos). *Surg Endosc.* 2014;28:1973.)

may originate from muscularis mucosae, from muscularis propria, or from submucosa of the esophagus.[32]

Grossly, a leiomyoma is a firm, rubbery, encapsulated lesion with intact overlying mucosa. It is usually uniform or it can be asymmetrically shaped. The size ranges from a few millimeters to up to 29 cm. Leiomyomas over 1000 g are considered "giant."[2] Half of all leiomyomas are less than 5 cm in diameter, 85% are less than 10 cm. Ninety-seven percent of esophageal leiomyomas are solitary, but leiomyomatosis involving the entire esophageal smooth muscle layer occurs in 2.4% of cases.[33] A leiomyoma has low malignant potential. Malignant behavior is most closely related to tumor size greater than 4 cm or rapid growth.[2] About 0.2% of leiomyomas undergo malignant transformation to leiomyosarcoma.[13]

Histologic features, immunohistochemical staining, and clinical characteristics of mesenchymal esophageal tumors are summarized in Table 46.1.[2] The cell of origin for the mesenchymal esophageal tumors is thought to be interstitial cells of Cajal, which regulate gut peristalsis. These cells retain the ability to differentiate into smooth muscle (leiomyoma), stromal (GIST), or neural sheath (schwannoma) cells. Histopathology shows fascicles or whorls, low to moderate cellularity, and eosinophilic cytoplasm with fibrillary or clumped appearance.[2,32] Immunohistochemical staining can be diagnostic for a leiomyoma, which is usually positive for smooth muscle actin (SMA), desmin, and estrogen receptors. Leiomyoma is usually negative for CD117 and CD34, differentiating it from GIST.[28,34,35]

Leiomyoma has been reported in association with other foregut disorders, including achalasia, other esophageal motility disorders, hiatal hernia, and epiphrenic diverticulum. Resection of the tumor has been shown to correct dysmotility in some cases.[36] Leiomyomatosis has been rarely identified in association with some genetic disorders. Li-Fraumeni syndrome, caused by a p53 mutation, is associated with sarcoma, breast cancer, brain cancer, and rarely esophageal leiomyomatosis.[30] Alport syndrome, an X-linked recessive syndrome with glomerular nephropathy, sensorineural deafness, and ocular abnormalities, has been reported in association with diffuse leiomyomatosis, including esophageal, gastric, vulvovaginal, and bronchial leiomyomas.[29,35] Symptomatic presentation may be similar to that of achalasia. If symptoms are severe in the case of diffuse leiomyomatosis, the only viable surgical option is esophagectomy.[35]

As with most SMTs, about 50% of leiomyomas are asymptomatic, and the development of symptoms is largely dependent on size.[37] Symptoms may include dysphagia related to intraluminal obstruction, substernal or epigastric pain or pressure, heartburn, or weight loss. Bleeding is rare except in lesions that involve the stomach, with associated mucosal erosion due to acid exposure. Cough, dyspnea, or other respiratory symptoms may rarely develop from large lesions causing airway obstruction.[2,33,38] Symptoms are usually chronic in nature, and generally progress with time, eventually prompting evaluation.

Both endoscopic and radiographic modalities can confirm the diagnosis and localize the extent of the esophageal leiomyoma. Contrast esophagram will usually show a smooth lesion with crisp margins that bulges into the lumen and impinges upon the column of esophageal contrast (Fig. 46.8).[2] Leiomyomas are rarely responsible for true obstruction or proximal esophageal dilation unless they are quite large or located at the GEJ.[2] CT is useful to evaluate the local involvement in larger tumors, and usually depicts an eccentric area of esophageal wall thickening (Fig. 46.9).[6] Positron emission tomography (PET) scans for leiomyoma may demonstrate abnormal 18-fluorodexoxyglucose (FDG) uptake (Fig. 46.10).[13] These tumors exhibit a broad spectrum of FDG avidity, with reports ranging from the standardized uptake value

TABLE 46.1 Esophageal Mesenchymal Tumors

Features	Schwannoma	Leiomyoma	GIST
Histology	Moderately cellular Peripheral lymphoid cuff Spindle cells	Eosinophilic cytoplasm	Highly cellular
Molecular genetic markers	+S-100, GFAP −CD117, CD34, SMA	+Desmin, SMA −CD117, CD34	+CD117, CD34
Gender ratio (M:F)	1:1	2:1	2:1
Mean age (y)	54	35	63
Malignant potential	Lowest	Mixed	Highest

GFAP, Glial fibrillary acidic protein; *GIST*, gastrointestinal stromal tumor; *SMA*, smooth muscle actin.

Data from Mansour KA, Hatcher CR, Haun CL. Benign tumors of the esophagus: experience with 20 cases. *South Med J.* 1977;70:461; Sweet RH, Soutter L, Valenzuela CT. Muscle wall tumors of the esophagus. *J Thorac Surg.* 1954;27:13, discussion 35; Nemir P Jr, Wallace HW, Fallahnejad M. Diagnosis and surgical management of benign diseases of the esophagus. *Curr Probl Surg.* 1976;13:1; Reed CE. Benign tumors of the esophagus. *Chest Surg Clin N Am.* 1994;4:769; Herrera JL. Benign and metastatic tumors of the esophagus. *Gastroenterol Clin North Am.* 1991;20:775; Avezzano EA, Fleischer DE, Merida MA, et al. Giant fibrovascular polyps of the esophagus. *Am J Gastroenterol.* 1990;85:299; Went PT, Dirnhofer S, Bundi M, et al. Prevalence of KIT expression in human tumors. *J Clin Oncol.* 2004;22:4514; Miettinen M, Sarlomo-Rikala M, Sobin LH, et al. Esophageal stromal tumors: a clinicopathologic, immunohistochemical, and molecular genetic study of 17 cases and comparison with esophageal leiomyomas and leiomyosarcomas. *Am J Surg Pathol.* 2000;24:211.

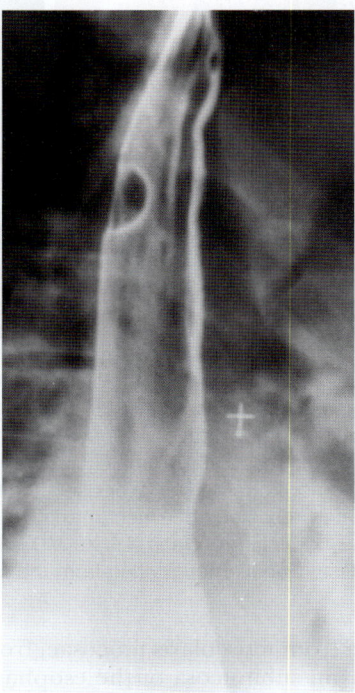

FIGURE 46.8 Contrast esophagram demonstrating the characteristic findings of a leiomyoma.

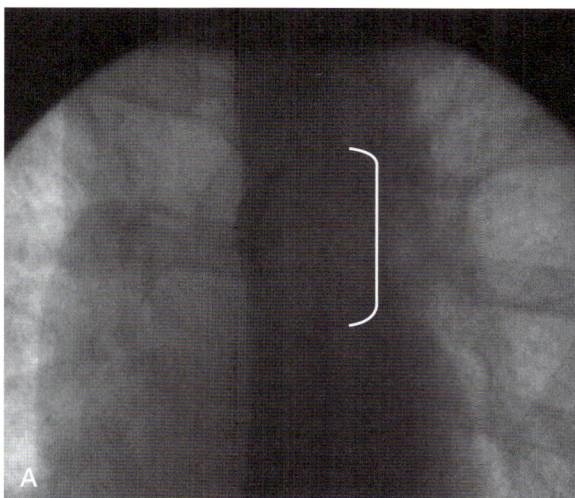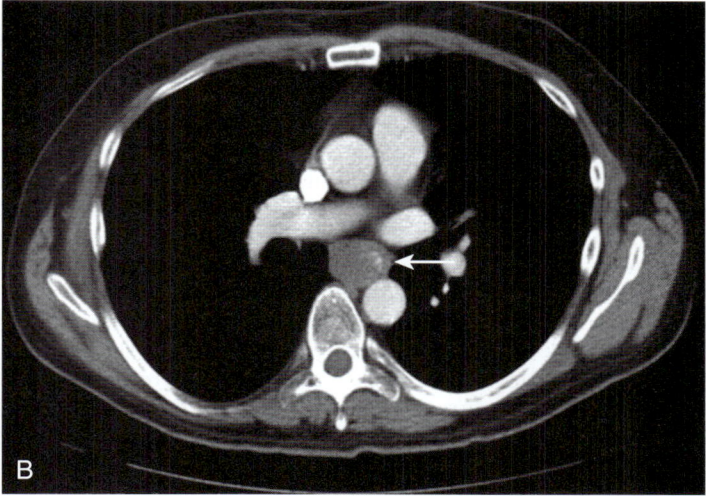

FIGURE 46.9 Barium swallow (A) and computed tomogram (B) reveal a large heterogeneous esophageal mass *(arrow)* measuring ~3.3 cm. (From Kernstine KH, Andersen ES, Falabella A, Ramirez NA, Anderson CA, Beblawi I. Robotic fourth-arm enucleation of an esophageal leiomyoma and review of literature. *Innovations [Phila]*. 2009;4:355.)

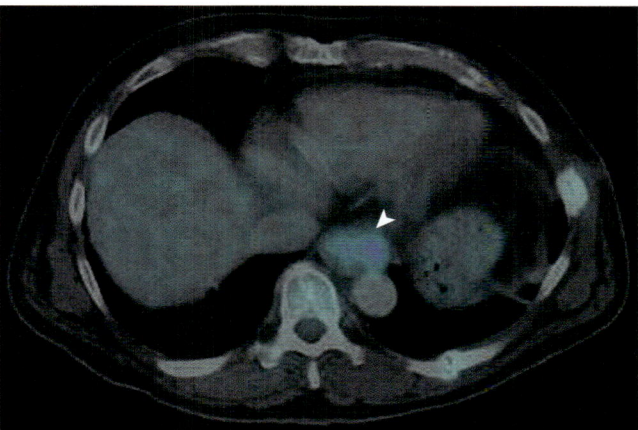

FIGURE 46.10 Positron emission tomography/computed tomography scan with abnormally increased fluorodeoxyglucose uptake *(arrowhead)* in an esophageal submucosal tumor. (From Haddad J, Bouazza F, Barake H, Liberale G, Flamen P, Nakadi IE. Surgical strategy in abnormally increased Fluorine-18 fluorodeoxyglucose uptake in an asymptomatic lower esophageal submucosal tumor—report of a case. *Int J Surg Case Rep.* 2014;5:590.)

maximum of 1.4 to 13.4. Clinicians should be aware of this finding in leiomyoma; however, it does not definitively indicate malignancy, nor does it reliably help in differentiating leiomyoma from GIST.[2,28,34,39,40] Similar FDG-PET avidity has been identified in gastroesophageal reflux disease (GERD), Barrett esophagus, and infectious and inflammatory conditions, and about 8.3% of FDG-avid esophageal lesions are malignant.[34]

Endoscopically, leiomyoma usually appears as a mobile bulge, with intact overlying mucosa, and may cause some luminal narrowing without obstruction (Fig. 46.11).[27] EUS can be helpful to identify the layer involved, and the extent of the lesion, the margins, and the size, and

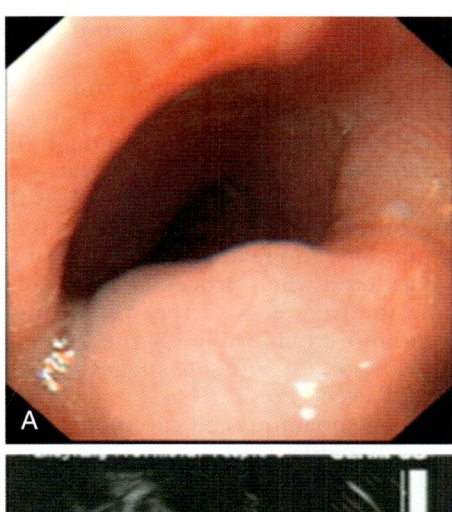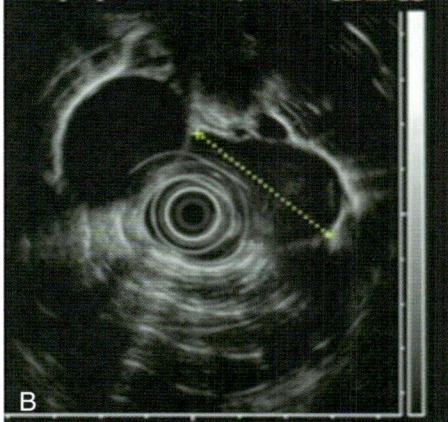

FIGURE 46.11 (A) Esophageal submucosal tumor. (B) Endoscopic ultrasonography imaging of the lesion arising from the muscularis mucosa. (With permission from Fei BY, Yang JM, Zhao ZS. Differential clinical and pathological characteristics of esophageal stromal tumors and leiomyomata. *Dis Esophagus*. 2014;27:32.)

can help predict histologic diagnosis.[4] An ultrasound of leiomyoma usually identifies a hypoechoic, homogeneous, well-demarcated lesion without locoregional lymphadenopathy (Fig. 46.11).[27] Large, irregular, heterogeneous, and locoregional lymphadenopathy are more suspicious for malignant tumor.[2,41] Endoscopic forceps or EUS-guided FNA biopsy of suspected leiomyoma is controversial. Traditionally, in the surgical literature, biopsy was condemned as a source of adhesions to mucosa, adding to the difficulty of operative resection and increasing the risk of mucosal injury, bleeding, leak, fistula, or mediastinitis.[8] However, others report no technical disadvantage after biopsy.[6,12,13,16,28,42,43] Proponents of biopsy suggest that EUS-guided needle biopsy is safe and is indicated in lesions with a diameter greater than 2 cm, growth during observation, or PET avidity to help guide management.[14,27] Immunohistochemistry is diagnostic, but adequate tissue may be difficult to obtain, with 50% to 80% of EUS-FNA samples being inadequate or pathologically inconclusive. Without biopsy, the accuracy of EUS predicting histologic diagnosis is about 80%, and the accuracy in predicting layer of origin of the tumor is 74.6%.[4] EUS with FNA biopsy sensitivity is 95%, specificity 100%, and diagnostic yield 85%, and it increases with three or more needle passes to improve diagnostic yield.[27,44]

In the case of a tumor with clinical and imaging characteristics consistent with a very small, benign leiomyoma, observation alone may be sufficient. Although there is not a definitive consensus, some experts in favor of surveillance suggest it is acceptable in lesions less than 2 cm in diameter; others suggest a cutoff of 4 to 5 cm.[21] Size, location, symptoms, and features of the tumor should be carefully considered when proceeding with observation to determine the frequency of repeat imaging. Patients should be monitored clinically for the development of symptoms, with some protocols suggesting endoscopy and EUS or CT every 6 months to 2 years.[10] At least one case of overlying squamous cell carcinoma and another of high-grade dysplasia associated with leiomyoma have been reported.[2,42] The underlying mechanism is thought to be increased stress and exposure of overlying mucosa due to mass effect.

LEIOMYOSARCOMA

Leiomyosarcoma, a malignant esophageal mesenchymal tumor, has a worse prognosis than other SMTs. Survival in the Chinese population at 1, 3, and 5 years is 60.2%, 42.8%, and 32.1%, respectively. Prognosis is better than other forms of esophageal cancer due to slow growth and relatively late presentation of metastatic disease. The treatment of leiomyosarcoma is primarily by surgical resection. Though this tumor is not typically radiosensitve, radiotherapy may be attempted in cases of unresectable disease.[45]

GASTROINTESTINAL STROMAL TUMOR

GIST is a mesenchymal tumor of the esophagus with specific molecular genetic features that differs from leiomyoma and schwannoma. GIST is the most common soft tissue sarcoma of the gastrointestinal tract, and develops as the result of mutations leading to the abnormal expression of c-KIT or platelet-derived growth factor

alpha. Of mesenchymal SMTs, GIST is less common than leiomyoma, but more common than schwannoma, and has greater malignant potential than either of these. GIST usually presents in older patients with the median age at presentation in the sixth decade, and rarely in patients under age 30.[46] The incidence of GIST is slightly higher in males than in females; the reported incidence from Surveillance, Epidemiology, and End Results (SEER) data was 54% in men and 46% in women between 1992 and 2000.[47] The incidence of GIST of all sites based on population studies is estimated to be about 10 cases per million, with only 1% of these being esophageal in origin.[46-48] Most esophageal GIST develops in the lower third, which is consistent with the increased distribution of interstitial cells of Cajal.[49]

The most common location for GIST is in the stomach, but they can develop anywhere in the gastrointestinal (GI) tract. Esophageal GIST symptoms are similar to leiomyoma, and may include dysphagia, globus, pain, or bleeding. Grossly, GIST is a firm, solid lesion. Histologically, GIST is a highly cellular lesion; the majority are spindle cell type, fewer are epithelioid type, and rarely, a combination of the two cellular patterns may be included.[46] Molecular genetic markers that can help to differentiate GIST from leiomyoma or schwanomma include positive KIT CD117 and CD34. Few GIST tumors (about 5%) are KIT negative, in which case DOG1, a calcium-dependent chloride channel protein may be tested and seems to be consistently expressed in GIST regardless of the type of mutation.[46]

Endoscopy is typically the first modality to identify esophageal GIST. GIST greater than 2 cm should prompt a staging work-up including CT of the abdomen/pelvis with contrast and chest CT.[50] PET may be useful to clarify ambiguous imaging findings or evaluate metastatic disease in consideration of resection, though some leiomyoma may be FDG avid as well.[46] EUS features may include increased echogenicity of GIST compared to leiomyoma, but this also has not been shown to be consistently reliable for diagnosis. EUS-guided FNA is generally included in the diagnostic algorithm when GIST is suspected, and is recommended in current National Comprehensive Cancer Network (NCCN) guidelines for management. EUS-FNA sensitivity is 95%, specificity 100%, and diagnostic yield 85%, and is increased with three or more needle passes to improve diagnostic yield.[27,44] In cases suspicious for esophageal GIST that are readily resectable, some experts have recommended avoiding preoperative FNA to avoid potential tumor rupture and dissemination, and for concerns of complicating resection margins with scar tissue.[8,46] However, biopsy results may change the management approach. Resection is recommended even for small GIST less than 2 cm with high-risk features, while GIST less than 2 cm with low-risk features may be considered for surveillance. The decision to obtain FNA biopsy should be individualized based on suspected tumor type and extent of disease.[50] For unresectable or metastatic tumors, tissue diagnosis is required to guide chemotherapy. We favor EUS with FNA biopsy of SMTs concerning for GIST to obtain precise measurement of the tumor size, mitotic activity in aspirated cells, and endoscopic features such as mucosal ulceration or erosion that may affect the surgical strategy.

Indications for the surgical resection of GIST generally include a size greater than 2 cm (though high-risk features may indicate resection for smaller GIST), development of symptoms, or growth while under surveillance. For GIST not meeting criteria for resection, surveillance by EUS every 6 to 12 months should be considered.[51] Techniques for surgical resection are similar to those for leiomyoma, but there is some controversy over the recommended extent of resection (as will be discussed later). Small, low-risk GIST can be enucleated with low risk for local recurrence as long as margins are negative.[17] More extensive resection or esophagectomy may be indicated for large, locally invasive, or recurrent GIST.[14]

Principles of any surgical resection for GIST include obtaining grossly and histologically negative margins, and avoiding violation of the tumor pseudocapsule, which can lead to bleeding, tumor rupture, and potential dissemination. GIST tends to be soft and friable and should be handled carefully, and the specimen should be extracted in a bag to avoid seeding peritoneum or port sites. Extended anatomic resection is rarely indicated as intramural extension is usually limited; therefore organ-sparing surgery in the case of the esophagus is recommended, and esophagectomy should be avoided when possible. Lymphadenectomy is generally not required unless there are pathologically positive nodes. If multiple organs are involved then extensive resection should not be first-line therapy. Re-resection of microscopically positive resection margins is generally not indicated.[50] Resection of distant metastases is not recommended except for palliation.[52]

Even in complete resection, about 50% of patients with malignant GIST at any site will develop recurrence or metastasis with median recurrence of about 2 years and 5-year survival of 50%.[50,53] Although surgical resection is still the primary treatment for GIST without metastatic disease, the standard of care has changed to include targeted drug therapy since the introduction of tyrosine kinase inhibitors because complete resection alone is commonly not curative. Evaluation of the risk of relapse is essential in determining the future prognosis of patients and tailoring multimodal treatment regimens, as well as a surgical approach.[54] Consideration for adjuvant therapy is based on risk stratification for recurrence.

Imatinib is a tyrosine kinase inhibitor that was originally used to treat leukemia. It was first found to be useful for metastatic GIST in 2000. In phase II and III trials, imatinib has been shown to be safe and effective for GIST, and is now used as adjuvant therapy to improve recurrence-free survival for localized GIST, based on significant improvement in recurrence-free survival in the Z9001 trial of adjuvant imatinib after complete surgical resection of GIST.[50,55] Imatinib is also indicated for GIST that is definitively unresectable, recurrent, or metastatic, prior to consideration of resection or re-resection. In patients with unresectable and/or metastatic GIST, imatinib has good overall response rates and progression-free survival, with an objective response in 50% of patients.[50] Neoadjuvant imatinib may be used to improve the resectability of GIST and to allow for a less invasive resection strategy. Imatinib is well tolerated and may be continued until just before surgery and resumed quickly in the adjuvant setting along

TABLE 46.2 National Institutes of Health Fletcher Criteria for Gastrointestinal Stromal Tumor Risk Assessment

Risk Category	Primary Tumor Size (cm)*	Mitotic Count (per 50 HPF)
Very low risk	<2	<5
Low risk	2–5	<5
Intermediate risk	<5	6–10
	5–10	<5
High risk	>5	>5
	>10	Any mitotic rate
	Any size	>10

HPF, High power field.
From Fletcher CD, Berman JJ, Corless C, et al. Diagnosis of gastrointestinal stromal tumors: a consensus approach. *Hum Pathol*. 2002;33(5):462.

with a postoperative diet. The testing of GIST for KIT and PDGFRA is strongly recommended. If these are missing, then further staining and mutation analysis, such as BRAF and SDH should be considered, as these tumor types are less likely to respond to imatinib. For GIST that does not respond or becomes resistant to imatinib, alternative therapies include sunitinib, and subsequently regorafenib kinase inhibitors. Adjuvant imatinib is recommended for at least 3 years for high-risk GIST.[50]

Previously, the majority of GIST were considered to be benign, but given the propensity for recurrence and metastases, more recently it has been accepted that any GIST has potential for malignant behavior. "The term *benign* has in general been replaced semantically with *very low risk*. Several risk classification systems have been developed; the National Institutes of Health (NIH) Fletcher criteria (Table 46.2) are simple and widely used. These criteria include tumor size (>5 cm) and mitotic rate (>5/HPF), and modified versions include other aggressive features. The modified NIH or Joensuu criteria also incorporate tumor rupture and nongastric primary tumor site as higher risk features that affect prognosis. Esophageal GIST is rare, but it does seem to have a worse prognosis than GIST in other areas of the GI tract. Feng et al. compared esophageal to gastric GIST in a case match series that matched tumor size, mitotic rate, and adjuvant imatinib therapy. For the 135 esophageal GIST in this series, disease-free survival and disease-specific survival were around 65%, which was significantly lower compared to gastric GIST. Of note, most of the esophageal cases were for high-risk GIST (57% were >5 cm large, and/or high mitotic rate) though only 28% received imatinib. Additionally, the type of surgical resection was not specified, and death related to esophagus-specific recurrence or distant metastases were not differentiated.[49]

The optimal surgical approach for GIST has not been definitively determined, and remains somewhat controversial. In general, GIST in any location requires only a margin negative resection as per the most recent consensus guidelines from the NCCN.[50] Specifically, esophagus-sparing surgery is recommended for GEJ GIST, where the goal is complete resection with minimal morbidity. However, historically, there is a trend for poorer overall prognosis for esophageal GIST compared to GIST of other organs. Theoretically, this may be due to the lack of serosalization of this organ, or the complexity of resection compared to intraabdominal serosalized organs. Some experts have suggested that esophagectomy for GIST is likely more oncologically sound, based on SEER data and on small series citing difficulty with enucleation due to large size, friability, and adherence of the GIST (all were high-risk GIST: >5 cm and >5 mitotic figures).[14,54] The data cited are limited, as esophageal GIST is a very rare tumor, with heterogeneous risk of malignancy. SEER data reviewed in 2005 reported an alarming 14% 5-year survival rate after diagnosis if it is an esophageal GIST, with better outcomes noted for "partial or total organ removal," though this included limited details of the surgical procedures and did not document the risk classification for esophageal GIST. Also, only 45% of esophageal GIST was localized at the time of diagnosis, probably representing a group of higher-risk GIST. Furthermore, the SEER data were for cases treated prior to 2002, before imatinib therapy was available and resection alone was the primary treatment.[47] These results are unlikely comparable to modern multimodal therapy. Locoregional recurrence of GIST is a known risk despite esophagectomy for high-risk tumors.[43]

More recent studies, since the onset of endoscopic enucleation of SMTs, include a small number of esophageal GIST. The results, although limited to short-term data in a few cases, are promising for a low rate of recurrence or metastasis. Of note, in general, these endoscopically resectable GISTs were of smaller size; therefore, they had a lower risk of malignancy than those in prior reports. Early results are encouraging for endoscopic resection by EMR, ESD, or submucosal tunneling techniques, though data are limited in number of cases and short-term follow-up.[4,24,32,56,57] Two cases of endoscopic resections that developed distant metastases were high-risk GIST primary tumors.[32] Results also have been favorable in many reports of open or minimally invasive enucleation for GIST, especially for low-risk tumors.[16,17,43,58-62]

It seems that small tumors with low-risk features are amenable to enucleation by endoscopic, minimally invasive, or open surgery with probable low risk of recurrence or metastatic disease. Esophagectomy may be considered for larger tumors with high mitotic rate, for a more thorough oncologic resection. However, in small series, even complete resection with esophagectomy did not prevent locoregional recurrence. The morbidity of esophageal resection is a significant concern. There is no definitive answer to the best surgical approach for esophageal GIST, so a multidisciplinary evaluation of any high-risk GIST is advisable, and close surveillance is necessary after any type of resection. We are unlikely to definitively answer this question due to the rarity and heterogeneity of this disease. This should be a case-by-case decision with the patient, surgeon, and oncologist.

SCHWANNOMA

Schwannoma is the least common of the esophageal mesenchymal SMTs. The majority of these tumors present between the fourth and sixth decade of life, and there is no apparent gender predominance. Like the other mesenchymal SMTs, schwannoma arises from interstitial cells of Cajal, and can present anywhere in the GI tract. Approximately 60% develop in the stomach, but only about 5% are esophageal. Grossly, schwannoma is a firm, irregular, rubbery, tan lesion.[63] Histologically, schwannoma is moderately cellular with spindle cells, a rim of lymphoid cells, and, in some cases, melanin pigmentation. S-100 and GFAP proteins are positive on immunohistochemical staining, while c-KIT, CD34, and SMA are negative (Fig. 46.12).

The presentation and work-up of schwannoma is similar to leiomyoma and GIST, depending on the size and location of the tumor. Dysphagia is the most typical presenting symptom. Endoscopy will show a submucosal protrusion with intact mucosa, and EUS shows hypoechoic tumors in the submucosa or muscularis propria.[62] Though typically benign, schwannomas may be FDG avid on PET, similar to leiomyoma or GIST.[64-66] Schwannoma tends to develop more proximally in the esophagus; therefore, tumors of larger size may present with tracheal compression or paresthesia in addition to esophageal obstruction.[65,67-69] Malignant potential is dependent upon tumor size and may rarely be associated with metastases to lymph nodes, with only a handful of malignant cases reported.[70-72] Chemotherapy and radiation are ineffective for schwannoma; the mainstay of treatment is resection, with similar guidelines as leiomyoma. Surgical options include endoscopic, minimally invasive, or open enucleation versus esophagectomy for very large or invasive tumors.[16,24,73,74] Postoperative outcome is dependent on the aggressiveness of the tumor, and negative margins of resection. Only one case of recurrence has been reported after resection.[65]

GRANULAR CELL TUMOR

Granular cell tumor (GCT) is an SMT that can be found in any organ system and is rare in the esophagus. It is most frequently found in the submucosa of the tongue (40%), skin (30%), and breast (15%), and less commonly the GI tract (5%), of which only one-third are esophageal.[75-79] Most esophageal GCTs are isolated, but may be multiple, and in 5% to 14% of cases may affect multiple organ systems.[75] Only about 2% to 3% of GCTs are malignant. A gender preponderance has not been reliably identified, and the average age of presentation is in the fourth decade.[75,80]

Grossly, a GCT appears as a submucosal bulge into the esophageal lumen and classically has a pale yellow coloration "molar-shaped" polypoid lesion, though this is not always present (Fig. 46.13).[79] Microscopically, GCT cells have small nuclei with abundant granular cytoplasm and overlying mucosa with pseudoepitheliomatous hyperplasia. GCT cells have electron microscopy features similar to schwannoma, and stain for neural proteins S-100 and neuron-specific enolase.[81] GCTs considered to be malignant may demonstrate aggressive histologic findings, such as increased cellularity and atypia; or aggressive clinical findings, such as large size (>4 cm), rapid growth, or recurrence.[79] Both local invasion and metastasis have been reported for malignant GCTs.[2]

The size of GCT correlates with the presentation of symptoms.[80] Only 50% are symptomatic, with presentation similar to other SMTs. The work-up is similar as well, with endoscopy as previously described. EUS can help to determine the layer of origin, and typically identifies

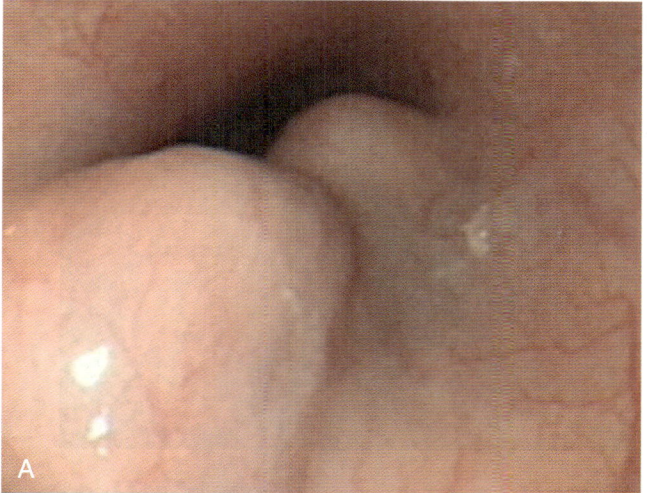

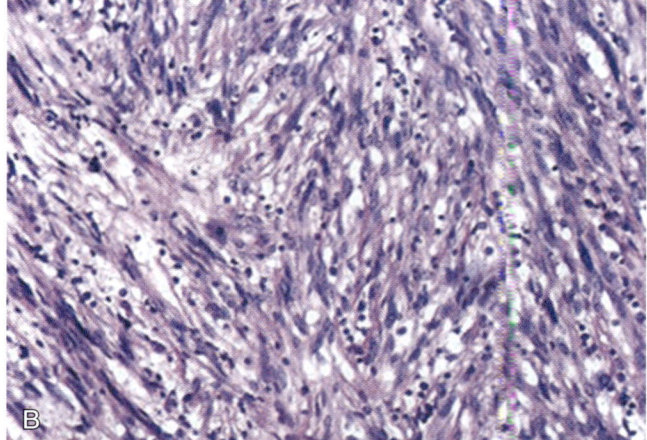

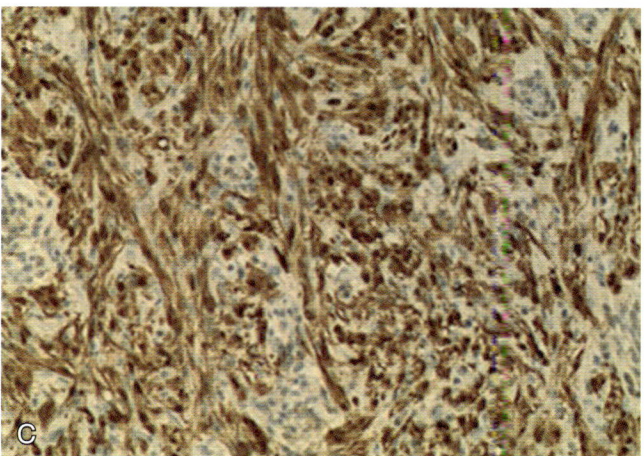

FIGURE 46.12 (A) Esophageal endoscopy of esophageal schwannoma showing two mucosal protrusions with normal esophageal mucosa. (B) Histopathologic findings reveal spindle-shaped cells in long fascicles. (C) Immunohistochemical staining reveals the tumor is positive for S-100 protein. (From Chen X, Li Y, Liu X, et al. A report of three cases of surgical removal of esophageal schwannomas. *J Thorac Dis*. 2016;8:E354, Fig. 1.)

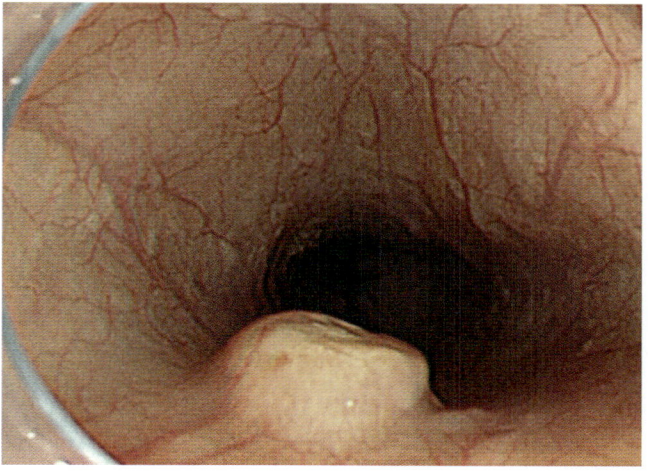

FIGURE 46.13 Endoscopic view of granular cell tumor of the esophagus. A yellow submucosal tumor is noted with normal overlying mucosa. (From An S, Jang J, Min K, et al. Granular cell tumor of the gastrointestinal tract: histologic and immunohistochemical analysis of 98 cases. *Hum Pathol*. 2015;46:815.)

a hyperechoic solid mass surrounded by hypoechoic submucosa without continuity to the muscularis propria.[82]

The ideal treatment for GCTs is somewhat controversial. Some authors advocate the resection of all tumors due to their unknown malignant potential; others suggest criteria for the resection of tumors that are relatively large or symptomatic. Selective surveillance for smaller, asymptomatic lesions is acceptable.[83] Ablative therapies, such as yttrium-aluminum-garnet (YAG) laser or alcohol injection, have been performed to avoid extensive surgical resection. The disadvantage of ablative techniques is the lack of histologic diagnosis and analysis.[78] There is a growing experience and acceptance of endoscopic resection for this group of SMTs, with success in a few series without evidence of increased risk of recurrence.[78,82,84-86]

HEMANGIOMA

Hemangioma is a rare, benign vascular tumor originating from esophageal submucosa. The prevalence of esophageal hemangiomas in the general population was 0.04% based upon autopsy series.[87] In a series of 99 cases, these accounted for 3% of all benign esophageal tumors.[1] Historically, only about 4% of all benign vascular tumors are located in the esophagus.[88] Of the few known cases, there is possibly a slight male predominance throughout a broad age range from children to elderly.[89] Multiple esophageal hemangiomatosis has been reported in association with Rendu-Osler-Weber syndrome.[3]

The presentation of symptoms may be similar to those of other SMTs, with the exception of the rare, massive hemorrhage of these vascular tumors. Rarely, very proximal lesions involving the larynx may present with stridor.[90] Endoscopically, hemangioma appears as a bluish polypoid lesion that is soft and compressible, arising from the submucosa with intact overlying mucosa (Fig. 46.14)[87] This may easily be misdiagnosed as esophageal varices. Suspected hemangioma should not be biopsied, due

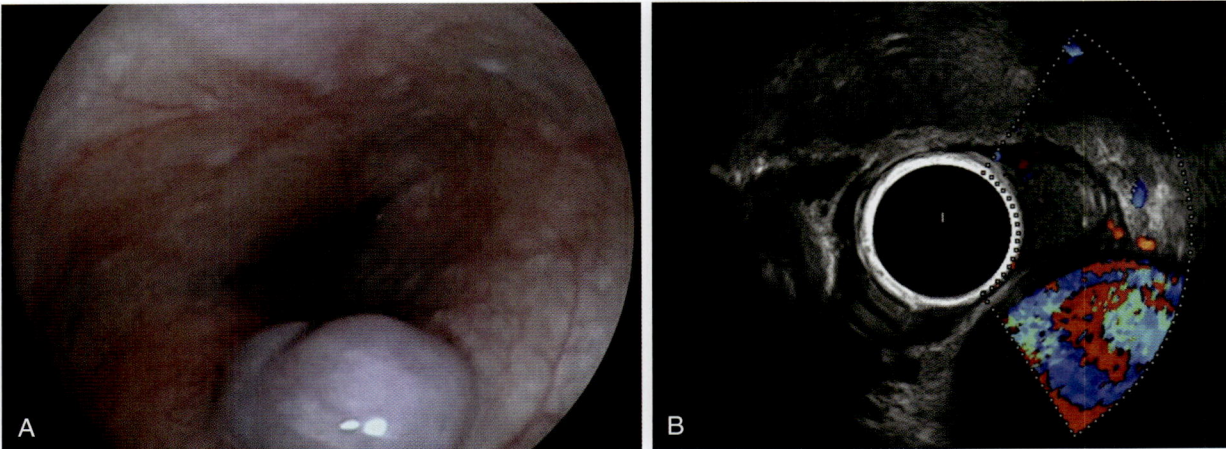

FIGURE 46.14 (A) Endoscopic image of esophageal submucosal lesion. (B) Endoscopic ultrasound image demonstrating no blood flow through the lesion. (From Chedgy FJ, Bhattacharyya R, Bhandari P. Endoscopic submucosal dissection for symptomatic esophageal cavernous hemangioma. *Gastrointest Endosc*. 2015;81:998.)

to risk of hemorrhage.[91] A hemangioma may be small and simple, or large and multinodular, and may appear anywhere along the length of the esophagus, though most are in the middle and distal thirds.[92] EUS with color Doppler may help to identify a vascularized lesion with continuity to major vascular structures, but may also show no flow.[93,94] Microscopically, hemangioma has a benign proliferation of cavernous vascular spaces, with fibrous septations. CT or magnetic resonance imaging (MRI) with intravenous contrast may be particularly helpful to define these vascular lesions for the purposes of diagnosis and surgical planning.

Incidentally identified hemangioma may be observed clinically without intervention.[90] The surgical approach for symptomatic hemangioma is variable, and techniques, including endoscopic, minimally invasive, or open enucleation or formal resection, depend on the extent of the tumor.[91,95,96] Careful dissection and hemostasis of the blood supply is critical to avoid significant bleeding, and has been successfully achieved recently with endoscopic tunneling techniques.[97] Mortality associated with resection is about 1%.[2] Ablative therapies, including YAG laser fulguration, injection sclerotherapy, and radiation therapy, are also available for esophageal hemangioma.[98,99]

FIBROVASCULAR POLYPS

A fibrovascular polyp is a rare tumor, but it is the most common intraluminal tumor of the esophagus.[100,101] There is a slight male preponderance and peak prevalence in the fifth through seventh decades.[100,102] These intraluminal polyps have a broad range of specific histologic types. It is hypothesized that fibrovascular polyps originate as a submucosal thickening in the proximal esophagus near the cricopharyngeus muscle that elongates into a polypoid shape due to esophageal peristalsis and luminal compression. Over time, fibrovascular polyps can reach impressive proportions, and may grow large enough to dilate the esophageal lumen, and long enough to reach the stomach before producing symptoms.[101] Presenting symptoms may include dysphagia, respiratory symptoms, bleeding (if the polyp is long enough to be exposed to

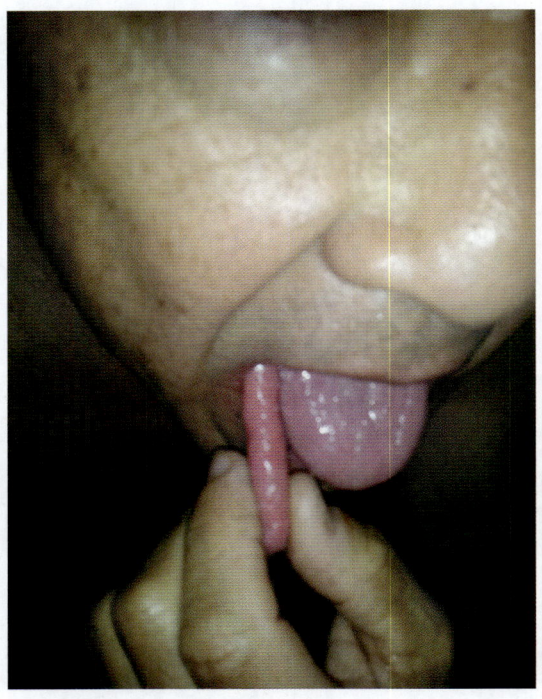

FIGURE 46.15 Regurgitation of a fibrovascular polyp.

gastric acid), and, most dramatically, regurgitation into the oropharynx. When the polyp is regurgitated, it may be reswallowed, captured, severed by the teeth, or aspirated (Fig. 46.15). Several cases of resultant asphyxiation have been reported.

Grossly, fibrovascular polyp is a cylindrical mass covered in intact mucosa and is attached by a stalk to the proximal esophageal wall. Fibrovascular polyps are usually solitary but may be multiple.[103] Histologically, they demonstrate mature fibrous tissue with varying amounts of vascularity and adipose tissue. The varying prominence of tissue type denotes the name for the polyp, which includes fibroma, fibrolipoma, myoma, myxofibroma, and fibroepithelial types. Biopsy of a fibrovascular polyp may be nondiagnostic

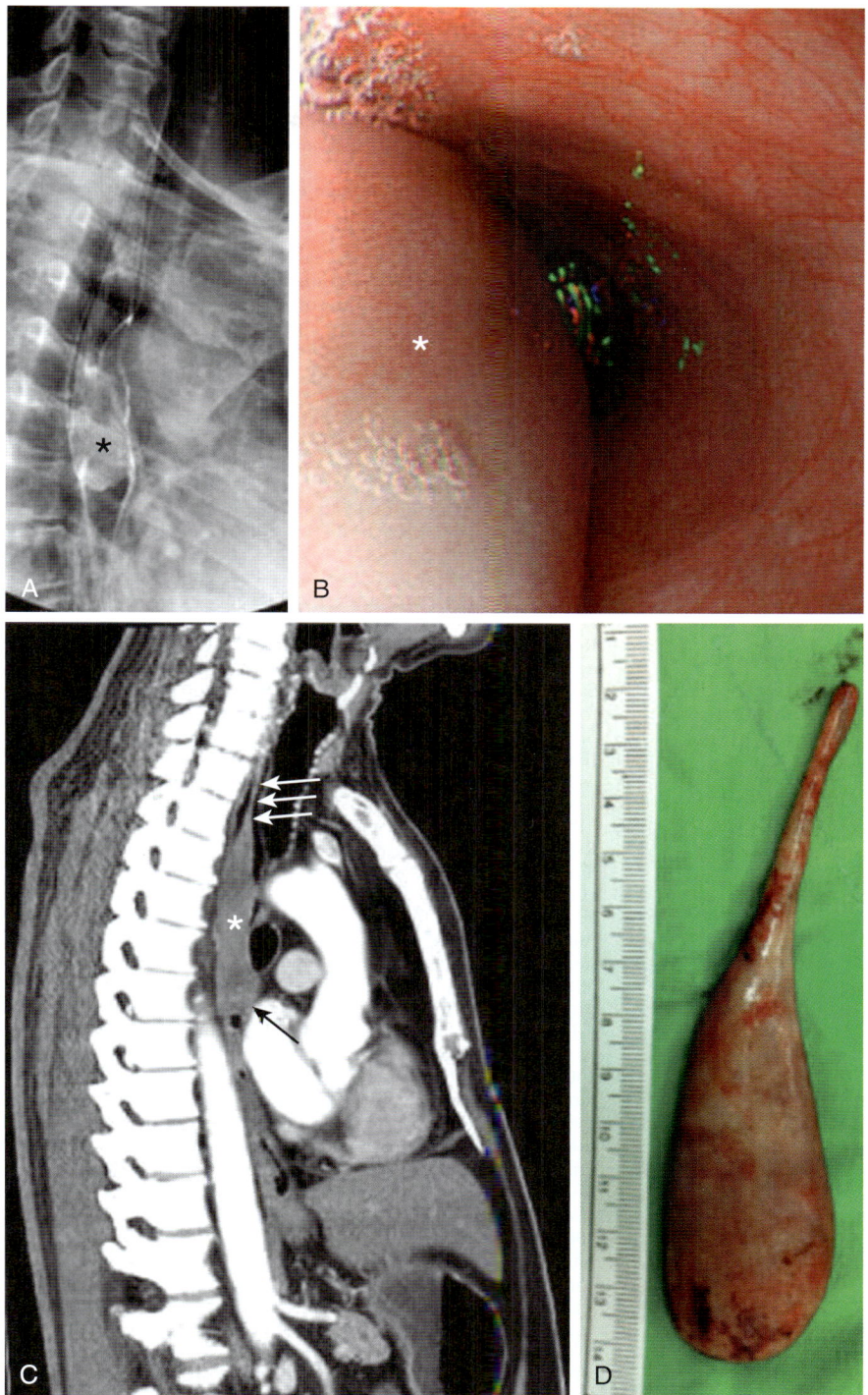

FIGURE 46.16 (A) Barium esophagram with a relatively smooth, sausage-shaped mass *(asterisk)* without mucosal destruction. (B) Endoscopy failed to detect this lesion *(asterisk)* because it almost filled the esophageal lumen and had a composition similar to that of the esophageal mucosa. (C) Computed tomography shows an intraluminal soft-tissue density mass *(asterisk)* arising in the cervical esophagus. The *black arrow* is the distal tip of the mass, and the *white arrows* show the proximal stalk. (D) Resected surgical specimen of the fibrovascular polyp. (From Shiau E. Giant fibrovascular polyp of the esophagus. *Am J Gastroenterol.* 2012;107:1473.)

due to normal overlying mucosa. One case of fibrovascular polyp harboring a well-differentiated liposarcoma has been reported.[104]

Barium esophagram of a fibrovascular polyp shows a filling defect that moves within the esophageal lumen. A fibrovascular polyp may be missed endoscopically or on esophagram, due to the proximal origin and normal overlying mucosa in up to one-third of cases.[100] Fibrovascular polyps are echo-dense on EUS. CT will show a heterogeneous mass, which may be confused with retained food or foreign material, or may suggest a leiomyoma or GIST (Fig. 46.16).[102,105] MRI may show a hyperintense mass on T1-weighted imaging, with decreased signal intensity on T2-weighted imaging.[106]

Resection is recommended for all fibrovascular polyps due to the potential for airway compromise. This has traditionally been performed with open surgery via a transcervical approach (Fig. 46.17) or thoracotomy in which the esophagus is opened opposite the origin of the polyp; the polyp and stalk is excised and the

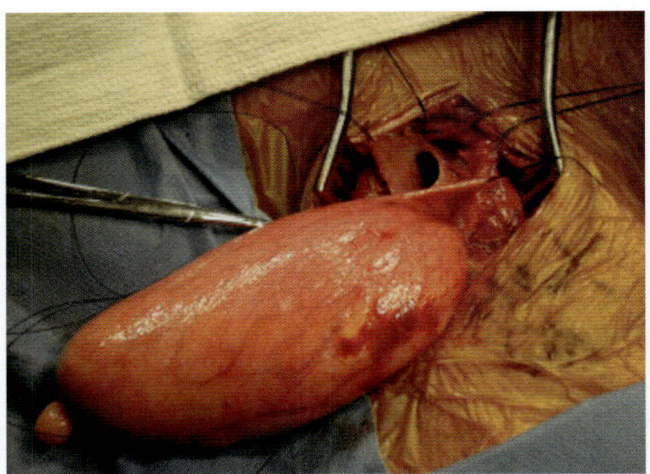

FIGURE 46.17 Delivery of giant fibrovascular polyp through the cervical esophagotomy. (From Peltz M, Estrera AS. Resection of a giant esophageal fibrovascular polyp. *Ann Thorac Surg.* 2010;90:1018.)

mucosal defect and esophagotomy closed.[107] Esophagectomy for fibrovascular polyp has only been required in a handful of cases. Kanaan and DeMeester reported a case of a particularly large polyp, with features initially suggestive of GIST or leiomyosarcoma, requiring transhiatal esophagectomy.[105] In other cases, endoscopic removal has been successful, though some authors raise concerns for the potential hemorrhage from the vascular stalk, or the potential for incomplete resection and a propensity for recurrence. Transorally, the fibrovascular polyp may be resected with open or endoscopic instruments, including polypectomy snare and cautery, or with energy devices, such as ultrasonic shears.[108,109] Regardless of approach, principles of surgical resection include complete removal of the base of the polyp to avoid the risk of local recurrence. EUS may be helpful intraoperatively to ensure complete endoscopic resection. No treatment deaths have been reported for either open surgical or endoscopic approach.[107] General anesthesia with careful protection of the airway is advisable for endoscopic interventions.[101,110]

CONCLUSION

SMTs of the esophagus and GEJ represent a heterogeneous group of neoplasms that provide unique surveillance and treatment challenges. Many are asymptomatic and require nothing more than reassurance and monitoring. Those that cause dysphagia, globus, and pain, those that present acutely with ulceration and hemorrhage, and those that are concerning for malignant behavior are appropriate for removal. The location of these tumors has prompted medical, endoscopic, and surgical improvements with decreasing invasiveness in the recent past. In severe cases, segmental resection and esophagogastric reconstruction is required. However, in many instances, enucleation via flexible endoscopy, thoracoscopy, or laparoscopy has allowed for short convalescence and organ-sparing return to baseline function for many patients.

REFERENCES

1. Plachta A. Benign tumors of the esophagus. Review of literature and report of 99 cases. *Am J Gastroenterol.* 1962;38:639-652.
2. Brock H. Benign tumors and cysts of the esophagus. In: Yeo CJ, ed. *Shackelford's Surgery of the Alimentary Tract.* Philadelphia: Saunders; 2012.
3. Choong CK, Meyers BF. Benign esophageal tumors: introduction, incidence, classification, and clinical features. *Sem Thorac Cardiovasc Surg.* 2003;15(1):3-8.
4. He G, Wang J, Chen B, et al. Feasibility of endoscopic submucosal dissection for upper gastrointestinal submucosal tumors treatment and value of endoscopic ultrasonography in pre-operation assess and post-operation follow-up: a prospective study of 224 cases in a single medical center. *Surg Endosc.* 2016;30(10):4206-4213.
5. Lee LS, Singhal S, Brinster CJ, et al. Current management of esophageal leiomyoma. *J Am Coll Surg.* 2004;198(1):136-146.
6. Kernstine KH, Andersen ES, Falabella A, Ramirez NA, Anderson CA, Beblawi I. Robotic fourth-arm enucleation of an esophageal leiomyoma and review of literature. *Innovations (Phila).* 2009;4(6):354-357.
7. Asteriou C, Konstantinou D, Lalountas M, et al. Nine years experience in surgical approach of leiomyomatosis of esophagus. *World J Surg Oncol.* 2009;7:102.
8. Bonavina L, Segalin A, Rosati R, Pavanello M, Peracchia A. Surgical therapy of esophageal leiomyoma. *J Am Coll Surg.* 1995;181(3):257-262.
9. Rendina EA, Venuta F, Pescarmona EO, et al. Leiomyoma of the esophagus. *Scand J Thorac Cardiovasc Surg.* 1990;24(1):79-82.
10. Samphire J, Nafteux P, Luketich J. Minimally invasive techniques for resection of benign esophageal tumors. *Sem Thorac Cardiovasc Surg.* 2003;15(1):35-43.
11. Jiang G, Zhao H, Yang F, et al. Thoracoscopic enucleation of esophageal leiomyoma: a retrospective study on 40 cases. *Dis Esophagus.* 2009;22(3):279-283.
12. Elli E, Espat NJ, Berger R, Jacobsen G, Knoblock L, Horgan S. Robotic-assisted thoracoscopic resection of esophageal leiomyoma. *Surg Endosc.* 2004;18(4):713-716.
13. Haddad J, Bouazza F, Barake H, Liberale G, Flamen P, Nakadi IE. Surgical strategy in abnormally increased Fluorine-18 fluorodeoxyglucose uptake in an asymptomatic lower esophageal submucosal tumor—Report of a case. *Int J Surg Case Rep.* 2014;5(9):589-593.
14. Blum MG, Bilimoria KY, Wayne JD, de Hoyos AL, Talamonti MS, Adley B. Surgical considerations for the management and resection of esophageal gastrointestinal stromal tumors. *Ann Thorac Surg.* 2007;84(5):1717-1723.
15. Jeon HW, Choi MG, Lim CH, Park JK, Sung SW. Intraoperative esophagoscopy provides accuracy and safety in video-assisted thoracoscopic enucleation of benign esophageal submucosal tumors. *Dis Esophagus.* 2015;28(5):437-441.
16. Kent M, d'Amato T, Nordman C, et al. Minimally invasive resection of benign esophageal tumors. *J Thorac Cardiovasc Surg.* 2007;134(1):176-181.
17. Mino JS, Guerron AD, Monteiro R, et al. Long-term outcomes of combined endoscopic/laparoscopic intragastric enucleation of presumed gastric stromal tumors. *Surg Endosc.* 2016;30(5):1747-1753.
18. Marshall MB, Haddad NG. Laparoscopic intragastric approach for gastroesophageal leiomyoma and cancer. *J Thorac Cardiovasc Surg.* 2015;149(4):1210-1212.
19. Xu X, Chen K, Zhou W, et al. Laparoscopic transgastric resection of gastric submucosal tumors located near the esophagogastric junction. *J Gastrointest Surg.* 2013;17(9):1570-1575.
20. Lamm SH, Steinemann DC, Linke GR, et al. Total inverse transgastric resection with transoral specimen removal. *Surg Endosc.* 2015;29(11):3363-3366.
21. Wang L, Ren W, Zhang Z, Yu J, Li Y, Song Y. Retrospective study of endoscopic submucosal tunnel dissection (ESTD) for surgical resection of esophageal leiomyoma. *Surg Endosc.* 2013;27(11):4259-4266.
22. Kinney T, Waxman I. Treatment of benign esophageal tumors by endoscopic techniques. *Sem Thorac Cardiovasc Surg.* 2003;15(1):27-34.
23. Sun S, Jin Y, Chang G, Wang C, Li X, Wang Z. Endoscopic band ligation without electrosurgery: a new technique for excision of small upper-GI leiomyoma. *Gastrointest Endosc.* 2004;60(2):218-222.

24. Liu BR, Song JT, Kong LJ, Pei FH, Wang XH, Du YJ. Tunneling endoscopic muscularis dissection for subepithelial tumors originating from the muscularis propria of the esophagus and gastric cardia. *Surg Endosc.* 2013;27(11):4354-4359.

25. Park YS, Park SW, Kim TI, et al. Endoscopic enucleation of upper-GI submucosal tumors by using an insulated-tip electrosurgical knife. *Gastrointest Endosc.* 2004;59(3):409-415.

26. Inoue H, Ikeda H, Hosoya T, et al. Submucosal endoscopic tumor resection for subepithelial tumors in the esophagus and cardia. *Endoscopy.* 2012;44(3):225-230.

27. Baysal B, Masri OA, Eloubeidi MA, Senturk H. The role of EUS and EUS-guided FNA in the management of subepithelial lesions of the esophagus: a large, single-center experience. *Endosc Ultrasound.* 2015;doi:10.4103/2303-9027.155772.

28. Dendy M, Johnson K, Boffa DJ. Spectrum of FDG uptake in large (>10 cm) esophageal leiomyomas. *J Thorac Dis.* 2015;7(12):E648-E651.

29. Burgos R, Muniz E, Rosa ER, Olivares CJ, Romaguera J. Comprehensive management of diffuse leiomyomatosis in a patient with Alport syndrome. *P R Health Sci J.* 2013;32(4):200-202.

30. Kazarin O, Vlodavsky E, Guralnik L, Kremer R, Lachter J, Bar-Sela G. Association between esophageal leiomyomatosis and p53 mutation. *Ann Thorac Surg.* 2013;95(4):1429-1431.

31. Hatch GF 3rd, Wertheimer-Hatch L, Hatch KF, et al. Tumors of the esophagus. *World J Surg.* 2000;24(4):401-411.

32. Fei BY, Yang JM, Zhao ZS. Differential clinical and pathological characteristics of esophageal stromal tumors and leiomyomata. *Dis Esophagus.* 2014;27(1):30-35.

33. Seremetis MG, Lyons WS, deGuzman VC, Peabody JW Jr. Leiomyomata of the esophagus. An analysis of 838 cases. *Cancer.* 1976;38(5):2166-2177.

34. Depypere L, Coosemans W, Nafteux P. Fluorine-18-fluorodeoxyglucose uptake in a benign oesophageal leiomyoma: a potential pitfall in diagnosis. *Interact Cardiovasc Thorac Surg.* 2012;14(2):234-236.

35. Sousa RG, Figueiredo PC, Pinto-Marques P, et al. An unusual cause of pseudoachalasia: the Alport syndrome-diffuse leiomyomatosis association. *Eur J Gastroenterol Hepatol.* 2013;25(11):1352-1357.

36. Amer KM, Payne HR, Jeyasingham K. The relevance of abnormal motility patterns in intra-mural oesophageal leiomyomata. *Eur J Cardio Thoracic Surg.* 1996;10(8):634-640.

37. Sweet RH, Soutter L, Valenzuela CT. Muscle wall tumors of the esophagus. *J Thorac Surg.* 1954;27(1):13-31, discussion 31-35.

38. Storey CF, Adams WC Jr. Leiomyoma of the esophagus; a report of four cases and review of the surgical literature. *Am J Surg.* 1956;91(1):3-23.

39. Shimada Y, Okumura T, Nagata T, et al. Successful enucleation of a fluorine-18-fluorodeoxyglucose positron emission tomography positive esophageal leiomyoma in the prone position using sponge spacer and intra-esophageal balloon compression. *Gen Thorac Cardiovasc Surg.* 2012;60(8):542-545.

40. Winant AJ, Gollub MJ, Shia J, Antonescu C, Bains MS, Levine MS. Imaging and clinicopathologic features of esophageal gastrointestinal stromal tumors. *AJR Am J Roentgenol.* 2014;203(2):306-314.

41. Todaro P, Crino SF, Ieni A, Pallio S, Consolo P, Tuccari G. Intraparietal esophageal leiomyomas diagnosed by endoscopic ultrasound-guided fine-needle aspiration cytology: Cytological and immunocytochemical features in two cases. *Oncol Lett.* 2014;8(1):123-126.

42. Ahn SY, Jeon SW. Endoscopic resection of co-existing severe dysplasia and a small esophageal leiomyoma. *World J Gastroenterol.* 2013;19(1):137-140.

43. Robb WB, Bruyere E, Amielh D, et al. Esophageal gastrointestinal stromal tumor: is tumoral enucleation a viable therapeutic option? *Ann Surg.* 2015;261(1):117-124.

44. Kim GH, Park DY, Kim S, et al. Is it possible to differentiate gastric GISTs from gastric leiomyomas by EUS? *World J Gastroenterol.* 2009;15(27):3376-3381.

45. Ma S, Bu W, Wang L, et al. Radiotherapy treatment of large esophageal leiomyosarcoma: a case report. *Oncology Lett.* 2015;9(5):2422-2424.

46. Demetri GD, von Mehren M, Antonescu CR, et al. NCCN Task Force report: update on the management of patients with gastrointestinal stromal tumors. *J Natl Compr Canc Netw.* 2010;8(suppl 2):S1-S41, quiz S42-S44.

47. Tran T, Davila JA, El-Serag HB. The epidemiology of malignant gastrointestinal stromal tumors: an analysis of 1,458 cases from 1992 to 2000. *Am J Gastroenterol.* 2005;100(1):162-168.

48. Lott S, Schmieder M, Mayer B, et al. Gastrointestinal stromal tumors of the esophagus: evaluation of a pooled case series regarding clinicopathological features and clinical outcome. *Am J Cancer Res.* 2015;5(1):333-343.

49. Feng F, Tian Y, Liu Z, et al. Clinicopathologic features and clinical outcomes of esophageal gastrointestinal stromal tumor: evaluation of a pooled case series. *Medicine (Baltimore).* 2016;95(2):e2446.

50. NCCN. Soft Tissue Sarcoma Version 2.2017; 2017. https://www.nccn.org/professionals/physician_gls/PDF/sarcoma.pdf.

51. Lok KH, Lai L, Yiu HL, Szeto ML, Leung SK. Endosonographic surveillance of small gastrointestinal tumors originating from muscularis propria. *J Gastrointest Liver Dis.* 2009;18(2):177-180.

52. Nunobe S, Sano T, Shimada K, Sakamoto Y, Kosuge T. Surgery including liver resection for metastatic gastrointestinal stromal tumors or gastrointestinal leiomyosarcomas. *Jpn J Clin Oncol.* 2005;35(6):338-341.

53. Rossi CR, Mocellin S, Mencarelli R, et al. Gastrointestinal stromal tumors: from a surgical to a molecular approach. *Int J Cancer.* 2003;107(2):171-176.

54. Pisters PW, Patel SR. Gastrointestinal stromal tumors: current management. *J Surg Oncol.* 2010;102(5):530-538.

55. DeMatteo RP, Ballman KV, Antonescu CR, et al. Adjuvant imatinib mesylate after resection of localised, primary gastrointestinal stromal tumour: a randomised, double-blind, placebo-controlled trial. *Lancet.* 2009;373(9669):1097-1104.

56. Guo J, Liu Z, Sun S, Liu X, Wang S, Ge N. Ligation-assisted endoscopic enucleation for treatment of esophageal subepithelial lesions originating from the muscularis propria: a preliminary study. *Dis Esophagus.* 2015;28(4):312-317.

57. Huang ZG, Zhang XS, Huang SL, Yuan XG. Endoscopy dissection of small stromal tumors emerged from the muscularis propria in the upper gastrointestinal tract: preliminary study. *World J Gastrointest Endosc.* 2012;4(12):565-570.

58. Isaka T, Kanzaki M, Onuki T. Long-term survival after thoracoscopic enucleation of a gastrointestinal stromal tumor arising from the esophagus. *J Surg Case Rep.* 2015;2015(2):doi:10.1093/jscr/rju155.

59. Coccolini F, Catena F, Ansaloni L, Lazzareschi D, Pinna AD. Esophagogastric junction gastrointestinal stromal tumor: resection vs enucleation. *World J Gastroenterol.* 2010;16(35):4374-4376.

60. Jiang P, Jiao Z, Han B, et al. Clinical characteristics and surgical treatment of oesophageal gastrointestinal stromal tumours. *Eur J Cardio Thorac Surg.* 2010;38(2):223-227.

61. Lee HJ, Park SI, Kim DK, Kim YH. Surgical resection of esophageal gastrointestinal stromal tumors. *Ann Thorac Surg.* 2009;87(5):1569-1571.

62. Chen X, Li Y, Liu X, et al. A report of three cases of surgical removal of esophageal schwannomas. *J Thorac Dis.* 2016;8(5):E353-E357.

63. Liu D, Yang Y, Qi YU, Wu K, Zhao S. Schwannoma of the esophagus: a case report. *Oncol Lett.* 2015;10(5):3161-3162.

64. Matsuki A, Kosugi S, Kanda T, et al. Schwannoma of the esophagus: a case exhibiting high 18F-fluorodeoxyglucose uptake in positron emission tomography imaging. *Dis Esophagus.* 2009;22(4):E6-E10.

65. Kassis ES, Bansal S, Perrino C, et al. Giant asymptomatic primary esophageal schwannoma. *Ann Thorac Surg.* 2012;93(4):e81-e83.

66. Makino T, Yamasaki M, Takeno A, et al. Thoracoscopic enucleation of esophageal schwannoma exhibiting (18)F-fluorodeoxyglucose uptake on positron emission tomography. *Dis Esophagus.* 2013;26(3):331-332.

67. Yoon HY, Kim CB, Lee YH, Kim HG. An obstructing large schwannoma in the esophagus. *J Gastrointest Surg.* 2008;12(4):761-763.

68. Chen HC, Huang HJ, Wu CY, Lin TS, Fang HY. Esophageal schwannoma with tracheal compression. *Thorac Cardiovasc Surg.* 2006;54(8):555-558.

69. Tomono A, Nakamura T, Otowa Y, et al. A case of benign esophageal schwannoma causing life-threatening tracheal obstruction. *Ann Thorac Surg.* 2015;21(3):289-292.

70. Murase K, Hino A, Ozeki Y, Karagiri Y, Onitsuka A, Sugie S. Malignant schwannoma of the esophagus with lymph node metastasis: literature review of schwannoma of the esophagus. *J Gastroenterol.* 2001;36(11):772-777.

71. Wang S, Zheng J, Ruan Z, Huang H, Yang Z, Zheng J. Long-term survival in a rare case of malignant esophageal schwannoma cured by surgical excision. *Ann Thorac Surg.* 2011;92(1):357-358.

72. Mishra B, Madhusudhan KS, Kilambi R, Das P, Pal S, Srivastava DN. Malignant schwannoma of the esophagus: a rare case report. *Korean J Thorac Cardiovasc Surg.* 2016;49(1):63-66.

73. Kitada M, Matsuda Y, Hayashi S, Ishibashi K, Oikawa K, Miyokawa N. Esophageal schwannoma: a case report. *World J Surg Oncol.* 2013;11:253.

74. Naus PJ, Tio FO, Gross GW. Esophageal schwannoma: first report of successful management by endoscopic removal. *Gastrointest Endosc.* 2001;54(4):520-522.

75. Giacobbe A, Facciorusso D, Conoscitore P, Spirito F, Squillante MM, Bisceglia M. Granular cell tumor of the esophagus. *Am J Gastroenterol.* 1988;83(12):1398-1400.

76. Sarma DP, Rodriguez FH Jr, Deiparine EM, Weilbaecher TG. Symptomatic granular cell tumor of the esophagus. *J Surg Oncol.* 1986;33(4):246-249.

77. Subramanyam K, Shannon CR, Patterson M, Davis M, Gourley WK. Granular cell myoblastoma of the esophagus. *J Clin Gastroenterol.* 1984;6(2):113-118.

78. Kahng DH, Kim GH, Park DY, et al. Endoscopic resection of granular cell tumors in the gastrointestinal tract: a single center experience. *Surg Endosc.* 2013;27(9):3228-3236.

79. An S, Jang J, Min K, et al. Granular cell tumor of the gastrointestinal tract: histologic and immunohistochemical analysis of 98 cases. *Hum Pathol.* 2015;46(6):813-819.

80. Coutinho DS, Soga J, Yoshikawa T, et al. Granular cell tumors of the esophagus: a report of two cases and review of the literature. *Am J Gastroenterol.* 1985;80(10):758-762.

81. Reed CE. Benign tumors of the esophagus. *Chest Surg Clin N Am.* 1994;4(4):769-783.

82. Tada S, Iida M, Yao T, Miyagahara T, Hasuda S, Fujishima M. Granular cell tumor of the esophagus: endoscopic ultrasonographic demonstration and endoscopic removal. *Am J Gastroenterol.* 1990;85(11):1507-1511.

83. Mineo TC, Biancari F, Francioni F, Trentino P, Casciani CU. Conservative approach to granular cell tumour of the oesophagus. Three case reports. *Scand J Thorac Cardiovasc Surg.* 1995;29(3):141-144.

84. Catalano F, Kind R, Rodella L, et al. Endoscopic treatment of esophageal granular cell tumors. *Endoscopy.* 2002;34(7):582-584.

85. Yasuda I, Tomita E, Nagura K, Nishigaki Y, Yamada O, Kachi H. Endoscopic removal of granular cell tumors. *Gastrointest Endosc.* 1995;41(2):163-167.

86. Esaki M, Aoyagi K, Hizawa K, et al. Multiple granular cell tumors of the esophagus removed endoscopically: a case report. *Gastrointest Endosc.* 1998;48(5):536-539.

87. Tsai SJ, Lin CC, Chang CW, et al. Benign esophageal lesions: endoscopic and pathologic features. *World J Gastroenterol.* 2015;21(4):1091-1098.

88. Gentry RW, Dockerty MB, Glagett OT. Vascular malformations and vascular tumors of the gastrointestinal tract. *Surg Gynecol Obstet.* 1949;88(4):281-323.

89. Riemenschneider HW, Klassen KP. Cavernous esophageal hemangioma. *Ann Thorac Surg.* 1968;6(6):552-556.

90. Rodrigues-Pinto E, Pereira P, Macedo G. Bluish discoloration of the esophagus: cavernous hemangioma of the pharynx and larynx with esophageal involvement. *Endoscopy.* 2015;47(suppl 1 UCTN):E213-E214.

91. Cantero D, Yoshida T, Ito T, Suzumi M, Tada M, Okita K. Esophageal hemangioma: endoscopic diagnosis and treatment. *Endoscopy.* 1994;26(2):250-253.

92. Govoni AF. Hemangiomas of the esophagus. *Gastrointest Radiol.* 1982;7(2):113-117.

93. Chedgy FJ, Bhattacharyya R, Bhandari P. Endoscopic submucosal dissection for symptomatic esophageal cavernous hemangioma. *Gastrointest Endosc.* 2015;81(4):998.

94. Ha C, Regan J, Cetindag IB, Ali A, Mellinger JD. Benign esophageal tumors. *Surg Clin N Am.* 2015;95(3):491-514.

95. Ramo OJ, Salo JA, Bardini R, Nemlander AT, Farkkila M, Mattila SP. Treatment of a submucosal hemangioma of the esophagus using simultaneous video-assisted thoracoscopy and esophagoscopy: description of a new minimally invasive technique. *Endoscopy.* 1997;29(5):S27-S28.

96. Kim AW, Korst RJ, Port JL, Altorki NK, Lee PC. Giant cavernous hemangioma of the distal esophagus treated with esophagectomy. *J Thorac Cardiovasc Surg.* 2007;133(6):1665-1667.

97. Kobara H, Mori H, Masaki T. Successful en bloc resection of an esophageal hemangioma by endoscopic submucosal dissection. *Endoscopy.* 2012;44(suppl 2 UCTN):E134-E135.

98. Shigemitsu K, Naomoto Y, Yamatsuji T, et al. Esophageal hemangioma successfully treated by fulguration using potassium titanyl phosphate/yttrium aluminum garnet (KTP/YAG) laser: a case report. *Dis Esophagus.* 2000;13(2):161-164.

99. Aoki T, Okagawa K, Uemura Y, et al. Successful treatment of an esophageal hemangioma by endoscopic injection sclerotherapy: report of a case. *Surg Today.* 1997;27(5):450-452.

100. Caceres M, Steeb G, Wilks SM, Garrett HE Jr. Large pedunculated polyps originating in the esophagus and hypopharynx. *Ann Thorac Surg.* 2006;81(1):393-396.

101. Peltz M, Estrera AS. Resection of a giant esophageal fibrovascular polyp. *Ann Thorac Surg.* 2010;90(3):1017-1019.

102. Levine MS, Buck JL, Pantongrag-Brown L, Buetow PC, Hallman JR, Sobin LH. Fibrovascular polyps of the esophagus: clinical, radiographic, and pathologic findings in 16 patients. *AJR Am J Roentgenol.* 1996;166(4):781-787.

103. Images of the month: Giant fibrovascular polyp of the esophagus. *Am J Gastroenterol.* 2012;107(10):1473.

104. Beylergil V, Simmons MZ, Ulaner G, Jurcic J, Hibshoosh H, Carrasquillo JA. FDG PET/CT findings in a rare case of giant fibrovascular polyp of the esophagus harboring atypical lipomatous tumor/well-differentiated liposarcoma. *Clin Nucl Med.* 2014;39(3):288-291.

105. Kanaan S, DeMeester TR. Fibrovascular polyp of the esophagus requiring esophagectomy. *Dis Esophagus.* 2007;20(5):453-454.

106. Goto A, Suzuki M, Iizuka K, et al. Regurgitation of a mass into the mouth: a fibrovascular polyp of the esophagus. *Endoscopy.* 2010;42(suppl 2):E248-E249.

107. Avezzano EA, Fleischer DE, Merida MA, Anderson DL. Giant fibrovascular polyps of the esophagus. *Am J Gastroenterol.* 1990;85(3):299-302.

108. Chauhan S, Draganov P. Endoscopic removal of two giant fibrovascular polyps of the esophagus using the "two channel, two devices technique." *Gastrointest Endosc.* 2011;73(5):1036-1037.

109. Lobo N, Hall A, Weir J, Mace A. Endoscopic resection of a giant fibrovascular polyp of the oesophagus with the assistance of ultrasonic shears. *BMJ Case Rep.* 2016;2016:doi:10.1136/bcr-2015-214158.

110. Pallabazzer G, Santi S, Biagio S, D'Imporzano S. Difficult polypectomy-giant hypopharyngeal polyp: case report and literature review. *World J Gastroenterol.* 2013;19(35):5936-5939.

Caustic Esophageal Injury

Daniel French | Suchir Sundaresan

A caustic esophageal ingestion involves damage to the wall of the esophagus, secondary to direct contact with an acid or base, through a well-described inflammatory response. Knowledge of the pathophysiology of caustic injuries guides complex management decisions through the multiple phases of these potentially life-threatening injuries.

EPIDEMIOLOGY

There are two etiologies of caustic ingestion: accidental and intentional. The age of the patient is predictive of the etiology. Accidental ingestions occur in pediatric patients younger than 5 years, whereas intentional ingestions occur in adults and adolescents as an act of self-harm.

The 2013 Annual Report of the American Association of Poison Control Centers' National Poison Data System found the majority of caustic ingestions occurred in children younger than 5 years,[1] thus the majority of the epidemiologic data is published in the pediatric literature. Retrospective studies consistently report low social economic status, low parental education, residence in low-income countries, and crowded living conditions as risk factors for accidental ingestion.[2-5] The majority of children ingest an alkaline substance, most commonly a household cleaning agent. Often the substance was not stored in a labeled container. Manufacturers in developing countries have poor compliance with the use of safety caps[2-5]; conversely, this injury appears to be declining in developed countries.[5]

PATHOPHYSIOLOGY

CHEMICAL FACTORS

The pathophysiology of caustic injuries is different for ingestion of acidic and alkali substances. In addition to pH, the severity of the injury depends on the following factors: viscosity, concentration, amount ingested, contact time, and comorbidities. Most studies report the substances consumed; however, the volume is not reported because this information cannot be gathered reliably from the patient. One study estimated the minimum consumption at 50 to 200 mL and attempted to predict the grade of injury based on volume and concentration of alkali substance consumed, acknowledging this inherent difficulty.[6] Not surprisingly, more severe esophageal injuries occur in adults attempting suicide compared with pediatric accidental ingestions, because larger quantities of the corrosive substance are ingested.[7] Substances with a pH < 2 or pH > 12 are known to cause significant damage.[8] Full-thickness injury to the esophagus occurs with 10 seconds of contact with 22.5% sodium hydroxide[9] or 1 second with 30%

sodium hydroxide.[10] Animal studies have shown variable degrees of injury with 10% sodium hydroxide exposed for 60 seconds.[11] The total alkalinity or acidity of a substance also appears to determine the depth of the injury.[12]

SUBSTANCES

The substances consumed are often household cleaners or hair products. In North America, alkalizing agents are more commonly used for cleaning, whereas in India strong acids are readily available and used for cleaning.[13,14] Commercially available drain cleaners (e.g., Liquid Plumr [Clorox, Oakland, California] and Drano [S.C. Johnson & Son, Inc., Racine, Wisconsin]) and oven cleaners contain varying concentrations of sodium hydroxide. Dishwasher detergents contain phosphates. Hair relaxers contain sodium or calcium hydroxide or ammonium hydroxide. *Lye* is a generic term used to describe high concentrations of sodium hydroxide or potassium hydroxide used for cleaning. Bleach is an alkali made of various chemical compounds and thus the pH varies by brand. Mister Plumber and Lysol toilet cleaners are acids. The majority of swimming pool cleaners are acids.

INFLAMMATORY RESPONSE

The pathophysiology differs for ingestion of acid (coagulation necrosis) and alkali (liquefaction necrosis).

There is a perception that acid injury is less severe. Acids cause instant burning when ingested, resulting in a lower quantity consumed compared with alkali substances. Esophageal mucosal exposure to acid also results in formation of a superficial and protective eschar; however, ingestion of a strong acid can still cause a transmural injury to the esophagus. One study reported more significant injuries and higher mortality with acid ingestion compared with alkali ingestion.[7] Acids are also thought to cause more significant injury to the stomach compared with the esophagus because of gastric retention of the substance due to pyloric spasm. However, a study focusing only on acidic ingestions reported a significantly higher grade of injury to the esophagus compared with the stomach.[13]

The pathophysiology resulting from an alkali ingestion is more complex than for acid ingestion. Animal studies in the 1950s and 1960s demonstrated that corrosive substances damage the esophagus through ischemia, thrombosis, and inflammation. Johnson studied 85 dogs after consumption of 10% sodium hydroxide and described three phases of injury based on the gross and histologic examination of the esophagus from the sacrificed dogs.[11,15] Haller et al. exposed cats to 10% sodium hydroxide for 1 minute, documenting similar findings to Johnson.[11] These phases of injury are described in Table 47.1.

The first phase, the acute necrotic phase, occurs during the first 72 hours of ingestion, featuring four findings:

TABLE 47.1 Histopathologic Phases of Caustic Injury to the Esophagus

Phase	Timing	Histopathologic Findings
Acute necrotic	<72 h	(1) Liquefaction necrosis of superficial layers of esophagus (2) Acute inflammation (3) Thrombosis of vasculature (4) Bacterial and hemorrhagic infiltration of underlying tissues
Ulcerative granular	3 days to 3 weeks	(1) Sloughing of superficial necrotic tissue (2) Ulceration (3) Development of fresh granulation tissue (4) Development of new blood vessels (5) Infiltration of fibroblasts (6) Early collagenous producing connective tissue
Cicatrization and stricturing	3 weeks to 3 months	(1) Ongoing formation of collagenous connective tissue (2) Submucosa and muscularis replaced with dense fibrosis (3) Decreasing inflammatory response (4) Reepithelialization with squamous cells

Data from Haller JA Jr, Andrews HG, White JJ, Tamer MA, Cleveland WW. Pathophysiology and management of acute corrosive burns of the esophagus: results of treatment in 285 children. *J Pediatr Surg.* 1971;6(5):578–584; and Johnson EE. A study of corrosive esophagitis. *Laryngoscope.* 1963;73:1651–1696.

(1) death of cells through coagulation of proteins, (2) an intense inflammatory response, (3) thrombosis of vessels, and (4) infiltration of the esophagus wall and underlying tissues with hemorrhage and bacteria. Johnson's studies showed that the submucosal layer and occasionally the muscularis were liquefied through a process called liquefaction necrosis.[11,15] Complete liquefaction of the esophagus and trachea and part of the lungs has been described with ingestion of a large quantity of alkaline substances.[16] Johnson described an intense but variable inflammatory response.[15] Interestingly, four decades later using a mouse model and intravital microscopy, Osman et al. reported minimal inflammatory cells in the early phases of the injury.[17] However, the same study did confirm thrombosis of the microcirculation.[17] Thrombosis inhibits blood flow contributing to necrosis in the compromised tissue and delays arrival of inflammatory cells. This concept is supported by a later study of esophageal injury in rats that showed increased free radicals after 24 hours and persisting for 72 hours.[18] The fourth finding results from the first: with necrosis of the protective layers of the esophagus, the muscularis propria is exposed to the contents of the esophagus, allowing bacterial invasion into the esophageal wall and surrounding mediastinal tissues.[11,15] Clinically, the majority of patients will present to medical attention in the first phase of the injury.

The second phase, the ulcerative/granular phase, spans 3 days to 3 weeks after ingestion. This phase begins with sloughing of the necrotic tissue produced in the first phase, resulting in ulcers throughout the damaged esophagus. Infiltration of fibroblasts and development of new blood vessels result in fresh granulation tissue and early collagen, producing very weak connective tissue. Clinically, it is at this time the healing esophagus is weakest and subject to hemorrhage or perforation.[15]

The third phase, cicatrization and stricturing phase, occurs between 3 weeks to 3 months after ingestion. Acute inflammatory cells are no longer present, replaced by dense fibrotic bands throughout the muscularis and submucosa. There is also reepithelialization of the mucosa with squamous cells. Clinically, it is during this third phase of the injury that deposition of dense connective tissue leads to esophageal narrowing due to annular fibrosis (stricture).[11,15]

The depth of injury is dependent on the pH of the substance and the duration of mucosal exposure. These factors ultimately determine the severity of the injury in all three phases, the patient's associated clinical condition, and risk of subsequent stricture formation. Therefore the degree of injury is an important predictor of long-term outcome, and attempts to improve outcomes have focused on interventions based on understanding the underlying pathophysiology. Despite the studies cited here describing separate pathophysiology for alkali and acid injuries, the initial clinical management of a patient with ingestion of a strong acid or alkali substance is similar.

CLINICAL FEATURES

It is important to obtain an accurate history and carefully assess the patient with special attention to their clinical stability. A combination of history, physical findings, laboratory studies, imaging, and endoscopic exams will be used to make management decisions for a patient with a caustic injury.

On history, it is important to characterize the substance ingested, including the name of the substance, texture (solid or liquid), quantity ingested, and the timing of the ingestion relative to time of presentation. In accidental ingestions the time passed since ingestion and quantity consumed are usually less than in intentional ingestions in the adult population. Patients must be questioned regarding dysphagia, odynophagia, refusal to drink, chest pain, vomiting, and epigastric pain. Dysphagia, odynophagia, refusal to drink in pediatric patients, and chest pain may represent esophageal injury. Vomiting is concerning for recurrent exposure of the esophagus to the caustic substance and risk of aspiration. Epigastric pain is concerning for gastric injury or perforation.

On physical exam, special attention to the patient's vital signs is essential to allow for early aggressive interventions that can be lifesaving. The mouth should be inspected for signs of mucosal injury. Drooling, hoarseness, and stridor must also be noted. The presence of oral mucosal injury and drooling has been reported to increase the

TABLE 47.2 Endoscopic Grading of Caustic Injuries

Grade	Endoscopic Finding
Grade 0	Normal
Grade 1	Superficial mucosal edema and erythema
Grade 2	Mucosal and submucosal ulcerations
Grade 2a	Superficial ulcerations, erosions, exudates
Grade 2b	Deep discrete or circumferential ulcerations
Grade 3	Transmural ulcerations with necrosis
Grade 3a	Focal necrosis
Grade 3b	Extensive necrosis
Grade 4	Perforations

From Zargar SA, Kochhar R, Mehta S, Mehta SK The role of fiberoptic endoscopy in the management of corrosive ingestion and modified endoscopic classification of burns. *Gastrointest Endosc.* 1991;37(2):165–169.

probability of significant esophageal injury.[13] Hoarseness and stridor can indicate injury to the larynx and airways. The abdomen should be examined because tenderness can represent a gastric injury or even perforation.

It has been recognized that correlating signs and symptoms of patients presenting with caustic ingestion can be difficult to correlate with severity of injury.[20] A detailed retrospective review of pediatric patients concluded no single or group of signs or symptoms can be used to determine the severity of the esophageal injury. However, they did report that all patients with grade 2 or 3 injury on endoscopic exam (Table 47.2) were symptomatic.[21] Another smaller retrospective review found that all patients with endoscopically proven injury were symptomatic, whereas all asymptomatic patients did not have endoscopic evidence of injury.[22] A more recent study assessed prospectively a series of 148 patients (majority adults) to create a model to predict severity of esophageal injury. Drooling, buccal mucosal burn, and elevated white blood cell count were useful parameters to predict significant esophageal injury.[19] Given these contradicting results, no single finding should be used to rule out a significant injury and all patients should undergo endoscopy for objective assessment.

The three clinical phases may be described as follows: acute, intermediate, and chronic. In the acute phase the priority and purpose of the clinical assessment is to guide resuscitation, assess for necrosis or perforation of the esophagus or stomach, and determine disposition. In the intermediate phase, repeated assessment is done to assess for necrosis or delayed perforation. The chronic phase requires attention to three common consequences of caustic injuries, which include stricture formation, dysmotility, and development of cancer.

INITIAL INVESTIGATIONS AND MANAGEMENT

A patient with a caustic injury should be managed as a critically ill patient, necessitating stabilization of the patient prior to completing all investigations. The priorities of airway, breathing, and circulation must be followed. A patient presenting with respiratory distress may require

a secure airway and/or drainage of large pleural effusions secondary to a perforation. Because of the intense inflammatory response the patient may also require management of septic shock with intravenous fluids and early administration of antibiotics.

Many studies have focused on applying data from initial investigations to predict the severity of injury, with outcomes including perforation and stricture rates. Although this is intriguing, it must be noted that these investigations may need to be repeated throughout a patient's clinical course to allow for ongoing reassessment. In addition to physical exam, routine blood work, chest radiography, endoscopy, and computed tomography (CT) scans of the chest and abdomen are fundamental in assessing a patient with a caustic injury.

Blood work including a complete blood count with differential, serum electrolyte, and renal function studies are important in the assessment of these patients. A multivariate retrospective analysis of 210 patients identified a white blood cell count greater than 20,000 on presentation as an independent predictor of death after caustic ingestion.[23] A retrospective study of 129 patients focusing on acid-base status determined that patients with a serum pH less than 7.22 or base excess less than 12 would require operative intervention.[24-26] Despite the results of these studies, it is highly unlikely a single laboratory value can fully characterize the severity of the injury.

IMAGING

Chest radiographs are helpful in the initial and ongoing assessment of patients with a caustic injury, paying particular attention for mediastinal air and pleural effusions that could suggest perforation. The role of a contrast esophagram to assess for esophageal perforation has been reviewed.[26] There is ongoing debate between the use of barium and water-soluble contrast: barium is felt to decrease pneumonitis in the setting of aspiration but irritate the peritoneal and pleural cavity if a perforation is present, whereas water-soluble contrast has the opposite effects.[27] Ultimately, with the availability of high-resolution endoscopy and cross-sectional imaging, esophagrams are not likely required in the initial assessment, and instead can be used very selectively in the later course to characterize strictures or assess for delayed perforations.

CT scans are used increasingly to assess these patients and for prognostic purposes. Fig. 47.1 shows images from a male who ingested toilet cleaner sustaining a serious caustic injury requiring urgent gastrectomy, subtotal esophagectomy, cervical esophagostomy, and feeding tube with delayed reconstruction with a colonic interposition graft. The grading system shown in Table 47.3 was developed based on a retrospective review of 49 patients who presented with a caustic injury. CT imaging done within 72 hours of the injury was used to assign a grade to the esophageal wall edema and inflammation of adjacent tissues. The grade system was designed to predict the subsequent development of a stricture as documented on esophagram completed at a later date.[28] Another study looked at the role of CT in guiding management of patients with grade 3b injuries on endoscopy. Seventy-two patients who had a CT scan were compared with 125 patients who did not. This study excluded patients who

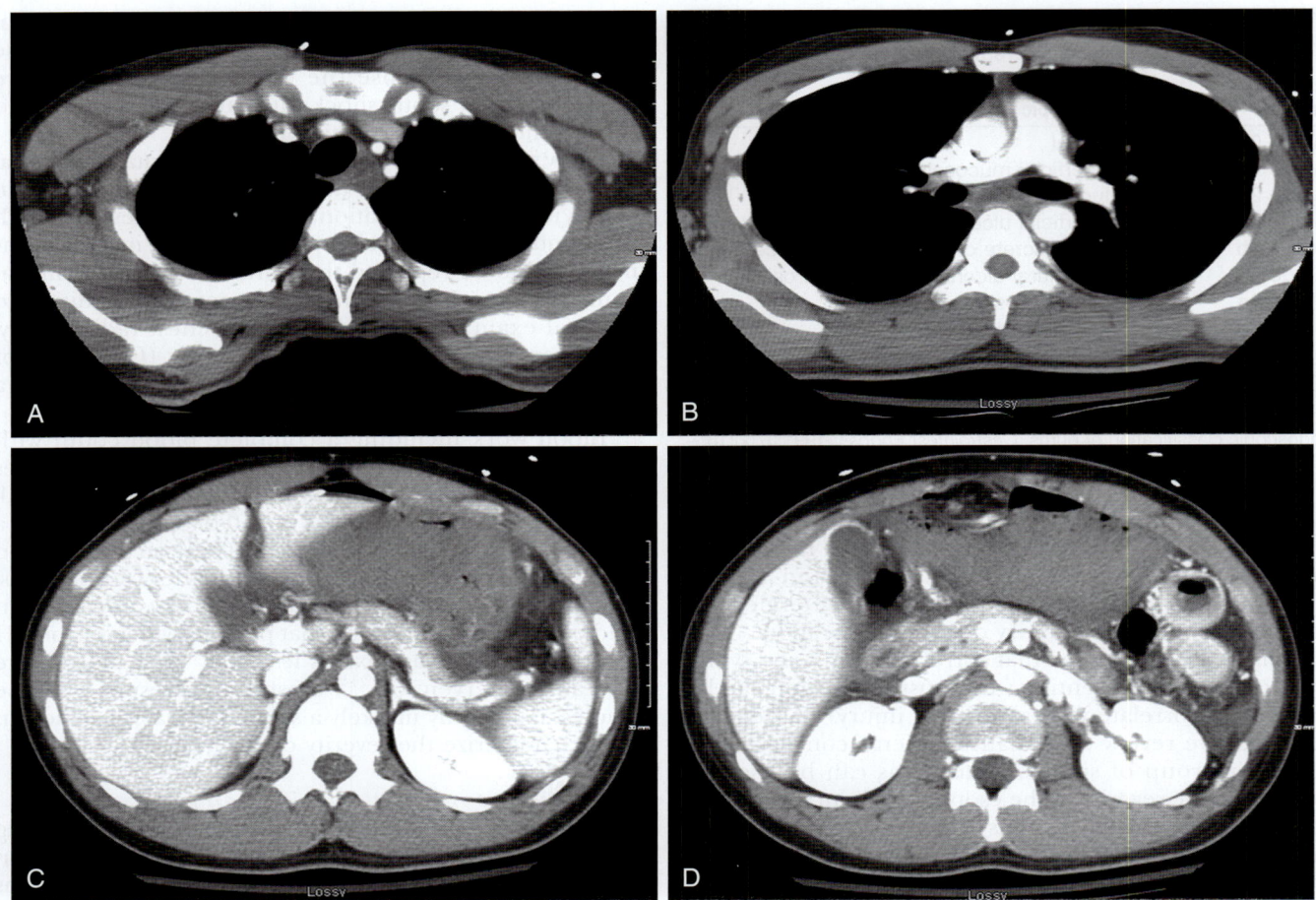

FIGURE 47.1 Computed tomography (CT) images of a male patient presenting with a severe caustic injury after ingestion of toilet cleaner. Images of the proximal (A) and distal (B) esophagus show inflammation of the esophageal wall with lack of enhancement. Abdominal images show inflammation and lack of enhancement in the proximal stomach (C) and pneumatosis and free air anterior to the liver suggesting gastric necrosis with perforation (D). The patient underwent a gastrectomy and subtotal esophagectomy with a cervical esophagostomy. He was eventually reconstructed with a colon interposition graft.

TABLE 47.3 Grading System for Computed Tomography Findings

Grade	CT Findings
Grade I	No definite swelling of esophagus wall (<3 mm within normal limits)
Grade II	Edematous wall thickening (>3 mm) without periesophageal soft tissue infiltration
Grade III	Edematous wall thickening with periesophageal soft tissue infiltration plus well-demarcated tissue interface
Grade IV	Edematous wall thickening with periesophageal soft tissue infiltration plus blurring of tissue interface or localized fluid collection around esophagus or descending aorta

CT, Computed tomography.
From Ryu HH, Jeung KW, Lee BK, et al. Caustic injury: can CT grading system enable prediction of esophageal stricture? *Clin Toxicol (Phila.).* 2010;48(2):137–142.

were hemodynamically unstable. They found a lower rate of esophagectomy in patients undergoing a CT scan without an increase in mortality.[29] A systematic review of the literature noted a lack of randomized controlled data but concluded that CT cannot replace endoscopy.[30] Essentially, the literature supports CT imaging as a useful adjunct to endoscopy in guiding management in hemodynamically stable patients.

ENDOSCOPY

Direct visualization of the esophageal mucosa has been considered the ideal means of evaluating a patient with a caustic injury. The grading system shown in Table 47.2 was developed based on 88 patients having a total of 381 endoscopy procedures.[6] Fig. 47.2 shows endoscopic images several hours after a male patient ingested sodium hydroxide. The injury was grade 2b, and he was ultimately managed without surgery. In contrast, the images in Fig. 47.3 were acquired 8 hours after a female ingested an unidentified quantity of Drano. These injuries are grade 3b, and the patient required emergent esophagogastrectomy. The final pathology revealed transmural necrosis with early

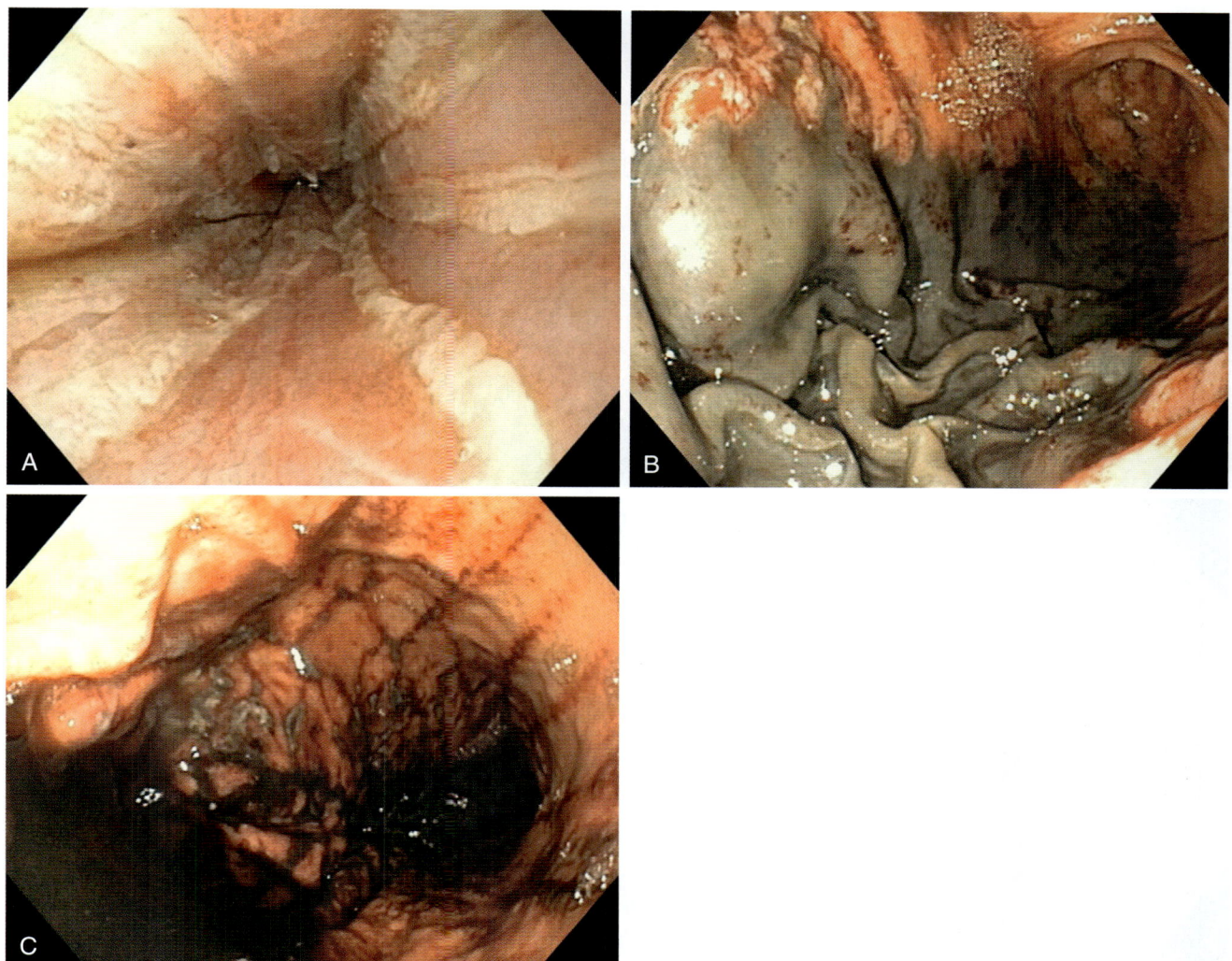

FIGURE 47.2 Endoscopic images of a male patient several hours after ingestion of a sodium hydroxide. Examination of the esophagus (A), body (B) and antrum (C) of the stomach show diffuse ulcerations of the esophagus and stomach consistent with a grade 2a caustic injury. The patient was managed without surgical intervention.

neutrophil infiltration. Despite the established utility of endoscopy, there are two persistent areas of debate: (1) the need to perform routine endoscopy on all patients presenting with a caustic ingestion; and (2) the role of advancing the endoscope through an area of injury to fully visualize the entire esophagus.

The first debate involves mainly pediatric patients because in adults there is a general consensus that all patients require endoscopic assessment of their esophagus. As noted, in the pediatric population most ingestions are accidental involving consumption of a small quantity of the caustic agent. A retrospective review of 28 pediatric patients reported that all four asymptomatic patients in the series had no findings at the time of endoscopy.[22] However, a larger study that reviewed 206 children with caustic injury found that 22 of 57 patients with normal clinical findings had abnormal endoscopic findings graded between 1 and 2b.[31] Another larger study found poor sensitivity and specificity of clinical findings, concluding endoscopy is mandatory in all pediatric patients. These

authors also emphasized that endoscopy allowed for early prognosis, early feeding, and earlier discharge in the setting of normal findings.[32] In summary, larger and current studies support the need to perform endoscopy in all patients to grade the esophageal injury.

The second debate involves the advancement of the endoscope through any area of injury. Although some authors argue that this increases the risk of perforation, others argue that a complete assessment of the esophagus is required to fully grade the injury and make treatment decisions. A recent report suggests that the opinion against full endoscopic assessment relates to the previous use of rigid endoscopy.[33] However, rigid esophagoscopy is rarely used currently and slimmer flexible endoscopes are now widely available. Thus, although there is a lack of clinical data to settle this debate, it is reasonable to predict a lower iatrogenic perforation rate with flexible endoscopy, and a complete endoscopic examination should be performed on all patients suspected to have a caustic ingestion.

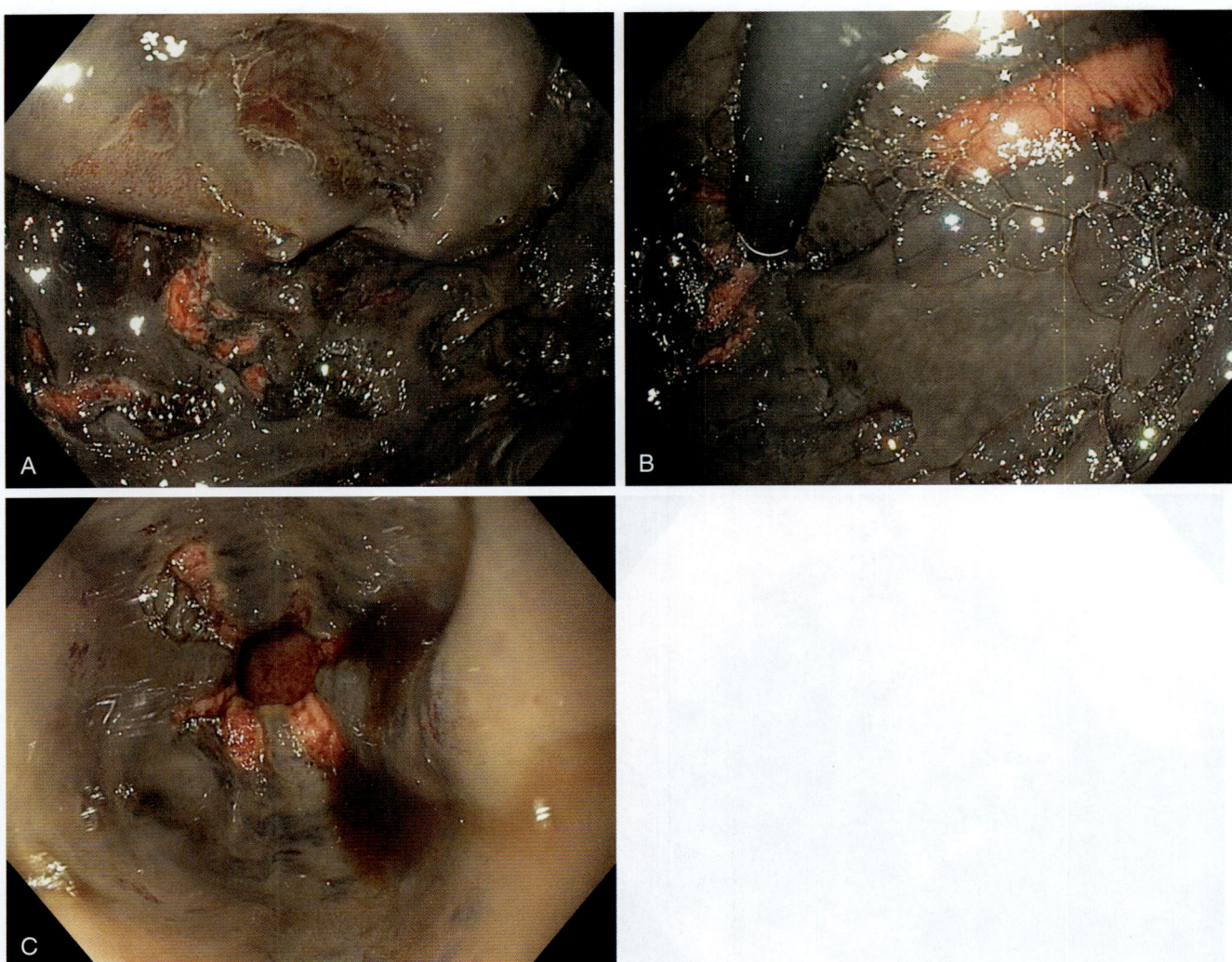

FIGURE 47.3 Endoscopic images of a female patient 8 hours after ingestion of Drano. Examination of the stomach body (A), fundus (B), and pylorus (C) show diffuse necrosis consistent with a grade 3b injury. The duodenal mucosa distal to the pylorus was not injured. The patient required emergent esophagogastrectomy where the final pathology revealed transmural necrosis with early neutrophil infiltration.

Endoscopic ultrasound (EUS) is a relatively new technology used for prognostication for caustic esophageal injuries. A retrospective review of 18 adult patients found that EUS can safely visualize the entire esophageal wall and demonstrate the depth of the injury. However, there was no added benefit to EUS when used in conjunction with endoscopy.[34] A smaller review of 11 adult patients reported that EUS can demonstrate injuries that penetrate the muscularis predicting the formation of strictures and concluded that EUS is useful for prognosticating.[35] In summary, EUS appears to be safe but has an undefined role in management of caustic injuries.

TREATMENT IN ACUTE PHASE

After a secure airway is confirmed and intravenous resuscitation has begun, the investigations noted earlier should be promptly initiated to grade the injury and guide management of the patient. In very general terms: grade 1 and 2a injuries can be given a trial of oral intake

and observed for 1 to 2 days; grade 2b and 3a injuries should be kept nil per os (NPO) and monitored in an intensive care unit, with follow-up endoscopy in 5 to 7 days to ensure improvement/healing before starting oral intake; and grade 3b or 4 injuries will require urgent operative intervention.[26,27,36-38] Although there is no high-level evidence to guide management of patients with grade 2b and higher injuries, there are data from multiple case series to guide medical and surgical treatments for individual patients.

MEDICAL MANAGEMENT

The goal of medical management has been to prevent acute perforation and chronic strictures. Evidence is lacking to clearly recommend interventions to achieve these goals, but there is evidence supporting avoidance of some common medical interventions.

Agents to induce emesis are contraindicated because emesis reexposes the esophagus to the caustic substance and a potential second insult. Ingestion of neutralizing agents has not been proven to benefit the patient but can lead to an exothermic reaction, further injuring the esophagus. Ingestion of milk and activated charcoal also have no proven benefit but can inhibit endoscopic examination of the esophagus.[26]

Antibiotics were originally used in conjunction with steroids. Data from prospective randomized controlled trials are lacking; however, many authors use broad-spectrum antibiotics in the management of caustic injuries.[24,37] However, other authors have published similar rates of mortality and morbidity without antibiotics,[33] and antibiotics have not been shown to prevent strictures.[39] Because the pathophysiology involves bacterial infiltration with higher-grade injuries, antibiotics can be justified and should be administered.

Although often used, the utility of proton pump inhibitors (PPIs) has not yet been clearly defined in prospective randomized controlled trials.[24,27] A prospective study of 13 patients with grades 1 to 3 injury receiving an infusion of omeprazole followed by omeprazole intravenously twice a day revealed significant healing on repeat endoscopy at 72 hours compared with a retrospective review of patients not receiving a PPI.[40] However, other authors have published similar rates of mortality and morbidity without acid suppression.[36] There is no basis for recommendation of routine use of PPIs in this setting.

Early administration of steroids has been a point of controversy for many years. Animal studies from the 1950s to 1960s suggested a benefit to steroids in reducing the acute inflammatory response in the esophagus and associated lung injuries.[15] This inhibition of the acute inflammatory response has also been proposed to decrease the incidence of stricture in the later phases of the injury. Unfortunately, this pharmacologic model has not been proven in two large meta-analyses. A systematic pooled analysis of 50 years of data showed no benefit from steroids in grade 2 injuries but did show an increased risk of perforation and infection, leading the authors to recommend against the use of steroids for grade 1 to 3 injuries.[41] A meta-analysis of 12 studies comparing patients with grades 2 and 3 injuries who received and did not receive steroids for longer than 8 days reported higher rates of strictures in patients who received steroids. The available evidence shows no benefit from steroids, and in fact a possible harm, to patients with a caustic injury.[42]

SURGICAL MANAGEMENT

Patients with grades 3b or 4 injuries on esophagoscopy, usually adults committing deliberate ingestion, require an operation.[38] Although surgery is not contraindicated in children, all efforts should be made to preserve their esophagus because of the challenges and long-term complications associated with restoring continuity of the gastrointestinal tract in a growing patient.[20]

The principles of damage control surgery apply in caustic injuries: careful assessment of the esophagus and stomach, removal of necrotic/nonviable tissue, preservation of hemostasis, and deferring definitive reconstruction. If the esophagus is nonviable, this will require esophagectomy with cervical esophagostomy. There is debate regarding the role of laparotomy versus laparoscopy to examine the stomach. Ultimately, this choice depends on the surgeon's

experience and preference. In grade 3a injuries a feeding jejunostomy should be considered to provide long-term enteral nutrition. Survival has been reported after upper abdominal exenteration including esophogastrectomy, total pancreatectomy, and duodenectomy.[43] Resection of the colon obviously limits later reconstructive options. If tissue viability is uncertain, a scheduled "second look" should be conducted in 12 to 24 hours.

TREATMENT IN INTERMEDIATE PHASE

It is patients with grade 2 to 3a injury who will require management in the intermediate phase. The majority of grade 1 injuries will not require any significant management, and grade 3b and 4 injuries will be recovering from removal of the esophagus and stomach. The two areas of focus of care include nutritional support and stricture prophylaxis.

NUTRITIONAL SUPPORT

A review of 315 patients managed with a nutritional protocol based on endoscopic grade revealed a 93% success rate with nonoperative management. Grade 0 and 1 injuries were allowed a normal diet and discharged home after 1 day of observation in hospital. Grade 2 to 3A injuries were placed on total parenteral nutrition (TPN) and had repeat endoscopy at 1 week. If the injury was improved or healed the patients were given a trial of oral intake; otherwise they were supported with TPN with repeat endoscopy after 3 weeks. Patients with grade 3a injury who were expected to have a prolonged course without oral intake had a feeding jejunostomy placed. All patients with grade 3b or 4 injuries were taken to the operating room for exploration.[38] A subsequent literature review recommended a similar approach.[27]

Placement of a nasogastric (NG) tube theoretically allows a route for enteral nutrition and a guide for future stricture dilation.[26,36,37] Risks include perforation during insertion, erosion, and exacerbating reflux secondary to stenting open natural sphincters. In one study, 53 patients had an NG tube safety placed endoscopically over a wire into the duodenum and fed through it for 8 weeks. When compared with 43 patients managed with jejunostomy feeds for 8 weeks, there was no difference in stricture rate or morbidity.[36] There is no evidence to support routine use of NG tubes in caustic injuries.

STRICTURE PROPHYLAXIS

Strictures predominantly affect grade 2 and 3 injuries.[41] As noted, there is not strong evidence to show that antibiotics or PPI in the acute phase of the injury prevent strictures. However, there is evidence to show steroids do not prevent strictures and may actually be harmful to the patient. In addition to these systemic therapies, there has been considerable effort to identify compounds that can be applied topically or injected into the esophageal wall to prevent stricture formation, progression, and recurrence. Several of these are summarized later; most have remained experimental. Therefore management of strictures involves mostly mechanical dilation or stenting.

Triamcinolone, a corticosteroid, has been injected into strictures to prevent progression.[44] Mitomycin C, a chemotherapy agent known to disrupt DNA, has been used in trials of topical application and injection.[45,46] In a prospective trial, mitomycin C was shown to reduce esophageal strictures in 18 pediatric patients with caustic injuries without systemic adverse events.[47] However, concerns regarding systemic absorption of this agent and the possibility of long-term secondary malignancy persist. The chemotherapy agent 5-fluorouracil (5-FU, an antimetabolite with antiproliferative effect through interference with pyrimidine metabolism) has been applied intraluminally in rats with caustic injuries and been shown to reduce esophageal strictures.[48]

Multiple antioxidant agents, the majority with antifibrotic and antiinflammatory properties, have been tried in animal models, but no human trials exist.[27] Pirfenidone, palifermin, tamoxifen, olmesartan, tenoxicam, and glucagon-like peptide 2 (GLP-2) have been shown in rats to decrease esophageal strictures after caustic injury.[49-54] There has also been an attempt to use mesenchymal stem cells to prevent strictures in rats following caustic injury.[55]

With lack of a medical means to prevent stricture formation, the predominant management has been dilatation of the strictures after they become evident. The role of early dilation to prevent clinically significant strictures has been debated for two reasons.[56] Firstly, stricture dilatation requires physically disrupting annular fibrosis, which will heal with further fibrosis; increased dilation is thus potentially associated with increased stricture rate. Secondly, it is not recommended to dilate between 7 and 21 days after the injury when necrotic tissue is sloughing and new collagen is forming, increasing the risk of esophageal perforation.[24,57,58] Savary dilators are safer than balloon dilatation because the operator can feel resistance to guide the dilation, thereby decreasing the perforation risk.[27,56] The overall rate of perforation has been reported to be between 5% and 32% depending on operator expertise.[58]

A retrospective review of 125 pediatric patients found early dilatation prevented the subsequent development of recalcitrant strictures.[57] Placement of a gastrostomy tube has been reported to facilitate retrograde dilatations.[58] Another author describes weekly scheduled dilatations with Savary dilators with injection of intralesional triamcinolone, reporting improvements in dysphagia scores and less on-demand dilatations after completing this regimen.[59]

Intraluminal stents have been advocated to avoid serial dilations; however, there is an absence of prospective and controlled data to provide clear evidence that stenting is superior to dilation. The majority of data come from the pediatric population in which a variety of stents have been used at different time intervals relative to the caustic injury.[56] Polypropylene stents covered with silicone were used in 10 pediatric patients with caustic strictures who failed 6 to 9 months of dilation. Stents were retained for 20 to 225 days, yielding a 50% cure rate.[60] In another study, customized polytetrafluoroethylene (PTFE) stents were placed for 9 to 14 months in 11 patients who previously failed 3 months of dilation. Eight of the 11 patients were eventually able to resume a normal diet.[61] A case series describing management of benign strictures (70% were secondary to caustic injuries) treated with silicon stents report fewer dilations with early stent placement. The authors concluded stents should be used for caustic injuries instead of serial dilation. In this series, one tracheoesophageal fistula is reported resulting from stent placement compared with six major complications from serial dilations.[62] Another study described antegrade insertion of stent for 2 to 3 months with success in 80% of patients.[63] A review of the literature quotes the efficacy of stenting at 50% to 72% with approximately a 10% migration rate. In summary, stenting is a reasonable option to avoid serial dilations in patients with strictures; however, timing and patient selection must be carefully individualized.

TREATMENT IN CHRONIC PHASE

The objective in the chronic phase of the injury is to restore functional gastrointestinal continuity. The patients who underwent emergent resection require a reconstructive operation, whereas those who did not often experience severe stricture formation or dysmotility.

Strictures are reported to occur in 6.3% to 13.8% and 23.1% to 71% of grade 2 and 3 injuries, respectively.[42] Because strictures start forming in the intermediate phase and continue to remodel in the chronic phase, the management of strictures crosses the two phases. As described previously, endoscopic dilation is the first line of therapy for strictures and some series report improved outcomes with early stent placement. Complications of stricture formation necessitating surgical intervention include obliteration of the lumen, nondilatable stricture (i.e., failure to achieve satisfactory patency despite multiple dilations), patient refusal to undergo serial dilatations, or perforation during dilatation.

There are two considerations in surgical management of patients in the chronic phase: (1) resection versus bypass of strictures, and (2) optimal conduits for reconstruction. For some patients the surgical options are dictated by the extent of resection in the earlier phases of the injury, or the location or pattern of the injury. In patients with intentional ingestions, establishment of psychiatric stability is vital prior to undertaking major reconstructive surgery.

RESECTION OR BYPASS OF STRICTURES

Resection has the benefit of preventing the formation of mucoceles and development of cancer in the injured organ. Esophageal carcinoma has been reported to occur in more than 30% of cases in both injured and noninjured portions of the esophagus, which has been used to justify performing total esophagectomy.[64] Arguments against esophageal resection include the risks of operating in a surgical field that has sustained a significant inflammatory response (e.g., injury to the airway or thoracic duct) and the long latent period until development of cancer (15 to 40 years).[65] Ultimately, there is a lack of high-level evidence and therefore a decision must be made on an individual basis considering the patient's life-expectance, comorbidities, ability to withstand a major procedure, and associated potential complications.

RECONSTRUCTION

Isolated injury to the esophagus allows for reconstruction with a gastric conduit or a colonic interposition graft. A gastric conduit is commonly used for reconstruction in oncologic resection and requires only a single anastomosis. Colon interposition involves greater operative time and complexity, with three anastomoses. A review of 28 patients treated on average 5 months after a caustic injury by transhiatal esophagectomy with cervical esophagogastrostomy reported good overall survival, but almost half of the patients developed strictures at the anastomosis requiring an average of three dilations.[66] Other authors implicate the increased incidence of reflux and aspiration associated with gastric conduits as the basis to recommend a colon graft instead—highlighting the colon as a straight and superior functioning conduit.[67]

Significant gastric injury mandates that a colon interposition graft be used. A review of 32 patients who had antesternal colonic interposition graft for persistent strictures or to restore gastrointestinal conduit after esophagogastrectomy report good functional outcomes.[65]

If the stomach and colon are both unavailable as conduits, more esoteric options must be considered. Jejunal interposition grafts are described but technically challenging, requiring microvascular anastomosis. Reverse gastric tubes are also described but known to be technically difficult.[68]

Severe strictures involving the pharynx and esophagus may require reconstruction with a colonic interposition graft or free jejunal graft. Pharyngocoloplasty does allow for restoration of gastrointestinal continuity with good survival outcomes, but patients do report significantly lower quality of life compared with patients who can undergo an esophagocoloplasty.[69] Free jejunal grafts have been described to reconstruct oropharyngeal injuries and after failure of colonic interposition grafts. Care must be taken to preserve the mesenteric vessels (which are divided near their origin); arterial and venous connections are later reestablished through anastomoses to the internal mammary artery and vein or a branch of the carotid artery and jugular vein.[70] Pedicled skin flaps have been described in case reports or small case series with limited success.[71,72] Supercharged reverse gastric tube with anastomosis to the superior thyroid artery and vein through a retrosternal tunnel has been described for caustic injuries requiring resection of diffuse laryngopharyngeal and esophageal stenosis.[68]

LONG-TERM CONSIDERATIONS

The most serious long-term complication after a caustic injury is the development of malignancy; benign complications such as esophageal stricture, dysmotility, gastroesophageal reflux disorder (GERD), and recurrent aspiration are far more common.

The incidence of adenocarcinoma and squamous cell carcinoma is 2% to 8% after esophageal caustic injury, with a latency of 15 to 40 years after the injury.[73] However, some series report a rate as high as 31.3%.[64] Standardized surveillance regimens are not established but should be considered on an individual basis as part of the patient's long-term care.

Tracheoesophageal fistula has been described after caustic injury to the esophagus and will require resection of the fistula and possibly the esophagus along with airway repair.[22] The incidence of GERD has been reported to be 63.5% in pediatric patients after a caustic injury. The length of stricture has been associated with an increased rate of GERD. It is possible that GERD promotes stricturing in addition to the underlying insult from the caustic injury. Prolonged and severe GERD, especially from a young age, may increase the risk of Barrett esophagus and eventual adenocarcinoma.[74]

SUMMARY

The majority of caustic injuries occur as accidental ingestions in children, whereas the minority is intentional ingestions in adolescents and adults. The pathophysiology is well described through animal models. Endoscopy is required to grade injuries and guide management. Clinical assessment, blood work and CT imaging are useful adjuncts to endoscopy. In general, grade 1 and 2a injuries are managed with a trial of oral intake, grade 2b and 3a injuries require close monitoring in hospital, and grade 3b and 4 injuries require emergent surgical intervention. In nonoperative patients, there is evidence to show steroids are not beneficial and controversies persist regarding other medical therapies. Ultimately, mechanical dilation is often required for management of strictures. Long-term complications of caustic injuries include an increased risk of malignancy, strictures, dysmotility, and GERD. Caustic injuries remain a surgical disease often requiring careful decision making regarding resection while planning for complex reconstructions to restore continuity of the gastrointestinal tract.

REFERENCES

1. Mowry JB, Spyker DA, Cantilena LR Jr, McMillan N, Ford M. 2013 Annual Report of the American Association of Poison Control Centers' National Poison Data System (NPDS): 31st Annual Report. *Clin Toxicol (Phila)*. 2014;52(10):1032-1283.
2. Bautista Casasnovas A, Estevez Martinez E, Varela Cives R, Villanueva Jeremias A, Tojo Sierra R, Cadranel S. A retrospective analysis of ingestion of caustic substances by children. Ten-year statistics in Galicia. *Eur J Pediatr*. 1997;156(5):410-414.
3. Sarioglu-Buke A, Corduk N, Atesci F, Karabul M, Koltuksuz U. A different aspect of corrosive ingestion in children: socio-demographic characteristics and effect of family functioning. *Int J Pediatr Otorhinolaryngol*. 2006;70(10):1791-1798.
4. Riffat F, Cheng A. Pediatric caustic ingestion: 50 consecutive cases and a review of the literature. *Dis Esophagus*. 2009;22(1):89-94.
5. Contini S, Swarray-Deen A, Scarpignato C. Oesophageal corrosive injuries in children: a forgotten social and health challenge in developing countries. *Bull World Health Organ*. 2009;87:950.
6. Zargar SA, Kochhar R, Mehta S, Mehta SK. The role of fiber-optic endoscopy in the management of corrosive ingestion and modified endoscopic classification of burns. *Gastrointest Endosc*. 1991;37(2):165-169.
7. Poley JW, Steyerberg EW, Kuipers EJ, et al. Ingestion of acid and alkaline agents: outcome and prognostic value of early upper endoscopy. *Gastrointest Endosc*. 2004;60(3):372-377.
8. Arevalo-Silva C, Eliashar R, Wohlgelernter J, Elidan J, Gross M. Ingestion of caustic substances: a 15-year experience. *Laryngoscope*. 2006;116(8):1422-1426.
9. Krey H. On the treatment of corrosive lesions in the oesophagus; an experimental study. *Acta Otolaryngol Suppl*. 1952;102:1-49.
10. Kirsh MM, Ritter F. Caustic ingestion and subsequent damage to the oropharyngeal and digestive passages. *Ann Thorac Surg*. 1976;21(1):74-82.
11. Haller JA Jr, Andrews HG, White JJ, Tamer MA, Cleveland WW. Pathophysiology and management of acute corrosive burns of

the esophagus: results of treatment in 285 children. *J Pediatr Surg.* 1971;6(5):578-584.

12. Hoffman RS, Howland MA, Kamerow HN, Goldfrank LR. Comparison of titratable acid/alkaline reserve and pH in potentially caustic household products. *J Toxicol Clin Toxicol.* 1989;27(4-5):241-246.

13. Zargar SA, Kochhar R, Nagi B, Mehta S, Mehta SK. Ingestion of corrosive acids. Spectrum of injury to upper gastrointestinal tract and natural history. *Gastroenterology.* 1989;97(3):702-707.

14. Lahoti D, Broor SL. Corrosive injury to the upper gastrointestinal tract. *Indian J Gastroenterol.* 1993;12(4):135-141.

15. Johnson EE. A study of corrosive esophagitis. *Laryngoscope.* 1963;73:1651-1696.

16. Emoto Y, Yoshizawa K, Shikata N, Tsubura A, Nagasaki Y. Autopsy results of a case of ingestion of sodium hydroxide solution. *J Toxicol Pathol.* 2016;29(1):45-47.

17. Osman M, Russell J, Shukla D, Moghadamfalahi M, Granger DN. Responses of the murine esophageal microcirculation to acute exposure to alkali, acid, or hypochlorite. *J Pediatr Surg.* 2008;43(9):1672-1678.

18. Gunel E, Caglayan F, Caglayan O, Akillioglu I. Reactive oxygen radical levels in caustic esophageal burns. *J Pediatr Surg.* 1999;34(3):405-407.

19. Havanond C, Havanond P. Initial signs and symptoms as prognostic indicators of severe gastrointestinal tract injury due to corrosive ingestion. *J Emerg Med.* 2007;33(4):349-353.

20. Gaudreault P, Parent M, McGuigan MA, Chicoine L, Lovejoy FH Jr. Predictability of esophageal injury from signs and symptoms: a study of caustic ingestion in 378 children. *Pediatrics.* 1983;71(5):767-770.

21. Gorman RL, Khin-Maung-Gyi MT, Klein-Schwartz W, et al. Initial symptoms as predictors of esophageal injury in alkaline corrosive ingestions. *Am J Emerg Med.* 1992;10(3):189-194.

22. Gupta SK, Croffie JM, Fitzgerald JF. Is esophagogastroduodenos-copy necessary in all caustic ingestions? *J Pediatr Gastroenterol Nutr.* 2001;32(1):50-53.

23. Rigo GP, Camellini L, Azzolini F, et al. What is the utility of selected clinical and endoscopic parameters in predicting the risk of death after caustic ingestion? *Endoscopy.* 2002;34(4):304-310.

24. Cheng HT, Cheng CL, Lin CH, et al. Caustic ingestion in adults: the role of endoscopic classification in predicting outcome. *BMC Gastroenterol.* 2008;8:31-230X-8-31.

25. Cheng YJ, Kao EL. Arterial blood gas analysis in acute caustic ingestion injuries. *Surg Today.* 2003;33(7):483-485.

26. Ramasamy K, Gumaste VV. Corrosive ingestion in adults. *J Clin Gastroenterol.* 2003;37(2):119-124.

27. Contini S, Scarpignato C. Caustic injury of the upper gastro-intestinal tract: a comprehensive review. *World J Gastroenterol.* 2013;19(25):3918-3930.

28. Ryu HH, Jeung KW, Lee BK, et al. Caustic injury: can CT grading system enable prediction of esophageal stricture? *Clin Toxicol (Phila).* 2010;48(2):137-142.

29. Chirica M, Resche-Rigon M, Pariente B, et al. Computed tomog-raphy evaluation of high-grade esophageal necrosis after corrosive ingestion to avoid unnecessary esophagectomy. *Surg Endosc.* 2015;29(6):1452-1461.

30. Bonnici KS, Wood DM, Dargan PI. Should computerised tomography replace endoscopy in the evaluation of symptomatic ingestion of corrosive substances? *Clin Toxicol (Phila).* 2014;52(9):911-925.

31. Temiz A, Oguzkurt P, Ezer SS, Ince E, Hicsonmez A. Predictability of outcome of caustic ingestion by esophagogastroduodenoscopy in children. *World J Gastroenterol.* 2012;18(10):1098-1103.

32. Boskovic A, Stankovic I. Predictability of gastroesophageal caustic injury from clinical findings: is endoscopy mandatory in children? *Eur J Gastroenterol Hepatol.* 2014;26(5):499-503.

33. Bosnali O, Moralioglu S, Celayir A, Pektas OZ. Is rigid endoscopy necessary with childhood corrosive ingestion? A retrospective comparative analysis of 458 cases. *Dis Esophagus.* 2016;30(3):1-7.

34. Chiu HM, Lin JT, Huang SP, Chen CH, Yang CS, Wang HP. Predic-tion of bleeding and stricture formation after corrosive ingestion by EUS concurrent with upper endoscopy. *Gastrointest Endosc.* 2004;60(5):827-833.

35. Kamijo Y, Kondo I, Kokuto M, Kataoka Y, Soma K. Miniprobe ultrasonography for determining prognosis in corrosive esophagitis. *Am J Gastroenterol.* 2004;99(5):851-854.

36. Kochhar R, Poornachandra KS, Puri P, et al. Comparative evaluation of nasoenteral feeding and jejunostomy feeding in acute corrosive injury: a retrospective analysis. *Gastrointest Endosc.* 2009;70(5):874-880.

37. Kay M, Wyllie R. Caustic ingestions in children. *Curr Opin Pediatr.* 2009;21(5):651-654.

38. Cabral C, Chirica M, de Chaisemartin C, et al. Caustic injuries of the upper digestive tract: a population observational study. *Surg Endosc.* 2012;26(1):214-221.

39. Salzman M, O'Malley RN. Updates on the evaluation and management of caustic exposures. *Emerg Med Clin North Am.* 2007;25(2):459-476.

40. Cakal B, Akbal E, Koklu S, et al. Acute therapy with intravenous omeprazole on caustic esophageal injury: a prospective case series. *Dis Esophagus.* 2013;26(1):22-26.

41. Fulton JA, Hoffman RS. Steroids in second degree caustic burns of the esophagus: a systematic pooled analysis of fifty years of human data: 1956–2006. *Clin Toxicol (Phila).* 2007;45(4):402-408.

42. Pelclova D, Navratil T. Do corticosteroids prevent oesophageal stricture after corrosive ingestion? *Toxicol Rev.* 2005;24(2):125-129.

43. Guarino S, Shobayo F, Qureshi YA, Daley F, Alaraimi B, Patel B. Upper abdominal exenteration: a life saving procedure following caustic ingestion. *Dig Liver Dis.* 2014;46(4):386-387.

44. Kochhar R, Ray JD, Sriram PV, Kumar S, Singh K. Intralesional steroids augment the effects of endoscopic dilation in corrosive esophageal strictures. *Gastrointest Endosc.* 1999;49(4):509-513.

45. Uhlen S, Fayoux P, Vachin F, et al. An alternative conservative treatment for refractory esophageal stricture in children? *Endoscopy.* 2006;38(4):404-407.

46. Berger M, Ure B, Lacher M. Mitomycin C in the therapy of recurrent esophageal strictures: hype or hope? *Eur J Pediatr Surg.* 2012;22(2):109-116.

47. El-Asmar KM, Hassan MA, Abdelkader HM, Hamza AF. Topical mitomycin C can effectively alleviate dysphagia in children with long-segment caustic esophageal strictures. *Dis Esophagus.* 2015;28(5):422-427.

48. Duman L, Buyukyavuz BI, Altuntas I, et al. The efficacy of single-dose 5-fluorouracil therapy in experimental caustic esophageal burn. *J Pediatr Surg.* 2011;46(10):1893-1897.

49. Orozco-Perez J, Aguirre-Jauregui O, Salazar-Montes AM, Sobrevilla-Navarro AA, Lucano-Landeros MS, Armendariz-Borunda J. Pir-fenidone prevents rat esophageal stricture formation. *J Surg Res.* 2015;194(2):558-564.

50. Numanoglu KV, Tatli D, Bektas S, Ebubekir E. Efficacy of keratinocyte growth factor (palifermin) for the treatment of caustic esophageal burns. *Exp Ther Med.* 2014;8(4):1087-1091.

51. Elmas O, Cevik M, Demir T, Ketani MA. Effect of oral tamoxifen on the healing of corrosive oesophageal burns in an experimental rat model. *Interact Cardiovasc Thorac Surg.* 2014;19(3):351-356.

52. Dereli M, Krazinski BE, Ayvaz S, et al. A novel approach for preventing esophageal stricture formation: olmesartan prevented apoptosis. *Folia Histochem Cytobiol.* 2014;52(1):29-35.

53. Tekin M, Topaloglu N, Kucuk A, Deniz M, Yildirim S, Erdem H. Protective effect of glucagon-like peptide-2 in experimental corrosive esophagitis. *Dis Esophagus.* 2015;28(3):258-261.

54. Erbas M, Kiraz HA, Kucuk A, et al. Effects of tenoxicam in experimen-tal corrosive esophagitis model. *Dis Esophagus.* 2015;28(3):253-257.

55. Kantarcioglu M, Caliskan B, Demirci H, et al. The efficacy of mes-enchymal stem cell transplantation in caustic esophagus injury: an experimental study. *Stem Cells Int.* 2014;2014:939674.

56. Bonavina L, Chirica M, Skrobic O, et al. Foregut caustic injuries: results of the World Society of Emergency Surgery consensus confer-ence. *World J Emerg Surg.* 2015;10:44. eCollection 2015.

57. Tiryaki T, Livanelioglu Z, Atayurt H. Early bougienage for relief of stricture formation following caustic esophageal burns. *Pediatr Surg Int.* 2005;21(2):78-80.

58. Contini S, Garatti M, Swarray-Deen A, Depetris N, Cecchini S, Scarpignato C. Corrosive oesophageal strictures in children: outcomes after timely or delayed dilatation. *Dig Liver Dis.* 2009;41(4):263-268.

59. Nijhawan S, Udawat HP, Nagar P. Aggressive bougie dilatation and intralesional steroids is effective in refractory benign esopha-geal strictures secondary to corrosive ingestion. *Dis Esophagus.* 2016;29(8):1027-1031.

60. Broto J, Asensio M, Vernet JM. Results of a new technique in the treatment of severe esophageal stenosis in children: poliflex stents. *J Pediatr Gastroenterol Nutr.* 2003;37(2):203-206.

61. Atabek C, Surer I, Demirbag S, Caliskan B, Ozturk H, Cetinkursun S. Increasing tendency in caustic esophageal burns and long-term polytetrafluorethylene stenting in severe cases: 10 years experience. *J Pediatr Surg.* 2007;42(4):636-640.

62. Foschia F, De Angelis P, Torroni F, et al. Custom dynamic stent for esophageal strictures in children. *J Pediatr Surg.* 2011;46(5):848-853.

63. Wang RW, Zhou JH, Jiang YG, et al. Prevention of stricture with intraluminal stenting through laparotomy after corrosive esophageal burns. *Eur J Cardiothorac Surg.* 2006;30(2):207-211.

64. Okonta KE, Tettey M, Abubakar U. In patients with corrosive oesophageal stricture for surgery, is oesophagectomy rather than bypass necessary to reduce the risk of oesophageal malignancy? *Interact Cardiovasc Thorac Surg.* 2012;15(4):713-715

65. Gvalani AK, Deolekar S, Gandhi J, Dalvi A. Antesternal colonic interposition for corrosive esophageal stricture. *Indian J Surg.* 2014;76(1):56-60.

66. Harlak A, Yigit T, Coskun K, et al. Surgical treatment of caustic esophageal strictures in adults. *Int J Surg.* 2013;11(2):164-168.

67. Boukerrouche A. Left colonic graft in esophageal reconstruction for caustic stricture: mortality and morbidity. *Dis Esophagus.* 2013;26(8):788-793.

68. Huang PM, Chen CN, Yang TL, Ko JY, Lee JM, Cheng NC. Supercharged reversed gastric tube technique: a microvascular anastomosis procedure for pharyngo-oesophageal reconstruction after total laryngopharyngo-oesophagectomy. *Eur J Cardiothorac Surg.* 2013;44(2):258-262.

69. Chirica M, Brette MD, Faron M, et al. Upper digestive tract reconstruction for caustic injuries. *Ann Surg.* 2015;261(5):894-901.

70. Kim SH, Kim HK, Kim K, Shim YM. Outcome of free jejunal transfer using the end-to-side arterial anastomosis technique as a pharyngo-oesophageal substitute: a 15-year experience. *Eur J Cardiothorac Surg.* 2013;44(3):520-524.

71. Sa YJ, Kim YD, Kim CK, Park JK, Moon SW. Recurrent cervical esophageal stenosis after colon conduit failure: use of myocutaneous flap. *World J Gastroenterol.* 2013;19(2):307-310.

72. Imaizumi A, Liem AA, Yang CF, Chen W, Chen SH, Chen HC. Long-term outcomes of simultaneous skin and bowel flaps for esophageal reconstruction. *Ann Plast Surg.* 2015;75(2):180-185.

73. Millar AJ, Cox SG. Caustic injury of the oesophagus. *Pediatr Surg Int.* 2015;31(2):111-121.

74. Iskit SH, Ozcelik Z, Alkan M, Turker S, Zorludemir U. Factors affecting the prevalence of gastro-oesophageal reflux in childhood corrosive oesophageal strictures. *Balkan Med J.* 2014;31(2):137-142.

Etiology and Management of Esophageal Perforation

Thomas J. Watson | Christian G. Peyre

Perforation of the esophagus is a potentially serious and life-threatening medical emergency. Given the diverse etiologies and wide variety in clinical presentations of the perforated esophagus, the managing physician must possess a thorough understanding of the principles behind its treatment, as well as have access to an array of therapeutic tools, to provide an optimal outcome. Surgical therapy has occupied a prominent place in the management armamentarium of esophageal perforation since Norman Barrett reported the first case of successful primary repair in 1946.[1] Over the subsequent decades, surgical techniques have been developed and refined, and improvements in antibiotics, critical care, radiologic imaging, and percutaneous interventions have evolved. More recently, nonoperative and endoscopic approaches have been introduced as alternatives to surgery in appropriately selected patients, further improving the ability to treat this condition.[2] Despite these advances, the morbidity and mortality following perforation of the esophagus remain high, especially in cases of diagnostic delay, underscoring the importance of prompt recognition and appropriate treatment of this malady. Therefore considerable clinical judgment is required on the part of the managing physician because treatment decisions may have a major impact on outcomes.

ETIOLOGY

The first report of spontaneous esophageal perforation was attributed to the Dutch physician Hermann Boerhaave in 1724. He described the demise of Barron van Wassenaer, the Grand Admiral of the Dutch fleet, after an episode of self-induced vomiting following a large meal. Spontaneous esophageal perforation, which has come to be known as Boerhaave syndrome, is due to an abrupt increase in the intraluminal pressure of the esophagus during forceful emesis leading to full-thickness rupture of the esophageal wall. The perforation is generally toward the left and may involve the thoracic or abdominal portion of the esophagus.

Fortunately, Boerhaave syndrome remains relatively uncommon, accounting for only 15% of esophageal perforations.[3] With the frequent utilization of flexible endoscopy and its adjuncts for esophageal diagnostics and therapeutics, the most common cause of esophageal perforation currently is iatrogenic injury following esophageal instrumentation, accounting for nearly 60% of all cases. Given the elective nature of most such interventions and the fact that the perforations are often both immediately recognized and occur with minimal initial contamination of surrounding tissues due to an empty stomach, the outcomes may be better than those following spontaneous perforation, where diagnosis may be delayed and extensive contamination may occur. Other contemporary etiologies of esophageal perforation include foreign body ingestion, blunt or penetrating trauma, iatrogenic operative injury, tumor, and tumor necrosis following cancer-related therapy, such as radiation or chemotherapy.

PRESENTATION

Esophageal perforations are quite variable in their manifestations and presentations depending upon multiple factors, including:
- Etiology
- Size
- Location
- Associated esophageal pathology
- Time interval since perforation
- Extent of neck, mediastinal, pleural or abdominal contamination
- Patient comorbidities

The most common presenting symptom is chest pain, although complaints of odynophagia, neck or abdominal pain, dyspnea, crepitus, fevers, and chills may occur in addition or in isolation. Symptoms may be mild, particularly if the perforation is contained or of recent onset. Within the first 8 to 24 hours following injury, frank sepsis with tachycardia, hypotension, altered mental status and respiratory failure may develop, particularly if the contamination is extensive. Given the potentially serious consequences of diagnostic delays, a high index of suspicion for esophageal perforation is necessary in any patient presenting with moderate to severe upper gastrointestinal symptoms of recent onset, especially following vomiting or a history of recent esophageal instrumentation.

During the initial evaluation, a thorough history focused on preexisting dysphagia, heartburn, or regurgitation, as well as prior esophageal surgery or known esophageal disorders, is important because concomitant esophageal pathology may have contributed to the perforation or may influence the treatment paradigm.

DIAGNOSIS

After a detailed clinical history and physical examination have been completed, the most useful and expeditious initial screening examination for evaluation of the patient with a suspected esophageal perforation is a plain upright chest radiograph. This quick, readily available, and inexpensive study may reveal a pleural effusion, pneumothorax, pneumoperitoneum, subcutaneous or mediastinal emphysema, or mediastinal widening suggestive of perforation. However, of importance, is the fact that a normal chest x-ray does not rule out the possibility of a leak, especially in the early time period after the suspected event, because it may be contained or inadequate

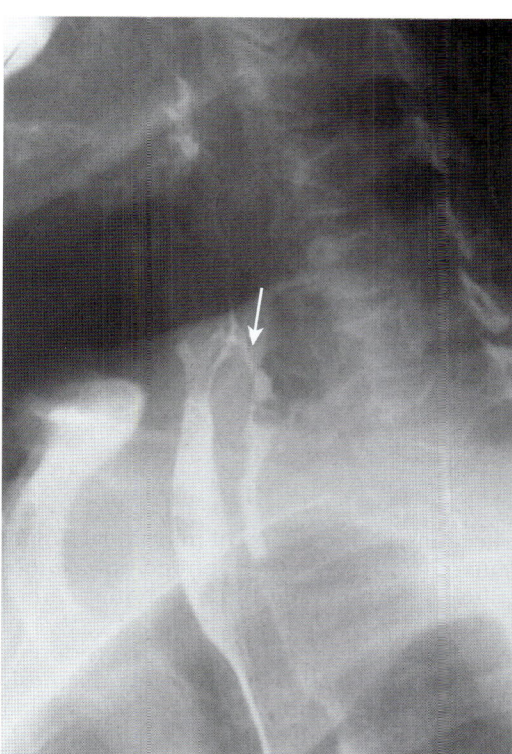

FIGURE 48.1 Lateral view of a Gastrografin esophagram demonstrating an esophageal perforation (arrow) with extravasation of contrast into the mediastinum. (From Soose RJ, Carrau RL. Esophagoscopy. In: Myers EN, ed. *Operative Otolaryngology: Head and Neck Surgery.* Philadelphia: Saunders; 2008:443–449.)

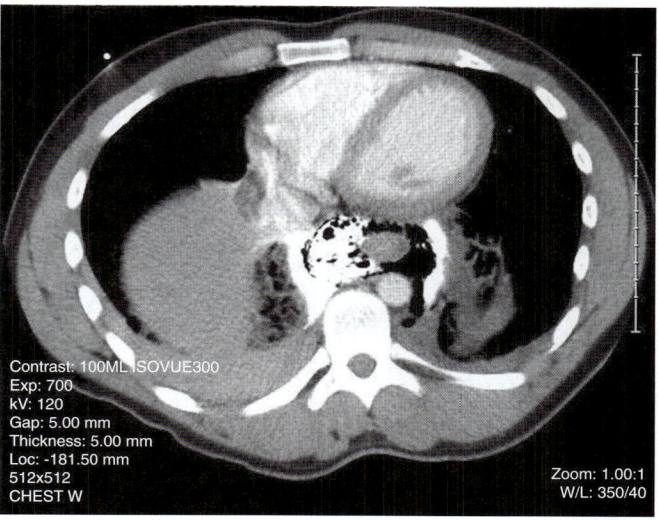

FIGURE 48.2 Computed tomography of the chest revealing a distal esophageal perforation with associated pleural effusion. Note the leakage of orally administered contrast.

time may have elapsed to allow for the development of a recognizable radiographic abnormality.

The most frequently used radiologic test specifically to assess for esophageal perforation has been the contrast esophagram (Fig. 48.1). The study traditionally is commenced with a water-soluble contrast agent, such as diatrizoate meglumine and diatrizoate sodium solution (Gastrografin), due to a concern for exacerbating mediastinal, pleural, or abdominal contamination if barium were used and leaked. However, contrast esophagography requires an alert and cooperative patient who is able to swallow without aspirating. In the intubated patient, contrast can be administered via a nasoesophageal tube. A risk of water-soluble contrast is the potential to induce a severe chemical pneumonitis if aspirated into the lung parenchyma. Therefore judgment must be exercised in using this study for the elderly patient or others considered at high risk for aspiration, because a resultant pulmonary injury could be a catastrophic insult added to the morbidity of the perforation.

The exam typically provides a reliable assessment of esophageal anatomy, the location and size of a perforation, and the presence of significant coexisting esophageal pathology, such as an esophageal stricture, malignancy, diverticulum, or motility disorder. In addition, a determination can be made as to whether the perforation is contained or freely leaking into the mediastinum, pleural spaces,

abdomen, or neck, as well as the size of associated fluid collections. A negative study with water-soluble contrast should be followed by one using thin barium to increase the sensitivity of the examination. Films also should be taken with the patient in both the left lateral and right lateral decubitus positions because proper positioning also may increase the sensitivity of the study in detecting a leak. However, a negative esophagram does not exclude a perforation because false-negative rates run in the range of 10% to 38%.[4,5]

Computed tomography (CT) has proven to be an extremely useful diagnostic modality for assessing esophageal perforations and guiding their management (Fig. 48.2). Findings on CT suggestive of perforation include pneumomediastinum, pneumoperitoneum, subcutaneous emphysema, mediastinal fluid or inflammation, pleural effusion, or abdominal abscess. Importantly, CT provides accurate information regarding the location and size of any extraesophageal fluid collections in need of operative intervention or percutaneous drainage.[5,6]

The finding of frank leakage of oral contrast is not sensitive and should not be the sole criterion to prove or disprove the diagnosis.

Flexible fiberoptic upper endoscopy serves a critical role in the assessment of a wide array of esophageal pathology, including perforations (Fig. 48.3). Not only does endoscopic assessment facilitate the determination of the location and size of a mucosal injury, it also allows identification of concomitant mucosal ischemia or ulceration, as well as more chronic or subacute pathology such as a stricture, diverticulum, or malignancy. Some perforations are subtle and do not demonstrate an obvious mucosal tear but rather only an ecchymotic or slightly disrupted mucosa that flutters with insufflation. Although concern may exist about the safety of flexible endoscopy in the setting of acute perforation, given the need for insufflation and the risk of inducing a tension pneumothorax or exacerbating pneumoperitoneum,

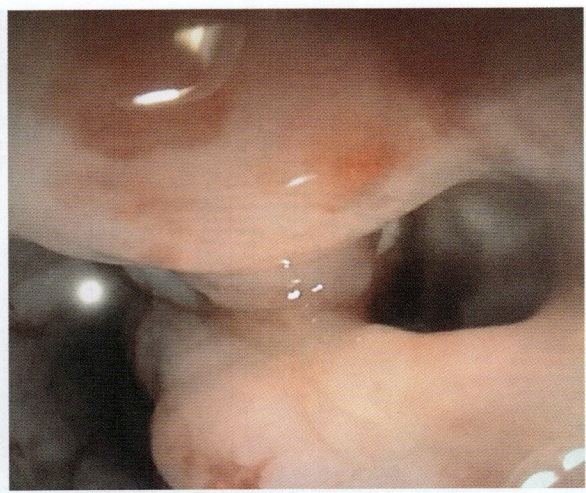

FIGURE 48.3 Flexible upper endoscopy revealing a full-thickness perforation of the esophagus after dilation of a stricture.

TABLE 48.1 Criteria for Nonoperative Management of Esophageal Perforation

- Small and contained leak with minimal extraluminal contamination
- Contrast drains into the esophageal lumen on esophagram
- Minimal symptoms
- Minimal signs of sepsis
- Absence of esophageal pathology (e.g., malignancy) or distal obstruction (e.g., stricture) that will impair healing

Modified from Cameron JL, Kieffer RF, Hendrix TR, et al. Selective nonoperative management of contained intrathoracic esophageal disruptions. *Ann Thorac Surg.* 1979;27:404–408; and Altorjay A, Kiss J, Voros A, Bohak A. Nonoperative management of esophageal perforations. Is it justified? *Ann Surg.* 1997;225:415–421.

the examination typically can be completed safely in experienced hands and with appropriate attention to detail. Insufflation should be kept to a minimum, and consideration should be given to placement of a chest tube prior to the procedure if concern exists about the consequences of a pneumothorax.

No single diagnostic study is absolutely reliable in the evaluation of esophageal perforation. Esophagography with water-soluble contrast agents is limited by its false negative rate and risk of aspiration pneumonitis, as well as by its relative insensitivity in assessing mucosal pathology. In addition, leaked barium risks exacerbating mediastinal, pleural, or abdominal sepsis. CT lacks sensitivity in locating the exact site of a perforation and detecting concomitant esophageal pathology. Endoscopy is invasive, requires sedation, risks exacerbating pneumothorax or pneumoperitoneum, and does not facilitate a determination of the extent of extraesophageal contamination.

As a result of the limitations of each of these diagnostic modalities, considerable judgment is required on the part of the managing physician to determine the sequence and optimal utilization of studies, taking into consideration the clinical suspicion for a leak, the information desired, patient comorbidities and performance status, and possible therapeutic alternatives. A point worthy of emphasis is that the location of a perforation and extent of contamination must be determined prior to surgical intervention because the location of incisions and the types of procedures chosen are dependent on the findings.

TREATMENT

PRINCIPLES OF INITIAL MANAGEMENT

The greatest threats from esophageal perforation are sepsis and death resulting from leakage of enteric contents. Accordingly, the focus of treatment should be the timely delivery of appropriate systemic antibiotics, elimination of the source of infection by repairing, occluding, diverting or exteriorizing the leak, adequate drainage of extraluminal

fluid collections, and provision of nutritional support. Any management strategy, whether nonoperative, endoscopic, or operative, must include these essential components of therapy.

After an esophageal perforation is considered in the differential diagnosis, prior to a definitive diagnosis being reached, initial interventions should include avoidance of food or liquids by mouth, administration of intravenous fluids, and initiation of broad-spectrum antibiotics. An extensive body of literature has shown a significant decrease in sepsis-related mortality with the expeditious administration of appropriate antibiotic therapy.[7,8] Leaked enteric contents cause a chemical burn in the surrounding tissues of the neck, mediastinum, pleural spaces, or peritoneal cavity and may lead to sequestration of large amounts of fluid, further exacerbating the hypotension that results from sepsis. Antibiotics should be directed toward enteric organisms, including gram-positive, gram-negative, and anaerobic bacteria, as well as fungi. Antifungal therapy is particularly relevant in individuals with a recent history of using proton pump inhibitors because they are known to increase the risk of fungal colonization in the stomach.[9] Closed tube thoracostomy should be considered early to drain large pleural effusions or treat a pneumothorax, even while preparations are made for definitive diagnosis and intervention.

NONOPERATIVE THERAPY

For many years, surgical intervention was considered a necessity for the majority of cases of esophageal perforation but was associated with high rates of morbidity and mortality. Based on the observation that patients with small, contained perforations and lacking evidence of systemic sepsis did well without surgery, a nonoperative treatment paradigm evolved. The criteria for nonoperative management in carefully selected patients were introduced by Cameron et al.[10] and subsequently refined by Altorjay et al. (Table 48.1).[11] With a nonoperative approach, the morbidity associated with major esophageal surgery in the emergent setting could be eliminated. The initial nonoperative experiences were for patients sustaining a spontaneous esophageal perforation, although the management principles have been extrapolated to other causes of perforation as well. Patients who meet the criteria can be treated with intravenous antibiotics and nothing by mouth with close observation in a monitored setting. The duration of therapy is dictated by the patient's clinical course. Follow-up endoscopy or radiographic imaging is useful in determining the resolution of the perforation and the timing of resumption of an oral diet. Of course, a clinical decline with the development of sepsis mandates an expeditious investigation and strong consideration of more invasive therapeutic measures.

ENDOSCOPIC MANAGEMENT

Advances in endoscopic technologies have led to novel techniques for management of esophageal perforations and their sequelae. Currently available endoscopic modalities used in the management of perforations include endoluminal suturing (OverStitch; Apollo Endosurgery, Inc., Austin, Texas), through-the-scope (TTS) clips, over-the-scope clips (OTSC System; Ovesco Inc., Tübingen, Germany), endoscopic vacuum therapy (EVT), and the placement of covered esophageal stents. These technologies have been used alone or in combination as part of an endoscopic treatment paradigm, and as either primary therapy or salvage after failed surgical repair of an esophageal rupture. The most extensive experience to date has been with stenting.

The first report of successful esophageal stent placement was by Symonds in 1887 using a prosthesis made of ivory and silver.[12] Multiple varieties of rigid, hollow prostheses placed with the assistance of transoral delivery systems were introduced much later by Mousseau et al., Celestin, and Atkinson et al., among others.[13-15] Because of their large diameter, bulk, and stiff construct, all of these stents were difficult and hazardous to place and extract. Rigid stents were used traditionally for palliation of dysphagia in patients with locoregionally advanced, obstructing esophageal neoplasms and a short life expectancy. Versions with a soft outer sponge encasing the main shaft also were created for occlusion of esophageal perforations and fistulas (Fig. 48.4).

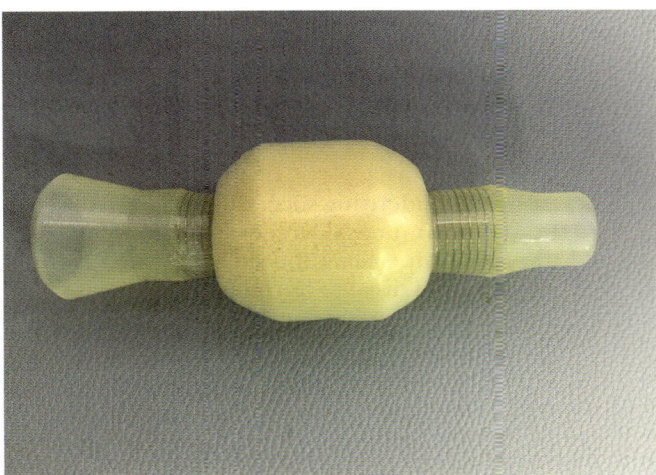

FIGURE 48.4 A rigid plastic esophageal stent with foam covering the shaft, intended for occlusion of an esophageal perforation or fistula.

Advances in engineering and manufacturing led to the development of self-expanding metallic stents (SEMSs) in the 1990s. These stents are constructed of steel alloys, such as nitinol (nickel and titanium) or elgiloy (cobalt, nickel, and chromium), and are woven, knitted, or cut into a mesh. They are introduced into the esophagus over a guidewire in a compressed state using a delivery system. Upon deployment, they are designed to self-expand up to a predetermined diameter. Advantages of such stents compared with prior versions include the ability to use flexible upper endoscopy for placement and the smaller esophageal luminal diameter requirements for insertion.

Subsequent versions of SEMSs incorporated a partial covering of polyurethane, silicone, or other polymers to prevent tumor ingrowth along most of the stent length. However, the proximal and distal 1.5 cm were left bare to facilitate better adherence to the mucosa and allow ingrowth of granulation tissue as a means to achieve stent fixation. This construct helps to prevent migration but also makes extraction at a later date difficult or impossible without risking significant injury to the esophagus and surrounding structures. Due to their potential for erosion when left in place for extended periods of time, partially covered stents are indicated only for cases of end-stage malignancy when life expectancy is short or in the preoperative setting for resectable cancer with the expectation that the esophagus and stent subsequently will be removed.

With advancements in materials, the next iteration in stent technology was the introduction of solid, collapsible, self-expanding plastic stents (SEPSs) coated with silicone. These devices can be inserted in a compressed state with minimal esophageal dilation, deployed within the esophageal lumen, and used to occlude esophageal perforations or fistulas. Because these stents are solid, ingrowth of tumor or granulation tissue is not a concern, although the decreased fixation increases the rate of stent migration.[16] However, they possess the advantage over partially covered SEMSs of being removable at a later date.

More recently, fully covered SEMSs and hybrid stents have been introduced that allow for later extraction yet are easier to introduce and require less dilation than SEPSs. These fully covered versions have broadened the indications for SEMSs to nonmalignant conditions such as strictures, perforations, and fistulas, including anastomotic complications arising after esophagectomy and foregut reconstruction.

Although a stent may be effective at controlling a leak, any extraluminal contamination that occurred prior to successful occlusion must also be addressed by appropriate drainage of the mediastinum, pleural spaces, or peritoneum.[17] Chest tubes or CT-guided pigtail catheters can be placed into small to moderate collections. A thoracotomy or minimally invasive video-assisted thoracic surgical (VATS) approach may be necessary for cases of more extensive contamination, facilitating washout and débridement of the mediastinal and pleural spaces, decortication of the lung, and placement of multiple drains under direct visualization.

Some perforations are not amenable to stenting. Examples include those high in the cervical esophagus where a stent would extend into the pharynx, causing

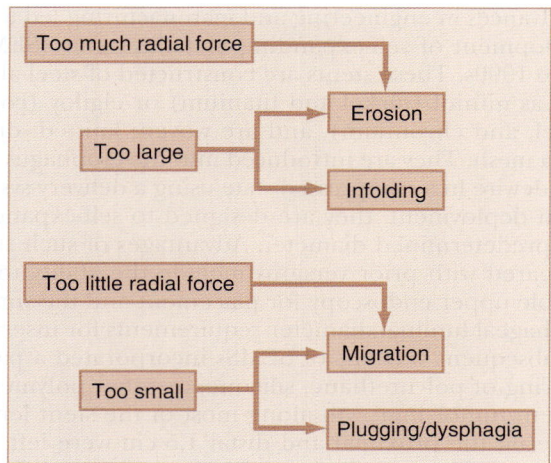

FIGURE 48.5 Considerations of appropriate esophageal stent design and sizing.

significant patient discomfort, or those spanning the gastroesophageal junction that are impossible to occlude due to the bulbous nature of the gastric cardia. A perforation occurring in a dilated esophagus, such as may be found in the setting of achalasia, may also prove impossible to occlude with a stent. Even in a normal esophagus, satisfactory occlusion of a leak may not be achieved, particularly if the stent is malpositioned or is of an inappropriate size or length.

Complications associated with esophageal stents include ongoing or recurrent esophageal leakage, migration, luminal obstruction, erosion, pain, bleeding, and inextractability at a later date (Fig. 48.5). In addition, for stents crossing the esophagogastric junction and compromising the lower esophageal high-pressure zone, the induction or exacerbation of gastroesophageal reflux is a significant concern. The endoscopist also must be alert to the possibility of isolating an extraluminal fluid collection, preventing it from draining back into the esophagus. The timing of stent removal is a matter of judgment, balancing the likelihood of healing of the perforation against potential complications, such as erosion or obstruction, which may arise the longer the stent is left in place.

Persistent or recurrent esophageal leaks after stenting can occur for a multitude of reasons, including malpositioning, incorrect size leading to inadequate proximal or distal stent apposition to the esophageal mucosa, tearing or degradation of the stent covering, leakage between two separate stents, and stent migration.[18] A number of techniques have been advocated to prevent "stent leaks" due to migration, including bridling and endoscopic clipping or suturing, although success rates have varied and reports proving efficacy are lacking.

Over the past few years, EVT has been advocated as a promising modality for managing esophageal perforations and contiguous fluid collections. Similar to vacuum therapy for superficial wound infections, EVT involves application of negative pressure in the region of the esophageal defect, administered via an electronically controlled vacuum device attached to a nasoesophageal tube-mounted polyurethane sponge. No commercially available system currently exists for EVT, so each setup must be customized. Continuous suction at a pressure of 125 mm Hg maintains the vacuum environment. The sponge can be exchanged every several days, using decreasing sizes as the wound cavity diminishes. An advantage of this technique compared with stenting or endoscopic mucosal closure is that the extraluminal fluid collection is controlled as well, obviating the need for another form of percutaneous or operative drainage. In addition, EVT can be used in all portions of the esophagus, including the cervical region and gastroesophageal junction, as well as in the pharynx. Of course, EVT makes sense only when an associated fluid collection is small and immediately adjacent to the enteric perforation.

OPERATIVE MANAGEMENT

Primary Surgical Repair

Historically, primary repair was the most frequently used therapy of the perforated esophagus; it remains the gold standard against which other forms of treatment should be measured. The traditional dogma was that repair should be undertaken only within the first 24 hours following a perforation, given concerns about tissue friability and poor healing in cases in which inflammation and infection were of a longer duration. Data from the 1980s and early 1990s suggested that leak rates following primary closure were higher when operation was delayed beyond 24 hours compared with earlier repair.[19] Over time, and with increasing experience, primary repair was advocated, in cases of treatment delayed beyond 24 hours, to avoid the morbidity associated with esophageal resection or exclusion and the need for a second, major reconstructive procedure at a later date.[20,21]

Primary surgical repair is best performed in two layers, the first consisting of the mucosa and submucosa and the second of the overlying circular and longitudinal muscle layers of the esophagus. In addition, buttressing of the suture lines with vascularized tissue such as pleura, pericardial fat, intercostal muscle, omentum, or gastric fundus is frequently added (Fig. 48.6). For perforations of the distal intrathoracic esophagus, a left thoracotomy via the seventh intercostal space is generally used. For perforations of the proximal to mid intrathoracic esophagus, a right thoracotomy via the fourth to sixth intercostal space is preferable. Of course, perforations of the cervical or intraabdominal esophagus require incisions in the neck or abdomen, respectively.

A key principle underlying successful esophageal repair is that the deeper mucosal defect commonly extends beyond the more superficial muscular one. A myotomy created proximal and distal to the injury is generally necessary to identify the mucosal edges and facilitate complete closure (Fig. 48.7). The mucosa, once adequately exposed, should be débrided back to healthy, noninflamed tissue and reapproximated with absorbable or nonabsorbable suture. The muscular layer can be closed more superficially with interrupted sutures. Care must be taken to prevent luminal narrowing in the process of closure; use of a transoral bougie is a consideration to ensure an adequate esophageal diameter. The repair can be buttressed with adjacent viable tissue, as described.

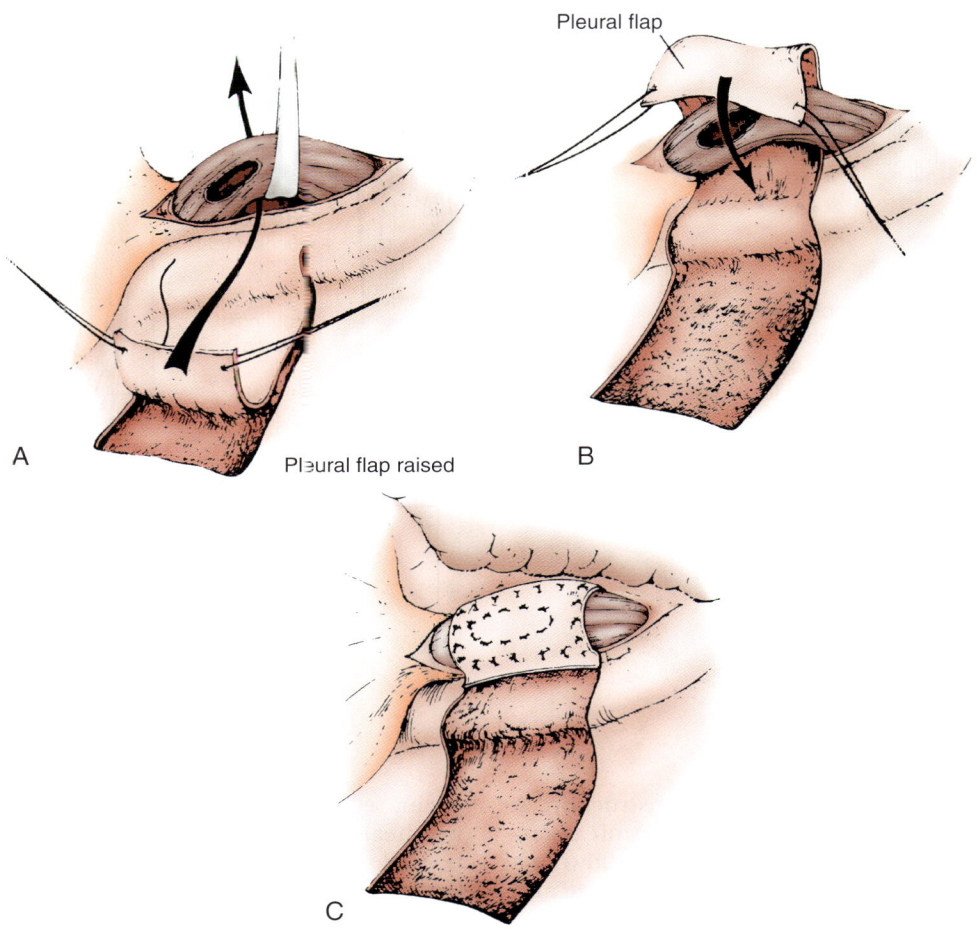

FIGURE 48.6 Pleural flap coverage of a large esophageal defect. (A) After mobilization of the esophagus, a pleural flap is raised. (B) The flap is wrapped around the esophagus, covering the perforation with or without primary repair of the esophageal defect. (C) The flap is sutured to itself. Sutures are placed proximally and distally at the margins of the flap, as well as to the perforation itself (if not primarily closed), to tack the pleura firmly to the esophageal musculature. (From Grillo HC, Wilkins FW. Esophageal repair following late diagnosis of intrathoracic perforation. *Ann Thorac Cardiovasc Surg*. 1975;20:337, by permission of the Society of Thoracic Surgeons.)

At the time of repair, washout with decortication, débridement, and drainage of the contaminated spaces is also important. A drain should be placed near, but not directly abutting, the esophageal suture line in case a recurrent leak develops in the early postoperative period. In addition, a feeding tube should be placed to facilitate nutritional support while the esophagus heals. The tube may be placed into the stomach or jejunum, either operatively (via laparotomy or laparoscopy) or using percutaneous techniques under endoscopic guidance, depending upon surgeon preference, available resources, and the clinical circumstances.

Esophagectomy

If clinical judgment determines that esophageal repair or stenting is not feasible, or the esophagus is deemed unsalvageable as in cases of end-stage achalasia, esophageal resection may be the best option in selected cases of esophageal perforation. A transthoracic approach, either open or performed with minimally invasive techniques, is commonly used because it allows for both the removal

of the perforated esophagus, as well as irrigation and drainage of the infected pleural and mediastinal spaces and decortication of the ipsilateral lung. Thus thoracotomy or thoracoscopy incisions generally are made on the side of a pleural effusion. During the abdominal phase of the operation, a gastric or jejunal feeding tube should be placed for postoperative nutritional support. A transhiatal resection may be the best choice in some cases, avoiding the morbidity of chest incisions and the need for single-lung ventilation when a transthoracic operation is undertaken.

If sepsis has arisen or is imminent because of a delay in diagnosis or the magnitude of extraluminal contamination, foregut reconstruction should be delayed due to concern of conduit ischemia from sepsis-related hypoperfusion and resultant anastomotic breakdown. In this situation a cervicothoracic end esophagostomy should be created to allow drainage of oral secretions. Important surgical details include a left neck approach to facilitate dissection of the cervical esophagus, protection of the recurrent laryngeal nerves, and preservation of as much proximal

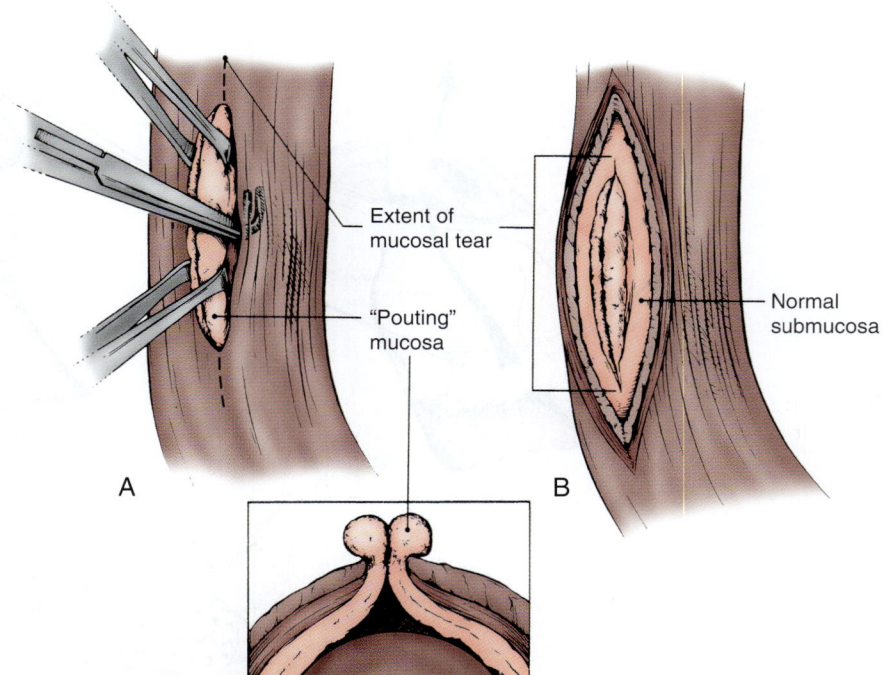

FIGURE 48.7 Primary repair of esophageal perforation illustrating exposure of the mucosal defect. (A) Extension of the muscular tear by a proximal and distal myotomy to facilitate complete exposure of the mucosal injury. The *inset* shows the damaged mucosa pouting between the muscle layers as initially assessed at surgery. (B) Mobilization in the submucosal plane to separate the mucosa from the muscularis propria, improving exposure of the limits of the mucosal defect. (From Whyte RI, Iannettoni MD, Orringer MB. Intrathoracic esophageal perforation: the merit of primary repair. *J Thorac Cardiovasc Surg.* 1995;109:140.)

esophagus as possible to aid in future reconstruction. A long length of esophageal remnant may permit placement of the esophagostomy on the chest wall, allowing a more secure application of an external drainage bag and increased patient comfort compared to a stoma placed on the neck. In such cases the esophagus should be tunneled superficial to the clavicle to reach the skin on the anterior chest. Care must be exercised in fashioning the tunnel so as to prevent compression and ischemia of the esophagus by the subcutaneous tissues or rigid clavicle. In our experience, stricturing or necrosis of the tip of the esophagostomy is not uncommon, leading to the need for dilation or surgical revision in a significant proportion of cases (unpublished data).

Esophageal Diversion

The most definitive method to divert the flow of gastrointestinal contents from the mediastinum is esophagectomy with end esophagostomy. However, some surgeons have advocated proximal and distal esophageal diversion without esophagectomy to facilitate foregut reconstruction after recovery. Proximal diversion is most commonly accomplished by end cervical esophagostomy,[22] although placement of an esophageal T-tube[23] and side cervical esophagostomy[24] have been described as alternatives. The latter option may be technically challenging, especially in the setting of obesity or when the patient's neck is otherwise thick. Distal diversion can be achieved by surgical division at the gastroesophageal junction using a linear cutting stapler or, alternatively, using a noncutting stapler without division of tissues. This latter technique for distal diversion has been touted to make future reconstruction easier, although it should be used with caution. Early recanalization of the stapled, undivided esophagus can

occur, resulting in ongoing soilage if the perforation has not healed. Esophageal diversion also runs the risk of pooled secretions within the esophageal lumen, leading to retching or nausea, and rarely should be necessary.

ADDITIONAL CONSIDERATIONS

LOCATION OF THE PERFORATION

Most perforations occur in the thoracic esophagus, although they may involve the cervical or intraabdominal portions as well. Cervical perforations are generally well tolerated because fascial investments surrounding the esophagus in the neck promote containment. Many pharyngeal or cervical esophageal leaks resolve with antibiotics alone. If the clinical condition deteriorates, a neck abscess develops, or fluid tracks into the mediastinum, surgical management should be pursued, including wide drainage through a cervical incision. In most operative situations, drainage is sufficient and attempts at direct visualization and repair of the perforation may prove difficult, unsuccessful, and unnecessary.

Because there are typically only a few centimeters of intraabdominal esophagus, perforations into the peritoneal cavity are less common than those occurring into the thorax. However, abdominal perforations can occur, particularly with endoscopic interventions aimed at the lower esophageal sphincter, such as pneumatic dilation or peroral endoscopic myotomy (POEM) for achalasia, balloon or rigid dilation for benign strictures or tumors, or a variety of endoscopic mucosal resective or ablative technologies. An important anatomic consideration in patients with sliding or paraesophageal hernias is that the hernia sac is bounded cranially by the phrenoesophageal ligament, rendering the herniated distal esophagus an intraabdominal structure. For all of these reasons, a distal esophageal perforation may need to be addressed by laparotomy or laparoscopy.

Preoperative CT imaging may assist in the decision as to whether a distal perforation is best approached through the chest or through the abdomen. When repair is performed below the diaphragm, the stomach can be used as a buttress by fashioning a partial or complete fundoplication to cover the repair site suture line. Although placing a fundoplication above the hiatus in the chest has been described, creating an iatrogenic hiatal hernia, common sense dictates that such repairs may lead to the problems inherent in any herniated fundic wrap including the potential for ischemia, pain, obstruction, or gastroesophageal reflux.

PREEXISTING ESOPHAGEAL PATHOLOGY

Esophageal perforation may occur due to, or in the face of, preexisting esophageal disease; both entities must be considered when devising a treatment plan. The concomitant pathology may influence the applicability of primary repair or esophageal stenting and whether esophageal resection is advisable.

A classic example is the patient with achalasia perforated at time of pneumatic dilation. Repair of the perforation alone will not ameliorate the dysphagia and regurgitation associated with the underlying disease. Of equal importance, the unrelieved distal esophageal obstruction imposed by a poorly relaxing or hypertensive lower esophageal sphincter may increase the risk of postoperative leak from the repair site. In this circumstance the best approach is to close the perforation in two layers, perform a distal esophageal (modified Heller) myotomy on the contralateral side of the esophagus away from the perforation, and create a partial fundoplication that serves as both an antireflux valve and a buttress of the mucosal repair. In patients with end-stage achalasia or a recalcitrant esophageal stricture, repair alone may lead to ongoing dysphagia or regurgitation; such individuals may benefit from esophagectomy.

Patients with esophageal malignancy should be considered for definitive surgical resection of their cancer at the time a perforation occurs, assuming clinical stability, lack of metastatic disease, and both a sufficient performance status and a reasonable life expectancy. Alternatively, a stent may be placed for temporary occlusion of the leak with the option of esophagectomy at a later date when the patient is more stable and a thorough preoperative evaluation has been completed. However, the presence of tumor will lead to nonhealing of a perforation, making subsequent stent extraction unfeasible without esophageal resection.

OUTCOMES

The results following therapy of esophageal perforation historically were poor with significant morbidity and mortality. A meta-analysis of 726 patients treated for a perforated esophagus between 1990 and 2003 revealed an overall mortality rate of 18%.[2] Delays in treatment clearly are associated with a worse outcome, with the first 24 hours after a perforation often cited as the critical window. Mortality rates in the setting of treatment occurring after 24 hours are quoted to be double of those recognized and managed earlier.[2,25,26] Similarly, the mortality following spontaneous perforations (36%) is almost double that from iatrogenic injuries (19%), likely representing the more rapid diagnosis in the latter cohort and the fact that such perforations typically occur in the setting of an empty stomach.[2]

Nonoperative approaches in carefully selected patients have shown superior outcomes to cohorts undergoing surgery, consistent with the less severe nature of the perforations in the former and the morbidity associated with operative intervention. Altorjay et al. reported on a series of 20 patients treated with an initial nonoperative paradigm.[11] Sixteen patients (80%) were managed successfully; four (20%) required operative intervention, after which two patients (10%) died. The morbidity rate was 20%. The authors commented that the mortalities resulted from an incorrect decision to manage in a nonoperative fashion; the patients were negatively impacted by the delays in operative intervention, underscoring the importance of appropriate patient selection. More recently, Keeling et al. reported on a series of 25 patients treated nonoperatively using strict criteria similar to those described in Table 48.1.[27] Their treatment algorithm resulted in a mortality of 8% and morbidity of 48%, with the two deaths occurring in patients with metastatic esophageal cancer who refused operative intervention.

Analyses of the surgical treatment of esophageal perforation have shown widely varied results. In a meta-analysis of 572 patients published in 2004 the mortality rates ranged from 0% to 80% among the case series reviewed.[2] For patients undergoing primary repair ($n = 322$) the average mortality was 12%. After esophagectomy ($n = 129$), mortality was 17%, whereas after esophageal exclusion ($n = 34$), mortality was 24%. Surgical drainage alone ($n = 88$) was associated with a 36% mortality rate.

Since the introduction of esophageal stents, enthusiasm for their application in the treatment of esophageal perforation has been increasing. Results from cohorts treated endoscopically compare favorably to surgical repair. A meta-analysis published in 2011 of 267 patients treated with esophageal stenting found a success rate of 85%.[28] Fifty-nine percent of patients required concurrent drainage of extraesophageal fluid collections. Mortality for stented patients was 13%, similar to patients undergoing surgical repair. Thirty-four percent of patients had a stent-related complication, including stent migration in 29%, bleeding in 2%, and tissue overgrowth in 5%. Surgical intervention for incomplete occlusion or stent-related complications was necessary in 13% of patients. Patients at increased risk for failure of endoscopic management include those with a perforation of the cervical esophagus or at the gastroesophageal junction, and those with esophageal injuries longer than 6 cm.[29]

The role of endoscopic clipping as therapy for esophageal perforation using either TTS clips or OTSCs was assessed in a literature review.[30] The analysis included 127 patients from 38 articles and concluded that TTS clips are effective in the treatment of early perforations (<24 hours old) with limited contamination and measuring less than 10 mm in length, whereas lesions up to 20 mm can be treated with OTS clipping.

Recent literature reviews of EVT for various types of upper gastrointestinal defects assessed data on more than 200 patients, with success rates ranging from 70% to 100%.[31,32] Although the results of both endoscopic clipping and EVT appear encouraging, they are limited to small case series and retrospective cohort studies from highly selected patient populations with limited extraluminal contamination. Lacking a control population undergoing expectant observation, the studies do not demonstrate the added value of these endoscopic interventions.

CONCLUSION

Esophageal perforation remains a challenging clinical problem and a potentially life-threatening emergency. Considerable skill, judgment, and creativity are necessary on the part of the managing physician in devising a treatment strategy that effectively addresses the perforation and its sequelae while minimizing morbidity.

The tools residing within the surgeon's armamentarium continue to evolve, although the principles underlying therapy remain constant and guide decision making. The basic tenets of closing, occluding, exteriorizing, or diverting proximal and distal to the esophageal defect, draining associated extraluminal fluid collections, alleviating distal esophageal obstruction, treating infection with antibiotics, and providing supportive care including nutrition are critical whether an operative, endoscopic, or noninvasive approach is pursued. A treatment plan must not only consider the specifics of the perforation, including its size and location, but also the time interval from onset, the extent of contamination, the presence of concomitant esophageal disease and the clinical condition of the patient, including comorbidities and performance status.

The introduction of fully covered, removable, self-expanding esophageal stents, both metal and plastic, as well as endoscopic clipping and EVT, has increased the utilization of endoscopy for definitive therapy, obviating the need for more invasive surgical intervention in many patients. The decision to proceed with surgery, whether it is for attempted primary repair and drainage, diversion, or esophageal extirpation, can be a difficult one, weighing the magnitude of the operation and the potential for perioperative and long-term morbidity against the risk of persistent leakage and sepsis from an ongoing esophageal defect.

The surgeon must be well versed in the treatment principles and the full spectrum of diagnostic and therapeutic modalities, including endoscopic techniques and operations involving the neck, thorax, and abdomen, to manage the various manifestations of the perforated esophagus in an optimal manner. Whichever approach is chosen, timely and appropriate intervention clearly plays a major role in achieving a successful outcome of this life-threatening condition.

REFERENCES

1. Barrett NR. Spontaneous perforation of the oesophagus; review of the literature and report of three new cases. *Thorax.* 1946;1:48-70.
2. Brinster CJ, Singhal S, Lee L, et al. Evolving options in the management of esophageal perforation. *Ann Thorac Surg.* 2004;77:1475-1483.
3. Sepesi B, Raymond DP, Peters JH. Esophageal perforation: surgical, endoscopic and medical management strategies. *Curr Opin Gastroenterol.* 2010;26:379-383.
4. Swanson JO, Levine MS, Redfern RO, Rubesin SE. Usefulness of high-density barium for detection of leaks after esophagogastrectomy, total gastrectomy, and total laryngectomy. *AJR Am J Roentgenol.* 2003;181:415-420.
5. Fadoo F, Ruiz DE, Dawn SK, et al. Helical CT esophagography for the evaluation of suspected esophageal perforation or rupture. *AJR Am J Roentgenol.* 2004;182:1177-1179.
6. White CS, Templeton PA, Attar S. Esophageal perforation: CT findings. *AJR Am J Roentgenol.* 1993;160:767-770.
7. Ferrer R, Martin-Loeches I, Phillips G, et al. Empiric antibiotic treatment reduces mortality in severe sepsis and septic shock from the first hour: results from a guideline-based performance improvement program. *Crit Care Med.* 2014;42:1749-1755.
8. Dellinger RP, Levy MM, Rhodes A, et al. Surviving sepsis campaign: international guidelines for management of severe sepsis and septic shock. *Crit Care Med.* 2012;2013(41):580-637.
9. Elsayed H, Shaker H, Whittle I, Hussein S. The impact of systemic fungal infection in patients with perforated oesophagus. *Ann R Coll Surg Engl.* 2012;94:579-584.
10. Cameron JL, Kieffer RF, Hendrix TR, et al. Selective nonoperative management of contained intrathoracic esophageal disruptions. *Ann Thorac Surg.* 1979;27:404-408.
11. Altorjay A, Kiss J, Voros A, Bohak A. Nonoperative management of esophageal perforations. Is it justified? *Ann Surg.* 1997;225:415-421.
12. Symonds CJ. The treatment of malignant stricture of the oesophagus by tubage or permanent catheterism. *Br Med J.* 1887;1:870-873.
13. Mousseau M, LeForestier J, Barbin J. Role of permanent intubation in palliative treatment of esophageal cancer. *Arch Mal Appar Dig Mal Nutr.* 1956;45:208-214.
14. Celestin LR. Permanent intubation in inoperable cancer of the oesophagus and cardia: a new tube. *Ann R Coll Surg Engl.* 1959;25:165-170.
15. Atkinson M, Ferguson R, Ogilvie AL. Management of malignant dysphagia by intubation at endoscopy. *J R Soc Med.* 1979;72:894-897.
16. Gelbmann CM, Ratiu NL, Rath HC, et al. Use of self-expandable plastic stents for the treatment of esophageal perforations and symptomatic anastomotic leaks. *Endoscopy.* 2004;36:695-699.
17. Vogel SB, Rout WR, Martin TD, Abbitt PL. Esophageal perforation in adults: aggressive, conservative treatment lowers morbidity and mortality. *Ann Surg.* 2005;241:1016-1021, discussion 1021–1013.
18. Stephens EH, Correa AM, Kim MP, Gaur P, Blackmon SH. Classification of esophageal stent leaks: leak presentation, complications, and management. *Ann Thorac Surg.* 2014;98:297-304.
19. Wang N, Razzouk AJ, Safavi A, et al. Delayed primary repair of intrathoracic esophageal perforation: is it safe? *J Thorac Cardiovasc Surg.* 1996;111:114-121.
20. Iannettoni MD, Vlessis AA, Whyte RI, Orringer MB. Functional outcome after surgical treatment of esophageal perforation. *Ann Thorac Surg.* 1997;64:1606-1610.
21. Barkley C, Orringer MB, Iannettoni MD, Yee J. Challenges in reversing esophageal discontinuity operations. *Ann Thorac Surg.* 2003;76:90-95.
22. Raymond DP, Watson TJ. Esophageal diversion. *Oper Tech Thorac Cardiovasc Surg.* 2008;13:138-146.
23. Linden PA, Bueno R, Mentzer SJ, et al. Modified T-tube repair of delayed esophageal perforation results in a low mortality rate similar to that seen with acute perforations. *Ann Thorac Surg.* 2007;83:1129-1133.
24. Urschel HC Jr, Razzuk MA, Wood RE, et al. Improved management of esophageal perforation: exclusion and diversion in continuity. *Ann Surg.* 1974;179:587-591.
25. White RK, Morris DM. Diagnosis and management of esophageal perforations. *Am Surg.* 1992;58:112-119.
26. Wright CD, Mathisen DJ, Wain JC. Reinforced primary repair of thoracic esophageal perforation. *Ann Thorac Surg.* 1995;60:245-248.
27. Keeling WB, Miller DL, Lam GT, et al. Low mortality after treatment for esophageal perforation: a single-center experience. *Ann Thorac Surg.* 2010;90:1669-1673, discussion 1673.
28. van Boeckel PG, Sijbring A, Vleggaar FP, Siersema PD. Systematic review: temporary stent placement for benign rupture or anastomotic leak of the oesophagus. *Aliment Pharmacol Ther.* 2011;33:1292-1301.

29. Freeman RK, Ascioti AJ, Giannini T, Mahidhara RJ. Analysis of unsuccessful esophageal stent placements for esophageal perforation, fistula, or anastomotic leak. *Ann Thorac Surg.* 2012;94:959-964, discussion 964–955.

30. Lázár G, Paszt A. Mán E. Role of endoscopic clipping in the treatment of oesophageal perforations. *World J Gastrointest Endosc.* 2016;8:13-22.

31. Kuehn F, Loske G, Schiffmann L, Gock M, Klar E. Endoscopic vacuum therapy for various defects of the upper gastrointestinal tract. *Surg Endosc.* 2017;doi:10.1007/s00464-016-5404-x; [Epub ahead of print].

32. Newton NJ, Sharrock A, Rickard R, Mughal M. Systematic review of the use of endo-luminal topical negative pressure in oesophageal leaks and perforations. *Dis Esophagus.* 2017;30:1-5.

Management of Esophageal Perforations and Leaks

Erin Gillaspie | Shanda H. Blackmon

The incidence of esophageal perforations is on the rise. Iatrogenic causes remain the most common and continue to increase in an era of frequent use of endoscopy for diagnostic and therapeutic procedures. Despite many advances in care, the mortality rate for an esophageal perforation remains high, with some series citing 12% to 50%.

The esophagus passes through the neck, chest, and abdomen, so surgeons managing perforations must be experienced with the unique anatomic considerations for approaching a perforation in any of these levels/locations. Many factors must be considered when managing these patients, including acuity of presentation, contamination, size of leak, cause of leak, and comorbid conditions. Those caring for esophageal perforation must be experienced in endoscopic procedures, esophageal resection, and complex esophageal reconstruction. Many of the current techniques involve a hybrid approach of stenting with a muscle buttress.

ANATOMIC CONSIDERATIONS

The esophagus is a long muscular tube that begins at the pharynx and ends at the gastroesophageal junction past the crura of the diaphragm, thus passing through three anatomic fields. The esophagus lacks a serosal layer, making it more susceptible to leak and less forgiving with surgical repair. The inner circular and outer longitudinal muscular layers are often weakened by perforation and do not hold sutures well. Perforations are often underestimated as the infection spreads through the submucosal plane and is covered by muscular tissue.

The cause of perforation often dictates the location. Important anatomic landmarks to appreciate, as they are common sites of perforation, are described in Table 49.1.

ETIOLOGY OF ESOPHAGEAL PERFORATIONS AND LEAKS

The most common cause of esophageal perforation remains iatrogenic, accounting for approximately 60% of all cases.[1] Most iatrogenic perforations are related to endoscopy. The risk of perforation is related to the indication of procedure—diagnostic carries a risk of 0.6% versus 6% for more complex interventional procedures.[2] Other less common causes include spontaneous perforation (15%), ingestion of foreign body (12%), trauma (9%), and malignancy (1%).[1] Table 49.2 presents a comprehensive list of causes and clinical findings associated with esophageal perforations.

Originally described by Herman Boerhaave, his eponymous esophageal perforation called Boerhaave syndrome results from a sudden increase in intraesophageal pressure. He described his findings in a 1724 pamphlet detailing postmortem observations of Baron de Wassenaer, the Grand Admiral of Holland, who suffered a fatal esophageal rupture as a result of self-induced vomiting in an attempt to relieve discomfort following unrestrained consumption of food.[3] Although most widely perceived to be associated with vomiting, spontaneous perforations may also be seen in situations of forceful valsalvae—weight lifting, child-birth, and defecation.

Esophageal disruption may occur in the setting of penetrating or, less frequently, blunt trauma. Gunshot wounds account for 75% of penetrating injury followed by stab wounds and other mechanisms.[4] The majority of injuries involve the cervical esophagus. Unfortunately these injuries continue to carry a very high mortality with a large series published in 2013 by Patel et al. citing 44%.[5]

Blunt trauma resulting in esophageal perforation is exceedingly rare with only about 100 cases reported in the literature. The mechanism of injury is debated and may be caused by anterior-posterior compression of the esophagus between the sternum and spine, severe hyperextension, increased intraluminal pressure, and chest compression with perforation occurring in a manner similar to Boerhaave's, or possibly ischemic injury from rapid deceleration with delayed perforation.[6]

Ingestion of caustic materials may result in severe esophageal injury and in some cases perforation. The extent of injury is dependent on a variety of factors including type of material, amount consumed, and length of time it is in contact with tissues. Caustic materials are generally categorized as acidic or alkali. Acids are generally poor to taste and irritating, resulting in smaller volume ingestion. They cause a coagulative necrosis, form an eschar, and have a lesser incidence of esophageal perforation. Lye or alkali liquids are tasteless and dense, and they cause liquefactive-type necrosis and have a propensity to full-thickness progression of esophageal injury.[7]

Infection is another important cause of esophageal perforation, particularly in immunocompromised patients. Eosinophilic esophagitis, which is characterized by inflammation, esophageal dysfunction, and eosinophil penetration into the esophageal wall, may result in spontaneous esophageal perforation as a complication of food impaction.[8,9]

Many diseases may result in esophageal stricture formation. Strictures may be grouped into several categories: intrinsic disease causing narrowing or extrinsic disease causing compression or invasion. Peptic strictures secondary to acid exposure are the most common cause of benign, intrinsic narrowing of the esophagus accounting for 70% to 75% of cases.[10] Disease processes that result

TABLE 49.1 Common Sites of Esophageal Perforations

Anatomic Landmark	Description
Piriform sinus	This sinus or recess flanks the laryngeal orifice. Trumpet players, manual laborers, and singers are prone to develop piriform sinus perforations. These can often result in massive subcutaneous emphysema and can often be treated by merely placing the patient NPO.
Killian triangle	A triangular region of the cervical esophagus formed by the oblique fibers of the inferior constrictor muscles of the pharynx and the transverse fibers of the cricopharyngeus muscles. Pharyngoesophageal diverticula occur here, and inadvertent cannulation of the diverticulum can result in perforation.
Cricopharyngeus muscle	The upper esophageal sphincter is a high-pressure zone at the proximal esophagus extending approximately 3–4 cm. It is comprised of the cricopharyngeus as the major contributor along with the inferior pharyngeal constrictor. This represents one of the most common sites of perforation. Spinal instrumentation can often protrude anteriorly toward the esophagus complicating endoscopy. Perforations at this level are often treated with mere drainage as long as the mediastinum does not become contaminated. Diversion is difficult for perforations in this location.
Aortic arch/ bronchus	The esophagus is in direct contact with the aortic arch and the bronchus, which both create a small indentation on esophagram. This angulation provides a potential location for food to become lodged. Unique problems specific to this location include complete vascular rings, a right-sided aortic arch, and the classic dysphagia lusoria (arteria lusoria), which is impairment in swallowing due to compression from an aberrant right subclavian artery.
Gastroesophageal junction	The lower esophageal sphincter is another location where iatrogenic injury often occurs; however, the most common etiology of perforation here remains Boerhaave's. This unfortunately can result in contamination of the mediastinum, bilateral pleural spaces, and the abdomen because of its location.

NPO, Nil per os.

in inflammation or perforation and leak may also result in stricture formation.

PATIENT PRESENTATION

The presenting symptoms vary largely by the anatomic location of the esophageal injury. Signs and symptoms common to all sites include fever, tachycardia, tachypnea, pain, leukocytosis, and varying grades of shock. *Mackler triad* describes the classic presenting syndrome of spontaneous esophageal rupture of a middle-aged man who consumes excessive food and alcohol, has active vomiting and retching, and develops chest pain and subcutaneous emphysema. The *Anderson triad* includes subcutaneous emphysema, rapid respirations, and abdominal rigidity.

Patients presenting with a high esophageal perforation—in the neck or piriform sinus—may describe neck pain, a change in their voice (generally a more nasal sound secondary to inflammation of the vocal cords), dysphagia, hemoptysis, or crepitus (a crunching sound or sensation when pushing on the skin secondary to the accumulation of subcutaneous emphysema; Fig. 49.1).

Intrathoracic perforations often present with symptoms such as chest or back pain, dysphagia, dyspnea, bleeding, vomiting, or signs and symptoms of sepsis. Signs of an intrathoracic perforation include pleural effusion, pneumopericardium, pneumomediastinum, or pneumothorax.

Intraabdominal perforations are more likely to present with abdominal pain and distention. Signs of an abdominal perforation of the esophagus include pneumoperitoneum, or free fluid detected by either exam or imaging (Fig. 49.2).

With an uncontained perforation, polymicrobial infection with bacteria such as *Staphylococcus, Pseudomonas, Streptococcus,* and *Bacteroides* typically occurs within the first 12 hours. Patients begin to develop tachycardia, fluid sequestration, fever, and a leukocytosis. In addition,

immunocompromised patients may fail to have a classic presentation and often warrant a more aggressive imaging approach with subtle signs such as a mere tachycardia, denoting infection.

EVALUATION

A high level of suspicion leading to early identification is essential in the management of esophageal perforations and leaks as timing of intervention correlates with outcome.

The work-up of any patient with suspected esophageal perforation begins with a detailed history and physical examination. Particular attention should be given to a history of instrumentation, trauma, food consumption, occupation, recent activity, and signs and symptoms of malignancy such as weight loss or dysphagia. In patients presenting with hemodynamic instability, this should be addressed immediately with placement of large bore IVs, fluid administration, and aggressive monitoring.

If esophageal perforation is suspected, an anteroposterior, lateral upright chest, and abdominal radiographs should be obtained promptly. Subcutaneous emphysema, pneumomediastinum, new effusion, pneumothorax, and pleural thickening are indicators of perforation. A plain radiograph may prove diagnostic in 80% of patients with suspected iatrogenic perforations. Radiographs are not only diagnostic but also assist in localizing the defect; midesophageal perforations manifest with right-sided efffusion, whereas distal esophageal injuries show left-sided effusion.

The gold standard diagnostic study remains a contrast swallow study with the treating surgeon present. The esophagram is performed fluoroscopically with the patient positioned obliquely in standing or semierect during swallowing of contrast. This facilitates the identification of subtle leaks (Fig. 49.3). The false-negative rate of

TABLE 49.2 Etiologies of Esophageal Perforations, Leaks and Strictures

Type	Causes	Clinical Findings
Anatomic	External compression from an aberrant right subclavian artery (Kommerell diverticulum) Schatzki ring	Dysphagia
Piriform sinus	Endoscopy, playing brass instruments, singing or yelling	Marked mediastinal and cervical subcutaneous emphysema
Anastomotic	Leakage at or near the site of a surgical anastomosis	History of surgically created esophageal anastomosis. May result in perforation, leak, or stricture.
Boerhaave's	Vomiting, straining, retching, weight lifting, hyperemesis, seizures causing a full-thickness tear at the gastroesophageal junction	Characteristic longitudinal tear on the left side of the esophagus, typically in the distal $\frac{1}{3}$ segment Mucosal defect typically longer than muscular defect
Iatrogenic	Endoscopic: Ablation, dilation, sclerotherapy, EMR, instrumentation, POEM Surgical: Esophageal surgery, pulmonary decortication, spine surgery	Recent history of surgery or endoscopy May occur secondary to nonesophageal surgery secondary to instrumentation
Traumatic	Penetrating or blunt trauma to neck or torso	Strong association with neck hyperextension
Cancer	Erosion of an esophageal tumor Extension of surrounding tumor through esophageal wall	Gas near or abutting the tumor on imaging
Paraesophageal hernia	Incarceration with necrosis of the distal esophagus	Evidence of left pleural effusion or abdominal fluid on imaging studies
Foreign body	Ingestion of a substance (i.e., chicken bone) that becomes lodged Esophageal webs Eosinophilic esophagitis	Upper esophageal impaction at the sphincter
Esophagitis	Inflammation and erosion of ulceration Peptic ulcers Zollinger–Ellison syndrome Barrett ulcer Infection (*Candida,* herpes simplex, viruses, CMV)	Immunocompromised patient
Ingestion	Ingestion of caustic substance Drug ingestion/impaction	Acid or base (lye) Tetracycline Potassium Quinidine NSAIDs Sustained-release formulations

CMV, Cytomegalovirus; *EMR,* endoscopic mucosal resection; *NSAIDs,* nonsteroidal antiinflammatory drugs; *POEM,* per oral endoscopic myotomy.

contrast radiography is about 10%. Consequently, we prefer to use angiography (Omnipaque) or low-osmolar water-soluble contrast solutions. Gastrografin has a higher false-negative rate—extravasating in only 50% to 80% of cases of esophageal perforation—and carries a risk of severe pneumonitis when aspirated. Barium has a higher diagnostic accuracy; however, it persists in the space after imaging and may complicate further imaging, making a closed perforation appear present after it has sealed.[11]

Patients who are unable to swallow or who are intubated may alternatively have a computed tomography (CT) scan performed (Fig. 49.4). CT is also helpful in cases of suspected perforation that are unable to be identified on upper gastrointestinal (GI) evaluation, and a nasogastric tube (NGT) should be placed under fluoroscopy to allow for contrast injection to better identify and delineate the leak. It is important to ensure that endotracheal tube cuff is inflated to prevent aspiration. CT scan is useful not only in identifying the site of leak, but also in delineating associated abscess of fluid collections that may require drainage.

Endoscopy is an important adjunct to imaging as it is diagnostic (Fig. 49.5) and therapeutic and allows irrigation and drainage of large perforations. Endoscopy in the setting of perforation must be approached cautiously by an expert endoscopist, but skilled thoracic surgeons are often more comfortable performing thoracic irrigation in the setting of a chronic esophageal perforation and can often immediately follow with appropriate surgical intervention while under the same anesthesia. Patient should be intubated and under general anesthesia in the operating room. In this setting, pleural effusions may also be sampled to determine if they are transudative or exudative effusions that could require additional treatment. Endoscopy is being used increasingly as an effective method for the treatment of some patients with perforation.[12]

Esophageal strictures, similarly, are worked up with an esophagram and endoscopy to denote the location and extent of esophageal involvement. Endoscopy is an important adjunct to the diagnosis to rule out malignancy as the cause of esophageal narrowing appreciated on a contrast study.

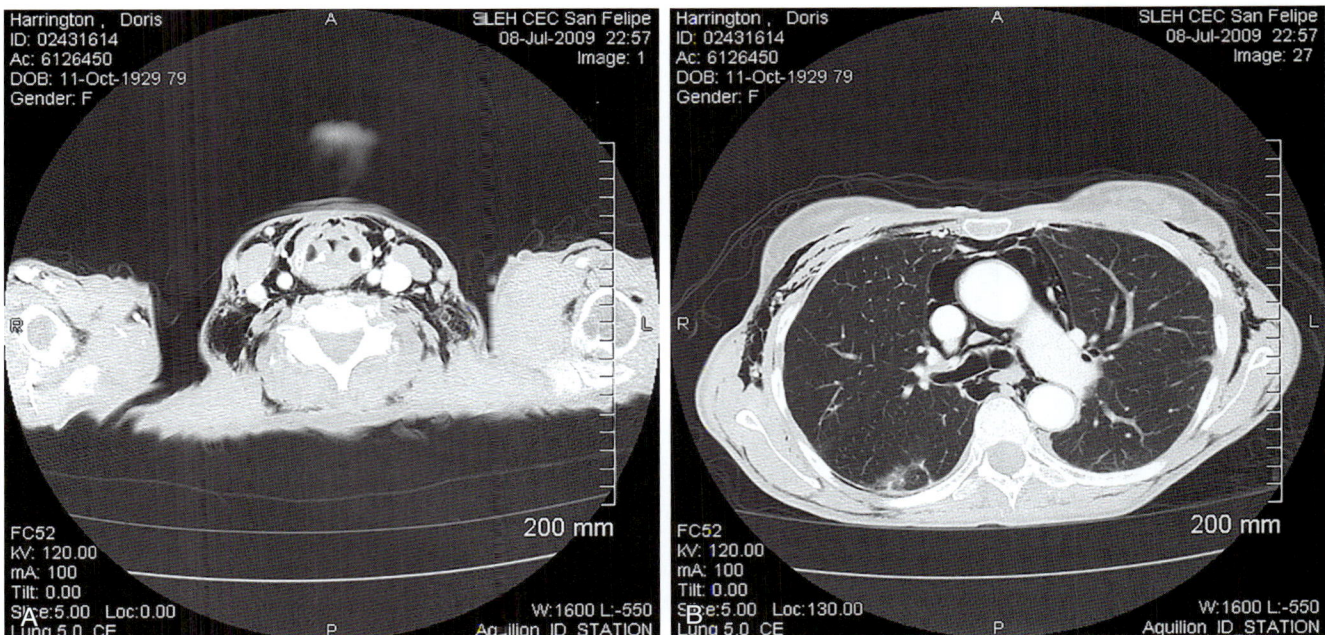

FIGURE 49.1 A patient presenting with a piriform sinus perforation manifesting with severe subcutaneous emphysema. Image (A) exhibits extensive subcutaneous emphysema at the level of the neck and (B) demonstrates the emphysema to have dissected down to the level of the mid-thorax.

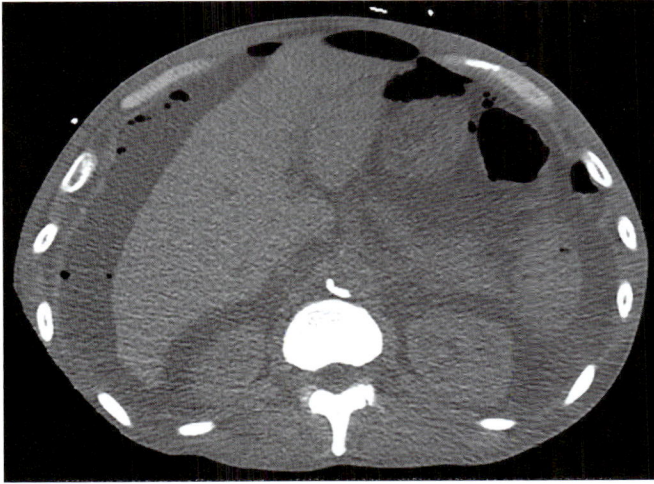

FIGURE 49.2 Patient presenting with a leak at the level of the gastroesophageal junction and was found to have peritonitis on physical examination and free air on computed tomographic scan.

MANAGEMENT

The treatment of esophageal perforations, leaks, and strictures continues to evolve, as traditional thoracotomy and repair versus diversion is now challenged by the less invasive endoscopy with stenting, dilation, and thoracoscopy.

Regardless of approach, the tenets of treatment remain the same for perforations and leaks: drainage of infection, timely intervention, prevention of progressive contamination, restoration of gastrointestinal continuity, and nutritional support.

One of the initial steps in patient management is determining whether or not the esophagus is salvageable. The traditional management of esophageal leaks and fistulas is currently being challenged by esophageal stents, which now may allow the surgeon to salvage a previously doomed esophagus. The use of temporary covered self-expanding metal and Silastic stents in the management of esophageal leakage is promising, but clinical trials in this area are being conducted for this sometimes off-label use.[11,13]

Refer to Fig. 49.6 for our algorithm for the management of esophageal perforations.

To Repair or Not to Repair

Most perforations and leaks that are identified acutely are amenable to treatment rather than diversion, while large perforations may not be amenable to repair. Perforations involving more than 50% of the circumference of the esophageal wall and longer than 3 cm are likely to become undilatable strictures once healed.

Nonviable tissue is debrided, and mucosal and muscle layers are closed separately. In some cases, the esophageal muscle must be opened additionally to adequately expose the mucosal defect and ensure adequate repair. The repair may be buttressed by well-vascularized tissue. Cervical perforations may be buttressed with sternocleidoastoid muscle, rhomboid, pectoralis, or intercostal muscle. Thoracic or abdominal perforations can use pedicled intercostal muscle flap, serratus, latissimus dorsi, pericardial fat pad, omentum, diaphragm, or gastric fundal flap.[14] Additionally, surgical repair is not typically recommended in patients with delayed presentation (>48 hours).

Alternative management strategies for complex, large, or delayed presentation include hybrid repairs, T-tube placement, temporary stenting, or diversion. Hybrid approach

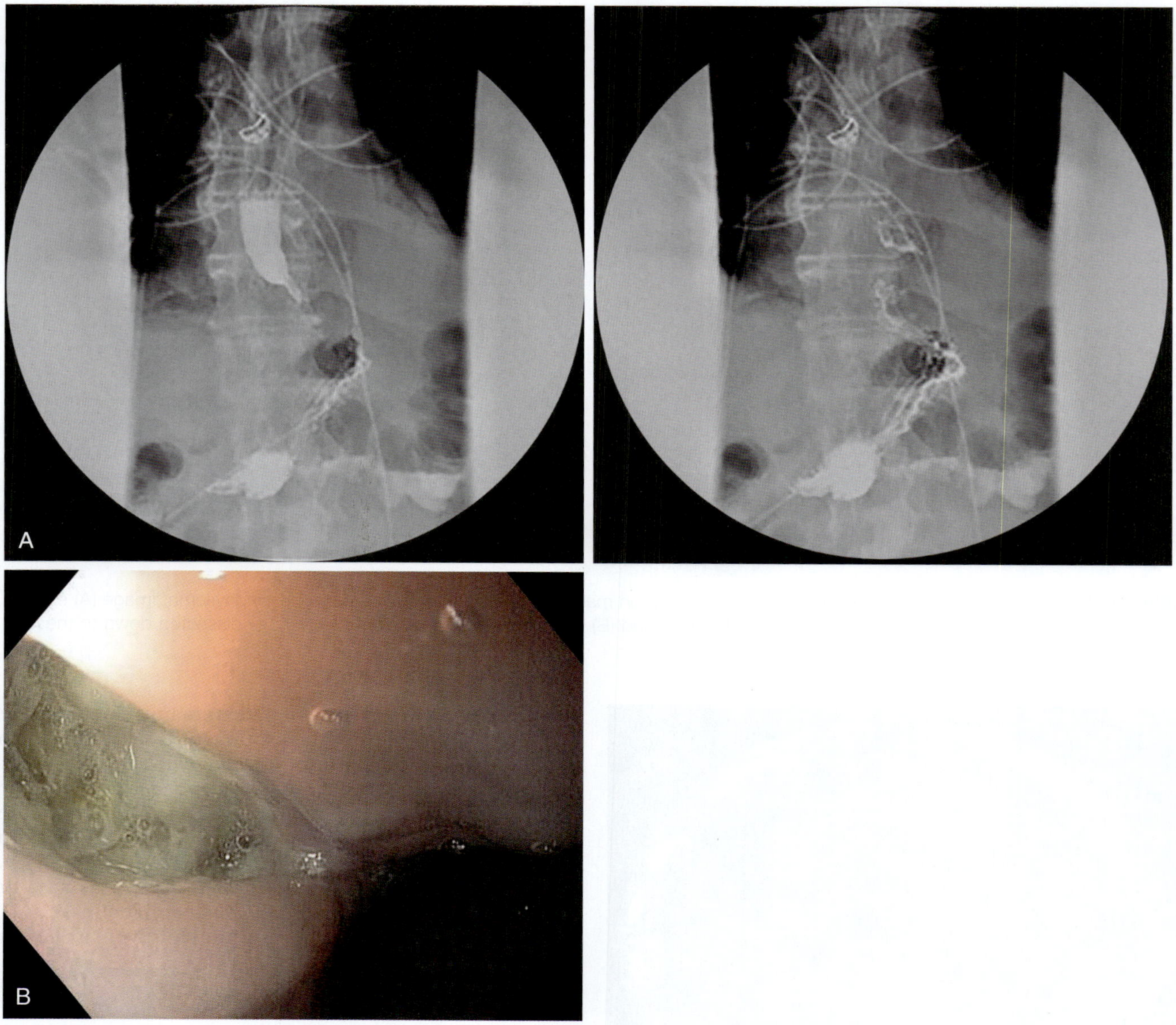

FIGURE 49.3 Patient with chronic distal esophageal stricture underwent attempted dilation resulting in contained perforation. The perforation was identified on esophagram (A). Endoscopy visualized the defect (B).

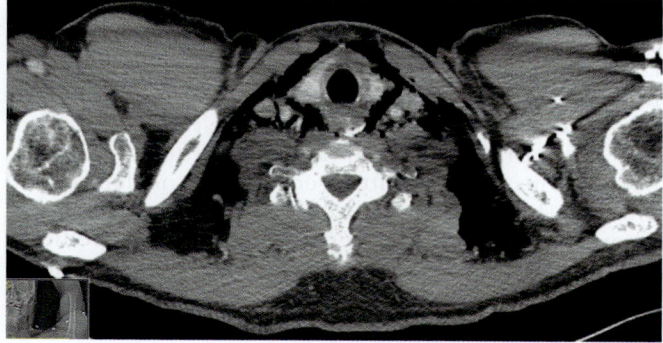

FIGURE 49.4 Computed tomography identification of esophageal perforation in a patient who was not able to swallow.

includes initial débridement and the placement of a buttressing muscle over the perforation to complement internal coverage with stenting, and it is essential to widely drain the region to prevent ongoing contamination. T-tubes can also be used to drain perforations and create a long, externalized fistula. However, these are unreliable means of ensuring fistula control and more frequently result in leakage around the tube than through the tube. Esophageal exclusion may also offer a proximal esophageal side diversion onto the neck and a temporary Vicryl suture tied distal to the diversion to eliminate salivary contamination of a severe, uncontrolled, distal esophageal perforation. A diverting esophagostomy may be a consideration with delayed reconstruction. In the case of very high cervical defects with insufficient length for diversion, a salivary bypass drainage tube may be required.

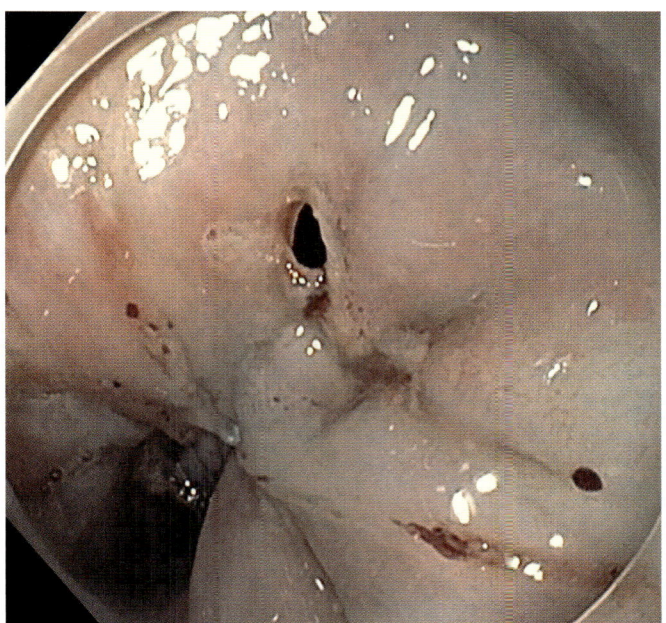

FIGURE 49.5 Esophageal perforation localized endoscopically. Removable stent was placed to cover the defect.

Surgical Approach

Cervical Perforations. The preferred surgical approach for cervical perforations is through a left neck, oblique incision along the anterior border of the sternocleidomastoid muscle. Small, contained perforations require only wide drainage and GI rest. Larger perforations may be repaired or require diversion. Despite our recommendation of placing a diversion below the level of the clavicle on the anterior chest wall, cervical perforations may have to be diverted onto the neck (Fig. 49.7).

Thoracic Perforations. Thoracic perforations must be divided into two categories based on proximal or distal thoracic esophagus. Perforations in the upper two-thirds of the thoracic esophagus can be approached surgically through a right posterolateral thoracotomy. We prefer a muscle-sparing thoracotomy in the fourth or fifth intercostal space, and an intercostal muscle can be harvested upon entry to provide a muscular flap for the repair (Fig. 49.8).

Ideally, a diverted ostomy should be brought out below the clavicle when the esophagus cannot be repaired. This type of anterior chest wall diversion provides a longer length of esophagus for future reconstruction and allows easier management of the ostomy device. Another benefit of a distal diversion is patient satisfaction, as patients find these devices are easily hidden under clothing and thereby less socially isolating.

Perforations of the lower third of the esophagus are approached through a left posterolateral thoracotomy through the sixth or seventh intercostal space. Similarly,

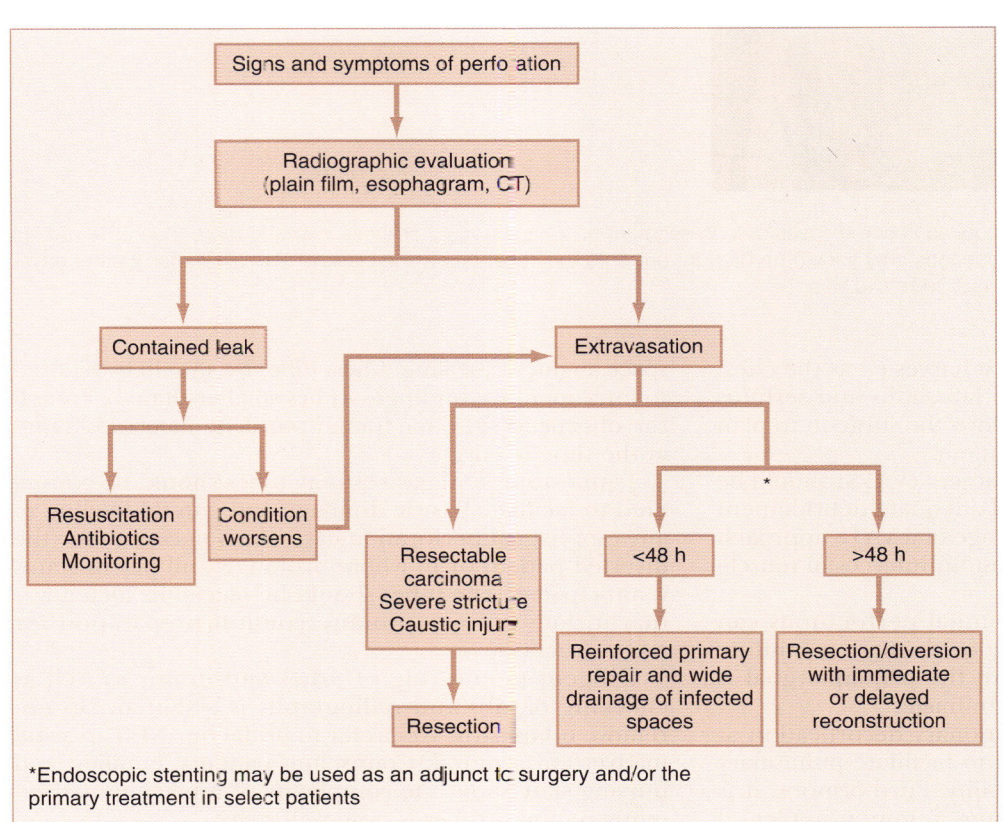

*Endoscopic stenting may be used as an adjunct to surgery and/or the primary treatment in select patients

FIGURE 49.6 Management of esophageal perforations. *CT,* Computed tomography.

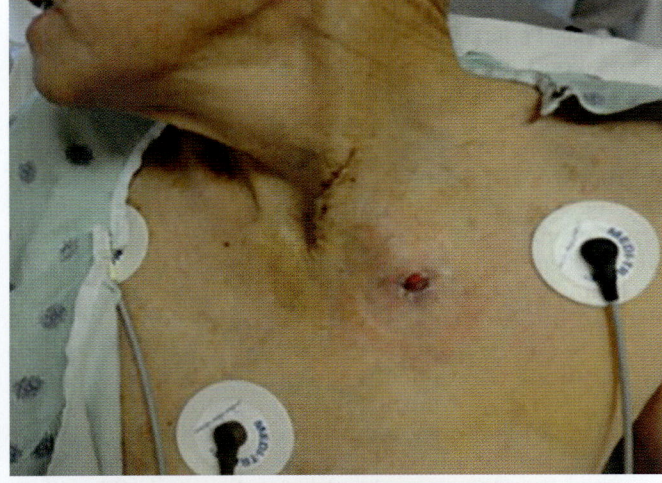

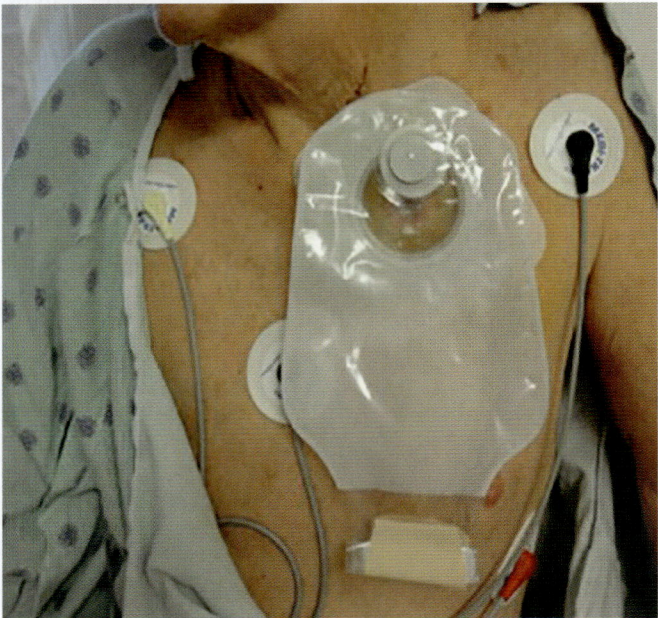

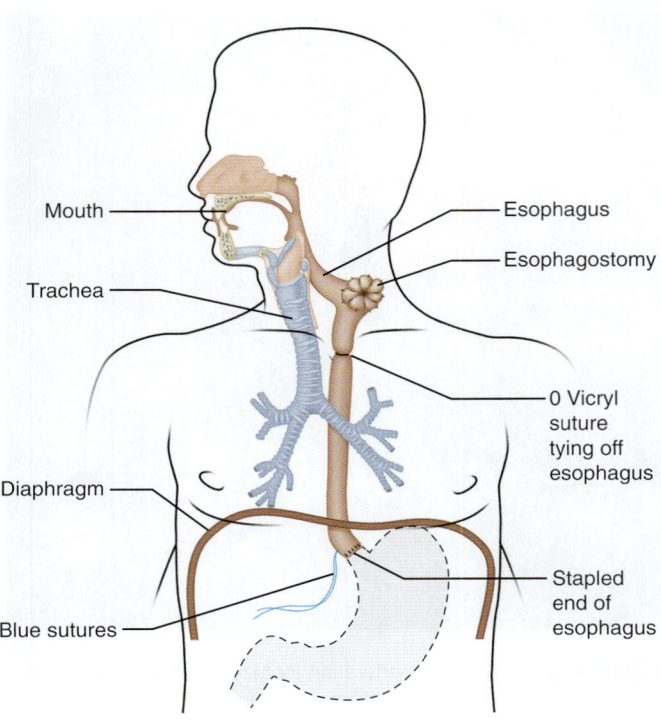

FIGURE 49.7 Esophageal diversion is required in some cases of long-segment esophageal injury or those involving more than 50% of the circumference. When possible, the esophagostomy should be brought out onto the chest below the clavicle. This allows for greater ease of care for the patient. *(Illustration courtesy Mike DeLaFlor.)*

intercostal muscle flaps should be harvested as the chest is entered and sparing both the latissimus and serratus each time the chest is entered allows the surgeon to plan for future complication management.

Video-assisted thoracoscopic surgery (VATS) should be reserved for early presentation if adequate débridement can be achieved.[15] The disadvantage of a VATS approach is the lack of the ability to harvest an intercostal muscle flap upon entry for buttressing.

Abdominal Perforations. Abdominal perforations can be approached laparoscopically or through a midline abdominal incision. Again, here the principal goal is débridement and repair versus drainage.

Adjunctive Considerations. Pulmonary decortication at the time of surgery is important to facilitate pulmonary reexpansion for respiratory stability. Furthermore, it is believed that expansion of the lung to minimize pleural

space augments healing. Chest tube size should be tailored to intraoperative findings—tubes smaller than 32 French can obstruct easily when frankly purulent material is found at the time of surgery.

Jejunostomy and gastrostomy tubes should be considered to facilitate gastric drainage and enteral feeding in any esophageal perforation case but is necessary for the diverted patient or in whom prolonged nil per os status is anticipated. The tubes should be placed in such a way that it does not compromise conduit preparation for reconstruction.

Diligent monitoring of tubes and drains as well as checking of labs and radiographs is essential. Do not remove tubes early. We prefer to bridal our NGT to avoid inadvertent removal. Counseling patients, families, and nursing staff about the complexity of replacing inadvertently removed tubes is time well spent.

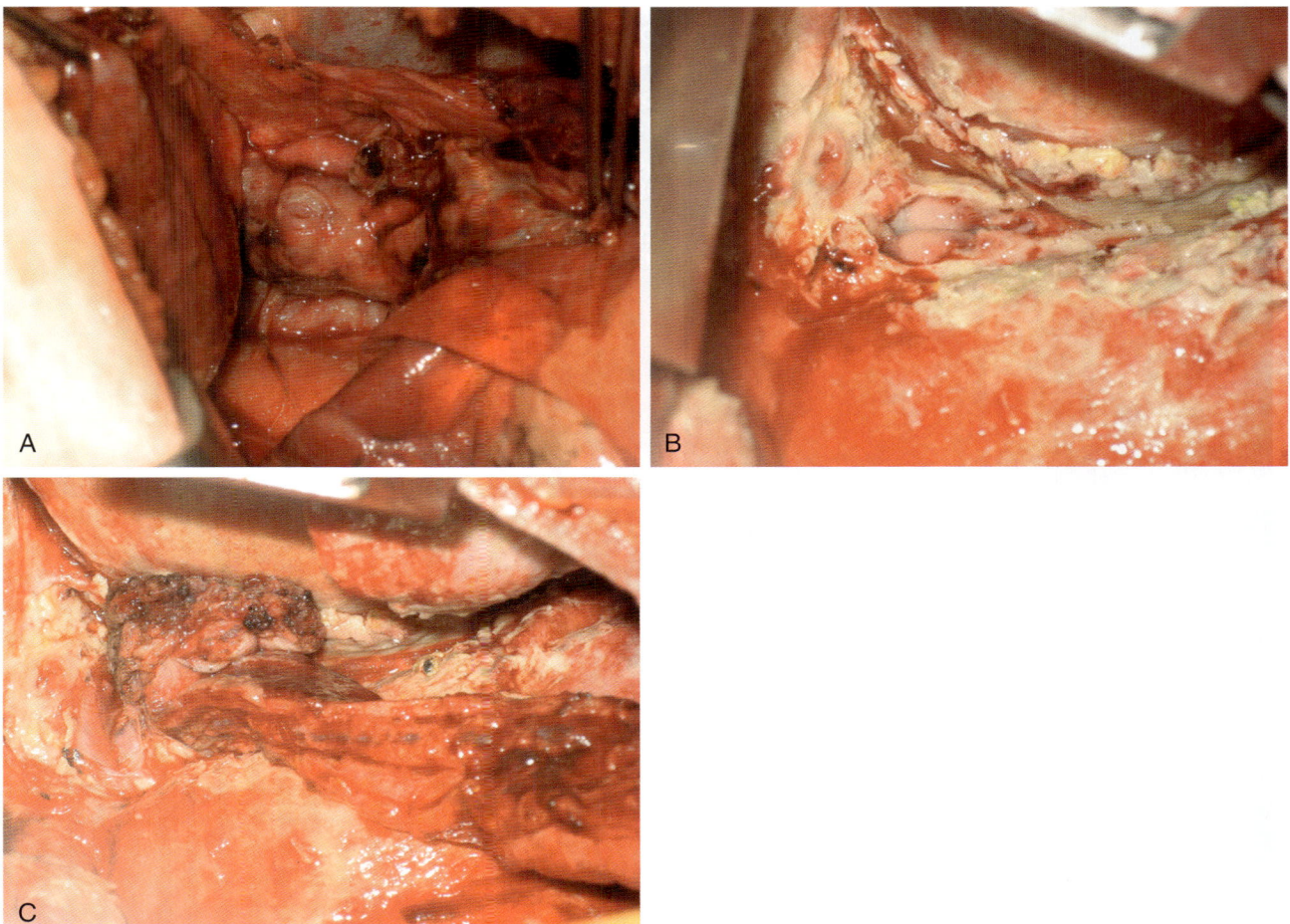

FIGURE 49.8 A patient who presented with a thoracic esophageal perforation just proximal to the gastroesophageal junction (A). Surgical approach was left thoracotomy, débridement of the esophagus (B) with primary repair, and buttressing with an intercostal muscle flap (C).

Broad-spectrum antibiotic therapy should be continued until the sensitivities of offending agents are confirmed. Microbes commonly responsible for infections related to esophageal perforations include *Staphylococcus*, *Pseudomonas*, *Streptococcus*, and *Bacteroides*, and adequate coverage for each of these species should be provided. We favor beginning with single-agent therapy such as piperacillin-tazobactam, which will cover gram positives, negatives, and anaerobes. This coverage can be extended with vancomycin, metronidazole (Flagyl), or antifungal agents as indicated. Therapy should continue until the patient has recovered fully from infection, and this typically takes 14 days.

ENDOSCOPIC MANAGEMENT OF ESOPHAGEAL PERFORATIONS AND LEAKS

Over the past decade, a number of centers have published on their experiences with endoscopic management of esophageal perforations and leaks. The use of endoscopic suturing, clipping, biologic glue, and endoluminal stenting has all been published in case series sharing institutional experiences. Although no large, multicenter trials have been published, the results have been promising in some circumstances with low procedural morbidity, low overall patient mortality, and high success in reestablishment of intestinal continuity.[16,17]

STENT SELECTION

Historically, stents were used principally to palliate malignant dysphagia. The introduction of removable stents helped to broaden the applications for stenting to include the treatment of tracheoesophageal fistulas,[18] corrosive burn injuries,[19] anastomotic leaks,[12,20] spontaneous and iatrogenic perforations,[12,21] strictures, and as a part of hybrid surgery to reinforce traditional repairs. One of the earliest reports by Mumtaz[22] in the *Annals of Thoracic Surgery* in 2002 described their experience in using a self-expanding metal stent (SEMS) to salvage the esophagus of a patient with iatrogenic perforation who had failed two surgical repairs.

There are two principal types of stents available for use: SEMS and self-expanding plastic stents (SEPS). Stents may be further classified as uncovered, fully covered, and partially covered. In addition, there are a variety of SEMS and SEPS available in the US market from Cook Medical,

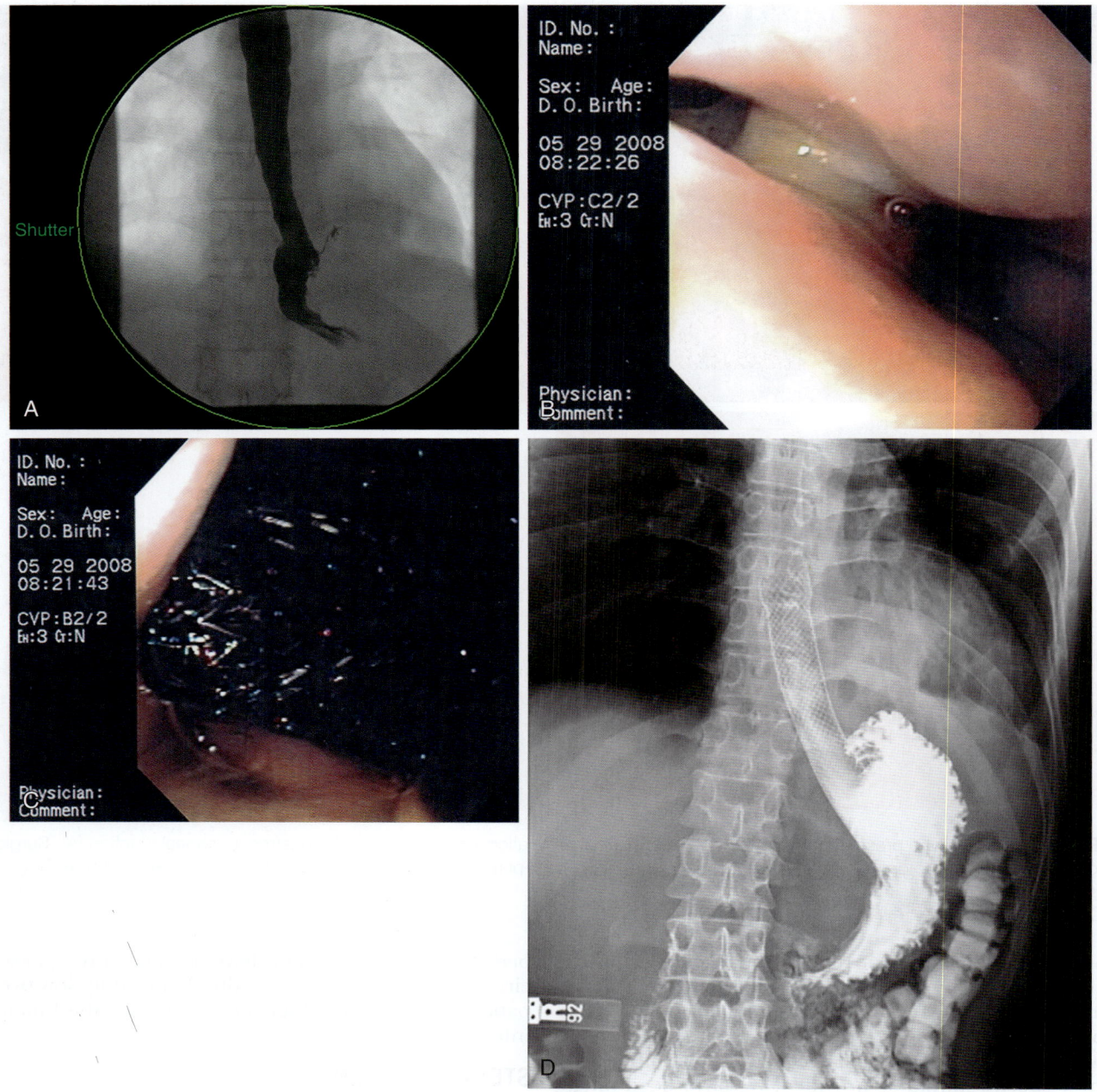

FIGURE 49.9 A patient who presented with an intrathoracic esophageal perforation. The perforation was visible on (A) esophagram and (B) endoscopically. Patient presented early with limited contamination. (C) A stent was deployed with good coverage and (D) no residual leak was noted on repeat radiographic study.

Boston Scientific, Merit Medical Endoteck, EndoChoice, and Taewoong Medical Company.

The original SEMS were uncovered stents (Fig. 49.9). These stents were generally left in situ and had significant tumor and tissue granulation and ingrowth. Once significant tissue ingrowth had occurred, these stents could not easily be removed. Covered stents were developed to prevent the tissue ingrowth. The metal framework of the stent is covered in polytetrafluoroethylene (most commonly) through the length of the entire stent for fully covered and the middle portion, leaving the proximal and distal ends uncovered for partially covered stents.[23]

Patient Selection for Endoscopic Management

Similar to any type of surgery, patient selection is of paramount importance. Identifying patients who are suitable for nonoperative management has not been well defined. However, Cameron[24] in 1979 proposed key considerations, and Altorjay[25] expanded on these two decades later. They included early diagnosis of an intramural perforation, transmural perforation within the neck or mediastinum with free drainage back into the esophagus on esophagram, the absence of benign or malignant obstructive esophageal disease, and minimal symptomatology without evidence of sepsis. Another commonly used indication for nonoperative therapy has been cases in which patients were deemed unsuitable for surgery secondary to significant comorbid conditions.

Endoluminal stenting has been highlighted to have the following benefits: less procedural morbidity than surgery and rapid closure of the perforation, which quickly eliminates ongoing soilage of the mediastinum and pleura and allows for earlier initiation of oral nutrition.

Our indications for stenting continue to expand. We use stenting most commonly in iatrogenic injuries that are discovered immediately with minimal contamination. Newer approaches include endoluminal suturing using the Apollo device or clipping with the resolution device or Ovesco clips. We find acute intentional incisions, similar to those created during per oral endoscopic myotomy (POEM), that are easily closed with the resolution clips. In addition, larger perforations or full-thickness perforations often require a larger clipping device such as the Ovesco. When clipping is not feasible, intraluminal suturing can always augment healing when the tissue is intact enough to hold the suture. Unfortunately, many esophageal perforations result in damage to the mucosa such that it becomes too friable to suture.

Esophageal Stenting for Perforations and Leaks

Essential components of nonoperative management for esophageal disruption remain the same as with an open strategy: drainage if required, prevention of ongoing contamination, and nutritional support while healing. In some cases, only endoscopic treatment may be required, and in others, it serves as an adjunct to surgical treatment as noted earlier.

Stents have been shown themselves to be highly successful in a few major arenas: iatrogenic perforations with early identification, esophageal anastomotic leaks, and gastric staple line leak after weight loss surgery.

Iatrogenic perforations with early identification are ideally suited for covered stent placement. The stent effectively occludes the leak preventing mediastinal contamination, allows for early institution of oral, enteral nutrition, and allows for accelerated patient recovery compared with open surgery. In their series of 17 patients, Freeman et al. demonstrated that with thoughtful patient selection, stents could be placed safely with a low morbidity, mortality, and high rate of success. See Fig. 49.9 for an example of endoscopic stenting for intrathoracic esophageal perforation.

More reports are emerging describing endoscopically placed stents for the treatment of anastomotic leaks. Most published series are small, but they cite good outcomes.[13,26] Stenting after esophagectomy is challenging, as the diameter of the esophagus is quite a bit smaller than the gastric conduit. This allows for more reflux up around the stent to the level of the anastomosis and makes the stent more prone to migration. D'Cunha et al.[27] reported one of the larger series in 2011. Their subgroup analysis of patients with anastomotic leak included 22 patients, and they had a 60% success rate with healing. It should be noted that the time to healing averaged 40 days and ranged from 22 to 120 days, and the mortality rate was 14%. The average time to per os (PO) intake was 6 days, and some patients were able to begin oral intake immediately. Importantly,

the group emphasized the importance of patient selection. Contraindications to esophageal stenting for anastomotic leak included nonviable conduit; leaks that were within 2 cm of the cricopharyngeus muscle to avoid significant patient discomfort; severe angulation of the conduit; and esophagojejunal conduits, as this resulted in obstruction and erosion.

Leak after laparoscopic bariatric surgery occurs in up to 7% of cases in some series. This severe complication is difficult to manage and can result in significant patient morbidity and cost. Covered SEMS have been shown to be effective in acute leaks when combined with drainage of associated collections. Simon et al.[28] in their series of nine patients with leaks after sleeve gastrectomy showed a 78% resolution of leak. Similarly, Eubanks et al.[29] showed a resolution of 84% in their 19 patients who were stented after gastric bypass. Importantly, symptomatic improvement was also seen in 90% of patients with oral feeding started immediately in 79%. Chronic leaks have a significantly reduced success rate in healing the chronic leak; however, they minimize ongoing sepsis and allow patients to continue enteral nutrition.[30]

Regardless of the indication, it is essential to couple stenting with adequate drainage of any associated infected space.[31] While once considered an indication for open surgery, mediastinal contamination is no longer a contraindication to endoscopic management, and drainage of small collections may be accomplished endoscopically with gentle aspiration and irrigation. In addition, double-pigtail stents may be placed through the esophageal wall into an abscess cavity temporarily to provide ongoing drainage for a few days. Larger abscesses and free pleural effusions often require the placement of additional surgical drains. In these cases, however, the utilization of a stent may help to avoid esophageal resection or diversion.

After stent deployment, it is important to assess for adequacy of coverage with an on-table contrast fluoroscopic examination. If there is no evidence of ongoing leak, the stent is sutured into place to prevent migration. If inadequate seal is perceived with ongoing leak, the stent is repositioned. Importantly, the contrast should also be seen to flow distally through the end of the stent. Distal obstruction leads to stasis, impairs proper healing, and may result in additional injury to the gastrointestinal tissues.

In some cases when no gastrostomy tube is present, we leave an NGT for ongoing decompression of the esophagus and stomach. The NGT is left to gravity drainage as active suction in the region of the stent can cause collapse and predispose to migration.

POSTSTENTING CONSIDERATIONS

Once a stent is placed, judicious ongoing management and surveillance is required. If a patient develops evidence of sepsis, the stent should be investigated for migration or failure to adequately seal the leak. In some cases, the stent can be repositioned with more effective coverage, while in other cases, surgical intervention must be pursued.[32]

Our protocol for management of patients after esophageal stenting is to obtain an esophagram within 24 hours. If no leak is present, the patient is initiated on a room-temperature liquid diet that is advanced to soft solids (essentially, anything you would feed a 1-year-old baby—nothing too hot or cold and nothing that does not dissolve into small pieces within a few minutes to prevent stent impaction). They receive special counseling regarding diet from our nutritionist as well as a handout to follow at home. They return within 2 weeks for repeat endoscopy, evaluation for healing, and ongoing leak. In some cases, the esophagus is fully healed, and the stent can be removed; in others, the stent is repositioned or exchanged to change the pressure points and resecured. In both cases, an esophagram is performed within another 24 hours to confirm the absence of leak. Once a stent has been removed, the soft diet is continued for a total of 2 to 6 weeks.

COMPLICATIONS OF STENTING

Early complications of stenting occur immediately or within 2 to 4 weeks of stent placement. These include patient discomfort, bleeding, acid reflux, perforation, stent leak, and most commonly stent migration.[33–37] Stent migration has been cited as the predominant problem in a number of series. New techniques and technology have been developed to mitigate this issue, including the use of partially covered stents, which allows some ingrowth of tissue proximally and distally to stabilize the stent, and suturing the stents into place.[13]

Stent leak is a feared complication of stent placement and has been reported in 10% to 40% of patients after stent placement. Stephens et al.[38] developed a classification system for the leaks (types 1 to 5) with recommendations on management of each type. Importantly, prompt recognition of a leak is essential to achieve good outcome. Knowledge of which factors may predispose to a stent leak led to a more timely identification and intervention for ongoing leaks.

Delayed complications may occur weeks to months after stent placement. These include stent migration, tumor ingrowth resulting in difficult extraction (Yoon), and perhaps the most feared complication, injury to surrounding structures. Case reports and institutional series detail esophageal fistulization and tumor erosion.[39–42]

Some of these complications may be avoided by earlier extraction. Studies have shown that extraction is not difficult if stents are removed within a 30-day window (Blackmon). Stent exchange should also be considered more frequently for stents located in the middle one-third of the esophagus. In this location, stents are intimately associated with the bronchus, and persistent pressure in a static location over a 4-week period may place a patient at risk for fistula formation. Resiting the stent every 2 weeks changes the pressure points and may reduce the incidence of fistula formation.

STENT-GUIDED REGENERATION AND REEPITHELIALIZATION

The boundaries and extent of endoscopic options continue to be tested. In 2009, Amrani et al.[43] shared their experience with treated completed anastomotic disunion with stenting. Their report on their nine cases launched the theory of "stent-guided regeneration and reepithelialization." They could show that by bridging gap and providing a scaffold, full reepithelialization can be accomplished.

The exciting future for esophageal surgery lies in the field of regenerative medicine. In 2012 Bradylak et al. published their experience, creating extracellular matrices, repopulating with autologous cells, and implanting into animal models. They observed that these biologic scaffolds provide a framework for structural and functional regeneration of tissues.

In 2016, Dua et al.[44] published their experience with in vivo regeneration for a 5-cm esophageal defect. They placed a stent as the framework to maintain the shape of the esophagus and wrapped it with a dermal matrix. Endoscopic monitoring over time revealed normal squamous mucosa ingrowth and endoscopic ultrasound showed the neoesophagus to have five layers, and peristalsis was seen on manometry. The neoesophagus demonstrated both structural and functional regeneration. Phase 1 and 2 clinical trials are needed, but this new technology could revolutionize all aspects of esophageal surgery.

CONCLUSION

The management of esophageal perforation is constantly evolving. With the increased use of endoscopy for both diagnostic and therapeutic interventions, it is a problem that should not expect a cure. Despite more minimally invasive approaches coming into vogue in the last 10 years, the basic principles of management remain unchanged: early identification, resuscitation, débridement, repair/diversion, drainage, and enteric access for feeding. A concern our group shares is the dissemination of endoluminal techniques used by those not surgically trained. This disconnected management strategy may often result in stenting without drainage of an adjacent abscess, placing a stent directly next to the aorta or adjacent drains, placing stents without a pexy resulting in migration, and excessive experimentation. The future of esophageal perforation may hold repair with the use of adjunctive techniques such as tissue regeneration, deploying matrices embedded with growth factors, and more advanced endoluminal techniques.

REFERENCES

1. Brinster CJ, Singhal S, Lee L, Marshall MB, Kaiser LR, Kucharczuk JC. Evolving options in the management of esophageal perforation. *Ann Thorac Surg.* 2004;77:1475-1483.
2. Tsao GJ, Damrose EJ. Complications of esophagoscopy in an academic training program. *Otolaryngol Head Neck Surg.* 2010;142:500-504.
3. Barrett NR. Spontaneous perforation of the oesophagus: review of the literature and report of three cases. *Thorax.* 1946;1:48-70.
4. Ascensio J, Chahwan S, Forno W, et al. Penetrating esophageal injuries: multicenter study of the American Association for the Surgery of Trauma. *J Trauma.* 2001;50(2):289-296.
5. Patel MS, Malinkoski DJ, Zhou L, Neal ML, Hoyt DB. Penetrating oesophageal injury: a contemporary analysis of the National Trauma Data Bank. *Injury.* 2013;44(1):48-55.
6. Monzon JR, Ryan B. Thoracic esophageal perforation secondary to blunt trauma. *J Trauma.* 2000;49(6):1129-1131.
7. Lupa M, Magne J, Guarisco JL, Amedee R. Update on the diagnosis and treatment of caustic ingestion. *Ochsner J.* 2009;9(2):54-59.
8. Lucendo AJ, Friginal-Ruiz AB, Rodriguez B. Boerhaave's syndrome as the primary manifestation of adult eosinophilic esophagitis. Two case reports and a review of the literature. *Dis Esophagus.* 2011;34:E11-E15.

9. Cohen MS, Kaufman A, DiMarino AJ, Cohen S. Eosinophilic esophagitis presenting as spontaneous esophageal rupture. *Clin Gastroenterol Hepatol.* 2007;5:24.

10. Ferguson DD. Evaluation and management of benign esophageal strictures. *Dis Esophagus.* 2005;18(6):359-364.

11. Madan R, Blair RJ, Chick JF. Complex iatrogenic esophageal injuries: an imaging spectrum. *AJR Am J Roentgenol.* 2015;204(2):W116-W125.

12. Freeman RK, Van Woerkom JM, Ascioti AJ. Esophageal stent placement for the treatment of iatrogenic intrathoracic esophageal perforation. *Ann Thorac Surg.* 2007;83(6):2003-2007.

13. Blackmon SH, Santora R, Schwarz P, Barroso A, Dunkin BJ. Utility of removable esophageal covered self-expanding metal stents for leak and fistula management. *Ann Thor Surg.* 2010;89(3):931-936.

14. Martin LW, Hofstetter W, Swisher SG, Roth JA. Management of intra-thoracic leaks following esophagectomy. *Adv Surg.* 2006;40:173-190.

15. Nguyen NT, Hinojosa MW, Fayad C, Wilson SE. Minimally invasive management of intrathoracic leaks after esophagectomy. *Surg Innov.* 2007;14(2):96-101.

16. Leers JM, Vivaldi C, Schafer H, et al. Endoscopic therapy for esophageal perforation or anastomotic leak with a self-expandable metallic stent. *Surg Endosc.* 2009;23:2258.

17. Kiev J, Amendola M, Bouhaidar D, Sandhu BS, Zhao X, Maher J. A management algorithm for esophageal perforation. *Am J Surg.* 2007;194:103.

18. Adler DG, Pleskow EK. Closure of a benign tracheoesophageal fistula by using a coated, self-expanding plastic stent in a patient with a history of esophageal atresia. *Gastrointest Endosc.* 2005;61:765-768.

19. Zhou JH, Jiang YG, Wang RW, et al. Management of corrosive esophageal burns in 149 cases. *J Thorac Cardiovasc Surg.* 2005;130:449-456.

20. Kauer WKH, Stein HJ, Dittler HJ, Siewert JR. Stent plantation as a treatment option in patients with thoracic anastomotic leaks after esophagectomy. *Surg Endosc.* 2002;22:50-53.

21. Fischer A, Thomusch O, Benz S, von Dobschuetz E, Baier P, Hopt UT. Nonoperative treatment of 15 benign esophageal perforations with self-expandable covered metal stents. *Ann Thorac Surg.* 2006;81:467-472.

22. Mumtaz H, Barone GW, Ketel BL, Ozdemir A. Successful management of a nonmalignant esophageal perforation with a coated stent. *Ann Thorac Surg.* 2002;74:1233-1235.

23. Hindy P, Hong J, Lam-Tsai Y, Gress F. A comprehensive review of esophageal stents. *Gastroenterol Hepatol.* 2012;8(8):526-534.

24. Cameron JL, Kieffer RF, Hendrix TR, Mehigan DG, Baker RR. Selective nonoperative management of contained intrathoracic esophageal disruptions. *Ann Thorac Surg.* 1979;27:404.

25. Altorjay A, Kiss J, Voros A, Bohák A. Nonoperative management of esophageal perforations: is it justified? *Ann Surg.* 1997;225:415.

26. Langer FB, Wenzl E, Prager G, et al. Management of postoperative esophageal leaks with the Polyflex self-expanding covered plastic stent. *Ann Thorac Surg.* 2005;79:398-404.

27. D'Cunha J, Rueth NM, Groth SS, Maddaus MA, Andrade RS. Esophageal stents for anastomotic leaks and perforations. *J Thorac Cardiovasc Surg.* 2011;142:39-46.

28. Simon F, Siciliano I, Gillet A, Castel B, Coffin B, Msika S. Gastric leak after laparoscopic sleeve gastrectomy: early covered self-expandable stent reduces healing time. *Obes Surg.* 2013;23:687-692.

29. Eubanks S, Edwards CA, Fearing NM, et al. Use of endoscopic stents to treat anastomotic complications after bariatric surgery. *J Am Coll Surg.* 2008;206(5):935-938.

30. Puig CA, Waked TM, Baron TH, et al. The role of endoscopic stents in the management of chronic anastomotic and staple line leaks and chronic strictures after bariatric surgery. *Surg Obes Relat Dis.* 2014;10(4):613-617.

31. Abbas G, Schuchert MJ, Pettiford BL, et al. Contemporaneous management of esophageal perforation. *Surgery.* 2009;146:749, discussion 755.

32. Dickinson KJ, Blackmon SH. Endoscopic techniques for the management of esophageal perforation. *Thorac Cardivasc Surg.* 2015;20(3):251-278.

33. Eubanks S, Edwards CA, Fearing NM. Use of endoscopic stents to treat anastomotic complications after bariatric surgery. *J Am Coll Surg.* 2008;206:935-938.

34. Ott C, Ratiu N, Endlicher E, et al. Self-expanding stents in esophageal disease: various indications, complications and outcomes. *Surg Endosc.* 2007;21:889-896.

35. Sabharwal T, Hamady MS, Chui S, Atkinson S, Mason R, Adam A. A randomised prospective comparison of the Flamingo Wallstent and Ultraflex stent for palliation of dysphagia associated with lower third oesophageal carcinoma. *Gut.* 2003;52:922-926.

36. Wang MQ, Sze DY, Wang ZP, Gao ZQ, Want YA, Dake MD. Delayed complications after esophageal stent placement for treatment of malignant esophageal obstruction and esophagorespiratory fistulas. *J Vasc Interv Radiol.* 2001;12:465-474.

37. Radecke K, Gerfen G, Trichel U. Impact of self-expanding plastic esophageal stent on various esophageal stenosis, fistulas and leakages: a single-center experience in 39 patients. *Gastrointest Endosc.* 2005;61:812-818.

38. Stephens EH, Correa AM, Kim MP, Gauer P, Blackmon SH. Classification of esophageal stent leaks: leak presentation, complication, and management. *Ann Thorac Surg.* 2014;98(1):297-304.

39. Tomaselli F, Maier A, Pinter H, Smolle-Juttner F. Management of iatrogenous esophageal perforation. *Thorac Cardiovasc Surg.* 2002;50:168-173.

40. Kennedy C, Steger A. Fatal hemorrhage in stented esophageal carcinoma: tumor necrosis of the aorta. *Cardiovasc Intervent Radiol.* 2001;24:443-444.

41. Yoon CJ, Shin JH, Song HY, Lim JO, Yoon HK, Sung KB. Removal of retrievable esophageal and gastrointestinal stents: experience with 113 patients. *Am J Roentgenol.* 2004;183:1437-1444.

42. Homan N, Nofts MR, Klingenberg–Noftz RD, Ludwig D. Delayed complications after placement of self-expanding stents in malignant esophageal obstruction: treatment strategies and survival rate. *Dig Dis Sci.* 2008;53(2):334-340.

43. Amrani L, Menard C, Berdah S, et al. From iatrogenic digestive perforation to complete anastomotic disunion: endoscopic stenting as a new concept of "stent-guided regeneration and re-epithelialization. *Gatrointest Endosc.* 2009;69(7):1282-1287.

44. Dua KS, Hoga WJ, Aadam AA, Gasparri M. In-vivo oesophageal regeneration in a human being by use of a non-biological scaffold and extracellular matrix. *Lancet.* 2016;388(10039):55-61. [Epub 08 April 2016].

PART NINE

Hernia

Basic Concepts and Factors Associated With Ventral Hernia Recurrence

Crystal F. Totten | J. Scott Roth

A hernia is described as a protrusion of an organ or tissue from its normal cavity. This protrusion may extend outside the abdominal wall or between body cavities. Hernias vary in presentation including congenital, umbilical and epigastric hernias, inguinal, traumatic flank hernias, and incisional hernias to name a few. In addition, hernia etiology may differ based upon type. A congenital hernia, present at birth, is the result of defective development of the abdominal wall; alternatively, hernias may be acquired later in life as the result of injury to the abdominal wall via trauma or surgery. An acquired hernia may be attributed to overexertion, weight lifting, jumping from a high distance, or violent coughing episodes, although underlying connective tissue disorders may also be a contributing factor. In recent years, the role of connective tissue disease such as Marfan syndrome, Ehlers-Danlos syndrome, and osteogenesis imperfecta have shown a predisposition for hernia development. Similarly, syndromes such as polycystic kidney disease, known for an abnormal extracellular matrix production, have been demonstrated to be associated with up to a 43% incidence of hernias. It is believed that abnormalities in collagen metabolism contribute to hernia formation and high recurrence rates in these populations. Multiple genomics projects are ongoing, looking at candidate genes responsible for the production of type I and III collagens as well as matrix metalloproteinases (MMPs).

The goal of ventral hernia repair generally includes closure of the midline without excess tension. Many risk factors influence the longevity of that repair including patient factors (increased intraabdominal pressure, diminished tissue integrity) and technical factors (infection, lateral mesh detachment, missed hernia). It is estimated that 75% of all recurrences are due to infection and inadequate repair material fixation and/or overlap.[1] Each type of hernia has specific hernia recurrence rates. Midline laparotomies for nonhernia surgery carry a 25% risk of developing an incisional hernia. Five-year reoperation rates for incisional hernia repairs have been reported at 24% following the first reoperation, 35% after the second, 39% after the third, with the 7-year rate after three operations nearing 50%. These data underscore the importance

of minimizing the risk for subsequent reoperations by employing the best evidence-based approach for the first hernia repair.[2] Multiple comorbidities have been identified to increase the risk of infection following hernia repair. A higher infection occurrence then augments the risk of recurrence. Comorbidities that increase rates of postoperative infections include smoking, diabetes, chronic corticosteroid use, immunosuppression, coronary artery disease, chronic obstructive pulmonary disease, low preoperative serum albumin levels, prolonged operative times, and use of absorbable synthetic mesh.[3]

Many classification systems have also been developed to categorize hernias to better understand who is at risk.

Global classifications for wound status include the Centers for Disease Control and Prevention (CDC) wound classification. This system categorized all surgeries into one of four groups: clean, clean-contaminated, contaminated, and dirty. Each CDC class was assigned a risk of postoperative wound infections by the CDC in 1985.[4] Clean wounds are known uninfected wounds without entry into any visceral tracts that carry a low risk of 1% to 5%. Clean-contaminated wounds are those in which the respiratory, alimentary, genital, or urinary tracts are entered under controlled conditions, increasing infection risk to 3% to 11%. Contaminated wounds include open, fresh, accidental wounds, those with major breaks in sterile technique, gross spillage from the gastrointestinal tract, and presence of nonpurulent inflammation. The risk of infection in a contaminated wound is 10% to 17%. Finally, dirty or infected wounds include those with old traumatic wounds, retained devitalized tissue, and those with an existing clinical infection or perforated viscus.[3] Their risk is expectedly elevated to greater than 27% for postoperative surgical site infection (SSI). The CDC updated the estimated SSI rates again in 1985 and 1991 following changes in antibiotic coverage and technique with 2.1% for clean, 3.3% for clean-contaminated, 10% to 17% for contaminated, and over 27% for dirty.[4] CDC classification focuses only on the characteristics of the wound at the time of repair.

The Ventral Hernia Working Group (VHWG) classification system developed a grading scale to predict

SSI based on characteristics of the individual and their hernia defect. Grade 1 represents patients considered low risk, no comorbidities, no history of prior wound infection, or current contamination. Grade 2 hernias include patients with comorbidities including smoking, obesity, diabetes, immunosuppression, chronic obstructive pulmonary disease, without current wound contamination or active infection. These patients are at increased risk of infection due to their associated comorbidities. Grade 3 hernias include those with a history of prior wound infection, presence of a stoma, or concurrent violation of the gastrointestinal tract. Grade 4 hernias are classified as infected with known mesh infections or septic dehiscence.[2] The awareness of risk factors and hernia grade allow for personalization of hernia repair, mesh selection, and risk optimization. The VHWG grading scale was not validated, however, due to lack of available data.

Published in 2012, the VHWG was modified following the review of 299 open ventral hernia repairs with determination of SSI rates for each grade. Following this analysis, the modified system was developed representing three grades. VHWG-M grade 1 includes low risk hernias with low risk of complications and no prior wound infections with a reported surgical site occurrence (SSO) rate of 14%. VHWG-M grade 2 hernias represent patients with significant comorbidities. VHWG-M grade 2 patients experience postoperative SSO rates of 27%. VHWG-M grade 3 includes hernias with all degrees of bacterial contamination including clean-contaminated, contaminated, and dirty procedures with SSO rates of 46%.[5]

The Ventral Hernia Risk Score (VHRS) was developed using a single-center data within a Veterans Affairs population to stratify SSI risk based upon wound classification, comorbid conditions, and technique. The VHRS assigns points ascribed to each of five clinical attributes: concomitant hernia repair (2 points), creation of skin flaps (2 points), American Society of Anesthesiologists (ASA) score 3 or greater (2 points), body mass index (BMI) 40 or more kg/m^2 (3 points), and incision class 4 or dirty (7 points). There are five VHRS subgroups with progressive associated risk for wound infection based upon the range of points accumulated group I (0 points), group II (2 to 3 points), group III (4 points), group IV (5 to 10 points), and group V (11 to 16 points). The risk of SSI development varied from group I at 7.8% compared with group V at 83.3%.[6] The VHRS was externally validated and found to have greater predictive accuracy compared with VHWG and CDC classification systems in determining risk of SSI at 30 days. Morbid obesity (odds ratio [OR] 2.4), elevated ASA class (OR 3.4), skin flap creation (OR 3.3), CDC wound class 4 (OR 4.7), and concomitant hernia repair (OR 1.7) are all risk factors for SSI. Smoking and diabetes mellitus were both associated with SSI development on univariable analysis but were not independent variables in the VHRS model. Several components of the VHRS are modifiable patient factors, allowing for identification of patients who will benefit from preoperative interventions.[7]

The European Hernia Society has developed a nomenclature system to facilitate the use of standardized terminology to describe hernias.[8] It was developed following a 2008 consensus conference in Belgium focusing on location of each hernia and width that can be attributed to midline

TABLE 50.1 European Hernia Society Classification of Incisional Hernia

Midline hernias	Subxiphoid	M1	From the xiphoid process to 3 cm caudally
	Epigastric	M2	From 3 cm below the xiphoid process to 3 cm above the umbilicus
	Umbilical	M3	3 cm above the umbilicus to 3 cm below the umbilicus
	Infraumbilical	M4	From 3 cm below umbilicus to 3 cm above pubis
	Suprapubic	M5	From the pubic bone to 3 cm caudally
Lateral hernias	Subcostal	L1	Between the coastal margin and the horizontal line 3 cm above the umbilicus
	Flank	L2	Lateral to the rectus sheath in the area 3 cm above and below the umbilicus
	Iliac	L3	Between a horizontal line 3 cm below the umbilicus and the inguinal region
	Lumbar	L4	Lateral and dorsal to the anterior axillary line

and lateral primary hernias as well as incisional hernias. The classification system allows for more specific discussion and comparison of hernias with a common nomenclature. Midline hernias are designated from the xiphoid process to the pubic bone and medial to the lateral margin of the rectus sheath on both sides. Lateral hernias occur from costal margin to inguinal region and from the lateral margin of the rectus sheaths to the lumbar region. Hernias are demarcated by size: W1, 1 to 4 cm; W2, 4 to 10 cm; and W3, greater than or equal to 10 cm as well as recurrent nature. Table 50.1, adapted from the European Hernia Society definitions, depicts the types of hernias that can occur on the abdominal wall.[8] A standardized classification for hernias should be used to allow for effective description of outcome measures as pertaining to hernia groups, recognizing that not all hernia repairs are associated with comparable results.

OPTIMIZING KNOWN RISK FACTORS

Multiple risk factors have been associated with increased ventral hernia recurrence following repair. It is important to optimize each one of these risk factors.

DIABETES MELLITUS

Diabetes mellitus has long been described as a risk factor for major morbidity and mortality after surgery.[9] Poorly regulated glucose metabolism due to insulin resistance or stress hyperglycemia after acute illness or trauma results in short-term glucose elevations associated with an increased SSI rate.[10] A recent study by Goodenough et al. reported the correlation of elevated preoperative HbA1c to perioperative glycemic control. Patients with normal preoperative HbA1c were more likely to have normal peak perioperative glucose, and similarly, patients with an elevated HbA1c experience a higher incidence of perioperative hyperglycemia, defined as glucose greater than 160 mg/dL. HbA1c was shown to be a stronger predictor of adverse events compared with preoperative diabetes mellitus status or perioperative glucose.[11] Other studies have identified a similar association between HbA1c and surgical outcomes. Although the optimal preoperative HbA1c has not been established, efforts should be made to optimize glycemic control and HbA1c prior to consideration of any elective hernia repair to enhance postoperative outcomes.

In 2001 Latham et al. reported a 7.9% SSI rate in patients with a HbA1c greater than 8, a twofold risk compared with patients with an HbA1c less than 8.[12] Endara et al. found that HbA1c greater than 6.5% was associated with increased rates of dehiscence after surgical wound closure similar to the finding by Goodenough et al. in which 6.5% was found to be the threshold HbA1c level at which complication rates increase.[11,13] Underwood et al. treated diabetic patients with HbA1c greater than 8% preoperatively, resulting in considerable blood glucose level improvements on the day of surgery.[14] The American Diabetes Association recommends that outpatient management of diabetes should ideally include a combination of target HbA1c less than 7%, preprandial blood glucose level of 90 to 130 mg/dL, and a peak postprandial blood glucose level of less than 180 mg/dL.[15] While no finite recommendation exists, most experts agree that attempts to obtain a HbA1c less than 8 should be made prior to elective hernia repair with a goal as close to 6.5% as feasible.

In Goodenough et al. publication, one-third of patients without a history of diabetes were found to have HbA1c greater than 6.5% on screening. These patients were more likely to have a BMI greater than 30, have additional comorbidities including coronary artery disease, and have chronic pulmonary obstructive disease, as well as categorized as non-Caucasian.[11] Based on these findings, we recommend obtaining HbA1c levels on all patients with BMI greater than 30 kg/m² presenting for elective ventral hernia repair.

SMOKING AND ALCOHOL CESSATION

Smoking and alcohol use have been shown to negatively impact postoperative outcomes. Current smokers have an increased risk of pulmonary and wound complications following operation. The effects of nicotine on a cellular level include vasoconstriction and tissue level hypoxia correlating with tissue nicotine levels, increased platelet aggregation, and reduced fibroblast migration. Carbon monoxide levels also reduce oxygen delivery to the tissues, leaving smokers who consume greater than 20 cigarettes hypoxic most of the day.[16] The additive effects of tissue hypoxia, reduced fibroblast proliferation, reduced collagen 1 to 3 ratios and reduced overall collagen deposition in smokers leads to increased wound infections and reduced tissue strength. Smoking one cigarette decreases cutaneous and subcutaneous blood flow by 38.1%.[17] Smoking cessation of 4 weeks preoperatively has been shown to reduce wound infection rates from 12% in 1 pack per day smokers to 1%, values comparable with patients who have never smoked. In that investigation, there was no difference between transdermal nicotine patch and placebo patches used for smoking cessation techniques. Specifically, in hernia patients, active smokers experience more frequent hernia recurrences and postoperative infections than comparable nonsmoking patients.[18] Smoking cessation efforts rank highly among the most challenging initiatives for patients and physicians. Smoking recidivism rates are not insignificant following attempts at smoking cessation. However, considering the increased morbidity and cost associated with hernia complications and recurrences, attempts at smoking cessation prior to elective ventral hernia repair should be attempted. Although extenuating circumstances may compel patients and surgeons to proceed with elective repair in patients using cigarettes, the risks should be carefully considered preoperatively, as each hernia recurrence carries a greater risk of recurrence than the prior repair. Patients with multiple recurrent hernias are generally not suitable for elective repair while smoking, but first-time repairs in smokers should be similarly discouraged to avoid the creation of recurrent-hernia patients.

Alcohol abuse is associated with an increased risk of bleeding, wound, and cardiopulmonary complications. Alcohol abuse is categorized as ingestion of five or more drinks (60 g of ethanol) a day. Abstinence from alcohol for 1 month preoperatively reduces postoperative morbidity with reduced responses to surgical stress, improved cardiac and immune dysfunction.[19]

WEIGHT OPTIMIZATION

BMI is considered a significant predictor for surgical site occurrence. Morbidly obese patients are at a higher risk for the development of abdominal wall defects and progression of the size of the defects due to increased intraabdominal pressure and poor wound healing potential.[20] The relationship between obesity and surgical complications including SSIs has been reported in colorectal surgery, and more recently, the association has been specifically related to ventral hernia repair.[21] BMI is considered a significant predictor for SSI when analyzed as a continuous variable, thus demonstrating that SSI risk increases with increasing BMI. These authors recommend optimization of comorbidities such as morbid obesity prior to surgical intervention.[6] While the ideal BMI for elective hernia repair is often debated, BMI should be evaluated in the context of individual patient and hernia characteristics when determining the best strategy for patient management. Other factors such as risk for incarceration, crescendo symptomatology, and rapidity of hernia progression may influence decision making. For example, patients with small defects with large volumes of incarcerated bowel may be at risk for significant intestinal loss in the event of strangulation. In such circumstances, elective repair may be appropriate in high BMI patients despite the increased perioperative risks.

Accordingly, patients amenable to a laparoscopic approach might be considered for an elective operation at higher BMI levels due to the reduced likelihood of postoperative infections in the morbidly obese compared with open hernia repairs. While conversion to an open procedure is always possible, conversion rates are low in many large laparoscopic ventral hernia repair series.

As the incidence of obesity in the adult population increases, surgeons are evaluating the outcomes of this patient subset to better understand the feasibility of hernia repair. One recent study reviewed the care of patients with BMI as high as 50 kg/m^2 in association with other patient characteristics that were deemed to be favorable for laparoscopic repair (gynecoid body habitus, reducible hernias found in a central location, abdominal wall thickness less than 4 cm, and the defect's largest diameter not exceeding 8 cm). In a short 2-year follow-up, there were minimal recurrences[22]; however, critics of this study state that hernia recurrence at later time intervals is eminent. A retrospective review of a prospectively maintained database of four hernia surgeons focused on patients with BMI greater than or equal to 40 kg/m^2 compared with patients with BMI less than 40 kg/m^2 undergoing laparoscopic ventral hernia repair. The authors found operative duration, length of hospital stay, and recurrence rate for a mean follow-up time of 19 months were significantly greater in the morbidly obese group than for patients with BMI less than 40 kg/m^2.[23] Other studies have found the laparoscopic approach to offer a safe alternative for obese patients but with apparent increased risk of recurrence of hernia for this subset of patients.[24–26]

Weight loss surgery is an effective method of weight loss, and ventral hernia repair can be safely combined with weight loss procedures such as Roux-en-Y gastric bypass and sleeve gastrectomy or performed in stages.[27–29] A large national database study showed that patients who underwent ventral hernia repair in conjunction with either laparoscopic Roux-en-Y gastric bypass or sleeve gastrectomy had increased incidence of SSI but not overall morbidity in the 30-day postoperative time period, again providing evidence of the seeming appropriateness of the combination of these procedures.[30] However, long-term outcome studies specifically addressing hernia recurrence rates in these populations are lacking.

As a patient's BMI approaches 30 kg/m^2, the risk of infection and recurrence reduce; however, an optimal cutoff BMI for ventral hernia repair in the obese population is still debatable. In general, a BMI of less than 40 kg/m^2 may be considered safe for repair supported by the work of Tsereteli et al.[23]

PRIOR WOUND INFECTIONS

Antecedent wound complications are not uncommon among patients presenting with incisional hernias as this is a significant risk factor for hernia formation. In a landmark study in the 1980s, a history of previous wound infection predicted a greater risk for subsequent wound infection following incisional hernia repair.[31] Houck et al. noted that 41% of patients with prior wound infections developed an infection following subsequent repairs compared with an infection rate of 12% in patients without previous infections ($P < .05$), thus emerging the concept that once an abdominal wall is infected, the risk for subsequent infections remains elevated.[31] Subsequent infections increase the risk of hernia recurrence by 80% with a relative risk of 4.3 compared with noninfected repairs.[32] Although the presence of prior infections represents a nonmodifiable risk factor for future complications, this increased risk associated with prior infections should heighten the awareness of other modifiable risk factors to facilitate optimal outcomes.

PREOPERATIVE RISK REDUCTION

Multiple enhanced recovery protocols have been developed to both optimize the risk factors previously discussed as well as optimize immediate nutritional and infectious factors to limit wound infections and complications. These enhanced recovery protocols strive to implement and standardize best practices to reduce perioperative risk, reduce hospital length of stay, and reduce the cost of care, thus enhancing health care value. Numerous measures are included in an enhanced recovery protocol, each of equal importance; thus, the implementation of the entirety of the program is essential in maximizing risk reduction.

IMMUNE MODULATORS AND PREOPERATIVE NUTRITION

Experimental studies have shown nutritional supplements containing L-arginine, omega-3 polyunsaturated fatty acids, and nucleotides boost immune responsiveness after surgery or trauma. L-Arginine is a semiessential amino acid and a precursor of nitric oxide, which is the most important endothelial vasodilator. L-arginine has been shown to improve wound healing, restore postoperative depressed macrophage function and lymphocyte responsiveness, and augment resistance to infections. Intake of additional omega-3 polyunsaturated fatty acids alters cell membrane phospholipid content and prostaglandin synthesis that is theorized as an important factor in suppression of the generalized inflammatory response and subsequent immunosuppression and capillary leakage after major surgery.[33] Elevated omega-3 levels also inhibit the metabolism of arginine. An oral immune-enhancing nutritional supplement taken for 5 days preoperatively has been shown to result in increased preoperative serum arginine concentration and decreased number of postoperative infections with preserved renal function.[34] Similarly, low albumin is also independently associated with major complications that can be improved with preoperative nutrition augmentation. As a component of our enhanced recovery protocol, patients undergoing ventral hernia repair are prescribed a 5-day course of an arginine-based supplement as an immune enhancing measure. Although the impact of this dietary regimen in ventral hernia repair has not been independently studied, the numerous studies demonstrating the benefits in other patient populations cannot be disregarded.[33,34]

Traditional surgical and anesthesia dogma has required patients to abstain from oral intake for at least 8 hours prior to an elective operation. Despite years of practice, no scientific evidence exists to support the basis for this fast, and in a Cochrane review, there was no evidence to suggest a shortened fluid fast results in an increased risk of aspiration, regurgitation, or morbidity compared with the standard fasting policy.[35] Patients following a standard fast present with depleted glycogen stores in the liver, which increases the demand for amino acids production resulting in protein catabolism following surgical stressors rather than tissue repair. Recent protocols have transitioned to providing a clear fluid that contains a relatively high concentration of complex carbohydrates

2 to 3 hours before induction of anesthesia allowing patients to undergo surgery in a metabolically fed state with adequate glycogen stores. As little as 400 mL of a 12.5% drink of mainly maltodextrins (e.g., Gatorade) reduces preoperative thirst, hunger, anxiety and postoperative insulin resistance, resulting in less postoperative losses of nitrogen and protein and better-maintained lean body mass and muscle strength.[36] Our enhanced recovery protocol includes administration of 32 ounces of a carbohydrate-rich, clear fluid 3 to 4 hours preoperatively as a method of ensuring euvolemia and adequate glycogen stores as elective hernia repair commences.

METHICILLIN-RESISTANT *STAPHYLOCOCCUS AUREUS* PROPHYLAXIS

Ventral hernia patients with a history of methicillin-resistant *Staphylococcus aureus* (MRSA) at any prior location (blood, urine, sputum, wound) experience increased wound infection rates compared with those patients without a history for MRSA.[37] In an effort to decolonize known MRSA carriers or reduce the risk of colony-forming units (CFU) of the skin flora with unknown MRSA status, the use of mupirocin intranasal ointment twice daily combined with chlorhexidine showers for 5 days preoperatively is considered effective with reports of a 44% reduction in SSI.[38,39] Although decontamination protocols have not been evaluated independently in hernia patients, MRSA decolonization has been investigated as a component of a hernia-enhanced recovery protocol.[40] Identification of patients with a history of MRSA infection often represents the greatest barrier to implementation. As a result, mupirocin and chlorhexidine showers may be prescribed preoperatively to all patients undergoing ventral hernia repair due to the low cost, infrequent side effects, and potential benefit in SSI reduction.

PREVENTION OF INTRAOPERATIVE HYPOTHERMIA

Patients becoming hypothermic (<36°C) have higher rates of wound infection, morbid cardiac events, and bleeding. The maintenance of a patient's temperature, rather than restoration following temperature decreases, is paramount. Normothermia may be accomplished with a suitable warming device and warmed intravenous fluids should be used routinely to keep body temperature greater than 36°C. Monitoring is essential to titrate warming devices and to avoid hyperpyrexia.[41] Warming devices such as forced-air heating blankets and warmed intravenous fluids should be routinely used to keep body temperature greater than 36°C.

EMERGENCY OPERATIONS

Emergency operations are known risk factors for postoperative complications and hernia recurrence. Patients presenting with surgical emergencies may not have the opportunity to be optimized through risk factor optimization and present with high levels of stress cortisol. Emergency and open operations both contribute to stress hyperglycemia by promoting a proinflammatory response.[11] Emergent conditions preclude the opportunity to perform patient optimization for modifiable risk factors. However, awareness of the inherent risk factors will allow for postoperative treatment of these modifiable conditions.

HERNIA PREVENTION

Incisional hernia formation occurs in a significant number of patients undergoing abdominal surgery and is the most common complication of a laparotomy. The rate of hernia occurrence after laparotomy approaches 25% by 3 years with no gold standard for prevention.[42] Two prospective studies evaluating incisional hernia rates have been conducted. While physical examination is the most common method for detecting incisional hernias, ultrasonography may be used as an adjunct to detect clinically occult hernias. Early detection of occult hernias may facilitate identification of patients at risk for hernia progression.[43] While neither ultrasonography nor examination has 100% specificity, incisional hernia rates are likely underreported.[44] While operation rates are often considered a surrogate for incisional hernia rates, minimally symptomatic hernias are often managed nonoperatively and further contribute to the underestimation of hernia incidence.

Hernia prophylaxis represents an opportunity to prevent the initial development of hernia, thus minimizing the subsequent morbidity associated with complications and recurrences. The optimal technique for laparotomy closure has been exhaustively investigated. Prior studies have evaluated suture choice, suture technique, stitch length, and mesh reinforcement at the time of laparotomy to reduce the risk of incisional hernia formation.

SUTURE SELECTION

Appropriate suture selection is paramount in preventing incisional hernias. There is no difference in the hernia rate between permanent versus absorbable sutures; however, wound sinuses and pain are more common with permanent suture. However, when long-lasting absorbable sutures are compared with short-acting ones (i.e., PDS vs. Vicryl), the differences become more apparent with higher rates of hernia formation associated with rapidly absorbable suture materials. Long-lasting absorbable sutures have the benefits of a permanent suture without suture site pain and development of wound sinuses and have become the standard over a permanent suture.[45]

STITCH LENGTH

Equally important to suture material is stitch length and suture size. Initial work evaluating at 4:1 suture–wound length ratio dates back to 1976 with Jenkins reporting suture-to-wound length ratio greater than 4:1 reducing laparotomy failure (e.g., abdominal burst wound).[46] This type of closure is based on the Pythagorean theorem in which 1 cm of travel along an abdominal closure will require approximately 4 cm of suture material. However, this only accounts for the length and width of suture required and does not account for the the thickness of the abdominal wall. Competing ideals debate the ideal suture-to-wound length ratio and whether it should incorporate the thickness of tissue and be as high as 6:1.[47]

In a prospective study of 450 patients undergoing laparotomy, the impact of suture-to-wound length ratios was compared. Hernia rates for closures with less than 4:1 suture-to-wound length ratio was 24% compared with 9% when the ratio was greater than 4:1. In a subsequent study, Israelsson et al. performed a single-site prospective trial comparing midline laparotomy closure with 2-0 polydiaxanone (PDS) running suture with 5 to 8 mm tissue bites and 5 to 8 mm advances (short stitch) compared with a No. 1 PDS with 1 cm bites and 1 cm advances (large stitch). The small stitch group experienced a reduced infection rate of 5.1% compared with 9.6% infection rate in the large stitch group. Furthermore, the small stitch hernia rate was reduced to one-third of that of the large stitch group, 4.7% compared with 17.1% for short stitch and long stitch, respectively.[48]

In a multicenter randomized controlled trial in Europe (STITCH trial), 609 patients were randomly assigned to undergo a large stitch or small stitch laparotomy closure, and were followed for a year with either physical examination or ultrasound. In these matched cohorts based upon age, gender, BMI, comorbid conditions, type of surgery including colorectal, upper GI, gynecologic, or vascular, the large stitch patients had fewer numbers of stitches (25 vs. 45) and shorter overall suture length used (95 vs. 110 cm) for equivalent laparotomy lengths. The ratio of suture to length of wound was longer in the small stitch (5 vs. 4.3), and the operative duration required to perform the short stich closure was 4 minutes longer in the small stitch cohort. Postoperative complications were no different, morbidity (ileus, cardiac, pneumonia), SSIs, rate of burst abdomen (1%), and hospital length of stay. Hernia rates were greater in the large stitch versus short stitch groups (21% vs. 12%). While the STITCH study demonstrated a reduction in hernia rates with the short stitch technique, no reduction in SSI rates were seen.[49] While this study clearly demonstrates the benefits of technique upon incisional hernia rates, the mean BMI of patients enrolled in the STITCH trial is 24 kg/m², and the technique has not been demonstrated to be effective in obese populations.

MESH REINFORCEMENT AS PREVENTION

Numerous studies have demonstrated the potential benefit of prophylactic mesh. In 2003, a prospective randomized controlled trial (RCT) of 100 patients who underwent laparotomy of at least 10 cm were closed with a permanent running suture and an onlay polypropylene mesh with 3 cm of overlap. In this study, there is 11% hernia formation in patients without mesh compared with 0% in those patients who did have mesh at 1-year follow-up. The seroma rate was higher in the nonmesh cohort with equal SSI rates and an increase in chronic pain scores for those with mesh placement.[50] A cohort of high-risk patients demonstrated one-third decreased hernia development following midline closure with prophylaxis mesh as reported in *Hernia* in 2009.[51] An RCT was published in 2014 that explored clean-contaminated or contaminated colorectal/gastric operations with a 20-cm laparotomy closed with either running

loop No. 1 PDS versus running closure with an onlay of lightweight polypropylene (3 cm of overlap). Hernia occurrence was determined by computed tomography (CT) imaging and physical exam at 12 months with 1.5% hernia rate in the mesh group versus 35.9% rate in the nonmesh group.[52] The technique of mesh prophylaxis and 4:1 closure was applied to patients undergoing emergent and elective colorectal surgery in an RCT published in *Annals of Surgery* in 2015. Fifty-four patients were closed with 4:1 technique alone compared with 53 patients reinforced with onlay polypropylene (PP) mesh, 2.5 cm overlap laterally. Suture only had a 31.5% rate of hernia development compared with 11.3% with mesh (P = .011), no difference in mesh in seroma, SSI, evisceration, or mortality.[53] The PRIMA trial is a double-blinded RCT ongoing to compare primary suture closure, glued onlay mesh augmentation (OMA), and sublay mesh augmentation (SMA). Initial 30-day results, published in 2015, showed no difference in SSI, hematoma, reintervention, or readmission; however, there was an increased OR of seroma formation using onlay low-weight PP mesh augmentation (OMA vs. primary suture [PS]: OR, 4.3; P = .004; OMA vs. SMA: OR, 2.09; P = .003).[54] Mesh augmentation for hernia prevention, even in high-risk patient populations, has been proven safe and effective; however, it has not become mainstream due to lack of acceptance or reimbursement.

MANAGEMENT OF A HERNIA

Once a hernia develops, there are multiple components involved in the optimal repair to avoid recurrence. Flum et al. reported that the 5-year reoperative rate following incisional hernia repair was 23.8% after the first reoperation, 35.3% after the second, and 38.7% after the third.[55] Many mechanisms of recurrence have been described in the literature including technical failures such as knot tying, suture pullout, inadequate mesh overall, lateral detachment of mesh, or inadequate choice of mesh or fixation as well as occurrence of infection, trauma, or increased intraabdominal pressure.[1] The goal of any hernia operation is approximation of the midline abdominal wall without tension. This goal is affected by the tissue integrity. Determining the degree of tension at the time of repair has been challenging. The use of tensiometers in the operating room to measure the force required to approximate midline is not only cumbersome, but also impractical, leading to reliance on clinical evidence such as tearing of tissues and elevated airway pressures as the mainstay of measurement.

Options for hernia repair include direct suture repair, repair using prosthetic material (synthetic, biologic, or composite mesh), using local fascial flaps, mobilization of anatomic layers, or a combined procedure of greater than one technique. This section will describe the literature regarding mechanisms of repair.

MESH VERSUS PRIMARY SUTURE CLOSURE

Open suture repair is the simplest and oldest method of hernia repair. It can be performed rapidly; however, it has a high recurrence rate. Luijendick et al. in 2000 reported recurrence rates following repair of primary or first-recurrence incisional hernias using either

No. 1 Prolene running suture closure or sublay PP mesh with 2 to 4 cm overlap and a midline closure if possible. The goal follow-up was 36 months; however, the average was only 26 months. In primary incisional hernias, the recurrence rate using suture alone was 43% compared with 24% in the group that used mesh ($P < .02$). This trend continued in patients undergoing repair of first recurrence, 58% suture alone versus 20% mesh. Pooled data often quoted reports 46% rate of hernia recurrence in suture alone and 23% rate following mesh repair ($P < .005$) with more patients in the suture-only arm developing hernia recurrences early around 12 months compared with mesh repairs.[32] The recurrence rate on this cohort of patients was updated by Burger et al. in 2004, with a 10-year cumulative rate of recurrence of 63% for suture repair and 32% for mesh ($P < .001$).[56] Using mesh repair of hernias less than 2 cm in size was debated until 2013. Christoffersen et al. reported results of a prospective cohort study using the Danish Ventral Hernia registry comparing elective open mesh versus suture-only repairs of small umbilical and epigastric hernias. A total of 4786 patients were included and followed up to 4 years with a reoperation rate for recurrence of 2.2% in the mesh group and 5.6% in the suture-alone group. Subset analysis in suture-alone group showed similar rates between non-, slow-, and fast-absorbable sutures. Rates of reoperation were also similar in regard to mesh position (inlay/plug 4.9%, sublay 2.5%, onlay 2.2%, and intraperitoneal 0.7%). The rates of reoperation cannot be correlated directly to recurrence rates; however, this paper does support the use of mesh reinforcement of hernias 2 cm or greater.[57]

PRINCIPLES OF MESH OVERLAP

Recommendations regarding the extent of overlap are often defined according to the size of the defect and vary from 2 to 5 cm, with a 5-cm mesh overlap in every direction from the defect generally accepted as an ideal.[58-60] Sufficient overlap depends on the location of the mesh, location of the defect, and limitations associated with adjacent osseous structures that can limit fixation. An important component of mesh selection is defect sizing. Ventral hernia defect area will increase with a rise in intraabdominal pressure (IAP); therefore a defect size is in constant flux during daily activities. For example, resting IAP is 2 to 4 mm Hg and is increased with activity such as jumping (IAP of 170 mm Hg), coughing (IAP of 100 mm Hg), Valsalva maneuver (IAP of 40 mm Hg), and standing (IAP of 20 mm Hg).[61]

Multiple models have been developed in attempts to answer the force required to displace the mesh-fascial interface. A recent dynamic in vivo study laparoscopically measured midline hernia defect sizes in the vertical and horizontal position at an IAP of 8 and 15 mm Hg to determine the defect area. Results confirm that increasing IAP increases defect area by an average of 25% when varying pressure between 8 and 15 mm Hg. When using a large mesh overlap of 5 cm or greater, precise measurement of the defect area becomes less important.[62]

MESH LOCATION

Multiple positions for mesh placement have been described, and the ideal mesh placement should allow for mesh-tissue integration, reduce wound complications, and have tissue coverage to minimize exposure to superficial SSIs as well as intraperitoneal contents. An onlay repair secures mesh to the anterior fascia, typically involving dissection of devascularizing skin flaps and primary closure of the fascia below the mesh.

Inlay repair places the mesh within the hernia defect, securing it circumferentially to the edges of the fascia without mesh-tissue integration. Sublay repair refers to retrorectus, commonly referred to as *Rives-Stoppa*, or preperitoneal mesh placement, with the mesh location beneath the rectus complex and primary closure of fascia over the mesh. This position allows for mesh-tissue integration to load-bearing tissues from both the posterior rectus sheath and the anterior myofascial complex while protecting the mesh from superficial exposure and minimizing skin flap creation. The underlay repair denotes an intraperitoneal position with mesh secured to the anterior abdominal wall, placed open, or laparoscopically. Advantages include mesh protection from superficial SSI and lack of skin flaps; however, there is an increased risk of deep/organ space infections and complications secondary to adjacent viscera.

The incidence of hernia recurrence due to mesh location is best described in Awad et al. in 2005, in which 119 papers were reviewed and the data were pooled to determine the cause of each hernia recurrence.[1] Criticisms of this paper include unreported length of follow-up, lower than previously reported hernia recurrence rates, and a heterogeneous patient population. Regardless, they were able to report a difference in hernia recurrence based on mesh location that is consistent with the understanding of mesh fixation to the abdominal wall and mechanisms allowing for recurrence. Regarding mesh location, the greatest risk of recurrence is associated with an inlay repair (12.7%). This is consistent with the mainstream understanding that a larger mesh-to-fascia interface allows for improved strength and longevity compared with an inlay, where the interface is completely dependent upon the suture strength approximating mesh to fascia. Onlay, sublay, and intraperitoneal repairs were similar in recurrence rates (5%, 4.4%, and 3.6%, respectively).[1] A meta-analysis regarding mesh placement in open ventral hernia repairs was published in 2016. Twenty-one studies reported on recurrence rates predominantly detected based on clinical exam during a 5- to 60-month follow-up. The pooled recurrence rate was 16.5% for onlay, 30.2% for inlay, 7.0% for sublay, and 14.7% for underlay. The rate of SSI based on mesh location was also reported based on 10 studies and had 16.9% for onlay, 31.3% for inlay, 3.7% for sublay, and 16.7% for underlay.[63] The recurrence rates in this meta-analysis were higher than those published by Awad et al.; however, the elongated duration of follow-up likely accounted for additional recurrence detection. Across all studies, mesh placed in an open sublay position (e.g., retrorectus, preperitoneal) is associated with the lowest risk of recurrence.

BRIDGE VERSUS BUTTRESS

The goal of any open ventral hernia repair is approximation of the midline discussed in the literature since the 1920s. Hernia repairs performed laparoscopically include primary fascial closure (PFC) of the defect via transfascial or intracorporeal suturing. Small underpowered studies have suggested lower recurrence rates with PFC repairs compared with bridged mesh repair alone.[34,65] In 2015, Wennergren et al. reported a multicenter retrospective review comparing PFC to bridging alone in laparoscopic ventral hernia repairs with no difference in patient outcomes in recurrence, SSI, readmission, or seroma rate. However, in subset analysis, there was a threefold increase in hernia recurrence, SSI, and seroma formation for bridging alone in hernias greater than 3 cm, which did not reach statistical significance ($P = .232$, $P = .247$, and $P = .077$, respectively).[63]

A common postoperative complaint of patients undergoing bridged repair of ventral hernias is tissue eventration, which results in the perception of an inadequate repair. Decreased tissue eventration associated with PFC reduces visible "bulging," enhances the aesthetic result, and increases cosmetic satisfaction.[67] Zeichen et al. demonstrated that the time required to close the fascia during laparoscopic hernia repairs did not significantly increase the total operative time, thus maintaining operative costs.[64] Differing results have been published regarding postoperative pain, with the most recent literature noting no difference.[67]

In the setting of open midline abdominal wall reconstruction, Booth et al. noted increased hernia recurrence with bridge repair (55.6% vs. 7.7%; $P < .001$) with an interval to recurrence 9 times quicker in bridged cohort. The bridged repair group experienced a sixfold higher overall complication rate than the mesh-reinforced group ($P < .001$).[68] Hernias larger than 15 cm repaired in a bridging fashion was an independent risk factor for recurrence. Criticisms include a high frequency of biologic mesh, majority using porcine acellular dermal matrix over synthetic, which had no recurrences in a bridge position. Booth et al. literature is used to support the statement that a biologic mesh should not be used in a bridge position due to a high rate of recurrence.

MESH MATERIAL: SYNTHETIC, BIOLOGIC, OR BIOABSORBABLE

The role of mesh in the repair of incisional hernia remains undisputed following the results of a landmark study by Luijendijk et al. in 1999 in which the rate of recurrence associated with primary ventral and incisional hernias was twofold greater in those repaired without the use of a prosthetic mesh.[32] In a subsequent publication of this trial, the 10-year recurrence rates for suture repair were 63%, while the recurrence rates associated with mesh repair were 32%.[56] These studies demonstrated for the first time the significant benefits associated with the use of a prosthetic mesh when repairing ventral hernias. However, these studies also highlighted the significant rate of recurrence associated with ventral hernia repair over time. Other authors have demonstrated similar trends in ventral hernia recurrence rates with increasing incidence of hernia recurrence and hernia reoperation rates over prolonged periods of time.[55,69]

Prosthetic mesh choices have evolved significantly since the time of the initial work by Luijendijk et al. with

TABLE 50.2 Characteristics of the Ideal Prosthetic Material

The ideal prosthetic material should:
1. Possess acceptable handling characteristics in the operating room
2. Invoke a favorable host response
3. Be strong enough to prevent recurrence
4. Place no restrictions on postimplantation function
5. Perform well in the presence of infection
6. Resist shrinkage or degradation over time
7. Make no restrictions on future access
8. Block transmission of infectious disease
9. Be inexpensive
10. Be easy to manufacture

the advent of many new mesh materials, designs, and configurations (Table 50.2). While favorable characteristics for the ideal mesh have been elucidated, no single mesh is considered the gold standard for all hernia repairs. Accordingly, many mesh materials are marketed for use in specific conditions based upon patient factors or choice of surgical technique.

Mesh materials can generally be classified based upon one of three categories: synthetic, biologic, or bioabsorbable. Synthetic mesh materials include those fabricated primarily from polypropylene, polyester, or polytetrafluoroethylene. Both polypropylene and polyester mesh materials are woven meshes with interstices to facilitate integration into the host tissues. These materials are generally the most cost-effective material for hernia repair, although there may be some limitations to their use.[70] Both polypropylene and polyester mesh materials are not suitable for placement within the peritoneal cavity adjacent to the intestines without the addition of an adhesion barrier. These synthetic meshes may be used as an onlay or in the retrorectus or preperitoneal space to avoid contact between the mesh and the viscera. Composite meshes that incorporate polypropylene or polyester with the addition of an adhesion barrier allow for the placement of mesh directly within the peritoneal cavity. Polytetrafluoroethylene meshes are commonly fabricated in two-sided fashion with a microporous surface that minimizes visceral adhesion and a surface with greater porosity to enhance tissue integration. Numerous studies have compared the characteristics of these materials from the standpoint of strength, contracture, and adhesion formation.[71–73] Polytetrafluoroethylene meshes may be advantageous in certain situations due to their dual-sided fabrication process, and the strength of integration is less than that of polypropylene.[71,74]

Synthetic mesh materials have historically been considered contraindicated in the presence of any degree of contamination due to concerns for mesh infection. In a study of over 30,000 ventral hernia repairs, patients undergoing ventral hernia repair in clean-contaminated or contaminated surgical fields were found to have increased risks for superficial SSI (2.53 vs. 3.84 OR), deep incisional SSI (3.09 vs. 5.33 OR) in clean-contaminated and contaminated wounds, respectively, compared with CDC class 1 wounds.[75] This study affirmed the beliefs of many surgeons that permanent synthetic meshes should be avoided in contaminated surgical fields. Although enterotomy or unplanned bowel resection at the time of hernia repair is relatively rare, the placement of a synthetic mesh at the time of these event is associated with a threefold increased incidence of complications, a fourfold increase in 30-day reoperations, and a 10-fold increased incidence of enterocutaneous fistula formation in a series of 1124 patients undergoing elective hernia repair.[76] In fact, the presence of an enterotomy is considered to be a significant predictor for the need for mesh explantation.[77]

The role of synthetic mesh in the setting of contaminated surgical fields has more recently been debated. In a series of 100 ventral hernia repairs in clean-contaminated or contaminated surgical fields, the incidence of mesh removal 10 months following initial operation was 4% with one patient developing an enterocutaneous fistula.[78] In this study, lightweight polypropylene mesh was placed in the retrorectus or preperitoneal space in all but one repair. This same group has more recently reported their outcomes with lightweight synthetic mesh hernia repairs in CDC class 1 wounds and noted an increased incidence of hernia recurrences with the use of lightweight meshes (22.9%) versus midweight polypropylene mesh (10.6%).[79] Further investigation into the role of synthetic meshes in contaminated fields will need to be conducted to appreciate the benefits, risks, and costs.

Biologic mesh emerged as an alternative to synthetic mesh hernia repair in the early 21st century as a class of materials derived from either human or animal sources. These materials provided an alternative to the use of synthetic mesh in complex hernia repair, although the cost associated with these materials was significantly greater than synthetic meshes.[70] Biologic mesh materials may be derived from numerous tissue sources including dermis, small intestine submucosa, urinary bladder, pericardium, and liver, to name a few. Each of these materials undergoes unique processing to remove cellular elements, leaving an intact extracellular matrix.[80]

Biologic grafts are typically used in surgical wounds with some level of contamination as a strategy to minimize the risk for mesh infection. However, similar to synthetic meshes, biologic grafts are not cleared by the US Food and Drug Administration for use in contaminated settings and many of these materials include warnings against use in the setting of infection within the instructions for use.[81]

Nevertheless, biologic grafts have been used with increasing frequency in contaminated surgical fields as an alternative to sutured repairs, synthetic mesh repairs, or the use of tissue flaps. Early experiences with biologic meshes demonstrated poor outcomes when these grafts were used as a bridging material to span a hernia defect with recurrence rates approaching 100%.[82] However, when biologic meshes are used in conjunction to a component separation in contaminated settings, reasonable outcomes can be expected with recurrence rates up to 31%.[83] Not dissimilar from outcomes with synthetic meshes, biologic mesh hernia repair outcomes are impacted by mesh location, with lower recurrence rates demonstrated with retrorectus mesh positioning.[84]

There is little evidence directly comparing outcomes with synthetic and biologic mesh materials in contaminated

surgical settings to support their use.[85] However, a meta-analysis from 2014 evaluating 1229 hernia repair patients among eight studies demonstrated no difference in hernia recurrence rates between biologic and synthetic mesh hernia repairs with statistically fewer wound infections in the biologic hernia repair group.[86] In a study of 761 ventral hernia repairs performed with suture, synthetic, or biologic mesh, there was no difference in SSI rates or hernia recurrence rates between groups.[87] Although this study was retrospective, the groups were similar in wound class, hernia size, comorbid conditions, use of fascial releases, and acuity of hernia presentation. These studies suggest that biologic mesh outcomes may rival that of synthetic mesh, but further studies directly comparing outcomes are needed prior to drawing definitive conclusions.

The greatest barrier to adoption of the use of biologic mesh materials for hernia repair is cost. In a value-based health care environment, the use of cost-efficient materials is paramount. The costs of biologic meshes are significantly greater than the cost of synthetic mesh.[70] In the United States, health care costs are generally reimbursed through a diagnosis-related group (DRG) payment. The choice of mesh material, biologic or synthetic, is unlikely to impact the facility reimbursement, and accordingly, the added costs associated with more expensive materials will directly impact a hospital's profit margin. Reynolds et al. reported average financial losses of $8370 with the use of biologic mesh during ventral hernia repair, while synthetic mesh repairs were associated with a positive contribution margin of $3110, and an overall profit of $60 inclusive of indirect costs.[70] Because of the cost differences between meshes with direct impact upon a hospital's finances, it is incumbent upon the surgeon to select appropriate materials based upon individual patient characteristics.

Biosynthetic meshes have emerged as a third class of mesh materials. This group of materials includes fabricated meshes derived from polylactic acid, polyglycolic acid, trimethylene carbonate, silk, and poly-4-hydroxybutyrate. This class of materials has emerged as a more cost-effective alternative to biologic mesh. These materials provide a scaffold to reinforce the abdominal wall while ultimately resorbing. Preclinical evidence with biosynthetic meshes have demonstrated predictable degradation and hernia repair strength in excess of the native abdominal wall strength.[88] A prospective observational trial of 107 patients undergoing ventral hernia repair with biosynthetic mesh demonstrated a clinical recurrence rate of 17.3% at 2 years.[89] Although several trials evaluating biosynthetic meshes are ongoing, there is inadequate evidence at this time to support widespread adoption.

Table 50.3 includes classification of prosthetic materials.

POSTOPERATIVE MANAGEMENT

Following effective preoperative and intraoperative decision making, critical postoperative management of risk factors and limiting infections are key to reducing hernia complications.

DIABETES MELLITUS CONTROL

The current guidelines from surgical societies recommend intraoperative glucose levels less than 180 mg/

TABLE 50.3 Classification of Prosthetic Materials

Type	Example	Notes
Noncomposite heavy weight plastic meshes	Polypropylene, polyester	Synthetic, nonabsorbable, more data available, most commonly used, scar tissue and adhesions can cause chronic pain and discomfort, direct contact with abdominal viscera can cause bowel obstruction or fistula formation
Noncomposite heavyweight membranes	Expanded polytetrafluoroethylene (ePTFE)	Has the longest safety history when placed in contact with intraabdominal viscera
Noncomposite lightweight plastic meshes	Polypropylene, polyester	Better abdominal wall compliance and decreased chronic pain. Long-term results are not available.
Composite prosthesis	Heavyweight 1. ePTFE + heavyweight polypropylene 2. ePTFE + lightweight polypropylene + PDS memory ring Lightweight ePTFE + lightweight polypropylene	Retains the advantages of the plastic mesh but can be placed intraabdominally because the ePTFE side faces the viscera
Coated prosthesis	a. Lightweight or midweight b. Absorbable or nonabsorbable coating Materials for coating: 1. Omega-3 fatty acid 2. Absorbable complex carbohydrate-oat beta glucan 3. Carboxymethylcellulose-sodium hyaluronate-polyethylene glycol 4. Oxidized regenerated cellulose 5. Titanium	Reduced chronic pain and recurrence, no need to close peritoneum in laparoscopic inguinal hernia repair, coating decreases the adherence of protein coagulum and inhibits partially the initiation of the inflammatory cascade
Biologic prosthesis	Types: Human dermis, porcine dermis, porcine small intestine submucosa, fetal bovine dermis, bovine pericardium	Used in contaminated fields, acutely incarcerated groin hernias associated with tissue necrosis and/or infection. Concept: possess the strength to withstand the physiologic and anatomic stresses of the abdominal wall, while simultaneously acting as a scaffold to support tissue regeneration by providing a matrix for native cells to populate. Theoretically, this latter property makes it more physiologic than synthetic prostheses, which heal by scar formation, and may influence the incidence of long-term complications, such as postherniorrhaphy groin pain that affects quality of life. Higher cost, higher recurrence risk.

dL while guidelines from nonsurgical societies recommend that glucose levels be no less than 140 mg/dL in noncritically ill hospitalized patients.[90] In addition, treatment of perioperative short-term hyperglycemia can improve outcomes. Kwon and colleagues reported that patients who experienced perioperative hyperglycemia were at increased risk of infection, reoperation, and death, but hyperglycemic patients who received insulin were at no greater risk than those with normal glucose levels.[91,92]

ANTIBIOTIC CHEMOPROPHYLAXIS

Antibiotic prophylaxis in clean surgery with implantation of prosthetic material is widely accepted; however, a recent prospective randomized control study evaluated the administration of single-dose cefazolin for prosthetic hernia repairs. This study group was compared with no antibiotic prophylaxis with no significant difference in

infection rate (1.27% no antibiotics, 2.53% antibiotic; P = .364). Critics of this study include low overall infection occurrences.[93] Ríos et al. in 2001 published results from 216 patients undergoing incisional hernia reconstruction using polypropylene mesh who met criteria for a clean operation. The surgical wound infection rate was 13.6% for antibiotic prophylaxis arm compared with 26.3% in those without preoperative antibiotic prophylaxis, which was statistically significant following multivariate analysis.[94] A retrospective study published in 2013 evaluating deep and superficial infection rates following hernia repair treated with either two doses, 2 days, or 4 days of antibiotic chemoprophylaxis with no significant difference in infection rates between groups during a 4- to 6-week follow-up.[95] Standard CDC-based recommendations for antibiotic chemoprophylaxis are recommended. Antibiotic prophylaxis duration for prior mesh infections is not available in the literature.

DRAINS

Often prophylactic routine use of subcutaneous drains reportedly decreases wound complications such as infection, seroma, or hematoma. However, the indication for the use of drains in ventral hernia repair is not studied. Although closed-suction surgical drains are used to remove fluids (seroma, lymph, blood, abscess) accumulating in the surgical field, the occurrence of postoperative seroma, hematoma, and abscess is independent of drain presence. Drains also have several disadvantages including patient discomfort, limitations of mobilization, and increasing inpatient and home nursing care. There are no RCTs comparing drains versus no drains after incisional hernia repair.[96] The use of subcutaneous drains following laparotomy closure has not shown a benefit.[8] In settings where drains are used per surgeon preference, prolonged drain duration for a goal of 40 mL/day effluent was linked to BMI of 35 or more and operations longer than 210 minutes. There was no relationship between the incidences of seroma and drain duration, but there was a direct linear relationship between wound complications and drain duration while adjusting for obesity.[97]

The use of retrorectus drains following Rives-Stoppa or transverse abdominis muscle release has not been published in the literature to date; however, postoperative seromas and hematomas in this location can be more difficult to access percutaneously and anecdotally supports the placement of postoperative drains. The effect of drain placement in this location needs to be researched further.

ACTIVITY RESTRICTIONS

No prospective studies were found on the restriction of physical activity after abdominal incisions. In questionnaires sent to surgeons in both 1998 and again in 2014, there were significant variations in duration of convalescence and lifting restrictions.[98] Nevertheless, it is advocated by some surgeons to limit lifting to decrease the risk of hernias, but there is no consensus on the level or the duration of the restriction.[99] Postoperative restriction might have an adverse impact on the return to normal activity and delay the return to work.

ABDOMINAL BINDER

Two systematic reviews are available in the literature regarding postoperative binder use. Bouvier et al. reported in 2014 that up to 94% of patients use their binder for postoperative support of the wound. No significant improvement for the short-term benefits was found by the small RCTs included in his review.[100] Rothman et al. reported also in 2014, following pooling 578 patients from multiple RCT and cohort studies. There was a nonsignificant tendency to reduce seroma formation after laparoscopic ventral hernia repair and a nonsignificant reduction in pain; however, binder use did reduce postoperative psychological distress.[101] Clay et al. reported a significant lower visual analog scale (VAS) score for pain at the fifth postoperative day.[102] However, none of these studies included endpoints of hernia formation. The duration of subjective benefit is unclear, and binders should be worn for patient comfort only.

CONCLUSION

The goal of a hernia operation is to optimize the current repair by preventing complications and recurrence. This is done by identifying the potential risk factors preoperatively, with appropriate optimizing of nutrition, blood glucose, weight, smoking, and contamination prior to operative repair. Surgery should include avoiding visceral injury, closing midline to the extent possible, using component separation, and reinforcing with prosthetic material appropriate for the situation. Perioperatively, expediting ambulation, nutrition, and mitigating risk factors for infection and complications are important steps to augment future hernia recurrence prevention.

REFERENCES

1. Awad ZT, Puri V, LeBlanc K, et al. Mechanisms of ventral hernia recurrence after mesh repair and a new proposed classification. *J Am Coll Surg.* 2005;201(1):132-140.
2. Breuing K, Bulter CE, Ferzoco S, et al. The Ventral Hernia Working Group. Incisional ventral hernias: review of the literature and recommendations regarding the grading and technique of repair. *Surgery.* 2010;148(3):544-558.
3. Hart D, Postlethwait RW, Brown IW Jr, Smith WW, Johnson PA. Postoperative wound infections: a further report on ultraviolet irradiation with comments on the recent (1964) national research council cooperative study report. *Ann Surg.* 1968;167(5):728-743.
4. Garner JS. CDC guideline for prevention of surgical wound infections, 1985. Supersedes guideline for prevention of surgical wound infections published in 1982. (Originally published in November 1985). Revised. *Infect Control.* 1986;7(3):193-200.
5. Kanters AE, Krpata DM, Biatnik JA, Novitsky YM, Rosen MJ. Modified hernia grading scale to stratify surgical site occurrence after open ventral hernia repairs. *J Am Coll Surg.* 2012;215(6):787-793.
6. Berger RL, Li LT, Hicks SC, Davila JA, Kao LS, Liang MK. Development and validation of a risk-stratification score for surgical site occurrence and surgical site infection after open ventral hernia repair. *J Am Coll Surg.* 2013;217(6):974-982.
7. Liang MK, Goodenough CJ, Martindale RG, Roth JS, Kao LS. External validation of the ventral hernia risk score for prediction of surgical site infection. *Surg Infect.* 2015;16(1):36-40.
8. Muysoms FE, Antoniou SA, Bury K, et al. European Hernia Society guidelines on the closure of abdominal wall incisions. *Hernia.* 2015;19(1):1-24.
9. Tebby J, Lecky F, Edwards A, et al. Outcomes of polytrauma patients with diabetes mellitus. *BMC Med.* 2014;12:111.
10. Dungan KM, Braithwaite SS, Preiser JC. Stress hyperglycemia. *Lancet.* 2009;373(9677):1798-1807.
11. Goodenough CJ, Liang MK, Nguyen MT, et al. Preoperative glycosylated hemoglobin and postoperative glucose together predict major complications after abdominal surgery. *J Am Coll Surg.* 2015;221(4):854-861.
12. Latham R, Lancaster AD, Covington JF, Pirolo JS, Thomas CS Jr. The association of diabetes and glucose control with surgical site infections among cardiothoracic surgery patients. *Infect Control Hosp Epidermiol.* 2001;22(10):607-612.
13. Endara M, Masden D, Goldstein J, Gondek S, Steinberg J, Attinger C. The role of chronic and perioperative glucose management in high-risk surgical closures: a case for tighter glycemic control. *Plast Reconstr Surg.* 2013;132(4):996-1004.
14. Underwood P, Askari R, Hurwitz S, Chamarthi B, Garg R. Preoperative A1C and clinical outcomes in patients with diabetes undergoing major noncardiac surgical procedures. *Diabetes Care.* 2014;37(3):611-616.
15. American Diabetes Association. Standards of medical care in diabetes—2009. *Diabetes Care.* 2009;32(suppl 1):S13-S61.
16. Sorensen LT, Karlsmark T, Gottrup F. Abstinence from smoking reduces incisional wound infection: a randomized controlled trial. *Ann Surg.* 2003;238(1):1-5.

17. Sorensen LT, Jorgensen S, Petersen LJ, et al. Acute effects of nicotine and smoking on blood flow, tissue oxygen, and aerobe metabolism of the skin and subcutis. *J Surg Res.* 2009;152(2):224-230.

18. Sorensen LT, Hemmingsen UB, Kirkeby LT, Kallehave F, Jørgensen LN. Smoking is a risk factor for incisional hernia. *Arch Surg.* 2005;140(2):119-123.

19. Tonnesen H, Rosenberg J, Nielsen HJ, et al. Effect of preoperative abstinence on poor postoperative outcome in alcohol misusers: randomized controlled trial. *BMJ.* 1999;318(7194):1311-1316.

20. Sugerman HJ, Kellum JM Jr, Reines HD, et al. Greater risk of incisional hernia with morbidly obese than steroid-dependent patients and low recurrence with prefascial polypropylene mesh. *Am J Surg.* 1996;171(1):80-84.

21. Wick EC, Hirose K, Shore AD, et al. Surgical site infections and cost in obese patients undergoing colorectal surgery. *Arch Surg.* 2011;146(9):1068-1072.

22. Eid MG, Mattar SG, Hamad G, et al. Repair of ventral hernias in morbidly obese patients undergoing laparoscopic gastric bypass should not be deferred. *Surg Endosc.* 2004;18(2):207-210.

23. Tsereteli Z, Pryor BA. Heniford BT, Park A, Voeller G, Ramshaw BJ. Laparoscopic ventral hernia repair (LVHR) in morbidly obese patients. *Hernia.* 2007;12(3):233-238.

24. Froylich D, Segal M, Weinstein A, Hatib K, Shiloni E, Hazzan D. Laparoscopic versus open ventral hernia repair in obese patients: a long-term follow-up. *Surg Endosc.* 2015;30(2):670-675.

25. Lee J, Mabardy A, Kermani R, Lopez M, Pecquex N, McCluney A. Laparoscopic vs open ventral hernia repair in the era of obesity. *JAMA Surg.* 2013;148(8):723-726.

26. Regner JL, Mrdutt MM, Munoz-Maldonado Y. Tailoring surgical approach for elective ventral hernia repair based on obesity and National Surgical Quality Improvement Program outcomes. *Am J Surg.* 2015;210(6):1024-1030.

27. Newcomb WL, Polhill JL, Chen AY, et al. Staged hernia repair preceded by gastric bypass for the treatment of morbidly obese patients with complex ventral hernias. *Hernia.* 2008;12(5):465-469.

28. Praveen Raj P, Senthilnathan P, Kumaravel R, et al. Concomitant laparoscopic ventral hernia mesh repair and bariatric surgery: a retrospective study from a tertiary care center. *Obes Surg.* 2012;22(5):685-689.

29. Raziel A, Sakran N, Szold A, Goitein D. Concomitant bariatric and ventral/incisional hernia surgery in morbidly obese patients. *Surg Endosc.* 2012;28(4):1209-1212.

30. Spaniolas K, Kasten K, Mozer A, et al. Synchronous ventral hernia repair in patients undergoing bariatric surgery. *Obes Surg.* 2015;25(10):1-5.

31. Houck JP, Rypins EB, Sarfeh IJ, et al. Repair of incisional hernia. *Surg Gynecol Obstet.* 1989;169(5):397-399.

32. Luijendijk RW, Hop WC, van den Tol MP, et al. A comparison of suture repair with mesh repair for incisional hernia. *N Engl J Med.* 2000;343(6):392-398.

33. O'Leary MJ, Coakley JH. Nutrition and immunonutrition. *Br J Anaesth.* 1996;77(1):18-27.

34. Tepaske R, Velthuis H, Oudemans-van Straaten HM, et al. Effect of preoperative oral immune-enhancing nutritional supplement on patients at high risk of infection after cardiac surgery: a randomized placebo-controlled trial. *Lancet.* 2001;358(9283):696-701.

35. Brady M, Kinn S, Stuar P. Preoperative fasting for adults to prevent perioperative complications. *Cochrane Database Syst Rev.* 2013;(4):CD004423.

36. Noblett SE, Watson DS, Huong H, Davison B, Hainsworth PJ, Horgan AF. Pre-operative oral carbohydrate loading in colorectal surgery: a randomized controlled trial. *Colorectal Dis.* 2006;8(7):563-569.

37. Ousley J, Baucom RB, Poulose BK, et al. Previous methicillin-resistant *Staphylococcus aureus* infection independent of body site increases odds of surgical site infection after ventral hernia repair. *J Am Coll Surg.* 2015;221(2):470-477.

38. Buehlmann M, Frei RM, Fenner LM, Dangel M, Fluckiger U, Widmer AF. Highly effective regimen for decolonization of methicillin-resistant *Staphylococcus aureus* carriers. *Infect Control Hosp Epidemiol.* 2008;29(6):510-516.

39. Bode LG, Kluytmans JA, Wertheim HF, et al. Preventing surgical-site infections in nasal carriers of *Staphylococcus aureus*. *N Engl J Med.* 2010;362(1):9-17.

40. Fayezizadeh M, Rosen MJ, Novitsky YW, Novitsky YW. Enhanced recovery after surgery pathway for abdominal wall reconstruction:

41. pilot study and preliminary outcomes. *Plast Reconstr Surg.* 2004;134(4 suppl 2):151S-159S.

41. Kurz A, Sessler D I, Lenhardt R. Perioperative normothermia to reduce the incidence of surgical-wound infection and shorten hospitalization. *N Engl J Med.* 1996;334(19):1209-1216.

42. Fink C, Baumann P, Wente MN, et al. Incisional hernia rate 3 years after midline laparotomy. *Br J Surg.* 2014;101(2):51-54.

43. Diener MK, Voss S, Jensen K, Buchler MW, Seiler CM. Elective midline laparotomy closure: the inline systematic review and meta-analysis. *Ann Surg.* 2010;251(5):843-856.

44. Young J, Gilbert AI, Graham MF. The use of ultrasound in the diagnosis of abdominal wall hernias. *Hernia.* 2007;11(4):347-351.

45. van 't Riet M, Steyerberg EW, Nellensteyn J, Bonjer HJ, Bonjer HJ, Jeekel J. Meta-analysis of techniques for closure of midline abdominal incisions. *Br J Surg.* 2002;89(11):1350-1356.

46. Jenkins TP. The burst abdominal wound: a mechanical approach. *Br J Surg.* 1976;63(11):873-876.

47. Varshney S, Manek P, Johnson CD. Six-fold suture: wound length ration for abdominal closure. *Ann R Coll Surg Engl.* 1999;81(5):333-336.

48. Israelsson LA, Jonsson T. Suture length to wound length ratio and healing of midline laparotomy incisions. *Br J Surg.* 1993;80(10):1284-1286.

49. Deerenberg EB, Harlaar JJ, Steyerberg EW, et al. Small bites versus large bites for closure of abdominal midline incisions (STITCH): a double-blind, multicentre, randomized controlled trial. *Lancet.* 2015;386(10000):1254-1260.

50. Gutierrez de la Pena C, Medina Achirica C, Dominguez-Adame E, Medina Diez J. Primary closure of laparotomies with high risk of incisional hernia using prosthetic material: analysis of usefulness. *Hernia.* 2003;7(3):134-136.

51. El-Khadrawy OH, Moussa G, Mansour O, Hashish MS. Prophylactic prosthetic reinforcement of midline abdominal incisions in high-risk patients. *Hernia.* 2009;13(3):264-274.

52. Caro-Tarrago A, Olona Casas C, Jimenez Salido A, Duque Guilera E, Moreno Fernandez F, Vicente Guillen V. Prevention of incisional hernia in midline laparotomy with an onlay mesh: a randomized clinical trial. *World J Surg.* 2014;38(9):2223-2230.

53. Garcia-Urena MA, Lopez-Monchus J, et al. Randomized controlled trial of the use of a large-pore polypropylene mesh to prevent incisional hernia in colorectal surgery. *Ann Surg.* 2015;261(5):376-381.

54. Timmermans L, Eker HH, Steyerberg EW, et al. Short-term results of a randomized controlled trial comparing primary suture with primary glued mesh augmentation to prevent incisional hernia. *Ann Surg.* 2015;261(2):276-281.

55. Flum DR, Horvath K, Koepsell T. Have outcomes of incisional hernia repair improved with time? A population-based analysis. *Ann Surg.* 2003;237(1):129-135.

56. Burger JW, Luijendijk RW, Hop WC, Halm JA, Verdaasdonk EG, Jeekel J. Long-term follow-up of a randomized controlled trial of suture versus mesh repair of incisional hernia. *Ann Surg.* 2004;240(4):278-283.

57. Christoffersen MW, Helgstrand F, Rosenberg J, Kehlet H, Bisgaard T. Lower reoperation rate for recurrence after mesh versus sutured elective repair in small umbilical and epigastric hernias. A Nationwide Register Study. *World J Surg.* 2013;37(11):2548-2552.

58. Conze J, Klinge U, Schumpelick V. Incisional hernia. *Chirurg.* 2005;76(9):897-909.

59. Binnebosel M, Rosch R, Junge K, et al. Biomechanical analyses of overlap and mesh dislocation in an incisional hernia model in vitro. *Surgery.* 2007;142(3):365-371.

60. Lambrecht J. Overlap-coefficient for the relationship between mesh size and defect size in laparoscopic ventral hernia surgery. *Hernia.* 2011;15(4):473-474.

61. Cobb WS, Burns JM, Kercher KW, Matthews BD, Norton J, Todd Heniford B. Normal intraabdominal pressure in healthy adults. *J Surg Res.* 2005;129(2):231-235.

62. Quandell H, O'Dwyer PJ. Relationship between ventral hernia defect area and intra-abdominal pressure: dynamic in vivo measurement. *Surg Endosc.* 2016;30(4):1480-1484.

63. Holihan JL, Bondre I, Askenasy EP, et al. Ventral Hernia Outcomes Collaborative (VHOC) Writing Group. Sublay versus underlay in open ventral hernia repair. *J Surg Res.* 2016;202:26-32.

64. Zeichen MS, Lujan HJ, Mata WN, et al. Closure versus non-closure of hernia defect during laparoscopic ventral hernia repair with mesh. *Hernia.* 2013;17(5):589-596.

65. Nguyen DH, Nguyen MT, Askenasy EP, Kao LS, Liang MK. Primary fascial closure with laparoscopic ventral hernia repair: systematic review. *World J Surg.* 2014;38:3097-3104.

66. Wennergren JE, Askenasy EP, Greenberg JA, et al. Laparoscopic ventral hernia repair with primary fascial closure versus bridged repair: a risk-adjusted comparative study. *Surg Endosc.* 2015;30(8):3231-3238.

67. Clapp ML, Hicks SC, Awad SS, Liang MK. Trans-cutaneous closure of central defects (TCCD) in laparoscopic ventral hernia repairs (LVHR). *World J Surg.* 2013;37(1):42-51.

68. Booth JH, Garvey PB, Baumann DP, et al. Primary fascial closure with mesh reinforcement is superior to bridged mesh repair in abdominal wall reconstruction. *J Am Coll Surg.* 2013;217(6):999-1009.

69. Helgstrand F, Rosenberg J, Kehlet H, Jorgensen LN, Bisgaard T. Nationwide prospective study of outcomes after elective incisional hernia repair. *J Am Coll Surg.* 2013;2016(2):217-228.

70. Reynolds D, Davenport DL, Korosec RL, Roth JS. Financial implications of ventral hernia repair: a hospital cost analysis. *J Gastrointest Surg.* 2013;17(1):159-166.

71. Iannitti DA, Hope WW, Tsikitis V. Strength of tissue attachment to composite and ePTFE grafts after ventral hernia repair. *JSLS.* 2007;11(4):415-421.

72. Burger JW, Halm JA, Wijsmuller AR, ten Raa S, Jeekel J. Evaluation of new prosthetic meshes for ventral hernia repair. *Surg Endosc.* 2006;20(8):1320-1325.

73. Young RM, Gustafson R, Dinsmore RC. Sepramesh vs. Dualmesh for abdominal wall hernia repairs in a rabbit model. *Curr Surg.* 2004;61(1):77-79.

74. Levy S, Plymale MA, Miller MT, Davenport DL, Roth JS. Laparoscopic parastomal hernia repair: no different than a laparoscopic ventral hernia repair? *Surg Endosc.* 2016;30(4):1542-1546.

75. Choi JJ, Palaniappa NC, Dallas KB, Rudich TB, Colon MJ, Divino CM. Use of mesh during ventral hernia repair in clean-contaminated and contaminated cases: outcomes of 33,832 cases. *Ann Surg.* 2012;255(1):176-180.

76. Gray SH, Vick CC, Graham LA, Finan KR, Neumayer LA, Hawn MT. Risk of complications from enterotomy or unplanned bowel resection during elective hernia repair. *Arch Surg.* 2008;143(6):582-586.

77. Hawn MT, Gray SH, Snyder CW, Graham LA, Finan KR, Vick CC. Predictors of mesh explantation after incisional hernia repair. *Am J Surg.* 2011;202(1):28-33.

78. Carbonell AM, Criss CN, Cobb WS, Novitsky YW, Rosen MJ. Outcomes of synthetic mesh in contaminated ventral hernia repairs. *J Am Coll Surg.* 2013;217(6):991-998.

79. Cobb WS, Warren JA, Ewing JA, Burnikel A, Merchant M, Carbonell AM. Open retromuscular mesh repair of complex incisional hernia: predictors of wound events and recurrence. *J Am Coll Surg.* 2015;220(4):606-613.

80. Bachman S, Ramshaw B. Prosthetic material in ventral hernia repair: how do I choose? *Surg Clin North Am.* 2008;88(1):101-112.

81. Primus FE, Harris HW. A critical review of biologic mesh use in ventral hernia repairs under contaminated conditions. *Hernia.* 2013;17(1):21-30.

82. Blatnik J, Jin J, Rosen M. Abdominal hernia repair with bridging acellular dermal matric—an expensive hernia sac. *Am J Surg.* 2008;196(1):47-50.

83. Rosen MJ, Krpata DM, Ermlich B, Blatnik JA. A 5-year clinical experience with single-staged repairs of infected and contaminated abdominal wall defects utilizing biologic mesh. *Ann Surg.* 2013;257(6):991-996.

84. Rosen MJ, Denoto G, Itani KM, et al. Evaluation of surgical outcomes of retro-rectus versus intraperitoneal reinforcement with bio-prosthetic mesh in the repair of contaminated ventral hernias. *Hernia.* 2013;17(1):31-35.

85. Huerta S, Varshney A, Patel PM, Mayo HG, Livingston E. Biological mesh implants for abdominal hernia repair: US Food and Drug Administration approval process and systematic review of its efficacy. *JAMA Surg.* 2016;151(4):374-381.

86. Darahzereshki A, Goldfarb M, Zehetner J, et al. Biologic versus nonbiologic mesh in ventral hernia repair: a systematic review and meta-analysis. *World J Surg.* 2014;38(1):40-50.

87. Bondre IL, Holihan JL, Askenasy EP, et al. Suture, synthetic, or biologic in contaminated ventral hernia repair. *J Surg Res.* 2016;200(2):488-494.

88. Deeken CR, Matthews BD. Characterization of the mechanical strength, resorption properties, and histologic characteristics of a fully absorbable material (poly-4-hydroxybutyrate-PHASIX Mesh) in a porcine model of hernia repair. *ISRN Surg.* 2013;28:238067.

89. Open Complex Ventral Incisional Hernia Repair Using Biosynthetic Material for Midline Fascial Closure Reinforcement (COBRA). ClinicalTrials.gov NCT01325792. Accessed 2015.

90. Qaseem A, Humphrey LL, Chou R, Snow V, Shekelle P, Clinical Guidelines Committee of the American College of Physicians. Use of intensive insulin therapy for the management of glycemic control in hospitalized patients: a clinical practice guideline from the American College of Physicians. *Ann Intern Med.* 2011;154(4):260-267.

91. Kwon S, Thompson R, Dellinger P, Farrohki E, Flum D. Importance of perioperative glycemic control in general surgery: a report from the surgical care and outcomes assessment program. *Ann Surg.* 2013;257(1):8-14.

92. Buchleitner AM, Martinez-Alonso M, Hernandez M, Solà I, Mauricio D. Perioperative glycemic control for diabetic patients undergoing surgery. *Cochrane Database Syst Rev.* 2012;(9):CD007315.

93. Mehrabi Bahar M, Jabbari Nooghabi A, Jabbari Nooghabi M, Jangjoo A. The role of prophylactic cefazolin in the prevention of infection after various types of abdominal wall hernia repair with mesh. *Asian J Surg.* 2015;38(3):139-144.

94. Ríos A, Rodríguez JM, Munitiz V, Alcaraz P, Pérez Flores D, Parrilla P. Antibiotic prophylaxis in incisional hernia repair using a prosthesis. *Hernia.* 2001;5(3):148-152.

95. Ioannidis O, Paraskevas G, Varnalidis I, et al. Hernia mesh repair of anterior abdominal wall and antibiotic chemoprophylaxis: multiple doses of antibiotics failed to prevent or reduce wound infection. *Chirurgia.* 2013;108(6):835-839.

96. Gurusamy KS, Allen VB. Wound drains after incisional hernia repair. *Cochrane Database System Rev.* 2013;(12):CD005570.

97. Plymale MA, Harris JW, Roth JS, Smith N, Levy S, Scott Roth J. Abdominal wall reconstruction: the uncertainty of the impact of drain duration upon outcomes. *Am Surg.* 2016;82(3):207-211.

98. Kehlet H, Callesen T. Recommendations for convalescence after hernia surgery. A questionnaire study. *Ugeskr Laeger.* 1998;160(7):1008-1009.

99. Pommergaard HC, Burcharth J, Danielsen A, et al. No consensus on restrictions on physical activity to prevent incisional hernias after surgery. *Hernia.* 2013;18(4):495-500.

100. Bouvier A, Rat P, Drissi-Chbihi F, et al. Abdominal binders after laparotomy: review of the literature and French survey of policies. *Hernia.* 2014;18(4):501-506.

101. Rothman JP, Gunnarsson U, Bisgaard T. Abdominal binders may reduce pain and improve physical function after major abdominal surgery—a systematic review. *Dan Med J.* 2014;61(11):A4941.

102. Clay L, Gunnarsson U, Franklin KA, Strigard K. Effect of an elastic girdle on lung function, intra-abdominal pressure, and pain after midline laparotomy: a randomized controlled trial. *Int J Colorectal Dis.* 2014;29(6):715-721.

Congenital Diaphragmatic Hernia

Craig Albanese | Chad M. Thorson

Ladd and Gross reported the first successful series of surgical repair for congenital diaphragmatic hernia (CDH) in 1940, followed by successful neonatal repair in 1946.[1] Gross subsequently reported the largest series of the time in 1953. The reported survival was 87%, but there was significant survivor bias, as many patients with rapid demise from severe lung hypoplasia and pulmonary hypertension were not included. From that time until the 1980s, it was believed that correction of the diaphragmatic defect could completely resolve the respiratory problems and should be performed urgently in the neonatal period. Subsequent investigations have shown that although the diaphragmatic defect requires surgical repair, success depends more on the preoperative and postoperative management of the associated physiological derangements.

In the last few decades, there have been numerous advances in prenatal diagnosis, neonatal care (ventilatory management, surfactant, inhaled nitric oxide [iNO], high-frequency oscillatory ventilation [HFOV], extracorporeal membrane oxygenation [ECMO]), and anesthetic and surgical techniques. Despite this, the mortality remains as high as 20% to 30%. The CDH Study Group is an international consortium of centers that contribute data into a registry from which participating centers may use to answer questions and monitor outcomes. Since 1995, 112 centers have participated, collecting data on more than 8000 children and has generated 35 manuscripts.[2] These investigations, along with others, have advanced our knowledge and ability to treat this once uniformly fatal neonatal disease.

EMBRYOLOGY, ANATOMY, AND PHYSIOLOGY

DIAPHRAGM DEVELOPMENT

The diaphragm is a musculotendinous partition that contains four embryonic components: (1) pleuroperitoneal membranes, (2) septum transversum, (3) dorsal mesentery of the esophagus, and (4) muscular ingrowth from lateral body walls.[3] The diaphragmatic precursors begin to form during the 4th week of gestation. The peritoneal fold develops from the lateral mesenchymal tissue, while the septum transversum also forms from the inferior portion of the pericardial cavity. In addition, the septum transversum eventually creates the central tendinous area of the diaphragm that separates the abdominal and thoracic cavities. The pleuroperitoneal folds extend from the lateral body wall and fuse with the septum transverse and dorsal mesentery of the esophagus during the 6th week. By the 8th week, the pleuroperitoneal membrane fully forms, with the right side occurring first.[3,4] Failure of complete formation of the pleuroperitoneal membrane is thought to contribute to the development of a CDH.

LUNG DEVELOPMENT

Normal lung development progresses along five distinct stages.[5,6] As will be discussed later in the chapter, these important phases of lung development are affected by the presence of a diaphragmatic hernia.

1. **Embryonic Phase**: during the 3rd week, a diverticulum forms off the caudal end of the laryngotracheal groove. By the 4th week, the trachea and two primary lung buds form.
2. **Pseudoglandular Phase**: defined lobar structures are present by week 6. From week 7 to 16, airways differentiate into bronchioles and terminal bronchioles.
3. **Canalicular Phase**: during week 16 to 24, crude air sacs and pneumocytes develop.
4. **Saccular Phase**: until term, continued remodeling of alveolar airspaces occurs, along with production of surfactant.
5. **Alveolar Phase**: shortly after birth, alveoli begin to appear, with maturation and multiplication taking place until the age of 8.

MIDGUT DEVELOPMENT

During the 4th week of gestation, the midgut grows rapidly; and due to the small capacity of the abdomen, it extends into the umbilical cord. At 10 weeks, the abdomen is large enough to accommodate the elongating loops of bowel, and they return while undergoing a counterclockwise rotation around the base of the mesentery.[3,4] If closure of the pleuroperitoneal canal has not occurred by the time the midgut returns to the abdomen, the viscera will be misplaced into the ipsilateral thoracic cavity. With this abnormal positioning, the midgut cannot undergo normal fixation, resulting in either malrotation or nonrotation.

FETAL CIRCULATION

The fetus preferentially shunts oxygenated blood from the placenta through the foramen ovale and ductus arteriosus (right-to-left shunt). In utero, the pulmonary vascular resistance remains elevated, resulting in very low cardiac output reaching the lungs. After birth, institution of breathing causes pulmonary vascular resistance to decrease, thus increasing pulmonary blood flow. As the systemic vascular resistance rises, the foramen closes, and increased arterial oxygen tension closes the ductus.[3,7]

Persistent fetal circulation occurs if the normal process is interrupted, which includes diaphragmatic hernia. Elevated pulmonary vascular resistance causes increased pulmonary artery pressures and decreased pulmonary blood flow. A right-to-left shunt may persist when blood crosses the foramen ovale (patent foramen ovale [PFO]) or ductus arteriosus (patent ductus arteriosus [PDA]).

This shunting results in delivery of unsaturated blood to the systemic circulation.

DIAPHRAGMATIC HERNIA

The presence of a diaphragmatic hernia results in abdominal contents (small bowel, colon, spleen, stomach, liver, and/or kidney) becoming relocated into the thoracic cavity. This space-occupying lesion results in detrimental effects on lung development. These include pulmonary hypoplasia from restricted lung growth and decreased alveolar development. Pulmonary hypoplasia is not strictly related to the herniated viscera, as muscularization around peripheral arterioles is also thought to contribute to the severe pulmonary hypertension.[8] Persistent fetal circulation ensues, leading to right-to-left shunting and progressive hypoxia after birth.

CLASSIFICATION

GENERAL

The overall incidence of CDH is 1:2000 to 1:5000 live births.[9,10] Left-sided defects are more common (80% to 85%), followed by right (15%) or bilateral (<5%) defects. In general, posterolateral left-sided hernias are more likely to be symptomatic and identified in the neonatal period, whereas anterior defects may go undetected.

BOCHDALEK (POSTEROLATERAL) HERNIA

The classic description of the congenital defect was by Bochdalek, for whom the defect was named. Typically, a 2- to 4-cm posterolateral diaphragmatic defect is present, through which the abdominal contents herniate into the thoracic cavity. The size of the defect is variable and may range from the classic small defect to complete diaphragmatic agenesis (Fig. 51.1). Most commonly, small bowel, spleen, stomach, liver, and/or colon may be in the chest. A nonmuscularized membrane forms a hernia sac in 10% to 20%.[11]

Right-sided posterolateral defects are rare. Patients with right-sided Bochdalek (non-Morgagni) type tend to have severely poor prognosis due to severe pulmonary hypotension/pulmonary hypoplasia. The large right lobe of the liver can occupy most of the hemithorax, and associated anomalous hepatic venous drainage is common. There is a high incidence of preterm complications, associated comorbidities, and frequent need for ECMO.[12] Bilateral congenital defects are rare (<5%) and are nearly always fatal due to arrest of bilateral lung development.[13]

MORGAGNI (ANTERIOR) HERNIA

Morgagni hernias account for less than 2% of diaphragmatic defects. They are typically located anteromedially on either side at the junction of the septum transversum and the anterior thoracic wall. They are most often asymptomatic, as the amount of pulmonary compression is minimal compared to posterolateral defects. In addition, patients typically have transverse colon herniation into the anterior mediastinum covered by a peritoneal sac. Most are discovered incidentally as an anterior chest mass or suspected pneumonia in an older child. Rarely,

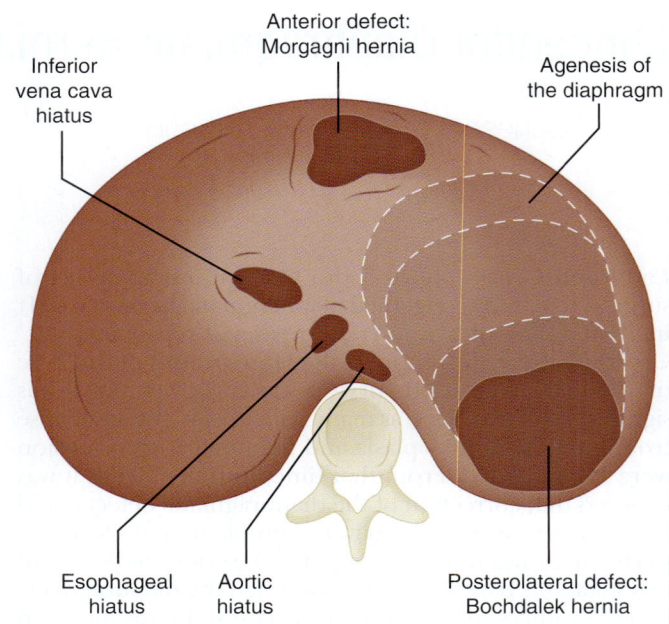

FIGURE 51.1 Location of diaphragmatic defect.

they may present with incarceration or strangulation.[14] Most often, there is low associated morbidity if they are repaired promptly. Surgical repair is most often performed via a transabdominal (open vs. laparoscopic) approach.

A rare form of anterior diaphragmatic hernia is included in the pentalogy of Cantrell.[15] The syndrome involves a ventral midline developmental defect resulting in anterior diaphragmatic hernia, epigastric omphalocele, sternal cleft, intracardiac defect (ventricular septal defect most commonly), and pericardial defect (usually results in ectopia cordis). Pentalogy is associated with an extremely high mortality.

ASSOCIATED ANOMALIES

The overall incidence of associated malformations is 20% to 60% and tend to be most often seen in those who present symptomatically within the first 6 hours of life.[16,17] Overall, cardiac anomalies are most common, affecting between 25% and 40%. They most commonly involve the cardiac outflow tract, including ventricular septal defects, tetralogy of Fallot, transposition, and coarctation.[18] Limb anomalies are seen in 30% and include limb shortening and costovertebral defects.[19] The most common airway anomalies are congenital tracheal stenosis and bronchial stenosis on the ipsilateral side.[20] Other reported defects are esophageal atresia, omphalocele, and cleft palate.[16]

Approximately 10% will have chromosomal anomalies such as trisomy (21, 18, 13) or other syndromes (Frey, Beckwith-Wiedemann, and Fryns). When CDH is associated with an abnormal karyotype, the outcome is poor.[21] Nearly all stillborn infants with CDH have associated lethal anomalies, with neural tube defects and cardiac anomalies being most common.

PRENATAL DIAGNOSIS AND PROGNOSTIC INDICATORS

DIAGNOSIS

Prenatal diagnosis was previously rare and associated with the highest mortality (~80%), as only the largest defects were identified on prenatal ultrasound.[22,23] With advances in prenatal imaging technology, prenatal detection rates are now greater than 60% and there does not appear to be an increased mortality simply with early detection.[24,25] Ultrasound most often demonstrates presence of the stomach in the fetal thorax at the same level as the heart. It may also demonstrate associated polyhydramnios, which occurs in 75% due to gastrointestinal obstruction.[22] Ultrasound allows for evaluation of the presence of liver herniation, mediastinal shift, gastric distention, and size of the ipsilateral lung. The diagnosis may not be detected with prenatal ultrasound, as intermittent herniation of viscera into the thoracic cavity may occur.[22] In addition, CDH may be confused with congenital cystic lung malformations.

When CDH is identified prenatally, it should prompt a search for associated anomalies, especially those affecting the cardiac and nervous systems. Fetal karyotyping should be offered with either chorionic villi sampling or amniocentesis, whichever is appropriate for gestational age at diagnosis. The parents should be encouraged to deliver in an appropriate tertiary care center with capabilities of advance respiratory care strategies and urgent pediatric surgical availability.

PRENATAL ULTRASOUND

The most often used prognostic indicator with prenatally diagnosed CDH is the lung-to-head ratio (LHR).[26] Ultrasound is used to measure the fetal lung area relative to the head circumference, therefore providing an indirect assessment of the contralateral lung volume and estimating the likelihood of pulmonary hypoplasia. In general, an LHR less than 1.0 is associated with low survival, while a ratio of more than 1.4 have improved outcomes.[23,26] Original cutoffs for LHR were between gestational age 24 to 26 weeks. Due to a more rapid growth of fetal lung compared to the head circumference that occurs during gestation, the observed-to-expected (O/E) LHR was introduced, as it is not dependent on gestational age at measurement. O/E LHR seems to be a useful predictor of subsequent survival, with severe left CDH characterized by a ratio of less than 25%.[27] Overall, there is no consensus as to what value of LHR should serve as a determinant of prognosis or when it should be calculated. Therefore, LHR should be used as a piece of information to estimate contralateral lung size, but it should not be used as a sole predictor of postnatal outcome or treatment.[23,26-28]

LIVER POSITION

Traditionally, the position of the liver has provided an estimate of CDH severity. Presence of liver in the chest ("liver-up") has not been consistently shown to predict mortality, although most studies suggest a decreased survival.[29,30] It is associated with worse prognosis, mainly due to the higher likelihood of requiring ECMO and need for patch repair of a larger defect.[29]

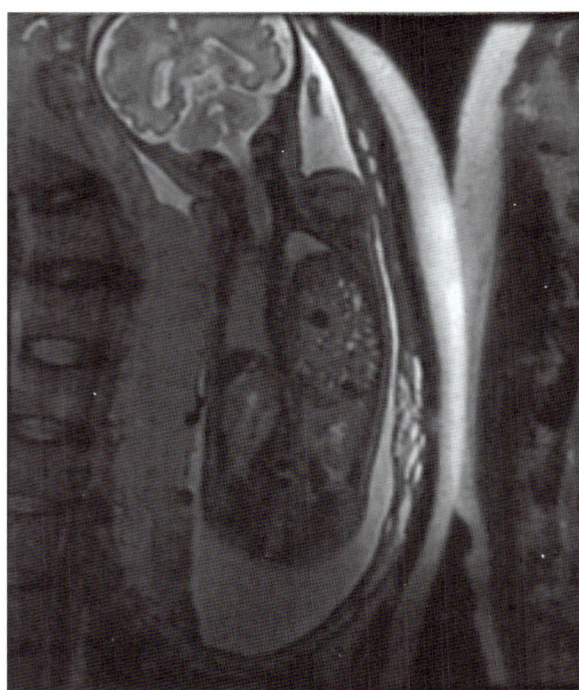

FIGURE 51.2 Fetal magnetic resonance imaging (coronal view) demonstrates presence of bowel in the left chest consistent with congenital diaphragmatic hernia.

FETAL MAGNETIC RESONANCE IMAGING

More recently, magnetic resonance imaging (MRI) has been used to characterize complex fetal anomalies (Fig. 51.2). Ultrafast MRI uses shorter acquisition times to eliminate issues with fetal movement. An additional benefit is reduced intraobserver variability of fetal lung volume measurements commonly seen with ultrasound techniques. It has proven superior to "liver-up" versus "liver-down," as it allows the exact quantification of the amount of liver herniated into the chest.[31] It appears from systematic reviews that measurement of fetal lung volumes, liver position, and side of defect identified with MRI correlates with neonatal survival.[32]

POSTNATAL DIAGNOSIS

The clinical presentation of the newborn with CDH depends on the degree of pulmonary hypoplasia and pulmonary hypertension. The most severely affected infants have respiratory distress immediately after birth, with associated hypoxemia, hypercarbia, and respiratory acidosis. Shunting of oxygenated blood may occur (persistent fetal circulation), which increases in proportion to the pulmonary hypertension. This is estimated by comparing preductal (right arm) and postductal (left arm or lower extremities) oxygen saturations, which will demonstrate decreased postductal readings.

The physical exam of a neonate with CDH classically demonstrates a scaphoid abdomen with decreased breath sounds on the ipsilateral chest. The chest may become asymmetrically distended as swallowed air distends the

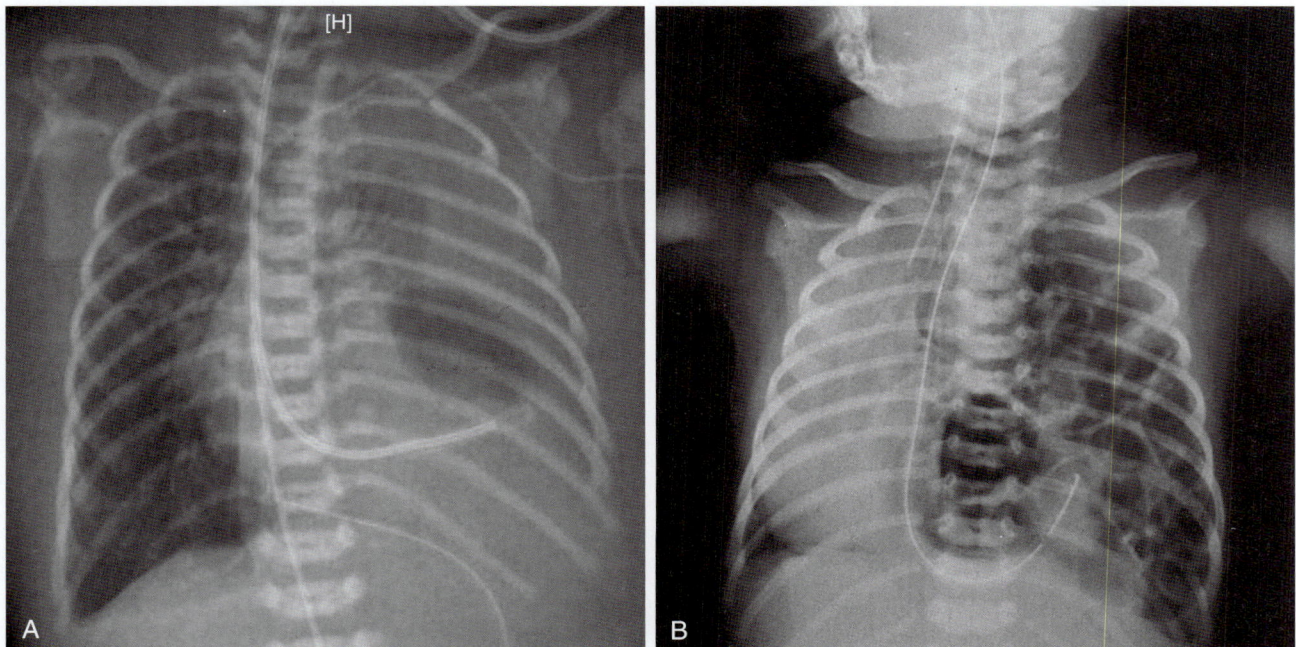

FIGURE 51.3 Chest radiograph demonstrating left diaphragmatic hernia immediately postnatally. Although the chest is opacified early (A), continued introduction of air results in eventual bowel distention (B).

intrathoracic viscera. Mediastinal compression may shift the trachea to the contralateral side or produce tension physiology with obstructed venous return. Pallor, cyanosis, sternal retractions, and grunting all signify increased work of breathing and impending deterioration.

A chest radiograph should be done soon after birth, which typically demonstrates loops of bowel located in the chest. The nasogastric tube location is useful for identifying the stomach position within the chest or abdomen. Lower chest opacification may be seen with initial radiographs, as the bowel has not yet accumulated with air (Fig. 51.3).

In addition to the chest x-ray, additional imaging studies include a transthoracic echocardiogram and head ultrasound. The echocardiogram is performed to rule out associated anomalies and assess ventricular function/pulmonary hypotension. This is best performed on day of life 2 to not overestimate the degree of pulmonary hypertension. Complex imaging such as a chest ultrasound, computerized tomography (CT), MRI, or upper gastrointestinal contrast study are not necessary to confirm presence of a diaphragmatic hernia. Right-sided defects may warrant MRI to rule out hepatopulmonary fusion and to assess the vascular anatomy of the mediastinum and liver.[33]

TREATMENT AND OUTCOMES

MEDICAL OPTIMIZATION

CDH was previously felt to constitute a surgical emergency, and infants typically underwent surgery in the first few hours of life. It was later understood that the majority of patients showed a deterioration in respiratory mechanics after a brief postoperative "honeymoon period" of adequate

gas exchange. Reduction of hernia contents into the abdomen rarely results in reexpansion of the lungs, as they are hypoplastic rather than atelectatic.[34] Due to these findings, the focus has now shifted to delayed repair after medical stabilization. CDH is now considered a physiologic emergency instead of a surgical one.

The resuscitation of a neonate with CDH starts with prompt endotracheal intubation, as ventilation by mask or Ambu bag may cause significant bowel distention and worsening ventilation.

A nasogastric tube should be inserted to allow gastric and intestinal decompression. Typically, umbilical venous and arterial catheters are placed along with oxygen saturation probes in the pre- and postductal locations to allow for shunt estimation. Excessive stimuli can easily exacerbate pulmonary pressures and lead to increased shunt flow/desaturations. For this reason, infants are kept sedated in beds/incubators with radiant warmers and external stimulation is limited. Muscle paralysis should only be used in extreme circumstances due to ventilatory consequences and added morbidity.

With advances in postnatal resuscitation and care, the survival rate has improved significantly. One of the most beneficial changes seems to be the idea of less aggressive ventilatory strategies. Previously, aggressive hyperventilation and induced alkalosis ($PaCO_2$ as low as 20 mm Hg) were used with the thought that this would minimize pulmonary hypertension and the associated shunting. To achieve these extremely low $PaCO_2$ levels, very high peak inspiratory pressures were used, which are potentially damaging to the lungs and may ultimately worsen chronic lung disease. In 1985, Wung and colleagues proposed permissive hypercapnia as a way to limit barotrauma and still achieve sufficient tissue oxygenation.[35] This concept has been widely applied, and hypercapnia ($PaCO_2$ 60 to 65 mm Hg) is tolerated (permissive hypercapnia) as long as the pH is greater than 7.2.[36,37]

VENTILATORY ADJUNCTS

Failure of conventional ventilation is suggested by worsening tachypnea (evidenced by retractions, paradoxical chest movement), inadequate oxygenation (preductal oxygen saturation <85%), severe hypercarbia ($PaCO_2$ >65 mm Hg), or worsening pulmonary hypertension (widened gap between pre- and postductal oxygen saturations). If customary measures cannot achieve adequate oxygenation and ventilation, then nonconventional ventilatory modes may be used. HFOV is one of the more popular modes due to its gentle ventilation properties and limitation of barotrauma.[38,39]

Persistent pulmonary hypertension is the major factor increasing pulmonary resistance and causing right-to-left shunting with hypoxemia. In theory, vasodilator therapy should lead to improvement, but it has shown to be unsuccessful due to inadequate pulmonary vasodilation and increased shunting from systemic hypotension. Nitric oxide, also known as endothelium-derived relaxing factor, directly stimulates cyclic GMP in vascular smooth muscle, causing relaxation. iNO diffuses across the alveoli to the vascular smooth muscle, allowing for selective pulmonary vasodilation. iNO has been shown to induce improvement in oxygenation when used at low doses (10 to 20 parts per million) and is now used as an adjunct to ventilatory strategies.[40] Unfortunately, clinical studies have been mixed; however, improved survival or decreased need for ECMO has been consistently demonstrated.[41,42]

EXTRACORPOREAL OXYGENATION

Despite the previous measures, overwhelming respiratory failure requiring ECMO is seen in 10% to 20% of infants with CDH. ECMO was first successfully used in infants in 1976,[43] and improved survival has been demonstrated in infants treated with extracorporeal oxygenation.[44] The goal of therapy is to meet tissue oxygen demands while providing a period of rest for the heart/lung during, which the persistent fetal circulation can resolve.

The most common parameter used to determine the need for ECMO is the oxygenation index (OI), derived from the formula: $OI = (FiO_2 \times Mean\ Airway\ Pressure) / PaO_2$. The indication for instituting ECMO is variable, but it is typically when OI is greater than 25 to 40.[44] Other indications are consistent preductal oxygen saturations less than 85%, persistent metabolic acidosis, or hypotension refractory to pressors. ECMO is contraindicated in prematurity (gestational age <34 weeks), head ultrasound demonstrating severe intraventricular hemorrhage, irreversible cardiac disease, or with another lethal congenital anomaly.[45]

ECMO can be accomplished via either a venoarterial (VA) or venovenous (VV) technique with cannulas placed in the carotid artery (VA) and internal jugular vein (VA/VV). Traditionally, VA bypass has been used due to the underlying pulmonary hypertension. The efficacy and survival with VV bypass has been found to be comparable to VA, with lower short-term neurologic sequelae due to avoidance of carotid ligation.[46,47] ECMO

requires systemic heparin anticoagulation to prevent thrombosis of the extracorporeal circuit and oxygenator. Hemorrhagic complications may be seen in up to 60% and include bleeding at the cannulation site, surgical site, head, chest, and gastrointestinal tract.[48] Due to hemorrhagic complications, surgical repair of CDH is typically delayed until ECMO decannulation.

TIMING OF REPAIR

Current management involves early stabilization and delayed repair, although the exact timing of surgery is not known.[49,50] The period of preoperative stabilization varies between institutions, but most allow ventilatory weaning and serial cardiac echocardiograms to evaluate improvement in pulmonary hypertension. For the stable infant without pulmonary hypertension, repair can be safely done after a 48-hour period of stabilization and adjustment to postnatal life.

Repair on ECMO poses a significant challenge due to systemic heparinization and difficulty in transportation to the operative suite. Outcomes appear to be improved for those who undergo surgical repair following ECMO, with significantly increased survival, lower rates of surgical bleeding, and decreased total duration of ECMO therapy compared to those repaired on pump.[51]

SUMMARY

In summary, there are a few major principles of initial preoperative CDH management.[35-48,52]
1. Minimizing the onset and impact of pulmonary hypertension.
2. Gentle ventilation with permissive hypercapnia minimizes iatrogenic injury. Unconventional modes of ventilation (HFOV, iNO, ECMO) may be used to achieve adequate cardiorespiratory support.
3. Imaging studies should be done to rule out associated anomalies.
4. Surgical repair should be ideally delayed until the patient is hemodynamically stable for at least 24 hours.

OPEN SURGICAL APPROACH

The traditional approach is through a subcostal incision on the side of the defect. Once the abdomen is entered, the bowel is reduced from the chest with gentle downward traction. Typically, the spleen and liver, if present, are the last organs to be reduced. Great care should be exercised during mobilization, as the spleen and liver may develop subcapsular hematomas and life-threatening hemorrhage with traumatic reduction. If a hernia sac is present, it should be excised to minimize the risk of recurrence. Although the anterior rim of diaphragm is usually prominent, the posterior rim is typically diminished and obscured in the retroperitoneal tissue. The posterior diaphragmatic tissue must then be mobilized from the retroperitoneum, revealing the size of the diaphragmatic defect. If adequate, a primary repair with interrupted nonabsorbable suture material is preferred (Fig. 51.4).

If the size of the defect precludes primary closure, use of prosthetic mesh is indicated (Fig. 51.5). The most commonly used mesh is Gore-Tex, although more recent biologic and absorbable mesh have also been used with no difference in recurrence or postoperative complications.[53]

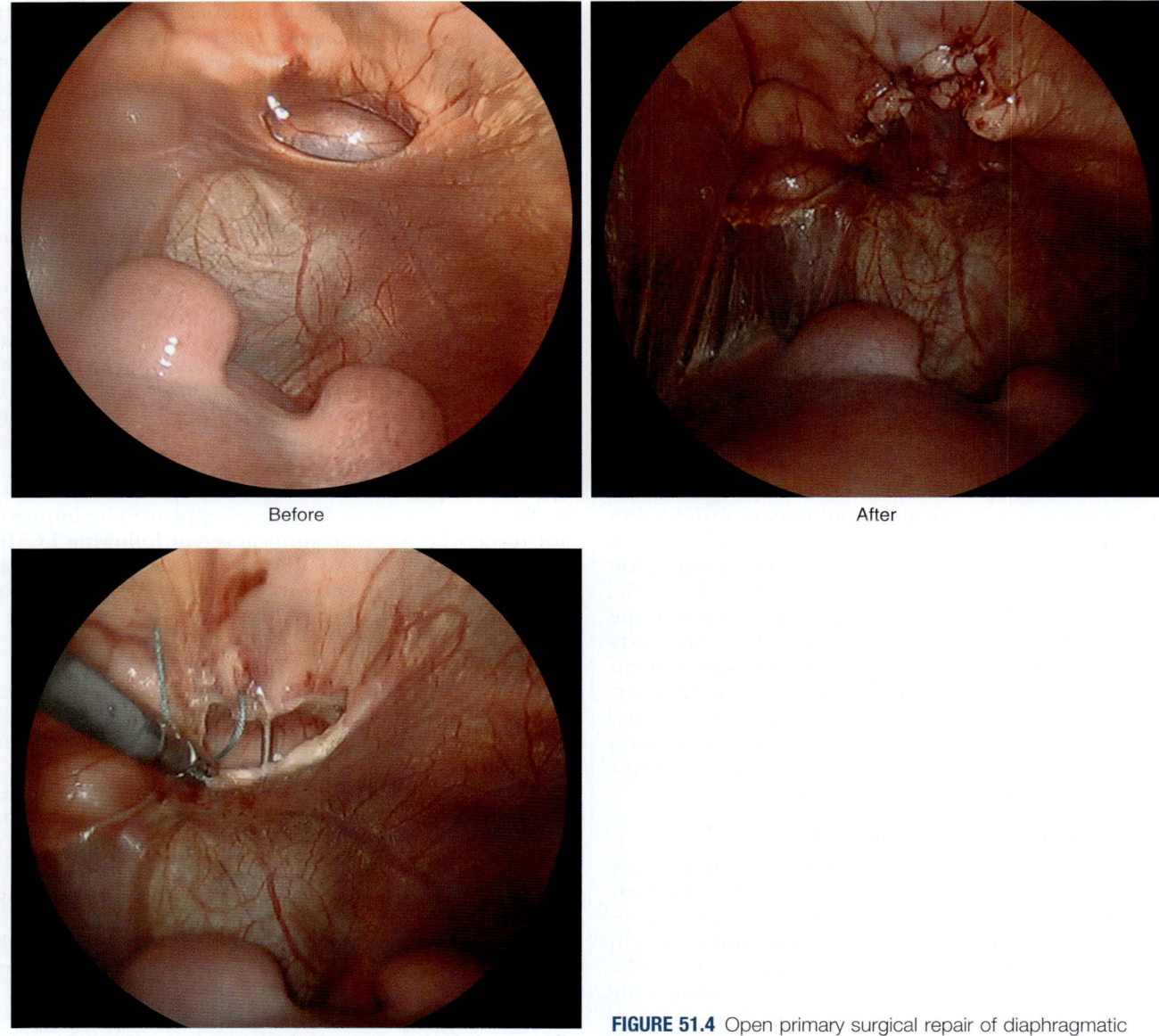

Before

After

During

FIGURE 51.4 Open primary surgical repair of diaphragmatic hernia.

Overall, use of prosthetic mesh is associated with a higher risk of recurrence, especially with a large initial defect or complete diaphragmatic agenesis.[54] With extremely large defects and loss of abdominal wall domain, return of viscera into the abdomen may result in inappropriately high intraabdominal pressures. A Silastic sheet can be used between fascial edges as a temporizing measure, with slow closure over the ensuing days-weeks. Eventual abdominal closure leads to a ventral hernia that can be dealt with outside the neonatal period. Additional techniques for repair of defects include internal oblique rotation flap or split abdominal wall muscle flap.[55]

THORACOSCOPIC APPROACH

Minimally invasive surgical techniques for repair of CDH are increasingly being used. The first successful thoracoscopic repair in an infant was reported in 1995.[56] Initial opposition for thoracoscopic repair was due to the concern that high end-tidal CO_2 requiring increasingly high inspiratory pressures would worsen pulmonary hypertension.[57] Potential advantages are improved cosmesis, improved surgical field visualization, and avoidance of thoracotomy-associated musculoskeletal deformities.

The operation is most often performed with a standard endotracheal tube. Due to the associated pulmonary hypoplasia, there is usually adequate room after the bowel is reduced into the abdomen. Contralateral mainstem intubation may also be used, if tolerated. The infant is then positioned transversely at the end of the bed in lateral decubitus positioning (Fig. 51.6). The Veress needle is inserted in the 5th intercostal space at the lower edge of the scapula (mid-posterior axillary line), and low pressure

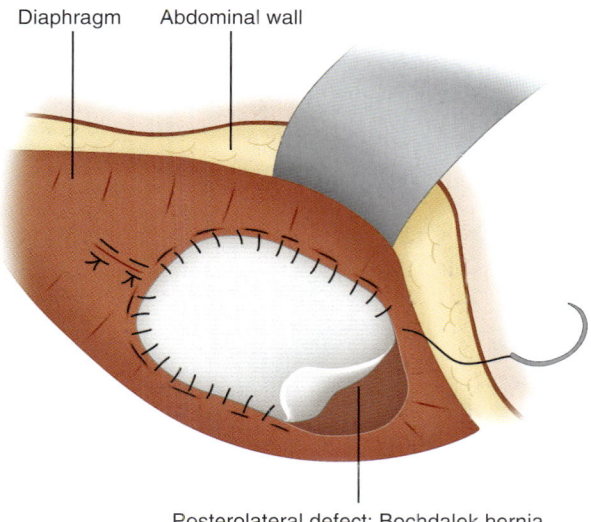

Diaphragm   Abdominal wall

Posterolateral defect: Bochdalek hernia
Repair with mesh

FIGURE 51.5 Open surgical repair with patch closure in large defects nonamenable to primary repair.

CO_2 insufflation (3 to 5 mm Hg) is used. Typically, three ports are used and include a 5-mm port in the site of the Veress insertion (4-mm camera), 3-mm port in the left anterolateral chest wall (bowel grasper), and 5/3-mm convertible port in the right posterolateral chest wall (bowel grasper, needle driver). The viscera are gently reduced with blunt graspers into the abdominal cavity. The posterolateral edge of the diaphragm is unfurled from the retroperitoneal tissue revealing the extent of the hernia, and needles can be introduced through the 3- to 5-mm port or through the chest wall. The defect is then closed with interrupted nonabsorbable sutures (2-0 Ethibond) beginning superior-medially and ending inferior-laterally (Fig. 51.7). Sutures are placed approximately 1 cm apart, and knots may be tied either intra- or extracorporeally. Some surgeons claim added benefit to "roughing up" the edge of the smooth diaphragmatic membrane using cautery.[58] The most difficult technical portion involves the lateral corner, where sutures must be placed around the rib and tied extracorporeally in a subcutaneous pocket.

Initial reports in 2003 suggested that although appropriate for Morgagni defects or those diagnosed outside the neonatal period, the minimally invasive surgery (MIS) approach for a newborn could not be recommended

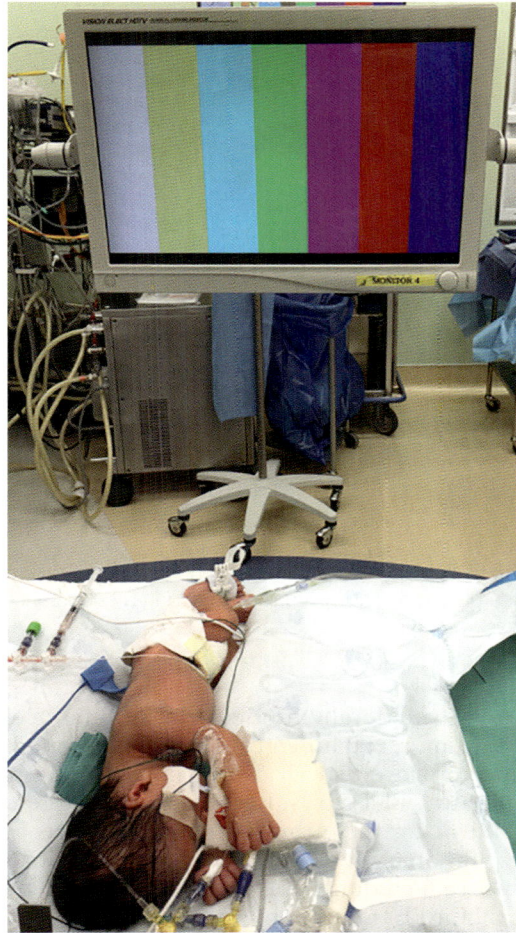

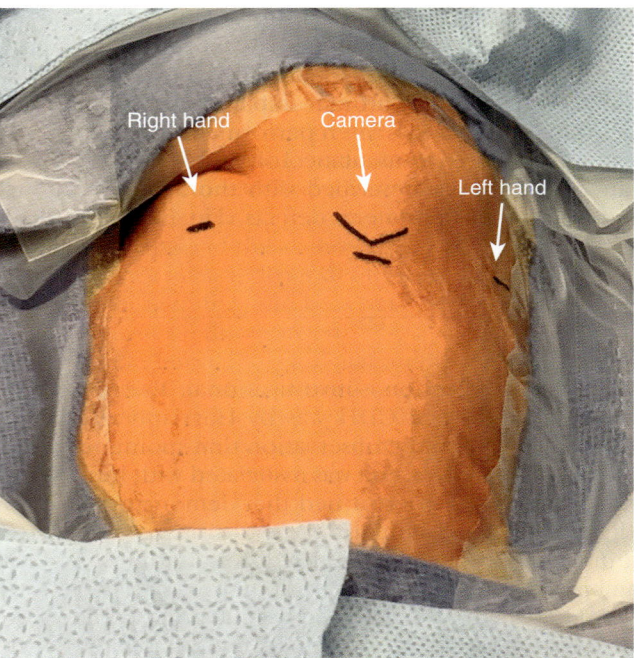

Right hand   Camera   Left hand

FIGURE 51.6 Operative positioning for thoracoscopic repair includes placing the patient transversely on the operative table with the surgeon standing at the neonate's head and monitors at the foot of the bed.

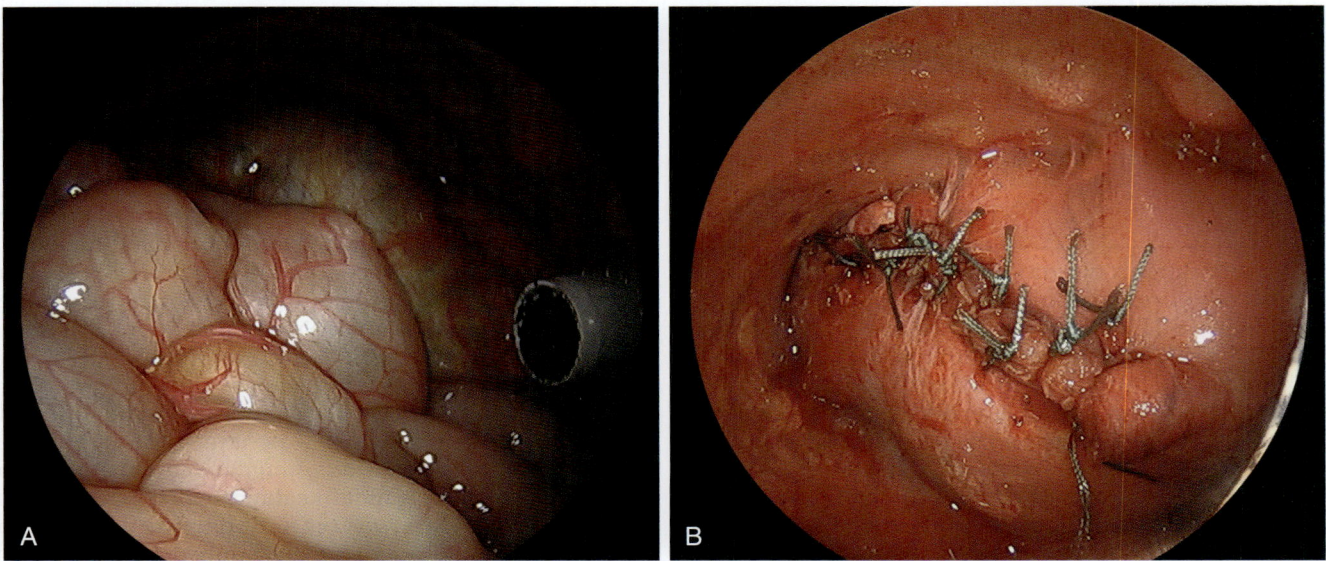

FIGURE 51.7 Thoracoscopic view of the chest before reduction (A) and with interrupted nonabsorbable sutures closing the diaphragmatic defect (B).

due to the high failure rate and frequent rise in PCO_2 levels.[59] Other reports also corroborated a high recurrence rate between 20% and 40%,[60,61] and more recent literature includes recurrence rates of 2% to 8%.[62,63] A recent meta-analysis including all nine published studies to date (507 patients) supports thoracoscopic repair due to lower postoperative morbidity/mortality.[64] From their data, it also appears that the majority of recurrences occur in those requiring patch repair for large defects.

MORGAGNI

Repair is recommended in children, but asymptomatic hernias in adults are often observed. Nearly all have a hernia sac, which can often only be partially removed due to dense adhesions to the pericardium. Laparoscopic repair with intracorporeal suturing is often performed, although sutures may also be placed transcutaneously and tied within a subcutaneous tunnel as described with thoracoscopic repair of congenital posterolateral defects (Fig. 51.8).

FUTURE DIRECTIONS

FETAL THERAPY

At this time, fetal intervention is investigational. The first successful repair of a fetal CDH was by Harrison and colleagues in 1990.[65] With the observation that spontaneously occurring laryngeal atresia was associated with lung hypertrophy, studies were performed that demonstrated tracheal ligation in fetal animals resulted in larger and more mature lungs at birth.[66] Based on these findings, a technique known as plug the lung until it grows (PLUG) was developed,[67] which ultimately led to fetal endoscopic tracheal occlusion (FETO).[68] The technique has been limited to extremely high-risk fetuses (LHR <1, signifying severe pulmonary hypoplasia), as those with less severe physiology will likely do well with conventional therapy.

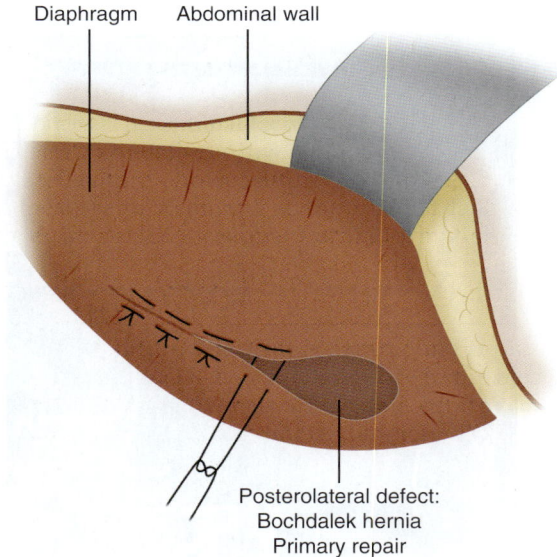

Diaphragm   Abdominal wall

Posterolateral defect:
Bochdalek hernia
Primary repair

FIGURE 51.8 Morgagni hernia repaired laparoscopically with sutures placed extracorporeally and tied in a subcutaneous tunnel.

An early, federally funded trial of fetal occlusion to promote antenatal lung growth was abandoned, as there was no improved survival over conventional postnatal treatment.[69] FETO resulted in lung enlargement, but this did not reverse the pathologic process associated with pulmonary hypoplasia. A recent systematic review from 2016 including five studies and 211 patients favored survival for FETO in those with isolated CDH and severe pulmonary hypoplasia.[70] Currently, an international randomized trial is ongoing in Europe, Australia, and Canada.[71]

REFERENCES

1. Gross RE. Congenital hernia of the diaphragm. *Am J Dis Child.* 1946;71:579-592.
2. Harting MT, Lally KP. The congenital diaphragmatic hernia study group registry update. *Semin Fetal Neonatal Med.* 2014;19(6):370-375.
3. Moore KL, Persaud TVN, Torchia MG, eds. *The Developing Human: Clinically Oriented Embryology.* 10th ed. Philadelphia: Saunders; 2016.
4. Moore KL, Persaud TVN, Torchia MG, eds. *Before We Are Born: Essentials of Embryology and Birth Defects.* 9th ed. Philadelphia: Saunders; 2016.
5. Davies G, Reid L. Growth of the alveoli and pulmonary arteries in childhood. *Thorax.* 1970;25(6):669-681.
6. Rottier R, Tibboel D. Fetal lung and diaphragm development in congenital diaphragmatic hernia. *Semin Perinatol.* 2005;29(2):86-93.
7. Rennie J. *Rennie & Roberton's Textbook of Neonatology.* 5th ed. Elsevier; 2012.
8. Yamataka T, Puri P. Pulmonary artery structural changes in pulmonary hypertension complicating congenital diaphragmatic hernia. *J Pediatr Surg.* 1997;32(3):387-390.
9. Langham MR Jr, Kays DW, Ledbetter DJ, Frentzen B, Sanford LL, Richards DS. Congenital diaphragmatic hernia. Epidemiology and outcome. *Clin Perinatol.* 1996;23(4):671-688.
10. Dott MM, Wong LY, Rasmussen SA. Population-based study of congenital diaphragmatic hernia: risk factors and survival in Metropolitan Atlanta, 1968-1999. *Birth Defects Res A Clin Mol Teratol.* 2003;67(4):261-267.
11. Zamora IJ, Cass DL, Lee TC, et al. The presence of a hernia sac in congenital diaphragmatic hernia is associated with better fetal lung growth and outcomes. *J Pediatr Surg.* 2013;48(6):1165-1171.
12. Hedrick HL, Crombleholme TM, Flake AW, et al. Right congenital diaphragmatic hernia: Prenatal assessment and outcome. *J Pediatr Surg.* 2004;39(3):319-323, discussion 319–323.
13. Neville HL, Jaksic T, Wilson JM. Bilateral congenital diaphragmatic hernia. *J Pediatr Surg.* 2003;38(3):522-524.
14. Kimmelstiel FM, Holgersen LO, Hilfer C. Retrosternal (Morgagni) hernia with small bowel obstruction secondary to a Richter's incarceration. *J Pediatr Surg.* 1987;22(11):998-1000.
15. Cantrell JR, Haller JA, Ravitch MM. A syndrome of congenital defects involving the abdominal wall, sternum, diaphragm, pericardium, and heart. *Surg Gynecol Obstet.* 1958;107(5):602-614.
16. Fauza DO, Wilson JM. Congenital diaphragmatic hernia and associated anomalies: their incidence, identification, and impact on prognosis. *J Pediatr Surg.* 1994;29(8):1113-1117.
17. Losty PD, Vanamo K, Rintala RJ, Donahoe PK, Schnitzer JJ, Lloyd DA. Congenital diaphragmatic hernia—does the side of the defect influence the incidence of associated malformations? *J Pediatr Surg.* 1998;33(3):507-510.
18. Cohen MS, Rychik J, Bush DM, et al. Influence of congenital heart disease on survival in children with congenital diaphragmatic hernia. *J Pediatr.* 2002;141(1):25-30.
19. Laudy JA, Van Gucht M, Van Dooren MF, Wladimiroff JW, Tibboel D. Congenital diaphragmatic hernia: an evaluation of the prognostic value of the lung-to-head ratio and other prenatal parameters. *Prenat Diagn.* 2003;23(8):634-639.
20. Nose K, Kamata S, Sawai T, et al. Airway anomalies in patients with congenital diaphragmatic hernia. *J Pediatr Surg.* 2000;35(11):1562-1565.
21. Benjamin DR, Juul S, Siebert JR. Congenital posterolateral diaphragmatic hernia: associated malformations. *J Pediatr Surg.* 1988;23(10):899-903.
22. Adzick NS, Harrison MR, Glick PL, Nakayama DK, Manning FA, deLorimier AA. Diaphragmatic hernia in the fetus: prenatal diagnosis and outcome in 94 cases. *J Pediatr Surg.* 1985;20(4):357-361.
23. Lipshutz GS, Albanese CT, Feldstein VA, et al. Prospective analysis of lung-to-head ratio predicts survival for patients with prenatally diagnosed congenital diaphragmatic hernia. *J Pediatr Surg.* 1997;32(11):1634-1636.
24. Wilson JM, Fauza DO, Lund DP, Benacerraf BR, Hendren WH. Antenatal diagnosis of isolated congenital diaphragmatic hernia is not an indicator of outcome. *J Pediatr Surg.* 1994;29(6):815-819.
25. Benachi A, Cordier AG, Cannie M, Jani J. Advances in prenatal diagnosis of congenital diaphragmatic hernia. *Semin Fetal Neonatal Med.* 2014;19(6):331-337.
26. Metkus AP, Filly RA, Stringer MD, Harrison MR, Adzick NS. Sonographic predictors of survival in fetal diaphragmatic hernia. *J Pediatr Surg.* 1996;31(1):148-151, discussion 151–152.
27. Jani J, Nicolaides KH, Keller RL, et al. Observed to expected lung area to head circumference ratio in the prediction of survival in fetuses with isolated diaphragmatic hernia. *Ultrasound Obstet Gynecol.* 2007;30(1):67-71.
28. Hedrick HL, Danzer E, Merchant A, et al. Liver position and lung-to-head ratio for prediction of extracorporeal membrane oxygenation and survival in isolated left congenital diaphragmatic hernia. *Am J Obstet Gynecol.* 2007;197(4):422 e1-422 e424.
29. Albanese CT, Lopoo J, Goldstein RB, et al. Fetal liver position and perinatal outcome for congenital diaphragmatic hernia. *Prenat Diagn.* 1998;18(11):1138-1142.
30. Mullassery D, Ba'ath ME, Jesudason EC, Losty PD. Value of liver herniation in prediction of outcome in fetal congenital diaphragmatic hernia: a systematic review and meta-analysis. *Ultrasound Obstet Gynecol.* 2010;35(5):609-614.
31. Lazar DA, Ruano R, Cass DL, et al. Defining "liver-up": does the volume of liver herniation predict outcome for fetuses with isolated left-sided congenital diaphragmatic hernia? *J Pediatr Surg.* 2012;47(6):1058-1062.
32. Mayer S, Klaritsch P, Petersen S, et al. The correlation between lung volume and liver herniation measurements by fetal MRI in isolated congenital diaphragmatic hernia: a systematic review and meta-analysis of observational studies. *Prenat Diagn.* 2011;31(11):1086-1096.
33. Katz S, Kidron D, Litmanovitz I, Erez I, Dolfin Z. Fibrous fusion between the liver and the lung: an unusual complication of right congenital diaphragmatic hernia. *J Pediatr Surg.* 1998;33(5):766-767.
34. Sakai H, Tamura M, Hosokawa Y, Bryan AC, Barker GA, Bohn DJ. Effect of surgical repair on respiratory mechanics in congenital diaphragmatic hernia. *J Pediatr.* 1987;111(3):432-438.
35. Wung JT, James LS, Kilchevsky E, James E. Management of infants with severe respiratory failure and persistence of the fetal circulation, without hyperventilation. *Pediatrics.* 1985;76(4):488-494.
36. Kays DW, Langham MR Jr, Ledbetter DJ, Talbert JL. Detrimental effects of standard medical therapy in congenital diaphragmatic hernia. *Ann Surg.* 1999;230(3):340-348, discussion 348–351.
37. Boloker J, Bateman DA, Wung JT, Stolar CJ. Congenital diaphragmatic hernia in 120 infants treated consecutively with permissive hypercapnea/spontaneous respiration/elective repair. *J Pediatr Surg.* 2002;37(3):357-366.
38. Reyes C, Chang LK, Waffarn F, Mir H, Warden MJ, Sills J. Delayed repair of congenital diaphragmatic hernia with early high-frequency oscillatory ventilation during preoperative stabilization. *J Pediatr Surg.* 1998;33(7):1010-1014, discussion 1014–1016.
39. Cacciari A, Ruggeri G, Mordenti M, et al. High-frequency oscillatory ventilation versus conventional mechanical ventilation in congenital diaphragmatic hernia. *Eur J Pediatr Surg.* 2001;11(1):3-7.
40. Kinsella JP, Neish SR, Shaffer E, Abman SH. Low-dose inhalation nitric oxide in persistent pulmonary hypertension of the newborn. *Lancet.* 1992;340(8823):819-820.
41. Finer NN, Barrington KJ. Nitric oxide for respiratory failure in infants born at or near term. *Cochrane Database Syst Rev.* 2001;(4):CD000399.
42. Finer NN, Sun JW, Rich W, Knodel E, Barrington KJ. Randomized, prospective study of low-dose versus high-dose inhaled nitric oxide in the neonate with hypoxic respiratory failure. *Pediatrics.* 2001;108(4):949-955.
43. Bartlett RH, Gazzaniga AB, Jefferies MR, Huxtable RF, Haiduc NJ, Fong SW. Extracorporeal membrane oxygenation (ECMO) cardiopulmonary support in infancy. *Trans Am Soc Artif Intern Organs.* 1976;22:80-93.
44. Does extracorporeal membrane oxygenation improve survival in neonates with congenital diaphragmatic hernia? The Congenital Diaphragmatic Hernia Study Group. *J Pediatr Surg.* 1999;34(5):720-724, discussion 724–725.
45. Annich G. *ECMO: Extracorporeal Cardiopulmonary Support in Critical Care.* 4th ed. Ann Arbor, MI: ELSO; 2012.
46. Dimmitt RA, Moss RL, Rhine WD, Benitz WE, Henry MC, Vanmeurs KP. Venoarterial versus venovenous extracorporeal membrane oxygenation in congenital diaphragmatic hernia: the Extracorporeal Life Support Organization Registry, 1990-1999. *J Pediatr Surg.* 2001;36(8):1199-1204.
47. Guner YS, Khemani RG, Qureshi FG, et al. Outcome analysis of neonates with congenital diaphragmatic hernia treated with venovenous vs venoarterial extracorporeal membrane oxygenation. *J Pediatr Surg.* 2009;44(9):1691-1701.

48. Vazquez WD, Cheu HW. Hemorrhagic complications and repair of congenital diaphragmatic hernias: does timing of the repair make a difference? Data from the Extracorporeal Life Support Organization. *J Pediatr Surg.* 1994;29(8):1002-1005, discussion 1005–1006.

49. Langer JC, Filler RM, Bohn DJ, et al. Timing of surgery for congenital diaphragmatic hernia: is emergency operation necessary? *J Pediatr Surg.* 1988;23(8):731-734.

50. West KW, Bengston K, Rescorla FJ, Engle WA, Grosfeld JL. Delayed surgical repair and ECMO improves survival in congenital diaphragmatic hernia. *Ann Surg.* 1992;216(4):454-460, discussion 460–462.

51. Partridge EA, Peranteau WH, Rintoul NE, et al. Timing of repair of congenital diaphragmatic hernia in patients supported by extracorporeal membrane oxygenation (ECMO). *J Pediatr Surg.* 2015;50(2):260-262.

52. Wilson JM, Lund DP, Lillehei CW, Vacanti JP. Congenital diaphragmatic hernia—a tale of two cities: the Boston experience. *J Pediatr Surg.* 1997;32(3):401-405.

53. Romao RL, Nasr A, Chiu PP, Langer JC. What is the best prosthetic material for patch repair of congenital diaphragmatic hernia? Comparison and meta-analysis of porcine small intestinal submucosa and polytetrafluoroethylene. *J Pediatr Surg.* 2012;47(8):1496-1500.

54. Moss RL, Chen CM, Harrison MR. Prosthetic patch durability in congenital diaphragmatic hernia: a long-term follow-up study. *J Pediatr Surg.* 2001;36(1):152-154.

55. Scaife ER, Johnson DG, Meyers RL, Johnson SM, Matlak ME. The split abdominal wall muscle flap—a simple, mesh-free approach to repair large diaphragmatic hernia. *J Pediatr Surg.* 2003;38(12):1748-1751.

56. Silen ML, Canvasser DA, Kurkchubasche AG, Andrus CH, Naunheim KS. Video-assisted thoracic surgical repair of a foramen of Bochdalek hernia. *Ann Thorac Surg.* 1995;60(2):448-450.

57. Bliss D, Matar M, Krishnaswami S. Should intraoperative hypercapnea or hypercarbia raise concern in neonates undergoing thoracoscopic repair of diaphragmatic hernia of Bochdalek? *J Laparoendosc Adv Surg Tech A.* 2009;19(suppl 1):S55-S58.

58. Davenport M, Rothenberg SS, Crabbe DC, Wulkan ML. The great debate: open or thoracoscopic repair for oesophageal atresia or diaphragmatic hernia. *J Pediatr Surg.* 2015;50(2):240-246.

59. Arca MJ, Barnhart DC, Lelli JL Jr, et al. Early experience with minimally invasive repair of congenital diaphragmatic hernias: results and lessons learned. *J Pediatr Surg.* 2003;38(11):1563-1568.

60. Cho SD, Krishnaswami S, Mckee JC, Zallen G, Silen ML, Bliss DW. Analysis of 29 consecutive thoracoscopic repairs of congenital diaphragmatic hernia in neonates compared to historical controls. *J Pediatr Surg.* 2009;44(1):80-86, discussion 86.

61. Gander JW, Fisher JC, Gross ER, et al. Early recurrence of congenital diaphragmatic hernia is higher after thoracoscopic than open repair: a single institutional study. *J Pediatr Surg.* 2011;46(7):1303-1308.

62. Liem NT. Thoracoscopic approach in management of congenital diaphragmatic hernia. *Pediatr Surg Int.* 2013;29(10):1061-1064.

63. Huang JS, Lau CT, Wong WY, Tao Q, Wong KK, Tam PK. Thoracoscopic repair of congenital diaphragmatic hernia: two centres' experience with 60 patients. *Pediatr Surg Int.* 2015;31(2):191-195.

64. Zhu Y, Wu Y, Pu Q, Ma L, Liao H, Liu L. Minimally invasive surgery for congenital diaphragmatic hernia: a meta-analysis. *Hernia.* 2016;20(2):297-302.

65. Harrison MR, Adzick NS, Longaker MT, et al. Successful repair in utero of a fetal diaphragmatic hernia after removal of herniated viscera from the left thorax. *N Engl J Med.* 1990;322(22):1582-1584.

66. Wilson JM, DiFiore JW, Peters CA. Experimental fetal tracheal ligation prevents the pulmonary hypoplasia associated with fetal nephrectomy: possible application for congenital diaphragmatic hernia. *J Pediatr Surg.* 1993;28(11):1433-1439, discussion 1439–1440.

67. Hedrick MH, Estes JM, Sullivan KM, et al. Plug the lung until it grows (PLUG): a new method to treat congenital diaphragmatic hernia in utero. *J Pediatr Surg.* 1994;29(5):612-617.

68. Chiba T, Albanese CT, Farmer DL, et al. Balloon tracheal occlusion for congenital diaphragmatic hernia: experimental studies. *J Pediatr Surg.* 2000;35(11):1566-1570.

69. Harrison MR, Keller RL, Hawgood SB, et al. A randomized trial of fetal endoscopic tracheal occlusion for severe fetal congenital diaphragmatic hernia. *N Engl J Med.* 2003;349(20):1916-1924.

70. Al-Maary J, Eastwood MP, Russo FM, Deprest JA, Keijzer R. Fetal tracheal occlusion for severe pulmonary hypoplasia in isolated congenital diaphragmatic hernia: a systematic review and meta-analysis of survival. *Ann Surg.* 2016;264:929-933.

71. Dekoninck P, Gratacos E, Van Mieghem T, et al. Results of fetal endoscopic tracheal occlusion for congenital diaphragmatic hernia and the set up of the randomized controlled TOTAL trial. *Early Hum Dev.* 2011;87(9):619-624.

Ventral Hernia and Abdominal Release Procedures

Heidi J. Miller | Yuri W. Novitsky

Ventral herniation presents a set of common, yet diverse and complex problems in the surgical world. It is a surgical disease with wide variation in management, variable outcomes, and high volumes. More than 2 million laparotomies are completed in the United States every year, and it is estimated that up to 28% of these will develop into ventral incisional hernias. Adding an additional 20% or more of primary congenital and acquired hernias,[1] this leads to an astounding incidence of ventral hernias in the United States alone. In 2006 more than 365,000 hernias were repaired in both inpatient and outpatient settings. The cumulative incidence of ventral hernias is increasing each year by an estimated 3%, which correlates with reported recurrence rates as high as 43%, even after mesh repair.[2] This leads to a calculation of nearly 500,000 ventral hernia repairs in the United States during 2015. The enormity of the ventral hernia problem corresponds with a high cost of care, with an estimated $3.2 billion spent in 2006 for ventral hernia repairs alone. Within this spending there is great variability in cost per patient or hernia because complex ventral hernias can lead to much higher costs, longer lengths of stay, and increased mortality rates in a small portion of patients compared with the majority.[1]

This disparity likely mirrors the complexity and variability that ventral herniation presents to surgeons, characteristics that lead to a lack of consensus in the literature and among hernia surgeons on the ideal repair technique. Traditional repair results have been fairly poor and the field of herniorrhaphy has finally been recognized by the surgical community as an important subspecialty.[3] It continues to be a rapidly changing field with innovations in mesh technology and surgical technique. Modern approaches include laparoscopy, open suture repair, mesh repair, component separation, and abdominal wall reconstruction. In the search for the ideal ventral hernia repair, the surgeon must consider cost-savings; risk adjustment by patient comorbidities; complexity of the hernia, such as recurrences and nonhealing wounds; improved mesh incorporation; and decreasing the risk of recurrence. Because there is no perfect repair for all ventral hernias, it is paramount for a surgeon to be familiar with a wide array of techniques and have a defined algorithm for evaluating and managing patients with ventral hernias.

DEFINITIONS

Hernia is derived from Latin meaning "rupture" or "protruding viscous" and a *ventral hernia* is a protrusion of viscera, usually intestine, through the layers of the anterior abdominal wall. A true hernia has a defect in the fascia of the abdominal wall and the formation of a hernia sac of peritoneum that contains visceral organs. Other bulges that may appear similarly, but are not true hernias, are diastasis recti and eventration. Diastasis recti is the thinning and broadening of the linea alba that leads to a bulge at the midline and is usually asymptomatic. An eventration is a bulge resulting from lack of muscle tone in the abdominal wall due to trauma, denervation, and surgical or congenital absence of the muscle. Neither diastasis recti nor eventration has a fascial defect and there is no hernia sac in either scenario.

Ventral hernia can be further defined by location and origin. An incisional hernia occurs at any previous surgical site of the anterior abdominal wall. Traumatic hernias occur due to injury of the fascia and musculature of the abdominal wall, and can be in any location. Lateral abdominal wall hernias, also known as flank hernias, are often caused by blunt trauma with disruption of the attachments of the lateral muscles of the abdominal wall. Subxiphoid hernias are located just inferior to the xiphoid at the midline. Epigastric hernias can be spontaneous or incisional at the midline between the xiphoid and the umbilicus. Umbilical hernias are located at the umbilicus and can be congenital or acquired spontaneously. Hypogastric hernias at the midline, inferior to the umbilicus are rare spontaneous occurrences. Suprapubic and parailiac hernias occur adjacent to the bony structures of the pelvis. Finally, spigelian hernias are spontaneous hernias that occur along the semilunar line, typically at its junction with the arcuate line of Douglas.

The European Hernia Society (EHS) has introduced a ventral and incisional hernia classification system in an attempt to create a common language for the evaluation and treatment of ventral hernias.[4] Primary and incisional hernias are separated in this classification system (Tables 52.1 and 52.2). A primary ventral hernia is divided by location between midline hernias (epigastric and umbilical) and lateral hernias (spigelian and lumbar). The size of primary ventral hernias is categorized into small (<2 cm), medium (2 to 4 cm), and large (>4 cm). Any weakness or protrusion at the site of a surgical scar defines an incisional hernia for the EHS, and because these hernias are more variable, the classification system is slightly more involved. First, incisional hernias are divided into medial or lateral, with the lateral edge of the rectus abdominis being the dividing line. Midline hernias are placed into one of five vertical zones (M1 to M5) ranging from subxiphoid to suprapubic. Lateral hernias are divided into four zones (L1 to L4) with subcostal, flank, and iliac stacked medial to the anterior axillary line and lumbar (L4) hernias arising anywhere dorsolateral to this line. Incisional hernias are divided into recurrent or not, and both length and width are taken into consideration. Hernias with multiple defects are measured at the point of greatest distance in

TABLE 52.1 European Hernia Society Classification System for Primary Ventral Hernias

	Diameter (cm)	Small <2 (cm)	Medium ≥2–4 (cm)	Large ≥4 (cm)
Midline	Umbilical Epigastric			
Lateral	Spigelian Lumbar			

Modified from Muysoms FE, Miserez M, Berrevoet F, et al. Classification of primary and incisional abdominal wall hernias. *Hernia*. 2009;13:407–414.

TABLE 52.2 European Hernia Society Classification System for Incisional Ventral Hernias

Midline	Subxiphoid	M1		
	Epigastric	M2		
	Umbilical	M3		
	Infraumbilical	M4		
	Suprapubic	M5		
Lateral	Subcostal	L1		
	Flank	L2		
	Iliac	L3		
	Lumbar	L4		
Recurrent?	Yes		No	
	Length: cm		Width: cm	
Width cm	W1 <4 cm		W2 ≥4–10 cm	W3 ≥10 cm

Modified from Muysoms FE, Miserez M, Berrevoet F, et al. Classification of primary and incisional abdominal wall hernias. *Hernia*. 2009;13:407–414.

either axis. Finally, width is divided into W1 (<4 cm), W2 (4 to 10 cm), and W3 (>10 cm). There was no consensus within the EHS on nomenclature for incisional hernias.[4]

Irrespective of the cause and location of the ventral hernia, current trends in repair are led by the philosophy of restoring a functional and anatomic abdominal wall, including the reconstruction of the tendinous insertion of the related muscles or re-creation of the linea alba.

ANATOMY

The anterior abdominal wall is a complex layering of muscle, fascia, and aponeuroses, all of which work symbiotically to fill a variety of functions (Fig. 52.1). The anterior abdominal wall protects and supports the viscera and aids with respiration by pulling down the rib cage in expiration. It also participates in a multitude of bodily functions, allows for rotation, bending, and flexion of the trunk, and protects the spine from hyperextension.

Laterally, the abdominal wall is constructed of three layered flat muscles. From superficial to deep these are the external oblique (EO), internal oblique (IO), and transversus abdominis muscles. The transversalis fascia is the deepest layer of fascia in the abdominal wall and separates the transversus abdominis muscle from the peritoneum. The EO muscle runs inferior-medially, originating at the lower costal margin and inserting at the linea alba, iliac crest, and pubic tubercle to form the inguinal ligament. The IO muscle runs perpendicular to the EO with its origination at the lateral half of the inguinal ligament, anterior iliac spine, and thoracolumbar fascia and inserting into the lower ribs and linea alba. Finally, the transversus abdominis muscle runs horizontally

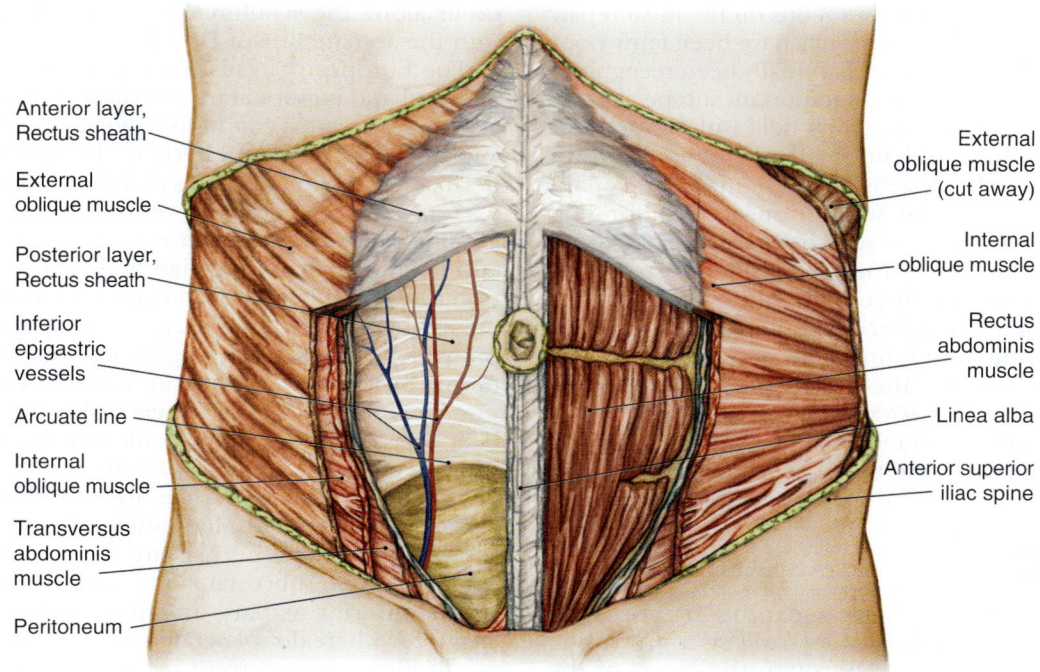

FIGURE 52.1 Muscles of the anterior abdominal wall.

from the iliac crest, lateral inguinal ligament, and costal cartilage to insert into the linea alba and joins the IO to form the conjoint tendon.

Each muscle body is surrounded by its relevant fascia and these laminal layers join to form aponeurotic connections for each flat muscle. Medially the three aponeuroses form the linea semilunaris, which lies at the lateral edge of the rectus abdominis muscle. The rectus abdominis is a vertically oriented muscle originating at the pubic symphysis and inserting into the fifth to seventh costal cartilages. In the upper third of the abdomen, the EO aponeurosis and anterior lamina of the IO aponeurosis fuse to form the anterior rectus sheath, while the posterior lamina of the IO overlies the transversus abdominis muscle body. The transversus abdominis muscle extends medially in the upper abdomen, just deep to the rectus muscle, and the posterior lamina eventually joins the transversus abdominis aponeurosis to form the posterior rectus sheath. In the middle third of the abdomen, the transversus abdominis muscle ends more laterally and the posterior rectus sheath is formed by the aponeurosis of the transversus abdominis and the posterior lamina of the IO aponeurosis. In the lower third of the abdomen, below the arcuate line, the IO and transversus abdominis aponeurosis fuse with the EO aponeurosis as part of the anterior rectus fascia, leaving only peritoneum deep to the rectus abdominis.

Medial to the body of the rectus abdominis muscle, all of the flat muscle aponeuroses fuse to create the linea alba and the midline of the anterior abdominal wall. The linea alba is widest at the xiphoid, where the rectus muscles diverge to insert into the costal cartilages and narrows to a thin line of fascia below the umbilicus until it reaches the pubic symphysis. The linea alba is weakest at the umbilicus, which lies at the midpoint between xiphoid and pubis and is a cicatricial remnant of the umbilical cord.

The spigelian fascia is a fusion of the IO and transversus abdominis aponeurosis that lies between the semilunar line and the lateral edge of the rectus abdominis muscle body. The spigelian fascia is weak inferior to the umbilicus as the aponeuroses of IO and TAMs run parallel in this location, so there is minimal crosslinking for strength. This weakness is worsened where the inferior epigastric arteries traverse the rectus abdominus muscle.

The vascular supply of the rectus abdominis enters the muscles laterally via branches of the inferior and superior epigastric arteries. The rectus abdominis is innervated segmentally via the thoracoabdominal (T7 to T11) nerves that also enter the muscle body at the lateral edge, just medial to the linea semilunaris. The vascular supply for the flat muscles of the abdomen are branches of intercostal arteries that run with thoracoabdominal nerves in the neurovascular space between the IO and transversus abdominis muscles. The skin and subcutaneous tissue of the anterior abdominal wall gets its blood supply from deep perforators that branch from the deep inferior and superior epigastric vessels.

ETIOLOGY AND EPIDEMIOLOGY

Ventral hernia formation is complex and multifactorial, and hernias may be congenital or acquired. Congenital hernias are present from birth and include complex entities such as omphalocele and gastroschisis, or more straightforward defects such as primary umbilical or epigastric hernias. More than 80% of primary congenital umbilical hernias will close spontaneously before the age of 5 and will not require repair. However, congenital epigastric hernias may be symptomatic with incarcerated preperitoneal fat and require surgical intervention.[5] Acquired ventral hernias are of the spontaneous or incisional variety. Spontaneous hernias most often occur at weaknesses of the abdominal wall, along the midline, or at the arcuate line or spigelian fascia. However, trauma to the abdominal wall may also lead to herniation in other locations. Incisional hernias are defined as any ventral herniation that is located at a previous surgical site or incision, including trocar sites. Spontaneous ventral hernias are diagnosed in adulthood and are usually the effect of increased abdominal pressure related to obesity, pregnancy, ascites, or other factors. Increased abdominal pressure leads to enlargement of the hernia defect as well as increased likelihood of incarceration. Fig. 52.2 shows the anatomic location of acquired and congenital hernias.

Epigastric hernias occur at the midline above the umbilicus where perforating neurovascular bundles travel through the fascial layers that interlace to create the linea alba. These defects are usually quite small but often have an incarcerated mushroom of preperitoneal fat that can be quite symptomatic for the patient.

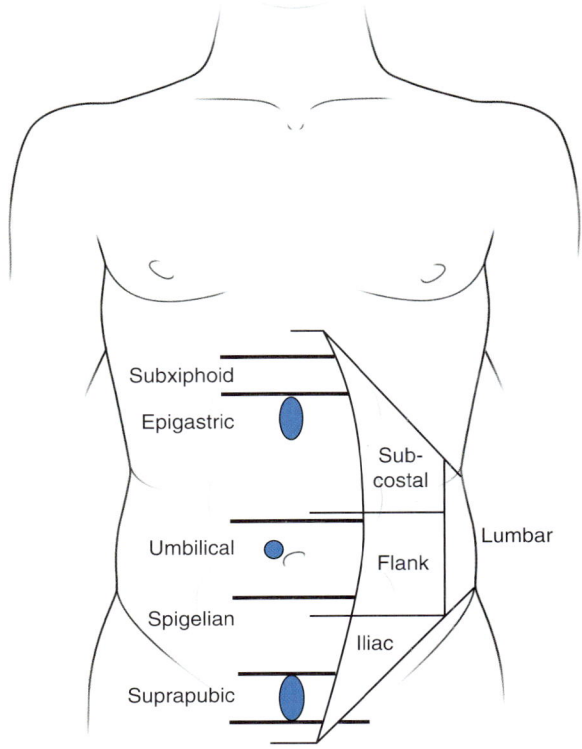

FIGURE 52.2 Anatomic locations of ventral hernias.

Umbilical hernias occur through the base of the umbilicus or in the surrounding tissue. The umbilical ring is formed as the flat discus of fetal cells begins its three-dimensional fold and is surrounded by the amniotic cavity. It eventually fuses with the linea alba and rectus complexes, and the umbilical cord is created. Here the linea alba is penetrated by the umbilical veins and arteries and after birth a cicatrix is formed as these vessels degenerate into the falciform and umbilical ligaments. It is thought that this is the weakest part of the abdominal wall; either the cicatrix itself or the tissues surrounding it are weak, allowing for vulnerability and the formation of umbilical or periumbilical hernias.[5] Other patient factors may add to the stress of the abdominal wall and contribute to the formation of ventral hernias, such as disorders of collagen formation, sleep apnea, steroid use, and smoking or chronic lung diseases. Whatever the etiology, umbilical hernias are a common problem and approximately 200,000 repairs are done in the United States every year.

Incisional hernias occur in up to 40% of patients after midline laparotomy. An innate problem with suture closure of laparotomy is that tension is required to approximate the rectus abdominis muscles and counter tension of the lateral abdominal wall musculature. Such tension may contribute to overtightening of sutures and ischemia to the midline tissues.[6]

There are three types of incisional hernias: acute wound dehiscence and evisceration due to sutures tearing through tissue, subacute with early gapping of the tissues approximated under tension, and chronic remodeling of the scar tissue causing "Swiss-cheese" or "cheese-cutting" hernias, formed as sutures cut through the weakened scar tissue. Thus, technical factors such as slipped knots, tension, and overtightened sutures can predispose to hernia development. Surgical site infection (SSI) has also been found to increase the risk of hernia by 50%.

Laparotomy closure should be done in a continuous fashion with a slowly absorbable monofilament suture with all midline layers en bloc.[7] Two recent randomized controlled trials have found that small stitches, incorporating about 5 mm of midline tissue and taken about 5 mm apart reduces the risk of infection, wound dehiscence, and incisional hernia development.[8,9] This is a change from historical surgical dogma where 1 cm was felt to be the proper amount of tissue and distance between stitches. Proper "small bite" technique should be confirmed at the time of closure by measuring the suture-to-wound-length ratio to be at least 4 to 1.[10] Although small bites may take longer to complete than the traditional larger bites, the added operating room time accounts only for a small increased cost and the cost savings with the reduced incidence of ventral hernia and complications is much greater.[11] There has also been some recent interest in exploring the use of prophylactic mesh at closure of primary laparotomy for incisional hernia prevention. A randomized controlled trial of mesh versus suture closure after abdominal aortic aneurysm repair found a fourfold reduction in hernia development with the use of prophylactic mesh. This study also showed a longer time to hernia development for those with mesh placement, and no increase in complications or mesh infections.[12]

A meta-analysis of prophylactic mesh placement during laparotomy in high-risk patients also found a significant decrease in incisional hernia development with prophylactic mesh placement, longer operating room (OR) times, and shorter hospital stays.[13] Therefore, prophylactic use of mesh during closure of laparotomy in high-risk patients can be considered to reduce the risk of incisional hernia, but no strong recommendations can be made for the general population.

Laparoscopic port site hernias are a growing problem within the incisional hernia category given the increasing use of laparoscopy and robotics, and the exploration of single-site minimally invasive approaches. The incidence of port site hernias has been shown to be between 0% and 5.2%. Ninety-six percent of port site hernias occur at 10-mm and larger port sites, and 86% occur at the umbilicus.[14] However, more recent studies have shown rates reaching 22% to 39%[15,16] after ventral hernia repair with large mesh and bariatric surgeries. It is generally believed that any port larger than 5 mm in diameter should be closed to prevent port site hernias. However, it remains controversial, and we believe that dilating, noncutting trocars less than 12 mm do not require closure.[17,18] Single-incision laparoscopic and robotic surgeries have been found to have slightly higher incidence of port site hernias of 3%, although this has improved over time and more recent studies have shown no difference.[19] Port site hernias may be difficult to diagnose because they may occur early, late, intrafascially, or as Richter-type hernias. Wound- and patient-related factors may also play a role in the formation of port site hernias: infection, delayed healing, steroids, collagen disorders, obesity, and increased abdominal pressure are all known to predispose to herniation.

PRESENTATION AND INDICATIONS FOR SURGERY

Most patients with ventral hernias present to the office with complaints of a bulge in their abdominal wall. The bulge may be more noticeable after physical activity, Valsalva maneuvers, coughing, or any other activities that increase intraabdominal pressure. Some patients will present with complaints of pain or discomfort along with the bulge, although about 25% of patients will be asymptomatic.[20] Pain associated with ventral hernias may be related to incarceration and at times relieved with rest, lying down, or reduction of the hernia contents. The most concerning presentations are incarcerated ventral hernias with signs of bowel obstruction or strangulation, which is more common with small defects. Other complaints that may accompany a ventral hernia are cosmetic, gastrointestinal or urinary symptoms, generalized pain, back pain, and respiratory difficulties.[20]

The mere presence of a ventral hernia is often considered a de facto indication for a surgical intervention. Other than incarceration and strangulation, generalized pain is the most common reasons surgeons choose to intervene on ventral hernias.[20] However, many ventral hernia patients have complex medical histories and the repairs are fraught with potential complications. Morbidity rates after ventral hernia repair can reach 60% and mortality rates can be as high as 5.3%.[21] Despite high complication and morbidity rates, surgery is often felt to be the primary treatment option for ventral hernias, largely because the natural history of ventral/incisional hernias is unstudied. A recent series of watchful waiting for ventral hernias showed no change in pain, functionality, or quality of life after 2 years of watchful waiting for minimally symptomatic ventral hernias larger than 9 cm.[21] The risk of incarceration or strangulation was less than 5% and another 8% of patients requested repair for symptoms within the 2 years.[21] This study is limited by a small sample size, but the low rates of complications and progression of disease mirrors the results of a randomized controlled trial for minimally symptomatic inguinal hernias that has shown that watchful waiting can be safe.[22] Also, although patients with symptomatic ventral hernias report improvement in pain and quality of life, patients with limited symptomatology report similar pain levels before and after repair.[20,23] However, follow-up data have shown a high rate of disease progression and although watchful waiting may be relatively safe, we believe most patients should be optimized and undergo repair in the earlier stages of the disease.

PATIENT EVALUATION

Initial intake begins with a thorough history and physical, which should identify comorbidities and risk factors for complications. The physical exam should delineate previous surgical scars, skin issues, the presence of stomas, fistulas, exposed mesh, or sinuses and hernia qualities such as location and defect size. As an adjunct to the physical exam, computed tomography (CT) of the abdomen and pelvis can help with operative planning. We routinely obtain a noncontrast CT for moderate and large ventral defects. Oral contrast may be useful in the presence of gastrointestinal or obstructive symptoms, and intravenous contrast may be helpful to identify soft tissue infections or delineate vasculature. Finally, a thorough review of the patient's operative history is necessary to identify any potential difficulties with the planned repair and to discover the type and location of any previous mesh placement. Based on this evaluation, we then decide on the type of repair most appropriate for the patient. We repair only very small (<2 cm) primary ventral hernias with a suture repair. Appropriate patients for laparoscopic hernia repair include recurrent ventral hernias with small defects and primary hernias that are larger than 2 cm but less than 10 to 12 cm in width. We usually make an exception for women of childbearing age and avoid the use of laparoscopy and/or permanent meshes. The defect size must also be considered in relation to the size of a patient, because a 10-cm defect in a large male patient is quite different than a 10-cm defect in a petite female patient. For larger or more complex hernias we use component separation strategies for abdominal wall reconstruction.

PREPARATION FOR SURGERY

To prepare the patient for surgery, we require smoking cessation of at least 4 weeks and will test for nicotine metabolites at preanesthesia testing. Weight loss counseling should also be provided for obese patients, with referral to bariatric surgery, if necessary, and agreement on set weight loss goals. In a recent retrospective review at our institution of over 800 ventral hernia repairs, we found that a body mass index (BMI) greater than 45 increased the risk of postoperative wound infection.[24] As a result, we have now set a BMI greater than 45 as an upper limit to qualify for an elective open ventral hernia repair. Pulmonary and cardiac problems must be addressed, and patients should be evaluated and treated for sleep apnea if they present with risk factors. Diabetes control should be optimized with a goal for an HbA1c below 7.5. Any age-appropriate screening, particularly a screening colonoscopy, is mandatory. Finally, preoperative counseling is important to set the patient up with appropriate expectations for the repair, results, postoperative care, and recovery. All possible outcomes should be discussed, including potential wound or mesh infections and recurrence. It is important to understand the patient's goals and their view of what outcomes may or may not be unacceptable.

PRINCIPLES OF VENTRAL HERNIA REPAIR

Tissue-based repairs of ventral hernias have been developed in an attempt to decrease recurrence rates; the Mayo repair used a "vest-over-pants" technique and mattress sutures to imbricate fascial edges and approximate healthy tissue. However, long-term follow-up found similar recurrence rates to fascial suture approximation. In the 1990s, a randomized controlled trial showed a 50% decrease in ventral hernia recurrence with the use of mesh compared to suture repair.[25] The decreased rate of recurrence was even more significant in smaller hernias, although with an associated increase in complications. Surgical site infections and the presence of abdominal aortic aneurysms increased the risk of hernia development. Patients randomized to mesh repair suffered more complications, but had lower levels of postoperative pain.[25]

The introduction of prosthetics has been a game changer in the repair of ventral hernias, and today the use of mesh reinforcement is recommended in the majority of ventral hernia repairs. Prosthetics used in hernia repair are in constant evolution and no "ideal" mesh has been discovered. The qualities of the ideal mesh include good tissue incorporation, limited foreign body reaction, and sufficient strength to withstand the forces of the abdominal wall along with good flexibility and compliance.[26,27]

Prosthetics are first divided by material type and can be synthetic, biologic, or biosynthetic. Synthetic meshes are usually made of polypropylene, polyester, or polytetrafluoroethylene (PTFE). Biologic meshes are either cadaveric allograft or xenograft tissue grafts that are processed to reduce host reaction and improve tissue integration. Finally, the newest category of biosynthetic meshes are made of slowly absorbable biodegradable synthetic polymers. Synthetic and biosynthetic meshes can be further divided into monofilament or multifilament construction, micro- or macroporous, and heavy, midweight, or lightweight types. Finally, to reduce visceral adhesion and fistula formation, there are covered meshes made for intraabdominal placement. It is important for the surgeon to be educated on the types of meshes available for hernia repair, the benefits and limitations of each mesh type, and to have an algorithm for choosing mesh in individual hernia repairs.

We prefer to use a macroporous, midweight monofilament polypropylene mesh for most extraperitoneal repairs. However, heavyweight polypropylene meshes are used in cases where more significant support of the repair is needed. Our use of biologic meshes is limited to actively infected fields and in cases of staged repair with a planned hernia. The role of slowly absorbable biosynthetics is currently evolving.

The most appropriate positioning of mesh within the abdominal wall is as big a question as which type of mesh to use. Neither of these questions has been answered in the literature, although 75% to 80% of hernia repairs involve mesh to reduce the risk of recurrence. Mesh can be placed as an onlay, sublay, underlay, or interposition (Fig. 52.3). Onlay mesh is placed above the anterior rectus sheath, whereas sublay mesh is positioned within the layers of the abdominal wall, typically retromuscular or in the preperitoneal plane. An underlay mesh is placed within the abdominal cavity underneath the peritoneum. Recurrence rates are lowest with sublay or retromuscular mesh placement, followed by underlay mesh placement.[28] Interposition mesh placement has the highest recurrence rate, reported to be as high as 80%.[28] Interposition mesh placement is fraught with complications and also holds the highest SSI rate, whereas sublay mesh placement has the lowest SSI rate and lowest rate of mesh excision.[28] However, there is significant discrepancy in the literature regarding outcomes related to mesh location, which accentuates the need for clinical decision making during ventral hernia repair. Mesh location, like mesh type, should be decided based upon patient characteristics, anticipated technique, and the characteristics of the hernia in question.

To help with clinical decision making in the repair of ventral hernias, as well as the ability to study and compare outcomes, the Ventral Hernia Working Group (VHWG) proposed a ventral hernia grading scale and recommendations for repair.[29] In 2010, the VHWG developed a four-grade scale of ventral hernias: Grade 1 includes healthy patients with no comorbidities or history of wound infections or contamination; grade 2 captures comorbid patients without infection or contamination; grade 3 includes higher-risk patients with potential for contamination with the presence of a stoma, history of wound infection, or opening of the intestinal tract; and grade 4 captures patients with active infections, fistulas, or contamination.[29] This grading scale was evaluated and modified 2 years later by Kanters et al., who found that increased grade correlated with increased risk of recurrence as well as surgical site occurrence (SSO).[30] However, they found significant difference between grades 2 and 3 with regard to SSO and proposed a modification of the grading scale to include only three grades. grade 1 remains the same low-risk group, grade 2 is mostly the same class of comorbid patients, with the added inclusion of a history of wound infection, and grade 3 is the contaminated group.[30] One of two major limitations of the modified grading system by Kanters et al. is that it segregated the groups based on often clinically irrelevant SSOs and not SSIs. Furthermore, there were not a sufficient number of patients with dirty (CDC wound class 4) wounds resulting in those patients being grouped together with patients with contamination and active infection in the grade 3 category.

The VHWG also provided guidance in the repair of ventral hernias with the first step including the evaluation of the hernia grade. The choice of repair technique and type of prosthetic used is then decided. For grade 3 and 4 hernias, the VHWG does not recommend the use of synthetic mesh and states that biologics can be considered. However, Carbonell and colleagues have found that synthetic mesh can be used in clean-contaminated and contaminated cases with favorable outcomes.[31] More recently Majumder and colleagues showed that the use of biologic mesh in clean-contaminated and contaminated ventral hernia repairs was associated with a markedly increased risk of surgical site events (SSEs), SSIs, and recurrence.[32] Therefore, the touted advantages of biologic grafts appear to have been exaggerated and their utilization continues to decline.

OPEN VENTRAL HERNIA REPAIR

Primary hernias that are less than 2 to 3 cm in width may be closed primarily with permanent or slowly absorbing monofilament suture. For any incisional hernias or primary hernias larger than 3 cm, mesh reinforcement with 4 to 5 cm of overlap is recommended. Open ventral hernia repair is done with closure of the defect to restore abdominal wall function and placement of a prosthetic of choice. Options for mesh placement include onlay, which requires some soft tissue dissection to clear the fascial plane for mesh fixation; underlay, which requires the use of intraperitoneal covered mesh and transfascial fixation; or sublay, which requires dissection between layers of abdominal wall or posterior component separation described later in this chapter. As mentioned above, interposition (inlay) mesh should be avoided except in circumstances of emergent or contaminated repair where hernia recurrence is an acceptable outcome within the balance of risks.

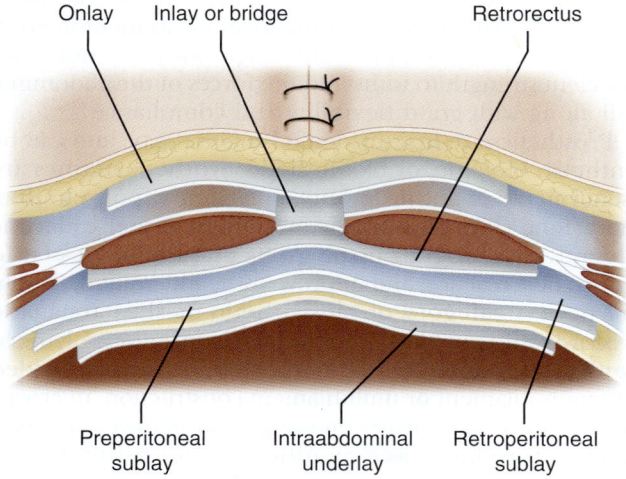

FIGURE 52.3 Mesh repair positioning options. (Based on Adrales G. Abdominal wall spaces for mesh placement: onlay, sublay, underlay. In: Novitsky Y, ed. *Hernia Surgery: Current Principles*. New York: Springer; 2016:80.)

MINIMALLY INVASIVE VENTRAL HERNIA REPAIR

Laparoscopic ventral hernia repair (LVHR) was described by Le Blanc and Booth in 1993 and was rapidly adopted by laparoscopic surgeons and used to repair all types of hernias.[33] In fact, LVHR had emerged as the preferred and even "gold standard" minimally invasive technique for many patients with small-to-medium-sized umbilical and ventral hernia defects. It has been touted for its low wound morbidity because it avoids large abdominal incisions, and results in a decreased length of stay.[34,35] Since then, the literature comparing open and laparoscopic ventral/incisional hernia repair is scarce and the debate over superiority continues. In 2011, a Cochrane review was only able to conclude that laparoscopy for incisional hernias was a promising approach with some emphasis on improvement of short-term outcomes.[36] This has been mirrored in a number of later studies that have compared laparoscopic to open ventral hernia repair and found no difference in recurrence rates and similar quality of life after 6 months.[33,37] The short-term improvements after laparoscopy include less postoperative pain, quicker rehabilitation and return to work, decreased wound infection rates, and better cosmetic outcomes. The frequently discussed downsides of laparoscopic ventral hernia repair are increased risk of incidental enterotomy during lysis of adhesions, increased seroma and hematoma development, and increased development of intraabdominal adhesions due to an intraperitoneal prosthetic; potentially longer operative times, and persistent bulging at the site of defects with bridged techniques.[33,35,37] In addition to these potential complications, traditional LVHR technique leaves mesh intraperitoneally, in close proximity to bowel, thus requiring the use of a covered mesh, which is more expensive and more likely to harbor infection due to the barrier coating. The overall impact of mesh placed in direct contact with bowel is unclear.

Even coated mesh confers increased risk for intraabdominal adhesions, with some studies showing one-third of patients having significant adhesions at reoperation, the potential for harboring infection, and increased cost.[38,39] Additionally, standard methods of fixation necessitate an expensive laparoscopic tacking device, and both permanent and absorbable tacks are correlated with increased postoperative and chronic pain.[40] Finally, intraperitoneal mesh is often anchored with transfascial sutures to stretch the mesh and limit shrinkage and hernia recurrence. Transfascial sutures have been shown to cause ischemia of the abdominal wall and are correlated with increased postoperative and prolonged pain and potentially incite recurrent hernias.[41]

Despite its myriad disadvantages, the LVHR technique has evolved very little since it initially gained acceptance and popularity in the early 1990s. More recently, however, it has been suggested that defect closure prior to mesh placement could alleviate some of the shortfalls of the traditional LVHR. Potential benefits of defect closure include reduced wound morbidity by reducing potential space for seroma and hematoma formation, lower rates of recurrence, improved abdominal wall functionality by reapproximation of linea alba, and better cosmesis.[42]

Additionally, the goal of avoiding intraperitoneal mesh in minimally invasive repairs has further motivated hernia specialists across the globe to innovate. Prasad et al. compared a laparoscopic transabdominal preperitoneal (TAPP) technique using simple polypropylene mesh for ventral hernia repair with LVHR and were able to show cost efficacy, decreased seroma formation, and decreased recurrence for the laparoscopic TAPP approach.[41] Predictably, this study showed equivalent pain scores across both groups, which was to be expected because the meshes were secured using both transfascial sutures and tacks for both groups. The laparoscopic TAPP approach to ventral hernia repair is a time-consuming and technically challenging procedure with a significant learning curve. Other innovations in laparoscopic hernia repair are the extended-view totally extraperitoneal (eTEP) hernia repair, originally developed by Daes for complex inguinoscrotal hernias and modified as an approach for ventral hernia.[43,44] eTEP for ventral hernias includes extraperitoneal balloon dissection in the subcutaneous, retromuscular, or preperitoneal planes, and allows for defect closure, component separation if needed, and wide prosthetic reinforcement in a sublay position. Yet another approach is the endoscopic-assisted transhernia mini-open sublay repair (MILOS) developed in Germany. MILOS achieves wide dissection using endoscopic or direct visualization with a lighted trocar through small incisions. The dissection is taken through the hernia sac and into the extraperitoneal plane allowing for closure of the defect and wide mesh overlap.[45,46] Furthermore, Belyansky and colleagues applied minimally invasive techniques for laparoscopic abdominal wall reconstruction with posterior component separation via TAR and extraperitoneal mesh reinforcement with very encouraging early results.[47] More recently, they used eTEP principles to perform retrorectus or posterior component separation, largely avoiding intraperitoneal dissection. Although the refinement of the technique is ongoing, this approach, coined *eTAR*, may evolve as one of the preferred, yet technically demanding, techniques for abdominal wall reconstructions.

With the advent of robotics in many surgical specialties, robotic-assisted ventral hernia repair has recently gained interest because it may confer the benefits of a minimally invasive approach while also allowing for a shorter learning curve. Surgeons are able to use a technique similar to an open approach (uncoated mesh in the extraperitoneal space, midline restoration, avoidance of transfascial sutures and tacks) through minimally invasive access. Detractors of the robotic approach cite heightened cost, although no comparative cost data on this subject currently exist. Moreover, it is important to point out that robotic repairs allow the surgeon to avoid expensive, and at times painful, tack fixation, and significantly more expensive composite meshes with antiadhesive coating, likely offsetting the costs of robotic instruments. To date, there has only been one retrospective study comparing laparoscopic ventral hernia repair to robotic ventral hernia repair, with both approaches using an intraperitoneal mesh (IPOM).[48] This study showed longer operative times for robotic cases and lower rates of complications and recurrences. The major technical differences were defect closure and circumferential suturing of the mesh in robotic cases.[48]

Several authors have also reported on feasibility of robotic ventral hernia repair and preperitoneal inguinal hernia repair concomitant with robotic prostatectomy.[49,50]

As surgeons become more comfortable with laparoscopy and mesh technologies evolve, there is potential for laparoscopic or robotic ventral hernia repair to grow into a place of superiority. As of now, it is one of many options for incisional hernia repair in the surgeon's armamentarium and should be deployed under an appropriate algorithm.

OPERATIVE TECHNIQUE—LAPAROSCOPIC VENTRAL HERNIA REPAIR

The patient is positioned supine on the operating table and the arms are tucked. Preoperative antibiotics and venothromboembolism (VTE) prophylaxis are given prior to incision. Orogastric tubes are placed, as we reserve nasogastric patients for those with an extensive adhesiolysis or bowel congestion from incarceration. A urinary catheter is placed in all patients; in those with infraumbilical extensions of the hernia defect, we place a three-way catheter to allow for instillation of saline to facilitate intraoperative bladder identification. The abdomen is sterilized and draped using an iodophor-impregnated drape (Ioban; 3M, St. Paul, Minnesota) as an extra layer of protection against mesh contamination. We typically enter the abdomen using an optical trocar in the subcostal region; however access should be individualized according to the surgeon's comfort. Additional 5-mm ports are placed laterally on the side of entry and another two 5-mm ports are placed on the contralateral side to aid in the placement and securing of the mesh. Adhesiolysis is carried out sharply, minimizing the use of electrocautery or energy devices to prevent burn injuries to underlying bowel. Contents

of the hernia are reduced using two atraumatic graspers, and the hernia sac is typically left intact. We then measure the defect intracorporeally using transabdominal spinal needles placed at each edge.

We routinely close fascial defects during laparoscopic hernia repairs. This is a widely debated topic among hernia surgeons and thus far the literature has shown a trend toward improved outcomes with primary fascial closure during laparoscopic hernia repair, citing lower recurrence rates, lower rates of seroma formation, and improved patient satisfaction.[51,52] However, the data are sparse and a randomized controlled trial comparing bridged laparoscopic repair to defect closure with synthetic mesh is ongoing. We use a laparoscopic "shoelacing" technique of figure-of-eight permanent sutures to close our defects.[42] Briefly, a vertical line is drawn down the middle of the defect, 3-cm intervals are marked (beginning at the upper edge of the defect), and stab wounds are created. The figure-of-eight transfascial sutures are placed using a suture passer with monofilament permanent sutures (Fig. 52.4A). Each suture incorporates 1 to 2 cm of fascial edge and the sac is left in situ. After all sutures are placed, the pneumoperitoneum is released and the sutures are tied from outside in, leaving buried subcutaneous knots. The abdomen is reinsufflated and the defect closure is confirmed.

The mesh is introduced through a 12-mm port placed near the midline and/or near the closed defect, in a location where it will be subsequently covered with mesh. We use a covered mesh in an underlay position and often have the luxury of a mesh deployment device. If this is unavailable, four monofilament sutures should be placed in four quadrants of the mesh prior to introduction into

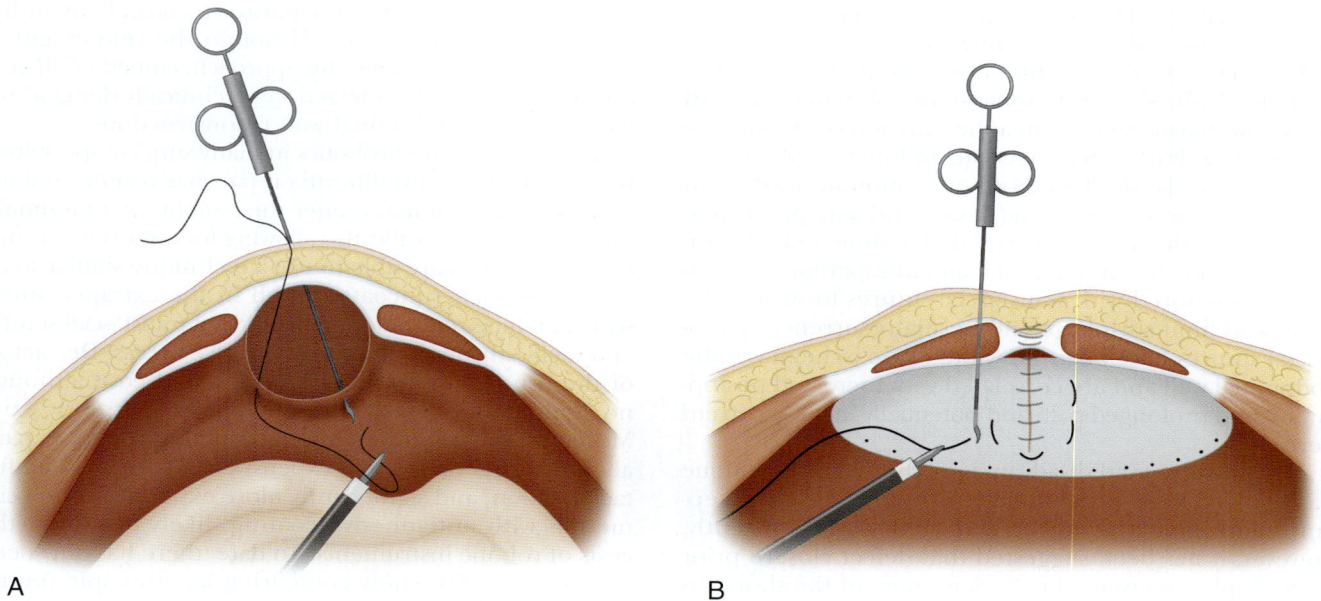

A   B

FIGURE 52.4 Laparoscopic ventral hernia repair (LVHR) technique with shoelacing technique defect closure. (A) Interrupted figure-of-eight sutures passed transfacially with a suture passer along the length of the defect. (B) LVHR repair with intraperitoneal mesh after defect closure showing circumferential tacks, lateral fixation sutures, and transfascial buttressing sutures just lateral to closure. (Based on Orenstein SB, Novitsky YW. Laparoscopic ventral hernia repair with defect closure. In: Novitsky YW, ed. *Hernia Surgery: Current Principles.* New York: Springer; 2016:235.)

the abdominal cavity. The mesh is unrolled and transfascial sutures are pulled through, keeping the mesh on stretch, with a suture passer. We recommend starting fixation by pulling the upper or lower stitch first, followed by the lateral ones. The edge of the mesh is secured with metal or absorbable tacks at 1-cm intervals. We then place transfacial stitches on either side of the closed defect (within 2 cm of the midline) to fix the mesh, take tension off our "primary" defect closure, and redistribute the tension on the mesh (see Fig. 52.4B). The ports are removed under direct vision, pneumoperitoneum is released, and the incisions are closed with subcutaneous sutures.

The most catastrophic potential complication of laparoscopic ventral hernia repair is small bowel injury during adhesiolysis, especially if they are missed.[53] Enterotomy has been reported in an average of 1.7% to 3.3% of patients in recent series of laparoscopic ventral hernia repairs.[54] If an enterotomy occurs, the mortality rate is reported to be 1.7% if it is recognized and repaired. However, if the enterotomy is missed, the mortality rate increases to 7.7%.[54] Management of a recognized intraoperative enterotomy varies according to the type and extent of the injured intestine and the type of mesh available. Small lacerations in the small intestine or bladder without significant contamination may not be an absolute contraindication to mesh placement either laparoscopically or by open means. In the event of fecal spillage, the bowel should be repaired and the adhesiolysis completed. A delayed hernia repair is generally warranted if a prosthetic is required. At times, the patient may be placed on antibiotics and returned to the operating room in 3 or 4 days for definitive repair. The safer option, however, is to perform a primary repair of the hernia defect or repair with a biologic mesh, but the long-term durability of these repairs is poor. We believe that placement of an intraperitoneal synthetic mesh in the presence of significant contamination is contraindicated. Another alternative that should be strongly considered is a conversion to laparotomy. This would include careful inspection of the entire bowel for other unrecognized injuries, and repair or resection of the involved segment followed by primary closure or extraperitoneal repair with mesh.

SPECIAL CONSIDERATIONS

UMBILICAL HERNIAS

Umbilical hernias are relatively common in the adult population and are another example of a spontaneous ventral hernia. More than 166,000 umbilical hernia repairs are performed annually in the United States, making it the second most prevalent abdominal wall hernia after inguinal hernia.[1] These umbilical hernias can be the result of a recurrence or persistent congenital umbilical hernia. In 90% of patients, it is an acquired defect that is a direct result of chronically increased abdominal pressure. Numerous factors have been linked to increased abdominal pressure including multiparous status, obesity, and cirrhosis with ascites.[4] Umbilical hernias tend to be more common in females and often develop in the fourth to fifth decade of life. The fascial ring that constitutes the neck of the hernia can be dense and is formed by gradual yielding of the cicatricial tissue closing the umbilical ring. In children younger than 2 years old, most umbilical hernias close spontaneously; however, in adults these hernias tend to enlarge with time.

Repair of an umbilical hernia, as described by William Mayo, using a vertical fascial overlap technique was discussed earlier. This operation (or simple fascial closure) is still performed frequently today by many surgeons. These repairs are effective and may be the preferred technique for small umbilical hernias with no tension after fascial approximation, but larger hernias have been shown to have a recurrence rate of up to 28%.[55]

The introduction of mesh prosthetics has appropriately had an impact on umbilical hernia repair. These tension-free repairs, which have been popularized for other ventral hernias, may have a role in umbilical hernia repair. The largest randomized controlled trial looking at mesh in umbilical hernia repair was completed in 2001 by Arroyo et al. This randomized controlled trial compared primary suture repair and mesh repair in 200 patients with umbilical hernias.[56] The two patient groups were comparable with regard to age, sex, hernia defect size, and American Society of Anesthesiologists (ASA) class. Operative times and complications were not statistically different. The mean follow-up was 64 months. The major difference was the recurrence rate of 11% in the suture repair group versus 1% in the mesh repair group ($P = .0015$). A review of all randomized controlled trials and observational studies found no difference in complication rates associated with mesh use, and an odds ratio of 0.09 in favor of mesh in randomized controlled trials and 0.40 in observational studies support the use of mesh in reducing umbilical hernia recurrence.[57]

The ideal technique for placement of a prosthetic during umbilical hernia repair remains debatable. Laparoscopic techniques have recently been proposed for umbilical hernias as well. The technical aspects are essentially the same as those applied to other ventral hernia defects. The laparoscopic approach takes longer to perform, tends to have fewer complications, and has no recurrences reported in a small retrospective series. Criticism of the laparoscopic approach includes the need for general anesthesia to establish pneumoperitoneum, and the increased length and cost of operating time. Conversely, placement of trocars around but not through the umbilicus has the potential to avoid the wound-related complications associated with an incision directly over the mesh.

There are many effective methods to repair umbilical hernias. Each patient must be evaluated individually, and one method of repair may not apply to all cases. Small primary umbilical defects in low-risk patients can probably be repaired with sutures alone and achieve acceptable results. As the defect size increases, particularly in obese patients or manual laborers, a mesh prosthetic should be considered. Whether the repair is better performed via an open or laparoscopic approach is controversial because prospective data are not available. Improvements in mesh prosthetics may continue to guide the ideal approach.

SPIGELIAN HERNIAS

Adriaan van der Spiegel, a Belgian anatomist, was the first to describe the semilunar line as a concave region at the lateral border of the rectus muscle formed by the aponeurosis of the IO. More than 100 years later, in 1764, Klinkosh identified the "hernia of the spigelian line" as a distinct entity.

Although spigelian hernias are rare (accounting for 0.1% to 2% of all abdominal wall hernias), its diagnostic incidence has been rising because of improved imaging technology and incidental identification during laparoscopy. Spigelian hernias usually occur in the sixth and seventh decades and affect both sexes and sides equally. Most are acquired, and nearly 50% of patients with spigelian hernias have a history of previous laparotomy or laparoscopy.[58] Other factors that have been implicated in contributing to the development of these hernias are alterations in compliance of the abdominal wall as a result of morbid obesity, multiple pregnancies, prostatic enlargement, chronic pulmonary disease, and rapid weight loss in obese patients.[58]

A spigelian hernia is a challenge to diagnose and requires a high index of suspicion. Pain is the most common initial complaint. The fascial defect is masked by the intact overlying EO aponeurosis, thus complicating physical examination.[59] In addition, a palpable mass (when present) may mimic an abdominal wall lipoma or desmoid tumor. Although abdominal imaging may be helpful, the findings of unusual abdominal complaints in the proper anatomic location should alert one to the possibility of a spigelian hernia. More than half of all spigelian hernias are diagnosed intraoperatively.[58]

Given the small neck of these hernias, 20% to 30% require emergency intervention.[58-60] Thus, even incidental spigelian hernias should be repaired electively to avoid incarceration. Surgical management of these hernias has typically been accomplished via a transverse incision and primary repair. Primary repairs have been associated with a low, but real recurrence rate of about 4%.[59] As expected, mesh repairs have been successfully applied to treat spigelian hernias. Few or no recurrences at long-term follow-up have been reported by investigators.[59] More recently, laparoscopic repair of spigelian hernias has also been reported and found to be safe and effective, although long-term recurrence outcomes are awaited.[60] Evidence-based surgical recommendations are limited by the rarity of this condition, and a recommendation regarding suture- or mesh-based repair (either open or laparoscopic) is not clear at present for the treatment of spigelian hernias.

SUPRAPUBIC HERNIAS

The abdominal oblique aponeurosis, rectus abdominis musculature, and rectus sheath insert on the symphysis pubis. Suprapubic hernias result from disruption of these musculotendinous elements of the lower abdominal wall and usually occur after blunt abdominal trauma or pelvic surgery. The origin of traumatic suprapubic hernias is often through a ruptured rectus muscle at or near its insertion to the pubic bone. In contrast, incisional suprapubic hernias develop as a result of apical pubic osteotomy or iatrogenic detachment of the rectus muscle from its pubic insertion to improve visualization during pelvic surgery. Inadequate tissue purchase inferiorly during closure may result in hernia formation, although infection and other

patient factors may also play a role. Radical prostatectomy is the most common operative procedure that leads to the development of a suprapubic defect. Similar defects are also seen after operations involving the uterus, urinary bladder, and sigmoid colon.

Suprapubic hernias may manifest as vague lower abdominal discomfort, urinary symptoms, or a palpable mass. The diagnosis of a suprapubic hernia may be missed because of the similarity of features with more common inguinal hernias. However, a thorough physical examination will demonstrate close proximity of the mass, defect, or both to the pubis and not the external inguinal ring. Although suprapubic hernias may be a source of significant abdominal pain, bowel incarceration requiring emergency repair is extremely rare.

Primary repair of traumatic suprapubic hernias may be a viable alternative if the herniorrhaphy is undertaken without delay. With time, the rectus muscle retracts and can lead to significant tension if primary repair is performed. Thus, a mesh repair is preferred for most traumatic and incisional suprapubic hernia repairs. Several approaches to mesh placement for suprapubic hernias have been described. The open preperitoneal approach provides excellent delineation of the bladder and pubis and allows for appropriate inferior fixation of the mesh in contrast to an onlay style of repair. The laparoscopic approach to suprapubic herniorrhaphy can also allow for a solid repair, provided that mobilization of the bladder is performed. This can be facilitated by using a three-way urinary catheter. The bladder is instilled with 300 mL of saline and can be clearly visualized for adequate mobilization to expose the entire pubis, Cooper ligament, and the iliac vessels. This is imperative to prevent inadequate overlap of the mesh and early recurrence. Regardless of the approach (open or laparoscopic), the dissection can be challenging because of the close proximity of these hernias to bony, vascular, and nerve structures, and to the bladder.

ABDOMINAL RELEASE PROCEDURES

Many complex and often multiply recurrent incisional hernias are not amenable to basic repairs or traditional laparoscopic techniques. Those patients frequently need more advanced reconstructive procedures to address their defects in order to provide a durable and functional repair. These patients require abdominal release or component separation procedures to provide for excessive-tension-free closure and reduce the risk of recurrence. Component separations include a variety of techniques wherein the layers of the abdominal wall are strategically divided and separated for the purpose of medialization of the rectus muscles and restoration of the linea alba. In other words, the redundancy of layers of anterior and lateral abdominal walls allows for sacrifice of one or several of its components to provide for myofasciocutaneous medialization aimed at restoring near-normal anatomy and physiology to the entire abdominal wall.

ANTERIOR COMPONENT SEPARATION

In 1990, Ramirez refined the technique of EO release that had been described in the early 20th century.[61] About a decade after its initial introduction, anterior component separation (ACS) became the most commonly employed reconstructive technique. Given the wide dissection required to reach the EO for division and separation, it also allows for wide mesh overlap. However, ACS is also fraught with a high potential for wound complications due to creation (and devascularization) of large skin flaps raised during dissection. In fact, wound morbidity of ACS has been reported to be 26% to 63%.[62] However, refinements that are described later, such as endoscopic ACS and perforator-sparing ACS, have successfully reduced the wound complication rates to 2% to 26%.[62]

Operative Technique

The patient is positioned supine on the operating table with arms out, and an orogastric tube and urinary catheter are placed. The abdomen is prepared with hair removal and sterilized widely. A laparotomy incision is made, and as needed can include teardrop or elliptical incisions to excise attenuated skin and scar tissue. A transverse incision can also be used and is often deployed when simultaneous panniculectomy or abdominoplasty is planned. Safe surgical access to the abdomen is imperative to avoid bowel injury and contaminating the field. In some cases, it is possible to remain extraperitoneal to avoid a hostile abdomen and the added time and morbidity of a long adhesiolysis. Once the abdomen is entered, a safe and complete adhesiolysis between the viscera and abdominal wall should be performed.

Next, the anterior fascia of the rectus abdominis muscle is identified and subcutaneous flaps are created. The skin and soft tissue are released from the anterior rectus fascia using electrocautery. These flaps are raised from the costal margin to the inguinal ligament and laterally to the midclavicular or anterior axillary line. The EO aponeurosis can be clearly identified by the directionality of its fibers and is incised 1 to 2 cm lateral to the semilunar line in a vertical fashion from the costal margin to just above the inguinal ligament. It is crucial to properly identify and protect the semilunar line. If this incision is made lateral enough to expose the muscle fibers of the EO, then the muscle fibers are divided using electrocautery and right angle dissector to avoid injury to the underlying IO aponeurosis (Fig. 52.5A). The muscle fibers should be divided along the length of the incision and can be extended above the costal margin to aid in the closure of subxiphoid or epigastric defects. Once the EO complex is divided, the EO muscle should be "separated" laterally from the underlying IO aponeurosis using blunt dissection along the avascular plane. Complete separation of the EO is critical to remove its contribution to the tension of the lateral abdominal wall, thus facilitating subsequent medialization of the rectus abdominis complex. If this release does not allow for sufficient medial advancement, a posterior rectus sheath release can also be performed. This release is accomplished by incising the posterior rectus sheath along the muscle body of the rectus to allow the rectus to be freed from its fascial encasement and facilitate its medialization. Both maneuvers were described by Ramirez et al.[61]

Once adequate release has been performed, mesh placement can be completed. The choice may depend on wound class, comorbidities, and other factors. Mesh positioning is also a choice the surgeon must make at

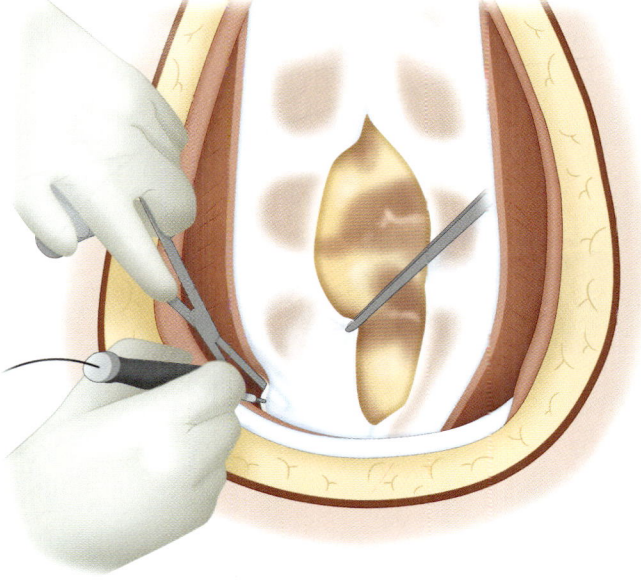

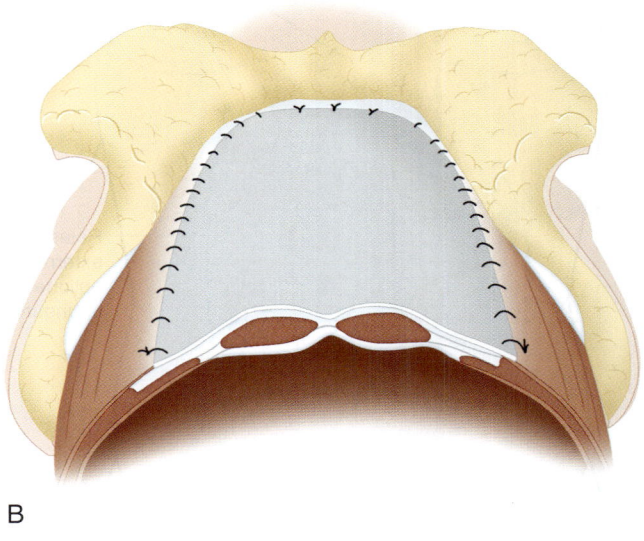

B

A

FIGURE 52.5 Anterior component separation (ACS) technique. (A) Skin flaps are raised laterally from midline, and bilateral external oblique fascia and muscle are cut to expose internal oblique muscle fibers to allow for midline closure of healthy anterior rectus sheath to re-create the linea alba. (B) Wide onlay mesh overlap after ACS with mesh fixed to the cut edges of the EO and re-created linea alba. (Based on Silverman R. Open component separation. In: Rosen M, ed. *Atlas of Abdominal Wall Reconstruction*. Philadelphia: Elsevier; 2012:131–138.)

this point. The mesh can be placed as an intraperitoneal underlay, as a sublay in the posterior rectus space, or as an onlay above the anterior rectus fascia (see Fig. 52.5B). Intraperitoneal mesh must be secured with circumferential transfascial sutures along the edge of the mesh, closing the space to abdominal contents. It must also be secured with some tension across the midline to allow for approximation of the fascia ventral to the taut mesh. To accomplish that, we measure half the width of the mesh from the midline closure to place our lateral sutures. Onlay mesh is placed after re-creation of the linea alba and is secured to the cut edges of the EO aponeurosis. Fibrin glue has also been used as an adjunct in mesh fixation for onlay meshes.[63] Large-bore closed-suction drains should be left ventral to the mesh, regardless of its position within the abdominal wall.

Midline fascial closure should be completed with absorbable monofilament suture either in a running fashion or using interrupted figure-of-eight sutures to achieve reconstruction of the linea alba and approximation of the rectus abdominis muscles. Soft tissue closure after ACS is of great importance because subcutaneous flaps can be a source of major wound and mesh morbidity. Dead space between subcutaneous tissue and fascia or mesh must be dealt with to avoid seroma and hematoma formation. This can be achieved with closed-suction drains or suturing the soft tissue back down to the fascia with progressive tension suture technique. Any old scars, as well as ischemic or devascularized, attenuated and redundant skin and soft tissue must be excised. We then suggest a layered closure of the soft tissue with absorbable sutures and skin staples.

PERIUMBILICAL PERFORATOR-SPARING ANTERIOR COMPONENT SEPARATION

The skin of the central abdominal wall gets its blood supply from the deep inferior and superior epigastric vessels. The deep epigastric vessels divide into a vast network of musculocutaneous perforating branches and are concentrated in the periumbilical region to provide the majority of vascularity to the central abdominal wall. Therefore, to combat the significant wound morbidity caused by the creation of the necessary large undermined subcutaneous flaps, Dumanian was first to develop a perforator-sparing component separation technique. The goal is to maintain pulsatile blood flow to the reapproximated tissue of the hernia repair and to release lateral tension at the midline.[64,65] Wound complications have been found to be reduced by 50% to 90% with techniques that allow for preservation of the periumbilical perforators of the abdominal wall.[64,65]

Perforator-sparing ACS can be completed via lateral incisions or via tunneling from the midline at the inferior and superior portions of the laparotomy incision (Fig. 52.6). If a lateral incision is used, a 6-cm incision should be made transversely at the costal margin and subcutaneous tissues divided until the EO fascia is identified. The EO fascia is incised and the EO muscle is bluntly separated from the underlying IO fascia. A tunnel in this plane is developed bluntly with finger dissection and the aid of a

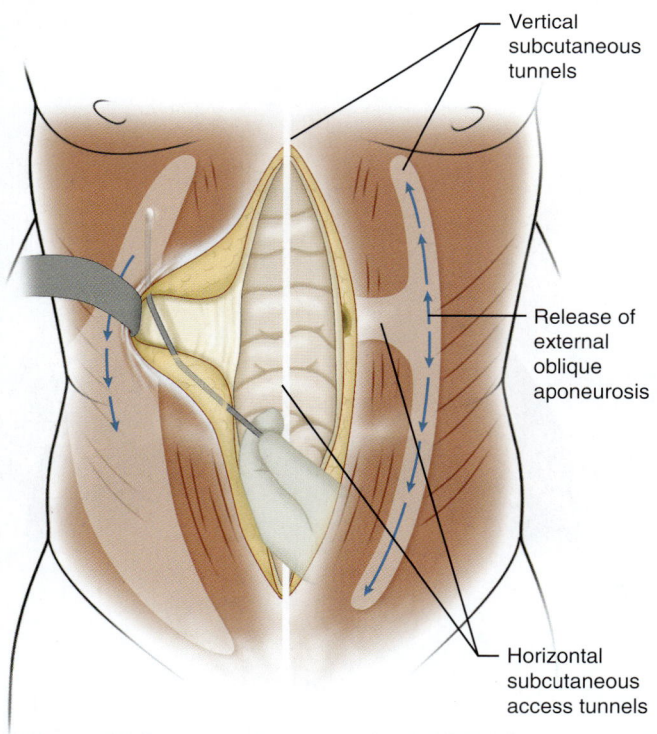

Vertical subcutaneous tunnels

Release of external oblique aponeurosis

Horizontal subcutaneous access tunnels

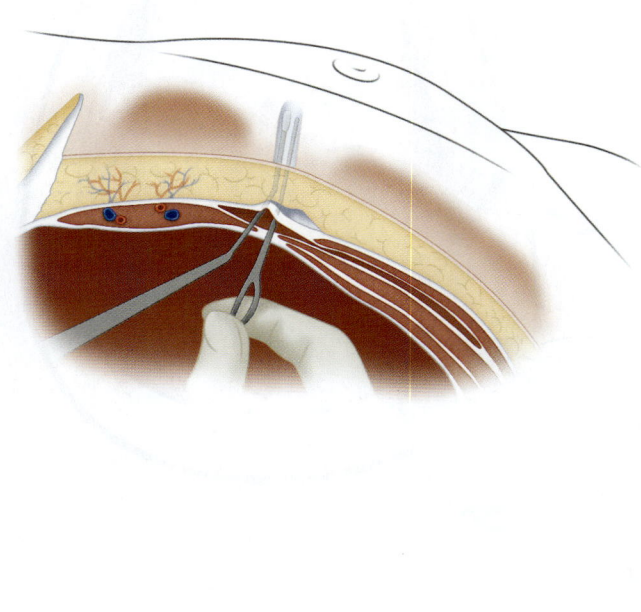

FIGURE 52.6 Perforator-sparing anterior component separation with lateral subcutaneous tunnel dissection. (Based on Dumanian GA. Open anterior component separation with perforator preservation. In: Novitsky YW, ed. *Hernia Surgery: Current Principles*. New York: Springer; 2016:150–158.)

lighted retractor for the length of the abdomen, spanning from inferior to the inguinal ligament to superior to the costal margin. The EO fascia and muscle is divided along the length of the tunnels and the external and IO muscles separated laterally in the avascular plane. Alternatively, subcutaneous tunnels can be created by lifting the soft tissue from the anterior rectus sheath starting at the midline and reaching laterally beyond the semilunar line. Superior and inferior such tunnels can be created until they meet in the middle lateral to the semilunar line, thus sparing the periumbilical perforators of the soft tissue dissection. Within this tunnel the EO fascia and muscles are divided and bluntly separated from the underlying IO fascia. Once the release is completed, the tunnels can be closed or drained and the hernia is repaired with mesh in the intraperitoneal underlay or retrorectus dissection.

ENDOSCOPIC SEPARATION OF COMPONENTS

In an effort to minimalize the morbidity of the ACS, a minimally invasive, endoscopic component separation technique (ECST) was described by Lowe et al. in 2000.[66] This was created to address the extensive lateral dissection required for EO release, thus creating large subcutaneous flaps and requiring ligation of perforating vessels and leading to wound infection rates of 25% to 57%. ECST provides the benefit of medialization of the abdominal wall allowing for tension-free closure during hernia repair, while limiting subcutaneous dissection and preserving deep periumbilical perforators.[67] It also allows for dissection and release within a clean plane, avoiding ostomy sites and infected prosthetics or midline processes.[68] ECST must be accompanied by midline closure and mesh reinforcement; options include open laparotomy at the midline with onlay mesh placement after raising subcutaneous flaps, open laparotomy with retrorectus dissection and sublay mesh placement, or laparoscopic ventral hernia repair with defect closure and intraperitoneal underlay mesh placement.

The patient is placed in the supine position with arms tucked. A 2- to 4-cm transverse incision is made near the costal margin at the tip of the 11th rib. The EO muscle fibers are identified and separated from the underlying IO fascia. A round balloon dissector is introduced between the EO muscle and IO fascia and pushed blindly toward the inguinal ligament medial to the anterior superior iliac spine. The balloon dissector is then inflated sequentially from distal to proximal, and then aimed toward the costal margin and inflated in the superior space. Three ports are placed and the EO insertion is divided sharply and with cautery along the subcutaneous tissue and fascia ventral to the dissection plane. Ventral hernia repair is then completed in the fashion chosen by the operating surgeon.

Advantages of ECST over open ACS include lower rates of wound necrosis, dehiscence, and infections, with wound complication rates reduced by almost 50%.[69] However, open ACS has shown a lower recurrence rate and lower rate of intraabdominal abscess formation.[67] Limitations of ECST include the possibility of inadvertent division of the linea semilunaris and creation of postoperative flank hernias with limited options for reinforcement of the area of release, limited options for mesh placement, and limited utility for nonmidline defects.

POSTERIOR COMPONENT SEPARATION

The French surgeons Jean Rives and Rene Stoppa revolutionized hernia repair by popularizing a retrorectus repair with a large prosthetic.[70,71] The prosthetic is placed in the preperitoneal space below the arcuate line or just superficial to the posterior rectus sheath above the umbilicus. Transfascial sutures are placed through the mesh to secure the prosthetic to the fascia and redistribute the forces of the abdominal wall away from the midline closure to the lateral abdominal wall.[72] In addition to mesh repair, the midline fascia is closed, which can restore the previously displaced abdominal muscle into a more anatomic position. In fact, Rives and Stoppa emphasized creation of "physiologic tension" at the midline to ensure a functional repair. Drains are then placed above the prosthetic. This method has a documented recurrence rate from 5% to 14%.[70,73] The advantages of a large mesh with significant overlap placed under the muscular abdominal wall can be explained by Pascal's principles of hydrostatics. Because the intraabdominal cavity functions as a cylinder, the pressure is distributed uniformly to all aspects of the system. Consequently, the same forces that are attempting to push the mesh through open hernia defects are also holding the mesh in place against the intact abdominal wall. In this manner, the prosthetic is held in place by intraabdominal pressure.

Operative Technique

A full laparotomy incision is made and adhesiolysis is carried out as needed. The posterior rectus release begins with the incision of the posterior rectus sheath at its most medial border, confirming the location of the rectus muscle ventral to the initial incision. This incision is taken along the full length of the rectus muscle, cranially to the xiphoid and caudally to the arcuate line and into the space of Retzius. The posterior sheath is dissected free from the rectus abdominus muscle medially to laterally using blunt dissection and electrocautery. This is a mostly avascular plane until the lateral edge of the rectus muscle is reached and deep perforating vessels are encountered. As the lateral edge is reached, the epigastric vessels can be visualized and should remain with the muscle body. The dissection is complete when the semilunar line has been reached. It is important to identify neurovascular bundles as they perforate the posterior rectus sheath just medial to the linea semilunaris. Superiorly this dissection leads into the subxiphoid space and the insertions of posterior sheath at the xiphoid can be incised to allow access into this plane across the midline. Inferiorly, the dissection leads into the space of Retzius; blunt dissection is performed to skeletonize the pubic symphysis and bilateral Cooper ligaments.

After bilateral retrorectus dissections are performed, posterior sheaths are reapproximated using running absorbable sutures. A mesh of choice is measured to fit the retrorectus space and is fixed with transfascial sutures at the lateral edges, ensuring sufficient overlap of the repaired hernia defect and physiologic tension of the mesh. Large-bore closed-suction drains may be placed ventral to the mesh if preferred. Finally, the linea alba is re-created ventral to the mesh by approximating anterior rectus fascia at the midline using slowly absorbable monofilament suture. Skin and soft tissue are closed in a layered fashion.

TRANSVERSUS ABDOMINIS RELEASE

We first performed the transversus abdominis release (TAR) procedure in 2006 with initial presentation of our early experience at the 2009 World Hernia Conference. Although it was originally met with skepticism, after subsequent publication of the technical description and outcomes in 2012, the TAR is rapidly becoming one of the fastest growing approaches to major abdominal wall reconstructions. The TAR procedure, a type of posterior component separation, is essentially an extension of the posterior rectus release described earlier. The TAR approach allows for significant medial advancement of the posterior rectus sheath, creates a large retromuscular pocket of vascularized tissue for placement of large meshes, and the reinforcement of the entire visceral sac. Moreover, it allows for the medialization of the rectus muscles and effective reconstruction of the linea alba.[74] The TAR technique has been shown to be durable and reliable in a number of series with recurrence rates between 3.7% and 5%.[75,76] It has also been found to be safe and effective for repairing recurrent ventral incisional hernias following ACS. Finally, TAR allows access to the space above the xiphoid and costal margins, aiding in repair of complex subcostal and subxiphoid hernias.

Operative Technique

The patient is positioned supine on the operating table with both arms out. A urinary catheter and orogastric tube are placed preoperatively, and the patient is prepped from nipples to thighs and laterally to the edge of the bed. The abdomen is draped using an iodoform-impregnated drape (Ioban; 3M, St. Paul, Minnesota). First, a generous midline incision is made and can be completed in linear, elliptical, or teardrop fashion for excision of old scar and excess soft tissue. Although some surgeons have advocated a completely extraperitoneal dissection,[77] we prefer a complete adhesiolysis to remove all visceral adhesions to the anterior abdominal wall. This reduces the risk of injury to underlying organs and allows for lateral retromuscular dissection and release. We reserve interloop adhesiolysis for patients who had obstructive symptoms in the preoperative period.

We then proceed with the posterior rectus sheath release and retrorectus dissection as described earlier, continuing this dissection laterally to the linea semilunaris and carefully identifying and preserving perforating neurovascular bundles (Fig. 52.7). Exposure and division of the transversus abdominis muscle (TAM) is begun by the incision of the posterior sheath 1 cm medial to the perforating vessels, as cephalad as possible. This incision exposes the muscular aspect of the TAM in the superior portion of the abdomen and the aponeurotic aspect in the inferior portion. The TAM fibers are then divided with electrocautery, using a right-angled dissector to isolate and lift the fibers from the underlying transversalis fascia and/ or peritoneum. This division is completed cranial-caudally until there is complete transection of the TAM and its aponeurosis. At the level of the arcuate line, the surgeon must make a transition into the preperitoneal space and divide the arcuate line laterally at its junction with the semilunar line.

Lateral and retroperitoneal dissections are then undertaken with the aid of a Kittner dissector using proper traction and counter-traction to separate the TAM from the underlying transversalis fascia. Once this plane is created, it can be continued laterally using blunt dissection until the retroperitoneum is reached and the psoas muscle is identified, if necessary. Dissection following the lateral edge of the psoas muscle caudally allows for identification of the entire myopectineal orifice and allows access to the space of Retzius and Cooper ligaments. In women, round ligaments are divided. In men, spermatic cord should be identified and protected.

The superior dissection is now undertaken, and depending on the location of the hernia, the cranial extent of the dissection may be in the epigastrium or the subxiphoid space. In the epigastrium, the posterior sheath must be disconnected from its insertion into the linea alba bilaterally to allow for sufficient mesh overlap cranially from the hernia defect. This is done by incising the insertion of the posterior sheath just lateral to the linea alba bilaterally, allowing intact linea alba to lift away and disconnecting either side of the posterior sheath. This should be done for at least 5 cm to allow for sufficient mesh overlap and prevent superior recurrences. For defects that already reach into the epigastrium, the subxiphoid and substernal spaces are entered to allow for sufficient dissection and mesh placement. To enter these spaces, the posterior sheath insertions to the xiphoid are divided. The most cranial transversus abdominis muscle fibers must be divided and the pretransversalis plane will lead into the retrosternal space. One must be careful not to divide the fibers of the anterior diaphragm because they interdigitate with the transversus abdominis at this level. Once this dissection into the pretransversalis plane is completed bilaterally, the two planes can be connected by dissecting above the subxiphoid fat pad. This dissection may be continued into the retrosternal space by separating transversalis fascia from the diaphragm until the central tendon of the diaphragm is exposed.

The next step is to reconnect medialized posterior layers and to re-create a continuous visceral sac with running absorbable sutures. Any small holes in the posterior layer may be closed with figure-of-eight or interrupted absorbable sutures, and any larger gaps in the posterior layer can be filled with an interposition of polyglactin (Vicryl Mesh; Ethicon, Somerville, New Jersey) or biologic mesh. Once the posterior sheath is closed, the abdominal contents are now excluded from the operative space. Generous irrigation of the retromuscular space is completed. We use antibiotic-laden irrigation (cephazolin 3 g, gentamicin 240 mg, Bacitracin 50,000 units per 3 L of normal saline) with a power irrigator in contaminated or clean-contaminated cases.

A mesh is then measured to fill the entire retromuscular space. We generally favor a midweight macroporous polypropylene mesh in most of our cases, although a heavier weight polypropylene may be used for unusual hernias such as flank hernias or in cases where the linea alba is either not restored or restored under significant tension.

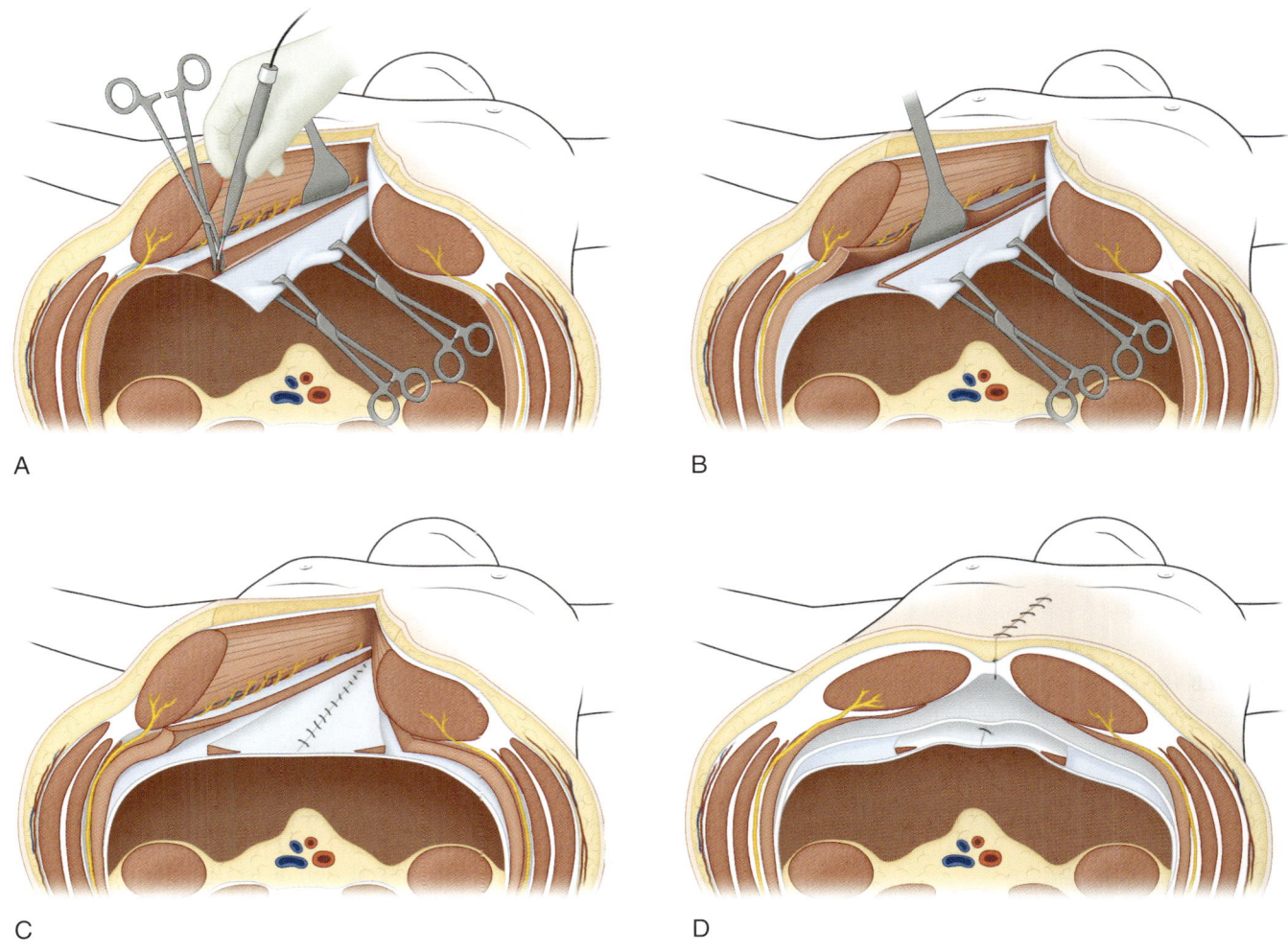

A

B

C

D

FIGURE 52.7 Transversus abdominis release (TAR) technique. (A) Incision of the transversus abdominis muscle after posterior rectus sheath release and incision. (B) Medialization of posterior sheath with TAR and lateral dissection. (C) Closure of the posterior sheath after bilateral TARs and exclusion of abdominal contents. (D) Reinforcement of visceral sac with large retromuscular mesh sublay and re-creation of the linea alba. (Based on Novitsky YW. Posterior component separation via transversus abdominis muscle release: the TAR procedure. In: Novitsky YW. *Hernia Surgery: Current Principles*. New York: Springer; 2016:117–136.)

Fixation of the mesh is done with long-lasting absorbable sutures to bilateral Cooper ligaments and transfascial sutures at the xiphoid. Lateral transfascial fixation can be done with a straight suture passer or a Reverdin needle, although recently we have found this to be superfluous, because the large mesh has limited mobility within the retromuscular space. Large closed-suction drains are placed ventral to the mesh and brought out laterally through the abdominal wall. Finally, the anterior fascia is closed with running or interrupted figure-of-eight sutures, and the skin and soft tissue are closed in layers after excision of any excess tissue.

Cautionary Note

Component separation procedures, including the TAR and ACS, should be used with care and only by surgeons who have been trained or are very familiar with the nuances of the procedures. It is possible to destabilize the entire abdominal wall by transecting the semilunar line or to create an iatrogenic Morgagni hernia during the TAR

dissection if the anatomy is unfamiliar. Similarly, there is a possibility of injury and destabilization of the lateral abdominal wall and resultant bulging/hernias, if the linea semilunaris or the IOs are injured during the ACS. Furthermore, there is a significant risk for soft tissue necrosis after raising soft tissue flaps to allow for EO release, which can be quite morbid, with possible exposure and infection of the underlying mesh. Component separations should be used for select patients only and indications for the procedure should be part of an algorithm for treatment of complex abdominal wall hernias.

HERNIA REPAIR ALGORITHM

As mentioned throughout the chapter, it is important to have a hernia repair algorithm and many possible approaches that can be tailored to individual cases. This algorithm takes into account patient and hernia characteristics to help with clinical decision making and technique selection. In Figs. 52.8 and 52.9 we have outlined

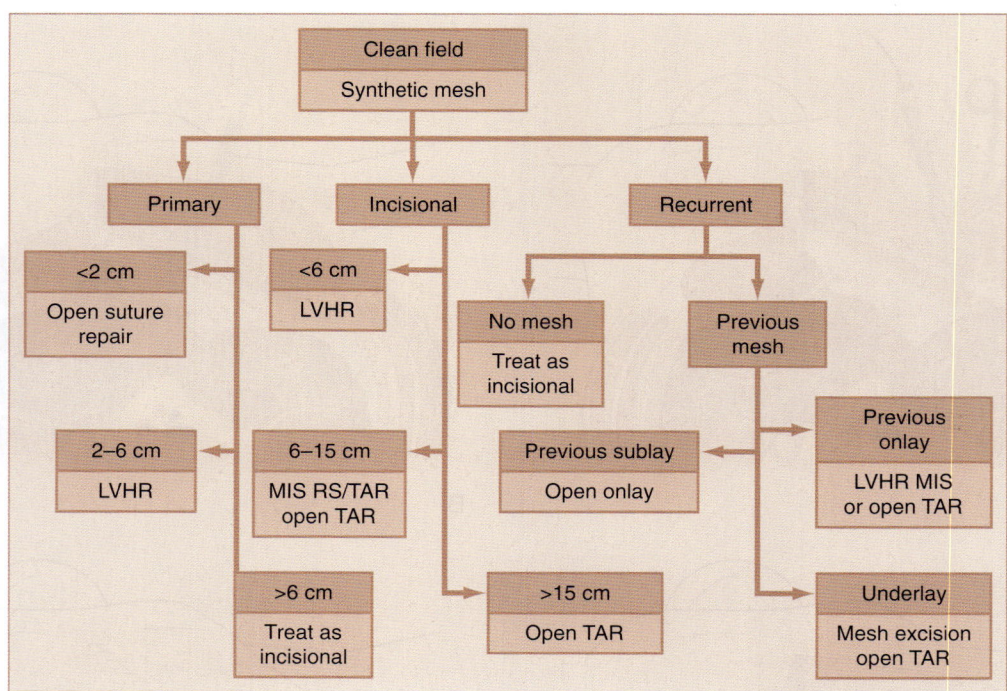

FIGURE 52.8 Hernia repair algorithm for clean fields. *LVHR*, Laparoscopic ventral hernia repair; *MIS,* minimally invasive surgery; *RS,* Rives-Stoppa; *TAR*, transversus abdominis release.

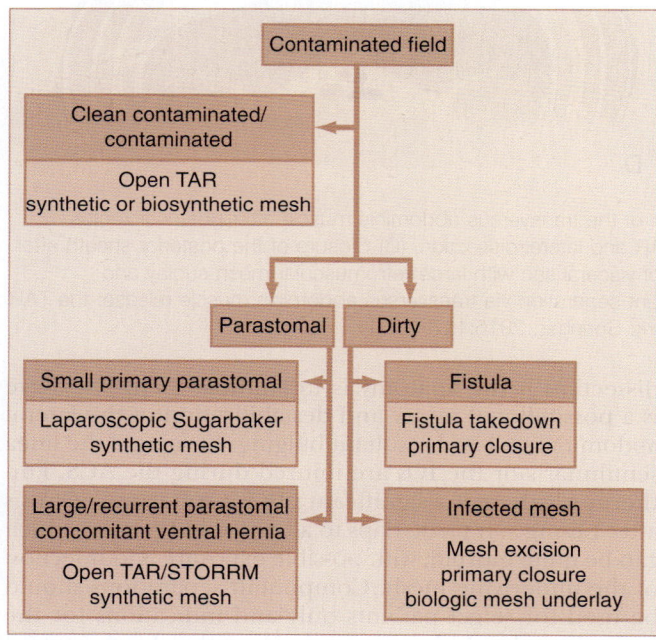

FIGURE 52.9 Hernia repair algorithm for contaminated fields. *TAR,* Transversus abdominis release; *STORRM,* Stapled transabdominal ostomy reinforcement with retromuscular mesh.

our hernia repair algorithm. Fig. 52.8 shows options for hernia repairs taking place in a clean field. Primary ventral hernias that are less than 2 cm in diameter we will close with an open suture repair using a permanent monofilament suture with tension-free closure. Any primary ventral hernia larger than 2 cm or incisional hernia less than 6 cm will receive an LVHR with defect closure and wide mesh overlap. We deploy the laparoscopic shoelacing technique described earlier and place transfascial sutures just lateral to the closed defect to distribute tension to the mesh. Incisional and primary ventral hernias that are larger than 6 cm are repaired via a retromuscular repair. For those patients who are conducive to minimally invasive repair, usually between 6 and 15 cm and without any skin defects or soft tissue issues, we may apply a laparoscopic, endoscopic, or robotic Rives-Stoppa (RS) or TAR procedure. Absolute contraindications to minimally invasive repairs include presence of significant skin/soft tissue issues, including thinned skin, history of skin grafts or wounds healed by secondary intention, and previous intraperitoneal mesh and/or a hostile abdomen. Patients presenting with any of these contraindications or hernias larger than 12 to 15 cm in width are approached with an open TAR. Recurrent hernias present a potentially more complex problem because of meshes used in previous repairs. In clean fields with no evidence of mesh complications we try to use an approach away from previous dissections. Patients with previous sublay such as RS, TAR, or preperitoneal mesh placement are best served with an open onlay repair with or without ACS, as needed. Failed onlay repairs are treated with retromuscular or LVHR approaches. Finally, for failed underlay or IPOM repairs we typically excise old mesh and employ an open TAR procedure.

Fig. 52.9 presents our decision-making algorithm for hernia repairs within contaminated fields. Clean-contaminated and contaminated fields may contain previous infections or draining sinuses or concomitant procedures such as colon resections or cholecystectomy.

There is limited use of minimally invasive hernia repair in contaminated fields; however we may consider a minimally invasive surgery (MIS) retromuscular repair for clean-contaminated cases with concomitant procedures. We generally approach contaminated fields with an open TAR and most often will use synthetic mesh. Biosynthetic or biologic meshes are used for patients with latent or active methicillin-resistant *Staphylococcus aureus* (MRSA) infections. Parastomal hernia repairs are described elsewhere in this book, but are included here within our algorithm. For small parastomal hernias, we use a laparoscopic mesh repair and prefer the Sugarbaker method. For large or recurrent parastomal hernias, or those with ventral hernia components, we use synthetic mesh in the retromuscular space using TAR with ostomy reinforcement with mesh. Finally, for dirty fields we will generally approach with planned staging and close primarily or reinforce with a biologic underlay. Grossly infected meshes are excised and primary repair is reinforced with an underlay biologic mesh to delay a hernia recurrence. This strategy allows us to leave the retromuscular space intact for future definitive reconstruction via TAR.

ENHANCED RECOVERY PATHWAYS AFTER ABDOMINAL WALL RECONSTRUCTION

Since 2013, our institution has implemented a multimodal enhanced recovery after surgery protocol, also known as the "pathway," to optimize abdominal wall reconstruction patients and outcomes. Our pathway begins at the initial evaluation and includes preoperative optimization that requires patient participation and buy-in. Weight loss counseling is provided and goals are set with the patient along with referrals to a medical weight loss or bariatric surgery program if necessary. Elimination of obesity remains our main goal; however, many patients are unable to achieve that, especially in the setting of significant abdominal discomfort or obstructive symptoms. With that in mind, we recently evaluated our data and identified a BMI of 45 as an upper cutoff for elective repairs, given a significant jump in postoperative wound complications in that cohort. Furthermore, diabetes management is extremely important. We require all patients to achieve better glycemic control and an HbA1c less than 7.5 is now mandated prior to scheduling surgery. Smoking cessation is also required for a minimum of 4 weeks and serum cotinine testing is undertaken at the patient's preanesthesia testing (PAT) appointment. Finally, as a part of nutritional optimization, we provide arginine and omega-3-rich supplementation (IMPACT Advanced Recovery; Nestle) shakes three times daily for 5 days). Finally, all patients are screened for obstructive sleep apnea (OSA) and MRSA. Perioperatively, patients receive subcutaneous heparin injections, a first-generation cephalosporin (those with positive MRSA screens also receive vancomycin), gabapentin, and alvimopan. Postoperatively, the pathway includes multimodal pain control with acetaminophen, gabapentin, intravenous and oral nonsteroidal antiinflammatory drugs (NSAIDS), and minimization of narcotics usage. Finally, enhanced gastrointestinal (GI) recovery includes limited use of nasogastric tubes, daily alvimopan, and a scheduled early diet advancement. We have found our outcomes greatly improved with the use of the pathway; as expected, patients have a quicker time to bowel function and advancement to regular diet. Furthermore, we have seen a shorter hospital length of stay, decreased to an average of 4 days from 6.1, and a lower 90-day readmission rate.[78] We also have integrated a nurse practitioner into the care of our abdominal wall reconstruction patients, allowing for better preoperative education, easier access to clinic appointments, and earlier intervention for potential problems.

CONCLUSION

Ventral hernia is a complex disease process that requires the general surgeon to have a wide armamentarium of repair techniques. An understanding of abdominal wall anatomy and physiology is key for restoration of abdominal wall function. Prevention of incisional hernias is still under evaluation, but proper closure of laparotomies and thoughtful use of prophylactic mesh may reduce the incidence of this costly and morbid disease. Utilization of advanced reconstructive techniques requires careful patient selection, preoperative optimization and intricate knowledge of abdominal wall anatomy and technical nuances. Surgical mishaps result in significant patient morbidity, need for reoperations, and significant negative impact on quality of life. Techniques for repair and technologies of prosthetics will continue to evolve as we search for the ideal repair with restoration of normal abdominal function and durable long-term results for patients with routine and complex hernias.

REFERENCES

1. Poulose BK, Beck WC, Phillips SE, Sharp KW, Nealon WH, Holzman MD. The chosen few: disproportionate resource use in ventral hernia repair. *Am Surg*. 2013;79:815-818.
2. Poulose BK, Shelton J, Phillips S, et al. Epidemiology and cost of ventral hernia repair: making the case for hernia research. *Hernia*. 2012;16:179-183.
3. Flum DR, Horvath K, Koepsell T. Have outcomes of incisional hernia repair improved with time? A population-based analysis. *Ann Surg*. 2003;237:129-135.
4. Muysoms FE, Miserez M, Berrevoet F, et al. Classification of primary and incisional abdominal wall hernias. *Hernia*. 2009;13:407-414.
5. Earle DB, McLellan JA. Repair of umbilical and epigastric hernias. *Surg Clin North Am*. 2013;93:1057-1089.
6. Klink CD, Binnebösel M, Alizai HP, et al. Tension of knotted surgical sutures shows tissue specific rapid loss in a rodent model. *BMC Surg*. 2011;11:36.
7. Diener MK, Voss S, Jensen K, Büchler MW, Seiler CM. Elective midline laparotomy closure: the INLINE systematic review and meta-analysis. *Ann Surg*. 2010;251:843-856.
8. McLeod RS, Brenneman FD, Rotstein OD, Bhanot P. Effect of stitch length on wound complications after closure of midline incisions: a randomized controlled trial. *J Am Coll Surg*. 2013;217:556-559.
9. Deerenberg EB, Harlaar JJ, Steyerberg EW, et al. Small bites versus large bites for closure of abdominal midline incisions (STITCH): a double-blind, multicentre, randomised controlled trial. *Lancet*. 2015;386:1254-1260.
10. Harlaar JJ, Deerenberg EB, van Ramshorst GH, et al. A multicenter randomized controlled trial evaluating the effect of small stitches on the incidence of incisional hernia in midline incisions. *BMC Surg*. 2011;11:20.
11. Millbourn D, Wimo A, Israelsson LA. Cost analysis of the use of small stitches when closing midline abdominal incisions. *Hernia*. 2013;18:1-6. doi:10.1007/s10029-013-1135-2.

12. Bevis PM, Windhaber RA, Lear PA, Poskitt KR, Earnshaw JJ, Mitchell DC. Randomized clinical trial of mesh versus sutured wound closure after open abdominal aortic aneurysm surgery. *Br J Surg.* 2010;97:1497-1502.

13. Bhangu A, Fitzgerald JE, Singh P, Battersby N, Marriott P, Pinkney T. Systematic review and meta-analysis of prophylactic mesh placement for prevention of incisional hernia following midline laparotomy. *Hernia.* 2013;17:445-455.

14. Helgstrand F, Rosenberg J, Bisgaard T. Trocar site hernia after laparoscopic surgery: a qualitative systematic review. *Hernia.* 2011;15:113-121.

15. Boldó E, Perez de Lucia G, Aracil JP, et al. Trocar site hernia after laparoscopic ventral hernia repair. *Surg Endosc.* 2007;21:798-800.

16. Scozzari G, Zanini M, Cravero F, Passera R, Rebecchi F, Morino M. High incidence of trocar site hernia after laparoscopic or robotic Roux-en-Y gastric bypass. *Surg Endosc.* 2014;28:2890-2898.

17. Johnson WH, Fecher AM, McMahon RL, Grant JP, Pryor AD. VersaStep trocar hernia rate in unclosed fascial defects in bariatric patients. *Surg Endosc.* 2006;20:1584-1586.

18. Chiong E, Hegarty PK, Davis JW, Kamat AM, Pisters LL, Matin SF. Port-site hernias occurring after the use of bladeless radially expanding trocars. *Urology.* 2010;75:574-580.

19. Agaba EA, Rainville H, Ikedilo O, Vemulapali P. Incidence of port-site incisional hernia after single-incision laparoscopic surgery. *JSLS.* 2014;18:204-210.

20. Evans KK, Chim H, Patel KM, Salgado CJ, Mardini S. Survey on ventral hernias: surgeon indications, contraindications, and management of large ventral hernias. *Am Surg.* 2012;78:388-397.

21. Bellows CF, Robinson C, Fitzgibbons RJ, Webber LS, Berger DH. Watchful waiting for ventral hernias: a longitudinal study. *Am Surg.* 2014;80:245-252.

22. Fitzgibbons RJ, Giobbie-Hurder A, Gibbs JO, et al. Inguinal hernia in minimally symptomatic men. *JAMA.* 2006;295:285-293.

23. Lauscher JC, Loh JC, Grone J, Buhr HJ, Ritz J-P, Rieck S. Oligosymptomatic vs. symptomatic incisional hernias—who benefits from open repair? *Langenbecks Arch Surg.* 2011;396:179-185.

24. Wen Y, Fayezizadeh M, Majumder A, Miller H, Novitsky Y. Analysis of ventral hernia repair in the obese: defining the goals of preoperative weight loss; 2016. In: *17th Annual Hernia Repair.*

25. Burger JW, Luijendijk RW, Hop WC, Halm JA, Verdaasdonk EG, Jeekel J. Long-term follow-up of a randomized controlled trial of suture versus mesh repair of incisional hernia. *Ann Surg.* 2004;240:578-583, discussion 583–585.

26. Brown CN, Finch JG. Which mesh for hernia repair? *Ann R Coll Surg Engl.* 2010;92:272-278.

27. Bringman S, Conze J, Cuccurullo D, et al. Hernia repair: the search for ideal meshes. *Hernia.* 2010;14:81-87.

28. Albino FP, Patel KM, Nahabedian MY, Sosin M, Attinger CE, Bhanot P. Does mesh location matter in abdominal wall reconstruction? A systematic review of the literature and a summary of recommendations. *Plast Reconstr Surg.* 2013;132:1295-1304.

29. Breuing K, Butler CE, Ferzoco S, et al. Incisional ventral hernias: review of the literature and recommendations regarding the grading and technique of repair. *Surgery.* 2010;148:544-558.

30. Kanters AE, Krpata DM, Blatnik JA, Novitsky YM, Rosen MJ. Modified hernia grading scale to stratify surgical site occurrence after open ventral hernia repairs. *J Am Coll Surg.* 2012;215:787-793.

31. Carbonell AM, Criss CN, Cobb WS, Novitsky YW, Rosen MJ. Outcomes of synthetic mesh in contaminated ventral hernia repairs. *J Am Coll Surg.* 2013;217:991-998.

32. Majumder A, Winder JS, Wen Y, Pauli EM, Belyansky I, Novitsky YW. Comparative analysis of biologic versus synthetic mesh outcomes in contaminated hernia repairs. *Surgery.* 2016;160:828-838.

33. Al Chalabi H, Larkin J, Mehigan B, McCormick P. A systematic review of laparoscopic versus open abdominal incisional hernia repair, with meta-analysis of randomized controlled trials. *Int J Surg.* 2015;20:65-74.

34. Schluender S, Conrad J, Divino CM, Gurland B. Robot-assisted laparoscopic repair of ventral hernia with intracorporeal suturing. *Surg Endosc.* 2003;17:1391-1395.

35. Misiakos EP, Patapis P, Zavras N, Tzanetis P, Machairas A. Current trends in laparoscopic ventral hernia repair. *JSLS.* 2015;19:e2015.00048.

36. Sauerland S, Walgenbach M, Habermalz B, Seiler CM, Miserez M. Laparoscopic versus open surgical techniques for ventral or incisional hernia repair. *Cochrane Database Syst Rev.* 2011;(3):CD007781, doi:10.1002/14651858.CD007781.pub2.

37. Basile F, Biondi A, Donati M. Surgical approach to abdominal wall defects: history and new trends. *Int J Surg.* 2013;11:S20-S23.

38. Franklin ME, Dorman JP, Glass JL, Balli JE, Gonzalez JJ. Laparoscopic ventral and incisional hernia repair. *Surg Laparosc Endosc.* 1998;8:294-299.

39. Brown CN, Finch JG. Which mesh for hernia repair? *Ann R Coll Surg Engl.* 2010;92:272-278.

40. Colavita PD, Tsirline VB, Belyansky I, et al. Prospective, long-term comparison of quality of life in laparoscopic versus open ventral hernia repair. *Ann Surg.* 2012;256:714-723.

41. Prasad P, Tantia O, Patle NM, Khanna S, Sen B. Laparoscopic ventral hernia repair: a comparative study of transabdominal preperitoneal versus intraperitoneal onlay mesh repair. *J Laparoendosc Adv Surg Tech A.* 2011;21:477-483.

42. Orenstein SB, Dumeer JL, Monteagudo J, Poi MJ, Novitsky YW. Outcomes of laparoscopic ventral hernia repair with routine defect closure using 'shoelacing' technique. *Surg Endosc.* 2011;25:1452-1457.

43. Daes J. The enhanced view–totally extraperitoneal technique for repair of inguinal hernia. *Surg Endosc.* 2012;26:1187-1189.

44. Daes J. Endoscopic subcutaneous approach to component separation. *J Am Coll Surg.* 2014;218:e1-e4.

45. Köckerling F, Botsinis MD, Rohde C, Reinpold W. Endoscopic-assisted linea alba reconstruction plus mesh augmentation for treatment of umbilical and/or epigastric hernias and rectus abdominis diastasis—early results. *Front Surg.* 2016;3:27.

46. Reinpold W. Neue Techniken in der Narben- und Bauchwandhernienchirurgie. *Chirurgische Allgemeine.* 2013;14:331-337.

47. Belyansky I, Zahiri HR, Park A. Laparoscopic transversus abdominis release, a novel minimally invasive approach to complex abdominal wall reconstruction. *Surg Innov.* 2016;23:134-141.

48. Gonzalez AM, Rabaza JR, Seetharamaiah R, Donkor C, Romero R, Kosanovic R, et al. Laparoscopic vs robotic ventral hernia repair: a single group experience. http://www.sages.org/wp-content/uploads/posters/2013/45846.jpg 2013 Accessed 6 January 16.

49. Tran H. Robotic single-port hernia surgery. *JSLS.* 2011;15:309-314.

50. Tayar C, Karoui M, Cherqui D, Fagniez PL. Robot-assisted laparoscopic mesh repair of incisional hernias with exclusive intracorporeal suturing: a pilot study. *Surg Endosc.* 2007;21:1786-1789.

51. Nguyen DH, Nguyen MT, Askenasy EP, Kao LS, Liang MK. Primary fascial closure with laparoscopic ventral hernia repair: systematic review. *World J Surg.* 2014;38:3097-3104.

52. Booth JH, Garvey PB, Baumann DP, et al. Primary fascial closure with mesh reinforcement is superior to bridged mesh repair for abdominal wall reconstruction. *J Am Coll Surg.* 2013;217:999-1009.

53. Berger D, Bientzle M, Müller A. Postoperative complications after laparoscopic incisional hernia repair. Incidence and treatment. *Surg Endosc.* 2002;16:1720-1723.

54. LeBlanc KA, Elieson MJ, Corder JM. Enterotomy and mortality rates of laparoscopic incisional and ventral hernia repair: a review of the literature. *JSLS.* 2007;11:408-414.

55. Celdran A, Bazire P, Garcia-Urena M, Marijuán JL. H-hernioplasty: a tension-free repair for umbilical hernia. *Br J Surg.* 1995;82:371-372.

56. Arroyo A, García P, Pérez F, Andreu J, Candela F, Calpena R. Randomized clinical trial comparing suture and mesh repair of umbilical hernia in adults. *Br J Surg.* 2001;88:1321-1323.

57. Aslani N, Brown CJ. Does mesh offer an advantage over tissue in the open repair of umbilical hernias? A systematic review and meta-analysis. *Hernia.* 2010;14:455-462.

58. Montes IS, Deysine M. Spigelian and other uncommon hernia repairs. *Surg Clin North Am.* 2003;83:1235-1253.

59. Larson DW, Farley DR. Spigelian hernias: repair and outcome for 81 patients. *World J Surg.* 2002;26:1277-1281.

60. Patle NM, Tantia O, Sasmal PK, Khanna S, Sen B. Laparoscopic repair of spigelian hernia: our experience. *J Laparoendosc Adv Surg Tech A.* 2010;20:129-133.

61. Ramirez OM, Ruas E, Dellon AL. 'Components separation' method for closure of abdominal-wall defects: an anatomic and clinical study. *Plast Reconstr Surg.* 1990;86:519-526.

62. Pauli EM, Rosen MJ. Open ventral hernia repair with component separation. *Surg Clin North Am.* 2013;93:1111-1133.

63. Shahan CP, Stoikes NF, Webb DL, Voeller GR. Sutureless onlay hernia repair: a review of 97 patients. *Surg Endosc.* 2015;30:3256-3261. doi:10.1007/s00464-015-4647-2.

64. Saulis AS, Dumanian GA. Periumbilical rectus abdominis perforator preservation significantly reduces superficial wound complications in 'separation of parts' hernia repairs. *Plast Reconstr Surg.* 2002;109:2275-2280, discussion 2281–2282.

65. Butler CE, Campbell KT. Minimally invasive component separation with inlay bioprosthetic mesh (MICSIB) for complex abdominal wall reconstruction. *Plast Reconstr Surg.* 2011;128:698-709.

66. Lowe JB, Garza JR, Bowman JL, Rohrich RJ, Strodel WE. Endoscopically assisted 'components separation' for closure of abdominal wall defects. *Plast Reconstr Surg.* 2000;105:720-729, quiz 730.

67. Switzer NJ, Dykstra MA, Gill RS, et al. Endoscopic versus open component separation: systematic review and meta-analysis. *Surg Endosc.* 2015;29:787-795.

68. Harth KC, Rosen MJ. Endoscopic versus open component separation in complex abdominal wall reconstruction. *Am J Surg.* 2010;199:342-347.

69. Ghali S, Turza KC, Baumann DP, Butler CE. Minimally invasive component separation results in fewer wound-healing complications than open component separation for large ventral hernia repairs. *J Am Coll Surg.* 2012;214:981-989.

70. Stoppa RE. The treatment of complicated groin and incisional hernias. *World J Surg.* 1989;13:545-554.

71. Rives J, Pire JC, Flament JB, Palot JP, Body C. [Treatment of large eventrations. New therapeutic indications apropos of 322 cases]. *Chirurgie.* 1985;111:215-225.

72. Wantz GE. Incisional hernioplasty with Mersilene. *Surg Gynecol Obstet.* 1991;172:129-137.

73. Iqbal CW, Pham TH, Joseph A, Mai J, Thompson GB, Sarr MG. Long-term outcome of 254 complex incisional hernia repairs using the modified Rives-Stoppa technique. *World J Surg.* 2007;31: 2398-2404.

74. Novitsky YW, Elliott HL, Orenstein SB, Rosen MJ. Transversus abdominis muscle release: a novel approach to posterior component separation during complex abdominal wall reconstruction. *Am J Surg.* 2012;204:709-716.

75. Novitsky YW, Fayezizadeh M, Majumder A, Neupane R, Elliott HL, Orenstein SB. Outcomes of posterior component separation with transversus abdominis muscle release and synthetic mesh sublay reinforcement. *Ann Surg.* 2016;264(2):226-232.

76. Jones CM, Winder JS, Potochny JD, Pauli EM. Posterior component separation with transversus abdominis release. *Plast Reconstr Surg.* 2016;137:636-646.

77. Johnson KC, Miller MT, Plymale MA, Levy S, Davenport DL, Roth JS. Abdominal wall reconstruction: a comparison of totally extraperitoneal and transabdominal preperitoneal approaches. *J Am Coll Surg.* 2016;222:159-165.

78. Majumder A, Fayezizadeh M, Neupane R, Elliott HL, Novitsky YW. Benefits of multimodal enhanced recovery pathway in patients undergoing open ventral hernia repair. *J Am Coll Surg.* 2016;222:1106-1115. doi:10.1016/j.jamcollsurg.2016.02.015.

Inguinal Hernia Repair: Laparoscopic

Namir Katkhouda | Kulmeet K. Sandhu | Kamran Samakar |

Evan Alicuben

Inguinal hernia repair is a frequently performed operation, and laparoscopic inguinal hernia repair has become increasingly prevalent, particularly for the repair of bilateral or recurrent hernias. The first described laparoscopic inguinal hernia repair was completed in 1990 by Ger in canines[1]; the procedure has since evolved to include the use of a prosthetic mesh to cover the myopectineal orifice. There are two commonly performed techniques: the transabdominal preperitoneal repair (TAPP) and the totally extraperitoneal repair (TEP). This chapter reviews the anatomy, technical considerations, benefits, and possible complications of laparoscopic inguinal hernia repair.

SURGICAL ANATOMY OF THE REGION

A comprehensive understanding of the anatomy of the preperitoneal space is critical to the performance of a safe and effective laparoscopic inguinal hernia repair.[2] The anterior approach to inguinal hernia repair involves recognition of the anatomy from a superficial to deep position; this is in contrast to laparoscopic repair, which requires identification of the critical structures from a reversed viewpoint.

The median umbilical ligament covers the urachus and travels from the umbilicus to the bladder (Fig. 53A.1). The paired medial umbilical ligaments are remnants of the fetal umbilical arteries. The inferior epigastric vessels originate from the external iliac vessels and have a peritoneal covering creating the paired lateral umbilical folds. These folds originate medial to the deep inguinal ring and travel to the arcuate line, where the inferior epigastric vessels enter the rectus sheath. The medial inguinal fossa is the space located between the medial umbilical ligament and lateral umbilical fold bilaterally. This is the space associated with direct inguinal hernias. The lateral inguinal fossa is the depression lateral to the lateral umbilical fold. Indirect inguinal hernias develop at this site. The pectineal (Cooper) ligament is formed from fascia and periosteum and travels along the pectineal line of the pubic bone. The iliopubic tract is a thickened band of fibers from the transversalis fascia that joins laterally to the iliac crest and inserts medially on the pubic tubercle and pectineal line.

The major vascular structures in this region are generally located medial to the deep inguinal ring. The inferior epigastric vessels branch from the external iliac vessels and travel to supply the anterior abdominal wall. A vascular connection may be noted in some patients between the obturator and external iliac vessels crossing the superior pubic ramus. This is known as the "corona mortis," or

crown of death, as injury due to dissection in this area can lead to significant hemorrhage. There are several other dangerous areas of dissection with laparoscopic hernia repair. The "triangle of doom" is located between the vas deferens medially and the gonadal vessels laterally. The external iliac vessels, deep circumflex iliac vein, genital branch of the genitofemoral nerve, and femoral nerve are located within this triangle.

The key nerves in this area are located lateral to the deep inguinal ring (Fig. 53A.2). In the laparoscopic approach, the following nerves with cutaneous innervation may be encountered from laterally to medially: the lateral femoral cutaneous nerve, the anterior femoral cutaneous nerve, femoral nerve, femoral branch of the genitofemoral nerve, and genital branch of the genitofemoral nerve. The area inferior to the iliopubic tract and lateral to the gonadal vessels is known as the "triangle of pain," where the lateral femoral cutaneous nerve and femoral branch of the genitofemoral nerve are found. Tacks placed in this area may injure either of these nerves. Together, the area between the vas deferens medially and the iliopubic tract superiorly and laterally constitutes "the square of doom," where tacks and electrocautery should never be applied to avoid nerve injury.

The previous anatomic discussion is required to understand the landmarks that define the three spaces associated with groin hernias (Fig. 53A.3):

1. Indirect inguinal hernia—lateral to the inferior epigastric vessels.
2. Direct inguinal hernia—medial to the inferior epigastric vessels and lateral to the border of the rectus abdominis muscle within the triangle of Hesselbach.
3. Femoral hernia—below the iliopubic tract, medial to the external iliac vein, and lateral to Cooper ligament.

All three of these spaces should be covered during the laparoscopic approach with an appropriately sized mesh.

LAPAROSCOPIC VERSUS OPEN REPAIR

The decision to perform an inguinal hernia repair via a laparoscopic versus an anterior approach remains difficult, complex, and nuanced. Tension-free anterior mesh repair has been the gold standard because of its low recurrence rate and lack of need for specialized equipment. Critiques of the laparoscopic approach include the higher in-hospital costs due to more expensive equipment, the possibility of intraabdominal organ or vascular injury, and the steep learning curve. Studies have indicated that greater than 250 operations are required to become experienced in this technically challenging operation.[3-5] In fact, a recurrence rate of greater than 10% has been reported for surgeons

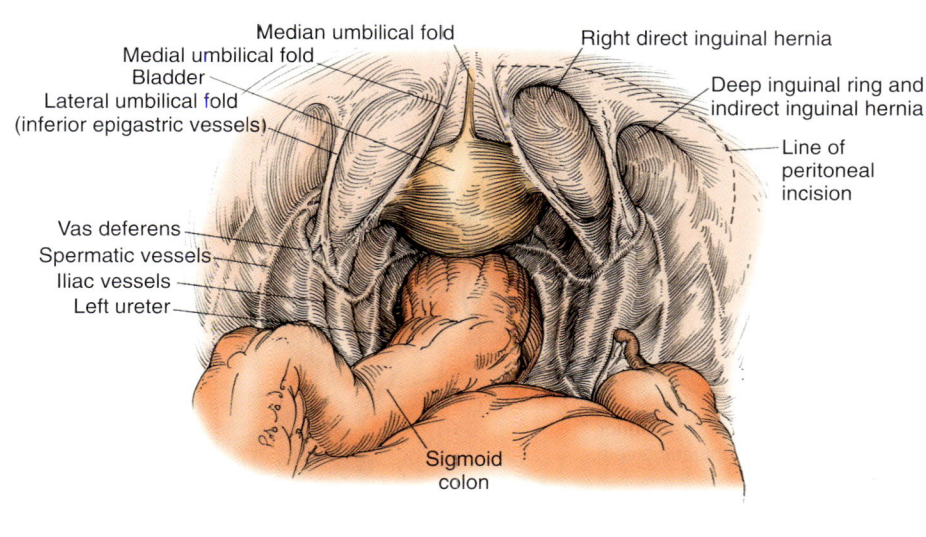

Median umbilical fold
Medial umbilical fold
Bladder
Lateral umbilical fold
(inferior epigastric vessels)

Right direct inguinal hernia

Deep inguinal ring and
indirect inguinal hernia

Line of
peritoneal
incision

Vas deferens
Spermatic vessels
Iliac vessels
Left ureter

Sigmoid
colon

FIGURE 53A.1 Laparoscopic view of the groin. (From Eubanks S. Hernias. In: Sabiston DC Jr, Lyerly HK, eds. *Sabiston Textbook of Surgery: The Biological Basis of Modern Surgical Practice.* 15th ed. Philadelphia: Saunders; 1997:1226.)

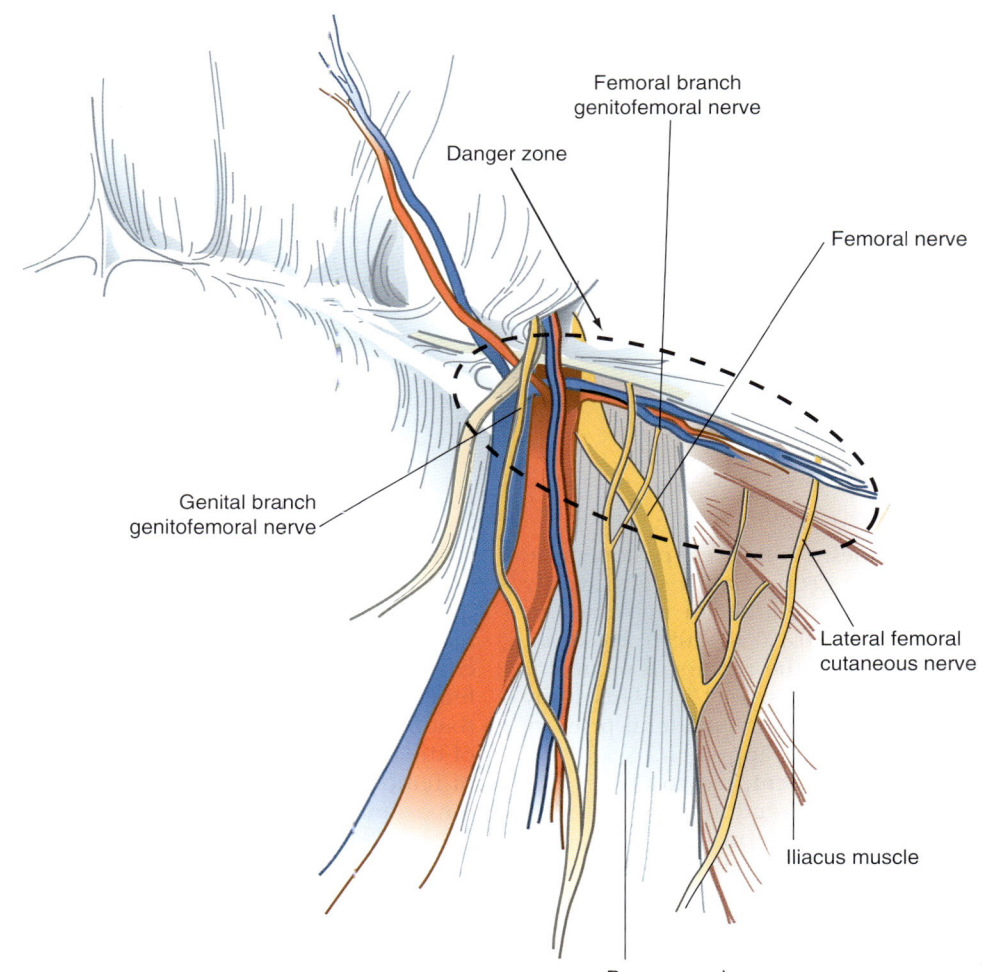

Femoral branch
genitofemoral nerve

Danger zone

Femoral nerve

Genital branch
genitofemoral nerve

Lateral femoral
cutaneous nerve

Iliacus muscle

Psoas muscle

FIGURE 53A.2 Nerves in the inguinal region.

who have performed fewer than 250 procedures.[3] For this reason, some have argued that the laparoscopic approach should be reserved for experienced centers. Conversely, many trials have shown significantly less early postoperative pain resulting in less narcotic use and swifter return to normal activity.[6,7]

Nevertheless, most large trials have failed to consistently show a difference in recurrence rates between the two approaches.[8-11] The biggest exception is a study out of the Veterans Administration (VA) system from 2004.[3] In this study, more than 2000 male patients within the VA system were randomized to an open or laparoscopic

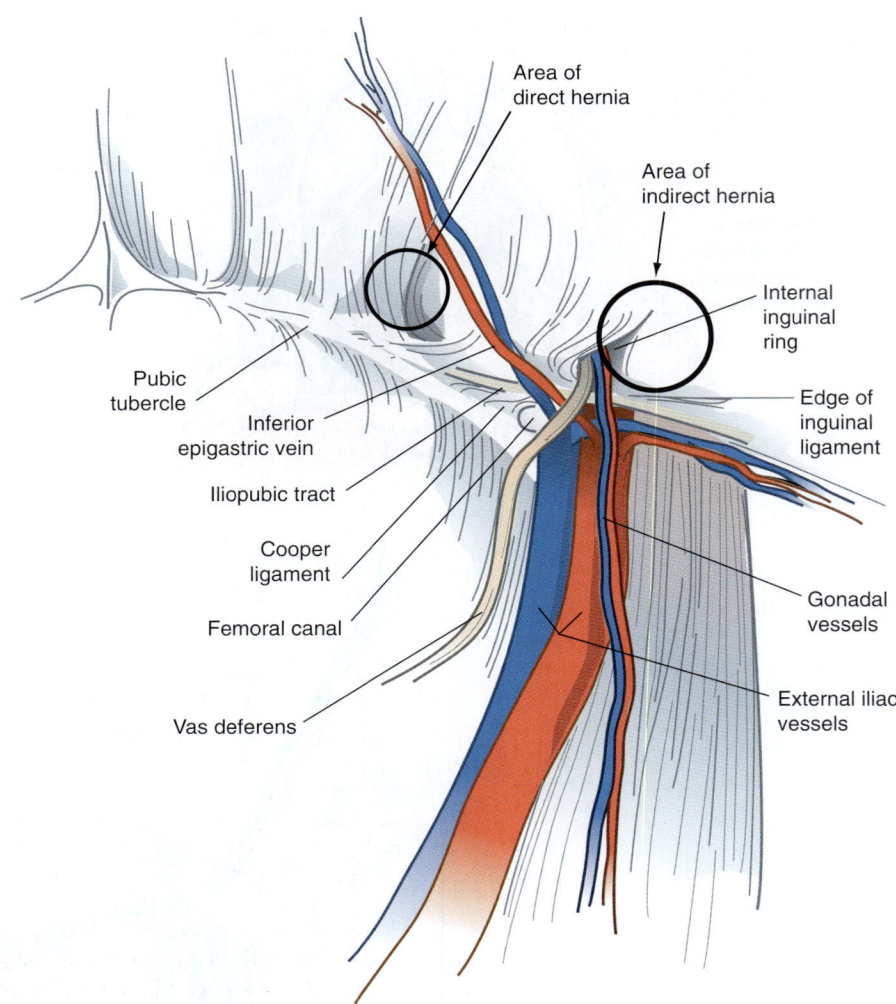

FIGURE 53A.3 Preperitoneal inguinal anatomy.

inguinal hernia repair with mesh. With 2-year postoperative follow-up, the laparoscopic group had a significantly higher recurrence rate than the anterior approach in the repair of primary hernias (10.1% vs. 4.0%). However, recurrence rates were similar if the repairs of recurrent hernias were compared (10.0% vs. 14.1%). This study has steered many surgeons to repair unilateral primary inguinal hernias through an open approach.

More recent research has attempted to clarify this dilemma. In a meta-analysis of 27 randomized controlled trials of primary unilateral inguinal hernia repair including 7161 patients, O'Reilly et al. found that the laparoscopic approach resulted in an increased risk of recurrence.[12] Interestingly, compared with open repair, TEP had increased rates of recurrence but TAPP had equivalent rates. Additionally, the laparoscopic approach was associated with higher perioperative complication risk. This was attributed to a higher complication risk with TAPP but equivalent risk with TEP. However, laparoscopic repair resulted in reduced risk of chronic groin pain and numbness compared with the anterior approach.

The laparoscopic repair technique may be better suited for bilateral or recurrent inguinal hernias and hernias in women. Bilateral hernias may be repaired through the same set of port sites and do not require additional incisions. In recurrent hernias, especially those with previous open repair, a posterior approach results in dissection through native tissue planes. Some studies have suggested this may lead to improved recurrence compared to redo anterior repair.[13] Inguinal hernias in females may be better performed laparoscopically given that the posterior placement of mesh allows for coverage of the femoral space, therefore addressing the incidence of femoral recurrence seen in Lichtenstein repair. The importance of this concept was illustrated in a series of hernia repairs in women which showed a 41.6% rate of femoral hernia found during operations for recurrences.[14]

OPERATIVE TECHNIQUE

TRANSABDOMINAL PREPERITONEAL REPAIR

The patient is placed in the supine position with both arms tucked. An indwelling catheter is placed in the bladder to prevent view obstruction and decrease the risk of injury to the bladder during dissection of the preperitoneal space. The monitor is placed at the foot of the table. The surgeon stands behind the shoulder opposite to the hernia, and the camera assistant stands on the other side of the patient. Steep Trendelenburg is

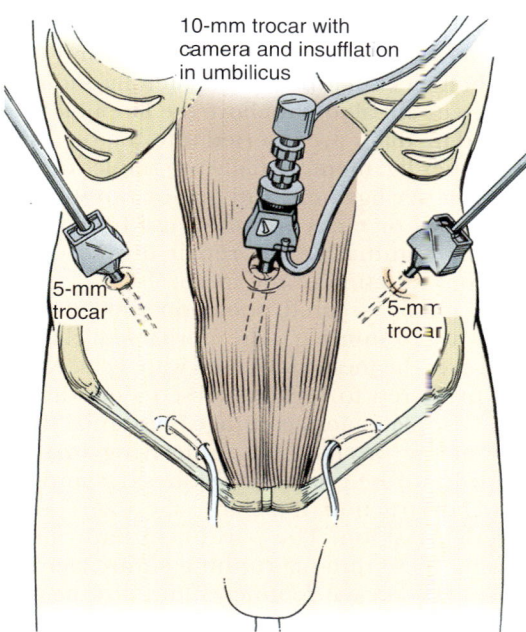

FIGURE 53A.4 Trocar placement for transabdominal preperitoneal hernia repair.

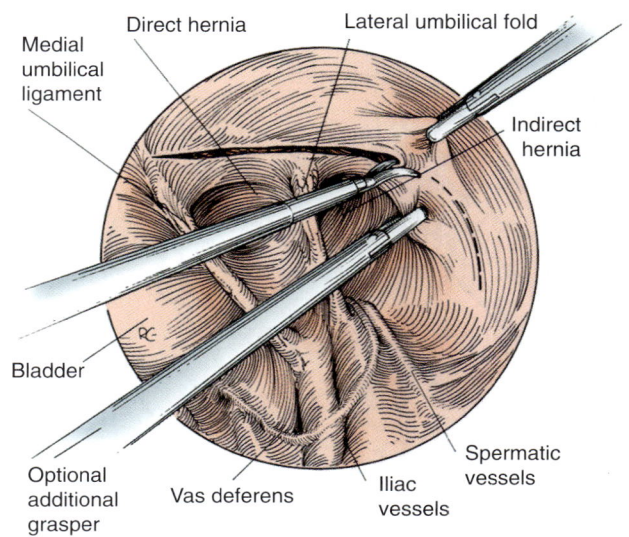

FIGURE 53A.5 Creation of the peritoneal flap. (From Eubanks S. Hernias. In: Sabiston DC Jr, Lyerly HK, eds. *Sabiston Textbook of Surgery: The Biological Basis of Modern Surgical Practice.* 15th ed. Philadelphia: Saunders; 1997:1226.)

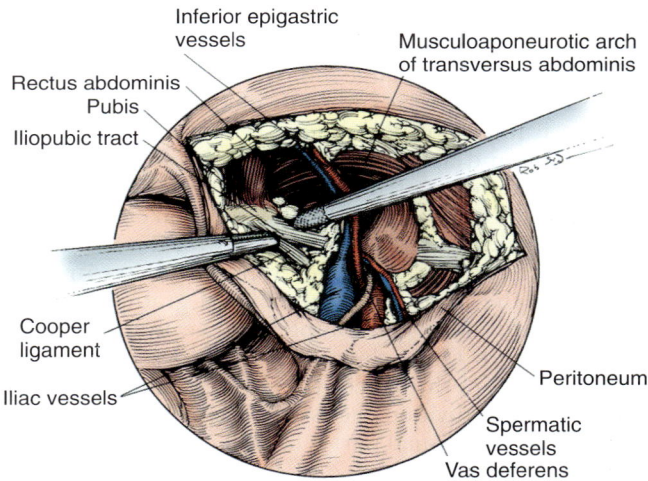

FIGURE 53A.6 Dissection of the inguinal region. (From Eubanks S. Hernias. In: Sabiston DC Jr, Lyerly HK, eds. *Sabiston Textbook of Surgery: The Biological Basis of Modern Surgical Practice.* 15th ed. Philadelphia: Saunders; 1997:1226.)

required to remove the small bowel from the pelvis and adequately visualize the area to be dissected.

Three ports are required for this operation. A 10-mm port for the laparoscope is placed at the umbilicus. Two additional 5-mm ports are placed lateral to the rectus muscle on either side at the junction of a line between the umbilicus and the anterior superior iliac spine (Fig. 53A.4). Alternately, the two 5-mm ports can be placed at the midline between the umbilicus and pubic bone for the TEP repair. A 30-degree laparoscope is required, as the oblique orientation of the inguinal canal makes it difficult to visualize small hernias and it is challenging to open the peritoneum at the anterior abdominal wall without the 30-degree angle.

Following the establishment of pneumoperitoneum— which is maintained at 15 mm Hg—and port introduction, attention is turned to raising the peritoneal flap. If the trocars are inserted too low, it can be very difficult to produce an adequately sized peritoneal flap or easily maneuver the tacking device or the fibrin glue sprayer. On the other hand, if they are placed too high, the small bowel may get in the way. Therefore optimal placement of trocars and a 30-degree laparoscope are essential to success.

The peritoneal flap may be incised from lateral to medial or medial to lateral. If a lateral-to-medial dissection is chosen, the incision begins medially to the anterior superior iliac spine (Fig. 53A.5). This then extends medially, staying at least 2 cm above the deep inguinal ring and hernia defect, and ends at the medial umbilical ligament. Blunt dissection is used to enlarge the peritoneal flap and expose the critical landmarks in the preperitoneal space, including the pubic tubercles, Cooper ligament, and the iliopubic tract (Fig. 53A.6). This dissection of the areolar tissue can be done with minimal hemostasis, and

electrocautery is used with care in this area to avoid nerve injury. The femoral nerve is present under the iliopubic tract at the lateral aspect of the dissection, but this nerve is not commonly visualized during this procedure. In thin patients, the lateral femoral cutaneous nerve and the genitofemoral nerve may be identified.

In males, the spermatic cord structures are dissected free of the peritoneal flap. This involves separating the cord structures, including the vas deferens, from the peritoneum and the hernia sac. The peritoneum must be dissected quite inferiorly, as inadequate mobilization can result in folding of the mesh after peritoneal closure and early recurrence. If the view of the operative site is obscured with blood, it can be irrigated and aspirated

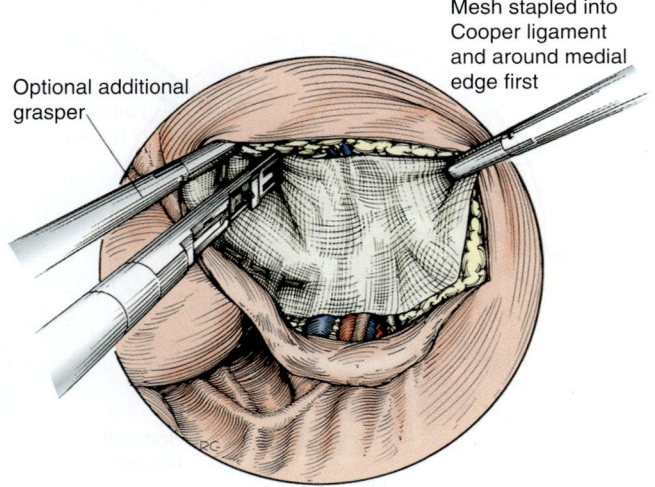

Mesh stapled into Cooper ligament and around medial edge first

Optional additional grasper

FIGURE 53A.7 Placement and fixation of the mesh. (From Eubanks S. Hernias. In: Sabiston DC Jr, Lyerly HK, eds. *Sabiston Textbook of Surgery: The Biological Basis of Modern Surgical Practice.* 15th ed. Philadelphia: Saunders; 1997:1226.)

or cleaned with gauze placed intraabdominally. Direct hernia sacs and small indirect hernia sacs can often be easily reduced during this dissection.

In the case of a very large indirect inguinoscrotal hernia, the distal part of the sac can be divided and left within the scrotum if it cannot be reduced. This dissection begins with gentle and atraumatic separation of the sac from the spermatic cord structures. As the sac is separated, it is divided, but care should always be taken to ensure that the vas deferens is not included with the sac. It may be easier to locate the vas deferens before starting the division of the hernia sac, but often a gradual division of the sac will allow for complete separation of the sac from the cord. Once the peritoneal sac is completely excised, the operation continues as usual. The distal portion of the divided sac is left open in the inguinal canal and the proximal part is ligated using an Endoloop or clips. This method is employed if the complete sac cannot be reduced as significant dissection at the distal sac in larger hernias can cause hematoma formation, ischemic orchitis, or atrophy of the testicle.

When the hernia sac has been completely reduced and dissection of the preperitoneal space is complete, the mesh is rolled and introduced through the umbilical port using a grasper (Fig. 53A.7). Mesh of an appropriate size should be used, typically a 15- by 10-cm piece will be adequate for one side. Once inside the abdominal cavity, the mesh is unrolled and positioned so that it covers the direct, indirect, and femoral spaces. Fixation is then performed with fibrin glue, tacks, or suture. Some surgeons feel that complications of fixation, and associated vascular or nerve entrapment can be avoided if a significantly large piece of mesh is placed. Our technique of choice currently is to use fibrin glue. The fibrin glue is sprayed over the mesh in a thin layer, especially over Cooper ligament and the lateral aspect of the mesh. However, if one chooses to use tacks, the mesh fixation can begin at the midportion, "three fingers" above the superior limit of the internal

ring to avoid nerve injury. Nerve injury can lead to severe chronic pain due to neuroma formation around the staple or tack. Then tacks may be placed laterally and medially; laterally, it is essential to stay above the iliopubic tract, but tacks placed medially are inserted into the rectus muscle and on Cooper ligament. Usually two staples or tacks are placed in Cooper ligament and one or two in the rectus muscle. Staples or tacks are often used for fixation in laparoscopic inguinal hernia repair due to the risk of shrinkage or migration of the mesh.

After the mesh is secured, pneumoperitoneum pressure is reduced to 10 mm Hg. The peritoneal flap is then positioned over the mesh and closed with tacks. Absorbable tacks are preferred to prevent subsequent adhesions to the tacks. Complete mesh coverage is essential to prevent exposure of the mesh to the underlying small bowel. This can lead to the creation of adhesions and possible small bowel obstruction. If possible, tacking is performed in an overlap fashion. The peritoneal flap can also be closed using a continuous running suture per surgeon preference. The fascia is routinely sutured at the umbilical port during closure.

TOTALLY PREPERITONEAL HERNIA REPAIR

The arcuate line of Douglas is a transitional line; above it, the rectus muscle has a defined anterior and posterior sheath composed of the aponeurotic fascia of the internal oblique and transversus abdominis muscles. Below the arcuate line, all fascial layers of the abdominal muscles are anterior to the rectus muscle, and behind the rectus muscle itself there is only the transversalis fascia. Preperitoneal dissection is performed below the arcuate line, which is located approximately midway between the umbilicus and pubis.

The operation is begun by making a 10-mm incision below the umbilicus. Two retractors are used to slide the incision to the right if the hernia is located on the right side, or to the left if the hernia is located on that side. The anterior rectus sheath on the side of the hernia is then opened under direct vision, and two stay sutures are placed on each edge. The rectus muscle is then bluntly separated using two retractors so that the posterior fascia can be visualized. At this point, it is essential not to open the posterior fascia of the rectus muscle but instead to dissect inferiorly toward the symphysis pubis in an oblique fashion, using either the index finger or a small peanut with an angulation of about 30 degrees. That will lead to the preperitoneal space below the arcuate line of Douglas.

The preperitoneal space is then dissected using a balloon space maker under direct vision with a 30-degree laparoscope (Fig. 53A.8). While the balloon is inflated, the rectus muscle should be seen anteriorly and superiorly, and the preperitoneal fat and peritoneum should be seen posteriorly. It is preferred that the inferior epigastric vessels stay anteriorly with the rectus muscle, as otherwise they may hamper dissection and possibly require ligation. The balloon should stay in place for approximately 15 seconds to tamponade any bleeding. The space-maker balloon is then removed and the Hasson port is introduced.

Two 5-mm ports are placed at the midline between the umbilicus and the symphysis pubis to allow for operating on both sides. The space created using this technique is small

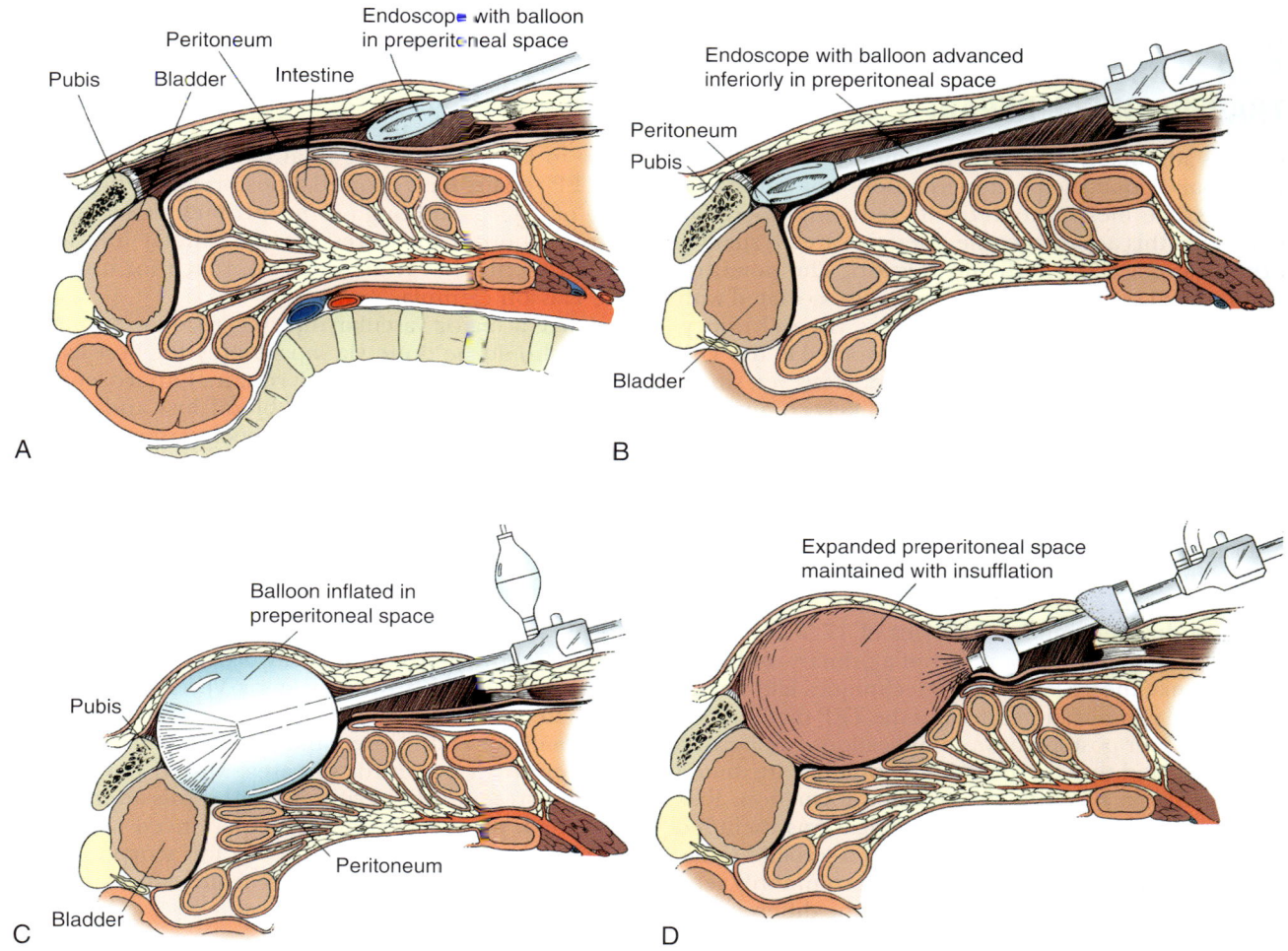

FIGURE 53A.8 Balloon dissection of the preperitoneal space. (A) A balloon dissector is introduced into the preperitoneal space. (B) The balloon dissector is advanced to the pubis in the preperitoneal space. (C) The balloon is inflated under direct vision with the laparoscope. (D) The balloon is removed and the preperitoneal space is insufflated with carbon dioxide. (From Shadduck PP, Schwartz LB, Eubanks WS. Laparoscopic inguinal herniorrhaphy. In: Pappas TN, Schwartz LB, Eubanks WS, eds. *Atlas of Laparoscopic Surgery*. Philadelphia: Current Medicine; 1996. Copyright 1996 by Current Medicine.)

and limits the movement of the laparoscopic instruments. Care should be taken to avoid perforating the peritoneum, since an opening in the peritoneum will allow CO_2 to escape into the abdominal cavity, which will subsequently compress the space and reduce it further. If this occurs, a Veress needle can be inserted into the abdomen to allow for the exit of CO_2. The perforation can be then be closed using an Endoloop or a 5-mm clip applier.

After the ports are in place, Cooper ligament is identified medially and the iliac vein's position is noted as well. These two structures are key anatomic landmarks in this procedure, as they aid in defining the inferior aspect of the dissection. It is possible to injure the iliac vein, and there have been reports of ligation of the iliac vein when it was mistaken for the hernia sac. Once the iliac vein is identified after careful dissection, the next step is locating the inferior epigastric vessels. This will help delineate the internal ring and Hesselbach triangle. The vas deferens is identified by following the internal ring medially and toward the iliac vein. Gentle, blunt dissection is then used to separate the sac from the cord structures and vas deferens. Small hernia sacs are usually easily reduced. If the hernia sac is large and dissection difficult, it may be prudent to amputate the sac, leave the distal part of the sac open, and close the proximal opening either with clips or an Endoloop. The mesh is then placed into the preperitoneal space and positioned as mentioned in the previous section. Once the mesh is in place, fibrin sealant or tacks can be used to fix the mesh in position. The fibrin sealant can be applied as an aerosol spray, which is attached to one of the open trocars to prevent excessive pressure inside the abdomen. This fibrin glue can be placed above or below the lightweight, large-pore mesh. It is important to use a lightweight, large-pore mesh to avoid or minimize the risk of mesh contraction and a foreign body reaction. The operation ends by desufflating the preperitoneal space and gradually removing the ports. A grasper is used to hold the mesh in place as the CO_2 is evacuated. After port removal, the anterior fascia is closed with the previously placed stay sutures.

TRANSABDOMINAL PREPERITONEAL REPAIR VERSUS TOTALLY EXTRAPERITONEAL REPAIR

An obvious advantage of the TEP technique over the TAPP hernia repair is that the peritoneum does not have to be closed over the mesh, theoretically reducing operative time. Despite this advantage, the operative area is smaller and the anatomy more difficult to grasp. The potential intraabdominal complications that may be associated with the transabdominal approach—such as visceral injury, adhesions, and trocar site hernias—are avoided in the TEP repair, as the peritoneum is not entered. However, small, unrecognized peritoneal violations are likely common in the TEP method, therefore making those complications possible with both techniques.

To date there have been no studies that have definitively shown an advantage of one approach over the other.[5,15-20] The largest published series is from the Herniamed registry, which is a multicenter Internet-based database with participating surgeons in Germany, Austria, and Switzerland. In their published series of 17,587 patients who underwent laparoscopic repair of a primary unilateral inguinal hernia, the TEP and TAPP techniques had similar intraoperative complication rates but the TEP method had significantly fewer postoperative complications.[21] Subgroup analysis indicated that these findings could be attributed to a difference in bleeding and seroma formation. Risk factors for the development of complications included increased defect size and the presence of a scrotal hernia. Of note, these characteristics were more commonly seen in the TAPP group, and this may explain the difference in complication rate. Nevertheless, the rate of reoperation for recurrence was equivalent between the two groups.

With regard to recurrent hernias, in a series of 1309 patients, the TEP approach was associated with a significantly increased rate of intraoperative complications (TEP 6.3% vs. TAPP 2.8%) and a longer operative time (TEP 80.3 minutes vs. TAPP 73.0 minutes), but the rates of postoperative complication were similar.[22] Overall these differences were felt to be clinically insignificant; therefore the procedures were deemed equivalent.

In a recent meta-analysis of 10 randomized controlled trials, Wei et al. reported no significant difference in operative time, cost, complications, or time to return to usual activities.[23] Given the failure to show benefit in the TEP group, this study suggested that the TAPP approach may be the preferred strategy, especially for nonexpert laparoscopic surgeons.

COMPLICATIONS

The incidence of complications following laparoscopic inguinal hernia repair has gradually declined and should continue to decline as the procedure becomes more prevalent. The reported rates of complications vary widely and reach as high as 25%, depending on the definition of morbidity put forth by the studies.[7,24]

Vascular Injuries

Significant vascular injury during the procedure is most likely to occur while gaining access to the peritoneal cavity. The risk of intraoperative bleeding has been reported at 2.3%, with the risk of major injury at 0.08%.[25] In a large series of Veress needle insertions, the rate of major vascular injury was 0.018% and most commonly involved injury to the iliac vessels and aorta.[26] Specifically to laparoscopic inguinal hernia repair, one series of TEP repairs has reported a postoperative hemorrhage rate of 0.4%.[27] Although some attribute these injuries to introduction of the Veress needle, similar injuries have been described with the open approach for insertion of the Hasson cannula.

Once a major vascular injury is recognized, management should be done via laparotomy for best exposure and preparation for vessel repair. Laparoscopy may underestimate the degree of blood loss and may limit retraction and exposure of the bleeding vessel. Significant abdominal wall hemorrhage is likely from injury to the epigastric vessels. Initial bleeding can be controlled with a cannula while preparations are made for suture ligation using transfascial sutures placed with fascial closure devices.

Bowel Injury

Injury to bowel most commonly occurs during entry into the abdomen with the trocar or Veress needle and is estimated to occur in 0.13% of cases.[28] Most frequently, the small bowel is injured and this can be detected intraoperatively in two-thirds of cases. Missed bowel injuries usually present with peritonitis and sepsis approximately one week postoperatively. An experienced laparoscopic surgeon may repair the injury via intracorporeal suturing or stapling, taking care to avoid narrowing of the intraluminal diameter.

Bladder Injury

Bladder injury is possible from placement of a suprapubic trocar or during dissection. Small injuries can be managed with urinary drainage, but larger defects require repair. If such an injury is recognized, laparoscopic repair is an option if the experience of the surgeon is sufficient. If unrecognized, injury may present later with hematuria, abdominal pain, or peritonitis.

Urinary Retention

The risk of developing urinary retention is significantly higher in laparoscopic repair compared with the anterior approach, given the use of general anesthesia compared with the possibility of local anesthesia for open repairs. The actual reported incidence varies widely up to 22%, and is higher in older patients with history of prostatic symptoms.[29-31] In one study, postoperative narcotic use of 6.5 mg or greater of morphine or morphine equivalent was an independent risk factor for the development of urinary retention.[31] Narcotic avoidance with the usage of antiinflammatory medications, acetaminophen, and regional nerve blocks may help to decrease the risk of retention. The amount of intraoperative fluids given, the presence of a urinary catheter during surgery, and operative time were not associated with increased risk. Intermittent catheterization or a temporary indwelling catheter usually resolves the symptoms.

Recurrence

The rate of recurrence has been reported to be between 0% and 13% with the VA trial showing a recurrence rate of 10% for primary unilateral hernias.[3] Diagnosing a recurrence may necessitate imaging studies, often ultrasound, magnetic resonance imaging (MRI), or computed tomography (CT). Anterior repair for recurrent hernias is a popular option given that the tissue planes have not been previously violated. However, if the initial laparoscopic repair was performed due to a recurrent hernia, dissection in either space can be difficult.

Ischemic Orchitis

Disruption of the vascular supply to the testis may cause pain, fever, and an enlarged, firm testicle associated with ischemic orchitis. This more commonly results from damage to the venous plexus as opposed to the testicular artery. Duplex ultrasound should be performed to evaluate for testicular torsion. Patients are managed expectantly with antiinflammatory agents for symptoms. Testicular necrosis may ensue and eventually result in testicular atrophy; however, this happens in a minority of cases.[24] Some believe that laparoscopic repair may result in less testicular ischemia due to a higher dissection on the spermatic cord. However, postoperative color Doppler ultrasonography has shown no measurable difference in blood flow.[32]

Groin Pain

The etiology and management of postinguinal groin pain following hernia repair remains poorly understood and reflects the complex nature of this problem. The incidence has varied greatly but has been reported to be as high as 53%, with 1% requiring referral to specialty pain clinic.[33,34] Laparoscopic repair causes significantly less early postoperative pain compared with the anterior approach. With long-term follow-up, overall rates of pain tend to equalize, but the laparoscopic approach has been shown to have less pain during strenuous activity.[35] It is difficult to make definitive recommendations given that pain is reported by a variety of scales. Etiology of the pain may be related to factors present prior to the hernia repair, including muscle strain, osteitis pubis, and other lumbosacral disorders. MRI offers the advantage of soft tissue and neural resolution for diagnosis and can serve to evaluate for hernia recurrence.

Neuropathic pain, which is most difficult to manage, is usually described by patients as sharp, originating close to the inguinal region or scar, and worsened with activity, especially movements around the hip joint. The pain may be related to entrapment or damage of the ilioinguinal, iliofemoral, or genital branch of the genitofemoral nerve due to suture, tacks, or mesh inflammation and scarring. Long-term studies have shown that the pain improves in the majority of patients. Until recently, there has been controversy with regard to neurectomy. A recently published meta-analysis showed that routine neurectomy in open inguinal hernia repair resulted in significantly less pain with no difference in sensation.[36]

Management of the pain should initially consist of nonoperative measures including antiinflammatory medications, nerve blocks, and physical therapy. Operative exploration should only be considered after all these measures have been exhausted. A popular option is laparoscopic exploration for mesh removal including securing devices (i.e., sutures, tacks, etc.), followed by open repair.

REFERENCES

1. Ger R, Monroe K, Duvivier R, Mishrick A. Management of indirect inguinal hernias by laparoscopic closure of the neck of the sac. *Am J Surg.* 1990;159:370.
2. Katkhouda N. Inguinal hernia repair. In: Karkhouda N: *Advanced Laparoscopic Surgery: Techniques and Tips.* 2nd ed. Heidelberg [u.a.]: Springer; 2010:149-168 [Chapter 10].
3. Neumayer L, Giobbie-Hurder A, Jonasson O, et al. Open mesh versus laparoscopic mesh repair of inguinal hernia. *N Engl J Med.* 2004;350:1819.
4. Neumayer LA, Gawande AA, Wang J, et al. Proficiency of surgeons in inguinal hernia repair. *Ann Surg.* 2005;242:344.
5. Wake BL, McCormack K, Fraser C, Vale L, Perez J, Grant AM. Transabdominal pre-peritoneal (TAPP) vs totally extraperitoneal (TEP) laparoscopic techniques for inguinal hernia repair. *Cochrane Database Syst Rev.* 2005;(1):CD004703.
6. Grant AM. Laparoscopic versus open groin hernia repair: meta-analysis of randomized trials based on individual patient data. *Hernia.* 2002;6:2.
7. Memon MA, Cooper NJ, Memon B, Memon MI, Abrams KR. Meta-analysis of randomized clinical trials comparing open and laparoscopic inguinal hernia repair. *Br J Surg.* 2003;90:1479.
8. Pikoulis E, Tsigris C, Diamantis T, et al. Laparoscopic preperitoneal mesh repair or tension-free mesh plug technique? A prospective study of 471 patients with 543 inguinal hernias. *Eur J Surg.* 2002;168:587.
9. Eklund A, Rudberg C, Smedberg S, et al. Short-term results of a randomized clinical trial comparing Lichtenstein open repair with totally extraperitoneal laparoscopic inguinal hernia repair. *Br J Surg.* 2006;93:1060.
10. Eklund AS, Montgomery AK, Rasmussen C, Sandbue RP, Bergkvist LA, Rudberg CR. Low recurrence rate after laparoscopic (TEP) and open (Lichtenstein) inguinal hernia repair. *Ann Surg.* 2009;249:33.
11. Langeveld HR, van't Riet M, Weidema WF, et al. Total extraperitoneal inguinal hernia repair compared with Lichtenstein (the LEVEL-trial). *Ann Surg.* 2010;251:819.
12. O'Reilly EA, Burke JP, O'Connell PR. A meta-analysis of surgical morbidity and recurrence after laparoscopic and open repair of primary unilateral inguinal hernia. *Ann Surg.* 2012;555:846.
13. Bisgaard T, Bay-Nielsen M, Kehlet H. Re-recurrence after operation for recurrent inguinal hernia. A nationwide 8-year follow-up study on the role of type of repair. *Ann Surg.* 2008;247:707.
14. Koch A, Edwards A, Haapaniemi S, Nordin P, Kald A. Prospective evaluation of 6895 groin hernia repairs in women. *Br J Surg.* 2005;92:1553.
15. Krishna A, Misra MC, Kumar Bansal V, Kumar S, Rajeshwari S, Chabra A. Laparoscopic inguinal hernia repair: transabdominal preperitoneal (TAPP) versus totally extraperitoneal (TEP) approach: a prospective randomized controlled trial. *Surg Endosc.* 2012;26:639.
16. McCormack K, Wake BL, Fraser C, Grant A. Transabdominal preperitoneal (TAPP) versus totally extraperitoneal (TEP) laparoscopic techniques for inguinal hernia repair: a systematic review. *Hernia.* 2005;9:109.
17. Gass M, Banz VM, Rosella L, Adamina M, Candinas D, Güller U. TAPP or TEP? Population-based analysis of prospective data on 4,552 patients undergoing endoscopic inguinal hernia repair. *World J Surg.* 2012;36:2782.
18. Bracale U, Melillo P, Pignata G, et al. Which is the best laparoscopic approach for inguinal hernia repair: TEP or TAPP? A systematic review of the literature with a network meta-analysis. *Surg Endosc.* 2012;26:3355.
19. Antoniou SA, Antoniou GA, Bartsch DK, et al. Transabdominal preperitoneal versus totally extraperitoneal repair of inguinal hernia: a meta-analysis of randomized studies. *Am J Surg.* 2013;206:245.

20. Sharma D, Yadav K, Hazrah P, Borgharia S, Lal R, Thomas S. Prospective randomized trial comparing laparoscopic transabdominal preperitoneal (TAPP) and laparoscopic totally extraperitoneal (TEP) approach for bilateral inguinal hernias. *Int J Surg.* 2015;22:110.

21. Kockerling F, Bittner R, Jacob DA, et al. TEP versus TAPP: comparison of the perioperative outcome in 17,587 patients with a primary unilateral inguinal hernia. *Surg Endosc.* 2015;29:3750.

22. Gass M, Scheiwiller A, Sykora M, Metzger J. TAPP or TEP for recurrent inguinal hernia? Population-based analysis of prospective data on 1309 patients undergoing endoscopic repair for recurrent inguinal hernia. *World J Surg.* 2016;40(10):2348-2352.

23. Wei FX, Zhang YC, Han W, Zhang YL, Shao Y, Ni R. Transabdominal preperitoneal (TAPP) versus totally extraperitoneal (TEP) for laparoscopic hernia repair: a meta-analysis. *Surg Laparosc Endosc Percutan Tech.* 2015;25:375.

24. Bittner R, Schmedt CG, Schwarz J, Kraft K, Leibl BJ. Laparoscopic transperitoneal procedure for routine repair of groin hernia. *Br J Surg.* 2002;89:1062.

25. Schafer M, Lauper M, Krahenbuhl L. A nation's experience of bleeding complications during laparoscopy. *Am J Surg.* 2000;180:73.

26. Azevedo JLMC, Azevedo OC, Miyahira SA, et al. Injuries caused by Veress needle insertion for creation of pneumoperitoneum: a systematic literature review. *Surg Endosc.* 2009;23:1428.

27. Tamme C, Scheidbach H, Hampe C, Schneider C, Kockerling F. Totally extraperitoneal endoscopic inguinal hernia repair (TEP). *Surg Endosc.* 2003;17:190.

28. Van der Voort M, Heijnsdijk EAM, Gouma DJ. Bowel injury as a complication of laparoscopy. *Br J Surg.* 2004;91:1253.

29. Koch CA, Grinberg GG, Farley DR. Incidence and risk factors for urinary retention after endoscopic hernia repair. *Am J Surg.* 2006;191:381.

30. Dulucq JL, Wintringer P, Mahajna A. Laparoscopic totally extraperitoneal inguinal hernia repair: lessons learned from 3,100 hernia repairs over 15 years. *Surg Endosc.* 2009;23:482.

31. Patel JA, Kaufman AS, Howard RS, Rodriguez CJ, Jessie EM. Risk factors for urinary retention after laparoscopic inguinal hernia repairs. *Surg Endosc.* 2015;29:3140.

32. Gurbulak EK, Gurbulak B, Algun IE, et al. Effects of totally extraperitoneal (TEP) and Lichtenstein hernia repair on testicular blood flow and volume. *Surgery.* 2015;158:1297.

33. Poobalan AS, Bruce J, Cairns W, et al. A review of chronic pain after inguinal herniorrhaphy. *Clin J Pain.* 2003;19:48.

34. Gitelis ME, Patel L, Deasis F, et al. Laparoscopic totally extraperitoneal groin hernia repair and quality of life at 2-year follow-up. *J Am Coll Surg.* 2016;223:153.

35. Singh AN, Bansal VK, Misra MC, et al. Testicular functions, chronic groin pain, and quality of life after laparoscopic and open mesh repair of inguinal hernia: a prospective randomized controlled trial. *Surg Endosc.* 2012;26:1304.

36. Barazanchi AWH, Fagan PVB, Smith BB, Hill AG. Routine neurectomy of inguinal nerves during open onlay mesh hernia repair. *Ann Surg.* 2016;264:64.

Inguinal Hernia Repair: Open

Kamran Samakar | Kulmeet K. Sandhu | Namir Katkhouda

Inguinal hernia repair is the most common general surgical procedure in the United States with approximately 800,000 performed annually. Throughout its long history, many techniques have been proposed for the repair of inguinal hernias. Modern-day repair of inguinal hernias is based on the tenets of minimizing tension and the use of mesh to provide a lasting repair. In this chapter, we review the most common techniques for the surgical repair of inguinal hernias, relevant anatomy, and the postoperative complications of herniorrhaphy.

BACKGROUND

A hernia is defined as an abnormal protrusion or bulge of an organ or tissue through the surrounding walls. The prevalence of inguinal hernias is estimated at 5% to 10% of the population of the United States. Inguinal hernia repair is the most common general surgery procedure in the United States, with approximately 800,000 performed annually.

Inguinal hernias have a variety of clinical manifestations, ranging from a painless groin bulge to pain without a bulge. Common symptoms include pain described as dull discomfort or pinching in the groin, which may or may not be accompanied by a noticeable bulge. Discomfort with activity such as lifting or coughing, pain extending to the scrotum or labia, and amelioration of symptoms while lying flat are all associated with inguinal hernias. The most common finding on physical examination in adults is a groin bulge. In most cases, diagnosis of an inguinal hernia can be made by history and physical examination alone.[1] When the diagnosis is not apparent, ultrasonography of the groin should be considered as the initial diagnostic modality.[2] Other imaging modalities include computed tomography (CT) and magnetic resonance imaging (MRI), both of which can aid in the evaluation of an inguinal hernia.

Consideration of hernia repair depends on the patient's symptoms and the potential for incarceration or strangulation. Common practice is to offer elective repair of symptomatic inguinal hernias for patients who are physically fit for surgery. Nonoperative management of asymptomatic or minimally symptomatic inguinal hernias has been shown to be a safe and acceptable approach.[3,4] Femoral hernias should be repaired at the time of diagnosis due to the increased risk of strangulation.

ANATOMY

The inguinal canal is formed by the aponeurosis of the external oblique muscle anteriorly, the transversalis fascia, and the transversus abdominis muscles posteriorly (Figs. 53B.1 and 53B.2). The canal is approximately 4 cm in length and is located cephalad to the inguinal ligament running between the internal (deep) inguinal and external (superficial) inguinal rings. In men, the inguinal canal contains the spermatic cord and, in women, it contains the round ligament. During open inguinal hernia repair, the iliohypogastric, ilioinguinal, and genital branches of the genitofemoral nerves are encountered (Fig. 53B.3). The ilioinguinal and iliohypogastric nerves can be identified as they pass between the external and internal oblique muscles. The genital branch of the genitofemoral nerve is generally found outside the area of dissection behind the cord structures.

Inguinal hernias are classified anatomically as direct or indirect. Indirect inguinal hernias are the most common type of hernia in both sexes. Indirect hernias are a protrusion of the hernia sac at the internal ring, lateral to the inferior epigastric vessels. Indirect inguinal hernias are the result of a patent processus vaginalis. In contrast, the sac of a direct inguinal hernia protrudes medial to the inferior epigastric vessels, within Hesselbach triangle. Hesselbach triangle is formed by the inguinal ligament (Poupart ligament) inferiorly, the inferior epigastric vessels laterally, and the rectus abdominis muscle medially. Direct hernias are a result of weakness in the floor of the inguinal canal.

SURGICAL TECHNIQUE

The open anterior approach to inguinal hernia repair remains the most common approach to primary unilateral hernias.[5] The exact choice of repair may vary depending on the use of mesh as well as operative technique. Based on multiple large systematic reviews, various hernia society guidelines generally advocate the use of mesh in a tension-free technique for hernia repair.[6-8] Hernia recurrence rates using mesh typically range from 1% to 5% and are estimated to be significantly lower than nonmesh repairs.[9] The ideal mesh used for inguinal hernia repair should be lightweight, macroporous, and inexpensive.[10] Still, the use of mesh in contaminated fields and complicated hernia repairs remains controversial with evidence to suggest that it may be done safely in certain circumstances.[11-16]

CONVENTIONAL ANTERIOR OPEN APPROACH

Open anterior inguinal hernia repairs generally follow the same initial steps: skin incision along the lines of Langer, deepening of the incision through Camper and Scarpa fascia to the external oblique aponeurosis, and incision of the external oblique through the external ring. Once the external oblique aponeurosis has been incised, the superior flap is created by bluntly sweeping off the internal oblique muscle. The ilioinguinal and iliohypogastric nerves are identified and preserved. Selective use of neurectomy is advocated in cases of inadvertent trauma or presumed injury due to mesh entrapment.[17-19] Inferiorly,

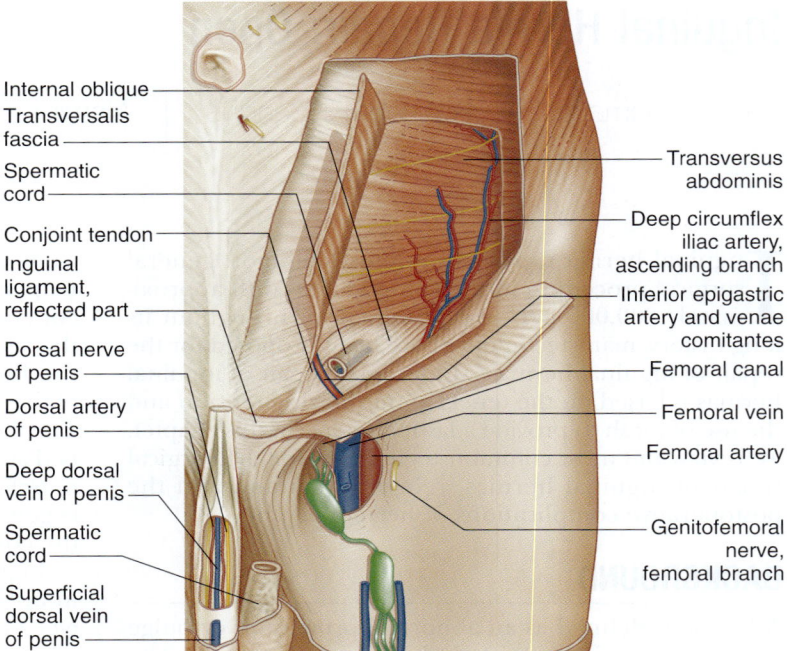

FIGURE 53B.1 Anterior view of the muscles of the groin area (parts of the external and internal oblique have been removed). (From Standring S, Ellis H, Healy JC, et al., eds. *Gray's Anatomy: The Anatomical Basis of Clinical Practice.* 40th ed. Philadelphia: Churchill Livingstone; 2008; Fig. 61.15.)

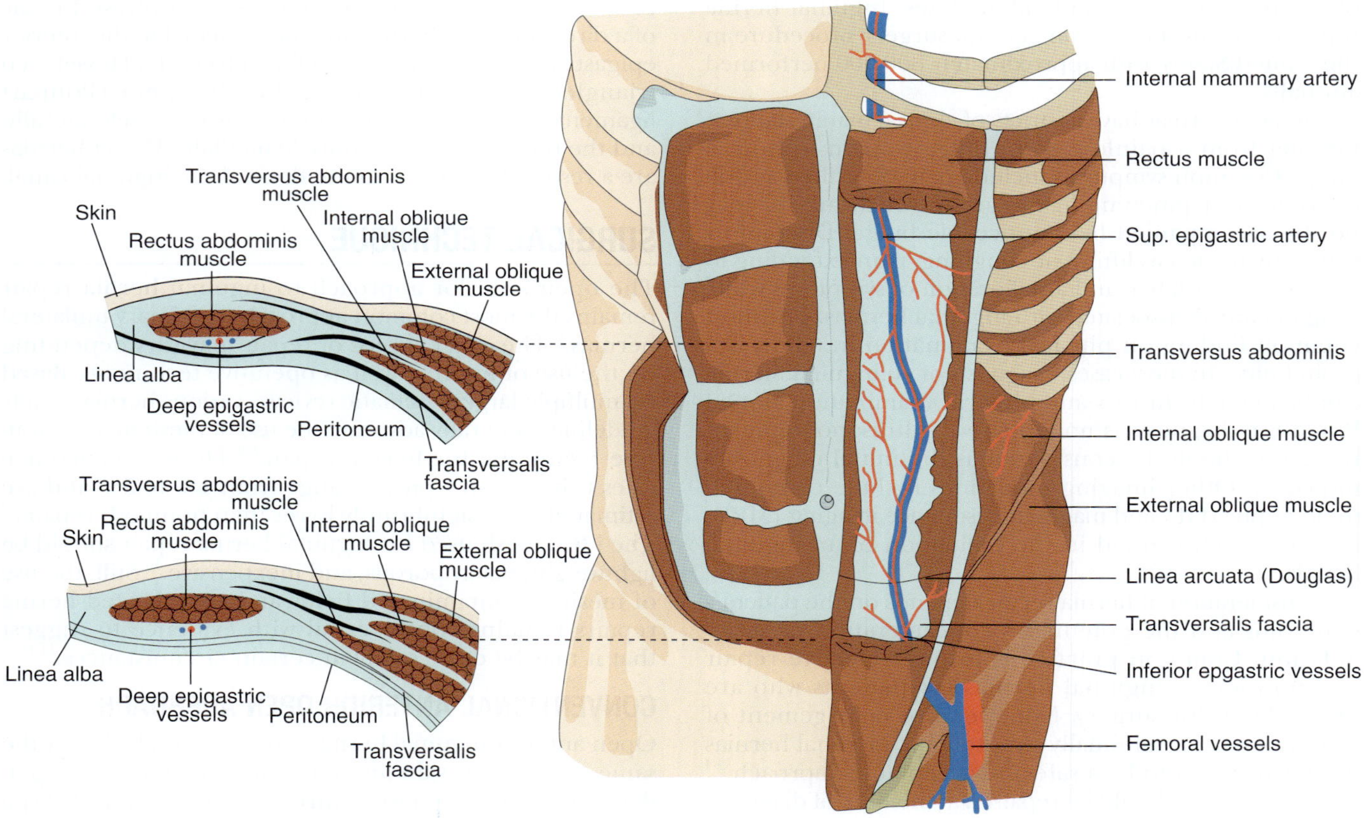

FIGURE 53B.2 Rectus abdominis muscle and rectus sheath.

the cord structures are separated from the inferior flap of the external oblique aponeurosis and blunt dissection is carried onto the pubic tubercle. Using both index fingers, the surgeon creates a window behind the cord structures at the pubic tubercle to allow for passage of a Penrose drain. Once the Penrose is placed for retraction, dissection of the cord is performed in order to identify an indirect hernia sac. The indirect hernia sac is then dissected free from the cord structures up to the level of the internal ring. The sac can either be high-ligated with

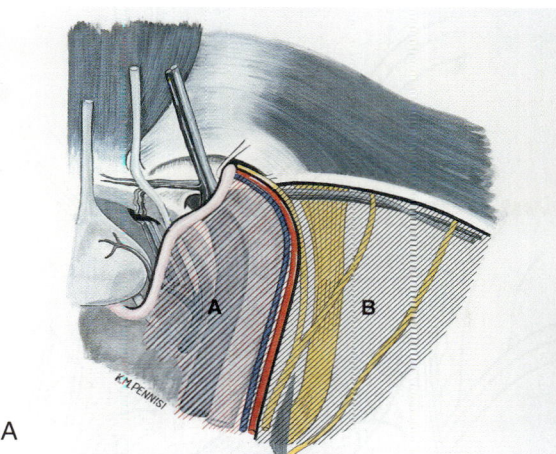

FIGURE 53B.3 (A) Preperitoneal view of the right groin depicting the so-called triangle of doom *(A)* and the triangle of pain or the electrical hazard zone *(B)*. (B) Cadaveric preparation that shows the structures included within these triangles that could be damaged during a preperitoneal herniorrhaphy. *AP,* Anterior pubic branch and iliopubic vein; *B,* bladder (reflected posteriorly); *CI,* common iliac artery; *CL,* Cooper ligament; *DC,* deep circumflex iliac vessels; *FB,* femoral branch of the genitofemoral nerve; *FN,* femoral nerve; *GB,* genital branch of the genitofemoral nerve; *GN,* genitofemoral nerve; *IA,* external iliac artery; *IE,* inferior epigastric vessels; *IL,* ilioinguinal nerve; *IM,* musculus iliacus; *IP,* iliopubic tract; *IPA,* iliopectineal arch; *IS,* internal spermatic vessels; *IV,* external iliac vein; *LC,* lateral femoral cutaneous nerve; *PB,* anastomotic pubic branch; *PM,* musculus psoas major; *RP,* retropubic vein; *U,* ureter; *UA,* umbilical artery; *VD,* vas deferens. (From Greene FL, Ponsky JL. *Endoscopic Surgery*. Philadelphia: Saunders; 1994:365.)

division and suture closure or it can simply be inverted and reduced into the preperitoneal space.[20] If a direct hernia is present, a purse-string suture can be placed in the transversalis fascia at the base of the hernia to allow for inversion and closure of the hernia.

LICHTENSTEIN REPAIR

Initial steps of the Lichtenstein repair are similar to the steps described previously (Fig. 53B.4). High ligation is performed after incising the cremasteric muscle longitudinally to fully mobilize the sac. Similarly, direct hernias are circumferentially dissected and reduced back into the preperitoneal space. A large mesh prosthesis is then tailored to the shape and size of the patient's anatomy to facilitate overlap of 2 cm onto the pubic tubercle, 4 cm above Hesselbach triangle, and 5 to 6 cm lateral to the internal ring. The mesh is sutured to the pubic tubercle on either side and then secured in a continuous fashion along the shelving edge of the inguinal ligament inferiorly until it is at least 1 cm lateral to the insertion of the internal oblique muscle into Poupart ligament. Similarly, the mesh is secured superiorly to the rectus sheath and subsequently to the internal oblique aponeurosis with interrupted sutures. Two tails are created in the mesh by incising it from the lateral edge to create a slit that encircles the spermatic cord and reconstructs the internal ring. The mesh tails encircling the cord are anchored in a fashion that overlaps the superior and inferior tails in a manner that creates a new internal ring fitting snugly around the spermatic cord. This is accomplished by suturing the tails together and tucking the ends of the tails under the external oblique aponeurosis. Creation of this shutter valve at the internal ring is a critical step for preventing indirect hernia recurrence. The superior and inferior tails can then be secured to the underlying internal oblique and

fascia. Care should be taken not to entrap the ilioinguinal, iliohypogastric, or genital branches of the genitofemoral nerves when placing sutures. The main limitation of this technique is that it does not address femoral hernias.

PLUG-AND-PATCH (RUTKOW–ROBBINS) REPAIR

The plug-and-patch technique begins in a similar fashion to the conventional anterior approach. For a direct hernia, a plug is fashioned from rolled mesh, or a prefabricated plug may be used, and the plug is inserted into the hernia defect and secured to the edges with suture (Fig. 53B.5). The plug can similarly be positioned within the indirect hernia and secured in place along the edges as well (Fig. 53B.6). In this way the plug can act as a preperitoneal underlay mesh. The patch is then positioned in a fashion similar to the Lichtenstein technique along the inguinal space. Limitations of this technique include the possibility of meshoma and pain requiring mesh explantation, mesh migration, and erosion of the mesh into adjacent organs/structures.[21-23]

PREPERITONEAL REPAIR

Preperitoneal mesh placement plays a central role in many hernia repair techniques, including those described by Nyhus-Condon, Wantz, Read, Rives, Stoppa, and Kugel.[24] The key component of the preperitoneal repair is placement of a large mesh in the preperitoneal space between the transversalis fascia and the peritoneum. The preperitoneal space is accessed anteriorly through the inguinal floor to allow for placement of the mesh. Subsequently, the mesh is secured with interrupted sutures and serves as reinforcement of the transversalis fascia. The external oblique is then closed in a continuous fashion. A limitation of this approach is the need for blunt dissection in the preperitoneal space, which can lead to structural injury,

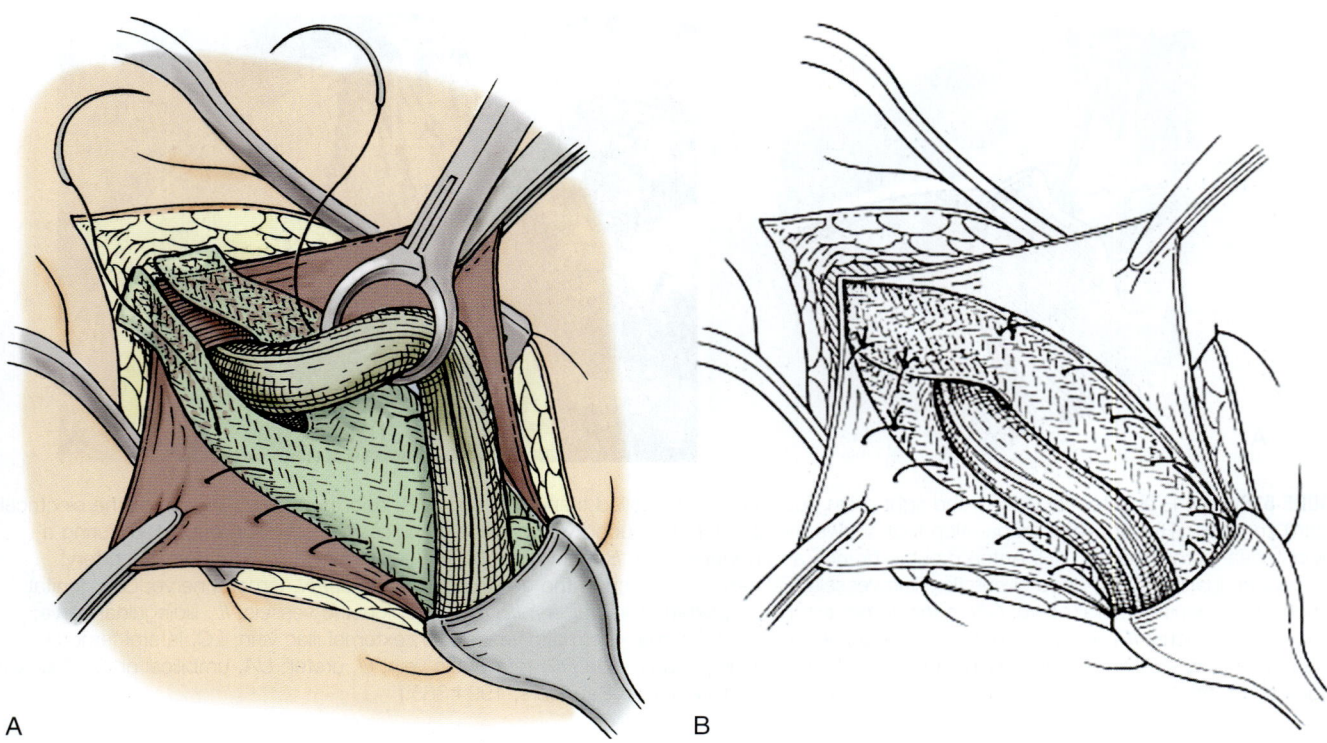

A   B

FIGURE 53B.4 Lichtenstein repair. (A) One of the sutures demonstrates the approximation of the inferior edge of the prosthesis to the inguinal ligament. The second suture will include the inferior surface of the superior tail and the inferior surface of the inferior tail just lateral to the internal ring as well as the inguinal ligament to create a "shutter" valve. (B) The shutter valve has been completed and the superior and medial surfaces have been sutured to the underlying internal oblique muscle and anterior rectus sheath, respectively. This older illustration shows continuous suture on the superomedial border of the prosthesis, but interrupted sutures are now preferred by most surgeons to minimize the incidence of nerve entrapment. (From Kurzer M, Belsham PA, Kark AE. The Lichtenstein repair for groin hernias. *Surg Clin North Am.* 2003;83:1110.)

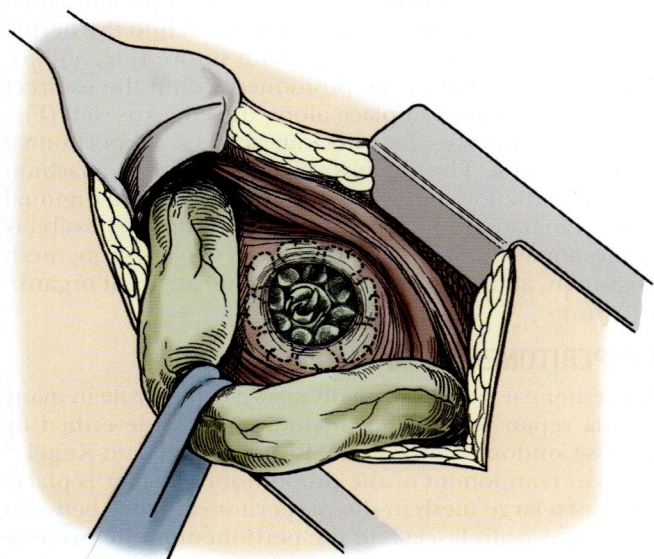

FIGURE 53B.5 Plug-and-patch technique. Plug placement for a direct inguinal hernia. (From Rutkow IM. The PerFix plug repair for groin hernias. *Surg Clin North Am.* 2003;83:1079.)

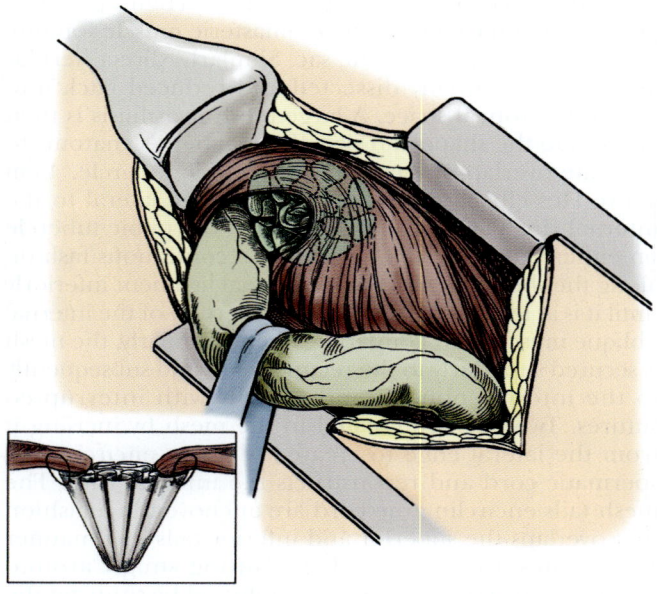

FIGURE 53B.6 Plug-and-patch technique. Plug placement for an indirect inguinal hernia. The *inset* shows a sagittal view of the implanted plug. (From Kurzer M, Belsham PA, Kark AE. The Lichtenstein repair for groin hernias. *Surg Clin North Am.* 2003;83:1099; Courtesy Gillian Lee.)

hematoma formation, and potential scar tissue formation, thus limiting future surgical dissection.

BILAYER MESH REPAIR

Bilayer mesh repair combines components of the Lichtenstein repair and the preperitoneal repair. The repair is performed by bluntly dissecting a pocket in the preperitoneal space for placement of the mesh deep to the transversalis fascia with a superficial layer placed in front of the transversalis fascia. Prefabricated mesh systems are available for this type of repair. Limitations of this repair are similar to those that apply to all preperitoneal repair techniques.

TISSUE (NONMESH) REPAIR

Numerous types of tissue repair are described in the surgical literature. The most commonly used tissue repairs in modern times are those of Shouldice, Bassini, and McVay. Among the nonmesh repairs, the Shouldice technique is preferred because it has the lowest associated recurrence rate.[25] Nonetheless, nonmesh repairs have a reported recurrence as high as 35% and have been shown to be clearly inferior to tension-free mesh repair through a number of randomized controlled trials.[26-28]

The Shouldice technique is an anterior approach that involves division of all the layers of the floor of the inguinal canal with reduction of the hernia followed by reconstruction of the inguinal canal. Once the transversalis fascia is split from the internal ring to the pubic crest, reconstruction of the canal is performed using a four-layer overlap technique and continuous suture. The repair starts at the pubic tubercle by approximating the iliopubic tract to the underside of the lateral edge of the rectus muscle. The suture line then continues by tacking the lateral flap of transversalis fascia to the medial flap, which is composed of the transversus abdominis, transversalis fascia, and internal oblique muscle. Reconstruction of the internal ring is performed by securing the transversalis fascia to the cremasteric muscle. Reversing back toward the pubic tubercle, this suture line approximates the medial flap tissue to the shelving edge of the inguinal ligament. The internal oblique and transversus abdominis are then approximated to the shelving edge of the inguinal ligament. The final suture line is then reversed; it runs laterally and secures the lower flap of the external oblique over the internal oblique in a similar fashion to the previous suture line. The major limitation of this technique is that it is technically difficult and hard to reproduce.

The Bassini repair strengthens the weakened inguinal floor by suturing the conjoined tendon to the inguinal ligament from the pubic tubercle to the area of the internal ring. This repair begins with the standard anterior approach and subsequently divides the transversalis fascia along the inguinal canal. Exposure of this space allows for inspection of possible femoral hernias. Once the hernia sac is high-ligated, reconstruction of the floor is performed by suturing the three layers of transversalis fascia, transversus abdominis, and internal oblique muscle to the inguinal ligament. Classic descriptions of this technique include an initial stitch of the three layers to the periosteum of the pubic tubercle and the rectus sheath. Laterally, the repair extends until closure of the internal ring.

The McVay repair is similar to the Bassini repair except for the use of Cooper ligament instead of the inguinal ligament for the medial portion of the repair. The conjoined tendon is sutured to Cooper ligament from the pubic tubercle and extends along the ligament until as far as the edge of the femoral sheath. The final stitch to the Cooper ligament is known as the transition stitch and includes the inguinal ligament and may include the medial aspect of the femoral sheath as well. This repair is commonly used to address femoral hernias by narrowing the femoral ring, but it can cause considerable tension and requires a relaxing incision to accomplish. The relaxing incision is performed by incising the anterior rectus sheath from the pubic tubercle cephalad for several centimeters along the fusion of the external oblique aponeurosis with the sheath.

FEMORAL HERNIAS

Femoral hernias are rare and typically seen in women. A femoral hernia occurs through the femoral canal, which is bound by the inguinal ligament anteriorly, the pectineal ligament posteriorly, the femoral vein laterally, and the lacunar ligament medially. Typically a femoral hernia will produce a bulge below the inguinal ligament; however, it may also present over the inguinal ligament. Femoral hernia repair can be performed by a preperitoneal approach, Cooper ligament repair (McVay), or laparoscopically. The essential components of a femoral hernia repair include dissection and reduction of the hernia sac and closure of the defect either through approximation of the iliopubic tract to Cooper ligament or through the use of mesh. Unlike inguinal hernias, all femoral hernias should be repaired once they are diagnosed due to the higher risk of strangulation.

COMPLICATIONS

There are myriad postoperative complications associated with open inguinal hernia repair. These include but are not limited to surgical site infection, urinary retention, orchitis, seroma, hematoma, injury to the vas deferens, hydrocele, testicular descent, bowel or bladder injury, osteitis pubis, prosthetic complications, and wound complications. Although some of these complications are related to underlying disease processes, others are directly related to technical aspects of the repair.

SURGICAL SITE INFECTION

Inguinal hernia repairs are generally considered clean operations except for instances of contamination, which may occur inadvertently or during the repair of strangulated hernias. The risk of surgical site infection is estimated to be up to 5% after open repair. The use of prophylactic preoperative antibiotics is controversial, with several studies concluding that there is no benefit to this practice.[29-31] Moreover, the use of prosthetic mesh does not confer a greater risk of infection or substantiate the need for prophylaxis. Surgical site infections can generally be managed with open drainage, local wound care, and oral antibiotics. Mesh infection may lead to a chronically draining sinus tract and ultimately require mesh explantation.

RECURRENCE

Recurrence rates after open tension-free inguinal hernia repair with mesh are generally low and estimated to range from 1% to 2%. Patients may present with a bulge upon examination, but occasionally the only symptom of a recurrence is pain. Hernia recurrences are usually caused by a variety of technical factors including excessive tension, improper mesh placement, missed hernias, failure to fully reduce the sac, inadequate closure of the internal ring, infection, and failure of the inguinal floor. Recurrences are most common with direct hernias and occur near the pubic tubercle at the medial border of the repair. Factors associated with increased hernia recurrence include increased intraabdominal pressure secondary to a chronic cough, morbid obesity, and impaired wound healing. Recurrences after mesh repair are best managed by performing a mesh repair from a different approach. In the case of anterior open approaches, many surgeons advocate the use of laparoscopic repair for recurrent hernias. Similarly, anterior repair may be best suited for recurrent hernias performed in a preperitoneal fashion. Recurrent hernias should almost always be managed with a mesh repair.

CHRONIC PAIN (INGUINODYNIA)

Nerve injury and chronic pain are often underrecognized and potentially debilitating complications of inguinal hernia repair. Nerve injury can occur from traction, mesh or suture entrapment, electrocautery, and transection. The nerves most commonly affected by open hernia repair are the ilioinguinal, iliohypogastric, and genital branch of the genitofemoral nerves. While chronic pain is often associated with nerve injury, it may also result from hernia recurrence, mesh-related problems, and infection. Chronic pain is defined as pain lasting longer than 3 months postoperatively and has been reported to range from 15% to 33%.[32] A subset of patients suffering from chronic pain, ranging from 2% to 4%, experience debilitating pain that does not allow them to return to a preoperative level of functioning and can be completely disabling.

The clinical presentation of chronic pain after hernia repair can be heterogeneous and variable. Careful evaluation of symptoms and physical findings should be performed to help identify the cause. Imaging may aid in the confirmation of hernia recurrence as well as inflammatory processes that may contribute to the problem. Variable treatment modalities ranging from early use of antiinflammatory agents, analgesics, and anesthetic nerve blocks may be attempted. Patients with suspected nerve entrapment may be best served by reexploration and neurectomy. Mesh removal in cases of meshoma or nerve entrapment may be required in some cases. Early recognition and treatment are central to appropriate care for patients suffering from chronic pain. Moreover, as part of the informed consent process, patients should be counseled on the risk of chronic pain complications in the preoperative setting.

CORD AND TESTICULAR INJURIES

Ischemic orchitis usually occurs between 1 and 5 days after surgery and results from the thrombosis of small veins of the pampiniform plexus. Presenting symptoms include a swollen and painful testis with possible low-grade fever. Management is supportive therapy with the addition of antiinflammatory medications, and the condition is usually self-limited. Ischemic orchitis may lead to testicular atrophy and is most commonly seen after the repair of a recurrent hernia.

Injury to the vas deferens may lead to dysejaculation syndrome, likely resulting from a stenotic lesion. Presenting symptoms include pain during ejaculation. Injuries to the vas deferens recognized during hernia surgery should be managed immediately and reanastomosis should be attempted. Ipsilateral vas deferens transection may lead to infertility resulting from the development of sperm antibodies as a consequence of extravasated sperm.

REFERENCES

1. Rosenberg J, Bisgaard T, Kehlet H, et al. Danish Hernia Database recommendations for the management of inguinal and femoral hernia in adults. *Dan Med Bull.* 2011;58:C4243.
2. Robinson A, Light D, Kasim A, Nice C. A systematic review and meta-analysis of the role of radiology in the diagnosis of occult inguinal hernia. *Surg Endosc.* 2013;27:11.
3. Fitzgibbons RJ Jr, Giobbie-Hurder A, Gibbs JO, et al. Watchful waiting vs. repair of inguinal hernia in minimally symptomatic men: a randomized clinical trial. *JAMA.* 2006;295:285.
4. O'Dwyer PJ, Norrie J, Alani A, Walker A, Duffy F, Horgan P. Observation or operation for patients with an asymptomatic inguinal hernia: a randomized clinical trial. *Ann Surg.* 2006;244:167.
5. Simons MP, Aufenacker T, Bay-Nielsen M, et al. European Hernia Society Guidelines on the treatment of inguinal hernia in adult patients. *Hernia.* 2009;13:343.
6. Society for Surgery of the Alimentary Tract. SSAT patient care guidelines. Surgical repair of groin hernias. *J Gastrointest Surg.* 2007;11:1228.
7. Scott NW, McCormack K, Graham P, Go PM, Ross SJ, Grant AM. Open mesh versus non-mesh for repair of femoral and inguinal hernia. *Cochrane Database Syst Rev.* 2002;(4):CD002197.
8. EU Hernia Trialists Collaboration. Repair of groin hernia with synthetic mesh: meta-analysis of randomized controlled trials. *Ann Surg.* 2002;235:322.
9. EU Hernia Trialists Collaboration. Mesh compared with non-mesh methods of groin hernia repair: systematic review of randomized controlled trials. *Br J Surg.* 2000;87:854.
10. Earle DB, Mark LA. Prosthetic material in inguinal hernia repair: how do I choose? *Surg Clin North Am.* 2008;88:179.
11. Ge BJ, Huang Q, Liu LM, Bian HP, Fan YZ. Risk factors for bowel resection and outcome in patients with incarcerated groin hernias. *Hernia.* 2010;14:259.
12. Hentati H, Dougaz W, Dziri C. Mesh repair versus non-mesh repair for strangulated inguinal hernia: systematic review with meta-analysis. *World J Surg.* 2014;38:2784.
13. Karatepe O, Adas G, Battal M, et al. The comparison of preperitoneal and Lichtenstein repair for incarcerated groin hernias: a randomized controlled trial. *Int J Surg.* 2008;6:189.
14. Elsebae MM, Nasr M, Said M. Tension-free repair versus Bassini technique for strangulated inguinal hernia: a controlled randomized study. *Int J Surg.* 2008;6:189.
15. Wsocki A, Kulawik J, Pozniczek M, Strzalka M. Is the Lichtenstein operation of strangulated groin hernia a safe procedure? *World J Surg.* 2006;30:2065.
16. Bessa SS, Katri KM, Abdel-Salam WN, Abdel-Baki NA. Early results from the use of the Lichtenstein repair in the management of strangulated groin hernia. *Hernia.* 2007;11:239.
17. Amid PK, Hiatt JR. New understanding of the causes and surgical treatment of postherniorrhaphy inguinodynia and orchalgia. *J Am Coll Surg.* 2007;205:381.
18. Amid PK. Causes, prevention, and surgical treatment of postherniorrhaphy neuropathic inguinodynia: triple neurectomy with proximal end implantation. *Hernia.* 2004;8:343.

19. Reinpold WM, Nehls J, Eggert A. Nerve management and chronic pain after open inguinal hernia repair: a prospective two phase study. *Ann Surg.* 2011;254:163.

20. Stylianidis G, Haapamaki MM, Sund M. Nilsson E, Nordin P. Management of the hernia sac in inguinal hernia repair. *Br J Surg.* 2010;97:415.

21. Chuback JA, Sing RS, Sills C, Dick LS. Small bowel obstruction resulting from mesh plug migration after open inguinal hernia repair. *Surgery.* 2000;127:475.

22. Kingsnorth AN, Hyland ME, Porter CA, Sodergren S. Prospective double-blind randomized study comparing Perfix plug-and-patch with Lichtenstein patch in inguinal hernia repair: one year quality of life results. *Hernia.* 2000;4:255-258.

23. Amid PK. Classification of biomaterials and their related complications in abdominal wall hernia surgery. *Hernia.* 1997;1:12-19.

24. Amid PK. Groin hernia repair: open techniques. *World J Surg.* 2005;29: 1046.

25. Amato B, Moja L, Panico S, et al. Shouldice technique versus other techniques for inguinal hernia repair. *Cochrane Database Syst Rev.* 2012;(4):CD001543.

26. Nordin P, Bartelmess P, Jansson C, Svensson C, Edlund G. Randomized trial of Lichtenstein versus Shouldice hernia repair general surgical practice. *Br J Surg.* 2002;89:45-49.

27. Danielsson P, Isacson S, Hansen MV. Randomized study of Lichtenstein compared with Shouldice inguinal hernia repair by surgeons in training. *Eur J Surg.* 1999;165:49-53.

28. McGillicuddy JE. Prospective randomized comparison of the Shouldice and Lichtenstein hernia repair procedures. *Arch Surg.* 1998;133:974-978.

29. Sanchez-Manuel FJ, Seco-Gil JL. Antibiotic prophylaxis for hernia repair. *Cochrane Database Syst Rev.* 2003;(2):CD003769.

30. Tzovaras G, Delikoukos S, Christodoulides G, et al. The role of antibiotic prophylaxis in elective tension-free mesh inguinal hernia repair: results of a single-centre prospective randomized trial. *Int J Clin Pract.* 2007;61(2):236-239.

31. Aufenacker TJ, van Geldere D, van Mesdag T, et al. The role of antiobiotic prophylaxis in prevention of wound infection after Lichtenstein open mesh repair of primary inguinal hernia: a multicenter double-blind randomized controlled trial. *Ann Surg.* 2004;240:955-966.

32. Towfigh S, Neumayer L. Inguinal hernia. In: Cameron JL, ed. *Current Surgical Therapy.* 11th ed. Philadelphia: Elsevier Saunders; 2014.

Lumbar, Pelvic, and Uncommon Hernias

Kais Rona | Nikolai A. Bildzukewicz

Aside from ventral and inguinal hernias, there are less common hernias of the abdominal wall and pelvis that may come to the attention of a general surgeon from time to time. It is important for the surgeon to have a general knowledge of these defects so that they may be included in the differential diagnosis and treated appropriately (and sometime expeditiously) if needed. These include hernias of the lumbar area in the lower back, as well as obturator, sciatic, and perineal hernias found within the pelvis. In this chapter, we will review the important anatomy, clinical presentation and evaluation, and surgical treatment of each one of these rare and unique entities.

LUMBAR HERNIA

ANATOMY AND CLASSIFICATION

Lumbar hernias are exceedingly rare, posterolateral, abdominal wall defects containing retroperitoneal fat or viscera. Lumbar hernias were first described several hundred years ago. Barbette suggested the entity of a lumbar hernia in 1672, but the first published case in the medical literature was in 1731 by DeGarangeot.[1] He reported the first incarcerated lumbar hernia on autopsy.[2] Twenty years later, Ravaton described the surgical reduction of a strangulated lumbar hernia.[3] The French surgeon Jean-Louis Petit in 1774 was the first to describe an inferior lumbar hernia through the anatomic boundary now often referred to as *Petit triangle*.[4] More than two centuries after its first description, Grynfelt and Lesshaft independently reported visceral herniation through a superior lumbar defect, now commonly known as a Grynfelt-Lesshaft hernia.[5,6]

Lumbar hernias occur through a parietal wall defect in the lumbar region whose boundaries are the 12th rib superiorly, the iliac crest inferiorly, the erector spinae muscle medially, and the posterior border of the external abdominal oblique laterally (Fig. 54.1). They can be classified anatomically into superior or inferior lumbar hernias based on two well-defined areas of weakness. The superior lumbar triangle is an inverted triangle bordered by the 12th rib superiorly, the internal abdominal oblique muscle anterolaterally, and the quadratus lumborum muscle posteromedially.[7] The latissimus dorsi and the aponeurosis of the transversalis muscle form the roof and the floor of the triangle, respectively. Areas of weakness include the region immediately below the costal margin where the transversalis fascia is not reinforced by the external abdominal oblique muscle, the area at which the 12th dorsal intercostal neurovascular bundle penetrates the fascia, and the area between the ligament of Henle and the inferior costal margin (Fig. 54.2).[8] The inferior

lumbar triangle, or Petit triangle, is an upright triangle bordered by the iliac crest inferiorly, the external abdominal oblique muscle anterolaterally, and the latissimus dorsi posteromedially. The floor is formed by the lumbodorsal fascia and transversalis muscle.[8] A medially displaced latissimus dorsi muscle, alterations in the origin of the external abdominal oblique muscle, and the presence of a Hartmann fissure at the vertex of the triangle may increase the likelihood of visceral protrusion through the inferior lumbar triangle (Fig. 54.3).[8] Herniation occurs more commonly in the superior triangle as it has a greater surface area, is a more vulnerable area of weakness (there is only transversalis fascia at its lower margin), and is not penetrated by neurovascular bundles.[7–9]

In addition to the anatomic classification, lumbar hernias can further be categorized as congenital or acquired based on etiology. Congenital defects of the lumbar region make up 10% to 20% of lumbar hernias.[9,10] Although often unilateral when presenting early in life, some patients may have bilateral hernias and develop symptoms in late adulthood as a result of progressive posterolateral abdominal muscle weakening.[11–13] Congenital lumbar hernias are most often associated with lumbocostovertebral syndrome, although it has been reported with vertebral anomalies, anal atresia, cardiac defects, tracheoesophageal fistulas, renal anomalies, and limb defects (VACTERL syndrome), congenital diaphragmatic hernia, and atrial septal defects, among other congenital malformations.[13,14]

Acquired lumbar hernias constitute the majority of lumbar defects encountered clinically and can be subdivided into primary or secondary acquired hernias.[9,10,15] Primary acquired hernias occur spontaneously, are often small in size, are confined to the borders of the superior or inferior lumbar triangles, and represent 55% of acquired lumbar hernias.[15] Risk factors for the development of a primarily acquired lumbar hernia include advanced age, chronic malnutrition or debilitation, obesity, chronic cough, and previous wound infections or a history of sepsis.[16] On the other hand, secondary acquired hernias are often the result of trauma or previous surgical procedures in the lumbar region.[9] These defects may be diffuse, extending beyond the margins of the lumbar triangle.[9,10] It is a rare complication of surgical procedures involving flank incisions. Examples include open partial or complete nephrectomy, adrenalectomy, and abdominal aortic aneurysm repair. It may also occur at previous bone graft donor sites.[9,17] The iliac crest is a common donor site for autogenous bone grafts given that it is easily accessible and supplies ample amounts of both cancellous and cortical bone.[18] Herniation of intraabdominal contents through the resulting bone defect is uncommon, occurring only in up to 5% of cases.[18–23] Blunt trauma is another rare cause of secondary acquired lumbar hernias, with less

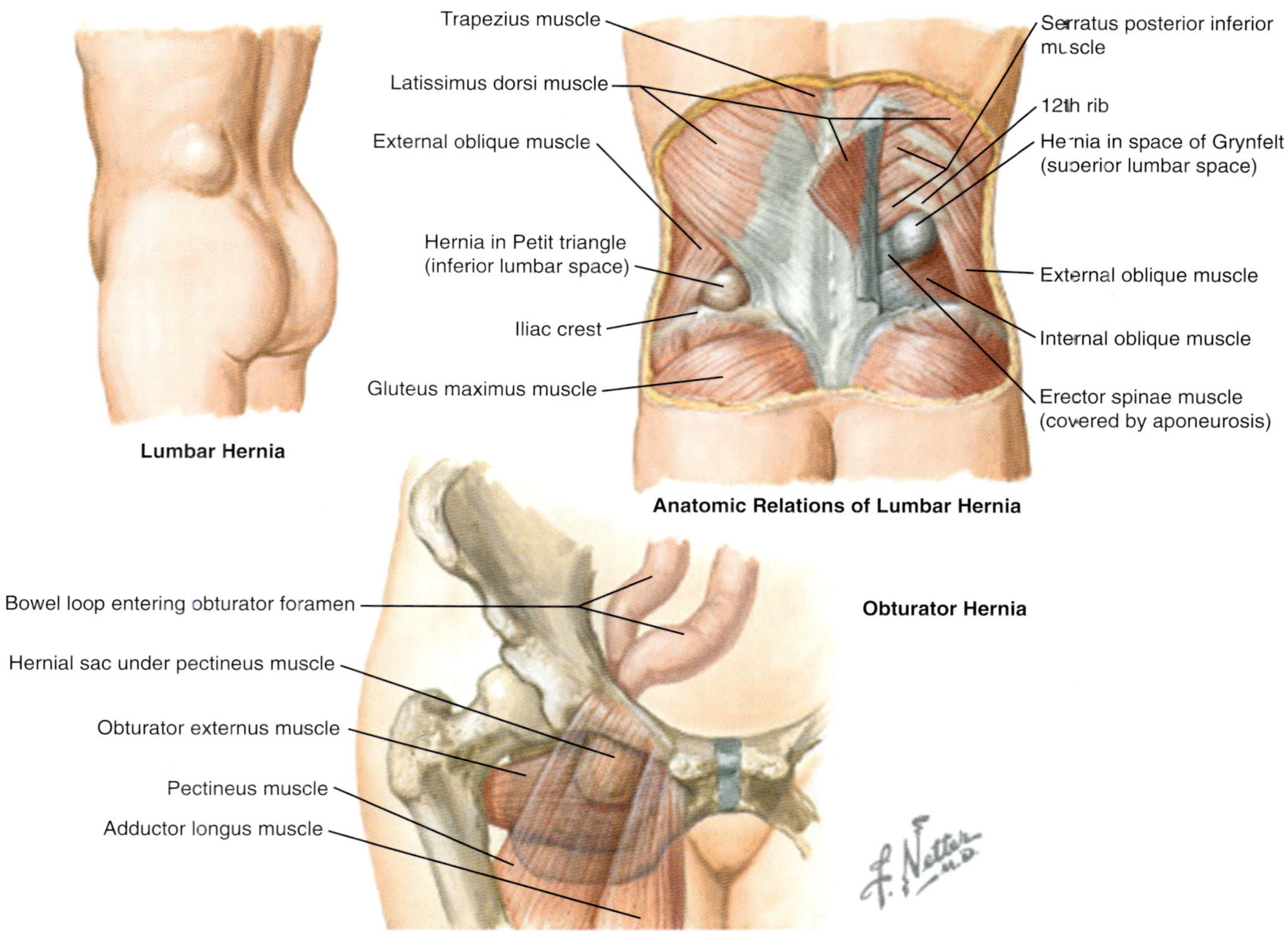

Trapezius muscle

Latissimus dorsi muscle

External oblique muscle

Hernia in Petit triangle
(inferior lumbar space)

Iliac crest

Gluteus maximus muscle

Lumbar Hernia

Serratus posterior inferior
muscle

12th rib

Hernia in space of Grynfelt
(superior lumbar space)

External oblique muscle

Internal oblique muscle

Erector spinae muscle
(covered by aponeurosis)

Anatomic Relations of Lumbar Hernia

Bowel loop entering obturator foramen

Hernial sac under pectineus muscle

Obturator externus muscle

Pectineus muscle

Adductor longus muscle

Obturator Hernia

FIGURE 54.1 Lumbar and obturator hernias. (From Yabara S, Rosenthal R. Lumbar, obturator, sciatic, and perineal hernias. In: Floch MH, ed. *Netter's Gastroenterology*. Philadelphia: Saunders; 2010:230–231.)

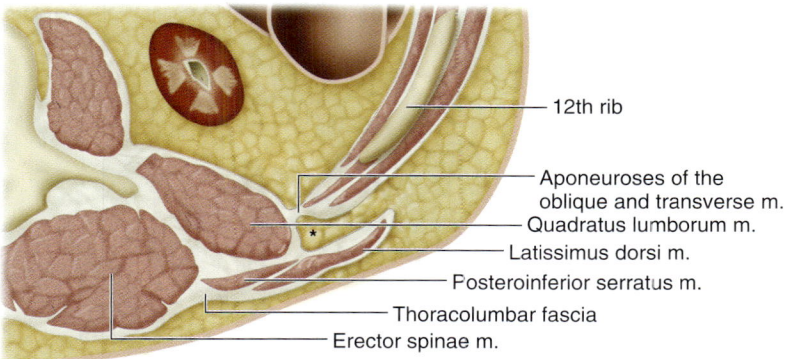

12th rib

Aponeuroses of the
oblique and transverse m.

Quadratus lumborum m.

Latissimus dorsi m.

Posteroinferior serratus m.

Thoracolumbar fascia

Erector spinae m.

FIGURE 54.2 Cross-sectional anatomy of the superior lumbar triangle. The *asterisk* denotes the area where a lumbar hernia may occur. (From Aguirre DA, Rivero OM, Martinez J. Normal anatomy of the abdominal wall. In: Sahani DV, ed. *Abdominal Imaging*. Philadelphia: Saunders; 2011:1439–1443.)

than 100 cases reported in the literature.[24] Traumatic lumbar hernias (TLHs) occur more commonly through the inferior lumbar triangle, and repair is often complex and challenging because there may be destruction of the surrounding muscle, leaving inadequate muscle or aponeurotic tissue for fascial reapproximation.[25]

CLINICAL PRESENTATION AND DIAGNOSIS

Patients usually present with a small protruding mass in the lumbar region that may be symptomatic or asymptomatic.[10,15,26] The majority of patients are males in their fifth or sixth decade of life.[7,15] The

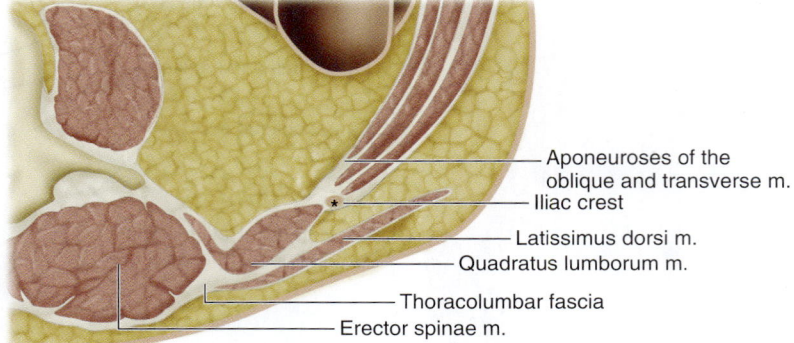

FIGURE 54.3 Cross-sectional anatomy of the inferior lumbar triangle. The *asterisk* denotes the area where a lumbar hernia may occur. (From Aguirre DA, Rivero OM, Martinez J. Normal anatomy of the abdominal wall. In: Sahani DV, ed. *Abdominal Imaging*. Philadelphia: Saunders; 2011:1439–1443.)

differential diagnosis includes but is not limited to a lipoma, rhabdomyoma, sarcoma and other malignant growths, abscess, hematoma, or a renal mass.[15,26] Pain is variable and can range from mild local discomfort to severe, diffuse intestinal colic.[15] Depending on the contents of the hernia, the pain can travel down the distribution of the sciatic nerve or be referred to the anterior abdomen, especially when incarceration or panniculitis is present.[15,17,27] Patients may also have gastrointestinal complaints such as nausea, vomiting, and/or bloating.[17,28] When a mass is palpated in the lumbar region, it is often soft and fluctuates in size. In addition, the mass may protrude with coughing or bearing down and even produce bowel sounds on auscultation based on the contents of the hernia.[28] Lumbar hernias may contain retroperitoneal fat, small and large intestine, omentum, appendix, stomach, cecum, ovary, spleen, and rarely the kidney.[29,30] Urinary obstruction or oliguria may be the presenting symptoms in patients having renal contents within the hernia sac.[8] Pain in the lumbar region accompanied by the signs and symptoms of intestinal obstruction is suggestive of an incarcerated or strangulated lumbar hernia.

Although the diagnosis can be made upon physical exam in the majority of cases, lumbar hernias may be less apparent when the hernia defects are smaller than 5 cm in diameter.[27,28] Computed tomography (CT) (Fig. 54.4) is the preferred diagnostic modality in patients who present with signs and symptoms concerning for a lumbar hernia.[9,15,28,29] It can provide useful information about the size of the fascial defect and allow for the assessment of hernia sac contents and regional anatomic relationships.[15,27] Magnetic resonance imaging (MRI) may also be performed to confirm the diagnosis of a lumbar hernia.[26] Ultrasonography is an alternative imaging modality that may be more appropriate in emergency settings. Although less accurate than CT in depicting anatomy, it is fastidious, less costly, effective, and does not expose the patient to ionizing radiation.[15,27,28] The diagnosis can be made with visualization of a hernia orifice in the posterolateral abdominal wall, which will appear as a defect in the echo line of the aponeurosis.[28] When identification of this orifice is difficult, the presence of a hernia may be suggested by the finding of an intraparietal sac or presence of abdominal contents. On

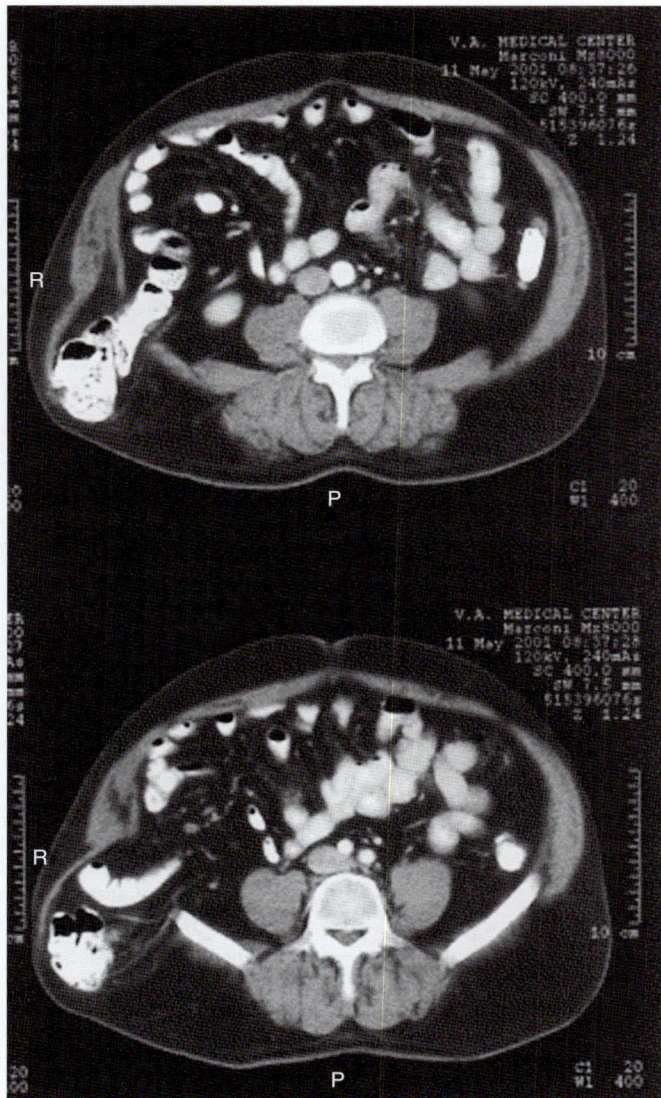

FIGURE 54.4 Intravenous and oral contrast-enhanced computed tomographic images of a right inferior lumbar hernia after iliac bone harvest. (From Patten LC, Awad SS, Berger DH, Fagan SP. A novel technique for the repair of lumbar hernias after iliac crest bone harvest. *Am J Surg.* 2004;188:85.)

ultrasound, this may be indicated by intraluminal gas, which projects as an area of focal dense echogenicity with acoustic shadowing.[28]

TREATMENT

The natural progression of lumbar hernias is a gradual increase in size over time.[15,26,27] Despite this, approximately 25% of patients will present with incarcerated bowel, and 10% to 18% will demonstrate evidence of strangulation.[9,15,27,31] Given the risk of associated complications and the increased complexity of repairing large hernias, surgical intervention upon diagnosis of a lumbar hernia is prudent when the patient's medical condition permits.[7,15,27] The repair of a lumbar hernia is challenging, and various techniques of repair have been described, including simple repair, musculofascial flaps, free grafts, and repair using synthetic mesh.[9,16,25,29,32] More recent studies have evaluated the efficacy of laparoscopic or retroperitoneoscopic repair.[15,27,33–35] Still, the rarity of lumbar hernias and lack of sufficient data preclude a standardized approach or optimal timing in the management of this condition.[15,27]

Lumbar hernias are traditionally approached through an open or anterior technique. In this approach the patient is placed in a lateral decubitus position contralateral to the side of the hernia. General or spinal anesthesia may be used based on the surgeon's discretion. A generous lumbar incision is made, and exploration of the hernia is performed (Fig. 54.5A).[26] The edges of the fascial defect are defined circumferentially. After the hernia sac is identified and its contents reduced, the sac may be excised or inverted.[26] If the defect is small, it may be repaired primarily with nonabsorbable sutures (see Fig. 54.5B–D), although larger defects require a mesh-enforced repair with reapproximation of the overlying muscle layers.[9,10,26,31–33,36] Nonabsorbable mesh may be secured in an extraperitoneal position with 3 to 5 cm of overlap.[7,10,12,26,34,36] In a case series by Cavallaro et al., seven patients with both Petit- and Grynfelt-type hernias underwent open repair with placement of an extraperitoneal mesh.[10] They reported no recurrences over a median of 25 months. Synthetic mesh was secured to the surrounding muscles and the 12th rib or iliac crest for superior and inferior defects, respectively. Solaini et al. described a separate case of open repair of a superior lumbar hernia with dart mesh (Bard Mesh Dart, a small monofilament knitted polypropylene) fixed to the 12th rib.[29] The mesh was fixed

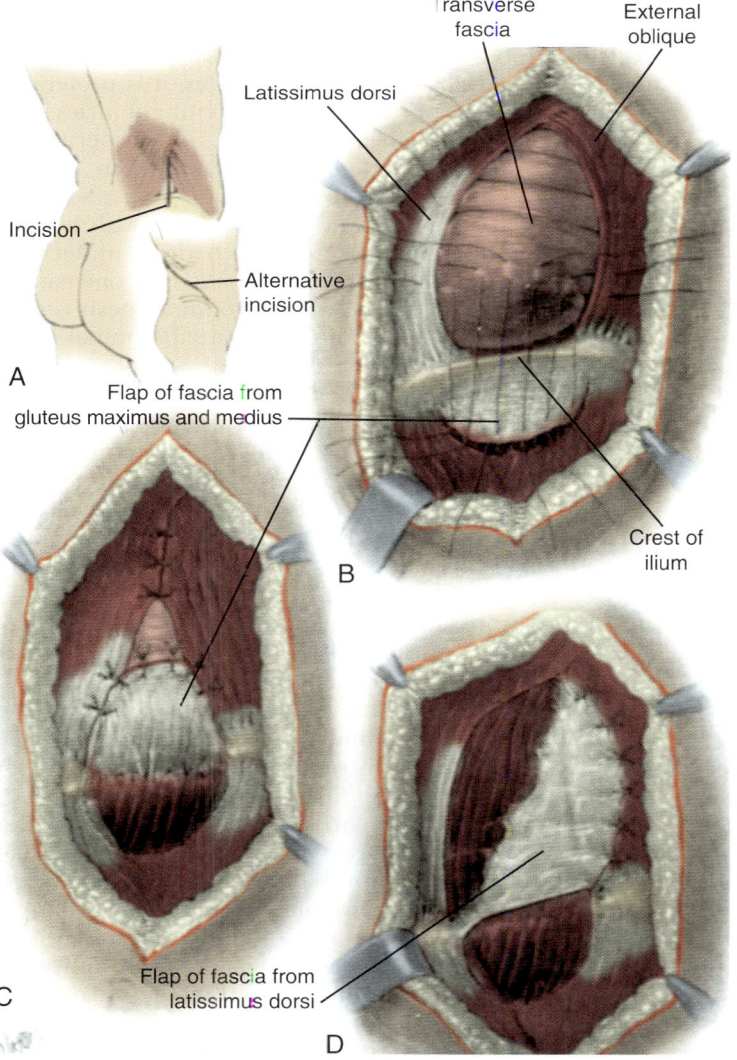

FIGURE 54.5 The Dowd operation for lumbar hernia. (A) Line of incision. (B) Turning up a flap of the fascia lata and aponeurosis of the gluteus maximus and medius muscles and suturing it to the lumbar fascia and external oblique and latissimus dorsi muscles. (C) The flap sutured. (D) Closing the remaining gap with a flap of fascia from the latissimus dorsi. (From Watson LF. *Hernia*. 3rd ed. St. Louis: Mosby; 1948.)

medially to the quadratus lumborum, externally to the internal oblique, and inferiorly to the serratus posterior. The patient was discharged on the first postoperative day and did not demonstrate a recurrence at 11 months of follow-up. The open or anterior approach may be preferable when the lumbar defect is small and well defined with adequate surrounding musculoaponeurotic tissue.[10] Interestingly, simple primary closure of lumbar hernias without mesh has demonstrated acceptable outcomes over a short follow-up period.[7] However, most authors agree that mesh reinforcement is an important component in ensuring the durability of the repair, particularly for larger hernia defects.[10,15,28,29,31,36,37]

The alternative to open repair is a laparoscopic repair. The laparoscopic technique may be performed through a transabdominal or retroperitoneoscopic approach. In the transabdominal approach, patient positioning is similar to that of the open approach. A lumbar roll may be placed to increase the distance between the inferior rib margin and the iliac crest.[27] Dissection occurs along the white line of Toldt. The colon is mobilized and the borders of the underlying lumbar defect are identified (Fig. 54.6).[26] The hernia sac and its contents are reduced. Mesh may then be secured with transabdominal full-thickness bites using a combination of nonabsorbable

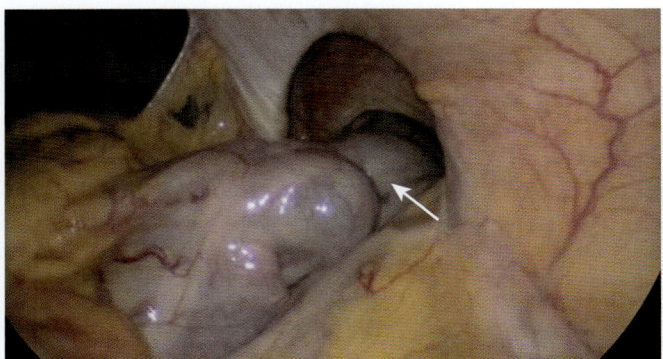

FIGURE 54.6 A lumbar hernia identified during laparoscopy containing incarcerated colon (From Varban O. Lumbar hernia after breast reconstruction. *Int J Surg Case Rep.* 2013, 4[10]: 869–871.)

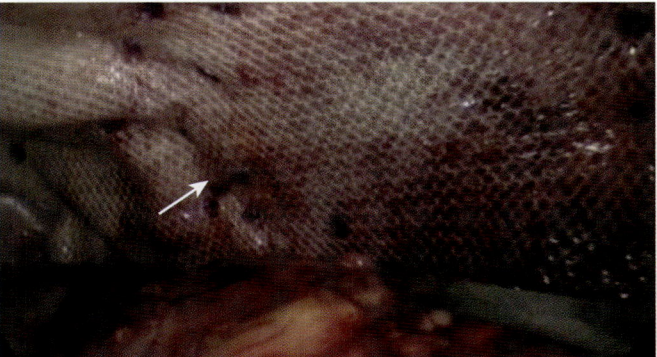

FIGURE 54.7 Completed laparoscopic mesh repair of a lumbar hernia. (From Varban O. Lumbar hernia after breast reconstruction. *Int J Surg Case Rep.* 2013;4[10]:869–871.)

sutures and tacks (Fig. 54.7).[27] The use of bone anchors has been described to secure mesh to the iliac crest in inferior lumbar hernias.[34] In a study of seven patients who underwent laparoscopic transabdominal incisional lumbar herniorrhaphy with polypropylene mesh reinforcement, there were no complications or recurrences over a mean follow-up of 34 months.[27] The laparoscopic transabdominal approach may also be preferable in patients with previous lumbar surgery.[27]

Unlike the transabdominal laparoscopic technique, the retroperitoneoscopic (or totally extraperitoneal [TEP]) repair avoids penetration into the abdominal cavity.[26,37,38] A flank incision is made and a balloon dissector is used to create a retroperitoneal plane and adequate operating space.[35,37,38] Nonabsorbable mesh is placed in an extraperitoneal position. Habib reported no recurrence out to 2 years in a patient who underwent tension-free retroperitoneoscopic repair of a superior lumbar hernia with polypropylene mesh.[38]

The management of TLH deserves special mention. The timing of the repair (early vs. delayed) and the surgical approach to those patients with TLH require individualization based on the patient's clinical status, presence of concomitant injuries, mechanism of injury, size of hernia, patient factors, and radiologic findings. Early repair is recommended in hemodynamically stable patients without major associated injuries.[25] In patients with extensive tissue loss and contamination, it is preferable to defer hernia repair until life-threatening injuries such as visceral injury have been addressed.[9] A transperitoneal approach is recommended by some authors in TLH to evaluate for concomitant bowel injuries.[9] In a case series by Chan et al., of four patients presenting with lumbar hernias following blunt trauma, two patients underwent delayed repair with mesh via a lumbar incision, one patient underwent a laparoscopic transabdominal mesh repair, and the last patient had an open transabdominal mesh repair.[25] In all of the patients, the mesh was placed in an extraperitoneal sublay position. There were no recurrences in their study, although one patient was lost to follow-up. A polytetrafluoroethylene or PTFE (Gore-Tex) tissue patch can be used for the coverage of large defects. It can also be used in the face of contamination because it is biologically inactive leading to decreased inflammation and adhesion formation, has good tensile strength, and may be resistant to infection.[9]

Although the laparoscopic transabdominal and retroperitoneoscopic approaches require less tissue dissection and provide an improved anatomic view in comparison to the open technique, there is no consensus regarding the preferred approach to lumbar hernias.[27,38] Moreno-Egea et al. performed the only reported comparative study of open versus laparoscopic lumbar hernia repair.[33] They demonstrated that a laparoscopic technique provides advantages such as decreased morbidity and length of stay, with quicker return to normal activity and no significant increase in cost.[33] A classification system has been proposed to help guide the management of lumbar hernias, which classifies them into four categories based on six individual criteria: size, location, contents within the hernia, the presence of muscular atrophy, origin, and a history of recurrence.[8] Although this classification system has yet to be validated, it may provide a basis to aid in the clinical management of lumbar hernias.

OBTURATOR HERNIA

ANATOMY AND CLASSIFICATION

The obturator hernia was first described at the Royal Academy of Sciences of Paris by Pierre Roland Arnaud de Ronsil in 1724.[39] More than 100 years later, Obre performed the first successful repair.[40] Currently, these rare defects represent only 0.05% to 1.4% of all hernias encountered by clinicians.[41–47] An obturator hernia occurs when intraabdominal viscera or extraperitoneal tissue project through the obturator canal, an osteofibrous tunnel that courses from the pelvis to the proximal thigh and is penetrated by the obturator neurovascular bundle (Figs. 54.8 and 54.9; see also Fig. 54.1). The foramen is created by the superior pubic ramus superiorly, the body and inferior ramus of the pubic bone interiorly, and the ramus and body of the ischium inferiorly.[46] Loss of the protective extraperitoneal areolar and adipose tissue overlying the obturator canal creates various anatomic pathways through which herniation can occur (Fig. 54.10).[42] In the most common pathway, the hernia sac protrudes through the external opening of the canal along the anterior division of the obturator nerve, with the sac lying beneath the pectineus muscle of the thigh. An alternative pathway is between the upper and middle fasciculi of the external obturator muscle along the posterior division of the obturator nerve. In this variation the sac can be found situated posterior to the adductor brevis muscle. Lastly, the least frequent pathway occurs with the entire sac penetrating and lying in between the internal and external obturator muscles.

CLINICAL PRESENTATION AND DIAGNOSIS

Often referred to as "the little old lady's hernia," obturator hernias are usually discovered in thin, elderly females in their seventh to eighth decade of life. Obturator hernias are 6 to 9 times more common in women.[42,48,49] This is likely secondary to differences in pelvic bone anatomy and angulation given females have a larger and wider pelvis with a horizontally inclined obturator canal.[49] Malnutrition and a thin body habitus are also significant risk factors.[40,50] Emaciation results in a loss of preperitoneal fat and connective tissue normally concealing the obturator canal.[40,43] Conditions that increase intraabdominal pressure and promote laxity of the pelvic floor, such as pregnancy and multiparity, may potentially predispose patients to herniation.[43] Of note, obturator hernias occur predominantly in the right pelvis due to the fact that the sigmoid colon often covers the left obturator foramen.[51] The hernia sac usually contains small bowel, although other organs, including the colon, appendix, Meckel diverticulum, bladder, and adnexa have been reported.[51]

The natural development of an obturator hernia occurs in three successive stages.[42] The first stage begins with

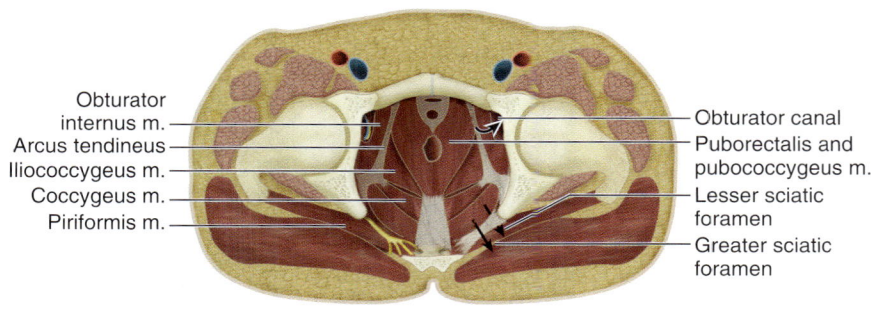

FIGURE 54.8 A diagram of normal pelvic floor anatomy showing the potential areas for obturator *(curved arrow)* and sciatic *(straight arrows)* herniation. (From Aguirre DA, Rivero OM, Martinez J. Normal anatomy of the abdominal wall. In: Sahani DV, ed. *Abdominal Imaging.* Philadelphia: Saunders; 2011:1439–1443.)

Labels (Fig. 54.8): Obturator internus m., Arcus tendineus, Iliococcygeus m., Coccygeus m., Piriformis m., Obturator canal, Puborectalis and pubococcygeus m., Lesser sciatic foramen, Greater sciatic foramen

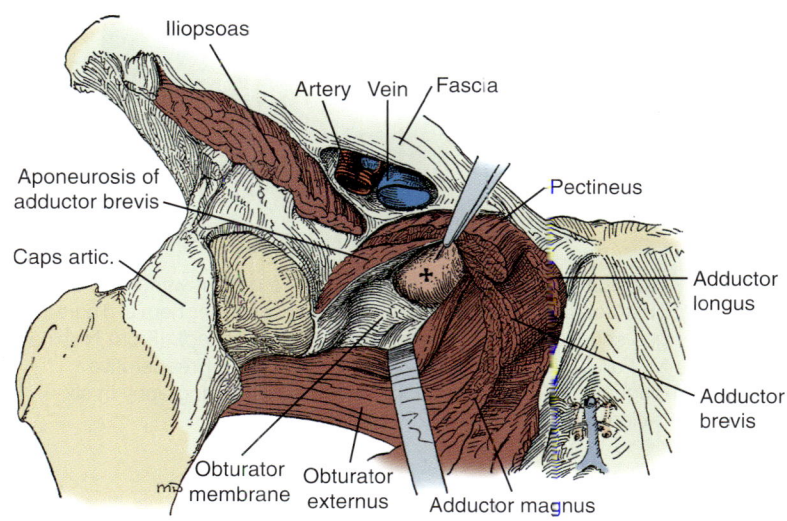

FIGURE 54.9 Anterior view of the obturator region with dissection carried to the level of the obturator membrane and obturator canal. The hernia sac can be seen protruding (marked by a *plus sign*). (From Watson LF. *Hernia.* 3rd ed. St. Louis: Mosby; 1948.)

Labels (Fig. 54.9): Iliopsoas, Artery, Vein, Fascia, Aponeurosis of adductor brevis, Caps artic., Pectineus, Adductor longus, Adductor brevis, Obturator membrane, Obturator externus, Adductor magnus

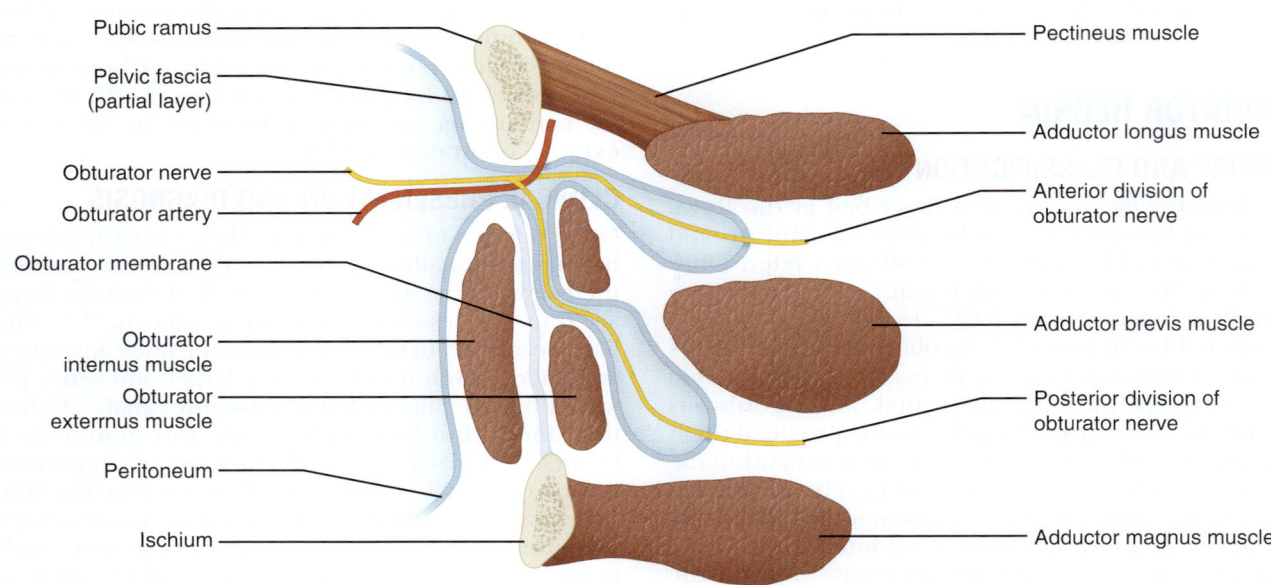

Pubic ramus
Pelvic fascia (partial layer)
Obturator nerve
Obturator artery
Obturator membrane
Obturator internus muscle
Obturator exterrnus muscle
Peritoneum
Ischium

Pectineus muscle
Adductor longus muscle
Anterior division of obturator nerve
Adductor brevis muscle
Posterior division of obturator nerve
Adductor magnus muscle

FIGURE 54.10 Side view of the anatomy of the obturator canal. A hernia can follow the path of either the anterior or posterior branch of the obturator nerve. (From Stamatiou D, Skandalakis LJ, Zoras O, et al. Obturator hernia revisited: surgical anatomy, embryology, diagnosis, and technique of repair. *Am Surg.* 2011;77:1147–1156.)

the bulging of preperitoneal fat through the obturator foramen. In the second, or developmental stage, prolongation of the peritoneum and formation of a true hernia sac occur. The third and final stage is marked by protrusion of viscera and the onset of clinical symptoms.

Diagnosis of an obturator hernia is challenging and requires a high clinical suspicion and an astute diagnostician because the condition is rare and often presents with nonspecific abdominal complaints.[52] The overwhelming majority of patients present with an acute small bowel obstruction.[42,44,51,53,54] A palpable mass in the groin is uncommon, but it may be appreciated upon a rectal or vaginal examination.[50] The Howship-Romberg sign, although considered pathognomonic of obturator herniation, is demonstrated in only 15% to 50% of cases.[53,55–57] This physical finding is confirmed by pain in the medial thigh from obturator nerve compression elicited by extension, abduction, and medial rotation of the ipsilateral lower extremity. The Hannington-Kiff sign, or an absent adductor reflex, may have increased specificity in comparison to the Howship-Romberg sign but occurs less frequently.[51,58] This maneuver is performed by percussing the medial thigh (over the adductor muscles) 5 cm above the patellar tendon. A positive sign is manifested by the absence of muscular contraction.

Abdominal radiography is often the first study performed in patients who present with findings suggestive of bowel obstruction. Plain radiographs may demonstrate dilated small bowel loops with an intraluminal gas shadow overlying the obturator foramen (Fig. 54.11), which should raise suspicion of an obturator hernia.[40] However, CT is the preferred diagnostic modality because it has greater than 90% accuracy and increased sensitivity for detecting an obturator hernia (Fig. 54.12).[46,51,53,54,56] Despite this, the

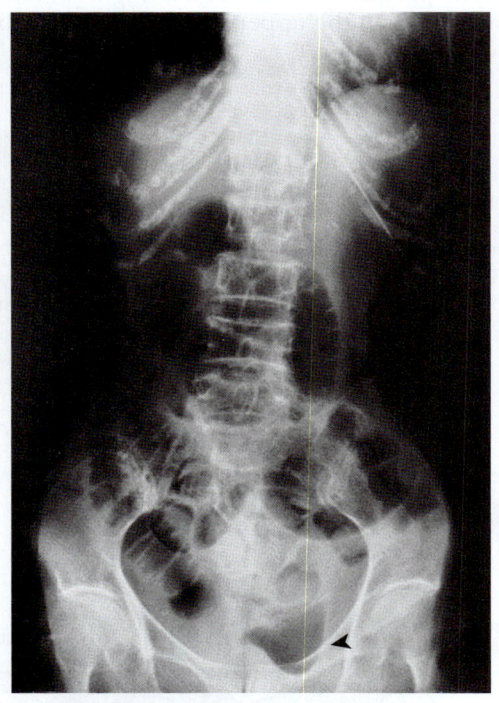

FIGURE 54.11 Abdominal radiograph in a patient with small bowel obstruction caused by an incarcerated obturator hernia. There is a gas shadow in the obturator foramen *(arrowhead).* (From Nishina M, Fujii C, Ogino R, Kobayashi R, Kohama A. Preoperative diagnosis of obturator hernia by computed tomography in six patients. *J Emerg Med.* 2001;20:277.)

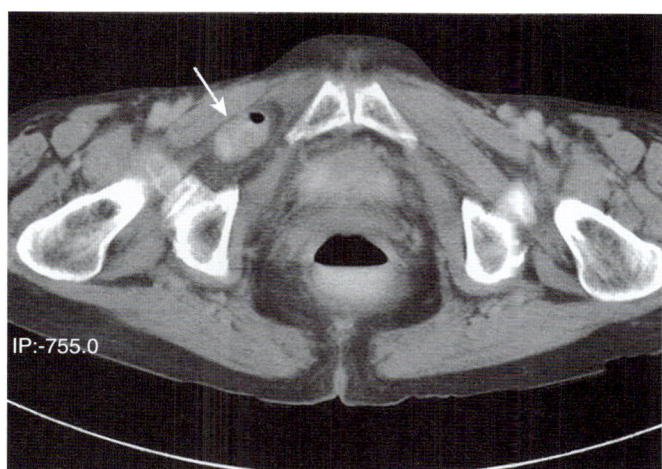

FIGURE 54.12 Pelvic computed tomographic scan showing bowel *(arrow)* protruding outside the right obturator foramen. (From Kim JJ, Jung H, Oh SJ, et al. Laparoscopic transabdominal preperitoneal hernioplasty of bilateral obturator hernia. *Surg Laparosc Endosc Percutan Tech.* 2005;15:106.)

clinical benefit of preoperative CT is controversial. Several previously published studies have reported a reduced rate of complications, need for small bowel resection, and mortality with the use of CT imaging.[42,51,56] However, more recent studies have been unable to demonstrate an added benefit with preoperative CT.[46,53,9] The role of CT may be important as it provides a prompt diagnosis of an obturator hernia and allows surgical planning, although it should never delay surgical intervention as any delay in treatment will significantly increase mortality.[56,57] Ultimately, CT is an incredibly valuable tool, but the diagnosis of an obturator hernia is best made in the operating room. The utility of other diagnostic modalities, such as contrast herniography and ultrasonography, have been described but their accuracy and relevance have yet to be determined.[52,50]

TREATMENT

A patient with an obturator hernia is typically female, elderly, frail, malnourished, has multiple comorbidities, and presents with an acute intestinal obstruction.[40,42] As a result, surgeons may prefer to conservatively manage such patients, given their inherently high surgical risk.[56] Despite this, urgent surgical intervention is crucial in the management of obturator hernias because the rate of strangulation reaches 50% to 75% and may increase further with any delay in treatment.[42,5] The classic surgical approach is through an exploratory laparotomy, although in recent years, inguinal and laparoscopic extraperitoneal techniques have been described.[40,61–63]

Exploration by laparotomy allows a complete assessment of intraabdominal viscera and pathology and evaluation of both obturator canals and facilitates bowel resection if required.[42] It is performed through a lower midline incision and preferred in patients with suspected intestinal perforation, strangulation, or peritoneal inflammation.[40] Laparoscopic transabdominal repair for obturator hernias has demonstrated good outcomes in both elective and emergency cases.[64,65] Although experience is limited, this approach shares the advantages of traditional exploratory laparotomy while potentially decreasing recovery time, hospital length of stay, and morbidity.[65] Both techniques allow for complete evaluation of intraabdominal pathology and evaluation for a contralateral defect. This is important because recent studies have reported an incidence of occult bilateral obturator hernias in 50% to 63%[64,66] of patients, despite a previously reported rate of 6%.[61] Alternative techniques of obturator hernia repair described in the literature include TEP, obturator, and inguinal routes.[63,67,68] These approaches may be appropriate in cases in which the preoperative diagnosis of an obturator hernia has been established and suspicion of necrotic bowel is absent.[42,53,67] Although unable to assess for bowel viability, the TEP technique provides the advantage of less surgical morbidity and a shorter recovery time.[67] Ultimately, the standard therapy remains an open transabdominal approach, and further studies are needed to elucidate the role of laparoscopic, extraperitoneal, and inguinal approaches in the management of an obturator hernia.[42]

After the obstructed segment of bowel is identified, reduction may be performed by simple gentle traction, if possible. In some instances, reduction of the herniated contents may be challenging and require incision of the obturator membrane, pubic osteotomy, or use of the "water pressure method" when incarcerated intestine is present.[42,64] In the water pressure method, an 8-French Nelaton catheter is inserted on the side of the hernia into the obturator foramen and water is injected into the hernia sac to promote intestinal reduction via water pressure.[64] After reduction of the hernia contents is achieved, the defect may be repaired using various methods. Small defects can be repaired by reapproximation of the hernia sac.[40,51] Larger defects require fascial closure (i.e., suturing the pectineus muscle to the periosteum of the pubic bone), coverage with local tissue (the round ligament, uterine fundus, ipsilateral ovary, or bladder), or prosthetic mesh reinforcement.[40,42,53,56] Although prosthetic mesh is contraindicated in cases with frank peritonitis or spillage of bowel contents, it may provide a more durable overall repair when its use is appropriate.[57] In a long-term study of 80 patients who underwent open abdominal and inguinal obturator hernia repair, recurrence rates at 3 years were significantly reduced (0% vs. 22%) with the use of prosthetic mesh.[57] Nevertheless, prospective long-term studies are needed to compare the efficacy and durability of the various repair techniques described.

SCIATIC HERNIA

ANATOMY AND CLASSIFICATION

Sciatic hernias are the rarest of the pelvic floor hernias. First described by Papen in 1750, only slightly more than 100 cases have been reported in the literature since then.[69] The sciatic notch is located between the posterior inferior iliac spine and ischial spine. Three distinctive anatomic spaces are created within the sciatic notch, and visceral herniation can occur through any one of these potential openings. The greater and lesser sciatic foramina are formed by the sacrospinous and sacrotuberous ligaments,

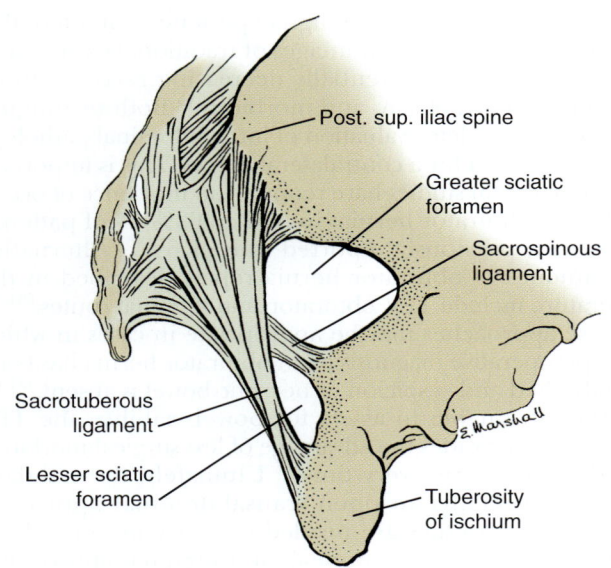

FIGURE 54.13 Posterolateral view of the pelvis showing the greater and lesser sciatic foramina and their ligamentous and osseous boundaries. (From Watson LF. *Hernia*. 3rd ed. St. Louis: CV Mosby; 1948.)

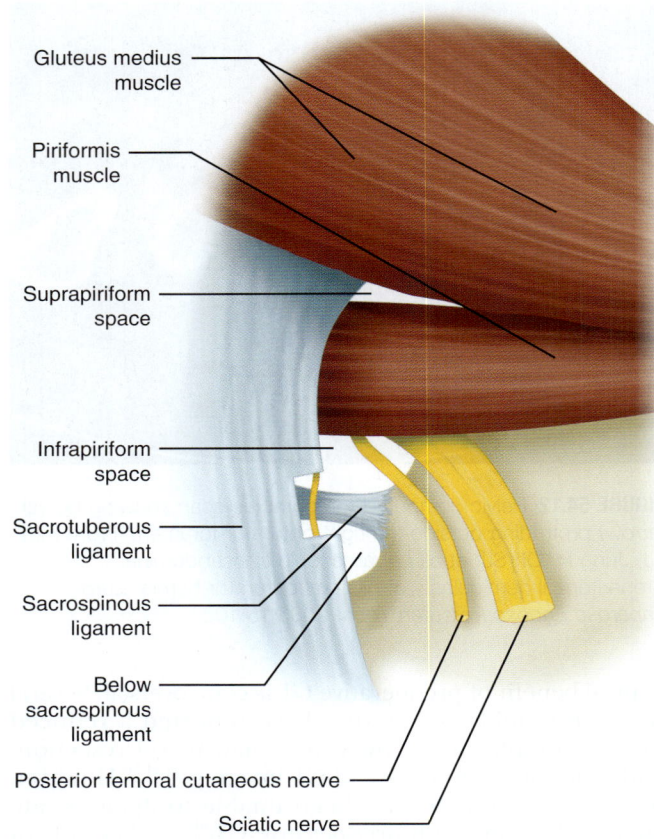

FIGURE 54.14 Anatomic locations for the three types of sciatic hernia on the right side. The gluteus maximus muscle is not shown. Sciatic hernias can occur through the suprapiriform space (1), through the infrapiriform space (2), or below the sacrospinous ligament (3). Also shown are the gluteus medius muscle (4), sacrospinous ligament (5), piriformis muscle (6), the sciatic nerve (7) and medial to it the posterior femoral cutaneous nerve, and the sacrotuberous ligament (8). (From Losanoff JE, Basson MD, Gruber SA, Weaver DW. Sciatic hernia: a comprehensive review of the world literature (1900–2008). *Am J Surg*. 2010;199[1] 52–59.)

respectively (Fig. 54.13; see also Fig. 54.8). The greater sciatic foramen is further subdivided by the piriformis muscle into the suprapiriform space and the infrapiriform space (Fig. 54.14). The precise mechanism by which a sciatic hernia forms has yet to be delineated, although atrophy of the piriformis muscle, sacrospinous ligament, and gluteus maximus muscle are associated pathologic findings.[70,71] Still, the etiology of sciatic hernias is likely more complex and involves interplay between different pathologic mechanisms.

CLINICAL PRESENTATION AND DIAGNOSIS

The clinical diagnosis of a sciatic hernia is extremely difficult because symptoms are usually limited to nonspecific pain and physical findings are often absent. Patients are more commonly female and may present with acute or chronic pain in the pelvis, buttock, or thigh.[72] Sciatica, or pain radiating down the posterior thigh, may be the presenting symptom in a patient with compression of the sciatic nerve by the hernia sac. Alternatively, sciatic hernias may present with acute intestinal obstruction or strangulation. An interesting variant described in the literature is a ureteric sciatic hernia.[73] In this type of hernia, the presence of a ureteral segment or bladder within the hernia sac can lead to obstructive uropathy. Small bowel, ovarian tissue, colon, and Meckel diverticulum may also protrude through the sciatic foramen.

There are no pathognomonic findings on physical exam that can facilitate the diagnosis of a sciatic hernia. Identification of a bulge or protrusion is exceedingly rare given the location of the hernia and the fact that the gluteus maximus muscle is disproportionately large and overlies the sciatic foramen. Therefore viscera protruding through the sciatic notch would be difficult to appreciate unless fairly large in size. Pelvic or rectal examination

may reveal a bulge in the sciatic region in some cases. Differential diagnoses include a gluteal abscess, arterial aneurysm, or a lipoma.[74]

The clinical diagnosis of a sciatic hernia requires high clinical suspicion and often adjunctive diagnostic imaging. The diagnosis of a sciatic hernia can be made using various imaging modalities including barium studies, transgluteal ultrasound, CT, and MRI.[69] The preferred diagnostic imaging is CT (Fig. 54.15) because it allows for a rapid diagnosis, delineates regional anatomy, and may provide information regarding intestinal viability. In the case of a ureteric sciatic hernia, diagnosis is traditionally achieved with an excretory or retrograde urogram, which will demonstrate a pathognomonic "curlicue ureter" (Fig. 54.16).[75]

TREATMENT

Sciatic hernias are treated surgically. The surgical approach may be abdominal transperitoneal, abdominal extraperitoneal, gluteal, or a combination of multiple techniques

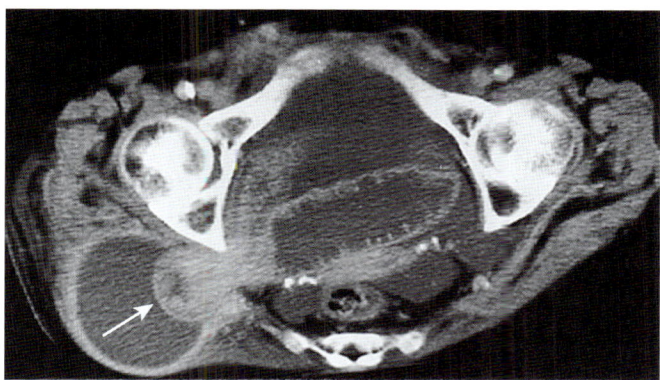

FIGURE 54.15 Computed tomographic scan showing incarcerated bowel *(arrow)* through the right sacral foramen and surrounding ascites in the right subgluteal region. (From Yu PC, Ko SF, Lee TY, Ng SH, Huang CC, Wan YL. Small bowel obstruction due to incarcerated sciatic hernia: ultrasound diagnosis. *Br J Radiol*. 2002;75:381.)

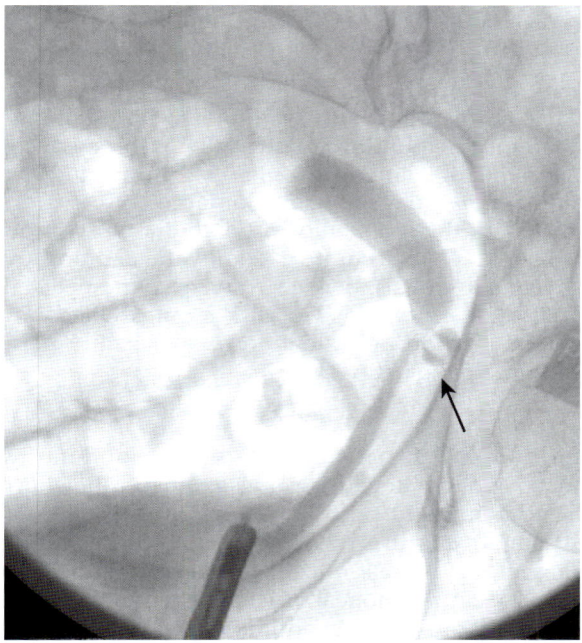

FIGURE 54.16 A retrograde pyelogram showing focal herniation of the left ureter *(arrow)* into the greater sciatic foramen causing ureteral obstruction. (From Zagoria RJ, Dyer R, Brady C. The renal sinus, pelvocalyceal system, and ureter. In: Zagoria RJ, ed. *Genitourinary Imaging: The Requisites*. Philadelphia: Elsevier; 2016:146–189.)

depending on patient factors and their presentation. Emergency laparotomy is preferred in patients who present with acute intestinal obstruction or strangulation because it permits complete evaluation of viscera and resection of bowel if necessary. The defect can be repaired with local tissue flaps or reinforced with prosthetic mesh when the defect is relatively large and bacterial contamination is absent. Prosthetic mesh is placed in an extraperitoneal position and secured to the periosteum of the pubis

centrally, the arcuate line of the ilium laterally, the levator ani muscle medially, and to the periosteum of the sacrum posteriorly.[69] One must be cautious to avoid injury to underlying nerves and vessels when suturing mesh to the surrounding tissue. The extraperitoneal or laparoscopic transabdominal approaches can be used to repair ureteric sciatic hernias.[69,76]

The gluteal approach avoids penetration of the peritoneum and can be pursued when a preoperative diagnosis of a sciatic hernia has been established and repair is elective. In this technique a muscle-splitting incision is made through the gluteus maximus in the orientation of the piriformis muscle. Although this technique can have a high risk of neurovascular injury in large complicated hernias, it may facilitate identification and reduction of the hernia.[69] Overall the surgical literature is scant and limited to case series and case reports. Thus a conclusive argument cannot be made to support one technique over another.

PERINEAL HERNIAS

ANATOMY AND CLASSIFICATION

Perineal hernias are rare hernias involving the pelvic floor. The first case of a perineal hernia was documented by De Garangeot in 1743, and the first surgical repair was reported by Moscowitz in 1916.[77] Perineal hernias are initially classified as congenital or acquired. Purely congenital perineal hernias are extremely rare, and only nine cases have been documented in the literature.[77] Acquired perineal hernias are classified as either primary or secondary. Primary acquired perineal hernias are also rare and occur most commonly in older, multiparous women. They have also been described in patients who have chronic conditions involving increased abdominal pressure, such as constipation or ascites.[78] They have also been described in cases of neurogenic atrophy of the pelvic floor.[79] Secondary perineal hernias are much more common and develop following extensive pelvic surgical procedures (and therefore are considered incisional hernias). These procedures include abdominoperineal resection (APR), pelvic exenteration, or hysterectomy.

Anatomically, perineal hernias can be further subclassified as anterior or posterior, based upon their location relative to the transverse perineal muscles (Fig. 54.17). Occurring in females only, anterior perineal hernias are caused by the passage of abdominal viscera (usually bladder and small or large intestine) through a defect in the urogenital diaphragm lateral to the vaginal vestibule. The anterior defects occur in a triangle bordered by the ischiocavernosus muscle laterally, the bulbospongiosus muscle medially, and the superficial transverse perineal muscle posteriorly. Anterior perineal hernias are extremely rare, with fewer than 17 cases reported in the literature.[80] In 1922 Chase reported a series of 13 cases of anterior peritoneal hernias, and this remains the largest reported series to date. Most cases reported are secondary by classification, having followed extensive or multiple pelvic procedures or prolonged labor.

Posterior perineal hernias occur posterior to the superficial transverse perineal muscle, either through the levator ani muscle (between the iliococcygeus and

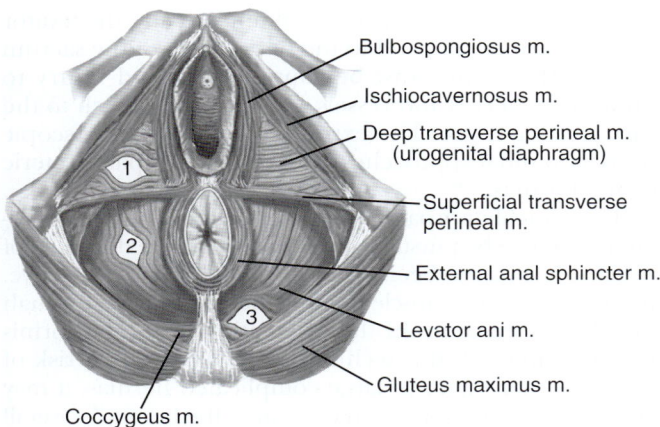

FIGURE 54.17 The anatomy of the perineum and typical locations of perineal hernias. (From Twiss C, Rosenblum N. Perineal hernia and perineocele. In: Raz S, ed. *Female Urology*. Philadelphia: Saunders Elsevier; 2008:743–750. Modified from Cali RL, Pitsch RM, Blatchford GJ, Thorson A, Christensen MA. Rare pelvic floor hernias. *Dis Colon Rectum*. 1992;35:604.)

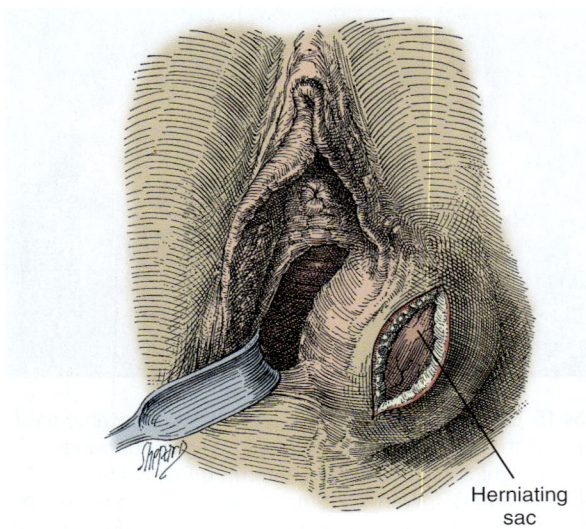

FIGURE 54.18 Anterior perineal hernia. When the hernia descends only into the posterior portion of the labium major, it is known as a pudendal or vaginolabial hernia. (From Watson LF. *Hernia*. 3rd ed. St. Louis: Mosby; 1948.)

pubococcygeus) or in a space between the levator ani and the coccygeus muscle. Most posterior perineal hernias are secondary, and the true incidence of primary posterior perineal hernias is unknown. Posterior hernias can be found in either sex, but they are 3 to 5 times more common in women.[81] Secondary posterior perineal hernias are incisional hernias through the pelvic floor that typically present within the first postoperative year.

CLINICAL PRESENTATION AND DIAGNOSIS

Patients with an anterior perineal hernia may be asymptomatic, but most will complain of a mass or heavy sensation within the labia. Because it is not uncommon for the anterior defects to contain portions of the bladder, patients may complain of difficulty with urination, including incontinence.[82] On physical exam, patients with anterior perineal hernias have a palpable mass in the posterior aspect of the labia (Fig. 54.18). This needs to be distinguished from other similar conditions, such as a Bartholin gland abscess, labial cysts, lipoma, hematoma, or inguinal hernia. An anterior perineal hernia can usually be reduced into the pelvic floor inferiorly or below the pubic ramus, whereas a true inguinal hernia will reduce by passing over or superior to the pubic ramus.

Patients with a posterior perineal hernia are usually asymptomatic, but when it causes symptoms, they usually complain of a perineal mass that produces pain and discomfort, especially upon sitting. Physical exam will reveal a soft, reducible mass between the anus and ischial tuberosity or occasionally ventral to the gluteus maximus muscle.[83]

Nausea, vomiting, and other signs of intestinal obstruction are rarely seen in perineal hernias due to the usually wide pelvic floor defect, as well as the laxity of the tissues. However, bowel obstruction and perineal skin breakdown have been reported in perineal hernias that occur following pelvic surgery.[84,85]

A thorough history and physical exam focusing on the vaginal, perineal, and rectal exams is important for all perineal hernias. If urinary symptoms are present, further work-up with cystourethrography and possibly cystoscopy is recommended. Plain radiographs or contrast studies (i.e., barium enema) may show small or large bowel within the hernia. With the availability of CT today, most clinicians will obtain a CT to accurately identify the contents within the hernia, as well as to assess the size of the pelvic floor defect. Furthermore, pelvic MRI is quickly becoming a preferred method of evaluation for pelvic and perineal pathology (Fig. 54.19A–D).

TREATMENT

As for most hernias, treatment is surgical and mostly on an elective basis. Repair is very similar to other hernias, with reduction and possible resection of the hernia sac and primary closure of the defect. It is important to remember that there is not always a clearly defined hernia sac because extraperitoneal structures can herniate through the pelvic floor defect. In addition, the size of the defect can be extensive, especially following pelvic exenteration.[80] Repair of such a large defect usually necessitates advanced reconstruction of the pelvic floor using mesh, free fascial grafts, or pedicled muscle flaps.[86–88]

Using a traditional open approach, the perineal hernia defect can be repaired via an abdominal, perineal, or a combined approach. Laparoscopic repair with mesh reinforcement has also been described and is becoming more common.[89,90] To date, there are no controlled trials or studies that have shown any approach to be superior to the others. The choice of approach is best determined by the size of the defect, the patient's comorbidities and previous surgical history, the condition of the pelvic tissues, and the experience and comfort level of the operating surgeon.

The abdominal approach via laparotomy allows for excellent exposure of the pelvic floor defect and hernia sac, especially for those cases where the defect is large requiring reconstruction with mesh.[86,91] The open abdominal

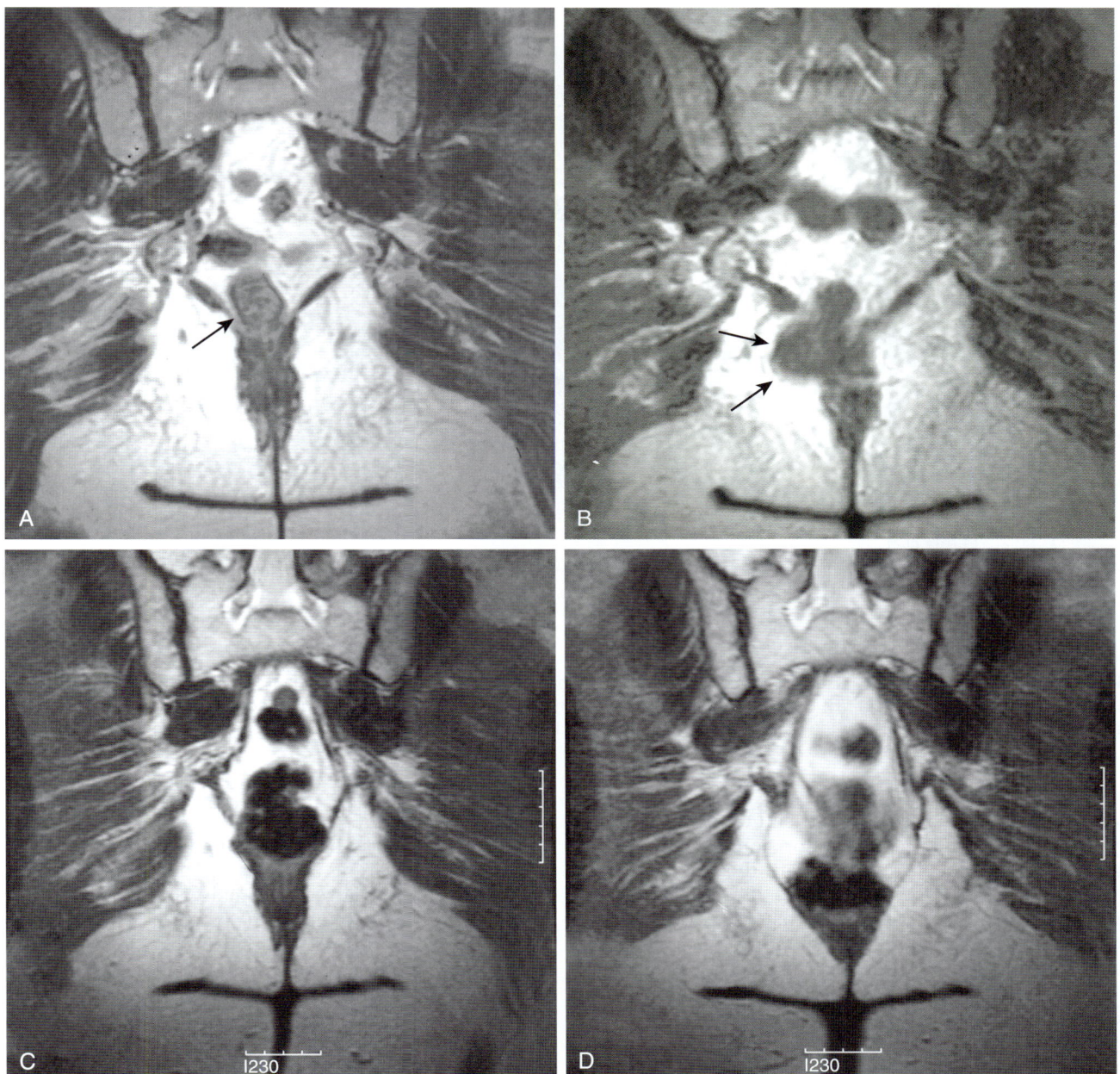

FIGURE 54.19 Coronal T2-weighted magnetic resonance images. (A) Rest image showing a midline rectum *(arrow)* in a patient with obstructed defecation. (B) Strain image demonstrating the rectum *(arrows)* herniating through a defect in the right levator ani complex. (C) Postoperative rest image after a combined abdominoperineal approach to simple levator hernia repair with no absorbable sutures. (D) The rectum remains midline after hernia repair, and the patient's symptoms of obstructed defecation were resolved. (From Kaufman HS, Buller JL, Thompson JR, et al. Dynamic pelvic MR imaging and cystocolpoproctography alter surgical management of pelvic floor disorders. *Dis Colon Rectum.* 2001;44:1575; discussion 1584.)

approach is necessary in cases involving strangulation to allow for possible resection of the hernia contents. Patients should be positioned in a modified lithotomy position to allow access to the perineum if needed. In addition, placing the patient in some degree of Trendelenburg will allow the viscera to fall out of the pelvis and therefore optimize visualization. In general, after obtaining adequate exposure, the hernia sac is identified, dissected out, and reduced. Small defects can be repaired primarily, whereas

larger defects (as seen following pelvic exenteration) require more complex reconstruction usually with mesh.

The perineal approach is the preferred initial approach, especially for small defects or otherwise straightforward cases. Advantages to this approach include less morbidity to the patient, as well as the ability to remove any excess or redundant skin accompanying larger hernias.[86] A notable disadvantage is limited exposure, making it difficult to lyse adhesions as well as to evaluate for recurrent cancer or

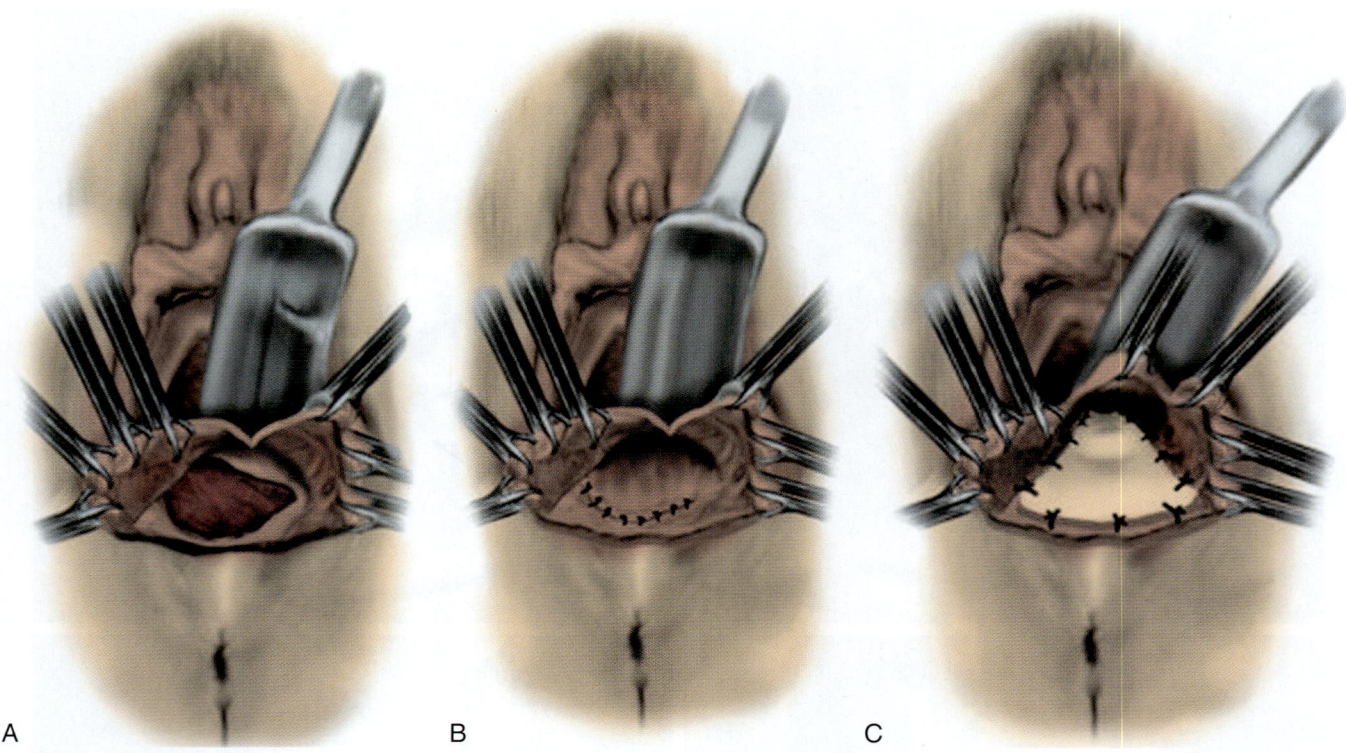

A   B   C

FIGURE 54.20 Site-specific rectocele repair of a distal defect with separation of the rectovaginal fascia from the perineal body. (A) Dissection of a discrete defect. (B) Repair of the defect to the perineal body. (C) Onlay dermal graft attached to the levators laterally, the rectovaginal fascia apically, and the perineal body distally. (From Kohli N, Miklos JR. Dermal graft-augmented rectocele repair. *Int Urogynecol J.* 2003;14:146.)

visceral injuries. It may also be difficult to properly fixate any mesh used in the reconstruction, and recurrences as high as 23% have been reported with this approach.[92]

For the perineal approach (Fig. 54.20A–C) the patient is generally positioned similar to that used for an open procedure (lithotomy and Trendelenburg position). The skin is carefully incised over the hernia sac. For anterior perineal hernias, this incision is made over or along the involved labia majora. The hernia sac is opened, its contents reduced, and then carefully dissected free from the margins of the defect and excised. The defect is then primarily repaired in layers using nonabsorbable suture with or without mesh reinforcement. A combined or abdominoperineal approach provides the benefits of each approach individually but is generally associated with increased morbidity.

Laparoscopic transabdominal repairs of perineal hernias are becoming more common as more experience is gained in the repair of these rare defects. The well-known benefits of less postoperative pain and quicker recovery have been documented following the repair of these pelvic hernias.[93] Laparoscopic repair almost always uses reinforcement with mesh, and repairs with both synthetic and biologic mesh have been performed successfully.[94] Combined laparoscopic approaches have also been described in the literature.[89,95] The hernia sac is generally mobilized and reduced laparoscopically, with subsequent primary suture repair of the defect performed via an open perineal approach. Even successful redo-laparoscopic mesh repair

of recurrent perineal hernias following previous repair with mesh has also been described.[96]

Despite the various approaches, recurrence rates following perineal hernia repair remain a significant concern. A recent study looked at 40 patients who underwent various techniques of perineal hernia repair following APR. A primary recurrence was noted in 13 patients, with a second recurrence in 3 patients.[97]

SUMMARY

Lumbar and pelvic hernias are unique hernias that are seldom seen in a surgeon's clinical practice. Presenting symptoms are often vague and underappreciated, which makes lumbar and pelvic hernias difficult to diagnose. However, the increased availability of CT and MRI has made it easier to make the diagnosis. These imaging modalities also allow clinicians to completely evaluate the size of the anatomic defect and the contents within the hernia sac. As with most hernias throughout the body, they can be repaired successfully via an open or laparoscopic approach, either with or without mesh reinforcement.

REFERENCES

1. Jeannel M. La hernie lombaire. *Arch Prov Chir Paris.* 1903;11:389-418.
2. DeGarangeot RJC. *Traite des Operations de Chirurgie.* 1731;1:369.
3. Cavallaro G, Sadighi A, Paparelli C, et al. Anatomical and surgical considerations on lumbar hernias. *Am Surg.* 2009;75(12):1238-1241.

4. Petit JL. Traité des maladies chirurgicales, et des operations qui leur convenient. *Didot.* 1774;2:256.
5. Grynfelt J. Quelque mots sur la hernie lombaire. *Montpellier Méd.* 1866;16:323.
6. Lesshaft P. Die lumbal gegend. *Anat Chirurgischer. Hinsicht Arch f Anat u Physiol u Wissensch Med Leipzig.* 1870;37:26–.
7. Zhou X, Nve JO, Chen G. Lumbar hernia: clinical analysis of 11 cases. *Hernia.* 2004;8:260-263.
8. Moreno-Egea A, Baena EG, Calle MC, Martínez JA, Albasini JL. Controversies in the current management of lumbar hernias. *Arch Surg.* 2007;142:82.
9. Esposito TJ, Federak I. Traumatic lumbar hernia case report and literature review. *J Trauma.* 1994;37:123-126.
10. Cavallaro G, Sadighi A, Miceli M, Burza A, Carbone G, Cavallaro A. Primary lumbar hernia repair: the open approach. *Eur Surg Res.* 2007;39:88-92.
11. Hickey M, Buick RG. Bilateral congenital lumbar hernia. *Ir J Med Sci.* 1982;151:388-389.
12. Lichtenstein IL. Repair of large diffuse lumbar hernias by an extraperitoneal binder technique. *Am J Surg.* 1986;151:501-504.
13. Vagholkar K, Dastoor K. Congenital lumbar hernia with lumbocostovertebral syndrome: a case report and review of the literature. *Case Rep Pediatr.* 2013;2013:532910. http://www.ncbi.nlm.nih.gov/pubmed/24159401. Accessed June 2016.
14. Harris K, Dorn C, Bloom B. Lumbocostovertebral syndrome with associated VACTERL anomalad: a neonatal case report. *J Perinatol.* 2009;29:826-827.
15. Heinford BT, Iannitti DA, Gagner M. Laparoscopic inferior and superior lumbar hernia repair. *Arch Surg.* 1997;132:1141-1144.
16. Sutherland RS, Gerow RR. Hernia after dorsal incision into lumbar region: a case report and review of pathogenesis and treatment. *J Urol.* 1995;153:382.
17. Stamatiou D, Skandalakis JE, Skandalakis LE, Mirilas P. Lumbar hernia: surgical anatomy, embryology and technique of repair. *Am Surg.* 2009;75:202.
18. Danikas D, Theodorou SJ, Stratoulias C, et al. Hernia through an iliac crest bone-graft donor site. *Plast Reconstr Surg.* 2007;120(131):61-63.
19. Prabhu R, Kumar N, Shenoy F. Iliac crest bone graft donor site hernia: not so uncommon. *BMJ Case Rep.* 2013;http://casereports.bmj.com/content/2013/bcr-2013-010386.long. Accessed June 2016.
20. Oldfield MD. Iliac hernia after bone grafting. *Lancet.* 1945;245(6357):810-812.
21. Kaushik R, Attri AK. Incisional hernia from iliac bone grafting sites—a report of two cases. *Hernia.* 2003;7(4):227-228.
22. Pyrtek LJ, Kelly CC. Management of herniation through large iliac bone defects. *Ann Surg.* 1960;152:998-1003.
23. Auleda J, Bianchi A, Tibau R, Rodriguez-Cano O. Hernia through iliac crest defects. A report of four cases. *Int Orthop.* 1995;19(6):367-369.
24. Burt BM, Afifi HY, Wantz GE, Barie PS. Traumatic lumbar hernia: report of cases and comprehensive review of the literature. *J Trauma.* 2004;57:1361-1370.
25. Chan K, Towsey K, Cavallucci D, Green B. Traumatic lumbar hernia: experience at the Royal Brisbane and Women's Hospital. *Hernia.* 2015;21(2):317-322.
26. Ahmed ST, Ranjan R, Saha SB, Singh B. Lumbar hernia: a diagnostic dilemma. *BMJ Case Rep.* 2014;doi:10.1136/bcr-2013-202085.
27. Yavuz N, Ersoy YE, Demirkesen O, Tortum OB, Erguney S. Laparoscopic incisional lumbar hernia repair. *Hernia.* 2009;13:281-286.
28. Losanov JE, Kjossev KT. Diagnosis and treatment of primary incarcerated lumbar hernia. *Eur J Surg.* 2002;168:193-195.
29. Solaini L, di Francesco F, Gourgiotis S, Solaini L. A very simple technique to repair Grynfelt-Lesshaft hernia. *Hernia.* 2010 14(4):439-441.
30. Salemis NS, Nisotakis K, Gourgiotis S, Tsohataridis E. Segmental liver incarceration through a recurrent incisional lumbar hernia. *Hepatobiliary Pancreat Dis Int.* 2007;6:442-444.
31. Schumpelick V. *Atlas of Hernia Surgery.* Philadelphia: BC Decker; 1990.
32. Geis WP, Saletta JD. Lumbar hernia. In: Nyhus LM, Condon RE, eds. *Hernia.* 3rd ed. London: Lippincott; 1989.
33. Moreno-Egea A, Torralba-Martinez JA, Morales G, et al. Open vs. laparoscopic repair of secondary lumbar hernias: a prospective nonrandomized study. *Surg Endosc.* 2005;19:184-187.
34. Links D, Berney C. Traumatic lumbar hernia repair: a laparoscopic technique for mesh fixation with an iliac crest suture anchor. *Hernia.* 2011;15:691-693.
35. Grauls A, Lallemand B, Krick M. The retroperitoneoscopic repair of a lumbar hernia of Petit. Case report and review of literature. *Acta Chir Belg.* 2004;104:330-334.
36. Carbonell AM, Kercher KW, Sigmon L, et al. A novel technique of lumbar hernia repair using bone anchor fixation. *Hernia.* 2005;9:22-25.
37. Arca MJ, Heniford BT, Pokorny R, et al. Laparoscopic repair of lumbar hernias. *J Am Coll Surg.* 1998;187:147-152.
38. Habib E. Retroperitoneoscopic tension-free repair of lumbar hernia. *Hernia.* 2003;7:150-152.
39. Gray SW, Skandalakis JE, Soria RE, et al. Strangulated obturator hernia. *Surgery.* 1974;75:20-27.
40. Stamatiou D, Skandalakis LJ, Zoras O, et al. Obturator hernia revisited: surgical anatomy, embryology, diagnosis, and technique of repair. *Am Surg.* 2011;77(9):1147-1157.
41. Kulkarni SR, Punamiya AR, Naniwadekar RG, et al. Obturator hernia: a diagnostic challenge. *Int J Surg Case Rep.* 2013;4:606-608.
42. Losanoff JE, Richman BW, Jones JW. Obturator hernia. *J Am Coll Surg.* 2002;194(5):657-663.
43. Bjork KJ, Mucha P, Cahill DR. Obturator hernia. *Surg Gynecol Obstet.* 1988;167:217-222.
44. Lo CY, Lorentz TG, Lau PWK. Obturator hernia presenting as small bowel obstruction. *Am J Surg.* 1994;167:396-398.
45. Skandalakis LJ. *Obturator Hernia.* 5th ed. New York: Lippincott Williams and Wilkins; 2002.
46. Yokoyama Y, Yamaguchi A, Isogai M, et al. Thirty-six cases of obturator hernia: does computed tomography contribute to postoperative outcome? *World J Surg.* 1999;23:214-216.
47. Maharaj D, Maharaj S, Young L, et al. Obturator hernia repair—a new technique. *Hernia.* 2002;6(1):45-47.
48. Cali RL, Pitsch RM, Blatchford GJ, et al. Rare pelvic floor hernias: report of a case and review of the literature. *Dis Colon Rectum.* 1992;35:604-612.
49. Temple DF, Miller RE. Incarcerated obturator hernia: two case reports and review of the literature. *J Natl Med Assoc.* 1980;72:513-515.
50. Tateno Y, Adachi K. Sudden knee pain in an underweight, older woman: obturator hernia. *Lancet.* 2014;384:206.
51. Rodriguez-Hermosa JI, Codina-Cazador A, Maroto-Genover A, et al. Obturator hernia: clinical analysis of 16 cases and algorithm for its diagnosis and treatment. *Hernia.* 2008;12:289-297.
52. Yokoyama T, Munakata Y, Ogiwara M, et al. Preoperative diagnosis of strangulated obturator hernia using ultrasonography. *Am J Surg.* 1997;174:76-78.
53. Nasir BS, Zendejas B, Ali SM, et al. Obturator hernia: the Mayo Clinic experience. *Hernia.* 2012;16(3):315-319.
54. Nazarian S, Narayanan A, Chang S. Diagnosis of an obturator hernia by CT. *BMJ Case Rep.* 2015;http://casereports.bmj.com/content/2015/bcr-2015-212239.long. Accessed June 2016.
55. Hodgins N, Cieplucha K, Conneally P, et al. Obturator hernia: a case report and review of the literature. *Int J Surg Case Rep.* 2013;4:889-892.
56. Kammori M, Mafune K, Hirashima T, et al. Forty-three cases of obturator hernia. *Am J Surg.* 2004;187:549-552.
57. Karasaki T, Nomura Y, Tanaka N. Long-term outcomes after obturator hernia repair: retrospective analysis of 80 operations at a single institution. *Hernia.* 2014;18(3):393-397.
58. Hannington-Kiff J. Absent thigh reflex in obturator hernias. *Lancet.* 1980;1:180.
59. Chan KV, Chan CKO, Yau KW, Fernández T, Girela E, Aguayo-Albasini JL. Surgical morbidity and mortality in obturator hernia: a 10-year retrospective risk factor evaluation. *Hernia.* 2014;18(3):387-392.
60. Carriquiry LA, Pineyro A. Pre-operative diagnosis of nonstrangulated obturator hernia: the contribution of herniography. *Br J Surg.* 1988;75:785.
61. Malik MU, Connelly TM, Hamid M, Pretorius F. Laparoscopic total extraperitoneal repair of preoperatively diagnosed bilateral obturator and incidental bilateral femoral herniae. *BMJ Case Rep.* 2016;doi:10.1136/bcr-2016-214978; http://casereports.bmj.com/content/2016/bcr-2016-214978.long. Accessed June 2016.
62. Wada Y, Ohtsuka H, Adachi K. Laparoscopic views of obturator hernia. *J Gastrointest Surg.* 2015;19:1925-1926.
63. Murai S, Akatsu T, Yabe N, Inoue Y, Akatsu Y, Kitagawa Y. Impacted obturator hernia treated successfully with a Kugel repair: report of two cases. *Surg Today.* 2009;39:821-824.
64. Hayama S, Ohtaka K, Takahashi Y, Ichimura T, Senmaru N, Hirano S. Laparoscopic reduction and repair for incarcerated obturator hernia: comparison with open surgery. *Hernia.* 2015;19:809-814.

65. Ng DCK, Tung KLM, Tang CN, Li M. Fifteen-year experience in managing obturator hernia: from open to laparoscopic approach. *Hernia.* 2014;18:381-386.

66. Yokoyama T, Kobayashi A, Kikuchi T, Hayashi K, Miyagawa S. Transabdominal preperitoneal repair for obturator hernia. *World J Surg.* 2011;35(10):2323-2327.

67. Karashima R, Kimura M, Taura N, Shimokawa Y, Nishimura T, Baba H. Total extraperitoneal approach for incarcerated obturator hernia repair. *Hernia.* 2016;20(3):479-482.

68. Shapiro K, Patel S, Choy C, Chaudry G, Khalil S, Ferzli G. Totally extraperitoneal repair of obturator hernia. *Surg Endosc.* 2004;18(6):954-956.

69. Losanoff JE, Basson MD, Gruber SA, Weaver DW. Sciatic hernia: a comprehensive review of the world literature (1900–2008). *Am J Surg.* 2010;199:52.

70. Gaffney LB, Schanno JF. Sciatic hernia. *Am J Surg.* 1958;95:974-975.

71. Ghahremani GG, Michael AS. Sciatic hernia with incarcerated ileum: CT and radiographic diagnosis. *Gastrointest Radiol.* 1991;16:120-122.

72. Miklos JR, O'Reilly MJ, Saye WB. Sciatic hernia as a cause of chronic pelvic pain in women. *Obstet Gynecol.* 1998;6:998-1001.

73. Rotchild TPE. Ureteral hernia: report of a case of herniation of the ureter into the sciatic foramen. *Arch Surg.* 1969;98:96-98.

74. Bernard AC, Lee C, Hoskins J, et al. Sciatic hernia: laparoscopic transabdominal extraperitoneal repair with plug and patch. *Hernia.* 2010;14:97.

75. Beck WC, Baurys W, Brochu J. Herniation of the ureter into the sciatic foramen ('curlicue ureter'). *JAMA.* 1952;179:441.

76. Gee J, Munson JL, Smith JJIII. Laparoscopic repair of ureterosciatic hernia. *Urology.* 1999;54:730-733.

77. Stamatiou D, Skandakakis JE, Skandalakis LJ, Mirilas P. Perineal hernia: surgical anatomy, embryology, and technique of repair. *Am Surg.* 2010;76(5):474-479.

78. Salameh JR. Primary and unusual abdominal wall hernias. *Surg Clin North Am.* 2008;88:45.

79. Rayhanabad J, Sassani P, Abbas MA. Laparoscopic repair of perineal hernia. *JSLS.* 2009;13:237.

80. Twiss CB, Rosenblum N. Perineal hernia and perineocele. In: Raz S, Rodriguz LV, eds. *Female Urology.* Vol. 76. Philadelphia: Elsevier; 2008:743-750.

81. Poon FW, Lauder JC, Finlay IG. Perineal herniation. *Clin Radiol.* 1993;47:49.

82. Anderson WR. Pudendal hernia. Unusual cause of labial mass. *Obstet Gynecol.* 1968;32:802.

83. Cali RL, Pitsch RM, Blatchford GJ, Thorson A, Christensen MA. Rare pelvic floor hernias. *Dis Colon Rectum.* 1992;35:604.

84. Ego-Aguirre E, Spratt JS, Butcher HR, Bricker EM. Repair of perineal hernia developing subsequent to pelvic exenteration. *Ann Surg.* 1964;159:66.

85. Kelly AR. Surgical repair of post-operative perineal hernia. *Aust N Z J Surg.* 1960;29:243.

86. Abdul Jabbar AS. Postoperative perineal hernia. *Hernia.* 2002;6:188.

87. Frydman GM, Polglase AL. Perineal approach for polypropylene mesh repair of perineal hernia. *Aust N Z J Surg.* 1989;59:895.

88. Brotschi E, Noe JM, Silen W. Perineal hernias after proctectomy. *Am J Surg.* 1985;149:301.

89. Franklin ME, Abrego D, Parra E. Laparoscopic repair of postoperative perineal hernia. *Hernia.* 2002;6:42.

90. Ghellai AM, Islam S, Stoker ME. Laparoscopic repair of postoperative perineal hernia. *Surg Laparosc Endosc Percutan Tech.* 2002;12:119.

91. Beck DE, Fazio VW, Jagelman DG, et al. Postoperative perineal hernia. *Dis Colon Rectum.* 1987;30:21.

92. So JB, Palmer MT, Shellito PC. Postoperative perineal hernia. *Dis Colon Rectum.* 1997;40:954.

93. Sorelli PG, Clark SK, Jenkins JT. Laparoscopic repair of primary perineal hernias: the approach of choice in the 21st century. *Colorectal Dis.* 2012;14(2):e72-e73.

94. Abbas Y, Garner J. Laparoscopic and perineal approaches to perineal hernia repair. *Tech Coloproctol.* 2014;18(4):361-364.

95. Gomes Portilla A, Cendoya I, Uzquiza E, et al. Giant perineal hernia. Laparoscopic mesh repair complemented by a perineal cutaneous approach. *Hernia.* 2010;13:199.

96. Goedhart-de Haan AM, Langenhoff BS, Petersen D, Verheijenet PM. Laparoscopic repair of perineal hernia after abdomino-perineal excision. *Hernia.* 2015;http://link.springer.com/articl e/10.1007%2Fs10029-015-1449-3. Accessed June 2016.

97. Mjoli M, Sloothaak DA, Buskens CJ, Bemelman WA, Tanis PJ. Perineal hernia repair after abdominoperineal resection: a pooled analysis. *Colorectal Dis.* 2012;e400-e406.

Mesh: Material Science of Hernia Repair

Samuel Wade Ross | David A. Iannitti

Mesh is defined as a network of interlaced material with a lattice-like structure, which in medicine has become synonymous with use for reinforcement of hernia repairs. Mesh use has become ubiquitous as inguinal hernia repair (IHR) is one of the most common procedures performed in the world.[1] Additionally, IHR is the most common type of hernia operation performed, with an estimated 700,000 performed annually in the United States alone.[1,2] The core principles of IHR remain the same regardless of which technique is performed (excision of the hernia sac tension, reduction of intraabdominal contents, and tension-free closure); however, the methods used between various surgical approaches and individual techniques differ significantly. An open approach via groin incision is still the most common IHR performed in the United States,[3] and the modified Lichtenstein repair has become the most common open repair type since its introduction in 1984.[4–6] In addition, the majority of repairs are now performed with a prosthetic mesh, as its use in an open repair has reduced hernia recurrence from 7% to 1%.[7] Laparoscopic repairs inherently require the use of mesh and have had an increasing utilization in the past 20 years as laparoscopic education and training have increased.[8,9]

Incisional and ventral hernia repair (VHR) is also one of the most common surgical procedures performed around the globe, with an estimated 350,000 performed in the United States and 300,000 performed in Europe per year.[10,11] Both IHR and VHR are one of the top five procedures performed by graduating general surgery residents consistently each year.[12] Mesh reinforcement of hernia defects was popularized by the work of Usher who first described the use of polypropylene (PP) mesh, and today, mesh use is ubiquitous in VHR.[13] However, few surgeons understand the inherent differences in the materials and properties of the mesh they use every day, the evolution of mesh technology and material science, different scenarios in which a certain mesh may be most effective, and most importantly, that mesh choice can effect critical patient outcomes.

Therefore the goal of this chapter is to describe the evolution and history of mesh for use for hernia repair, the physical properties on which we evaluate mesh, the underlying materials used to construct them, the classification schemas used to differentiate mesh, the nonmesh adjuncts being used in combination with and used to fixate mesh, new technologies used to construct mesh (especially biologic and absorbable synthetic mesh), as well as the inherent risks and complications that can result due to mesh implantation. Additionally, we hope to focus on evidence-based scenarios and recommendations on when and what type of mesh is appropriate.

HISTORY

Hernias have been recognized as medical problems since the time of the Egyptians in 1500 BC and have gone through a long evolution of treatment.[14] The Greeks and Romans were the first to realize that inadequate technique in surgical abdominal closure was linked to incisional hernias, and Galen was the first to describe mass closure techniques in the second century AD. Galen also advocated for use of the paramedian incision to prevent incisional hernia, a technique now proven to reduce hernia rates.[15] In the 18th and 19th centuries, hernias were described and differentiated in detail by anatomists, but not much headway was made in the operative repair of hernias until after the advancements in anesthesia and antisepsis in the late 19th century that allowed for modern aseptic and general anesthetic techniques. This allowed for complex tissue repair techniques such as the Bassini repair, which is still in use today.[16]

Modern hernia repair is characterized by the use of mesh reinforcement, which was popularized in 1958 by the work of Usher who first described the use of PP mesh.[13] Lesser known was that the first artificial mesh implant was actually performed in 1900 by Goepel and Witzel using a silver wire braided weave, which resulted in stiff, nonfunctional abdominal walls, which also had the deleterious side effect of toxic sulfur silver buildup.[14] Subsequently, stainless steel or tantalum gauze was used in the early 20th century, but these were plagued with high infection and complication rates. It was not until the dawn of plastic science after World War II and the creation of PP, polyester, and polyfluoroethylene (PTFE) and expanded polyfluoroethylene (ePTFE) that suitable materials were present for the creation of malleable, pliable, and durable meshes with relatively low complication rates.[14]

In 1968, Rives and Stoppa described broad mesh reinforcement of groin hernias using Dacron grafts[17] and then applied this technique to large abdominal wall defects with mesh in the retrorectus position, which was popularized in the 1980s.[18,19] The onlay technique was first described by Chevrel in 1979, which involves mesh being placed superficial to the anterior rectus fascia following suture repair of the fascial defect.[20,21] Another mesh technique, intraperitoneal mesh placement, was previously looked upon unfavorably due to the risk of mesh erosion into viscera and formation of fistulas. However, with creation of barrier-coated meshes and use of biologic and absorbable synthetic meshes, intraperitoneal mesh placement is now ubiquitous and the way most laparoscopic VHR is performed.[22,23] The first laparoscopic VHR repair was described by LeBlanc in 1993,[22] and recently, the field of robotic surgery has provided an opportunity to explore advanced minimally invasive techniques; the first robotic VHR was described in 2003.[24]

Perhaps even more significant than minimally invasive techniques, the introduction of biologic-derived mesh and absorbable synthetic mesh has changed the playing field for hernia repair. Interestingly, the first biologic reinforcements for hernia repair were with frozen cadaveric dermis, tensor fasciae latae, and dural mater tissues in the 1930s and 1940s, but these had poor results.[14] The renaissance of the biologic mesh came about in the early 2000s when acellular dermal matrix (AlloDerm; Allergan, Dublin, Ireland) was created from cadaveric human dermis for use in reconstructive and burn procedures. Later it was studied for potential use in VHR in contaminated fields first in a pig model[25] and then for use in stoma site hernias in humans.[26] With the use in hernia repair solidified, the number and type of biologic mesh developed has exploded in the last decade with various tissue sources, xenografts, allografts and now even absorbable synthetic, and biosynthetic created meshes. Where in previous years there were only a handful of mesh options, now the number of meshes available gives surgeons a plethora of options in how best to repair hernias tailored to specific patients.[27]

EVIDENCE FOR MESH REPAIR

Mesh reinforcement for hernia repair is a much less debated topic than in prior decades, and it is currently standard of care in developed nations given the high rate of hernia recurrence with primary tissue repairs. IHR with mesh has been studied for longer than VHR, with the first randomized control trial dating from the 1990s, and several meta-analyses showing that the risk of hernia recurrence is reduced 50% to 75% with mesh reinforcement compared with tissue repair alone.[28,29] The landmark study on this topic in VHR by Luijendijk et al. in 2000 described a 43% hernia recurrence rate at 3 years with suture repair compared with a 24% rate for mesh repair,[30] which increased to 63% recurrence at 6 years.[31] Numerous studies have verified these results, and a recent meta-analysis clearly demonstrated that mesh repair results in less recurrence.[32] Most surgeons acknowledge that it is standard of care to perform VHR with mesh.[7,31,33] Despite this, there have been some proponents of performing primary VHR with component separation alone without the use of a prosthetic mesh to buttress the repair.[34–37] However, recurrence after VHR with component separation alone can result in inferior outcomes and is reported to occur anywhere from 5% to 23% in short-term follow-up of 2 years.[38–40]

MESH CATEGORIES

Materials science for mesh has come a long way since the time of silver wire weaves, and in the past 15 years, the market for number and types of mesh has multiplied exponentially. The original synthetic plastic mesh repair described by Usher was with a Marlex mesh composed of PP,[13] and since that time, hernia mesh has evolved from this single synthetic material to three broad classes of materials: permanent synthetic, biologic, and absorbable synthetic. Each category of mesh has its own benefits and

drawbacks that make it ideal in certain situations. To guide the use of mesh selection, the Ventral Hernia Working Group published a grading scale for hernias by level of hernia and patient complexity and contamination: grade 1 hernias are clean fields in low-risk patients without significant comorbidities; grade 2 are clean fields but with patient comorbidities including diabetes, smoking, and obesity; grade 3 are potential contamination such as the presence of an ostomy, enterotomy, prior wound infection; and grade 4 are mesh infection present or a septic wound.[41]

In general, synthetic mesh is ideal in lower grade hernias, and biologic mesh should be used in higher-grade hernias. The use of these meshes to avoid mesh infection of synthetic mesh should be balanced with the much higher financial cost associated with biologic mesh, as well as the higher hernia recurrence rate, as these meshes stretch over time. Indeed, in lower risk, lower grade hernias, synthetic mesh has been found to be more cost effective than biologic mesh.[42] For this reason, mesh companies have developed new mesh materials that have biochemical scaffolds that will dissolve over time and allow for tissue ingrowth: so-called absorbable synthetic, resorbable, or biosynthetic mesh (terms vary in literature).

SYNTHETIC

MATERIAL

The first plastic synthetic mesh was originally composed of PP, which is a permanent monofilament carbon polymer that is flexible and biologically inert.[43] PP is composed of hydrophobic polymer with alternating methyl moieties. The monofilament nature allows for large pores, which facilitates tissue ingrowth and less interstices for bacteria to set up biofilms, which are more likely the smaller the pore and in multifilamentous mesh.[44] The majority of commercially available mesh is still made from PP, but various evolutions of the original monofilament large-pore mesh have been created. An in situ image of a PP knit mesh for IHR is displayed in Fig. 55.1. The body uses the PP as a lattice to build scar tissue on, which is the process for tissue reinforcement, but it is also a drawback if it is placed in direct contact with the viscera. Adhesion formation can be severe if placed intraperitoneally, resulting in bowel obstructions and mesh erosion into bowel.[45,46] Therefore, coatings have been added to PP to prevent visceral adhesion formation when it is placed in body cavities.[47,48]

After the introduction of PP meshes, PTFE and ePTFE meshes were synthesized. PTFE is a sheet of hydrophobic inert fluoropolymer that the body does not incorporate into but encapsulates around as a foreign body. One reason for this is that the material is highly negatively charged, so water and oils will not adhere to the material. PTFE is generally not currently used since the introduction of ePTFE. This material is more microporous than PTFE but still does not allow for tissue ingrowth when made as a flat sheet.[46] The principal advantage of ePTFE is that it can be placed directly onto viscera and not form adhesions, as depicted in Fig. 55.2. This must be balanced with the fact that it is highly susceptible to bacterial colonization in addition to seroma formation.

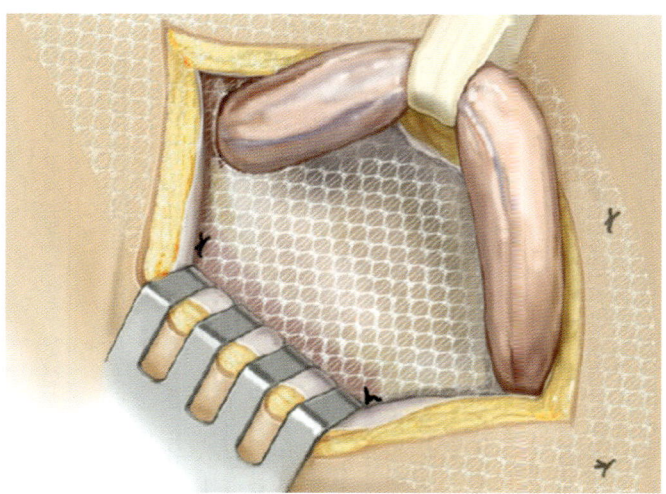

FIGURE 55.1 In situ image of a wide-pore lightweight polypropylene mesh for onlay Lichtenstein-type repair for inguinal hernia repair. (Copyright 2016 Davol, Inc. All rights reserved. Used with the permission of Davol, Inc.)

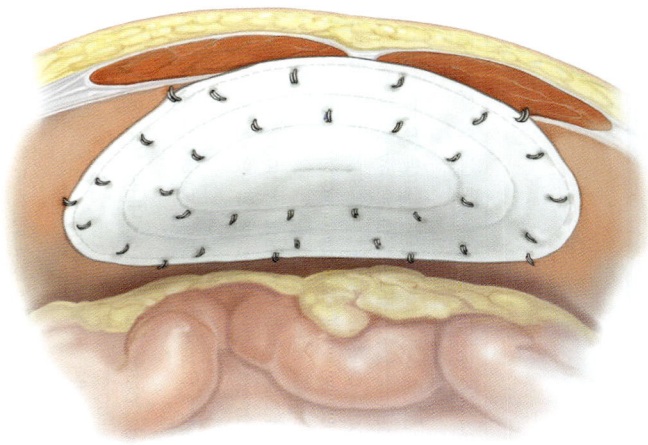

FIGURE 55.3 Intraperitoneal sublay placement of biologically inert expanded polyfluouroethylene mesh that resists adhesion formation and can be placed directly next to viscera. (Copyright 2016 Davol, Inc. All rights reserved. Used with the permission of Davol, Inc.)

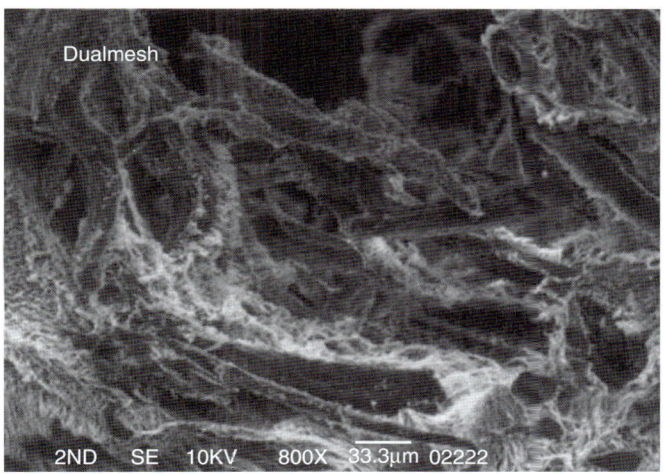

FIGURE 55.2 Scanning electron microscope image of the rough side of DualMesh expanded polyfluouroethylene, designed to increase surface area to facilitate better tissue incorporation. (Copyright 2016 Davol, Inc. All rights reserved. Used with the permission of Davol, Inc.)

FILAMENT, WEAVE, KNIT

Mesh can differ significantly in how the strands of material, usually PP, are arranged, from very simple one-to-one knits to intricate and complicated weaves. The choice in the configuration can affect bursting pressure, tensile strength, and elasticity of the mesh.[43] In addition, mesh can have a multifilament, braided, or almost ropelike structure that can then be knitted or woven. Multiple filaments can increase tensile strength, but they obligate a decreased pore size that can decrease tissue ingrowth while increasing mesh surface area, which can decrease ability to clear bacteria colonization.[52] One advantage of multiple filaments is that an absorbable polymer such as Vicryl or Monocryl (Ethicon, Somerville, New Jersey) can be woven into the mesh to help facilitate tissue incorporation. Just as in fabric, knit mesh involves creating loops of material using multiple needles with one thread. Woven mesh involves a similar process but with multiple threads at right angles.

In general, knit mesh will have larger pore size, elasticity, and will stretch in all directions, called isotropic stretch.[53] However, woven mesh will only stretch in a direction oblique to the intersection of the thread weaves, called anisotropic stretch, which is a little understood but vitally important aspect to consider when orienting mesh for implantation.[54] Mesh placed with the greatest direction of force on the vector oblique from the weave will stretch more than if oriented in the direction of the weave threads. A closeup of a monofilament woven PP mesh is displayed in Fig. 55.4. These factors of filament number, size of the filament, and knit versus weave are what contribute mostly to mesh weight, tensile strength, and burst strength.

MESH WEIGHT AND BURST STRENGTH

Synthetic mesh varies by weight with three broad categories: lightweight, midweight, and heavyweight mesh, which have different inherent tensile strengths depending on their weave and material composition.[55] The weight of the

Most surgeons would recommend that infected ePTFE must always be explanted.[46,49] To combat the issue of poor tissue incorporation, different-sided ePTFE mesh has become available in DualMesh (Gore Medical, Flagstaff Arizona), which allows textures of ePTFE with a corduroy side for more surface area for tissue incorporation and a smooth side for visceral contact.[50] An electronic microscope image of the corduroy side is seen in Fig. 55.3.

Polyester mesh was created after PP and ePTFE, but while available, is not generally used in the United States, since it has similar properties to PP mesh. It is created from polymers of terephthalic acid, which is hydrophilic and can be degraded by hydrolysis.[51] Commonly available synthetic mesh categorized by physical properties are displayed in Table 55.1.

TABLE 55.1 Synthetic Mesh

Material	Barrier Strategy	Weight Category	Filament	Structure	Pore Size	Mesh Brand Name	Additional Comments
Polypropylene	None	Light	Mono	Knit	Macro	Bard Soft	For all hernia repair types, Soft is lighter weight, larger pore, Plug version available
		Light	Mono	Knit	Macro	Prolene Soft	For all hernia repair types, Soft is lighter weight, larger pore
		Light	Mono	Weave	Macro	Progrip	Self-gripping mesh for laparoscopic IHR facilitated by polylactic acid mesh component, absorbs over 18 months, tacking not required
		Light	Mono	Weave	Macro	3D Max Light	Contoured mesh for laparoscopic IHR, Light version is lighter weight
		Light	Mono	Knit	Macro	Prolite, Prolite Ultra	For IHR, Ultra is lighter weight, larger pore
		Light	Mono	Weave	Macro	VitaMesh Blue	For all hernia repairs, dyed blue for better visualization
		Light	Multi	Knit	Macro	Ultrapro, Ultrapro Advanced	Monocryl as one of the filaments, absorbs over 2 weeks, leaving 70% of mesh
		Light	Multi	Weave	Macro	Vypro, Vypro II	Polyglactin 910 as one of the filaments, absorbs over 4 weeks, leaving 70% of mesh
		Mid	Mono	Knit	Macro	Bard	For all hernia repairs, Kugel patch for IHR and UHR, Visilex for LVHR, Plug version available
		Mid	Mono	Knit	Macro	Prolene	For all hernia repair types, Soft is lighter weight
		Mid	Mono	Weave	Macro	VitaMesh	For all hernia repairs
		Mid	Mono	Weave	Macro	3D Max	Contoured mesh for laparoscopic IHR, Light version is lighter weight
		Mid	Mono	Knit	Macro	Prolite	For all hernia repairs
		Heavy	Mono	Knit	Intermediate	Marlex	Original PP mesh, for all hernia repairs
	O3FA	Mid	Mono	Knit	Macro with barrier	C-QUR, C-QUR V-patch, C-QUR CentriFX	PP coated in O3FA, V-patch for UHR, CentriFX for IHR
	Titanium	Mid	Mono	Weave	Macro	TiMesh, TiLene, TiSure	Titanium oxide bonded to PP filaments in titanization process, no actual barrier, for all hernia types
	ORC	Mid	Mono	Knit	Macro with barrier	Proceed	UHR and VHR versions, ORC layer absorbed in unknown time period
	Seprafilm	Mid	Mono	Weave	Macro with barrier	Sepramesh	For VHR and UHR, Seprafilm absorbs within 30 days, replaced by Ventralight mesh
	Hydrogel	Mid	Mono	Weave	Macro with barrier	Ventrio, Ventralex ST, Ventralight ST	Ventrio and Ventralex ST for UHR, Ventralight for VHR, similar to Sepramesh technology, absorbs over 30 days
	ePTFE	Heavy	Mono	Sheet	Micro	Composix, Ventralex, Ventrio	Ventralex for UHR, Composix for VHR, PP abdominal side to facilitate ingrowth, ePTFE for visceral side
Polyester	None	Heavy	Mono	Knit	Intermediate	Dacron	Outdated, not routinely used
		Heavy	Mono	Knit	Intermediate	Mersilene	Outdated, not routinely used
	Collagen	Mid	Mono	Knit	Macro	Symbotex	3D coated monofilament, for intraperitoneal placement
		Mid	Multi	Knit	Macro	Parietex	Collagen-coated polyester mesh to prevent adhesion formation
ePTFE	None	Heavy	N/A	Sheet	Micro	Gore-Tex	Original ePTFE mesh
		Heavy	N/A	Dual sided sheet	Macro/Micro	Dulex	Larger pores on the abdominal side, microporous on the visceral side to inhibit adhesions
		Heavy	N/A	Dual sided sheet	Micro	DualMesh	Corduroy microporous abdominal side and smooth microporous visceral side

ePTFE, Expanded poly(tetrafluoroethylene); *IHR*, inguinal hernia repair; *LVHR*, laparoscopic ventral hernia repair; *Macro*, macroporous; *Micro*, microporous; *O3FA*, omega 3 fatty acid; *ORC*, oxidized regenerated cellulose; *PP*, polypropylene; *UHR*, umbilical hernia repair; *VHR*, ventral hernia repair.

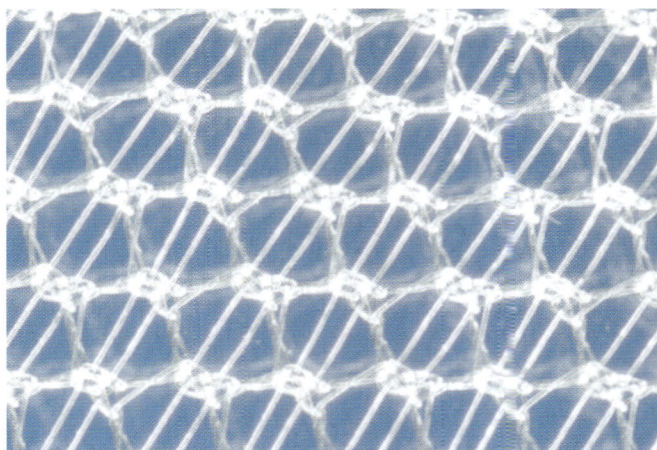

FIGURE 55.4 Micrograph of a lightweight polypropylene woven mesh. (Copyright 2016 Davol, Inc. All rights reserved. Used with the permission of Davol, Inc.)

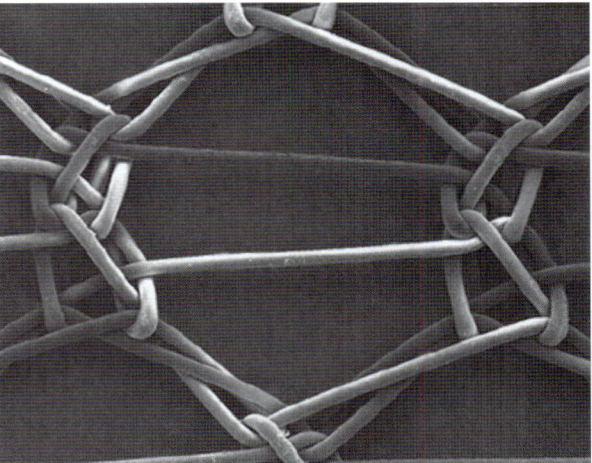

Open pore mesh design, 35x magnification

FIGURE 55.5 Micrograph of large-pore polypropylene mesh. (Copyright 2016 Davol, Inc. All rights reserved. Used with the permission of Davol, Inc.)

mesh actually refers to the mass of the material in a set area, which is in actuality density. Lightweight mesh is also considered less than 35 g/m^2, and these PP meshes are usually monofilament, smaller caliber woven meshes with large pores of up to 4 mm.[56] Midweight mesh is between 35 and 60 g/m^2 and has larger caliber filaments, is woven, and has larger pores. Heavyweight mesh has a density of 60+ g/m^2, and a knitted, monofilament PP mesh such as Marlex has a weight of 95 g/m^2.[55] Heavyweight mesh has higher tensile strength in the range of 1200 N compared with light (540 N) and midweight mesh (560 N). However, given the concern for mesh sensation, stiffness, and ability to clear bacterial infection, in the past decade there has been trend away from using heavyweight for lighter weight mesh. Recently data have suggested that quality of life does not suffer with heavyweight mesh[57] and that lightweight mesh can suffer catastrophic central failure due to shearing forces, which can result in inordinately high hernia recurrence rates of 8% at 1 year.[58] Therefore the use of midweight and heavyweight mesh, especially for VHR, has had a resurgence.

POROSITY

Multiple filaments, increased caliber of polymers, and therefore increased mesh weight, result in decreased pore size in PP mesh. This is important because pores must be greater than 75 mm in diameter to allow infiltration by macrophages, fibroblasts to create neovascularization, and tissue ingrowth. It is because of the lack of this feature that ePTFE mesh gets such poor tissue ingrowth.[43] In addition, pore size affects the ability of the immune system to penetrate the mesh and clear bacterial infection, and it has been demonstrated in multiple studies that narrow-pore meshes do not clear bacteria as well as wide-pore lightweight mesh.[44,59] Coated meshes with absorbable layers blocking the pores on both sides of the mesh would also potentially have problems with tissue ingrowth. Heavyweight PP mesh typically has a 1-mm or less pore size, while lightweight mesh has a 3- to 4-mm pore diameter. A micrograph of a large-pore mesh is displayed

in Fig. 55.5. The long-term strength of the mesh repair is not from the mesh itself but in creating tissue ingrowth and fibrosis, and there is some data to suggest that too small of a pore size prevents fibrosis from occurring through the mesh. This "bridging fibrosis" is key to sustained tissue strength.[56] Given the need for balance between bridging fibrosis and early mesh failure in lightweight mesh and decreased porosity and bacterial clearance in heavyweight mesh, midweight mesh may theoretically be the ideal uncoated synthetic mesh. However, there is no randomized clinical data to support midweight mesh as superior, and surgeons should be knowledgeable about mesh materials so they can choose the most appropriate mesh for each clinical situation.

SHAPED MESH

The first mesh, and the majority of mesh since that time, was a flat sheet of metal or plastic. But in recent years shaped mesh technology has become available to create mesh designed to fulfill certain roles and contoured to specific body spaces. Shaping mesh involves either creating seams in the mesh on which the direction changes or through heat annealing, which is a more recent process. One of the first shaped meshes originally described by Lichtenstein was simply the creation of a hernia plug to perform femoral and IHR, which at the time was simply suturing a flat mesh into a three-dimensional (3D) shape.[60] Since that time, specifically designed mesh plugs have been created for the same purpose, as can be seen in Fig. 55.6. Lichtenstein also popularized the tension-free onlay mesh hernia repair,[4] which has been modified to incorporate a sublay and an onlay mesh with the introduction of mesh hernia systems. These incorporate a preperitoneal sublay that is attached via a mesh cone to an onlay portion of mesh. Although this has theoretical advantages in providing a sandwiched repair of the hernia, a head-to-head analysis of two mesh systems and a simple Lichtenstein repair shows the same hernia recurrence rate and quality of life.[61]

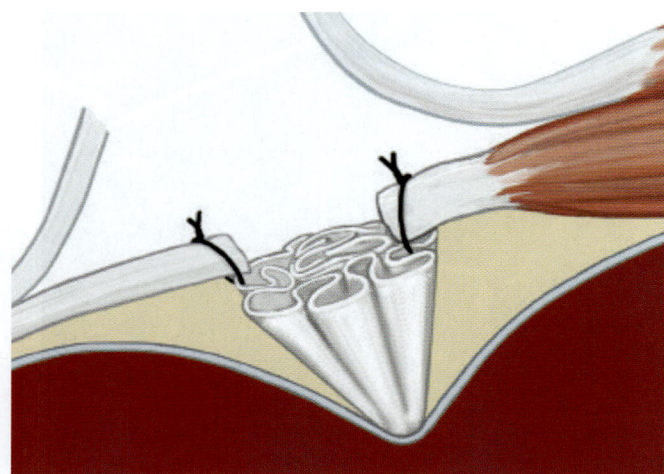

FIGURE 55.6 Shaped polypropylene hernia mesh plug in the indirect inguinal space. (Copyright 2016 Davol, Inc. All rights reserved. Used with the permission of Davol, Inc.)

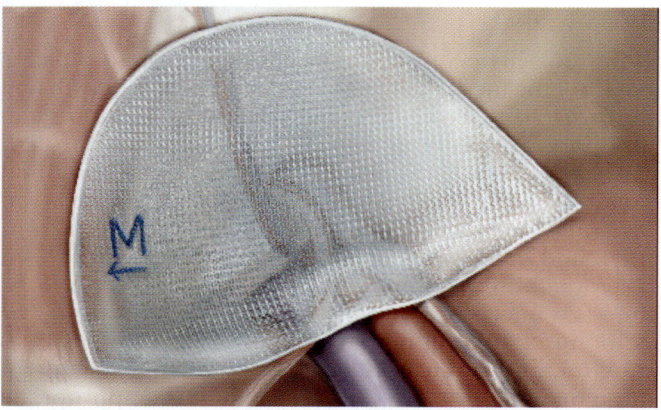

FIGURE 55.7 Shaped and anatomically contoured three-dimensional mesh placed in the preperitoneal inguinal space for laparoscopic transabdominal preperitoneal hernia repair. (Copyright 2016 Davol, Inc. All rights reserved. Used with the permission of Davol, Inc.)

Although many repairs involve cutting the mesh in two dimensions to try to fit the 3D patient anatomy, a unique mesh was created for laparoscopic IHR that conforms to the anatomy in all three dimensions. The original creator of the 3D contoured inguinal hernia mesh measured the common anatomic measurements of the preperitoneal inguinal region from cadavers and were able to create a design for a contoured mesh to fit the typical anatomy.[62] Technology at the time could not create the contour; therefore a new process was developed of heat annealing a flat piece of lightweight PP mesh over a mold and then rapidly cooling it led to a stable 3D contoured mesh. Fig. 55.7 displays an in vivo image of the 3D mesh.

COATED AND COMPOSITE VERSUS UNCOATED

PP is the most common prosthetic mesh used in VHR and IHR,[57] mostly due to the properties described previously,

which result in a strong, durable, and flexible repair that promotes excellent tissue ingrowth. While biologically inert, the mesh is designed to stimulate an inflammatory response resulting in fibrosis and scar formation. When placed in the peritoneum, the mesh will create visceral adhesions. These adhesions may lead to bowel obstruction, mesh erosion into the bowel, and enterocutaneous fistula formation.[63,64] These concerns have driven the development of coated forms of PP and composite prosthetics with PP fixated to other mesh such as ePTFE to protect one side of the mesh from visceral adhesion development. These materials are most frequently used in laparoscopic repairs where intraperitoneal mesh is used, but they are also used in open VHR and umbilical hernia repair (UHR) and have theoretical use for laparoscopic IHR.

Composite meshes are made of PP embedded on or attached to another synthetic material less prone to adhesions, most commonly ePTFE.[65] These meshes were the precursors to absorbable coated mesh and are designed to facilitate tissue ingrowth into the PP side and have an inert ePTFE side to prevent visceral attachments. These are still on the market today, but they have all the drawbacks associated with ePTFE mesh and have been associated with increased propensity to infections (particularly methicillin-resistant *Staphylococcus aureus* [MRSA]), and low rates of mesh salvage after infection.[66–68] The high degree of contraction and stiffening of combined permanent materials have led to patient discomfort and the mesh pulling free of the abdominal wall with subsequent hernia recurrence.[59] Difficulty with laparoscopic handling of composite meshes has also been noted by surgeons.[69] The problems associated with the use of permanent composite meshes have also led to increased demand for meshes with a bioabsorbable barrier. In addition, these meshes are coated with an absorbable substance on one side that acts as a barrier between PP and the visceral organs to reduce adhesion formation.[45,70]

Coated, absorbable prosthetics are an alternative to permanent composite meshes. Many different types of coated PP mesh are commercially available, including omega-3 fatty acid coatings (O3FA),[71] hyaluronate-carboxymethylcellulose (HCMC) hydrogel,[72] and oxidized regenerated cellulose (ORC).[73] HCMC is interesting in that the hydrogel layer is absorbable but bound to the PP mesh structure with additional polyglycolic acid fibers. This keeps the layer bound to the mesh with a substance that also dissolves over time. An electron micrograph of HCMC-coated mesh is displayed in Fig. 55.8, and a closeup demonstrating the difference in layers is displayed in Fig. 55.9. Although these coated prosthetics have been demonstrated to reduce adhesions with intraabdominal placement, concerns arise in regard to other complications associated with the use of these substances.[74] Specifically, there is some concern that tissue ingrowth could be impeded due to initial blockage of the pores and reduced ability to clear bacterial infection due to bacteria setting up biofilms.[75] The risk of these complications, however, are not outweighed by the risk of mesh erosion and enterocutaneous fistula formation, and these meshes represent the best option when intraperitoneal mesh is required. Great care should be taken to ensure that the correct side is placed toward the viscera and, especially in

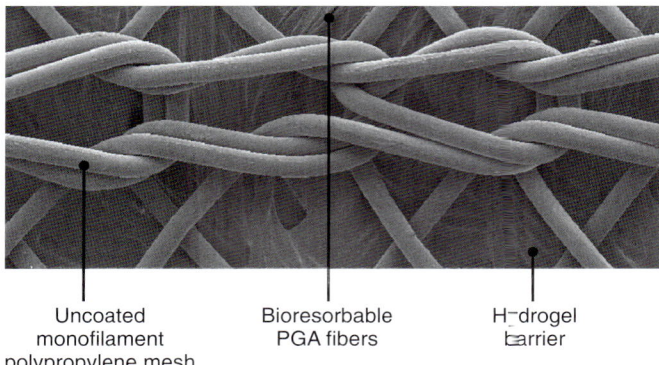

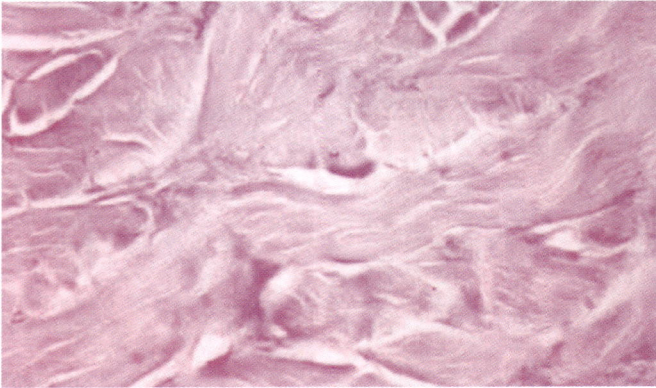

FIGURE 55.8 Scanning electron micrograph of Ventralight-coated polypropylene mesh. *PGA,* Polyglycolic acid. (Copyright 2016 Davol, Inc. All rights reserved. Used with the permission of Davol, Inc.)

FIGURE 55.10 Micrograph using hematoxylin and eosin stain of porcine-derived orcine derived acellular dermal matrix showing collagen deposition. (Copyright 2016 Davol, Inc. All rights reserved. Used with the permission of Davol, Inc.)

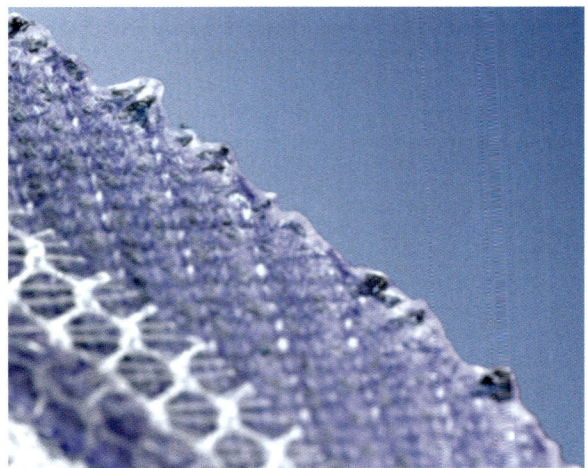

FIGURE 55.9 Closeup of coated polypropylene mesh showing the hydrogel coating and underlying polypropylene mesh. (Copyright 2016 Davol, Inc. All rights reserved. Used with the permission of Davol, Inc.)

laparoscopic surgery, that fixation devices and handling do not rub off the coated layer.

BIOLOGIC MESH

Since the introduction of AlloDerm, biologic mesh has exploded in number and type.[76] These are derived from decellularized, collagen-rich animal or human tissue and vary widely in source, durability, and cost. A microscopic cross section of the acellular collagen structure is displayed in Fig. 55.10. Allografts are derived from human tissue and xenografts from animal sources. Xenografts are typically porcine, bovine, or equine sources.[43] Dermis is most commonly used, although pericardium and intestinal submucosa are available. After the first generation of biologics was noted to stretch significantly, developers started performing collagen cross-linkage of the mesh to increase tensile strength. It was soon realized that cross-linking limited early native tissue ingrowth.[77] In general, biologic meshes cost much more than synthetic meshes

per square centimeter given the cost of procuring and processing the tissues from cadaveric or animal donors. Regardless of cross-linkage, these meshes are limited in their durability as they lose their strength as the body degrades and incorporates the collagen scaffold of the mesh. Human studies of biologic mesh use in contaminated fields has elucidated that these hernias have an exceedingly high hernia recurrence rate of 31.3% at 5 years[78] and 56% or higher when a biologic bridge repair is performed.[79]

Most hernia specialists reserve biologic mesh for contaminated and dirty scenarios where the risk of synthetic mesh infection outweighs the risk of hernia recurrence and increased cost of a biologic mesh. A recent large study of biologic mesh placement has shown that with an average of 18 months, follow-up hernia recurrence can be anywhere from 15% to 60% depending on the mesh placed, but this results in an exceedingly expensive repair with average mesh costs being almost $30,000.[80] Additionally, it was possible for biologic mesh to become chronically infected and require explantation. These meshes should be reserved for the Ventral Hernia Working Group (VHWG) grade 3 or 4 hernias and may likely be replaced in the future with absorbable synthetic mesh given their high cost and recurrence rate. Biologic mesh categorized by physical characteristics is displayed in Table 55.2.

ABSORBABLE SYNTHETIC MESH

Biosynthetic or absorbable synthetic mesh is constructed from biologically derived or absorbable synthetic polymers that form a temporary scaffold for tissue ingrowth. These materials have become available over the past decade and function similar to permanent mesh in creating a scaffold for tissue incorporation, but they are hydrolyzed and eventually replaced by native tissue.[81] While many of these materials are on the cutting edge of biochemistry and bioengineering, the first mesh in this class has been available for decades, polyglactin 910. More commonly known as Vicryl mesh, polyglactin 910 has a half-life on the order of 2 to 4 weeks and is completely absorbed by 3 months. This has mostly been used to allow for

TABLE 55.2 Biologic Mesh

Graft Source	Tissue Source	Cross-Linkage	Mesh Brand Name	Additional Comments
Human	Dermis	No	AlloDerm	Small sizes, requires refrigeration and subsequent rehydration, highly elastic
			Allomax	Acellular, sterilized by gamma radiation
			FlexHD	No refrigeration or rehydration, reduced elasticity
Porcine	Dermis	Yes	Permacol	Acellular, sterilized by gamma radiation, no refrigeration necessary
			CollaMend	Acellular and lyophilized
		No	Strattice	Acellular, available in large sizes, fenestrated versions available to facilitate ingrowth
			XenMatrix, XenMatrix AB	Acellular, available in large sizes, AB has drug elution of minocycline and rifampin for 7 days
	Intestinal submucosa		Surgisis	Acellular, no refrigeration but does require rehydration
Bovine	Dermis	No	SurgiMend	Fetal bovine derived, requires rehydration
	Pericardium		Veritas	Initially used for staple line reinforcement, now for VHR
			Tutopatch	Fenestrated mesh also available, 5-year shelf life
		Yes	Periguard	Can be used in multiple scenarios where patch is needed, less studied for hernia repair, requires rehydration

VHR, Ventral hernia repair.

granulation tissue ingrowth in open abdomens and chronic wounds.[82] Unfortunately, there is a high fistula rate of 9% to 17%.[72,83,84]

The first modern mesh in this class was Gore Bio-A, which is constructed from 67% polyglycolic acid and 33% trimethylene carbonate, and was first marketed for hernia repair in the early 2010s.[85,86] However, the material has been used for years previously as polyglyconate in orthopedic repairs and in SeamGuard (Gore Medical) for staple line reinforcement.[81] This material forms an absorptive web for tissue ingrowth and has been described for use in inguinal,[85] paraesophageal,[87] and VHR.[88] The scaffold dissolves completely by 6 months and promotes fibrovascular replacement of the mesh. The largest study to date in VHR with biosynthetic placement is the COBRA study, which was performed in 104 clean contaminated or contaminated cases. There was a high rate of ostomy reversal, enterocutaneous fistula takedown, and/or current mesh infection, and at 2 years there was only a 17% recurrence rate.[88]

A newer material that is truly a biosynthetic product is poly-4-hydroxybutyrate (P4HB), which is created using genetically engineered *Escherichia coli* to produce a protein substrate. This is then refined and polymerized and knitted into a mesh pattern, which has a much longer absorption period, 12 to 18 months.[89] Mechanically, this mesh has properties similar to an uncoated light- to midweight PP mesh. A micrograph of a P4HB mesh is pictured in Fig. 55.11. However, unlike Bio-A or biologic mesh, this mesh will cause significant adhesion formation; therefore a hydrogel-coated version has become available, and early animal data show that it functions similar to a coated synthetic PP mesh.[90] The only current human data on this mesh are from reconstructive surgery after deep inferior epigastric perforator flap creation, which showed decreased abdominal bulge when P4HB was used as an onlay.[91] There are many other materials coming to market in this category, and in general, this is the fastest growing

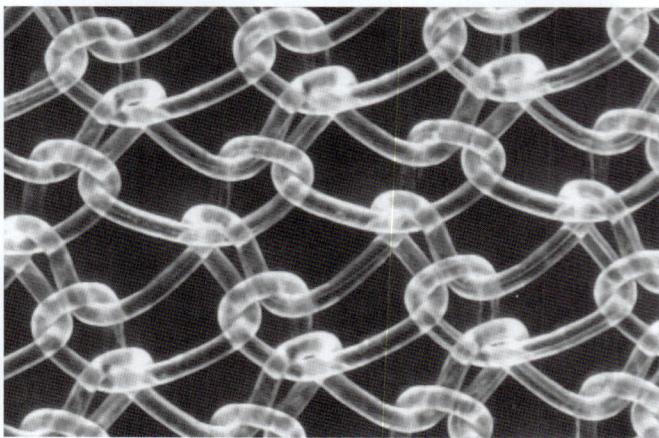

FIGURE 55.11 Scanning electron micrograph of poly-4-hydroxybutyrate knit mesh (brand name Phasix). (Copyright 2016 Davol, Inc. All rights reserved. Used with the permission of Davol, Inc.)

area in mesh science and may offer more durable options than biologic mesh. Currently, however, there have been no head-to-head comparisons of biologic, synthetic, and biosynthetic mesh. Available absorbable synthetic mesh categorized by physical properties is displayed in Table 55.3.

MESH FIXATION

The technology for securing mesh to the abdominal wall has not evolved as rapidly as the prostheses themselves, and most surgeons still use simple suture to secure mesh in open IHR, VHR, and UHR. Laparoscopic IHR brought about the need for new fixation methods given the small space, and the first tacking devices appeared soon after the introduction of the technique. The initial design for these, which has continued today, was permanent titanium tackers

TABLE 55.3 Biologic Mesh

Material	Structure	Absorption Time	Brand Name
Polyglactin 910	Knit and weave forms available	3 months	VICRYL
Polyglycolic acid/trimethylene carbonate	Web	6 months	GORE BIO-A Tissue Reinforcement
Poly-4-hydroxybutyrate (P4HB)	Knit, ST version has a hydrogel layer to prevent intestinal adhesions	18 months	Phasix, Phasix ST
Copolymer: fast dissolving glycolide, lactide, and trimethylene carbonate; slow dissolving glycolide and trimethylene carbonate	Knit, first polymer rapidly absorbed to allow for larger pores for long term ingrowth	4 months for first polymer, 36 months for second	TIGR Matrix

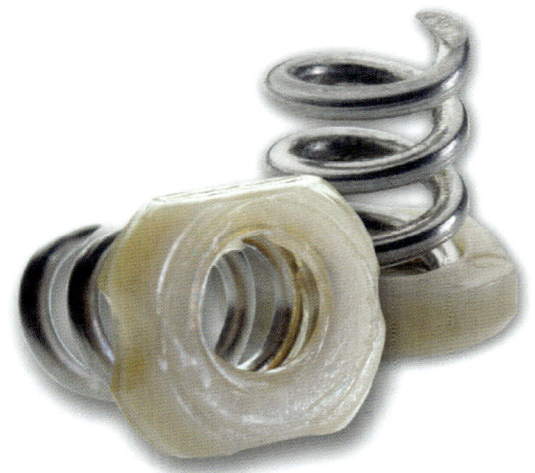

FIGURE 55.12 Titanium spiral coil with polymer cap for mesh fixation. (Copyright 2016 Davol, Inc. All rights reserved. Used with the permission of Davol, Inc.)

with a spiral coil pattern. Originally these were uncovered tacks that could stimulate adhesion formation leading to bowel obstructions[92] or even erode into other structures,[93] but later designs have added a plastic cap to prevent this, pictured in Fig. 55.12. Since titanium is permanent, some have theorized chronic pain after laparoscopic IHR could be due to the continued presence of the tack. Therefore absorbable tacks have also been designed and are available in arrow, spiral, and spike shapes. However, the only study to date to compare permanent and absorbable tacks has shown no pain or hernia recurrence difference between the two.[94] Given the same concern for nerve injury and chronic pain, others have advocated for glue fixation of mesh using fibrin-thrombin biologic glue, which will not penetrate the abdominal wall but merely hold the mesh in place long enough for tissue to incorporate. Two recent meta-analyses have verified that there is less chronic pain with glue fixation compared with tacks with no difference in hernia recurrence.[95,96]

MESH-SPECIFIC COMPLICATIONS

Analogous to other prosthetic utilization surgeries, such as vascular graft and orthopedic joint insertion,

mesh can become colonized and result in long-term infection, especially if it has eroded into the abdominal viscera, creating enterocutaneous fistulas. Mesh erosion is highest in uncoated PP mesh placed directly into the peritoneum adjacent to the viscera and can erode into the small intestine, colon, and even bladder.[97–99] However, ePTFE and polyester can erode as well and, in severe uncontrolled fistulas, can even result in necrotizing fasciitis of the abdominal wall.[100] These complications are often underreported since patients may present to physicians other than the index surgeon and since presentation can occur very delayed from the original surgery. These complications are disabling, both financially and in terms of patient quality of life. Surgical repair of the erosion is usually mandated to explant the mesh and resect the fistula track.

Similarly, infection of the mesh without fistula formation can be a debilitating condition requiring multiple procedures, long-term antibiotics, and ultimately mesh explantation. A recent abstract at the American College of Surgeons meeting reported 161 patients with mesh infection. Examination of different techniques to salvage the mesh found that if there was an enterocutaneous fistula or a MRSA infection present, if the patient was a smoker, or if there was a coated, ePTFE, or composite mesh, the patients had 100% need for mesh resection. Patients with a lightweight, PP mesh did best, and some were able to be managed with antibiotics and percutaneous drain placement.[101]

ANTIMICROBIAL COATINGS

Since surgical site infection can occur in 5% to 60% of abdominal wall reconstruction procedures and mesh infection has an incidence of 0.5% to 5%, mesh developers have tried to prevent infection by coating the mesh itself with antimicrobial material. Soaking mesh in antibiotic or antimicrobial solution during the case prior to implantation is one possible mechanism to improve infection rates and has shown promise in vivo.[102] However, this strategy will not likely provide a durable effect, as the antimicrobial simply washes out, and the only human study of the type using vancomycin showed no reduction in surgical site infection with antibiotic-soaked mesh.[103]

Therefore a more productive line of inquiry seems to be bonding mesh with materials that will repel or kill bacteria. Since ancient times, silver has been known to have antimicrobial properties, and silver has had a resurgence in wound care, dressing, and even endotracheal tubes to prevent pneumonia. Studies have shown that mesh bonded with nanoparticles of silver can decrease bacterial load by greater than 99% when inoculated with *Staphylococcus aureus* and *E. coli*.[104] Similarly, gold-palladium nanoparticles bound to mesh have demonstrated 0% surgical site infection when inoculated with *Staphylococcus epidermidis*.[105] However, given the rarity of these materials widespread use of these technologies may be cost prohibitive. Lysostaphin is an antistaphylococcal protein that has been shown to decrease bacterial loads and increase survival in rat models when applied to PP mesh and could be a cheaper alternative.[106,107] Actual antibiotics have been combined with drug-eluting particles that are then bound to mesh. In addition, vancomycin,[108] ofloxacin,[109] and rifampin/minocycline[110] have been studied in vitro and animals, but no human studies have been performed.

SUMMARY AND RECOMMENDATIONS

Mesh science has come a long way since the days of hand weaving together silver threads, and with the incidence and number of hernia repairs increasing every year, the technology and capital investment in mesh hernia repair will likely continue to escalate. Synthetic meshes, especially large-pore midweight PP, continue to offer the most robust repairs when performed in clean cases, but the surgeon should use discretion in the choice of mesh for contaminated and dirty fields. While biologic mesh has been well studied over the last decade, newer biosynthetic materials will likely supplant biologic mesh, and biosynthetics and antimicrobials will likely be the fastest changing area of mesh science in the immediate years to come. Ultimately, hernia surgeons should use their best judgment and select the mesh and the approach that is most likely to optimize patient outcomes.

REFERENCES

1. Rutkow IM. Demographic and socioeconomic aspects of hernia repair in the United States in 2003. *Surg Clin North Am.* 2003;83(5):1045-1051, v–vi.
2. Masukawa K, Wilson SE. Is postoperative chronic pain syndrome higher with mesh repair of inguinal hernia? *Am Surg.* 2010;76(10):1115-1118.
3. Saleh F, Okrainec A, D'Souza N, Kwong J, Jackson TD. Safety of laparoscopic and open approaches for repair of the unilateral primary inguinal hernia: an analysis of short-term outcomes. *Am J Surg.* 2014;208(2):195-201.
4. Lichtenstein IL, Shulman AG, Amid PK, Montllor MM. The tension-free hernioplasty. *Am J Surg.* 1989;157(2):188-193.
5. Amid PK. The Lichtenstein repair in 2002: an overview of causes of recurrence after Lichtenstein tension-free hernioplasty. *Hernia.* 2003;7(1):13-16.
6. Smietanski M, Bigda J, Zaborowski K, Worek M, Sledzinski Z. Three-year follow-up of modified Lichtenstein inguinal hernioplasty using lightweight poliglecaprone/polypropylene mesh. *Hernia.* 2009;13(3):239-242.
7. Vrijland WW, van den Tol MP, Luijendijk RW, et al. Randomized clinical trial of non-mesh versus mesh repair of primary inguinal hernia. *Br J Surg.* 2002;89(3):293-297.
8. Zendejas B, Ramirez T, Jones T, et al. Trends in the utilization of inguinal hernia repair techniques: a population-based study. *Am J Surg.* 2012;203(3):313-317, discussion 317.
9. Heniford BT, Matthews BD, Box EA, et al. Optimal teaching environment for laparoscopic ventral herniorrhaphy. *Hernia.* 2002;6(1):17-20.
10. Poulose BK, Shelton J, Phillips S, et al. Epidemiology and cost of ventral hernia repair: making the case for hernia research. *Hernia.* 2012;16(2):179-183.
11. Sauerland S, Walgenbach M, Habermalz B, Seiler CM, Miserez M. Laparoscopic versus open surgical techniques for ventral or incisional hernia repair. *Cochrane Database Syst Rev.* 2011;(3):CD007781.
12. Accreditation Council for Graduate Medical Education. Case Log Statistical Reports; 2013. http://www.acgme.org/acgmeweb/tabid/274/DataCollectionSystems/ResidentCaseLogSystem/CaseLogsStatisticalReports.aspx Accessed 15 September 2016.
13. Usher FC, Ochsner J, Tuttle LL Jr. Use of marlex mesh in the repair of incisional hernias. *Am Surg.* 1958;24(12):969-974.
14. Sanders DL, Kingsnorth AN. From ancient to contemporary times: a concise history of incisional hernia repair. *Hernia.* 2012;16(1):1-7.
15. Muysoms FE, Antoniou SA, Bury K, et al. European Hernia Society guidelines on the closure of abdominal wall incisions. *Hernia.* 2015;19(1):1-24.
16. McClusky DA 3rd, Mirilas P, Zoras O, Skandalakis PN, Skandalakis JE. Groin hernia: anatomical and surgical history. *Arch Surg.* 2006;141(10):1035-1042.
17. Rives J, Stoppa R, Fortesa L, Nicaise H. [Dacron patches and their place in surgery of groin hernia. 65 cases collected from a complete series of 274 hernia operations]. *Ann Chir.* 1968;22(3):159-171.
18. Stoppa RE. The treatment of complicated groin and incisional hernias. *World J Surg.* 1989;13(5):545-554.
19. Rives J, Pire JC, Flament JB, Palot JP, Body C. [Treatment of large eventrations. New therapeutic indications apropos of 322 cases]. *Chir Mem Acad Chir.* 1985;111(3):215-225.
20. Alexandre JH. Jean-Paul Chevrel (1933–2006). *Hernia.* 2007;11(4):293-296.
21. Stoikes N, Webb D, Powell B, Voeller G. Preliminary report of a sutureless onlay technique for incisional hernia repair using fibrin glue alone for mesh fixation. *Am Surg.* 2013;79(11):1177-1180.
22. LeBlanc KA, Booth WV. Laparoscopic repair of incisional abdominal hernias using expanded polytetrafluoroethylene: preliminary findings. *Surg Laparosc Endosc.* 1993;3(1):39-41.
23. Heniford BT, Park A, Ramshaw BJ, Voeller G. Laparoscopic repair of ventral hernias: nine years' experience with 850 consecutive hernias. *Ann Surg.* 2003;238(3):391-399, discussion 399–400.
24. Ballantyne GH, Hourmont K, Wasielewski A. Telerobotic laparoscopic repair of incisional ventral hernias using intraperitoneal prosthetic mesh. *JSLS.* 2003;7(1):7-14.
25. Silverman RP, Li EN, Holton LH 3rd, Sawan KT, Goldberg NH. Ventral hernia repair using allogenic acellular dermal matrix in a swine model. *Hernia.* 2004;8(4):336-342.
26. Kish KJ, Buinewicz BR, Morris JB. Acellular dermal matrix (AlloDerm): new material in the repair of stoma site hernias. *Am Surg.* 2005;71(12):1047-1050.
27. Ramaswamy A. Biologic Mesh; 2016. http://www.sages.org/wiki/biologic-mesh/. Accessed 18 September 2016.
28. Scott NW, McCormack K, Graham P, Go PM, Ross SJ, Grant AM. Open mesh versus non-mesh for repair of femoral and inguinal hernia. *Cochrane Database Syst Rev.* 2002;(4):CD002197.
29. Collaboration EUHT. Repair of groin hernia with synthetic mesh: meta-analysis of randomized controlled trials. *Ann Surg.* 2002;235(3):322-332.
30. Luijendijk RW, Hop WC, van den Tol MP, et al. A comparison of suture repair with mesh repair for incisional hernia. *N Engl J Med.* 2000;343(6):392-398.
31. Burger JW, Luijendijk RW, Hop WC, Halm JA, Verdaasdonk EG, Jeekel J. Long-term follow-up of a randomized controlled trial of suture versus mesh repair of incisional hernia. *Ann Surg.* 2004;240(4):578-583, discussion 583–575.
32. den Hartog D, Dur AH, Tuinebreijer WE, Kreis RW. Open surgical procedures for incisional hernias. *Cochrane Database Syst Rev.* 2008;(3):CD006438.
33. Mathes T, Walgenbach M, Siegel R. Suture versus mesh repair in primary and incisional ventral hernias: a systematic review and meta-analysis. *World J Surg.* 2016;40(4):826-835.
34. DiCocco JM, Fabian TC, Emmett KP, Magnotti LJ, Goldberg SP, Croce MA. Components separation for abdominal wall reconstruction: the Memphis modification. *Surgery.* 2012;151(1):118-125.

35. Vargo D. Component separation in the management of the difficult abdominal wall. *Am J Surg.* 2004;188(6):633-637.

36. de Vries Reilingh TS, van Goor H, Charbon JA, et al. Repair of giant midline abdominal wall hernias: "components separation technique" versus prosthetic repair : interim analysis of a randomized controlled trial. *World J Surg.* 2007;31(4):756-763.

37. Espinosa-de-los-Monteros A, Dominguez I, Zamora-Valdes D, Castillo T, Fernandez-Diaz OF, Luna-Torres HA. Closure of midline contaminated and recurrent incisional hernias with components separation technique reinforced with plication of the rectus muscles. *Hernia.* 2013;17(1):75-79.

38. Fischer PE, Fabian TC. Decreasing the reherniation rate using a modified components separation technique. *World J Surg.* 2007;31(11):2266, author reply 2267–2268.

39. Jernigan TW, Fabian TC, Croce MA, et al. Staged management of giant abdominal wall defects: acute and long-term results. *Ann Surg.* 2003;238(3):349-355, discussion 355–347.

40. Ko JH, Wang EC, Salvay DM, Paul BC, Dumanian GA. Abdominal wall reconstruction: lessons learned from 200 "components separation" procedures. *Arch Surg.* 2009;144(11):1047-1055.

41. Ventral Hernia Working G, Breuing K, Butler CE, et al. Incisional ventral hernias: review of the literature and recommendations regarding the grading and technique of repair. *Surgery.* 2010;148(3):544-558.

42. Fischer JP, Basta MN, Mirzabeigi MN, Kovach SJ 3rd. A comparison of outcomes and cost in VHWG grade II hernias between Rives-Stoppa synthetic mesh hernia repair versus underlay biologic mesh repair. *Hernia.* 2014;18(6):781-789.

43. Bilsel Y, Abci I. The search for ideal hernia repair; mesh materials and types. *International J Surg.* 2012;10(6):317-321.

44. Blatnik JA, Krpata DM, Jacobs MR, Gao Y, Novitsky YW, Rosen MJ. In vivo analysis of the morphologic characteristics of synthetic mesh to resist MRSA adherence. *J Gastrointest Surg.* 2012;16(11):2139-2144.

45. Borrazzo EC, Belmont MF, Boffa D, Fowler DL. Effect of prosthetic material on adhesion formation after laparoscopic ventral hernia repair in a porcine model. *Hernia.* 2004;8(2):108-112.

46. Matthews BD, Pratt BL, Pollinger HS, et al. Assessment of adhesion formation to intra-abdominal polypropylene mesh and polytetrafluoroethylene mesh. *J Surg Res.* 2003;114(2):126-132.

47. Vrijland WW, Tseng LN, Eijkman HJ, et al. Fewer intraperitoneal adhesions with use of hyaluronic acid-carboxymethylcellulose membrane: a randomized clinical trial. *Ann Surg.* 2002;235(2):193-199.

48. van 't Riet M, de Vos van Steenwijk PJ, Bonthuis F, et al. Prevention of adhesion to prosthetic mesh: comparison of different barriers using an incisional hernia model. *Ann Surg.* 2003;237(1):123-128.

49. Petersen S, Henke G, Freitag M, Faulhaber A, Ludwig K. Deep prosthesis infection in incisional hernia repair: predictive factors and clinical outcome. *Eur J Surg Acta Chir.* 2001;167(6):453-457.

50. Dolce CJ, Keller JE, Stefanidis D, et al. Evaluation of soft tissue attachments to a novel intra-abdominal prosthetic in a rabbit model. *Surg Innov.* 2012;19(3):295-300.

51. Novitsky YW, Harrell AG, Hope WW, Kercher KW, Heniford BT. Meshes in hernia repair. *Surg Technol Int.* 2007;16:123-127.

52. Harrell AG, Novitsky YW, Kercher KW, et al. In vitro infectability of prosthetic mesh by methicillin-resistant Staphylococcus aureus. *Hernia.* 2006;10(2):120-124.

53. Tomaszewska A. Mechanical behaviour of knit synthetic mesh used in hernia surgery. *Acta Bbioeng Biomech.* 2016;18(1):77-86.

54. Cordero A, Hernandez-Gascon B, Pascual G, Bellon JM, Calvo B, Pena E. Biaxial mechanical evaluation of absorbable and nonabsorbable synthetic surgical meshes used for hernia repair: physiological loads modify anisotropy response. *Ann Biomed Eng.* 2016;44(7):2181-2188.

55. Cobb WS, Burns JM, Peindl RD, et al. Textile analysis of heavy weight, mid-weight, and light weight polypropylene mesh in a porcine ventral hernia model. *J Surg Res.* 2006;136(1):1-7.

56. Cobb WS, Kercher KW, Heniford BT. The argument for lightweight polypropylene mesh in hernia repair. *Surg Innov.* 2005;12(1):63-69.

57. Ladurner R, Chiapponi C, Linhuber Q, Mussack T. Long term outcome and quality of life after open incisional hernia repair—light versus heavy weight meshes. *BMC Surg.* 2011;11:25.

58. Petro CC, Nahabet EH, Criss CN, et al. Central failures of lightweight monofilament polyester mesh causing hernia recurrence: a cautionary note. *Hernia.* 2015;19(1):155-159.

59. Novitsky YW, Harrell AG, Cristiano JA, et al. Comparative evaluation of adhesion formation, strength of ingrowth, and textile properties of prosthetic meshes after long-term intra-abdominal implantation in a rabbit. *J Surg Res.* 2007;140(1):6-11.

60. Lichtenstein IL, Shore JM. Simplified repair of femoral and recurrent inguinal hernias by a "plug" technic. *Am J Surg.* 1974;128(3):439-444.

61. Magnusson J, Nygren J, Gustafsson UO, Thorell A. UltraPro Hernia System, Prolene Hernia System and Lichtenstein for primary inguinal hernia repair: 3-year outcomes of a prospective randomized controlled trial. *Hernia.* 2016;20(5):641-648.

62. Bell RC, Price JG. Laparoscopic inguinal hernia repair using an anatomically contoured three-dimensional mesh. *Surg Endosc.* 2003;17(11):1784-1788.

63. Leber GE, Garb JL, Alexander AI, Reed WP. Long-term complications associated with prosthetic repair of incisional hernias. *Arch Surg.* 1998;133(4):378-382.

64. Halm JA, de Wall LL, Steyerberg EW, Jeekel J, Lange JF. Intraperitoneal polypropylene mesh hernia repair complicates subsequent abdominal surgery. *World J Surg.* 2007;31(2):423-429, discussion 430.

65. Koehler RH, Begos D, Berger D, et al. Minimal adhesions to ePTFE mesh after laparoscopic ventral incisional hernia repair: reoperative findings in 65 cases. *JSLS.* 2003;7(4):335-340.

66. Cobb WS, Carbonell AM, Kalbaugh CL, Jones Y, Lokey JS. Infection risk of open placement of intraperitoneal composite mesh. *Am Surg.* 2009;75(9):762-767, discussion 767–768.

67. Cobb WS, Harris JB, Lokey JS, McGill ES, Klove KL. Incisional herniorrhaphy with intraperitoneal composite mesh: a report of 95 cases. *Am Surg.* 2003;69(9):784-787.

68. Greenberg JJ. Can infected composite mesh be salvaged? *Hernia.* 2010;14(6):589-592.

69. Gal I, Balint A, Szabo L. [Results of laparoscopic repair of abdominal wall hernias using an ePTFE-polypropylene composite mesh]. *Zentralbl Chir.* 2004;129(2):92-95.

70. Deeken CR, Faucher KM, Matthews BD. A review of the composition, characteristics, and effectiveness of barrier mesh prostheses utilized for laparoscopic ventral hernia repair. *Surg Endosc.* 2012;26(2):566-575.

71. Pierce RA, Perrone JM, Nimeri A, et al. 120-day comparative analysis of adhesion grade and quantity, mesh contraction, and tissue response to a novel omega-3 fatty acid bioabsorbable barrier macroporous mesh after intraperitoneal placement. *Surg Innov.* 2009;16(1):46-54.

72. van't Riet M, de Vos van Steenwijk PJ, Bonjer HJ, Steyerberg EW, Jeekel J. Mesh repair for postoperative wound dehiscence in the presence of infection: is absorbable mesh safer than non-absorbable mesh? *Hernia.* 2007;11(5):409-413.

73. Harrell AG, Novitsky YW, Peindl RD, et al. Prospective evaluation of adhesion formation and shrinkage of intra-abdominal prosthetics in a rabbit model. *Am Surg.* 2006;72(9):808-813, discussion 813–804.

74. Deerenberg EB, Mulder IM, Grotenhuis N, Ditzel M, Jeekel J, Lange JF. Experimental study on synthetic and biological mesh implantation in a contaminated environment. *Br J Surg.* 2012;99(12):1734-1741.

75. Kathju S, Nistico L, Melton-Kreft R, Lasko LA, Stoodley P. Direct demonstration of bacterial biofilms on prosthetic mesh after ventral herniorrhaphy. *Surg Infect (Larchmt).* 2015;16(1):45-53.

76. Kolker AR. Multilayer reconstruction of abdominal wall defects with acellular dermal allograft (AlloDerm) and component separation. *Ann Plast Surg.* 2005;55(1):36-41, discussion 41–32.

77. Deeken CR, Melman L, Jenkins ED, Greco SC, Frisella MM, Matthews BD. Histologic and biomechanical evaluation of crosslinked and non-crosslinked biologic meshes in a porcine model of ventral incisional hernia repair. *J Am Coll Surg.* 2011;212(5):880-888.

78. Rosen MJ, Krpata DM, Ermlich B, Blatnik JA. A 5-year clinical experience with single-staged repairs of infected and contaminated abdominal wall defects utilizing biologic mesh. *Ann Surg.* 2013;257(6):991-996.

79. Booth JH, Garvey PB, Baumann DP, et al. Primary fascial closure with mesh reinforcement is superior to bridged mesh repair for abdominal wall reconstruction. *J Am Coll Surg.* 2013;217(6):999-1009.

80. Huntington CR, Cox TC, Blair LJ, et al. Biologic mesh in ventral hernia repair: outcomes, recurrence, and charge analysis. *Surgery.* 2016;160(6):1517-1527.

81. Kim M, Oommen B, Ross SW, et al. The current status of biosynthetic mesh for ventral hernia repair. *Surg Technol Int.* 2014;25:114-121.

82. Levasseur JC, Lehn E, Rignier P. [Experimental study and clinical use of a new material in severe postoperative evisceration of the abdomen (author's transl). *Chirurgie*. 1979;105(7):577-581.

83. Fabian TC, Croce MA, Pritchard FE, et al. Planned ventral hernia. Staged management for acute abdominal wall defects. *Ann Surg*. 1994;219(6):643-650, discussion 651–643.

84. Greene MA, Mullins RJ, Malangoni MA, Feliciano PD, Richardson JD, Polk HC Jr. Laparotomy wound closure with absorbable polyglycolic acid mesh. *Surg Gynecol Obstet*. 1993;176(3):213-218.

85. Negro P, Gossetti F, Dassatti MR, Andreuccetti J, D'Amore L. Bioabsorbable Gore BIO-A plug and patch hernia repair in young adults. *Hernia*. 2012;16(1):121-122.

86. Burgess PL, Brockmeyer JR, Johnson EK. Amyand hernia repaired with Bio-A: a case report and review. *J Surg Educ*. 2011;68(1):62-66.

87. Priego Jimenez P, Salvador Sanchis JL, Angel V, Escrig-Sos J. Short-term results for laparoscopic repair of large paraesophageal hiatal hernias with Gore Bio A(R) mesh. *International J Surg*. 2014;12(8):794-797.

88. Rosen MJ, Bauer JJ, Harmaty M, et al. Multicenter, prospective, longitudinal study of the recurrence, surgical site infection, and quality of life after contaminated ventral hernia repair using biosynthetic absorbable mesh: the COBRA study. *Ann Surg*. 2017;265:205-211.

89. Deeken CR, Matthews BD. Characterization of the mechanical strength, resorption properties, and histologic characteristics of a fully absorbable material (Poly-4-hydroxybutyrate-PHASIX Mesh) in a porcine model of hernia repair. *ISRN Surg*. 2013;2013:238067.

90. Scott JR, Deeken CR, Martindale RG, Rosen MJ. Evaluation of a fully absorbable poly-4-hydroxybutyrate/absorbable barrier composite mesh in a porcine model of ventral hernia repair. *Surg Endosc*. 2016;30(9):3691-3701.

91. Wormer BA, Clavin NW, Lefaivre JF, et al. Reducing postoperative abdominal bulge following deep inferior epigastric perforator flap breast reconstruction with onlay monofilament poly-4-hydroxybutyrate biosynthetic mesh. *J Reconstr Microsurg*. 2016;33(1):8-18.

92. Withers L, Rogers A. A spiral tack as a lead point for volvulus. *JSLS*. 2006;10(2):247-249.

93. Reynvoet E, Berrevoet F. Pros and cons of tacking in laparoscopic hernia repair. *Surg Technol Int*. 2014;25:136-140.

94. Colak E, Ozlem N, Kucuk GO, Aktimur R, Kesmer S, Yildirim K. Prospective randomized trial of mesh fixation with absorbable versus nonabsorbable tacker in laparoscopic ventral incisional hernia repair. *Int J Clin Exp Med*. 2015;8(11):21611-21616.

95. Shah NS, Fullwood C, Siriwardena AK, Sheen AJ. Mesh fixation at laparoscopic inguinal hernia repair: a meta-analysis comparing tissue glue and tack fixation. *World J Surg*. 2014;38(10):2558-2570.

96. Kaul A, Hutfless S, Le H, et al. Staple versus fibrin glue fixation in laparoscopic total extraperitoneal repair of inguinal hernia: a systematic review and meta-analysis. *Surg Endosc*. 2012;26(5):1269-1278.

97. Chand M, On J, Bevan K, Mostafid H, Venkatsubramaniam AK. Mesh erosion following laparoscopic incisional hernia repair. *Hernia*. 2012;16(2):223-226.

98. Riaz AA, Ismail M, Barsam A, Bunce CJ. Mesh erosion into the bladder: a late complication of incisional hernia repair. A case report and review of the literature. *Hernia*. 2004;8(2):158-159.

99. Foda M, Carlson MA. Enterocutaneous fistula associated with ePTFE mesh: case report and review of the literature. *Hernia*. 2009;13(3):323-326.

100. Moussi A, Daldoul S, Bourguiba B, Othmani D, Zaouche A. Gas gangrene of the abdominal wall due to late-onset enteric fistula after polyester mesh repair of an incisional hernia. *Hernia*. 2012;16(2):215-217.

101. Augenstein VA, Cox TC, Hlavacek C, et al. Treatment of 161 Consecutive Synthetic Mesh Infections: Can Mesh Be Salvaged? 2016. Washington, DC: Americas Hernia Society.

102. Perez-Kohler B, Garcia-Moreno F, Brune T, Pascual G, Bellon JM. Preclinical bioassay of a polypropylene mesh for hernia repair pretreated with antibacterial solutions of chlorhexidine and allicin: an in vivo study. *PLoS ONE*. 2015;10(11):e0142768.

103. Yabanoglu H, Arer IM, Caliskan K. The effect of the use of synthetic mesh soaked in antibiotic solution on the rate of graft infection in ventral hernias: a prospective randomized study. *Int Surg*. 2015;100(6):1040-1047.

104. Kumar V, Jolivalt C, Pulpytel J, Jafari R, Arefi-Khonsari F. Development of silver nanoparticle loaded antibacterial polymer mesh using plasma polymerization process. *J Biomed Mater Res A*. 2013;101(4):1121-1132.

105. Saygun O, Agalar C, Aydinuraz K, et al. Gold and gold-palladium coated polypropylene grafts in a S. epidermidis wound infection model. *J Surg Res*. 2006;131(1):73-79.

106. Belyansky I. The addition of lysostaphin dramatically improves survival, protects porcine biomesh from infection, and improves graft tensile shear strength. *J Surg Res*. 2011;171(2):409-415.

107. Belyansky I, Tsirline VB, Montero PN, et al. Lysostaphin-coated mesh prevents staphylococcal infection and significantly improves survival in a contaminated surgical field. *Am Surg*. 2011;77(8):1025-1031.

108. Harth KC, Rosen MJ, Thatiparti TR, et al. Antibiotic-releasing mesh coating to reduce prosthetic sepsis: an in vivo study. *J Surg Res*. 2010;163(2):337-343.

109. Guillaume O, Lavigne JP, Lefranc O, Nottelet B, Coudane J, Garric X. New antibiotic-eluting mesh used for soft tissue reinforcement. *Acta Biomater*. 2011;7(9):3390-3397.

110. Majumder A, Scott JR, Novitsky YW. Evaluation of the antimicrobial efficacy of a novel rifampin/minocycline-coated, noncrosslinked porcine acellular dermal matrix compared with uncoated scaffolds for soft tissue repair. *Surg Innov*. 2016;23(5):442-455.

Stomach and Small Intestine

Anatomy and Physiology of the Stomach

Rickesha L. Wilson | Christina E. Stevenson

The stomach is a remarkable organ that aids in digestion, regulating nutrition, and controlling appetite. The complex physiologic processes by which the stomach exerts its endocrine and nutritional functions have been researched for decades and there is still much to be learned. This chapter on the anatomy and physiology of the stomach aims to equip the surgeon with the detailed knowledge of not only the gross anatomy and vascular supply of the stomach, but also the physiologic properties behind the complex process of gastric acid secretion and hormonal regulation related to digestion.

EMBRYOLOGIC DEVELOPMENT

The stomach arises from the embryonic endoderm and comprises a portion of the foregut along with the esophagus, the first portion of the duodenum, as well as the liver, bile ducts, and pancreas. During the fourth week of gestation, the foregut is oriented as a craniocaudal tube with the primitive stomach and first portion of the duodenum forming the caudal end. The ventral mesogastrium and the dorsal mesogastrium are attached to the stomach anteriorly and posteriorly and suspend the stomach in the peritoneal cavity. The greater and lesser curvatures of the stomach are formed because the dorsal portion of the gastric wall grows at a faster rate than the ventral portion.[1] At approximately weeks 7 and 8, as the foregut develops, it rotates 90 degrees clockwise on its long axis so that the ventral mesogastrium is positioned to the right of the stomach and the dorsal mesogastrium is to the left (Fig. 56.1). The ventral mesogastrium forms the lesser omentum comprised of the gastrohepatic and hepatoduodenal ligaments and contains the liver, which grows rapidly and pushes the stomach to the left portion of the peritoneal cavity. The dorsal mesogastrium develops into the greater omentum, comprised of the gastrophrenic, gastrosplenic, and gastrocolic ligaments and is where the spleen is located during development. This rotation also positions the left vagal nerve trunk anterior to the stomach and the right vagal nerve trunk in the posterior position. The stomach descends as cephalad structures grow and is eventually located between T10 and L3 in the adult.

GROSS ANATOMY AND ANATOMIC RELATIONSHIPS OF THE STOMACH

The stomach is a dilated cylindrical J-shaped organ that rests in the epigastric and left hypochondrial region of the abdomen at the level of the first lumbar vertebra (Fig. 56.2). It is bordered anteriorly by the left hemidiaphragm, the left lobe of the liver and a portion of the right lobe, and the parietal portion of the anterior abdominal wall. Posteriorly, the pancreas (neck, body, and tail), left kidney, and adrenal grand border the stomach. The spleen sits posterolaterally and the transverse colon inferiorly. The two points of attachment are at the gastroesophageal junction superiorly and the retroperitoneal duodenum. Ligamentous attachments also help to further anchor the stomach to surrounding organs: gastrophrenic (diaphragm), hepatogastric or lesser omentum (liver), gastrosplenic or gastrolienal (spleen), and the gastrocolic or greater omentum (transverse colon).

The anatomic regions of the stomach can be distinguished based on surgical landmarks (Fig. 56.3). Beginning superiorly from the abdominal portion of the esophagus and the gastroesophageal junction, the cardiac portion of the stomach follows just inferiorly and the fundus of the stomach is superior and to the left extending above the gastroesophageal junction, forming a sharp angle with the distal esophagus known as the cardiac notch. The corpus or body of the stomach extends and curves inferiorly as a distensible reservoir and forms a sharp medial border called the lesser curvature to the right and a lateral border called the greater curvature on the left. The gastric antrum of the stomach is not anatomically distinguishable but is estimated to be a region from the angular notch along the distal lesser curvature to a point along an inferior line to the distal greater curvature. The gastric antrum empties into the pyloric canal leading to the pyloric sphincter, a palpable thickened ring of smooth muscle that empties into the first portion of the duodenum.

The visceral peritoneum covering the stomach forms its outermost serosal layer, which is contiguous with the lesser and greater omenta anteriorly and the anterior wall of the lesser sac posteriorly. The muscularis externa of the stomach wall comprises three layers: the outermost longitudinal muscle layer, the middle circular muscle layer, and the innermost oblique muscle layer (Fig. 56.4). The longitudinal muscle layer of the stomach is concentrated proximally at the gastroesophageal junction and along the greater and lesser curvatures, and subsequently spreads unevenly over the corpus until joining more densely near the pylorus. Deep to the longitudinal muscle fibers, the circular muscle layer covers the stomach completely and is contiguous with the lower esophageal sphincter muscle proximally and forms a thickened band at the pylorus distally. The innermost oblique muscle layer is blended proximally with the circular muscle layer at the collar of Helvetius and splays incompletely over the anterior and posterior gastric walls. The submucosa, which is also the strength layer of the gastric wall, is the next layer deep to the muscle layers followed by the muscularis mucosae, and finally the mucosa, which contains the

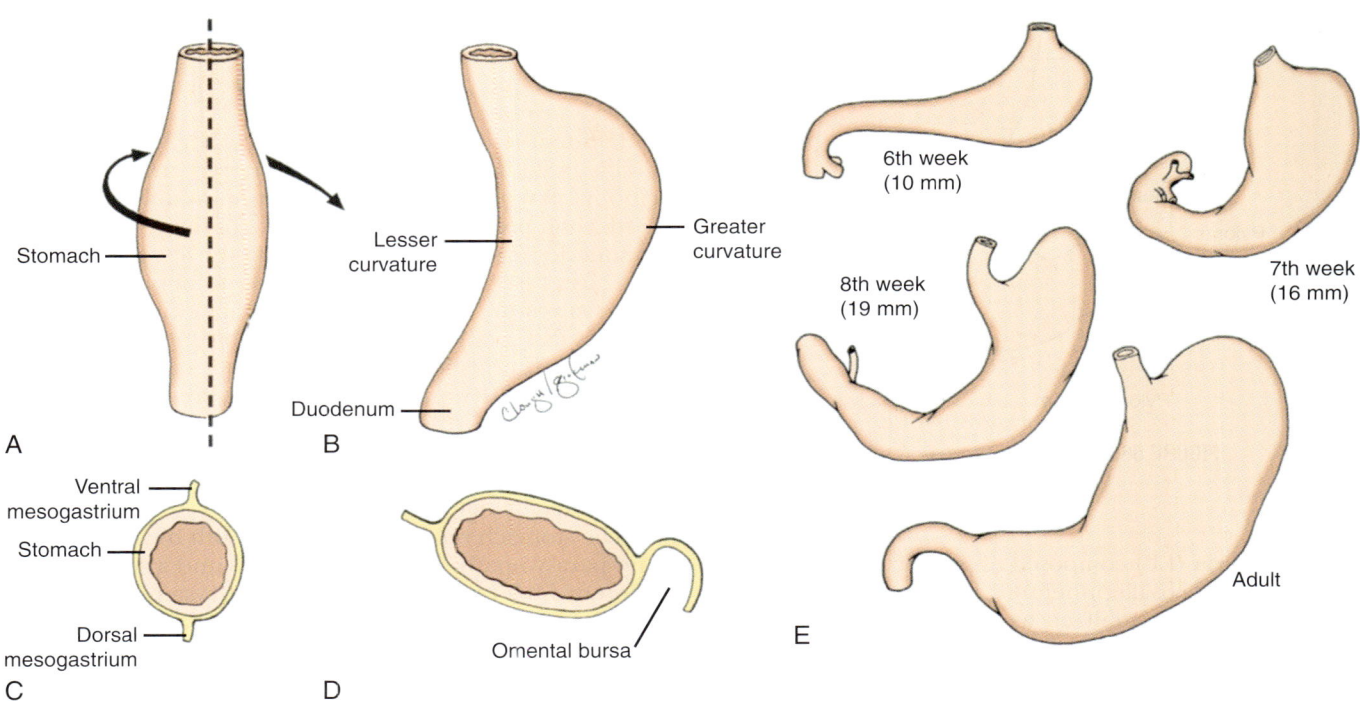

FIGURE 56.1 Positional changes of the developing stomach. (A and B) Anterior view of the stomach rotating on its longitudinal axis. (C and D) Transverse section of peritoneal attachments during rotation of the stomach. (E) Shape of the stomach at various prenatal stages and in the adult. ([A–D] Based on Sadler TW. *Langman's Medical Embryology*. 5th ed. Baltimore: Williams & Wilkins; 1985. In Skandalakis LJ, et al. Stomach. In: Skandalakis JE, et al, eds. *Skandalakis' Surgical Anatomy*. New York: McGraw-Hill; 2004 [Chapter 15]. [E] From Lewis FT. The development of the stomach. In: Keibel WP, Mall FP, eds. *Manual of Human Embryology*. Philadelphia: JB Lippincott; 1912. In Skandalakis LJ, et al. Stomach. In: Skandalakis JE, et al, eds. *Skandalakis' Surgical Anatomy*. New York: McGraw-Hill; 2004 [Chapter 15].)

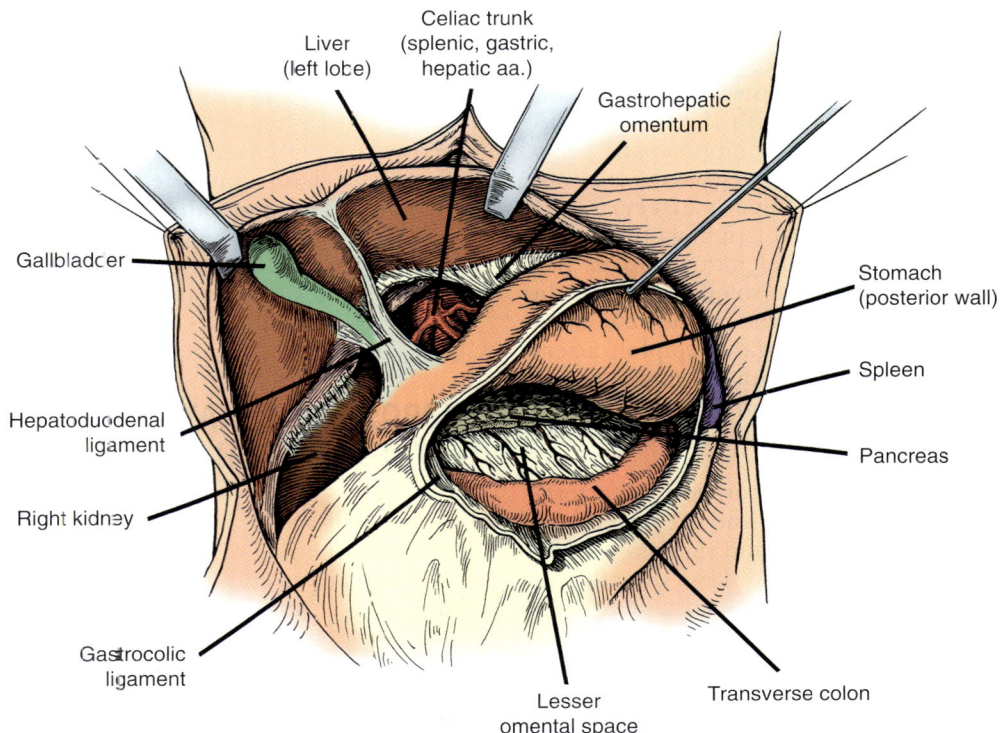

FIGURE 56.2 The stomach in situ.

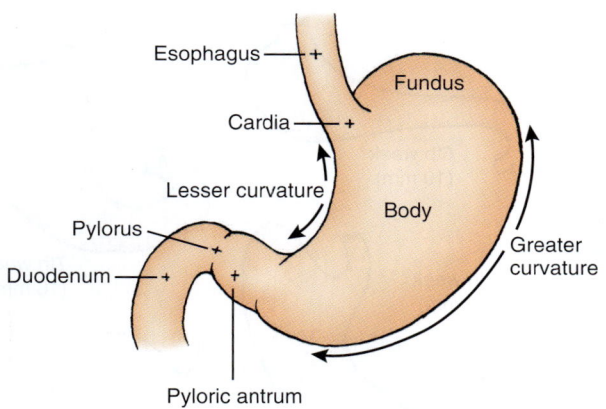

FIGURE 56.3 Regions of the stomach.

lamina propria (LP) composed of connective tissue, blood vessels, and mucosal epithelium. The inner surface of the stomach can be visualized as multiple irregular folds, termed *rugae*, which help to increase surface area of the stomach and flatten out to allow the stomach to expand and accommodate meals.

VASCULAR, LYMPHATIC, AND NEURAL SUPPLY TO THE STOMACH

The vasculature of the stomach contains a well-developed network of anastomosing vessels that stem from the celiac trunk (Fig. 56.5). This rich blood supply makes ischemia of the stomach rare and can make control of gastric hemorrhage a significant challenge. The greater and lesser omenta contain the majority of the blood vessels supplying the stomach. The left gastric artery is a direct branch from the celiac trunk and courses along the lesser curvature to anastomose distally with the right gastric artery, most often a branch of the common hepatic artery. The gastroduodenal artery also branches from the common hepatic (proximal to the right hepatic artery) and it supplies the greater curvature with the right gastroepiploic (right gastro-omental) artery. The left gastroepiploic (left gastro-omental) branches from the splenic artery at the superior and proximal portion of the greater curvature before anastomosing with the right gastroepiploic artery. The short gastric arteries supply the fundus and proximal body of the stomach by branching from the splenic hilum, unlike the other vessels that course through the greater and lesser omenta.

Venous drainage of the stomach parallels the arterial blood supply with eventual drainage into the portal vein. The left gastric vein (coronary vein) and right gastric vein course along the lesser curvature and drain directly into the portal vein. The greater curvature is drained by the right gastroepiploic vein into the superior mesenteric vein and by the left gastroepiploic vein, which empties into the splenic vein. The splenic vein also drains the short gastric veins and the inferior mesenteric vein and finally joins the superior mesenteric vein to form the portal vein. In cases of portal hypertension, portal venous drainage may be redirected to lower resistance paths, especially via the left gastric vein and esophageal tributaries and also the short gastric vein, resulting in gastric varices.

Lymphatic drainage of the stomach can also vary as much as the arterial and venous supply, and gastric carcinoma may spread to multiple lymph node groups. The cardia and proximal lesser curvature of the stomach drain to superior gastric lymph nodes near the left gastric artery and gastroesophageal junction. The distal portion of the lesser curvature drains into the suprapyloric lymph node region. Pancreaticosplenic nodes near the splenic hilum drain the fundus and proximal greater curvature of the stomach, and lymph from the distal greater curvature, antrum, and pylorus drains to the subpyloric lymph nodes. Ultimately, lymph drains to the celiac axis nodal basin, which then drains to the cisterna chyli nodes and into the thoracic duct.

The stomach receives input from both the sympathetic and parasympathetic nervous systems and also originates afferent fibers of the enteric nervous system (ENS) that provide input to the sympathetic (via splanchnic nerves) and parasympathetic systems (via the vagus). The ENS is considered the third branch of the autonomic nervous system (the other two being the sympathetic and parasympathetic) and although it is relatively poorly understood, it is recognized that it contains as many neurons as the spinal cord and can function autonomously.[2]

Presynaptic efferent parasympathetic neurons originate in the dorsal motor nucleus and travel in the left and right vagus nerves that enter the abdomen through the esophageal hiatus on the anterior and posterior surfaces of the esophagus, respectively (Fig. 56.6). These fibers synapse with postsynaptic neurons located between the circular and longitudinal muscle layers—the myenteric (Auerbach) plexus—and within the submucosal (Meissner) plexus. Afferent fibers originating in the stomach travel in the vagus and synapse with cell bodies in the nucleus of the solitary tract of the brainstem.[3]

Presynaptic efferent sympathetic fibers travel in the sympathetic chain alongside the eighth to tenth thoracic vertebrae and synapse with neurons located in the splanchnic (celiac) ganglia before terminating in the gastric neuronal plexuses. Sympathetic afferents from the stomach have cell bodies located in the dorsal root ganglia of the thoracic spinal nerves.[3]

MICROSCOPIC ANATOMY AND PHYSIOLOGY OF THE STOMACH

GASTRIC MUCOSA

The mucosal lining of the stomach is characterized by a simple columnar epithelium (SCE) that uniformly lines the stomach. Surface mucous cells (SMs) make up the gastric pits (GPs), which lead to long, branched, tubular glands, giving the gastric mucosa a leafy appearance, termed the *gastric foveolae*. Each gland has distinct regions from the surface down: the gastric pit, isthmus, neck, and base (Fig. 56.7). The stomach can be divided into three glandular regions and these glands are composed of

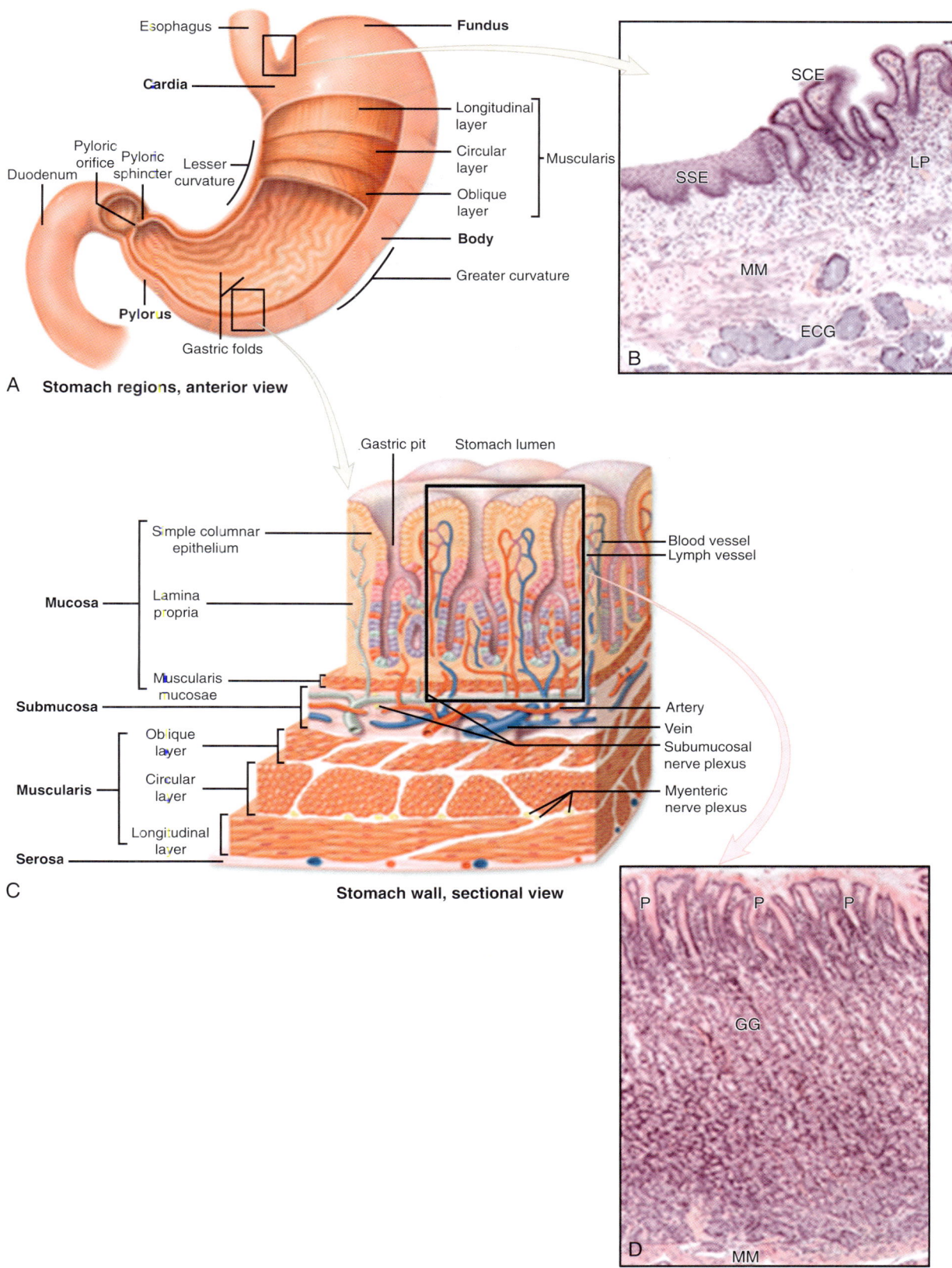

FIGURE 56.4 The stomach wall: (A) Anterior view of the stomach regions and the muscle layers. (B) Transitional epithelium between the esophagus and the stomach. Stratified squamous epithelium *(SSE)* in the esophagus becomes simple columnar epithelium *(SCE)* in the proximal stomach. The lamina propria *(LP)* underlies the epithelium and the muscularis mucosa *(MM)* is deep to the LP with esophageal cardiac glands *(ECG)* pictured. (C) The simple columnar epithelium of the gastric mucosa contains gastric pits leading to gastric glands with various cell types. Additional layers of the stomach wall are illustrated. (D) Histologic section of the gastric mucosa illustrating the relation of the gastric pits *(F)* leading into the gastric glands *(GG)* inferiorly bordered by muscularis mucosa *(MM)*. (Modified from Mescher AL. Digestive tract. In: Mescher AL, ed. *Junqueira's Basic Histology*. 14th ed. New York: McGraw-Hill; 2016.)

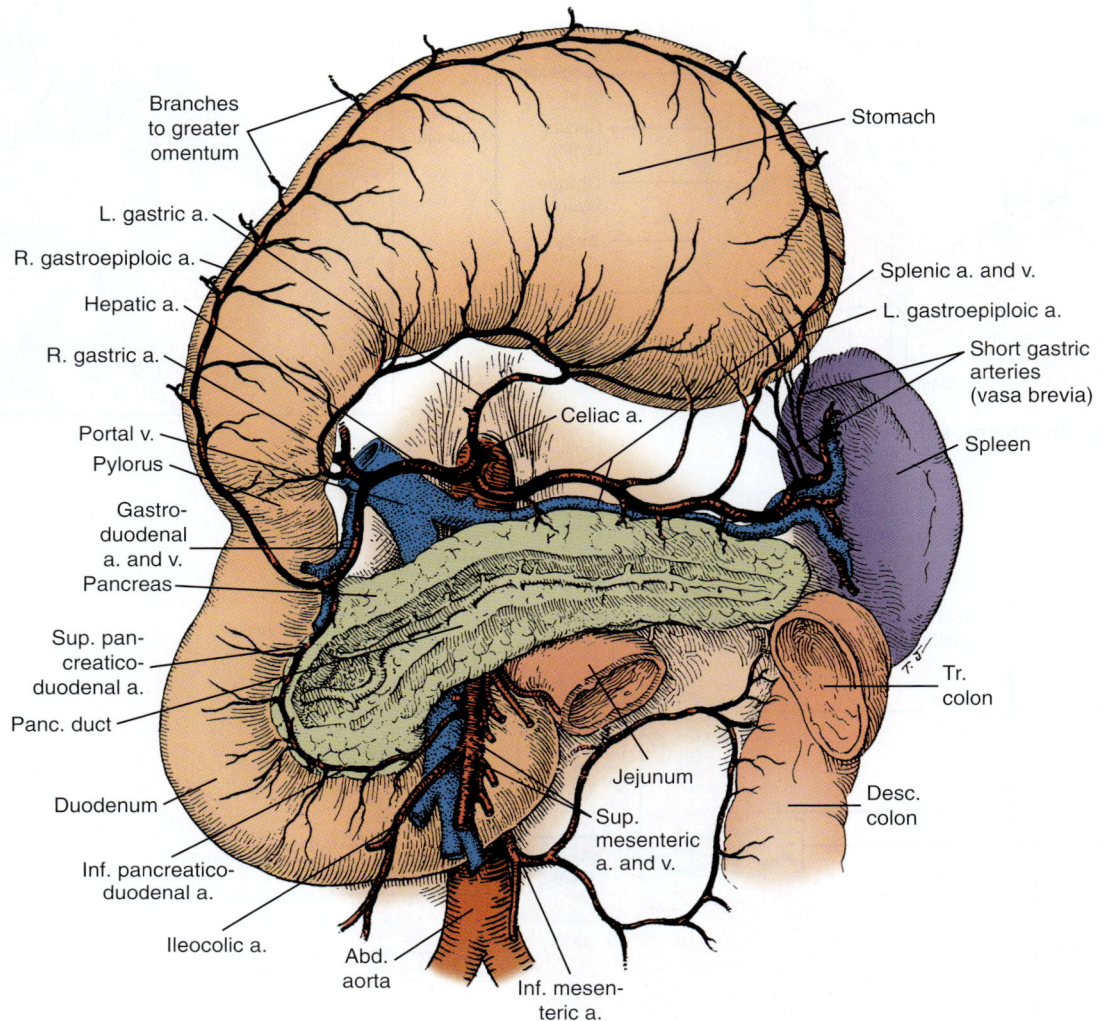

FIGURE 56.5 Vascular supply of the foregut. The stomach is shown reflected cephalad and the pancreatic duct is exposed.

various cell types: cardiac glands in the cardia, oxyntic glands in the fundus and body, and antral glands in the pyloric portion of the stomach.[4]

Cardiac glands are chiefly comprised of mucous cells along with a few scattered parietal cells, undifferentiated cells in the neck, and a majority of endocrine cells at the base of the glands. The cardiac glands make up the 10- to 30-mm transition zone between the squamous epithelium of the distal esophagus and the oxyntic glands of the fundus, and have a primary function of producing mucus. Although thought to be congenital, the expression of these glands varies among ethnic populations.[5] When the basal half of these glands expresses more parietal cells, they are termed *oxyntocardiac glands.*

Oxyntic glands are located in the fundus and body of the stomach and are appropriately named for their acid-producing functions, based on the Greek *oxynein,* meaning "acid-forming." The main cell types are the surface epithelial cells, the mucous cells located in the GPs and in the isthmus and neck, the parietal cells that secrete hydrochloric acid (HCl) and intrinsic factor

and are heavily concentrated in the neck, the basal chief (zymogenic) cells that secrete pepsinogen, and enterochromaffin-like (ECL) cells that produce histamine—a powerful stimulus for parietal cell acid production—located throughout the gland.

The antral mucosa is distinct from fundus/body mucosa in its lack of acid-producing cells and greater proportion of gastrin-secreting G cells. Gastric mucosal cells secrete an electrolyte-rich solution that aids in churning, mixing, and lubricating food. Gastric fluid also acts as a vehicle for proteolytic enzymes that are active in the fluid phase. The volume and electrolyte composition of gastric fluid depend on stimuli such as vagal/cholinergic tone and hormonal/paracrine factors (i.e., gastrin, histamine). In healthy individuals, the basal secretory rate of the stomach is more than 60 mL of fluid hourly, which, in experimental studies, can increase to more than double that when stimulated by histamine. Total average daily fluid production is more than 1.5 L. The electrolyte composition of gastric fluid is similarly dependent on external stimuli and is summarized in Table 56.1.

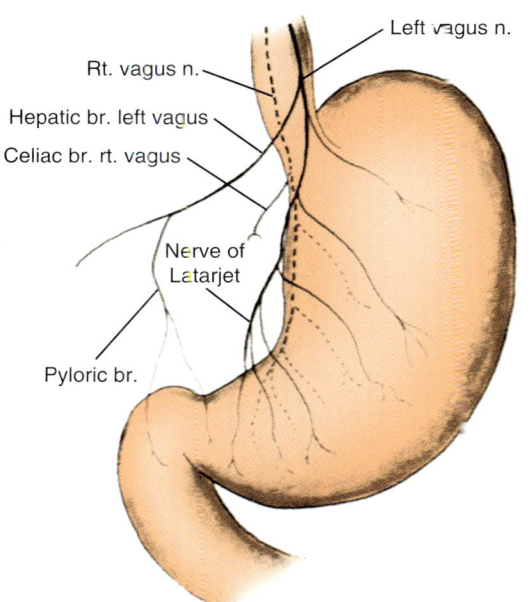

FIGURE 56.6 Diagram of the vagal innervation of the human stomach. (From Menguy R: *Surgery of Peptic Ulcer*. Philadelphia: Saunders; 1976.)

TABLE 56.1 Gastric Fluid Volume and Electrolyte Composition in 200 Healthy Volunteers

	Basal	Histamine
Volume (mL/h)	67.9 ± 27.0	149.1 ± 18.3
H⁺ (mEq/L)	27.1 ± 13.8	95.0 ± 20.6
Na⁺ (mEq/L)	48.1 ± 15.7	23.4 ± 6.1
K⁺ (mEq/L)	13.4 ± 3.1	15.2 ± 2.2
Cl⁻ (mEq/L)	93.5 ± 20.1	139.9 ± 16.3

From Meeroff JC, Rofrano JA, Meeroff M. Electrolytes of the gastric juice in health and gastroduodenal diseases. *Am J Dig Dis*. 1975;18:865.

GASTRIC CELLS AND PHYSIOLOGY OF SECRETORY PRODUCTS

Knowing the various secretory products produced by gastric cells is important in understanding the grand scheme of the stomach's complex role in digestion (Table 56.2).[4,6]

Mucous Cells

Mucous cells are located on the surface and in the neck of the gastric glands (GGs). SMs that line the stomach lumen and the GPs have a columnar shape and secrete an alkaline, highly viscous mucous substance rich in bicarbonate ions that helps to protect the stomach mucosa from abrasive food particles and erosive gastric acid. The mucous cells located deeper in the isthmus and neck of the GGs secrete a more acidic mucin substance and have a rounded nuclei with apical secretory granules. These mucous neck cells (MNs) are the anchored pluripotent stem cells that divide to replace all other cell types in the gastric gland. The SMs have a 4- to 7-day turnover rate,

TABLE 56.2 Important Gastric Secretory Products

Product	Source	Functions
HCl	Parietal cell	Hydrolysis; sterilization of meal
Intrinsic factor	Parietal cell	Vitamin B₁₂ absorption
Pepsinogen	Chief cell	Protein digestion
Mucus, bicarbonate	SM	Gastroprotection
Trefoil factors	SM	Gastroprotection
Histamine	ECL cells	Regulation of gastric secretion
Gastrin	G cells	Regulation of gastric secretion
Gastrin-releasing peptide	Nerves	Regulation of gastric secretion
ACh	Nerves	Regulation of gastric secretion
Somatostatin	D cells	Regulation of gastric secretion

Ach, Acetylcholine; *ECL*, enterochromaffin-like; *HCl*, hydrochloric acid; *SM*, surface mucous cells.

Modified from Barrett KE. Gastric secretion. In: Barrett KE, et al., eds. *Gastrointestinal Physiology*. 2nd ed. New York: McGraw-Hill; 2014 [chapter 3].

whereas deeper secretory cells turn over at a much slower rate.

Parietal Cells

Parietal (oxyntic) cells are located in the neck and deeper parts of the GGs and secrete HCl and intrinsic factor. This cell has a rounded or pyramidal appearance with a round nucleus and a highly eosinophilic cytoplasm due to the mitochondrial density (30% to 40% cell volume) needed to operate the cells' H⁺/K⁺ pump. Water is converted to a hydrogen ion (H⁺) and a hydroxide ion (OH⁻) (Fig. 56.8). The H⁺ is pumped into the gastric lumen in exchange for K⁺, which is maintained in the cytosol above chemical equilibrium by the basolateral Na⁺/K⁺ ATPase and the sodium/potassium/chloride cotransporter (NKCC1). Research in recent years has proposed that more regulatory apical membrane channels participate in the critical process of pumping K⁺ back into the cell from the gastric lumen.[7,8] An OH⁻ combines with CO₂ to form a bicarbonate ion (HCO₃⁻), which is transported across the basolateral membrane into the bloodstream. This process is catalyzed by the carbonic anhydrase II enzyme. A chloride ion is simultaneously transported across the basolateral membrane into the parietal cell lumen and across the apical membrane to combine with H⁺ to form HCl. When the parietal cell is stimulated by acetylcholine (Ach), histamine, or gastrin to secrete gastric acid, important intracellular events take place as the cell shifts from a resting to a secretory state. In particular, intracellular canaliculi and tubulovesicles that house the H⁺/K⁺ proton pumps fuse together and with the apical membrane of the cell. This amplifies the working surface area of the cell 5- to 10-fold and the concentration of proton pumps to the apical membrane increases as well as the parietal cell's power to produce HCl.[4]

Proton pump inhibitors (PPIs) block acid secretion by directly inhibiting the H⁺/K⁺ exchange ATPase at the apical membrane. Inhibitors such as omeprazole are weak bases and become protonated in the highly acidic

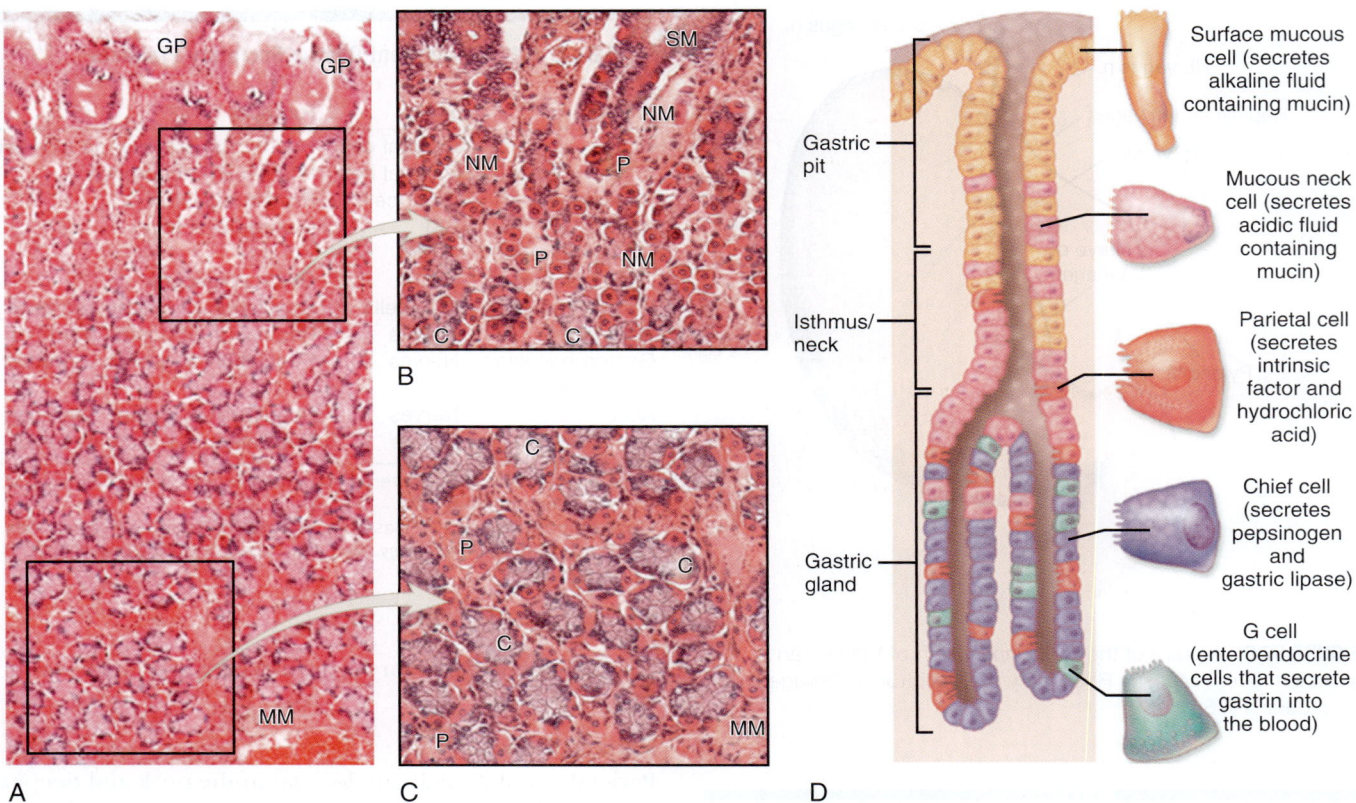

FIGURE 56.7 Gastric glands (GG): (A) The long, coiled GGs penetrate the complete thickness of the mucosa, from the gastric pits *(GP)* to the muscularis mucosae *(MM)*. (B) In the neck of a gastric gland, below the surface mucous cells *(SM)* lining the gastric pit, are small mucous neck cells *(NM)*, scattered individually or clustered among parietal cells (P) and stem cells that give rise to all epithelial cells of the glands. The numerous parietal cells are large distinctive cells often bulging from the tubules, with central nuclei surrounded by intensely eosinophilic cytoplasm with unusual ultrastructure. Chief cells *(C)* begin to appear in the neck region. Around these tubular glands are various cells and microvasculature in connective tissue. (C) Near the MM, the bases of these glands contain fewer parietal cells *(P)* but many more zymogenic chief cells *(C)*. Chief cells are found in clusters, with basal nuclei and basophilic cytoplasm. From their apical ends chief cells secrete pepsinogen, the zymogen precursor for the major protease pepsin. Zymogen granules are often removed or stain poorly in routine preparations. (Both x200; H&E stain) (D) Diagram showing general morphology and functions of major gastric gland cells. (Modified from Mescher AL. Digestive tract. In: Mescher AL, ed. *Junqueira's Basic Histology.* 14th ed. New York: McGraw-Hill; 2016.)

environment immediately surrounding the parietal cell membrane and subsequently form a covalently linked mercapto complex that inactivates the enzyme.[9] By blocking the final step in the acid-secretion pathway, PPIs are able to attenuate acid secretion stimulated by gastrin/histamine and vagal/cholinergic pathways.

Intrinsic factor is a 45-kDa glycoprotein that is secreted by parietal cells and is required for cobalamin (vitamin B_{12}) uptake in the terminal ileum. Secretion of intrinsic factor is independent of acid secretion and is unaffected by PPIs and histamine receptor blockers, although a higher gastric pH may inhibit absorption of food-bound vitamin B_{12}. Although intrinsic factor is synthesized and secreted in the acidic environment of the stomach, it binds with cobalamin at an optimum pH of approximately 7 and is fairly resistant to breakdown by acid and proteolytic enzymes in the stomach. Vitamin B_{12} is initially bound by haptocorrin (R factor), after which, exposure to the higher pH and proteolytic enzymes of the duodenum dissociates the haptocorrin–B_{12} complex and allows for intrinsic

factor binding. Upon reaching the terminal ileum, the intrinsic factor–B_{12} complex is endocytosed by specialized epithelial cells. Patients undergoing proximal gastric resection or total gastrectomy and those with pernicious anemia require parenteral injections of vitamin B_{12}.

Chief Cells

Chief (zymogenic) cells are predominantly located in the basal regions of the GGs. These protein-secreting cells have an abundance of rough endoplasmic reticulum and apical granules containing pepsinogen, an inactive precursor protein secreted into the gastric lumen by a compound exocytosis. Pepsinogen is a 42-kDa proenzyme that undergoes catalytic cleavage in the acidic environment of the stomach and is converted to pepsin, which can activate additional molecules of pepsinogen and effectively degrades collagen. At higher pH, proteolytic activity is diminished because of denaturation, with irreversible loss of proteolytic function above pH 7.2. Stimuli for the secretion of pepsinogen are similar to that of gastric acid

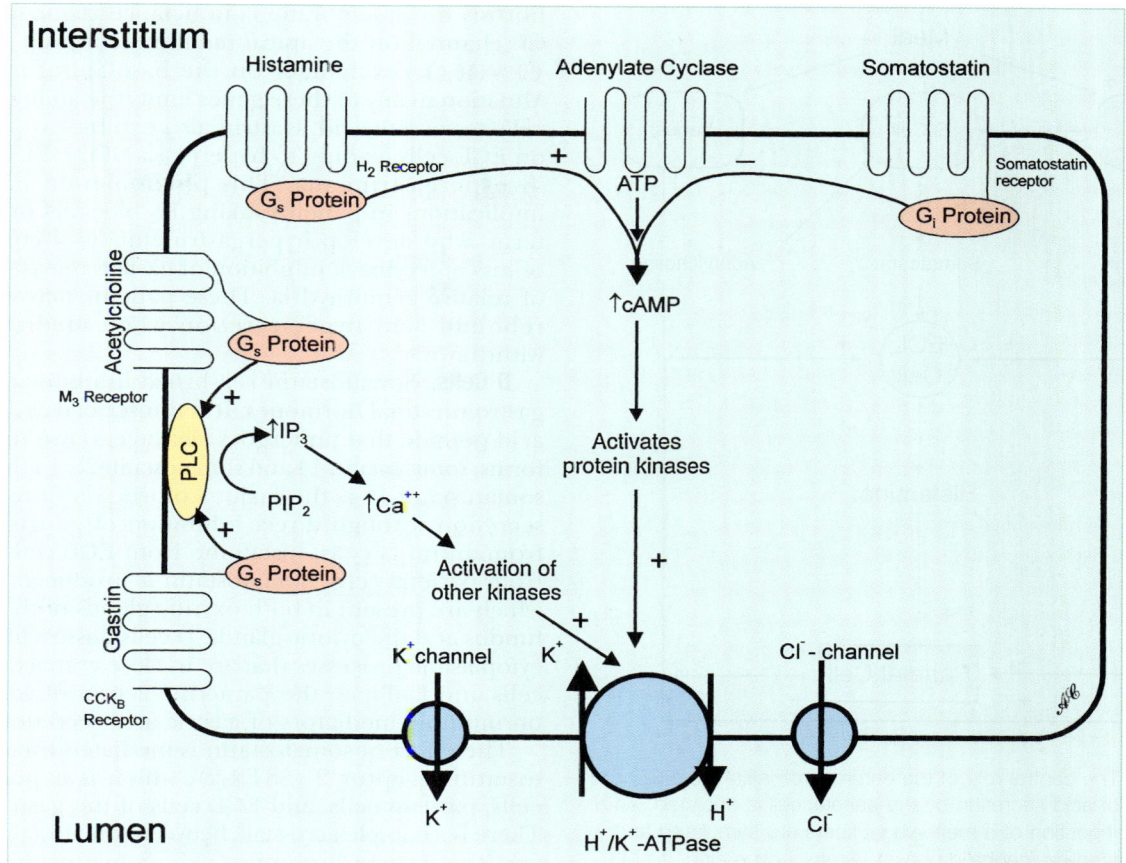

FIGURE 56.8 Molecular mechanics of parietal cell acid production. The intracellular events after ligand binding to the parietal cell are depicted. Gastrin binds to the type B CCK receptor and acetylcholine binds to M3 receptors to stimulate phospholipase C *(PLC)* through a G protein–linked mechanism. Activated PLC converts membrane-bound phospholipids into inositol triphosphate *(IP$_3$)*, which stimulates the release of intracellular calcium from intracellular calcium stores. The increase in intracellular calcium leads to the activation of protein kinases, which activate H$^+$/K$^+$-ATPase. Histamine binds to its H$_2$ receptor to stimulate adenylate cyclase, which also occurs through a G protein–linked mechanism. Activation of adenylate cyclase leads to an increase in intracellular cyclic adenosine monophosphate *(cAMP)* levels, which activates protein kinases. Activated protein kinases stimulate a phosphorylation cascade that results in increased levels of phosphoproteins, which activate the proton pump. Activation of the proton pump leads to extrusion of cytosolic hydrogen in exchange for extracytoplasmic potassium. In addition, chloride is secreted through a chloride channel located at the luminal side of the membrane. *ATP,* Adenosine triphosphate; *ATPase,* adenosine triphosphatase; *G$_s$,* stimulatory guanine nucleotide protein; *G$_i$,* inhibitory guanine nucleotide protein; *PIP$_2$,* phosphatidylinositol 4,5-diphosphate.

and include Ach, gastrin, gastrin-releasing peptide (GRP), cholecystokinin, and nitric oxide. Increasing intracellular calcium is the primary cellular mechanism by which exocytosis of pepsinogen occurs.

Enteroendocrine Cells

Enteroendocrine cells are epithelial cells distributed along the mucosa of the entire digestive tract that release hormones in a paracrine or endocrine fashion. These cells are part of the diffuse neuroendocrine system (DNES) and can be categorized as "closed" if the cellular apex is surrounded by neighboring cells and "open" if the apical portion of the cell is open to the gastric gland lumen with chemoreceptors to sample luminal contents. The various enteroendocrine cells of the stomach are the enterochromaffin cells (closed), which secrete serotonin and substance P to increase gut motility; the D cells of the pylorus, which secrete somatostatin and act on other DNES cells; and G

cells (open) of the pylorus, which secrete gastrin promoting gastric acid secretion.

G Cells. Gastrin is produced by G cells located primarily in the antral mucosa. It is a crucial stimulus for gastric acid secretion. Gastrin undergoes post-translational cleavage and modification prior to its release into the circulation, resulting in several isoforms of the peptide with varying biologic activities and half-lives. Gastrin-17 is the predominant active form, although varying amounts of gastrin-34 and gastrin-71 are produced in healthy and hypersecretory disease states, such as gastrinoma. Stimuli for gastrin release include Ach from vagal efferent fibers, luminal peptides and amino acids, alkaline gastric pH, and calcitonin. Gastrin release is inhibited by somatostatin and acidic pH.

The effect of gastrin on acid secretion is indirect and involves ECL cells, which express the cholecystokinin-2 (CCK-2) receptor (a G protein–coupled transmembrane

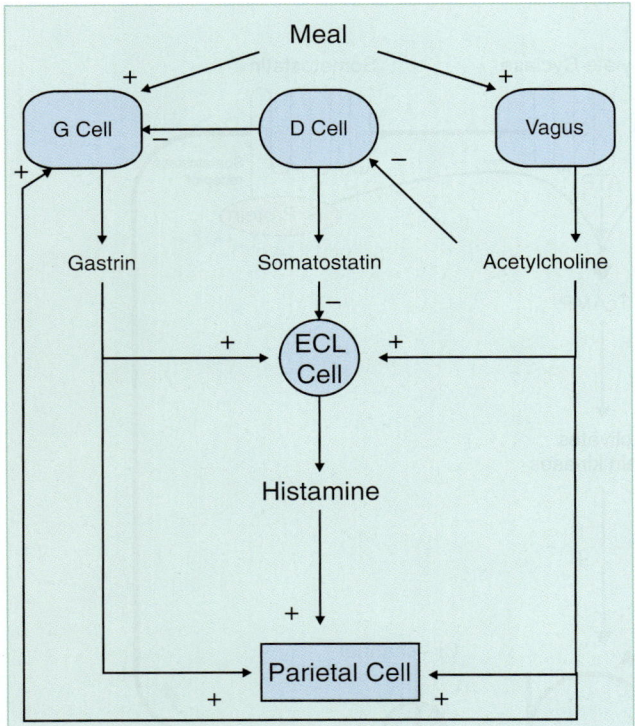

FIGURE 56.9 The central role of the enterochromaffin-like (ECL) cell in regulation of acid secretion by the parietal cell is depicted. As shown, after ingestion of a meal, vagal fibers are stimulated and release acetylcholine (cephalic phase). Acetylcholine binds to M3 receptors located on the ECL cell, parietal cell, and G cell to cause the release of histamine, hydrochloric acid, and gastrin, respectively. Acetylcholine also interacts with M3 receptors located on the D cell to inhibit somatostatin release. Food within the gastric lumen also stimulates the G cell to release gastrin, which, in turn, binds to type B cholecystokinin receptors located on the ECL cell and parietal cell and causes the release of histamine and hydrochloric acid, respectively (gastric phase). Somatostatin released from the D cell inhibits histamine release from the ECL cell and gastrin release from the G cell. Somatostatin also inhibits acid secretion by the parietal cell (not shown). The principal stimulus for activation of the D cell is antral luminal acidification (not shown).

receptor) and serve as intermediaries between G cells and parietal cells (Fig. 56.9). No physiologically functional CCK-2 receptor has been identified on parietal cells. In response to gastrin binding, there is activation of phospholipase C (PLC) and elevation of intracellular calcium in the ECL cell, leading to release of histamine that acts in a paracrine manner on parietal cells.

ECL Cells. Histamine is produced by ECL cells by decarboxylation of l-histidine and is stored in intracellular secretory vesicles. Histamine binding to the histamine (H_2) receptor on parietal cells activates adenylate cyclase causing a rise in cyclic adenosine monophosphate (cAMP), which induces translocation of the H^+/K^+ exchange ATPase pump to the apical membrane, thus increasing proton secretion into the gastric lumen and lowering the gastric pH.[10] To maintain electroneutrality, parietal cells must also have functional voltage-gated K^+ channels and cystic

fibrosis transmembrane conductance regulator (CFTR) Cl^- channel on the apical membrane as well as the Ae2 Cl^-/HCO_3^- exchanger on the basolateral membrane. Mutation in any of these genes limits the ability of parietal cells to secrete acid. Gastrin also exhibits trophic effects on ECL cells leading to hyperplasia of the ECL cell mass in hypergastrinemia. This phenomenon has clinical implications in patients taking H_2 blockers or PPIs long term, who develop hypergastrinemia as a consequence of loss of feedback inhibition of gastrin release as a result of relative achlorhydria. These patients may experience rebound acid hypersecretion when medications are withdrawn.

D Cells. Somatostatin is a broad inhibitor of multiple gastrointestinal hormones. It is transcribed as a 92-amino-acid peptide that undergoes cleavage to two major active forms, somatostatin-14 and somatostatin-28. In the stomach, somatostatin-14 is the major isoform and it inhibits acid secretion through direct inhibition of gastrin secretion from antral G cells, histamine from ECL cells, and acid from parietal cells. Somatostatin is produced by D cells, which are present in both oxyntic glands of the body and fundus and the pyloric glands. D cells possess intercalating cytoplasmic processes that are in close contact with target cells and facilitate the paracrine action of somatostatin on multiple mediators of gastric acid secretion.

The effect of somatostatin is mediated through somatostatin receptor 2 (SSTR-2), which is expressed in G cells, parietal cells, and ECL cells of the gastric mucosa. There is a complex crosstalk between somatostatin signaling and the gastrin-histamine axis. Somatostatin binding blunts histamine-stimulated translocation of the H^+/K^+ exchange ATPase to the apical membrane in parietal cells. Somatostatin also prevents gastrin-induced histamine release in ECL cells by the same G protein–inhibitory mechanism.

Somatostatin release is partly regulated by cholinergic (vagal) neurons. Ach inhibits somatostatin release, which disinhibits gastrin signaling and acid production. Histamine released by ECL cells also inhibits somatostatin release through a distinct receptor, the H3 receptor. Increased gastrin levels and low gastric pH exert a negative feedback effect that increases somatostatin levels and serves to blunt acid secretion. Finally, there is a baseline level of somatostatin secretion that exerts a tonic inhibition on gastric acid production in the resting state. However, there appear to be redundant pathways for baseline inhibition of gastric acid production because of the observation that knockout of somatostatin does not result in hypergastrinemia or acid hypersecretion. Instead there is a compensatory increase in galanin receptor 1 (GAL1) on gastric ECL cells that inhibits histamine release. Inhibition of Gal1 in conjunction with somatostatin knockout produces the expected hypergastrinemic/acid hypersecretory phenotype.

Ghrelin Cells. In the late 1970s, synthetic factors called growth hormone secretagogues (GHSs) were being produced based on the finding that they could stimulate the release of growth hormone from the pituitary by a distinctly different mechanism from the hypothalamic growth hormone–releasing hormone (GHRH). These GHSs work through a receptor (growth hormone secretagogue receptor [GHS-R]) and a Japanese research group first isolated the endogenous ligand for GHS-R from a rat stomach extract and named it *ghrelin*.[11] *Ghre* is the Proto-Indo-European root for "growth" and the suffix *rhelin* means "to release substances." Ghrelin is secreted by the X/A-like cells located in the mucosal layer of the gastric body, particularly in oxyntic glands. Ghrelin is a 28-amino-acid peptide with a unique octanoyl group on its serine-3 position that is important for its biologic activity, but it is found in other areas of the gastrointestinal tract as well as organs.[12] It is synthesized in two major forms by a process of alternative splicing. The active form undergoes acylation of serine-3 and is responsible for the majority of hormonal activity, whereas desacyl ghrelin comprises up to 90% of circulating ghrelin, but accounts for little of its biologic activity. The ghrelin receptor (GHS-R) is expressed in the hypothalamus and in nerve fibers of the ENS. Acylated ghrelin acts primarily via a central mechanism by increasing vagal tone—and, subsequently histamine release—thereby augmenting gastric acid production. However, ghrelin levels peak prior to meals and drop sharply in the postprandial period, indicating that ghrelin has a primary role in basal rather than inducible acid secretion. Ghrelin is also known to be a stimulant of gastric motility and the ghrelin peptide exhibits marked sequence homology with another gastrointestinal hormone, motilin, which is discussed in Gastric Motility, later in this chapter. Finally, ghrelin has been linked with the stimulation of appetite and feeding, as well as increased adiposity.

PROTECTIVE FACTORS OF THE GASTRIC MUCOSA

The acidic pH and proteolytic enzymes present in the gastric lumen combine to facilitate the breakdown of dietary proteins, enhance the absorption of nutrients such as iron and vitamin B_{12}, and minimize the threat posed by pathogenic microbes. This environment also poses a risk of damage to the gastric mucosa itself. Various protective factors are necessary to prevent injury to and breakdown of the gastric mucosa (Table 56.3).

Mucous cells located throughout the stomach provide a physical barrier between the luminal contents and the cells of the mucosa. Mucus consists of mucin glycoproteins, surface phospholipids, and water. Disulfide bonds crosslink adjacent mucin molecules and their oligosaccharides provide a viscoelastic structure that expands with hydration. The mucin layer is further stabilized by trefoil factors, which are small peptides that interact with the carbohydrate side chains. The hydrophobicity of the mucous layer can be attributed to phospholipids, and bicarbonate ions secreted at the base of the mucous layer provide an additional layer of protection from an injuriously low pH by neutralization.

Gastric mucosal blood flow is critical to mucosal health. Prostaglandins are important regulators of mucosal blood flow and crucial mediators of mucosal health. As an example, nonsteroidal antiinflammatory drugs cause altered prostaglandin synthesis and can lead to erosive gastritis and gastrointestinal bleeding. Prostaglandins are a family of long-chain fatty acid derivatives of arachidonic acid with vasoactive and neurohormonal properties. The mechanisms of prostaglandin-induced mucosal protection are varied and include enhancement of blood flow,

TABLE 56.3 Mucosal Protective Factors

	Function	Source
Blood flow	Buffering effect minimizes effect of luminal acid. Delivery of nutrients allows rapid turnover of epithelium.	—
Bicarbonate Mucus	Acid buffering Creates an "unstirred layer," a physical barrier between luminal contents and epithelium. Concentrates bicarbonate creating an alkaline layer.	Epithelial cells Surface and gland mucous cells
Prostaglandins (PGE_2, PGI_2)	Increase mucosal blood flow and reduce acid production locally.	COX-1- and COX-2- expressing epithelial cells
Neuropeptides (Bombesin)	Increase prostaglandin production (induce expression of COX-2)	Nonadrenergic, noncholinergic efferent neurons

COX, Cyclooxygenase.

prevention of gastric mucosal barrier disruption, stimulation of mucus secretion, and stimulation of nonparietal alkaline secretion.[13]

Neurohormonal peptides are also involved in gastric mucosal protection. There is a neural reflex arc involving autonomic sensory neurons and noncholinergic afferent neurons that secrete bombesin in response to noxious chemical stimuli such as capsaicin. Bombesin, in turn, mediates an increase in mucosal blood flow both directly and through stimulation of cyclooxygenase (COX), leading to increased production of prostaglandins.

PHASES OF DIGESTION

Gastric acid production is maintained at a low basal rate in the fasting state by the tonic inhibition of acid secretion by somatostatin from gastric D cells. Somatostatin acts in a paracrine manner on G cells in the antrum, along with ECL and parietal cells in the fundus and body of the stomach to suppress gastrin, histamine, and acid secretion. Gastric acid secretion as it relates to a meal occurs in three phases: cephalic, gastric, and the intestinal phase. Most gastric acid secretion occurs in the gastric phase.[10]

Prior to the ingestion of food, olfactory, gustatory, cephalic, and visual stimuli begin to increase gastric acid production and stimulate gastric motility.[14,15] Higher brain centers send information to the dorsal vagal complex in response to the premeal stimuli. Subsequently, vagal output activates enteric nerves to release GRP and Ach. GRP stimulates the antral G cells to release gastrin, which activates parietal and chief cells in an endocrine fashion. Ach inhibits somatostatin release from D cells resulting in disinhibition of gastrin, histamine, and acid release, as well as the direct stimulation of antral G cells and parietal cells.

Once feeding begins and the meal enters the gastric lumen, chemical and mechanical factors add to the continued vagal stimulation from the cephalic phase to promote continued gastric secretion. Luminal amino acids and short peptides, released from dietary protein by the action of pepsin from chief cells, activate receptors on G cells to release gastrin. Alcoholic beverages, coffee, and dietary calcium also activate gastrin release.[16] The stomach distends as it receives a meal (receptive relaxation) and stretch receptors active long and short reflex arcs that stimulate vagal nerves to release Ach to activate parietal cells directly, or release Ach to activate ECL cells to secrete histamine and GRP to activate G cells to secrete gastrin for indirect gastric acid secretion. Distention and the presence of luminal peptides produce continued gastric acid secretion and increased motility.[17,18]

Finally, in the intestinal phase, gastric acid secretion is returned to its basal level by several mechanisms. Decreased sensory stimuli and gastric distention following a meal lead to a tapering of the cephalic and gastric phase responses. The gastrin released during the cephalic and gastric phases exerts negative feedback through D cells in the antrum, which releases somatostatin leading to inhibition of gastrin release.[19] Food entering the duodenum leaves the gastric mucosa exposed to the full acidifying effect of parietal cell proton production leading to chemoreceptor activation and neural reflex release of calcitonin gene-related peptide (CGRP) near D cells to release somatostatin. This results in restoration of the tonic inhibition of somatostatin upon acid secretion and a return to basal acid production. The marked increase in gastric blood flow during this phase boosts gastric cell secretory function.

NEUROPHYSIOLOGY OF THE STOMACH

Parasympathetic and sympathetic reflex arcs are important modulators of gastric acid secretion and gastric motility. Additionally, parasympathetic afferent input from the stomach provides important information on gastric pH, secretion, and emptying along with visceral sensory input relating to nausea and satiety. Highlighting the importance of afferent signals from the stomach is the finding that 75% to 90% of vagal neurons are afferent fibers.[20] Nociceptive stimuli travel primarily through the sympathetic afferents. There does appear to be crossover with vagal parasympathetic afferents that may produce clinically confusing pain syndromes as a result of similar sensory pathways for the heart, esophagus, and stomach. This can lead to the mislabeling of upper gastrointestinal pathology such as gastritis or gastroesophageal reflux as anginal heart pain.[21]

Acetylcholine

Presynaptic vagal efferent neurons synapse with neurons of the myenteric and submucosal plexuses that, in turn, stimulate gastrin release from antral G cells, leading to increased acid secretion. Postsynaptic fibers also provide direct stimulation to parietal cells. Redundancy in this pathway makes pharmacologic suppression of acid secretion incomplete when targeting only one pathway, as with H_2 receptor blockers. Ach binds to the M3 muscarinic receptors located on G cells, parietal, and chief cells, causing activation of PLC and increases in intracellular calcium. M2 and M4 receptors located on D cells mediate the decreased somatostatin release seen with increased vagal tone.

Neuropeptides

The ENS is increasingly recognized as a complex and dynamic system. As mentioned earlier, there is a complex interaction between the ENS and the parasympathetic and sympathetic autonomic nervous systems. Although efferent signals are primarily conducted via the cholinergic neurotransmitter Ach, preganglionic afferents and postganglionic fibers of the ENS utilize a variety of peptide neurotransmitters including Ach, GRP, vasoactive intestinal polypeptide, pituitary adenylate cyclase-activating polypeptide, nitric oxide, substance P, and neuropeptide Y.[22] These substances may have direct effects on acid secretion as in the case of Ach on parietal cells or indirect effects through modulation of gastrin, histamine, or somatostatin release.[23] Many have important implications in gastric mucosal health and response to, and/or prevention of, mucosal injury.[24]

GASTRIC MOTILITY

The stomach has a salient role in initiating important events in digestion relating to its powerful secretory function but also because of its complex motility properties. The stomach is a great homogenizer and helps to mechanically break down food to small particles making digestion easier. It also serves as a reservoir with the ability for controlled release of food distally to the small intestine depending on the content and consistency of meals for ease of assimilation downstream. Approximately 200 kcal/h is released to the small intestines from the stomach. Finally, the stomach is able to move indigestible items in its lumen further along in the gastrointestinal tract. The migrating motor complex (MMC) is the term that describes this complex process.[16]

The proximal portion of the stomach, consisting of the cardia, fundus, and proximal body, serve as a reservoir, whereas the distal body and antrum mix gastric contents. The pylorus acts as a sphincter to control the rate at which ingested material exits the stomach and its relaxation is key for the proper functioning of the MMC. Smooth muscle in the different regions of the stomach determine the type of contractions that take place as part of the MMC, namely, phasic or tonic contractions. Phasic contractions occur in the distal stomach and are initiated and terminated in a matter of seconds. Tonic contractions, on the other hand, occur proximally in the stomach and last for several minutes at a time. Each type of contraction is important in the stomach carrying out its primary function in each region.

There are three major phases of gastric motility: fasting, accommodation, and postprandial. Fasting motility occurs between meals and is characterized by stereotypical movements that last about 100 minutes. This process is known as the MMC, where the stomach is able to do "housekeeping" and ensure that any indigestible materials do not remain in the stomach and potentially obstruct the lumen, causing pathologic conditions such as bezoars. Fasting motility consists of three phases: phase I, motor quiescence;

phase II, irregular contractility; and phase III, organized strong propulsive contractions occurring every 90 to 120 minutes and lasting 5 to 10 minutes.[25] A majority of propagated MMCs originate in the stomach, although areas of the small intestine may also serve as the pacemaker for phase III contractions.[26] The location of the initiation of MMCs (i.e., stomach vs duodenum and jejunum) affects the periodicity and duration of contractions, as well as the relative proportion of phase I, II, or III contractions that occur. MMCs originating in the stomach are more often phase III and are more likely to propagate distally than those originating in the small bowel.[27] There is a high degree of variability in the pattern of MMC activity between persons and even in the same individual at different times. Phase III contractions serve to propel air, digestive fluids, debris, and gut flora distally, thus preventing stasis and bacterial overgrowth that would occur otherwise.

During feeding, MMCs disappear and the stomach acts as a reservoir, although not in a passive capacity. Feeding is characterized by adaptive and receptive relaxation of gastric smooth muscle in the body and fundus, allowing expansion of the stomach to several times its resting volume with minimal increases in intragastric pressure. Adaptive relaxation involves a local reflex arc with activation of stretch receptors in the gastric wall in response to elevation of intragastric pressure. Mechanoreceptors relay impulses via afferent sensory neurons in the myenteric plexus that lead to release of nitric oxide and relaxation of smooth muscle fibers.[28] The adaptive relaxation reflex remains largely intact following proximal vagotomy and functions maximally at higher gastric volumes. Alternatively, receptive relaxation is triggered by passage of food through the gastroesophageal junction and is transmitted by cholinergic vagal efferent fibers originating in the nucleus of the solitary tract. Interruption of vagal innervation to the stomach as in proximal (truncal) vagotomy abolishes receptive relaxation and leads to decreased emptying time of liquids as a result of increased intragastric pressure during feeding.

Postprandial gastric motility serves to triturate and mix stomach contents and empty the meal in a manner that maximizes the digestive and absorptive capacity of the small intestine. Solids and liquids are handled differently by the stomach as reflected by distinct physiologic mechanisms and rates of emptying for each. Liquids tend to empty rapidly following the initiation of a meal, whereas solids experience a lag period where emptying is minimal for a period of time.[29] Human and animal studies have identified several important aspects of differential emptying of solids and liquids: gastric distention and activation of inhibitory and excitatory reflex arcs modulate intragastric pressure and rate of emptying of liquids[28]; antral propulsive and triturating contractions regulate the emptying of solids[29]; pyloric and fundal pressure affect emptying of solids by acting as a peristaltic pump and preventing the passage of large particles to the duodenum[30]; and the anatomic configuration of the stomach leads to sedimentation of solids in the dependent portion of the stomach, whereas liquids preferentially flow toward the pylorus leading to rapid emptying of liquids during the lag phase.

Neural Control

Gastric slow waves are rhythmic depolarizations of gastric smooth muscle that originate within interstitial cells of Cajal (ICC), "pacemakers" of gastrointestinal peristalsis, and propagate via action-potential-like and phase wave mechanisms that are dependent on intercellular calcium fluxes.[31] Slow waves propagate rapidly circumferentially and slowly along the longitudinal axis of the stomach, generating a propulsive wave that propagates in the oral-anal direction. Two distinct populations of ICC exist and reside within the myenteric plexus and the intramuscular plane. In general, ICCs in the myenteric plexus act as pacemakers, whereas ICCs in the intramuscular network are targets for neural input.

Vagal efferent fibers releasing CGRP are important inhibitors of gastric motility and are thought to be primary mediators of gastrointestinal ileus following abdominal operation, although they do not appear to influence gastrointestinal motility in the physiologic state.[32] A reflex arc involving sensory afferent neurons throughout the gastrointestinal tract, interacting with noncholinergic, nonadrenergic efferent neurons, produces the global hypomotility seen following manipulation of the stomach or intestine during surgery. These discoveries have important implications for the treatment of postoperative ileus, a major cause of prolonged hospitalization, increased costs, and morbidity following surgery.

Motilin

Motilin is a 22-amino-acid peptide synthesized by M cells of the proximal small intestine and is the principal stimulant of MMCs. It is a close homologue of another gastrointestinal peptide hormone, ghrelin, which is cosecreted along with motilin and exhibits 50% sequence homology.[33] Motilin plasma level peaks correspond closely to periods of high MMC activity and drop quickly following initiation of a meal when phase III contractions are abolished. Motilin acts in an endocrine fashion on both gastric smooth muscle and nerves of the myenteric plexus through binding with the motilin receptor GPR 38, a G protein–coupled receptor.[34,35] Macrolide antibiotics such as erythromycin act as motilin receptor agonists resulting in the promotility qualities that are employed in patients with delayed gastric emptying.

Ghrelin

As mentioned earlier, ghrelin is a closely related peptide hormone secreted by X/A-like cells of the oxyntic gland of the stomach.[36] Despite their close relation, ghrelin acts at a separate receptor from motilin and there is no evidence that the two receptors exhibit cross reactivity to the two ligands. Ghrelin's role in regulating gastrointestinal motility is not completely understood but evolving, and evidence exists for promotility actions similar to motilin.

ACKNOWLEDGMENTS

The authors would like to acknowledge Jonathan C. King and O. Joe Hines for their contributions to the previous edition's chapter.

REFERENCES

1. Skandalakis LJ, Colborn GL, Weidman TA, Kingsnorth AN, Skandalakis JE, Skandalakis PN. Stomach. In: Skandalakis JE, Colburn GL, Weidman TA, et al., eds. *Skandalakis' Surgical Anatomy*. New York: McGraw-Hill; 2004 [chapter 15].
2. Furness JB, Costa M. Types of nerves in the enteric nervous system. *Neuroscience*. 1980;5(1):1-20.
3. Scharoun SL, Barone FC, Wayner MJ, Jones SM. Vagal and gastric connections to the central nervous system determined by the transport of horseradish peroxidase. *Brain Res Bull*. 1984;13(4):573-583.
4. Barrett KE. Gastric secretion. In: *Gastrointestinal Physiology*. 2nd ed. New York: McGraw-Hill; 2014 [chapter 3].
5. Huang Q. Controversies of cardiac glands in the proximal stomach: a critical review. *J Gastroenterol Hepatol*. 2011;26(3):450-455.
6. Mescher AL. Digestive tract. In: *Junqueira's Basic Histology*. 14th ed. New York: McGraw-Hill; 2016.
7. Kaufhold MA, Krabbenhoft A, Song P, et al. Localization, trafficking, and significance for acid secretion of parietal cell Kir4.1 and KCNQ1 K^+ channels. *Gastroenterology*. 2008;134(4):1058-1069.
8. Heitzmann D, Warth R. No potassium, no acid: K^+ channels and gastric acid secretion. *Physiology (Bethesda)*. 2007;22:335-341.
9. Tutunji MF, Qaisi AM, El-Eswed BI, Tutunji LF. Reactions of sulfenic acid with 2-mercaptoethanol: a mechanism for the inhibition of gastric (H^+-K^+)-adenosine triphosphate by omeprazole. *J Pharm Sci*. 2007;96(1):196-208.
10. Di Mario F, Goni E. Gastric acid secretion: changes during a century. *Best Pract Res Clin Gastroenterol*. 2014;28(6):953-965.
11. Kojima M, Hosoda H, Date Y, Nakazato M, Matsuo H, Kangawa K. Ghrelin is a growth-hormone-releasing acylated peptide from stomach. *Nature*. 1999;402(6762):656-660.
12. Wang G, Lee HM, Englander E, Greeley GH Jr. Ghrelin—not just another stomach hormone. *Regul Pept*. 2002;105(2):75-81.
13. Miller TA. Protective effects of prostaglandins against gastric mucosal damage: current knowledge and proposed mechanisms. *Am J Physiol*. 1983;245(5 Pt 1):G601-G623.
14. Rogers J, Raimundo AH, Misiewicz JJ. Cephalic phase of colonic pressure response to food. *Gut*. 1993;34(4):537-543.
15. Katschinski M. Nutritional implications of cephalic phase gastrointestinal responses. *Appetite*. 2000;34(2):189-196.
16. Barrett KE. Gastric motility. In: *Gastrointestinal Physiology*. 2nd ed. New York: McGraw-Hill; 2014 [chapter 8].
17. Schiller LR, Walsh JH, Feldman M. Distention-induced gastrin release: effects of luminal acidification and intravenous atropine. *Gastroenterology*. 1980;78(5 Pt 1):912-917.
18. Yeo CJ, Bastidas JA, Schmieg RE Jr, Zinner MJ. Meal-stimulated absorption of water and electrolytes in canine jejunum. *Am J Physiol*. 1990;259(3 Pt 1):G402-G409.
19. Meshkinpour H, Dinoso VP Jr, Lorber SH. Effect of intraduodenal administration of essential amino acids and sodium oleate on motor activity of the sigmoid colon. *Gastroenterology*. 1974;66(3):373-377.
20. Berthoud HR, Neuhuber WL. Functional and chemical anatomy of the afferent vagal system. *Auton Neurosci*. 2000;85(1-3):1-17.
21. Qin C, Chandler MJ, Miller KE, Foreman RD. Responses and afferent pathways of C(1)-C(2) spinal neurons to gastric distension in rats. *Auton Neurosci*. 2003;104(2):128-136.
22. Smith VC, Dhatt N, Buchan AM. The innervation of the human antro-pyloric region: organization and composition. *Can J Physiol Pharmacol*. 2001;79(11):905-918.
23. Schubert ML, Peura DA. Control of gastric acid secretion in health and disease. *Gastroenterology*. 2008;134(7):1842-1860.
24. Gyires K. Neuropeptides and gastric mucosal homeostasis. *Curr Top Med Chem*. 2004;4(1):63-73.
25. Szurszewski JH. A migrating electric complex of canine small intestine. *Am J Physiol*. 1969;217(6):1757-1763.
26. Dooley CP, Di Lorenzo C, Valenzuela JE. Variability of migrating motor complex in humans. *Dig Dis Sci*. 1992;37(5):723-728.
27. Luiking YC, van der Reijden AC, van Berge Henegouwen GP, Akkermans LM. Migrating motor complex cycle duration is determined by gastric or duodenal origin of phase III. *Am J Physiol*. 1998;275(6 Pt 1):G1246-G1251.
28. Desai KM, Sessa WC, Vane JR. Involvement of nitric oxide in the reflex relaxation of the stomach to accommodate food or fluid. *Nature*. 1991;351(6326):477-479.
29. Camilleri M, Malagelada JR, Brown ML, Becker G, Zinsmeister AR. Relation between antral motility and gastric emptying of solids and liquids in humans. *Am J Physiol*. 1985;249(5 Pt 1):G580-G585.
30. Haba T, Sarna SK. Regulation of gastroduodenal emptying of solids by gastropyloroduodenal contractions. *Am J Physiol*. 1993;264(2 Pt 1):G261-G271.
31. van Helden DF, Laver DR, Holdsworth J, Imtiaz MS. Generation and propagation of gastric slow waves. *Clin Exp Pharmacol Physiol*. 2010;37(4):516-524.
32. Plourde V, Wong HC, Walsh JH, Raybould HE, Tache Y. CGRP antagonists and capsaicin on celiac ganglia partly prevent postoperative gastric ileus. *Peptides*. 1993;14(6):1225-1229.
33. Poitras P, Peeters TL. Motilin. *Curr Opin Endocrinol Diabetes Obes*. 2008;15(1):54-57.
34. Takeshita E, Matsuura B, Dong M, Miller LJ, Matsui H, Onji M. Molecular characterization and distribution of motilin family receptors in the human gastrointestinal tract. *J Gastroenterol*. 2006;41(3):223-230.
35. Xu L, Depoortere I, Tomasetto C, et al. Evidence for the presence of motilin, ghrelin, and the motilin and ghrelin receptor in neurons of the myenteric plexus. *Regul Pept*. 2005;124(1-3):119-125.
36. De Vriese C, Delporte C. Ghrelin: a new peptide regulating growth hormone release and food intake. *Int J Biochem Cell Biol*. 2008;40(8):1420-1424.

Diagnostic and Therapeutic Endoscopy of the Stomach and Small Bowel

Chao Li | James Ellsmere

Endoscopy is the gold standard for providing visual access to the endoluminal space of the gastrointestinal (GI) tract for diagnostic and therapeutic purposes. As a diagnostic tool, it allows for direct visualization of the mucosal surface and permits the identification of abnormalities including mucosal changes, polyps, strictures, and external compression. As a therapeutic tool, the included instrument channel allows passage for instruments that can sample mucosa for pathologic examination, treat bleeding, dilate strictures, and access other organ pathologies through the wall of the GI tract. Upper GI endoscopy allows for examination of the esophagus, stomach, and proximal duodenum down to the ligament of Treitz. The small bowel between the ligament of Treitz and the ileocecal valve is more difficult to access although techniques such as video capsule endoscopy and balloon endoscopy have expanded the roles of endoscopic evaluation and therapy. Endoscopy is a growing domain and a majority of GI pathology either involves the mucosa directly or can be identified indirectly from within the lumen of the GI tract.

INDICATIONS AND CONTRAINDICATIONS

General indications for endoscopy include persistent upper abdominal symptoms despite appropriate medical therapy or have associated worrisome symptoms such as vomiting, weight loss, anorexia, dysphagia, and odynophagia. Other indications include chronic or iron-deficiency anemia without a source on colonoscopy, evaluation of suspicious radiographic abnormalities, or surveillance for premalignant lesions or conditions such as familial adenomatous polyposis. Indications for therapy include tissue sampling and excision, treatment of acute upper GI bleeding (UGIB), foreign body retrieval, dilation or stenting of strictures or leaks, and placement of feeding tubes.[1]

Relative contraindications for endoscopy under conscious sedation include inability to tolerate the procedure or sedation, inadequate patient cooperation, and suspicion of perforated viscus. It is possible to perform endoscopy in these cases under general anesthesia, although the risks and benefits must be weighed carefully and that the potential result of the endoscopy should change future management. Endoscopy in patients with a suspicion of perforation is best done with carbon dioxide insufflation and the ability to quickly decompress pneumoperitoneum surgically if required. Surgical anastomoses are considered safe to be evaluated endoscopically. Patients with recent myocardial infarction, stroke, or pneumonia should be assessed independently for risk of worsening their existing comorbidity. Coagulopathy or inhibition of platelet aggregation is a relative contraindication for therapeutic procedures.

EQUIPMENT

ENDOSCOPY TOWER

An endoscopy tower is used to concentrate and organize the equipment needed to perform endoscopy within a compact and portable unit. It generally includes a digital video processor, which allows connection of the endoscope electronics to provide signal-to-video and post-processing capabilities. It should also allow capture and saving of still pictures and video for documentation purposes. A light source is also important, interfacing with the light-guide cables of the scope to provide illumination that travels to the tip of the endoscope. Finally, a video monitor provides a display capability that allows the endoscopist and assistant(s) to directly visualize the magnified picture produced by the camera at the tip of the scope.

Most common optional equipment includes a foot pedal–activated auxiliary water pump, which allows the production of a water jet for lavage through the auxiliary water channel. A radiofrequency generator or other source of energy is usually also bundled, allowing the delivery of monopolar cautery and bipolar/thermal energy. Finally, an accessory insufflator can be used to allow luminal distention with carbon dioxide.

ENDOSCOPE

The modern endoscope includes an objective lens and a charge-coupled device (CCD) camera at the tip. A light-guide system enables transmission of illumination from the light source. Cables allow for angulation and deflection of the instrument tip. The endoscope also supplies channels for insufflation and optionally an auxiliary water channel. Importantly, there is also an instrument channel through which therapeutic modalities can be delivered (Fig. 57.1). The size of the instrument channel can vary from scope to scope, with diagnostic scopes having smaller channels and therapeutic scopes with larger or even double channels. Mini-scopes also exist to facilitate passage through tight strictures. Moreover, the objective and instrument channels can be placed at the tip of the instrument (end viewing) or to the side of the instrument (side viewing), which are adapted to visualization of specific regions of the GI tract.

PREPARATION

Prior to endoscopy, an assessment of general medical condition, medication allergies, the patient's ability to

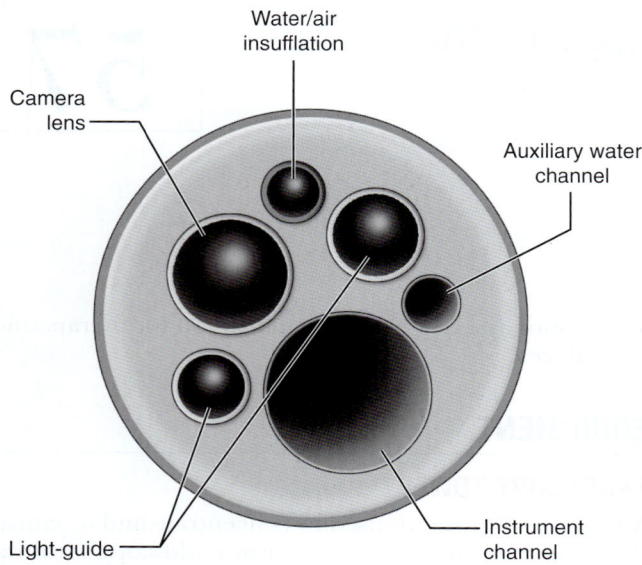

FIGURE 57.1 Example layout of the distal end of the endoscope.

tolerate the procedure, and prior reactions to sedation should be undertaken. Prior airway issues should be explored. In case of therapeutic intervention, an up-to-date coagulation panel and platelet count should be checked to ensure it is within safe ranges. If fluoroscopy is considered, pregnancy testing should be considered for women of childbearing age. Informed consent should be taken detailing the risks and benefits of the procedure.

For routine upper GI endoscopy, the last oral intake of solids should be 6 hours and clear liquids 2 hours prior to intervention.[2] This helps prevent regurgitation and aspiration and improves endoscopic visualization. In cases of known gastroparesis or obstruction, a longer fasting period or the prior insertion of a nasogastric tube to empty the stomach may be appropriate. In GI bleeding, lavage may be performed through a nasogastric tube both as a diagnostic tool and to help clear clots and blood, thereby improving visualization.

SEDATION

Typically, patients are first anesthetized using a topical solution of local anesthetic spray or gargle, to decrease the gag reflex. Removable partial and complete dentures are removed. Adequate monitoring must be maintained throughout the procedure for safety of conscious sedation. It includes the use of pulse oximetry, a blood pressure cuff, and visual cues of respiratory rate and effort. Certain patients with knowledge of the procedure and low anxiety may be able to tolerate an unsedated short diagnostic procedure.

For the majority of patients, the procedure is more comfortable with conscious sedation. Sedation protocols usually include a combination of a short-acting narcotic with a benzodiazepine delivered intravenously (e.g., a combination of fentanyl and midazolam), with a dose titrated to previous history of sedation, gender, and age.[3] For older patients, it is recommended to start with a lower dose and to supplement sedation as required. Adjunctive

sedation medication such as promethazine can also be given as supplementation. Sedation can also be achieved with intravenous propofol. Propofol has a quick onset and emergence, but requires a dedicated anesthesiologist or trained practitioner to titrate the drug as required. Patients who are oversedated with slow breathing and dropping oxygen saturation can often be incited to take additional deep breaths with coaching. Furthermore, reversal agents for both classes of agents, flumazenil for benzodiazepines and naloxone for narcotics, should be ready at all times if required.

TECHNIQUE

The patient is placed in the left lateral decubitus position. A bite block is placed to protect the teeth and to allow easy gliding of the endoscope with limited impedance. The endoscope is initially passed along, following the surface of the tongue and curved to view the epiglottis. Passing under the epiglottis allows visualization of the vocal cords. It is important to inspect the vocal cords to rule out any lesions, polyps, cord paresis, or reflux laryngitis. Passing the scope under and to the side of the arytenoid cartilages, the endoscope is then advanced back toward the midline with gentle pressure and air insufflation. It is important not to forcefully advance the endoscope blindly in this location, especially in older patients. The presence of a pulsion (Zenker) diverticulum or cervical osteophytes may impede the passage of the scope. Asking the patient to swallow with a flexed neck position, or performing a jaw-thrust can help pass the endoscope beyond the upper esophageal sphincter.

The mucosa of a healthy esophagus is glistening white, representing the squamous epithelium. The esophagus is usually straight, narrow, devoid of remnant liquid or solid particles, and shows active peristalsis. It can, however, become tortuous in older patients. In achalasia, the esophagus may become dilated and even sigmoid shaped. There can be presence of mid and lower esophageal diverticula. Further information about the endoscopy of the esophagus can be found in Chapter 7. The gastroesophageal junction is found approximately 40 cm from the incisors. Passing the lower esophageal sphincter signals a change from the squamous epithelium of the esophagus to the columnar epithelium of the stomach. This transition is identified with a change in color from glistening white to a pinkish-brown. The body and fundus of the stomach also display rugae, a series of ridges and folds along the internal surface of the stomach. The stomach can be distended to flatten the rugae at this juncture to allow for complete inspection of its mucosal surface.

Upon entering the stomach, it is important to note whether there is any liquid or solid food particles present, especially in the fundus situated to the left side of the field of view. A large, distended stomach may signify a downstream obstruction or poor emptying. It is wise to use the suction channel of the scope to aspirate as much of the liquid contents in the fundic pool of the stomach as possible before proceeding further, especially if there is higher risk of regurgitation and aspiration. Pushing the endoscope forward with a slight clockwise rotation places it along the greater curve of the stomach. As the endoscope is advanced into the antrum, the rugae disappear and the color of the mucosa turns to a lighter pink. The pylorus is usually in view at this point. Continued advancement of the endoscope in the long position through the pyloric channel is possible with proper alignment and gentle pressure.

Once the pylorus is passed, the scope falls into the duodenal bulb. It is important to obtain adequate circumferential examination of the first part of the duodenum at this point in the long position because the short position achieved on withdrawing later is unstable in the first portion of the duodenum because the endoscope will have a tendency to fall back into the stomach. To pass from the first part to the second part, the endoscope tip is flexed upward and given a gentle clockwise turn, revealing the second part of the duodenum. Further advancement into the second part is possible by transitioning from a long, greater curve position to a short, lesser curve position (Fig. 57.2). This is accomplished by pulling the endoscope back, which reduces the gastric loop, and paradoxically advances the scope to the second and third parts of the duodenum. Examination of the ampulla can be difficult with a straight viewing scope because it is situated on the medial curve of the second part of the duodenum. This area can sometimes be seen on the right-hand side as the endoscope is pulled back in the short position. A side viewing scope allows an en face position toward the ampullary complex and is the best method for obtaining visualization and access to ampulla.

Once the duodenum is thoroughly examined, it is possible to pull back into the stomach and perform retroflexion, flexing the scope such that it looks back onto itself. This allows visualization of the incisura, which is the most often overlooked area of the stomach. Pulling back and rotating the endoscope in the retroflexed position will then show the cardia and hiatus of the stomach, allowing identification of hiatal hernias and lesions in the proximal stomach. It is essential to suction any remaining fluid in the fundus to prevent aspiration and to ensure there is no hidden pathology behind fluid pools. Once the examination of the stomach is complete, the distended stomach is suctioned to decrease discomfort and the scope is pulled back into the esophagus.

GASTRIC PATHOLOGY

The most common variety of benign gastric pathology is inflammatory disease. Acute inflammation of the stomach, otherwise termed gastritis, can be caused by a variety of inciting factors.[4] Nonatrophic gastritis is usually caused by *Helicobacter pylori* infection and presents as inflammation that predominantly affects the antrum of the stomach. Chronic *H. pylori* infection can also cause a multifocal atrophic gastritis with patchy atrophy and metaplasia beginning at the incisura and the transitional zone between antrum and body and affecting predominantly the antrum.[5] Atrophic gastritis due to pernicious anemia is of autoimmune origin and results in the destruction of parietal cell mass (Fig. 57.3). This usually affects the body of the stomach with relative sparing of the antrum. Patients with atrophic gastritis are considered at higher risk for gastric adenocarcinoma. A chemical gastritis can also occur where

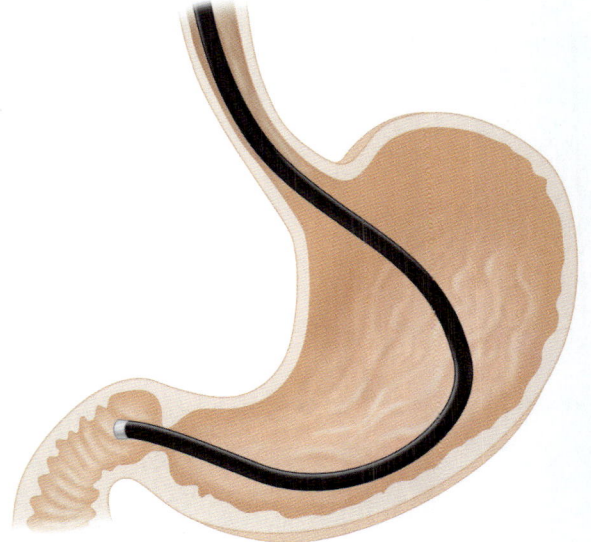

Long position

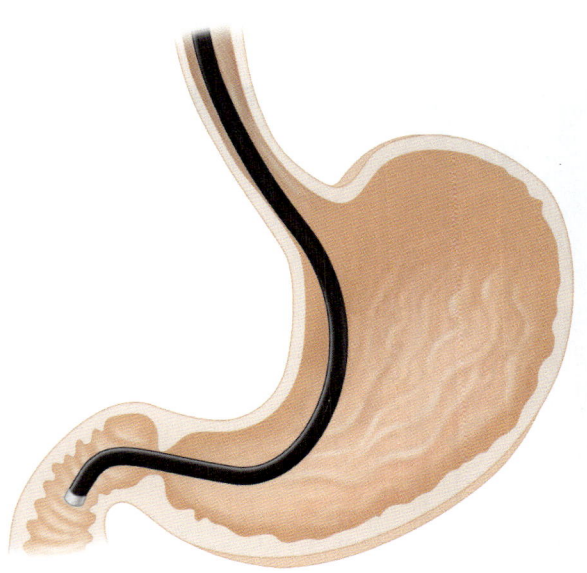

Short position

FIGURE 57.2 Initial entry past the pylorus is made in the long or greater curve position. Pulling back on the endoscope after passing the duodenal cap paradoxically advances the endoscope to the short or lesser curve position.

irritation results from nonsteroidal antiinflammatory drugs (NSAIDs), bile reflux, or alcohol.

Peptic ulcer disease may also result from *H. pylori* infection. An ulcer is an erosive defect in the wall of the stomach or duodenum mucosa, exposing the underlying submucosa or muscularis. Ulcers can be identified in the antrum, body, or fundus of the stomach and the first to second portions of the duodenum (Fig. 57.4). Gastric ulcers should be biopsied when encountered

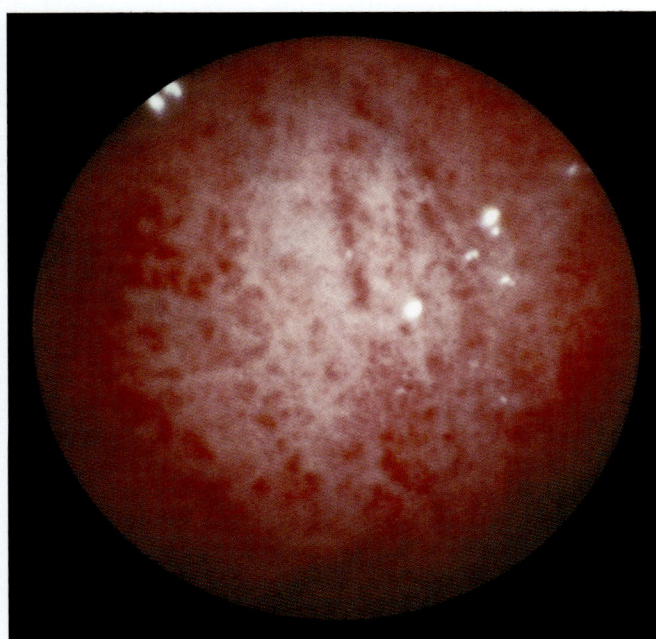

FIGURE 57.3 Diffuse gastritis in the body of the stomach. Testing for *Helicobacter pylori* must always be done in this situation.

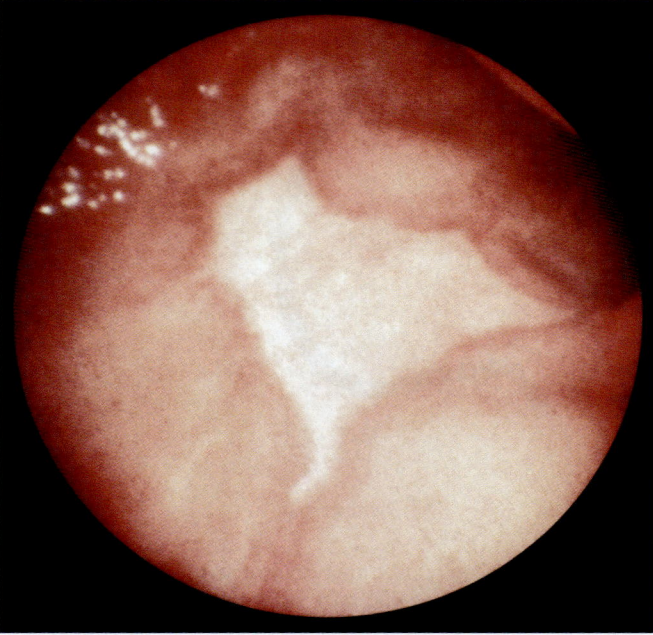

FIGURE 57.4 Large benign gastric ulcer seen on the greater curvature of the stomach.

endoscopically due to their risk of malignancy. Features suspicious for malignancy include an associated mass, irregular or heaped edges, a deep ulcerated base, or diffusely irregular adjacent mucosal folds. Repeat endoscopy and rebiopsy is warranted despite a benign initial biopsy if any visual features were suspicious for malignancy or if the patient remains symptomatic. If the ulcer is refractory and fails to heal despite appropriate medical

treatment, surveillance endoscopy should be continued until healing of the ulcer is documented. Persistent nonhealing gastric ulcers should be considered for surgical excision. Up to 80% of duodenal ulcers are associated with concurrent infection with *H. pylori* infection. These ulcers do not require sampling because they are overwhelmingly benign.

Endoscopic testing for *H. pylori* involves biopsy of the antrum and body of the stomach for identification of organisms on histology, polymerase chain reaction, or rapid urease test. Culture and sensitivity can also be obtained for resistant strains. Other nonendoscopic options for *H. pylori* testing include the carbon urea breath test, serologic antibody tests, and fecal antigen test. *H. pylori* has been implicated in the pathogenesis of gastritis, gastric and duodenal ulcers, gastric adenocarcinoma, and gastric mucosa-associated lymphoid tissue (MALT) lymphoma. As such, when it is identified, it should be eradicated with pharmacotherapy and its eradication should be documented with repeat testing.[6]

Vascular abnormalities may also be identified and treated on upper endoscopy. Gastric varices are similar to, and may be present with or independently from, esophageal varices. They are usually located in the fundal area of the stomach. Presence of both esophageal and gastric varices usually implies portal hypertension, whereas isolated gastric varices are often caused by splenic venous hypertension alone. This is often due to splenic vein thrombosis associated with pancreatitis or pancreatic malignancy. Varices appear as serpentine dilated submucosal veins that cross over existing gastric rugae and are easily compressible with the tip of a blunt endoscopic instrument. Incidentally found nonbleeding gastric varices do not require prophylactic endoscopic therapy.

A Dieulafoy lesion is a single ectatic submucosal arteriole that erodes through the mucosa and becomes exposed. These lesions can be present anywhere in the GI tract but are most commonly seen in the proximal stomach along the lesser curvature. They often come to attention due to massive UGIB and can be difficult to identify when not actively bleeding. Angiodysplasia are dilated vessels that develop in association with systemic diseases such as renal failure, heart failure, and cirrhosis. They appear as reddish discolorations with surrounding small tortuous vessels and are usually multiple and multicentric. A subset of angiodysplasia, gastric antral vascular ectasia (GAVE) or watermelon stomach, refers to the presence of vascular ectasia in a linear fashion in the antrum of the stomach.[7] This gives the antrum a striped appearance similar to that of a watermelon (Fig. 57.5). Vascular abnormalities are a significant cause of acute or chronic GI blood loss.

Hiatal hernias are herniations of the stomach above the diaphragmatic hiatus. These can be seen in the forward position and in the retroflexed view. Hiatal hernias can be associated with gastroesophageal reflux disease and dysphagia, but are often asymptomatic when incidentally found (Fig. 57.6). Cameron lesions, linear erosions found near or at the level where the herniated stomach meets the diaphragmatic hiatus, are caused by mechanical trauma from constriction of the diaphragm and may represent a source for blood loss. Paraesophageal hernias represent herniations of the gastric fundus through the hiatus beside

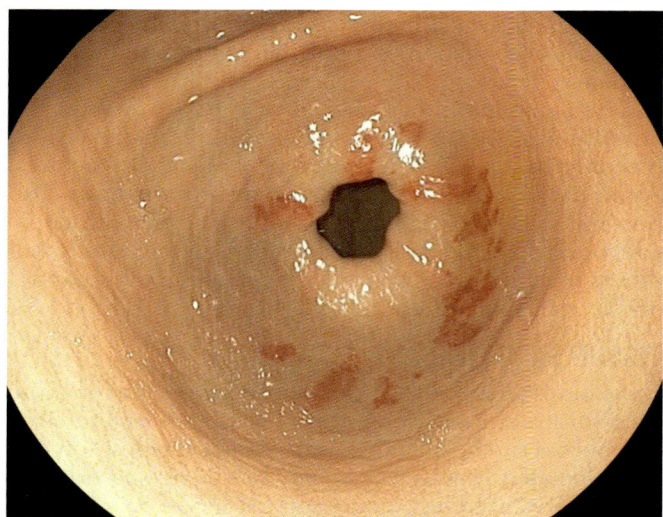

FIGURE 57.5 Mild gastric antral vascular ectasia.

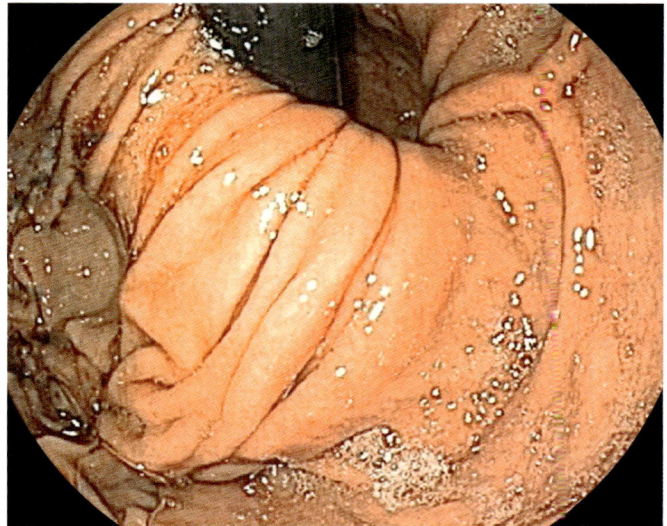

FIGURE 57.6 Full retroflex view of the gastroesophageal junction showing a hiatal hernia.

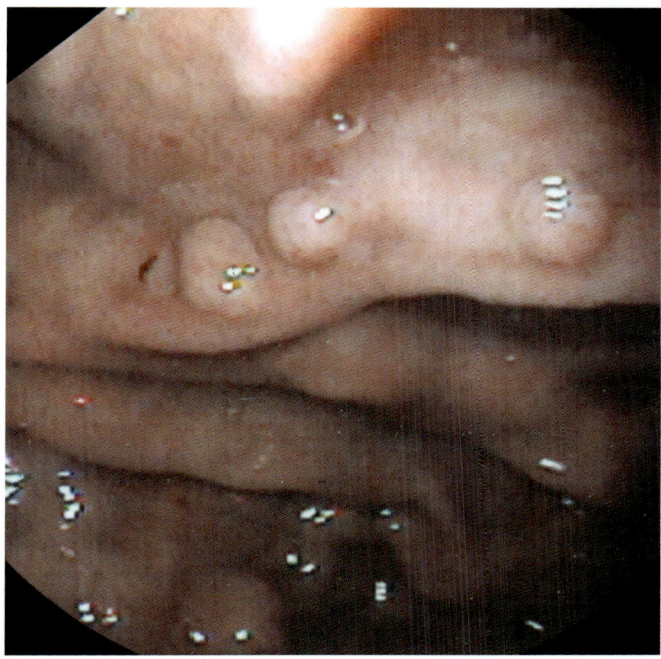

FIGURE 57.7 Multiple fundic gland polyps seen in the proximal part of the stomach.

the esophagus. The position of the squamocolumnar junction and diaphragmatic hiatus can be measured from the incisors and used to size the herniated stomach. Symptomatic hiatal and paraesophageal hernias may be considered for surgical repair. Other rare congenital lesions include antral webs that mimic the appearance of the pylorus but occur in the more proximal part of the antrum. Congenital pyloric stenosis usually presents in childhood, but can also be identified in adults. Pancreatic rests, typically found in the antrum or duodenum, appear as a 5- to 10-mm raised donut-shaped lesion with a punctate center and are benign.

Polypoid lesions of the stomach can be classified as benign, potentially malignant, and malignant. By order of prevalence, these include fundic gland polyps, hyperplastic polyps, adenomatous polyps, and malignancies.[8] The most common type of gastric polyp is the fundic gland polyp, which are usually numerous, sessile polyps found in the fundus of the stomach (Fig. 57.7). They do not have a stalk, have the same color as the gastric mucosa, and may show glandular hyperplasia. Fundic gland polyps can develop in the context of familial adenomatous polyposis, Zollinger-Ellison syndrome, or chronic proton pump inhibitor use, and though they may show signs of metaplasia, they are not considered premalignant.[9] Hyperplastic polyps are caused by inflammation and can grow extremely large. They typically have a reddish appearance and are more common in the antrum of the stomach. They are often associated with inflammation of the surrounding mucosa. Hyperplastic polyps are not classically considered malignant, but they often arise in the context of metaplastic chronic gastritis and may contain metaplasia or dysplasia.[10] Polyps greater than 1 cm and with pedunculated morphology have been associated with dysplasia. Biopsy or excision of hyperplastic polyps often results in bleeding. Adenomatous polyps are relatively rare but should be endoscopically removed when possible. Adenomatous polyps can also be found in the duodenum in the periampullary region, especially seen in patients with familial adenomatous polyposis (Fig. 57.8).

Gastric adenocarcinoma is the most common form of gastric malignancy and can take on various endoscopic appearances. It may present as an exophytic mass lesion, a nonhealing gastric ulcer, or an infiltrative process in the submucosa termed linitis plastica. Diagnosis is made with multiple mucosal biopsies. Once diagnosis is made, further staging and management is discussed in Chapter 61. Leiomyomas and gastrointestinal stromal tumors (GISTs) are the most common mesenchymal tumor of the stomach. They are rounded submucosal lesions that can present anywhere in the stomach but most commonly

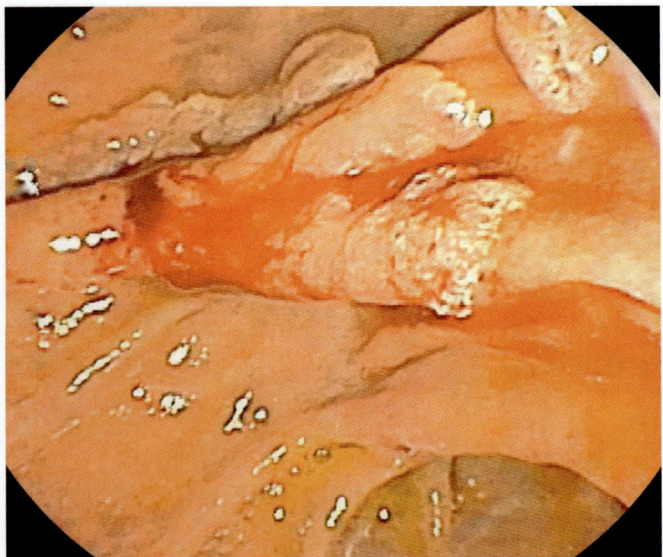

FIGURE 57.8 A large sessile duodenal periampullary polyp. The ampulla is visible to the right of the polyp.

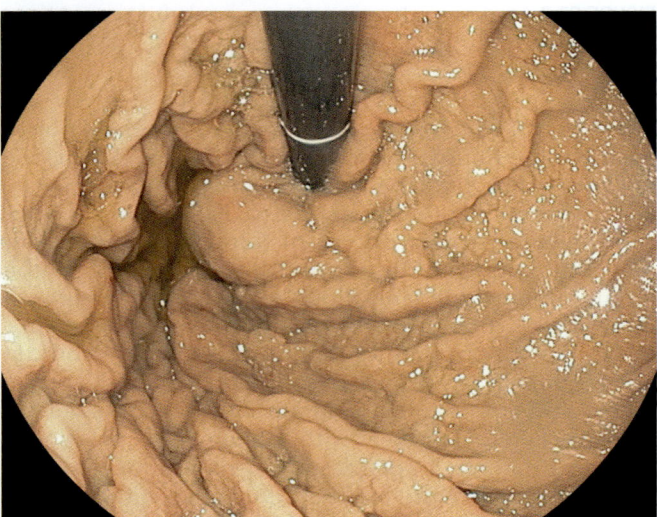

FIGURE 57.9 Full retroflex view of the gastroesophageal junction showing a small submucosal tumor at the angle of His.

found in the cardia or fundus adjacent to the gastroesophageal junction (Fig. 57.9). Malignant potential is determined by the size, irregular borders, and mitotic index. Due to their submucosal location, tissue may be difficult to obtain without an endoscopic ultrasound assessment and core biopsy.[11]

THERAPEUTIC ENDOSCOPY

Although the endoscope itself is a purely diagnostic instrument, it is possible to pass a variety of small instruments through the scope in the included instrument channel. Larger instruments are also available, with most of these needing to be loaded as a cap on the end of the scope or beside the scope. Therapeutic endoscopy consists of combining the use of these instruments with endoscopic guidance, and sometimes supplemented with fluoroscopic guidance.

The most common therapeutic interventions in the endoluminal space are tissue sampling and excision, bleeding control, and dilatation or stenting of strictures. Some transluminal therapeutic interventions have also become standard, including percutaneous endoscopic gastrostomy (PEG) and endoscopic cystogastrostomy, but others remain in the experimental phase, notably natural orifice transluminal endoscopic surgery (NOTES).

TISSUE SAMPLING AND EXCISION

Basic biopsy methods for upper endoscopy mirror those used for lower endoscopy. Superficial biopsies limited to the mucosa can be obtained using standard biopsy forceps. Pedunculated lesions can be excised using snare polypectomy. Advanced techniques such as endoscopic mucosal resection (EMR) and endoscopic submucosal dissection (ESD) allow for the excision of larger lesions in a piecemeal or en bloc fashion at a deeper submucosal plane.

Standard biopsy forceps are an excellent and easy-to-use tool for obtaining tissue. For example, forceps can be used for obtaining random specimen to rule out celiac disease in the duodenum or *H. pylori* organisms in the stomach. They can also be used to obtain partial samples from larger lesions or complete samples of very small lesions. The most common model of biopsy forceps today is the double-bite model. These forceps feature two closable metal cups and a central needle spike. The central spike provides deeper purchase by impaling the tissue to be biopsied. It also allows for this type of biopsy forceps to hold up to two bites at a time. Other models include jumbo biopsy forceps, which have a larger capacity and require a larger instrument channel. The increased surface area of the metal cups allows collection of a specimen 2 to 3 times larger than with standard biopsy forceps.

For polypoid lesions, the instrument of choice is a polypectomy snare. Snare polypectomy can also be performed for larger sessile lesions, and is an integral step in EMR. The standard snare is a wire loop device that can be slipped over the lesion to be excised. Closure of the wire over the lesion allows cutting of the lesion. For larger lesions or lesions at risk for bleeding, cutting through can be facilitated by the passage of monopolar energy from a radiofrequency generator through the snare, thereby decreasing the risk of bleeding. For smaller lesions or lesions at low risk for bleeding, closure of the snare without cautery allows for less architectural distortion and a better pathology specimen. Snares come in various sizes, oval or hexagonal shapes, and braided or unbraided wires. A hexagonal snare keeps its shape and stays open better than the standard snare. A braided wire allows for increased drag and friction, thereby improving tissue purchase.

EMR is a technique used to obtain deeper and larger biopsies of benign masses as well as for the staging and treatment of premalignant and superficial malignant lesions. There are two techniques for performing EMR. The first method, well adapted to sessile lesions, is a saline lift EMR (Fig. 57.10). A needle injector is used to instill saline or a starch based volume-expander mixed with blue dye into the submucosal space, under and around the

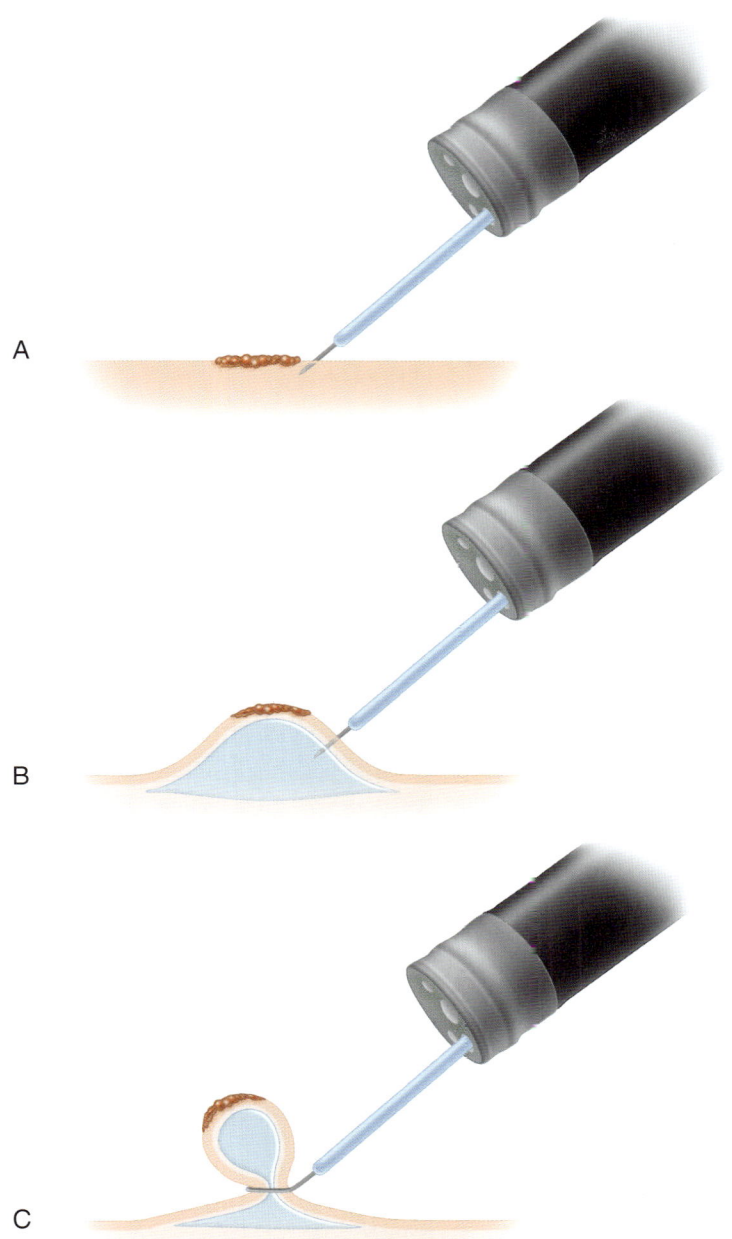

FIGURE 57.10 Steps of a saline-lift endoscopic mucosal resection. (A) A needle injector is positioned under the lesion. (B) Saline mixed with blue dye is injected to lift the lesion. (C) A polypectomy snare is used to excise the lifted lesion.

lesion, thereby lifting it. Failure of the saline lift is a worrisome sign of deeper invasion of the lesion. The lifted lesion can then be excised using a snare in standard fashion. The second method is EMR with a cap-and-snare technique, which allows for the excision down into the submucosa and enables accurate examination of the depth of invasion of malignant lesions (Fig. 57.11). The distal end of the endoscope is fitted with a cap that is preloaded with elastic bands, similar to a variceal bander. The tissue to be excised is centered and suctioned into the cap until it fills the cap completely. The band is then fired over the suctioned tissue, trapping the tissue into a pseudopolyp. A polypectomy snare is then used to remove the trapped lesion at its "stalk," at or above the level of the elastic

band. EMR can be considered curative for malignant lesions that are completely excised with negative margins, are limited to the mucosa (T1a), are well-differentiated, and do not have lymphovascular invasion.[12] Risks associated with EMR include bleeding, perforation, and stricturing. Post-EMR, patients are typically placed on proton pump inhibitors until reassessment of the EMR site at repeat endoscopy confirms appropriate healing (Fig. 57.12).

Larger lesions that are beyond the size of the EMR cap-and-band device can be removed by ESD. In this technique, the margins of the tumor are marked with cautery. A lift is then performed in the submucosal space with a starch-based volume expander mixed with blue dye. An incision along the premarked margin is made

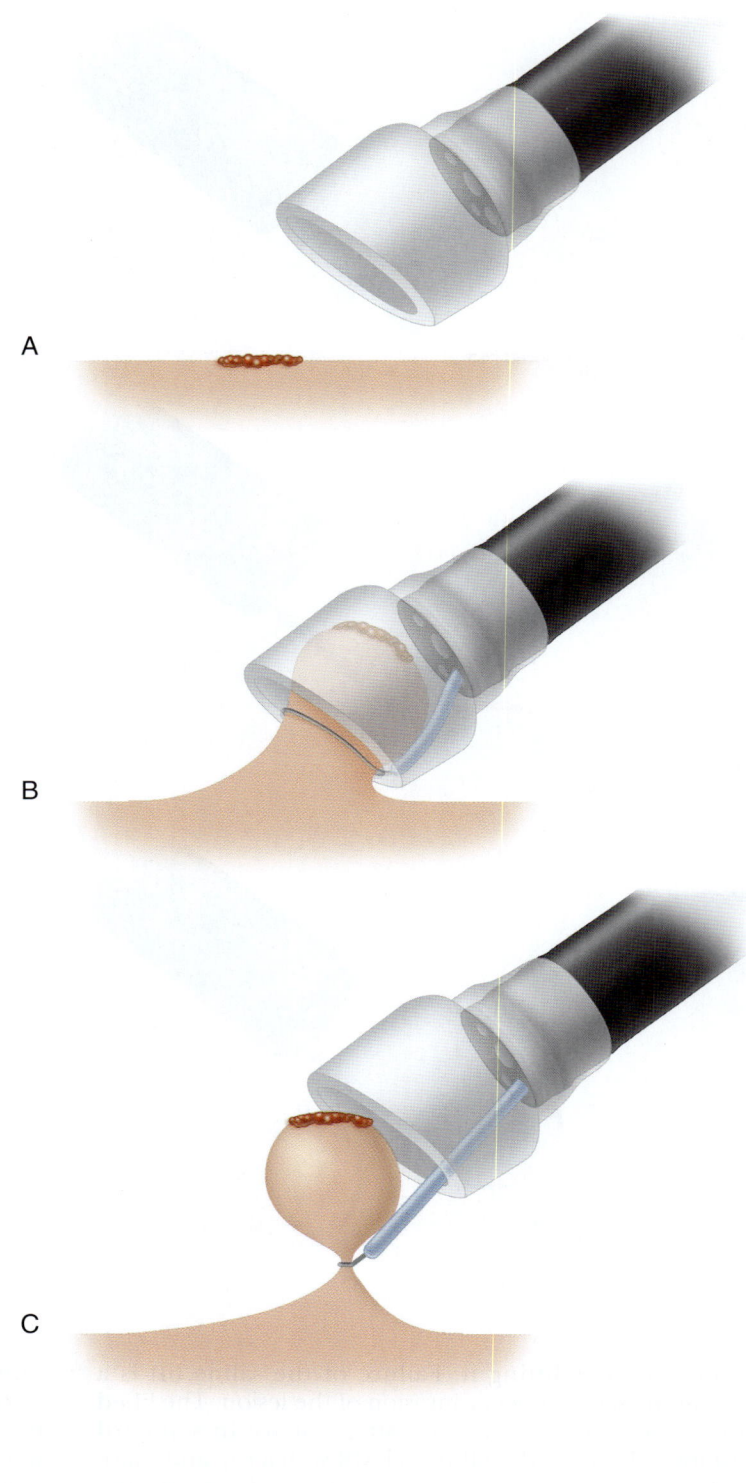

A

B

C

FIGURE 57.11 Steps of a cap-and-snare endoscopic mucosal resection. (A) A cap fitted with elastic bands is advanced onto the lesion. (B) The lesion is suctioned up into the cap and the elastic band is fired, creating a pseudopolyp. (C) A polypectomy snare is used to excise the pseudopolyp at the elastic band.

with a needle knife and a cap-fitted endoscope. The cap is then used as a retraction device to continue dissection along the submucosal plane using the needle knife. This enables precise dissection in the proper submucosal plane, direct control over the margins of the lesions, and results in a higher en bloc resection specimen rate.[13] ESD is, however, far more technically challenging, has a higher risk of perforation, and is time consuming to perform.

CONTROL OF GASTROINTESTINAL BLEEDING

UGIB is one of the most common indications for therapeutic intervention in upper endoscopy. Timing of

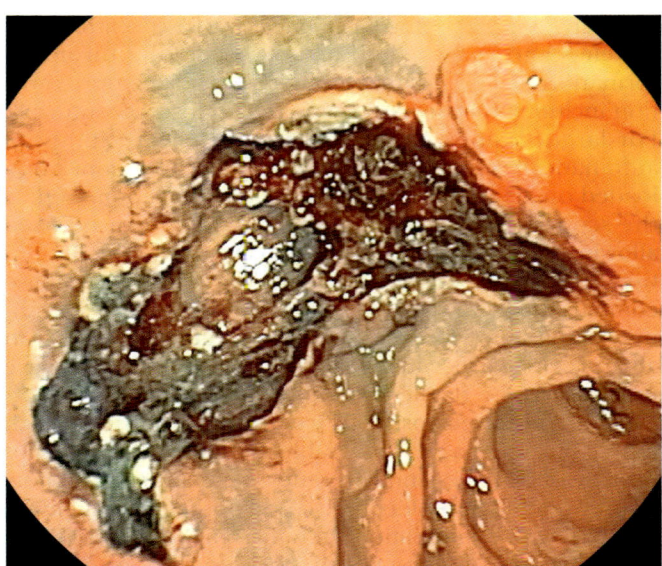

FIGURE 57.12 Previously seen sessile duodenal polyp in Fig. 57.8 has been excised with a saline-lift endoscopic mucosal resection technique.

intervention is determined by the clinical scenario and patients can be categorized as requiring early endoscopy, surveillance, or discharge. Patients considered to be at a higher risk for severe UGIB include those older than 60 years, patients with known concomitant liver disease including varices, patients with witnessed hematemesis or hematochezia, which are signs of ongoing bleeding, or patients with tachycardia or hypotension on presentation.[14] These patient characteristics are associated with higher mortality from a bleeding episode and benefit from early endoscopic management. A low threshold should be maintained for use of early endoscopy because the consequences of missing a severe UGIB are significantly higher than the morbidity of additional nontherapeutic endoscopies.

There are several important considerations for patient preparation prior to safe performance of endoscopy. Proton pump inhibitors should be started prior to endoscopy, which reduces the severity of the bleeding and the requirement of therapy at endoscopy, but does not change clinical outcomes and mortality.[15] Patients with ongoing UGIB may require volume repletion and blood product transfusion. Careful monitoring in an intensive care unit may be required. Coagulation parameters must be obtained and any anticoagulant should be reversed but should not delay endoscopy. These patients may be at high risk of aspiration and may benefit from airway control and protection using endotracheal intubation. It is possible to perform lavage of the stomach by instilling warm saline in a large-bore naso- or orogastric tube as a diagnostic tool and to facilitate future endoscopic visualization. An aspirate yielding blood confirms UGIB, but a negative sample does not preclude bleeding and can miss up to 20% of bleeding. Promotility agents such as intravenous erythromycin can also be used prior to endoscopy to improve clearance of the upper GI tract but has not been shown to improve clinical outcomes.[16]

The most common cause of UGIB remains peptic ulcer disease, which accounts for 40% to 50% of UGIBs. Predominant causes for peptic ulcer disease include infection with *H. pylori* organisms and chronic use of NSAIDs. During endoscopy, a lesion can be classified according to its risk for rebleeding. Major stigmata of recent hemorrhage have a high risk of rebleeding without endoscopic therapy and include active arterial bleeding and a non-bleeding visible vessel.[17] Endoscopic treatment in these cases significantly reduces rates of rebleeding, blood transfusions, and need for surgical intervention but have not been shown to improve mortality, which is generally driven by comorbidities. Any clot on an ulcer bed should warrant focused irrigation to dislodge the clot for proper assessment of the underlying lesion. Endoscopic treatment of adherent clots is controversial and should be combined with other considerations such as patient comorbidities, size of the ulcer (greater than 2 cm) and ulcer location along the posterior gastric lesser curve or posterior duodenal wall.[18] Lesions with lower risk for rebleeding include clean-based ulcer with minor oozing and black or red spots. Lower-risk lesions have a good prognosis and do not require endoscopic treatment.

Multiple tools can be used for endoscopic treatment and can be categorized as injection, thermal, and mechanical therapy.[19] The goal of injection therapy is to provide hemostasis through a combination of the tamponade effect due to the volume of the injection itself and vasoconstricting or sclerosing effect due to the injected compound. The most commonly used compound for injection of nonvariceal bleeding sources is dilute 1:10,000 epinephrine, which provides local compression and adds a vasoconstrictive effect. Other compounds include normal saline solution, which provides local compression alone, and ethanol or sodium morrhuate, which have sclerosing effect. Thrombin, fibrin, or cyanoacrylate glues may provide primary tissue sealing. Injection therapy alone has been shown to be suboptimal and insufficient to prevent rebleeding. Injection therapy with dilute epinephrine is best used as a method to gain initial control and hemostasis, but should be used in combination with either thermal therapy, mechanical clipping, or sclerosant or sealant injection.[20] Complications from injection are usually related to the injected compound itself; epinephrine rarely causing arrhythmias or hypertension, whereas sclerosants have a higher rate of local effects such as tissue necrosis, strictures, bleeding, and perforation.

Thermal options include contact methods and non-contact methods and are based on delivery of energy-inducing direct tissue coagulation, contraction, and desiccation. Contact methods include the delivery of monopolar and bipolar energy and require the use of a radiofrequency generator. Monopolar energy completes a circuit through an active electrode and a grounding pad. Multiple instruments such as hot biopsy forceps and snares can serve as the active electrode. Bipolar energy includes both electrodes at the tip of the instrument, completing the circuit locally. Bipolar energy can be used directly by completing the circuit at the level of the tissue to be treated itself or can be used as part of a heater probe, using thermocoupling to generate a constant temperature and induce coagulation through direct heat transfer. Contact probes are advantageous in allowing for direct pressure tamponade of bleeding using the probe itself and cause a deeper burn than noncontact methods. This deeper burn does increase the risk, albeit rare, of peptic ulcer perforations and precipitation of bleeding. Some contact probes are combined with an injection needle allowing for delivery of combination therapy using a single instrument. Noncontact methods include argon plasma coagulation, which uses the flow of argon gas from the tip of the instrument.[21] The argon gas is ignited using an electrode, turning it into argon plasma, which travels to the nearest conductive tissue, and is often used for creating a superficial burn. The superficiality of the burn renders complications rare, but the argon gas itself can create overdistention of the GI tract, subcutaneous emphysema, and pneumoperitoneum.

The most commonly deployed mechanical hemostatic device is the endoscopic clip. Standard through-the-scope endoscopic clips are loaded through the instrument channel and are generally made of a two-pronged metal clip attached to a deployment handle that allows opening, closing, and firing of the clip. Their handles often allow rotation of the clip to facilitate positioning. Endoscopic clips provide direct tissue approximation and superficial vessel closure and can also be used for closure of perforation (Fig. 57.13). Through-the-scope clips generally dislodge within a week. Other methods for mechanical hemostasis include detachable loops, which are similar to loop ligature devices. These are most useful in controlling the stalk of a lesion to be snared, thereby preventing bleeding once the lesion is excised. Endoscopic band ligators were initially created to band esophageal varices and consist of elastic bands loaded onto a cap, but can also be used to ligate gastric varices and Dieulafoy lesions.

Emerging methods for hemostasis include Hemospray (Cook Medical, Winston-Salem, North Carolina), an inorganic mineral powder that is sprayed onto the bleeding lesion using a carbon dioxide cartridge.[22] The adherent powder achieves hemostasis by acting as a scaffold for platelets and coagulation factors, promoting thrombus formation. Investigational methods for tissue approximation include over-the-scope clips and endoscopic suturing. For larger lesions, a "bear-claw" type clip includes an automatically closing spring mechanism and comes preloaded on an applicator cap in the open position.[23] Once the scope is properly positioned, the clip can be fired allowing the two parts of the clip to close onto the desired tissue. Over-the-scope clips lead to a deeper purchase compared to standard endoscopic clips and may remain in position much longer. Endoscopic suturing devices can also provide direct mechanical approximation but are unwieldy to use in the context of UGIB.

After initial endoscopic treatment of patients with high-risk stigmata, it is advisable to monitor the patient for at least 72 hours and continue proton pump inhibitors to prevent risk of rebleeding.[24] Appropriate management of UGIB with combination therapy is highly effective and initial hemostasis is achieved in up to 95% of cases. If appropriate initial management was performed, routine repeat endoscopy in 24 hours is not necessary. Nonetheless, there is a risk for rebleeding in 5% to 10% of all cases. Patients with rebleeding should undergo a second endoscopic assessment and treatment if appropriate. If endoscopic hemostasis fails, second-line options include percutaneous embolization and surgical treatment, which is further described in Chapter 59. In patients with peptic ulcer disease, *H. pylori* testing should be carried out. A negative *H. pylori* test during an episode of bleeding is considered to have lower sensitivity and further testing should be repeated at a later time. *H. pylori* infections should be eradicated and eradication should be documented to reduce the recurrence rate of peptic ulcer disease. In patients with ulcer complications due to NSAIDs, their cessation must be considered. If NSAIDs cannot be discontinued, concomitant use of a proton pump inhibitor may decrease risk of recurrent bleeding, although there is still associated risk.

Other common causes of UGIB include esophagitis, stress gastritis, varices, Mallory-Weiss tears, malignancy, and angiodysplasia. Bleeding from esophagitis and Mallory-Weiss tears is usually self-limited with proper medical management. Vascular abnormalities such as angiodysplasia and GAVE are classically treated using argon plasma coagulation (APC). Gastric varices can be treated preferably with cyanoacrylate injection or using a variceal band ligator (Fig. 57.14).[25] Dieulafoy lesions can be treated optimally with clips or ligated.[26] Bleeding malignancies are challenging to treat endoscopically and friable masses inevitably rebleed over time. Surgical resection or radiotherapy may be the best option for persistent bleeding from a malignancy.

DILATION AND STENTING OF BENIGN AND MALIGNANT STRICTURES

Gastric outlet obstruction can be caused by benign lesions such as congenital or peptic ulcer–induced pyloric stenosis or malignant lesions such as direct invasion by gastric or periampullary carcinoma or extrinsic compression by pancreatic cancer. Endoscopic treatment of strictures is minimally invasive and can act as a primary treatment, as

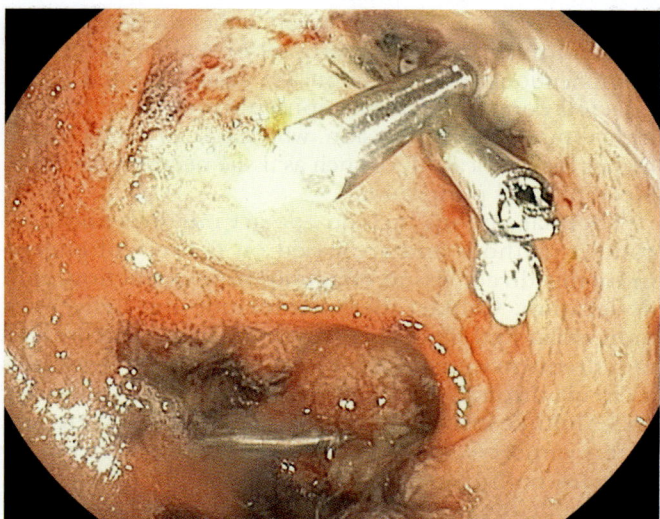

FIGURE 57.13 A large duodenal ulcer is seen along the posterior aspect of the first stage of the duodenum. Three endoscopic clips are placed on a visible vessel.

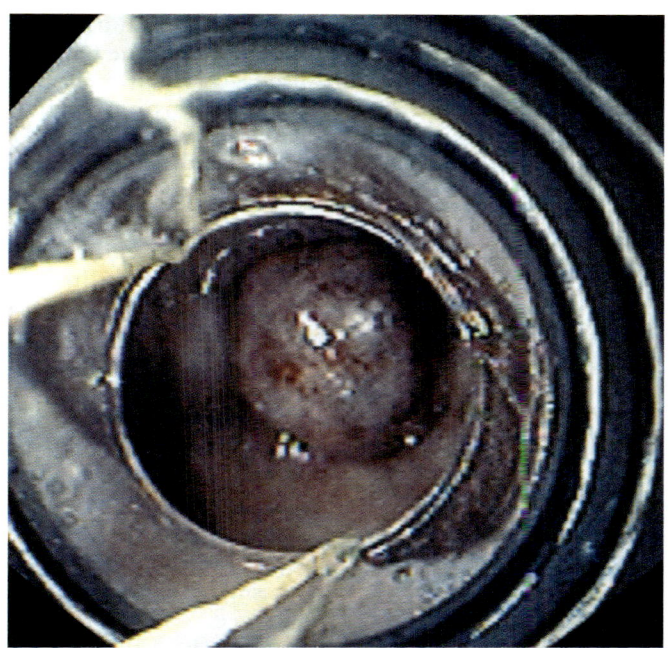

FIGURE 57.14 Image through an endoscopic band ligator after placement of a band. This technique can also be used as first step in the cap-and-snare technique for endoscopic mucosal resection.

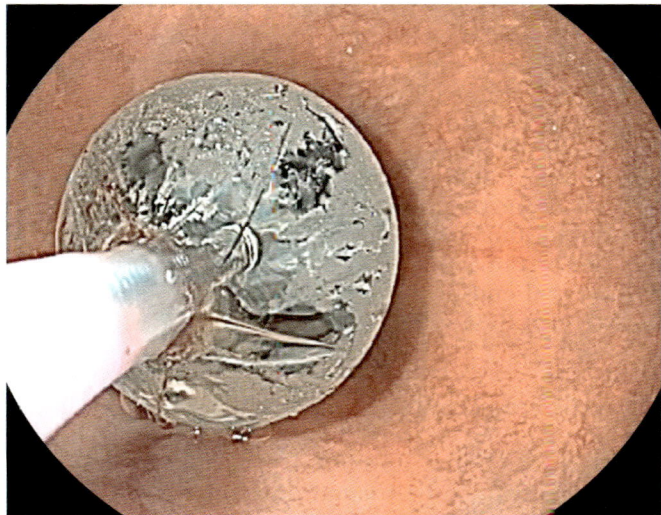

FIGURE 57.15 View of a hydrostatic balloon dilator as it dilates a stricture.

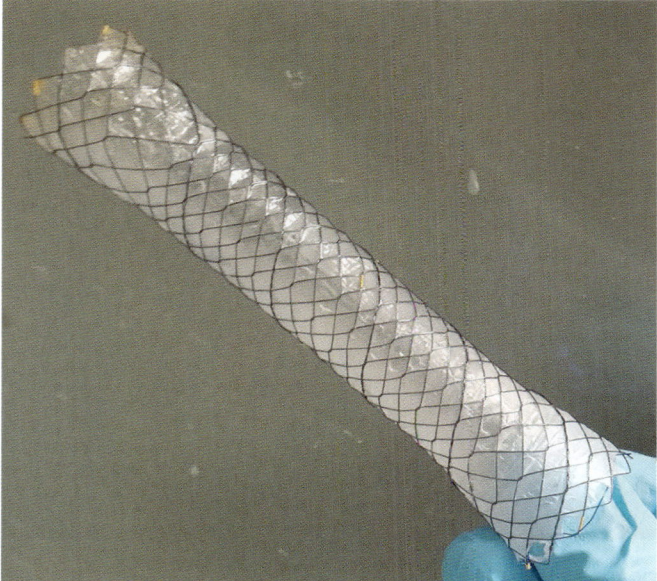

FIGURE 57.16 Example of a covered self-expanding metal stent. The stent flares out at both ends to decrease risk of migration.

a bridge to surgery, or as a palliative replacement for surgery altogether.

For benign strictures, the use of balloon dilatation often results in at least temporary improvement in symptoms.[27] Balloon dilators are catheters with a channel for injection into a balloon affixed to the tip (Fig. 57.15). The shape of the balloon is cylindrical and comes in various diameters. Balloon dilators are passed through the endoscope instrument channel. A specially made inflation device with pressure indicator allows inflation and pressurization of the balloon through the catheter to specific pressures and sizes. It is not uncommon to require multiple balloon dilations. It is recommended to size the initial dilation to the tightness of the stricture and use successively larger balloon sizes over time to progressively dilate and avoid perforation. Once adequate dilation is achieved, up to 80% of patients achieve long-lasting effect.[28] In the case of a peptic stricture, it is important to eliminate the root cause by treating *H. pylori* infections, discontinuing NSAIDs, and use proton pump inhibitors. Adjunctive therapy can increase efficacy of dilation, including local injection of long-acting steroids and cutting any permanent suture materials or knots at tight anastomoses using endoshears. Patients failing multiple dilations and having recurrent stricturing disease may require surgery.

For malignant strictures, tissue regrowth is of concern and balloon dilation therefore has little value in providing a long-lasting solution. In patients with resectable disease, the proper treatment is attempt at oncologic surgery with curative intent. In patients with unresectable or metastatic disease, the preferred endoscopic treatment is the placement of a self-expanding metal stent (SEMS) with palliative intent.[29,30] SEMS are available as uncovered, partially covered, or fully covered stents (Fig. 57.16). They are made using nitinol, a nickel-titanium metal alloy that has shape memory and super elasticity. These properties allow the stent to be compressed into the size of a deployment catheter and to then recover its original shape over time once deployed. Covered stents add a coating of silicone on the exterior and/or interior surface of the stent, whereas uncovered or bare-metal stents do not. This covering prevents the ingrowth of tumor between the metal wires of the stent, with the disadvantage of a higher rate of migration. Fully covered stents also allow the exclusion of food from the wall of the GI tract and can

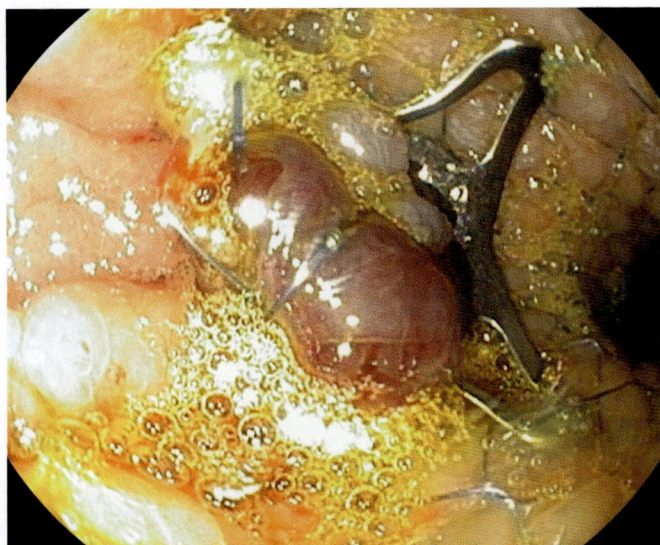

FIGURE 57.17 Picture of an over-the-scope clip placed to help prevent migration of a fully covered stent placed across a strictured gastrojejunostomy.

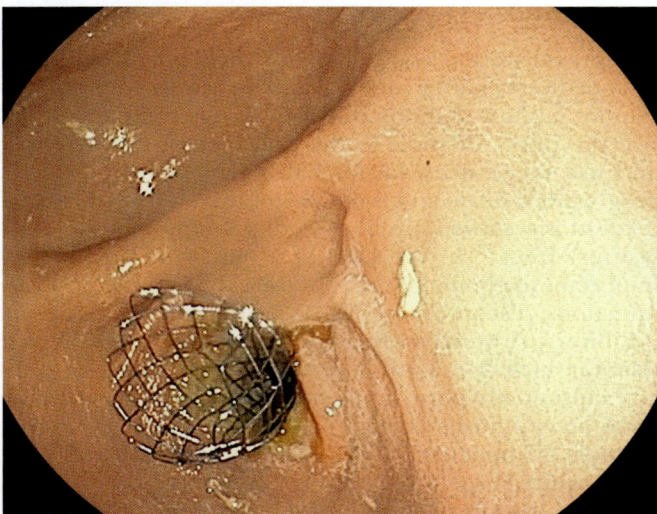

FIGURE 57.18 View of the antrum after deployment of an uncovered duodenal stent with prepyloric position of the proximal end of the stent for palliative treatment of duodenal obstruction by pancreatic cancer.

be useful in treating fistulas, anastomotic leaks, and perforations (Fig. 57.17). They are also easier to reposition and remove after insertion. Uncovered stents, on the other hand, allow tissue ingrowth that prevents migration, but can ultimately lead to stent occlusion due to ingrowth (Fig. 57.18). Both types of stent usually also feature flared ends to further increase the radial holding pressure and decrease risk of migration. SEMS placed across a malignant stricture will gradually dilate the stricture as the stent returns to its original shape. Optimal placement of a SEMS is centered on the stricturing lesion as the stent undergoes a certain amount of foreshortening as it expands.

The main challenge with dilation and stenting of strictures is the identification and passage of the balloon or stent through the stricture itself, especially with very tight strictures where distal visualization is impossible. When the endoscope is able to pass the stricture itself, it becomes simple to deploy the balloon or stent at the level of the stricture. If the endoscope is unable to pass the stricture, multiple options exist to ascertain the positioning of the balloon or stent introducer prior to deployment. Typically, a catheter and guidewire can be used through the instrument channel to intubate the stricture and pass beyond it using fluoroscopic guidance. Injection of contrast material through the catheter can then confirm intraluminal location of the distal guidewire. Alternatively, a small-diameter endoscope or mini-scope can be used to traverse a stricture that a regular-sized endoscope could not, thereby enabling a guidewire to be placed beyond the stricture safely. The balloon or stent can then be loaded onto the guidewire for delivery through the stricture either through the scope or beside the scope. Dilation or deployment can then proceed using a combination of fluoroscopic and endoscopic guidance.

Endoscopic treatment of stricturing lesions is not without risk. Balloon dilation of tight strictures or larger (>15 mm) balloon sizes carries a non-negligible risk of perforation and peritonitis. Tearing of the mucosa and submucosa at the site of dilation may also induce bleeding. A stent during its expansion phase also causes abdominal pain and a potential risk for perforation, especially if the stent is positioned across a corner and there is pressure on the edges of the stent. Placement of a duodenal stent over the ampulla prior to metal stenting of the biliary tree may also cause biliary obstruction or inability to access the ampulla for further biliary therapy (Fig. 57.19).[31] A stent may migrate into the small bowel and cause obstruction and perforation, classically at existing adhesions or stenosis downstream. An uncovered stent may become blocked by tumor ingrowth. A covered stent may become blocked by tumor overgrowth either at the proximal or at the distal end of the stent. Finally, food may become impacted in the lumen of the stent.

TRANSLUMINAL THERAPY

Although endoscopy is best adapted to treat lesions inside the lumen of the GI tract, the proximity of other organs to the stomach and duodenum allows pathologies in adjacent organs to be treated transluminally. The most common example of this is a percutaneous gastrostomy, which is described in Chapter 58. Another example is the drainage of pancreatic pseudocysts by creating an endoscopic cystogastrostomy.

In general, we wait 6 to 8 weeks after the episode of pancreatitis to allow for the pseudocyst wall to mature before drainage of large symptomatic non-resolving pseudocysts.[32] This image-guided endoscopic technique is usually done under endoscopic ultrasound guidance. Assessment of patient tolerance is important because the procedure can be uncomfortable and it is often better performed under general anesthesia. Preprocedure antibiotics are given. If gallstone pancreatitis is suspected, prior clearance of the biliary tract with standard endoscopic retrograde cholangiopancreatography is recommended.

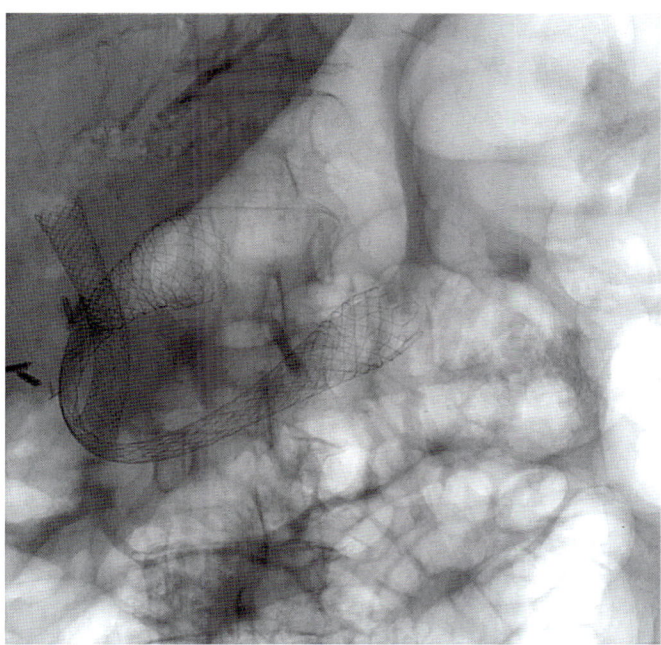

FIGURE 57.19 A fluoroscopic view after insertion of two self-expanding metal stents, a biliary and duodenal stent for palliation of pancreatic cancer. There is external compression on the duodenum as seen from the narrowing of the duodenal stent. This malignant stricture will be expanded as the stent regains its shape over the course of the next 2 days.

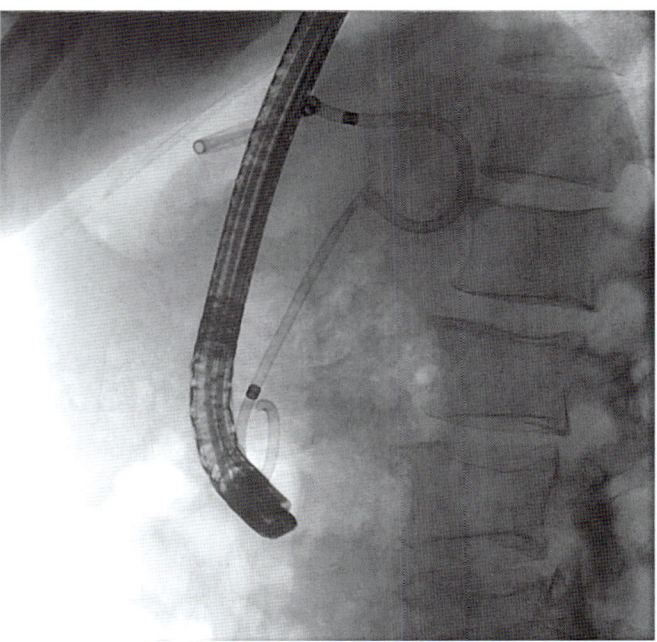

FIGURE 57.20 A fluoroscopic view after insertion of a double pigtail stent serving as cystogastrostomy for pseudocyst drainage. A transpapillary stent is also seen draining the same pseudocyst.

Cannulation of the pancreatic duct may also allow assessment of the potential for transpapillary drainage of the pseudocyst with a pancreatic stent (Fig. 57.20).[33]

A survey of the posterior stomach or duodenum often reveals a prominent bulge associated with the pseudocyst. Endoscopic ultrasound is used to ensure an avascular plane is present prior to puncture. A needle puncture is made, fluid sampled, and a guidewire is advanced into the pseudocyst. The size and shape of the pseudocyst are assessed by contrast injection and confirmation of successful cannulation of the pseudocyst by the endoscopic guidewire is achieved on fluoroscopy. The tract is dilated using a hydrostatic balloon dilator. Care must be taken on removal of the balloon dilator as large pseudocysts will drain under pressure, may preclude visualization, and can cause aspiration. Dilation of the stomach wall is also uncomfortable and appropriate sedation is required prior to this step. Once the tract is dilated, soft double pigtail stents are inserted into the pseudocyst to allow free drainage of pseudocyst contents into the stomach. Multiple double pigtails stents beside each other cause friction against each other, reduce stent blockage, and enable increased drainage around the stents (Fig. 57.21). Most pseudocysts will resolve with stent drainage within 2 weeks.

Novel lumen-apposing covered SEMS have recently been introduced to facilitate creation of anastomoses through the GI tract and can be used for creation of cystogastrostomies and cholecystogastrostomies.[34,35] This specially designed SEM has two deployable flanges, one that can be deployed inside the structure to be drained,

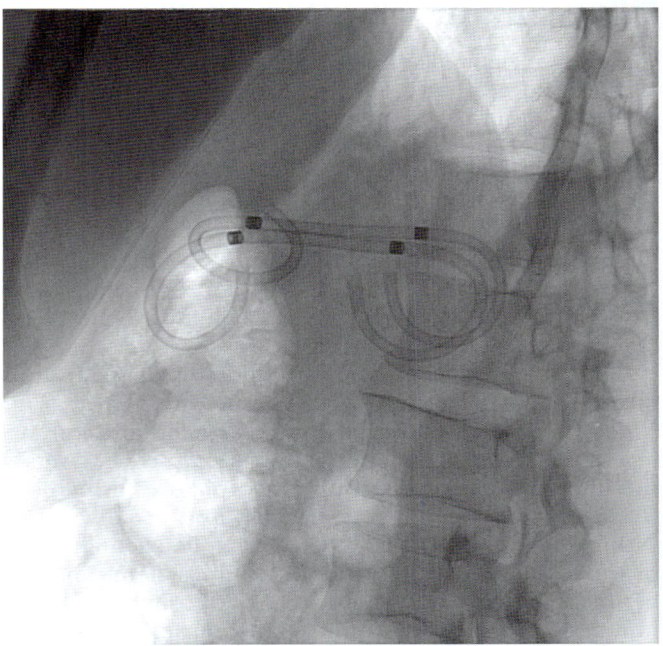

FIGURE 57.21 Two double pigtail stents are placed in the same cystogastrostomy. The friction between the stents helps keep the cystogastrostomy open.

and the other inside the lumen of the stomach. These two flanges allow the covered stent to create a watertight seal by apposing the lumen of the two cavities. This allows a simpler one-instrument cystogastrostomy procedure and creates a larger channel for drainage with the possibility

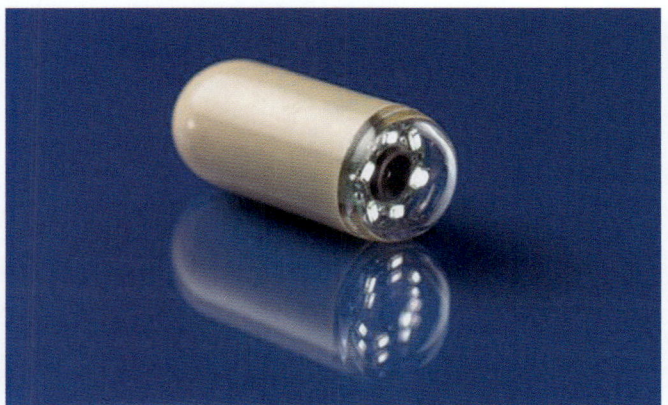

FIGURE 57.22 A capsule used for wireless video capsule endoscopy.

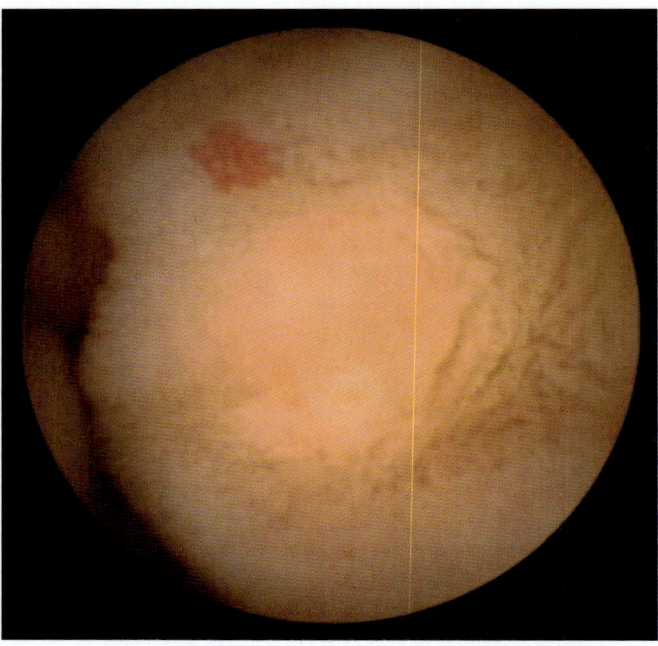

FIGURE 57.23 Angiodysplasia as seen from a video capsule. This is a common cause for obscure gastrointestinal bleeding in the small intestine.

for easier future pancreatic debridement. More investigational transluminal therapies include the potential for leaving the luminal space altogether by creating a gastrostomy and entering the peritoneal cavity. This experimental branch of minimally invasive surgery is termed NOTES and features "scarless" abdominal operations such as cholecystectomy and appendectomy, which are done through the wall of the stomach or vagina.

ENDOSCOPY OF THE SMALL BOWEL

The midgut, defined as small intestine between the ampulla and the ileocecal valve, is a challenging area to investigate due to its length and the relatively long distance away from natural orifices. The most common indication for investigation of the midgut is to find a source for obscure GI bleeding, defined as bleeding that persists despite negative colonoscopy and esophagogastroduodenoscopy. Other indications include evaluation for Crohn disease, surveillance of small bowel polyposis syndromes, and investigation of tumors such as lymphomas or carcinoids.

The preferred technique for endoscopic visualization of the small intestine is video capsule endoscopy (Fig. 57.22). A camera and light source are contained in an ingested pill-sized capsule. The capsule endoscope traverses the intestinal tract, collecting timed pictures, which are wirelessly transferred to a receiver, and usually passes within a day (Figs. 57.23 and 57.24). The sequence of pictures, time recording, and navigation system can then be used to visually assess and situate abnormalities in the lumen of the small intestine. Video capsule endoscopy has a significantly higher diagnostic yield than enteroclysis.[36] Video capsule endoscopy is safe and easily tolerated, which makes it ideal to use as initial diagnostic modality. Unfortunately, there is no potential for tissue sampling or providing therapy because capsule endoscopy is only a diagnostic tool and must be carefully used in patients with suspected small bowel obstruction or strictures. This deficiency has now been addressed with the progression to deep bowel enteroscopy.

Deep bowel enteroscopy consists of the use of an enteroscope with a fitted overtube and balloon(s) to

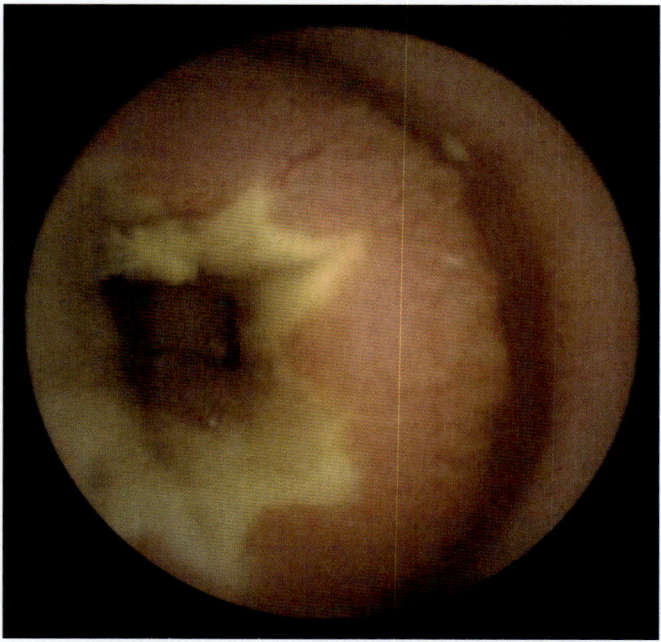

FIGURE 57.24 Small bowel ulceration and stricture secondary to Crohn disease.

examine the small intestine either from the oral route and the ileocecal route. Two competing technologies exist: double-balloon and single-balloon enteroscopy.[37] The mechanism for both technologies is similar. It consists in the inflation of the balloon on the overtube with a balloon-pump system that allows the plication of the small bowel onto itself as the enteroscope is advanced through a push-and-pull technique. In selected patients, it is possible to combine antegrade and retrograde balloon endoscopy to examine the entire small bowel.[38] However, it is more common to use video capsule endoscopy to identify and situate the lesion first followed by balloon enteroscopy to perform therapy.[39] Therapy can be delivered through the instrument channel with specialized long instruments. This enables tissue sampling, hemostasis, injection, stricture dilation, and foreign body removal in the small intestine. Balloon enteroscopy can also be used to access the duodenum and ampulla in patients with surgically altered anatomy.[40] However, balloon enteroscopy requires advanced endoscopic skill, is particularly time consuming, and may be poorly tolerated by patients without general anesthesia. Potential complications include perforation, deep mucosal tears, and acute pancreatitis.

With the advances in deep enteroscopy, the use of intraoperative enteroscopy has been reduced. Despite balloon endoscopy, total endoscopy is not feasible in all patients and there often remains a part of the small bowel that cannot be accessed by deep enteroscopic techniques. This is especially the case for patients with previous abdominal surgery, bowel obstruction, or coagulopathy.[41] Intraoperative enteroscopy is associated with a higher rate of complications, including wound infection and intestinal ischemia. As such, it should not be used as a first-line diagnostic tool to limit negative surgical explorations.

CONCLUSION

Upper endoscopy has become a cornerstone in providing diagnostic capabilities for diseases of the stomach and the small bowel. Continued development in the field of therapeutic endoscopy has provided the skilled GI surgeon with an increasing variety of techniques and novel instruments. These endoscopic techniques are often improvements on conventional surgical therapy and are increasingly becoming standard of care. As surgery becomes increasingly minimally invasive, advanced endoscopic treatments are a new frontier where exponential future growth is to be expected.

ACKNOWLEDGMENT

The authors would like to acknowledge Jeffrey L. Ponsky and Chike V. Chukwumah for the excellent version of this chapter in the seventh edition.

REFERENCES

1. Early DS, Ben-Menachem T, Decker GA, et al. Appropriate use of GI endoscopy. *Gastrointest Endosc.* 2012;75(6):1127-1131.
2. Committee ASoA. Practice guidelines for preoperative fasting and the use of pharmacologic agents to reduce the risk of pulmonary aspiration: application to healthy patients undergoing elective procedures: an updated report by the American Society of Anesthesiologists Committee on Standards and Practice Parameters. *Anesthesiology.* 2011;114(3):495-511.
3. Vargo JJ, DeLegge MH, Feld AD, et al. Multisociety sedation curriculum for gastrointestinal endoscopy. *Gastrointest Endosc.* 2012; 76(1):e1-e25.
4. Dixon MF, Genta RM, Yardley JH, Correa P. Classification and grading of gastritis. The updated Sydney System. International Workshop on the Histopathology of Gastritis, Houston 1994. *Am J Surg Pathol.* 1996;20(10):1161-1181.
5. Marshall B, Warren JR. Unidentified curved bacilli in the stomach of patients with gastritis and peptic ulceration. *Lancet.* 1984;323 (8390):1311-1315.
6. Chey WD, Wong BC. American College of Gastroenterology guideline on the management of *Helicobacter pylori* infection. *Am J Gastroenterol.* 2007;102(8):1808-1825.
7. Jabbari M, Cherry R, Lough JO, Daly DS, Kinnear DG, Goresky CA. Gastric antral vascular ectasia: the watermelon stomach. *Gastroenterology.* 1984;87(5):1165-1170.
8. Carmack SW, Genta RM, Schuler CM, Saboorian MH. The current spectrum of gastric polyps: a 1-year national study of over 120,000 patients. *Am J Gastroenterol.* 2009;104(6):1524-1532.
9. Genta RM, Schuler CM, Robiou CI, Lash RH. No association between gastric fundic gland polyps and gastrointestinal neoplasia in a study of over 100,000 patients. *Clin Gastroenterol Hepatol.* 2009;7(8):849-854.
10. Jain R, Chetty R. Gastric hyperplastic polyps: a review. *Dig Dis Sci.* 2009;54(9):1839-1846.
11. Hiki N, Yamamoto Y, Fukunaga T, et al. Laparoscopic and endoscopic cooperative surgery for gastrointestinal stromal tumor dissection. *Surg Endosc.* 2008;22(7):1729-1735.
12. Ono H, Kondo H, Gotoda T, et al. Endoscopic mucosal resection for treatment of early gastric cancer. *Gut.* 2001;48(2):225-229.
13. Oka S, Tanaka S, Kaneko I, et al. Advantage of endoscopic submucosal dissection compared with EMR for early gastric cancer. *Gastrointest Endosc.* 2006;64(6):877-883.
14. Blatchford O, Murray WR, Blatchford M. A risk score to predict need for treatment for upper-gastrointestinal haemorrhage. *Lancet.* 2000;356(9238):1318-1321.
15. Sreedharan A, Martin J, Leontiadis GI, et al. Proton pump inhibitor treatment initiated prior to endoscopic diagnosis in upper gastrointestinal bleeding. *Cochrane Database Syst Rev.* 2010;(7):CD005415.
16. Barkun AN, Bardou M, Martel M, Gralnek IM, Sung JJ. Prokinetics in acute upper GI bleeding: a meta-analysis. *Gastrointest Endosc.* 2010;72(6):1138-1145.
17. Rockall TA, Logan RF, Devlin HB, Northfield TC. Risk assessment after acute upper gastrointestinal haemorrhage. *Gut.* 1996;38(3): 316-321.
18. Barkun AN, Bardou M, Kuipers EJ, et al. International consensus recommendations on the management of patients with nonvariceal upper gastrointestinal bleeding. *Ann Intern Med.* 2010;152(2):101-113.
19. Hwang JH, Fisher DA, Ben-Menachem T, et al. The role of endoscopy in the management of acute non-variceal upper GI bleeding. *Gastrointest Endosc.* 2012;75(6):1132-1138.
20. Calvet X, Vergara M, Brullet E, Gisbert JP, Campo R. Addition of a second endoscopic treatment following epinephrine injection improves outcome in high-risk bleeding ulcers. *Gastroenterology.* 2004;126(2):441-450.
21. Grund KE, Storek D, Farin G. Endoscopic argon plasma coagulation (APC) first clinical experiences in flexible endoscopy. *Endosc Surg Allied Technol.* 1994;2(1):42-46.
22. Sung JJ, Luo D, Wu JC, et al. Early clinical experience of the safety and effectiveness of Hemospray in achieving hemostasis in patients with acute peptic ulcer bleeding. *Endoscopy.* 2011;43(4):291-295.
23. Kirschniak A, Subotova N, Zieker D, Königsrainer A, Kratt T. The Over-The-Scope Clip (OTSC) for the treatment of gastrointestinal bleeding, perforations, and fistulas. *Surg Endosc.* 2011;25(9):2901-2905.
24. Lau JY, Sung JJ, Lee KK, et al. Effect of intravenous omeprazole on recurrent bleeding after endoscopic treatment of bleeding peptic ulcers. *N Engl J Med.* 2000;343(5):310-316.
25. Garcia-Tsao G, Bosch J. Management of varices and variceal hemorrhage in cirrhosis. *N Engl J Med.* 2010;362(9):823-832.
26. Chung I-K, Kim E-J, Lee M-S, et al. Bleeding Dieulafoy's lesions and the choice of endoscopic method: comparing the hemostatic efficacy of mechanical and injection methods. *Gastrointest Endosc.* 2000;52(6):721-724.
27. DiSario JA, Fennerty MB, Tietze CC, Hutson WR, Burt RW. Endoscopic balloon dilation for ulcer-induced gastric outlet obstruction. *Am J Gastroenterol.* 1994;89(6):868-871.
28. Miller A. Endoscopic options for benign and malignant gastric outlet obstruction. *Curr Surg Rep.* 2014;2(4):1-7.
29. Adler DG, Baron TH. Endoscopic palliation of malignant gastric outlet obstruction using self-expanding metal stents: experience in 36 patients. *Am J Gastroenterol.* 2002;97(1):72-78.
30. Tringali A, Didden P, Repici A, et al. Endoscopic treatment of malignant gastric and duodenal strictures: a prospective, multicenter study. *Gastrointest Endosc.* 2014;79(1):66-75.

31. Maire F, Hammel P, Ponsot P, et al. Long-term outcome of biliary and duodenal stents in palliative treatment of patients with unresectable adenocarcinoma of the head of pancreas. *Am J Gastroenterol.* 2006;101(4):735-742.

32. Bergman S, Melvin WS. Operative and nonoperative management of pancreatic pseudocysts. *Surg Clin North Am.* 2007;87(6):1447-1460, [ix].

33. Varadarajulu S, Bang JY, Sutton BS, Trevino JM, Christein JD, Wilcox CM. Equal efficacy of endoscopic and surgical cystogastrostomy for pancreatic pseudocyst drainage in a randomized trial. *Gastroenterology.* 2013;145(3):583-590.e1.

34. Shah RJ, Shah JN, Waxman I, et al. Safety and efficacy of endoscopic ultrasound-guided drainage of pancreatic fluid collections with lumen-apposing covered self-expanding metal stents. *Clin Gastroenterol Hepatol.* 2015;13(4):747-752.

35. Widmer J, Singhal S, Gaidhane M, Kahaleh M. Endoscopic ultrasound-guided endoluminal drainage of the gallbladder. *Dig Endosc.* 2014;26(4):525-531.

36. Triester SL, Leighton JA, Leontiadis GI, et al. A meta-analysis of the yield of capsule endoscopy compared to other diagnostic modalities in patients with obscure gastrointestinal bleeding. *Am J Gastroenterol.* 2005;100(11):2407-2418.

37. Khashab MA, Pasha SF, Muthusamy VR, et al. The role of deep enteroscopy in the management of small-bowel disorders. *Gastrointest Endosc.* 2015;82(4):600-607.

38. Xin L, Liao Z, Jiang YP, Li ZS. Indications, detectability, positive findings, total enteroscopy, and complications of diagnostic double-balloon endoscopy: a systematic review of data over the first decade of use. *Gastrointest Endosc.* 2011;74(3):563-570.

39. Pasha SF, Leighton JA, Das A, et al. Double-balloon enteroscopy and capsule endoscopy have comparable diagnostic yield in small-bowel disease: a meta-analysis. *Clin Gastroenterol Hepatol.* 2008;6(6): 671-676.

40. Itoi T, Ishii K, Sofuni A, et al. Single-balloon enteroscopy–assisted ERCP in patients with Billroth II gastrectomy or Roux-en-Y anastomosis (with video). *Am J Gastroenterol.* 2010;105(1):93-99.

41. Bonnet S, Douard R, Malamut G, Cellier C, Wind P. Intraoperative enteroscopy in the management of obscure gastrointestinal bleeding. *Dig Liver Dis.* 2013;45(4):277-284.

Access and Intubation of the Stomach and Small Intestine

David S. Shapiro | Stephanie C. Montgomery

Intubation of the gastrointestinal (GI) tract occurs frequently in the course of patient care. Enteral access, whether via the nasal or percutaneous route, is procured in the majority of instances for decompression or nutrition. Intestinal access is indicated for diagnostic and therapeutic reasons in a variety of disorders, including bowel obstruction, gastric outlet obstruction, gastroesophageal reflux, GI bleeding, and disorders of motility (Table 58.1). Despite the frequent need and indication for gastric and small intestinal intubation in modern medical and surgical practices, the means of access and the access devices themselves carry innate risks that must be considered. Serious, even potentially fatal, complications may result from the placement or management of enteral tubes. Feasibility, appropriateness, timing, and route of access must all be considered to determine the proper patient and procedure.

Providers who are intubating the stomach and small intestine should always consider potential complications of tube placement when examining possible indications. The routine use of postoperative gastric decompression has been a matter of contention, but current evidence suggests that routine postoperative nasogastric tubes are unnecessary. Further, early postoperative enteral nutrition is an important goal in most enhanced recovery efforts, and an indwelling tube may compromise this goal as a result of common in-place protocols and patient interest. Two meta-analyses of more than 3000 patients support decompression in selective postoperative settings only (extensive adhesiolysis, known gastroparesis, mechanically ventilated patients, etc.), and these authors suggest that other routine postoperative use should be abandoned.[1] Any benefit of gastric decompression carries a concomitant risk of aspiration, sinusitis, and pressure-related skin and soft tissue ulceration, as described. There are also inherent procedural risks, including nasopharyngeal injury, epistaxis, and even pneumothorax. Significantly more pulmonary complications occurred in patients with nasogastric tubes placed routinely, although there was no difference in wound-related complications when compared with selective placement of tubes for vomiting and gastric distention.[2]

Patients undergoing laparotomy or other surgical procedures may be intolerant of intragastric nutrition or medication administration in the early postoperative period. Akin to GI intubation for decompression, the benefit of accessing the GI tract for nutritive and/or pharmaceutical reasons must be weighed against the potential risks. Further, the addition of a surgically created enteral access must be considered if the patient is anticipated to be unable to take sufficient calories by mouth in the longer postoperative period (see the decision tree in Fig. 58.1). The feasibility of placement, potential duration of use, and route of enteral access are equally important considerations in determining the optimal intestinal intubation for nutrition. Gastric access for feeding may be of little value or even detrimental in patients with a high risk for aspiration or impaired gastric emptying. Decisions should be based on consideration of underlying medical and comorbid conditions, the anticipated length of time that enteral access will be required, and the setting in which it will occur. Some conditions may offer relative contraindications or completely preclude enteral intubation. Obstructions of the nasopharynx, esophagus, or proximal stomach are absolute contraindications to nasoenteric intubations, and usually contraindicate any endoscopically placed tubes. Coagulopathy, ascites, obesity, previous abdominal surgery, and gastroesophageal varices are all relative contraindications to enteral tube placement by any method.

NASOGASTRIC AND NASOENTERIC INTUBATION

GI intubation is a well-established diagnostic and therapeutic modality with a long record of experience. Early descriptions of nasogastric tubes and intestinal intubation date from the 17th century.[3] Modern tubes are known eponymously for the individual who introduced them into clinical practice. In 1921, Levin described a single lumen catheter fenestrated at the distal end for decompression with low intermittent suction or gravity drainage, or feeding.[4] A modification of the Levin tube is now widely used and known as a *Salem sump*.[4a] The Salem sump tube has a second lumen that permits air to be withdrawn into the stomach, or sump, during suctioning, thereby avoiding adherence of the tube to the gastric mucosa, and possible injury. This tube is used most commonly today for GI decompression in the setting of gastroparesis, mechanical bowel obstruction, or functional inertia of the bowel or ileus.

In 1934, Miller and Abbott first introduced a long, balloon-tipped intestinal tube designed to pass into the intestine via gentle advancement and peristalsis; subsequent modifications included percutaneous, weighted, multilumen, and silicone models. Temporary placement of a long tube into the small intestine for decompression was described by White in 1956 and was later popularized by Baker, who devised his own eponymous tube.[5–7] Generally, long tubes have weighted or balloon-tipped ends and are intended to pass distally to provide intestinal or gastric decompression.

TABLE 58.1 Enteral Access: Common Methods With Indications and Contraindications

Route	Dx	Tx	Indication	Contraindications
Nasogastric	X	X	Decompression, ileus, obstruction, upper GI bleeding, toxic ingestion	Nasopharyngeal obstruction, esophageal varices, coagulopathy, thrombocytopenia, craniofacial trauma, profound neutropenia
Nasoenteric	X	X	Enteral nutrition, medication administration, traumatic brain injury	Long-term nutritional need >14 days, craniofacial injury
Gastric (PEG)		X	Malnutrition, head and neck cancer, cerebrovascular accident, traumatic brain injury, prolonged intubation or coma, respiratory failure	Delayed gastric emptying, gastroparesis, gastric outlet obstruction, recent foregut surgery
Gastric (open)		X	Same as PEG, plus inability to perform endoscopy	Same as PEG
Intestinal (jejunal)		X	Concomitant surgery with other indications, gastric outlet obstruction, severe malnutrition, gastroparesis, pancreatitis, fistula	Short bowel syndrome, distal obstruction, inability to provide continuous infusion

Dx, Diagnostic; *GI,* gastrointestinal; *PEG,* percutaneous endoscopic gastrostomy; *Tx,* therapeutic.
Modified from Ponsky JL, Chukwumah CV. Intubation of the stomach and small intestine. In: Yeo CJ, ed. *Shackelford's Surgery of the Alimentary Tract.* 7th ed. Philadelphia: Saunders; 2013.

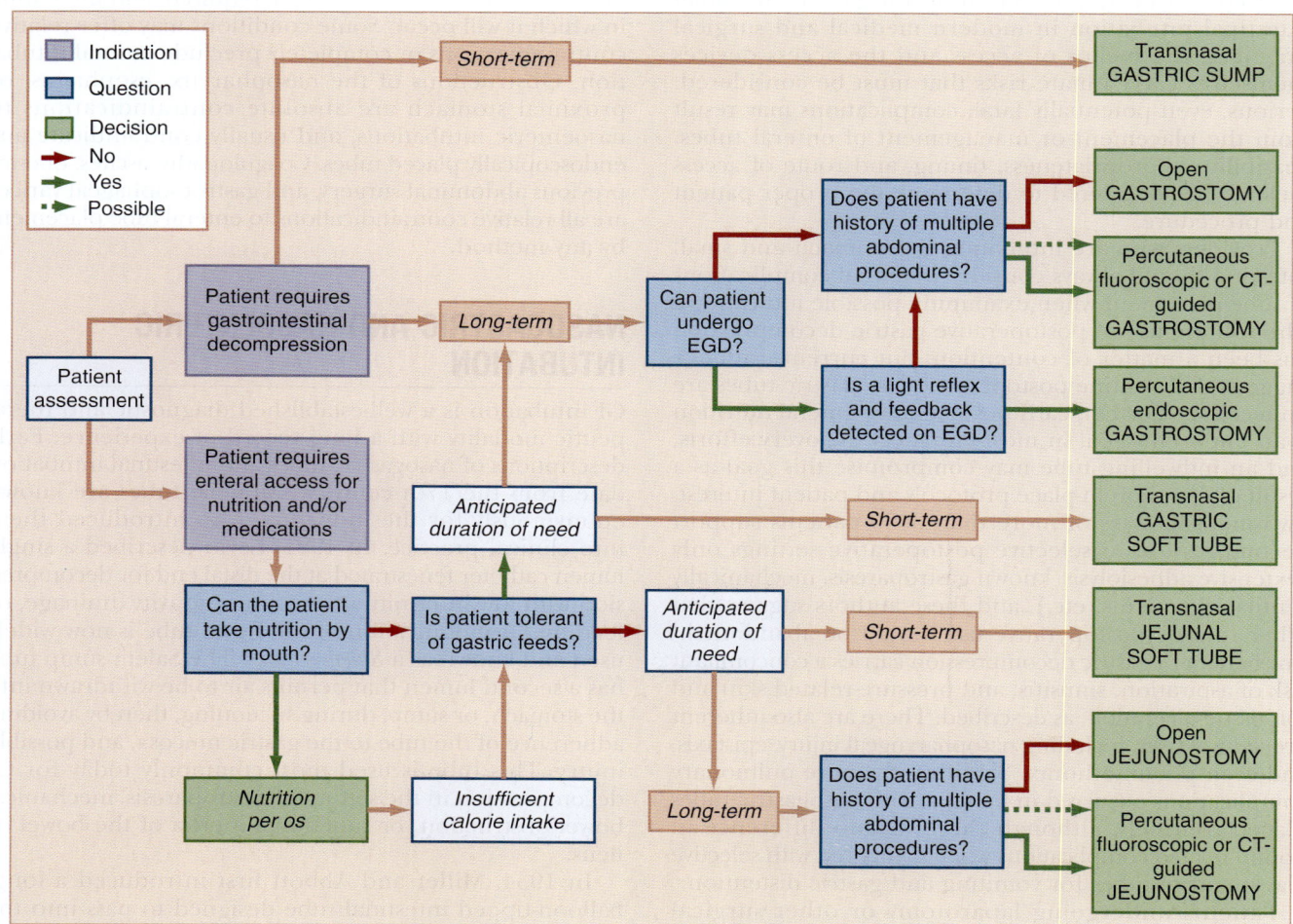

FIGURE 58.1 Decision tree for gastric/small intestine intubation and methodologies for possible techniques and devices. *CT,* Computed tomography; *EGD,* esophagogastroduodenoscopy; *per os,* by mouth. (Created by David S. Shapiro, MD.)

Nasoenteric tubes designed for feeding are similar to long tubes and are intended to traverse the pylorus, but unlike decompressive tubes, they are generally of smaller caliber and made of softer materials than standard sump or long tubes. These tubes often require a stiffening stylus for passage and manipulation. The most widely used of these tubes, introduced by Dobbie and Hoffmeister in the 1970s, is now recognized as the *Dobbhoff tube.* The tip of this tube is slightly larger and heavier than the remainder of the catheter, which may or may not facilitate passage with the pylorus.[8] Unassisted bedside placement into a postpyloric position can be simple, and a multitude of methodologies have been suggested. Promotility agents, patient positioning, insufflation of air, and other methods have been advocated to assist with advancement into a postpyloric position, but results are mixed. Endoscopic, radiologic, magnetic, and electromagnetic methods have been described, and will be discussed later.

INDICATIONS

Obstruction and the need for decompression are the most common indications for nasogastric and nasoenteric intubation. Less commonly, intubation of the stomach or small intestine is used for diagnostic or therapeutic means, including gastric lavage and evacuation of gastric contents in the initial management of upper GI bleeding or toxic ingestion. Diagnostic uses are numerous and include aspiration to determine the presence of drugs or toxins, measurement of gastric secretions, volume of output, or pH, and for the procurement of specimens for culture of *Mycobacterium* or *Helicobacter pylori*. Therapeutic uses for gastric and enteral intubation are well defined. Decompression of air or enteric contents is very common, and is often used in the setting of ileus, mechanical bowel obstruction, gastric dilation, perioperative gastric drainage, or reduction of aspiration risk in select patients. The routine use of postoperative nasogastric decompression after abdominal surgery has fallen out of favor. The evidence does suggest that selective use in patients with the indications listed earlier, including chronic nausea and vomiting, is associated with more frequent pulmonary complications than routine postoperative tube decompression.[9] Decompression is integral to the management of intestinal obstruction; it relieves any advancement of fluid or gas from the stomach and can be used to determine improvement because the volume of output will decrease if the obstruction improves.

In terms of decompressive treatment of intestinal obstruction, nasogastric decompression was often sufficient to relieve the obstruction from the influx of air and fluid. In the case of partial intestinal obstruction, decompression may effect relief of obstruction within 48 hours. Persistent obstructions will warrant further diagnostic investigation and possible operative management. In patients with suspected complete intestinal obstruction, nasogastric intubation is important in the preoperative resuscitative period to decompress the stomach and minimize aspiration, but surgical management remains the mainstay of therapy.

Intraluminal plication of at-risk bowel following extensive adhesiolysis using a long tube (Baker, Cantor, others) has been described and evaluated in the literature. Although the technique is encouraged by some, it has gradually fallen out of favor because complications associated with an enterostomy-placed Baker tube are prohibitive. Nasally introduced tubes have been suggested as having efficacy in decompression of partially obstructed bowel, but the results are mixed. However, without gastric decompression, symptomatic relief from nausea and/or emesis may not be achieved. One randomized control study comparing short and long decompressive tubes demonstrated no advantage.[10] Although others have described long tubes as a secondary treatment and have anecdotally noted value in this legacy therapy, most have abandoned it.

CONTRAINDICATIONS

Soft feeding tubes (Dobbhoff, Keofeed, Cortrak and similar tubes) are smaller bore and useful for gastric or postpyloric feeding and may be placed at bedside transnasally. Nasoenteric access is a simple, useful, and reasonably comfortable means of enteral access when desired in patients with indications. Contraindications to nasoenteral access include nasopharyngeal obstruction, esophageal obstruction or perforation, recent foregut manipulation or surgery, and craniofacial trauma. While orogastric intubation is the preferred route for access in the presence of craniofacial trauma, it may not be practical in the patient without a secured airway. Coagulopathy is also an important contraindication when intubation is placed for nonurgent purposes to avoid epistaxis or other bleeding.

METHODS OF BEDSIDE INTUBATION

Nasoenteric intubation is easily done at the bedside, but despite the simplicity of the procedure, it can have several pitfalls leading to complications. Patients vary in their level of cooperation, alertness, and cognitive capacity. Consent should be obtained according to institutional requirements, and should include an assessment of benefits, risks, and experience.

For patients who are awake, alert, and cooperative, Fowler position is helpful with a 90-degree angle preferred. A chair may be used, but a stretcher or bed may provide better patient comfort. The patient's neck should be slightly flexed to avoid endotracheal placement. The patient should be in a quiet room because distractions can be problematic. The patient should understand the reason for the procedure, the steps involved, and be prepared for the uncomfortable nature of nasogastric intubation. Parenteral anxiolytic and analgesic agents are usually not necessary, and can complicate appropriate passage.

Assessment for nasal passage patency is important, especially in a patient with a history of septum abnormality. An emesis basin and protective barrier (towel, drape) may be helpful to the patient. Inhalation through the nose with each nostril sequentially obstructed can help decide which passage to use.

The tube should be warmed by sliding it repeatedly through gloved hands to soften the structure and create a slight curve in the tube. Most tubes are marked with centimeter indicators to identify the length of the indwelling section, but some may be unlabeled. The correct distance of insertion should be about 50 cm for intragastric placement, and usually more than 65 cm for postpyloric placement.

Prior to insertion, a water-based lubricant with or without local topical anesthetic (2% lidocaine, viscous) should be applied to the tube and to the nasal passages. Anesthetic sprays (benzocaine, butamben) may also be used, but will not offer any lubrication.

The tube is inserted into the nostril with a trajectory toward the posterior nasopharynx, parallel to the patient's ipsilateral angle of the jaw or pinnae. The tube should not be inserted in the cephalad direction because this will result in the tube curling in the nasopharynx or trauma to the nasal mucosa. Maintaining the tube along the floor of the nasal passage may facilitate entry into the posterior pharynx. As the tube reaches the posterior nasopharynx and some mild resistance is met, gentle pressure will facilitate the tip of the tube turning caudally to descend into the oropharynx.

The patient may be given a cup of water with a straw and permitted to sip steadily and swallow water (once the tube is inserted and the first resistance is met), which facilitates closing the epiglottis and allowing directed passage into the upper esophagus. Patients who experience severe pain, gagging, anxiety coughing, respiratory distress, or significant resistance noted by the inserter should be permitted respite before subsequent attempts are made. Gagging, coughing, or other respiratory distress may be signs of laryngeal passage and should prompt the provider to remove the tube and restart.

Once passage into the esophagus is successful, the tube should continue to advance until the desired depth is reached. Once in the stomach, at about 50 to 55 cm, the tube's position should be assessed. Confirmation of tube placement should be accomplished prior to using the tube for any indication, and many methods have been described.

Insufflation with auscultation alone is an unreliable technique, and although it may be helpful in the distal tube position for some providers, it should not be the only method used to confirm location. Aspiration of enteric or gastric material may also offer confidence in some settings, but the tube contents are unclear during passage and there is no proof of tip location. Radiographic evidence remains the mainstay for tip location confirmation and should be performed routinely after intubation. Contrast may be required in some settings to determine the course of the tube, and thinned solutions of barium are likely the least expensive and simplest to use. Devices currently exist that use electromagnetic sensors at the tube tip (Cortrak, CORPAK MedSystems, Buffalo Grove, Illinois), and have been reviewed (Fig. 58.2). Retrospective and prospective studies exist demonstrating reliable use of an active positioning detection system to follow the tube as it is passed by the provider. Systems using real-time imaging to provide gastric or small bowel intubation are useful bedside adjuvants to the provider, and provide a level of confidence. Resistance, patient symptoms, and training of personnel should be considered when deciding how best to confirm location. In experienced hands, electromagnetic detection is useful and provides cost savings with respect to radiographic imaging, but is not yet the gold standard.[11] Placement in the respiratory system occurred in up to 3.2% of patients in one study, and pneumothorax occurred in up to 1.2%, with an associated mortality.[12-14] These authors advocate a simple multimodality method for confirmation, including an experienced procedurist, accurate reporting regarding ease of passage, patient symptoms and signs, and the use of routine electromagnetic detection with selective radiographic imaging or with routine radiographic imaging. The risk of pneumothorax, intrapleural placement (and

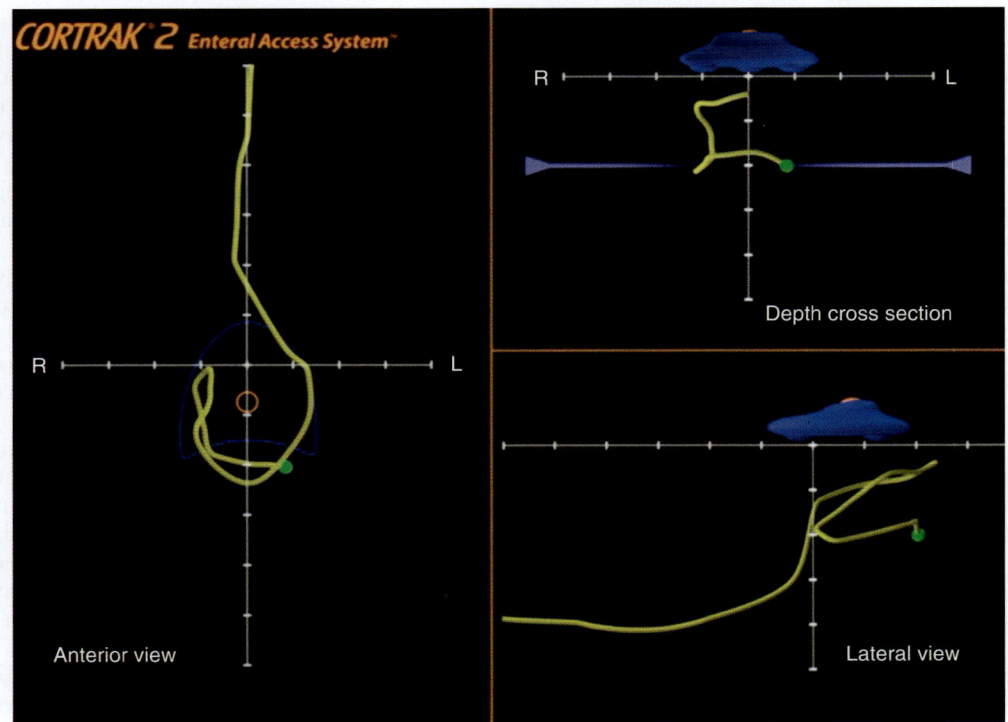

FIGURE 58.2 The Cortrak2 Enteral Access System provides direct feedback from an electromagnetic tip in an enclosed tube system. The device is followed in real time and provides a map of tube passage.

subsequent administration of nutrition), or other complications, although low, has dramatic and morbid complications that should be regarded as "never events" in the realm of patient safety.

ACCESS TO THE STOMACH OR SMALL INTESTINE

Access to the stomach or small intestine may be provided by any number of interventions or devices. Access may be endeavored for either enteral nutritional support or decompression and other therapeutics. Access for nutrition may include multiple methods. Tube access can provide a route for cyclic bolus feedings, which are physiologically more advantageous because they mirror normal daily functional eating. This type of bolus nutrition is sometimes impractical in the inpatient setting, and therefore continuous enteral support is provided by intragastric or postpyloric continuous feeding. Although these may be provided by nasoenteric routes as described earlier, the duration of need should be part of the decision tree to select the nasoenteric route versus nonnasoenteric, or more invasive, methods. Decision making should include discussions of feeding technique as well. Cyclic bolus feedings into the stomach result in variations in blood insulin levels, resulting in lipolysis and the preferred anabolic state.[15] Gastric atony and cholestasis may also be improved by intragastric nutrition. Gastric intubation is also more simply accomplished than postpyloric or jejunal access because it can be performed at the bedside without sedation or special equipment in most situations. Pharyngeal obstruction, foregut surgery, hiatal hernia, esophageal pathology including varices, and other sequelae of portal hypertension, among other concerns, may be contraindications to direct transnasal or transoral access. Furthermore, long-term nutritional support, especially in skilled nursing facilities and centers for rehabilitation, may preclude the temporary nature of the nasogastric or orogastric route. These patients may require a more appropriate surgical or procedure-based method of providing enteral nutrition (see Fig. 58.1, Decision Tree). Short-term versus long-term needs may be arbitrary in some settings, but if enteral nutrition is required for more than 14 days in a patient who cannot tolerate sufficient nutrition orally, more definitive tube-based nutrition is indicated. In addition, anesthetic risk assessments, anatomic limitations, body habitus, prior abdominal surgery, gastroparesis or gastric obstruction, insufficient absorptive intestinal surface, and inflammatory bowel disease may be contraindications to particular methodologies.

PROCEDURES FOR INTUBATION OF THE STOMACH AND SMALL INTESTINE

GASTROSTOMY

A gastrostomy is an opening created in the wall of the stomach that connects to the skin through the abdominal wall. The wall of the anterior stomach is apposed directly to the parietal peritoneum by sutures and/or by the tube itself. This leads to the existence of a planned gastrocutaneous fistula, and is the most common form of long-term enteral access performed by surgeons. This form of enteral access is preferred because it minimizes patient discomfort in the long term, eliminates the nasal passage irritation associated with transnasal enteral access devices, and obviates the need for frequent changes because of clogging or inadvertent removal of the tube. Multiple surgical techniques have been described for the insertion of gastrostomies including open techniques, endoscopically placed tubes, and laparoscopic maneuvers.

Open Gastrostomy

The open approach for gastrostomy tube placement is performed most commonly in the technique described by Martin Stamm in 1894. The procedure is performed under operating room conditions and via a small upper midline incision. The greater omentum and transverse colon are identified and gently retracted downward to identify the stomach. The stomach is grasped and manual traction is applied upward to identify a relatively avascular site along the anterior aspect of the greater curvature to place the tube. This area ideally should be away from the pylorus and antrum and without undue tension on the stomach. Once the site is chosen, a stab incision is made in the left upper quadrant of the abdomen away from the course of the epigastric vessels and approximately 2 to 3 finger breadths below the costal margin. The tract is made by passage of a blunt clamp through the skin incision and into the peritoneal cavity using firm but controlled pressure with attention to avoid visceral injury. Electrocautery can be useful to assist the surgeon by making an opening in the peritoneal layer at the point of contact with the clamp. Many different tubes may be used, but a 22- or 24-French tube with a balloon or mushroom tip is commonly selected. The tube is passed through the abdominal wall using the in situ clamp. The surgeon may create a single or double purse string at the chosen site with permanent suture. The purse strings should accommodate the chosen tube's diameter without redundant serosa and should be placed before the gastrostomy is made. These sutures are left untied for tying after the tube has been passed. A gastrostomy is made in the center of the purse-string suture using electrocautery, and the tube is passed through the gastrostomy and advanced several centimeters into the gastric lumen (Fig. 58.3). If the tube has a balloon, it is now inflated and the purse-string sutures are carefully tied to secure the tube. Careful attention must be used to avoid balloon puncture during fixation. Four to six stay sutures are placed around the gastrostomy (Fig. 58.4) to affix the anterior wall of the stomach to the anterior wall entry site on the parietal peritoneum (Figs. 58.5 and 58.6). These are usually silk sutures. The tube is secured to the skin using nylon sutures. The abdominal incision is closed in the customary manner.

Percutaneous Endoscopic Gastrostomy

The percutaneous endoscopic gastrostomy (PEG), an endoscopically placed gastrostomy tube, has allowed for safe and efficient placement of long-term feeding access without the requirement of prolonged general anesthesia or a laparotomy incision. Few contraindications exist for PEG, but include upper abdominal surgery, patients with

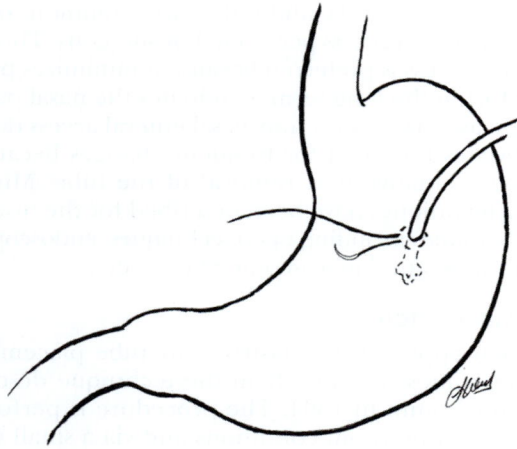

FIGURE 58.3 A single purse string is left untied as the gastrostomy tube is passed into the stomach. (Illustration by Jacob Wood, MD.)

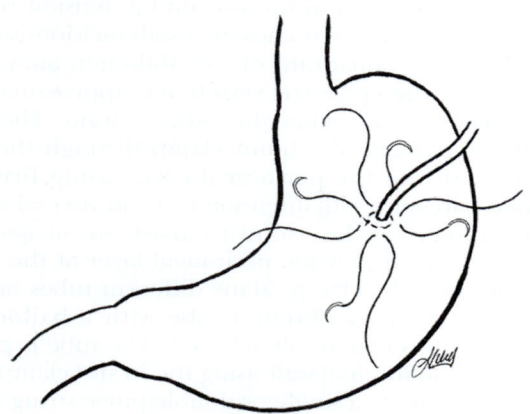

FIGURE 58.4 The stay sutures are placed circumferentially around the tied purse-string sutures, ready for gastropexy. (Illustration by Jacob Wood, MD.)

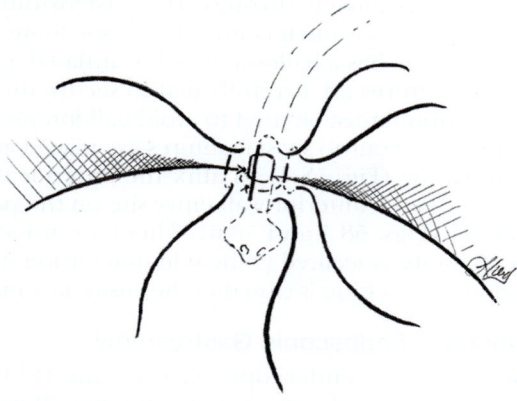

FIGURE 58.5 The stomach is advanced toward the parietal peritoneum near the entry site of the gastrostomy tube. As the stomach and abdominal wall become apposed, the lateral-most suture should be secured first. (Illustration by Jacob Wood, MD.)

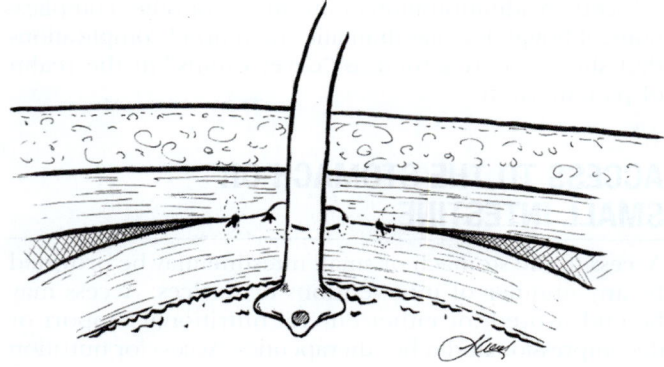

FIGURE 58.6 The completed Stamm gastrostomy, with gastropexy sutures secured and the tube in good intragastric position. (Illustration by Jacob Wood, MD.)

ascites, or other recent abdominal surgical procedures. The two most frequently used techniques for PEG placement include the "push" and the "pull" methods. Both approaches may be performed in the operating room, in the endoscopy suite, or at the bedside with careful monitoring of vital signs and procedural tolerance. Appropriate anesthesia is usually obtained with conscious sedation and infiltration of local anesthesia at the surgical site just prior to incision. The patient's upper abdominal hair is clipped, the abdomen is prepared with surgical preparatory solution, and sterile draping is applied. Both the push and pull methods use esophagogastroscopy and air insufflation of the stomach. The gastroscope is carefully advanced into the stomach once the patient is appropriately sedated. Careful inspection of the esophagus and stomach should be performed prior to the procedure to assess any pathologic findings or contraindications. The endoscopist then looks toward the anterior gastric wall with the scope. At this point, the surgeon inspects the anterior abdominal wall for transillumination from the endoscope. Transillumination settings are usually available on most gastroscopic apparatus and should be used to assist in visualization. The area that is brightly transilluminated is then palpated by a single finger on the abdominal wall to assess for a prominent indentation seen in the interior of the stomach (Fig. 58.7). This maneuver, sometimes referred to as "finger feedback" continues until the area that corresponds to the best gastric indentation and bright transillumination is noted. Careful consideration and time spent at this stage of the procedure may help reduce procedural complications such as transcolonic passage. The chosen area is anesthetized with local anesthetic while the endoscopist places a snare through the gastroscope channel and maneuvers into position, ready for deployment. The assistant makes a small, usually transverse, skin incision measuring approximately 1 cm and passes the PEG kit catheter-over-needle cannula through the incision and into the gastric lumen. This should be done in one swift motion to decrease the incidence of the needle displacing the stomach away from the anterior abdominal wall, and it should be performed under scope visualization. The snare is maneuvered to encircle the cannula and is tightened around it. The cannula inner needle is

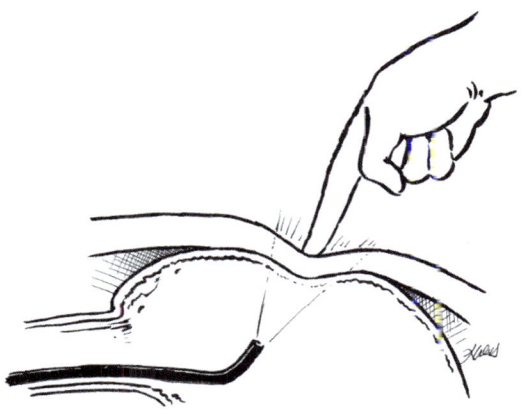

FIGURE 58.7 The "light reflex" or transillumination step and "finger feedback" step during a percutaneous endoscopic gastrostomy identifying the stomach to be immediately apposed to the abdominal wall. (Illustration by Jacob Wood, MD.)

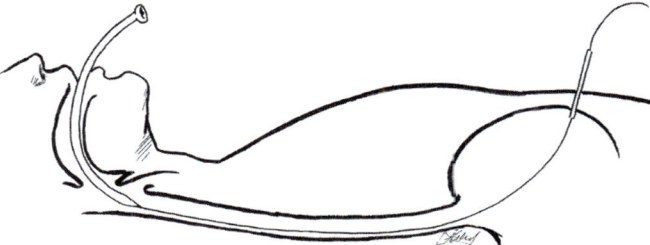

FIGURE 58.9 The guidewire has been passed through the abdominal wall, into the stomach, and pulled up through the mouth. Here, the percutaneous endoscopic gastrostomy tube is advanced to just beyond the oropharynx into the esophagus, and can be pushed or pulled along the guidewire. (Illustration by Jacob Wood, MD.)

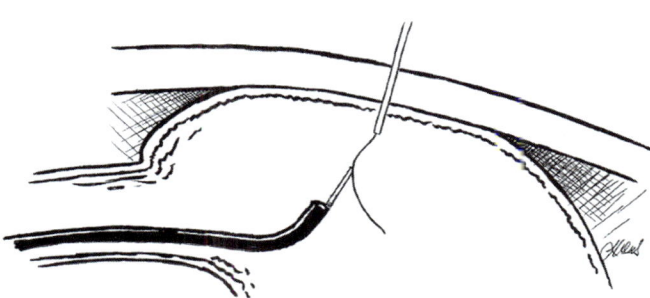

FIGURE 58.8 During a percutaneous endoscopic gastrostomy, the snare is used to grasp the guidewire. (Illustration by Jacob Wood, MD.)

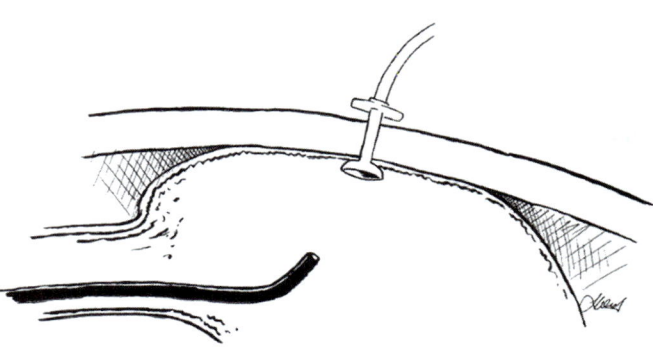

FIGURE 58.10 The completed percutaneous endoscopic gastrostomy (PEG) in good position. Note the securing bolster is not immediately against the skin, but instead limits the movement of the PEG tube. (Illustration by Jacob Wood, MD.)

subsequently removed and a guidewire is passed through in a Seldinger-like technique, into the gastric lumen. After several centimeters of the wire have been advanced, the snare is loosened slightly to allow the cannula to be pulled from the stomach. The snare is retightened to firmly grasp the wire alone (Fig. 58.8). The endoscopist then withdraws the scope from the patient and the wire is pulled along with the snare. The assistant must ensure that the wire is easily advanced. Using the most common pull method, the gastroscope is removed and the gastrostomy tube, equipped with a wire loop, is affixed to the guidewire exiting the patient's mouth and the assistant exerts gentle traction on the wire traversing the abdominal wall (Fig. 58.9). This gentle pulling moves the gastrostomy tube down the patient's esophagus and into the stomach and finally exits the skin incision. In the push method, the gastrostomy tube is threaded over the guidewire withdrawn through the patient's mouth. The gastroscope is removed and the wire is passed through the gastrostomy tube until it is completely through the tube. The tube is gently pushed along the wire until the long, tapered tip passes through the incision. This is somewhat facilitated by slight tension being exerted on the abdominal side of the guidewire. Of note, the tubes are often equipped with a stiffened, disposable end that exits first through the skin. The junction of the soft tube and the stiffened end usually

is the largest diameter, and the skin incision must accommodate this easily. In either method, once the tube emerges from the skin incision, it is grasped and pulled gently upward until the intraluminal button is in contact with the gastric mucosa. During the placement, the intragastric end of the tube or "button" will reach the patient's mouth prior to being passed into the patient. At this point, we advocate the reintroduction of the gastroscope to inspect the placement of the tube and to verify that it is in proper position without undue tension (Fig. 58.10). The button should be in close but sufficiently loose contact with the mucosa. These authors advocate spinning the tube on its axis; if the mucosa is seen to move with the button, it is too tight. At this point, the outer bolster is affixed to the tube and pushed carefully to rest at skin level to maintain this position. The bolster should not be advanced to the point that it applies pressure to the skin and a distance of 2 to 3 mm from the skin is appropriate. The bolster may be sutured to the skin, but this step is unnecessary with contemporary tubes. The use of occlusive dressings is universally discouraged because it encourages infection. Routine and uncomplicated insertion of PEGs can be done immediately following the procedure.

Jejunostomy

The most common operative approach for the open jejunostomy is the Witzel technique, named for Friedrich

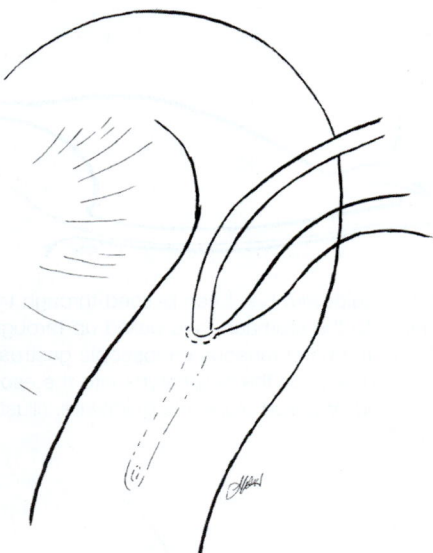

FIGURE 58.11 A single purse string is placed in the small intestine wall, and left untied as the tube is placed into the lumen. (Illustration by Jacob Wood, MD.)

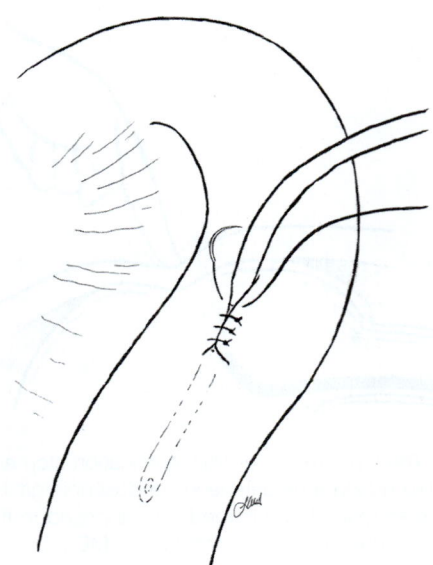

FIGURE 58.12 Prior to the enteropexy, a "tunnel" is created in a Witzel enterostomy, imbricating serosa of the small intestine to secure the tube, and creating a functional "one-way valve." Should the tube become dislodged, the likelihood of leakage of succus entericus is decreased. (Illustration by Jacob Wood, MD.)

Witzel (1865–1925). During a laparotomy, the surgeon must first identify the ligament of Treitz and then progress along the jejunum until a point 15 to 20 cm distally. This chosen area should be sufficiently mobile to allow for tension-free apposition to the anterior abdominal wall. A silk purse string is placed around the desired point of entry of the tube. A small stab incision is made in the center of the purse-string suture. The chosen catheter (usually a 12- to 18-French catheter) is then threaded into the lumen of the jejunum and care is taken to ensure that the catheter tip is directed distally (Fig. 58.11). The purse string is gently secured. A tunnel is created by imbricating the serosa over the tube for approximately 6 to 8 cm (Fig. 58.12) using the Lembert technique and silk suture. Once completed, the loop of intestine is anchored to the parietal peritoneum using silk suture (Fig. 58.13). The surgeon should continually assess and reassess the enterostomy to ensure that it is securely anchored. The enteropexy should be secure and be sufficiently broad to help decrease the likelihood of tube rotation around the newly created fixed point, resulting in an obstruction.

Combination or Multilumen Tubes

In a specific set of patients, it is necessary to provide postpyloric enteral nutrition at the same time that gastric decompression is indicated. In this case, a multilumen tube is very useful. These tubes may be assisted fluoroscopically via the endoscope, or at laparotomy. The operative technique is identical to the Stamm gastrostomy tube, but prior to securing the purse strings, the tube is advanced into the jejunum by hand or using a commercially available device guide. Whichever method is chosen, transgastric jejunal tubes usually pass through the pylorus, or through a newly created gastrojejunostomy. This can sometimes be difficult. The surgeon must ensure that care is taken

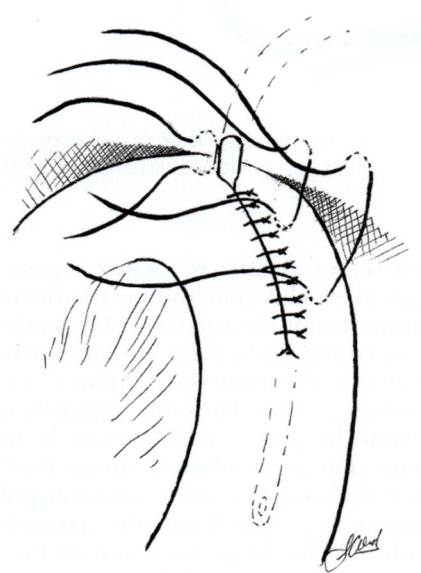

FIGURE 58.13 The Witzel enterostomy is secured to the abdominal wall with separate silk sutures, creating a broad-based enteropexy to avoid obstruction or twisting. (Illustration by Jacob Wood, MD.)

not to cause jejunal or duodenal perforation during the procedure. If clinically warranted, an existing gastrostomy may have a fluoroscopy-assisted conversion to a multilumen tube in a similar manner.

Other Devices

In addition to fluoroscopy assistance in tube placement, percutaneous methods exist via our interventional radiology colleagues. Occasionally, computed tomography or sonography is used to achieve access. This may be facilitated by the use of effervescent material given by mouth or via nasogastric or nasoenteric means. The tubes placed percutaneously are usually of smaller caliber, and are subject to occlusion with medications, nutritional material, or other means.

MANAGEMENT AND COMPLICATIONS OF INTESTINAL TUBES

Recent literature has diminished concern raised on the safety of early enteral feeding of newly placed intestinal tubes and instead highlighted its benefits, including shorter hospital length of stay, with no increase in the risk of anastomotic leak, pneumonia, readmission, reoperation, or mortality.[16] Typically, surgeons choose to begin feeds within 24 hours after tube placement, regardless of the method that was chosen to place the tube. It is common practice to begin feeding at a low rate and increase as tolerated until the goal rate is reached; however some surgeons advocate beginning at the goal rate if the patient was tolerating the goal rate preoperatively.

Reported rates of gastrostomy complications vary from 0.4% to 22.5% of patients.[17,18] Most of these complications are minor, but life-threatening complications can and do occur. The surgeon should remain vigilant and treat them assertively. Infection of the gastrostomy site is a common complication and an infection is reported to occur once for every 2.1 years that a gastrostomy is in situ.[19] Signs of a gastrostomy site infection include leakage of feeds, erythema of the site, purulent drainage, and induration of the skin. Local wound care usually suffices; however, patients sometimes require a local incision-and-drainage procedure if abscess formation has occurred. Antibiotics may also be indicated.

Undue tension on a gastrostomy tube can cause the internal fixation device (the button or balloon) to migrate through the tract and cause "buried bumper" syndrome and eventually a larger gastrocutaneous fistula. Excessive compression of the tissue between the external bumper and the internal fixation device is the main causative factor, but any force that acts to pull the tube away from the patient, as when the tube is placed for gravity drainage or with frequent pulling or manipulation by the patient or provider, can also cause problems. Care should be taken at initial operation to avoid unnecessarily tight bolster placement, and caution should be exercised over the lifetime of the tube to regularly ensure its position, avoid slippage of the bolster, and avoid any excess compression of the skin. Additionally, if the bolster becomes loose, the internal fixation device on the tube may migrate too far *into* the lumen. This could result in luminal obstruction of the intestine. In this case, simply pulling the tube back to the proper position and re-securing the bolster is all that is required.

Inadvertent removal of the intestinal tube is a common complication that occurs in 2.5% to 12.8% of patients.[18,20,21] If the tube has been in place for a period of time that supports permanent tract formation (>10 to 14 days), a replacement tube may be reinserted along the tract, but a contrast study to confirm placement in the lumen is imperative. This process can be time consuming and costly and care should be taken to avoid this preventable issue. If the tube has been in place for fewer than 10 to 14 days, immediate laparotomy and replacement of the tube is indicated. Some providers advocate for an abdominal binder or girdle to secure transabdominal tubes. Caution must be used to avoid pressure, shear injury, or other phenomena, but this can keep patients without sufficient motor control from unintentional dislodgement of their access.

SUMMARY

Many indications exist for enteral access in surgical patients, including nutritional support and decompression of the GI tract. Practicing surgeons should be well versed in the indications, techniques, and complications associated with each method and carefully consider the options for their patients.

REFERENCES

1. Nelson R, Tse B, Edwards S. Systematic review of prophylactic nasogastric decompression after abdominal operations. *Br J Surg.* 2005;92(6):673-680.
2. Cheatham ML, Chapman WC, Key SP, Sawyers JL. A meta-analysis of selective versus routine nasogastric decompression after elective laparotomy. *Ann Surg.* 1995;221(5):469-476, [discussion 476–468].
3. Boyes RJ, Kruse JA. Nasogastric and nasoenteric intubation. *Crit Care Clin.* 1992;8(4):865-878.
4. Levin A. A new gastroduodenal catheter. *J Am Med Assoc.* 1921;76:1007.
4a. McConnell EA. Ensuring safer stomach suctioning with the Salem sump tube. *Nursing.* 1977;7(9):54-57.
5. Baker JW. A long jejunostomy tube for decompressing intestinal obstruction. *Surg Gynecol Obstet.* 1959;109:518-520.
6. Baker JW. Stitchless plication for recurring obstruction of the small bowel. *Am J Surg.* 1968;116(2):316-324.
7. White RR. Prevention of recurrent small bowel obstruction due to adhesions. *Ann Surg.* 1956;143(5):714-719.
8. Levenson R, Turner WW Jr, Dyson A, Zike L, Reisch J. Do weighted nasoenteric feeding tubes facilitate duodenal intubations? *JPEN J Parenter Enteral Nutr.* 1988;12(2):135-137.
9. Wolff BG, Pemberton JH, van Heerden JA, et al. Elective colon and rectal surgery without nasogastric decompression. A prospective, randomized trial. *Ann Surg.* 1989;209(6):670-673, [discussion 673–675].
10. Fleshner PR, Siegman MG, Slater GI, Brolin RE, Chandler JC, Aufses AH Jr. A prospective, randomized trial of short versus long tubes in adhesive small-bowel obstruction. *Am J Surg.* 1995;170(4):366-370.
11. Metheny NA, Meert KL. Effectiveness of an electromagnetic feeding tube placement device in detecting inadvertent respiratory placement. *Am J Crit Care.* 2014;23(3):240-247, [quiz 248].
12. Koopmann MC, Kudsk KA, Szotkowski MJ, Rees SM. A team-based protocol and electromagnetic technology eliminate feeding tube placement complications. *Ann Surg.* 2011;253(2):287-302.
13. October TW, Hardart GE. Successful placement of postpyloric enteral tubes using electromagnetic guidance in critically ill children. *Pediatr Crit Care Med.* 2009;10(2):196-200.
14. Powers J, Luebbehusen M, Spitzer T, et al. Verification of an electromagnetic placement device compared with abdominal radiograph to predict accuracy of feeding tube placement. *JPEN J Parenter Enteral Nutr.* 2011;35(4):535-539.
15. Davidson P, Kwiatkowski CA, Wien M. Management of hyperglycemia and enteral nutrition in the hospitalized patient. *Nutr Clin Pract.* 2015;30(5):652-659.
16. Willcutts KF, Chung MC, Erenberg CL, Finn KL, Schirmer BD, Byham-Gray LD. Early oral feeding as compared with traditional timing of oral feeding after upper gastrointestinal surgery: a systematic review and meta-analysis. *Ann Surg.* 2016;264:54-63.

17. Cyrany J, Rejchrt S, Kopacova M, Bures J. Buried bumper syndrome: a complication of percutaneous endoscopic gastrostomy. *World J Gastroenterol.* 2016;22(2):618-627.

18. Vanis N, Saray A, Gornjakovic S, Mesihovic R. Percutaneous endoscopic gastrostomy (PEG): retrospective analysis of a 7-year clinical experience. *Acta Inform Med.* 2012;20(4):235-237.

19. Clarke E, Pitts N, Latchford A, Lewis S. A large prospective audit of morbidity and mortality associated with feeding gastrostomies in the community. *Clin Nutr.* 2016;doi:10.1016/j.clnu.2016.01.008.

20. Rosenberger LH, Newhook T, Schirmer B, Sawyer RG. Late accidental dislodgement of a percutaneous endoscopic gastrostomy tube: an underestimated burden on patients and the health care system. *Surg Endosc.* 2011;25(10):3307-3311.

21. Ao P, Sebastianski M, Selvarajah V, Gramlich L. Comparison of complication rates, types, and average tube patency between jejunostomy tubes and percutaneous gastrostomy tubes in a regional home enteral nutrition support program. *Nutr Clin Pract.* 2015;30(3):393-397.

Surgery for Peptic Ulcer Disease

Abubaker Ali* | Bestoun H. Ahmed | Michael S. Nussbaum

Gastroduodenal peptic ulcer disease (PUD) is a common problem with significant geographic variation in prevalence. In Western countries the incidence of PUD has steadily declined. Recent population-based studies have shown a prevalence rate of 4% with 20% of patients having asymptomatic ulcers.[1] In developing countries, the prevalence is much higher. In a recent population-based study from China, 17.2% of the population had endoscopically documented duodenal or gastric ulcers; however, more than 70% of these patients were asymptomatic. Such variations are likely related to the prevalence of *Helicobacter pylori*, smoking, and use of ulcerogenic drugs, such as nonsteroidal antiinflammatory drugs (NSAIDs). In a systematic review of the literature covering developed countries, the annual incidence of PUD ranged from 0.1% to 0.19% for physician-diagnosed PUD and 0.01% to 0.17% when based upon hospitalized patients.[1] In a 1996 Veterans Affairs study the prevalence of PUD in *H. pylori*–positive patients was found to be 2%.[2]

In the United States, there has been a decrease in the prevalence and number of hospitalizations for PUD. Between 1993 and 2006 the rate of PUD-related admissions decreased by 30%, with a larger decrease in duodenal ulcer–related admissions than gastric ulcers. Such preferential decreases in duodenal versus gastric ulcer disease likely relate to testing for *H. pylori* and introduction of more potent and successful therapeutic regimens.[3] The advent of histamine H_2-receptor antagonists (H_2 blockers) in the 1970s was responsible for an initial 40% decrease in incidence of ulcer operations. The later development of proton pump inhibitors (PPIs) in the late 1980s led to further acid reduction and faster, more efficient healing of active ulcer disease. The development of PPIs has not only influenced elective medical management but also has had an effect in the emergency setting. When combined, PPIs and endoscopic treatment have further decreased the need for emergency operation.

PUD complications include bleeding, perforation, and gastric outlet obstruction. There has been a significant downward trend in the incidence of these complications. Although older studies demonstrated a stable or even an increase in the number of patients admitted with one of these complications, recent studies demonstrated that the rate of perforation and bleeding has been decreasing in the United States.[4] Complications of PUD vary depending on the geographic location, with bleeding being the most common in the United States, whereas obstruction may be more common in other locations in the world.[5,6]

Risk factors for peptic ulcer complications and their recurrence included NSAID and/or acetylsalicylic acid use, *H. pylori* infection, and ulcer size greater than or equal to 1 cm. PPI use has reduced the risk of peptic ulcer hemorrhage.[7]

Current indications for surgical intervention are as follows:
1. Protracted bleeding despite endoscopic therapy. Bleeding is the most common complication of PUD in the United States, with an incidence of approximately 100 per 100,000 population.
2. Perforation is the second most common with an annual incidence of 11 operations per 100,000 population. Perforations are associated with the highest rate of mortality.[5]
3. Obstruction occurs as a consequence of scarring following healing of prepyloric and/or duodenal ulcers.
4. Intractability despite maximum medical therapy is an uncommon indication for operation.
5. Inability to rule out cancer when an ulcer remains despite treatment and negative endoscopic biopsies. This is of particular importance with gastric ulcers.

The goals of surgical procedures are to
1. Permit ulcer healing
2. Prevent or treat ulcer complications
3. Address the underlying ulcer etiology
4. Minimize postoperative digestive consequences

No single procedure satisfies all of these objectives. To choose the best operation, the surgeon must consider the characteristics of the ulcer (location, chronicity, type of complication), the likely etiology (acid hypersecretion, drug induced, possible role of *H. pylori*), the patient (age, nutrition, comorbid illnesses, condition on presentation), and the operation (mortality rate, side effects). In some respects, all ulcer operations represent a compromise: The morbidity of ulcer disease is replaced by the morbidity of the operation. Finally, surgeon experience must play a role in the choice of operation; nowadays, most surgical residents complete their training with little experience with the more complex procedures. Undoubtedly this influences their choices for both elective and emergent operations.

HISTORY OF SURGICAL TREATMENT OF PEPTIC ULCER DISEASE

PHYSIOLOGIC DISCOVERY

Initial operations for ulcer disease were based on local control without a good understanding of the physiology involved. As the physiology of digestion and acid production was delineated, the operations changed and were subsequently shifted toward addressing the current understanding of the cause of PUD.

Benjamin Brodie, an English physiologist and surgeon, in 1814, described the vagus nerves and their connection

*Supported by a grant from the Foundation for Surgical Fellowships.

with the production of gastric acid. Then in 1822, William Beaumont, an army surgeon, cared for Alexis St. Martin, a man who sustained a shotgun wound to the abdomen. Beaumont treated his wound but expected him to die; however, the patient survived and was left with a gastrocutaneous fistula. In 1825 Beaumont began to study the patient's digestive process by tying food to a string and inserting it through the fistula into the stomach and observe how it had been digested. He also studied the gastric fluid from the fistula. In 1833 Beaumont published his findings as *Experiments and Observations on the Gastric Juice, and the Physiology of Digestion.*[8]

The discovery of the three separate, yet related, phases of gastric secretion and its involvement in the consumption and digestion of a meal defined the surgical treatment of PUD. The cephalic, gastric, and to a lesser extent the intestinal phases are examples of physiologic discovery molding surgical practice. Ivan Pavlov, a Russian physiologist and physician, described the cephalic phase of gastric secretion. Through his physiologic studies with dogs, Pavlov showed that stimulation of the vagus nerves resulted in the secretion of gastric acid. His discovery earned him the 1904 Nobel Prize in Physiology and Medicine.

The gastric or antral phase of secretion revolves around the work of the physiologist John Edkins, who injected an extract of pyloric mucus membrane "activated by hydrochloric acid or boiling" into the jugular vein of cats. He noted a marked increase in the gastric acid and pepsin secretion. In 1905 he named the active agent "gastrin." Further study led to the understanding that gastric distention stimulates the release of gastrin from the antrum, resulting in the release of gastric acid.[9] This knowledge was applied directly to the treatment of PUD and became the basis for antrectomy.

The intestinal phase of gastric secretion refers to specific situations when a food bolus, which has not been exposed to gastric acid, comes in contact with the duodenal mucosa. In this situation the stomach is stimulated to secrete acid. Physiologically, food boluses are acidified and upon contact with the duodenal mucosa stimulate an inhibitory response.

SURGICAL TREATMENT

In 1881 the Prussian surgeon, Ludwik Rydygier, performed the first successful resection for a gastric ulcer.[10] In the early 1900s the standard operation performed for the treatment of gastric and duodenal ulcers was either a pyloroplasty without vagotomy or a gastroenterostomy. These operations were performed regardless of the presence or absence of obstructive symptoms, and many patients had resolution of their symptoms.

Gastroenterostomy soon surpassed pyloroplasty as the treatment of choice. Charles Mayo presented the Mayo Clinic data on gastroenterostomy for treatment of both gastric ulceration and duodenal ulceration. His data from 647 patients with gastric ulcers showed a mortality rate of 3.2% after gastroenterostomy and less than 2% in the 2734 patients with duodenal ulceration.[11] Eventually, recurrence rates and marginal ulcer formation were recognized, and surgical management began to change. Gastric resection gained favor, and the use of gastroenterostomy alone declined. In 1941 the Mayo Clinic data on the use of subtotal gastrectomy in the treatment of benign gastric ulcer were presented. The data showed a mortality rate of only 2.2% and that other, previously used operations were being performed with much less frequency.[10]

In 1921 Andre Latarjet described the anatomy of the vagus nerves and applied that knowledge clinically by performing an anatomically complete vagotomy for dyspepsia. Subsequently, he observed postoperative issues with inadequate gastric emptying and included a gastrojejunostomy.[12] Despite the improved understanding in vagal anatomy and physiology, therapeutic vagotomy remained an obscure treatment option for PUD. Lester Dragstedt, a physiologist and surgeon at the University of Chicago and later at the University of Florida, was paramount in the development of vagotomy for the treatment of peptic ulcers. Through his animal research, he elucidated the role of acid hypersecretion in the development of ulcers and stated "pure gastric juice as it is secreted by the fundus of the stomach has the capacity to destroy and digest all living tissue, including the wall of the jejunum, duodenum, and even the stomach itself."[13,14] Despite his understanding of the physiology, he was reluctant to perform a vagotomy on a human because he was unsure that a person could withstand the operation. However, in 1943 he managed a 35-year-old man with ulcer disease who had failed medical therapy. The patient was offered a subtotal gastrectomy and the patient promptly declined. The patient stated that both his father and his brother had undergone subtotal gastrectomies and that his father had died and his brother was miserable as a result of the operation.[12,15] Dragstedt performed a bilateral vagotomy through a left thoracotomy. The patient had immediate relief of his symptoms postoperatively. By 1945 Dragstedt had performed vagotomies on 60 patients and, as other surgeons had noted, he began to see postvagotomy "pyloric stenosis." Although he initially performed a drainage operation only for patients who were symptomatic from the impaired gastric emptying, he later modified his operation and performed abdominal truncal vagotomies (TVs) with a pyloroplasty concomitantly (Fig. 59.1).

Vagotomy and drainage was gradually accepted because of its relatively equal results in regard to resolution of symptoms and a lower mortality when compared with resective procedures. Dragstedt considered his vagotomy surgical technique "the most important contribution of his career." George Crile reported the Cleveland Clinic data: gastrectomy was associated with an ulcer recurrence rate and a mortality rate approximately three times higher than that in the vagotomy group.[16] Goligher et al. compared vagotomy and pyloroplasty with other operations for duodenal ulceration and found that vagotomy and pyloroplasty had a recurrence rate at 2 years of 6.3%, vagotomy and enterostomy of 3.6%, whereas gastric resection had 0% recurrence.

The surgical dictum of the time was that the treatment of ulcer disease was directed at reducing acid secretion. Vagotomy was used to eliminate the cephalic phase of acid secretion, which was considered to be the major contributor in duodenal ulceration. Antrectomy was the solution to eliminating the gastric phase of acid secretion, considered to be a major cause of gastric ulceration. Incorporating both vagotomy and antrectomy would

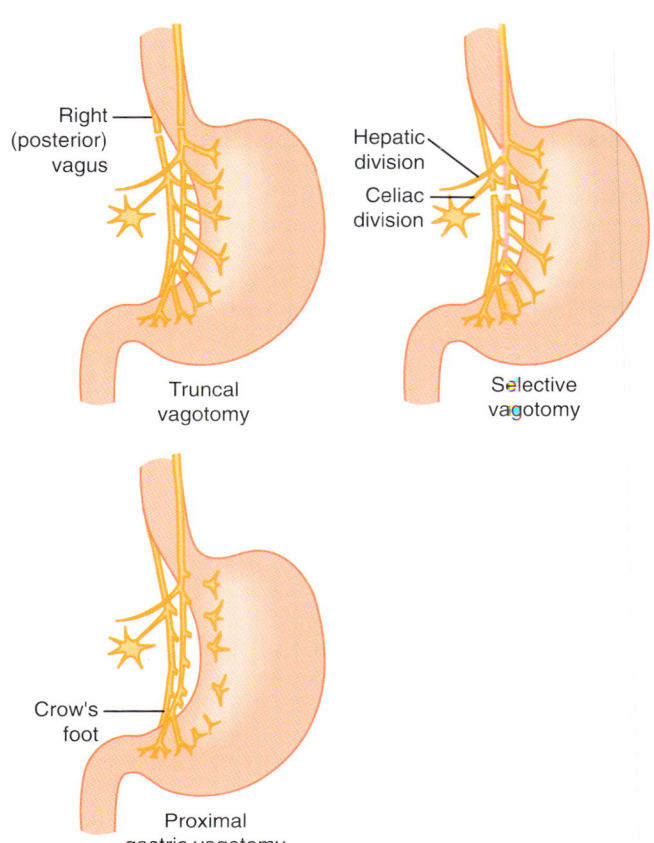

FIGURE 59.1 Schematic representation of the three standard forms of vagotomy. (From Sleisenger MH, Fordtran JS. Operations for peptic ulcer disease and early postoperative complications. In: Sleisenger MH, Fordtran JS, eds. *Gastrointestinal Disease*. 5th ed. Philadelphia: Saunders; 1993.)

effectively reduce, if not eradicate, acid production, thus continuing the "no acid, no ulcer" dogma of the time, and eradicated the need for a drainage procedure.

Hubert et al. from the Mayo Clinic presented their results for vagotomy with antrectomy with a mean 17-year follow-up. They showed an operative mortality rate of 1.1% and an ulcer recurrence rate of 0.7%; the incidence of major postoperative complications was less than 1%.[17] Extensive controversy revolved around the decision to perform a vagotomy and pyloroplasty versus a vagotomy with antrectomy. The idea that the two procedures both had a place in the treatment of ulcer disease was gradually accepted. At the time it was well established that for recurrent disease the optimal operation was vagotomy with resection. It was believed that, although both operations had equivalent results as to resolution of symptoms, vagotomy with antrectomy was associated with a lower recurrence rate, whereas vagotomy with drainage was associated with a lower mortality rate.

The selective vagotomies (SVs) were thought to be the answer to the question of how to decrease acid secretion and at the same time limit the known and occasionally debilitating postoperative morbidity of the previously discussed operations. The basis behind the more SVs was

the work done by Griffith and Harkins in 1957. They showed that fibers originating from the vagal trunks along the lesser curvature of the stomach innervate small groupings of parietal cells and as they approach the pylorus, they have a primary motor function.

The goal of selective gastric vagotomy (SGV), first performed in the 1960s, was to limit the side effects encountered with other operations. However, gastric stasis was still a factor. In response to the motor denervation, a pyloroplasty or other drainage procedure was needed. Siim et al. followed 105 patients for up to 13 years and showed satisfactory resolution of symptoms in only 77% of those with low-grade ulcerations. In the individuals with high-grade/severe ulcer disease, only 19% had good results. In addition to the poor clinical results, there was a 15% recurrence rate. Ultimately, they concluded that "selective gastric vagotomy has no place in elective treatment."[18]

Proximal gastric vagotomy (PGV), also referred to as a parietal cell vagotomy or highly SV, does not affect the distal motor function and thus does not impede gastric emptying. In the 1970s PGV became the most popular operation for elective treatment of PUD because of its lower mortality and morbidity rates and the omission of a drainage procedure.[18] van Heerden et al. reported the data on 223 patients from 1973 to 1977 at the Mayo Clinic. With a 39-month mean follow-up, the incidence of postoperative adverse effects was less than 3%, with 0% deaths and a 4.9% recurrence rate. At the end of their study, they concluded that "proximal gastric vagotomy is an effective, safe, and satisfactory option."[19]

Hoffmann et al. compared TV to SGV and PGV in a randomized controlled study of 248 patients with an 11- to 15-year follow-up. They found recurrence rates of 28.5% (TV), 37.4% (SGV), and 39.3% (PGV). Although there was a trend with lower recurrence in the TV group, the difference between the three groups failed to show statistical significance. Overall, the patient satisfaction for the three groups was similar, with approximately two-thirds of the patients being satisfied. The findings led to the conclusion that "none of the three forms of vagotomy can be recommended as the standard operative treatment."[20]

As the discovery of H_2 blockers and PPIs emerged, surgical indications decreased. The improved understanding of the pathogenesis of ulcer disease with the discovery of *H. pylori* and understanding the impact of NSAIDs further decreased the need for operation. Management became primarily medical in nature, with operation reserved for the emergency treatment of bleeding and perforation. This chapter discusses elective operations for intractable peptic ulcers and emergency procedures for complications.

PATHOPHYSIOLOGY OF PEPTIC ULCER DISEASE

The decades of surgical therapy dominating the treatment of PUD have been followed by a period of potent acid-reducing medication use that has now been replaced with a short-term regimen targeting the elimination of *H. pylori* infection. Discussions of the best operation have been

---

BOX 59.1 **Classification of Gastric and Duodenal Ulcers**

Helicobacter pylori infection
Drug induced
Nonsteroidal antiinflammatory drugs
Low-dose aspirin
Acid hypersecretory state
    Zollinger-Ellison syndrome
    Retained gastric antrum
Anastomotic ulcer following gastric surgery
Severe physiologic stress
Tumors

---

replaced with a discussion of the best drug combination to treat the various manifestations of both gastric and duodenal peptic ulceration. A 10-day to 2-week course of drug therapy directed against *H. pylori* has an ulcer recurrence rate equivalent to TV with pyloroplasty. Although emergency operations for both peptic ulcer bleeding and perforation are still occasionally required, even their incidences are on the wane.[21]

The introduction of histamine H_2-receptor antagonists in 1977 radically changed the need for elective surgical therapy of PUD. Yet, it was the discovery of the association of *Campylobacter pyloridis* (renamed *H. pylori* in 1989) with peptic ulceration by Warren and Marshall in 1982 that truly revolutionized our understanding of ulcer pathogenesis and its treatment.[22] They received the Nobel Prize for this work in 2005. Epidemiology studies revealed a strong association between *H. pylori* infection and both gastric and duodenal ulcer disease. Treatment of the infection resulted in long-term cure of peptic ulcers. Despite the development of potent antisecretory drugs and treatment for *H. pylori* infection, PUD remains an important clinical problem because of the widespread use of NSAIDs. The cause of peptic ulcers is complex and multifactorial, as they result from the interplay of the effects of gastric acid and pepsin and the gastric mucosal barrier. Any entity that either increases acid and pepsin secretion or weakens the mucosal barrier can result in ulcers (Box 59.1).

HELICOBACTER PYLORI AND PEPTIC ULCER DISEASE

H. pylori is the most common chronic bacterial infection in humans. Once acquired, infection persists and may or may not produce gastroduodenal disease. A number of factors determine whether *H. pylori* infection causes disease: the pattern of histologic gastritis induced; changes in homeostasis of gastrin and acid secretion; gastric metaplasia in the duodenum; interaction of *H. pylori* with the mucosal barrier; and the strain of *H. pylori* present. There is a great deal of variation in the virulence of different strains of *H. pylori*. Some genotypes of *H. pylori* appear to be particularly toxic and are more common in patients with peptic ulcers. These are vacA and cagA positive.[23] There is also a genetic predisposition to acquire *H. pylori* infection.

H. pylori colonizes the entire gastric epithelium. However, the severity of the chronic mucosal inflammation is variable and the resultant clinical scenario is dependent on the distribution of the inflammation. The incidence of *H. pylori* in the setting of gastric ulcers is between 80% and 90% and up to 100% in the setting of duodenal ulcers.[24] In patients with duodenal ulcer, density of infection and severity of inflammation are greatest in the distal antral region with sparing of the acid-secreting body mucosa. After *H. pylori* eradication, the gastric mucosal changes revert to normal.

In gastric ulcers, the body and antrum are affected to a similar degree. In this case, gastric acid secretion can be decreased because of the more severe involvement of the parietal cell region. In response to the same stimulation with gastrin, duodenal ulcer patients with *H. pylori* produce more acid than infected patients without ulcers. This may result from an impaired acid-secreting ability of the nonulcer *H. pylori*-infected patient's more diseased acid-secreting fundus mucosa. Increased gastric acid can lead to the development of gastric metaplasia in the duodenal bulb. This is a necessary forerunner to colonization of the duodenal epithelium with *H. pylori*, because *H. pylori* exclusively binds to the gastric epithelium. The metaplastic, *H. pylori*-colonized, duodenal epithelium then becomes more susceptible to acid and pepsin effects and ulceration. After the eradication of *H. pylori* infection, gastric metaplasia in the duodenum does not revert to normal, but with the elimination of the infection, the risk of ulcer recurrence is eliminated.[24]

H. pylori infection impairs the negative feedback of gastrin release by somatostatin secreted by antral D cells. Somatostatin causes inhibition of gastrin release through a paracrine effect. Production of alkaline ammonia by the bacteria on both the surface epithelium and in the antral glands prevents the D cells from properly interpreting the level of acid present. This leads to improperly low levels of somatostatin, and thus loss of gastrin inhibition. Chronic hypergastrinemia caused by *H. pylori* exerts a trophic effect and hyperplasia of the acid-secreting parietal cells.[25]

Infection with *H. pylori* also interferes with the neural connections between the antrum and fundus that downregulate acid production. This impaired neural control, coupled with hypergastrinemia, leads to further increases in acid production. With *H. pylori* eradication, the hypergastrinemia rapidly resolves. Resolution of acid hypersecretion occurs much more slowly.[26]

The inflammatory response caused by *H. pylori* infection of the gastric mucosa leads to cytokine production, mainly, interleukin (IL)-8.[27] IL-8 acts as a potent chemotactic and attracts neutrophils and acute inflammatory cells into the submucosa. Other cytokines include IL-17 and IL-18. In a recent animal model, increased serum level of IL-17 was found to correlate with severity of gastritis; this correlation was not observed with changes in serum level of IL-8 and IL-18.[28]

Complex interactions occur between *H. pylori* and host defense mechanisms that affect the occurrence of peptic ulceration. Duodenal ulcers appear to be predominantly related to increased acid production, whereas in gastric ulceration, defense mechanism breaches appear to prevail. Despite these differences in mechanisms, *H. pylori* eradication effectively cures PUD and prevents relapses. In addition, the rate of ulcer healing is accelerated if antibiotics effective against *H. pylori* are given in addition to drugs that suppress acid.

NONSTEROIDAL ANTIINFLAMMATORY DRUGS AND ULCER DISEASE

NSAIDs increase the risk of peptic ulcers. NSAIDs are the most commonly identified risk factor for peptic ulcer bleeding, especially in older adults; the risk is drug specific and dose dependent. NSAIDs decrease the mucosal defense by suppression of prostaglandin synthesis in gastric and duodenal mucosa.[29] Controlled trials with cyclooxygenase-2 (COX-2)-selective inhibitors have demonstrated a reduction in the risk of gastroduodenal ulcers and their associated complications.[30]

The presence of gastric acid contributes to NSAID injury by converting superficial mucosal lesions to deeper ulcers. In addition, acid interferes with platelet aggregation and impairs ulcer healing.[31] Acid suppression is the mainstay in the therapy of NSAID-associated ulcer disease. Risk factors that influence PUD in NSAID users include history of ulcer; advancing age; high-dose NSAIDs; steroids; aspirin; anticoagulants; and *H. pylori* infection.[32] The use of COX-2 inhibitor and PPI can significantly reduce complications associated with NSAID intake.

LOW-DOSE ASPIRIN AND ULCER DISEASE

Even at very low doses (75 mg daily), aspirin decreases gastric mucosal prostaglandin levels and can cause significant gastric lesions. The effect of aspirin is dose dependent, and ulcer complications are twofold to fourfold higher in patients taking 75 to 300 mg daily compared with controls.[33] PPIs, given with low-dose aspirin, can significantly decrease the risk of developing peptic ulceration.[34]

ACID HYPERSECRETORY STATES AND ULCER DISEASE

Both Zollinger-Ellison (ZE) syndrome as a consequence of gastrinoma, and retained gastric antrum after antrectomy with gastrojejunal anastomosis (so-called retained excluded antrum) result in peptic ulceration secondary to high levels of gastrin secretion. In cases of retained excluded gastric antrum, the residual gastric antral tissue is constantly bathed in a fluid with a high pH (nonacid), resulting in continuous secretion of gastrin. Fortunately, because of the infrequency of antrectomy in current surgical practice, this clinical situation is rarely encountered. In both disease states, high levels of serum gastrin result in gastric acid hypersecretion and resultant peptic ulceration. Serum gastrin elevations are also seen in chronic atrophic gastritis as a consequence of the lack of gastric acid secretion (typically achlorhydria) causing chronic G-cell stimulation.

SEVERE SYSTEMIC DISEASE (STRESS ULCER)

The pathophysiology of stress ulceration is multifactorial and undefined. A breakdown of the gastroduodenal mucosal barrier, often a result of severe physiologic stress and splanchnic hypoperfusion, combined with gastric acid may lead to ulceration and bleeding. After splanchnic perfusion is restored, a reperfusion injury can further

exacerbate the condition. It can develop within hours in critically ill patients, typically starting in the fundus and spreading distally. Prior to the development of effective medical therapy to reduce or eliminate gastric acid, this was a feared and highly lethal condition, often requiring total or near-total gastrectomy for control in extremely ill patients. Even with such heroic measures, mortality was extremely high. With the advent of histamine H_2-receptor antagonists and PPI therapy, the primary goal of stress ulcer therapy has been to prevent clinically important bleeding by identifying those patients at risk for the development of stress ulceration (Box 59.2) and administering appropriate prophylactic measures. Fortunately, acid-reducing medication effectively prevents significant bleeding in nearly all patients at risk for stress ulceration. Esophagogastroduodenoscopy (EGD) is the first line of intervention. It aids with the diagnosis. However, treatment is usually unsuccessful secondary to the diffuse nature of the bleeding. Angiography should be considered in patients who fail endoscopic intervention. Angiography can facilitate embolization of the bleeding vessel(s), which is usually the left gastric artery, or can help reduce the rate of bleeding by selective vasopressin infusion. Operative intervention is considered as the last resort in patients.

INDICATIONS FOR THE SURGICAL TREATMENT OF PEPTIC ULCER DISEASE

ELECTIVE OPERATION FOR INTRACTABLE DUODENAL ULCER DISEASE

The treatment of PUD has undergone a significant change. The previous use of elective surgical means to treat PUD has faded into history, and medical therapy has moved to the forefront of current treatment. Elective surgical procedures for PUD are limited these days to patients with gastric outlet obstruction because of long-standing, untreated or poorly treated ulcer disease. These patients are rare, and many are treatable with endoscopic dilation with or without stenting.

In a meta-analysis including 2102 patients with PUD, the 12-month ulcer remission rates for gastric and duodenal ulcers were significantly higher in patients who were successfully eradicated of *H. pylori* infection when compared

---

BOX 59.2 Risk Factors for Stress Ulcer–Related Bleeding

Respiratory failure requiring mechanical ventilation >48 h
Coagulopathy or anticoagulation
Acute renal insufficiency
Acute hepatic failure
Sepsis
Hypotension
Brain or spinal cord injury
History of gastrointestinal bleeding
Low intragastric pH
Burn involving >35% of body surface area
Major operation (>4 h)
High-dose corticosteroids (>250 mg/day hydrocortisone or equivalent)

with those with a persistent infection (97% and 98% vs. 61% and 65%, respectively).[35] *H. pylori* eradication even without concurrent acid suppression therapy heals greater than 85% of duodenal ulcers.[36] Confirmation of *H. pylori* eradication should be strongly considered for all patients receiving treatment because of the availability of accurate, relatively inexpensive, and noninvasive tests. All patients with duodenal ulcer(s) should receive antisecretory therapy to facilitate ulcer healing; however, the duration of therapy will vary depending upon ulcer characteristics, risk factors for recurrent PUD, and the presence of ulcer complications. In patients with uncomplicated duodenal ulcer who test positive for *H. pylori*, PPI, given for 10 to 14 days, along with the antibiotic regimen to eradicate *H. pylori*, is usually adequate to induce healing, and additional PPI therapy is not needed as long as they are asymptomatic following therapy.[37] Thus medical therapy for duodenal ulcer has shifted away from an antisecretory/antacid or surgical approaches to an antimicrobial strategy.

Most peptic ulcers respond to medical treatment. However, in some individuals the ulcer is either refractory to conventional therapy or recurs following successful initial treatment. A refractory peptic ulcer is defined as an endoscopically proven ulcer greater than 5 mm in diameter that does not heal after 12 weeks of treatment with a PPI. On the other hand, a recurrent peptic ulcer is defined as an endoscopically proven ulcer greater than 5 mm in diameter that develops within 12 months following complete ulcer healing documented by repeat endoscopy. Prior to labeling the ulcer disease as intractable, it is important to rule out the following:

- Cancer by performing endoscopy with adequate biopsy of the ulcer edge and base.
- Gastrinoma by measuring fasting serum gastrin.
- Total serum calcium should be measured to screen for hyperparathyroidism.
- Ulcerogenic medication (e.g., NSAIDs, aspirin).
- Persistent *H. pylori* infection by undergoing additional tests to confirm eradication. Ideally patients should be off of the PPI for at least 2 weeks to reduce false-negative results.[38]
- Chronic smoking, although smoking does *not* appear to be a risk factor for ulcer relapse after *H. pylori* has been eradicated.

After these have been ruled out and when operative intervention is being considered, the strategy continues to be based on reduction of acid secretion. Gastric distention is an important stimulant of gastrin release by G cells, which are mainly located in the antrum; thus decompressing the stomach in patients with bleeding ulcers and gastric outlet obstruction secondary to ulcer is important to reduce gastrin and hence acid release. Acid release can surgically be reduced by dividing the vagus (cephalic phase), and eliminating hormonal stimulation from the antrum (gastric phase). Each of these maneuvers has consequences in terms of the normal physiology of the upper gastrointestinal tract that tend to be amplified when the procedures are combined, such as with vagotomy and antrectomy. In the past, the choice of operation involved weighing the risk of recurrent ulceration with the possibility of postoperative complications and long-term sequelae (postgastrectomy syndromes). This decision

dilemma prompted a large number of trials comparing these procedures in the surgical literature. Improvements in medical therapy, particularly treatment of *H. pylori*, have markedly reduced the risk of ulcer recurrence, rendering much of these data obsolete. Thus surgical decision-making has become confusing with little quality data available from the post–*H. pylori* era. The choices for surgical intervention for intractable duodenal ulcer disease include either a vagotomy with or without a drainage procedure or with a gastric resection.

VAGOTOMY

The rationale for vagotomy is the elimination of direct cholinergic stimulation of gastric acid secretion. The released acetylcholine stimulates acid secretion via a specific receptor on the parietal cell. Vagotomy also renders the acid-producing parietal cells less responsive to histamine and gastrin. The distal portion of the anterior and posterior trunks send branches to the antrum and pylorus that serve a primarily motor function. Gastric motility is affected by the antral and pyloric branches of the vagus that stimulate peristaltic activity of the antrum and relaxation of the pylorus. The celiac branch of the posterior vagus mediates small intestine motility, whereas the hepatic branch mediates bile flow and gallbladder motility.

TV results in a variety of physiologic alterations in the stomach. Acid secretion is drastically reduced because of diminished cholinergic stimulation of parietal cells, and the cephalic phase of gastric secretion is essentially eliminated. There is a 75% decrease in basal acid secretion and a 50% decrease in maximum acid output. The increased intraluminal stomach pH leads to elimination of the negative feedback on gastrin secretion; therefore, this results in increased serum gastrin levels and gastrin cell hyperplasia. As a result of loss of reflex relaxation of the gastric fundus, there is rapid emptying of liquids. Similarly, TV affects distal gastric motility, resulting in difficulty in emptying solids. Because of the latter alterations, approximately 20% to 30% of patients develop gastric atony, which leads to stasis and chronic abdominal pain and distention. For that reason, it is recommended that after a TV patients should undergo a drainage procedure to counteract the nonrelaxing pylorus, which acts as an obstruction. The various drainage procedures available are discussed later. There are four types of vagotomy to consider: *truncal, selective, proximal gastric,* and *supradiaphragmatic.* Truncal and proximal gastric are commonly used to treat PUD, whereas selective and supradiaphragmatic vagotomies are used infrequently.

TRUNCAL VAGOTOMY

TV (see Fig. 59.1) involves division of the anterior and posterior vagal trunks after they emerge below the diaphragm. The first step is to incise the peritoneal covering of the gastroesophageal junction. The peritoneum is opened horizontally, from the lesser curvature to the cardiac notch at the greater curvature. The surgeon uses thumb and right index finger for blunt dissection to encircle the esophagus. A Penrose drain is placed around the lower esophagus to place more effective downward traction on the gastroesophageal junction. When encircling the esophagus, the surgeon stays wide of the esophagus to prevent inadvertent entry into the lumen and to include the vagal trunks. In the course of this maneuver, the posterior vagal trunk usually will be palpated as a taut cord anterior to the aorta. A single anterior vagal trunk is usually identified in the anterior midportion of the esophagus, 2 to 4 cm above the gastroesophageal junction. It is not uncommon for vagal fibers to be distributed among two or three smaller cords at this level. These trunks are individually lifted up, and 2- to 4-cm segments of each are separated from surrounding tissues. A 1- to 2-cm length of nerve is resected and a clip is applied to the cut ends of the nerve. The "criminal nerve" of Grassi also may be identified wrapping around the cardiac notch from its origin in the posterior trunk and is a common cause of incomplete vagotomy.

The posterior vagal trunk is usually identified along the right edge of the esophagus. If the anterior vagus has already been divided, the esophagus is more mobile. This mobility allows downward traction on the gastroesophageal junction, causing the posterior vagus to "bowstring" and making it easier to identify. A 2- to 4-cm segment is separated from surrounding tissues, its margins marked with clips, and resected. The resected portions of the anterior and posterior vagal trunks should be sent to pathology for frozen section. This procedure completely denervates the stomach and eliminates vagal innervation to the pancreas, small intestine, proximal colon, and hepatobiliary tree. Although this procedure significantly reduces acid secretion, it also markedly alters gastric motility. As discussed earlier, some form of gastric emptying procedure should be performed.

SELECTIVE VAGOTOMY

The SV procedure (see Fig. 59.1) was developed in an attempt to decrease the incidence of postvagotomy diarrhea and ameliorate the increased incidence of gallbladder stasis, which may lead to increased gallstone formation. The vagal fibers are divided distal to the takeoff of the hepatic branch(es) from the anterior vagus and the celiac branch(es) from the posterior vagus. This procedure is technically more demanding than TV and requires a more careful and meticulous dissection. This technique spares vagal innervation to the gallbladder and intestine while completely denervating the stomach. Because the vagal pyloric innervation is also eliminated, a drainage procedure is still required. The primary reason for the development of this technique was its presumed lower side-effect profile. However, a prospective randomized study failed to show substantial benefit for SV over TV.[8] The incidence of diarrhea following an SV was no different when compared with TV. The introduction of PGV with its lower side-effect profile and the elimination of the need for a drainage procedure resulted in a limited use of SV as a therapeutic option.

PROXIMAL GASTRIC VAGOTOMY

PGV is also known as parietal cell vagotomy and highly SV (see Fig. 59.1). The rationale for PGV is to eliminate the vagal stimulation to the acid-secreting portion of the stomach without interrupting motor innervation to the antrum and pylorus. The operation involves severing all branches of the vagus nerve along the lesser curvature that innervate the corpus and fundus of the stomach, while preserving the hepatic and celiac branches, as well as the distal vagal branches extending to the antrum and pylorus. The end result of this procedure is the same reduction in acid secretion that occurs after TV (basal and stimulated acid secretion are reduced by more than 75% and 50%, respectively) but without the troublesome stasis and gastric atony. Because the distal motor nerves are preserved, emptying of solids is normal; however, the nerves affecting receptive relaxation are divided, and some rapid emptying of liquids may occur. The alteration in liquid emptying is usually minimal. This procedure is associated with the lowest morbidity rate of all vagotomy procedures and became the operation of choice in many centers despite a reported ulcer recurrence rate of between 5% and 20%. A meta-analysis of 12 trials confirmed that PGV has the highest recurrence rate when compared with TV with pyloroplasty, but fewer long-term side effects.[39] PGV also has been compared with TV in a randomized trial, in which it was shown to have a lower incidence of dumping syndrome and weight loss. Although the ulcer recurrence rates were higher with PGV, this was not significant when prepyloric ulcers (for which PGV is not an adequate operation) were excluded.[40]

PGV is a complex and lengthy procedure, and, to help to simplify the procedure, several variations have been described. They usually consist of a posterior TV and a more selective ablation of the anterior vagal fibers to the gastric fundus and body. Hill and Baker performed a posterior TV with an anterior PGV (Hill-Baker procedure). Taylor combined the posterior TV with anterior lesser-curve seromyotomy (Taylor procedure). Randomized studies confirm the superiority of the Taylor procedure to TV[41] and document equal outcomes to PGV with a shorter operative time.[42] With the decreased incidence of elective ulcer surgery, such operations are not commonly used. However, such approaches are popular for laparoscopic treatment of ulcer disease.

SUPRADIAPHRAGMATIC VAGOTOMY

This procedure is performed primarily for patients for whom attempts at complete vagotomy via an abdominal approach have failed; it is thought that further attempts to find the missed trunks in the reoperated abdomen may be difficult, and thus a thoracic approach is advised. This operation involves performing a thoracotomy or thoracoscopy, identifying the two large nerve trunks, and performing a TV.

DRAINAGE PROCEDURES

Any patient who undergoes a truncal, selective, or supradiaphragmatic vagotomy should undergo a drainage procedure to facilitate gastric emptying. Drainage procedures fall into two categories: pyloroplasties and gastrojejunostomy (Fig. 59.2). Pyloroplasty is the preferred approach because it perpetuates the original anatomy, is a simple procedure, and is associated with less bile reflux than gastrojejunostomy. More than 90% of all drainage procedures currently performed are variations of pyloroplasty.

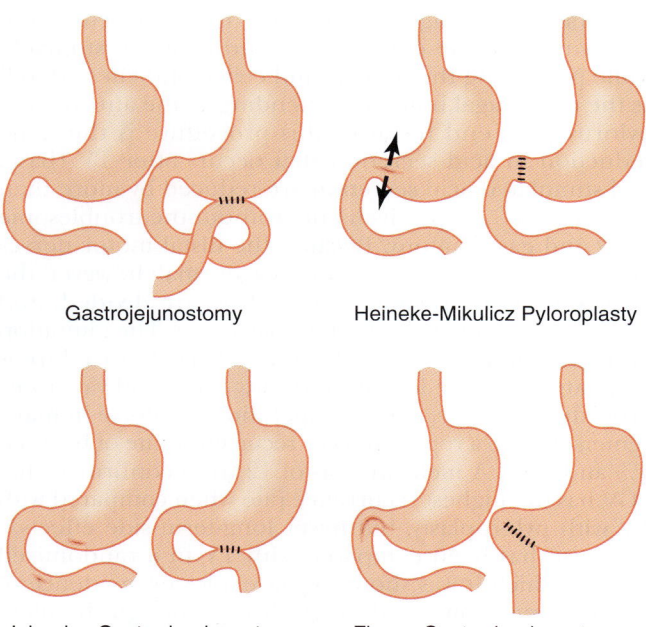

Gastrojejunostomy

Heineke-Mikulicz Pyloroplasty

Jaboulay Gastroduodenostomy

Finney Gastroduodenostomy

FIGURE 59.2 Drainage procedures used with truncal or selective vagotomy. (From Matthews JB, Silen W. Operations for peptic ulcer disease and early operative complications. In: Sleisenger MH, Fordtran JS, eds. *Gastrointestinal Disease*. 5th ed. Philadelphia: Saunders; 1993.)

PYLOROPLASTY

Heineke-Mikulicz Pyloroplasty

In 1888 the Heineke-Mikulicz procedure (see Fig. 59.2) was described independently by two surgeons, Heineke and Mikulicz. The technique is popular because it is technically straightforward, applicable to many clinical ulcer scenarios, and associated with few complications. The Heineke-Mikulicz pyloroplasty is the most commonly performed drainage procedure, and when conducted carefully and in a technically sound fashion, obstruction or leakage is rare. Patients who are candidates for this procedure include those who have a mobile, uninvolved anterior pylorus; those who have no evidence of a severely distorted or edematous pylorus; and those with small, minimally deforming pyloric perforations (massive perforations make pyloroplasty difficult and somewhat treacherous). The procedure may be performed using a single- or double-layer closure. After the pylorus is identified and the duodenum is mobilized with a Kocher maneuver, two traction sutures are placed in the anterior surface of the pylorus at the 12 and 6 o'clock positions; efforts should be made to include the pyloric vein of Mayo in these sutures, which is typically found in the inferior-anterior position on the pylorus (the vein may be used as a marker to identify the pylorus location, which is especially useful during laparoscopic procedures) to partially control the subsequent bleeding. The sutures are elevated, placing gentle tension on the anterior surface of the pylorus. A full-thickness longitudinal (horizontal) incision through the anterior wall of the pylorus (thus interrupting the circular muscle of the sphincter) is made, starting on the anterior surface of the stomach 2 to 3 cm proximal to the pylorus and extending through the pylorus and approximately the same distance onto the anterior surface of the duodenum. In the presence of marked deformity, it may be advisable to incise the midportion of the duodenum and then one can use a curved clamp, such as a hemostat, directed up through the constricted pyloric canal as a guide. Traction on the angle sutures draws the longitudinal incision apart until it becomes diamond shaped; with the pylorus widely open one can ensure that there is no evidence of obstruction. The longitudinal incision is then closed in a transverse fashion. Typically this is done in either a two- or one-layer fashion (Fig. 59.3). The goal is complete inversion with good serosa-to-serosa approximation. Care is taken not to narrow the lumen by incorporating too much tissue into the closure. The thumb and index finger are used to palpate the newly formed lumen by invaginating the gastric and duodenal walls on each side of the transverse closure.

Finney Pyloroplasty

The Finney pyloroplasty (Fig. 59.4; see also Fig. 59.2) is indicated in the setting of extensive scarring and narrowing of a significant portion of the duodenal bulb, making a Heineke-Mikulicz pyloroplasty untenable. The pylorus is identified and mobilized with a generous Kocher maneuver. Traction sutures are placed along the pylorus as described for the Heineke-Mikulicz pyloroplasty. Then a single inverted U- or V-shaped incision is made though the prepyloric antrum, the pylorus, and the first part of the duodenum for a distance of approximately 7 cm in each direction. The reconstruction starts at the pylorus, in the middle of the incision, along the incised inferior aspect. The inferior leaf of the stomach is sutured to the inferior leaf of the anterior duodenal wall and continues to the extent of the incisions laterally on the stomach and duodenum. This is done with a running absorbable suture, and after the inferior leaflet has been approximated to the extent of the incision, it is continued back toward the pylorus, approximating the superior leaflets in the same fashion. A layer of Lembert sutures is then placed to invert the inner layer. The use of this drainage procedure makes a larger lumen possible but is more technically demanding compared with the Heineke-Mikulicz technique, involving a great deal more suturing, and has greater potential for complications.

Jaboulay Gastroduodenostomy

The Jaboulay drainage procedure (Fig. 59.5; see also Fig. 59.2) is the only one of the three described here that does not transect the pyloric muscle. The procedure involves an anastomosis of the distal stomach to the first and second portions of the duodenum, thus bypassing the pylorus. The procedure is indicated primarily for the severely scarred or deformed pylorus or duodenal bulb that would be too difficult and treacherous to incise. After carrying out a very extensive Kocher maneuver with thorough mobilization of the second and third portions of the duodenum, an area of the duodenum distal to the stenotic/scarred area is chosen, as is an area of the distal stomach just proximal to the pylorus. The duodenum is rolled anteriorly onto the stomach, and a posterior row

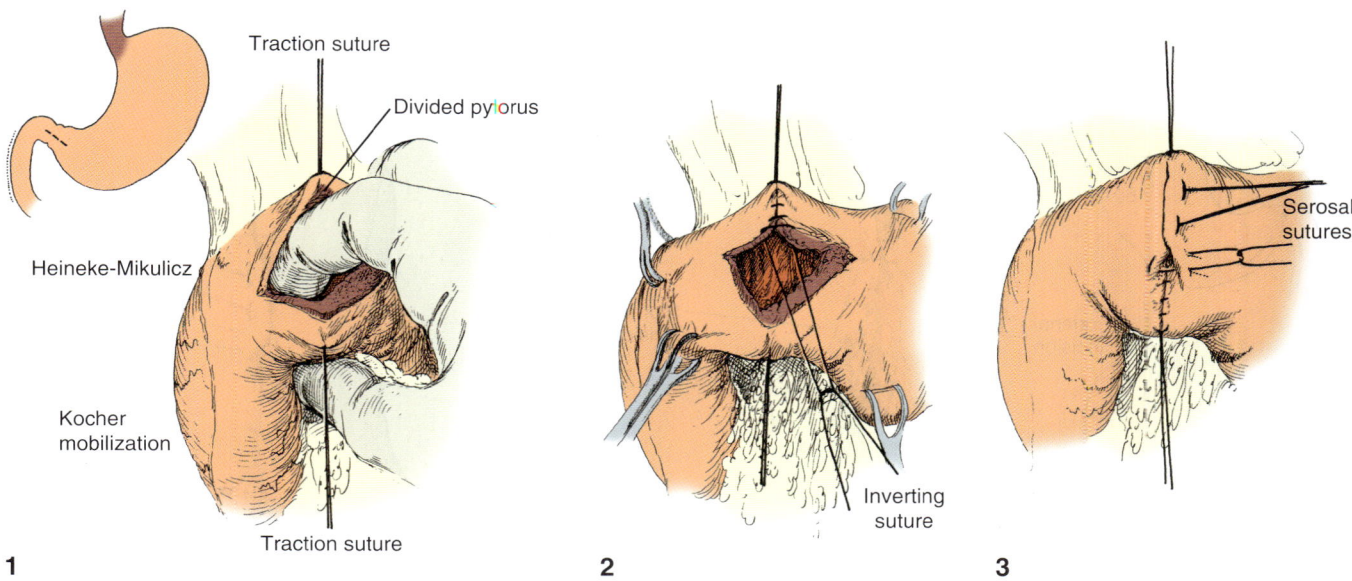

FIGURE 59.3 Schematic representation of Heineke-Mikulicz pyloroplasty. While lifting up on the traction sutures, a longitudinal incision is made through the pyloric muscles and extended 2 to 3 cm proximally into the stomach and distally into the duodenum *(part 1)*. If the duodenum is soft, pliable, and minimally deformed, a running closure of the inside layer is begun with absorbable suture in an inverting fashion *(part 2)*. An outside layer of Lembert silk sutures in an interrupted fashion completes the procedure *(part 3)*. (From Zollinger RM. *Atlas of Surgical Operations*. New York: Macmillan; 1975.)

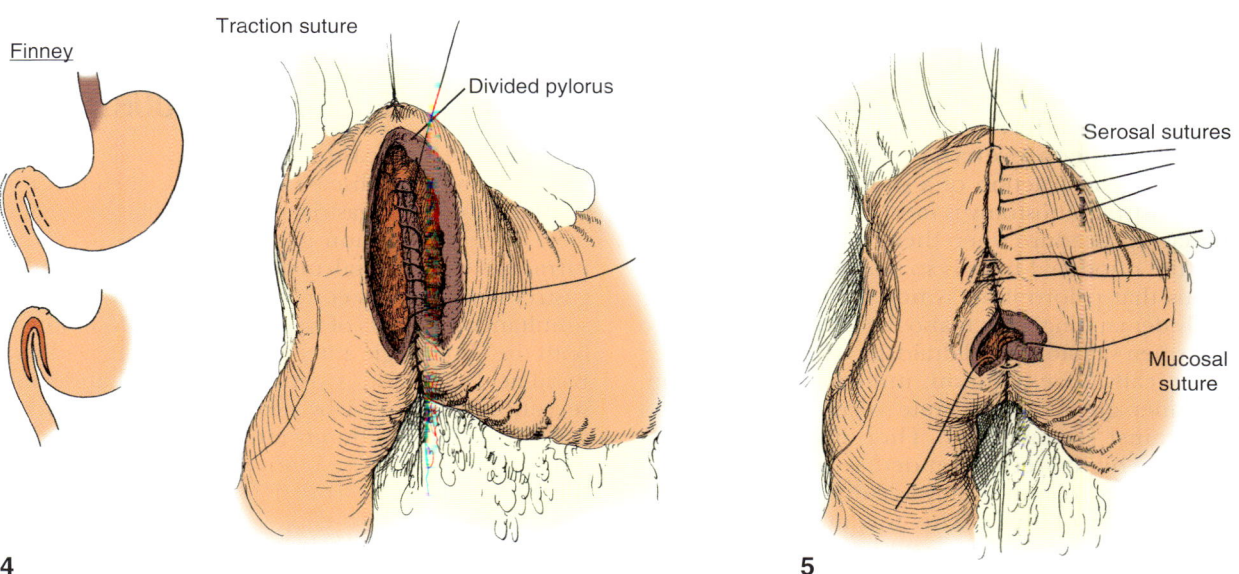

FIGURE 59.4 Schematic of the Finney pyloroplasty. After the careful exploration, closure is initiated by using absorbable suture to begin a running closure *(part 4)*. A final, interrupted row of silk sutures is then placed in Lembert fashion to complete the pyloroplasty *(part 5)*. (From Zollinger RM. *Atlas of Surgical Operations*. New York: Macmillan; 1975.)

of Lembert sutures are placed. Two separate incisions are made through the previously chosen sites on the prepyloric antrum and the first portion of the duodenum. The posterior inner layer of the gastroduodenal anastomosis is completed with a continuous full-thickness absorbable suture; the anterior inner layer is completed with a continuous inverting Connell suture. Finally, anterior Lembert interrupted sutures are placed. The anastomosis can also be performed in a single layer. Use of the Jaboulay procedure has been associated with increased bile reflux as the anastomosis is close to the ampulla of Vater.

GASTROJEJUNOSTOMY

Gastrojejunostomy (see Fig. 59.2) was first performed alone in 1881 and was plagued by two problems: marginal ulcers (because no vagotomy was performed) and vomiting,

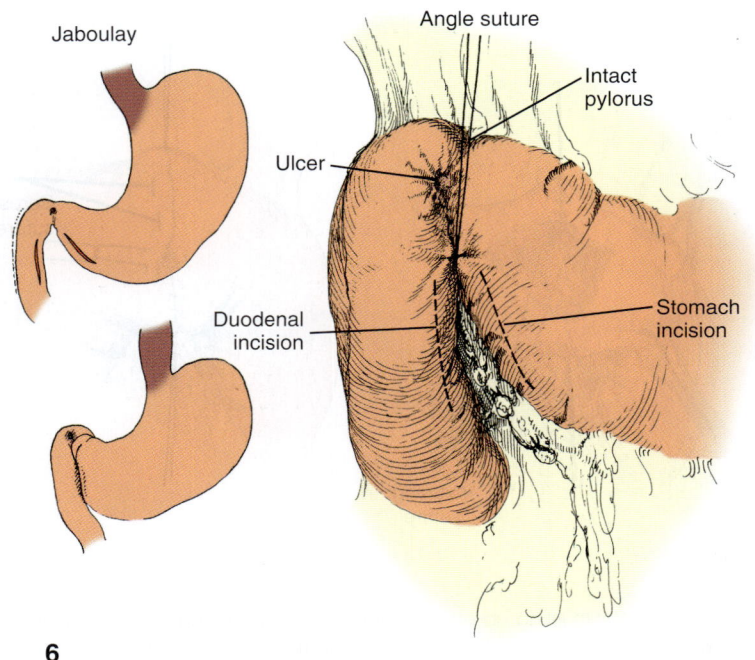

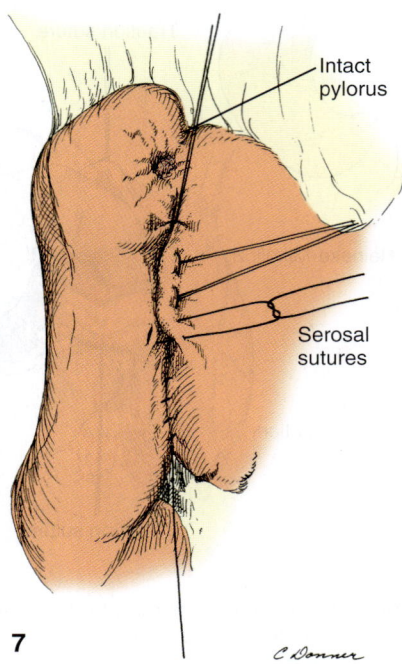

FIGURE 59.5 Schematic of the Jaboulay gastroduodenostomy. Equal-size incisions are made in the distal stomach and proximal duodenum approximately 4 to 5 cm in length *(part 6)*. A final anterior, outside layer of interrupted Lembert silk sutures is then placed to complete the gastroduodenostomy *(part 7)*. (From Zollinger RM. *Atlas of Surgical Operations*. New York: Macmillan; 1975.)

which was thought to be caused by kinking with an excessive length of the afferent limb of jejunum. The two problems have been overcome with the addition of vagotomy and construction of a shorter afferent jejunal segment. Gastrojejunostomy is most commonly indicated as a drainage procedure when there is duodenal obstruction and the duodenal bulb is so scarred, inflamed, and edematous that pyloroplasty is not safe or is excessively technically demanding. This is also the drainage procedure of choice when vagotomy and drainage is being performed laparoscopically. The jejunum, unlike the duodenum, lacks Brunner glands that secrete alkaline solution and protect against stomach pH. Therefore, historically, vagotomy was highly recommended as an adjunct when performing a gastrojejunostomy as a drainage procedure in the treatment of PUD. This was mainly to reduce the incidence of marginal ulcers; however, in the era of PPIs, we have learned that lifelong PPI can significantly reduce this complication without the morbidity associated with vagotomy.[43] Older patients with achlorhydria and atrophic gastritis make little acid, and a vagotomy may not be necessary, especially in the setting of malignant obstruction.

A variety of postgastrectomy complications may occur after pyloroplasty or gastroenterostomy, including dumping, diarrhea, alkaline reflux gastritis, anemia, and marginal ulceration. These may be seen in up to 50% of patients after operation on a temporary basis, but they resolve within 6 to 8 months in most, and only 5% to 7% of patients have a persistent, symptomatic postoperative complication such as dumping.

GASTRIC RESECTION PROCEDURES

Although subtotal gastrectomy was used for the treatment of duodenal ulcer disease in the past, currently it is most commonly used for gastric ulcer and distal gastric malignancies. A more common gastric resection performed for intractable duodenal ulcer is antrectomy (40% distal gastrectomy) that is combined with a TV or an SV. The simultaneous effects of vagotomy and antrectomy remove both the cholinergic and gastrin stimulus to acid secretion. Basal acid secretion is virtually abolished and stimulated secretion is reduced by nearly 80%. After antrectomy, gastrointestinal continuity must be restored by some form of reconstruction. The remnant is anastomosed either to the duodenum (Billroth I [B I]) or, after closing the duodenal stump, to the jejunum distal to the ligament of Treitz (Billroth II [B II]) (Fig. 59.6). B I reconstruction has several theoretical advantages:

1. Restoring normal GI continuity
2. Leaving specialized duodenal mucosa next to the gastric mucosa
3. Avoiding problems with an afferent and efferent limb
4. Allowing easier performance of endoscopic retrograde cholangiopancreatography (ERCP) and endoscopic examination of the bowel
5. Reduced incidence of gastric cancer in the remnant stomach.[44]

Despite the theoretical physiologic advantages, no important functional differences have ever been demonstrated between these reconstructions. Although studies show a larger fecal fat loss following a B II procedure, this is unlikely to be of any significance. The difference in cancer risk is real but significant only after a long follow-up period (>15 years).[45,46] The choice is typically based on the degree of scarring of the duodenum and the ease with which the duodenum and gastric remnant can be brought together. Several variations of the B I and B II operations have been described, and these are summarized in Figs. 59.7 and 59.8.

Both Billroth reconstructions can lead to bile reflux, which can result in disabling symptoms. To avoid such complications, some favor a Roux-en-Y reconstruction. The long-term results (12 to 21 years) of a study in which patients were randomized to B II or 60-cm Roux-en-Y reconstruction confirm improved patient satisfaction and endoscopic appearance of the esophagus and the gastric remnant after Roux-en-Y reconstruction.[47] Unfortunately, the Roux-en-Y reconstruction can be plagued with a Roux stasis syndrome. Studies show that the Braun variation of B II (see Fig. 59.8) has a lower incidence of bile reflux; consequently, some authors recommend this as the standard reconstruction technique.[48] However, other authors promote the "uncut" Roux-en-Y reconstruction[49] (Fig. 59.9).

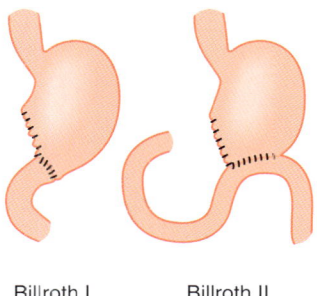

Billroth I   Billroth II

FIGURE 59.6 Reconstruction techniques after partial gastrectomy: Billroth I gastroduodenostomy and Billroth II gastrojejunostomy. (From Matthews JB, Silen W. Operations for peptic ulcer disease and early operative complications. In: Sleisenger MH, Fordtran JS, eds. *Gastrointestinal Disease*. 5th ed. Philadelphia: Saunders; 1993.)

PARTIAL GASTRECTOMY WITH BILLROTH I RECONSTRUCTION

An antrectomy removes the acid-secreting portion of the stomach, which contains the G cells that are responsible for secreting gastrin. To adequately remove all the G cells, 35% of the distal stomach should be removed. This correlates to removing 45% of the lesser curve (approximately 7 cm from the pylorus); the incisura is a reasonable proximal margin along the lesser curve. Fifteen percent of the distal greater curve should be removed; this correlates to the terminal portion of the right gastroepiploic artery. First, the greater curvature is mobilized along its distal portion by incising the gastrocolic ligament in an avascular plane. The dissection begins at the pylorus with ligation of the right gastroepiploic artery and proceeds cephalad along the greater curvature. It is important to take special care to avoid injury to the mesocolon and middle colic artery (Fig. 59.10). The dissection should be carried approximately 1 cm past the pylorus if a B I reconstruction is anticipated. If B II is anticipated, the dissection need only be carried far enough to comfortably place the transverse linear stapler past the pylorus or to close the duodenum by a handsewn technique. Next, the lesser curvature is mobilized (Fig. 59.11). The flimsy tissues of the lesser omentum are divided along the lesser curvature starting at the incisura and working toward the pylorus. The right gastric artery is divided and ligated. The posterior wall of the duodenal bulb is then carefully dissected off the pancreas. A Kocher maneuver should be performed prior to distal gastrectomy to minimize tension on the anastomosis. For handsewn gastroduodenostomy reconstruction first, the lower portion of the gastric staple line is removed. The length of the staple line to be removed is the same as the width of the duodenal stump. The duodenum and the stomach are then apposed through the placement of a posterior serosal layer of interrupted silk sutures (Fig. 59.12). An inner mucosal closure is initiated with a continuous absorbable suture (Fig. 59.13). The mucosal suture continues anteriorly (Fig. 59.14). Finally, an anterior serosal layer is placed with interrupted silk seromuscular sutures (Fig. 59.15).

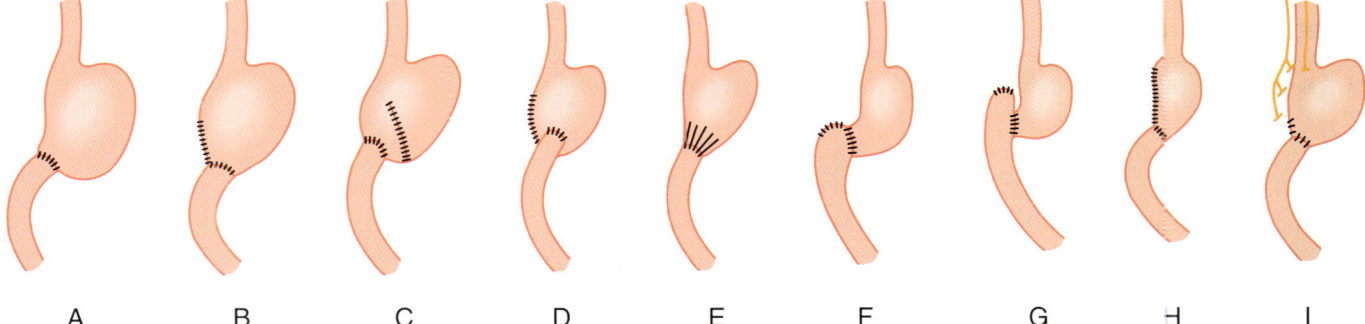

A   B   C   D   E   F   G   H   I

FIGURE 59.7 Variations of Billroth I reconstructions. (A) Billroth (1881). (B) Billroth (1881). (C) Kocher (1890). (D) Kutscha-Lissberg (1925). (E) v. Haberer (1920). (F) v. Haberer (1920), Finney (1923). (G) Winkelbauer (1927). (H) Schoemaker (1911). (I) Harkins, Nyhus (1960). (From Siewert JR, Bumm R. Billroth I gastrectomy. In: Baker RJ, Fischer JE, eds. *Mastery of Surgery*. Philadelphia: Lippincott Williams & Wilkins; 2001.)

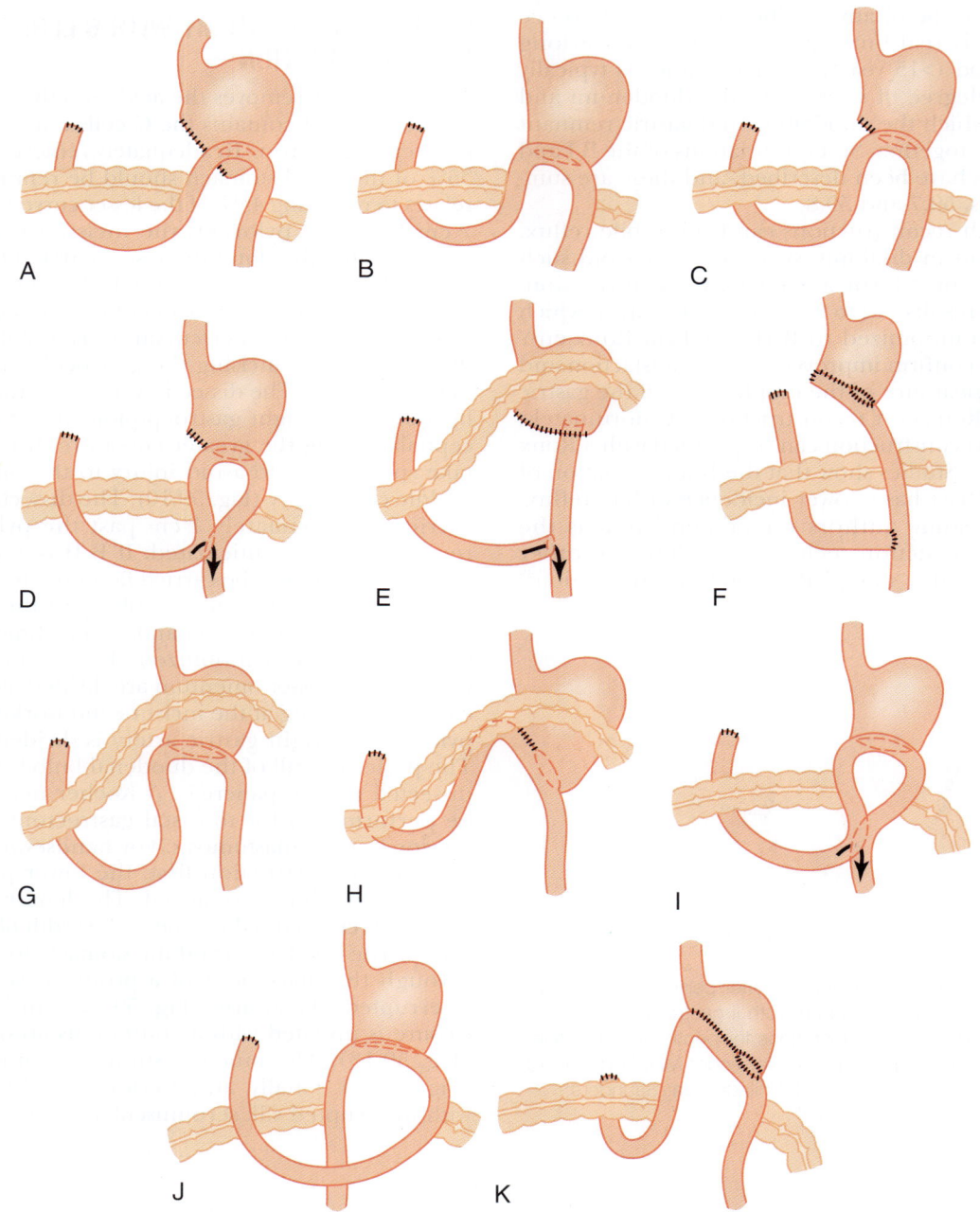

FIGURE 59.8 Variations of Billroth II reconstruction. (A) Billroth II. (B) Kronelin. (C) von Eiselberg. (D) Braun. (E) Roux. (F) Roux-en-Y. (G) Ploy and Reichel. (H) Finsterer-Hofmeister. (I) Balfour. (J) Moynihan. (K) Tanner. (From Wastell C, Davis PA. Billroth II gastrectomy. In: Baker RJ, Fischer JE, eds. *Mastery of Surgery*. Philadelphia: Lippincott Williams & Wilkins; 2001.)

For a stapled gastroduodenostomy, a gastrotomy is created with electrocautery on the anterior surface of the stomach at least 3 cm proximal to the staple closure (Fig. 59.16). The end-to-end stapling device, without the anvil, is passed into the anterior gastrotomy with the rod advancing through the posterior gastric wall, again 3 cm proximal to the stapled edge. The anvil is introduced into the duodenum after placement of a purse-string suture in the end of the duodenum (Fig. 59.17). The end-to-end anastomotic (EEA) stapler is closed, fired, and withdrawn.

The anastomosis is inspected to ensure adequate hemostasis. The anvil is then removed and checked to ensure that tissue doughnuts from both the duodenum and the stomach are present. The gastrotomy is closed by the application of a TA stapling device or sutured closed in two layers (Fig. 59.18). Laparoscopic partial gastrectomy with B I reconstruction has been described using many different surgical techniques. It can be performed using linear or end-to-end stapling devices depending on the surgeon's preference and mobility of the duodenum.

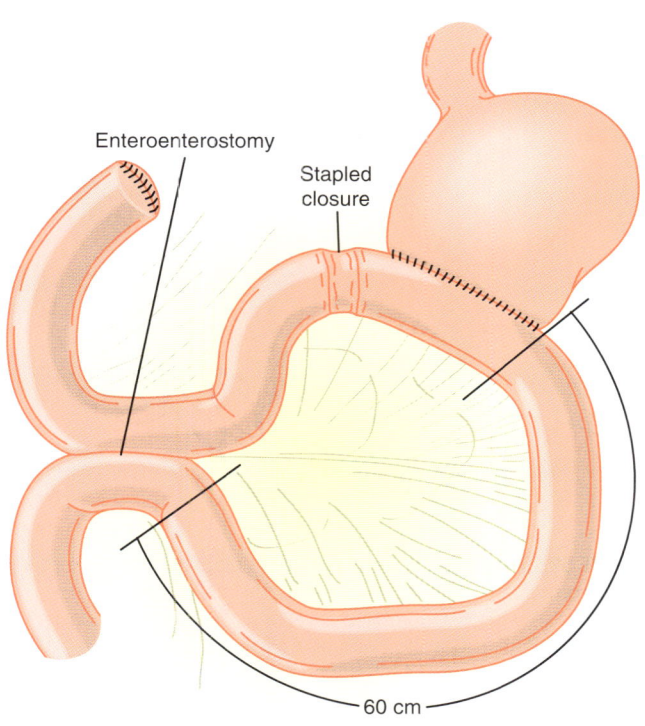

FIGURE 59.9 "Uncut" Roux-en-Y reconstruction after partial gastrectomy. A jejunoduodenostomy with a 60-cm efferent limb is constructed. The afferent limb is occluded with a staple line. (From van Stiegmann G, Goff JS. An alternative to Roux-en-Y for treatment of bile reflux gastritis. *Surg Gynecol Obstet.* 1988;166:69.)

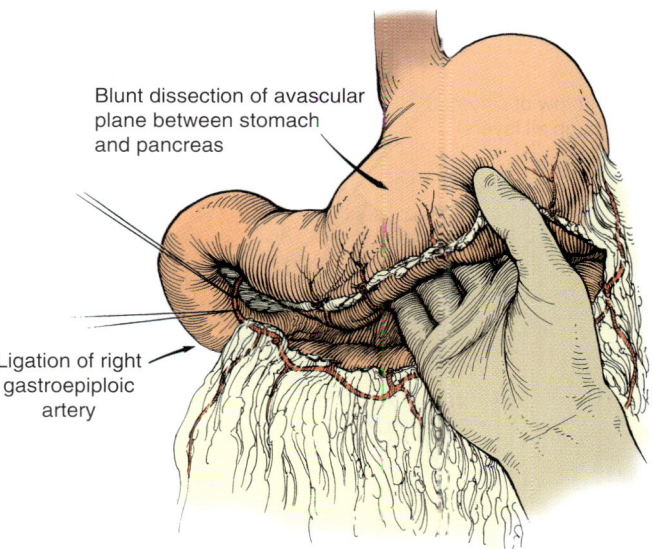

FIGURE 59.10 The gastrocolic omentum is dissected from the stomach. The dissection begins at the pylorus with ligation of the right gastroepiploic artery and proceeds cephalad along the greater curvature. The posterior antrum is then separated from the anterior pancreas and base of the transverse mesocolon by division of fine connective tissue attachments. (From Jones RS. Gastric resection: Billroth I anastomosis. In: Sabiston DC Jr, ed. *Atlas of General Surgery*. Philadelphia: Saunders; 1994:263.)

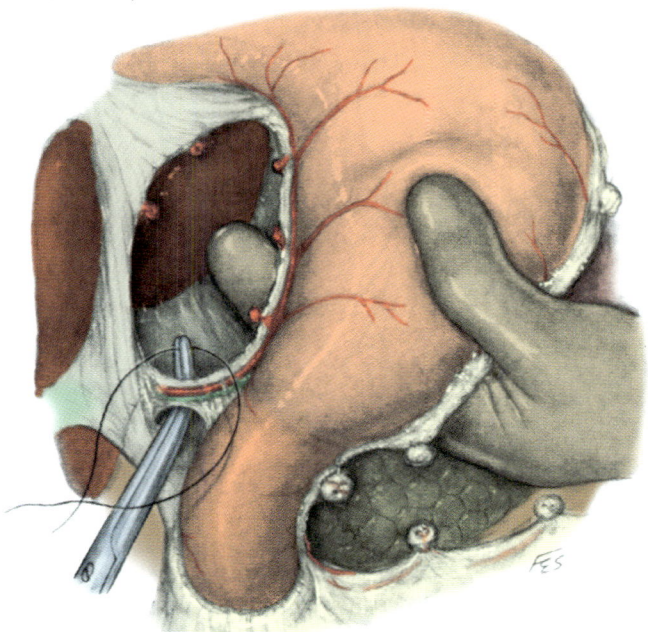

FIGURE 59.11 The gastrohepatic ligament is incised, and the lesser curvature is dissected. The right gastric vessels are ligated close to the stomach. In patients with pyloric inflammation, care must be taken to avoid injury to both the hepatic artery and the common bile duct. (From Sedgewick C. Gastrectomy. In: Braasch JW, Sedgewick CE, Veidenheimer MC, Ellis FH Jr, eds. *Atlas of Abdominal Surgery*. Philadelphia: Saunders; 1991:37.)

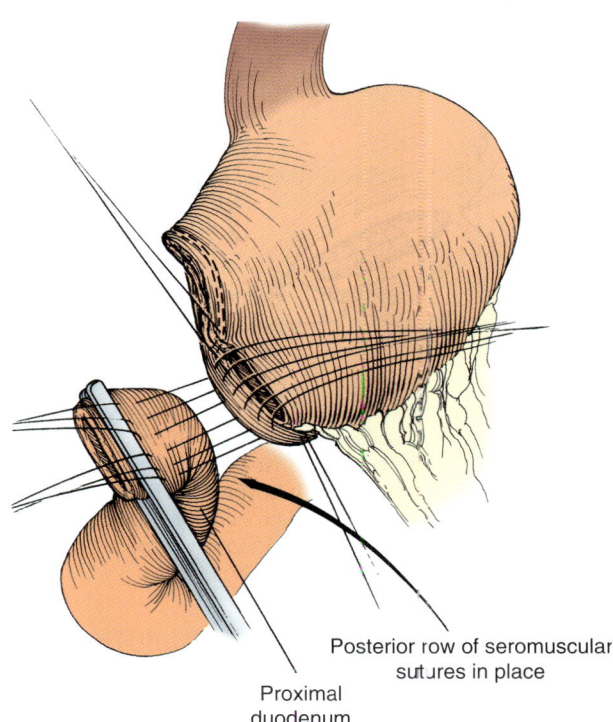

FIGURE 59.12 For gastroduodenostomy reconstruction, the duodenum and the inferior gastric staple line are apposed through the placement of a posterior serosal layer of interrupted silk sutures. (From Jones RS. Gastric resection: Billroth I. In: Sabiston DC Jr, ed. *Atlas of General Surgery*. Philadelphia: Saunders; 1994:267.)

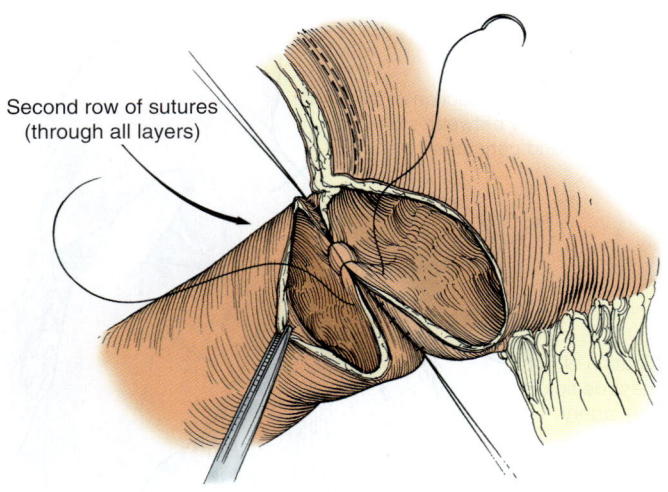

FIGURE 59.13 An inner mucosal closure is initiated with a continuous absorbable suture. (From Jones RS: Gastric resection: Billroth I. In: Sabiston DC Jr, ed. *Atlas of General Surgery*. Philadelphia: Saunders; 1994:268.)

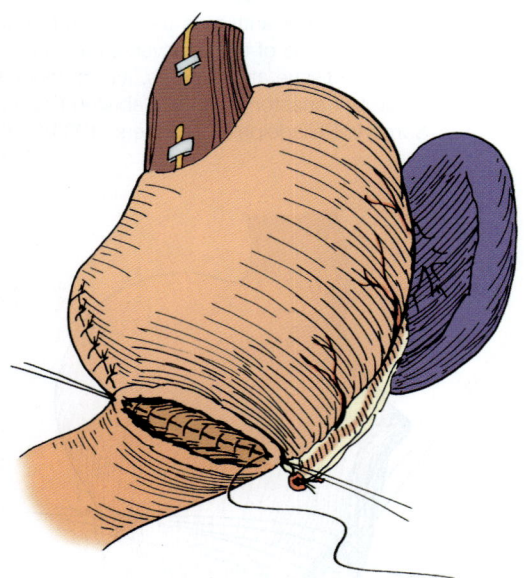

FIGURE 59.14 The mucosal suture continues anteriorly. (From Zinner MJ. *Atlas of Gastric Surgery*. New York: Churchill Livingstone; 1992. After Gloege. In: Soybel DI, Zinner MJ: Stomach and duodenum: operative procedures. In: Zinner MJ, Schwartz SI, Ellis H, eds. *Maingot's Abdominal Operations*. Stamford, CT: Appleton and Lange; 1997:1105.)

PARTIAL GASTRECTOMY WITH A BILLROTH II RECONSTRUCTION

Antrectomy is carried out as described previously. The proximal end of the stomach is divided with a TA 90 stapling device or can also be accomplished with two applications of a gastrointestinal anastomotic (GIA) stapling device. The proximal duodenum is divided with care to avoid injury to the common bile duct. The duodenal closure can be reinforced with interrupted 3-0 silk sutures. The gastric staple line is oversewn superiorly with either

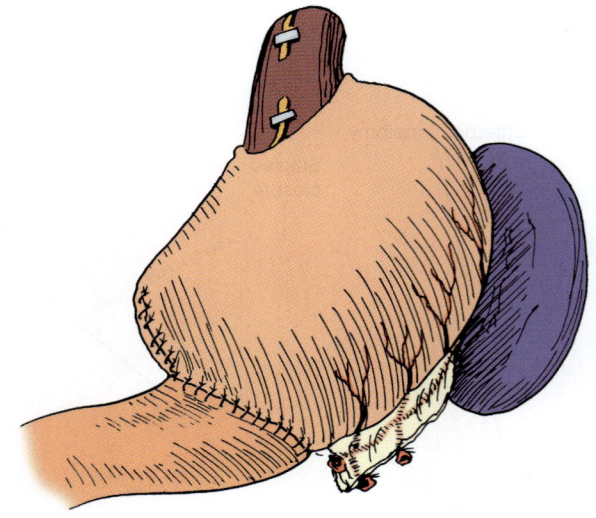

FIGURE 59.15 An anterior serosal layer is placed with interrupted silk seromuscular sutures. (From Zinner MJ. *Atlas of Gastric Surgery*. New York: Churchill Livingstone; 1992. After Gloege. In: Soybel DI, Zinner MJ: Stomach and duodenum: operative procedures. In: Zinner MJ, Schwartz SI, Ellis H, eds. *Maingot's Abdominal Operations*. Stamford, CT: Appleton and Lange; 1997:1105.)

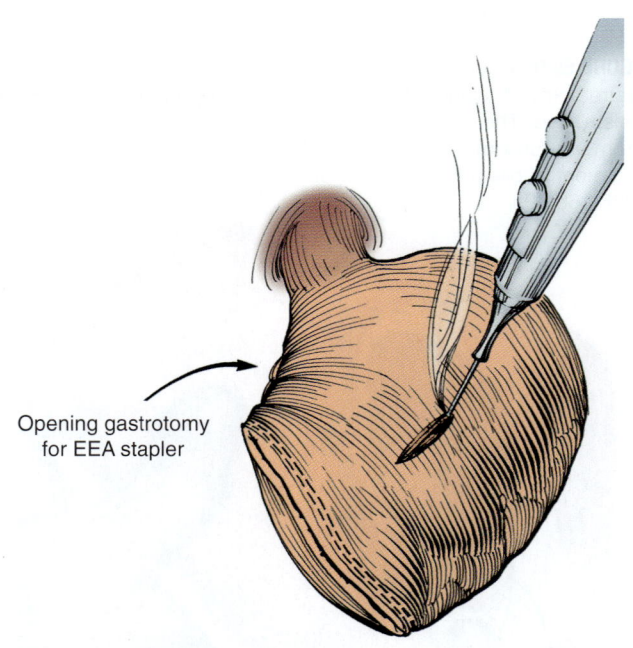

Opening gastrotomy for EEA stapler

FIGURE 59.16 For a stapled gastroduodenostomy, a gastrotomy is created with electrocautery on the anterior surface of the stomach at least 3 cm proximal to the staple closure. *EEA*, End-to-end anastomotic. (From Siegler HF. Gastric resection: Billroth I anastomosis [stapler]. In: Sabiston DC Jr, ed. *Atlas of General Surgery*. Philadelphia: Saunders; 1994:274.)

continuous or interrupted suture (Fig. 59.19). Traction sutures are useful to steady the remnant within the operative field. A proximal loop of jejunum is chosen and apposed to the stomach. The jejunum can be delivered through an incision in the transverse mesocolon or anterior to the transverse colon. As long as the anastomosis will

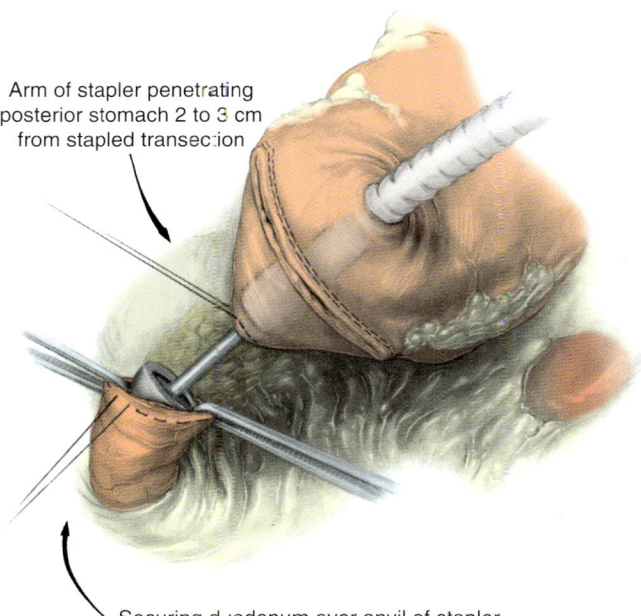

Arm of stapler penetrating posterior stomach 2 to 3 cm from stapled transection

Securing duodenum over anvil of stapler

FIGURE 59.17 The end-to-end stapling device, without the anvil, is passed into the anterior gastrotomy with the rod advancing through the posterior gastric wall, again 3 cm proximal to the stapled edge. The anvil is introduced into the duodenum after placement of a purse-string suture with an automatic device. The end-to-end anastomotic stapler is closed, fired, and withdrawn. (From Siegler HF. Gastric resection: Billroth I anastomosis [stapler]. In: Sabiston DC Jr, ed. *Atlas of General Surgery.* Philadelphia: Saunders; 1994:275.)

not be under tension, the antecolic position will permit emptying as effective as the retrocolic anastomosis. For malignant disease, some surgeons favor an antecolic anastomosis to avoid disease recurrence and subsequent gastric outlet obstruction. If a retrocolic position is chosen, the window in the transverse mesocolon should be closed following construction of the anastomosis to prevent kinking and obstruction of the jejunal limbs. Interrupted sutures are placed in seromuscular fashion between the posterior gastric wall and the antimesenteric border of the jejunum (Fig. 59.20). Matching incisions are made with electrocautery in the jejunum and stomach, with the latter involving partial excision of the stapled gastric closure (Fig. 59.21). The posterior full-thickness suture line is initiated with a continuous suture of absorbable material on a double arm. Corner sutures include the anterior gastric wall, the posterior gastric wall, and the jejunum. The inner layer, full-thickness suture is continued along the length of the anterior aspect of the anastomosis. An anterior layer of interrupted silk sutures completes the anastomosis (Fig. 59.22).

For stapled gastroenterostomy, the jejunal limb is placed next to gastric stapled line. Traction sutures are placed. A linear stapler is placed through a small gastrotomy and small enterotomy to create gastrojejunostomy. The enterotomy sites are closed either by TA stapler or handsewn. Similar to the open technique, a laparoscopic partial gastrectomy and B II reconstruction procedure is conducted in the same order as previously described.

TABLE 59.1 Ulcer Recurrence Rates for the Three Common Acid-Reducing Procedures

Surgical Procedure	Ulcer Recurrence Rate (%)	Risk of Side Effects
Truncal vagotomy with drainage	10	Highest
Truncal vagotomy with antrectomy	2	High
Proximal gastric vagotomy	5	Low

PARTIAL GASTRECTOMY WITH A ROUX-EN-Y RECONSTRUCTION

After antrectomy and duodenal closure, reconstruction with the Roux-en-Y gastrojejunostomy is performed by dividing the jejunum approximately 40 cm distal to the ligament of Treitz. The mesentery is divided in a straight line down to the origin to allow more mobility of the Roux limb. A 50- to 70-cm Roux limb is created and a side-to-side jejunojejunal anastomosis is constructed. The mesenteric defect is closed using a running 2-0 silk suture to prevent internal hernias. A mesocolic window large enough to accommodate the Roux limb is created to the left of the middle colic vessels. The Roux limb is then advanced through the window up to the proximal stomach. Care must be taken not to twist the mesentery of the Roux limb when performing this maneuver. Alternatively the Roux limb may be placed in an antecolic position. The gastrojejunostomy can be performed via handsewn, an EEA- or a side-to-side linear-stapled anastomosis.

CHOICE OF OPERATION FOR INTRACTABLE DUODENAL ULCER

As can be seen from the earlier descriptions, a variety of surgical operations are available for patients with intractable duodenal ulcer. Reliable data on the results of the various procedures for duodenal ulcer were generated by a series of trials during the latter half of the 20th century. Published series generally used different criteria for patient selection and for estimating the incidence of side effects. Table 59.1 summarizes the data on the three most commonly performed procedures: TV and antrectomy, TV and drainage, and PGV. Mortality and early morbidity were highest for the resection procedures and lowest for PGV, which avoids opening the gastrointestinal tract. Recurrence rates were significantly lower for vagotomy and antrectomy. TV with pyloroplasty is virtually never indicated as an elective procedure because it has both the disadvantages of a high incidence of postgastrectomy complications and a high ulcer recurrence rate (10% to 15%).

Historically, an important factor when considering the choice of operation was the ulcer recurrence rate. However, with identification of *H. pylori*, it is believed that recurrences are for the most part eliminated, although no data in this setting have yet been generated. Because of this, PGV, which is associated with fewer postoperative sequelae, is the preferred acid-reducing procedure in patients with intractable ulcer symptoms. One trial randomized 248

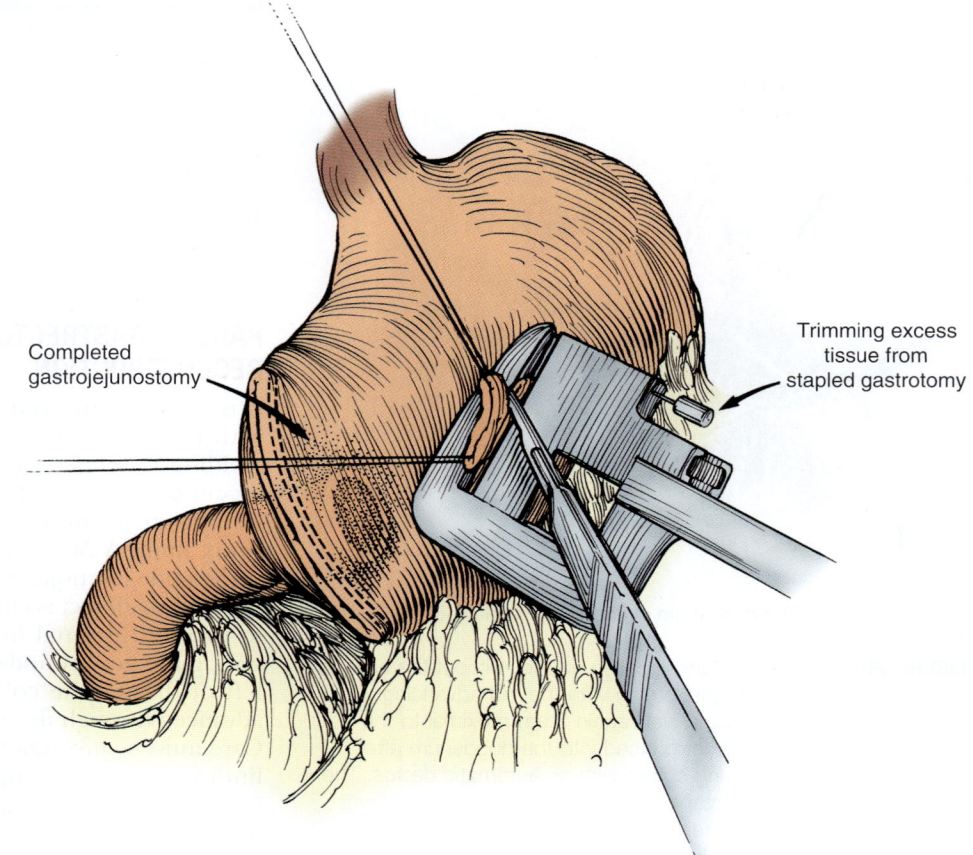

FIGURE 59.18 The anastomosis is inspected to ensure adequate hemostasis. The anvil is then removed and checked to ensure that tissue doughnuts from both the duodenum and the stomach are present. The gastrotomy is closed by the application of a TA stapling device. (From Siegler HF. Gastric resection: Billroth I anastomosis [stapler]. In: Sabiston DC Jr, ed. *Atlas of General Surgery*. Philadelphia: Saunders; 1994:276.)

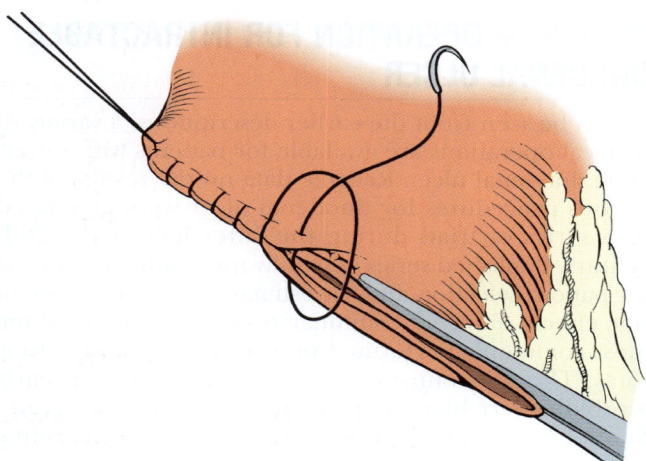

FIGURE 59.19 The gastric staple line is oversewn superiorly. (Modified from Townsend CM, Evers BM. *Atlas of General Surgical Techniques*. Philadelphia: Elsevier; 2010; [Fig. 27.6B and C].)

patients with stable PUD to TV and drainage, SV and drainage, or PGV. At 11 to 15 years after surgery, PGV was associated with reductions in the incidence of severe postvagotomy symptoms, such as dumping, diarrhea, and dyspepsia. Interestingly, this study did not show a significant difference in the ulcer recurrence rates among the three groups.[20] Although this would more strongly favor PGV,

current experience with this more complex procedure is limited.

GIANT DUODENAL ULCER

Giant duodenal ulcer (GDU) is defined as a duodenal ulcer that is benign and measures at least 2 cm in diameter. The size of the ulcer makes it difficult to treat because the ulcer, by definition, involves the full circumference of the duodenal wall, leading to scarring and deformity of the duodenal bulb. GDU is seen in up to 1% to 2% of all duodenal ulcer.[47] When compared with standard-size duodenal ulcers, GDUs are less often associated with *H. pylori* infection, and NSAID use plays a more prominent role.[50]

Patients usually present with epigastric pain that can radiate to the back, particularly when the ulcer penetrates into the pancreas. In complicated cases, patient can present with a combination of bleeding, perforation, and/or obstruction. Diagnosis is established via upper endoscopy. It is important to measure the ulcer so as not to misdiagnose it as a simple peptic ulcer. The ulcer usually involves more than 50% of the duodenal bulb circumference. It is essential to rule out cancer as the cause of ulcer formation with biopsy in the setting of GDUs, because the risk of malignancy in such a setting is approximately 19%.[47]

The first line of treatment for an uncomplicated GDU after ruling out cancer is PPI with eradication of *H. pylori* and discontinuation of NSAIDs. It is very important to confirm *H. pylori* eradication through a noninvasive test such as urea breath test and repeat endoscopy to confirm healing in 8 to 12 weeks. If the ulcer is partially healed,

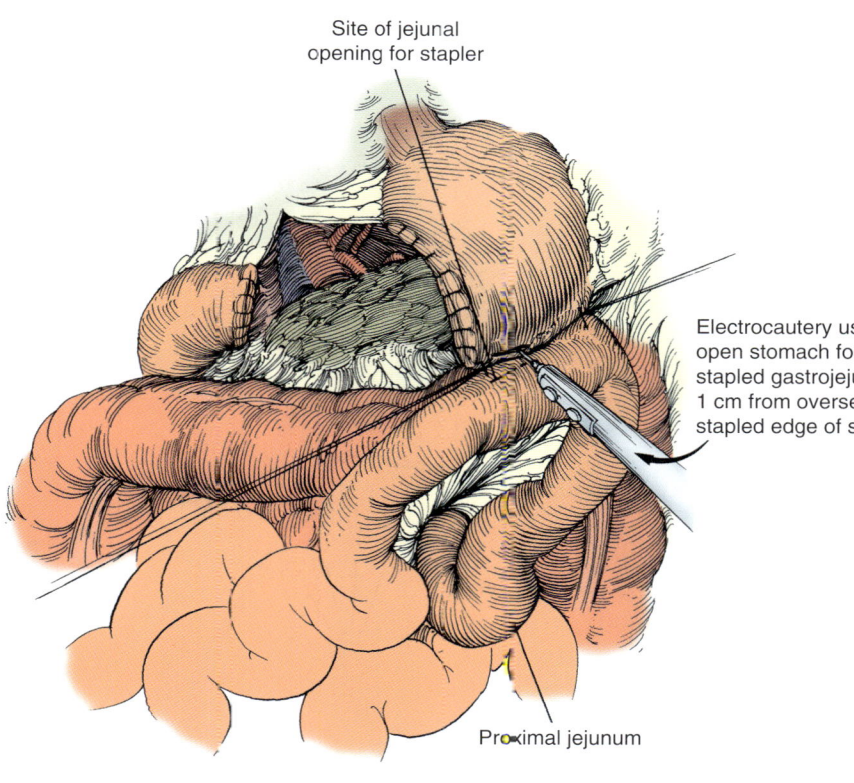

Site of jejunal
opening for stapler

Electrocautery used to
open stomach for
stapled gastrojejunostomy
1 cm from oversewn
stapled edge of stomach

Proximal jejunum

FIGURE 59.20 A proximal loop of
jejunum is apposed to the stomach.
Interrupted sutures are placed in
seromuscular fashion between the
posterior gastric wall and the
antimesenteric border of the jejunum.
(From Jones RS. Gastric resection:
Billroth II. In: Sabiston DC Jr, ed. *Atlas
of General Surgery*. Philadelphia:
Saunders; 1994:284.)

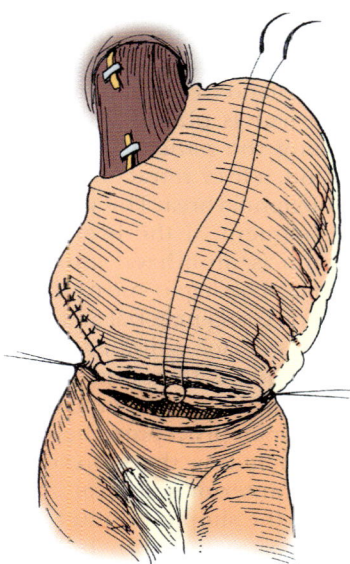

FIGURE 59.21 Matching incisions are made in the jejunum and
stomach, with the latter involving partial excision of the stapled
gastric closure. The posterior mucosal closure is initiated with a
continuous suture of absorbable material. Corner sutures include
the anterior gastric wall, the posterior gastric wall, and the
jejunum. (From Zinner MJ. *Atlas of Gastric Surgery*. New York:
Churchill Livingstone; 1992. After Gloege. In: Soybel DI, Zinner
MJ: Stomach and duodenum: operative procedures In: Zinner
MJ, Schwartz SI, Ellis H, eds. *Maingot's Abdominal Operations*.
Stamford, CT: Appleton and Lange; 1997:1112.)

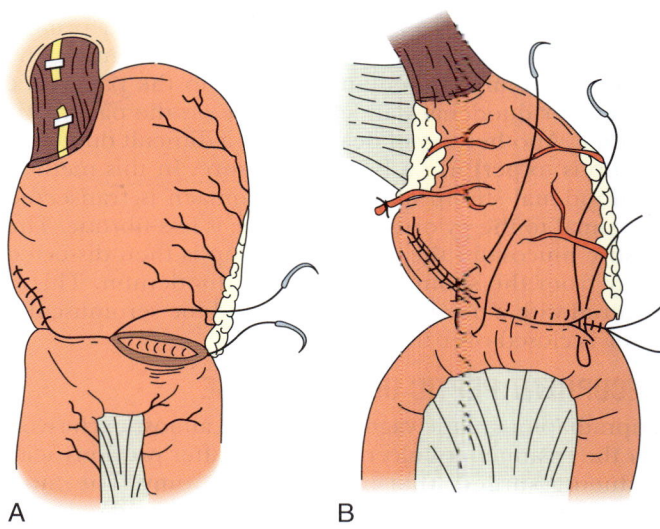

A   B

FIGURE 59.22 (A) The mucosal suture is continued along the
length of the anterior aspect of the anastomosis. (B) An anterior
layer of interrupted silk sutures completes the anastomosis.

medical treatment should continue for another 8 to 12 weeks, with repeat endoscopy afterward to confirm complete healing.

Because of the large, penetrating nature of these ulcers, when not recognized and treated promptly, complications such as hemorrhage and perforation can occur, resulting in high rates of morbidity and mortality.

Operative intervention for GDU is indicated for patients who present with

1. Hemorrhage in spite of maximum endoscopic intervention
2. Perforation
3. Gastric outlet obstruction
4. Intractability or recurrent disease in spite of maximum medical therapy

The chronic inflammatory changes associated with this condition often make the operations technically challenging. A definitive acid-reducing operation should be performed in addition to removing the involved duodenum whenever possible. If the inflammation and edema of the duodenum is not a factor, a B I reconstruction can occasionally be performed. However, dissection and anastomosis can be hazardous, and it is best to leave the ulcer bed in situ and perform a B II. In such cases, duodenal stump leak is a major source of morbidity and mortality postoperatively. The use of a duodenostomy tube is known to be a safe and effective means in dealing with a difficult duodenal stump. This involves insertion of a tube through the second portion of the duodenum to encourage formation of a controlled fistula; by doing so, this takes off the pressure from the stump and allows healing.

In situations in which the duodenum is scarred to the pancreatic capsule, a Nissen closure can be performed. This is performed by first transecting the duodenum. The duodenal stump is then anastomosed to the pancreatic capsule or duodenal wall left in place on the pancreatic capsule. Another way of dealing with a difficult duodenal stump is to perform a Bancroft closure. In this method of duodenal stump closure, the stomach is transected proximal to the pylorus, where tissue is less fibrotic. The gastric mucosa in the duodenal stump is then dissected away from the submucosa into the duodenum. This is secured with a purse-string suture, and the seromuscular layer is closed over the stump.

RECURRENT PEPTIC ULCER DISEASE

Supradiaphragmatic vagotomy is used almost exclusively for the treatment of ulcer recurrence after previous acid-reducing surgery that included vagotomy. The most common cause for ulcer recurrence after an acid-reducing procedure is an incomplete vagotomy. Attempting to find the missed nerve through the densely scarred upper abdomen is fraught with difficulty and can be hazardous. Transthoracic TV may be successfully used. The procedure can now be performed with minimally invasive thoracoscopic techniques.

LAPAROSCOPIC SURGERY

An increasing number of reports indicates the feasibility of laparoscopic and robotic assisted approaches to operations for PUD. When performing a laparoscopic partial gastrectomy, the abdomen is entered at the left subcostal area using an optical trocar. The camera port is placed

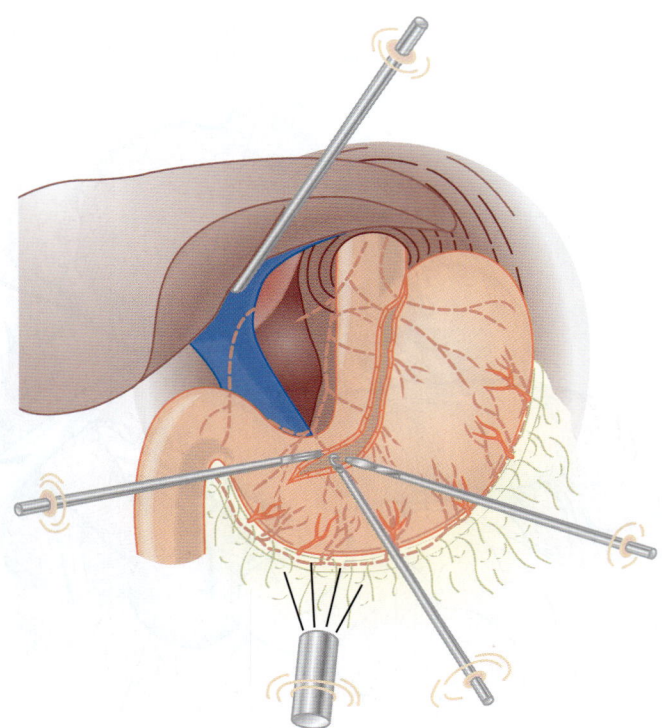

FIGURE 59.23 Laparoscopic anterior seromyotomy as part of the Taylor procedure. (From Dubois F. New surgical strategy for gastroduodenal ulcer: laparoscopic approach. *World J Surg.* 2000;24:270.)

approximately 15 cm from the xiphoid process, slightly to the left of the midline. A 12-mm trocar is used for the surgeon's right hand to accommodate a linear stapler. A third 5-mm trocar is placed in the right subcostal area. After placing the patient in steep reverse Trendelenburg position, a liver retractor is placed via a 5-mm incision in the subxiphoid area. This will elevate and retract the left lateral segment of the liver. The first portion of the duodenum is mobilized and divided using a laparoscopic stapler. The staple line can be reinforced with suture or staple-buttressing material at the surgeon's discretion. The proximal stomach is divided using a laparoscopic stapler. Reconstruction is then performed either with a B II gastrojejunostomy or a Roux-en-Y gastrojejunostomy.

Although most open procedures have been attempted laparoscopically, including the more difficult PGV, the Taylor procedure (anterior seromyotomy with posterior TV) appears to be the simplest option (Fig. 59.23). The Taylor procedure was reported in 1982 as an open procedure. Although the open approach is not widely performed, the technique is very suitable for a laparoscopic procedure. This procedure starts with a posterior TV followed by a seromyotomy that should start approximately 6 cm proximal to the pylorus. The circular muscle is incised 1.5 cm from the lesser curve and the muscle fibers divided using a hook coagulator. The dissection is continued caudally as far as the gastroesophageal junction. Along the length of the myotomy all of the circular muscle fibers are divided. It is not necessary to divide the deeper thin layer of the oblique muscle. Air is injected through a nasogastric tube to make sure there are no leaks. The seromyotomy is then closed with an overlapping running suture.[51]

ELECTIVE OPERATION FOR INTRACTABLE GASTRIC ULCER DISEASE

Although both gastric and duodenal ulcers are peptic lesions, fundamental differences between these entities affect surgical strategy. The most important difference is that gastric ulcers more commonly may harbor malignancy and thus must be excised or generously biopsied. Acid hypersecretion, which is important in pathogenesis of duodenal ulcers, does not have a role in pathogenesis of many gastric ulcers. In 1965 Dr. H.D. Johnson published a classification system that subsequently was adopted and, with little modification, is still currently in use. In his 1965 paper, he discusses Dragstedt's theory that the cephalic phase of acid secretion is responsible for duodenal ulceration and that the gastric phase was responsible for gastric ulceration. He observed that his theory disregards the findings that less than half of patients with gastric ulcers are acid hypersecreters. He argues for a multifactorial pathogenesis for ulcers beyond the hypersecretion of gastric acid.[52] The Johnson classification system, which is based upon anatomic location and acid-secretory potential, provides a useful basis for considering operative treatment of gastric ulcer (Table 59.2 and Fig. 59.24).

TYPE I GASTRIC ULCER

Type I ulcers are the most common form and are responsible for up to 60% of gastric ulcers. These typically occur along the lesser curvature at the junction of the fundic and antral mucosa near the area of the incisura and occur in the setting of acid hyposecretion. Distal gastrectomy with B I or II reconstruction is recommended for most patients because this approach removes the ulcer and the diseased antrum. Partial gastrectomy also eliminates the risk of missing a malignancy associated with a biopsy and reduces the acid secretory potential. Another option is to perform distal gastrectomy with Roux-en-Y gastrojejunostomy; as compared with B I and II, there is decreased dumping syndrome and patients do not get bile reflux gastritis.[53,54] However, patients who undergo Roux-en-Y reconstruction are at higher risk of delayed gastric emptying. A randomized study evaluating patients who underwent B I versus Roux-en-Y reconstruction following distal gastrectomy for cancer found no difference in long-term quality of life.[55] Earlier recommendations of performing a biopsy of the ulcer combined with vagotomy and drainage are now outdated because of the high ulcer recurrence rates.[56] Addition of a TV to gastric resection offers no additional benefit to the patient.[57] Low recurrence rates (5%) and excellent symptomatic relief are usually achieved with a distal gastrectomy alone.

TYPE II GASTRIC ULCER

Type II gastric ulcers occur in the pyloric channel synchronously with ulceration in the duodenum or metachronously with scarring in the duodenum. Therefore patients presenting with a pyloric channel ulcer and history of duodenal ulcer classifies the gastric ulcer as type II and should be treated as such. They tend to be large, deep ulcers with poorly defined margins. They frequently occur in younger men and are associated with increased acid secretion. Preoperative endoscopic examination of such ulcers must include biopsy of the lesion to rule out an underlying malignancy. Treatment is similar to duodenal ulcer, with vagotomy and antrectomy as the preferred approach. PGV alone in type II gastric ulcer is

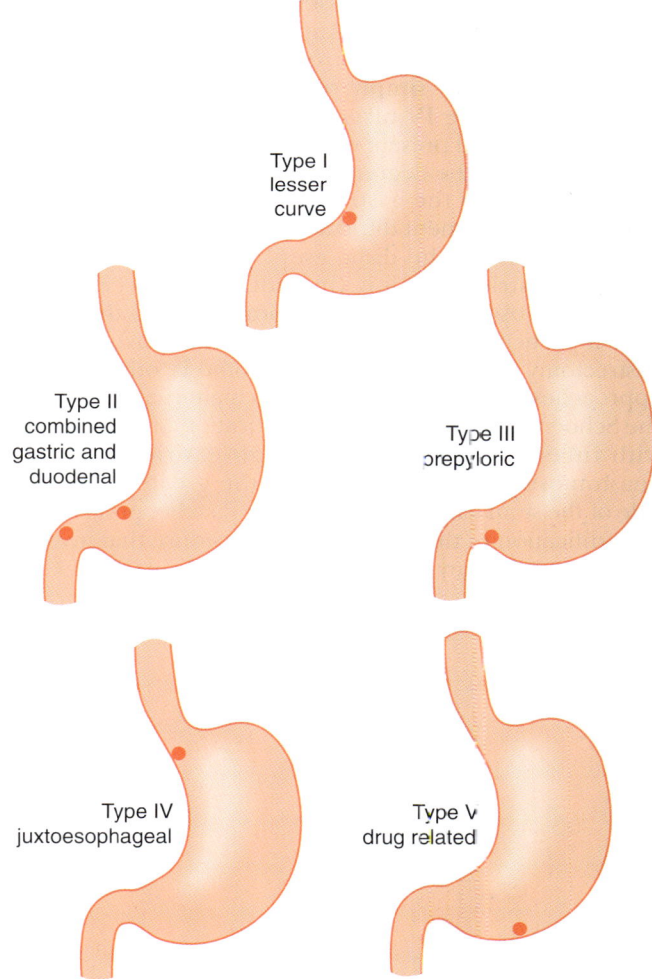

FIGURE 59.24 Classification of gastric ulcers based on their anatomic location. (From Matthews JB, Silen W. Operations for peptic ulcer disease and early operative complications. In: Sleisenger MH, Fordtran JS, eds. *Gastrointestinal Disease.* Philadelphia: Saunders; 1993.)

TABLE 59.2 Modified Johnson Classification of Gastric Ulcers

Type	Location	Acid Secretion
I	Lesser curvature	Low
II	Body of stomach and duodenum	High
III	Prepyloric (within 2–3 cm of pylorus)	High
IV	High on lesser curve, near gastroesophageal junction	Low
V	Anywhere, induced by medication	Low

discouraged because it leaves the gastric ulcer behind, which can harbor malignancy.

TYPE III GASTRIC ULCER

Type III ulcers are prepyloric or pyloric channel ulcers. They occur in the setting of increased acid secretion and are also approached in a manner similar to duodenal ulcer and type II gastric ulcer. Type III ulcers are particularly resistant to both medical therapy and PGV, with recurrence rates ranging from 16% to 44% in various series.[39] This finding, plus the observation that these lesions may harbor gastric malignancy, makes vagotomy and antrectomy the most prudent approach. Early consideration for surgical referral is advisable for resistant ulcers or those that present with obstructive symptoms. Ulcers associated with acid hypersecretion are responsible for approximately 45% of gastric ulcer disease, with type II accounting for 25% and type III for 20%.

TYPE IV GASTRIC ULCER

Type IV gastric ulcer is distinguished by its anatomic location high along the lesser curvature, close to the gastroesophageal junction. Antral mucosa may extend to within 1 to 2 cm of the gastroesophageal junction; thus type IV ulcers may simply represent a subset of type I gastric ulcer. Type IV ulcers are associated with gastric hyposecretion and present early with dysphagia and reflux. Large ulcer size, the degree of surrounding inflammation, and proximity to the gastroesophageal junction render operative management difficult and potentially dangerous. If the integrity of the distal esophagus can be ensured, subtotal gastric resection (including the ulcer bed) is considered optimal. However, lesions close to the cardia pose a particular challenge, and, to help to avoid a total gastrectomy and an esophageal anastomosis, other surgical approaches have been described. Such alternatives include the Schoemaker procedure (a modification of B I resection with tube-shaped resection of high gastric ulcers and anastomosis of the duodenum to the greater curvature side of the stomach; see Fig. 59.7), the Pauchet procedure,[58] a modification of the Schoemaker procedure that involves a lower gastrectomy and excision of the ulcer (Fig. 59.25),

or nonresective procedures in which the ulcer itself is not excised, the Kelling-Madlener procedure, or vagotomy with pyloroplasty, which has a high ulcer recurrence rate. The risk of malignant transformation or missed malignancy (despite biopsies) is small but real, and thus the nonresective procedures are not recommended in this setting.

Although there is no consensus in the literature, some have suggested that for ulcers 5 cm below the cardia, the Pauchet procedure should be used, whereas for those lesions within 2 cm of the cardia, the Csendes procedure should be attempted (see Fig. 59.25).[59] The Csendes procedure involves a near-total gastrectomy and a Roux-en-Y esophagogastrojejunostomy for reconstruction. The principle of this operation is to remove the high gastric ulcer such that the circumference of the esophageal mucosa remains intact.

TYPE V GASTRIC ULCER

These lesions can occur anywhere in the stomach and are induced by the use of medications, such as NSAIDs. Prophylactic regimens that have been shown to dramatically reduce the risk of ulcers, especially if the NSAID treatment cannot be stopped, include the use of PPI and/or prostaglandin analogue.[60,61] A definitive antisecretory operation (TV and antrectomy) should be considered if medical treatment fails or if the NSAID treatment cannot be stopped.

GASTRIC OUTLET OBSTRUCTION

More than half of gastric outlet obstruction cases are caused by malignant disease rather than by chronic PUD. Consequently, a careful work-up with biopsy should be done to clarify the diagnosis. Gastric outlet obstruction represents 5% to 8% of ulcer-related complications and results in an estimated 2000 operations per year in the United States.[62] Patients with gastric outlet (pyloric) obstruction because of a duodenal ulcer typically present with symptoms of gastric retention, including early satiety, bloating, indigestion, anorexia, nausea, vomiting, epigastric pain, and weight loss. They are frequently malnourished and dehydrated and have a metabolic alkalosis, which are factors that increase the operative risk. Operation in these

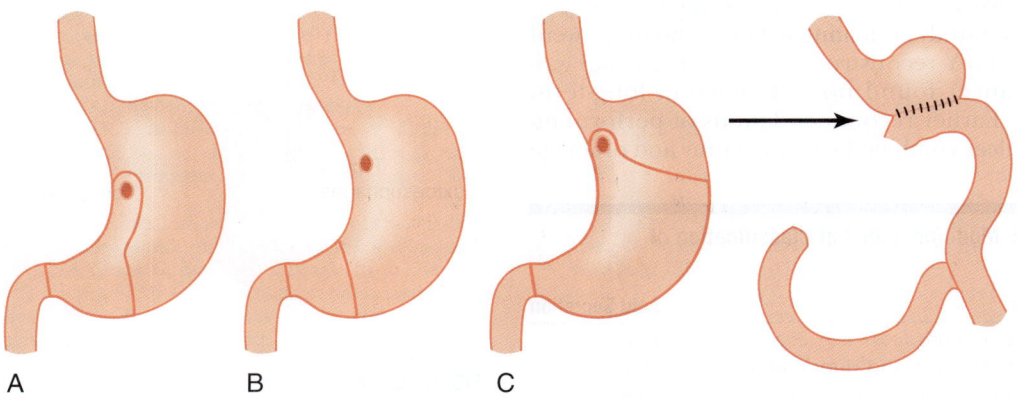

FIGURE 59.25 Operations for a type IV gastric ulcer. (A) Pauchet procedure. (B) Kelling-Madlener procedure. (C) Csendes procedure (esophagogastrojejunostomy). (Modified from Seymour NE. Operations for peptic ulcer and their complications. In: Feldman M, Scharschmidt BF, Sleisenger MH, eds. *Gastrointestinal Disease*. Philadelphia: Saunders; 1998.)

cases is almost never emergent and should be performed only after the patient has been stabilized and nutritional and electrolyte abnormalities have been corrected. Nasogastric decompression is helpful in decreasing gastric atony and hastening the time to resumption of postoperative oral intake. Nevertheless, operation is generally indicated if obstruction fails to resolve despite 48 to 72 hours of adequate intravenous fluid replenishment, antisecretory therapy, and nasogastric tube decompression. In a less acute setting in which the obstruction is incomplete, balloon dilation of the scarred pylorus may be attempted. Approximately 65% of patients experience sustained relief, but many require more than one dilation session. In patients who fail endoscopic dilation, operation is a reasonable option. The most serious complication of dilation is a perforation. Whenever balloon dilation is being attempted, it is important to rule out an underlying malignancy.

TV with antrectomy is the ideal procedure for this condition. Placement of a feeding jejunostomy tube at the time of operation is usually recommended, both because of preoperative malnutrition and because the chronic gastric outlet obstruction predisposes to delayed postoperative gastric emptying. Furthermore, addition of either a retrograde jejunogastrostomy or gastrostomy tube is also beneficial. As a result of the extensive scarring present in the duodenum, pyloroplasty of various types are usually not possible. The Jaboulay side-to-side duodenoplasty may be used in this setting. In one report of 19 patients treated with this procedure combined with PGV, there was a high degree of patient satisfaction (100% modified Visick grade I or II), universal weight gain, and no operative mortality or ulcer recurrence at mean follow-up of 31 months.[63] However, these benefits have not been noted in all reports. One trial randomized 90 consecutive patients with gastric outlet obstruction secondary to duodenal ulcer to PGV with gastrojejunostomy, PGV with Jaboulay duodenoplasty, or SV with antrectomy. Although there were no differences in the postoperative course or the reduction in gastric acid secretion, both PGV with gastrojejunostomy and SV with antrectomy produced a superior clinical result to PGV with Jaboulay pyloroplasty.[64] Although the need for pyloric reconstruction or bypass would theoretically negate several advantages of PGV over other options, preservation of antropyloric innervation may preserve controlled gastric emptying and minimize bile reflux.[65] In the past, simple gastrojejunostomy was not recommended because of a nearly 50% recurrence rate of ulcer disease.[66] It should be noted that these data preceded the era of effective acid-reducing medication. With the increased adaptation of minimally invasive approaches, gastrojejunostomy with either vagotomy or lifelong proton pump inhibitor medication has gained resurgence in the management of gastric outlet obstruction.

The role of *H. pylori* in the pathogenesis of gastric outlet obstruction has also been evaluated. Studies show that the incidence of *H. pylori* infection in this population is low (33% to 57%).[62] However, in those infected with the organism, eradication therapy and balloon dilation may result in long-term symptomatic relief and alleviate the need for operation. In general, operation should be

the standard of therapy in this group (in particular, *H. pylori*–negative patients) until further studies define the role of nonoperative therapy in the *H. pylori*–positive patients.

EMERGENCY OPERATION FOR COMPLICATED PEPTIC ULCER DISEASE

Approximately two-thirds of operations for complicated PUD are required because of bleeding and approximately one-third are because of perforations.[21] Emergency operations for complicated PUD are most often performed in older adults and the sick. Patients may present with bleeding, perforation, or obstruction. The objectives of operation in these cases are to

1. Deal with the complication that necessitated surgical intervention
2. Reduce the risk of future ulcer recurrence
3. Perform a safe, quick, and effective operation
4. Minimize long-term effects on the gastrointestinal tract
5. Establish the *H. pylori* status of the patient

The major intraoperative dilemma is whether to proceed with a definitive antiulcer operation (to reduce the risk of recurrence) in addition to addressing the specific ulcer complication. This issue has received considerable attention over the past several decades but remains unsettled. Shifting ulcer epidemiology, recognition of the role of *H. pylori*, and improvements in medical therapy have confused this issue considerably, and the decision must be individualized. However, studies show a trend toward favoring of less complex procedures in the setting of emergencies (patching or oversewing of ulcers) and of avoiding vagotomy or gastric resections.[67]

Omission of an acid-reducing ulcer procedure carries a risk of recurrent ulcer symptoms and complications; this risk is variable in the literature but not negligible. Evidence suggests that this risk may be considerably reduced by treatment for *H. pylori* postoperatively but obviously only if the patient is *H. pylori* positive. Unfortunately, there is no reliable, rapid test for *H. pylori* at the time of operation to help guide this decision making. A definitive procedure is always more appropriate in the setting of NSAIDs, especially if the patient is unlikely to be able to stop the treatment because of an underlying medical condition. A definitive procedure is also recommended if patient has been on antisecretory therapy and developed an ulcer complication despite acid suppression. On the other hand, inclusion of an acid-reducing ulcer procedure may result in serious gastrointestinal sequelae in patients who may not have required the intervention. Definitive operation is generally avoided during emergency procedures with major underlying medical illness or intraoperative hemodynamic instability.

BLEEDING

Two-thirds of the emergency operations performed for PUD are carried out for uncontrolled hemorrhage. However, as endoscopic abilities improved, the indication for surgical treatment continued to decrease. As the indications for surgical interventions have changed dramatically, so have the operations. Eighty to 85% of bleeding

TABLE 59.3 The Forrest Classification for Endoscopic Findings and Rebleeding Risks

Classification	Rebleeding Risk
Grade Ia: active, pulsatile bleeding	High
Grade Ib: active, nonpulsatile bleeding	High
Grade IIa: nonbleeding visible vessel	High
Grade IIb: adherent clot	Intermediate
Grade IIc: black dot	Low
Grade III: no signs of recent bleeding	Low

ulcers stop bleeding spontaneously.[66] Of the remaining patients, 85% to 95% can be effectively treated by endoscopic means.[68,69] Currently many surgeons choose a limited surgical approach followed by medical management instead of the historical aggressive resections and gastric denervation procedures. Most patients who present with a bleeding upper gastrointestinal lesion have an endoscopic examination of the stomach, the first and second part of the duodenum. This procedure enables identification of the site of bleeding and allows therapeutic attempts at stopping the bleeding. Despite endoscopic advances, the mortality rate following ulcer bleeding has remained stable at 5% to 10%. Indeed, recent epidemiologic data suggest that the incidence and mortality rate of bleeding duodenal ulcers may be increasing in older women.[3] However, an estimated 10% to 20% of patients admitted with bleeding peptic ulcers fail medical therapy and require urgent surgical intervention. Thus the ability to predict the risk of rebleeding is important to the endoscopist and the surgeon because this permits closer monitoring of high-risk patients and early involvement of the surgical team in their management. High recurrent bleeding rates are associated with a spurting vessel, a visible arterial vessel in the ulcer bed, adherent clot, or a large ulcer bed. The Forrest classification was developed in an attempt to assess the risk of rebleeding based on endoscopic findings (Table 59.3).

Of those patients who have recurrent bleeding, a second endoscopic attempt at control of bleeding will fail in 25%, requiring an emergency operation. This has stimulated some debate as to the timing of operation for a bleeding peptic ulcer and the role of a second attempt at endoscopic therapy. Randomized prospective studies have shown no increase in mortality rate in patients who undergo a second therapeutic endoscopy versus surgery after the first failed endoscopy. Consequently, most clinicians would encourage a second attempt at endoscopic control.[70]

Current indications for operation for peptic ulcer hemorrhage include

1. Hemodynamic instability despite vigorous resuscitation (>4 units or >6 units taking into consideration the patient's age, with more transfusion tolerated for the younger patient)
2. Failure of endoscopic techniques to arrest hemorrhage
3. Recurrent hemorrhage after initial stabilization (with up to two attempts at obtaining endoscopic hemostasis)
4. Shock associated with recurrent hemorrhage
5. Continued slow bleeding with a transfusion requirement exceeding 3 units per day
6. GDU

Secondary or relative indications include a rare blood type or difficult crossmatch, refusal of transfusion, shock on presentation, advanced age, severe comorbid disease, and bleeding chronic gastric ulcer. The surgical threshold may have to be lowered in elderly patients who poorly tolerate prolonged resuscitation, large-volume transfusion, and periods of hypotension.

The mortality rate for bleeding PUD is approximately 6%, with most patients dying of non–bleeding-related causes, such as multiple organ system failure. Thus further improvements in endoscopic or pharmacologic therapy are unlikely to lower the mortality rate, and our focus should be on appropriate management of these patients to avoid organ failure.[71]

Operation for Bleeding Duodenal Ulcer

The first priority during an emergency operation for a bleeding duodenal ulcer is control of the bleeding site. If EGD has failed to identify the source of hemorrhage, a longitudinal pyloroduodenotomy is necessary to inspect the duodenal bulb and gastric antrum. The gastroduodenal artery is the usual source of bleeding, which should be controlled by placement of suture ligatures. After the bleeding has been addressed, a definitive acid-reducing operation may be performed. With the identification of *H. pylori*, the utility of a vagotomy has been questioned. However, the data suggest that, even in the era of *H. pylori* and our ability to eradicate it, a TV perhaps should be performed in those patients with a bleeding duodenal ulcer. There are several reasons for this recommendation:

1. Only 40% to 70% of patients with a bleeding duodenal ulcer are positive for *H. pylori*.
2. *H. pylori* testing in the setting of an acute hemorrhage is less reliable, with the CLO (*Campylobacter*-like organism) test having a false-negative rate of 18% versus 1% in those not actively bleeding.[72]
3. If an acid-reducing procedure is not performed, up to 50% of patients are at risk of recurrent bleeding.
4. Conflicting evidence that *H. pylori* treatment changes the risk of recurrent bleeding.

Our inability to determine the *H. pylori* status in the case of acute bleeding and the lack of evidence that treatment of *H. pylori* alters the risk of rebleeding reinforces the need to perform an acid-reducing operation at the time of initial operation; however, if the patient is unstable, addition of an acid-reducing procedure to the hemorrhage control aspect of the operation adds to the operative time and should be avoided. In the latter case, postoperative long-term PPI therapy and eradication of *H. pylori* is the more appropriate course of action.

Because it is simple to open the pylorus in a longitudinal fashion, TV with pyloroplasty is the most frequently used operation for bleeding duodenal ulcer. In most cases the bleeding will be localized in the first part of the duodenum and the bleeding vessel can be controlled at the time through the pyloroplasty incision. Upon entering the duodenum, the duodenal mucosa is inspected for any evidence of active bleeding, ulceration, or induration. If active bleeding is encountered, this is controlled by digital pressure. This controls the bleeding and gives time for fluid resuscitation of the patient. The bleeding vessel is then ligated. This vessel is often the gastroduodenal artery,

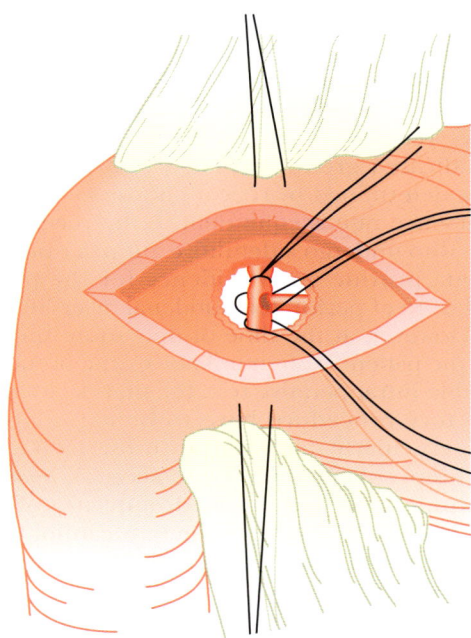

FIGURE 59.26 Technique of suture control of a bleeding duodenal ulcer. After a longitudinal pyloric incision and identification of the bleeding vessel, figure-of-eight sutures are placed at the cephalic and caudal aspects of the ulcer deep enough to occlude the gastroduodenal artery. An additional U stitch is placed to control small transverse pancreatic branches from the main vessel. (From Debas HT, Mulvihill SJ. Complications of peptic ulcer. In: Zinner MJ, Schwartz SJ, Ellis H, eds. *Maingot's Abdominal Operations.* Stamford, CT: Appleton & Lange; 1997.)

which can be ligated both through the lumen as well as extraluminally. This vessel at the level of the posterior duodenal wall has a T or three-vessel junction. It is important to suture ligate the gastroduodenal artery superiorly and inferiorly, followed by ligation of the medial transverse pancreatic branches using a U stitch (Fig. 59.26). Care should be taken to avoid injury to the common bile duct during suture placement. If no bleeding is encountered upon opening the lumen, the mucosa should be carefully inspected for an ulcer. If identified, the ulcer base should be cleaned to help to identify a visible vessel, which if seen should be ligated. In situations in which no active bleeding is seen, it is important to carry out a careful inspection of the mucosa, looking for other potential bleeding ulcers, even if a nonbleeding ulcer is identified. This inspection can be done by manual palpation of the lumen using a finger. In cases in which the preoperative endoscopy failed to identify a specific location, it is reasonable to start with a duodenotomy, which can be extended proximally or distally to allow further exploration. On occasion, a second gastrotomy near the esophageal junction is needed to inspect the proximal stomach. After gaining control of the bleeding, the pyloroplasty is performed. Most often this is done as a Heineke-Mikulicz pyloroplasty. Performing a TV then completes the procedure.

Bleeding Gastric Ulcer

For bleeding gastric ulcers, distal gastrectomy with ulcer excision and B I or II reconstruction is preferred. This permits excision and histologic evaluation of the ulcer to rule out malignancy. In high-risk patients or in case of ulcers that are due to high acid secretion (types II and III), a vagotomy may be added.

PERFORATION

Smoking and NSAIDs are important etiologic factors for ulcer perforations, and epidemiologic studies have documented an increasing rate of perforation, particularly in older women. The outcome of patients presenting with a perforated ulcer depends on the following:

1. Time delay to presentation and treatment—data suggest increasing delays for surgical treatment, in part as a consequence of more extensive diagnostic work-up
2. Site of perforation—gastric perforation is associated with a poorer prognosis
3. Patient's age—older patients who often have associated comorbidities have a worse outcome
4. Presence of hypotension at presentation (systolic blood pressure <100 mm Hg)

Recent studies comparing nonoperative treatment with surgical treatment in perforated PUD showed no decrease in morbidity or mortality with surgical treatment in carefully selected groups of patients. The nonoperative approach should be considered only if a water-soluble contrast study has confirmed that the ulcer is sealed with no extravasation of contrast into the peritoneal cavity. Such patients should be followed closely with regular physical exams and, if their abdominal exam or laboratory findings indicate progressive sepsis, they should undergo prompt operation. This approach is generally used for individuals who have a perforation of greater than 24 hours' duration, are stable, and often have significant comorbidities that increase the risk of surgical intervention. It should be noted that, although this approach is often used for the older patient with comorbidities, studies show that the risk of nonoperative treatment failure is highest in older adults and thus close observation of such patients is recommended. Because perforated gastric ulcers have a higher rate of reperforation and complications, nonoperative therapy in situations in which the source of the perforation is known to be gastric is not recommended.

Perforated Duodenal Ulcer

An acute perforation is estimated to occur in 2% to 10% of patients with a duodenal ulcer. Operation for this indication should be directed at closing the perforation and cleansing the abdomen of debris. This can be done either as an open procedure or laparoscopically. There appears to be little difference in outcome between the two techniques. Surgeons have traditionally performed either simple patch closure or TV with pyloroplasty (incorporating the perforation). The natural history of those treated by a simple repair has been documented in a paper that followed the course of 122 such patients over a 25-year period. In total, 48% of the original study population required further ulcer treatment in the form of prolonged medical therapy or further surgery.[74] Consequently, a TV with pyloroplasty had been recommended as the minimal therapy required. A study reported the outcomes in 159 patients who were followed more than

10 years after vagotomy with pyloroplasty for perforated duodenal ulcer.[75] The perioperative mortality was 5.5%, ulcers recurred in 8.8%, and postoperative digestive sequelae, notably diarrhea and dumping, developed in 16%. Nevertheless, the overall results were good to excellent in almost 90% of cases. PGV with patch closure does at least as well. Boey et al., in a prospective study of 101 patients randomized to simple closure, TV with pyloroplasty, or PGV, showed 39-month recurrence rates of 63.3%, 11.8%, and 3.8%, respectively. The operative time was significantly more for the PGV, but there were no mortalities in any group. However, the study excluded older adults (older than age 70 years) and patients with preoperative shock; this may account for the low mortality rates.[76] Another randomized study by the same group, comparing PGV with simple closure, documented recurrence rates of 10.6% and 36.6% (half requiring surgical intervention) at 3 years. Again there was a sample bias in the group because the unstable and older patients were excluded.[77] Another series of 107 patients with perforated pyloroduodenal ulcers documented minimal morbidity, low mortality, and excellent patient satisfaction for omental patching and PGV, with a recurrence rate of 3.7% for duodenal ulcer; the recurrence rate for pyloric and prepyloric ulcer was substantially higher at 16%.[78] Chronic pyloroduodenal scarring is considered a relative contraindication to PGV in this setting because it may be associated with delayed gastric emptying after surgery.

With the identification of *H. pylori*, the ideal surgical approach has again been questioned. A study showed that 81% of patients with a perforated duodenal ulcer are *H. pylori* positive. In this study, all patients underwent a simple closure of the perforation. The *H. pylori*-positive patients were then randomized postoperatively to a 4-week course of PPIs alone versus *H. pylori* eradication therapy. The ulcer recurrence rate at 1 year was 5% in the *H. pylori*-eradicated group versus 38% in the PPI-treated group, as determined by repeat endoscopy. Notably, the 5% recurrence rate is equivalent to the recurrence rate for those who undergo a definitive antiulcer procedure.[79] These data provide good evidence for the practice of simple closure of perforated duodenal ulcers in the acute setting. However, at the time of operation, the *H. pylori* status of the patient is often unknown and, in the absence of a reliable intraoperative test, the merits of a definitive antisecretory procedure have to be considered. This may be particularly important in those patients with a previous history of peptic ulcer operation, *H. pylori* eradication, chronic ulcer symptoms despite use of PPIs, or those on NSAIDs in whom this therapy cannot be discontinued. In general, simple patch closure is appropriate for patients with

1. Acute NSAID-related perforation (provided that the drugs can be discontinued postoperatively) and for patients who have never been treated for PUD but who can be treated with PPIs and *H. pylori* eradication
2. Perforation in the setting of ongoing shock, delayed presentation, considerable comorbid disease, or marked peritoneal contamination

Fig. 59.27 summarizes the recommended approach to a perforated duodenal ulcer. To perform the patch procedure, a midline laparotomy is performed and the

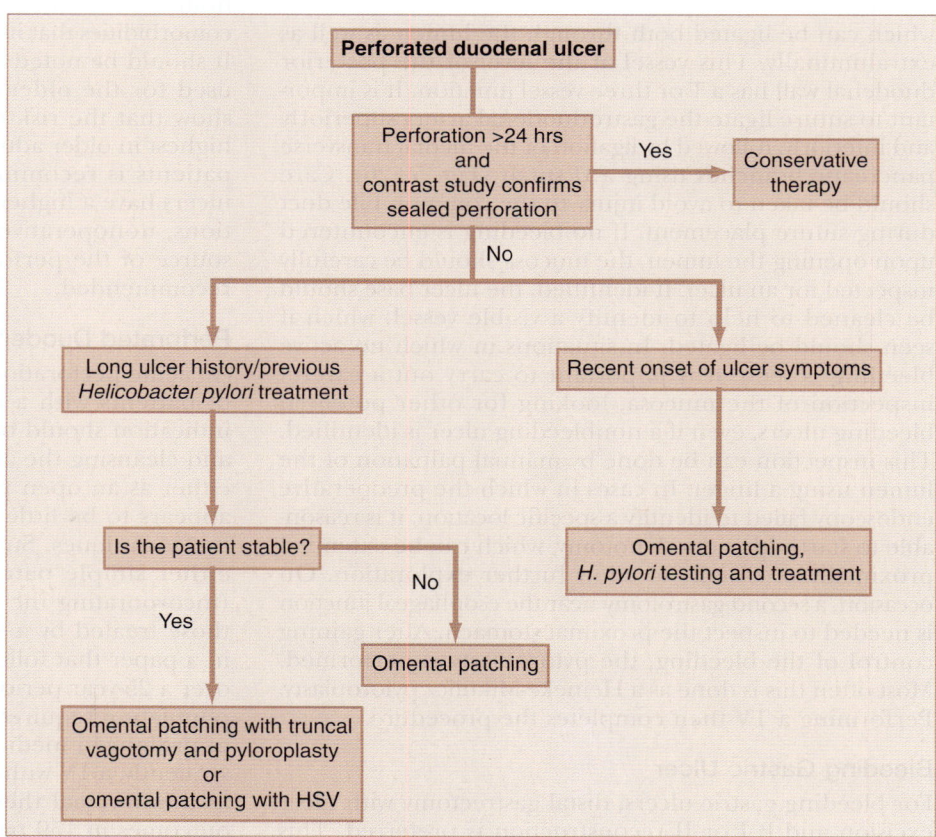

FIGURE 59.27 Treatment algorithm for surgery for perforated duodenal ulcers. *HSV,* Highly selective vagotomy.

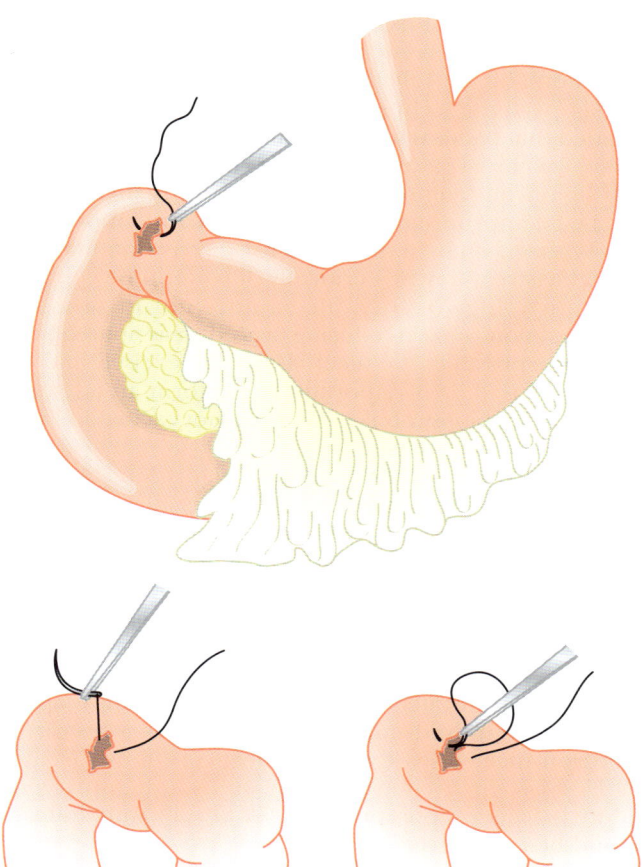

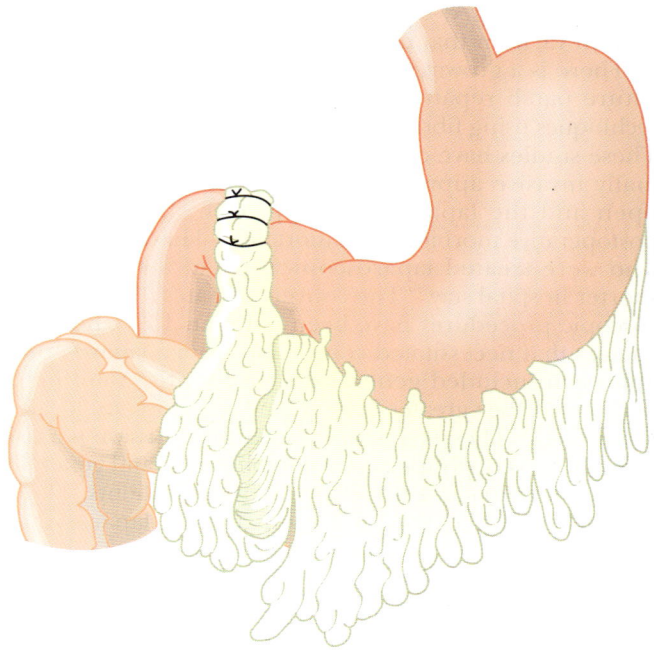

FIGURE 59.29 The omentum, which has been mobilized on a vascular pedicle, is secured in place with sutures tied loosely enough to prevent tissue strangulation. This technique allows effective closure of the perforation without narrowing the duodenal lumen. (From Baker RJ. Perforated duodenal ulcer. In: Baker RJ, Fischer JE, eds. *Mastery of Surgery*. Philadelphia: Lippincott Williams & Wilkins; 2001.)

FIGURE 59.28 Perforated duodenal ulcers. Repair is begun by placing sutures through the full thickness of the bowel wall in two steps. This allows the use of smaller, tapered needles, and reduces the risk of inadvertent penetration of the posterior duodenal wall. (From Baker RJ. Perforated duodenal ulcer. In: Baker RJ, Fischer JE, eds. *Mastery of Surgery*. Philadelphia: Lippincott Williams & Wilkins; 2001.)

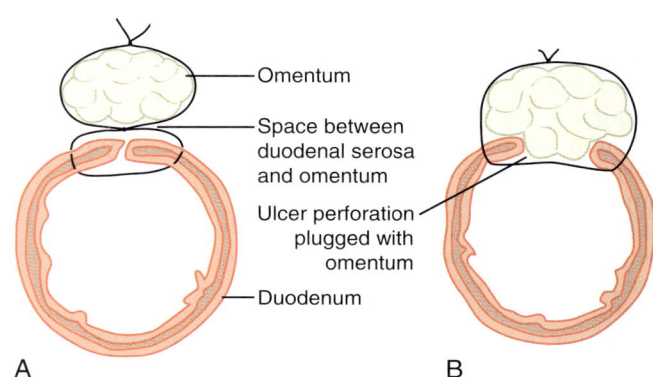

FIGURE 59.30 When the sutures are initially tied to approximate the edges of the ulcer and the omentum is placed above those knots (A), there is less intimate apposition of the duodenal serosa to the omentum. By performing the procedure as described, the omentum plugs the hole (B) and is closely applied to the serosa, ensuring watertight closure. (From Baker RJ. Perforated duodenal ulcer. In: Baker RJ, Fischer JE, eds. *Mastery of Surgery*. Philadelphia: Lippincott Williams & Wilkins; 2001.)

intraabdominal organs are inspected. The presence of bilious fluid in the peritoneal cavity suggests an upper gastrointestinal perforation. After a duodenal perforation has been confirmed, pads are placed around the perforation to contain any further spillage. Next, 3-0 silk or polydioxanone sutures are placed across the perforation. Usually three to four sutures are needed. It is important to take bites of appropriate length (0.5 to 1 cm) to prevent the sutures cutting through the inflamed duodenal tissue. To ensure bites that are full thickness, it is recommended that one pass the needle through the wall of duodenum on one side of the ulcer, retrieving the needle through the perforation, and then passing it through the wall on the other side of the perforation (Fig. 59.28). These sutures should not be tied to approximate the ulcer; rather, the adjacent omentum should be mobilized on an intact vascular pedicle and brought up. The sutures are tied over this omental pedicle to secure this in place. These sutures should not be tied too tightly, to avoid strangulation of the omental patch (Fig. 59.29). Sewing the ulcer closed before placing the omental pedicle over

the perforation is discouraged because it reduces the surface contact of the omentum with the duodenal mucosa (Fig. 59.30). Following closure of the ulcer, a thorough irrigation of the peritoneal cavity should be done with warm saline irrigation. Drains are not needed, and their use is discouraged because it tends to create a negative suction vacuum that can interfere with the repair.

There is a growing body of literature on laparoscopic suture patch repair, as well as laparoscopic sutureless techniques using fibrin glue to repair the perforated ulcer. These studies have demonstrated the feasibility of minimally invasive approaches.[80] A comparison of primary open and the laparoscopic approach showed similar postoperative morbidity and mortality.[81] However, patients who were treated laparoscopically had a significantly shorter hospital stay.[80] The conversion rates for such laparoscopic procedures have been between 15% and 20%. Factors that necessitated conversion from a laparoscopic approach included generalized peritonitis, Mannheim peritonitis index greater than 21, and a perforation located posteriorly.[81] The presence of shock on admission is a risk factor for severe postoperative complications and generally an open approach is preferable in these patients. There are no absolute contraindications for the laparoscopic approach.

To perform laparoscopic repair of a duodenal ulcer, the patient should be supine. The operating surgeon can stand either on the patient's left or between the patient's legs, with the patient placed in split leg position. The patient is then placed in reverse Trendelenburg position. Initially, a diagnostic laparoscopy is performed. After the ulcer size is carefully measured with reference to the 5-mm–diameter working laparoscopic instrument, the perforation is patched in similar fashion as described for the open approach with polydioxanone, polyglactin, or silk sutures. The perforation is closed by intracorporeal or extracorporeal knotting (depending on the surgeon preference) with an omental patch (omentopexy) directly applied to the perforation site. This approach avoids tension on the inflamed ulcer margin and cutting through the tissue. It is critical during the process to avoid anchoring the posterior duodenal wall. This can be avoided by pulling the needle through the perforation and reinserting it through the perforation to complete the next half of the stitch. It is important when tying the knots down to pay attention so as not to strangulate the omental pedicle. A leak test can be performed via a nasogastric tube; however, this step is not necessary. Suctioning of the peritoneal fluid is then performed with special attention directed to potential spaces for fluid collection. The fluid collected can be sent for Gram stain and culture in case the patient develops an abscess during recovery; however, this should not extend antibiotic coverage beyond 24 hours. Some surgeons advocate the performance of lavage of the abdominal cavity using 3 to 5 L of warm normal saline with the patient in various positions. Drains are not necessary.

Perforated Gastric Ulcer

A perforated gastric ulcer carries a greater overall mortality that ranges from 10% to 40%, and increases significantly with age (>65 years).[82] There has been debate in cases of perforated types I and IV gastric ulcers over whether to perform a partial gastrectomy or proceed with a simple patching of the perforation. Partial gastrectomy is the preferred approach unless the patient is at unacceptably high risk because of advanced age, comorbid disease, intraoperative instability, or severe peritoneal soilage.[83]

Even in patients in this high-risk group, who may present with shock, there is increasing evidence that definitive operation can be tolerated as well as the simpler and quicker patching technique.[84,85] Consequently, it is recommended that patients with a perforated type I gastric ulcer undergo a partial gastrectomy unless the patient is unstable with significant comorbidities. Biopsy and patch closure may be an appropriate approach for treatment of a high type IV ulcer, where a more extensive resection may lead to total gastrectomy in a critically ill patient. Because the pathophysiology of such ulcers does not involve acid hypersecretion, an acid-reducing procedure is not required. Whenever possible, the ulcer should be excised and the stomach closed. It is important to perform an adequate four-quadrant biopsy of ulcers that are not excised followed by patch closure.[86]

For type II ulcers, the treatment algorithm should be similar to that for perforated duodenal ulcers because the pathophysiology of the disease is very similar. This means that the ulcers should be patched, *H. pylori* status of the patient determined with an intraoperative biopsy, and the patient treated appropriately. In addition, it is important to obtain an intraoperative biopsy to rule out malignancy that can be associated with such gastric ulcers. Similar to a perforated duodenal ulcer, a definitive operation is not required unless the patient has a history of recurrent ulcer disease and has been previously treated for *H. pylori*. In circumstances in which a definitive procedure is deemed appropriate, a PGV or a TV with drainage should be considered.

Type III ulcers are also thought to have a similar pathogenesis to duodenal ulcers; however, their treatment in the case of an acute perforation deserves particular attention. Patch repair of such prepyloric ulcers is associated with a high incidence of gastric outlet obstruction,[86] and PGV is associated with a high recurrence rate for these ulcers. Therefore antrectomy with vagotomy is the best surgical approach in this setting. Fig. 59.31 summarizes the proposed surgical approach to a perforated gastric ulcer. Gastric ulcers can be managed laparoscopically as described previously for duodenal ulcers; however, these patients should have a follow-up EGD to rule out cancer as the cause of the ulcer.

ACKNOWLEDGMENTS

The authors acknowledge these authors of chapters from the seventh edition of Shackelford's Surgery of the Alimentary Tract:

Tavakkolizadeh A, Ashley SW. Operations for peptic ulcer. In: Yeo CJ, McFadden DW, eds. *Shackelford's Surgery of the Alimentary Tract.* Vol. I. 7th ed. Philadelphia: Elsevier; 2013:701-719.

Postier RG, Havron WS III. Vagotomy and drainage. In: Yeo CJ, McFadden DW, eds. *Shackelford's Surgery of the Alimentary Tract.* Vol. I. 7th ed. Philadelphia: Elsevier; 2013:720-730.

Ben-David K, Caban AM, Behrns KE. Gastric resection and reconstruction. In: Yeo CJ, McFadden DW, eds. *Shackelford's Surgery of the Alimentary Tract.* Vol. I. 7th ed. Philadelphia: Elsevier; 2013:731-748.

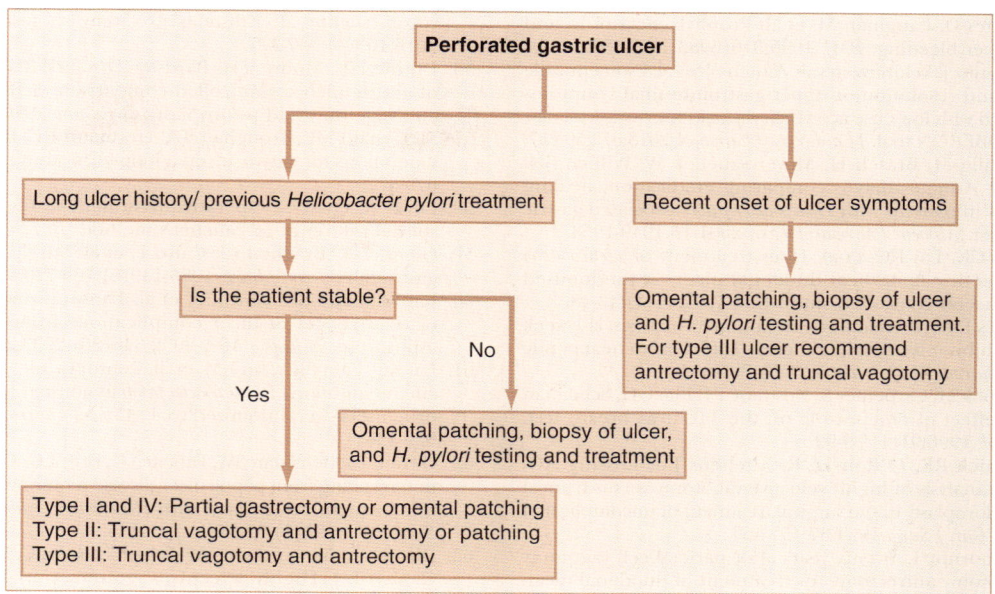

FIGURE 59.31 Recommended treatment algorithm for surgical management of perforated gastric ulcers.

REFERENCES

1. Sung JJ, Kuipers EJ, El-Serag HB. Systematic review: the global incidence and prevalence of peptic ulcer disease. *Aliment Pharmacol Ther.* 2009;29(9):938-946.
2. Anand BS, Raed AK, Malaty HM, et al. Low point prevalence of peptic ulcer in normal individuals with *Helicobacter pylori* infection. *Am J Gastroenterol.* 1996;91(6):1112-1115.
3. Groenen MJ, Kuipers EJ, Hansen BE, Ouwendijk RJ. Incidence of duodenal ulcers and gastric ulcers in a Western population: back to where it started. *Can J Gastroenterol.* 2009;23(9):604-608.
4. Bashinskaya B, Nahed BV, Redjal N, Kahle KT, Walcott BP. Trends in peptic ulcer disease and the identification of *Helicobacter pylori* as a causative organism: population-based estimates from the US nationwide inpatient sample. *J Glob Infect Dis.* 2011;3(4):366-370.
5. Wang YR, Richter JE, Dempsey DT. Trends and outcomes of hospitalizations for peptic ulcer disease in the United States, 1993 to 2006. *Ann Surg.* 2010;251(1):51-58.
6. Irabor DO. An audit of peptic ulcer surgery in Ibadan, Nigeria. *West Afr J Med.* 2005;24(3):242-245.
7. Lau JY, Sung J, Hill C, Henderson C, Howden CW, Metz DC. Systematic review of the epidemiology of complicated peptic ulcer disease: incidence, recurrence, risk factors and mortality. *Digestion.* 2011;84(2):102-113.
8. Beaumont W. Nutrition classics. *Experiments and Observations on the Gastric Juice, and the Physiology of Digestion.* By William Beaumont, Plattsburgh. Printed by F. P. Allen. 1833.
9. Modlin IM, Kidd M, Marks IN, Tang LH. The pivotal role of John S. Edkins in the discovery of gastrin. *World J Surg.* 1997;21(2):226-234.
10. Paulino F, Netto AP. Evolution of the surgical treatment of duodenal ulcer. *Rev Assoc Med Bras.* 1963;9:268-272.
11. Herrington JL Jr. Gastroduodenal ulcer. Overview of 150 papers presented before the Southern Surgical Association 1888-1986. *Ann Surg.* 1988;207:754-769.
12. Modlin IM, Darr U. The centenary of Lester Dragstedt—fifty years of therapeutic vagotomy. *Yale J Biol Med.* 1994;67(3-4):63-80.
13. Gustafson J, Welling D. "No acid, no ulcer" 100 years later: a review of the history of peptic ulcer disease. *J Am Coll Surg.* 2010;210:110-116.
14. Dragstedt LR. Vagotomy for gastroduodenal ulcer. *Ann Surg.* 1945;122:973-989.
15. Woodward ER. The history of vagotomy. *Am J Surg.* 1987;153(1):9-17.
16. Stempien SJ, Temkin E, Dagradi A. Duodenal ulcer; gastrectomy versus vagotomy with accessory procedures. *Calif Med.* 1956;84(3):168-171.
17. Hubert JP Jr, Kiernan PD, Beahrs OH, ReMine WH. Truncal vagotomy and resection in the treatment of duodenal ulcer. *Mayo Clin Proc.* 1980;55:19-24.
18. Siim C, Lublin HK, Jensen HE. Selective gastric vagotomy and drainage for duodenal ulcer: a 10-13-year follow-up study. *Ann Surg.* 1981;194(6):687-691.
19. van Heerden JA, Kelly KA, Dozois RR, et al. Proximal gastric vagotomy. Initial experience. *Mayo Clin Proc.* 1980;55(1):10-13.
20. Hoffmann J, Jensen HE, Christiansen J, Olesen A, Loud FB, Hauch O. Prospective controlled vagotomy trial for duodenal ulcer. Results after 11–15 years. *Ann Surg.* 1989;209(1):40-45.
21. Zittel TT, Jehle EC, Becker HD. Surgical management of peptic ulcer disease today—indication, technique and outcome. *Langenbecks Arch Surg.* 2000;385(2):84-96.
22. Marshall BJ, Warren JR. Unidentified curved bacilli in the stomach of patients with gastritis and peptic ulceration. *Lancet.* 1984;1(8390):1311-1315.
23. Rauws EA, Tytgat GN. Cure of duodenal ulcer associated with eradication of *Helicobacter pylori*. *Lancet.* 1990;335(8700):1233-1235.
24. Kokoska ER, Kauffman GL Jr. *Helicobacter pylori* and the gastroduodenal mucosa. *Surgery.* 2001;130(1):13-16.
25. Graham DY, Go MF, Lew GM, Genta RM, Rehfeld JF. *Helicobacter pylori* infection and exaggerated gastrin release. Effects of inflammation and progastrin processing. *Scand J Gastroenterol.* 1993;28(8):690-694.
26. McColl KE, Gillen D, El-Omar E. The role of gastrin in ulcer pathogenesis. *Baillieres Best Pract Res Clin Gastroenterol.* 2000;14(1):13-26.
27. Kim JM, Kim JS, Jung HC, Oh YK, Kim N, Song IS. Inhibition of *Helicobacter pylori*-induced nuclear factor-kappa B activation and interleukin-8 gene expression by ecabet sodium in gastric epithelial cells. *Helicobacter.* 2003;8(5):542-553.
28. Zhao YR, Zhou Y, Lin G, Hu WJ, Du JM. Association between IL-17, IL-8 and IL-18 expression in peripheral blood and *Helicobacter pylori* infection in mongolian gerbils. *Jundishapur J Microbiol.* 2015;8(8):e21503.
29. Wallace JL. Prostaglandins, NSAIDs, and gastric mucosal protection: why doesn't the stomach digest itself? *Physiol Rev.* 2008;88(4):1547-1565.
30. Lanas A, Baron JA, Sandler RS, et al. Peptic ulcer and bleeding events associated with rofecoxib in a 3-year colorectal adenoma chemoprevention trial. *Gastroenterology.* 2007;132(2):490-497.
31. Wallace JL, McKnight GW. The mucoid cap over superficial gastric damage in the rat. A high-pH microenvironment dissipated by nonsteroidal antiinflammatory drugs and endothelin. *Gastroenterology.* 1990;99(2):295-304.
32. Melcarne L, Garcia-Iglesias P, Calvet X. Management of NSAID-associated peptic ulcer disease. *Expert Rev Gastroenterol Hepatol.* 2016;10(6):723-733.

33. Weil J, Colin-Jones D, Langman M, et al. Prophylactic aspirin and risk of peptic ulcer bleeding. *BMJ.* 1995;310(6983):827-830.

34. Scheiman JM, Herlitz J, Veldhuyzen van Zanten SJ, et al. Esomeprazole for prevention and resolution of upper gastrointestinal symptoms in patients treated with low-dose acetylsalicylic acid for cardiovascular protection: the OBERON trial. *J Cardiovasc Pharmacol.* 2013;61:250-257.

35. Leodolter A, Kulig M, Brasch H, Meyer-Sabellek W, Willich SN, Malfertheiner P. A meta-analysis comparing eradication, healing and relapse rates in patients with *Helicobacter pylori*-associated gastric or duodenal ulcer. *Aliment Pharmacol Ther.* 2001;15:1949-1958.

36. Lam SK, Ching CK, Lai KC, et al. Does treatment of *Helicobacter pylori* with antibiotics alone heal duodenal ulcer? A randomised double blind placebo controlled study. *Gut.* 1997;41(1):43-48.

37. Gisbert JP, Pajares JM. Systematic review and meta-analysis: is 1-week proton pump inhibitor-based triple therapy sufficient to heal peptic ulcer? *Aliment Pharmacol Ther.* 2005;21(7):795-804.

38. Chey WD, Spybrook M, Carpenter S, Nostrant TT, Elta GH, Scheiman JM. Prolonged effect of omeprazole on the 14C-urea breath test. *Am J Gastroenterol.* 1996;91(1):89-92.

39. Chan VM, Reznick RK, O'Rourke K, Kitchens JM, Lossing AG, Detsky AS. Meta-analysis of highly selective vagotomy versus truncal vagotomy and pyloroplasty in the surgical treatment of uncomplicated duodenal ulcer. *Can J Surg.* 1994;37:457-464.

40. Jordan PH Jr, Thornby J. Twenty years after parietal cell vagotomy or selective vagotomy antrectomy for treatment of duodenal ulcer. Final report. *Ann Surg.* 1994;220(3):283-293; discussion 293-296.

41. Taylor TV, Lythgoe JP, McFarland JB, Gilmore IT, Thomas PE, Ferguson GH. Anterior lesser curve seromyotomy and posterior truncal vagotomy versus truncal vagotomy and pyloroplasty in the treatment of chronic duodenal ulcer. *Br J Surg.* 1990;77(9):1007-1009.

42. Oostvogel HJ, van Vroonhoven TJ. Anterior lesser curve seromyotomy with posterior truncal vagotomy versus proximal gastric vagotomy. *Br J Surg.* 1988;75(2):121-124.

43. Coblijn UK, Lagarde SM, de Castro SM, Kuiken SD, van Tets WF, van Wagensveld BA. The influence of prophylactic proton pump inhibitor treatment on the development of symptomatic marginal ulceration in Roux-en-Y gastric bypass patients: a historic cohort study. *Surg Obes Relat Dis.* 2016;12(2):246-252.

44. Tersmette AC, Offerhaus GJ, Tersmette KW, et al. Meta-analysis of the risk of gastric stump cancer: detection of high risk patient subsets for stomach cancer after remote partial gastrectomy for benign conditions. *Cancer Res.* 1990;50(20):6486-6489.

45. Moller H, Toftgaard C. Cancer occurrence in a cohort of patients surgically treated for peptic ulcer. *Gut.* 1991;32(7):740-744.

46. La Vecchia C, Negri E, D'Avanzo B, Moller H, Franceschi S. Partial gastrectomy and subsequent gastric cancer risk. *J Epidemiol Community Health.* 1992;46:12-14.

47. Rathi P, Parikh S, Kalro RH. Giant duodenal ulcer: a new look at a variant of a common illness. *Indian J Gastroenterol.* 1996;15(1):33-34.

48. Vogel SB, Drane WE, Woodward ER. Clinical and radionuclide evaluation of bile diversion by Braun enteroenterostomy: prevention and treatment of alkaline reflux gastritis. An alternative to Roux-en-Y diversion. *Ann Surg.* 1994;219(5):458-465; discussion 465-466.

49. Park JY, Kim YJ. Uncut Roux-en-Y reconstruction after laparoscopic distal gastrectomy can be a favorable method in terms of gastritis, bile reflux, and gastric residue. *J Gastric Cancer.* 2014;14(4):229-237.

50. Fischer DR, Nussbaum MS, Pritts TA, et al. Use of omeprazole in the management of giant duodenal ulcer: results of a prospective study. *Surgery.* 1999;126(4):643-648; discussion 648-649.

51. Croce E, Olmi S, Russo R, Azzola M, Mastropasqua E, Golia M. Laparoscopic treatment of peptic ulcers. A review after 6 years experience with Hill-Barker's procedure. *Hepatogastroenterology.* 1999;46(26):924-929.

52. Johnson HD. Gastric ulcer: classification, blood group characteristics, secretion patterns and pathogenesis. *Ann Surg.* 1965;162(6):996-1004.

53. Csendes A, Burgos AM, Smok G, Burdiles P, Braghetto I, Díaz JC. Latest results (12–21 years) of a prospective randomized study comparing Billroth II and Roux-en-Y anastomosis after a partial gastrectomy plus vagotomy in patients with duodenal ulcers. *Ann Surg.* 2009;249(2):189-194.

54. Nunobe S, Okaro A, Sasako M, et al. Billroth 1 versus Roux-en-Y reconstructions: a quality-of-life survey at 5 years. *Int J Clin Oncol.* 2007;12(6):433-439.

55. Nakamura M, Nakamori M, Ojima T, et al. Randomized clinical trial comparing long-term quality of life for Billroth I versus Roux-en-Y reconstruction after distal gastrectomy for gastric cancer. *Br J Surg.* 2016;103(4):337-347.

56. Duthie HL, Moore TH, Bardsley D, Clark RG. Surgical treatment of gastric ulcers. Controlled comparison of Billroth-I gastrectomy and vagotomy and pyloroplasty. *Br J Surg.* 1970;57(10):784-787.

57. McDonald MP, Broughan TA, Hermann RE, Philip RS, Hoerr SO. Operations for gastric ulcer: a long-term study. *Am Surg.* 1996;62(8):673-677.

58. Lewis A, Qvist G. Operative treatment of high gastric ulcer with special reference to Pauchet's method. *Br J Surg.* 1972;59(1):1-4.

59. Csendes A, Braghetto I, Calvo F, et al. Surgical treatment of high gastric ulcer. *Am J Surg.* 1985;149(6):765-770.

60. Lai KC, Lam SK, Chu KM, et al. Lansoprazole for the prevention of recurrences of ulcer complications from long-term low-dose aspirin use. *N Engl J Med.* 2002;346(26):2033-2038.

61. Lai KC, Lam SK, Chu KM, et al. Lansoprazole reduces ulcer relapse after eradication of *Helicobacter pylori* in nonsteroidal anti-inflammatory drug users—a randomized trial. *Aliment Pharmacol Ther.* 2003;18(8):829-836.

62. Gibson JB, Behrman SW, Fabian TC, Britt LG. Gastric outlet obstruction resulting from peptic ulcer disease requiring surgical intervention is infrequently associated with *Helicobacter pylori* infection. *J Am Coll Surg.* 2000;191(1):32-37.

63. Dittrich K, Blauensteiner W, Schrutka-Kolbl C, Hoffer F, Armbruster C, Vavrik J. Highly selective vagotomy plus Jaboulay: a possible alternative in patients with benign stenosis secondary to duodenal ulceration. *J Am Coll Surg.* 1995;180(6):654-658.

64. Csendes A, Maluenda F, Braghetto I, Schutte H, Burdiles P, Diaz JC. Prospective randomized study comparing three surgical techniques for the treatment of gastric outlet obstruction secondary to duodenal ulcer. *Am J Surg.* 1993;166(1):45-49.

65. Donahue PE, Griffith C, Richter HM. A 50 year perspective upon selective vagotomy. *Am J Surg.* 1996;172:9-12.

66. Stabile BE, Passaro E Jr. Surgery for duodenal and gastric ulcer disease. *Adv Surg.* 1993;26:275-306.

67. Smith BR, Wilson SE. Impact of nonresective operations for complicated peptic ulcer disease in a high-risk population. *Am Surg.* 2010;76(10):1143-1146.

68. Kapetanakis AM, Kyprizlis EP, Tsikrikas TS. Efficacy of repeated therapeutic endoscopy in patients with bleeding ulcer. *Hepatogastroenterology.* 1997;44(13):288-293.

69. Wang BW, Mok KT, Chang HT, et al. APACHE II score: a useful tool for risk assessment and an aid to decision-making in emergency operation for bleeding gastric ulcer. *J Am Coll Surg.* 1998;187(3):287-294.

70. Lau JY, Sung JJ, Lam YH, et al. Endoscopic retreatment compared with surgery in patients with recurrent bleeding after initial endoscopic control of bleeding ulcers. *N Engl J Med.* 1999;340(10):751-756.

71. Lanas A. Editorial: upper GI bleeding-associated mortality: challenges to improving a resistant outcome. *Am J Gastroenterol.* 2010;105(1):90-92.

72. Behrman SW. Management of complicated peptic ulcer disease. *Arch Surg.* 2005;140(2):201-208.

73. Deleted in review.

74. Griffin GE, Organ CH Jr. The natural history of the perforated duodenal ulcer treated by suture plication. *Ann Surg.* 1976;183:382-385.

75. Robles R, Parrilla P, Lujan JA, et al. Long-term follow-up of bilateral truncal vagotomy and pyloroplasty for perforated duodenal ulcer. *Br J Surg.* 1995;82(5):665.

76. Boey J, Lee NW, Koo J, Lam PH, Wong J, Ong GB. Immediate definitive surgery for perforated duodenal ulcers: a prospective controlled trial. *Ann Surg.* 1982;196(3):338-344.

77. Boey J, Branicki FJ, Alagaratnam TT, et al. Proximal gastric vagotomy. The preferred operation for perforations in acute duodenal ulcer. *Ann Surg.* 1988;208(2):169-174.

78. Jordan PH Jr, Thornby J. Perforated pyloroduodenal ulcers. Long-term results with omental patch closure and parietal cell vagotomy. *Ann Surg.* 1995;221(5):479-486; discussion 486-488.

79. Ng EK, Lam YH, Sung JJ, et al. Eradication of *Helicobacter pylori* prevents recurrence of ulcer after simple closure of duodenal ulcer perforation: randomized controlled trial. *Ann Surg.* 2000;231(2):153-158.

80. Byrge N, Barton RG, Enniss TM, Nirula R. Laparoscopic versus open repair of perforated gastroduodenal ulcer: a National Surgical

Quality Improvement Program analysis. *Am J Surg.* 2013;206(6):957-962; discussion 962-963.

81. Muller MK, Wrann S, Widmer J, Klasen J, Weber M, Hahnloser D. Perforated peptic ulcer repair: factors predicting conversion in laparoscopy and postoperative septic complications. *World J Surg.* 2016;40(9):2186-2193.

82. Hewitt PM, Krige J, Bornman PC. Perforated gastric ulcers: resection compared with simple closure. *Am Surg.* 1993;59(10):669-673.

83. McGee GS, Sawyers JL. Perforated gastric ulcers. A plea for management by primary gastric resection. *Arch Surg.* 1987;122(5):555-561.

84. Hodnett RM, Gonzalez F, Lee WC, Nance FC, Deboisblanc R. The need for definitive therapy in the management of perforated gastric ulcers. Review of 202 cases. *Ann Surg.* 1989;209(1):36-39.

85. Di Quinzio C, Phang PT. Surgical management of perforated benign gastric ulcer in high-risk patients. *Can J Surg.* 1992;35(1):94-97.

86. Turner WW Jr, Thompson WM Jr, Thal ER. Perforated gastric ulcers. A plea for management by simple closures. *Arch Surg.* 1988;123(8):960-964.

Zollinger-Ellison Syndrome

Mary E. Dillhoff | E. Christopher Ellison

Zollinger-Ellison syndrome (ZES) was initially described in two index cases of refractory ulcer disease and diarrhea in 1955 at the Ohio State University.[1] The index patients had recurrent peptic ulceration after multiple gastric operations, requiring complete gastrectomy to control their symptoms.[2] ZES is a rare cause of peptic ulcer disease for which a high index of suspicion is required to make the diagnosis. The syndrome is characterized by severe peptic ulcer disease caused by gastrin-secreting neuroendocrine tumors, most commonly located in the duodenum and pancreas. Frequently gastrinomas are not recognized at initial clinical presentation and are often mistreated. Symptoms that should raise suspicion of a gastrinoma include idiopathic peptic ulcer disease or long-standing refractory diarrhea. The term *gastrinoma* is interchangeably used with ZES.

Pancreatic neuroendocrine tumors (PNETs) are rare cancers occurring in approximately 1000 patients per year in the United States, representing 3% of all pancreatic tumors.[3] The incidence has increased over the last three decades, likely from improvement in imaging modalities and increased frequency of imaging.[4-6] The incidence has increased from 17 per 100,000 population in 1973 to 47 per 100,000 population in 2007.[7] There is a male predominance (60%) and the mean age at diagnosis is 50 years with most diagnosed between the age of 20 and 60 years. Survival is significantly longer than those with pancreatic adenocarcinoma; however, patients with metastatic disease are not likely to be cured. Surgery plays a critical role in palliation of symptoms of hormone-producing tumors and for cure if only localized disease is present. Endocrine tumors of the pancreas originate from islet cells, hence the traditional name of islet cell tumor. The tumors are broadly classified as functional and nonfunctional. Nonfunctional tumors compose 60% to 90% of all PNETs and are more common than functional tumors. Nonfunctional tumors are more likely to present with metastatic disease because there is a lack of symptoms, leading them to present late in the disease course.[8,9] Functional tumors cause symptoms from the hormone that the tumor produces. Approximately half of pancreatic endocrine tumors are functional, and of these, about 50% are gastrinomas.

Gastrinomas can be encountered in a familial pattern in the setting of multiple endocrine neoplasia type 1 (MEN1 or Wermer syndrome), or rarely (10% to 15%) with von Hippel-Lindau (VHL) syndrome,[10] both autosomal dominant inherited diseases.[10] MEN1 is characterized by nearly complete penetrance with variable expressivity; it typically involves the parathyroid glands, pituitary gland, and pancreas. Ninety to 100% of MEN1 patients will develop primary hyperparathyroidism, and 50% to 75% of patients develop symptoms from functioning neoplasms

of the pancreas. Gastrinoma is the most common pancreatic islet cell tumor in patients with MEN1, followed by insulinomas. Those with MEN-associated gastrinomas typically present at a younger age. Pituitary adenomas occur less commonly (20% to 65%) as do adrenal tumors (10% to 73%) and thyroid adenomas (0% to 10%).[11,12] Pancreatic tumors occurring in patients with MEN1 are commonly multiple, often requiring different treatment strategies than those used for patients with sporadic pancreatic endocrine tumors, which tend to be solitary. Thus MEN1-associated gastrinomas are rarely cured with surgery.

ANATOMY, PATHOPHYSIOLOGY, AND MOLECULAR BIOLOGY

Endocrine tumors of the pancreas originate from islet cells. The islets arise from neural crest cells or embryonic foregut endoderm. Histologically PNETs appear similar to carcinoid tumors of the gastrointestinal tract. Gastrin is synthesized in the G cells, found predominantly in the gastric antrum and in smaller numbers in the duodenal mucosa. Gastrin release is controlled by chemical, neural, or mechanical stimuli. Gastrin release is stimulated by ingested protein and gastric distention. Calcium, epinephrine, and achlorhydria are also potent stimuli for gastrin secretion. Gastrin release is inhibited by beta-blockade and atropine.[2] Pernicious anemia, atrophic gastritis, and the use of proton pump inhibitors (PPIs) all can cause elevation of serum gastrin and achlorhydria. Acid hypersecretion and hypergastrinemia may be found with many conditions such as *Helicobacter pylori* infection, gastric outlet obstruction associated with peptic ulcer, retained antrum, short gut syndrome, or renal failure. Despite several advances in the understanding of gastrinomas, the cell of origin remains uncertain. Duodenal gastrinomas contain many well-differentiated gastrin-containing G cells, and their origin may be the gastrin cells in the duodenal crypts and Brunner glands. Pancreatic gastrinomas are more pleomorphic, with more heterogeneous cell arrangements. Although G cells are not normally present in the adult pancreas, it has been proposed that multipotent, endocrine-programmed stem cells undergoing differentiation toward G cells are responsible for pancreatic gastrinomas.[13-15]

Although gastrinomas tend to be slow growing, 60% to 90% of them will have aggressive biology. The liver is the most common site of metastasis with 70% to 80% of patients diagnosed with liver metastasis at the time of diagnosis. Liver metastasis is considered to be the most important predictor for long-term survival, as these patients tend to have a worse prognosis.[16,17]

CLINICAL PRESENTATION: SYMPTOMS AND SIGNS

Frequently the symptoms of gastrinomas are not recognized at initial clinical presentation, which means that they are often underdiagnosed. Nonspecific symptoms of elevated gastric acid output include a long course of reflux, abdominal pain, and diarrhea. Idiopathic peptic ulcer disease or long-standing diarrhea should raise suspicion for gastrinoma. The high acid load delivered to the duodenum causes diarrhea and the inactivation of pancreatic enzymes causes malabsorption. These symptoms are relieved by nasogastric suction. Diarrhea can be the sole initial complaint in as many as 20% of patients. In 261 patients treated at the National Institutes of Health (NIH) Digestive Disease Branch,[18] abdominal pain and diarrhea were the most common symptoms, occurring in more than 70%, followed by heartburn (44%), nausea (33%), vomiting (25%), and weight loss (17%). Patients who present late may have signs and symptoms of the metastatic disease, such as right upper quadrant pain secondary to liver disease or bone pain secondary to metastatic deposits. Occasionally, patients will present with complications of high acid output, such as bleeding and perforation secondary to severe peptic ulcer disease. However, widespread use of potent acid suppression medication has decreased the incidence of such complications. Zollinger and Grant reported in 1964 that bleeding was a major finding in 45% of patients and in 20% it was considered massive.[19] In contrast, the 2000 NIH study reported bleeding in only 24% of patients; the incidence of complications related to ulcer disease was 44% before 1980, decreasing to 11% between 1990 and 1999.[18] Nevertheless, despite widespread awareness of ZES, delay in diagnosis still persists; a mean delay to diagnosis of 5.2 years was seen in this series.[18]

DIAGNOSIS AND MEDICAL THERAPY

Although ZES is rare, a patient should be referred for prompt workup if exhibiting refractory peptic ulcer disease, long-standing diarrhea, absence of *H. pylori* infection, or failure to improve after treatment for *H. pylori* and acid suppression therapy. In addition, the presence of nephrolithiasis and hypercalcemia should raise suspicion of possible MEN1. In addition, a careful family history should be elucidated to evaluate for MEN1 or other inherited conditions related to MEN or VHL.

Fasting serum gastrin is the appropriate initial diagnostic test for patients with suspected ZES; however it is not sufficient alone to establish the diagnosis as several medical conditions may cause hypergastrinemia. Conditions that cause acid hypersecretion and suppression may cause hypergastrinemia, all of which are more likely to be the cause of hypergastrinemia than ZES. Most commonly, pernicious anemia, atrophic gastritis, and pharmacologic acid suppression may cause achlorhydria or reduced acid suppression, which can cause hypergastrinemia not due to ZES. Other conditions that may cause fasting hypergastrinemia associated with increased acid hypersecretion include *H. pylori* infection, gastric outlet obstruction associated with peptic ulcer, antral G-cell hyperplasia, retained antrum, short bowel syndrome, and renal failure. Pernicious anemia and atrophic gastritis and the associated achlorhydric state are the most common cause of hypergastrinemia. Indeed, fasting gastrin level may and frequently does exceed 1000 pg/mL in this group of patients. Hence a fasting serum gastrin greater than 1000 pg/mL is not diagnostic for ZES unless there is marked acid production (gastric pH <2). Determination of gastric pH and verification of acid production is essential to confirm ZES. Gastrin is determined by a rapid immunoassay, a technique that is readily available. The patient should be off pharmacologic acid suppression for 72 hours (ideally 7 days) prior to testing. Fasting gastrin levels tend to be greater in patients with extensive disease; however, patients with ZES associated with MEN1 and hyperparathyroidism have comparable levels to sporadic gastrinoma patients.[2]

In ZES, a normal fasting gastrin is very rare, occurring in 1% to 3% of patients. This renders serum gastrin measurement a very good screening test for ZES, with a sensitivity that approaches 99%. Several authors indicate that levels greater than 500 pg/mL, or more than fivefold normal, are highly suggestive of gastrinoma in the presence of increased gastric acid production.[2] Berna et al. studied 2229 cases from the literature, finding that 57% to 63% of ZES patients had gastrin levels in this range.[20] However, two-thirds of gastrinoma patients had fasting serum gastrin levels that overlapped with levels seen in more common conditions.

Of particular interest when evaluating hypergastrinemia is a condition referred to as retained excluded antrum syndrome. This rarely occurs in patients who have had a partial distal gastrectomy with Billroth II reconstruction. In this condition, a portion of antrum is left attached to the duodenum. Because it is disconnected from the proximal stomach and is not exposed to gastric acid, there is no inhibition of the normal gastrin production in the residual antrum. This leads to chronic hypertrophy of the gastrin-producing cells in the retained excluded distal stomach and chronic hypergastrinemia. This may result in very high gastric acid output if parietal cells have been preserved in the proximal stomach. These patients have elevated fasting gastrin levels, elevated acid production, and a negative secretin provocation test and may have medically refractory ulcer disease. This condition may require surgical intervention for removal of the retained antrum.

All patients with hypergastrinemia and suspected ZES should undergo confirmation with provocative gastrin testing. In addition, those patients with normal fasting gastrin levels but still with symptoms suspicious for ZES should also undergo provocative gastrin screening. Provocative testing can be performed with secretin, calcium, or meal stimulation. Results of these tests are given in a relative rise in gastrin over the baseline value. Secretin was first reported to cause stimulation of gastrin in ZES patients by Hansky et al. in 1971 and was clearly elucidated by Isenberg et al. in 1972.[21,22] Its effect is mediated through secretin receptors that are present on gastrinoma cells. Following an overnight fast, patients are given an intravenous (IV) bolus injection of secretin of 0.4 µg/kg of body weight over 1 minute. Serial serum gastrin levels are then obtained. Importantly, it is not necessary to discontinue PPIs or histamine-2 (H_2) blockers for this test. Minimal side effects of secretin infusion may include flushing and nausea. Blood draws for determination of gastrin levels are collected and analyzed at 0, 2, 5, 10, 20, and 30 minutes following the administration. Multiple definitions for a positive test exist based on the absolute change in gastrin concentration.[2] Based on the absolute change in gastrin concentration, four definitions of a positive test exist: greater than 100 pg/mL, greater than 110 pg/mL, greater than 120 pg/mL, and greater than 200 pg/mL. Percentage of change can also be used, either greater than 50% or greater than 100%, and maximum gastrin after secretion greater than 186 pg/mL or greater than 335 pg/mL have also been used. To maximize the sensitivity and specificity of the test, the following change in gastrin concentrations are best used: greater than 100 pg/mL (95%, 99.8%), greater than 110 pg/mL (94%, 100%), greater than 120 pg/mL (94%, 100%), and greater than 200 pg/mL (87%, 100%).[23] At the Ohio State University, we use the 110 pg/mL threshold, as proposed by Deveney et al.,[24] a level of increase that we have found to be accurate in nearly 100% of patients.[2] Most patients with ZES will experience this increase from their basal level within 5 minutes of injection. Rarely, false-negative or false-positive tests may occur. The false-positive rate is 0% in nonachlorhydric patients when greater than 110 pg/mL or greater than 120 pg/mL criteria are used.[23]

Alternatively, a calcium stimulation test may be used, as a second-line test in the rare patient with a negative secretin test in whom there is a high degree of suspicion for ZES, or if secretin is not available. The patient is given a 12-mg/kg infusion of elemental calcium (calcium gluconate or calcium chloride) over 3 hours. Gastrin levels are measured at 0 and 30 minutes and then at 1, 2, 3, 4, and 5 hours following administration of calcium. Levels increased by 100% yield a sensitivity and specificity of 68% and 90%, respectively.[2] Unfortunately, multiple side effects including abdominal pain, nausea, vomiting, headache, phlebitis, and significant risk of cardiac arrhythmias occur, so it is rarely used today.

Other less common modalities previously described for possible diagnosis include meal stimulation or glucagon stimulation. Ingestion of food stimulates release of gastrin from the antrum and duodenum. This test has not been shown to be accurate for discrimination of hypergastrinemia in ZES. Attempts were made to use glucagon stimulation when secretin was in short supply because it is in the same family of GI peptides. In a report of Shibata et al. after injecting glucagon, patients reportedly had decrease in serum gastrin levels.[25] However this test needs to be further explored to be a viable diagnostic option.

Once the diagnosis of gastrinoma has been confirmed biochemically and physiologically, the next immediate step in management is medical control of the excessive acid output. Historically, the treatment for ZES was total removal of all acid-secreting tissue by total gastrectomy. Trying to avoid total gastrectomy led to recurrence, often with life-threatening complications. With the advent of potent acid-reducing medications (first H_2-receptor antagonists and now PPIs), the most critical step in the initial management of patients with ZES is the adequate suppression of gastric acid output. With current medical options, it is possible to control the gastric acid secretion very effectively with PPIs. The doses to achieve symptom relief will be much greater than with typical ulcer disease or dyspepsia. Alternatively, the H_2-receptor antagonists such as cimetidine, ranitidine, and famotidine can be used; however, they are less effective than PPIs and require larger and more frequent doses. PPI dosing should be titrated based on symptoms and documented ulcer healing. Resolution of symptoms may not be a good guide to gauge treatment response. Documentation of ulcer healing, with serial upper endoscopies is necessary. Alternatively, determination of basal acid output (BAO) was suggested in the past as a method to individualize the dose of PPI. The recommended goal is to achieve a BAO less than 10 mEq/h in men and 5 mEq/h in women. Many recent studies have brought attention to the safety of long-term PPI use. Many long-term consequences include hypomagnesemia, osteoporosis and bone fractures, increased cardiovascular events in patients taking antiplatelet therapy, community-acquired pneumonia, *Clostridium difficile* infection, and iron absorption.[26-30] Obviously these risks are mitigated by the importance of controlling acid production in this patient population. However, the risks should be recognized so that preventive measures may be taken to prevent some of these side effects when possible. Another potential drawback of PPIs is a delay in diagnosis of ZES in the patient who has not had a definitive diagnosis.[31] Finally, somatostatin analogues, such as octreotide, were seen to cause significant and long-lasting inhibition of both tumor gastrin release and gastric acid secretion, and more recently shown to prolong progression-free survival and believed to stabilize tumor growth.[32,33] These properties render them useful in the management of tumors refractory to conventional acid suppression regimens.[34]

MEASUREMENT OF OTHER GASTROINTESTINAL HORMONES

It has been recommended that patients undergo plasma biochemical evaluation of fasting pancreatic polypeptide (PP), pancreastatin, and chromogranin A (CgA) in addition to glucagon and gastrin levels.[35] In the past CgA has been shown to have modest value in the diagnosis of sporadic PNETs with modest sensitivity and specificity. Recently chromogranin has been shown to be an unreliable tumor marker for neuroendocrine tumors (NETs).[36-39] CgA is recommended by the recent European Neuroendocrine Tumor Society (ENETS) and North American Neuroendocrine Tumor Society (NANETS) in the most recent guidelines as a practical and useful serum marker, despite the mixed data.[40,41] PP levels are not typically elevated in sporadic gastrinoma. Initially, markedly elevated fasting plasma PP level in MEN1 patients was 95% sensitive and 88% specific for the presence of pancreatic islet cell tumors detected by imaging, and thus it was thought that PP may be a marker for MEN1 in patients with ZES.[42] However, more recently CgA and PP were not found to be independent prognostic markers for overall survival in a study by Walter et al. These findings were confirmed by two other studies in which CgA did not appear to be an independent predictor of mortality.[43–45]

GENETICS AND ASSESSMENT FOR MULTIPLE ENDOCRINE NEOPLASIA SYNDROMES

MEN1 is an autosomal dominant inherited disease.[10] Of patients with MEN1 90% to 100% have primary hyperparathyroidism. PNETs are the next most common manifestation of the syndrome and can be functional or nonfunctional. Most commonly they are nonfunctional but when functional, gastrinomas are most common.[46] Pituitary adenomas, adrenal tumors, and thyroid adenomas occur less commonly.[11,12] Work-up of patients with suspected MEN1 syndrome should include biochemical screening for gastrin, insulin, PP, glucagon, and CgA. In addition, calcium levels should be obtained and hyperparathyroidism should be treated first before treatment of any pancreatic endocrine tumor. Hyperparathyroidism should be treated with subtotal thyroidectomy or total parathyroidectomy with autotransplant of parathyroid tissue. This helps reduce gastrin by removing the stimulation from the elevated calcium.

Suspicion for MEN1 should be considered in patients with a family history consistent with endocrine tumors of the pancreas, family members with pituitary or thyroid disease, kidney stones, young age at diagnosis, endocrine tumor associated with hypercalcemia, multiple NETs, or any patient with ZES.[47]

Several authors have attempted to describe biologic markers and link them to the clinical behavior of endocrine pancreatic tumors and their outcome. Several markers have been indicated as potential predictors of aggressive biology or metastatic disease such as increased *HER2/neu* expression,[17,18] tumor size larger than 2 cm, p16/MTS1 tumor suppressor gene inactivation,[19] Ki67 proliferative index, and cytokeratin (CK) 19 expression.[13] Recently, a study identified chromosomal instability and specific chromosomal alterations to be reliable indicators for metastatic disease and poor tumor-free survival.[13] Mutations in the MEN1 gene are found with considerable variations in PNETS, and approximately 37% of gastrinomas harbor this mutation.[48] The menin gene and its role in the carcinogenesis of the syndrome has been well defined.[49,50] The MEN1 tumor suppressor gene encodes for a 610-amino-acid nuclear protein product called menin. Germline mutations in the menin gene include nonsense, missense, deletions, or RNA splicing defects.[51] These discoveries hold promise because they shed light on the molecular underpinnings of carcinogenesis of gastrinoma. Future goals include developing novel diagnostic and perhaps therapeutic tools that will exploit these molecular targets.

TUMOR LOCALIZATION

The initial localization test should be cross-sectional imaging with computed tomography (CT) of the abdomen and pelvis, with fine cuts through the pancreas. Neuroendocrine tumors are hypervascular and therefore

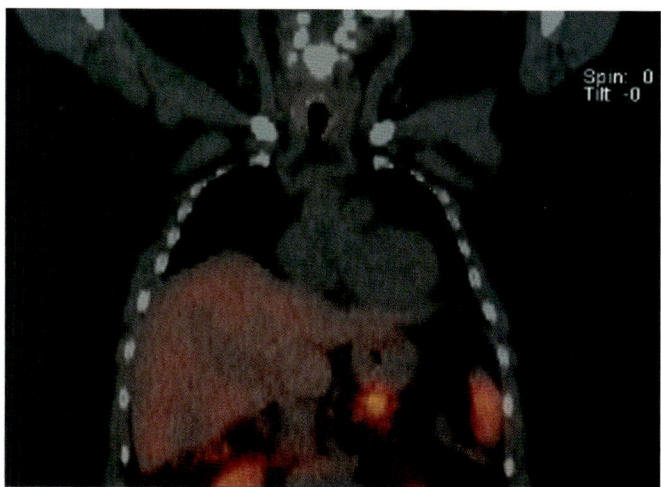

FIGURE 60.1 Octreotide scan (somatostatin receptor scintigraphy) shows an avid lesion at the tail of the pancreas in this female patient with Zollinger-Ellison syndrome. Somatostatin receptor scintigraphy can be combined with computed tomography scanning. Digital reconstruction of the images provides additional information regarding the lesion and its surrounding organs that may assist in preoperative planning.

demonstrate a greater degree of enhancement than the normal pancreas during the arterial and capillary phases of the contrast bolus. This is helpful in identification and differentiation of PNETs from other pancreatic tumors or cancer. Dual-phase magnetic resonance imaging (MRI) of the abdomen with delayed images may also be helpful to delineate the primary tumor or metastatic burden to the liver. An octreotide scan (somatostatin receptor scintigraphy [SRS]) can be of great value in the preoperative localization of gastrinoma (Fig. 60.1). A prospective study from the NIH compared the imaging methods in the localization of gastrinomas in 80 consecutive patients with ZES. The authors compared ultrasonography, CT, MRI, selective angiography, and SRS performed using a radiolabeled octreotide colloid solution. The authors concluded that SRS was significantly better than all of the conventional imaging methods in the identification of gastrinomas later found at surgery, but that scintigraphy still missed 20% of gastrinomas.[52] Several studies have confirmed these findings, whose authors advocated that octreotide scan should be the initial imaging study in ZES.[52–54] Nevertheless, based on current imaging modalities, the overall success of preoperative localization approaches 70% to 80%. Endoscopic ultrasound (EUS) is an alternative imaging technique when cross-sectional imaging and SRS have not revealed the location of the tumor. In addition, biopsy can be accomplished at the time of EUS. The sensitivity of EUS to localize small PNETs is excellent (as high as 97%) compared with CT (85%) or MRI (70%).[55] The majority of these tumors are found at the gastrinoma triangle, first described by Stabile et al.[56] This anatomic area is defined by the junction of the cystic duct to the common bile duct, the transition of the head of the pancreas to the neck of the pancreas, and the transition

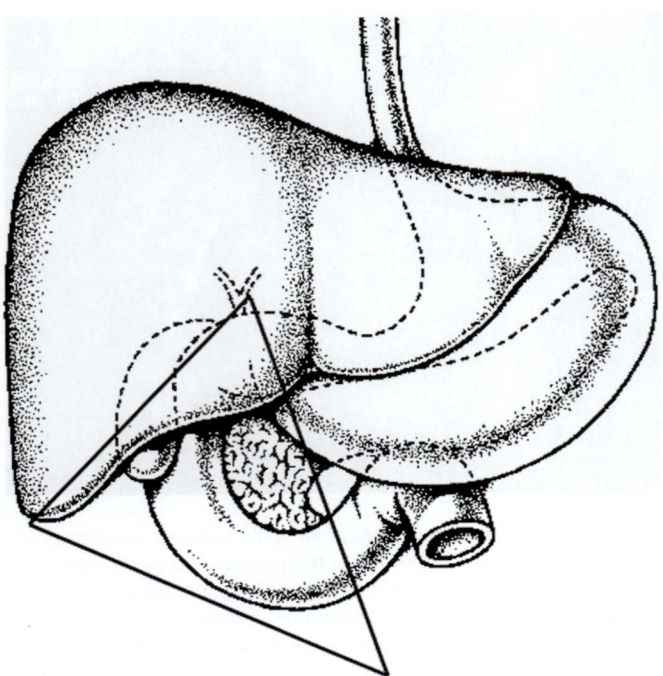

FIGURE 60.2 Gastrinoma triangle. The majority of gastrinomas are found at an anatomic area that is defined by the junction of the cystic duct and the common bile duct, the transition of the head of the pancreas to the neck of the pancreas, and the transition of the second portion of the duodenum to the third.

of the second portion of the duodenum to the third (Fig. 60.2).

Alternatively, selective secretin arteriography may be employed when CT, MRI, SRS, or EUS fail to localize the tumor. This can localize up to 70% of small tumors (<5 mm) with a characteristic blush. Selective portal sampling can also be performed by cannulation of the right hepatic vein for sampling of serum for gastrin. Very small doses of secretin are selectively administered intra-arterially into the gastroduodenal artery, the splenic artery, the superior mesenteric artery, and the proper hepatic artery with sampling at 0, 20, 40, and 60 seconds. A step-up in hepatic vein gastrin will indicate the dominant blood supply of the tumor and its likely location.

New on the horizon is the ^{68}Ga-DOTATATE positron emission tomography (PET)/CT. With the availability of PET in recent years, PET tracers labeled with somatostatin analogues have developed rapidly. With the help of [68]Ge/^{68}Ga generators, which immobilize the parent isotope germanium, the PET radiolabeled tracers can be made less expensively for clinical practice.

PNETs, including gastrinomas, are slow growing and hence ^{18}F-fluorodeoxyglucose (FDG) PET/CT is not commonly used for initial evaluation. Due to the slow metabolic activity of PNETs in the initial stages, they are not extremely avid on ^{18}F-FDG PET/CT. Conversely, they are avid for ^{68}Ga-DOTATATE, which demonstrate high uptake because neuroendocrine tumors express significant somatostatin 2 receptor. Srirajaskanthan et al.[57] were the first to compare the ^{68}Ga-DOTATATE to octreotide scan. They evaluated the diagnostic and management role of ^{68}Ga-DOTATATE PET imaging in patients with neuroendocrine tumors and negative or equivocal findings on ^{111}In-diethylenetriaminepentaacetic acid (DTPA)-octreotide scintigraphy. They showed that ^{68}Ga-DOTATATE PET was positive in 41 of 47 patients (87.2%). No false-positive lesions were identified. ^{68}Ga-DOTATATE PET identified significantly more lesions than ^{111}In-DTPA-octreotide scintigraphy (168 vs. 27 respectively, $P < .001$). ^{68}Ga-DOTATATE is not yet approved by the US Food and Drug Administration (FDA).

INTRAOPERATIVE IMAGING

Few advances in imaging techniques over the past several decades have advanced the surgical management of PNETs. Even with current cross-sectional imaging, preoperative localization can be difficult. Thus intraoperative imaging techniques have been developed. Hall et al. combined an intraoperative portable large-field-of-view gamma camera and a handheld gamma detection probe for ^{111}In-pentetreotide radioguided localization and confirmation of gastrinoma in five patients.[58]

The algorithm for the diagnosis and localization of gastrinoma is summarized in Fig. 60.3. Localization of primary gastrinoma will be possible in 60% to 70% of ZES patients with sporadic gastrinoma. Patients with negative localization tests may be recommended to have exploration as well, but there is a possibility that no tumor may be identified in as many as 15% to 30% of image-negative patients. The principles of exploration are summarized in the following section. Patients with MEN-associated ZES with negative imaging should not undergo exploration because cure is rare and because of metachronous primary tumors as a result of the underlying endocrinopathy.

SURGICAL THERAPY AND PRINCIPLES OF SURGERY

The ultimate goal of surgery is to provide a biochemical cure, prevent disease progression, and prolong survival. These patients benefit from a multidisciplinary team that includes surgeons, gastroenterologists, endocrinologists, medical oncologists, and interventional radiologists. Sporadic gastrinomas without metastatic disease are most amenable to surgical resection and cure. The main principle is to perform a low-morbidity, complete resection of the disease with preservation of the maximum amount of normal pancreas. Patients who have a positive preoperative localization should be offered surgical exploration. Twenty to 30% of patients will have negative localization tests; these patients may be offered exploration as well, accepting the possibility that no tumor will be identified in as many as 15% of imaging-negative patients. When unable to locate the tumor preoperatively, the surgeon should perform a thorough intraoperative search to locate the gastrinoma. The principles of exploration include (1) a wide Kocher maneuver to permit careful examination of the head of the pancreas and uncinate process, (2) mobilization of the body and tail of the pancreas to permit bimanual palpation, (3) intraoperative ultrasound,

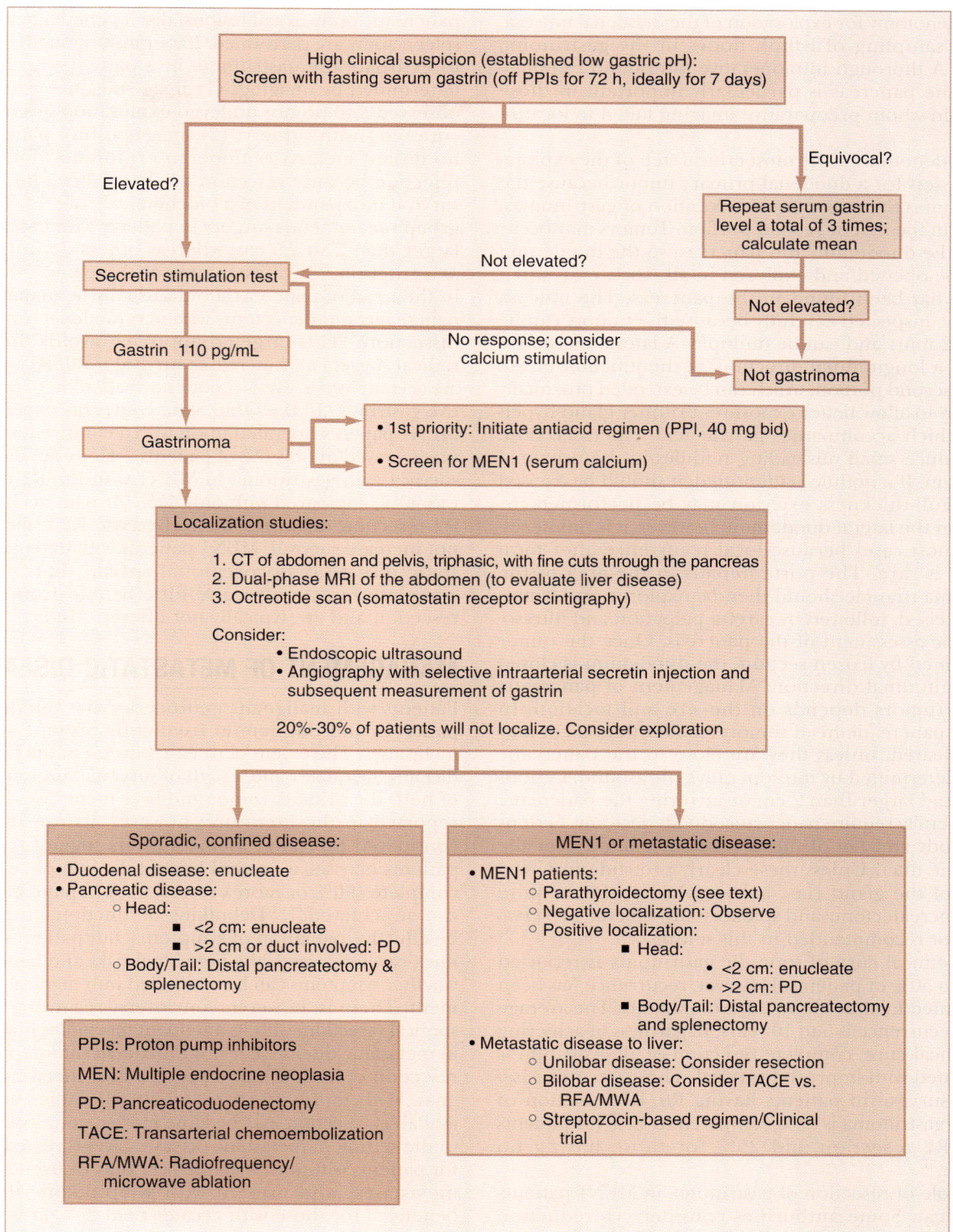

FIGURE 60.3 Flow chart depicting the diagnosis and management of Zollinger-Ellison syndrome. *CT,* Computed tomography; *MRI,* magnetic resonance imaging.

(4) duodenotomy for exploration of the duodenal mucosa, and (5) sampling of lymph nodes in the gastrinoma triangle. A thorough intraoperative ultrasound examination of the pancreas is particularly important in those patients in whom preoperative imaging failed to localize a tumor.

A duodenotomy is the most critical step of the exploration to assess for a duodenal primary tumor because the duodenum is the most common location of gastrinomas, typically in the first or second portion. Tumors may occur in both the duodenum and pancreas, so the duodenum should be opened and explored in all cases, even when a tumor has been found in the pancreas. The mucosa should be inspected carefully because the tumors can be small (<2 mm) and can be multiple. A lateral incision is made in a longitudinal direction, at the junction of the first and second portion, which can be extended proximally or distally to allow better exposure. Brunner gland hyperplasia, which accompanies gastric acid hypersecretion, may produce small misleading nodules in the proximal duodenum. If a nodule is identified, it should be excised locally. Full-thickness excision may be performed for lesions on the lateral duodenum; however, it is not necessary in most cases because local recurrence after local excision is rare. The porta hepatis in the area of the gastrinoma triangle should then be explored and lymph nodes excised, followed by careful palpation and ultrasonographic assessment of the pancreas. Once the tumor is confirmed by frozen section, the duodenum is closed in a longitudinal direction. Management of pancreatic primary tumors depends on the size and location. In general, pancreatic head tumors smaller than 2 cm may be enucleated, unless they are close to the pancreatic duct as determined by intraoperative ultrasound. Lesions in the head larger than 2 cm or involving the pancreatic duct generally require pancreaticoduodenectomy. Lesions in the body and tail of the pancreas are often near the pancreatic duct. Unless these clearly protrude from the surface of the gland (i.e., are exophytic), they require distal pancreatectomy and splenectomy. Splenic preservation is not recommended in this setting.

Biochemical cure of sporadic gastrinoma is reported in 30% to 50% of patients. However, recurrence has been documented in almost one-third of patients. The average time to recurrence is 5 to 10 years. Regardless of achieving biochemical cure, complete resection of all gross tumor is associated with improved survival. The 10-year disease-specific survival in patients having R0/R1 resection of sporadic gastrinoma is 85% compared to 40% for patients having R2 resection and 25% for those having no resection.[57]

The role of resection of gastrinoma in MEN1 patients is less clear. Some authorities consider cytoreduction important in improving survival and preventing metastatic disease gastrinoma in MEN1, even though long-lasting biochemical cure is rare. However, this recommendation is largely based on individual experience and there are no level I or level II data to support radical surgery in ZES in MEN1. Considering the rarity of cure and the indolent natural history of the disease, a targeted approach with enucleation of tumors, while preserving the head of the pancreas and duodenum, seems more prudent. For pancreatic body or tail lesions, distal pancreatectomy and splenectomy are performed. In our institution, the decision to extirpate the gastrinoma in a patient with MEN1 is determined by imaging: (1) image-negative patients are observed and do not undergo exploration given the low cure rates with surgery; (2) image-positive patients with no distant metastases undergo exploration for surgical resection because resection has been shown to improve survival independent of a biochemical cure.[38,39] The NIH group recommends surgery in patients with index lesions larger than 2 to 2.5 cm, whereas others do not use size as a criterion.[40] Invasive tumors or those more than 2 cm in the head of pancreas should usually be managed by a pancreaticoduodenectomy with periduodenal lymph node dissection.[8] This targeted approach avoids the risk of radical surgery and increases survival if R0/R1 resections are accomplished, even without normalization of postoperative gastrin.[2,38] In the Ohio State University experience of MEN1 patients operated upon with a curative intent, cure was achieved in only 6% of patients.[38] However, the 10-year survival with gastrinoma in MEN1 with R0/R1 resection was 90%, compared with only 45% for patients having an R2 resection or no resection. Because R2 resections do not increase survival, MEN1 patients with extensive metastatic disease or locoregional spread that precludes complete resection receive little benefit from surgical resection and are typically not offered surgery.[57,59]

MANAGEMENT OF METASTATIC DISEASE

Patients with malignant neuroendocrine tumors of the pancreas and duodenum frequently present with liver metastases. The extent of disease burden in the liver often dictates the quality and length of survival. Surgical excision of both the primary tumor and liver metastases has been reported in the literature; however, its use should be considered carefully.[60] Some authors suggest that select patients may see a survival benefit if a complete or near-complete (90% or more) resection of hepatic metastases can be achieved.[61,62] Debulking of functional tumors can be effective palliation of symptoms, but patient selection must carefully weigh the individual risks and benefits and whether symptoms can be controlled with medical management. There is, however, controversy regarding whether surgical resection, with its attendant morbidity, is warranted in metastatic disease. For nonfunctional tumors, complete resection of both the primary and liver metastases is the goal. With more effective systemic therapies becoming available, resection may become more commonplace even in the setting of metastatic disease. Liver-directed therapy for patients with unresectable liver only or liver-dominant metastases, who present with symptomatic disease is beneficial for those with greater than 25% liver burden. Transarterial chemoembolization (TACE), radionuclide-laden spheres (yittrium-90), or local ablative therapy (radiofrequency or microwave ablation) are all effective liver-directed therapies.[63–65] These modalities will not cure the patient, but they may provide effective cytoreduction of liver metastases, alleviate symptoms attributable to metastatic disease, and possibly extend survival. However, these modalities have not been compared to one another or to best supportive care. Hence, these patients are best served in the context of a multidisciplinary team and perhaps in the framework of a clinical trial. Caution is advised when performing resection, ablation, or intraarterial therapies after pancreaticoduodenectomy because these patients are at higher risk for hepatic abscess and septic complications because of the contaminated biliary tree.

SYSTEMIC TREATMENTS

CYTOTOXIC CHEMOTHERAPY

Trials using chemotherapeutic drugs including doxorubicin, streptozocin, 5-fluorouracil (5-FU), temozolomide, and dacarbazine have established cytotoxic effects in pancreatic endocrine tumors.[66,67] A study from the NIH showed that the growth rate of metastatic gastrinoma varies markedly in different patients and 26% demonstrate no growth.[68] This growth rate needs to be considered in determining when and in whom antitumor therapy is initiated, as well as in the assessment of response to tumoricidal therapies. In comparison with targeted therapies, the objective response rates with cytotoxic therapies are greater. Capecitabine and temozolomide have been shown to have a high and durable response in PNETs in a small study.[69] Seventy percent of patients had a radiographic response with median progression-free survival of 18 months. Given this radiographic response, this regimen has also been reported in the neoadjuvant setting.[70]

TARGETED THERAPY

There has recently been progress in developing agents that exploit the molecular underpinnings of neuroendocrine pathophysiology. Everolimus and sunitinib are both FDA-approved treatments for advanced pancreatic endocrine tumors.[71] A randomized controlled trial of everolimus, an oral inhibitor of mammalian target of rapamycin (mTor), showed an increase in progression-free survival from 4.6 months to 11.0 months.[72] Sunitinib, a multitargeted tyrosine kinase inhibitor, has also been shown to increase progression-free survival to 11.4 months from 5.5 months and increase in overall survival in patients with metastatic unresectable disease.[73] Although both have been shown to increase progression-free survival, response rates by Response Evaluation Criteria In Solid Tumors (RECIST) criteria are low. Thus, when response is needed prior to resection, targeted therapies are not always the best choice given their low radiologic response rate. There is no current data for the use of these agents in the adjuvant setting. Continued investigation of these agents should offer a better understanding of their role in patients with advanced neuroendocrine tumors and could additionally illuminate the molecular basis of these tumors, thus expanding the therapeutic armamentarium.

SOMATOSTATIN ANALOGUES

Both octreotide and lanreotide have been shown to prolong progression-free survival; however overall survival has not been significantly increased. These drugs are thought to stabilize tumor growth in addition to relieving symptoms associated with functional tumors.[32,33]

SURVEILLANCE

There is no level I or II evidence outlining the best approach to the follow-up of the surgically treated patient with gastrinoma. A reasonable approach is to do yearly gastrin determinations in the patient who is thought to have achieved cure. If the gastrin level was normal after the operation and is noted to increase, then a secretin provocative test is necessary. If this confirms gastrinoma, then repeat imaging is needed to guide an individualized approach to the patient. It should be noted that following successful curative gastrinoma resection, up to 40% of patients may still require antisecretory therapy.[74] This is presumably secondary to hypertrophy of the parietal cell mass secondary to prolonged exposure to gastrin. It often subsides with time.

For patients with residual or unresectable disease, enrolling in a clinical trial is encouraged and follow-up dictated by the protocol. If the patient is not enrolled in a clinical trial, then gastrin levels should be determined biannually and imaging ordered if there is a significant increase in the gastrin level. Repeat secretin provocative tests are not necessary in this group of patients because it provides no additional diagnostic or prognostic information. If there is progression of disease, then consultation with a medical oncologist is advised and a treatment plan determined with a multidisciplinary team regarding systemic and regional therapies.

PROGNOSIS

Comparisons of predictors of disease-specific survival show that the odds of death from gastrinoma are equivalent in sporadic and MEN1 patients.[58] Lymph node metastases do not affect survival because its occurrence is not associated with poorer disease-specific survival or disease-free survival. Tumor size is independently predictive of disease survival.[58] Tumor size is also highly predictive of distant metastases, with the likelihood of such noted to be nearly 60% for primary tumors larger than 3 cm. In addition, primary tumor location affects outcomes: patients with duodenal tumors have a better prognosis than those with pancreatic or combined pancreatic and duodenal primaries. In terms of completeness of resection, patients with R0 and R1 resection do far better than those with R2 resection or those who cannot undergo resection. In other words, patients who undergo surgical exploration resulting in R2 resection do not survive longer compared with patients not undergoing resection.[58]

REFERENCES

1. Zollinger RM, Ellison EH. Primary peptic ulcerations of the jejunum associated with islet cell tumors of the pancreas. *Ann Surg.* 1955;142(4):709-723 [discussion 724-748].
2. Ellison EC, Johnson JA. The Zollinger-Ellison syndrome: a comprehensive review of historical, scientific, and clinical considerations. *Curr Probl Surg.* 2009;46(1):13-106.
3. Davies K, Conlon KC. Neuroendocrine tumors of the pancreas. *Curr Gastroenterol Rep.* 2009;11(2):119-127.
4. Modlin IM, Lye KD, Kidd M. A 5-decade analysis of 13,715 carcinoid tumors. *Cancer.* 2003;97(4):934-959.
5. Cheema A, Weber J, Strosberg JR. Incidental detection of pancreatic neuroendocrine tumors: an analysis of incidence and outcomes. *Ann Surg Oncol.* 2012;19(9):2932-2936.

6. Yao JC, Eisner MP, Leary C, et al. Population-based study of islet cell carcinoma. *Ann Surg Oncol.* 2007;14(12):3492-3500.

7. Lawrence B, Gustafsson BI, Chan A, Svejda B, Kidd M, Modlin IM. The epidemiology of gastroenteropancreatic neuroendocrine tumors. *Endocrinol Metab Clin North Am.* 2011;40(1):1-18 [vii].

8. Halfdanarson TR, Rabe KG, Rubin J, Petersen GM. Pancreatic neuroendocrine tumors (PNETs): incidence, prognosis and recent trend toward improved survival. *Ann Oncol.* 2008;19(10):1727-1733.

9. Metz DC, Jensen RT. Gastrointestinal neuroendocrine tumors: pancreatic endocrine tumors. *Gastroenterology.* 2008;135(5):1469-1492.

10. Jensen RT, Berna MJ, Bingham DB, Norton JA. Inherited pancreatic endocrine tumor syndromes: advances in molecular pathogenesis, diagnosis, management, and controversies. *Cancer.* 2008;113(7 suppl):1807-1843.

11. Burgess JR, David R, Parameswaran V, Greenaway TM, Shepherd JJ. The outcome of subtotal parathyroidectomy for the treatment of hyperparathyroidism in multiple endocrine neoplasia type 1. *Arch Surg.* 1998;133(2):126-129.

12. Skogseid B, Rastad J, Gobl A, et al. Adrenal lesion in multiple endocrine neoplasia type 1. *Surgery.* 1995;118(6):1077-1082.

13. Solcia E, Capella C, Buffa R, Usellini L, Frigerio B, Fontana P. Endocrine cells of the gastrointestinal tract and related tumors. *Pathobiol Annu.* 1979;9:163-204.

14. Jonkers YM, Claessen SM, Perren A, et al. DNA copy number status is a powerful predictor of poor survival in endocrine pancreatic tumor patients. *Endocr Relat Cancer.* 2007;14(3):769-779.

15. Klöppel G, Willemer S, Stamm B, Häcki WH, Heitz PU. Pancreatic lesions and hormonal profile of pancreatic tumors in multiple endocrine neoplasia type I. An immunocytochemical study of nine patients. *Cancer.* 1986;57(9):1824-1832.

16. Abood GJ, Go A, Malhotra D, Shoup M. The surgical and systemic management of neuroendocrine tumors of the pancreas. *Surg Clin North Am.* 2009;89:249-266 [x].

17. Gibril F, Jensen RT. Advances in evaluation and management of gastrinoma in patients with Zollinger-Ellison syndrome. *Curr Gastroenterol Rep.* 2005;7(2):114-121.

18. Roy PK, Venzon DJ, Shojamanesh H, et al. Zollinger-Ellison syndrome. Clinical presentation in 261 patients. *Medicine (Baltimore).* 2000;79:379-411.

19. Zollinger RM, Grant GN. Ulcerogenic tumor of the pancreas. *J Am Med Assoc.* 1964;190:181-184.

20. Berna MJ, Hoffmann KM, Serrano J, Gibril F, Jensen RT. Serum gastrin in Zollinger-Ellison syndrome: I. Prospective study of fasting serum gastrin in 309 patients from the National Institutes of Health and comparison with 2229 cases from the literature. *Medicine (Baltimore).* 2006;85(6):295-330.

21. Hansky J, Soveny C, Korman MG. Effect of secretin on serum gastrin as measured by immunoassay. *Gastroenterology.* 1971;61(1):62-68.

22. Isenberg JI, Walsh JH, Passaro E Jr, Moore EW, Grossman MI. Unusual effect of secretin on serum gastrin, serum calcium, and gastric acid secretion in a patient with suspected Zollinger-Ellison syndrome. *Gastroenterology.* 1972;62(4):626-631.

23. Berna MJ, Hoffmann KM, Long SH, Serrano J, Gibril F, Jensen RT. Serum gastrin in Zollinger-Ellison syndrome: II. Prospective study of gastrin provocative testing in 293 patients from the National Institutes of Health and comparison with 537 cases from the literature. Evaluation of diagnostic criteria, proposal of new criteria, and correlations with clinical and tumoral features. *Medicine (Baltimore).* 2006;85:331-364.

24. Deveney CW, Deveney KS, Jaffe BM, Jones RS, Way LW. Use of calcium and secretin in the diagnosis of gastrinoma (Zollinger-Ellison syndrome). *Ann Intern Med.* 1977;87(6):680-686.

25. Shibata C, Funayama Y, Fukushima K, et al. The glucagon provocative test for the diagnosis and treatment of Zollinger-Ellison syndrome. *J Gastrointest Surg.* 2008;12(2):344-349.

26. Hoorn EJ, van der Hoek J, de Man RA, Kuipers EJ, Bolwerk C, Zietse R. A case series of proton pump inhibitor-induced hypomagnesemia. *Am J Kidney Dis.* 2010;56(1):112-116.

27. Melloni C, Washam JB, Jones WS, et al. Conflicting results between randomized trials and observational studies on the impact of proton pump inhibitors on cardiovascular events when coadministered with dual antiplatelet therapy: systematic review. *Circ Cardiovasc Qual Outcomes.* 2015;8(1):47-55.

28. Lambert AA, Lam JO, Paik JJ, Ugarte-Gil C, Drummond MB, Crowell TA. Risk of community-acquired pneumonia with outpatient proton-pump inhibitor therapy: a systematic review and meta-analysis. *PLoS One.* 2015;10(6):e0128004.

29. Biswal S. Proton pump inhibitors and risk for *Clostridium difficile* associated diarrhea. *Biomed J.* 2014;37(4):178-183.

30. Ngamruengphong S, Leontiadis GI, Radhi S, Dentino A, Nugent K. Proton pump inhibitors and risk of fracture: a systematic review and meta-analysis of observational studies. *Am J Gastroenterol.* 2011;106:1209-1218 [quiz 1219].

31. Corleto VD, Annibale B, Gibril F, et al. Does the widespread use of proton pump inhibitors mask, complicate and/or delay the diagnosis of Zollinger-Ellison syndrome? *Aliment Pharmacol Ther.* 2001;15(10):1555-1561.

32. Caplin ME, Pavel M, Ćwikła JB, et al. Lanreotide in metastatic enteropancreatic neuroendocrine tumors. *N Engl J Med.* 2014;371(3):224-233.

33. Rinke A, Müller HH, Schade-Brittinger C, et al. Placebo-controlled, double-blind, prospective, randomized study on the effect of octreotide LAR in the control of tumor growth in patients with metastatic neuroendocrine midgut tumors: a report from the PROMID Study Group. *J Clin Oncol.* 2009;27(28):4656-4663.

34. Ellison EC, O'Dorisio TM, Sparks J, et al. Observations on the effect of a somatostatin analog in the Zollinger-Ellison syndrome: implications for the treatment of apudomas. *Surgery.* 1986;100(2):437-444.

35. Thakker RV, Newey PJ, Walls GV, et al. Clinical practice guidelines for multiple endocrine neoplasia type 1 (MEN1). *J Clin Endocrinol Metab.* 2012;97(9):2990-3011.

36. Kidd M, Bodei L, Modlin IM. Chromogranin A: any relevance in neuroendocrine tumors? *Curr Opin Endocrinol Diabetes Obes.* 2016;23(1):28-37.

37. Paik WH, Ryu JK, Song BJ, et al. Clinical usefulness of plasma chromogranin A in pancreatic neuroendocrine neoplasm. *J Korean Med Sci.* 2013;28(5):750-754.

38. Hijioka M, Ito T, Igarashi H, et al. Serum chromogranin A is a useful marker for Japanese patients with pancreatic neuroendocrine tumors. *Cancer Sci.* 2014;105(11):1464-1471.

39. Qiao XW, Qiu L, Chen YJ, et al. Chromogranin A is a reliable serum diagnostic biomarker for pancreatic neuroendocrine tumors but not for insulinomas. *BMC Endocr Disord.* 2014;14:64.

40. O'Toole D, Grossman A, Gross D, et al. ENETS Consensus Guidelines for the Standards of Care in neuroendocrine tumors: biochemical markers. *Neuroendocrinology.* 2009;90(2):194-202.

41. Vinik AI, Woltering EA, Warner RR, et al. NANETS consensus guidelines for the diagnosis of neuroendocrine tumor. *Pancreas.* 2010;39(6):713-734.

42. Mutch MG, Frisella MM, DeBenedetti MK, et al. Pancreatic polypeptide is a useful plasma marker for radiographically evident pancreatic islet cell tumors in patients with multiple endocrine neoplasia type 1. *Surgery.* 1997;122:1012-1019 [discussion 1019-1020].

43. Walter T, Chardon L, Chopin-laly X, et al. Is the combination of chromogranin A and pancreatic polypeptide serum determinations of interest in the diagnosis and follow-up of gastro-entero-pancreatic neuroendocrine tumours? *Eur J Cancer.* 2012;48(12):1766-1773.

44. Massironi S, Conte D, Sciola V, et al. Plasma chromogranin A response to octreotide test: prognostic value for clinical outcome in endocrine digestive tumors. *Am J Gastroenterol.* 2010;105(9):2072-2078.

45. Ahmed A, Turner G, King B, et al. Midgut neuroendocrine tumours with liver metastases: results of the UKINETS study. *Endocr Relat Cancer.* 2009;16(3):885-894.

46. Gibril F, Schumann M, Pace A, Jensen RT. Multiple endocrine neoplasia type 1 and Zollinger-Ellison syndrome: a prospective study of 107 cases and comparison with 1009 cases from the literature. *Medicine (Baltimore).* 2004;83(1):43-83.

47. Waldmann J, Fendrich V, Habbe N, et al. Screening of patients with multiple endocrine neoplasia type 1 (MEN-1): a critical analysis of its value. *World J Surg.* 2009;33(6):1208-1218.

48. Duerr EM, Chung DC. Molecular genetics of neuroendocrine tumors. *Best Pract Res Clin Endocrinol Metab.* 2007;21(1):1-14.

49. Starker LF, Carling T. Molecular genetics of gastroenteropancreatic neuroendocrine tumors. *Curr Opin Oncol.* 2009;21(1):29-33.

50. Lairmore TC, Chen H. Role of menin in neuroendocrine tumorigenesis. *Adv Exp Med Biol.* 2009;668:87-95.

51. Lairmore TC, Quinn CE, Martinez MJ. Neuroendocrine tumors of the pancreas: molecular pathogenesis and current surgical management. *Translation Gastrointest Cancer.* 2013;3:29-43.

52. Gibril F, Reynolds JC, Doppman JL, et al. Somatostatin receptor scintigraphy: its sensitivity compared with that of other imaging

methods in detecting primary and metastatic gastrinomas. A prospective study. *Ann Intern Med.* 1996;125(1):26-34.

53. Cadiot G, Bonnaud G, Lebtahi R, et al. Usefulness of somatostatin receptor scintigraphy in the management of patients with Zollinger-Ellison syndrome. Groupe de Recherche et d'Etude du Syndrome de Zollinger-Ellison (GRESZE). *Gut.* 1997;41:107-114.

54. Jensen RT, Gibril F, Termanini B. Definition of the role of somatostatin receptor scintigraphy in gastrointestinal neuroendocrine tumor localization. *Yale J Biol Med.* 1997;70(5-6):481-500.

55. Fujimori N, Osoegawa T, Lee L, et al. Efficacy of endoscopic ultrasonography and endoscopic ultrasonography-guided fine-needle aspiration for the diagnosis and grading of pancreatic neuroendocrine tumors. *Scand J Gastroenterol.* 2016;51(2):245-252.

56. Stabile BE, Morrow DJ, Passaro E Jr. The gastrinoma triangle: operative implications. *Am J Surg.* 1984;147(1):25-31.

57. Srirajaskanthan R, Kayani I, Quigley AM, Soh J, Caplin ME, Bomanji J. The role of 68Ga-DOTATATE PET in patients with neuroendocrine tumors and negative or equivocal findings on 111In-DTPA-octreotide scintigraphy. *J Nucl Med.* 2010;51(6):875-882.

58. Hall NC, Nichols SD, Povoski SP, et al. Intraoperative use of a portable large field of view gamma camera and handheld gamma detection probe for radioguided localization and prediction of complete surgical resection of gastrinoma: proof of concept. *J Am Coll Surg.* 2015;221(2):300-308.

59. Ellison EC, Sparks J, Verducci JS, et al. 50-Year appraisal of gastrinoma: recommendations for staging and treatment. *J Am Coll Surg.* 2006; 202(6):897-905.

60. Bloomston M, Muscarella P, Shah MH, et al. Cytoreduction results in high perioperative mortality and decreased survival in patients undergoing pancreatectomy for neuroendocrine tumors of the pancreas. *J Gastrointest Surg.* 2006;10(10):1361-1370.

61. Norton JA, Warren RS, Kelly MG, Zuraek MB, Jensen RT. Aggressive surgery for metastatic liver neuroendocrine tumors. *Surgery.* 2003;134:1057-1063 [discussion 1063–1065].

62. Chamberlain RS, Canes D, Brown KT, et al. Hepatic neuroendocrine metastases: does intervention alter outcomes? *J Am Coll Surg.* 2000;190(4):432-445.

63. Chen H, Hardacre JM, Uzar A, Cameron JL, Choti MA. Isolated liver metastases from neuroendocrine tumors: does resection prolong survival? *J Am Coll Surg.* 1998;187:88-92 [discussion 92–93].

64. Rhee TK, Lewandowski RJ, Liu DM, et al. 90Y Radioembolization for metastatic neuroendocrine liver tumors: preliminary results from a multi-institutional experience. *Ann Surg.* 2008;247(6):1029-1035.

65. Mazzaglia PJ, Berber E, Milas M, Siperstein AE. Laparoscopic radiofrequency ablation of neuroendocrine liver metastases: a 10-year experience evaluating predictors of survival. *Surgery.* 2007;142(1):10-19.

66. Martin RC, Scoggins CR, McMasters KM. Safety and efficacy of microwave ablation of hepatic tumors: a prospective review of a 5-year experience. *Ann Surg Oncol.* 2010;17(1):171-178.

67. Moertel CG, Lefkopoulo M, Lipsitz S, Hahn RG, Klaassen D. Streptozocin-doxorubicin, streptozocin-fluorouracil or chlorozotocin in the treatment of advanced islet-cell carcinoma. *N Engl J Med.* 1992;326(8):519-523.

68. Ramanathan RK, Cnaan A, Hahn RG, Carbone PP, Haller DG. Phase II trial of dacarbazine (DTIC) in advanced pancreatic islet cell carcinoma. Study of the Eastern Cooperative Oncology Group-E6282. *Ann Oncol.* 2001;12(8):1139-1143.

69. Sutliff VE, Doppman JL, Gibril F, et al. Growth of newly diagnosed, untreated metastatic gastrinomas and predictors of growth patterns. *J Clin Oncol.* 1997;15(6):2420-2431.

70. Strosberg JR, Fine RL, Choi J, et al. First-line chemotherapy with capecitabine and temozolomide in patients with metastatic pancreatic endocrine carcinomas. *Cancer.* 2011;117(2):268-275.

71. Devata S, Kim EJ. Neoadjuvant chemotherapy with capecitabine and temozolomide for unresectable pancreatic neuroendocrine tumor. *Case Rep Oncol.* 2012;5(3):622-626.

72. Oberstein PE, Saif MW. Update on novel therapies for pancreatic neuroendocrine tumors. *JOP.* 2012;13(4):372-375.

73. Pavel ME, Hainsworth JD, Baudin E, et al. Everolimus plus octreotide long-acting repeatable for the treatment of advanced neuroendocrine tumours associated with carcinoid syndrome (RADIANT-2): a randomised, placebo-controlled, phase 3 study. *Lancet.* 2011;378(9808): 2005-2012.

74. Raymond E, Dahan L, Raoul JL, et al. Sunitinib malate for the treatment of pancreatic neuroendocrine tumors. *N Engl J Med.* 2011;364(6):501-513.

75. Metz DC, Benya RV, Fishbeyn VA, et al. Prospective study of the need for long-term antisecretory therapy in patients with Zollinger-Ellison syndrome following successful curative gastrinoma resection. *Aliment Pharmacol Ther.* 1993;7(3):247-257.

Gastric Adenocarcinoma

Kevin E. Behrns | Jessica L. Cioffi

Gastric surgery for benign and malignant diseases has decreased significantly over the last few decades, but the multimodal management of gastric cancer requires that the surgeon be well-versed in the medical and surgical facets of care. The purpose of this work is to provide an overview of the management of gastric cancer with specific emphasis on the perioperative care.

EPIDEMIOLOGY

In 2016, the American Cancer Society estimated that in the United States 26,370 people will be diagnosed with gastric cancer with 10,730 deaths.[1] Worldwide, however, gastric cancer remains the fifth most common cancer and a leading cause of cancer mortality. The incidence of gastric cancer has considerable geographic variability with a significantly higher occurrence in Asia and Latin America than in North America and Europe.[2]

The average age of diagnosis in the United States is 69 years of age with the majority of patients diagnosed in the seventh decade of life and later. Men are more likely to have gastric cancer than women, and Hispanic Americans, African Americans, and Asian/Pacific Islanders are more frequently affected than non-Hispanic whites. Individuals with lower socioeconomic status are more likely to be affected in both the United States and in developing countries.[1]

Since 1930, the incidence of gastric cancer has decreased significantly, although the reasons for this change are unclear. The incidence of tumors located distally within the stomach have decreased, whereas the incidence of more proximal gastric tumors has increased. Despite the decreasing incidence, gastric cancer remains highly lethal in the United States with an anticipated overall 5-year survival rate of 29%.[1,3]

RISK FACTORS

Known risk factors for gastric adenocarcinoma include *Helicobacter pylori* infection, a history of mucosa-associated lymphoid tissue (MALT) lymphoma, the presence of adenomatous gastric polyps, previous gastric operations, pernicious anemia, atrophic gastritis, intestinal metaplasia, exposure to nitrosamines from cured or smoked foods, tobacco use, and family history. A relationship between obesity and gastric cancer has not been identified definitively, although a hypothesis exists that increasing rates of gastroesophageal reflux disease (GERD) associated with obesity may predispose individuals to more proximal tumors. In addition, lower rates of gastric cancer are observed in individuals with a diet high in fresh fruits and vegetables.[1–4]

Certain ethnicities are at risk for the development of gastric adenocarcinoma. Japanese, Koreans, Vietnamese, Native Americans, and people of Pacific Island descent are at the greatest risk. In contrast, Filipinos and Caucasians are at the lowest risk, and Chinese, Latinos, and people of African descent are at intermediate risk.[2]

Familial syndromes such as Peutz-Jeghers and familial adenomatous polyposis (FAP) harbor an increased risk of gastric cancer. Mutations in proteins such as E-cadherin, p53, and BRCA2 have also been shown to increase the potential for the development of gastric adenocarcinoma.[1] A complete list of risk factors is presented in Table 61.1.

PATHOLOGY

Ninety to 95% of gastric cancers are adenocarcinoma with the remainder being attributed to lymphoma, gastrointestinal stromal tumors, and carcinoid tumors.[1] Although several histopathology classification systems exist, the most frequently used is the Lauren classification. This classifies gastric adenocarcinomas as intestinal (well differentiated) and diffuse (poorly differentiated).

Intestinal-type adenocarcinomas are derived from the gastric mucosa and form glands. They are more frequently associated with hematogenous metastases and are observed in elderly patients, men, or those individuals in high-risk populations. They are also more common in the distal portion of the stomach. This type of adenocarcinoma is associated with the risk factors of *H. pylori* infection, chronic atrophic gastritis, intestinal metaplasia, and diets high in nitrosamines.[5–6]

Diffuse-type adenocarcinoma arises from the lamina propria and spreads through the submucosa. Lymphatic metastases are more common with diffuse-type cancers, which are more predominant in younger patients and women. In contrast to intestinal type, diffuse-type adenocarcinomas are not gland-forming and are more frequently observed in the proximal stomach. In addition, diffuse-type cancers may have transmural extension, develop peritoneal metastases, and are more aggressive overall. *Linitis plastica*, involvement of the entire stomach, is a rare and aggressive form of diffuse-type cancer that constitutes less than 10% of all gastric adenocarcinomas.[5,6]

DIAGNOSIS

The early signs and symptoms of gastric cancer are nonspecific and include nausea and epigastric pain. As a result, the majority of cancers are diagnosed at advanced stages. Physical exam findings are also nonspecific, but may include palpable lymph nodes such as the Sister Mary Joseph node in the periumbilical region, the Virchow

TABLE 61.1 Risk and Protective Factors for Gastric Adenocarcinoma

ACQUIRED
High-salt diet
High-nitrate diet
Smoked/cured foods
Low vitamin A and C
Well water
Cigarette smoking
Helicobacter pylori
Epstein-Barr virus
Radiation exposure
Previous gastric surgery
Coal workers
Rubber workers

GENETIC
Type A blood
Pernicious anemia
Family history
Hereditary nonpolyposis colorectal cancer
Li-Fraumeni syndrome
Peutz-Jeghers syndrome
Familial adenomatous polyposis

PRECURSORS
Adenoma
Atrophic gastritis
Dysplasia
Intestinal metaplasia
Ménétrier disease

PROTECTIVE
Raw vegetables
Citrus fruits
Antioxidants
Selenium, zinc, iron
Green tea

node in the left supraclavicular region, or the Blumer shelf, which is a palpable prerectal drop metastases that may be evident on digital rectal exam. Development of a palpable abdominal mass or ascites are findings of advanced disease.[7]

As with all suspected malignancies, a complete history and physical examination are essential. Laboratory values including a complete blood count and chemistry and nutritional parameters should be obtained. Many tumor markers may be elevated in the setting of gastric cancer, including carcinoembryonic antigen (CEA), CA-125, CA 19-9, and β-HCG. These biomarkers, however, lack sufficient sensitivity and specificity to establish a diagnosis. Imaging with computed tomography (CT) of the chest, abdomen, and pelvis with oral and intravenous contrast should be obtained, but the diagnosis is established definitively with an upper endoscopy and biopsy confirmation of an adenocarcinoma. Endoscopic ultrasound (EUS) accurately assesses the depth of tumor invasion and enlargement of perigastric lymph nodes, although this technology may not be available in all facilities.[7-11]

Cross-sectional imaging with CT scan or magnetic resonance imaging (MRI) is useful for the evaluation of metastatic disease. Positron emission tomography (PET)

may also be used, as most gastric cancers are PET avid. Both MRI and PET scans, however, may be cost-prohibitive, not universally available, and unnecessary in the presence of a high-quality CT. If metastatic disease is identified, human epidermal growth factor receptor 2 (HER2-neu) testing is recommended. In addition, screening for family history and smoking cessation are important points of assessment during the initial diagnosis.[11]

Diagnostic laparoscopy and peritoneal washings may be useful in identifying small-volume metastatic disease that is not obvious with other diagnostic modalities. In recent studies, it was reported that 30% of patients were upstaged after diagnostic laparoscopy, thereby changing the overall management. National Comprehensive Cancer Network (NCCN) recommendations include the use of diagnostic laparoscopy and peritoneal washings for cytology for all tumors stage IB or higher when resection is considered.[10-12]

Gastric cancers and esophageal cancers are managed differently with respect to neoadjuvant, adjuvant, and surgical therapy. Esophagogastric junction (EGJ) tumors are assessed using the Siewert classification, which for gastric adenocarcinoma includes only the Siewert type III lesions. These tumors are defined as subcardial carcinomas with the tumor epicenter located 2 to 5 cm below the EGJ with infiltration of the EGJ and esophagus from below. Siewert type I and II lesions are considered esophageal cancers and their management is beyond the scope of this chapter.[11]

Endoscopic screening programs in endemic areas are recommended and have been shown to diagnose tumors at an earlier stage. This practice is not applicable to areas where the incidence of gastric cancer is low, and thus, screening is not currently recommended in the United States.

STAGING

The American Joint Committee on Cancer (AJCC) TNM system is the most widely used staging system for gastric cancer. The system assesses the primary tumor (T), the presence of lymph node involvement (N), and the presence of metastatic disease (M). T stage is based on the depth of invasion of the tumor. N stage identifies lymph node involvement and requires assessment of at least 15 lymph nodes. Metastatic disease is identified as distant metastasis including positive cytology from peritoneal washings. Complete descriptions of all TNM levels and stages are presented in Tables 61.2 and 61.3.[13]

TUMOR MANAGEMENT

Despite significant advances in the multimodal treatment of gastric cancer, operative resection remains the best chance for cure. Survival varies greatly based upon the stage of the tumor at the time of resection (Fig. 61.1).[11] Preoperative staging with EUS and cross-sectional imaging is recommended. Once diagnosis and staging are complete, formal multidisciplinary evaluation should be performed to determine the optimal treatment strategy.

Stage IA tumors may be managed endoscopically with endoscopic mucosal resection (EMR) or endoscopic

TABLE 61.2 American Joint Committee on Cancer Staging of Gastric Adenocarcinoma

TUMOR

Tx	Primary tumor cannot be assessed
T0	No evidence of primary tumor
Tis	Carcinoma in situ; intraepithelial tumor without invasion of the lamina propria
T1	Tumor invades lamina propria, muscularis mucosa, or submucosa
T1a	Tumor invades lamina propria or muscularis mucosa
T1b	Tumor invades submucosa
T2	Tumor invades muscularis propria
T3	Tumor penetrates subserosal connective tissue without invasion of visceral peritoneum or adjacent structures
T4	Tumor invades serosa (visceral peritoneum) or adjacent structures
T4a	Tumor invades serosa (visceral peritoneum)
T4b	Tumor invades adjacent structures

LYMPH NODES

Nx	Regional lymph nodes cannot be assessed
N0	No regional lymph node metastasis
N1	Metastasis in 1–2 regional lymph nodes
N2	Metastasis in 3–6 regional lymph nodes
N3	Metastasis in 7 or more regional lymph nodes

METASTASES

Mx	Distant metastases cannot be assessed
M0	No distant metastases
M1	Distant metastases (includes peritoneal cytology)

Modified from *AJCC Cancer Staging Manual*. 7th ed. 2009.

TABLE 61.3 TNM Staging of Gastric Adenocarcinoma

Stage	T	N	M
Stage 0	Tis	N0	M0
Stage IA	T1	N0	M0
Stage IB	T2	N0	M0
	T1	N1	M0
Stage IIA	T3	N0	M0
	T2	N1	M0
	T1	N2	M0
Stage IIB	T4a	N0	M0
	T3	N1	M0
	T2	N2	M0
	T1	N3	M0
Stage IIIA	T4a	N1	M0
	T3	N2	M0
	T2	N3	M0
Stage IIIB	T4b	N0	M0
	T4b	N1	M0
	T4a	N2	M0
	T3	N3	M0
Stage IIIC	T4b	N2	M0
	T4b	N3	M0
	T4a	N3	M0
Stage IV	Any T	Any N	M1

TNM, Tumor, node, metastasis.
Modified from *AJCC Cancer Staging Manual*. 7th ed. 2009.

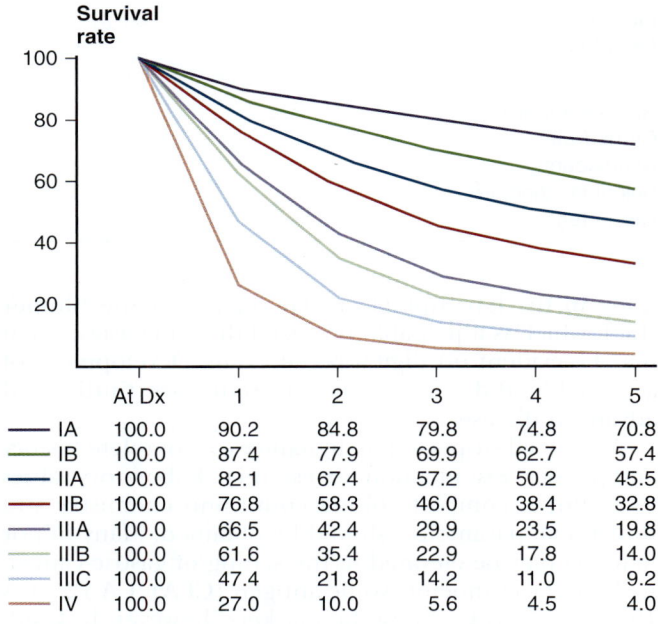

	At Dx	1	2	3	4	5
—— IA	100.0	90.2	84.8	79.8	74.8	70.8
—— IB	100.0	87.4	77.9	69.9	62.7	57.4
—— IIA	100.0	82.1	67.4	57.2	50.2	45.5
—— IIB	100.0	76.8	58.3	46.0	38.4	32.8
—— IIIA	100.0	66.5	42.4	29.9	23.5	19.8
—— IIIB	100.0	61.6	35.4	22.9	17.8	14.0
—— IIIC	100.0	47.4	21.8	14.2	11.0	9.2
—— IV	100.0	27.0	10.0	5.6	4.5	4.0

FIGURE 61.1 Observed survival rates for surgically resected gastric adenocarcinoma based on SEER database, 1973–2005. *Dx,* Diagnosis. (Modified from *AJCC Cancer Staging Manual*. 7th ed. 2009. Fig. 11.1.)

submucosal dissection (ESD), whereas stage IB to stage IIIC tumors are potentially curable with multimodality therapy.[13] All patients with these clinically staged tumors should be reviewed and discussed at a multidisciplinary tumor board.

Tumors that appear locoregionally advanced on cross-sectional imaging are not candidates for surgical resection for curative intent. Findings consistent with locoregionally advanced tumors exhibit disease infiltration at the root of the mesentery, have paraaortic lymph node involvement on imaging or biopsy, and invasion or encasement of major vascular structures excluding the splenic vessels.

In addition, the presence of distant metastases or peritoneal seeding (stage IV tumors) negates the potential for operative cure, and these patients should receive chemotherapy.

MULTIMODALITY THERAPY

Many clinical trials and meta-analyses have evaluated the role of perioperative chemotherapy, preoperative chemoradiation, and postoperative chemotherapy or chemoradiation with conflicting results. Overall, survival in patients with stage IB or higher gastric cancer is significantly improved with the addition of adjuvant therapy following resection. Both the Macdonald protocol, 5-fluorouracil (5-FU)-based adjuvant chemoradiotherapy, and the Medical Research Council Adjuvant Gastric Cancer Infusional Chemotherapy (MAGIC) trial protocol, with pre- and postoperative chemotherapy for resectable cancers, demonstrated significant improvement in overall survival and disease-free survival. Patient factors, including the ability to tolerate the aggressive neoadjuvant protocol prescribed in the MAGIC trial or the ability to tolerate radiation as in the Macdonald protocol should be individualized. Tumor-specific factors, including nodal involvement and location within the stomach, should also guide perioperative planning and the appropriateness of operative resection. Institutional approaches to the treatment of gastric cancer may vary significantly, and the treatment plan should be developed in a multidisciplinary setting prior to initiating any treatment.[14]

NEOADJUVANT THERAPY

The MAGIC trial evaluated the role of pre- and postoperative chemotherapy for patients with resectable gastroesophageal cancers. A total of 503 patients with stage II or higher gastric and esophageal cancer were randomized in two groups. One group received three cycles of chemotherapy (5-FU, epirubicin, and cisplatin) prior to surgery with curative intent, followed by an additional three cycles of chemotherapy, whereas the other group was treated with surgery alone. There was a significant improvement in 5-year survival (36% vs 23%, $P = .009$), a longer interval of progression-free survival, and a decrease in local recurrence rates with pre- and postoperative chemotherapy compared to surgery alone. In addition, tumor downstaging was observed.[15]

These results were comparable to the Actions Concertées dans les Cancer Colorectaux et Digestifs (ACCORD) 07 trial, which demonstrated downsizing of tumor and nodal stages with pre- and postoperative chemotherapy.[16] In both of these trials, however, 50% or less of the patients completed all cycles of chemotherapy. Thus, the effects observed are likely due to the preoperative chemotherapy, thereby demonstrating the significant role of neoadjuvant chemotherapy.[17]

SURGICAL THERAPY

Overall survival is improved significantly with complete surgical resection. Curative intent gastrectomy requires an R0 resection. To achieve margin-negative resection, intragastric margins of 5 cm are recommended; however, a margin of this distance may need to be increased for diffuse-type cancers. In addition, an omentectomy and lymph node dissection should be conducted.[11] Intraoperative frozen section must be performed on the proximal margin, and intraoperative analysis of the distal margin is highly recommended to ensure the presence of duodenal mucosa.

Proximal tumors of the cardia, including Siewert type III lesions, are best managed with total gastrectomy with Roux-en-Y esophagojejunostomy reconstruction. This is preferred over a proximal gastrectomy with pyloroplasty due to the incidence of alkaline reflux esophagitis. Distal lesions, including those in the body and antrum, should be extirpated via subtotal (or near total) gastrectomy to achieve negative margins as total gastrectomy, despite presumed greater margins, does not demonstrate a survival benefit, and patients report improved quality of life with a subtotal gastrectomy versus total gastrectomy.[18] Reconstruction with a Billroth I gastroduodenostomy is the reconstruction of choice because it preserves natural enteric flow. Loop gastrojejunostomy (Billroth II) is an alternative reconstruction that is performed frequently. Roux-en-Y gastrojejunostomy is another preferred method of anastomotic reconstruction; however it is associated with the Roux stasis syndrome and poor gastric remnant function.

Placement of a temporary jejunal feeding tube to assist in postoperative nutritional recovery is recommended for all patients. Nasogastric tube decompression may be beneficial following partial gastrectomy but is not recommended for total gastrectomy. Prophylactic drain placement has not been shown to be beneficial, but it is employed frequently, especially following total gastrectomy with esophagojejunostomy.

Laparoscopic resection for early gastric cancer has been performed for more than a decade with excellent results. Several trials have demonstrated its benefits when compared to the open approach, including decreased pain, length of hospital stay, blood loss, and complications.[19] Most recently, the Korean Laparoscopic Gastrointestinal Surgery Study (KLASS)-01 trial demonstrated decreased morbidity and wound infections with the laparoscopic approach without compromising overall survival for stage I gastric cancers.[20]

LYMPHADENECTOMY

The extent of lymphadenectomy associated with gastrectomy has long been controversial. Gastric adenocarcinoma is accompanied by lymph node metastases in more than half of patients at the time of initial presentation or resection. Lymphadenectomy at the time of gastrectomy has been shown to improve staging accuracy and is the standard of care. In 1988, 16 stations of lymph node drainage for the stomach were first described (Table 61.4) and subsequently expanded by the Japanese.[21] Dissection of stations 1 to 6, a D1 lymphadenectomy, refers to dissection of the perigastric lymph nodes. A D2 lymphadenectomy includes stations 1 to 11 and involves removal of the perigastric lymph nodes as well as the lymph nodes extending along the hepatic, left gastric, celiac, and splenic arteries. Traditionally, this has also included a distal

TABLE 61.4 Lymph Node Stations According to the Japanese Classification of Gastric Carcinoma

Station	Description of Lymph Node Location
1	Right cardia
2	Left cardia
3	Lesser curvature of stomach
4sa	Short gastric vessels
4sb	Left gastroepiploic vessels
4d	Right gastroepiploic vessels
5	Suprapyloric
6	Infrapyloric
7	Left gastric artery
8a	Common hepatic artery (anterosuperior group)
8p	Common hepatic artery (posterior group)
9	Celiac artery
10	Splenic hilum
11p	Proximal splenic artery
11d	Distal splenic artery
12a	Hepatoduodenal ligament (along the hepatic artery)
12b	Hepatoduodenal ligament (along the bile duct)
12p	Hepatoduodenal ligament (behind the portal vein)
13	Posterior surface of pancreatic head
14v	Superior mesenteric vein
14a	Superior mesenteric artery
15	Middle colic vessels
16a1	Aortic hiatus
16a2	Abdominal aorta (from celiac trunk to left renal vein)
16b1	Abdominal aorta (from left renal vein to inferior mesenteric artery)
16b2	Abdominal aorta (from inferior mesenteric artery to aortic bifurcation)
17	Anterior surface of pancreatic head
18	Inferior margin of pancreas
19	Infradiaphragmatic
20	Esophageal hiatus of diaphragm
110	Paraesophageal in lower thorax
111	Supradiaphragmatic
112	Posterior mediastinal

pancreatectomy and splenectomy, but this component of the operation is no longer performed regularly. A D3 lymphadenectomy includes stations 1 to 16 and removes the nodal stations listed previously as well as the periaortic and porta hepatic lymph nodes (Fig. 61.2).[21]

Extended lymphadenectomy or a D2 lymph node dissection has been advocated to more accurately stage the disease extent, which, in turn, will minimize stage migration and ensure removal of all tumor-laden lymph nodes. However, this procedure has been associated with higher morbidity and mortality, primarily due to the morbidity associated with a distal pancreatectomy and splenectomy. In addition, the initial Dutch trial found no significant difference in overall survival with extended lymphadenectomy. Similarly, no benefit has been observed with a D3 lymphadenectomy.[21–23]

More recently, 15-year follow-up of the Dutch trial demonstrated a long-term survival benefit of D2 lymphadenectomy with improved disease-specific survival. Current NCCN guidelines recommend D2 lymphadenectomy in the "hands of experienced surgeons with expertise in the field, at tertiary centers where gastrectomies are often performed." To decrease morbidity associated with this extended lymphadenectomy, a separate retroperitoneal lymphadenectomy may be performed after removal of the gastric and omental specimens. Splenectomy and distal pancreatectomy are performed only when necessary based on tumor involvement.[11,24]

Sentinel lymph node biopsy has been proposed by several Japanese authors to determine the need for lymphadenectomy in early gastric cancers. The relevance of this procedure to Western gastric cancers has been questioned. Early gastric cancers may harbor lymph node metastases in 10% to 15% of cases, thus making endoscopic resection a poor choice of management. However, this practice has yet to transition to clinical practice here in the United States.[25]

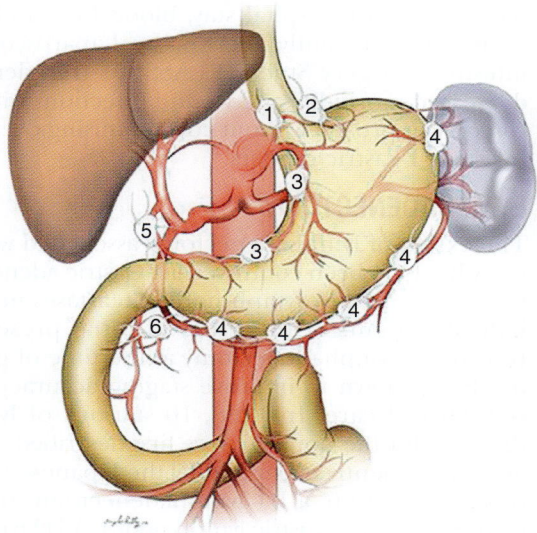

D1 lymphadenectomy

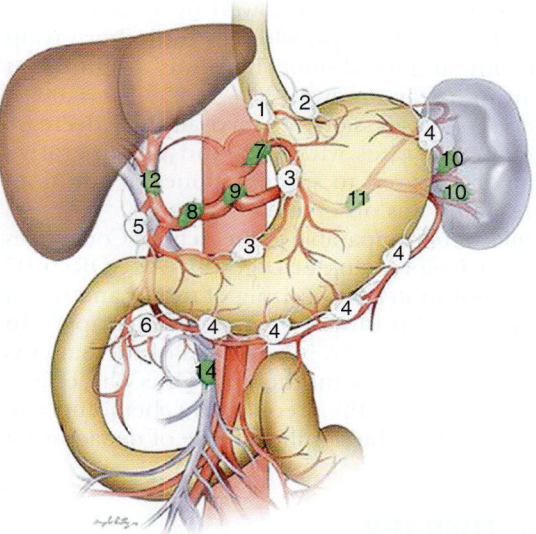

D2 lymphadenectomy

FIGURE 61.2 D1 vs D2 lymphadenectomy. Numbers reference lymph node stations as listed in Table 61.4. *White* numbers refer to D1 lymphadenectomy. *Green* numbers are additional stations included in D2 lymphadenectomy. *(Courtesty Dr. Steven J. Hughes.)*

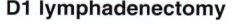

ADJUVANT THERAPY

Adjuvant chemotherapy following surgical resection is strongly advocated despite multiple trials with modest results. When compared to surgery alone, adjuvant chemotherapy with 5-FU-based regimens has not shown a significant difference in overall survival; however, these studies have been underpowered and include a variety of chemotherapeutic agents. The Global Advanced/Adjuvant Stomach Tumor Research International Collaboration (GASTRIC) group evaluated 31 trials and demonstrated a modest advantage for overall survival and disease-free survival in the adjuvant chemotherapy group.[26] More recently, the Capecitabine and Oxaliplatin Adjuvant Study in Stomach Cancer (CLASSIC) trial proposed the use of postoperative chemotherapy including capecitabine and oxaliplatin with significantly improved disease-free survival for all stages. This treatment was performed in conjunction with a D2 lymphadenectomy. Thus, adjuvant chemotherapy does not confer a distinct survival benefit.[27]

Gastric cancer is generally radioresistant, and radiation therapy is therefore rarely indicated. However, concomitant adjuvant chemotherapy and radiation have shown a significant survival advantage. The Macdonald protocol, a regimen of 5-FU-based chemoradiotherapy, improves disease-free and overall survival when compared to observation alone. A significant criticism of this trial is the lack of appropriate lymphadenectomy at the time of surgical resection because more than one-half of patients did not even have a D1 resection. Nonetheless, due to the significant increase in survival, adjuvant chemoradiation is recommended.[28,29]

Recurrence of gastric adenocarcinoma occurs frequently in the peritoneal cavity. Systemic chemotherapy has poor response rates with peritoneal carcinomatosis. Cytoreductive surgery and intraperitoneal chemotherapy have been studied in select patients with mixed results and currently are not recommended as the standard of care.[30]

MANAGEMENT OF ADVANCED DISEASE

Locoregionally advanced or metastatic gastric cancer does not benefit from surgical resection. Obstruction and bleeding tend to be the most common symptoms. Palliative-intent gastrectomy is rarely performed, but may be beneficial for uncontrolled bleeding after failure of radiation therapy, which is the preferred management for tumor-related bleeding. Gastric bypass with gastrojejunostomy may be performed for obstruction in an attempt to palliate symptoms. However, recent advances in endoscopic management, including the use of stents, may allow for sufficient symptom control without the need for invasive procedures.

Palliative chemotherapy may reduce symptoms and improve survival and quality of life in the setting of advanced disease. Multiagent chemotherapy with cisplatin and fluoropyrimidine are recommended as the first-line chemotherapy. Trastuzumab may be added in HER2-positive cancers. Second-line agents include irinotecan and docetaxel. The best supportive care to prevent, reduce, and relieve suffering and improve the quality of life is always indicated.[11]

SURVEILLANCE

Close monitoring of nutritional status is required following gastric resection. Specific attention should be paid to vitamin B_{12} and iron levels, which may require supplementation. Supplemental tube feeding through a jejunostomy feeding tube is recommended until completion of adjuvant therapy. NCCN guidelines recommend a complete history and physical examination every 3 to 6 months for the first 2 years, followed by evaluation every 6 to 12 months for years 3 through 5, and annually thereafter. Laboratory studies, cross-sectional imaging, and endoscopic evaluation are performed if clinically indicated.[11]

PROGNOSIS

Although survival rates for gastric cancer have slowly improved, the overall 5-year survival rate remains poor at 29%. Prognosis correlates with the stage of disease at initial presentation (see Fig. 61.1). Neoadjuvant chemotherapy significantly improves survival and utilization of the previously discussed protocols is strongly advocated. Patients presenting with advanced disease may benefit from palliative chemotherapy; however, this has not been shown to dramatically alter life expectancy.[1,11]

PROPHYLACTIC GASTRECTOMY

Overall, 1% to 3% of gastric cancers are hereditary in nature, with the most common type being hereditary diffuse gastric cancer. This is characterized by an autosomal dominant inheritance pattern and diffuse signet ring cells due to a germline mutation in CDH1 (E-cadherin). Guidelines for screening include:
- a known mutation in a gastric cancer susceptibility gene within the family,
- gastric cancer in one family member before age 40,
- gastric cancer in two first-degree or second-degree relatives with at least one case diagnosed before age 50,
- gastric cancer in three or more first-degree or second-degree relatives regardless of the age of onset,
- gastric cancer and breast cancer in one patient with one diagnosis before age 50, or
- gastric cancer in one patient and breast cancer in one first-degree or second-degree relative with one diagnosis before age 50.

Once the mutation has been diagnosed, prophylactic gastrectomy is recommended for asymptomatic carriers between the ages of 18 and 40. Annual surveillance endoscopy with biopsy should be performed for those patients who elect not to undergo prophylactic gastrectomy, although the efficacy of this practice is not well established due to the diffuse nature of these malignancies.[11,31]

SUMMARY

Although the incidence of gastric cancer is declining, it remains a highly lethal disease. Eradication and treatment of *H. pylori* has assisted in this decline. A high index of suspicion is necessary to diagnose gastric adenocarcinoma at an early stage. Diagnosis and staging require endoscopy with biopsy, EUS, and CT scan to evaluate for locoregionally advanced or metastatic disease. Diagnostic laparoscopy and peritoneal cytology are important components of staging for advanced tumors. Surgery remains the only chance for cure, but it must be accompanied by perioperative chemotherapy or postoperative chemoradiation. Palliation with radiation, chemotherapy, endoscopic stenting, or surgery is indicated for appropriate patients with advanced or metastatic disease. Prophylactic gastrectomy is indicated for all patients with hereditary diffuse-type gastric cancer.

REFERENCES

1. American Cancer Society. *Cancer Facts and Figures 2016*. Atlanta, GA: American Cancer Society; 2016.
2. Siegel RL, Miller KD, Jemal A. Cancer statistics, 2016. *CA Cancer J Clin*. 2016;66(1):7-30.
3. Salvon-Harman JC, Cady B, Nikulasson S, Khettry U, Stone MD, Lavin P. Shifting proportions of gastric adenocarcinomas. *Arch Surg*. 1994;129(4):381-388, [discussion 388–389].
4. Fock KM, Talley N, Moayyedi P, et al. Asia-Pacific consensus guidelines on gastric cancer prevention. *J Gastroenterol Hepatol*. 2008;23(3):351-365.
5. Lauren P. The two histological main types of gastric carcinoma: diffuse and so-called intestinal-type carcinoma. An attempt at a histo-clinical classification. *Acta Pathol Microbiol Scand*. 1965;64:31-49.
6. Werner M, Becker KF, Keller G, Höfler H. Gastric adenocarcinoma: pathomorphology and molecular pathology. *J Cancer Res Clin Oncol*. 2001;127(4):207-216.
7. Gore RM. Gastric cancer. Clinical and pathologic features. *Radiol Clin North Am*. 1997;35(2):295-310.
8. Kodera Y, Yamamura Y, Torii A, et al. The prognostic value of preoperative serum levels of CEA and CA 19-9 in patients with gastric cancer. *Am J Gastroenterol*. 1996;91(1):49-53.
9. Willis S, Truong S, Gribnitz S, Fass J, Schumpelick V. Endoscopic ultrasonography in the preoperative staging of gastric cancer: accuracy and impact on surgical therapy. *Surg Endosc*. 2000;14(10):951-954.
10. D'Ugo DM, Pende V, Persiani R, Rausei S, Picciocchi A. Laparoscopic staging of gastric cancer: an overview. *J Am Coll Surg*. 2003;196(6):965-974.
11. Gastric cancer. Clinical Practice Guidelines in Oncology. National Comprehensive Cancer Network 2016. http://www.nccn.org/professionals/physician_gls/pdf/gastric.pdf.
12. Karanicolas PJ, Elkin EB, Jacks LM, et al. Staging laparoscopy in the management of gastric cancer: a population based analysis. *J Am Coll Surg*. 2011;213(5):544-551.
13. Washington K. 7th edition of the AJCC cancer staging manual: stomach. *Ann Surg Oncol*. 2010;17(12):3077-3079.
14. Knight G, Earle CC, Cosby R, et al. Neoadjuvant or adjuvant therapy for resectable gastric cancer: a systematic review and practice guidelines for North America. *Gastric Cancer*. 2013;16(1):28-40.
15. Cunningham D, Allum WH, Stenning SP, et al. Perioperative chemotherapy versus surgery alone for resectable gastroesophageal cancer. *N Engl J Med*. 2006;355(1):11-20.
16. Ychou M, Boige V, Pignon JP, et al. Perioperative chemotherapy compared with surgery alone for resectable gastroesophageal adenocarcinoma: an FNCLCC and FFCD multicenter phase III trial. *J Clin Oncol*. 2011;29(13):1715-1721.
17. Matuschek C, Bolke E, Peiper M, et al. The role of neoadjuvant and adjuvant treatment for adenocarcinoma of the upper gastrointestinal tract. *Eur J Med Res*. 2011;16(6):265-274.
18. Davies J, Johnston D, Sue-Ling H, et al. Total or subtotal gastrectomy for gastric carcinoma? A study of quality of life. *World J Surg*. 1998;22(10):1048-1055.
19. Lee JH, Han HS, Lee JH. A prospective randomized study comparing open vs laparoscopy-assisted distal gastrectomy in early gastric cancer: early results. *Surg Endosc*. 2005;19(2):168-173.
20. Kim W, Kim HH, Han SU, et al. Decreased morbidity of laparoscopic distal gastrectomy compared with open distal gastrectomy for stage I gastric cancer: short-term outcomes from a multi-center randomized controlled trial (KLASS-01). *Ann Surg*. 2016;263(1):28-35.
21. Schwarz RE, Smith DD. Clinical impact of lymphadenectomy extent in resectable gastric cancer of advanced stage. *Ann Surg Oncol*. 2007;14(2):317-328.
22. Bonenkamp JJ, Hermans J, Sasako M, et al. Extended lymph-node dissection for gastric cancer. *N Engl J Med*. 1999;340(12):908-914.
23. Wu CW, Hsiung CA, Lo SS, et al. Nodal dissection for patients with gastric cancer: a randomized controlled trial. *Lancet Oncol*. 2006;7:309-315.
24. Songun I, Putter H, Kranenbarg EM, Sasako M, van de Velde CJ. Surgical treatment of gastric cancer: 15-year follow up results of the randomized nationwide Dutch D1D2 trial. *Lancet Oncol*. 2010;11:439-449.
25. Tani T, Sonoda H, Tani M. Sentinel lymph node navigation surgery for gastric cancer: does it really benefit the patient? *World J Gastroenterol*. 2016;22(10):2894-2899.
26. Paoletti X, Oba K, Burzykowski T, et al. Benefit of adjuvant chemotherapy for resectable gastric cancer: a meta-analysis. *JAMA*. 2010;303(17):1729-1737.
27. Bang YJ, Kim YW, Yang HK, et al. Adjuvant capecitabine and oxaliplatin for gastric cancer after D2 gastrectomy (CLASSIC): a phase 3 open-label randomized controlled trial. *Lancet*. 2012;379:315-321.
28. Macdonald JS, Smalley SR, Benedetti J, et al. Chemoradiotherapy after surgery compared with surgery alone for adenocarcinoma of the stomach or gastroesophageal junction. *N Engl J Med*. 2001;345(10):725-730.
29. Kozak KR, Moody JS. The survival impact of the intergroup 0116 trial on patients with gastric cancer. *Int J Radiat Oncol Biol Phys*. 2008;72(2):517-521.
30. Seshadri RA, Glehen O. Cytoreductive surgery and hyperthermic intraperitoneal chemotherapy in gastric cancer. *World J Gastroenterol*. 2016;22(3):1114-1130.
31. Chen Y, Kingham K, Ford JM, et al. A prospective study of total gastrectomy for CDH1-positive hereditary diffuse gastric cancer. *Ann Surg Oncol*. 2011;18(9):2594-2598.

Postgastrectomy Syndromes

Kristoffel Dumon | Daniel T. Dempsey

U p to 30% of patients who have had operations on the stomach are afflicted with chronic symptoms that have been relegated to the category of *postgastrectomy syndromes*. This convenient classification is somewhat of a misnomer because some of these patients have not had a gastrectomy (e.g., dumping after a pyloroplasty or fundoplication), and not infrequently the symptom complex for the individual patient does not fit a stereotypical "syndrome." Most patients with an identifiable postgastrectomy syndrome have one or more of the following problems: diarrhea, vomiting, abdominal pain, and malnutrition or nutritional deficiency. These patients have had operations on the stomach for peptic ulcer, cancer, obesity, or gastroesophageal reflux disease (GERD) and represent the subset of gastric surgery patients with a variety of chronic symptoms that range from annoying to life altering. The evaluation of the most common postgastrectomy symptoms and the associated generally recognized postgastrectomy syndromes are outlined in Figs. 62.1 to 62.3.[1–3]

Because operations on the stomach are frequently performed, postgastrectomy syndromes are not uncommon. The indications for gastric surgery worldwide have changed significantly over the past five decades. Elective gastric surgery for peptic ulcer disease has all but disappeared, whereas bariatric surgery in many countries has increased dramatically.[4,5] Worldwide, gastric cancer is the third leading cause of cancer death. Gastrectomy remains the only potentially curative treatment for most patients, and cancer is the most frequent indication for gastric resection worldwide.[6] Therapeutic vagotomy for peptic ulcer is rarely performed, but partial or complete "inadvertent" vagotomy is still quite common during gastric surgery for obesity and cancer. Laparoscopic fundoplication is commonly performed in children and adults for GERD and hiatal hernia. It is the most common cause of dumping syndrome (DS) in children.

The frequency with which postgastrectomy symptoms and syndromes are found depends on how hard they are sought. For instance, some studies indicate that after partial gastrectomy, the majority of patients suffer from one or more upper abdominal symptoms, but clinical experience teaches that only a small percentage of these patients are truly debilitated; most do quite well. The incidence of clinically significant chronic postgastrectomy complications in patients who undergo subtotal gastrectomy and Billroth II reconstruction for gastric adenocarcinoma is low (<5%). The incidence is substantially higher in the first postoperative year, but most patients report improvement within 1 year after surgery.[7] Thus long-term survivors after gastrectomy for gastric cancer usually have normal body weight and lean body mass and satisfactory gastrointestinal (GI) quality of life.

However, a small percentage (<5%) of patients after a variety of gastric operations have persistent debilitating symptoms due to the postgastrectomy syndromes discussed in this chapter. It is important for the managing physician and surgeon to understand the pathophysiology and treatment options for these conditions. The management of patients with severe postgastrectomy symptoms can be challenging, but appropriate therapy can have a significant impact on the patient's long-term outcome.

DUMPING SYNDROME

DS is a constellation of GI and vasomotor symptoms, which present postprandially due to rapid gastric emptying. It is caused by loss of pyloric regulation of gastric emptying and/or decreased gastric compliance.[8] The human stomach possesses the remarkable capability of adapting to large volumes of orally administered liquids and solids through vagally mediated accommodation and receptive relaxation.[9] These intragastric contents, usually hypertonic, are then acted on by secreted acid and pepsin along with muscular churning to prepare an isosmotic gastric chyme that is slowly discharged into the duodenum for further digestion and absorption. If there has been a vagotomy, or a portion of the stomach has been removed, or the normal pyloric sphincter has been disrupted or bypassed, the ingested meal may be incompletely processed by the stomach and/or prematurely discharged into the proximal small intestine. The flow of liquid out of the stomach is determined partly by intragastric pressure and partly by pyloric resistance. Procedures that alter the normal intragastric pressure/volume relationship (proximal gastric vagotomy, sleeve gastrectomy, fundoplication) or outflow resistance (pyloroplasty, gastrojejunostomy [GJ]) predispose to DS. Procedures that alter both have the highest incidence of dumping (gastrectomy, Roux-en-Y gastric bypass [RYGBP]). Dumping symptoms have been reported in up to 70% of Billroth II patients and up to 75% of patients after RYGBP for obesity.[10] Similarly, after gastrectomy for cancer, 67% of patients present with early dumping symptoms and 38% with late dumping.[11] Depending on the speed of liquid emptying and the osmolarity of the contents being discharged, a variety of symptoms may result that have been referred to as the *dumping syndrome*. Both an early and late form of this disorder have been identified. The role of surgically induced microbiome changes in the etiology of DS is unknown.

Early dumping is more common and includes systemic and abdominal symptoms. Systemic manifestations include palpitations, tachycardia, fatigue, a need to lie down following meals, flushing or pallor, diaphoresis, lightheadedness, hypotension, headache, and possibly syncope. Abdominal symptoms include early satiety, epigastric fullness or pain,

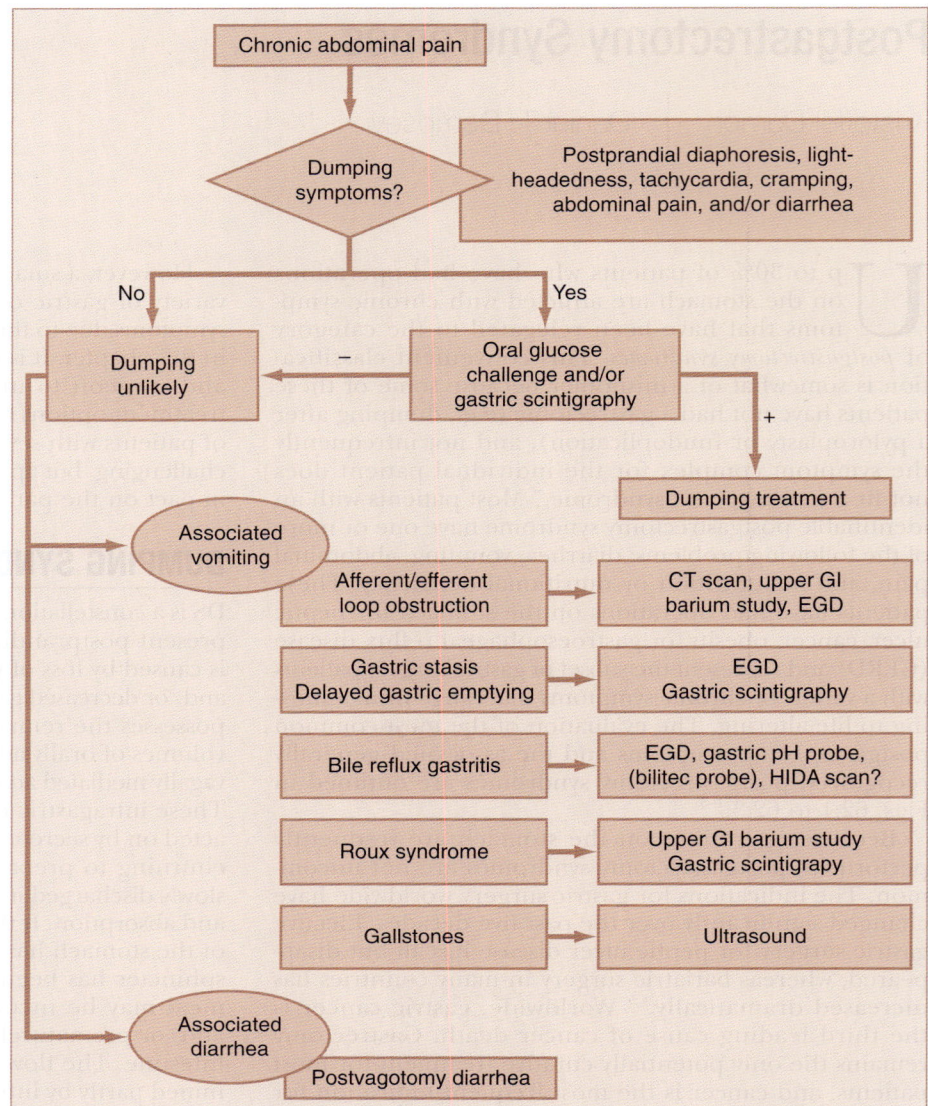

FIGURE 62.1 Chronic abdominal pain. The evaluation of abdominal pain and the associated generally recognized postgastrectomy syndromes. *CT,* Computed tomographic; *EGD,* esophagogastroduodenoscopy; *GI,* gastrointestinal; *HIDA,* hepatobiliary iminodiacetic acid.

diarrhea, nausea, cramps, bloating, and borborygmi. Early dumping begins within 30 minutes following a meal and is attributable to bowel distention, relative hypovolemia, GI hormone hypersecretion, and autonomic dysregulation.[12,13] Late dumping is characterized by symptoms that occur 1 to 3 hours postprandially. Symptoms of late dumping consist of perspiration, faintness, decreased concentration, and altered levels of consciousness, among others. These symptoms are related to a reactive hypoglycemia that occurs 1 to 3 hours postprandially. Patients with late dumping often have early dumping as well.[14]

Most patients with DS have mild to moderate symptoms, but some patients have disabling symptoms that may be severe enough to cause protein-energy malnutrition.[15] The differential diagnosis of DS includes gastroparesis, partial small bowel obstruction, anastomotic stricture, postvagotomy diarrhea, inflammatory bowel disease, irritable bowel disease, and bacterial overgrowth. Dumping symptoms are triggered by rapid gastric emptying of hyperosmolar voluminous chyme that causes bowel

distention, hypermotility, and splanchnic blood pooling. This leads to both the GI and vasomotor symptoms that characterize early DS.[16,17] Hormones play an important role as mediators of this pathophysiologic response (e.g., vasoactive intestinal peptide [VIP], serotonin, bradykinin, norepinephrine).[18,19] Late dumping involves a reactive hypoglycemia brought on by the rapid and high initial glucose load presented to and absorbed by the small intestine, leading to a GLP-1–mediated inappropriately high insulin response and hypoglycemia.

An oral glucose challenge will confirm the diagnosis of DS. Patients fast for 10 hours overnight and then ingest 50 g of glucose. It is reported to have a sensitivity and specificity of up to 100% and 94%, respectively.[20] The diagnosis of early DS in a patient with clinical symptomatology may also be confirmed with a scintigraphic gastric emptying study, in which greater than 50% of an isotope-labeled solid meal has emptied within 1 hour.

A variety of gastric procedures may give rise to early dumping. More than half of the patients who have had RYGBP for obesity or total gastrectomy experience early

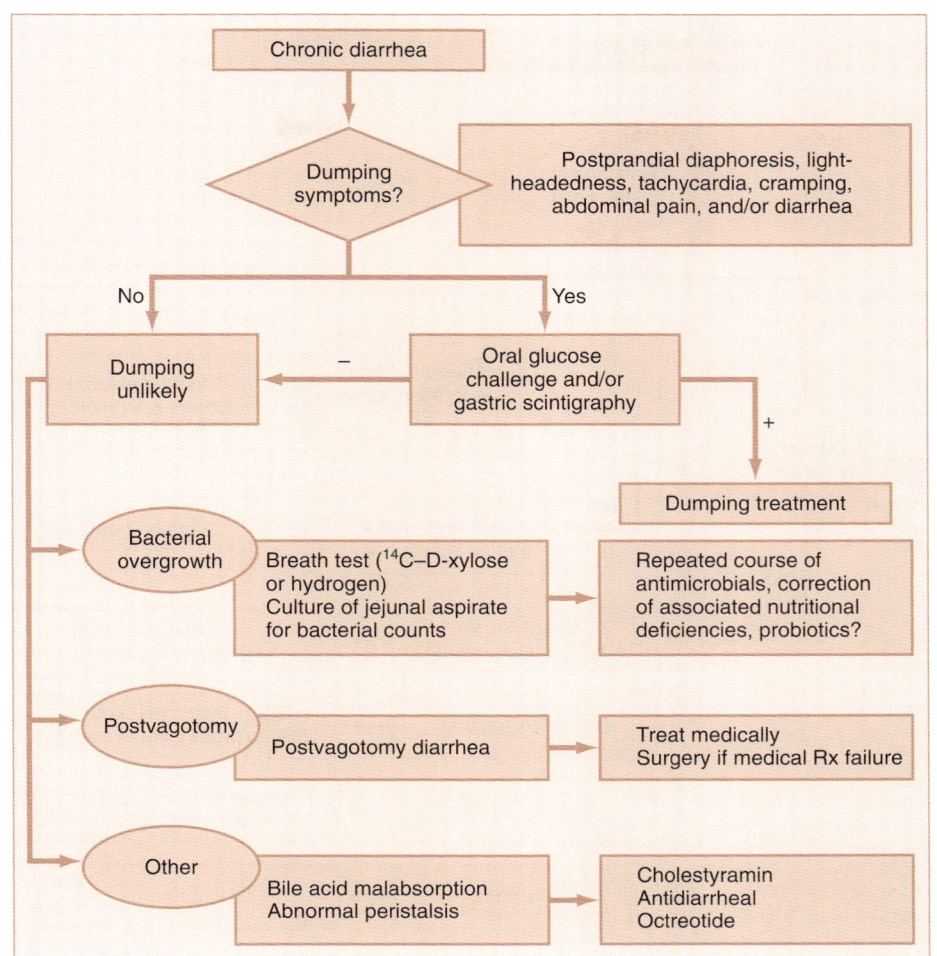

FIGURE 62.2 Chronic diarrhea. The evaluation of diarrhea and the associated generally recognized postgastrectomy syndromes.

dumping symptoms, and approximately 30% of those with partial gastrectomy have early dumping. The risk of problematic dumping after sleeve gastrectomy is low (1.6%), although up to 30% to 40% of patients may have very mild symptoms.[21,22] Up to 15% of patients with pyloroplasty or simple GJ experience early dumping, as do 2% of patients with proximal gastric vagotomy and fundoplication. The type of GI reconstruction after distal gastrectomy influences the risk of DS because Roux-en-Y GJ (11%) has a lower rate of dumping than either Billroth I (B1) or Billroth II (B2). DS after B1 (17%) is less than after B2, (70%), perhaps because B1 gastric effluent enters the duodenum and triggers a neuroendocrine response that slows gastric emptying (duodenal brake). The risk of dumping with pyloroplasty and loop GJ are similar, but the latter gastric drainage procedure is easily reversible. Dumping symptoms tend to improve with time in most patients.[7,24]

Late dumping, less common than the early variant, is caused by hyperinsulinemic hypoglycemia and occurs 2 to 3 hours postprandially. In late dumping the rapid delivery of monosaccharides and disaccharides into the small intestine causes hyperglycemia. The pancreas is subsequently triggered to release insulin by glucagon-like peptide 1 (GLP-1) and in the process actually "overshoots" so that marked hypoglycemia is induced. This insulin shock condition stimulates the adrenal glands to release catecholamines, which cause a constellation of symptoms, including tachycardia, tachypnea, diaphoresis, and light-headedness. Late DS is more frequent in patients who had early DS.[21] Late DS has been reported in more than 50% of bariatric patients after gastric bypass. In some of these patients, late DS developed 1 to 8 years after the surgery and was significantly more common in patients with type 2 diabetes mellitus (44.9% vs. 5.6%). One must rule out an unrelated islet cell tumor as the cause of a severe refractory hypoglycemia by documenting the fasting plasma glucose, serum insulin, and C-peptide level. A prolonged oral glucose tolerance test will also confirm the diagnosis of late dumping.[25] Early dumping tends to improve with time, whereas late dumping tends to persist or exacerbate.

In most patients with DS, symptoms are not severe and medical management is successful. Consultation with an experienced dietitian is helpful. Dietary modification is the first-line treatment for DS. Daily intake should be divided into at least 6 meals. Liquids and solids should be separated. Diets should be high in protein and fat, and simple sugars should be avoided. Vasomotor symptoms can often be ameliorated if the patient lies down for 30 minutes after meals. Elimination of milk and dairy products has been successful in many patients.[26] Another simple therapy is adding dietary fiber. Guar gum and pectin are useful in increasing the viscosity of the food,

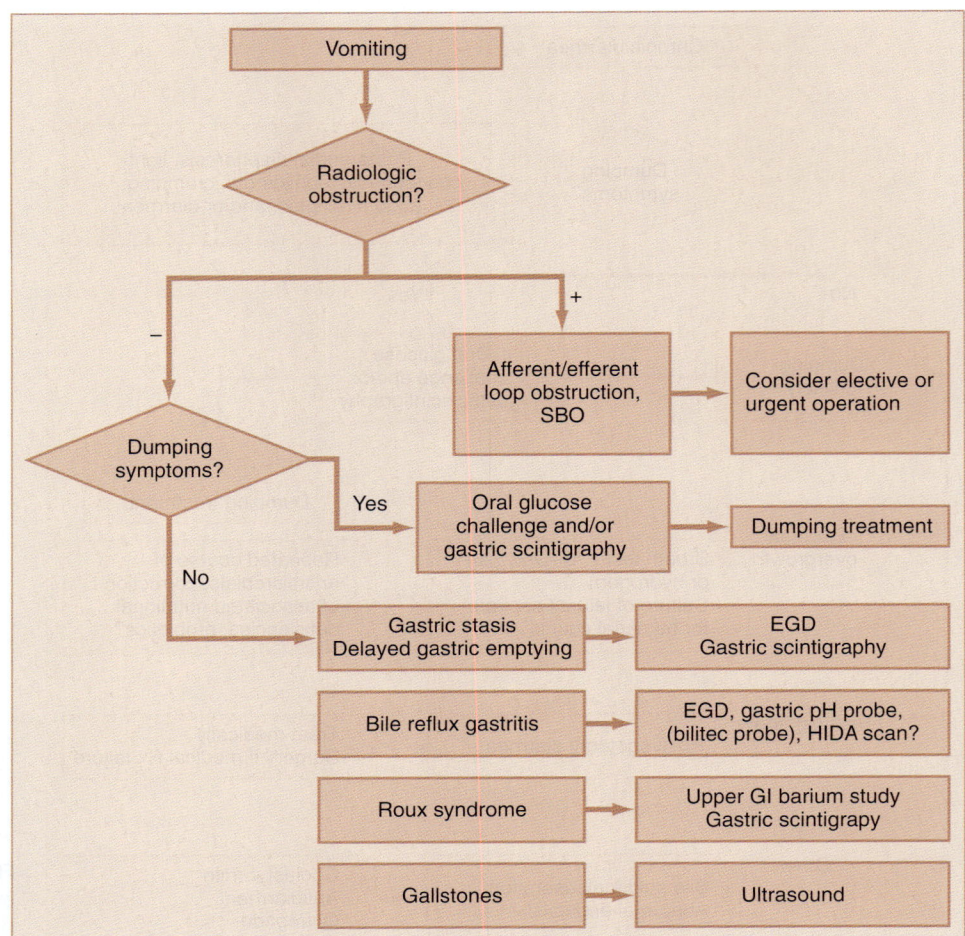

FIGURE 62.3 Vomiting. The evaluation of vomiting and the associated generally recognized postgastrectomy syndromes. *EGD,* Esophagogastroduodenoscopy; *GI,* gastrointestinal; *HIDA,* hepatobiliary iminodiacetic acid; *SBO,* small bowel obstruction.

but their poor taste limits patient compliance.[27] Hard candy can be consumed to abort the hypoglycemia of late DS. Acarbose is an α-glycosidase hydrolase inhibitor that delays carbohydrate digestion and absorption[28–30] and is efficient in the treatment of late dumping. Side effects include excess flatulence[31] and hypoglycemia if carbohydrate absorption is excessively inhibited.[25,26,28,29]

A number of pharmacologic options exist for the treatment of the DS. Tincture of opium is especially effective in relieving diarrhea associated with DS.[33] Symptomatic treatment of DS may be addressed with over the counter medications. Treatment for diarrhea (e.g., Imodium), nausea (e.g., meclizine, promethazine, proton pump inhibitors [PPIs]), or antigas measures may be helpful. Inadequate digestion of nutrients can cause gas and bloating when they reach colonic bacteria; therefore probiotics may be a useful adjunct. Anticholinergic agents, such as dicyclomine, hyoscyamine, and propantheline, slow gastric emptying and are also antispasmodic, thus decreasing abdominal pain related to small bowel motility.[34] Diazoxide is a potassium channel activator that inhibits the secretion of insulin. Thus diazoxide has showed success in recent studies in treating late dumping hypoglycemia and can be used when acarbose and lifestyle modifications are insufficient.[35,36]

Octreotide, a somatostatin analogue, should be considered for patients with severe postgastrectomy DS refractory to diet therapy. Octreotide can markedly improve the quality of life in DS patients,[37] but the data are limited for long-term efficacy. Octreotide alleviates both early and late dumping symptoms through inhibition of hormone mediators. It also delays gastric emptying time and inhibits splanchnic vasodilation.[38,39] Short-acting and long-acting octreotide are equally effective in blunting dumping symptoms, but the long-acting preparation scored significantly better on quality-of-life measures.[13] Long-term octreotide therapy loses its efficacy because side effects such as diarrhea and steatorrhea as well as cost lead to lack of compliance.[26,38,39]

Only a small percentage of patients with dumping symptoms ultimately require surgery. Most patients improve with time (months and even years), dietary management, and medication. Therefore the surgeon should not rush to reoperate on the patient with DS. Multidisciplinary nonsurgical management must be optimized first. Before reoperation, a period of in-hospital observation is useful to define the severity of the patient's symptoms, and patient compliance with prescribed dietary and medical therapy. The results of remedial operation for dumping are variable and unpredictable. There are a variety of surgical approaches, none of which work consistently well. In addition, there is not a great deal of experience reported in the literature with any of these methods. Long-term follow-up is rare.

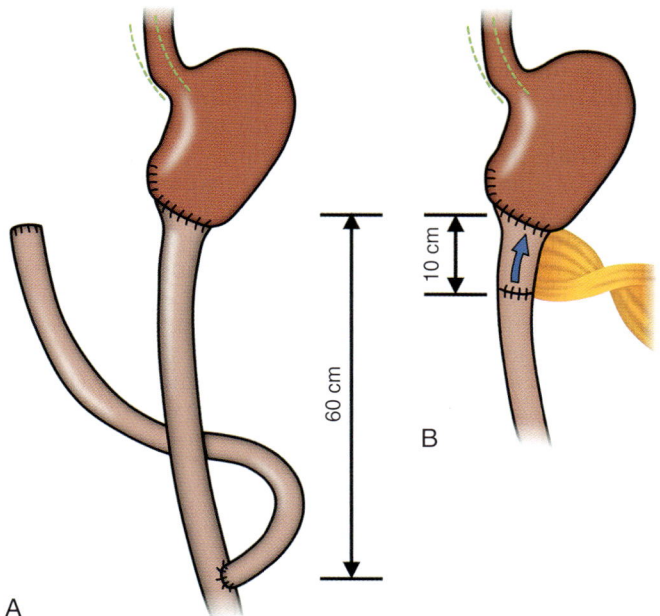

FIGURE 62.4 Surgical approaches to treat dumping syndrome. (A) Long-limb Roux-en-Y anastomosis in which the jejunojejunostomy is fashioned approximately 60 cm from the gastrojejunostomy. (B) A 10-cm loop of jejunum is twisted 180 degrees on its mesentery so that its distal end is anastomosed to the stomach and its proximal end to the small intestine in an antiperistaltic fashion. (Modified from Miller TA, Mercer DW. Derangements in gastric function secondary to previous surgery. In: Miller TA, ed. *Modern Surgical Care: Physiologic Foundations and Clinical Applications.* 2nd ed. St. Louis: Quality Medical; 1998:400.)

Patients with disabling refractory dumping after GJ can be considered for simple takedown of this anastomosis provided that the pyloric channel is patent endoscopically. For dumping following pyloroplasty, pyloric reconstruction is described, but modern day experience with this is rare and today's surgeon should view pyloroplasty as irreversible. Distal gastrectomy with Roux reconstruction (Fig. 62.4A), or a "duodenal switch" with division of the postbulbar duodenum and anastomosis to a Roux jejunal limb, is currently the best option for the uncommon patient with refractory postpyloroplasty dumping. For severe dumping after Billroth I or II gastrectomy, conversion to Roux-en-Y GJ should be considered because the motility of the Roux limb tends to slow gastric emptying. However, gastric stasis and/or marginal ulceration may result particularly in the presence of a large gastric remnant. Lifelong acid suppression should be considered. The reversed intestinal interposition is rarely used currently for DS—and rightly so. This operation interposes a 10-cm reversed segment of intestine between the stomach and the proximal small bowel (see Fig. 62.4B). This slows gastric emptying but often leads to obstruction, requiring reoperation. Isoperistaltic interposition (Henley loop) between the gastric remnant and the duodenum has not been successful in sustained improvement of DS. Because pyloric ablation is a dominant factor in the etiology of postgastrectomy dumping, it is not surprising that conversion of Billroth

II to Billroth I anastomosis cannot ensure resolution of dumping symptoms.[34,40,41] Newer surgical techniques, such as pylorus-preserving segmental gastrectomy for early cancer of the midbody of the stomach, have been reported and may significantly decrease the incidence of postoperative dumping.[42–44]

POSTVAGOTOMY DIARRHEA

Truncal vagotomy is associated with clinically significant diarrhea in 5% to 10% of patients. It occurs soon after surgery and usually is not associated with other GI or systemic symptoms, a fact that helps to distinguish it from dumping. The diarrhea may be a daily occurrence, or there may be significant periods of relatively normal bowel function. The symptoms tend to improve over the months and years after the index operation, and long-term significant postvagotomy diarrhea occurs in only 1% to 2% of vagotomy patients. The cause of postvagotomy diarrhea is unclear. Although rare, it can even occur after proximal gastric vagotomy or fundoplication, suggesting that intestinal vagal denervation may not be the sole cause. Factors contributing to postvagotomy diarrhea include intestinal dysmotility and accelerated transit, bile acid malabsorption, rapid gastric emptying, altered microbiome, and bacterial overgrowth. The latter problem is facilitated by decreased gastric acid secretion and (even small) blind loops. Although bacterial overgrowth can be confirmed with the hydrogen breath test, a simpler test is an empirical trial of oral antibiotics and/or probiotics. Some patients with postvagotomy diarrhea respond to cholestyramine, whereas in others codeine or loperamide may be useful. It has been shown experimentally that the total bile acid content in the stools of patients with postvagotomy diarrhea, although not significantly greater than in those without this problem, has more than twice the amount of chenodeoxycholic acid.[45] Such findings lend support to the hypothesis that bile acid malabsorption may contribute to postvagotomy diarrhea in some patients.

Fat malabsorption should also be considered in the differential diagnosis of postvagotomy diarrhea. This can be caused by acid inactivation of pancreatic enzymes, poorly coordinated mixing of food and digestive juices, or bacterial overgrowth. This can be confirmed with a qualitative test for fecal fat. It is best treated with acid suppression and pancreatic enzyme supplements, and if appropriate oral antibiotics. Postvagotomy diarrhea usually does not respond to these modalities.

In the rare patient who is debilitated by postvagotomy diarrhea unresponsive to maximal medical management for at least 1 year, operation might be considered but outcomes can be problematic. The operation of choice is probably a 10-cm reversed jejunal interposition placed in continuity 100 cm distal to the ligament of Treitz (Fig. 62.5). Another option is the onlay antiperistaltic distal ileal graft. Both operations can cause obstructive symptoms and/or bacterial overgrowth.[10]

GASTRIC STASIS

In the rare patient with *acute gastric stasis* after gastric surgery, persistent nausea and vomiting prevent removal

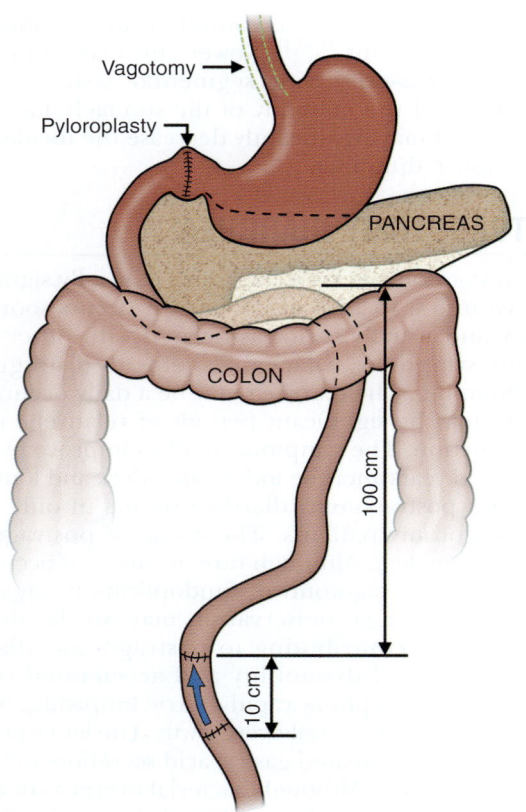

FIGURE 62.5 Surgical management of postvagotomy diarrhea: A 10-cm loop of jejunum is rotated 180 degrees on its mesentery. (Modified from Miller TA, Mercer DW. Derangements in gastric function secondary to previous surgery. In: Miller TA, ed. *Modern Surgical Care: Physiologic Foundations and Clinical Applications.* 2nd ed. St. Louis: Quality Medical; 1998:407.)

of the nasogastric tube. If the nasogastric tube cannot be removed within a period of 7 to 10 days after surgery, a gastrostomy may be placed either laparoscopically or endoscopically. Alimentation can then be given via a J tube extension placed during one of these procedures. If the gastric remnant is not of sufficient size to accommodate these approaches, a decompressing gastric tube can often be passed retrograde through the efferent limb and exited through the skin via a Witzel technique. Distal to this placement, another tube may be placed antegrade as a Witzel feeding jejunostomy. In patients in whom these enteral approaches to alimentation are not possible, total parenteral nutrition is an alternative. In any event, reoperative surgery should generally be delayed for at least 3 months as the majority of patients will regain satisfactory GI function without surgery. Only after this period should reexploration be considered.

Chronic gastric stasis[46] following gastric surgery may be due to a problem with gastric motor function or be caused by an obstruction. The gastric motility abnormality may have been preexisting and unrecognized by the operating surgeon. More commonly it is secondary to some aspect of the operation, such as deliberate or unintentional vagotomy or resection of the dominant gastric pacemaker. Truncal vagotomy is more likely to cause chronic gastric stasis

than proximal gastric (parietal cell) vagotomy because it denervates the antropyloric pump mechanism. Obstruction may be mechanical (e.g., anastomotic stricture, efferent limb kink from adhesions or constricting mesocolon, or a proximal small-bowel obstruction) or functional (e.g., retrograde peristalsis in a Roux limb).

Chronic gastric stasis presents with vomiting (often of undigested food), bloating, epigastric pain, and weight loss. Symptoms are usually improved by a liquid diet and always improved by prolonged fasting. Differential diagnosis includes primary gastroparesis, chronic small bowel obstruction, anastomotic stricture, afferent loop syndrome, internal hernia, GERD, and achalasia. The evaluation includes esophagogastroduodenoscopy (EGD), upper GI series, gastric emptying scan (scintigraphy), and gastric motor testing. Endoscopy shows gastritis and retained food or bezoar in the stomach. The gastroenteric anastomosis and efferent limb should be evaluated for stricture or narrowing. A dilated efferent limb suggests chronic stasis, either from a motor abnormality (e.g., Roux syndrome) or mechanical small bowel obstruction (e.g., chronic adhesion). If the problem is thought to be primarily a disorder of intrinsic motor function, newer techniques, such as electrogastrography and GI manometry, should be considered. However, it should be recognized that chronic distal mechanical obstruction may result in disordered motility in the proximal organ.

After mechanical obstruction has been ruled out, medical treatment is successful in most cases of gastric motor dysfunction following gastric surgery. Management consists of dietary modification and promotility agents. One of several gastrokinetic agents, such as metoclopramide, domperidone, and erythromycin, will generally prove efficacious in a given patient. Metoclopramide is a dopamine antagonist that works on the stomach by facilitating acetylcholine release from enteric cholinergic neurons.[47] It may cause irreversible movement disorder if used more than 3 months and/or at high doses. Domperidone works on both the stomach and the intestine by facilitating acetylcholine release from the mesenteric plexus of the gut.[48] Erythromycin is a motilin agonist that works on both the stomach and intestine by binding to motilin receptors on GI smooth muscle.[49] One of these agents is usually sufficient to enhance gastric tone so that improved gastric emptying results. Intermittent oral antibiotic therapy may be helpful in treating bacterial overgrowth, with its attendant symptoms of bloating, flatulence, and diarrhea. Probiotics should be tried because alterations in gut microbiome are likely.

Surgery should be considered when chronic postoperative gastric stasis is severe and resistant to medical management. At operation small bowel obstruction and efferent limb obstruction should always be ruled out. Gastroparesis following vagotomy and drainage procedures may be treated with subtotal (75%) gastrectomy. Billroth II anastomosis with Braun enteroenterostomy (Fig. 62.6A) may be preferable to Roux-en-Y reconstruction after subtotal gastrectomy in this setting because Roux reconstruction may result in persistent gastric emptying problems (Roux syndrome) ultimately necessitating near-total or total gastrectomy, a nutritionally unattractive option. Delayed gastric emptying following vagotomy and

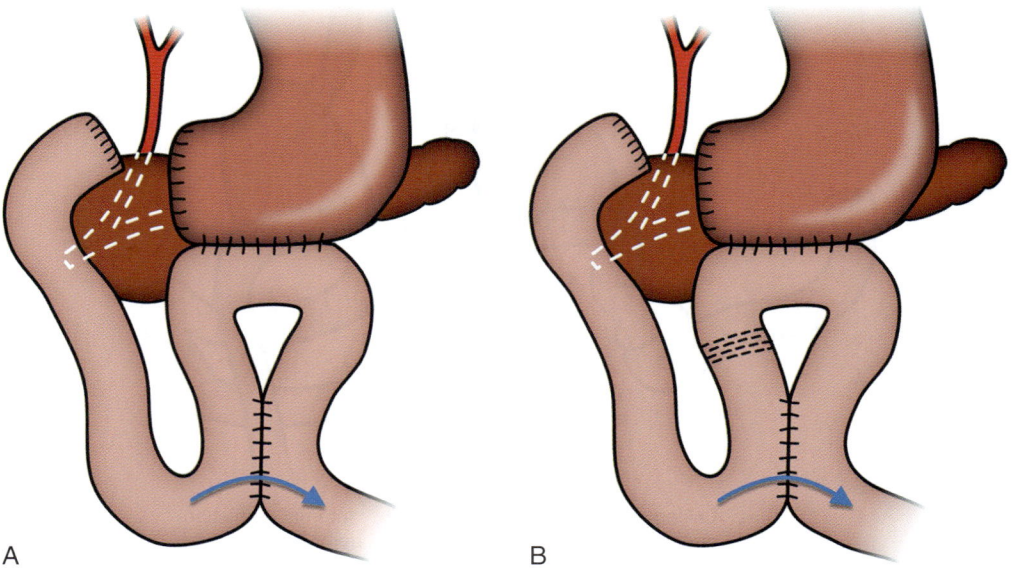

FIGURE 62.6 (A) The Braun procedure is one of the oldest attempts at bile diversion. The figure on the *left* shows the original procedure with Billroth II gastrojejunostomy and "downstream" enteroenterostomy to divert bile distally. (B) A more recent modification (on the *right*) adds a staple line distal to the enteroenterostomy in an effort to more completely divert the duodenal contents distally. It has been designated the "uncut" Roux-en-Y. (Modified from Madura JA. Postgastrectomy problems: remedial operations and therapy. In: Cameron JL, ed. *Current Surgical Therapy.* 7th ed. St. Louis: Mosby; 2001.)

drainage or vagotomy and antrectomy may represent an anastomotic stricture due to recurrent (marginal) ulcer, or proximal small bowel obstruction. Recurrent ulcer may respond to medical therapy with PPI and abstinence from nonsteroidal antiinflammatory drugs (NSAIDs), aspirin, and smoking. Endoscopic dilation is occasionally helpful. Gastroparesis following subtotal gastric resection is best treated with near-total (95%) or total gastric resection and Roux-en-Y reconstruction. High-frequency gastric electrical stimulation (GES) may be an effective treatment for patients with postsurgical gastroparesis who failed standard medical therapy,[50] but long-term follow-up and randomized controlled trials (RCTs) are lacking.

AFFERENT LOOP OBSTRUCTION

Afferent loop obstruction, also called afferent loop syndrome, is a mechanical complication that infrequently occurs following construction of a GJ. The creation of a GJ leaves a segment of proximal small bowel (duodenum and proximal jejunum) upstream from the anastomosis. With Billroth II or loop GJ the afferent limb conducts bile, pancreatic juices, and other proximal intestinal secretions toward the GJ[51]; with Roux-en-Y the afferent limb conducts the succus toward the jejunojejunostomy and is also called the biliopancreatic limb. The operations most commonly associated with afferent loop obstruction are Billroth II and Roux-en-Y GJ (distal gastrectomy or gastric bypass), and Roux-en-Y esophagojejunostomy (total gastrectomy).[52] The incidence of significant afferent loop obstruction after these procedures is low (0.3% to 1.0%) and is similar after open and laparoscopic surgery.

The etiologies of afferent loop obstruction include: (1) entrapment, compression, and kinking of the afferent loop by postoperative adhesions; (2) internal herniation, volvulus, and intussusception of the afferent loop; (3) scarring due to marginal ulceration of the GJ; (4) locoregional recurrence of cancer (lymph nodes, peritoneum, gastric remnant, anastomotic sites); (5) radiation enteritis of the afferent loop; and (6) enteroliths, bezoars, and foreign bodies impacted in the afferent loop (Fig. 62.7). In patients with Billroth II anastomoses, afferent loop syndrome is seen more commonly in patients with redundant (longer than 30 to 40 cm) and antecolic afferent loops, which are more prone to kinking, volvulus, and entrapment by adhesions. Improperly closed mesocolic defects may predispose to internal herniation of the retrocolic afferent limb.[53] In contrast, it is more common to find an obstruction or internal herniation of the Roux limb in the retrocolic retrogastric position than in the antecolic antegastric positioning after RYGBP. The role of closing the mesenteric defect remains unclear.[54]

Although both acute and chronic forms of afferent loop syndrome have been described, chronic partial obstruction is the more common clinical manifestation.[55] The classic presentation of chronic afferent loop syndrome is postprandial abdominal pain relieved by bilious vomiting, but the latter may be lacking with Roux-en-Y GJ.

A meal elicits pancreatic, biliary, and duodenal secretion into the obstructed afferent limb. As the volume of these secretions increases, the obstructed duodenum and proximal jejunum become more distended. Eventually the pressure in the partially obstructed afferent limb overcomes the obstruction (usually 30 to 60 minutes postprandially), delivering a large volume of bilious secretions into the stomach or Roux limb. This leads to bilious vomiting and prompt relief of the pain, which was caused by the afferent limb distention. Weight loss and anemia are common.

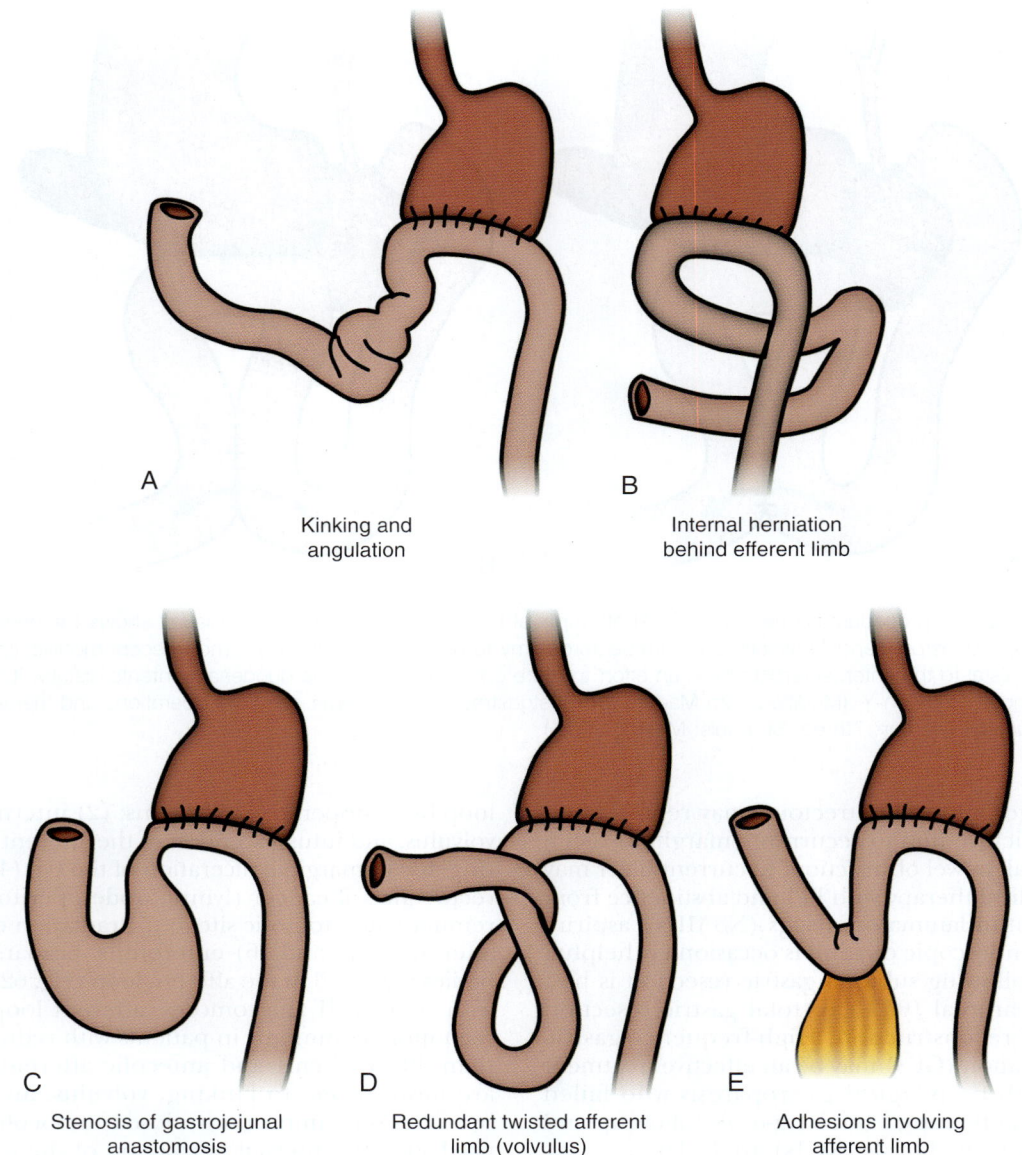

A

Kinking and
angulation

B

Internal herniation
behind efferent limb

C

Stenosis of gastrojejunal
anastomosis

D

Redundant twisted afferent
limb (volvulus)

E

Adhesions involving
afferent limb

FIGURE 62.7 Causes of afferent loop syndrome include (A) kinking and angulation of the afferent limb, (B) internal herniation of the afferent limb behind the efferent limb, (C) stenosis of the gastrojejunal anastomosis, (D) redundancy of the afferent limb leading to volvulus, or (E) adhesions involving the afferent limb. (Modified from Miller TA, Mercer DW. Derangements in gastric function secondary to previous surgery. In: Miller TA, ed. *Modern Surgical Care: Physiologic Foundations and Clinical Applications.* 2nd ed. St. Louis: Quality Medical; 1998:402.)

Bacterial overgrowth secondary to afferent limb stasis may contribute to these problems due to malabsorption of fat and other nutrients, such as vitamin B_{12} or iron.

If the obstruction is high grade or complete, the distended afferent loop may not sufficiently decompress. In this scenario, vomiting, if present, will be nonbilious, and a clinical picture of "closed loop obstruction" manifested as an acute abdomen will result. If this condition is not recognized early, the afferent loop may actually perforate and result in peritonitis. Urgent surgery is necessary to correct this problem.

Depending on the acuity and severity of the afferent loop obstruction, physical examination can reveal one or more of the following findings: weight loss, upper abdominal distention, upper abdominal mass, and abdominal tenderness. Peritoneal findings or pain out of proportion to physical findings are ominous. Rarely jaundice, cholangitis, or pancreatitis can confuse the clinical picture.

Abdominal multiple detector computed tomography (CT) is the diagnostic study of choice. CT appearance of the obstructed afferent loop consists of a C-shaped, fluid-filled tubular mass located in the midline between the abdominal aorta and the superior mesenteric artery (c-loop sign) with valvulae conniventes projecting into the lumen (keyboard sign).[56] Adhesions are suspected when a point of transition from a dilated to a normal-caliber loop is observed without other apparent cause. An internal hernia is suspected when crowding, stretching, and crossover of mesenteric vessels and the whirl sign are observed. Local recurrence and radiation enteritis are suspected when focal and diffuse bowel wall thickening are observed. Carcinomatosis is suspected when ascites and peritoneal enhancement are present and bowel wall thickening around the level of obstruction is absent.[57] Barium upper GI, contraindicated in patients with an acute abdomen, can be helpful in patients with chronic intermittent symptoms. Suggestive findings of afferent limb obstruction on this study include nonfilling of the afferent loop and/or retention of barium in the dilated afferent loop. However, these findings cannot be deemed conclusive because 20% of normal afferent loops are not filled after a barium meal. Although balloon dilation and/or stenting may be useful in special cases, the cornerstone of treatment for afferent loop obstruction in patients with curable cancer or benign disease is surgery. At operation the primary cause of afferent loop obstruction should be confirmed and treated. This may include resection for tumor or marginal ulcer, lysis of adhesions, or repair of internal hernia. Procedures to consider include addition of a Braun anastomosis in a former Billroth II reconstruction, excision of the redundant loop and conversion of Billroth II to Roux-en-Y GJ or Billroth I, and excision of the redundant loop and reconstruction of the former Roux-en-Y jejunojejunostomy (Fig. 62.8). Endoscopic interventions and percutaneous approaches (percutaneous endoscopic gastrostomy [PEG], balloon dilation, double-pigtail stents traversing the afferent loop strictured area) have an important role in the management of patients with stage IV cancer. These techniques may also be useful as temporizing measures in high-risk patients.

In contrast to the relatively stereotypical manifestation of afferent loop obstruction, efferent loop obstruction generally mimics proximal small bowel obstruction. It is most commonly caused by adhesions, but internal hernia must also be considered.

ALKALINE (BILE) REFLUX GASTRITIS

Alkaline reflux gastritis is presumably caused by the long-standing presence of an abnormal amount of duodenal content in the stomach or gastric remnant, a situation that often occurs in patients after pyloroplasty or loop GJ with or without gastric resection. A distinction must be made between *histologic* bile gastritis, which is present in many patients after gastric surgery (up to 85% in Billroth II patients), most of whom are asymptomatic, and the presence of *clinical* bile gastritis leading to significant symptoms, a much more unusual situation. Although both histologic and clinical bile gastritis can occur without previous gastric operation (primary bile reflux gastritis), it is much more common after gastric surgery. Histologic bile gastritis is more common after Billroth II (40% to 85%) than Billroth I anastomosis (29% to 48%) or gastric drainage operations (pyloroplasty or loop GJ, 15%). Rarely cholecystectomy is associated with the clinical syndrome,[58,59] possibly due to the loss of bile reservoir function, resulting in a continuous flow of bile into the duodenum with

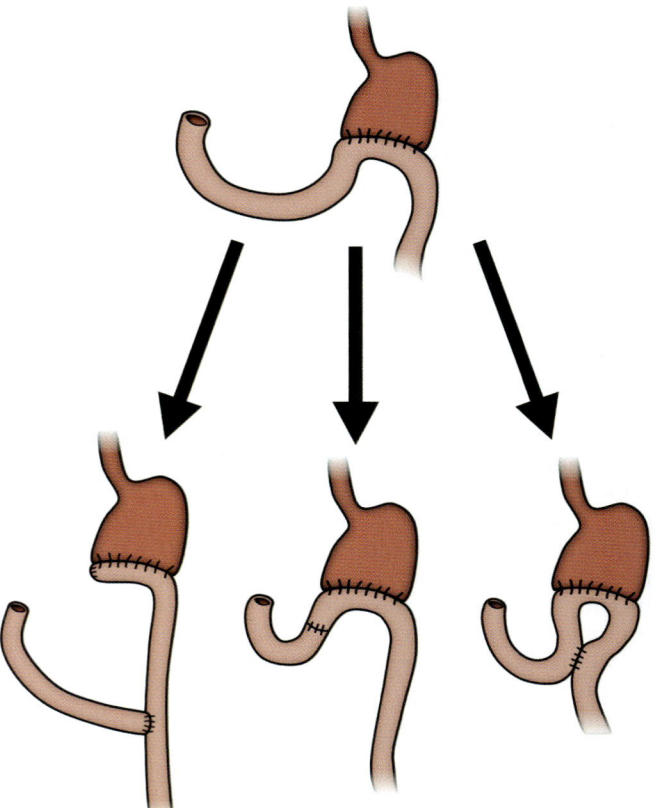

FIGURE 62.8 Surgical management of afferent loop syndrome. (From Miller TA, Mercer DW. Derangements in gastric function secondary to previous surgery. In: Miller TA, ed. *Modern Surgical Care: Physiologic Foundations and Clinical Applications*. 2nd ed. St. Louis: Quality Medical; 1998:404.)

the potential for duodenogastric reflux in the setting of pyloric dysfunction.[60,61] Postgastrectomy gastric stasis may potentiate the damaging effects of duodenal contents on the gastric mucosa. Smoking and NSAIDs also may contribute. The role of gastric acid in the pathophysiology of chronic bile gastritis is unclear. In laboratory models, luminal hydrochloric acid potentiates the mucosal damage caused by bile salts but acidic pH also inactivates pancreatic enzymes in duodenal refluxate. In a subset of patients, bile gastritis leads to dysplasia and some of these patients progress to gastric cancer ("stump cancer").

Clinically significant bile reflux gastritis is not common. Although many patients have histologic gastritis, the relationship of chronic gastric mucosal inflammation to symptoms in this setting is problematic. The most common symptoms attributed to chronic bile gastritis are abdominal pain and bilious vomiting. Although the surgeon can almost always eliminate bile from the vomitus, pain and vomiting may persist after remedial operation, particularly in patients on chronic narcotics preoperatively. The pain is midepigastric burning abdominal pain, often associated with nausea, and characteristically unrelieved by antacids or acid suppressive medication. Unlike afferent limb syndrome, the pain does not resolve after vomiting. Weight loss and anemia are common.

The diagnosis of alkaline reflux gastritis is essentially a diagnosis of exclusion and is largely based on symptomatology. The first step in patient evaluation is endoscopy. Inflammatory changes in the stomach involving more than just the peristomal area are suggestive of excessive enterogastric reflux.[62] Mucosal biopsies will show the characteristic histologic features of reflux: *foveolar hyperplasia, glandular cystic degeneration, edema of the lamina propria, and vasocongestion of the mucosal capillaries, all in association with minimal inflammatory cell infiltration.*[63] However, the endoscopic and histologic features of gastritis do not correlate well with the severity of symptoms.[61,63] These changes are frequently observed in asymptomatic patients and are therefore considered supportive but not specific. It is not possible to accurately evaluate the degree of reflux and the severity of symptoms by endoscopy. Upper GI barium study provides useful information regarding postoperative anatomy, stomach patency, size of the residual gastric pouch, and the status of the afferent and efferent limbs. Hepatobiliary iminodiacetic acid (HIDA) scans can provide a semiquantitative assessment of bile reflux/stasis in the stomach. Ultrasound and CT scanning may be useful to exclude pancreatic or biliary causes of symptoms.

Medical management has limited success in relieving symptoms. Suggested treatment modalities include the administration of cholestyramine, antacids, H_2 blockers, PPIs, sucralfate, or promotility agents to enhance clearance of refluxate from the gastric remnant. When these measures fail, surgery is considered for patients with incapacitating symptoms, a reasonably secure clinical diagnosis, and realistic expectations. Preoperative nutritional support may be required, and jejunostomy tube placement should be considered strongly during remedial operation, the aim of which is diversion of duodenal contents away from the stomach.

The Roux-en-Y GJ is the surgical reconstruction most frequently chosen to treat patients with alkaline reflux gastritis (Fig. 62.9).[41] Conversion of Billroth I or II to Roux-en-Y GJ with a 60-cm Roux limb reliably diverts intestinal contents from the gastric remnant and improves symptoms in up to 85% of patients.[61,62,65–67] This procedure also results in significant improvement of endoscopic findings.[68] Vagotomy at the time of reoperation may be considered to reduce the risk of marginal ulceration,[62] but chronic PPI might be equally efficacious and preferred given the gastric emptying issues seen with vagotomy. Although Roux-en-Y GJ achieves satisfactory symptom relief following surgery, during long-term follow-up epigastric pain can recur in up to 30% of patients.[62] The only symptom that is consistently relieved is bilious vomiting.

Other less commonly used procedures are the Henley operation (interposition of an isoperistaltic jejunal loop between residual stomach and intestine),[69] the Tanner 19 procedure, the biliary diversion,[60] and the suprapapillary duodenojejunostomy (duodenal switch).[70] The Roux-en-Y Tanner 19, which is a modification of the original Roux-en-Y GJ, has some theoretical advantages, but in clinical practice there is no evidence that the Tanner procedure is better than the classical Roux-en-Y reconstruction. The Henley procedure is an infrequently used technique for the management of alkaline reflux gastritis (Fig. 62.10). This technique was first described by Henley in 1952[71] as

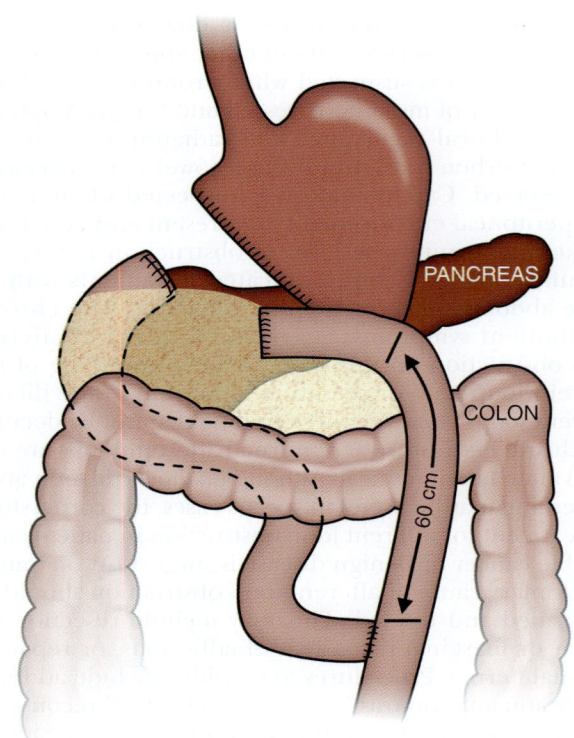

FIGURE 62.9 Roux-en-Y gastrojejunostomy for the treatment of alkaline reflux gastritis. Note the generous distal gastrectomy. Adequate Roux length minimizes bile reflux. (From Fromm D. Ulceration of the stomach and duodenum. In: Fromm D, ed. *Gastrointestinal Surgery*. New York: Churchill Livingstone; 1985.)

a gastrojejunoduodenostomy (i.e., isoperistaltic jejunal interposition between the gastric remnant and the duodenum following revision of prior Billroth I or II). The jejunal segment should be approximately 40 cm in length to minimize enterogastric reflux. Reported advantages of the Henley procedure include the duodenal passage of chyme, with the possibility of improving mixing and synchronization of pancreaticobiliary secretion, as well as improved iron and nutrient absorption, and the theoretical avoidance of peristaltic dyskinesis and the stasis syndrome.[69] Although this method achieved satisfactory results in up to 70% of patients,[69,72] most authors prefer the Roux-en-Y GJ because of its technical simplicity.[67]

Other procedures described for the management of alkaline reflux gastritis are the biliary diversion and the suprapapillary duodenojejunostomy. During biliary diversion, previous gastric procedures are converted to a gastroduodenal anastomosis (a Billroth I configuration). All patients then undergo a choledochojejunostomy with a 35- to 40-cm newly created or preexisting Roux-en-Y limb. Biliary diversion achieves complete elimination of bile salts from the gastric/duodenal lumen by the choledochojejunostomy, and therefore symptoms associated with enterogastric reflux are alleviated.[60]

The suprapapillary duodenojejunostomy—the so-called duodenal switch—proposed by DeMeester et al.[73] achieved good results without altering gastric emptying[70,74] in patients with primary bile reflux gastritis, a rare entity (Fig. 62.11).

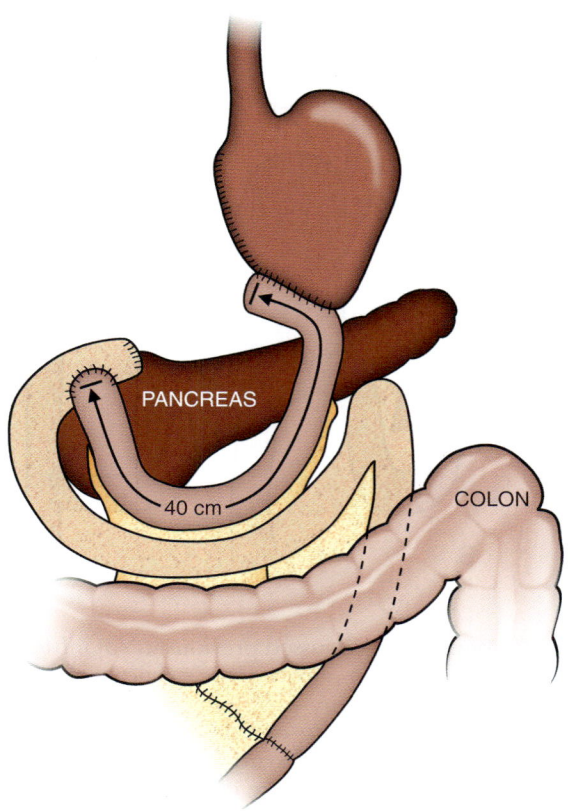

FIGURE 62.10 Interposition of a 40-cm isoperistaltic jejunal segment between the stomach and duodenum to treat alkaline reflux gastritis (Henley loop). (From Aronow JS, Matthews JB, Garcia-Aquilar J, Novak G, Silen W. Isoperistaltic jejunal interposition for intractable postgastrectomy alkaline reflux gastritis. *J Am Coll Surg.* 1995;180:648.)

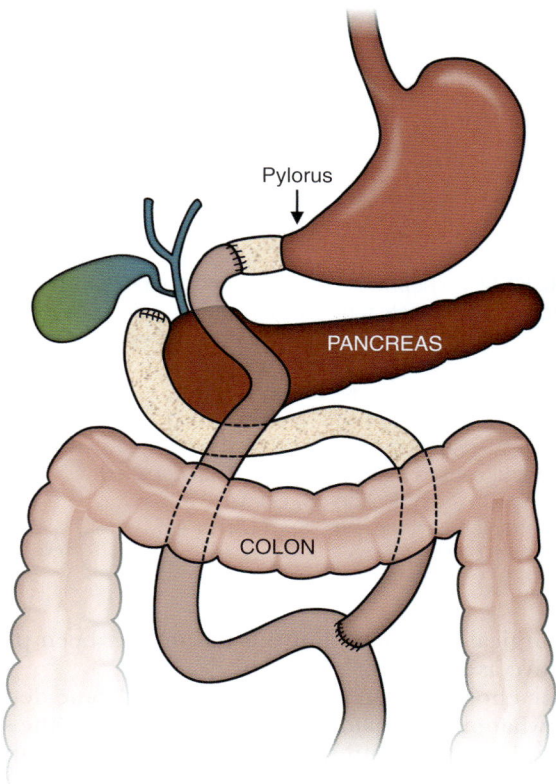

FIGURE 62.11 Duodenal switch procedure as described by Demeester et al. as a treatment for primary bile reflux gastritis. The postbulbar duodenum is divided and a 60-cm retrocolic Roux limb is anastomosed to the proximal duodenum. (Modified from Strignano P, Collard JM, Michel JM, et al. Duodenal switch operation for pathologic transpyloric duodenogastric reflux. *Ann Surg.* 2007;245:247–253.)

Advantages of the technique include the avoidance of extensive tissue dissection and the maintenance of the normal gastric reservoir and normal foregut physiology. It may be prudent to add proximal gastric vagotomy or chronic PPI treatment to minimize the risk of marginal ulcer with duodenal switch for primary bile gastritis. In summary, remedial gastric surgery can be effective in ameliorating symptoms of bile reflux gastritis in the majority of patients, but careful patient selection is essential to achieve satisfactory results.

ROUX STASIS SYNDROME

After distal gastrectomy with Roux-en-Y reconstruction, some patients experience symptomatic delayed gastric emptying of solids. This phenomenon has been termed the *Roux syndrome* or *Roux stasis syndrome* because it has generally been attributed to measurable abnormalities in Roux limb motility. Peristalsis is abnormal in a Roux limb, with a significant number of propulsive contractile waves proceeding in the proximal direction (i.e., toward the stomach). Presumably this slows gastric emptying, particularly solid emptying. Interestingly, Roux syndrome is more common in the presence of a large gastric remnant or after vagotomy and quite uncommon after RYGBP.

Preoperative delayed gastric emptying is also a risk factor. These clinical observations suggest that the gastric pouch plays a significant role in the etiology of the Roux syndrome, and these factors undoubtedly account for the reported variability in the incidence of this problem.[75] When performing a distal gastrectomy, the surgeon should be cognizant of the factors that predispose to Roux syndrome.

Symptoms of Roux syndrome include abdominal pain and distention, postprandial bloating, nausea, and vomiting.[76] Typically the vomitus contains solid food and is nonbilious. Bacterial overgrowth, with diarrhea and nutrient malabsorption, may result. Endoscopically, the gastric remnant may be dilated with retained food and mucosal irritation. The anastomosis is patent and the Roux limb may also be dilated. There is no evidence of mechanical obstruction on CT or upper GI series. Scintigraphy shows markedly delayed emptying of solids. Liquid emptying is usually not delayed.

Most patients with the Roux syndrome can be successfully managed conservatively with dietary manipulations and use of prokinetic agents,[77] but some patients require revisional operation in an attempt to relieve debilitating symptoms and improve nutritional status. Pacing of the intestine and/or stomach has been investigated as potential

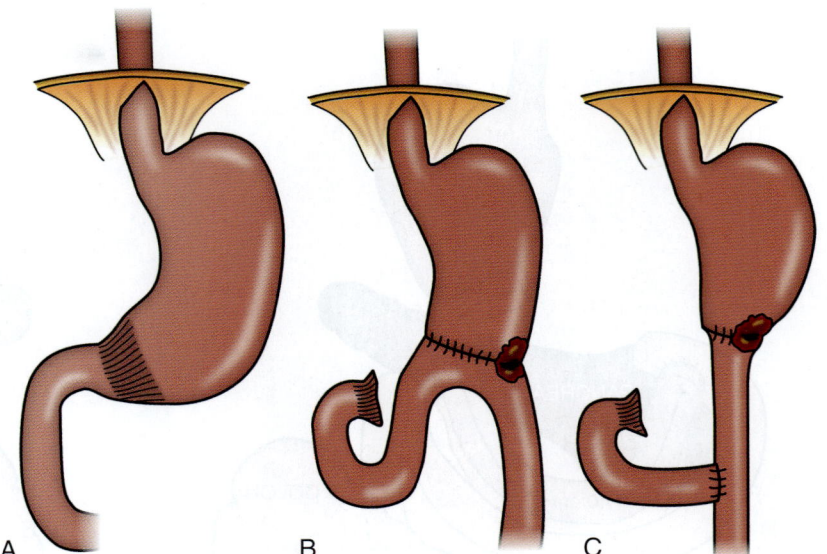

FIGURE 62.12 Pathophysiology of retained antrum syndrome. (A) Normal stomach with antrum. A segment of incompletely resected antrum bathed in the alkaline environment of the adjoined duodenum during distal gastrectomy with (B) Billroth II or (C) Roux-en-Y reconstruction results in intense gastrin secretion by the retained antrum and causes marginal ulceration as depicted in (B) and (C). (From Bolton JS, Corway WC, Postgastrectomy syndromes. *Surg Clin N Am.* 2011;91:1105–1122.)

nonsurgical treatment, but this has not yet been proven effective as long-term treatment.[78]

The choice of operation for Roux syndrome depends somewhat on the anatomy of the gastric pouch, the status of the Roux limb, and the condition of the patient. The addition of a feeding jejunostomy is usually prudent. In general, if the original gastrectomy removed less than half the stomach, consideration can be given to subtotal gastrectomy with anastomosis to a new Roux limb (usually the original Roux should be resected), or with B2 reconstruction and Braun enteroenterostomy. However, bile reflux gastritis and esophagitis remain a risk with the latter procedure. Although the addition of a "TA" staple line in the afferent limb distal to the Braun anastomosis and proximal to the B2 GJ preserves normal small bowel motility in the efferent limb and eliminates bile from the stomach (the "uncut Roux" procedure [see Fig. 62.6B]), the latter effect is transient because the staple line inevitably opens up.[79–81]

If the original gastrectomy removed more than half the stomach, consideration should be given to total gastrectomy with Roux reconstruction. In this setting, if the left gastric artery is intact, equally good results might be achieved with 95% gastrectomy, leaving a small, vertically oriented lesser curvature gastric pouch analogous to that used for the Roux-en-Y gastric bypass bariatric procedure. A small, horizontally oriented residual gastric pouch should be avoided because of the potential for dilation and stasis. Since the frequency of Roux stasis symptoms may be higher when Roux-en-Y limbs are longer, the Roux should be limited to 50 cm long in revisional operation for Roux syndrome.[62,68,79,80]

MARGINAL ULCERS

Marginal ulceration (i.e., juxtaanastomotic ulceration) is a well-described complication of GJ. Although not typically considered as one of the postgastrectomy syndromes, it is not uncommon and thus must be considered as part of the differential diagnosis for many of the more

traditional syndromes discussed previously. Not infrequently it contributes to the complexity of the surgical management of these postgastrectomy problems. For example, it is not unusual to find acute or chronic ulceration when operating for afferent loop syndrome, bile gastritis, and Roux syndrome. The incidence of marginal ulcer ranges from 0.6% to 25%. It is more common after Roux-en-Y anastomosis (Fig. 62.12C) than after Billroth II (see Fig. 62.12B) because the former arrangement lacks the buffering afferent limb contents that counteract the noxious effect of gastric acid on the jejunal mucosa (usually the ulceration is on the jejunal side of the anastomosis). Chronic ischemia and permanent suture material may also be contributing factors. NSAIDs (including aspirin) and smoking predispose to marginal ulcer. Incomplete vagotomy, *Helicobacter* infection, and hypergastrinemia must also be considered.[81,82] Presentation may be acute (usually perforation) or chronic. Symptoms include abdominal pain, vomiting, and various signs and symptoms of chronic or acute blood loss. In most cases, marginal ulcers can be adequately treated with PPIs, the elimination of NSAIDs, *Helicobacter* treatment, and smoking cessation.

If medical treatment fails and if incomplete vagotomy is diagnosed by history or the sham feeding pancreatic polypeptide test, thoracoscopic truncal vagotomy may be an option.[83] Hypergastrinemia after distal gastrectomy can be caused by gastrinoma or retained antrum. In the latter there is residual antral tissue left in continuity with the duodenal stump after gastric resection with Billroth II anastomosis. The G cells in this retained antral tissue are not exposed to luminal acid, resulting in continuous secretion of gastrin and intense stimulation of acid production by parietal cells in the proximal gastric remnant. The exposure of the unbuffered jejunum to this high acid level at the Billroth II GJ results in marginal ulcer (see Fig. 62.12B). Clinical suspicion of retained antrum may be confirmed by review of previous operative and pathology reports, barium upper GI study, and/or technetium 99m scan. Reexcision is curative. Gastrinoma is suspected when secretin infusion leads to significant further elevation of gastrin level. CT, endoscopic ultrasound (EUS), and octreotide scan may be helpful, but exploration by an experienced surgeon is the best way to find the tumor(s) if operation is indicated.

After operation for marginal ulcer, eventual recurrence is almost inevitable if both smoking and NSAIDs cannot be eliminated. Vagotomy and/or lifelong PPI should also be considered, as well as empiric *Helicobacter* treatment.[84–96]

GALLSTONES

Gallstone formation following gastric surgery is not uncommon. It occurs in 10% to 20% of patients and typically presents within 3 years after surgery.[97] The pathophysiology of increased gallstone formation after gastrectomy is not completely clear. The type of gastrectomy, the extent of lymph node dissection, and the method of digestive reconstruction seem to influence the rate of postgastrectomy gallstone formation. Vagal denervation is the most thoroughly studied mechanism. Denervation of the gallbladder can occur through truncal vagotomy or selective division of the hepatic branches of the left vagus. Also, nodal dissection can lead to transection of the nerves controlling gallbladder motility. This may explain the higher risk and earlier occurrence of gallstone formation after total gastrectomy than after distal gastrectomy[98] and after extended lymphadenectomy compared to more limited perigastric lymphadenectomy.[86,98] Other factors that affect gallstone formation include changes in the secretions of gut hormones, including cholecystokinin (CCK). The exclusion of food passage through the duodenum after Roux-en-Y reconstruction results in decreased secretion of CCK with a resultant decrease in gallbladder motility, which explains the higher incidence of stone formation when Roux-en-Y reconstruction is performed.[98] Other contributing factors include weight loss, leading to mobilization of cholesterol stores and supersaturation of biliary cholesterol, and the presence of edema or inflammation around the bile ducts with resultant biliary stasis.[100–102]

Following gastrectomy for cancer, 25% of patients will develop cholelithiasis within 2 years[100] and 6% will ultimately undergo cholecystectomy for symptoms.[103] It is more likely to occur after radical gastrectomy (30%) than after simple gastrectomy (5%).[104] A Roux-en-Y reconstruction increases the risk of gallstone development compared with techniques that do not exclude the duodenum (28%).[86,98,105,106] In the first 2 years after gastric bypass, the risk of cholelithiasis rises to 5.8 times that of the general population. Of note, the incidence of cholelithiasis in the obese female patient is as high as 21% to 38%.[107] Gastric bypass with Roux-en-Y GJ is intrinsically more lithogenic than adjustable gastric banding.[108] The incidence of gallstones after sleeve gastrectomy has not been well studied but seems to be similar to that after gastric bypass.[109] For all types of bariatric surgery, the rapid rate of weight loss[110] and the extent of the weight loss[111,112] lead to the development of cholesterol stones in supersaturated bile.

There is currently no consensus regarding the need for prophylactic cholecystectomy during gastric operation. Although routine incidental cholecystectomy is unwise, cholecystectomy may be considered if preoperative or intraoperative evaluation reveals sludge, gallstones, or an abnormal gallbladder, especially if subsequent cholecystectomy is likely to be difficult. Unless the gallbladder is symptomatic, prophylactic cholecystectomy should only be considered if it is likely to be straightforward and the gastric operation has gone well. Studies have shown that the morbidity of cholecystectomy performed concurrently with upper abdominal surgery is higher than that of cholecystectomy alone performed at a subsequent intervention. In addition, the results of controlled studies and meta-analyses comparing prophylactic cholecystectomy to no cholecystectomy remain inconclusive.

NUTRITIONAL ABNORMALITIES

WEIGHT LOSS

Weight loss is common in patients who have had a gastric operation for tumor or ulcer. The degree of weight loss tends to parallel the magnitude of the operation. It may be insignificant in the large person or devastating in the asthenic female. The surgeon should always consider the possible nutritional consequences before performing a gastric resection for benign disease in a thin female. The causes of weight loss after gastric surgery generally fall into one of two categories: altered dietary intake or malabsorption. Chronic nausea, vomiting, and/or pain frequently lead to decreased food consumption and/or change in meal composition. Postoperative "blind loops" can lead to bacterial overgrowth and alteration in the small bowel (resection and/or Roux limb) can decrease absorptive surface area, both leading to malabsorption of protein, fat, and vitamins.

Chronic postgastrectomy weight loss is most likely due to decreased intake if a stool stain for fecal fat is negative. This is the most common cause of weight loss after gastric surgery and may be due to a combination of specific factors such as small gastric pouch, postoperative gastric stasis, anorexia due to loss of ghrelin, or self-imposed dietary modification because of symptoms. If bacterial overgrowth is suspected, a lactulose breath test and/or trial of oral antibiotics or probiotics should be considered. Consultation with an experienced dietitian may prove invaluable. Prolonged enteral or parenteral nutritional support may be necessary in the worse cases.

ANEMIA

Anemia is a common finding in postgastrectomy patients, occurring in up to one-third of patients. This is generally secondary to nutrient malabsorption but can also be caused by decreased nutrient intake or chronic blood loss due to ulcer, tumor, or mucosal inflammation. Iron, vitamin B_{12}, and folate deficiencies are the most common cause of chronic nutritional anemia after gastric surgery. Iron absorption takes place primarily in the duodenum and proximal jejunum and is facilitated by an acidic environment in the stomach. Intrinsic factor, essential for the enteric absorption of vitamin B_{12}, is made by the parietal cells of the stomach. Vitamin B_{12} bioavailability also is facilitated by an acidic gastric environment. Folate-rich foods (e.g., green leafy vegetables, fresh fruit, enriched bread) may be problematic in patients with a small or hypomotile gastric pouch.

With this as background, it is easy to understand why many patients who have had a gastric operation are at risk for anemia. Iron deficiency is the most common cause of anemia after gastric surgery, but vitamin B_{12} and/or folate deficiency are common. Although patients who have had a total gastrectomy will all develop life-threatening B_{12} deficiency without supplemental B_{12}, it may be prudent to monitor all patients after gastric operation for these three nutrient deficiencies. Routine supplementation with oral iron, oral folic acid, and oral or parenteral B_{12} should be done after gastric bypass and total gastrectomy.

CHRONIC CALCIUM DEFICIT AND OSTEOPOROSIS

Chronic calcium deficit and osteoporosis may occur after gastric operation. Calcium absorption occurs primarily in the duodenum, so any gastric operation that diverts the food stream away from the duodenum will disturb calcium homeostasis. This includes simple GJ, distal gastrectomy with Billroth II, and Roux-en-Y GJ (including gastric bypass) or Roux-en-Y esophagojejunostomy. Furthermore, any gastric procedure that predisposes to bacterial overgrowth or inadequate mixing of food and digestive enzymes may interfere with the absorption of fat-soluble vitamins, including vitamin D. Thus it is likely that both calcium and vitamin D malabsorption contribute to metabolic bone disease in patients following gastric surgery. The problems usually manifest as pain and/or fractures years after the index operation. Musculoskeletal symptoms should prompt a study of bone density. Oral calcium and vitamin D supplementation may be useful in preventing these complications and should be considered in all patients in whom the duodenum is bypassed. Routine skeletal monitoring of high-risk patients (women > 50 years, men > 65 years, smokers, fracture history) may prove useful in identifying early reversible skeletal deterioration.

REFERENCES

1. Kitagawa Y, Dempsey DT, et al. Stomach. In: Brunicardi FC, Andersen DK, Billiar TR, eds. *Schwartz's Principles of Surgery*. New York: Mc Graw Hill; 2015.
2. Dempsey DT. Reoperative gastric surgery and postgastrectomy syndromes. In: Zuidema GD, Yeo CJ, eds. *Shackleford's Surgery of the Alimentary Tract*. Philadelphia, PA: Saunders; 2002:161.
3. Meilahn JE, Dempsey D. Postgastrectomy problems: remedial operations and therapy. In: Cameron JL, ed. *Current Surgical Therapy*. Phladelphia, PA: Elsevier Mosby; 2004.
4. Gustavsson S, Kelly KA, Melton LJ 3rd, Zinsmeister AR. Trends in peptic ulcer surgery. A population based study in Rochester, Minnesota, 1956–1985. *Gastroenterology*. 1988;94(3):688-694.
5. Bardhan KD, Royston C. Time, change and peptic ulcer disease in Rotherham, UK. *Dig Liver Dis*. 2008;40(7):540-546.
6. Wainess RM, Dimick JB, Upchurch GR Jr, Cowan JA, Mulholland MW. Epidemiology of surgically treated gastric cancer in the United States, 1988–2000. *J Gastrointest Surg*. 2003;7(7):879-883.
7. Pedrazzani C, Marrelli D, Rampone B, et al. Postoperative complications and functional results after subtotal gastrectomy with Billroth II reconstruction for primary gastric cancer. *Dig Dis Sci*. 2007;52(8):1757-1763.
8. Le Blanc-Louvry I, Savoye G, Maillot C, Denis P, Ducrotté P. An impaired accommodation of the proximal stomach to a meal is associated with symptoms after distal gastrectomy. *Am J Gastroenterol*. 2003;98(12):2642-2647.
9. Abrahamsson H, Jansson G. Vago-vagal gastro-gastric relaxation in the cat. *Acta Physiol Scand*. 1973;88(3):289-295.
10. Abell TL, Minocha A. Gastrointestinal complications of bariatric surgery: diagnosis and therapy. *Am J Med Sci*. 2006;331(4):214-218.
11. Mine S, Sano T, Tsutsumi K, et al. Large-scale investigation into dumping syndrome after gastrectomy for gastric cancer. *J Am Coll Surg*. 2010;211(5):628-636.
12. Tack J, Arts J, Caenepeel P, De Wulf D, Bisschops R. Pathophysiology, diagnosis and management of postoperative dumping syndrome. *Nat Rev Gastroenterol Hepatol*. 2009;6(10):583-590.
13. Arts J, Caenepeel P, Bisschops R, et al. Efficacy of the long-acting repeatable formulation of the somatostatin analogue octreotide in postoperative dumping. *Clin Gastroenterol Hepatol*. 2009;7(4):432-437.
14. Berg P, Hall M, McCallum RW, Sarosiek I. Dumping syndrome: updated perspectives on etiologies and diagnosis. *Pract Gastroenterol*. 2014;38:30-38.
15. Behrns KE, Sarr M. Diagnosis and management of gastric emptying disorders. *Adv Surg*. 1994;27:233-255.
16. Gulsrud PO, Taylor IL, Watts HD, Cohen MB, Elashoff J, Meyer JH. How gastric emptying of carbohydrate affects glucose tolerance and symptoms after truncal vagotomy with pyloroplasty. *Gastroenterology*. 1980;78:1463-1471.
17. Lipsitz LA, Ryan SM, Parker JA, Freeman R, Wei JY, Goldberger AL. Hemodynamic and autonomic nervous system responses to mixed meal ingestion in healthy young and old subjects and dysautonomic patients with postprandial hypotension. *Circulation*. 1993;87(2):391.
18. Yamamoto H, Mori T, Tsuchihashi H, Akabori H, Naito H, Tani T. A possible role of GLP-1 in the pathophysiology of early dumping syndrome. *Dig Dis Sci*. 2005;50(12):2263-2267.
19. Ukleja A. Dumping syndrome: pathophysiology and treatment. *Nutr Clin Pract*. 2005;20(5):517-525.
20. van der Kleij FG, Vecht J, Lamers CB, Masclee AA. Diagnostic value of dumping provocation in patients after gastric surgery. *Scand J Gastroenterol*. 1996;31(12):1162-1166.
21. Papamargaritis D, Koukoulis G, Sioka E, et al. Dumping symptoms and incidence of hypoglycaemia after provocation test at 6 and 12 months after laparoscopic sleeve gastrectomy. *Obes Surg*. 2012;22(10):1600-1606.
22. Ramadan M, Loureiro M, Laughlan K, et al. Risk of dumping syndrome after sleeve gastrectomy and Roux-en-Y gastric bypass: early results of a multicentre prospective study. *Gastroenterol Res Pract*. 2016;2016:2570237.
23. Deleted in review.
24. Berg P, McCallum R. Dumping syndrome: a review of the current concepts of pathophysiology, diagnosis, and treatment. *Dig Dis Sci*. 2016;61(1):11-18.
25. Hejazi RA, Patil H, McCallum RW. Dumping syndrome: establishing criteria for diagnosis and identifying new etiologies. *Dig Dis Sci*. 2010;55(1):117-123.
26. Didden P, Penning C, Masclee AA. Octreotide therapy in dumping syndrome: analysis of long-term results. *Aliment Pharmacol Ther*. 2006;24(9):1367-1375.
27. Leeds AR, Ralphs DN, Ebied F, Metz G, Dilawari JB. Pectin in the dumping syndrome: reduction of symptoms and plasma volume changes. *Lancet*. 1981;317(8229):1075-1078.
28. Imhof A, Schneemann M, Schaffner A, Brändle M. Reactive hypoglycaemia due to late dumping syndrome: successful treatment with acarbose. *Swiss Med Wkly*. 2001;131(5-6):81-83.
29. Yamada M, Ohrui T, Asada M, et al. Acarbose attenuates hypoglycemia from dumping syndrome in an elderly man with gastrectomy. *J Am Geriatr Soc*. 2005;53(2):358-359.
30. De Cunto A, Barbi E, Minen F, Ventura A. Safety and efficacy of high-dose acarbose treatment for dumping syndrome. *J Pediatr Gastroenterol Nutr*. 2011;53(1):113-114.
31. Hasegawa T, Yoneda M, Nakamura K, et al. Long-term effect of α-glucosidase inhibitor on late dumping syndrome. *J Gastroenterol Hepatol*. 1998;13(12):1201-1206.
32. Deleted in review.
33. Parrish CR. The clinician's guide to short bowel syndrome. *Pract Gastroenterol*. 2005;29:67.
34. Berg P, Hall M, Sarosiek I, McCallum RW. Understanding the etiologies, clinical spectrum, and diagnostic challenge of dumping syndrome. *Gastroenterology*. 2013;144:S-734.

35. Thondam SK, Nair S, Wile D, Gill GV. Diazoxide for the treatment of hypoglycaemic dumping syndrome. *QJM.* 2013;106(9):855.

36. Spanakis E, Gragnoli C. Successful medical management of status post-Roux-en-Y- gastric-bypass hyperinsulinemic hypoglycemia. *Obes Surg.* 2009;19(9):1333-1334.

37. Li-Ling J, Irving M. Therapeutic value of octreotide for patients with severe dumping syndrome—a review of randomised controlled trials. *Postgrad Med J.* 2001;77:441-442.

38. Hasler WL, Soudah HC, Owyang C. Mechanisms by which octreotide ameliorates symptoms in the dumping syndrome. *J Pharmacol Exp Ther.* 1996;277(3):1359.

39. Vecht J, Lamers CB, Masclee AA. Long-term results of octreotide-therapy in severe dumping syndrome. *Clin Endocrinol (Oxf).* 1999;51(5):619-624.

40. Richards WO, Golzarian J, Wasudev N, Sawyers JL. Reverse phasic contractions are present in antiperistaltic jejunal limbs up to twenty-one years postoperatively. *J Am Coll Surg.* 1994;178(6):557-563.

41. Sawyers JL, Herrington JL Jr. Superiority of antiperistaltic jejunal segments in management of severe dumping syndrome. *Ann Surg.* 1973;178(3):311-319.

42. Nunobe S, Sasako M, Saka M, Fukagawa T, Katai H, Sano T. Symptom evaluation of long-term postoperative outcomes after pylorus-preserving gastrectomy for early gastric cancer. *Gastric Cancer.* 2007;10(3):167-172.

43. Ishikawa K, Arita T, Ninomiya S, Bandoh T, Shiraishi N, Kitano S. Outcome of segmental gastrectomy versus distal gastrectomy for early gastric cancer. *World J Surg.* 2007;31(11):2204-2207.

44. Katsube T, Konno S, Murayama M, et al. Gastric emptying after pylorus-preserving gastrectomy: assessment using the 13C-acetic acid breath test. *Hepatogastroenterology.* 2007;54(74):639-642.

45. Duncombe VM, Bolin TD, Davis AE. Double-blind trial of cholestyramine in post-vagotomy diarrhoea. *Gut.* 1977;18(7):531-535.

46. Forstner-Barthell AW, Murr MM, Nitecki S, et al. Near-total completion gastrectomy for severe postvagotomy gastric stasis: analysis of early and long-term results in 62 patients. *J Gastrointest Surg.* 1999;3(1):15-21 [discussion 21–23].

47. McClelland RN, Horton JW. Relief of acute, persistent postvagotomy atony by metoclopramide. *Ann Surg.* 1978;188(4):439-447.

48. Davis RH, Clench MH, Mathias JR. Effects of domperidone in patients with chronic unexplained upper gastrointestinal symptoms: a double-blind, placebo-controlled study. *Dig Dis Sci.* 1988;33(12):1505-1511.

49. Tack J, Janssens J, Vantrappen G, et al. Effect of erythromycin on gastric motility in controls and in diabetic gastroparesis. *Gastroenterology.* 1992;103(1):72-79.

50. McCallum R, Lin Z, Wetzel P, Sarosiek I, Forster J. Clinical response to gastric electrical stimulation in patients with postsurgical gastroparesis. *Clin Gastroenterol Hepatol.* 2005;3(1):49-54.

51. Woodfield CA, Levine MS. The postoperative stomach. *Eur J Radiol.* 2005;53(3):341-352.

52. Bolton JS, Conway WC 2nd. Postgastrectomy syndromes. *Surg Clin North Am.* 2011;91(5):1105-1122.

53. Kimura H, Ishikawa M, Nabae T, et al. Internal hernia after laparoscopic gastrectomy with Roux-en-Y reconstruction for gastric cancer. *Asian J Surg.* 2017;40(3):203-209.

54. Al Harakeh AB, Kallies KJ, Borgert AJ, Kothari SN. Bowel obstruction rates in antecolic/antegastric versus retrocolic/retrogastric Roux limb gastric bypass: a meta-analysis. *Surg Obes Relat Dis.* 2016;12(1):194-198.

55. Mitty WF Jr, Grossi C, Nealon TF Jr. Chronic afferent loop syndrome. *Ann Surg.* 1970;172(6):996-1001.

56. Zissin R. CT findings of afferent loop syndrome after a subtotal gastrectomy with Roux-en-Y reconstruction. *Emerg Radiol.* 2004;10(4):201-203.

57. Zissin R, Osadchy A, Gayer G. Abdominal CT findings of delayed postoperative complications. *Can Assoc Radiol J.* 2007;58:200-211.

58. Perdikis G, Wilson P, Hinder R, et al. Altered antroduodenal motility after cholecystectomy. *Am J Surg.* 1994;168(6):609-615.

59. Hubens A, Van de Kelft E, Roland J. The influence of cholecystectomy on the duodenogastric reflux of bile. *Hepatogastroenterology.* 1989;36(5):384-389.

60. Madura JA, Grosfeld JL. Biliary diversion: a new method to prevent enterogastric reflux and reverse the roux stasis syndrome. *Arch Surg.* 1997;132(3):245-249.

61. Ritchie WP. Alkaline reflux gastritis: a critical reappraisal. *Gut.* 1984;25(9):975-987.

62. Ritchie WP. Alkaline reflux gastritis. *Gastroenterol Clin North Am.* 1994;23:281-294.

63. Dixon MF, O'Connor HJ, Axon AT, King RF, Johnston D. Reflux gastritis: distinct histopathological entity? *J Clin Pathol.* 1986;39(5):524-530.

64. Deleted in review.

65. Davidson ED, Herish T. The surgical treatment of bile reflux gastritis. *Ann Surg.* 1986;192:175-187.

66. Ritchie WP Jr, Dempsey DT. Postgastrectomy syndromes. In: Moody FG, ed. *Surgical Treatment of Digestive Disease.* Chicago: Year Book Medical Publishers; 1990:236-248.

67. Cabrol J, Navarro X, Sancho J, Simo-Deu J, Segura R. Bile reflux in postoperative alkaline reflux gastritis. *Ann Surg.* 1990;211(2):239-243.

68. McAlhany JC, Hanover TM, Taylor SM, Sticca RP, Ashmore JD Jr. Long-term follow-up of patients with Roux-en-Y gastrojejunostomy for gastric disease. *Ann Surg.* 1994;219(5):451-457.

69. Aranow JS, Matthews JB, Garcia-Aguilar J, Novak G, Silen W. Isoperistaltic jejunal interposition for intractable postgastrectomy alkaline reflux gastritis. *J Am Coll Surg.* 1995;180(6):648-653.

70. Klingler PJ, Perdikis G, Wilson P, Hinder RA. Indications, technical modalities and results of the duodenal switch operation for pathologic duodenogastric reflux. *Hepatogastroenterology.* 1999;46(25):97-102.

71. Henley FA, Hudson RV. Gastrectomy with replacement. A preliminary communication with an introduction. *Br J Surg.* 1952;40(160):118-128.

72. Herrington JL, Sawyers JL, Whitehead WA. Surgical management of reflux gastritis. *Ann Surg.* 1974;180(4):526-535.

73. DeMeester TR, Fuchs KH, Ball CS, Albertucci M, Smyrk TC, Marcus JN. Experimental and clinical results with proximal end-to-end duodenojejunostomy for pathologic duodenogastric reflux. *Ann Surg.* 1987;206(4):414-426.

74. Hinder RA. Duodenal switch: a new form of pancreaticobiliary diversion. *Surg Clin North Am.* 1992;72(2):487-499.

75. Kojima K, Yamada H, Inokuchi M, Kawano T, Sugihara K. A comparison of Roux-en-Y and Billroth-I reconstruction after laparoscopy-assisted distal gastrectomy. *Ann Surg.* 2008;247(6):962-967.

76. Miedema BW, Kelly KA. The Roux stasis syndrome: treatment by pacing and prevention by use of an uncut Roux limb. *Arch Surg.* 1992;127(3):295-300.

77. Janssens J, Peeters TL, Vantrappen G, et al. Improvement of gastric emptying in diabetic gastroparesis by erythromycin. *N Engl J Med.* 1990;322(15):1028-1031.

78. Verne GN, Sninsky CA. Chronic intestinal pseudo-obstruction. *Dig Dis.* 1995;13(3):163-181.

79. Le Blanc-Louvry IL, Ducrotté P, Lemeland JF, Metayer J, Denis P, Ténière P. Motility in the Roux-Y limb after distal gastrectomy: relation to the length of the limb and the afferent duodenojejunal segment—an experimental study. *Neurogastroenterol Motil.* 1999;11(5):365-374.

80. Hinder RA, Esser J, DeMeester TR. Management of gastric emptying disorders following the Roux-en-Y procedure. *Surgery.* 1988;104(4):765-772.

81. Turnage RH, Sarosi G, Cryer B, Spechler S, Peterson W, Feldman M. Evaluation and management of patients with recurrent peptic ulcer disease after acid-reducing operations: a systematic review. *J Gastrointest Surg.* 2003;7(5):606-626.

82. Gurusamy KS, Pallari E. Medical versus surgical treatment for refractory or recurrent peptic ulcer. *Cochrane Database Syst Rev.* 2016;(3):CD011523.

83. Ingvar C, Adami HO, Enander LK, Enskog L, Rydberg B. Clinical results of reoperation after failed highly selective vagotomy. *Am J Surg.* 1986;152(3):308-312.

84. Tolin RD, Malmud LS, Stelzer F, et al. Enterogastric reflux in normal subjects and patients with Billroth II gastroenterostomy. Measurement of enterogastric reflux. *Gastroenterology.* 1979;77(5):1027-1033.

85. Natomi H, Sugano K, Iwamori M, Takaku F, Nagai Y. Region-specific distribution of glycosphingolipids in the rabbit gastrointestinal tract: preferential enrichment of sulfoglycolipids in the mucosal regions exposed to acid. *Biochim Biophys Acta.* 1988;961(2):213-222.

86. Akatsu T, Yoshida M, Kubota T, et al. Gallstone disease after extended (D2) lymph node dissection for gastric cancer. *World J Surg.* 2005;29(2):182-186.

87. Arlt G, Schumpelick V, Kloppel G. [Ulcer risk in the Roux-Y stomach. An animal experiment study]. *Langenbecks Arch Chir.* 1984;362(1):43-52.

88. Oliver JV. Effect of vagus section and isolation of the pyloric antrum on the development of the Mann-Williamson ulcer in the dog. *Surg Forum.* 1953;4:336-338.

89. Kalaiselvan R, Exarchos G, Hamza N, Ammori BJ. Incidence of perforated gastrojejunal anastomotic ulcers after laparoscopic gastric bypass for morbid obesity and role of laparoscopy in their management. *Surg Obes Relat Dis.* 2012;8(4):423-428.

90. Patel RA, Brolin RE, Gandhi A. Revisional operations for marginal ulcer after Roux-en-Y gastric bypass. *Surg Obes Relat Dis.* 2009;5(3):317-322.

91. Rasmussen JJ, Fuller W, Ali MR. Marginal ulceration after laparoscopic gastric bypass: an analysis of predisposing factors in 260 patients. *Surg Endosc.* 2007;21(7):1090-1094.

92. Suggs WJ, Kouli W, Lupovici M, Chau WY, Brolin RE. Complications at gastrojejunostomy after laparoscopic Roux-en-Y gastric bypass: comparison between 21- and 25-mm circular staplers. *Surg Obes Relat Dis.* 2007;3(5):508-514.

93. Felix EL, Kettelle J, Mobley E, Swartz D. Perforated marginal ulcers after laparoscopic gastric bypass. *Surg Endosc.* 2008;22(10):2128-2132.

94. Higa KD, Boone KB, Ho T. Complications of the laparoscopic Roux-en-Y gastric bypass: 1,040 patients—what have we learned? *Obes Surg.* 2000;10(6):509-513.

95. Bendewald FP, Choi JN, Blythe LS, Selzer DJ, Ditslear JH, Mattar SG. Comparison of hand-sewn, linear-stapled, and circular-stapled gastrojejunostomy in laparoscopic Roux-en-Y gastric bypass. *Obes Surg.* 2011;21(11):1671-1675.

96. Capella JF, Capella RF. Gastro-gastric fistulas and marginal ulcers in gastric bypass procedures for weight reduction. *Obes Surg.* 1999;9(1):22-27 [discussion 28].

97. Kodama I, Yoshida C, Kofuji K, Ohta J, Aoyagi K, Takeda J. Gallstones and gallbladder disorder after gastrectomy for gastric cancer. *Int Surg.* 1996;81(1):36-39.

98. Kobayashi T, Hisanaga M, Kanehiro H, Yamada Y, Ko S, Nakajima Y. Analysis of risk factors for the development of gallstones after gastrectomy. *Br J Surg.* 2005;92(11):1399-1403.

99. Deleted in review.

100. Fukagawa T, Katai H, Saka M, Morita S, Sano T, Sasako M. Gallstone formation after gastric cancer surgery. *J Gastrointest Surg.* 2009;13(5):886-889.

101. Chiloiro M, Pezzolla F, Riezzo G, Maselli MA, Lorusso D. Gallbladder motility before and after Billroth II gastric resection. *Neurogastroenterol Motil.* 1995;7(3):145-149.

102. Masclee AA, Jansen JB, Driessen WM, Geuskens LM, Lamers CB. Effect of truncal vagotomy on cholecystokinin release, gallbladder contraction, and gallbladder sensitivity to cholecystokinin in humans. *Gastroenterology.* 1990;98(5 Pt 1):1338-1344.

103. Gillen S, Michalski CW, Schuster T, Feith M, Friess H, Kleeff J. Simultaneous/incidental cholecystectomy during gastric/esophageal resection: systematic analysis of risks and benefits. *World J Surg.* 2010;34(5):1008-1014.

104. Wu CC, Chen CY, Wu TC, Iiu TJ, P'eng PK. Cholelithiasis and cholecystitis after gastrectomy for gastric carcinoma: a comparison of lymphadenectomy of varying extent. *Hepatogastroenterology.* 1995;42(6):867-872.

105. Nunobe S, Okaro A, Sasako M, et al. Billroth 1 versus Roux-en-Y reconstructions: a quality-of-life survey at 5 years. *Int J Clin Oncol.* 2007;12(6):433-439.

106. Csendes A, Larach J, Godoy M. Incidence of gallstones development after selective hepatic vagotomy. *Acta Chir Scand.* 1978;144(5):289-291.

107. Veyrie N, Servajean S, Berger N, Loire P, Basdevant A, Bouillot JL. [Gallbladder complications after bariatric surgery]. *Gastroenterol Clin Biol.* 2007;31(4):378-384.

108. Fobi M, Lee H, Igwe D, et al. Prophylactic cholecystectomy with gastric bypass operation: incidence of gallbladder disease. *Obes Surg.* 2002;12(3):350-353.

109. Li VK, Pulido N, Martinez-Suartez P, et al. Symptomatic gallstones after sleeve gastrectomy. *Surg Endosc.* 2009;23(11):2488-2492.

110. Iglezias Brandao de Oliveira C, Adami Chaim E, da Silva BB. Impact of rapid weight reduction on risk of cholelithiasis after bariatric surgery. *Obes Surg.* 2003;13(4):625-628.

111. Li VK, Pulido N, Fajnwaks P, Szomstein S, Rosenthal R, Martinez-Duartez P. Predictors of gallstone formation after bariatric surgery: a multivariate analysis of risk factors comparing gastric bypass, gastric banding, and sleeve gastrectomy. *Surg Endosc.* 2009;23(7):1640-1644.

112. Tarantino I, Warschkow R, Steffen T, Bisang P, Schultes B, Thurnheer M. Is routine cholecystectomy justified in severely obese patients undergoing a laparoscopic Roux-en-Y gastric bypass procedure? A comparative cohort study. *Obes Surg.* 2011;21(12):1870-1878.

Operations for Morbid Obesity

Bruce Schirmer

Bariatric surgery had its beginnings in the 1950s when malabsorptive operations were performed upon patients with severe hyperlipidemia and obesity. Edward Mason was undoubtedly the father of American bariatric surgery, having first described the gastric bypass in 1969[1] and later the vertical banded gastroplasty (VBG)[2] in 1981. In between, unfortunately, the field suffered a major initial setback from which it took decades to recover. The culprit was the performance of the jejunoileal bypass. The operation was originally designed for hyperlipidemia and obesity together and was frequently performed in the 1970s before its untoward side effects, especially hepatic failure in a small percentage of patients, were described and appreciated.[3] The subsequent two decades involved reversing these operations for many of the patients who had received them, as they manifested problems with malabsorption of protein, calories, or essential minerals such as magnesium. Liver failure in 2% of patients, however, was the true insurmountable danger of this procedure.

Restriction, rather than malabsorption, was then felt to be the optimal approach for patients with morbid obesity. Various stapling operations of the stomach were performed to try to limit food intake. Many of these suffered from the lack of understanding that a staple line in an intact stomach will, in a high percentage of cases, break down and allow passage of luminal contents. This is the principle used in pyloric exclusion for duodenal injury. Thus many of the patients who had these stapling procedures experienced initial excellent weight loss but subsequent regain after the staple line broke down.[4]

Mason then championed the VBG, which proved to have more durability than simple stapled operations.[2] The lesser curvature of the stomach, which is resistant to dilation with pressure, was used for the restrictive pouch. The pouch outlet was reinforced with a circular piece of permanent mesh material. Due to its relative technical ease of performance, the operation became immensely popular in the 1980s and was for a period of time the most popular bariatric procedure performed. This trend continued until the last decade of the 20th century. By that time the limitations of the VBG had become apparent. Patients could not eat a normal healthy diet of vegetables and fruits, due to the restriction of the band and pouch, and turned instead to a diet of high-calorie liquids and junk food. Weight regain followed. In addition, a percentage experienced severe gastric outlet obstruction due to progressive hypertrophy around the band, requiring revisional surgery.

The operation that the VBG was revised to was most often the gastric bypass. Since its introduction in 1969, it had evolved quickly from a loop gastrojejunostomy to a Roux-en-Y gastrojejunostomy, due to complications of bile acid reflux esophagitis from the loop. Griffen et al.

popularized this modification.[5] The Roux-en-Y gastric bypass (RYGB) proved to be a very effective operation for weight loss, as well as treatment of comorbidities associated with obesity. Major proponents of the procedure during the 1980s included Sugerman, who described its efficacy in treating hypertension, diabetes,[6] pseudotumor cerebri,[7] and venous stasis ulcers.[8] Pories and his group from East Carolina University were the first to emphasize the beneficial effect of RYGB on the treatment of type 2 diabetes.[9] Improvements in life expectancy, degree of comorbid medical problems, and cost effectiveness of the procedure were soon shown in large studies by Christou and MacLean's group,[10,11] Buchwald,[12] and Adams.[13]

Bariatric surgery experienced its only major change in operative approach, through the advent of laparoscopy, slightly later than most general surgery procedures. Wittgrove and Clark[14] described the first laparoscopic gastric bypass in 1995. Soon thereafter, Schauer[15] and later Nguyen and Wolfe[16] confirmed the efficacy and benefits of performing RYGB using this approach. Patients voted rather quickly for adopting this new approach, with the incidence of RYGB in the United States increasing exponentially during the years 1999–2004 (Fig. 63.1).[17] Since then, the incidence of performance of all bariatric operations in the United States has risen only by 25% in the past 10 to 12 years. However, the spectrum of procedures and their relative safety of performance have changed significantly since the introduction of laparoscopy in the first few years of the 21st century.

Although the RYGB was the predominant procedure performed in the United States at the start of the 21st century, internationally the laparoscopic adjustable gastric band (LAGB), introduced by Belachew in 1994,[18] was taking the European and Australian continents by storm. LAGB's popularity blossomed in the 15 years following its introduction, to the point where in 2009 in the United States it rivaled RYGB as the most popular operation performed for morbid obesity. Its safety profile was excellent, and it proved effective in settings where careful and available follow-up for adjustments to the band existed.[19] Patients viewed it as a less invasive procedure, and its popularity increased accordingly. However, by 2010 the long-term efficacy of the LAGB had proven poor in many centers. Patients had experienced problems with poor weight loss, frequent prolapse of the band requiring multiple adjustments, and overall lack of satisfaction with the amount of weight loss versus the symptoms, cost, and inconvenience of maintaining the band in exactly the correct range of restriction. Centers began reporting a high incidence of band removal, with long-term follow-up showing more than 50% of bands removed in one center.[20] Many patients lost insurance coverage for adjustments, further decreasing the efficacy of the band. By 2012 the operation was clearly

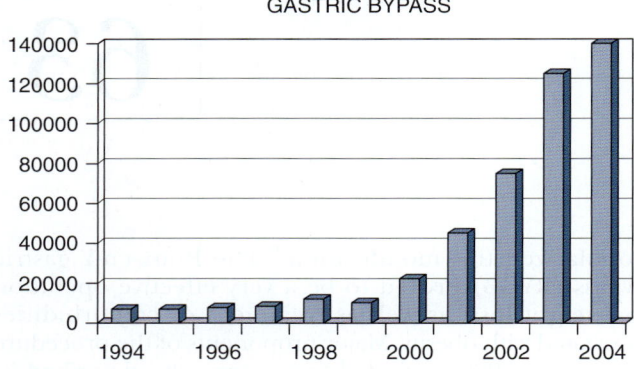

FIGURE 63.1 The rising exponential curve of bariatric operations performed during the Bariatric Revolution.

TABLE 63.1 American Society of Metabolic and Bariatric Surgery Estimate of Numbers of Bariatric Procedures in United States

	2011	2012	2013	2014	2015
Total	158,000	173,000	179,000	193,000	196,000
RYGB	36.7	37.5	34.2	26.8	23.1
Sleeve	17.8	33	42.1	51.7	53.8
Band	35.4	20.2	14	9.5	5.7
DS	0.9	1	1	0.4	0.6
Revisions	6	6	6	11.5	13.6
Other	3.2	2.3	2.7	0.1	3.2

DS, Duodenal switch; *RYGB,* Roux-en-Y gastric bypass.

on the way out, and its use has declined precipitously in the United States since then (Table 63.1).

Part of the reason for the LAGB decline has been the evolution of the laparoscopic sleeve gastrectomy (LSG). Initially described by Gagner and his group as being an effective first step in the two-stage performance of the laparoscopic duodenal switch (LDS) procedure,[21] the patients who had this first stage performed experienced good weight loss and often refused to have the second stage of the duodenal switch (DS) performed. Performance of the sleeve gastrectomy as a stand-alone operation then became more popular in the years 2004–2008, and by 2009 there was considerable evidence for its efficacy.[22] By 2011, through considerable efforts from the American Society of Metabolic and Bariatric Surgery (ASMBS), the procedure received approval as a standard operation by most insurance companies. Since then its popularity has risen to where by 2015 it had become the most commonly performed bariatric procedure in the United States (see Table 63.1). Patients often perceive this procedure as being less invasive, and surgeons certainly have found it to be a less technically difficult procedure than either laparoscopic RYGB (LRYGB) or LDS.

Malabsorptive procedures have never been very popular in most areas for the treatment of morbid obesity. Scopinaro and his group[23] championed the performance of the biliopancreatic diversion (BPD) in Italy in the late 1970s and early 1980s. Its long-term efficacy in producing durable weight loss and resolution of comorbidities such as hyperlipidemia, type 2 diabetes, and hypertension has been excellent. However, it had the disadvantage of a high incidence of marginal ulcers, leading Hess[24] and Marceau[25] to independently and virtually simultaneously devise the DS procedure. LDS remains the internationally most commonly performed metabolic and bariatric malabsorptive operation. However, it accounts for only 2% or less of overall procedures done. Despite LDS being the best procedure for long-term weight loss,[12] its higher incidence of significant metabolic complications, its need for more vitamin supplements, including parenteral fat-soluble vitamins, and its limitations of lifestyle, in terms of diarrhea and frequent bowel movements after eating, have limited its popularity to those patients who are in need of the most severe restriction of caloric absorption or reversal of metabolic diseases.

The safety of performance of bariatric procedures during the past 15 years has improved dramatically. In 2000 the literature reflected the fact that open RYGB had an accepted mortality rate approaching 1%, with 2% being seen in higher-risk patient populations.[26] The profession then did an outstanding job of quality improvement through several means. Laparoscopic procedures proved less morbid, especially for long-term wound complications and incisional hernias. They also were less morbid for short-term complications, length of hospital stay, and mortality.[27] The ASMBS and the American College of Surgeons (ACS) adopted the concept of centers of excellence, and self-review, peer pressure, and external auditing all combined to produce centers that achieved improved outcomes for bariatric procedures.[28] By 2014 the reported national mortality rate for a LRYGB was 0.15% and even lower for LSG.

Currently, the main procedures performed in the United States and internationally are the LSG and the LRYGB. The LAGB is rapidly declining in popularity, and within a year may be as infrequently performed as LDS, which has consistently represented 1% to 2% of procedures for the past several years.

LAPAROSCOPIC ADJUSTABLE GASTRIC BAND

The LAGB was very popular 10 to 13 years ago, and there are a large number of patients who have the device in place. Even though its popularity has decreased recently, it is still important for surgeons to understand the procedure and how it is done to be able to offer it to appropriate selected candidates, as well as treat its complications.

Patients who have had the best success with the LAGB are those whose weight loss goals do not exceed 100 pounds, who have successfully dieted in the past, and who are physically active and will remain so after the procedure. It is also quite helpful and important that patients have ongoing insurance coverage that will allow visits for adjustments of the band, as well as treatment of any complications of the band, to be covered and thus not a financial burden for the patient. Otherwise compliance and follow-up, important for the long-term success of the LAGB, will be severely compromised.

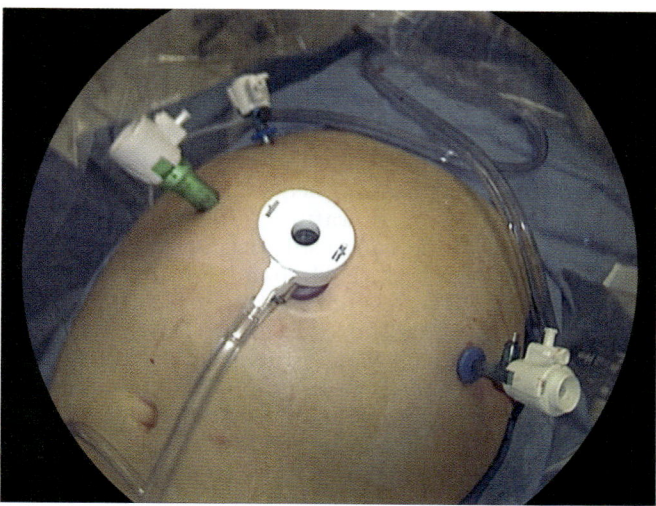

FIGURE 63.2 Port placement for lap band.

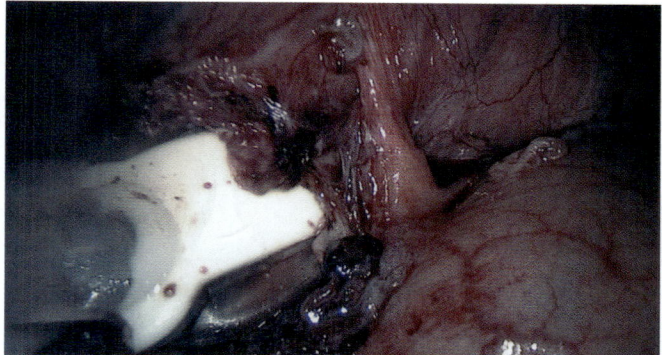

FIGURE 63.4 Suturing fundus over lap band.

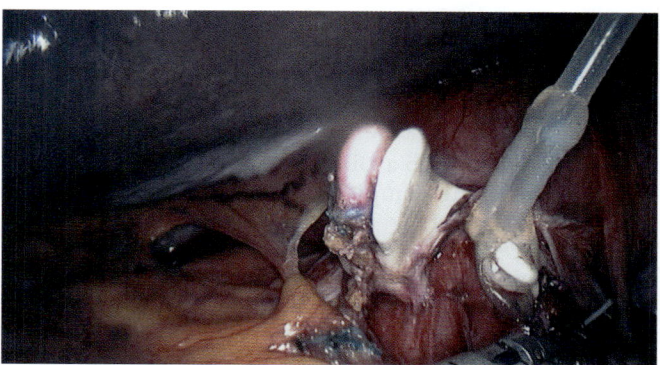

FIGURE 63. 3 Buckle for lap band.

Relative contraindications to an LAGB would be a high body mass index (BMI) of more than 50, poor mobility, lack of ability to exercise, failure to have successfully dieted and lost more than 25 pounds, small hiatal hernia, and previous gastric surgery. Absolute contraindications include previous antireflux surgery, large hiatal hernias, and esophageal motility disorders.

OPERATIVE STEPS

Ports for surgery are generally located above the umbilicus, within 15 to 18 cm of the xiphoid. A 15-mm and 5-mm port are placed in the right upper quadrant for the surgeon's right and left hands, respectively, with the surgeon standing on the patient's right side. The assistant, standing on the patient's left side, can optimally help with two left upper quadrant 5-mm ports. The camera port (12 mm) is placed just to the left and above the umbilicus. A liver retractor is placed in the xiphoid region (Fig. 63.2).

After port placement, the surgeon opens the gastrohepatic ligament in its avascular region proximally. This *pars flaccida* area has been used to describe this technique of band placement. The right crus is identified, and an area approximately 2 to 3 cm below the gastroesophageal junction on the medial border of the right crus is opened with a Harmonic scalpel or similar energy device to allow the beginning of a tunnel for the lap band posterior to the stomach. This tunnel is then developed by the surgeon's left hand, gently passing a grasper from the right to left crus area posterior to the proximal stomach, hugging the surface of the crura. There is a fair amount of fibrous tissue in this area, and the goal is to develop a tunnel within this tissue that allows for some posterior security of the band, preventing migration in either direction. Once the grasper has emerged in the area of the angle of His, the band itself is introduced into the abdomen via the 15-mm port. The tubing end of the band system is then grasped by the grasper and pulled back to the patient's right crus, through the previously developed tissue tunnel. The tubing is pulled through until the band is partially around the stomach.

The band is then placed around the proximal stomach, 2 cm below the gastroesophageal junction, and with just that small amount of stomach above the top of the band. It is locked onto itself, securing it in place. The band has a locking buckle mechanism that allows it to self-secure in this location (Fig. 63.3). The buckle of the band is positioned above the lesser curvature of the stomach.

The fundus is now brought up over the left lateral and anterior portions of the band to cover the band and secure it further into position. Several sutures are required to secure the fundus in this location (Fig. 63.4). Care should be taken to avoid placing the fundus over the buckle of the band because erosion may occur.

The tubing is now brought out through the abdominal wall in a location where the port will be sited. We have favored placing the port just below the costal margin in the epigastric region. This location makes the port more easily palpable for adjustments. An incision is made on the abdominal wall in the desired area of the port. The tubing is brought out from the abdomen through a stab wound on the medial side of this incision, as far to the end of the incision as possible. This allows the tubing to emerge through the fascia and take a natural slow bend medially to be joined to the port. Securing the tubing to the port and then the port to the fascia in the incision site completes the operation except to visually confirm that addition of saline to the system causes the band to expand and not leak. The band is normally placed without any

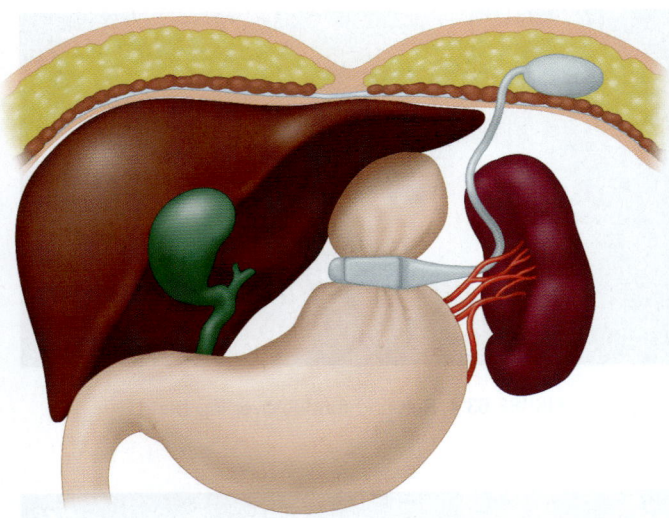

FIGURE 63.5 Fundus imbricated over lap band.

saline in the system to avoid initial excessive obstruction. Fig. 63.5 shows the completed LAGB.

BAND ADJUSTMENTS

Postoperative adjustments to the band are necessary to provide an optimal amount of restriction. When such adjustments are made, a good rule of thumb is to have the patient drink several swallows of water quickly after the adjustment is made. If the patient feels the water stop and give a sensation of partial blockage, then the adjustment is too tight and must be loosened. Optimal restriction varies from patient to patient, but in general a goal of restriction to one cup of food or less at a meal and production of satiety for at least a few hours after eating are the goals of an optimal adjustment.

Probably more so than any of the other procedures, the success of LAGB is dependent on patient understanding of diet recommendations and compliance. The LAGB should help promote healthy eating habits, and nutritional counseling on a frequent basis, especially early after the procedure, is important.

OUTCOMES

The LAGB has produced some excellent initial results in patients. O'Brien and colleagues probably had the best overall international experience with the band.[29] Ren and Fielding published a large experience with good results in the United States.[30] Optimal weight loss at 3 years after LAGB was approximately 50% of excess weight in these series. Dixon et al.[31] showed the efficacy of the LAGB in treating type 2 diabetes. Long-term results have been less overall good and more controversial. There are published reports of a high incidence of band removal after 10 years.[20] A combination of patient frustration with the lack of progressive weight loss with the band, recurrent prolapse or other adjustment issues, and the need for ongoing readjustments have caused an increasing number of patients to seek band removal with or without a second bariatric operation. More attractive outcomes from sleeve gastrectomy have caused most surgeons to drastically decrease placement of the LAGB in favor of other procedures such as the sleeve gastrectomy.

COMPLICATIONS

Early postoperative complications after band placement are rare, and discharge the same day is the norm. However, complications can occur, and these have been well described in the literature.[32] Inaccurate or poor dissection technique can result in gastric perforation and postoperative leak. Early band erosion occurs in approximately 1% or less of cases.

Stenosis at the band site, or excessive band restriction, will produce nausea and vomiting in most situations but can also present as new-onset gastroesophageal reflux disease (GERD) in less stenotic situations. Any such symptoms of new onset need to be investigated promptly for either simple excessive restriction or, more commonly, prolapse of the band. Prolapse occurs when the stomach below the band herniates up into the central lumen of the band and too much stomach is forced into this space. Complete or partial obstruction results. In severe cases the prolapse can lead to ischemia and gangrene of the prolapsed portion of the stomach. Chronic prolapse is seen at times with surprisingly large protrusions of the distal stomach up and over the edge of the gastric band. Technically prolapse is when the stomach herniates up through the band. Slippage is when the band slips down onto the stomach. Both produce the same end result mechanically and symptomatically. Prolapse can occur at any time after the procedure, and its incidence slowly rises with duration of the band being in place. Recurrent prolapse has been a common reason for band removal among patients.

Diagnosis of prolapse is a clinical and, if necessary, radiographic one. The signs and symptoms are of obstruction or GERD, with obstruction present in most cases. A plain film of the abdomen will reveal the band position, normally at a 7 o'clock to 1 o'clock orientation, flattened to horizontal on the film. This is diagnostic for prolapse. If doubt exists, a low-volume Gastrografin or barium swallow will confirm the diagnosis.

Treatment for prolapse initially is removal of all fluid in the system. This will, in most cases of acute prolapse, provide enough reduction in the restriction of the prolapsed stomach to allow it to slip back down through the band and resume its normal position. However, if removal of all fluid does not produce immediate relief of symptoms by the patient, a swallow study is indicated. If the swallow shows a large and persistent prolapse, emergent surgical therapy is indicated to laparoscopically reduce the prolapse and prevent gastric ischemia. A laparoscopic approach to freeing the buckle of the band, unbuckling the system, reducing the prolapse to its appropriate location, and repositioning and rebuckling the band is quite feasible.

Other complications are less common. Chronic stenosis or band placement too high onto the distal esophagus may produce esophageal obstruction and dilation. This must be corrected when diagnosed. Resolution of the obstruction will usually result in the esophagus regaining its normal size. Failure to secure the port to the fascia can result in the port turning in the subcutaneous space and being unable to be accessed for further adjustments. An outpatient procedure under local anesthesia can correct this problem.

LAPAROSCOPIC ROUX-EN-Y GASTRIC BYPASS

The gold standard operation for bariatric surgery has been the RYGB. It achieved initial popularity in the mid 1970s and has remained a standard operation since that time. The operation was first described by Mason and Itoh in 1969.[1] Griffen published the first large experience after revising it to a Roux limb.[3] It stood the test of time as the VBG came and went in the 1980s and 1990s. As described previously, Wittgrove's description of its performance laparoscopically[14] and Schauer and others' reports[15] soon championed the laparoscopic approach. LRYGB was the most common procedure performed in the early part of the 21st century, when bariatric centers of excellence were formulated and when greater attention to quality outcomes produced significant improvements in the safety of the procedure.

As with many popular operations, there are considerable variations on the theme as to how to best perform LRYGB. The technique of creating the gastrojejunostomy and the length and location of the Roux limb has varied from surgeon to surgeon. No optimal technique or configuration has emerged, although some differences have been shown. Its performance using a laparoscopic approach has clearly been an improvement over the open approach, as with all other operations where minimal access has been used. Elimination of incisional hernias, decreased pain and recovery time, and decreased overall complication rates and mortality have all been confirmed with using the laparoscopic approach.

Indications for performing LRYGB follow the general guidelines for metabolic and bariatric surgery as outlined in the National Institutes of Health (NIH) Consensus conference of 1990.[33] A BMI greater than 40 or greater than 35 with comorbid medical problems associated with obesity are the indications. Failure of a trial of dieting and mental stability are also considered standard criteria. Other criteria vary among surgeons and institutions, including upper and lower age limits, size limits, and requirements of cessation of addictive habits. Patients who have significant symptoms from GERD or who have insulin-dependent type 2 diabetes remain optimal candidates for LRYGB in our practice. LRYGB has been shown to give superior results in treating GERD[34] and insulin-dependent diabetes.[35] Another factor that favors LRYGB over other operations is its known durability (when considering the younger patient). It also produces the overall best weight loss and resolution of comorbid medical problems of all the restrictive operations, although sleeve gastrectomy has been shown to have close to comparable results in some studies in which GERD and type 2 diabetes are not factors.

Absolute contraindications to LRYGB include failure to meet NIH criteria, psychiatric instability, ongoing drug or alcohol addiction, and excessively morbid medical problems precluding safe surgery. Relative contraindications include age younger than 15 or older than 65 to 70, weight greater than 600 pounds (our cutoff), persistent smoking, lack of mobility, and severe medical problems.

OPERATIVE STEPS

We use a similar port placement for LRYGB as we do for LAGB. Many surgeons do not use as many ports for LAGB. However, for LRYGB, we find the assistant having two available hands to assist is very helpful to essential in many steps of the operation. The superior left upper quadrant port is a 12-mm one in this procedure as we perform it, because we do a double-stapled enteroenterostomy technique and the stapler angle is optimal from that location for the second firing (Fig. 63.6).

After ports are placed, I prefer to create the Roux limb as the first step. The ligament of Treitz is clearly identified, after which the proximal jejunum is divided with a white load of the GIA stapler (Covidien-Medtronic, Dublin, Ireland) at approximately 45 to 50 cm distal to the ligament (Fig. 63.7). The mesentery is then further divided with the Harmonic scalpel to obtain as deep a division of the mesentery as possible without encountering the very large vessels at the base of the mesentery. The proximal end of the Roux limb is then marked by suturing a small Penrose drain to it. The Roux limb length is now estimated and

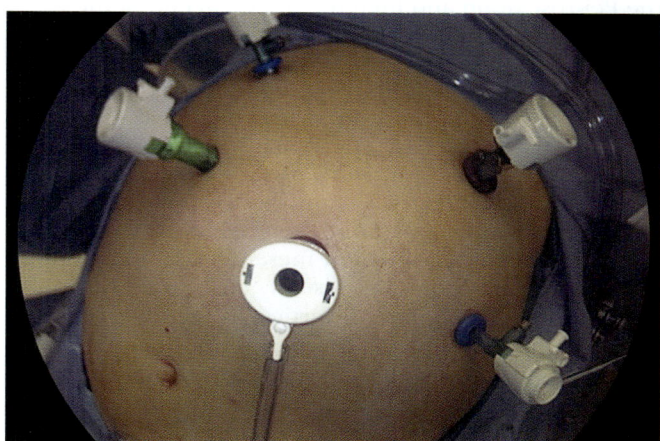

FIGURE 63.6 Port placement for lap gastric bypass.

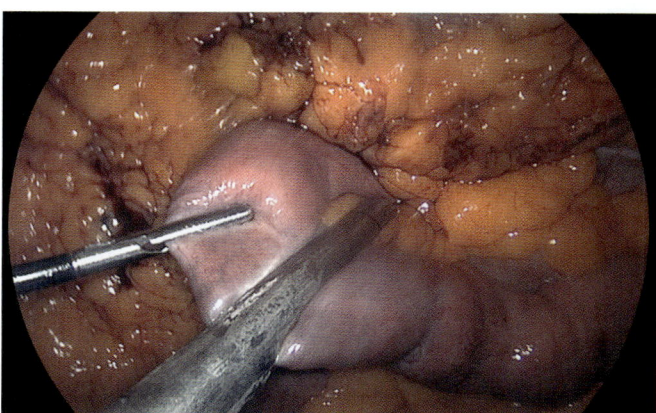

FIGURE 63.7 Dividing jejunum.

measured. I usually prefer a 150-cm Roux limb for patients with a BMI greater than 50. As the limb is being measured, it is pulled to the left upper quadrant. The jejunum at the desired distance is then placed adjacent to the proximal jejunum, with the distal end of the proximal jejunum facing to the patient's right and the proximal end of the Roux limb with the Penrose on it facing up and to the left. A double-stapled enteroenterostomy is now created with two white loads of the GIA stapler. The stapler defect is sewn closed with running absorbable suture. Then the mesenteric defect at the enteroenterostomy is closed with a running permanent suture.

The transverse colon mesentery is now grasped and elevated, exposing the lower portion of the mesentery near the ligament of Treitz. A defect is made in the mesentery to the left and a few centimeters above the ligament of Treitz. This location usually avoids major vessels, but the surgeon must be aware of the vascular anatomy, if visible, and cautious not to disrupt it unnecessarily. Openings between mesenteric vessels are easier to find than dealing with bleeding from major mesenteric vessels. Once the mesentery has been opened to expose the lesser sac, the posterior surface of the stomach can be seen. It is grasped and pulled out of the mesenteric defect a few centimeters, after which the plane below the stomach is confirmed with a grasper. Adhesions, if present, are divided to now allow the Penrose drain and then the proximal end of the Roux limb to be placed into the retrogastric space (Fig. 63.8). Usually if one can pass 4 cm of bowel or more past the cut edge of the mesentery, that will suffice for later retrieval. Perhaps one of the most important technical issues now must be strictly obeyed. The Roux limb mesentery must not have any twists in it. It is very easy to have the bowel twisted a full 180 degrees or more between first passing it to the left upper quadrant then retrieving it to pass it through the transverse colon mesentery. The mesentery of the Roux limb must be visually confirmed without a doubt as being straight and vertical as the limb is passed superiorly through the transverse colon mesentery.

Now attention is shifted to the stomach. The left lobe of the liver is retracted with a laparoscopic liver retractor of the surgeon's choice. The Harmonic scalpel is used to create an opening in the mesentery along the lesser curvature of the stomach. For most patients, this can be done a centimeter or two above the incisura. However, for very large patients, creating this opening at the incisura is advisable because the longer gastric pouch is often needed to allow the Roux limb to easily reach the proximal stomach without tension. Once the opening is created, a green load of the GIA stapler is fired from the lesser curvature of the stomach to partially divide the stomach body. Then I prefer to size the pouch with an Ewald tube (30 French) and place the stapler close to but not directly adjacent to the tube, which is visible by the contour it creates on the gastric surface. The stapler, now firing directly cephalad parallel to the lesser curvature, is fired several times until the stomach is divided up to the angle of His (Fig. 63.9). It is important to exclude the fundus from the proximal part of the newly created gastric pouch. Care should be taken not to catch the Penrose drain in the stapler. Similarly, the anesthesiologist needs to double confirm there are no temperature probes or orogastric tubes in the stomach other than the Ewald tube.

The Penrose drain is now usually visible in the retrogastric space. If it is not, the inferior surface of the transverse colon mesentery must again be exposed and the Roux limb passed into the retrogastric space again. I continue to use a retrogastric retrocolic location of the Roux limb due to the fact this is the shortest distance from between jejunum and proximal stomach. A more popular approach is to bring the Roux limb directly anterior to both transverse colon and distal stomach and create the gastrojejunostomy. This approach is technically easier, except when the mesentery of the Roux limb is short and there is difficulty in stretching the Roux limb to reach the proximal gastric pouch. For the retrocolic retrogastric approach, I now place the proximal suture line of the Roux limb directly adjacent to the distal part of the proximal gastric pouch. The distal 5 cm of gastric pouch is then tacked to the side of the proximal 5 cm of the Roux limb with a running absorbable suture.

The gastrojejunostomy is created using a linear stapling device. We have found that the linear stapler is associated with an insignificant incidence of postoperative stenosis, whereas the circular stapler in our experience yielded a 10% or higher stenosis rate. The Ewald tube serves as a good backstop against which to make a gastrotomy in the end of the pouch. An enterotomy in the Roux

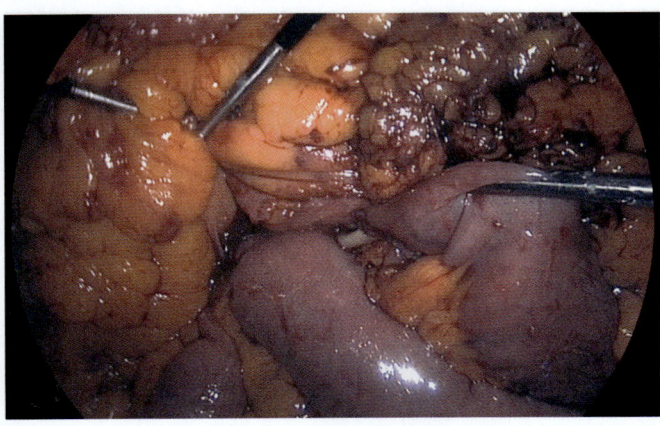

FIGURE 63.8 Passing Roux limb.

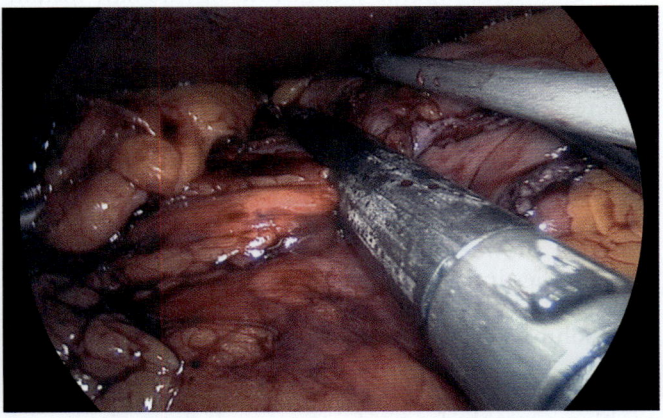

FIGURE 63.9 Creating gastric pouch.

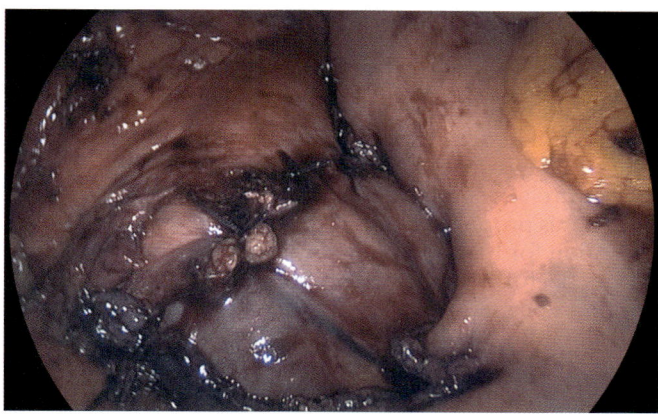

FIGURE 63.10 Gastrojejunostomy.

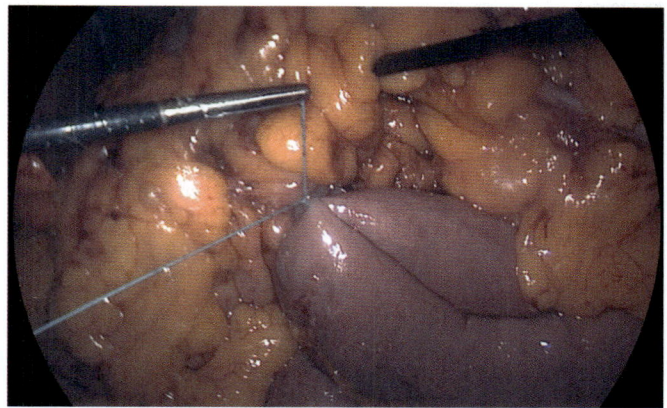

FIGURE 63.11 Closing mesenteric defect.

limb is less difficult. Having pulled the Ewald tube back, the stapler is advanced into the two lumens to its full extent and fired (Fig. 63.10). We have not found that restricting the anastomotic size has any relationship to long-term postoperative weight loss. The gastric pouch size must be small, but the anastomosis need not be very small. The staple defect is closed with a running layer of absorbable suture and reinforced with a second such layer. An intraoperative leak test is now performed by having the anesthesiologist forcefully inject a methylene blue dye solution into the lumen of the proximal pouch, after having readvanced the tip of the Ewald tube to that level.

Closure of the mesenteric defects with permanent suture is now performed. For this procedure, the Roux limb must be secured to the jejunum at the ligament of Treitz to prevent the Roux limb from telescoping up into the retrogastric space and becoming kinked and obstructed. I use a short four-bite purse-string suture between those two loops of bowel at the ligament of Treitz area and two bites of the transverse colon mesentery above the pieces of bowel (Fig. 63.11). Further sutures between the two limbs are placed, as well as sutures to close the space between the left lateral side of the Roux limb and the transverse colon mesentery. Fig. 63.12 shows the completed LRYGB.

Port sites 12 mm or larger are closed with laparoscopically passed sutures for the fascia. I do not routinely use drains or nasogastric tubes after this operation.

Postoperative care includes providing adequate analgesia, early ambulation, liquids on postoperative day 1, and discharge on postoperative day 2 on our phase 2 gastric bypass diet (blenderized food). A Foley catheter is used and removed on the first postoperative day. This may be unnecessary. I still perform a Gastrografin swallow on the first postoperative day to confirm no distal obstruction, as well as no obvious leak.

OUTCOMES

LRYGB is associated with excellent weight loss and resolution of comorbid medical problems. We have recently published our 10-year outcomes for patients undergoing RYGB. Some of these patients had an open procedure, but most had a laparoscopic one. At 10 years the overall excess

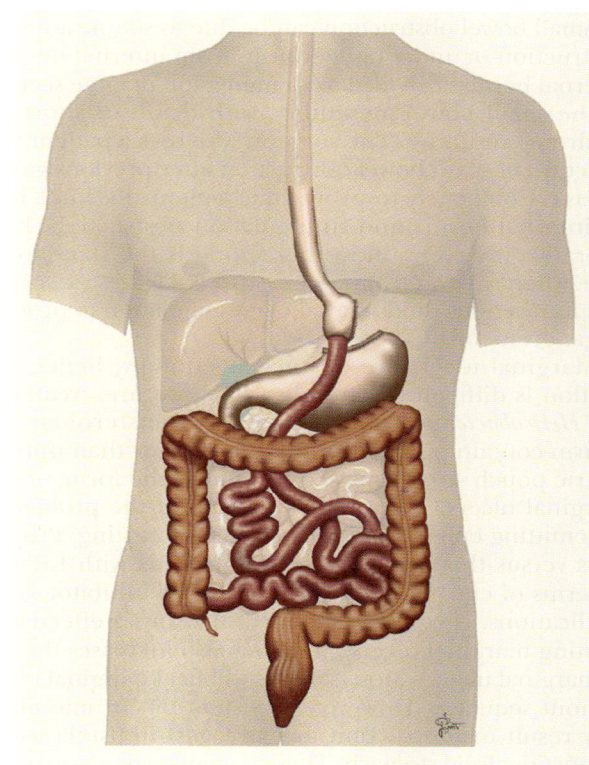

FIGURE 63.12 Configuration of lap gastric bypass. (Courtesy Inamed Health, Santa Barbara, California.)

BMI loss was 52%. There was a significant improvement in obesity-related comorbid medical problems for all problems assessed after 10 years. This was true even in patients who had regained weight after initial weight loss. Excess BMI loss was maximal at approximately 70% for the first 3 years after surgery but by year 5 had decreased to closer to approximately 65%.[36] Type 2 diabetes remained in remission in 60% of patients, hypertension in 45%, and obstructive sleep apnea in 65%. Data from national databases show that the incidence of mortality in recent years after LRYGB is now 0.14%, with complication rates being in the 5.9% range at 30 days.[27]

COMPLICATIONS

Early

Complications within the first month after LRYGB include an anastomotic leak rate of approximately 1%, gastrointestinal bleeding rate requiring intervention of less than 1%, venous thromboembolism rate of approximately 1%, and pulmonary embolism rate of 0.3%. Early small bowel obstruction may be in the 2% range and can be associated with major staple line disruptions.

Late

Late complications after LRYGB include anastomotic stenosis (under 2% with a linear stapling technique), small bowel obstruction (estimated at 4% to 5%), and marginal ulcer (incidence varies widely among series, from 2% to 15%). Stenosis is usually amenable to endoscopic or fluoroscopic balloon dilation.[37]

Small bowel obstruction can be due to simple adhesive obstruction or, more dangerously, from internal hernias. Internal hernias can lead to strangulation of large sections of the small bowel mesentery, with death or short gut syndrome resulting. The surgeon who sees a patient with a picture of small bowel obstruction after previous gastric bypass is obligated to prove that patient does not have an internal hernia and strangulation obstruction. Early operative intervention in this setting is the standard of care, whereas conservative therapy with nasogastric suction and intravenous fluids may allow strangulation to proceed to gangrene of the bowel.

Marginal ulcers are of unclear etiology; hence prevention is difficult. Use of absorbable suture, treatment for *Helicobacter pylori*, avoidance of nonsteroidal and aspirin-containing medications, and larger than optimal gastric pouch size all may contribute to the formation of marginal ulcers. The classic symptom of the problem is unremitting epigastric pain, unrelated to eating. Prophylaxis versus this problem among patients with LRYGB, in terms of chronic use of proton pump inhibitor (PPI) medications, is controversial. PPI therapy is effective in treating marginal ulcers. Smoking also increases the risk of marginal ulcer.[38] Most patients will heal marginal ulcers without sequelae. However, persistent or chronic ulcers may result in obstruction or gastrogastric fistula to the defunctionalized stomach. These patients require operative revision. In most cases, re-creation of the gastrojejunostomy and resection of the ulcer and any fistula is performed. However, in selected cases of chronic or repeated ulcers, takedown of the gastrojejunostomy and performance of a gastrogastrostomy, with gastric narrowing (converting to sleeve gastrectomy) or without gastric narrowing, may be the best option.

The most common adverse long-term result after LRYGB is weight regain. For approximately one-third of patients, this is an unfortunate development. For some patients, situational stresses result in weight gain. Others never establish a firm enough change in eating and exercise habits to sustain the initial weight loss produced by the operation. Options for revisional surgery include performing further restrictive measures endoscopically or surgically or adding a malabsorptive component to the anatomy. Revisional surgery will be discussed in more detail later.

SLEEVE GASTRECTOMY

A vertical parietal cell gastrectomy was first performed as a modification of the DS procedure in the early 1990s with the goal of reducing the adverse side effects associated with distal gastrectomy. Patients who underwent the new procedure were noted to have increased weight loss.[39] In 2003 it was proposed that LSG be performed as a first-stage operation for high-risk patients, with a laparoscopic gastric bypass performed after an initial period of weight loss.[40] Surgeons began to notice good and prolonged weight loss with LSG only, and it became a stand-alone procedure.[41] Currently, it is the most commonly performed bariatric procedure at many centers in the United States.

The sleeve gastrectomy involves resection of the greater curvature of the stomach, leaving a small, tubular stomach based on the lesser curvature blood supply. The operation removes approximately 80% of the stomach. The popularity of the procedure is not surprising. It is easy for patients to understand and relatively straightforward for surgeons to perform. Because there is no malabsorptive component, patients are less likely to develop nutrient deficiencies. In addition, because the operation does not bypass any intestinal segments, there are no potential spaces for internal herniation. Sleeve gastrectomy also leaves open the possibility of revision to a full BPD with DS or a gastric bypass if weight loss is inadequate.

The indications, patient preparation, and positioning are similar to gastric bypass. Eligible patients should have a BMI of 40 or a BMI of 35 with obesity-related comorbidity, have failed prior attempts at weight loss, and have undergone psychologic evaluation.

OPERATIVE STEPS

Antibiotic and venous thromboembolic prophylaxis are administered in the preoperative area or at least prior to induction. The patient is positioned supine or split leg (French position). A footboard is used to allow for steep reverse Trendelenburg.

Port placement is also similar to gastric bypass, although fewer 12-mm ports are needed because stapling is done through only one or two ports. Four or five ports are used, as well as a stab incision for the liver retractor. We use one 15-mm port and one 12-mm port, with the remainder being 5 mm. The 15-mm site is later used to extract the specimen (Fig. 63.13).

Retraction of the left lobe of the liver provides exposure of the proximal stomach and the gastroesophageal junction. The patient is placed in reverse Trendelenburg position. The pylorus is identified, and a position on the greater curvature of the stomach 4 cm from the pylorus is selected for the initial dissection.

This 4-cm margin preserves the antral pump mechanism. Alternatively, dissection is begun on the greater curvature in the mid-body and carried back to this point. Entrance to the lesser sac is easier in this position.

Ultrasonic shears or a bipolar energy device is used to enter the lesser sac and divide the gastroepiploic arcade proximally from the point of entry along the entire greater curvature of the stomach, including the short gastric vessels. Dissection stays very close to the greater curve, dividing gastroepiploic vessels attached to it (Fig. 63.14). This

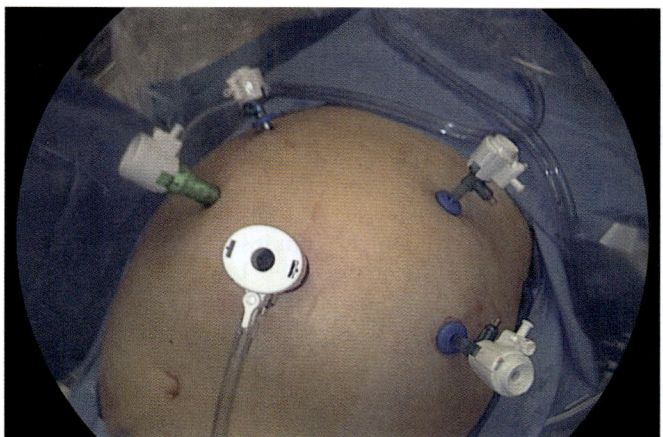

FIGURE 63.13 Port placement for sleeve gastrectomy.

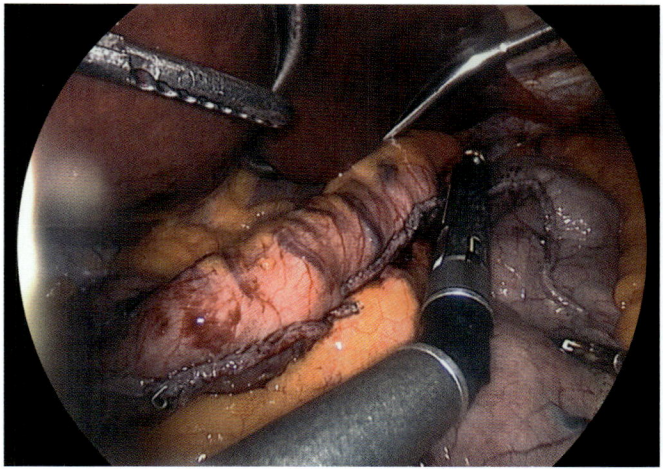

FIGURE 63.15 Firing stapler to make sleeve.

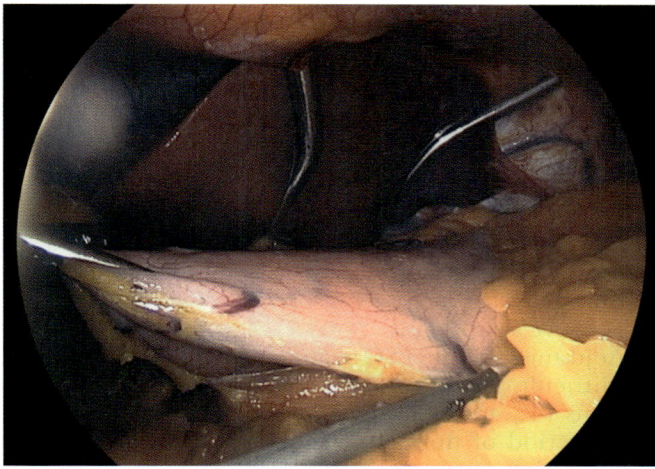

FIGURE 63.14 Dividing tissue along greater curvature.

minimizes the amount of fat attached to the gastrectomy specimen and facilitates easier extraction. Division of the phrenoesophageal ligament completes mobilization of the fundus and allows for detection of a hiatal hernia. If one is discovered, the distal esophagus is freed of mediastinal attachments and brought into the abdomen. The crura are approximated posteriorly with permanent suture. Dissection of posterior gastric adhesions to the body of the pancreas and retroperitoneum completes mobilization of the body of the stomach.

Prior to stapling, any previously placed orogastric tubes are removed and the anesthesiologist inserts a bougie. With the assistance and guidance of the surgeon, it is positioned along the lesser curve and directed to the pylorus. The size of the bougie dilator varies from 32 to 50 French, but 36 French is the most common size.[42] I use a large-bore gastric lavage tube (Ewald), which measures 34 French and is excellent for subsequent leak testing with methylene blue. It is important when using a smaller-diameter bougie to leave a 1- to 2-mm distance between the bougie and the stapler (Fig. 63.15). This is evaluated by the surgeon with the tip of a grasper. An initial linear stapler load is introduced through a right

upper quadrant port, and the sleeve resection is begun at a point 4 to 5 cm proximal to the pylorus. Black (2.3 mm closed height) or green (2 mm) 60-mm stapler cartridges are used for the initial fires, transitioning to blue (1.5 mm) as the tissue thickness decreases at the fundus. We feel that matching the staple height to the thickness of the tissue aids in hemostasis. Care is taken not to staple too close to the incisura angularis because stenosis is common at this level. Equal portions of anterior and posterior wall are taken to avoid twisting or spiraling of the staple line. This is facilitated by stretching the greater curvature as the stapler is positioned. Six to seven stapler fires are generally needed. Fig. 63.16 shows the completed sleeve gastrectomy.

Staple line reinforcement is controversial. Approximately 80% of surgeons use some form of reinforcement, with 60% of those using absorbable buttressing material, and the remainder oversewing the staple line.[42] A meta-analysis in 2016 found that use of buttressing material was associated with a lower risk of staple line hemorrhage, but there was not a significant decrease in the rate of leaks. Oversewing the staple line showed no clear advantages.[43]

The integrity of the staple line may be tested with an air leak or instillation of 50 to 100 mL of methylene blue in saline solution. Intraoperative endoscopy may also be used, which further facilitates the detection of stenosis or intraluminal bleeding. Although common, there are no current data supporting the ability of routine intraoperative leak testing to detect leaks.[44]

Some surgeons perform omentoplasty, suturing the gastric omentum to the staple line or buttressing material in an effort to reproduce the natural orientation of the stomach, reduce spiraling of the sleeve, and further buttress the staple line. Data are lacking to support this practice. Drains are not routinely used. The specimen is removed through one of the port sites. Use of a 15-mm port site generally eliminates the need to dilate the site. We close all port sites 12 mm in size or larger. We generally place two sutures in the 15-mm port site and a single suture in the 12-mm site, using a transfascial suture passer. Closure of the 12-mm sites is optional when noncutting trocars are used.

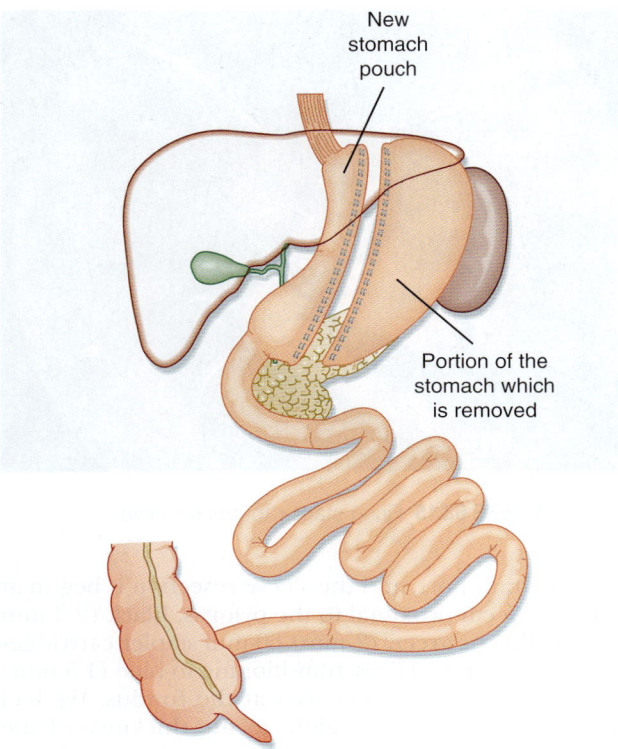

New
stomach
pouch

Portion of the
stomach which
is removed

FIGURE 63.16 Final configuration of sleeve gastrectomy. (From Poirier RF. Complications of bariatric surgery. In: Adams JG, Barton ED, Collings J, eds. *Emergency Medicine.* Philadelphia: Saunders; 2008.)

OUTCOMES

LSG is associated with excellent durable weight loss and resolution of comorbid medical problems. Weight loss is slightly lower than that seen after gastric bypass but greater than after lap band.[27] Excess weight loss varying from 51% to 71% at 1 year has been reported in the literature after LSG.[42,45,46]

LSG has been shown to improve comorbid medical problems in a comparable way as gastric bypass. Hutter et al.[27] showed that resolution of comorbid medical problems for LSG was not significantly different than seen after LRYGB, with the notable exception of GERD. GERD is apparently the Achilles heel of the LSG. One report suggested that patients with preoperative GERD did significantly less well after LSG than patients without GERD, even to the point where morbidity and reoperation rates were affected.[47] There have been two large consensus conferences among experts in the field regarding sleeve gastrectomy, with results published in the literature. The first consensus conference[42] confirmed the operation was effective for producing weight loss of from 59% excess weight loss at 1 year to 50% at 6 years. Mortality was 0.33% and serious complications of leak (1.1%), bleeding (1.8%), and stenosis (0.9%) occurred rarely. The second consensus conference showed that experts felt GERD needed to be thoroughly evaluated prior to sleeve gastrectomy but did not necessarily represent a total contraindication. It also showed experts were much more likely to consider

GERD a contraindication to performing LSG than were nonexpert surgeons.[48]

Prospective randomized studies have demonstrated that LSG can produce excellent resolution of medical problems and weight loss. The STAMPEDE study at 5 years showed that LSG produced resolution of type 2 diabetes in 24% of patients versus 5% in the medical treatment arm.[49] The Swiss randomized trial[46] confirmed LSG produces comparable weight loss to LRYGB. A recent review of the literature suggested LSG can achieve the same remission for type 2 diabetes as LRYGB,[49] although prospective trials still show an advantage of LRYGB for this disease.

COMPLICATIONS

LSG is associated with a very low incidence of morbidity and mortality. One large database recently reported the incidence of 30-day mortality as 0.1% and serious morbidity as 3.8%. Reoperation rates were 1.6%.[50]

The most common complications that occur after LSG are staple line leaks and staple line bleeding. Staple line bleeding is generally reported in the 1% range, with the use of buttress material decreasing the rate from 1.0% to 0.75%. Staple line leak rate is similarly reported in the 1% range, with buttressing actually potentially increasing the incidence of leakage from 0.65% to 0.96%.[51]

Stenosis of the staple line is the only other major commonly reported complication after LSG. Its incidence is in the 1% to 2% range generally, with reoperation being required if dilation does not produce adequate relief of obstructive symptoms.

Adjustment to the LSG anatomy can, for some patients, be difficult. We have observed a small percentage of patients (4% to 6%) who experience persistent nausea, for a period of up to 3 months after surgery, despite confirmation of no obstructive anatomy postoperatively.

After a patient is more than a few months out from an LSG, the incidence of later complications is relatively low. This is especially true when compared with LRYGB, which has long-term problems of bowel obstruction and marginal ulcers. New-onset GERD may arise after LSG, with an estimated incidence of 8%.[47]

Data on weight regain after LSG are just now being appreciated with most series nearing their 10-year mark from the start of performing cases. The early data do not suggest the incidence will be that much higher than LRYGB.

DUODENAL SWITCH

Marceau[24] and Hess[25] performed and described this operation in response to the high marginal ulceration rate seen both after the BPD operation popularized by Scopinaro[23] and his followers. The BPD involved the creation of a partial distal gastrectomy, leaving a generous proximal gastric pouch. The ileum, at a point 200 cm proximal to the ileocecal valve, was divided and anastomosed to the gastric pouch. The remaining proximal bowel was anastomosed to the ileum either 50 or 100 cm proximal to the ileocecal valve, depending on the demographics of the patient population. In northern Italy, where the Italian population ate more protein, Scopinaro created the anastomosis at 50 cm, whereas for southern Italians, who ate more pasta and less protein, he created a 100-cm common channel. Marceau and Hess both used the same distal bowel design but advocated the longer common channel. However, for the DS the stomach was decreased in size by creating a sleeve of the lesser curvature of the stomach, which was the first performance of sleeve gastrectomy. The duodenum was instead divided in the distal first portion, to which the distal ileum was connected to create the shortened alimentary tract.

The performance of the DS laparoscopically was and remains challenging. Initial reports by Gagner's group[21] showed an increased morbidity and mortality for these patients, who were typically heavier with correspondingly more associated medical problems, warranting the performance of a malabsorptive operation. The separation of the sleeve gastrectomy as a first-stage procedure prior to later performance of the malabsorptive component of the operation led to the recognition by patients and surgeons that the sleeve gastrectomy operation was an effective stand-alone procedure.

Variations on the DS have been described that include longer length alimentary tract limbs and longer common channels. Fig. 63.17 shows the most commonly performed version of the DS. Indications for performance of DS include the same parameters as for any standard bariatric and metabolic operation. DS has not proven to be a popular option for patients, whether done open in the past or laparoscopically as at present. Current statistics show that DS represents no more than approximately 1% of bariatric operations performed annually in the United States. Patients who may be candidates for this type of procedure in preference to other more popular ones could include those who have failed a restrictive procedure, are particularly large, or have severe metabolic syndrome or hyperlipidemia or diabetes. Patients who wish to be less restricted in terms of their eating but who understand will have more bowel activity due to the malabsorption component of the operation would also be good candidates for DS.

Malabsorptive operations require careful follow-up to monitor for potential nutritional complications. DS patients also optimally need significant vitamin and mineral supplementation annually, which can represent a significant out-of-pocket cost. The patient should be aware of this potential expense and be willing and able to meet it.

OPERATIVE STEPS

The operation begins with the creation of the sleeve gastrectomy. Ports are placed in the mid to upper abdomen, as well as a liver retractor placed in the epigastric region. A sleeve gastrectomy is first performed, as described previously in this chapter. After the sleeve gastrectomy is completed, the duodenum is carefully dissected at a location several centimeters distal to the pylorus. An instrument such as a Harmonic scalpel is helpful for dividing tissue hemostatically. Creation of a tunnel underneath the duodenum is then followed by placement of a stapler across the duodenum, which staples and divides it securely.

Attention is now turned to the distal ileum and the ileocecal area. The distal ileum is then measured backward from the cecum, and the desired distance of the alimentary tract, usually 250 cm but for some surgeons 300 cm, is determined. At that point the ileum is divided with a linear stapler and the distal end of that bowel marked for connection to the duodenum.

The enteroenterostomy of the proximal end of the divided bowel to a point 100 to 150 cm proximal to the ileocecal valve is now performed. A standard side-to-side stapled anastomosis is performed. This can be either a single fire or double fire staple technique, with care being taken to avoid any stenosis of the anastomosis. The stapler defect is closed with sutures. The mesenteric defect is also then closed.

The ileum is now brought up to the first part of the duodenum. Most surgeons amputate the staple line of the duodenum and perform an end-to-side duodenum to ileum handsewn anastomosis. A circular stapled anastomosis is also feasible. A linear stapled anastomosis is only feasible if the duodenal stump is at least 5 cm in length, which is often not the case. After the anastomosis is completed and tested for security, the operation is completed except for closure of port sites.

Although not advocated by all surgeons, most surgeons who perform DS also offer the patient a simultaneous laparoscopic cholecystectomy as prophylaxis against likely postoperative gallstone formation. The decreased bile salt pool coupled with rapid weight loss makes this operation one that is associated with a high incidence of postoperative cholelithiasis. The performance of laparoscopic cholecystectomy with DS has not been well reviewed in terms of the additional morbidity it might create. However, our group has shown that the additional morbidity of

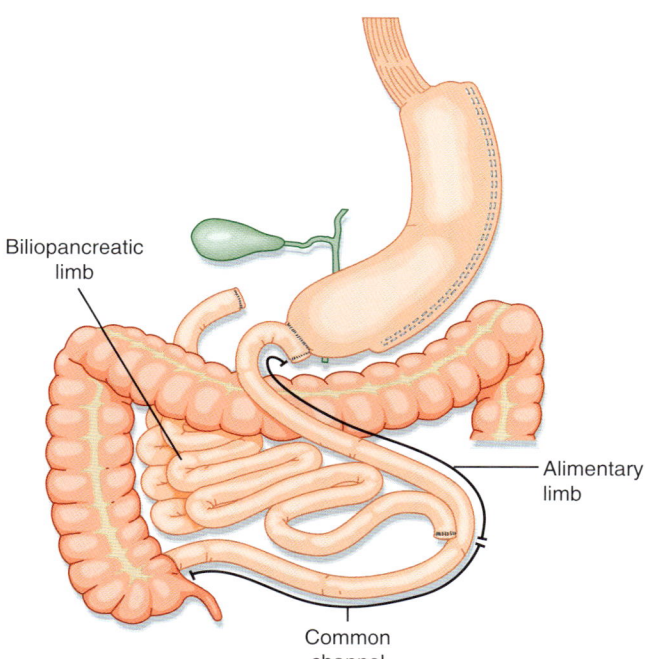

FIGURE 63.17 Configuration of duodenal switch. (From Poirier RF. Complications of bariatric surgery. In: Adams JG, Barton ED, Collings J, eds. *Emergency Medicine.* Philadelphia: Saunders; 2008.)

Biliopancreatic limb

Alimentary limb

Common channel

laparoscopic cholecystectomy when performed with LRYGB is quite low.[52]

OUTCOMES

DS provides the most durable, largest, long-term weight loss when compared with other bariatric operations.[12] Patients do ingest more calories per day, but the malabsorptive component of the operation produces the greater weight loss. Excess weight loss of 70% after 5 years or longer is commonly reported. Resolution or comorbidities of type 2 diabetes and hyperlipidemia are also optimal with this procedure. Resolution of other less metabolically related conditions, such as obstructive sleep apnea, are as good as or better than with LRYGB. In general, GERD resolution is comparable to that seen after SG, which is less optimal than after LRYGB.

COMPLICATIONS

Patients who undergo laparoscopic DS have similar risks for early postoperative complications as do those who undergo LRYGB. The potential for staple line leak, bleeding, and anastomotic stenosis and early obstruction are comparable and are seen in similar incidence. Late small bowel obstruction is as frequent after this procedure as after LRYGB, which has an incidence of from 3% to 7% in most series. Most surgeons will consider simultaneous cholecystectomy when performing DS. However, if the gallbladder is not removed, the incidence of gallstone formation postoperatively is significantly increased due to the decrease in bile salt pool. A high incidence of cholecystectomy is seen in this patient population long-term after DS.

Nutritional issues are of greater concern after DS than after the other operations described in this chapter because it is the only major malabsorptive operation currently performed in the United States. Length of the common channel is important in determining the risk of protein-calorie malnutrition. For common channel lengths less than 100 cm, this incidence is appreciable and greater than 5%. However, most surgeons rely on a common channel length of greater than 100 cm, most often in the 150-cm range. The overall incidence of protein-calorie malnutrition, the most concerning of the nutritional complications seen after DS, is between 0.5% and 4.9% for most published series in which this complication required operative intervention.[53] Less severe protein deficiencies likely occur more frequently. Episodes of mild protein-calorie malnutrition may be adequately treated with total parenteral nutrition to reverse the symptoms. However, repeated need for such treatments is an indication for reoperation and lengthening of the common channel. Few data exist as to how much lengthening is appropriate and likely varies from case to case. Assurance of an adequate length of absorptive bowel is the goal if reoperation is required. Standard prophylaxis for prevention of nutritional complications after DS includes parenteral replacement of fat-soluble vitamins, as well as supplementation of iron, vitamin B_{12}, and calcium. Patients who are contemplating DS should be aware of the potential out-of-pocket expense for full compliance with this regimen, which can be more than $1000 per year.

NOT YET STANDARDIZED PROCEDURES

SINGLE ANASTOMOSIS GASTRIC BYPASS

Initially described in the literature as the "mini gastric bypass," this operation has undergone some modification over the years and is now enjoying increased popularity. It has not yet been recognized as a standard operation for insurance reimbursement to date, although the numbers of patients successfully treated using the procedure continues to accumulate in the literature. The International Federation of Societies for Obesity (IFSO) has recently adopted the term *one-anastomosis gastric bypass (OAFB)* for this procedure. This procedure was introduced by Rutledge[54] and subsequently modified by others to increase the length of the gastric pouch to prevent bile reflux esophagitis (Fig. 63.18).

Indications for the SAGB are similar to those for gastric bypass. The operation confers slightly more malabsorption than LRYGB but is not associated with any significant incidence of protein-calorie malnutrition. Patients with metabolic comorbidities appear to be well served with this operation. Previous bowel resection, malabsorptive bowel diseases, and significant liver disease may all be contraindications to this operation.

OPERATIVE STEPS

The procedure begins with creation of a proximal gastric pouch that is longer than that created for a gastric bypass. The lesser curvature of the stomach is used in its entirety for the pouch. Adequate length of the pouch to prevent

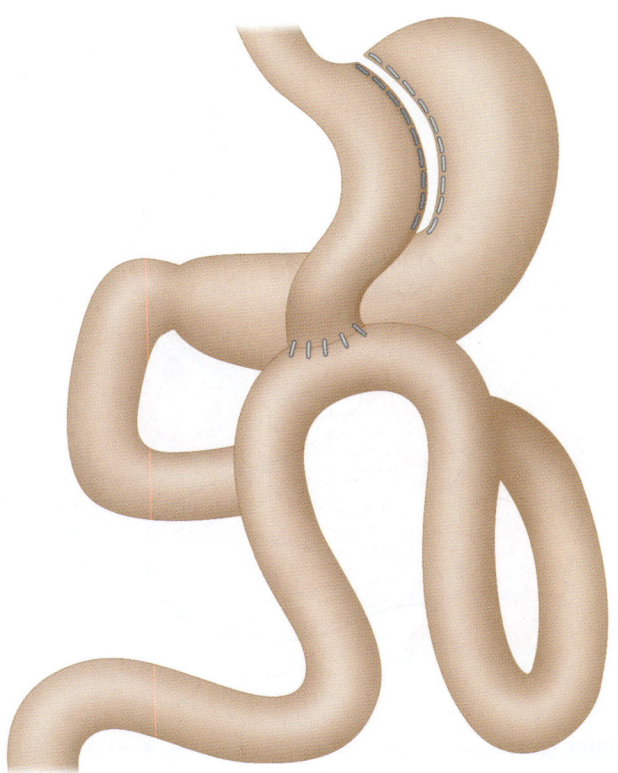

FIGURE 63.18 Configuration of one-anastomosis gastric bypass.

bile reflux to the esophagus is important and was a weakness of the initial operative procedure described.[54] The lesser curvature is important for use of the pouch due to its resistance to dilation postoperatively. A gastrojejunostomy is then performed at 200 cm distal to the ligament of Treitz. This may be created using a stapled or a handsewn anastomotic technique.

OUTCOMES

In a prospective randomized trial of mini gastric bypass versus standard gastric bypass, the weight loss for groups was slightly in favor of the mini gastric bypass.[55] More recent descriptions of outcomes of the operation show good weight loss as well as resolution of comorbid medical problems in a comparable manner as seen after LRYGB. The initial concern of biliary reflux esophagitis seen after this operation has been reduced with changes in the technique of lengthening the gastric pouch. Other complication rates for the procedure are generally similar to those seen after LRYGB. Kim et al. have shown good efficacy for the procedure.[56] A recently published 12-year experience with this operation for 1200 patients showed a 70% long-term excess weight loss and mortality of only 0.16%, with no reported long-term metabolic complications.[57]

Currently there are strong advocates for the adoption of this procedure as a standardized operation for metabolic and bariatric surgery, but as of yet the accumulated data have not swayed the general opinion of experts and societies sufficiently to include it as a standard procedure. However, the prognosis for its inclusion is improving with improving accumulated data.

SINGLE ANASTOMOSIS DUODENAL SWITCH

A somewhat analogous modification of the standard DS is the single anastomosis DS. A single duodenoileal anastomosis 200 cm proximal to the ileocecal valve has yielded excellent weight loss (>90% excess weight at 5 years) and excellent control of type 2 diabetes (HgbA1c <6.0 in 70% of insulin-dependent diabetics and 84% of those on oral medications at 5 years).[58] These results are from a single center, and review of the operation by the ASMBS Clinical Issues Committee concluded there was inadequate evidence to recommend the operation as a standard one.[59]

ENDOSCOPIC PROCEDURES

Endoscopic procedures may become very important in the near future as part of the overall treatment of obesity and its medically related conditions. Currently only 1% to 2% of eligible patients have surgery to treat morbid obesity. The only major increase in the number of such operative procedures performed over the past 4 decades occurred when laparoscopic procedures were introduced. Introduction of endoscopic treatment options may promote a similar increase in the use of procedures by patients to help them overcome the issues and problems of morbid obesity. Furthermore, endoscopic procedures may also have a potentially larger audience than standard surgical procedures because their indication is to date for the patient population with a BMI of 30 to 40, a larger group than that with a BMI greater than 40.

INTRAGASTRIC BALLOONS

Two brands of intragastric balloons received US Food and Drug Administration (FDA) approval for use in the United States in the summer of 2015. The Obera balloon is a single balloon system, whereas the Reshape balloon has two smaller balloons joined together. Both work on the principle of creating a large space-occupying object to fill the diameter of much of the lumen of the stomach.[60] There has been much experience in the past 15 years in other countries using the Bioenterics Intragastric Balloon. Meta-analysis shows that system produces an average 15 kg weight loss or 32% of excess weight after 1 year in patients.[61] However, the few long-term studies that have looked at outcomes after intragastric balloon show a high incidence of weight regain by 5 years.[62] These balloon systems all use endoscopy for balloon placement and withdrawal 6 months later. Balloon systems that are placed without endoscopy in the office are currently being trialed in the United States.

OTHER ENDOSCOPIC SUTURING PROCEDURES

The potential for performing a standard bariatric and metabolic operative procedure using a totally endoscopic approach has now arrived. Over the past decade, a number of endoscopic procedures have been trialed to reproduce the restriction or malabsorption of standard bariatric surgical procedures. Unfortunately, most of these have been abandoned or the instrumentation used to perform them removed from the market. Restrictive operative procedures using the EndoCinch procedure proved ineffective at maintaining suture integrity, and it has been removed from the market. Diversion of food from duodenal absorption was achieved with the EndoBarrier, an endoscopic sleeve procedure,[63] which has been removed from the market due to an increased incidence of hepatic abscess. The AspireAssist device, FDA approved, is essentially a gastrostomy tube that is opened postprandially to allow gastric contents to drain out.[64]

The most promising of all the current endoscopic procedures is the endoscopic sleeve gastrectomy, or ESG procedure. Performed by using the Overstitch device, the procedure reproduces approximately the configuration of a sleeve gastrectomy by performing a sutured gastroplasty with a limited-size lumen for gastric contents. Published data to date have shown a mean total body weight loss at 18 months of 20% with an excellent safety profile.[65]

Although none of the endoscopic procedures has yet proven as effective or durable as standard metabolic and bariatric surgical procedures, it remains that only approximately 1% of eligible patients elect to undergo metabolic and bariatric surgery. This is despite the recent very safe track record for standard operations. It is hoped that the less invasive aspect of these endoscopic procedures may prove more acceptable to patients who then will begin the process of using endoscopic then perhaps later surgical procedural assistance to combat their disease of severe obesity.

CONCLUSION

The most commonly performed operations both in the United States and worldwide are the LSG and the

LRYGB. Both are associated with excellent durable weight loss and resolution of associated medical comorbidities. These operations are furthermore done with increasing safety, such that they are associated with lower morbidity and mortality than all intraabdominal operations except appendectomy. The LAGB is rapidly losing popularity due to poor long-term efficacy, whereas the DS and other malabsorptive operations are chosen infrequently by patients. Finally, new endoscopic and minimally invasive procedures offer potentially less invasive mechanisms of producing weight loss, although their long-term efficacy and durability still are not established.

REFERENCES

1. Mason EE, Ito C. Gastric bypass in obesity. *Surg Clin North Am.* 1969;47:1345-1351.
2. Mason EE, Doherty C, Cullen JJ, Scott D, Rodriguez EM, Maher JW. Vertical gastroplasty: evolution of vertical banded gastroplasty. *World J Surg.* 1998;22:919-924.
3. Griffen WO, Young VL, Stevenson CC. A prospective comparison of gastric and jejunoileal bypass procedures for morbid obesity. *Ann Surg.* 1977;186:500-509.
4. Deitel M. Overview of operations for morbid obesity. *World J Surg.* 1998;22:913-918.
5. Griffen WO, Bivins MA, Bell RM, Jackson KA. Gastric bypass for morbid obesity. *World J Surg.* 1981;5:817-822.
6. Sugerman HJ, Wolfe LG, Sica DA, Clore JN. Diabetes and hypertension in severe obesity and effects of gastric bypass-induced weight loss. *Ann Surg.* 2003;237:751-758.
7. Sugerman HJ, Felton WL 3rd, Sismanis A, Kellum JM, DeMaria EJ, Sugerman EL. Gastric surgery for pseudotumor cerebri associated with severe obesity. *Ann Surg.* 1999;229:634-642.
8. Sugerman HJ, Sugerman EL, Wolfe L, Kellum JM Jr, Schweitzer MA, DeMaria EJ. Risks and benefits of gastric bypass in morbidly obese patients with severe venous stasis disease. *Ann Surg.* 2001;234:41-46.
9. Pories WJ, MacDonald KG, Flickinger EG, et al. Is type II diabetes mellitus (NIDDM) a surgical disease? *Ann Surg.* 1992;215:633-643.
10. Christou NV, Sampalis JS, Liberman M, et al. Surgery decreases long-term mortality, morbidity, and health care use in morbidly obese patients. *Ann Surg.* 2004;240:416-424.
11. Sampalis JS, Liberman M, Auger S, Christou NV. The impact of weight reduction surgery on health-care costs in morbidly obese patients. *Obes Surg.* 2004;14:939-947.
12. Buchwald H, Avidor Y, Braunwald E, et al. Bariatric surgery. A systematic review and meta-analysis. *JAMA.* 2004;292:1724-1737.
13. Adams TD, Gress RE, Smith SC, et al. Long-term mortality after gastric bypass surgery. *N Engl J Med.* 2007;357(8):753-761.
14. Wittgrove AC, Clark WG, Tremblay LJ. Laparoscopic gastric bypass, Roux en-Y: preliminary report of five cases. *Obes Surg.* 1994;4:353-357.
15. Schauer PR, Ikramuddin S, Gourash W, Ramanathan R, Luketich J. Outcomes after laparoscopic Roux-en-Y gastric bypass for morbid obesity. *Ann Surg.* 2000;232:515-529.
16. Nguyen NT, Goldman C, Rosenquist CJ, et al. Laparoscopic versus open gastric bypass: a randomized study of outcomes, quality of life, and costs. *Ann Surg.* 2001;234:279-289.
17. Santry H, Gillen DL, Lauderdale DS. Trends in bariatric surgical procedures. *JAMA.* 2005;294:1909-1917.
18. Belachew M, Legrand MJ, Defechereux TH, Burtheret MP, Jacquet N. Laparoscopic adjustable silicone gastric banding in the treatment of morbid obesity. A preliminary report. *Surg Endosc.* 1994;8:1354-1356.
19. Dixon JB, O'Brien PE. Laparoscopic adjustable gastric banding: outcomes. In: Schauer PR, Schirmer BD, Brethauer SA, eds. *Minimally Invasive Bariatric Surgery.* New York: Springer; 2007:189-196.
20. Aarts EO, Dogan K, Koehestanie P, Aufenacker TJ, Janssen IM, Berends FJ. Long-term results after laparoscopic adjustable gastric banding: a mean fourteen-year follow-up study. *Surg Obes Relat Dis.* 2014;4:633-640.
21. Ren CJ, Patterson E, Gagner M. Early results of laparoscopic biliopancreatic diversion with duodenal switch: a case series of 40 consecutive patients. *Obes Surg.* 2000;10:514-524.
22. Brethauer SA, Hammel JP, Schauer PR. Systematic review of sleeve gastrectomy as staging and primary bariatric procedure. *Surg Obes Relat Dis.* 2009;5:469-475.
23. Scopinaro N, Gianetta E, Civalleri D, Bonalumi U, Bachi V. Biliopancreatic bypass for obesity. Initial experience in man. *Br J Surg.* 1979;66:618-620.
24. Marceau P, Hould FS, Simard S, et al. Biliopancreatic diversion with a duodenal switch. *World J Surg.* 1998;22:947-954.
25. Hess DS, Hess DW. Biliopancreatic diversion with a duodenal switch. *Obes Surg.* 1998;8:267-282.
26. Flum DR, Dellinger EP. Impact of gastric bypass operation on survival: a population-based analysis. *J Am Coll Surg.* 2004;199:543-551.
27. Hutter MM, Schirmer BD, Jones DB, et al. First report of the American College of Surgeons Bariatric Surgery Center Network: laparoscopic sleeve gastrectomy has morbidity and effectiveness positioned between the band and the bypass. *Ann Surg.* 2011;254:410-422.
28. Morton JM, Garg T, Nguyen N. Does hospital accreditation impact bariatric surgery safety? *Ann Surg.* 2014;260:504-509.
29. O'Brien PE, Dixon JB, Brown W, et al. The laparoscopic adjustable gastric banding (Lap-Band): a prospective study of medium-term effects on weight, health, and quality of life. *Obes Surg.* 2002;12:652-660.
30. Carelli AM, Youn HA, Kurian MS, Ren CJ, Fielding GA. Safety of the laparoscopic adjustable gastric band: 7-year data from a U.S. center of excellence. *Surg Endosc.* 2010;24:1819-1823.
31. Dixon JB, O'Brien PE, Playfair J, et al. Adjustable gastric banding and conventional therapy for type 2 diabetes: a randomized controlled trial. *JAMA.* 2008;279:316-323.
32. Allen JW. Laparoscopic gastric band complications. *Med Clin North Am.* 2007;9:485-497.
33. National Institutes of Health Consensus Conference. Gastrointestinal surgery for severe obesity, Consensus Development Conference Panel. *Ann Intern Med.* 1991;115:956-961.
34. Kindel TL, Oleynikov D. The improvement of gastroesophageal reflux disease and Barretts after bariatric surgery. *Obes Surg.* 2016;26:718-720.
35. Schauer PR, Bhatt DL, Kiwan JP, et al. Bariatric surgery versus intensive medical therapy for diabetes—3-year outcomes. *N Engl J Med.* 2014;370:2002-2013.
36. Mehaffey JH, LaPar DJ, Clement KC, et al. 10-Year outcomes after Roux-en-Y gastric bypass. *Ann Surg.* 2016;264:121-126.
37. Schirmer B, Erenoglu C, Miller A. Flexible endoscopy in the management of patients undergoing Roux-en-Y gastric bypass. *Obes Surg.* 2002;12:634-638.
38. Azagury DE, Abu Dayyeh BK, Greenwalt IT, Thompson CC. Marginal ulceration after Roux-en-Y gastric bypass surgery: characteristics, risk factors, treatment, and outcomes. *Endoscopy.* 2011;43:950-954.
39. Marceau P, Biron S, Bourque RA, Potvin M, Hould FS, Simard S. Biliopancreatic diversion with a new type of gastrectomy. *Obes Surg.* 1993;3:29-35.
40. Regan JP, Inabnet WB, Gagner M, Pomp A. Early experience with two-stage laparoscopic Roux-en-Y gastric bypass as an alternative in the super-super obese patient. *Obes Surg.* 2003;13:861-864.
41. D'Hondt M, Venneste S, Pottel H, Devriendt D, Van Rooy F, Vansteenkiste F. Laparoscopic sleeve gastrectomy as a single-stage procedure for the treatment of morbid obesity and the resulting quality of life, resolution of comorbidities, food tolerance, and 6-year weight loss. *Surg Endosc.* 2011;25:2498-2504.
42. Gagner M, Deitel M, Erickson AL, Crosby RD. Survey on laparoscopic sleeve gastrectomy (LSG) at the Fourth International Consensus Summit on Sleeve Gastrectomy. *Obes Surg.* 2013;23:2013-2017.
43. Wang Z, Dai X, Xie H, Feng J, Li Z, Lu Q. The efficacy of staple line reinforcement during laparoscopic sleeve gastrectomy: a meta-analysis of randomized controlled trials. *Int J Surg.* 2016;25:145-152.
44. Bingham J, Lallemand M, Baron M, et al. Routine intraoperative leak testing for sleeve gastrectomy: is the leak test full of hot air? *Am J Surg.* 2016;211:943-947.
45. Wang S, Li P, Sun XF, Ye NY, Xu ZK, Wang D. Comparison between laparoscopic sleeve gastrectomy and laparoscopic adjustable gastric banding for morbid obesity: a meta-analysis. *Obes Surg.* 2013;23:980-986.
46. Peterli R, Wolnerhanssen BK, Vetter D, et al. Laparoscopic sleeve gastrectomy versus Roux-en-Y gastric bypass for morbid obesity—3-year outcomes of the prospective randomized Swiss multicenter bypass or sleeve study (SM-BOSS). *Ann Surg.* 2017;265:466-473.
47. DuPree CE, Blair K, Steele SR, Martin MJ. Laparoscopic sleeve gastrectomy in patients with preexisting gastroesophageal reflux disease: a national analysis. *JAMA Surg.* 2014;149:328-334.

48. Gagner M, Hutchinson C, Rosenthal R. Fifth international consensus conference: current status of sleeve gastrectomy. *Surg Obes Relat Dis.* 2016;12:750-756.

49. Cho JM, Kim HJ, Lo Menzo E, Park S, Szomstein S, Rosenthal RJ. Effect of sleeve gastrectomy on type 2 diabetes as an alternative treatment modality to Roux-en-Y gastric bypass: systemic review and meta-analysis. *Surg Obes Relat Dis.* 2015;11:1273-1280.

50. Young MT, Gebhart A, Phelan MJ, Nguyen NT. Use and outcomes of laparoscopic sleeve gastrectomy vs. laparoscopic gastric bypass: analysis of the American College of Surgeons NSQIP. *J Am Coll Surg.* 2015;220:880-885.

51. Berger ER, Clements RH, Morton JM, et al. The impact of different surgical techniques on outcomes in laparoscopic sleeve gastrectomies. First report from the Metabolic and Bariatric Surgery Accreditation and Quality Improvement Program (MBSAQIP). *Ann Surg.* 2016;264:464-473.

52. Kim JJ, Schirmer B. Safety and efficacy of simultaneous cholecystectomy at the time of Roux-en-Y gastric bypass. *Surg Obes Relat Dis.* 2009;5:48-53.

53. Phillipe A, Topart MD, Becouam G. Revision and reversal for biliopancreatic diversion for excessive side effects or ineffective weight loss: a review of the current literature on indications and procedures. *Surg Obes Relat Dis.* 2015;11:965-972.

54. Rutledge R. The mini-gastric bypass: experience with the first 1,274 cases. *Obes Surg.* 2001;11:276-280.

55. Lee WJ, Ser KH, Lee YC, Tsou JJ, Chen SC, Chen JC. Laparoscopic Roux-en-Y vs. mini-gastric bypass for the treatment of morbid obesity: a 10-year experience. *Obes Surg.* 2012;22:1827-1834.

56. Lee WJ, Lin YH. Single-anastomosis gastric bypass (SAGB): appraisal of clinical evidence. *Obes Surg.* 2014;24:1749-1756.

57. Carbajo MA, Luque-de-Leon E, Jiminez JM, Ortiz-de-Solórzano J, Pérez-Miranda M, Castro-Alija MJ. Laparoscopic one-anastomosis gastric bypass: technique, results, and long-term follow-up in 1200 patients. *Obes Surg.* 2017;27(5):1153-1167.

58. Sanchez-Pernaute A, Angel Rubio M, Cabrerizo L, Ramos-Levi A, Pérez-Aguirre E, Torres A. Single-anastomosis duodenoileal bypass with sleeve gastrectomy (SADI-S) for obese diabetic patients. *Surg Obes Relat Dis.* 2015;11:1092-1098.

59. Kim J, ASMBS Clinical Issues Committee. ASMBS statement on single anastomosis duodenal switch. *Surg Obes Relat Dis.* 2016;12:944-945.

60. Bazerbachi F, Vargas Valls EJ, Abu Dayyeh BK. Recent clinical results of endoscopic bariatric therapies as an obesity intervention. *Clin Endosc.* 2017;50:42-50.

61. Imaz I, Martinez-Cervell C, Sendra-Gutierrez JM, Gonzalez-Enriquez J. Safety and effectiveness of intragastric balloon for obesity. A meta analysis. *Obes Surg.* 2008;7:841-846.

62. Dastis NS, Francois E, Deviere J. Intragastric balloon for weight loss: results in 100 individuals followed for at least 2.5 years. *Endoscopy.* 2009;41:575-580.

63. ASGE Bariatric Endoscopy Task Force and ASGE Technology Committee, Abu Dayyeh BK, Kumar N, et al. ASGE Bariatric Endoscopy Task Force systematic review and meta-analysis assessing the ASGE PIVI thresholds for adopting endoscopic bariatric therapies. *Gastrointest Endosc.* 2015;82:425-438.

64. Thompson CC, Abu Dayyeh BK, Kushner R, et al. Percutaneous gastrostomy device for the treatment of class II and Class III obesity: results of a randomized controlled trial. *Am J Gastroenterol.* 2017;112(3):447-457.

65. Lopez-Nava G, Sharaiha RX, Neto M, et al. Endoscopic sleeve gastroplasty for obesity: a multicenter study of 242 patients with 18 months follow-up. *Gastroenterology.* 2016;150(4 suppl 1):S26.

Foreign Bodies and Bezoars of the Stomach and Small Intestine

Stephanie Scurci | Robert Kozol

FOREIGN BODY INGESTION

Foreign body ingestion is an unusual occurrence. Foreign body ingestion may be intentional or unintentional. There are several ways to classify and consider foreign body ingestion. One way is by type of object (size and shape). Foreign body ingestion may also be considered according to age groups. It is well established that 80% to 90% of ingested foreign objects will pass through the gastrointestinal (GI) tract without intervention. Endoscopic removal is required in 10% to 20% of cases and about 1% will require surgical intervention.[1]

FOREIGN BODY INGESTION IN CHILDREN

Witnessed foreign body ingestion in small children is generally addressed rapidly. In cases where the ingestion was both unintentional and not realized, clinical presentation will depend on where the foreign object becomes lodged. For example, in the pharynx, symptoms are usually immediate and include choking and hypersalivation. In the esophagus, dysphagia or odynophagia usually occur early after ingestion. The treatment is urgent endoscopic removal of the foreign object. Detailed algorithms for endoscopic therapy in children have been published by the North America Society for Pediatric Gastroenterology, Hepatology, and Nutrition.[2] Foreign objects in the stomach most commonly pass into the small bowel. However, if a foreign object lodges in the stomach, it may cause nausea and/or vomiting but also may remain without presenting symptoms for a considerable time. Foreign objects in the small bowel frequently pass into the colon. Objects in the small bowel may cause injury at any point, but often become lodged in the distal ileum due to its small caliber. Injuries in the small bowel include perforation and fistula formation. These situations are discussed in detail in this chapter.

EXPLORATORY INGESTION

Exploratory ingestion is the term used when small children ingest substances while exploring their environment.[3] These cases are usually not witnessed. The age group most at risk is from 6 months to 3 years of age. Common objects ingested include coins, batteries, pills, and pins. Based on their size and shape, almost all coins, pebbles, and small stones pass spontaneously. Rarely, such an object will lodge in the terminal ileum causing small bowel obstruction. As mentioned, any object lodged in the esophagus should be removed urgently via endoscopy. This is because neglected foreign bodies in the esophagus may lead to esophageal perforation requiring thoracotomy and repair.[4] Once an object enters the stomach it will likely pass spontaneously. However, sharp, long (>6 cm), or large (wider than 2.5 cm) objects in the stomach should be removed endoscopically. Once in the small bowel, even sharp objects can be watched vigilantly via imaging. These patients must be observed as inpatients because perforation occurs in 15% to 35% of cases.[1] Signs of obstruction or perforation indicate emergency operation.

MAGNETS

Several foreign body ingestion types in children require special attention. Ingestion of multiple magnets is rare but dangerous. This foreign body ingestion puts a child at risk for perforation and/or fistula formation.[5] A solitary magnet will almost always pass spontaneously. Multiple magnets seen on radiographs in the esophagus or stomach should be removed endoscopically. Multiple magnets in the small bowel in an asymptomatic child may be followed with serial plain films. Magnets in adjacent bowel loops or a single magnet with another metallic foreign object may erode the adjacent loops, resulting in perforation or fistula formation (Fig. 64.1). These cases require surgical intervention.

LAUNDRY PODS

Colorful laundry pods are new items causing problems in small children. The pods look like candy. In this patient group, 4% to 5% require hospitalization.[6] Ingestion may cause metabolic acidosis with an increased anion gap. Symptoms may include nausea, vomiting, and somnolence. These patients may require endotracheal intubation and ventilator support. At least one death has been reported.[7]

BATTERIES

Although ingestion of cylindrical batteries is usually harmless, ingestion of modern disc batteries are of grave concern. These batteries contain alkaline electrodes capable of causing rapid liquefaction necrosis of tissue. Injuries may be due to leakage of battery content or by the generation of an electrical current. It has been reported that 85% of these batteries pass spontaneously without causing problems.[8] However, larger disc batteries may lodge in the esophagus. The combination of both larger size and lithium cell seems to be important, because outcomes for lithium ingestions less than 20 mm are comparable to other cell types.[9] This has resulted in perforation, tracheoesophageal fistula, mediastinitis, erosion into a carotid artery, and death.[10] These batteries are usually apparent on plain films. Batteries lodged in the esophagus must be treated with emergency endoscopic

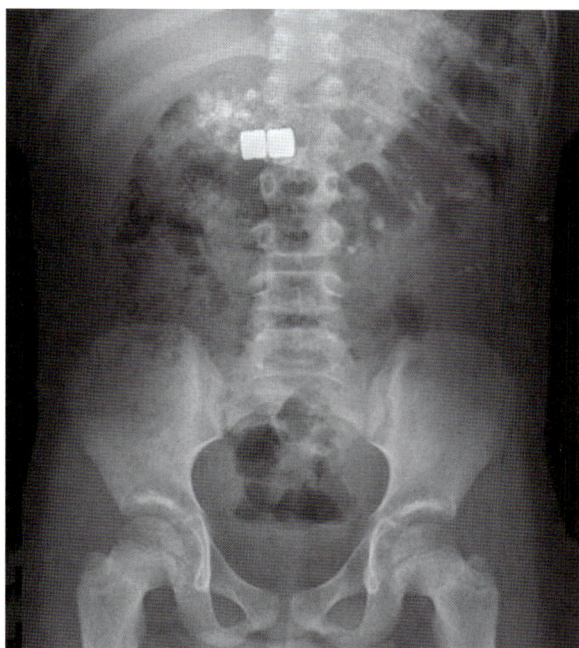

FIGURE 64.1 A 7-year-old boy who had two groups of magnets surgically removed from the small bowel. Radiograph reveals a central gap between two magnet conglomerates, suggesting entrapment of the bowel wall. (With kind permission from Guelfguat M, Kaplinskiy V, Reddy SH, DiPoce J. Clinical guidelines for imaging and reporting ingested foreign bodies. *AJR Am J Roentgenol*. 2014;203:37.)

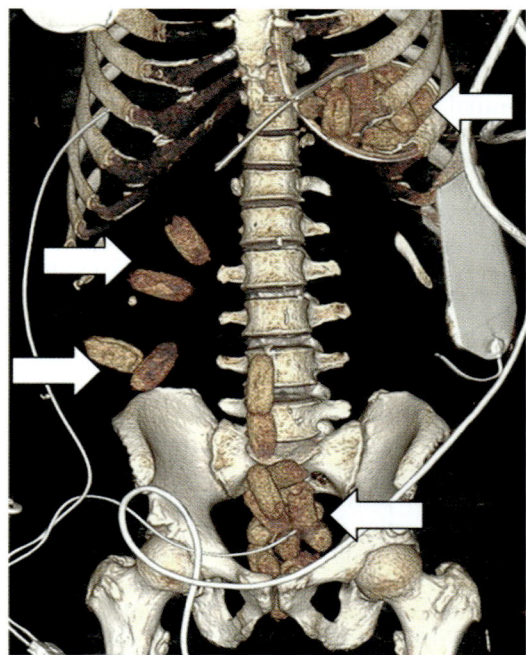

FIGURE 64.2 Three-dimensional volume rendered computed tomography image highlighting the burden of foreign material in the stomach, ascending colon, and rectosigmoid (arrows), most of which was obscured on plain radiography. (From Esterson YB, Vihas P, Nicastro J, Friedman B. Plain radiography may underestimate the burden of body packer ingestion: a case report. *Clin Imaging*. 2017;44:57-60.)

removal. Batteries distal to the esophagus will most frequently pass spontaneously.

ADOLESCENTS

In adolescents, esophageal food impaction is most common.[11] These may be precipitated by a sudden event like a motor vehicle accident. Intentional ingestions may be secondary to mental illness or may occur for secondary gain. One well-recognized example of the former is trichophagia, the chronic ingestion of their own hair, usually seen in teenage girls. This may result in a trichobezoar, which is covered in detail later in this chapter.

ADULTS

Intentional Ingestion

An example of intentional ingestion for secondary gain is that of a prisoner who dismantles his toilet and ingests toilet parts in order to be transferred to a medical facility. The senior author of this chapter treated such a patient on multiple occasions. The toilet parts were lodged in the stomach and removed via flexible endoscopy. Another clever ploy seen in prisoners or patients with Munchausen syndrome is to ingest razor blades wrapped in thick paper. On radiographs, the wrap is not seen and the patients are operated upon.

Illicit Drugs: Drug Packers

Body packing is the transportation of illicit drugs by internal concealment, which has increased in recent

years as a result of increased border security since 9/11.[12] Most commonly the drugs are heroin, cocaine, and amphetamines. Body packers may use antimotility drugs (loperamide) during transit and promotility agents (metoclopramide) once they arrive at their destination. Many drug packers are asymptomatic. In symptomatic patients, symptoms range from nausea and vomiting to abdominal pain and obstruction. Computed tomography (CT) scanning is most sensitive for diagnosis; however plain films may be used to monitor the progress of packets (Fig. 64.2).

In most cases, patients can be given a bowel regimen and observed until the passage of all packets.[13] This is in part because of more sophisticated packet production, which has reduced the risk of rupture. When rupture does occur, it can be fatal, so endoscopic retrieval should not be attempted in most cases. Surgical intervention is required if packets rupture, cause small bowel obstruction, or fail to progress through the GI tract. A final on-table radiograph should be obtained to confirm that all packets have been successfully removed.

Unintentional Ingestion

Toothpicks. In adults, a common unintentional foreign body ingestion is seen with toothpicks.[14,15] A common situation concerns people who chronically chew on toothpicks. The patient will likely recognize such an ingestion. A second scenario is seen with a diner eating an hors d'oeuvre or sandwich fixed by a toothpick. Alcoholic beverages usually accompany this. These patients usually do not recognize the ingestion. Long sharp objects such as toothpicks and animal bones are prone to cause perforation of the GI tract. The most common sites are the terminal ileum and the rectosigmoid. These patients present with abdominal pain and may have sepsis. On radiographs, they may have free air under the diaphragm or adjacent to the injury. Perforations at the terminal ileum, on CT scan, often have fat stranding and thickening of the bowel and mesentery. The differential diagnosis on CT may include perforated appendicitis, Crohn disease, or lymphoma. Often the precise diagnosis is only made at operation. If the foreign body perforation is recognized on radiographs in the rectum or in rare cases in the terminal ileum, some cases may be treated with endoscopic removal and antibiotics.

Dentures. In the elderly population, dentures account for the most commonly ingested foreign body.[16] The radiolucency of polymethylmethacrylate (PMMA), the base of most partial denture prosthetics, can also make diagnosis challenging. Metallic struts frequently allow identification on imaging. Patients may present with nonspecific symptoms or may be unable to provide an accurate history. The most common site of impaction is the esophagus, for which endoscopy is the treatment of choice.[17] Surgical intervention is required for dentures that perforate, obstruct, or fail to pass with observation.

Noningested Foreign Bodies. The modern use of biliary and pancreatic stents represents foreign bodies intentionally placed by physicians. The use of stents for obstructive biliary and pancreatic disorders has increased dramatically over the past few decades. Stents may be metallic or plastic. Stents may be permanent in patients with a short life expectancy but are more frequently removed when the disorder has resolved. Distal stent migration occurs in 5% to 10% of cases.[18] Most such cases can be managed expectantly, because the stents pass through the GI tract. However, small bowel obstruction or perforation as a result of the stent mandates surgical intervention. Endoscopic removal of proximally migrated biliary stents is successful in more than 80% of patients.[19] With distal biliary migration, the stent often passes naturally through the GI tract, although it may become lodged, resulting in possible obstruction or perforation.[20]

GASTRIC BEZOARS

Bezoars are aggregates of indigestible material that accumulate in the GI tract. The word *bezoar* is derived from the Arabic *bazahr* or *badzehr*, which means "antidote" or "counter-poison." For centuries, animal bezoars, bezoar stones, were believed to have the ability to soak up poison. Their pharmaceutical use was abandoned in the 19th century.

Gastric bezoars are rare, with an incidence of about 0.5%.[21] Bezoars may be found anywhere in the GI tract, but the stomach is the most common location. The curved shape of the stomach and narrow pyloric outlet contribute to the accumulation of bezoars.

Several risk factors predispose patients to the development of bezoars including gastroparesis, psychiatric disorders like pica, wearing of dentures, and the use of

TABLE 64.1   Contents of Various Bezoars

Phytobezoar	Trichobezoar	Pharmacobezoar
Celery	Hair	Nifedipine
Pumpkin	Carpet fibers	Procainamide
Grape skins	String	Verapamil
Prunes	Clothing	Theophylline
Raisins		Cholestyramine
Leeks		Meprobamate
Beets		Sucralfate
Persimmons		Kayexalate resin
		Guar gum
		Enteral feeding formulas
		Vitamin C tablets
		Vitamin B$_{12}$
		Lecithin
		Ferrous sulfate

From Pfau PR, Ginsberg GG. Foreign bodies and bezoars. In: Feldman M, Friedman LS, Sleisenger MH, et al, eds. *Gastrointestinal and Liver Disease*. Philadelphia: Saunders; 2002:386.

anticholinergics and opiates. Gastric surgery, most commonly gastrectomy, vagotomy, and restrictive bariatric procedures including Roux-en-y gastric bypass and sleeve gastrectomy, may also contribute to the development of gastric bezoars.

Bezoars are characterized by their composition as phytobezoars, pharmacobezoars, trichobezoars, or lactobezoars (Table 64.1). Phytobezoars are most common and develop from poorly digested fibrous plant or fruit material (Fig. 64.3). One subtype of phytobezoars that is particularly hard and difficult to treat forms from the persimmon fruit and is named the diospyrobezoar.[21]

Pharmacobezoars are composed of medications, especially those with extended release enteric coatings designed to resist digestion. Trichobezoars are composed of human hair, which is difficult to digest as a result of the enzyme-resistant cuticle. These are most commonly found in young female patients with psychiatric illnesses.

DIAGNOSIS

Most bezoars do not cause a complete obstruction and are therefore asymptomatic. The cases that do produce symptoms tend to be nonspecific and present insidiously. Presenting symptoms include abdominal pain, nausea, vomiting, early satiety, weight loss, and anorexia. Late presenting symptoms may include GI bleeding due to concomitant gastric ulcers.[22]

Gastric outlet obstruction is rare for gastric bezoars. However, the patient may present with a small bowel obstruction if the bezoar passes into the small intestine. Physical exam is often normal, although occasionally a palpable mass may be found. Plain film or upper GI contrast studies may be used to identify large, obstructing lesions.

CT scan is more sensitive and can more specifically detect bezoars by the appearance of trapped air bubbles and surrounding mottled appearance.[23] Endoscopy remains the gold standard for both the diagnosis and treatment of bezoars and can also rule out malignancy.

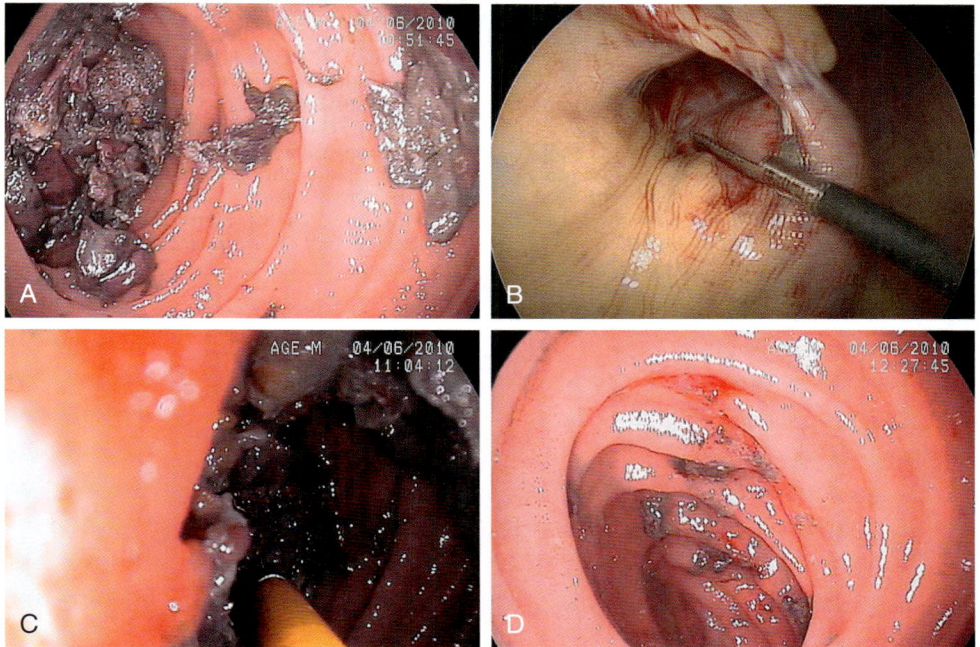

FIGURE 64.3 (A) Phytobezoar distal to gastrojejunal anastomosis. (B) Patent mesocolic window. (C) Endoscopy showing endoscopic fragmentation of bezoar using biopsy forceps. (D) Patent Roux limb after endoscopic fragmentation of bezoar. (From Powers WF, Miles DR: Phytobezoar causing small bowel obstruction seven years after laparoscopic Roux-en-Y bypass. *Surg Obes Related Dis*. 2011;7:e3-e5.)

MANAGEMENT

Once a diagnosis is made, treatment may consist of medical management, endoscopic removal, or surgery. Bezoars that are minimally symptomatic may initially be treated with chemical dissolution. Treatment with cola, cellulase, papain, and N-acetylcysteine has been described with variable results. A 40% to 70% success rate has been reported, and most treatments are well tolerated.[24]

The addition of promotility agents such as metoclopramide (Reglan) has been found to reduce time to dissolution.[25] On occasion, bezoars that are only partially digested may pass into the small bowel and cause obstruction, which often needs to be treated with surgery.

Most gastric bezoars require endoscopic therapy to mechanically fragment the bezoar. A water jet is commonly used, followed by removal with suction, snare, or forceps. Success rates approach 80% to 90% with endoscopic therapy alone.[23] When chemical dissolution and endoscopic therapy fail, surgery is required. Associated complications may include refractory bleeding, obstruction, or perforation. A laparoscopic approach is often initially attempted and intraoperative endoscopy may be considered to improve localization. Once a bezoar has been cleared, therapy aimed at prevention of recurrence should be instituted including consideration for psychiatric assessment, if appropriate.

REFERENCES

1. Webb WA. Management of foreign bodies of the upper gastrointestinal tract: update. *Gastrointest Endosc.* 1995;41:36.
2. Kramer RE, Lerner DG, Lin T, et al. Management of ingested foreign bodies in children: a clinical report of the NASPGHAN Endoscopy Committee. *J Pediatr Gastroenterol Nutr.* 2015;60(4):562-574.
3. Fontane E. Ingestion of concentrated laundry detergent pods. *J Emerg Med.* 2015;49(1):e37-e38.
4. Peters NJ, Mahajan JK, Bawa M, Chabbra A, Garg R, Rao KLN. Esophageal perforations due to foreign body impaction in children. *J Pediatr Surg.* 2015;50(8):1260-1263.
5. Romine M, Ham PB, Yon JR, Pipkin WL, Howell CG, Hatley RM. Multiple magnet ingestion in children. *Am Surg.* 2014;80(7):e189-e191.
6. Valdez AL, Casavant MJ, Spiller HA, Chounthirath T, Xiang H, Smith GA. Pediatric exposure to laundry detergent pods. *Pediatrics.* 2014;134(6):1127-1135.
7. Hernández AR. Infant dies after ingesting detergent pod. *Orlando Sentinel.* 2013.
8. Chang YJ, Chao HC, Kong MS, Lai MW. Clinical analysis of disc battery ingestion in children. *Chang Gung Med J.* 2004;27(9):673-677.
9. Litovitz T, Whitaker N, Clark L, White NC, Marsolek M. Emerging battery-ingestion hazard: clinical implications. *Pediatrics.* 2010;125(6):1168-1177.
10. Centers for Disease Control and Prevention (CDC). Injuries from batteries among children aged <13 years—United States, 1995–2010. *MMWR Morb Mortal Wkly Rep.* 2012;61(34):661.
11. Sahn B, Mamula P, Ford CA. Review of foreign body ingestion and esophageal food impaction management in adolescents. *J Adolesc Health.* 2014;55(2):260-266.
12. Traub SJ, Hoffman RS, Nelson LS. Body packing—the internal concealment of illicit drugs. *N Engl J Med.* 2003;349:2519.
13. Bulstrode N, Banks F, Shrotria S. The outcome of drug smuggling by "body packers"—the British experience. *Ann R Coll Surg Engl.* 2002;84:35.
14. Steinbach C, Stockmann M, Jara M, Bednarsch J, Lock JF. Accidentally ingested toothpicks causing severe gastrointestinal injury: a practical guideline for diagnosis and therapy based on 136 case reports. *World J Surg.* 2014;38(2):371-377.
15. Zouros E, Oikonomou D, Theoharis G, Bantias C, Papadimitropoulos K. Perforation of the cecum by a toothpick: report of a case and review of the literature. *J Emerg Med.* 2014;47(6):e133-e137.

16. Haidary A, Leider J, Silbergleit R. Unsuspected swallowing of a partial denture. *AJNR Am J Neuroradiol.* 2007;28:1734.

17. Gachaboyov M, Isaev M, Orujova L, Isaev E, Yaskin E, Neronov D. Swallowed dentures: two cases and a review. *Ann Med Surg.* 2015;4:407.

18. Diller R, Senninger N, Kautz G, Tübergen D. Stent migration necessitating surgical intervention. *Surg Endosc.* 2003;17:1803.

19. Tarnasky PR, Cotton PB, Baillie J, et al. Proximal migration of biliary stents: attempted endoscopic retrieval in forty-one patients. *Gastrointest Endosc.* 1995;42(6):513-519.

20. Mistry BM, Memon MA, Silverman R, et al. Small bowel perforation from a migrated biliary stent. *Surg Endosc.* 2001;15:1043.

21. Andrus CH, Ponsky JL. Bezoars: classification, pathophysiology, and treatment. *Am J Gastroenterol.* 1988;83:476.

22. Byrne WJ. Foreign bodies, bezoars, and caustic ingestion. *Gastrointest Endosc Clin N Am.* 1994;4:99.

23. Iwamuro M, Okada H, Matsueda K, et al. Review of the diagnosis and management of gastrointestinal bezoars. *World J Gastrointest Endosc.* 2015;7:336.

24. Ladas D, Kamberoglou D, Karamanolis G, Vlachogiannakos J, Zouboulis-Vafiadis I. Systematic review: Coca-Cola can effectively dissolve gastric phytobezoars as a first-line treatment. *Aliment Pharmacol Ther.* 2013;37:169.

25. Winkler W, Saleh J. Metoclopramide in the treatment of gastric bezoars. *Am J Gastroenterol.* 1983;78:403.

Motility Disorders of the Stomach and Small Intestine

Justin Barr | Rebekah R. White

GASTRIC MOTILITY

ANATOMY AND PHYSIOLOGY

The gastric fundus, body, antrum, and pylorus must contract and relax in a coordinated manner to produce satisfactory gastric function and emptying (Figs. 65.1 and 65.2). The thinner fundus receptively relaxes to store food and liquids and then contracts to empty liquids from the stomach. The gastric pacemaker, which is located in the body along the greater curvature, stimulates both the filling and mixing of food in the body and antrum. The antrum strongly and periodically contracts against the closed pylorus to grind solid food particles down to a small size. The antrum peristalses at a frequency of three cycles per minute and propels small particles and liquids into the duodenum as the pylorus opens. Consequently, the stomach has three motile regions that coordinate to empty the stomach. The fundus receptively relaxes and subsequently contracts, and the body then fills and mixes. The antropyloroduodenal complex triturates and then empties into the duodenum as the pyloric sphincter opens.

Noncontractile gastric slow waves originate from the gastric pacemaker at a frequency of three waves per minute and propagate in both circumferential and longitudinal directions.[1] The network of interstitial cells of Cajal (ICCs) in the myenteric plexus initiates the slow wave and then conducts it to the smooth muscle layer by inducing depolarization. A deeper region of intramuscular ICCs is located in the muscularis propria. These serve to amplify the gastric slow wave signal to reach an action potential level through activation of calcium channels resulting in muscle contractions. Thus the ICCs in the myenteric plexus initiate the slow wave frequency in the smooth muscle, and the intramuscular ICCs propagate the slow wave and permit peristalsis.[2]

Gastric emptying comes under neural and hormonal control. The enteric nervous system (ENS; the "second brain") runs along the course of the stomach and intestines, contains over 100 million neurons, and can function independently of the central nervous system (CNS). It consists of two plexuses, submucosal (Meissner) and myenteric (Auerbach), which help direct the smooth muscle. The vagus nerve connects the ENS and the CNS. Several hormones, such as gastrin, cholecystokinin (CCK), glucagon-like peptide (GLP)-1 and GLP-2, peptide YY, and others, also influence gastric motility; a full review of these hormones is beyond the scope of this chapter and is described elsewhere.[3]

GASTROPARESIS

Gastroparesis is objectively delayed gastric emptying in the absence of organic causes such as stricture, ulcer, tumor, or mechanical obstruction, and in the absence of other causes such as functional dyspepsia, rumination syndrome, cyclic vomiting syndrome, or bulimia/anorexia nervosa. Official diagnosis requires both objectively confirmed delayed gastric emptying and associated symptoms of nausea, vomiting, bloating, and pain.

Mechanisms

Recent research has demonstrated the synergistic effect of multiple mechanisms in causing gastroparesis. With gastroparesis, both abnormal peristaltic contractile activity and abnormal electrical slow waves are usually present. Antral hypomotility, likely a neuropathic process reflecting the loss of ICCs, commonly occurs in diabetic patients, with evidence linking it to those with Parkinson disease as well.[4] Although the fundus has minimal contractile activity, its normally firm tone facilitates food movement to the body; a lax fundus—shown to result from both vagotomy and diabetes—delays passage of chyme. In contrast, impaired pyloric relaxation, seen primarily in type 1 diabetics, can trap contents in the stomach. The stomach and duodenum must act together, with the pylorus and duodenum relaxing as the antrum contracts. Disruptions in this concert or the various neurohormonal factors that coordinate the process also lead to gastric dysmotility.

Epidemiology and Etiology

Gastroparesis has an overall prevalence of 24 per 100,000 Americans. The disease affects females more often than males (4:1), with the onset of symptoms beginning at an average age of 34 years. There were 16,736 primary hospitalizations for gastroparesis in 2009 (up 18-fold from 1994), at a cost of an average $25,000 per hospitalization.[5]

The most common etiology of gastroparesis is, unfortunately, idiopathic, representing half of all cases. Diabetes causes about 25% of cases. Gastroparesis typically develops after 10 or more years of diabetes; patients almost always present with various symptoms of autonomic dysfunction as well as increased incidence of microvascular disease.[6,7] In the community, around 5% of type 1 diabetics and 1% of type 2 diabetics develop gastroparesis (numbers from patients with more advanced disease receiving care at tertiary centers are much higher: 40% and 15%, respectively).[7] Improved glycemic control does not appear to relieve gastroparesis, with symptoms and emptying time unchanged in patients despite better management of blood sugars.[8] Gastroparesis does not appear to cause increased mortality in diabetic patients but does serve as a marker for increased morbidity and mortality, likely due to shared effects of microvascular disease.

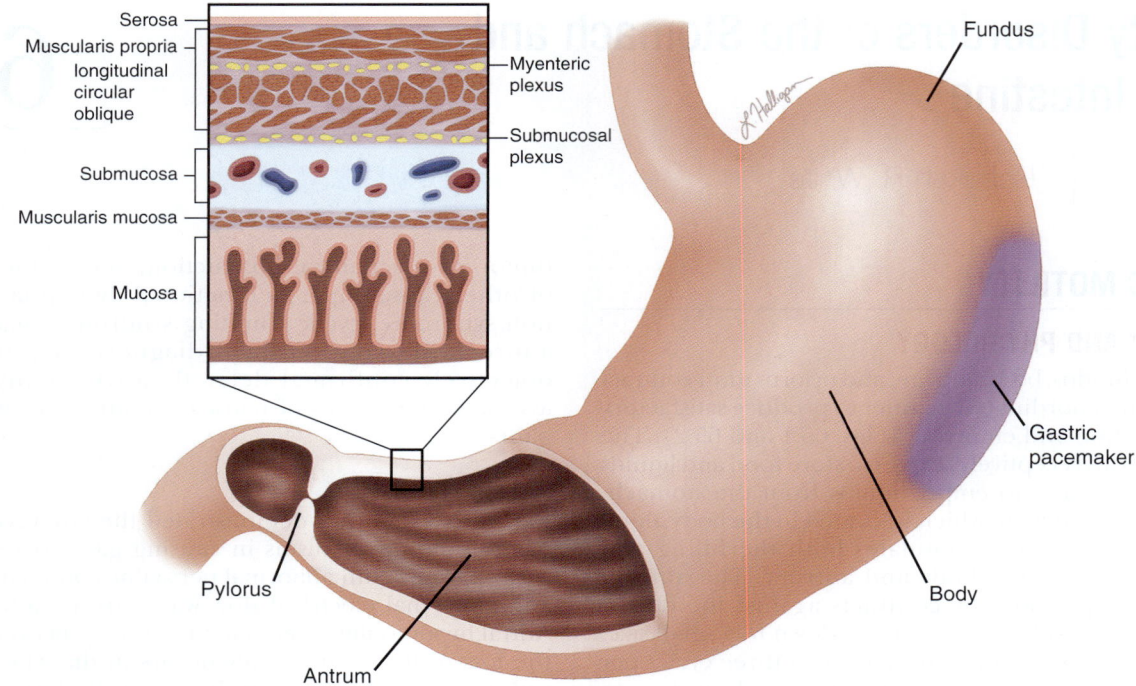

FIGURE 65.1 Anatomy and histology of the stomach. *(Illustrated by Lauren Halligan, MSMI; copyright Duke University 2016.)*

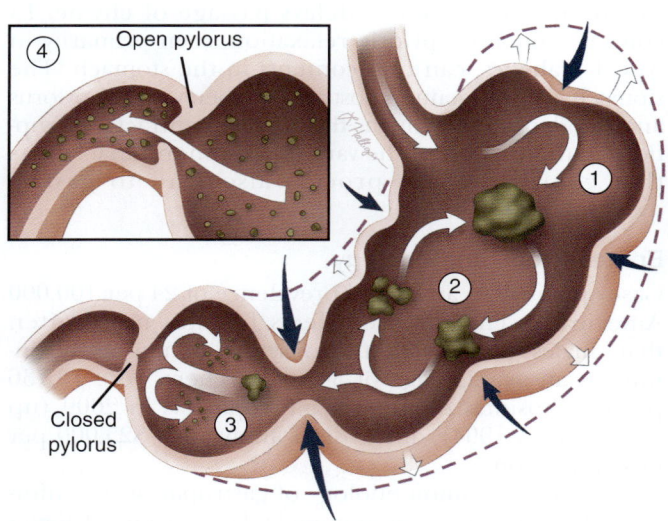

FIGURE 65.2 Peristalsis of the stomach. *1,* Fundus relaxes to accept food. *2,* Body of stomach fills and mixes the food. *3,* Antrum contracts against closed pylorus, aiding the digestive process. *4,* Pylorus periodically opens in rhythm with antral contractions to allow contents into the duodenum. *(Illustrated by Lauren Halligan, MSMI; copyright Duke University 2016.)*

Postsurgical sequelae (especially with intended or inadvertent vagotomy) cause approximately 13% of gastroparesis cases. The remaining patients suffer from a variety of less common causes: radiation, viral disease (e.g., Norwalk), connective tissue disorders (e.g., scleroderma), paraneoplastic syndromes, infiltrative diseases (e.g., amyloidosis), and neurologic disorders (e.g., Parkinson disease, ~7.5% of cases).[9] Specific therapies for these rare etiologies are not addressed in this chapter.

Clinical Presentation

The predominant symptoms are similar regardless of etiology: nausea (80% to 92%) and vomiting (66% to 85%), abdominal bloating (55% to 75%) and early satiety (54% to 60%).[10] Previously underestimated, epigastric abdominal pain is present in almost 90% of patients, is worsened by eating (72%), occurs nocturnally (74%), and often disturbs sleep (66%). Abdominal pain is not usually treated satisfactorily by gastric electrical stimulation or by prokinetic drugs.[11] Some studies suggest diabetic patients have more vomiting and idiopathic patients have more satiety, but the differences are not significant enough to affect diagnosis or management. Symptoms frequently overlap with functional dyspepsia, a condition that shares similar pathophysiology and presentation and can be difficult to distinguish even with objective testing.[12] The Gastroparesis Cardinal Symptom Index (GCSI) is a validated tool used to assess patients' severity of symptoms.[13] Differential diagnoses for these symptoms include gastroparesis, dumping syndrome, functional dyspepsia, ulcer disease, malignancy, gastroesophageal reflux disease, rumination syndrome, cyclic vomiting syndrome, bulimia, and mechanical gastric outlet obstruction.

Diagnosis

The diagnosis of gastroparesis is usually made after extensive testing to rule out other organic causes. Upper endoscopy with biopsy and an upper gastrointestinal (GI) contrast radiography with or without a small bowel follow-through are usually performed to rule out an organic cause. If these are inconclusive, a gastric emptying scan may diagnose gastroparesis. The nuclear medicine solid-phase gastric emptying test is the current gold standard for the diagnosis of gastroparesis, in the absence of gastric outlet obstruction. Diagnosis is probable if more than 50% of a solid meal is retained 2 hours after ingestion, or more than 10% of a solid meal is retained at 4 hours. Liquid emptying is less accurate for diagnosis of gastroparesis because liquids may empty normally even with an abnormal solid-emptying scan; recent studies have shown that delayed emptying of liquids relative to solids can increase the sensitivity of the test, especially in non-diabetic patients, although the clinical implications are unclear.[14] A radionuclide eggbeater meal (250 kcal and low fat) is used as a test meal for the solid-emptying scan.[15] Patients should avoid medicines such as promotility agents, anticholinergics, and opioids 48 hours prior to testing. Diabetic patients should have their blood sugar controlled; blood glucose greater than 275 is a contraindication for proceeding.[16]

Although not commonly used in clinical settings, breath testing for gastroparesis can be performed with ^{13}C-labeled octanoate or the blue-green algae, *Spirulina platensis*, in a solid meal, which is absorbed in the small bowel after gastric emptying. It is metabolized to $^{13}CO_2$, and then removed by respiration and available for breath testing.[6,11]

Gastric antral, pyloric, and duodenal motility may also be assessed with antroduodenal manometry. This procedure is available at tertiary medical centers, and does require fluoroscopy, catheter placement, and some patient discomfort. The wireless motility capsule has also been used to characterize the number of contractions as well as the motility index in the antrum and the duodenum.[6] Diabetic patients with gastroparesis show significantly lower numbers of contractions in both the stomach and small bowel compared with normal patients, whereas idiopathic gastroparetic patients do not show significant differences.[17]

Pharmacologic Treatment

Gastroparesis is initially treated by correcting fluid and electrolyte abnormalities, nutritional deficiencies, identifying and treating underlying causes, and suppressing the symptoms of nausea and vomiting. Diets are changed, using softer solid foods, more liquid supplements, and smaller, more frequent meals. Low-fat and low-fiber diets also help, as does avoidance of carbonated beverages, alcohol, and smoking.[18,19] In a diabetic patient, tight glucose control should be achieved because hyperglycemia has been shown to worsen gastroparetic symptoms, although long-term benefit is controversial and some antidiabetic medications (e.g., GLP-analogs and amylin analogs) can prolong gastric transit time. The mainstay of medical treatment for gastroparesis is the use of both antiemetic and prokinetic medications.[11] Regrettably, many of the current recommendations rest on studies performed several decades ago.

Symptom management includes controlling nausea, vomiting, and pain. Useful antiemetic agents include prochlorperazine (Compazine) and trimethobenzamide (Tigan), which antagonize dopamine receptors. Antihistamines with histamine (H_1)-receptor antagonist properties include diphenhydramine (Benadryl), promethazine, ondansetron (Zofran), granisetron (Kytril), and dolasetron

(Anzemet). Other agents include scopolamine, an anticholinergic, and aprepitant (Emend), a substance P/neurokinin-1 receptor antagonist. Dronabinol has also proven effective in subsets of patients.[20] Ideally, opioids should be avoided or limited for pain control given their effect on slowing gastrointestinal motility. Selective serotonin reuptake inhibitors (SSRIs) and tricyclic antidepressants (TCAs) have been used with the latter also demonstrating some relief of nausea and vomiting, although amitriptyline has significant anticholinergic side effects that delay gastric emptying.[21] All these medications are used empirically with little level I evidence to support one over another.

Metoclopramide remains the only US Food and Drug Administration (FDA)-approved medication to treat gastroparesis and should be the first motility agent tried. It functions as a dopamine D_2 receptor antagonist and serotonin 5-HT_4 receptor agonist, increases gastric motility through acetylcholine release, and relieves nausea via receptors in the brainstem (see later in this chapter for more on dopamine and serotonin). The drug carries a risk of serious side effects, including acute dystonias (incidence 0.2%), of which 1% are tardive dyskinesia. Less severe complications include CNS side effects, such as drowsiness, insomnia, and fatigue, in 20% of patients. Higher doses, longer courses of treatment, and female sex were all associated with increased risk of adverse effects.[22–24]

Multiple studies over the last few decades, including placebo-controlled randomized clinical trials, have proven the efficacy of metoclopramide.[25,26] Resulting papers have consistently demonstrated faster gastric emptying times and improved nausea and vomiting among patients. However, due to the risk of side effects, most studies terminated after 4 weeks, leaving longer-term use under investigated and essentially empirical.[27] Recent investigation into nasally administered metoclopramide has shown promise with symptom control and ability to use long-term with diminished risk of side effects.[28]

Domperidone is another option that also functions as a D2 receptor antagonist. It has similar ability to control symptoms of nausea and vomiting as metoclopramide, demonstrated through placebo-controlled and head-to-head clinical trials.[29,30] The starting dose is 10 mg three times per day (TID), increasing to 20 mg TID and at bedtime (qHS). Because domperidone does not cross the blood-brain barrier, patients are not at risk for the CNS side effects that limit metoclopramide use. However, domperidone does prolong the QTc interval and has been associated with sudden cardiac death.[31] The drug is not FDA approved and thus not for sale at most US pharmacies; providers may write a prescription for the drug, allowing patients to fill it at a compounding or international pharmacy.

Erythromycin works on the motilin receptors located in the gastric antrum and proximal duodenum. Although studies show short-term improvement in gastric motility, no long-term benefit has been demonstrated. The antibacterial properties of the drug potentially alter gut flora, with variable consequences on motility; cardiac side effects (lengthening repolarization time) also complicate the use of the drug.[32] Mitemcinal, an erythromycin-derived motilin agonist, has been tested in patients with idiopathic and diabetic gastroparesis. Although it did improve gastroparetic symptoms, there was no statistically significant improvement over the prominent placebo effect.[33]

Ghrelin is expressed primarily by neuroendocrine cells in the gastric fundus and the duodenum. It structurally resembles motilin, and its receptor resembles the motilin receptor. Ghrelin and motilin are coproduced in the same cells in the duodenum and proximal jejunum.[34] Basic science investigations have clearly shown its ability, in high doses, to stimulate gastric motility, increase gastric tone, and increase activity of migrating motor complexes (MMCs) in small bowel.[35] Ghrelin itself has too short a half-life for clinical utility, leading researchers to create various synthetic analogs. Early randomized double-blinded clinical studies failed to demonstrate superiority over placebos.[36] However, new formulations (RM-131) have shown early promise in symptom management, and this remains a very active area of research.[37]

Intrapyloric Botulinum Injections

Pylorospasm has been indicted as a possible cause for delayed gastric emptying. Injected into the pylorus, botulinum toxin works as a neuroinhibitor, preventing muscle contraction. Although nonrandomized trials have reported patient improvement, two prospective, blinded randomized clinical trials demonstrated faster gastric emptying but no relief of symptoms.[38] Thus, there is no good evidence to support this practice; the demonstration of benefit in open-label trials suggests a component of placebo effect, recognized as important in functional gastrointestinal illness.[39]

Gastric Electrical Stimulation

Gastric electrical stimulation seeks to induce gastric motility by inducing muscle contraction. The evidence for gastric electrical stimulation has been conflicting. Initial attempts used high-energy, low-frequency electricity to capture and regulate slow waves, normalizing intrinsic gastric electrical and, ideally, motor function. Subsequent studies later demonstrated subjective benefit but no evidence of changes in gastric motor function.[40] More recently, technique has shifted to low-energy, high-frequency stimulation, which does not influence slow waves but does appear to modulate gastric nerve activity. In 2000, the FDA approved a Medtronic (Minneapolis, Minnesota) device for treating gastroparesis using these parameters.

The stimulator package consists of a Medtronic Enterra stimulator (sized similar to a cardiac pacemaker) and two insulated wire electrodes with an uninsulated metal tip electrode that is connected to a monofilament suture on a straightened needle (Fig. 65.3). The two electrodes are positioned along the anterior greater curvature of the stomach using partial-thickness penetration into the muscularis.[41] Placement may be accomplished laparoscopically or via a small upper midline incision.[42] Upper endoscopy is performed at the time of electrode placement to exclude full-thickness gastric wall penetration by the electrode. The stimulator is placed in a subcutaneous pocket on the abdominal wall in a location consistent with the patient's wishes, previous surgical procedures, and the potential need for future feeding tubes. Both electrodes are then brought through the abdominal wall

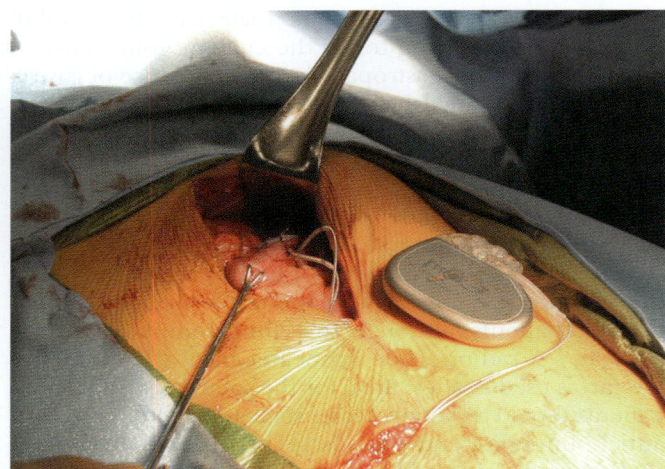

FIGURE 65.3 Enterra gastric electric stimulator system, with two Enterra leads, an introducer rod, plastic disks, and Enterra stimulator.

and are connected to the stimulator. Next, the electrical resistance of the circuit through the gastric wall is measured. A typical impedance value of less than 800 ohms is satisfactory. If the impedance is greater, the electrodes may need to be repositioned.

Risks associated with the gastric electrical stimulator include full-thickness electrode penetration of the gastric wall at the time of placement or subsequent erosion into the gastric lumen with infection or abscess, for which the electrodes should be removed.[43] The presence of two looping wire electrodes within the abdomen can lead to small bowel obstruction, particularly in patients with a history of prior abdominal surgeries. Infection or abscess at the skin pocket stimulator site mandates its removal. Erosion of the stimulator through the skin, even without cellulitis, is also treated by removal. Magnetic resonance imaging (MRI) is not possible after stimulator placement. In hospital, mortality after implantation ranges from 0.8% to 2.4%. Tracked over 10 years, the reoperation rate following stimulator implantation for problems specific to the device is 11.1%, with device removal in 8.4%.[44]

Evidence regarding efficacy varies. The initial trials underlying FDA approval included an open-label study reporting broad symptomatic improvement and an underpowered double-blind randomized crossover trial (enrolling only 50% of desired participants) that reported some improvement in weekly vomiting frequency, although not in patients with idiopathic disease.[41] Most subsequent trials have been open label and/or lacked controls. These have nonetheless demonstrated consistent symptomatic improvement among patients, particularly those with diabetic gastroparesis. Studies have most consistently demonstrated decreased incidence of weekly vomiting.

However, a metaanalysis of clinical trials evaluating gastric electrical stimulation did not find any persistent symptom relief.[44] Five randomized clinical trials with 185 patients formed the foundation for this analysis, which the authors recognized as differing substantially from conclusions reached in open-label trials. The authors attribute these differences to placebo effect and regression to the mean, noting that those with the most severe symptoms reported the most subjective benefit. Other studies have demonstrated surgery exerting a more powerful placebo effect than medications, perhaps partially explaining the reported superiority of gastric electrical stimulation to pharmacologic management.[45] Given the 11% risk of reoperation, these results give pause to reflexive implantation. Additional studies are needed.

Other Surgical Interventions

When prokinetic and antiemetic medications are insufficient to maintain body weight, then venting and feeding tubes are used. A percutaneous gastrostomy tube alone may reduce the incidence of vomiting through intermittent venting or by setting the tube at continuous external drainage. A combination transgastric gastrojejunal tube can vent the stomach and also enable proximal jejunal tube feeding. Placement of a feeding jejunostomy tube allows both adequate nutrition and fluids, and it can reduce the need for hospitalization for intravenous repletion of fluids; it does not improve symptoms. Placement of both a gastrostomy tube for venting and a jejunostomy tube for fluids and nutrition allows some gastroparetics to manage symptoms and improve quality of life. Enteral feeding is preferred over parenteral nutrition, with lower overall cost and avoidance of complications from central intravenous access. Enteral feeding via the jejunostomy tube may be maintained for months or years. Potential complications of a feeding jejunostomy include tube dislodgement with closure of the opening, infection and cellulitis, and leakage from the site as the tract enlarges, which then requires a larger-diameter feeding tube. If small bowel dysmotility accompanies gastroparesis, tube feed rates may need to be limited secondary to nausea, pain, or bloating. If ongoing weight loss then occurs, total parenteral nutrition (TPN) may be required via a percutaneous indwelling central venous catheter line or tunneled central venous catheter.

More aggressive surgical interventions have also been studied, including gastrojejunostomy, pyloromyotomy, and completion or subtotal gastrectomy. Drainage procedures include pyloroplasty or pyloromyotomy, and a retrospective review of prospectively collected data on 28 patients demonstrated marked improvement of symptoms ranging from nausea to bloating to pain at 3 months. Gastric transit time decreased from an average of 320 to 112 minutes. Diabetic patients saw less improvement than other patient populations.[46] With minimally invasive techniques and shorter lengths of stay minimizing morbidity, this method merits more thorough investigation. Completion or subtotal gastrectomy is most often performed for postsurgical gastroparesis. With a near-total gastrectomy, a small proximal gastric pouch, via a vertical staple line, may be constructed similar to a gastric bypass procedure. A large gastrojejunostomy with a short Roux limb and a feeding jejunostomy should be performed.[47]

INTESTINAL MOTILITY

In the fasting state, small intestinal motility is controlled by the MMC, which exhibits three phases. Phase I is a quiescent period and represents 20% to 30% of the total cycle length. Phase II accounts for 40% to 60% of the total cycle length and is characterized by intermittent and irregular contractions. In phase III, intense, rhythmic contractions develop and propagate from the proximal to the distal portion of the intestine over a 5- to 10-minute period. The MMC cycle occurs approximately every 90 minutes during the interdigestive period. However, after a meal, this fasting pattern of intestinal motility is changed to a postprandial pattern, with intermittent phasic contractions of irregular amplitude that are similar to the phase II contractions of the MMC.[48] Peristalsis occurs when a segment of circular muscle contracts as a result of excitatory motor neurons while the intestinal segment aboral to the contracted segment is simultaneously relaxed by inhibitory neurons.[49]

The ICCs are known to be essential regulators of GI motility and seem to serve as pacemaker cells in the GI tract and mediators of neural regulation in GI motility. They lie in close proximity to smooth muscle cells and elements of the ENS. The generation of slow waves occurs within the Auerbach plexus and is an intrinsic property of the ICC network; both circumferential intestinal contractions and longitudinal contractions are produced.[49] ICC abnormalities are increasingly being recognized in a number of GI tract disorders, such as chronic intestinal pseudoobstruction, with findings of decreased ICCs or an abnormal ICC network.[50,51] Surgical procedures involving the small intestine disrupt ICC networks at the level of the myenteric and deep muscular plexuses, with resultant loss of slow waves and phasic contractions. This loss of intestinal motility, however, partially recovers within 24 hours after surgery.[52]

Because intestinal motility is controlled by interactions among smooth muscle, enteric nerves, extrinsic nerves, and humoral factors, abnormalities in any of these areas may result in intestinal dysmotility. Small intestinal dysmotility symptoms include abdominal bloating, distention, pain, nausea, and vomiting. Primary disorders causing small intestinal dysmotility include inherited familial visceral myopathies, characterized by smooth muscle degeneration, and familial visceral neuropathies, characterized by the degeneration of enteric nerves. Secondary causes of small intestinal dysmotility include myopathic processes (scleroderma, muscular dystrophies, amyloidosis), neurologic diseases (Parkinson disease, neurofibromatosis, Chagas disease), endocrine disorders (diabetes mellitus, hyperthyroidism, hypothyroidism, hypoparathyroidism), celiac disease, and pharmacologic agents (anti-Parkinson medications, phenothiazines, TCAs, narcotics).[53]

Smooth muscle disease, such as scleroderma, frequently affects the GI tract, and small intestinal dysmotility develops in approximately 40% of such patients. Proximal involvement leads to megaduodenum or wide-mouth diverticula of the small bowel, with resulting delayed transit, bacterial overgrowth, and malabsorption. Octreotide is useful in treating stasis and the resultant bacterial overgrowth. Muscular dystrophies affect motility of the entire gut; although barium studies may be normal, small intestinal manometry may reveal a myopathic pattern. Amyloidosis produces infiltration of both smooth muscle and the autonomic nerves and affects the motility of the entire GI tract.[53]

Neurologic disease is most commonly seen with Parkinson disease, with degeneration of the ENS and inhibition of intestinal motility by anti-Parkinson medications. Neurofibromatosis may produce dysmotility as a result of mechanical obstruction with GI tract tumor formation, but it is also associated with neuronal dysplasia of the ENS. Chagas disease (infection with *Trypanosoma cruzi*) results in neuronal injury and is manifested as megaduodenum, megajejunum, or pseudoobstruction.[53] Hirschsprung disease or its allied disorders hypoganglionosis and intestinal neuronal dysplasia may produce small intestinal dysmotility.[54]

Endocrine disorders may also give rise to intestinal dysmotility. Hypothyroidism produces delayed transit, constipation, and pseudoobstruction, which is reversible with thyroid hormone replacement. Hypoparathyroidism may be associated with small intestinal dysmotility and pseudoobstruction, which improve with calcium repletion. Small intestinal complications of diabetes with autonomic neuropathy include delayed transit with bacterial overgrowth and diarrhea. Celiac sprue produces abdominal pain, distention, and malabsorption, with delayed intestinal transit, bacterial overgrowth, and pseudoobstruction.[55] Both villous damage and small intestinal dysmotility improve with a gluten-free diet.[53]

GI motility is enhanced by the stimulation of distinct serotonin (5-hydroxytryptamine [5-HT]) receptors on intestinal sensory nerves. 5-HT is released from mucosal enterochromaffin cells in response to mechanical and chemical stimuli within the intestine. 5-HT activates $5-HT_4$ receptors on nerves synapsing in the myenteric plexus, which results in motor responses and increased peristalsis and intestinal transit.[52] Tegaserod, a selective $5-HT_4$ partial agonist, significantly accelerates small bowel transit time and gastric emptying.[56]

DIAGNOSIS OF INTESTINAL DYSMOTILITY

After the history, physical examination, and conventional radiographic studies suggest the possibility of intestinal dysmotility, an upper GI study with small bowel follow-through should be performed. This study may demonstrate the possibility of obstructing lesions, such as tumor, stricture, diverticula, or adhesions, and in their absence may identify general small bowel dysmotility. Evaluation of small intestinal transit then may be done by small bowel scintigraphy, with imaging up to 6 hours after ingestion of a radiolabeled meal. Scintigraphy has a specificity of up to 75% for the diagnosis of dysmotility, but it does not differentiate between myopathic and neuropathic causes.

Small bowel manometry may be performed if abnormal small bowel transit is found to be present. In the interdigestive period, the MMC is monitored to examine the cycle duration (interval between phase III events), the duration of each phase including the amplitude and propagation velocity of phase III, and the rate of contraction of phase III. A motility disorder is present with abnormal bursts of phasic activity, low-amplitude contractions, poorly coordinated activity, or absent, incomplete, or retrograde phase III activity. With eating, a change in typical postprandial activity is expected, with irregular, phasic contractions of variable amplitude as the intestinal contents are mixed and propelled distally. This postprandial period

lasts for about 4 hours, and then a return to the interdigestive pattern should be noted. Whereas short-duration (2-hour) manometry studies may diagnose abnormalities while a patient is in the fed or postprandial state, longer study periods facilitate study in the interdigestive period as well. This concept has been extended to ambulatory study systems in an attempt to improve diagnostic accuracy. Manometry may also help distinguish myopathic causes of dysmotility from neuropathic causes.

POSTOPERATIVE ILEUS

One of the most common etiologies for intestinal dysmotility is postoperative ileus, defined as the lack of intestinal motility after abdominal or pelvic surgery. Ambiguity surrounding the distinction between physiologic postoperative gastrointestinal tract dysfunction and pathologic postoperative ileus problematizes its conception and hampers clinical and epidemiologic investigation of the condition. The precise pathophysiology also remains unclear, and it is thought that inflammatory mediators, interruption of neurotransmitters, and iatrogenic factors, such as anesthesia and opioids, synergistically inhibit bowel peristalsis.[57] Increased bowel manipulation and bowel irritation by blood or fecal spillage increase the incidence and severity of the disorder[58]; incision length does not.[59] The small bowel recovers most rapidly after surgery (12–24 hours), followed by the stomach (24–48 hours), and lastly the large bowel (3–5 days).

Despite theoretical confusion, most surgeons can readily identify the condition in their patients. Postoperative ileus presents with a lack of bowel function and intolerance to oral intake in the absence of any mechanical obstruction. Clinical presentation varies from asymptomatic dysmotility to crampy pain, nausea, and vomiting. On exam, patients are often distended with tympanic abdomens; bowel sounds, previously heralded as a specific sign of ileus, have recently not demonstrated correlation with the condition or its resolution.[60] No objective test can definitively diagnose postoperative ileus. Plain radiographs often show dilated loops of intestine, a nonspecific finding. Computed tomography (CT) scans with contrast can help distinguish between mechanical obstruction and ileus.[61]

Treatment for postoperative ileus remains limited and essentially unchanged for the last 100 years. Early 20th-century management involved enterostomies, with high mortality rates around 40%. In the 1930s, Owen Wangensteen advocated using nasogastric tubes to decompress the GI tract and expedite healing, a modality that became increasingly popular and routine.[62] Later prospective studies demonstrated the futility of intraoperative placement in preventing ileus, but it remains a common intervention to manage the condition postoperatively in symptomatic patients. Every known promotility drug has been tested with the hope of a pharmaceutical cure, but none consistently demonstrated a more rapid return of bowel function. Recently, several studies have demonstrated the benefit of chewing gum. A Cochrane Review found that chewing gum decreased time to flatus and first bowel movement by about 12 hours, and decreased total length of hospital stay by almost a day, with more dramatic effects seen (and better studied) in colorectal patients.[63]

The risk of postoperative ileus has complicated decisions over when to feed patients after surgery. For most of the 20th century, most clinicians waited for bowel function to return in the form of either flatus or stool before advancing the patient's diet.[64] More recently, prospective, randomized clinical trials have demonstrated that early enteral feeding is not only safe but actually hastens return of bowel functions and is associated with a decreased risk in anastomotic leaks, at least in rectal surgery.[65] Early feeding has become the standard of care in colorectal patients through enhanced recovery after surgery (ERAS) pathways and is rapidly extending to other patient populations.

PHARMACOLOGIC TREATMENT

Pharmaceutical treatment for intestinal dysmotility largely parallels that for gastric dysmotility. The addition of erythromycin, a motilin agonist, stimulates both gastric emptying and intestinal contractions at low doses. Tegaserod, a $5\text{-}HT_4$ partial agonist, accelerates small bowel transit time and increases both gastric emptying and colonic transit.[53,56] Some agents have benefits specifically targeted at pathologies afflicting the small bowel. Octreotide, for example, has been demonstrated as especially effective in scleroderma-induced dysmotility.[67] Alvimopan (Entereg) is a novel agent designed to prevent opioid-induced ileus by blocking μ-opioid receptors in the gastrointestinal tract; its limited systemic absorption and inability to cross the blood-brain barrier allow narcotics to continue to treat pain. It must be given to a patient prior to surgery to be effective. Multiple randomized clinical trials have proven that alvimopan reduces time to return of bowel function.[68,69] A recent large study demonstrated the clinical utility of the drug in colorectal cases, showing shortened (by 1 day) and cheaper (by approximately $600) postoperative hospital stays.[70] Methylnaltrexone (Relistor), which similarly works by blocking peripheral μ receptors, is FDA approved for the treatment of opioid-induced constipation in patients receiving palliative care when other laxatives have failed.[71] There does not appear to be any benefit—and there is risk of significant harm—to using alvimopan for opioid-induced constipation in terminal patients or methylnaltrexone to treat acute, postoperative ileus.[72]

SURGICAL TREATMENT

Surgical options for the treatment of nonmechanical small intestine dysmotility are limited. Conversely, mechanical pathologies respond readily to operative intervention. Thus, a thorough investigation for mechanical causes ought to be pursued, including both axial imaging and barium swallow studies as needed. Endoscopy can also be informative while simultaneously harvesting biopsy samples from the gastric, duodenal, and proximal jejunal mucosa for pathological investigation. Small intestinal manometry allows assessment of the MMC. If all the above fail to elicit a diagnosis, surgeons may be asked to perform a diagnostic laparoscopy or, more rarely, laparotomy. The operation must examine the entire course of the bowel. Surgeons can also collect full-thickness jejunal biopsies to assess for visceral myopathy or neurogenic causes of small bowel dysmotility and chronic intestinal pseudoobstruction.[73]

Small bowel resection is uncommonly performed, although localized findings may justify segmental resection. Isolated megaduodenum (type I familial visceral myopathy) has been treated by drainage or subtotal duodenal resection, with the posterior biliopancreatic duodenal wall left intact and the proximal jejunum used as an onlay patch.[53,74] Primary amyloidosis confined to the small intestine has been reported in the setting of persistent pseudoobstruction and has been treated by partial jejunectomy.[75]

TRANSPLANTATION

In some situations, small intestine transplant is the only curative remedy. Most commonly used in mechanical short-gut patients, transplantation should be considered in any patient permanently dependent on parenteral nutrition for intestinal dysmotility. This includes conditions such as chronic intestinal pseudoobstruction, a heterogeneous group of neuropathic or myopathic pathologies, such as Hirschsprung disease, that result in ineffective smooth muscle contraction and intestinal dysmotility . It most commonly presents in children but can also occur in adults.[76]

Early referral for transplantation should be considered once permanent TPN has become necessary. About half of such patients require decompressive gastrostomies/jejunostomies for symptomatic management. Among children with the disorder, over 70% required TPN for more than 5 years, a substantially higher rate than for mechanical short gut. In one series of such patients, none successfully weaned from TPN without transplant.[77] In another small series, intestinal transplantation permitted cessation of TPN and increased survival in these patients.[78] Adult patients with chronic intestinal pseudoobstruction similarly benefit from small bowel transplantation, often as a part of a multivisceral transplant operation given common involvement of the stomach in adults. In one study, graft and patient survival at 5 years was 60% and 70%, respectively, and at 10 years, 45% and 56% respectively.[79]

SUMMARY

Disorders of gastric and small intestinal motility are challenging for clinicians and particularly for patients. A wide array of conditions with overlapping clinical presentations and few unique objective signs prevents facile diagnosis. The physician must carefully assemble the history, context, and judiciously chosen tests to identify the malady. Once recognized, many of these conditions resist simple treatment. Most pharmacologic interventions date back decades and have either limited efficacy and/or severe side effects, although recent research is identifying novel regimens. Surgical interventions, through implantable devices or alteration of normal anatomy, have limited efficacy in many cases and carry significant risks of their own. Despite these challenges, gastric and intestinal dysmotility affect several thousand patients and carry substantial morbidity. They remain an area of active research.

ACKNOWLEDGMENTS

The authors are grateful to John E. Meilahn for his work on a prior version of this chapter that formed the foundation for the current iteration.

REFERENCES

1. Sanjeevi A. Gastric motility. *Curr Opin Gastroenterol*. 2007;23(6):625-630.
2. Forster J, Damjanov I, Lin Z, Sarosiek I, Wetzel P, McCallum RW. Absence of the interstitial cells of Cajal in patients with gastroparesis and correlation with clinical findings. *J Gastrointest Surg*. 2005;9(1):102-108.
3. Khoo J, Rayner CK, Feinle-Bisset C, Jones KL, Horowitz M. Gastrointestinal hormonal dysfunction in gastroparesis and functional dyspepsia. *Neurogastroenterol Motil*. 2010;22(12):1270-1278.
4. Marrinan S, Emmanuel AV, Burn DJ. Delayed gastric emptying in Parkinson's disease. *Mov Disord*. 2014;29(1):23-32.
5. Nusrat S, Bielefeldt K. Gastroparesis on the rise: incidence vs awareness? *Neurogastroenterol Motil*. 2013;25(1):16-22.
6. Parkman HP, Camilleri M, Farrugia G, et al. Gastroparesis and functional dyspepsia: excerpts from the AGA/ANMS meeting. *Neurogastroenterol Motil*. 2010;22(2):113-133.
7. Camilleri M, Bharucha AE, Farrugia G. Epidemiology, mechanisms, and management of diabetic gastroparesis. *Clin Gastroenterol Hepatol*. 2011;9(1):5-12; quiz e7.
8. Jones KL, Russo A, Berry MK, Stevens JE, Wishart JM, Horowitz M. A longitudinal study of gastric emptying and upper gastrointestinal symptoms in patients with diabetes mellitus. *Am J Med*. 2002;113(6):449-455.
9. Stein B, Everhart KK, Lacy BE. Gastroparesis: a review of current diagnosis and treatment options. *J Clin Gastroenterol*. 2015;49(7):550-558.
10. Nguyen LA, Snape WJ Jr. Clinical presentation and pathophysiology of gastroparesis. *Gastroenterol Clin North Am*. 2015;44(1):21-30.
11. Parkman HP, Hasler WL, Fisher RS. American Gastroenterological Association technical review on the diagnosis and treatment of gastroparesis. *Gastroenterology*. 2004;127(5):1592-1622.
12. Talley NJ, Ford AC. Functional dyspepsia. *N Engl J Med*. 2015;373(19):1853-1863.
13. Revicki DA, Rentz AM, Dubois D, et al. Development and validation of a patient-assessed gastroparesis symptom severity measure: the Gastroparesis Cardinal Symptom Index. *Aliment Pharmacol Ther*. 2003;18(1):141-150.
14. Sachdeva P, Malhotra N, Pathikonda M, et al. Gastric emptying of solids and liquids for evaluation for gastroparesis. *Dig Dis Sci*. 2011;56(4):1138-1146.
15. Reddymasu SC, Singh S, Sankula R, Lavenbarg TA, Olyaee M, McCallum RW. Endoscopic pyloric injection of botulinum toxin-A for the treatment of postvagotomy gastroparesis. *Am J Med Sci*. 2009;337(3):161-164.
16. Camilleri M, Parkman HP, Shafi MA, Abell TL, Gerson L. Clinical guideline: management of gastroparesis. *Am J Gastroenterol*. 2013;108(1):18-37; quiz 38.
17. Kloetzer L, Chey WD, McCallum RW, et al. Motility of the antro-duodenum in healthy and gastroparetics characterized by wireless motility capsule. *Neurogastroenterol Motil*. 2010;22(5):527-533, e117.
18. Camilleri M. Appraisal of medium-and long-term treatment of gastro paresis and chronic intestinal dysmotility. *Am J Gastroenterol*. 1994;89(10):1769-1774.
19. Sanaka M, Anjiki H, Tsutsumi H, et al. Effect of cigarette smoking on gastric emptying of solids in Japanese smokers: a crossover study using the 13C-octanoic acid breath test. *J Gastroenterol*. 2005;40(6):578-582.
20. McCallum RW, Sunny J. Status of pharmacologic management of gastroparesis: 2014. *Pract Gastroenterol*. 2014;38(9):20-42.
21. Sawhney MS, Prakash C, Lustman PJ, Clouse RE. Tricyclic antidepressants for chronic vomiting in diabetic patients. *Dig Dis Sci*. 2007;52(2):418-424.
22. Bateman DN, Rawlins MD, Simpson JM. Extrapyramidal reactions with metoclopramide. *Br Med J (Clin Res Ed)*. 1985;291(6500):930-932.
23. Heeley E, Riley J, Layton D, Wilton LV, Shakir SA. Prescription-event monitoring and reporting of adverse drug reactions. *Lancet*. 2001;358(9296):1872-1873.
24. Miller LG, Jankovic J. Metoclopramide-induced movement disorders. Clinical findings with a review of the literature. *Arch Intern Med*. 1989;149(11):2486-2492.
25. Snape WJ Jr, Battle WM, Schwartz SS, Braunstein SN, Goldstein HA, Alavi A. Metoclopramide to treat gastroparesis due to diabetes mellitus: a double-blind, controlled trial. *Ann Intern Med*. 1982;96(4):444-446.
26. Parkman HP, Misra A, Jacobs M, et al. Clinical response and side effects of metoclopramide: associations with clinical, demographic, and pharmacogenetic parameters. *J Clin Gastroenterol*. 2012;46(6):494-503.
27. Lata PF, Pigarelli DL. Chronic metoclopramide therapy for diabetic gastroparesis. *Ann Pharmacother*. 2003;37(1):122-126.
28. Parkman HP, Carlson MR, Gonyer D. Metoclopramide nasal spray is effective in symptoms of gastroparesis in diabetics compared to conventional oral tablet. *Neurogastroenterol Motil*. 2014;26(4):521-528.
29. Patterson D, Abell T, Rothstein R, Koch K, Barnett J. A double-blind multicenter comparison of domperidone and metoclopramide in the treatment of diabetic patients with symptoms of gastroparesis. *Am J Gastroenterol*. 1999;94(5):1230-1234.
30. Heer M, Müller-Duysing W, Benes I, et al. Diabetic gastroparesis: treatment with domperidone—a double-blind, placebo-controlled trial. *Digestion*. 1983;27(4):214-217.
31. van Noord C, Dieleman JP, van Herpen G, Verhamme K, Sturkenboom MC. Domperidone and ventricular arrhythmia or sudden cardiac death: a population-based case-control study in the Netherlands. *Drug Saf*. 2010;33(11):1003-1014.
32. Acosta A, Camilleri M. Prokinetics in gastroparesis. *Gastroenterol Clin North Am*. 2015;44(1):97-111.
33. McCallum RW, Cynshi O. Clinical trial: effect of mitemcinal (a motilin agonist) on gastric emptying in patients with gastroparesis—a randomized, multicentre, placebo-controlled study. *Aliment Pharmacol Ther*. 2007;26(8):1121-1130.
34. Wierup N, Bjorkqvist M, Westrom B, Pierzynowski S, Sundler F, Sjolund K. Ghrelin and motilin are cosecreted from a prominent endocrine cell population in the small intestine. *J Clin Endocrinol Metab*. 2007;92(9):3573-3581.
35. Camilleri M, Papathanasopoulos A, Odunsi ST. Actions and therapeutic pathways of ghrelin for gastrointestinal disorders. *Nat Rev Gastroenterol Hepatol*. 2009;6(6):343-352.
36. McCallum RW, Lembo A, Esfandyari T, et al. Phase 2b, randomized, double-blind 12-week studies of TZP-102, a ghrelin receptor agonist for diabetic gastroparesis. *Neurogastroenterol Motil*. 2013;25(11):e705-e717.
37. Shin A, Wo JM. Therapeutic applications of ghrelin agonists in the treatment of gastroparesis. *Curr Gastroenterol Rep*. 2015;17(2):1-9.
38. Bai Y, Xu MJ, Yang X, et al. A systematic review on intrapyloric botulinum toxin injection for gastroparesis. *Digestion*. 2010;81(1):27-34.
39. Enck P, Klosterhalfen S. The placebo response in functional bowel disorders: perspectives and putative mechanisms. *Neurogastroenterol Motil*. 2005;17(3):325-331.
40. Hasler WL. Methods of gastric electrical stimulation and pacing: a review of their benefits and mechanisms of action in gastroparesis and obesity. *Neurogastroenterol Motil*. 2009;21(3):229-243.
41. Abell T, McCallum R, Hocking M, et al. Gastric electrical stimulation for medically refractory gastroparesis. *Gastroenterology*. 2003;125(2):421-428.
42. Mason RJ, Lipham J, Eckerling G, Schwartz A, Demeester TR. Gastric electrical stimulation: an alternative surgical therapy for patients with gastroparesis. *Arch Surg*. 2005;140(9):841-846; discussion 847–848.
43. Liu RC, Sabnis AA, Chand B. Erosion of gastric electrical stimulator electrodes: evaluation, management, and laparoscopic techniques. *Surg Laparosc Endosc Percutan Tech*. 2007;17(5):438-441.
44. Levinthal DJ, Bielefeldt K. Systematic review and meta-analysis: gastric electrical stimulation for gastroparesis. *Auton Neurosci*. 2017;202:45-55.
45. Meissner K, Fässler M, Rücker G, et al. Differential effectiveness of placebo treatments: a systematic review of migraine prophylaxis. *JAMA Intern Med*. 2013;173(21):1941-1951.
46. Hibbard ML, Dunst CM, Swanström LL. Laparoscopic and endoscopic pyloroplasty for gastroparesis results in sustained symptom improvement. *J Gastrointest Surg*. 2011;15(9):1513-1519.
47. Hejazi RA, McCallum RW. Treatment of refractory gastroparesis: gastric and jejunal tubes, botox, gastric electrical stimulation, and surgery. *Gastrointest Endosc Clin N Am*. 2009;19(1):73-82, vi.
48. Xing J, Chen JD. Alterations of gastrointestinal motility in obesity. *Obes Res*. 2004;12(11):1723-1732.
49. Thomson AB, Drozdowski L, Iordache C, et al. Small bowel review: normal physiology, part 2. *Dig Dis Sci*. 2003;48(8):1565-1581.
50. Kubota M, Kanda E, Ida K, Sakakihara Y, Hayashi M. Severe gastrointestinal dysmotility in a patient with congenital myopathy: causal relationship to decrease of interstitial cells of Cajal. *Brain Dev*. 2005;27(6):447-450.

51. Feldstein AE, Miller SM, El-Youssef M, et al. Chronic intestinal pseudoobstruction associated with altered interstitial cells of Cajal networks. *J Pediatr Gastroenterol Nutr.* 2003;36(4):492-497.
52. Yanagida H, Yanase H, Sanders KM, Ward SM. Intestinal surgical resection disrupts electrical rhythmicity, neural responses, and interstitial cell networks. *Gastroenterology.* 2004;127(6):1748-1759.
53. Kuemmerle JF. Motility disorders of the small intestine: new insights into old problems. *J Clin Gastroenterol.* 2000;31(4):276-281.
54. Tomita R, Ikeda T, Fujisaki S, Shibata M, Tanjih K. Upper gut motility of Hirschsprung's disease and its allied disorders in adults. *Hepatogastroenterology.* 2003;50(54):1959-1962.
55. Tursi A. Gastrointestinal motility disturbances in celiac disease. *J Clin Gastroenterol.* 2004;38(8):642-645.
56. Degen L, Petrig C, Studer D, Schroller S, Beglinger C. Effect of tegaserod on gut transit in male and female subjects. *Neurogastroenterol Motil.* 2005;17(6):821-826.
57. Mattei P, Rombeau JL. Review of the pathophysiology and management of postoperative ileus. *World J Surg.* 2006;30(8):1382-1391.
58. Doorly MG, Senagore AJ. Pathogenesis and clinical and economic consequences of postoperative ileus. *Surg Clin North Am.* 2012;92(2): 259-272, viii.
59. Cali RL, Meade PG, Swanson MS, Freeman C. Effect of morphine and incision length on bowel function after colectomy. *Dis Colon Rectum.* 2000;43(2):163-168.
60. Felder S, Margel D, Murrell Z, Fleshner P. Usefulness of bowel sound auscultation: a prospective evaluation. *J Surg Educ.* 2014;71(5): 768-773.
61. Vather R, Trivedi S, Bissett I. Defining postoperative ileus: results of a systematic review and global survey. *J Gastrointest Surg.* 2013;17(5):962-972.
62. Wangensteen OH. The early diagnosis of acute intestinal obstruction with comments on pathology and treatment: with a report on successful decompression of three cases of mechanical small bowel obstruction by nasal catheter siphonage. *West J Surg Obstet Gynecol.* 1932;40:1-17.
63. Short V, Herbert G, Perry R, et al. Chewing gum for postoperative recovery of gastrointestinal function. *Cochrane Database Syst Rev.* 2015;(2):CD006506, doi:10.1002/14651858.CD006506.pub3.
64. Livingston EH, Passaro EP Jr. Postoperative ileus. *Dig Dis Sci.* 1990;35(1):121-132.
65. Boelens PG, Heesakkers FF, Luyer MD, et al. Reduction of postoperative ileus by early enteral nutrition in patients undergoing major rectal surgery: prospective, randomized, controlled trial. *Ann Surg.* 2014;259(4):649-655.
66. Reference deleted in review.
67. Soudah HC, Hasler WL, Owyang C. Effect of octreotide on intestinal motility and bacterial overgrowth in scleroderma. *N Engl J Med.* 1991;325(21):1461-1467.
68. Wolff BG, Michelassi F, Gerkin TM, et al. Alvimopan, a novel, peripherally acting mu opioid antagonist: results of a multicenter, randomized, double-blind, placebo-controlled, phase III trial of major abdominal surgery and postoperative ileus. *Ann Surg.* 2004;240(4):728-734; discussion 734–735.
69. Delaney CP, Weese JL, Hyman NH, et al. Phase III trial of alvimopan, a novel, peripherally acting, mu opioid antagonist, for postoperative ileus after major abdominal surgery. *Dis Colon Rectum.* 2005;48(6): 1114-1125; discussion 1125–1126; author reply 1127–1129.
70. Ehlers AP, Simianu VV, Bastawrous AL, et al. Alvimopan use, outcomes, and costs: a report from the Surgical Care and Outcomes Assessment Program Comparative Effectiveness Research Translation Network Collaborative. *J Am Coll Surg.* 2016;222(5):870-877.
71. Brenner DM, Chey WD. An evidence-based review of novel and emerging therapies for constipation in patients taking opioid analgesics. *Am J Gastroenterol Suppl.* 2014;2:38-46.
72. Rodriguez RW. Off-label uses of alvimopan and methylnaltrexone. *Am J Health Syst Pharm.* 2014;71(17):1450-1455.
73. Arslan M, Bayraktar Y, Oksuzoglu G, et al. Four cases with chronic intestinal pseudo-obstruction due to hollow visceral myopathy. *Hepatogastroenterology.* 1999;46(25):349-352.
74. Endo M, Ukiyama E, Yokoyama J, Kitajima M. Subtotal duodenectomy with jejunal patch for megaduodenum secondary to congenital duodenal malformation. *J Pediatr Surg.* 1998;33(11):1636-1640.
75. Deguchi M, Shiraki K, Okano H, et al. Primary localized amyloidosis of the small intestine presenting as an intestinal pseudo-obstruction: report of a case. *Surg Today.* 2001;31(12):1091-1093.
76. Bond GJ, Reyes JD. Intestinal transplantation for total/near-total aganglionosis and intestinal pseudo-obstruction. *Semin Pediatr Surg.* 2004;13(4):286-292.
77. Hukkinen M, Merras-Salmio L, Sipponen T, et al. Surgical rehabilitation of short and dysmotile intestine in children and adults. *Scand J Gastroenterol.* 2015;50(2):153-161.
78. Pakarinen MP, Kurvinen A, Koivusalo AI, et al. Surgical treatment and outcomes of severe pediatric intestinal motility disorders requiring parenteral nutrition. *J Pediatr Surg.* 2013;48(2):333-338.
79. Lauro A, Zanfi C, Pellegrini S, et al. Isolated intestinal transplant for chronic intestinal pseudo-obstruction in adults: long-term outcome. *Transplant Proc.* 2013;45(9):3351-3355.

Miscellaneous Benign Lesions and Conditions of the Stomach, Duodenum, and Small Intestine

David B. Adams | Katherine A. Morgan

Benign disorders of the foregut originate in the genes and the environment of the stomach, duodenum, and small intestine. Embryologic events orchestrate anatomic and cellular variations that predispose the adult foregut to obstructive and neoplastic conditions. Webs, stenosis, duplications, and a variety of ectopic and heterotopic cellular occurrences are uncommon and may remain asymptomatic until adulthood. Genetic mutations and environmental stressors have a relationship with hyperplasia and benign tumors. Environmental factors such as drugs, alcohol, and smoking cause foregut inflammation and mucosal injury. For the most part, these benign foregut conditions do not need operative management, and most commonly are found incidentally on endoscopic or radiologic examination. On occasion, benign conditions are discovered at the time of surgery for other disorders of the foregut, and require an operative decision about how and why to perform an excisional biopsy. Diagnostic upper gastrointestinal endoscopy, capsule endoscopy, and widespread utilization of abdominal computed tomography (CT) uncover many of these benign conditions. Management of foregut disorders has improved with endoscopic ultrasound (EUS), which provides a diagnosis by ultrasound image-defined criteria, ultrasound-directed aspiration biopsy, and when indicated by endoscopic mucosal or submucosal resection.

Inflammatory gastropathies will be covered in other chapters, as will gastrointestinal polyposis syndromes, gastrointestinal stromal tumors (GISTs), and carcinoid tumors. Foregut intussusception, congenital webs, and duplications are discussed in another chapter but figure prominently in any discussion of miscellaneous conditions of the stomach, duodenum, and small intestine in adults. Rare in children, these congenital variations in foregut anatomy are rarer in adults and typically present with vague symptoms and difficulty in diagnosis with modern as well as traditional imaging techniques.

BENIGN LESIONS OF THE STOMACH, DUODENUM, AND SMALL INTESTINE

BENIGN LESIONS OF THE STOMACH

Benign lesions of the stomach include heterotopic pancreas, pancreatic acinar metaplasia, gastric adenomyoma, chronic gastritis, acute gastritis, collagenous gastritis, eosinophilic gastritis, granulomatous gastritis, malakoplakia, cytomegalovirus infection, fungal infection, graft-versus-host disease, peptic ulcer, duplication, diverticula, cysts, hyperplastic polyp, adenoma, lipoma, fundic gland polyp, polyposis syndrome, inflammatory fibroid polyp,

Ménétrier disease, gastric antral vascular ectasia (GAVE), telangiectasia, neurogenic tumors, glomus tumor, and many others. In a study of a 12-year experience with 10,000 gastric specimens accumulated over 12 years, 8579 benign gastric conditions were described (Table 66.1).[1] The most common inflammatory conditions of the stomach are chronic gastritis and peptic ulcer disease with *Helicobacter pylori* seen in the majority of specimens. Foveolar hyperplastic polyps are notable for harboring malignant foci and dysplastic glands in 2% to 3% of cases, demonstrating the potential they have in the transition from dysplasia to carcinoma. Fundic gland polyps are benign lesions that have neither clinical relevance nor risk of malignant transformation. Heterotopic pancreas has a characteristic endoscopic appearance that may be mistaken for adenocarcinoma unless deep biopsies are taken. Pancreatic acinar metaplasia is an incidental microscopic lesion that is problematic when misdiagnosed as cancer. Gastric amyloidosis is a manifestation of systemic disease often related to multiple myeloma and chronic inflammatory disease.

BENIGN LESIONS OF THE DUODENUM

Benign lesions of the duodenum include heterotopic pancreas, heterotopic gastric mucosa, duplication, atresia, diverticulum, celiac disease, tropical sprue, Whipple disease, amyloidosis, parasite infestation, duodenal ulcer, duodenitis, acquired immune deficiency syndrome (AIDS)-related inflammatory disease, fungal infection, cytomegalovirus infection, radiation duodenitis, Brunner gland hyperplasia, Brunner gland adenoma, adenoma, hamartomatous polyp, endometriosis, inflammatory fibroid polyp, lipoma, hemangioma, lymphangioma, telangiectasia, neurofibroma, ganglioneurofibroma, and congenital fibromatosis. In a review of pathologic reports of 615 duodenal specimens collected over 10 years, 567 benign lesions and 48 malignant lesions were identified.[2] The benign lesions were identified as chronic nonspecific duodenitis in 334 cases (60.0%), duodenal ulcer in 101 cases (17.8%), heterotopic gastric mucosa in 81 cases (14.3%), hyperplastic polyp in 16 cases (2.8%), Brunner gland hyperplasia in 14 cases (2.5%), Brunner gland adenoma in 8 cases (1.4%), lymphoid polyp in 5 cases (0.8%), tubular adenoma in 4 cases (0.7%), lymphangioma in 2 cases (0.4%), endocrine cell micronests in 1 case (0.2%), and amyloidosis in 1 case (0.2%).

Similar to the stomach, duodenitis and ulcer disease are the most common benign duodenal conditions. Heterotopic gastric mucosa is a rare disorder that may be congenital or acquired and consists of two types: foveolar epithelium and fundic glands. Surgical awareness is

TABLE 66.1 Prevalence of Various Lesions Among 8570 Benign Gastric Lesions[1]

Benign Lesions	No. of Cases (%)
Almost normal stomach	74 (0.9)
Chronic gastritis	4374 (51.0)
Benign peptic gastric ulcer	2195 (25.6)
Foveolar hyperplastic polyp	1004 (11.7)
Fundic gland polyp	421 (4.9)
Adenoma	487 (5.6)
Heterotopic pancreas	9 (0.1)
Pancreatic acinar metaplasia	8 (0.1)
Amyloidosis	7 (0.1)

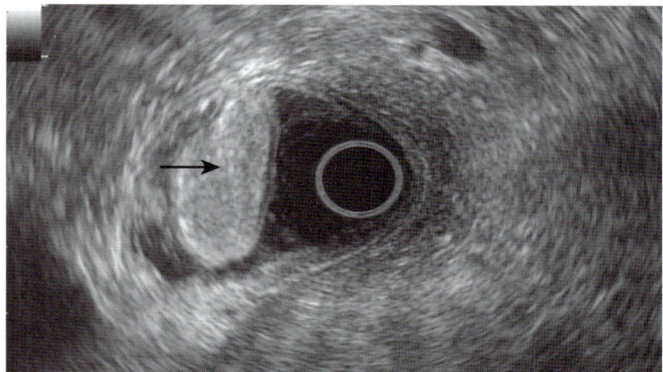

FIGURE 66.1 Endoscopic ultrasound image of submucosal gastric lipoma *(arrow)*.

important because adenoma and adenocarcinoma on rare occasion arise in heterotopic gastric mucosa. Hyperplastic polyps are usually in the first and second portions of the duodenum, and they too may very rarely undergo malignant transformation. Brunner gland hyperplasia is usually seen in the first and second portion of the duodenum. Adenoma and carcinoma arising in Brunner gland hyperplasia occurs but is almost as rare as hen's teeth.[2] Lymphoid polyps are uncommon and are important only in their differentiation from lymphoma.

BENIGN LESIONS OF THE SMALL INTESTINE

Benign tumors of the small intestine are not common but are being identified with increasing frequency via wireless capsule endoscopy and prograde push enteroscopy. Benign small intestinal tumors may uncommonly develop malignant changes. Small intestinal tumors are frequently difficult to diagnose given the challenge of identifying them by endoscopic means or by axial imaging. They may present with hemorrhage or intestinal obstruction but are often asymptomatic, and often remain undiagnosed until found incidentally at the time of laparotomy for other indications. The major types of benign tumors of the small bowel include adenomas, leiomyomas, and lipomas. These increase in frequency moving distally within the small bowel. In general, adenomas are removed endoscopically when accessible, and push enteroscopy increases the opportunity for endoscopic resection of small proximal tumors.[3] Larger lesions or those not amenable to endoscopic resection should be excised laparoscopically.

DIAGNOSIS AND TREATMENT OF SUBMUCOSAL TUMORS OF THE STOMACH, DUODENUM, AND SMALL INTESTINE

Submucosal tumors (SMTs) are a class of gastrointestinal lesions that originate below the mucosal layer from the muscularis mucosa, submucosa, and muscularis propria. SMTs include leiomyoma, stromal tumors, lipomas, and neurogenic tumors. Neoplastic SMTs are typically nonepithelial tumors. Nonepithelial tumors are subdivided into mesenchymal tumors and lymphomas, such as mucosa-associated lymphoid tissue (MALT) and malignant lymphomas. Mesenchymal tumors include GISTs, myogenic tumors such as leiomyoma and leiomyosarcoma, neurogenic

tumors including schwannoma and neurofibroma, vascular tumors, and others. Patients with SMTs may present with bleeding or obstruction, but usually display no specific symptoms, and in most cases they are discovered incidentally during endoscopic examination. Gastrointestinal SMTs are usually benign, and only a small portion are malignant. The characteristic endoscopic appearance of an SMT is a protuberant lesion covered with intact mucosa. The nature of the lesion may be evident endoscopically based on the size, shape, firmness, surface color, and overall appearance, but histologic diagnosis is limited. EUS is capable of determining the nature of a lesion based on the originating layer, size, and internal echoes of the lesion (Fig. 66.1). Endoscopic ultrasound-guided fine-needle aspiration (EUS-FNA) plays a key role in management of SMTs.[4,5]

Endoscopic submucosal resection (ESR) is the treatment for most gastrointestinal SMTs in the stomach and duodenum under 2 cm in diameter. Some specialized centers use endoscopic knife technology to perform endoscopic full-thickness resection (EFTR) and endoscopic closure to excise early gastrointestinal cancer and precancerous lesions. EFTR competes at times at a disadvantage with laparoscopic-assisted full-thickness and partial-thickness resections.[6]

Because EUS and EUS-FNA are not available for managing and following small intestinal SMTs, operative excision is recommended even if small. Most benign SMTs can be excised with minimally invasive techniques. The majority of SMTs are resected without preoperative diagnosis. High-risk features of SMTs include irregular border, inhomogeneous internal echo, and heterogeneous enhancement with contrast media. Symptomatic SMTs should undergo surgery. SMTs increasing in size should undergo surgical resection even if asymptomatic and small.[4] Gastric SMTs not amenable to ESR or EFTR due to size or location are good candidates for traditional laparoscopic excision with endoscopic guidance. The technique involves identification of the lesion intraoperatively with an endoscopic view, and full-thickness intraperitoneal excision of the lesion with a laparoscopic cutting and stapling device. For large lesions and lesions that are not readily resected without compromise of the gastric lumen, combined transgastric and endoscopic approaches work well. Similarly, lesions at the gastro-esophageal junction are difficult to address endoscopically and lend themselves to a combined endoscopic and transgastric laparoscopic approach.[7,8] The technique involves endoscopic placement of three 5-mm transgastric balloon-secured ports, which allow access to the gastric lumen for submucosal resection of the tumor with laparoscopic techniques. Although the endoscope can identify the tumor, resection is easier if a 5-mm transgastric laparoscope is used for the resection. Mucosa is reapproximated with transgastric laparoscopic suturing and the tumor is retrieved transorally with an endoscopic retrieval device.

BENIGN CONDITIONS OF THE STOMACH, DUODENUM, AND SMALL INTESTINE

INTUSSUSCEPTION OF THE STOMACH, DUODENUM, AND SMALL INTESTINE

Gastrointestinal intussusception in adults is a rare condition, representing only 5% of all intussusceptions. Intussusception can evolve from any pathologic lesion that alters peristalsis. About 90% of cases of adult intussusception have an identifiable pathologic lesion as a lead point, usually a tumor. Intussusception has been noted in patients with celiac disease, abdominal trauma, during the postoperative period, and with acquired immunodeficiency syndrome–related gut disease. Unlike intussusception in children, intussusception in adults usually presents with vague signs and symptoms and is rarely diagnosed preoperatively.[9]

Gastroduodenal intussusception is an uncommon condition usually caused by the prolapse of a benign gastric tumor into the duodenum with subsequent invagination of a portion of the stomach wall. Adenoma, leiomyoma, lipoma, hamartoma inflammatory polyp, adenocarcinoma, and leiomyosarcoma are known to cause gastroduodenal intussusception. Clinical manifestations may mimic many other disease entities and are nonspecific. Diagnosis is best accomplished with CT or magnetic resonance imaging (MRI). Treatment involves reduction of the intussusception and surgical excision of the lead point, either endoscopically or with laparotomy.[10]

Duodenal intussusception is a rare entity because of the fixed, retroperitoneal position of the duodenum. Most of the cases of intussusception involving the duodenum are gastroduodenal or distal duodenojejunal intussusceptions. Diagnosis of duodenal intussusception is usually delayed because of its long-standing, intermittent, and nonspecific symptoms, and most cases are diagnosed at emergency laparotomy. Duodenal intussusception remains in the differential diagnosis of gastric outlet obstruction, pancreatitis, and obstructive jaundice in adults.[11]

The clinical presentation in adult intussusception of the small intestine is often chronic, and most patients present with nonspecific symptoms that are suggestive of intestinal obstruction. Abdominal pain is the most common symptom followed by vomiting and rectal bleeding. Radiologic studies are frequently used to evaluate patients with intussusception. The plain abdominal radiograph is rarely diagnostic and often demonstrates nonspecific signs of intestinal obstruction, and CT imaging is more useful.

The dense nature of the intussuscepted mass, comprised of edematous bowel wall and mesentery in the lumen, gives it the characteristic "target" sign or sausage-shaped appearance.[12]

The optimal management of adult intestinal intussusception remains controversial. Most of the debate focuses on the issue of primary en bloc resection versus initial reduction followed by a more limited resection. The inability to preoperatively or intraoperatively differentiate malignant from benign causes suggests that small bowel intussusception be resected without reduction. A selective approach to resection is recommended when taking into consideration the influence of the site of intussusception or the likelihood of a malignant lead point. Simple reduction is acceptable in post-traumatic and idiopathic intussusceptions where no pathologic cause is identified.[12] Benign, incidental small intestine intussusception is noted with increasing frequency in patients on CT imaging. Usually unrelated to the indication for the CT scan, there is neither an associated lead point nor an indication for operation when reduction of the intussusception occurs spontaneously and symptoms resolve. Capsule endoscopy may be indicated in this situation but is not likely to identify a lead point.

STENOSIS AND WEBS OF THE DUODENUM

There are several varieties of congenital duodenal webs due to embryonic duodenal atresia. When atresia is complete, diagnosis is made in infancy. When atresia is incomplete, patients may remain asymptomatic until adulthood when misdiagnosis of an acquired acid-peptic stricture is made. The tipoff to the correct diagnosis is the location of the stenosis in the descending duodenum (Fig. 66.2). In adults, webs are perforated centrally or eccentrically, and because of the juxtaampullary position, surgical or endoscopic extirpation is a potentially

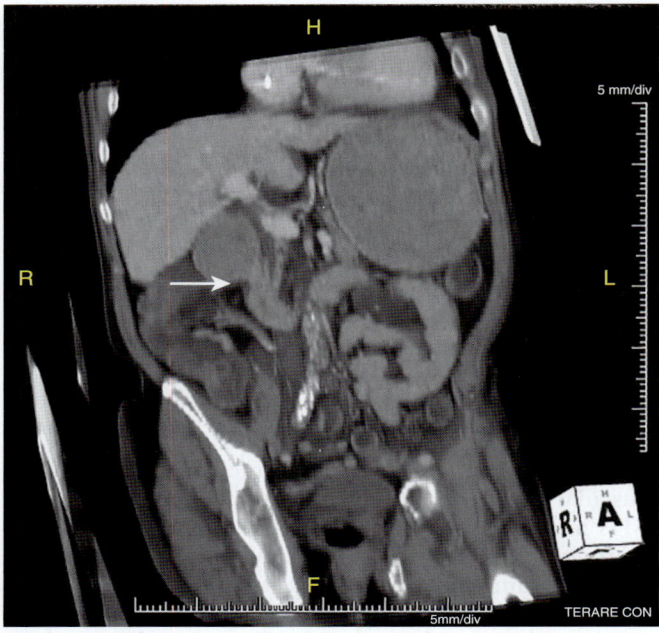

FIGURE 66.2 Computed tomography image of adult duodenal web (*arrow*) in a juxtaampullary position.

dangerous procedure. Sutton's law states: "Congenital obstruction and narrowing of the alimentary canal is always found in the situation of embryological events,"[13] and is a reminder that when duodenal webs are present, anomalous pancreato-biliary union may coexist. When duodenal stenosis is diagnosed in the adult, the question arises as to why symptoms did not develop in infancy or childhood. The answer is that the propulsive force of the stomach is strong and symptoms do not develop until there is decompensation of the peristaltic force of the stomach and proximal duodenum.[14] Associated gastro-duodenal dilation develops, and the web itself can stretch and produce what is called a windsock deformity, which may present a polypoid appearance endoscopically.

The conventional treatment of duodenal webs is longitudinal duodenotomy with partial or near-complete excision of the web and transverse closure of the duodenum. When web excision is performed, careful attention should be given to protection of the biliopancreatic sphincter mechanism by avoiding resection of the juxta-ampullary portion of the web or intubating the common duct to protect the ducts. The duodenum should be inspected for distal webs by passing a Foley catheter distally and withdrawing it with the balloon. Endoscopic incision and excision of a web are options as is a laparoscopic approach, provided the biliary and pancreatic duct union with the duodenum is safeguarded.[15]

DUPLICATION CYSTS OF THE STOMACH, DUODENUM, AND SMALL INTESTINE

Gastrointestinal duplication cysts, which occur from the mouth to the anus, are rare in children and rarely symptomatic in adults, presenting diagnostic and treatment dilemmas. Duplication cysts are located in or immediately adjacent to the wall of the gastrointestinal tract on the mesenteric side, and typically do not show luminal communication.[14] They have a muscular wall and may contain gastric, pancreatic, and respiratory tissue. When respiratory tissue is present, the cyst does not fit the strict criteria of a gastrointestinal duplication cyst but follows similar management principles.[16]

Gastric duplications and foregut cysts are usually asymptomatic, rarely presenting as a mass on physical examination. In the adult patient, complications of bleeding, obstruction, and perforation may indicate the need for operation. As a result of the cyst location within the gastric muscular layer and a lack of communication with the gastric lumen, many lesions are preoperatively misdiagnosed as intramural GIST or leiomyoma. CT can detect the presence of the abdominal mass, but it frequently fails to recognize its cystic nature due to the thick cyst wall. EUS is helpful in identifying the intramural or extramural relation of the gastrointestinal tract (Fig. 66.3). CT, MRI, and ultrasonography identify the mass but cannot specify the diagnosis. EUS-FNA can provide cytologic information. Expectant management of asymptomatic cysts is recommended, though most patients come to attention because they are symptomatic. Cysts that communicate with the gastric lumen can be associated with perforation, bleeding, obstruction, and malignant transformation and are managed with partial gastrectomy. For cysts that do not communicate with the stomach, cyst

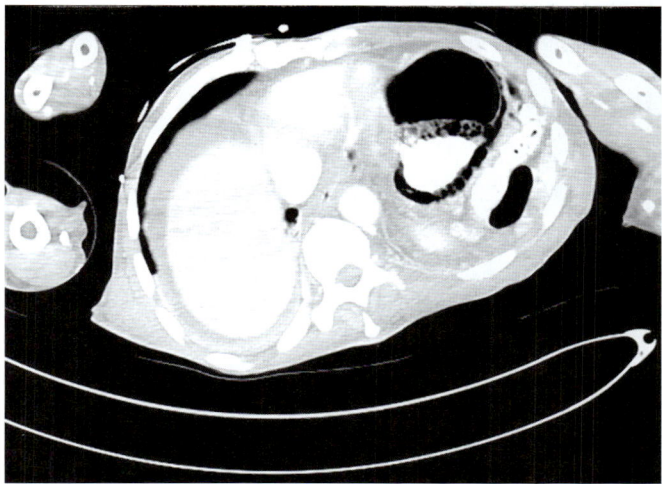

FIGURE 66.3 Endoscopic ultrasound image of adenocarcinoma arising is a duodenal duplication cyst.

excision without opening the stomach is indicated and can be done laparoscopically.[16]

Duodenal duplication cysts usually present in children, although it is important to know that duodenal duplications may remain asymptomatic until adulthood. More than one-third are diagnosed after the age of 20. Duodenal duplication cysts are usually located posteromedially in the descending duodenum and are closely associated with the pancreatobiliary duct system. Duodenal duplication cysts are usually spherical and noncommunicating and have a well-developed smooth muscle coat. They share a common wall with the native duodenum with luminal communication in the minority of cases. The most common presenting symptoms are nonspecific abdominal pain, nausea, and vomiting. Other presenting symptoms include gastrointestinal hemorrhage, intussusception, obstruction, jaundice, and pancreatitis. Complications of duodenal duplication cysts include bowel obstruction, bile duct obstruction, and pancreatitis, bleeding, intussusception, and malignancy. Duodenal duplication cysts may be lined by ectopic gastric epithelium, predisposing to ulceration, bleeding, and perforation.[17,18]

Intestinal duplication in adults is rare and most commonly comes to surgical attention when obstruction, perforation, or bleeding occurs. In patients with nonspecific symptoms, ultrasound, CT scan, and MRI are useful in making a diagnosis. Carcinomas arising in duplication cysts are rare and include carcinoid tumors, squamous cell carcinoma, and adenocarcinoma. The indications for surgery for intestinal duplications are the same as those of the stomach and duodenum: bleeding, obstruction, perforation, intractability, or suspicion of malignancy. Open or laparoscopic sleeve resection is the preferred treatment.

PNEUMATOSIS OF THE STOMACH AND SMALL INTESTINE

Gastric pneumatosis represents a spectrum of conditions ranging from benign disease to septic shock and death.

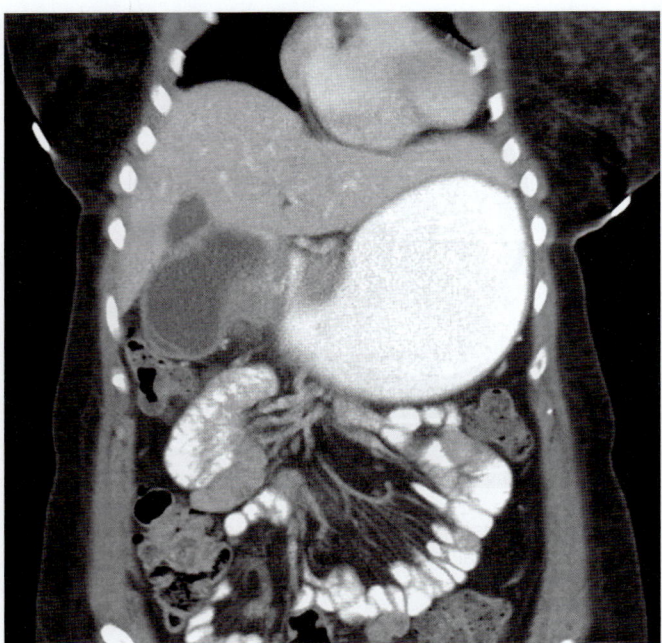

FIGURE 66.4 Computed tomography image in a patient with benign gastric pneumatosis.

Pneumatosis is identified radiographically and grossly when small mucosal, submucosal, or subserosal air-filled cysts develop in benign and life-threatening conditions. When associated with hepatoportal venous gas, it can indicate the need for emergent surgical exploration.[19] With widespread use of CT imaging, an increasing number of benign causes of gastric pneumatosis have been reported (Fig. 66.4). There exist two types of gastric pneumatosis, emphysematous gastritis and gastric emphysema. Emphysematous gastritis may occur by direct inoculation of gas-producing bacteria into the gastric mucosa or by hematogenous spread. *Clostridium perfringens, Escherichia coli, Pseudomonas aeruginosa,* streptococci, staphylococci, and *Enterobacter* species are the most frequent pathogens. Immunosuppression, diabetes mellitus, ingestion of corrosive substances, alcoholism, and nonsteroidal antiinflammatory drug ingestion are common predisposing factors.[19] Affected patients are very ill with severe abdominal pain, peritoneal signs, and leukocytosis, often resulting in fulminant sepsis. Gastric emphysema is noninfectious in origin and occurs primarily due to entry of intraluminal air into the wall of the stomach from traumatic, obstructive, and pulmonary origins.

Traumatic gastric emphysema caused by transmural diffusion of air after a mucosal injury, can occur after esophagogastroduodenoscopy, severe vomiting, and cardiopulmonary resuscitation. Obstructive gastric emphysema has been reported in patients with gastric outlet obstruction due to gastric cancer, gastric volvulus, duodenal obstruction, and hypertrophic pyloric stenosis. Pulmonary gastric emphysema is theoretically caused by alveolar rupture and air tracking through the mediastinum to the gastric wall. Clinical manifestations of gastric emphysema are usually nonspecific. Patients may present with nausea, vomiting, epigastric discomfort, or abdominal pain, and if the diagnosis is correct they will follow a benign course that resolves spontaneously without sequelae.[19]

Pneumatosis can affect any portion of the gastrointestinal tract and more commonly involves the small intestine than the stomach. Different mechanisms are associated with different mechanical, bacterial, or biochemical pathologic conditions. Pneumatosis intestinalis, which typically presents in adults in the fifth to eighth decade, is idiopathic in 15% of patients and secondary in 85%. Pneumatosis can be reproduced experimentally by insufflating air into a segment of bowel in which mucosal incisions have been made. Alternatively, gas-forming organisms that invade the submusosa can produce pneumatosis. CT scans are much more sensitive than plain abdominal radiographs, and may suggest an underlying cause. The clinical quandary is to differentiate benign pneumatosis from acute surgical problems: intestinal ischemia, infarction, obstruction, and perforation. In patients who have a history, physical exam, and laboratory findings of an acute abdomen, exploration of the abdomen is indicated. In those with benign findings, CT variables may indicate the need for exploration. Worrisome CT findings are thickening of the bowel wall, free peritoneal fluid, periintestinal soft tissue stranding, and extensive pneumatosis. The location of pneumatosis and the presence of free peritoneal air may not indicate severity of disease. Feeding jejunostomy, gastrostomy, esophagogastroduodenoscopy (EGD), colonoscopy, and endoscopic retrograde cholangiopancreatography (ERCP) may all cause benign pneumatosis. Other diseases and conditions associated with pneumatosis include infection, pulmonary disease, mechanical ventilation, asthma, cystic fibrosis, immune compromise, inflammatory bowel disease, peptic ulcer disease, cancer, diabetes, scleroderma, Hirschsprung disease, intestinal pseudoobstruction, amyloidosis, and collagen vascular disease. Most patients with idiopathic pneumatosis do not come to the attention of the clinician.[20] They do so when identified on radiographic studies for nonspecific gastrointestinal symptoms. However, in patients who present to the emergency department with pneumatosis, bowel ischemia is the most likely diagnosis. The critical decision in patient management is whether to treat the patient conservatively or proceed with emergent exploratory laparotomy. In patients whose clinical findings are inconsistent with an acute abdominal catastrophe, conservative management and a search for other causes should be undertaken.

CONCLUSIONS

Benign lesions of the stomach and small bowel are varied. A general knowledge of the potential diagnoses and management implications of these disorders is essential to the armamentarium of the general surgeon. Given the uncommon nature of many of these lesions, experience and the art of medicine are often required for successful management. Appropriate caution for malignant potential should be observed, although overtreatment of incidental conditions should be avoided.

REFERENCES

1. Terada T. Histopathological study using computer database of 10 000 consecutive gastric specimens: (1) benign conditions. *Gastroenterol Rep (Oxf)*. 2015;3:238.
2. Terada T. Pathologic observations of the duodenum in 615 consecutive duodenal specimens in a single Japanese hospital: II. Malignant lesions. *Int J Clin Exp Pathol*. 2012;5:52.
3. Song HJ, Shim KN. Current status and future perspectives of capsule endoscopy. *Intest Res*. 2016;14:21.
4. Nishida T, Kawai N, Yamaguchi S, Nishida Y. Submucosal tumors: comprehensive guide for the diagnosis and therapy of gastrointestinal submucosal tumors. *Dig Endosc*. 2013;25:479.
5. Papanikolaou IS, Triantafyllou K, Kourikou A, Rösch T. Endoscopic ultrasonography for gastric submucosal lesions. *World J Gastrointest Endosc*. 2011;3:86.
6. Zhang J, Huang K, Ding S, et al. Clinical applicability of various treatment approaches for upper gastrointestinal submucosal tumors. *Gastroenterol Res Pract*. 2016;2016:9430652. doi:10.1155/2016/9430652; [Epub 2016 Jan 11].
7. Barajas-Gamboa JS, Acosta G, Savides TJ, et al. Laparo-endoscopic transgastric resection of gastric submucosal tumors. *Surg Endosc*. 2015;29:2149.
8. Conrad C, Nedelcu M, Ogiso S, Aloia TA, Vauthey JN, Gayet B. Techniques of intragastric laparoscopic surgery. *Surg Endosc*. 2015;29:202.
9. Eisen LK, Cunningham JD, Aufses AH Jr. Intussusception in adults: institutional review. *J Am Coll Surg*. 1999;188:390.
10. Lin F, Setya V, Signor W. Gastroduodenal intussusception secondary to a gastric lipoma: a case report and review of the literature. *Am Surg*. 1992;58:772.
11. Pradhan D, Kaur N, Nagi B. Duodenoduodenal intussusception: report of three challenging cases with literature review. *J Cancer Res Ther*. 2015;11:1031.
12. Azar T, Berger DL. Adult intussusception. *Ann Surg*. 1997;226:134.
13. Sutton JB. Imperforate ileum. *Am J Med Sci*. 1889;98:457.
14. Adams DB. Management of the intraluminal duodenal diverticulum: endoscopy or duodenotomy? *Am J Surg*. 1986;151:524.
15. Ladd AP, Madura JA. Congenital duodenal anomalies in the adult. *Arch Surg*. 2001;136:576.
16. Geng YH, Wang CX, Li JT, Chen QY, Li XZ, Pan H. Gastric foregut cystic developmental malformation: case series and literature review. *World J Gastroenterol*. 2015;21:432.
17. Tsai SD, Sopha SC, Fishman EK. Isolated duodenal duplication cyst presenting as a complex solid and cystic mass in the upper abdomen. *J Radiol Case Rep*. 2013;7:32.
18. Chen JJ, Lee HC, Yeung CY, Chan WT, Jiang CB, Sheu JC. Meta-analysis: the clinical features of the duodenal duplication cyst. *J Pediatr Surg*. 2010;45:1598.
19. Parikh MP, Sherid M, Ganipisetti V, Gopalakrishnan V, Habib M, Tripathi M. Vomiting-induced gastric emphysema and hepatoportal venous gas: a case report and review of the literature. *Case Rep Med*. 2015;2015:413230. doi:10.1155/2015/413230; [Epub 2015 Feb 11].
20. Khalil PN, Huber-Wagner S, Ladurner R, et al. Natural history, clinical pattern, and surgical considerations of pneumatosis intestinalis. *Eur J Med Res*. 2009;14:231.

Surgical Disease of the Stomach and Duodenum in Infants and Children

Paul M. Jeziorczak | Alice King | Brad W. Warner

The spectrum of diseases of the stomach and duodenum in the pediatric population is broad. Surgical treatment of the pediatric patient requires a thorough understanding and knowledge of developmental biology, in addition to the unique physiologic and pathologic processes. Many congenital anomalies of the stomach and duodenum are identified prenatally or in the neonatal period, while other lesions are acquired and may manifest later in childhood and adolescence.

This chapter discusses the evaluation and management of some of the more common surgical disease in infants and children within the first two decades of life.

EMBRYOLOGY

Rapid growth of the foregut occurs during the fourth week of gestation. The proximal aspect dilates to become the stomach. Over the next few weeks, the posterior wall of the foregut grows faster than the anterior wall to form the greater and lesser curves of the stomach. Concurrently, the proximal foregut rotates around both longitudinal and anteroposterior (AP) axes. Rotation around the AP axes brings the caudal position to the right and superiorly to the normal position of the pylorus and the cephalic portion to the left and inferiorly.

The duodenum arises at the junction between the foregut and midgut. The lumen of the duodenum is obliterated at the fifth week of gestation by the proliferation of growing epithelial cells. Recanalization through vacuolization occurs around the eighth week with patency typically restored by 11 weeks. Errors in this recanalization process may result in proximal small bowel obstruction.

During the 5th to 11th week of gestation, the duodenum shifts from a midline, freely mobile structure to the normal position in the upper retroperitoneum. The development of the duodenum is closely associated with the pancreas. The pancreas is formed by dorsal and ventral pancreatic buds that originate from the endodermal lining of the duodenum just distal to the forming stomach. The ventral pancreas rotates around the duodenum toward the dorsal pancreas. As the pancreas increases in size and the stomach completes its rotation, the duodenum shifts toward the left and results in the characteristic C-shaped loop.[1]

Malrotation or nonrotation of the intestines occurs in approximately one in 500 live births. Infants presenting with bilious emesis should have a high index of suspicion for malrotation and possible volvulus. An expedient upper gastrointestinal (UGI) contrast study is crucial to identify the characteristic C loop of the duodenum and the position of the ligament of Treitz crossing left of the midline and returning to the level of the pylorus. Malrotation is the anatomic anomaly that predisposes infants to volvulus because of a narrow mesenteric pedicle that can lead to intestinal infarction. Midgut volvulus is a surgical emergency (Fig. 67.1).

PRENATAL DIAGNOSIS

The fetal stomach is visible beginning at 9 weeks of gestation on the prenatal sonogram as a cystic structure in the left upper quadrant of the abdomen. The bowel appears uniformly echogenic until the third trimester, when more prominent meconium-filled large bowel may become apparent.

Multiple developmental abnormalities may become apparent antenatally on ultrasound or magnetic resonance imaging (MRI). Proximal obstructions, such as duodenal atresias may be visualized with abnormal cystic structures identified between 20 and 25 weeks' gestation. These obstructions are commonly associated with polyhydramnios as the fetus is incapable of swallowing and absorbing sufficient amniotic fluid.

The rate of associated anomalies will vary depending on the underlying developmental abnormality. However, antenatal diagnosis of foregut pathology should generally prompt further evaluation of associated anomalies. For instance, approximately half of patients with duodenal atresia will have associated anomalies including trisomy 21, malrotation, skeletal and other gastrointestinal abnormalities.[1]

CONGENITAL LESIONS

STOMACH AND DUODENUM

Enteric Duplication

Incidence and Etiology. Enteric duplications may occur anywhere along the gastrointestinal tract. Gastric and duodenal duplications represent ~15% in a series spanning 31 years by Iyer and Mahour, with the remainder of enteric duplications occurring in the distal small bowel, colon, and rectum. Multiple mechanisms have been proposed, including persistent fetal enteric diverticula, incomplete recanalization following obliteration of the lumen during duodenal development, and the "split notocord" theory, whereby abnormal adhesions persist between the ectoderm and endoderm leading to herniation of the yolk sac between the vertebra, resulting in local duplication of the gut. Duplications may be saccular or tubular in morphology

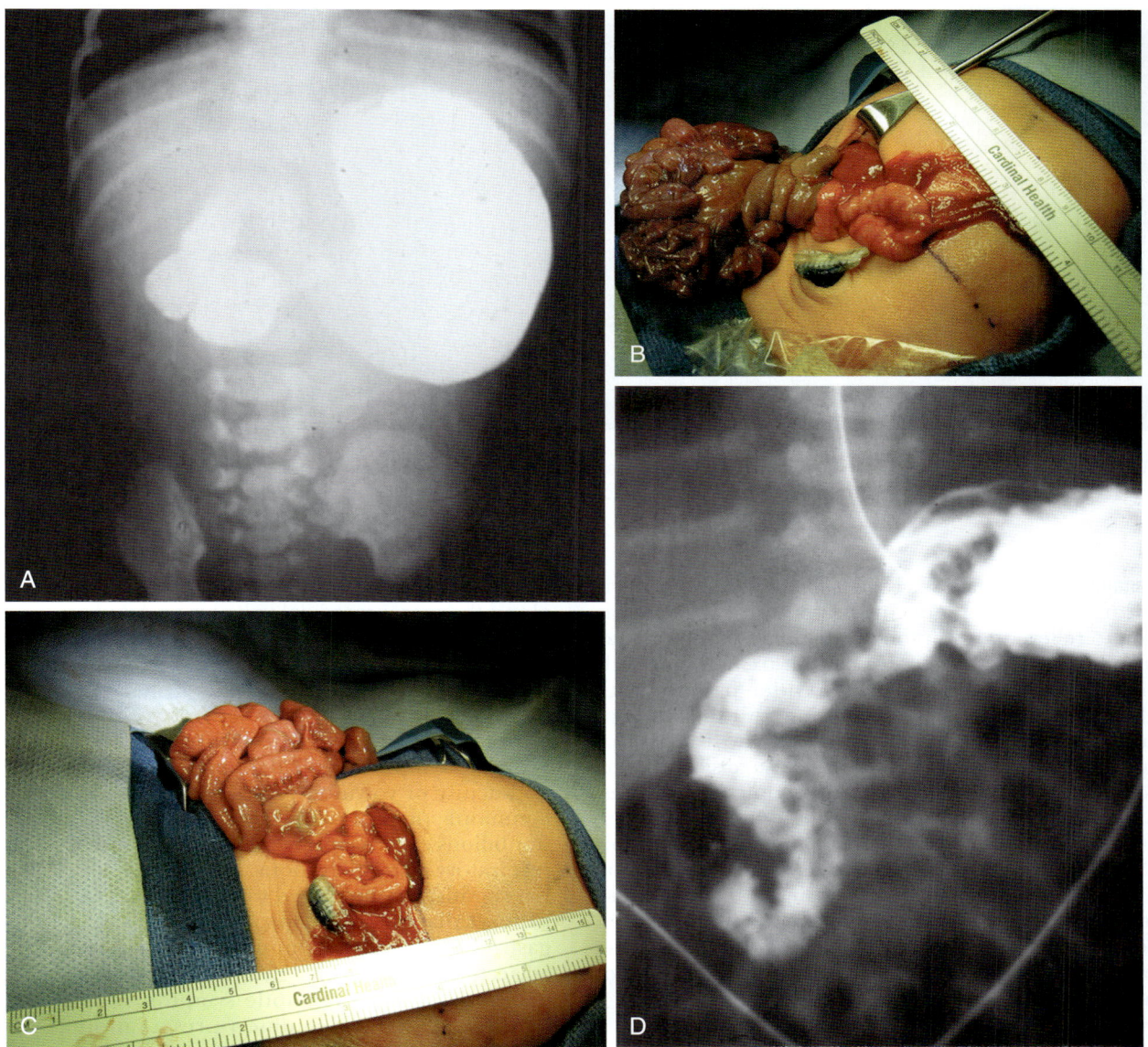

FIGURE 67.1 (A) Upper gastrointestinal (UGI) study showing malrotation with midgut volvulus. (B) Operative photograph showing intestinal malrotation with midgut volvulus. (C) Operative photograph showing intestinal malrotation after reduction of torsion. (D) UGI study showing malrotation, with the ligament of Treitz to the right of the midline and no evidence of volvulus.

and may be located in the intermuscular, submucosal, or subserosal layers of the intestinal wall. They primarily occur on the mesenteric side of the involved segment and have variable communication with the lumen of adjacent bowel. Histology will demonstrate smooth muscle within the wall and a mucosal lining.[1,2]

Presentation and Diagnosis. Two-thirds of patients are diagnosed within the first year of life, while many asymptomatic patients or patients with mild symptoms may remain undiagnosed until adulthood. Many of the symptoms are a result of a mass effect as the duplication grows in size from accumulating mucosal secretions. Patients may present relatively asymptomatic with a mobile mass or increasing abdominal girth. Enteric duplications may result in visceral pain or obstruction from compression of adjacent structures. Duodenal and gastric duplications

can result in gastric outlet obstruction. Almost one-half of enteric duplications contain gastric mucosa, which can lead to ulceration and gastrointestinal bleeding. Pancreatitis and perforation may occur from peptic ulceration within duodenal duplications. Malignancy has been described in rare case reports.[2]

Diagnosis of enteric duplication can be detected with enteric contrast studies. In the advent of routine antenatal imaging, increasing numbers of patients are diagnosed before birth. Both prenatal ultrasound and MRI have been used in detecting these lesions. MRI is valuable in the evaluation of associated anomalies such as cardiac, pulmonary, and spinal defects. Once the lesion is prenatally diagnosed, surveillance is important to monitor for rapid growth leading to mass effect on neighboring structures in utero (Fig. 67.2A).[3-5]

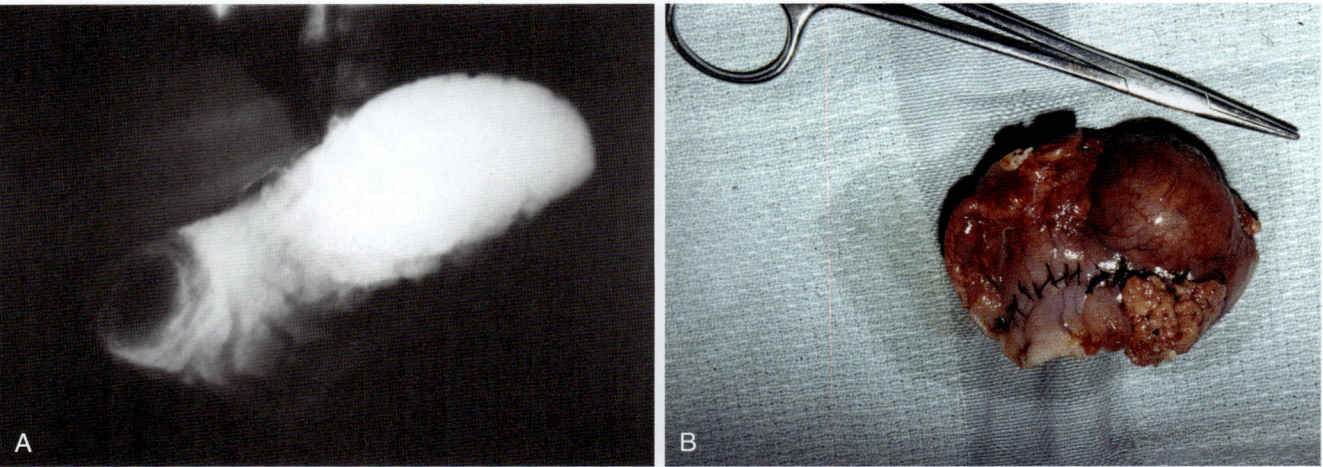

FIGURE 67.2 (A) Upper gastrointestinal (UGI) study showing a gastric duplication in the antral region of the stomach. (B) Resected specimen of a gastric duplication from the antral region of the stomach as seen on the UGI study.

Management. Surgical excision is the mainstay of enteric duplication management and is required in a timely fashion to relieve the symptomatic patient. Asymptomatic, prenatally diagnosed neonates can be treated electively within the first 6 months of life. Older patients with incidental diagnosis found on imaging for other reasons should undergo elective resection due to the risk of complications over a lifetime. Surgical excision can be performed through open or laparoscopic approaches. The enteric duplication may be excised alone; however, care must be taken to preserve the common blood supply with the adjacent bowel. Selective excision of duodenal duplications is particularly challenging at times because of proximity to hepatobiliary and pancreatic structures. Mucosal stripping and cyst excision or Roux-en-Y cyst-jejunostomy have been described in surgical management of these potentially difficult lesions (see Fig. 67.2B).[6,7]

STOMACH

Gastric Volvulus

Incidence and Etiology. Gastric volvulus is rare in the pediatric population with only 581 cases described in 78 years. Nonetheless, it continues to be an important pathology that must be recognized early to ensure a good outcome. The stomach is normally anchored by a number of fixation points. The gastrocolic, gastrosplenic, gastrohepatic, and gastrosplenic ligaments, along with the esophagogastric junction and pylorus, normally prevent abnormal rotation of the stomach. Failure of usual fixation can result from agenesis, laxity, or disruption of these ligaments and can lead to pathologic rotation of the stomach. Gastric volvulus may also result from gastric neoplasm, intestinal malrotation, and abnormal development of the diaphragm, spleen, transverse colon, and liver.[8]

The stomach may rotate along two planes. Organoaxial volvulus occurs along the longitudinal axis, when the stomach rotates around the plane between the esophagogastric junction and the pylorus. The stomach will appear upside-down, with the greater curvature located superior to the lesser curve. The stomach may also rotate along the mesenteroaxial volvulus or AP plane, resulting in the antrum and pylorus anterior and superior to the esophagogastric junction. Gastric volvulus around both planes has also been diagnosed.[9]

Presentation and Diagnosis. Gastric volvulus in pediatric population can present in either an acute or chronic fashion. Symptoms will depend on degree of twisting and acuity of volvulus. Acute gastric volvulus will most commonly present in children less than 5 years old with nonbilious emesis, epigastric pain, abdominal distention, respiratory distress, cyanosis, and hematemesis. Mortality has significantly improved with increasing awareness and prompt diagnosis with survival more than 90%. Acute gastric volvulus is commonly associated with abnormal adjacent organs. Chronic gastric volvulus is a more difficult diagnosis, with more subtle symptoms of intermittent volvulus. The most common presentation of chronic gastric volvulus is in an infant less than 1 year old with nonbilious emesis, feeding intolerance, abdominal pain, and respiratory distress.[8,9]

Plain radiographs may show a dilated gastric silhouette at or above the level of the diaphragm. The orientation of the stomach may be horizontal if twisted along the organoaxial axis or vertical if volvulized along the mesenteroaxial axis. Definitive diagnosis is confirmed by a UGI study.[8]

Management. The underlying etiology of the gastric volvulus directs medical versus surgical treatment. Acute gastric volvulus is potentially life-threatening and must be managed expediently. Fluid resuscitation and gastric decompression via nasogastric or orogastric decompression must be initiated. The goals of surgery are to reduce the volvulus, and gastropexy, and any associated intraabdominal factors predisposing to volvulus are repaired.

Chronic primary gastric volvulus may be treated nonoperatively with prone or right lateral positioning following feeding. However, in the United States, most chronic volvulus is managed surgically with gastric fixation by gastropexy or gastrostomy tube placement.[8]

Hiatal Hernia

Incidence and Etiology. While paraesophageal hernia may occur as a complication following fundoplication, congenital paraesophageal hernia is a rare pathology and accounts for less than 5% of all hiatal hernias. Approximately one-third of patients will have an associated anomaly, such as intestinal malrotation, microgastria, or trisomy 21. Hiatal hernias can be classified into four types. Type I hiatal hernias are sliding hernias involving the gastric cardia. Types II, III, and IV are paraesophageal hernias. In type II, the gastroesophageal junction remains in the normal position with herniation of the gastric fundus alongside. In type III hernias, the gastroesophageal junction herniates into the thoracic cavity with the gastric fundus, and type IV hernia involves herniation of any additional intraabdominal organs, such as the colon, spleen, small intestine, or omentum.[10]

Presentation and Diagnosis. Hiatal hernia most commonly presents with emesis and is concomitantly diagnosed with gastroesophageal reflux disease. In approximately 70% of patients with type III and IV hernias, respiratory distress will accompany gastrointestinal symptoms. Diagnosis can be suggested on chest x-ray with lateral films to differentiate between Bochdalek and Morgagni hernia. The diagnosis is confirmed on UGI study or CT scan.[11,12]

Management. Congenital hiatal hernias are managed surgically with the reduction of stomach and gastroesophageal junction to the abdominal cavity and repair of the hiatus with fundoplication. The hernia sac may be redundant and adherent to thoracic structures. However, efforts to excise the hernia should be attempted, as the sac may tether intraabdominal contents and prevent successful reduction. Repair may be performed laparoscopically or through an open approach. Most often in pediatrics, the hiatal defect may be closed primarily without the use of biologic or mesh material. The esophagus may be stented with a bougie during hiatal closure and fundoplication to avoid excessive narrowing.[10,13]

Agastria and Microgastria

Incidence and Etiology. Congenital microgastria is a rare anomaly with only 63 reported cases. Microgastria is defined by a small, underdeveloped stomach with agastria representing the extreme of the spectrum with the complete absence of the stomach. Microgastria most often occurs with other anomalies, including asplenia, esophageal atresia, intestinal malrotation, cardiac defects, renal malformations, central nervous system abnormalities, laryngotracheal stenosis, bronchial clefts, and limb irregularities.[14]

Presentation and Diagnosis. The underdeveloped stomach is unable to serve as a reservoir, leading to feeding intolerance with frequent emesis, failure to thrive, gastroesophageal reflux, and recurrent respiratory infections from aspiration. Diagnosis is confirmed with a UGI study that demonstrates a small tubular stomach in a transverse orientation and may be associated with a proximally dilated esophagus.[14]

Management. Microgastria is initially managed medically with small-volume nasogastric feeds and medical control of associated reflux. Failure of medical management results in both short-term and long-term sequelae, including poor growth, cognitive delay, and dumping syndrome. Definitive management of microgastria has not been defined, as it is most frequently associated with other conditions. The initial goals of surgical management are to optimize nutrition and growth such as creation of a gastrojejunostomy, a feeding jejunostomy, or a Roux-en-Y feeding jejunostomy. These efforts are met with limited success with persistent poor growth and development, as well as a high occurrence of dumping syndrome. Definitive surgical treatment for congenital microgastria with improvement of dumping syndrome was initially demonstrated in 1980 with the description of the jejunal Hunt-Lawrence pouch as a Roux-en-Y limb.[14,15]

Congenital Gastric Outlet Obstruction

Incidence and Etiology. There are several lesions that may lead to primary congenital gastric outlet obstruction including mass effect from adjacent enteric duplications or tumors. Congenital pyloric atresia is a rare cause of gastric outlet obstruction with an incidence of 1 in 100,000 births. Pyloric atresia is classified into three types. Type I is a simple luminal web or membrane. Type II is a complete atresia separated by a fibrous band. Type III involves a complete separation with a resultant gap. Forty percent of congenital pyloric atresia is accompanied by other disorders, most commonly intestinal atresia and epidermolysis bullosa (Fig. 67.3).[16,17]

Presentation and Diagnosis. Congenital gastric outlet obstructions will most often present with nonbilious emesis as neonates. Prenatal diagnosis is often possible with the identification of a dilated stomach on ultrasound or MRI and associated polyhydramnios as early as 24 weeks' gestation. Plain radiographs of the infant will show a dilated stomach with air with relative paucity of distal gas (Fig. 67.4). The diagnosis can be confirmed with a UGI study.[16,18]

Management. Pyloric atresia is managed surgically, including assessing and addressing associated disorders. Gastric decompression is initially accomplished through nasogastric or orogastric tube placement and fluid resuscitation is initiated to correct any electrolyte abnormalities. The membranous web in type I pyloric atresia is a fenestrated diaphragm comprised of two layers of mucosa. The membrane is excised circumferentially with a Heineke-Mikulicz pyloroplasty if the lesion is within 1 cm of the pylorus. Type II pyloric atresia is best treated by resection of the obstructed, fibrous segment and creation of a gastroduodenostomy. Type III pyloric atresia can be treated with a gastrogastrostomy or gastroduodenostomy.[19]

Dextrogastria

Incidence and Etiology. Dextrogastria is a rare finding with only 80 cases described in the literature. Dextrogastria is always associated with additional anomalies. Most commonly, it occurs in the setting of heterotaxy, situs inversus, or with significant cardiac anomalies such as transposition of great arteries, pulmonary atresia, total anomalous pulmonary venous return, and hypertrophic cardiomyopathy. Asplenia has also been associated with dextrogastria.[20,21]

Presentation and Diagnosis. Generally, dextrogastria is asymptomatic and identified as an incidental finding.

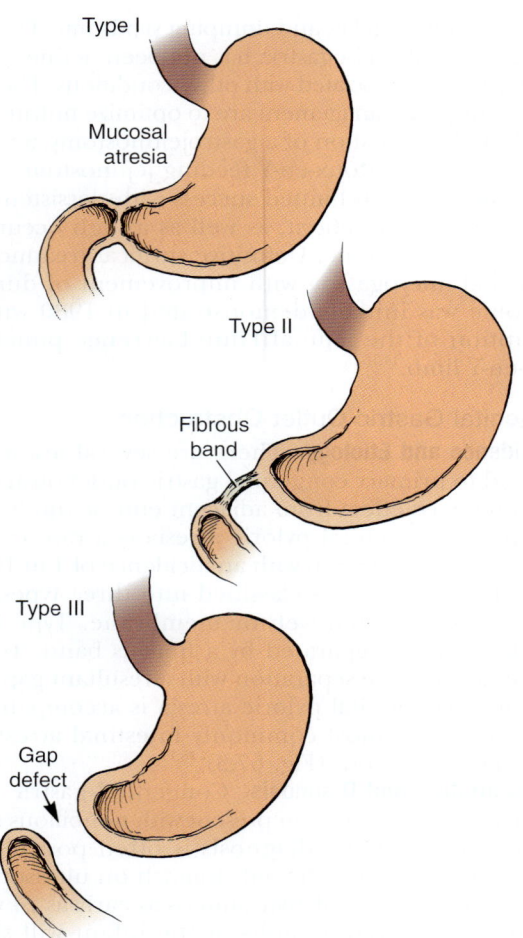

FIGURE 67.3 Illustration showing the different types of congenital pyloric atresia. (From O'Neil JA Jr, ed. *Principles of Pediatric Surgery*. 2nd ed. St. Louis: Mosby; 2003:486.)

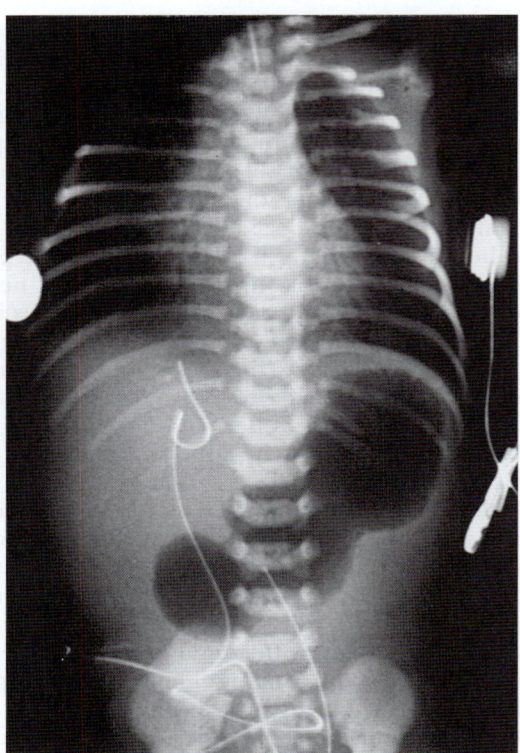

FIGURE 67.4 Classic plain film radiograph showing gastric outlet obstruction.

Diagnosis may be made on antenatal ultrasound and should prompt further investigation for associated cardiac and splenic anomalies with echocardiography and abdominal imaging, respectively.[18,20,21]

Management. The need for elective investigation for malrotation and subsequent elective surgical correction is an area of active controversy. In light of the significant risks with the commonly associated cardiac comorbidities, Versteegh et al. have advocated a more expectant management with treatment of only symptomatic malrotation. The significance of asplenia or polysplenia with dextrogastria is unknown with some centers empirically initiating vaccination and antibiotic prophylaxis.[21]

DUODENUM

Duodenal Atresia

Incidence and Etiology. Congenital duodenal atresia occurs one in 10,000 live births and was first reported by Ladd in 1931. Duodenal atresia is an isolated finding in up to one-half of patients. The remaining patients may present with associated cardiac and renal defects. Approximately 30% of patients with duodenal atresia have an associated chromosomal abnormality, most commonly Down syndrome. Conversely, only 2.5% of patients with Down syndrome will have duodenal stenosis. Duodenal atresia is thought to be secondary to failure of recanalization of the solid cord stage of the duodenum. This proposed mechanism contrasts with more distal jejunoileal intestinal atresia, thought to result from vascular disruption in utero. Duodenal atresia is classified into three types. Type I is the most common and accounts for approximately two-thirds of patients. The duodenal wall is intact, but the lumen is obstructed with an obstructing web. A common "windsock" variant occurs when the duodenal web balloons and extends intraluminally so that the point of obstruction appears distal to the point of origin. In type II duodenal atresia, the proximal and distal ends are separated by a fibrous cord, whereas in type III, proximal and distal ends are completely separated with a mesenteric defect (Fig. 67.5).[22,23]

Presentation and Diagnosis. The majority of patients with duodenal atresia are diagnosed early in the postnatal period with emesis and feeding intolerance. Prenatal diagnosis can be made on ultrasound with identification of the characteristic "double bubble" sign (Fig. 67.6). This sign is also shown on abdominal plain films and is due to dilation of the stomach and the first part of the duodenum proximal to the obstruction. Maternal polyhydramnios on ultrasound is commonly identified and occurs in more than 50% of patients with duodenal atresia. In cases of complete atresia, the remainder of the abdomen will have a paucity of gas. Duodenal atresias from a perforated web

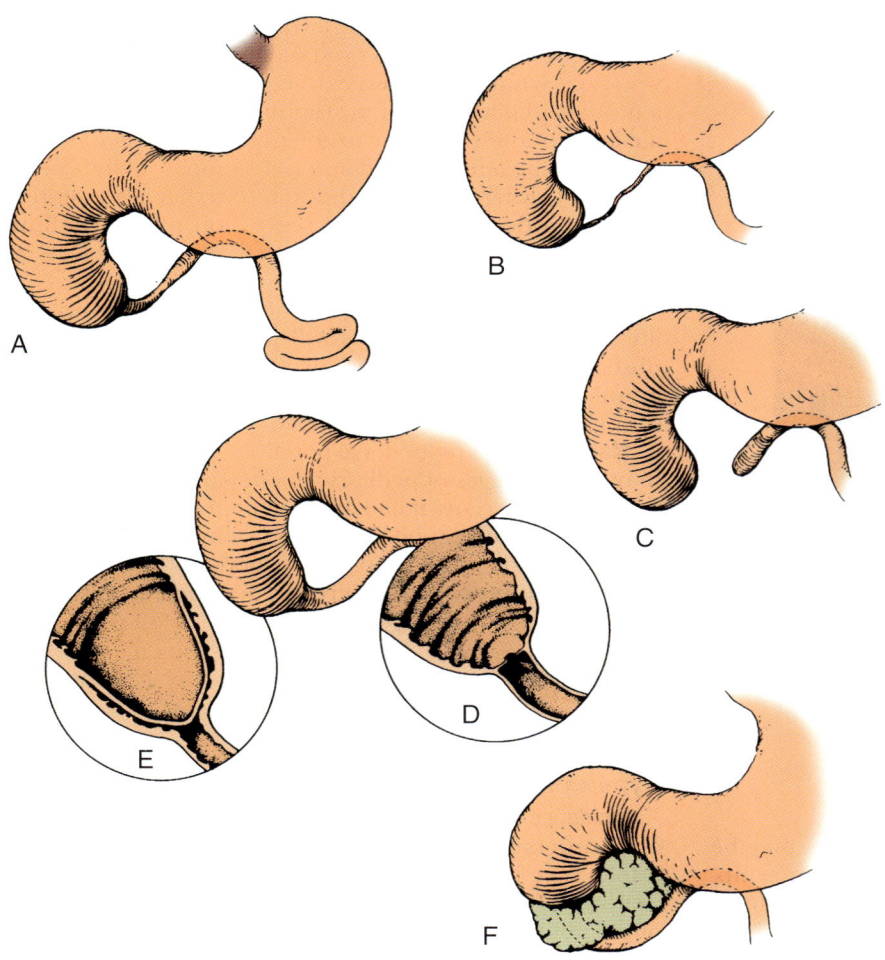

FIGURE 67.5 Classification of anomalies causing duodenal obstruction. (A) Type I atresia with intact membrane producing marked discrepancy in size between proximal and distal segments. (B) Blind ends (type II) of duodenum connected by a fibrous cord. (C) Blind ends (type III) are separated, and the mesentery is absent at the separation. (D) Intraluminal membrane with a perforation. (E) Windsock anomaly. An incision in the distal portion of the dilated segment is still beyond the obstruction. (F) Annular pancreas. (From O'Neil JA Jr, ed. *Principles of Pediatric Surgery*. 2nd ed. St. Louis: Mosby; 2003:472.)

or stenosis will demonstrate the area of partial obstruction with passage of some air or contrast distal on UGI study.[23]

Management. Duodenal atresia is managed surgically; however the presence of associated anomalies must first be identified and addressed prior to surgical repair. Echocardiogram and renal ultrasound are useful modalities, in addition to chromosomal studies. A nasogastric or orogastric tube is inserted to decompress the stomach and fluid resuscitation is started to correct electrolyte abnormalities. An open approach through a transverse right upper quadrant is most commonly used to repair duodenal atresias. The duodenum is mobilized using a Kocher maneuver. The entire small bowel is inspected for evidence of other sites of atresia. A catheter may be passed into the distal segment and injected with saline. Passage of saline into the colon is observed to rule out additional stenoses or atresias. A small balloon-tipped catheter may then be passed with the balloon inflated on withdrawal to identify a perforated web in an effort to identify and repair "windsock" variants of duodenal atresia (Fig. 67.7). Duodenal atresia can be repaired through duodenoduodenostomy as described by Kimura. A transverse duodenotomy is made in the proximal dilated segment and approximated with a longitudinal duodenotomy along the distal limb to form a diamond shape. Side-to-side duodenoduodenostomy, as well as duodenojejunostomy have also been described as safe techniques. Care must also be taken to avoid injury to the pancreatic or common bile duct (Fig. 67.8).[24]

Laparoscopic approaches have also been described to repair duodenal atresia. Multiple retrospective cohort studies have been conducted. These studies have cumulatively demonstrated no differences in operative times, timing to initial enteral feeding, or full enteral feeding, and length of hospital stay. The studies cumulatively suggest laparoscopic repair is feasible and safe in the repair of duodenal atresia with operator skill; however further study with a larger sample size is needed to determine whether open or laparoscopic technique is superior (Fig. 67.9).[24,25]

Annular Pancreas

Incidence and Etiology. The exact incidence of annular pancreas is unknown, as many individuals are asymptomatic. In autopsy series, annular pancreas is present in up to 15 per 100,000 adults. Annular pancreas is a possible etiology of congenital duodenal obstruction and is associated with other congenital anomalies such as Down syndrome, duodenal atresia, and imperforate anus. This anomaly results from failure of the ventral pancreatic bud to rotate behind the duodenum leading to pancreatic tissue fully encircling the second portion of the duodenum.[26,27]

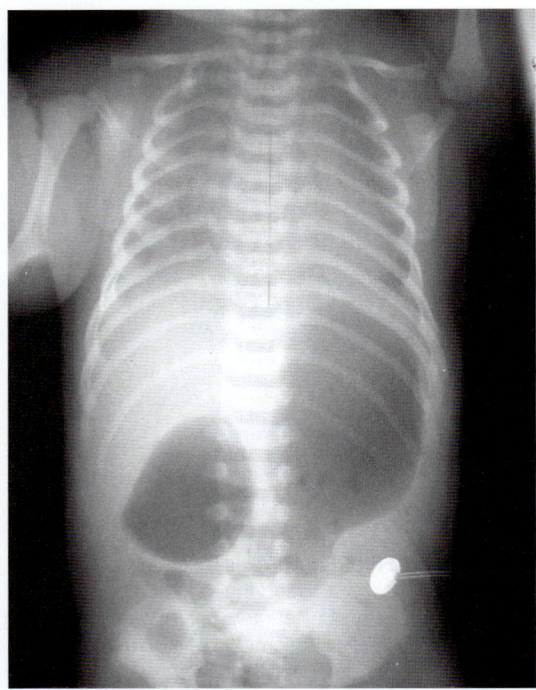

FIGURE 67.6 Classic plain film radiograph showing the "double bubble" in a patient with duodenal atresia. (Courtesy Dr. Polly Kochan.)

Presentation and Diagnosis. Annular pancreas may be asymptomatic in many patients; however, when symptomatic, it presents with vague gastrointestinal symptoms with a differential diagnosis of duodenal atresia, pyloric stenosis, and intestinal malrotation. Patients will present with feeding intolerance including frequent emesis to complete proximal obstruction with gastric distention and vomiting. Obstruction may occur postampullary (80%) or preampullary (20%); as such, emesis may be bilious or nonbilious. Diagnostic imaging in the neonate will suggest annular pancreas but typically will not definitively differentiate pathology from duodenal atresia. A "double bubble" sign may be apparent on ultrasound and plain abdominal films may demonstrate a "double bubble" sign. UGI study will demonstrate a narrowing at the second portion of the duodenum. However, as all neonates with partial or complete duodenal obstruction require surgical management, diagnosis is made definitively at the time of exploration.[26,27]

Management. Symptomatic annular pancreas is managed surgically. Associated anomalies are identified and addressed, the stomach is decompressed with an orogastric or nasogastric tube, and electrolytes are corrected with fluid resuscitation. The pancreas is left intact to avoid potential injury to biliopancreatic drainage and the obstruction is bypassed with a duodenoduodenostomy as described previously with duodenal atresia (Fig. 67.10).[26]

Preduodenal Portal Vein

Incidence and Etiology. Preduodenal portal vein is a rare anomaly that may lead to duodenal obstruction as the portal vein crosses anteriorly to the duodenum as opposed to posteriorly. First described in 1921, this anomaly is thought to occur from aberrant development of the vitelline veins. At 6 weeks' gestation, two parallel vitelline veins are connected by two extrahepatic communications: a more cephalad branch posterior to the duodenum and a caudal branch anterior to the duodenum. As the fetus develops, the left cephalad and right caudal vitelline veins involute leaving an S-shaped portal vein that lies posterior to the duodenum. Aberrant regression of the vitelline veins can lead to an anterior portal vein that results in duodenal obstruction.[28,29]

Presentation and Diagnosis. Patients may be asymptomatic. Symptomatic patients will present with duodenal obstruction with differential diagnoses of duodenal web, annular pancreas with possible "double bubble" sign on sonogram and on abdominal plain film.[30]

Management. Preduodenal portal vein is managed similar to other etiologies of pediatric duodenal obstruction. The patient is fluid resuscitated and decompressed with orogastric or nasogastric tube. The portal vein is left intact and the obstruction is bypassed with a duodenoduodenostomy to avoid injury to biliopancreatic drainage as described earlier (Fig. 67.11).[28]

ACQUIRED LESIONS

STOMACH

Hypertrophic Pyloric Stenosis

Incidence and Etiology. When considering the spectrum of disorders that result in nonbilious emesis and feeding intolerance in the neonatal period, hypertrophic pyloric stenosis (HPS) remains the most common acquired lesion of the stomach and duodenum. This disease has a tendency to be more common among Caucasian and Hispanic infants compared to African Americans and Asians. There is a male predominance of 4:1 with an incidence of approximately two per 1000 live births. There is no identified genetic mechanism of HPS, but there are trends toward increased risk among families with affected infants.[31]

From an anatomic standpoint, this disease process leads to an acquired gastric outlet obstruction. Progressive concentric and longitudinal hypertrophy of the pyloric muscle is thought to be responsible for the disease process. There have been many theories about the nature of this disease process. There have been a number of studies looking at environmental factors contributing to the development of HPS. It has been shown in both animal models and in infants receiving erythromycin both directly and indirectly through breastfeeding mothers on the medication that it can induce pyloric stenosis, the mechanism of which remains unclear.[32]

Additionally, dysregulation of nitric oxide (NO) synthase within the pyloric muscle has been proposed as one theory for this disease process. There has been a plethora of work in the NO pathway and loss of smooth-muscle relaxation in a number of disease processes. A deficiency of NO in HPS is thought to lead to pylorospasm. The remaining theories about the disease have focused on dysregulation of the multiple hormonal pathways that regulate digestion and the passage of material from the stomach into the duodenum such as gastrin, secretin, cholecystokinin, and somatostatin. Finally, signaling pathways and the interstitial

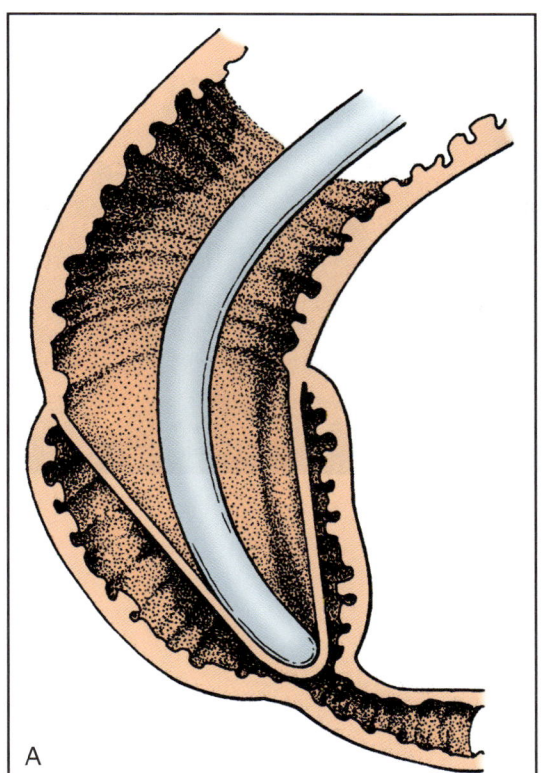

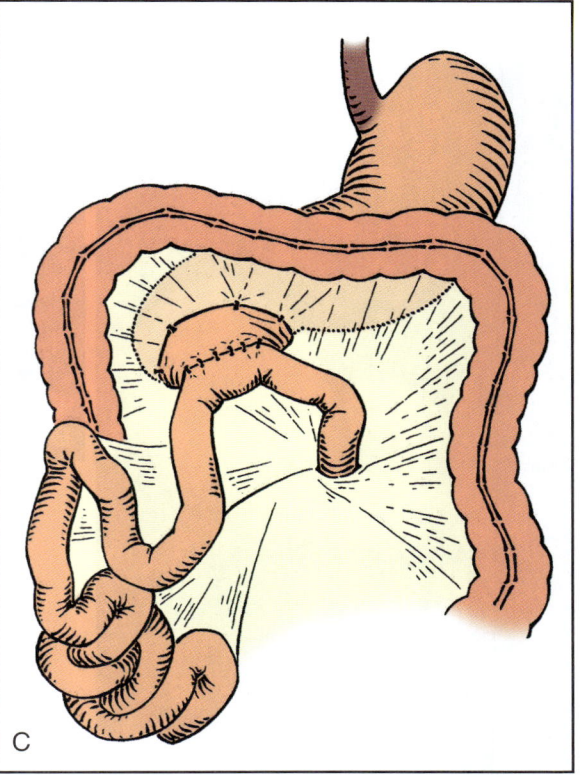

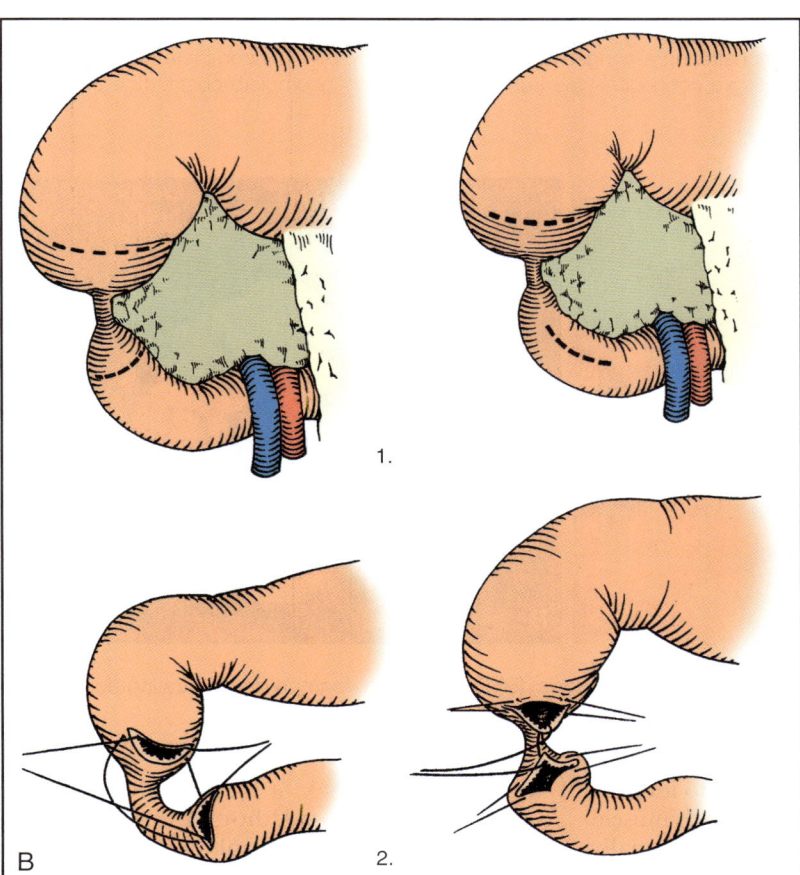

FIGURE 67.7 (A) Pressure on the tube at the bottom of the web produces an indentation in the duodenal wall, indicating the point apex of the web. The incision should be placed at that point. (B) Duodenoduodenostomy. (1) Standard side-to-side anastomosis. (2) Diamond-shaped duodenoduodenostomy. (C) Duodenojejunostomy. A loop of proximal jejunum is brought through an opening in the transverse mesocolon and anastomosed to the most dependent portion of the obstructed duodenum. This approach now is used only when direct duodenal anastomosis is not feasible. (From O'Neil JA Jr, ed. *Principles of Pediatric Surgery*. 2nd ed. St. Louis: Mosby; 2003:474.)

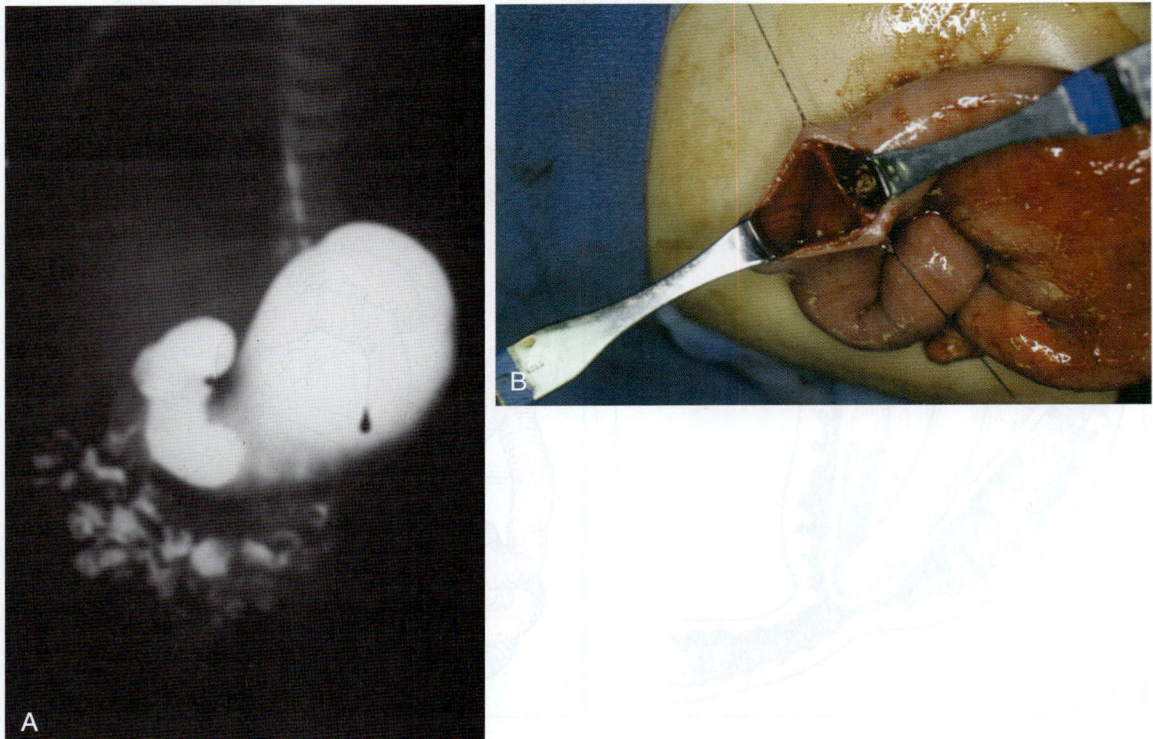

FIGURE 67.8 (A) Upper gastrointestinal study demonstrating a congenital type I duodenal web with incomplete obstruction of the duodenum. (B) Operative photograph demonstrating a congenital type I duodenal web with incomplete obstruction of the duodenum visualized through the duodenotomy.

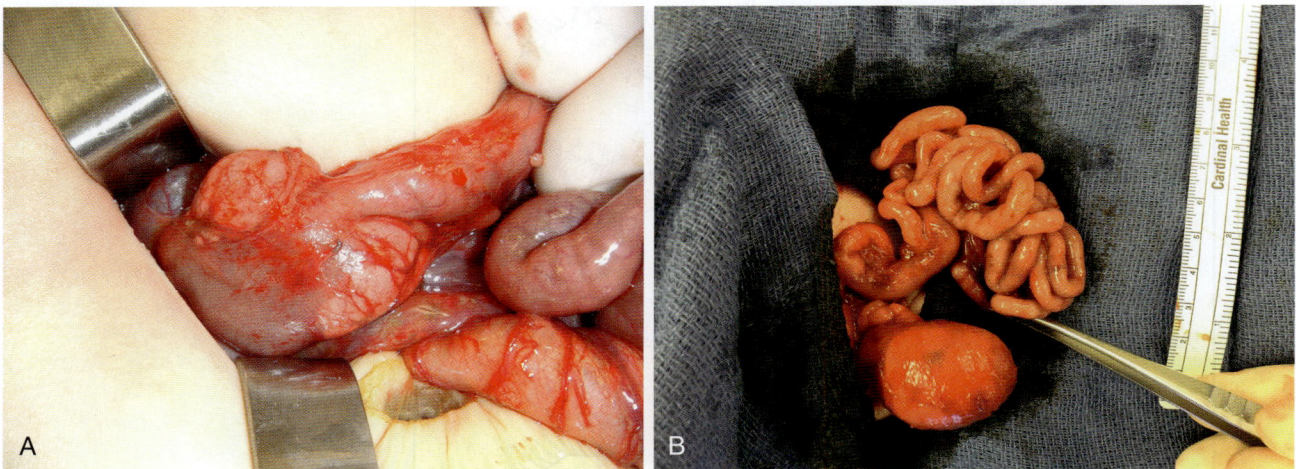

FIGURE 67.9 (A) Operative photograph demonstrating duodenal stenosis. (B) Operative photograph demonstrating duodenal atresia with an "apple peel" distal jejunum.

cells of Cajal have also been studied extensively to identify disorders in the complex innervation of the smooth muscle complex. The number of pathways that can potentially play a role in the development of HPS highlights the likely multifactorial nature of this disease process.[32]

Presentation and Diagnosis. Many infants struggle with feeding issues that can cause a significant amount of stress for families. The classic described presentation is projectile, nonbilious postprandial emesis. Children can develop HPS

within the first week of life, usually with a peak around 6 to 8 weeks of life. Although rare, HPS has also been described in children of older age. In infancy, parents usually describe multiple attempts to change formula as well as the addition of acid-suppressing medications to treat reflux. Despite these measures the child continues to have progressive emesis.[33]

On exam, children can present with poor skin turgor and sunken fontanelles. Children who present in a delayed

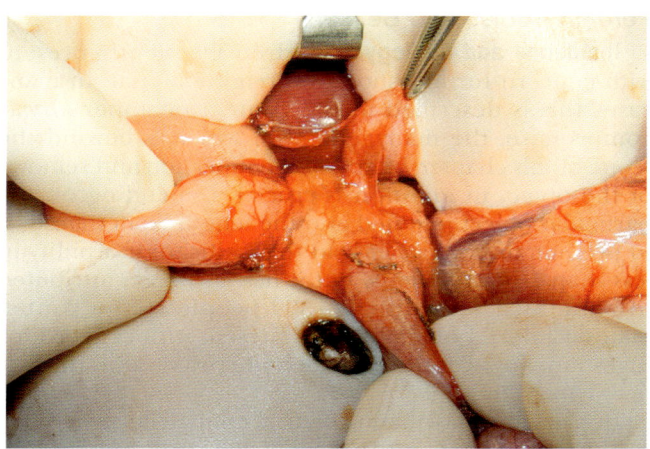

FIGURE 67.10 Operative photograph demonstrating annular pancreas.

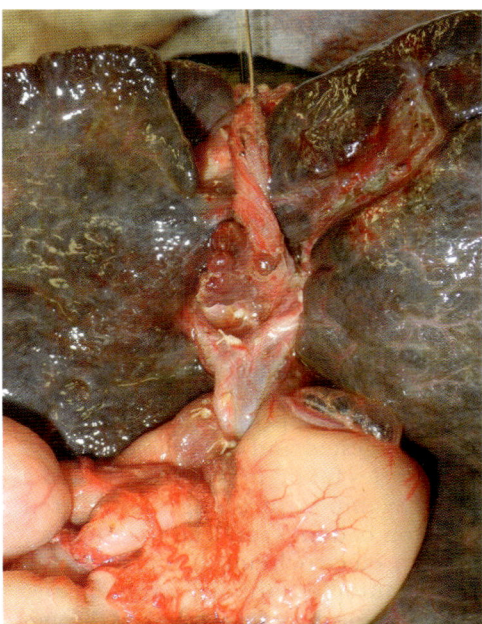

FIGURE 67.11 Operative photograph demonstrating preduodenal portal vein.

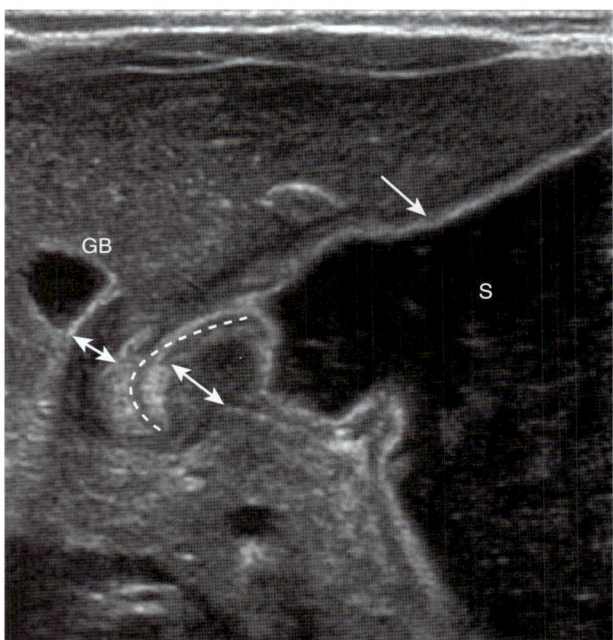

FIGURE 67.12 Ultrasound showing hypertrophic pyloric stenosis. The *arrows* demonstrate the muscle thickness on either side of the pyloric mucosa. The *upper arrow* points to the stomach mucosa. *GB,* Gallbladder; *S,* stomach. (From Lichtor JL, Shiveley TJ, Wallace EC. Images in anesthesiology: pyloric stenosis. *Anesthesiology.* 2010;112:1270.)

fashion often look emaciated and lethargic. In these children, it is often easier to palpate the pyloric muscle, which has been described as "palpating the olive." This is often due to a loss of abdominal muscle tone in a lethargic infant and the thought that the pyloric muscle is often more hypertrophied. A high index of suspicion must be maintained about the severe electrolyte abnormalities that are associated with ongoing gastric losses.

The diagnostic modality of choice is a transabdominal ultrasound of the pyloric muscle at the hands of a skilled operator with a high level of institutional experience diagnosing this disease process. Positive measurements for HPS are generally a muscle thickness greater than 3.5 mm and a channel length greater than 14 mm in a child 6 to 8 weeks of age. Additionally, ultrasound can be helpful in identifying multiple peristaltic waves and a loss of contents traversing the pyloric channel. Other imaging adjuncts include plain radiographic identification of a large gastric bubble and a formal upper gastrointestinal contrast evaluation that similarly shows failure of contents passing into the duodenum and a prominence of the antral pyloric border referred to as shouldering (Fig. 67.12).[34-36]

Management. While there is often concern about the anatomic problem with HPS, preoperative correction of the electrolyte abnormalities is paramount. Children present with a hypokalemic hypochloremic metabolic alkalosis with a paradoxical aciduria. Initial management includes establishment of IV access and a 20-mL/kg bolus of normal saline. Electrolytes should be drawn to evaluate the severity of derangement and assess appropriateness of the resuscitation attempts. After the initial bolus, an infusion of 1.5 times the maintenance rate of 5% dextrose in 0.45 normal saline without potassium should be started. The child should be closely monitored and a telemetry or critical care bed should be considered in extreme cases. The child's vitals and urine output should be used to guide endpoints of resuscitation. A goal of normalizing electrolytes and decreasing the bicarbonate level to less than 30 mEq/L decreases the potential for perioperative complications such as cardiac arrhythmias and postoperative apnea.[37]

There have been many approaches used in the surgical management of this disease. The modern approach was based on the work of Conrad Ramsted, who described a procedure in which the mucosa was left exposed after a longitudinal incision. The Ramsted pyloromyotomy, classically performed through a right upper quadrant

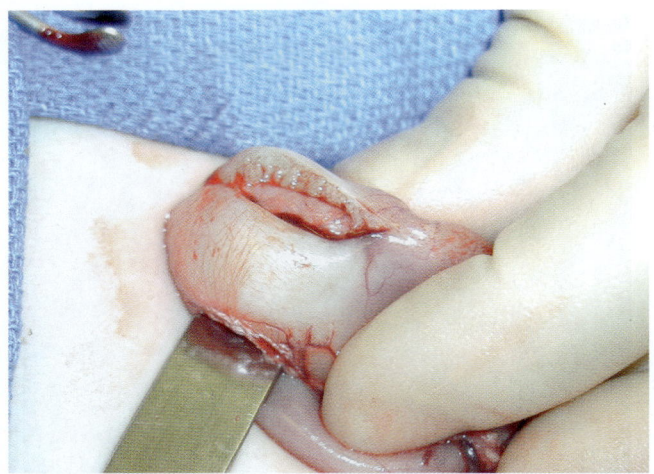

FIGURE 67.13 Operative photograph demonstrating an open pyloromyotomy.

incision, is still a safe approach to this disease process (Fig. 67.13). Modifications have included a circumumbilical open approach, and after a successful series in the early 1990s by Alain et al. in 1991, laparoscopic.[38]

Several different studies have evaluated the optimal approach in treatment of pyloric stenosis. Perger et al. compared the outcomes of 622 patients treated with each of the three approaches over an 8-year period. Significant differences were noted in the circumumbilical group in terms of wound complications and length of operation. There was a trend toward fewer episodes of emesis in the laparoscopic group. Importantly, the length of hospital stay did not differ between the three groups.[39]

Despite many prospective trials and meta-analyses, no significant differences have been revealed between the groups in terms of postoperative complications or feeding intolerance. The laparoscopic approach has a steep learning curve with approximately 30 cases required before the operator is facile with the operation. This learning curve likely accounts for descriptions of incomplete pyloromyotomy and increased duration of anesthesia in the laparoscopic group (91 vs. 82 minutes, $P = .02$; 30 vs. 23 minutes, $P = .0001$, respectively). Furthermore, there continues to be evidence of increased wound complications with the open approach. These complications, however, do not appear to have long-term morbidity and do not significantly affect the length of stay.

A recent double-blinded randomized multicenter international trial in 2009 compared open and laparoscopic pyloromyotomy in 180 patients. Median time to achieve full enteral feeds was significantly shorter in the laparoscopic group, as was postoperative length of stay. Differences measured in postoperative vomiting and perioperative complications did not achieve statistical significance.[40-42]

While there has been much work done in identifying the best approach, both open and laparoscopic operations can be performed safely and effectively. The approach should be selected based on the individual surgeon's experience. Consideration of transfer to a facility with pediatric surgical capability should be made in the absence of a capable surgeon (Fig. 67.14).

Foreign Bodies and Bezoars

Incidence and Etiology. Children frequently present with concern for ingestion of foreign material. In many cases this is described in the context of upper airway compromise, the management of which is beyond the scope of this chapter, but rapid identification and removal of the object in question is crucial. Depending on the particular object ingested and the length from ingestion to presentation, this can lead to significant morbidity in less than 1% of patients, but it has also been attributed to an annual mortality of 1500 people in the United States. Children of all ages can present with concern for ingestion; however there is a definite peak within the first few years of life.[43,44]

Bezoars are a fascinating clinical entity. The term refers to the concretions created from ingested foreign and intrinsic materials in the stomach and bowel. Bezoars are named based on their composing material: trichobezoar (most common), consisting of hair; phytobezoar, consisting of fibers, seeds, and vegetable skin; or lithobezoar made of rocks and dirt. Trichobezoars are seen in children with psychiatric disorders, more commonly in girls. It is associated with trichotillomania, a disorder of hair pulling and subsequent ingestion. The consumed hair collects in the stomach and creates a mass of hair. As this accumulates, the stomach is unable to expel the mass, leading to a gastric outlet obstruction.[45,46]

Presentation and Diagnosis. Most patients come in for evaluation after a witnessed ingestion event. Often there are minimal or no symptoms. Depending on the type of foreign material ingested, many can be safely observed. However, if they present with concerns for airway compromise, ongoing dysphagia, or peritoneal signs, rapid identification and intervention is necessary. A thorough history and physical is a prudent guide to identifying the type of object ingested and the time course.

Button batteries found in many household goods and magnets are examples of foreign bodies that require removal. Button batteries can lead to significant mucosal burns through electrochemical injury. Magnets, when swallowed in multiples, are also problematic. Multiple magnets can become magnetically linked through adjacent loops of bowel, leading to a pressure necrosis and fistula formation. Therefore, ingestion of either object should prompt attempts at removal.[47]

Plain radiographs and ultrasonography can be useful adjuncts in identifying the location of the object. Most objects that make it into the stomach will continue into the remainder of the gastrointestinal (GI) tract and require little intervention. In cases where there is continuing concern for injury, radiolucent objects, or ongoing symptoms, endoscopy can be diagnostic and therapeutic.

Treatment. Foreign bodies that are felt to be able to pass unimpeded through the GI tract can be safely observed in the outpatient setting. To date, there are no data to support the use of laxatives or other cathartics in an attempt to speed the expulsion process. The remainder of proximal foreign bodies can be removed through flexible or rigid esophagoscopy. In the case of objects that have gone into the third portion of the duodenum, a decision must be made about ongoing surveillance versus operative removal.

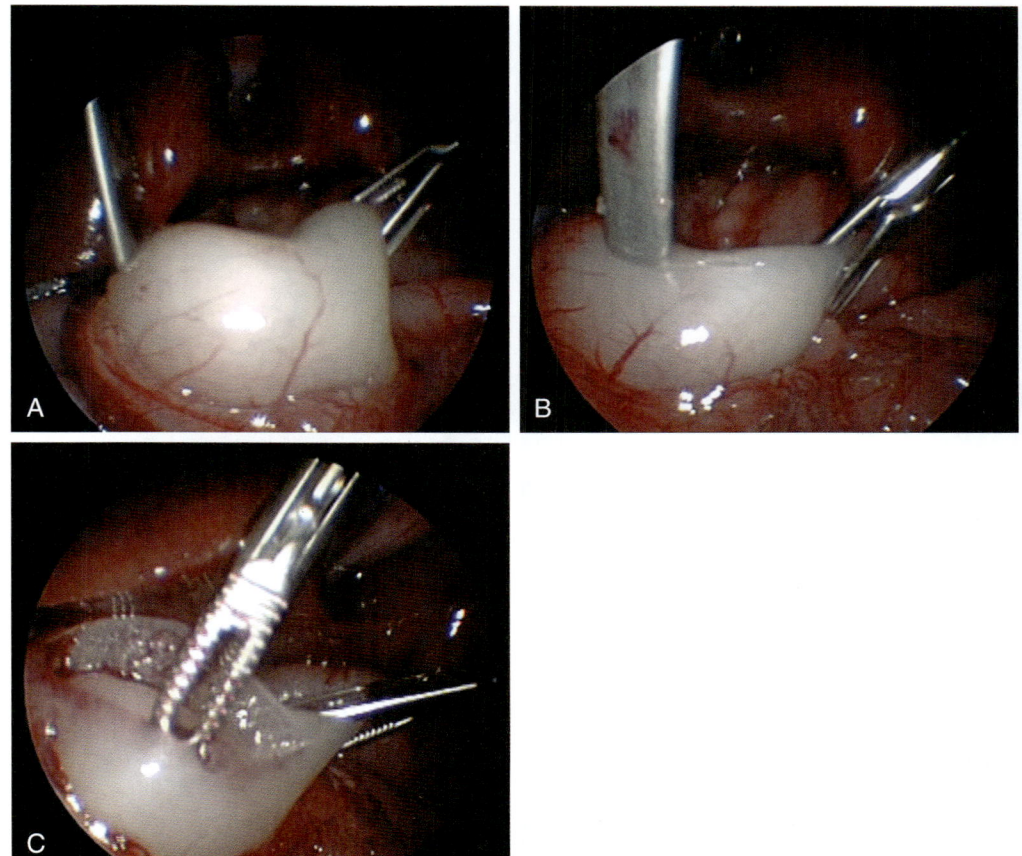

FIGURE 67.14 (A) Laparoscopic view of hypertrophic pylorus. (B) Laparoscopic seromuscular incision along the length of the pylorus. (C) Laparoscopic pyloromyotomy. Note the submucosa bulging from within the spread incision.

Children should be monitored for development of obstructive or peritoneal symptoms. Most distal obstructions occur at the level of the ileocecal valve and even at the appendicular orifice. These objects can be safely removed using laparoscopy.

Attempts can be made to remove bezoars via endoluminal approaches; however, surgical removal is often required (Fig. 67.15).[43,47,48]

Gastric Perforation

Incidence and Etiology. There has been debate in the literature about gastric perforation in the neonatal period as either spontaneous or secondary to an underlying process such as necrotizing enterocolitis (NEC). As with NEC, gastric perforation is seen in a higher frequency in preterm infants and can be associated with gastric pneumatosis. Gastric perforation in the neonatal period can occur secondary to both iatrogenic and noniatrogenic causes. Gastric perforation can occur during endotracheal intubation and placement of nasoenteric tubes. It can also be seen in infants with NEC, those who receive steroids or NSAIDs, and in neonates with an obstructive process such as an atresia, internal hernia, or volvulus; this can lead to overdistention and perforation, especially in gavage-fed infants.[49]

Presentation and Diagnosis. Gastric perforation, as in the adult population, in extreme cases, presents with a neonate in shock and thrombocytopenia. Additionally there is concomitant abdominal distention, feeding intolerance, lethargy, abdominal wall erythema, bloody stool, or nasogastric output, and respiratory distress. Plain abdominal radiographs are sufficient in diagnosing a gastric perforation. The adjunct of a lateral decubitus view with identification of free air and extraluminal air-fluid levels makes the diagnosis. In addition, this can highlight concomitant intestinal NEC. As with any septic picture, early goal-directed resuscitation is paramount.[49]

Treatment. Depending on the status of the neonate, current weight, and comorbidities, an appropriate route for source control can be chosen. For those children who would clinically not tolerate a laparotomy or an open abdomen, a bedside drainage procedure is indicated. This involves placing a Penrose or other similar drain through the abdominal wall to allow the egress of air and succus. Neonates who undergo laparotomy should have a thorough evaluation of the stomach and intestines. Upon identification of a gastric perforation, care should be taken to ensure viable surrounding tissue for repair. Unlike in adults, the omentum in neonates is rudimentary and has limited ability to act as a patch material. Débridement of the edges of the perforation with primary repair and washout is usually sufficient. If there is concern of an ongoing process, the abdomen should be left open with a temporary closure or silo for a second-look laparotomy.[49]

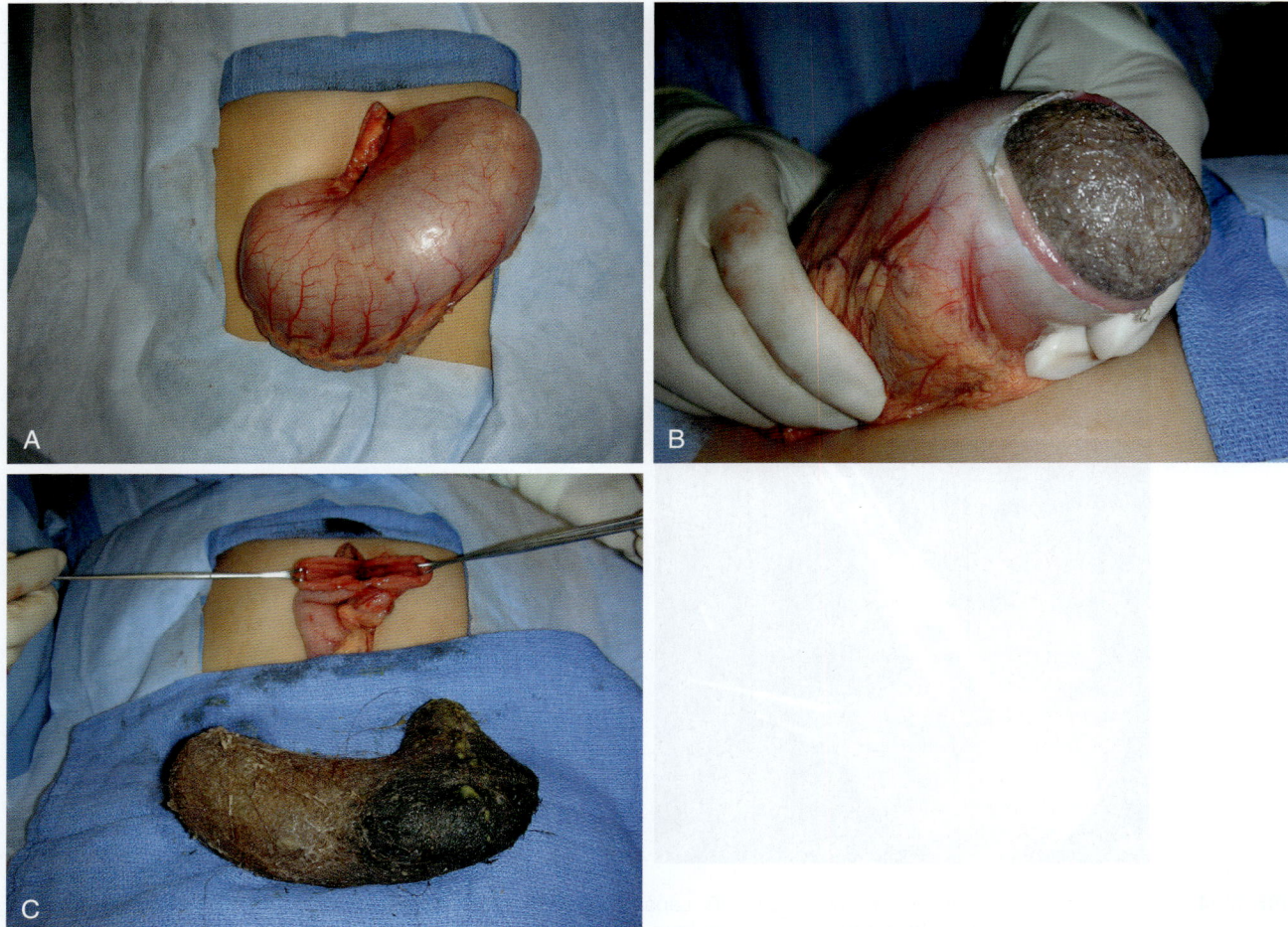

FIGURE 67.15 (A) Operative photograph demonstrating a stomach containing a large trichobezoar. (B) Operative photograph of a partially delivered trichobezoar after gastrotomy. (C) A large trichobezoar that caused gastric obstruction removed surgically.

Gastric Tumors

This clinical entity is extremely rare in the pediatric population. Mortality and incidence of gastric cancer has continued to decline due to improved food handling and preservation. Gastric cancer in children less than 18 years of age accounts for less than 0.5% of all gastric cancer cases. Other tumors that can be associated with the stomach include gastric lymphoma secondary to *Helicobacter pylori* infection, gastrointestinal stromal tumors, teratomas, schwannomas, and rhabdomyosarcomas.[50,51]

Presentation and Diagnosis. Most children present with nonspecific symptoms. This can include a constellation of vague epigastric discomfort, weight loss, and poor appetite. In some cases there is a report of change in bowel habits with ongoing nausea and emesis.

In addition to a history and physical exam, laboratory evaluation can lead to an identification of anemia. Children with a history of peptic ulcer disease, or prior *Helicobacter pylori* infection, should be screened for resolution of the infection in cases of gastric lymphoma. Plain radiographs can be helpful in identifying gastric outlet obstruction with or without administration of oral contrast. Additional information can be obtained via cross-sectional imaging. The most definitive exam is endoscopy to visualize the tumor, take biopsies, and evaluate any potential ongoing hemorrhage.[50,52]

Treatment. The mainstay of treatment for most tumors is surgical excision with wide margins. Prognosis depends on the initial pathology, disease stage, and the response to treatment. As this continues to be a rare clinical entity in the pediatric population, most treatment algorithms are based on adult data (Fig. 67.16).[50,53]

Superior Mesenteric Artery Syndrome

Incidence and Etiology. Superior mesenteric artery syndrome was first described by Carl von Rokitansky in 1842. It is a cause of UGI obstruction from the compression of the third portion of the duodenum between the aorta and SMA leading to duodenal obstruction. It has a prevalence of approximately 0.3% and is seen more frequently in females. There is a higher peak of this disease between 10 and 18 years of age. Other names for this disease process include Wilkie syndrome, aortomesenteric duodenal compression, and Cast syndrome. Its development is thought to be secondary to rapid weight loss seen in patients with eating disorders, hyperthyroidism, during chemotherapy, and profound gastroenteritis. It has also been described following orthopedic and neurosurgical

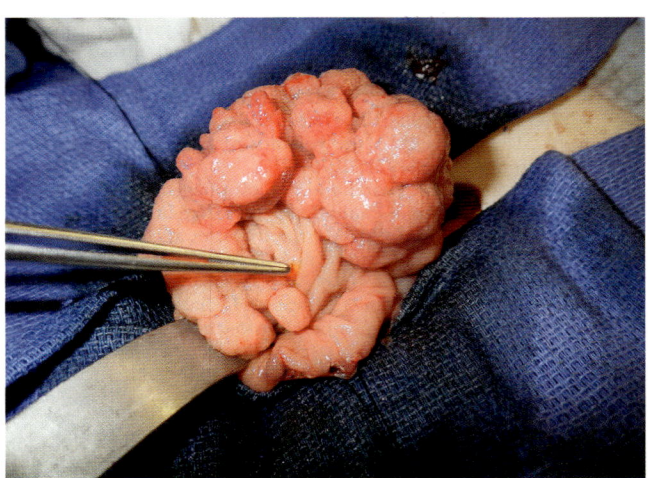

FIGURE 67.16 Operative photograph demonstrating gastric polyposis.

operations after operative correction of scoliosis and hip-spica cast application.[54,55]

Presentation and Diagnosis. The presentation of SMA syndrome is varied. A high index of suspicion should be kept in children who have recently experience rapid weight loss. Presenting symptoms can also be vague epigastric pain as well as nausea and emesis. The emesis is most frequently bilious. Often there is a description of either intermittent or postprandial abdominal discomfort. Some patients can have symptomatic relief by bringing their knees up to their chest or lying on their stomach, which is thought to open the aortomesenteric angle.[54]

Diagnosis can be made by symptomatology and imaging. Upper GI fluoroscopy can point to an obstruction of the duodenum. A CT angiogram with or without oral contrast is the definitive imaging modality. The syndrome is defined by radiographic evidence of the superior mesenteric artery compressing on the third portion of the duodenum with an aortomesenteric angle less than 22 degrees (normal 38 to 65 degrees) and an aortomesenteric distance less than 8 mm (normal 10 to 28 mm).[54,56]

Treatment. Conservative management is the treatment of choice for this disease process in the absence of a pathologic condition that requires surgical intervention such as a mass or vascular aneurysm. Children are kept NPO (nil per os) and in the immediate period can be decompressed with a nasogastric tube if there is significant emesis. As stated in the section on pyloric stenosis, correction of electrolyte abnormalities is paramount. Children should be provided with nutritional support. Preferential nasojejunal feeding should be initiated when possible with total parenteral nutrition reserved for select cases.[54]

A number of procedures have been described both open and laparoscopically in the event of conservative management failure. The goal of each procedure is to improve the narrow aortomesenteric angle. Strong's procedure involves mobilization of the fourth portion of the duodenum and division of the ligament of Treitz. This procedure is advantageous because it does not require a bowel anastomosis. The remaining operative approaches

create a surgical bypass with a duodenojejunostomy or a gastrojejunostomy.[57]

Paraduodenal Hernia

Incidence and Etiology. Paraduodenal hernias are the most common congenital internal hernia (pericecal being second). Internal hernias, as opposed to external hernias, remain within the thoracoabdominal cavities. The majority of internal hernias are the result of congenital abnormalities of intestinal rotation and peritoneal attachment. Paraduodenal hernia is due to incomplete rotation of the midgut. Failure of rotation results in entrapment of the duodenum in the mesocolon traversing through Waldeyer fossa at the root of the small bowel mesentery. Seventy-five percent of paraduodenal hernias occur on left side and 25% on right side.[58,59]

Presentation and Diagnosis. Most children remain asymptomatic and the paraduodenal hernia is often an incidental finding during other evaluation. However, this can also present with intermittent midabdominal discomfort as well as acute intestinal obstruction and even strangulation.

An ongoing history of chronic abdominal symptoms can point to intermittent obstruction of the herniated intestine. As with any hernia, rapid identification is important to prevent strangulation and loss of intestine.[60,61]

The preoperative diagnosis of paraduodenal hernia can be established only via radiography. The most sensitive test is cross-sectional imaging, with a higher yield of identification during a symptomatic period. Plain radiographs can show concern for proximal intestinal obstruction that should then prompt UGI studies. Radiologic examination shows concern for a closed-loop obstruction with both afferent and efferent loops trapped with a mesenteric pedicle. In a right-sided paraduodenal hernia, there is reversal of the normal left-sided jejunal arteries. The major CT findings include the abnormal course of the jejunal arterial branches and venous tributaries as well as a collection of small bowel loops in the midabdomen.[62]

Treatment. In cases of uncertainty, diagnostic laparoscopy or laparotomy can be useful. The mainstay of treatment once identified is the same as with any hernia. The surgical principles require reduction of the herniated contents, thorough examination to assess for viability, and closure of the hernia defect. Any compromised bowel should be excised, gross spillage controlled, and depending on the patient's status, a decision should be made in proceeding with a primary anastomosis or coming back for a second-look operation after adequate resuscitation. In cases of left-sided paraduodenal hernia, the bowel often can be easily reduced and the peritoneal defect can be easily reapproximated. Right-sided paraduodenal hernias are often more challenging as the herniated contents can be fixed into the retroperitoneum. Careful dissection and derotation is paramount. A lateral to medial approach is the safest option to avoid injury to the superior mesenteric artery, the ileocolic artery, and the right colic vein.[63-65]

Inflammatory Bowel Disease

Incidence and Etiology. Inflammatory bowel disease and the spectrum of ulcerative colitis to Crohn disease is typically located in the distal small intestine, colon, and rectum. Within the spectrum of this disease gastritis, gastroduodenal ulceration, dudodentitis, and villous atrophy have been described. Many studies have attempted to identify the environmental and genetic factors that lead to the abnormal immunomodulatory response that leads to this chronic inflammatory process. However, clinically significant gastroduodenal disease is more frequently described with Crohn disease with an incidence of 0.5% to 4%. Most patients will have continuous disease involving the distal portion of the stomach, pylorus, and duodenum.[66,67]

Presentation and Diagnosis. Most children who present with Crohn disease will have classic symptoms of changes in bowel pattern and unexplained weight loss. In the subset who have gastroduodenal involvement, epigastric pain with or without blood-tinged emesis can be common presenting symptoms. Laboratory evaluation of these patients is reflective of a protein-losing enteropathy and nutritional deficiency. Endoscopy remains the cornerstone of treatment. Evaluation of the stomach and duodenum with multiple biopsies is important for diagnosis. Irregularity of the evaluated mucosa with the classic cobblestone appearance and subsequent histologic identification of noncaseating granulomas is diagnostic.[67]

Treatment. The mainstay of treatment for inflammatory bowel disease remains immunomodulatory therapy. For those children with gastroduodenal Crohn disease, many studies have shown a benefit of intense acid suppression as well as eradication of any concomitant *Helicobacter pylori* infection. This can often lead to significant healing when used in conjunction with standard therapies for Crohn disease. After induction corticosteroid regimens, most children are subsequently transitioned to aminosalicylates, immune suppressants such as 6-MP, methotrexate, or monoclonal antibody therapy against the proinflammatory cytokine tumor necrosis factor.[68,69]

Surgical intervention is reserved for cases of stricture, obstruction, or hemorrhage. In some cases strictures can be managed with endoscopic balloon dilation with an acceptably low rate of perforation. Operative approaches for the treatment of stricture include duodenal strictureplasty and formal bypass via duodenoduodenostomy or gastrojejunostomy. Postoperative complications include anastomotic leak, proximal high-output enterocutaneous fistula, intraabdominal abscess, and recurrent stricture. In all cases continued enteral feeding and nutritional support is important.[70,71]

REFERENCES

1. Sadler TW. *Langman's Medical Embryology.* 13th ed. Baltimore, MD: Lippincott Williams & Wilkins, a Wolters Kluwer business; 2015.
2. Iyer CP, Mahour GH. Duplications of the alimentary tract in infants and children. *J Pediatr Surg.* 1995;30:1267-1270.
3. Bentley JFR, Smith JR. Developmental posterior enteric remnants and spinal malformations: the split notochord syndrome. *Arch Dis Child.* 1960;35:76-86.
4. Ribaux C, Meyer P. Adenocarcinoma in an ileal duplication. *Ann Pathol.* 1995;15:443-445.
5. Brink DA, Balsara ZN. Prenatal ultrasound detection of intraabdominal pulmonary sequestration with postnatal MRI correlation. *Pediatr Radiol.* 1991;21:227.
6. Laje P, Flake AW, Adzick NS. Prenatal diagnosis and postnatal resection of intraabdominal enteric duplications. *J Pediatr Surg.* 2010;45:1554-1558.
7. Ford WDA, Guelfand M, López PJ, Furness ME. Laparoscopic excision of a gastric duplication cyst detected on antenatal ultrasound scan. *J Pediatr Surg.* 2004;39:e8-e10.
8. Cribbs RK, Gow KW, Wulkan ML. Gastric volvulus in infants and children. *Pediatrics.* 2008;122:e752-e762.
9. Cole BC, Dickinson SJ. Acute volvulus of the stomach in infants and children. *Surgery.* 1971;70:707-717.
10. Garvey EM, Ostlie DJ. Hiatal and paraesophageal hernia repair in pediatric patients. *Semin Pediatr Surg.* 2017;26:61-66.
11. Scarpato E, D'Armiento M, Martinelli M, et al. Impact of hiatal hernia on pediatric dyspeptic symptoms. *J Pediatr Gastroenterol Nutr.* 2014;59:795-798.
12. Namgoong JM, Kim DY, Kim SC, Hwang JH. Hiatal hernia in pediatric patients: laparoscopic versus open approaches. *Ann Surg Treat Res.* 2014;86:264-269.
13. Gorenstein A, Cohen AJ, Cordova Z, Witzling M, Krutman B, Serour F. Hiatal hernia in pediatric gastroesophageal reflux. *J Pediatr Gastroenterol Nutr.* 2001;33:554-557.
14. Jones VS, Cohen RC. An eighteen year follow-up after surgery for congenital microgastria—case report and review of literature. *J Pediatr Surg.* 2007;42:1957-1960.
15. Neifeld JP, Berman WF, Lawrence W, Kodroff MB, Salzberg AM. Management of congenital microgastria with a jejunal reservoir pouch. *J Pediatr Surg.* 1980;15:882-885.
16. Al-Salem AH. Congenital pyloric atresia and associated anomalies. *Pediatr Surg Int.* 2007;23:559-563.
17. Achiron R, Hamiel-Pinchas O, Engelberg S, Barkai G, Reichman B, Mashiach S. Aplasia cutis congenita associated with epidermolysis bullosa and pyloric atresia: the diagnostic role of prenatal ultrasonography. *Prenat Diagn.* 1992;12:765-771.
18. Inaoka T, Sugimori H, Sasaki Y, et al. VIBE MRI for evaluating the normal and abnormal gastrointestinal tract in fetuses. *Am J Roentgenol.* 2007;189:W303-W308.
19. Dessanti A, Di Benedetto V, Iannuccelli M, Balata A, Cossu Rocca P, Di Benedetto A. Pyloric atresia: a new operation to reconstruct the pyloric sphincter. *J Pediatr Surg.* 2004;39:297-301.
20. Ardill W. Dextrogastria. *J Am Coll Surg.* 2002;194:676.
21. Versteegh HP, Adams SD, Boxall S, Burge DM, Stanton MP. Antenatally diagnosed right-sided stomach (dextrogastria): a rare rotational anomaly. *J Pediatr Surg.* 2016;51:236-239.
22. Ladd WE. Congenital obstruction of the duodenum in children. *N Engl J Med.* 1932;206:277-283.
23. St. Peter SD, Little DC, Barsness KA, et al. Should we be concerned about jejunoileal atresia during repair of duodenal atresia? *J Laparoendosc Adv Surg Tech.* 2010;20:773-775.
24. Kimura K, Mukohara N, Nishijima E, Muraji T, Tsugawa C, Matsumoto Y. Diamond-shaped anastomosis for duodenal atresia: an experience with 44 patients over 15 years. *J Pediatr Surg.* 1990;25:977-979.
25. Spilde TL, St. Peter SD, Keckler SJ, Holcomb GW, Snyder CL, Ostlie DJ. Open vs laparoscopic repair of congenital duodenal obstructions: a concurrent series. *J Pediatr Surg.* 2008;43:1002-1005.
26. Komuro H, Gotoh C, Urita Y, Fujishiro J, Shinkai T. A pediatric case of an unusual type of annular pancreas presenting with duodeno-pancreatic reflux. *Pediatr Surg Int.* 2012;28:715-717.
27. Merrill JR, Raffensperger JG. Pediatric annular pancreas: twenty years' experience. *J Pediatr Surg.* 1976;11:921-925.
28. Weber WF, Draus JM Jr. Preduodenal portal vein: a rare cause of neonatal bowel obstruction. *Am Surg.* 2016;82:775-776.
29. Baglaj M, Gerus S. Preduodenal portal vein, malrotation, and high jejunal atresia: a case report. *J Pediatr Surg.* 2012;47:e27-e30.
30. Choi SO, Park WH. Preduodenal portal vein: a cause of prenatally diagnosed duodenal obstruction. *J Pediatr Surg.* 1995;30:1521-1522.
31. Golladay ES. Pyloric stenosis—a timed perspective. *Arch Surg.* 1987;122:825.
32. Panteli C. New insights into the pathogenesis of infantile pyloric stenosis. *Pediatr Surg Int.* 2009;25:1043-1052.
33. Boybeyi Ö, Karnak İ, Ekinci S, et al. Late-onset hypertrophic pyloric stenosis: definition of diagnostic criteria and algorithm for the management. *J Pediatr Surg.* 2010;45:1777-1783.
34. Keller H, Waldmann D, Greiner P. Comparison of preoperative sonography with intraoperative findings in congenital hypertrophic pyloric stenosis. *J Pediatr Surg.* 1987;22:950-952.
35. van der Schouw YT, van der Velden MT, Hitge-Boetes C, Verbeek AL, Ruijs SH. Diagnosis of hypertrophic pyloric stenosis: value of sonography when used in conjunction with clinical findings and laboratory data. *AJR Am J Roentgenol.* 1994;163(4):905-909.

36. Cohen HL, Chism PB, Radtke I. Excessive bright echoes sign for hypertrophic pyloric stenosis suggest the diagnosis: gastric pneumatosis and portal venous gas in infants suggest HPS. *J Ultrasound Med.* 2017;36:1059-1063.
37. Yanchar NL. Rangu S. Corrected to uncorrected? The metabolic conundrum of hypertrophic pyloric stenosis. *J Pediatr Surg.* 2017;52:734-738.
38. Alain JL, Moulies D, Longis B, Grousseau D, Lansade A, Terrier G. Pyloric stenosis in infants. New surgical approaches. *Ann Pediatr (Paris).* 1991;38:630-632.
39. Perger L, Fuchs JR, Komidar L, Mooney DP. Impact of surgical approach on outcome in 622 consecutive pyloromyotomies at a pediatric teaching institution. *J Pediatr Surg.* 2009;44:2119-2125.
40. Leclair MD, Plattner V, Mirallie E, et al. Laparoscopic pyloromyotomy for hypertrophic pyloric stenosis: a prospective, randomized controlled trial. *J Pediatr Surg.* 2007;42:692-698.
41. Lansdale N, Al-Khafaji N, Green P, Kenny SE. Population-level surgical outcomes for infantile hypertrophic pyloric stenosis. *J Pediatr Surg.* 2017;doi:10.1016/j.jpedsurg.2017.05.018.
42. Hall NJ, Pacilli M, Eaton S, Reblock K, Gaines BA, Pastor A, et al. Recovery after open versus laparoscopic pyloromyotomy for pyloric stenosis: a double-blind multicentre randomised controlled trial. *Lancet.* 2009;373(9661):390-398.
43. Eisen GM, Baron TH, Dominitz JA, et al. Guideline for the management of ingested foreign bodies. *Gastrointest Endosc.* 2002;55:802-806.
44. Uyemura MC. Foreign body ingestion in children. *Am Fam Physician.* 2005;72:287-291.
45. Bhargava P, Phillips G. Giant gastric bezoar presenting as an acute abdominal emergency. *Pediatr Radiol.* 2010;40(suppl 1):S99.
46. Lung D, Cuevas C, Zaid U, Ancock B. Venlafaxine pharmacobezoar causing intestinal ischemia requiring emergent hemicolectomy. *J Med Toxicol.* 2011;7:232-235.
47. Dutta S, Barzin A. Multiple magnet ingestion as a source of severe gastrointestinal complications requiring surgical intervention. *Arch Pediatr Adolesc Med.* 2008;162:123.
48. Wong KK, Fang CX, Tam PK. Selective upper endoscopy for foreign body ingestion in children: an evaluation of management protocol after 282 cases. *J Pediatr Surg.* 2006;41:2016-2018.
49. Abadir J, Emil S, Nguyen N. Abdominal foregut perforations in children: a 10-year experience. *J Pediatr Surg.* 2005;40:1903-1907.
50. Curtis JL, Burns RC, Wang L, Mahour GH, Ford HR. Primary gastric tumors of infancy and childhood: 54-year experience at a single institution. *J Pediatr Surg.* 2008;43:1487-1493.
51. Wong KKY, Chung PHY, Lan LCL, Lin SCL, Tam PKH. Trends in the prevalence of *Helicobacter pylori* in symptomatic children in the era of eradication. *J Pediatr Surg.* 2005;40:1844-1847.
52. Bethel CAI, Bhattacharyya N, Hutchinson C, Ruymann F, Cooney DR. Alimentary tract malignancies in children. *J Pediatr Surg.* 1997;32:1004-1009.
53. Subbiah V, Varadhachary G, Herzog CE, Huh WW. Gastric adenocarcinoma in children and adolescents. *Pediatr Blood Cancer.* 2011;57:524-527.
54. Mosalli R, El-Bizre B, Farooqui M, Paes B. Superior mesenteric artery syndrome: a rare cause of complete intestinal obstruction in neonates. *J Pediatr Surg.* 2011;46:e29-e31.
55. Ricca RL, Kasten J, Javid PJ. Superior mesenteric artery syndrome after minimally invasive correction of pectus excavatum: impact of post-operative weight loss. *J Pediatr Surg.* 2012;47:2137-2139.
56. Santer R, Young C, Rossi T, Riddlesberger MM. Computed tomography in superior mesenteric artery syndrome. *Pediatr Radiol.* 1991;21:154-155.
57. Alsulaimy M, Tashiro J, Perez EA, Sola JE. Laparoscopic Ladd's procedure for superior mesenteric artery syndrome. *J Pediatr Surg.* 2014;49:1533-1535.
58. Teng BP, Yamout SZ. Left paraduodenal hernia causing small bowel obstruction in an adolescent patient. *J Pediatr Surg.* 2009;44:2417-2419.
59. Shinohara T, Okugawa K, Furuta C. Volvulus of the small intestine caused by right paraduodenal hernia: a case report. *J Pediatr Surg.* 2004;39:e8-e9.
60. Lam G, Clifton MS, Bhatia AM. Right paraduodenal hernia leading to bowel strangulation. *J Pediatr Surg.* 2011;46:2032-2034.
61. Moran JM, Salas J, Sanjuan S, et al. Paramesocolic hernias: consequences of delayed diagnosis. Report of three new cases. *J Pediatr Surg.* 2004;39:112-116.
62. Prada-Arias M, Sanchis-Solera L, Perez-Candela V, Wiehoff-Neumann A, Alonso-Jimenez L, Beltra-Pico R. Computed tomography diagnosis of symptomatic right paraduodenal hernia associated with enteric duplication cyst. *J Pediatr Surg.* 2007;42:1938-1941.
63. Dengler WC, Reddy PP. Right paraduodenal hernia in childhood: a case report. *J Pediatr Surg.* 1989;24:1153-1154.
64. Parmar BP, Parmar RS. Laparoscopic management of left paraduodenal hernia. *J Minim Access Surg.* 2010;6:122-124.
65. Bittner JG. Laparoscopic right paraduodenal hernia repair. *J Minim Access Surg.* 2010;6:89.
66. Van Limbergen J, Russell RK, Drummond HE, et al. Definition of phenotypic characteristics of childhood-onset inflammatory bowel disease. *Gastroenterology.* 2008;135:1114-1122.
67. Sauer CG, Kugathasan S. Pediatric inflammatory bowel disease: highlighting pediatric differences in IBD. *Med Clin North Am.* 2010;94:35-52.
68. Griffiths AM, Alemayehu E, Sherman P. Clinical features of gastroduodenal Crohn's disease in adolescents. *J Pediatr Gastroenterol Nutr.* 1989;8:166-171.
69. Tobin JM, Sinha B, Ramani P, Saleh ARH, Murphy MS. Upper gastrointestinal mucosal disease in pediatric Crohn disease and ulcerative colitis: a blinded, controlled study. *J Pediatr Gastroenterol Nutr.* 2001;32:443-448.
70. Alkhouri RH, Bahia G, Smith AC, Thomas R, Finck C. Sayej W. Outcome of medical management of intraabdominal abscesses in children with Crohn's disease. *J Pediatr Surg.* 2017;doi:10.1016/j.jpedsurg.2017.03.059.
71. Amil-Dias J, Kolacek S, Turner D, et al. Surgical management of Crohn disease in children: guidelines from the paediatric IBD Porto Group of ESPGHAN. *J Pediatr Gastroenterol Nutr.* 2017;64:818-835.

Anatomy and Physiology of the Duodenum

Brian Shames

Although spanning only 20 to 30 cm, from the pylorus to the ligament of Treitz, the duodenum is the "gate" that controls the passage of food from the stomach to the jejunum.[1] The name is derived from the Latin phrase *intestinum duodenum digitorum,* or "intestine of twelve digits." This Latin phrase may have derived from the writings of the Greek physician Herophilus (334–280 BC).

Although it is the shortest segment of small bowel, the duodenum is the initial site of contact for gastric secretions, bile, and digestive enzymes from the common bile duct and the pancreas. Thus it plays an important role in the regulation of digestion, absorption of essential micronutrients and macronutrients, and bowel motility. Its relationships to the major structures of the upper abdomen lend it to exposure during a large number of gastrointestinal (GI) surgical interventions. As such, it is important to understand both the structure and function of the duodenum as it relates to alimentary surgery.

EMBRYOGENESIS

In the adult the duodenum's position in the upper abdomen follows the normal development and rotation of the embryonic gut. This process starts at the beginning of the third week of embryonic development with primitive foregut demarcation from the midgut and hindgut. Early in the second month of gestation, the embryologic midgut migrates ventrally to descend into the yolk sac. The apex of this loop is marked by the omphalomesenteric duct (yolk sac) with an axis around the superior mesenteric artery, the proximal portion of the yolk sac's primitive blood supply (vitelline artery). Over the next several weeks, the midportion of the intestine elongates faster than the abdominal cavity expands, thereby enlarging the midgut loop, which continues to push into the umbilical cord. As this occurs, the midgut undergoes a counterclockwise 90-degree rotation around the superior mesenteric artery, forming "prearterial" and "postarterial" halves. Following this rotation, the cranial ("prearterial") segment of midgut (future duodenum and proximal small bowel) lies to the right of the caudal ("postarterial") segment (future colon). The cranial ("prearterial") segment continues to elongate into the umbilical cord until the tenth gestational week, after which the midgut returns into the abdomen. The cranial limb migrates back into the abdomen first, causing the duodenum to pass behind the superior mesenteric artery. The caudal limb follows with the cecum and terminal ileum entering last. During its return, the midgut rotates another 180 degrees (total rotation = 270 degrees).

At the completion of these movements, the colon is situated anterior to the superior mesenteric artery, and the cecum is located at the level of the iliac crest. From the twelfth week of gestation until after birth, the colon elongates while the cecum remains in its original position. This colonic growth effectively produces an "ascent" of the hepatic flexure toward the right upper quadrant that seems like a cecal "descent."[2]

Anatomic relations between the duodenum, liver, and pancreas are also dictated by early development. The future duodenum lies between the transverse septum of the ventral mesentery (the future primordium of the liver, the bile ducts, and the ventral pancreatic bud) and the dorsal mesentery (the future dorsal pancreatic bud). After midgut rotation is complete, the hepatic parenchyma and the intestines proliferate and the dorsal and ventral pancreatic buds fuse, establishing the duodenum's final anatomic location (Fig. 68.1).

Initially, the duodenum is composed of a single layer of endodermal cells surrounded by undifferentiated mesenchymal cells. By the end of the fourth week of gestation, the duodenal mucosa begins to proliferate along the ventral wall near the origin of the hepatic diverticulum. During midgut rotation, mesenchymal tissue beyond the first portion of the duodenum increases along the dorsal aspect of the duodenum, fixing it to the retroperitoneum beyond this point. During fixation, this dorsal mesentery transforms into an avascular plane of loose connective tissue known as the fascia of Treitz (not to be confused with the ligament of Treitz). This plane is entered when lifting the duodenum medially during a Kocher maneuver.[3]

At the end of the third gestational week, the liver primordium, gallbladder, and biliary duct (both originating from the gallbladder bud) arise as a ventral outgrowth from the distal end of the foregut. Later (fifth gestational week) the connecting elements between the hepatic diverticulum and the duodenum form the bile duct and, ultimately, the cystic duct and the gallbladder. Around the ninth week of gestation, rapid hepatic growth occurs secondary to the hematopoietic function of the liver and the formation of multiple hepatic sinusoids. This hepatic growth, combined with the midgut's elongation, pushes the duodenum below the liver. At this time, the ventral mesentery produces the lesser omentum, the falciform ligament, and the hepatoduodenal ligament; these structures envelop the portal triad as it extends from the liver.

Other structures within the portal triad include the hepatic artery and the portal vein. Spatially, the portal vein is complexly related to the duodenum during the latter's development. The portal vein develops from the primitive paired vitelline veins that arise in the yolk sac and pass up the body stalk to enter the developing heart. Two extrahepatic cross-connections develop between the paired vessels: The cranial anastomosis lies behind the duodenum and the caudal anastomosis passes in front of the duodenum. Normally the cranial retroduodenal

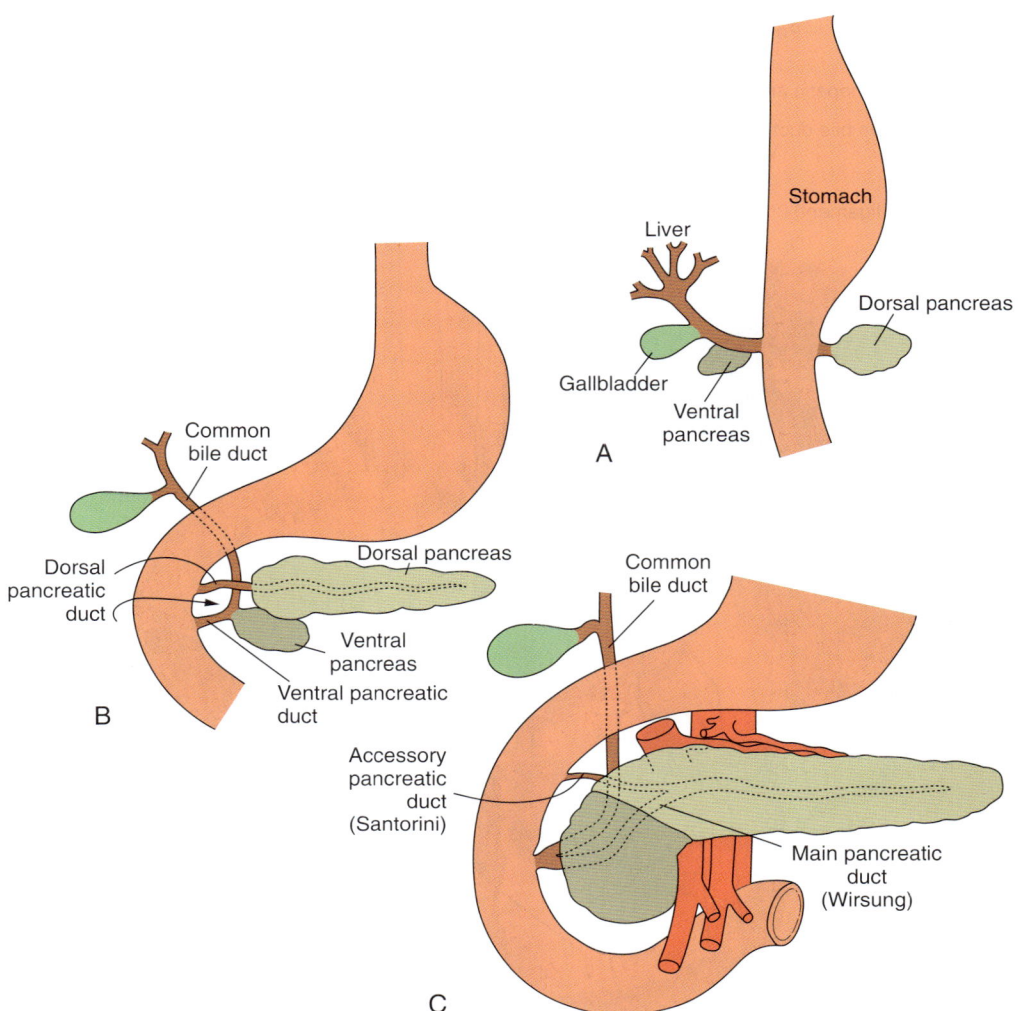

FIGURE 68.1 Embryonic relations of pancreas and duodenum. (A) Formation of dorsal and ventral pancreatic primordial. (B) Rotation of ventral pancreas. (C) Fusion of primordial to form adult pancreas. (Redrawn from Androulakis J, Colborn GL, Skandalakis PN, Skandalakis LJ, Skandalakis JE. Embryologic and anatomic basis of duodenal surgery. *Surg Clin North Am*. 2000;80:172, figure 1.)

anastomosis persists as the portal vein and the caudal anastomosis disappears. This preduodenal caudal anastomosis can persist as the portal vein, leading to the rare congenital anomaly known as a preduodenal portal vein.[4,5]

At the end of the fourth gestational week (see Fig. 68.1), the developing duodenum is joined by a dorsal pancreatic primordium. One week later the ventral pancreatic primordial bud arises at the base of the hepatic diverticulum. At the end of the sixth week, these two primordia fuse as the ventral pancreas migrates below and behind the dorsal pancreatic segment; these changes form portions of the adult pancreatic head and uncinate process. After fusion, the principal pancreatic ducts fuse, typically with the ventral duct fusing at the midportion of the dorsal pancreatic duct. The combination of the ventral duct and the fused mid- to distal dorsal duct becomes the duct of Wirsung. This duct connects to the common bile duct, contributing to the ampulla of Vater at the site of the common bile duct's entry into the duodenum. After fusion, the proximal portion of the dorsal pancreatic duct (the duct of Santorini) typically regresses as the duct of Wirsung assumes dominance. As the midgut expands and rotates, the duodenum achieves its final location along the retroperitoneum with the first and second portion located laterally while the remainder traverses inferiorly to the fused pancreatic primordia (Fig. 68.2).[6]

Failure of the pancreatic primordia to fuse results in a condition known as pancreatic divisum. In this situation the ducts of Wirsung and Santorini drain separately into the duodenum. Annular pancreas may also develop after anomalous pancreatic fusion; in this developmental anomaly, a thin flat band of normal pancreatic tissue surrounds the second portion of the duodenum and connects to either side of the pancreatic head. The ring that forms around the duodenum can cause duodenal stenosis. Although this anomaly is described in children, it may be entirely asymptomatic until discovered as an incidental finding on necropsy.[7]

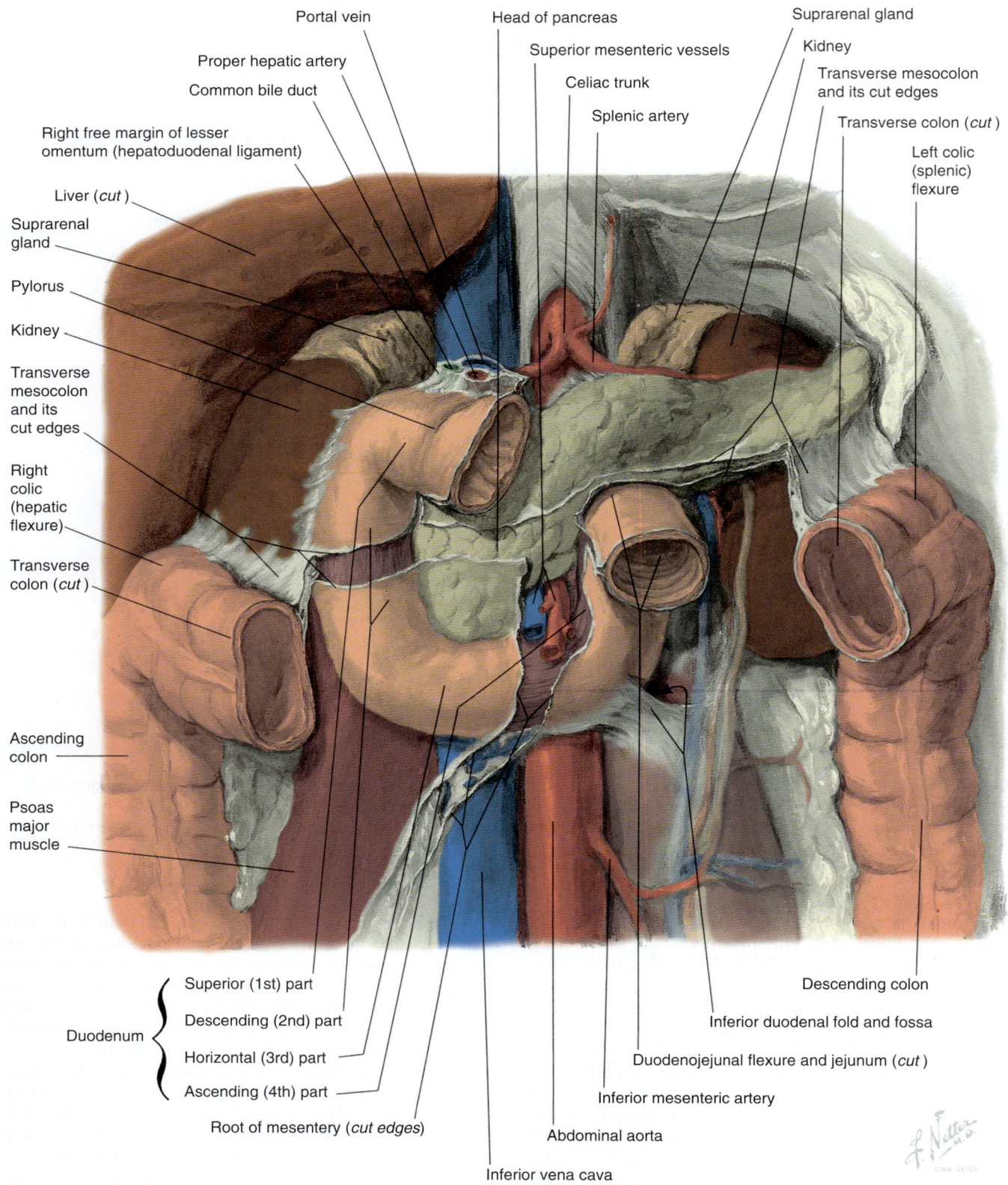

FIGURE 68.2 The abdominal contents as seen after removal of the stomach, jejunum, and ileum. The branches of the superior and inferior mesenteric arteries are shown. (From Netter FH. *Atlas of Human Anatomy*. East Hanover, NJ: Novartis Medical Education; 1989, Ciba-Geigy, plate 261. Copyright 1999, ICON Learning Systems, LLC, a subsidiary of Havas MediMedia USA Inc. Reprinted with permission from ICON Learning Systems, LLC, illustrated by Frank H Netter, MD. All rights reserved.)

GROSS ANATOMY AND TOPOGRAPHIC RELATIONS

The duodenum is divided into four segments: the duodenal bulb or cap; the second vertical or descending portion; the third horizontal or transverse portion; and the fourth oblique or ascending portion (Fig. 68.3). The duodenum begins at the end of the gastric pylorus, in the plane of the first lumbar vertebra. Starting at the second portion, it descends in a C-shaped curve around the pancreatic head. The third part of the duodenum lies inferior to the superior mesenteric artery at the level of the second lumbar vertebra; it is situated in the angle formed by the superior mesenteric artery and the aorta where it crosses the midline to join the fourth duodenal segment and later the jejunum.

The duodenum is related anteriorly to the liver and gallbladder; superiorly to the epiploic foramen; laterally (second portion) and inferiorly (third portion) to the pancreatic head; and posteriorly to the common bile duct, portal vein, inferior vena cava, and gastroduodenal artery. It is separated laterally from the inferior vena cava by a small amount of connective tissue.

FIRST DUODENAL SEGMENT (APPROXIMATELY 5 CM LONG)

The first portion of the duodenum passes superiorly from the gastric pylorus to the neck of the gallbladder. The proximal half, the duodenal bulb or cap, is mobile; the distal half is fixed. Most (90%) duodenal ulcers occur in the duodenal bulb. Clinically, the mobility of the duodenal bulb facilitates operations on the pylorus and duodenum, particularly after a Kocher maneuver. Its longitudinal muscle folds can be appreciated on upper endoscopy and used as a landmark prior to entering the second portion where transverse folds can be seen.

The hepatoduodenal portion of the lesser omentum attaches to the superior duodenal border within the initial 2.5 cm of this segment; the greater omentum attaches to this segment's inferior border. The distal 2.5 cm is covered by peritoneum anteriorly, resulting in the posterior surface closely contacting the portal triad and the gastroduodenal artery. This segment's relationship to the gastroduodenal artery explains the artery's susceptibility to bleeding when posterior peptic ulcers erode. When encountering this condition, surgeons should remember that the gastroduodenal artery arises 15 to 30 mm above the superior border of the first part of the duodenum, and the distance between the artery's origin and the pylorus can range from 5 to 50 mm.[8] Finally, the duodenum's proximity to the gallbladder facilitates cholecystoduodenal fistulas and the passage of gallstones into the intestinal tract after severe bouts of cholecystitis.

SECOND DUODENAL SEGMENT (APPROXIMATELY 7.5 CM LONG)

This portion of the duodenum extends from the gallbladder neck to the upper border of L4. It joins the first portion of the duodenum on the right side of the first lumbar vertebra, behind the costal margin slightly superior and medial to the ninth costal cartilage's tip. Beyond this junction, the duodenum becomes a retroperitoneal structure through fusion of its lateral visceral peritoneum to the posterolateral abdominal wall. After forming an acute angle with the superior duodenal flexure, the second portion descends from the gallbladder with a loop that passes over the right renal hilum, the adrenal gland, the psoas major, and the edge of the inferior vena cava. Concurrently, it passes under the right hepatic lobe, the colonic hepatic flexure, and parts of the transverse colon and the jejunum. Peritoneal folds pass above and below this duodenal segment to form the mesocolon. The relationship between the duodenum, hepatic flexure, and mesocolon must be considered when mobilizing the hepatic flexure during surgical interventions on the proximal colon.

Medially, the pancreatic head is intimately related to the duodenal C-loop. The superior pancreaticoduodenal branch of the gastroduodenal artery runs in the groove between the two structures. At about the midpoint of the C-loop, the pancreaticobiliary tract opens into the papilla of Vater, on the second duodenal segment's concave posteromedial side.

THIRD DUODENAL SEGMENT (APPROXIMATELY 12 TO 13 CM LONG)

The third portion of the duodenum extends from the right side of L3 or L4 to the left side of the aorta. As this segment passes from right to left across the midline anterior to the ureter, the psoas muscles, the inferior vena cava and the aorta, it remains posterior to the superior mesenteric vessels. Superiorly, the pancreatic head and uncinate processes are separated from this part of the duodenum by a groove containing the inferior pancreaticoduodenal artery. This segment ends to the left of the third or fourth lumbar vertebra, next to the root of the small intestine's mesentery.

FOURTH DUODENAL SEGMENT (APPROXIMATELY 2.5 CM LONG)

The fourth portion of the duodenum starts at the left upper border of L2. After an upward and oblique ascent, it travels to the duodenojejunal angle at the root of the transverse mesocolon, approximately 4 cm below and medial to the ninth costal cartilage's tip. It then descends leftward to form the duodenojejunal flexure where the duodenum's suspensory ligament attaches to the mesentery (ligament of Treitz). This ligament, a remnant of the dorsal mesentery, extends from the duodenojejunal flexure to the right diaphragmatic crus. Its termination closely approximates the terminal part of the inferior mesenteric vein, the left ureter, and the left kidney.[9]

ARTERIAL SUPPLY

The first portion of the duodenum is supplied by the posterior superior pancreaticoduodenal branch of the gastroduodenal artery, and variably by the supraduodenal and retroduodenal arteries (either separately or in variable combinations). In some patients, branches of the right gastric artery also supply the first centimeter of the duodenum. The gastroduodenal artery descends between the first part of the duodenum and the pancreatic head,

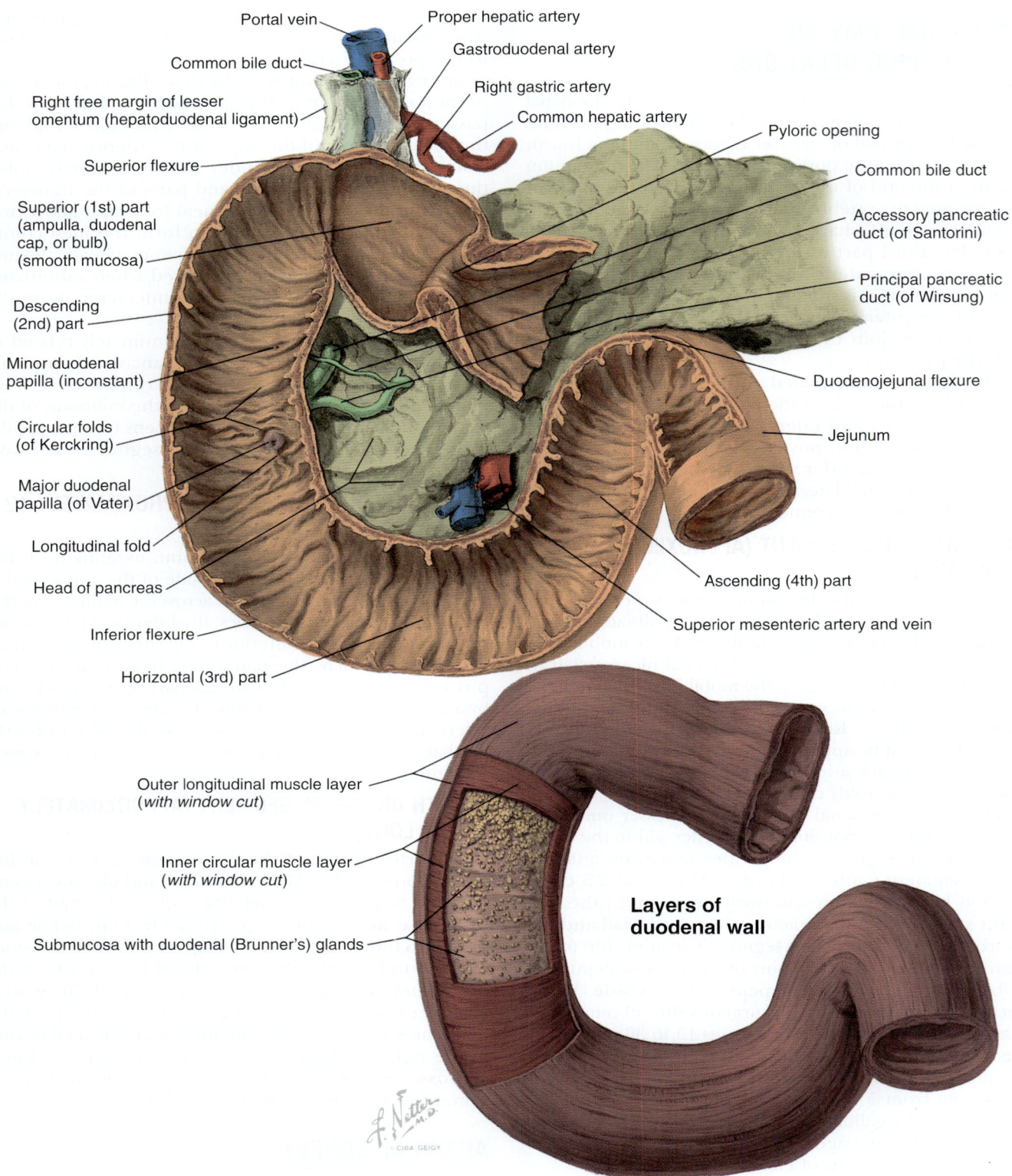

Layers of duodenal wall

Portal vein

Proper hepatic artery

Common bile duct

Gastroduodenal artery

Right gastric artery

Right free margin of lesser omentum (hepatoduodenal ligament)

Common hepatic artery

Pyloric opening

Superior flexure

Common bile duct

Superior (1st) part (ampulla, duodenal cap, or bulb) (smooth mucosa)

Accessory pancreatic duct (of Santorini)

Principal pancreatic duct (of Wirsung)

Descending (2nd) part

Minor duodenal papilla (inconstant)

Duodenojejunal flexure

Circular folds (of Kerckring)

Jejunum

Major duodenal papilla (of Vater)

Longitudinal fold

Head of pancreas

Ascending (4th) part

Inferior flexure

Superior mesenteric artery and vein

Horizontal (3rd) part

Outer longitudinal muscle layer (*with window cut*)

Inner circular muscle layer (*with window cut*)

Submucosa with duodenal (Brunner's) glands

FIGURE 68.3 The duodenum, the four portions, and their relationship to the bile duct and pancreas. (From Netter FH. *Atlas of Human Anatomy*. East Hanover, NJ: Novartis Medical Education; 1989, Ciba-Geigy, plate 262. Copyright 1999, ICON Learning Systems, LLC, a subsidiary of Havas MediMedia USA Inc. Reprinted with permission from ICON Learning Systems, LLC, illustrated by Frank H Netter, MD. All rights reserved.)

terminating into the right gastroepiploic artery and the anterior superior pancreaticoduodenal artery.[10] This rich periduodenal arterial anastomotic network often frustrates attempts to control bleeding from posterior duodenal ulcers.

The arterial supply to the remainder of the duodenum is derived from major arterial anastomoses between the celiac and superior mesenteric arterial circulations. As noted earlier, the anterior superior pancreaticoduodenal artery arises from the gastroduodenal artery on the pancreas' ventral surface. The posterior superior pancreaticoduodenal artery crosses in front of the common bile duct and then spirals posteriorly to the pancreatic head. The anterior and posterior inferior pancreaticoduodenal arteries arise from the superior mesenteric artery or its first jejunal branch, either separately or through a common origin. These two arteries split and run in posterior and anterior grooves between the descending and transverse portions of the duodenum and the pancreatic head, where they join to form continuous anterior and posterior arcades. Through these arterial arcades, the duodenum shares its blood supply with the proximal pancreas (Fig. 68.4). As such, resection of either the duodenum or the pancreas alone is technically challenging and potentially hazardous.

VENOUS SUPPLY

Pancreaticoduodenal veins parallel the pancreaticoduodenal arteries, accompanying them in anterior and posterior pancreaticoduodenal arcades (Fig. 68.5). Surgeons usually encounter these veins superficial to their arterial analogues. The lower portion of the proximal duodenal bulb drains into the right gastroepiploic veins; the upper part drains into the portal vein or posterior superior pancreaticoduodenal vein via several suprapyloric veins. The posterior arcade ends in the portal vein above and the superior mesenteric vein below. The posterior superior pancreaticoduodenal vein may follow its companion artery anterior to the bile duct, although it usually runs behind the duct. This vein terminates inferiorly on the superior mesenteric vein's left border. Here it may be joined by a jejunal vein or by the anterior inferior pancreaticoduodenal vein.

LYMPHATIC DRAINAGE

The lymphatic drainage of the duodenum generally parallels its vasculature. Anterior lymphatic channels drain to anterior pancreatic nodal basins and posterior channels drain to basins posterior to the pancreatic head. Although primary duodenal carcinomas may invade the pancreas via direct extension or lymphatic infiltration, they usually spread to the periduodenal lymph nodes and liver first.

INNERVATION

The duodenum's extrinsic innervation (Fig. 68.6) is parasympathetic, arising from the anterior and celiac vagal branches, and sympathetic, arising from the splanchnic nerves of the celiac ganglion (T6 to T12). Intrinsic innervation arises from the Auerbach myenteric and the Meissner submucosal plexuses. Processes from these neurons innervate their targets (e.g., smooth muscle, secretory and absorptive cells) but also connect to sensory receptors and interdigitate with other neural processes arising from both inside and outside the plexuses.

HISTOLOGY

The duodenal wall is made up of four layers: the *serosa*: an outer peritoneal coat; the *muscularis*: a muscular coat made up of longitudinal and circular fibers; the *submucosa*; and the *mucosa* that forms its inner lining (Fig. 68.7). The serosa is an extension of the peritoneum. It consists of a single layer of flattened mesothelial cells overlying loose connective tissue. The portions of the posterior and lateral duodenal walls that are retroperitoneal lack this peritoneal or serosal coat.

The muscularis is composed of two layers of smooth muscle: an outer (longitudinal) layer and an inner (circular) layer. The myenteric plexus of Auerbach lies between these two layers. The Meissner plexus is found in the submucosa along with a network of loose connective tissue rich in lymphatics and small blood vessels (see Fig. 68.7).

The glands of Brunner, a characteristic histologic feature of the mammalian duodenum, are found in the submucosa; these glands empty into the crypts of Lieberkühn through small secretory ducts (Fig. 68.8). Brunner gland secretion is viscous, alkaline (pH 8.2 to 9.3), and clear. These mucoid, viscous, alkaline secretions help to protect the duodenal mucosa against the corrosive action of gastric juice.

The intestinal mucosa forms numerous fingerlike projections, or villi, that greatly increase the mucosal surface area (see Fig. 68.7). Columnar cells containing mucus and HCO_3^--secreting surface cells as well as absorptive cells line the villi's epithelium. The mucosa lining the crypts and villi can be divided into three layers: the muscularis mucosae (deep); the lamina propria (middle); and an inner layer consisting of a continuous sheet of columnar epithelial cells.

The crypt epithelium's main functions include (1) cell renewal; (2) exocrine, endocrine, water, and ion secretion; and (3) absorption of salt, water, and specific nutrients. The crypt epithelium is composed of at least four distinct cell types: Paneth, goblet, undifferentiated, and endocrine cells.

PHYSIOLOGY

The main functions of the duodenum are to (1) alkalinize acidic chyme, thereby protecting its mucosa and facilitating digestion; (2) absorb calcium and iron; (3) further the breakdown of food products; and (4) exert neuroendocrine control of upper GI motility and secretion.

ALKALINIZATION AND DUODENAL MUCOSAL DEFENSE

Duodenal luminal pH can fluctuate rapidly between pH 2 and 7 as secreted bicarbonate and gastric acid mix.[11] Prevention of mucosal damage requires a coordinated defense via regulated premucosal, mucosal, and submucosal components. These components include mucus and bicarbonate (HCO_3^-) secretion, intracellular buffering, neuronal activation, and increased blood flow.

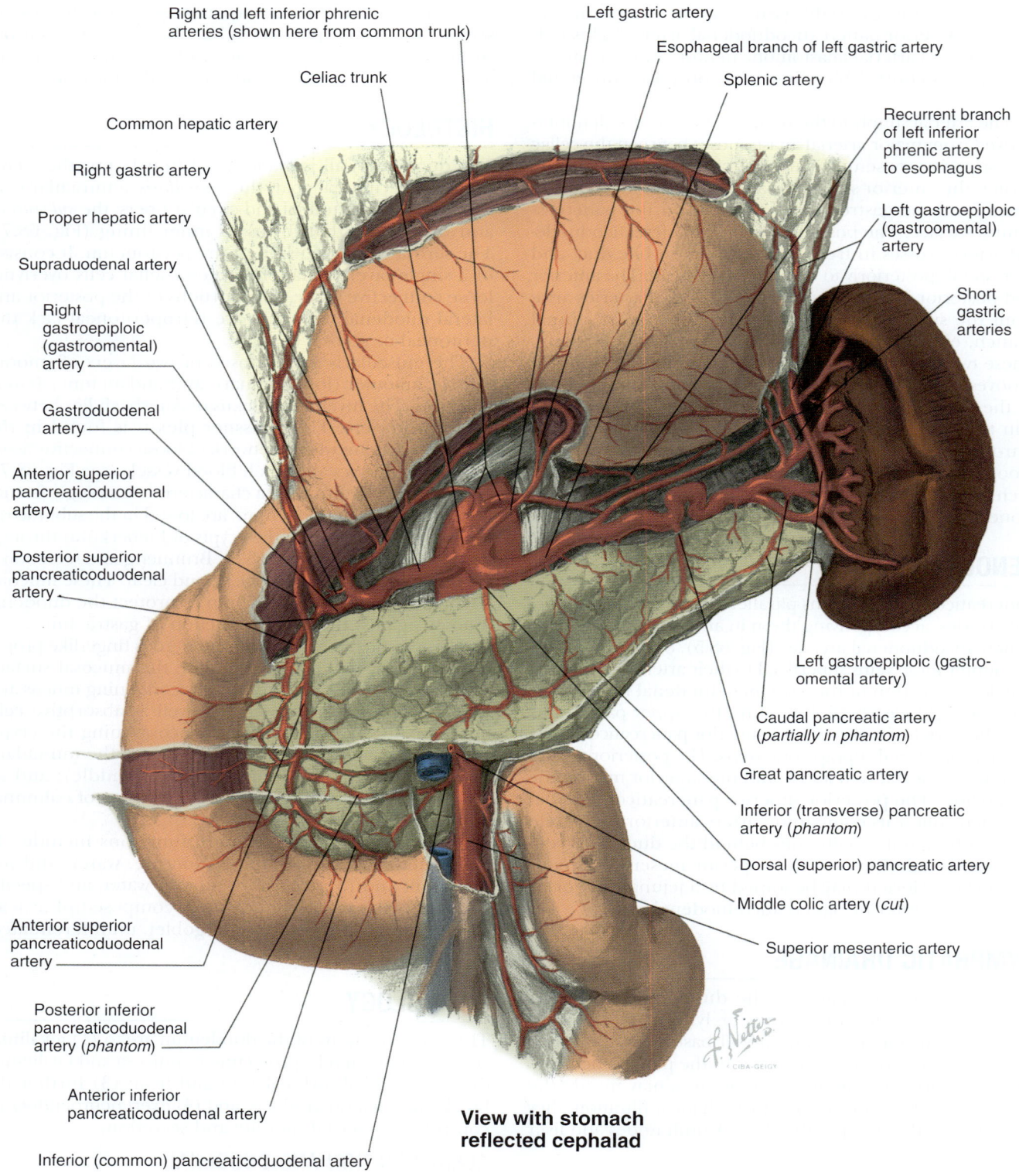

Right and left inferior phrenic arteries (shown here from common trunk)

Left gastric artery

Esophageal branch of left gastric artery

Celiac trunk

Splenic artery

Common hepatic artery

Recurrent branch of left inferior phrenic artery to esophagus

Right gastric artery

Proper hepatic artery

Left gastroepiploic (gastroomental) artery

Supraduodenal artery

Short gastric arteries

Right gastroepiploic (gastroomental) artery

Gastroduodenal artery

Anterior superior pancreaticoduodenal artery

Posterior superior pancreaticoduodenal artery

Left gastroepiploic (gastro-omental artery)

Caudal pancreatic artery (*partially in phantom*)

Great pancreatic artery

Inferior (transverse) pancreatic artery (*phantom*)

Dorsal (superior) pancreatic artery

Middle colic artery (*cut*)

Superior mesenteric artery

Anterior superior pancreaticoduodenal artery

Posterior inferior pancreaticoduodenal artery (*phantom*)

Anterior inferior pancreaticoduodenal artery

Inferior (common) pancreaticoduodenal artery

View with stomach reflected cephalad

FIGURE 68.4 View of the arteries of the duodenum and pancreas, with the stomach reflected cephalad. (From Netter FH. *Atlas of Human Anatomy*. East Hanover, NJ: Novartis Medical Education; 1989, Ciba-Geigy, plate 283. Copyright 1999, ICON Learning Systems, LLC, a subsidiary of Havas MediMedia USA Inc. Reprinted with permission from ICON Learning Systems, LLC, illustrated by Frank H Netter, MD. All rights reserved.)

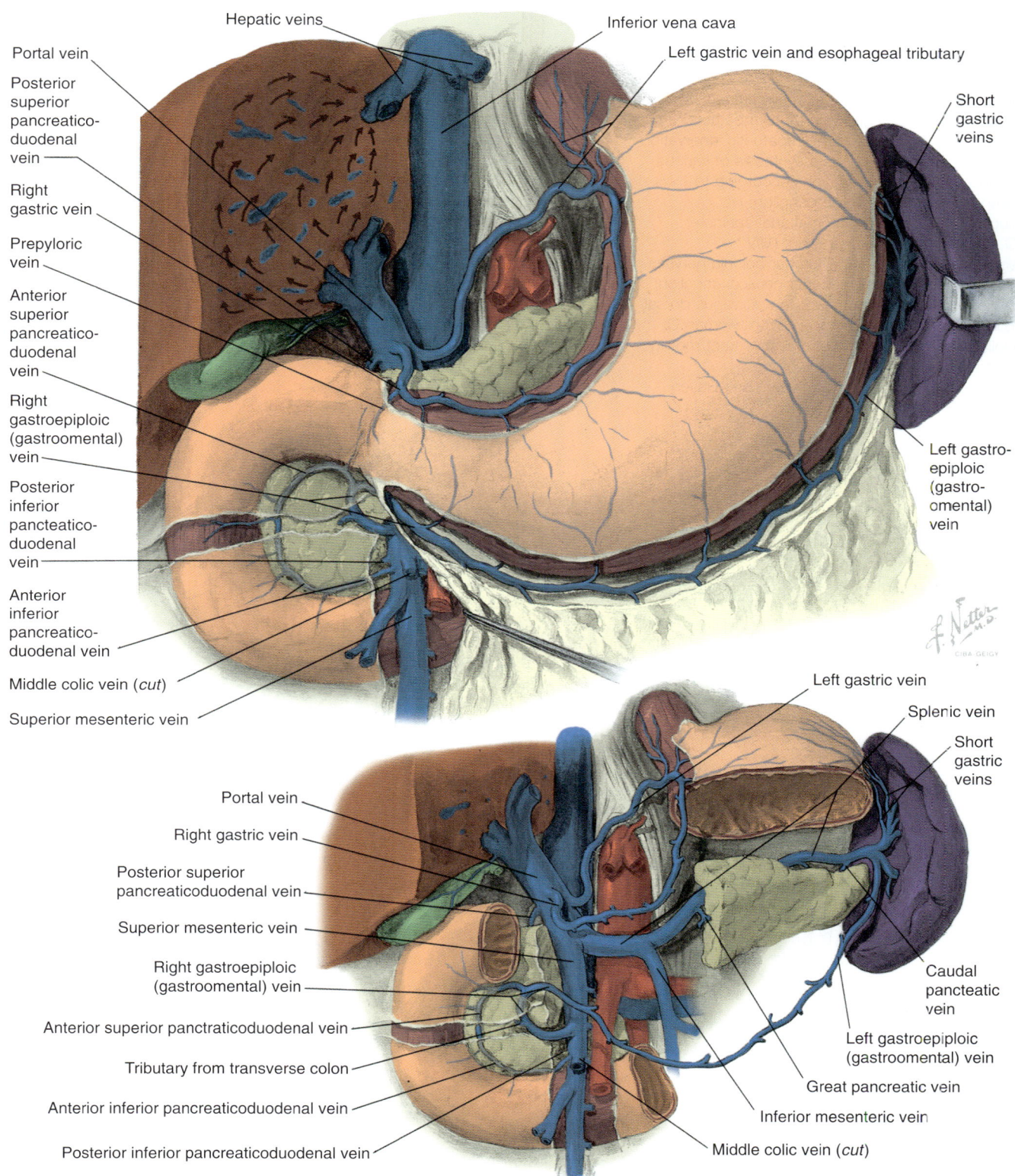

Hepatic veins

Inferior vena cava

Portal vein

Left gastric vein and esophageal tributary

Posterior superior pancreaticoduodenal vein

Short gastric veins

Right gastric vein

Prepyloric vein

Anterior superior pancreaticoduodenal vein

Right gastroepiploic (gastroomental) vein

Posterior inferior pancteaticoduodenal vein

Left gastroepiploic (gastroomental) vein

Anterior inferior pancreaticoduodenal vein

Middle colic vein (*cut*)

Superior mesenteric vein

Left gastric vein

Splenic vein

Short gastric veins

Portal vein

Right gastric vein

Posterior superior pancreaticoduodenal vein

Superior mesenteric vein

Right gastroepiploic (gastroomental) vein

Anterior superior panctraticoduodenal vein

Tributary from transverse colon

Anterior inferior pancreaticoduodenal vein

Posterior inferior pancreaticoduodenal vein

Caudal pancteatic vein

Left gastroepiploic (gastroomental) vein

Great pancreatic vein

Inferior mesenteric vein

Middle colic vein (*cut*)

FIGURE 68.5 View of the veins of the duodenum and pancreas, with the stomach removed. (From Netter FH. *Atlas of Human Anatomy.* East Hanover, NJ: Novartis Medical Education; 1989, Ciba-Geigy, plate 294. Copyright 1999, ICON Learning Systems, LLC, a subsidiary of Havas MediMedia USA Inc. Reprinted with permission from ICON Learning Systems, LLC, illustrated by Frank H Netter, MD. All rights reserved.)

FIGURE 68.6 Schema of the extrinsic efferent innervation of the gut showing the sympathetic innervation *(left)* and the parasympathetic innervation *(right).* This representation is a synthesis of various data and may present variations according to different species. *CG,* Celiac ganglion; *HN,* hypogastric nerves; *IAS,* internal anal sphincter; *IMG,* inferior mesenteric ganglion; *IMN,* intermesenteric nerve; *LCN,* lumbar colonic nerves; *PN,* pelvic nerves; *SCG,* superior cervical ganglion; *SMG,* superior mesenteric ganglion; *X,* vagus dorsal motor nucleus and vagus nerve. (From Roman C, Gonella J. Extrinsic control of digestive tract motility. In: Johnson LR, ed. *Physiology of the Gastrointestinal Tract.* 2nd ed. New York: Raven Press; 1987:507.)

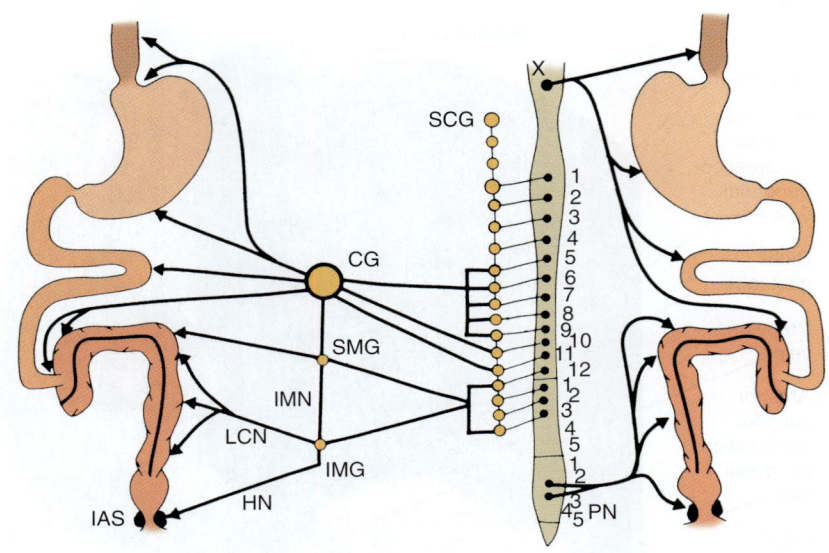

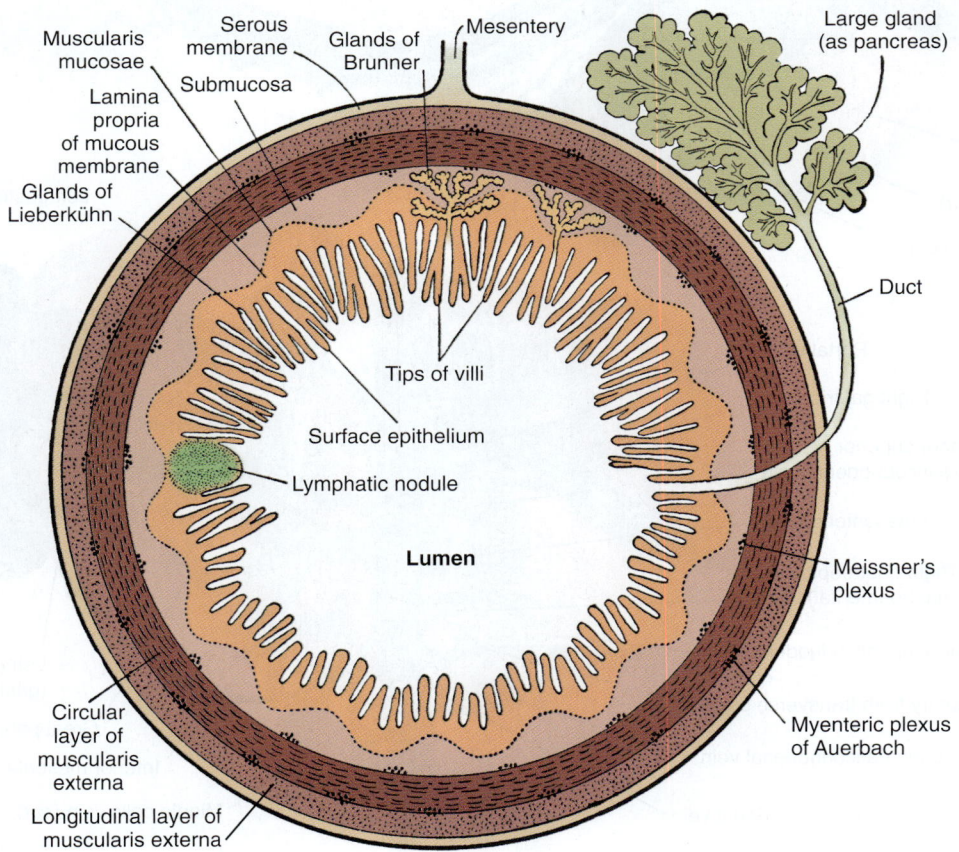

FIGURE 68.7 Schematic of a cross section of the intestinal tract. (From Bloom WN, Fawcett DW. *A Textbook of Histology.* Philadelphia: Saunders; 1968.)

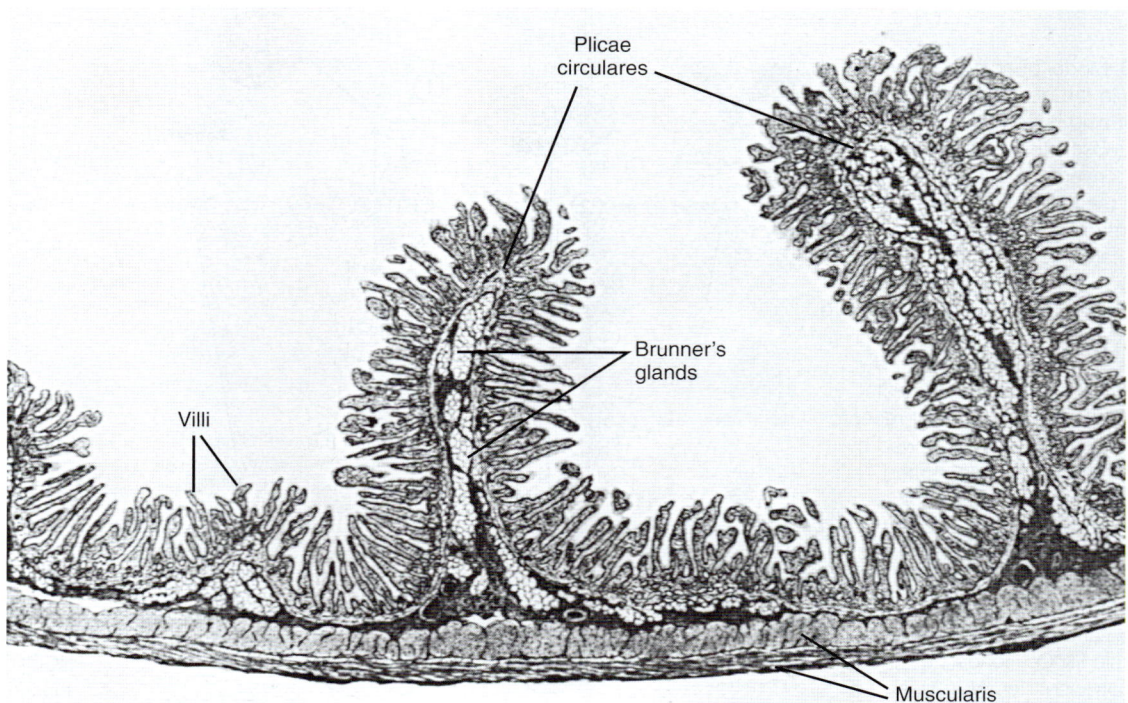

FIGURE 68.8 Drawing of a longitudinal section through the wall of the duodenum of an adult human showing the plicae circulares (valves of Kerckring), the villi, and the submucosal glands of Brunner. (From Bargmann W. *Histologie und Mikroskopische Anatomie des Menschen*. 6th ed. Stuttgart, Germany: Georg-Thieme Verlag; 1962.)

The duodenum has a unique luminal chemosensing capacity that allows the mucosa to respond to acid. After duodenal luminal acidification, a number of compounds stimulate bicarbonate secretion from the liver, pancreas, and duodenum including secretin, vagally produced acetylcholine, vasoactive intestinal polypeptide (VIP), pituitary adenylate cyclase–activating polypeptide (PACAP), melatonin,[12] and motilin.[13] This process may also be mediated by a feedback loop involving luminal adenosine triphosphate and intestinal alkaline phosphatase activity.[14] However, the principal components contributing to duodenal mucosal defense involve HCO_3^- secretion from the epithelium within the duodenal bulb.[15]

Duodenal mucosal bicarbonate secretion is stimulated by a complex array of mediators that lead to a net influx of acid from the duodenal lumen into the extracellular space, and a net efflux of extracellular HCO_3^- into the lumen (Fig. 68.9). The process is thought to start with neutralization of luminal H^+ by secreted HCO_3^-. This process is facilitated by extracellular, membrane-bound carbonic anhydrase.[16] A decrease in intracellular pH promotes H^+ extrusion into the subepithelial space via basolateral Na^+/H^+ exchanger 1 (NHE1) activity and movement of extracellular bicarbonate into the cell through basolateral Na^+/HCO_3^- transporter channels (NBC). This new intracellular HCO_3^- is then secreted into the duodenal lumen via brush border Cl^-/HCO_3^- anion exchangers in conjunction with cystic fibrosis transmembrane conductance regulators (CFTRs) (Fig. 68.10).[14,17,18]

Although duodenal mucosal bicarbonate secretion is believed to be one of the primary duodenal mucosal

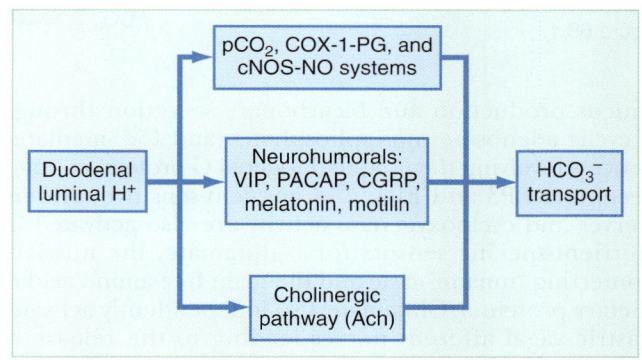

FIGURE 68.9 The mechanism of duodenal HCO_3^- secretion in response to gastric H^+ involves a variety of neurotransmitters, pCO_2, cyclooxygenase-1-prostaglandin *(COX-1-PG)*, and the constitutive nitric oxide synthase–nitric oxide *(cNOS-NO)* system. *Ach*, Acetylcholine; *CGRP*, calcitonin gene-related peptide; *PACAP*, pituitary adenylate cyclase–activating polypeptide; *VIP*, vasoactive intestinal polypeptide. (From Konturek PC, Konturek SJ, Hahn EG. Duodenal alkaline secretion: its mechanisms and role in mucosal protection against gastric acid. *Dig Liver Dis*. 2004;36:505.)

protective mechanisms, additional mechanisms are beginning to emerge, including the receptor potential vanilloid 1 ion channels (TRPV1). Activation causes the release of enteroglucagon, calcitonin gene–related peptide, and nitric oxide (NO), all of which act to simulate mucus secretion and increase blood flow. Concurrently, increased cyclooxygenase activity leads to a delayed increase in

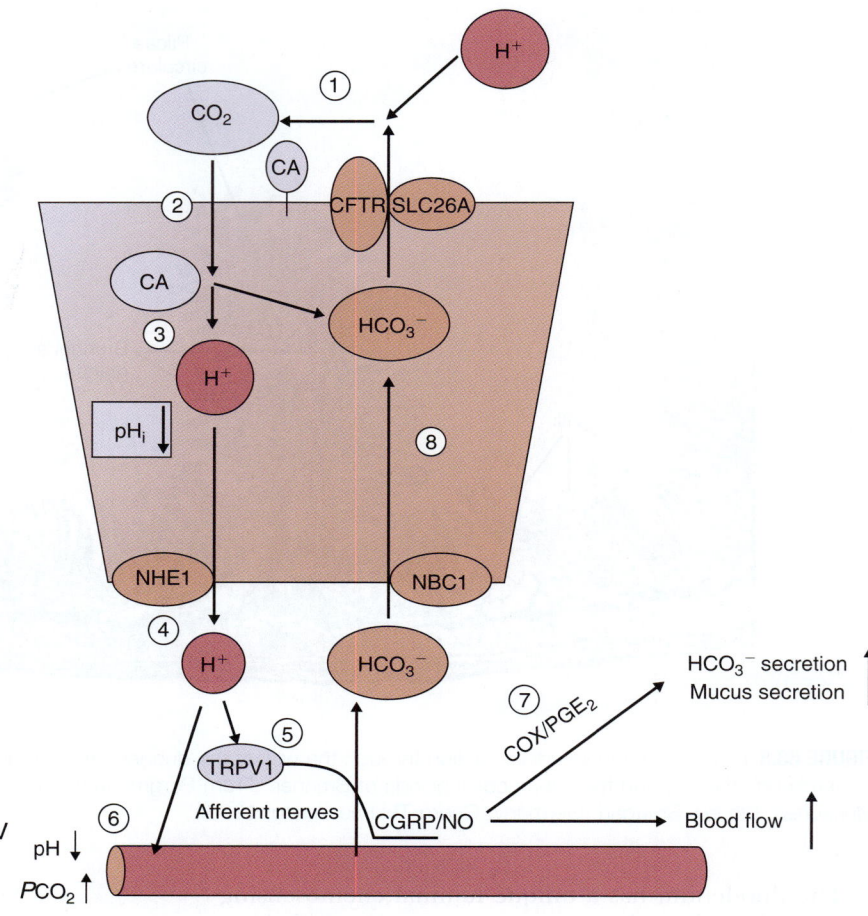

FIGURE 68.10 Model of acid/CO_2-sensing mechanisms in the duodenum. The net movement of acid is from the lumen to the mucosa (absorption), whereas net bicarbonate movement is from the mucosa to the lumen (secretion). *(1)* Luminal H^+ from the stomach is neutralized by extracellular carbonic anhydrase *(CA)*, generating CO_2. *(2)* CO_2 traverses the apical membrane. *(3)* CO_2 is converted into H^+ and HCO_3^- by cytosolic CA. *(4)* H^+ acidifies cells and is extruded into the subepithelium via Na^+/H^+ exchanger 1 *(NHE1)*. *(5)* H^+ stimulates transient receptor potential vanilloid 1 *(TRPV1)*, followed by the release of calcitonin gene-related peptide *(CGRP)* and nitric oxide *(NO)*, increasing blood flow. *(6)* H^+ acidifies portal vein *(PV)* blood. *(7)* Concurrently, cyclooxygenase *(COX)* produces prostaglandin E_2 *(PGE$_2$)*, which signals HCO_3^- and mucus secretion. *(8)* Cytoplasmic HCO_3^-, loaded via the Na^+/HCO_3^- cotransporter *(NBC1)*, is secreted through an apical solute carrier family 26Ax *(SLC26A)* anion exchanger or cystic fibrosis transmembrane conductance regulator *(CFTR)*. (Redrawn from Akiba Y, Kaunitz JD. Luminal chemo sensing and upper-gastrointestinal mucosal defenses. *Am J Clin Nutr.* 2009;90:S827, figure 68.1.)

mucus production and bicarbonate secretion through a cyclic adenosine monophosphate– and Ca^{2+}-mediated process involving the unique duodenal G protein–coupled receptors EP3 and EP4.[13,19] Capsaicin-sensitive afferent nerves and cyclooxygenase activity are also activated by nutrient-specific sensors for L-glutamate, the nutrient conferring "umami" taste and the main free amino acid in dietary protein. L-Glutamate also independently activates gastric vagal afferent nerves leading to the release of NO and 5-hydroxytryptamine or serotonin (5-HT), both of which increase luminal mucous gel thickness and intracellular pH.[16]

Cumulatively, these factors stabilize the pH gradient, increase NO-mediated vasodilation and subsequent regional blood flow, and increase mucus production by goblet cells and Brunner glands. The latter effect creates a thickened mucous gel lining composed of water, mucin glycoproteins, bicarbonate, and trefoil factor family peptides. This thickened mucous lining creates a zone of low turbulence that buffers the duodenal lumen, allowing a small amount of bicarbonate to help neutralize a large amount of gastric acid.[15,17]

CALCIUM ABSORPTION

Calcium balance depends on the net absorption of calcium across the intestine and the regulated loss of calcium via renal, cutaneous, and osseous mechanisms. Absorption is a function of two systems: a saturatable active transport

(transcellular) system that can absorb up to 80% to 100% of calcium intake when oral intake is low, and a nonsaturable passive diffusion (paracellular) system that dominates during high calcium intake. The duodenum is the primary site for active transport, whereas passive transport occurs primarily in the jejunum.

The duodenal active transport system is mediated by the vitamin D endocrine system and involves three stages.[20] Activated vitamin D [cholecalciferol, $1\alpha,25(OH)2D_3$] triggers the vitamin D receptor that upregulates the mediators involved in all three steps (TRPV5 and 6, CaBP, and PMCA1b) (Fig. 68.11). Calciferol interaction with nuclear vitamin D receptors takes 6 to 8 hours to develop effector proteins and almost 12 hours to impact calcium homeostasis.[21]

Researchers also have discovered a vitamin D receptor that can affect calcium levels within minutes to hours. This receptor evokes responses that induce rapid intestinal absorption of calcium (also known as transcaltachia); this process may be activated by interaction of different cholecalciferol ligands with receptors found on caveolae-enriched plasma membranes.[22]

Although calcium can also be absorbed via paracellular pathways throughout the small intestine, this mechanism is less efficient and can accommodate only 20% to 60% of oral calcium intake. This process is time and concentration gradient dependent; it is most effective with high levels of dietary calcium intake or slow intestinal transit time.[23]

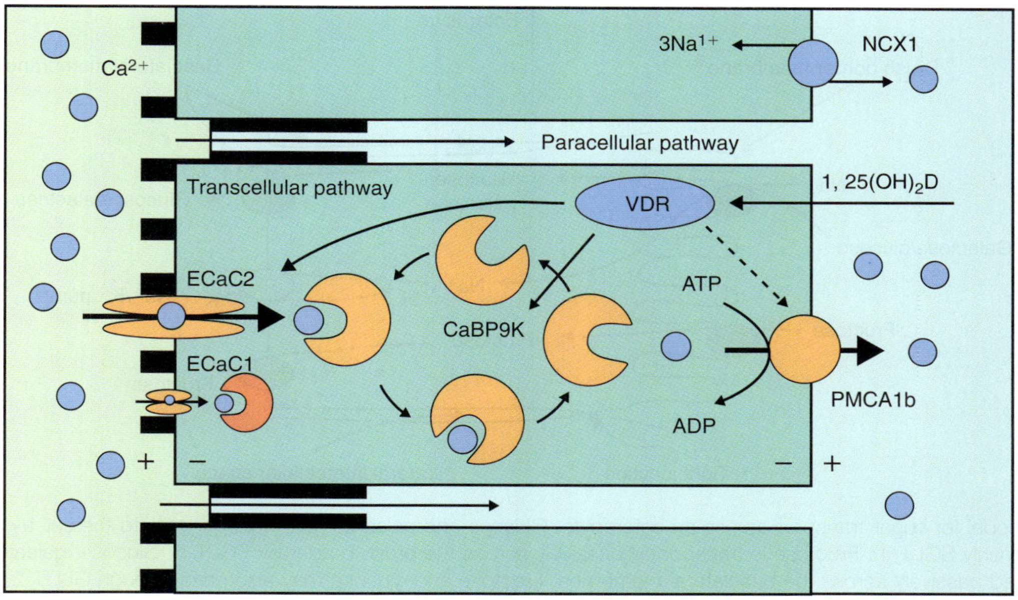

FIGURE 68.11 Molecular model for intestinal calcium absorption. Paracellular and transcellular mechanisms are depicted. Specifically, the transcellular pathway involves entry through specialized calcium channels (ECaC2, ECaC1), intracellular transport while attached to the Calbindin-D9K binding protein, and extrusion through PMCA1b through an adenosine triphosphate (ATP)-driven mechanism. (From Bouilon R, Van Cromphaut S, Carmeliet G. Intestinal calcium absorption: molecular vitamin D mediated mechanisms. *J Cell Biochem.* 2003;88:333, figure 68.1.)

However, the existence of this paracellular system ensures calcium absorption in the absence of vitamin D.

IRON ABSORPTION

Nearly all absorption of dietary iron occurs within the duodenum (1 to 2 mg/day). Iron absorption from both heme (10%) and nonheme (90%) dietary sources occurs at the duodenocyte's apical membrane.[24] Iron attached to hemoglobin is the most bioavailable form, followed in decreasing order by reduced (ferrous [Fe^{2+}] state) and nonreduced (ferric [Fe^{3+}] state) iron, respectively.

Heme iron is absorbed via a membrane-bound protein (likely heme carrier protein 1). Absorbed heme iron is either directly available as heme or released inside the cell as ferrous iron by heme oxygenase activity. Nonheme iron, initially in the Fe^{3+} form, is first reduced to Fe^{2+} by a ferrireductase enzyme (Dcytb) before being transported across the apical membrane by a divalent metal transporter-1 (DMT-1). In both cases, once Fe^{2+} is inside the cell, it is either stored within ferritin or exported across the basolateral membrane by ferroportin-1. The latter process is facilitated by conversion of ferrous iron back to Fe^{3+} by a multicopper oxidase protein called hephaestin (Fig. 68.12). Once in the extracellular space, the iron is bound by plasma transferrin for eventual transport to erythroid cells, immune cells, and hepatocytes.[24]

The absorption of nonheme iron can be diminished by gastric hypoacidity (e.g., proton pump inhibitor administration, antacids), high-fiber diets, and by coffee and tea consumption. *Helicobacter pylori* infection produces gastric atrophy that can also lead to profound iron-deficiency anemia.

The body has no effective means of excreting iron; iron losses occur only through intestinal sloughing,

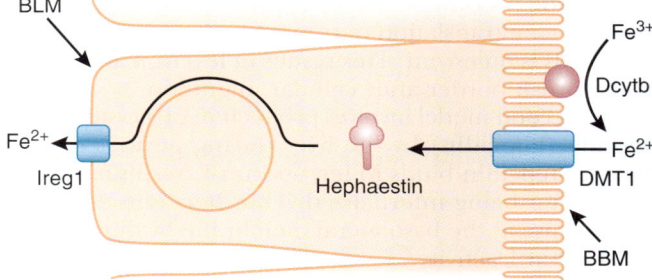

FIGURE 68.12 Components of the intestinal iron absorption pathway. (1) Luminal Fe^{3+} is reduced to Fe^{2+} by Dcytb. (2) Fe^{2+} is transported intracellularly across the brush border membrane (BBM) by the divalent metal transporter DMT-1. (3) Hephaestin facilitates Fe^{2+} transport and oxidation at the basolateral membrane (BLM). (4) Fe^{2+} is transferred across the BLM into the body by Ireg1. (From Frazer DM, Anderson GJ. The orchestration of body iron intake: how and where do enterocytes receive their cues? *Blood Cells Mol Dis.* 2003;30:288.)

menstruation, or other forms of blood loss. As such, the duodenum plays a crucial role in iron hemostasis, particularly in meeting the bone marrow requirements for erythropoiesis (20 to 30 mg/day) while avoiding absorption of excess iron. There are two proposed mechanisms for duodenal iron regulation: the crypt programming model and the hepcidin model. The crypt programming model involves a feedback mechanism regulating the iron absorptive capacity of crypt enterocytes as they migrate from the duodenal crypts to the absorptive brush border. Intracellular iron stores within crypt cells correspond to storage levels within the body. In a low iron state, iron regulatory proteins within the duodenal crypt cells increase

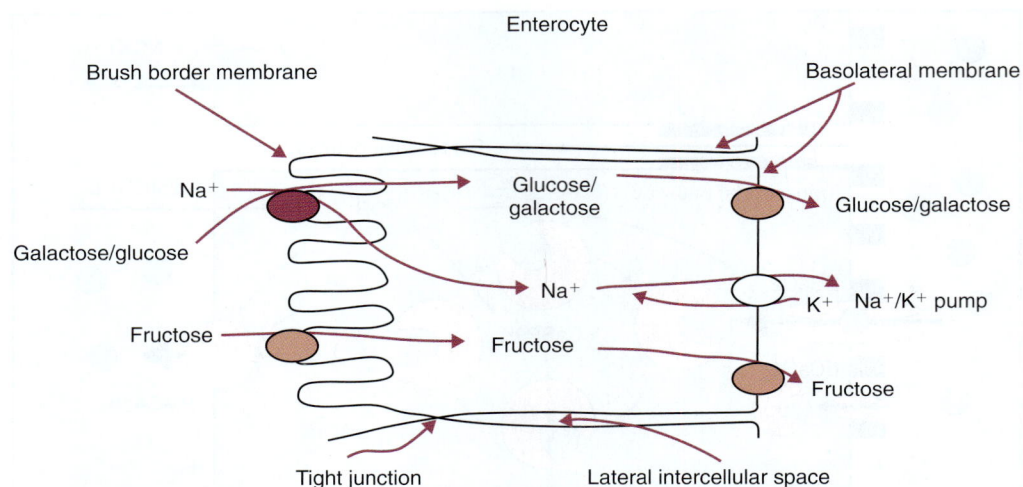

FIGURE 68.13 A model for sugar transport across an enterocyte. Glucose and galactose are transported into the cell by a sodium glucose cotransporter (primarily SGLT-1). Fructose is transported passively across the brush border by SGLT-5. Glucose, galactose, and fructose are also transported passively across the basolateral membrane. Fructose and glucose may also pass through GLUT-2, and fructose also passes through GLUT-5. (From Wright EM, Martin MG, Turk E. Intestinal absorption in health and disease: sugars. *Best Pract Res Clin Gastroenterol.* 2003;17:954, figure 68.1.)

the translation of several effectors of iron transport, thereby increasing the cells' iron absorptive capacity.[25] Eventually, as these cells migrate upward to become absorptive cells on the brush border, these potentiated cells absorb more dietary iron.[26] Conversely, during periods where iron stores are high, the translation of transport effectors within the crypt cells is quiescent. This results in less iron absorption at the brush border after cellular migration.

The second model involves production of a cysteine-rich peptide (hepcidin) by the liver during periods of iron excess. Hepcidin binds to ferroportin-1, resulting in this transporter being internalized. Thus hepcidin decreases iron release at the basolateral membrane by diminishing ferroportin-1 activity.[27]

Hepcidin likely affects more mature enterocytes, whereas crypt programming occurs at the apical membrane of younger crypt cells. It is likely that both control mechanisms are needed to allow acute (hepcidin) as well as delayed (crypt programming) regulation of iron absorption.[25]

NUTRIENT ABSORPTION AND DIGESTION

The duodenocyte's brush border begins nutrient absorption of largely undigested food particles emptied from the stomach. As the initial site for interaction between a food bolus and pancreaticobiliary secretions, the duodenum helps initiate starch hydrolysis, protein digestion, and fat absorption.

Carbohydrates

Humans consume carbohydrates as starches (amylose and amylopectin) and disaccharides (sucrose and lactose). Amylose is a polysaccharide consisting of α-1,4-glycosidic bonds; amylopectin is a polysaccharide consisting of α-1,4 linkages and branch point α-1,6-glycosodic bonds that occur every 20 to 25 glucose units. In the duodenum, chyme mixes with pancreatic α-amylase, which hydrolyzes starches at the interior α-1,4 bonds, yielding maltose, maltotriose, and α-limit dextrin. This breakdown process is

nearly completed once the carbohydrate load reaches the early jejunum.[28] Maltose, maltotriose, and α-limit dextrins, along with the dietary disaccharides, are then further broken down into monosaccharides (glucose, galactose, and fructose) by brush border enzymes in the villus cells of the jejunum and upper ileum. Final absorption of glucose and galactose is mediated by carrier proteins (sodium-dependent glucose transporters [SGLT-1]) that actively transport these sugars; facilitative diffusion via glucose transport (GLUT) carriers is also involved. Unlike glucose and galactose, fructose absorption requires facilitative diffusion through interaction with GLUT-5. Intracellular monosaccharides are then delivered across the basolateral membrane to enter the systemic system either via GLUT-2 (all three sugars) or through exocytosis (glucose exclusively) (Fig. 68.13).[29]

Proteins

Proteins contain long-chain amino acids bound by peptide linkages. Up to 20% of peptide bonds are cleaved in the stomach. The remainder of peptide bonds are cleaved within the proximal intestine by pancreatic endopeptidases (trypsin, chymotrypsin, and elastase). The duodenocyte brush border enzyme enteropeptidase (enterokinase) converts trypsinogen into trypsin, which, in turn, activates all other pancreatic zymogens.[30] After proteolysis, the majority of amino acid digestion occurs through dipeptide and tripeptide proton-coupled cotransporters (PepT1), which are found in the duodenum and jejunum.[31] As much as 50% of ingested protein is digested and absorbed in the duodenum.

Lipids

Most dietary fat is absorbed in the duodenum and upper jejunum. Fat entering the duodenum stimulates secretion of cholecystokinin (CCK), which, in turn, promotes pancreatic lipase release. Duodenal hydrolysis of dietary lipids and biliary phospholipids and cholesterol is carried out by pancreatic lipase and colipase. Biliary phospholipids and cholesterol are hydrolyzed through phospholipase A_2 and cholesterol esterase activity. These processes are facilitated by bile acid solubilization, which starts in the duodenum, yielding mixed micelles and liposomes. Once these are delivered to the brush border, their lipid contents passively diffuse via fatty acid transport proteins.

ENDOCRINE PHYSIOLOGY

The duodenum produces a diverse group of GI hormones that are critical for coordinated digestion and absorption of nutrients throughout the small intestine. In conjunction with the central and peripheral neural system, these neuro-endocrine agents initiate a complex cascade of physiologic processes in the duodenum and distal small intestine. Although the biologic effects of some GI hormones are well established, others' roles in the duodenal and small bowel remain unclear. What follows is a brief description of the major GI hormones associated with the duodenum. Table 68.1 provides a complete list of these and other GI hormones found in the duodenum.

Secretin is produced by secretin-containing cells (S cells) in the duodenum and proximal jejunum. S cells release secretin in response to passage of gastric acid into the duodenal lumen; this effect is mediated by secretin-releasing peptide and controlled by the afferent vagal system.[32] Target cells expressing secretin receptor are distributed along multiple organs but mainly expressed in the pancreas (both ductal and acinar cells), stomach, liver, kidney, and colon.

Secretin's major physiologic actions include stimulation of pancreatic secretion of water and bicarbonate in synergy with CCK. In addition, secretin inhibits gastric secretion and emptying, stimulates biliary secretion, and enhances production of pepsin and mucus in gastric and intestinal mucosa.

CCK is secreted by duodenal and small intestinal I cells. Ingestion of lipids and proteins and duodenal luminal acidification initiate CCK release. Together with secretin, CCK stimulates pancreatic enzymatic secretion and sphincter of Oddi relaxation via a VIP- and NO-regulated pathway. CCK activates gallbladder contraction via an acetylcholine-mediated mechanism.[33] In the small bowel, CCK primarily regulates motility by relaxing the lower esophageal sphincter, enhancing gastric emptying, and inhibiting intestinal transit by interruption of the

---

TABLE 68.1 Physiologic Functions of Gastrointestinal Hormones

Active Agent	Origin/Distribution	Target Organ	Function	Clinical Significance
Secretin	S cells Duodenum, small and large intestine	Pancreas Stomach Liver Esophagus Colon	Stimulates pancreatic exocrine secretion Inhibits gastric secretion and motility Stimulates gastric pepsin release Stimulates biliary secretion of bicarbonate, chloride, and water Decreases bile salt concentration Decreases LES tone and colonic motility	Diagnosis of Zollinger-Ellison syndrome Pancreatic stimulation in MRCP/ERCP Localization of gastrinomas
CCK	I cells Duodenum and small intestine	Gallbladder Pancreas Esophagus Small bowel Stomach Brain	Stimulates gallbladder contraction Stimulates pancreatic enzyme secretion Induces relaxation of sphincter of Oddi Stimulates pancreatic growth Decreases LES tone Inhibits gastric emptying Induces satiety Slows intestinal transit Neurotransmitter	CCK antagonists used in treatment of obesity, anorexia, and bulimia Treatment of PUD
Gastric inhibitory polypeptide (glucose-dependent insulinotropic peptide)	K cells (GIP) L cells (GLP-1) Duodenum and proximal small intestine	Pancreas Heart Bone Stomach Hypothalamus	Enhances insulin secretion Regulates stomach emptying	Potential treatment target for DM, HTN, myocardial infarction, osteoporosis, Parkinson and Alzheimer diseases
Somatostatin	D cells δ cells Intramural enteric nervous system of duodenum and small bowel	Stomach Duodenum Small bowel Pancreas Gallbladder Colon	Inhibits motility and secretion of gastrin and pepsin Inhibits absorption of amino acids Inhibits secretion of water and electrolytes Inhibits secretion of pancreatic enzymes Inhibits gallbladder contractions Prolongs large bowel transit time	Treatment of cirrhosis, variceal bleeding, peptic ulcer disease, pancreatic fistulas, pancreatitis, and others
Motilin	Nonargentaffin cells Small bowel mucosa	Stomach Pancreas Gallbladder	Initiates phase III contraction of MMC Stimulates gastric emptying and pepsin secretion Activates secretion of pancreatic enzymes Stimulates contraction of gallbladder	Motilin receptor agonist used in the treatment of gastroparesis

Continued

TABLE 68.1 Physiologic Functions of Gastrointestinal Hormones—cont'd

Active Agent	Origin/Distribution	Target Organ	Function	Clinical Significance
5-HT	Enterochromaffin cells Duodenum, proximal small bowel	Stomach Small bowel	Induces stomach relaxation Increases intestinal motility	5-HT antagonists are used as antiemetics 5-HT receptor agonists are used for treatment of diarrhea, IBS
Nitric oxide	Myenteric plexus Duodenum, small bowel	Esophagus Stomach Small bowel Gallbladder	Relaxes LES Relaxes smooth muscle cells of GI tract and biliary system	Potential application in PUD as a protector of gastric mucosa
Vasoactive intestinal polypeptide	Nerve plexus of the bowel	Stomach Small bowel Gallbladder Biliary system Liver	Inhibits pepsin production Enhances secretion of water and electrolytes Inhibits intestinal absorption Induces relaxation of gallbladder Glycogenolytic effect in the liver	Potential benefit in treatment of IBD, immunosuppression, and respiratory diseases such as asthma and COPD
Neurotensin	N cells Duodenum, small bowel, brain	Stomach Pancreas Colon Hypothalamus	Decreases stomach motility Increases pancreatic secretion Stimulates colonic contraction Stimulates CNS	Potential role in treatment of substance abuse, schizophrenia, Parkinson disease
Substance P	Terminals of sensory nerves of the bowel	Stomach Small bowel Biliary system Pancreas	Increases motility of GI tract Stimulates CCK release Increases contraction of gallbladder Increases bile flow Reduces pancreatic flow	Blocks substance P receptors Has potential role in treatment of chronic inflammatory diseases and pain
Gastrin-releasing peptide	Postganglionic fibers of vagus	Stomach Small bowel Hypothalamus	Modulates acid, gastrin, and peptide secretion in GI tract Stimulates CCK release Regulates circadian signals	Involved in carcinogenesis of tumors of the lung, colon, stomach, pancreas, breast, and prostate
Ghrelin	P/D1 cells Gastric mucosa and pancreas	Stomach Hypothalamus	Increases gastric acid secretion Accelerates food intake	Potential role of agonists and antagonists of ghrelin in treatment of cachexia and obesity
Endorphins and enkephalins	Myenteric plexus of bowel	Stomach Small bowel Large bowel	Decrease motility	Antagonists used for treatment of postoperative ileus
Peptide YY and pancreatic polypeptide	Endocrine cell L cells Ileum, colon	Stomach Small bowel Pancreas Biliary system	Stimulate secretion of stomach, pancreas, and liver Increase motility of GI tract Cause satiety	Peptide YY is being investigated as weight-loss drug
Melatonin	EC cells Bowel, pineal gland	Duodenum Small bowel	Stimulates secretion of HCO_3^- Antioxidant	Potential role in treatment of various GI conditions, including peptic ulcers, esophagitis, and gastritis
Gastrin	G cells Stomach	Stomach Small bowel Pancreas Biliary system	Stimulates acid secretion Promotes gastric motility Relaxes ileocecal valve Induces pancreatic secretion and gallbladder emptying	Pentagastrin is used in diagnosis of hypergastrinemia

5-HT, 5-Hydroxytryptamine or serotonin; *CCK,* cholecystokinin; *CNS,* central nervous system; *COPD,* chronic obstructive pulmonary disease; *DM,* diabetes mellitus; *ERCP,* endoscopic retrograde cholangiopancreatography; *GI,* gastrointestinal; *GIP,* gastric inhibitory polypeptide; *HTN,* hypertension; *IBD,* inflammatory bowel disease; *IBS,* irritable bowel syndrome; *LES,* lower esophageal sphincter; *MMC,* migrating motor complex; *MRCP,* magnetic resonance cholangiopancreatography; *PUD,* peptic ulcer disease.

migrating motor complex. CCK may be involved in the induction of satiety.[34]

Gastric inhibitory polypeptide (GIP; also referred to as glucose-dependent insulinotropic peptide) is a polypeptide structurally similar to secretin. Together with glucagon-like peptide 1 (GLP-1), GIP enhances insulin secretion after a meal. Intraluminal glucose and lipids in the duodenum and proximal small intestine directly interact with K cells and L cells in the bowel mucosa to induce secretion of GIP and GLP-1, respectively. These endocrine peptides stimulate insulin secretion in a glucose-dependent manner; as such, they are referred to as incretins. Impaired incretin function may be involved in the development of type 2 diabetes mellitus.[35] GIP and GLP-1 also enhance pancreatic β-cell proliferation and resistance to apoptosis.[36]

Somatostatin is produced by intramural enteric neural cells and D cells in the duodenum, proximal jejunum, and stomach. Somatostatin secretion is stimulated by ingested fat and proteins in the distal stomach and duodenum together with calcitonin gene–related peptide and catecholamines. Somatostatin's release is inhibited by an acetylcholine-mediated mechanism.

Somatostatin influences a variety of GI processes. In the stomach, it inhibits gastrin and pepsin expression. In the duodenum, somatostatin decreases absorption of amino acids and attenuates water and electrolyte secretion. In the pancreas, it inhibits enzyme release and antagonizes secretin and CCK.

Somatostatin analogues are used in treating multiple conditions, including cirrhosis, variceal bleeding, peptic ulcer disease, pancreatic fistulas, acute and chronic pancreatitis, dumping syndrome, small bowel fistulas, psoriasis, and autonomic hypotension.[37,38]

Motilin is a polypeptide secreted by endocrine cells located in the duodenal and proximal jejunal mucosa. Motilin's primary function is to initiate phase III of the migrating motor complex in the stomach. Less importantly, motilin also stimulates pepsin and exocrine pancreatic secretion, stimulates gallbladder contraction and sphincter of Oddi tone, and increases serum concentrations of pancreatic polypeptide and insulin. The presence of fat in the duodenum inhibits motilin secretion, slowing the upper GI tract. Erythromycin's prokinetic effect on the GI tract is believed to be mediated via motilin receptors. The nonantibiotic motilin receptor agonist mitemcinal has been reported to reduce symptoms of gastroparesis.[39,40]

Serotonin (5-HT) is secreted by enterochromaffin cells located on mucosal villous tips in the duodenum, small bowel, and rectum. Serotonin functions as a neurotransmitter and signaling molecule, regulating interactions among mucosal cells. Its release is evoked by duodenal distention and the presence of nutrients in the bowel. Serotonin relaxes the stomach and enhances intestinal secretion and motility.

Several infectious agents and chemotherapeutic regimens (particularly those involving cisplatinum and cyclophosphamide) act via 5-HT$_3$ receptors resulting in diarrhea, nausea, and emesis. For this reason, 5-HT$_3$ receptor antagonists can markedly reduce nausea and emesis associated with cisplatinum and cyclophosphamide. 5-HT receptor antagonists are also widely used as antiemetic (5-HT$_3$) or antidiarrheal (5-HT$_4$) agents in treatment of several GI disorders, including carcinoid and irritable bowel syndrome.[41]

NO is one of the major nonadrenergic, noncholinergic neurotransmitters in the GI tract. It is produced by the conversion of L-arginine to L-citrulline by NO synthase, an enzyme that exists as inducible and constitutive isoforms.[42] Released in response to stimulation of the myenteric plexus and vagal stimulation, NO relaxes gastric and intestinal smooth muscles and is important in the neuronal regulation of the intestinal tract. In addition, NO regulates the physiologic tone of the lower esophageal sphincter, sphincter of Oddi, pyloric sphincter, gallbladder, and anus.[42]

MOTILITY

Regulation of duodenal motility is the end result of intrinsic and extrinsic paracrine, endocrine, and neuronal regulation. Duodenal motility involves a combination of multiple motility patterns including peristalsis and the interdigestive motor cycle/migratory motor complex.

Intrinsic Control

The fibrous septum separating the gastric antrum and the pylorus from the duodenum prevents most antropyloric electrical stimuli from reaching the duodenum or small bowel. Thus the enteric nervous system is an essential regulator of duodenal and small bowel motility. The duodenum has an autonomous electrical pacemaker that differs from that of the pylorus; this pacemaker has a dominant contraction frequency of approximately 12 cycles per minute (cpm) and a slow-wave propagation velocity of 15 cm/min. The duodenum's contraction pattern also differs from the pattern found in the distal jejunum (approximately 10 cm/min). These divergent contraction patterns facilitate rapid propulsion of large nutrient boluses along the duodenum and a longer propulsion time within the distal intestine, enhancing digestion.

The enteric nervous system contains up to 100 million neurons—many more fibers than either the vagus or splanchnic nerves. It consists of two neural networks: the myenteric and submucosal plexuses. The myenteric (Auerbach) plexus provides inhibitory and stimulatory signals to circular and longitudinal muscle layers within the bowel wall. In addition, ascending and descending interneurons provide regulatory intercellular signaling along the GI tract. In the submucosal (Meissner) plexus, secretory motor neurons regulate fluid and electrolyte secretion, blood flow, and contraction of the muscularis mucosae.

Neuroendocrine regulation of duodenal motility is complex. Duodenal smooth muscle cells express large number of neuroendocrine receptors involved in duodenal contraction; these include receptors for CCK, gastrin, substance P, bombesin, acetylcholine, and others. Other agents have been identified as smooth muscle relaxants, including VIP and adenosine triphosphate (Table 68.2).[43,44]

Extrinsic Control

Extrinsic control of duodenal motility is primarily regulated by the autonomic nervous system.[45] Afferent and efferent vagal fibers innervate the entire small intestine, including the duodenum. The sympathetic innervation consists

TABLE 68.2 Major Neurohormones Involved in the Regulation of Duodenal Motility

DUODENAL MOTILITY	
Stimulatory	**Inhibitory**
Acetylcholine	Calcitonin gene–regulated peptide
Bombesin	Neurotensin
Cholecystokinin	Peptide YY
Gastrin-releasing	Somatostatin
polypeptide	Secretin
Motilin	Vasoactive intestinal polypeptide
Serotonin	Nitric oxide
Substance P	

of preganglionic neuronal processes originating from T9 and T10. These run in the splanchnic nerves and synapse with the celiac ganglia. Thus the duodenum derives its sympathetic innervation from both celiac (proximal duodenum) and superior mesenteric (distal duodenum) ganglia. These fibers consist of both cholinergic and noradrenergic neurons; however, the sympathetic innervation of the stomach and duodenum is largely inhibitory.

The preganglionic vagal efferent neurons have cholinergic excitatory and inhibitory interneuronal connections before intestinal innervation. Therefore the vagus nerve can elicit several responses in the stomach and duodenum.

There is a delicate interplay between net stimulatory and inhibitory effects in response to vagal activity. In the stomach, vagal stimulation causes gastric acid secretion; truncal vagotomy causes incoordination of antral contractions, loss of receptive relaxation, and rapid gastric emptying. In the duodenum, vagal stimulation inhibits duodenal motility.

ACKNOWLEDGMENT

The author thanks and acknowledges David A. McClusky III, Max Yezhelyev, and Aaron S. Fink for their previous contributions to this textbook on this subject, from which this chapter was significantly borrowed.

REFERENCES

1. Benedetti A. *Historia Corporis Humani Sive Anatomice*. Venice: Impressum Venetis; 1502.
2. Skandalakis JE, Gray SW, Ricketts RR, Richardson DD. Small intestines. In: Skandalakis JE, Gray SW, eds. *Embryology for Surgeons*. 2nd ed. Baltimore: Williams & Wilkins; 1994:184.
3. Androulakis JA, Skandalakis LJ, Kingsnorth AN, et al. Small intestine. In: Skandalakis JE, ed. *Surgical Anatomy: The Embryologic and Anatomic Basis of Modern Surgery*. Athens: Paschalidis Medical Publications; 2004:789.
4. Knight HO. An anomalous portal vein with its surgical dangers. *Ann Surg*. 1921;74:697.
5. Skandalakis JE, Branum GD, Colborn GL, et al. Extrahepatic biliary tract and gallbladder. In: Skandalakis JE, ed. *Surgical Anatomy: The Embryologic and Anatomic Basis of Modern Surgery*. Athens: Paschalidis Medical Publications; 2004:1093.
6. Skandalakis JE, Gray SW, Ricketts RR, et al. Pancreas. In: Skandalakis JE, Gray SW, eds. *Embryology for Surgeons*. 2nd ed. Baltimore: Williams & Wilkins; 1994:366.
7. Lloyd-Jones W, Mountain JC, Warren KW. Annular pancreas in the adult. *Ann Surg*. 1972;176:163.
8. Bonnel F, Pujol J, Barthélémy M, Carabalona P, Rabischong P. Topographical relationships of the first part of the duodenum, gastroduodenal artery and bile duct. *Anat Clin*. 1982;4:289.
9. Androulakis JA, Colborn GL, Skandalakis PN, Skandalakis LJ, Skandalakis JE. Embryologic and anatomic basis of duodenal surgery. *Surg Clin North Am*. 2000;80:171.
10. Hentati N, Fournier H, Papon X, Aube C, Vialle R, Mercier P. Arterial supply of the duodenal bulb: an anatomoclinical study. *Surg Radiol Anat*. 1999;21:159.
11. Kaunitz JD, Akiba Y. Duodenal carbonic anhydrase: mucosal protection, luminal chemosensing, and gastric acid disposal. *Keio J Med*. 2006;55:96.
12. Bubenik GA. Localization, physiological significance and possible clinical implication of gastrointestinal melatonin. *Biol Signals Recept*. 2001;10:350.
13. Konturek PC, Konturek SJ, Hahn EG. Duodenal alkaline secretion: its mechanisms and role in mucosal protection against gastric acid. *Dig Liver Dis*. 2004;36:505.
14. deFoneska A, Kaunitz JD. Gastroduodenal mucosal defense. *Curr Opin Gastroenterol*. 2010;26:604.
15. Allen A, Flemstrom G. Gastroduodenal mucus bicarbonate barrier: protection against acid and pepsin. *Am J Physiol Cell Physiol*. 2005;288:C1.
16. Akiba Y, Kaunitz JD. Luminal chemosensing and upper gastrointestinal mucosal defenses. *Am J Clin Nutr*. 2009;90:826S.
17. Ham M, Kaunitz JD. Gastroduodenal mucosal defense. *Curr Opin Gastroenterol*. 2008;24:665.
18. Nayeb-Hashemi H, Kaunitz J. Gastroduodenal mucosal defense. *Curr Opin Gastroenterol*. 2009;25:537.
19. Takeuchi K, Koyama M, Hayashi S, Aihara E. Prostaglandin EP receptor subtypes involved in regulating $HCO_3(-)$ secretion from gastroduodenal mucosa. *Curr Pharm Des*. 2010;16:1241.
20. Bronner F. Mechanisms of intestinal calcium absorption. *J Cell Biochem*. 2003;88:387.
21. Norman AW. Intestinal calcium absorption: a vitamin D-hormone-mediated adaptive response. *Am J Clin Nutr*. 1990;51:290.
22. Norman AW. Minireview: vitamin D receptor: new assignments for an already busy receptor. *Endocrinology*. 2006;147:5542.
23. Heller HJ. Calcium hemostasis. In: Griffin JE, Ojeda SR, eds. *Textbook of Endocrine Physiology*. 5th ed. New York: Oxford University Press; 2004:362.
24. Muñoz M, Villar I, García-Erce J. An update on iron physiology. *World J Gastroenterol*. 2009;15:4617.
25. Siah CW, Obiga J, Adams LA, Trinder D, Olynyk JK. Normal iron metabolism and the pathophysiology of iron overload disorders. *Clin Biochem Rev*. 2006;27:5.
26. Roy CN, Enns CA. Iron hemostasis: new tales from the crypt. *Blood*. 2000;96:4020.
27. Nemeth E, Ganz T. Hepcidin and iron-loading anemias. *Haematologica*. 2006;91:727.
28. Chung DH, Evers BM. The digestive system. In: O'Leary JP, Capote LR, eds. *The Physiologic Basis of Surgery*. 3rd ed. Philadelphia: Lippincott Williams & Wilkins; 2002:457.
29. Wright E, Martín M, Turk E. Intestinal absorption in health and disease—sugars. *Best Pract Res Clin Gastroenterol*. 2003;17:943.
30. Jeno P, Green JR, Lentze MJ. Specificity studies on enteropeptidase substrates related to the N-terminus of trypsinogen. *Biochem J*. 1987;241:721.
31. Ogihara H, Saito H, Shin BC, et al. Immuno-localization of H+/peptide cotransporter in rat digestive tract. *Biochem Biophys Res Commun*. 1996;220:848.
32. Chey WY, Chang TM. Neural control of the release and action of secretin. *J Physiol Pharmacol*. 2003;54:105.
33. Rehfeld J. Clinical endocrinology and metabolism: cholecystokinin. *Best Pract Res Clin Endocrinol Metab*. 2004;18:569.
34. Little TJ, Horowitz M, Feinle-Bisset C. Role of cholecystokinin in appetite control and body weight regulation. *Obes Rev*. 2005;6:297.
35. Fonesca VA, Zinman B, Nauck MA, Goldfine AB, Plutzky J. Confronting the type 2 diabetes epidemic: the emerging role of incretin-based therapies. *Am J Med*. 2010;123:S2.
36. Kim SJ, Winter K, Nian C. Glucose-dependent insulinotropic polypeptide (GIP) stimulation of pancreatic beta-cell survival is dependent on phosphatidylinositol-3-kinase (P13K)/protein kinase B (PKB) signalling, inactivation of the forkhead transcription factor Foxo1, and down-regulation of bax expression. *J Biol Chem*. 2005;280:22297.

37. Bang UC, Semb S, Nøjgaard C. Pharmacological approach to acute pancreatitis. *World J Gastroenterol.* 2008;14:2968.

38. Corleto VD. Somatostatin and the gastrointestinal tract. *Curr Opin Endocrinol Diabetes Obes.* 2010;17:63.

39. Smet BD, Mitselos A, Depoortere I. Motilin and ghrelin as prokinetic drug targets. *Pharmacol Ther.* 2009;123:207.

40. Sanger GJ. Motilin, ghrelin and related neuropeptides as targets for the treatment of GI diseases. *Drug Discov Today.* 2008;13:234.

41. Spiller R. Serotonin and GI clinical disorders. *Neuropharmacology.* 2008;55:1072.

42. Bredt DS, Snyder SH. Isolation of nitric oxide synthetase, a calmodulin-requiring enzyme. *Proc Natl Acad Sci USA.* 1990;87:682.

43. Hansen MB. Neurohumoral control of gastrointestinal motility. *Physiol Res.* 2003;52:1.

44. Shuttleworth CW, Keef KD. Roles of peptides in enteric neuromuscular transmission. *Regul Pept.* 1995;56:101.

45. Roman C, Gonella J. Extrinsic control of digestive tract motility. In: Johnson L, ed. *Physiology of the Gastrointestinal Tract.* New York: Raven Press; 1987:507.

Adenocarcinoma of the Small Intestine

Shrawan G. Gaitonde | Anton J. Bilchik

Although the small intestine is an infrequent site of gastrointestinal (GI) cancer, the incidence of small intestinal cancer has increased considerably in the past several decades, primarily due to an increase in adenocarcinoma and particularly small bowel neuroendocrine tumors; together, these cancers account for two-thirds of all small bowel malignancies. In 2016, an estimated 10,090 Americans will be diagnosed with small intestinal cancer, about one-third of which will be adenocarcinoma.[1] Recent advances have been made in the treatment of gastric and other GI malignancies,[2,3] but the biological behavior of and optimal treatment strategies for small intestinal adenocarcinoma remain poorly understood.

PATHOGENESIS AND RISK FACTORS

The small intestine and large intestine share similarities in structure as well as function but can display dramatically different patterns of malignancy. The duodenum and small intestine account for more than 90% of the absorptive surface of the GI system and about 75% of its length, yet malignancy is about 50 times less common in this region than in the colorectum.[4] Several hypotheses have been presented to explain this disparity. First, as the small intestine is traversed, bacterial concentrations increase but remain substantially lower than those in the colon. This variation in gut microbiota confers different carcinogenic potential.[5] Additionally, in healthy individuals, transit time is faster through the small intestine than the large intestine, which decreases exposure of the mucosa to potentially harmful bacteria. Although digestive enzymes are protective in portions of the GI tract,[6] the highest concentration of digestive enzymes is in the proximal small intestine, namely the duodenum, which has the highest incidence of small intestinal adenocarcinoma. The interaction of pancreatic, biliary, and gastric secretions has been implicated in the higher incidence of adenocarcinoma of the duodenum, possibly through the development of reactive oxygen species during activation of bile acid receptors. Although this occurs throughout the small intestine, the large variations in acid content in the duodenum make it less able to repair cell damage, as compared with the jejunum and ileum.[7]

Dietary and behavioral risk factors have also been examined. Heavy alcohol intake increases the risk of small intestinal adenocarcinoma in some cohorts.[8] Smoking, obesity, dietary fiber intake, and dietary fat intake have been investigated with varying results.[9]

Analyses of national and multi-institutional databases suggest that Crohn disease increases the risk of developing small intestinal cancer by about 60-fold.[10] In one review of more than 12,000 patients with Crohn disease, the mean interval between onset of Crohn symptoms and diagnosis of carcinoma was 9 years, yet the absolute risk of small intestinal cancer was only marginally higher for Crohn patients than for non-Crohn patients.[11]

Familial adenomatous polyposis (FAP) reflects a germline mutation in the adenomatous polyposis coli (APC) gene. Virtually all patients with FAP will develop duodenal polyps, and polyps carry a 100- to 330-fold higher risk of duodenal cancer in FAP patients than in non-FAP patients.[12] In fact, FAP patients with duodenal polyps have a 5% to 10% estimated cumulative risk of developing duodenal cancer by 60 years of age. These neoplasms are adenocarcinomas or desmoid tumors. Increased awareness of the link between FAP and colon cancer has increased the number of prophylactic colectomies; as a result, duodenal cancer now confers the highest risk of death in FAP.[13] Several management strategies have been proposed for patients with FAP. Upper endoscopy screening increases identification of polyps but does not improve overall survival because the optimal treatment strategy is still controversial.[14] Several issues exist in this regard primarily because most duodenal polyps are broad-based and thus are not as amenable to endoscopic resection as are colonic polyps. As such, many clinicians are left to determine whether a duodenal resection is needed in the absence of a proven malignancy. The Spigelman classification[15] scores the severity of duodenal polyposis on a scale of 0 to IV. According to this scoring system, the risk of duodenal malignancy is 2.3%, 2.4%, and 36% for patients with stage II, III, and IV polyposis, respectively.

Other high-risk factors include celiac sprue; however, the exact magnitude of the increased risk is unclear. In a collaborative study performed more than 30 years ago, Rampertab et al.[16] determined that the risk of small bowel adenocarcinoma in patients with celiac disease was equivalent to the risk of colon cancer in normal populations. However, many patients in this study might have been noncompliant with their gluten-free diets. Nevertheless celiac disease remains a widely accepted risk factor for adenocarcinoma development.

DUODENAL ADENOCARCINOMA

CLINICAL PRESENTATION

The clinical presentation of duodenal lesions often consists of obstructive symptoms including nausea, vomiting, and abdominal pain. Anemia secondary to bleeding can also be encountered. The duodenum is the most common site of adenocarcinoma of the small intestine, and most duodenal lesions are in the mid and distal duodenum; only 15% are in the duodenal bulb and postpyloric channel.[4] If lesions are in the periampullary region, symptoms consistent with biliary or pancreatic duct obstruction can occur, specifically jaundice and/or pancreatitis.

WORKUP

The diagnostic modality of choice for duodenal tumors is an upper endoscopy, which allows visualization and biopsy of these lesions. Although contrast-enhanced imaging including cross-sectional imaging and dynamic swallow studies can show filling defects, tissue diagnosis is needed before making treatment decisions. Tumor markers are elevated in only one-third of patients with duodenal lesions, with an equal incidence of elevations in both serum carbohydrate associated antigen (CA 19-9) and carcinoembryonic antigen (CEA).[17] Recent studies have failed to demonstrate novel markers specific to duodenal cancer.

Metastatic workup mirrors that for most other adenocarcinomas of the GI tract, and includes contrast computed tomography (CT) imaging of the chest, abdomen, and pelvis to rule out distant metastatic disease. Endoscopic ultrasound is suggested if there is a possibility that the tumor has invaded local vascular structures and to evaluate resectability.

In high-risk patients, such as those with FAP, endoscopic screening is recommended to allow for early diagnosis. The frequency of screening endoscopy can be based on the Spigelman stage: every 4 years for stage 0, every 2 to 3 years for stages I and II, and every 6 months for stage III polyposis, with consideration given to early surgical intervention. In the absence of absolute surgical contraindications, patients with stage IV polyposis should undergo resection and further screening is not recommended.[15]

TREATMENT

Surgical resection of duodenal adenocarcinoma is the treatment of choice and is usually recommended at diagnosis. Five-year survival rates are as high as 45% to 71% in certain cohorts, more favorable than those associated with other periampullary malignancies.[17]

The extent of surgical resection is determined by the exact anatomic location of the tumors. Most proximal and mid-duodenal lesions will require a pancreaticoduodenectomy. Distal lesions that that can be resected without sacrificing the ampulla have equivalent long-term oncologic outcomes.[18] Prognosis after resection depends on the extent of nodal involvement; perineural/perivascular invasion, tumor differentiation, margin status after resection, and tumor site or depth of invasion (T stage) are not independently associated with survival.[19,20] The largest reported study of duodenal adenocarcinoma, which examined records from 122 patients, found that the number of tumor-involved lymph nodes predicted survival; an adequate specimen contained at least 10 lymph nodes.[17] This is in contrast to the current American Joint Committee on Cancer (AJCC) staging system, which suggests that adequate lymph node sampling should examine at least 6 lymph nodes.[21] See Table 69.1 for survival estimates based on stage. Small studies have shown equivalence in outcomes between pylorus-sparing and classic pancreaticoduodenectomy, but these studies were not limited to extraampullary neoplasms. In patients with

TABLE 69.1 Incidence and 5-Year Survival by Stage of Small Bowel Adenocarcinoma

Stage[21]	Incidence (%)[4]	5-Year Survival (%)[21]
I	11.8	55
II	30.1	35–49
III	26.9	18–31
IV	32.2	5

FAP, pylorus preservation should not be undertaken because the duodenal bulb remains at risk for new polyp formation.[22]

No randomized trials have examined the efficacy of chemotherapy specifically for duodenal adenocarcinoma. ESPAC 3 was a randomized phase III study to determine whether adjuvant chemotherapy (gemcitabine or fluorouracil based) conferred an overall survival advantage over observation. This trial included periampullary adenocarcinoma but not extraampullary lesions.[23] Adjuvant chemotherapy for periampullary adenocarcinoma was not associated with improved overall survival on primary analysis, but after correcting for prognostic factors, a survival benefit was demonstrated on multivariate subset analysis. Several small-scale studies have examined commonly used regimens such as leucovorin + fluorouracil + oxaliplatin (FOLFOX) and other platinum- and gemcitabine-based strategies used for proximal GI tract and hepatobiliary malignancies.[17,24,25] These studies have shown that chemotherapy for advanced disease slows disease progression and improves overall survival. In the adjuvant setting, systemic therapy is most helpful for patients with later stage disease. A recent study based on the National Cancer Database found that postoperative adjuvant therapy significantly improved the survival of patients with stage III disease.[26]

Advances in molecular medicine have identified alterations in cellular pathways of carcinogenesis in several other GI malignancies and have resulted in successful targeted therapies for these cancers. Their specific sites of action on neoplastic cells should make these treatments more effective and less toxic. Current phase II studies are examining therapies such as ceritinib, an anaplastic lymphoma kinase (ALK) inhibitor, and dabrafenib, a BRAF inhibitor in rare GI malignancies.[27,28] As with other low-incidence malignancies, a multidisciplinary approach and consideration for clinical trial are indicated.

JEJUNAL AND ILEAL ADENOCARCINOMA

CLINICAL PRESENTATION

Unlike duodenal cancer, adenocarcinoma distal to the ligament of Treitz is often asymptomatic at an early stage. Even when symptomatic, the symptoms associated with early disease usually are nonspecific (abdominal pain, malaise, bloating). Thus diagnosis can be delayed months to years; in the meantime, patients are often misdiagnosed with nonspecific colitis and irritable bowel syndromes.[29] Untreated patients will become symptomatic, usually in the sixth and seventh decades of life. Advanced disease

TABLE 69.2 Chemotherapy in Small Intestinal Adenocarcinoma—Studies Published in the Last 10 Years

Author	Country	Year	No. of Pts	Study Type	Stage	Chemotherapy Regimen	RR (%)	Median OS (Months)
Czaykowski[24]	Canada	2007	16	Retrospective	Advanced	Fluopyrimidine based	6	15.6
Fishman[36]	Canada	2006	44	Retrospective	Advanced	Various regimens	36	18.6
Overman[37]	US	2008	29	Retrospective	Advanced	Fluoropyrimidine + platinum	41	14.8
			51			Other regimens	16	12
Overman[38]	US	2009	30	Prospective - phase II	Advanced	Capecetabine + oxaliplatin	50	20.4
Ono[39]	Japan	2008	10	Retrospective	Advanced	Cisplatin + irinotecan	12.5	17.3
Suenaga[40]	Japan	2009	10	Retrospective	Advanced or recurrent	Fluoropyrimidine based	10	12
Zaanan[41]	France	2010	6	Retrospective	Advanced	Leucovorin+ 5-fluorouracil	0	13.5
			38	—	—	FOLFOX	34	17.8
			11	—	—	FOLFIRI	9	10.6
			13	—	—	Leucovorin + cisplatin	31	9.3
Koo[42]	Korea	2011	40	Retrospective	Advanced	Fluoropyrimidine based	11.1	11.8
Tsushima[43]	Japan	2012	60	Retrospective	Unresectable or recurrent	Fluoropyrimidine monotherapy	NR	13.9
			17	—	—	Fluoropyrimidine + cisplatin	NR	12.6
			22	—	—	Fluoropyrimidine + oxaliplatin	NR	22.2
			11	—	—	Fluoropyrimidine + irinotecan	NR	9.4
			22	—	—	Other regimens	NR	8.1

NR, Not reported; *OS*, overall survival; *RR*, response rate; *FOLFOX*, fluorouracil + oxaliplatin + leucovorin; *FOLFIRI*, fluorouracil + leucovorin + irinotecan.

generally produces obstructive symptoms, GI bleeding, or perforation.[30]

WORKUP

Unlike malignancies of the upper GI tract, not all jejunoileal lesions are accessible to early endoscopic identification. Screening strategies include contrast-enhanced follow-through studies, plain radiographs, and CT or magnetic resonance (MR) enterography. The overall sensitivity of CT approaches 45% but depends on tumor size and stage.[31] For higher-risk patients, such as those with Crohn disease, an aggressive approach to screening should be taken, with a high index of suspicion for occult small intestine malignancy in patients with long-standing disease and nonspecific GI complaints. This can include balloon-assisted enteroscopy and capsule endoscopy. In patients with occult GI bleeding, balloon enteroscopy will often identify lesions missed on capsule endoscopy and is recommended if capsule investigations are nondiagnostic.[32,33] Given the relative rarity of jejunal and ileal adenocarcinoma, no accepted screening timelines exist.

TREATMENT

Once a diagnosis is made or suspected, treatment consists of surgical resection with lymphadenectomy. Curative resection is possible in 45% to 70% of patients; the remaining patients may have extensive local disease, extensive lymphatic involvement, and/or distant spread.[34] Because jejunoileal adenocarcinoma is considered radioresistant, radiation therapy is restricted to the palliative setting.

A recent review of almost 30 years of cases from a single institution assessed 54 patients who underwent surgical resection with negative margins; those who received chemotherapy usually received 5-fluorouracil-based regimens, often in combination with other treatments. Adjuvant therapy improved disease-free but not overall survival.[35] Several retrospective studies have examined the effect of chemotherapy for patients with locally advanced or unresectable disease (Table 69.2). Most demonstrate an overall survival advantage as compared with observation alone.

SUMMARY

Because small intestinal adenocarcinomas are uncommon as compared with proximal GI and colorectal adenocarcinoma, diligent workup of high-risk patients with suggestive symptomatology is important. Optimal treatment remains unclear, but when resection is possible, every effort should be made to achieve adequate operative margins and lymphatic sampling. Although adjuvant therapies are limited, a coordinated multidisciplinary approach provides the best chance for prolonged survival. Fig. 69.1 demonstrates a stepwise algorithmic approach to consider in these cases. The increase in molecular/genetic screening tools should allow development of better diagnostic modalities and risk stratification guidelines. Immunophenotyping of small intestine adenocarcinoma has yielded promising results. ERBB2, KRAS, VEG-F, and Her2 are mutated and may represent opportunities for future targeted therapies.[44,45] Beclin-1 is overexpressed in about 50% of duodenal adenocarcinomas, and its overexpression is associated with a higher response rate to chemotherapy and improved overall survival.[46] These novel discoveries provide direction for future studies to improve the treatment of these uncommon but often devastating malignancies.

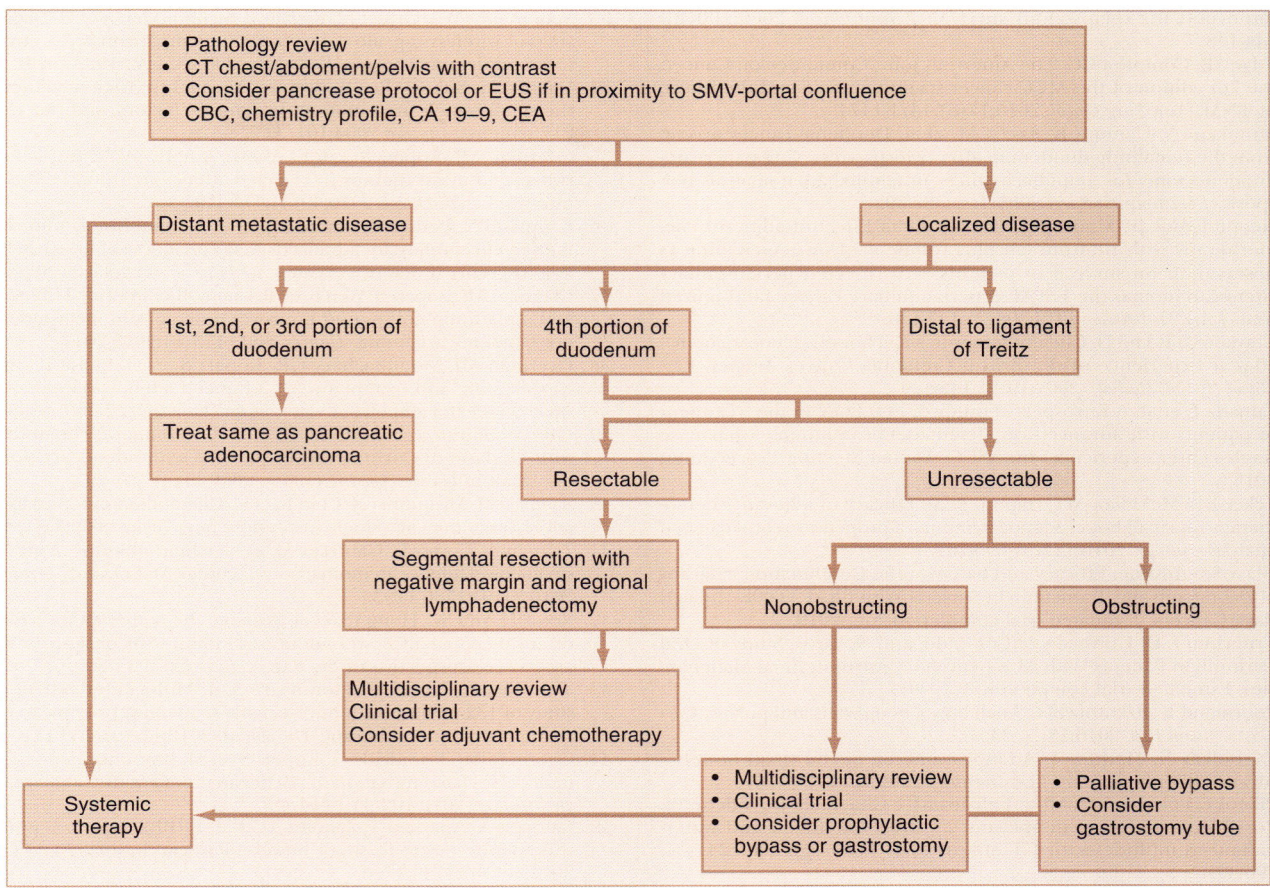

FIGURE 69.1 Small intestinal mass suspicious for invasive cancer: stepwise algorithmic approach. *CBC,* Complete blood count; *CEA,* carcinoembryonic antigen; *CT,* computed tomography; *EUS,* endoscopic ultrasound; *SMV,* superior mesenteric vein.

REFERENCES

1. Smith RA, Andrews K, Brooks D, et al. Cancer screening in the United States, 2016: a review of current American Cancer Society guidelines and current issues in cancer screening. *CA Cancer J Clin.* 2016;66(2):95-114.
2. Choi AH, Kim J, Chao J. Perioperative chemotherapy for resectable gastric cancer: MAGIC and beyond. *World J Gastroenterol.* 2015; 21(24):7343-7348.
3. Wu Q, Li G, Xu F. Resected gastric cancer with D2 dissection: advances in adjuvant chemoradiotherapy and radiotherapy techniques. *Expert Rev Anticancer Ther.* 2015;15(6):703-713.
4. Bilimoria KY, Bentrem DJ, Wayne JD, Ko CY, Bennett CL, Talamonti MS. Small bowel cancer in the United States: changes in epidemiology, treatment, and survival over the last 20 years. *Ann Surg.* 2009;249(1): 63-71.
5. Hold GL. Gastrointestinal microbiota and colon cancer. *Dig Dis.* 2016;34(3):244-250.
6. Donaldson MS. Nutrition and cancer: a review of the evidence for an anti-cancer diet. *Nutr J.* 2004;3:19.
7. Bernstein H, Bernstein C, Payne CM, Dvorakova K, Garewal H. Bile acids as carcinogens in human gastrointestinal cancers. *Mutat Res.* 2005;589(1):47-65.
8. Bennett CM, Coleman HG, Veal PG, Cantwell MM, Lau CC, Murray LJ. Lifestyle factors and small intestine adenocarcinoma risk: a systematic review and meta-analysis. *Cancer Epidemiol* 2015;39(3): 265-273.
9. Schatzkin A, Park Y, Leitzmann MF, Hollenbeck AR, Cross AJ. Prospective study of dietary fiber, whole grain foods, and small intestinal cancer. *Gastroenterology.* 2008;135(4):1163-1167.
10. Cahill C, Gordon PH, Petrucci A, Boutros M. Small bowel adenocarcinoma and Crohn's disease: any further ahead than 50 years ago? *World J Gastroenterol.* 2014;20(33):11486-11495.
11. Shaukat A, Virnig DJ, Howard D, Sitaraman SV, Liff JM, Lederle FA. Crohn's disease and small bowel adenocarcinoma: a population-based case-control study. *Cancer Epidemiol Biomarkers Prev.* 2011; 20(6):1120-1123.
12. Bulow S, Björk J, Christensen IJ, et al. Duodenal adenomatosis in familial adenomatous polyposis. *Gut.* 2004;53(3):381-386.
13. Brosens LA, Keller JJ, Offerhaus GJ, Goggins M, Giardiello FM. Prevention and management of duodenal polyps in familial adenomatous polyposis. *Gut.* 2005;54(7):1034-1043.
14. Syngal S, Brand RE, Church JM, et al. ACG clinical guideline: genetic testing and management of hereditary gastrointestinal cancer syndromes. *Am J Gastroenterol.* 2015;110(2):223-262 [quiz 263].
15. Groves CJ, Saunders BP, Spigelman AD, Phillips RK. Duodenal cancer in patients with familial adenomatous polyposis (FAP): results of a 10 year prospective study. *Gut.* 2002;50(5):636-641.
16. Rampertab SD, Forde KA, Green PHR. Small bowel neoplasia in coeliac disease. *Gut.* 2003;52(8):1211-1214.
17. Poultsides GA, Huang LC, Cameron JL, et al. Duodenal adenocarcinoma: clinicopathologic analysis and implications for treatment. *Ann Surg Oncol.* 2012;19(6):1928-1935.
18. Cloyd JM, Norton JA, Visser BC, Poultsides GA. Does the extent of resection impact survival for duodenal adenocarcinoma? Analysis of 1611 cases. *Ann Surg Oncol.* 2015;22(2):573-580.
19. Cloyd JM, George E, Visser BC. Duodenal adenocarcinoma: advances in diagnosis and surgical management. *World J Gastrointest Surg.* 2016;8(3):212-221.
20. Struck A, Howard T, Chiorean EG, Clarke JM, Riffenburgh R, Cardenes HR. Non-ampullary duodenal adenocarcinoma: factors

important for relapse and survival. *J Surg Oncol.* 2009;100(2): 144-148.

21. Edge SB, Compton CC. The American Joint Committee on Cancer: the 7th edition of the AJCC cancer staging manual and the future of TNM. *Ann Surg Oncol.* 2010;17(6):1471-1474.

22. Murakami Y, Uemura K, Sasaki M, et al. Duodenal cancer arising from the remaining duodenum after pylorus-preserving pancreato-duodenectomy for ampullary cancer in familial adenomatous polyposis. *J Gastrointest Surg.* 2005;9(3):389-392.

23. Neoptolemos JP, Moore MJ, Cox TF, et al. Effect of adjuvant chemotherapy with fluorouracil plus folinic acid or gemcitabine vs observation on survival in patients with resected periampullary adenocarcinoma: the ESPAC-3 periampullary cancer randomized trial. *J Am Med Assoc.* 2012;308(2):147-156.

24. Czaykowski P, Hui D. Chemotherapy in small bowel adenocarcinoma: 10-year experience of the British Columbia Cancer Agency. *Clin Oncol (R Coll Radiol).* 2007;19(2):143-149.

25. Yamada I, et al. A retrospective study of FOLFOX in the treatment of patients with advanced duodenal adenocarcinoma: a Japanese single-center experience. In: ASCO Annual Meeting Proceedings; 2015.

26. Ecker BL, McMillan MT, Datta J, et al. Efficacy of adjuvant chemotherapy for small bowel adenocarcinoma: a propensity score-matched analysis. *Cancer.* 2016;122(5):693-701.

27. GlaxoSmithKline. Efficacy and Safety of the Combination Therapy of Dabrafenib and Trametinib in Subjects With BRAF V600E-Mutated Rare Cancers; Estimated trial completion Aug 2019.

28. Criterium I, D. University of Colorado, and Novartis, Study of Oral Ceritinib in Patients With ALK-Activated Gastrointestinal Malignancies; Estimated trial completion Aug 2017.

29. Pourmand K, Itzkowitz SH. Small bowel neoplasms and polyps. *Curr Gastroenterol Rep.* 2016;18(5):23.

30. Vagholkar K, Mathew T. Adenocarcinoma of the small bowel: a surgical dilemma. *Saudi J Gastroenterol* 2009;15(4):264-267.

31. Pilleul F, Penigaud M, Milot L, Saurin JC, Chayvialle JA, Valette PJ. Possible small-bowel neoplasms: contrast-enhanced and water-enhanced multidetector CT enteroclysis. *Radiology.* 2006;241(3): 796-801.

32. Ross A, Mehdizadeh S, Tokar J, et al. Double balloon enteroscopy detects small bowel mass lesions missed by capsule endoscopy. *Dig Dis Sci.* 2008;53(8):2140-2143.

33. Voderholzer WA, Ortner M, Rogalla P, Beinhölzl J, Lochs H. Diagnostic yield of wireless capsule enteroscopy in comparison with computed tomography enteroclysis. *Endoscopy.* 2003;35(12):1009-1014.

34. Dabaja BS, Suki D, Pro B, Bonnen M, Ajani J. Adenocarcinoma of the small bowel: presentation, prognostic factors, and outcome of 217 patients. *Cancer.* 2004;101(3):518-526.

35. Overman MJ, Kopetz S, Lin E, Abbruzzese JL, Wolff RA. Is there a role for adjuvant therapy in resected adenocarcinoma of the small intestine? *Acta Oncol.* 2010;49(4):474-479.

36. Fishman PN, Pond GR, Moore MJ, et al. Natural history and chemotherapy effectiveness for advanced adenocarcinoma of the small bowel: a retrospective review of 113 cases. *Am J Clin Oncol.* 2006;29(3):225-231.

37. Overman MJ, Kopetz S, Wen S, et al. Chemotherapy with 5-fluorouracil and a platinum compound improves outcomes in metastatic small bowel adenocarcinoma. *Cancer.* 2008;113(8):2038-2045.

38. Overman MJ, Varadhachary GR, Kopetz S, et al. Phase II study of capecitabine and oxaliplatin for advanced adenocarcinoma of the small bowel and ampulla of Vater. *J Clin Oncol.* 2009;27(16):2598-2603.

39. Ono M, Shirao K, Takashima A, et al. Combination chemotherapy with cisplatin and irinotecan in patients with adenocarcinoma of the small intestine. *Gastric Cancer.* 2008;11(4):201-205.

40. Suenaga M, Mizunuma N, Chin K, et al. Chemotherapy for small-bowel adenocarcinoma at a single institution. *Surg Today.* 2009;39(1):27-31.

41. Zaanan A, Costes L, Gauthier M, et al. Chemotherapy of advanced small-bowel adenocarcinoma: a multicenter AGEO study. *Ann Oncol.* 2010;21(9):1786-1793.

42. Koo DH, Yun SC, Hong YS, et al. Systemic chemotherapy for treatment of advanced small bowel adenocarcinoma with prognostic factor analysis: retrospective study. *BMC Cancer.* 2011;11:205.

43. Tsushima T, Taguri M, Honma Y, et al. Multicenter retrospective study of 132 patients with unresectable small bowel adenocarcinoma treated with chemotherapy. *Oncologist.* 2012;17(9):1163-1170.

44. Overman MJ, Pozadzides J, Kopetz S, et al. Immunophenotype and molecular characterisation of adenocarcinoma of the small intestine. *Br J Cancer.* 2010;102(1):144-150.

45. Laforest A, Aparicio T, Zaanan A, et al. ERBB2 gene as a potential therapeutic target in small bowel adenocarcinoma. *Eur J Cancer.* 2014;50(10):1740-1746.

46. Wu XY, Chen J, Cao QH, et al. Beclin 1 activation enhances chemosensitivity and predicts a favorable outcome for primary duodenal adenocarcinoma. *Tumour Biol.* 2013;34(2):713-722.

Reoperations on the Stomach and Duodenum

Morgan Bonds | Alessandra Landmann | Russell Postier

Operations on the stomach and duodenum are performed for six primary reasons: neoplasia, gastroesophageal reflux disease (GERD), obesity, peptic ulcer disease, trauma, and congenital defects. Any operation done for these reasons, whether laparoscopic or open, can result in long-term complications requiring reoperation. This chapter describes how these complications can be avoided by attention to the details of the first operation and how they are managed by laparoscopic or open techniques. Reoperations for obesity-related procedures will be covered in the chapters dealing with bariatric surgery.

One of the challenges of reoperative surgery is reentry into the abdomen. This can be made easier if the initial procedure was done laparoscopically or if a bioresorbable barrier was placed beneath the incision in open surgery. The relative infrequency of reoperative surgery and the high cost of these barriers have limited their use.[1-4]

Certain principles can be applied in reoperative surgery to facilitate a safe procedure. If the dissection is started just below the xiphoid process in the midline, reentry of the peritoneal cavity is less likely to cause injury to underlying small bowel or colon. The liver and stomach underlie this area and are both less susceptible to injury and easier to repair than small bowel or colon. Meticulous sharp dissection is essential to obtaining adequate exposure. Lysis of all intraabdominal adhesions is unnecessary and may increase the likelihood of iatrogenic small bowel or colonic injury. The dissection should be limited to the exposure needed to complete the planned procedure. Early reoperation will result in the most difficulty due to the presence of adhesions, which are most intense in the first few weeks after the initial procedure. Over time, many of these adhesions resorb, and thus waiting at least 6 months between the index operation and the reoperation, if possible, is advisable.

Prior to performing reoperations, it is essential to obtain as much information regarding the initial operation as possible. The dictated operative report should be obtained and reviewed to allow a good understanding of the altered anatomy to be encountered. This can be further enhanced by reviewing previously done imaging or endoscopic studies or obtaining additional studies if necessary. An accurate understanding of the anatomy to be encountered, including the placement of intestinal limbs, will greatly aid in designing an efficient and successful reoperation.

Many complications of operations on the stomach and duodenum that require reoperation result in significant malnutrition. It is essential that this be corrected prior to the repeat operation if at all possible. This can be done with total parenteral nutrition in nearly all cases; however, if access to the small bowel can be obtained, enteral nutrition has some advantages. In any case, measuring prealbumin levels and other nutritional assessment parameters, and delaying operation until they return to normal or close to normal values, can lead to lower morbidity, faster recovery, and overall better outcomes.

PEPTIC ULCER DISEASE

RECURRENT ULCER DISEASE

Recurrent ulcer disease is most commonly caused by continued use of ulcerogenic medications, *Helicobacter pylori* infection, or an incomplete vagotomy at the initial operation.[1] In the United States, nonsteroidal antiinflammatory drug (NSAID) usage and *H. pylori* infection are the predominant causes of peptic ulcer disease, 24% and 48% of cases respectively. In the setting of recurrent ulcer disease or persistence of symptoms after an initial operation, it is important to rule out similar causes as the underlying etiology.[5]

In the absence of NSAID usage or *H. pylori* infection, incomplete vagotomy may explain recurrent ulcer disease. The relationship between persistent acid production and recurrent ulcers is supported by measurement of increased acid production through pH probe monitoring.[1] For NSAID-induced ulcers, however, there may be normal or decreased acid production because the medication produces the ulcers irrespective of acid production. This can be demonstrated by ulcer formation in patients using NSAIDs with suppressed acid secretions.[1] Continued NSAID use places 80% to 90% of patients at risk for repeat ulceration.[6]

In the absence of continued NSAID use, incomplete vagotomy, or recurrent *H. pylori*, a search for unusual causes of increased acid secretion should be undertaken. Possible causes include retained antrum or gastrinoma. Retained antrum should be suspected in patients with hypergastrinemia after antrectomy with Billroth II gastrojejunostomy. In this scenario, the remaining stump of antrum is continuously bathed in alkaline secretions from the duodenum and pancreas, resulting in increased gastrin secretion. When this diagnosis is suspected, a fasting serum gastrin level should be measured. If elevated, a secretin stimulation test will show a decrease in gastrin levels after administration of secretin, which confirms the diagnosis. Additionally, sodium 99m-technetium scans can facilitate identification of remaining antrum.

Another uncommon cause of hypergastrinemia and recurrent ulceration is gastrinoma, which can also present after an adequate acid-reducing operation. Patients may complain of diarrhea and abdominal pain. They may also have reflux symptoms, gastrointestinal (GI) bleeding, or weight loss. Family history may also provide diagnostic clues. Testing of fasting serum gastrin or total serum calcium (in the case of multiple endocrine neoplasia type 1 [MEN1] hyperparathyroidism) should be performed. A secretin stimulation test should be performed to exclude other causes of hypergastrinemia. In the case of gastrinoma, secretin stimulates a dramatic rise in serum gastrin; this is inhibited by secretin in normal gastric cells. On endoscopy, rugal hypertrophy may be present and prominent. Diagnosis is made with fasting serum gastrin and fasting pH levels. Confirmatory testing can be done with secretin stimulation if the previous studies are ambiguous.[1] Treatment involves resection of the gastrinoma when possible; if not, then lifelong, high-dose proton pump inhibitors (PPIs) are required.

The initial step in the workup for recurrent peptic ulcer disease involves endoscopic evaluation of the esophagus, remnant stomach, and duodenum. This allows identification of multiple ulcers, anastomotic strictures, or bezoars. It is important to obtain adequate biopsy specimens of any ulcers because neoplastic disease can present as recurrent ulceration, with many reports of increased risk of neoplastic transformation in patients with a history of gastric surgery.[6]

Upper GI contrast imaging can be beneficial in identifying motility or emptying disorders; however, gastric outlet obstruction in the presence of recurrent ulcer disease is often a product of, and not the cause of, the underlying problem. In the case of uncertain anatomy or unknown previous operation, contrast studies are essential.[6]

Treatment of recurrent ulcer disease begins with cessation of any offending medications, including all NSAIDs, and smoking. Antisecretory medications, such as PPIs or H$_2$ blockers, should be initiated for a minimum of 12 weeks.[7] *H. pylori* testing is warranted, with confirmation based on biopsy, serology, or urea breath testing, to be followed by appropriate treatment.[6] Medical management has the potential to resolve recurrent ulceration in these patients, with one report demonstrating improvement in 40% of patients on secretory therapy. However, most studies were performed before the development of PPIs.[8] Once there is evidence of a healed ulcer on endoscopy, patients can resume acetaminophen or non-NSAIDs, as needed.[6]

In patients with persistent symptoms, additional testing should be performed to exclude other causes. Surgical intervention, for the most part, is limited to patients with gastric outlet obstruction (discussed later). However, for patients with recurrent ulcer symptoms despite maximal medical therapy, an inability to comply with medical therapy, or after an elimination of causative factors, surgical intervention will depend on the initial index operation.

- Antrectomy or partial gastrectomy: The traditional approach to repeat operation in patients with a previous antrectomy or partial gastrectomy is a subtotal or total gastrectomy.[1] This should be reserved for those patients who fail to improve despite maximal medical therapy, because morbidity and mortality are significantly higher than at index operation; 20% to 40% have significant symptoms after revision surgery.[6]
- Retained antrum: The treatment for retained antrum is revision surgery to excise the remaining tissue. Frozen

section should be performed to look for Brunner glands or duodenal glands at the distal resection margin, and to ensure that any retained antrum is removed prior to performing the anastomosis.[6]
- Gastrinoma: In the case of gastrinoma from Zollinger-Ellison syndrome or MEN syndrome, operation should be performed to remove the gastrin-producing tumor when possible.
- Failed vagotomy: In the case of a failed or incomplete vagotomy with pyloroplasty and adequate gastric drainage, many patients can be treated with antisecretory medications. However, for the rare subset of patients for whom medical management is unsuccessful or who cannot tolerate the medical management protocols, reoperation may be performed for completion vagotomy. This can be approached through the abdomen or the chest, depending on the surgeon's comfort level. Frozen section demonstrating nerve tissue should be performed prior to leaving the operating room.

GASTRIC OUTLET OBSTRUCTION AFTER PYLORIC OR DUODENAL ULCER SURGERY

Gastric outlet obstruction after pyloric or duodenal surgery can occur months to years after the index operation. The presentation and timing will be largely reflective of the primary operation, and this will also determine the treatment: antrectomy with or without a vagotomy with Billroth I, Billroth II, or Roux-en-Y reconstruction. Initial, nonoperative management includes nasogastric decompression, fluid resuscitation, and antisecretory therapy.[9]

Occasionally, gastric outlet obstruction may occur due to hypertrophy at the pylorus. This may occur in patients who did not undergo a gastric drainage procedure with their acid-reducing operation, such as vagotomy with or without an omental patch. Endoscopic balloon dilation can provide modest short-term results with minimal pain and recovery time. This can allow passage of gastric contents through a strictured pylorus, at least temporarily. However, most patients will have recurrence of symptoms and will require surgery for adequate gastric emptying.[10]

In situations where patients have a gastric anastomosis at the index operation, such as a Roux-en-Y or Billroth II, the underlying cause may be an anastomotic stricture, which will be discussed later in this chapter.

GASTRIC OUTLET OBSTRUCTION AT THE SITE OF A GASTROJEJUNOSTOMY

Anastomotic stricture at the site of a gastrojejunostomy can result in gastric outlet obstruction due to incomplete gastric emptying with symptoms of bloating, nausea, and nonbilious vomiting.[11] This has a reported frequency of up to 20% of patients undergoing a Roux-en-Y and may be higher in Billroth II reconstructions because these anastomoses are more prone to stricture formation.[12] Diagnosis is made with upper GI contrast studies, with emphasis on both head-on and profile images to assess the width and length of the anastomotic stricture.[11] Conservative management begins with nasogastric decompression and intravenous hydration. Patients may be offered balloon dilation, with reports of success in up to 89% of patients.[13] However, frequent recurrence and limited response to dilation are indications for surgical revision.

GASTRIC OUTLET OBSTRUCTION FROM GASTRIC BEZOARS

The physiologic changes in the operated stomach may result in decreased acid secretion and stasis resulting in bezoar formation from ingested fibrous material.[8] This large mass has the potential to cause gastric outlet obstruction from mass effect, or rarely, result in small bowel obstruction if the fibrous material is unable to pass distally. These lesions can be distinguished from gastric tumors based on their free-floating appearance on upper GI imaging, in addition to air trapping within the mass and speculated surface. Treatment involves removal of the offending mass. Removal at endoscopy is often successful, but surgical excision may be required.[11]

ANASTOMOTIC (MARGINAL) ULCER

Ulceration at a gastroenteric anastomosis can occur due to multiple causes, including those associated with recurrent ulcer disease (discussed earlier) and those associated with altered anatomy, such as ischemia, presence of a foreign body (such as permanent suture or staples), or high acid content from gastric reservoir.[14] Antrectomy with Roux-en-Y gastrojejunostomy is an ulcerogenic operation. In such patients, an ulcer may occur in the jejunum just distal to the gastric anastomosis. This is due to the jejunum being continually bathed in acid without alkaline bile present.[12,15] Adequate gastric drainage and a small gastric remnant can help minimize symptoms. Patients may remain asymptomatic for many years; in one study, the mean time to development of symptoms was 12 years.[16] A comprehensive evaluation including upper endoscopy is warranted, in which the location, size, and depth of the ulcer is noted, and the possible presence of a foreign body is investigated.[14] Additionally, causes of recurrent ulceration, such as those discussed earlier, including NSAID use, *H. pylori* infection, retained antrum, and gastrinoma, should be ruled out. It is important to also assess the patient for possible remnant gastric carcinoma, which can have many different presentations.

Medical management is the primary treatment and includes antisecretory therapy with PPI, sucralfate, and smoking cessation.[14] Surgical therapy is recommended for patients with continued upper GI bleeding and those with nonhealing ulcers despite maximal medical therapy. The operative approach involves resection of the ulcer and creation of a gastroenteric anastomosis.

POSTGASTRECTOMY DUMPING AND DIARRHEA

DUMPING

Postgastrectomy dumping refers to a constellation of symptoms and signs that gastric content is reaching the small bowel too quickly, causing large fluid shifts into the intestinal lumen with resultant rapid small bowel distention.[17] First described by Hertz in 1913,[18] 10% to 50% of patients report symptoms consistent with dumping after gastrectomy in the early postoperative period.[17] The frequency is even higher, up to 75%, in bariatric surgery patients and is considered to be a desired side effect to facilitate weight loss in this subset of patients.[19] This syndrome is divided into early dumping, occurring 10 to 30 minutes after a meal, and late dumping, occurring 2 to 3 hours after eating.[17] Early dumping symptoms include abdominal pain, diarrhea, bloating, and nausea. Patients frequently also complain of vasomotor symptoms, such as flushing, palpitations, perspiration, tachycardia, hypotension, or syncope. Late dumping symptoms include hypotension, perspiration, palpitations, hunger, weakness, confusion, tremor, and syncope and are due to oversecretion of insulin in response to a carbohydrate-rich meal with subsequent hypoglycemia.[18] Early dumping syndrome is much more common than late dumping.[17] Dumping can often be diagnosed based on history and symptoms. An oral glucose tolerance test can be performed as an adjunct to diagnosis, using 75 g of glucose and observation for the development of symptoms.[17,18] The glucose dosage is important in this situation because a higher dose can mimic dumping even in nondumpers.[20] Treatment for dumping syndrome involves dietary modification, with six small meals per day, limited carbohydrate intake, and lying down after eating.[18] Despite dietary modifications, 3% to 5% of patients will continue to have severe symptoms. Octreotide, administered 30 minutes before or immediately following a meal has allowed improvement of symptoms in select patients.[17] Before consideration of revisional surgery, an inpatient observation of the severity of dumping symptoms is warranted. This will also allow direct observation of patient compliance with diet. A trial of 1 year of conservative measures, with medical, dietary, and behavioral modifications, is recommended before a repeat operation may be considered.[21] Because the stomach serves as a reservoir of food, with delayed passage through the pylorus in normal anatomy, surgical intervention that delays the transit of food contents into the small intestine will improve symptoms. Interventions include narrowing of an anastomosis, conversion of a Billroth II to a Billroth I, and conversion to a Roux-en-Y. If an intact pylorus exists, a pylorus reconstruction procedure can also be performed, which may be technically easier than creating another anastomosis.[22] In addition, a 10-cm antiperistaltic limb of jejunum can be placed to delay transit.[18,20,21] In patients with refractory symptoms despite revisional operation, a salvage feeding jejunostomy can be placed to allow hydration and nutrition.[18]

DIARRHEA

Postgastrectomy diarrhea can occur in conjunction with dumping, due to increased transit of food from the stomach into the small intestine, or as a separate disease entity. When occurring alone, this syndrome is due to the increased presence of unconjugated bile salts in the small intestine, which stimulate colonic secretions and result in diarrhea. Present in up to 30% of patients, this is often self-limited but can be treated with oral cholestyramine, which facilitates bile salt binding. For refractory causes of life-limiting diarrhea, an antiperistaltic jejunal limb may slow GI transit and may improve symptoms.[12]

GASTROPARESIS AND IMPAIRED MOTILITY

GASTROPARESIS

Normal gastric emptying involves a complex interplay of hormones, muscle contraction, neural input, meal content, and functional relaxation of the duodenum.[23] Gastroparesis occurs with delayed gastric emptying in the absence of mechanical causes.[24] Patients with gastroparesis complain of nausea, vomiting, early satiety, abdominal pain, and fullness.[23] Patients commonly describe a characteristic pain shortly after eating, localized to the left upper quadrant at or above the costal margin.[15] Gastroparesis is confirmed with a solid-phase gastric emptying study and likely has an underlying element of chronic gastric atony and lack of parasympathetic tone as an underlying cause.[25] Critical in the diagnosis is the confirmation of abnormal gastric emptying, a cornerstone of this syndrome, because these symptoms can be caused by a variety of other postgastrectomy problems.[23] As interventions are not benign procedures, adequate documentation of decreased transit time is important.[26] Operations known to result in some element of gastroparesis include Nissen fundoplication, vagotomy for ulcer disease, Billroth I and II reconstructions and operations for gastric cancer, and pancreaticoduodenectomy.[27] Vagal denervation of a gastric remnant has been shown to decrease emptying.[28] During evaluation, endoscopy should be used to confirm appropriate functioning of the pylorus or the absence of an anatomic or mechanical explanation for delayed emptying. In addition, hypothyroidism should be investigated as a possible medical cause for delayed gastric emptying. If endoscopy and radionucleotide scintigraphy fail to identify an etiology, a small bowel contrast study should be used to evaluate appropriate forward propulsion of meals and to exclude other rare causes such as jejunogastric intussusception or efferent limb obstruction. Because many gastric operations result in a transient delay in gastric emptying, most authors recommend at least 1-year trial of conservative medical management prior to reoperation.[25] The general principle is to maintain hydration and nutrition and improve glycemic control in diabetics.[23]

PROKINETICS

A trial of prokinetic therapy can be attempted in most patients, such as erythromycin or metoclopramide, although the recommended use should not exceed 12 weeks.

Side effects of metoclopramide therapy, including dystonia, tardive dyskinesia, and hyperprolactinemia, can be troublesome in up to 20% of patients and results in cessation of therapy.[23]

ENTERAL NUTRITION

In patients unable to tolerate adequate per os intake to maintain hydration and nutrition, placement of a jejunostomy tube may be indicated. These are much better tolerated in patients with frequent emesis compared to gastrojejunal tubes, the latter of which can be dislodged with frequent vomiting.[23,26] Patients can be placed on a trial of nasojejunal feeds, and in those patients who tolerate goal feeds, a jejunostomy tube is placed.[26]

GASTRIC ELECTRICAL STIMULATION

Gastric electrical stimulation is currently under investigation in nonrandomized case series.[23]

Many series report short-term improvement; however studies have failed to demonstrate a functional improvement in gastric emptying.[26]

OPERATIVE THERAPY

Surgical management is reserved for patients with severe symptoms refractory to medical management.[29] Operative intervention consists of total or near-total gastrectomy with gastroduodenal or gastrojejunal reconstruction.[25,26] In several studies, 40% to 67% of patients reported symptom improvement with near-total gastrectomy.[26,27,30] Predictors of poor outcome include the need for total parenteral nutrition (TPN) before surgery and retained food on endoscopy. These patients rarely benefit from a revision of their previous surgery or a limited gastric resection.[25] Near-total gastrectomy has been reported with success in 40% to 78% of patients.[25,30,31] However, we recommend placement of a jejunostomy tube at revisional operation, if not placed previously, to allow for maintenance of nutrition.

ROUX LIMB SYNDROME

Roux limb syndrome is a constellation of symptoms of severe nausea, vomiting, abdominal pain, and bezoar formation in patients who have previously undergone a Roux-en-Y operation. Incidence may be as high as 30% to 50%.[25,32] The cause is unknown, but is believed to be related to delayed transit through the stomach and Roux limb due to lack of vagal drive, atonic gastric remnant, and/or motor abnormalities through the Roux limb.[25,29] Many hypotheses exist, such as acid production causing disturbed motility[32] and loss of GI pacemakers.[33] This condition is believed to arise from Roux limbs that are longer than 45 cm,[22,32] with reports of successfully eliminating symptoms with Roux limbs as short as 20 cm to minimize obstruction and angulation. A wide-mouth, end-to-side anastomosis has also been advocated for appropriate drainage to avoid this syndrome.[19]

The underlying cause is thought to be the net propulsion of food toward, instead of away from, the stomach,[12] resulting in the constellation of signs and symptoms that characterize this condition. There is some argument for maintaining vagal input to the gastric remnant to facilitate forward conduction and GI pacemakers.[19] Medical treatment includes the use of prokinetics such as metoclopramide or erythromycin.[12] Surgical revision is indicated in failure to respond to medical management, and includes near-total gastrectomy to remove the atonic portion of the stomach and shortening of the Roux limb.[19,23]

GASTROESOPHAGEAL REFLUX DISEASE

GERD is a common GI disorder in the United States. The number of antireflux procedures performed increased during the mid-1990s, but have declined in the past 10 years as bariatric procedures have become more prominent.[34] However, surgeons continue to see a significant number of patients who are experiencing symptoms after undergoing antireflux procedures. It is imperative to understand the anatomic cause for the failure of the fundoplication to effectively revise these patients.

What constitutes a failed antireflux procedure is controversial. Some surgeons define postoperative anatomic abnormality on imaging as a failure regardless of symptoms present, whereas others rely solely on the presence of symptoms. In our opinion, a combination of subjective and objective evidence is necessary prior to judging the efficacy of a previous procedure. The most common symptoms that prompt patients to seek reevaluation after initial antireflux procedures are (1) persistent reflux or pyrosis, (2) dysphagia, and (3) gas bloat.[35–39] Papasavas et al. found that the median time to repeat procedure was 12.5 months, with 85% of patients undergoing repeat procedure before 2 years.[35] This suggests that most patients who are dissatisfied with their antireflux procedure will present with symptoms within the first 2 years, making this time point a reasonable minimal follow-up interval.

The preoperative evaluation for a patient with complaints after antireflux surgery is similar to the initial evaluation of a patient with reflux. An upper GI contrast study is generally the initial step in evaluation; it is useful in determining the location of the fundoplication and identifying whether the wrap hinders passage of fluid into the stomach. Esophagogastroduodenoscopy (EGD) should be performed prior to reoperation, particularly if esophagitis is a possible cause of symptoms. Should these first two tests prove nondiagnostic, it would then be appropriate to obtain a pH study to prove that reflux of acidic contents is occurring in the esophagus.[40] Importantly, if patients are having difficulty with dysphagia and/or pain, repeat manometry is indicated. Hunter et al. discovered that 10% of referrals for revision of fundoplication were actually suffering from achalasia.[41] It is recommended that esophageal and gastric dysmotility be excluded as reasons for presenting symptoms prior to repeat surgical intervention, especially if upper GI contrast studies, EGD, and pH studies are normal, because revision of fundoplication will not improve symptoms in these situations.

After the decision to revise an antireflux procedure has been made, it is important to determine why the first procedure failed. There are four major reasons for failure of a fundoplication procedure[37]:

1. Herniation into the mediastinum: This would result from incomplete reduction of a hiatal hernia or breakdown of the crural repair. Transdiaphragmatic herniation can be remedied by ensuring complete dissection of the hiatal hernia sac and tension-free approximation of the crura.
2. Shortened esophagus: A short esophagus creates upward traction on the gastroesophageal (GE) junction, disrupting the positive pressure zone created by the diaphragm. Preoperative evaluation, particularly manometry, can help determine the location of the GE junction. Intraoperatively, identification of the GE junction fat pad will assist in evaluating esophageal length. Any esophagus deemed too short to remain in the peritoneal cavity without tension should be lengthened surgically.
3. Poorly constructed fundoplication: Once again, correct identification of the GE junction is necessary to construct a functional fundoplication. Dysphagia is generally caused by a fundoplication that is too tight or too long, while reflux is caused by wraps being constructed too loosely. These findings can be seen on an upper GI contrast study to assist in planning for revisional surgery.
4. Other: This category includes vagal injury during the previous procedure resulting in poor gastric emptying as well as esophageal dysmotility.

At the time of revisional surgery, four anatomic abnormalities will be found. The most frequently documented causes for failure of a previous antireflux procedure were transdiaphragmatic migration of the wrap, misplaced wrap, disrupted fundoplication, and a fundoplication that is too tight.[35,41,42]

The surgical approach for a revisional antireflux procedure is controversial. Some believe that laparoscopy should be attempted only if the primary procedure was minimally invasive. However, a systematic review of 20 studies investigating revision of antireflux surgeries found that 92.8% of these cases could be completed laparoscopically, although they took significantly longer to complete.[43] Additionally, a study from Emory University confirmed that previous open fundoplication does not prohibit attempting a laparoscopic redo antireflux procedure.[41] The discovery of dense adhesions between the left lobe of the liver and the stomach should be anticipated, and the approach technique including handling this obstacle will depend on surgeon experience. It is our belief that a minimally invasive approach should be attempted initially if the operating surgeon is experienced or comfortable with this approach.

Performing revisional antireflux surgery requires the same steps, whether it is done open or laparoscopically. Once the intraperitoneal cavity has been entered, the previous fundoplication should be identified. The reason for dysfunction of the primary antireflux surgery is usually readily apparent, as described earlier. If a significant hiatal hernia exists, the hernia should be reduced and the hernia sac completely excised. The fundoplication should be completely taken down and normal anatomy restored to evaluate for causes of failure; this includes complete dissection of the fundus to perform the redo fundoplication. After all anatomy has been identified, abdominal esophageal length at rest should be assessed. There should be a minimum of 2 cm of tension-free esophagus in the abdomen. Should there be any difficulty in identifying the GE junction, intraoperative endoscopy can be helpful. Collis gastroplasty is one option that can be used to lengthen the intraabdominal esophagus and increase the likelihood of success of the revisional antireflux procedure but is used rarely. Finally, the crura are reapproximated without tension and fundoplication is performed over a bougie (54- to 60-French). The most important principles of revisional antireflux surgery are presented in Box 70.1.

Recurrent hiatal hernias pose unique challenges in repair. Large, recurrent hernias can be difficult to repair and can be approached through the chest or abdomen, with an open or minimally invasive technique. Haider

BOX 70.1 Major Principles of Reoperative Antireflux Surgery

1. Prepare for adhesions between the left lobe of the liver and stomach.
2. Identify the source of the previous antireflux procedure failure: disruption of the wrap, recurrent diaphragmatic hernia, misplaced wrap, or a combination.
3. Reestablish normal anatomy by taking down the previous fundoplication.
4. Confirm 2-cm length of intraabdominal esophagus.
5. Reconstruct the diaphragm crura and perform fundoplication.
6. Check for leaks and organ injury.

et al. found that symptom outcomes were equivalent between laparotomy and laparoscopy repair of recurrent hiatal hernia, but they also noted that selection bias between the two groups did exist.[44] In the case of multiple previous upper abdominal procedures, the transthoracic approach may allow for an easier repair. An approach via left thoracotomy or thoracoscopy will allow resection of the hernia sac and repair of the diaphragmatic defect. The principles remain the same for thoracic repair as for abdominal repair.

Biologic mesh has been used in the repair of large recurrent hernias in a selected group of patients.[45] In this group there were no episodes of mesh erosion and no increase in surgical site adhesions from the mesh. However, the use of hiatal mesh has been associated with complications, such as erosion, requiring esophagectomy.[46] An alternative to mesh is to create a counter ("relaxing") incision lateral to the hiatus to mobilize the crura for simple suture repair. Regardless of the technique chosen, the most important aspect of hiatal repair is that it is completed without tension.

At times, an unconventional antireflux procedure should be considered at time of revisional surgery. This decision should be made using the preoperative study results described earlier. Patients without relaxation of the lower esophageal sphincter on manometry will require a GE myotomy to relieve their symptoms. Others may find improvement with a more extensive procedure. One study demonstrated that Roux-en-Y reconstruction provides better symptom outcomes in the subset of patients with esophageal dysmotility, delayed gastric emptying, and morbid obesity compared with redo fundoplication.[46] It is important to discuss these alternatives with patients presenting for revisional antireflux surgery because the postoperative complication profiles are significantly different.

As with most revisional procedures, redo antireflux surgeries are more complicated than the index surgery. The complication profile for redo fundoplication is similar to those seen in primary fundoplication, but they occur with more frequency. In a series from University of Wisconsin, the complication rate of revisional fundoplications was 18.4% as compared to a rate of 0% in the primary fundoplication procedures.[47] The most frequent complications include stomach and esophagus injury, pneumothorax, persistent postoperative nausea, and postoperative dysphagia. Additionally, laparoscopic revisional antireflux procedures are more likely to necessitate conversion to open procedures and have longer hospital stays than those undergoing primary laparoscopic fundoplication.[48]

Outcomes of revisional antireflux surgery are generally quite good. However, they tend to fall short of outcomes achieved with primary antireflux procedures. In a retrospective study of 275 patients, the probability of successful redo fundoplication was 95%, 93%, and 84% at 1 year, 2 years, and 5 years, respectively; they also demonstrated a trend of multiple redo operations being associated with failure.[42] When comparing open to laparoscopic revisions, rates of reflux control were slightly better in the open group (91% vs. 87%), but freedom from dysphagia was more common in the laparoscopic group (91% vs. 70%).[41] Papasavas et al. demonstrated improvement in patient quality of life and activity scores after patients had undergone redo antireflux surgery for failed fundoplications, and furthermore, the majority of patients were able to stop medical therapy for reflux.[35] These findings suggest that attempting to revise a failed fundoplication is a worthy endeavor because it is highly successful in improving patient symptoms and productivity.

In conclusion, reoperation for failed antireflux surgery can be performed with good outcomes, despite having lower success rates than the primary procedure. Revisional surgery can be undertaken safely and successfully from either an open or laparoscopic approach. It is important to consider referring these cases to higher-volume centers because they have fewer complications, including mortality and shorter length of stay.[34] Finally, adequate preoperative workup and choosing the appropriate procedure are imperative to achieving satisfactory results.

BILE REFLUX GASTRITIS

The gastric mucosa is designed to accommodate a certain amount of bile reflux without development of gastritis. When this capacity to accommodate is overcome, symptoms tend to develop. Patients who have had previous operations on the stomach and/or duodenum are more susceptible to bile reflux gastritis due to alterations in anatomy or disruption of neural input. The most common symptoms of bile reflux gastritis are epigastric pain, nausea, and bilious vomiting, and quality of life is often impacted significantly enough to require reoperation.

Limiting the amount of bile that refluxes into the stomach may prevent the development of gastric cancer. A study in 1993 demonstrated a positive association between high bile concentrations in the stomach and intestinal metaplasia of gastric mucosa, as well as mucosal atrophy.[49] A later study containing 2283 subjects confirmed these findings; however, it was noted that metaplasia and mucosal atrophy were only associated with the upper quartile of gastric bile concentrations (over 330 nmol/mL).[50] Intestinal metaplasia is believed to be part of the progression to malignancy, and steps should be taken to limit this potentially carcinogenic exposure. This evidence suggests that revision may be indicated in patients with significant enterogastric reflux as well as those with symptoms.

A detailed history and physical exam will generally lead to the diagnosis of bile reflux gastritis. However, confirming this diagnosis objectively can be challenging. Other causes for the presenting symptoms must be ruled out first. Processes that mimic enterogastric reflux are afferent loop syndrome (discussed later), obstructed efferent loop, distal small bowel obstruction, and gastroparesis, particularly if the vagal nerve has been disrupted. Initial examination should include (1) an upper GI with small bowel follow-through to evaluate gastric emptying and rule out possible obstruction, and (2) upper endoscopy with biopsy to evaluate the gastric mucosa for metaplasia, and intragastric bile measurements to quantify enterogastric reflux. Hepatobiliary scintigraphy can be used to evaluate the quantity of bile reflux. Chen et al. compared scintigraphy to intragastric bile concentrations and found scintigraphy to be the more sensitive and specific test.[51] The cause of a patient's symptoms should be found with this battery of tests, and appropriate action can then be taken.

Once the diagnosis for true bile reflux gastritis has been made, surgical intervention is dependent on existing anatomy. A previous gastrojejunostomy allows for the creation of a Braun enteroenterostomy for drainage of bile directly from the afferent limb. This technique has been shown to cause objective and subjective improvements in duodenogastric reflux when compared with controls.[52] The Braun enteroenterostomy is constructed approximately 30 cm from the gastrojejunostomy and can be done with a hand-sewn anastomosis or a GI stapler. Another surgical treatment option is conversion to Roux-en-Y drainage. Bile reflux has been measured in the proximal organ with Roux limbs measuring 60 cm, with some patients being symptomatic. Lengthening the previous limb to 110 cm has been shown to improve bile reflux in patients with bile reflux and existing Roux limb reconstruction.[53] Care should be taken to avoid creating the enteroenterostomy too distal in the alimentary tract because this could lead to significant weight loss.

AFFERENT LOOP SYNDROME

Afferent loop syndrome is a rare occurrence caused by obstruction of the afferent, or biliopancreatic, loop of a gastrojejunostomy reconstruction. The syndrome is produced by retention of bile and pancreatic secretions in the afferent loop. Once pressure builds in the afferent limb to allow decompression into the stomach, bilious vomiting ensues. This physiology corresponds with the symptoms that are associated with this syndrome. Patients will experience epigastric pain after meals as bile and pancreatic juices accumulate, followed by bilious emesis that relieves the pain and bloating. Chronic diarrhea can also develop from bacterial overgrowth in the obstructed afferent limb.

Obstruction of the afferent limb can be the result of malignant or benign causes. Prevention of this problem is best achieved by making the afferent limb as short as possible, limiting the likelihood that adhesive obstruction of the limb will occur. Early presentations of afferent limb syndrome are likely due to technical failure in creating the gastrojejunostomy. Late presentation could be from a number of causes including but not limited to adhesions, radiation enteropathy, chronic volvulus, internal herniation with obstruction, or recurrent malignancy. Afferent loop

syndrome from these causes has been demonstrated in pancreaticoduodenectomy patients with median time to occurrence being 1.2 years.[54] In such cases, recurrent cancer is often the cause. Roux-en-Y reconstructions can also develop afferent limb syndrome, although it occurs at lower rates than in Billroth II reconstructions (0.2% vs. 1.0%).[55]

Diagnosis of afferent limb syndrome is generally clinical. Some patients will demonstrate elevated serum bilirubin and amylase secondary to stasis of bile and pancreatic secretions in the afferent limb. If there is any doubt concerning the source of symptoms, abdominal CT with oral contrast or upper GI radiograph can be performed. Abdominal CT will reveal a large fluid-filled loop of bowel with small amounts of air in the right upper quadrant. Plain radiographs tend to miss this finding because the obstruction prohibits bowel gas from collecting in the affected loop.

The diagnosis of afferent loop syndrome requires prompt operative revision. Simple adhesiolysis may be all that is required in some cases to relieve the obstruction. Adhesiolysis and shortening of the afferent limb is the revisional procedure of choice.

REFERENCES

1. Ellis H. The cause and prevention of postoperative intraperitoneal adhesions. *Surg Gynecol Obstet.* 1971;133:497.
2. Ellis H, Moran BJ, Thompson JN, et al. Adhesion-related hospital readmissions after abdominal and pelvic surgery: a retrospective cohort study. *Lancet.* 1999;353:1456.
3. Cohen Z, Cohen Z, Senagore AJ, et al. Prevention of postoperative abdominal adhesions by a novel, glycerol/sodium hyaluronate/carboxymethylcellulose-based bioresorbable membrane: a prospective, randomized, evaluator-blinded multicenter study. *Dis Colon Rectum.* 2005;48:1130.
4. Becker JM, Dayton MT, Fazio VW, et al. Prevention of postoperative abdominal adhesions by a sodium hyaluronate-based bioresorbable membrane: a prospective, randomized, double-blind multicenter study. *J Am Coll Surg.* 1996;183:406.
5. Lagoo J, Pappas TN, Perez A. A relic or still relevant: the narrowing role for vagotomy in the treatment of peptic ulcer disease. *Am J Surg.* 2014;207:120-126.
6. Turnage RH, Sarosi G, Cryer B, Spechler S, Peterson W, Feldman M. Evaluation and management of patients with recurrent peptic ulcer disease after acid-reducing operations: a systematic review. *J Gastrointest Surg.* 2003;7(5):606-626.
7. Hopkins RJ, Girardi LS, Turney EA. Relationship between *Helicobacter pylori* eradication and reduced duodenal and gastric ulcer recurrence: a review. *Gastroenterology.* 1996;110(4):1244.
8. Ingvar C, Adami HO, Enander LK, Enskog L, Rydberg B. Clinical results of reoperation after failed highly selective vagotomy. *Am J Surg.* 1986;152:308-312.
9. Barksdale AR, Schwartz RW. The evolving management of gastric outlet obstruction from peptic ulcer disease. *Curr Surg.* 2002;59(4):404-409.
10. Cherian PT, Cherian S, Singh P. Long-term follow up of patients with gastric outlet obstruction related to peptic ulcer disease treated with endoscopic balloon dilation and drug therapy. *Gastrointest Endosc.* 2007;66(3):491-497.
11. Woodfield C, Levine MS. The post-operative stomach. *Eur J Radiol.* 2005;53:341-352.
12. Bolton JS, Conway WC. Postgastrectomy syndromes. *Surg Clin North Am.* 2011;91(5):1105-1122.
13. Kim JH, Song HY, Park SW, et al. Early symptomatic strictures after gastric surgery: palliation with balloon dilation and stent placement. *J Vasc Interv Radiol.* 2008;19(4):565-570.
14. Nguyen NT, Hinojosa MW, Gray J, Fayad C. Reoperation for marginal ulceration. *Surg Endosc.* 2007;21:1919-1921.

15. Speicher JE, Thirlby RC, Burggraaf J, Kelly C, Levasseur S. Results of completion gastrectomies in 44 patients with postsurgical gastric atony. *J Gastrointest Surg.* 2009;13:874-880.

16. Jordan G. Recurrence after highly selective vagotomy should be treated by gastric resection. *Am J Surg.* 1986;152:312-313.

17. Li-Ling J, Irving M. Therapeutic value of octreotide for patients with severe dumping syndrome—a review of randomized control trials. *Postgrad Med J.* 2001;77:441-442.

18. Tack J, Arts J, Canenpeel P, De Wulf D, Bisschops R. Pathophysiology, diagnosis and management of postoperative dumping syndrome. *Nat Rev Gastroenterol Hepatol.* 2009;6:583-590.

19. Midema BW, Kelly KA. The Roux operation for postgastrectomy syndromes. *Am J Surg.* 1991;161:256-261.

20. Ukleja A. Dumping syndrome: pathophysiology and treatment. *Nutr Clin Pract.* 2005;20:5.

21. Berg P, McCallum R. Dumping syndrome: a review of current concepts of pathophysiology, diagnosis and treatment. *Dig Dis Sci.* 2016;61:11-18.

22. Cheadle WG, Baker PR, Cuschieri A. Pyloric reconstruction for severe vasomotor dumping after vagotomy and pyloroplasty. *Ann Surg.* 1985;202(5):568-572.

23. Bouras EP, Roque MI, Aranda-Michel J. Gastroparesis: from concept to management. *Nutr Clin Pract.* 2013;28(4):437-447.

24. Cameilleri M, Parkman HP, Shafi MA, Abell TL, Gerson L. Clinical guideline: management of gastroparesis. *Am J Gastroenterol.* 2013;108(1):18-37.

25. Eckhauser FE, Conrad M, Knol JA, Mulholland MW, Colletti LM. Safety and long-term durability of completion gastrectomy in 81 patients with postsurgical gastroparesis syndrome. *Am Surg.* 1998;64(8):711-716.

26. Jones MP, Maganti K. A systematic review of surgical therapy for gastroparesis. *Am J Gastroenterol.* 2003;98(10):2122-2129.

27. Sarosiek I, Davis B, Eichler E, McCallum RW. Surgical approaches to treatment of gastroparesis: gastric electrical stimulation, pyloroplasty, total gastrectomy and enteral feeding tubes. *Gastroenterol Clin North Am.* 2015;44:151-167.

28. Van der Mijle HCJ, Beehuis H, Bleichrody RP, Kleibeuker JH. Transit disorders of the gastric remnant and Roux limb after Roux-en-Y gastrojejunostomy: relation to symptomatology and vagotomy. *Br J Surg.* 1993;80(1):60-64.

29. Bouras EP, Scolapio JS. Gastric motility disorders: management that optimizes nutritional status. *J Clin Gastroenterol.* 2004;38(7):549-557.

30. Forstner-Barthell AW, Murr MM, Nitecki S, et al. Near-total completion gastrectomy for severe postvagotomy gastric stasis: analysis of early and long-term results in 62 patients. *J Gastrointest Surg.* 1999;3(1):15021.

31. Williams JA. The place of surgery in the treatment of postgastrectomy syndromes. *Acta Gastroenterol Belg.* 1964;27:610-617.

32. Gustavsson S, Ilstrup DM, Morrison P, Kelly KA. Roux-Y stasis syndrome after gastrectomy. *Am J Surg.* 1988;155:490-494.

33. Tu BLN, Kelly K. Surgical treatment of Roux stasis syndrome. *J Gastrointest Surg.* 1999;3(6):612-617.

34. Wang YR, Dempsey DT, Richter JE. Trends and perioperative outcomes of inpatient antireflux surgery in the United States, 1993–2006. *Dis Esophagus.* 2011;24:215-223.

35. Papasavas PK, Yeaney WW, Landreneau RJ, et al. Reoperative laparoscopic fundoplication for the treatment of failed fundoplication. *J Thorac Cardiovasc Surg.* 2004;128:509-516.

36. Makdisi G, Nichols F, Cassivi S, et al. Laparoscopic repair for failed antireflux procedures. *Ann Thorac Surg.* 2014;98:1261-1266.

37. Pennathur A, Awais O, Luketich J. Minimally invasive redo antireflux surgery: lessons learned. *Ann Thorac Surg.* 2010;89:S2174-S2179.

38. Hatch KF, Daily MF, Christensen BJ, Glasgow RE. Failed fundoplications. *Am J Surg.* 2004;188:786-791.

39. Engstrom C, Cai W, Irvine T, et al. Twenty years of experience with laparoscopic antireflux surgery. *Br J Surg.* 2012;99:1415-1421.

40. Stefanidis D, Hope W, Kohn G, Reardon P, Richardson W, Fanelli R. Guidelines for surgical treatment of gastroesophageal reflux disease. *Surg Endosc.* 2010;24:2647-2669.

41. Hunter JG, Smith CD, Branum GD, et al. Laparoscopic fundoplication failures: patterns of failure and response to fundoplication revision. *Ann Surg.* 1999;230(4):595-606.

42. Awais O, Luketich J, Schuchert M, et al. Reoperative antireflux surgery for failed fundoplication: an analysis of outcomes in 275 patients. *Ann Thorac Surg.* 2011;92:1083-1090.

43. Symons N, Purkayastha S, Dillemans B, et al. Laparoscopic revision of failed antireflux surgery: a systematic review. *Am J Surg.* 2011;202:336-343.

44. Haider M, Iqbal A, Salinas V, Karu A, Mittal S, Filipi C. Surgical repair of recurrent hiatal hernia. *Hernia.* 2006;10:13-19.

45. Bell R, Fearon J, Freeman K. Allograft dermal matrix hiatoplasty during laparoscopic primary fundoplication, paraesophageal hernia repair, and reoperation for failed hiatal hernia repair. *Surg Endosc.* 2013;27:1997-2004.

46. Mittal S, Legner A, Tsuboi K, Juhasz A, Bathla L, Lee T. Roux-en-Y reconstruction is superior to redo fundoplication in a subset of patients with failed antireflux surgery. *Surg Endosc.* 2013;27:927-935.

47. Musunuru S, Gould J. Perioperative outcomes of surgical procedures for symptomatic fundoplication failure: a retrospective case-control study. *Surg Endosc.* 2012;26:838-842.

48. Funch-Jensen P, Bendixen A, Iversen M, Kehlet H. Complications and frequency of redo antireflux surgery in Denmark: a nationwide study, 1997–2005. *Surg Endosc.* 2008;22:627-630.

49. Sobala GM, O'Connor HJ, Dewar EP, King RG, Axon AR, Dixon MF. Bile reflux and intestinal metaplasia in gastric mucosa. *J Clin Pathol.* 1993;46:235-240.

50. Matsuhisa T, Arakawa T, Watanabe T, et al. Relation between bile acid reflux into the stomach and the risk of atrophic gastric and intestinal metaplasia: a multicenter study of 2283 cases. *Dig Endosc.* 2013;25(5):519-525.

51. Chen TF, Yadav PK, Wu RJ, et al. Comparative evaluation of intragastric bile acids and hepatobiliary scintigraphy in the diagnosis of duodenogastric reflux. *World J Gastroenterol.* 2013;19(14):2187-2196.

52. Vogel SB, Drane WE, Woodward ER. Enteroenterostomy: prevention and treatment of alkaline reflux gastritis. An alternative to Roux-en-Y diversion. *Ann Surg.* 1994;219(5):458-466.

53. Collard JM, Romagnoli R. Roux-en-Y jejunal loop and bile reflux. *Am J Surg.* 2000;179:298-303.

54. Pannala R, Brandabur J, Gan SI, et al. Afferent limb syndrome and delayed GI problems after pancreaticoduodenectomy for pancreatic cancer: single-center 14-year experience. *Gastrointest Endosc.* 2011;74(2):295-302.

55. Aoki M, Saka M, Morita S, Fukagawa T, Katai H. Afferent loop obstruction after distal gastrectomy with Roux-en-Y reconstruction. *World J Surg.* 2010;34:2389-2392.

Anatomy and Physiology of the Small Intestine

Jacob Campbell | James Berry | Yu Liang

The small intestine is the longest organ in the gastrointestinal (GI) tract. It is responsible for the absorption of nutrients, maintaining water and electrolyte balance, providing an immunologic barrier, and endocrine secretion.

EMBRYOLOGY

During the fourth week of gestation, the flat embryonic endoderm folds and fuses in the midline to create the gut tube. The tube consists of the foregut, midgut, and hindgut. The midgut, which will give rise to the distal duodenum, jejunum, and ileum, is located in the middle of this tube and is open to the yolk sac. During development, the connection between the midgut and the yolk sac will close and become only a thin stalk known as the vitelline duct. A Meckel diverticulum is the persistent remnant of this structure. The endoderm will form the epithelial lining of the digestive tract, and the splanchnic mesoderm will give rise to the muscle, connective tissue, and peritoneal components of the gut wall.

Throughout gestation, the small intestine will lengthen and rotate. By the fifth to seventh weeks, the midgut will have outgrown the capacity of the abdominal cavity, forcing it into a hairpin loop configuration and then herniating into the umbilical cord. As it herniates, the loop rotates 90 degrees counterclockwise. This rotation places the ileum in the left quadrant of the abdomen. Between the tenth and twelfth weeks, the midgut retracts back into the abdomen and will rotate an additional 180 degrees. By the end of the twelfth week, the midgut has rotated 270 degrees counterclockwise. The superior mesenteric artery is the axis of this rotation (Fig. 71.1). The rotation of the intestines is important for establishing the permanent location of the abdominal organs. The proximal jejunum is positioned on the left side of the abdomen and the remaining loops of intestine will be displaced to the right. Errors in midgut rotation result in congenital malrotation. Omphalocele results from mistakes in the midgut returning to the abdominal cavity.

The location of the duodenum is affected by stomach rotation and pancreas development. As the stomach rotates during gestation, the duodenum will move to the right of the abdomen and up against the dorsal wall, and it will become retroperitoneal. The fusion of the ventral and dorsal pancreatic buds displaces the duodenum laterally creating the characteristic C-loop.[1,2]

CELL DIFFERENTIATION

It is known that the gut develops along four different axes: (1) anterior-posterior, (2) dorsal-ventral, (3) left-right, and (4) radial. The development and differentiation of different regions of the gut are dependent on reciprocal interaction between the endoderm and the splanchnic mesoderm. In the initial stages of formation, the intestinal tract is lined by simple columnar endodermal epithelium that is surrounded by splanchnopleuric mesoderm. During the sixth week, the endodermal epithelium proliferates and occludes the lumen completely. Over the next 2 weeks, vacuoles will develop and coalesce to create a hollow tube. This process is known as recanalization. Duplication cysts and intestinal stenosis are the result of errors in recanalization. After this process is complete, the mucosal layer will develop villi as aggregates of mesoderm push through the epithelium. The submucosal connective tissue and smooth muscle layers arise from the mesodermal coating of the gut tube.

During the creation of the villi, pitlike intestinal crypts form at the base of the villi. Epithelial stem cells reside within the crypt and undergo a high rate of mitosis, which gives rise to the epithelial cells for the entire intestine. The epithelial cells within each crypt are of monoclonal origin. The stem cell divides into daughter cells, leaving one daughter cell anchored in the crypt, whereas the other continues to divide and migrate up the side of the crypt and onto the villus. This division and migration is responsible for renewing the intestinal lining in a rapid manner. While in utero, the stem cells will differentiate into one of the four major epithelial cell types: Paneth, enteroendocrine, goblet, or enterocyte (the function of each cell will be discussed in a later section) (Fig. 71.2).

At 12 weeks of gestation, cell differentiation has begun but maturation will continue during the fetal period and through the first months of life. The cells will not develop digestive function until exposed to food. The first stool, meconium, is actually lanugo, a mixture of vernix caseosa from the skin, desquamated cells from the gut, and bile.

ANATOMY

The small intestine is approximately 7 meters in length, starting at the pylorus and ending at the ileocecal valve (ICV). It is divided into three sections: the duodenum, jejunum, and ileum. The majority of the duodenum is located in the retroperitoneum, whereas the jejunum and ileum are intraperitoneal structures.

The lumen of the small intestine is a complex arrangement of structures that aid in nutrient absorption. Each structure is responsible for increasing the surface area of the intestine to enhance digestion and absorption of nutrients. The net result is a 600- to 1000-fold increase in surface area for a total of 250 to 400 m². The epithelium of the small intestine is replaced every 3 to 6 days and can be influenced by a variety of factors. The rapid turnover and high mitotic rate of the cells makes the intestinal

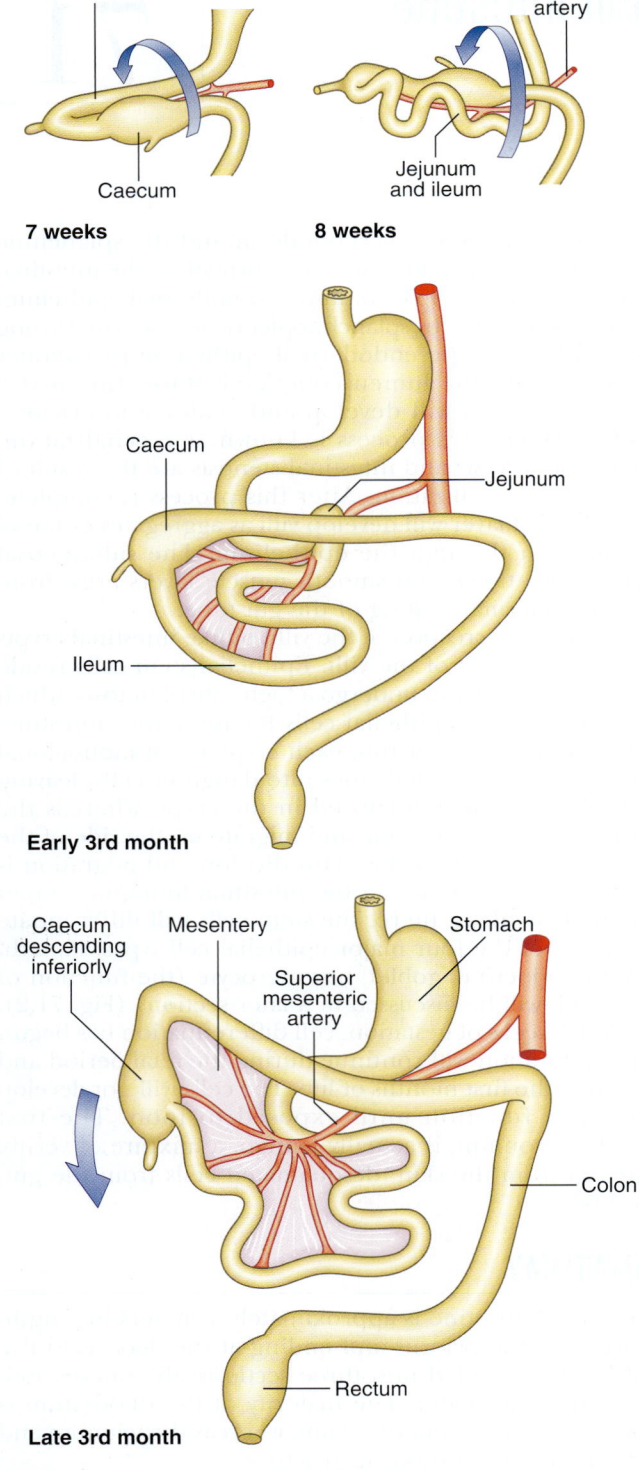

Small intestine

Caecum

7 weeks

Superior mesenteric
artery

Jejunum
and ileum

8 weeks

Caecum

Jejunum

Ileum

Early 3rd month

Caecum
descending
inferiorly

Mesentery

Superior
mesenteric
artery

Stomach

Colon

Rectum

Late 3rd month

FIGURE 71.1 During gestation the midgut outgrows the capacity of the abdominal cavity and herniates into the umbilicus, rotating 90 degrees counterclockwise. The midgut will rotate an additional 180 degrees as it retracts back into the abdomen around the 10th to 12th week of gestation for a total rotation of 270 degrees. (From Mitchell B. *Embryology: An Illustrated Color Text.* 2nd ed. Oxford: Churchill-Livingstone; 2005, Fig. 7.11, p. 45.)

lining susceptible to the effects of radiation and chemotherapy.

The wall of the small intestine is made up of four main layers: the mucosa, submucosa, muscularis propria, and serosa. The innermost layer is the mucosa. It is composed of three separate layers: epithelium, lamina propria, and muscularis mucosae. The mucosa is the site of absorption of nutrients and water from the intestinal lumen. The submucosa is the strength layer of the bowel wall and is composed of dense connective tissue. When completing a bowel anastomosis, it is important to incorporate suture through this layer of tissue to ensure integrity of the anastomosis. Blood vessels and lymphatics, including Peyer patches and Brunner glands, are found in this layer of the bowel wall. The Meissner, or submucosal plexus, is also located in the submucosa and is an integral component of the enteric nervous system (ENS). It is responsible for regulating bowel motility and secretion in the mucosal layer. The muscularis propria is composed of two smooth muscle layers, an outer longitudinal layer, and an inner circular layer. The myenteric, or Auerbach plexus, is situated between these two muscle layers and, like the Meissner plexus, helps control bowel motility and secretion. The serosa is the outermost layer of the bowel wall and is a single layer of mesothelial cells (Fig. 71.3).

Plicae circulares are transverse folds of mucosa and submucosa that aid in absorption of nutrients by increasing the surface area of the small intestine threefold. These folds are deep and visible on gross inspection and on radiographic imaging, even when the small intestine is distended.

Villi are fingerlike projections of the mucosa that are present along the entire length of the small intestine. The villi are longest in the duodenum, where most of the digestion and absorption occurs, and shortest in the distal ileum. They increase the absorptive area 10-fold. The villus is coated with a single layer of columnar epithelial cells, called enterocytes. Between the enterocytes are goblet cells that secrete mucin. The mucin will lubricate and protect the intestinal wall as chyme and undigested food passes. Goblet cells become more prominent throughout the length of the small intestine.

At the base of each villus are 0.3- to 0.5-mm invaginations of intestinal mucosa called intestinal crypts or crypts of Lieberkühn. Crypt cells are responsible for mitosis and secretion of fluid and electrolytes. Each crypt is monoclonal and contains only one stem cell type. The stem cell divides into daughter cells, leaving one daughter cell anchored in the crypt, whereas the other continues to divide and migrate up the side of the crypt and onto the villus. On the villus, the daughter cell may differentiate into a goblet cell, an enterocyte, or an enteroendocrine cell. The enterocyte will continue to mature as it migrates toward the apical end of the villus and take on increased digestive and absorptive ability. Enteroendocrine cells produce hormones that modulate the digestive process by altering secretion and motility. Other cells may migrate to the bottom of the crypt to become Paneth cells. The purpose of the Paneth cell is discussed in detail in the immunology section.

Within each villus is a rich vascular supply from an arteriole and a venule that contribute to a network of

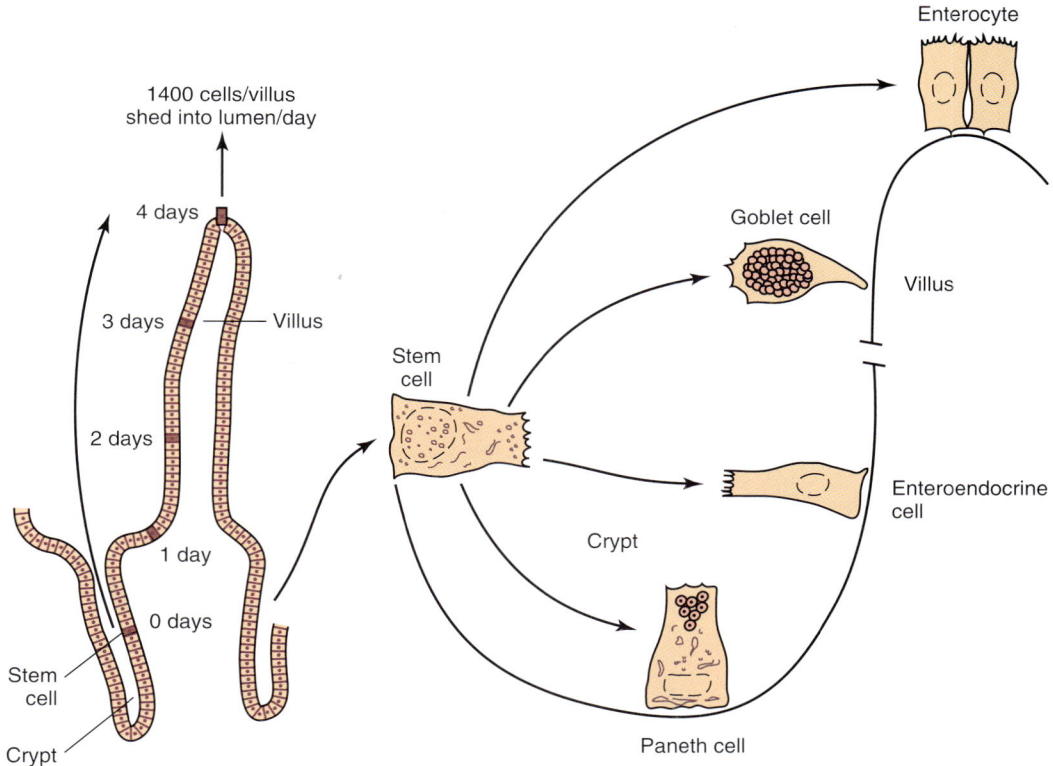

FIGURE 71.2 Stem cells differentiate in utero into one of four major epithelial cell types: Paneth, enteroendocrine, goblet, or enterocyte. (From Carlson B. *Human Embryology and Developmental Biology*. 2nd ed. St Louis: Mosby; 2004, Fig. 14.10, p. 331.)

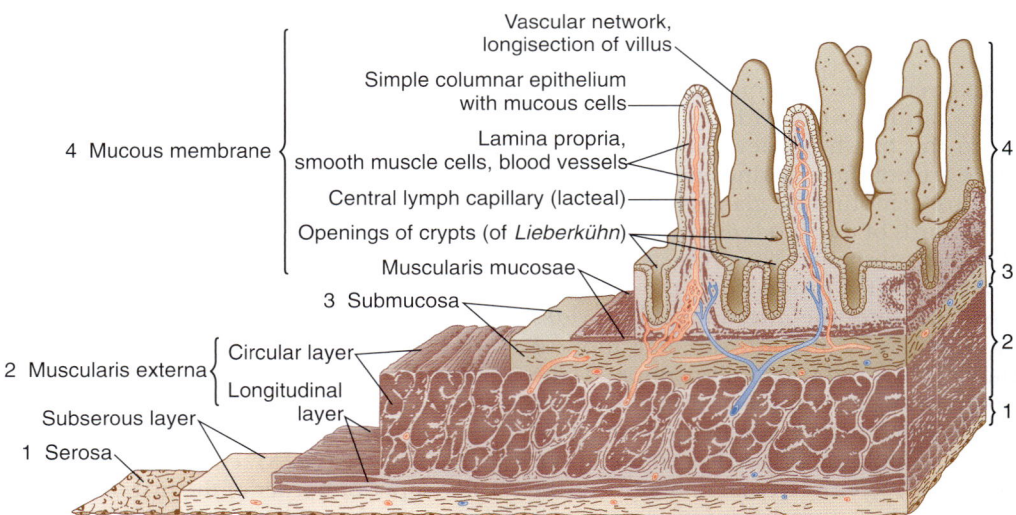

FIGURE 71.3 There are four main layers of the small intestine. The outermost layer is the serosa followed by the subserosa. Next is the muscularis externa, which is made up of an outer longitudinal and an inner circular layer. The submucosa layer is next and the innermost layer is the mucous membrane, which consists of the intestinal villi. (From Sobotta J, Figge FHJ, Hild WJ. *Atlas of Human Anatomy*. New York: Hafner; 1974.)

capillaries. There is also a lacteal, a lymphatic capillary that runs the length of the villus. The lacteal can absorb larger particles containing lipids and lipid-soluble vitamins (Fig. 71.4). These particles are known as chylomicrons, which are generated by neighbor enterocytes as they absorb and process lipid.

Microvilli are tiny projections of the plasma membrane that line the apical border of the enterocyte. The microvilli are coated with a thick glycocalyx that aids in nutrient absorption and serves as a protective barrier. In addition, many enzymes necessary for digestion and absorption, collectively referred to as the *brush border enzymes*, are

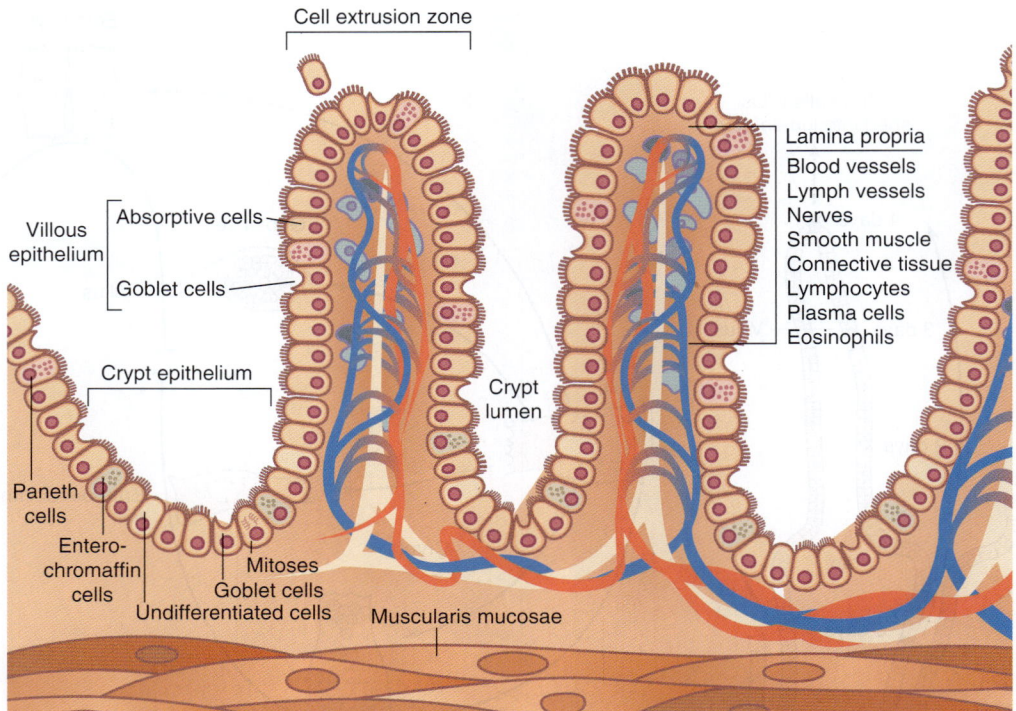

FIGURE 71.4 Schematic representation of small intestinal mucosa. (From Townsend C, Beauchamp RD, Evers BM, et al., eds. *Sabiston Textbook of Surgery*. 18th ed. Philadelphia: Saunders; 2008. Modified from Keljo DJ, Gariepy CE. Anatomy, histology, embryology, and developmental anomalies of the small and large intestine. In: Feldman M, Scharschmidt BF, Sleisenger MH, eds. *Sleisenger & Fordtran's Gastrointestinal and Liver Disease: Pathology/Diagnosis/Management*. Philadelphia: Saunders; 2002:1646.)

released within this layer. These enzymes include nucleosidases, peptidases, and disaccharidases. Millions of microvilli make up the brush border and function to increase the surface area of the intestine another 20-fold.

Brunner glands are acinotubular glands found mostly in the proximal two-thirds of the duodenum. They secrete an alkaline mucus-like substance that protects the duodenum from the acidic chyme produced by the stomach. The substance also lubricates the intestine and provides an alkaline environment essential for the activation of enzymes important for digestion and absorption. Many protective factors have been identified within Brunner gland secretions including human epidermal growth factor (beta urogastrone), an inhibitor of gastric acid secretion. Lysozyme and pancreatic secretory trypsin inhibitor (PSTI) have been identified in these secretions as well.[3]

Peyer patches are specialized aggregates of lymphoid follicles in the lamina propria. They are found along the antimesenteric border and are most abundant in the ileum. Peyer patches play an important role in mucosal immunity by recognizing and processing antigens. The germinal centers contain B lymphocytes, and T lymphocytes are in the interfollicular area. A specialized immune cell, the microfold cell or M cell, can be found in the epithelium overlying the lymphoid follicles. These cells are important in passive immunity by transporting antigens from the luminal surface to antigen-presenting cells into the lymphoid follicle.

DUODENUM

The duodenum is the first section of the small intestine. It begins at the pylorus and ends at the ligament of Treitz and is approximately 25 cm in length. The duodenum is largely retroperitoneal and has an intimate anatomic relationship with the pancreas. It is divided into four sections: first (bulb), second (descending), third (transverse), and fourth (ascending).

The first section, or the bulb, begins at the pylorus, which is demarcated by the prepyloric vein, and is approximately 5 cm in length. The posterior wall of this portion of the duodenum is in direct contact with the gastroduodenal artery (GDA), common bile duct, and portal vein. The superior border of the first segment of the duodenum is attached to the porta hepatis by the hepatoduodenal ligament, which envelops the portal triad. This portion of the duodenum begins the C-loop around the head of the pancreas (Fig. 71.5).

The second, descending, section is retroperitoneal and is approximately 10 cm in length. This segment is anterior to the right kidney and ureter and the lateral border of the inferior vena cava. The medial border is in direct contact with the head of the pancreas. Evaluation of the posterior surface of the descending duodenum, the posterior surface of the pancreatic head, and the common bile duct requires medial rotation of the descending duodenum using the Kocher maneuver. The main

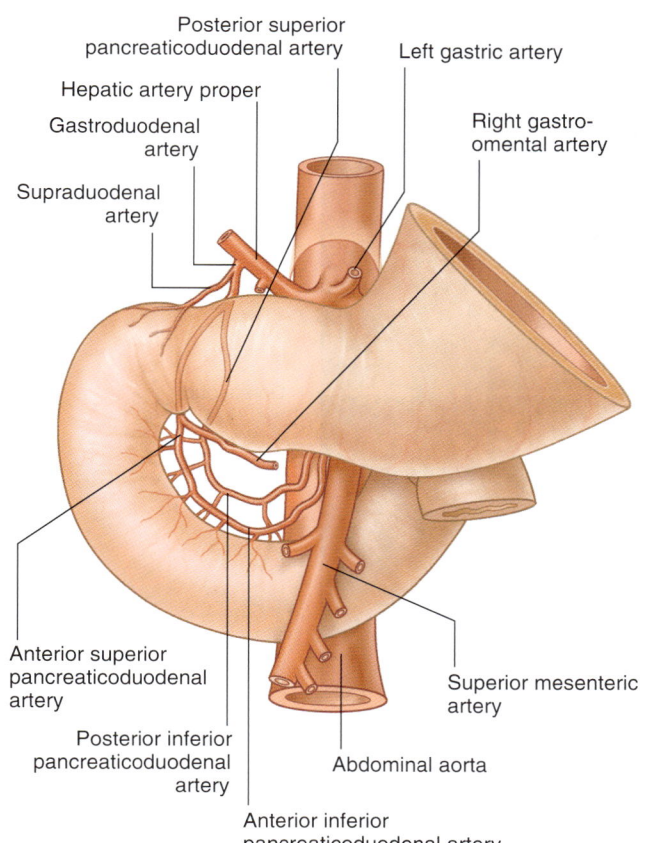

FIGURE 71.5 Arterial supply to the duodenum. (From Drake RL, Vogl AW, Mitchel AWM. *Gray's Anatomy for Students*. 2nd ed. Philadelphia: Churchill Livingstone; 2009, Fig. 4.64.)

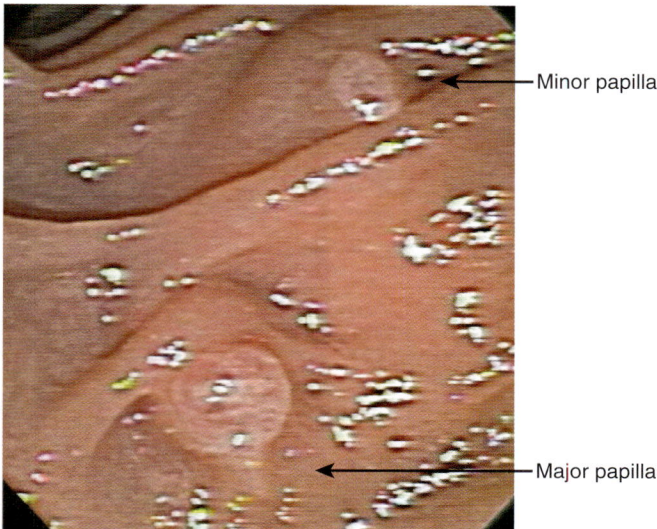

FIGURE 71.6 Endoscopic image of the major papilla and proximal minor papilla.

pancreatic duct, the duct of Wirsung, and the common bile duct join and empty into the posteromedial wall of the midportion of the descending duodenum. This opening is known as the ampulla of Vater. The minor pancreatic duct, the duct of Santorini, may also empty into the duodenum as the minor papilla (Figs. 71.6 and 71.7).

The third, transverse, section is also retroperitoneal and is bordered by the uncinate process of the pancreas superiorly and the hepatic flexure of the colon anteriorly. The relationship of the duodenum to the colon is important during mobilization of the hepatic flexure during colon resection. Care must be taken to avoid injury to the duodenum. The superior mesenteric vessels run anterior to the transverse duodenum. The right ureter, right gonadal vessels, inferior vena cava, and aorta are posterior to the transverse duodenum.

The fourth portion of the duodenum courses in a cephalad direction to the left of the aorta and inferior to the neck of the pancreas. The end of the fourth portion is marked by the ligament of Treitz. The ligament serves as a point of fixation during intestinal rotation and runs from the right crus of the diaphragm and attaches to the intestinal wall at the duodenojejunal flexure.

JEJUNUM AND ILEUM

The jejunum and ileum lie within the peritoneal cavity and are anchored to the retroperitoneum by a broad-based mesentery. The average length of the jejunum and ileum is 5 meters: 40% jejunum, 60% ileum. The jejunum begins at the ligament of Treitz and the ileum ends at the ICV. The jejunum is located centrally in the abdomen, whereas the ileum lies mostly in the hypogastric region and pelvic cavity. There is no clear anatomic landmark that marks the transition from the end of the jejunum to the beginning of the ileum; they are instead distinguished by other anatomic characteristics. The jejunum has a thicker mucosal lining, thicker wall, larger diameter, less fatty mesentery, and longer and straighter vasa recta. Another distinguishing feature is the plicae circulares, also known as the valvulae conniventes, in the mucosa. Plicae circulares are transverse folds of mucosa and submucosa that aid in absorption of nutrients by increasing the surface area of the small intestine. These folds are deep and are visible on gross inspection even when the small intestine is distended (Fig. 71.8). They are prominent in the proximal intestine and diminish throughout the length of the small intestine. The plicae circulares are also visible radiographically, thus differentiating the small intestine from the large intestine, which is devoid of this feature.

ILEOCECAL VALVE

The ICV is a distinct feature of the small intestine and operates independently of the ileum or colon. It prevents the fecal contents in the colon from entering the small intestine and controls the flow of contents from the small intestine into the colon. The ability of the ICV to control the flow of digested contents may also help to prevent malabsorption and diarrhea. The valve is triggered by distention in the small intestine or the colon. If the ileum becomes distended, the valve will relax and allow the passage of contents from the small intestine into the

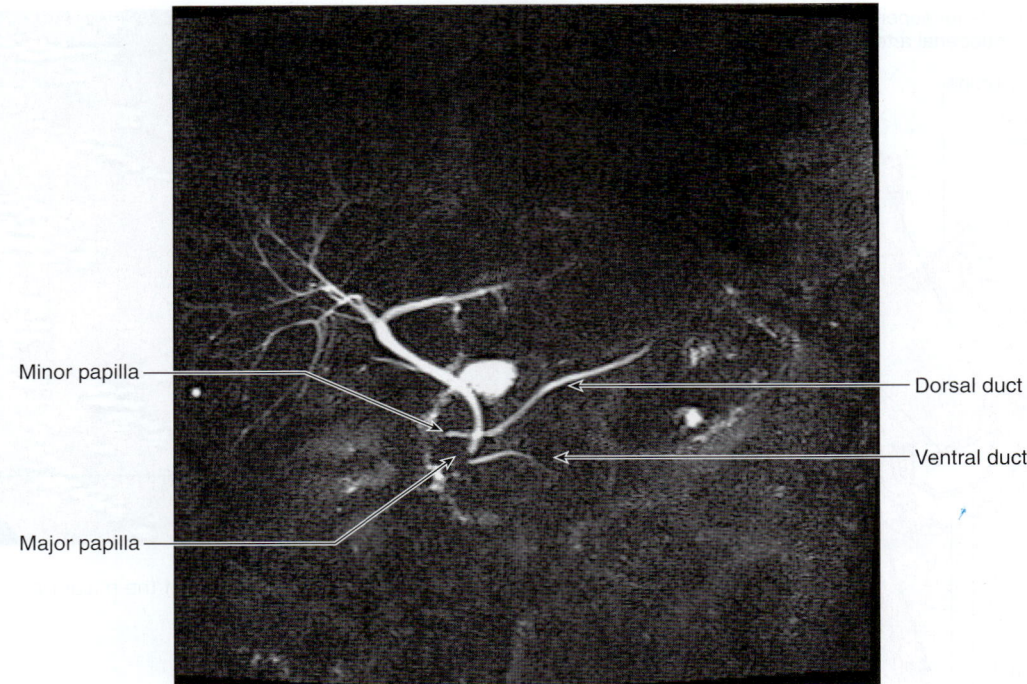

Minor papilla — Dorsal duct

Major papilla — Ventral duct

FIGURE 71.7 Magnetic resonance cholangiopancreatographic image demonstrating pancreas divisum with drainage of the dorsal duct through the minor papilla.

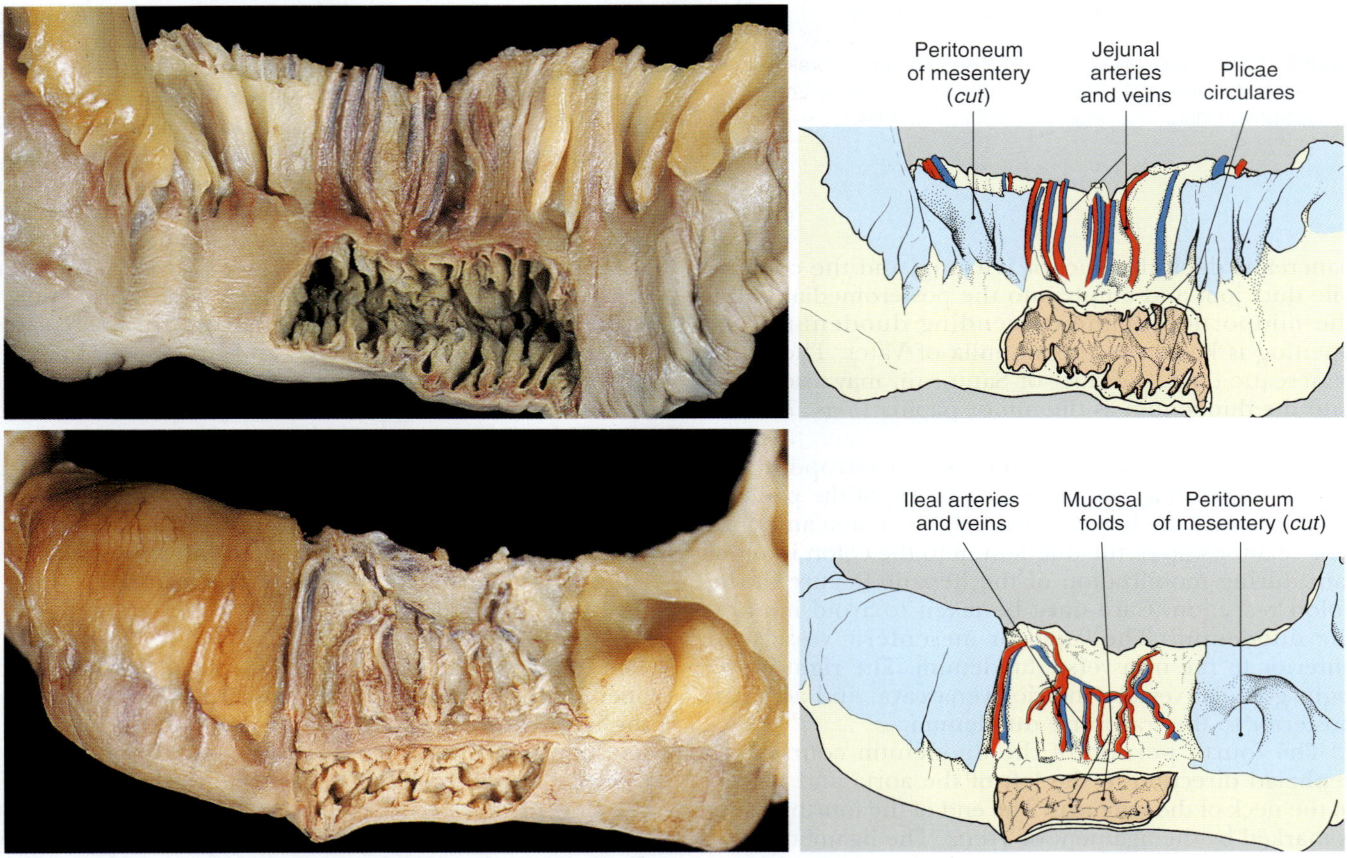

Peritoneum of mesentery (*cut*)   Jejunal arteries and veins   Plicae circulares

Ileal arteries and veins   Mucosal folds   Peritoneum of mesentery (*cut*)

FIGURE 71.8 Plicae circulares are transverse folds of mucosa and submucosa that aid in absorption. These folds are deep and are visible on gross inspection. (From Gosling JA. *Human Anatomy Color Atlas and Textbook*. 5th ed. Philadelphia: Mosby; 2009, Fig. 4.64, p. 176.)

colon. If the colon becomes distended, however, the valve will close by increasing its tone to prevent the passage of contents from the colon into the ileum.

The structure and neural control of the ICV are still being investigated. Recent work suggests that the valve forms from an intussusception of the ileum into the cecum and that the myenteric and submucosal plexuses are present within the valve along with interstitial cells of Cajal. Three muscle layers, an external circular, inner circular, and a longitudinal muscle layer, are continuous between the ileum and cecum, suggesting the mechanism for the propagation of motor activity from the ileum into the cecum.[4]

VASCULATURE ARTERIAL SUPPLY

The small intestine is derived from the embryonic gut tube regions of the foregut and midgut. The celiac artery supplies the foregut and the superior mesenteric artery (SMA) supplies the midgut. The duodenum is both a foregut and midgut structure and thus receives dual blood supply. The jejunum and ileum are midgut structures and receive arterial blood from the SMA only (Fig. 71.9).

The celiac trunk gives rise to the common hepatic artery, which divides into the proper hepatic artery and the GDA. The GDA supplies branches to the duodenum, stomach, and pancreas. The anterior superior and posterior superior pancreaticoduodenal arteries arise from the GDA and supply blood to the second and third portions of the duodenum as well as the pancreas.

The SMA branches directly off of the aorta and supplies blood to the pancreas and to the second half of the duodenum to the mid transverse colon. The SMA gives rise to several branches that are important surgically. The posterior inferior and anterior inferior pancreaticoduodenal arteries anastomose with the superior pancreaticoduodenal arteries from the GDA to supply blood to the duodenum and pancreas. The intestinal arteries are branches from the SMA that create a unique network of arteries known as an arcade that supply the jejunum and ileum. Arterial branches known as vasa recta course from the arcade to the intestinal wall. These arteries then bifurcate and travel along the intestinal wall to provide adequate blood flow. The vasa recta represent another anatomic variant to help distinguish the jejunum from the ileum. The vasa recta of the jejunum are straight and long, whereas those supplying blood to the ileum are arborized and short (refer to Fig. 71.8). The ileocolic artery supplies blood to the ileum, cecum, right colon, and appendix.

VENOUS DRAINAGE

The venous drainage of the small intestine mirrors the arterial supply. The duodenum empties into the pancreaticoduodenal, the right gastroepiploic, and the portal vein. The jejunum and ileum are drained by the superior mesenteric vein, which joins with the splenic vein to drain into the portal vein (Fig. 71.10).

LYMPHATICS

There are several levels of lymphatic drainage of the small intestine that follow the vasculature. The lymph drains into the nodal chain adjacent to the bowel wall and then into the nodes of the mesenteric arcade. From there the lymphatic vessels follow along the trunk of the SMA and join with the two lumbar lymphatic trunks to drain into the cisterna chyli. The cisterna chyli is located below the level of the diaphragm at the end of the thoracic duct anterior to the lumbar spine and posterior to the aorta. Once lymph collects in this dilated sac, it will then pass through the aortic opening of the diaphragm and flow into the main thoracic duct. The thoracic duct runs parallel with the aorta and empties into the left subclavian vein where it joins the jugular vein (Fig. 71.11).

INNERVATION

The innervation of the small intestine is composed of two separate systems that function independently. The autonomic nervous system (ANS) is derived from the central nervous system (CNS). The ENS is a specialized nervous system found only in the GI tract. This system is composed of neurons that lie within the bowel wall that respond to local and systemic stimulation. Parasympathetic and sympathetic nerve fibers connect the ENS to the CNS and can modulate the activity of the ENS in response to external stimuli. The ENS also functions independently, regulating its own function in response to intrinsic stimuli. There are also sensory neurons in the bowel wall that provide feedback to the ENS, the sympathetic system, the spinal cord, and the brainstem.

AUTONOMIC NERVOUS SYSTEM

The ANS is composed of sympathetic and parasympathetic nerve fibers. The sympathetic innervation to the intestine is derived from nerve fibers located in the thoracolumbar spinal cord between segments T5 and L2. The paravertebral ganglia are located along either side of the vertebral column and span the length of the spinal cord. The prevertebral ganglia include the celiac, mesenteric, and hypogastric ganglia and are located along the aorta and its branches. The sympathetic innervation travels via preganglionic and postganglionic fibers. The sympathetic system secretes norepinephrine, which results in a direct inhibition of the smooth muscle. It also works indirectly by stimulating an inhibitory response from the ENS. Stimulation of the sympathetic system results in decreased intestinal motility, decreased secretion, and vasoconstriction.

The parasympathetic system is composed of nerve fibers that leave the CNS via the cranial nerves and the sacral spinal nerves. The paired vagus nerve (cranial nerve X) provides parasympathetic innervation to the thoracic and abdominal viscera, which includes the pyloric sphincter and small intestine. The parasympathetic nervous system, like the sympathetic system, has preganglionic and postganglionic neurons. The length and location of these nerve fibers and neurons is a distinguishing feature between the parasympathetic and sympathetic systems. The preganglionic parasympathetic fibers are relatively long and often pass uninterrupted from the CNS to the viscera. In the small intestine, the postganglionic neurons are located within the bowel wall as part of the myenteric and submucosal plexuses. The postganglionic nerve fibers are very short because they have only a minimal distance

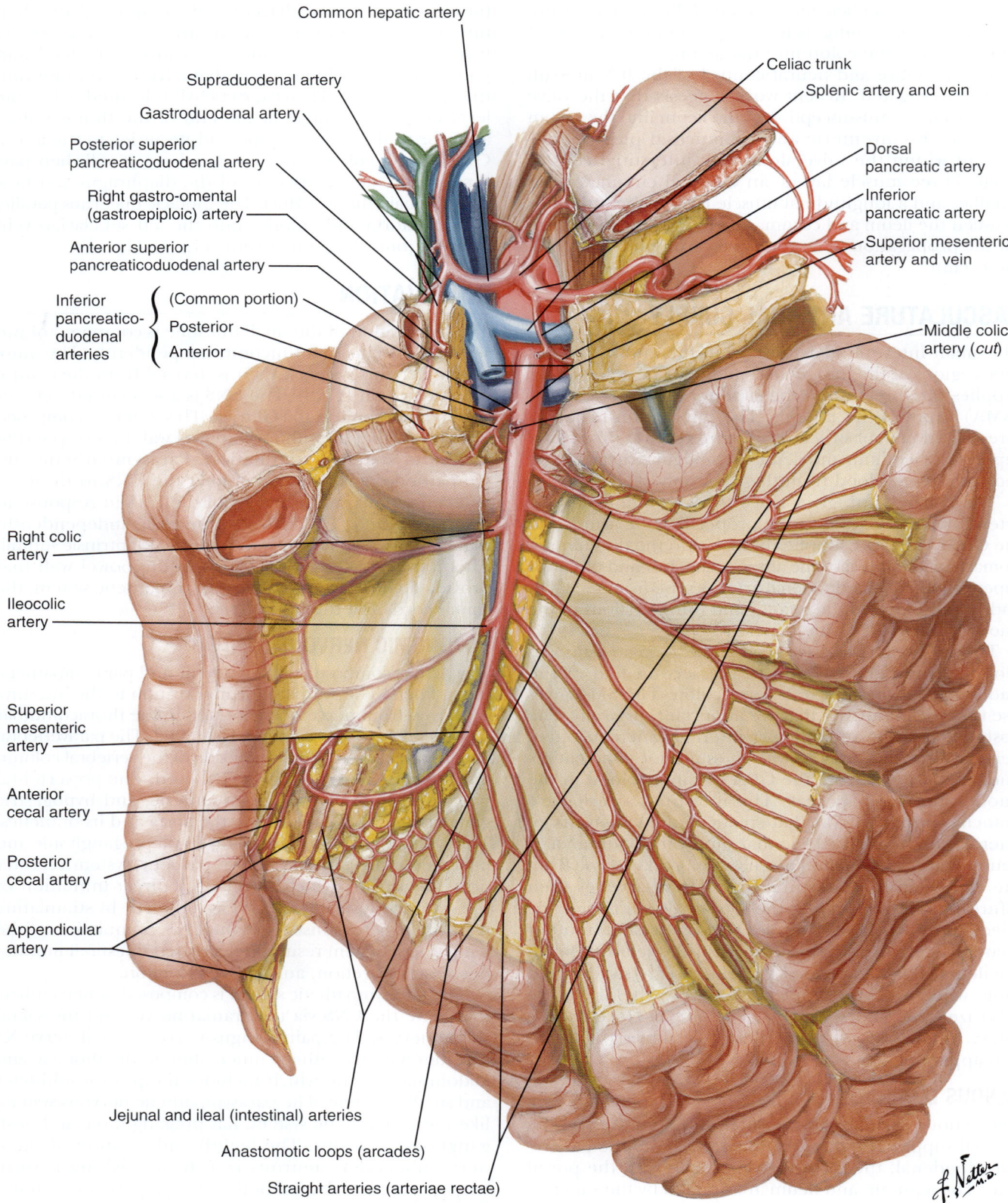

Common hepatic artery

Supraduodenal artery

Gastroduodenal artery

Posterior superior
pancreaticoduodenal artery

Right gastro-omental
(gastroepiploic) artery

Anterior superior
pancreaticoduodenal artery

Inferior
pancreatico-
duodenal
arteries
{ (Common portion)
Posterior
Anterior

Celiac trunk

Splenic artery and vein

Dorsal
pancreatic artery

Inferior
pancreatic artery

Superior mesenteric
artery and vein

Middle colic
artery (cut)

Right colic
artery

Ileocolic
artery

Superior
mesenteric
artery

Anterior
cecal artery

Posterior
cecal artery

Appendicular
artery

Jejunal and ileal (intestinal) arteries

Anastomotic loops (arcades)

Straight arteries (arteriae rectae)

FIGURE 71.9 Arterial anatomy of the small intestine. (Netter illustration from http://www.netterimages.com. Copyright Elsevier Inc. All rights reserved.)

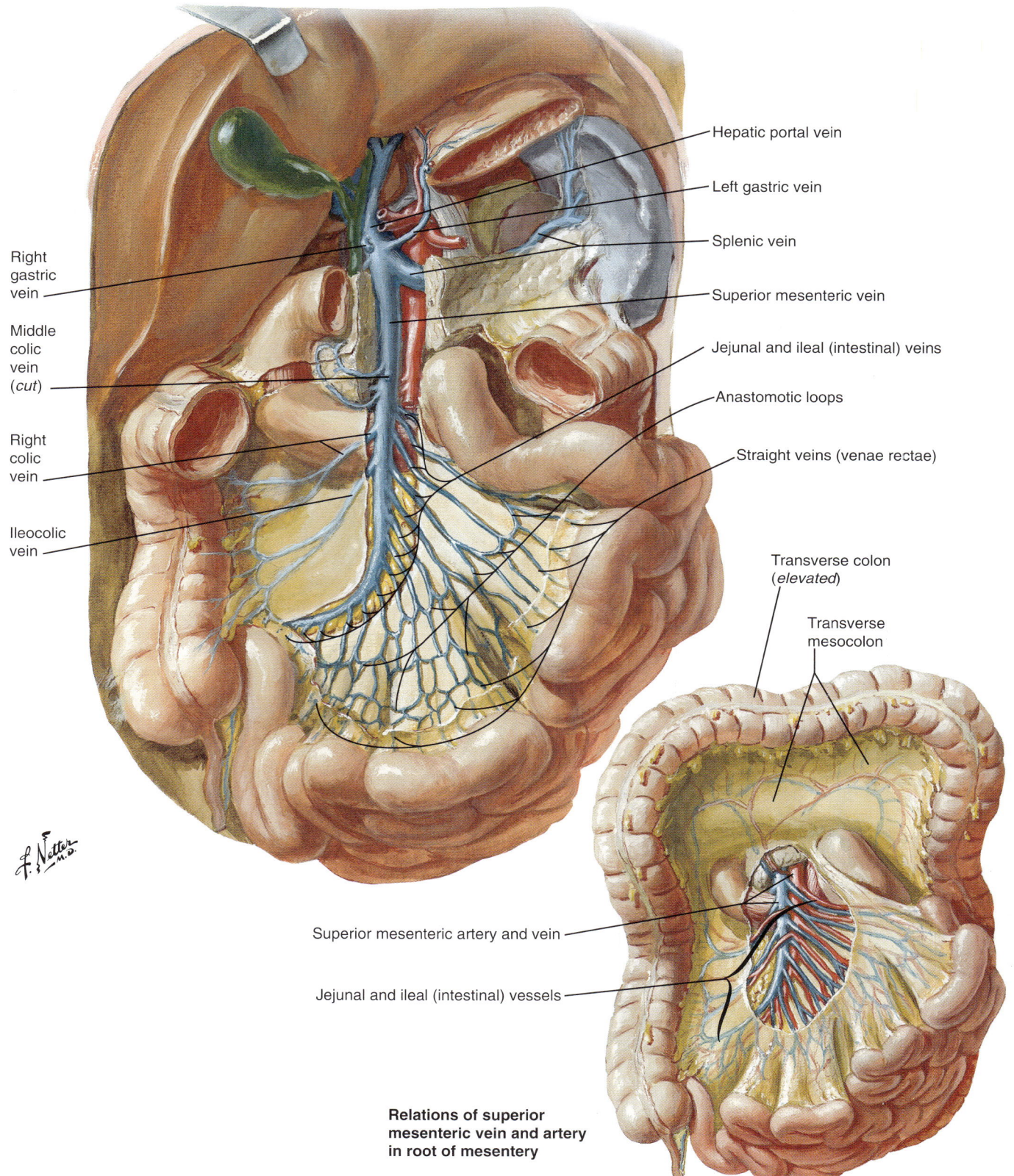

Hepatic portal vein

Left gastric vein

Splenic vein

Superior mesenteric vein

Jejunal and ileal (intestinal) veins

Anastomotic loops

Straight veins (venae rectae)

Right gastric vein

Middle colic vein (*cut*)

Right colic vein

Ileocolic vein

Transverse colon (*elevated*)

Transverse mesocolon

Superior mesenteric artery and vein

Jejunal and ileal (intestinal) vessels

Relations of superior mesenteric vein and artery in root of mesentery

FIGURE 71.10 Venous anatomy of the small intestine. (Netter illustration from http://www.netterimages.com. Copyright Elsevier Inc. All rights reserved.)

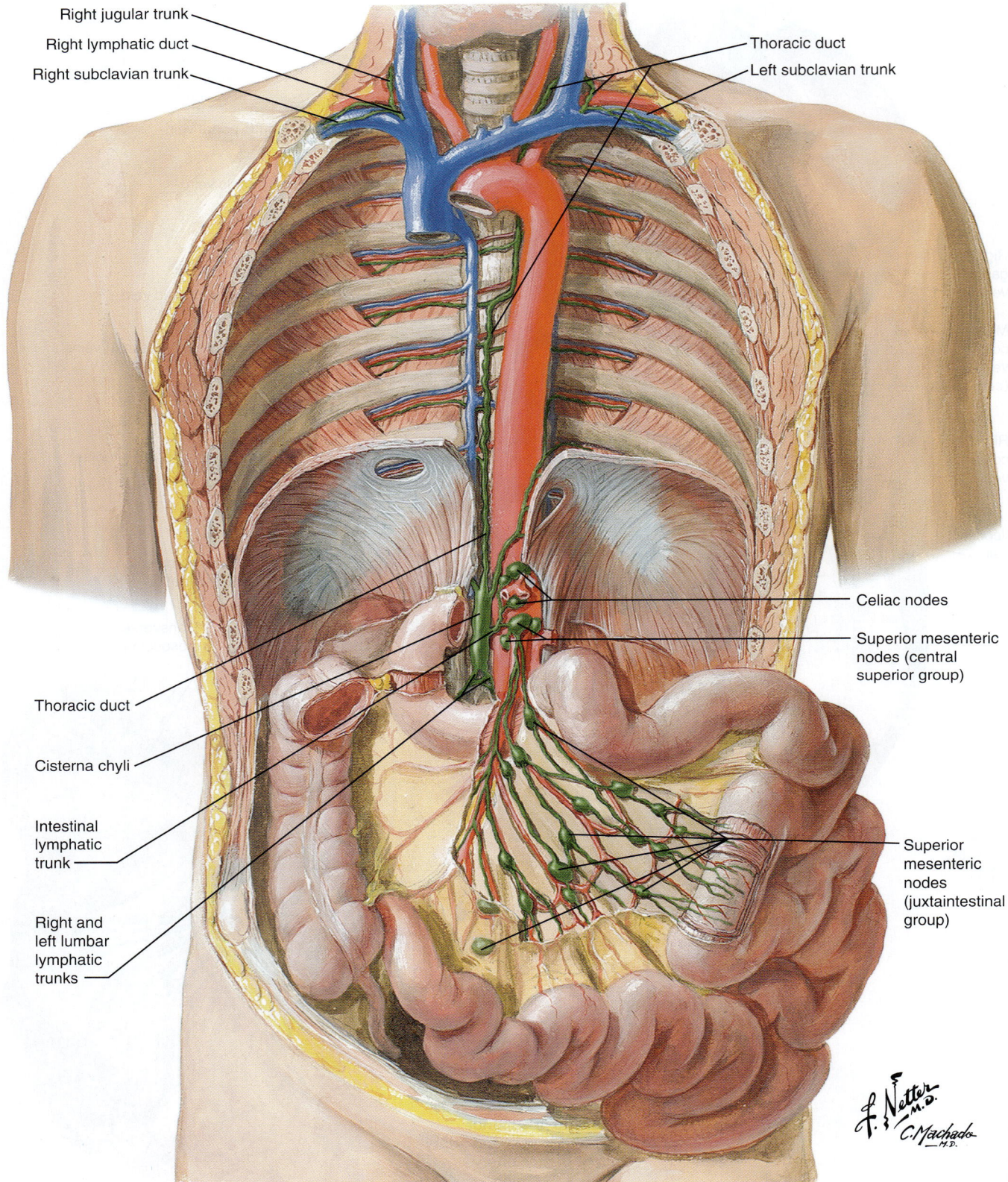

Right jugular trunk

Right lymphatic duct

Right subclavian trunk

Thoracic duct

Left subclavian trunk

Celiac nodes

Superior mesenteric nodes (central superior group)

Thoracic duct

Cisterna chyli

Intestinal lymphatic trunk

Right and left lumbar lymphatic trunks

Superior mesenteric nodes (juxtaintestinal group)

FIGURE 71.11 Lymphatic anatomy of the small intestine. (Netter illustration from http://www.netterimages.com. Copyright Elsevier Inc. All rights reserved.)

to travel to innervate the surrounding tissue. When the intestine is under the influence of parasympathetic stimulation, there is increased intestinal motility and secretion.

ENTERIC NERVOUS SYSTEM

The ENS is an independently functioning system that can affect motility, secretion, vascular tone, and hormone release in the small intestine. The system, derived from the neural crest, is made up of more than 100 million neurons. The vagal neural crest is the source of the precursors that give rise to the ENS.[5] Sacral neural crest cells also play a role in populating the distal gut; however their purpose is less well understood. Neural crest cells populate the gut via two main pathways: the RET/GFRα1/GDNF pathway and the EDNRB/Endothelin-3 pathway. This is significant because while loss-of-function mutations in the RET gene are associated with Hirschsprung disease, gain-of-function mutations are associated with neuroendocrine neoplasms.[6] The cell bodies lie within the bowel wall and reside within two named plexuses. The myenteric, or Auerbach, plexus is located between the longitudinal and circular muscle layers. The submucosal, or Meissner, plexus is located in the submucosa of the bowel wall between the circular muscle layer and mucosa. Once the myenteric plexus is populated with neural crest cells, they migrate inward to populate the submucosal plexus. This process is driven by netrins.[7]

The myenteric plexus runs the entire length of the intestinal wall and provides innervation to the muscular layers. Its main function is to control motor activity of the intestine. Stimulation of the myenteric plexus can result in excitatory or inhibitory effects. Excitatory effects include increased intestinal wall tone, increased intensity and rate of rhythmic contractions, and increased velocity of excitatory waves resulting in increased peristalsis. When inhibitory peptides are released, they act at the pyloric valve and ICV.

The submucosal plexus provides innervation to intestinal glands, endocrine cells, and blood vessels. It works at a local level to control the secretion, absorption, and contraction within each segment of the intestine.[8]

SMALL INTESTINAL MOTILITY

Small intestinal motility is regulated through a combination of myogenic, neural, and hormonal factors. Of these three, myogenic factors are the most important. Neural and hormonal factors act to modify myogenic-initiated motor patterns. Intestinal motor activity can persist even with complete blockade of neural signals.

Intestinal motor activity exists in two phases: a fed state and a fasting, or interdigestive, state. During the fed state, food is moved along the intestine via segmentation and peristalsis. Segmentation is characterized by a pattern of pressure waves traveling short distances that serve to mix chyme and enhance its contact with the villous surfaces. The peristaltic pattern moves food along the intestine by a muscular contraction proximal to the food bolus and relaxation distal to the bolus.[9]

Motor activity continues during the interdigestive state via the migratory motor complex (MMC). The purpose of this activity is to propel undigested material through

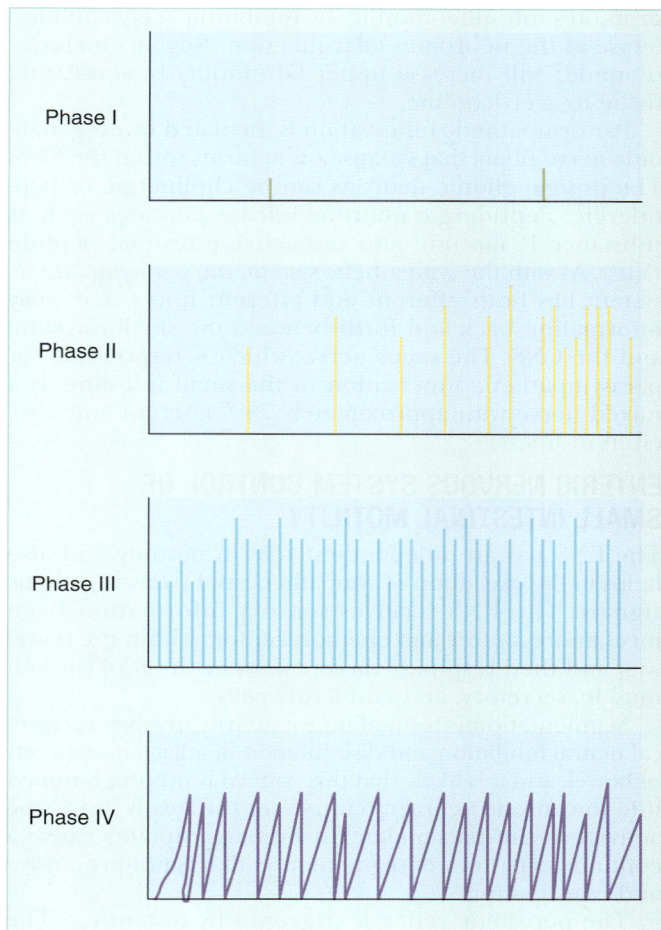

FIGURE 71.12 Diagrammatic representation of the four phases of the migratory motor complex. Amplitudes versus time are displayed.

the small intestine and into the colon. It also prevents reflux of bacteria from the colon into the terminal ileum. The MMC begins in the stomach and moves distal. Peristalsis occurs when these MMC electrical spikes are superimposed on intrinsic pacemaker potentials.[10] There are three phases of the MMC. Phase I is characterized by an absence of motor activity, phase II consists of disorganized high-pressure waves that are accelerating in rate and occur intermittently, phase III is characterized by a continuous high rate of rhythmic contractions, and in phase IV the contractions once again become intermittent. This cycle repeats every 1.5 to 2 hours (Fig. 71.12).

AUTONOMIC NERVOUS SYSTEM CONTROL OF MOTILITY

Sympathetic control of the small bowel synapses on the ENS and directly innervates smooth muscle, endocrine, and secretory cells. When the sympathetic system is stimulated, digestive and secretory functions are inhibited. Studies suggest that sympathetic tone primarily acts to lower propulsive force. α-Adrenoreceptors, with $α_1$ being most important, have been well demonstrated to inhibit intestinal motility in humans and animals.[11,12] Neostigmine promotes intestinal motility by inhibiting acetylcholinesterase at the neuromuscular junction. Reglan (metoclopramide) will increase upper GI motility by sensitizing tissue to acetylcholine.

Parasympathetic innervation is mediated by preganglionic nerve fibers that synapse on neurons within the ENS. The postganglionic neurons can be cholinergic or peptidergic. Peptidergic neurons release peptides such as substance P, motilin, and vasoactive intestinal peptide (VIP). As with the sympathetic system, the parasympathetic system has both efferent and afferent fibers that relay information back and forth between the small intestine and the CNS. The vagus nerve, which is responsible for parasympathetic innervation to the small intestine, is a mixed nerve with approximately 75% afferent and 25% efferent fibers.

ENTERIC NERVOUS SYSTEM CONTROL OF SMALL INTESTINAL MOTILITY

The ENS has an independent role in motility and also helps in the execution of sympathetic and parasympathetic signals. The ENS receives sensory information from mechanoreceptors and chemoreceptors within the bowel wall and then responds via direct innervation of smooth muscle, secretory, and endocrine cells.

Segmentation intestinal motor activity involves reciprocal neural inhibition and disinhibition of adjacent segments of bowel, and it is likely that this pattern is preprogrammed into the enteric neural circuitry with the steady burst-type activity as the pacemaker. In humans, opiates cause a continuous pattern of segmentation that is nonpropulsive and constipating.

The peristaltic reflex is triggered by distention. The peristaltic reflex consists of a reciprocal action that propels chyme along the small intestine. Immediately behind the bolus, longitudinal muscle relaxes and lengthens, whereas circular muscle contracts. Ahead of the bolus, the longitudinal muscle contracts, expanding the lumen, and circular muscle relaxes (Fig. 71.13). The precise sequential nature of this motor pattern compared to segmentation suggests that the neural pattern required for this is more complex. The contraction is thought to be mediated by acetylcholine and substance P, whereas the relaxation is mediated by VIP and nitric oxide. Several lines of evidence suggest serotonin and substance P are involved in initiating and maintaining peristalsis.[13] Infusion of partially digested triglycerides into the ileum has an inhibitory effect on jejunal motility and increases small intestinal transit time, the *ileal brake reflex*. This allows more time for nutrient absorption when the absorptive capacity of the more proximal small intestine is limited by accelerated transit or mucosal disease. Peptide YY released from ileal endocrine cells has been suggested as a possible effector of this reflex, and was found experimentally to be significantly correlated with lowering of jejunal peristalsis.[14]

HORMONAL CONTROL OF SMALL INTESTINE MOTILITY

Multiple hormones have a role in modifying motor activity in the small intestine. All act through modification of the electrical and contractile patterns. The pacemaker activity of the small intestine is consistent with a pacemaker focus

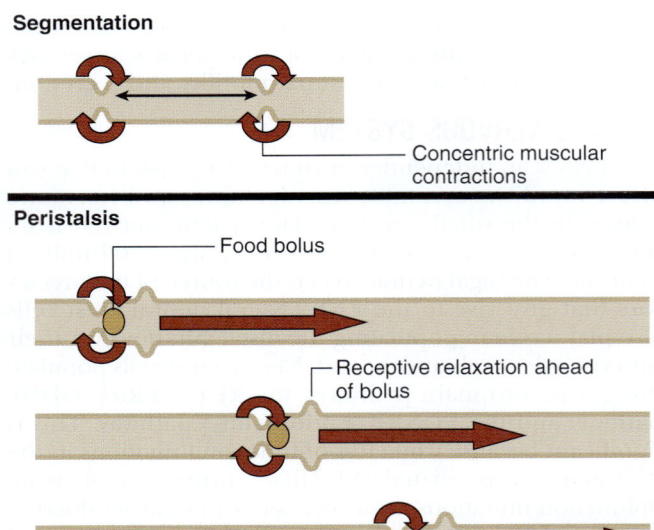

Segmentation

Concentric muscular contractions

Peristalsis

Food bolus

Receptive relaxation ahead of bolus

FIGURE 71.13 Mechanisms of peristalsis. The peristaltic pattern moves food along the intestine by a muscular contraction proximal to the food bolus and relaxation distal to the bolus. (Modified from http://leavingbio.net/Human%20Nutrition/Human%20Nutrition_files/image018.jpg.)

TABLE 71.1 Hormonal Control of Small Intestinal Motility

Hormone	Actions
PROMOTILITY	
Gastrin	Increased contraction rate
CCK	Smooth muscle contraction; increased mixing of intestinal contents, increased intestinal transit
Motilin	Increased intestinal transit
VIP	Duodenal contractions; increased motility
ANTIMOTILITY	
Secretin	Reduced contractility, more pronounced in duodenum
Glucagon	Inhibitory effect globally

CCK, Cholecystokinin; *VIP,* vasoactive intestinal peptide.

in the proximal duodenum. The periodic rate of the proximal pacemaker operates at a higher frequency than do pacemaker cells more distally, and thereby override and drive distal pacemaker activity at this higher rate. Distally in the distal jejunum and ileum, there is a declining ability to overdrive pacemaker activity at a higher rate, setting up a gradient of gradual distal slowing of pacemaker activity.

How GI hormones modulate the intrinsic small intestinal pacemaker has been a subject of much study. The pharmacodynamics of many GI hormones, including gastrin, cholecystokinin (CCK), and secretin, are similar in that they show a rapid rise up to a peak level within approximately 20 to 40 minutes and thereafter a fall (Table 71.1).

Most experimental evidence is in agreement that gastrin increases the number of contractions of the small intestine. Its effect on intestinal transit time is less clear; however, findings from a study of serum levels of GI hormones on patients with functional bowel diseases clearly demonstrated that gastrin peak levels and total response were impaired in those patients with constipation-predominant symptoms.[15]

CCK increases action potentials in smooth muscle occurring in line with pacemaker potentials. Overall this increases mixing of intraluminal contents and speeds propulsion through the small intestine. However, there is one region of the small intestine where this does not hold true; in the region of the sphincter of Oddi, CCK relaxes intestinal smooth muscle.[16]

The effect of motilin is similar to the effects of gastrin and CCK. Motilin increases small bowel action potentials without increasing the rate of pacemaker activity; however, its stimulatory activity is greatest proximally and diminishes beyond the duodenum progressively. Motilin does accelerate small intestinal transit through an increase of small bowel propulsive contractions, but its potency is only about half of that of CCK.

Vasoactive intestinal peptide has been shown to cause duodenal muscle contraction in some experiments, but its overall effect is unclear. Small doses appear to cause a muscular reaction, whereas larger doses result in a biphasic response, where an initial relaxation is followed by increased muscle tone and sustained contractions. Experimental evidence is consistent with VIP having a stimulatory effect on motility.

In contrast to motilin, secretin reduces contractility and action potentials in the small bowel without having a significant effect on the duodenal pacemaker. This inhibitory effect on contractility is greatest proximally and steadily decreases distally. Secretin also opposes the action of CCK and can prevent CCK-induced contractions, but this can be overcome by large amounts of CCK.

Glucagon has generally been found to have an inhibitory effect on small intestinal motility; however, it does stimulate small intestinal action potentials in low doses.[16,17]

Prostaglandin E_1 has also been found to speed GI motility. Oral ingestion has led to rapid development of abdominal colic and diarrhea.[18]

Hormonal Effects on Integrated Patterns of Small Bowel Motility

Motilin is believed to be the initiating factor of the MMC motor pattern, with CCK and gastrin opposing it. Plasma motilin levels have been found to be elevated during the initiation of bursts of action potentials and contractions in the stomach and duodenum, with levels falling as the bursts travel distally through the small intestine. Exogenous CCK disrupts the initiation and propagation of this motor pattern, whereas secretin delays the initiation of burst-type electrical activity and reduces the number of action potentials without affecting the distal propagation of electrical activity (Fig. 71.14).[16]

Serotonin is stored in the small intestine and secreted from it in large amounts, both prandially and postprandially. There are serotonin receptors on neurons, endothelial cells, and smooth muscle cells. Serotonin has an important

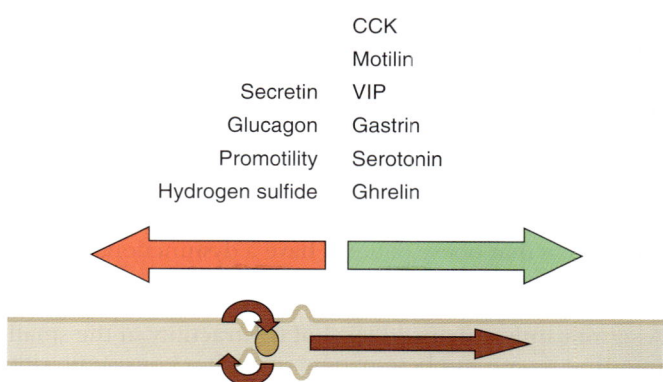

FIGURE 71.14 Hormonal effects on integrated patterns of small bowel motility. The *green arrow* indicates promotility and the *red arrow* indicates inhibition of motility. *CCK,* Cholecystokinin; *ViP,* vasoactive intestinal peptide.

physiologic effect during digestion by causing intestinal hyperemia, motility, and secretion. In patients with irritable bowel syndrome, modulation of serotonin levels with selective serotonin receptor agonists or antagonists has been demonstrated to successfully treat patients with constipation and diarrhea-predominant disease.[19,20]

Ghrelin, a protein with 50% homology to motilin, stimulates the MMC and causes increased motility in the small intestine.[21,22]

FACTORS AFFECTING SMALL BOWEL MOTILITY

Systemic Disease

It is well recognized that certain patients with digestive diseases have altered small intestinal motility. It was recognized in 1977 that patients with small intestinal bacterial overgrowth also had small intestinal dysmotility.[23] A high proportion of patients with irritable bowel syndrome were initially identified as having small intestinal bacterial overgrowth; however, this is controversial because of the low sensitivity of the lactulose breath test that was used for diagnosis. Disordered small intestine motility has been demonstrated in patients with liver disease and portal hypertension, and in patients with nonalcoholic steatohepatitis (NASH). A subsequent study identified small intestinal bacterial overgrowth in approximately one-third of cirrhotic patients. NASH patients in a separate study were found to have a higher baseline level of hydrogen by the lactulose breath test. Abnormal small intestinal motility has also been demonstrated in patients with chronic renal failure.[24]

Colonic Distention

Patients with functional bowel disorders have an association between disordered upper GI motility and colorectal dysfunction. This may reflect inappropriate activation of visceral reflexes. In one human study, rectal distention during the fasting state increased the incidence of the MMC and decreased duodenal contractility, whereas in the fed state the effect on decreasing motility was even more profound and the rate of small intestinal transit was significantly slowed.[25]

Obesity

Obesity has also been suggested as a factor that modulates the rate of small bowel transit. Considering that the rate of small intestinal transit plays a critical role in determining the rate of food intake, satiety, digestion, and absorption of nutrients, it has been questioned whether there is an association between obesity and small intestinal dysmotility. This, however, has not been thoroughly studied. There are reports that obese patients have a dysfunctional MMC, with the result that contractile action of the small intestine is more prominent in the fasting state in obese subjects. A significantly enhanced level of contractility in the small intestine is seen in obese patients, which is consistent with a neutrally mediated etiology. Such increased contractility may lead to more rapid nutrient absorption and loss of postprandial satiety.[26,27]

Circadian Rhythm Disruption

Circadian rhythms drive cell proliferation as well as motor and secretory activity in the GI tract and liver. Disruption of the sleep-wake cycle has been demonstrated to result in many GI pathologies including irritable bowel syndrome (IBS), gastroesophageal reflux disease (GERD), and peptic ulcer disease (PUD). Circadian disruption also accelerates aging and promotes tumorgenesis in the GI tract. Treatment with melatonin has shown a protective effect on GI mucosa and improves symptoms in patients with functional GI disorders.[10]

SMALL INTESTINAL SECRETION

The small intestine has a multitude of tightly regulated secretory functions, and their disruption is prominent in certain GI disease states. Secretion may be through passive or active transport. Passive transport is driven by an existing electrochemical gradient, whereas active transport is an energy-requiring process that acts against a gradient. Small intestinal secretions include mucin, bicarbonate, and water.

MUCIN SECRETION

The mucin layer, produced by goblet cells, is a vital part of the innate immunity of the GI tract. Its production is regulated by immune mediators: leukotrienes, interferon, interleukin (IL)-9, IL-13.[28] The mucin layer in the stomach and duodenum is approximately 80 to 280 μm thick and creates a pH gradient that protects the mucosa (Fig. 71.15). The mucin also creates an antimicrobial barrier. The mucin glycoproteins are toxic to many bacteria and the mucin lattice provides an anchor for immunoglobulin A (IgA) and antimicrobial peptides.[28] Other protective measures include the production of potent vasodilators, nitric oxide, and prostaglandins, as well as angiogenic growth factors to help maintain adequate blood flow to the intestinal mucosa.[29,30] Along with mucin, intestinal bicarbonate is the first line of defense against mucosal damage by acid and pepsin. The duodenum secretes the highest rate of bicarbonate per unit of area. Duodenal

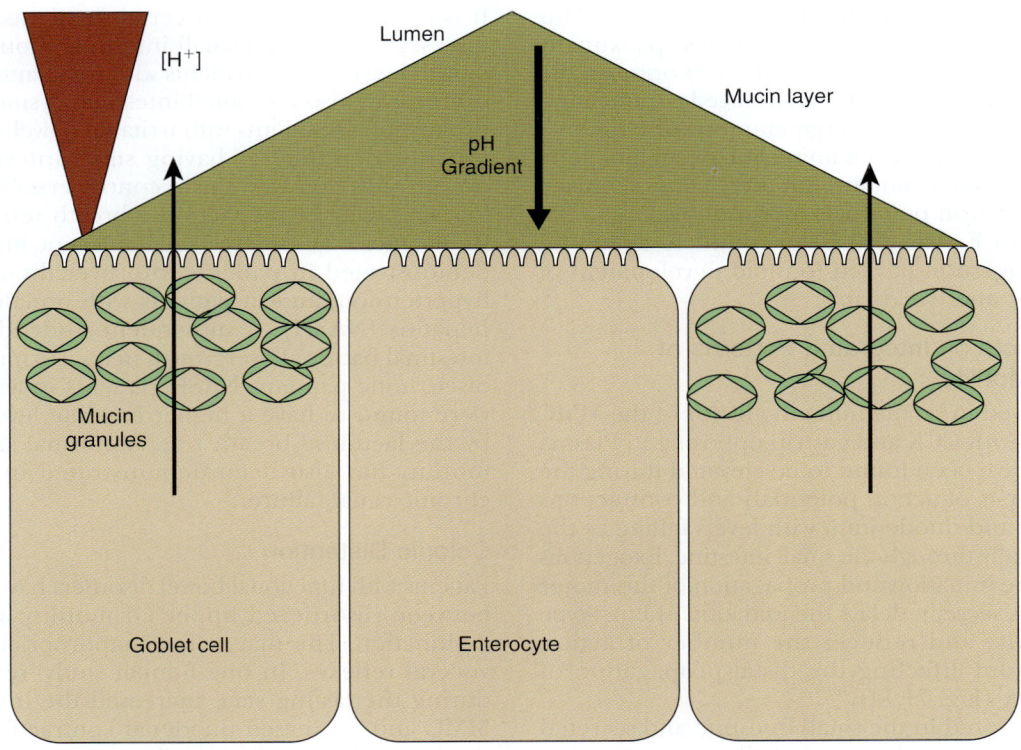

FIGURE 71.15 Mucin secretion in the proximal small intestine. Mucin combined with bicarbonate secretion establishes a pH gradient that protects the mucosal surface from damage by acidic luminal contents.

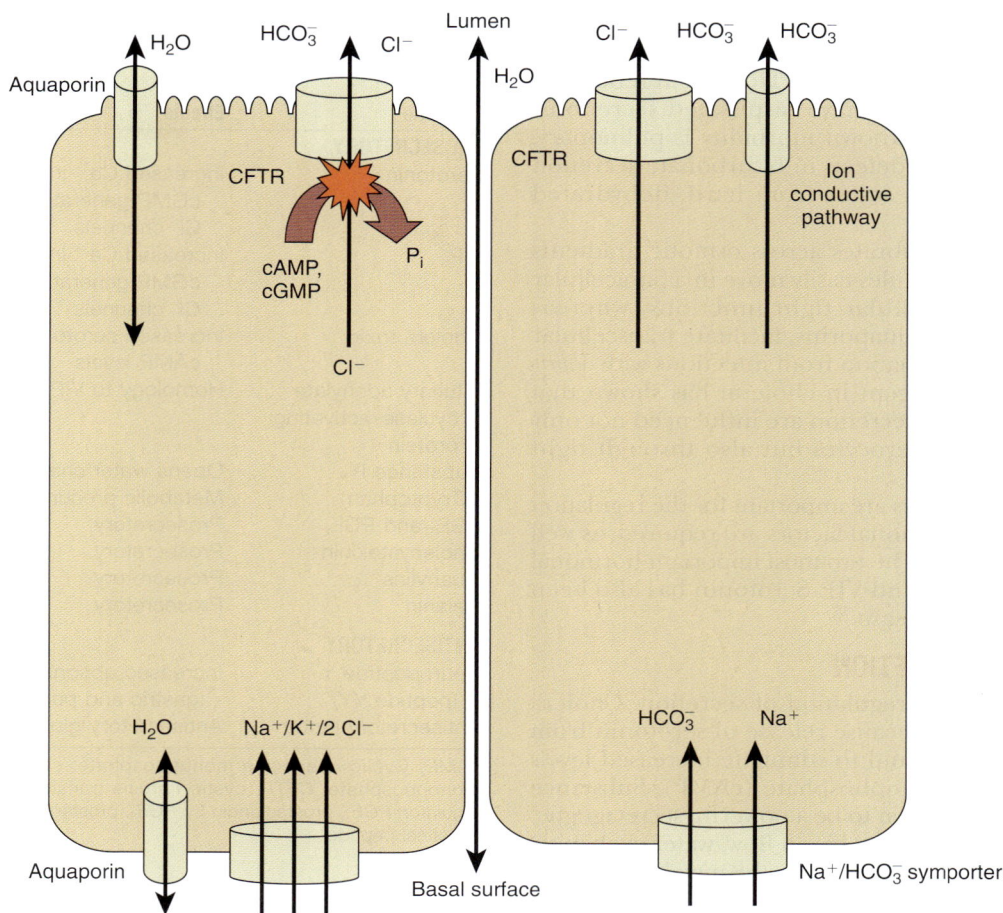

FIGURE 71.16 Movement of water and bicarbonate through small intestinal enterocytes by transcellular and paracellular methods. *cAMP*, Cyclic adenosine monophosphate; *CFTR*, cystic fibrosis transmembrane conductance regulator; *cGMP*, cyclic guanosine monophosphate.

bicarbonate production is estimated to neutralize approximately 40% of the total postprandial acid load to ensure that the pH in duodenal mucus is maintained at neutral under all conditions of gastric acidities. The precise mechanism that senses duodenal acid remains unknown.

Duodenal bicarbonate secretion is driven by the cystic fibrosis transmembrane conductance regulator (CFTR) and by an apical anion conductive pathway (Fig. 71.16). The CFTR transport process requires energy, and the action of carbonic anhydrase is also required for efficient HCO_3^- transport. Duodenal HCO_3^- secretion is under paracrine, hormonal, and neural control of the ENS and CNS. Despite their proximity to the stomach, these two organs achieve secretory control in important and different ways. Duodenal bicarbonate secretion markedly increases in response to the presence of duodenal acid. This is mediated by both neural reflexes and prostaglandin activity. The neural effectors are believed to include VIP and acetylcholine.

The peptides guanylin and uroguanylin have an important role in the local control of bicarbonate secretion. These endogenous proteins are secreted by enterochromaffin cells of the duodenum. They both markedly increase HCO_3^- secretion by increasing cellular cyclic guanosine monophosphate (cGMP) and thereby driving the action of CFTR. Uroguanylin is most abundant in the proximal small intestine, and its release is stimulated by low pH in the duodenum. Dopamine also controls HCO_3^- secretion. D_1, but not D_2, receptor stimulation has been demonstrated to lead to HCO_3^- secretion in both animal models and human studies.

The action of the sympathetic nervous system is also important in modulating duodenal HCO_3^- secretion. Overall, the sympathetic nervous system appears to have a potent inhibitory effect on HCO_3^- secretion by the duodenum, which likely influences the ability of the mucosal lining to protect itself from acid-mediated injury.[29]

WATER SECRETION IN THE SMALL INTESTINE

Although the small intestine has a net absorptive balance of water transit, it concurrently secretes water to solubilize and dilute intraluminal nutrients and maintain intraluminal fluidity. The movement of water is both transcellular and paracellular. It is generally accepted, although not conclusively proven, that water movement into the lumen is dependent on a Cl^- gradient established by CFTR.[31] Recent studies in mice have further supported the role of CFTR in establishing this anion gradient.[32] Certain disease states associated with abnormal chloride transport provide evidence for this hypothesis. Patients with cystic fibrosis, in which there is a defect in the CFTR protein rendering it hypo- or nonfunctional, have inspissated secretions. Although the most well-known morbidity is pulmonary, these patients also have defects in bicarbonate secretion from the pancreas and suffer from hard, dehydrated stools.

Water passively equilibrates across osmotic gradients in two ways. Water molecules easily move in a paracellular route through intercellular tight junctions, whereas water channels, called aquaporins, facilitate transcellular water movement. Information from infections with *Vibrio cholerae*, the causative agent in cholera, has shown that water permeability and secretion are influenced not only by ion channels in enterocytes but also through tight junctions.[31,33,34]

A multitude of effectors are important for the regulation of water secretion. Hormonal factors are required, as well as signaling by the ENS. The two most important hormonal effectors are serotonin and VIP. Serotonin has also been found to trigger VIP release.[35]

REGULATION OF SECRETION

The ENS is involved in regulation of secretion. Cholera toxin has been found to cause release of serotonin from enterochromaffin cells and to stimulate increased levels of cyclic adenosine monophosphate (cAMP). Substance P has also been long known to be a powerful secretagogue. Substance P causes increased blood flow, water exchange, and intestinal motility. L-Tryptophan, the metabolic precursor of serotonin, also stimulates secretion. Histamine affects H_2 receptors in the small intestine that are known to control secretion. Prostaglandins are also involved, specifically prostaglandin $(PG)E_1$ and PGE_2. Several other molecules, including CCK, guanylins, and galanin, are all prosecretory.

Peptide YY is the major antisecretory hormone. It has a range of effects, including slowing motility to lengthen contact time of intraluminal contents with the absorptive epithelial lining, and has been associated with the ileal brake, the primary inhibitory feedback mechanism that slows transit of a meal through the gut.[36] It also inhibits gastric and pancreatic secretions as well as chloride secretion. A more recently discovered neuropeptide called antisecretory factor is another potent effector and can be induced by certain types of partially hydrolyzed complex carbohydrates. This has important clinical application in patients with inflammatory bowel disease. In trials where patients are given cereal made with partially hydrolyzed complex carbohydrates, the antisecretory factor synthesis is triggered and most patients report subjective improvement (Table 71.2, Fig. 71.17).[34,35,37–39]

Small intestinal secretion and absorption must be tightly regulated because any derangement in this tight balance may have major physiologic consequences, as in the case of cholera infection. The degree of regulation is highlighted by the handling of nitric oxide (NO) in the small intestine. It behaves chemically as a free radical but its effects persist for only seconds. This makes for an ideal mechanism of regulation by nervous or hormonal signaling because its action can be quickly switched on and off.

TABLE 71.2 Hormonal Control of Small Intestinal Secretion

Hormone	Effects
PROSECRETORY	
Serotonin	Increased Ca^{2+} influx, cAMP and cGMP generation, opening of Cl^- channels
VIP	Increased Ca^{2+} influx, cAMP and cGMP generation, opening of Cl^- channels
Cholera toxin	Increased serotonin levels, increased cAMP levels
Pituitary adenylate cyclase–activating protein	Homology to VIP; receptors in ileum
Substance P	Opens water channels; affects CFTR
L-Tryptophan	Metabolic precursor of serotonin
PGE_1 and PGE_2	Prosecretory
Cholecystokinin	Prosecretory
Guanylins	Prosecretory
Galanin	Prosecretory
ANTISECRETORY	
Neuropeptide Y (peptide YY)	Increased absorptive time, decreased gastric and pancreatic secretions
Antisecretory factor	Antisecretory globally in small intestine

cAMP, Cyclic adenosine monophosphate; *cGMP*, cyclic guanosine monophosphate; *CFTR*, cystic fibrosis transmembrane conductance regulator; PGE_1, prostaglandin E_1; PGE_2, prostaglandin E_2; *VIP*, vasoactive intestinal peptide.

Control of NO synthesis is arguably the point where multiple signaling pathways converge, including neurohormones, cytokines, and cyclic nucleotides. Evidence indicates that a careful balance of NO synthesis in the small intestine may be responsible for the overall preabsorptive state. Experimental manipulation of levels of L-arginine, the biochemical precursor of NO, shows its effect on secretion. Low luminal levels of L-arginine are associated with increased absorption of water, glucose, and electrolytes, whereas higher levels cause reduced exchanges of fluid. Cathartics such as magnesium sulfate and bisacodyl cause increases in NO synthesis, in addition to osmotic effects. Decreased luminal levels of NO due to scavenging or sequestration may be responsible for the antisecretory effects of soluble and poorly soluble fibers, as well as bismuth subsalicylate and kaolin. NO is also closely associated with cyclic nucleotide metabolism.[31]

SMALL INTESTINAL MUCOSAL IMMUNITY

The small intestine provides the largest immune barrier between the epithelial surface of the body and the body interior. It comes into heavy and constant contact with foreign proteins, viruses, bacteria, and bacterial toxins as well as harmful chemical compounds from the environment. Accordingly, the mucosal surfaces of the body have an immune complement to match. Taken together, the mucosa-associated lymphoid tissues (MALT) include approximately 80% of all immune cells in a healthy human being, with the majority, or 70% of the overall total number

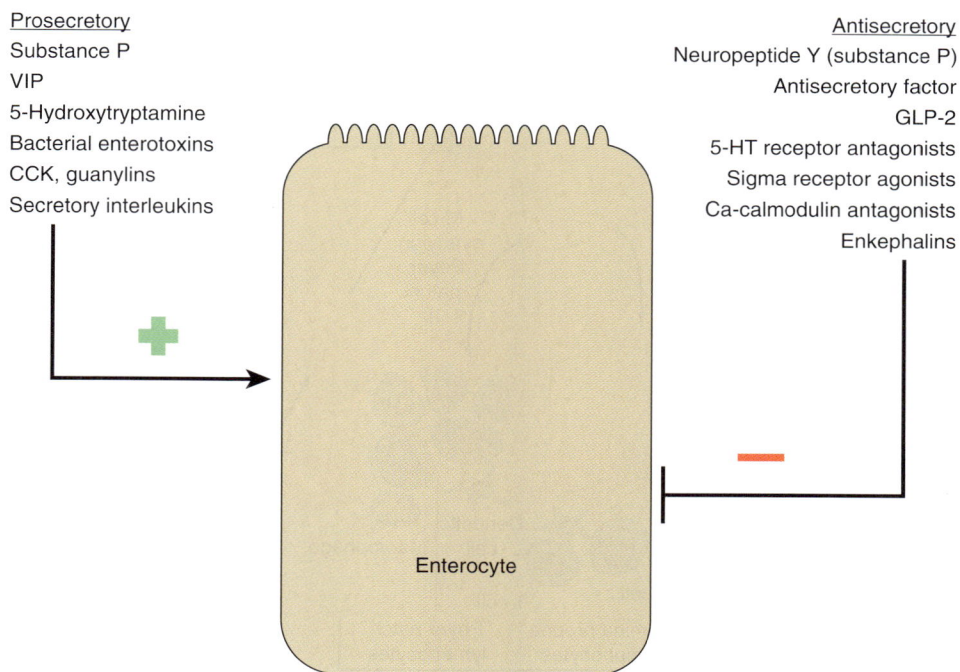

Prosecretory
Substance P
VIP
5-Hydroxytryptamine
Bacterial enterotoxins
CCK, guanylins
Secretory interleukins

Antisecretory
Neuropeptide Y (substance P)
Antisecretory factor
GLP-2
5-HT receptor antagonists
Sigma receptor agonists
Ca-calmodulin antagonists
Enkephalins

Enterocyte

FIGURE 71.17 Regulators of small intestinal secretion. *CCK*, Cholecystokinin; *GLP-2*, glucagon-like peptide 2; *5-HT*, 5-hydroxytrpyamine; *VIP*, vasoactive intestinal peptide. (Modified from Wapnir RA, Teichberg S. Regulation mechanisms of intestinal secretion: implications in nutrient absorption. *J Nutr Biochem.* 2002;13:190.)

of immunocytes, belonging to the gut-associated lymphoid tissues (GALT).

The mucosal immune system of the small intestine has three main functions: (1) protect mucosal surfaces against colonization or invasion by harmful microbes; (2) provide a barrier to undigested foreign antigens including those from ingested material and those produced by nonpathogenic commensal flora; and (3) prevent the development of immune responses to these antigens, which may be potentially harmful to the host. Most of the other areas of the body under immune surveillance are sterile. The mucosal surfaces, however, are surrounded by a milieu of foreign material at all times. Thus MALT must select appropriate effector mechanisms and the intensity of response to foreign antigens to avoid self-harm from the response.[40]

The mucosal immune system of the small intestine is composed of multiple elements of innate and adaptive immunity. IgA secretion may be the best recognized component of mucosal immunity. It is diverse and includes specialized antigen-presenting cells, mucosal macrophages, antibacterial proteins released from the epithelium, and specialized B and T cells (Fig. 71.18).

PANETH CELLS

Paneth cells provide strong innate mucosal immunity by the exocytosis of bactericidal granules in response to inflammatory signals (Fig. 71.19). Paneth cells originate from crypt stem cells. After differentiation, they migrate down into the crypt of Lieberkühn and reside adjacent to the stem cells. The Paneth cell also produces proepidermal growth factor and signal molecules essential for the maintenance of crypt stem cell activity.[41] The Paneth

cell has an average life span of 20 days. Their distribution in the small intestine is heterogeneous and increases distally, resulting in a high concentration in the terminal ileum. Their appearance elsewhere in the large intestine is considered Paneth cell metaplasia and is a recognized feature of inflammatory bowel disease (IBD). The granules of Paneth cells contain several antimicrobial proteins including lysozyme, α-defensins, and phospholipase. Lysozyme inhibits bacterial growth by attacking and hydrolyzing glycosidic bonds found in bacterial cell wall peptidoglycans. It is found in cytoplasmic granules and is directly exocytosed in response to bacteria.

The α-defensins comprise the majority of the secretory granules from the Paneth cell. Their function is to attack intraluminal bacterial and fungal pathogens. In humans, there are only two α-defensins: HD5 and HD6. Recombinant HD5 is effective against *Candida albicans* and several species of bacteria. HD5 disrupts the cell membrane of target microbes. HD6 self-assembles to form fibrils and nanonets that entangle bacteria. In vivo studies have shown that HD5 plays an important role in shaping the composition of the gut flora. Studies in humans have shown that a reduced expression of HD5/6 is a central feature of ileal Crohn disease. This link is thought to be due to a weakened mucosal defense and an altered group of commensal bacteria.[42]

Secretory phospholipase A_2 type IIA (sPLA2-IIA) is another important product released by Paneth cells, macrophages, and vascular smooth muscle cells. Luminal sPLA2-IIA degrades bacterial membrane phospholipids, stimulates leukocytes, and modifies circulating phospholipids. Its expression is markedly increased by proinflammatory signals such as bacterial lipopolysaccharide, IL-1,

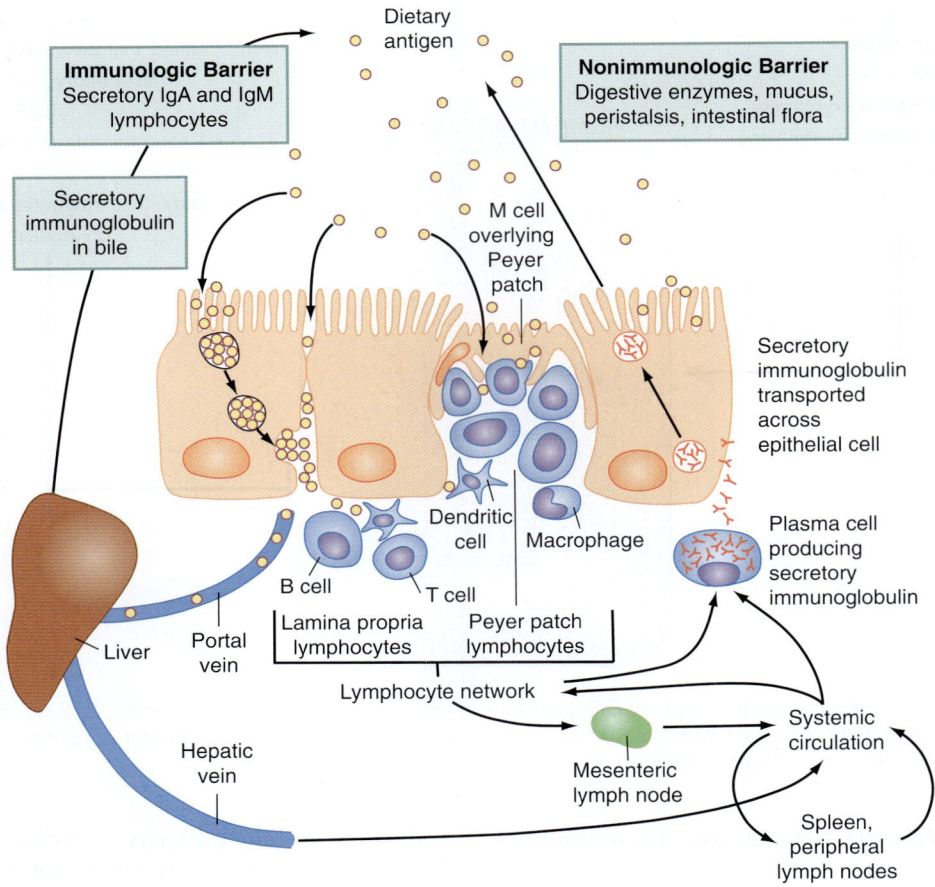

FIGURE 71.18 Schematic representation of the small intestine immunologic defenses. (From Townsend C, Beauchamp RD, Evers BM, et al, eds. *Sabiston's Textbook of Surgery*. 18th ed. Philadelphia: Saunders; 2008, Fig. 48.11; Modified from Duerr RH, Shanahan F. Food allergy. In: Targan SR, Shanahan F, eds. *Immunology and Immunopathology of the Liver and Gastrointestinal Tract*. New York: Igaku-Shoin; 1990, p. 510.)

tumor necrosis factor-α (TNF-α), and interferon (IFN)-γ. sPLA2-IIA knockout mice, a model of human familial adenomatous polyposis coli (FAP), are more susceptible to colorectal tumorigenesis. This suggests that sPLA2-IIA is involved in intestinal tumor suppression.[43,44]

Paneth cells also express TNF-α, the pleiotropic inflammatory mediator, in an inducible fashion. Its specific function in Paneth cells is unknown. There is some evidence to suggest that it plays a role in crypt regeneration and is induced following damage to Paneth or crypt cell populations. Interestingly, transgenic mice with constitutive TNF-α expression will develop lesions that resemble Crohn disease and rheumatoid arthritis. Antibodies against TNF-α (Infliximab) are a very effective treatment for Crohn disease and rheumatoid arthritis.

Nucleotide oligomerization domain 2 (*NOD2*), a part of an intracellular signaling molecule, binds peptidoglycan from bacteria and activates the inflammatory cascade. It may be regarded as an intracellular sensor of microbial patterns similar to Toll-like receptors. *NOD2* was the first gene identified to be correlated with a risk of developing Crohn disease. Individuals with homozygous *NOD2* mutation have an increased risk of developing Crohn disease by 40-fold. The possibility that Crohn disease pathogenesis is related to disordered mucosal defense highlights the importance of interrelation among physiologic processes of the small intestine.[45–47]

MICROFOLD CELLS

Microfold (M) cells are specialized cells that form an essential part of the host mucosal defense by sampling intraluminal contents for pathogens and foreign antigens. They are located in the follicle-associated epithelium surrounding Peyer patches, and in isolated follicles, the appendix, and extraintestinal MALT. M cells are so named because of the presence of microfolds on the apical surface. M cells originate from stem cells in intestinal crypts, and share a common precursor with enterocytes, goblet cells, enteroendocrine cells, and Paneth cells. M cells have a characteristic morphology of the basolateral surface. They possess a marked concavity that allows close contact with antigen-presenting cells.[28]

The function of M cells is transcellular transport. They internalize substances from the intestinal lumen and transport them across the epithelial barrier to the basal membrane, where interaction with immune cells can take place. M cells have been demonstrated to transport a variety of particulates, from inert substances such as latex beads to microorganisms. The precise method by which M cells internalize various molecules and microbes varies with the size, pH, chemical nature, and presence or absence of a specific M cell receptor to the material. Although internalized substances traverse the M cell cytoplasm, they do not undergo major processing.

The avidity of M cells for foreign molecules and organisms and their rapid transepithelial transport may be exploited by a variety of pathogens, which target M cells for host invasion. Many of these pathogens use M cells preferentially or even almost exclusively. Foremost among them, and most studied, are *Salmonella*. M cells comprise the major route of entry for this pathogen, and its uptake is associated with extensive damage to the follicular area, leading to unrestricted invasion and ulcer formation. *Yersinia, Shigella, Vibrio cholerae*, the pathogenic strain of *Escherichia* (O157:H7), poliovirus, human immunodeficiency virus 1 (HIV-1), and prion disease all exploit M cells for ease of entry. Additionally, some pathogens can increase M cell density by promoting M cell differentiation.[48,49]

INTESTINAL MACROPHAGES

Macrophages are ubiquitous in the body and play a prominent role in the immune response. Functionally,

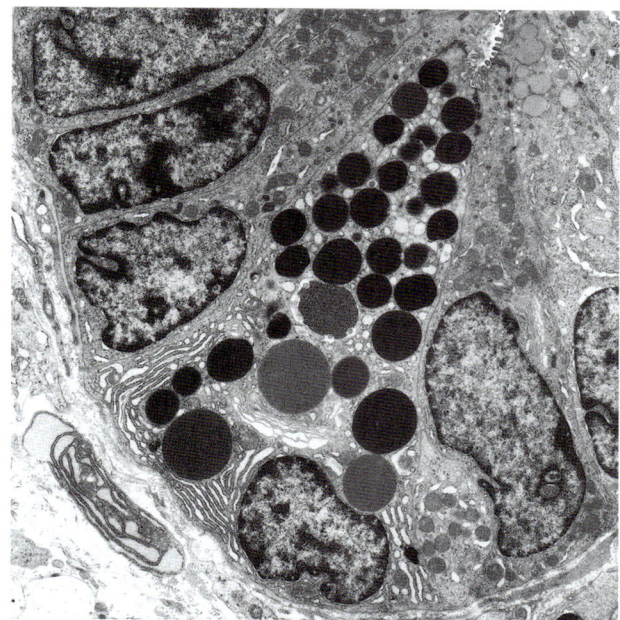

FIGURE 71.19 Histologic representation of a Paneth cell. (From Gartner LP. *Color Textbook of Histology*. 3rd ed. Philadelphia: Saunders; 2007, Fig. 17.18, p. 404.)

mucosal macrophages have important effects on bacterial clearance, maintaining homeostasis, and protective immunity. The small intestine is replete with resident macrophages that can be found in the lamina propria and within Peyer patches. Small-intestine macrophages are derived from the common bone marrow myeloid precursor that produces monocytes, macrophages, and dendritic cells (DCs). The small-intestine macrophages differ from circulating macrophages by expressing surface markers unique to their role in mucosal defense (Table 71.3). It is known that mediators in the mucosal environment are capable of modifying and conditioning DCs in the intestine as well as giving regulatory T cells gut-homing properties, and it is suspected that the same is true in the development of mucosal macrophages.

Intestinal macrophages are strongly phagocytic like their hematopoietic counterparts. Their position adjacent to the lamina propria makes them well suited to encounter luminal bacteria that have crossed the intestinal epithelial barrier. Intestinal macrophages may also encounter pathogens that have been transferred by epithelial cells.

Mucosal macrophages prevent pathologic inflammation in the intestine. They are highly phagocytic and exhibit strong bactericidal activity to clear out bacteria without activating the inflammatory pathway. Mucosal macrophages do not secrete proinflammatory signals such as IL-12, IL-23, TNF-α, or IL-1. They do not express or upregulate costimulatory molecules such as cluster of differentiation (CD)40, CD80, or CD86. Additionally, mucosal macrophages constitutively release antiinflammatory cytokine IL-10. Deletion or inhibition of IL-10 results in spontaneous colitis in mice. Finally, they produce the transcription factor peroxisome proliferator-activated receptor-γ (PPAR-γ) to suppress the expression of proinflammatory genes.[50,51]

DENDRITIC CELLS IN THE SMALL INTESTINE

DCs in the small intestine play an important and interconnected role in promoting a tolerogenic environment to commensal bacteria while still allowing for robust immune activation due to pathogens. They exist in several areas, notably in Peyer patches of the small intestine, in isolated lymphoid follicles, and in mesenteric lymph nodes. On encountering foreign material, the Peyer patches and lamina propria DCs migrate to mesenteric lymph nodes, where they present antigen to T cells.

The origin of DCs in the small intestine appears to be from a monocyte precursor. The basic subtypes of DCs in small intestinal GALT are similar to other lymphoid organs in the body with a population of conventional DCs and plasmacytoid DCs. Retinoic acid produced by DCs appears important in maintaining homeostasis in the

TABLE 71.3 Differences Between Circulating and Small Intestinal Macrophages

Type of Macrophage	Toll-Like Receptor	CD14 (LPS Recognition)	FcαR (IgA Recognition)	FcγR1 and FcγRIII (IgG Recognition)	Complement Receptors CR 3, CR 4
Small intestine macrophage	+ or Absent	Absent	Absent	Absent	Absent
Circulating macrophage	++++	+++	+	+	+

Ig, Immunoglobulin; *LPS,* lipopolysaccharide.

small intestine immune environment. NO also appears to have a role as a transmitter in the pathways influenced by DCs. NO is important in DC migration within MALT.

T CELLS IN THE SMALL INTESTINE

T cells circulate in the small intestine and have important distinct properties and differences from the T cells circulating in other areas of the body. T cells have specific tropism, which is imprinted by DCs. T cells are found in different anatomic levels of the small intestine. There are, broadly speaking, two populations: intraepithelial lymphocytes and lamina propria lymphocytes. Lamina propria T lymphocytes consist of a largely equal percentage of CD4+ and CD8+ cells. Intraepithelial T lymphocytes are primarily CD8+ and are composed of two populations: CD8 αβ cells with the αβ T-cell receptor (TCR), and a smaller CD8 αα population. These relatively less numerous CD8 αα cells are only rarely found in other tissues and are thought to be resident in the small intestine.[52]

IMMUNOGLOBULIN A IN THE SMALL INTESTINE

IgA is the most prevalent immunoglobulin in the human body. IgA synthesis and secretion by the gut is likely one of the most recognized features of small intestinal mucosal immunity. In steady-state conditions, approximately 40 to 60 mg/kg/day of IgA are produced and it is estimated that about 80% of all IgA is produced in the gut. Human IgA consists of two forms: IgA1 and IgA2. IgA1 is the predominant form in the small intestine, and IgA2 is prevalent in the colon.

IgA production only takes place in MALT. The majority of B cells that produce it are found in the lamina propria but migrate to Peyer-patch germinal centers for IgA synthesis. However, there is also extrafollicular IgA synthesis that has been reported in isolated lymphoid follicles as well as in the lamina propria.

IgA has a variety of functions. In general, low-affinity IgA antibodies produced by T-cell–independent pathways function in immune exclusion, or containing commensal bacteria in the intestinal lumen. High-affinity antibodies resulting from T-cell–dependent production are thought to prevent pathogenic microbes from colonizing or invading the epithelial lining. However, neither of these is absolute. IgA mediates transcytosis of certain antigens across M cells and intestinal epithelial cells; this controlled entry may be critical in initiating immune responses. In addition, depending on the type of IgA bound to antigen, an antiinflammatory or proinflammatory response is driven. IgA also has a role in maintaining intestinal homeostasis. IgA interaction with commensal bacteria can prevent their internalization and also regulate their surface expression of inflammatory signals, promoting host tolerance. IgA antibodies to commensal bacteria can limit the inflammatory response of intestinal epithelial cells. IgA can shape the overall composition of intestinal bacteria.[52–55]

DIGESTION AND ABSORPTION

The small intestine is the site of absorption of nutrients, water, and vitamins from food. Although digestion of proteins and carbohydrates has begun by the time food

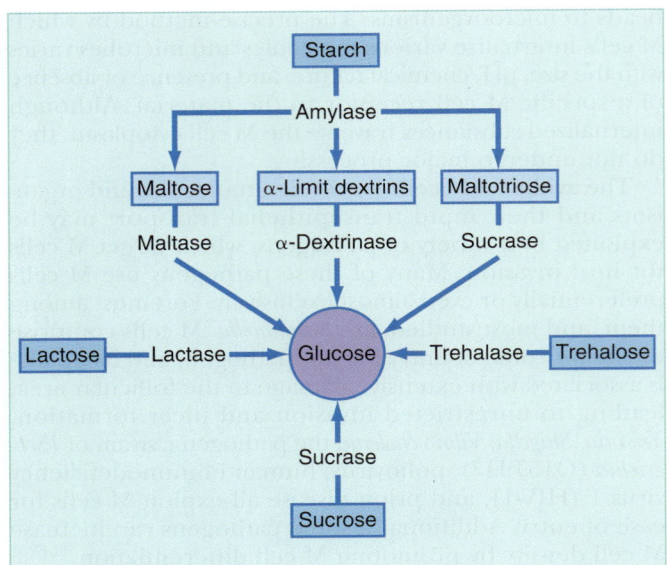

FIGURE 71.20 Carbohydrate digestion. The oligosaccharides (starch) and disaccharides (lactose, trehalose) are digested via hydrolytic cleavage to monosaccharides by saccharidases located in the brush border.

reaches the duodenum, the small intestine is completely responsible for fat digestion. This process of digestion and absorption usually takes 3 to 6 hours.

CARBOHYDRATE DIGESTION

Carbohydrates constitute the majority of the human diet. Complex starches, disaccharides, and monosaccharides (simple sugars) are the sources of digestible carbohydrates. Starch is the most abundant form of carbohydrate consumed and exists as amylose or amylopectin. Amylose is a linear polymer of glucose, and amylopectin is a branched form of amylose. Sucrose and lactose are commonly consumed disaccharides. Sucrose is a glucose-fructose dimer and lactose is a glucose-galactose dimer. Glucose, galactose, and fructose are monosaccharides and when ingested do not require any further digestion for absorption.

Starches and disaccharides must be broken down into monosaccharides before they can be absorbed in the small intestine. Digestion of starch begins immediately in the mouth via salivary amylase. This period of digestion is short as salivary amylase is quickly inactivated by gastric acid. The majority of carbohydrate digestion takes place in the small intestine with the help of pancreatic amylase. Amylase breaks the starches down into short-chain sugars called oligosaccharides. The most common oligosaccharides are maltotriose, maltose, and α-limit dextrins, which are digested via hydrolytic cleavage to monosaccharides by saccharidases located in the brush border. The family of saccharidases includes lactase, maltase, sucrase-isomaltase, and trehalase. They break down the short-chain sugars into glucose, galactose, and fructose (Fig. 71.20).

The absorption of monosaccharides requires active transport. A low intracellular Na+ concentration provides the gradient for active transport from the intestinal lumen into the enterocyte. The transport of glucose and galactose can be the rate-limiting step in absorption because they compete for the same sodium-coupled carrier. Fructose is absorbed via carrier-mediated facilitated diffusion. The enterocyte can use the monosaccharides for energy or transport them into the venous system.

PROTEIN DIGESTION

There are three main sources of protein: dietary, endogenous secretions, and desquamated cells. Protein digestion begins in the stomach via pepsin and continues in the small intestine. Pancreatic fluid is also necessary for protein digestion (Fig. 71.21). Proteases secreted by the pancreas enter the duodenum in inactive states as proenzymes. The proenzymes are activated by brush border enzymes. The two main classes of enzymes are endopeptidase and exopeptidase. The endopeptidase cleaves internal bonds, whereas the exopeptidase cleaves bonds on the carboxyl terminal. One of the most important proenzymes is trypsinogen. Once released into the duodenum, trypsinogen is converted to the active enzyme trypsin by the endopeptidase, enterokinase. Once active, trypsin converts several other proenzymes into their active forms (chymotrypsinogen to chymotrypsin, proelastase to elastase, and procarboxypeptidase to carboxypeptidase). In addition, trypsin can activate trypsinogen molecules. Proteins are broken down in the intestinal lumen by the proteases into short oligopeptides and amino acids. The brush border enzymes, peptidases, further hydrolyze the oligopeptides into free amino acids, dipeptides, and tripeptides, which can all be absorbed by enterocytes.

Dipeptides and tripeptides are more easily absorbed by the enterocyte because they are transported via a transmembrane H^+ gradient. Amino acids require active transport that is Na^+ dependent. Once in the cell, dipeptides and tripeptides are broken down into amino acids by cytosolic peptidases. Amino acids, specifically glutamine, can be used by the cell for energy. Other amino acids will be used for protein synthesis or will pass into the portal circulation. The majority of protein absorption occurs in the jejunum (Fig. 71.22).

FAT DIGESTION

Fats are ingested as triglycerides, phospholipids, cholesterol, and cholesterol esters. Triglycerides make up 90% of ingested fat in the Western diet. It is composed of three fatty acids and one glycerol. Pancreatic enzymes are integral in the digestive process of fat. Fat digestion also requires bile from the liver for emulsification, which is the process by which large fat globules are broken down into smaller sizes that are easier targets for water-soluble enzymes. Bile salts and lecithin are amphiphilic and are important in the breakdown of large fat molecules into small molecules. The fat-soluble portion absorbs into the fat globules, leaving the water-soluble end projecting outward to dissolve in the aqueous solution in the intestinal lumen. Once they become part of the aqueous solution in the lumen, the fat globules are more susceptible to fragmentation by mechanical agitation and enzymatic cleavage. Pancreatic lipase breaks down the triglycerides into free fatty acids and 2-monoglycerides. The fat components are transported to the brush border for absorption via micelles. Micelles are composed of bile salts and lecithin that are oriented with their fat-soluble end forming a sterol nucleus and the water-soluble end projecting outward. Digested fats

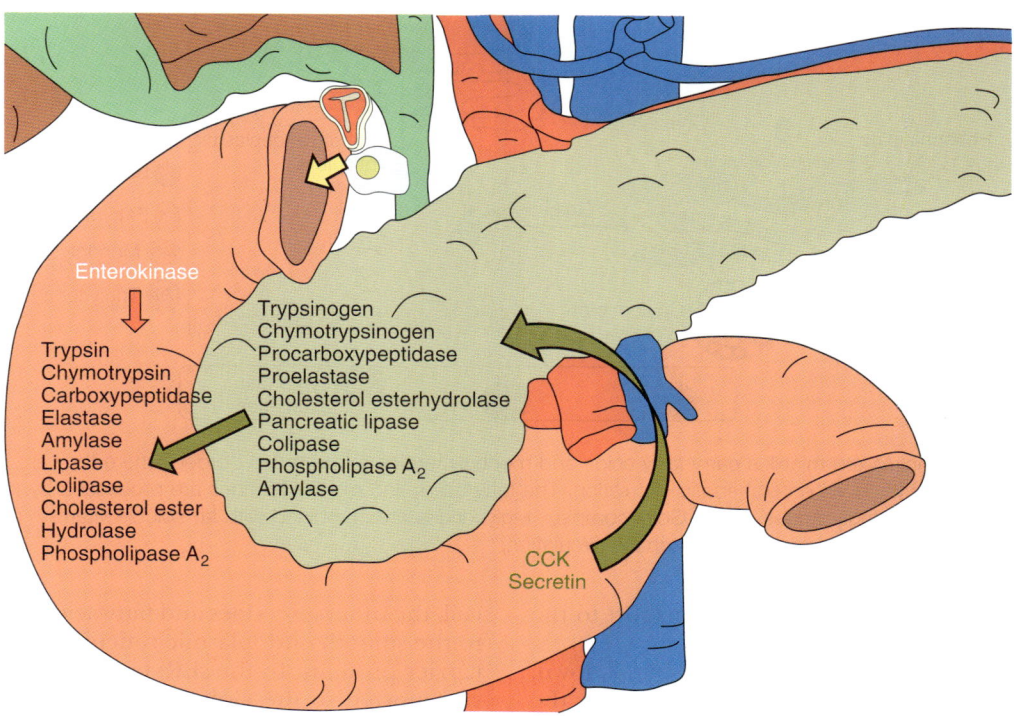

FIGURE 71.21 Protein digestion in the small intestine requires enzymes secreted from the pancreas. These enzymes are secreted as proenzymes and are activated by brush border enzymes in the small intestine. *CCK,* Cholecystokinin.

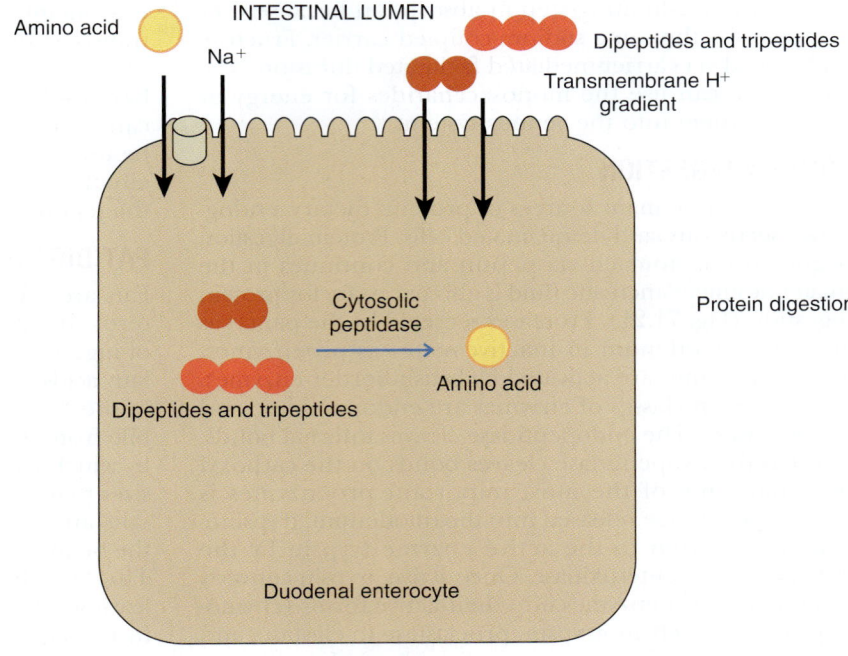

FIGURE 71.22 Protein digestion. Amino acids require Na$^+$-dependent active transport. Dipeptides and tripeptides diffuse via transmembrane H$^+$ gradient and are subsequently degraded to amino acids by cytosolic peptidase.

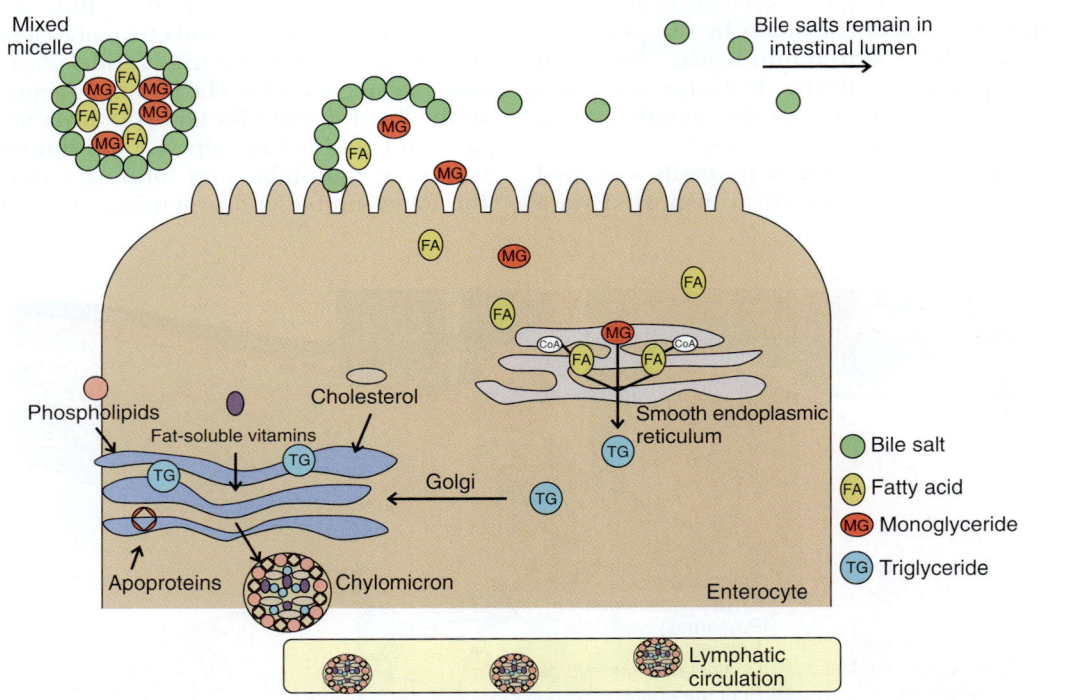

FIGURE 71.23 Lipid digestion. Mixed micelles carry fatty acids and monoglycerides to the brush border, where they are absorbed into the enterocyte. Bile salts are recycled via enterohepatic circulation. The fatty acids and monoglycerides are processed by the smooth endoplasmic reticulum to form triglycerides. In the Golgi complex, triglycerides are combined with fat-soluble vitamins and apoproteins to form chylomicrons, which are transported in the lymphatic circulation.

are easily absorbed into the micelles for transport to the brush border (Fig. 71.23).

Once at the brush border, the micelle will break down, allowing the fatty acids and monoglycerides to enter the cell and the bile salts to remain in the intestinal lumen, where they will join with new monoglycerides and fatty acids to repeat the same transport process. Once in the

cell, the monoglycerides and fatty acids will be transported to the smooth endoplasmic reticulum (sER) via cytosolic carrier proteins. In the sER, triglycerides reform and are transported to the Golgi apparatus to be packaged for exocytosis. In the Golgi, the triglycerides will be combined with cholesterol, phospholipids, and apoproteins to become a chylomicron. The core of the chylomicron contains the triglycerides, cholesterol, phospholipids, and fat-soluble vitamins, making it hydrophobic. Phospholipids and apoproteins line the chylomicron's surface. The chylomicrons are then packaged into secretory vesicles and exit the cell and enter the central lacteal via exocytosis. Once in the lacteal, the chylomicrons are part of the lymphatic circulation. Short- and medium-chain fatty acids may be absorbed directly into the portal blood. This is only a small portion, however, and the majority of fat is absorbed as chylomicrons and is transported in the intestinal lymphatics to the thoracic duct. Cholesterol is also absorbed in the small intestine as very-low-density lipoproteins (VLDLs). The VLDL particle contains a high ratio of cholesterol to triglyceride and is taken up into the lymphatic system.

ENTEROHEPATIC CIRCULATION

The majority of fat is absorbed in the duodenum and proximal jejunum. The bile salts involved in fat absorption are actively absorbed in the ileum and passively absorbed in the jejunum.[56] The average bile salt pool in humans is 2 to 3 g. Approximately 95% of bile salts are reabsorbed into the portal circulation for transport back to the liver. Once in the liver, the bile salts are resecreted and stored in the gallbladder until the next meal stimulates their release. This process of absorption from the intestine with transport back to the liver and resecretion from the gallbladder is known as enterohepatic circulation. This process occurs about six times in a 24-hour period.

Bile salts can be absorbed passively or actively. Bile salts that are unconjugated easily diffuse into the circulation in the jejunum. Conjugated bile salts are absorbed in the terminal ileum by an Na^+-dependent active transport system. Regardless of the mechanism, the majority of the bile salts are recycled back to the liver via the portal circulation. A minimal amount, less than 0.5 g, of bile salts is not reabsorbed and passes into the colon for excretion. A small amount of bile salt in the colon is not clinically significant; however, a large amount may produce diarrhea. Patients who have undergone an ileal resection lose the ability to reabsorb conjugated bile salts, and the high concentration of bile salts in the colon may impair sodium and water absorption, causing diarrhea. Cholestyramine is a bile salt–binding resin that can be used to treat patients with this condition.

VITAMIN ABSORPTION

The small intestine is the site of absorption of both water-soluble and fat-soluble vitamins. The fat-soluble vitamins A, D, E, and K are transported and absorbed similarly to dietary fats. They are taken up by micelles and transported into the enterocyte, where they are packaged into chylomicrons and then taken up into the lymphatic system. The water-soluble vitamins are absorbed in the jejunum and ileum by active or passive transport (Table 71.4). Vitamin B_{12} (cobalamin) is absorbed in a unique fashion. First, intrinsic factor, secreted from gastric parietal cells, couples with vitamin B_{12}. The complex then binds to a membrane receptor at the terminal ileum and is absorbed. Once in the cell, the complex dissociates and vitamin B_{12} enters the portal circulation. Diseases that alter the availability of intrinsic factor or membrane receptor in the

TABLE 71.4 Vitamins and Method of Intestinal Absorption

Vitamin	Method of Absorption
Fat soluble: A, D, E, K	Chylomicrons
Vitamin C (ascorbic acid)	Na^+-dependent brush border carriers
Biotin	Na^+-dependent brush border carriers
Nicotinic acid	Passive diffusion
Folic acid	Na^+-independent brush border carriers
B_2 (riboflavin)	Na^+-dependent brush border carriers
B_1 (thiamine)	Na^+-independent brush border carriers
B_6 (pyridoxine)	Passive diffusion
B_{12} (cobalamin)	Translocation with intrinsic factor

terminal ileum can cause vitamin B_{12} deficiency. Proximal or total gastrectomy, gastric bypass, and distal ileal resection can all result in vitamin B_{12} deficiency.

WATER AND ELECTROLYTE ABSORPTION

On average, 8 to 10 L of fluid will flow through the small intestine in a 24-hour period. The sources of water are dietary intake, salivary fluid, and gastric, biliary, pancreatic, and intestinal secretions. The small intestine is the greatest site of water and electrolyte absorption, and less than a liter of fluid is presented to the colon for absorption. The colon will absorb the rest of the water, allowing only a small amount to be excreted in the stool. Water is absorbed in the small intestine by passive diffusion or as a result of osmotic pressure differences due to electrolyte absorption.

The absorption of water is tightly regulated by the absorption of electrolytes. Water will follow the flow of electrolytes to maintain an isotonic environment between the tissue and intestinal lumen. In the proximal small intestine, water freely flows into the cell through permeable tight junctions between enterocytes. The tight junctions become less permeable in the distal intestine, where water requires active transport to enter the cell. This process usually requires coupling with electrolytes.

Electrolyte absorption occurs by active transport or coupling. Sodium, chloride, bicarbonate, calcium, and iron are all absorbed in the small intestine. Potassium, magnesium, phosphate, and other ions are also absorbed through the intestinal mucosa. Sodium enters the enterocyte via solute-coupling or electroneutral sodium chloride absorption and is then released into the circulation by an Na^+/K^+-ATPase pump. Solutes such as glucose, amino acids, short-chain peptides, and bile acids are absorbed via cotransport with Na^+. Na^+ enters the cell with the solute and then exits at the basolateral membrane via the Na^+/K^+-ATPase pump. This in turn creates an electrochemical gradient across the cell that allows for the accumulation of solutes (Fig. 71.24). The absorption of Cl^- is also facilitated by this gradient. The absorption of Na^+ leaves the luminal contents electronegative and the cell and paracellular space electropositive. The negatively charged Cl^- ions can then freely diffuse across the cell. Most of the Cl^- absorption occurs in the duodenum and jejunum.

Bicarbonate is absorbed in the duodenum and jejunum. A large portion of the bicarbonate found in the intestinal

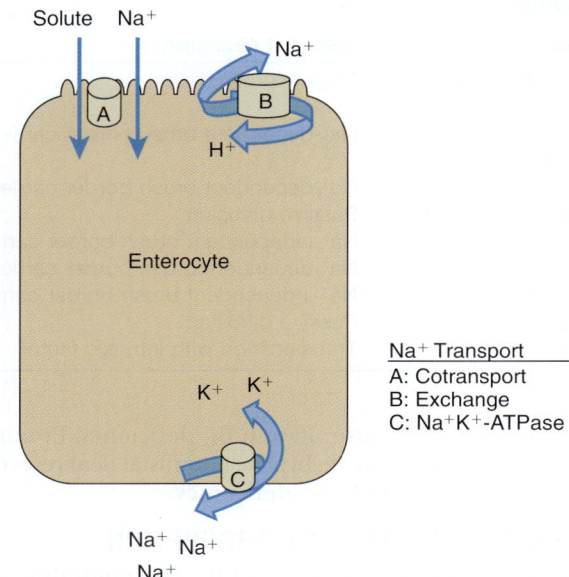

INTESTINAL LUMEN

Solute   Na$^+$

Na$^+$

A

B

H$^+$

Enterocyte

K$^+$ K$^+$

C

Na$^+$ Na$^+$
Na$^+$

Na$^+$ Transport
A: Cotransport
B: Exchange
C: Na$^+$K$^+$-ATPase

FIGURE 71.24 Sodium transport in the enterocyte via the three primary mechanisms of cotransport, exchange, and Na$^+$/K$^+$-ATPase.

chyme is a result of pancreatic secretion and bile. The process of bicarbonate absorption involves two indirect steps. First, H$^+$ ions are secreted into the lumen in exchange for Na$^+$ entering the cell. The H$^+$ in the intestinal lumen combines with the bicarbonate ions to form carbonic acid (H$_2$CO$_3$). The carbonic acid dissociates into carbon dioxide (CO$_2$) and water (H$_2$O). The H$_2$O remains in the intestinal lumen and the CO$_2$ is taken up into the circulation and then exhaled.

Calcium is actively absorbed in the duodenum and jejunum. The absorption of calcium is dependent on parathyroid hormone and vitamin D. Parathyroid hormone activates vitamin D by stimulating the conversion of 25-hydroxycholecalciferol to 1,25-dihydroxycholecalciferol, which is the active form of vitamin D. 1,25-Dihydroxycholecalciferol increases the availability of calcium-binding protein located in the brush border. Calcium will bind to this specific protein and be absorbed into the cell. Calcium ions move out of the cell into the circulation by facilitated diffusion. In the presence of activated vitamin D, approximately 35% of ingested calcium is absorbed in the small intestine.

The absorption of iron from dietary sources takes place in the duodenum in the presence of bile. Bile contains apotransferrin, a molecule that binds with free iron, hemoglobin, and myoglobin. Once bound to the iron product, the apotransferrin becomes transferrin. Transferrin molecules, with their iron product, bind to membrane receptors on the intestinal epithelium and are absorbed into the cell via pinocytosis. Once in the cell, the transferrin and iron product will pass into the circulation as plasma transferrin.

The small intestine is responsible for many functions that are necessary for human life. Disorders of these functions can result in debilitating disease states and even death. There is much that is known about the mechanisms by which these disease states occur, but further understanding of the molecular and genetic organization of the small intestine will serve to enhance clinical care.

ACKNOWLEDGMENT

The authors would like to thank Andrea M. Abbott, Leonard Armstrong, and Eric H. Jensen for their contributions to the previous version of this chapter.

REFERENCES

1. Larsen W. *Human Embryology.* New York: Chuchill Livingstone; 1997.
2. Skandalakis JE, Colborn GL, Weidman TA. *Skandalakis' Surgical Anatomy: The Embryologic and Anatomic Basis of Modern Surgery—2 Volumes.* 1st ed. Athens, Greece: Paschalidis Medical Publications, Ltd.; 2004.
3. Bohe H, Bohe M, Lindstrom C, Ohlsson K. Pancreatic secretory trypsin inhibitor in human Brunner's glands. *J Gastroenterol.* 1995; 30(1):90-95.
4. Cserni T, Paran S, Kanyari Z, et al. New insights into the neuromuscular anatomy of the ileocecal valve. *Anat Rec (Hoboken).* 2009;292(2): 254-261.
5. Gonella J, Bouvier M, Blanquet F. Extrinsic nervous control of motility of small and large intestines and related sphincters. *Physiol Rev.* 1987;67(3):902-961.
6. Burns AJ, Thapar N. Advances in ontogeny of the enteric nervous system. *Neurogastroenterol Motil.* 2006;18(10):876-887.
7. Lake JI, Heuckeroth RO. Enteric nervous system development: migration, differentiation, and disease. *Am J Physiol Gastrointest Liver Physiol.* 2013;305(1):G1-G24.
8. Burns AJ, Roberts RR, Bornstein JC, Young HM. Development of the enteric nervous system and its role in intestinal motility during fetal and early postnatal stages. *Semin Pediatr Surg.* 2009;18(4):196-205.
9. Bortoff A. Myogenic control of intestinal motility. *Physiol Rev.* 1976;56(2):418-434.
10. Konturek PC, Brzozowski T, Konturek SJ. Gut clock: implication of circadian rhythms in the gastrointestinal tract. *J Physiol Pharmacol.* 2011;62(2):139-150.
11. Ahluwalia NK, Thompson DG, Barlow J, Heggie L. Beta adrenergic modulation of human upper intestinal propulsive forces. *Gut.* 1994;35(10):1356-1359.
12. Thollander M, Svensson TH, Hellstrom PM. Stimulation of beta-adrenoceptors with isoprenaline inhibits small intestinal activity fronts and induces a postprandial-like motility pattern in humans. *Gut.* 1997;40(3):376-380.
13. Wood JD. Intrinsic neural control of intestinal motility. *Annu Rev Physiol.* 1981;43:33-51.
14. Spiller RC, Trotman IF, Adrian TE, Bloom SR, Misiewicz JJ, Silk DB. Further characterisation of the 'ileal brake' reflex in man—effect of ileal infusion of partial digests of fat, protein, and starch on jejunal motility and release of neurotensin, enteroglucagon, and peptide YY. *Gut.* 1988;29(8):1042-1051.
15. Preston DM, Adrian TE, Christofides ND, Lennard-Jones JE, Bloom SR. Positive correlation between symptoms and circulating motilin, pancreatic polypeptide and gastrin concentrations in functional bowel disorders. *Gut.* 1985;26(10):1059-1064.
16. Thomas PA, Akwari OE, Kelly KA. Hormonal control of gastrointestinal motility. *World J Surg.* 1979;3(5):545-552.
17. Harvey RF. Hormonal control of gastrointestinal motility. *Am J Dig Dis.* 1975;20(6):523-539.
18. Misiewicz JJ, Waller SL, Kiley N. Effect of oral prostaglandin E1 on intestinal transit in man. *Lancet.* 1969;1(7596):648-651.
19. Hansen MB, Arif F, Gregersen H, Bruusgaard H, Wallin L. Effect of serotonin on small intestinal contractility in healthy volunteers. *Physiol Res.* 2008;57(1):63-71.
20. Aros SD, Camilleri M. Small-bowel motility. *Curr Opin Gastroenterol.* 2001;17(2):140-146.
21. Gallego D, Clave P, Donovan J, et al. The gaseous mediator, hydrogen sulphide, inhibits in vitro motor patterns in the human, rat and

mouse colon and jejunum. *Neurogastroenterol Motil.* 2008;20(12): 1306-1316.

22. Charoenthongtrakul S, Giuliana D, Longo KA, et al. Enhanced gastrointestinal motility with orally active ghrelin receptor agonists. *J Pharmacol Exp Ther.* 2009;329(3):1178-1186.

23. Vantrappen G, Janssens J, Hellemans J, Ghoos Y. The interdigestive motor complex of normal subjects and patients with bacterial overgrowth of the small intestine. *J Clin Invest.* 1977;59(6):1158-1166.

24. Jones MP, Wessinger S. Small intestinal motility. *Curr Opin Gastroenterol.* 2006;22(2):111-116.

25. Kellow JE, Gill RC, Wingate DL. Modulation of human upper gastrointestinal motility by rectal distension. *Gut.* 1987;28(7):864-868.

26. Gallagher TK, Geoghegan JG, Baird AW, Winter DC. Implications of altered gastrointestinal motility in obesity. *Obes Surg.* 2007;17(10): 1399-1407.

27. Gallagher TK, Baird AW, Winter DC. Constitutive basal and stimulated human small bowel contractility is enhanced in obesity. *Ann Surg Innov Res.* 2009;3:4.

28. Mowat AM, Agace WW. Regional specialization within the intestinal immune system. *Nat Rev Immunol.* 2014;14(10):667-685.

29. Flemstrom G, Isenberg JI. Gastroduodenal mucosal alkaline secretion and mucosal protection. *News Physiol Sci.* 2001;16:23-28.

30. Yandrapu H, Sarosiek J. Protective factors of the gastric and duodenal mucosa: an overview. *Curr Gastroenterol Rep.* 2015;17(6):24.

31. Wapnir RA, Teichberg S. Regulation mechanisms of intestinal secretion: implications in nutrient absorption. *J Nutr Biochem.* 2002;13(4):190-199.

32. Collaco AM, Jakab RL, Hoekstra NE, Mitchell KA, Brooks A, Ameen NA. Regulated traffic of anion transporters in mammalian Brunner's glands: a role for water and fluid transport. *Am J Physiol Gastrointest Liver Physiol.* 2013;305(3):G258-G275. doi:10.1152/ajpgi.00485.2012.

33. Fasano A, Uzzau S, Fiore C, Margaretten K. The enterotoxic effect of zonula occludens toxin on rabbit small intestine involves the paracellular pathway. *Gastroenterology.* 1997;112(3):839-846.

34. Kaper JB, Morris JG Jr, Levine MM. Cholera. *Clin Microbiol Rev.* 1995;8(1):48-86.

35. Thiagarajah JR, Verkman AS. CFTR pharmacology and its role in intestinal fluid secretion. *Curr Opin Pharmacol.* 2003;3(6):594-599.

36. Van Citters GW, Lin HC. The ileal brake: a fifteen-year progress report. *Curr Gastroenterol Rep.* 1999;1(5):404-409.

37. Ma T, Verkman AS. Aquaporin water channels in gastrointestinal physiology. *J Physiol.* 1999;517(Pt 2):317-326.

38. Turvill JL, Farthing MJ. Water and electrolyte absorption and secretion in the small intestine. *Curr Opin Gastroenterol.* 1999;15(2):108-112.

39. Thomson AB, Drozdowski L, Iordache C, et al. Small bowel review: normal physiology, part 1. *Dig Dis Sci.* 2003;48(8):1546-1564.

40. Holmgren J, Czerkinsky C. Mucosal immunity and vaccines. *Nat Med.* 2005;11(4 suppl):S45-S53.

41. Sato T, van Es JH, Snippert HJ, et al. Paneth cells constitute the niche for Lgr5 stem cells in intestinal crypts. *Nature.* 2011;469(7330): 415-418.

42. Bevins CL. Innate immune functions of alpha-defensins in the small intestine. *Dig Dis.* 2013;31(3-4):299-304.

43. Murakami M, Taketomi Y, Girard C, Yamamoto K, Lambeau G. Emerging roles of secreted phospholipase A2 enzymes: lessons from transgenic and knockout mice. *Biochimie.* 2010;92(6):561-582.

44. Murakami M, Taketomi Y, Miki Y, Sato H, Yamamoto K, Lambeau G. Emerging roles of secreted phospholipase A2 enzymes: the 3rd edition. *Biochimie.* 2014;107(Pt A):105-113.

45. Keshav S. Paneth cells: leukocyte-like mediators of innate immunity in the intestine. *J Leukoc Biol.* 2006;80(3):500-508.

46. Ouellette AJ. IV. Paneth cell antimicrobial peptides and the biology of the mucosal barrier. *Am J Physiol.* 1999;277(2 Pt 1): G257-G261.

47. Salzman NH, Underwood MA, Bevins CL. Paneth cells, defensins, and the commensal microbiota: a hypothesis on intimate interplay at the intestinal mucosa. *Semin Immunol.* 2007;19(2):70-83.

48. Corr SC, Gahan CC, Hill C. M-cells: origin, morphology and role in mucosal immunity and microbial pathogenesis. *FEMS Immunol Med Microbiol.* 2008;52(1):2-12.

49. Mabbott NA, Donaldson DS, Ohno H, Williams IR, Mahajan A. Microfold (M) cells: important immunosurveillance posts in the intestinal epithelium. *Mucosal Immunol.* 2013;6(4):666-677.

50. Platt AM, Mowat AM. Mucosal macrophages and the regulation of immune responses in the intestine. *Immunol Lett.* 2008;119(1-2):22-31.

51. Chassaing B, Kumar M, Baker MT, Singh V, Vijay-Kumar M. Mammalian gut immunity. *Biomed J.* 2014;37(5):246-258.

52. Johansson-Lindbom B, Agace WW. Generation of gut-homing T cells and their localization to the small intestinal mucosa. *Immunol Rev.* 2007;215:226-242.

53. Cerutti A, Rescigno M. The biology of intestinal immunoglobulin A responses. *Immunity.* 2008;28(6):740-750.

54. Fagarasan S. Evolution, development, mechanism and function of IgA in the gut. *Curr Opin Immunol.* 2008;20(2):170-177.

55. Mora JR, von Andrian UH. Differentiation and homing of IgA-secreting cells. *Mucosal Immunol.* 2008;1(2):96-109.

56. Ridlon JM, Kang DJ, Hylemon PB. Bile salt biotransformations by human intestinal bacteria. *J Lipid Res.* 2006;47(2):241-259.

Small Bowel Obstruction

Lily E. Johnston | John B. Hanks

Descriptions of patients with small bowel obstruction (SBO) date back to the earliest medical literature. It was not until the 19th century and the advent of anesthesia and antisepsis, however, that surgery became a recognized and effective treatment. At the same time, physiologic studies of fluid shifts, electrolyte imbalances, intravenous resuscitation, and antibiotics allowed even safer surgical approaches to patients with obstruction. Despite advances in treatment, SBO remains a common clinical problem, accounting for as many as 400,000 admissions annually in the United States, with between 30% and 40% requiring operative exploration.[1] Moreover, these admissions are costly both in terms of time and money: the average length of stay for patients requiring operative exploration is 6 days following a laparoscopic lysis of adhesions and 11 days following a laparoscopic bowel resection, with mean hospital charges of $38,669 and $71,218 respectively,[1] with a national burden of $2.1 billion.[2]

At the time of initial evaluation for SBO, it is critical to determine whether a true mechanical obstruction or pseudoobstruction (dysmotility/ileus) is the cause of symptoms; this distinction will guide all subsequent treatment. Clinical judgment must also be employed to determine illness severity, resuscitation requirements, and the urgency of operative intervention. Patients may present acutely, or with a chronic and relapsing problem with symptoms ranging from modest discomfort to critical illness and shock (Fig. 72.1).

PATHOPHYSIOLOGY

The earliest response of the proximal gut to obstruction is to increase bowel wall contractility to overcome the blockage. This increase in contractility, which may occur proximal or distal to the obstruction, may result in early symptoms of diarrhea or enhanced output; however, if the obstruction persists, ultimately the contractions become less efficient and may cease altogether. At this point, proximal bowel dilatation may occur. Dilatation and the lack of contractility may allow water and electrolytes to accumulate proximal to the obstruction. Significant third-space losses in addition to vomiting may result in marked dehydration and hypovolemia. Metabolic derangement may be significant, and depends on the level of the obstruction. Proximal obstruction may result in hypochloremia, hypokalemia, and metabolic alkalosis. Concurrent, persistent vomiting can exacerbate these alterations. Obstruction of the distal small bowel results in a larger capacitance effect with enhanced volume loss. Electrolyte disturbances may be somewhat less severe; however, significant hypovolemia and even renal damage can occur. If obstruction is not relieved and these processes continue, volume loss and abdominal distention will result in decreased venous return, diaphragmatic elevation, and perhaps compromised ventilation, all of which will exacerbate the symptoms of an acute abdomen.

Under normal circumstances, the luminal content of the small bowel contains very few bacteria; up to one-third of jejunal aspirates in healthy volunteers will be sterile.[3] Interestingly, obstruction provokes a profound change in the flora of the small intestine, with stasis permitting overgrowth of the few native species as well as being populated by reverse peristalsis from the colonic microbiota. These are most commonly *Escherichia coli*, *Streptococcus faecalis*, and *Klebsiella* species. Overgrowth can occur rapidly. Even prior to frank perforation with gross contamination, there is evidence that bacteria can translocate through the intestinal wall and may well contribute to a deteriorating sepsis picture if the treatment of initial obstruction is delayed.[4]

CLASSIFICATION AND ETIOLOGY

SBO can be classified by mechanism. The patient's symptoms and presenting signs may be caused by a functional obstruction from dysmotility, or a true mechanical obstruction. Mechanical SBO may be further classified as partial or complete obstruction, with the etiology of mechanical SBO divided into three main categories: extrinsic, intrinsic/ intramural, and intraluminal.

DYSMOTILITY

Dysmotility or ileus can be caused by a wide range of insults (see Fig. 72.1), and the recognition and diagnosis of pseudoobstruction is critical to avoiding an unnecessary, unhelpful operation that is likely to worsen rather than improve the clinical picture. A comprehensive, thorough history including all medications, comorbid conditions, and social history often points to a diagnosis favoring dysmotility over mechanical obstruction. The case of postoperative ileus following recent abdominal or pelvic surgery is reasonably straightforward. However, other causes including blunt trauma, pancreatitis, kidney stones, mesenteric ischemia, and retroperitoneal hematoma can also lead to ileus. Additionally, many classes of medications including opioids, some psychotropic medications, chemotherapeutic agents, and anticholinergic drugs are known to slow motility and may cause or contribute to a diagnosis of dysmotility. In select cases, pharmacologic agents such as alvimopan or methylnaltrexone may play a role in preventing or mitigating ileus.[5] Although commonly used, there is little data to support the use of prokinetic agents such as erythromycin or metoclopramide in the setting of postoperative ileus.[6]

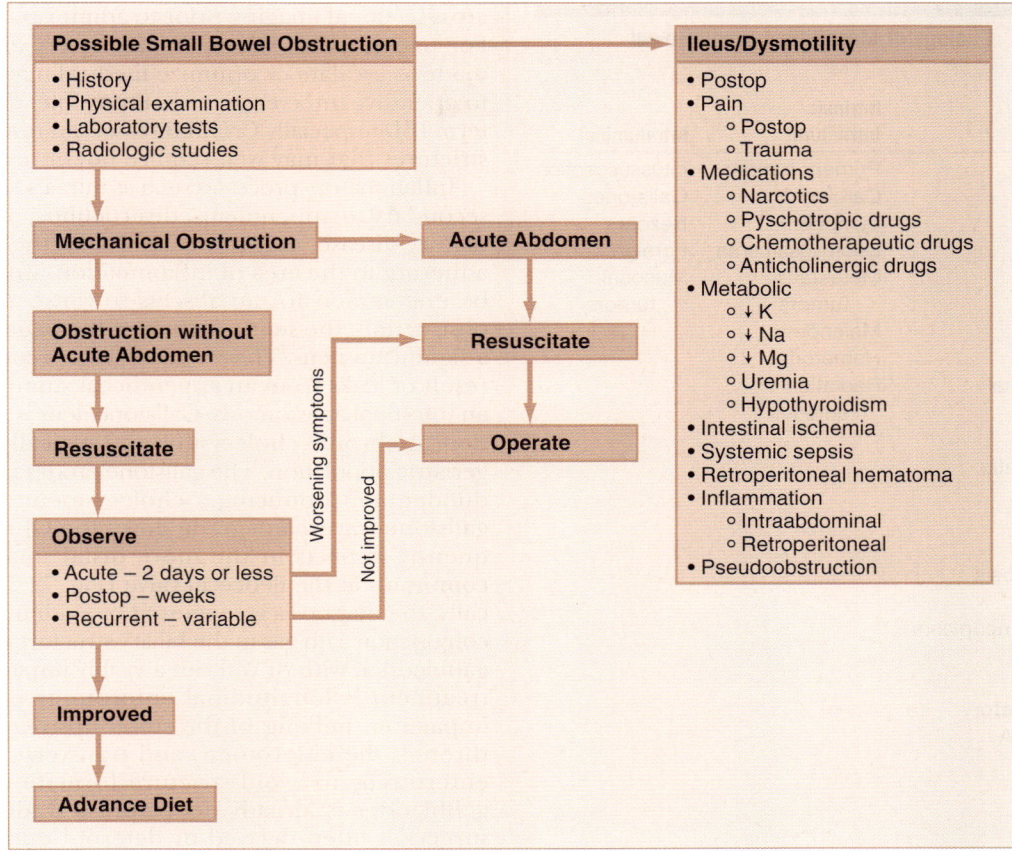

FIGURE 72.1 This algorithm suggests an organized approach to small bowel obstruction. Common causes for ileus or dysmotility are seen on the right side of the chart and need to be considered prior to the assumption of a mechanical obstruction.

MECHANICAL OBSTRUCTION

Mechanical SBO can be divided into three main categories: extrinsic, intramural, and intraluminal (Table 72.1). The vast majority of SBOs are caused by postsurgical adhesions. Adhesions caused by previous gynecologic or colorectal or intestinal resection have been reported as causing more than 50% of mechanical SBOs.[7–9] Additionally, adhesions in the lower abdominal quadrants and pelvis are far more frequent than in the upper abdomen. The advent of laparoscopy has been thought to lower the rate of SBO due to decreased traumatization of both the visceral and parietal peritoneal surfaces, resulting in reduced inflammation and subsequent fibrin deposition.[7]

Hernias, including ventral, incisional, internal, and groin hernias, are the second most common cause of SBO.[10,11] In addition to standard anatomic hernias, internal hernias through mesenteric defects are increasingly common: the rate of internal hernias through the Peterson space in antecolic, antegastric Roux-en-Y gastric bypass has been reported to occur in 6.2% of patients without closure of the mesenteric defect. Internal hernias can be much more difficult to detect radiographically, especially in the absence of an accurate history. The index of suspicion for an internal hernia in gastric bypass patients with unexplained abdominal pain, nausea, or vomiting, or evidence of SBO must be high, and laparoscopic exploration may be indicated even in the setting of negative or ambiguous imaging.[12]

Malignancy appears to cause up to 20% of SBOs, and is typically thought of as the third most common reason for SBO. Both benign and malignant tumors can cause obstruction, and they may be found within, or extrinsic to, the small bowel. Extrinsic compression can occur from the small bowel or, more commonly, colonic tumors that impinge on the small bowel, thereby causing obstruction proximal to the tumor. Intraabdominal carcinomatosis can also obstruct by peritoneal seeding and bowel entrapment. The most common sources for these are gastric or ovarian primaries, although colorectal cancer may act in a similar fashion. While large intrinsic tumors may obstruct the small bowel, smaller tumors can still cause obstruction by serving as the lead point of an intussusception. Tumors associated with SBO include metastatic melanoma, lipomas, gastrointestinal stromal tumors, adenomas, adenocarcinomas, and carcinoid tumors. Gastrointestinal carcinoids, which account for approximately 25% of all small bowel tumors, occur most frequently in the small intestine, and symptoms generally reflect local invasion or tumor-induced fibrosis due to the relatively slow, indolent nature of the tumor growth. In fact, many patients are diagnosed incidentally at the time of surgery for what was thought to be an idiopathic SBO. If the diagnosis is suspected preoperatively, biochemical studies such as plasma

TABLE 72.1 Etiology of Mechanical Small Bowel Obstruction

Extrinsic	Intrinsic/ Intramural	Intraluminal
Adhesions	Primary tumors	Intussusception
Hernias	Carcinoid	Gallstones
External	Lymphoma	Bezoars
Inguinal	Leiomyosarcoma	Foreign body
Femoral	Metastatic	Mucosal
Incisional	tumors	tumors
Obturator	Melanoma	
Internal	Hematoma	
Paraduodenal	Radiation	
Epiploic	enteritis	
Foramen		
Diaphragmatic		
Tumors		
Peritoneal		
Metastasis		
carcinomatosis		
Desmoid		
Extraintestinal neoplasm		
Abscess		
Diverticulitis		
Pelvic inflammatory disease/TOA		
Inflammation		
Crohn disease		
Tuberculosis		
Endometriosis		

TOA, Tuboovarian abscess.

chromogranin A, serotonin, or urinary 5-hydroxyindoleacetic acid (5-HIAA) can be helpful in confirming the diagnosis. Imaging of these tumors and their metastases using receptor-targeted radiolabeled somatostatin analogues, commonly referred to as octreotide scanning, can also be a useful adjunct. Small intestinal carcinoids have a 5-year survival of approximately 60%.[13] Primary small bowel tumors are exceedingly rare, although they can occasionally present in a middle-aged patient with recurrent SBO and no history of previous surgery. Such a patient should be carefully worked up for this rare, and if missed, fatal disease.

Inflammatory bowel disease (IBD), particularly Crohn disease, is an important diagnostic consideration when evaluating SBO. Obstruction can be caused by extraluminal compression or acute inflammation of the bowel wall. However, it generally does not produce an acute obstruction; chronic or relapsing-remitting obstructions are more common. Acute onset of symptoms is usually secondary to a food impaction in an area of stenotic or strictured bowel, or a complication of the disease, such as an abscess. In the case of obstruction secondary to food, intravenous steroids to decrease the swelling around the impaction along with rehydration and *nil per os* may resolve the acute SBO without operative intervention. An abscess or phlegmon that may require percutaneous drainage and intravenous antibiotics should be ruled out with

cross-sectional imaging prior to administration of steroids. For patients with Crohn disease, every effort should be made to escalate or optimize medical management prior to operative intervention when possible. Chronic or long-term IBD, especially Crohn disease, can result in significant strictures that may well require bowel resection.

Inflammatory processes such as intraabdominal abscesses secondary to appendicitis, diverticulitis, or pelvic inflammatory disease, may cause an SBO as the result of bowel adhering to the area of inflammation. Although it might be uncommon for an abscess to cause an extraluminal obstruction, the septic picture of the patient may include a significant ileus. These circumstances could be a clinical result of leaks from an appendiceal stump or leak within an intestinal anastomosis. Gallstone ileus is a rare complication of chronic cholecystitis and typically occurs in the geriatric population. The gallstone erodes into the adjacent duodenum, producing a cholecystoenteric fistula. The gallstone travels antegrade down the GI tract and subsequently impacts in the more distal small bowel, most commonly at the ileocecal valve (Fig. 72.2). Radiographically, the diagnosis is suggested by evidence of an SBO in conjunction with gas in the biliary structures or a contracted gallbladder, with or without a visibly impacted stone. The treatment is longitudinal enterotomy proximal to the impaction, milking of the stone upstream and delivery through the enterotomy, and transverse closure of the enterotomy to avoid stricture formation; because the gallbladder is already decompressed, definitive biliary surgery is often delayed or deferred until acute inflammatory processes have resolved.

All surgeons should also be aware of the more unusual causes of SBO, which may still mandate operative intervention. These entities include intussusception, which is more common in children, but can occur in adults where a lead point such as a tumor or polyp is encountered; foreign bodies, including those ingested and those migrating from other areas in the abdomen or pelvis (e.g., stents, intrauterine devices); bezoars; spontaneous intramural hematoma in patients on chronic anticoagulation or at high risk for bleeding; and superior mesenteric artery syndrome, which typically presents as a partial obstruction with postprandial nausea, vomiting, and weight loss with radiographic evidence of compression of the third portion of the duodenum. Finally, it is worth noting that in the developing world, helminths are a leading cause of bowel obstruction. In endemic areas this should be suspected as a cause of SBO, and initial management should be antihelminthic therapy with operative intervention reserved for abdominal emergencies such as perforation or volvulus, or those patients who cannot tolerate medical therapy.

CLINICAL PRESENTATION AND DIAGNOSIS

CLINICAL FINDINGS

The clinical presentation and decision making for operative intervention or nonoperative treatment is, in the majority of cases, straightforward. Clearly, situations arise where confounding factors occur and may cloud the picture, including ileus, metabolic abnormalities, and multiple previous abdominal surgeries. Although these factors

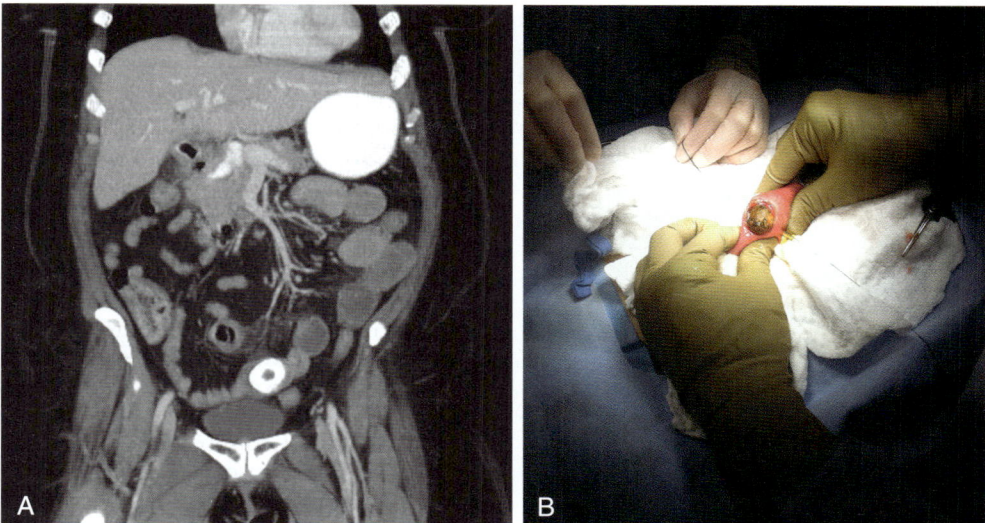

FIGURE 72.2 (A) Axial multidetector computed tomography image in a patient with a small bowel obstruction caused by a gallstone. A cholecystoenteric fistula is suggested by the air visible in an inflamed subhepatic structure most consistent with the gallbladder. The gallstone is visible as a brightly radioopaque structure in the pelvis. (B) The gallstone extracted from the small bowel at the time of surgery.

must be weighed against the ultimate decision to operate, they must not impede the decision to proceed if the indications warrant exploration. Operation for relief of obstruction is generally considered to fall into two categories: unrelenting mechanical obstruction and/or progression of a septic picture caused by vascular compromise to the gut and necrosis, or leakage due to perforation or anastomotic failure. The first scenario—complete obstruction—classically presents in a patient with a history of previous abdominal surgery, progressive abdominal swelling with or without tenderness, and failure to pass flatus or bowel movements. For more proximal obstruction, vomiting is more common, which might result in a hypochloremic alkalosis. Distention might not be so marked. For lower small bowel or colonic obstruction, more distention and abdominal swelling is present. Third-space, intraluminal collection of fluid might present as dehydration as demonstrated by lab values and clinical findings. Interestingly, in early stages, as the obstruction increases, diarrhea may be present and might confuse the clinical picture. Bowel sounds may initially be hyperactive, then decrease.

A septic picture raises the more ominous diagnosis of strangulated bowel or leak. Both result in a more seriously ill patient whose complication rate and mortality can be worsened by a delay in diagnosis. Bowel wall integrity can be compromised by a folding or knuckling of the bowel from adhesion or hernia. Additionally, patients prone to arterial emboli can have mesenteric ischemia and present with an ileus/obstruction picture. In patients with strangulation or leakage, the white blood count can be elevated along with serum lactate levels. Abdominal tenderness and rebound are usually more pronounced than in simple mechanical obstruction. Bowel sounds are usually diminished or absent. In all cases where obstruction or strangulation is suspected, a rectal exam must be performed. This gives important information including mass effect in the pelvis, presence of stool, and possibly blood suggesting malignancy.

IMAGING

Radiologic imaging plays a crucial role in the diagnosis and management of patients with suspected SBO. Whether the stable patient can be managed by medical therapy (nasogastric decompression, intravenous [IV] fluid hydration, and electrolyte replacement) or needs surgical intervention hinges on whether intestinal strangulation can be excluded.[14–16] The radiologic assessment of these patients must focus on several important questions: (1) Is the small bowel obstructed? (2) What is the severity of the bowel obstruction? (3) Where is the obstruction located (is there a point of transition)? (4) What is the etiology of the obstruction? (5) Is there a closed-loop obstruction? (6) Is bowel ischemia or strangulation present?[17] A myriad of radiologic investigations are available, and the evaluating physician must choose in a reliable, cost-effective way.

Historically, the initial radiographic study, after a thorough history and physical exam, would be plain abdominal radiographs in standing and supine positions. These studies can classically show distended loops of bowel, intestinal wall thickening, air-fluid levels, and radiopaque objects, which might be the cause of the obstruction (Fig. 72.3). Obviously, any or all of these findings may be present, but the skilled clinician should be able to correlate these radiograph findings with the clinical picture. A recent study evaluating plain radiographs in patients with suspected SBO demonstrated good accuracy, with a mean sensitivity of 83% in correctly identifying an SBO.[18] One major reason that abdominal radiography has a low specificity in diagnosing an SBO is that both mechanical obstruction and functional bowel disorders may appear identical.

Recent guidelines have a level 1 recommendation for the use of computed tomography (CT) scans in patients suspected of having an SBO. This is based on several studies that demonstrate improved sensitivity in CT scans compared to radiographs to detect obstruction and ischemia, and cross-sectional imaging provides valuable information regarding the level and often the cause of

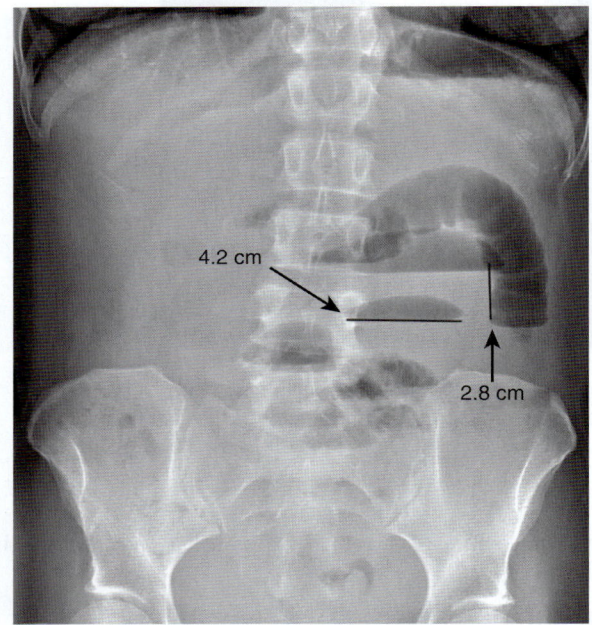

FIGURE 72.3 Upright plain radiograph of a patient with a high-grade distal small bowel obstruction demonstrating multiple dilated small bowel loops (>3 cm in diameter), more than two air-fluid levels, an air-fluid level wider than 2.5 cm *(horizontal black line),* and air-fluid small bowel levels differing more than 5 mm from one another in the same bowel loop *(vertical black line).*

the obstruction (Fig. 72.4).[19] A CT scan with intravenous and oral contrast can give more detailed information about the point of obstruction, abdominal masses including malignancy or abscess, and the likelihood of closed-loop obstruction or bowel ischemia. Vascular anatomy can be more carefully evaluated as well. The most important finding of SBO on cross-sectional imaging is the presence of dilated proximal small bowel (diameter >2.5 cm) loops, with decompressed or normal-caliber distal small bowel.[20,21] Patients should be evaluated after the administration of IV contrast when possible, remembering that the use of IV contrast mandates evaluation of renal function and appropriate hydration. IV contrast is essential for discriminating normal bowel wall enhancement from areas of abnormal enhancement caused by intrinsic small bowel abnormalities (Crohn disease, infectious enteritis, small bowel neoplasms, vasculitis, hematoma, or intussusception), extrinsic causes (adhesions, hernias, endometriosis, or metastatic intraperitoneal tumor), or bowel wall ischemia or infarction from strangulation or closed-loop obstruction. Consideration of both contrast-enhanced and unenhanced bowel wall may improve sensitivity.[22] An obstruction is considered a closed-loop type when a loop of bowel is obstructed at two points at a single site.[21] The site of obstruction may involve a single or multiple loops of small bowel; an incarcerated hernia is a classic example (Fig. 72.5). The closed loop is able to rotate on its axis along with its mesentery, potentially producing a small bowel volvulus classically associated with a "swirl sign" (Fig. 72.6). If the obstruction is severe enough or volvulus occurs, bowel ischemia ensues with subsequent infarction and/or perforation. Closed-loop obstructions should be considered an indication for urgent surgical intervention in most cases because they are exceedingly unlikely to resolve with nonoperative therapy and the potential for bowel

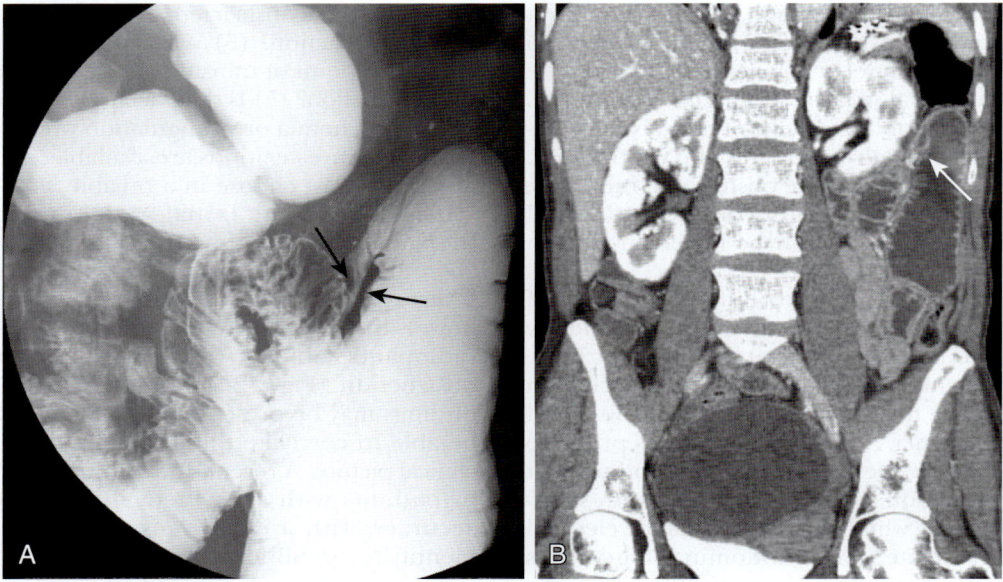

FIGURE 72.4 (A) Image from small bowel follow-through after administration of water soluble contrast medium in a patient with a proximal high-grade small bowel obstruction demonstrating extrinsic compression from an adhesive band *(arrows).* (B) Coronal reformatted multidetector computed tomography image of the same patient demonstrating proximal dilated loops of small bowel leading up to an abrupt transition zone *(arrow).*

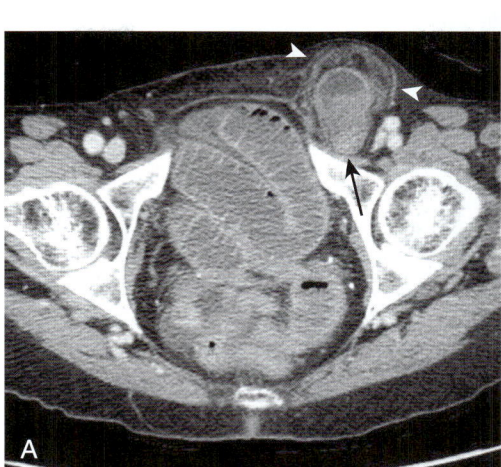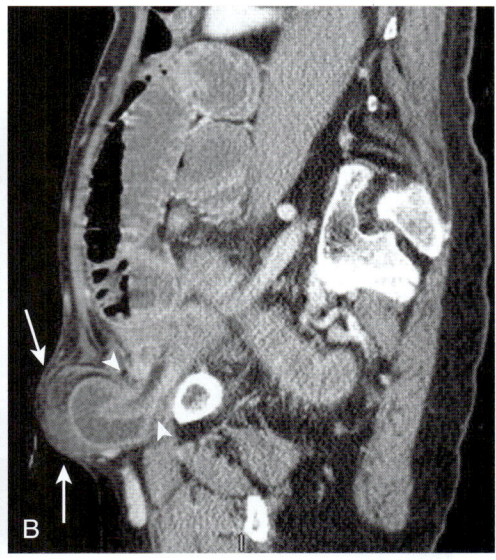

FIGURE 72.5 (A) Axial multidetector computed tomography image in a patient with a closed-loop small bowel obstruction produced by an incarcerated left inguinal hernia with ischemia demonstrating an edematous herniated small bowel loop *(arrow)* with infiltrating fluid in subcutaneous fat *(arrowheads)*. (B) Sagittal reformatted multidetector computed tomography image of the same patient better demonstrates the incarcerated herniated small bowel loop *(arrowheads)* and infiltrated subcutaneous fluid *(arrows)*.

ischemia is high and increases with delay in definitive therapy. In one recent series, 23 of 24 patients (95.8%) with closed-loop obstruction identified on CT scan required bowel resection for ischemia or necrosis.[23] The use of water-soluble contrast (Gastrografin) may be a therapeutic intervention as well as a diagnostic one. The purported therapeutic value of water-soluble contrast agents is related to their high osmolality, which is approximately 6 times that of extracellular fluid.[24,25] As a result, fluid from the edematous bowel wall may shift into the lumen, both reducing the constriction of the bowel wall and diluting the luminal contents, hopefully thus permitting their passage through a partially obstructed area. It may be a predictor of whether a patient will need operative intervention, as well. Failure of contrast to reach the colon within 24 hours correctly predicts the need for surgery 96% of the time.[24,26] This technique decreased the time to operation and subsequent length of stay in the hospital by more rapidly determining who needs an operation.[24,27–29] Consequently, the Eastern Association for the Surgery of Trauma recommends that all patients who fail to improve after 48 hours of nonoperative management should undergo a water-soluble contrast study for both therapeutic and diagnostic purposes (level 2 recommendation).[19]

Instillation of barium and small bowel follow-through studies have largely been supplanted by CT with oral contrast. That said, it may well be that barium small bowel follow-through studies remain an option for patients with uncertain diagnosis of low-grade, recurrent obstructive patterns. Primary small bowel malignancy, though rare, can be investigated using this study or capsule endoscopy.

Other studies are available, but of limited applicability. Magnetic resonance imaging (MRI) may be used as an alternative to CT in patients for whom the radiation exposure is an issue, as in pregnancy. However, there are no good data that MRI offers any advantage under routine circumstances, and in fact, is both more costly and more cumbersome in terms of time to acquire and read the images. Ultrasound is also an alternate modality, but really of limited use, especially when intestinal dilation is present and air-fluid levels limit the effectiveness of the study.

In summary, the approach to the patient with SBO should be initiated with a thorough, cost-effective strategy. History and physical exam are important, and necessarily thorough and inclusive of a wide range of presenting symptoms. Laboratory studies should be directed toward evaluation of electrolyte imbalance, dehydration, and renal function. In more severe cases, sepsis should be considered and treated if identified. Imaging should also be expeditious and directed at a specific cause and location. This workup needs to be done in a thorough and timely manner to avoid deterioration of a patient from a simple obstruction picture into a more complex septic scenario with loss of bowel integrity.

TREATMENT

As emphasized previously, the diagnosis of SBO offers a wide spectrum of complexity. Decision making for surgery can be equally challenging. The most straightforward reasoning, however, is that persistent mechanical obstruction would dictate operative intervention, for two reasons: failure of conservative management and/or prevention of serious deterioration to a septic picture due to strangulation. During the time of preoperative decision making, optimization of the patient's clinical status should be undertaken. Fluid status and electrolyte disturbances should be corrected. Foley catheterization can be used to monitor fluid output. Any cardiac or pulmonary issues should be addressed. Strict input and output measurements

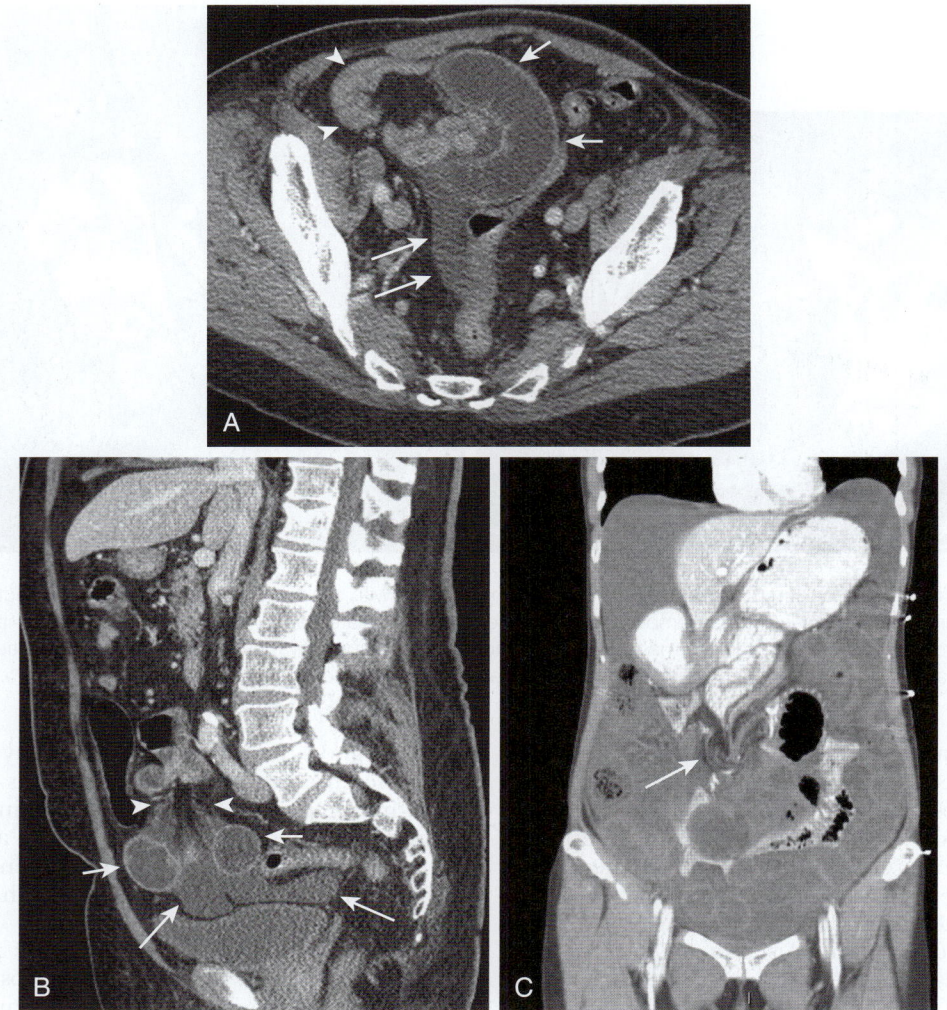

FIGURE 72.6 (A) Axial multidetector computed tomography image in a patient with a closed-loop small bowel obstruction with ischemia caused by an internal hernia demonstrating a dilated C-shaped loop *(short arrows)*, decompressed distal small bowel *(arrowheads)*, and fluid adjacent to the incarcerated loop of the small bowel *(long arrows)*. (B) Sagittal reformatted multidetector computed tomography image of same patient better demonstrates the incarcerated small bowel loop *(short arrows)*, with convergence of mesenteric vessels at the internal hernia site *(arrowheads)* and adjacent fluid indicating bowel wall ischemia *(long arrows)*. (C) A coronal view of a different patient clearly demonstrates the swirl sign *(arrow)*, indicative of bowel rotated on its mesenteric axis.

should be kept and deficiencies dealt with preoperatively. Prophylactic antibiotics should be administered as the clinical situation dictates. For more complicated preoperative situations, consultations with the anesthesia or cardiology services can be helpful, particularly if there are intraoperative events needing related care.

Several recent studies have evaluated possible predictors for increased risk for surgical intervention that might aid decision making. Miller et al. reviewed more than 400 patients with SBO, of whom 36% underwent operations. They found that among patients with SBO and previous laparotomies, colorectal and gynecologic operations were the two most common antecedant procedure types.[30] O'Leary et al. reviewed more than 200 patients and identified independent predictors for surgery. Multivariable analysis showed that persistent abdominal pain, persistent distention, fever at 48 hours, and high-grade obstruction on CT scans were significant predictors of the need for

operative management. Eighty-five percent of patients who had none of these findings were managed nonoperatively.[31] Bilderback and colleagues evaluated the admitting service for patients with SBO. They reported that patients evaluated on a surgical service when compared to a hospitalist service showed decreased length of stay (LOS) and reduced cost in preoperative workup if management was ultimately operative in nature.[32]

Decision making necessarily includes timing of intervention. Except under the most unusual circumstances, surgery need not be an emergency. Adequate time must be taken for fluid resuscitation as discussed previously. However, these are also consequences of inappropriate delay. Two recent studies using the American College of Surgeons National Surgical Quality Improvement Program (NSQIP) evaluated "early" versus "delayed" intervention for SBO. Keenan's group evaluated more than 9000 patients and reported an increased 30-day overall morbidity, though not mortality, for patients who received operation after 3 days in the hospital as compared with those receiving operation earlier in their stay.[33] Teixeira's group studied more than 4000 patients using the same NSQIP database. They reported that a delay of greater than 24 hours in surgery was associated with significantly higher mortality, surgical site infections, sepsis, and septic shock. Early intervention had a significantly shorter LOS.[34]

The advent of laparoscopy has added a new technology while leaving all the elements of decision making intact. Recent literature reports the effect that this technique has had on outcomes. Kelly evaluated NSQIP data for more than 9000 patients with "adhesive SBO" from 2005 to 2011. They compared patients receiving laparoscopic versus open procedures. Patients undergoing laparoscopic procedures had significantly shorter operative times and shorter postoperative LOS. They were less likely to develop major complications or incisional complications. Thirty-day mortality was 1.3% compared to the open group's 4.7%, a significant reduction.[35] Lombardo's group also evaluated NSQIP data on more than 6000 patients from 2005 to 2009. In contrast, their propensity-matched analysis of almost 450 patients did not show any differences in operative time, reoperation within 30 days, or mortality when comparing laparoscopic versus open procedures; however, they did show significantly lower rates of postoperative morbidity with the laparoscopic group.[36] However, it is critical to recognize that NSQIP and other such registry data do not reliably capture the conversion rate from laparoscopic to open, which ranges from 20% to 50% in some series.[37,38] Many other studies are emerging evaluating the use of laparoscopy, documenting its arrival and acceptance as a technologic addition, and possibly improvement, in the treatment of SBO.[1,39] These and other reports emphasize at least two important factors that remain paramount in dealing with the clinical evaluation of the patient with SBO:

- First, the capability of using laparoscopy does not change decision making about the need for operation.
- Second, technical expertise is needed for the procedure and willingness to convert to open should not be regarded as a failure.

Intraoperative considerations during the course of exploration of the patient with SBO are the same whether done as an open procedure or laparoscopically. First, care must be employed when entering the abdomen. In fact, the opening may well be the critical part of the case. Adhesions are often present along the previous incision (or port) site. Careful visualization and dissection are important. Upon entering the abdomen, it is important to determine the cause of the obstruction and be prepared to deal with it. These include adhesive band or bands, matted adhesions, tumors requiring resection or colostomy, gallstone ileus, or diffuse carcinomatosis requiring proximal decompression. Whether or not these procedures can be done with confidence by the operating surgeon requires his or her own frank assessment of both the findings and his or her own technical abilities. Finally, upon completion of the procedure, it should be the goal of the operating surgeon to evaluate the entire GI tract and abdominal contents and have confidence that no small tears, bowel wall rents, or ischemic areas are left behind. Inadvertent tears or electrocautery burns can occur outside the field of vision in both open and laparoscopic cases, and can have devastating postoperative consequences.

SUMMARY

There have been substantial improvements recently in both the quality and quantity of imaging and surgical techniques available for the treatment of SBO. Although these have somewhat changed current practice for evaluation and treatment, the key to successful management of SBO remains selecting the right patient for the right procedure at the right time to minimize morbidity and time to recovery.

ACKNOWLEDGMENT

This chapter is based on a previous version written by Klinger, Sudakoff, and Otterson.

REFERENCES

1. Jafari MD, Jafari F, Foe-Paker JE, et al. Adhesive small bowel obstruction in the United States: has laparoscopy made an impact? *Am Surg.* 2015;81(10):1028-1033.
2. Ray N. Abdominal adhesiolysis: inpatient care and expenditures in the United States in 1994. *J Am Coll Surg.* 1998;186(1):1-9. doi:10.1016/S1072-7515(97)00127-0.
3. Bures J. Small intestinal bacterial overgrowth syndrome. *World J Gastroenterol.* 2010;16(24):2978-2990. doi:10.3748/wjg.v16.i24.2978.
4. MacFie J. Current status of bacterial translocation as a cause of surgical sepsis. *Br Med Bull.* 2004;71(1):1-11. doi:10.1093/bmb/ldh029.
5. Becker G, Plum HE. Novel opioid antagonists for opioid-induced bowel dysfunction and postoperative ileus. *Lancet.* 2009;373(9670):1198-1206. doi:10.1016/S0140-6736(09)60139-2.
6. Traut U, Brügger L, Kunz R, et al. Systemic prokinetic pharmacologic treatment for postoperative adynamic ileus following abdominal surgery in adults. *Cochrane Database Syst Rev.* 2008;(1):CD004930. doi:10.1002/14651858.CD004930.pub3.
7. Schnüriger B, Barmparas G, Branco BC, Lustenberger T, Inaba K, Demetriades D. Prevention of postoperative peritoneal adhesions: a review of the literature. *Am J Surg.* 2011;201(1):111-121. doi:10.1016/j.amjsurg.2010.02.008.
8. Menzies D, Ellis H. Intestinal obstruction from adhesions—how big is the problem? *Ann R Coll Surg Engl.* 1990;72(1):60-63. doi:10.2307/40719809?ref=search-gateway:82bdb86a102bea3c725a93e5df4fe9b7.
9. Weibel MA, Majno G. Peritoneal adhesions and their relation to abdominal surgery. *Am J Surg.* 1973;126(3):345-353. doi:10.1016/S0002-9610(73)80123-0.
10. Fevang BT, Fevang J, Stangeland L, Søreide O, Svanes K, Viste A. Complications and death after surgical treatment of small bowel obstruction. *Ann Surg.* 2000;231(4):529-537. doi:10.1097/00000658-200004000-00012.
11. Miller G, Boman J, Shrier I, Gordon PH. Etiology of small bowel obstruction. *Am J Surg.* 2000;180(1):33-36. doi:10.1016/S0002-9610(00)00407-4.
12. Bauman RW, Pirrello JR. Internal hernia at Petersen's space after laparoscopic Roux-en-Y gastric bypass: 6.2% incidence without closure—a single surgeon series of 1047 cases. *Surg Obes Relat Dis.* 2009;5(5):565-570. doi:10.1016/j.soard.2008.10.013.
13. Modlin IM, Kidd M, Latich I, Zikusoka MN, Shapiro MD. Current status of gastrointestinal carcinoids. *Gastroenterology.* 2005;128(6):1717-1751. doi:10.1053/j.gastro.2005.03.038.
14. Maglinte DDT, Heitkamp DE, Howard TJ, Kelvin FM, Lappas JC. Current concepts in imaging of small bowel obstruction. *Radiol Clin North Am.* 2003;41(2):263-283. doi:10.1016/S0033-8389(02)00114-8.

15. Tingstedt B, Isaksson J, Andersson R. Long-term follow-up and cost analysis following surgery for small bowel obstruction caused by intra-abdominal adhesions. *Br J Surg.* 2007;94(6):743-748. doi:10.1002/bjs.5634.

16. Snyder CL, Ferrell KL, Goodale RL, Leonard AS. Nonoperative management of small-bowel obstruction with endoscopic long intestinal tube placement. *Am Surg.* 1990;56(10):587-592.

17. Silva AC, Pimenta M, Guimaraes LS. Small bowel obstruction: what to look for. *Radiographics.* 2009;29(2):423-439. doi:10.1148/rg.292085514.

18. Thompson WM, Kilani RK, Smith BB, et al. Accuracy of abdominal radiography in acute small-bowel obstruction: does reviewer experience matter? *Am J Roentgenol.* 2007;188(3):W233-W238. doi:10.2214/AJR.06.0817.

19. Maung AA, Johnson DC, Piper GL. Evaluation and management of small-bowel obstruction: an Eastern Association for the Surgery of Trauma practice management guideline. *J Trauma Acute Care Surg.* 2012;73(5 suppl 4):S362-S369.

20. Nicolaou S, Kai B, Ho S, Su J, Ahamed K. Imaging of acute small-bowel obstruction. *Am J Roentgenol.* 2005;185(4):1036-1044. doi:10.2214/AJR.04.0815.

21. Furukawa A, Yamasaki M, Furuichi K, et al. Helical CT in the diagnosis of small bowel obstruction. *Radiographics.* 2001;21(2):341-355. doi:10.1148/radiographics.21.2.g01mr05341.

22. Chuong AM, Corno L, Beaussier H, et al. Assessment of bowel wall enhancement for the diagnosis of intestinal ischemia in patients with small bowel obstruction: value of adding unenhanced CT to contrast-enhanced CT. *Radiology.* 2016;280(1):98-107. doi:10.1148/radiol.2016151029.

23. Makar RA, Bashir MR, Haystead CM, et al. Diagnostic performance of MDCT in identifying closed loop small bowel obstruction. *Abdom Radiol.* 2016;41(7):1253-1260. doi:10.1007/s00261-016-0656-4.

24. Burge J, Abbas SM, Roadley G, et al. Randomized controlled trial of Gastrografin in adhesive small bowel obstruction. *ANZ J Surg.* 2005;75(8):672-674. doi:10.1111/j.1445-2197.2005.03491.x.

25. Pickleman J, Lee RM. The management of patients with suspected early postoperative small bowel obstruction. *Ann Surg.* 1989;210(2):216-219. doi:10.1097/00000658-198908000-00013.

26. Di Saverio S, Catena F, Ansaloni L, Gavioli M, Valentino M, Pinna AD. Water- soluble contrast medium (Gastrografin) value in adhesive small intestine obstruction (ASIO): a prospective, randomized, controlled, clinical trial. *World J Surg.* 2008;32(10):2293-2304. doi:10.1007/s00268-008-9694-6.

27. Fevang T, Jensen D, Fevang J, et al. Upper gastrointestinal contrast study in the management of small bowel obstruction—a prospective randomised study. *Eur J Surg.* 2000;166(1):39-43. doi:10.1080/110241500750009681.

28. Choi H-K. Value of Gastrografin in adhesive small bowel obstruction after unsuccessful conservative treatment: a prospective evaluation. *World J Gastroenterol.* 2005;11(24):3742. doi:10.3748/wjg.v11.i24.3742.

29. Branco BC, Barmparas G, Schnüriger B, Inaba K, Chan LS, Demetriades D. Systematic review and meta-analysis of the diagnostic and therapeutic role of water-soluble contrast agent in adhesive small bowel obstruction. *Br J Surg.* 2010;97(4):470-478. doi:10.1002/bjs.7019.

30. Miller G, Boman J, Shrier I, Gordon PH. Natural history of patients with adhesive small bowel obstruction. *Br J Surg.* 2000;87(9):1240-1247. doi:10.1046/j.1365-2168.2000.01530.x.

31. O'Leary EA, Desale SY, Yi WS, et al. Letting the sun set on small bowel obstruction: can a simple risk score tell us when nonoperative care is inappropriate? *Am Surg.* 2014;80(6):572-579.

32. Bilderback PA, Massman JD, Smith RK, La Selva D, Helton WS. Small bowel obstruction is a surgical disease: patients with adhesive small bowel obstruction requiring operation have more cost-effective care when admitted to a surgical service. *J Am Coll Surg.* 2015;221(1):7-13. doi:10.1016/j.jamcollsurg.2015.03.054.

33. Keenan JE, Turley RS, McCoy CC, Migaly J, Shapiro ML, Scarborough JE. Trials of nonoperative management exceeding 3 days are associated with increased morbidity in patients undergoing surgery for uncomplicated adhesive small bowel obstruction. *J Trauma Acute Care Surg.* 2014;76(6):1367-1372. doi:10.1097/TA.0000000000000246.

34. Teixeira PG, Karamanos E, Talving P, Inaba K, Lam L, Demetriades D. Early operation is associated with a survival benefit for patients with adhesive bowel obstruction. *Ann Surg.* 2013;258(3):459-465. doi:10.1097/SLA.0b013e3182a1b100.

35. Kelly KN, Iannuzzi JC, Rickles AS, Garimella V, Monson JRT, Fleming FJ. Laparotomy for small-bowel obstruction: first choice or last resort for adhesiolysis? A laparoscopic approach for small-bowel obstruction reduces 30-day complications. *Surg Endosc.* 2014;28(1):65-73. doi:10.1007/s00464-013-3162-6.

36. Lombardo S, Baum K, Filho JD, Nirula R. Should adhesive small bowel obstruction be managed laparoscopically? A National Surgical Quality Improvement Program propensity score analysis. *J Trauma Acute Care Surg.* 2014;76(3):696-703. doi:10.1097/TA.0000000000000156.

37. Tasselli S, Zerman G, Pedrazzani C, Manzoni G, Borzellino G. Laparoscopic approach to postoperative adhesive obstruction. *Surg Endosc.* 2004;18(4):686-690. doi:10.1007/s00464-003-9106-9.

38. Wullstein C, Gross E. Laparoscopic compared with conventional treatment of acute adhesive small bowel obstruction. *Br J Surg.* 2003;90(9):1147-1151. doi:10.1002/bjs.4177.

39. Byrne J, Saleh F, Ambrosini L, Quereshy F, Jackson TD, Okrainec A. Laparoscopic versus open surgical management of adhesive small bowel obstruction: a comparison of outcomes. *Surg Endosc.* 2015;29(9):2525-2532. doi:10.1007/s00464-014-4015-7.

Volvulus of the Stomach and Small Bowel

Riaz Cassim

The term *volvulus* derives from the Latin word *volvere*, meaning to turn or roll. Clinically, *volvulus* refers to a greater than 180-degree twisting of a hollow organ about its mesentery, resulting in luminal obstruction, impaired venous return, and eventually ischemia and perforation. Although much less common than volvulus of the cecum and sigmoid colon, small bowel volvulus (SBV) and gastric volvulus (GV) are clinical problems that, when not recognized promptly, can lead to necrosis of the involved organ with resultant high morbidity and mortality.

SMALL BOWEL VOLVULUS

EPIDEMIOLOGY

Volvulus of the small bowel is more common in children and is most often secondary to malrotation. The incidence of SBV in adults varies considerably in different parts of the world, being uncommon in Western countries but more of a health care burden in Central Africa, Middle East, Asia, and the Indian subcontinent.[1–24] No population-based studies have been reported from European, African, or Asian countries, making an assessment of the true incidence difficult. Retrospective studies dating back several decades suggest that the annual occurrence of SBV is 1.7 to 5.7 in North America and Western Europe, as compared with 6 to 37.5 patients diagnosed with SBV/year in Africa, Middle East, and Asia.[1,9–12,16,19–24] Case series from the Western countries estimate that SBV accounts for 1.7% to 8% of all bowel obstructions and 4% to 13% of all small bowel obstructions.[2,17,23] In Nepal, Uganda, Iran, and India 3.5% to 37% of all obstructions and 18.5% to 51.5% of all small bowel obstructions are attributable to SBV.[5,7,9,11,14,19,20,24]

Coe et al. published results from a US population-based study using the Nationwide Inpatient Sample (1998–2010), a 20% stratified sample of US hospitals. Of the 2.065 million hospitalizations for bowel obstruction (representing an estimated 10.33 million hospitalizations across the United States) there were 20,680 cases of SBV, representing an incidence of 1%.[4] Females were more often affected (56.6%), with the mean age of the patient population being 66 years, which is similar to previous studies reported from the Western countries.[2,3,15,16] In contrast, the overwhelming majority of patients presenting with SBV in Nepal, India, Iran, and Afghanistan were young males.[5–12,14,19,20,24]

ETIOLOGY

SBV is categorized as primary or secondary.[14,18] Primary SBV occurs without predisposing factors or underlying anatomic abnormalities. In the African, Asian, and Middle Eastern countries 31% to 100% of patients with SBV have no other underlying pathology, whereas less than 30% (10% to 30%) of patients with SBV in the Western world and Far East share this etiology.[1–3,13,16,17,19–24] The underlying cause of primary SBV is poorly understood, and several anatomic and dietary factors have been implicated. Primary SBV in developing nations correlates with lower socioeconomic status, with a vast majority of affected individuals being laborers and farmers. The consumption of large infrequent meals consisting of vegetables and high-fiber along with manual labor in an upright position has been postulated to account for this condition.[6–11] SBV has been observed in Afghanistan during the month of Ramadan, when Muslims ingest large quantities of high-fiber food after prolonged fasting.[6] De Souza reported 12 cases of primary SBV over a 2-year period in a Ugandan tribe who consumed a large amount of a beer rich in serotonin.[25] A recent review from Spain noted an association of primary SBV with diabetic neuropathy and its altered small bowel motility.[16]

Anatomically, the small bowel in high-risk populations has been observed to have a longer mobile mesentery with a narrower insertion and a lack of mesenteric fat. Patients with SBV in the Eastern countries have firm, muscular abdomens, theoretically limiting the mobility of bowel in the anteroposterior plane. It is thus postulated that females are less often diagnosed with primary SBV in the developing countries, their abdominal wall laxity from childbearing conferring an advantage.[8,14,19,20] These observations support a popular theory that rapid filling of a segment of proximal intestine with high-bulk chyme pulls the heavier loops down into the left pelvis where there is little resistance and displaces the empty distal bowel loops upward toward the right upper abdomen, thereby initiating the torsion around the superior mesenteric vessels.[13,14,18]

In contrast, secondary SBV is caused by predisposing factors, either congenital or acquired, and is more common than primary SBV in North America and Western Europe. In secondary SBV the intestine is twisted around an underlying point of fixation, and as the loop fills with fluid, peristalsis exacerbates the torsion, causing a closed-loop obstruction. By far the most common cause of secondary SBV are postoperative adhesions.[4] Case reports have described a number of other lead points, including small bowel and mesenteric tumors,[21,26–29] mesenteric lymph nodes,[30] Meckel diverticulum,[2,23] malrotation,[4,23] small intestinal diverticula,[21,22] ascariasis,[20,31] tuberculous adhesions,[20] and stomas.[3] In pregnancy, SBV is the second most common cause of small bowel obstruction after adhesions.[21,32]

In 56% to 80% of cases of primary SBV the intestinal torsion is clockwise, as it is for neonatal midgut volvulus associated with congenital malrotation.[8,14] However, congenital malrotation causing volvulus rarely manifests in delayed fashion. Among all patients hospitalized for

TABLE 73.1 Modern Series of Small Bowel Volvulus

Author	Roggo[2]	Ruiz-Tovar[16]	Gurleyik[23]	Ghebrat[19]	Demissie[20]	Ray[24]
Country	USA	Spain	Turkey	Ethiopia	Ethiopia	Nepal
Study period	1980–1990	1977–2007	1985–1995	1995–1997	1992–1996	1996–2000
Number of patients	35	129	38	51	98	35
Male-to-female ratio	1:1.2	1:1.15	6.6:1	12:1	8.8:1	4.8:1
Average age	67	55	30	37	34	41
Primary small bowel volvulus	14%	30.2%	47%	92%	95%	100%
Gangrenous small bowel	46%	46.5%	32%	18%	27.5%	34%
Mortality overall	9%	9.3%	2.6%	12%	13.3%	8%
Mortality from gangrene	17%	Not stated	8.3%	Not stated	25.9%	25%

SBV (20,680), Coe et al. identified only 169 adult patient with malrotation (0.82%).[4] In most case series the ileum was most often affected segment of small bowel.[3,9,13,16,17]

Table 73.1 compares six case series of SBV, illustrating some of the differences between primary and secondary SBV between the Western countries and parts of Africa and Asia.

DIAGNOSIS

Clinically, the findings in patients with SBV are nonspecific, making preoperative diagnosis difficult. Ruiz-Tovar et al. preoperatively diagnosed only 18.6% of their cases (24/129). Most patients present emergently (89%) with signs and symptoms of acute small bowel obstruction, with 19% presenting with an acute abdomen.[4] Central abdominal pain is the cardinal symptom.[1,2,19,21] Patients also have other frequent symptoms of acute bowel obstruction, including nausea, emesis, abdominal distention, and constipation/obstipation. In some cases a previous history of intermittent obstructive symptoms, such as crampy epigastric or periumbilical abdominal pain signifying chronic intermittent SBV may be elicited. Although not specific or sensitive, pain out of proportion to the physical findings should raise suspicion of vascular compromise and bowel ischemia, as should fever, tachycardia, peritoneal signs, acidosis, and leukocytosis. Ray et al. from Nepal reported that 80% of patients presenting with tachycardia greater than 100/minute, fever of greater than 38°C, involuntary guarding and rebound, and a white cell count of greater than 15,000/mm³ had gangrenous bowel.[24]

Plain abdominal radiographs are usually nonspecific and may demonstrate dilated loops of bowel or air-fluid levels. As volvulus is a closed-loop obstruction, the bowel loops may be filled with fluid and have little or no air and plain abdominal films may reveal a gasless lower abdomen. If the small bowel is gangrenous, pneumatosis or portal venous gas may be seen. Gastrointestinal contrast studies may show a corkscrew pattern or an abrupt "bird beak" at the point of obstruction, and angiography may demonstrate a spiraling pattern of the mesenteric vessels described as the "barber pole" sign.[30] In the acute setting, computed tomography (CT) has largely replaced these modalities for the evaluation of acute small bowel obstruction because it is widely available, rapid, noninvasive, and can rule out other causes of obstruction and intraabdominal pathology. In SBV the classic CT finding is the "whirl" sign (Fig. 73.1). The superior mesenteric vein (SMV) is displaced,

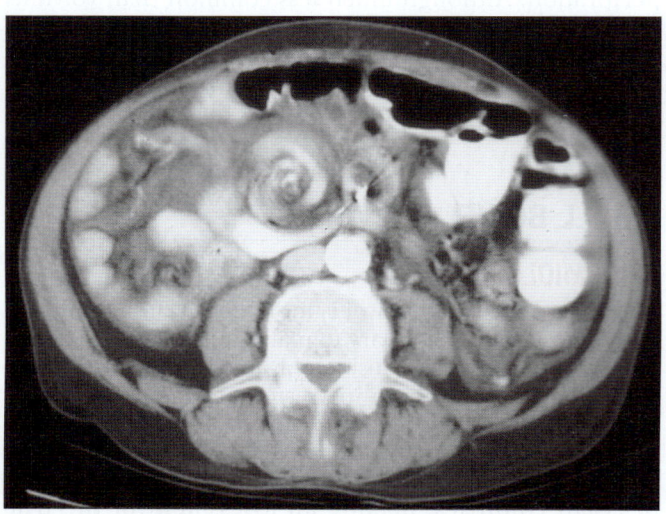

FIGURE 73.1 Abdominal computed tomography scan with a "whirl" sign in a patient with small bowel volvulus secondary to postoperative adhesions. (Courtesy William M. Thomson, MD.)

lying anterior to the superior mesenteric artery (SMA) rather than in its normal right-sided position, along with a twist of the mesentery.[33] The latter can be seen in other intraabdominal condition such as adhesions and previous hemicolectomy, and the sensitivity of the CT "whirl" sign is between 27% and 64%.[21,33,34] The abrupt termination of the dilated bowel segments in the vicinity of the mesenteric whirl is another important sign. The proximal afferent loop of bowel leading into the closed loop dilates, and the departing efferent segment collapses. Thus there are three dilated loops: two formed by the closed loop and the third by the proximal afferent loop, with all three loops tapering abruptly at the point of torsion, giving rise to the "bird beak" sign.[33] Small bowel wall thickening, pneumatosis, portal venous gas, and free intraperitoneal fluid suggest small bowel ischemia. The accuracy of CT imaging in SBV is estimated at 83%.[16]

TREATMENT

Acute SBV is a surgical disease, and early diagnosis and treatment are essential to avoid intestinal necrosis. Gangrenous bowel requires the appropriate segmental resection, with most series advocating primary anastomosis. In Western series, up to 50% of patients with SBV require resection for gangrenous small bowel.[2,3,16] The rarity of SBV in North America and Europe may lead to a delay in diagnosis and a higher incidence of gangrenous small bowel than in Asian and African countries.

For patients without ischemic bowel, the optimal surgical treatment is less clear. Most case series describe simple detorsion of the volvulus without resection, although no long-term follow-up is available to determine recurrence rate. To prevent recurrent volvulus, some authors have described bowel resection in the absence of gangrene while others have performed intestinopexy of long segments of bowel. These procedures run the risk of short gut syndrome and increased risk of adhesive bowel obstruction and must be used with caution. No prospective studies have addressed the issue of recurrence. Two series have reported recurrence rates of 3.9% to 5.4% associated with simple detorsion in primary SBV.[16,35]

The outcome of SBV likely depends on early diagnosis, patient's age and physiologic status, associated illnesses, presence of infarcted bowel, and time to surgical intervention. Overall mortality in patients undergoing exploration for SBV ranges from 10% to 35%.[1]

The mortality for SBV with viable bowel ranges from 0% to 26%,[2,7,24,25] whereas it can rise to 40% to 100% in cases of gangrenous bowel.[6,8,13,20,24,25] Coe et al. in their population-based study from the United States reported an overall mortality of 7.92% (operative and nonoperative cases). If surgery was performed on the day of admission, the mortality was 4.78%, rising to 6.65% if surgical treatment was delayed to the second day of admission.[4]

GASTRIC VOLVULUS

ETIOLOGY AND EPIDEMIOLOGY

Similar to SBV, GV occurs when the stomach or a portion of the stomach is rotated at least 180 degrees along its longitudinal or transverse axes. The normal stomach is a very mobile intraabdominal organ and intermittently rotates without symptoms or sequelae. The correct orientation of the stomach is maintained by its four anchoring ligaments (gastrohepatic, gastrocolic, gastrophrenic, and gastrosplenic) together with the gastroesophageal junction and the retroperitoneal duodenum. Failure of these gastric attachments may be the result of agenesis, elongation, or disruption and may predispose the stomach to volvulize.[36–46] In cadaveric experiments, Dalgaard showed that gastric rotation greater than 180 degrees could not be achieved unless the gastrosplenic and/or the gastrocolic ligaments were divided.[47] Acute GV was first described by Ambroise Pare in a patient with a strangulated diaphragmatic hernia following a sword wound.[48] Berti in 1866 further detailed postmortem descriptions in a 60-year-old woman.[49]

Three classification systems exist for GV and are often used in combination. GV can be classified according to anatomy, onset (acute or chronic), and etiology (primary or secondary). The anatomic classification as proposed by Singleton[50] in 1940 is composed of (1) organoaxial rotation, (2) mesenteroaxial rotation, or (3) mixed—combination of the two. Organoaxial rotation accounts for two-thirds of cases and occurs when the stomach rotates around its longitudinal axis—a transverse line

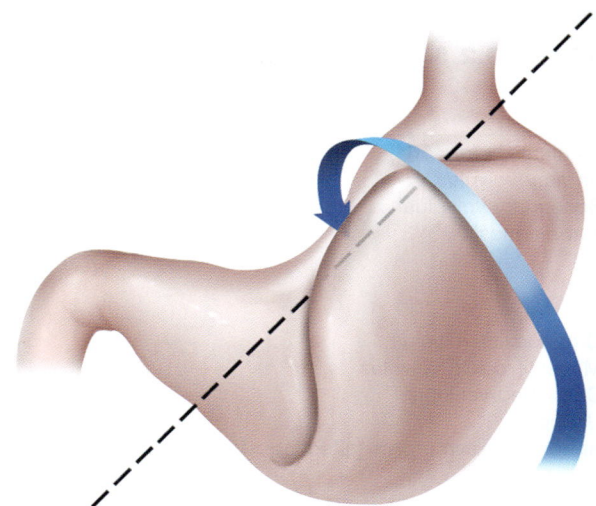

FIGURE 73.2 Organoaxial rotation occurs when the stomach rotates around its longitudinal axis—a transverse line between the pylorus and gastroesophageal junction.

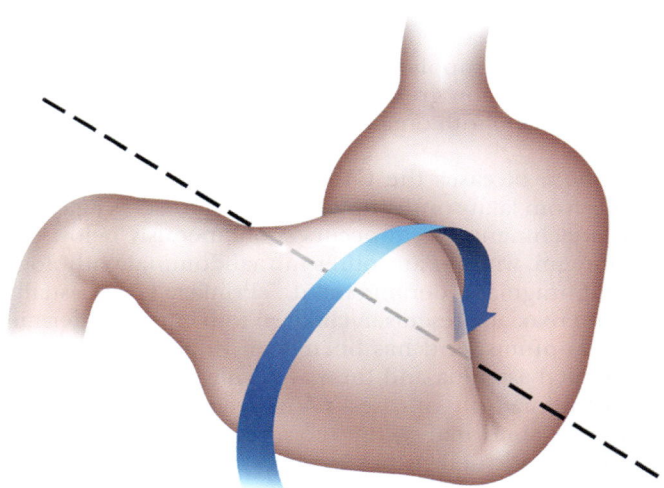

FIGURE 73.3 Mesenteroaxial rotation occurs when the stomach rotates around its short axis—a longitudinal line parallel to the gastrohepatic omentum.

between the pylorus and the gastroesophageal junction (Fig. 73.2). In most cases the antrum rotates anteriorly and superiorly and the fundus posteriorly and inferiorly, twisting the greater curvature, which comes to lie superior to the lesser curvature. Mesenteroaxial rotation is less common, accounting for one-third of cases. In this form the stomach rotates around its short axis—a longitudinal line connecting the middle of the lesser and greater curvatures and running parallel to the gastrohepatic omentum (Fig. 73.3). The pylorus rotates anteriorly and superiorly (more common) or posteriorly from right to left so that the posterior surface of the stomach lies anterior. Rarely the fundus rotates around the same axis. As the stomach fills with fluid the torsion is exacerbated. Despite

TABLE 73.2 Summary of Data in Children Worldwide With Gastric Volvulus

	Acute Gastric Volvulus	Chronic Gastric Volvulus
% Total cases (n = 584)	43	57
% Primary volvulus	31	74
% Secondary volvulus	69	26
Age at diagnosis	0–12 months (58%)	0–12 months (71%)
	1–5 years (27%)	1–5 years (16%)
	6–12 years (10%)	6–12 years (7%)
	13–18 years (4%)	13–18 years (5%)
% Organoaxial volvulus	54	85
% Mesenteroaxial volvulus	41	10
% Combined volvulus	2	3
% Unknown	3	2
Most common symptoms (affecting >10%)	Nonbilious vomiting (75%)	Nonbilious vomiting (71)
	Epigastric distention (47%)	Epigastric distention (34%)
	Abdominal pain (34%)	Failure to thrive (30%)
	Acute respiratory distress (11%)	Abdominal pain (12%)
	Cyanosis (10%)	GERD (12%)
		Colic (10%)
% Treated surgically	89	40
Overall mortality rate	7.1%	2.7%

Modified from Gerstle JT, Chiu P, Emil S. Gastric volvulus in children: lessons learned from delayed diagnoses. *Semin Pediatr Surg.* 2009;18:98–103.

the rich blood supply of the stomach, strangulation can occur with torsion greater than 180 degrees and is much more common with organoaxial than with mesenteroaxial volvulus.[38]

In 30% of cases the GV is considered primary and results from laxity or disruption of the stomach's ligamentous attachments.[36–46] It occurs spontaneously below the diaphragm, without any other intraabdominal pathology or diaphragmatic derangement.[38] Primary GV is usually mesenteroaxial, presents in children with chronic intermittent symptoms, and has been seen in association with congenital asplenia and the wandering spleen.[36,51–54]

In the majority of cases, GV is secondary to another anatomic abnormality, the most common of which are diaphragmatic defects predisposing the rotated stomach to lie in the thoracic cavity. Paraesophageal hernia is the most common cause of secondary GV in adults, whereas diaphragmatic eventration accounts for the majority of cases in children.[36,38] Intrathoracic GV has also been described in association with congenital diaphragmatic hernias (Morgagni and left-sided Bochdalek).[36,38] Most cases of secondary GV are organoaxial, with the greater curvature rotating up into the chest either anteriorly (more common) or posteriorly, giving rise to the intrathoracic "upside-down" stomach. Although secondary GV is typically intrathoracic and occurs as a result of diaphragmatic dysfunction, secondary intraabdominal GV has also been reported to occur as a result of abdominal bands and adhesions[36,37,55] and gastric tumors,[56] after sleeve gastrectomy and laparoscopic gastric banding,[57,58] and after adult living-donor liver transplantation.[59] Gastric hypermobility and volvulus is also seen in patients with severe postural deformities, such as kyphoscoliosis and patients with Down syndrome.[39,60]

The true prevalence and incidence of GV is unknown. Shriki et al.[55] estimated that more than 350 cases of GV

have been reported in the literature. No studies have estimated the actual occurrence in the adult population. In newer published series the mean age in adults with GV is 70 years, with a male preponderance (74% to 84%).[40,42] In a review article Cribbs et al. searched for all cases of GV in children published in the English literature between 1929 and 2007 (Table 73.2). A total of 581 cases of GV were identified, and 55% of children affected were males, 43% (252) presented in an acute fashion, and 69% of these cases were secondary to an associated pathologic abnormality—diaphragmatic eventration (25%), Morgagni hernia (17%), paraesophageal hernia (7%), intestinal malrotation (7%), wandering spleen (6%), asplenism (6%), and hiatal hernia (5%).[36]

DIAGNOSIS

The clinical manifestations can vary depending on the acuteness of the onset, the anatomic orientation, degree of rotation, and amount of obstruction. In 1904 Bouchardt[61] described the triad of severe epigastric pain and distention, vomiting followed by retching with an inability to vomit, and difficulty or inability to pass a nasogastric tube. This triad indicates an initial block at the pylorus, then at the cardia and later gastric distention as closed-loop obstruction develops. The Bouchardt triad can be seen in up to 70% of adult acute organoaxial GV.[39,61] The gastroesophageal junction is open in acute mesenteroaxial volvulus, and nasogastric tube placement should not be difficult. For patients with intrathoracic GV, the abdominal findings may be minimal, with predominant complaints being chest pain, shortness of breath, and symptoms secondary to mediastinal compression, including arrhythmia and tamponade.[38,55] In contrast, children with the acute form of GV do not exhibit the Bouchardt triad and present with nonbilious vomiting, epigastric distention, and abdominal pain.[36,43] Ischemia leading to gangrene can occur in 5% to 28% of cases of acute GV and is more likely to occur in organoaxial than in mesenteroaxial volvulus.[37,38] When gastric strangulation or perforation has occurred with either intraabdominal or intrathoracic GV, signs of gastrointestinal bleeding and septic shock may be evident.

In contrast, the signs and symptoms of chronic GV may be vague and intermittent,[40] or it may be an incidental finding on an imaging study. Symptoms of chronic primary GV include upper abdominal discomfort, vomiting, early satiety, dysphagia, heartburn, weight loss, and hiccups. In addition to these obstructive symptoms, patients with chronic intrathoracic GV may describe postprandial chest pain, shortness of breath, and dysphagia. The clinical diagnosis of chronic GV can be difficult because symptoms mimic gastroesophageal reflux disease and peptic ulcer disease.

Radiographic diagnosis of chronic primary GV may be difficult because the volvulus can be intermittent.[39] In the acute setting, plain abdominal films may demonstrate a spherical stomach on supine views and a double air-fluid level on upright views: one in the fundus (lower) and one in the antrum (upper). A retrocardiac air-fluid level on a lateral chest radiograph is highly suggestive of secondary intrathoracic GV. Fluoroscopy (barium swallow) has been the standard for diagnosis of GV in older reported series. Findings on upper gastrointestinal contrast study most predictive of volvulus include a paucity of distal bowel gas, gastric air-fluid level above the diaphragm, reversal of relative position of the greater to the lesser curvatures of the stomach, and a downward pointing pylorus (Fig. 73.4).[62]

CT scan is often the diagnostic modality of choice for acutely ill patients who may not be able to tolerate oral contrast for fluoroscopic examination. In addition, CT will detect other intraabdominal predisposing factors for GV (e.g., diaphragmatic defects, wandering spleen, malrotation, and gastric pneumatosis suggestive of ischemia). CT signs of GV include a transition point at the pylorus, antropyloric junction above the gastroesophageal junction, herniation of the antrum into the left hemithorax, reversed position of the greater and lesser gastric curvatures, and stenosis of the gastric segments through the stretched hiatus. The presence of the first two findings as diagnostic criteria for GV had 100% sensitivity and specificity.[63] Light et al. reported that the CT scan was diagnostic in all of their 26 patients (Fig. 73.5).[42]

In hemodynamically stable patients, endoscopy can aid in the diagnosis, with difficulty in passing the pylorus being the principal finding. Teague et al. showed that out of 18 patients who underwent upper GI endoscopy, 5 procedures were diagnostic and 6 suggestive of GV.[44]

TREATMENT

Acute GV is a surgical emergency. Mortality rates as high as 30% to 50% have been reported for this condition, with the major cause of death being sepsis secondary to gastric strangulation.[37,38,42,60] The goals of surgery are reduction of the volvulus, gastric fixation to prevent recurrence, and repair of any predisposing factors. Partial gastrectomy, gastrojejunostomy, fundoantral gastrogastrostomy (Opolzer operation), Tanner gastropexy with colonic displacement (complete division of gastrocolic omentum), and Grey's Ghimenton gastropexy (transverse mesocolic defect created

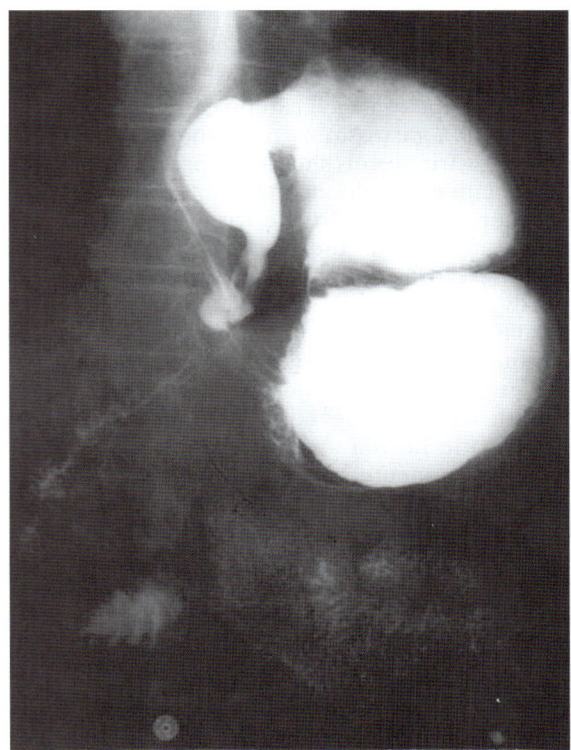

FIGURE 73.4 Upper gastrointestinal contrast study demonstrating a paraesophageal hernia with organoaxial volvulus. The greater curvature is intrathoracic, and the pylorus is in close proximity to the normally positioned gastroesophageal junction. (Courtesy William M. Thompson, MD.)

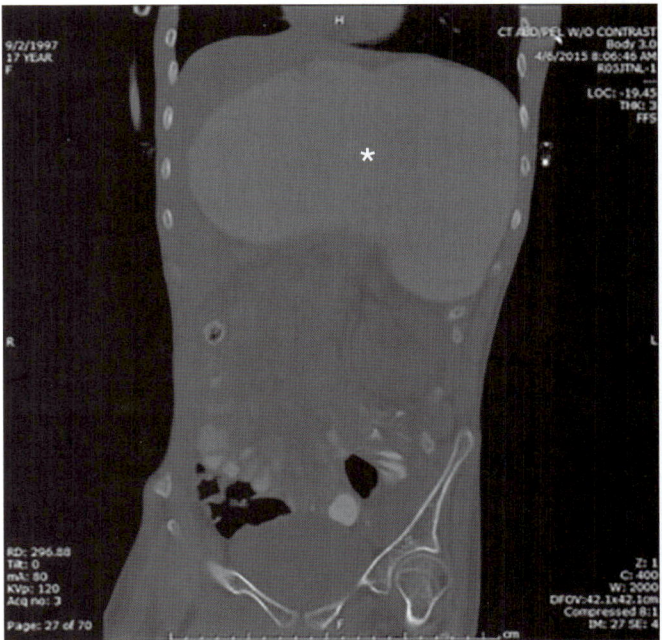

FIGURE 73.5 Computed tomography scan shows a displaced stomach with the greater curvature displaced superior to the lesser curvature, consistent with organoaxial volvulus (From Samko T, Ho CH, Ford HR. Upside-down. *J Pediatr.* 2016;169:329.)

and sutured to anterior stomach) have been described as ways to stabilize the stomach.[64,65] The most common procedure performed in adults and children is the open anterior gastropexy, which can be easily accomplished by placement of a gastrostomy tube and may be sufficient. The short gastric vessels should be preserved, if possible, both to retain their blood supply and to help to anchor the greater curvature. In the case of GV secondary to diaphragmatic hernia the diaphragmatic defect should be repaired with removal of the hernia sac. In septic or medically high-risk patients, reduction and gastropexy alone may be safer and sufficient, particularly in those with limited life expectancy.

The etiology of chronic GV dictates treatment. It is difficult to know the percentage of patients with a diaphragmatic hernia and intrathoracic stomach who will progress to acute gastric strangulation. Hsu et al.[40] reported on 44 patients with chronic GV, of whom 26 had secondary GV treated conservatively with no severe complications, with an average follow-up of 16 months. However, the high morbidity and mortality associated with strangulation justify expeditious repair, even in asymptomatic patients. In contrast, chronic primary GV is often intermittent and is much less likely to become strangulated. In the pediatric population, chronic primary GV volvulus has been successfully managed nonoperatively (positioning child right side down/prone with head elevated) in 43% of cases worldwide with good success.[36,66,67]

Upper endoscopy can be diagnostic and therapeutic for both acute and chronic GV. In selected cases of acute GV without gastric necrosis, gastric decompression, either by placement of a nasogastric tube or endoscopically, may convert an emergency to an urgent operation or even avoid an operation altogether. After the stomach has been reduced, gastropexy can be achieved by placement of a percutaneous endoscopic gastrostomy tube. However, purely endoscopic techniques are best reserved for high-risk patients because these techniques do not address the underlying pathology.

Laparoscopic and combined laparoscopic and endoscopic approaches have the potential to combine minimally invasive techniques with repair of the diaphragmatic defect.[68–72] Recent case series report minimally invasive techniques to be safe and associated with a shorter hospital stay.

REFERENCES

1. Iwuagwu O, Deans GT. Small bowel volvulus: a review. *J R Coll Surg Edinb.* 1999;44:150.
2. Roggo A, Ottinger LW. Acute small bowel volvulus in adults. A sporadic form of strangulating intestinal obstruction. *Ann Surg.* 1992;216:135.
3. Frazee RC, Mucha P Jr, Farnell MB, van Heerden JA. Volvulus of the small intestine. *Ann Surg.* 1988;208:565.
4. Coe TM, Chang DC, Sicklick JK. Small bowel volvulus in the adult populace of the United States: results from a population-based study. *Am J Surg.* 2015;210:201.
5. Saidi F. The high incidence of intestinal volvulus in Iran. *Gut.* 1969;10:838.
6. Duke JH Jr, Yar MS. Primary small bowel volvulus: cause and management. *Arch Surg.* 1977;112:685.
7. Gulati SM, Grover NK, Tagore NK, Taneja OP. Volvulus of the small intestine in India. *Am J Surg.* 1973;126:661.
8. Agrawal RL, Misra MK. Volvulus of the small intestine in Northern India. *Am J Surg.* 1970;120:366.
9. Tiwari VS, Gupta HC, Varma MM, et al. Volvulus of the small intestine. *Int Surg.* 1982;67:476.
10. Parkes G. Primary small bowel volvulus in rural Nepal. *Trop Doct.* 1997;27:156.
11. McDonald IO, Hawker DB. Small bowel volvulus—the commonest abdominal emergency in Nepal. *Bristol Med Chir J.* 1980;95:355.
12. Tegegne A. Small intestinal volvulus in adults of Gonder Region, northwestern Ethiopia. *Ethiop Med J.* 1992;30:111.
13. Moretz WH, Morton JJ. Acute volvulus of small intestine: analysis of 36 cases. *Ann Surg.* 1950;132:899.
14. Vaez-Zadeh K, Dutz W, Nowrooz-Zadeh M. Volvulus of the small intestine in adults: a study of predisposing factors. *Ann Surg.* 1969;169:265.
15. Welch GH, Anderson JR. Volvulus of the small intestine in adults. *World J Surg.* 1986;10:496.
16. Ruiz-Tovar J, Morales V, Sanjuanbenito A, Lobo E, Martinez-Molina E. Volvulus of the small bowel in adults. *Am Surg.* 2009;75:1179.
17. Juler GL, Stemmer EA, Connolly JE. Preoperative diagnosis of small bowel volvulus in adults. *Am J Gastroenterol.* 1971;56:235.
18. Svane S. Volvulus of the entire small intestine. Four cases without anomalies of intestinal rotation. *Acta Chir Scand.* 1965;129:649.
19. Ghebrat K. Trend of small intestinal volvulus in north western Ethiopia. *East Afr Med J.* 1998;75:549.
20. Demissie M. Small intestinal volvulus in Southern Ethiopia. *East Afr Med J.* 2001;78:208.
21. Huang JC, Shin JS, Huang YT, et al. Small bowel volvulus among adults. *J Gastroenterol Hepatol.* 2005;20:1906.
22. Chou CK, Mark CW, Wu RH, Chang JM. Large diverticulum and volvulus of the small bowel in adults. *World J Surg.* 2005;29:80.
23. Gurleyik E, Gurleyik G. Small bowel volvulus: a common cause of mechanical intestinal obstruction in our region. *Eur J Surg.* 1998;164:51.
24. Ray D, Harishchandra B, Mahapatra S. Primary small bowel volvulus in Nepal. *Trop Doct.* 2004;34:168.
25. De Souza LJ. Volvulus of the small bowel. *Br Med J.* 1976;1:1055.
26. Werner TA, Kropil F, Schoppe MO, Kröpil P, Knoefel WT, Krieg A. Small bowel volvulus as a complication of von Recklinghausen's disease: a case report. *World J Gastroenterol.* 2014;20:7979.
27. Lachhab I, Traore BZ, Saoud O, et al. Small bowel volvulus with intussusception: an unusual revelation of neuroendocrine tumor. *Pan Afr Med J.* 2015;22:6.
28. Devillers A, Vitellius M, Brandicourt P, Labat J, Savoye-Collet C. An atypical acute small-bowel obstruction. *Diagn Interv Imaging.* 2016;97:133.
29. Jang JH, Lee SL, Ku YM, An CH, Chang ED. Small bowel volvulus induced by mesenteric lymphangioma in an adult: a case report. *Korean J Radiol.* 2009;10:319.
30. Qayyum A, Cowling MG, Adam EJ. Small bowel volvulus related to a calcified mesenteric lymph node. *Clin Radiol.* 2000;55:483.
31. Madiba TE, Hadley GP. Surgical management of worm volvulus. *S Afr J Surg.* 1996;34:33.
32. Dilbaz S, Gelisen O, Caliskan E. Small bowel volvulus in pregnancy. *Eur J Obstet Gynecol Reprod Biol.* 2003;111:204.
33. Loh YH, Dunn GD. Computed tomography features of small bowel volvulus. *Australas Radiol.* 2000;44:464.
34. Gollub MJ, Yoon S, Smith LM, Moskowitz CS. Does the CT whirl sign really predict small bowel volvulus?: experience in an oncologic population. *J Comput Assist Tomogr.* 2006;30:25.
35. Inberg MV, Havia T, Davidsson L, Salo M. Acute intestinal volvulus. A report of 238 cases. *Scand J Gastroenterol.* 1972;7:209.
36. Cribbs RK, Gow KW, Wulkan ML. Gastric volvulus in infants and children. *Pediatrics.* 2008;122:e752.
37. Wasselle JA, Norman J. Acute gastric volvulus: pathogenesis, diagnosis, and treatment. *Am J Gastroenterol.* 1993;88:1780.
38. Carter R, Brewer LA 3rd, Hinshaw DB. Acute gastric volvulus. A study of 25 cases. *Am J Surg.* 1980;140:99.
39. Rashid F, Thangarajah T, Mulvey D, Larvin M, Iftikhar SY. A review article on gastric volvulus: a challenge to diagnosis and management. *Int J Surg.* 2010;8:18.
40. Hsu YC, Perng CL, Chen CK, Tsai JJ, Lin HJ. Conservative management of chronic gastric volvulus: 44 cases over 5 years. *World J Gastroenterol.* 2010;16:4200-4205.
41. Jacob CE, Lopasso FP, Zilberstein. Gastric volvulus—a review of 38 cases. *Arq Bras Cir Dig.* 2009;22:96.

42. Light D, Links D, Griffin M. The threatened stomach: management of the acute gastric volvulus. *Surg Endosc.* 2016;30:1847.

43. Chang SW, Lee HC, Yeung CY. Gastric volvulus in children. *Acta Paediatr Taiwan.* 2006;47:18.

44. Teague WJ, Ackroyd R, Watson DI, Devitt PG. Changing patterns in the management of gastric volvulus over 14 years. *Br J Surg.* 2000;87:358.

45. Gourgiotis S, Vougas V, Germanos S, Baratsis S. Acute gastric volvulus: diagnosis and management over 10 years. *Dig Surg.* 2006;23:169.

46. Ogunbiyi OA. Gastric volvulus: more common than previously thought? *Afr J Med Sci.* 1994;23:379.

47. Dalgaard JB. Volvulus of the stomach. *Acta Clir Scand.* 1952;103:131.

48. Hamby WB, ed. *The Case Reports and Autopsy Records of Ambriose Pare.* Translated from JP Malgiagne's "Ouevres Completes d'Ambroise Pare." Paris, 1840. Springfield, IL: Charles C. Thomas; 1960.

49. Berti A. Singolare attortigliamento dele'esofago col duodeno seguita da rapida morte. *Gazz Med Ital.* 1866;9:139.

50. Singleton AC. Chronic gastric volvulus. *Radiology.* 1940;34:53.

51. Uc A, Kao SC, Sanders KD, Lawrence J. Gastric volvulus and wandering spleen. *Am J Gastroenterol.* 1998;93:1146.

52. Spector JM, Chappell J. Gastric volvulus associated with wandering spleen in a child. *J Pediatr Surg.* 2000;35:641.

53. Ooka M, Kohda E, Iizuka Y. Wandering spleen with gastric volvulus and intestinal non-rotation in an adult male patient. *Acta Radiol Short Rep.* 2013;2:2047981613499755.

54. Lianos G, Vlachos K, Papakonstantinou N, Katsios C, Baltogiannis G, Godevenos D. Gastric volvulus and wandering spleen: a rare surgical emergency. *Case Rep Surg.* 2013;2013:561752.

55. Shriki JE, Nguyen K, Rozo JC. Rare chronic gastric volvulus associated with left atrial and mediastinal compression. *Tex Heart Inst J.* 2002;29:324.

56. Deevaguntla CR, Prabhakar B, Prasad GR. Gastric leiomyoma presenting as gastric volvulus. *Indian J Gastroenterol.* 2003;22:230.

57. Del Castillo Déjardin D, Sabench Pereferrer F, Hernàndez Gonzàlez M. Gastric volvulus after sleeve gastrectomy for morbid obesity. *Surgery.* 2013;153:431.

58. Bortul M, Scaramucci M, Tonello C. Gastric wall necrosis from organo-axial volvulus as a late complication of laparoscopic gastric banding. *Obes Surg.* 2004;14:285.

59. Shirouzu Y, Sakurai K, Asonuma K. Gastric volvulus as a complication in the recipients after adult living donor liver transplantation. *Surgery.* 2010;147:581.

60. Gerstle JT, Chiu P, Emil S. Gastric volvulus in children: lessons learned from delayed diagnoses. *Semin Pediatr Surg.* 2009;18:98.

61. Bouchardt M. Zun pathologie and therapie des magnevolvulus. *Arch Klin Chir.* 1904;74:243.

62. Al-Balas H, Hani MB, Omari HZ. Radiological features of acute gastric volvulus in adult patients. *Clin Imaging.* 2010;34:344.

63. Millet I, Orliac C, Alili C. Computed tomography findings of acute gastric volvulus. *Eur Radiol.* 2014;24:3115.

64. Tanner NC. Chronic and recurrent volvulus of the stomach with late results of "colonic displacement". *Am J Surg.* 1968;115:505.

65. Mangray H, Latchmanan NP, Govindasamy V, Ghimenton F. Grey's Ghimenton gastropexy: an anatomic make-up for management of gastric volvulus. *J Am Coll Surg.* 2008;206:195.

66. Al-Salem AH. Acute and chronic gastric volvulus in infants and children: who should be treated surgically? *Pediatr Surg Int.* 2007;23:1095.

67. Elhalaby EA, Mashaly EM. Infants with radiologic diagnosis of gastric volvulus: are they over-treated? *Pediatr Surg Int.* 2001;17:596.

68. Katkhouda N, Mavor E, Achanta K, et al. Laparoscopic repair of chronic intrathoracic gastric volvulus. *Surgery.* 2000;128:784.

69. Palanivelu C, Rangarajan M, Shetty AR. Laparoscopic suture gastropexy for gastric volvulus: a report of 14 cases. *Surg Endosc.* 2007;21:863.

70. Yates RB, Hinojosa MW, Wright AS. Laparoscopic gastropexy relieves symptoms of obstructed gastric volvulus in high operative risk patients. *Am J Surg.* 2015;209:875.

71. Channer LT, Squires GT, Price PD. Laparoscopic repair of gastric volvulus. *JSLS.* 2000;4:225.

72. Jeong SH, Ha CY, Lee YJ. Acute gastric volvulus treated with laparoscopic reduction and percutaneous endoscopic gastrostomy. *J Korean Surg Soc.* 2013;85:47.

Internal Hernias: Congenital and Acquired

Justin Wilkes | Joseph J. Cullen

Intestinal obstruction is a commonly encountered surgical condition. The diagnosis is made with a history of nausea, vomiting, abdominal pain, signs of abdominal distention and tenderness, and imaging displaying dilated bowel with air-fluid levels. Adhesive disease is the etiology of approximately 50% to 75% of small bowel obstructions, with Crohn obstruction, neoplasm, and abdominal wall hernia completing the differential diagnosis in most cases. Internal hernias, defined as a protrusion of viscus through an intraabdominal aperture without traversing fascial planes, cause 0.6% to 5.8% of small bowel obstructions.[1,2] The aperture can be acquired or congenital and often presents with symptoms of intermittent small bowel obstruction or vague abdominal pain. The diagnosis may be elusive, even in its acute state.

Mortality associated with acute internal hernia is reported to be as high as 31% to 50%, which may be an overestimation because the increasing use of Roux-en-Y gastric bypass (RYGB) to treat morbid obesity has heightened the awareness of this condition.[3] Appropriate management of small bowel obstruction is consistent with appropriate internal hernia management; high suspicion, early diagnosis, and early operative intervention are key in limiting morbidity and mortality. This chapter will discuss acquired and congenital forms of internal hernias, their diagnosis, and management.

ACQUIRED INTERNAL HERNIA

An acquired internal hernia requires the formation of an intraabdominal aperture through which bowel and other viscera may pass.[3] Any rearrangement of intraabdominal organs creates a potential space through which bowel may herniate. These include the mesenteric defect created in a bowel anastomosis, hepaticojejunostomy during liver transplantation or Whipple procedures, and even ostomy formation. The most common site for internal hernia after liver transplantation is through the transverse mesocolon.[2] Most notably, and more common, are the multiple defects formed during an RYGB. Due to the remarkable increase in the use of bariatric surgery for weight loss, and the importance of this complication, this chapter highlights the procedure's propensity for internal hernia, subsequent work-up, and management.

ROUX-EN-Y GASTRIC BYPASS

With the increasing incidence of morbid obesity in developed countries, its surgical management has increased steadily over the last 50 years. Although multiple restriction and malabsorption operations have been devised and implemented, the RYGB provides profound lasting excess weight loss of 65% to 85%.[4–6] The nadir in patient weight is typically between 18 and 24 months, with an average of 20% weight regain between 2 and 6 years postoperatively.[7,8] From a public health perspective, the resolution of significant comorbidities associated with obesity is more important than the weight loss itself. Comorbidities, including degenerative joint disease (DJD), hypercholesterolemia, hypertension, gastroesophageal reflux disease (GERD), depression, hypertriglyceridemia, sleep apnea and obesity-related hypoventilation, fatty liver disease, urinary stress incontinence, type 2 diabetes mellitus, cholelithiasis, and asthma, are resolved in as many as 96% of patients.[4,6–8] Most importantly, large retrospective and prospective trials of bariatric surgery have shown approximately 35% decreased overall death rate and decreased obesity-related risk of death in long-term follow-up. These effects are even more pronounced in patients with a body mass index (BMI) greater than 45.[8,9,9a]

In 1994, the laparoscopic Roux-en-Y gastric bypass (LRYGB) was introduced with the advantages of fewer wound infections, incisional hernias, splenic injuries, and clinically significant adhesions, as well as lower mortality and less postoperative pain. The disadvantage of the laparoscopic approach is the increased incidence of gastrojejunal anastomotic stricture and internal hernia. The increased incidence of internal hernia after laparoscopic bypass is due to the lack of adhesion formation and the resulting mobility of the bowel. A similar increased incidence of internal hernia is seen in immunosuppressed patients, and is also thought to be due to decreased adhesion formation.[10,11]

The reoperation rate after LRYGB has been reported at 6.9% to 13%, with early studies showing reoperation rates as high as 42%. The most common secondary operations are cholecystectomy, lysis of adhesions, liver biopsies, and umbilical hernia repairs. Reoperations may be classified as early or late reoperations. Early operation, defined as within 90 days of the initial operation, accounts for 18% of all reoperations. The most common indication for early reoperation is bowel obstruction or obstructive symptoms due to gastrojejunal stricture, obstruction at the jejunojejunal (JJ) anastomosis, malorientation, or adhesive disease. Late reoperation, occurring after 90 days, is most commonly done for exploration secondary to pain, nausea, or vomiting of unclear etiology, but can also be due to adhesive obstruction or internal hernia. Although studies vary, the incidence of internal hernia after LRYGB is somewhere between 1.8% and 7.6%. Internal hernia is the indication for less than half of reoperations after LRYGB. The median time to reoperation for internal hernia ranges from 15 to 33.5 months. The drastic weight loss leading up to this time frame results in increased intraabdominal space, bowel mobility, and widening of previous mesenteric defects due to mesenteric fat loss. The average excess weight loss at time of reoperation is 54% to 90%. Due to this relatively delayed complication after surgery, studies reporting internal hernia rates prior to at least 2 years' median follow-up may have a misleadingly low incidence.[4,5,12–18]

PRESENTATION

As with abdominal wall hernias, symptoms of obstruction predominate with internal hernia. The lack of overt visual cues makes the diagnosis difficult, so suspicion must be high. In LRYGB, there are three potential segments of bowel that may become obstructed, and it is important to understand the complex anatomy defining an RYGB to understand variance in presentation. Roux limb obstruction most commonly results in ill-defined epigastric and left upper quadrant pain temporarily relieved with emesis. Signs of high-grade obstruction will be present in 50% of patients, and 40% of patients will have abdominal pain. Common channel obstruction presents in much the same fashion; however, bilious emesis indicates that obstruction is beyond the JJ anastomosis. Finally, herniation of the biliopancreatic limb, a rare event, may result in pain, remnant gastric distention, tachycardia, and hiccoughs.[16–18]

Physical exam findings are generally nonspecific; however warning signs of bowel ischemia include tachycardia, fever, and tenderness to palpation. Laboratory examinations are generally nondiagnostic, but patients with internal hernia may present with amylasemia and leukocytosis. Leukocytosis, accompanying the physical exam findings described earlier, necessitates early diagnostic laparoscopy if an alternative diagnosis is not clear by imaging. The lack of a hernia sac in LRYGB, which may be present in some forms of congenital internal hernia, allows herniation of long segments of bowel and may lead to catastrophic ischemia.[3,19]

ANATOMY OF THE ROUX-EN-Y

Before attempting interpretation of imaging or operative exploration, it is paramount to thoroughly understand the anatomy of an RYGB. Knowledge of the specifics of a patient's index operation is as important here as for any other operation. The typical RYGB has a 100- to 150-cm Roux limb anastomosed to a 15-mL gastric pouch. The Roux limb may be passed anterior or posterior to the transverse mesocolon (antecolic or retrocolic, respectively) and remnant stomach (Fig. 74.1). Distally, the Roux limb will be anastomosed to the biliary limb, commonly called the JJ anastomosis. Distal to the anastomosis, the bowel is called the common channel or limb. The biliary limb includes the length of the duodenum and approximately 30 cm of jejunum measured from the ligament of Treitz. There are two potential sites of herniation in any RYGB. A defect in the mesentery at the JJ anastomosis (Brolin space) may occur. When the Roux limb traverses the transverse colon, the aperture created by the crossing of the two bowels' mesenteries creates what is known as a Petersen defect. Retrocolic passage of the Roux limb at the index operation creates a third potential aperture in the transverse mesocolon, where bowel may herniate alongside the Roux limb. Closure or nonclosure of all of these defects at the index operation has been described. There is evidence of decreased incidence of internal

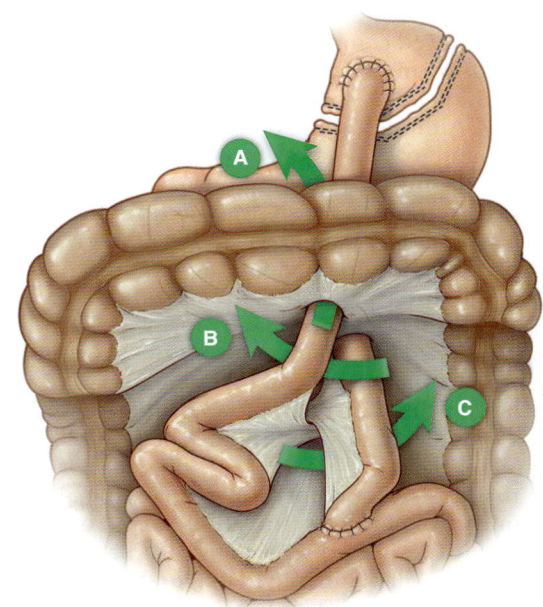

FIGURE 74.1 Potential mesenteric opening that could lead to an internal hernia after a Roux-en-Y gastric bypass. *A,* Transverse mesocolon defect. *B,* Space between the Roux limb mesentery and the transverse mesocolon (Petersen hernia). *C,* Jejunojejunostomy mesenteric defect.

hernia with closure of every defect at initial operation. This is preferably performed with nonabsorbable suture in a running fashion. Reported closure of the defects does not rule out the potential for internal hernia in these locations because closure breakdown or massive weight loss can widen spaces that were once thought to be obliterated.[6,20]

Most closely studied with regard to internal hernia is the antecolic versus the retrocolic approach to LRYGB. The retrocolic approach was originally favored due to fear of excess stretch on the gastrojejunal anastomosis with an antecolic approach. Most studies report an increased incidence of internal hernia in the retrocolic approach compared to the antecolic approach of 2.3% to 8.5% versus 0.3% to 3.8%, respectively. The variability in these studies is likely due to the variability in time to follow-up. Studies with shorter follow-up time report a lower incidence of internal hernia. This is likely due to mesenteric fat loss that is inadequate to significantly widen mesenteric defects. The increased incidence of internal hernia with the retrocolic approach appears to be due to herniation through the transverse mesocolic defect. Routine closure of this defect significantly reduces the occurrence of herniation to 0.2% to 0.7%, with recent studies showing internal hernia rates similar to the antecolic approach. Because closure of the mesentery at the JJ anastomosis has become standard, the Petersen defect is the most common site of herniation in the antecolic approach to gastric bypass. Data are conflicting, but there appears to be a trend toward decreased incidence of internal hernia with routine closure of the Petersen space as well.[13,15,16–18,20–22]

Imaging

Contrast-enhanced computed tomography (CT) has largely replaced any form of plain film studies with oral contrast due to its availability, speed, and multiplanar formatting capabilities. Although small bowel follow-through studies and ultrasound may aid in diagnosis, this section will focus on the CT diagnosis of internal hernia. Because internal hernias often spontaneously reduce, it is important to image the *symptomatic* patient with signs of internal hernia. Oral contrast may help elucidate the etiology of obstruction; however, internal hernias in this setting are typically proximal obstructions without a pylorus to slow filling of the small bowel. Thus, small amounts of oral contrast are sufficient if the patient cannot tolerate the typical dosage. Simply having the patient swallow a tolerable amount of contrast on the table immediately before scanning is adequate.[19]

The diagnosis of any form of internal hernia on CT scan requires experience and high suspicion. Medical centers with experienced radiologists with a suspicion for internal hernia will be unable to diagnose internal hernia on imaging in 16% to 20% of cases. Despite a reportedly normal CT, concerning signs and symptoms in a patient with history of RYGB requires diagnostic laparoscopy. Generally speaking, the CT findings indicating potential internal hernia include aberrant vascular arrangement, clustering of bowel loops, and signs of obstruction. A swirl sign occurs when tension on the small bowel mesentery causes the mesenteric vessels to twist around in a whorl-like fashion and occurs in 55% of patients with internal hernia. This may be a sign of intestinal volvulus and is concerning for ischemia. Any abrupt changes in the direction of mesenteric vessels or vascular engorgement are also concerning findings. When possible, attempting to trace bypass anatomy from its origin will uncover the etiology of the patient's symptoms. Specifically, clustering of bowel loops in aberrant locations is indicative of obstruction. Lateral clustering with displacement of the colon, mass effect on the stomach, or abnormal location of the omentum (if it is known where its ultimate location was at the end of the index operation) are all signs of potential internal hernia. CT signs of obstruction in a patient with potential for internal hernia necessitate diagnostic laparoscopy. Small bowel dilation is found in 25% of patients, and mesenteric edema and free fluid are found in 11%.[15–17,19,23,24]

Repair

Because there are multiple potential spaces for herniation and altered anatomy, it is important to have an orderly approach to operating on suspected internal hernias. The laparoscopic approach to exploration has been shown to be safe. This is likely aided by the massive weight loss, which increases abdominal domain, and the lead time to typical presentation of this complication allowing adhesions to diminish. Laparoscopic access can typically be safely gained through the prior laparoscopic port sites. With the patient in supine or lithotomy position, access is achieved through the left-sided port sites initially. After insufflation, the bowel anatomy should be delineated either proximal to distal or vice versa. Identification of the gastrojejunal anastomosis is first, with atraumatic laparoscopic graspers working distally to define the Roux limb, mesocolic defects, Petersen space, and the JJ anastomosis. An alternative approach is to start distally, at the terminal ileum, and work proximally toward the JJ anastomosis. Some prefer the latter approach because the decompressed distal bowel is less tenuous to handle. It is critical to be able to perform either approach because the anatomy can be disorienting. Also, while tracing the bowel, at times the surgeon will be placing uncomfortable tension on a loop of bowel diving into a yet undefined space. Approaching from the opposite end will occasionally free up a loop of previously trapped bowel, inexplicably and unexpectedly relieving the obstruction. It is also important to note that whether or not an internal hernia is found, the presence of a defect itself is indication for closure of the defect. Closure should be performed with nonabsorbable suture in a running fashion. Signs of obstruction status–post spontaneous reduction include dilated bowel, thickened mesentery, and chylous ascites. Necrotic bowel is found in 8.1% of operations for internal hernia. If extensive bowel of questionable viability is encountered, temporary closure with plans for return to the operating room in 24 to 48 hours is indicated.[15]

INTERNAL HERNIA IN PREGNANCY

LRYGB is commonly performed in women of childbearing age. At times, the procedure itself is performed to increase fertility that has been repressed by polycystic ovarian syndrome (PCOS). Although the general consensus is to delay pregnancy until 1 to 2 years after LRYGB, studies have shown no difference in neonatal or maternal outcome regardless of whether pregnancy is attained during or after the period of maximal weight loss. Pregnant patients who present after LRYGB with abdominal pain are a particular diagnostic challenge, and obstetricians need to be aware of the potential complications of LRYGB. Right upper quadrant ultrasound should be performed to assess for gallbladder pathology. Imaging that suggests remnant stomach dilation could be a potential sign of biliary limb obstruction. The threshold for operative exploration in these patients is low. With the relatively low negative predictive value of CT and the risk of radiation to the fetus, CT is not mandatory prior to exploration. Laparoscopy is safe up to 31 weeks' gestation. After this period, an open approach is preferred, with some sources recommending mandatory cesarian section after 36 weeks for both fetal safety and ease of exploration.[25–28]

CONGENITAL INTERNAL HERNIAS

Due to their incredible infrequency, congenital internal hernias are rarely suspected preoperatively and are frequently diagnosed intraoperatively. There are multiple types of congenital internal hernias, each with unique anatomy and pathogenesis. The most common congenital internal hernias are the paraduodenal, pericecal, foramen of Winslow, transmesenteric, supravesical or perivesical, and omental types. The term congenital is not synonymous with childhood in this instance because these hernias are often diagnosed later in life.[28a] The rest of this chapter focuses on the presentation, pathology, radiographic findings, and treatment of congenital internal hernias. Mortality associated with congenital internal hernias is inevitably due to delayed diagnosis and the septic complications of bowel ischemia. Due to the rarity of each individual type and their varying presentations, mortality rates vary greatly.[2]

PARADUODENAL HERNIA

Paraduodenal hernias comprise 50% of all congenital internal hernias. They are more common in men at a 3:1 ratio, and despite their congenital nature, they most commonly present in the third or fourth decades of life. They are either left (75%) or right sided (25%), and distinct in their pathogenesis[3,19,29–32]

Left Paraduodenal Hernia

A left paraduodenal hernia is defined as bowel herniation into the potential space known as the Landzert fossa. The space is typically obliterated during the 5th to 10th weeks of gestation as the left colonic mesentery, inferior mesenteric vein (IMV), and ascending left colic artery fuse with the retroperitoneum while the small bowel is simultaneously undergoing its 270-degree counterclockwise rotation around the superior mesenteric artery (SMA). However, in 1% to 2% of the population, it is believed that bowel invagination into the avascular plane posterior to the named vessels, behind the left mesocolon, perpetuates the fossa. Thus, the anterior border of this aperture, the IMV, and the ascending left colic artery are displaced anteriorly, and the anterior wall of this hernia is left colon mesentery. The splenic flexure, pancreas, and descending colon may be displaced anteriorly. The afferent limb of these hernias is typically the fourth portion of the duodenum, and the efferent limb can be as distal as the ileum if substantial herniation occurs.[29–31]

The presentation is variable, but it is not uncommon for a patient with a left paraduodenal hernia to report a lifetime history of intermittent, self-resolving, postprandial abdominal pain with extensive negative work-up. The average age of diagnosis is 38.5 years. Up to 70% of patients will have a history of chronic abdominal pain.

CT findings of left paraduodenal hernia include clustering of small bowel in the left upper quadrant with mass effect on the posterior stomach and transverse colon, and inferomedial displacement of the duodenojejunal junction. Clustering of vessels associated with loops of small bowel entering the sac may also be apparent. Anterior displacement of the IMV and ascending colic artery are also described, but often difficult to visualize.[2,19,30,31,33]

Awareness of the vascular anterior border of the aperture during repair of a left paraduodenal hernia is imperative. Ideally, simple reduction of bowel and obliteration of the aperture with nonabsorbable suture prevents future herniation. In the event that bowel is not easily reduced, herniotomy of the sac lateral to the vessels may relieve edema, allowing reduction of bowel. With the relatively high likelihood of adhesions involved in this intermittently inflamed sac of small bowel, some advocate for ligation of the IMV and ascending colic artery involved in forming the aperture because this does not increase the risk for left colonic ischemia in otherwise healthy patients. Prognosis and recovery depend on the degree

of herniation, strangulation, and ischemia of the involved bowel.[3,30,32]

Right Paraduodenal Hernia

A right paraduodenal hernia is defined as bowel herniation into a potential space known as the Waldeyer fossa. This space is typically obliterated as the SMA and right colon mesentery fuse with the retroperitoneum after passing over the third portion of the duodenum during the third stage of intestinal rotation. However, in approximately 1% of the population, failure of the prearterial portion of bowel to complete more than 90 degrees of rotation leaves it on the right side of the abdomen to be covered by the postarterial segment (namely the cecum) as it completes its 270 degrees of rotation. With small bowel interfering, the right colonic mesentery does not fuse to the posterior abdominal wall, perpetuating the space known as the Waldeyer fossa. Thus, the anterior border of this aperture, the SMA, the hepatic flexure, and the ascending colon may be displaced anteriorly. The afferent limb of these hernias is typically the first segment of the jejunum, and the efferent limb can be as distal as the ileum if a large herniation occurs.[19,30,31]

CT may show clustering of small bowel loops in the right upper quadrant with displacement of the descending duodenum superiorly and the transverse and ascending mesocolon anteriorly. Jejunal arterial branches may course superior and posterior to the SMA in this space. Other findings of malrotation, such as incomplete leftward and cephalic rotation of the ligament of Treitz may also be seen.[19]

Repair is similar to repair of the left paraduodenal hernia, with reduction and obliteration of the space. If unable to reduce the bowel, takedown of the hepatic flexure will expose the hernia sac allowing herniotomy and potential decompression of the trapped bowel. Again, awareness of the vascular nature of the anterior border of the aperture is imperative. A second type of repair, which avoids potential damage to the SMA, may be beneficial for very large right paraduodenal hernias. It is very similar to the Ladd procedure, essentially leaving the bowel in a nonrotated state. This involves takedown of the lateral ascending colon peritoneal attachments with reflection of the right colon to the left side of the abdomen, placing the entirety of the small bowel in the right side of the abdomen. Removal of the appendix should be strongly considered given the iatrogenic aberrant anatomy.[31]

FORAMEN OF WINSLOW HERNIA

Internal hernias involving the foramen of Winslow comprise approximately 5% to 10% of all congenital internal hernias. Approximately 160 cases in adults and 4 in children are described in the literature. The aperture in this case is the natural entrance to the lesser sac itself. The borders are the caudate lobe, inferior vena cava, duodenum, and hepatoduodenal ligament (containing the portal triad). As in the case of right paraduodenal hernias, it is common for these patients to have some element of malrotation. Small bowel alone is contained in the sac in two-thirds of patients. One-third of patients will have a mobile ascending colon that has failed to fuse to the abdominal side wall herniating into this space along with terminal ileum. Gallbladder, transverse colon, and omental herniation have all been described.[19,34-36]

Patients will typically present with symptoms of proximal small bowel obstruction. A local mass effect can cause decreased gastric volume or even gastric outlet obstruction. Given its association with the common bile duct, patients may also present with jaundice. Because the bowel is isolated from the peritoneum in the lesser sac, frankly necrotic bowel may not present with peritonitis. Children may display a tendency to draw their knees to their chest in this condition, which theoretically reduces tension across the hepatoduodenal ligament.[19,34,35]

CT findings are relatively intuitive with foramen of Winslow hernias. Loops of small bowel will be clustered posterior to the stomach with anterior displacement of the stomach. Stretched mesenteric vessels entering the lesser sac may be apparent. This can be confused with left paraduodenal hernia on imaging, but the herniated bowel is more superiorly located in the right upper quadrant with displacement of the stomach instead of the transverse colon.[16] Again, as with other congenital internal hernias, treatment involves reduction of the contents into the peritoneal cavity with possible aid from a counterincision, this time to the left of the hepatoduodenal ligament into the lesser sac with awareness of a possible replaced left hepatic artery. The vital surrounding structures afford little leeway with widening of the foramen, although the Kocher maneuver has been used. If a malrotated cecum is present in the hernia, resection is recommended, as it would be with cecal volvulus. Opinions are mixed as to whether the defect should be closed. There are no reports of recurrence of this rare internal hernia. Case reports exist that describe suturing of the open aperture to the retroperitoneum, or pexy of the omentum, hepatic flexure, or duodenum into the foramen to block the aperture.[35,37]

TRANSMESENTERIC HERNIA

Transmesenteric internal hernias are aptly named because they involve herniation through a gap in the mesentery. Although surgeons are well aware of the acquired type of transmesenteric hernia after bowel anastomosis, the congenital form is quite rare. It is most likely due to failure of proper mesenteric development secondary to ischemic insult in utero, similar to the pathogenesis of intestinal atresia. This is supported by the most common associated anomaly, intestinal atresia, which is found in 50% of infants presenting with transmesenteric hernia. Although this may occur anywhere along the length of the mesentery, the most commonly encountered locations involve the pericecal mesentery, the sigmoid mesentery, and the duodenojejunal junction. Approximately 30% of cases will remain symptomatic throughout life.[19,33,36-38]

PERICECAL HERNIA

Pericecal internal hernias comprise 10% to 15% of all congenital internal hernias, and are the most common congenital transmesenteric internal hernia. As described earlier, failure of proper development of the pericecal mesentery, likely due to an ischemic event in utero, allows the presence of an aperture through which small bowel may herniate. Not unexpectedly, this can easily be mistaken for appendicitis clinically, and indeed, many cases are discovered intraoperatively. Because this aperture usually does not involve a peritoneal covering, or sac, significant lengths of small bowel may herniate, which can quickly lead to strangulation. CT findings show loops of small bowel clustering lateral to the cecum with anterior displacement of the cecum. Treatment involves reduction of the herniated contents, closure of the aperture, and resection of necrotic bowel, if necessary.

INTERSIGMOID HERNIA

Intersigmoid hernias comprise approximately 5% of all congenital internal hernias. Improper development can lead to varying degrees of defects in the sigmoid mesentery. Simply redundant sigmoid colon may also have redundant sigmoid mesentery, which can form a pseudo sac into which bowel may herniate and be trapped. A defect in one leaf of the mesocolon may create a true sac which bowel can fill, blocked by the other leaf of mesentery. Lastly, a through-and-through mesenteric defect can obviously allow sizeable lengths of bowel to herniate. Diagnosis on imaging is difficult, but loops of small bowel in the left lower quadrant that displace the sigmoid colon anteriorly or medially may be apparent.[19,39]

CONCLUSION

Internal hernias are rare, but must persist in the surgeon's differential diagnosis of small bowel obstruction and abdominal pain of unknown etiology. The increasing prevalence of patients with gastric bypass anatomy makes awareness more imperative. Diagnosis in a patient with acute abdominal pain requires prompt surgical response because bowel ischemia and necrosis can develop rapidly, as with other hernias.

REFERENCES

1. Miller G, Boman J, Shrier I, Gordon PH. Etiology of small bowel obstruction. *Am J Surg.* 2000;180(1):33-36.
2. Blachar A, Federle MP. Internal hernia: an increasingly common cause of small bowel obstruction. *Semin Ultrasound CT MR.* 2007;23(2):174-183.
3. Newsom BD, Kukora JS. Congenital and acquired internal hernias: unusual causes of small bowel obstruction. *Am J Surg.* 1986;152(3):279-285.
4. Schauer PR, Ikramuddin S, Gourash W, Ramanathan R, Luketich J. Outcomes after laparoscopic Roux-en-Y gastric bypass for morbid obesity. *Ann Surg.* 2000;232(4):515-529.
5. Nguyen NT, Goldman C, Rosenquist CJ, et al. Laparoscopic versus open gastric bypass: a randomized study of outcomes, quality of life, and costs. *Ann Surg.* 2001;234(3):279-289; discussion 289–291.
6. Wittgrove AC, Clark GW. Laparoscopic gastric bypass, Roux-en-Y- 500 patients: technique and results, with 3–60 month follow-up. *Obes Surg.* 2000;10(3):233-239.
7. NIH conference. Gastrointestinal surgery for severe obesity. Consensus Development Conference Panel. *Ann Intern Med.* 1991;115(12):956-961.
8. Adams TD, Davidson LE, Litwin SE, et al. Health benefits of gastric bypass surgery after 6 years. *J Am Med Assoc.* 2012;308(11):1122-1131.
9. Sjostrom L, Narbro K, Sjöström CD, et al. Effects of bariatric surgery on mortality in Swedish obese subjects. *N Engl J Med.* 2007;357(8):741-752.
9a. Adams TD, Gress RE, Smith SC, et al. Long-term mortality after gastric bypass surgery. *N Engl J Med.* 2007;357(8):753-761.
10. Longitudinal Assessment of Bariatric Surgery (LABS) Consortium, Flum DR, Belle SH, et al. Perioperative safety in the longitudinal assessment of bariatric surgery. *N Engl J Med.* 2009;361(5):445-454.

11. Huang YM, Chou AS, Wu YK, et al. Left paraduodenal hernia presenting as recurrent small bowel obstruction. *World J Gastroenterol.* 2005; 11(41):6557-6559.
12. Thompson E, Ferrigno L, Grotts J, et al. Causes and timing of nonelective reoperations after bariatric surgery: a review of 1304 cases at a single institution. *Am Surg.* 2015;81(10):969-973.
13. Zak Y, et al. Laparoscopic Roux-en-Y gastric bypass patients have an increased lifetime risk of repeat operations when compared to laparoscopic sleeve gastrectomy patients. *Surg Endosc.* 2015;30:1833-1838.
14. Karcz WK, Zhou C, Daoud M, et al. Modification of internal hernia classification system after laparoscopic Roux-en-Y bariatric surgery. *Wideochir Inne Tech Maloinwazyjne.* 2015;10(2):197-204.
15. Al-Mansour MR, Mundy R, Canoy JM, Dulaimy K, Kuhn JN, Romanelli J. Internal hernia after laparoscopic antecolic Roux-en-Y gastric bypass. *Obes Surg.* 2015;25(11):2106-2111.
16. Obeid A, McNeal S, Breland M, Stahl R, Clements RH, Grams J, et al. Internal hernia after laparoscopic Roux-en-Y gastric bypass. *J Gastrointest Surg.* 2014;18(2):250-255; discussion 255-256.
17. Higa KD, Ho T, Boone KB. Internal hernias after laparoscopic Roux-en-Y gastric bypass: incidence, treatment and prevention. *Obes Surg.* 2003;13(3):350-354.
18. Koppman JS, Li C, Gandsas A. Small bowel obstruction after laparoscopic Roux-en-Y gastric bypass: a review of 9,527 patients. *J Am Coll Surg.* 2008;206(3):571-584.
19. Martin LC, Merkle EM, Thompson WM, et al. Review of internal hernias: radiographic and clinical findings. *AJR Am J Roentgenol.* 2006;186(3):703-717.
20. Steele KE, Prokopowicz GP, Magnuson T, Lidor A, Schweitzer M. Laparoscopic antecolic Roux-en-Y gastric bypass with closure of internal defects leads to fewer internal hernias than the retrocolic approach. *Surg Endosc.* 2008;22(9):2056-2061.
21. Rondelli F, Bugiantella W, Desio M, et al. Antecolic or retrocolic alimentary limb in laparoscopic roux-en-Y gastric bypass? A meta-analysis. *Obes Surg.* 2016;26:182-195.
22. Al Harakeh AB, Kallies KJ, Borgert AJ, Kothari SN. Bowel obstruction rates in antecolic/antegastric versus retrocolic/retrogastric Roux limb gastric bypass: a meta-analysis. *Surg Obes Relat Dis.* 2016;12:194-198.
23. Blachar A, Federle MP, Brancatelli G, Peterson MS, Oliver JH 3rd, Li W. Radiologist performance in the diagnosis of internal hernia by using specific CT findings with emphasis on transmesenteric hernia. *Radiology.* 2001;221(2):422-428.
24. Blachar A, Federle MP, Dodson SF. Internal hernia: clinical and imaging findings in 17 patients with emphasis on CT criteria. *Radiology.* 2001;218(1):68-74.
25. Wax JR, Cartin A, Wolff R, Lepich S, Pinette MG, Blackstone J. Pregnancy following gastric bypass for morbid obesity: effect of surgery-to-conception interval on maternal and neonatal outcomes. *Obes Surg.* 2008;18(12):1517-1521.
26. Wax JR, Wolff R, Cobean R, Pinette MG, Blackstone J, Cartin A. Intussusception complicating pregnancy following laparoscopic Roux-en-Y gastric bypass. *Obes Surg.* 2007;17(7):977-979.
27. Gudbrand C, Andreasen LA, Boilesen AE. Internal hernia in pregnant women after gastric bypass: a retrospective register-based cohort study. *Obes Surg.* 2015;25:2257-2262.
28. Antedomenico E, Singh NN, Zagorski SM, Dwyer K, Chung MH. Laparoscopic repair of a right paraduodenal hernia. *Surg Endosc.* 2004;18(1):165-166.
28a. Abu-Jaish W, Forgione P. Internal hernia—congenital and acquired. In: Yeo CJ, DeMeester SR, McFadden DW, et al., eds. *Shackelford's Surgery of the Alimentary Tract.* 7th ed. Philadelphia: Saunders; 2013.
29. Tong RS, Sengupta S, Tjandra JJ. Left paraduodenal hernia: case report and review of the literature. *ANZ J Surg.* 2002;72(1):69-71.
30. Mboyo A, Goura E, Massicot R, et al. An exceptional cause of intestinal obstruction in a 2-year-old boy: strangulated hernia of the ileum through Winslow's foramen. *J Pediatr Surg.* 2008;43(1):e1-e3.
31. Bartlett MK, Wang C, Williams WH. The surgical management of paraduodenal hernia. *Ann Surg.* 1968;168(2):249-254.
32. Al-Khyatt W, Aggarwal S, Birchall J, Rowlands TE. Acute intestinal obstruction secondary to left paraduodenal hernia: a case report and literature review. *World J Emerg Surg.* 2013;8(1):5.
33. Malit M, Burjonrappa S. Congenital mesenteric defect: description of a rare cause of distal intestinal obstruction in a neonate. *Int J Surg Case Rep.* 2012;3(3):121-123.
34. Ray K, Snowden C, Khatri K, McFall M. Gastric outlet obstruction from a caecal volvulus, herniated through epiploic foramen: a case report. *BMJ Case Rep.* 2009;2009.
35. Tauro LF, Vijaya G, D'Souza CR, et al. Mesocolic hernia: an unusual internal hernia. *Saudi J Gastroenterol.* 2007;13(3):141-143.
36. Osvaldt AB, Mossmann DF, Bersch VP, Rohde L. Intestinal obstruction caused by a foramen of Winslow hernia. *Am J Surg.* 2008;196(2):242-244.
37. Bandawar MS, Nayak P, Shaikh IA, Sakthivel MS, Yadav TD. Strangulated small bowel obstruction secondary to a transmesosigmoid hernia. *Indian J Surg.* 2014;76(2):148-149.
38. ur Rehman Z, Khan S. Large congenital mesenteric defect presenting in an adult. *Saudi J Gastroenterol.* 2010;16(3):223-225.
39. Podnos YD, Jimenez JC, Wilson SE, Stevens CM, Nguyen NT. Complications after laparoscopic gastric bypass: a review of 3464 cases. *Arch Surg.* 2003;138(9):957-961.

Crohn Disease and Its Surgical Management

Christy Cauley | Richard Hodin

Crohn disease is an incurable, chronic disease of unknown etiology, which along with ulcerative colitis comprises inflammatory bowel disease (IBD). Crohn disease is characterized by transmural inflammation that can involve any part of the gastrointestinal tract, from mouth to anus, and presentations of the disease vary widely. Although there is no cure for Crohn disease at this time, great advances in medicine and surgery have aided in reducing the symptoms and suffering of these patients. As such, a multidisciplinary team approach to care, including specialized experts in gastroenterology, surgery, and radiology is essential to ensure these patients receive current, appropriate, and high-quality care.

EPIDEMIOLOGY

The exact number of Crohn disease cases is not known due to variability in reporting and diagnostic criteria. The estimated incidence in North America is 3.1 to 20.2 cases per 100,000 person-years.[1,2] Current estimates of Crohn disease in a large cohort study of 9 million health insurance claims estimate prevalence to be 201 cases per 100,000 people.[3] The prevalence of Crohn disease appears to be increasing despite steady annual incidence rates[2]; this could be due to improved survival from advances in medical and surgical therapies.

RISK FACTORS

Although the etiology of Crohn disease is unclear, the most common explanation is that a genetically predisposed individual comes into contact with an environmental trigger.[4–7] Several important risk factors should be considered when a patient presents with an illness that could be Crohn disease. There is an overall female predominance in Crohn disease; however, there is no current evidence that there is a hormonal effect on disease expression.[8] In addition, there is a bimodal distribution to the age at diagnosis with the highest peak between the second or third decade of life and a second peak in the sixth or seventh decade.[9] Researchers have proposed that this bimodal distribution might be due to environmental factors, differences in disease presentation over time, or a delay in diagnosis until a relapse of the disease occurs.[1,9] There is also a predominance of Crohn disease among certain ethnic and racial groups, with the highest incidence in Jewish and white populations compared with non-Jewish and black or Hispanic populations.[10–14] These differences between racial and ethnic groups could be due to genetic or environmental factors.

Environmental Factors

The microbial environment of the gastrointestinal tract, including commensal and pathologic organisms, is important to maintaining intestinal health. An imbalance in this system is thought to play a role in the pathophysiology of Crohn disease.[15–19] Therefore medications (including antibiotics, nonsteroidal antiinflammatory drugs, and oral contraceptive pills)[20–22] and diet are thought to impact the development of Crohn disease. Specifically, a Western style diet including processed, fried, low-fiber, and sugary foods has been implicated in the development of Crohn disease.[23–25] Previous studies suggest that improved hygiene is also associated with Crohn disease.[26] Smoking is associated with an increased risk of Crohn disease and increased risk of disease recurrence and has been suggested to contribute to disease severity.[27–29]

GENETIC FACTORS

Breakthroughs in the field of genetics have aided in our understanding of Crohn disease. Although only 15% of patients with Crohn disease have a family history of IBD, patients with a first-degree relative with IBD are 3 to 20 times more likely to develop the disease compared with the general population.[30–33] IBD appears to follow a nonmendelian pattern of inheritance. Monozygotic twins have a higher rate of disease (44%) than dizygotic twins (3.8%).[34] This less than complete penetrance leads researchers to believe that environmental factors play a key role in disease development. In addition to the overall risk of developing Crohn disease within families, there appears to be concordance in the location (e.g., colonic vs. ileal) and phenotype (e.g., fistulizing vs. fibrostenotic) of the disease.[35] Genetic anticipation is also observed in susceptible families with the development of earlier onset and more severe disease in the offspring of affected parents in subsequent generations.[36,37]

Animal models have also aided in our understanding of the pathophysiology of the disease. A variety of genes affecting the adaptive and innate immune systems and epithelial function can all lead to colitis, and a single gene alteration can lead to variable clinical presentations depending on the mouse strain.[38,39] In addition, a germ-free environment is protective against IBD development in some animal strains.

Genome-wide association studies have found more than 100 distinct susceptibility loci for IBD.[40–43] Studies analyzing the function of proteins encoded by these genes have provided insights into underlying mechanisms for disease development. The *IBD1* gene encodes for the nucleotide-binding oligomerization domain-containing protein 2 (NOD2) (also known as caspase recruitment domain-containing protein 15 [CARD15]) protein, which is associated with ileal Crohn disease.[44] Mutations in this protein lead to problems with intracellular innate immune pathways involved in recognizing microbial products in the cytoplasm. *ATG16L1*, *IRGM*, and *LRRK* genes regulate the autophagy pathway, which recycles intracellular organelles and removes intracellular microorganisms.[45] Problems with regulating adaptive immune function have been found with alterations in the *IL23R, IL12B, STAT3, JAK2, TYK2, IL27,* and *TNFSF15* genes.[46] In addition to alterations in immune function, Crohn disease is associated with mutations in proteins important to epithelial cell function, such as the *XBP1* and *NOD2* genes.[47] Although these gene alterations are found in some patients with Crohn disease, there is no current standard for genetic testing of patients or their family members if a Crohn diagnosis is being considered.

NATURAL HISTORY AND PATHOPHYSIOLOGY

Experts agree that both environmental and genetic factors contribute to alteration in mucosal integrity of the gastrointestinal tract. In addition, complex alterations in local and systemic immune response lead to varying presentations of Crohn disease. There are two distinct phases of Crohn disease: active disease and remission. Disease severity varies widely from asymptomatic, post-treatment remission to asymptomatic, mild, moderate, or severe active disease.

Cohort studies have found that only 10% to 20% of patients with Crohn disease have prolonged remission after their initial presentation with active disease.[48,49] If a patient has a year-long remission of their disease, there is an 80% chance that they will remain in remission for subsequent years. Unfortunately, the majority of patients (53%) develop strictures or penetrating disease by 10 years of follow-up, as demonstrated in Fig. 75.1.[49] Patients who present at a younger age (<40 years old), have perianal or rectal lesions, smoke, have low education level, or require steroids for their initial treatment course are at risk of having a severe course of disease over their lifetime.[50,51] The majority of patients with perianal fistulas who receive medical or surgical therapy recur at a rate of 59% to 82%.[52]

Up to 80% of patients with Crohn disease will require a surgical intervention during their disease course. Surgical care is reserved for patients who do not respond to medical therapy or those who develop complications (e.g., abscess, fistula, or stricture). Less than 2% of patients have been reported to undergo an intestinal operation within the first year of diagnosis; however, this rate increases over time to up to 17% at 5 years and 28% at 10 years after diagnosis. The relapsing and remitting course of Crohn disease requires that patients understand the need to seek medical attention if they are having symptoms requiring urgent attention. With improved medical therapies, multidisciplinary specialty teams who understand the disease course and improvements in therapy with tailored treatments to achieve the best outcome given the profile of the patient's disease course, Crohn specialists might reduce the need for invasive surgical treatments.[53]

Long-term survival of patients with Crohn disease is very good, with 20-year survival reported at 93% to 94%; however, quality of life scores in patients with Crohn disease are worse than healthy individuals and worse than patients with ulcerative colitis.[54] Several studies have found that there are disease-independent factors that influence the quality of life perceived by Crohn disease patients, including gender, smoking status, perceived stress, psychiatric comorbid disease, social support, coping mechanisms, and patient personality. Importantly, remission of the disease improves quality of life, whether it is achieved through medical or operative management.[55] Long-term, longitudinal quality of life assessments comparing surgical and medical treatment modalities are needed to understand the durability of these findings.

The cost of this chronic disease should also be understood by clinicians in an effort to understand the burden placed on patients. As a chronic disease, Crohn disease is very costly due to the direct expenses of medical and surgical treatments and hospitalizations. However, one should not overlook the indirect and opportunity costs from the disease due to days missed at work by the patient, as well as their caretakers. Similar to other chronic diseases, being aware of this cost is important because the financial hardship placed on patients and families can affect compliance with treatment or cause delays in presentation for medical care leading to poorer outcomes.

CLINICAL PRESENTATION

Crohn disease is a heterogeneous problem in its disease presentation and course. There are a variety of gastrointestinal and extraintestinal manifestations, which can make each patient's presentation unique. This variability in disease presentation makes diagnosis difficult in some patients. The majority of patients (70%) are diagnosed within 1 year of symptom onset; however, 14% of patients have a delay in diagnosis of 5 years. This is especially true in older patients who are less likely to be referred to specialty clinics.[56]

The majority of patients present with complaints consistent with small bowel or colonic disease, and many patients have pain at the same location over time. In contrast, the behavior of the disease tends to progress over the course of the patient's disease from inflammatory to stricturing or penetrating lesions. Patients with ileocolonic or colonic disease tend to progress to penetrating

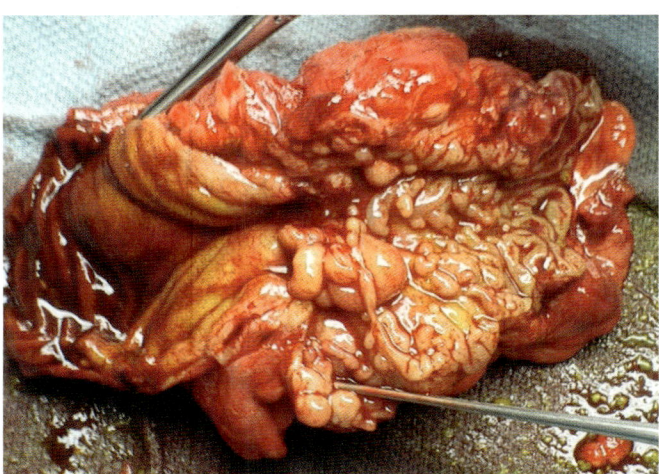

FIGURE 75.1 Crohn disease of the small bowel with evidence of stricture.

disease over time, whereas patients with small bowel disease tend to progress to stricturing disease. Complications are common long term, with 94% of terminal ileal disease patients and 78% of colonic disease patients experiencing a complication at 20 years.[57]

The symptoms expressed by the patient are related to the pathology of the disease (i.e., inflammation, stenosis, abscess, or fistula). Abdominal pain is usually mild and diffuse with inflammation but can be colicky with underlying obstruction of the small or large bowel. Patients with obstruction often also present with nausea, vomiting, and abdominal distention.

Diarrhea is a common complaint in patients with Crohn disease and can have several etiologies. Impaired fluid absorption by inflamed bowel segments can lead to diarrhea from excessive intraluminal fluid content. Terminal ileal inflammation or resection can lead to bile salt malabsorption and subsequent diarrhea. Finally, patients who have lost a large portion of their small bowel through disease and/or surgical resection can exhibit steatorrhea due to bile salt deficiency, leading to fat malabsorption.

Fistula formation is a common complaint in patients, with Crohn disease with one-third of patients developing a fistula within 10 years of disease presentation and half of patients developing a fistula within 20 years of disease presentation. The most common sites for fistulas in Crohn disease are enterovesical (intestine to bladder), enterocutaneous (intestine to skin), enteroenteric (intestine to intestine), and enterovaginal (intestine to vagina). However, not all sinus tracts turn into fistulas. Many sinus tracts develop into phlegmons or abscesses.

Severe, acute hemorrhage in patients with Crohn disease is rare (<10% of patients). However, occult bleeding is reported in up to 24% of patients with Crohn disease. Bleeding most commonly occurs in patients with colon disease, but it can occur in patients with inflammation in any location of the gastrointestinal tract.[58]

Perianal disease is frequently seen in patients with Crohn disease. This problem is addressed elsewhere in this book; however, it is important to note that perianal involvement occurs in 10% of patients as the initial symptom of disease and is the sole location of disease in approximately 5% of patients. Approximately 30% of Crohn patients will experience perianal disease at some point in their disease course.[59]

Due to the systemic nature of this inflammatory disease, there is often a general prodrome associated with active Crohn disease. Weight loss can occur due to malnutrition from malabsorption of diseased bowel segments or due to anorexia from the systemic immune response. It is important to be mindful of this potential problem when considering resection of the small bowel in operative management of this disease. This is especially important in patients who present with Crohn disease requiring surgical interventions at a young age. Fatigue and malaise are also common complaints that are thought to occur due to an imbalance in inflammatory mediators and immune cells in the systemic circulation. Fever can occur due to ongoing inflammation and dysregulation of the immune system; however, it is important to note that high fevers could be due to active infections, such as uncontrolled abscesses.

Extraintestinal manifestations of Crohn disease are reported with wide overall incidence (6% to 40%), depending on the study population. They occur due to the inflammatory nature of Crohn disease. The most common extraintestinal manifestations are arthritis (20%), eye involvement (e.g., iritis/uveitis; 5%), skin disorders (e.g., pyoderma gangrenosum and erythema nodosum; 10%), primary sclerosing cholangitis (5%), secondary amyloidosis (rare), and thromboembolic disease due to hypercoagulability.[60]

DISEASE CLASSIFICATION

There are several ways to categorize Crohn disease: by age of onset, disease location, and disease behavior (phenotype). Variations in the natural history and clinical features of the disease affect our understanding of the patient's prognosis and treatment options. The Vienna classification system is used to objectively classify Crohn disease patient subgroups by considering the patient's age (<40 or ≥40), disease location (terminal ileum, colon, ileocolon, upper gastrointestinal), and disease behavior (inflammatory, stricturing, penetrating).[61] Ongoing research using this classification scheme could improve our understanding of patient outcomes in more detail, allowing us to better tailor future therapies to specific patient subgroups.

TESTING

The goal of testing in Crohn disease is to (1) confirm the diagnosis, (2) identify the location, extent, and severity of lesions, (3) evaluate for extraintestinal manifestations, and (4) determine the most appropriate course of treatment. The differential diagnosis of Crohn disease includes a wide range of disorders of the gastrointestinal tract, including other IBDs (i.e., ulcerative colitis), irritable bowel syndrome, lactose intolerance, infectious colitis, appendicitis, diverticulitis, diverticular colitis, ischemic colitis, carcinoma, lymphoma, chronic ischemia, endometriosis, and carcinoid. Diagnosis requires the clinician to evaluate the patient's clinical history and physical exam, laboratory studies, endoscopy, radiographic findings, and histopathologic findings.

LABORATORY STUDIES

Blood tests that are useful in the evaluation of patients with possible Crohn disease include testing for general inflammatory markers and anemia. Standard tests that are routinely obtained for patients being considered for Crohn disease diagnosis include complete blood count, blood chemistry (including electrolytes, renal function tests, liver enzymes, and blood glucose), erythrocyte sedimentation rate, C-reactive protein, serum iron, and vitamin B_{12} levels. In addition, there are some unique serum antibodies that can be measured.

General laboratory findings in patients with active inflammation include an elevated white blood cell count, platelet count, erythrocyte sedimentation rate, and C-reactive protein. All of these studies lack specificity but can be helpful in monitoring patients for changes in the level of inflammation of the disease over time.

There are a number of antibodies that have been used in testing for IBD; however, these antibodies have low specificity for Crohn disease. For example, anti-*Saccharomyces cerevisiae* antibodies are found in 48% to 69% of patients with Crohn disease and 5% to 15% of patients with ulcerative colitis. Perinuclear antineutrophil cytoplasmic antibodies are found in only 5% to 20% of patients with Crohn disease and 48% to 82% of patients with ulcerative colitis. In addition, the anti-OmpC antibody has been identified in 46% of patients with Crohn disease. Although these antibodies might be more suggestive of one IBD over another, no serologic test has been identified that can discriminate between these diseases.[62,63] Therefore caution should be used in recommending the use of these tests and in interpretation of their findings.

Other tests that are currently under investigation are genetic and stool markers. Genetic testing for the *IBD1* gene, which encodes the NOD2/CARD15 protein, is not currently recommended by any clinical society. Mutations in this gene are infrequent in patients with Crohn disease, and the inheritance pattern of the gene is not strictly mendelian. Stool markers for intestinal inflammation, including fecal calprotectin and lactoferrin, have shown promise for identification of patients with IBD. These are increasingly being used in clinical practice, especially as an indication of acute inflammatory activity.[64]

ENDOSCOPY

There are advantages to both endoscopy and radiography, depending on the clinical scenario. Endoscopy allows the clinician to observe mucosal lesions with very good resolution so that even subtle mucosal lesions with mild inflammation can be appreciated. The upper gastrointestinal tract can be evaluated with esophagogastroduodenoscopy, and the lower intestinal tract can be evaluated with ileocolonoscopy. Endoscopy also affords the examiner the ability to perform biopsies to obtain tissue for histologic examination and allows for intraluminal therapeutic interventions, such as endoscopic balloon dilation with or without steroid injections for intestinal strictures. In addition, patients with long-standing colitis from Crohn disease are at risk for cancer formation; therefore colonoscopic cancer surveillance should be performed in these patients.

When chronic diarrhea is the presenting complaint and the clinical evaluation is suggestive of IBD, ileocolonoscopy is a good first line choice for evaluation. It allows the examiner to evaluate the extent, severity, and location of mucosal changes throughout the colon and distal ileum. In addition, biopsies can be obtained throughout the colon and ileum to evaluate for histologic changes consistent with IBD. The colonoscopic findings that are most consistent with Crohn disease rather than ulcerative colitis are aphthous ulcers, cobblestoning, and skip or discontinuous lesions. Rectal sparing and involvement of the terminal ileum also suggest Crohn disease rather than ulcerative colitis, which classically starts in the rectum with continuous inflammation moving proximally. However, there are caveats to these findings in both diseases.

Patients with Crohn disease who have upper gastrointestinal symptoms should undergo esophagogastroduodenoscopy to evaluate for proximal lesions. Although Crohn disease was historically thought to infrequently involve the proximal gastrointestinal tract, there are increasing numbers of reports of concurrent and isolated Crohn disease in this location.

There are endoscopic scoring systems that have been developed to describe the severity of Crohn disease as seen on endoscopy. One such score is the Crohn's Disease Endoscopic Index of Severity (CDEIS) score; however, it is a complex scoring system, which limits its usefulness in daily practice. The Simplified Endoscopic Activity Score for Crohn's Disease (SES-CD) is a simpler scoring system, which rates the (1) presence and size of ulcers, (2) extent of ulcerated surface, (3) extent of affected surface, and (4) presence and type of narrowing. These four characteristics are scored from 0 to 3 in each area of the large intestine (rectum, left colon, transverse colon, or right colon) and ileum. This scoring system has been found to be reproducible among providers; however, there is no agreement on a cutoff score to define disease remission. Another scoring system, the Rutgeerts score, is used to grade lesions recurring at the site of an anastomosis or neoterminal ileum. This score is meant to predict the likelihood of symptomatic recurrence of Crohn disease after curative resection.[65]

Wireless Video Capsule Endoscopy

Wireless video capsule endoscopy is being increasingly used to evaluate for small bowel Crohn disease, which is present in 70% of patients. During the course of this 8-hour study, two images are acquired every second, yielding around 50,000 images in total. Patients are able to continue their normal daily activities while the images are being obtained. Movement of the capsule through the gastrointestinal tract relies upon peristalsis and complete evaluation of the small intestine is achieved in 65% to 80% of patients. Patients with suspected intestinal strictures are recommended not to undergo this study because the capsule may not be able to pass through the narrowing, necessitating surgical removal. Patency capsules to test for severe narrowing due to strictures can be used prior to use of this technology to ensure that it will not become lodged during the examination. Actual reported rates of surgical or endoscopic retrieval of wireless endoscopy capsules due to stricture are as low as 0% to 15% in studies of Crohn disease patients. Although this examination might continue to improve and evolve with new advances in technology, current cost-effectiveness studies have recommended against the use of this study as a third examination if ileocolonoscopy and computed tomography (CT) enterography or small bowel follow-through are found to be negative.[66]

RADIOGRAPHIC STUDIES

Gastrointestinal imaging studies in Crohn disease have been very useful in documenting the length and location of strictures in areas not easily accessible by endoscopy, especially the small intestine. Many preferences regarding imaging in gastrointestinal disorders reflect local experience and are hospital specific. Traditionally, barium contrast studies, including barium enema or upper gastrointestinal series with small bowel follow-through were performed to assess for narrowing in the gastrointestinal lumen. The current standard of care has evolved with most centers using CT or magnetic resonance (MR) enterography to evaluate for gastrointestinal changes related to Crohn disease.

Due to the chronic nature of Crohn disease, clinicians should take note of the amount of ionizing radiation provided to these patients. This is especially important in patients who are diagnosed with Crohn disease at a young age. Contrast-enhanced ultrasound and MR imaging (MRI) techniques should be considered to reduce the lifetime cumulative exposure to ionizing radiation.

Ultrasound

Transabdominal ultrasound is an infrequently used imaging modality for Crohn disease in the United States compared with European health care settings. It has many reported advantages, including lower cost, wider availability, non-invasiveness, and lack of ionizing radiation. Intraluminal and intravenous contrast agents have been used in some clinical settings with reports of improved image quality of Crohn disease intestinal lesions. Drawbacks to the use of transabdominal ultrasound as a diagnostic study for intestinal lesions include its poor visualization in patients who are obese or with intraluminal gas. In addition, image quality is dependent on the technical ability of the operator, which can lead to poor reproducibility of images in different settings.

Small Bowel Follow-Through and Enteroclysis

Enteroclysis is an imaging study that uses a barium contrast suspension that is directly introduced into the small intestine using a tube. It is similar to the small bowel follow-through study, which uses the same barium contrast suspension that is swallowed by the patient. Evaluation of the two techniques have found that enteroclysis is more uniform in contrast delivery; however, this is at the cost of discomfort to the patient. Although enteroclysis appears to provide better mucosal detail, it does not allow for evaluation of the stomach or duodenum. Preference for either technique appears to be due to institutional support and provider preferences. Evaluation of the small intestine using these techniques can reveal several features of Crohn disease, including ulcers, fissures, fistulas, sinus tracts, cobblestoning, thickened mucosal folds, wall thickening, ileocecal valve enlargement, extent and location of intestinal narrowing and dilation, and skip lesions (Fig. 75.2). The diagnostic sensitivity and specificity of small bowel enteroclysis for Crohn disease has been reported to be as high as 100% and 98%, respectively.[67]

Traditional Computed Tomography and Computed Tomography Enterography

Traditional CT and CT enterography can both be used in the diagnosis of Crohn disease lesions and their complications. Traditional CT uses barium contrast solution and cannot evaluate subtle mucosal lesions associated with early inflammatory Crohn disease. However, this traditional imaging study can be used to identify trans-mural, extramural, or extraintestinal disease (Fig. 75.3). Intravenous and intraluminal contrast agents should be used to improve clinician's ability to see lesions and the intestinal anatomy in this cross-sectional imaging study. A variety of intraluminal contrast agents have been used in CT (e.g., diatrizoate meglumine and methylcellulose)

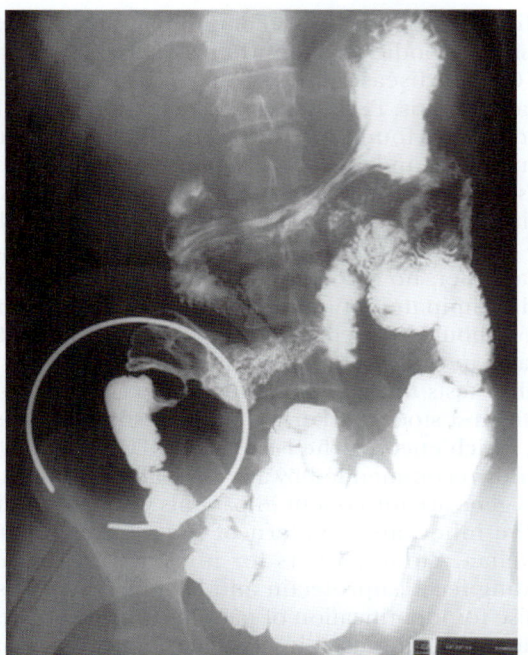

FIGURE 75.2 Small bowel follow-through revealing postoperative recurrence of Crohn disease 18 months after initial presentation requiring ileocolectomy. Stenosis of the diseased bowel creates an obstruction causing dilation of the proximal bowel segment.

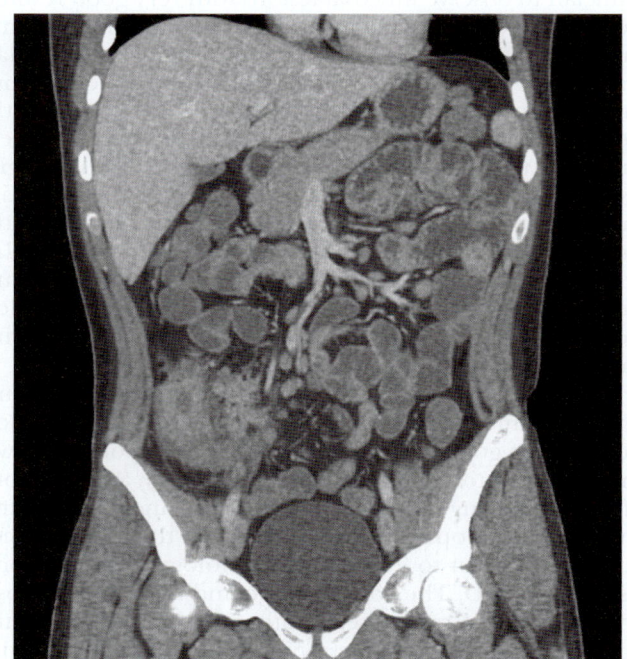

FIGURE 75.3 Computed tomography with contrast in a male patient with right lower quadrant pain due to ileocecal Crohn disease.

to distend the bowel lumen. It is important to note that for all of these studies, if the bowel lumen is not completely distended, the flattened loops could be mistaken for abscesses, masses, strictures, or thickened segments of bowel. CT enterography is a newer radiographic technique that uses a neutral contrast agent. This allows for better evaluation of the wall of the small bowel, leading to higher accuracy in detection of inflammation associated with Crohn disease.[68–70]

Traditional Magnetic Resonance Imaging and Magnetic Resonance Enterography

Similar to the limitations of traditional CT, traditional MRI cannot evaluate for subtle mucosal lesions associated with early Crohn disease. However, MRI is effective in delineating transmural, extramural, or extraintestinal disease. Similar to other cross-sectional imaging techniques, intravenous and intraluminal contrast agents can be used to improve clinician's ability to see lesions and the intestinal anatomy. Isoosmolar polyethylene glycol solution and dilute barium have been used in traditional MRI contrast studies. MR enterography using a neutral contrast agent has the advantage of improved visualization of the small bowel.[71]

Both MRI and CT can provide information regarding: the length of involved segments, presence of skip lesions, wall thickening (>2 mm for small intestine and >3 mm for colon), areas of enhancement (active lesions) and attenuation (target sign), stenotic lesions (intraluminal diameter of <2.5 cm with possible proximal dilation), abscess, phlegmon, fistula (less sensitive than traditional enteroclysis), creeping fat in the mesentery, increased vascularity of vasa recta (comb sign), and mesenteric adenopathy (3 to 8 mm are inflammatory; >10 mm concerning for carcinoma or lymphoma).

Early lesions are not usually able to be identified using traditional CT or MRI. The sensitivity and specificity of both CT and MRI for the diagnosis of Crohn disease are reported to be 94% and 95%, respectively. Studies have found that CT and MR enterography have similar accuracy in the identification of disease location, wall thickening and enhancement, enlarged lymph nodes, and involvement of mesenteric fat; however, MR enterography has demonstrated improved accuracy in the detection of strictures related to Crohn disease. In addition, MRI has the added advantage of being free of ionizing radiation. This is an important consideration for patients who will have multiple imaging studies over their lifetime due to the chronic, recurrent nature of Crohn disease. MR enterography has been touted for its ability to distinguish active inflammation from more chronic fibrosis, an important distinction when deciding the best treatment for individual patients. Refinements in imaging modalities in the future will hopefully provide better ways for the clinician to determine the degree of active inflammation versus chronic scar in patients with Crohn disease.[69,70]

PATHOLOGY

Full-thickness inflammatory lesions can arise from any part of the gastrointestinal tract, from the mouth to the anus. The most common site of Crohn disease is the ileocecal area, with the majority of patients (80%) having some small bowel involvement. Approximately one-third of patients have disease confined to the small intestine, and 20% have disease confined to the colon. Approximately one-third of patients have perianal disease. Involvement

of the upper gastrointestinal tract was historically thought to be rare in Crohn disease; however, increased rates of upper endoscopy and biopsy in these patients reveal a high disease prevalence. As many as 50% of patients have active disease on biopsy despite lacking reported symptoms. Involved tissue is most commonly identified in the gastric antrum or duodenum. The esophagus and other regions of the stomach are rarely affected.

GROSS FEATURES

There are two distinct phases of Crohn disease, which can be seen on pathologic examination. The active phase of the disease is identified when inflammatory changes are present in the tissue. Active lesions begin as small, flat, soft aphthous ulcers with a pale, white center and surrounding erythema. These lesions deepen into transmural inflammatory lesions, leading to abscesses and fistulae. When the tissue heals and scars, strictures can form obstructive lesions at the site of previous inflammation. In contrast to other IBD, Crohn disease lesions can occur as scattered "skip" lesions with islands of normal mucosa between, leading to a cobblestone appearance (Fig. 75.4). It is important to note that these lesions can coalescence into a continuous pattern similar to that seen with ulcerative colitis. In addition to the cobblestone appearance, other classic descriptions of intestinal lesions include bowel wall and mesenteric thickening, in some patients resulting in narrowing of the lumen. A distinctive feature of Crohn disease is "creeping" of the mesenteric fat, a feature best seen grossly at the time of surgical exploration (Fig. 75.5). In addition, mesenteric thickening from fat thickening and enlarged lymph nodes are also common features of Crohn disease. The remission phase occurs after the inflammatory phase and is identified by healing and fibrosis of the previously inflamed tissue. As the tissue heals, fibrosis can lead to stenosis of the intestinal lumen.

MICROSCOPIC FEATURES

On microscopy, inflammatory cell aggregates form microabscesses under aphthous ulcerations. These microabscesses are associated with intestinal crypts and can lead to fissure formation (Fig. 75.6). The classic microscopic finding of

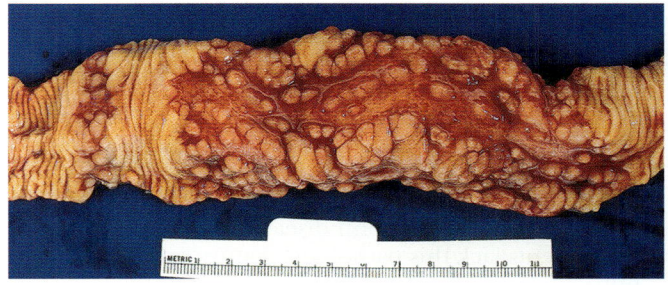

FIGURE 75.4 Small bowel resection revealing cobblestoning ulcerations. (From Hart J. Non-neoplastic diseases of the small and large intestine. In: Silverberg SG, DeLellis RA, Frable WJ, et al., eds. *Silverberg's Principles and Practice of Surgical Pathology and Cytopathology*. Vol 2. 4th ed. Edinburgh: Churchill Livingstone; 2006:1391.)

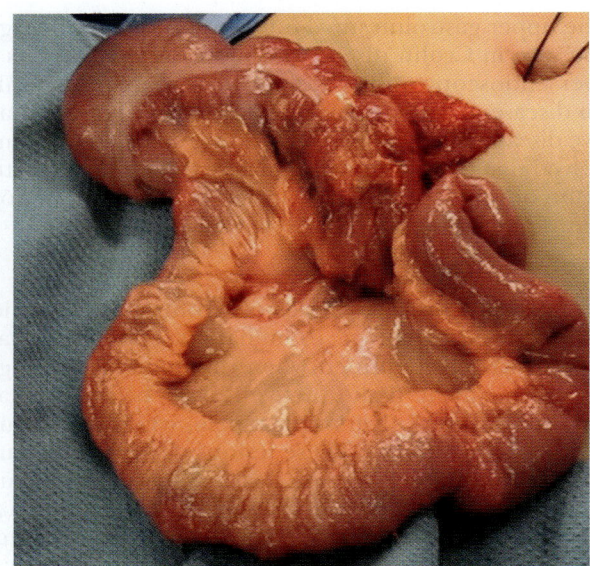

FIGURE 75.5 Small bowel specimen with active Crohn disease demonstrating extension of the mesenteric fat onto the serosal surface of the bowel, also known as creeping fat.

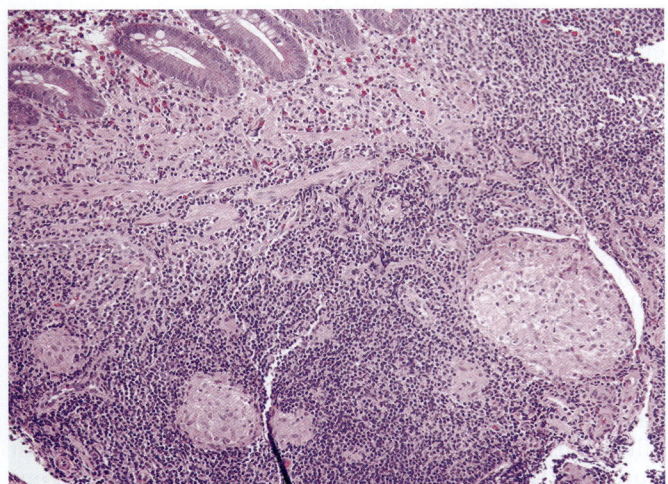

FIGURE 75.7 Multiple submucosal noncaseating granulomas, which are pathognomonic for Crohn disease (ileal biopsy, hematoxylin and eosin stain). (From Dilworth HP, Montgomery E, Iacobuzio-Donahue CA. Non-neoplastic and inflammatory disorders of the small intestine. In: Iacobuzio-Donahue CA, Montgomery E, eds. *Gastrointestinal and Liver Pathology*. Philadelphia: Churchill Livingstone; 2005:170.)

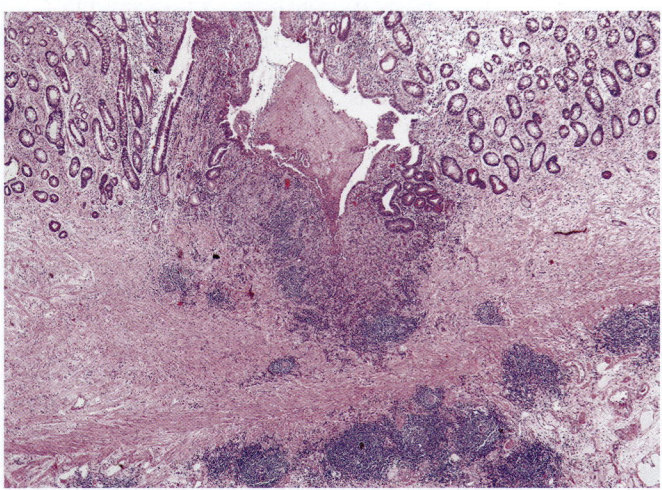

FIGURE 75.6 Classic Crohn disease ulcer with extension into the submucosa and surrounding chronic inflammation (hematoxylin and eosin stain). (From Dilworth HP, Montgomery E, Iacobuzio-Donahue CA. Non-neoplastic and inflammatory disorders of the small intestine. In: Iacobuzio-Donahue CA, Montgomery E, eds. *Gastrointestinal and Liver Pathology*. Philadelphia: Churchill Livingstone; 2005:172.)

noncaseating granulomas with multinucleated giant cells is pathognomonic for Crohn disease (Fig. 75.7); however, many patients lack this pathologic feature on examination (approximately 50% of Crohn patients will display granulomas on histology).

TREATMENT

The goal of all treatments for Crohn disease is to reduce symptoms and improve the patient's quality of life, while minimizing side effects of the treatment being provided. Patients are diagnosed with Crohn disease due to the presence of active symptoms; therefore the clinician must first treat the active disease in an attempt to achieve remission and then focus on finding a treatment that will maintain remission over the long term.

MEDICAL THERAPY

Medical treatment regimens should be tailored to the severity of inflammation (mild, moderate, or severe) and the location of the active lesions. Formal grading systems used to describe disease severity include the Crohn's Disease Activity Index (CDAI) and the Harvey-Bradshaw Index (a simplified version of the previous system).[52,72] The CDAI takes into account several factors, including patient-reported stool pattern, average abdominal pain rating over the past 7 days, general well-being each day over 7 days, presence of complications, findings of an abdominal mass, presence of anemia, and weight change. Both of these scales can be simplified to identify four grades of disease: asymptomatic remission, mild to moderate Crohn disease, moderate to severe Crohn disease, and severe-fulminant disease (Table 75.1). Asymptomatic patients who require continued use of steroids are referred to as "steroid-dependent" and are not considered to be in remission. In addition to the severity of symptoms and location of lesions, the patient's previous responsiveness to different medical therapies should be taken into account for treating recurrent flares of the disease.

There are two distinct treatment strategies in treating patients with mild to moderate Crohn disease: the step-up approach and top-down approach. The step-up approach starts with the least potent therapies and moves on to more potent therapies if they are ineffective. The less potent therapies generally have fewer side effects; therefore this was traditionally how this disease was treated. More

TABLE 75.1 Crohn Disease Activity Index

Symptom	Severity	Categories
General well-being	Well, slightly poor, poor, very poor, extremely poor	0–4
Abdominal pain	None, mild, moderate, severe	0–3
Diarrhea	—	1 for each liquid stool per day
Abdominal mass	None, dubious, definite, definite + tenderness	0–3
Complications	Arthralgia, uveitis, erythema nodosum, pyoderma gangrenosum, aphthous ulcer, anal fissure, new fistula, or abscess	1 for each item

recently, clinicians seem to favor the top-down approach, starting with the more potent therapies, such as biologic or immunomodulator therapies. Many patients now receive biologic and immunomodulator therapies before they are given glucocorticoids in an effort to avoid glucocorticoid dependence.

Medical therapies that are commonly used in Crohn disease include:

- Conventional glucocorticoids: prednisone
- Nonsystemic glucocorticoids: budesonide
- Oral 5-aminosalicylates: sulfasalazine, mesalamine
- Antibiotics: ciprofloxacin, metronidazole
- Immunomodulators: azathioprine, 6-mercaptopurine, methotrexate
- Biologic therapies: infliximab, adalimumab

Corticosteroids have historically been used in the treatment of active disease in an effort to induce remission. Although steroids appear to be effective in the short term, some patients become intolerant to steroids due to serious side effects and others might see little or no improvement in their symptoms after multiple treatments (steroid-resistant patients). Still other patients might become dependent on steroids, exhibiting disease flares when tapering off the drug. To avoid these effects of conventional steroids, budesonide can be used. Due to its extensive first-pass liver metabolism, budesonide has less systemic steroidal effects compared with the standard oral corticosteroid, prednisone. However, this medication is effective only in up to 70% of patients and has been found to be less effective in patients with left-sided colonic disease.[73,74] Due to the long-term side effects of steroids, these medications are not recommended for long-term maintenance therapy.

Although oral 5-aminosalicylates, including mesalamine and sulfasalazine, have historically been used to induce remission in patients with Crohn disease, studies evaluating their efficacy have produced mixed results. Experts agree that these medications are not very effective in maintaining remission, and there is disagreement on whether they are useful in inducing remission with active disease.[75,76]

Antibiotics have been used for induction of remission in mild to moderate Crohn disease as single agents or in combination. Metronidazole and ciprofloxacin are the two most commonly used antibiotics currently. A trial comparing metronidazole to placebo found that it is superior in inducing remission[77]; however, its efficacy and safety compared with other agents has not been as positive.[78] Similarly ciprofloxacin has been found to be superior to placebo in inducing remission, but when compared with active agents the outcomes are not as promising.[79,80] At many institutions these agents are provided in combination in an attempt to induce remission; however, concern for antibiotic-resistance of gastrointestinal bacteria is growing. The use of these agents in patients with mild symptoms is recommended by some experts only as a second line therapy if there is concern for an undetected pathogen, bacterial overgrowth, or unsuspected microperforation that is contributing to active symptoms.

Patients who fail to improve with the aforementioned treatments are categorized as having refractory Crohn disease and require more aggressive therapy with immunomodulators or biologic agents. In addition, patients who present with severe Crohn disease might warrant treatment with these more aggressive medical treatments early on in the disease course (top-down approach). Patients presenting with severe symptoms should first be hospitalized and provided intravenous glucocorticoids in addition to bowel rest, parenteral nutrition, and hydration. If these patients have an abdominal mass, broad-spectrum antibiotics are indicated to treat for potential abscess or microperforation, which can be evaluated through cross-sectional imaging, usually CT scan.

Immunomodulators used in Crohn disease include azathioprine, 6-mercaptopurine, and methotrexate. 6-Mercaptopurine and its prodrug, azathioprine, reduce the number of active lymphocytes, thereby decreasing inflammation. They are precursors to purine antimetabolites, which block proliferation of mitotically active lymphocytes. Multiple studies have proven the efficacy of these medications; however, their effect is reported to take 3 to 6 months. Side effects of both of these medications include bone marrow suppression, increased risk of infection, allergic reactions, and pancreatitis.[81]

Methotrexate is another immunomodulator, which acts as a competitive inhibitor to the enzyme dihydrofolate reductase. Inhibition of this enzyme blocks purine and pyrimidine synthesis, impairing DNA synthesis. It has been shown to be effective in inducing remission in Crohn disease compared with placebo and is used in patients who have resistance or intolerance to treatment with steroids and other immunomodulators. This medication is reported to take 1 to 3 months to take effect. Side effects of methotrexate include liver toxicity and nausea; it is also a teratogen.

The main biologic agents used in the treatment of Crohn disease in the United States include infliximab, adalimumab, and certolizumab pegol.[82] All of these drugs have the same mechanism of action; they are antibodies against tumor necrosis factor-α (TNF-α).[83] Infliximab was the first biologic agent to be used in Crohn disease, and its success led to wider use and development of new agents. A meta-analysis revealed that patients treated with anti-TNF biologic agents were more likely to achieve remission compared with placebo.[84] The number of patients who need to be treated to achieve one remission is eight, and an estimate of the number of patients who need to be treated to prevent one relapse is four.[85] No head to head randomized controlled trials have been performed to compare these three agents; however, anecdotal evidence supports the belief that infliximab and adalimumab have similar efficacy, whereas certolizumab may be less effective in inducing remission.

Other biologic agents that are being developed and increasingly used in the treatment of Crohn disease include natalizumab, ustekinumab, and vedolizumab. Natalizumab is a humanized monoclonal antibody directed against $\alpha 4$ integrin; however, its side effect profile currently limits its use. Ustekinumab is a human immunoglobulin IgG_{1k} (IgG_{1k}) monoclonal antibody that blocks the biologic activity of interleukin (IL)-12 and IL-23 by inhibiting receptors on T cells, natural killer cells, and antigen presenting cells.[86] Finally, vedolizumab is a humanized anti-$\alpha 4$-$\beta 7$ integrin monoclonal antibody, which was approved by the US Food and Drug Administration in 2014 for moderate to severe Crohn disease.[87]

Maintaining Remission

After induction of remission is achieved, the next goal of medical therapy is to maintain remission. This can be achieved with a variety of medications; however, it is important to consider the possible side effects of each of the medications from long-term use. Daily azathioprine and 6-mercaptopurine have proven efficacy in maintaining remission after medical induction compared with placebo. There are mixed results on the rates of relapse after withdrawal of these medications from no relapses over a 5-year period to a 2- to 3-fold increased relapse risk compared with continued therapy.[88] Methotrexate can also be used to maintain remission after it is used for induction of remission. This medication is given on a weekly basis, and patients should be assessed for risk of liver disease and desire to become pregnant prior to initiation of long-term therapy.

Biologic agents are increasingly being used as maintenance therapy.[88,89] However, patients may form antibodies to these medications, which can lead to acute and delayed hypersensitivity reactions. Infusion centers should be equipped to deal with these potentially life threatening side effects. In addition, patients have been reported to develop resistance to infliximab infusions. Medical therapies that are not recommended for maintenance therapy include steroids and 5-aminosalicylates. Due to their long-term side effect profile, steroids are not recommended in maintaining remission of Crohn disease. Budesonide has been found to prolong the time to relapse; however, studies have shown that it is not effective for long-term maintenance beyond 6 months.[90] 5-Aminosalicylates have limited efficacy in maintaining remission in medically treated patients.

When determining the right maintenance therapy for a given patient, the clinician must consider efficacy, adverse effects, and cost. The biologic agents are generally much more expensive than immunomodulator therapies; however, all of these therapies have toxicities.[91] Some clinicians support one or more trials off medication to see if symptoms recur; however, in such cases the patients should be given strict instructions for follow-up with the understanding that disease recurrence is likely.

NUTRITION

Nutrition is an important part of maintaining the health of patients with Crohn disease. The goal of nutritional interventions in Crohn disease includes maximizing nutritional status, maintaining adequate intake, and avoiding foods that seem to contribute to flares of symptoms. The first step to determining the nutritional health of the patient is to perform a nutritional assessment. This assessment should include a focused history, physical exam, and measurement of dietary intake, energy expenditure, body composition, and serum studies (e.g., albumin, prealbumin, and iron studies).

Malnutrition

Malnutrition is common in patients with Crohn disease and can be related to reduced nutritional intake due to anorexia, abdominal pain and bowel obstructions, malabsorption, drug effects, and increased metabolic requirements including vitamin B_{12} (cobalamin), calcium, fat-soluble vitamins, folate, iron, selenium, and zinc. In addition, patients with extensive terminal ileal disease or resection could suffer from fat malabsorption. Consequences of malnutrition in these patients are growth failure and pubertal delay in children, bone loss, delayed healing of fistulas and wounds, and increased susceptibility to infection.

Nutrition supplementation with protein, calories, and micronutrients can be provided to patients through oral, enteral, or parenteral routes. In general, the most optimal way to provide nutrients to patients is by oral route, then enteral feeding, and finally parenteral routes due to complications associated with placement of feeding tubes and intravenous access. However, if patients are unable to tolerate oral feedings, nutrition should be provided by the available route. Total parenteral nutrition is expensive and has the greatest risk for complications; therefore its use should be limited to patients with bowel obstruction or high-output fistulas, with the goal of using it for limited time periods. Exceptions to this are patients with short-gut syndrome, who cannot achieve the caloric intake needed to support themselves by oral and enteral methods alone. Some studies have shown that preoperative parenteral nutrition can correct nutritional deficiencies and improve surgical outcomes; the utility of total parenteral nutrition in the preoperative setting is limited.[92] Patients with severe malnutrition should undergo close monitoring of their electrolytes, especially phosphate levels, to avoid refeeding syndrome.

Nutrition as Primary Therapy

Many patients with Crohn disease can identify types of food that seem to precipitate flares of their disease. As such, many clinicians propose that patients undergo an elimination diet to identify other potential at risk foods that can be avoided long term.[93] In contrast, some clinicians support the use of restrictive diets to reduce intake of carbohydrates, lactose, sucrose, and processed foods; however, results of studies of dietary restriction are mixed.

A Cochrane review of randomized controlled trials reports that elemental formulations of enteral feedings are not more efficacious than nonelemental formulas in inducing remission of active Crohn disease.[94] In addition, enteral nutrition is not as effective as steroids at inducing remission; however, it does appear to have more efficacy than placebo in inducing remission of active disease. There is currently no convincing evidence that high-fiber diets, probiotics, omega-3 polyunsaturated fatty acids, glutamine supplementation, or antioxidants affect the disease course of patients with Crohn disease.

SURGICAL THERAPY

In this chapter, we will focus on surgical therapy for Crohn disease involving the small intestine. As stated earlier, the majority of patients with Crohn disease have small bowel involvement; therefore surgeons caring for patients with Crohn disease should understand the indications for surgical intervention in small bowel Crohn disease and the techniques currently used to ensure that patients receive appropriate care (Box 75.1). The presence of adhesions, malnutrition, and medical therapy with immunosuppressive agents are factors that can impact surgical decision making, but most important is the understanding that Crohn disease is a chronic condition with high recurrence rates after surgery.

The majority of patients with Crohn disease will need input from a surgeon who understands the nature of their disease. A cohort study of patients with Crohn disease found that 57% of patients require at least one surgical resection. Interestingly, a more historical cohort study found that 78% of patients required surgery by 20 years after symptom onset.[53,95] The recent drop in surgical intervention rate might reflect improvements in surgical decision-making or medical therapies with more aggressive use of immunomodulators and biologic therapies.

Indications

There is no operation that will cure Crohn disease. The purpose of all operations is to treat the complications that cannot be treated by less invasive means (medical or endoscopic therapy). All operations should be performed with the goal of conserving as much small intestinal length as possible due to the potential for recurrence and need for reoperation. The following are indications for operative intervention:

- Obstruction due to fibrotic stricture: It is important to examine the entire length of the small bowel to ensure that all obstructive strictures are identified to avoid recurrence of symptomatic obstruction due to missed segments of disease. The number, length, and location of strictures should inform surgical decision making when considering stricturoplasty versus resection. All patients with high-grade small bowel obstruction should undergo decompression and resuscitation prior to surgical intervention.
- Perforation: Free perforation is a rare complication of Crohn disease, but it is a surgical emergency. Contained perforations resulting in abscess formation are usually best addressed initially using interventional radiology drainage and systemic antibiotics, but subsequent surgical intervention is often required.
- Fistulas resistant to medical therapy: Small bowel fistulas related to Crohn disease tend to be resistant to medical therapies and therefore surgery to close the fistula and remove the underlying diseased bowel is often required.
- Failure of medical therapy: Medical therapy has failed if (1) maximal medical therapy cannot control symptoms of active disease, (2) induction of remission is followed by failure of maintenance therapy to retain remission, or (3) significant medication-associated complications develop. Rates of medical therapy failure may be decreasing with the development of more effective biologic agents.
- Other complications: Massive gastrointestinal hemorrhage, cancer, toxic megacolon, and growth retardation are less common indications for surgery.

Preoperative Preparation

Thorough preoperative preparation is imperative to ensure the best outcome for patients presenting for surgical intervention in Crohn disease. Each patient should undergo a history and physical exam to assess for comorbid medical conditions. Appropriate ancillary testing should be performed prior to nonurgent surgical interventions to ensure appropriate risk stratification. As previously stated, the patient's nutritional status should be assessed to determine if malnutrition needs to be corrected prior to intervention. If the patient has an albumin level less than 3.0 g/dL, they are at increased risk for postoperative complications, such as wound infection. Oral and enteral supplementation are the preferred routes to optimize nutrition prior to surgery; however, total parenteral nutrition can be helpful in severely malnourished patients. Patients who smoke should be counseled about smoking cessation to reduce their cardiovascular risk, as well as decrease their risk for disease recurrence after the operation.

Complete evaluation of the gastrointestinal tract using a combination of endoscopy and cross-sectional imaging, such as MR or CT enterography, might be warranted to localize all areas affected by disease preoperatively to aid

---

BOX 75.1 Indications for Surgery in Crohn Disease

- Obstruction due to fibrotic stricture
- Perforation resulting in free perforation or contained perforation not resolved using interventional radiology techniques
- Fistulas resistant to medical therapy
- Failure of medical therapy:
  - Maximal medical therapy cannot control symptoms of active disease
  - Induction of remission is followed by failure of maintenance therapy to retain remission
  - Or, significant medication-associated complications develop
- Other rare indications:
  - Massive gastrointestinal hemorrhage
  - Cancer
  - Toxic megacolon
  - Growth retardation

in surgical planning. However, regardless of the preoperative testing results, the surgeon should examine the entire small intestine at the time of operation to ensure that no skip lesions are left untreated. In addition, it is useful to directly measure the amount of remaining small bowel in each patient since this may be important to future surgical decision making. It is important to note that all patients undergoing surgical interventions should be provided with adequate resuscitation, antibiotics (for treatment or prophylaxis), and thromboembolic prophylaxis. Mechanical bowel preparation is not needed for small bowel surgery.

The impact of preoperative immunosuppressive drugs on surgical outcomes is controversial. Most of these medications can be safely discontinued prior to surgery without any side effects with the exception of corticosteroids. Patients on long-term corticosteroid therapy should be given preoperative stress-dose steroid coverage and should have their steroids gradually tapered postoperatively.[96]

When obtaining consent from patients undergoing operations for Crohn disease, the surgeon should consider if an intestinal stoma will be necessary. Always err on the side of disclosure, especially in emergency operations. For elective or less urgent operations, patients should meet with an enterostomal therapist to have stoma site markings placed and receive education on stoma care. Inappropriate stoma placement can make postoperative management difficult and in some cases increase the likelihood of leakage of bowel contents onto the peristomal skin and/or into the surgical wound.

OPERATIVE STRATEGIES AND TECHNIQUES

ABDOMINAL INCISION

Many patients will be appropriate candidates for a laparoscopic approach, but, regardless of whether the approach is laparoscopic, laparoscopically assisted, or open, the surgeon should be mindful of the placement of any and all abdominal incisions, recognizing that future reoperation is likely. Midline laparotomy incisions or low, transverse Pfannenstiel incisions are the most appropriate in Crohn patients. When combined with laparoscopic bowel mobilization, the low Pfannenstiel incision allows good access to the small intestine and pelvic structures while at the same time providing excellent cosmetic outcomes and low hernia rates (0% to 3.7% vs. up to 42% with a standard midline laparotomy).[97,98]

ABDOMINAL EXPLORATION AND IDENTIFICATION OF DISEASED SEGMENTS

Assessment of the entire abdominal cavity should be performed to identify all diseased segments of the gastrointestinal tract, including areas of stenosis, perforation, abscesses, masses, and fistulae. Active Crohn lesions might be easily identified due to thickening of the bowel wall and adjacent mesentery, serosal hyperemia, and creeping fat (extension of mesenteric fat onto the serosal surface of the bowel wall). However, subtle lesions might be more difficult to identify, requiring careful visual inspection, palpation, and in some cases passage

of an intraluminal balloon to rule out subtle areas of narrowing.

MANAGEMENT OF STENOTIC BOWEL SEGMENTS: RESECTION VERSUS STRICTUROPLASTY

Patients who present with obstructive symptoms due to fibrostenotic lesions commonly require surgical intervention to achieve symptom relief. Surgical techniques for relieving these obstructive lesions are broadly classified as those involving bowel resection and those not involving resection. Because these lesions can recur, the surgeon must consider the best way to relieve the patient's symptoms while preserving bowel length. The fear of iatrogenic short bowel syndrome has led surgeons to develop techniques to spare the bowel in this clinical setting. This mindfulness for retaining bowel length has led to excellent outcomes, with only 5% of patients being left with less than 180 cm of residual intestine and only 1.5% of patients requiring home total parenteral nutrition in a cohort study.[99]

The use of stricturoplasty in Crohn disease was first described in 1982 by Lee and Papaioannou.[100] Multiple clinical series using this technique have established that it is both safe and effective in the treatment of Crohn strictures (Fig. 75.8). In addition, the risk of disease recurrence appears to be unchanged in this technique compared with resection, which was a previous concern of many clinicians.[101]

Stricturoplasty is generally considered the preferred approach to a Crohn stricture but is inappropriate in the setting of active inflammation/infection, large phlegmon, when the length or number of strictures within a given segment makes resection a better option, or when there is concern about carcinoma.

Stricturoplasty Techniques

The two main types of stricturoplasty are the Heineke-Mikulicz technique and the techniques involving a side-to-side anastomosis. When deciding what technique to use, one must consider the stricture length. Short strictures

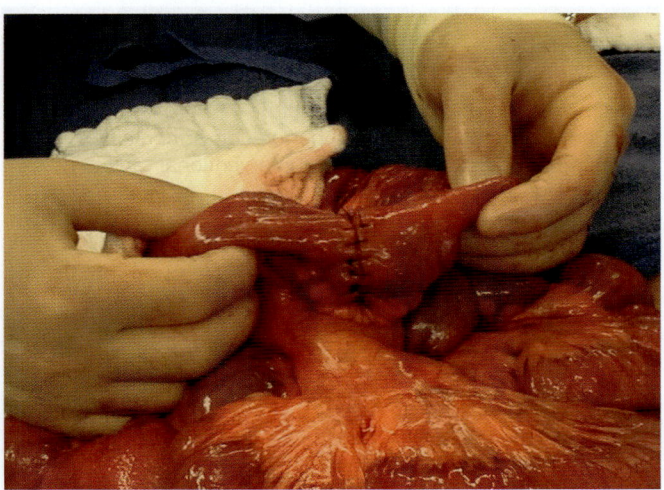

FIGURE 75.8 Completed stricturoplasty for small bowel stenosis due to Crohn disease.

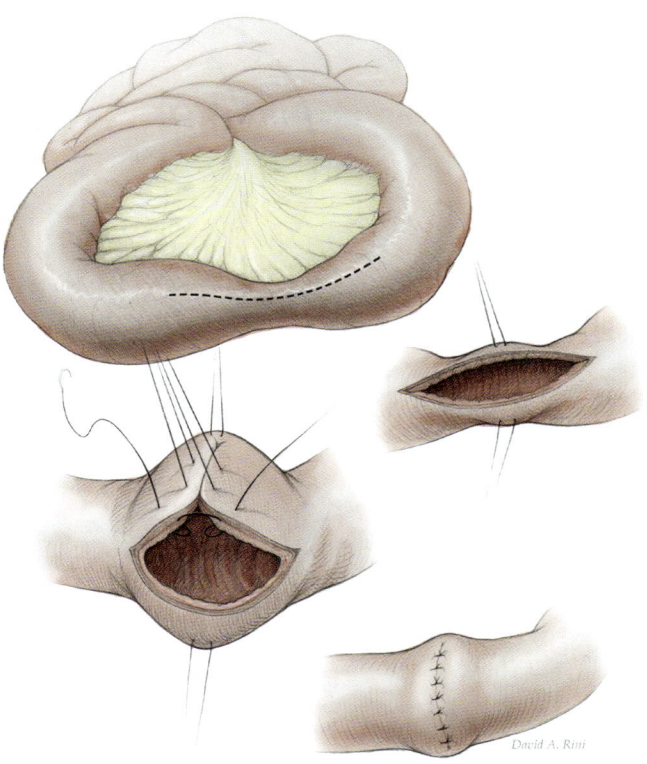

FIGURE 75.9 Heineke-Mikulicz stricturoplasty technique: longitudinal enterotomy over the stricture followed by transverse closure. (From Talamini M. Stricturoplasty in Crohn's disease. In: Cameron JL, ed. *Current Surgical Therapy*. 8th ed. Philadelphia: Mosby; 2004:117.)

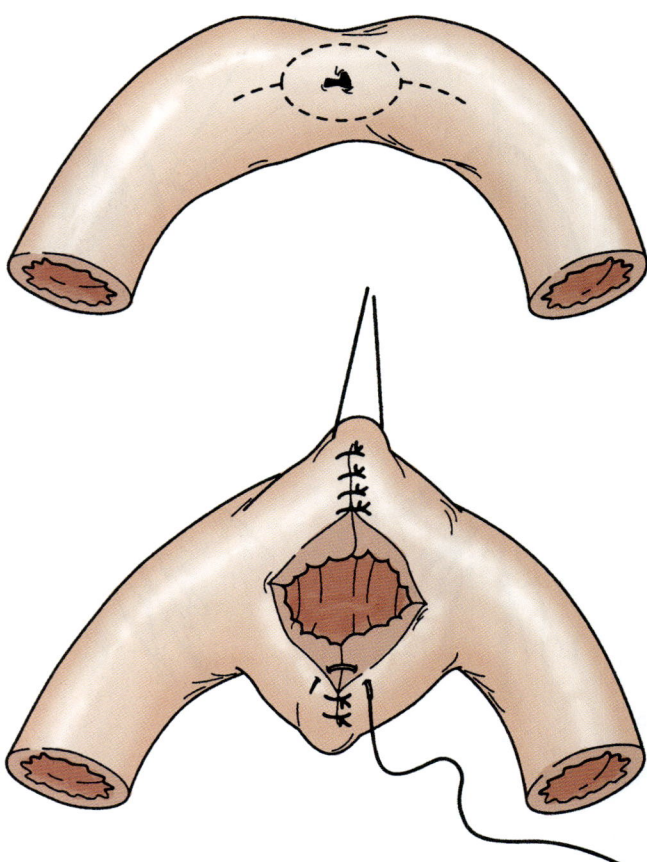

FIGURE 75.10 Judd stricturoplasty technique: longitudinal enterotomy with transverse closure. (From Michelassi F, Hurst RD. Stricturoplasty in Crohn's disease. In: Cameron JL, ed. *Current Surgical Therapy*. 8th ed. Philadelphia: Mosby; 2004:134.)

(<10 cm long) are more suited to the Heineke-Mikulicz technique. Longer strictures (>10 cm long) or lesions with many short strictures in close proximity are more suited to a side-to-side technique. The Finney stricturoplasty is usually recommended for strictures between 10 and 15 cm long, whereas the Michelassi technique is usually performed for longer diseased segments.[101–103]

The following is a summary of the Heineke-Mikulicz stricturoplasty and its variations:

- Heineke-Mikulicz stricturoplasty: This technique involves longitudinal transmural opening of the antimesenteric wall of the strictured bowel and reorientation of the incision so that it is closed transversely to widen the luminal narrowing. It is closed with seromuscular interrupted or running absorbable suture (Fig. 75.9).
- Judd stricturoplasty: A longitudinal elliptical resection of a small portion of bowel wall is performed. The bowel wall is then closed transversely to widen the luminal narrowing. This technique is most useful when there is a small area of penetration or damaged wall within a short stricture (Fig. 75.10).
- Moskel-Walske-Neumayer stricturoplasty: A Y-shaped enterotomy is made, and the bowel wall is closed transversely. This reduces the tension of the suture line and is most useful when there is a mismatch of diameters, such as lesions with prestenotic dilation (Fig. 75.11).

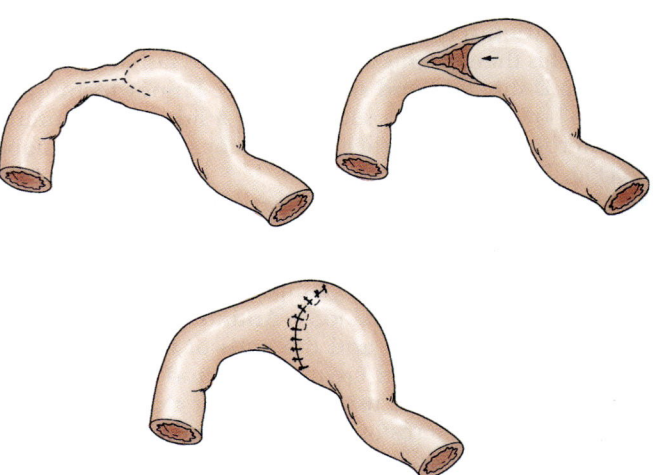

FIGURE 75.11 Moskel-Walske-Neumayer stricturoplasty technique: Y-shaped enterotomy with transverse closure. (From Michelassi F, Hurst RD. Stricturoplasty in Crohn's disease. In: Cameron JL, ed. *Current Surgical Therapy*. 7th ed. St Louis: Mosby; 2001:134.)

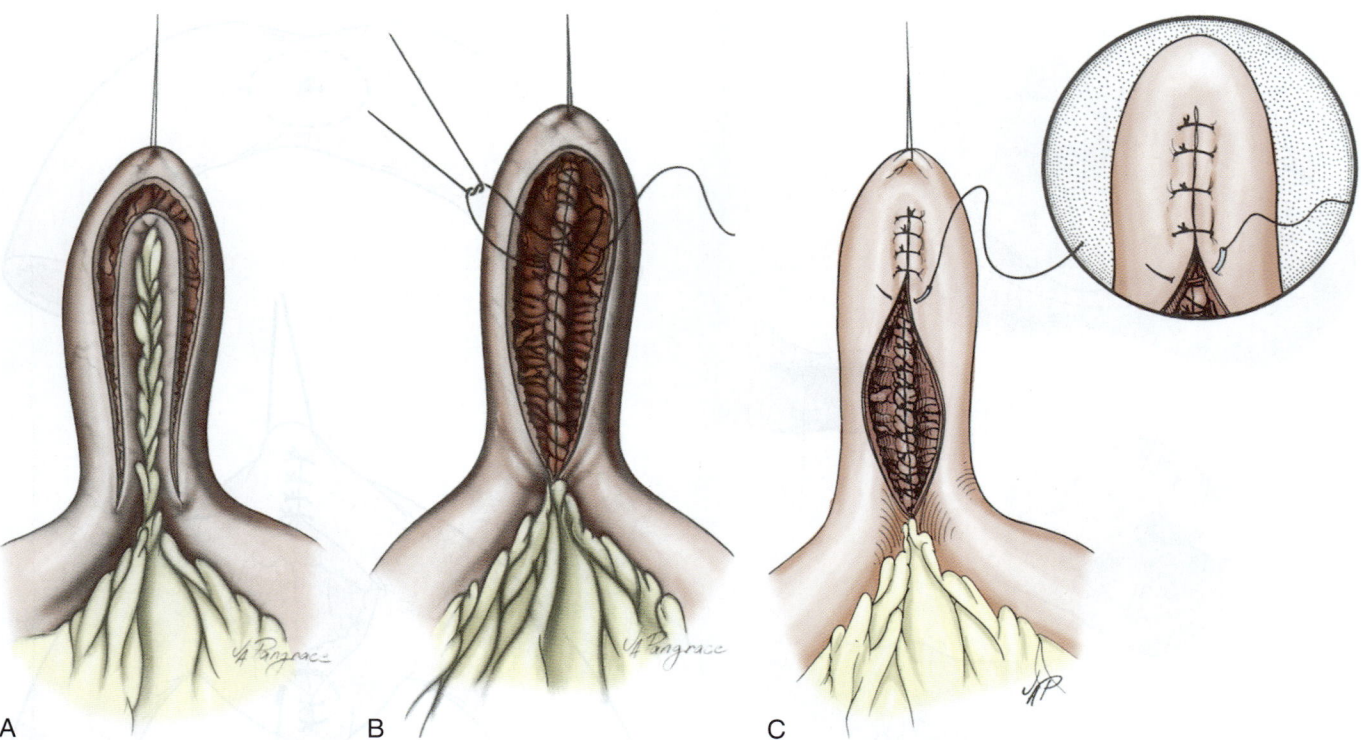

A   B   C

FIGURE 75.12 Finney stricturoplasty technique: Enteroenterostomy U-shaped configuration. (A) Longintudinal enterotomy is performed. (B) The posterior wall of the bowel is closed using a standard suturing technique. (C) The anterior wall is closed to completely close the enterotomy. (From Talamini M. Stricturoplasty in Crohn's disease. In: Cameron JL, ed. *Current Surgical Therapy*. 8th ed. Philadelphia: Mosby; 2004:118.)

Side-to-side anastomosis techniques are most useful for long strictures:

- Finney stricturoplasty: A single antimesenteric longitudinal enterotomy is performed, and the bowel is oriented in a side-to-side fashion by creating a U-shaped bend. The bowel is then closed beginning with the posterior wall using a standard suturing technique, although linear stapling devices can also be used (Fig. 75.12).
- Jaboulay stricturoplasty: Two separate antimesenteric longitudinal enterotomies are performed, leaving the most strictured portion of the bowel unopened. The bowel is then oriented in a side-to-side fashion by creating a U-shaped bend similar to the Finney technique. The bowel is then closed creating a side-to-side enteroenterostomy using either a sutured or stapling technique (Fig. 75.13).
- Michelassi (or side-to-side isoperistaltic) stricturoplasty: First the small bowel mesentery is divided at the midpoint of the affected segment. Next, the bowel is divided using atraumatic bowel clamps and the proximal loop is placed over the distal loop. Antimesenteric enterotomies are then made and the ends of the small bowel are tapered to avoid creation of blind pouches. The bowel is then closed using a two-layer closure, creating a long enteroenterostomy. This nontraditional technique should be used only when there is major concern about short bowel syndrome (Fig. 75.14).

Bowel Resection and Anastomotic Techniques

When the surgeon identifies a segment of diseased bowel that requires resection, they must first identify the proximal

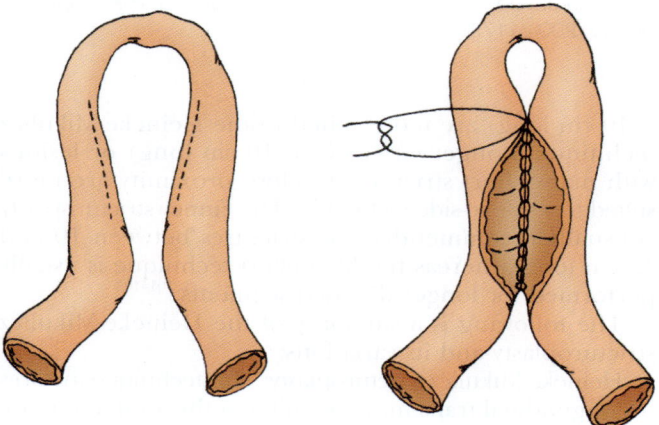

FIGURE 75.13 Jaboulay stricturoplasty technique: two separate enterotomies side-to-side closure. (Modified from Tichansky D, Cagir B, Yoo E, Marcus SM, Fry RD. Strictureplasty for Crohn's disease: meta-analysis. *Dis Colon Rectum*. 2000;43:911.)

and distal extent of the disease. Prospective, randomized trials have clearly shown that wide margin resections beyond the area of grossly diseased bowel provide no benefit in regard to disease recurrence and therefore should be avoided. The diseased bowel segment can be divided between clamps or with a linear cutting gastrointestinal stapler. Decompression of the intestine might be necessary prior to dividing the bowel if it is dilated from an obstructing lesion. To decompress the bowel, the

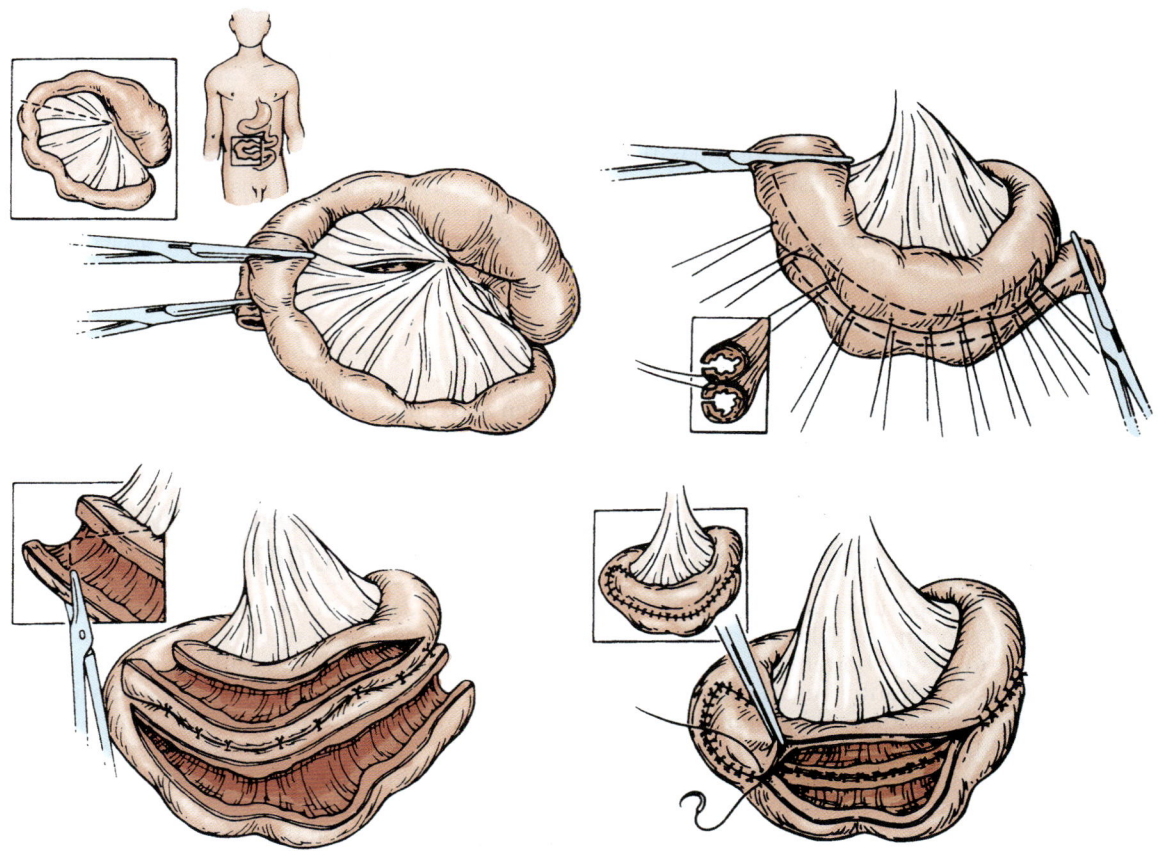

FIGURE 75.14 Michelassi stricturoplasty technique: side-to-side isoperistaltic stricturoplasty performed as a long side-to-side enteroenterostomy. (From Michelassi F, Hurst RD. Stricturoplasty in Crohn's disease. In: Cameron JL, ed. *Current Surgical Therapy*. 7th ed. St Louis: Mosby; 2001:136.)

intestinal contents should be milked away from the area of disease and kept in place using atraumatic bowel clamps. A controlled enterotomy should then be performed followed by vacuum suction of the intestinal contents. After the diseased bowel has been stapled, care should be used in dividing it away from the mesentery. Active Crohn lesions tend to be associated with thickened, shortened, and hyperemic mesentery and will often require suture ligation rather than simple surgical ties.

After resecting the diseased segment of bowel, the surgeon must decide whether it is most appropriate to perform a primary anastomosis with or without diverting loop stoma versus an end stoma. This decision depends on several factors including: the stability of the patient, their nutritional status, their use of steroids and other medications, the condition of the bowel that would be used in the anastomosis and the condition of the abdomen in general. All of these factors affect the likelihood that the patient will suffer a septic complication, such as abscess or anastomotic leak. In general, the risks associated with small bowel to small bowel or ileocolonic anastomoses are quite low, so it is only in rare cases that a stoma will be required.

If the surgeon decides to perform an anastomosis, the considerations for anastomoses for small bowel disease in Crohn disease are similar to the considerations for all intestinal anastomoses: ensure adequate blood supply, ensure the anastomosis is tension-free, consider the proximal and distal bowel diameter, and avoid distal obstruction. This last factor is of particular importance in Crohn disease, where distal lesions could place a proximal anastomosis at risk for leak due to increased intraluminal pressure in the postoperative period. The decision to perform a stapled versus handsewn anastomosis is generally based on operator preference; however, there are some reports that a functional end-to-end stapled anastomosis is superior to other stapled or handsewn anastomotic techniques. Additional support for this technique includes its ability to be performed on bowel of varying caliber.

STOMA FORMATION

As discussed previously, it is best to prepare patients for the possibility of needing a stoma before the operation. Having patients meet with an enterostomal therapist can help them to understand what stoma care entails and will provide stoma site marking, which can avoid misplacement in the operating room. The majority of stomas created in patients with Crohn disease are temporary; however, a poorly placed stoma can cause daily inconvenience to the patient and could increase the risk of wound complications.

Stomas should be located within the rectus muscle to reduce the risk of hernia formation. The site should ideally be free of scar and located at a distance from the ribs and iliac crest. Most enterostomal therapists will provide a few markings of ideal stoma sites; it is up to the surgeon to choose a site that is appropriate for the patient taking into account the surgical incision that will be required for the operation. If there is not time for the patient to meet with an enterostomal therapist prior to the operation, the surgeon should consider optional sites while the patient is able to sit up and lie down. This is especially important in obese individuals, to avoid skin creases or protrusions that can affect the adherence of the stoma appliance.

The techniques for creating and maturing stomas for patients with Crohn disease are the same as for other patients. An approximate 2-cm disk of skin is sharply excised, and the subcutaneous fat is opened to the level of the rectus fascia. A cruciate incision is then made in the anterior rectus sheath, and the rectus muscle is spread to expose the posterior sheath, which is then opened to reveal the peritoneum. The peritoneum is opened with a cruciate incision and the tract is dilated to create an opening large enough to fit the bowel through with its mesentery. The mesentery should be oriented in the cephalad position after the abdominal incision is closed; the stoma is matured with absorbable sutures in a Brooke fashion, making certain to have at least 2 to 3 cm of everted bowel projecting from the abdominal wall to minimize the chances of skin exposure to enteric contents.

BYPASS PROCEDURES

Intestinal bypass operations are rarely used in the treatment of Crohn disease lesions of the jejunum or ileum. However, gastrojejunostomy or duodenojejunostomy bypass operations are frequently used to treat duodenal Crohn lesions.

MINIMALLY INVASIVE SURGERY IN CROHN DISEASE

The pathology associated with Crohn disease can present unique challenges to surgeons attempting to use minimally invasive surgical techniques, including laparoscopic, robotic, and natural orifice surgical techniques. Intense inflammation leads to friable tissues, which can be difficult to handle with laparoscopic instruments, thickened mesentery can provide challenges in mobilization of the bowel, and previous operations can make safe entry into the abdominal cavity challenging. Despite these challenges, the improved outcomes of minimally invasive surgery seen in other abdominal operations, including less postoperative pulmonary complications, postoperative ileus, shorter hospital stay, and improved cosmetic outcomes, should not be ignored. Similar to other abdominal operations, the surgeon must keep the patient's safety in mind when using minimally invasive techniques and be ready for conversion to an open operation if the approach does not seem feasible or is not in the patient's best interest. Contraindications to minimally invasive surgical approaches in Crohn disease are evolving as surgeons feel more comfortable in their technical ability using these approaches. Some contraindications that have been agreed upon by experts in the field include: uncorrected

---

> **BOX 75.2** **Contraindications to Minimally Invasive Surgery in Crohn Disease**
>
> - Uncorrected coagulopathy
> - Intraabdominal varices from portal hypertension
> - Dense intraabdominal adhesions or history of multiple open abdominal operations
> - Diffuse peritonitis
> - Severe obstruction with massively dilated intestine

coagulopathy, intraabdominal varices from portal hypertension, dense intraabdominal adhesions or history of multiple open abdominal operations, diffuse peritonitis, and severe obstruction with massively dilated intestine (Box 75.2).[104]

TREATMENT OF SMALL BOWEL CROHN DISEASE COMPLICATIONS

As discussed earlier in the chapter, the Vienna classification system groups Crohn disease patients into subcategories based on disease behavior (inflammatory, stricturing, and penetrating), age (<40 or ≥40), and disease location (terminal ileum, colon, ileocolonic, upper gastrointestinal).[61] This classification scheme allows clinicians and researchers to better understand the natural course and treatment outcomes for this disease in better detail. The need for surgical therapy appears to be most dependent on disease behavior involving the stricturing and penetrating subgroups. Complications of these two high-risk subgroups will be the focus of the next section.

STRICTURING DISEASE

Stricturing disease leads to a range of symptom severity from chronic low-grade obstructions to acute high-grade or complete obstructions. Because of this, patients can present with either chronic intermittent symptoms of intolerance to solids and then liquids or acute symptoms with abdominal pain, nausea, vomiting, distention, and potentially obstipation. A chronic stricture is more likely to lead to food avoidance, weight loss, failure to thrive, and malnourishment over time. Hospital admission might be required for either disease course for medical and/or surgical therapy. If there is no evidence of bowel compromise or peritonitis on examination, patients with obstructive symptoms should initially be treated with bowel rest, nasogastric decompression, and resuscitation. Endoscopy or contrast imaging studies should be performed to assess for inflammation in the area of stricture. If inflammation is contributing to the stenosis, aggressive medical therapy could avoid the need for operative intervention. Patients with intermittent low-grade obstructive symptoms can be counseled on eating a low-residue diet to reduce the incidence of partial bowel obstruction. However, many of these patients will require operative intervention in the long term. Patients with complete bowel obstruction also require surgical intervention.

As discussed in the previous section, intestinal stenosis can be treated with bowel resection or stricturoplasty. The surgeon should consider the health of the bowel surrounding the stenosis, the total length of bowel that will remain, the patient's nutritional health, recent steroid or biologic therapy use, and presence of other lesions (e.g., phlegmon, abscess, or fistula).

PENETRATING DISEASE: ENTERIC FISTULAS AND PERFORATION

Patients with a penetrating pattern of Crohn disease are at risk of forming fistulas and perforations. This chapter will focus on the treatment of small bowel Crohn disease fistulas; however, perianal fistulas are even more common in this disease. Fistulas are named for the organs that they connect, for example: small intestine to small intestine (enteroenteric); small intestine to colon (enterocolonic); small intestine to any part of the urogenital tract, including the bladder (enterovesical), ureters (enteroureteral), and vagina (enterovaginal); and small intestine to skin (entero-cutaneous fistula). Population-based cohort studies have found that fistulas develop in 35% of patients with Crohn disease, approximately two-thirds of which are perianal fistulas.[105,106] Some fistulas are asymptomatic or can heal over with conservative management. Fistulae can lead to complications, including diarrhea or malabsorption (due to either bacterial overgrowth or bypassing large segments of the intestine) or infection (from communication with the genitourinary systems). Fistulae can also lead to significant decrement in quality of life due to external drainage, which can be difficult for patients to manage.

Treatment of fistulae historically involved supportive care by optimizing nutrition for healing, and wound care around externally draining fistulas. With the introduction of immunomodulator therapies and biologic agents, great improvements in the treatment of this disease have been made. Infliximab, azathioprine, and 6-mercaptopurine have all been established as standard treatment for Crohn disease-related fistulae. A meta-analysis comparing biologic therapy to placebo found a significant improvement in healing of fistula over the trial period.[85] However, it should be noted that most of the data on biologic treatments for Crohn fistulae involve perianal, rather than small bowel fistulae. It is also important to note that stenotic lesions causing obstruction distal to a fistula site will contribute to nonhealing of fistulae.

Enteroenteric Fistulas

Simple enteroenteric fistulae between short segments of bowel are usually asymptomatic and are identified incidentally on imaging studies or during abdominal exploration (Fig. 75.15). These fistulae do not require any specific intervention in and of themselves but often exist due to severe underlying disease that will require surgical intervention. Rarely enteroenteric fistulae lead to malabsorption and diarrhea due to bypass of lengthy segments of normal bowel. The surgical approach to small bowel fistulae is to resect the diseased segments and primarily repair the "innocent bystander" bowel that is involved in the fistulizing process. Ileocecal fistulae behave similarly and should be treated in the same manner.

Ileosigmoid Fistulas

Fistulas between the small bowel (usually terminal ileum) and sigmoid colon occur in up to 6% of patients with

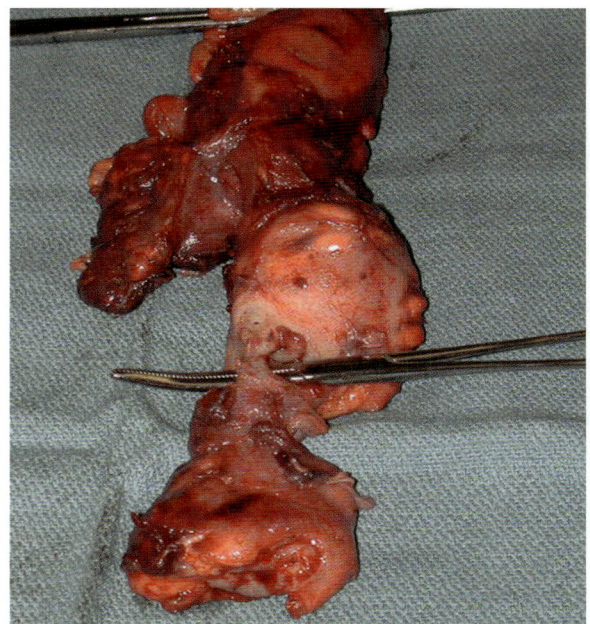

FIGURE 75.15 Enteroenteric fistula identified in a small bowel specimen of a patient with active Crohn disease.

Crohn disease, and these can be asymptomatic or lead to such symptoms as abdominal pain, diarrhea, and malabsorption. These fistulae may be difficult to detect on endoscopic or imaging studies. Treatment of these fistulas involves separation of the small bowel from the sigmoid colon, resection of the diseased ileum, and primary closure of the colon as long as it is not affected by intrinsic active Crohn disease. Rarely the sigmoid will have active Crohn disease with rigid thickening of the colonic wall and in such cases resection will be needed. If the sigmoid is resected, primary anastomosis can usually be performed with or without temporary proximal diversion. The decision to perform proximal diversion should be based on the same factors discussed previously.

Enterovesical and Enteroureteral Fistulas

Fistulas from the ileum, colon, or rectum to the genito-urinary system occur at a rate of 1% to 8% in patients with Crohn disease. Unlike enteroenteric fistulas, these fistulas are usually symptomatic and rarely close without surgery. Patients usually present with dysuria, urinary urgency, urinary frequency, suprapubic discomfort, pneumaturia, or fecaluria after a well-established diagnosis of Crohn disease. Diagnosis is usually made using cystoscopy or radiography (e.g., small bowel follow-through, CT enteroclysis, or MR enteroclysis). The bladder dome is the most common site involved, and definitive treatment usually requires surgical therapy. First, the connection between the bladder and the intestine is divided and the diseased bowel is resected. The opening in the bladder is then débrided and closed primarily. A Foley catheter is left in place postoperatively (usually for 10 to 14 days) to drain the bladder and reduce tension on the repair.[106,107]

Enterogenital Fistulas

Enterogenital fistulas are more common in women than men and usually occur between the rectum and vagina, but enterovaginal, enterosalpingeal, and enterouterine fistulas can also develop in some patients. Symptoms include malodorous vaginal discharge and passage of air or stool from the vagina. As with other small bowel fistulae, the fistulous tract is first divided, and the opening in the genital tract is débrided and primarily closed, assuming this is technically feasible. Any decision to resect the involved genital organ should bear in mind the potential reproductive, endocrine, and sexual dysfunction that could occur. This is especially important in treating women of childbearing age and should be part of the informed consent discussion. The diseased small bowel is removed and anastomoses performed, unless a stoma is deemed necessary.[105]

Enterocutaneous Fistulas

Spontaneous enterocutaneous fistulas rarely occur in Crohn disease, but when they do they are generally associated with a very aggressive and severe disease phenotype. The majority of enterocutaneous fistulas occur as postoperative complications, commonly draining through the surgical wound. Such fistulas are usually the result of anastomotic leaks but could be due to an unrecognized bowel injury. The natural history and treatment recommendations between these two types of fistula vary greatly. Spontaneous fistulas due to penetrating Crohn disease rarely close spontaneously. Immunomodulators and biologic agents may be of some benefit; however, operative intervention is frequently needed to achieve closure. It is important to note that operative therapy should not be delayed if there are complicating factors, such as distal obstruction, high fistula output, or difficult to manage wounds.

In contrast, enterocutaneous fistulas secondary to surgical complications tend to respond well to conventional treatment of fistulae, especially if the involved bowel is intrinsically normal and not affected by active Crohn disease. Long, low-output fistulas are likely to close with nonoperative, conservative management, whereas short, high-output fistulae are more likely to require operative therapy. Similar to the previous surgical interventions for fistula disease, operative management includes division of the fistula, resection of the diseased bowel, and débridement of the fistula tract.[108]

PERFORATIONS: ABSCESSES AND FREE PERFORATION

The perforating subtype of Crohn disease usually presents in the acute setting with abdominal pain and fever. Adequate resuscitation and source control are the goals of treatment in these patients.

Abscesses

Up to one-third of patients with Crohn disease will have an abscess at some point during their disease course. Unlike other surgical patients with abscesses, Crohn disease patients may have few symptoms due to their use of steroids, immunomodulators, and biologic agents. However, some patients will exhibit the classic signs and symptoms of an

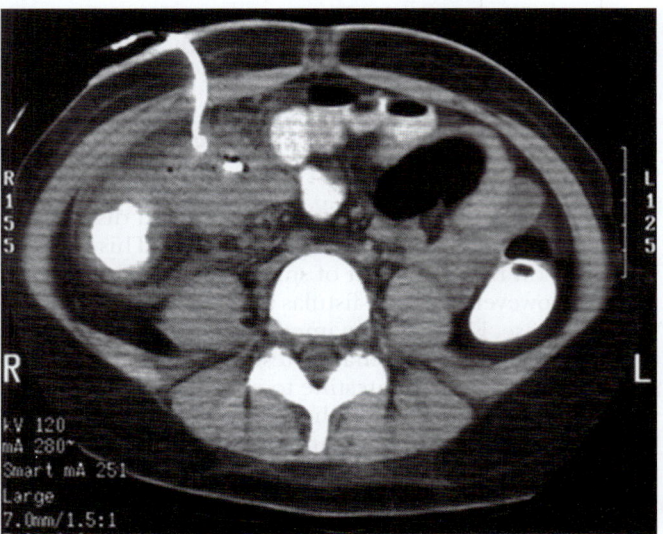

FIGURE 75.16 Successful drain placement for intraabdominal abscess using interventional radiology.

intraabdominal infection: abdominal pain and tenderness, fever, ileus or obstruction, and potentially a palpable mass. Cross-sectional imaging should be used to aid diagnosis. Percutaneous drainage of the abscess should be performed depending on the location of the abscess and the comfort of the interventional radiographer. Open surgical drainage of an intraabdominal abscess related to Crohn disease is rarely needed in this era of advanced interventional radiology (Fig. 75.16). Medical therapy should be initiated for the patient's active Crohn disease and treatment with adequate resuscitation, antibiotics, and nutritional support with close monitoring for signs of systemic infection.[109]

Free Perforation

Although a rare event, free perforation in patients with Crohn disease does occur. It is most common in patients who present with concurrent toxic colitis, distal obstruction, or cancer or as a complication after surgical or endoscopic intervention. Patients who are on chronic immunosuppression, such as steroids, immunomodulators, and biologic therapy, might present with minimal symptoms. A high index of suspicion is required in patients taking these agents. A plain abdominal radiograph might reveal free air and in some cases may be the only imaging study needed as the patient is best served by urgent laparotomy. In other cases, cross-sectional imaging may be appropriate to better define the disease process and to determine if urgent exploration is needed.

Emergent surgical exploration is usually required when free perforation is suspected, and these patients should also receive adequate resuscitation, timely broad-spectrum antibiotics, and stress-dose steroids if appropriate. Prior to incision, the surgeon should mark the patient for possible stoma placement. Upon entry of the abdominal cavity, the source of perforation should be identified. Débridement and primary repair of gastric or duodenal perforations are usually sufficient, and resection with primary anastomosis can be performed for most jejunal or ileal perforations. Proximal diversion with a loop or end stoma should be considered if the patient is on chronic immunosuppression, malnourished, or if the patient is hemodynamically unstable.

OTHER ISSUES IN THE SURGICAL MANAGEMENT OF SMALL BOWEL CROHN DISEASE

CROHN DISEASE OF THE DUODENUM

Symptomatic duodenal Crohn disease is rare. Patients with duodenal lesions present with symptoms of dyspepsia or epigastric pain, anorexia, and obstructive symptoms (e.g., early satiety, nausea, vomiting, and weight loss). Duodenal disease can include inflammatory lesions, strictures, and fistulas, and long-standing disease increases the risk of duodenal cancer. Because it is a rarer entity, medical treatment of duodenal Crohn disease is less well studied; however, recommendations are similar to those for more distal disease: (1) initiate medical therapy for active Crohn disease, (2) provide nutritional support, and (3) drain any abscess for source control usually via percutaneous approach. Duodenal fistulas should be approached by taking down the fistula tract, resecting the other diseased bowel, and then by addressing the duodenal opening. Longitudinal primary closure of the duodenum might lead to stenosis. As such, closure of the duodenum after division of fistulas or stenosis operations should employ the Heineke-Mikulicz technique and, if needed, a bypass using a duodenojejunostomy, gastrojejunostomy, or Roux-en-Y anastomosis.[110]

URETERAL OBSTRUCTION

Ureteral obstruction in patients with Crohn disease can occur due to stone formation after resection of the terminal ileum, but it is more frequently due to acalculous obstructions due to involvement by a nearby inflammatory process. Symptoms of acalculous obstructions include urinary frequency and urgency, flank pain, and fever. Patients might also present with a palpable abdominal or flank mass. Urinalysis and urine culture should be obtained but are often normal. Axial imaging of the genitourinary system will reveal ureteral stenosis with upstream dilation. It frequently occurs concurrently with ileocecal disease (i.e., right-sided obstruction is more common). Treatment includes initiation of medical therapy for Crohn disease and ureteral stenting if a significant obstruction is present, as well as percutaneous drainage of any abscesses. Resection of the diseased bowel and ureterolysis should be performed if nonoperative management fails.[107]

POSTOPERATIVE CARE

Postoperative care of patients who have undergone surgery for Crohn disease is similar to management of other gastrointestinal surgical patients. Specifically, there are no clear benefits of routine use of nasogastric suction for distal procedures, and use of enteric suction in upper gastrointestinal operations is surgeon dependent. Perioperative coverage with stress-dose steroids should be used in patients who have been on long-term systemic steroids and then should be tapered as soon as possible in a gradual fashion.

LONG-TERM MANAGEMENT

Patients should be counseled regarding the chronic, recurrent nature of their disease. Up to 80% of patients will have endoscopic evidence of disease recurrence 1 year after intestinal resection, and the majority of patients (60%) will have symptomatic recurrence 10 years after their initial operation. In patients with a diverting stoma, there is an increased likelihood that they will have a recurrence after intestinal flow is restored. Preventing disease recurrence is preferable to trying to treat active disease; therefore patients should undergo risk stratification and be treated with medical therapies appropriate to their risk profile. Fig. 75.17 provides a treatment algorithm for decreasing recurrence risk.

Postoperative therapy should be tailored to each individual patient based on the profile of their disease course. There are three risk categories that patients with Crohn disease fall into: low, intermediate, or high risk. It is imperative that patients are given clear follow-up instructions to ensure that treatment is monitored and modified based on clinical symptoms or endoscopic evidence of recurrence. Endoscopic surveillance should be performed at 6- to 12-month intervals, with objective evaluation of endoscopic findings using current scoring modalities as described in the previous sections (Fig. 75.18). In postoperative patients, the Rutgeerts score should be used to risk-stratify patients endoscopically over their postoperative course (Table 75.2). A Rutgeerts score less than 2 predicts a disease recurrence of less than 10%, whereas scores of 3 and 4 predict higher recurrence rates (50% or 100%).[65]

RISK FACTORS FOR RECURRENCE

Risk factors that are associated with disease recurrence include early age at onset, penetrating disease phenotype, current smoking, and extensive disease (>100 cm and/or multiple disease sites). There are indications that certain genetic mutations (such as the *NOD2/CARD15* gene) have an increased risk for recurrence; however, this is not routinely tested in the clinical setting. The Rutgeerts endoscopic recurrence score also correlates with the likelihood of future clinical and surgical recurrence.[65] All of these factors should be considered by the surgeon and gastroenterologist when recommending a patient's therapeutic course. In terms of modifiable factors, smoking postoperatively carries a 2.5-time increased risk of postoperative disease recurrence according to a meta-analysis of Crohn disease patients, and therefore smoking cessation should be recommended to all patients with Crohn disease.[111,112]

MEDICATIONS TO PREVENT RECURRENCE

A Cochrane review has found a significant decrease in the relative risk of postoperative recurrence with the use of 5-aminosalicylates and 6-mercaptopurine/azathioprine when compared with placebo, but strong evidence is mounting that biologic agents are more effective in the prevention of postoperative recurrence.[113,114] A cohort

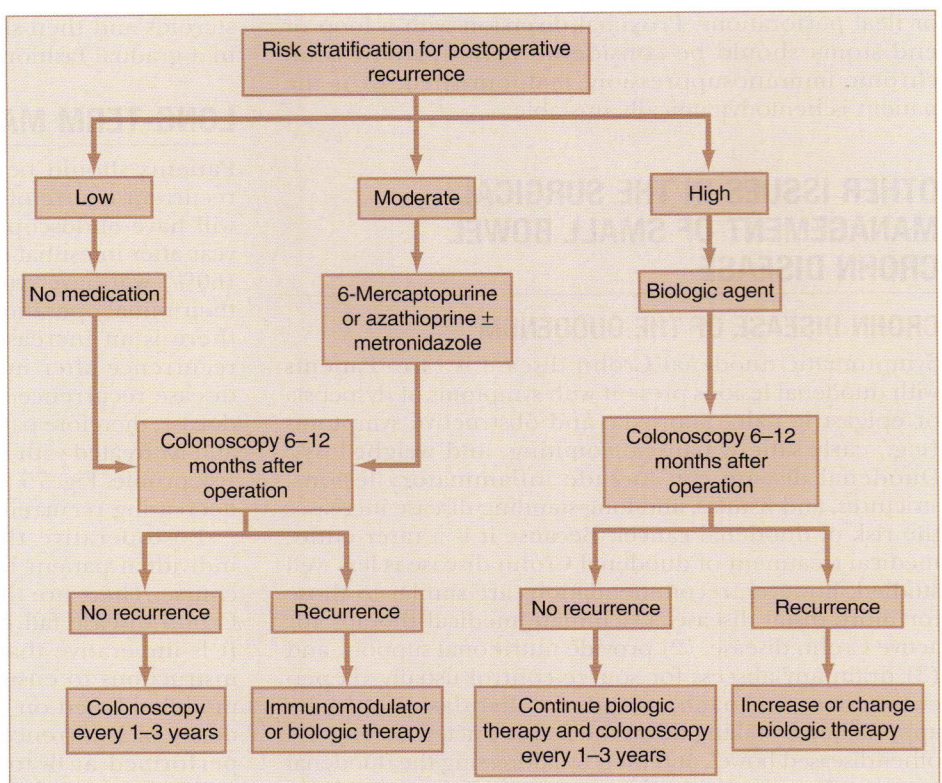

FIGURE 75.17 Postoperative follow-up and treatment algorithm.

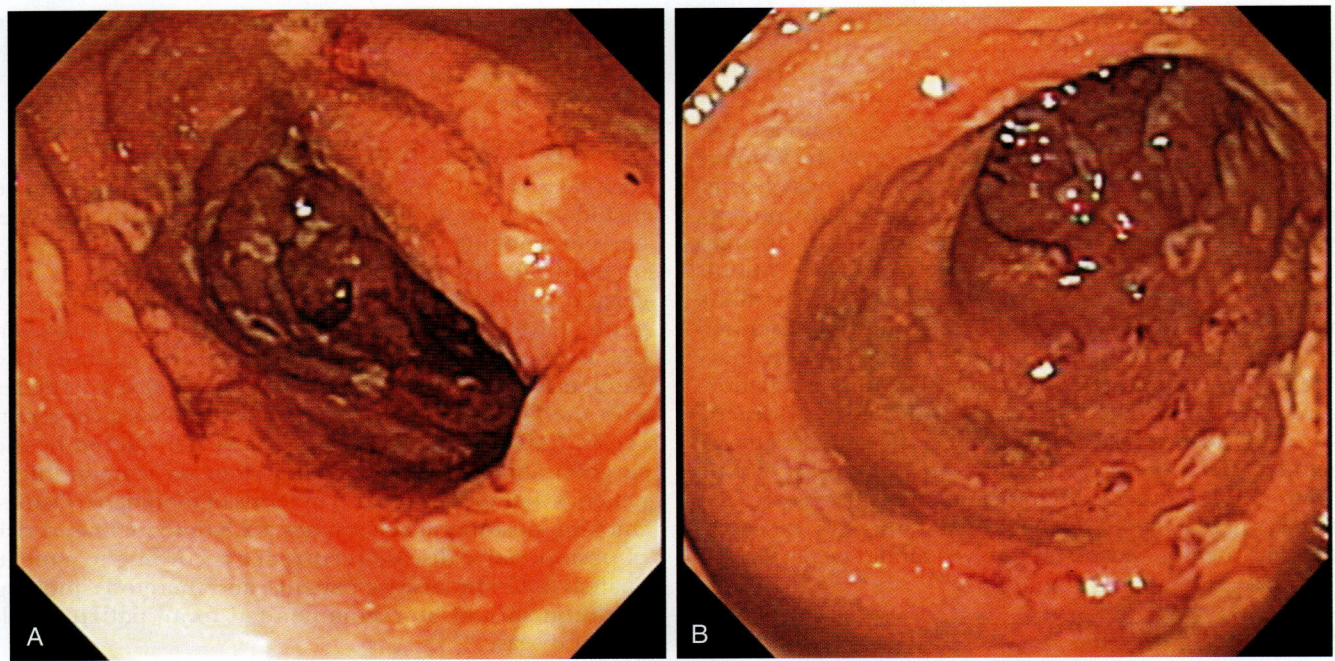

FIGURE 75.18 Recurrent Crohn disease identified on endoscopy with multiple ulcerations in the neoterminal ileum identified 3 months after initial resection. (A) Multiple ulcerations identified on endoscopy. (B) Recurrence of Crohn disease in the neoterminal ileum seen on endoscopy. (From Krok KL, Lichtenstein GR. Inflammatory bowel disease. In: Ginsberg GG, Kochman ML, Norton ID, et al., eds. *Clinical Gastrointestinal Endoscopy*. Philadelphia: Saunders; 2005:317.)

TABLE 75.2 Rutgeerts Score for Endoscopic Risk Stratification

Grade	Definition	Estimated 3-Year Recurrence Risk (%)
i0	No lesions	<10
i1	≤5 aphthous lesions	<10
i2	>5 aphthous lesions with normal intervening mucosa or skip areas of larger lesions or lesions confined to the ileocolonic anastomosis (i.e., <1 cm long)	15–20
i3	Diffuse aphthous ileitis with diffusely inflamed mucosa	40
i4	Diffuse inflammation with enlarged ulcers, nodules, and/or narrowing	90

study of 33 patients found that no patients (0 of 17) recurred at 2 years when treated with infliximab and methotrexate compared with 75% of patients (12 of 16) who received mesalamine alone. Another randomized trial of 24 patients found significantly less recurrence at 1 year on histologic and endoscopic examination with postoperative prophylactic infliximab.

CANCER SURVEILLANCE

There is a clear association between cancer formation in areas of chronic inflammation associated with Crohn disease, including both the small intestine and colon. In addition, squamous cell carcinoma of the anus and skin, duodenal neoplasia, and testicular cancer are the most commonly reported cancers with increased incidence in the Crohn disease patient population. In addition, thiopurines, a common treatment for IBD, are associated with an increased risk of developing lymphoproliferative disorders.[115,116]

REFERENCES

1. Loftus EV Jr. Clinical epidemiology of inflammatory bowel disease: incidence, prevalence, and environmental influences. *Gastroenterology.* 2004;126(6):1504-1517.
2. Molodecky NA, Soon IS, Rabi DM, et al. Increasing incidence and prevalence of the inflammatory bowel diseases with time, based on systematic review. *Gastroenterology.* 2012;142(1):46-54.e42; quiz e30.
3. Kappelman MD, Rifas-Shiman SL, Kleinman K, et al. The prevalence and geographic distribution of Crohn's disease and ulcerative colitis in the United States. *Clin Gastroenterol Hepatol.* 2007;5(12):1424-1429.
4. Birrenbach T, Bocker U. Inflammatory bowel disease and smoking: a review of epidemiology, pathophysiology, and therapeutic implications. *Inflamm Bowel Dis.* 2004;10(6):848-859.
5. Ekbom A, Montgomery SM. Environmental risk factors (excluding tobacco and microorganisms): critical analysis of old and new hypotheses. *Best Pract Res Clin Gastroenterol.* 2004;18(3):497-508.
6. Korzenik JR. Past and current theories of etiology of IBD: toothpaste, worms, and refrigerators. *J Clin Gastroenterol.* 2005;39(4 suppl 2):S59-S65.
7. Sanders DS. Mucosal integrity and barrier function in the pathogenesis of early lesions in Crohn's disease. *J Clin Pathol.* 2005;58(6):568-572.
8. Munkholm P, Langholz E, Nielsen OH, Kreiner S, Binder V. Incidence and prevalence of Crohn's disease in the county of Copenhagen, 1962-87: a sixfold increase in incidence. *Scand J Gastroenterol.* 1992;27(7):609-614.
9. Ekbom A, Helmick C, Zack M, Adami HO. The epidemiology of inflammatory bowel disease: a large, population-based study in Sweden. *Gastroenterology.* 1991;100(2):350-358.
10. Acheson ED. The distribution of ulcerative colitis and regional enteritis in United States veterans with particular reference to the Jewish religion. *Gut.* 1960;1:291-293.
11. Mayberry JF, Judd D, Smart H, Rhodes J, Calcraft B, Morris JS. Crohn's disease in Jewish people—an epidemiological study in south-east Wales. *Digestion.* 1986;35(4):237-240.
12. Calkins BM, Lilienfeld AM, Garland CF, Mendeloff AI. Trends in incidence rates of ulcerative colitis and Crohn's disease. *Dig Dis Sci.* 1984;29(10):913-920.
13. Roth MP, Petersen GM, McElree C, Feldman E, Rotter JI. Geographic origins of Jewish patients with inflammatory bowel disease. *Gastroenterology.* 1989;97(4):900-904.
14. Sonnenberg A, McCarty DJ, Jacobsen SJ. Geographic variation of inflammatory bowel disease within the United States. *Gastroenterology.* 1991;100(1):143-149.
15. Feller M, Huwiler K, Stephan R, et al. *Mycobacterium avium* subspecies paratuberculosis and Crohn's disease: a systematic review and meta-analysis. *Lancet Infect Dis.* 2007;7(9):607-613.
16. Jones P, Fine P, Piracha S. Crohn's disease and measles. *Lancet.* 1997;349(9050):473.
17. Montgomery SM, Morris DL, Pounder RE, Wakefield AJ. Paramyxovirus infections in childhood and subsequent inflammatory bowel disease. *Gastroenterology.* 1999;116(4):796-803.
18. Porter CK, Tribble DR, Aliaga PA, Halvorson HA, Riddle MS. Infectious gastroenteritis and risk of developing inflammatory bowel disease. *Gastroenterology.* 2008;135(3):781-786.
19. Thompson NP, Montgomery SM, Pounder RE, Wakefield AJ. Is measles vaccination a risk factor for inflammatory bowel disease? *Lancet.* 1995;345(8957):1071-1074.
20. Ananthakrishnan AN, Higuchi LM, Huang ES, et al. Aspirin, nonsteroidal anti-inflammatory drug use, and risk for Crohn disease and ulcerative colitis: a cohort study. *Ann Intern Med.* 2012;156(5):350-359.
21. Card T, Logan RF, Rodrigues LC, Wheeler JG. Antibiotic use and the development of Crohn's disease. *Gut.* 2004;53(2):246-250.
22. Cornish JA, Tan E, Simillis C, Clark SK, Teare J, Tekkis PP. The risk of oral contraceptives in the etiology of inflammatory bowel disease: a meta-analysis. *Am J Gastroenterol.* 2008;103(9):2394-2400.
23. Glassman MS, Newman LJ, Berezin S, Gryboski JD. Cow's milk protein sensitivity during infancy in patients with inflammatory bowel disease. *Am J Gastroenterol.* 1990;85(7):838-840.
24. Persson PG, Ahlbom A, Hellers G. Diet and inflammatory bowel disease: a case-control study. *Epidemiology.* 1992;3(1):47-52.
25. Tragnone A, Valpiani D, Miglio F, et al. Dietary habits as risk factors for inflammatory bowel disease. *Eur J Gastroenterol Hepatol.* 1995;7(1):47-51.
26. Lopez-Serrano P, Perez-Calle JL, Perez-Fernandez MT, Fernández-Font JM, Boixeda de Miguel D, Fernández-Rodríguez CM. Environmental risk factors in inflammatory bowel diseases. Investigating the hygiene hypothesis: a Spanish case-control study. *Scand J Gastroenterol.* 2010;45(12):1464-1471.
27. Calkins BM. A meta-analysis of the role of smoking in inflammatory bowel disease. *Digest Dis Sci.* 1989;34(12):1841-1854.
28. Mahid SS, Minor KS, Soto RE, Hornung CA, Galandiuk S. Smoking and inflammatory bowel disease: a meta-analysis. *Mayo Clin Proc.* 2006;81(11):1462-1471.
29. Tobin MV, Logan RF, Langman MJ, McConnell RB, Gilmore IT. Cigarette smoking and inflammatory bowel disease. *Gastroenterology.* 1987;93(2):316-321.
30. Fielding JF. The relative risk of inflammatory bowel disease among parents and siblings of Crohn's disease patients. *J Clin Gastroenterol.* 1986;8(6):655-657.
31. Laharie D, Debeugny S, Peeters M, et al. Inflammatory bowel disease in spouses and their offspring. *Gastroenterology.* 2001;120(4):816-819.
32. Orholm M, Munkholm P, Langholz E, Nielsen OH, Sørensen TI, Binder V. Familial occurrence of inflammatory bowel disease. *N Engl J Med.* 1991;324(2):84-88.
33. Roth MP, Petersen GM, McElree C, Vadheim CM, Panish JF, Rotter JI. Familial empiric risk estimates of inflammatory bowel disease in Ashkenazi Jews. *Gastroenterology.* 1989;96(4):1016-1020.
34. Hume G, Radford-Smith GL. The pathogenesis of Crohn's disease in the 21st century. *Pathology.* 2002;34(6):561-567.

35. Henckaerts L, Van Steen K, Verstreken I, et al. Genetic risk profiling and prediction of disease course in Crohn's disease patients. *Clin Gastroenterol Hepatol.* 2009;7(9):972-980.e2.

36. Grandbastien B, Peeters M, Franchimont D, et al. Anticipation in familial Crohn's disease. *Gut.* 1998;42(2):170-174.

37. Satsangi J, Grootscholten C, Holt H, Jewell DP. Clinical patterns of familial inflammatory bowel disease. *Gut.* 1996;38(5):738-741.

38. Mizoguchi A, Mizoguchi E. Animal models of IBD: linkage to human disease. *Curr Opin Pharmacol.* 2010;10(5):578-587.

39. Saleh M, Elson CO. Experimental inflammatory bowel disease: insights into the host-microbiota dialog. *Immunity.* 2011;34(3):293-302.

40. Bianco AM, Girardelli M, Tommasini A. Genetics of inflammatory bowel disease from multifactorial to monogenic forms. *World J Gastroenterol.* 2015;21(43):12296-12310.

41. Cleynen I, Vermeire S. The genetic architecture of inflammatory bowel disease: past, present and future. *Curr Opin Gastroenterol.* 2015;31(6):456-463.

42. Gordon H, Trier Moller F, Andersen V, Harbord M. Heritability in inflammatory bowel disease: from the first twin study to genome-wide association studies. *Inflamm Bowel Dis.* 2015;21(6):1428-1434.

43. McGovern DP, Kugathasan S, Cho JH. Genetics of inflammatory bowel diseases. *Gastroenterology.* 2015;149(5):1163-1176.e2.

44. Hampe J, Grebe J, Nikolaus S, et al. Association of NOD2 (CARD 15) genotype with clinical course of Crohn's disease: a cohort study. *Lancet.* 2002;359(9318):1661-1665.

45. McCarroll SA, Huett A, Kuballa P, et al. Deletion polymorphism upstream of IRGM associated with altered IRGM expression and Crohn's disease. *Nat Genet.* 2008;40(9):1107-1112.

46. Duerr RH, Taylor KD, Brant SR, et al. A genome-wide association study identifies IL23R as an inflammatory bowel disease gene. *Science.* 2006;314(5804):1461-1463.

47. Kaser A, Lee AH, Franke A, et al. XBP1 links ER stress to intestinal inflammation and confers genetic risk for human inflammatory bowel disease. *Cell.* 2008;134(5):743-756.

48. Farmer RG, Whelan G, Fazio VW. Long-term follow-up of patients with Crohn's disease. Relationship between the clinical pattern and prognosis. *Gastroenterology.* 1985;88(6):1818-1825.

49. Solberg IC, Vatn MH, Hoie O, et al. Clinical course in Crohn's disease: results of a Norwegian population-based ten-year follow-up study. *Clin Gastroenterol Hepatol.* 2007;5(12):1430-1438.

50. Beaugerie L, Seksik P, Nion-Larmurier I, Gendre JP, Cosnes J. Predictors of Crohn's disease. *Gastroenterology.* 2006;130(3):650-656.

51. Cosnes J, Bourrier A, Nion-Larmurier I, Sokol H, Beaugerie L, Seksik P. Factors affecting outcomes in Crohn's disease over 15 years. *Gut.* 2012;61(8):1140-1145.

52. Lichtenstein GR, Hanauer SB, Sandborn WJ. Management of Crohn's disease in adults. *Am J Gastroenterol.* 2009;104(2):465-483; quiz 464, 484.

53. Loftus EV Jr, Schoenfeld P, Sandborn WJ. The epidemiology and natural history of Crohn's disease in population-based patient cohorts from North America: a systematic review. *Aliment Pharmacol Ther.* 2002;16(1):51-60.

54. Card T, Hubbard R, Logan RF. Mortality in inflammatory bowel disease: a population-based cohort study. *Gastroenterology.* 2003; 125(6):1583-1590.

55. Huppertz-Hauss G, Lie Hoivik M, Jelsness-Jorgensen LP, et al. Health-related quality of life in patients with inflammatory bowel disease 20 years after diagnosis: results from the IBSEN study. *Inflamm Bowel Dis.* 2016;22(7):1679-1687.

56. Zankel E, Rogler G, Andus T, Reng CM, Schölmerich J, Timmer A. Crohn's disease patient characteristics in a tertiary referral center: comparison with patients from a population-based cohort. *Eur J Gastroenterol Hepatol.* 2005;17(4):395-401.

57. Cosnes J, Cattan S, Blain A, et al. Long-term evolution of disease behavior of Crohn's disease. *Inflamm Bowel Dis.* 2002;8(4):244-250.

58. Berg DF, Bahadursingh AM, Kaminski DL, Longo WE. Acute surgical emergencies in inflammatory bowel disease. *Am J Surg.* 2002; 184(1):45-51.

59. Schwartz DA, Pemberton JH, Sandborn WJ. Diagnosis and treatment of perianal fistulas in Crohn disease. *Ann Intern Med.* 2001;135(10): 906-918.

60. Turkcapar N, Toruner M, Soykan I, et al. The prevalence of extraintestinal manifestations and HLA association in patients with inflammatory bowel disease. *Rheumatol Int.* 2006;26(7):663-668.

61. Gasche C, Scholmerich J, Brynskov J, et al. A simple classification of Crohn's disease: report of the Working Party for the World Congresses of Gastroenterology, Vienna 1998. *Inflamm Bowel Dis.* 2000;6(1):8-15.

62. Peeters M, Joossens S, Vermeire S, Vlietinck R, Bossuyt X, Rutgeerts P. Diagnostic value of anti-*Saccharomyces cerevisiae* and antineutrophil cytoplasmic autoantibodies in inflammatory bowel disease. *Am J Gastroenterol.* 2001;96(3):730-734.

63. Mow WS, Vasiliauskas EA, Lin YC, et al. Association of antibody responses to microbial antigens and complications of small bowel Crohn's disease. *Gastroenterology.* 2004;126(2):414-424.

64. Sipponen T. Diagnostics and prognostics of inflammatory bowel disease with fecal neutrophil-derived biomarkers calprotectin and lactoferrin. *Dig Dis.* 2013;31(3-4):336-344.

65. Rutgeerts P, Geboes K, Vantrappen G, Beyls J, Kerremans R, Hiele M. Predictability of the postoperative course of Crohn's disease. *Gastroenterology.* 1990;99(4):956-963.

66. Levesque BG, Cipriano LE, Chang SL, Lee KK, Owens DK, Garber AM. Cost effectiveness of alternative imaging strategies for the diagnosis of small-bowel Crohn's disease. *Clin Gastroenterol Hepatol.* 2010;8(3):261-267, 267.e1-4.

67. Maglinte DD, Kelvin FM, O'Connor K, Lappas JC, Chernish SM. Current status of small bowel radiography. *Abdom Imaging.* 1996; 21(3):247-257.

68. Barlow JM, Goss BC, Hansel SL, et al. CT enterography: technical and interpretive pitfalls. *Abdom Imaging.* 2015;40(5):1081-1096.

69. Bruining DH, Bhatnagar G, Rimola J, Taylor S, Zimmermann EM, Fletcher JG. CT and MR enterography in Crohn's disease: current and future applications. *Abdom Imaging.* 2015;40(5):965-974.

70. Morris MS, Chu DI. Imaging for inflammatory bowel disease. *Surg Clin N Am.* 2015;95(6):1143-1158, v.

71. Yoon K, Chang KT, Lee HJ. MRI for Crohn's disease: present and future. *Biomed Res Int.* 2015;2015:786802.

72. Harvey RF, Bradshaw JM. A simple index of Crohn's-disease activity. *Lancet.* 1980;1(8167):514.

73. Mowat C, Cole A, Windsor A, et al. Guidelines for the management of inflammatory bowel disease in adults. *Gut.* 2011;60(5):571-607.

74. Hanauer SB, Sandborn W. Management of Crohn's disease in adults. *Am J Gastroenterol.* 2001;96(3):635-643.

75. Travis SP, Stange EF, Lemann M, et al. European evidence based consensus on the diagnosis and management of Crohn's disease: current management. *Gut.* 2006;55(suppl 1):i16-i35.

76. Sandborn WJ, Feagan BG, Lichtenstein GR. Medical management of mild to moderate Crohn's disease: evidence-based treatment algorithms for induction and maintenance of remission. *Aliment Pharmacol Therapeut.* 2007;26(7):987-1003.

77. Sutherland L, Singleton J, Sessions J, et al. Double blind, placebo controlled trial of metronidazole in Crohn's disease. *Gut.* 1991;32(9): 1071-1075.

78. Ursing B, Alm T, Barany F, et al. A comparative study of metronidazole and sulfasalazine for active Crohn's disease: the cooperative Crohn's disease study in Sweden. II. Result. *Gastroenterology.* 1982; 83(3):550-562.

79. Arnold GL, Beaves MR, Pryjdun VO, Mook WJ. Preliminary study of ciprofloxacin in active Crohn's disease. *Inflamm Bowel Dis.* 2002; 8(1):10-15.

80. Colombel JF, Lemann M, Cassagnou M, et al. A controlled trial comparing ciprofloxacin with mesalazine for the treatment of active Crohn's disease. Groupe d'Etudes Therapeutiques des Affections Inflammatoires Digestives (GETAID). *Am J Gastroenterol.* 1999;94(3):674-678.

81. Siegel CA, Sands BE. Review article: practical management of inflammatory bowel disease patients taking immunomodulators. *Aliment Pharmacol Ther.* 2005;22(1):1-16.

82. Peyrin-Biroulet L, Deltenre P, de Suray N, Branche J, Sandborn WJ, Colombel JF. Efficacy and safety of tumor necrosis factor antagonists in Crohn's disease: meta-analysis of placebo-controlled trials. *Clin Gastroenterol Hepatol.* 2008;6(6):644-653.

83. Lawson MM, Thomas AG, Akobeng AK. Tumour necrosis factor alpha blocking agents for induction of remission in ulcerative colitis. *Cochrane Database Syst Rev.* 2006;(3):CD005112.

84. Kawalec P, Mikrut A, Wisniewska N, Pilc A. Tumor necrosis factor-alpha antibodies (infliximab, adalimumab and certolizumab) in Crohn's disease: systematic review and meta-analysis. *Arch Med Sci.* 2013;9(5):765-779.

85. Ford AC, Sandborn WJ, Khan KJ, Hanauer SB, Talley NJ, Moayyedi P. Efficacy of biological therapies in inflammatory bowel disease:

systematic review and meta-analysis. *Am J Gastroenterol.* 2011;106(4): 644-659; quiz 60.

86. Sandborn WJ, Gasink C, Gao LL, et al. Ustekinumab induction and maintenance therapy in refractory Crohn's disease. *N Engl J Med.* 2012;367(16):1519-1528.

87. Sandborn WJ, Feagan BG, Rutgeerts P, et al. Vedolizumab as induction and maintenance therapy for Crohn's disease. *N Engl J Med.* 2013;369(8):711-721.

88. Egan LJ, Sandborn WJ. Advances in the treatment of Crohn's disease. *Gastroenterology.* 2004;126(6):1574-1581.

89. Brookes MJ, Green JR. Maintenance of remission in Crohn's disease: current and emerging therapeutic options. *Drugs.* 2004;64(10): 1069-1089.

90. Ford AC, Bernstein CN, Khan KJ, et al. Glucocorticosteroid therapy in inflammatory bowel disease: systematic review and meta-analysis. *Am J Gastroenterol.* 2011;106(4):590-599; quiz 600.

91. Dretzke J, Edlin R, Round J, et al. A systematic review and economic evaluation of the use of tumour necrosis factor-alpha (TNF-alpha) inhibitors, adalimumab and infliximab, for Crohn's disease. *Health Technol Assess.* 2011;15(6):1-244.

92. Evans JP, Steinhart AH, Cohen Z, McLeod RS. Home total parenteral nutrition: an alternative to early surgery for complicated inflammatory bowel disease. *J Gastrointest Surg.* 2003;7(4):562-566.

93. Riordan AM, Hunter JO, Cowan RE, et al. Treatment of active Crohn's disease by exclusion diet: East Anglian multicentre controlled trial. *Lancet.* 1993;342(8880):1131-1134.

94. Akobeng AK, Thomas AG. Enteral nutrition for maintenance of remission in Crohn's disease. *Cochrane Database Syst Rev.* 2007;(3): CD005984.

95. Mekhjian HS, Switz DM, Watts HD, Deren JJ, Katon RM, Beman FM. National Cooperative Crohn's Disease Study: factors determining recurrence of Crohn's disease after surgery. *Gastroenterology.* 1979; 77(4 Pt 2):907-913.

96. Brown CJ, Buie WD. Perioperative stress dose steroids: do they make a difference? *J Am Coll Surg.* 2001;193(6):678-686.

97. Kisielinski K, Conze J, Murken AH, Lenzen NN, Klinge U, Schumpelick V. The Pfannenstiel or so called "bikini cut": still effective more than 100 years after first description. *Hernia.* 2004; 8(3):177-181.

98. Luijendijk RW, Jeekel J, Storm RK, et al. The low transverse Pfannenstiel incision and the prevalence of incisional hernia and nerve entrapment. *Ann Surg.* 1997;225(4):365-369.

99. Hurst RD, Molinari M, Chung TP, Rubin M, Michelassi F. Prospective study of the features, indications, and surgical treatment in 513 consecutive patients affected by Crohn's disease. *Surgery.* 1997;122(4):661-667; discussion 667–668.

100. Lee EC, Papaioannou N. Minimal surgery for chronic obstruction in patients with extensive or universal Crohn's disease. *Ann R Coll Surg Engl.* 1982;64(4):229-233.

101. Roy P, Kumar D. Strictureplasty. *Br J Surg.* 2004;91(11):1428-1437.

102. Michelassi F, Upadhyay GA. Side-to-side isoperistaltic strictureplasty in the treatment of extensive Crohn's disease. *J Surg Res.* 2004;117(1): 71-78.

103. Tichansky D, Cagir B, Yoo E, Marcus SM, Fry RD. Strictureplasty for Crohn's disease: meta-analysis. *Dis Colon Rectum.* 2000;43(7): 911-919.

104. Stocchi L, Milsom JW, Fazio VW. Long-term outcomes of laparoscopic versus open ileocolic resection for Crohn's disease: follow-up of a prospective randomized trial. *Surgery.* 2008;144(4):622-627; discussion 627–628.

105. Schwartz DA, Loftus EV Jr, Tremaine WJ, et al. The natural history of fistulizing Crohn's disease in Olmsted County, Minnesota. *Gastroenterology.* 2002;122(4):875-880.

106. Levy C, Tremaine WJ. Management of internal fistulas in Crohn's disease. *Inflamm Bowel Dis.* 2002;8(2):106-111.

107. Pardi DS, Tremaine WJ, Sandborn WJ, McCarthy JT. Renal and urologic complications of inflammatory bowel disease. *Am J Gastroenterol.* 1998;93(4):504-514.

108. Poritz LS, Gagliano GA, McLeod RS, MacRae H, Cohen Z. Surgical management of entero and colocutaneous fistulae in Crohn's disease: 17 year's experience. *Int J Colorectal Dis.* 2004;19(5):481-485; discussion 486.

109. Jawhari A, Kamm MA, Ong C, Forbes A, Bartram CI, Hawley PR. Intra-abdominal and pelvic abscess in Crohn's disease: results of noninvasive and surgical management. *Br J Surg.* 1998;85(3):367-371.

110. van Hogezand RA, Witte AM, Veenendaal RA, Wagtmans MJ, Lamers CBHW. Proximal Crohn's disease: review of the clinicopathologic features and therapy. *Inflamm Bowel Dis.* 2001;7(4):328-337.

111. Ryan WR, Allan RN, Yamamoto T, Keighley MRB. Crohn's disease patients who quit smoking have a reduced risk of reoperation for recurrence. *Am J Surg.* 2004;187(2):219-225.

112. Yamamoto T. Factors affecting recurrence after surgery for Crohn's disease. *World J Gastroenterol.* 2005;11(26):3971-3979.

113. Qiu Y, Mao R, Chen BL, He Y, Zeng ZR, Chen MH. Systematic review with meta-analysis of prospective studies: anti-tumour necrosis factor for prevention of postoperative Crohn's disease recurrence. *J Crohn's Colitis.* 2015;9(10):918-927.

114. Behm BW, Bickston SJ. Tumor necrosis factor-alpha antibody for maintenance of remission in Crohn's disease. *Cochrane Database Syst Rev.* 2008;(1):CD006893.

115. Garg SK, Loftus EV Jr. Risk of cancer in inflammatory bowel disease: going up, going down, or still the same? *Curr Opin Gastroenterol.* 2016;32(4):274-281.

116. Jauregui-Amezaga A, Vermeire S, Prenen H. Use of biologics and chemotherapy in patients with inflammatory bowel diseases and cancer. *Ann Gastroenterol.* 2016;29(2):127-136.

Gastric, Duodenal, and Small Intestinal Fistulas

Michael S. Nussbaum | David W. McFadden

A fistula is an abnormal communication between two epithelialized surfaces. Over the past half century, the mortality associated with gastrointestinal fistulas has decreased from 40% to 60% to approximately 15% to 20% of patients.[1] This improvement in prognosis is attributable to advances in fluid and electrolyte/acid-base knowledge and therapy, blood administration, critical care, antibiotic regimens, and nutritional management. Formerly, malnutrition and electrolyte imbalance were the major causes of death in affected patients. Currently, mortality is principally attributable to uncontrolled sepsis and its associated malnutrition. Sepsis is responsible for 80% of all deaths in fistula patients.[2]

Spontaneous fistulas account for 15% to 25% of gastrointestinal fistulas and causes include radiation, inflammatory bowel disease, diverticular disease, appendicitis, ischemic bowel, perforation of gastric or duodenal ulcers, pancreatic and gynecologic malignancies, and intestinal actinomycosis or tuberculosis. The majority (75% to 85%) of gastrointestinal fistulas are iatrogenic as a result of technical complications of surgical procedures and trauma. Etiologies include anastomotic dehiscence, intraoperative injury to the bowel or its blood supply, erosion from indwelling tubes, retention sutures or prosthetic mesh, and misplacement of a suture through the bowel during abdominal closure. Other complications that may cause a fistula include intraperitoneal bleeding and abscess formation with or without suture line dehiscence. Fistulas may develop after percutaneous abscess drainage.

The critical tenets in successful management of gastrointestinal fistulas are recognition of the fistula, control of infection and further contamination, restoration of fluid and electrolyte losses, and reestablishment of a positive nutritional balance before undertaking major definitive corrective procedures.

GENERAL PRINCIPLES

Gastrointestinal fistulas are a consequence of perforations that communicate with adjacent organs or intestine (internal fistulas) or externally with the abdominal wall (enterocutaneous fistulas [ECFs]). Enteroatmospheric fistulas are a specific type of ECF that occur in an open abdomen. Several factors make gastrointestinal fistulas complex and potentially lethal. First, the patients are usually systemically ill. Sepsis is a recognized antecedent risk factor for the development of a gastrointestinal fistula, and the high metabolic requirement of the septic state can prevent spontaneous closure. Sepsis is often secondary to the factor leading to the fistula itself. Malnutrition is also common and results both from the hypermetabolic state of the septic, postoperative patient and from the large volume of protein-rich fluid produced and lost through the

fistula. Fluid and electrolyte abnormalities (hypovolemia, hypokalemia, hypomagnesemia, metabolic acidosis) are common and result from the sustained loss of intestinal fluid. Such losses are not limited to ECF because internal fistulas, such as enterocolic fistulas, bypass normal intestinal continuity and may overwhelm the absorptive capacity of the recipient organ. Malabsorption and malnutrition from bacterial overgrowth may occur in gastrocolic or enterocolic fistulas. Local wound excoriation and discomfort from the intestinal effluent can thwart potential abdominal wall reconstruction and recovery after operation to repair a fistula. Finally, operating on a fistula before control of sepsis and nutritional optimization can lead to increased mortality and operative failure.

ETIOLOGY

GASTRIC AND DUODENAL FISTULAS

The majority of gastric and duodenal fistulas occur after surgical, endoscopic, or interventional procedures. Anastomotic or suture line failures account for 80% to 85% of all such fistulas. Before 1950, greater than 60% mortality was observed in patients with gastric and duodenal fistulas, but in the 21st century the incidence has decreased to less than 3% and the mortality rate has decreased to less than 15%.[3] Comparisons of sutured versus stapled anastomoses show no obvious superiority of either. Postoperative leaks from gastric staple or suture lines after ulcer surgery accounted for most perforations in the past. However, the decline in gastric resection for ulcer disease, along with the broad application of new endoscopic and laparoscopic techniques for other diseases, contributes to other newer causes of perforation, albeit at a lower incidence.

Surgical Causes

Any of the available gastric operations for morbid obesity may result in gastric staple line disruption in the early or late postoperative period. Early anastomotic or staple line leaks in this patient population are highly morbid and often lethal. For gastric bypasses, the 10% to 30% incidence rate of internal fistula formation after simple stapling has been reduced to 3% to 6% by either gastric division after stapling or up to three applications of the stapler without division.[4,5]

In a series of 318 partial gastrectomies, Pickleman reported a 1.3% anastomotic leak rate, all from the gastrojejunostomy. After total gastrectomy with Roux-en-Y esophagojejunostomy, anastomotic leaks occurred in 4.8%.[6] A perforation rate of 1.5% has been reported after vertical banded gastroplasty for morbid obesity,[7] and leak rates as high as 6% have been reported after gastric bypass, again from the gastrojejunostomy.[8] The risk of leakage at gastric staple lines may be increased with the use of cautery to control bleeding at the stapled edge, intersecting staple lines within an anastomosis, and the use of a thin tissue stapler on a thickened or edematous gastric wall, which may cause overcompression, tearing, and devascularization. In such tissue a handsewn closure may be preferable.

Duodenal stump leakage has declined because of the decreased use of antrectomy for ulcer disease.[3] Duodenal stump leakage is more common after difficult gastric resections. In a high-risk patient, morbidity and mortality can be decreased and possibly prevented by placement of a duodenostomy tube along with closed suction drains external to the duodenum.

The ongoing extension of laparoscopic techniques to gastric surgery has not eliminated the risk of perforation or fistula formation. The incidence of esophageal or gastric perforation during fundoplication ranges from 0.3% to 1.9%, with a large retrospective review of 2453 procedures by Perdikis et al. showing an overall incidence of 1%.[9] Laparoscopic fundoplication may also result in delayed gastric perforation along the greater curvature from inadvertent thermal or cautery injury during division of the short gastric arteries. If the diaphragmatic crura are not approximated adequately, the fundoplication can herniate into the chest during postoperative straining, vomiting, or heavy lifting, with subsequent gastric ischemia and perforation. Laparoscopic revision of a previous fundoplication requires more gastric traction and division of adhesions, with a 3% risk for gastric laceration.[10] The laparoscopically placed adjustable silicone gastric band, positioned around the proximal part of the stomach for the treatment of morbid obesity, has also resulted in gastric perforation in less than 1% of patients.[11]

Laparoscopic cholecystectomy may produce duodenal injury if the duodenum and gallbladder are densely adherent to one another as a result of either direct cutting action or cautery and thermal injury. Laparoscopic cholecystectomy may also result in colonic injury by the same mechanisms. In addition, improperly insulated instruments may cause electrical arcing to the duodenum, small bowel, or colon with resultant perforation. These injuries are usually apparent within 24 to 72 hours and fistulas are rare.

Endoscopic Causes

The capacity and compliance of the stomach make endoscopic examination routine, with a low incidence of injury. However, endoscopic polypectomy or attempts at tumor removal with a snare, cautery, or endomucosal resection may cause either immediate full-thickness perforation or deep penetration with thermal injury and subsequent delayed perforation and fistula. Percutaneous endoscopic gastrostomy tube placement has also resulted in perforation, either from dislodgement of the tube before complete gastric adhesion to the abdominal wall or from trauma during placement. Tube insertion may perforate the adjacent jejunum or transverse colon and result in a persistent gastrojejunal or gastrocolic fistula, even after the gastrostomy tube has been removed. Gastrostomy tube placement may cause a persistent gastrocutaneous fistula that enlarges through erosion or infection of fascia

and skin. These fistulas may be difficult to control, with continued drainage of gastric fluid onto the surrounding skin. The substitution of a larger gastrostomy tube will not control the leakage and usually results in enlargement of the opening. Persistent drainage may require either tube removal or placement of a smaller tube, along with direct or nasogastric suction until the tract contracts down around the tube. Surgical closure is required for a persistent gastrocutaneous fistula that does not respond to such measures. Endoscopic clipping of the gastric opening has been described and is effective in a select group of affected patients.[12]

Because many endoscopic duodenal procedures involve the second portion of the duodenum, perforation is usually retroperitoneal. Failure to recognize an injury or a delay in treatment markedly increases morbidity and mortality. Perforation after endoscopic retrograde cholangiopancreatography (ERCP) with ampullary sphincterotomy for stone extraction or biliary stent placement is one of the more frequent postendoscopic indications for urgent surgical intervention. Repair of the distal bile duct, as well as repair of the duodenum, may be required. Controlled leaks confined to the retroperitoneum can often be monitored with very close clinical observation in stable patients. Retroperitoneal perforation is more common during therapeutic ERCP, with an incidence of 0.6% to 1.8% and a mortality rate of up to 25%.[12] Delayed duodenal perforation from the biliary stent itself may be caused by partial extrusion and impingement of the end of the stent on the distal second or proximal third portion of the duodenum, with eventual erosion and perforation. Proximal stent migration into the common bile duct may cause a choledochoduodenal fistula to subsequently form if the stent reenters the duodenum away from the papilla. Similarly, pancreatic duct stents may produce a pancreaticogastric fistula with proximal migration of the stent into the gastric antrum. Other procedures at risk for the development of duodenal perforation include endoscopic polyp or tumor removal, push enteroscopy, endoscopic ultrasound with transduodenal biopsy, and endoscopically assisted transgastric jejunal feeding tube placement.

Inflammatory Causes

Crohn disease is a rare cause of gastrocolic, duodenocolic, or duodenocutaneous fistulas. Primary gastric or duodenal involvement is reported in less than 1% of patients with Crohn disease; duodenocutaneous fistulas may develop from the first or second portion of the duodenum. However, most gastric or duodenal fistulas are internal and result from involvement of primary Crohn disease of the transverse colon or, more commonly, from recurrence at the ileocolic anastomosis after previous resection. Those with gastrocolic fistulas have a 40% incidence of vomiting, which may be feculent; duodenocolic fistulas are often asymptomatic, with only a 4% incidence of vomiting, which is not usually feculent.[13]

Neoplastic causes of internal fistulas are uncommon. Gastrocolic fistulas have resulted from gastric ulcer erosion and invasion of the transverse colon by gastric adenocarcinoma or lymphoma. In rare instances, primary hepatic flexure or transverse colon adenocarcinoma may invade and create a fistula to the duodenum or stomach.[14,15]

SMALL INTESTINAL FISTULA

Small intestinal fistulas can arise in a number of ways. The small intestine's length, as well as its elaborate anatomy, predisposes it to association in a variety of diseases. Any surgical procedure involving the abdomen can result in iatrogenic injury to the small intestine and later fistula formation. The development of a fistula between the small intestine and an internal structure can be a life-threatening event, as with exsanguination from an aortoenteric fistula. Other fistulas, particularly enteroenteric fistulas may be asymptomatic. External small intestinal fistulas (enterocutaneous fistulas, or ECFs) are the most prevalent of small intestinal fistula. ECFs most commonly follow postoperative complications and are often the result of technical errors at the time of an abdominal procedure. ECF mandates careful management to avoid further complicating the well-being of the patient.[1,2] Of 35 fistulas originating in the jejunum or ileum reported in one study, 75% drained externally.[16] The ileum is the most common site of origin of an ECF.[1] ECF can be classified according to the daily volume of drainage. A high-output fistula drains 500 mL/day or more of fluid. In general, a high-output fistula is associated with greater morbidity and mortality. Polk et al. found that patients with high-output fistulas had a greater incidence of malnutrition and fluid and electrolyte disturbances.[2] Mortality was increased, and the rate of fistula closure was low. In contrast, excellent results with high-output fistulas were reported in Graham's series in which 35 of 39 consecutive patients underwent spontaneous fistula closure with a 3% mortality rate.[17] High-output fistulas usually originate from a proximal portion of the small intestine. Independent conditions, such as previous intestinal irradiation, intraabdominal sepsis, or the presence of diseased or ischemic intestine, can also cause external fistulas. Enteroenteric or enterocolic fistulas develop almost exclusively from the transmural inflammation associated with Crohn disease.

Webster and Carey proposed five general mechanisms for small intestinal fistula formation[16]:

1. **Congenital**. A rare form of congenital small bowel fistula involves failure of the vitellointestinal duct to obliterate, resulting in an ECF to the umbilicus. The diagnosis should be suggested by the appearance of fecal material at the umbilicus after postnatal slough of the umbilical cord.

2. **Trauma**. Traumatic injury to the small intestine that results in fistula formation usually occurs from an internal source, such as a swallowed fish bone, toothpick, magnet, or metallic object. Erosion of these objects into an adjacent loop of small intestine results in an internal enteroenteric fistula. Major penetrating trauma without damage-control laparotomy rarely results in fistula formation because these cases are explored surgically and the intestinal injuries repaired. Patients treated with damage-control laparotomy techniques have an increased risk for delayed formation of intestinal fistulas caused by prolonged exposure and desiccation of multiple intestinal loops.[18]

3. **Infection**. An abscess or invasive intestinal infection may erode through the intestine and create a fistula. Amebiasis, tuberculosis, coccidioidomycosis, actinomycosis, and salmonellosis may cause intestinal fistulas. Intestinal perforation at the ileum from tuberculosis and typhoid fever is still occasionally seen in the Third World. *Actinomyces* is a rare cause of after appendectomy.

4. **Perforation or Injury with Abscess**. Perforation of the intestinal wall by tumor, inflammation, or operative injury may result in the local formation of an abscess. A fistula may develop if this abscess subsequently erodes into an adjacent structure. An ECF rarely develops spontaneously—most develop after an abdominal operation. Most ECFs develop as a result of injury to the small intestine during surgery. They also arise from exposure of the bowel to an abdominal defect or prosthetic mesh used to repair such defects. Abdominal wall dehiscence with evisceration and strangulation of a hernia with infarction and perforation have been implicated in the development of external fistulas. In most large series, 60% to 90% of ECFs were caused by operative complications.[12] In addition, ECFs are caused by leakage from an intestinal anastomosis or enterotomy closure. Fistulas may also develop as a result of percutaneous drainage of an intraabdominal abscess.

5. **Inflammation, Irradiation, or Tumor**. The small intestine and an adjacent structure can become densely adherent from chronic inflammatory conditions, abdominal radiation injury, or tumor erosion. Subsequent degeneration of the common wall results in fistula formation. Inflammatory bowel disease, particularly Crohn disease, is well known to create fistulas in this fashion. In Crohn disease the disease makes fistula formation after anastomosis more likely. Although a spontaneous external fistula can develop as a direct result of Crohn disease, most occur only after a previous operation has caused the affected intestine to adhere to the abdominal wall. Postoperative fistulas in the setting of Crohn disease are as likely to develop after simple exploration, bypass, or appendectomy as after primary resection. Fistula formation after laparotomy is usually an early complication, especially when arising from an anastomosis, whereas a late fistula generally indicates recurrent Crohn disease. Fistula formation is particularly apt to occur after irradiation of a pelvic malignant lesion. Fistulas that arise secondary to radiation injury rarely, if ever, close spontaneously. Laparoscopy has been found to decrease the incidence of fistula in Crohn disease.[19]

DIAGNOSIS OF PERFORATIONS AND FISTULAS

Acute intraoperative perforations are best handled by maintaining a strong index of suspicion for technical errors, recognizing the injury before the end of the procedure, and immediately repairing, suturing, or reinforcing weakened tissues. The tendency for potential injuries must be recognized and overcome, especially during prolonged laparoscopic cases. Serosal injuries should be carefully examined. Intraluminal instillation of methylene blue and saline or direct endoscopic examination can demonstrate a small perforation or provide reassurance that an area of concern is not a full-thickness injury. During repeat laparotomy for an open abdomen secondary to damage-control laparotomy, the urge to break up interloop adhesions to search for interloop abscesses and reaffirm "normal" small intestinal anatomy should be suppressed because the dense inflammation between the viscera leads to the development of serosal injuries and possible future fistulas.[20]

Postoperatively, unrecognized perforations or leaks that develop at suture or staple lines are manifested as instability or failure to improve as expected. A gastrointestinal fistula can be obvious in some patients and extremely difficult to identify in others. Fistula formation is frequently heralded by fever and abdominal pain until gastrointestinal contents discharge through an abdominal incision. Spontaneous fistulas from neoplasm or inflammatory disease usually develop in a more indolent manner. ECFs often have intestinal contents or gas exiting from a drain site or through the abdominal incision after an operation. The drainage fluid is usually typical of intestinal contents, with obvious bile staining, and intestinal gas may accompany the effluent. At times the initial fistula drainage may appear clear rather than yellow or green, and the fistula may be misdiagnosed as a seroma or wound infection. At other times a heavy purulent component may also mask the enteric communication and instead suggest a wound infection. If the drainage persists and the diagnosis is uncertain, the patient may be given activated charcoal or indigo carmine by mouth and the drainage inspected for these substances.

STAGING AND CLASSIFICATION

Gastrointestinal fistulas are classified by their anatomic characteristics and are either internal or external (enterocutaneous). Typically the name of a fistula is derived from the involved and connected organs or structures. Examples include gastrocolic, jejunoileal, and aortoenteric fistulas. The anatomy of a fistula will suggest the cause and help to predict whether spontaneous closure will occur. Fistulas can be classified physiologically in terms of output over a 24-hour period. They can be classified as low (<200 mL/day), moderate (200 to 500 mL/day), and high (>500 mL/day).[2] An accurate measure of fistula output, as well as the chemical makeup of the effluent, assists in preventing and treating metabolic deficits and correcting ongoing fluid, electrolyte, and protein losses. The anatomic and etiologic factors are more important in predicting spontaneous closure than the actual output of the fistula. The underlying disease process helps to forecast both the closure rate and mortality.

ECFs are the most common type of small intestinal fistula and are usually recognizable. In contrast, internal fistulas that communicate between the intestine and another hollow viscus may not be suspected for some time because the symptoms may be minimal or mimic the underlying disease process.

COMPLICATIONS

FLUID AND ELECTROLYTE ABNORMALITIES

Fluid and electrolyte disturbances occur commonly in patients with ECFs. The salivary glands, stomach, duodenum, pancreas, liver, and small intestine secrete 8 to 10 L/day of a fluid rich in sodium, potassium, chloride, and bicarbonate. The degree of volume loss and electrolyte imbalance depends on the anatomic location of the fistula and may exceed 3000 mL/day.[2] Duodenal fistulas are particularly prone to volume and electrolyte loss.[3] High-output duodenal or jejunal fistulas continue to carry a mortality rate of approximately 35%.[2] A distal fistula, such as one arising from the terminal ileum in a patient with Crohn disease, is associated with smaller fluid losses because of proximal absorption.

The most common abnormalities seen are hypovolemia, hypokalemia, and metabolic acidosis. Hypokalemia occurs primarily from potassium loss in the fistula effluent; hypovolemia contributes by causing renal retention of sodium in exchange for potassium secretion. Sepsis contributes to the hypovolemic state by raising the metabolic rate and increasing insensible water loss. Metabolic acidosis results from the loss of pancreatic juice rich in bicarbonate and is more common with proximal fistulas. Gastric fistulas may cause a hypokalemic, hypochloremic metabolic alkalosis secondary to the loss of a large volume of hydrochloric acid.

Patients with fistulas causing fluid and electrolyte abnormalities have a higher mortality rate. Advances in critical care, invasive monitoring, and aggressive fluid and electrolyte management can reduce this early mortality considerably, as evidenced by data from the Massachusetts General Hospital.[2,21]

MALNUTRITION

The small intestine contains fluid replete with ingested nutrients and endogenous proteins, such as enzymes and albumin. Protein–calorie malnutrition and mineral and micronutrient depletion develop in almost all patients with a small intestinal fistula when an extensive absorptive surface is bypassed or enteric contents are lost externally. Loss of luminal nutrients has a large effect on gut growth and function. Luminal nutrients improve mucosal cell sloughing and provide local nutrition to the enterocytes. Nutrients in the gut lumen also have trophic effects, such as increasing gastrointestinal hormone and growth factor release that then stimulate the paracrine, endocrine, and autocrine effects of the growth factors. Indirect effects of intraluminal nutrients include increasing motility and gastrointestinal secretions. Magnesium, selenium, and zinc depletion are common in patients with high-output fistulas and should be monitored. Nutritional deficiencies are worsened by the increased metabolic demands of sepsis or additional surgery. Before the introduction of total parenteral nutrition (TPN), 74% of patients with intestinal fistulas exhibited malnutrition, and 59% of these patients died.

SEPSIS

With advances in fluid and electrolyte replacement and nutritional support, sepsis is currently the major determinant of mortality in fistula patients. Abscesses can cause and complicate fistulas. Abdominal sepsis may lead to bacteremia, local and distant infection, and multisystem organ failure. Local extension often results in wound infection and abdominal wall defects predispose the patient to additional sepsis episodes and a high mortality rate. In a large series by Schein and Decker, the fistula mortality rate associated with sepsis doubled to 60%[22] when a large abdominal wall defect was present.

ABDOMINAL WALL AND WOUND ABNORMALITIES

Skin erosion and excoriation commonly result from an ECF. The digestive effects of the gastrointestinal secretions, particularly pancreatic enzymes, result in considerable patient discomfort. The magnitude of the local skin excoriation depends on the output and contents of the effluent and is most severe with proximal intestinal fistulas. Malnutrition aggravates this process by delaying the formation of granulation tissue and scar. Those fistulas that occur in large open abdominal wall defects are particularly difficult to control because the effluent soils the entire gut surface. Use of novel therapies to isolate these enteroatmospheric fistulas from the neighboring granulating loops of bowel, such as the use of ostomy appliances, DuoDERM (ConvaTec, Bridgewater, New Jersey), paste, and hemivacuum therapies, are valuable.[20] Isolation of the fistula may require coverage of the remaining wound with a split-thickness skin graft allowing expeditious correction of nutritional, fluid, and electrolyte deficits.[23]

OTHER COMPLICATIONS

Other complications of small intestinal fistulas occur less frequently. Gastrointestinal hemorrhage can result from the formation of a fistula between the small intestine and a blood vessel. One or more "herald bleeds" may precede hemorrhage. More commonly, anemia develops chronically and is associated with slow blood loss from a friable fistula tract. Colonization and small intestine overgrowth by colonic bacteria can occur with enterocolic fistulas and result in malabsorption and severe, malodorous diarrhea. Distal obstruction beyond the fistula tract from adhesions or other disease can develop and result in an increase in fistula output or failure of the proximal tract to close. Finally, carcinoma has been reported in chronic fistulas, especially those associated with Crohn disease.

MANAGEMENT

Management of a gastrointestinal fistula is a difficult and complex process. However, a systematic approach can lead to treatment that is effective and potentially rewarding. In general, management can be compartmentalized into five stages: stabilization, investigation, decision, definitive therapy, and healing.[1,24]

The goal when treating gastrointestinal fistulas is to restore continuity of the gastrointestinal tract. However, fistulas usually are not treated simply by a return to the operating room. Instead, many weeks and perhaps months of care are often required. Management can be seen as a series of steps to control life-threatening abnormalities rapidly and then to intervene in a timely and controlled manner with convalescent or surgical care. Although these steps address the physical well-being of the patient, one should not undervalue the impact of a fistula on mental and emotional health. A gastrointestinal fistula puts a great deal of stress on a patient's self-esteem. Therefore family members, social workers, and mental health professionals play salient roles during the prolonged convalescence that is typical with this disease process.

STABILIZATION

The first step in the management of an intestinal fistula is stabilization of the patient within the first 24 to 48 hours. These patients are often in a vulnerable state of health. They may be febrile and septic from a presumed wound infection treated by opening the wound. Alternatively, they may be immunocompromised secondary to ongoing therapy (e.g., steroids, cancer radiation treatment, chemotherapy) or additional infectious processes. Therefore the most important priority is to resuscitate and stabilize the patient. Patients require correction of obligate third-space losses, as well as emesis, fistula output, and urine output. Initial efforts should be directed toward intravenous fluid resuscitation, control of infection, ongoing measurement of fistula and urine output, and protection of the surrounding skin. The incision should be examined for fascial integrity, and any subcutaneous collections should be drained. Only after these steps are addressed should attention be shifted to identification of the fistulous source, the nature of the tract, and associated fluid collections or abscesses.

Resuscitation

Restoration of a normal circulating blood volume and correction of electrolyte and acid-base imbalances are a priority. Rehydration usually requires isotonic fluid until the patient is euvolemic. High-output fistulas, greater than 500 mL/day, continue to have the highest mortality rate, up to 35%.[2] Moderate- and low-output fistulas are associated with low mortality rates and higher spontaneous closure rates. Small bowel, pancreatic, and biliary losses are isotonic. Colonic losses may be hypotonic, and gastric fistulas may be associated with the classic hypokalemic, hypochloremic metabolic alkalosis. Although certain patterns can be predicted, electrolyte levels in an aliquot of the fistula output, as well as electrolyte levels in the patient's serum, should be measured. Because most patients require considerable volume replacement, close monitoring is essential to ensure the safety and efficacy of therapy.

Initial management should address any existing hypovolemia, anemia, hypoalbuminemia; electrolyte depletion; bile salt losses; and acid-base disorders. Strict intake and output measurements, central venous pressure monitoring, and urinary catheterization are especially helpful with high-output fistulas. The patient's urine output should be restored to greater than 0.5 mL/kg per hour, assuming that renal function is normal. In patients with cardiovascular impairment or evidence of shock, a pulmonary artery catheter may guide ongoing fluid repletion.

Potassium, calcium, phosphorus, and magnesium deficits should be corrected. These electrolyte deficits take time to correct because the measured serum levels incompletely reflect the massive depletion of intracellular ions. Sodium bicarbonate administration may be required to correct the metabolic acidosis that develops with a high-output or proximal fistula. Because the deficit in circulating blood volume is caused by extracellular fluid losses, replacement should be in the form of an isotonic solution. Normal saline or lactated Ringer solution is preferred. However, specific parenteral fluids may be selected on the basis of the initial electrolyte levels. Transfusion may be necessary. There is no specific hemoglobin or hematocrit level that requires transfusion; rather, transfusion should be based on the patient's overall hemodynamic status, oxygen-carrying capacity, and oxygen delivery.

Often, these patients are in a severe catabolic state and have very low protein and albumin levels. This is important for several reasons. First, patients will have low capillary oncotic pressure, which may contribute to profound edema, especially after resuscitation has begun. Severe hypoalbuminemia will take weeks to correct. Short-term supplemental intravenous salt-poor albumin administration will help to increase oncotic pressure and minimize edema and may improve wound healing.[25] However, more importantly, the patient is in a state of nutritional emergency. For this patient to be stabilized and to potentially heal the fistula, positive nitrogen balance must be achieved.

Nutrition

Ongoing nutritional assessment and institution of nutritional support have improved the overall outcome in patients with small intestinal fistulas. The study in 1964 by Chapman et al. emphasized that the key to successful management was to "get control of fistula," combat sepsis, and from the very beginning maintain adequate nutritional support.[26] They reported a decreased mortality rate of 14% from 55% in patients treated with an excess of 3000 calories per day via a combination of intravenous (peripheral administration of protein hydrolysates) and tube feedings. In 1971 Sheldon et al. documented the success of such a treatment regimen and noted that most patients could be given adequate nutrition by standard methods, such as tube and enterostomy feedings.[27] Roback and Nicholoff reported closure of 73% of enteric fistulas in patients with adequate caloric supplementation, versus 19% when nutritional support was inadequate.[28]

With the widespread advent of parenteral nutrition in the 1970s, the overall reduction in mortality to a range of 15% to 20% was achieved consistently in a variety of reports, while improving the spontaneous closure rate. However, parenteral nutrition had no impact on fistula mortality; maintenance of adequate nutrition with more conventional methods was equally effective.[1,2] Despite aggressive nutritional support, malnutrition continues to be a major clinical problem in 55% to 90% of patients.[1] Parenteral nutrition has greatly simplified the nutritional management of patients with gastrointestinal fistulas. Even though these patients often have abdominal abscesses and bacteremia, parenteral nutrition is safe and the overall incidence of catheter-related septic complications is no greater than that in other clinical situations.[21]

It is advised to begin nutritional support as soon as the patient is stabilized. Full caloric and nitrogen replacement can be provided within a few days.[25] Nutrition can be given by several routes. Usually, either enteral tube feeding or parenteral nutrition will be required. The choice depends on the fistula anatomy. It is better to provide at least a portion of the calories through the enteral route as the gastrointestinal tract is a much more efficacious way of providing nutrition, maintaining the intestinal mucosal barrier and immunologic integrity and stimulating hepatic protein synthesis.[29] Thus, whenever possible, enteral nutrition is preferable to parenteral nutrition and may decrease the incidence of multisystem organ failure and sepsis if administered appropriately.[30]

The principles for reduction of fistula output are similar to those used in the management of short bowel syndrome. When oral intake is possible, intake of hypotonic fluids should be restricted and electrolyte solution containing high concentrations of both sodium and glucose, such as the World Health Organization's oral rehydration solution, substituted. This solution contains 40 g/L of glucose, 90 mEq/L of sodium, and 20 mEq/L potassium and has an osmolality of 311 mOsm. In patients with proximal fistulas the intake of hypotonic fluids such as water will make effluent increase, worsening dehydration and electrolyte imbalances. The use of an optimal oral rehydration solution may facilitate the use of the oral route in patients desirous of oral intake.

However, enteral nutrition is not without complications, and the process should be monitored closely. Complications such as diarrhea, aspiration, and bowel ischemia are not uncommon without careful clinical monitoring. Enteral nutrition can be given for upper gastrointestinal fistulas, especially when the feeding tube can be placed beyond the fistula (e.g., a feeding tube placed beyond the ligament of Treitz for a gastric, duodenal, or pancreatic fistula). In general, feeding tubes should be placed beyond the ligament of Treitz to decrease the potential risk for aspiration. If at least four feet of functional bowel exists between the ligament of Treitz and the external site of the fistula, enteral feedings of highly absorbable, low-residue nutrients should be administered. The initial volume and concentration administered may be low and then subsequently increased over several days to full strength as tolerated. During the time the enteral nutrition is increasing the patient should be supplemented with TPN. In the face of a proximal fistula, if the intestine distal to the fistula can be intubated, enteral nutrition can be instituted (fistuloclysis).[31,32] Enteral feeding should also be used for distal fistulas (e.g., a colonic fistula), as long as feedings do not significantly increase fistula output. Parenteral nutrition can be a valuable tool in the long-term treatment of fistulas as well. Patients with small bowel fistulas may not be able to tolerate enteral nutrition without increasing fistula output. In these cases and in others in which patients cannot tolerate enteral feeding, parenteral nutrition is indicated. In patients with a persistent adynamic ileus and before the fistula tract is well established, parenteral nutrition is very useful. Parenteral nutrition techniques and advantages are well known, although complications occur in almost one-third of patients.[31]

The presence of a gastric or duodenal fistula will not usually permit oral alimentation, unless it is of low output and eating does not markedly worsen losses. If a feeding tube beyond the ligament of Treitz or a tube jejunostomy is in place, enteral nutrition should be started; with normal small and large intestinal function, all nutritional needs can be met. Those with low-output fistulas require 30 to 35 kcal/kg per day, with 1 to 2 g protein per kilogram body weight per day. Those with high-output fistulas require more calories—up to 1.5

to 2 times normal energy expenditure, with a protein supply of 1.5 to 2.5 g/kg per day.[25] This is especially the case with duodenal fistulas because of the loss of gastric, duodenal, biliary, and pancreatic exocrine protein-rich secretions. Short-turnover protein (prealbumin, retinol-binding protein, transferrin) levels should be measured at least weekly to assess the adequacy of protein delivery. Serum C-reactive protein (CRP) has been shown to be a predictor of success.[33] An ongoing catabolic state will adversely affect short-turnover protein levels, even with maximal protein delivery. Those with high-output fistulas may benefit from twice the recommended daily allowance of vitamins, trace elements, and zinc and up to 10 times the daily requirement for vitamin C.[25] The daily delivered volume should include both maintenance fluids and ongoing fistulous losses.

Historically, high output from a fistula was a relative contraindication to enteral nutrition. However, both human and animal data suggest that even these complicated fistulas can be adequately managed with enteral nutrition, although the parenteral route may still succeed in further reducing fistula output. Enteral nutrition, both orally and by tube feeding,[32] has been used increasingly when treating small intestinal fistulas because of its trophic effect on the intestine. The overall success with nutritional supplementation by the enteric route rivals that of parenteral nutrition. Indications for enteral supplementation depend on the site of the fistula and the extent of the remaining small intestine that can be used for absorption. As little as 20% to 25% of the nutrition supplied enterally is usually sufficient to provide the advantages of enteral nutrition, and the remainder can be supplied via parenteral nutrition.[31] Contrariwise, the decreased fistula output that accompanies parenteral nutrition can simplify the management of high-output fistulas. In addition to this adjunctive role with parenteral nutrition, tube feeding continues to be an important measure in the complete nutritional management of some fistula patients with distal and low-output fistulas, when the fistulas are nearly healed, or when parenteral nutrition is difficult or impossible to institute.

Because both enteric and parenteral feeding have advantages and disadvantages, the source of nutritional supplementation should depend on the individual patient and the surgeon's preference and experience. In most cases, parenteral nutrition should be instituted as soon as possible. Thereafter, steps are taken to localize the fistula and control infection. Normal intestinal motility and function generally return once abdominal sepsis is controlled and fluid and electrolyte imbalances are corrected. If the fistula location is such that enteric access and alimentation are possible, enteral nutrition can be instituted and parenteral nutrition phased out. By using a combination of approaches, adequate nutrition can be maintained throughout the patient's course.

Control of Sepsis (and Control of Fistula Effluent)

Uncontrolled sepsis remains the major factor contributing to mortality in patients with small intestinal fistulas. Aggressive management of ongoing infections and careful surveillance for new septic foci are necessary for successful management. Tachycardia, persistent fever, and leukocytosis predict inadequate control of the fistula or abscess formation. Frequent physical examination and judicious use of ultrasonography and computed tomography (CT) are mandatory.

Malnutrition in the presence of uncontrolled sepsis cannot be treated without effective drainage of the septic source. The stabilization phase often involves control of a septic source. Typically, drainage of an intraabdominal abscess is required, which is ideally accomplished in an image-guided, percutaneous fashion. In addition, fistula drainage must be controlled and the skin of the abdominal wall protected. Local control is an extremely important component of the early management of a fistula. Discontinuation of oral intake and initiation of parenteral nutrition are important first steps. Suction aspiration via placement of a nasogastric tube or a nasoenteric tube positioned proximal to the fistula may be helpful with enteric fistulas involving the duodenum or proximal jejunum. Egress of the fistula output from the abdominal cavity must be facilitated with an immature ECF as inadequate external drainage results in internal loculation, abscess formation, or peritonitis. It is important to prevent the severe local skin excoriation that develops around the site of an ECF. Fistulas that have been controlled with a tube should cause minimal injury to fascia, subcutaneous tissue, and skin. Such injuries typically include perforations with abscesses that have been percutaneously drained or have been converted at surgery to a controlled fistula with an indwelling tube or an adjacent drain.

Drainage should be collected to measure the output and provide guidance for fluid and electrolyte replacement. The method of controlling fistula drainage is individualized. Precautionary steps should be instituted early because once excoriation is present, healing is difficult in the presence of ongoing drainage. A fistula should be exteriorized on a flat portion of the abdominal wall with avoidance of bony prominences and skin folds. This permits secure application of an ostomy bag or other device to collect and monitor fluids and protect the skin. Specialized nursing assistance by an enterostomal therapist or wound care specialist is necessary in the management of these complex wounds. Drainage with a single catheter placed into the site generally fails because the catheter becomes occluded or the volume of fluid expelled with peristalsis exceeds the capacity of the catheter. In some instances, a sump suction catheter can be placed through the external opening and gentle continuous suction applied to control fistula drainage.[1] One useful modification of fistula wound management was described by Suripaya and Anderson (Fig. 76.1). A disposable ileostomy bag with adhesive backing is fitted to the fistula site.[34] The opening in the ileostomy bag is cut to fit the fistula as exactly as possible. Two 18-French or larger catheters with multiple side perforations are tied together and passed into the fistula through the open end of the bag. All perforations are placed within the fistula below skin level. A third 18-French catheter with multiple perforations is placed in the ileostomy bag, and the open end of the bag is tied securely around all three catheters. One of the two catheters within the fistula and the catheter lying free in the bag are set for continuous suction at a minimum of 40 mm Hg of negative pressure. The adjacent catheter

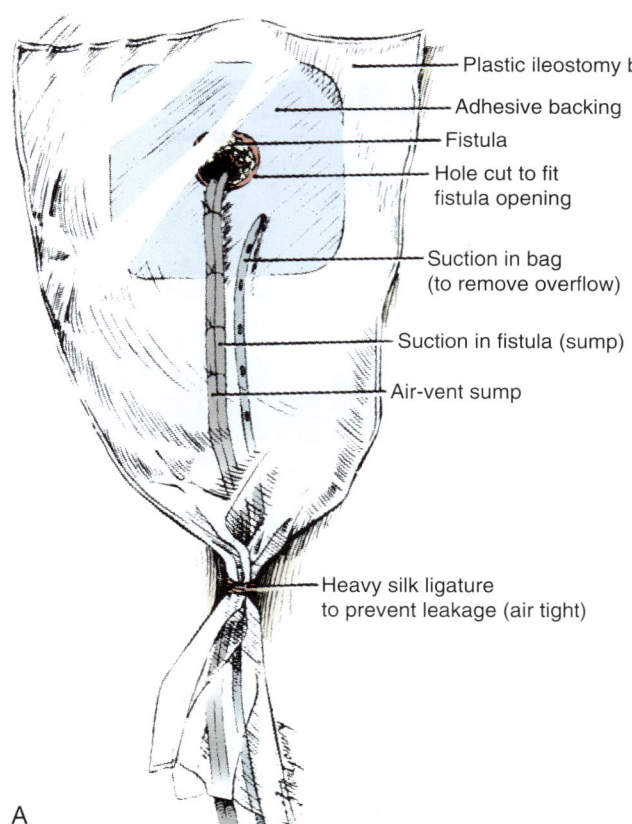

- Plastic ileostomy bag
- Adhesive backing
- Fistula
- Hole cut to fit fistula opening
- Suction in bag (to remove overflow)
- Suction in fistula (sump)
- Air-vent sump
- Heavy silk ligature to prevent leakage (air tight)

A

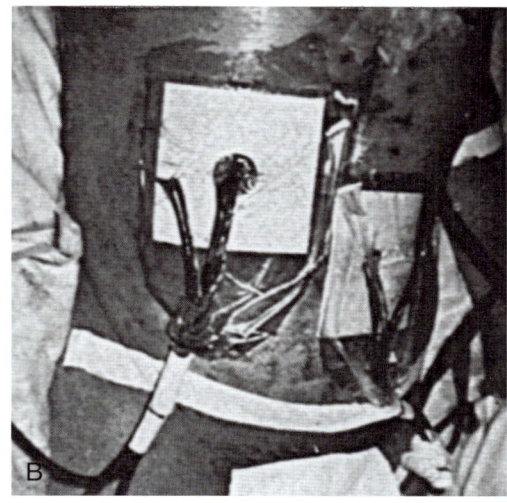

B

FIGURE 76.1 Enterocutaneous fistula drainage device. (A) Components of the suction device. (B) Bag collapsed by negative suction. (From Suriyapa C, Anderson MC. A simple device to control drainage from enterocutaneous fistulas. *Surgery.* 1971;70:456.)

in the fistula serves as an air vent. When functioning, the bag is completely collapsed, and fluid leaking from the tract is immediately aspirated away. The surrounding skin can be protected with Stomahesive paste, karaya gum powder, aluminum paste, tincture of benzoin, or zinc oxide/menthol cream.

Alternatively, a wound vacuum (vacuum-assisted closure [VAC] device) drainage system works very well to control fistula drainage and protect the skin (Fig. 76.2). With negative pressure application to the wound, the VAC apparatus allows for excellent control of drainage, minimizes the size of the abdominal wound, simplifies management by decreasing the frequency of dressing changes, and may actually promote healing of the fistula.[23] By simplifying wound care and control of output, patients can be discharged sooner and the VAC can be managed in a home care or extended care setting. For many ECFs, this has become our method of choice for controlling fistula drainage and protecting the surrounding skin.

Once intraabdominal sepsis is present, the use of antibiotics does not eliminate the need for surgical treatment or percutaneous drainage. Adequate drainage of an abscess must be accomplished. If possible, general anesthesia and major surgical procedures should be avoided or postponed until the patient is stabilized. Ultrasound and CT are most often used to search for peritonitis or an intraabdominal abscess. These two modalities localize

such processes and permit image-guided percutaneous drainage, an invaluable procedure in a critically ill patient who may not tolerate an operative procedure (Fig. 76.3). Abdominal exploration may be required in septic patients who are losing ground, even if diagnostic studies have not pinpointed an abscess. In the rare case that exploratory laparotomy is required for drainage, one should avoid the temptation of definitive repair of the fistula, as it is prone to failure. In addition, such failure may make subsequent attempts more difficult and possibly result in infection of previously uninvolved areas of the abdomen. Control of the fistula should be established during the operation by allowing complete drainage to the skin surface or by exteriorizing the fistula.

The fistula effluent should be cultured for both bacteria and fungi. Sputum, urine, wound, and blood cultures, including those from central venous lines, should also be obtained. Wound or drain site collections should be evacuated. The wound should be débrided of all grossly infected and necrotic tissue. Culture results and the patient's systemic response should modify subsequent antibiotic therapy, particularly if *Enterococcus,* resistant gram-negative bacteria, or fungus is cultured.

After sepsis is controlled, parenteral/enteral nutrition should result in improved nutritional status, allow skin lesions to heal, and the future operative field to become quiescent. Early operative intervention in the presence

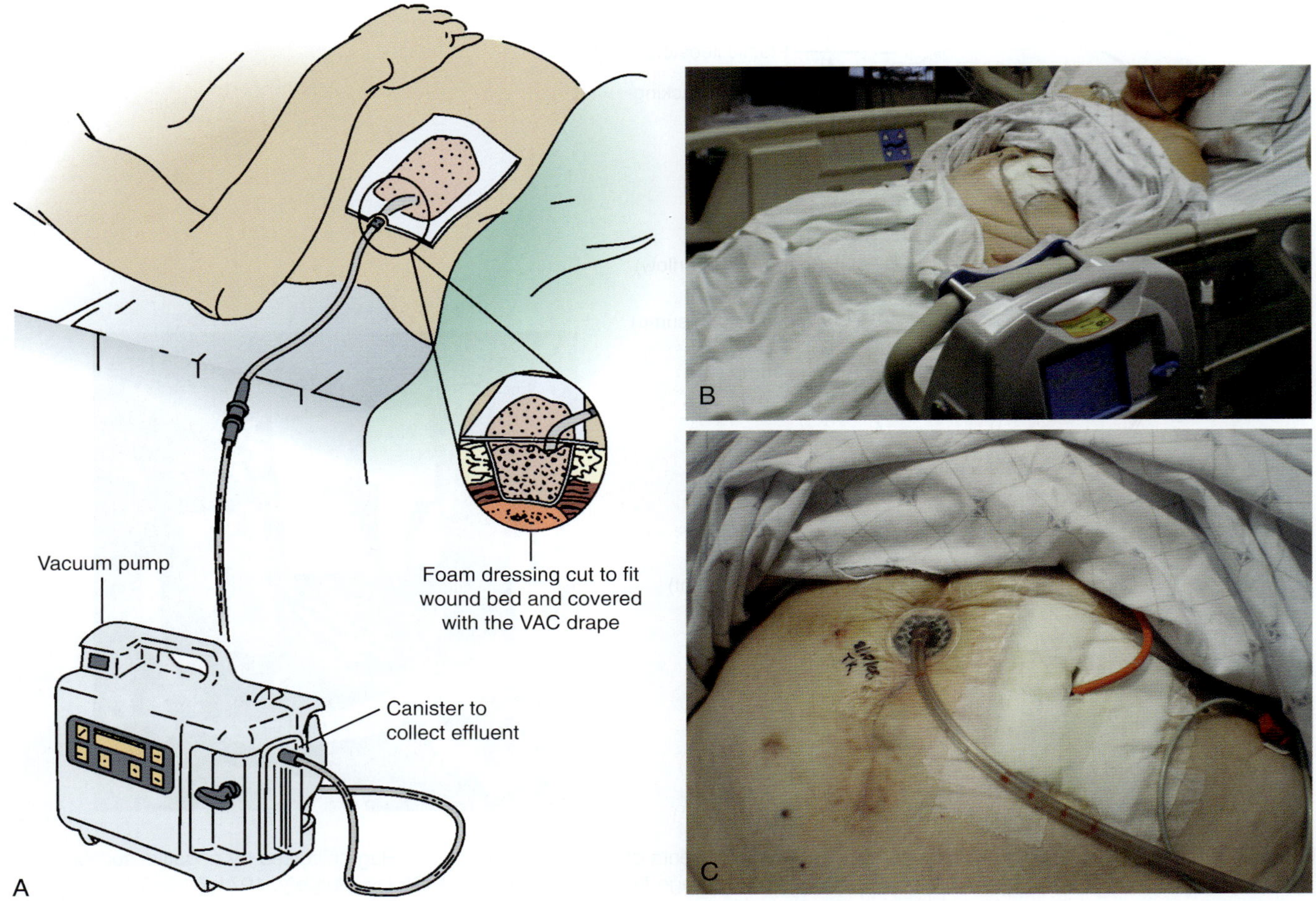

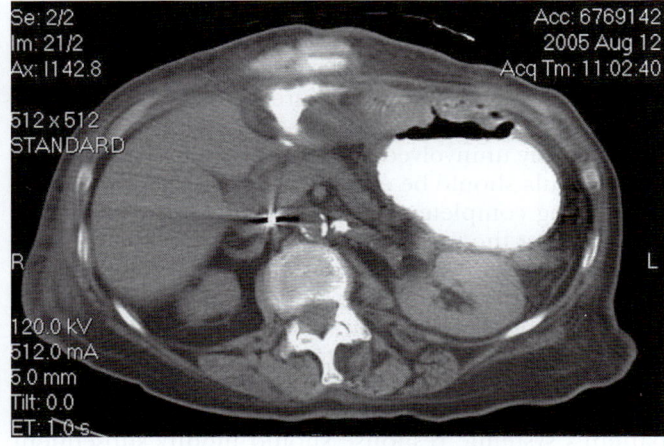

FIGURE 76.2 (A) The wound vacuum-assisted closure *(VAC)* apparatus allows for excellent control of drainage, minimizes the size of the abdominal wound, and simplifies management. (B) Wound VAC on a patient with a gastrocutaneous fistula (see Fig. 76.3). (C) Control of gastrocutaneous fistula with the wound VAC apparatus. ([A] From Cro C, George KJ, Donnelly J, Irwin S, Gardiner K. Vacuum assisted closure system in the management of enterocutaneous fistulae. *Postgrad Med J.* 2002;78:364.)

FIGURE 76.3 Computed tomography scan demonstrating free air and contrast extravasation from the stomach into an anterior intraabdominal abscess after vagotomy, antrectomy, and Billroth II gastrojejunostomy for a giant duodenal ulcer.

of malnutrition is unnecessary and may be detrimental. Even if the regimen of bowel rest in conjunction with intravenous and enteral nutrition does not lead to successful spontaneous fistula closure, the patient is generally in better nutritional and metabolic condition to tolerate a definitive operation.

Pharmacologic Support

The concept of using somatostatin to inhibit pancreatic exocrine secretion in the treatment of gastrointestinal fistulas was first introduced in 1979 by Klempa et al.[35] Somatostatin, a 14-amino-acid peptide, is a well-established inhibitor of gastrointestinal secretion, inhibiting both endocrine and exocrine pancreatic secretion and reducing pancreatic blood flow. Use of the long-acting somatostatin analogue octreotide for decreasing pancreatic and ECF output was popularized during the 1990s. An inhibitory effect on gastric, biliary, and pancreatic secretions is generally observed in clinical use. With typical subcutaneous dosages of 100 to 250 µg every 8 hours, fistulous output is reduced by 40% to 60% after the first day, regardless of fistula site or volume of output.[36] Side effects are not usually severe and include hyperglycemia, decreased bowel motility, and elevated cholesterol levels. Placebo-controlled studies indicate that octreotide decreases fistula-related complications, reduces fistulous output, and decreases fistula healing time and the time required for TPN.[37] Octreotide promotes fistula closure within a significantly shorter time than TPN alone, even with malignant enterocutaneous disease, and is particularly helpful in decreasing secretions in high-output fistulas to a manageable level.[38] However, the mortality rate, hospitalization time, and overall fistula closure rate has not been improved. It has been suggested that if fistula output is not decreased within 48 hours of treatment with somatostatin-14 or octreotide, then treatment should be discontinued.[37] A positive effect on fluid balance is seen in trials of octreotide in 50% to 60% of patients; otherwise, withdrawal should be considered. Evidence suggests that a first-day response of a greater than 50% reduction in output in response to somatostatin-14 in combination with TPN is a prognostic indicator for spontaneous closure.[38] Somatostatin-14 and its analogues are not intended as a replacement for conservative treatment. Instead, when used in combination, somatostatin-14 and TPN appear to exert a synergistic effect on the reduction of gastrointestinal secretions and improve fistula closure rates.[39] The use of local fibrin glue has recently been shown to improve closure rates in low-output ECFs.[40]

Proton pump inhibitors or histamine H_2-receptor antagonists are advised to reduce gastric acid production, slow transit, and reduce gastric secretions. These medications may be useful in decreasing fistula output, particularly with proximal fistulas or when gastric secretion is high. Other agents that are helpful in reducing intestinal transit times and decreasing intestinal volume losses include antiperistaltic agents such as loperamide at a dose of 8 to 16 mg/day or more, diphenoxylate at 10 to 20 mg/day or more, paregoric at 20 to 40 mL/day, or tincture of opium at 2.4 mL/day. Most failures of these medications occur when suboptimal doses are used by practitioners and, in the case of patients attempting oral nutrition, when medications are timed incorrectly. It is best to administer these drugs 20 to 30 minutes before a meal.

Patients with refractory fistulas related to Crohn disease have been successfully treated with short courses of cyclosporine and other immunosuppressive drugs. In five patients with a total of 12 fistulas, Hanauer and Smith used an infusion of 4 mg/kg per day for 6 to 10 days, followed by oral dosing at 8 mg/kg per day adjusted to maintain serum cyclosporine levels of 100 to 200 ng/mL.[41] All fistulas responded to cyclosporine infusion with decreased drainage and improvement in both local inflammation and patient comfort. Complete resolution occurred in 10 of the 12 fistulas after a mean of 8 days. Therapy was continued for a mean of 6 months, with five recurrences, two of which were related to inadequate cyclosporine serum levels. Similar results with cyclosporine were reported by Present and Lichtiger.[42] Although useful for short-term treatment, long-term administration of cyclosporine is generally avoided because of the potentially septic complications of immunosuppression, as well as hypertension and nephrotoxicity.

In the past decade, infliximab, a chimeric monoclonal antibody to tumor necrosis factor-α, was developed as treatment for Crohn disease. Infliximab is effective in closing fistulas in patients with Crohn disease. In a randomized, multicenter trial investigating infliximab administered intravenously at 0, 2, and 6 weeks and dosed at 5 mg/kg for the treatment of 94 adult Crohn disease patients with chronic fistulas, partial resolution of multiple lesions occurred in 68% and complete closure occurred in 55% of patients.[43] Other studies also support the efficacy of infliximab in treating Crohn disease–related small bowel fistulas.[44,45] Complications of this therapy occur in more than 60% of patients and include headache, abscess, upper respiratory tract infection, and fatigue.

INVESTIGATION

Investigation is the next phase of management. Stabilization is accomplished in the first 24 to 48 hours; investigation usually occurs over the following 7 to 10 days. Investigation includes a thorough evaluation of the gastrointestinal tract, definition of the anatomy of the fistula, and identification of any complicating features such as abscess, stricture, or distal obstruction.[20] Investigative studies should be designed to determine the presence and location of the fistula and to provide information regarding its cause. This objective can be accomplished by several methods. Early on, oral administration of indigo carmine or charcoal can be used to demonstrate the presence of a connection between the gastrointestinal tract and the abdominal wall or urinary bladder. These tests prove only the presence of a fistula and do not identify its site or source. Probably the most important first test is a fistulogram, which will define the length and width of the fistula, as well as its anatomic location. A fistulogram can be performed by inserting a small catheter through the drainage site into the fistula tract and then slowly injecting water-soluble contrast under fluoroscopy (Fig. 76.4). It is best performed by the responsible surgeon in collaboration with the radiologist. The value of the procedure is enhanced by close involvement of the surgeon and the radiologist as the study is performed.

Fistulography performed early in the course of the disease will help to determine (1) the site of the fistula, (2) intestinal continuity with the fistula, (3) the presence or absence of distal intestinal obstruction, (4) the nature of the intestine immediately adjacent to the fistula, and possibly (5) the presence or absence of an intraabdominal abscess. Performing the fistulogram first is prudent as contrast from an upper gastrointestinal series, contrast enema, or CT may make it difficult to interpret a fistulogram. Fistulography should be followed by a complete contrast study of the gastrointestinal tract either orally or through existing intraluminal tubes. Such study is valuable both for identifying the internal source of the fistula, the presence of additional fistulas, and for defining its size and complicating factors such as distal obstruction.

Additional useful tests in the early stage of investigation are CT and ultrasonography. These tests can define the anatomy of the vicinity of the fistula and evaluate for any ongoing or unrecognized intraabdominal processes or abscesses, as well as distal obstruction. A CT scan will be required in almost all patients for these reasons,

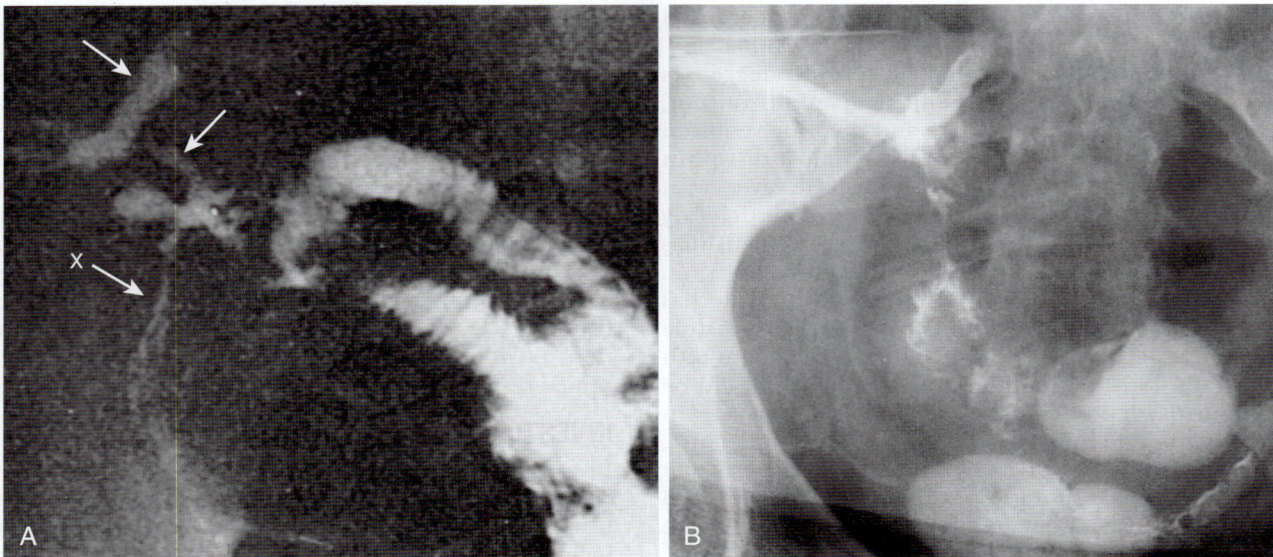

FIGURE 76.4 (A) Fistulogram. Injection of a cutaneous fistula demonstrates several tracts *(arrows)* leading to the ileum. Crohn disease is present in one loop *(arrow with X).* (B) Fistulogram demonstrating an enterocutaneous fistula in a patient after appendectomy for acute perforated appendicitis. ([A] From Goldfarb WB, Monafo W, McAlister WH. Clinical value of fistulography. *Am J Surg*. 1964;108:902.)

especially to rule out any undrained fluid collections. CT scanning with oral and intravenous contrast media is highly sensitive and specific for intraabdominal free air and will assist in locating the fistula and identifying adjacent fluid collections and concomitant bowel obstruction. However, the use of CT within the first week after surgery is associated with the expected presence of postoperative air within the abdominal cavity and thus may be difficult to interpret. Obviously, extravasation of intraluminal contrast on CT examination is diagnostic of perforation. CT and ultrasound are useful adjuncts when an intraabdominal abscess is suspected (Fig. 76.5). If found, significant fluid collections should be drained and an indwelling catheter left in the cavity. This permits subsequent examination of the cavity under fluoroscopy with water-soluble contrast to assist in delineation of the fistula tract. Although the site of perforation may not be identified on initial injection because of inflammation, subsequent examinations after several days of drainage will often show the site of the fistula. In general, CT is the most sensitive study for identifying a colovesical or enterovesical fistula. Endoscopic evaluation, including colonoscopy, esophagogastroduodenoscopy, and ERCP, may be helpful in certain specific clinical situations. However, endoscopy is not usually advisable if an acute perforation is suspected and should generally be delayed until the acute inflammatory process has resolved. Endoscopic examination of the stomach and duodenum may occasionally be used to identify a fistulous source and to take biopsy samples of adjacent tissue for exclusion of malignancy. For suspected gastrocolic or duodenocolic fistulas, colonoscopy may identify the involved site and enable a biopsy to be performed to diagnose inflammatory bowel disease or malignancy. Two recent large studies also have shown the therapeutic benefit of endoscopic fistula management.[12,46]

In the rare circumstance when perforation has not been excluded by noninvasive tests and the patient's condition is not improving or is worsening, diagnostic laparotomy should be considered. Morbidity and mortality rates are only increased by a delay under these circumstances. Diagnostic laparoscopy may be useful to rule out perforation after a previous laparoscopic procedure or after an endoscopic procedure. It is not usually appropriate in a septic, hypotensive patient and does not enable a satisfactory examination of the retroperitoneal duodenum. Early laparoscopy for tachycardia or unexplained fever is essential to prevent mortality from an anastomotic leak after gastric bypass surgery.

DECISION

The next step in fistula management is a decision on management and the timing of such management. When making these decisions, the likelihood of spontaneous closure must be estimated. The likelihood of closure depends on several factors. The first is anatomic location. In general, anatomic locations that are favorable for closure are the oropharynx, esophagus, duodenal stump, pancreas, biliary tree, and jejunum. Alternatively, unfavorable locations include the stomach, lateral duodenum, ligament of Treitz, and the ileum. Patients with poor nutritional status are much less likely to close a fistula no matter what the anatomic location.[39] More importantly, if a patient's nutritional status is poor, the mortality rate is higher. Another important factor is the presence or absence of sepsis. The absence of sepsis has a positive predictive value for closure, whereas the converse is true in the presence of sepsis. Elimination of sepsis is a necessity for spontaneous closure. The cause of the fistula is also predictive of closure. Postoperative fistulas and fistulas secondary to appendicitis or diverticulitis are likely to close. Fistulas associated with active Crohn disease are unlikely

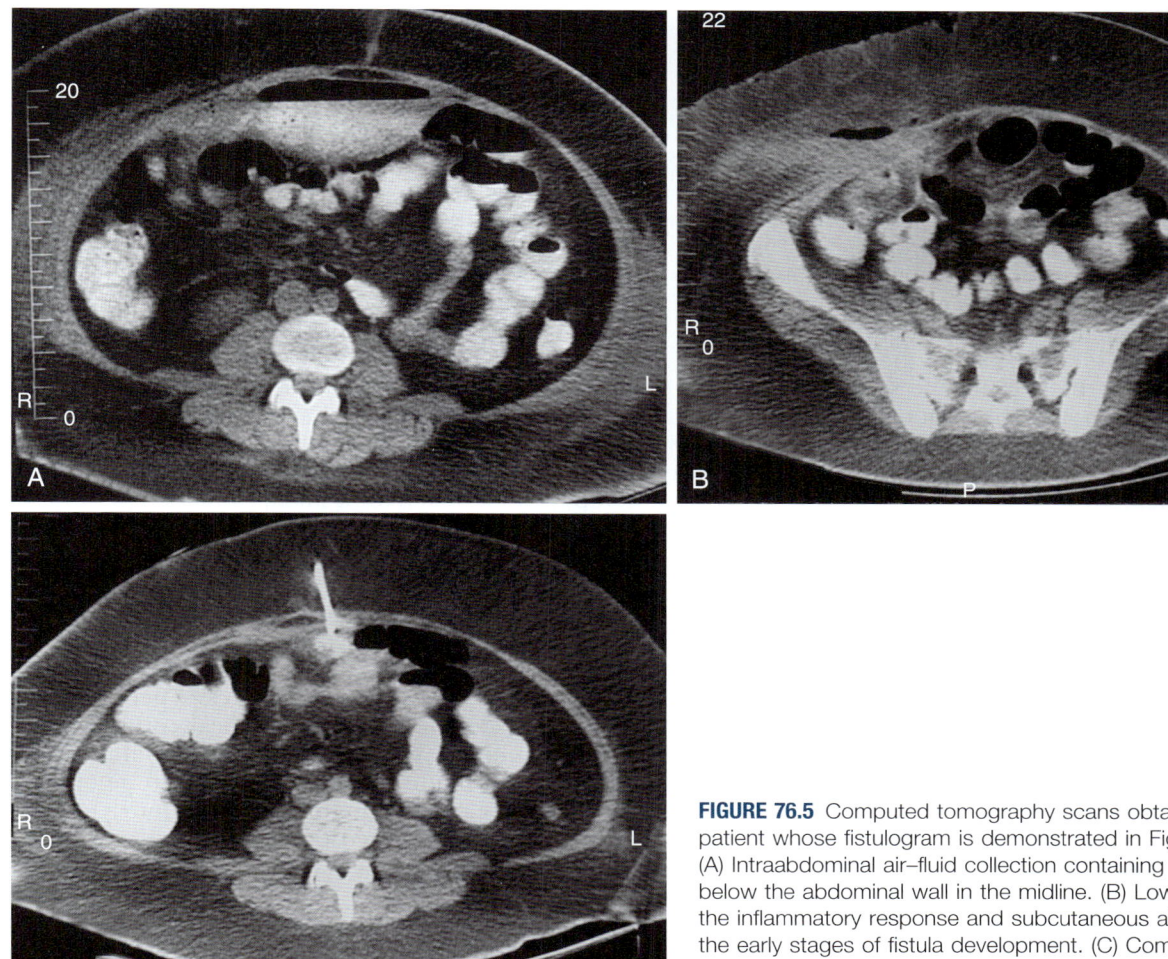

FIGURE 76.5 Computed tomography scans obtained in the patient whose fistulogram is demonstrated in Fig. 76.4B. (A) Intraabdominal air–fluid collection containing contrast just below the abdominal wall in the midline. (B) Lower cuts showing the inflammatory response and subcutaneous air representing the early stages of fistula development. (C) Computed tomography scan demonstrating resolution of an intraabdominal abscess after percutaneous catheter drainage.

to close until the Crohn disease is quiescent. Fistulas associated with cancer will usually require excision of the tumor along with the fistula. In addition, the presence of a foreign body will prevent closure of the fistula without operative intervention.

After sepsis has been controlled and diagnostic studies have been completed, management of a fistula should follow a conservative course. An opportunity for spontaneous healing should be permitted. It is important to provide adequate nutritional support and to aggressively investigate any new onset of signs of sepsis during this convalescent period. The duration of conservative treatment must be individualized. If a positive nitrogen balance is maintained, fistula output decreases, and no septic complications develop, nonoperative management may be continued. The spontaneous closure rate of ECF in several large series ranged from 32% to 80%,[2,17] with more than 90% of small intestinal fistulas that closed did so within a month. Less than 10% closed after 2 months, and none closed spontaneously after 3 months. Thus a reasonable management plan may consist of at least 1 month of nonoperative management, with reasonable extensions should the fistula show signs of slow but continued healing. Delaying operation allows peritoneal reaction and

inflammation to subside, thus making a definitive surgical procedure easier and safer. Delaying repair also permits nutritional optimization, thereby decreasing the likelihood of postoperative wound complications. A postoperative ECF usually extends hospitalization by 2 to 3 months, but this period may shorten somewhat with refinements in TPN, administration of somatostatin analogue, VAC usage, and wider availability of outpatient nursing care. In fact, many patients are candidates for discharge home or to a skilled nursing facility during the convalescent period because of the availability of these agents in such settings.

The condition of the bowel or other organs involved in the fistula is also important. Healthy adjacent tissue is a favorable factor, as are small fistulas, quiescent disease, and the absence of an abscess. Total disruption of the bowel negates closure, as does distal obstruction, abscess, malignancy, irradiation (or both), epithelialization of the fistula tract, and active disease. Typically, a long fistula tract (longer than 2 cm) is more likely to close than a short fistula tract. Similarly, a thin, narrow tract is a favorable prognostic indicator (i.e., less than 1 cm^2). Therefore short, wide tracts are unlikely to close spontaneously.[20] In general, a fistula with an everted or ostomized appearance is unlikely to spontaneously close and will require repair.

Failure of an ECF to close spontaneously is associated with a number of factors that are represented by the acronym *FRIENDS*: the presence of a *foreign body* within the tract or adjacent to it, previous *radiation* exposure of the site, ongoing *inflammation* (most commonly from Crohn disease) or *infection* that contributes to a catabolic state, *epithelialization* of the fistula tract (particularly if the fistula tract is less than 2 cm long), *neoplasm, distal intestinal obstruction,* and pharmacologic doses of *steroids.* Fistulas associated with a concurrent pancreatic fistula also have a low rate of spontaneous closure, as do those occurring in the presence of malnutrition or adjacent infection. Vigorous attempts to identify each of these confounding factors and to modify their influence may increase the success of nonoperative strategies, but operative intervention is generally necessary when they are present.

Campos et al. analyzed prognostic factors for closure of external duodenal fistulas and found that the odds of spontaneous closure were (1) three times greater with low-output fistulas than with high-output fistulas, (2) five times greater with postoperative fistulas than with fistulas associated with inflammatory bowel disease or trauma, and (3) two times greater with duodenal fistulas than with jejunoileal fistulas.[47] For duodenal fistulas, spontaneous closure was observed in 33% of patients, with an overall mortality rate of 36%. Williams et al. found that even high-output lateral duodenal fistulas spontaneously closed in 63% of patients with TPN and eradication of sepsis.[48] Their median output was 1480 mL/day, with a median time to closure of 29 days and an overall mortality rate of 15%. Kuvshinoff et al. found that seven of eight gastric fistulas closed spontaneously, but only one of four duodenal fistulas did so; approximately 50 days was required for closure.[29]

After considering all of the aforementioned factors, one determines whether to observe the fistula for spontaneous closure or plan early operation after stabilization. General wisdom holds that a fistula that has not closed by 4 to 6 weeks is unlikely to do so and operation is indicated. The decision to operate is tempered by the patient's condition and the state of the abdomen. In particular, when faced with a firm, indurated abdomen, it is better to stabilize the infection, nutrition, and fluid balance in this circumstance, and wait until the abdomen is soft, without significant induration, to maximize the chance for operative success and minimize the risk of creating new ECF. In certain cases, then, the period of waiting may be greater than 6 weeks.[48] One must also be aware of the quality of life, social, and psychological condition of the fistula patient. Härle et al.'s excellent study revealed that fistula patients have profound restrictions in daily life, approaches to illness, emotions, dependence, and need of support. A constant fear of leakage from the fistula appliance, being dependent on intravenous fluids and being dependent on health care professionals caused isolation and social restriction.[49]

DEFINITIVE THERAPY

The next important decision is to determine whether definitive operative therapy is necessary and the timing of such therapy. When operative therapy has been chosen, the operation must be carefully planned. Whenever possible, the operation should not take place until the patient is stable, not septic, and in an adequate nutritional state. The most favorable time to reoperate on patients is either within 10 days of diagnosis or after 4 months.[20,34] This prolonged treatment period is associated with prolonged morbidity, risk of mortality, and significant psychological stress.[49] It is important to discuss healing times and realistic expectations with patients to provide them with a framework to deal with the outcomes.

Gastric and Duodenal Perforations and Fistulas

Bell et al. reported 12 retroperitoneal perforations in a series of 2769 ERCP procedures; six were treated nonoperatively, with one death.[50] From a surgical standpoint, they warned that patients with perforations diagnosed within 24 hours of surgery had a mortality rate of 13%, whereas delay beyond 24 hours increased mortality rates to 43% because of sepsis or multiorgan failure. If medical therapy is undertaken for a small, contained perforation, close monitoring should be performed with surgical exploration initiated within 24 hours for perforations that do not improve or that worsen.

With both laparoscopic and open procedures, anastomotic leaks will frequently occur later, approximately 1 week after surgery. The decision to operate will be influenced by the ability to drain associated abscesses percutaneously and the presence of peritonitis. Focal collections that are adequately drained with a good systemic response and only local tenderness may continue to be observed for eventual closure. Ongoing sepsis, poorly drained collections, or generalized peritoneal signs may require reexploration, débridement, drainage, and management of the perforation.

A leaking gastroduodenostomy may be treated by distal gastric resection with conversion to a Billroth II gastrojejunostomy. Perforations that are recognized in the first several days postoperatively should usually be treated by reoperation and closure or by anastomotic revision. More typically, nearly 1 week after surgery, the onset of fever, tachycardia, respiratory failure, and acidosis with ileus and pain will suggest a leak or abscess. After CT-guided percutaneous drainage, with appropriate antibiotic therapy, the perforation will often heal. Failure to resolve shifts the focus to management of a fistula. Gastroduodenal fistulas that develop in association with necrotizing pancreatitis and necrosectomy may be treated during laparotomy or by subsequent percutaneous drainage. Duodenal fistulas may be treated with tube duodenostomy or Roux-en-Y duodenojejunostomy; late-developing duodenal fistulas may be treated by percutaneous drainage.[21]

If the gastric or duodenal defect is too large to allow primary closure or the fistula originates in conjunction with the ampulla and pancreatic duct, a Roux-en-Y gastrojejunostomy or duodenojejunostomy is a flexible and valuable technique for dealing with such difficult gastric or duodenal fistulas. It is best used in the absence of ongoing infection, when sufficient time has been allowed, and the jejunum is pliable and not edematous. Although mucosa-to-mucosa apposition is best, handsewing the end of the Roux limb, even with the chronically thickened tissue around a fistula, often results in healing. A feeding jejunostomy distal to the enteroenterostomy should be considered.

Treatment of a duodenal stump fistula is based on the condition of the stump and surrounding tissue and the surgeon's judgment. Options include primary suture closure, mobilization of the stump with resuture or stapling, lateral tube duodenostomy for duodenal decompression, direct tube drainage through the fistula, a serosal patch, or the use of a Roux jejunal limb. Duodenal fistulas that are associated with recurrence of Crohn disease at an ileocolic anastomosis are managed by resection of the recurrent disease with reanastomosis. The duodenal end of the fistula is débrided and primarily closed, and omentum is interposed to separate it from the new anastomosis. Difficult duodenal closure has been managed by either a jejunal serosal patch or duodenojejunostomy. Primary colonic Crohn disease with either a gastric or duodenal fistula is similarly treated by resection of the primary source and closure of the fistula, with duodenojejunostomy reserved for large residual defects.[3,5,13]

Internal gastrocolic or duodenocolic fistulas from colon carcinoma are generally managed by partial colon resection, as well as by resection of the involved stomach or duodenum, along with primary closure. Large duodenal defects require a patch or duodenojejunostomy. A gastro-jejunocolic fistula is treated by a partial gastrectomy with excision of the involved jejunum and colon, including the anastomosis. Reconstruction may be performed by either reanastomosis of the jejunum with a more distal loop gastrojejunostomy (to include truncal vagotomy if ulcer related) or conversion to a Roux-en-Y gastrojejunostomy. The colon may be anastomosed, or a proximal colostomy may be performed if extensive local inflammation is present.

For repair of both perforations and fistulas, the use of fibrin sealant as an adjunct should be considered.[40] Lau et al. compared sutured repair and fibrin sealant with a gelatin sponge for the treatment of perforated ulcers and also compared laparoscopic and open techniques.[51] They did not find any significant differences between sutured and fibrin sealant repair. These results, combined with successful reports of nonoperative fistula closure with the use of fibrin sealant, suggest a broader role in operative management.

Enterocutaneous Fistulas

Many ECFs close spontaneously if infection is controlled, nutrition is adequate, and distal obstruction is not present. Definitive operative correction remains the final step in the management of nonhealing small intestinal fistulas. As with the duration of medical management, the surgical procedure needs to be individualized. Direct suture closure of the fistula is associated with a high incidence of breakdown and fistula recurrence.[1,2] In most cases, the preferred operation is resection of the involved segment of intestine and primary end-to-end anastomosis. In the setting of extensive sepsis, primary anastomosis may not be appropriate. In these circumstances, exteriorization of both the proximal and distal ends of the intestine may be performed. It is critical that the proximal end be constructed as a standard everted Brooke stoma so that a proper appliance can be fitted and the subsequent effluent adequately managed.

If the fistula is not deemed appropriate for resection, such as when it develops as a complication of a deep pelvic procedure, staged approaches involving bypass should be considered. A simple side-to-side anastomosis proximal and distal to the fistula is inadequate, as is unilateral (proximal or distal) exclusion of the involved segment. Bilateral exclusion with isolation of both the proximal and distal portions of the involved intestine is necessary for effective defunctionalization of the fistula. In a staged procedure, the fistulous segment is left in situ, or the ends are exteriorized as mucous fistulas; the afferent and efferent bowel loops are anastomosed to restore intestinal continuity. Alternatively, if the efferent loop cannot be mobilized, the intestine proximal to a distal ileal fistula can be divided and anastomosed to the transverse colon. The fistulous segment is again returned to the pelvis or exteriorized as a mucous fistula. This technique is not as satisfactory as complete exclusion but works reasonably well if the ileocecal valve is competent. Optimally, the staged procedure is completed when the fistula segment is removed at a later date, although this is not always possible.

Gastrointestinal fistulas associated with large abdominal defects, termed *enteroatmospheric fistulas*, are not only the most difficult to manage surgically, but also the most likely to result in mortality. These fistulas often require multiple staged operations, with mortality rates of 20% to 60%.[20] As the principles of damage-control laparotomy have developed, the complications associated with the posttraumatic open abdomen have also been delineated. The incidence of fistula formation in this population varies between 2% and 25%. The etiology of fistulas is expanded from those described earlier in the more traditional surgical settings to include the development of fistulas from exposure of the bowel to atmospheric air for prolonged periods of time resulting in desiccation, the presence of packs and dressings that adhere to the bowel causing erosion of the serosa, and from the repeated trauma of abdominal washouts and reexplorations. Further complicating the disease in these patients is that the original inciting event for the fistula (i.e., desiccation as a consequence of a large volume of bowel exposed to atmospheric air for prolonged periods) places the patient at risk for more than one fistula. Frequently, these patients are found to have several fistulous openings develop over the period of their debility.

The wound VAC device works well to keep these wounds controlled, both in terms of overall wound size and volume of effluent. The VAC frequently closes even large abdominal wall defects when used appropriately and aggressively to counter the loss of domain associated with the chronically open abdomen. The VAC protects the bowel, preserves the fascia, limits loss of domain, reduces need for dressing changes, removes excess fluid, decreases bacterial counts, and increases the vascularity of the wound.[20,23,34]

The fistulas located in the midst of a fixed visceral block should not be intubated as, in general, the tubes placed into the openings result in further damage and generally are not useful. The VAC may be coupled with the use of isolative techniques to wall off the fistula from the large granulating abdominal wound (Fig. 76.6). Placement of ostomy pouches may then capture the fistula effluent while the VAC allows the remainder of the wound to be covered.[23]

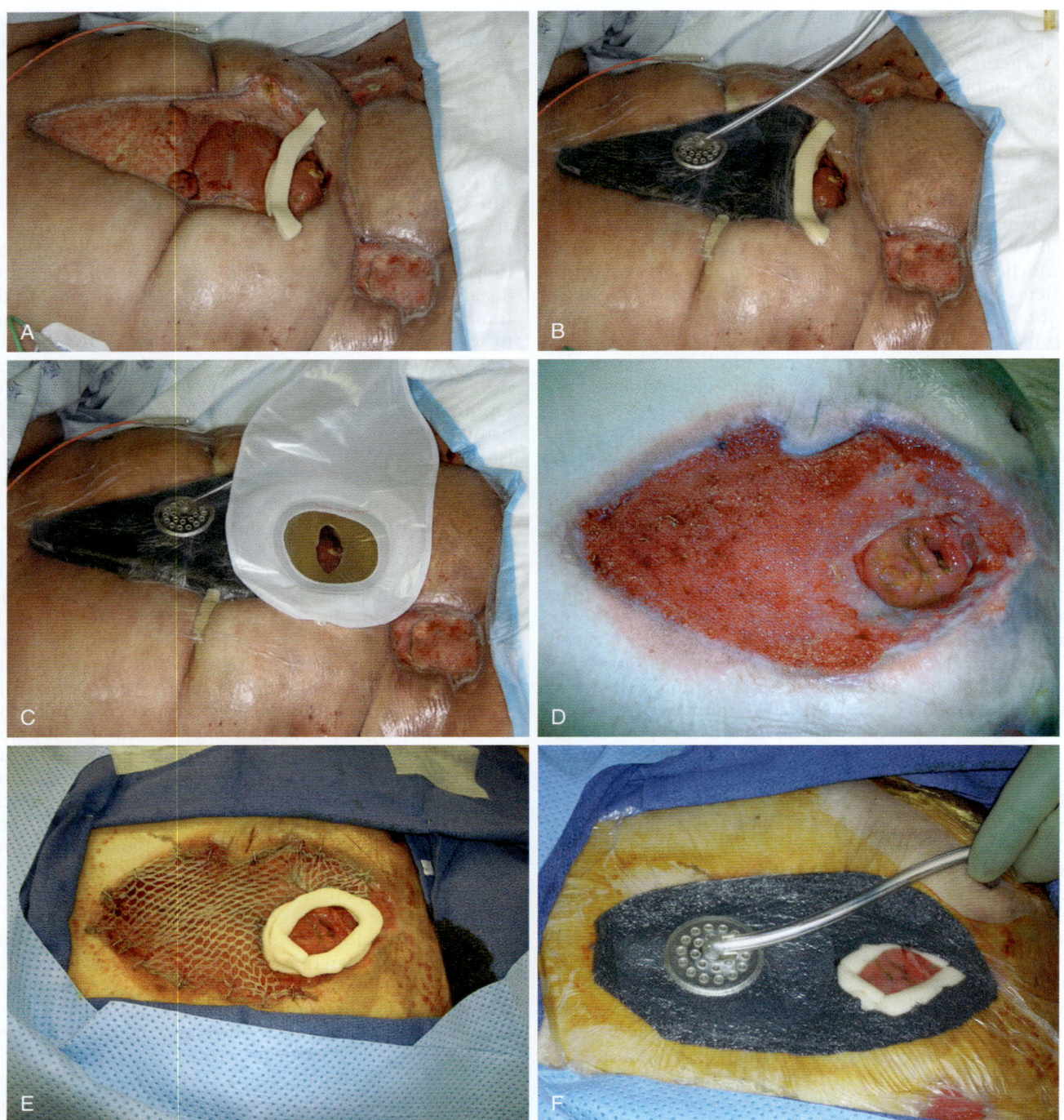

FIGURE 76.6 (A) The vacuum-assisted closure (VAC) may be coupled with the use of isolative techniques to (B) wall off the fistula from the large granulating abdominal wound. (C) Placement of ostomy pouches may then capture the fistula effluent while the VAC allows the remainder of the wound to be covered. (D) If local control of the wound can thus be established and nutrition has been appropriately optimized, (E) the patient may be a candidate for a split-thickness skin graft over the controlled granulated portion of the wound while (F) the fistula remains walled off.

If local control of the wound can thus be established and nutrition has been appropriately optimized, the patient may be a candidate for a split-thickness skin graft over the controlled granulated portion of the wound while the fistula remains walled off (see Fig. 76.6E and F). In this manner, the larger wound is closed, decreasing the catabolic demands associated with a large wound, and the fistula becomes easier to control. After a 6- to 12-month recovery time to replenish protein and calorie stores and regain muscle strength and mobility, successful abdominal wall reconstruction coupled with resection of the fistula(s) may be performed.

Musculocutaneous flaps and the application of abdominal wall reconstruction techniques involving component separation and prosthetic materials may be required to obtain adequate coverage.[23] The use of synthetic prosthetic materials is relatively contraindicated; rather the use of a biologic or biosynthetic prosthesis in patients with large wounds in the presence of a resection of a fistula should be considered. Long-term data regarding the recurrence rates of abdominal wall hernia and laxity in patients with the use of biologics are needed. However, as coverage of the large open wound is critical to prevent future new fistulas from forming, biologics are a necessary part of the surgical armamentarium used to help close the open abdomen.

Enteroenteric Fistulas

An internal fistula refers to a communication between the small intestine and some other organ or structure within the peritoneal cavity. An enteroenteric fistula occurs when the small intestine joins with either another segment of small intestine or the colon. Most enteroenteric fistulas are caused by Crohn disease, although colonic diverticulitis and colon cancer can also be causative. Symptoms develop in proportion to the length of the involved intestine. Ileocecal fistulas are most common because of the high percentage of patients with Crohn disease who have chronic inflammation of the terminal ileum. The jejunum and duodenum are involved less frequently.

Careful evaluation is needed to diagnose an enteroenteric fistula because abnormalities may be subtle, reported as generalized complaints, or even absent. Symptoms such as diarrhea, abdominal pain, weight loss, and fever are not specific and are frequently caused by the underlying disease process, as well as the fistula. Enteroenteric fistulas are often serendipitously diagnosed on a small bowel series or barium enema obtained for evaluating vague abdominal discomfort or dysfunction (Fig. 76.7). Sometimes the fistula is not discovered until laparotomy. In other patients with Crohn disease, long-term parenteral nutrition, bowel rest, and the use of pharmacologic therapy have been successful.[41-45] This outcome contrasts greatly with the natural history of these fistulas before such pharmacologic innovation. Surgical intervention is still necessary in many patients because of refractory disease or intolerance to medications and their side effects.

When surgical intervention is warranted, the operative procedure of choice is en bloc resection of the diseased intestine in continuity with the fistula tract. If inflammation or an abscess is present, primary resection may be unwise. In such a situation, proximal diversion or percutaneous drainage of any associated abscess cavity is prudent. Resection of the diseased intestine and fistula should be delayed for 6 weeks, if possible, to allow the inflammatory process to subside. Nutritional support during this time is essential.

Any resection, whether primary or as part of a staged procedure, should be confined to the involved segment of intestine to conserve overall bowel length. Extensive resection does not appear to protect against further complications and only increases the likelihood of subsequent malabsorption. This is particularly true in Crohn disease, in which repeat laparotomy, intestinal resection, and

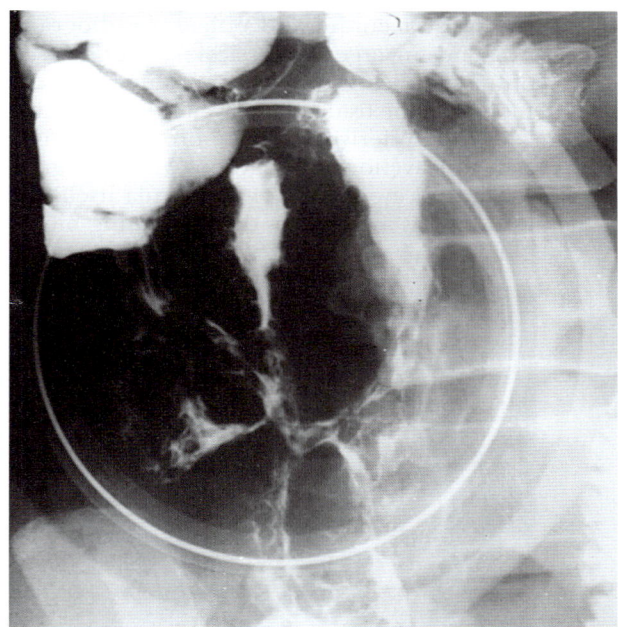

FIGURE 76.7 Small bowel series demonstrating a complex "starburst" enteroenteric fistula.

subsequent absorptive loss are common and could result in short gut syndrome.

Enterovesical Fistulas

Colonic communication with the urinary bladder caused by diverticulitis or colon cancer is seen more frequently. Fistula formation between the small intestine and the bladder is rare. More than half of all enterovesical fistulas occur as a complication of Crohn disease; however, radiation injury to the small bowel can also result in fistula formation. An ileovesical fistula develops in 2% to 4% of patients with regional enteritis, usually as a late manifestation of their disease. Such fistulas tend to be long, narrow, and tortuous (Fig. 76.8). Many fistulas seem to maintain patency only intermittently. The fistula frequently tracks downward from the ileum in the right iliac fossa. The uterus does not function as an anatomic barrier to such fistula tracts as it does with the short, localized fistulas resulting from diverticulitis or rectosigmoid cancer. Thus enterovesical fistulas have an even distribution among the sexes.

More than 80% of patients with enterovesical fistulas have urinary symptoms such as fecaluria or pneumaturia.[52] Evidence of bladder irritability and subsequent dysuria are common. In a few patients, fulminant sepsis may develop because of contamination of the urine with intestinal organisms. The presence of an internal fistula involving the urinary tract can be confirmed by the appearance of charcoal or indigo carmine in the urine after oral administration, or even using the "poppy seed" test. Cystoscopy is helpful in establishing or confirming the diagnosis. The most consistent finding is an area of bullous edema, usually on the posterior lateral wall or the fundus of the bladder. In some patients, the fistula opening can be directly visualized. Biopsy should be performed to evaluate for unusual causes such as tuberculosis or cancer.

CT is the most accurate and efficient radiographic means for diagnosing an enterovesical fistula (Fig. 76.9). Barium contrast studies of the gastrointestinal tract often do not demonstrate the fistula but may help in determining the nature of the underlying disease process and assessing its extent. Intravenous pyelography and cystography are rarely useful in evaluation of the fistula itself. They may be important as a means of demonstrating bilateral renal function and evaluating abnormalities of the upper urinary tract.

In the absence of obstruction, inflammation, or abscess, the preferred treatment of an enterovesical fistula is resection of the diseased intestine and involved portion of the bladder. Removal of the fistula is particularly important to prevent continued contamination of the urinary tract. A primary anastomosis is used to restore intestinal continuity, and the bladder wall is closed. We prefer operative ureteral stenting during these procedures. As with other fistulas, if an inflamed intestine or mass makes resection unsafe, transection plus cutaneous diversion of the proximal and distal intestinal segments is recommended.

Enterovaginal Fistulas

Fistulas from the small intestine to the vagina are rare. As with colovaginal fistulas, enterovaginal fistulas are more likely to occur in women who have undergone a hysterectomy. Enterovaginal fistulas are usually caused by regional enteritis, radiation enteritis, granulomatous disease, or rarely, malignant tumors. They can also occur rarely as a complication of an ileoanal pouch procedure for ulcerative colitis.

Most patients have a purulent or feculent vaginal discharge. Gas may also be intermittently expelled from the vagina. Associated intraabdominal sepsis is common and may cause fever, chills, and abdominal pain. Enterovaginal fistulas can lead to hypovolemia and severe fluid and electrolyte abnormalities, particularly when the drainage is profuse. Speculum examination generally confirms the diagnosis by revealing vaginal erosion and drainage of intestinal contents. CT scanning, as well as contrast studies of the small intestine or vagina, is diagnostic. In more subtle cases, a suspected fistula between the intestine and the vagina may be identified by placing a tampon in the vagina before the oral administration of charcoal or indigo carmine.

Management of an enterovaginal fistula is similar to that for an ECF. Local drainage through sump drains placed through the vagina may allow adequate control of sepsis and fistula output. If sepsis is eradicated, fistula output is low, and adequate nutrition is provided, an

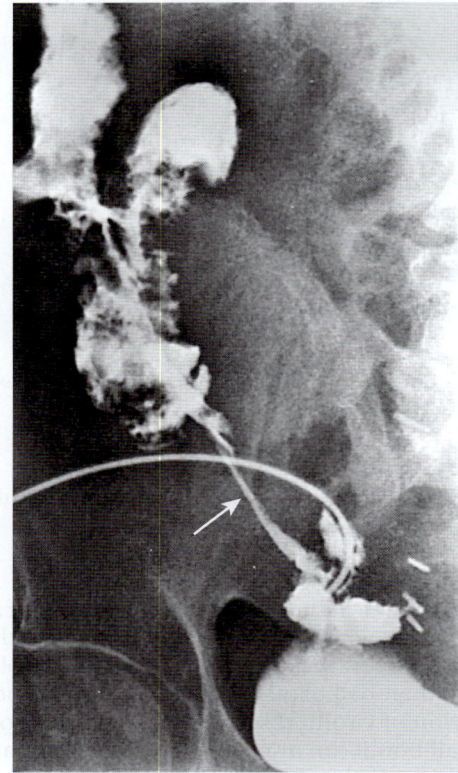

FIGURE 76.8 Fistulogram demonstrating an enterovesical fistula in a patient with long-standing ileal Crohn disease (*arrow* indicates a fistula tract). (From Tassiopoulos AK, Baum G, Halverson ID. Small bowel fistulas. *Surg Clin North Am.* 1996;76:1175.)

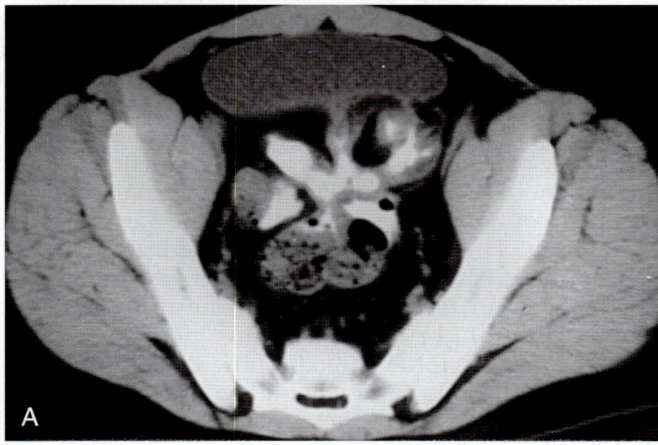
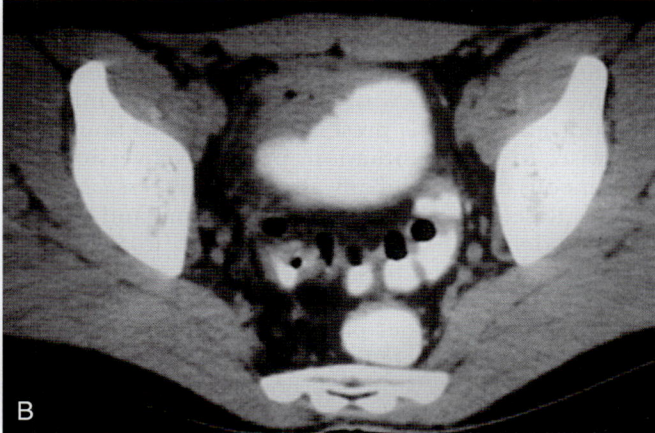

FIGURE 76.9 Computed tomographic scans in patients with enterovesical fistulas. (A) Complex enteroenteric and enterovesical fistula. (B) A loop of small intestine is adherent and causing significant inflammation on the wall of the bladder with subsequent fistula formation.

enterovaginal fistula may close without an operation. However, spontaneous closure of a fistula associated with Crohn disease is rare. Resection of a cuff of vaginal tissue along with the fistula and involved intestine is the preferred surgical approach. A primary intestinal anastomosis should be performed if the surrounding inflammation permits. The vaginal defect may be left open to allow external drainage of the pelvis postoperatively.

Vascular Enteric Fistulas

Enteric fistulas involving the vascular system, whether arterial or venous, are potentially lethal and often require urgent correction. True enterovenous and colovenous fistulas are rare but potentially lethal entities. The most commonly reported causes of duodenocaval fistula include migration of vena caval filters, right nephrectomy, peptic ulcer disease, and ingestion of a foreign body.[53] These fistulas are often detected unexpectedly on barium studies by observing extravasation of the contrast agent. Substantial barium extravasation reportedly carries a high mortality rate.[54]

The aorta lies proximal to the gastrointestinal tract for much of its thoracic and abdominal course. Consequently, aortoenteric fistulas potentially can involve the gut anywhere from the esophagus to the colon. The most common fistula between the arterial tree and the small intestine arises from the aorta. Complications of aortic aneurysms and their repair are by far the most frequent cause of this entity, although such fistulas have occurred after other abdominal procedures. Spontaneous or primary aortoenteric fistulas usually occur when the plaque of an atherosclerotic aortic aneurysm ruptures into the intestine. On rare occasion, mycotic, tubercular, or traumatic aneurysms may also rupture into the small bowel. The duodenum is most often involved when a spontaneous fistula develops. Reckless et al. reviewed 131 spontaneous aortoenteric fistulas and found that rupture into the third portion of the duodenum occurred in 57.6% of cases, whereas the remainder of the small intestine was involved in only 8%.[55]

Secondary aortoenteric fistulas complicate 2% to 4% of all aortic reconstructions and generally involve aortoiliac or aortofemoral prosthetic grafts. The fistulas usually occur at the level of the proximal aortic anastomosis, and most rupture into the duodenum. If the fistula occurs at the anastomosis between the prosthesis and the iliac arteries, the ileum is the most commonly involved segment of intestine.

Two processes can cause secondary aortoenteric fistulas and result in different clinical manifestations. A direct communication between the intestine and the arterial lumen ultimately leads to massive gastrointestinal hemorrhage. Initially, bleeding is intermittent and is rarely exsanguinating, the "herald" or "sentinel bleed."[56] Such episodic bleeding is generally painless and may cause chronic anemia. Melena or hematemesis in any patient with an aortic prosthesis should be assumed to be from an aortoenteric fistula until proved otherwise. Several months may elapse between the initial bleeding episode and the inevitable massive hemorrhage. The second form of secondary fistula is known as a *paraprosthetic enteric fistula*. In this type of aortoenteric fistula, the intestine communicates with a perigraft abscess or aneurysm and not directly with the arterial lumen. Most of these patients have manifestations of sepsis. Although a distinct clinical entity, a paraprosthetic fistula ultimately leads to a direct communication with the arterial lumen and subsequent hemorrhage if untreated.[57]

These patients should be prepared for an urgent operation, but there is generally enough time to perform further diagnostic investigation. Upper gastrointestinal endoscopy should be performed initially to exclude common causes of hemorrhage, such as peptic ulcer disease or esophageal varices. The actual erosion into the intestinal wall can often be seen if the endoscopist is instructed to examine the third portion of the duodenum. Biopsy of the erosion is contraindicated. CT is sensitive in evaluating the retroperitoneum for suspected aortoenteric fistulas. CT has the advantages of rapid imaging and wide availability (Fig. 76.10). Because it is a noninvasive study, CT does

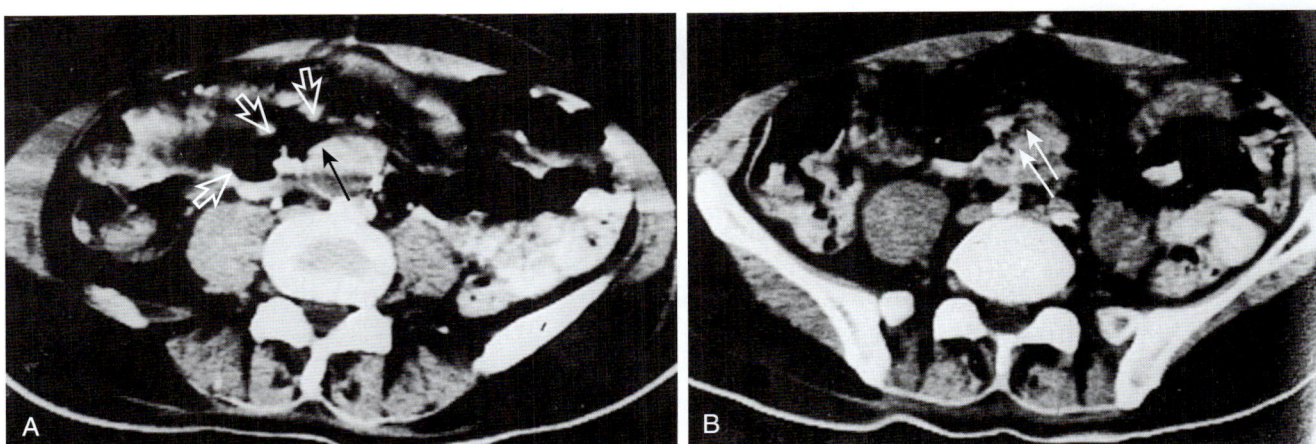

FIGURE 76.10 Computed tomographic scan of aortoenteric erosion. (A) Apparent erosion of an aortic graft *(black arrow)* into the overlying duodenum *(open arrows)*. (B) Perigraft air *(arrows)*. (From Bernhard VM. Aortoenteric fistulas. In: Rutherford RB, ed. *Vascular Surgery*. Philadelphia: Saunders; 1989:530.)

not require technical expertise and does not cause patient discomfort, thereby avoiding the potentially disastrous consequences of raising the patient's blood pressure. CT may demonstrate loss of the normal fatty plane between the aortic graft and the duodenum, a finding indicative of a probable fistula. It may also reveal a false aneurysm at the anastomosis or the presence of a periaortic gas or fluid collection.

Management of an aortoenteric fistula, once confirmed, consists of early and aggressive operative intervention.[57] Removal of the prosthesis and extraanatomic bypass should be coupled with broad-spectrum antibiotics appropriate for the multiple enteric organisms usually present. Conventional wisdom holds that the presence of infection at the prosthetic site precludes less involved procedures such as local closure of the fistula or replacement of the prosthesis without extraanatomic bypass.[57] The survival rate in patients with aortoenteric fistulas is poor, often because of exsanguinating hemorrhage or associated cardiovascular or renal impairment. The mortality rate has been reported to be as high as 50%.

General Considerations

When planning the operation for fistula patients, the surgeon should allow adequate time for a difficult and prolonged procedure. Depending on the complexity of the abdominal wound, component release and other reconstructive maneuvers may be required to achieve closure of the abdominal wall. It is frequently helpful to enlist the expertise of a plastic surgeon for closure of the abdominal wound (Fig. 76.11A). The component separation release technique is useful for the reconstruction of

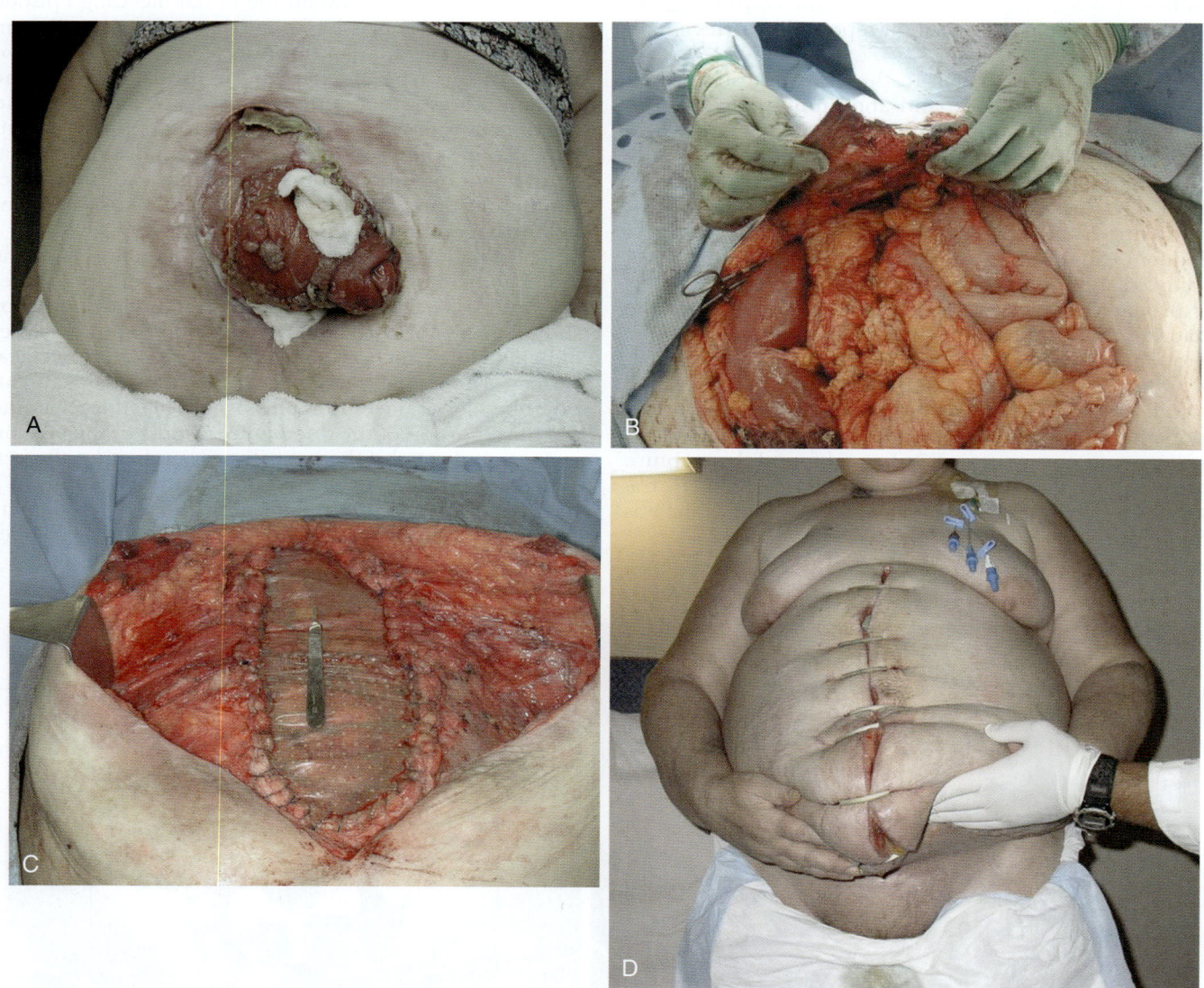

FIGURE 76.11 (A) Enterocutaneous fistula with epithelialization of the tract and a large abdominal wall defect. (B) The entire intestinal tract has been mobilized and complete enterolysis performed. (C) The large abdominal wall defect is closed with a combination of abdominal wall and small intestinal submucosa (Surgisis Gold). (D) Completed resection of the fistula and abdominal wall closure with loose closure of the skin and the use of retention sutures.

large abdominal wall defects, especially when contaminated conditions exist in which the use of prosthetic material may be contraindicated. Thus preoperative consultation and evaluation by the plastic and reconstructive surgery team should be considered. Preoperative preparation should include mechanical bowel preparation whenever feasible and perioperative antibiotics directed toward bowel and skin flora, as well as any specific organisms identified by recent culture and sensitivity information.

Whenever possible, a new incision or extension of the previous incision over "virgin" abdominal wall will make reentry into the abdominal cavity easier and safer. Once the peritoneal cavity is entered, the entire intestinal tract should be mobilized, and complete enterolysis should be performed if possible, especially if there is any question of distal obstruction (see Fig. 76.11B). A useful adjunct during this portion of the operation is to use laparotomy pads soaked in saline solution to "rehydrate" the adhesions before attempting adhesiolysis. By using a combination of gentle compression and palpation with one hand and sharp dissection with either scissors or a scalpel in conjunction with the use of copious amounts of saline-soaked sponges, one can usually carry out complete mobilization of the involved intestine. In general, an intestinal fistula cannot be repaired primarily; such repair usually results in recurrence. Fistulas require complete resection back to healthy tissue with enteroenterostomy. If the anastomosis is performed on healthy bowel, the choice between a stapled or handsewn anastomosis does not matter. More importantly, the anastomosis should be under no tension, there must be adequate blood supply, and distal obstruction cannot be present. A feeding jejunostomy or nasoenteric tube should be placed. Ongoing nutritional repletion is an extremely important constituent of a successful outcome, and most patients will not be able to take enough calories by mouth during the postoperative recovery period. A gastrostomy tube may also be a useful adjunct in the postoperative period to provide mid- to long-term gastric decompression in patients and obviate the need for a nasogastric tube. Depending on the state of the intestinal tract, the extent of enterolysis required, and the underlying process that led to fistula formation, prolonged postoperative ileus commonly occurs, and decompression via a gastrostomy tube, while downstream enteral nutrition is given, may be very beneficial and more comfortable for the patient. Because of the usual extensive nature of the dissection during such operations, the formation of intraabdominal adhesions is likely. Methods for decreasing intraabdominal adhesions, such as the use of hyaluronic acid–carboxymethylcellulose membrane (Seprafilm), may be beneficial in preventing postoperative complications.[58] Omental wrapping of suture lines has been shown recently to be beneficial as well.[59] Finally, abdominal wall closure is extremely important to allow the best chance for success and to prevent recurrent fistulization. It is essential that the abdominal wall be closed with autologous tissue (using component separation or musculocutaneous flaps) or an absorbable bioprosthesis consisting of either human acellular dermal matrix, porcine dermal collagen, bovine pericardium, porcine small intestinal submucosa, or a biosynthetic web scaffold (see Fig. 76.11C). In those patients with a previously open abdomen that has been left to heal by skin grafts or by secondary intention, there may be insufficient skin left over the abdominal wall to close. In the patient who has had a bioprosthesis placed, the use of a wound VAC device to prevent desiccation of exposed grafts is invaluable. The placement of preoperative tissue expanders over the lateral abdominal walls may allow expansion of the skin and subsequently allow skin closure at operation (see Fig. 76.11D).

HEALING

Most postoperative fistula patients are in a profoundly catabolic state in the early postoperative period and are at risk for nutritional complications. Optimal nutrition is as important postoperatively as preoperatively. Supplemental nutrition via enteral, parenteral, or a combination is frequently required, and with time, the patient can be transitioned to complete intake by mouth. Even when a patient cannot tolerate full caloric intake via the enteral route, providing a portion of the nutrition enterally remains an important objective. It may be useful to cycle tube feeding at night after the patient is eating, in an attempt to stimulate appetite. Meals from home also occasionally help with appetite stimulation. Consultation with a dietitian can be very helpful. A period of home tube feeding or, if necessary, home parenteral nutrition is not unreasonable in these patients as reestablishing normal eating habits may be a long process. The final phase of the treatment of fistulas, then, is healing, and this phase is highly dependent on good nutrition after a well-performed operation. If the patient cannot tolerate at least 1500 kcal/day enterally, parenteral nutrition should be continued until this goal is achieved. After enteral intake approaches this range, the patient can be weaned from parenteral nutrition.

The overall mortality rate, if one includes all fistulas, is approximately 20%. Mortality with a postoperative fistula is not as high. Postoperative fistulas are associated with less than 2% mortality and approximately 12% morbidity. Delayed complications may include short bowel syndrome, depending on the extent of the intestinal resection, previous resections, and the underlying disease state (i.e., Crohn disease). In patients with a marginal amount of bowel remaining, some intestinal adaptation may occur, and with time, it may be possible to wean the patient off parenteral nutrition. As a general guide, approximately 90 cm of small intestine with an intact ileocecal valve may be adequate to prevent short bowel syndrome, whereas 150 cm may be necessary when the ileocecal valve has been resected. The surgeon must be vigilant for recurrent fistulas postoperatively. These patients are also highly susceptible to adhesive small bowel obstruction. It is generally prudent to manage early postoperative small bowel obstruction in these patients with long-tube decompression and TPN, rather than risk further complications with another operation in the early postoperative period.

SUMMARY

Management of intestinal fistulas provides a surgeon with multiple challenges. Careful attention must be paid to the physiologic, metabolic, and immunologic derangements in these patients. An organized and tolerant approach to the stabilization, investigation, planning and implementation of medical and surgical therapy, and healing phase should allow for a successful outcome in the majority of patients.

REFERENCES

1. Ortiz LA, Zhang B, McCarthy MW, et al. Treatment of enterocutaneous fistulas, then and now. *Nutr Clin Pract.* 2017;884533617701402.
2. Polk TM, Schwab CW. Metabolic and nutritional support of the enterocutaneous fistula patient: a three-phase approach. *World J Surg.* 2012;36(3):524-533.
3. Paik HJ, Lee SH, Choi CI, et al. Duodenal stump fistula after gastrectomy for gastric cancer: risk factors, prevention, and management. *Ann Surg Treat Res.* 2016;90(3):157-163.
4. Cucchi SG, Pories WJ, MacDonald KG, Morgan EJ. Gastrogastric fistulas: a complication of divided gastric bypass surgery. *Ann Surg.* 1995;221:387.
5. Girard E, Messager M, Sauvanet A, et al. Anastomotic leakage after gastrointestinal surgery: diagnosis and management. *J Visc Surg.* 2014;151(6):441-450.
6. Pickleman J, Watson W, Cunningham J, Fisher SG, Gamelli R. The failed gastrointestinal anastomosis: an inevitable catastrophe? *J Am Coll Surg.* 1999;188:473.
7. Papakonstantinou A, Alfaras P, Komessidou V, Hadjiyannakis E. Gastrointestinal complications after vertical banded gastroplasty. *Obes Surg.* 1998;8:215.
8. Kirkpatrick JR, Zapas JL. Divided gastric bypass: a fifteen-year experience. *Am Surg.* 1998;64:62.
9. Perdikis G, Hinder RA, Lund RJ, Raiser F, Katada N. Laparoscopic Nissen fundoplication: where do we stand? *Surg Laparosc Endosc.* 1997;7:17.
10. Hunter JG, Smith CD, Branum GD, et al. Laparoscopic fundoplication failures: patterns of failure and response to fundoplication revision. *Ann Surg.* 1999;230:595.
11. Watkins BM, Montgomery KF, Ahroni JH. Laparoscopic adjustable gastric banding: early experience in 400 consecutive patients in the USA. *Obes Surg.* 2005;15:82.
12. Talbot M, Yee G, Saxena P. Endoscopic modalities for upper gastrointestinal leaks, fistulae and perforations. *ANZ J Surg.* 2017;87(3):171-176.
13. Spirt M, Sachar DB, Greenstein AJ. Symptomatic differentiation of duodenal from gastric fistulas in Crohn's disease. *Am J Gastroenterol.* 1990;85:455.
14. Forbes N, Al-Dabbagh R, Lovrics P, Morgan D. Gastrocolic fistula: a shortcut through the gut. *Can J Gastroenterol Hepatol.* 2016;614-617.
15. Huttenhuis JM, Kouwenhoven EA, van Zanten RA, Veneman TF. Malignant gastrocolic fistula: review of the literature and report of a case. *Acta Chir Belg.* 2015;115(6):423-425.
16. Webster NW, Carey LC. *Fistulae of the Intestinal Tract.* Vol. 13. No 6. Chicago: Year Book; 1976.
17. Graham JA. Conservative treatment of gastrointestinal fistulas. *Surg Gynecol Obstet.* 1977;144:512.
18. Reinisch A, Liese J, Woeste G, et al. A retrospective, observational study of enteral nutrition in patients with enteroatmospheric fistulas. *Ostomy Wound Manage.* 2016;62(7):36-47.
19. Ren J, Liu S, Wang G, et al. Laparoscopy improves clinical outcome of gastrointestinal fistula caused by Crohn's disease. *J Surg Res.* 2016;200(1):110-116.
20. Di Saverio S, Tarasconi A, Walczak DA, et al. Classification, prevention and management of entero-atmospheric fistula: a state-of-the-art review. *Langenbecks Arch Surg.* 2016;401(1):1-13.
21. Jiang W, Tong Z, Yang D, et al. Gastrointestinal fistulas in acute pancreatitis with infected pancreatic or peripancreatic necrosis: a 4-year single-center experience. *Medicine (Baltimore).* 2016;95(14):e3318.
22. Schein M, Decker GA. Gastrointestinal fistula associated with large abdominal wall defects: experience with 43 patients. *Br J Surg.* 1990;77:97.
23. Misky A, Hotouras A, Ribas Y, Ramar S, Bhan C. Systematic literature review on the use of vacuum assisted closure for enterocutaneous fistula. *Colorectal Dis.* 2016;(9):846-851.
24. Pritts TA, Fischer DR, Fischer JE. Postoperative enterocutaneous fistula. In: Holzheimer RG, Mannick JA, eds. *Surgical Treatment—Evidence-Based and Problem-Oriented.* New York: W Zucksschwerdt Verlag; 2001:134.
25. Dudrick SJ, Maharaj AR, McKelvey AA. Artificial nutritional support in patients with gastrointestinal fistulas. *World J Surg.* 1999;23:570.
26. Chapman R, Foran R, Dunphy JE. Management of intestinal fistulas. *Am J Surg.* 1964;108:157.
27. Sheldon GF, Gardiner BN, Way LW, Dunphy JE. Management of gastrointestinal fistulas. *Surg Gynecol Obstet.* 1971;133:385.
28. Roback SA, Nicholoff DM. High output enterocutaneous fistulas of the small bowel. *Am J Surg.* 1972;123:317.
29. Kuvshinoff BW, Brodish RJ, McFadden DW, Fischer JE. Serum transferrin as a prognostic indicator of spontaneous closure and mortality in gastrointestinal cutaneous fistulas. *Ann Surg.* 1993;217:615.
30. Atema JJ, Mirck B, Van Arum I, Ten Dam SM, Serlie MJ, Boermeester MA. Outcome of acute intestinal failure. *Br J Surg.* 2016;103(6):701-708.
31. Thibault R, Picot D. Chyme reinfusion or enteroclysis in nutrition of patients with temporary double enterostomy or enterocutaneous fistula. *Curr Opin Clin Nutr Metab Care.* 2016;19(5):382-387.
32. Picot D, Layec S, Dussaulx L, Trivin F, Thibault R. Chyme reinfusion in patients with intestinal failure due to temporary double enterostomy: a 15-year prospective cohort in a referral center. *Clin Nutr.* 2017;36(2):593-600.
33. Martinez JL, Luque-de-León E, Ferat-Osorio E. Predictive value of preoperative serum C-reactive protein for recurrence after definitive surgical repair of enterocutaneous fistula. *Am J Surg.* 2017;213(1):105-111.
34. Suriyapa C, Anderson MC. A simple device to control drainage from enterocutaneous fistulas. *Surgery.* 1971;70:455.
35. Klempa J, Schwedes U, Usadel KH. Verhütung von postoperativen pankreatitischen Komplikationen nach Duodenopankreatektomie durch Somastatin. *Chirurg.* 1979;50:427.
36. Paran H, Neufeld D, Kaplan O, et al. Octreotide for treatment of postoperative alimentary tract fistulas. *World J Surg.* 1995;19:430.
37. Dorta G. Role of octreotide and somatostatin in the treatment of intestinal fistulae. *Digestion.* 1999;60:53.
38. Ayache S, Wadleigh RG. Treatment of a malignant enterocutaneous fistula with octreotide acetate. *Cancer Invest.* 1999;17:320.
39. Di Costanzo J, Cano N, Martin J, et al. Treatment of external gastrointestinal fistulas by a combination of total parenteral nutrition and somatostatin. *J Parenter Enteral Nutr.* 1987;11:465.
40. Wu X, Ren J, Gu G, et al. Autologous platelet rich fibrin glue for sealing of low-output enterocutaneous fistulas: an observational cohort study. *Surgery.* 2014;155(3):434-441.
41. Hanauer SB, Smith MB. Rapid closure of Crohn's disease fistulas with continuous intravenous cyclosporine A. *Am J Gastroenterol.* 1993;88:646.
42. Present DH, Lichtiger S. Efficacy of cyclosporine in treatment of fistula of Crohn's disease. *Dig Dis Sci.* 1994;39:374.
43. Present DH, Rutgeerts P, Targan S, et al. Infliximab for the treatment of fistulas in patients with Crohn's disease. *N Engl J Med.* 1999;340:1398.
44. Ricart E, Sandborn WJ. Infliximab for the treatment of fistulas in patients with Crohn's disease. *Gastroenterology.* 1999;117:1247.
45. Lichtenstein GR, Yan S, Bala M, et al. Infliximab maintenance treatment reduces hospitalizations, surgeries, and procedures in fistulizing Crohn's disease. *Gastroenterology.* 2005;128:862.
46. Rogalski P, Daniluk J, Baniukiewicz A, Wroblewski E, Dabrowski A. Endoscopic management of gastrointestinal perforations, leaks and fistulas. *World J Gastroenterol.* 2015;21(37):10542-10552.
47. Campos AC, Andrade DF, Campos GM, Matias JE, Coelho JC. A multivariate model to determine prognostic factors in gastrointestinal fistulas. *J Am Coll Surg.* 1999;188:483.
48. Williams NM, Scott NA, Irving MH. Successful management of external duodenal fistula in a specialized unit. *Am J Surg.* 1997;173:240.
49. Härle K, Lindgren M, Hallböök O. Experience of living with an enterocutaneous fistula. *J Clin Nurs.* 2015;24(15-16):2175-2183.
50. Bell RC, Van Stiegman G, Goff J, Reveille M, Norton L, Pearlman NW. Decision for surgical management of perforation following endoscopic sphincterotomy. *Am Surg.* 1991;57:237.
51. Lau WY, Leung KL, Kwong KH, et al. A randomized study comparing laparoscopic versus open repair of perforated peptic ulcer using suture or sutureless technique. *Ann Surg.* 1996;224:131.
52. Kirsh GM, Hampel N, Shuck JM, Resnick MI. Diagnosis and management of vesicoenteric fistulas. *Surg Gynecol Obstet.* 1991;173:91.
53. Guillem PG, Binot D, Dupuy-Cuny J, et al. Duodenocaval fistula: a life-threatening condition of various origins. *J Vasc Surg.* 2001; 33:643.

54. Vitellas KM, Stone JA, Bennett WF, Mueller CF. The hyperdense liver and spleen: a CT manifestation of barium embolization through a duodenocaval fistula. *AJR Am J Roentgenol.* 1997;169:915.

55. Reckless JP, McColl I, Taylor GW. Aortoenteric fistulas: an uncommon complication of abdominal aortic aneurysms. *Br J Surg.* 1972;59:461.

56. Deijen CL, Smulders YM, Coveliers HM, et al. The importance of early diagnosis and treatment of patients with aortoenteric fistulas presenting with herald bleeds. *Ann Vasc Surg.* 2016;36:28-34.

57. Kakkos SK, Bicknell CD, Tsolakis IA, Bergqvist D. Hellenic Co-operative Group on Aortic Surgery. Editor's choice—management of secondary aorto-enteric and other abdominal arterio-enteric fistulas: a review and pooled data analysis. *Eur J Vasc Endovasc Surg.* 2016;52(6):77-83.

58. Vrijland WW, Tseng LN, Eijkman HJ, et al. Fewer intraperitoneal adhesions with use of hyaluronic acid–carboxymethylcellulose membrane: a randomized clinical trial. *Ann Surg.* 2002;235:193.

59. Nasiri S, Mirminachi B, Taherimehr R, Shadbakhsh R, Hojat M. The effect of omentoplasty on the rate of anastomotic leakage after intestinal resection: a randomized controlled trial. *Am Surg.* 2017;83(2):157-161.

Small Bowel Diverticula

Hadley K.H. Wesson | Karen R. Natoli | James E. Harris Jr. |

Michael E. Zenilman

Small bowel diverticular disease occurs in 0.3% to 20% of the population and is much less common than large bowel diverticular disease, which is present in 15% to 40% of adults. Of those with small bowel diverticula, only 4% will develop symptoms. Despite these relatively low statistics, it is nevertheless important for the general surgeon to have a firm understanding of small bowel diverticular disease when considering the broad differential diagnoses of abdominal pain and gastrointestinal bleeding. Three types of small bowel diverticula warrant particular consideration: duodenal diverticula, jejunoileal diverticula, and Meckel diverticula. The most frequently encountered diverticula are duodenal (45%), compared to jejunoileal (25%) and Meckel diverticula (25%), and jejunoileal diverticula are most often symptomatic. This chapter discusses each type of diverticulum as it relates to its epidemiology, pathogenesis, clinical presentation, diagnosis, and management.

Two key distinctions exist among these types of diverticula. The first is whether they are congenital or acquired. In general, Meckel diverticula are congenital and not associated with other types of diverticula. Most duodenal and jejunoileal diverticula are acquired, with the exception of intraluminal duodenal diverticula. The second distinction is whether they are true or false diverticula. Meckel diverticula are true diverticula containing all three layers of bowel. Duodenal and jejunoileal diverticula are false, or pseudodiverticula, and most result from pulsion due to increased intraluminal pressure and intestinal dysmotility.

DUODENAL DIVERTICULA

EPIDEMIOLOGY

Duodenal diverticula are the most common type of small bowel diverticula and are found in up to 23% of autopsies and in as many as 27% of patients undergoing upper endoscopy procedures.[1] Duodenal diverticula are intraluminal or extraluminal, with the former being congenital and quite rare. Extraluminal duodenal diverticula are much more common, second in incidence only to large bowel diverticula. Unlike intraluminal diverticula that develop in utero, the extraluminal type usually develop in the fifth decade of life or later.

PATHOGENESIS

An intraluminal duodenal diverticulum begins to form in utero as a duodenal web, most often in the second portion of the duodenum. This web becomes stretched over time by peristaltic flow creating a saclike shape within the lumen of the duodenum that becomes a false diverticulum. If the apex of the diverticulum does not have an opening and remains closed, neonatal duodenal obstruction will occur.

An extraluminal diverticulum, like those most commonly seen in the colon, is acquired. It is most often located within 2 cm of the ampulla of Vater. It is a false diverticulum that contains only the mucosa and submucosa that herniated between the muscle at sites of weakness in the bowel wall. These areas of weakness are usually where the blood supply to the bowel creates small structural defects, allowing the mucosa and submucosa to herniate outward.[2]

CLINICAL PRESENTATION

Although duodenal diverticula are relatively common, only 12% of patients will develop symptoms. The most commonly reported symptoms are postprandial epigastric pain, bloating, nausea, vomiting, and gastrointestinal bleeding. Because most of these symptoms can be caused by other more common gastrointestinal problems, the diagnosis is often delayed or missed.[1]

Like diverticular disease of the colon, duodenal diverticula can lead to complications that include perforation, bleeding, infection, and obstruction. The incidence of obstruction from an intraluminal diverticulum is much more common given its anatomic location within the lumen of the duodenum. There have even been case reports of duodenal diverticula causing obstruction of the ampulla of Vater that resulted in biliary obstruction and pancreatitis.[1] For the far more common extraluminal type, perforation and bleeding are more often seen.

DIAGNOSIS

Duodenal diverticula can be diagnosed under direct visualization with esophagogastroduodenoscopy (EGD) or endoscopic retrograde cholangiopancreatography (ERCP), which can also be used for therapeutic treatment. Radiographic means of diagnosis are less invasive and are considered more appropriate initial methods of evaluation. Fluoroscopy can reliably identify duodenal diverticula with an upper GI study and small bowel follow-through. The classic "wind-sock" sign describes the saclike projection of an intraluminal duodenal diverticulum outlined by oral contrast within the duodenum. Extraluminal duodenal diverticula can be similar in appearance to those seen in the colon as an outpouching. Computed tomography (CT) with oral and intravenous (IV) contrast along with magnetic resonance cholangiopancreatography can also be helpful diagnostic modalities.[2]

MANAGEMENT

Less than 1% of patients with duodenal diverticula require invasive endoscopic or surgical interventions. Among those who require surgery, the morbidity and mortality can be quite high. Endoscopy is an appropriate means of controlling hemorrhage and ERCP is often effective in relieving biliary and pancreatic obstruction with sphincterotomy and stent placement, although there is a risk of perforation if a sphincterotomy is performed and the diverticulum is in close proximity to the ampulla of Vater.[1]

Perforation, if not contained, must be managed surgically. The morbidity and mortality are higher for diverticula in close proximity to the ampulla. During surgical exploration, a Kocher maneuver is performed to allow thorough evaluation of the duodenum (Fig. 77.1). Diverticulectomy may be feasible if there is adequate distance from the ampulla. If the diverticulum is close, the ampulla should be cannulated to avoid injury. Once the diverticulum is resected, the duodenum should be closed in two layers transversely to avoid stricture and can be buttressed with an omental or jejunal patch.

Biliary and enteric diversions have been described if the diverticulum is very close to or involves the ampulla. Even more invasive means such as pancreaticoduodenectomy have been reported with a relatively low risk of complications, but there is not adequate data at this time to justify its use in all cases. In the setting of perforation where diverticulectomy cannot be safely performed or if the patient is not a surgical candidate, wide drainage and antibiotics can sometimes serve as definitive management.[1,3]

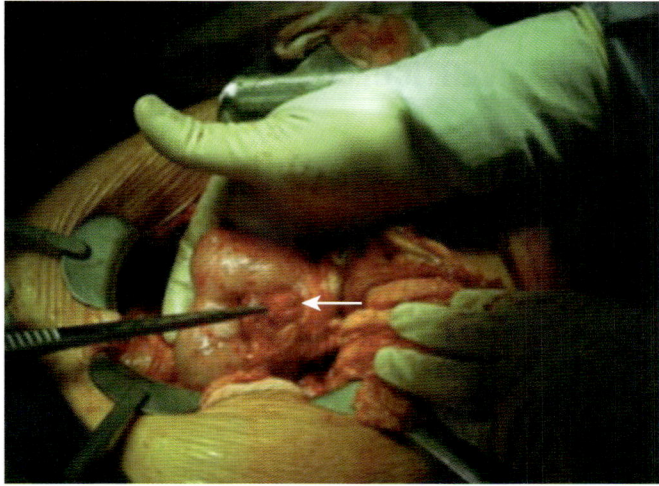

FIGURE 77.1 Intraoperative findings of a duodenal diverticulum (*arrow*) in relation to the head of the pancreas after the duodenum has been mobilized. (From Teven CM, Grossman E, Roggin KK, Mathews JB. Surgical management of pancreaticobiliary disease associated with juxtapapillary duodenal diverticula: case series and review of the literature. *J Gastrointest Surg.* 2012;16:1436–1441.)

JEJUNOILEAL DIVERTICULA

EPIDEMIOLOGY

Jejunal and ileal diverticula are the least common small bowel diverticula, with an incidence of 0.2% to 5% based on imaging and autopsy data. The incidence peaks around the sixth or seventh decade of life. Jejunal diverticula are seven to eight times more common than ileal diverticula.[4] Most patients will have numerous diverticula in the jejunum with a decrease in frequency moving distally toward the ileum. It is estimated that 60% to 70% of patients with jejunoileal diverticula are asymptomatic. Of those patients who develop chronic symptoms or acute complications, only 10% will require surgery.[5]

PATHOGENESIS

Jejunoileal diverticula are false diverticula that penetrate through the mesenteric side of the bowel. They are considered to be acquired rather than congenital, and while the exact pathogenesis is unknown, it is thought to be a result of smooth muscle dysfunction or a defect in the myenteric plexus. Similar to extraluminal duodenal diverticula, this results in irregular bowel contractions, increased intraluminal pressure, and subsequent pulsion of the mucosa and submucosa at weakened areas where the vasa recta enter the small intestine.[5] Because jejunoileal diverticula are usually buried within the mesentery, they are often overlooked during surgical exploration.

CLINICAL PRESENTATION

Although jejunoileal diverticula are the least common small bowel diverticula, they are the most likely to be symptomatic as a result of complications that include diverticulitis with or without perforation, hemorrhage, and obstruction. Diverticulitis is the most common presentation, accounting for up to 55% of complications. Clinically, patients have localized or diffuse abdominal pain, fever, and leukocytosis. Imaging may reveal an inflammatory mass, abscess, fat stranding, or air within the mesentery. Most perforations will be walled off by the surrounding mesentery or small bowel. The presentation and imaging may be suspicious for perforated colonic diverticulitis or appendicitis depending on the location of the abscess. The mortality rate for perforated diverticulitis can reach 50% due to the difficulty, and subsequent delay, in diagnosis.[5,6]

Hemorrhage from a jejunoileal diverticulum can be seen in 5% to 33% of patients with acute symptomatic disease. Bleeding results from inflammation of a diverticulum near a mesenteric vessel that erodes into the vessel. These patients often present with painless bright red blood per rectum, although they may also present with melena or hematemesis. Due to the location of the diverticula, endoscopic intervention is unsuccessful at controlling the hemorrhage. Colonoscopy and upper endoscopy can be helpful to rule out proximal and distal sources of gastrointestinal hemorrhage. If bleeding has not been identified on endoscopy, a radiolabeled red blood cell scan or angiography may be performed to better delineate the location of bleeding. The mortality associated with massive hemorrhage from jejunoileal diverticula is approximately 80%, but decreases with early diagnosis and prompt surgical resection of the diseased segment of small bowel.[4,7] Bowel obstruction due to jejunoileal diverticulosis is the least common complication and results from a broad array of etiologies. Strictures and adhesions from prior diverticulitis, an inflammatory mass causing extrinsic compression of the bowel, volvulus of a segment with large diverticula, and pseudoobstruction due to function dysmotility can all lead to symptoms of abdominal distention, nausea, and vomiting. A diverticulum can also act as a lead point for intussusception. Finally, enteroliths can form within a diverticulum due to stasis. The enterolith can obstruct the bowel lumen when it is dislodged from the diverticulum. If surgical intervention is indicated due to a complete obstruction, the enterolith may be milked into the distal bowel and removed through an enterotomy in a healthy segment of bowel. Alternatively, it can be resected along with the diverticular disease, especially in the setting of associated inflammation.[4]

DIAGNOSIS

Diagnosing jejunoileal diverticular disease is challenging. Often the diagnosis is made intraoperatively. Different imaging modalities have been used with varying success over the years. Occasionally, plain films will show air–fluid levels within diverticula. An upper gastrointestinal series with small bowel follow-through and enteroclysis can be both diagnostic and therapeutic. Although enteroclysis is a more sensitive diagnostic test, it is expensive and can cause discomfort for the patient. The diagnosis can also be made on delayed images where contrast is retained within a diverticulum even after the enteric contrast has moved through the small bowel lumen. In the acute presentation, CT is useful to assess for complications related to jejunoileal diverticulosis and rule out other etiologies (Fig. 77.2).[5] Capsule endoscopy and double balloon enteroscopy can visualize diverticula as well; their use, however, is often limited in the setting of acute inflammation.

MANAGEMENT

Asymptomatic jejunoileal diverticula should be left alone when discovered incidentally. However, patients who experience complications related to small bowel diverticular disease should undergo segmental resection with primary anastomosis. There is no role for invagination of diverticula or simple diverticulectomy because this results in poor blood flow, ischemia, and a high leak rate. Nonoperative management may be pursued in more chronic cases that present with vague abdominal pain, bloating, or symptoms of bacterial overgrowth and malnutrition. Antibiotics and vitamin supplementation may provide benefit for these patients. A conservative approach is also indicated for patients with extensive disease where surgical resection would result in short gut syndrome. Select cases of uncomplicated diverticulitis are successfully managed with antibiotics as well, but appropriate patient selection remains paramount. If there are any signs of hemodynamic instability, sepsis, or peritonitis, surgical resection is recommended.

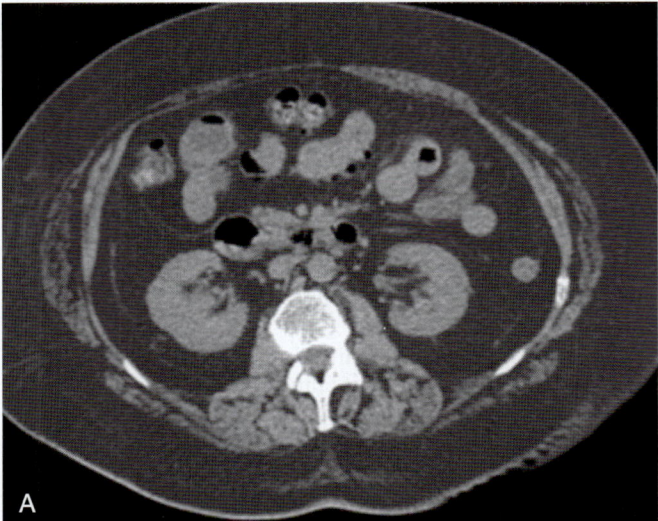

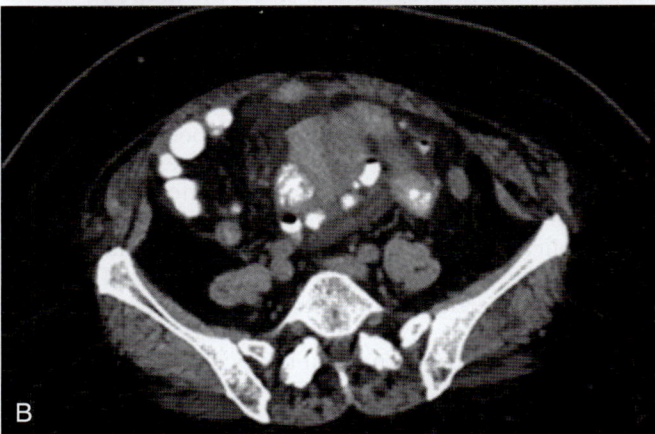

FIGURE 77.2 (A) Computed tomography of a jejunoileal diverticulum in a patient treated with antibiotics and (B) elective resection 4 weeks later.

MECKEL DIVERTICULUM

EPIDEMIOLOGY

Named after the German anatomist and embryologist Johann Meckel, a Meckel diverticulum is the most common congenital anomaly of the small intestine. We are taught to think of a Meckel diverticulum in terms of the *Rule of 2s*: located 2 feet (60 cm) from the terminal ileum, 2 inches in length, affecting 2% of the general population, occurring twice as often in males, containing one or two types of heterotopic mucosa (most commonly gastric or pancreatic), and presenting in the first 2 decades of life, most commonly in the first 2 years of life. While this catchy phase is easy to remember and captures the most common presentations of Meckel diverticula, it does not expand on how the diagnosis is made, the indications for surgical intervention, and what surgery entails. This section will focus on these issues.

PATHOGENESIS

To understand what a Meckel diverticulum is and why, unlike duodenal and jejunoileal diverticula, it is a true diverticulum, we must revisit our embryology. In the third week of gestation, the vitelline duct, also called the omphalomesenteric duct, is widely patent allowing the yolk sac to communicate with the gut. Between the fifth and ninth week of gestation, the duct will obliterate and the placenta replaces the yolk sac as the source of fetal nutrition. If the vitelline duct fails to obliterate, a Meckel diverticulum can result. This is why a Meckel diverticulum is a true diverticulum—and the only true diverticulum—of the small intestine that contains all layers of the small bowel.

Interestingly, failure of the vitelline duct to obliterate can result in other anomalies, although these are much less common than a Meckel diverticulum. Such anomalies include an ileal umbilical fistula, which occurs if the entire duct remains patent; a vitelline duct cyst, which results from the failure of the umbilical side of the duct to obliterate; and a fibrous cord connecting the ileum to the umbilicus. A Meckel diverticulum is by far the most common, representing 90% of vitelline duct anomalies.[8]

Up to 60% of Meckel diverticula have heterotopic mucosa. Although pancreatic tissue is the most common type of heterotopic tissue, gastric tissue is the most common type in a symptomatic Meckel diverticulum, as later discussed. A Meckel diverticulum is usually positioned within 100 cm of the ileocecal valve, although the mean distance varies with age: the older the patient, the farther away the Meckel diverticulum is from the ileocecal valve. In children less than 2 years of age, the mean distance is 34 cm, compared to 46 cm in children aged 3 to 21 years old and 67 cm in people older than 21 years.

CLINICAL PRESENTATION

It is rare for a Meckel diverticulum to be symptomatic. Symptoms only occur in 2% to 4% of cases.[9] Patients can present with colicky abdominal pain, vomiting, and diarrhea from a broad range of complications that include obstruction, intussusception, diverticulitis, and perforation. Patients can also present with gastrointestinal bleeding, although this is more common in children. Bleeding can present as bright red rectal bleeding or painless, slow, intermittent melena.

In adults, the most common type of complication is intestinal obstruction, accounting for approximately one-third of complications (Table 77.1). Mechanisms of obstruction include enlargement of the small bowel around a fibrous band attached to the umbilicus, entrapment of an intestinal loop within a mesodiverticular band, intussusception with a free diverticulum acting as a lead point, volvulus around an umbilical band, and stenosis secondary to chronic diverticulitis.

Diverticulitis occurs in approximately 20% of patients with a symptomatic Meckel diverticulum and is arguably indistinguishable from acute appendicitis in both presentation and potential complications, including necrosis and perforation.[9] A Meckel diverticulum may also be present in an inguinal or femoral hernia sac resulting in a Littre hernia. Between 0.5% and 3.2% of symptomatic Meckel diverticula are tumors, of which the most common are carcinoid.[10]

In children, bleeding is one of the more common complications of symptomatic Meckel diverticula. A review

TABLE 77.1 Adult Complications From a Meckel Diverticulum

Type of Complication	Incidence (%)
Intestinal obstruction	37
Intussusception	14
Diverticulitis	13
Hemorrhage	12
Perforation	7
Component of hernia sac	5
Volvulus	3
Neoplasm	3

From Yamaguchi M, Takeuchi S, Awazu S. Meckel's diverticulum investigation of 600 patients in the Japanese literature. *Am J Surg.* 1978;136:247–249.

TABLE 77.2 Pediatric Complications From a Meckel Diverticulum in Children Younger Than 18 Years of Age

Type of Complication	Incidence (%)
Intestinal obstruction	30.0
Hemorrhage	27.0
Intussusception	19.0
Omphalitis	0.4

From Ruscher KA, Fisher JN, Hughes CD, et al. National trends in the surgical management of Meckel's diverticulum. *J Pediatr Surg.* 2011;46:893–896.

of 815 children with Meckel diverticula conducted by Ruscher et al. found that bleeding occurred in 27% of symptomatic cases (Table 77.2), whereas other studies have cited this to be as much as 50% of all complications.[9,11] Bleeding occurs when gastric heterotopic mucosa is present in a Meckel diverticulum. The ectopic gastric mucosa can produce gastric acid and pepsin, which can cause ileal ulceration and subsequent bleeding. This is rare in patients older than 30 years of age because after this age, the gastric mucosa usually atrophies.

Several risk factors are associated with increased complication rates including age, gender, and anatomic variants of Meckel diverticula. The risk of complications is inversely related to age, with a 4% to 5% risk at 2 years of age and 1% at 40 years. By 75 years of age, there is a near zero percent risk of complication from a Meckel diverticulum.[12] It is estimated that 50% of patients who develop symptoms are younger than 10 years of age. Symptomatic Meckel diverticula are more common in men than women with a male-to-female ratio ranging from 2:1 to 5:1. Anatomically, longer, narrow-based diverticula are more likely to cause obstruction or inflammation as compared to short, large-based diverticula, which are more prone to entrapment.

DIAGNOSIS

Less than 10% of symptomatic Meckel diverticula are diagnosed preoperatively.[9] Radiographic imaging, such as CT and ultrasound, is limited because it is often difficult to distinguish between a diverticulum and intestinal loops of bowel. A Meckel diverticulum should be considered in patients with right lower quadrant pain or signs of acute appendicitis and intraoperatively are found to have a normal-appearing appendix. In this case, the recommended surgical practice is to examine the small bowel for a Meckel diverticulum.

If gastrointestinal bleeding is present, a ^{99m}Tc-pertechnetate scintigraphy (also referred to as a Meckel scan) may be obtained. On imaging, a Meckel diverticulum is identified as a focus of activity in the lower abdomen or upper pelvis that generally appears at the time the stomach is visualized and increases as the stomach activity increases. ^{99m}Tc-pertechnetate is the radiopharmaceutical of choice because it localizes to gastric mucosa.[13] Because the scan requires heterotopic gastric mucosa to take up the radiotracer, it is only useful when gastric tissue is present; in adults with atrophic gastric mucosa, the scan has a much lower sensitivity (60% to 85%) compared to its specificity (95% to 96%).[14,15]

If there is a high clinical suspicion for a Meckel diverticulum with a negative Meckel scan, a hybrid single photon emission computed tomography/computed tomography (SPECT/CT) may be useful. A SPECT/CT allows precise localization of activity at an abnormal anatomic structure and has become more favorable in recent years.[16] However, most symptomatic Meckel diverticula are still diagnosed at the time of exploration. Operative intervention is arguably the gold standard in making the diagnosis compared to an expensive, and at times, low-yield radiographic workup.

MANAGEMENT

For a symptomatic Meckel diverticulum, surgical resection is indicated. In the asymptomatic patient, indications for surgical intervention have been the subject of many studies, but despite these studies, the topic remains controversial. Part of the controversy is that older, retrospective reviews cite high rates of morbidity and mortality following diverticular resection. Historically, studies from the 1950s reported a mortality rate of 20% from a diverticulectomy.[17] In the 1970s, this decreased to an average of 7%. Since the 1980s, studies have repeatedly reported a near-zero mortality rate, changing the dogma on surgical management.

The current recommendation is that unless there are strong contraindications, an incidentally discovered Meckel diverticulum should be removed.[18] Specially, if found incidentally, resection is indicated for any of the following criteria: patients younger than 50 years of age, a Meckel diverticulum longer than 2 cm, the presence of a fibrous band, or evidence of heterotopic mucosa (Table 77.3). Strong contraindications include Crohn disease.

The principles of resection are similar for symptomatic and asymptomatic Meckel diverticula: the diverticulum and any associated bands should be removed with an ileal resection or a simple diverticulectomy. The decision of which treatment option to pursue lies in whether the patient presents with bleeding. Bleeding usually results

from an ulcer in the heterotopic gastric mucosa and the ulcer along with the Meckel diverticulum should be excised with an ileal resection. This can be achieved using a stapler to divide the small bowel just proximal and distal to the diverticulum (Fig. 77.3). A primary anastomosis is then performed and the small bowel mesenteric rent is closed.

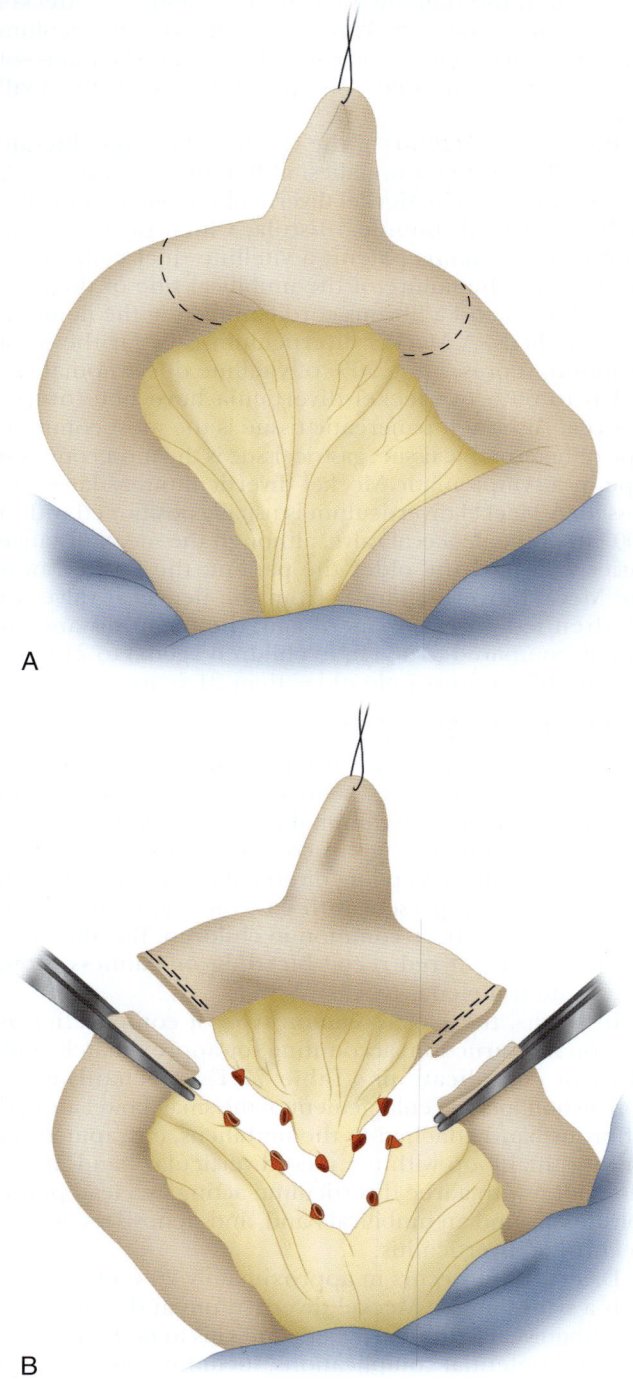

A

B

FIGURE 77.3 For a bleeding Meckel diverticulum, an ileal resection is performed (A) with control of the proximal and distal bowel content using bowel clamps (B) prior to creating an anastomosis. (From Chung DH. Meckel's diverticulectomy. In: Townsend CM Jr, Evers BM, eds. *Atlas of General Surgery Techniques*. Philadelphia: Saunders; 2010.)

TABLE 77.3 Indications to Resect an Incidentally Found Meckel Diverticulum

Patient <40 years of age
Meckel diverticulum longer than 2 cm
Presence of a fibrous band
Evidence of heterotopic mucosa

In the absence of bleeding, a V-shaped diverticulectomy can be performed with a transverse closure to avoid narrowing of the lumen (Fig. 77.4). A two-layer closure is often used with an inner running layer of absorbable suture followed by an outer layer of silk Lembert sutures. Additionally, several studies in children with symptomatic Meckel diverticula show that a laparoscopic approach is safe, feasible, and may improve outcomes.[11,19]

CONCLUSION

Small bowel diverticula are rarely symptomatic because they are in continuity with the lumen and function as part of the small bowel lumen. However, when they are symptomatic, diverticula can become inflamed, perforate, obstruct, and bleed. Bleeding from a duodenal or jejunoileal diverticulum results from blood vessels associated with the vasa recta. Bleeding from a Meckel diverticulum is a result of ulceration from the acid secretion from heterotopic gastric mucosa. A duodenal diverticulum can present a unique surgical challenge given its close proximity to the ampulla of Vater. Jejunoileal diverticula are the least common type of small bowel diverticula, but are most likely to produce symptoms. It is for these reasons that the general surgeon should be well versed in the diagnosis and management of small bowel diverticula.

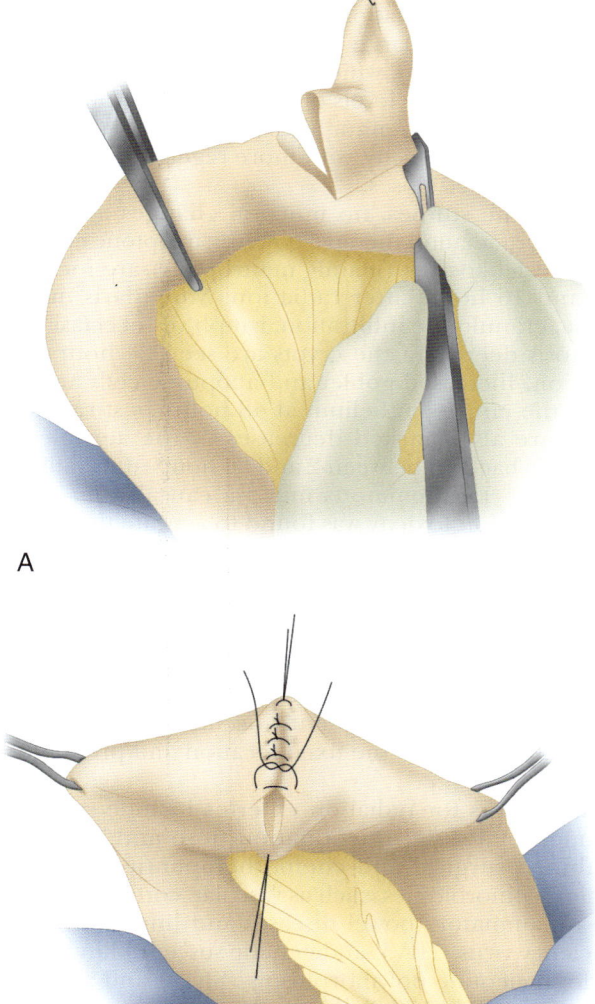

FIGURE 77.4 For a nonbleeding Meckel diverticulum, a V-shaped diverticulectomy (A) is performed with a two-layer transverse closure (B). (From Chung DH. Meckel's diverticulectomy. In: Townsend CM Jr, Evers BM, eds. *Atlas of General Surgery Techniques*. Philadelphia: Saunders; 2010.)

REFERENCES

1. Teven CM, Grossman E, Roggin KK, Mathews JB. Surgical management of pancreaticobiliary disease associated with juxtapapillary duodenal diverticula: case series and review of the literature. *J Gastrointest Surg*. 2012;16:1436-1441.
2. Schroeder TC, Hartman M, Heller M, Klepchick P, Ilkhanipour K. Duodenal diverticula: potential complications and common imaging pitfalls. *Clin Radiol*. 2014;69:1072-1076.
3. Kouraklis G, Glinavou A, Mantas D, Kouskos E, Karatzas G. Clinical implications of small bowel diverticula. *Isr Med Assoc J*. 2002;4:431-433.
4. Makris K, Tsiotos GG, Stafyla V, Ponsky J, Shuck JM. Small intestinal nonmeckelian diverticulosis. *J Clin Gastroenterol*. 2009;43:201-207.
5. Woods K, Williams E, Melvin W, Sharp K. Acquired jejunoileal diverticulosis and its complications: a review of the literature. *Am Surg*. 2008;74:849-854.
6. Kassahun WT, Fangmann J, Harms J, Bartels M, Hauss J. Complicated small-bowel diverticulosis: a case report and review of the literature. *World J Gastroenterol*. 2007;13:2240-2242.
7. Yen HH, Chen YY, Yang CW, Soon MS. Diagnosis and management of jejunoileal diverticular hemorrhage: a decade of experience. *J Dig Dis*. 2012;13:316-320.
8. Turgeon DK, Barnett JL. Meckel's diverticulum. *Am J Gastroenterol*. 1990;85:777-781.
9. Yahchouchy EK, Marano AF, Etienne JC, Fingerhut AL. Meckel's diverticulum. *J Am Coll Surg*. 2001;192:658-662.
10. Caracappa D, Gulla N, Lombardo F, et al. Incidental finding of carcinoid tumor on Meckel's diverticulum: case report and literature review, should prophylactic resection be recommended? *World J Surg Oncol*. 2014;12:144.
11. Ruscher KA, Fisher JN, Hughes CD, et al. National trends in the surgical management of Meckel's diverticulum. *J Pediatr Surg*. 2011; 46:893-896.
12. Leijonmarck CE, Bonman-Sandelin K, Frisell J, Räf L. Meckel's diverticulum in the adult. *Br J Surg*. 1986;73:146-149.
13. Ziessman H, O'Malley J, Thrall J. *Nuclear Medicine: The Requisites*. Philadelphia: Elsevier Saunders; 2013.
14. Sfakianakis GN, Conway JJ. Detection of ectopic gastric mucosa in Meckel's diverticulum and in other aberrations by scintigraphy: ii. Indications and methods—a 10-year experience. *J Nucl Med*. 1981; 22:732-738.
15. Swaniker F, Soldes O, Hirschl RB. The utility of technetium 99m pertechnetate scintigraphy in the evaluation of patients with Meckel's diverticulum. *J Pediatr Surg*. 1999;34:760-764, [discussion 765].
16. Dillman JR, Wong KK, Brown RK, Frey KA, Strouse PJ. Utility of SPECT/CT with Meckel's scintigraphy. *Ann Nucl Med*. 2009;23:813-815.
17. Wansbrough RM, Thomson S, Leckey RG. Meckel's diverticulum: a 42-year review of 273 cases at the Hospital for Sick Children, Toronto. *Can J Surg*. 1957;1:15-21.
18. Cullen JJ, Kelly KA, Moir CR, et al. Surgical management of Meckel's diverticulum. An epidemiologic, population-based study. *Ann Surg*. 1994;220:564-568, [discussion 568–569].
19. Chan KW, Lee KH, Mou JW, Cheung ST, Tam YH. Laparoscopic management of complicated Meckel's diverticulum in children: a 10-year review. *Surg Endosc*. 2008;22:1509-1512.

Radiation Enteritis

Asish D. Patel | Jon S. Thompson

The first record of radiation enteritis was described in 1897 and involved transient symptoms of pain and diarrhea that correlated with radiation exposure. The symptoms did not return after a lead shield was used during the experiments.[1] Fifty to 70% of patients with malignancy undergo radiation therapy.[2,3] Symptoms of acute radiation enteritis (ARE) are reported in a majority of patients. The incidence of chronic radiation enteritis (CRE) is reported between 1.2% and 15% of patients undergoing radiation therapy and appears within months and up to decades after completion of treatment.[4-6] Because more patients are receiving radiation treatment and living longer, an increasing number of patients are at risk for CRE. The scope of this chapter will include radiation injury to the small intestine and colon. Radiation injury to the rectum, referred to as radiation proctitis, will not be discussed here.

ETIOLOGY

Ionizing radiation (IR) consists of photon-based (x-rays and gamma rays) or particle radiation. Photon radiation is used most commonly for cancer treatment. High-energy photons create ionizing electrons that then directly break chemical bonds. X-rays or gamma rays create 1000 ionization tracks per Gray (Gy) and mainly produce reactive oxygen species from water, such as hydroxyl radicals, singlet oxygen, superoxide, and hydrogen peroxide that indirectly cause damage within cells.[7] The role of oxygen is critical for the effects of free radicals to be effective. Oxygen not only can participate in the cascade of free radical generation, but it can also "fix" damage in biologic molecules and so prevent its repair. Hypoxia is one cause of radiation treatment failure.[7]

DNA damage is the hallmark of radiation therapy. Most DNA damage from daily environmental exposure occurs in the form of single-strand breaks and base damage, which is repaired by base excision repair. However, IR causes complex damage consisting of 15 to 20 double-strand breaks per cell per Gy. Double-strand breaks can also be repaired through nonhomologous end joining and homologous recombination; however, the complex damage of IR may overwhelm these repair mechanisms.[7]

CLINICAL FEATURES AND PATHOPHYSIOLOGY OF INJURY

Radiation can cause acute and chronic gastrointestinal toxicity (Table 78.1). Acute effects secondary to radiation therapy in the gastrointestinal tract occur due to depletion of the radiation-sensitive progenitor cells from which the mature cells are derived. ARE can occur with doses as low as 5 to 12 Gy.[8] Tissue function is then maintained by the nonproliferating differentiated cells until they are also depleted after normal cell turnover. Despite depletion of dividing crypt cells within days of irradiation in the small bowel, symptoms of acute toxicity will take approximately 2 weeks to manifest because the nonproliferative villi do not show immediate depletion following irradiation but rather slough into the lumen over time. The quiescent stem cell population is few in number and gives rise to the progenitor population. Lethal toxicity may occur due to depletion of the large progenitor population, not the stem cell population, which is considered radioresistant possibly due to high levels of antioxidants. However, the regeneration of progenitor and stem cells determines the severity of acute toxicity, with more regeneration allowed with fractionated doses.[7]

In murine studies, no mucosal changes are seen 2 hours after radiation therapy; however, apoptotic epithelial cells and leukocytes (mainly neutrophils) are increased at 6 and 16 hours after radiation. Muscularis mucosa edema, granulocyte infiltration, lymph vessel ectasia, and apoptosis deeper in the crypts are seen 24 hours after radiation. Increased goblet and apoptotic cells are seen across the entire epithelium at 48 hours post radiation. There are also marked decreases in the aerobic and anaerobic bacteria between 2 and 24 hours after radiation treatment.[9] Erythematous mucosa can also be seen.[10] Acute radiation toxicity was found to activate the Fas and glycolysis pathways in mice, both pathways that can induce cell apoptosis and activate inflammation.[11]

CRE is characterized by fibroblast and collagen proliferation, as well as obliterative vasculitis causing transmural injury.[4,5] Fibrosis is the end result, and transforming growth factor beta (TGF-β) plays a critical role in the mechanism.[5,12,13] CRE most frequently occurs in the ileum and ileocecal valve, given the fixed location and proximity to the pelvis.

Risk factors for radiation enteritis include treatment volume; total dose; fractionation dose and schedules; combined surgical and chemotherapeutic modalities; medical comorbidities, such as vascular, connective tissue, and inflammatory bowel diseases and human immunodeficiency virus (HIV); and genetic susceptibility, such as single nucleotide polymorphisms (SNPs) and ataxia telangiectasia (Table 78.2).[14] Prior laparotomy is also a risk factor for CRE, and studies have shown a 4.25 increased rate of late gastrointestinal complications in irradiated patients.[15] The majority of patients requiring surgical intervention for CRE have undergone radiation due to gynecologic (62%) and rectal cancers (22% to 36%).[16,17]

The degree of normal tissue toxicity in the small bowel depends not only on the dose of radiation but also on the amount of bowel irradiated. However, studies trying

TABLE 78.1 Features of Acute and Chronic Radiation Enteritis

Acute	Chronic
INCIDENCE	
75%–80%	1.2%–15%
TIMING	
2–4 weeks	6–24 months
HISTOLOGY	
Inflammatory infiltrate	Obliterative endarteritis
Reduced crypt mitosis	Fibrosis
Crypt microabscesses	Lymphatic dilation
Ulceration	Tissue ischemia and necrosis
CAUSES OF SYMPTOMS	
Malabsorption	Obstruction(stricture, adhesions)
Bacterial overgrowth	Fistula
	Intestinal failure (malabsorption, short bowel syndrome)
	Neoplasia (recurrent or new)

TABLE 78.2 Risk Factors for Radiation Enteritis

Risk Factors

Volume of small bowel in field
Radiation dose and fractionation
Radiation technique
Concomitant chemotherapy
Prior intestinal surgery
Medical comorbidities

to determine toxicity to small bowel have used inconsistent methods of measuring the small bowel. Predictive models of toxicity show that the volume of small bowel receiving greater than 15 Gy should be restricted to less than 120 mL if individual bowel loops are delineated; however, if the entire peritoneal cavity that the small bowel can move is delineated, radiation greater than 45 Gy should be limited to 195 mL.[15] Radiation doses are generally limited to 4500 to 5000 cGy due to small bowel toxicity.

Other risk factors include euthyroid sick syndrome, which consists of low triiodothyronine (T_3) levels.[18] A multivariate analysis found that chemotherapy was associated with CRE (odds ratio [OR] = 3.59, 1.20 to 10.73).[19] ARE has also been associated with the development of subsequent CRE.[19,20]

CRE accounts for the major morbidity of IR. Twenty percent of patients were found to have CRE in a survey study of 100 patients who received radiation therapy due to prostate, cervical, endometrial, or rectal cancer. Three percent reported requiring hospitalization due to diarrhea or bowel obstruction.[19] Radiation enteritis accounted for 11% of cases in a review of 688 adults with chronic intestinal failure from benign disease resulting in long-term parenteral nutrition (PN). These patients suffered from short bowel syndrome (SBS), motility disorders, and extensive parenchymal disease.[21] Patients with SBS on PN with a history of irradiation had significantly higher rates of cirrhosis and portal hypertension compared

with nonirradiated SBS patients on PN.[22] A prospective longitudinal study of 27 patients undergoing pelvic and/or abdominal irradiation with follow-up time of 2 years found that at least one parameter of bowel function was abnormal in 16 of 18 patients who completed all measurements. Significantly changed parameters included increased stool frequency, decreased bile acid absorption, and more rapid small intestinal transit time.[23] Malabsorption of carbohydrates and bile salts occurs from loss of villi, and fat malabsorption occurs due to bacterial overgrowth. Kong et al. reported a significant increase in the etiology of SBS secondary to radiation enteritis in recent years in China (17% of SBS cases from 2004 to 2009 vs. 26% from 2009 to 2010; $P < .05$).[24] Neoadjuvant chemoradiotherapy has become standard for rectal cancer. Zakaria et al. reported two cases of efferent loop terminal ileum obstruction secondary to radiation enteritis discovered after takedown of ileostomy after proctectomy due to rectal cancer.[25]

Intestinal failure can be due to malabsorption secondary to anatomic SBS or functional SBS secondary to mucosal damage.[26] Anatomic SBS is secondary to surgical resection or fistula that can bypass segments of small bowel. Functional SBS is characterized by mucosal damage in the setting of adequate small bowel length.[26] Intestinal failure secondary to CRE has a worse prognosis (approximately 70% survival rate at 5 years) compared with other causes of SBS.[27] In their analysis, death secondary to recurrent cancer was censored, and so the underlying pathology of CRE-induced intestinal failure truly affected survival. Various studies have reported that between 3% and 14% of patients requiring home PN do so because of CRE.[26]

DIAGNOSIS

Radiation enteritis is characterized by a multitude of symptoms.[28] Manifestations of ARE include abdominal pain, nausea, vomiting, and diarrhea and typically resolves in 2 to 6 weeks. Small intestinal bacterial overgrowth may play a role in ARE, and lab tests to help to confirm this etiology of diarrhea include serum erythrocyte sedimentation rate or C-reactive protein, duodenal aspirate, or glucose hydrogen methane breath test.[28,29] CRE will manifest with more severe symptoms of malabsorption, such as debilitating diarrhea requiring replacement, steatorrhea, anorexia, and weight loss. It can also present with gastrointestinal hemorrhage and ulceration.[14,28] Investigation for radiation enteritis depends upon the symptoms and will involve either esophagogastroduodenoscopy, colonoscopy, or computed tomography/magnetic resonance of the abdomen with or without enteroclysis.[8] Capsule endoscopy can be used to identify mucosal atrophy, mucosal edema, stricturing, and bleeding for CRE.[30]

Recurrence of malignancy must always be ruled out with worsening symptoms and increasing malnutrition. Twelve percent of patients with weight loss and nonspecific abdominal complaints after prior radiation for pelvic malignancies were found to have recurrent cancer.[26] Regimbeau reported a 14% mortality rate due to recurrent cancer in 107 patients who underwent surgical intervention for CRE.[16] Boland et al. reported a mortality rate of 35% in patients with resultant SBS secondary to CRE due to underlying malignancy.[17]

A major challenge in diagnosing radiation injury is the lack of signs prior to symptom onset. Biomarkers for signs of radiation injury are being investigated; however, none have been used in clinical practice. Gut barrier function and enterocyte transport have been assessed by measuring absorption of bile acids, vitamin B_{12}, glucose, and isotope nuclear scintography. Other markers studied include diamine oxidase, fatty acid binding proteins, and calprotectin; however, these have also not proved clinically useful due to low sensitivity, specificity, or inability to localize the injury.[31]

A clinically useful biomarker for radiation enteritis must be tissue specific, have a dose and volume response relationship, not be affected by other medical conditions, and be easily accessible. Plasma citrulline, an end product of enterocyte glutamine metabolism, is one such marker that has been studied in a variety of conditions affecting the small bowel, rejection following small bowel transplant, celiac disease, and viral enteritis. Plasma citrulline in patients receiving myeloablative therapy for hematologic malignancies demonstrated that the marker correlated with mucosal damage and recovery.[32]

PREVENTION

Medical and surgical methods have been attempted at preventing radiation enteritis (Table 78.3). A randomized control trial looking at glutamine and the prevention of CRE did not find any difference in the rate of CRE development at 1 year, compared with placebo (relative risk ratio [RR] = 1.33, 0.35 to 5.03).[33] Triamcinolone was effective at preventing and treating grade 1 and 2 ARE ($P = .022$).[34] Pectin treatment before radiation was shown to increase intestinal stem cells by twofold.[35] Radioprotective agents, such as cysteine, amifostine, and L-carnitine, have also been used to reduce mucosal toxicity.[29] A randomized, double blind, placebo-controlled trial including gynecologic cancer patients receiving abdominal radiation therapy reported that prebiotics administration trended toward fewer days of watery diarrhea (3.3 vs. 2.2 days; $P = .08$).[36] Nutritional modifications have also been studied extensively in the prevention of radiation enteritis and have shown mixed results. A Cochrane systematic review found that fat restriction, lactose restriction, and fiber supplementation during pelvic radiotherapy were able to reduce diarrhea (RR = 0.66, 0.51 to 0.87).[37] However, a systemic review did not find enough evidence to support nutritional intervention during pelvic radiation to counteract ARE.[38]

Physical methods to reduce small bowel exposure to radiation include mesh slings to displace the small bowel out of the pelvis, supine versus prone positioning, tilting, bladder distention, shields, and belly board.[29] A case report also described that laparoscopic insertion of a pelvic expander allowed a patient with prostate cancer and loops of bowel low in the pelvis to receive radiotherapy without developing radiation enteritis.[39] Safety and efficacy of inserting a pelvic sling for radiotherapy in patients with pelvic malignancies and excessive small bowel in the pelvis were demonstrated in six patients.[40,41] Other surgical methods for prevention include reperitonealization, omental transposition flaps, abdominopelvic omentopexy, absorbable mesh slings, and occlusion of the pelvis with prosthetics, bladder, or uterus.[29]

TREATMENT

MEDICAL

Treatment of radiation enteritis depends on the etiology of the symptoms.[28] Conservative treatment includes antidiarrheals to decrease motility, cholestyramine for bile salt malabsorption, and antibiotics if bacterial overgrowth is identified.[29,42] Dietary modifications, such as fiber, fat reduction, and probiotics, may also help symptom management.

Hyperbaric oxygen increases angiogenesis in irradiated tissue.[43,44] A systematic review of this therapy demonstrated that a majority of studies had positive results for treatment or prevention of delayed radiation injury.[43,45]

SURGICAL

Approximately a third of patients with CRE require an operation. CRE requiring surgical intervention can present in four major ways: intestinal obstruction (65% to 80%), fistula (10% to 30%), perforation (1% to 10%), and intestinal failure (20%) (Figs. 78.1 and 78.2).[6,24,46] Surgical intervention can consist of bypass, resection/reanastomosis, or resection/ostomy. Given the challenges of resecting fibrosed and friable bowel, conventional teaching has favored bypass. However, current studies have shown the effectiveness of resection in appropriately selected patients, with results demonstrating improved morbidity and mortality, reoperative rates, and dependence on PN.

Surgical intervention for obstruction, fistula, perforation, or hemorrhage has a mortality between 0% and 5% and Clavien-Dindo grades II–IV morbidity between 20% and 40%.[16,47,48] Complications include recurrent obstruction, fistula, dehiscence, and PN dependence. Li et al. reported that 12% of patients undergoing resection were permanently dependent on PN and 6% of patients developed recurrent obstruction after surgery with a follow-up time of 3 to 128 months.[47] Zhang et al. reported significantly reduced hospital stay, stoma rate, and postoperative moderate to severe complications with the use of a clinical pathway to treat CRE patients.[49] One-fourth of CRE cases are emergent, with a reported mortality rate of 11%, which highlights the importance of preoperative preparation and appropriate patient selection.[16,17]

TABLE 78.3 Preventive Methods for Radiation Enteritis

Therapy Modifications	Medical	Surgical
Positioning (supine, prone, Trendelenburg)	Glutamine	Mesh slings
	Triamcinolone	Pelvic expander
	Pectin	Pelvic sling
Bladder distention	Cysteine	Reperitonealization
Shields (belly board)	Pentoxifylline/ tocopherol	Omental transposition flaps
	Amifostine	Abdominopelvic omentopexy
	L-Carnitine	
	Prebiotics	Occlusion of the pelvis with bladder/uterus

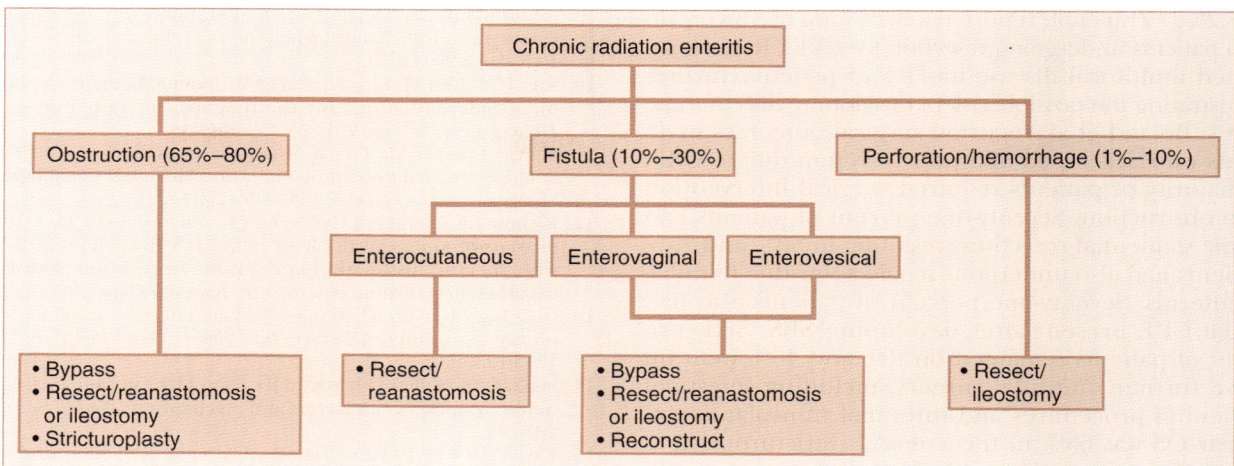

FIGURE 78.1 Surgical presentation of chronic radiation enteritis and treatment algorithm.

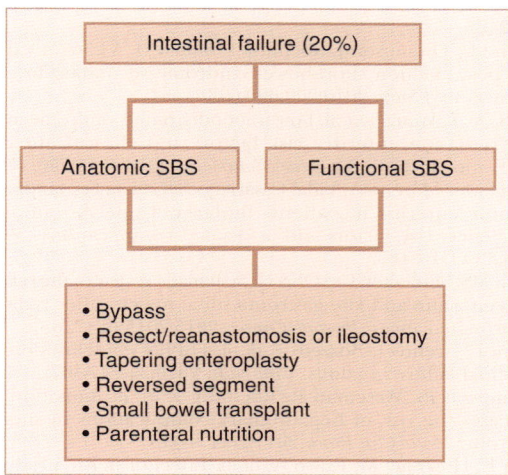

FIGURE 78.2 Treatment options for intestinal failure secondary to chronic radiation enteritis. *SBS*, Short bowel syndrome.

Retrospective studies comparing the outcomes of resection with conservative surgical treatment have demonstrated comparable or improved outcomes with resection. Reported stoma rates are also not significantly different between resection and conservative groups, with approximately half of patients receiving a stoma.[16,17] Even malnourished patients recovered well after preoperative nutrition and subsequent resection/reanastomosis.[6] The rate of complications has also been shown to be lower in groups undergoing resection-anastomosis compared with other procedures.[50] Perrin et al. found a significantly reduced reoperation rate in patients who underwent resection (47%) compared with conservative management (adhesiolysis, bypass, diverting stoma) (86%).[51] Lefevre et al. reported outcomes in 107 patients requiring surgical intervention for CRE, and the patients who did not undergo ileocecal resection had a significantly higher rate of reoperation (OR = 4.48, 2.52 to 8.31).[46] Zhu et al. reported 100% symptom resolution in 13 patients who underwent resection of a previously bypassed segment that had persistent obstruction, perforation, and

anastomotic dehiscence.[6] Stricturoplasty has also been used successfully to treat CRE patients with long segment strictures.[52] Historical dogma has always been to bypass when there is doubt. However, resection has comparable or improved outcomes compared with a more conservative approach of bypass for obstruction due to CRE. One possible reason for increased failure with bypass may be the formation of blind loop syndrome.[5]

Wound healing is also affected by radiation. A transverse incision had better outcomes than vertical, likely due to radiation-induced skin damage hindering healing.[5,6] Minimally invasive surgery is also an option to avoid wound problems, and laparoscopic surgery for intestinal stenosis secondary to radiation enteritis is a safe option. Wang et al. compared laparoscopic with open ileocolic resection and found no significant difference in postoperative morbidity.[53] However, laparoscopy should be used cautiously because the conversion rate was 23%.[53]

Enterovaginal fistulas are a rare complication of an irradiated pelvis. Lillemoe et al. reported significant morbidity and mortality in four patients who underwent resection for enterovaginal fistulas.[54] Deaths occurred within 2 years of the operation and secondary to sepsis, SBS, and worsening radiation enteritis. The surviving patient required reoperation due to ileostomy necrosis. Shafer et al. reported successful repair of recurrent enterovaginal fistulas in three women using a rectus abdominis muscle flap.[55] There is no consensus on the repair of enterovaginal fistulas; however, given the debilitating nature of the disease and the high morbidity, mortality, and recurrence associated with resection, both patient and surgeon will need to be prepared for postoperative complications.

Intestinal failure due to CRE is another indication for surgical intervention (see Fig. 78.2). Kalaiselvan et al. reported that 3.8% of intestinal failure cases were secondary to CRE over a 13-year period. They found that 96% of those intestinal failure patients had undergone laparotomy due to their CRE and that 56% still required home PN. Patients were admitted for intestinal failure due to obstruction, intractable weight loss, and/or high-output fistulas/stomas. The 10-year overall survival (OS) of the group was 48.2%.[56] Zhu et al. reported a 3.7% rate of SBS occurring in patients undergoing resection for CRE.[6] Regimbeau reported multifocal disease in 41% of patients, further demonstrating the possible risk of developing SBS in these patients. Boland et al. reported surgical outcomes in 48 patients who developed SBS post resection due to CRE. The majority of patients required surgical intervention due to obstruction. Seventy-one percent of patients had multiple sequential resections resulting in SBS, and 75% of patients had also undergone a colectomy due to radiation enteritis. Seventy-one percent of patients also had residual CRE present after developing SBS. Sixty-two percent of patients remained on PN, and 48% went on to have further intestinal surgery, including intestinal lengthening procedures and intestinal transplantation. Five-year OS was 68% in this cohort.[17] Stricturoplasty is also an effective option for PN-dependent patients with SBS secondary to chronic obstruction.[52] Amiot et al. reported the long-term outcomes of 107 patients who had undergone intestinal resection due to CRE with resultant SBS and concluded that survival was dependent upon existing comorbidities of residual neoplastic disease, American Society for Anesthesiologists class, and age at CRE diagnosis. They reported a 43% probability of dependence on home PN at 3 years post surgery, and dependence on PN significantly decreased with residual small bowel length greater than 100 cm, adaptive hyperphagia, and the absence of a permanent stoma.[4]

CONCLUSION

As the use of radiation for treatment of malignancy continues to increase, surgical intervention for the complications of CRE will increasingly be encountered. The safety and efficacy of resection has been established and is the preferred surgical intervention. However, the appropriate surgical method will depend on the patient's symptoms, nutritional state, remaining functional small bowel, and remission of cancer.

REFERENCES

1. Walsh D. Deep tissue traumatism from roentgen ray exposure. *Br Med J.* 1897;2:272-273.
2. Shadad AK, Sullivan FJ, Martin JD, Egan LJ. Gastrointestinal radiation injury: prevention and treatment. *World J Gastroenterol.* 2013;19:199-208.
3. Vidal-Casariego A, Calleja-Fernández A, de Urbina-González JJ, Cano-Rodríguez I, Cordido F, Ballesteros-Pomar MD. Efficacy of glutamine in the prevention of acute radiation enteritis: a randomized controlled trial. *JPEN J Parenter Enteral Nutr.* 2014;38:205-213.
4. Amiot A, Joly F, Lefevre JH, et al. Long-term outcome after extensive intestinal resection for chronic radiation enteritis. *Dig Liver Dis.* 2013;45:110-114.
5. Hogan NM, Kerin MJ, Joyce MR. Gastrointestinal complications of pelvic radiotherapy: medical and surgical management strategies. *Curr Probl Surg.* 2013;50:395-407.
6. Zhu W, Gong J, Li Y, Li N, Li J. A retrospective study of surgical treatment of chronic radiation enteritis. *J Surg Oncol.* 2012;105:632-636.
7. McBride WH, Withers HR. Biologic basis of radiation therapy. In: Halperin EC, Wazer DE, Perez CA, Brady LW, eds. *Perez & Brady's Principles and Practice of Radiation Oncology.* 6th ed. Philadelphia: Lippincott Williams & Wilkins; 2013.
8. Theis VS, Sripadam R, Ramani V, Lal S. Chronic radiation enteritis. *Clin Oncol (R Coll Radiol).* 2010;22:70-83.
9. Johnson LB, Riaz AA, Adawi D, et al. Radiation enteropathy and leucocyte-endothelial cell reactions in a refined small bowel model. *BMC Surg.* 2004;4:10.
10. Kim HM, Kim YJ, Kim HJ, Park SW, Bang S, Song SY. A pilot study of capsule endoscopy for the diagnosis of radiation enteritis. *Hepatogastroenterology.* 2011;58:459-464.
11. Song S, Chen D, Ma T, et al. Molecular mechanism of acute radiation enteritis revealed using proteomics and biological signaling network analysis in rats. *Dig Dis Sci.* 2014;59:2704-2713.
12. Richter KK, Langberg CW, Sung CC, Hauer-Jensen M. Association of transforming growth factor beta (TGF-beta) immunoreactivity with specific histopathologic lesions in subacute and chronic experimental radiation enteropathy. *Radiother Oncol.* 1996;39:243-251.
13. Coia LR, Myerson RJ, Tepper JE. Late effects of radiation therapy on the gastrointestinal tract. *Int J Radiat Oncol Biol Phys.* 1995;31:1213-1236.
14. Shadad AK, Sullivan FJ, Martin JD, Egan LJ. Gastrointestinal radiation injury: symptoms, risk factors and mechanisms. *World J Gastroenterol.* 2013;19:185-198.
15. Kavanagh BD, Pan CC, Dawson LA, et al. Radiation dose-volume effects in the stomach and small bowel. *Int J Radiat Oncol Biol Phys.* 2010;76:S101-S107.
16. Regimbeau JM, Panis Y, Gouzi JL, Fagniez PL, French University Association for Surgical Research. Operative and long term results after surgery for chronic radiation enteritis. *Am J Surg.* 2001;182:237-242.
17. Boland E, Thompson J, Rochling F, Sudan D. A 25-year experience with postresection short-bowel syndrome secondary to radiation therapy. *Am J Surg.* 2010;200:690-693.
18. Fan S, Ni X, Wang J, et al. Low triiodothyronine syndrome in patients with radiation enteritis: risk factors and clinical outcomes an observational study. *Medicine (Baltimore).* 2016;95:e2640.
19. Hernández-Moreno A, Vidal-Casariego A, Calleja-Fernández A, et al. Chronic enteritis in patients undergoing pelvic radiotherapy: prevalence, risk factors and associated complications. *Nutr Hosp.* 2015;32:2178-2183.
20. Peach MS, Showalter TN, Ohri N. Systematic review of the relationship between acute and late gastrointestinal toxicity after radiotherapy for prostate cancer. *Prostate Cancer.* 2015;2015:624736.
21. Pironi L, Arends J, Bozzetti F, et al. ESPEN guidelines on chronic intestinal failure in adults. *Clin Nutr.* 2016;35:247-307.
22. Thompson JS, Weseman R, Rochling F, et al. Radiation therapy increases the risk of hepatobiliary complications in short bowel syndrome. *Nutr Clin Pract.* 2011;26:474-478.
23. Yeoh E, Horowitz M, Russo A, et al. Effect of pelvic irradiation on gastrointestinal function: a prospective longitudinal study. *Am J Med.* 1993;95:397-406.
24. Kong W, Wang J, Ni X, et al. Transition of decade in short bowel syndrome in China: yesterday, today, and tomorrow. *Transplant Proc.* 2015;47:1983-1987.
25. Zakaria Z, Toomey D, Deasy J. Radiation-induced distal ileal obstruction complicating ileostomy closure. *Tech Coloproctol.* 2014;18:195-198.
26. Webb GJ, Brooke R, De Silva AN. Chronic radiation enteritis and malnutrition. *J Dig Dis.* 2013;14:350-357.
27. Vantini I, Benini L, Bonfante F, et al. Survival rate and prognostic factors in patients with intestinal failure. *Dig Liver Dis.* 2004;36:46-55.
28. Andreyev HJ, Muls AC, Norton C, et al. Guidance: the practical management of the gastrointestinal symptoms of pelvic radiation disease. *Frontline Gastroenterol.* 2015;6:53-72.
29. Harb AH, Abou Fadel C, Sharara AI. Radiation enteritis. *Curr Gastroenterol Rep.* 2014;16:383.
30. Schembri J, Azzopardi M, Ellul P. Small bowel radiation enteritis diagnosed by capsule endoscopy. *BMJ Case Rep.* 2014;2014. doi:10.1136/bcr-2013-202552.
31. Lutgens L, Lambin P. Biomarkers for radiation-induced small bowel epithelial damage: an emerging role for plasma citrulline. *World J Gastroenterol.* 2007;13:3033-3042.
32. Lutgens LC, Blijlevens NM, Deutz NE, Donnelly JP, Lambin P, de Pauw BE. Monitoring myeloablative therapy-induced small bowel toxicity by serum citrulline concentration: a comparison with sugar permeability tests. *Cancer.* 2005;103:191-199.
33. Vidal-Casariego A, Calleja-Fernández A, Cano-Rodríguez I, Cordido F, Ballesteros-Pomar MD. Effects of oral glutamine during abdominal radiotherapy on chronic radiation enteritis: a randomized controlled trial. *Nutrition.* 2015;31:200-204.

34. Cetin E, Ozturk AS, Orhun H, Ulger S. Role of triamcinolone in radiation enteritis management. *World J Gastroenterol.* 2014;20:4341-4344.

35. Sureban SM, May R, Qu D, et al. Dietary pectin increases intestinal crypt stem cell survival following radiation injury. *PLoS One.* 2015;10:e0135561.

36. Garcia-Peris P, Velasco C, Hernandez M, et al. Effect of inulin and fructo-oligosaccharide on the prevention of acute radiation enteritis in patients with gynecological cancer and impact on quality-of-life: a randomized, double-blind, placebo-controlled trial. *Eur J Clin Nutr.* 2016;70:170-174.

37. Henson CC, Burden S, Davidson SE, Lal S. Nutritional interventions for reducing gastrointestinal toxicity in adults undergoing radical pelvic radiotherapy. *Cochrane Database Syst Rev.* 2013;(11):CD009896.

38. Wedlake LJ, Shaw C, Whelan K, Andreyev HJ. Systematic review: the efficacy of nutritional interventions to counteract acute gastrointestinal toxicity during therapeutic pelvic radiotherapy. *Aliment Pharmacol Ther.* 2013;37:1046-1056.

39. McKay GD, Wong K, Kozman DR. Laparoscopic insertion of pelvic tissue expander to prevent radiation enteritis prior to radiotherapy for prostate cancer. *Radiat Oncol.* 2011;6:47.

40. Joyce M, Thirion P, Kiernan F, et al. Laparoscopic pelvic sling placement facilitates optimum therapeutic radiotherapy delivery in the management of pelvic malignancy. *Eur J Surg Oncol.* 2009;35: 348-351.

41. Devereux DF, Kavanah MT, Feldman MI, et al. Small bowel exclusion from the pelvis by a polyglycolic acid mesh sling. *J Surg Oncol.* 1984;26:107-112.

42. Wedlake L, Thomas K, McGough C, Andreyev HJ. Small bowel bacterial overgrowth and lactose intolerance during radical pelvic radiotherapy: an observational study. *Eur J Cancer.* 2008;44:2212-2217.

43. Stacey R, Green JT. Radiation-induced small bowel disease: latest developments and clinical guidance. *Ther Adv Chronic Dis.* 2014;5:15-29.

44. Bennett MH, Feldmeier J, Hampson NB, et al. Hyperbaric oxygen therapy for late radiation tissue injury. *Cochrane Database Syst Rev.* 2016;(4):CD005005.

45. Feldmeier JJ, Hampson NB. A systematic review of the literature reporting the application of hyperbaric oxygen prevention and treatment of delayed radiation injuries: an evidence based approach. *Undersea Hyperb Med.* 2002;29:4-30.

46. Lefevre JH, Amiot A, Joly F, Bretagnol F, Panis Y. Risk of recurrence after surgery for chronic radiation enteritis. *Br J Surg.* 2011;98:1792-1797.

47. Li N, Zhu W, Gong J, et al. Ileal or ileocecal resection for chronic radiation enteritis with small bowel obstruction: outcome and risk factors. *Am J Surg.* 2013;206:739-747.

48. Perrakis N, Athanassiou E, Vamvakopoulou D, et al. Practical approaches to effective management of intestinal radiation injury: benefit of resectional surgery. *World J Gastroenterol.* 2011;17:4013-4016.

49. Zhang L, Gong JF, Dong JN, Zhu WM, Li N, Li JS. Effectiveness of a clinical pathway for inpatients undergoing ileal/ileocecal resection for chronic radiation enteritis with intestinal obstruction. *Am Surg.* 2015;81:252-258.

50. Parlakgumus A, Caliskan K, Parlakgumus HA, et al. Emergent surgical treatment of radiation-induced enteropathies for patients with urogynecological and colorectal carcinomas. *Clin Exp Obstet Gynecol.* 2011;38:63-66.

51. Perrin H, Panis Y, Messing B, Matuchanski C, Valleur P. Aggressive initial surgery for chronic radiation enteritis: long-term results of resection vs non-resection in 44 consecutive cases. *Colorectal Dis.* 1999;1:162-167.

52. Dietz DW, Remzi FH, Fazio VW. Strictureplasty for obstructing small-bowel lesions in diffuse radiation enteritis—successful outcome in five patients. *Dis Colon Rectum.* 2001;44:1772-1777.

53. Wang J, Yao D, Zhang S, Mao Q, Li Y, Li J. Laparoscopic surgery for radiation enteritis. *J Surg Res.* 2015;194:415-419.

54. Lillemoe KD, Brigham RA, Harmon JW, Feaster MM, Saunders JR, d'Avis JA. Surgical management of small-bowel radiation enteritis. *Arch Surg.* 1983;118:905-907.

55. Shafer KE, Cohen AC, Wiebke EA. Novel approach to surgical repair of enterovaginal fistula in the irradiated pelvis. *Plast Reconstr Surg.* 2012;130:385e-386e.

56. Kalaiselvan R, Theis VS, Dibb M, et al. Radiation enteritis leading to intestinal failure: 1994 patient-years of experience in a national referral centre. *Eur J Clin Nutr.* 2014;68:166-170.

Short Bowel Syndrome

Magesh Sundaram | John Kim

The "normal" length of an adult human's small intestine has been estimated between 20 and 22 feet, or 609 and 670 cm. Past estimates of normal small intestine length have been between 300 and 800 cm, and this variability is based on measurements from surgical, radiologic, or autopsy measurements.[1,2] Short bowel syndrome (SBS) occurs when there is less than 200 cm of small intestine remaining. The minimal length of small intestine necessary to prevent lifelong dependence on parenteral nutrition (PN) is approximately 100 cm if the colon is absent and 60 cm with a completely functional colon present. The etiology of SBS may be congenital or acquired and may be functional or related to surgical resection (Table 79.1).[3] In the pediatric population, intestinal atresia (jejunal or ileal) is the congenital etiology, whereas small bowel resection for the diagnoses of necrotizing enterocolitis, gastroschisis, and volvulus are the common acquired etiologies. In adults, SBS is the sequelae of massive or multiple resections of the small intestine. Approximately 15% of all adults who undergo bowel resection exhibit sequelae of SBS, from either massive resection (76%) or multiple resections (24%).[4] SBS is seen after multiple intestinal resections performed for the diagnoses of Crohn disease, trauma, malignancy, radiation enteritis, or ischemia and gangrene associated with late-stage small bowel obstruction. Of note, a vascular event of the intestine, such as mesenteric arterial embolism or venous thrombosis, may lead to a single massive resection done as a life-saving maneuver for an apparent intraabdominal catastrophe. Functional SBS is seen without intestinal resection with physiologic loss of function or persistent malabsorption syndromes. Diagnoses that may lead to functional SBS include radiation enteritis, low-grade or indolent malignancies (e.g., pseudomyxoma peritonei), refractory sprue, congenital villous atrophy, and chronic intestinal pseudoobstruction syndrome.

SBS is a disabling intestinal condition that reduces the quality and length of life and limits the social integration of the affected individual. The hallmark of SBS is severe nutrient and fluid malabsorption leading to chronic imbalances of micronutrient, fluid, protein, electrolyte, and carbohydrate stores. Quality of life is limited in these patients due to persistent manifestations of SBS via failure to thrive, diarrhea, dehydration, malnutrition, and long-term dependence on alternate means of nutritional support. Frequent medical care episodes for nutritional maintenance, as well as acute management of associated complications, interferes with social integration. Historically SBS patients have been on long-term, if not lifelong, PN. However, newer concepts of SBS management, including intestinal rehabilitation (IR), surgical optimization of absorption, and transplantation, are leading SBS patients to enteral autonomy and an improved quality of life.

INCIDENCE AND DEMOGRAPHICS OF SHORT BOWEL SYNDROME

The true incidence of SBS in the United States has not been accurately identified because there are no reliable national registries or patient databases. In addition, on review of surveys of managing gastroenterologists and nutritionists, the accurate diagnosis of SBS is often not identified in the prescription of long-term home parenteral use. The Oley Registry of home parenteral use in North America in 1992 identified 40,000 patients with the broader category of *intestinal failure* as the diagnosis, with only approximately 26% of cases attributed to SBS.[5] Some patients receiving PN in the Oley Registry carried the diagnosis of radiation enteritis or malignancy, and these patients could be reclassified with SBS due to those diagnoses. In 1995, an estimate of 10,000 to 20,000 patients receiving home PN for SBS was made by Byrne et al.[6]

It is estimated that the number of SBS patients may be in the range of 2 per million, based on extrapolation of home parenteral use for SBS patients in the United Kingdom.[7] A more recent European survey from 1997 identified the incidence of home total parenteral nutrition (TPN) use at close to 3 per million and the prevalence greater than 4 per million.[8] It would seem that the prevalence of SBS is lower in regions where access to specialized nutritional care is lacking, and this is likely due to underreporting, lack of recognition of the disease process, and a resultant shorter life expectancy. The prevalence of SBS is noted to be 0.4 per million in Poland, whereas it is noted to be 30 per million in Denmark, and this may be attributed to the development of a leading IR center (IRC) in Denmark that has led to a twofold increase in the number of patients listed as receiving PN or intravenous (IV) fluid support over the past 40 years.[9] Further underreporting of SBS incidence in both the United States and Europe can be realized when there is no accounting of patients with SBS who do not require home PN/IV support or who have been weaned off PN/IV support.

Historically, characterizing the demographics of patients with SBS is limited without a prospective national registry or database. A survey of 688 patients awaiting intestinal transplants and receiving PN/IV support revealed the diagnosis of chronic intestinal failure and 75% also had SBS identified. The age of these patients was 52.9 ± 1.52 (range, 18.5 to 88.0), with 57% women. The most common etiologies were mesenteric ischemia (27%), Crohn disease (23%), and radiation enteritis (11%).[10] Similar findings of a median age of 52.5, a majority of females (52%), and a body mass index (BMI) of 20.7 kg/m^2 was identified in a study limited to 268 SBS patients. Mesenteric infarction (43%), radiation enteritis (23%), surgical complications (12%), and Crohn disease (6%) were the common

TABLE 79.1 Etiologies of Short Bowel Syndrome

CONGENITAL
Intestinal atresia

ACQUIRED
Surgical resection of bowel
Recurrent Crohn disease
Massive enterectomy secondary to a catastrophic vascular
   event, such as a mesenteric arterial embolism or venous
   thrombosis, volvulus, trauma, or tumor resection
Gastroschisis
Necrotizing enterocolitis
Intestinal atresias
Extensive aganglionosis
Chronic intestinal pseudoobstruction syndrome
Refractory sprue
Radiation enteritis
Congenital villous atrophy

Modified from DeLegge M, Alsolaiman MM, Barbour E, Bassas S, Siddiqi MF, Moore NM. Short bowel syndrome: parenteral nutrition versus intestinal transplantation. Where are we today? *Dig Dis Sci*. 2007;52(4):876–892.

etiologies identified.[11] Better recognition of SBS is now being seen with cooperative transplant registry data collection. SBS was identified as the most common primary indication for intestinal transplantation when 61 intestinal transplant programs in 19 countries provided data on 989 transplants in 923 patients.[12]

PROGNOSTIC FACTORS IN SHORT BOWEL SYNDROME

SBS is associated with short- and long-term complications that lead to significant morbidity and mortality. Historically the prime determinant of mortality in SBS patients was nutritional failure, as seen with a case-fatality rate of 37.5% in neonates, among an SBS incidence of 24.5 per 100,000 live births.[13] The advent of effective long-term PN and indwelling central venous access in the late 1960s led to good nutritional rehabilitation with low complication rates in SBS patients. In the two decades following, widespread adoption of PN support led to a reduction in SBS mortality from nutritional failure. The current era of SBS management includes pharmacologic medical therapies, multidisciplinary IRCs, and surgical intestinal optimization and transplant procedures. These management principles have led to improvement in both morbidity and mortality rates in SBS patients. Fifty percent to 70% of patients who require PN after the initial diagnosis of SBS can be weaned off PN within 2.5 years of the referral to a specialized center. Up to 70% of pediatric SBS patients can now be discharged from the hospital and are alive 1 year after diagnosis.[14]

The prognosis of SBS is dependent on several factors, including the remaining length of functional intestine, the active presence of underlying etiologic diseases (Crohn, radiation enteritis, vasculopathy), the presence or functional continuity of the colon, and the ileocecal valve (ICV). Previously, it was felt that the ICV carried a greater role in gate-keeping transit times of intestinal loads to the colon, as well as preventing colonic reflux. However, when subsets of SBS patients are matched for length of intestinal resection, the value of the ICV appears to be primarily a marker of greater ileal or colon resection.[15] The patient's age at presentation and the chronicity of enteral dependence are also contributing prognostic factors. Buchman reports the overall survival rate after 6 years of enteral dependence to be 65% in patients with at least 50 cm of intestine, but survival rates are much lower in patients with less than 50 cm of intestine.[16] These patients with less residual intestine are more likely to develop PN-related complications, such as liver and kidney failure if not being permanently dependent on PN. The mortality in SBS patients with well-established PN dependence and with adequate residual intestine is less likely to be due to PN-related complications and more likely to be due to complications of their underlying disease, such as Crohn disease, cancer, and heart failure.

NORMAL INTESTINAL PHYSIOLOGY AND PATHOPHYSIOLOGY OF SHORT BOWEL SYNDROME

The normal intestinal physiology of an intact digestive system is notable for a progressively decreasing absorptive gradient from proximal to distal. The absorptive surface area of the duodenum and jejunum is greater than that of the ileum. The proximal jejunum contains plicae circulares in greater number and thickness and with longer villi than the ileum. The absorptive surface area is also larger in the proximal intestine because the luminal diameter decreases as the gastrointestinal (GI) tract progresses from duodenum to ileum. Direct proximity to biliary and pancreatic enzymatic activity in the duodenum and jejunum is a major driver of nutrient digestion and absorption, more so than what is seen in the ileum, where bile acid resorption is a more prominent function.

The absorption of nutrients, minerals, vitamins, and amino acids is carefully distributed to preferential areas along the GI tract, as described in Chapter 71 (Fig. 79.1).[17]

The anatomy, length, and reconfiguration of the GI tract that remains after intestinal resection in the setting of SBS directly affect the proximal to distal gradient of digestion and absorption of nutrients and fluids. The small intestine has a large functional reserve capacity, and resection of up to 50% of intestinal length can be well tolerated. However, crossing the threshold of less than 200 cm of residual intestine leads to some of the clinical sequelae of SBS in at least 50% of these patients. The progression to massive intestinal loss leads to the full manifestation of SBS via the pathophysiology of loss of absorptive surface area and an increase in intestinal transit times. The clinical consequences of SBS are a result of the loss of intestinal absorption surface, the loss of site-specific absorptive areas, the loss of the ICV, and the decrease in intestinal hormone production. After major intestinal resection, larger volumes of undigested nutrients result in hyperosmotic loads entering the distal GI tract sooner, resulting in a response of increased luminal water. The resulting intense diarrhea is one of the major

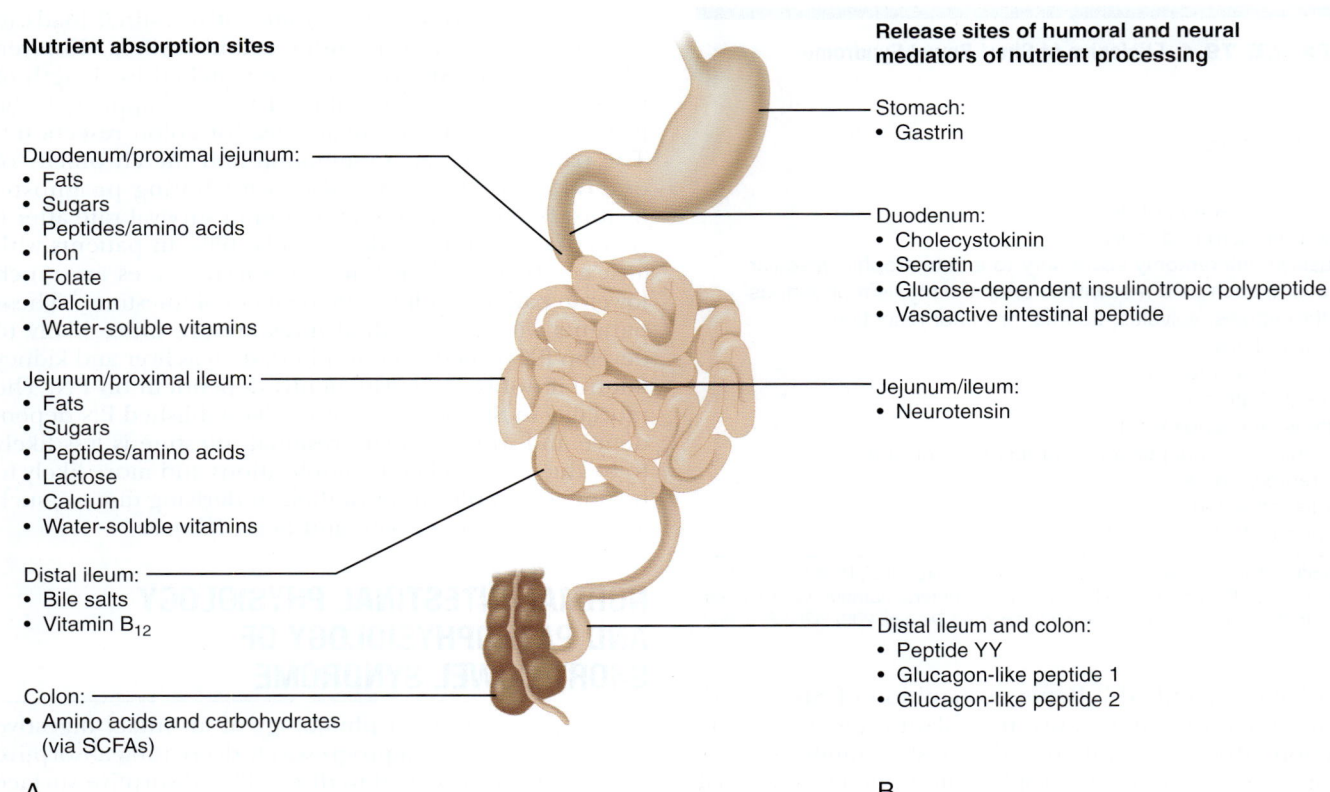

Nutrient absorption sites

Duodenum/proximal jejunum:
- Fats
- Sugars
- Peptides/amino acids
- Iron
- Folate
- Calcium
- Water-soluble vitamins

Jejunum/proximal ileum:
- Fats
- Sugars
- Peptides/amino acids
- Lactose
- Calcium
- Water-soluble vitamins

Distal ileum:
- Bile salts
- Vitamin B_{12}

Colon:
- Amino acids and carbohydrates (via SCFAs)

Release sites of humoral and neural mediators of nutrient processing

Stomach:
- Gastrin

Duodenum:
- Cholecystokinin
- Secretin
- Glucose-dependent insulinotropic polypeptide
- Vasoactive intestinal peptide

Jejunum/ileum:
- Neurotensin

Distal ileum and colon:
- Peptide YY
- Glucagon-like peptide 1
- Glucagon-like peptide 2

A   B

FIGURE 79.1 Nutritional absorption (A) and hormonal release sites (B) across the gastrointestinal tract. *SCFAs,* Short-chain fatty acids. (From Tappenden KA. Pathophysiology of short bowel syndrome: considerations of resected and residual anatomy. *J Parenter Enteral Nutr.* 2014;38[suppl 1]:14S–22S.)

TABLE 79.2 Anatomic Subtypes of Short Bowel Syndrome

Subtype	Resection/Remnant	Avoidance Permanent PN Dependence	GI Tract Pathophysiology	Clinical Manifestations
1. Jejunal-ileal anastomosis	Majority of jejunum resected. 10+ cm of ileum, ICV, colon remain	Usually good but poor if <40 cm jejunum remains	Impaired digestion, increased gastric acid secretion	Diarrhea
2. Jejunal-colic anastomosis	All/most ileum resected. Parts of jejunum, colon may also be resected	Variable but poor if <65 cm jejunum remains	Deficiencies in vitamin B_{12}, bile salts, fat-soluble vitamins. Fat malabsorption	Diarrhea, steatorrhea
3. End jejunostomy	Some jejunum retained. Ileum, ICV colon removed. End jejunal ostomy	Variable but poor if <100 cm jejunum remains	Deficiencies in vitamin B_{12}, bile salts, magnesium. Fluid and nutrient malabsorption	Excessive ostomy output, dehydration

GI, Gastrointestinal; *ICV,* ileocecal valve; *PN,* parenteral nutrition.

symptoms of the initial phase of SBS manifestation. The consequence is decreased digestion and absorption of lipids and fat-soluble vitamins, as well as emulsification and processing of cholesterol and complex fats.

Intestinal resection and reconstruction of the GI tract in the setting of SBS can be categorized into three anatomic subtypes (Table 79.2). Type I is associated with significant jejunal resection and GI tract reconstruction via a jejunal-ileal anastomosis. The remnant GI tract includes at least 10 cm of terminal ileum, the ICV, and the entire colon. Type II is associated with resection of most or all of the ileum, frequently the ICV, and possibly part of the colon,

usually the proximal or right colon. The GI tract in type II SBS patients is frequently reconstructed via a jejunocolic anastomosis. Type III SBS occurs with resection of all of the ileum, ICV, and the colon, with variable resection of the jejunum. The GI tract output is via an end jejunostomy, without connection to the rectum and anus.

Type I SBS patients have the greatest chance of nutritional recovery over time. Although there is initial loss of the proximal to distal gradient associated with the proximal jejunum, there is greater potential for the development of functional adaptation by the ileum to reduce the severity of nutritional losses long term. The possibility of intestinal adaptation is good with type I, and the permanent need for PN is low. In type I SBS, intestinal failure and the need for permanent PN or transplant consideration occur more commonly when only less than 40 cm of jejunum (or <10% of expected intestine for gestational age in infants) remains to form the jejunal-ileal anastomosis. Clinical manifestations may be seen due to changes in intestinal endocrine regulation. Loss of cholecystokinin production in the postresection state leads to increased gastric acid hypersecretion and rapid intestinal transit time of fluids. Alteration of the intestinal pH from increased acid load can lead to reduced pancreatic enzymatic digestive capabilities. Fortunately, the acid hypersecretion postresection state can be corrected in a few weeks to months, with the addition of a proton pump inhibitor or H_2-blocker regimen.[18] Type I SBS patients tend not to have dehydration issues long term because the intact colon can serve as a water reservoir and absorptive conduit. When the duodenum and at least 40 cm of jejunum are preserved, deficiencies of water-soluble vitamins are less typical because these areas of the proximal intestine can slow down water-soluble vitamin absorption times.

Type II patients typically exhibit more severe clinical manifestations of SBS due to the loss of the adaptive capacity of the ileum and the colon. More extensive ileal resections are associated with worse outcomes. When less than 65 cm of jejunum remains and no ileum, the avoidance of permanent PN dependence is poor in these type II SBS patients. Clinical manifestations occuring with ileal resections are due to disruption of the vitamin B_{12} and enterohepatic bile salt systems. Without the site-specific ileal B_{12} receptors, long-term maintenance with vitamin B_{12} supplements is needed. Lacking bile salt reabsorption, steatorrhea from fat malabsorption is a frequent manifestation. The persistence of unabsorbed bile salts in the colon stimulates colonic motility and secretion, further exacerbating the steatorrhea. Chronic deficiencies of the fat-soluble vitamins will lead to the expected clinical presentations—dry skin, night blindness and xerophthalmia (vitamin A), pediatric rickets and adult osteomalacia and osteoporosis (vitamin D), macular degeneration (vitamin E), and spontaneous hemorrhage and poor clotting ability (vitamin K).

Type III patients with an end jejunostomy are the most challenging to manage because they have high fluid output losses. Without both the ileum and the colon, they will have the greatest malabsorptive issues as compared with the other patients. End jejunostomy patients no longer have the water reservoir and absorptive potential of the colon but also lose ileal site-specific nutritional deficiencies. When end jejunostomy patients have less than 100 cm of jejunum remaining, there is the added issue of loss of gastric acid and intestinal secretions, resulting in a chronic net-secretory state of high fluid output. The type III patients with less than 100 cm of jejunum typically will need permanent PN/IV support.

Water losses become less of a permanent issue with an intact ileum and colon. Permeability to water is less in the ileum than jejunum because the ileum has tighter junctions and a narrower luminal surface area. Therefore less water enters the ileal lumen than the jejunal lumen in response to a hyperosmotic-loaded meal. In adaptation,

the colon is capable of increasing its fluid absorption capability from approximately 1.8 to 5 L a day, or up to 400% of normal.[19] However, patients with a resected colon (type II SBS) or with an end jejunostomy (type III SBS) may have significant water and sodium losses that may lead to acute hypotension and chronic kidney insufficiency states. Hypomagnesemia in particular may lead to muscle fatigue, cardiac dysrhythmia, and neurologic impacts from depression to seizures.

INTESTINAL ADAPTATION

Intestinal adaptation is the mechanism of GI tract functional recovery that occurs in the postresection state of SBS patients. This adaptive process begins within 24 hours of significant intestinal resection and continues over a 2-year period. The degree or success of intestinal adaptation depends on anatomic factors, such as the extent and site of intestinal resections, the patient's health and existent underlying disease processes, the mechanism of nutritional support, and regaining the endocrine regulatory mechanisms of the GI tract. Keller[20] has identified three phases of intestinal adaptation:

- Acute phase—postresection to 4 weeks. The goal is stabilization of the patient's sequelae of diarrhea, malabsorption, and dysmotility.
- Adaptive phase—1 to 2 years. The goal is achieving maximal intestinal adaptation with a gradual increase of nutritional exposure.
- Maintenance phase—long term. Optimizing fluid balance and individualized dietary regimen. Management of acute exacerbations.

Successful intestinal adaptation depends on morphologic changes in the residual intestine's microanatomy. The absorptive capacity may be increased by several hundred percent from increased mucosal surface, as well as increased absorption per surface area. In the postresection state the acute phase is marked by hyperemia of the bowel wall. Increased blood flow to the remnant intestine may be seen for up to 4 weeks after resection.[21] Hyperemic changes promote mucosal hyperplasia, with resulting increased number and size of crypts and villi in the ileum. The normal ileum is typically exposed to fewer luminal nutrients than the jejunum. Taking advantage of the ileum's adaptive capability, therapeutic stimulation via planned and gradual exposure of macronutrients to ileal intestinal mucosa leads to a net increase in the absorptive surface area.[22] Intestinal wall lengthening, luminal diameter increase, and wall thickening can occur in the ileum. Such adaptive growth of intestinal length and diameter is most prominent in premature babies with SBS.[23] After morphologic changes occur over the initial 2-year period, there is evidence of retention of these features—Joly has reported that there is a 35% increase in crypt depth and a 22% increase in cell numbers and crypts in type II jejunocolic anastomosis patients up to 9.8 years after resection, as compared with healthy controls.[24]

Functional changes in intestinal enterocytes are further key elements of increasing absorptive capacity. Differentiation of specialized mucosal cells may occur, thereby optimizing electrolyte (sodium, calcium) transport and exchange processing.[25] Such differentiation occurs at the microvilli level. Functional adaptation occurs in the remnant colon through the process of hyperfermentation of undigested carbohydrates by colonic bacteria.[26] Carbohydrate conversion to short-chain fatty acids (SCFAs), which are then absorbed in the colon, has proved to be an energy preservation mechanism.[27]

Slowing small bowel transit time and thereby lengthening the time of contact between nutrients and the absorptive surface area is a change that improves quality of life. Although diarrhea is a prominent feature of the acute phase, long-term success in fluid, electrolyte, and nutritional balance can be achieved during the adaptive phase with deceleration in intestinal transit time.[28]

Although calorie maintenance can be achieved with PN, the intestinal structural integrity can only be maintained via enteral stimulation. Lack of enteral nutrition leads to mucosal atrophy, blunting of villi and crypts, changes in brush border integrity, and increased fluid permeability. Intestinal adaptation is highly dependent on the luminal presence of nutrients. Increased complexity of nutrients seen by the remnant intestine promotes greater adaptation, by promotion of pancreaticobiliary secretions, stimulation of neurohormonal endocrine release, and ongoing use of the absorptive surface area. For example, long-chain triglycerides induce intestinal hyperplasia to a greater extent than medium-chain triglycerides.[29] Certain nutrients are more valuable in the promotion of intestinal adaptation.

Glutamine is the primary energy source for enterocyte growth and metabolism. Studies that have examined the utility of glutamine in intestinal adaptation show modest benefit clinically. Glutamine added as a supplement to PN does reduce the severity of PN-induced intestinal atrophy. In contrast, glutamine added as part of a nutritional dietary regimen does not seem to yield measurable structural intestinal changes, such as villous growth. The lack of glutamine-driven effect may be due to the greater complexity of the luminal nutrients of the existing dietary regimen. The combination of glutamine with growth hormone (GH) is perhaps more valuable clinically. Studies of SBS patients receiving GH plus glutamine show greater long-term fluid and electrolyte maintenance as well as reductions in PN/IV volume requirements compared with patients receiving GH alone.[30] A Cochrane meta-analysis of human trials indicated that GH, with or without glutamine, improves energy absorption and weight gain in SBS patients, but such benefits were lost when GH therapy was discontinued.[31]

MEDICAL MANAGEMENT

The main goals of medical management of SBS are the optimization and maintenance of
- nutritional absorption
- fluid and electrolyte balance
- vitamin and trace element retention
- nutritional and weight maintenance

In the acute phase after intestinal resection, attention must be paid to the dominant clinical issue of massive diarrhea and attendant fluid and electrolyte loss. The first few postoperative days require IV fluid replacement of losses, preferably using lactated Ringer with glucose

TABLE 79.3 Drug Therapy Recommendations in the Acute Phase of Short Bowel Syndrome Management

Drug	Dose per Day
Cholestyramine	4–16 g
Famotidine	40–80 mg
Loperamide	4–16 mg
Metronidazole	800–1200 mg
Pancreatic enzyme	25,000–40,000 U per meal
Octreotide	50–100 µg 2–3 times
Omeprazole	20–40 mg
Ranitidine	300–600 mg

solution (dextrose 5% [D5]). A schedule of replacement of water-soluble vitamins and trace elements must be instituted. Gastric acid hypersecretion should be controlled with proton pump inhibitor and H_2-blocker therapy for the first 6 months. Occasionally, the somatostatin analogue octreotide is useful to reduce the intraluminal fluid load, especially in the type III patients with end jejunostomies. Diarrhea may be controlled with the judicious use of intestinal motility inhibition agents, such as loperamide. Cholestyramine is useful in promoting bile salt retention and should be used to reduce cholerheic diarrhea. Sepsis control and correction of postoperative infection is critical to preventing ileus and early intestinal atrophy. Metronidazole is useful in the prevention of small bowel bacterial overgrowth (SBBO). A regular schedule of maintenance drug therapy is recommended in the acute phase for SBS patients (Table 79.3).

Enteral nutrition should begin by postoperative day 4 to 5, via a low continuous infusion via nasal/percutaneous feeding tube, or by oral intake. The institution of early enteral feeding may be tempered by surgical concerns about ongoing ischemic changes in the massive vascular accident patient or for anastomotic integrity, peritoneal infection, or septic shock. Initial assessment of the adequacy of early enteral nutrition may be difficult because initial use of the remnant GI tract will lead to apparent worsening of diarrhea. The nutritional load will typically exceed immediate remnant absorptive capacity. A goal of 30 to 40 kcal/kg per day should be sought, but, given potential malabsorption rates of 30%, up to 45 to 60 kcal/kg per day may be the input level of enteral nutrition.

Enteral nutrition over the first 3 to 4 weeks after resection should progress with a structured program of increasing nutrient loads, first with isotonic salt-glucose solutions. Similarly, the nutritional program should introduce elemental level amino acids early on, including glutamine. Medium-chain triglycerides are preferred in the acute phase, for patients with a preserved colon, but not in type II or III SBS patients. For type II or III patients, a dietary balance of 40% to 50% carbohydrates and 30% to 40% lipids is recommended (Table 79.4).[32]

In the beginning of the adaptive phase, past the 4-week point, dietary expansion begins with long-chain triglycerides, free fatty acids, and carbohydrates such as maltose, saccharose, and pectin. Proteins should comprise approximately 20% of the diet. In patients with an intact colon, soluble dietary fibers can be degraded by colonic bacteria to yield SCFAs and provide a supplementary

TABLE 79.4 Dietary Recommendations in Maintenance Phase of Recovery

Nutrient	Small Bowel Ostomy	Colonic Continuity
Carbohydrates	50% of total energy; complex carbohydrates including soluble fiber, limit simple sugars	50%–60% of total energy; complex carbohydrates, including soluble fiber
Proteins	20%–30% of total energy	20%–30% of total energy
Fats	40% of total energy	20%–30% of total energy
Fluids	ORS important; minimize fluids with meals, sipping of fluids between meals	Minimize fluids with meals, sipping of fluids between meals
Vitamins	Daily multiple vitamin with minerals; monthly vitamin B_{12}; possibly vitamins A, D, and E supplements	Daily multiple vitamin with minerals; possibly vitamin B_{12}; possibly vitamins A, D, and E supplements
Minerals	Generous use of sodium chloride on food; calcium 1000–1500 mg daily; possibly iron, magnesium, and zinc supplements	400–600 mg calcium with meals; possibly iron, magnesium, and zinc supplements; reduced oxalate
Meals	4–6 small meals	3 small meals plus 2–3 snacks

ORS, Oral rehydration solution.
Modified from Wall E. An overview of short bowel syndrome management: adherence, adaptation and practical recommendations. *J Acad Nutr Diet.* 2013;113:1200–1208.

energy supply of up to 500 to 1000 kcal/day.[33] These patients benefit from a carbohydrate-rich diet but should avoid lipids. Soluble fibers also promote better formed stool production as opposed to insoluble fibers, which can promote diarrhea.

Steadfast attention and maintenance of elemental levels, particularly magnesium and calcium, is also required at the early adaptive stage. Calcium supplementation should be at the 800- to 1200-mg/daily oral. Oxalates in the diet should be avoided to prevent the development of oxalate nephrolithiasis. Development of metabolic acidosis may be treated with addition of bicarbonate during the first few months of the adaptation phase. Oral magnesium supplementation may not be possible, due to the laxative effect of enteral magnesium.

A generic formula of PN may be started in the early postoperative period, with tailoring to an individual PN formula after the first week, dependent on review of electrolyte levels. In the first two phases of SBS recovery, the desired PN balance consists of 3 to 5 g/kg per day carbohydrates, 1.5 g/kg per day protein, and 1 g/kg per day lipids. Progression to the maintenance phase is with an emphasis of reduction/termination of PN. If intestinal adaptation is mature and the balance between delivery and loss of nutrients is equilibrated, these patients may regain substantial quality of life. The widespread adoption of PN led to significant reduction in morbidity and mortality in SBS patients in the 1970s. One-year survival of SBS adult patients on PN was recognized to be 91%, but leveling off at 86% at 5 years.[34] The long-term utility of PN is counterbalanced by PN-related complications, such as indwelling catheter–associated septic and venous thrombotic events, as well as the development of PN-associated liver disease (PNALD). Fifteen percent of PN-dependent patients will develop end-stage liver disease, which carries a 100% mortality rate within 2 years of diagnosis.[35]

Oral nutrition in the stable SBS patient should consist of many small meals, with an emphasis on a high-fat diet and moderate fluid intake with meals. Accounting for chronic malabsorption rate reduction from the acute 30% potential, the maintenance diet should still be balanced to achieve target absorption rate of 30 to 40 kcal/kg per day. The transition to the high-fat diet of the maintenance phase may yield recurrence of steatorrhea symptoms for which the patient should be prospectively counseled and managed appropriately.

Novel drug therapy for SBS includes the use of teduglutide for PN-dependent patients. Teduglutide is the recombinant human analogue of glucagon-like peptide 2 (GLP-2). Both GLP-1 and GLP-2 are intestine-trophic hormones released by the endocrine L cells in the ileum and colon. Upregulation of GLP-1 and GLP-2 synthesis is seen after ileal resection if there is remaining colon in a jejunocolic configuration. These GLP hormones promote villous height and crypt cell mass increase. In a randomized placebo-controlled phase III trial, the use of 0.05 mg/kg/day SQ of teduglutide led to a significant decrease in weekly PN volume requirements of 32% versus 21% in the placebo group ($P < .001$) by 24 weeks.[36] Teduglutide-associated PN volume reduction also led to improved quality-of-life scores among SBS patients.[37] The increased crypt cell mass growth caused by teduglutide raises the concern for promotion of neoplastic growth, and therefore a prospective colonoscopy prior to teduglutide therapy is recommended to exclude active intestinal malignancy.

MULTIDISCIPLINARY INTESTINAL REHABILITATION

Although the population of SBS patients may be small, they have complex pathophysiology and require an intense focus of care to lead successful lives without morbidity and mortality. A newer paradigm in the care of SBS patients is multidisciplinary IR at a specialized intestinal care center. These IRCs offer SBS patients a comprehensive management approach that recognizes the nutritional management challenges and short- and long-term complications and transitions patients from medical/pharmacologic management to surgical interventions of intestinal reconstruction or transplant.

Clinical pathways are triggered with an SBS patient from the initial postsurgical phase, the IR phase, with monitoring for complications (Fig. 79.2).[38] An IR program's well-established clinical pathways are tailored to the individual

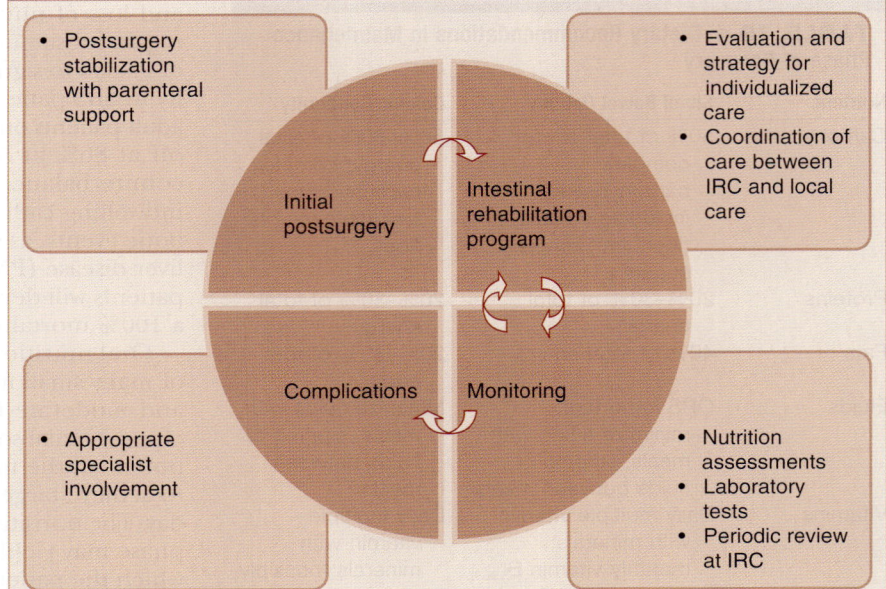

FIGURE 79.2 Clinical pathways of short bowel syndrome patients at intestinal rehabilitation center (IRC). (From Matarese LE, Jeppesen PB, O'Keefe SJ. Short bowel syndrome in adults: the need for an interdisciplinary approach and coordinated care. *J Parenter Enteral Nutr.* 2014;38[suppl 1]:60S–64S.)

SBS patient with an emphasis on patient education. In addition to the fluid, nutritional, and medical management in the initial postsurgical phase of SBS, educational counseling is oriented toward the patient's understanding of the major lifestyle changes ahead, as well as broadening familiarity of the program's services and capabilities of support. Understanding the intestinal remnant and configuration, as well as the patient's underlying health, leads to the formulation of a detailed nutritional assessment of the degree of short- and long-term nutritional deficits.

Specialized IRCs typically have a gastroenterology program director with nutritional, medical, pharmacy, surgical, interventional radiology, and social work team members (Fig. 79.3).[38] Pathways are developed in a coordinated fashion to seamlessly hand off the SBS patient from one major transition point to the next—for example, specialist referral for an acute complication, or surgical referral for transplantation in the setting of intestinal failure (Table 79.5).[38] One such important transition point is the first discharge from the hospital to a home care environment. A specialized IR program will have established protocols of communication between the patient, the nutrition specialist (PN/enteral nutrition/fluid support), the pharmacist (for relevant medications), and the social worker. Patient recognition of symptom exacerbations (e.g., dehydration, diarrhea, cramping) is prospectively co-managed to reduce severity or minimize hospital readmissions.

Studies indicate that IRCs are capable of delivering improved outcomes in SBS patients. Nehme[39] compared 211 patients whose PN was managed by a dedicated nutritional support team (NST) against 164 patients whose PN was managed by a variety of individual physician providers, over a 2-year period. The NST group had a catheter complication rate of 3.7% versus 33.5% in the non-NST group. Catheter sepsis rates were 1.3% in the NST group and 26.2% in the non-NST group.[39] NST management led to a 50% decrease in complication rates when compared with the group managed by individual physicians ($P < .001$).[40] Such coordinated care of the SBS patient on PN may yield cost savings of $4.20 for every $1.00 assigned to the use of a NST.[40]

COMPLICATIONS OF SHORT BOWEL SYNDROME

In addition to the specific nutritional, metabolic, and fluid deficiencies associated with SBS, there are several notable and specific complications that arise in the management of these patients.

SMALL BOWEL BACTERIAL OVERGROWTH

SBBO is a common complication associated with SBS. The inherent bacterial load in the GI tract is primarily in the oropharyngeal and colorectal domains. In the normal GI tract, bacterial contamination in the small intestine is limited by the bactericidal action of gastric acid, enzymatic digestion, antegrade peristalsis, and the ICV. However, the alterations of the GI tract's structure and function in SBS can lead to overabundance of bacterial contamination in the remnant small intestine. The pathophysiologic changes that lead to bacterial overgrowth include villous atrophy, loss of the gut-associated lymphoid tissue, reflux of colon bacteria in the absence of the ICV, and rapid intestinal transit time.

SBBO is recognized as the symptomatic presence of more than 10^5 colony-forming units (CFU)/mL in the intestine. Symptoms include dyspepsia, abdominal cramping, bloating, and diarrhea acutely. Persistence of SBBO may lead to chronic nutritional malabsorption and weight loss. The definitive diagnosis of SBBO is made with endoscopic capture and culture of small intestinal fluid, with identification of 10^5 + CFU/mL of bacteria. Hydrogen breath testing is a simple, noninvasive alternative means of diagnosis wherein the hydrogen produced by bacterial metabolism of intestinal carbohydrates can be measured from the patient's breath. Colonic bacterial fermentation

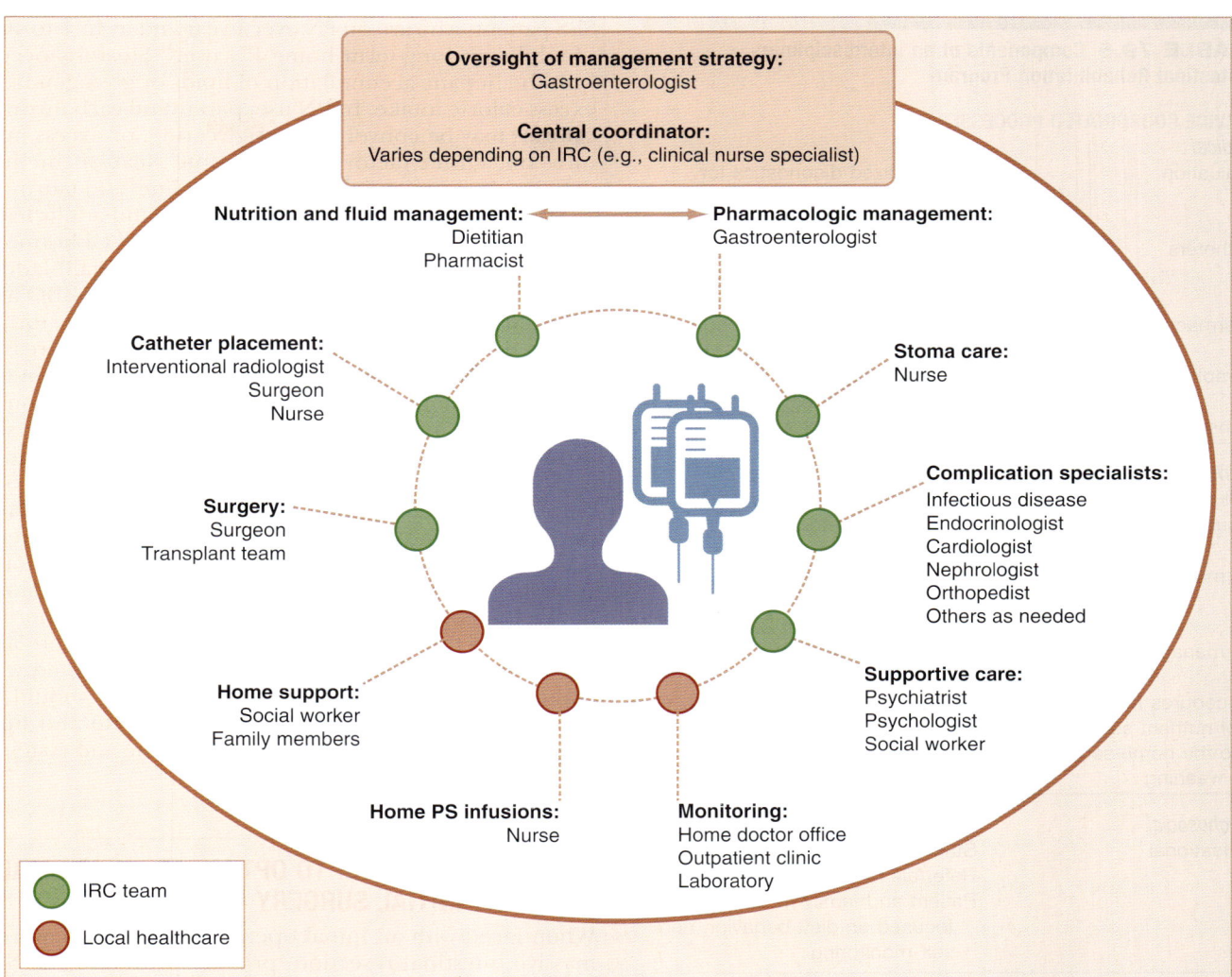

FIGURE 79.3 The framework of intestinal rehabilitation. *IRC*, Intestinal rehabilitation center. (Modified from Matarese LE, Jeppesen P, O'Keefe SJ. Short bowel syndrome in adults: the need for an interdisciplinary approach and coordinated care. *J Parenter Enteral Nutr.* 2014;38[Suppl 1]:60S–64S.)

of simple carbohydrates may not only lead to increased hydrogen load orally but eventually metabolic acidosis with a high anion gap.

Treatment of an acute SBBO state depends on the precipitating factors, bacterial species involved, and the severity of symptoms. Most commonly, empiric treatment for SBBO is with the regular use of broad-spectrum oral antibiotics or the regular regimented use of metronidazole. In addition, recognition of contributory anatomic abnormalities such as fistulas, strictures, and diverticula is valuable; surgical correction of these issues may provide immediate relief from the SBBO load. Altering the dietary composition away from carbohydrate loads will ameliorate the etiology of colonic bacterial fermentation. Antimotility agents should not be used to control diarrhea when the diagnosis of SBBO is made.

Probiotic (*Lactobacillus* and *Bifidobacterium*) therapy may be effective in reducing the use of antibiotics and controlling symptoms of bacterial overgrowth. Probiotic bacteria demonstrate a mucosal barrier–enhancing capability with their adherence to intestinal villi, therein displacing pathogenic bacteria into the intestinal lumen for discard. Probiotics offer resistance to pathogenic bacterial colonization by direct competition to attachment sites and for nutrients. GI tract intestinal immune functions, such as the secretion of antibacterial peptides (defensins), are enhanced by probiotics.[41]

CATHETER-RELATED INFECTIONS

The long-term use of central venous catheters (CVCs) is a central feature of the management of SBS patients. CVCs are needed to maintain hydration and nutritional status, as well as antibiotic and pharmacologic agent delivery. A common morbidity associated with CVCs is catheter-related infection (CRI) with an incidence of 3% to 60% over the life span of the CVC.[42] At least one hospitalization a year for SBS patients is from CRIs. CVC sepsis is a dominant cause of mortality in SBS patients, with up to one-third of SBS patient deaths from this issue, with a 50% 5-year mortality rate.[14] CVC infection in the SBS patient population is commonly from coagulase-negative *Staphylococcus* spp., *S. aureus*, or gram-negative bacilli.

TABLE 79.5 Components of an Interdisciplinary Intestinal Rehabilitation Program

SERVICE COORDINATED PROCESSES

Medical

Evaluation	Standardized diagnostics for physical and biochemical assessments
Catheters	Protocols with interventional radiologists, surgeons, and nurse team
Pharmacologic	Review options and protocols with nutrition team
Complications	Protocols for referral to appropriate specialists
Transplantation option	Referral to transplant team

Nutrition

Diet modifications support	Protocols for optimized fluid, macronutrients, and micronutrients
EN management	Protocols for initiation, transitioning, and discontinuation of EN
PN management	Protocols for fluid, macronutrients, and micronutrients support
Procedures for delivery of nutrient solutions to the home setting	—
PN weaning	

Psychosocial

Educational	Standardized assessments
	Referrals for emotional support
	Patient and family material focused on diet, behavior, and self-monitoring

EN, Enteral nutrition; *PN,* parenteral nutrition.
Modified from Matarese LE, Jeppesen PB, O'Keefe SJ. Short bowel syndrome in adults: the need for an interdisciplinary approach and coordinated care. *J Parenter Enteral Nutr.* 2014;38(suppl 1):60S–64S.

An integrated team approach to the management of CVCs is needed with SBS patients. A popular means of prevention and treatment of CRIs with these patients is the use of antibiotic or ethanol locks of the catheters. Mouw et al. describe the daily use of a 70% ethanol lock method that reduced the rate of CRIs from 11.15 per 1000 catheter-days to 2.06 per 1000 catheter-days.[43]

LIVER DISEASE

Liver disease may result from either long-term PN use (PNALD) or from progressive intestinal failure (intestinal failure–associated liver disease [IFALD]). SBS patients may progress along a spectrum of liver disease from cholestasis to steatosis (fatty liver) and then fibrosis/cirrhosis and end-stage liver failure. The cholestatic changes are more prominent in long-term pediatric SBS patients, whereas steatosis is more prominent in adult SBS patients. Factors found to promote fibrosis and cirrhosis leading to end-stage liver disease include use of PN over 1 year, central line infections, cholecystectomy, and intestinal length less than 60 cm. Liver disease is seen in up to 40% to 60% of pediatric

SBS patients who are on PN over 1 year and in 15% to 40% of adults on long-term home PN use.[34] Steatosis occurs with the hepatic accumulation of lipids or glycogen from excess caloric intake. In PN use, parenteral carbohydrate calories may be converted to triglyceride, or excess lipid infusion. Other factors that promote steatosis include deficiencies in essential fatty acids, choline, and taurine.[44]

Lack of enteral intake in both infants and adults leads to decreased levels of GI hormones. Reduced GI hormone levels result in intestinal stasis and loss of gallbladder contractility. Transient subclinical episodes of SBBO and bacterial translocation lead to cholestasis and stone formation in the liver and gallbladder, with associated increased levels of lithocholic acid. A subclinical septic state in the GI tract promotes IFALD because of the combination of reduction of bile flow, increased lithocholic bile salt production, and decreased enterohepatic bile salt cycling.

The contemporary prevention of liver disease in SBS patients is primarily prophylactic or monitoring and intervention to prevent progression. Routine enteral feeding in the maintenance phase for SBS patients should consist of at least 20% to 30% of the total daily caloric intake, thereby promoting GI hormonal release and normal function of the enterohepatic bile salt cycle. Acute and subclinical episodes of SBBO should be prevented with maintenance antibiotic therapy. PN mixtures should be carefully balanced in terms of carbohydrate and lipid loads in addition to maintenance of taurine and cysteine.

SURGICAL MANAGEMENT

SURGICAL APPROACH TO OPTIMIZATION OF SMALL BOWEL AT INITIAL SURGERY

When faced with an initial operation that may require a massive intestinal resection, primary prevention of SBS should be a high priority. Early surgical intervention is paramount in avoiding extensive bowel resection in cases of intestinal ischemia, mesenteric emboli or thrombi, or complete bowel obstruction.[45] The goal of resection should be to preserve as much bowel length possible, including the ICV. This difficult intraoperative decision is challenging.[46] After final resection, accurate documentation of the length of bowel remaining with or without ICV is important. If a stoma is required, consideration to maturing a stoma next to a mucus fistula may aid in restoring intestinal continuity while avoiding a full laparotomy and an extensive lysis of adhesions. Specific disease processes such as Crohn should prompt a conservative bowel-preserving approach focused on the judicious use of stricturoplasties and minimal bowel resection. Even if SBS is likely after the index case, adjunctive procedures should not be performed at the time of initial surgery. In almost 75% of patients with SBS, intestinal adaptation is sufficient enough to sustain growth and long-term survival and precludes the need for surgical therapy.[47]

SURGICAL APPROACH TO OPTIMIZATION OF THE REMNANT SMALL BOWEL AT REOPERATION

Operation for SBS is a complicated surgical challenge. With enteral autonomy as a goal, each surgical option must be carefully weighed and individualized. Often promotility agents (i.e., metoclopramide, cisapride, or erythromycin base) are used to aid in propulsion to improve tolerance.[48] In cases with persistent vomiting refractory to antiemetic medication, a jejunal tube can also be used to gain access for distal feeds. Bowel functions are documented and carefully monitored for infectious etiologies (i.e., *Clostridium difficile*, rotavirus) in the advent of increased stool output. Stool studies are sent, and pathogens are treated with antibiotics if appropriate. Once ruled out, antidiarrheal agents (i.e., loperamide) can be added to slow bowel transit.[49] PN is weaned as the enteral tolerance is optimized.

Ultimately, patients who fail to achieve PN independence and are burdened with these associated complications are offered autologous intestinal reconstruction surgery (AIRS) or transplantation. In determining which operation to perform, a small bowel follow-through is essential in the preoperative planning process.[50,51] Additional questions include whether a stricture will require a stricturoplasty or resection, or if any isolated nonfunctional dilated loops need to be tapered. If hepatic synthetic function is concerning for failure, a liver biopsy is helpful in determining whether a patient has end-stage liver disease, in which case a multivisceral (both small bowel and liver) transplantation should be considered.[52] If not performed preoperatively, a liver biopsy should be obtained at the time of surgery. If the results show cholestasis as a consequence of PN, then a prophylactic cholecystectomy may be considered at the time of surgery.[53]

AUTOGENOUS INTESTINAL RECONSTRUCTION SURGERY

The concepts for surgical procedures for SBS revolve around resolving the major functional problems associated with adapted small bowel, namely disordered motility and stasis that leads to bacterial overgrowth.[51] Therefore the primary objective for AIRS is to improve intestinal function, optimize bowel motility, and increase the mucosal absorptive surface area.

PROCEDURES TO IMPROVE INTESTINAL FUNCTION

Stricturoplasty, Lysis of Adhesions, and Segmental Resection

At reoperation, the surgeon must recognize the need to maximize the remnant bowel. In patients with a history of Crohn disease, necrotizing enterocolitis, or multiple abdominal surgeries, the risk of mechanical obstruction secondary to stenosis from inflammation or ischemia or dense adhesions or anastomotic stricture, respectively, is to be anticipated. Adding to this complexity is that dilated proximal bowel due to distal mechanical obstruction is difficult to distinguish from dilated bowel from SBS adaptation. All sources of mechanical obstructions must be sought and corrected to improve intestinal function. All pathologic adhesions are lysed and stricturoplasty is performed over resection if the affected segment of bowel length is short.[44] If resection is required, then resection should be kept as short in length as possible with consideration to perform multiple end-to-end anastomoses over large segmental resections with blind loops to optimize the remainder of the remnant bowel.

Stoma Takedown and Reestablishing Intestinal Continuity

In patients with abdominal catastrophes, stomas are often required in the initial management of patients who subsequently develop SBS. Stoma takedown and reestablishing intestinal continuity offers clear advantages to improving bowel function. In particular, the colon reabsorbs water and prolongs transit time, particularly if the ICV is intact. In addition, the colon regains the major absorptive function of deriving 5% to 10% of daily caloric energy from SCFAs.[54] Restoring colonic continuity is functionally equivalent to adding another foot of small bowel.[55] If possible, early stoma closure is recommended to enhance adaptation and help in weaning from PN.[56] Finally, stoma reversal may offer an improved quality of life for the patient.

Although the benefits are evident, the uncertain response of the colon to intestinal continuity should prompt careful patient selection. Unabsorbed bile acids can cause irritation of the colon, resulting in a debilitating secretory diarrhea. In patient with severe malabsorption, diarrhea can develop into perineal complications. In addition, because the bile acids prevent the excretion of oxalate in the stool, the oxalate is absorbed in the colon and the patients become at risk for developing calcium oxalate nephrolithiasis. Therefore the decision for stoma reversal and intestinal continuity should be carefully considered and made on an individual basis. At least 3 feet of small intestine is required to prevent diarrhea and perineal complications.[54] The length and location of intestinal remnant, the presence of the ICV, and the patient's overall condition must all be considered and weighed.

Procedures to Prolong Transit or Improve Motility

Procedures to slow intestinal transit are applicable to only a small subset of patients with SBS. There is very limited clinical experience, hence the following procedures should be cautiously applied to patients who have near-adequate remnant length and demonstrate rapid transit. Because these procedures have historically been performed during the adaptive phase after massive surgery or at the time when additional bowel is being recruited into the intestinal tract, the efficacy is difficult to track.[55] Thompson et al. recommend that these procedures be considered after the patient has had maximum SBS adaptation of bowel.[55]

Reversal of Intestinal Segment

Conceptually, creating a distal antiperistaltic segment generates retrograde peristalsis and disrupts coordinated antegrade propulsion of the proximal intestine. Furthermore, the disruption of the intrinsic nerve plexus slows the myoelectrical activity in the distal remnant, thereby prolonging transition time and improving absorption. The largest case series to date of 38 SBS patients treated with a distally placed reverse segment of 10 to 12 cm concluded that this procedure was a safe alternative to small bowel transplantation in patients with permanent PN dependency, with a minimum small bowel length of 25 cm and without chronic liver failure.[57] The literature suggests clinical improvement in slowed intestinal transit and increased absorption in 70% to 80% of patients, although the methods of assessment and follow-up are variable. The length of reversed small intestinal segment ranges from 5 to 15 cm. The challenge has been to determine how long the reversed segment should be because long segments could potentiate an interstitial obstruction. The optimal length appears to be approximately 10 cm in adults and 3 cm in children. Children are generally less favorable candidates.[58]

Colonic Interposition

The colonic segment can be positioned in either the isoperistaltic or antiperistaltic orientation to slow transit time. Colonic interposition into small bowel relies on the premise that colonic peristaltic contractions are lower in frequency than the adjoining small bowel. Therefore proximally placed isoperistaltic interposition serves to slow down the rate of nutrient delivery to the distal small bowel. Alternatively, antiperistaltic interpositions are placed distally and function in a similar fashion as the reversed small bowel intestinal segment. The colon also adds the benefit of reabsorption of water, electrolytes, and nutrients, in addition to delaying transit and having an increased effect on absorption. The length of the colonic segment used does not appear to be as critical as in reversed intestinal segments and ranges from 8 to 24 cm in the literature. There also appears to be fewer obstructive complications with isoperistaltic interposition. Complications include colonic dilation and enterocolitis within the transposed segment.[59]

Intestinal Tapering and Plication

Tapering or plication of functionally dysmotile segments have shown to reduce the diameter of the bowel, thereby improving peristalsis and decreasing the bacterial overgrowth. In tapering enteroplasty, the dilated segment of the antimesenteric border is tapered to match the diameter of the intestinal loop. An appropriate-size chest tube can be used as a guide in resection of the excess bowel along the edge of the tube using a stapler or freehand then sutured.[46] Unfortunately optimization of the bowel caliber comes at the expense of losing significant absorptive surface. Therefore ideal candidates are those who have stasis and malabsorption in dilated bowel yet have adequate intestinal length. The main advantage of this procedure is that the arterial supply from the mesenteric border is left unaffected. As a result, tapering enteroplasty should also be considered when vascular anatomy of the dilated bowel is not amenable for division for a lengthening procedure (Figs. 79.4 and 79.5).[59]

Intestinal plication is also designed to improve motility by decreasing the diameter of the dilated lumen, but, by folding the redundant antimesenteric wall into the lumen and imbricated along the serosal edge, no bowel is resected and therefore no mucosal absorptive surface area is lost. In addition, this procedure avoids the concerns of a long anastomotic suture line leak.[60] Complications reported include development of bowel obstruction from inverted bowel and suture line breakdown, resulting in redilatation and dysmotility.[61]

Procedures to Increase Absorption

The longitudinal intestinal lengthening and tailoring (LILT) and serial transverse enteroplasty (STEP) have gained widespread acceptance as primary AIRS procedures

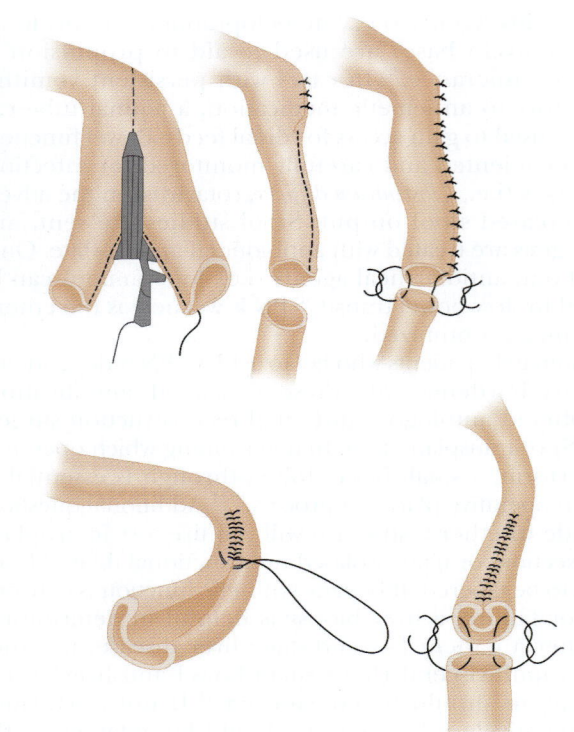

FIGURE 79.4 Intestinal tapering and imbrication. (From Thompson J, Sudan D. Intestinal lengthening for short bowel syndrome. *Adv Surg.* 2008;42:49–61.)

among surgeons. King et al. published a systematic literature review of the LILT and STEP procedures and reported overall survival of 89%, citing no significant difference between the two procedures. Interestingly, LILT has been found to have higher rate of weaned patients, 55% versus 48%, but has been associated with a higher rate of patients receiving transplantations, at 10% versus 6%.[62]

LONGITUDINAL INTESTINAL LENGTHENING AND TAILORING

In 1980 Bianchi reported the LILT procedure in seven pigs and ushered in a new era in SBS management. His technique doubled the length of a loop of small intestine while concurrently reducing the lumen diameter.[63] This novel approach combined the benefits of lengthening, as well as intestinal tapering, which delayed transit time without compromise of mucosal surface loss needed for absorption. In 1981 the first clinical application was reported by Boeckman et al., when LILT was used successfully on 50 cm of dilated bowel in a 4-year-old male with gastroschisis and intrauterine bowel necrosis.[64] Within 10 weeks, the patient was weaned off TPN and was able to obtain enteral autonomy.[65]

LILT was designed on the premise that a bifurcated blood supply exists within the mesentery. This anatomy allows for the two layers of mesentery containing the blood vessels to be separated bluntly on the mesenteric side and bowel divided longitudinally along each parallel lumen. The bowel can be divided using staplers or opened

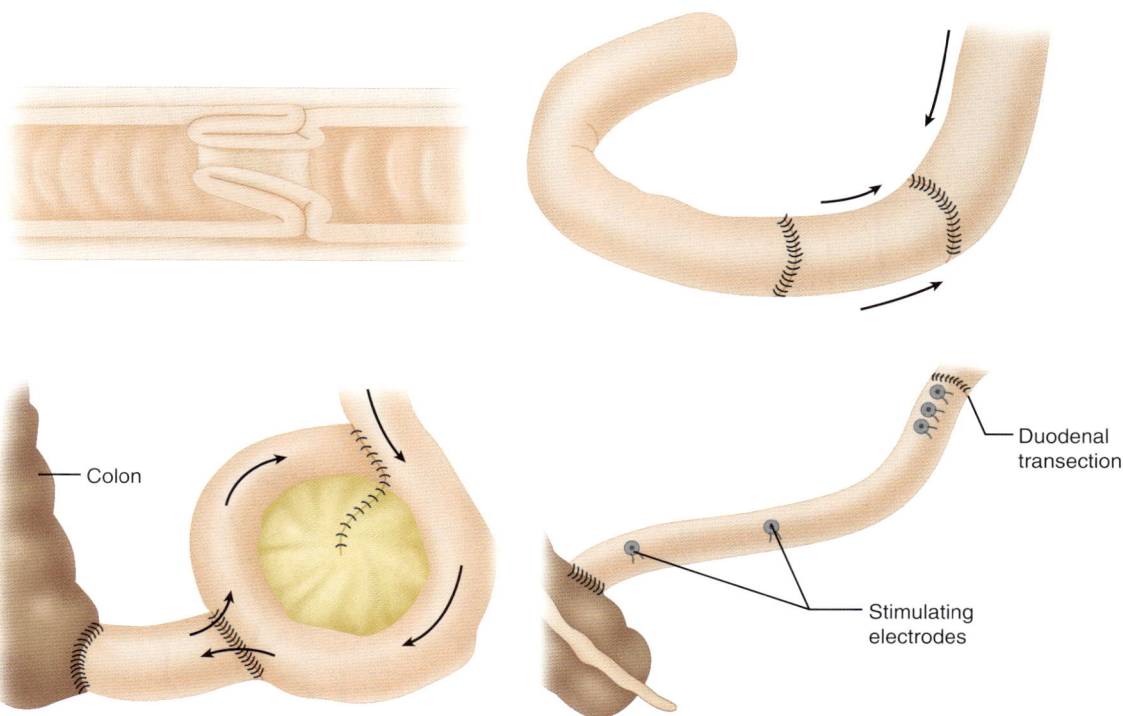

FIGURE 79.5 Creation of intestinal valves, retrograde intestinal pacing, and loop recirculation. (From Thompson JS, Rikkers LF. Surgical alternatives for the short bowel syndrome. *Am J Gastroenterol.* 1987;82:97–106.)

and hemiloops created using suture closure. The end result is two isopropulsive "neo" small bowel lumina, each with its individual blood supply. These two fully vascularized small bowel segments are anastomosed isoperistaltically in a gentle S loop, effectively tapering and doubling the length of the original segment (Fig. 79.6).[62] Anatomic criteria for patient selection include (1) intestinal diameter greater than 3 cm, (2) length of residual small bowel greater than 40 cm, and (3) length of dilated bowel greater than 20 cm.[66] However, regardless of the length, SBS patients with substantial bowel adaptive dilatation secondary to intestinal failure or with life-threatening complications of TPN mentioned previously should receive consideration for LILT.[67]

The surgeon must also be cognizant that anatomic variations, such as predominant blood supply to one side of the intestinal wall, exist that will limit potential success of the procedure.[68] Furthermore, careful consideration is warranted in patients whose mesentery is thickened and scarred due to inflammation or adhesions. For bowel mesentery that is shortened or when the only short gut remaining is a dilated duodenum, the Iowa procedure might be an alternative to the LILT. The Iowa two-step elongation procedure was developed by Kimura et al. and reported in 1993. The initial surgery consists of deseromyotomizing the antimesenteric surface of the dilated segment of bowel to a host organ, such as deperitonealized abdominal wall (Iowa model I),[69] decapsulized liver (Iowa model II),[70] and adjacent bowel with incised serosa (Iowa model III).[71] The concept is to allow vessel collaterals to coapt onto the attached segment of bowel where the two raw and exposed surfaces are reapproximated. After

collaterals have developed, then the second stage consists of a longitudinal split of the parasitized antimesenteric bowel with its own developed blood supply and the mesenteric bowel with the native blood supply. Then an end-to-end anastomosis is created to reestablish intestinal continuity, having created more bowel length.[68] The major disadvantage is that multiple laparotomies are required and weeks are needed for the process of coaptation to develop. For these reasons, the Iowa procedure has not had widespread acceptance as a primary means for bowel lengthening but has a place in specific patients when the mesentery is not favorable (Fig. 79.7).[59]

Bianchi's review of the worldwide published series of 150 patients for LILT reveals a survival percentage ranging from 30% to 100% and reports that the ability to wean from TPN also varies from 28% to 100%.[64] Multiple complications associated with LILT are anastomotic stenosis, interloop abscess and fistula formation, staple line leakage, and hemiloop necrosis resulting from vascular compromise.[65,72] Recurrent dilatation of the lengthened bowel is a common problem that may require additional tapering. Disadvantages to the LILT are that it is a technically challenging procedure that cannot be repeated on the same intestinal segment. In patients unable to wean from PN after LILT, a small bowel transplant (SBTx) was used as a rescue procedure.[52]

SERIAL TRANSVERSE ENTEROPLASTY

In 2003 Kim et al. published a description of the STEP technique in six pigs.[73] He then followed up this animal study with a first human case report later that year after

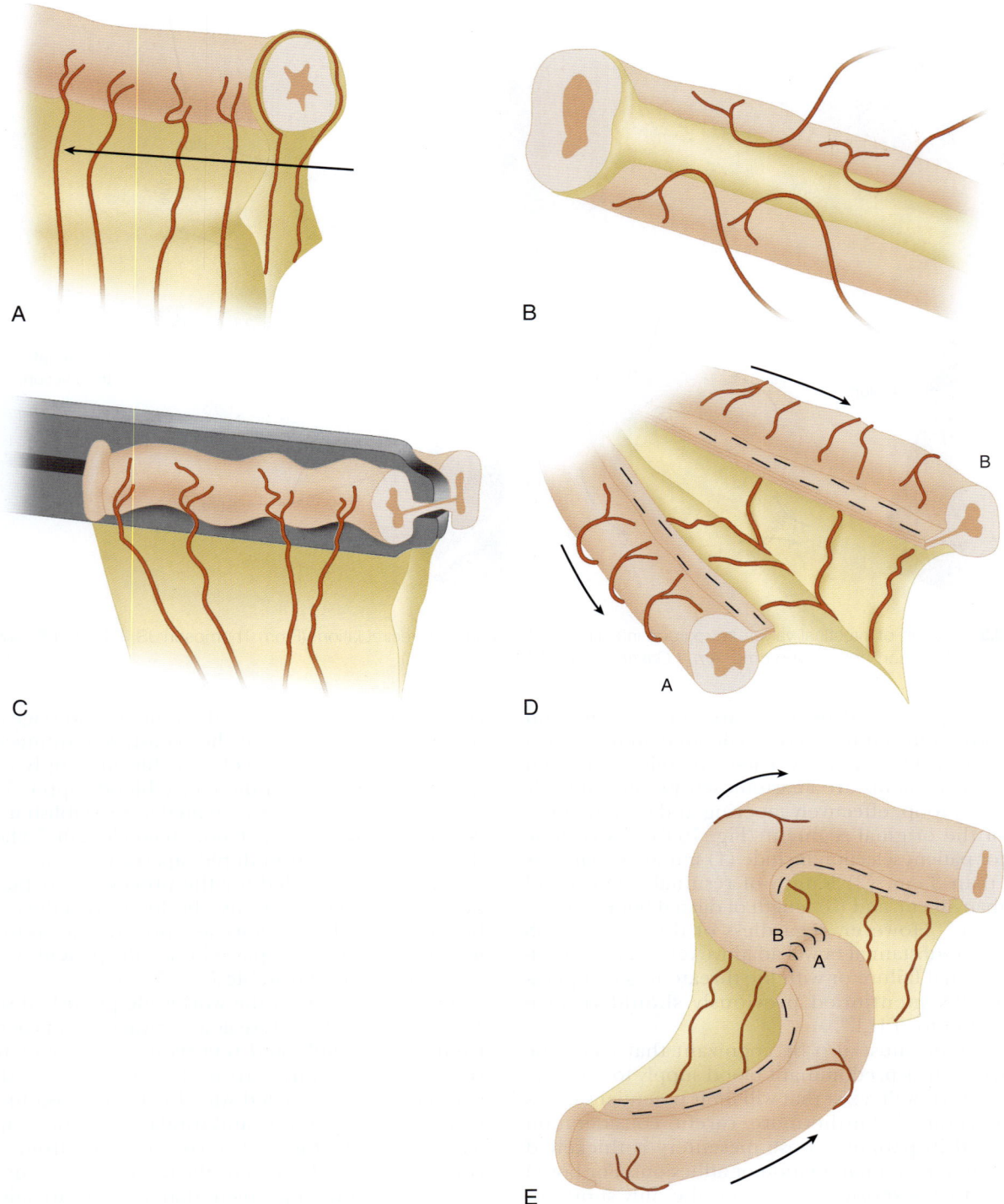

FIGURE 79.6 Bianchi procedure. (From Bianchi A. Intestinal loop lengthening—a technique for increasing small intestinal length. *J Pediatr Surg.* 1980;15:145–151).

performing a successful STEP procedure on a 2-year-old male born with gastroschisis and a complication of dilated surgically lengthened bowel after a Bianchi LILT. The operation successfully increased 83 cm of dilated and previously lengthened bowel to 147 cm.[74]

The STEP relies on the anatomic premise that the small bowel blood supply from the mesentery runs perpendicular to the long axis of the small bowel. Therefore placing alternating and opposite transverse staple fires parallel to the mesentery along the length of the dilated bowel results in a zig zag–shaped elongated bowel with minimal vascular compromise. Several technical considerations are to properly orient the small bowel by marking the antimesenteric border so as to prevent twisting and performing

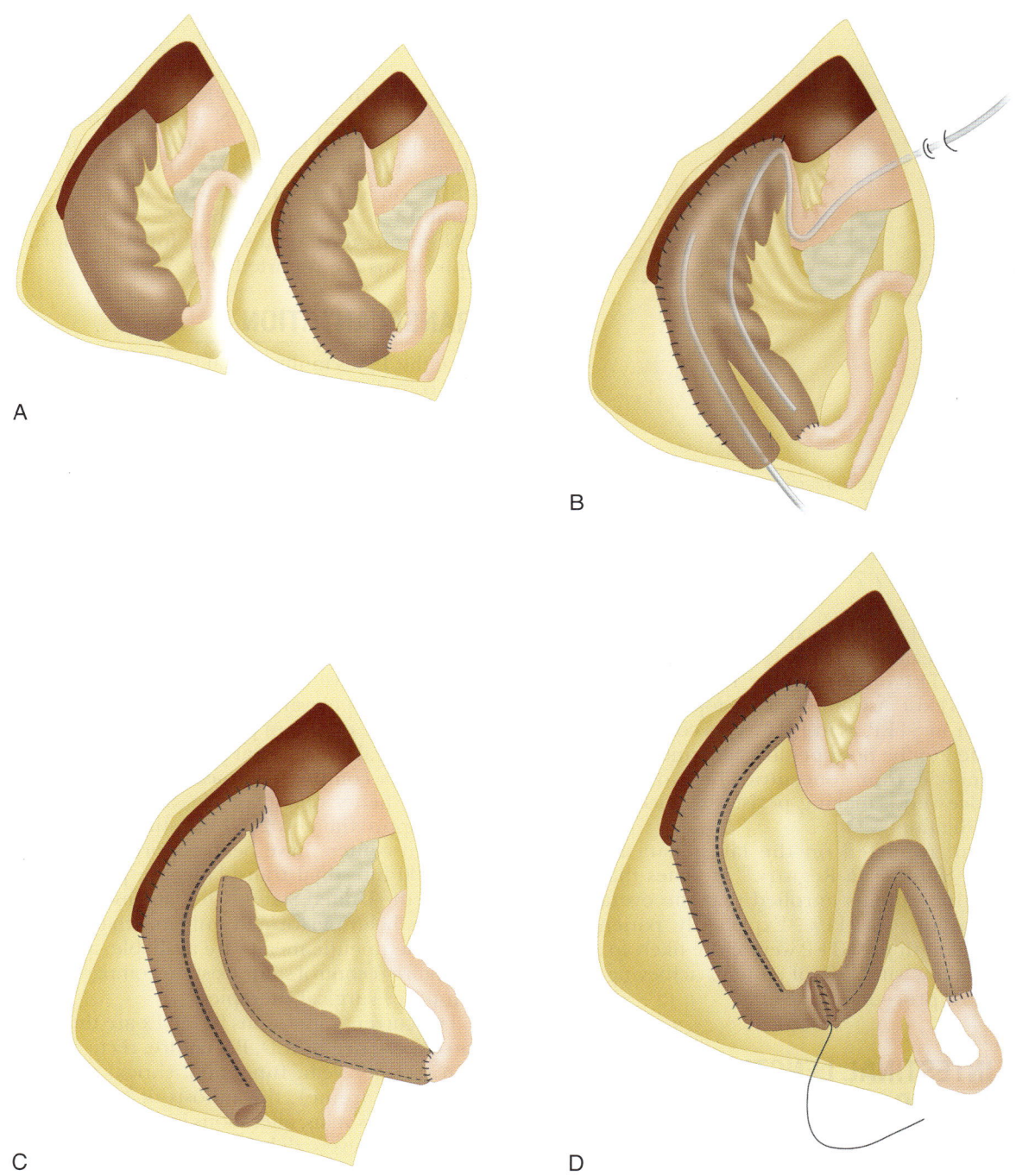

A

B

C

D

FIGURE 79.7 Iowa procedure. (From Kimura K, Soper RT. A new bowel elongation technique for the short-bowel syndrome using the isolated bowel segment Iowa models. *J Pediatr Surg.* 1993;28:792–794.)

partial division of the bowel so as not to cause obstruction. The distance between the staple lines is typically 1.5 times the diameter of the remaining lumen. An average of 10 to 20 staple lines are used, reducing the average dilated diameter of 5 to 6 cm to 2 cm and increasing the ultimate length to 1.5- to 2-fold. The length gained will depend on the original length and width of the bowel and number of staple fires. The crotch or apex of the staple line can be reinforced with suture (Fig. 79.8).[75]

The advantage with the STEP is that it is a simpler bowel lengthening procedure, easily reproducible with minimal manipulation to the mesentery, and no associated bowel anastomosis required. The STEP procedure has been ideal for asymmetrical bowel dilatation and segments of dilated bowel with complicated intricacies such as duodenum with associated pancreas and biliary system, as well as the jejunum and its association near the ligament of Treitz. The significant benefit of the STEP is that it

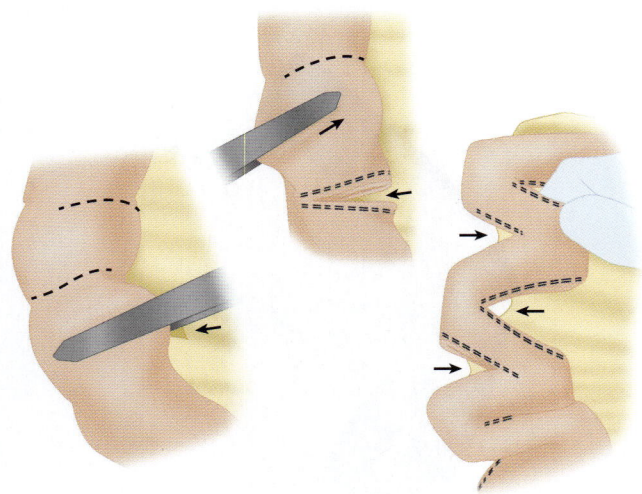

FIGURE 79.8 Serial transverse enteroplasty procedure. *Arrows* indicate direction of stapler (open jaw) placement onto bowel. (From Kim HB, Fauza D, Garza J, Oh JT, Nurko S, Jaksic T. Serial transverse enteroplasty [STEP]: a novel bowel lengthening procedure. *J Pediatr Surg.* 2003;38:425–429.)

can be performed as a primary index lengthening procedure or be repeated on patients who develop dilatations after LILT or STEP operations.[76,77] However, several disadvantages also exist. Asymmetrical postoperative redilation can also occur in STEP, as in LILT. This complication has been attributed to the postoperative alterations in orientation of the muscles from concentric fibers to longitudinal fibers and vice versa, making peristalsis uncoordinated, resulting in dilation.[78,79]

Jones et al. reported on the latest data from the International STEP Data Registry.[80] He cites that of the 111 consecutive patients enrolled that the overall postoperative mortality was 11%. Expectedly, patients with longer bowel length pre-STEP were more likely to achieve enteral autonomy, with 47% of patients achieving enteral autonomy post procedure.[80]

SPIRAL INTESTINAL LENGTHENING AND TAILORING

The latest innovation in the bowel lengthening is the spiral intestinal lengthening and tailoring (SILT). In 2013 Cserni et al. published the description of SILT successfully performed on six Vietnamese minipigs.[81] This new technique entails cutting the bowel and its associated mesentery along a 45- to 60-degree spiral line, then longitudinally tightening the spiral and lengthening the bowel. The bowel edges are approximated with suture. The advantages reported are minimal manipulation to the mesentery and no changes to the orientation of the bowel fibers, which have been attributed to cause redilation after STEP (Fig. 79.9).[78] The potential complications are intestinal leakage and abscess formation. No long-term data exist on this procedure because the first two applications on human patients were reported in 2014. Cserni followed his in vivo case report with the first human application on a

3-year-old female with 22 cm of small bowel remaining, resulting from a midgut volvulus. SILT was able to lengthen 11 cm of her dilated 22 cm of small bowel an additional 20 cm, with the total bowel length of 31 cm. The patient was able to wean off TPN with improvement in liver functions but still remained on gastrostomy tube feeds.[81] Alberti et al. also reported on the successful application of SILT on a 10-month-old who, at 1-year follow-up, was on the 15 to 25 percentile on 82% oral calories and 18% TPN.[82] Long-term data should follow as more successful applications are reported (Fig. 79.10).

TRANSPLANTATION

Since the 1960s multivisceral transplantation (MVTx) has been complicated by challenges of graft rejection, infection, and progression of underlying disease. Tacrolimus was introduced in 1989 and drastically reduced the rates of allograft rejection, hence improving surgical outcomes.[83] With steady improvements in immunosuppression strategies and surgical techniques, survival rates have also improved. For intestinal and MVTx, the 1- and 3-year survival rates are reported to be 78% and 66%, respectively, with the intestinal graft survival of 80% in adults.[84] In addition, Abu-Elmagd et al. report a patient survival rate after a 15-year follow-up to be as high as 61%.[85] More than 90% of patients undergoing intestinal transplantation are reported to have been liberated off of TPN.[86] This level of success has elevated small bowel transplantation as a final curative option in patients with intestinal failure and futile medical and surgical rehabilitation attempts, offering relief from complications associated with TPN and ultimately, a better quality of life. Since its inception in the 1990s, approximately 2887 intestinal transplants from 87 different centers have been reported. Since 2001 more than 100 intestinal transplants are performed per year, 75% in the United States.[86] To date, intestinal transplantation has been performed only in situations in which no other therapeutic means are available, and as a result no randomized control study exists to compare transplantation with other surgical therapies.[3]

The current indications for SBTx are those SBS patients who experience IFALD, PN failure, recurrent CRIs (more than two per year, fungemia, shock, acute respiratory distress syndrome), thrombosis of two of the six major central access veins, alterations in growth and development in children, severe dehydration with refractory electrolyte changes, and impending liver failure or established liver disease with cirrhosis and portal hypertension.[87,88]

Depending on other associated organs needing replacement, intestinal transplantation has a number of variations. An isolated SBTx is offered in irreversible intestinal failure in the absence of concomitant liver failure proven by liver biopsy. The entire jejunum and ileum is transplanted with or without the colon, in efforts to maintain as much functional bowel as possible. Intestinal continuity is established 8 to 10 cm distal to the ligament of Treitz via side-to-side graft to native jejunojejunal anastomosis. Then a side-to-side graft ileum to native colon anastomosis approximately 15 cm from the ileostomy is created to reestablish continuity. In all of these transplant procedures, an allograft end ileostomy is performed so as to be used

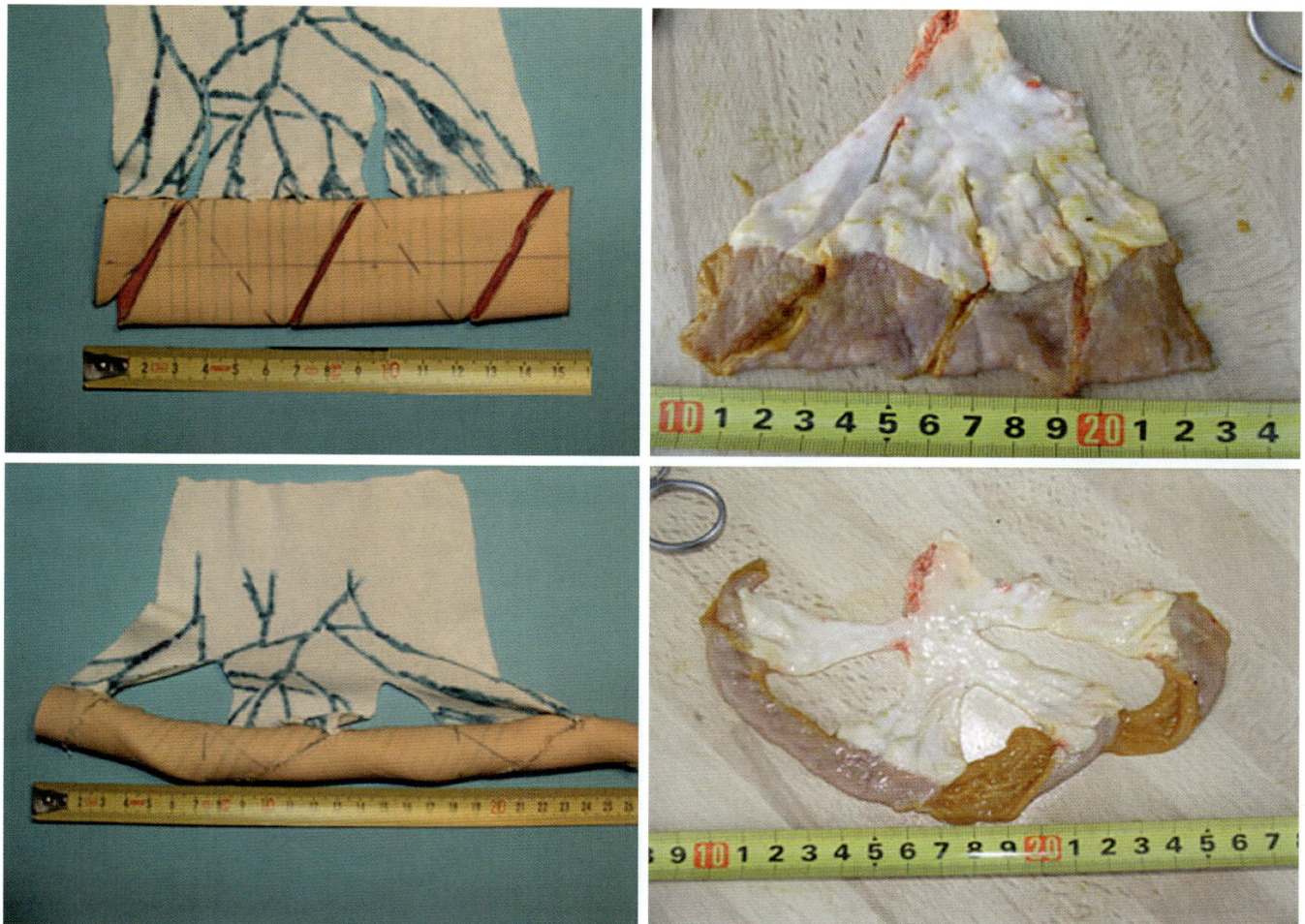

FIGURE 79.9 Spiral intestinal lengthening and tailoring procedure. (From Cserni T, Takayasu H, Muzsnay Z, et al. New idea of intestinal lengthening and tailoring. *Pediatr Surg Int*. 2011;27:1009–1013.)

for graft surveillance for allograft rejection via repeated biopsies if needed.[59] A combined liver-intestinal transplant (SB-LTx) is performed when patients with intestinal failure also have a coexisting irreversible liver disease. A MVTx is reserved for cases in which abdominal catastrophes (i.e., extensive intestinal resection, severe abdominal trauma, multiple enterocutaneous fistulas, chronic diffuse mesenteric vascular thrombosis) necessitate a complete replacement of all abdominal organs.[89] MVTx requires the removal and transplantation of both foregut and midgut. Variations include replacement of liver, kidneys, and large intestine, as well depending on the need.[59]

Complications associated with intestinal transplantation are vast, complex, and life-threatening and beyond the scope of this chapter. The most common complications include postoperative hemorrhage, biliary or vascular complications, and GI leaks. Biliary leak often occurs in the early postoperative period at the Roux-en-Y choledo-chojejunostomy in SB-LTx. Vascular complications are rare but devastating. Necrosis of the tissues results from arterial thrombosis and may necessitate graft removal. Venous thrombosis of the superior mesenteric vein or portal vein access can result in an outflow obstruction and also compromise the intestinal graft. GI leaks from

the proximal and distal anastomosis usually occur in the first postoperative week. Bleeding is the most common GI complication, and rejection of the intestinal graft must be investigated and distinguished from infection. Endoscopy is performed through the end ileostomy, and biopsies are taken to assess for rejection.[90–94]

Infectious etiologies of bleeding include Epstein-Barr virus (EBV) or cytomegalovirus (CMV), which can also be identified as bleeding ulcers via endoscopy. EBV infection remains one of the most serious consequences after intestinal transplantation. EBV-associated posttransplant lymphoproliferative disorder (PTLD) presents as a constellation of disorders ranging from a nonspecific, self-limiting mononucleosis to serious PTLD leading to lymphoma. PTLD incidence is higher with intestinal transplant at 20% as compared with other types of organ transplants.[3] CMV is the most common viral infection after intestinal transplant and also has significant morbidity and mortality. The overall incidence is 34%, primarily involving the allograft intestine.[3] CMV is diagnosed by monitoring CMV polymerase chain reaction (PCR) or culture and treated with intravenous ganciclovir or valganciclovir as first-line and foscarnet as second-line therapy.[95]

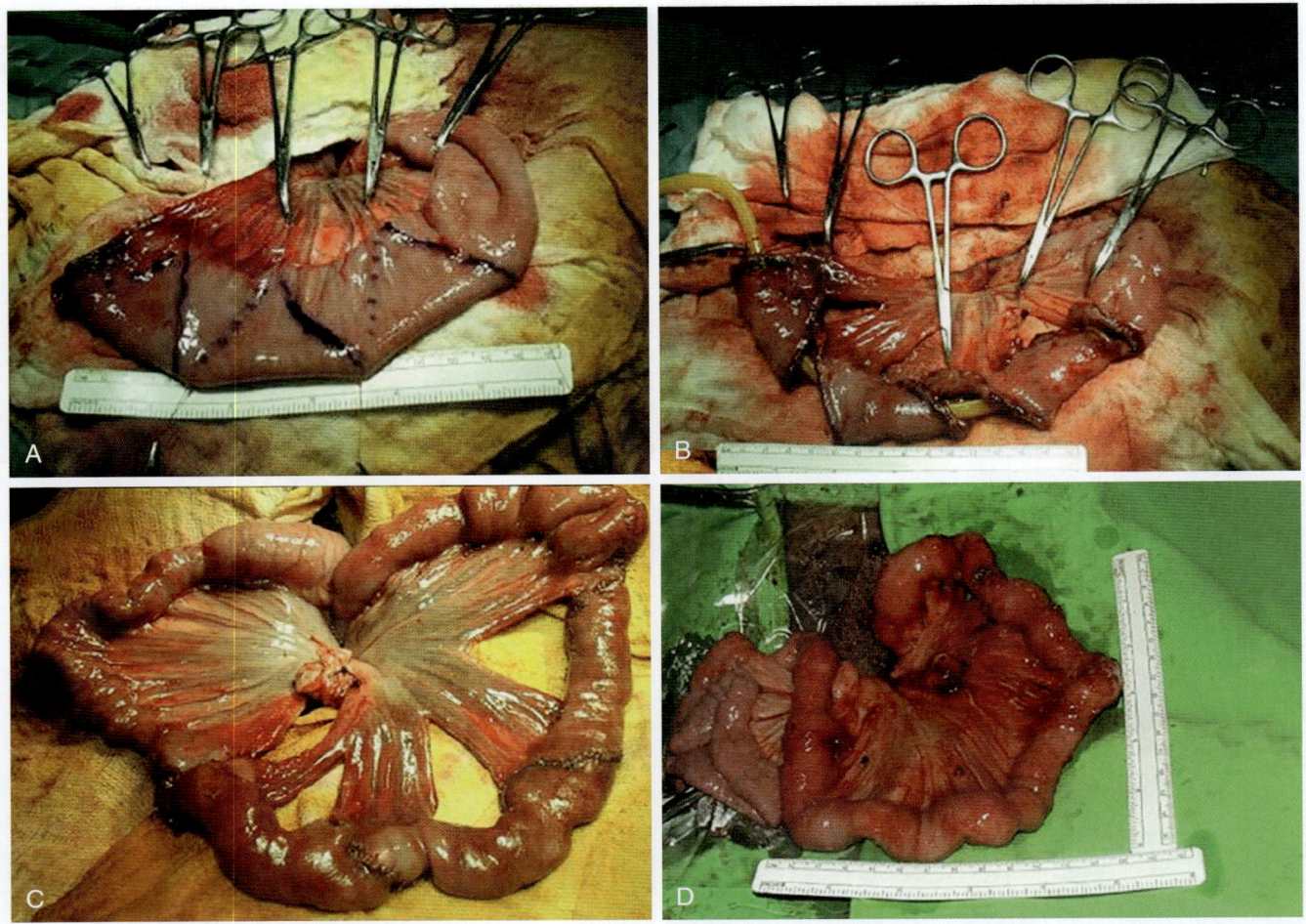

FIGURE 79.10 Spiral intestinal lengthening and tailoring in vivo. (From Cserni T, Varga G, Erces D, et al. Spiral intestinal lengthening and tailoring—first in vivo study. *J Pediatr Surg.* 2013;48:1907–1913.)

Interestingly, although the survival rates mentioned previously are higher for isolated SBTx than MVTx, the risk of acute cellular rejection (ACR) is higher in SBTx (79%) when compared with combined SB-LTx (71%) or MVTx (59%), respectively.[89,96] This immunologic reaction has been attributed to the highly immunogenic small bowel allograft, which contains a large amount of gut-associated lymphoid tissue, as well as donor dendritic cells that propagate an ACR.[97] It has been postulated that the MVTx and the SB-LVTx have protective effects from the liver. ACR can occur any time with 48% presenting within 30 days and 66% presenting within the first 100 post-transplantation.[98] Induction therapy with IL-2 blocker has become the standard of care in over 75% of intestine transplant recipients, leading to decreased incidence of acute rejection and improved patient survival.[99] Proto-colized surveillance endoscopies through the graft ileos-tomy are usually performed twice weekly for the first 4 to 6 weeks then in decreasing frequency in the following weeks following transplantation; therefore most acute rejections are discovered.[100] ACR presents with diarrhea resulting in damage to the gut mucosal barrier. This barrier compromise leads to bacterial sepsis and fever. Once endoscopy and biopsies confirm the diagnosis, the patient is initially treated with a cumulative steroid dose of 30 mg/kg methylprednisolone given in three divided doses for three days or a 10 mg/kg bolus followed by tapered doses of 5, 4, 3, and 2 mg/kg each day after. Posttreatment biopsies are performed until symptoms resolve or pathology shows histologic improvement. Steroid refractory rejection manifests as ongoing exfoliation of mucosa and persistent crypt loss on histology and will require the addition of antilymphocyte antibodies (i.e., murine anti-CD3 monoclonal antibody [OKT3]). Five to seven doses are used. Other antibody agents used are anti-CD52 humanized monoclonal antibodies (alemtu-zamab) and rabbit antihuman thymocyte globulin (rATG).[87] Sepsis remains the leading cause of graft loss in 50% of cases, followed by graft-related causes including rejection at 13% and cardiovascular events at 8%.

CONCLUSION

Patients with SBS are a small part of the population; however, these patients have complex pathophysiologies that demand intensive long-term health care. Great progress in the survival of SBS patients occurred with the development and adoption of PN, but with raised secondary costs of an iatrogenic nature (PN-related catheter complications, nutritional deficiencies, and liver failure). The success in optimizing the life span and the quality of life for SBS patients is delivered with the optimization of fluid and dietary management, education and psychosocial support, metabolic management, innovative pharmacologic nutritional additives (teduglutide), and the transition to focused surgical interventions (intestinal surgical rehab or transplantation). Better understanding of both the loss and adaptation capacity of small intestine also means an individualized program of support for each SBS patient. Further progress in the management of these patients will likely occur at the expansion of IRCs with the established clinical pathways and programmatic orientation toward these patients.

REFERENCES

1. Crenn P, Hanchie M, Valleur P, Hautefeuille P, Rambaud JC, Messing B. Surgical versus radiological evaluation of remaining small bowel length in short bowel syndrome. *Gastroenterology.* 1996;110:A321.
2. Nightingale JMD, Bartram CI, Lennard-Jones JE. Length of residual small bowel after partial resection: correlation between radiographic and surgical measurements. *Gastrointest Radiol.* 1991;16(1):305-306.
3. DeLegge M, Alsolaiman MM, Barbour E, Bassas S, Siddiqi MF, Moore NM. Short bowel syndrome: parenteral nutrition versus intestinal transplantation. Where are we today? *Dig Dis Sci.* 2007; 52(4):876-892.
4. Thompson J. Comparison of massive vs. repeated resection leading to short bowel syndrome. *J Gastrointest Surg.* 2000;4(1):101-104.
5. Chopy K, Winkler M, Schwartz-Barcott D, Melanson K, Greene G. A qualitative study of the perceived value of membership in the Oley Foundation by home parenteral and enteral nutrition consumers. *JPEN J Parenter Enteral Nutr.* 2014;39(4):426-433.
6. Byrne TA, Persinger RL, Young LS, Ziegler TR, Wilmore DW. A new treatment for patients with short-bowel syndrome. Growth hormone, glutamine, and a modified diet. *Ann Surg.* 1995;222(3):243-255.
7. Mughal M. Home parenteral nutrition in the United Kingdom and Ireland. *Lancet.* 1986;328(8503):383-387.
8. Bakker H, Bozzetti F, Staun M, et al. Home parenteral nutrition in adults: a European multicentre survey in 1997. ESPEN-Home Artificial Nutrition Working Group. *Clin Nutr.* 1999;18(3):135-140.
9. Brandt CF, Bangsgaard L, Jess T, et al. Mo1179 the evolution of treatment of patients with intestinal failure with home parenteral nutrition. *Gastroenterology.* 2012;142(5):S-613-S-614.
10. Pironi L, Hébuterne X, Van Gossum A, et al. Candidates for intestinal transplantation: a multicenter survey in Europe. *Am J Gastroenterol.* 2006;101(7):1633-1643.
11. Amiot A, Messing B, Corcos O, Panis Y, Joly F. Determinants of home parenteral nutrition dependence and survival of 268 patients with non-malignant short bowel syndrome. *Clin Nutr.* 2013;32(3):368-374.
12. Grant D, Abu-Elmagd K, Reyes J, et al. 2003 Report of the intestine transplant registry. *Ann Surg.* 2005;241(4):607-613.
13. Wales PW, de Silva N, Kim J, Lecce L, To T, Moore A. Neonatal short bowel syndrome: population-based estimates of incidence and mortality rates. *J Pediatr Surg.* 2004;39(5):690-695.
14. Messing B, Crenn P, Beau P, Boutron-Ruault MC, Rambaud JC, Matuchansky C. Long-term survival and parenteral nutrition dependence in adult patients with the short bowel syndrome. *Gastroenterology.* 1999;117(5):1043-1050.
15. Wales PW, Christison-Lagay ER. Short bowel syndrome: epidemiology and etiology. *Semin Pediatr Surg.* 2010;19(1):3-9.
16. Buchman AL. The medical and surgical management of short bowel syndrome. *MedGenMed.* 2004;6:12.
17. Tappenden KA. Pathophysiology of short bowel syndrome: considerations of resected and residual anatomy. *JPEN J Parenter Enteral Nutr.* 2014;38(1 suppl):14S-22S.
18. Kumpf V. Pharmacological management of diarrhea in patients with short bowel syndrome. *JPEN J Parenter Enteral Nutr.* 2014;38 (suppl 1):38S-44S.
19. Debongnie JC, Phillips SF. Capacity of the human colon to absorb fluid. *Gastroenterology.* 1978;74:698-703.
20. Keller J, Panter H, Layer P. Management of the short bowel syndrome after extensive small bowel resection. *Best Pract Res Clin Gastroenterol.* 2004;18(5):977-992.
21. Ulrich-Baker MG, Höllwarth ME, Kvietys PR, Granger DN. Blood flow response to small bowel resection. *Am J Physiol.* 1986;251:G815-G822.
22. Tappenden K. Intestinal adaptation following resection. *JPEN J Parenter Enteral Nutr.* 2014;38(suppl 1):23S-31S.
23. Spencer AU, Neaga A, West B, et al. Pediatric short bowel syndrome: redefining predictors of success. *Ann Surg.* 2005;242:403-412.
24. Joly F, Mayeur C, Messing B, et al. Morphological adaptation with preserved proliferation/transporter content in the colon of patients with short bowel syndrome. *Am J Physiol Gastrointest Liver Physiol.* 2009;297:G116-G123.
25. Doldi S. Intestinal adaptation following jejuno-ileal bypass. *Clin Nutr.* 1991;10:138-145.
26. Royall D, Wolever TM, Jeejeebhoy KN. Evidence for colonic conservation of malabsorbed carbohydrate in short bowel syndrome. *Am J Gastroenterol.* 1992;87:751-756.
27. Nordgaard I, Hansen BS, Mortensen PB. Importance of colonic support for energy absorption as small-bowel failure proceeds. *Am J Clin Nutr.* 1996;64:222-231.
28. Nightingale JM, Kamm MA, van der Sijp JR, Ghatei MA, Bloom SR, Lennard-Jones JE. Gastrointestinal hormones in short bowel syndrome: peptide YY may be the "colonic brake" to gastric emptying. *Gut.* 1996;39:267-272.
29. Chen WJ, Yang CL, Lai HS, Chen KM. Effects of lipids on intestinal adaptation following 60% resection in rats. *J Surg Res.* 1995;58:253-259.
30. Byrne TA, et al. Growth hormone, glutamine, and an optimal diet reduces parenteral nutrition in patients with short bowel syndrome. *Ann Surg.* 2005;242(5):655-661.
31. Wales PW, Nasr A, de Silva N, Yamada J. Human growth hormone and glutamine for patients with short bowel syndrome. *Cochrane Database Syst Rev.* 2010;(6):CD006321.
32. Wall E. An overview of short bowel syndrome management: adherence, adaptation and practical recommendations. *J Acad Nutr Diet.* 2013;113:1200-1208.
33. Nordgaard I, Hansen BS, Mortensen PB. Colon as a digestive organ in patients with short bowel. *Lancet.* 1994;343:373-376.
34. Torres C, Vanderhoof JA. Chronic complications of short bowel syndrome. *Curr Paediatr.* 2006;16(5):291-297.
35. Cavicchi M. Prevalence of liver disease and contributing factors in patients receiving home parenteral nutrition for permanent intestinal failure. *Ann Intern Med.* 2000;132(7):525.
36. Jeppesen PB, Pertkiewicz M, Messing B, et al. Teduglutide reduces need for parenteral support among patients with short bowel syndrome with intestinal failure. *Gastroenterology.* 2012;143:1473-1481.
37. Jeppesen PB, Pertkiewicz M, Forbes A, et al. Quality of life in patients with short bowel syndrome treated with the new glucagon-like peptide-2 analogue teduglutide—analyses from a randomised, placebo-controlled study. *Clin Nutr.* 2013;32:713-721.
38. Matarese LE, Jeppesen PB, O'Keefe SJ. Short bowel syndrome in adults: the need for an interdisciplinary approach and coordinated care. *JPEN J Parenter Enteral Nutr.* 2014;38(suppl 1):60S-64S.
39. Nehme A. Nutritional support of the hospitalized patient: the team concept. *JAMA.* 1980;243(19):1906-1908.
40. Hassell JT, Games AD, Shaffer B, Harkins LE. Nutrition support team management of enterally fed patients in a community hospital is cost-beneficial. *J Am Diet Assoc.* 1994;94(9):993-998.
41. Reddy VS, Patole SK, Rao S. Role of probiotics in short bowel syndrome in infants and children—a systematic review. *Nutrients.* 2013;5:679-699.
42. Mermel LA, Farr BM, Sherertz RJ, et al. Guidelines for the management of intravascular catheter-related infections. *Infect Control Hosp Epidemiol.* 2001;22(4):222-242.
43. Mouw E, Chessman K, Lesher A, Tagge E. Use of an ethanol lock to prevent catheter-related infections in children with short bowel syndrome. *J Pediatr Surg.* 2008;43(6):1025-1029.
44. Drongowski RA, Coran AG. An analysis of factors contributing to the development of total parenteral nutrition-induced cholestasis. *JPEN J Parenter Enteral Nutr.* 1989;13(6):586-589.
45. Thompson J. Surgical considerations in the short bowel syndrome. *Surg Gynecol Obstet.* 1993;176(1):89-101.

46. Wales PW. Surgical therapy for short bowel syndrome. *Pediatr Surg Int.* 2004;20(9):647-657.

47. Anagnostopoulos D, Valioulis J, Sfougaris D, Maliaropoulos N, Spyridakis J. Morbidity and mortality of short bowel syndrome in infancy and childhood. *Eur J Pediatr Surg.* 1991;1(5):273-276.

48. Puntis JWL, Booth IW, Buick R. Cisapride in neonatal short gut. *Lancet.* 1986;328(8498):108-109.

49. Nightingale JMD. Management of patients with a short bowel. *Nutrition.* 1999;15(7-8):633-637.

50. Barksdale EM, Stanford A. The surgical management of short bowel syndrome. *Curr Gastroenterol Rep.* 2002;4(3):229-237.

51. Warner BW, Chaet MS. Nontransplant surgical options for management of the short bowel syndrome. *J Pediatr Gastroenterol Nutr.* 1993;17(1):1-12.

52. Jones BA, Hull MA, McGuire MM, Kim HB. Autologous intestinal reconstruction surgery. *Semin Pediatr Surg.* 2010;19(1):59-67.

53. Thompson JS. The role of prophylactic cholecystectomy in the short-bowel syndrome. *Arch Surg.* 1996;131(5):556.

54. Scolapio JS, Fleming CR. Short bowel syndrome. *Gastroenterol Clin North Am.* 1998;27(2):467-479.

55. Thompson JS. Surgical rehabilitation of intestine in short bowel syndrome. *Surgery.* 2004;135(5):465-470.

56. Andorsky DJ, Lund DP, Lillehei CW, et al. Nutritional and other postoperative management of neonates with short bowel syndrome correlates with clinical outcomes. *J Pediatr.* 2001;139(1):27-33.

57. Beyer-Berjot L, Joly F, Maggiori L, et al. Segmental reversal of the small bowel can end permanent parenteral nutrition dependency: an experience of 38 adults with short bowel syndrome. *Ann Surg.* 2012;256(5):739-745.

58. Vernon AH, Georgeson KE. Surgical options for short bowel syndrome. *Semin Pediatr Surg.* 2001;10(2):91-98.

59. Rege A. The surgical approach to short bowel syndrome—autologous reconstruction versus transplantation. *Viszeralmedizin.* 2014;30(3):179-189.

60. de Lorimier AA, Harrison MR. Intestinal plication in the treatment of atresia. *J Pediatr Surg.* 1983;18(6):734-737.

61. Thompson JS, Langnas AN, Pinch LW, Kaufman S, Quigley EM, Vanderhoof JA. Surgical approach to short-bowel syndrome. *Ann Surg.* 1995;222(4):600-607.

62. King B, et al. Intestinal bowel lengthening in children with short bowel syndrome: systematic review of the Bianchi and STEP procedures. *World J Surg.* 2012;37(3):694-704.

63. Bianchi A. Intestinal loop lengthening—a technique for increasing small intestinal length. *J Pediatr Surg.* 1980;15(2):145-151.

64. Boeckman CR, Traylor R. Bowel lengthening for short gut syndrome. *J Pediatr Surg.* 1981;16(6):996-997.

65. Bianchi A. From the cradle to enteral autonomy: the role of autologous gastrointestinal reconstruction. *Gastroenterology.* 2006;130(2):S138-S146.

66. Goulet O, Sauvat F. Short bowel syndrome and intestinal transplantation in children. *Curr Opin Clin Nutr Metab Care.* 2006;9(3):304-313.

67. Thompson J, Sudan D. Intestinal lengthening for short bowel syndrome. *Adv Surg.* 2008;42:49-61.

68. Thompson JS, Vanderhoof JA, Antonson DL. Intestinal tapering and lengthening for short bowel syndrome. *J Pediatr Gastroenterol Nutr.* 1985;4(3):495-497.

69. Kimura K, Soper RT. A new bowel elongation technique for the short-bowel syndrome using the isolated bowel segment Iowa models. *J Pediatr Surg.* 1993;28(6):792-794.

70. Yamazato M, Kimura K, Yoshino H, Soper RT. The isolated bowel segment (Iowa model II) created in functioning bowel. *J Pediatr Surg.* 1991;26(7):780-783.

71. El-Murr M, Kimura K, Ellsberg D, Yamazato M, Yoshino H, Soper RT. Motility of isolated bowel segment Iowa model III. *Dig Dis Sci.* 1994;39(12):2619-2623.

72. Weber TR. Isoperistaltic bowel lengthening for short bowel syndrome in children. *Am J Surg.* 1999;178(6):600-603.

73. Kim HB, Fauza D, Garza J, Oh JT, Nurko S, Jaksic T. Serial transverse enteroplasty (STEP): a novel bowel lengthening procedure. *J Pediatr Surg.* 2003;38(3):425-429.

74. Kim HB, Lee PW, Garza J, Duggan C, Fauza D, Jaksic T. Serial transverse enteroplasty for short bowel syndrome: a case report. *J Pediatr Surg.* 2003;38(6):881-885.

75. Sigalet D. STEP procedure. *Oper Tech Gen Surg.* 2007;9(1):39-42.

76. Ehrlich PF, Mychaliska GB, Teitelbaum DH. The 2 STEP: an approach to repeating a serial transverse enteroplasty. *J Pediatr Surg.* 2007;42(5):819-822.

77. Andres AM, Thompson J, Grant W, et al. Repeat surgical bowel lengthening with the STEP procedure. *Transplantation.* 2008;85(9):1294-1299.

78. Cserni T, Takayasu H, Muzsnay Z, et al. New idea of intestinal lengthening and tailoring. *Pediatr Surg Int.* 2011;27(9):1009-1013.

79. Kang KH, Gutierrez IM, Zurakowski D, et al. Bowel re-dilation following serial transverse enteroplasty (STEP). *Pediatr Surg Int.* 2012;28(12):1189-1193.

80. Jones BA, Hull MA, Potanos KM, et al. Report of 111 consecutive patients enrolled in the International Serial Transverse Enteroplasty (STEP) Data Registry: a retrospective observational study. *J Am Coll Surg.* 2013;216(3):438-446.

81. Cserni T, Varga G, Erces D, et al. Spiral intestinal lengthening and tailoring—first in vivo study. *J Pediatr Surg.* 2013;48(9):1907-1913.

82. Alberti D, Boroni G, Giannotti G, et al. "Spiral intestinal lenghtening and tailoring (SILT)" for a child with severely short bowel. *Pediatr Surg Int.* 2014;30(11):1169-1172.

83. Tocci MJ, Matkovich DA, Collier KA, et al. The immunosuppressant FK506 selectively inhibits expression of early T cell activation genes. *J Immunol.* 1989;143(2):718-726.

84. Smith JM, Skeans MA, Horslen SP, et al. OPTN/SRTR 2012 Annual Data Report: Intestine. *Am J Transplant.* 2014;14(S1):97-111.

85. Abu-Elmagd KM, Kosmach-Park B, Costa G, et al. Long-term survival, nutritional autonomy, and quality of life after intestinal and multivisceral transplantation. *Ann Surg.* 2012;256(3):494-508.

86. Abu–Elmagd KM. Intestinal transplantation for short bowel syndrome and gastrointestinal failure: current consensus, rewarding outcomes, and practical guidelines. *Gastroenterology.* 2006;130(2):S132-S137.

87. Vianna RM, Mangus RS, Tector AJ. Current status of small bowel and multivisceral transplantation. *Adv Surg.* 2008;42:129-150.

88. Sudan D. The current state of intestine transplantation: indications, techniques, outcomes and challenges. *Am J Transplant.* 2014;14(9):1976-1984.

89. Nishida S, Hadjis NS, Levi DM, et al. Intestinal and multivisceral transplantation after abdominal trauma. *J Trauma.* 2004;56(2):323-327.

90. Fishbein TM, Gondolesi GE, Kaufman SS. Intestinal transplantation for gut failure. *Gastroenterology.* 2003;124(6):1615-1628.

91. Farmer DG, McDiarmid SV, Yersiz H, et al. Outcomes after intestinal transplantation: a single-center experience over a decade. *Transplant Proc.* 2002;34(3):896-897.

92. Reyes J, Bueno J, Kocoshis S, et al. Current status of intestinal transplantation in children. *J Pediatr Surg.* 1998;33(2):243-254.

93. Reyes J, Abu-Elmagd K. Small bowel transplantation in children. In: Kelly DA, ed. *Diseases of the Liver and Biliary System in Children.* Oxford: Wiley-Blackwell; 1999:402-420.

94. Langnas AN, Shaw BW Jr, Antonson DL, et al. Preliminary experience with intestinal transplantation in infants and children. *Pediatrics.* 1996;97(4):443-448.

95. Florescu DF, Abu-Elmagd K, Mercer DF, Qiu F, Kalil AC. An international survey of cytomegalovirus prevention and treatment practices in intestinal transplantation. *Transplantation.* 2014;97(1):78-82.

96. Donohoe CL, Reynolds JV. Short bowel syndrome. *Surgeon.* 2010;8(5):270-279.

97. Nayyar N, et al. Pediatric small bowel transplantation. *Semin Pediatr Surg.* 2010;19(1):68-77.

98. Lee RG, et al. Pathology of human intestinal transplantation. *Gastroenterol.* 1996;110(6):1820-1834.

99. Israni AK, et al. OPTN/SRTR 2011 annual data report: deceased organ donation. *Am J Transplant.* 2012;13:179-198.

100. Garau P, et al. Pancreatitis associated with olsalazine and sulfasalazine in children with ulcerative colitis. *J Pediatr Gastroenterol Nutr.* 1994;18(4):481-485.

Gastrointestinal Carcinoid Tumors

Linda Barry | David W. McFadden

In 1867 Theodor Langhans reported the first description of a carcinoid tumor in a 50-year-old woman with a mushroom-shaped small bowel tumor that contained nesting glandular structures within a fibrous stroma.[1] Otto Lubarsch subsequently described autopsy findings of two patients with ileal tumors in 1888, making the astute observation that they were unlikely to be carcinomas.[2] Soon thereafter, William Ransom described the first case of carcinoid syndrome[3] in a 50-year-old woman with severe diarrhea and attacks of wheezing, whose autopsy revealed multiple ileal and hepatic tumors. Like Lubarsch, he commented upon their peculiar biologic behavior and noted that these tumors appeared to "demonstrate very slight, local malignancy."

Siegfried Oberndorfer coined the term *karzinoide* (carcinoid, meaning carcinoma-like) in 1907 during a presentation at the German Pathological Society.[4] He emphasized salient differences between carcinomas of the ileocecal junction and those more benign-behaving and often multifocal tumors of the ileum. Although initially he viewed these as benign, he later came to realize that these tumors could have malignant phenotypes and the ability to metastasize.[5]

In 1914 Gosset and Masson suggested that carcinoid tumors might arise in the Kulchitsky cells in the glands of Lieberkühn. The serum vasoconstrictor serotonin (5-hydroxytryptamine) was isolated and named by Rapport in 1948.[6] Two years later, it was determined that the Kulchitsky cell produced serotonin. Lembeck soon thereafter confirmed that serotonin was produced by an ileal carcinoid and was responsible for the carcinoid syndrome.[7]

In contrast to many other malignancies, the story of carcinoid tumors is unfinished. The first tumor-node-metastasis (TNM) staging system for organ-specific neuroendocrine tumors (NETs) was not published until 2010, and the discussion of the nomenclature surrounding these enigmatic tumors currently continues. There continue to be unresolved issues in our understanding of their pathobiology, which will be resolved in the future.

BIOLOGY OF THE NEUROENDOCRINE SYSTEM

The neuroendocrine system consists of a glandular (solid) system and a diffuse system (DNES). The glandular system is composed of the pituitary, parathyroids, paraganglia, and adrenal medulla. The diffuse system comprises cells dispersed throughout the skin, thyroid, lung, thymus, pancreas, gastrointestinal (GI) tract, biliary tree, and the urogenital system. The multiplicity of neuroendocrine cells in the GI tract makes it the largest single endocrine organ.

A characteristic feature of neuroendocrine cells is the production of a diversity of biogenic amines, peptides, prostaglandins, and tachykinins. These secretory products are stored in both large dense-core vesicles and small synaptic-like vesicles. Among other functions, it appears that the protein, chromogranin A (CgA), is essential in the genesis of vesicles and regulates the biogenesis of the dense-core granules.[8] Such granules are then secreted under control of a complex variety of stimuli. The type of secretory granule produced depends in part on the cell type. Currently there are 16 different types of endocrine cells, producing more than 100 secretory products, that have been described.[9] Although some of these cell types are present throughout the GI tract, others have a more restricted topography (Table 80.1). Some cell types are located in one organ and produce specific products that result in well-described clinical syndromes (e.g., beta cells in the pancreas and insulinomas), whereas others produce a spectrum of disease states and are in a variety of locations (e.g., enterochromaffin [EC] cells and somatostatin in the stomach, small bowel, and colon). Curiously, the common nonfunctional NET, frequently found in the pancreas, has no clear cell of origin and no obvious secretory product.

There has been significant debate and misunderstanding about the developmental origin of gut neuroendocrine cells. Gut endocrine cells have many similarities to neural cells—they produce substances with transmitter functions, have secretory granules, and have similar cellular antigens (synaptophysin and neuron-specific enolase). For this reason, it was initially postulated that they were of neuroectodermal origin and were thus initially termed *neuro*endocrine cells.[10] However, it has since been convincingly demonstrated that these cells come not from the ectoderm but rather have endodermal origins.[11,12] Furthermore, it has been demonstrated more recently that all four intestinal epithelial cell types (enteroendocrine cells, goblet cells, Paneth cells, and enterocytes) differentiate from common pluripotent stem cells in the intestinal crypts.[13,14] These enteroendocrine cells renew themselves from a large reservoir of stem cells and continue the process of differentiation throughout life. The regulatory controls for this process of enteroendocrine cell differentiation are under active investigation and are incompletely understood. Interestingly, it appears that the regulation of differentiation of enteroendocrine cells is similar to that for cells within the nervous system. Both cell types are controlled by similar genes encoding basic helix-loop-helix (bHLH) transcription factors under the

TABLE 80.1 Distribution of Enteroendocrine Cells

Cell Type	Primary Location	Secondary Locations	Product	Tumor Type
A	Pancreas		Glucagon	Glucagonoma
B	Pancreas		Insulin	Insulinoma
D	Stomach, jejunum, pancreas	Ileum, appendix, colon, rectum	Somatostatin	Somatostatinoma
EC	Stomach, jejunum, ileum, appendix, colon	Rectum, pancreas	Serotonin	Carcinoid
ECL	Stomach		Histamine	Gastric carcinoid
G	Stomach (antrum)		Gastrin	Gastrinoma
I	Duodenum, jejunum	Ileum, rectum	Cholecystokinin	CCKoma
L	Small intestine		Glucagon-like peptide, peptide YY, neuropeptide Y	Neuroendocrine tumor NOS
N	Jejunum, ileum	Duodenum	Neurotensin	
PP	Pancreas		Pancreatic polypeptide	PPoma
S	Duodenum, jejunum		Secretin	
VIP	Pancreas	Stomach, small bowel, colon, rectum	Vasoactive intestinal polypeptide	VIPoma
Unknown	Pancreas	Small bowel	None known	Nonfunctional NET

Modified from Schimmack S, Svejda B, Lawrence B, Kidd M, Modlin IM. The diversity and commonalities of gastroenteropancreatic neuroendocrine tumors. *Langenbecks Arch Surg.* 2011;396:273; and Modlin IM, Oberg K, Chung DC, et al. Gastroenteropancreatic neuroendocrine tumours. *Lancet Oncol.* 2008;9:64.

control of the Notch signaling pathway, which may have potential therapeutic implications for NETs.[15]

NOMENCLATURE

The term *carcinoid* was coined before there was a full understanding of the tumor type. However, this term has remained in use clinically and is in part responsible for the confusion surrounding the terminology of NETs. First, the term *neuroendocrine* is not entirely accurate. As described previously, this term was used because it was assumed these cells derived from the neuroectoderm. Because it has since been shown that this is not the case, many have suggested the term be abandoned in favor of *enteroendocrine.* However, because there are many shared structural and regulatory properties between neural cells and endocrine cells, the term *neuroendocrine tumor, or NET,* seems appropriate, and most international groups have accepted its use.

An older term used for these enteroendocrine tumors was APUDoma (amine precursor uptake and decarboxylation), which describes a common biologic function of the cell type. These cells also have been referred to as EC or argentaffin cells because of their staining affinity for chromium and silver salts, respectively. Furthermore, those cells that required a reducing agent to stain with silver salts were termed argyrophilic cells. Those tumors that produce an active product are often referred to by the specific term for each product (glucagonoma, insulinoma, etc.) or by the term for the group that produces these products most often—islet cell tumors.

The number of terms in use for this cell type and their respective tumor types has served to generate significant confusion in the field. In fact, a group of experts participating in a summit of the National Cancer Institute identified this as one of the major hurdles to progress and commented "semantic issues continue to obfuscate the field."[16] For example, the term *carcinoid* unfortunately continues to give the inaccurate impression of the relative benignity of these lesions although many do not behave as such. The more accurate term for this group of tumors currently advocated by the World Health Organization (WHO), the European Neuroendocrine Tumor Society (ENETS), and the North American Neuroendocrine Tumor Society (NANETS) is gastroenteropancreatic neuroendocrine tumors (GEP-NETs).[17] However, the term *carcinoid* continues to be in use and is best understood as a synonym for well-differentiated neuroendocrine neoplasms of the luminal GI tract.

INCIDENCE

The clinical incidence of NETs ranges from approximately 1.3 per 100,000[17] to 5.25 per 100,000 in a study using the 2004 data from Surveillance, Epidemiology and End Results (SEER).[18] However, detailed autopsy studies have shown that the majority of carcinoid tumors are discovered after death from another cause. A Swedish study, from 1958 to 1969, demonstrated that only 10% of all cases were identified on surgical specimens, with 90% discovered incidentally at autopsy. In fact, 1.2% of people had a carcinoid tumor at autopsy.[19] A second smaller but more recent autopsy study in Japan demonstrated that a similar fraction (1.6%) of patients had endocrine tumors in their pancreas on random sectioning, but when the pancreas was more carefully examined with serial sections, a full 10% of patients had endocrine tumors.[20]

Multiple studies have documented a significantly increasing incidence of NETs over the past several decades, with an estimated 3% to 10% increase per year over the past 35 years. The lack of consensus in nomenclature results in differences in classification and incidence reports. Although a fraction of this rise may be related to a true increase in disease frequency, much of this is probably more because of the improvements in clinical awareness of the disease, the improvement in diagnostic and imaging technology, and the changing classification systems. For example, because databases such as SEER included malignant disease only, lower-grade carcinoid tumors were not reported until 1986. Furthermore, the distribution of the primary sites of tumor has changed with time as well. For example, rectal carcinoids represented only 9% of tumors in the early SEER cohort (1973 to 1991) compared with 18% in the later cohort (1992 to 1999). Similarly, 7% of the early cohort had appendiceal carcinoids compared with 2% in the later cohort.[21] These changes could reflect the increase in the use of sigmoidoscopy and the decrease in incidental appendectomies, respectively, rather than a true change in the sites of disease.

Although carcinoid tumors are often considered rare, they are actually the second most prevalent GI cancer, after colorectal cancer. The estimated 29-year limited-duration prevalence of NETs in 2004 was approximately 103,000, making them significantly more common than esophageal, gastric, pancreatic, and hepatobiliary cancers.[18]

RISK FACTORS

The risk factors for the development of sporadic NETs are still unknown. Not surprisingly, the risk factor shown to be most significantly associated with development of a NET is the parental history of a carcinoid tumor in an extrapulmonary site. A similar pattern was seen with history of carcinoid tumor in a sibling.[22] In addition, there was an increase in the incidence of carcinoid tumors in the offspring of parents with cancers of the brain, breast, liver, endocrine system, and urinary tract.[22] This finding of an excess number of cases of carcinoid tumors in offspring of parents with any history of cancer was also demonstrated in a US case-control series. In addition, this study demonstrated that a long-term history of diabetes mellitus was a risk factor for the development of gastric carcinoids, especially in women.[23] For environmental exposures, the bulk of the evidence suggests that there is not a strong association with cigarette smoking. A large European population-based case-control study suggested an increased risk of small bowel carcinoid with occupational exposure to organic solvents and rust-preventive paint containing lead, although more evidence is needed.[24]

Although little is known about the risk of sporadic NETs, there are four well-established genetic disorders that are strongly associated with the development of pancreatic neuroendocrine tumors (PNETs).[25] The most recognized is multiple endocrine neoplasia type 1 (MEN1), which is associated with PNETs in approximately 65% of cases; 7% have gastric carcinoids. The PNETs in MEN1 patients are most commonly nonfunctional, but gastrinomas and insulinomas are frequently reported. The treatment strategies in these patients are complicated given the multifocality of pancreatic tumors and the need to balance a morbid operation against the potential for benefit in the context of multiple other competing medical issues.

The second genetic disorder known to be associated with PNETs is the von Hippel-Lindau (VHL) syndrome, caused by a mutation in the VHL tumor suppressor gene. Pancreatic cysts and tumors develop in the majority of

patients. PNETs develop in approximately 15% of patients with VHL, are usually nonfunctional, and asymptomatic. In general, the tumors in VHL patients show indolent growth and rarely metastasize if less than 3 cm in size. For these reasons, many authors recommend routine resection only when tumors are larger than 3 cm.[26] The third genetic disorder associated with PNETs is von Recklinghausen syndrome (neurofibromatosis 1). These patients are affected in only 10% of cases, with nearly all patients having a duodenal somatostatinoma. These generally are large periampullary tumors and generally require resection to treat local complications. The final genetic association with PNETs is tuberous sclerosis. Only a small fraction of these patients are affected, and both functional and nonfunctional tumors occur.

STAGING AND CLASSIFICATION SCHEMES

A large part of the difficulty in arriving at a standard classification scheme for GEP-NETs has been their widely variable biologic behavior coupled with their locations throughout the GI tract. To further complicate the situation, until recently the WHO classification for NETs used a system that incorporated both grading and staging information in a single system. Although it provided some prognostic information, this schema did not allow for more advanced tumor stages with metastatic disease to benefit from the significant amount of clinical information that derives from grade alone. The 2000 version of the WHO classification used the terms *well-differentiated NET with benign behavior, well-differentiated NET with uncertain behavior, well-differentiated NE carcinoma with low-grade malignancy,* and *poorly differentiated NE carcinoma.*[27] In contrast, the 2004 version described *well-differentiated endocrine tumor, well-differentiated neuroendocrine carcinoma,* and *poorly differentiated carcinoma.* These terms are still encountered in pathology reports because the protocols for NET specimen examination published from the College of American Pathologists in 2010 still advocate the use of these earlier staging systems.[28]

TUMOR GRADING

The most important distinction for classifying NETs is to separate those that are well differentiated from those that are poorly differentiated. This degree of differentiation is reflected by tumor grade. In general, well-differentiated tumors include low and intermediate grades, whereas poorly differentiated tumors are high grade. The grading scheme, now accepted by the WHO, ENETS, and NANETS, is determined by markers of the tumor's proliferative index: the mitotic rate and the Ki67 labeling index (Table 80.2).[29-31] The mitotic rate is reported as the number of mitoses per 10 high-power fields (HPFs). The Ki67 antigen is an important marker of cellular proliferation and mitotic activity and is detected in all phases of the cell cycle except G0. A monoclonal antibody (MIB-1) that binds to the Ki67 nuclear antigen is used to estimate the percentage binding to 2000 cells in the area of highest nuclear activity.

TUMOR STAGING

No formal TNM staging system existed for NETs until the American Joint Committee on Cancer (AJCC) published

TABLE 80.2 Grading Proposal for Gastroenteropancreatic Neuroendocrine Tumors

Grade	Differentiation	Descriptor	Mitotic Count (Per 10 High-Power Field)		Ki67 Index (%)
Low grade	Well differentiated	Neuroendocrine tumor OR neoplasm	<2	AND	≤2
Intermediate grade	Well differentiated	Neuroendocrine tumor OR neoplasm	2–20	OR	3–20
High grade	Poorly differentiated	Neuroendocrine carcinoma small or large cell	>20	OR	>20

Modified from Kloppel G, Couvelard A, Perren A, et al. ENETS consensus guidelines for the standards of care in neuroendocrine tumors: towards a standardized approach to the diagnosis of gastroenteropancreatic neuroendocrine tumors and their prognostic stratification. *Neuroendocrinology*. 2009;90:164 (and later erratum); and Klimstra DS, Modlin IR, Coppola D, Lloyd RV, Suster S. The pathologic classification of neuroendocrine tumors: a review of nomenclature, grading, and staging systems. *Pancreas*. 2010;39:710.

one for each anatomic site in 2010,[32] in parallel to the TNM system published under the Union for International Cancer Control (UICC). Prior to this publication, ENETS had made recommendations for a staging system, already in use in Europe. These two systems have considerable overlap but there are important differences as well, particularly for pancreatic and appendiceal primaries.[33] For the AJCC system in general, stage I disease includes small tumors (≤1 cm for small bowel and stomach; ≤2 cm for colon and appendix) without invasion beyond the submucosa. Stage II disease includes local disease only but with larger tumors and deeper depth of invasion. Stage III disease includes advanced local disease with T4 tumors (those that have penetrated the serosa in gastric and small bowel tumors; those that are growing into nearby structures in appendiceal and colon tumors) and locoregional tumors with nodal disease. Stage IV disease requires evidence of distant metastasis.[32] The College of American Pathologists protocols recommend continued use of the older classification schemes and terminology on clinical pathology reports.[28,34]

DIAGNOSIS OF NEUROENDOCRINE TUMORS

CARCINOID SYNDROME

The carcinoid syndrome is a well-described constellation of symptoms that results from an excess of the neurohumoral factors released by some NETs. Symptomatically, it is characterized by episodic flushing, which primarily involves the face and torso, lasting only minutes. It is often described as having a dark red to purple hue and can be accompanied by a burning sensation of the skin. These episodes can include bronchospastic symptoms of wheezing and dyspnea. Another characteristic and more debilitating symptom is the presence of a secretory diarrhea and associated abdominal pain and cramping.

From a mechanistic standpoint, these symptoms result in part from serotonin excess that occurs from the conversion of dietary tryptophan to serotonin and subsequently 5-hydroxyindoleacetic acid (5-HIAA). Excess serotonin results in hypoalbuminemia and nicotinic acid deficiency from an effective tryptophan deficiency, diarrhea as a result of stimulation of intestinal motility and secretion, and fibrotic processes in the bowel mesentery and the cardiac valves. In addition, there is an excess of histamine production that can lead to flushing and pruritus. Excessive bradykinin production can lead to vasodilation and flushing, and other polypeptides, such as neurokinin A, may contribute to both flushing and diarrhea. The carcinoid syndrome requires the presence of liver metastases as the portal venous circulation permits the liver to clear the bioactive products before they can arrive in the systemic circulation, although it has been described in patients with retroperitoneal invasion.

CLINICAL PRESENTATION

Although the carcinoid syndrome is a dramatic and well-known presentation of NETs, it is uncommon and occurs in only 10% to 20% of patients. The most common presentations of GI NETs are periodic abdominal pain and cramping, intermittent small bowel obstruction, and GI bleeding. Up to one-third of patients are asymptomatic and have their tumor detected incidentally.[35] The most difficult group of patients and those with the longest delay in diagnosis are those who present with more protean symptoms, such as psychiatric disorders, depression, food allergy, lactose intolerance, and menopausal symptoms.[36] It is the very nature of carcinoid disease that makes it so difficult to diagnose, namely, that it is located in the segment of the GI tract that is not easily accessed endoscopically, that it is submucosal in nature and grows extrinsically, and that it causes symptoms that may not be easily referable to the abdomen, such as flushing. The most important aspect of making the diagnosis in these cases is the suspicion of its presence, without which the patient will have delays in diagnosis and treatment.

LABORATORY EVALUATION

In the evaluation of the patient with a suspected carcinoid tumor, it is essential to consider the differential diagnosis so as not to miss other more common alternative diagnoses. This should include considering infectious causes (such as appendicitis or terminal ileitis), vascular causes (mesenteric ischemia or vasculitis), mechanical causes (adhesions, volvulus), neoplastic causes (adenocarcinoma, lymphoma), and inflammatory causes (Crohn disease, celiac disease).[37] Other causes of flushing should also be considered and evaluated when this is a predominant symptom. These include such diverse etiologies as renal cell carcinoma, mastocytosis, panic attack, menopause, autonomic neuropathy, medications, and pheochromocytoma.[38]

In patients in whom other diagnoses have been ruled out or those in whom the likelihood of a GEP-NET seems particularly high, we proceed first with measurement of a 24-hour urine sample for 5-HIAA. This has a sensitivity

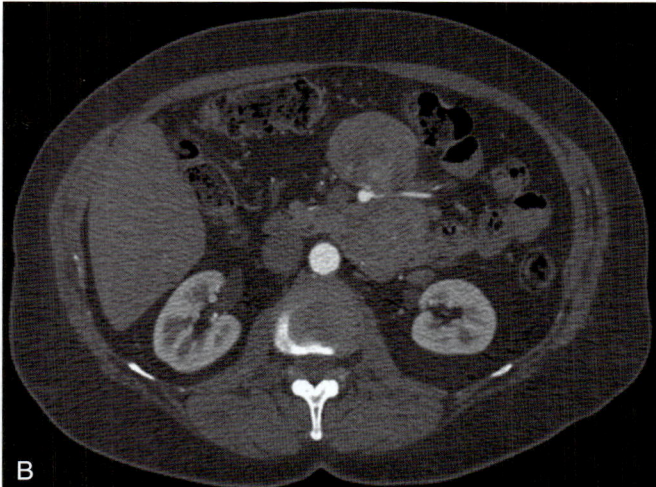

FIGURE 80.1 (A) Sagittal view from a computed tomography (CT) angiogram in a patient with a large neuroendocrine tumor of the proximal jejunum. The superior mesenteric artery can be seen to be enveloped by this bilobed tumor. (B) Axial view from the same CT angiogram showing the intimate anatomic relationship between the mesenteric vasculature and the neuroendocrine tumor of the proximal jejunum.

of 75% and specificity of more than 90%, but it requires adequate preparation to achieve these statistics. Specifically, foods with high tryptophan content, such as avocados, bananas, and walnuts, are proscribed. Some medications can disrupt the test and lead to either falsely high (e.g., acetaminophen, guaifenesin, nicotine) or falsely low (e.g., heparin, aspirin, isoniazid) values. Measurement of urine 5-HIAA is useful mainly for midgut tumors and is much less helpful for tumors from the foregut and hindgut.[39]

The measurement of serum CgA is a useful test in patients with suspected NETs. This can be elevated in both functional and nonfunctional tumors, and its sensitivity varies according to the NET site and tumor burden. This test is particularly sensitive to the assay technique, and it is advised that serial measurements be performed. In addition, there are many nonneoplastic causes of elevated CgA that should be considered, including impaired renal and hepatic function, hypergastrinemia secondary to proton pump inhibitors or atrophic gastritis, and inflammatory bowel disease.

Blood serotonin measurements can also be useful in making the diagnosis of a GEP-NET, particularly when the urinary 5-HIAA yields equivocal results. Other pancreatic peptides should be measured as indicated by the clinical picture, including gastrin, vasoactive intestinal peptide, somatostatin, insulin, and glucagon. Other tests that can be helpful in the diagnosis, in rare cases, include pancreatic polypeptide, neuron-specific enolase, pancreastatin, and neurokinin A.[38]

RADIOGRAPHIC EVALUATION

If clinically suspected, a gastric, duodenal, or rectal carcinoid is best evaluated endoscopically, both with standard techniques and endoscopic ultrasound. However, standard axial imaging with computed tomography (CT) and magnetic resonance imaging (MRI) remains the mainstay of the evaluation of intraabdominal complaints. Although routine abdominopelvic CT imaging may detect

large NETs, it is much less sensitive for the detection of small bowel luminal lesions. However, this can be improved by performing CT enterography, magnetic resonance (MR) enterography, or enteroclysis. The value of CT and MRI is that they can simultaneously detect hepatic metastases, examine regional lymph node basins, and specify the mesenteric vasculature that is often involved (Fig. 80.1). Their ability to detect PNETs is also excellent, with hypervascular masses often being seen best on arterial phase imaging. For these reasons, contrast-enhanced CT scan is the imaging modality of choice for the majority of intraabdominal NETs.[35]

Somatostatin receptor scintigraphy (Octreoscan) involves the use of ^{111}In–diethylenetriaminepentaacetic acid (DTPA)-labeled octreotide to locate small tumors that overexpress somatostatin receptors (particularly subtypes 2 and 5). This is most useful for PNETs, with the exception of insulinomas. This has more recently been coupled with CT imaging to provide improved localization of areas of uptake. It is thought to be the most sensitive imaging modality for detecting metastatic disease. Other imaging modalities to consider include the use of intraoperative or endoscopic ultrasound for difficult-to-locate pancreatic lesions.

NEUROENDOCRINE TUMORS BY THE ORGAN OF ORIGIN

GASTRIC NEUROENDOCRINE TUMORS

Background

Gastric carcinoid tumors arise from histamine-containing enterochromaffin-like (ECL) cells. This category is inclusive of a wide spectrum of disease biology and has four types. Type I gastric carcinoids are defined by their association with chronic hypergastrinemia as a result of chronic atrophic gastritis. It is presumed that the chronic state of hypergastrinemia provides the stimulus for ECL cell hyperplasia and subsequent development of carcinoid tumors. Type I tumors account for approximately 75% of all gastric carcinoids. These tumors often are small, multiple, well differentiated, and associated with prolonged survival.

Type II gastric carcinoids are similar to type I in that they also arise from a hypergastrinemic stimulus on ECL cells. However, in contrast to type I tumors, the stimulus is excessive production of gastrin and occurs as a result of the presence of a gastrinoma, either with Zollinger-Ellison syndrome or MEN1. Type II tumors comprise only approximately 5% of gastric carcinoids and in general are similar to type I tumors in that they are usually well differentiated, small, and multiple. However, they are more often associated with distant disease and their course is influenced more by the presence of MEN than by the carcinoid itself.

Type III gastric carcinoids account for approximately 20% of gastric carcinoids and are associated with more morbidity. These sporadic tumors are usually large, singular, and not associated with hypergastrinemia. They are much more often metastatic and have a worse prognosis. These tumors produce 5-hydroxytryptophan and can be associated with the development of an atypical carcinoid crisis (flushing, hypotension, lacrimentation, edema, and bronchoconstriction).

Type IV gastric carcinoids have been introduced more recently, and they are usually a solitary large tumor, which is a non-ECL cell tumor, and is associated with parietal cell hyperplasia. Its phenotype is similar to type III tumors in that it tends to be more locally invasive and have metastatic potential. They can be located anywhere in the stomach, whereas types I to III carcinoid tumors are most common in the body and fundus.

Incidence

Gastric carcinoids have long been considered rare lesions, but with an increasing use of upper endoscopy and the increasing use of proton pump inhibitors, their incidence is increasing. Over a period of 50 years, the proportion of gastric carcinoids among all carcinoid tumors has increased from 2.4% to 8.7%. Furthermore, although still quite uncommon, they are also increasing in frequency relative to other gastric malignancies—from 0.3% to 1.8%.[21]

Diagnosis

A large fraction of these tumors are asymptomatic and are found incidentally at screening endoscopy. However, they can also be symptomatic and most commonly cause abdominal pain, GI bleeding, and anemia.[40] In addition, these tumors occur most often in female patients. The diagnosis is made at gastroscopy by biopsies, which should be taken of the largest polyps as well as from the antrum (two biopsies) and fundus (four biopsies). The purpose of biopsies is to confirm that the polyps represent carcinoid rather than more benign (inflammatory polyps or hyperplastic polyps) or more malignant pathologies (adenocarcinoma). In addition, the normal mucosa is sampled so that the diagnosis of associated atrophic gastritis can be confirmed.[41] In addition, serum gastrin and chromogranin levels should be measured and gastric pH tested. Endoscopic ultrasound and cross-sectional imaging should be considered for tumors larger than 1 cm.

Treatment

The treatment for types III and IV gastric carcinoids is the most straightforward and is similar to that for standard gastric adenocarcinoma. The principles of treatment include resection with widely negative margins, formal lymphadenectomy, and assessment of metastatic disease. Those with metastatic disease can be considered for either surgical or percutaneous treatment of hepatic metastases in conjunction with resection of the primary, whereas those with widely metastatic disease should have gastric surgery only as a means of symptom control.

The treatment of type II gastric carcinoids has much more to do with the assessment of the advisability of proceeding with resection of the gastrinoma, usually in the setting of MEN. This is a more difficult decision and is discussed in Chapter 60.

The treatment of patients with type I gastric carcinoids is controversial because there are very little data about their natural history and how it is influenced by various treatment strategies. Furthermore, because they are relatively indolent tumors, large numbers of patients would be required, over longer periods of time, to definitively determine the best treatment strategy.

Nearly 400 patients undergoing treatment for type I gastric carcinoid have been cumulatively reported by several groups. The overall disease-specific survival in most series was 100%, with a follow-up on the order of 5 years. Furthermore, a mixture of conservative and aggressive strategies was used, making it difficult to sort out natural history from treatment effect.[42] However, what is clear is that some type I gastric carcinoids are associated with lymph node and distant metastases. This occurred in nearly 8% of those reported by Borch et al. and was seen even for one lesion confined to the submucosa.[40] That figure appears consistent with the literature that estimates the rate of lymph node metastases to be 10% overall. The ideal treatment strategy would of course be able to identify those at highest risk for locoregional disease and treat them accordingly. Unfortunately, at present, this cannot be achieved with precision, so size and depth of the primary tumor are used as surrogates for poor tumor biology.

ENETS, NANETS, and several individual authors have made recommendations for treatment of gastric carcinoids. When taken together, it is clear that there is significant confusion about the optimal treatment strategy for these patients. Guidelines from ENETS suggest observation alone with annual surveillance for tumors smaller than 1 cm. For tumors larger than 1 cm, endoscopic mucosal resection (EMR) is advocated for tumors that do not penetrate the muscularis propria. Surgical intervention is advocated for those with positive margins after EMR or lesions that penetrate the gastric wall more deeply. Antrectomy and local resection is advised with lymphadenectomy added only for patients with positive nodes.[41] Guidelines from NANETS suggest that endoscopic resection be considered only in patients with lesions smaller than 2 cm and fewer than six in number. Surgical intervention is advised for those lesions more than 2 cm, those with more than six lesions, and those with recurrent tumors. Local resection is advocated, with antrectomy to be considered.[43]

The group from Memorial Sloan Kettering has advocated surgical resection primarily in those patients with enlarging or persistent solitary lesions and those with pathologic features suggestive of malignant gland transformation. Although they express agreement with the threshold of 1 cm for surgical therapy, more than half of the patients who underwent resection in their series had tumors less than 1 cm. They specifically disagree that the number of lesions should guide a decision with regard to surgical therapy.[44]

At the present time, it is reasonable to assume that the new AJCC staging scheme for gastric carcinoids will assist in determining the outcomes of similar groups of patients with differing treatment strategies. As more data accumulate, we will be able to determine which patients would most benefit from surgical intervention, what the proper place of antrectomy is for these patients, and how large the benefit of surgical therapy will be for patients with a relatively indolent disease process.

SMALL INTESTINAL NEUROENDOCRINE TUMORS

Small intestinal NETs are most commonly serotonin-producing tumors. They can occur anywhere from the duodenum to the terminal ileum. They can present in a protean fashion, with the symptoms most commonly being vague abdominal pain, bloating, diarrhea, weight loss, and intermittent bowel obstruction. The occurrence of the carcinoid syndrome occurs in less than 10% of patients with GI NETs overall, but it is distinctly more common in patients with tumors in the jejunoileum and ileocecum (36% and 24%, respectively).[45] In more than 95% of patients with the carcinoid syndrome, evidence of extensive hepatic disease is present but in a small fraction of patients, metastases to the ovaries or other retroperitoneal structures can be the source of serotonin in the systemic circulation.[46]

Although some patients present with minimal symptomatology, others present with overt bowel obstruction, ischemia, or bleeding. This can occur either as a direct consequence of the tumor itself, with either luminal compromise or as a lead point for intussusception. However, it is more often the effect of local tissue change from presumed neurohormonal effectors. This can lead to extensive fibrosis and kinking of the small bowel, with resultant obstruction. Alternatively, mesenteric ischemia can occur and is related to either mechanical compromise of arterial inflow or venous outflow, or alternatively to elastic vascular sclerosis and vasospasm that is potentially related to the effects of tissue levels of serotonin.

These tumors are multifocal in 25% of affected patients, particularly in the ileum. They can be present both in the submucosa and the mucosa. Importantly, clonality studies have suggested that multiple tumors are metastases from the primary tumor rather than distinct primaries.[47] When these cases have been carefully examined, endocrine cell hyperplasia in the adjacent mucosa has not been seen, making the etiology of the multiplicity likely to be quite different than that which occurs in type I gastric carcinoids.[48] Although there are limited data, it appears

TABLE 80.3 Frequency of Metastases in Small Bowel and Colorectal Carcinoids

Metastases Location	RORSTAD (2005) Lymphatic (%)	Distant (%)	SUTTON ET AL. (2003) Lymphatic (%)	Distant (%)
SMALL INTESTINE				
≤1 cm	12	5	40	10
1–2 cm	70	19	60	25
≥2 cm	85	47	85	60
APPENDIX				
≤1 cm	0	0	<0.1	<0.1
1–2 cm	8	4	<5	<5
≥2 cm	33	2	30	20
COLON				
≤1 cm	18	18	10	5
1–2 cm			20	15
≥2 cm	55	39	80	40

From Rorstad O. Prognostic indicators for carcinoid neuroendocrine tumors of the gastrointestinal tract. *J Surg Oncol*. 2005;89:153; and Sutton R, Doran HE, Williams EM, et al. Surgery for midgut carcinoid. *Endocr Relat Cancer*. 2003;10:472.

that patients with solitary tumors have a less aggressive phenotype than those with multiple tumors.[48]

Another striking feature of small bowel carcinoids is their propensity toward both regional and distant metastasis. At presentation, only 31% of small bowel tumors are localized, 37% are regional, and 27% are distant.[49] Notably, they have a tendency to metastasize even when they are less than 1 cm in size (Table 80.3). The estimates for lymphatic metastases from small bowel tumors less than 1 cm in size range from 11% to 44%. The 5-year survival of the most favorable group of patients with small bowel carcinoids (T1, N0) is only 86%, suggesting that early tumors can still behave aggressively.[32]

Of all GI tract NETs, 38% are of small bowel origin.[21] Carcinoids are the most common small bowel tumor and represent 35% of the total, with adenocarcinomas being the second most common at 31%.[49] Of all small bowel carcinoids, at least 50% are located in the ileum.[49]

Diagnosis

Because of their vague symptoms, small bowel carcinoids often present already metastatic. This often occurs when liver lesions are detected by ultrasound and then further imaging is undertaken. However, when patients present with symptoms suggestive of small bowel NETs, laboratory evaluation should be undertaken. Both urinary 5-HIAA and serum chromogranin are particularly useful for midgut tumors, when compared with foregut or hindgut tumors. The sensitivity of 5-HIAA for midgut carcinoids is on the order of 75%, whereas the specificity is even higher at 88% to 100%. Serum chromogranin is also a sensitive but less specific marker of midgut NETs. Chromogranin appears to be the best marker to follow to screen for recurrence in patients having undergone complete resection of midgut NETs.[50]

Imaging studies that assist in diagnosing and staging a midgut NET include plain chest films, cross-sectional abdominal imaging (CT or MRI), and octreotide scanning.[51]

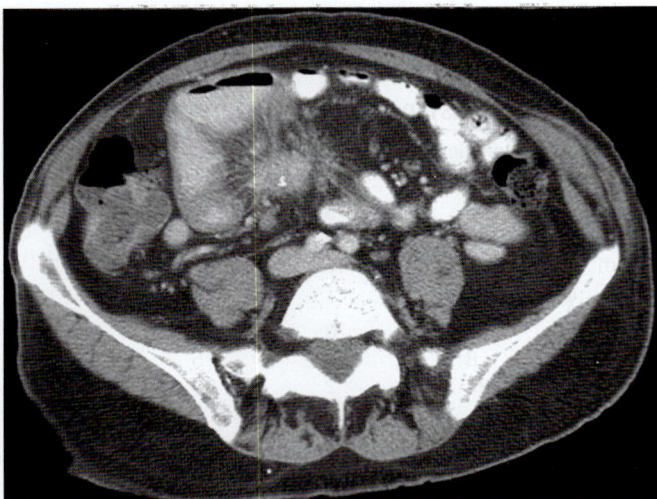

FIGURE 80.2 Axial view from a computed tomography scan of a patient with a classic mass in the small bowel mesentery, demonstrating retraction of the involved small bowel loop.

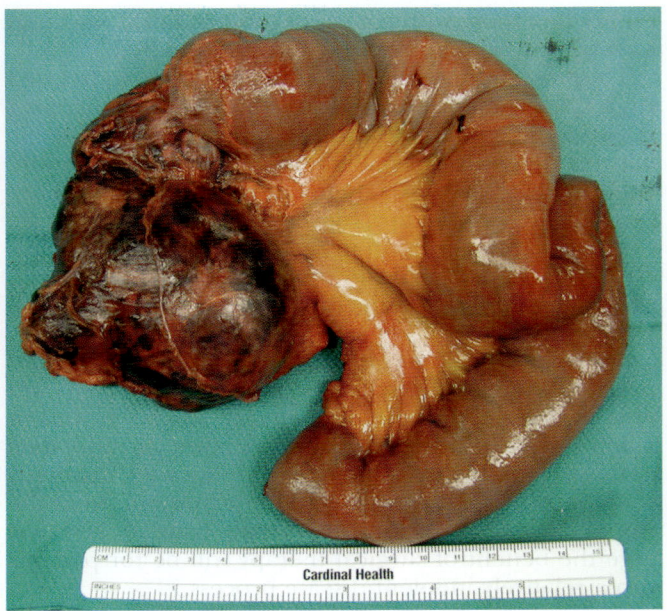

FIGURE 80.3 Photograph of the resected specimen of the patient with the proximal jejunal tumor shown in Fig. 80.1. Note the puckering of the small bowel into the area of the mesenteric mass.

Because these tumors are particularly vascular, CT imaging with both arterial- and portal-phase imaging is helpful in differentiating the tumor from surrounding tissues. CT enterography may also be helpful for the elusive small bowel mass. With cross-sectional imaging, the bowel, liver, and peritoneal cavity can all be adequately evaluated. The appearance of a mesenteric tumor with radiating spokes is pathognomonic for a mesenteric midgut tumor (Fig. 80.2). Octreotide scanning is very useful for disease staging and is positive in more than 80% of patients with small bowel carcinoids. Its limitations are for small lesions and those tumors lacking types 2 and 5 somatostatin receptors. When these routine imaging studies are unrevealing, it can be necessary to consider adjunctive testing, such as small bowel contrast studies, gallium-DOTA-octreotide positron emission tomography (PET), and diagnostic laparoscopy. Capsule endoscopy should be used only with caution given that, in patients with significant small bowel tethering and luminal disease from carcinoid, it may lead to obstruction.

Treatment

It is essential in all cases of small bowel carcinoid to consider the possibility of other concomitant malignancies, reported to occur in 12% to 46% of cases.[52] Given that the majority of these secondary tumors are GI in origin, preoperative upper and lower endoscopy should be considered for any patient undergoing elective operation for small bowel carcinoid. Furthermore, at exploration, a thorough search of the abdominal cavity should always be undertaken.

Resection of small bowel carcinoids entails segmental resection with wide mesenteric lymphadenectomy. It is important to resect malignant lymphadenopathy at the mesenteric root because this disease, if left behind, can result in subsequent mesenteric vascular compromise, a primary source of morbidity and mortality for these patients (Fig. 80.3). Often ileocolic resections are required for more distal ileal tumors. These patients often have significantly foreshortened mesenteries and extensive fibrotic changes throughout the mesentery that can make this procedure difficult and hazardous. These difficult cases can be approached by mobilizing the right colon and small bowel mesenteries off of the retroperitoneum and isolating the mesenteric vessels as they exit near the pancreatic neck. The vessels can then be dissected from the root out into the mesentery, peeling the nodes carefully away from the vasculature. This technique requires delaying the bowel resection until after the mesenteric dissection is completed to preserve a maximum length of well-perfused bowel.[53] Because of the rarity of this condition and the technical difficulty associated with resections in these patients, some have advocated that these patients be evaluated and treated by an experienced and multidisciplinary surgical team.[51] Laparoscopic approaches are also reported.

COLON AND RECTAL NEUROENDOCRINE TUMORS

Most colonic carcinoids present in older patients. Weight loss or abdominal pain are the usual chief complaints. Colonic carcinoids are larger tumors with an average size of 5 cm at diagnosis and are metastatic in 40% of patients at presentation. In contrast, rectal carcinoids are most often detected incidentally or with symptoms of rectal bleeding or pain. Approximately 80% of rectal carcinoids are localized at presentation, and they are most often less than 1 cm in size. Colonic NETs make up only 12% of all GI carcinoids and are most commonly located in either the cecum/right colon (48%) or in the rectosigmoid

(43%).[21,54] Rectal carcinoids are nearly twice as common as colonic and constitute 21% of all GI NETs.[21]

DIAGNOSIS

The laboratory evaluation is limited in utility because these tumors rarely produce amines or other measurable hormones. In contrast, serum chromogranin is highly sensitive and should be measured routinely. The primary method of diagnosis in both the colon and rectum is endoscopy. These tumors have a typical appearance, as sessile, submucosal tumors with a discolored, yellowed mucosal covering. The diagnosis is most often made when a polyp is examined histologically. The margins should be carefully examined to determine if further treatment is needed. Endoscopic ultrasound also plays a role in the evaluation of rectal carcinoids to assist in staging and determining suitability for endoscopic resection. For high-grade colonic lesions, a metastatic evaluation should be undertaken with cross-sectional imaging of the chest and abdomen and an octreotide scan. Some poorly differentiated colonic NETs do not label with octreotide, and traditional fluorodeoxyglucose (FDG)-PET scanning may be useful for those patients.[55]

TREATMENT

The operative approach to colonic carcinoids is similar to colonic adenocarcinomas. For small, incidentally detected colonic carcinoids completely removed with polypectomy, endoscopic surveillance alone should be considered. However, for tumors that are larger than 2 cm and invade the muscularis propria, formal colectomy with lymphadenectomy should be undertaken.

Rectal tumors should be carefully staged with endoscopic ultrasound or endorectal MRI prior to resection. If a rectal polyp is removed and the pathology unexpectedly reveals a NET, strong consideration should be given for prompt repeat endoscopy so that the area of interest can be tattooed for later reexcision or reevaluation. In general, it is recommended that rectal tumors that are larger than 2 cm, invade the muscularis propria (regardless of size), or have evidence of mesorectal lymphadenopathy should be managed by standard rectal resection techniques.[56] The management of tumors in the rectum less than 2 cm in size is controversial. For tumors less than 10 mm in size, some suggest that endoscopic resection alone is adequate,[55] but it has been shown that the incidence of lymph node positivity in subcentimeter rectal carcinoids may be as high as 7%. It has therefore been suggested that rectal carcinoids less than 2 cm in size be considered for formal resection if the tumor penetrates the muscularis or has adverse features such as a high proliferative index, lymphovascular invasion, or gross ulceration.[57] For tumors that are incompletely removed by polypectomy or have positive margins, submucosal endoscopic resection or full-thickness transanal excision should be considered.

APPENDICEAL NEUROENDOCRINE TUMORS

Appendiceal carcinoids represent 18% of all GI NETs. They are found incidentally after appendectomy in 0.3% to 0.9% of patients. Carcinoid tumors of the appendix rarely cause symptoms and are most often detected incidentally at the time of appendectomy. Approximately three-fourths of appendiceal carcinoids are located in the tip of the appendix, and 95% of appendiceal carcinoids are less than 2 cm in diameter.

DIAGNOSIS

It is unusual to find or suspect an appendiceal carcinoid prior to operative intervention. At the time of operative inspection, if concern for an appendiceal mass is raised, it is helpful to resect as much mesoappendix as possible and to ensure that the base of the appendix is included in the specimen. Careful pathologic evaluation of the appendix is required and should include tumor dimensions, depth of invasion, mitotic rate, and the presence or absence of lymphovascular invasion.[34]

TREATMENT

Appendiceal carcinoids can be considered cured with appendectomy alone if they are less than 1 cm in size, are confined to the tip, are well differentiated, have no evidence of lymphovascular invasion, and do not invade the mesoappendix. Formal right hemicolectomy is currently recommended for any one of the following: tumors greater than 2 cm in size, invasion at the appendiceal base, evidence of lymphovascular invasion, any invasion of the mesoappendix, mixed histology (goblet cell carcinoids, adenocarcinoids), and intermediate- to high-grade tumors.[51] Although small appendiceal tumors are considered benign, it is important to recall that even for 1-cm appendiceal tumors, there is a mortality rate of 5% at 5 years and for those with regional disease, the 5-year survival is 78%.

METASTATIC DISEASE

Given that a significant portion of patients with GI NETs will present with metastatic disease, it is essential to understand the optimal therapies in this subgroup. Patients with jejunoileal carcinoids present with metastatic disease in 30% of cases, whereas those with cecal and pancreatic primaries present with metastatic disease in 44% and 64%, respectively.[18]

ROLE OF SOMATOSTATIN ANALOGUES

The somatostatin analogue octreotide is an effective treatment for patients with symptomatic carcinoid disease, and it has been used broadly for symptomatic relief with excellent results. A recent randomized trial (PROMID) was completed in 2009 by a German consortium and randomized patients with locally inoperable or metastatic, well-differentiated midgut carcinoids to either long-acting octreotide or placebo.[58] The data suggested a significant difference in time to tumor progression from 6 months in the placebo group to 14 months in the treatment group. Although some methodologic questions have been raised, the general consensus of the neuroendocrine community has been that there is now clear evidence of somatostatin's antiproliferative activity and its use is now advocated in patients with asymptomatic metastatic NETs. In December 2014 the US Food and Drug Administration (FDA) approved lanreotide, a long-acting somatostatin analogue, for the treatment of patients with unresectable, well or moderately differentiated, locally advanced or metastatic GEP-NETs. This drug requires only monthly injections.

TREATMENT OF HEPATIC METASTATIC DISEASE

Resectable Metastatic Disease

Patients with untreated hepatic metastatic disease from well-differentiated NETs have a 5-year survival of 30% and may be very symptomatic. Patients who have undergone resection of liver metastases have 45% to 60% 5-year survival rates.[59,60] For this reason, resection should be recommended to patients with resectable hepatic metastases if the tumor is well differentiated, no peritoneal or extraabdominal disease is present, and the patient can tolerate the planned procedure with an acceptable morbidity and mortality.[61] The primary goal in patients with metastatic disease is to remove all evidence of disease and to leave the patient with a liver remnant sufficient for synthetic function.

Unresectable Metastatic Disease

Debulking procedures should be considered if the extent of metastatic disease in the liver is such that complete resection cannot be accomplished. Although there are little objective data to suggest that this strategy yields a survival benefit, it should be considered in patients who are symptomatic despite somatostatin therapy. Of symptomatic patients with functioning tumors, 90% report significant symptomatic improvement postoperatively.[60] Unfortunately the response is not durable; recurrence of symptoms occurs at a median of 20 to 25 months postoperatively. An alternative strategy for patients with symptomatic unresectable hepatic disease is hepatic arterial embolization. Case series have suggested a symptomatic relief and prolonged survival in patients who show appropriate decrement in serum markers posttreatment.[62] Unfortunately, this procedure has a mortality rate of nearly 2%.[62] Even in asymptomatic patients with unresectable metastatic disease, surgical debulking may have a role. Some surgeons have advocated if resection of more than 90% of the tumor burden can be accomplished, that hepatic debulking should be considered with the goal of prolonging survival.[63]

A final, albeit controversial, treatment option for patients with unresectable hepatic metastatic disease is liver transplantation. This option has been studied in a limited number of well-selected patients in only a handful of centers, but the available data suggest that there is significant prolongation of survival in patients with favorable disease biology. These features include: resection of primary tumor, isolated hepatic metastatic disease, low proliferative index (Ki67 less than 5% and staining for E-cadherin), absence of significant hepatomegaly, and primary tumor not of pancreatic or rectal origin.[61,64,65]

ROLE OF RESECTION OF PRIMARY TUMOR IN THE SETTING OF METASTATIC DISEASE

For the symptomatic patient with a well-differentiated small bowel primary, resection of the primary tumor should be considered even in the presence of metastatic disease. The more difficult question is how to approach the primary tumor in the asymptomatic patient with unresectable metastatic disease. Several lines of evidence suggest that resection of the primary may be beneficial in this setting. A case series of 84 patients demonstrated a significant prolongation of progression-free survival in those patients who had resection of their primary tumor (56 vs. 25 months).[66] In addition, a retrospective multicenter trial demonstrated in a multivariate analysis that resection of the primary tumor was an independent predictor of survival in patients with metastatic NET of midgut origin.[67] Finally, in the PROMID study, it was demonstrated that the antiproliferative effects of octreotide were most pronounced in the patients in whom the primary tumor had been resected.[58] The clinical decisions in this subset of patients clearly need to be individualized, but consideration should at least be given to resection of the primary tumor even in the setting of asymptomatic unresectable metastatic disease.

SYSTEMIC CHEMOTHERAPY

The use of systemic chemotherapy in patients with advanced, well-differentiated NETs has been the subject of much research because few effective therapeutic options are available. To summarize, both interferon and various alkylating agents have had a place in clinical care for patients with progressive disease. However, these therapies are associated with significant side effects and have limited effectiveness. Targeted therapies have recently shown promise in the treatment of patients with PNETs. Sunitinib, a tyrosine kinase inhibitor, and everolimus, a mammalian target of rapamycin (mTOR) inhibitor, have both been shown in randomized placebo-controlled trials to result in a significant improvement in progression-free survival.[68,69] These two trials and others in progress have brought promise to the field of NETs that has long been lacking in effective systemic therapies.

PERIOPERATIVE AND SURGICAL ISSUES

AVOIDANCE OF CARCINOID CRISIS

For patients with NETs, there are several important issues to consider before proceeding with any planned operative intervention. Most important is the avoidance of a carcinoid crisis, which can be provoked by the induction of general anesthesia as well as by manipulation of the tumor. This life-threatening complication can be avoided by pretreating the patient with octreotide (200 µg subcutaneously 3 times a day) for 2 to 3 weeks prior to surgery and with continuous intravenous therapy intraoperatively (50 µg per hour). Should a carcinoid crisis occur, it is essential to avoid adrenergic drugs to treat the hypotension as they may exacerbate the crisis. As always, careful preoperative planning and effective communication between the surgeon and anesthesiologist is essential to providing optimal care for these patients.[70]

EVALUATION FOR CARCINOID HEART DISEASE

Carcinoid heart disease is only present in 3% to 4% of patients with NETs but is seen in 40% to 50% of patients with the carcinoid syndrome. It is postulated that the systemic exposure to serotonin and other vasoactive amines results in fibrosis of the right-sided cardiac structures, similar to their effect on the mesentery of the small bowel. Specifically, tricuspid valve disease occurs in 90% of cases, with pulmonary valve stenosis occurring in 50%. These defects can cause right heart dysfunction that complicates any abdominal surgery, particularly hepatic surgery. It is therefore recommended that patients with carcinoid syndrome undergo routine echocardiography prior to abdominal exploration.[71] In case correctable and hemodynamically significant disease is found, valve replacement should be considered prior to abdominal surgical intervention.

CONSIDERATION OF PROPHYLACTIC CHOLECYSTECTOMY

Because the use of octreotide appears to result in an increase in biliary complications, it has been recommended that prophylactic cholecystectomy be considered during abdominal exploration for midgut carcinoid tumors. In a study of 235 patients, gallbladder complications occurred in 15% of those patients receiving octreotide therapy compared with only 6% of those not receiving it.[72] An additional consideration is that the later use of hepatic arterial embolization can lead to an increase in the rates of biliary complications.

FUTURE CHALLENGES IN THE TREATMENT OF NEUROENDOCRINE TUMORS

As discussed, much progress has recently been made in the recognition and classification of NETs, but there is room for progress. In 2007 Modlin reviewed the previous three decades and noting no change in survival, aptly termed it "the rapid pace of no progress."[49] To avoid such an assessment three decades from now, many challenges in the treatment of these patients must be addressed.

First, there are significant limitations in our understanding of the basic cellular biology and the mechanisms of tumorigenesis in NETs. This limits the ability to develop novel therapies and hinders progress. Furthermore, reliable surrogates for tumor biology in individual patients are not available, making it difficult to predict prognosis and select patients with a higher likelihood of disease progression for more aggressive therapies. The appreciation on the part of providers for the early signs and symptoms of carcinoid, the variability of disease biology, and the potential for more aggressive treatment strategies is limited by their past experience and should be improved with educational efforts.

Although both the new staging and grading standards are a step forward, it is essential that these are widely implemented and data accumulated so that prognosis can be more accurately determined for each disease site. Most importantly, collaborative efforts among the neuroendocrine community, both nationally and internationally, will continue to allow for novel therapies to be efficiently studied in important patient subsets.

REFERENCES

1. Langhans T. Uber einen drsenpolyp im ileum. *Virchows Arch Pathol Anat.* 1867;38:550.
2. Lubarsch O. Uber dem primaren Krebs des Ileum nebst Bemerkungen ber das gleichzeitige Vorkommen von Krebs und Tuberculose. *Virchows Arch Pathol Anat.* 1888;111:280.
3. Ransom W. A case of primary carcinoma of the ileum. *Lancet.* 1890;2:1020.
4. Oberndorfer S. Karzinoide tumoren des dunndarms. *Frankf Zschr Pathol.* 1907;1:426.
5. Oberndorfer S. Karzinoide. In: *Handbook of Pathological Anatomy.* Berlin, Germany: Verlag von Julius Springer; 1929.
6. Rapport MM, Green AA, Page IH. Serum vasoconstrictor, serotonin: isolation and characterization. *J Biol Chem.* 1948;176:1243.
7. Lembeck F. 5-Hydroxytryptamine in a carcinoid tumor. *Nature.* 1953;172:910.
8. Schimmack S, Svejda B, Lawrence B, Kidd M, Modlin IM. The diversity and commonalities of gastroenteropancreatic neuroendocrine tumors. *Langenbecks Arch Surg.* 2011;396:273.
9. Basuroy R, Srirajaskanthan R, Ramage J. Neuroendocrine tumors. *Gastroenterol Clin North Am.* 2016;45:487-507.
10. Pearse AG. The cytochemistry and ultrastructure of polypeptide hormone-producing cells of the APUD series and the embryologic, physiologic and pathologic implications of the concept. *J Histochem Cytochem.* 1969;17:303.
11. Pictet RL, Rall LB, Phelps P, Rutter WJ. The neural crest and the origin of the insulin-producing and other gastrointestinal hormone-producing cells. *Science.* 1976;191:191.
12. Le Douarin NM. On the origin of pancreatic endocrine cells. *Cell.* 1988;53:169.
13. Cheng H, Leblond CP. Origin, differentiation and renewal of the four main epithelial cell types in the mouse small intestine. V. Unitarian theory of the origin of the four epithelial cell types. *Am J Anat.* 1974;141:537.
14. Ponder BA, Schmidt GH, Wilkinson MM, Wood MJ, Monk M, Reid A. Derivation of mouse intestinal crypts from single progenitor cells. *Nature.* 1985;313:689.
15. Greenblatt DY, Vaccaro AM, Jaskula-Sztul R, et al. Valproic acid activates notch-1 signaling and regulates the neuroendocrine phenotype in carcinoid cancer cells. *Oncologist.* 2007;12:942.
16. Modlin IM, Moss SF, Chung DC, Jensen RT, Snyderwine E. Priorities for improving the management of gastroenteropancreatic neuroendocrine tumors. *J Natl Cancer Inst.* 2008;100:1282.
17. Jayasena C, Dhillo W. Carcinoid syndrome and neuroendocrine tumours. *Endocr Cancer.* 2013;41:566-569.
18. Yao JC, Hassan M, Phan A, et al. One hundred years after "carcinoid": epidemiology of and prognostic factors for neuroendocrine tumors in 35,825 cases in the United States. *J Clin Oncol.* 2008;26:3063.
19. Berge T, Linell F. Carcinoid tumours. Frequency in a defined population during a 12-year period. *Acta Pathol Microbiol Scand [A].* 1976;84:322.
20. Kimura W, Kuroda A, Morioka Y. Clinical pathology of endocrine tumors of the pancreas. Analysis of autopsy cases. *Dig Dis Sci.* 1991;36:933.
21. Modlin IM, Lye KD, Kidd M. A 5-decade analysis of 13,715 carcinoid tumors. *Cancer.* 2003;97:934.
22. Hiripi E, Bermejo JL, Sundquist J, Hemminki K. Familial gastrointestinal carcinoid tumours and associated cancers. *Ann Oncol.* 2009;20:950.
23. Fraenkel M, Kim MK, Faggiano A, Valk GD. Epidemiology of gastroenteropancreatic neuroendocrine tumours. *Best Pract Res Clin Gastroenterol.* 2012;26:691-703.
24. Kaerlev L, Teglbjaerg PS, Sabroe S, et al. Occupational risk factors for small bowel carcinoid tumor: a European population-based case-control study. *J Occup Environ Med.* 2002;44:516.
25. Jensen RT, Berna MJ, Bingham DB, Norton JA. Inherited pancreatic endocrine tumor syndromes: advances in molecular pathogenesis, diagnosis, management, and controversies. *Cancer.* 2008;113:1807.
26. Blansfield JA, Choyke L, Morita SY, et al. Clinical, genetic and radiographic analysis of 108 patients with von Hippel-Lindau disease (VHL) manifested by pancreatic neuroendocrine neoplasms (PNETs). *Surgery.* 2007;142:814.
27. Solcia E, Kloppel G, Sobin LH. *Histological Typing of Endocrine Tumors (World Health Organization: International Classification of Tumours).* 2nd ed. Heidelberg: Springer-Verlag; 2000.
28. Washington MK, Tang LH, Berlin J, et al. Protocol for the examination of specimens from patients with neuroendocrine tumors (carcinoid tumors) of the small intestine and ampulla. *Arch Pathol Lab Med.* 2010;134:181.

29. Klimstra DS, Modlin IR, Coppola D, Lloyd RV, Suster S. The pathologic classification of neuroendocrine tumors: a review of nomenclature, grading, and staging systems. *Pancreas.* 2010;39:707.

30. Bosman FT, Carneiro F, Hruban RH, eds. *Classification of Tumors of the Digestive System.* 4th ed. Lyon: IARC; 2010.

31. Kloppel G, Couvelard A, Perren A, et al. ENETS Consensus Guidelines for the Standards of Care in Neuroendocrine Tumors: towards a standardized approach to the diagnosis of gastroenteropancreatic neuroendocrine tumors and their prognostic stratification. *Neuroendocrinology.* 2009;90:162.

32. Edge S, Byrd D, Carduci M. *AJCC Cancer Staging Manual.* 7th ed. New York, NY: Springer; 2010.

33. Liszka L, Pajak J, Mrowiec S, Zielińska-Pająk E, Gołka D, Lampe P. Discrepancies between two alternative staging systems (European Neuroendocrine Tumor Society 2006 and American Joint Committee on Cancer/Union for International Cancer Control 2010) of neuroendocrine neoplasms of the pancreas. A study of 50 cases. *Pathol Res Pract.* 2011;207(4):220-224.

34. Washington MK, Tang LH, Berlin J, et al. Protocol for the examination of specimens from patients with neuroendocrine tumors (carcinoid tumors) of the appendix. *Arch Pathol Lab Med.* 2010;134:171.

35. Sundin A. Radiological and nuclear medicine imaging of gastroenteropancreatic neuroendocrine tumours. *Best Pract Res Clin Gastroenterol.* 2012;26:803-818.

36. Toth-Fejel S, Pommier RF. Relationships among delay of diagnosis, extent of disease, and survival in patients with abdominal carcinoid tumors. *Am J Surg.* 2004;187:575.

37. Knigge U, Hansen CP. Surgery for GEP-NETs. *Best Pract Res Clin Gastroenterol.* 2012;26:819-831.

38. Maxwell J, O'Dorisio T, Howe J. Biochemical diagnosis and preoperative imaging of gastroenteropancreatic neuroendocrine tumors. *Surg Oncol Clin N Am.* 2016;25:171-194.

39. O'Toole D, Grossman A, Gross D, et al. ENETS consensus guidelines for the standards of care in neuroendocrine tumors: biochemical markers. *Neuroendocrinology.* 2009;90:194.

40. Sato Y. Clinical features and management of type I gastric carcinoids. *Clin J Gastroenterol.* 2014;7:381-386.

41. Kidd M, Gustafsson B, Modlin IM. Gastric carcinoids (neuroendocrine neoplasms). *Gastroenterol Clin North Am.* 2013;42:381-397.

42. Massironi S, Sciola V, Spampatti MP, Peracchi M, Conte D. Gastric carcinoids: between underestimation and overtreatment. *World J Gastroenterol.* 2009;15:2177.

43. Kulke MH, Anthony LB, Bushnell DL, et al. NANETS treatment guidelines: well-differentiated neuroendocrine tumors of the stomach and pancreas. *Pancreas.* 2010;39:735.

44. Gladdy RA, Strong VE, Coit D, et al. Defining surgical indications for type I gastric carcinoid tumor. *Ann Surg Oncol.* 2009;16:3154.

45. Vinik A, Chaya C. Clinical presentation and diagnosis of neuroendocrine tumors. *Hematol Oncol Clin North Am.* 2016;30:21-48.

46. Ramage JK, Ahmed A, Ardill J, et al. Guidelines for the management of gastroenteropancreatic neuroendocrine (including carcinoid) tumours (NETs). *Gut.* 2012;61:6-32.

47. Guo Z, Li Q, Wilander E, Pontén J. Clonality analysis of multifocal carcinoid tumours of the small intestine by X-chromosome inactivation analysis. *J Pathol.* 2000;190:76.

48. Yantiss RK, Odze RD, Farraye FA, Rosenberg AE. Solitary versus multiple carcinoid tumors of the ileum: a clinical and pathologic review of 68 cases. *Am J Surg Pathol.* 2003;27:811.

49. Strosberg J. Neuroendocrine tumours of the small intestine. *Best Pract Res Clin Gastroenterol.* 2012;26:755-773.

50. Kanakis G, Kaltsas G. Biochemical markers for gastroenteropancreatic neuroendocrine tumours (GEP-NETs). *Best Pract Res Clin Gastroenterol.* 2012;26:791-802.

51. Boudreaux JP, Klimstra DS, Hassan MM, et al. The NANETS consensus guideline for the diagnosis and management of neuroendocrine tumors: well-differentiated neuroendocrine tumors of the jejunum, ileum, appendix, and cecum. *Pancreas.* 2010;39:753.

52. Ito T, Igarashi H, Jensen RT. Pancreatic neuroendocrine tumors: clinical features, diagnosis and medical treatment: advances. *Best Pract Res Clin Gastroenterol.* 2012;26:737-753.

53. Ohrvall U, Eriksson B, Juhlin C, et al. Method for dissection of mesenteric metastases in mid-gut carcinoid tumors. *World J Surg.* 2000;24:1402.

54. Murray S, Lloyd RV, Sippel RS, Chen H. Clinicopathologic characteristics of colonic carcinoid tumors. *J Surg Res.* 2013;184:183-188.

55. Ramage JK, Goretzki PE, Manfredi R, et al. Consensus guidelines for the management of patients with digestive neuroendocrine tumours: well-differentiated colon and rectum tumour/carcinoma. *Neuroendocrinology.* 2008;87:31.

56. Anthony LB, Strosberg JR, Klimstra DS, et al. The NANETS consensus guidelines for the diagnosis and management of gastrointestinal neuroendocrine tumors (NETs): well-differentiated NETs of the distal colon and rectum. *Pancreas.* 2010;39:767.

57. Konishi T, Watanabe T, Kishimoto J, et al. Prognosis and risk factors of metastasis in colorectal carcinoids: results of a nationwide registry over 15 years. *Gut.* 2007;56:863.

58. Narayanan S, Kuntz P. Role of somatostatin analogues in the treatment of neuroendocrine tumors. *Hematol Oncol Clin North Am.* 2016;30:163-177.

59. Norton JA, Kivlen M, Li M, Schneider D, Chuter T, Jensen RT. Morbidity and mortality of aggressive resection in patients with advanced neuroendocrine tumors. *Arch Surg.* 2003;138:859.

60. Kennedy A. Hepatic-directed therapies in patients with neuroendocrine tumors. *Hematol Oncol Clin North Am.* 2016;30:193-207.

61. Steinmuller T, Kianmanesh R, Falconi M, et al. Consensus guidelines for the management of patients with liver metastases from digestive (neuro)endocrine tumors: foregut, midgut, hindgut, and unknown primary. *Neuroendocrinology.* 2008;87:47.

62. Sward C, Johanson V, Nieveen van Dijkum E, et al. Prolonged survival after hepatic artery embolization in patients with midgut carcinoid syndrome. *Br J Surg.* 2009;96:517.

63. Saxena A, Chua TC, Sarkar A, et al. Progression and survival results after radical hepatic metastasectomy of indolent advanced neuroendocrine neoplasms (NENs) supports an aggressive surgical approach. *Surgery.* 2011;149:209.

64. Le Treut YP, Gregoire E, Belghiti J, et al. Predictors of long-term survival after liver transplantation for metastatic endocrine tumors: an 85-case French multicentric report. *Am J Transplant.* 2008;8:1205.

65. Chung H, Chapman W. Liver transplantation for metastatic neuroendocrine tumors. *Adv Surg.* 2014;48:235-252.

66. Givi B, Pommier SJ, Thompson AK, Diggs BS, Pommier RF. Operative resection of primary carcinoid neoplasms in patients with liver metastases yields significantly better survival. *Surgery.* 2006;140:891, discussion 897.

67. Ahmed A, Turner G, King B, et al. Midgut neuroendocrine tumours with liver metastases: results of the UKINETS study. *Endocr Relat Cancer.* 2009;16:885.

68. Raj N, Reidy-Lagunes D. Systemic therapies for advanced pancreatic neuroendocrine tumors. *Hematol Oncol Clin North Am.* 2016;30:119-133.

69. Berardi R, Rinaldi S, Torniai M, et al. Gastrointestinal neuroendocrine tumors: searching the optimal treatment strategy—a literature review. *Crit Rev Oncol Hematol.* 2016;98:264-274.

70. Akerstrom G, Falconi M, Kianmanesh R, et al. ENETS consensus guidelines for the standards of care in neuroendocrine tumors: pre- and perioperative therapy in patients with neuroendocrine tumors. *Neuroendocrinology.* 2009;90:203.

71. Plockinger U, Gustafsson B, Ivan D, et al. ENETS consensus guidelines for the standards of care in neuroendocrine tumors: echocardiography. *Neuroendocrinology.* 2009;90:190.

72. Norlen O, Hessman O, Stalberg P, Akerström G, Hellman P. Prophylactic cholecystectomy in midgut carcinoid patients. *World J Surg.* 2010;34:1361.

Gastrointestinal Stromal Tumors

Bruce M. Brenner

EPIDEMIOLOGY

Gastrointestinal stromal tumors (GISTs) are the most common mesenchymal, or nonepithelial, neoplasms of the gastrointestinal (GI) tract. GISTs may be found anywhere in the GI tract, from the esophagus to the internal anal sphincter. The most common GI location is the stomach (56%), as reported in a 2015 review of multiple population-based studies, followed by the small intestine (32%), colon and rectum (6%), and esophagus (<1%).[1] The remaining 5% of lesions occur in other less common locations, including the mesentery, pelvis, pancreas, liver, omentum, and genitourinary tract. Occurrence of these extragastrointestinal lesions, or EGISTs, is described predominantly in case reports and small series.

GISTs were historically thought to be of smooth muscle origin and therefore categorized as leiomyomas or leiomyosarcomas. Prior to 1983, when the term stromal tumor was first used, they remained largely unrecognized as a separate class of neoplasms.[2] The development of specific pathologic criteria has allowed for more accurate categorization of mesenchymal tumors and reclassification of many of these tumors as GISTs. The exact incidence of GISTs was initially unclear because many studies included data from the era prior to their recognition as a distinct disease entity. In a review of population-based studies including more recent data from 19 countries, the incidence ranged from 7 to 15 cases per million people in most studies.[1] A study published in 2015 based on Surveillance, Epidemiology, and End Results (SEER) data estimated the incidence to be approximately 6.8 cases per million, or approximately 2100 total cases in the United States.[3] This study also reported 5-year overall and disease-specific survivals of 65% and 79%, respectively. The true incidence of GISTs may be underreported because SEER requires reporting of these tumors only if they are classified as malignant or metastatic.[4] As the recognition of these tumors has grown, several groups are in the process of developing databases to better estimate the true incidence of GISTs.

PATHOLOGY AND DIAGNOSIS

HISTOLOGY

GISTs are diagnosed based on morphologic features supported by immunohistochemical (IHC) studies. Histologically, GISTs can occur in three different types: spindle cell, which accounts for approximately 70% of tumors, epithelioid, and mixed, which contains a variable combination of spindle cells and epithelioid cells (Fig. 81.1). Rarely, GISTs may have myxoid stroma, neuroendocrine features, signet ring variant, or marked lymphocytic infiltrate. The pathologic distinction may still be difficult to conclusively define in individual cases, with fibromatosis and leiomyosarcomas still being mistaken for GISTs.

IDENTIFICATION OF CELLS OF ORIGIN OF GASTROINTESTINAL STROMAL TUMORS

In 1983 the term stromal tumor was first used to describe a series of gastric tumors that appeared to arise not from smooth muscle but rather from nerve sheath cells that did not resemble typical Schwann cells.[2] This initial distinction was based on IHC and electron microscopic analysis that demonstrated lack of desmin, positivity for the s100 protein, and lack of ultrastructural features typical of smooth muscle or Schwann cells.

Numerous studies were subsequently performed in an attempt to identify the cells of origin of these tumors. In the early 1990s it was found that the majority of (but not all) GISTs were positive for the myeloid progenitor cell antigen CD34, which is not typically seen in leiomyomas or Schwannomas.[5] The identification of IHC staining for the CD117 protein, which is the tyrosine kinase receptor known as *KIT*, was a critical step in better classifying these tumors.[6] This led to the hypothesis that GISTs arise from the interstitial cells of Cajal (ICC), which also express both CD34 and CD117.

The ICC were identified in 1893 by Santiago Ramon y Cajal, who aptly named them "interstitial" cells given their interposition between nerve endings and smooth muscle cells in the gut wall. These cells have very few contractile elements (unlike smooth muscle cells) and have a greater proportion of mitochondria. They arise from mesenchymal cells and are thought to play an integral role in the propagation of intrinsic slow-wave gut peristalsis. ICC, although primarily known for their role in gut motility, are also found outside of the GI tract, including the genitourinary system, portal vein, and pancreas. The higher frequency of tumors confined to the GI tract likely represents the increased proportion of ICC in the GI tract because no clear histologic distinction has been elucidated among the ICC of various locations.

MOLECULAR MECHANISM OF CARCINOGENESIS

After the IHC and phenotypic distinction of GISTs were established, significant attention was directed to the molecular mechanism of carcinogenesis. The basic underlying pathophysiology in the majority of lesions appears to involve a gain of function mutation leading to increased activity of the *KIT* tyrosine kinase receptor on the cell membrane.[7] Normal physiology consists of a monomeric tyrosine kinase receptor that binds to an extracellular

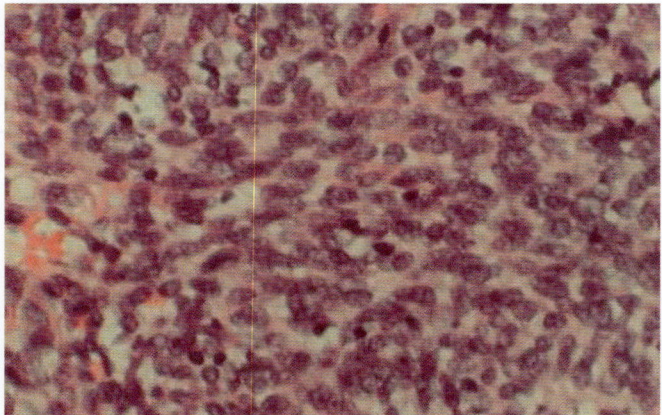

FIGURE 81.1 Typical gastrointestinal stromal tumor histopathology.

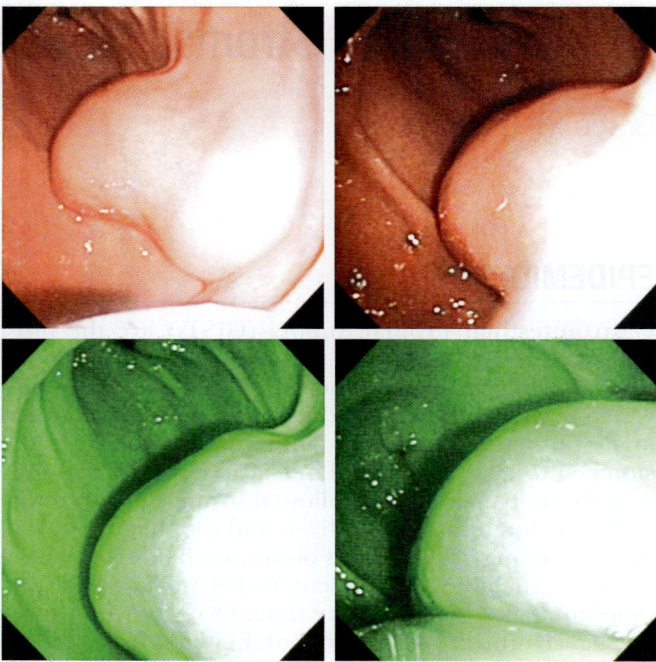

FIGURE 81.2 Gastrointestinal stromal tumor in stomach exhibiting typical smooth, protuberant appearance on endoscopy.

ligand, stem cell factor (SCF), which then causes dimerization of the receptor. This dimerization allows for subsequent autophosphorylation, activating downstream intracellular signaling pathways, and leads to increased cell proliferation. Some lesions may also develop due to gain of function mutations in platelet-derived growth factor receptor A (PDGFRA), another tyrosine kinase receptor, or BRAF, a protooncogene serine/threonine kinase, each of which may contribute to the development of approximately 10% of GISTs.

IMMUNOHISTOCHEMICAL STAINING

CD117 IHC staining has now been widely accepted as the primary criterion for a pathologic diagnosis of GIST,[7] with a reported sensitivity greater than 95% and a high specificity. PDGFRA staining has also been identified as a marker of GIST, with a frequency of up to 15%. PDGFRA may be used in combination with c-Kit or as a marker for GISTs that lack the c-Kit mutation.[8] An additional IHC marker, DOG1, which stands for discovered on GIST, also has utility in the diagnosis of tumors that lack c-Kit or PDGFRA mutations. DOG1 has an overall sensitivity of 95%, similar to Kit.[9] There is growing evidence of a significant correlation between immunophenotype and histology, as well as other features of GISTs.[10]

CLINICAL PRESENTATION OF GASTROINTESTINAL STROMAL TUMORS

GISTs are often asymptomatic and discovered only as incidental findings on imaging studies or endoscopy performed for other indications. Patients with a symptomatic GIST often have symptoms that are related to the size and location of the tumor. Early in disease progression, symptoms may be very nonspecific, such as mild pain, bloating, or dyspepsia. More significant symptoms generally do not occur until much later in the course of the disease, when they have grown quite large. This is likely due to their submucosal location, exophytic growth, and propensity to displace rather than invade adjacent organs. Patients presenting with large GISTs may have palpable tumors and present with pressure or pain or symptoms related to compression of adjacent organs. Patients may also present with acute GI blood loss or symptoms of chronic anemia and associated fatigue resulting from overlying mucosal ulceration, or with peritonitis related to tumor perforation.

IMAGING AND DIAGNOSIS

The increased awareness of GISTs has improved preoperative diagnosis. Suspected GISTs should be evaluated with contrast-enhanced computed tomography (CT) and/or magnetic resonance imaging (MRI). Typical findings are variable, depending on the size and aggressiveness of the lesion.[11] Large GISTs appear as hypervascular, enhancing masses and are often heterogeneous because of necrosis, hemorrhage, or cystic degeneration. They often displace but rarely invade adjacent organs. Smaller GISTs are usually more homogeneous and polypoid in appearance.

Many GISTs are also identified during endoscopy for evaluation of upper GI symptoms. A submucosal mass (Fig. 81.2) may be seen that is smooth in appearance and often appears to form a bulge into the lumen of the stomach (Fig. 81.3). Ulceration may be seen in lesions that present with bleeding or anemia. Cross-sectional imaging should be performed on all patients with suspected GIST identified endoscopically because endoscopic findings may underestimate the full extent of disease.

Biopsy of a suspected GIST is not required if it appears surgically resectable. However, if neoadjuvant or palliative therapy is being considered for large, unresectable, or metastatic tumors, a tissue diagnosis is needed. Endoscopic biopsies are preferable, if possible, to percutaneous techniques because of the risk of bleeding and tumor rupture.

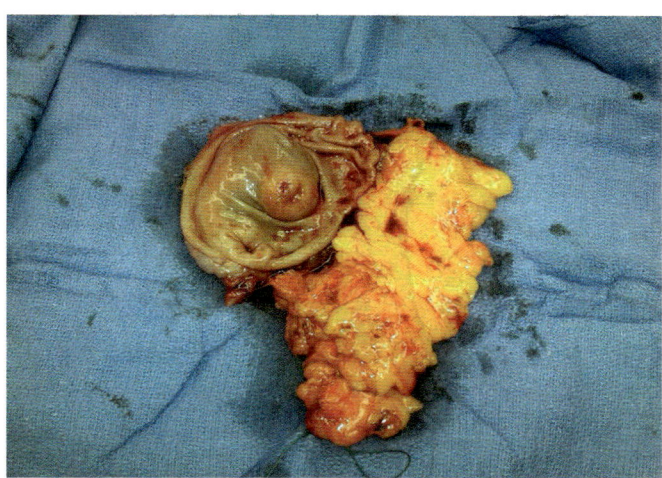

FIGURE 81.3 Resected gastrointestinal stromal tumor bulging outward from lumen.

TABLE 81.1 Joensuu Modification of National Institutes of Health Consensus Classification for Selecting Patients With Gastrointestinal Stromal Tumors for Adjuvant Therapy

Risk Category	Tumor Size (cm)	Mitotic Index (per 50 HPFs)	Primary Tumor Site
Very low risk	<2.0	≤5	Any
Low risk	2.1–5.0	≤5	Any
Intermediate risk	2.1–5.0	>5	Gastric
	<5.0	6–10	Any
	5.1–10.0	≤5	Gastric
High risk	Any	Any	Tumor rupture
	>10 cm	Any	Any
	Any	>10	Any
	>5.0	>5	Any
	2.1–5.0	>5	Nongastric
	5.1–10.0	≤5	Nongastric

HPF, High-power field.
From Joensuu H. Risk stratification of patients diagnosed with gastrointestinal stromal tumor. *Hum Pathol.* 2008;39(10):1411–1419.

Endoscopic ultrasound (EUS) may also aid in the differentiation of a submucosal gastric mass versus impingement from surrounding organs (i.e., pancreatic mass, pseudocyst). EUS is also useful in biopsy of these lesions due to their submucosal location. EUS is particularly important in the management of very small (<2 cm) gastric GISTs. In these patients, EUS is indicated to evaluate for high-risk features. These include irregular borders, cystic spaces, ulceration, echogenic foci, and internal heterogeneity.[12] EUS–fine-needle aspiration may be performed on these lesions to confirm the diagnosis of GIST.

Chest imaging should be considered for staging of patients with GISTs. Positron emission tomography (PET) scans may also have utility in preoperative staging. PET/CT scans have already been shown to be useful in the early determination of the response of GISTs to systemic therapy.[13] Ring-shaped uptake on preoperative PET scan has recently been shown to be an independent adverse prognostic factor for postoperative recurrence.[14]

MALIGNANT POTENTIAL AND STAGING

Initially it was thought that the malignant potential of GISTs covered a broad spectrum from benign tumors to aggressive malignancies, with a high risk for distant metastases. As longer-term data have accumulated, it appears that most GISTs have some potential to metastasize and should not be considered truly benign. The major exception to this rule is very small (< 2 cm) gastric GISTS that also lack high-risk histologic features.[12] Gastric GISTs generally seem to behave less aggressively than tumors that arise in other locations.

Current American Joint Committee on Cancer (AJCC) staging of GISTs includes tumor size, presence of nodal metastases, distant metastases, and grade (high grade is > 5 mitoses/50 high-power field).[15] GISTs rarely metastasize to lymph nodes, but distant metastases, particularly to the liver and peritoneum, are not uncommon. Separate stage groupings are used for gastric and extragastric lesions, reflecting the less aggressive behavior of gastric GISTs. Several studies have been published that attempt to better delineate criteria that predict the malignant potential of GIST. The first widely cited criteria were developed at a National Institutes of Health workshop and are commonly referred to as the Fletcher criteria.[16] The two best predictors of disease recurrence in this study were tumor size and number of mitotic figures per high-power field, both of which demonstrated statistical significance. The Joensuu criteria are a modification of the Fletcher criteria that include mitotic index, tumor size, tumor location, and tumor rupture[17] (Table 81.1) and were validated in a later study.[18] Another study supported the addition of tumor anatomic site as a predictor of disease recurrence and developed a nomogram for predicting the risk of disease recurrence.[19] A more recent study that included data from a multiinstitutional cohort of patients treated in North America developed a nomogram that incorporates patient sex, tumor site, tumor size, and mitotic rate.[20] This nomogram was found to perform better than the other criteria previously used.

As mentioned previously, a recent study demonstrated that preoperative PET scanning may provide additional information on recurrence risk after surgery. In this study, ring-shaped uptake on PET and Joensuu high-risk score were shown to be independent adverse prognostic indicators for postoperative recurrence.[14]

TREATMENT OF GASTROINTESTINAL STROMAL TUMORS

SURGICAL THERAPY

Complete surgical resection remains the mainstay of treatment for primary GISTs and is the only potentially curative therapy. Important considerations for surgical planning include the feasibility of obtaining a complete resection with maximal organ preservation. GISTs have the beneficial feature of growing exophytically without submucosal spread (Fig. 81.4) and also rarely invade adjacent organs. Based on these anatomic features, complete surgical resection of all gross tumor at initial surgery is often possible without the need for more extensive or multiorgan resections to achieve wide margins. Care must be taken not to violate the tumor pseudocapsule or rupture the tumor because

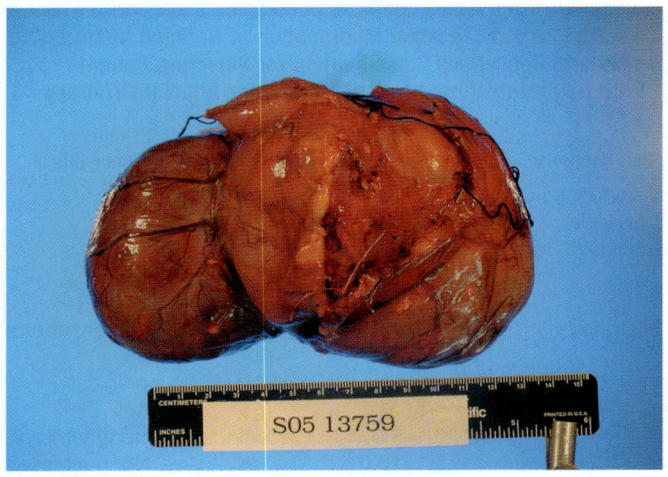

FIGURE 81.4 Resected gastrointestinal stromal tumor displaying lobulated, exophytic characteristics.

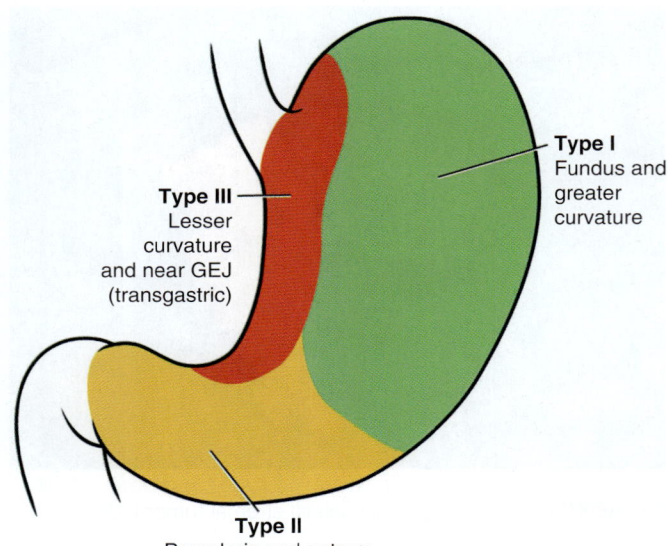

FIGURE 81.5 Tumor locations and corresponding surgical technique as reported by Privette et al. (From Privette A, McCahill L, Borrazzo E, Single RM, Zubarik R. Laparoscopic approaches to resection of suspected gastric gastrointestinal stromal tumors based on tumor location. *Surg Endosc.* 2008;22:487 [Fig. 1].)

violation of the tumor pseudocapsule causes risk for subsequent tumor seeding into the peritoneum.[21] Lymphadenectomy is not indicated unless enlarged or pathologic nodes are seen on imaging or intraoperatively because GISTs rarely spread to regional nodes.

Interestingly, the presence of microscopically positive margins (R1) after macroscopic total resection may not confer a worse prognosis. In a review of data from more than 800 patients enrolled in two large North American multiinstitutional trials, there was no difference in recurrence-free survival in those who had R1 versus R0 resections.[22] This was true with or without the addition of systemic therapy. If a pathologic specimen is found to have microscopically positive margins, optimal management is still not well defined and may include re-resection, watchful waiting, and/or systemic therapy. This decision must be individualized to and discussed with each patient.

EXTENT OF SURGICAL RESECTION

Complete resection with at least a 1- to 2-cm gross margin should be the goal of surgical treatment. Gastric tumors, the most common location for GIST, typically require only a partial gastrectomy or even gastric wedge resection to achieve these margins. Partial gastrectomy confers the same progression-free survival (PFS) as total gastrectomy but spares the perioperative and postoperative morbidity of the more extensive surgery. Small bowel GISTs are treated with segmental resection. Surgical therapy of rectal GISTs depends on location in the rectum and size of the lesion and can range from radical resection with low anterior resection or abdominoperineal resection to transanal excision.[23]

MINIMALLY INVASIVE APPROACHES

There is a growing body of data that minimally invasive resection of GISTs is comparable to open techniques. The same oncologic principles should be applied to minimally invasive approaches as to open surgery, including obtaining adequate margins and avoiding violation of the tumor pseudocapsule. Studies have shown that laparoscopic resections of GISTs are associated with decreased blood loss and shorter hospital stays when compared with open surgery.[24,25]

Laparoscopic resection of GISTs was initially reserved for small gastric tumors that could be mobilized easily and were amenable to wedge resection. Initially, guidelines suggested limiting this approach to gastric tumors less than 2 cm in diameter.[26] Many of these tumors are now classified as very small or micro-GISTs and may be managed differently than larger tumors. Multiple subsequent studies proved the feasibility of resecting larger gastric and some small bowel tumors with excellent oncologic outcomes.[27–29] Current guidelines do not generally recommend laparoscopic resection for tumors greater than 5 cm in diameter. A key feature unique to successful laparoscopic resection of GIST is the removal of the specimen within a closed system, such as a retrieval bag to avoid tumor spillage or seeding of port sites.

A 2008 study proposed a classification schema (Fig. 81.5) to identify three distinct minimally invasive approaches to resecting gastric GISTs based on tumor location in the stomach.[30] Type I tumors were located in the fundus or greater curvature and were treated using a laparoscopic stapled partial gastrectomy. Type II tumors were located in the antrum/prepyloric region and were approached using laparoscopic distal gastrectomy. Type III tumors were located in the lesser curvature near the gastroesophageal junction and were resected by laparoscopic transgastric resection (Fig. 81.6). Simultaneous intraoperative endoscopy was also used in select cases to aid in obtaining grossly negative margins.

MANAGEMENT OF VERY SMALL GASTRIC GASTROINTESTINAL STROMAL TUMORS

Gastric GISTs behave less aggressively than small bowel, colorectal, or GISTs in other locations. Gastric GISTs that

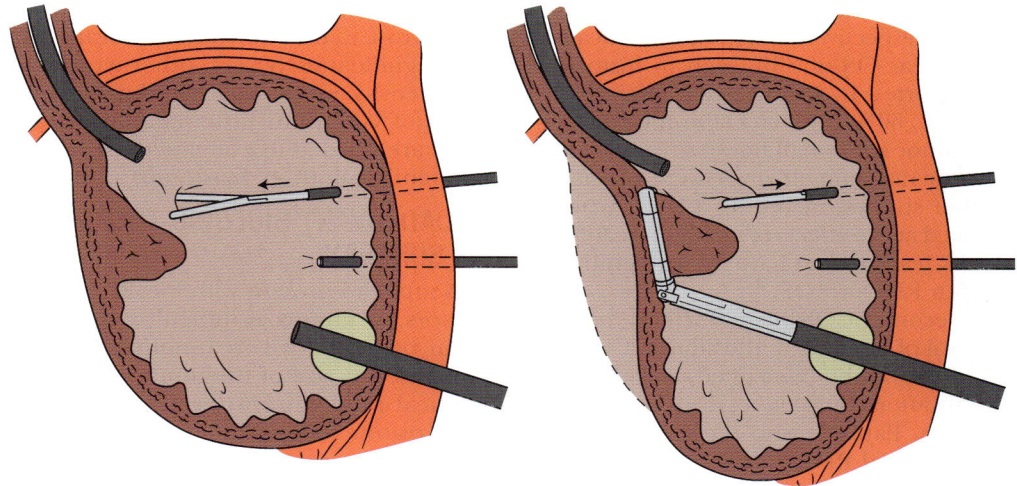

FIGURE 81.6 Transgastric resection of gastrointestinal stromal tumor on lesser curvature using simultaneous endoscopy as depicted by Privette et al. (From Privette A, McCahill L, Borrazzo E, Single RM, Zubarik R. Laparoscopic approaches to resection of suspected gastric gastrointestinal stromal tumors based on tumor location. *Surg Endosc*. 2008;22:487 [Fig. 1].)

are less than 2 cm in diameter and asymptomatic are currently referred to as very small, mini- (1 to 2 cm), or micro- (<1 cm) GISTs. Many of these are found only incidentally at endoscopy, in pathologic specimens after gastric resection, or at autopsy. They generally demonstrate benign clinical behavior. Only those lesions that are found to have high-risk features on EUS described previously are felt to be at risk for progression. Current recommendations include initial evaluation with EUS for micro-GISTs and EUS with or without CT for mini-GISTs and subsequent follow-up with serial EUS.[12] Surgery is reserved for lesions with high-risk features or those that progress on follow-up imaging. Principles of surgical resection are similar to those for other gastric GISTs described previously, and these lesions are often amenable to minimally invasive approaches.

FOLLOW-UP AND RECURRENCE AFTER SURGICAL RESECTION

Follow-up after surgical resection of GISTs generally consists of history and physical exam every 3 to 6 months for 5 years, then annually, as well as serial CT scans every 3 to 6 months for 3 to 5 years, then annually. Approximately 40% to 50% of GISTs will recur or develop metastases, even after potentially curative resection. As discussed previously, several groups have proposed criteria and/or nomograms to better predict risk of recurrence after surgical resection. Use of these criteria can improve the ability to identify patients who would potentially benefit from adjuvant systemic therapy to decrease recurrence.

SYSTEMIC THERAPY WITH BIOLOGIC AGENTS

Several factors contributed to the importance of developing alternative treatments for GISTs. First and foremost was the high disease recurrence rate after surgical resection alone and the resulting need for effective adjuvant therapy. Second, the lack of benefit of cytotoxic chemotherapy

limited treatment options for those patients with recurrent disease or those who presented with metastatic or unresectable disease. Improved understanding of the molecular mechanism of GIST carcinogenesis allowed for the development and testing of targeted biologic agents in their treatment. Several biologic agents are currently available for the treatment of GISTs (see later). Genotyping should be performed when medical therapy is planned. This may add some prognostic information but more importantly can predict response to tyrosine kinase inhibitors. For example, wild-type GISTs, which lack *KIT* and *PDGFRA* mutations, may not be sensitive to imatinib. Certain specific mutations in the *KIT* gene may also predict aggressiveness or response to therapy. For example, exon 11 deletions are associated with a high risk of recurrence.

IMATINIB (GLEEVEC)

Imatinib mesylate (Gleevec) is an oral medication that binds to tyrosine kinase receptors, preventing phosphorylation. It was initially developed for the treatment of chronic myelogenous leukemia, targeting the bcr-abl kinase that is responsible for its pathogenesis. Given the similarities between bcr-abl and *KIT* signaling, it was soon applied to the treatment of advanced GISTs in small phase I and II trials. An early case report published in 2001 highlighted the dramatic effect of imatinib on achieving metastatic GIST shrinkage.[31] The US Food and Drug Administration (FDA) rapidly approved the use of imatinib in 2002 for recurrent, locally invasive, or metastatic GIST. The drug is generally well tolerated, with the most common side effects being diarrhea and fatigue.

The American College of Surgeons Oncology Group (ACOSOG) soon initiated two landmark trials in the adjuvant therapy of GISTs. ACOSOG Z9000 was designed to evaluate the impact of imatinib on overall survival (OS) in localized, high-risk lesions after complete gross surgical resection.[32] This included patients with tumor diameter greater than 10 cm, intraperitoneal tumor rupture, or up to four peritoneal implants. All patients received 1 year of therapy. Long-term results of this trial, with a median follow-up of 7.7 years demonstrated 1-, 3-, and 5-year OS of 99%, 97%, and 83%, respectively, which was significantly improved from the 5-year OS of 35% seen in historical controls. They also reported 1-, 3-, and 5-year relapse-free survivals (RFSs) of 96%, 60%, and 40%. On multivariate analysis, increasing tumor size, small bowel site, *KIT* exon 9 mutation, high mitotic rate, and older age were associated with lower RFS. Other studies, including a large Scandinavian trial, have looked at the effects of imatinib treatment in GISTs with high-risk features and have shown significant improvements in both RFS and OS.[33]

The results of the second ACOSOG trial, Z9001, helped to lead to FDA approval of imatinib in the adjuvant setting. This was a randomized, placebo-controlled trial of 1 year of imatinib treatment after complete resection of GISTs ≥3 but less than 10 cm. Patients who received imatinib had a significantly improved RFS, which was maintained on long-term follow-up.[34] There was no difference in OS. On multivariate analysis, small bowel tumors had worse outcomes than gastric tumors, as did tumors with high mitotic rates. A European trial confirmed the benefit of imatinib in the adjuvant setting, again with significantly improved RFS but no change in OS.[35]

Imatinib has also been shown to improve survival in patients with metastatic or unresectable GISTs. In this setting, response rates of up to 70% have been seen, with a median PFS of nearly 2 years and OS of up to 57 months.[36,37] These results are particularly important in that these patients had no effective treatment options prior to the development of imatinib. The National Comprehensive Cancer Network (NCCN) and other treatment guidelines have advocated the use of imatinib as first-line therapy for metastatic or unresectable GIST, establishing imatinib therapy as the standard of care for patients with advanced disease.

SUNITINIB (SUTENT) AND REGORAFENIB (STIVARGA)

Despite overall favorable response rates for GISTs, some tumors are refractory to imatinib therapy or progress while on treatment and some patients do not tolerate imatinib therapy. Sunitinib is a multitargeted tyrosine kinase receptor inhibitor that has activity against *KIT*, as well as *PDGFR*, *BRAF*, and other receptors. A randomized trial of patients with imatinib-resistant GISTs demonstrated a median time to tumor progression of 27 weeks for patients treated with sunitinib compared with 6 weeks for patients receiving placebo.[38] This trial was unblinded early due to the significant difference in survival between the two groups. Median OS nearly doubled to 73 weeks from a calculated time of 39 weeks in untreated patients. Other trials have demonstrated similar results. The FDA approved sunitinib for GIST patients either refractory to or unable to tolerate imatinib in 2006.

Regorafenib is another multitargeted tyrosine kinase receptor inhibitor that is active against *KIT*. Several studies have shown efficacy of regorafenib in patients who have failed standard tyrosine kinase inhibitor therapy with imatinib and sunitinib. In a recent study looking at long-term results of patients who had failed standard tyrosine kinase inhibitor therapy, treatment with regorafenib resulted in a median PFS of 13 months and a median OS of 25 months.[39] Regorafenib is currently FDA approved and advocated as third-line therapy in the NCCN and other guidelines. Several other tyrosine kinase inhibitors with activity against *KIT* have been discussed in the treatment of GIST, but little data are available and clinical trials are needed to evaluate these agents. These include sorafenib, nilotinib, masitinib, and others.

NEOADJUVANT BIOLOGIC THERAPY FOLLOWED BY SURGERY

Patients who present with locally advanced disease, large tumors, or tumors at difficult anatomic sites may benefit from preoperative treatment with imatinib. This may decrease the size of the tumors, allowing a more limited surgical procedure to be performed, improving organ preservation and enabling complete resection. It can also decrease the risk of tumor rupture and spillage into the peritoneal cavity.

In a study of 161 patients with locally advanced, nonmetastatic GISTs who received neoadjuvant imatinib, 80% demonstrated a tumor response and 83% were able to undergo R0 resections.[40] Only two patients had disease progression during neoadjuvant therapy. Five-year disease-free survival in this study was 65%, and median OS was 104 months. In another study of 57 patients with locally advanced GISTs, median tumor size was reduced from 12 to 6 cm before surgery.[41] No tumor perforation occurred, and R0 resection was achieved in 84% of patients. Five-year PFS and OS were 77% and 88%, respectively.

These and other studies support the use of neoadjuvant therapy in locally advanced GISTs. Surgical resection can be accomplished in these patients, with acceptable morbidity and high R0 resection rates. The duration of preoperative therapy generally ranges from 4 to 12 months and response is monitored with serial imaging studies. Surgery should be carefully timed to occur when maximal response to imatinib has occurred. Continued therapy with imatinib for 1 to 2 years is generally recommended postoperatively to reduce recurrence rates.

ROLE OF RADIATION THERAPY

Historically, GISTs have been considered resistant to radiation therapy. Current guidelines mainly advocate the use of radiation only in the palliation of bone metastases from GISTs. However, a recent study evaluated the treatment of intraabdominal or liver metastases from GISTs with external beam radiation.[42] Eight percent of patients achieved partial remission, 80% had stable disease, and 12% progressed with a median follow-up time of 19 months. Of note, the median time to progression in the radiated lesions was 4 times as long as the median time to progression at any site (16 vs. 4 months). Clearly, more data are needed to fully elucidate the role of radiation therapy in the treatment of intraabdominal GIST metastases.

TREATMENT OF RECURRENT AND METASTATIC DISEASE

Imatinib remains the primary treatment for recurrent or metastatic GISTs. Multiple trials have shown partial or complete response rates of approximately 45% to 55%

in these patients,[37,43] with significant improvements in PFS and OS compared with historical controls. There has been an ongoing debate regarding the benefit of high-dose imatinib (up to 800 mg/day), which substantially increases toxicity compared with the standard dose (400 mg/day). In a large meta-analysis including patients from two large, randomized trials, there was a small but significant difference in PFS that was maintained for only up to 2 years and no difference in OS.[44] Of note, the exon 9 *KIT* mutation was the only predictive factor for improved PFS, and the authors therefore advocate using high-dose treatment only in patients whose tumors harbor this mutation.

The optimal duration of therapy with imatinib has not been conclusively established. An ACOSOG study examining the benefit of continuing imatinib therapy beyond 1 year of treatment concluded that interruption of therapy led to rapid disease progression.[45] This has been confirmed in other studies even up to 3 years after initiation of treatment.[46] Discontinuation of imatinib is therefore not recommended unless the patient develops significant toxicity. Other tyrosine kinase inhibitors, including sunitinib, regorafenib, and nilotinib have been shown to significantly improve PFS, but not OS, in patients resistant to or intolerant of imatinib.[47]

Surgical resection may also have a role in the treatment of patients with advanced GISTs. Some studies have shown improved survival in patients who have R0 or R1 resections of GIST metastases in combination with imatinib therapy.[48,49] Debulking or R2 resection does not appear to lead to the same survival benefit.[50] Surgery for advanced GISTs should be reserved for patients treated with imatinib who can undergo complete gross resection without incurring significant morbidity.

PEDIATRIC GASTROINTESTINAL STROMAL TUMORS

Pediatric GISTs are exceptionally rare and appear to demonstrate significantly different genetic features and disease behavior than do adult GISTs. These tumors are more often epithelioid or mixed rather than spindle cell morphology and have a predilection for females. Approximately 85% occur in the stomach, and the most common presenting symptom is GI bleeding. There is a higher rate of metastases and local recurrence, yet they tend to follow a more indolent course and have a more favorable long-term prognosis than do adult GISTs.[51]

The molecular characteristics of pediatric GISTs also differ from those of the adult population. Despite *KIT* expression in the majority of lesions, few have *KIT* or *PDGFR* mutations. Wild-type GISTs, which lack *KIT* and *PDGFRA* mutations, are the predominant type of GISTs in children but are rare in adults. These harbor mutations in a variety of other genes, including *IGF1R, BRAF, SDH,* and *NF1*.[52]

Because of their rarity, little has been published on the treatment of pediatric GISTs. Pediatric patients with *KIT* mutations are considered to have the adult form of the disease and are treated based on adult guidelines. For others, surgery is indicated for lesions that can be resected with minimal morbidity or for debulking lesions as a means of palliation. The lack of *KIT* mutations suggests that treatment with tyrosine kinase receptor inhibitors may have limited efficacy in these patients. Treatment with imatinib or sunitinib is generally reserved for unresectable lesions that are symptomatic or progress during observation.[53] Mutations in other genes, such as *IGF1R* and *BRAF*, may serve as targets for therapeutic agents, but little or no data exist on GIST treatment with such agents.

HEREDITARY GASTROINTESTINAL STROMAL TUMORS

The vast majority of GISTs are sporadic, with only approximately 5% considered to be familial in origin. Syndromes associated with GISTs include *NF1* mutation, the Carney triad (GIST, pulmonary chondroma, and pheochromocytoma/paraganglioma), familial GIST syndrome (*c-Kit/PDGFRA* mutation), and the Carney-Stratakis syndrome (GIST and paraganglioma; *SDHD, SDHC,* and *SDHB* mutations). The genetic defect leading to the Carney triad is unknown. A familial GIST should be suspected in patients with multiple GISTs or other findings compatible with one of these syndromes. Confirmatory genetic testing should be performed and genetic testing of family members considered if a syndrome is identified. Specific guidelines for the treatment of syndromic GISTs are lacking. However, they tend to be indolent and behave like pediatric GISTs, and therefore treatment recommendations may be similar to those in pediatric GISTs.

SUMMARY

GISTs are rare but represent the most common mesenchymal tumor of the GI tract. They are often found incidentally on imaging studies or endoscopy performed for other indications. Biopsy is only necessary in lesions that are unresectable, metastatic, or locally advanced with an indication for preoperative systemic therapy. Complete surgical resection remains the mainstay of treatment. Very small gastric GISTs without high-risk features may be managed with observation. Systemic therapy with imatinib is indicated in the adjuvant, neoadjuvant, and metastatic setting. Second- and third-line systemic therapy is available with sunitinib and regorafenib. Given these treatment modalities, patients with GISTs can be treated in a multidisciplinary fashion with vastly improved outcomes than were possible in the past.

REFERENCES

1. Søreide K, Sandvik OM, Søreide JA, Giljaca V, Jureckova A, Bulusu VR. Global epidemiology of gastrointestinal stromal tumours (GIST): a systematic review of population-based cohort studies. *Cancer Epidemiol.* 2015;40:39-46.
2. Mazur M, Clark H. Gastric stromal tumors. Reappraisal of histogenesis. *Am J Surg Pathol.* 1983;7(6):507-519.
3. Ma G, Murphy J, Martinez M, Sicklick J. Epidemiology of gastrointestinal stromal tumors in the era of histology codes: results of a population-based study. *Cancer Epidemiol Biomarkers Prev.* 2015;24(1): 298-302.

4. Choi A, Hamner J, Merchant S, et al. Underreporting of gastro-intestinal stromal tumors: is the true incidence being captured? *J Gastrointest Surg.* 2015;19(9):1699-1703.

5. Miettinen M, Virolainen M, Maarit-Sarlomo R. Gastrointestinal stromal tumors—value of CD34 antigen in their identification and separation from true leiomyomas and schwannomas. *Am J Surg Pathol.* 1995;19(2):207-216.

6. Hirota S, Isozaki K, Moriyama Y, et al. Gain-of-function mutations of c-kit in human gastrointestinal stromal tumors. *Science.* 1998;279(5350):577-580.

7. Corless CL, Fletcher JA, Heinrich MC. Biology of gastrointestinal stromal tumors. *J Clin Oncol.* 2004;22(18):3813-3825.

8. Zheng S, Chen LR, Wang HJ, Chen SZ. Analysis of mutation and expression of c-kit and PDGFR-alpha gene in gastrointestinal stromal tumor. *Hepatogastroenterology.* 2007;54(80):2285-2290.

9. Miettinen M, Wang Z, Lasota J. DOG1 antibody in the differential diagnosis of gastrointestinal stromal tumors: a study of 1840 cases. *Am J Surg Pathol.* 2009;33(9):1401-1408.

10. Chetty R, Serra S. Molecular and morphological correlation in gastrointestinal stromal tumours (GISTs): an update and primer. *J Clin Pathol.* 2016;69(9):754-760.

11. Hong X, Choi H, Loyer EM, Benjamin RS, Trent JC, Charnsangavej C. Gastrointestinal stromal tumor: role of CT in diagnosis and in response evaluation and surveillance after treatment with imatinib. *Radiographics.* 2006;26(2):481-495.

12. Nishida T, Goto O, Raut CP, Yahagi N. Diagnostic and treatment strategy for small gastrointestinal stromal tumors. *Cancer.* 2016;122(20):3110-3118.

13. Van den Abbeele AD. The lessons of GIST–PET and PET/CT: a new paradigm for imaging. *Oncologist.* 2008;13(suppl 2):8-13.

14. Miyake KK, Nakamoto Y, Mikami Y, et al. The predictive value of preoperative 18 F-fluorodeoxyglucose PET for postoperative recurrence in patients with localized primary gastrointestinal stromal tumour. *Eur Radiol.* 2016;26(12):4664-4674.

15. Edge SB. *AJCC Cancer Staging Manual.* 7th ed. New York: Scribner; 2010.

16. Fletcher CD. Clinicopathologic correlations in gastrointestinal stromal tumors. *Hum Pathol.* 2002;33(5):455.

17. Joensuu H. Risk stratification of patients diagnosed with gastro-intestinal stromal tumor. *Hum Pathol.* 2008;39(10):1411-1419.

18. Rutkowski P, Bylina E, Wozniak N, et al. Validation of the Joensuu risk criteria for primary resectable gastrointestinal stromal tumour—the impact of tumour rupture on patient outcomes. *Eur J Surg Oncol.* 2011;37(10):890-896.

19. Gold JS, Gönen M, Gutiérrez A, et al. Development and validation of a prognostic nomogram for recurrence-free survival after complete surgical resection of localised primary gastrointestinal stromal tumour: a retrospective analysis. *Lancet Oncol.* 2009;10(11):1045-1052.

20. Bischof D, Kim A, Behman Y, et al. Anomogram to predict disease-free survival after surgical resection of GIST. *J Gastrointest Surg.* 2014;18(12):2123-2129.

21. Demetri GD, von Mehren M, Antonescu CR, et al. NCCN task force report: update on the management of patients with gastrointestinal stromal tumors. *J Natl Compr Canc Netw.* 2010;8(suppl 2):S1-S41.

22. McCarter MD, Antonescu CR, Ballman KV, et al. Microscopically positive margins for primary gastrointestinal stromal tumors: analysis of risk factors and tumor recurrence. *J Am Coll Surg.* 2012;215(1):53-59.

23. Chen CW, Wu CC, Hsiao CW, et al. Surgical management and clinical outcome of gastrointestinal stromal tumor of the colon and rectum. *Z Gastroenterol.* 2008;46(8):760-765.

24. MacArthur KM, Nicholl MB, Baumann BC. Laparoscopic versus open resection for Gastrointestinal Stromal Tumors (GISTs). *J Gastrointest Cancer.* 2016 Aug 5;[Epub ahead of print].

25. Hu J, Or BH, Hu K, Wang ML. Comparison of the post-operative outcomes and survival of laparoscopic versus open resections for gastric gastrointestinal stromal tumors: a multi-center prospective cohort study. *Int J Surg.* 2016;33:65-71.

26. Nguyen SQ, Divino CM, Wang JL, Dikman SH. Laparoscopic management of gastrointestinal stromal tumors. *Surg Endosc.* 2006;20(5):713-716.

27. Nguyen S, Divino Q, Wang C, Dikman M. Laparoscopic management of gastrointestinal stromal tumors. *Surg Endosc.* 2006;20(5):713-716.

28. Nakamori M, Iwahashi M, Nakamura M, et al. Laparoscopic resection for gastrointestinal stromal tumors of the stomach. *Am J Surg.* 2008;196(3):425-429.

29. Bischof D, Kim A, Dodson Y, et al. Open versus minimally invasive resection of gastric GIST: a multi-institutional analysis of short- and long-term outcomes. *Ann Surg Oncol.* 2014;21(9):2941-2948.

30. Privette A, McCahill L, Borrazzo E, Single RM, Zubarik R. Laparo-scopic approaches to resection of suspected gastric gastrointestinal stromal tumors based on tumor location. *Surg Endosc.* 2008;22(2):487-494.

31. Joensuu H, Roberts PJ, Sarlomo-Rikala M, et al. Effect of the tyrosine kinase inhibitor STI571 in a patient with a metastatic gastrointestinal stromal tumor. *N Engl J Med.* 2001;344(14):1052-1056.

32. DeMatteo RP, Ballman KV, Antonescu CR, et al. Long-term results of adjuvant imatinib mesylate in localized, high-risk, primary gastrointestinal stromal tumor: ACOSOG Z9000 (Alliance) intergroup phase 2 trial. *Ann Surg.* 2013;258(3):422-428.

33. Joensuu H, Eriksson M, Sundby Hall K, et al. Adjuvant imatinib for high-risk GI stromal tumor: analysis of a randomized trial. *J Clin Oncol.* 2016;34(3):244-250.

34. Corless C, Ballman K, Antonescu C, et al. Pathologic and molecular features correlate with long-term outcome after adjuvant therapy of resected primary GI stromal tumor: the ACOSOG Z9001 trial. *J Clin Oncol.* 2014;32(15):1563-1570.

35. Casali PG, Le Cesne A, Poveda Velasco A, et al. Time to definitive failure to the first tyrosine kinase inhibitor in localized GI stromal tumors treated with imatinib as an adjuvant: a European Organisation for Research and Treatment of Cancer Soft Tissue and Bone Sarcoma group intergroup randomized trial in collaboration with the Aus-tralasian gastro-intestinal trials group, UNICANCER, French Sarcoma Group, Italian Sarcoma Group, and Spanish Group for Research on Sarcomas. *J Clin Oncol.* 2015;33(36):4276-4283.

36. Blanke CD, Demetri GD, von Mehren M, et al. Long-term results from a randomized phase II trial of standard- versus higher-dose imatinib mesylate for patients with unresectable or metastatic gastrointestinal stromal tumors expressing KIT. *J Clin Oncol.* 2008;26(4):620-625.

37. Blanke C, Rankin C, Demetri G, et al. Phase III randomized, intergroup trial assessing imatinib mesylate at two dose levels in patients with unresectable or metastatic gastrointestinal stromal tumors expressing the kit receptor tyrosine kinase: S0033. *J Clin Oncol.* 2008;26(4):626-632.

38. Demetri G, Garrett C, Schöffski P, et al. Complete longitudinal analyses of the randomized, placebo-controlled, phase III trial of sunitinib in patients with gastrointestinal stromal tumor following imatinib failure. *Clin Cancer Res.* 2012;18(11):3170-3179.

39. Ben-Ami E, Barysauskas CM, von Mehren M, et al. Long-term follow-up results of the multicenter phase II trial of regorafenib in patients with metastatic and/or unresectable GI stromal tumor after failure of standard tyrosine kinase inhibitor therapy. *Ann Oncol.* 2016;27(9):1794-1799.

40. Rutkowski P, Gronchi A, Hohenberger P, et al. Neoadjuvant imatinib in locally advanced Gastrointestinal Stromal Tumors (GIST): the EORTC STBSG experience. *Ann Surg Oncol.* 2013;20(9):2937-2943.

41. Tielen R, Verhoef C, van Coevorden F, et al. Surgical treatment of locally advanced, non-metastatic, gastrointestinal stromal tumours after treatment with imatinib. *Eur J Surg Oncol.* 2013;39(2):150-155.

42. Joensuu H, Eriksson M, Collan J, et al. Radiotherapy for GIST progressing during or after tyrosine kinase inhibitor therapy: a prospective study. *Radiother Oncol.* 2015;116(2):233-238.

43. Demetri GD, Von Mehren M, Blanke CD, et al. Efficacy and safety of imatinib mesylate in advanced gastrointestinal stromal tumors. *N Engl J Med.* 2002;347(7):472-480.

44. Gastrointestinal Stromal Tumor Meta-Analysis Group (MetaGIST). Comparison of two doses of imatinib for the treatment of unresectable or metastatic gastrointestinal stromal tumors: a meta-analysis of 1,640 patients. *J Clin Oncol.* 2010;28(7):1247-1253.

45. Blay JY, Le Cesne A, Ray-Coquard I, et al. Prospective multicentric randomized phase III study of imatinib in patients with advanced gastrointestinal stromal tumors comparing interruption versus continuation of treatment beyond 1 year: the French Sarcoma Group. *J Clin Oncol.* 2007;25(9):1107-1113.

46. Le Cesne A, Ray-Coquard I, Bui BN, et al. Discontinuation of imatinib in patients with advanced gastrointestinal stromal tumours after 3 years of treatment: an open-label multicentre randomised phase 3 trial. *Lancet Oncol.* 2010;11(10):942-949.

47. Wu L, Zhang Z, Yao H, Liu K, Wen Y, Xiong L. Clinical efficacy of second-generation tyrosine kinase inhibitors in imatinib-resistant

gastrointestinal stromal tumors: a meta-analysis of recent clinical trials. *Drug Des Devel Ther.* 2014;8:2061-2067.

48. Bauer S, Rutkowski P, Hohenberger P, et al. Long-term follow-up of patients with GIST undergoing metastasectomy in the era of imatinib—analysis of prognostic factors (EORTC-STBSG collaborative study). *Eur J Surg Oncol.* 2014;40(4):412-419.

49. Rutkowski P, Andrzejuk J, Bylina E, et al. What are the current outcomes of advanced gastrointestinal stromal tumors: who are the long-term survivors treated initially with imatinib? *Med Oncol.* 2013;30(4):765.

50. An H, Ryu M, Ryoo B, et al. The effects of surgical cytoreduction prior to imatinib therapy on the prognosis of patients with advanced GIST. *Ann Surg Oncol.* 2013;20(13):4212-4218.

51. Pappo AS, Janeway KA. Pediatric gastrointestinal stromal tumors. *Hematol Oncol Clin North Am.* 2009;23(1):15-34.

52. Patil DT, Rubin BP. Genetics of gastrointestinal stromal tumors: a heterogeneous family of tumors? *Surg Pathol Clin.* 2015;8(3):515-524.

53. Pappo A, Janeway K, Laquaglia M, Kim SY. Special considerations in pediatric gastrointestinal tumors. *J Surg Oncol.* 2011;104(8):928-932.

Gastrointestinal Lymphomas

Nathan Bolton | William Conway | John Bolton

The incidence of non-Hodgkin lymphoma (NHL) increased significantly in the United States and worldwide in the last two decades of the 20th century; most of this increase has been attributed to the HIV epidemic. The incidence of NHL appeared to reach a plateau around the turn of the 21st century,[1] both in the human immunodeficiency virus (HIV)-infected and the non–HIV-infected population, and according to some reports[2] may be decreasing in the HIV-infected population, presumably as a result of better antiviral therapy. Moreover, the 5-year cancer-specific survival rate for some major subtypes of NHL is improving, reflecting better cancer therapy, with current 5-year survival rates of 66% for diffuse large B-cell lymphoma (DLBCL), 84% for chronic lymphocytic leukemia/small lymphocytic lymphoma, and 82% for follicular lymphoma.[3]

Approximately 30% of patients with NHL present as extranodal disease,[4] and among these patients, the gastrointestinal (GI) tract is the most common site of presentation.[5] Within the GI tract, the stomach is the most common site (65%), followed by the small intestine (18%), and colon and rectum (15%), while the liver, gallbladder, and pancreas collectively account for only 2%.[5]

There has been debate over the years about the definition of primary GI tract NHL (PGINHL). Strict criteria were proposed by Dawson in 1961,[6] who considered patients to have PGINHL only if no palpable superficial lymphadenopathy was found at first examination, chest radiograph showed no obvious enlargement of mediastinal lymph nodes, and the white blood cell count was within normal limits. Furthermore, upon laparotomy, the bowel lesion had to be shown to be dominant, and only involvement of lymph nodes in the immediate vicinity of the primary lesion was acceptable. Patients were excluded from analysis when distant abdominal lymph nodes, spleen, or liver were involved. A liberal definition of primary extranodal NHL has been proposed[5] that includes all patients who present with NHL that apparently originated at an extranodal site, even in the presence of disseminated disease, as long as the extranodal component is clinically dominant. Use of strict criteria for PGINHL selects patients with earlier stage disease and, probably for this reason, for many years patients with GI tract NHL were thought to have a better prognosis than patients with nodal or disseminated NHL. However, the overall survival with treatment for extranodal NHL, including NHL of the GI tract, is similar to that for nodal NHL when patients with similar International Prognostic Index (Table 82.1)[7] and malignancy grade are compared.[5]

BIOLOGY AND EPIDEMIOLOGY

NHLs of the GI tract are a heterogeneous group of entities; there are multiple subtypes with different cells of origin, at different stages of maturation, and with different natural histories, biologic behavior, and prognosis. Ninety percent of PGINHL is of B-cell lineage; the two most common subtypes are DLBCL, which comprises approximately 60% of PGINHL,[8] and mucosa-associated lymphoid tissue (MALT) lymphoma, primarily occurring in the stomach, which accounts for approximately 30% of all PGINHL. These two entities are the main focus of this chapter. Several other uncommon B-cell PGINHLs occur, including follicular lymphoma presenting typically in the duodenum, mantle cell lymphoma presenting typically in the terminal ileum, and Burkitt lymphoma, associated with Epstein-Barr virus infection, and typically presenting in the terminal ileum in children and young adults. These will not be discussed in detail in this chapter.

The only T-cell PGINHL of significance is the enteropathy-associated T-cell lymphoma (ETL), which accounts for approximately 5% of PGINHL and occurs most often in the jejunum but may affect multiple segments of small intestine.[9,10] ETL can arise in the setting of refractory celiac disease (RCD), defined as celiac disease that does not respond histologically to at least 12 months of strict gluten-free diet,[11] or in patients without a known history of celiac disease (primary ETL). In the setting of RCD, it often presents as an exacerbation with abdominal pain, diarrhea, and weight loss; as a de novo entity, it often presents acutely as GI perforation, obstruction, or hemorrhage. RCD can be classified based on intraepithelial lymphocyte (IEL) populations into two distinct subtypes; RCD type II, which involves clonal expansion of abnormal IELs lacking surface cluster of differentiation (CD)3, CD8, and T-cell receptor markers, but expresses intracellular CD3, is the subtype which evolves into ETL in 60% to 80% of patients within 5 years.[12] Patients with ETL have a poor prognosis with less than 30% of patients alive at 2-year follow-up, and ETL that occurs in the setting of RCD has a worse prognosis.[13]

Risk factors for the development of gastrointestinal lymphoma include *Helicobacter pylori* infection, immunosuppression after solid organ transplantation, celiac disease, Epstein-Barr viral infection, inflammatory bowel disease, and HIV infection.[14–16]

DIFFUSE LARGE B-CELL LYMPHOMA

The most common histologic subtype of PGINHL, DLBCL accounts for slightly less than 50% of primary gastric lymphomas and the great majority of PGINHL occurring in the small bowel, colon, and rectum. DLBCLs of the GI tract are morphologically similar to DLBCLs at other sites. Histologically, tumors consist of diffuse sheets of large, blastic lymphoid cells, 2 to 4 times larger than normal lymphocytes, often infiltrating and destroying the gastric glandular architecture.[17] Vesicular nuclei, prominent

TABLE 82.1 International Prognostic Index

Risk factors	Ann Arbor stage III to IV (advanced disease) >1 extranodal site Age >60 years High LDH Performance status ≥2 (ECOG)
RISK ASSESSMENT	
Low risk	0 to 1 risk factors
Low intermediate risk	2 risk factors
High intermediate risk	3 risk factors
High risk	4 to 5 risk factors

ECOG, Eastern Cooperative Oncology Group; LDH, lactate dehydrogenase. Modified from Koniaris LG, Drugas G, Katzman PJ, Salloum R. Management of gastrointestinal lymphoma. J Am Coll Surg. 2003;197(1):127–141.

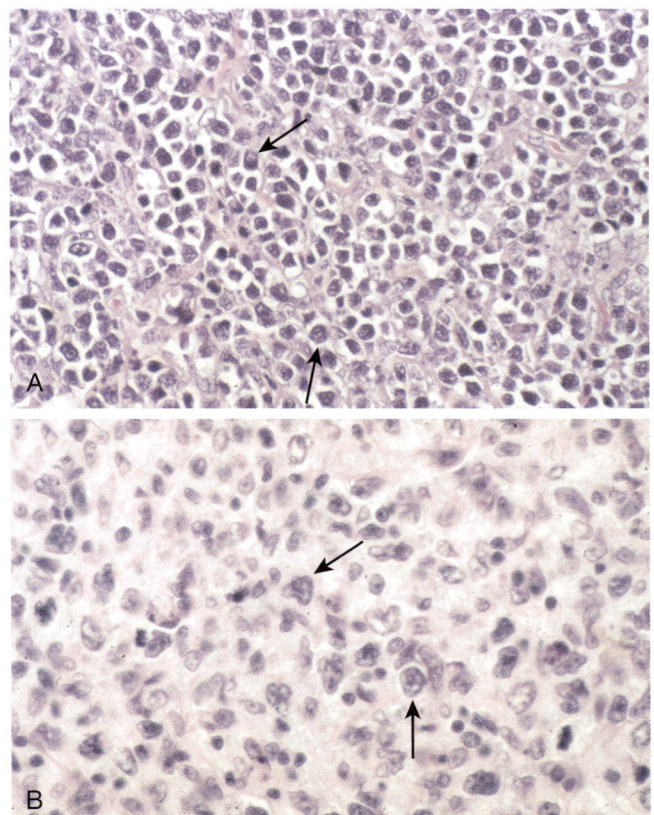

FIGURE 82.1 Diffuse large B-cell lymphoma of the stomach showing a monotonous high-grade infiltrate of large centroblast-like cells (arrows) under low- (A) and high-power (B) magnification. (Courtesy Mary R. Schwartz, MD, Baylor College of Medicine.)

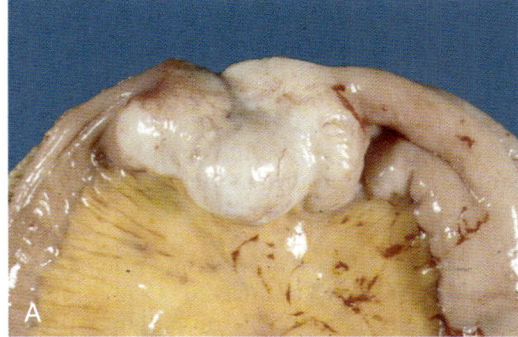

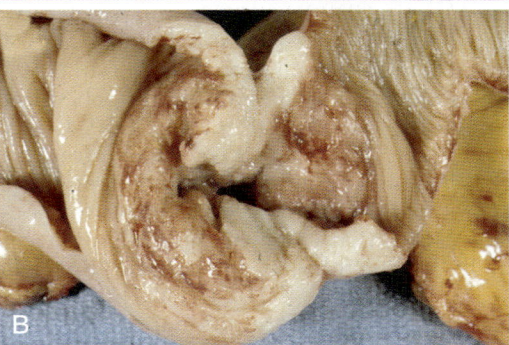

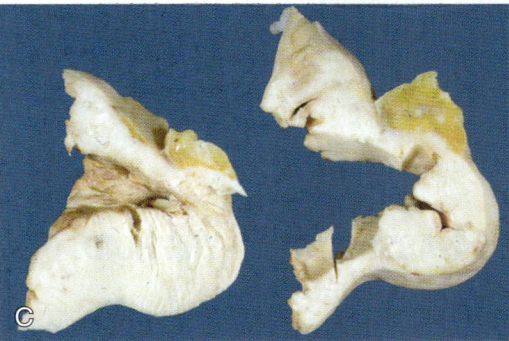

FIGURE 82.2 Diffuse large B-cell lymphoma of the jejunum, demonstrating the external aspect (A), the mucosal aspect (B), and cross sections showing transmural involvment and expansion of the wall by lymphoma (C). (Courtesy Mary R. Schwartz, MD, Baylor College of Medicine.)

nucleoli, a basophilic cytoplasm, and a moderate to high proliferation fraction may also be noted (Figs. 82.1 and 82.2).[18] A variety of cell types may be observed but the most common cell appears as a large noncleaved cell, an immunoblast, or a mixture of these two types.[19] Approximately 30% to 50% of primary gastric DLBCLs have

components of MALT lymphoma,[20–22] but the extent of this low-grade component varies from only small residual foci to dominant MALT lymphoma with only a small proportion of solid or sheet-like transformed blasts. In gastric DLBCLs with a component of MALT lymphoma, the tumor should be diagnosed as a DLBCL, noting the presence of accompanying MALT lymphoma, and the term high-grade MALT lymphoma should not be used for this entity.

DLBCL has recently been found to be a heterogeneous disease, with different prognoses for different subtypes. It may be subdivided into germ-center B-cell and activated B-cell subtypes.[23] Germ-center subtypes typically exhibit a translocation in the antiapoptotic BCL2 gene (t[14;18]) and amplification of REL (chromosome 2p). Although germ-center variants will exhibit downregulation of factors influencing cellular growth, such as nuclear factor-κB (NF-κB), activated B-cell subtypes exhibit upregulation.[24] DLBCL is frequently the result of a mutation in *BCL6* (involved in T-cell–dependent antigen responses), which may be associated with longer disease-free survival.[25,26] Overall survival prognostication may require more integrative modeling of multiple factors and may need to account for multiple underlying genetic mutations.[24,27]

The neoplastic cells are of B-cell phenotype, expressing pan B-cell antigens (CD19, CD20, CD22, and CD79a) but may lack one or more of these. The typical immunophenotype is CD20+, CD45+, and CD3−. Adequate immunophenotyping to establish the diagnosis and to differentiate germinal center B-cell–like (GCB) vs. non-GCB origin requires an immunohistochemical (IHC) panel including CD20, CD3, CD5, CD10, CD45, B-cell lymphoma 2 *(BCL2), BCL6, Ki-67*, interferon regulatory factor 4 *(IRF4)*/melanoma associated antigen (mutated) 1 *(MUM1)*, v-myc avian myelocccytomatosis viral oncogene homolog *(MYC)*, with or without cell surface marker analysis by flow cytometry to include kappa/lambda, CD45, CD3, CD5, CD19, CD10, CD20.[28] Also useful under certain circumstances are additional studies to establish lymphoma subtype, including IHC staining for cyclin D1, kappa/lambda, CD30, CD138, Epstein-Barr virus in situ hybridization, anaplastic lymphoma receptor tyrosine kinase (ALK), human herpesvirus-8 *(HHV8)*, SRY-box 11 *(SOX11)*, and karyotype or fluorescence in situ hybridization (FISH) analysis for *MYC, BCL2*, and *BCL6* rearrangements.

MUCOSA-ASSOCIATED LYMPHOID TISSUE LYMPHOMA

MALT lymphomas comprise about 50% of all primary lymphomas of the stomach. Interestingly, the stomach is normally devoid of lymphoid tissue, but it is the most common site for MALT lymphoma. Lymphoid follicles develop in the presence of chronic inflammation and gastritis associated with *H. pylori* infection, as evidenced by a rate of *H. pylori* infection of greater than 90% in patients with MALT lymphoma.[29] These lymphoid follicles resemble lymph node tissue and are composed of reactive T cells, activated plasma cells, and B cells. It is the B cells that undergo clonal expansion and subsequently develop into a MALT lymphoma.[27,30] The neutrophilic response to the bacterial infestation promotes neutrophil migration and the release of reactive oxygen free radicals that may induce genetic mutations secondary to the oxidative stress.[31]

Histologically, the characteristic marginal zone B cells are of intermediate size with pale cytoplasm and a slightly irregular nucleus.[17] The most significant finding is the presence of a variable number of lymphoepithelial lesions defined by evident invasion and partial destruction of mucosal glands by the tumor cells (Figs. 82.3 and 82.4). MALT lymphoma shows the immunophenotype of B cells in the normal marginal zone of spleen, Peyer patches, and lymph nodes. The tumor B cells can express the surface immunoglobulin and pan-B antigens (CD19, CD

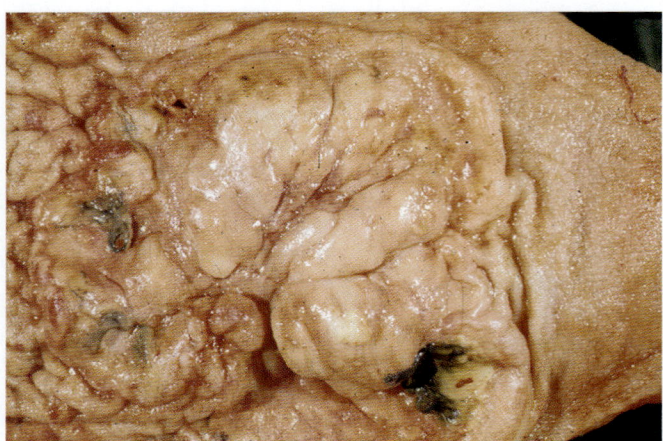

FIGURE 82.3 Gastric mucosa-associated lymphoid tissue lymphoma, gross photograph. (Courtesy Mary R. Schwartz, MD, Baylor College of Medicine.)

20, and CD79a), the marginal zone–associated antigens (CD35 and CD21, and lack CD5, CD10, CD23), and cyclin D1. MALT lymphoma can be divided into *H. pylori* positive or negative based on the presence of *H. pylori. H. pylori*–negative MALT lymphomas have a higher positive rate for t(11;18)(q21;q21) translocation than *H. pylori*–positive MALT lymphoma.[14,32]

Adequate immunophenotyping to establish the diagnosis of MALT lymphoma includes an IHC panel consisting of CD20, CD3, CD5, CD10, BCL2, kappa/lambda, CD21 or CD23, cyclin D1, and BCL6, with or without cell surface marker analysis by flow cytometry including kappa/lambda, CD19, CD20, CD5, CD23, CD10.[28] Also, *H. pylori* staining (gastric) of biopsy tissue should be obtained; if positive, then PCR or FISH for t(11:18). If *H. pylori* staining is negative by histopathology, then use noninvasive *H. pylori* testing (stool antigen, urea breath, or blood antibody test).

Several genetic alterations may promote the pathogenesis of MALT lymphoma. One translocation (t[11:18]) joins the inhibitor of apoptosis gene-2 (IAP2) to the MALT-1 gene (MLT).[33] The resultant fusion protein not only has proapoptotic and transforming functions via the Bcl-10 protein, but also activates the NF-κB pathway, further promoting growth.[30] Approximately 21% to 60% of MALT lymphoma may be attributed to this genetic alteration,[33] and this particular translocation may portend a more aggressive underlying tumor biology.[34] A second translocation (t[1;14]) occurs in less than 5% of MALT lymphomas and results in the constitutive activation of the bcl-10 gene as a result of the transfer of the immunoglobulin heavy chain promoter.[33] Although differing in the locus of translocation, this genetic mutation shares the final common pathway of antiapoptosis, activation of NF-κB, and progression of disease. Because the possibilities of these genetic alterations exist and, when present, affect the biologic behavior and treatment responsiveness of gastric MALT lymphomas, cytogenetics or FISH analysis for t(1:14), t(11:14), t(11:18), and t(3:4) may be useful in selected cases.[28]

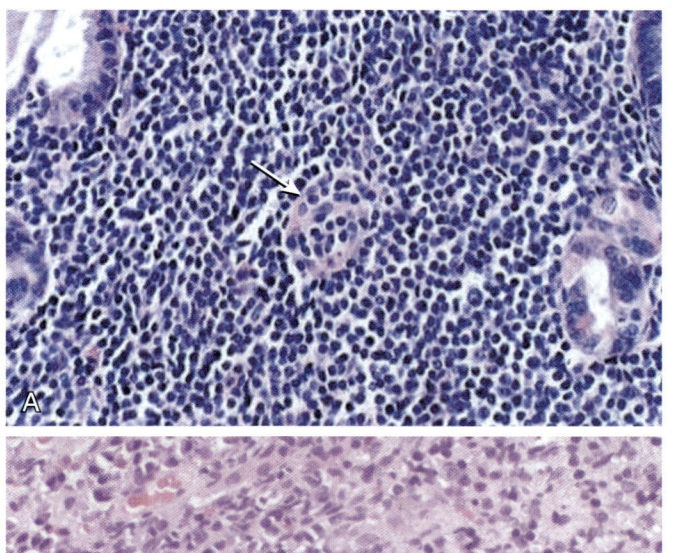

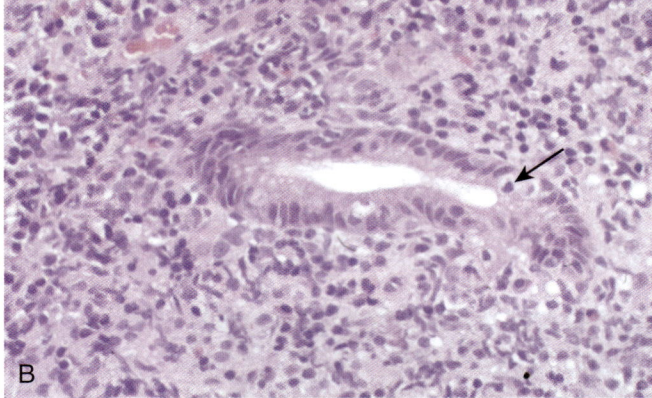

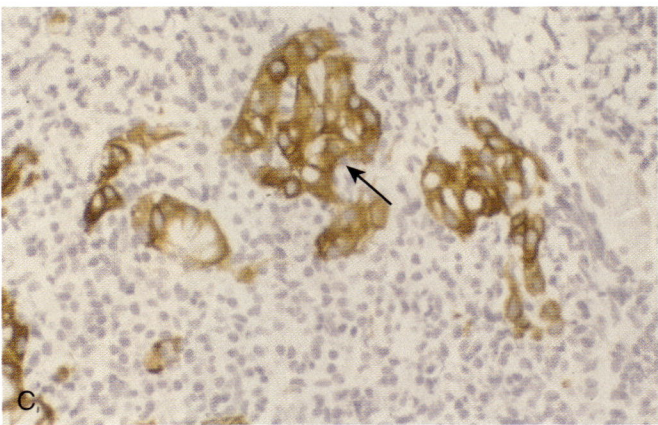

FIGURE 82.4 Histopathologic characteristics of mucosa-associated lymphoid tissue (MALT) lymphoma. (A) Monocytoid, lymphocytic infiltrate with lymphocytes infiltrating the epithelial component (lymphoepithelial lesion) *(arrow)*. (B) Low-grade MALT lymphoma of the stomach demonstrating lymphoepithelial lesions *(arrow)*, and (C) keratin immunohistochemical stain demonstrating lymphoepithelial lesions with infiltration and partial destruction of glandular structures by lymphocytes *(arrow)*. ([A], Courtesy Suimin Qiu, MD, The University of Texas Medical Branch; [C], Courtesy Mary R. Schwartz, MD, Baylor College of Medicine.)

ROLE OF SURGERY IN THE TREATMENT OF GASTROINTESTINAL LYMPHOMA

There are very few situations, if any, where a surgeon will be the primary manager of a patient with GI lymphoma and make unilateral decisions about the overall treatment plan. In general, a specialist in hematology or medical oncology is the "quarterback" of the multidisciplinary team managing these patients. Generally, there are few, if any, indications for elective primary resection of an NHL of the stomach, small bowel, or colon in patients with no or mild symptoms. This strategy of nonsurgical management has been established in two randomized controlled trials evaluating the role of surgery in the management of early Lugano system (Table 82.2)[35] (stage I and II) high-grade gastric MALT lymphoma[36] and gastric DLCBL[37]; in these studies, initial complete surgical resection prior to chemotherapy did not confer any survival benefit compared with chemotherapy alone, and late toxicity was more frequent and severe in patients who underwent surgery. Although randomized controlled trials evaluating the role of initial surgical resection for PGINHL of the small bowel and colon are not available, similar

TABLE 82.2 Lugano Classification for Staging*

LUGANO STAGING SYSTEM	
Stage I	Confined to GI tract (single primary or noncontiguous lesions)
Stage I₁	Confined to mucosa
Stage I₂	Infiltrates the submucosa, muscularis propria, subserosa or penetrates serosa
Stage II	Extends to abdominal lymph nodes
Stage II₁	Involvement of local (paragastric) lymph nodes
Stage II₂	Involvement of distant (mesenteric, paraaortic, paracaval, pelvic, inguinal) lymph nodes
Stage IIₑ	Infiltration of adjacent organs or tissues by direct infiltration
Stage IV (extranodal involvement or concomitant supradiaphragmatic nodal involvement)	Spread to extraabdominal lymph nodes
	Noncontinuous involvement of separate site in GI tract (e.g., stomach and rectum)
	Noncontinuous involvement of other organs (e.g., tonsils, parotid gland, ocular adnexa, liver, and spleen) or tissues (e.g., peritoneum and pleura)
	Bone marrow not involved
DESIGNATIONS	
A	Absence of systemic symptoms
B	Presence of systemic symptoms (fever, night sweats, and weight loss >10% body weight)
X	Bulky mass (lesion of 10 cm or more in the longest diameter)

*This system of staging does not have a stage III.
GI, Gastrointestinal.
Modified from Armitage JO. Staging non-Hodgkin lymphoma. *CA Cancer J Clin.* 2005;55:368.

treatment principles may be applicable; however, the currently available surgical literature does not provide firm guidelines. A recent collected review of 1658 patients with PGINHL of the small and large intestines found that a substantial majority of patients (60.7%) were treated with a combination of surgery and chemotherapy, although nearly half of these patients underwent emergent surgery for perforation, obstruction, bleeding, or complications of treatment,[38] so the therapeutic benefit of routine elective resection for patients not presenting with emergency indications for surgery is not addressed by this review. Perhaps the worst outcome in patients undergoing primary resection is the occasional patient who incurs serious postoperative complications such as intraabdominal abscess, enterocutaneous fistula, prolonged sepsis, and inanition, which greatly delay or impair the delivery of adequate chemoimmunotherapy.

Nonetheless, there are several clinical situations where a surgeon may encounter and be involved in the management of a GI tract lymphoma. Examples of these situations and general guidelines for management follow:

- Acute obstruction, intussusception, GI bleed, or perforation as the presenting symptom of a GI lymphoma, requiring urgent surgical intervention: resection of all grossly involved bowel segment(s) is desirable if it can be done in a reasonably safe manner. It is *not* necessary to achieve microscopically negative margins.

- As an unexpected finding when proceeding with elective major resection for what is presumed to be some other histologic type of neoplasm, most commonly an intraabdominal sarcoma or gastrointestinal stromal tumor (Fig. 82.5): Suspicion of lymphoma might arise if prominent regional adenopathy, perhaps even extending outside of the planned operative field, is found in the course of the procedure. In such an event, a node can be sampled and a frozen section obtained to confirm the surgeon's suspicion. If a lymphoma is confirmed, the surgeon must make a decision about whether to proceed with the planned resection. In general, if a safe, low-risk resection will remove all grossly involved bowel, this would be the preferred course; however, if the surgical procedure is nonemergent and resection would be complex, high-risk, multivisceral, and/or include major vascular resection, it should be avoided and the procedure terminated after adequate tissue for diagnostic studies is obtained.

- In a situation where a presumptive clinical diagnosis, supported by endoscopic biopsy, fine-needle aspiration cytology obtained by endoscopic ultrasound- or computed tomography (CT)-guidance exists: In this case

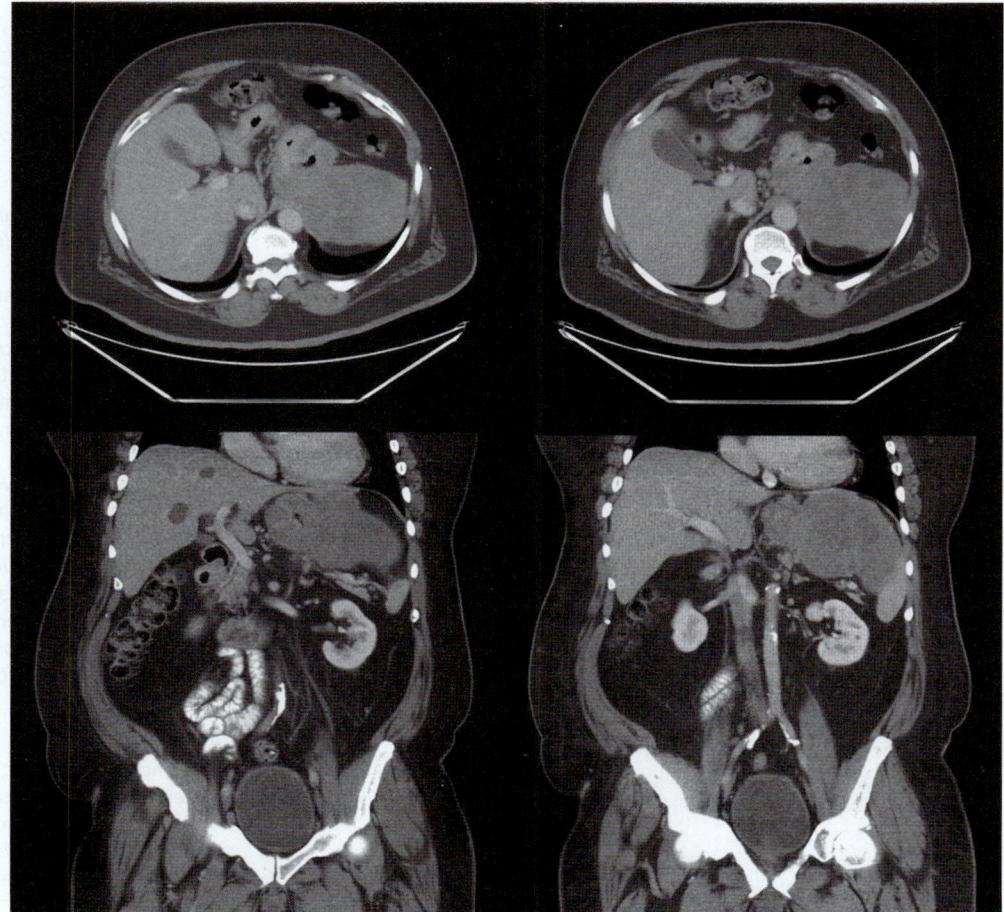

FIGURE 82.5 Computed tomography images showing a large intraabdominal tumor involving the upper stomach and spleen. The radiology diagnosis was angiosarcoma, but this proved to be a diffuse large B-cell lymphoma.

the primary objective is to obtain adequate tissue for accurate diagnosis, classification, and treatment decision making. If adequate tissue sampling can be obtained from an enlarged node or bulky tumor without undertaking a complex resection of the GI tract segment involved, this would be the preferred course of action.

- Rare instance of bleeding or perforation in a patient receiving antineoplastic therapy: Emergency resection is required and may be complicated by recent chemotherapy with low blood counts and immunosuppression.
- As an incidental finding of chronic lymphocytic leukemia (CLL) or small lymphocytic lymphoma (SLL) in a patient undergoing GI surgery for another indication: Occasionally, the presence of CLL/SLL may be apparent because of the presence of multiple rounded, enlarged, slightly firm nodes in the bowel mesentery or porta hepatis. In this situation, the surgeon should proceed with the primary operation, but also obtain adequate nodal tissue to allow for accurate diagnosis of the CLL/SLL.

PATHOLOGIC, IMMUNOLOGIC, MOLECULAR, AND CLINICAL WORKUP FOR GASTROINTESTINAL LYMPHOMA

Although the number of available tests in use for the diagnosis and subtyping of lymphoma appears baffling initially, the process can be broken down into three steps:

1. Routine surgical pathology including evaluation of frozen section and fixed hematoxylin and eosin sections which, combined with clinical correlation (site of presentation, age, predisposing factors), provide a tentative diagnosis.
2. Immunophenotyping with a panel of IHC stains including CD20, CD3, CD5, CD10, CD45, BCL2, BCL6, Ki-67, IRF/MUM1, MYC with or without cell surface marker analysis by flow cytometry to include kappa/lambda, CD45, CD3, CD5, CD19, CD10, CD20 for suspected DLBCL. For suspected MALT lymphoma, IHC for CD21 or CD23 and for cyclin D1 (CCND1) should be added, with CD23 also added to the flow cytometry panel. These tests establish the cell lineage and monoclonality of the abnormal cell population and confirm or modify the initial pathologic diagnosis.
3. Performing selected molecular studies (FISH, IHC, polymerase chain reaction [PCR], gene expression profiling [GEP], cytogenetics/karyotyping or gene rearrangement analysis) to subclassify the neoplasm, often to add prognostic insight or to suggest modifications in treatment. Examples would be analysis for t(11:18) gene rearrangement in a gastric MALT, or MYC amplification in a DLBCL (the so-called *double-hit* variant of DLBCL).

When a surgeon resects tissue in a known or suspected case of lymphoma, communication with the pathologist on duty is important to make sure that adequate tissue is obtained and handled properly to allow the full range of diagnostic testing. For example, flow cytometry requires fresh tissue, so if a diagnosis of lymphoma is suspected clinically and/or on a frozen section of surgical biopsy but is not definitively established, fresh, nonfixed tissue should be set aside in appropriate tissue media and kept

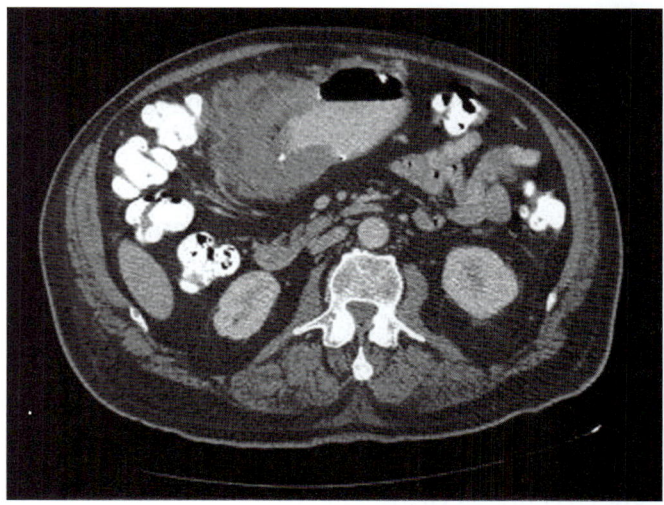

FIGURE 82.6 Computed tomography (CT) scan of an 80-year-old male who initially presented with weakness, fatigue, weight loss, decreased appetite, and vague epigastric pain. He reported nausea and reflux symptoms without emesis. CT scan shows a large mass of the gastric antrum, which proved to be a gastric lymphoma.

until the initial histopathology determines whether flow cytometry is needed. Especially when the surgical procedure is being performed solely for the purpose of obtaining tissue for diagnostic purposes, it is best to confirm with the pathologist that adequate tissue of good diagnostic quality has been obtained before concluding the surgical procedure.

The clinical evaluation of a patient with GI lymphoma includes a good general exam with emphasis on performance status, presence or absence of "B" symptoms (fever, night sweats, weight loss, pruritus), and coexisting conditions that might affect the safety of specific treatments (e.g., rituximab may reactivate hepatitis B). Nutritional evaluation with development of a plan for ensuring adequate nutrition during the period of induction therapy is uniquely important in the evaluation of the patient with PGINHL, who often presents with difficulty maintaining adequate nourishment. Complete blood count, a comprehensive metabolic panel including lactate dehydrogenase (LDH) and uric acid, and hepatitis B testing are also required. Positron emission tomography (PET) scan or CT (Fig. 82.6) of the chest/abdomen/pelvis and bone marrow biopsy are required in most but not all cases (for example, a low-grade gastric MALT stage I). In addition, a multigated acquisition (MUGA) scan or echocardiogram is needed if an anthracycline-based chemotherapy regimen is needed, and pregnancy testing should be done in women of childbearing age. Finally, the International Prognostic Index (see Table 82.1) should be calculated.

TREATMENT OF GASTROINTESTINAL LYMPHOMAS

There has been an explosion of new, targeted therapies for lymphoma in the past 5 years (see next section) and clinical trials are underway to evaluate several strategies to incorporate evolving new therapies into the upfront paradigm. To date, however, the initial or upfront therapy for most GI tract lymphomas has not changed dramatically. Current therapeutic recommendations for the two most common types of PGINHL are covered in this section.

MUCOSA-ASSOCIATED LYMPHOID TISSUE

Recent analysis from the Surveillance, Epidemiology, and End Results (SEER) database[39] shows 89% 5-year survival for MALT lymphoma at all sites; however, patients with MALT lymphoma of gastrointestinal or pulmonary origin had inferior survival compared to MALT lymphoma arising in ocular, cutaneous, or endocrine sites. *H. pylori* infection plays a key role in the pathogenesis of gastric MALT lymphoma and its eradication can lead to tumor remission.[40,41] However, *H. pylori* infection is not evident in 5% to 10% of gastric MALT lymphomas and a high proportion of these will harbor the t(11:18) translocation, which fuses the AP12 gene to the MALT1 gene.[42–44] This translocation has been associated with disseminated disease and resistance to antibiotic treatment in patients with gastric MALT lymphoma,[34,45] so molecular analysis for t(11:18) by FISH or PCR is recommended.

Using the Lugano classification system (see Table 82.2), which has been widely adopted for use in patients with PGINHL, current initial therapy for gastric MALT lymphoma is as follows[34]:

- For stages I_{E1}, I_{E2}, or II_E in patients who are *H. pylori* positive, initial therapy consists of currently acceptable antibiotic therapy for eradication of *H. pylori* and follow-up endoscopy at 3 months to confirm *H. pylori* eradication and tumor remission. For patients who are *H. pylori* negative and lymphoma-free at 3 months, continue observation; if *H. pylori* persists, second-line antibiotic treatment is given. If at 3 months the *H. pylori* is eradicated but lymphoma persists as a stable or partially responsive disease with no clinical symptoms, observation can continue with repeat endoscopy in 3 months because some time can be required for disease response. If, at 3 months, a patient has progressive or symptomatic disease, radiation therapy (RT, 30 gray [Gy]) is begun along with second-line antibiotic treatment if *H. pylori* persists.
- For patients who are *H. pylori* positive but also t(11:18) positive, initial therapy for symptomatic patients consists of antibiotic therapy for eradication of infection and involved site radiation therapy (ISRT) or rituximab if ISRT is contraindicated. If the patient has early I_E disease and is asymptomatic, an initial trial of antibiotic therapy only may be considered, but the patient should be closely followed with the expectation that additional therapy will likely be needed.
- For patients with stage I_E or II_E gastric MALT lymphoma who are *H. pylori* negative, initial therapy consists of ISRT (or rituximab if ISRT is contraindicated) with follow-up endoscopy 3 months after RT with rebiopsy.
- For the rare patient with stage IV disease requiring treatment, induction chemoimmunotherapy (rituximab, cyclophosphamide, hydroxydaunomycin, Oncovin, prednisolone [RCHOP] or other first-line regimen for

follicular lymphoma) or, in the elderly or infirm who cannot tolerate chemotherapy, four doses of rituximab can be given with or without RT.

For nongastric MALT lymphoma involving small bowel or colon at Lugano stage I or II, ISRT is the preferred initial therapy for most patients, with rituximab or surgical resection (if possible) as other alternatives if RT is contraindicated. For Lugano stage IV MALT lymphoma of the small bowel or colon, initial management in most patients is chemoimmunotherapy (RCHOP or other first-line therapy for advanced follicular lymphoma).

For gastric or nongastric MALT lymphoma with concurrent large cell transformation, initial therapy follows the principles for DLBCL (see the subsequent section Diffuse Large B-Cell Lymphoma).

DIFFUSE LARGE B-CELL LYMPHOMA

For patients with good performance status who have Ann Arbor stages[46] I or II disease and no contraindications to therapy, standard first-line therapy is six cycles of RCHOP[28] with the addition of ISRT for bulky disease (defined as >7.5 cm in maximal diameter) (see Table 82.3). For disease that is *nonbulky*, standard upfront therapy is three cycles of RCHOP plus RT or six cycles of RCHOP without radiation. These recommendations do not apply to patients who are very elderly (>80 years old), frail, or with poor left ventricular function. Patients identified with double-hit DLBCL (defined as having MYC rearrangement in addition to BCL2 or BCL6 rearrangement) have inferior outcomes with RCHOP and are treated with a more intense regimen such as dose-adjusted etoposide, prednisone, vincristine, cyclophosphamide, doxorubicin, and rituximab (DA-EPOCH-R).[47,48] Higher-stage disease (Ann Arbor III and IV) may be considered for clinical trial or high-dose therapy with autologous stem cell rescue. A discussion of salvage therapy for relapsed or nonresponsive DLBCL is beyond the scope of this chapter.

TABLE 82.3 Ann Arbor Classification for Staging

Stage	Features
I	Single lymph node region or structure (e.g., spleen, thymus)
II	Two or more lymph node regions on same side of diaphragm
III	Two or more lymph node regions on both sides of diaphragm
IV	Extranodal involvement beyond "E" designation
DESIGNATIONS	
A	No symptoms
B	Fever (>38°C), drenching sweats, unintentional weight loss (>10% body weight over 6 months)
E (stages I to III only)	Involvement of a single, extranodal site contiguous or proximal to known nodal site

Modified from Armitage JO. Staging non-Hodgkin lymphoma. *CA Cancer J Clin.* 2005;55:368.

EVOLVING THERAPIES

No current discussion of NHL would be complete without acknowledging the recent exciting developments for the treatment of hematologic malignancies including NHL. These include an array of therapies targeted at precise points of the tumor cell's signaling pathways, surface antigens, or microenvironment. Among these are small-molecule inhibitors, monoclonal antibodies, and immune therapies including programmed cell death protein 1 (PD1) inhibitors and chimeric antigen receptor T cells (CARTs). In fact, the explosion of new agents has opened up a daunting number of possibilities for future research,[49] which will take some time to come into focus. Although a comprehensive discussion is beyond the scope of this chapter, the following will provide a current overview for the reader, who is also referred to a number of current reviews on these topics.[49–51]

The B-cell receptor pathway (BCRP) is important in multiple cellular processes including cell proliferation, differentiation, and apoptosis. Ibrutinib is a small-molecule, irreversible inhibitor of Bruton tyrosine kinase, an important constituent of the BCRP, and has shown impressive response rates in relapsed/refractory mantle cell lymphoma and DLBCL with non-GCB cell of origin.[52] Idelalisib is a selective inhibitor of the delta isoform of the p110 subunit of phosphatidyl-inositol-3-kinase (P13k), another constituent of the BCRP, and has shown good activity in heavily pretreated, indolent B-cell lymphoma,[53] but use of this agent may be limited by GI and pulmonary toxicity.

The Bcl-2 family of proteins are key regulators of apoptosis in cancer cells. Venetoclax is a small-molecule, orally dosed BH-3 mimetic that interacts with the pro-apoptotic Bax and Bak members of the Bcl-2 family to stimulate apoptosis and may be most useful in combination with rituximab and bendamustine.[54] An alternative approach to targeting Bcl-2 is the use of DNA oligonucleotides to hybridize to the BCL2 gene but not to other Bcl-2 family members. Based on promising phase I data for this approach,[55] phase II trials in relapsed/refractory DLBCL are ongoing.

Next-generation anti-CD20 monoclonal antibodies, such as obinutuzumab, are being developed that have higher affinity for the CD20 antigen and enhanced antibody-dependent cellular cytotoxicity (ADCC) activity.[56] Monoclonal antibodies to CD19, the expression of which is mostly limited to B cells and is maintained when CD20 activity has been downregulated, are also under development and may have use both as a single agent[57] and in combination with rituximab.

The PD1 receptor is an inhibitory receptor expressed by antigen-stimulated T lymphocytes. Interactions between PD1 and its ligand, programmed death-ligand 1 (PD-L1), which is expressed by many tumors including B-cell lymphomas, activate signaling pathways that inhibit T-cell activity and thus block the antitumor immune response. Antibodies targeting PD1 or PD-L1 block the PD1 pathway and reactivate T-cell activity.[58] Pidilizumab,[59] pembrolizumab,[60] and nivolumab[61] are humanized or fully human anti-PD1 monoclonal antibodies with demonstrated antitumor activity against a variety of subtypes of NHL, including DLBCL. Phase II studies of these drugs in multiple histologic subtypes are ongoing.

Another promising technology in patients with relapsed/refractory B-cell malignancies including DLBCL is the development of anti-CD19 CART therapy.[62,63] Autologous T cells are gene modified to carry antigen specificity for CD19. Cyclophosphamide and fludarabine are also administered as conditioning chemotherapy. In a trial at the National Cancer Institute,[64] six of seven assessable patients with DLBCL, and all patients with indolent NHL, achieved a response to therapy. CART cells reached a peak in the peripheral blood 7 to 17 days after infusion and rapidly declined thereafter. Despite this, nine patients remained in ongoing remission at last follow-up, with the longest remission at 23 months from therapy. A second study[65] evaluated 38 patients with relapsed/refractory NHL including 21 with DLBCL. The conditioning regimen varied depending on the histologic subtype and past treatment history. Cytokine release syndrome and neurologic toxicity occurred in 16 and 3 patients, respectively; the objective response rate was 68% overall and 43% for the patients with DLBCL, with progression-free survival at a median follow-up of 11.7 months of 62%.

REFERENCES

1. Shiels MS, Engels EA, Linet MS, et al. The epidemic of non-Hodgkin lymphoma in the United States: disentangling the effect of HIV, 1992–2009. *Cancer Epidemiol Biomarkers Prev.* 2013;22:1069.
2. Silverberg MJ, Lau B, Achenbach CJ, et al. Cumulative incidence of cancer among persons with HIV in North America: a cohort study. *Ann Intern Med.* 2015;163:507.
3. Howlader N, Morton LM, Feuer EJ, Besson C, Engels EA. Contributions of subtypes of non-Hodgkin lymphoma to mortality trends. *Cancer Epidemiol Biomarkers Prev.* 2016;25:174.
4. Glass AG, Karnell LH, Menck HR. The National Cancer Data Base report on non-Hodgkin's lymphoma. *Cancer.* 1997;80:2311.
5. Krol ADG, Le Cessie S, Snijder S, Kluin-Nelemans JC, Kluin PM, Noordijk EM. Primary extranodal non-Hodgkin's lymphoma (NHL): the impact of alternative definitions tested in the Comprehensive Cancer Centre West population-based NHL registry. *Ann Oncol.* 2003;14:131.
6. Dawson IP, Cornes JS, Morson BC. Primary malignant lymphoid tumours of the intestinal tract. Report of 37 cases with a study of factors influencing prognosis. *Br J Surg.* 1961;49:80.
7. The International Non-Hodgkin's Lymphoma Prognostic Factors Project. A predictive model for aggressive non-Hodgkin's lymphoma. *New Engl J Med.* 1993;329:987.
8. Shannon EM, MacQueen IT, Miller JM, Maggard-Gibbons M. Management of primary gastrointestinal non-Hodgkin lymphomas: a population-based survival analysis. *J Gastrointest Surg.* 2016;20:1141.
9. Swerdlow SH, Camppo E, Harris NL, et al. *WHO Classification of Tumours of Haematopoietic and Lymphoid Tissues.* Lyon: IARC; 2008.
10. Gale J, Simmonds PD, Mead GM, Sweetenham JW, Wright DH. Enteropathy-type T-cell lymphoma: clinical features and treatment of 31 patients in a single institution. *J Clin Oncol.* 2000;18:795.
11. Biagi F, Corazza GR. Defining "gluten refractory enteropathy". *Eur J Gastroenterol Hepatol.* 2001;13:561.
12. Al-Toma A, Verbeek WH, Hadithi M, von Blomberg BM, Mulder CJ. Survival in refractory celiac disease and enteropathy-associated T-cell lymphoma: retrospective evaluation of single-centre experience. *Gut.* 2007;56:1373.
13. Delabie J, Holte H, Vose JM, et al. Enteropathy-associated T-cell lymphoma: clinical and histological findings from the international peripheral T-cell lymphoma project. *Blood.* 2011;118:148.
14. Ghimire P, Wu GY, Zhu L. Primary gastrointestinal lymphoma. *World J Gastroenterol.* 2011;17:697.

15. Müller AM, Ihorst G, Mertelsmann R, Engelhardt M. Epidemiology of non-Hodgkin's lymphoma (NHL): trends, geographic distribution, and etiology. *Ann Hematol.* 2005;84:1.

16. Ghai S, Pattison J, Ghai S, O'Malley ME, Khalili K, Stephens M. Primary gastrointestinal lymphoma: spectrum of imaging findings with pathologic correlation. *Radiographics.* 2007;27:1371.

17. Nakamura S, Muller-Hermelink HK, Delabie J, Ko YH, Van Krieken JH, Jaffe ES. Lymphoma of the stomach. In: Bosman FT, Carneiro F, Hruban RH, Theise ND, eds. *WHO Classification of Tumours of the Digestive System.* Lyon: International Agency for Research on Cancer (IARC); 2010.

18. Harris NL, Jaffe ES, Stein H, et al. A revised European-American classification of lymphoid neoplasms: a proposal from the International Lymphoma Study Group. *Blood.* 1994;84:1361.

19. Feller AC, Diebold J. *Histopathology of Nodal and Extranodal Non-Hodgkin's Lymphomas.* 3rd ed. New York: Springer-Verlag; 2004.

20. Kock P, del Valle F, Berdel WE, et al. Primary gastrointestinal non-Hodgkin's lymphoma: I. Anatomic and histologic distribution, clinical features, and survival data of 371 patients registered in the German Multicenter Study GIT NHL 01/92. *J Clin Oncol.* 2001;19:3861.

21. Nakamura S, Matsumoto T, Iida M, Yao T, Tsuneyoshi M. Primary gastrointestinal lymphoma in Japan: a clinicopathologic analysis of 455 patients with special reference to its time trends. *Cancer.* 2003;97: 2462.

22. Papaxoinis G, Papageorgiou S, Rontogianni D, et al. Primary gastrointestinal non-Hodgkin's lymphoma: a clinicopathologic study of 128 cases in Greece. A Hellenic Cooperative Oncology Group study (HeCOG). *Leuk Lymphoma.* 2006;47:2140.

23. Boot H. Diagnosis and staging in gastrointestinal lymphoma. *Best Pract Res Clin Gastroenterol.* 2010;24:3.

24. Rosenwald A, Wright G, Chan WC, et al. Lymphoma/leukemia molecular profiling project: the use of molecular profiling to predict survival after chemotherapy for diffuse large-B-cell lymphoma. *N Engl J Med.* 2002;346:1937.

25. Lossos IS, Jones CD, Warnke R, et al. Expression of a single gene, BCL-6, strongly predicts survival in patients with diffuse large B-cell lymphoma. *Blood.* 2001;98:945.

26. Uccella S, Placidi C, Marchet S, et al. Bcl-6 protein expression, and not the germinal centre immunophenotype, predicts favourable prognosis in a series of primary nodal diffuse large B-cell lymphomas: a single centre experience. *Leuk Lymphoma.* 2008;49:1321.

27. Li L. Survival prediction of diffuse large-B-cell lymphoma based on both clinical and gene expression information. *Bioinformatics.* 2006; 22:466.

28. NCCN Clinical Practice Guidelines in Oncology, Non-Hodgkin's Lymphoma, National Comprehensive Cancer Network v2. https://www.nccn.org/professionals/physician_gls/f_guidelines.asp.

29. Ahmad A, Govil Y, Frank BB. Gastric mucosa-associated lymphoid tissue lymphoma. *Am J Gastroenterol.* 2003;98:975.

30. Kahl BS. Update: gastric MALT lymphoma. *Curr Opin Oncol.* 2003;15:347.

31. Du MQ, Isaacson PG. Gastric MALT lymphoma: from aetiology to treatment. *Lancet Oncol.* 2002;3:97.

32. Nakamura S, Matsumoto T, Nakamura S, et al. Chromosomal translocation t(11;18)(q21;q21) in gastrointestinal mucosa associated lymphoid tissue lymphoma. *J Clin Pathol.* 2003;56:36.

33. Nardone G, Morgner A. *Helicobacter pylori* and gastric malignancies. *Helicobacter.* 2003;8:44.

34. Liu H, Ye H, Ruskone-Fourmestraux A, et al. T(11;18) is a marker for all stage gastric MALT lymphomas that will not respond to *H. pylori* eradication. *Gastroenterology.* 2002;122:1286.

35. Rohatiner A, D'Amore F, Coiffier B. Report on a workshop convened to discuss the pathologic and staging classification of gastrointestinal tract lymphoma. *Ann Oncol.* 1994;5:397.

36. Avilés A, Neri N, Nambo MJ, Huerta-Guzman J, Cleto S. Surgery and chemotherapy versus chemotherapy as treatment of high-grade MALT gastric lymphoma. *Med Oncol.* 2006;23:295.

37. Avilés A, Nambo MJ, Neri N, et al. The role of surgery in primary gastric lymphoma: results of a controlled clinical trial. *Ann Surg.* 2004;240:44.

38. Lightner AL, Shannon E, Gibbons MM, Russell MM. Primary gastrointestinal non-Hodgkin's lymphoma of the small and large intestines: a systematic review. *J Gastrointest Surg.* 2016;20:827.

39. Olszewski AJ, Castillo JJ. Survival of patients with marginal zone lymphoma: analysis of the survival, epidemiology, and end-results database. *Cancer.* 2013;119:629.

40. Wotherspoon AC. Gastric lymphoma of mucosa-associated lymphoid tissue and *Helicobacter pylori.* *Annu Rev Med.* 1998;49:289.

41. Isaacson PG, Spencer J. Gastric lymphoma and *Helicobacter pylori.* *Important Adv Oncol.* 1996;111-121.

42. Auer IA, Gascoyne RD, Connors JM, et al. t(11;18)(q21;q22) is the most common translocation in MALT lymphomas. *Ann Oncol.* 1997;8:979.

43. Murga Penas EM, Hinz K, Röser K, et al. Translocations t(11;18)(q21;q21) and t(14;18)(q32;q21) are the main chromosomal abnormalities involving MLT/MALT1 in MALT lymphomas. *Leukemia.* 2003;17:2225.

44. Ye H, Liu H, Raderer M, et al. High incidence of t(11;18)(q21;q21) in *Helicobacter pylori*-negative gastric MALT lymphoma. *Blood.* 2003;101:2547.

45. Morgner A, Bayerdorffer E, Neubauer A, Stolte M. *Helicobacter pylori* associated gastric B cell MALT lymphoma: predictive factors for regression. *Gut.* 2001;48:290.

46. Armitage JO. Staging non-Hodgkin's lymphoma. *CA Cancer J Clin.* 2005;55:368.

47. de Jonge AV, Roosma TJ, Houtenbos I, et al. Diffuse large B-cell lymphoma with MYC gene rearrangements: current perspective on treatment of diffuse large B-cell lymphoma with MYC gene rearrangements; case series and review of the literature. *Eur J Cancer.* 2016;55:140.

48. Lamar ZS, Fino N, Palmer J, et al. Dose-adjusted Etoposide, Prednisone, Vincristine, Cyclophosphamide, and Doxorubicin (EPOCH) with or without rituximab as first-line therapy for aggressive non-Hodgkin lymphoma. *Clin Lymphoma Myeloma Leuk.* 2016;16:76.

49. Armand P. Checkpoint blockade in lymphoma. *Hematolgy Am Soc Hematol Educ Program.* 2015;2015:69-73. doi:10.1182/asheducation-2015.1.69.

50. Blum K. B-cell receptor pathway modulators in NHL. *Hematology Am Soc Hematol Educ Program.* 2015;2015:82-91. doi:10.1182/asheducation-2015.1.82.

51. Cheah C, Fowler N, Wang M. Breakthrough therapies in B-cell non-Hodgkin lymphoma. *Ann Oncol.* 2016;27:778.

52. Wilson WH, Young RM, Schmitz R, et al. Targeting B cell receptor signaling with ibrutinib in diffuse large B cell lymphoma. *Nat Med.* 2015;21:922.

53. Flinn IW, Kahl BS, Leonard JP, et al. Idelalisib, a selective inhibitor of phosphatidylinositol 3-kinase-delta, as therapy for previously treated indolent non-Hodgkin lymphoma. *Blood.* 2014;123:3406.

54. de Vos S, Swinnen L, Kozloff M, et al. A dose-escalation study of venetoclax (ABT-199/GDC-0199) in combination with bendamustine and rituximab in patients with relapsed or refractory non-Hodgkin's lymphoma. *Blood.* 2015;126:255.

55. Harb WA, Lakhani N, Logsdon A, et al. The BCL2 targeted deoxyribonucleic acid inhibitor (DNAi) PNT2258 is active in patients with relapsed or refractory non-Hodgkin's lymphoma. *Blood.* 2014;124: 1716.

56. Morschhauser FA, Cartron G, Thieblemont C, et al. Obinutuzumab (GA101) monotherapy in relapsed/refractory diffuse large B-cell lymphoma or mantle-cell lymphoma: results from the phase II GAUGUIN study. *J Clin Oncol.* 2013;31:2912.

57. Jurczak W, Bryk AH, Mensah P, et al. Single-agent MOR208 salvage and maintenance therapy in a patient with refractory/relapsing diffuse large B-cell lymphoma: a case report. *J Med Case Rep.* 2016; 14:123.

58. Farkona S, Diamandis EP, Blasutig IM. Cancer immunotherapy: the beginning of the end of cancer? *BMC Med.* 2016;14:73.

59. Westin JR, Chu R, Zhang M, et al. Safety and activity of PD1 blockade by pidilizumab in combination with rituximab in patients with relapsed follicular lymphoma: a single group, open-label, phase 2 trial. *Lancet Oncol.* 2014;15:69.

60. Zinzani PL, Ribrag V, Moskowitz CH, et al. Phase 1b study of PD-1 blockade with pembrolizumab in patients with relapsed/refractory primary mediastinal large B-cell lymphoma (PMBCL). *Blood.* 2015; 126:3986.

61. Lesokhin AM, Ansell SM, Armand P, et al. Preliminary results of a phase I study of nivolumab (BMS-936558) in patients with relapsed or refractory lymphoid malignancies. *Blood.* 2014;124:291.

62. Porter DL, Levine BL, Kalos M, Bagg A, June CH. Chimeric antigen receptor-modified T cells in chronic lymphoid leukemia. *N Engl J Med.* 2011;365:725.

63. Kochenderfer JN, Dudley ME, Kassim SH, et al. Chemotherapy-refractory diffuse large B-cell lymphoma and indolent B-cell

malignancies can be effectively treated with autologous T cells expressing an anti-CD19 chimeric antigen receptor. *J Clin Oncol.* 2015;33:540.

64. Schuster SJ, Svoblda J, Dwivedy Nasta A, et al. Sustained remissions following chimeric antigen receptor modified T cells directed against CD19 (CTL019) in patients with relapsed or refractory CD19[+] lymphomas. *Blood.* 2015;126:183.

65. Turtle CJ, Berger C, Sommermeyer D, et al. Anti-CD19 chimeric antigen receptor-modified T cell therapy for B cell non-Hodgkin lymphoma and chronic lymphocytic leukemia: fludarabine and cyclophosphamide lymphodepletion improves in vivo expansion and persistence of CAR-T cells and clinical outcomes. *Blood.* 2015; 126:184.

Surgical Conditions of the Small Intestine in Infants and Children

Yue-Yung Hu | Todd Jensen | Christine Finck

In infants and children, small intestinal disorders encompass a wide spectrum of congenital and acquired conditions distinct from those seen in adults. Congenital lesions, such as rotational anomalies, duodenal or jejunoileal atresia, meconium ileus, omphalomesenteric remnants, and duplication cysts, are more likely to present in infancy, if not prenatally. Acquired pediatric small intestinal diseases include necrotizing enterocolitis (NEC) and intussusception.

MALROTATION

Intestinal malrotation represents one of the most common congenital anomalies of the gastrointestinal tract encountered by surgeons. Although 90% of cases manifest during the first year of life (with 50% to 75% presenting within the first month of life),[1] patients may present with midgut volvulus and/or obstruction at any age, making an understanding of the embryology, diagnosis, and treatment of malrotation essential for all abdominal surgeons.

The embryologic steps of intestinal rotation have been well described (Fig. 83.1). At gestational week 5, the midgut herniates out of the abdomen into the umbilicus and rotates 90 degrees counterclockwise around the axis of its primary blood supply, the superior mesenteric artery (SMA). At week 10, the midgut returns to the abdomen, rotating another 180 degrees counterclockwise.[2] Ultimately, the duodenum passes under the SMA and crosses over the spine such that the duodenojejunal junction is anchored in the left upper abdomen, while the cecum is fixed in the right lower quadrant.[3,4] As a result, the mesentery of the small intestine runs obliquely across the long axis of the abdomen from the ligament of Treitz to the right paracolic gutter; this broad fixation anchors the small bowel and prevents it from volvulizing. The right and left colons are anchored to the posterior abdominal wall by mesenteric attachments. Those anchoring the right colon—Ladd bands—attach to the cecum regardless of the cecum's position.[5]

Classic malrotation, also known as nonrotation, is the most common form. Complete nonrotation implies both duodenojejunal malrotation (the duodenojejunal junction does not cross the spine to lay left of midline) and cecocolic malrotation (the cecum is found in the midabdomen, rather than in the right lower quadrant) and results in suspension of the small intestine on a narrow mesentery that is prone to volvulize (Fig. 83.2A).[3,4] Isolated duodenojejunal malrotation (see Fig. 83.2B) may present with duodenal obstruction secondary to Ladd bands. In isolated cecocolic malrotation, the cecum is extremely mobile and prone to cecal volvulus (see Fig. 83.2C). In addition, Ladd

bands extending from the right paracolic region to the malpositioned cecum may obstruct the duodenum. Reverse rotation, in which the duodenum and SMA are antecolic, rather than retrocolic, may present with transverse colon obstruction (see Fig. 83.2D).[6]

In 30% to 60% of patients with malrotation, additional congenital anomalies, such as duodenal atresia, imperforate anus, Meckel diverticulum, annular pancreas, preduodenal portal vein, biliary atresia, cardiac anomalies, heterotaxia, trisomy 21, and 16q24 chromosomal deletion syndrome, are seen.[7–9] Because the pancreas and hepatobiliary tract develop concurrently with intestinal rotation, the association of malrotation with annular pancreas and/or persistent preduodenal portal vein is unsurprising. Congenital diaphragmatic hernias and abdominal wall defects (omphaloceles and gastroschisis) interfere with or abrogate normal rotation before the 10th week of gestation; as such, infants with these conditions are malrotated by definition.[1]

The hallmark of malrotation with midgut volvulus is an infant with bilious emesis. Forty to 60% of neonatal bilious emesis is attributable to surgical bowel obstructions, of which malrotation is the most common cause.[10] As ischemia progresses in midgut volvulus, the infant may develop abdominal distention, hematemesis, hematochezia, peritonitis, and shock. However, it should be noted that volvulized patients may never develop abdominal distention because the point of obstruction may be as proximal as the ligament of Treitz. Malrotation without volvulus may manifest as chronic abdominal pain and/or failure to thrive. It may also be completely asymptomatic and found incidentally during work-up for an unrelated condition.

Early diagnosis of malrotation with volvulus is paramount to prevent potentially life-threatening bowel ischemia. Children with suspected midgut volvulus who show signs of bowel ischemia should undergo emergent surgical exploration without radiologic evaluation. If the child is clinically stable, imaging should be obtained. There are no plain film findings that are pathognomonic for malrotation with volvulus; x-rays may demonstrate a gasless abdomen, a high-grade bowel obstruction, or an essentially normal bowel gas pattern.[5] Ultrasound has gained some degree of acceptance as a screening tool for malrotation. Reversal of the normal anatomic relationship between the SMA and superior mesenteric vein (SMV) is suggestive of malrotation. An ultrasonographic *whirlpool sign* is consistent with midgut volvulus. However, caution is warranted because false-positive rates of up to 21% are reported with ultrasonographic diagnoses. Therefore, if an ultrasound demonstrates SMA/SMV reversal, malrotation should be confirmed with an upper gastrointestinal contrast study (UGI).[11] UGI remains the criterion standard

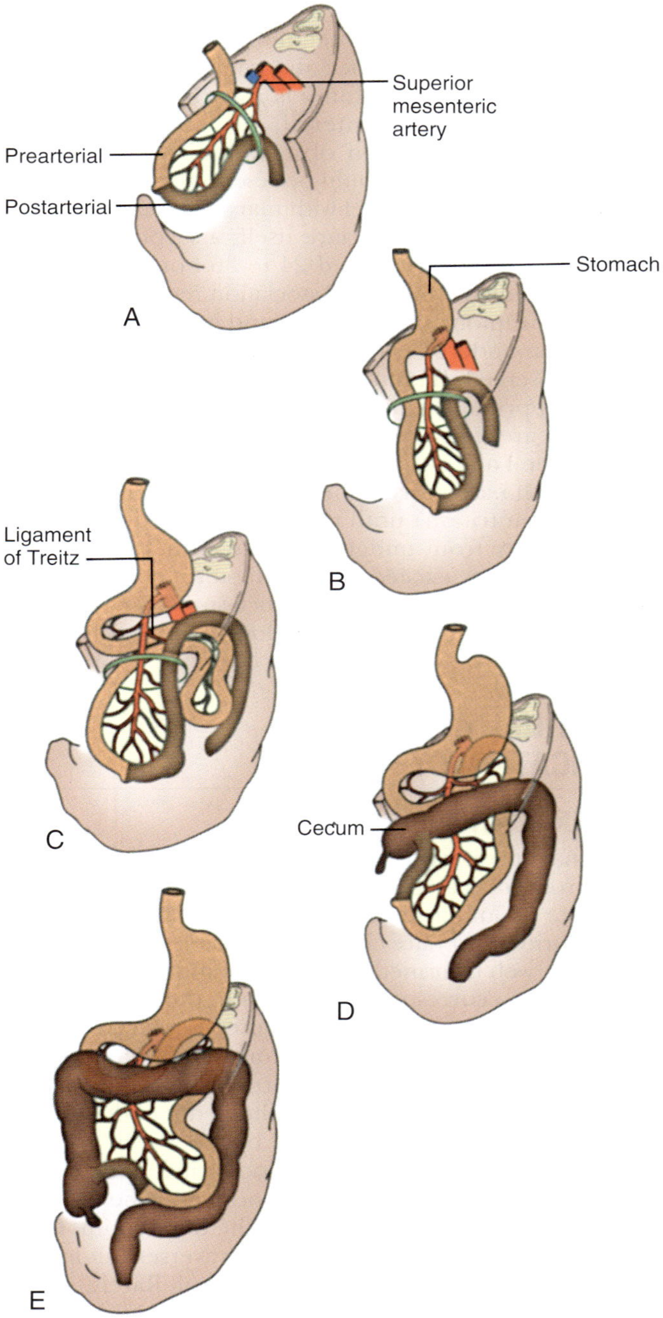

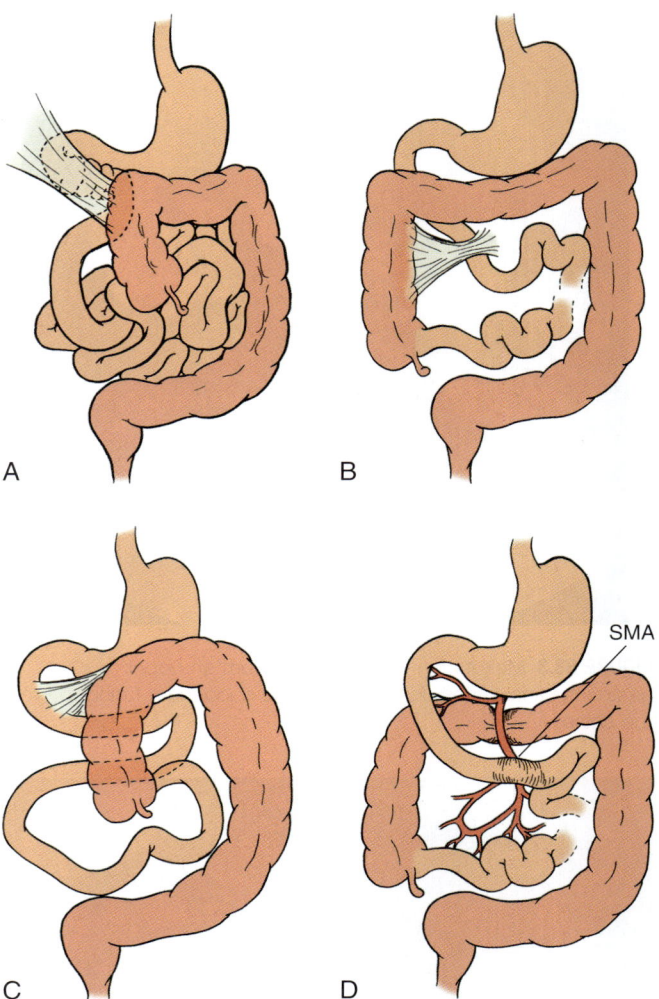

FIGURE 83.1 Normal midgut rotation is shown beginning in the fifth gestational week (A) through completion of the process in the twelfth week (E). (From Ashcraft KW, Holder TM, eds. *Pediatric Surgery*. Philadelphia: Saunders; 1999.)

FIGURE 83.2 (A) Complete nonrotation of the midgut. Neither the duodenojejunal junction nor the cecum has rotated around the superior mesenteric artery (SMA). All of the small bowel lies to the right of the SMA, and all of the colon lies to the left. This anomaly is the most frequent type of malrotation, and the risk for midgut volvulus is ever present. (B) Nonrotation of the duodenojejunal junction with normal rotation of the cecum. This abnormality may be manifested clinically as duodenal obstruction secondary to abnormal mesenteric (Ladd) bands from the colon across the anterior duodenum. (C) Normal rotation of the duodenojejunal junction with nonrotation of the cecum. These patients are at risk for midgut volvulus. (D) Reverse rotation with the duodenojejunal junction passing ventral rather than dorsal to the SMA, followed by reverse rotation of the colon with the cecum rotating dorsal rather than ventral to the SMA. This abnormality may be manifested clinically as obstruction of the transverse colon. (From Oldham KT, Colombani PM, Foglia RP, eds. *Surgery of Infants and Children: Scientific Principles and Practice*. Philadelphia: Lippincott-Raven; 1997.)

test for the diagnosis of malrotation.[12] On a normal UGI, the duodenum should cross to the left of the vertebral column and posterior to the stomach. With duodenojejunal malrotation, the duodenum remains to the right of the spine (Fig. 83.3). In midgut volvulus, the small intestine assumes a corkscrew configuration (Fig. 83.4). Contrast enema is rarely used in the work-up for malrotation because the presence of a normally located cecum in the right lower quadrant does not exclude duodenojejunal

malrotation and infants often have mobile cecum that may result in false-positive results.[1] Computed tomography (CT) scans may demonstrate twisting of the mesenteric vessels, bowel obstruction, and malposition of the ligament of Treitz and/or cecum.[11] However, the radiation exposure that CT engenders is not without risk. A high-quality UGI

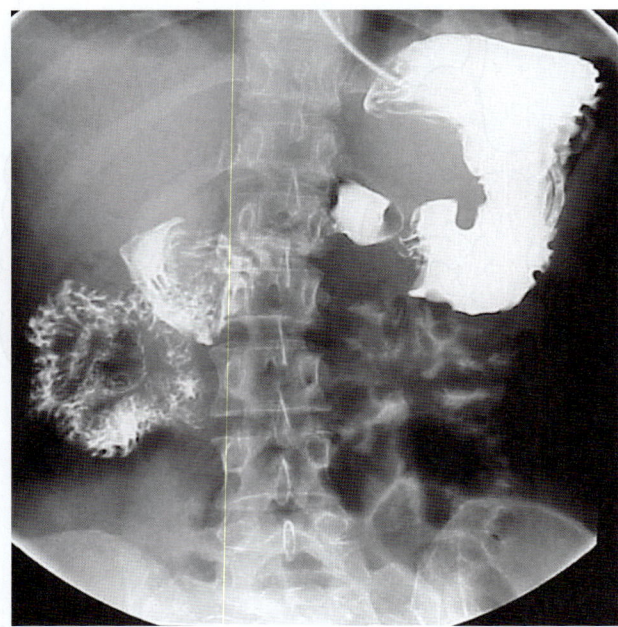

FIGURE 83.3 Malrotation on a spot film from an upper gastrointestinal series demonstrates the duodenum failing to cross the spine.

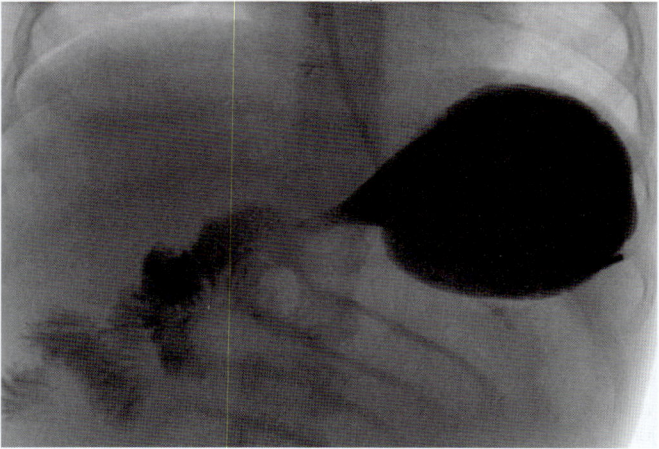

FIGURE 83.4 A spot film from an upper gastrointestinal series demonstrates a corkscrew configuration of the proximal small bowel consistent with volvulus.

conducted by an experienced pediatric radiologist may obviate the need for cross-sectional imaging altogether.

Prompt surgical exploration should be undertaken if midgut volvulus is suspected. In 1936 William Ladd described the surgical procedure for correction of malrotation and midgut volvulus that continues to be used currently.[4] The Ladd procedure is usually done through a right upper quadrant transverse incision in infants and a midline laparotomy in older children and adults. The bowel is inspected and, if volvulized, detorsed in a counterclockwise direction (one may remember to "turn back the hands of time") (Fig. 83.5C). Ladd bands (peritoneal bands crossing from the right paracolic gutter over the duodenum) are lysed (see Fig. 83.5D), and the base of the mesentery is widened. The bowel is replaced in the abdomen with the small bowel in the right abdomen and the cecum in the left upper abdomen (see Fig. 83.5E). An incidental appendectomy is usually performed. If ischemic bowel is encountered, its viability should be assessed after a period of observation. Small areas of frankly necrotic bowel should be resected with or without primary anastomosis. Bowel with marginal viability should be left and allowed to declare itself; a second-look procedure should be performed 24 to 36 hours later.[1] The American Pediatric Surgical Association recommends that younger asymptomatic children found incidentally to have malrotation undergo Ladd procedure whereas older ones may be observed. If an operation is electively pursued, it may be approached laparoscopically; the steps of the operation are the same.[12]

After the Ladd procedure, patients should be decompressed with nasogastric tubes (and possibly receive total parenteral nutrition) until their bowel function returns. The mortality from midgut volvulus with severe bowel compromise may exceed 30%. Long-term complications include adhesive small bowel obstruction (10%), recurrent volvulus, and, if significant bowel loss has been sustained, short gut syndrome.

INTESTINAL ATRESIA AND DUPLICATION CYSTS

DUODENAL ATRESIA

Duodenal atresia occurs in 1 in 6000 to 10,000 births. It arises from a recanalization error; the gut tube fails to obliterate its lumen in the sixth week of gestation. The vast majority (92%) are classified as type I: an obstructing septum or web is formed by either the mucosa or submucosa without a corresponding defect in the muscularis or the mesentery (Fig. 83.6A). Type II atresias, which comprise only 1% of all duodenal atresias, consist of two blind ends of duodenum connected by a short fibrous cord (see Fig. 83.6B). Type III atresias, with two blind ends of duodenum that are completely disconnected but overlie a V-shaped mesenteric defect (see Fig. 83.6C), occur in 7%. Eighty-five percent of duodenal atresias are located at the junction of the first and second portions of the duodenum. Commonly, the distal common bile duct traverses the medial septum, to which the ampulla is proximal. Rarely, a bifid common bile duct with both proximal and distal ampullae is found.[13]

The presentation of duodenal atresia is variable. Polyhydramnios may be detected on prenatal ultrasound in 30% to 65% of cases. Neonates will demonstrate bilious emesis. Upper abdominal fullness may be appreciated on exam. A *double bubble sign*, representing the stomach and the obstructed duodenum, on radiography of the abdomen is pathognomonic for the diagnosis (Fig. 83.7); however, distal gas may be seen in patients with incomplete obstructions or bifid common bile ducts. Type I duodenal atresias may be incompletely obstructing and therefore remain undetected until solid foods are introduced. UGI may reveal a rounded end representing the windsocking web.

If duodenal atresia is suspected or diagnosed, the stomach should be decompressed and the infant

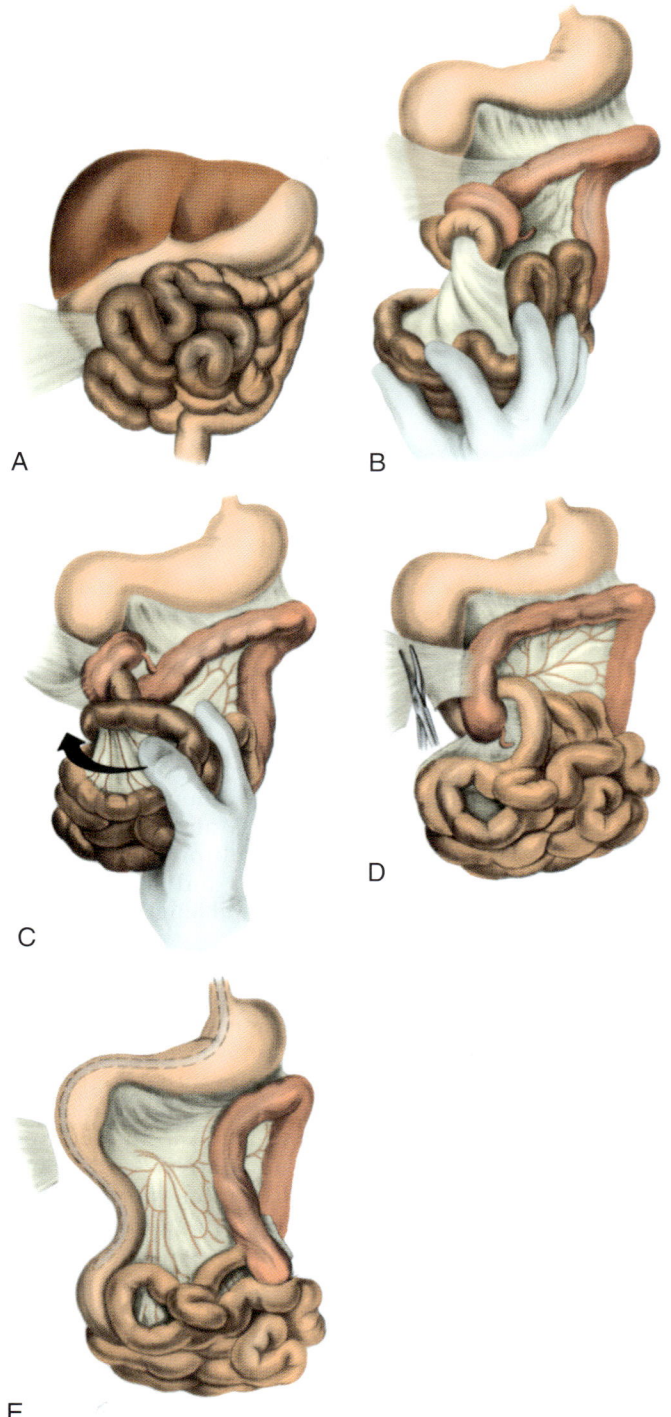

FIGURE 83.5 Malrotation of the intestine. (A) Appearance of the viscera as the abdominal cavity is opened. The small intestines are seen at once and seem to hide the colon. Vascular compromise of the intestine may be obvious. (B) The entire intestinal mass is delivered out of the wound and drawn downward to reveal the base of the mesentery. Coils of intestine or ascending colon are wrapped around the root of an incompletely anchored mesentery. The volvulus has taken place in a clockwise direction. The descending duodenum is dilated because of extrinsic pressure from Ladd bands or peritoneal folds that cross it. (C) The volvulus is reduced by taking the entire intestinal mass in the hand and rotating it counterclockwise (in most cases). (D) With reduction of the volvulus, the cecum lies in the right paravertebral gutter. The peritoneal folds from the cecum obstruct the duodenum. The folds are incised close to the lateral serosal border of the duodenum. The underlying superior mesenteric pedicle is identified and carefully preserved. (E) Appearance of the intestines and ascending colon at the end of surgery. The duodenum descends along the right gutter. The small intestines lie on the right side of the abdomen, and the cecum and ascending colon are in the midline or left side of the abdomen. The superior mesenteric artery and its branches are left exposed as shown. A nasogastric tube has been passed into the jejunum to exclude intrinsic obstruction. (From O'Neill JA Jr, Rowe MI, Grosfeld JL, et al., eds. *Pediatric Surgery*. St Louis: Mosby-Year Book; 1998.)

it may balloon ("windsock") distally; caution is advised in placing the duodenotomy because it may be difficult to reach the proximal origin of the web if the bowel is opened at the point of the externally apparent obstruction. Two blind ends may be reapproximated with a diamond-shaped anastomosis, in which the proximal end is opened transversely and the distal longitudinally (Fig. 83.8). Alternatively, duodenojejunostomy or gastrojejunostomy may be performed, although the latter carries the risks of marginal ulceration and blind loop syndrome.[14] When performed open, a catheter should be passed distally to ensure there are no distal atresias; however, this occurrence is rare. In fact, when performed laparoscopically, this step is skipped.

JEJUNOILEAL ATRESIA

Jejunoileal atresia is one of the most common causes of neonatal intestinal obstruction, with a reported incidence of 1 in every 2000 to 3000 live births.[15] The site of the defect is nearly equally distributed between the jejunum (51%) and the ileum.[16] In contrast to duodenal atresia, jejunoileal atresia is thought to result from an in utero vascular accident leading to necrosis and resorption of the affected bowel segments.[17] This mechanism explains the association between small bowel atresias and conditions causing mechanical constriction of the mesentery and bowel (e.g., volvulus, intussusception, internal hernia, gastroschisis),[18] as well as the use of vasoactive medications (pseudoephedrine, ergotamine, and caffeine) during pregnancy.[19] Jejunoileal atresias are categorized according to the modified Louw classification scheme. In type I atresias, the bowel and mesentery are in continuity but there is an intraluminal diaphragm (Figs. 83.9A and

resuscitated. A work-up should be undertaken to look for associated anomalies: 28% have Down syndrome, 23% annular pancreas, 23% congenital heart disease, and 20% malrotation. After the patient is stable, operative repair may be attempted. Thin webs may be excised through a longitudinal duodenotomy that is started near the point of obstruction, carried proximally over the web, and later closed transversely. The base of these lesions is typically found in the second portion of the duodenum, although

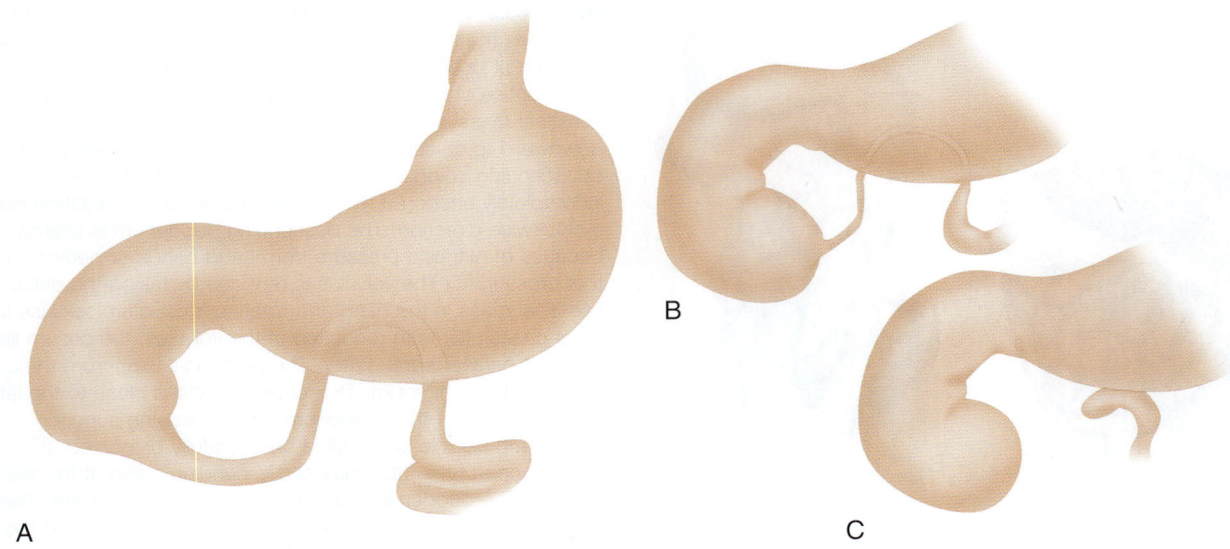

FIGURE 83.6 Classification of duodenal atresia. (A) Type I: an obstructing septum or web is formed by either the mucosa or submucosa without a defect in the muscularis or the mesentery. (B) Type II: two blind ends of duodenum connected by a short fibrous cord. (C) Type III: two blind ends of duodenum, completely disconnected with an underlying V-shaped mesenteric defect (From Coran A, Adzick NS, Krummel TM, et al. eds. *Pediatric Surgery.* 7th ed. Philadelphia: Mosby; 2012.)

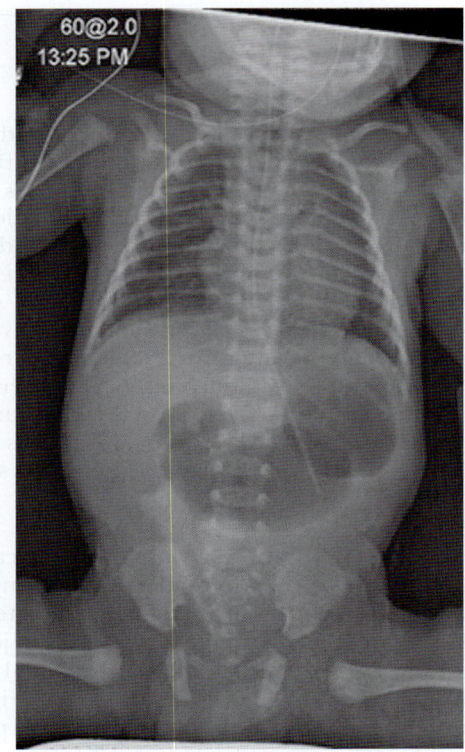

FIGURE 83.7 The double bubble sign indicating duodenal atresia on plain abdominal film.

83.10A). Type II atresias consist of two blind ends connected by a fibrotic cord and supplied by an intact mesentery (see Figs. 83.9B and 83.10B). Type IIIa atresias have two blind ends separated by a V-shaped mesenteric defect (see Fig. 83.9C). In type IIIb atresias, also called

apple peel lesions or *Christmas tree deformities,* a significant amount of proximal bowel is missing and the remaining short distal atretic segment is wrapped around a retrograde blood supply (see Fig. 83.9D). Type IV atresias ("string of sausages") are characterized by multiple small atretic segments (see Fig. 83.9E). Type IIIb and IV atresia are associated with significant loss of bowel length and worse outcomes.[17]

The diagnosis of jejunoileal atresia may be suggested by a prenatal ultrasound demonstrating dilated loops of fluid-filled bowel.[20] Polyhydramnios is seen in up to 50% of cases. The postnatal presentation is usually that of an infant who develops bilious emesis and progressive abdominal distention. The frequency of the emesis and the degree of distention vary in relation to the location of the atresia; infants with proximal atresias will vomit frequently and display minimal distention, whereas those with distal atresias will exhibit more distention but later-onset emesis. One-third of infants will pass meconium in the first 24 hours of life. Ten percent of patients present with meconium peritonitis from in utero bowel perforation. Concomitant congenital anomalies may occur in more than one-third of infants.[18] Ten to 20% of children with atresias have cystic fibrosis (CF).[21]

The postnatal radiographic evaluation for suspected congenital bowel obstructions begins with plain radiographs, which may show dilated loops of small bowel without distal air. Contrast studies are generally not required to make the diagnosis of jejunoileal atresia, but a contrast enema may be helpful, particularly for differentiating it from colonic atresia or meconium ileus. In jejunoileal atresia, contrast enema will demonstrate microcolon and a small-caliber terminal ileum with an abrupt end to the passage of contrast in the small bowel (Fig. 83.11). Similarly, in colonic atresia, contrast will stop progressing; it will not fill the cecum or ileocecal valve.

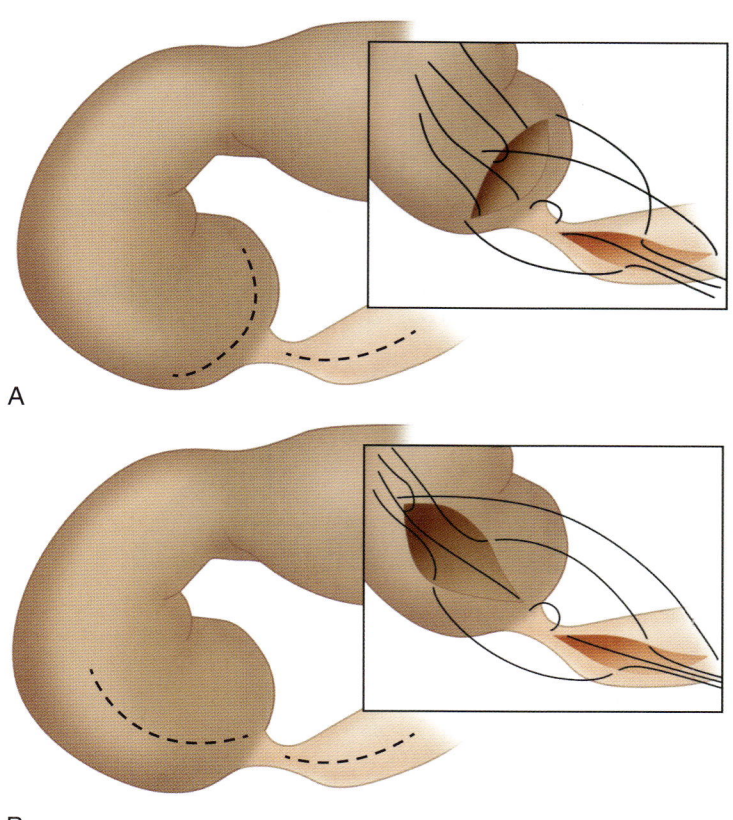

FIGURE 83.8 Anastomosis between a transverse proximal duodenotomy and a longitudinal distal duodenotomy results in a diamond duodenostomy. (From Coran A, Adzick NS, Krummel TM, et al, eds. *Pediatric Surgery*. 7th ed. Philadelphia: Mosby; 2012.)

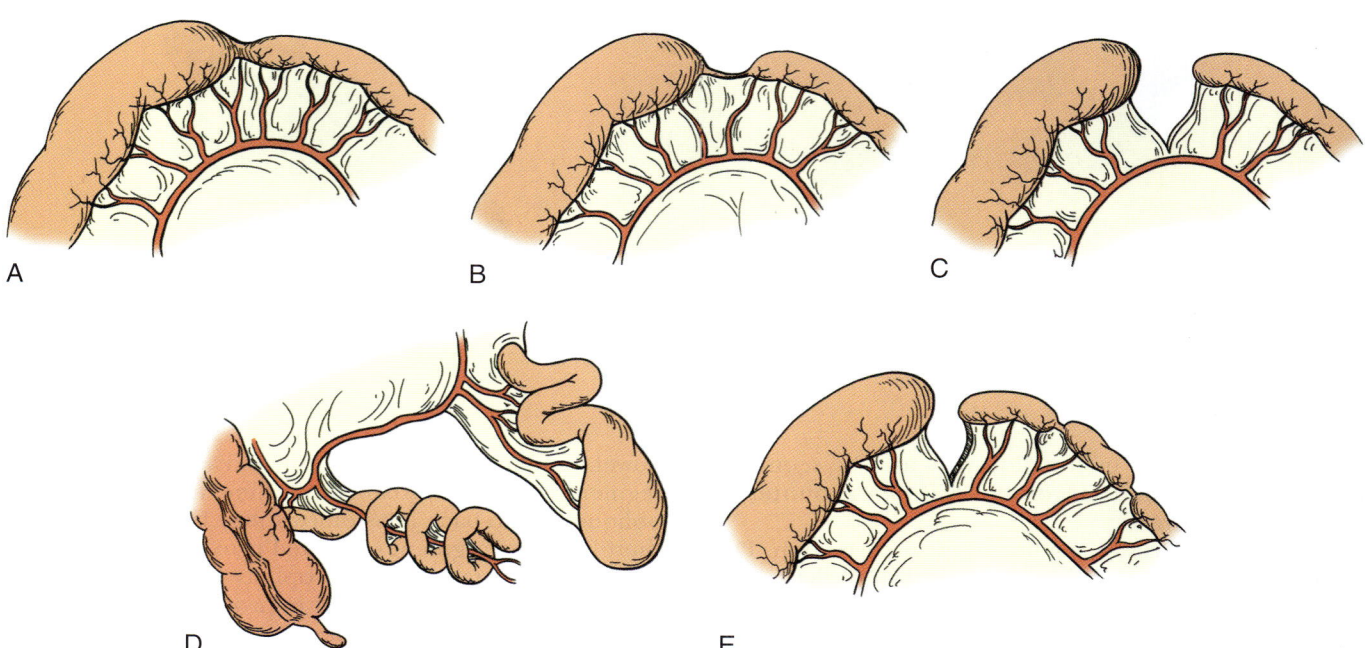

FIGURE 83.9 Classification of jejunoileal atresia. (A) Type I, membranous atresia with intact bowel and mesentery. (B) Type II, blind ends separated by a fibrous cord. (C) Type IIIa, blind ends separated by a V-shaped mesenteric defect. (D) Type IIIb, "apple peel" atresia. (E) Type IV, multiple atresias ("string of sausages"). (From Oldham KT, Colombani PM, Foglia RP, eds. *Surgery of Infants and Children: Scientific Principles and Practice*. Philadelphia: Lippincott-Raven; 1997.)

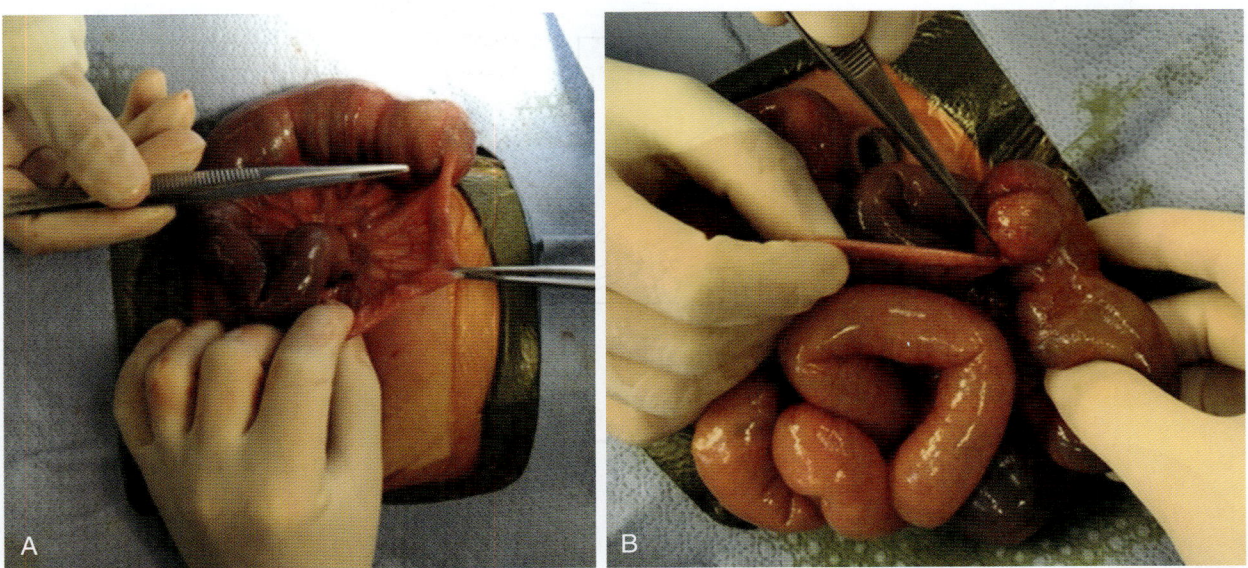

FIGURE 83.10 Intraoperative photos of ileal atresia. (A) Type I. (B) Type II.

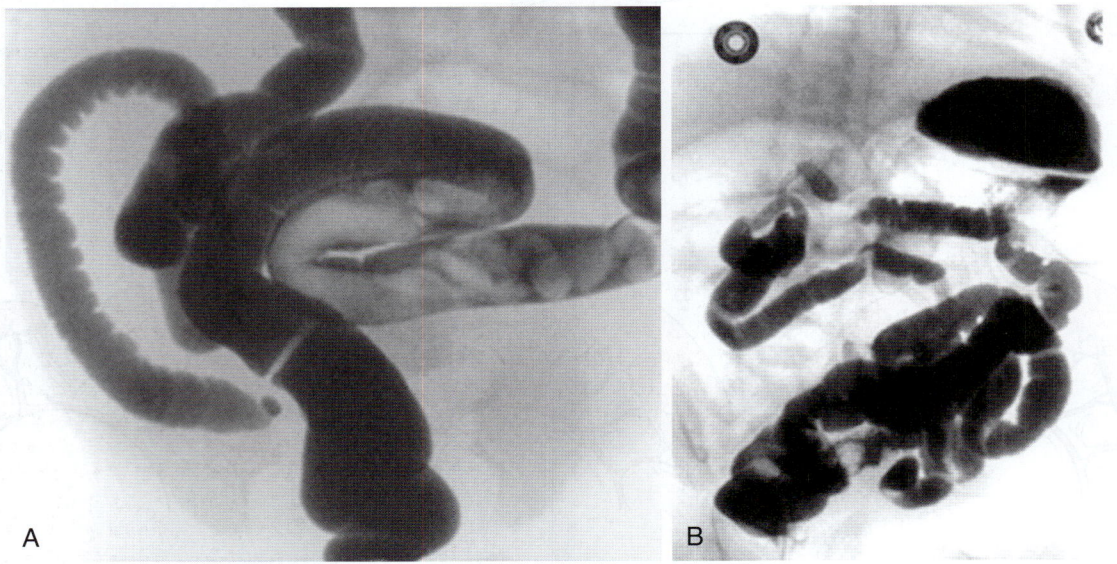

FIGURE 83.11 (A and B) Intraoperative photograph from patient in Fig. 83.10 demonstrating meconium within bowel and a blind-ending ileum.

In meconium ileus, microcolon may also be seen, but pellets of inspissated meconium will be encountered, outlined by contrast.[22]

Small bowel atresias require surgical correction. Preoperative management includes fluid and electrolyte resuscitation, gastric decompression, and antibiotic administration. Operative interventions for jejunoileal atresias should be directed at restoring bowel continuity while preserving functional intestinal length; resection and primary anastomosis should be performed in most cases. Saline should be injected in the distal segment to evaluate for additional distal atresias. Often the proximal atretic segment will be quite dilated and atonic; it should be resected if there is adequate length of the remaining bowel. In infants who have an isolated atresia and a short segment of dilated proximal intestine, an end-to-end or oblique end-to-back anastomosis may be performed. If there is a long segment of dilated proximal intestine, an antimesenteric tapering enteroplasty may be performed to preserve bowel length and improve peristalsis in the proximal segment.[13,18] To reduce the size mismatch between the proximal and distal bowel, the distal segment may be opened obliquely or the enterotomy may be extended with a Cheatle slit.[6,23] In type IIIb atresias, the dilated proximal bowel is anastomosed to the tenuous distal atretic segment. Type IV atresias often require staged repairs.[18] In cases with meconium peritonitis or bowel ischemia, a diverting ostomy may be required. Infants are

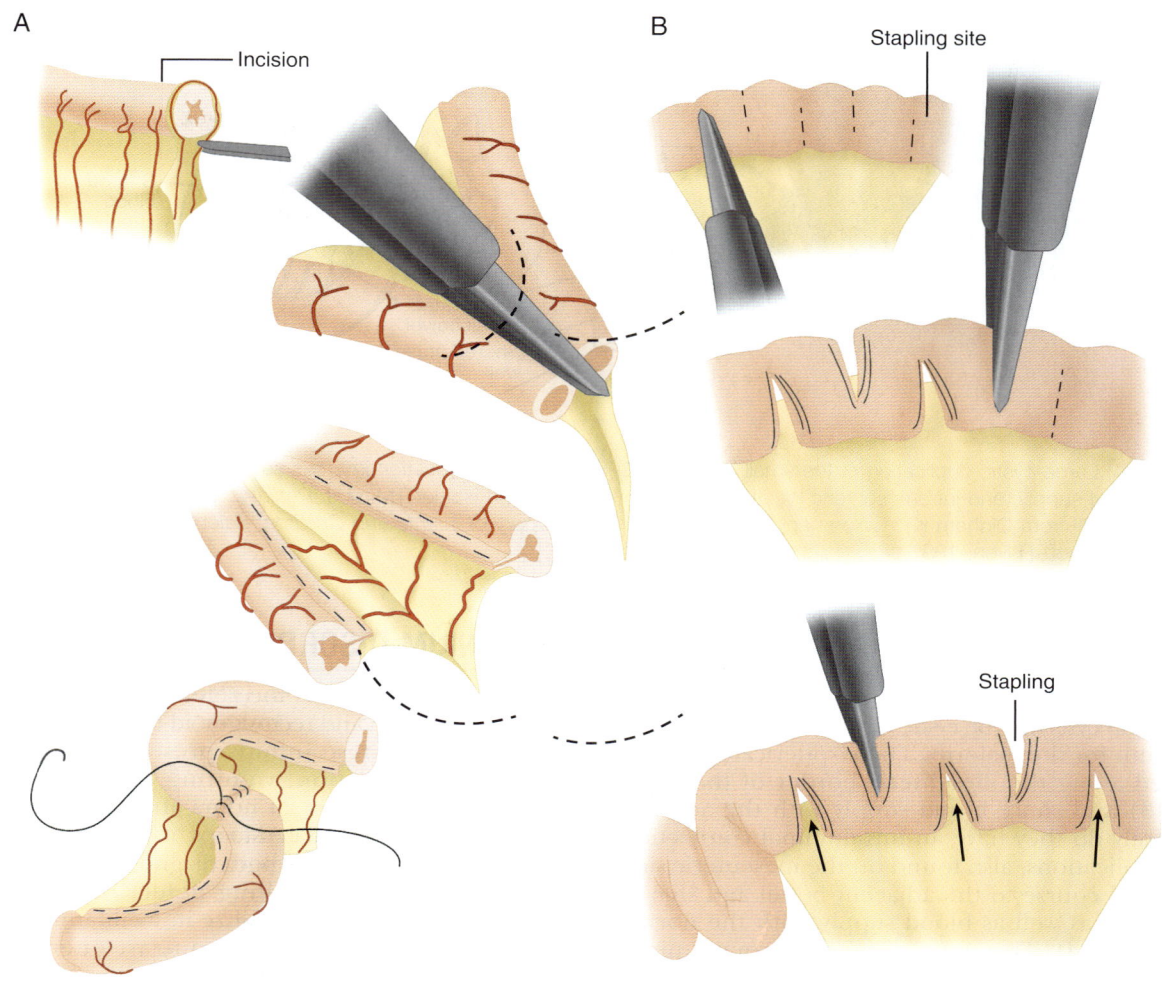

A

Incision

B

Stapling site

Stapling

FIGURE 83.12 (A) Bianchi procedure. (B) Serial transverse enteroplasty procedure. ([A] From Bianchi A. Intestinal loop lengthening—a technique for increasing small intestine length. *J Pediatr Surg.* 1980;15:145–151; [B] from Kim HB, Fauza D, Garza J, Oh JT, Nurko S, Jaksic T. Serial transverse enteroplasty [STEP]: a novel bowel lengthening procedure. *J Pediatr Surg.* 2003;38:425–429.)

managed postoperatively with gastrointestinal tract decompression and total parenteral nutrition until there is return of bowel function, which is often delayed; in one series, the median time to full feeding was 20 days.[13,24]

Overall survival rates for infants with jejunoileal atresia have improved from 30% to 50% in the 1950s to more than 90% in current series.[13] This improvement in survival has been attributed to advances in neonatal critical care, nutrition, and surgical techniques. Mortality is dependent on the length of the remaining small bowel; in those with 40 cm or more, survival reaches 95%, whereas in those with 14 to 40 cm, survival decreases to 50%.[16] Postoperative complications include anastomotic leak or stricture (7% to 15%) and adhesive small bowel obstruction (10%).[13,18,25] Infants with type IIIb and type IV atresias or those who undergo extensive bowel resections may develop short bowel syndrome, requiring prolonged parenteral nutrition. These children may be candidates for subsequent bowel lengthening procedures.[13] In the Bianchi procedure, also known as the longitudinal intestinal lengthening and tailoring (LILT) procedure, the bowel is longitudinally divided and corresponding mesentery is split into dorsal and ventral leaves such that each half remains perfused. The two longitudinal halves are then anastomosed end-to-end (Fig. 83.12A).[23] In the serial transverse enteroplasty (STEP), dilated bowel is partially transected perpendicular to the longitudinal access of the bowel, creating a zig-zag channel, (see Fig. 83.12B).[23]

Duplication Cysts

The incidence of duplication cysts is 1 in 100,000 births.[16] According to Ladd's definition, duplication cysts have (1) a well-developed coat of smooth muscle, (2) an epithelial lining representing gastrointestinal mucosa, and (3) an intimate anatomic association with a portion of the gastrointestinal tract.[19] They may occur anywhere in the gastrointestinal tract between the mouth and the anus; the most common sites, in descending order, are the ileum, esophagus, jejunum, colon, stomach, appendix, and rectum.[26] Ten to 20% of patients with duplication cysts have multiple.[23] Often, they share a muscular wall and blood supply with the adjacent bowel. Up to 25%

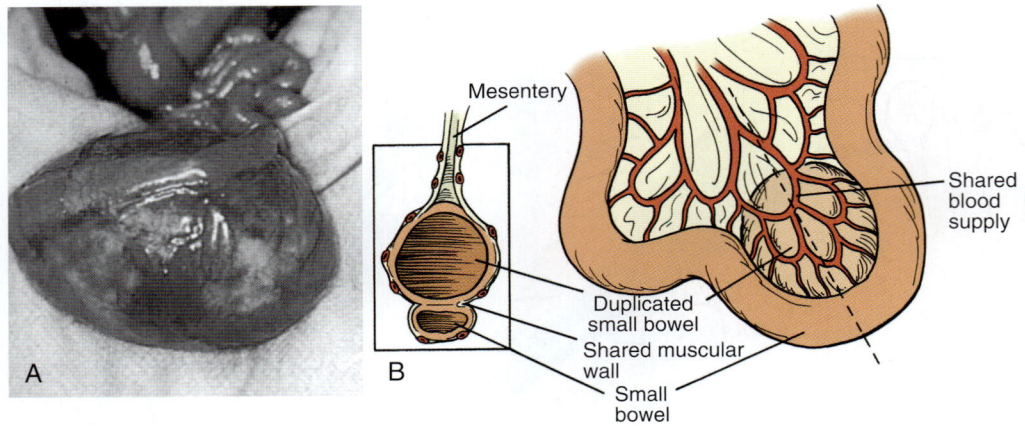

FIGURE 83.13 (A) Large cystic duplication of the small intestine. (B) Small bowel duplication in cross section demonstrating the common wall, shared blood supply, and intramesenteric location. ([A] From Ashcraft KW, Holder TM, eds. *Pediatric Surgery*. Philadelphia: Saunders; 1999; [B] from Oldham KT, Colombani PM, Foglia RP, eds. *Surgery of Infants and Children: Scientific Principles and Practice*. Philadelphia: Lippincott-Raven; 1997.)

may communicate with the lumen of this intestine. Gastric or pancreatic mucosa is found in approximately 25% and may cause ulceration, bleeding, and/or perforation.[23]

Duplication cysts may be cystic or tubular. Cystic duplications account for the majority. These spherical structures are located along the mesenteric border of the bowel (Fig. 83.13) and share blood supply with the adjacent bowel. Rarely do they have an intraluminal connection. Tubular duplications, also found on the mesenteric side, run a parallel course to the adjacent bowel and share a common wall, as well as blood supply, with the normal bowel (Fig. 83.14). They more frequently communicate with the lumen of the normal intestine and have a significant incidence of ectopic gastric mucosa.[26]

Ultrasonography is sometimes able to identify these cysts during prenatal screening.[16] The majority become symptomatic during infancy; symptoms are rarely seen after 12 years of age.[26] Children may present with abdominal distention, bowel obstruction (secondary to compression, intussusception, or volvulus), gastrointestinal bleeding, abdominal pain, and a palpable abdominal mass. Ultrasound is the most common imaging modality used for diagnosis.[27] Upper gastrointestinal contrast series with small bowel follow-through, oral contrast-enhanced CT scans, or magnetic resonance enterography may provide additional information. Technetium 99m sodium pertechnetate scans may demonstrate duplication cysts containing ectopic gastric mucosa.[27,28]

When feasible, duplication cysts should be completely excised. The presence of a shared common wall and blood supply usually necessitates segmental bowel resection encompassing both the duplication cyst and the adjacent bowel; to minimize bowel loss, resection should be reserved for cystic and short (<20 cm) tubular duplications.[29] Several options exist for extensive tubular duplications that cannot be resected without major bowel loss. Bowel may be opened along the longitudinal axis for cyst mucosectomy (mucosal stripping if ectopic gastric mucosa is present), drained into a Roux-en-Y loop of small bowel, or marsupialized to adjacent intestine both proximally and distally.[23]

MECONIUM DISORDERS

Meconium plug syndrome refers to obstruction of the descending colon and rectosigmoid by a plug of inspissated meconium.[30] These infants present with progressive abdominal distention, vomiting, and failure to pass meconium in the first 24 hours after birth. Plain radiographs demonstrate dilated loops of bowel. A water-soluble contrast enema is usually both diagnostic and therapeutic; it will demonstrate a filling defect representing the meconium plug, and solubilize it, facilitating its passage (Fig. 83.15).[30–32] Repeated contrast enemas may be required. Often included under the rubric of meconium plug is small left colon syndrome, often occurring in infants born to diabetic mothers. These infants have small-caliber descending colons and rectosigmoids. As with meconium plug syndrome, administration of contrast enemas usually relieves the obstruction.[32,33]

Meconium plug syndrome is associated with maternal magnesium tocolysis,[33] as well as Hirschsprung disease (incidence 3% to 38%) and CF (incidence 0% to 43%).[22,32] Infants who continue to experience difficulty with stooling after passage of the meconium plug should undergo rectal biopsy to exclude Hirschsprung disease.[33] Infants with small left colon syndrome do not appear to have an increased risk of Hirschsprung disease.[32]

Meconium ileus refers to obstruction of the small bowel and colon with inspissated meconium. It is almost universally associated with CF and is the presenting symptom in 6% to 20% of these children.[22] Prenatal pancreatic exocrine deficiency results in abnormally thick and tenacious meconium that becomes impacted in the ileum. The obstructed ileum becomes dilated as meconium builds up behind the obstruction. Fluid is absorbed from the meconium in the ileum distal to the obstruction, resulting in hard pellets of inspissated meconium and microcolon (Figs. 83.16 and 83.17).[23]

Meconium ileus may be suspected prenatally if fetal ultrasounds show dilated loops of bowel with echogenic debris. Postnatally, meconium ileus usually presents as

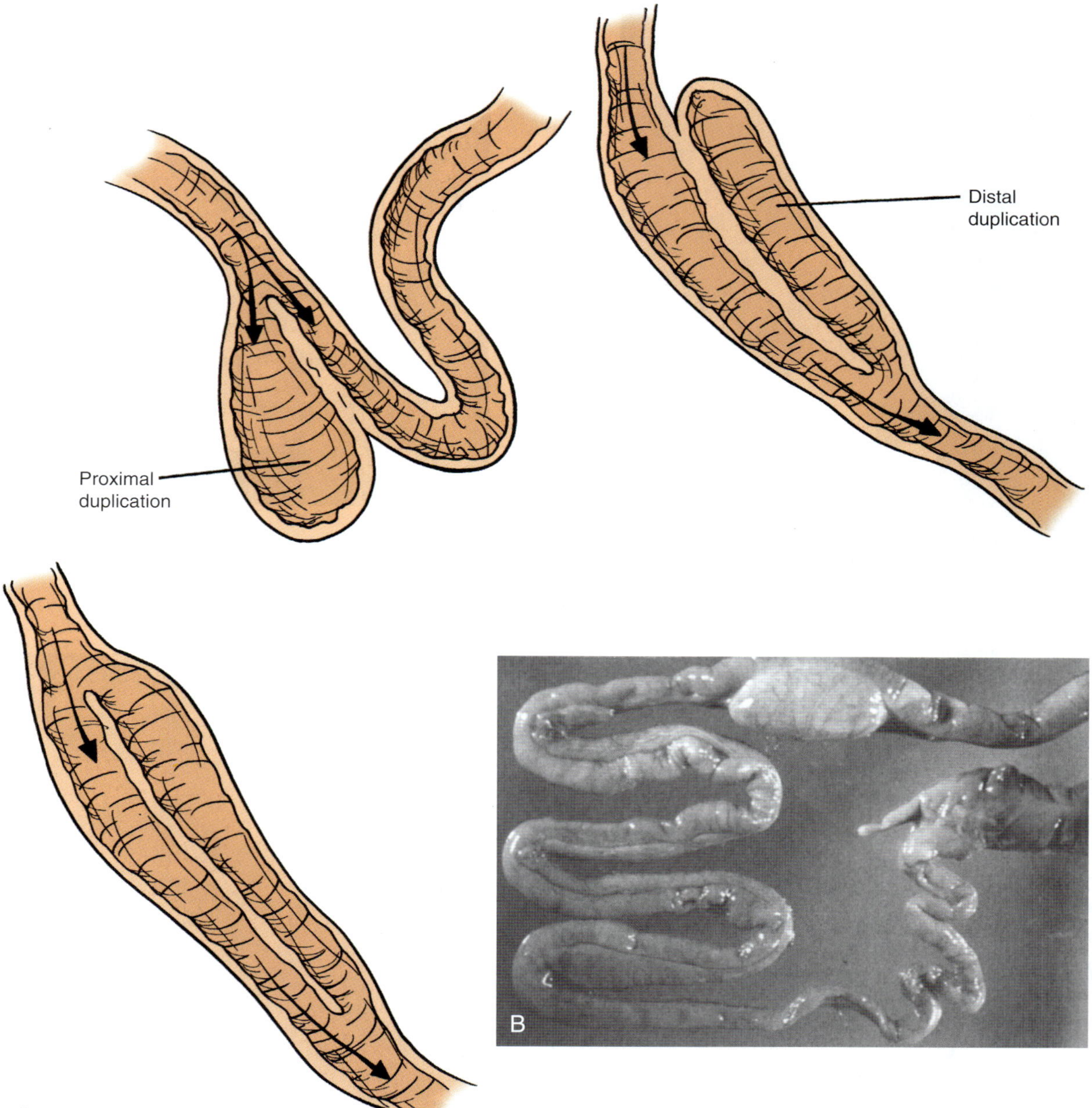

FIGURE 83.14 (A) Schematic depiction of the various forms of communicating tubular duplications: duplication communicating proximally and forming a bulbous mass, duplication communicating distally and remaining clinically asymptomatic, and duplication communicating proximally and distally. *Arrows* depict direction of intestinal flow. (B) Autopsy specimen showing a tubular small bowel duplication involving a portion of the ileum and much of the jejunum. (From Oldham KT, Cclombani PM, Foglia RP, eds. *Surgery of Infants and Children: Scientific Principles and Practice*. Philadelphia: Lippincott-Raven; 1997.)

abdominal distention and bilious vomiting. Plain abdominal radiographs demonstrate dilated bowel loops with a ground-glass appearance in the right lower quadrant (Fig. 83.18).[22] In the absence of clinical signs of complicated meconium ileus (i.e., meconium ileus associated with perforation, volvulus, or atresia), a water-soluble contrast enema should be performed. Classically, microcolon is seen with meconium pellets in the distal ileum and dilated proximal small bowel. As with meconium plug syndrome, the study may be therapeutic as well as diagnostic; the

contrast may loosen the impacted meconium and allow it to be evacuated. Multiple enemas may be administered over several days in an attempt to clear all of the inspissated meconium. Meticulous attention to the infant's hydration status is critical to prevent dehydration as a result of the enemas. The success rate for contrast enemas is 50% to 60%, but it is dependent on the length of bowel affected by meconium,[34,35] as well as the underlying pathophysiology. Failure of enemas to relieve the obstruction is an indication for exploratory laparotomy. When associated with CF, the

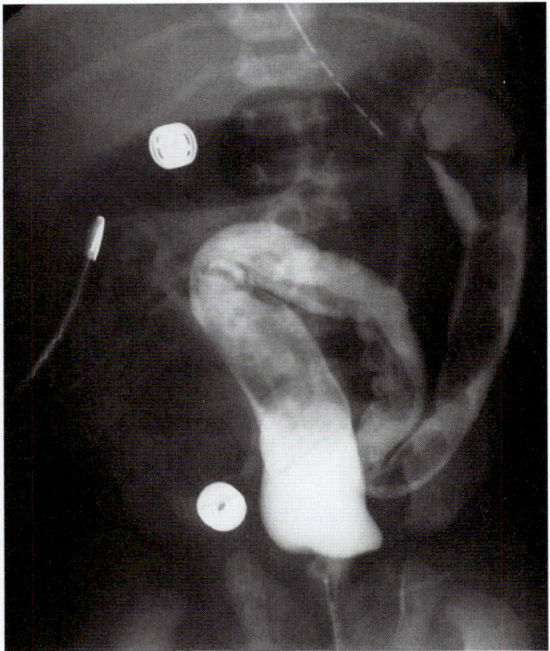

FIGURE 83.15 Image from a water-soluble contrast enema demonstrating an intraluminal meconium plug extending from the transverse colon to the rectum, as well as a small left colon. (Courtesy A.B. Campbell, MD, St. Christopher's Hospital for Children.)

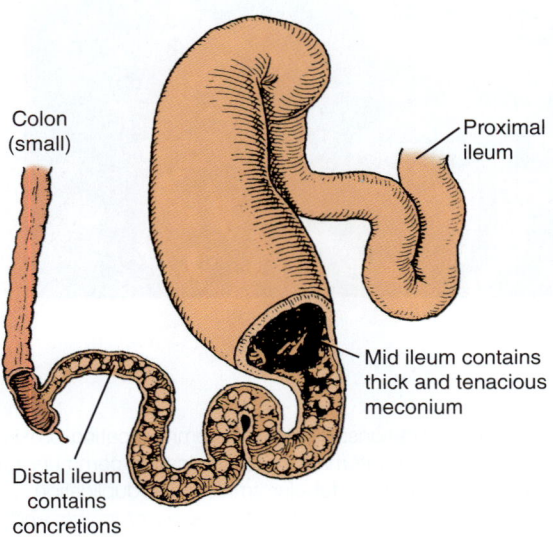

FIGURE 83.16 Schematic of meconium ileus. (From Lloyd DA: Meconium ileus. In: Welch KJ, ed. *Pediatric Surgery*. Chicago: Mosby Year Book; 1986.)

Colon (small)

Proximal ileum

Mid ileum contains thick and tenacious meconium

Distal ileum contains concretions

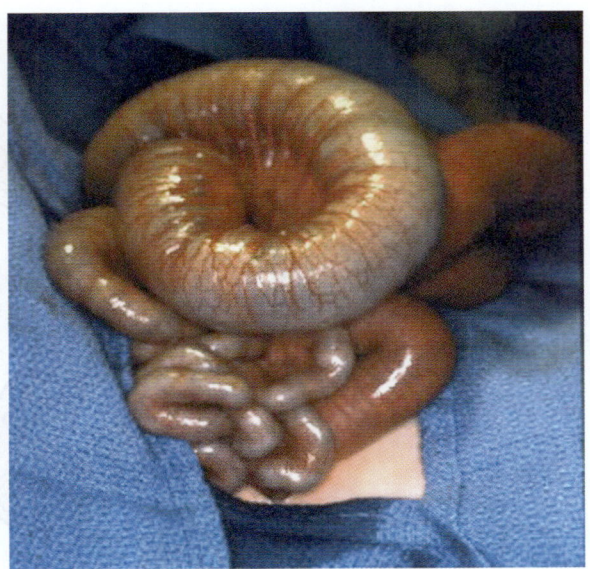

FIGURE 83.17 Operative photograph of an infant with meconium ileus showing dilated bowel impacted with meconium and distal ileum with inspissated meconium pellets.

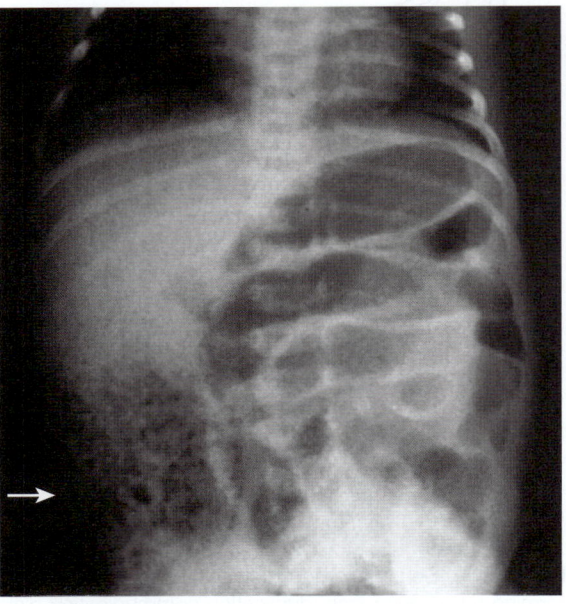

FIGURE 83.18 Plain abdominal radiograph of meconium ileus with distended loops of bowel and a mass of meconium *(arrow)* with a ground-glass appearance from mixed air and stool. (From Ashcraft KW, Holder TM, eds. *Pediatric Surgery*. Philadelphia: Saunders; 1999.)

incidence of complex meconium ileus is high; in one series, more than 90% of these children required laparotomy.[36]

A variety of surgical approaches have been used to clear meconium obstructions. Enterotomy with irrigation with either saline or 4% acetylcysteine solution and manual evacuation of meconium is usually effective. In cases in which the distal obstruction cannot be cleared, a T tube or an ostomy (Bishop-Koop, Santulli) for distal irrigation may be placed. Bowel resection with primary anastomosis may be necessary to remove the area of impacted meconium. In complicated meconium ileus, resection of the damaged bowel with ostomy formation is often necessary due to the inflammation of the bowel and surrounding tissue.[35] Infants are managed postoperatively with gastrointestinal tract decompression and total parenteral nutrition until return of bowel function.

OMPHALOMESENTERIC REMNANTS

In utero the omphalomesenteric duct serves as a nutritive conduit between the yolk sac and the gut of the developing fetus. During the eighth week of gestation, the placenta develops and replaces the yolk sac as the source of fetal nutrition, with subsequent regression of the omphalomesenteric duct. Failure of the omphalomesenteric duct to obliterate completely is estimated to occur in 1% to 4% of infants and may result in a wide spectrum of omphalomesenteric anomalies, including a patent omphalomesenteric (vitelline) duct, omphalomesenteric cysts and bands, and Meckel diverticulum (Fig. 83.19).[37,38]

Approximately 5% of omphalomesenteric duct remnants are patent omphalomesenteric ducts—persistent connections between the distal ileum and the umbilicus. These disorders usually present following separation of the umbilical cord with intermittent drainage of small bowel contents from the umbilicus. A sinus tract may be apparent at the base of the umbilicus. Ultrasound may demonstrate a tubular structure beneath the umbilicus. If a sinus tract is present, it may be cannulated and contrast injected to demonstrate communication with the small bowel. Ectopic gastric mucosa is identified in approximately a third of patients with a complete fistula. Treatment consists of resection of the entire omphalomesenteric remnant (Fig. 83.20).[23]

Omphalomesenteric duct cysts are lined with mucosa and may be located in the intraperitoneal or the preperitoneal space. They result from obliteration of the omphalomesenteric duct at the umbilical and ileal ends. They may become quite large, get infected, or cause bowel obstruction, and therefore should be excised.[23]

Omphalomesenteric bands are the result of fibrosis of the omphalomesenteric duct or the associated vitelline blood vessels with failure of involution. A fibrous cord tethers the bowel to the umbilicus. Bowel may volvulize around or become obstructed by these bands.[39]

Meckel diverticulum represents 90% of omphalomesenteric duct remnants. In fact, it is the most common congenital anomaly of the gastrointestinal tract,[37] occurring in 1% to 2% of the population. Symptoms develop in 4% to 6% of affected individuals; of those, 50% do so by 3 years of age and 75% by 10 years. Males are twice as likely to develop symptoms as females.[38]

Meckel diverticula contain all three layers of the intestinal wall and therefore are true diverticula, typically measuring 3 to 6 cm in length. They are located on the antimesenteric border of the ileum, usually within 50 to 100 cm from the ileocecal valve. They arise from incomplete degeneration of the intestinal end of the yolk stalk and are supplied by a persistent vitelline vessel.[37] Approximately 50% have heterotopic mucosa, of which 60% is gastric and 15% pancreatic. A fibrous connection from the Meckel diverticulum to the umbilicus occurs in up to 25% of patients.[37]

Painless lower gastrointestinal bleeding is the most common complication and usually occurs in children. It is the consequence of ectopic gastric acid–induced mucosal

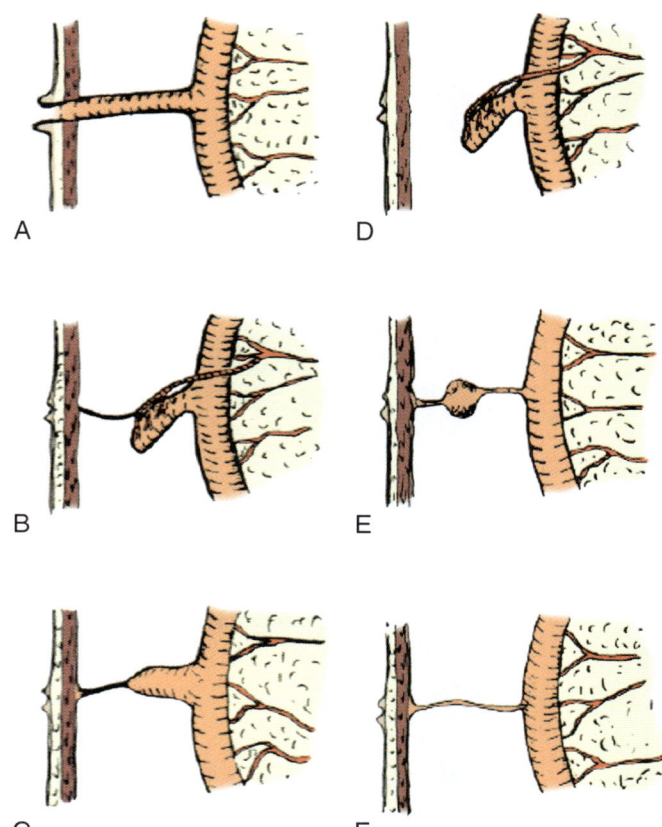

FIGURE 83.19 Illustrated are some of the more common residual congenital abnormalities that result from the embryonic yolk sac. (A) Patent omphalomesenteric duct representing a communication from the terminal ileum to the umbilicus. (B) Meckel diverticulum with a patent right vitelline artery illustrated as a cord to the undersurface of the umbilicus. (C) Meckel diverticulum with a cord connecting the tip of the diverticulum to the undersurface of the umbilicus. The cord (band) represents the distal residual of the omphalomesenteric duct. (D) Typical appearance of Meckel diverticulum with persistence of the vitelline artery. (E) Involution of the proximal and distal ends of the omphalomesenteric duct with a residual cord or band and central preservation of the omphalomesenteric duct resulting in a mucosa-lined cyst. (F) Intraperitoneal band from the ileum to the undersurface of the umbilicus representing involution without resolution of the omphalomesenteric duct. (From Wyllie R, Hyams J, eds. *Pediatric Gastrointestinal Disease*. Philadelphia: Saunders; 1999.)

ulceration or ectopic pancreatic secretions eroding into the submucosal artery, either at the junction of ileal and ectopic mucosa in the diverticulum or in the mesenteric ileal wall opposite the opening of the diverticulum into the lumen. *Helicobacter pylori* plays no pathogenic role in Meckel-related ulceration.[37] The gastric mucosa in a Meckel diverticulum may take up technetium 99m pertechnetate; thus a Meckel scan may be used to diagnose a Meckel diverticulum in patients presenting with painless bleeding. However, the sensitivity and specificity of the Meckel scan are only 89% and 98%, respectively.[40] Alternatively, double-balloon enteroscopy or capsule endoscopy may be performed.[41]

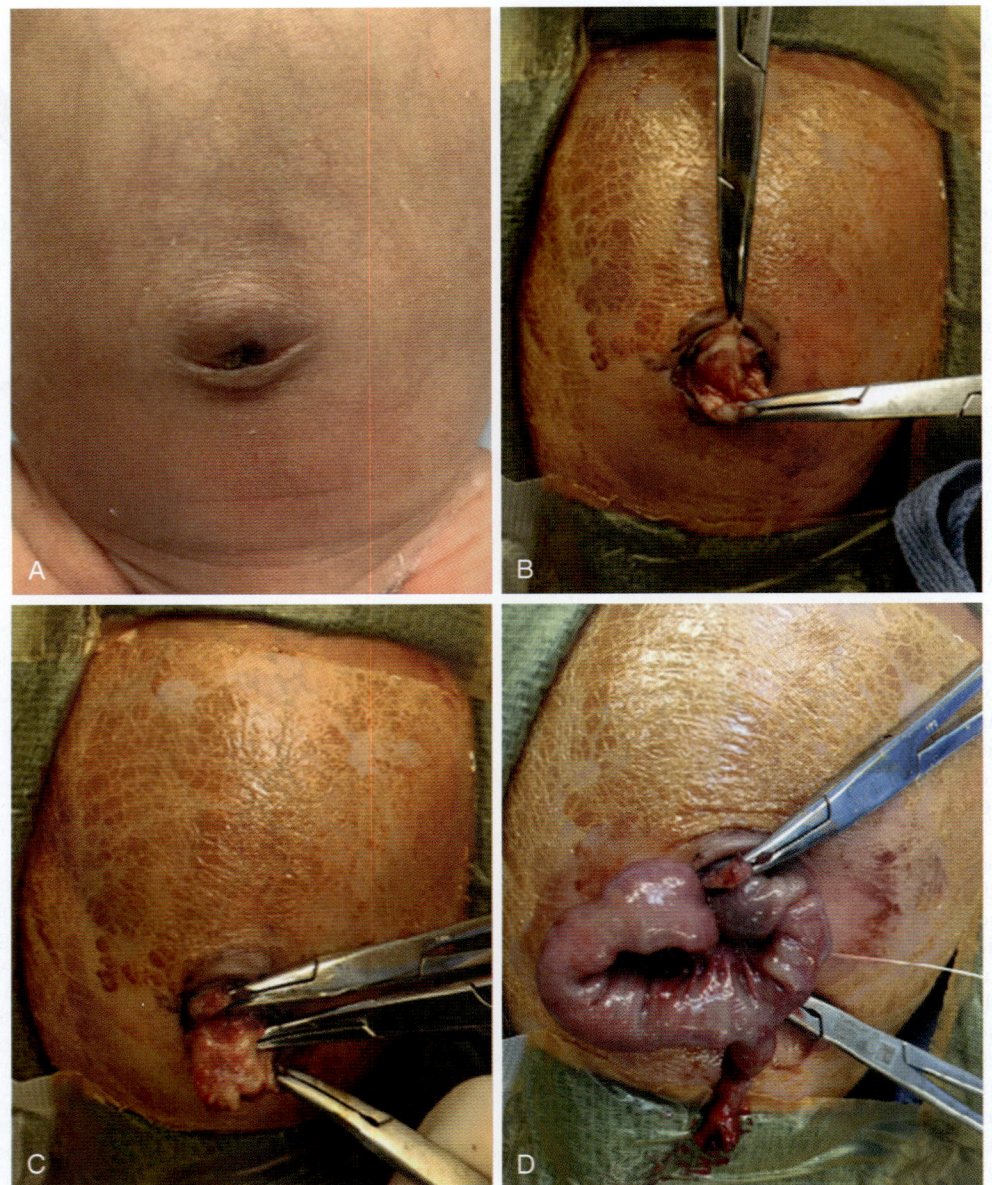

FIGURE 83.20 (A) A patent omphalomesenteric duct that became apparent upon drainage of small bowel contents. (B to D) Dissection of the duct from the umbilicus down to its connection with the small bowel.

Bowel obstruction is the second most common complication of Meckel diverticulum. In adults, it is the most common source of related morbidity. Symptomatic bowel obstructions may occur from intussusception of the diverticulum (Fig. 83.21), herniation of a loop of bowel under the extramesenteric vitelline artery that supplies the Meckel (Fig. 83.22), or volvulus of a loop of bowel around a fibrous band tethering the Meckel to the umbilicus. Meckel diverticulum should be considered in patients presenting with small bowel obstruction but no history of previous abdominal surgery.[37]

Meckel diverticulitis is often clinically indistinguishable from acute appendicitis and is usually diagnosed during the radiologic or operative evaluation and management of suspected appendicitis. The diverticulum becomes inflamed and may become gangrenous and/or perforate. Heterotopic gastric or pancreatic mucosa is frequently present in the inflamed diverticulum.[37]

Malignancies within Meckel diverticula—usually lymphomas or carcinoid tumors—are rare and account for only 0.5% to 2% of Meckel complications.[37]

Symptomatic Meckel diverticula require surgical excision, which may be accomplished by either open or laparoscopic approaches.[42] Amputation of the diverticulum from the antimesenteric border of the bowel is suitable when the diverticulum is narrow, but resection of the diverticulum with a segment of the adjoining ileum may be preferable if the diverticulum is short and broad based. When resecting a Meckel diverticulum for bleeding, examination of the lumen of the Meckel diverticulum and the ileum may be performed to ensure that the ulcerated area is removed.[38] However, some surgeons advocate diverticulectomy even if ulcerations are found in the mesenteric bowel, given the additional morbidity of bowel resection and the fact that diverticulectomy alone removes the source of caustic secretions and therefore should allow any ileal ulcers to heal.[38]

The management of an asymptomatic, incidentally found Meckel remains controversial. The surgeon must weigh the risk of complications from resection against the risk of Meckel-related complications. Many surgeons have used anatomic criteria to decide whether to resect. Most surgeons opt to resect a narrow Meckel diverticulum with a bandlike vitelline vessel that poses a risk for obstruction or a diverticulum with thickened tip consistent with the presence of ectopic mucosa (Fig. 83.23). A 2008 systematic review of 244 published studies demonstrated a significantly higher postoperative complication rate with

resection of incidentally detected Meckel diverticula than leaving them intact; 758 patients would have to undergo resection of an asymptomatic Meckel diverticulum to prevent one Meckel-related death.[43]

NECROTIZING ENTEROCOLITIS

NEC, the most common gastrointestinal tract emergency in neonates, is an inflammatory disorder that produces various degrees of ischemic necrosis in affected bowel. The inflammation may be limited to the mucosa or may be transmural. Perforation secondary to full-thickness necrosis occurs in approximately one-third of infants with NEC. The distribution of involved bowel is often patchy, but the terminal ileum and colon are particularly prone to involvement. The entire small bowel is involved in 10% of cases of NEC.[44]

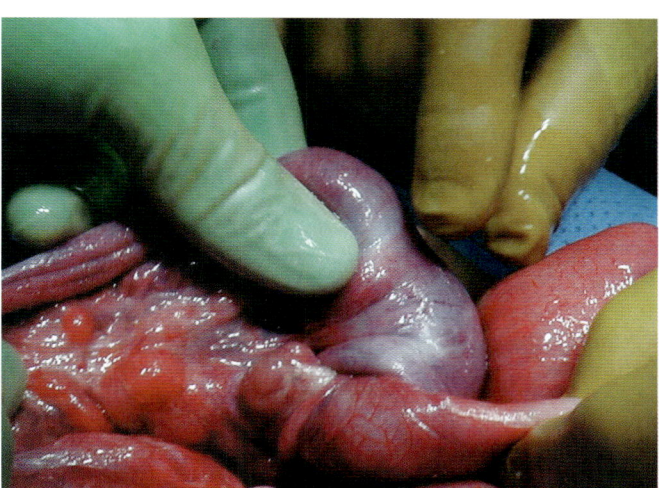

FIGURE 83.21 Intussusception caused by Meckel diverticulum as a lead point. Note the hypertrophied mesenteric lymph nodes.

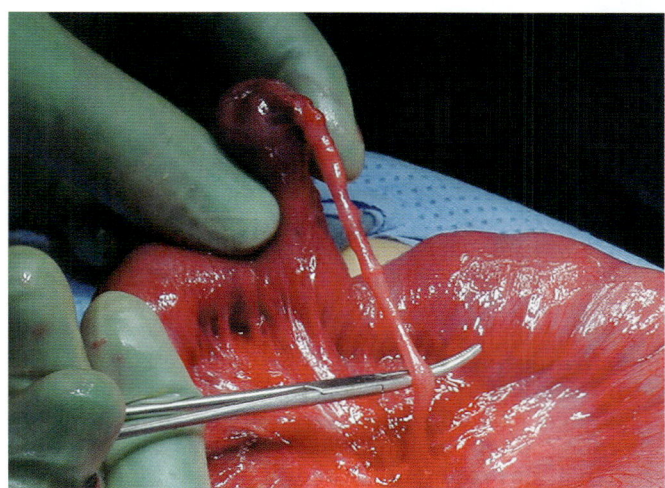

FIGURE 83.22 Reduced Meckel from Fig. 83.11 showing the extramesenteric vitelline vessel feeding the Meckel that may cause an internal hernia.

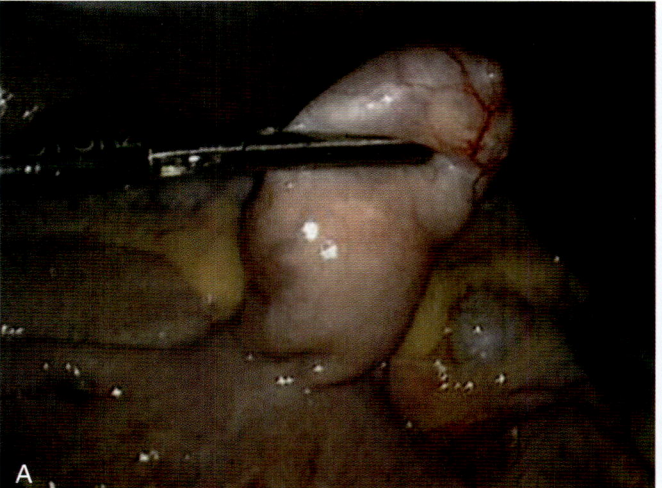
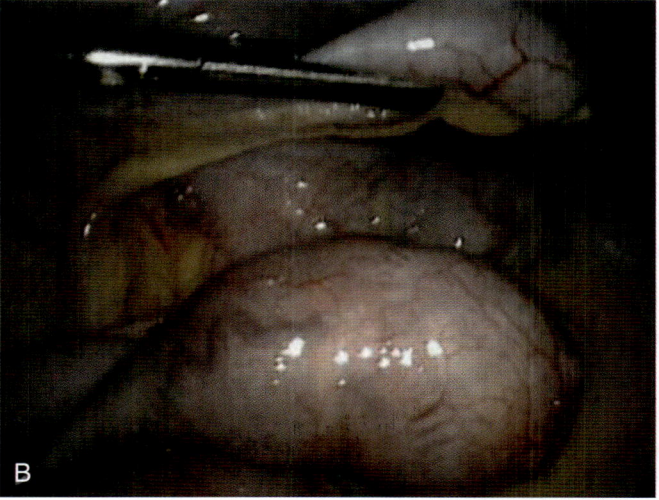

FIGURE 83.23 (A) Meckel diverticulum with a thickened tip that contained heterotopic gastric mucosa. Note that it emanates from the antimesenteric small bowel. (B) The appendix is held near the Meckel for comparison.

NEC is primarily a disease of prematurity, with only 10% of cases occurring in full-term infants.[45] As such, the recognition of NEC as a distinct disease process did not occur until the late 1960s, paralleling the development of neonatal intensive care units (NICUs).[44] Since its description, the morbidity and mortality of NEC have remained largely unchanged, in part because advances in neonatal critical care have increased the survival of extremely low birth weight (ELBW) premature infants (<1000 g). NEC is estimated to occur in 7% of NICU infants weighing 1500 g or less.[45]

A subset of premature infants develop isolated perforation of the intestine without significant bowel inflammation, a condition called spontaneous intestinal perforation (SIP) or focal intestinal perforation (FIP). Controversy exists as to whether SIP is a form of NEC or a distinct pathologic entity. SIP occurs primarily in ELBW babies (<1000 g) and at an earlier age than NEC. Unlike NEC, infants usually have not been fed. Often they have received indomethacin or systemic postnatal steroids. Plain films show free air, but pneumatosis intestinalis and portal venous air are rarely seen. At surgical exploration, an isolated perforation of the antimesenteric ileum with minimal surrounding bowel inflammation is found.[46]

Despite decades of experience with and research into NEC, the causes of this disorder are not yet fully elucidated. The pathogenesis of NEC appears to be multifactorial; prematurity, enteral feeding, and the gut immune response to bacterial colonization are major contributors to its development.[45] Premature infants, especially those with low birth weights, are prone to perinatal stress that may impair intestinal perfusion. This relative ischemia, in addition to their gut dysmotility, higher gut pH, and weakened immune systems may predispose them to microbial colonization by nosocomial bacteria present in the NICU environment. Moreover, they exhibit an inappropriate inflammatory response to intraluminal gut bacteria.[47] Formula-fed infants have an increased susceptibility to NEC as compared with those fed breast milk. Breast milk contains immunoglobulins, lactoferrin, lysozymes, oligosaccharides, glycoconjugates, and various white cells that appear to protect the immature gut.[48] Mounting evidence implicates the alterations in the gut microbiome in the development of NEC; studies show a bloom of Proteobacteria, specifically Enterobacteriaceae species,[49] and *Clostridium perfringens*[50] in the intestinal flora prior to the onset of NEC. Transfusion of packed red blood cells may increase the risk of developing NEC.[37] Full-term infants who develop NEC usually have comorbidities predisposing them to decreased mesenteric perfusion, such as congenital cardiac disease, sepsis, congenital bowel anomalies, or maternal drug use.[49-51] Infants who develop SIP are thought to have impaired intestinal perfusion secondary to the vasoconstricting effects of indomethacin and glucocorticoids.[52]

NEC typically presents with feeding intolerance, abdominal distention, and heme-positive or grossly bloody stool in a 7- to 14-day-old premature infant. Other early signs of NEC include apnea, bradycardia, lethargy, temperature instability, and hyperglycemia. As NEC progresses, acidosis, thrombocytopenia, leukopenia, abdominal discoloration, peritonitis, and shock may develop.[45] Plain

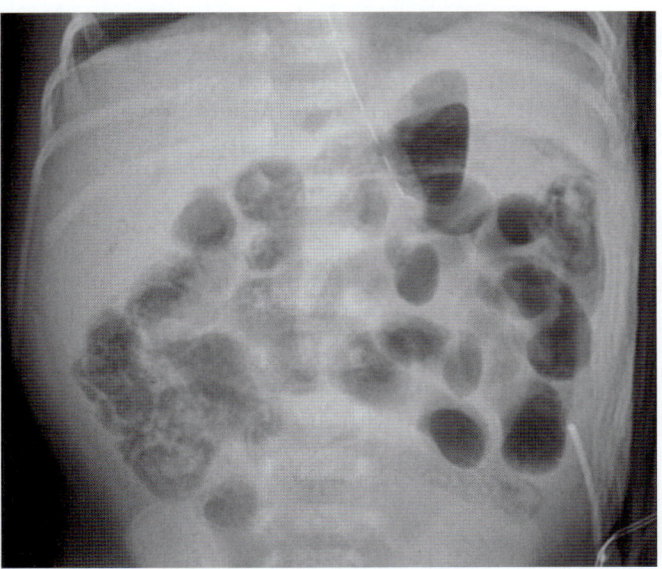

FIGURE 83.24 An abdominal radiograph in a neonate with necrotizing enterocolitis demonstrates pneumatosis and portal venous gas.

radiographs may show dilated loops of bowel, pneumatosis intestinalis, portal venous gas, or free air (Fig. 83.24). There is growing use of ultrasound to diagnose and manage NEC: findings of echogenic ascites, thin-walled aperistaltic bowel, and bowel with minimal Doppler blood flow suggest necrotic or perforated bowel.[52]

Medical management usually includes cessation of enteral feeds, gastrointestinal decompression, broad-spectrum antibiotics, and total parenteral nutrition. Serial abdominal radiographs, complete blood counts, and blood gases should be obtained every 8 hours to monitor for the development of free intraabdominal air, thrombocytopenia, and acidosis while the infant remains ill. With these measures, 60% to 70% of infants will recover.[45]

The decision making regarding the need for and timing of surgical interventions on these fragile, critically ill infants is complex. The only absolute indication for surgical intervention is the radiologic finding of intraabdominal free air signifying bowel perforation. An operation should be considered for infants with NEC who fail to improve despite maximal medical therapy, as indicated by persistent or progressive metabolic acidosis, thrombocytopenia, and hemodynamic instability.[53] Other "relative" indications for surgery include a palpable abdominal mass, abdominal wall erythema, portal venous gas, persistent hyponatremia, and a static loop of dilated bowel on serial abdominal films. Although suggestive of a need for intervention, none of these signs alone is an indication for surgery.[45,54] Hackam et al. developed a scoring system to predict the development of NEC totalis in premature infants: thrombocytopenia, hyperphosphatemia, elevated creatinine, and older age at diagnosis were all associated with increased risk.[53]

In the surgical treatment of NEC, the goal is to remove necrotic bowel while preserving maximal bowel length. The two most common surgical procedures for NEC are laparotomy and peritoneal drainage (PD). For infants weighing more than 1500 g, laparotomy is preferred over PD. A number of techniques have been used to manage the diseased bowel during laparotomy. The operative approach is predicated on the extent and location of the involved intestine. When an isolated area of intestinal necrosis is found at exploration, resection of the area of necrosis and creation of an ostomy should be performed.[55] Although resection with primary anastomosis for perforated NEC has been described, it has not been widely used or accepted. When multiple areas of inflamed bowel that are not frankly necrotic are encountered, closure with a planned second-look reexploration 24 to 48 hours later or a proximal diverting enterostomy with or without a second-look procedure have been advocated.[39] In the "clip and drop back" technique, necrotic bowel is resected, surgical clips placed on the blind ends, and the bowel is dropped back into the abdomen in discontinuity. The infant is reexplored in 24 to 48 hours, at which time either bowel continuity is restored or diversion is performed. The "patch, drain, and wait technique" was developed in an attempt to preserve bowel length in cases of extensive intestinal involvement. The areas of necrosis are débrided, imbricated, and drained with Penrose drains. The infant is then treated with antibiotics and total parenteral nutrition.[55,56]

The treatment of perforated NEC in very low birth weight (VLBW) infants (<1500 g) and ELBW infants (<1000 g) is an area of active controversy. In these extremely fragile infants, laparotomy has been associated with a 35% mortality rate and a 25% incidence of neurodevelopmental impairment.[54,57] The use of bedside PD under local anesthesia for the management of perforated NEC was first reported in 1977.[58] Although initially described as a temporizing measure to stabilize critically ill VLBW infants with perforated NEC until laparotomy could be tolerated, investigators have reported that PD without laparotomy may serve as the definitive procedure.[58,59] PD has become many surgeons' preferred initial intervention in ELBW infants with perforated NEC, although most survivors will ultimately require a laparotomy.[59] Several multicenter randomized controlled trials (RCTs) have compared laparotomy with PD for the management of perforated NEC.[59,60] Moss et al. were unable to demonstrate any difference in survival, duration of total parenteral nutrition, or length of stay between PD and laparotomy in a multicenter RCT of 117 VLBW infants; mortality was 35% in each group, and 38% of the PD group ultimately required laparotomy.[60] In a European multicenter RCT, Rees et al. were not able to demonstrate any advantage in survival for either laparotomy or PD for ELBW infants with perforated NEC, although 74% of infants randomized to PD ultimately underwent a delayed laparotomy. They also found that the use of PD did not result in any immediate improvement in clinical status, challenging the utility of PD as a temporizing measure in critically ill infants.[59] In a 2010 systematic review of published studies comparing PD versus laparotomy, PD was associated with a 55% excess mortality compared with laparotomy.[61] On late follow-up (18 to 22 months), infants who had PD for NEC had a higher late mortality rate and a higher incidence of neurodevelopmental impairment compared with children who underwent

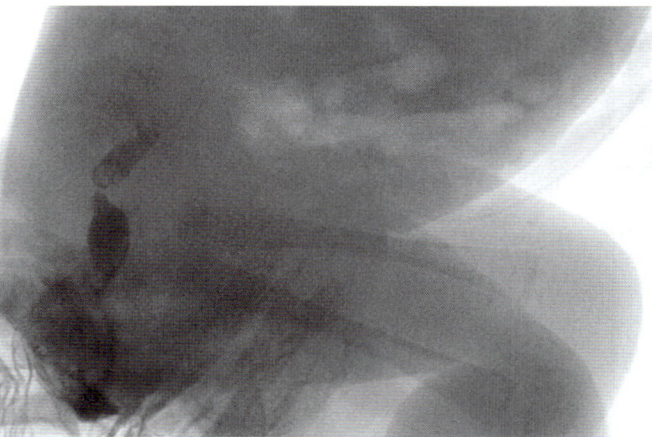

FIGURE 83.25 The infant pictured in Fig. 83.24 underwent small bowel and proximal colon resection with an end ostomy. Prior to ostomy takedown, a contrast enema was done, demonstrating a stricture at the rectosigmoid junction.

laparotomy.[56] The difficulty demonstrating any advantage to either laparotomy or PD underscores that the need for any type of surgical intervention for NEC in infants is associated with significant morbidity and mortality. Both laparotomy and PD have a role in the management of perforated NEC in these critically ill infants; the decision as to which approach to use must be individualized to each patient. The role of PD is similarly debated in infants with SIP.[55,56,62,63]

The mortality rate for NEC is 20% to 35% and is highest for infants requiring surgical intervention.[54] Gastrointestinal morbidity is significant and includes bowel strictures and short bowel syndrome. Approximately one-third of infants who recover from medically or surgically treated NEC develop strictures of the small bowel or colon. Strictures most commonly develop at watershed areas of intestinal blood flow: the terminal ileum, splenic flexure, and the proximal sigmoid colon. Strictures may present as partial bowel obstructions, feeding intolerance, or persistently dilated loops of bowel on abdominal radiographs.[55,56] If a stricture is suspected, a contrast enema should be performed (Fig. 83.25). All infants with stomas should have a contrast enema or ostomy study prior to stoma closure. All NEC-related strictures should be resected. Finally, survivors of NEC are prone to the development of nongastrointestinal diseases as well; infants who recover from NEC have a 25% incidence of neurodevelopmental impairment.[57]

INTUSSUSCEPTION

Intussusception, one of the most common causes of bowel obstruction in infants and toddlers, results from the invagination of a portion of proximal intestine (intussusceptum) into another more distal segment of bowel (intussuscipiens; Figs. 83.26 and 83.27). The progressive intussusception of the bowel leads to compression and angulation of the mesenteric vessels and lymphatics of the invaginated bowel with subsequent obstruction, ischemia, and eventually necrosis. More than 80% of

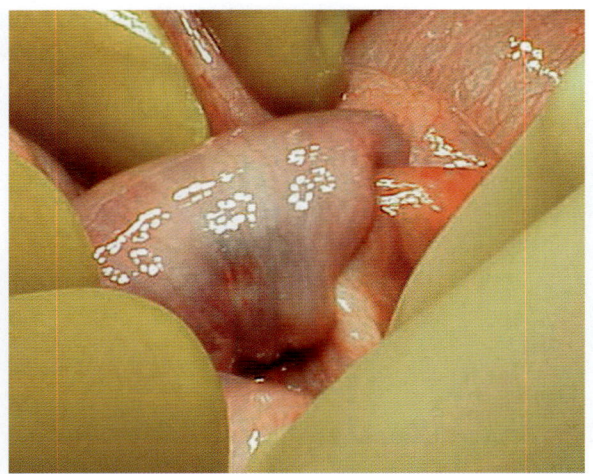

FIGURE 83.26 An ileocolic intussusception prior to manual reduction.

intussusceptions are ileocolic. Small bowel–to–small bowel intussusceptions also occur but are generally transient and self-resolving; they are often an incidental finding, especially in the setting of hypermotility, as with gastroenteritis. One notable exception is Henoch-Schönlein purpura (HSP), in which submucosal hematomas may act as lead points.[23]

Intussusception occurs most commonly during the first year of life, beginning at approximately 4 months of age and peaking at 8 months. Although intussusception may occur throughout childhood, less than 15% of cases occur beyond 36 months of age. Most intussusceptions in infants and toddlers are idiopathic; they lack a clear lead point. Children with idiopathic intussusception often have a history of current or antecedent upper respiratory tract infections or gastrointestinal illnesses. Adenoviruses and rotavirus have been implicated in the development of up to 50% of cases of idiopathic intussusception. Hypertrophy of Peyer patches is universally seen at surgery and has been speculated to contribute to the development of intussusception. True anatomic lead points occur in only 2% to 10% of cases and include Meckel diverticulum (most frequent), polyps, benign and malignant tumors, duplication cysts, lymphomas, foreign bodies, and submucosal hemorrhage from HSP.[64] The chances of finding an anatomic lead point underlying an intussusception increase with age. Children older than age 3 years should be suspected of having a lead point.

The typical presentation for intussusception is an infant or toddler with episodes of cyclical, severe abdominal pain, each lasting 5 to 15 minutes. During these episodes of pain, the child is often described as inconsolable. He or she frequently draws his or her knees up to the chest. Between episodes, the child may be normal or lethargic. In some cases, profound lethargy may be the only symptom. As the intussusception progresses, the child may develop bilious vomiting and pass maroon currant jelly stool. If left untreated, bowel necrosis and shock will develop. Between 1979 and 1997 there were 323 intussusception-related deaths reported to the US Centers for Disease Control and Prevention.[65]

Physical examination of a child with an intussusception may reveal a palpable sausage-shaped mass in the right upper quadrant of the abdomen. Grossly bloody or occult heme-positive stool may be present on rectal examination. Overt peritonitis is seen in advanced intussusception and mandates immediate operative intervention. Abdominal plain films may show dilated loops of small bowel with a paucity of air in the right lower quadrant. With a sensitivity of 98% to 100% and a specificity of 88% to 100%, ultrasound has become the primary modality of diagnosing intussusception. The presence of a kidney-shaped mass in the longitudinal view or a "target sign" in the transverse view is diagnostic (Fig. 83.28). A contrast enema had traditionally been the criterion standard for diagnosis and may still be useful as a diagnostic, as well as therapeutic, tool when ultrasound is not available or is equivocal.[65]

After intussusception has been confirmed, fluids and antibiotics should be administered. Reduction via air or contrast enema should be attempted in children with intussusception without evidence of peritonitis. Success rates of 60% to 80% have been reported for air or hydrostatic contrast enemas.[65–67] Ultrasound-guided saline enema reductions have also been reported. Successful reduction is confirmed by reflux of air or contrast into the terminal ileum (Fig. 83.29). Bowel perforation rates from air or contrast enemas are less than 1%, but require emergency surgery if they occur.[65]

Failure to reduce the intussusception via air or contrast enema and/or the presence of peritonitis mandates operative intervention. Both the open and laparoscopic approach may be used.[67,68] The open approach is done through a transverse right lower quadrant incision. Gentle retrograde pressure is applied in a distal-to-proximal direction, effectively milking the intussusceptum out of the intussuscipiens (Fig. 83.30). The appendix is often removed. Laparoscopic reduction is accomplished by gently pulling the intussusceptum from the intussuscipiens. Care must be taken to avoid vigorous pulling that may tear the bowel.

After operative reduction, the bowel is carefully inspected for viability and the presence of a lead point. The ileocecal valve will often be edematous and thickened and may be mistaken for a lead point and unnecessarily resected. Assessment for a lead point is somewhat more difficult with the laparoscopic approach. If the lead point is a Meckel diverticulum or a polyp, it should be resected. If the intussusception is not reducible or nonviable bowel is found after reduction, it should be resected (Fig. 83.31). A primary anastomosis may usually be performed. Recurrence rates are 5% to 10% and 1% to 4% following successful air/hydrostatic reduction or operative reduction, respectively.[65,67] Recurrence is usually managed by hydrostatic reduction. Repeated episodes of intussusception necessitate an upper gastrointestinal series with small bowel follow-through or magnetic resonance enterography to investigate for a lead point. Following reduction of an intussusception, children are admitted to the hospital to monitor for signs of recurrence. Fevers are not uncommon following reduction. Oral intake is resumed quickly, and most children are able to be discharged from the hospital in 12 to 24 hours.[13,23]

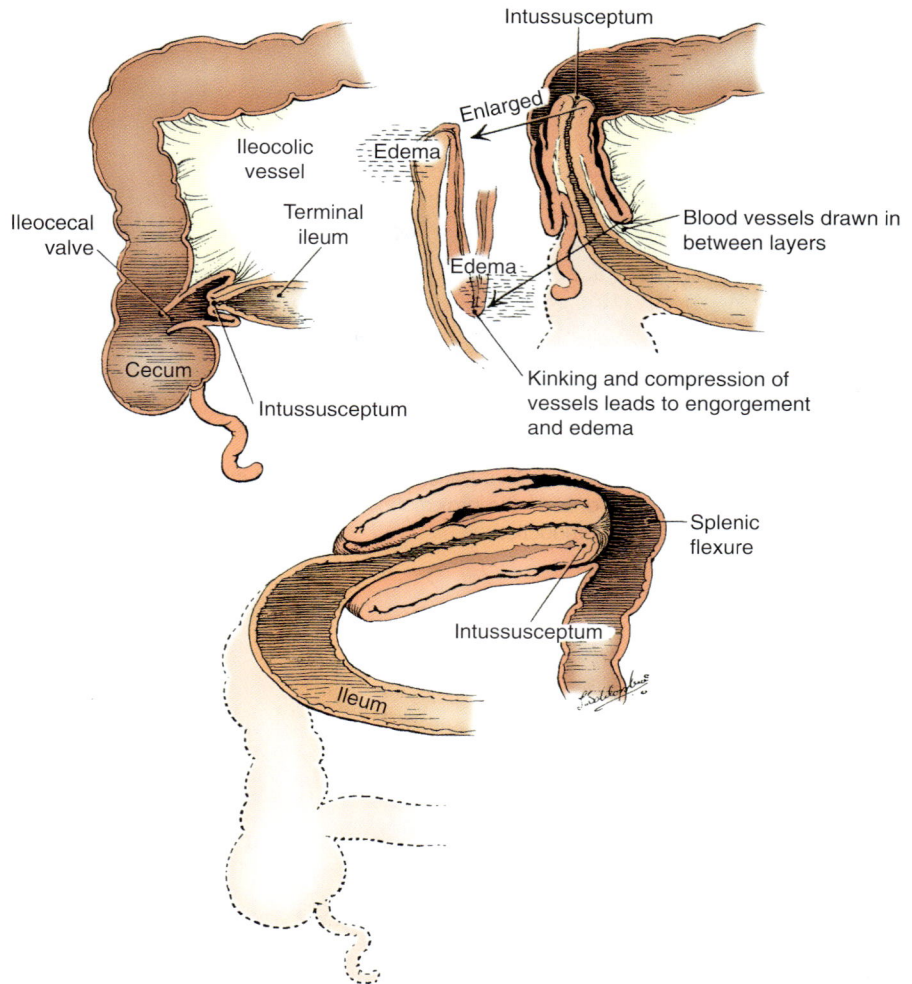

FIGURE 83.27 Development of an intussusception. Most intussusceptions in infants and children are of the kind shown here. The intussusception begins at or near the ileocecal valve without an obvious local anatomic lesion to cause it. From the first moment, there is simultaneous interference with patency of the alimentary canal and with the vascular supply of the intussusceptum. The drawings indicate the manner in which the mesenteric vessels are drawn between the layers of the intussusception and compressed. The slight interference with lymphatic and venous drainage that occurs almost immediately results in edema and an increase in tissue pressure. This further increases resistance to the return of venous blood, the venules and capillaries become enormously engorged, and bloody edema fluid drips into the lumen. The mucosal cells swell into goblet cells and discharge mucus, which, after mixing in the lumen with the bloody transudate, forms a "currant jelly" stool. Edema increases until venous inflow is completely obstructed. As arterial blood continues to pump in, tissue pressure rises until it is higher than arterial pressure, and gangrene ensues. The drawings indicate the sharp U-shaped turns of the intestine and mesenteric vessels at either end of the intussusceptum. The outer coat of the intussusceptum (middle layer of the intussusception) is isolated between the two sharp bends and understandably is the first to become gangrenous. Gangrene appears in this coat near the tip of the intussusceptum and progresses back toward the neck of the intussusceptum. Rarely, the intussuscipiens is damaged. (From Ravitch MM, Welch KJ, Benson CD, et al., eds. *Pediatric Surgery*. 3rd ed. Chicago: Year Book; 1979.)

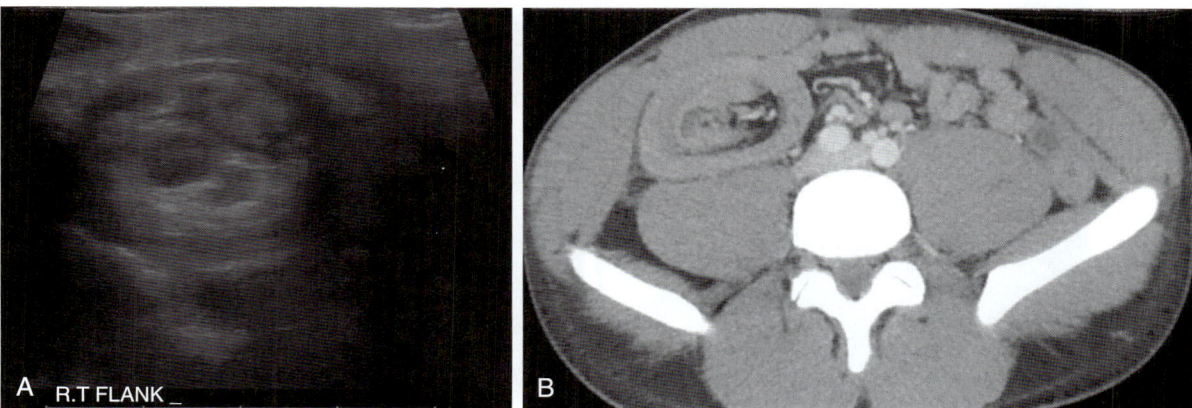

FIGURE 83.28 (A) Ultrasound appearance of an intussusception demonstrating the concentric "target sign" of intussuscepted bowel. (B) Computed tomography scan demonstrating the "target sign" of intussusception. Mesentery and mesenteric vessels may be seen in between the walls of the intussuscipiens (colon) and the intussusceptum (small bowel).

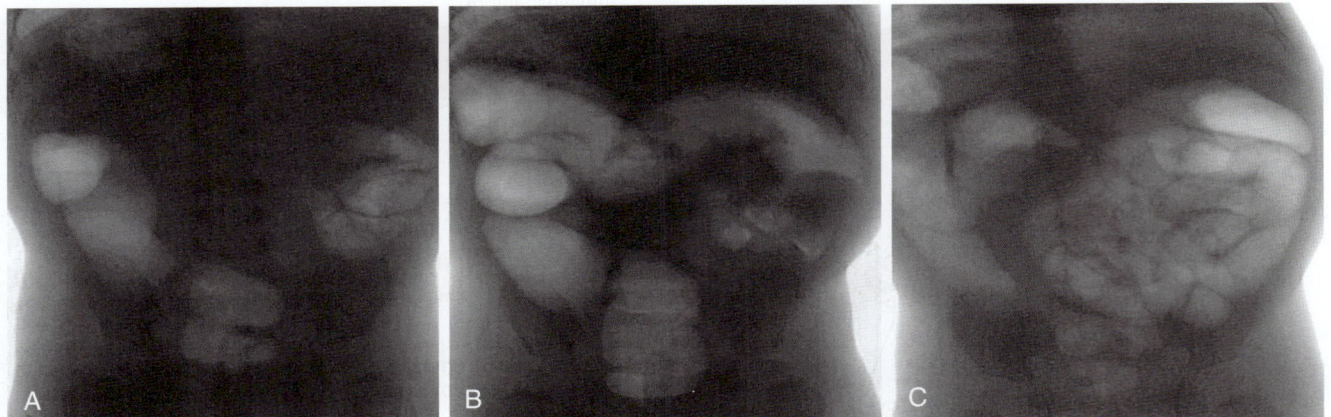

FIGURE 83.29 Reduction of ileocolic intussusception by air enema. Patient is prone. (A) At initiation of the air enema, air is seen to progress up the descending colon. There is a paucity of air in the proximal colon. (B) The intussusception is seen outlined by air. (C) Reflux of air into the terminal ileum confirms successful reduction.

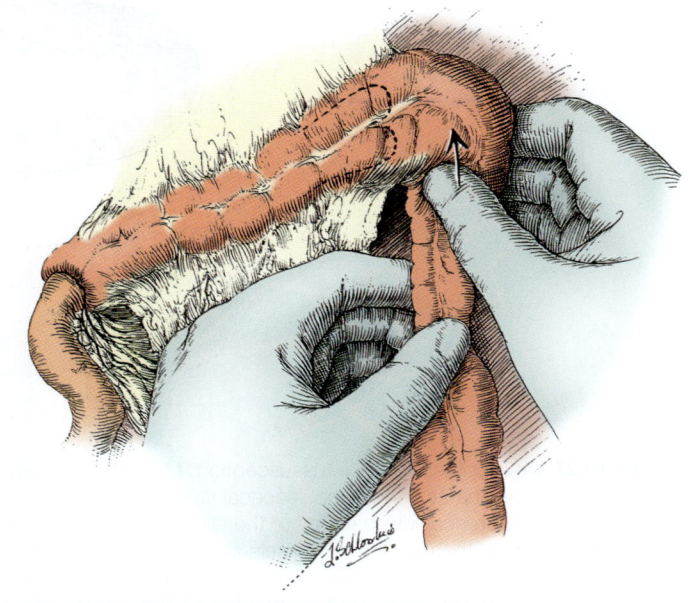

FIGURE 83.30 Manual reduction of intussusception. If a barium enema fails or intussusception is encountered during laparotomy for intestinal obstruction, manual reduction is required. The intestine is occluded immediately distal to the intussusception with the fingers of one hand and stripped proximally with the fingers of the other. In effect, this maneuver increases intraluminal pressure just as an enema does. The intestine should not be pulled. If reduction is not readily achieved, resection and anastomosis should be performed. *Arrow* depicts direction of proximal reduction of intussusception. (From Ravitch MM, Welch KJ, Benson CD, et al., eds. *Pediatric Surgery*. 3rd ed. Chicago: Year Book; 1979.)

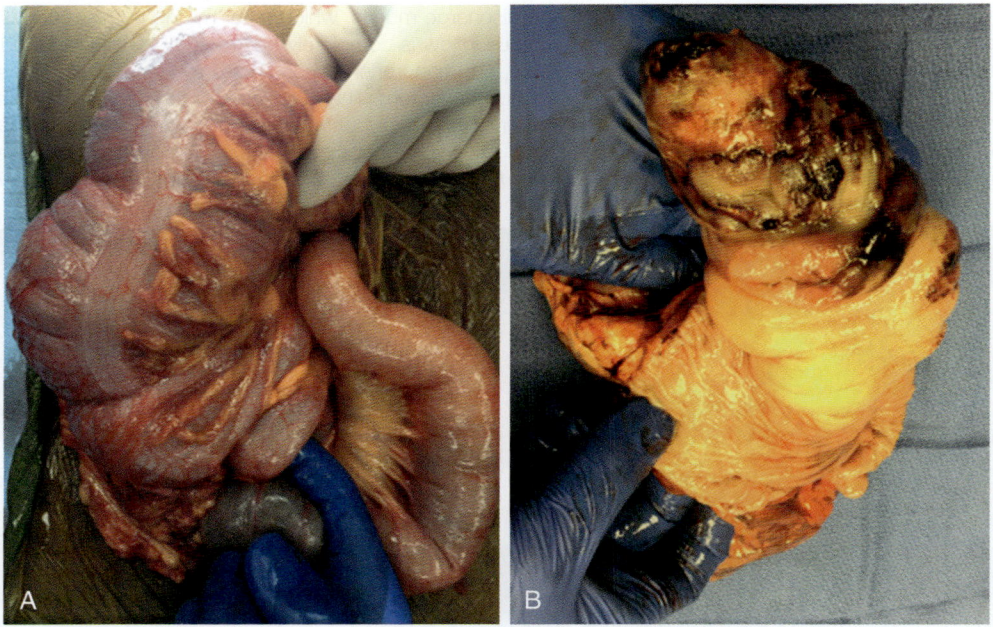

FIGURE 83.31 (A) Intraoperative photograph of ileocolic intussusception. The white-gloved hand marks the distal end of the intussusception. The blue-gloved finger is inside the proximal invagination of the intussusception. (B) Resection specimen with the intussuscipiens incised to reveal a necrotic intussusceptum.

REFERENCES

1. Applegate KE. Evidence-based diagnosis of malrotation and volvulus. *Pediatr Radiol.* 2009;39(suppl 2):S161-S163.
2. Skandalkis J, Gray S, Ricketts R. *Embryology for Surgeons.* Baltimore: Williams & Wilkins; 1994.
3. Mall FP. Development of the human intestine and its position in the adult. *Bull Johns Hopkins Hosp.* 1898;9:197.
4. Ladd WE. Surgical diseases of the alimentary tract in infants. *N Engl J Med.* 1936;215:705.
5. Skandalakis JE, Gray SW, Ricketts R, Richardson DD. The small intestines. In: Skandalakis JE, Gray SW, eds. *Embryology for Surgeons: The Embryological Basis for the Treatment of Congenital Anomalies.* 2nd ed. Baltimore: Williams & Wilkins; 1994:184.
6. Warnber B. *Surgery of Infants and Children: Scientific Principles and Practice.* Philadelphia: Lippincott-Raven; 1997.
7. Martin V, Shaw-Smith C. Review of genetic factors in intestinal malrotation. *Pediatr Surg Int.* 2010;26(8):769-781.
8. Warner BW. Malrotation. In: Oldham KT, Colombani PM, Foglia RP, eds. *Surgery of Infants and Children: Scientific Principles and Practice.* Philadelphia: Lipincott-Raven; 1997:1229.
9. Seashore JH, Touloukian RJ. Midgut volvulus. An ever-present threat. *Arch Pediatr Adolesc Med.* 1994;148(1):43-46.
10. Godbole P, Stringer MD. Bilious vomiting in the newborn: how often is it pathologic? *J Pediatr Surg.* 2002;37(6):909-911.
11. Penco JM, Murillo JC, Hernandez A, De La Calle Pato U, Masjoan DF, Aceituno FR. Anomalies of intestinal rotation and fixation: consequences of late diagnosis beyond two years of age. *Pediatr Surg Int.* 2007;23(8):723-730.
12. Graziano K, Islam S, Dasgupta R, et al. Asymptomatic malrotation: diagnosis and surgical management: an American Pediatric Surgical Association outcomes and evidence based practice committee systematic review. *J Pediatr Surg.* 2015;50(10):1783-1790.
13. Burjonrappa S, Crete E, Bouchard S. Comparative outcomes in intestinal atresia: a clinical outcome and pathophysiology analysis. *Pediatr Surg Int.* 2011;27(4):437-442.
14. Applebaum H, Sydorak R. Duodenal atresia and stenosis - annular pancreas. In: Coran AG, Adzick NS, Krummel TM, Laberge JM, Shamberger RC, Caldamone AA, eds. *Pediatric Surgery.* Vol. 2. 7th ed. Philadelphia: Elsevier; 2012:1051-1057.
15. Forrester MB, Merz RD. Population-based study of small intestinal atresia and stenosis, Hawaii, 1986–2000. *Public Health.* 2004;118(6): 434-438.
16. Morris G, Kennedy A Jr, Cochran W. Small bowel congenital anomalies: a review and update. *Curr Gastroenterol Rep.* 2016;18(4):16.
17. Davies MR, Louw JH, Cywes S, Rode H. The classification of congenital intestinal atresias. *J Pediatr Surg.* 1982;17(2):224.
18. Gosche JR, Vick L, Boulanger SC, Islam S. Midgut abnormalities. *Surg Clin North Am.* 2006;86(2):285-299, viii.
19. Ladd W. Surgical diseases of the alimentary tract in infants. *N Engl J Med.* 1936;215:705.
20. Phelps S, Fisher R, Partington A, Dykes E. Prenatal ultrasound diagnosis of gastrointestinal malformations. *J Pediatr Surg.* 1997;32(3): 438-440.
21. Roberts HE, Cragan JD, Cono J, Khoury MJ, Weatherly MR, Moore CA. Increased frequency of cystic fibrosis among infants with jejunoileal atresia. *Am J Med Genet.* 1998;78(5):446-449.
22. Hussain SM, Meradji M, Robben SG, Hop WC. Plain film diagnosis in meconium plug syndrome, meconium ileus and neonatal Hirschsprung's disease. A scoring system. *Pediatr Radiol.* 1991;21(8):556-559.
23. Coran A, Adzick S, Krummel T, Laberge J-M, Chamberger R, Caldamon A, eds. *Pediatric Surgery.* 7th ed. Philadelphia: Mosby; 2012.
24. Wang J, Du L, Cai W, Pan W, Yan W. Prolonged feeding difficulties after surgical correction of intestinal atresia: a 13-year experience. *J Pediatr Surg.* 2014;49(11):1593-1597.
25. Calisti A, Olivieri C, Coletta R, Briganti V, Oriolo L, Giannino G. Jejunoileal atresia: factors affecting the outcome and long-term sequelae. *J Clin Neonatol.* 2012;1(1):38-41.
26. Holcomb GW 3rd, Gheissari A, O'Neill JA Jr, Shorter NA, Bishop HC. Surgical management of alimentary tract duplications. *Ann Surg.* 1989;209(2):167-174.
27. Kurtz RJ, Heimann TM, Holt J, Beck AR. Mesenteric and retroperitoneal cysts. *Ann Surg.* 1986;203(1):109-112.
28. Hur J, Yoon CS, Kim MJ, Kim OH. Imaging features of gastrointestinal tract duplications in infants and children: from oesophagus to rectum. *Pediatr Radiol.* 2007;37(7):691-699.
29. O'Donnell PL, Morrow JB, Fitzgerald TL. Adult gastric duplication cysts: a case report and review of literature. *Am Surg.* 2005;71(6):522-525.
30. Clatworthy HW Jr, Howard WH, Lloyd J. The meconium plug syndrome. *Surgery.* 1956;39(1):131-142.
31. Keckler SJ, St Peter SD, Spilde TL, et al. Current significance of meconium plug syndrome. *J Pediatr Surg.* 2008;43(5):896-898.
32. Burge D, Drewett M. Meconium plug obstruction. *Pediatr Surg Int.* 2004;20(2):108-110.
33. Cuenca AG, Ali AS, Kays DW, Islam S. "Pulling the plug"—management of meconium plug syndrome in neonates. *J Surg Res.* 2012;175(2):e43-e46.
34. Kao SC, Franken EA Jr. Nonoperative treatment of simple meconium ileus: a survey of the Society for Pediatric Radiology. *Pediatr Radiol.* 1995;25(2):97-100.
35. Winfield RD, Beierle EA. Pediatric surgical issues in meconium disease and cystic fibrosis. *Surg Clin North Am.* 2006;86(2):317-327, viii-ix.
36. Farrelly PJ, Charlesworth C, Lee S, Southern KW, Baillie CT. Gastrointestinal surgery in cystic fibrosis: a 20-year review. *J Pediatr Surg.* 2014;49(2):280-283.
37. Yahchouchy EK, Marano AF, Etienne JC, Fingerhut AL. Meckel's diverticulum. *J Am Coll Surg.* 2001;192(5):658-662.
38. Cullen JJ, Kelly KA, Moir CR, Hodge DO, Zinsmeister AR, Melton LJ 3rd. Surgical management of Meckel's diverticulum. An epidemiologic, population-based study. *Ann Surg.* 1994;220(4):564-568; discussion 568-569.
39. Gaisie G, Curnes JT, Scatliff JH, Croom RD, Vanderzalm T. Neonatal intestinal obstruction from omphalomesenteric duct remnants. *AJR Am J Roentgenol.* 1985;144(1):109-112.
40. Suh M, Lee HY, Jung K, Kim SE. Diagnostic accuracy of Meckel scan with initial hemoglobin level to detect symptomatic Meckel diverticulum. *Eur J Pediatr Surg.* 2015;25(5):449-453.
41. Sinha CK, Pallewatte A, Easty M, et al. Meckel's scan in children: a review of 183 cases referred to two paediatric surgery specialist centres over 18 years. *Pediatr Surg Int.* 2013;29(5):511-517.
42. Ruscher KA, Fisher JN, Hughes CD, et al. National trends in the surgical management of Meckel's diverticulum. *J Pediatr Surg.* 2011;46(5):893-896.
43. Zani A, Eaton S, Rees CM, Pierro A. Incidentally detected Meckel diverticulum: to resect or not to resect? *Ann Surg.* 2008;247(2):276-281.
44. Touloukian RJ, Berdon WE, Amoury RA, Santulli TV. Surgical experience with necrotizing enterocolitis in the infant. *J Pediatr Surg.* 1967;2:389.
45. Neu J, Walker WA. Necrotizing enterocolitis. *N Engl J Med.* 2011;364(3):255-264.
46. Gordon PV. Understanding intestinal vulnerability to perforation in the extremely low birth weight infant. *Pediatr Res.* 2009;65(2):138-144.
47. Neu J, Chen M, Beierle E. Intestinal innate immunity: how does it relate to the pathogenesis of necrotizing enterocolitis. *Semin Pediatr Surg.* 2005;14(3):137-144.
48. Goldman AS, Ogra PL. Anti-infectious and infectious agents in human milk. In: Ogra PL, Mestecky J, Lamm ME, eds. *Mucosal Immunology.* Vol. 1. San Diego: Academic Press; 1999:72.
49. Elgin TG, Kern SL, McElroy SJ. Development of the neonatal intestinal microbiome and its association with necrotizing enterocolitis. *Clin Ther.* 2016;38(4):706-715.
50. Heida FH, van Zoonen AG, Hulscher JB, et al. A necrotizing enterocolitis-associated gut microbiota is present in the meconium: results of a prospective study. *Clin Infect Dis.* 2016;62(7):863-870.
51. Martinez-Tallo E, Claure N, Bancalari E. Necrotizing enterocolitis in full-term or near-term infants: risk factors. *Biol Neonate.* 1997;71(5):292-298.
52. Dilli D, Suna Oguz S, Erol R, Ozkan-Ulu H, Dumanli H, Dilman U. Does abdominal sonography provide additional information over abdominal plain radiography for diagnosis of necrotizing enterocolitis in neonates? *Pediatr Surg Int.* 2011;27(3):321-327.
53. Sho S, Neal MD, Sperry J, Hackam DJ. A novel scoring system to predict the development of necrotizing enterocolitis totalis in premature infants. *J Pediatr Surg.* 2014;49(7):1053-1056.
54. Fitzgibbons SC, Ching Y, Yu D, et al. Mortality of necrotizing enterocolitis expressed by birth weight categories. *J Pediatr Surg.* 2009;44(6):1072-1075; discussion 1075-1076.
55. Hunter CJ, Chokshi N, Ford HR. Evidence vs experience in the surgical management of necrotizing enterocolitis and focal intestinal perforation. *J Perinatol.* 2008;28(suppl 1):S14-S17.

56. Blakely ML, Gupta H, Lally KP. Surgical management of necrotizing enterocolitis and isolated intestinal perforation in premature neonates. *Semin Perinatol*. 2008;32(2):122-126.

57. Hintz SR, Kendrick DE, Stoll BJ, et al. Neurodevelopmental and growth outcomes of extremely low birth weight infants after necrotizing enterocolitis. *Pediatrics*. 2005;115(3):696-703.

58. Ein SH, Shandling B, Wesson D, Filler RM. A 13-year experience with peritoneal drainage under local anesthesia for necrotizing enterocolitis perforation. *J Pediatr Surg*. 1990;25(10):1034-1036; discussion 1036-1037.

59. Rees CM, Eaton S, Kiely EM, Wade AM, McHugh K, Pierro A. Peritoneal drainage or laparotomy for neonatal bowel perforation? A randomized controlled trial. *Ann Surg*. 2008;248(1):44-51.

60. Moss RL, Dimmitt RA, Barnhart DC, et al. Laparotomy versus peritoneal drainage for necrotizing enterocolitis and perforation. *N Engl J Med*. 2006;354(21):2225-2234.

61. Sola JE, Tepas JJ 3rd, Koniaris LG. Peritoneal drainage versus laparotomy for necrotizing enterocolitis and intestinal perforation: a meta-analysis. *J Surg Res*. 2010;161(1):95-100.

62. Jakaitis BM, Bhatia AM. Definitive peritoneal drainage in the extremely low birth weight infant with spontaneous intestinal perforation: predictors and hospital outcomes. *J Perinatol*. 2015;35(8):607-611.

63. Rao SC, Basani L, Simmer K, Samnakay N, Deshpande G. Peritoneal drainage versus laparotomy as initial surgical treatment for perforated necrotizing enterocolitis or spontaneous intestinal perforation in preterm low birth weight infants. *Cochrane Database Syst Rev*. 2011; (6):CD006182.

64. Meier DE, Coln CD, Rescorla FJ, OlaOlorun A, Tarpley JL. Intussusception in children: international perspective. *World J Surg*. 1996;20(8):1035-1039; discussion 1040.

65. Applegate KE. Intussusception in children: evidence-based diagnosis and treatment. *Pediatr Radiol*. 2009;39(suppl 2):S140-S143.

66. Guo JZ, Ma XY, Zhou QH. Results of air pressure enema reduction of intussusception: 6396 cases in 13 years. *J Pediatr Surg*. 1986;21(12): 1201-1203.

67. Liu KW, MacCarthy J, Guiney EJ, Fitzgerald RJ. Intussusception—current trends in management. *Arch Dis Child*. 1986;61(1):75-77.

68. Bonnard A, Demarche M, Dimitriu C, et al. Indications for laparoscopy in the management of intussusception: a multicenter retrospective study conducted by the French Study Group for Pediatric Laparoscopy (GECI). *J Pediatr Surg*. 2008;43(7):1249-1253.

Ileostomy

Vikram B. Reddy | Walter E. Longo

Ileostomy is an intestinal stoma fashioned from the distal small intestine. Although the creation of an ileostomy can be the smallest part of a larger surgery, the stoma can have the most significant physical and psychosocial effect on a patient.[1-6] Despite an eventual return to a prior quality of life and activity level, body image and sexual function do not change over time. A well-constructed ileostomy can be lifesaving with minimal adverse effect on the quality of life, when constructed after careful counseling of the patient, preoperative planning, excellent technique, and valuable postoperative enterostomal therapy. Even after a well-constructed ileostomy, recognition and prevention of postoperative dehydration due to the liquid output is imperative to prevent pouching problems, electrolyte abnormalities, and even renal failure.

HISTORY

Stoma is derived from the Greek word *stomat,* meaning mouth or opening. Spontaneous small bowel stomas from abdominal trauma or incarcerated hernias with subsequent survival ensured the possibility of stomas as lifesaving procedures. Although reports of colostomies existed throughout the 18th century with the first report by Littre in 1710,[7] small intestinal stomas were successfully applied more commonly in the 20th century. Baum in Germany recorded the first ileostomy in 1879 in a patient with an obstructing right colon cancer. In 1888 Maydl from Vienna reported on the successful use of exteriorization of a loop of small or large bowel and suspension over the abdominal wall by a rubber rod through a defect in the mesentery.[8]

Both in Europe and the United States the successful role of enterostomy to relieve abdominal distention gained acceptance. Initially, ileostomies, as described by Brown in 1913,[9] were primarily associated with surgical relief from ulcerative colitis, dysentery, tuberculosis, and large bowel obstruction. However, the use of an ileostomy, even for ulcerative colitis, was met with disdain, whereas other procedures, even those involving ileosigmoid anastomoses, were favored.[10] It was not until the 1940s that the justified and inevitable role of an ileostomy in the management of ulcerative colitis was accepted at major institutions.[11-15] In 1931 Rankin described staged proctocolectomy with ileostomy for the management of ulcerative colitis and polyposis.[16] The initial staged ileostomy was created through a McBurney incision, division of the ileum close to the ileocecal valve, and exteriorization of the proximal end with a clamp on the end for 2 days. Bargen et al.,[17] working on Rankin's technique, replaced the clamp with a small drainage catheter in the exteriorized ileostomy. Although he noted immediate convalescence, significant fluid losses from the ileostomy requiring drastic fluid resuscitation were required. Similar fluid and electrolyte losses were noted by Cattell and Sachs[18] and Cave and Nickel,[19] with the latter reporting a 33% mortality following an ileostomy. Despite the initial success, ileostomy creation was associated with significant morbidity due to the peristomal skin irritation from the small bowel effluent. Lahey later described the morbidity and the mortality associated with ileostomies.[13]

Warren and McKittrick of Massachusetts General Hospital reported in 1951 on the outcome of 210 patients with ulcerative colitis managed by an ileostomy between 1930 and 1949.[20] They coined ileostomy dysfunction and characterized it as "cramp-like pain and, paradoxically, increase in the volume of ileostomy discharge," which in severe cases can lead to emesis and watery diarrhea with significant loss of fluids and electrolytes leading to a shocklike state. Unfortunately, these symptoms were noted in 62% of the patients. They also observed that early dysfunction was due to the peristaltic activity against the rigid abdominal wall, whereas late dysfunction was due to cicatrizing granulation tissue on the serosa of exteriorized ileostomy. Symptomatic relief was achieved with catheter decompression, which was required in a third of all ileostomy patients and in more than half of all patients with ileostomy dysfunction.

Crile and Turnbull summarized ileostomy dysfunction as the sequelae of peritonitis of the protruding ileostomy that causes a functional obstruction.[21] They noted spontaneous maturation over 4 to 6 weeks by eversion of the mucosa to the abdominal wall. Several procedures to combat the serositis, and thus ameliorate ileostomy dysfunction, were proposed: skin grafting the ileostomy as described by Dragstedt et al.,[22] fasciocutaneous grafting by Monroe and Olwin,[23] and mucosal grafting by Turnbull and Crile.[24] However, the most technically facile procedure was described by chance by Brooke of the University of Birmingham in 1952 and involved the evagination of the ileal end and suturing of the mucosa to the skin.[15] To this day, the so-called Brooke ileostomy remains the standard technique for constructing an ileostomy.

INDICATIONS

Although ileostomies were initially used after proctocolectomy (for ulcerative colitis and polyposis) or the relief of obstruction, their use has evolved over the years in numerous disease processes. Etiologies include functional, hemorrhagic, infectious, inflammatory, ischemic, malignant, or mechanical. Their indications are better described by their permanence: permanent, temporary, or protecting, as shown in Table 84.1.

PERMANENT

An end ileostomy is usually indicated in situations in which the disease process affects the entire colon and

TABLE 84.1 Indications for Ileostomy

Type	Surgical Procedure and Disease Process
Permanent	Proctocolectomy with end ileostomy
	• Crohn disease
	• Ulcerative colitis
	• Polyposis (familial adenomatous polyposis, Lynch syndrome, etc.)
	Total colectomy or proctocolectomy with end ileostomy
	• Colonic dysmotility with poor anorectal function
	• Neurogenic bowel
Temporary	Colectomy with ileostomy
	• Crohn disease with subsequent ileorectal anastomosis
	• Ulcerative colitis as the first stage of ileal pouch anal anastomosis
	• *Clostridium difficile* colitis
	• Gastrointestinal hemorrhage
	Partial colectomy with ileostomy
	• Right colon perforation/obstruction in immunocompromised or morbidly ill
	• Ileocolonic ischemia
Diverting	Colorectal anastomosis
	• Low anastomosis
	• Radiation
	• High-risk patient
	Ileal pouch anal anastomosis

rectum or the functional status of a patient precludes an anastomosis. Currently, a permanent ileostomy is used in the management of severe proctocolitis due to ulcerative colitis[25,26] or Crohn disease (especially with significant perianal disease),[27] familial adenomatous polyposis (FAP), and functional disorders, such as colonic dysmotility (with poor anorectal function)[28,29] and neurogenic bowel.[30]

TEMPORARY

A functional end ileostomy is fashioned after a segmental or total colectomy for a disease process that spares the distal colon or rectum and allows for a delayed reestablishment of intestinal continuity. This is encountered in patients with fulminant or toxic Crohn colitis or ulcerative colitis, *Clostridium difficile* colitis,[31] uncontrolled lower gastrointestinal bleeding without a clear source, ischemia involving the ileocolic pedicle, or malignant obstruction involving the ascending colon or small bowel in the setting of immunosuppression where an anastomosis may not be prudent.

DIVERTING

In some disease processes, a proximal diversion with a loop ileostomy may be necessary as the first of a series of staged interventions or for protection of a distal anastomosis. The role of diverting loop ileostomies have been extensively studied with low anastomoses in rectal cancer[32] and with ileal pouch anal anastomoses.[33–36]

Diverting loop ileostomies have been used to diminish the complications of a distal anastomotic leak, especially in the pelvis or in high-risk patients. In immuno-compromised or malnourished patients, anastomoses that can otherwise be safely performed may also need fecal diversion. Although fecal diversion with an ileostomy may not diminish the risk of an anastomotic leak, the septic complications are significantly diminished and may avoid reoperation.[37]

Loop transverse colostomies were traditionally used for fecal diversion. This trend changed when Williams et al. performed a randomized controlled trial to compare the outcomes of a loop colostomy with a loop ileostomy and demonstrated that the incidence of prolapse, leakage, skin irritation, odor, and surgical site infection at the time of the ostomy closure were significantly lower with a loop ileostomy.[38] Multiple other meta-analyses have confirmed the significantly lower incidence of prolapse with a loop ileostomy and lower chance of wound infection and hernia formation after closure of a loop ileostomy as opposed to a loop colostomy.[39–43]

PHYSIOLOGY

In the absence of any intestinal disorders or resection, the small intestine is able to absorb most of the fluid that it is exposed to. Ninety percent of the nutrients and nearly 6 L of fluid are absorbed in the jejunum while the ileum can absorb the remaining 2.5 L, leading to a concentrated effluent into the colon, where an additional 1.5 L are absorbed. The transport of water is passive and requires movement of solutes. The rate of water absorption in different portions of the intestine is a function of the solute absorption in that segment of the bowel. Sodium absorption is more complex and involves both active and passive transport. In the jejunum, sodium is transferred out of the lumen by cotransport with active uptake of both carbohydrates and amino acids, whereas it is actively transported against an electrochemical gradient in the ileum. Bicarbonate ions facilitate the active transport of sodium out of the lumen against the electrochemical gradient. Bicarbonate uptake in the jejunum is by active transport, whereas its trafficking in the ileum depends on the intraluminal concentration. The majority of chloride ions follow sodium transport passively down the electrochemical gradient. Potassium ion movement into the lumen is also passive down the electrochemical gradient.

Vitamin B_{12} and bile salts are absorbed in the terminal ileum. Without ileal reabsorption, hepatic synthesis of bile salts would not be sufficient for fat digestion. Lack of absorption of bile salts can lead to profound diarrhea by causing fluid and electrolyte secretion into the lumen and impairing colonic absorption of water and sodium. Serum vitamin B_{12} levels remain normal unless more than 100 cm of terminal ileum has been removed.

Interestingly, the ileum aids in slowing the transit and allows for absorption proximally. The transit time of the first 50% is one-third of the ileum.[44] Consequently ileal resection can lead to shortened transit time and increased output, whereas resection of an equivalent segment of jejunum may not have an effect on transit time.

Ileostomy volume in the absence of proximal bowel loss can vary among individuals with output greater than 1.5 L, concerning for diarrhea and possibly fluid and electrolyte derangement. Ileostomies empty in small volumes constantly, with increase in output after meals. Different foods have different transit times, and this may vary even among individuals, even for the same food.

Normal ileostomy output is almost isotonic with normal saline, and sodium loss is significantly more than with normal stool. Fluctuations in sodium resorption with food intake are also noted. With intake of hypotonic solutions, fluid output in the ileostomy decreases to allow for sodium reabsorption, whereas excessive salt intake causes watery effluent.[45] Water intake has no effect on output, with increased intake increasing urine output only.

In addition, normal ileostomy effluent carries a significantly higher quantity of bacteria, mainly coliform organisms.[46] The effluent also contains a significant quantity of proteolytic enzymes that can damage exposed skin.

The incidence of cholelithiasis increases from 5% at 5 years after ileostomy formation to approximately 50% after 15 years. This worsens in the presence of ileal resection and by decreased solubility of cholesterol with a reduction in the bile salt pool.[47] The situation is further worsened in patients with ileal Crohn disease.[48] Renal conservation of sodium and water in the setting of an ileostomy leads to acidic urine, which may contribute to a high incidence of uric acid and calcium stones.[49]

PREOPERATIVE CONSIDERATIONS

An ileostomy can be a very effective method of fecal diversion and is compatible with an excellent quality of life. However, the placement of the ileostomy is paramount. The ileostomy should be placed in a location that is convenient for the patient to see and manage with minimal hindrance of movement and difficulty in disguising it with clothing (Fig. 84.1). Counseling and consultation with an enterostomal therapist or an ostomate of similar age, gender, and disease process may need to be arranged. The United Ostomy Association (www.ostomy.org) has extensive material that may be a helpful resource.

There are several factors to consider when marking a stoma site preoperatively: the patient's occupation, clothing style, belt line, flexibility, abdominal wall contour in different positions, any physical disabilities, location of previous abdominal scars, bony prominences, and abdominal girth. The ideal location for most ileostomies is in the right lower quadrant away from any skin creases, bony prominences, or the midline incision. It is particularly important to avoid any location that will disrupt the skin-appliance seal with change in body position. Most often, the ideal location is in the infraumbilical fat mound overlying the rectus sheath. The ostomy site should be marked with the patient standing or supine, bending, and sitting.[50] Location of the stoma at the belt line should be avoided. Although desirable, creation of an ileostomy below the belt line to facilitate hiding of the stoma may not be feasible in the obese or those with a history of prior ostomies. In the obese patient, a stoma in the upper quadrants where there will be less abdominal wall fat may be a more suitable location. In patients with a history of prior abdominal procedures, several stoma sites should be marked with notation made of the most to least preferred sites. The sites should be noted with a marking pen, making an "X"

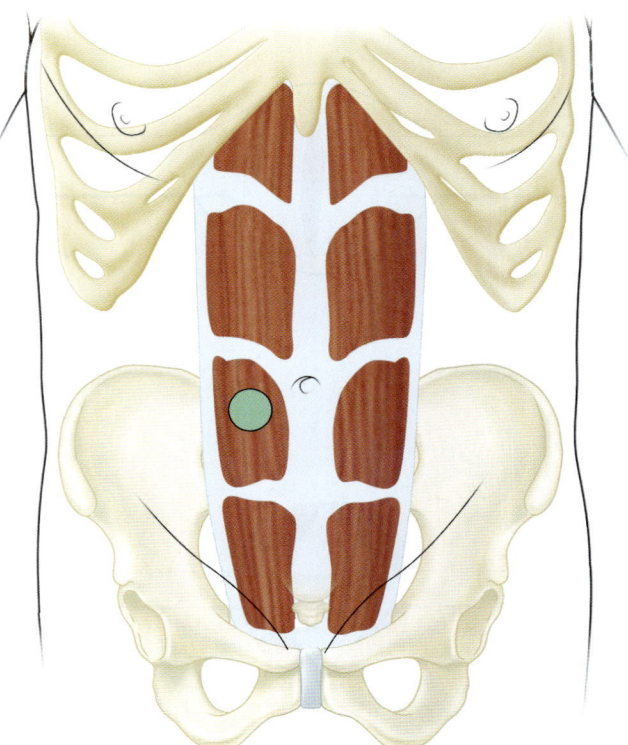

FIGURE 84.1 Siting of an ileostomy.

and a number next to it indicating the preference of the site. This should be covered with a translucent occlusive dressing. Alternatively, subcutaneous injection of methylene blue can be used to achieve a more permanent marking of the abdominal wall, although this is seldom needed. After the patient has been anesthetized for the surgery, a 27-gauge needle can be used to mark the skin at the site of the "X" after removing the occlusive dressing.

SURGICAL TECHNIQUE

Creation of an ileostomy (Fig. 84.2), irrespective of the nature of the stoma, begins with mobilization of the selected segment of bowel to reach beyond the abdominal wall at the site of the stoma marking. Corresponding to the size of the bowel to be used for the stoma, a 1.5- to 2-cm circumferential incision is placed in the skin and extended through the subcutaneous tissues, down to the anterior rectus fascia. During open surgery, Kocher clamps are placed on the edge of the fascia to allow alignment of the layers of the abdominal wall during stoma creation. A vertical incision is then placed; the underlying rectus muscle fibers are visualized and split along the length of the fibers to expose the posterior rectus sheath. Care is taken to avoid any injury to the epigastric vessels, which, if unintentionally injured, can be ligated. A transverse incision is placed on the anterior rectus sheath to create a cruciate opening. The posterior rectus sheath and the underlying peritoneum are divided as one while avoiding any injury to the underlying bowel. In open surgery, a laparotomy pad can be placed underneath the peritoneum

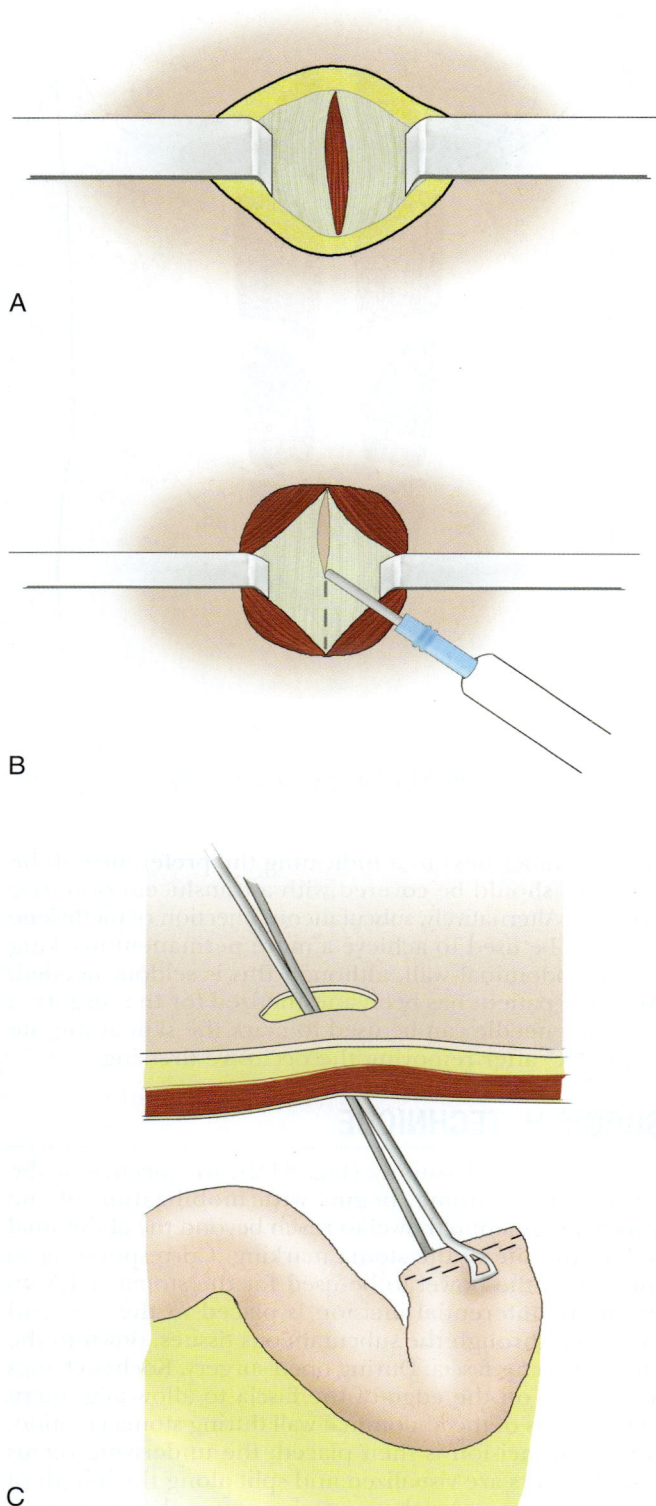

during its division, while in a laparoscopy, pneumoperitoneum can be maintained while entry is made into the abdominal cavity. The created hole should allow passage of two fingers. However, this may vary with the habitus of the patient and the edema of the bowel wall. A larger opening may lead to a parastomal hernia but may be preferable with edematous bowel or with hemodynamic instability. A tight opening may cause ischemia and obstruction of the ileostomy. At this point, the mobilized small bowel should be exteriorized and examined for viability and tension. Care should be taken to avoid twisting of the mesentery. If the mesentery is floppy and appears to twist around the luminal axis, it should be tacked to the anterior abdominal wall with absorbable sutures. Viability of the exteriorized bowel can be entertained by visualizing the pink serosa, palpating the pulsatile flow in the immediate vicinity, examining the viable mucosa of the stoma, or by trimming the ileostomy edge to confirm bleeding. After adequate length to avoid creation of a flat stoma has been ensured, the abdominal wall can be closed and the stoma can be matured depending on the type of ileostomy. Absorbable sutures are commonly used to mature the stoma, and bites should be placed in the subcuticular area rather than the epidermis to prevent ectopic mucosal implants at the suture sites on the dermis, which can lead to mucous production and break in the appliance-skin seal.

END ILEOSTOMY

An end ileostomy is technically the easiest small bowel stoma to create due to the mobility of the small bowel mesentery (Fig. 84.3). The mobilized, well-vascularized stapled end of the small bowel is everted through the abdominal wall while avoiding any twisting of the mesentery. Thick or bulky mesentery may need debulking to facilitate eversion. The staple line is completely removed. Three to four full-thickness sutures (depending on the peristomal fat) can be placed through the edge of the stoma, a more proximal seromuscular bite approximately 4 to 6 cm proximal to the edge, and into the subcuticular area of the skin opening (tripartite bites). After the sutures are placed, they can be tied to evert the ileostomy. Multiple other absorbable sutures can then be placed between the full-thickness edge of the ileostomy and the subcuticular layer to complete the mucocutaneous junction. Some surgeons prefer to not place any sutures in the seromuscular layer and are still able to evert the stoma without difficulty. The finished end ileostomy should protrude approximately 2 to 3 cm above the skin surface to increase the distance of the effluent egress from the skin-appliance interface, thereby diminishing leaks and peristomal skin irritation.[51] Because most end ileostomies are often permanent or long term, care should be taken to avoid stomas that are flush or barely protrude above the skin because short ileostomies tend to leak ostomy effluent under the stoma flange and cause severe skin excoriation and weeping wounds with resultant pain and difficulty with pouching the stoma.[52]

DIVERTING LOOP ILEOSTOMY

A diverting loop ileostomy (Fig. 84.4) is typically used for fecal diversion after a proctectomy with ileoanal

FIGURE 84.2 Construction of an ileostomy. (A) Incising the fascia. (B) Splitting the rectus and dividing the posterior sheath and peritoneum. (C) Exteriorizing the small bowel.

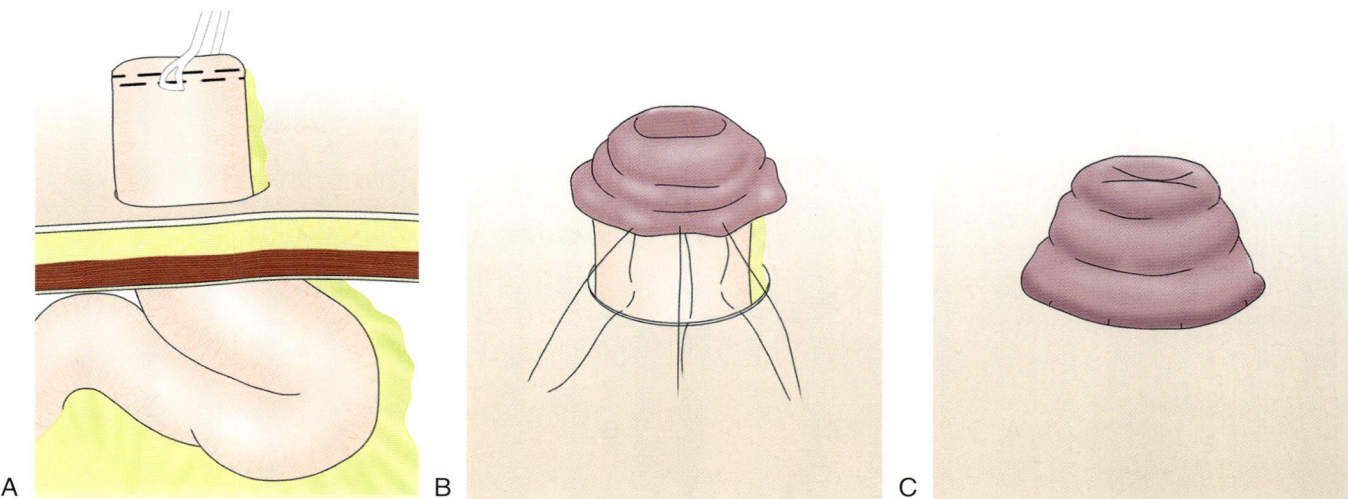

FIGURE 84.3 End ileostomy. (A) Configuration of the end ileostomy. (B) Eversion with tripartite sutures. (C) Completed end Brooke ileostomy.

pouch or a low anterior resection with a low colorectal or coloanal anastomosis. Compared with a loop colostomy, a loop ileostomy has a higher risk of dehydration and obstruction after takedown but a lower risk of prolapse or wound infection at the time of takedown.[42] The takedown of a loop ileostomy is also technically much easier (Fig. 84.5).

The loop stoma is created by mobilizing a loop of ileum, making an opening in the abdominal wall slightly larger than would be anticipated for an end ileostomy, and subsequently exteriorizing the mobilized loop with knowledge of the direction of luminal flow (this can be marked with sutures or with ink on the antimesenteric border). A mesenteric defect is made, and a stoma rod is then placed. This defect can also be made prior to the mobilization, and a Penrose drain or umbilical tape can be placed to aid in the externalization of the loop for maturation as a stoma. The remaining fascial openings and skin are closed prior to proceeding with the maturation of the ileostomy. Cautery is used to divide the antimesenteric wall of the ileum close to the efferent limb at the level of the stoma bridge. This opening is created from one mesenteric edge to the other. The defunctional limb is matured first with interrupted sutures between the edge of the ileostomy and less than a third of the circumference of the subcuticular layer of the abdominal opening. The proximal limb is matured by taking a full-thickness bite through the edge of the stoma and attaching it to the subcuticular layer (with or without a proximal seromuscular bite) to create an everted bud. The functional limb should occupy the majority (75%) of the skin opening, and a well-constructed loop ileostomy can completely divert the fecal stream while allowing reflux of the downstream secretions via the defunctionalized limb. Interrupted absorbable sutures can be placed in between the tripartite everting sutures to complete the mucocutaneous junction. Wrapping the ileostomy with a sheet of sodium hyaluronate can decrease the adhesions at the time of the ileostomy takedown.[53,54]

END-LOOP ILEOSTOMY

Indications for a loop-end ileostomy include obese patient with a short mesentery or a thick abdominal wall, or conversion of a loop ileostomy to an end ileostomy (Fig. 84.6). The bowel is mobilized to the maximal extent possible, and the bowel is transected with a stapler. While the vascularity of the mobilized loop is maintained, a segment of bowel on the mobilized loop attaining the maximal elevation above the skin is selected. The orientation of the bowel and the mesentery is maintained similar to the technique of a loop ileostomy. The stoma is matured in a similar fashion to the loop ileostomy with the functional limb occupying most of the abdominal wall circumference. A support rod can also be placed under the bowel, and this can alleviate the tension at the mucocutaneous junction, which would otherwise be noted with an end ileostomy.

LAPAROSCOPY

Laparoscopic loop ileostomy was first described by Khoo et al. in 1993.[55] The technique is similar to open surgery. After pneumoperitoneum has been attained and the resection, if needed, has been carried out, an abdominal wall opening is created at a preselected site. Often, a port can be placed at the preselected site, and this can be enlarged. A wound retractor is placed, and with the aid of a laparoscopic locking atraumatic bowel grasper, the selected loop of bowel is directed to the opening. A Babcock clamp is used to externalize the selected bowel while maintaining orientation and avoiding any twisting of the mesentery. The stoma is matured as previously described. Single-port surgery is also feasible and will avoid additional incisions.[56,57]

DIFFICULT ILEOSTOMY

Patient characteristics that predict a difficult ileostomy include obesity, emergency surgery, inflammatory bowel disease, or a history of multiple abdominal surgeries.

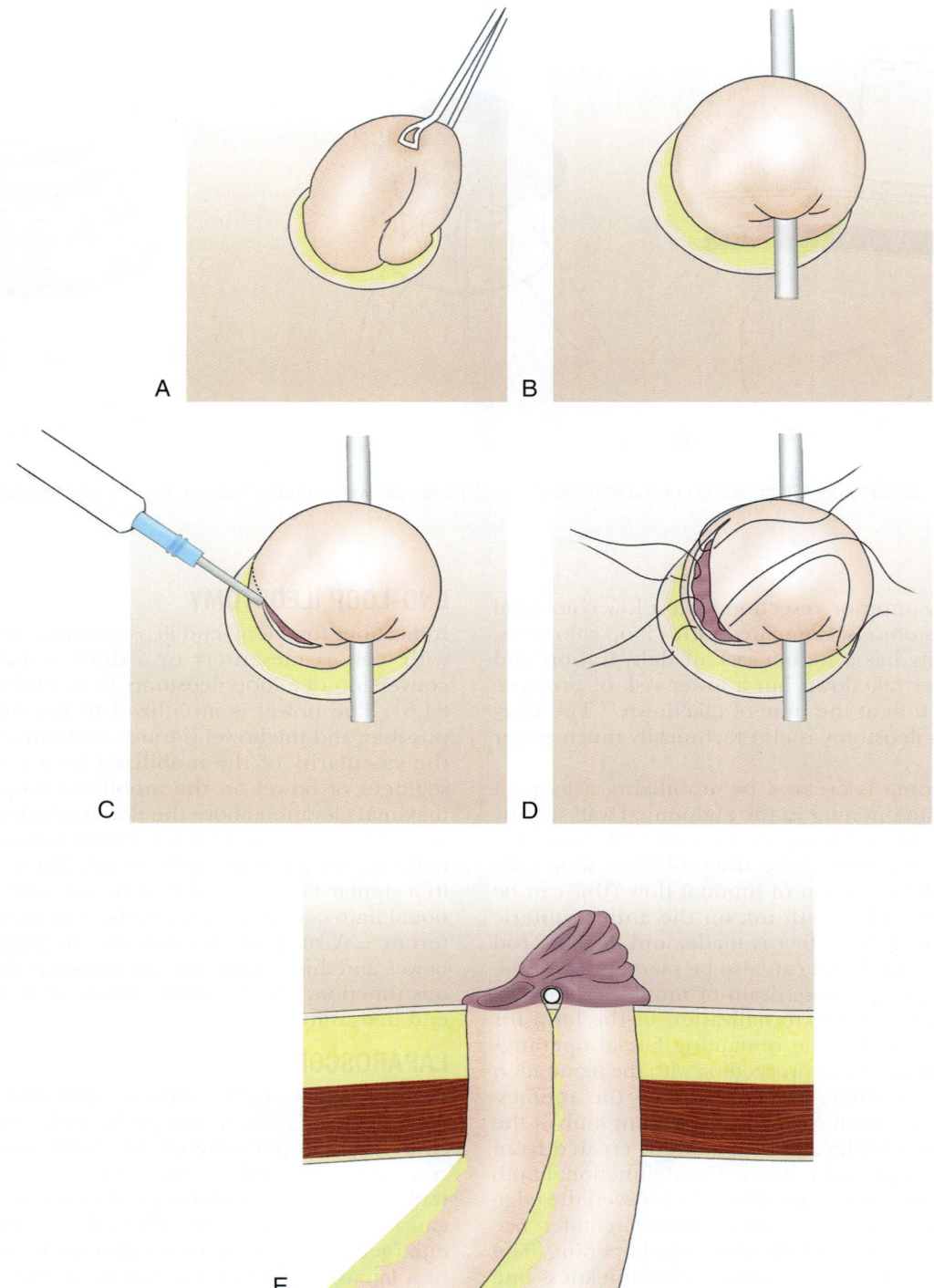

FIGURE 84.4 Loop ileostomy. (A) Exteriorization of a loop. (B) Placement of a bridge in the mesentery. (C) Incising the bowel. (D) Maturation of the limbs (simple for the defunctionalized limb, and tripartite for the functional Brooke ileostomy). (E) Completed loop ileostomy.

Intraoperatively, length and quality of the bowel and the associated mesentery dictates the ease of construction of an ileostomy. Elevated body mass index (BMI), large pannus, foreshortened or thickened mesentery (inflammatory bowel disease), mesenteric fibrosis, intraabdominal adhesions, or inflammation, and extent of the residual small bowel will have an impact on the ease of stoma creation.

The most common problem encountered in a difficult stoma is the reach of the terminal portion of the small bowel to and beyond the abdominal wall. The following maneuvers may be attempted to allow for reach:

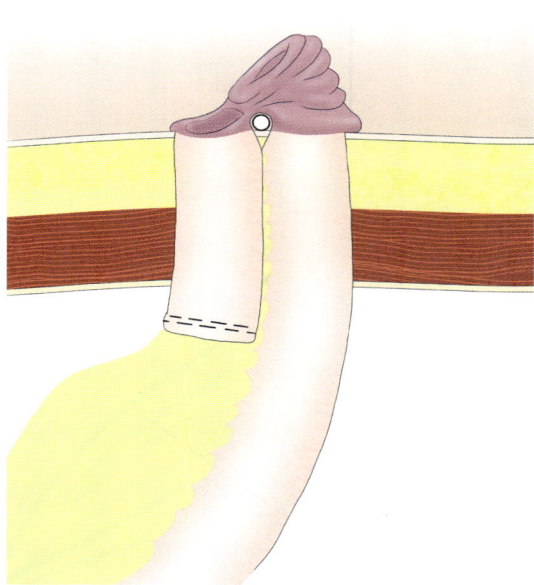

FIGURE 84.5 End-loop ileostomy.

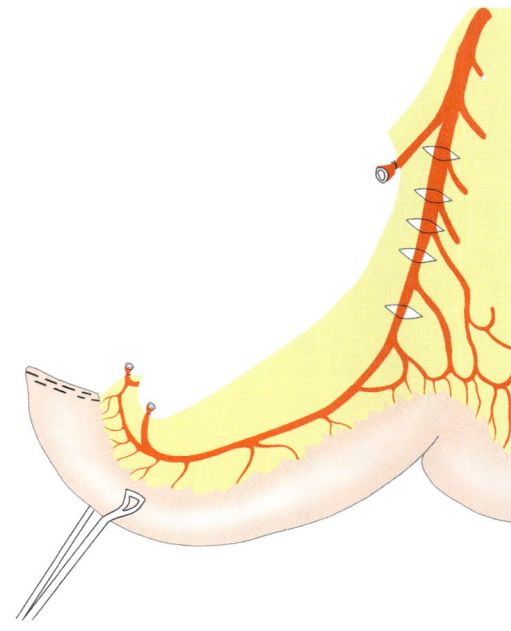

FIGURE 84.7 Pedicled ileostomy.

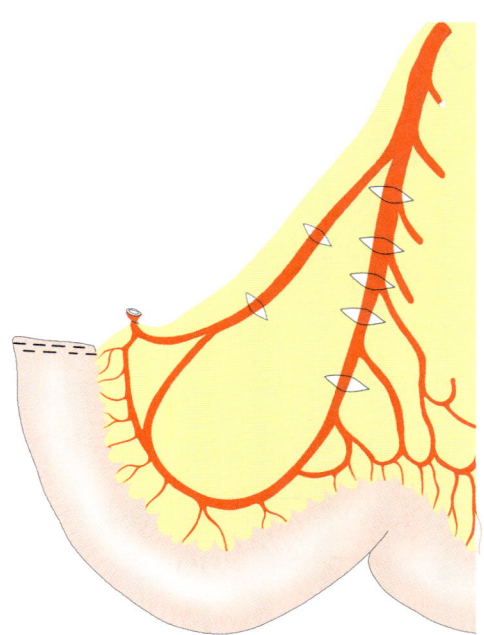

FIGURE 84.6 Mesenteric lengthening.

- Division of the terminal ileum close to the ileocecal valve.
- Division of the ileocolic pedicle at its origin while carefully avoiding damage to the ileal branches.
- Mobilization of the ileal mesentery to and over the duodenum. Further length can be obtained by kocherizing the duodenum.
- Placement of the ileostomy in the upper abdominal wall where the subcutaneous adiposity is generally lower and may also facilitate better visualization of the stoma.

- Exteriorization of the mobilized bowel through a lubricated wound retractor (Alexis wound retractor, Applied Medical, Rancho Santa Margarita, California) to avoid any traction injury on the vasculature of the bowel or accidental trauma to the bowel wall.
- Incising the peritoneal lining of the mesentery perpendicular to the mesenteric vessels on both sides of the mesentery (Fig. 84.7). In a bulky mesentery, clearing the mesenteric fat while avoiding the vascular pedicles may provide a little more length.
- The stoma can be pedicalized (Fig. 84.8) by dividing the arcade off the superior mesenteric artery while maintaining the collateral flow and the branches close to the wall of the bowel.
- Creation of an end-loop ileostomy as described before.
- A loop-end ileostomy may be advisable rather than a loop ileostomy.[58] The mobilized bowel loop is delivered through the abdominal wall trephine, and the bowel is divided at the most mobile ileal site. The afferent limb is then matured in the usual fashion after dividing the mesentery. The efferent limb can be brought out through the same opening or through another smaller opening on the skin, and the antimesenteric portion of the staple line is removed, and this is sutured to the subcuticular area. If this is not feasible, the afferent limb can be left stapled off below the fascia as long as there is no risk of a distal obstruction.[59]
- Use of mesenteric support rods at the fascia. Usually support rods are placed in the mesenteric defect above the skin but, with a difficult ileostomy, may not prevent retraction or splitting the ileostomy. A mesenteric support rod can be placed below the subcutaneous tissues at the level of the anterior rectus sheath while maintaining the support rod exit sites lateral to the stoma appliance interface on the skin.

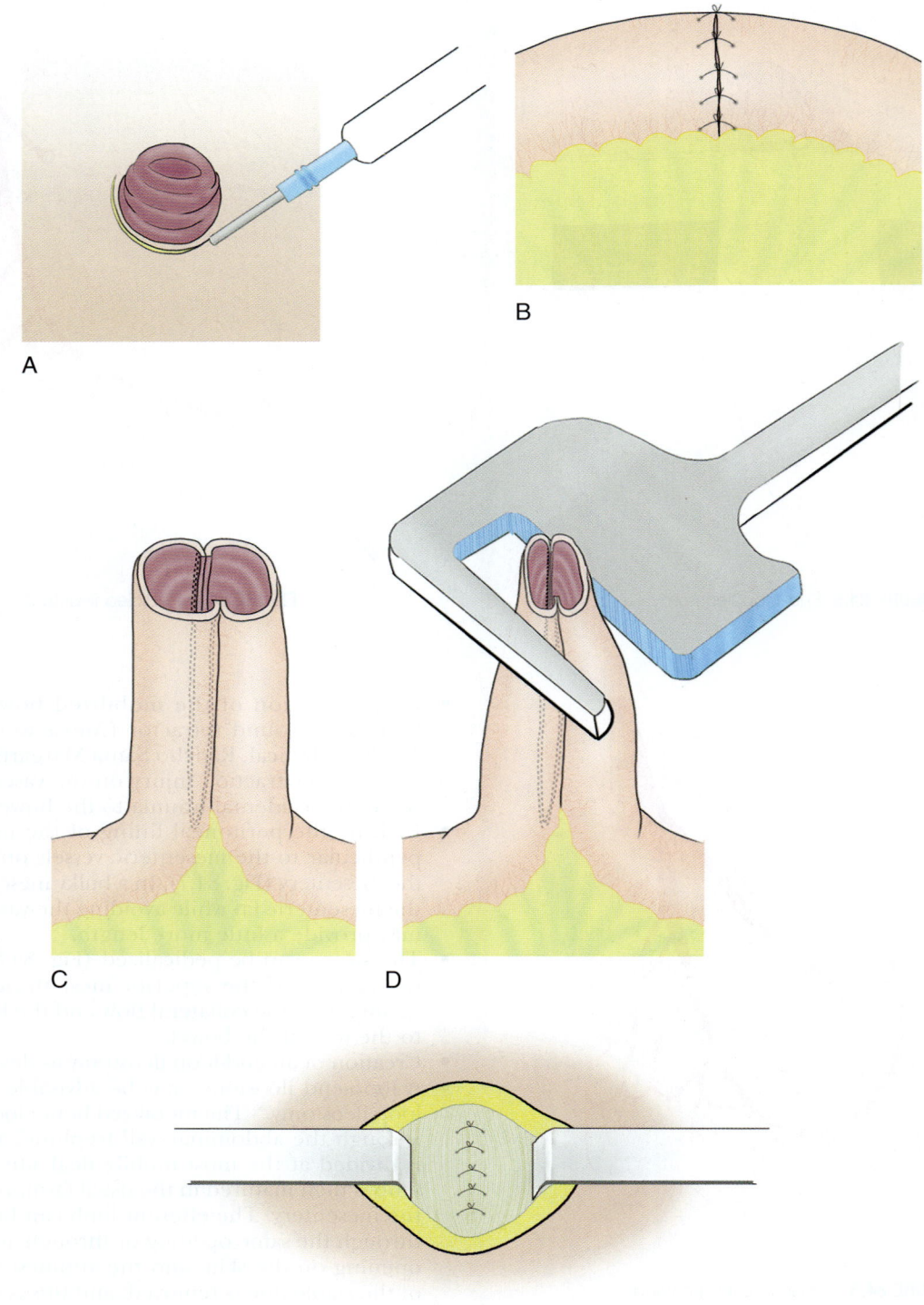

FIGURE 84.8 Loop ileostomy closure. (A) Taking down the mucocutaneous junction. (B) Handsewn closure. (C) Stapled side-to-side anastomosis. (D) Closure of the common channel. (E) Fascial closure.

- Modified abdominoplasty or abdominal wall contouring may be used in the morbidly obese.[60,61]

Another difficulty that could be encountered is with the eversion and maturation of the stoma. The following solutions may be applicable:

- Suture the seromuscular wall to the subcuticular area without exerting the ileal mucosa. The resulting serositis will eventually constrict the stoma, but this can be eventually revised.
- Crile and Turnbull technique for construction of the ileostomy.[24] The serosa and the muscularis of the distal portion of the ileostomy are dissected off, and the resulting mucosal cuff is everted and sutured to the subcuticular layer of the opening.

POSTOPERATIVE CARE

A newly created ileostomy is often edematous and will shrink over the next 4 to 6 weeks. Initially, the stoma output is serosanguinous, lacks any particulate matter, and has been traditionally called *bowel sweat*. As the stoma starts to function, dark green bilious output is noted, and as the diet is advanced, particulate matter appears in the effluent. The exodus of the retained bowel contents from the postoperative ileus can lead to initial voluminous output, which slowly tapers over time. Dehydration is of concern in the early postoperative period and studies have shown readmission rates of 17% to 20%,[62,63] with one study showing renal failure in 8.9%[62] of those with ileostomies. Patient education, visiting nurse care, stoma output logs, and early follow-up have shown to decrease the incidence of readmissions for dehydration.[51]

Patient and caregiver education to manage the stoma and troubleshoot the appliance should be undertaken as soon as possible in the postoperative period. However, most ostomates are only able to empty their appliances at the time of discharge and will require education and troubleshooting with assistance from visiting nurse care. Postoperative education is crucial to care for the stoma, troubleshoot problems with the stoma and the appliance, and improve quality of life with the stoma. Enlisting a Wound, Ostomy and Continence Nurses (WOCN)-certified nurse to assist in the perioperative care of the patient will decrease ostomy-related distress and improve quality of life.[51] Over the long term, periodic consultation with an enterostomal therapist and attendance at support groups will improve the quality of life of the patients.

COMPLICATIONS

Complications from the construction of an ileostomy can be numerous, as was described by numerous authors in the surgical evolution of stoma formation. Complications in ileostomy patients can be noted in more than 70%.[64] Stoma height (<2 cm), female gender, advanced BMI, young age, loop ileostomy, malignancy, and emergent surgery have been associated with increase in postoperative complications.[52] They can be classified as early (within 30 days) or late. Most early complications are due to technical issues with the construction of the ileostomy that can result in peristomal skin irritation, ischemia, retraction, or mucocutaneous separation. Unfortunately, significant diarrhea despite a perfectly constructed ileostomy is often prevalent (20%) in the early postoperative period. Prolapse, stenosis, and parastomal hernia are late complications, which often require operative revision.

The primary determinant of output is the length and quality of the bowel proximal to the stoma, rather than the amount of bowel resected. Clinically significant diarrhea is noted in up to 20% of patients.[65] The highest risk is seen in the first week when the patients are still not able to match the stoma output with fluid intake and small bowel adaption has not completed. Removal of smaller segments of bowel over a long period of time has less impact on output rather than resection of an equivalent length at one sitting. Diarrhea associated with limited ileal resection, even up to 100 cm, is secretory with minimal nutritional losses rather than the osmotic diarrhea noted with greater resection (and resultant decreased fat reabsorption due to disruption of the enterohepatic circulation).[66] Increased gastric acid secretion may contribute to increased ileostomy output, and proton pump inhibitors can play a role in decreasing the volume output in patients with extensive small bowel resection.[67] This effect is mediated by the lack of peptide YY, which acts as an intestinal brake, especially in patients with extensive bowel resection.[68]

Antimotility agents, fiber supplements, bile acid–binding agents, and intravenous hydration with appropriate electrolytes may be needed to counter the fluid losses and to decrease transit times (Table 84.2).[69–71]

Peristomal skin irritation, especially in the immediate postoperative period, is the most common complaint.[72] Up to 70% of new ileostomates have unrecognized peristomal skin irritation.[73,74] Most of the peristomal complications are due to ill-fitting appliances or a large aperture on the flange that allows the ileal effluent to contact the skin. This irritated peristomal skin then weeps exudative fluid, which in turn weakens the seal with ostomy appliance and causes more skin irritation. To compound this further, leakage also causes more frequent appliance changes, which further disrupts the already damaged skin, setting up a vicious cycle. Consultation with an enterostomal therapist for appraisal of the type of appliance and aperture on the flange is necessary.

Care should be taken to fit the stoma flange aperture to the mucocutaneous junction. The peristomal skin should be protected with skin barrier wipes. If weeping skin is encountered, stoma powder or nystatin powder

TABLE 84.2 Causes of High Output

Extensive resection
Discontinuation of steroids, narcotics, and antimotility agents
Crohn disease
Stricture
Intestinal ischemia
Infectious enteritis
Radiation enteritis
Bacterial overgrowth
Food intolerance
Dietary indiscretion
Anxiety

should be used. If a retracted or flat stoma is noted, a convex pouching system may be indicated. Peristomal contour abnormalities should be caulked with stoma paste to prevent any leakage underneath the flange. If peristomal satellite lesions are noted under the area of the appliance flange, fungal infections should be suspected. Topical nystatin powder is applied, excess powder is brushed off, and an adhesive barrier is applied followed by placement of the stoma appliance.

Ischemia of the ileostomy is suspected when the mucosa of the newly matured ileostomy appears dusky. Its incidence ranges from 1% to 21%.[64,75–77] Causes include poor vascular supply or a small abdominal wall opening that can lead to congestion and compression of the vasculature supplying the ileostomy. Loop ileostomies, with their preserved arcades and collateral flow across an intact and undivided mesentery, are less prone to arterial insufficiency. Palpation of the arterial flow in the mesentery, bleeding from the edge of small bowel, and mucosal evaluation are paramount to prevent stomal ischemia. Frequently the distal edge of the stoma, which is the segment most susceptible to ischemia, will show mucosal changes and, with time, can even show demarcation where the vascular supply is tenuous. Usually the mesentery can be trimmed to the bowel edge for 2 to 5 cm without any decreased perfusion of the mucosa.[78] Trimming the bowel to the area of the demarcation can minimize the need for a future stoma revision. If an adequately vascularized segment of bowel is exteriorized, and the stoma becomes ischemic, venous engorgement should be suspected. The opening in the wall may need to be enlarged, and, if this is not feasible, the mesenteric fat may need debulking to allow venous dilation.

The extent of ischemia can be variable, and scoring the mucosa with a needle to assess for perfusion facilitates assessment or preferably by shining light through a lubricated test tube placed in the os of the stoma. Stomal ischemia is suspected when changes are noted in the mucosa: they can vary from pallor to petechiae to dusky and almost gray necrosis. With mild ischemia, the mucosal surface can slough, but the deeper layers will be viable, and this can be observed without the need for reintervention. If the ischemia extends below the fascia, exploration and revision of the ileostomy is needed to prevent progression to intraperitoneal perforation.[79] If the ischemia is confined to the bowel above the fascia and a permanent ileostomy was fashioned, revision should be entertained depending on the patient's clinical condition because distal ischemia can lead to necrosis and a flat stoma that may be difficult to pouch. Oftentimes, as the edema decreases and the abdominal wall opening stretches, mild ischemia can resolve. In conservatively managed mucosal ischemia, a fibrotic ring of the mucocutaneous junction can develop with eventual stenosis that will need revision.

Retraction of the stoma is another late consequence of ischemia. This can occur with separation of the mucosa from the skin surface. Most common etiologies include tension at the anastomosis or use of diseased bowel for the maturation of the stoma. Operative intervention is not needed, and it can be managed by covering the separation with stoma adhesive powder and placing the appliance on top. The separation heals by secondary intention and will eventually lead to stenosis. Stoma retraction has been previously defined as a stoma that is 0.5 cm or more below the skin surface, usually due to tension.[77] Late retraction is usually due to an ischemic insult. Retraction in the early postoperative phase, even in a well-constructed ileostomy, can be noted in obese patients due to an inadequately mobilized stoma with a large hanging pannus.

Obstruction can be mechanical or functional. Mechanical causes include obstruction due to a tight abdominal aperture, twisting around the mesenteric axis, or a misplaced stitch during maturation. Postoperative ileus is the most common cause of early functional obstruction. In the presence of an ileus, the stoma output can be green or yellow, watery fluid with no odor or gas. The other symptoms of ileus may also be present. Distinguishing between the two etiologies of obstruction will need an ileoscopy or a retrograde contrast study via the stoma. Although mechanical causes will need operative intervention, ileus can be managed expectantly and should eventually resolve.

Peristomal abscess, which presents due to contamination at the time of the ostomy formation or due to a fistula, presents with surrounding erythema, warmth, and increasing tenderness in the vicinity of the peristomal skin. Management involves drainage of the collection at a site that will not interfere with the pouching or at the mucocutaneous junction. Common causes of a fistula include Crohn disease, unrecognized suprafascial enterotomy during stoma formation, or accidental incorporation of the dermis when placing the tripartite sutures during the eversion of the ileostomy. Rarely, an intraabdominal process can present as a fistula or peristomal abscess, and these will need operative management. Late peristomal abscess should raise the suspicion of underlying Crohn disease.

LATE COMPLICATIONS

Late complications are more prone to occur after the patient has recovered from the initial surgery and has become quite familiar with the everyday life of their ileostomy. Involving these patients with an enterostomal therapist in a dedicated enterostomal therapy clinic with regularly scheduled visits can be very rewarding for the patient and ameliorate some of these patients' anxiety when complications occur and thereby improve the outcome and quality of life. These late complications generally bother patients with permanent ileostomies because most temporary stomas are reversed within 3 to 6 months. Late complications include bleeding, stoma prolapse and retraction, stenosis, small bowel obstruction, and parastomal hernia.

Lower gastrointestinal bleeding manifested by blood in the ileostomy bag is rarely a complication unless it is a result of preexisting inflammatory bowel disease or bleeding from the foregut. Such entities as bleeding from small bowel diverticulosis, arteriovenous malformations, or small bowel tumors must always be considered. That being said, major bleeding from the stoma exclusive of the aforementioned causes remains uncommon. There is a subset of patients with advanced liver disease and portal hypertension who are prone to develop stomal varices.[80] This may specifically be seen in patients with ulcerative colitis in the setting of primary sclerosing cholangitis and in alcoholic cirrhosis. These stomal varices remain a challenge to manage. Local treatment using mucocutaneous separation or ligation may be effective; however, transjugular intrahepatic portosystemic shunting at times is often required.[81-83] Not uncommonly encountered is bleeding secondary to excoriation from the mucocutaneous junction secondary to inadequate pouching. This presents as bright red blood per os. This is easily diagnosed and treated in conjunction with the enterostomal therapist.

Ileostomy prolapse occurs in approximately 5% to 10% of patients when reported but in reality is most likely underestimated. This can be an annoying complication that may be difficult to resolve. Complications from the prolapse, such as incarceration or strangulation, may occur in less than 10% of prolapsed stomas. Uncomplicated ileostomy prolapse can be managed conservatively with manual reduction or the use of osmotic agent facilitated by table sugar or even honey.[84] In the setting of complicated prolapse with ischemia or incarceration that is unable to be reduced, the ileostomy requires surgery. This involves full-thickness resection of the prolapsed segment. This is accompanied by construction of the stoma at the original site.[65]

Ileostomy stenosis is often due to a technical complication that has occurred early on with subsequent ischemia or mucocutaneous separation.[85] This results in scarring and may pose difficulty in both evacuation and pouching and narrowing of the stoma sufficient to interfere with normal bowel function. Because the effluent from the ileostomy is liquid, intestinal obstruction is uncommon, unless the stenosis involves a segment of the ileum instead of stenosis only at the skin level. The patient should be evaluated for other causes of stenosis, such as primary or recurrent Crohn disease or malignancy. Dilation, either digital or endoscopic, may be entertained; however, care must be taken to avoid perforation. Simple revision is required in this setting, unless it extends to the fascial or subfascial level where a segmental bowel resection may be required. At times, enlargement of the skin opening is required. A local revision involving a Z-plasty can also be effective.[86]

Parastomal herniation of an ileostomy is an extremely challenging problem for the patient and physician.[87] Often your conduct at the initial operation when the stoma is created is your best opportunity to make all efforts to prevent this complication. Regardless, patient morbidity, such as obesity, diabetes, liver and pulmonary disease, chronic steroid usage, malnutrition, advanced cancer, and age, are some of the factors that predispose patients to this. Not all parastomal hernias require surgical repair. Asymptomatic patients need assurance, but at the same time, instruction on signs and symptoms of incarceration should be provided. Once again, involving the enterostomal therapist in their care is paramount. Abdominal binders and stoma belts may be worn to aid in promoting hernia reduction and appliance fitting. Surgical repair will be required in a small group of patients.[88] Choice of surgical procedure depends on many factors. Procedures include repair by direct fascial reapproximation, local repair with prosthetic mesh, or stoma relocation. There should be a

low threshold to involve plastic surgery when recurrent or complex parastomal hernias are present. One must be quite frank with patients and their families that recurrence rates approach 50%. An open or laparoscopic approach when feasible should be entertained. Mesh complications occur in a variable rate.

Small bowel obstruction in the setting of an ileostomy will occur just as in any patient who has had previous abdominal or pelvic surgery. The etiologies of intestinal obstruction include adhesions, volvulus, internal hernia, recurrent Crohn disease, food bolus obstruction, and stomal stenosis. Patients will classically describe minimal to absent ileostomy output, distention, anorexia, and vomiting. Pain may be a presenting symptom and, when present, should alert the clinician to the possibility of threatened bowel and impending ischemia. The aperture lends to advantages in diagnosis and therapeutics, such as ileoscopy and retrograde contrast enema. It is often advantageous to involve the enterostomal therapist in treatment because food impaction will respond to enemas and irrigations and dietary modifications, especially if recurrent. Intestinal obstruction in the setting of an ileostomy is managed similar to other bowel obstructions. Initial correction of dehydration and electrolyte abnormalities is paramount, followed by a detailed physical examination and diagnostic imaging, which currently is often a double-contrast computed tomography scan. In the absence of writhing pain and/or peritonitis, nonoperative management is instituted, which may involve nasogastric decompression. After eliminating a bolus obstruction, failure to resolve the obstruction within a short period of time may require surgery. A minimally invasive approach, if possible, is preferred.

Other less common complications may also occur. Dermatitis can result in severely denuded skin due to the nature of the ileostomy effluent. With chronic irritation and wetness, acanthotic changes develop in the peristome skin. Allergy to pouching products should always be suspected and may require a change in the brand and type of appliance, along with topical steroids. Treatment, in conjunction with an enterostomal therapist, involves correction of causative factors, skin barriers, and antifungals.

Peristomal pyoderma gangrenosum (characterized by painful ulcers with violaceous undermining borders and thin bridges of epidermis bridging the ulcer) can be seen at the stoma site in patients with inflammatory bowel disease. It is often associated with female gender, obesity, and inflammatory bowel disease.[89,90] At times difficult to diagnose because of inadvertent suspicion of other entities such as contact dermatitis, extension of Crohn disease, or stitch abscess, these lesions are best managed by systemic, intralesional or topical antiinflammatory agents, including steroids[91] and tacrolimus.[92,93] Pyoderma parallels inflammatory bowel disease activity, and use of immunomodulators and biologics have been associated with resolution. Ultimately, stoma repositioning may be needed for managing refractory pyoderma, but relocation cannot guarantee against recurrence at the new stoma site.

Adenocarcinoma arising in an ileostomy has been described.[94-99] Etiology can be chronic irritation or association with inflammatory bowel disease. Unfortunately, it is often diagnosed late. Treatment is similar to other instances of adenocarcinoma of the small intestine and involves resection and preferably resiting of the stoma.

ILEOSTOMY CLOSURE

A loop ileostomy is generally closed 2 to 3 months after its creation, provided remission of distal pathology or adequate healing of a distal anastomosis is established. Studies have suggested the possibility of closure within 2 weeks of the creation. The initial study showed that two-thirds of patients could have their ileostomies closed during the same admission as their index surgery without any increase in complications.[100] Since then, other studies have confirmed the low morbidity of an early closure.[101–106] A multicenter randomized controlled trial showed the safety of closure within 2 weeks as opposed to 12 weeks.[107]

In the setting of chemotherapy, closure can be undertaken a month after completion of therapy. Ileostomy closure is generally not advisable prior to or during chemotherapy to mitigate any delay in therapy should a complication arises as a result of the stoma closure.[108]

Prior to the closure of a loop ileostomy, a water-soluble contrast enema study is used to assess the bowel distal to the ileostomy for any structural abnormalities or anastomotic leak.[109] Due to the liquid effluent from the ileostomy, most patients may not need a bowel preparation prior to the ileostomy closure. In a majority of the cases, the loop ileostomy takedown can be achieved with a circumferential incision placed approximately 1 to 2 mm from the mucocutaneous edge. Both limbs of the ileostomy are then dissected free off the subcutaneous tissues and the fascial edges and prolapsed out of the abdominal cavity. Only in a few selective cases, where prohibitive adhesions are encountered, should the takedown be undertaken with a midline laparotomy. Any serosal tears encountered, especially to the fascial edges or the rectus muscle, should be addressed immediately to prevent their progression to enterotomies due to retraction. Any occult enterotomies can be ascertained by insufflating the bowel loops with povidone-iodine (Betadine) solution. The loop ileostomy can be closed by apposing the antimesenteric edges of the ileostomy or by a side-to-side anastomosis, which can be fashioned either hand sewn or stapled. No differences in outcomes have been noted with either technique,[110] and individual surgeon preference and comfort should dictate the operative approach. After the anastomosis has been fashioned and reduced into the abdominal cavity, the fascia is approximated. The subcutaneous tissues are irrigated and approximated to decrease the dead space. The skin can be partially reapproximated. Several approaches to skin closure have been described.

REFERENCES

1. Sutherland AM, Orbach CE, Dyk RB, Bard M. The psychological impact of cancer and cancer surgery. I. Adaptation to the dry colostomy: preliminary report and summary of findings. *Cancer.* 1952;5(5):857-872.
2. Nilsson LO, Kock NG, Kylberg F, Myrvold HE, Palselius I. Sexual adjustment in ileostomy patients before and after conversion to continent ileostomy. *Dis Colon Rectum.* 1981;24(4):287-290.
3. Follick MJ, Smith TW, Turk DC. Psychosocial adjustment following ostomy. *Health Psychol.* 1984;3(6):505-517.
4. Walsh BA, Grunert BK, Telford GL, Otterson MF. Multidisciplinary management of altered body image in the patient with an ostomy. *J Wound Ostomy Continence Nurs.* 1995;22(5):227-236.
5. Nugent KP, Daniels P, Stewart B, Patankar R, Johnson CD. Quality of life in stoma patients. *Dis Colon Rectum.* 1999;42(12):1569-1574.
6. Krouse RS, Grant M, Wendel CS, et al. A mixed-methods evaluation of health-related quality of life for male veterans with and without intestinal stomas. *Dis Colon Rectum.* 2007;50(12):2054-2066.
7. Littre A. Diverses observations anatomiques. *Histoire de l'Académie R Sci Paris.* 1710.
8. Maydl K. Zur technik der kolotomie. *Zentralbl Chir.* 1888.
9. Brown JY. The value of complete physiological rest of the large bowel in the treatment of certain ulcerative and obstructive lesions of this organ. *Surg Gynecol Obstet.* 1913;16:610-613.
10. Arn ER. Chronic ulcerative colitis: surgical treatment of refractory cases. *Ohio State Med J.* 1931;27:121-127. doi:10.1046/j.1440-1622.2000.01773.x/abstract.
11. Bargen JA, Lindahl WW, Ashburn FS, Pemberton JD. Ileostomy for chronic ulcerative colitis (end results and complications in 185 cases). *Ann Intern Med.* 1943;18:43-56.
12. Corbett RS. A review of the surgical treatment of chronic ulcerative colitis: president's address. *Proc R Soc Med.* 1945;38:277-290.
13. Lahey FH. Indications for surgical intervention in ulcerative colitis. *Ann Surg.* 1951;133(5):726-742.
14. Brooke BN. The surgery of ulcerative colitis. *Ann R Coll Surg Eng.* 1951;8(6):440-456.
15. Brooke BN. The management of an ileostomy, including its complications. *Lancet.* 1952;2(6725):102-104.
16. Rankin FW. Total colectomy: its indication and technic. *Ann Surg.* 1931;94(4):677-704.
17. Bargen JA, Brown PW, Rankin FW. Indications for and technique of ileostomy in chronic ulcerative colitis. *Surg Gynecol Obstet.* 1932;55:196-202.
18. Cattell RB, Sachs E Jr. Surgical treatment of ulcerative colitis. *JAMA.* 1948;137(11):929-935.
19. Cave HW, Nickel WF. Ileostomy. *Ann Surg.* 1940;112(4):747-762.
20. Warren R, McKittrick LS. Ileostomy for ulcerative colitis: technique, complications, and management. *Surg Gynecol Obstet.* 1951;93(5):555-567.
21. Crile G Jr, Turnbull RB Jr. The mechanism and prevention of ileostomy dysfunction. *Ann Surg.* 1954;140(4):459-466.
22. Dragstedt LR, Dack GM, Kirsner JB. Chronic ulcerative colitis: a summary of evidence implicating bacterium necrophorum as an etiologic agent. *Ann Surg.* 1941;114(4):653-662.
23. Monroe CW, Olwin JH. Use of an abdominal flap graft in construction of a permanent ileostomy. *Arch Surg.* 1949;59(3):565-577.
24. Turnbull RB Jr, Crile G Jr. Mucosal-grafted ileostomy in the surgical treatment of ulcerative colitis. *JAMA.* 1955;158(1):32-34.
25. Pemberton JH, Phillips SF, Ready RR, Zinsmeister AR, Beahrs OH. Quality of life after Brooke ileostomy and ileal pouch-anal anastomosis. Comparison of performance status. *Ann Surg.* 1989;209:620-626; discussion 626–628.
26. Dozois EJ. Proctocolectomy and Brooke ileostomy for chronic ulcerative colitis. *Clin Colon Rectal Surg.* 2004;17(1):65-70.
27. Goligher JC. Surgical treatment of Crohn's disease affecting mainly or entirely the large bowel. *World J Surg.* 1988;12(2):186-190.
28. Kamm MA, Hawley PR, Lennard-Jones JE. Outcome of colectomy for severe idiopathic constipation. *Gut.* 1988;29(7):969-973.
29. Hasegawa H, Radley S, Fatah C, Keighley MRB. Long-term results of colorectal resection for slow transit constipation. *Colorectal Dis.* 1999;1:141-145.
30. Furlan JC, Urbach DR, Fehlings MG. Optimal treatment for severe neurogenic bowel dysfunction after chronic spinal cord injury: a decision analysis. *Br J Surg.* 2007;94(9):1139-1150.
31. Sailhamer EA, Carson K, Chang Y, et al. Fulminant *Clostridium difficile* colitis: patterns of care and predictors of mortality. *Arch Surg.* 2009;144:433-439; discussion 439–440.
32. Hüser N, Michalski CW, Erkan M, et al. Systematic review and meta-analysis of the role of defunctioning stoma in low rectal cancer surgery. *Ann Surg.* 2008;248(1):52-60.
33. Tjandra JJ, Fazio VW, Milsom JW, Lavery IC, Oakley JR, Fabre JM. Omission of temporary diversion in restorative proctocolectomy—is it safe? *Dis Colon Rectum.* 1993;36(11):1007-1014.
34. Gorfine SR, Gelernt IM, Bauer JJ, Harris MT, Kreel I. Restorative proctocolectomy without diverting ileostomy. *Dis Colon Rectum.* 1995;38(2):188-194.

35. Farouk R, Dozois RR, Pemberton JH, Larson D. Incidence and subsequent impact of pelvic abscess after ileal pouch-anal anastomosis for chronic ulcerative colitis. *Dis Colon Rectum.* 1998;41(10):1239-1243.

36. Remzi FH, Fazio VW, Gorgun E, et al. The outcome after restorative proctocolectomy with or without defunctioning ileostomy. *Dis Colon Rectum.* 2006;49:470-477.

37. Matthiessen P, Hallböök O, Rutegård J, Simert G, Sjödahl R. Defunctioning stoma reduces symptomatic anastomotic leakage after low anterior resection of the rectum for cancer: a randomized multicenter trial. *Ann Surg.* 2007;246(2):207-214.

38. Williams NS, Nasmyth DG, Jones D, Smith AH. De-functioning stomas: a prospective controlled trial comparing loop ileostomy with loop transverse colostomy. *Br J Surg.* 1986;73(7):566-570.

39. Gooszen AW, Geelkerken RH, Hermans J, Lagaay MB, Gooszen HG. Quality of life with a temporary stoma: ileostomy vs. colostomy. *Dis Colon Rectum.* 2000;43(5):650-655.

40. Edwards DP, Leppington-Clarke A, Sexton R, Heald RJ, Moran BJ. Stoma-related complications are more frequent after transverse colostomy than loop ileostomy: a prospective randomized clinical trial. *Br J Surg.* 2001;88(3):360-363.

41. Guenaga KF, Lustosa SA, Saad SS, Saconato H, Matos D. Ileostomy or colostomy for temporary decompression of colorectal anastomosis. *Cochrane Database Syst Rev.* 2007;(1):CD004647. doi:10.1002/14651858.CD004647.pub2.

42. Rondelli F, Reboldi P, Rulli A, et al. Loop ileostomy versus loop colostomy for fecal diversion after colorectal or coloanal anastomosis: a meta-analysis. *Int J Colorectal Dis.* 2009;24:479-488.

43. Chen J, Wang DR, Zhang JR, Li P, Niu G, Lu Q. Meta-analysis of temporary ileostomy versus colostomy for colorectal anastomoses. *Acta Chir Belg.* 2013;113(5):330-339.

44. Connel AM. Propulsion in the small intestine. *Rendic R Gastroenterol.* 1970;2:38-46.

45. Kramer P. The effect of varying sodium loads on the ileal excreta of human ileostomized subjects. *J Clin Invest.* 1966;45(11):1710-1718.

46. Gorbach SL, Nahas L, Weinstein L, Levitan R, Patterson JF. Studies of intestinal microflora. IV. The microflora of ileostomy effluent: a unique microbial ecology. *Gastroenterology.* 1967;53(6):874-880.

47. Kurchin A, Ray JE, Bluth EI, et al. Cholelithiasis in ileostomy patients. *Dis Colon Rectum.* 1984;27(9):585-588.

48. Bluth EI, Merritt CR, Sullivan MA, Kurchin A, Ray JE. Inflammatory bowel disease and cholelithiasis: the association in patients with an ileostomy. *South Med J.* 1984;77(6):690-692.

49. Christie PM, Knight GS, Hill GL. Comparison of relative risks of urinary stone formation after surgery for ulcerative colitis: conventional ileostomy vs. J-pouch. A comparative study. *Dis Colon Rectum.* 1996;39(1):50-54.

50. Brand MI, Dujovny N. Preoperative considerations and creation of normal ostomies. *Clin Colon Rectal Surg.* 2008;21(1):5-16.

51. Hendren S, Hammond K, Glasgow SC, et al. Clinical practice guidelines for ostomy surgery. *Dis Colon Rectum.* 2015;58(4):375-387.

52. Cottam J, Richards K, Hasted A, Blackman A. Results of a nationwide prospective audit of stoma complications within 3 weeks of surgery. *Colorectal Dis.* 2007;9(9):834-838.

53. Tang CL, Seow-Choen F, Fook-Chong S, Eu KW. Bioresorbable adhesion barrier facilitates early closure of the defunctioning ileostomy after rectal excision: a prospective, randomized trial. *Dis Colon Rectum.* 2003;46(9):1200-1207.

54. Salum M, Wexner SD, Nogueras JJ, et al. Does sodium hyaluronate- and carboxymethylcellulose-based bioresorbable membrane (Seprafilm) decrease operative time for loop ileostomy closure? *Tech Coloproctol.* 2006;10:187-190; discussion 190-191.

55. Khoo RE, Montrey J, Cohen MM. Laparoscopic loop ileostomy for temporary fecal diversion. *Dis Colon Rectum.* 1993;36(10):966-968.

56. Atallah S, Albert M, Larach S. Technique for constructing an incisionless laparoscopic stoma. *Tech Coloproctol.* 2011;15(3):345-347.

57. Shah A, Moftah M, Hadi Nahar Al-Furaji H, Cahill RA. Standardized technique for single port laparoscopic ileostomy and colostomy. *Colorectal Dis.* 2014;16:O248-O252.

58. Prasad ML, Pearl RK, Orsay CP, Abcarian H. Rodless ileostomy. A modified loop ileostomy. *Dis Colon Rectum.* 1984;27(4):270-271.

59. Sitzmann JV. A new alternative to diverting double barreled ileostomy. *Surg Gynecol Obstet.* 1987;165(5):461-464.

60. Evans JP, Brown MH, Wilkes GH, Cohen Z, McLeod RS. Revising the troublesome stoma: combined abdominal wall recontouring and revision of stomas. *Dis Colon Rectum.* 2003;46(1):122-126.

61. Beck DE. Abdominal wall modification for the difficult ostomy. *Clin Colon Rectal Surg.* 2008;21(1):71-75.

62. Paquette IM, Solan P, Rafferty JF, Ferguson MA, Davis BR. Readmission for dehydration or renal failure after ileostomy creation. *Dis Colon Rectum.* 2013;56(8):974-979.

63. Hayden DM, Pinzon MC, Francescatti AB, et al. Hospital readmission for fluid and electrolyte abnormalities following ileostomy construction: preventable or unpredictable? *J Gastrointest Surg.* 2013;17:298-303.

64. Leong AP, Londono-Schimmer EE, Phillips RK. Life-table analysis of stomal complications following ileostomy. *Br J Surg.* 1994;81(5):727-729.

65. Shabbir J, Britton DC. Stoma complications: a literature overview. *Colorectal Dis.* 2010;12(10):958-964.

66. Lennard-Jones JE. Review article: practical management of the short bowel. *Aliment Pharmacol Ther.* 1994;8(6):563-577.

67. Jeppesen PB, Staun M, Tjellesen L, Mortensen PB. Effect of intravenous ranitidine and omeprazole on intestinal absorption of water, sodium, and macronutrients in patients with intestinal resection. *Gut.* 1998;43(6):763-769.

68. Nightingale JM, Kamm MA, van der Sijp JR, Ghatei MA, Bloom SR, Lennard-Jones JE. Gastrointestinal hormones in short bowel syndrome. Peptide YY may be the 'colonic brake' to gastric emptying. *Gut.* 1996;39(2):267-272.

69. Newton CR. Effect of codeine phosphate, Lomotil, and Isogel on ileostomy function. *Gut.* 1978;19(5):377-383.

70. King RF, Norton T, Hill GL. A double-blind crossover study of the effect of loperamide hydrochloride and codeine phosphate on ileostomy output. *Aust N Z J Surg.* 1982;52(2):121-124.

71. DuPont AW, Sellin JH. Ileostomy diarrhea. *Curr Treat Options Gastroenterol.* 2006;9(1):39-48.

72. Salvadalena G. Incidence of complications of the stoma and peristomal skin among individuals with colostomy, ileostomy, and urostomy: a systematic review. *J Wound Ostomy Continence Nurs.* 2008;35(6):596-607.

73. Herlufsen P, Olsen AG, Carlsen B, et al. Study of peristomal skin disorders in patients with permanent stomas. *Br J Nurs.* 2006;15(16):854-862.

74. Nybaek H, Bang Knudsen D, Nørgaard Laursen T, Karlsmark T, Jemec GB. Skin problems in ostomy patients: a case-control study of risk factors. *Acta Derm Venereol.* 2009;89(1):64-67.

75. Duchesne JC, Wang Y-Z, Weintraub SL, Boyle M, Hun JP. Stoma complications: a multivariate analysis. *Am Surg.* 2002;68:961-966; discussion 966.

76. Park JJ, Del Pino A, Orsay CP, et al. Stoma complications: the Cook County Hospital experience. *Dis Colon Rectum.* 1999;42(12):1575-1580.

77. Arumugam PJ, Bevan L, Macdonald L, et al. A prospective audit of stomas—analysis of risk factors and complications and their management. *Colorectal Dis.* 2003;5(1):49-52.

78. Wu JS, Fazio VW. Difficult stomas. *Persp Colon Rectal Surg.* 1998;10:33-60.

79. Kann BR. Early stomal complications. *Clin Colon Rectal Surg.* 2008;21(1):23-30.

80. Roberts PL, Martin FM, Schoetz DJ Jr, Murray JJ, Coller JA, Veidenheimer MC. Bleeding stomal varices. The role of local treatment. *Dis Colon Rectum.* 1990;33(7):547-549.

81. Fitzgerald JB, Chalmers N, Abbott G, et al. The use of TIPS to control bleeding caput medusae. *Br J Radiol.* 1998;71(845):558-560.

82. Shibata D, Hyland W, Busse P, et al. Immediate reconstruction of the perineal wound with gracilis muscle flaps following abdominoperineal resection and intraoperative radiation therapy for recurrent carcinoma of the rectum. *Ann Surg Oncol.* 1999;6(1):33-37.

83. Pennick MO, Artioukh DY. Management of parastomal varices: who re-bleeds and who does not? A systematic review of the literature. *Tech Coloproctol.* 2013;17(2):163-170.

84. Shapiro R, Chin EH, Steinhagen RM. Reduction of an incarcerated, prolapsed ileostomy with the assistance of sugar as a desiccant. *Tech Coloproctol.* 2010;14(3):269-271.

85. Robertson I, Leung E, Hughes D, et al. Prospective analysis of stoma-related complications. *Colorectal Dis.* 2005;7(3):279-285.

86. Pemberton JH. Management of conventional ileostomies. *World J Surg.* 1988;12(2):203-210.

87. Williams JG, Etherington R, Hayward MW, Hughes LE. Paraileostomy hernia: a clinical and radiological study. *Br J Surg.* 1990;77(12):1355-1357.

88. Safadi B. Laparoscopic repair of parastomal hernias: early results. *Surg Endosc.* 2004;18(4):676-680.

89. Poritz LS, Lebo MA, Bobb AD, Ardell CM, Koltun WA. Management of peristomal pyoderma gangrenosum. *J Am Coll Surg.* 2008;206(2):311-315.

90. Wu XR, Mukewar S, Kiran RP, Remzi FH, Hammel J, Shen B. Risk factors for peristomal pyoderma gangrenosum complicating inflammatory bowel disease. *J Crohns Colitis.* 2013;7(5):e171-e177.

91. Kiran RP, O'Brien-Ermlich B, Achkar J-P, Fazio VW, Delaney CP. Management of peristomal pyoderma gangrenosum. *Dis Colon Rectum.* 2005;48:1397-1403.

92. Khurrum Baig M, Marquez H, Nogueras JJ, Weiss EG, Wexner SD. Topical tacrolimus (FK506) in the treatment of recalcitrant parastomal pyoderma gangrenosum associated with Crohn's disease: report of two cases. *Colorectal Dis.* 2004;6:250-253.

93. Vidal D, Alomar A. Successful treatment of periostomal pyoderma gangrenosum using topical tacrolimus. *Br J Dermatol.* 2004;150(2):387-388.

94. Carter D, Choi H, Otterson M, Telford GL. Primary adenocarcinoma of the ileostomy after colectomy for ulcerative colitis. *Dig Dis Sci.* 1988;33(4):509-512.

95. Smart PJ, Sastry S, Wells S. Primary mucinous adenocarcinoma developing in an ileostomy stoma. *Gut.* 1988;29(11):1607-1612.

96. Roberts PL, Veidenheimer MC, Cassidy S, Silverman ML. Adenocarcinoma arising in an ileostomy. Report of two cases and review of the literature. *Arch Surg.* 1989;124(4):497-499.

97. Gadacz TR, McFadden DW, Gabrielson EW, Ullah A, Berman JJ. Adenocarcinoma of the ileostomy: the latent risk of cancer after colectomy for ulcerative colitis and familial polyposis. *Surgery.* 1990;107(6):698-703.

98. Metzger PP, Slappy AL, Chua HK, Menke DM. Adenocarcinoma developing at an ileostomy: report of a case and review of the literature. *Dis Colon Rectum.* 2008;51(5):604-609.

99. Annam V, Panduranga C, Kodandaswamy C, Suresh DR. Primary mucinous adenocarcinoma in an ileostomy with adjacent skin invasion: a late complication of surgery for ulcerative colitis. *J Gastrointest Cancer.* 2008;39(1-4):138-140.

100. Bakx R, Busch OR, van Geldere D, Bemelman WA, Slors JF, van Lanschot JJ. Feasibility of early closure of loop ileostomies: a pilot study. *Dis Colon Rectum.* 2003;46(12):1680-1684.

101. Menegaux F, Jordi-Galais P, Turrin N, Chigot JP. Closure of small bowel stomas on postoperative day 10. *Eur J Surg.* 2002;168(12):713-715.

102. Krand O, Yalti T, Berber I, Tellioglu G. Early vs. delayed closure of temporary covering ileostomy: a prospective study. *Hepatogastroenterology.* 2008;55(81):142-145.

103. Worni M, Witschi A, Gloor B, Candinas D, Laffer UT, Kuehni CE. Early closure of ileostomy is associated with less postoperative nausea and vomiting. *Dig Surg.* 2011;28(5-6):417-423.

104. Perdawid SK, Andersen OB. Acceptable results of early closure of loop ileostomy to protect low rectal anastomosis. *Dan Med Bull.* 2011;58(6):A4280.

105. Memon S, Heriot AG, Atkin CE, Lynch AC. Facilitated early ileostomy closure after rectal cancer surgery: a case-matched study. *Tech Coloproctol.* 2012;16(4):285-290.

106. Omundsen M, Hayes J, Collinson R, Merrie A, Parry B, Bissett I. Early ileostomy closure: is there a downside? *ANZ J Surg.* 2012;82(5):352-354.

107. Danielsen AK, Park J, Jansen JE, et al. Early closure of a temporary ileostomy in patients with rectal cancer: a multicenter randomized controlled trial. *Ann Surg.* 2016;1:doi:10.1097/SLA.0000000000001829.

108. Phatak UR, Kao LS, You YN, et al. Impact of ileostomy-related complications on the multidisciplinary treatment of rectal cancer. *Ann Surg Oncol.* 2014;21(2):507-512.

109. Dolinsky D, Levine MS, Rubesin SE, Laufer I, Rombeau JL. Utility of contrast enema for detecting anastomotic strictures after total proctocolectomy and ileal pouch-anal anastomosis. *AJR Am J Roentgenol.* 2007;189(1):25-29.

110. Wong KS, Remzi FH, Gorgun E, et al. Loop ileostomy closure after restorative proctocolectomy: outcome in 1,504 patients. *Dis Colon Rectum.* 2005;48(2):243-250.

Suturing, Stapling, and Tissue Adhesion

David Giles | Ethan Talbot

Surgical procedures typically involve excision, resection, or transection to address a pathologic situation. Subsequent reconstruction, which includes maneuvers to secure a restoration of function, often allows the choice of a variety of methods. Surgical and general medical principles, safeguards, and prophylactic measures require planning, vigilance, and support across the health care spectrum to facilitate a completely successful result. Preoperative planning should be anticipatory, perioperative monitoring appropriate, surgical technique thoughtful and carefully executed, and postoperative care robust.[1] Frequently during the course of a gastrointestinal (GI) or abdominal operation, whether for benign or malignant disease, a resection of a hollow viscus with subsequent reconstruction is required. The anastomosis often anchors the procedure. Successful healing influences the outcome positively. Conversely, anastomotic failures not only increase morbidity and permanent stoma rates but delay adjunctive therapy, increase the intensity and duration of hospital care, and are associated with increased rates of distal recurrence (of malignancy) and mortality (short-term and long-term all cause).[2] Because a majority of the factors influencing an anastomosis's subsequent behavior are determined by the time a patient leaves the operating room, attention must first include the timing and choice of procedure, as well as the technique itself.

Wound healing proceeds in a stepwise, time-dependent fashion. Healing a GI anastomosis has parallels but important differences.[3–5] No chronic wound exists in a healing anastomosis, a situation in which repair must allow for rapid recovery of tensile strength and function. The goal of eliminating anastomotic leaks is challenged by our poor understanding of this pathophysiology. The multilayered architecture, the heavy colonization of the lumen, the influence of the different bowel layers, the vasoactive vascular supply, and variations in the rate and process of healing set the GI tract apart from subcutaneous tissues.

When the bowel is surgically transected, there is an immediate inflammatory response elicited by activation of the clotting cascade and by recruitment of platelets. The inflammatory cascade is propagated via the release of inflammatory mediators stored in platelet granules. Neutrophils are subsequently mobilized into the wound. At this time, the collagen matrix is degraded by collagenases and metalloproteinases. Collagenolysis is necessary to create a local pool of amino acids, especially those unique to collagen—proline and lysine. The newly formed collagen "recycles" these amino acids. The extent of collagenolysis varies among tissue, proceeding along the sides of the wound for variable distances. These tissues undergoing collagenolysis around the wound become weaker than normal tissue and are the site most susceptible to failure in the early phases of wound healing. It is during this initial phase that the integrity of the anastomosis depends almost entirely on the mechanical sealing of the lumen by sutures or staples.[4]

Between the third and fifth postoperative day there is a transition from the inflammatory phase to the proliferative phase of wound healing. With the proliferation of fibroblasts and smooth muscle cells, there is a shift from collagen degradation to collagen deposition. Once collagen deposition predominates over collagenolysis, the approximation of the two ends of bowel is no longer dependent on sutures or staples but on the cellular matrix surrounding the collagen fibers. Although bursting strength is 50% of normal in small bowel anastomoses (35% to 75% of normal in large bowel anastomoses) at 2 to 3 days post procedure, it approaches 100% by 7 days.

It is important to recognize that the time frames of tissue healing stages are shifted by factors impairing wound healing, potentially with catastrophic consequences. Corticosteroids, chemotherapeutics, and antirejection medications attenuate and prolong the inflammatory phase. Antiangiogenic drugs and nutrient deficiencies extend collagenolysis and blunt collagen synthesis, as does hypoxia. Similarly, the presence of local infection intensifies collagenolysis. Consequently, the selection of materials, sutures, and/or staples should be made with consideration to these factors.[5–7]

Successful gastrointestinal anastomosis (GIA) healing relies on a good blood supply to the bowel that is not under tension as it is accurately ("watertight") anastomosed. Adequate vascular supply includes local anatomy as well as systemic perfusion. Ischemia inhibits collagen deposition and maturation in particular. Tension leads to ischemia in addition to loss of closure (of the defect), especially with stapled anastomoses. Although the submucosa is the strongest layer of the bowel wall and must be included in all anastomoses, all layers of the bowel wall contribute to wound healing. Closure in the process of creating anastomoses must be watertight/airtight, involving healthy and "clean" bowel edges. Distal obstruction, whether mechanical or not, leads to increasing bowel diameter, with increasing wall tension resulting in local ischemia. Hypoalbuminemia represents a marker of a much broader physiologic derangement than just malnutrition. Animal experiments have demonstrated that the body prioritizes visceral wound healing over most other sources of protein consumption, including parietal wound healing.

As a GIA is created, the tolerance for anastomotic leak is essentially zero. Multiple approaches have been shown to be effective, including surgical stapling as equally secure to suturing under many conditions. The indications to staple are generally the same as those to suture. Given that surgical stapling or suturing is not equally applicable in every situation, the surgeons' facility with both techniques may vastly improve the outcome of an operation requiring an intestinal anastomosis. A number of older studies looked at differences between handsewn and stapled bowel anastomoses. In general, no differences were noted in the leak rate, morbidity, mortality, and cancer recurrence.[8,9] A meta-analysis of the emergency laparotomy setting suggested, in the context of sparse evidence and high bias, neither technique was favored.[10] Preference for handsewn repair of small bowel injuries in trauma settings remains strong.[11,12]

SURGICAL SUTURING AND TECHNIQUE

As with any other skill, handsewing an intestinal anastomosis requires practice. Having observed or done a few handsewn intestinal anastomoses under direct supervision does not necessarily allow for the development of the skills necessary to perform an anastomosis, particularly in critical situations (i.e., any situation where a stapler cannot be used). Therefore it may be to everyone's benefit (patient, surgeon, and operating team) to perform handsewn anastomoses, particularly in straightforward cases.

The ideal suture material for intestinal anastomosis is one that produces the smallest amount of tissue reaction while providing maximal strength during the lag or inflammatory phase of wound healing. All sutures result in some degree of tissue inflammation because the act of pulling the suture thread through the bowel wall causes some tissue injury. This inflammatory reaction affects levels of activated collagenases and matrix metalloproteinases leading to decreased tensile strength of the healing wound. It is critical to avoid this strength imbalance during the critical lag period (days 1 to 5) as the wound transitions from the inflammatory phase to the proliferative phase. Similarly, other factors that foster inflammation (e.g., necrotic tissue, debris, and infection) will delay healing of the anastomosis, and should be minimized.[13]

In current clinical practice, most handsewn colorectal anastomoses are constructed with polydioxanone sutures.[14] These possess most of the qualities of the ideal suture for this purpose. As a monofilament suture, coupled with an appropriate needle, it allows for the least amount of tissue injury from the act of suturing. It is slowly absorbed with good retention of strength for up to 6 weeks, well past the critical lag period.[15]

With the pathophysiology of wound healing in mind, other types of suture and coatings have been experimented with. Application of basic fibroblast growth factor (bFGF) on the rat anastomosis was shown to significantly increase neovascularization, fibroblast infiltration, and collagen production around the anastomotic site, along with significant increases in the bursting pressure.[16] Coating suture with a matrix metalloproteinase inhibitor (in this case, doxycycline) resulted in higher breaking strength in rat intestinal anastomosis.[17] Using a knotless barbed suture for intestinal anastomosis has also been shown to be safe and reproducible.[18,19] These adjuncts have variably reached clinical use, but warrant further research.

The adherence of bacteria to the suture material has been postulated as a possible explanation for bacterial infection and weakening of the intestinal anastomosis. Polydioxanone has been shown to have the lowest affinity to adherence of bacteria among the absorbable sutures.[13] This same group of researchers showed that bacterial adherence is 5 to 8 times higher for braided versus monofilament sutures. Others showed the degree of infection in mice in the presence of suture correlated with the adherence properties of that suture for bacteria.[20] A different group of researchers showed that polyglycolic acid suture had the highest rate of bacterial adherence, concluding that absorbable braided suture should not be used in closure of contaminated wounds or wounds at risk for developing infection.[21]

With this evidence of suture potentiating wound infection, it is not surprising that research has focused on the effects of coating suture with antibiotic. Coating suture with an antibacterial agent (triclosan) significantly reduces adherent bacteria to polyglactin, is associated with decreased microbial viability and significantly increased bursting pressure in colonic anastomoses.[22,23] PVDF (polyvinylidene fluoride; a permanent suture) coated with gentamicin was shown to increase the stability and bursting strength of colonic anastomosis in the rat.[24] In summary, polydioxanone suture has low affinity for bacterial adherence, furthering its position as the suture of choice for intestinal anastomosis. Although there are animal data supporting the use of antibacterial-coated suture for this purpose, it will require human study before this becomes routine clinical practice.

SUTURE METHODS

Suture lines can be created either in an interrupted fashion or in a continuous, running manner. The continuous suture has the advantage of being more watertight with the disadvantage that the integrity of the entire suture line is based on one stitch. Although hemostasis is also improved with a continuous suture, the converse effect, that continuous suture may constrict anastomotic blood flow leading to ischemia and anastomotic dehiscence, is also true. Most human studies indicate that a continuous anastomosis can be performed safely and quickly, with no significant difference between continuous and interrupted suture pattern.[25,26]

Intestinal anastomosis can be constructed in a single-layer or double-layer method. Single-layer anastomosis consists of one layer of interrupted or continuous absorbable sutures, whereas a double-layer typically consists of an inner full-thickness layer of absorbable suture and an outer layer of interrupted absorbable or nonabsorbable sutures.[27] Single-layer does not differ from double-layer anastomosis in terms of rates of anastomotic leak, perioperative complications, length of hospital stay, and mortality, while also shortening operative time and total cost.[27–29] These findings were confirmed in a Cochrane review encompassing seven randomized controlled trials and 842 patients.[30] Anastomosis in the trauma setting gravitates toward the double-layer anastomosis.

Anastomoses with the inverted technique heal faster[31] with superior bursting pressure and more prompt return to normal bowel architecture.[32] The majority of both animal and human studies indicate the superiority of the inverting anastomotic technique. Everted anastomoses are associated with increased rates of adhesion formation, anastomotic leak, wound infection, peritonitis, and fecal

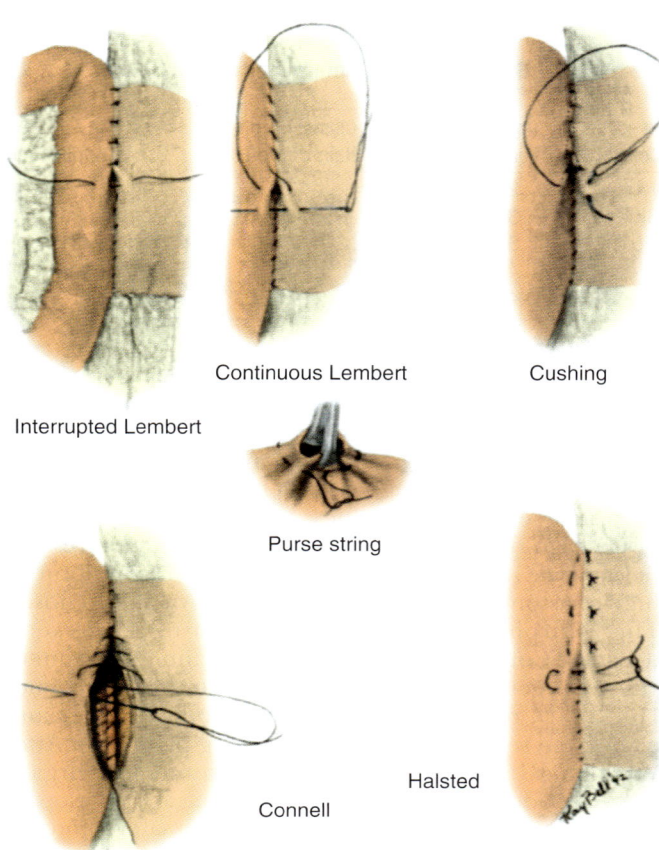

Interrupted Lembert — Continuous Lembert — Cushing — Purse string — Connell — Halsted

FIGURE 85.1 Intestinal suture methods. (From Orr TG. *Operations of General Surgery*. 2nd ed. Philadelphia: Saunders; 1949.)

fistulation.[33–35] Regardless of the suture particulars, a bowel anastomosis must adhere to the following principles (in addition to those articulated earlier): the anastomosis must be watertight and have mucosal apposition; the submucosa, which supplies much of the strength to a bowel anastomosis, must be incorporated into the closure; and care must be taken not to strangulate or instrument the edges of the bowel during closure to avoid stricture or necrosis and subsequent anastomotic leakage.

The Lembert suture is the most commonly used suture in GI surgery (Fig. 85.1). It is used as the outer layer of a two-layer bowel anastomosis and is also used to repair seromuscular tears in the bowel wall. The stitch is started approximately 3 to 4 mm lateral to the incision and placed at a right angle to the long axis of the incision ("follow the curve of the needle"). It incorporates only the seromuscular layer; care must be taken to not incorporate the full thickness of the bowel wall. The tip of the needle is brought out close to the edge of the incision and is then reinserted in the apposing wound edge and brought out 3 to 4 mm lateral to the wound edge. The suture is then tied down to a tension that approximates the tissue but not tight enough to tear the tissue. The most commonly used material for a Lembert suture is either (3-0) silk or PDS. This stitch can be performed in an interrupted or continuous manner.

A horizontal mattress suture, or Halsted suture, is predominantly used for seromuscular apposition in multilayer bowel anastomoses (see Fig. 85.1). The suture is passed through the seromuscular layer 2 to 3 mm lateral to the wound edge and brought out at the wound edge; the needle is then passed through the opposing edge of the wound and brought out 2 to 3 mm lateral. On that same side of the wound, approximately 2 mm distal, the suture is passed through both edges of the wound to create two free ends of the suture on one side of the wound edge with the loop of the suture on the other side. This stitch is particularly useful in damaged, inflamed, or abnormal tissue where a Lembert suture pulls through the tissue. Because the horizontal mattress stitch distributes tension in a plane perpendicular to that of a Lembert suture, it allows for apposition of tissues with less crushing effect.

A purse-string suture is used to invert appendiceal stumps or to secure feeding tubes or drainage tubes in place. It is basically a circular continuous Lembert suture about a fixed point or opening in the GI tract. It is most commonly performed with nonabsorbable suture (see Fig. 85.1).

The Connell suture is a full-thickness, usually continuous, suture that allows for the mucosa to be inverted into the lumen of a bowel anastomosis (see Fig. 85.1). The suture is started at the edge of the anastomosis and brought, full thickness, from inside to out on one side and then outside to in on the opposite side. The suture is tied so that the knot is inside the lumen. The suture is then passed through the tissues from inside to out on one side to begin the Connell stitch. On the other limb of the anastomosis the suture is driven through the tissues, full thickness, from outside to in. On the inside of the bowel lumen the stitch is advanced 2 to 3 mm along the wall and then driven through the (transmural) bowel wall from inside to out on the *same* side. With the suture now on the outside of the bowel, the next pass is performed on the opposite side in an identical manner. This creates a U-shaped, full-thickness, running inverted suture line. It usually serves as an inner layer of a two-layer anastomosis. Absorbable sutures are generally used for these applications. The Cushing suture is the same as the Connell, except the suture does not enter the lumen, rather it exits through the submucosa.

The Gambee suture is an interrupted single-layer suture that inverts the mucosa into the lumen (Fig. 85.2). The suture is brought full thickness from outside to in and then passed back through the mucosa to exit through the submucosal layer on the same side. It is then passed from the submucosa through the mucosa on the opposite limb. The final pass is a full-thickness one from inside to out on this side. The suture is tied extraluminally. This creates a full-thickness, inverting suture line. Absorbable sutures are typically used for this type of anastomosis. Some surgeons prefer the Gambee stitch for closure of a pyloroplasty; it is rarely used elsewhere.[36]

A double-layer closure, also known as the Czerny-Lembert suture, is still considered by some as the "gold standard" of bowel anastomoses. This technique features an inner, full-thickness, continuous, absorbable suture layer surrounded by an outer layer of interrupted, often permanent, seromuscular (Lembert) sutures. Typically the deep or posterior outer layer is placed first, after (seromuscular) stay sutures of the lateral aspects of this

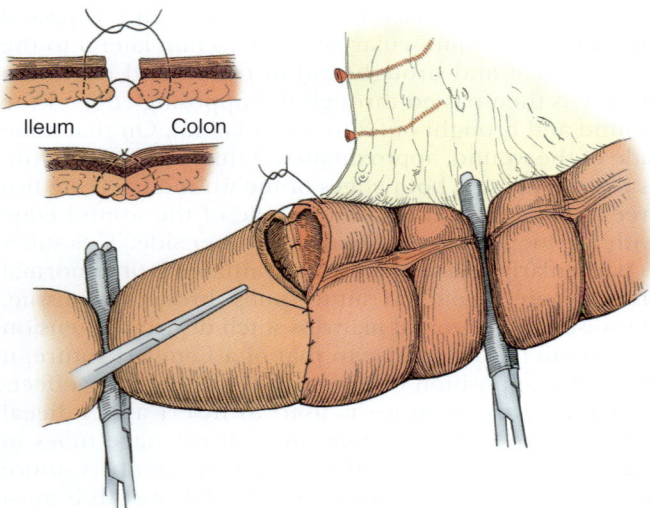

FIGURE 85.2 The Gambee method of intestinal suturing. (From Gambee LP, Gamjobst W, Hardwick CE. 10 years experience with a single layer anastomosis in colon surgery. *Am J Surg.* 1956;92:222.)

layer had been placed to allow the bowel to be aligned. With the deep, outer layer completed between the stay sutures, a simple running suture of all layers commences in both directions of the posterior wall, converting to running Connell, or Cushing, on the anterior surface to meet in closure on the antimesenteric aspect. The anterior aspect of the second layer is completed last. The outer layer might be constructed with 3-0 silk, the inner transmural layer with 3-0 polyglycolic acid, polyglactic acid, or chromic gut suture.

A single-layer anastomosis begins at the mesenteric border and sequentially moves in both directions to the antimesenteric aspect. This can be done as interrupted or continuous suture. The interrupted approach described by Gambee used permanent suture (cotton or silk originally). The continuous suture described by others starts on the outside of the lumen at the mesentery. Using a double-armed suture to sew in both directions, it includes all layers except mucosa and will end on the antimesenteric border. Being on the outside, the two ends are tied to produce watertight/airtight anastomosis without compromising the luminal diameter. Polypropylene or polydiaxonone (3-0) are typically used.[37]

STAPLERS AND STAPLING TECHNIQUE

Staplers permit or facilitate surgical techniques, specifically resection, transection, and/or anastomosis, in a rapid, accurate, and reproducible fashion. Part of the attraction (historically) was the need to generate high-quality surgical work by individuals who did not possess the skills (training and/or experience) to successfully complete surgical maneuvers. The continued refinement of the stapler has allowed their widespread deployment and adaptation (to open, laparoscopic, or robotic uses) by all members of the surgical community. Although not a replacement for sound surgical judgment or competence, staplers enlarge

the spectrum of approaches available to address problems, situations, pathologies, and/or locations.[1]

Almost 200 years ago the Belgian surgeon Dr. Henroz DeMarche devised a ring for small bowel anastomoses that he tested successfully in dogs. In 1892 John B. Murphy of Chicago developed a sutureless metallic compression device for GIA. Both inventions were in recognition of high anastomotic leak rates with handsewn anastomoses. The "Murphy button" enjoyed human use for several decades. Concerned with spillage at a time of frequent gastric surgeries (resections, partial or complete), Húmer Hültt, MD, of Budapest developed a bulky stapler and elaborated several fundamental stapling principles. After World War II, the USSR's Scientific Institute for Surgical Devices made a major step forward studying and developing a number of staplers, thereby promoting safe, standardized surgical treatment nationwide. A visiting American surgeon from Johns Hopkins, Mark Ravitch, MD, brought a stapler to the United States in 1958, eventually leading to the founding of the United States Surgical Corporation and much research into and development of surgical stapling.[38]

The principles underlying surgical stapling began with Húmer Hültt. He stressed compression of the tissue, placing (metal) staples in a closed "B" shape, with two rows of staples in a staggered formation. Similar to a standard office stapler, a B-shaped staple is formed from the interaction with an anvil. This action allows maintenance of the compression, with its hemostasis and watertight/airtight sealing, while encouraging viability, minimizing tissue damage, and stabilizing the new configuration. Formed in the tissue at the time of deployment, each staple, individually and collectively, contributes to these goals. The promotion of compression, accurate staple formation, and desired tissue configuration must underlie the methods needed in deployment of the stapler.[7,38]

TYPES OF STAPLERS

Intestinal tissue is biphasic, with both solid and liquid components in varying ratios (dependent on the type of tissue, and the milieu). Staples are therefore of varying sizes, as good compression enhances the results of stapling (lower leak notes, improved hemostasis, minimized wound contraction, and decreased stricture rates).[7] Historically, staplers have either used predetermined (uniform) staple heights or variable staple height (Table 85.1). With time, manufacturers are modifying the technology of stapling with changes that include varying the predetermined heights of the staples, using rectangular wires (instead of

TABLE 85.1 Defined/Predetermined Staple Heights

Color	Open Staple Length (mm)	Closed Staple Height (mm)	Usage Application
White	2.5–2.6	1.0	Thin/Mesentery
Blue	3.5–3.8	1.5	Regular use
Gold	3.8	1.8	Regular/thick
Green	4.1–4.8	2.0	Thick (stomach)
Black	4.2	2.3	Very thick

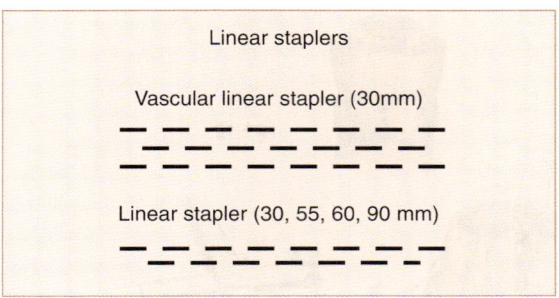

FIGURE 85.3 (Modified from Feil W, Lippert H, Lozac'h P, Palazzini G, Amaral J. *Atlas of Surgical Stapling*. Heidelberg, Germany: Johann Ambrosius Barth; 2000.)

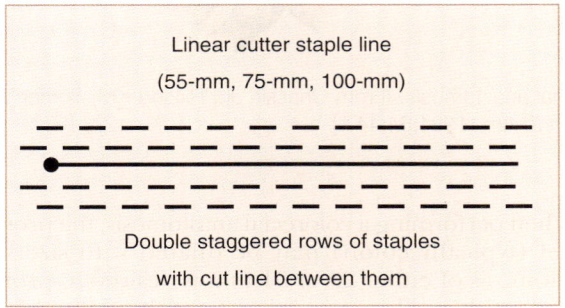

FIGURE 85.4 (Modified from Feil W, Lippert H, Lozac'h P, Palazzini G, Amaral J. *Atlas of Surgical Stapling*. Heidelberg, Germany: Johann Ambrosius Barth; 2000.)

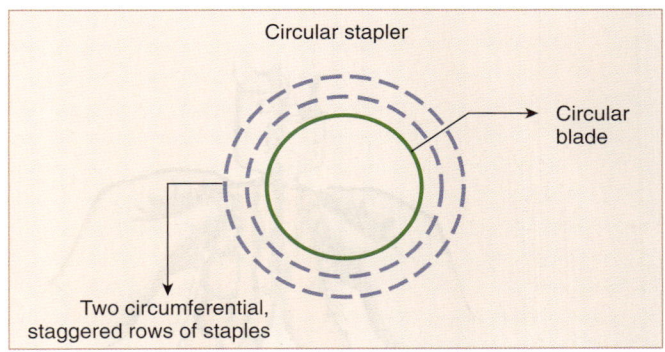

FIGURE 85.5 Circular stapler.

round), using gripping surface technologies, and adjusting the closure and anvil mechanisms.

In brief, skin staplers are popular for their ease of use, enhanced comfort (especially during removal), and rapid application. Clip applicators have a wide range of clip sizes, clip numbers, and working lengths. LDS (ligating, dividing, and stapling device) was historically used to divide omental and mesenteric tissue in open operations. This stapler is infrequently used today.

Linear (noncutting) staplers (e.g., thoracoabdominal [TA] staplers) deliver a double-staggered row of staples (Fig. 85.3). They are used in a wide variety of situations, including closure of a hollow viscus and incisions (enterotomies and others), and ligation of large vessels. Staple length/height is fixed, but various lengths and heights are available. The stapler mechanism/head comes in four lengths and can be articulating or nonarticulating. A third row of staples is found on the vascular subtype.

Linear cutting staplers (e.g., GIA) both close and transect hollow viscera by first delivering two (historically) double-staggered rows of staple lines and then deploying a knife to divide the tissue between the staple lines (newer versions may use triple-staggered rows) (Fig. 85.4). GIA staplers were used to transect tubular structures, create side-to-side anastomosis (both functional end-to-end and otherwise), and resect solid organs. These versatile instruments, in open, laparoscopic, and robotic varieties, feature varying fixed lengths and widths, articulating and nonarticulating heads, straight and newer curved (only nonarticulating) types.

Circular staplers (e.g., creating an end-to-end anastomosis [EEA] with intraluminal [staple] deployment) are used for inverted end-to-end, end-to-side, and occasional side-to-side anastomoses (Fig. 85.5). These staplers have a detachable head/anvil and place a circular, double-staggered row of staples of varying diameters (21, 25, 29, and 33 mm). The staples can be variably tightened to a closed staple height of 1 to 2.5 mm, depending on the desire of the surgeon.

The creativity displayed in the deployment of staplers is remarkable. Several atlases have been dedicated to surgical stapling techniques.[38,39] Two of the more prominent maneuvers follow.

FUNCTIONAL END-TO-END ANASTOMOSIS

A functional EEA (Fig. 85.6), first described in the 1960s, is the most frequent side-to-side anastomosis created with the GIA stapler. Antimesenteric surfaces of two segments of bowel are apposed. Enterotomies in each segment allow one arm of the GIA stapler to be placed in each lumen. The stapler is fired to create a common lumen.[40] The lumen is examined and the staple lines checked for hemostasis. Bleeding points along the staple line in the lumen may be controlled with fine suture, but the application of cautery on the staple lines should be discouraged (because the current can be transmitted along the length of the staple line due to the metal of the staples and thereby harm otherwise healthy tissue). The common enterotomy (involving both limbs of the bowel) is grasped, full thickness, at its edges, usually transversely, with Allis clamps to ensure that all layers are closed. A single firing of the TA stapler is used to close this common enterotomy. Before firing the TA across the common enterotomy, an important technical point is to ensure that the anterior termination and posterior termination of the GIA staple lines are staggered to avoid the crossing of three staple lines.[41] When multiple staple lines cross at the same point, the staples may not close properly, which could lead to anastomotic leakage (see Fig. 85.6). This staple line is an everting one. Placing seromuscular sutures to cover the staple line may attenuate the propensity to form adhesions. Alternatively, the common enterotomy may be closed in an inverting (one- vs. two-layer) handsewn fashion.

Hocking et al. demonstrated in a canine model that creation of a functional EEA alters small bowel motility

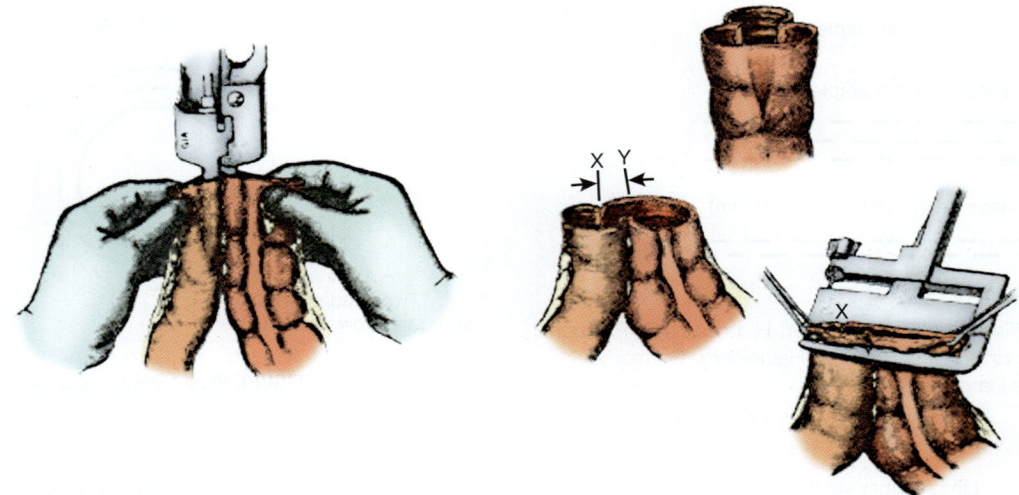

FIGURE 85.6 Example of a side-to-side, functional end-to-end stapled intestinal anastomosis. (From Chassin JL, Rifkind KM, Turner JW. Errors and pitfalls in stapling gastrointestinal tract anastomoses. *Surg Clin North Am*. 1984;64:447.)

to a greater degree than an EEA does and that this may predispose to bacterial overgrowth.[42] Even 2 years after surgery, only 50% of the myoelectrical impulses crossed the functional EEA. Case reports have also shown that this dysmotility and bacterial overgrowth can lead to massive luminal dilation and subsequent volvulus.

STAPLED END-TO-END ANASTOMOSIS

This type of anastomosis is performed with a circular stapler (e.g., EEA) and is commonly used for the creation of esophagogastrostomy, esophagoenterostomy, gastroenterostomy, and coloproctostomy. After resection of the pathology, the anvil is typically placed in the mid or distal esophagus, the small bowel that is to be anastomosed to the stomach, or the proximal bowel to be anastomosed to the rectum. With the use of the anvil, an integral part of using the EEA stapling device, a monofilament purse-string suture is placed in the open lumened bowel, cinched around the rod of the anvil and tied tightly. If there are any gaps in the purse-string suture, the suture line might be incomplete and a leak may ensue. A mattress suture may be tied around the rod to reinforce the purse-string suture. Care must be taken to dissect free any fat that may be incorporated into the staple lines because this may predispose the anastomosis to leakage. The blood supply should not be too close to the ends of the involved bowel for fear of intraluminal bleeding after the stapler is fired. Once the pin is advanced, the anvil and stapler are engaged, the device is closed tightly, and the stapler deployed.

The cervical esophageal anastomosis is typically hand-sewn with or without the use of a GIA; the EEA is often used in the mid to distal esophagus. To ensure the purse string involves all the layers of the esophagus and the anvil is placed appropriately, the mucosa is grasped and exteriorized (prior to the placement of the purse-string suture and the anvil). Supporting sutures to affix the anastomosing stomach or small bowel to the mediastinal pleura, diaphragm, and/or hiatus are used to diminish the tension on the completed esophageal anastomosis.

When performing a colorectal anastomosis, the proximal bowel (typically colon) may be dilated with sizers. An anastomosis of either 29 or 31 mm is desired to promote a good result and less stricturing. Care should be taken to avoid creating serosal or muscular tears during dilatation, relaxing the smooth muscle with intravenous glucagon (1 mg) to help prevent these tears if needed. Placing the stapling device into the rectum transanally, care is taken to follow the contour of the rectum and the sacrum as it is advanced to the end of the rectal cuff. The pin should be advanced to come out in the middle of the staple line rather than advancing the pin at any other point through the mesorectum, or incorporating bladder or the vaginal wall in females.

STAPLING PRINCIPLES

Important steps in the use of staplers include the following:

1. For each device you plan to use, familiarize yourself with the "IFU" (instructions for use) document generated by the (device) manufacturer.[43]
2. Following standard surgical principles, ensure the viability and reasonable condition of the tissue to be manipulated. Exclude a distal obstruction and carefully evaluate areas that have experienced radiation, peritonitis, and local changes (including swelling, fistula, inflammatory-based disease and cancer).[41]
3. Avoid tension on staple lines.
4. Precisely dissect tissues included in the anticipated stapling to avoid incorporating extraneous, vascular, or necrotic-prone tissue.[1]
5. Use adequate compression to cause hemostasis and prevent leakage, but avoid excessive compression leading to tissue damage. Stapler configuration/choice may need to be adjusted even within the same organ when multiple firings are indicated (especially the stomach).[43–46]
6. Ensure that the stapler is properly loaded and configured. Leave the safety mechanism engaged until ready to deploy the stapler.

7. Allow 15 (plus) seconds of compression before deploying the stapler. This allows for more accurate formation of staples and more stable and hemostatic configuration.[45,46]
8. If stapler appears to function abnormally, do not force the stapler to deploy. If creating a long staple line, check for a crotch staple.[43]
9. Be prepared to oversew or repair/reanastomose stapled material. Consider prophylactically addressing staple line crossings. When completed, check the anastomosis for integrity.[47]

SURGICAL ADJUNCTS

With the severity of complications that can result from anastomotic dehiscence, much research has gone into development and testing of adjuncts for intestinal anastomosis, including novel techniques that have yet to reach wide clinical practice. Wrapping omentum around an intestinal anastomosis to reinforce the anastomosis and foster the natural process of healing theoretically allows the omentum to mechanically seal the anastomosis in adhesions and play a role in angiogenesis.[48,49] These theories were confirmed by several early animal studies,[50–52] which led many surgeons to use an omental wrap when worried about the integrity of an anastomosis. Called into question in 1998 by the French Association for Surgical Research, their study showed no significant difference in the rates of anastomotic leakage or death between patients who did or did not have an omental wrap of a colorectal anastomosis.[53] It remains commonplace for surgeons to use an omental wrap for anastomoses they are worried about, despite conflicting clinical evidence regarding the benefit from this practice.

Tissue adhesives are fibrin glues that are commonly used for hemostasis, bone sealing, and other straightforward tissue repairs. They rely on the conversion of fibrinogen to cross-linked fibrin to aid in hemostasis and the reinforcement of tissue strength. A systematic review of tissue adhesives applied to GIA (published since 2000), the majority being animal studies, demonstrated mixed results with colonic anastomoses and largely positive results more proximally.[54] In experimental studies in the rat, the use of fibrin sealant for intestinal anastomosis is associated with increased adhesion formation, lower anastomotic bursting pressure, and lower hydroxyproline concentrations.[55] Sealing a "high-risk" colonic anastomosis with fibrin glue (human or bovine derived) is also associated with higher rates of anastomotic leak, excessive perianastomotic adhesion formation, and poor clinical outcome.[56–58] This may result from the fibrin glue impairing the ingrowth of vascular granulation tissue during the early stages of healing. In conclusion, the routine clinical use of tissue adhesives for the reinforcement of bowel anastomoses has to be made with consideration. Further research is needed to clarify the influence on anastomotic healing.

Adhesion barriers are hyaluronic acid–based absorbable films whose goal is to reduce adhesion formation during the normal healing process. They mechanically separate adhesiogenic tissue by becoming a hydrated gel and then absorbing over the course of approximately a week. Although there is some evidence that it may be beneficial in healing ischemic colonic anastomosis in the rat,[59] there is a preponderance of evidence against its use with an intestinal anastomosis. Use of a hyaluronic acid–based film has been shown to increase the rate of fistula formation and peritonitis in patients undergoing intestinal anastomosis. Furthermore, in a subgroup of patients who had the film wrapped around a fresh anastomosis, anastomotic leak, fistula, peritonitis, abscess, and sepsis occurred significantly more frequently.[60] Therefore use of adhesion barriers cannot be recommended when performing intestinal anastomosis; wrapping a fresh anastomosis in an adhesion barrier should be avoided.

In 1985 a biofragmentable anastomotic ring was developed with the intention to facilitate sutureless intestinal anastomosis. The device consists of two identical circular rings composed of Dexon and 12% barium sulfate. Prolene sutures are used to create purse-string stitches at the two cut ends of the bowel, and the sutures are tightened around the rings after the rings are placed inside the bowel lumens. The device is closed by applying pressure to both sides of the anastomosis. The device is broken down and passed in stool at some later time. The feasibility and safety of this device was confirmed in a dog model.[61] The safety and efficacy of the device for human use was examined in a prospective, randomized, multicenter clinical study, with confirmation by a different research group.[62,63] There was no significant difference in the morbidity, mortality, and clinical course of the patients, including anastomotic leak, fistula, hemorrhage, wound infection, ileus, small bowel obstruction, length of stay, diet, or return to bowel function. Further study has shown this device to be safe for use also in emergency anastomosis.[64,65]

A newer novel intestinal anastomotic device, the compression anastomosis clip, has been shown to be safe and efficacious in humans.[66] It can be used during open or laparoscopic surgery but requires counterincisions on both sides of their anastomosis. Both of these devices likely need long-term follow-up before they will be considered in clinical practice for replacement of traditional anastomotic techniques.

Animal studies using a bovine pericardium patch to reinforce intestinal anastomosis have shown promising results. Use of a porcine model indicates the patch is safe and effective and demonstrated improvement in mitochondrial function and normalization of mucosal transport after wrapping the anastomosis with the patch.[67] Other results indicate its safety of use, some promotion of microscopic wound healing, but without a change in anastomotic strength at 30 days in the pig.[68] This anastomotic adjunct also requires further research. Although these results are promising, future research will have to focus on human results before either patch can enter routine clinical practice.

Prophylactic placement of an abdominal drain after GI surgery has the theoretical advantage of early detection of postoperative complications. Early results indicate no significant difference in terms of outcome, leak rate, or infection for patients with intestinal anastomosis.[69,70] Retrospective studies demonstrate a drain increases the risk of anastomotic leak in rectal anastomoses[71] even as an independent predictor of anastomotic leak (in intestinal anastomoses) (odds ratio, 8.9).[72] Thus there is no strong clinical evidence showing a benefit of prophylactic drainage after intestinal anastomosis,[73] and with the evidence of increased leak rate, the routine use of prophylactic drainage after intestinal anastomosis is not recommended.

The ideal time to resume oral feeding after intestinal anastomosis has been the subject of much debate. Traditional teaching centered around keeping the patient *nil per os* (NPO) until resolution of intestinal ileus. The preponderance of evidence points to the lack of harm, and often the benefit, of early oral feeding. A number of studies indicate there is no clear advantage to keeping patients NPO post operation, especially after colorectal surgeries, and that early feeding is safe, tolerated by the majority of patients, and may provide some benefits.[74–78] Data from the pediatric population also affirm the safety of early oral feeding after intestinal anastomosis, along with increased patient satisfaction and reduction in hospital stay and cost.[79,80] In conclusion, early oral feeding after intestinal anastomosis is generally safe and may benefit the patient and the health system.

CONCLUSION

A number of principles regarding GI anastomoses have been discovered. Despite their articulation and the appreciated importance of a number of preoperative and postoperative maneuvers, the ideal technique appears to vary by location, patient factors, general context, and surgeon perspective, skill, and experience. Because of the biology involved in this activity, the creation of an anastomosis remains something of an art form.

REFERENCES

1. Steichen FM, Wolsch RA. *Mechanical Sutures in Operations on the Small & Large Intestine & Rectum.* Woodbury, CT: Ciné-Med; 2008.
2. Kraup PM, Nordholm-Cartsensen A, Jorgensen LN, Harling H. Anastomotic leak increases distant recurrence and long-term mortality after curative resection for colonic cancer. *Ann Surg.* 2014;259(5):930-938.
3. Thonton FJ, Barbul A. Healing in the gastrointestinal tract. *Surg Clin North Am.* 1997;77(3):549-573.
4. Thompson SK, Chang EY, Jobe BA. Clinical review: healing in gastrointestinal anastomoses, Part I. *Microsurgery.* 2006;26(3):131-136.
5. Phillips B. Reducing gastrointestinal anastomotic leak rates: review of challenges and solutions. *Open Access Surg.* 2016;9:5-14.
6. Witte MB, Barbul A. Repair of full-thickness bowel injury. *Crit Care Med.* 2003;31(8 suppl):S538-S546.
7. Chekan E, Whelan R. Surgical stapling device–tissue interactions: what surgeons need to know to improve patient outcomes. *Med Devices (Auckl).* 2014;7:305-318.
8. Macrae HM, Mcleod RS. Handsewn vs. stapled anastomoses in colon and rectal surgery. *Dis Colon Rectum.* 1998;41(2):180-189.
9. Docherty JG, Mcgregor JR, Akyol AM, Murray GD, Galloway DJ. Comparison of manually constructed and stapled anastomoses in colorectal surgery. *Ann Surg.* 1995;221(2):176-184.
10. Naumann DN, Bhangu A, Kelly M, Bowley DM. Stapled versus handsewn intestinal anastomosis in emergency laparotomy: a systemic review and meta-analysis. *Surgery.* 2015;157(4):609-618.
11. Goulder F. Bowel anastomoses: the theory, the practice and the evidence base. *World J Gastrointest Surg.* 2012;4(9):208.
12. Mattox KL, Moore EE, Feliciano DB, eds. *Trauma.* 7th ed. New York: McGraw-Hill; 2013.
13. Chu C, Williams DF. Effects of physical configuration and chemical structure of suture materials on bacterial adhesion. *Am J Surg.* 1984;147(2):197-204.
14. Slieker JC, Daams F, Mulder IM, Jeekel J, Lange JF. Systematic review of the technique of colorectal anastomosis. *JAMA Surg.* 2013;148(2):190-201.
15. Ethicon. *Wound Closure Manual.* Somerville, NJ: Ethicon, Inc.; 2007:11-16.
16. Hirai K, Tabata Y, Hasegawa S, Sakai Y. Enhanced intestinal anastomotic healing with gelatin hydrogel incorporating basic fibroblast growth factor. *J Tissue Eng Regen Med.* 2013;10(10):E433-E442.
17. Pasternak B, Rehn M, Andersen L, et al. Doxycycline-coated sutures improve mechanical strength of intestinal anastomoses. *Int J Colorectal Dis.* 2007;23(3):271-276.
18. Facy O, Blasi VD, Goergen M, Arru L, Magistris LD, Azagra J. Laparoscopic gastrointestinal anastomoses using knotless barbed sutures are safe and reproducible: a single-center experience with 201 patients. *Surg Endosc.* 2013;27(10):3841-3845.
19. Blanc P, Lointier P, Breton C, Debs T, Kassir R. The hand-sewn anastomosis with an absorbable bidirectional monofilament barbed suture Stratafix® during laparoscopic one anastomosis loop gastric bypass. Retrospective study in 50 patients. *Obes Surg.* 2015;25(12):2457-2460.
20. Katz S, Izhar M, Mirelman D. Bacterial adherence to surgical sutures. *Ann Surg.* 1981;194(1):35-41.
21. Masini BD, Stinner DJ, Waterman SM, Wenke JC. Bacterial adherence to suture materials. *J Surg Educ.* 2011;68(2):101-104.
22. Edmiston CE, Seabrook GR, Goheen MP, et al. Bacterial adherence to surgical sutures: can antibacterial-coated sutures reduce the risk of microbial contamination? *J Am Coll Surg.* 2006;203(4):481-489.
23. Arikanoglu Z, Cetinkaya Z, Akbulut S, et al. The effect of different suture materials on the safety of colon anastomosis in an experimental peritonitis model. *Eur Rev Med Pharmacol Sci.* 2013;17(19):2587-2593.
24. Schoeb DS, Klink CD, Lambertz A, et al. Influence of gentamicin-coded PVDF suture material on the healing of intestinal anastomosis in a rat model. *Int J Colorectal Dis.* 2015;30(11):1571-1580.
25. Law WL, Bailey RH, Max E, et al. Single-layer continuous colon and rectal anastomosis using monofilament absorbable suture (Maxon®). *Dis Colon Rectum.* 1999;42(6):736-740.
26. Koruda MJ, Rolandelli RH. Experimental studies on the healing of colonic anastomoses. *J Surg Res.* 1990;48(5):504-515.
27. Chen C. The art of bowel anastomosis. *Scand J Surg.* 2012;101(4):238-240.
28. Garude K, Tandel C, Rao S, Shah NJ. Single layered intestinal anastomosis: a safe and economic technique. *Indian J Surg.* 2012;75(4):290-293.
29. Shikata S, Yamagishi H, Taji Y, Shimada T, Noguchi Y. Single- versus two-layer intestinal anastomosis: a meta-analysis of randomized controlled trials. *BMC Surg.* 2006;6(1):2.
30. Sajid M, Siddiqui M, Baig MK. Single layer versus double layer suture anastomosis of the gastrointestinal tract. *Cochrane Database Syst Rev.* 2012;(1):CD005477.
31. Ortiz H, Azpeitia D, Casalots J, Sitges A. [Comparative experimental study of inverting and everting sutures in the colon]. *J Chir (Paris).* 1975;109(5-6):691-696. [French].
32. Trueblood HW, Nelsen TS, Kohatsu S, Oberhelman HA Jr. Wound healing in the colon: comparison of inverted and everted closures. *Surgery.* 1969;65(6):919-930.
33. Gill W, Fraser SJ, Carter DC, Hill R. Everted intestinal anastomosis. *Surg Gynecol Obstet.* 1969;128(6):1297-1303.
34. Abramowitz HB. Everting and inverting anastomoses. An experimental study of comparative safety. *Rev Surg.* 1971;28(2):142.
35. Goligher JC, Morris C, Mcadam WA, Dombal FT, Johnston D. A controlled trial of inverting versus everting intestinal suture in clinical large-bowel surgery. *Br J Surg.* 1970;57(11):817-822.
36. Gambee LP, Garnjobst W, Hardwick CC. Ten years' experience with a single layer anastomosis in colon surgery. *Am J Surg.* 1956;92(2):222-227.
37. Burch JM, Franciose RJ, Moore EE, Biffl WL, Offner PJ. Single-layer continuous versus two-layer interrupted intestinal anastomosis. *Ann Surg.* 2000;231(6):832-837.
38. Barth JA. *Atlas of Surgical Stapling.* Heidelberg: Barth; 2000.
39. Rubio PA. Contraindications and precautions. In: Rubio PA, Phelps TH, eds. *Atlas of Stapling Techniques.* Rockville, MD: Aspen Publishers; 1986:13-15.
40. Steichen FM. The use of staplers in anatomical side-to-side and functional end-to-end enteroanastomoses. *Surgery.* 1968;64(5):948-953.
41. Chassin JL, Rifkind KM, Turner JW. Errors and pitfalls in stapling gastrointestinal tract anastomoses. *Surg Clin North Am.* 1984;64(3):441-459.
42. Hocking M, Carlson R, Courington K, Bland KI. Altered motility and bacterial flora after functional end-to-end anastomosis. *Surgery.* 1990;108(2):384-391.

43. Baker RS, Foote J, Kemmeter P, et al. The science of stapling and leaks. In: *Obesity Surgery.* New York, NY: Springer Science + Business Media; 2013:1290-1298.

44. Mery C, Shafi B, Binyamin G, Morton JM, Gertner M. Profiling surgical staplers: effect of staple height, buttress, and overlap on staple line failure. *Surg Obes Relat Dis.* 2008;4(3):416-422.

45. Nakayama S, Hasegawa S, Nagayama SA, et al. *The Importance of Precompression Time for Secure Stapling With a Linear Stapler.* New York: Springer Science + Business Media; 2011:2382-2386.

46. Myers SR, Rothermel WS, Shaffer L. The effect of tissue compression on circular stapler line failure. *Surg Endosc.* 2011;25(9):3043-3049.

47. Offodile AC, Feingold DL, Nasar A, Whelan RL, Arnell TD. High incidence of technical errors involving the EEA circular stapler: a single institution experience. *J Am Coll Surg.* 2010;210(3):331-335.

48. Genzini T, D'Alburquerque LA, de Miranda MP, Scafuri AG, de Oliveira e Silva A. Intestinal anastomoses. *Rev Paul Med.* 1992;110:183-192.

49. Enestvedt CK, Thompson SK, Chang EY, Jobe BA. Clinical review: healing in gastrointestinal anastomoses, Part II. *Microsurgery.* 2006;26(3):137-143.

50. Mclachlin A, Denton D. Omental protection of intestinal anastomoses. *Am J Surg.* 1973;125(1):134-140.

51. Katsikas D, Sechas M, Antypas G, Floudas P, Moshovos K, Gogas J, et al. Beneficial effect of omental wrapping of unsafe intestinal anastomoses. An experimental study in dogs. *Int Surg.* 1977;62(8):435-437.

52. Adams W, Ctercteko G, Bilous M. Effect of an omental wrap on the healing and vascularity of compromised intestinal anastomoses. *Dis Colon Rectum.* 1992;35(8):731-738.

53. Merad F, Hay J, Fingerhut A, Flamant Y, Molkhou J, Laborde Y. Omentoplasty in the prevention of anastomotic leakage after colonic or rectal resection. *Ann Surg.* 1998;227(2):179-186.

54. Vakalopoulos KA, Daams F, Wu Z, et al. Tissue adhesives in gastrointestinal anastomosis: a systematic review. *J Surg Res.* 2013;180(2):290-300.

55. Haukipuro KA, Hulkko OA, Alavaikko MJ, Laitinen ST. Sutureless colon anastomosis with fibrin glue in the rat. *Dis Colon Rectum.* 1988;31(8):601-604.

56. Ham AC, Kort WJ, Weijma IM, Van Den Ingh HFGM, Jeekel H. Healing of ischemic colonic anastomosis. *Dis Colon Rectum.* 1992;35(9):884-891.

57. van der Ham AC, Kort WJ, Weijma IM, van den Ingh HF, Jeekel J. Effect of fibrin sealant on the healing colonic anastomosis in the rat. *Br J Surg.* 1991;78(1):49-53.

58. Byrne DJ, Wood H, McIntosh R, Hopwood D, Cuschieri A. Adverse influence of fibrin sealant on the healing of high-risk sutured colonic anastomoses. *J R Coll Surg Edinb.* 1992;37(6):394-398.

59. Erturk S, Yuceyar S, Temiz M, et al. Effects of hyaluronic acid-carboxymethylcellulose antiadhesion barrier on ischemic colonic anastomosis. *Dis Colon Rectum.* 2003;46(4):529-534.

60. Beck DE, Cohen Z, Fleshman JW, Kaufman HS, van Goor H, Wolff BG. Adhesion Study Group Steering Committee. A prospective, randomized, multicenter, controlled study of the safety of Seprafilm adhesion barrier in abdominopelvic surgery of the intestine. *Dis Colon Rectum.* 2003;46(10):1310-1319.

61. Hardy TG Jr, Pace WG, Maney JW, Katz AR, Kaganov AL. A biofragmentable ring for sutureless bowel anastomosis. An experimental study. *Dis Colon Rectum.* 1985;28(7):484-490.

62. Corman ML, Prager ED, Hardy TG, Bubrick MP. Comparison of the Valtrac biofragmentable anastomosis ring with conventional suture and stapled anastomosis in colon surgery. *Dis Colon Rectum.* 1989;32(3):183-187.

63. Dyess L, Curreri PW, Ferrara J. A new technique for sutureless intestinal anastomosis. A prospective, randomized, clinical trial. *Am Surg.* 1990;56(2):71-75.

64. Ghitulescu GA, Morin N, Jetty P, Belliveau P. Revisiting the biofragmentable anastomotic ring: is it safe in colonic surgery? *Can J Surg.* 2003;46(2):92-98.

65. Choi HJ, Kim HH, Jung GJ, Kim SS. Intestinal anastomosis by use of the biofragmentable anastomotic ring. *Dis Colon Rectum.* 1998;41(10):1281-1286.

66. Lee H, Woo J, Park S, Kang N, Park K, Choi H. Intestinal anastomosis by use of a memory-shaped compression anastomosis clip (Hand CAC 30): early clinical experience. *J Korean Soc Coloproctol.* 2012;28(2):83. doi:10.3393/jksc.2012.28.2.83.

67. Testini M, Gurrado A, Portincasa P, et al. Bovine pericardium patch wrapping intestinal anastomosis improves healing process and prevents leakage in a pig model. *PLoS One.* 2014;9(1):e86627. doi:10.1371/journal.pone.0086627.

68. Hoeppner J, Crnogorac V, Marjanovic G, et al. Small intestinal submucosa for reinforcement of colonic anastomosis. *Int J Colorectal Dis.* 2009;24(5):543-550.

69. Johnson CD, Lamont PM, Orr N, Lennox M. Is a drain necessary after colonic anastomosis? *J R Soc Med.* 1989;82(11):661-664.

70. Rolph R, Duffy JM, Alagaratnam S, Ng P, Novell R. Intra-abdominal drains for the prophylaxis of anastomotic leak in elective colorectal surgery. *Cochrane Database Syst Rev.* 2004;(4):CD002100.

71. Vignali A. Factors associated with the occurrence of leaks in stapled rectal anastomoses: a review of 1,014 patients. *J Am Coll Surg.* 1997; 185(2):105-113.

72. Morse BC, Simpson JP, Jones YR, Johnson BL, Knott BM, Kotrady JA. Determination of independent predictive factors for anastomotic leak: analysis of 682 intestinal anastomoses. *Am J Surg.* 2013;206(6):950-956.

73. Samaiya A. To drain or not to drain after colorectal cancer surgery. *Indian J Surg.* 2015;77(S3):1363-1368.

74. Lewis SJ, Egger M, Sylvester PA, Thomas S. Early enteral feeding versus "nil by mouth" after gastrointestinal surgery: systematic review and meta-analysis of controlled trials. *BMJ.* 2001;323(7316):773-776.

75. Reissman P, Teoh T, Cohen SM, Weiss EG, Nogueras JJ, Wexner SD. Is early oral feeding safe after elective colorectal surgery? A prospective randomized trial. *Ann Surg.* 1995;222(1):73-77.

76. Hartsell PA, Frazee R, Harrison J, Smith R. Early postoperative feeding after elective colorectal surgery. *Arch Surg.* 1997;132(5):518.

77. Ortiz H, Armendariz P, Yarnoz C. Is early postoperative feeding feasible in elective colon and rectal surgery? *Int J Colorectal Dis.* 1996; 11(3):119-121.

78. Dag A, Colak T, Turkmenoglu O, Gundogdu R, Aydin S. A randomized controlled trial evaluating early versus traditional oral feeding after colorectal surgery. *Clinics (Sao Paulo).* 2011;66(12):2001-2005.

79. Mamatha B, Alladi A. Early oral feeding in pediatric intestinal anastomosis. *Indian J Surg.* 2013;77(S2):670-672.

80. Amanollahi O, Azizi B. The comparative study of the outcomes of early and late oral feeding in intestinal anastomosis surgeries in children. *Afr J Paediatr Surg.* 2013;10(2):74.

Anatomy and Physiology of the Mesenteric Circulation

Pamela Zimmerman | Khumara Huseynova | Lakshmikumar Pillai

The focus of this chapter is limited to describing the embryology, anatomy, and physiology of the mesenteric circulation. The terms *mesenteric circulation* and *splanchnic circulation* are sometimes used interchangeably; however, they have distinct meanings. The mesenteric circulation refers specifically to the vasculature of the intestines, whereas the splanchnic circulation provides blood flow to the entire abdominal portion of the digestive system that includes the hepatobiliary system, spleen, and pancreas.[1] The primitive gut comprises the foregut, midgut, and hindgut. The foregut is further divided into upper foregut (embryonic pharynx) and lower foregut, which includes the esophagus, stomach, and the descending portion of the duodenum together with the hepatobiliary derivatives. By convention, the boundaries of the specific segments of the gut are determined by the three unpaired abdominal aortic trunks. The celiac axis supplies the abdominal foregut and its accessory organs, which include the abdominal esophagus, stomach, and proximal duodenum, along with the hepatobiliary, pancreatic structures and spleen. The superior mesenteric artery (SMA) supplies the midgut, which begins just distal to the ampulla of Vater and extends to the proximal two-thirds of the transverse colon. The inferior mesenteric artery (IMA) supplies the hindgut, which includes the distal third of the transverse colon, the descending colon, and the rectum, and extends to the upper part of the anal canal. However, studies have shown that demarcation of these specific segments of the gut occurs well before the development of these vessels and depends on specific gene expression within the gut.[2]

EMBRYOLOGY

ARTERIAL CIRCULATION

The mesenchymal angioblastic tissue covering the yolk sac within the connecting stalk and in the chorionic sac wall give rise to the rudimentary embryonic vessels.[3] By necessity, the cardiovascular arcade and organs are the first system to function in the embryo. Vitelline arteries arising in the yolk sac wall give rise to the arterial supply of the gastrointestinal tract (Fig. 86.1). They connect in the form of plexuses with the ventral surface of the aorta. By the end of week 4, they lose connection with the yolk sac and reduce in number to five cranial and three caudal to the diaphragm, to supply specific regions of the developing abdominal gut.

The celiac axis, which is the most superior of the three abdominal vitelline arteries, initially joins the aorta at the C7 level but with the developing gut descends to the T12

level. In addition to the foregut, it supplies branches to the embryologic outgrowths of the foregut, including the liver, gallbladder, pancreas, and spleen.

The midgut is supplied by the second abdominal vitelline artery, the SMA. This vessel initially joins the aorta at the T2 level but later migrates to the L1 level. At approximately week 5, the midgut, with its mesentery, elongates more rapidly than does the abdominal cavity, leading to formation of a primary intestinal loop with the SMA running down its long axis. By approximately week 10, the midgut completes a 270-degree counterclockwise rotation around the SMA, as shown in Fig. 86.2. As a consequence, the proximal duodenal branches arise on the right side of the SMA, branches to the small bowel arise on the left side, and those to the colon arise from the right side of the SMA.

The blood supply to the hindgut is via the third and final abdominal vitelline artery, the IMA. The cloaca, which is an expansion of the primitive gut just superior to the cloacal membrane, is divided into an anterior portion (urogenital sinus) and a posterior portion (anorectal canal) by the urorectal septum. The distal one-third of the anorectal canal develops from an ectodermal invagination called the anal pit. Therefore, the upper two-thirds of the anorectal canal (endodermal origin) is supplied by the IMA and the lower one-third (ectodermal origin) by the systemic circulation.[2,4]

VENOUS CIRCULATION

The vitelline veins, like the vitelline arteries, arise from the vascular plexuses of the yolk sac. The vitelline venous system initially starts as paired veins that drain into the sinus horns of the heart, as shown in Fig. 86.3A, and anastomose.[5] The veins subsequently develop plexuses in the septum transversum, within which the liver cords grow to form the liver sinusoids, as shown in Fig. 86.3B. The left vitelline vein regresses and disappears by the third month, except for a few transverse anastomoses between the liver and the abdominal foregut (see Fig. 86.3C). The blood from the vitelline system now drains to the heart by the right vitelline vein, which enlarges and becomes the hepatocardiac channel, the cranial portion of which becomes the proximal inferior vena cava (IVC). The right vitelline vein, caudal to the liver, also regresses, except for the portion just caudal to the liver together with a few proximal left to right vitelline anastomoses (see Fig. 86.3B). This segment close to the liver becomes the portal vein (PV) and the superior mesenteric vein (SMV; see Fig. 86.3C and D). The left to right vitelline anastomoses differentiate into the splenic vein (SV) and the inferior mesenteric vein (IMV). Many of the commonly

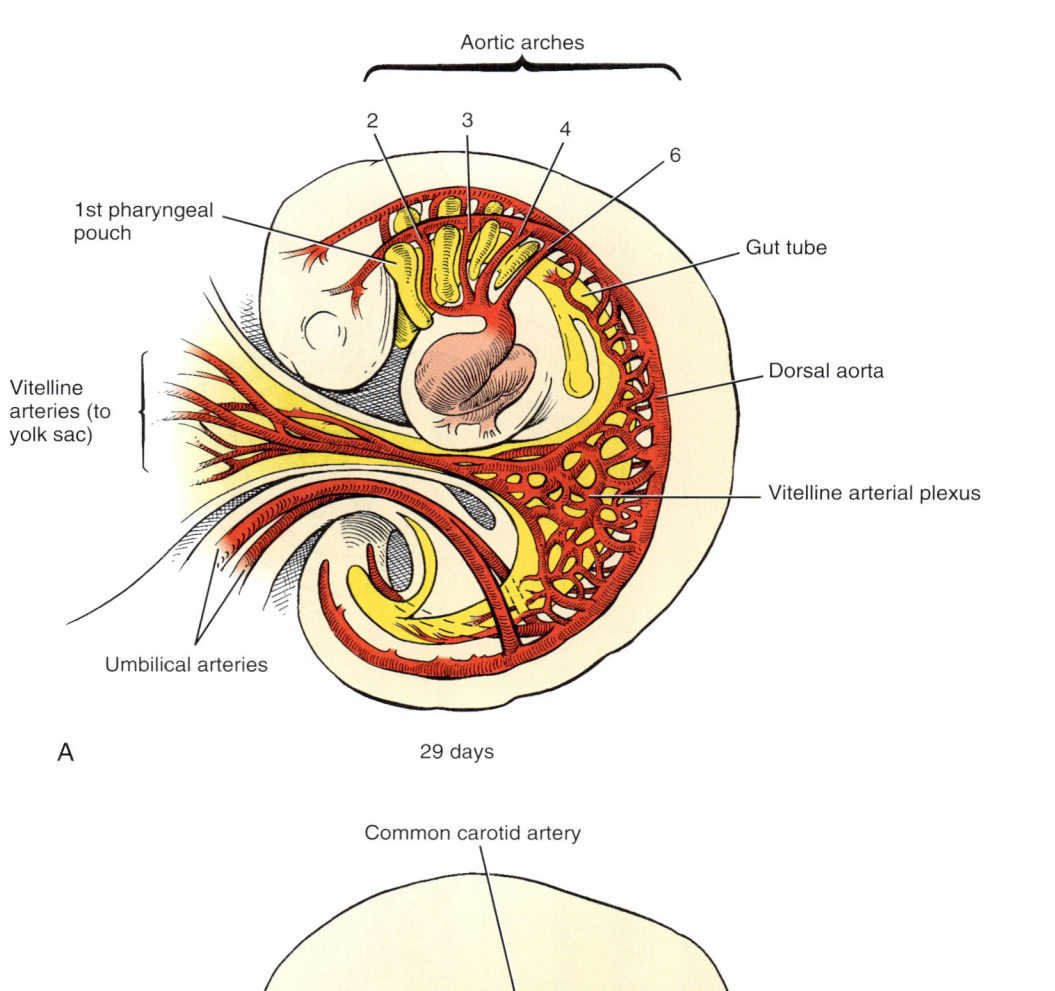

A   29 days

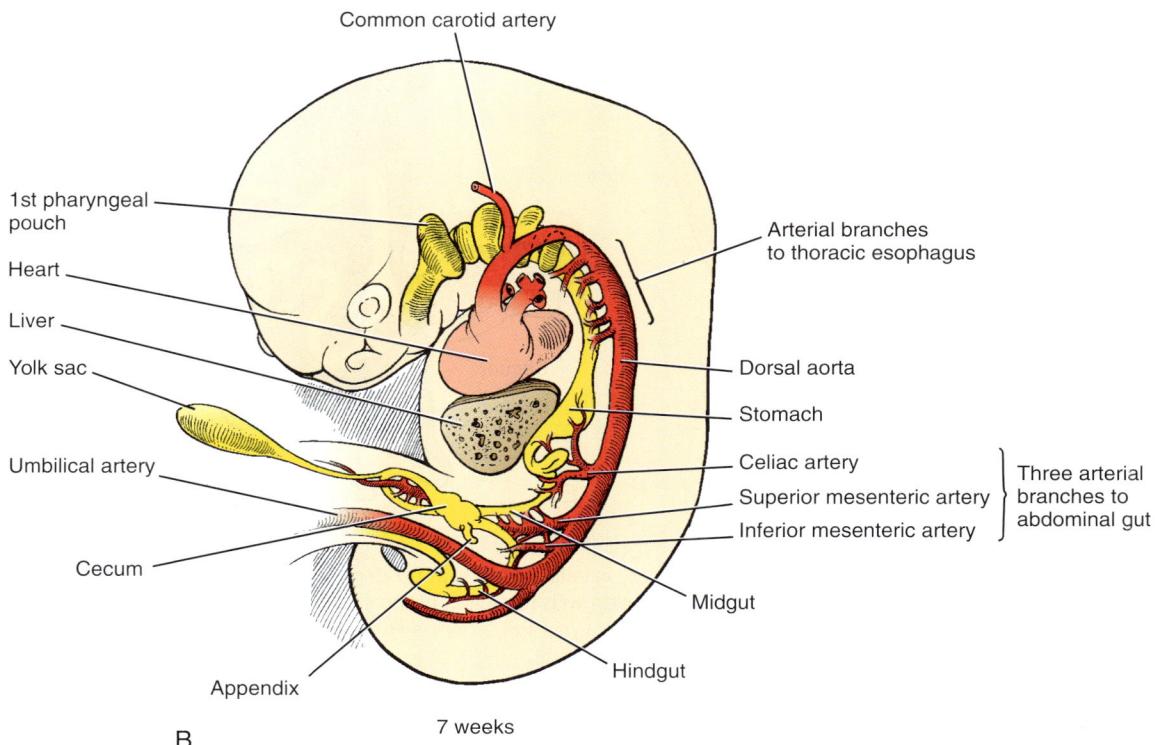

B   7 weeks

FIGURE 86.1 Development of the three arterial trunks. (A) Several vitelline arteries between the aorta and the yolk sac. (B) Vitelline arteries reduced in number to approximately five in the thoracic region and three in the abdominal region. (From Schoenwolf GC, Bleyl SB, Brauer PR, Francis-West PH, Philippa H. *Larsen's Human Embryology*. 4th ed. Philadelphia: Churchill Livingstone Elsevier; 2009:409, Fig. 13.19.)

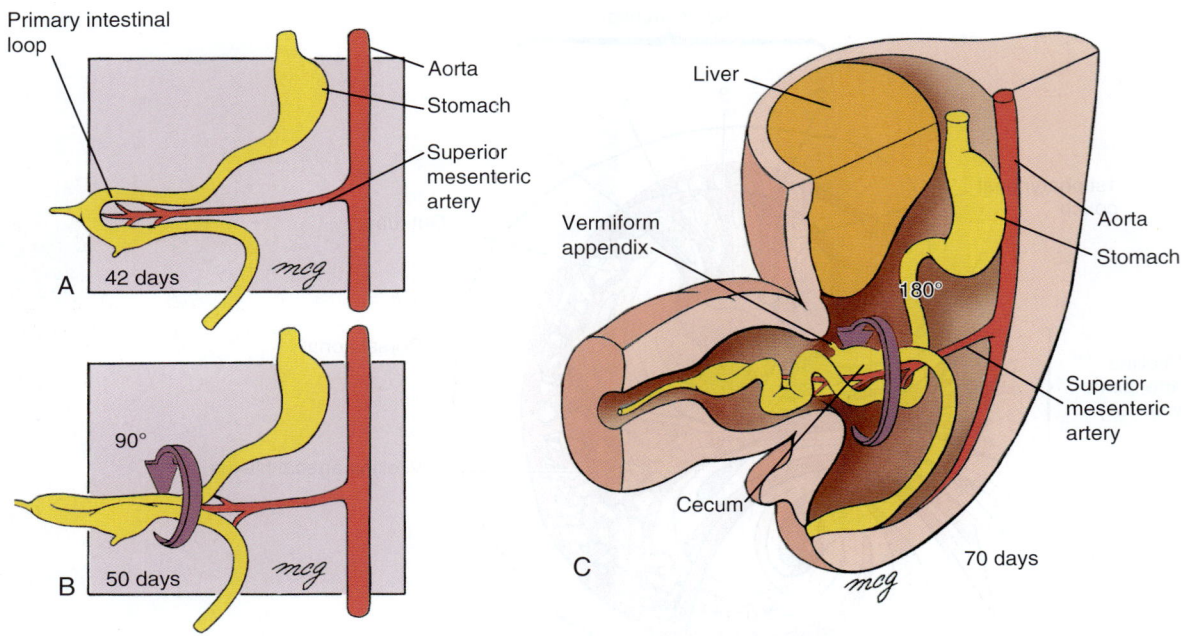

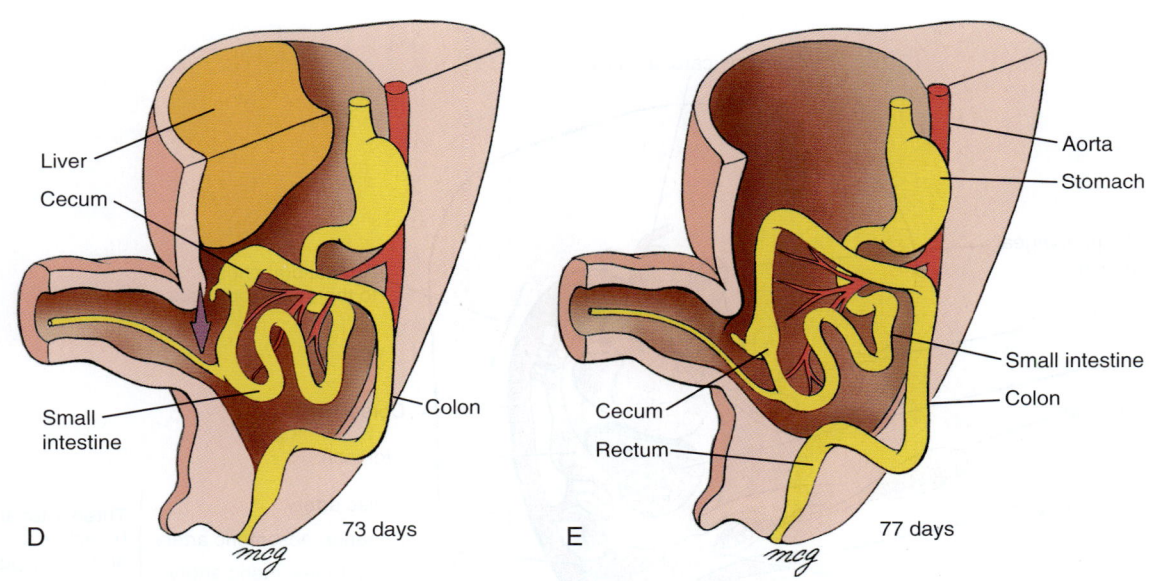

FIGURE 86.2 A 270-degree rotation of the midgut. (A–B) Primary intestinal loop with 90-degree rotation. (C) The gut elongates with an additional 180-degree rotation. (D–E) Completion of the rotation with retraction of the gut within the abdominal cavity to assume the final position. (From Schoenwolf GC, Bleyl SB, Brauer PR, Francis-West PH, Philippa H. *Larsen's Human Embryology.* 4th ed. Philadelphia: Churchill Livingstone Elsevier; 2009:457, Fig. 14.15.)

encountered anomalies of the mesenteric circulation can be attributed to incomplete regression (or persistence) of the early vitelline vessels.

ANATOMY

The arterial and venous circulation of the abdominal viscera form an intricate vascular network marked by a large number of collateral pathways offering ample protection against ischemic events. As noted, the three major aortic branches are responsible for the arterial supply to the intestines and include the celiac axis, SMA, and IMA. The mesenteric venous drainage mirrors the arterial system to a certain extent and includes the SMV and IMV.

ARTERIAL ANATOMY

Celiac Axis

The celiac axis, one of the largest branches of the aorta, originates at the level of the T12 or L1 vertebral body at

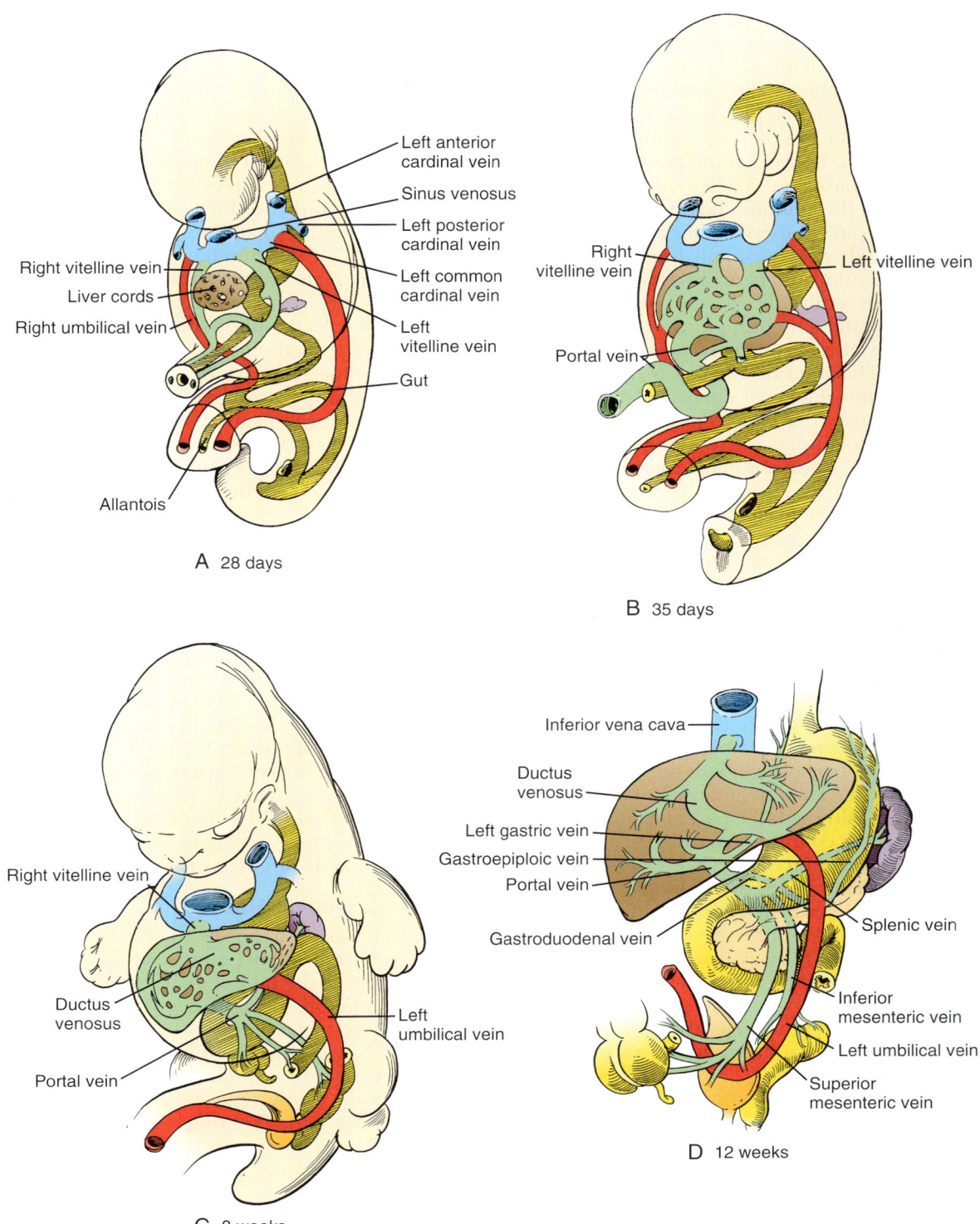

FIGURE 86.3 (A–D) Differentiation of the vitelline veins into mesenteric venous circulation. (From Schoenwolf GC, Bleyl SB, Brauer PR, Francis-West PH, Philippa H. *Larsen's Human Embryology*. 4th ed. Philadelphia: Churchill Livingstone Elsevier; 2009:420, Fig. 13.28.)

a relatively acute angle, traveling for 1 to 2 cm before trifurcating into the left gastric, common hepatic, and splenic arteries. The left gastric artery supplies the distal portion of the esophagus and superior portion of the stomach, then follows the lesser curvature to anastomose with the right gastric artery, which emanates from the common hepatic artery (CHA).

The CHA gives off the right gastric artery and the gastroduodenal artery before becoming the proper hepatic artery. The proper hepatic artery branches into the right and left hepatic arteries. As mentioned earlier, the right gastric artery follows the lesser curvature of the stomach to anastomose with the left gastric artery to supply the lesser curve of the stomach. The gastroduodenal artery descends posterior to the first portion of the duodenum, anterior to the head of the pancreas, and to the left of the common bile duct. It gives off the posterior superior pancreaticoduodenal artery (also called the retroduodenal artery) that supplies the common bile duct, then divides into the right gastroepiploic artery and the anterior superior pancreaticoduodenal artery to supply the antrum of the stomach, the duodenum, and pancreas. The right gastroepiploic artery runs along the greater curvature of the stomach in the greater omentum and eventually communicates with the left gastroepiploic artery, a branch of the splenic artery. The anterior superior pancreaticoduodenal artery divides into duodenal and pancreatic branches.

The splenic artery is the largest branch of the celiac axis and follows a tortuous course along the superior aspect of the pancreas. During its initial course, the splenic artery is a retroperitoneal structure. It then enters the lienorenal ligament before reaching the spleen. The short gastric and left gastroepiploic arteries supplying the greater curvature of the stomach arise from the splenic artery before it enters the hilum. The left gastroepiploic artery continues to join with the right gastroepiploic artery along the inferior aspect of the greater curvature. In addition, the splenic artery gives rise to the dorsal pancreatic artery, which lies posterior to the confluence of the splenic and SMVs.

Anatomic Variants. The classic celiac axis anatomy as described previously is seen in only 55% of patients. A common aortic trunk from which both the celiac axis and the SMA originate, the celiomesenteric artery, occurs in only 1% of patients. Although the potential for individual anatomic variations is countless, common patterns with important clinical relevance have been described. An anomalous right or left hepatic artery has been reported in almost 50% of patients. The right hepatic artery may arise from the SMA in 20% of these cases, the gastroduodenal artery in 2%, and directly from the celiac axis in 1% (also called a replaced right hepatic artery). In addition, the left hepatic artery has been reported to arise from the left gastric artery in 17%, the gastroduodenal artery in 1%, and the celiac trunk in 2% (also called a replaced left hepatic artery).[6]

Hiatt et al., in the largest report to date on the surgical anatomy of the hepatic arteries, observed six arterial patterns as follows: type 1, normal anatomy; type 2, a replaced or accessory left hepatic artery arising from the left gastric artery; type 3, a replaced or accessory right hepatic artery originating from the SMA; type 4, both the right and left hepatic artery arising from the superior mesenteric and left gastric arteries, respectively; type 5, the entire CHA arising as a branch of the SMA; and type 6, the CHA originating directly from the aorta (Fig. 86.4).[7] The presence of a replaced right hepatic artery is particularly significant when pancreaticoduodenectomy or liver transplantation is being considered. In addition to anomalous origins, hepatic arteries have been shown to follow anomalous courses. For example, a replaced or accessory right hepatic artery originating from the SMA may follow a retropancreatic path or remain anterior to the pancreatic neck.

Superior Mesenteric Artery

The SMA arises from the anterior surface of the aorta at the level of the first lumbar vertebral body and passes posterior to the neck of the pancreas and SV and follows a course medial and anterior to the uncinate process of the pancreas and the third part of the duodenum. It supplies the entire small intestine, with the exception of the first part of the duodenum. Its first branch is the inferior pancreaticoduodenal artery that divides into the anterior inferior pancreaticoduodenal and posterior inferior pancreaticoduodenal arteries. These arteries anastomose with the anterior and posterior superior pancreaticoduodenal arteries originating from the gastroduodenal artery to form two robust arterial arcades supplying the head of the pancreas and the duodenum (Fig. 86.5). After crossing the third portion of the duodenum anteriorly, the SMA enters the root of the mesentery. The second branch of the SMA is the middle colic artery that supplies the majority of the transverse colon. The middle colic further divides into right and left branches that anastomose with the right colic artery. The right colic artery commonly arises from the SMA as a common trunk with the middle colic artery, separately from SMA in 38%, is absent in 2%, from the ileocolic artery in 8%, and rarely from the left colic artery.[8] The SMA further divides into multiple jejunal and ileal branches. There are approximately 4 to 6 jejunal and 10 to 14 ileal arteries that originate from the left side of the SMA that run within the mesentery to form a series of arcades before reaching the intestinal wall. Finally, the ileocolic artery arises from the right side of the SMA and supplies the terminal ileum, the cecum, and ascending colon. The ileocolic artery further divides into superior and inferior branches. The appendiceal artery commonly originates from its inferior branch.

Inferior Mesenteric Artery

The IMA arises from the left anterior surface of the aorta at the level of the third lumbar vertebral body. Initially retroperitoneal, the IMA branches as it enters the sigmoid mesocolon before giving rise to the left colic, sigmoidal, and superior rectal vessels. The IMA branches perfuse the large bowel from the mid-distal transverse colon to the upper rectum, including the sigmoid colon. Several rich, clinically significant, and highly variable collateral networks exist between branches of the left colic vessels and the SMA, including at the splenic flexure (Griffith point) and sigmoidal arteries and the superior rectal vessels (Sudek point). These collateral pathways are particularly important when rectosigmoid or splenic flexure resection is performed.

Collateral Pathways

Natural collateral pathways between these mesenteric vessels can circumvent chronic vascular occlusive disease, provided the efficiency of this collateral network adequately meets the metabolic demand. The mesenteric circulation is well known for its rich collateral network and resilience to chronic ischemia. However, these pathways may not be sufficient in acute ischemic events.

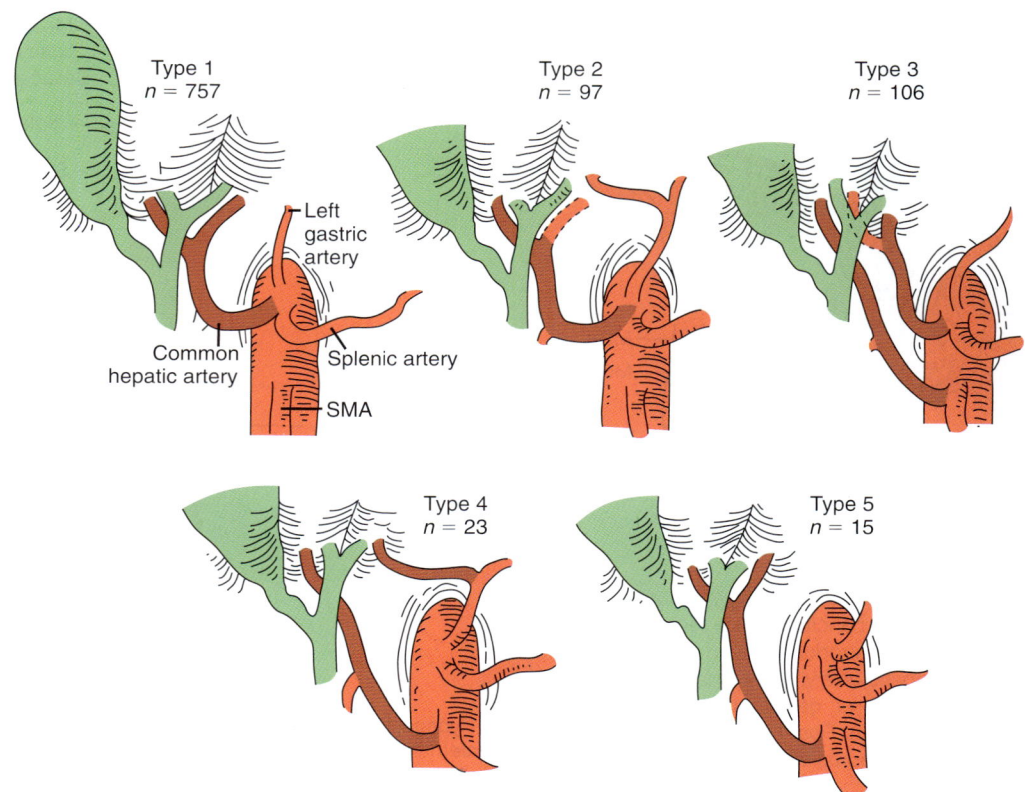

FIGURE 86.4 Hepatic arterial anatomy in 998 cases. *Dotted lines* indicate that the variant artery may be accessory (if branch shown by *dotted line* is present) or replaced (if absent). Type 1, normal; type 2, replaced (accessory) left hepatic artery from left gastric; type 3, replaced (accessory) right hepatic artery from superior mesenteric artery (SMA); type 4, double replaced system; and type 5, common hepatic artery from SMA. In two patients (not shown), the common hepatic artery arose directly from the aorta. (Redrawn from Hiatt JR, Gabbay J, Busuttil RW. Surgical anatomy of the hepatic arteries in 1000 cases. *Ann Surg.* 1994;220:50.)

Celiac Axis—Superior Mesenteric Artery. The major collateral pathway of critical importance, especially in the presence of occlusive disease affecting the celiac axis or the SMA, is between the superior pancreaticoduodenal vessels, from the gastroduodenal artery, and the inferior pancreaticoduodenal vessels, from the SMA. Additional important collateral channels can also exist between the dorsal pancreatic artery and the SMA (Fig. 86.6; see also Fig. 86.5).[9]

Superior Mesenteric Artery—Inferior Mesenteric Artery

The marginal artery of Drummond, the arc of Riolan, and the meandering artery of Moskowitz comprise the major collateral pathways between the SMA and IMA. The marginal artery of Drummond consists of interconnections between the middle colic, right colic, and ileocolic vessels and runs along the periphery of the colonic mesentery (Fig. 86.7). Unless there is significant mesenteric occlusive disease, this vessel is usually small in caliber. Notably, both the arc of Riolan and the meandering mesenteric artery (Moskowitz) are seen only in the presence of significant mesenteric occlusive disease.[8,10] These two collateral pathways consist of IMA-SMA connections through either the proximal branches of the middle colic artery with the ascending branch of the left colic artery (Moskowitz) or the middistal branches of the middle colic artery with the left colic artery (Riolan). Hence they are distinguishable by the more central mesenteric location of the former versus the more peripheral mesenteric location of the latter. IMA reimplantation is usually not required for most patients undergoing open abdominal aortic aneurysm repair because of chronic thrombotic occlusion. However, reimplantation of a patent IMA should be considered during open aortic aneurysm repair, especially in the presence of a known large mesenteric collateral pathway. In addition, in this instance, endovascular aneurysm repair should not be undertaken without assessing the status of the celiac axis and SMA.

Inferior Mesenteric Artery—Hypogastric Artery. A rich and sometimes important collateral pathway exists between the mesenteric circulation and the systemic circulation because of the anastomosing channels between the superior rectal and middle and inferior rectal vessels (see Fig. 86.6). The superior rectal vessels supply circulation to the upper two-thirds of the rectum, and the middle and inferior rectal vessels supply the remaining one-third with the inferior rectal vessels also supplying the anal canal.

VENOUS ANATOMY

The mesenteric venous anatomy grossly mirrors the arterial system. The IMV drains the rectum via the valveless superior

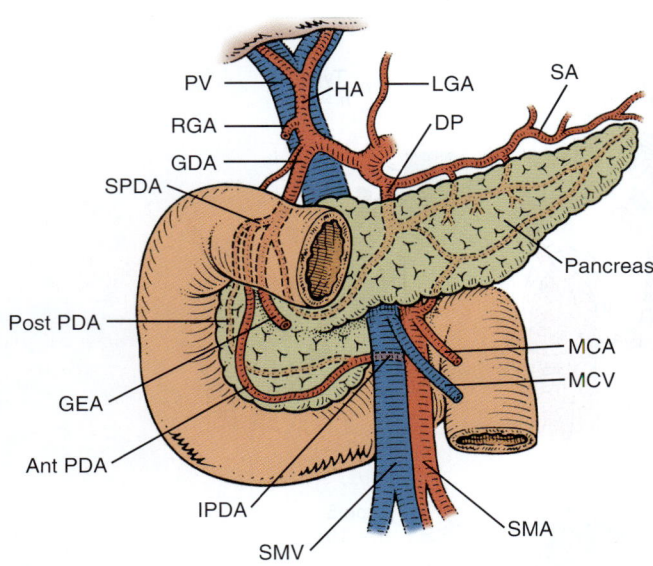

FIGURE 86.5 Arterial vascular arcades supplying the duodenum and pancreas. *Ant PDA,* Anterior pancreaticoduodenal artery; *DP,* dorsal pancreatic artery; *GDA,* gastroduodenal artery; *GEA,* right gastroepiploic artery; *HA,* hepatic artery; *IPDA,* inferior pancreaticoduodenal artery; *LGA,* left gastric artery; *MCA,* middle colic artery; *MCV,* middle colic vein; *Post PDA,* posterior pancreaticoduodenal artery; *PV,* portal vein; *RGA,* right gastric artery; *SA,* splenic artery; *SMA,* superior mesenteric artery; *SMV,* superior mesenteric vein; *SPDA,* superior pancreaticoduodenal artery. (From Blumgart LH, Hann LE. Surgery of the liver and biliary tract. In: Blumgart LH, Fong Y, eds. *Surgical and Radiologic Anatomy of the Liver and Biliary Tract.* 3rd ed. London: Saunders, 2000.)

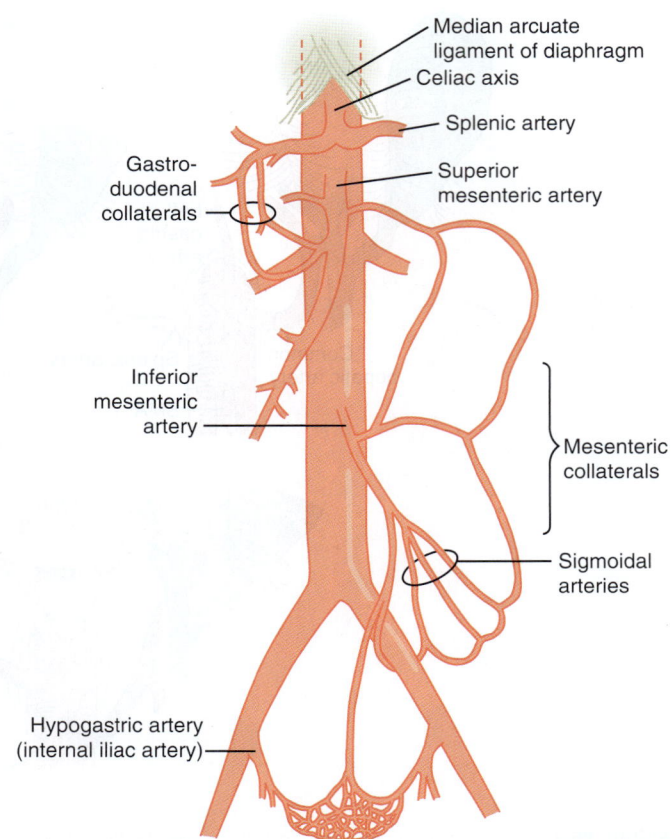

FIGURE 86.6 Schematic depiction of the major visceral vessels and collateral pathways. (Modified from Hanson KJ. Mesenteric ischemia syndromes. In: Dean RH, Yao JST, Brewster DC, eds. *Current Diagnosis and Treatment in Vascular Surgery.* Englewood Cliffs, NJ: Appleton & Lange/Prentice Hall; 1995:264.)

hemorrhoidal vein; more proximally it is joined by the sigmoid and left colic veins that respectively drain the sigmoid and descending colon. The SMV is formed by the confluence of the ileocolic vein (which receives the appendiceal, distal ileal, and right colic veins), segmental ileal and jejunal veins, and gastrocolic trunk anterior to the pancreatic head. The gastrocolic trunk drains the omentum, the distal stomach, and part of the head of the pancreas via the right gastroepiploic, middle colic, and anterior superior pancreaticoduodenal veins. The SV drains the spleen and is joined by the IMV, the left gastric vein, the short gastric veins, multiple pancreatic veins, and the left gastroepiploic vein. Finally, the superior mesenteric and splenic veins join to form the PV.

Intramural Vessels and Microcirculation

Eventually all branches of the major mesenteric arteries terminate into arcades that give rise to vasa recta intestinalis, which divides into short and long branches to supply the circumference of the intestine (Fig. 86.8).

Typical anatomic patterns can be recognized following mesenteric ischemic events. In cases of SMA embolism, the emboli usually land distal to the origin of the middle colic artery, thereby sparing the proximal jejunum and colon. In contrast, in patients with mesenteric arterial thrombosis who have diffuse atherosclerotic disease, where the plaque originates from the aortic wall and progresses

through the ostium of the mesenteric vessel, the mesenteric vessels occlude at their origin. In cases of nonocclusive mesenteric ischemia, the low-flow state is the result of vasoconstriction of the distal jejunal and ileal branches. A similar pattern may be recognized in case of mesenteric venous thrombosis and is associated with dilation of the SMV often observed on computed tomography (CT) angiography.

PHYSIOLOGY

MESENTERIC CIRCULATION

The splanchnic circulation consists of the blood supply to the gastrointestinal tract, liver, spleen, and pancreas. It consists of two large capillary beds partially in series. The small splanchnic arterial branches supply the capillary beds, and then the efferent venous blood flows into the PV. The PV and hepatic artery supply blood flow to the liver.[12]

The mesenteric circulation refers to the vasculature of the intestines. Small mesenteric arteries form an extensive vascular network in the intestinal submucosa. The arterial branches penetrate the longitudinal and circular muscle layers of the intestines and give rise to arterioles. In an

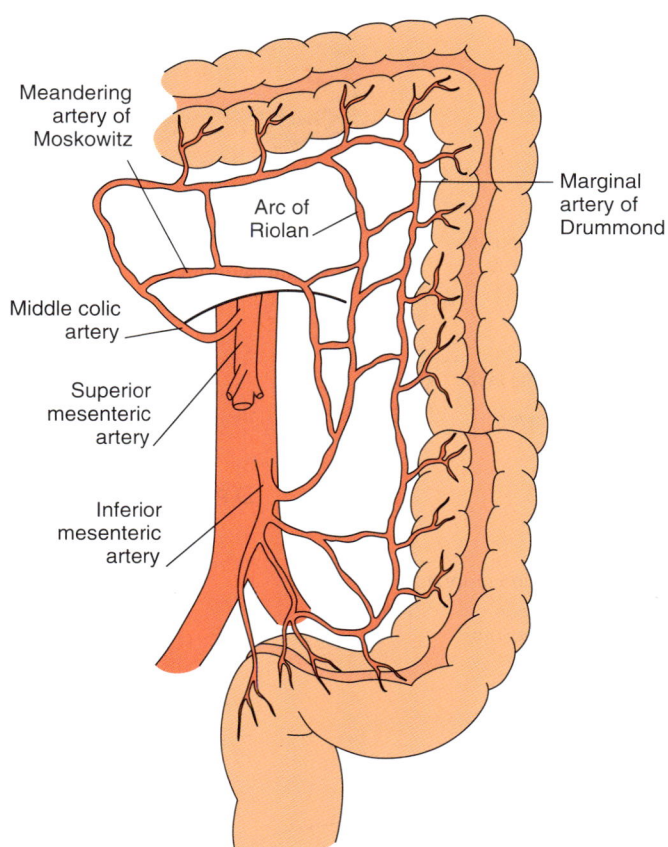

FIGURE 86.7 The collateral vessels between the superior mesenteric and inferior mesenteric arteries. (From Lin PH, Chaikof EL. Embryology, anatomy, and surgical exposure of the great abdominal vessels. *Surg Clin N Am.* 2000;80:417.)

Labels on figure: Meandering artery of Moskowitz; Arc of Riolan; Middle colic artery; Superior mesenteric artery; Inferior mesenteric artery; Marginal artery of Drummond

intestinal villus, blood flows in the opposite direction in the capillaries and venules compared with that of the main arterioles. This creates a countercurrent exchange system in which sodium and water can be absorbed while oxygen diffuses from arterioles to tissues to venules.[12]

Blood flow regulation in the gastrointestinal tract is maintained within narrow limits and changes in response to various intrinsic and extrinsic controls. There are intrinsic vasoregulatory control systems, such as pressure-flow autoregulation, and functional hyperemia. Pressure-flow autoregulation of the intestines is not as developed as in other vascular beds, such as the kidney and brain, and is still incompletely understood. Internal regulation of blood flow by splanchnic vessels occurs when there is a reduction in perfusion. To preserve tissue perfusion, arteriolar smooth muscles relax in response to adenosine or other metabolites that accumulate in tissue injury or ischemia.[13] The most metabolically active region of the intestine is the mucosa, and it has the greatest autoregulation ability within the intestine.[14] Although blood flow is not perfectly regulated with an arterial pressure varying between 100 and 50 mm Hg, oxygen consumption remains within normal limits over the same range of pressures.[15,16] In in vitro human intestinal studies, oxygen consumption remains constant until flow decreases to a critical level of

30 mL/minute per 100 g.[17] Tissue oxygenation, rather than blood flow, is thought to be the trigger for autoregulation within the intestine. Adenosine concentration in mesenteric venous blood also rises after arterial occlusion. Adenosine is a potent vasodilator in the mesenteric vascular bed and may also be a major metabolic mediator of autoregulation.[12]

Hyperemia is an engorgement or excess of blood. Arterial hyperemia is due to local or general relaxation of arterioles. Postprandial hyperemia is an increase in blood flow that occurs in response to a meal. During ingestion of food, the gastrointestinal blood flow remains unchanged. In animal studies, blood flow to the stomach and proximal bowel increases 30 to 90 minutes after ingestion of a meal.[18–21] Blood flow to the ileum increases 45 to 120 minutes postprandially. Colonic blood flow does not increase. Blood flow in the SMA of conscious animals typically increases by 25% to 130% after ingestion of a meal.[18–20,22] Depending on the type and quantity of a meal, the splanchnic vasodilation may last for 4 to 7 hours.[23,24]

Hyperemia in the human intestines is demonstrated on duplex examination. Normal duplex examination of SMA flow shows an increase in vessel diameter that peaks 45 minutes after a 1000-calorie meal. At the same time, flow velocity increases from a mean velocity of 22 to 57 cm/second.[25] The Doppler waveform changes from a high-resistance, triphasic signal in the preprandial state to a low-resistance pattern with high end-diastolic flow postprandially.[26] Blood flow is continuously required after eating.[26] An abnormal mesenteric duplex result is when the postprandial pattern of blood flow in the SMA and IMA continues to have high resistance. This is suggestive of a stenosis or mesenteric ischemia. The blood flow pattern in the celiac artery is not affected postprandially, but it still needs to be examined for proximal stenosis. Normal peak systolic velocity in the celiac artery is less than 160 cm/second, with end-diastolic velocities of less than 55 cm/second. An abnormal fasting peak systolic velocity of greater than 200 cm/second is predictive of a greater than 70% to 99% diameter reduction.[27] Normal peak systolic velocities in the SMA are less than 175 cm/second. Abnormal fasting peak systolic velocities of greater than 275 cm/second are predictive of a greater than 70% to 99% diameter reduction.[27]

Food ingestion and absorption also increases intestinal blood flow. Much research has been done to define luminal stimuli that are responsible for postprandial hyperemia. Some mechanical stimulation of mucosa elicits a hyperemia response, but chyme does not produce enough mechanical stimulation necessary to increase intestinal blood flow. Undigested food does not increase blood flow, although digested food does.[28] It has been proposed that hydrolytic products of food digestion may initiate hyperemia. Osmolality of a meal can dilate vasculature if luminal osmolalities exceed 1500 mOsm/kg, but there is no response at lower osmolalities. Gut blood flow also increases when luminal pH is less than 2.5. Bile causes glucose and long-chain fatty acids to become vasoactive[29,30] but does not increase jejunal blood flow. Bile acids double blood flow in the ileum.[28,31] Protein meals in humans also increase splanchnic blood flow. Glucose within the lumen produces only slight hyperemia in animal models.[28,32] Long-chain fatty acids

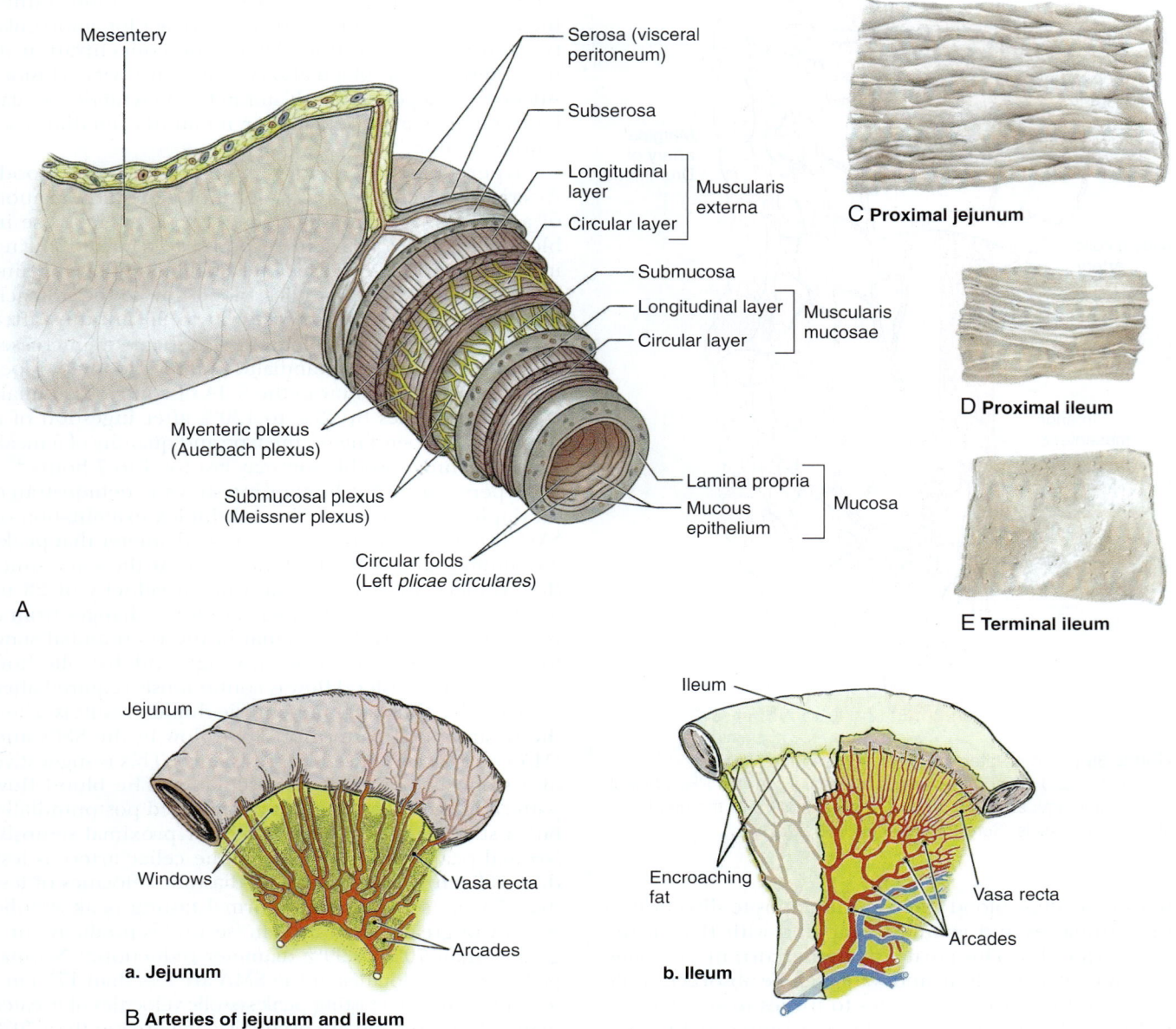

Characteristic	Jejunum (Ba & C)		Ileum (Bb, D, & E)	
Color	Deeper red		Paler pink	
Caliber	2-4 cm		2-3 cm	
Wall	Thick and heavy		Thin and light	
Vascularity	Greater		Less	
Vasa recta	Long	Ba	Short	Bb
Arcades	A few large loops		Many short loops	
Fat in mesentery	Less		More	
Circular folds (L. *plicae circulares*)	Large, tall, and closely packed (C)		Low and sparse (D); absent in distal part (E)	
Lymphoid nodules (Peyer patches)	Few		Many (E)	

FIGURE 86.8 Distinguishing characteristics of the jejunum and ileum in the living body. (From Moore KL, Dalley AF II. *Clinically Oriented Anatomy*. 5th ed. Baltimore, MD: Lippincott Williams & Wilkins, 2006: 266, Table 2.9.)

appear to be the most potent luminal stimulus of post-prandial intestinal hyperemia.[29,32] Lipids, protein, and carbohydrates may act synergistically to stimulate intestinal hyperemia. Intestinal absorption of nutrients is required to initiate a vasomotor response that leads to an intestinal hyperemia.[33] Nonabsorbed substances or water has little effect on mesenteric blood flow.

Extrinsic neurohumoral mechanisms also contribute to the control of intestinal blood flow. These mechanisms include the sympathetic nervous system, the renin-angiotensin system (RAS), and vasopressin. Splanchnic organs receive 25% of cardiac output and contain 25% of total blood volume at rest.[34] Changes in the resistance of mesenteric arterioles cause fluctuation in splanchnic blood flow. The percentage of cardiac output to the intestines varies from 10% to 35%.[35,36] Most of the variability of mesenteric blood flow is accounted for by changes in flow to the small intestine. Neural regulatory control of the mesenteric circulation is mostly sympathetic and is mediated by alpha receptors. This response causes constriction of the mesenteric arterioles and capacitance vessels. Preganglionic cholinergic fibers of the greater splanchnic nerves synapse at the celiac ganglia. Postganglionic adrenergic fibers of the celiac ganglia cause mesenteric artery and arteriolar vasoconstriction. An infusion of β-receptor agonists results in vasodilation. During a fight-or-flight response, vasoconstriction occurs in the mesenteric vascular bed. This shifts blood flow from the temporarily less important intestinal circulation to the more crucial areas of the heart and brain. Parasympathetic fibers of the vagi innervate the intestine but exert little effect on the mesenteric vasculature.[37] When extracellular volume decreases, the RAS is stimulated and causes selective mesenteric vasoconstriction directly through angiotensin II and indirectly through adrenergic potentiation.[38] Loss of blood volume and increase in hyperosmolarity also results in stimulation of the neurohypophysis axis, and pituitary release of vasopressin (antidiuretic hormone) occurs. This causes mesenteric vasoconstriction and venorelaxation.

INTESTINAL ISCHEMIA

Ischemic damage to the intestine occurs when mesenteric blood flow decreases to a level at which delivery of oxygen and nutrients cannot maintain oxidative metabolism. Cell integrity becomes compromised and infarction and cell death occur. Blood flow to the gastrointestinal tract may be compromised by a generalized nonocclusive mesentery ischemia (low-flow state) or from an occlusive disorder (embolism, thrombosis, atherosclerosis, and nonatherosclerotic lesion) that primarily involves the mesenteric circulation.

At low-flow rates, a substantial fraction of oxygen may be shunted from arterioles to venules near the base of the villus. This limits the supply of oxygen to the mucosal cells at the tip of the villus. When intestinal blood flow is reduced, shunting of oxygen occurs, which may cause necrosis of the intestinal villi. The response to the decreased blood flow can range from no damage to transmural necrosis.[39] An alteration of intestinal morphology starts to occur within 30 to 60 minutes of mesenteric artery occlusion. Compromise of the mucosa occurs first, within 30 minutes, with subepithelial edema, and at 1 hour the mucosal lesions progress to loss of epithelial cells along the villus. By 2 hours of occlusion, there is total loss of villi.[39-41]

Changes in vascular and mucosal permeability also occur with an ischemic event. Capillary filtration and microvascular permeability increase in the small intestine.[42] The increase in permeability can occur within 1 hour of ischemia and reperfusion and is dependent on the duration and severity of the ischemic insult. Ischemic injury to the intestine occurs when blood flow is reduced to levels at which oxygenation and nutrients to the tissue are compromised. Correlation of tissue PO_2, mucosal blood flow, and mucosal injury needs further investigation, but reduction of blood flow to levels that do not affect oxygen uptake are not associated with any evidence of mucosal damage in adult animals.[43]

Collateral flow is important in preventing intestinal ischemia.[44-46] It occurs through anastomotic connections of the celiac, superior mesenteric, and inferior mesenteric arteries, arcades, and marginal arteries.[44,47] The collaterals provide a network of flow around occluded vessels. Newborns' intestines may be at greater risk for ischemic injury than an adult because of poorly developed collateral blood vessels.

CLINICAL CORRELATION

ACUTE MESENTERIC ISCHEMIA

Although covered in another chapter, a brief review of intestinal ischemic events is included in this discussion. The mortality of acute mesenteric ischemia (AMI) in adults has been reported at 70% to 90%.[48] It has been reported at 40% in infants with necrotizing enterocolitis (NEC).[49,50] Mortality in the adult is high because of the difficulty of making a diagnosis before bowel death occurs. Single-vessel disease is more likely to cause ischemia if it represents a complete, sudden SMA occlusion or if there is an SMA stenosis combined with previously interrupted collateral pathways. Acute mesenteric ischemic syndrome etiologies in the adult include occlusive disease (embolic or thrombotic), nonocclusive disease, and mesenteric venous thrombosis. In the premature infant, AMI occurs from NEC. Acute occlusion of the celiac artery or IMA generally is asymptomatic in an otherwise normal person; acute occlusion of the SMA, if untreated, results in intestinal infarction and death.

The best clinical indicator of the presence of acute intestinal ischemia is severe abdominal pain that is out of proportion to physical findings. The patient has abdominal pain that is sudden, severe, diffuse, and on examination is without rebound[1] tenderness.[51] Nearly half of the patients have had prior symptoms consistent with chronic mesenteric ischemia (CMI). Vomiting, diarrhea, and occult gastric or rectal blood may be present. Late findings of peritoneal signs and acidosis are usually indicative of dead bowel. The diagnosis is made based on clinical index of suspicion. Diagnosis can be confirmed with computed tomography angiography (CTA) or less commonly now standard catheter angiography. CTA shows SMA occlusion or bowel ischemia signs, such as bowel wall thickening, bowel dilation, ileus, or pneumatosis intestinalis.[52] It can delineate anatomy and guide therapy and should be used cautiously based on clinical judgment.

Initial therapy is geared toward judicious fluid resuscitation to avoid volume overload, using vasopressors only if necessary in hemodynamically unstable patients not responding to fluid therapy, and anticoagulation.[52] Administration of intravenous antibiotics is associated with reduced infection rates due to bacterial translocation.[53]

Surgical interventions (embolectomy, bypass, intestinal resection, transplantation) are used to treat AMI, but mortality continues to be significant. It is difficult to predict reversibility of ischemia; therefore revascularization should precede resection. If the etiology is an embolic event, treatment consists of embolectomy; if a thrombotic event, bypass is performed for revascularization. A second- and third-look laparotomy may be necessary to determine bowel viability.[51] There is a limited role for endovascular therapy with angioplasty and stenting and thrombolysis.[54] Endovascular approach should be reserved for patients with less severe ischemia and for patients with prohibitively high comorbidities precluding open surgery.[52] Nearly one-third of patients who had endovascular intervention for AMI were able to avoid laparotomy in one study.[55] There is insufficient evidence for hybrid therapy including open surgical thrombectomy and retrograde angioplasty/stenting of the mesenteric artery for AMI.[56]

Nonocclusive mesenteric ischemia occurs when intestinal gangrene occurs with patent arteries. Low-flow states are responsible. Examples include hypovolemia or hemorrhagic shock, drugs (digitalis or cocaine), hemodialysis, cardiopulmonary bypass, congestive heart failure, arrhythmias, pancreatitis, and vasopressor agents. Angiography shows a "string of sausages." Treatment is to address the underlying cause. Selective SMA infusion of a vasodilator, such as papaverine, has been reported to relieve vasospasm. Patients need exploration for peritonitis. Generally speaking, patients have poor outcomes because of the underlying cause and comorbidities.

Mesenteric venous thrombosis occurs most commonly because of hypercoagulable states. Other causes include low-flow states from congestive heart failure, cirrhosis with portal hypertension, Budd-Chiari syndrome, intraabdominal inflammatory processes, malignancy, smoking, prior deep venous thrombosis, or unknown etiology. Treatment consists of systemic anticoagulation. Mortality and recurrence rates are lower in patients who receive anticoagulation. Approximately 5% of patients continue to get worse even after anticoagulation and may require intervention in the form of percutaneous or transhepatic thrombectomy with thrombolysis or intraarterial thrombolysis.[52] In general, there is a poorly defined role for thrombectomy and operative thrombolysis. Exploration is reserved for peritonitis and to resect nonviable bowel. Multiple looks at bowel viability may be necessary. Again, outcomes are poor from mesenteric venous thrombosis.

CHRONIC MESENTERIC ISCHEMIA

CMI is relatively uncommon, and like AMI, requires a clinically high index of suspicion. It usually involves two- or three-vessel disease of the mesenteric vessels because collateral vessels permit gradual occlusion of one vessel to be tolerated. The SMA must be one of the two vessels involved. It typically occurs in younger women, smokers, and those with a history of other vascular disease. The most reliable sign or symptom when making the clinical diagnosis of CMI is abdominal pain 30 to 60 minutes after eating. Other classic symptoms include weight loss and "food fear." Diagnosis is made with arterial duplex, CTA, magnetic resonance angiography, or angiography. Treatment is needed when the patient becomes symptomatic, but clinical manifestations are rare due to the extensive collateral circulation.

Open revascularization (OR) for CMI was first performed in 1958 and is still considered the gold standard.[57] There is still debate about optimal reconstruction method (endarterectomy, antegrade or retrograde bypass), completeness of revascularization (one-vessel or two-vessel reconstruction), optimal graft configuration, and optimal conduit.[58-60] In 1980 endovascular repair of visceral vessels was first performed and has now become the preferred treatment for older patients and/or with multiple comorbidities who are poor candidates for OR.[57] Endovascular treatment of CMI with balloon angioplasty and stent has been reported for patients with high risk for operative complications.[61,62] Advantages of endovascular treatment include initial success rate of 95%, lower rate of serious complications, and shorter hospital stay compared with open repair.[52] Restenosis rate and patency is significantly less if angioplasty alone is used.[58,59]

Overall, many more patients are now having treatment with endovascular techniques. A retrospective study from 2008 to 2012 was performed at Albany, New York with 161 consecutive patients with CMI. Outcomes of OR and endovascular revascularization (ER) were compared and outcome analysis and predictors of endovascular failure were performed. Overall mortality was 6.8%. Perioperative mortality (30 day) was not statistically significant between open and endovascular groups (5% vs. 11%), but long-term survival was higher in the endovascular treatment group. A subgroup analysis between patients with successful ER and failure of ER was performed. Patients who required operative intervention after ER failure had higher perioperative mortality than either primary open or endovascular techniques. Failure of endovascular techniques occurred with extensive aortic occlusive disease and lesions greater than 2 cm in length. Although endovascular therapy is now more commonly used than OR, patient selection for each procedure is important to avoid unsuccessful treatment of CMI.[57]

CONCLUSION

Intestinal ischemic disorders are uncommon but are clinically important causes of abdominal pain. Their lethal nature requires vigilance to avoid patient death. Acute occlusive mesenteric ischemia requires a high index of suspicion, and a rapid preoperative evaluation is imperative. Revascularization with open surgical techniques is the gold standard, with resection of nonviable bowel and liberal use of second-look laparotomy. However, an endovascular first approach in conjunction with laparoscopy/laparotomy may be preferred in the high-risk patient. In addition, timely revascularization of symptomatic patients with CMI may reduce the incidence and subsequent high morbidity and mortality of AMI.

REFERENCES

1. Jacobson ED. Physiology of the mesenteric circulation. *Physiologist.* 1982;25:439.
2. Schoenwolf GC, Bleyl SB, Brauer PR, Francis-West PH, Philippa H. *Larsen's Human Embryology.* 4th ed. Philadelphia: Churchill Livingstone Elsevier; 2009.
3. Moore KL. *The Developing Human.* 3rd ed. Philadelphia: Saunders; 1982:298.
4. Sadler TW. *Langman's Medical Embryology.* 10th ed. Baltimore: Lippincott Williams & Wilkins; 2006.
5. Collardeau-Frachon S, Scoazec JY. Vascular development and differentiation during human liver organogenesis. *Anat Rec.* 2008;291:614.
6. Winston CB, Lee NA, Jarnagin WR, et al. CT angiography for delineation of celiac and superior mesenteric artery variants in patients undergoing hepatobiliary and pancreatic surgery. *AJR Am J Roentgenol.* 2007;188:W13.
7. Hiatt JR, Gabbay J, Busuttil RW. Surgical anatomy of the hepatic arteries in 1000 cases. *Ann Surg.* 1994;220:50.
8. Douard R, Chevallier JM, Delmas V, Cugnenc PH. Clinical interest of digestive arterial trunk anastomoses. *Surg Radiol Anat.* 2006; 28:219.
9. Ferrari R, De Cecco CN, Iafrate F, Paolantonio P, Rengo M, Laghi A. Anatomical variations of the coeliac trunk and the mesenteric arteries evaluated with 64-row CT angiography. *Radiol Med.* 2007;112:988.
10. Lange JF, Komen N, Akkerman G, et al. Riolan's arch: confusing, misnomer, and obsolete. A literature survey of the connection(s) between the superior and inferior mesenteric arteries. *Am J Surg.* 2007;193:742.
11. Reference deleted in review.
12. Berne RM, Levy MN. Splanchnic circulation. In: *Physiology.* St. Louis: Mosby; 1993:524.
13. Rosenblum JD, Boyle CM, Schwartz LB. The mesenteric circulation: anatomy and physiology. *Surg Clin North Am.* 1997;77:289.
14. Lundgren O, Svanvik J. Mucosal hemodynamics in the small intestine of the cat during reduced perfusion pressure. *Acta Physiol Scand.* 1973;88:551.
15. Kvietys PR, Granger DN. Regulation of colonic blood flow. *Fed Proc.* 1982;41:2106.
16. Kvietys PR, Miller T, Granger DN. Intrinsic control of colonic blood flow and oxygenation. *Am J Physiol.* 1980;128:G478.
17. Desai TR, Sisley AC, Brown S, Gewertz BL. Defining the critical limit of oxygen extraction in the human small intestine. *J Vasc Surg.* 1996;23:832.
18. Fronek K, Fronek A. Combined effect of exercise and digestion on hemodynamics in conscious dogs. *Am J Physiol.* 1970;218:555.
19. Fronek K, Stahlgren LH. Systemic and regional hemodynamic changes during food intake and digestion in non-anesthetized dogs. *Circ Res.* 1968;23:687.
20. Vatner SF, Franklin D, Van Citters RL. Mesenteric vasoactivity associated with eating and digestion in the conscious dog. *Am J Physiol.* 1970;219:170.
21. Vatner SF, Franklin D, Van Citters RL. Coronary and visceral vasoactivity associated with eating and digestion in conscious dogs. *Am J Physiol.* 1970;219:1380.
22. Snape WJ Jr, Wright SH, Battle WM, Cohen S. The gastrocolic response: evidence for a neural mechanism. *Gastroenterology.* 1979;77:1235.
23. Chou CC. Splanchnic and overall cardiovascular hemodynamics during eating and digestion. *Fed Proc.* 1983;42:1658.
24. Fara JW. Postprandial mesenteric hyperemia. In: Shepherd AP, Granger DN, eds. *Physiology of the Intestinal Circulation.* New York: Raven Press; 1984:99.
25. Jager K, Bollinger A, Valli C, Ammann R. Measurement of mesenteric blood flow by duplex scanning. *J Vasc Surg.* 1986;3:462.
26. Rumwell C, McPharlin M. Arterial evaluation. In: *Vascular Technology.* Pasadena, CA: Davies Publishing, Inc.; 2006:104.
27. Moneta GL, Yeager RA, Dalman R, Antonovic R, Hall LD, Porter JM. Duplex ultrasound criteria for diagnosis of splanchnic artery stenosis or occlusion. *J Vasc Surg.* 1991;14:511.
28. Chou CC, Kvietys PR, Post J, Sit SP. Constituents of chyme responsible for postprandial intestinal hyperemia. *Am J Physiol.* 1978;235:H677.
29. Kvietys PR, Gallavan RH, Chou CC. Contribution of bile to postprandial intestinal hyperemia. *Am J Physiol.* 1980;238:G284.
30. Kvietys PR, Gallavan RH, Chou CC. Contribution of bile to postprandial intestinal hyperemia. *Am J Physiol.* 1980;238:G284.
31. Kvietys PR, Mclendon JM, Granger DN. Postprandial intestinal hyperemia: role of bile salts in the ileum. *Am J Physiol.* 1981;241:G469.
32. Chou CC, Burns TD, Hsieh CP, Dabney JM. Mechanism of local vasodilation with hypertonic glucose in the jejunum. *Surgery.* 1972;71:380.
33. Qamar MI, Read AE, Skidmore R, Evans JM, Williamson RC. Transcutaneous Doppler ultrasound measurement of celiac axis blood flow in man. *Br J Surg.* 1985;72:391.
34. Rowell LB, Johnson JM. Role of the splanchnic circulation in reflex control of the cardiovascular system. In: Shepherd AP, Granger DN, eds. *Physiology of the Intestinal Circulation.* New York: Raven Press; 1984:153.
35. Rapp JH, Reilly LM, Qvarfordt PG, Goldstone J, Ehrenfeld WK, Stoney RJ. Durability of endarterectomy and antegrade grafts in the treatment of chronic visceral ischemia. *J Vasc Surg.* 1986;3:799.
36. Schwartz LB, Purut CM, O'Donohoe MK, Smith PK, Hagen PO, McCann RL. Quantitation of vascular outflow by measurement of impedance. *J Vasc Surg.* 1991;14:353.
37. Granger DN, Richardson PD, Kvietys PR, Mortillaro NA. Intestinal blood flow. *Gastroenterology.* 1980;78:837.
38. Reilly PM, Bulkley GB. Vasoactive mediators and splanchnic perfusion. *Crit Care Med.* 1993;21:S55.
39. Chiu CJ, McArdle AH, Brown R, Scott HJ, Gurd FN. Intestinal mucosal lesions in low-flow states. I. A morphological, homodynamic and metabolic reappraisal. *Arch Surg.* 1970;101:478.
40. Haglund U, Lundgren O. Reactions within consecutive vascular sections of the small intestine of the cat during prolonged hypotension. *Acta Physiol Scand.* 1972;84:151.
41. Robinson JWL, Mirkovitch V. The roles of intraluminal oxygen and glucose in the protection of the rat intestinal mucosae from the effects of ischemia. *Biomedicine.* 1977;27:60.
42. Granger DN, Sennett M, McElearney P, Taylor AE. Effect of local arterial hypotension on cat intestinal capillary permeability. *Gastroenterology.* 1980;79:474.
43. Bohlen HG. Intestinal mucosal oxygenation influences absorptive hyperemia. *Am J Physiol.* 1980;239:H489.
44. Michels NA, Siddharth P, Kornblith PL, Parke WW. Routes of collateral circulation of the gastrointestinal tract as ascertained in a dissection of 500 bodies. *Int Surg.* 1968;49:8.
45. Meyers MA. Griffiths' point: crucial anastomosis at the splenic flexure. *AJR Am J Roentgenol.* 1976;126:77.
46. Saegesser F, Loosli H, Robinson JWL, Roenspies U. Ischemic diseases of the large intestine. *Int Surg.* 1981;66:103.
47. Cho KJ, Schmidt RW, Lenz J. Effects of experimental embolization of superior mesenteric artery branch on the intestine. *Invest Radiol.* 1979;14:207.
48. Boley SJ, Brandt LJ. Selective mesenteric vasodilators: a future role in acute mesenteric ischemia? *Gastroenterology.* 1986;91:247.
49. Kliegman RM, Fanaroff AA. Necrotizing enterocolitis. *N Engl J Med.* 1984;310:1093.
50. Holzman IR, Brown DR. Necrotizing enterocolitis: a complication of prematurity. *Semin Perinatol.* 1986;10:208.
51. Park MM, Gloviczki P, Cherry KJ Jr, et al. Contemporary management of acute mesenteric ischemia: factors associated with survival. *J Vasc Surg.* 2002;35:445.
52. Clair DG, Beach JM. Mesenteric ischemia. *N Engl J Med.* 2016;374(10):959-968.
53. Silvestri L, van Saene HK, Zandstra DF, Marshall JC, Gregori D, Gullo A. Impact of selective decontamination of the digestive tract on multiple organ dysfunction syndrome: systematic review of randomized controlled trials. *Crit Care Med.* 2010;38(5):1370-1376.
54. Wyers MC. Acute mesenteric ischemia: diagnostic approach and surgical treatment. *Semin Vasc Surg.* 2010;23:9.
55. Arthurs ZM, Titus J, Bannazadeh M, et al. A comparison of endovascular revascularization with traditional therapy for the treatment of acute mesenteric ischemia. *J Vasc Surg.* 2011;53(3):698-704.

56. Blauw JT, Meerwaldt R, Brusse-Keizer M, Kolkman JJ, Gerrits D, Geelkerken RH. Multidisciplinary study group of mesenteric ischemia. Retrograde open mesenteric stenting for acute mesenteric ischemia. *J Vasc Surg*. 2014;60(3):726-734.

57. Zacharias N, Eghbalich S, Change B, et al. Chronic mesenteric ischemia outcome analysis and predictors of endovascular failure. *J Vasc Surg*. 2016;63:1582-1587.

58. Oderich GS, Bower TC, Sullivan TM, Bjarnason H, Cha S, Gloviczki P. Open versus endovascular revascularization for chronic mesenteric ischemia: risk-stratified outcomes. *J Vasc Surg*. 2009;49(6):1472-1479.

59. Mateo RB, O'Hara PJ, Hertzer NR, Mascha EJ, Beven EG, Krajewski LP. Elective surgical treatment of symptomatic chronic mesenteric occlusive disease: early results and late outcomes. *J Vasc Surg*. 1999;29:821.

60. McMillan WD, McCarthy WJ, Bresticker MR, et al. Mesenteric artery bypass: objective patency determination. *J Vasc Surg*. 1995;21:729.

61. van Petersen AS, Kolkman JJ, Beuk RJ, Huisman AB, Doelman CJ, Geelkerken RH. Multidisciplinary study group of splanchnic ischemia. Open or percutaneous revascularization for chronic splanchnic syndrome. *J Vasc Surg*. 2010;51(5):1309-1316.

62. Peck MA, Conrad MF, Kwolek CJ, LaMuraglia GM, Paruchuri V, Cambria RP. Intermediate-term outcomes of endovascular treatment for symptomatic chronic mesenteric ischemia. *J Vasc Surg*. 2010;51: 140.

Mesenteric Ischemia

Adam Cloud | John N. Dussel | Carissa Webster-Lake | Jeffrey Indes

Mesenteric ischemia represents insufficient perfusion of the mesentery to meet the metabolic demands of the splanchnic system. Understanding the etiology and presentation of the different forms of mesenteric ischemia is pivotal to the prompt diagnosis and treatment of this often life-threatening condition, with mortality rates that can range from 24% to 94%.[1] This chapter will separate the forms of mesenteric ischemia based on the acuity of their presentation and the nature of the underlying pathology. Mesenteric ischemia is divided into acute mesenteric ischemia (AMI) and chronic mesenteric ischemia (CMI). The four commonly identified causes of AMI include arterial embolism (AE), arterial thrombosis (AT), venous thrombosis (VT), and nonocclusive mesenteric ischemia (NOMI).[2] CMI is attributed to atherosclerotic disease in 95% of cases, with all major mesenteric arteries demonstrating stenosis or occlusion.[1] Other causes include forms of dissection, vasculitis, radiation, and malignancy. Findings of CMI often precede AMI, as regions of chronic narrowing are susceptible to acute chronic thrombosis, a progression that is associated with greater than 50% mortality.[3]

Symptoms manifest in different ways based on the degree and acuity of ischemia. Each form of ischemia has its defining characteristics that affect the regions of mesentery affected, and define the treatments that are appropriate and available. AMI is frequently evaluated in the emergency department, where the patient presents after the sudden onset of abdominal pain that is classically described as "pain out of proportion" with examination. Acute presentations require rapid diagnosis to decrease mortality.[3] Despite the best efforts of modern medicine, mortality still exceeds 50%.[4] Factors that contribute to this high mortality rate include patient demographics and the catastrophic impact that the disease process has on multiple organ systems. Acute presentations can be difficult to identify as symptoms overlap with other conditions, and there are several disease processes that can lead to AMI. CMI is far more likely to be seen in patients who have experienced symptoms of postprandial abdominal pain, nausea, and weight loss over an extended period of time. This constellation of symptoms, frequently provoked by oral intake, results in the classically described phenomenon of *food fear*. CMI can be a challenging diagnosis to make, as multiple areas of arterial obstruction do not necessarily relate to degree of symptoms. Often patients with CMI have undergone evaluation by other specialists and have had prior imaging for evaluation of abdominal pain that was insufficient to identify mesenteric ischemia. Imaging, laboratory studies, and clinical examination do not have findings exclusive to either form of mesenteric ischemia, and the constellation of evaluation studies and clinical examination must be combined with an appropriately focused history and physical to guide in further assessment and care. Historically one of the earliest successful surgically treated presentations of mesenteric ischemia described in the medical literature dates back to 1895. In a remarkable case series of two surgically treated patients, Dr. Elliott[5] became the first physician to demonstrate the utility of surgical intervention in the treatment of mesenteric ischemia. Litton, who had been cited in Elliott's work, had specifically concluded that acute occlusion by emboli would result in necrosis, whereas gradual narrowing and occlusion had previously been demonstrated by Virchow to be tolerable, and even asymptomatic, in some patients.

The standard of surgical intervention that persisted for many years involved only resection of gangrenous bowel. No attempt at restoration of perfusion had been made until 1951, when the use of surgical embolectomy was reported in the treatment of superior mesenteric artery (SMA) occlusion due to embolus from atrial fibrillation.[6] This proved that vascular intervention decreased morbidity and mortality in a previously unsalvageable condition. Once established, options for revascularization were developed and continue to expand as modern modalities of less invasive procedures become available. Now alternatives such as stent placement and catheter directed lytic therapy are available, and the focus of clinical inquiry turns to which modality is best for each specific patient.[7]

ANATOMY

Blood flow to the mesentery is dependent on integrity of the three main vessels providing perfusion to the end organs of the viscera. These vessels include the celiac artery (CA), the SMA space, and the inferior mesenteric artery (IMA) space; Fig. 87.1). The CA supplies the foregut and originates as the first of these branches just above the renal arteries on the anterior aspect of the abdominal aorta. Flow bifurcates early and supplies portions of the stomach, pancreas, spleen, and liver. Multiple smaller branches collateralize and provide flow to portions of the duodenum and pancreas as they connect with the SMA, which is the second branch from the aorta providing flow to the mesentery. The SMA has multiple branches that provide flow to the midgut, composed of the small bowel and first portion of the colon. Importantly an early branch supplies the pancreas, duodenum, and first portion of jejunum, a crucial fact in the viable bowel left after an embolic event, as opposed to its chronic thrombotic

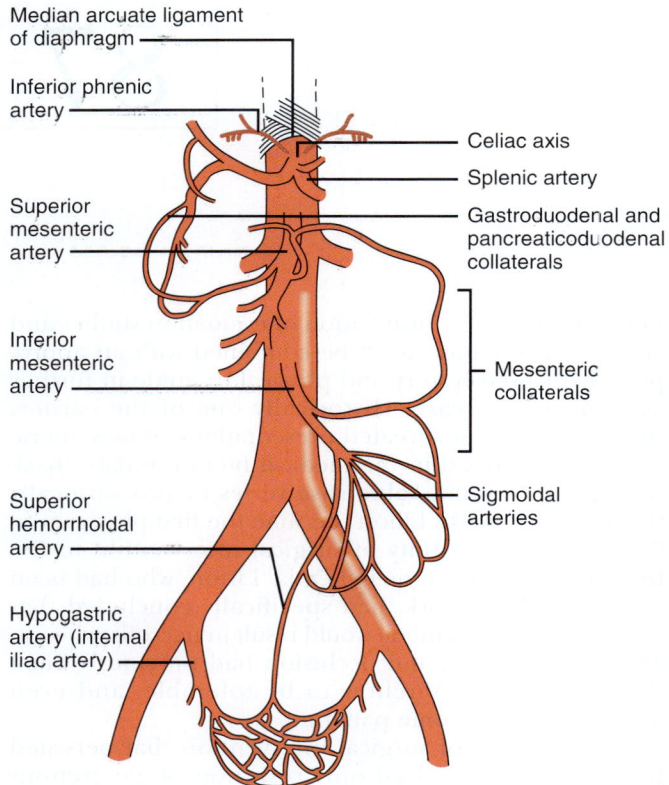

Median arcuate ligament of diaphragm

Inferior phrenic artery

Superior mesenteric artery

Inferior mesenteric artery

Superior hemorrhoidal artery

Hypogastric artery (internal iliac artery)

Celiac axis

Splenic artery

Gastroduodenal and pancreaticoduodenal collaterals

Mesenteric collaterals

Sigmoidal arteries

FIGURE 87.1 Anatomy of the arterial tree of the mesenteric vessels.

angiographically and represents a dilated central anastomotic artery or arc of Riolan. Chronically occluded vessels may result in retrograde flow through alternate pathways, which maintain end-organ perfusion. This expansion of collaterals takes place within the periphery as well as in response to gradual occlusion of primary flow channels. The venous system also has the ability to dilate, as flow is reestablished when a primary pathway has been occluded. Venous occlusions as observed in cirrhosis and mesenteric VT, if tolerated, can eventually develop profound alternate flow pathways.

Mesenteric blood flow is significantly influenced by autoregulation (see Chapter 86). Factors that diminish cardiac output may also affect mesenteric perfusion. Several medications have also been implicated for contributing to diminished mesenteric flow. Alpha antagonists frequently used within the intensive care unit to preserve blood pressure do so by vasoconstriction. In combination with poor cardiac output, they can decrease mesenteric flow to a critical level. Autoregulation and other factors decreasing flow can result in conditions such as NOMI. As the name implies, nonocclusive mesenteric ischemia does not require a fixed defect to be present for acute ischemia to develop. Understanding and recognizing the many factors that contribute to different presentations of mesenteric ischemia will aid in diagnosis and treatment.[8]

ACUTE MESENTERIC ISCHEMIA

The distinct causes of AMI include arterial and venous occlusion, and NOMI. Arterial occlusion is categorized based on the inciting cause of occlusion, embolus, or thrombosis.

ARTERIAL EMBOLI

AE arises frequently from cardiac sources, previously considered the most common cause of AMI, though recent studies show that AT is responsible for at least 50% of arterial AMI.[2,9] Typical embolic causes include thrombus, which has accumulated in the atria due to mitral stenosis, atrial fibrillation, or within the ventricle after infarction. Septic emboli from endocarditis as well as thrombi from aneurysms, atheromatous plaques, and intravascular devices can occur. The embolic material causing AMI is most likely to lodge within the SMA due to its acute origin and high flow state. Females, who have a greater incidence of AMI due to AE, are observed to have a more acute SMA takeoff angle compared with males, which may contribute to their higher susceptibility to this condition. One-half of emboli lodge distal to the origin of the middle colic artery.[10] This contributes to the ischemia frequently isolated to the jejunum, ileum, and ascending colon with preservation of the duodenum, and portions of proximal jejunum. Ischemia of the duodenum and proximal jejunum may also be found with emboli as 15% lodge at the SMA origin.[10] Onset of symptoms is sudden and may be associated with a history of cardiac arrhythmias or recent myocardial infarction. Patients often describe the time or activity associated with the onset of symptoms. On physical examination, these patients are less likely to be malnourished or have other signs of CMI. The pain described is periumbilical and constant, and palpation of

counterpart. The IMA originates significantly lower on the aorta and brings flow to the remainder of the colon and hindgut.

Venous drainage of the mesentery runs in parallel with the arterial system although final outflow within each region drains into the portal system. Interruption in flow is affected by stenosis, hepatic resistance, intravascular devices, and thrombosis resulting from inflammation or hypercoagulable states.

Collateral blood flow provides multiple alternate pathways for perfusion of the mesentery to be preserved despite occlusions within other mesenteric vessels. Abundant collateral circulation to the stomach, duodenum, and rectum accounts for the paucity of ischemic events in these areas. The major anastomosis between the CA and the SMA is formed from the superior pancreaticoduodenal branch of the CA and the inferior pancreaticoduodenal branch of the SMA. These vessels constitute the pancreaticoduodenal arcade and provide blood to the duodenum and the pancreas. The splenic flexure and sigmoid colon have limited anastomoses, and ischemic damage is more common in these locations. There are three potential paths of communication between the SMA and IMA: the marginal artery of Drummond, which is closest to and parallel with the wall of the intestine; the central anastomotic artery or meandering mesenteric artery, a larger and more centrally placed vessel; and the arc of Riolan, an artery in the base of the mesentery. In the presence of SMA or IMA occlusion, a large collateral termed the *meandering artery* may be identified

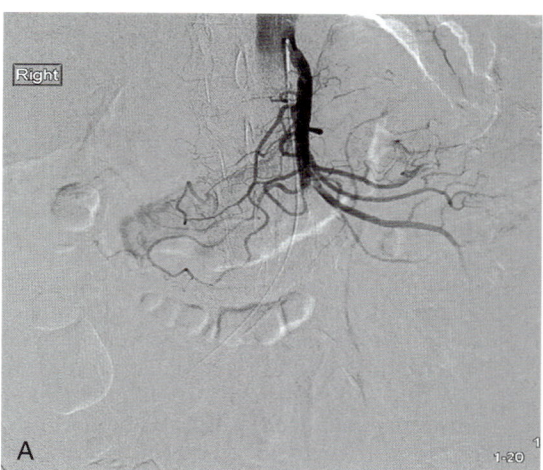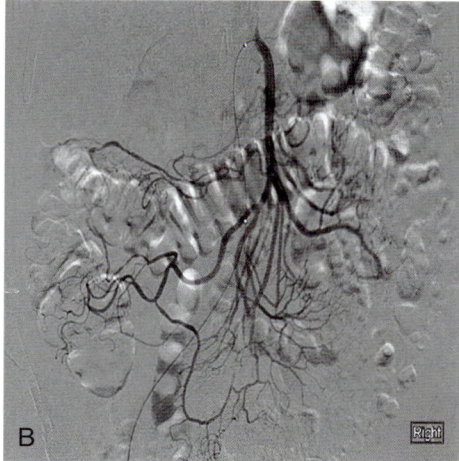

FIGURE 87.2 Computed tomography angiography showing superior mesenteric artery occlusion by embolus.

the abdomen is more severe than anticipated for the exam. This fits the classic description of pain out of proportion with exam. Although the appearance of rebound tenderness may be present, true peritoneal signs are a late marker of severe ischemia resulting from full-thickness ischemia or perforation. A thorough physical examination is mandatory, as other associated complications from emboli may be present, and other sources of mesenteric ischemia may have severe sequelae if not identified and addressed.

Diagnosis

Convincing clinical examination may be enough evidence to initiate therapy in cases where laparotomy is required. Often further work-up is indicated. Laboratory studies are universally obtained and nonspecific leukocytosis is the most common early finding. Late findings include acidosis and elevated lactate levels. Multiple imaging modalities have been used to assess the acute abdomen. Abdominal plain films and ultrasounds are readily obtained in the emergency room. These studies are capable of demonstrating gross findings, but they are rarely specific. Magnetic resonance imaging (MRI) is frequently available but has longer acquisition times, overestimates stenosis, and lacks the resolution of computed tomography angiography (CTA) (Fig. 87.2).[10] Conventional angiography remains the gold standard as a diagnostic study, but its use is primarily relegated to cases where percutaneous catheter based intervention is anticipated and in the diagnosis of CMI. Conventional angiography is limited due to the availability of equipment and personnel to obtain the study in a timely fashion, and its invasive nature. For those reasons, CTA, which is readily available and has a sensitivity and specificity of 94% and 95%, respectively, has become the imaging modality of choice.[11]

Treatment

AE is a surgical emergency. Delay in intervention has a direct negative impact on patient survival. Open surgical intervention remains the standard of care for any patient who has an acute abdomen, as it permits both treatment of the inciting problem and complete evaluation of the

bowel integrity. AE most frequently lodge within the SMA distal to the middle colic artery, sparing jejunal branches, and single-vessel embolectomy is capable of restoring perfusion (Fig. 87.3). Full-thickness ischemia and nonviable bowel must be resected following revascularization. Bowel that is frankly perforated mandates treatment before revascularization to decrease abdominal contamination; otherwise bowel is reassessed once perfusion is restored. Minimizing bowel loss is paramount, and in many cases leaving the bowel in discontinuity with second look laparotomy is indicated to ensure bowel viability and reestablish enteric continuity more safely. Bowel reperfusion can be assessed during laparotomy by restoration of palpable pulses within the mesentery, Doppler signals along the antimesenteric border of the bowel, and overt color change observed in tissue that had been previously underperfused (Fig. 87.4).

There are reports of successful catheter based interventions for restoration of perfusion with both embolectomy and catheter directed thrombolytic therapy. These interventions may be most appropriate for patients who are unable to tolerate open intervention and are unlikely to have full-thickness mesenteric injury. Endovascular intervention is limited in its ability to assess bowel viability. At this time there has been no proven mortality advantage with endovascular treatment.[12] Studies without selection bias have not been performed, and further understanding of the appropriateness of endovascular intervention in all but selected cases is limited. A second consideration is the duration of time required for thrombolytic intervention, which could potentially perpetuate ischemia.

ARTERIAL THROMBOSIS

Thrombosis of the mesenteric vessels resulting in AMI frequently occurs within areas of arteriosclerotic narrowing at the proximal origin of the major mesenteric vessels. Patients with AT frequently have had symptoms of CMI due to progressive narrowing of the three primary mesenteric blood vessels. As occlusions are frequently an orificial process, ischemic injury is likely to affect branch vessels that embolic injury spares, resulting in more devastating bowel infarction. Ischemia may involve the

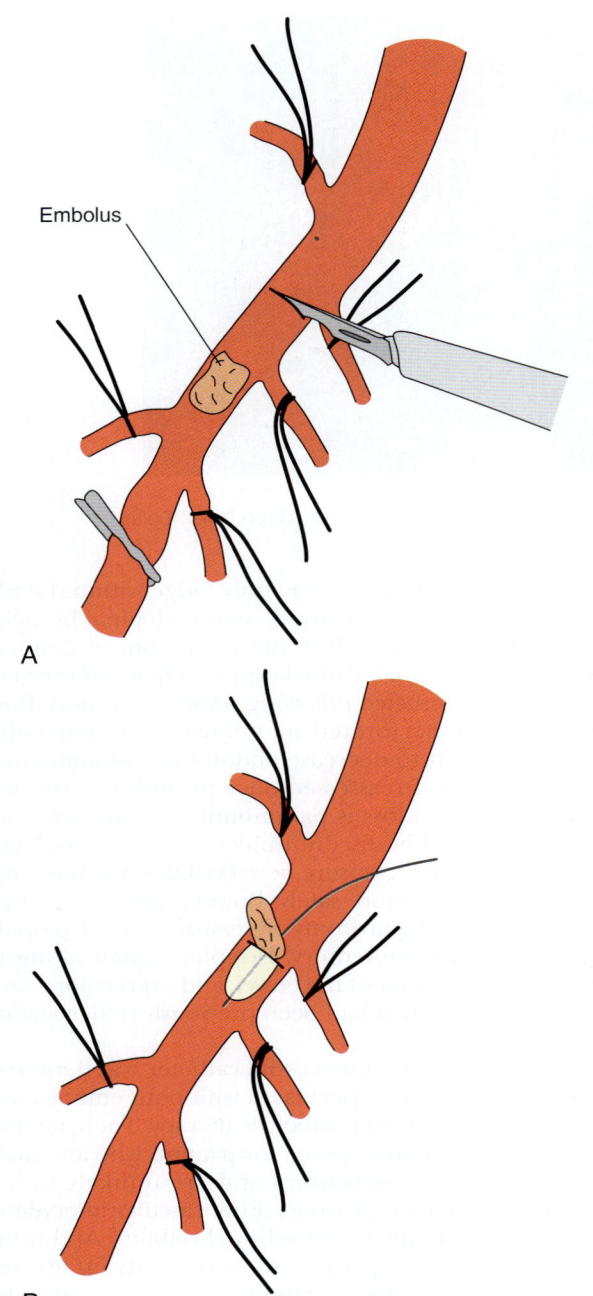

Embolus

A

B

FIGURE 87.3 Embolectomy of superior mesenteric artery. ([B] From Moore EM, Endean ED. Treatment of acute intestinal ischemia caused by arterial occlusions. In: Rutherford RB, ed. *Vascular Surgery*. 6th ed. Philadelphia: Elsevier Saunders; 2005:1725.)

duodenum and the first portion of jejunum, and result in pulselessness of the entire SMA. Distinct from embolic injury, thrombosis requires revascularization bypass around or treatment of the inflow stenosis, along with any necessary embolectomy of the distal vasculature. Multiple bypass options exist, including antegrade, retrograde, and direct aortic. These may be constructed with autogenous tissue or with prosthetic. The choice of technique and conduit

used must be tailored to patient specific considerations: calcification of vessels, comorbidities, and autogenous conduit options are important factors. Full-thickness ischemia and bowel contamination would suggest the use of an autogenous conduit, but this has not been shown to change outcomes. Affected patients frequently have had little preoperative evaluation due to the acuity of their illness, so factors such as shock, myocardial dysfunction, and the physiologic stress of the procedure favor minimally invasive techniques to have an attractive role in treatment. Embolectomy techniques with retrograde stent have the potential to decrease physiologic insult and negate the need for vascular graft placement (Fig. 87.5). The lower long-term effectiveness of stent placement should be balanced against its benefit in rapid restoration of blood flow during acute intervention when compared with surgical bypass options.

NONOCCLUSIVE MESENTERIC ISCHEMIA

NOMI is a condition of decreased mesenteric flow due to contraction of the otherwise normal vessel lumen. Luminal obstructions due to preexisting conditions are not present. This arterial spasm may be elicited by a combination of pharmacotherapy, stress response to sepsis, myocardial dysfunction, or shock. Impediment of blood flow can precipitate ischemia and thrombosis. Often this process is insidious and progressive. Critically ill patients frequently are unable to express their discomfort. History and physical examination may be of limited productivity, and more common diagnoses for abdominal pain are generally considered before NOMI. As with all forms of AMI, early diagnosis portends improved outcomes. A critically ill patient with persistent midabdominal pain, sepsis, hypotension, cardiac dysfunction, renal failure, or alpha-antagonist administration should raise the suspicion for NOMI.

Although plain films, ultrasound, and MRI may have suggestive findings, the most useful studies for revealing severe small vessel arterial spasm are CTA and conventional diagnostic angiography. In this condition conventional angiography has the highest sensitivity and provides the best avenue for therapeutic intervention. Goals of care are directed at increasing bowel perfusion and resolving arterial spasm. Techniques for maximizing cardiac output, appropriate resuscitation, anticoagulation, and discontinuation of potentiating medications are components of therapy. Diagnostic angiography is frequently necessary to make the diagnosis of NOMI, and once established can permit administration of spasmolytic agents. Papaverine administered directly into the SMA through catheter placement is maintained until clinical improvement. Close follow-up angiography to demonstrate effectiveness is indicated, although clinical improvement may be readily observed.

MESENTERIC VEIN THROMBOSIS

Mesenteric venous thrombosis (MVT) is the cause of 2.9% to 15% of all AMI cases.[8,13,14] Recent reviews have demonstrated that the number of AMI cases caused by MVT have declined considerably over time.[15] MVT constitutes only 0.38% of all patients explored operatively for acute abdominal pain.[16] Mortality rates for MVT are lower than

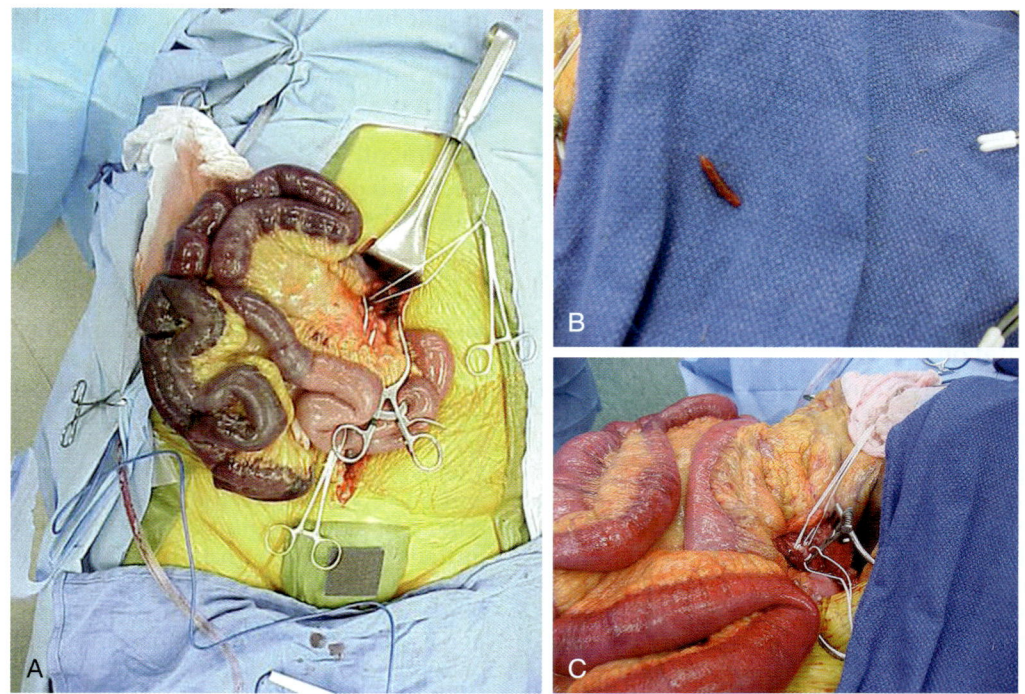

FIGURE 87.4 Ischemic segment of bowel caused by embolus to the superior mesenteric artery.

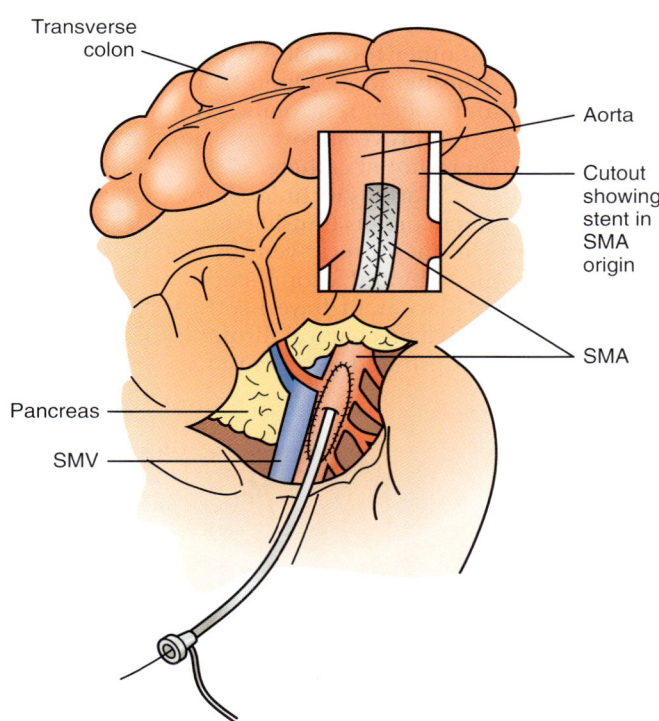

FIGURE 87.5 Retrograde stenting of superior mesenteric artery *(SMA)*. *SMV*, Superior mesenteric vein. (From Wyers MC. Mesenteric vascular disease: acute ischemia. In: Rutherford RB, ed. *Vascular Surgery*. 7th ed. Philadelphia; Elsevier Saunders; 2010:2301.)

those of arterial origin. The superior mesenteric vein is most commonly involved. Extension of thrombus into the portal vein is not uncommon. The clinical presentation of AMI due to MVT is significantly different from arterial-based pathologies. The demographics of patients with MVT are unique from other forms of AMI. Patients tend to be younger and do not have predisposing arteriosclerotic risk factors. Distribution by gender is biased toward males. Patients with procoagulant conditions make up this patient population. MVT is recognized earlier secondary to the availability of highly sensitive imaging modalities, which has led to a distinction between acute, subacute, and chronic subtypes. Acute MVT is defined as new-onset symptomatic thrombosis of the superior mesenteric vein or its branches without evidence of collateralization.[15] Subacute and chronic MVT are frequently diagnosed incidentally, especially in evaluation of bleeding secondary to portal hypertension.

MVT is associated with hematologic and nonhematologic procoagulant states. The most prevalent hematologic inherited or acquired conditions are protein C and protein S deficiencies, antithrombin III deficiency, and factor V Leiden. Other hematologic conditions such as polycythemia vera, paroxysmal nocturnal hemoglobinuria, hyperfibrinogenemia, and myeloproliferative disorders are also associated. Nonhematologic, low-flow, or inflammatory states that contribute to VT include cirrhosis with portal hypertension, congestive heart failure, pancreatitis, intraabdominal trauma, and intraabdominal inflammatory processes. Previous episodes of deep venous thrombosis (DVT) are reported in 20% to 40% of patients with MVT.[15] Up to 54% of patients with MVT have inherited hypercoagulable states, which is more frequent than those with DVT.[17]

Intestinal ischemia from MVT results as venous congestion inhibits arteriolar perfusion at the capillary level. Thrombosis of larger veins is frequently the result of vascular trauma or inflammation. Hypercoagulable states often result in clot formation within venous arcades and may be more likely to cause infarction, as there are fewer collaterals present in the periphery.[15] Bowel wall swelling and edema also frequently lead to the formation of bloody ascites. Venous collateral drainage frequently spares upper abdominal viscera (stomach and duodenum) and the colon from the development of ischemic injury.

Clinical Presentation

The onset of symptoms from MVT is frequently slower than arterial AMI, and patients often have had pain for days before seeking medical attention. Over 75% of patients report at least 2 days of pain; the average duration ranges from 5 to 14 days.[15] Frequently patients present with complaints of nausea, abdominal pain, diarrhea, or bleeding that are nonspecific. The most common laboratory abnormality from MVT is mild leukocytosis. Late findings of peritoneal signs and other markers of full-thickness intestinal ischemia may be present. Chronic MVT manifests very differently, with complications of portal hypertension, including variceal bleeding and ascites. These patients, who have dilated collateral vessels and features of chronic thrombosis, are unlikely to complain of abdominal pain.[18]

Diagnosis

Abdominal CT with appropriate venous phase contrast is highly sensitive and specific. It is the most reliable modality to diagnose MVT. Multiple findings indicative of venous thrombus can be appreciated, including vein wall enhancement, distended venous lumen, and noncontrast opacified thrombus (Fig. 87.6).[15] Other findings include bowel wall thickness greater than 3 mm, indistinct bowel wall margins, new or unexplained ascites, and thickened mesentery.[15] Late findings with 90% sensitivity for transmural infarction include homogeneous enhancement and decreased density of infarcted bowel. Large amounts of ascites and indistinct outer intestinal wall margins are extremely specific for transmural infarction.[19]

Treatment

Therapy is dependent on the clinical severity of the disease process. Standard resuscitation practices should be initiated. The cornerstone of treatment is anticoagulation; heparinization should be started upon diagnosis of MVT. Several studies have demonstrated the ability of heparin to decrease the recurrence of thrombosis and decrease mortality.[15,19,20] As with all forms of mesenteric ischemia, prompt surgical resection of all frankly gangrenous bowel is indicated.[14] Some authors suggest that wider margins are required for resection of VT than with arterial AMI, and most would agree that anticoagulation intraoperatively and postoperatively is indicated in spite of the increased risk of bleeding complications. Both fractionated and unfractionated heparin are appropriate. Conversion to warfarin and 3 to 6 months therapy is indicated unless persistent hypercoagulability or idiopathic thrombosis occurred, which may indicate lifelong therapy. MVT patients who require laparotomy will have markedly different intraoperative findings than those with AT or AE. The bowel is likely to have severe edema, and bloody ascites are frequently present. Resected edges must be evaluated for thrombus and only accepted where margins are without thrombus (Fig. 87.7).

As opposed to other forms of AMI, vessel clearance is not a routine consideration. Open SMV thrombectomy is associated with frequent rethrombosis and has not been demonstrated to improve survival.[21] There are growing reports in the literature of catheter directed lytic therapy to resolve MVT.[21–24] Various techniques for catheter placement include percutaneous transhepatic and transjugular placement in the mesenteric venous system. Catheter placement in the SMA and a combination of arterial and venous catheter placement have been used, sometimes in conjunction with a mechanical thrombectomy.[23] Several studies have demonstrated excellent technical success at

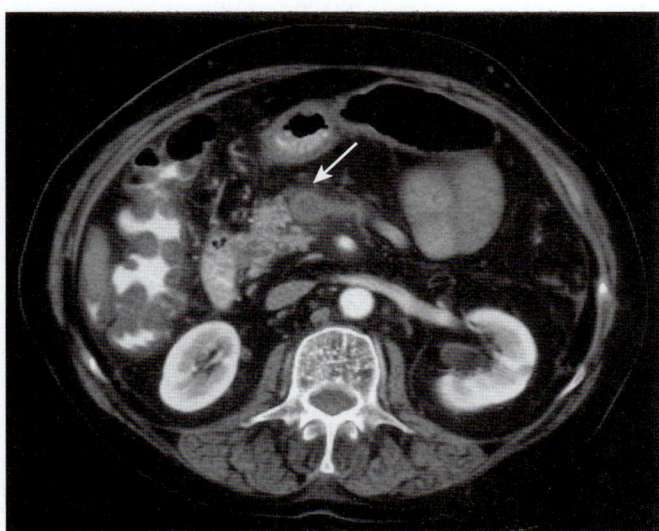

FIGURE 87.6 Mesenteric vein thrombosis with associated bowel wall edema.

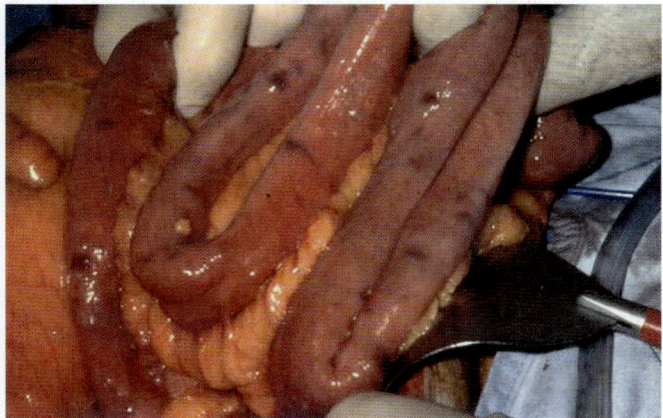

FIGURE 87.7 Bowel of questionable viability requiring careful evaluation and possible second look to ensure adequate perfusion.

accessing the mesenteric venous system and resolving thrombus. Debate still remains as to which patients are appropriate for this form of intervention. The majority of patients will experience rapid symptom relief with anticoagulation alone, and it is yet to be determined which patients will not respond to anticoagulation and eventually require other interventions. Of patients receiving thrombolytic medication, some studies have demonstrated that up to 60% experience major complications and incomplete lysis frequently occurs.[24] Routine thrombectomy and lytic therapy are not recommended.[25]

The mortality of MVT patients is 25% to 30%, and in those who require bowel resection approaches 50%.[15,17] As opposed to other forms of AMI, where cardiac complications are responsible for the majority of mortalities in MVT patients, sepsis with resultant multisystem organ failure is the most common cause. In survivors, short-gut syndrome is common. Long-term therapy should include lifetime anticoagulation for those patients with documented hypercoagulable states. For those with inflammatory states, 3 to 6 months of anticoagulation following resolution of the abdominal process is recommended. For idiopathic MVT, long-term anticoagulation should be considered.

CHRONIC MESENTERIC ISCHEMIA

CMI refers to the constant hypoperfusion of the small bowel that occurs when two or more major mesenteric vessels are stenosed or occluded.[26] This process is relatively uncommon because of the rich collateral mesenteric circulation. The true incidence of mesenteric arterial disease is unknown.[27] Most patients with mesenteric atherosclerotic disease are asymptomatic. Ultrasound imaging from one study demonstrated that 17.5% of asymptomatic patients over the age of 65 years had critical stenosis of more than one mesenteric vessel.[28] However, CMI is estimated to account for less than 2% of hospital admissions for gastrointestinal disease.[29] Because of this relative infrequency, other more common clinical entities are investigated and sometimes treated before CMI is considered.

The most common cause of CMI is ostial atherosclerotic disease. Less common causes include fibromuscular dysplasia, median arcuate ligament compression, vasculitides such as Takayasu disease, or coarctation. The typical patient with CMI is a female smoker in her seventh decade with long-standing abdominal pain. Men are less commonly affected with a male-to-female ratio of 1 : 4.

CMI is characterized by crampy periumbilical abdominal pain that occurs within 30 minutes of meals. Initially pain may be felt only after large meals. As the atherosclerotic burden of the mesenteric vessels becomes more pronounced, the severity and frequency of symptoms increase. The duration and severity of the pain response depend on the size of the meal as well as the food composition. Foods that are thought to precipitate symptoms are avoided, and unintentional weight loss can result. This aversion to food is classically described as *food fear*. The evolution of symptoms is typically gradual (over months) and progressive. The presence of all three classic symptoms (postprandial pain, food fear, and significant weight loss) is almost pathognomonic for CMI. Without these three

elements of the symptom complex, other disease processes should be considered. Other gastrointestinal symptoms including bloating, nausea, vomiting, and diarrhea can accompany the hallmark signs.

There is no single characteristic physical finding for patients with CMI. The abdomen is usually flat or scaphoid, and bruits may be present. Many have an extensive smoking history and other risk factors for atherosclerotic disease. Signs of peripheral vascular disease including diminished or absent pulses and scars from prior vascular surgery may be seen.

Because CMI is rare, it may go unrecognized for a long period of time. Most patients referred to vascular surgeons have undergone a thorough work-up for gastrointestinal complaints. Radiologic and endoscopic studies are frequently used to evaluate for malignancy during this process. Not uncommonly, lack of symptom improvement following ulcer treatment or cholecystectomy leads the clinicians to investigate less common sources of abdominal pain.

In the unfed, unstressed state, the circulatory demands of the resting bowel are easily met and there is no pain. After eating, in times of high demand, pain occurs. These symptoms develop when fixed mesenteric vascular obstructions limit blood flow to the intestine during the increased metabolic demands of the postprandial state. Flow differences in the resting and postprandial state are significant and necessary for digestion to occur. Blood flow increases two to three times following the consumption of a meal and is necessary for effective digestion. Typical maximal circulatory increases occur within 1 hour following food consumption. Ischemic pain occurs when this circulatory demand cannot be met. The extensive collateral circulation among the mesenteric vessels is usually able to compensate for stenosis in one or two mesenteric arteries. Provided there are no acute-on-chronic events, chronic, progressive vessel stenosis with chronic occlusion of a mesenteric artery is frequently a clinically silent event.

DIAGNOSIS

Multiple imaging studies are available to physicians to assist in making the diagnosis of CMI. These include both noninvasive and invasive methods. The decision on which modality to use is based on patient body habitus, degree of suspicion for CMI, and availability of various modalities.

Duplex is a good initial study. Patients need to be studied in the fasting state. Experience of the noninvasive laboratory is extremely important to the routine use of this modality. Typically, patients with CMI have lost extensive weight, have not eaten large meals, and are usually ideal patients to study. There are two commonly used criteria for noninvasive mesenteric investigation. The Wisconsin criteria are based on the peak systolic velocity in the CA and SMA. Flow velocities greater than 200 cm/s in the celiac and greater than 275 cm/s in the SMA correspond to a stenosis higher than 70%. Alternatively the Dartmouth criteria use end-diastolic velocity to determine the degree of stenosis. An end-diastolic velocity greater than 55 cm/s in the CA and greater than 45 cm/s in the SMA are indicative of more than 50% stenosis. Both systems (criteria) have been validated in independent trials.[30,31]

Advances in the capability of multirow detectors have allowed CTA to become an important diagnostic tool when evaluating patients for CMI. Although this study does require both radiation exposure and contrast load, it gives accurate information regarding mesenteric vessel stenosis as well as information regarding perfusion to solid organs and the condition of the bowel. This noninvasive modality has surpassed angiography as the diagnostic modality of choice.

Similar to CTA, MRI has greatly improved over the past decade with the addition of open magnets and decreased acquisition times. Gadolinium contrast with MRI has yielded image resolution similar to that of CTA. Initially there was enthusiasm for the use of magnetic resonance angiography (MRA) with gadolinium in patients with renal dysfunction. However, reports of significant complications, specifically nephrogenic systemic fibrosis, in patients with renal disease have limited the use of MRA. The specificity and sensitivity of MRA is comparable to CTA.

Angiography has historically been considered the gold standard for the evaluation of mesenteric occlusive disease. However, with the advancement of CTA and MRA, this invasive modality is used more often to deliver specific therapy than to diagnose the disease. Disadvantages of this imaging modality include not only its invasive nature but also the resources necessary (angiography suite or operating room) to perform the test. Risks of angiography include arterial trauma, dissection, or pseudoaneurysm formation. Additional risks include contrast-induced nephropathy and radiation exposure.

TREATMENT

The goals of therapy in treating CMI are to relieve symptoms, restore normal digestion, and prevent bowel infarction. Revascularization is warranted in symptomatic patients. Treatment should not be delayed in symptomatic patients, as more than 40% of patients with AMI have had symptoms of CMI. Prophylactic intervention is seldom performed, as there is minimal risk of ischemia in asymptomatic patients.

Open revascularization was the only treatment option for many years. Over the past two decades, percutaneous and hybrid procedures have provided a less invasive alternative to open therapies. The choice of therapy should be individualized to the patient, accounting for the patient's overall health, degree of malnutrition, and anatomic pattern of disease.

Open Surgery

Open surgical techniques for mesenteric revascularization include antegrade or retrograde aorto-mesenteric and/or celiac bypass grafting, endarterectomy, and mesenteric reimplantation. For patients deemed to be candidates for open surgery, the choice of procedure depends primarily on the presenting anatomy, as indicated by the preoperative imaging and intraoperative findings. Heavily diseased and calcific arterial segments are technically difficult to work with and are typically avoided.

Antegrade Bypass. Antegrade bypass can be performed through either a midline or bilateral subcostal chevron incision (Fig. 87.8). The abdomen should be expeditiously

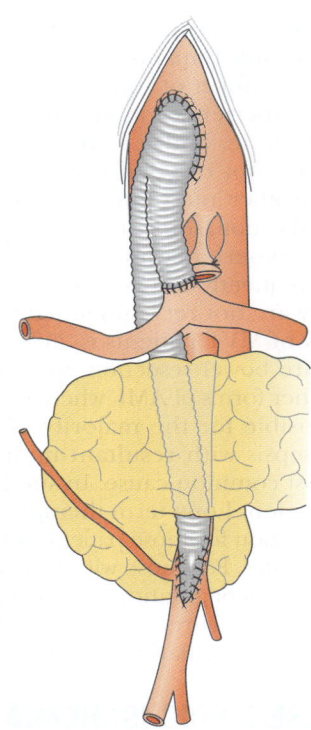

FIGURE 87.8 Bifurcated aorto-celiac and aorto–superior mesenteric artery bypass. (From Huber TS, Lee WA. Mesenteric vascular disease: chronic ischemia. In: Rutherford RB, ed. *Vascular Surgery*. 7th ed. Philadelphia: Elsevier Saunders; 2010. Fig. 148.6.)

explored on entry and the viability of the bowel assessed. Subsequently, the supraceliac aorta should be exposed by division of the left triangular ligament of the liver and retraction of the left lateral lobe. The use of a self-retaining retractor can facilitate exposure. The esophagus is identified by the presence of a nasogastric tube and is retracted to the patient's left along with the stomach. The lesser sac is entered. Here the possibility of an accessory left hepatic artery should be considered. The aorta is then exposed by incising the median arcuate ligament and separating the diaphragmatic crura. During this process, phrenic arteries may be encountered, and these should be ligated. Lateral connective tissue bands posterior to the diaphragm drape over the aorta. These must be cleared to appropriately prepare the aorta for clamping. If left intact, these bands can result in clamp slippage during reconstruction. The celiac axis is then exposed by dissecting caudally along the anterior surface of the aorta.

The SMA can be exposed through a number of approaches, depending on the location of the stenoses. More commonly, the proximal 3 to 5 cm of the SMA is heavily diseased, and the vessel can be approached at the base of the transverse colon mesentery. Alternatively, with the small bowel swept to the right of the midline, the more proximal SMA can be approached laterally by mobilizing the distal duodenum and longitudinally dividing the ligament of Treitz. After preparing proximal inflow and distal target sites, a tunnel must be made. An anatomic, retropancreatic tunnel is created using bimanual blunt

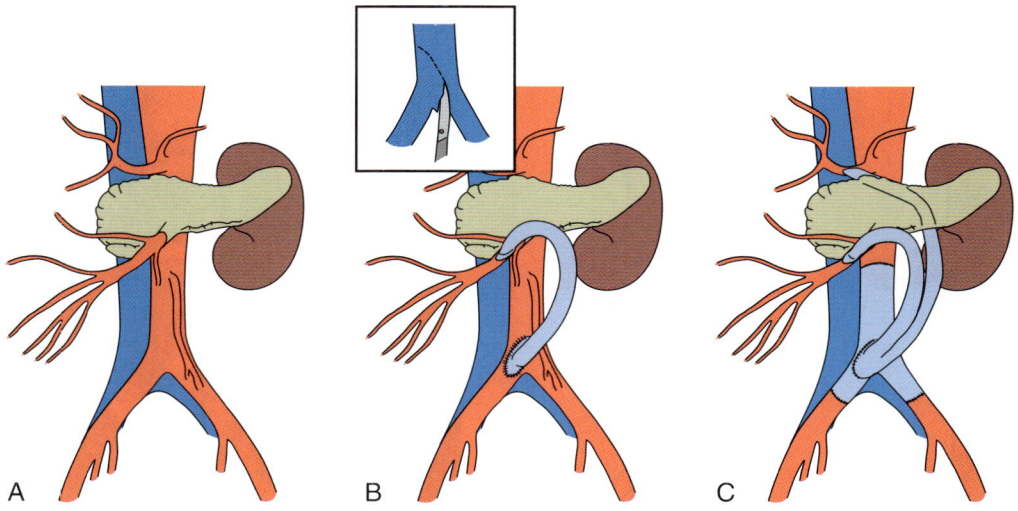

FIGURE 87.9 Infrarenal bypass options.

dissection from the supraceliac aorta to the SMA. Extreme care must be taken, as this tunnel is adjacent to the splenic and portal veins. A Penrose drain or straight aortic clamp can be left in place to assist passage of the bypass limb. If extensive retroperitoneal fibrosis is encountered and tunneling is considered hazardous, a more ventral tunnel over the pancreas through the transverse colon mesentery is acceptable. In this case, the angle of the bypass will frequently necessitate selection of a more distal SMA segment as a target.

The proximal anastomosis is performed with clamps, allowing for partial occlusion. The patient is systemically heparinized and an arteriotomy is performed. A 4-mm aortic punch is helpful in creating a more anatomic aortotomy. If a single artery is to be bypassed, saphenous vein or a 6- to 8-mm prosthetic graft is used. If two vessels are to be bypassed, a 12 × 6 mm bifurcated prosthesis is chosen. The grafts are tunneled and the distal anastomoses are completed in either end-to-end or end-to-side fashion. Graft patency and technical adequacy can then be assessed by handheld Doppler or intraoperative duplex ultrasound analysis.[32,33] The mesenteric peritoneum should then be closed over the graft, and the abdominal cavity closed in standard fashion.

Retrograde Bypass. Infrarenal mesenteric bypasses are advantageous for two reasons (Fig. 87.9). Most importantly, clamp placement is below the renal arteries and less stressful for the patient. Second, the exposure is more familiar than the upper abdominal aorta. This approach is useful when the patient has had extensive adhesions from upper abdominal surgery or needs simultaneous infrarenal aortic reconstruction, or if one is performing the bypass in an urgent situation, due to a quicker revascularization time from a less extensive exposure. The inflow anastomosis can be completed at the infrarenal aorta or either iliac artery (preferably the right iliac). The selection site should be based on the intraoperative ease of clamp placement in the absence of severe calcification. The infrarenal aorta and iliac bifurcation are exposed by retracting the transverse colon cranially and the small

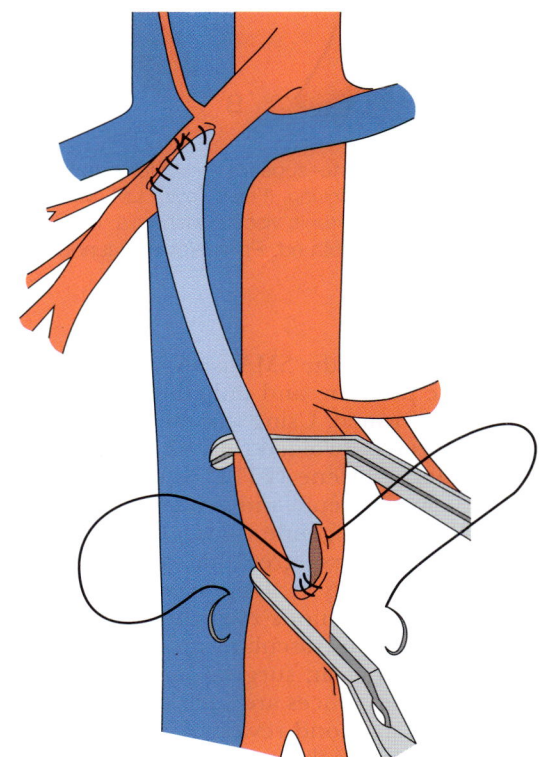

FIGURE 87.10 Infrarenal aorto–superior mesenteric artery bypass.

bowel to the right side of the abdominal cavity. The retroperitoneum is entered, and the aorta and iliac arteries are dissected free and palpated for appropriate clamp positions.

The SMA is exposed by longitudinal dissection of the ligament of Treitz and mobilization of the distal duodenum. Here the choice of conduit is important. If the autogenous vein is used, the SMA anastomosis (distal) is performed first (Fig. 87.10). On completion of the distal anastomosis,

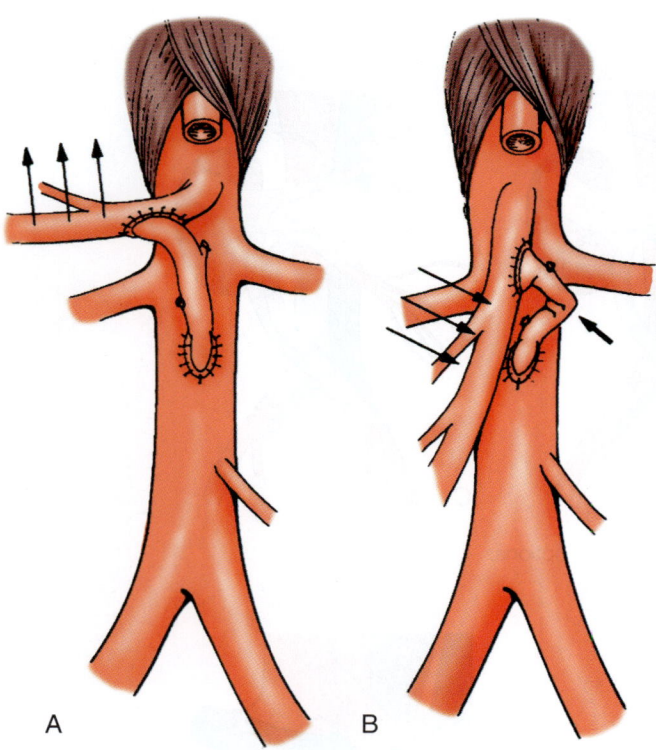

FIGURE 87.11 Infrarenal aorto–superior mesenteric artery bypass with malposition causing kinking. (From Taylor LM, Moneta GL, Porter JM. Treatment of chronic visceral ischemia. In: Rutherford RB, ed. *Vascular Surgery*. 5th ed. Philadelphia: Saunders; 2000:1536.)

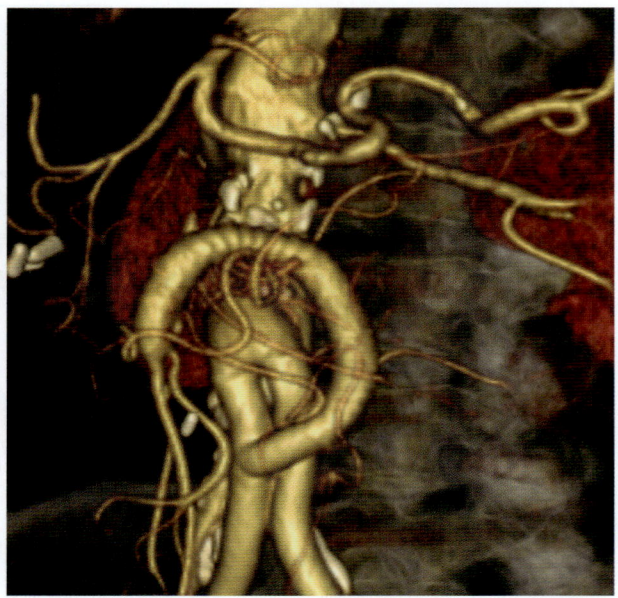

FIGURE 87.12 Right iliac–to–superior mesenteric artery bypass on computed tomography reconstruction.

retractors are relaxed, the SMA is allowed to return to a more anatomic position, and only then is the proximal anastomosis performed. Using this method, kinking of a short vein graft can be avoided (Fig. 87.11). When Dacron or polytetrafluoroethylene (PTFE) is used, the graft traverses the retroperitoneum and swings back through the ligament of Treitz in a gentle C-loop.

Although all authors agree that revascularizing the SMA should be a priority in all-open procedures for CMI, there are differing opinions regarding either single[34,35] or multiple[36,37] vessel revascularization. Because the literature is less than clear, surgical judgment should be employed. If circumstances are such that the procedure is going well and a second revascularized vessel will not add to the morbidity of the procedure, this should likely be performed. It is not an uncommon observation that several years after multivessel mesenteric revascularization, one limb is occluded and the patient has remained asymptomatic.

Similarly, some discussion in the literature exists as to the proper selection of conduit.[38,39] In general, if any abdominal contamination is suspected or encountered, short vein conduits should be used. However, in most cases of CMI, contamination is not an issue. Similar long-term patencies are noted, with both autogenous and prosthetic conduits. Ease of use without the trauma of vein harvest speaks for the use of prosthetic material. However, in some cases, small-diameter mesenteric vessels

and calcified distal targets may demand the use of an autogenous conduit.

Bypass. Open surgical repair provides excellent long-term outcomes with primary intermediate (1- to 3-year) graft patencies reported to be 80% to 100%. Long-term open revascularization is a durable repair with 5-year recurrence-free survival rates of 91%.[40–42] Combined primary and secondary patency rates at 5 years are significantly higher with open techniques (88% and 97%) when compared with endovascular methods.[42] The durability of open repair is offset by the accompanying 3% to 6% perioperative mortality and significant hospital stay and recovery. In general, operative repair is favored in patients who can tolerate surgery, and in those patients where percutaneous revascularization is not feasible. In modern series, with low-risk patients, operative mortalities are less than 2%.

Early postoperative CTA is helpful in evaluating both the bypass graft and the abdominal contents following surgery (Fig. 87.12). This baseline study can be used for future comparison when and if abdominal complaints occur. Duplex ultrasound is an excellent modality for routine graft imaging. In the first year, this should be done twice and once yearly thereafter.

In all patients with bulky mesenteric plaque, antiplatelet agents should be considered for life. Further, long-term risk factor management involves smoking cessation, hypertension control, and considerations for statin therapy.

Endarterectomy. Stoney et al. popularized the use of paravisceral aortic endarterectomy in the 1970s.[43] Bypassing and stenting mesenteric disease are far more common in the modern era.[44] Circumstances do exist when endarterectomy is useful. If there is gross contamination of the abdominal cavity and an autogenous conduit is not available, endarterectomy allows for revascularization without the use of a conduit. Exuberant aortic plaque of the "coral reef" type involving the paravisceral segment does not

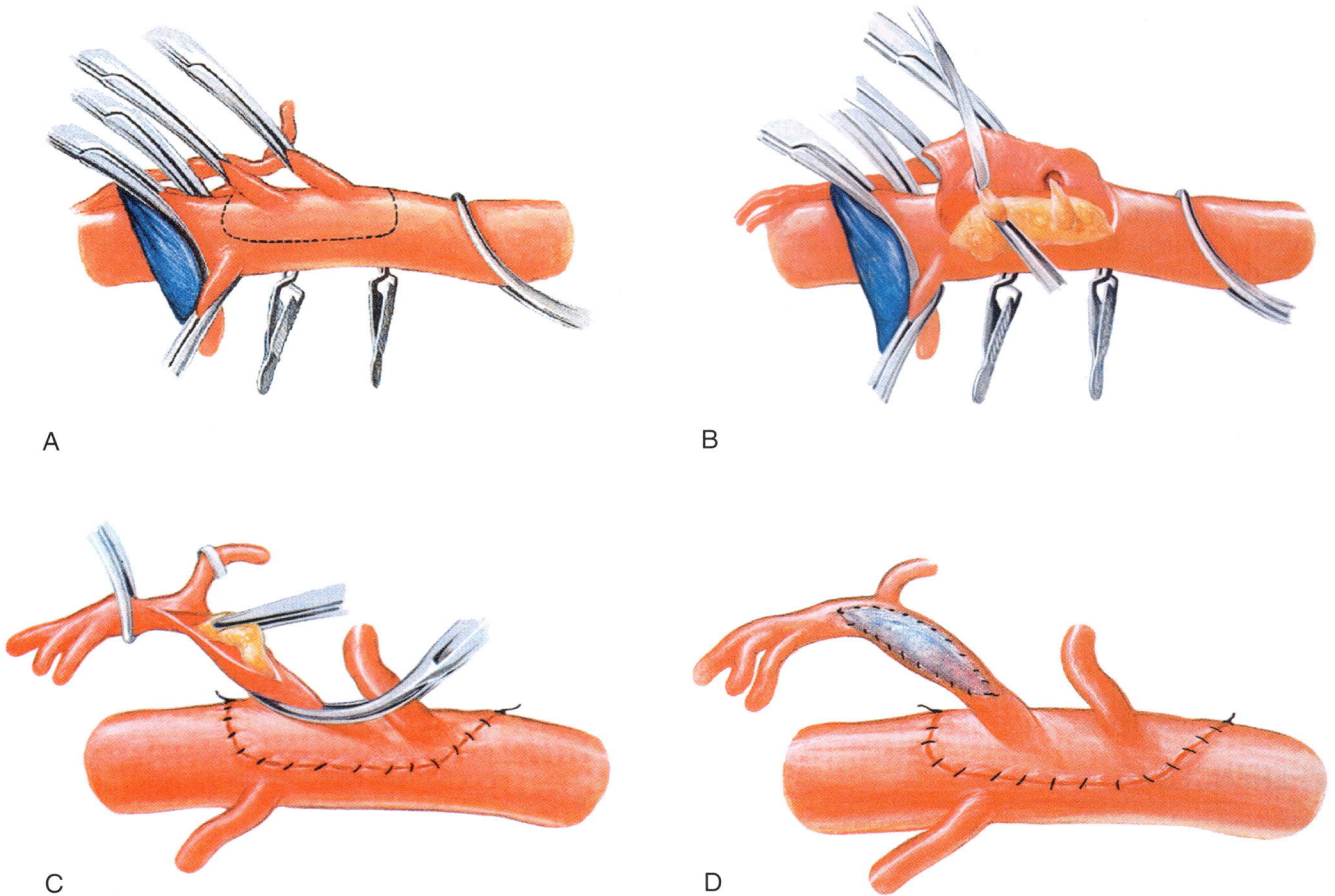

A

B

C

D

FIGURE 87.13 Aortomesenteric endarterectomy. (From Wylie EJ, Stoney RJ, Ehrenfeld WK. *Manual of Vascular Surgery*. Vol 1. New York: Springer-Verlag; 1980:215.)

respond well to endovascular methods but can be well treated with endarterectomy. Lastly, when disease of both the supraceliac aorta and infrarenal aorta prevents using these two segments for inflow and surgical bypass, end-arterectomy is an excellent tool.

Technically, optimal exposure of the SMA involves leaving the left kidney in place unless the left renal artery is to be treated as well. Proximal clamp position is developed above the CA where the diaphragmatic attachments require division. The infrarenal aorta is controlled via standard technique. Both the celiac and SMA should be dissected at their origins. If a long posterior-wall SMA plaque is palpated or seen preoperatively, the first 4 to 6 cm of the SMA should be dissected to prepare for separate SMA endarterectomy if necessary.

Right-angled aortic clamps are helpful in optimizing the utilization of exposed space. Once clamps are in position, a trapdoor-type incision is used (Fig. 87.13) to access the area of interest. Endarterectomy of the aorta and proximal mesenteric vessels is then performed. The aorta then should be closed primarily with 4-0 monofilament polypropylene. Celiac plaque is frequently solely orificial; however, SMA plaque may extend. In these cases, plaque should be everted and divided well into the vessel and the aortic endarterectomy closed. With the aorta

closed and distal perfusion restored, the remaining SMA disease can then be controlled separately and a second endarterectomy of the distal plaque performed to reach a satisfactory end point. Patch closure is used to prevent recurrence of SMA disease. Standard closure is then performed.

Endovascular Therapy. Endovascular therapy formerly was reserved for chronically debilitated patients who were unable to tolerate general anesthesia and open revascularization. In the last decade, however, it has become the first-line therapy for patients with CMI, relegating open surgical revascularization to patients who failed endovascular therapy or have unsuitable anatomy.

Endovascular revascularization of high-grade stenosis or occlusion of the SMA in particular is technically successful in reducing the stenosis to less than 50% of luminal diameter in 90% of cases, and provides immediate symptomatic relief in 75% to 100% of patients.[45–47] Although there are no randomized comparisons between different types of endovascular techniques, most experts agree that primary stenting should be performed because rates of restenosis are high for angioplasty alone, and covered stents are associated with less restenosis, recurrences, and reinterventions when compared with bare metal stents.[48]

Though less physiologically upsetting for the patient, revascularization by endovascular means may be made more challenging by severe calcifications, occlusions, long lesions, small vessel diameter, and multiple tandem lesions.[26] The preoperative CT scan may be helpful for allowing the surgeon to identify those challenges and create an appropriate strategic approach.

While most of these interventions are performed using a femoral approach, a left brachial approach may be required in some patients.[31,49] Use of a 6-french sheath or smaller enables a percutaneous brachial approach. If a larger than 6-french sheath is needed, an open exposure of the brachial or axillary arteries is another option. If the lesions are amenable to endovascular treatment, heparin is administered and the lesion is crossed using a series of preshaped catheters and hydrophilic wires. After crossing the lesion with the wire, the catheter should be advanced past the lesion and luminal position confirmed. Stiffer wires can be substituted at this point for better tracking of a balloon or stent.

Because of the high restenosis rate, routine duplex surveillance is recommended particularly in the first year. However, duplex evidence of restenosis may or may not correlate with symptom development, and the clinical symptomatology should guide further decisions about surveillance and therapy.[50]

REFERENCES

1. Mastoraki A, Mastoraki S, Tziava E, et al. Mesenteric ischemia: pathogenesis and challenging diagnostic and therapeutic modalities. *World J Gastrointest Pathophysiol.* 2016;7(1):125-130.
2. Corcos O, Nuzzo A. Gastro-intestinal vascular emergencies. *Best Pract Res Clin Gastroenterol.* 2013;27(5):709-725.
3. Wilkins LR, Stone JR. Chronic mesenteric ischemia. *Tech Vasc Interv Radiol.* 2015;18(1):31-37.
4. Carver TW, Vora RS, Taneja A. Mesenteric ischemia. *Crit Care Clin.* 2016;32(2):155-171.
5. Elliott JW. Operative relief of gangrene of the intestine due to occlusion of the mesenteric vessels. *Ann Surg.* 1895;73:128.
6. Klass AA. Embolectomy in acute mesenteric occlusion. *Ann Surg.* 1951;134:913.
7. Roussel A, Castier Y, Nuzzo A, et al. Revascularization of acute mesenteric ischemia after creation of a dedicated multidisciplinary center. *J Vasc Surg.* 2015;62(5):1251-1256.
8. Schoots IG, Koffeman GI, Legemate DA, Levi M, van Gulik TM. Systematic review of survival after acute mesenteric ischaemia according to disease aetiology. *Br J Surg.* 2004;91(1):17-27.
9. Ryer EJ, Kalra M, Oderich GS, et al. Revascularization for acute mesenteric ischemia. *J Vasc Surg.* 2012;55(6):1682-1689.
10. Wyers MC. Acute mesenteric ischemia: diagnostic approach and surgical treatment. *Semin Vasc Surg.* 2010;23(1):9-20.
11. Cudnik MT, Darbha S, Jones J, Macedo J, Stockton SW, Hiestand BC. The diagnosis of acute mesenteric ischemia: a systematic review and meta-analysis. *Acad Emerg Med.* 2013;20(11):1087-1100.
12. Björck M, Orr N, Endean ED. Debate: whether an endovascular-first strategy is the optimal approach for treating acute mesenteric ischemia. *J Vasc Surg.* 2015;62(3):767-772.
13. Abdu RA, Zakhour BJ, Dallis DJ. Mesenteric venous thrombosis—1911 to 1984. *Surgery.* 1987;101:383-388.
14. Kamar S, Sarr MG, Kamath PS. Mesenteric venous thrombosis. *N Engl J Med.* 2001;345:1683-1688.
15. Harnik IG, Brandt LJ. Mesenteric venous thrombosis. *Vasc Med.* 2010;15(5):407-418.
16. Rius X, Escalante JF, Llaurado MJ, Jover J, Puig La Calle J. Mesenteric infarction. *World J Surg.* 1979;3:489.
17. Morasch MD, Ebaugh JL, Chiou AC, Matsumura JS, Pearce WH, Yao JS. Mesenteric venous thrombosis: a changing clinical entity. *J Vasc Surg.* 2001;34:680.
18. Orr DW, Harrison PM, Devlin J, et al. Chronic mesenteric venous thrombosis: evaluation and determinants of survival during long-term follow-up. *Clin Gastroenterol Hepatol.* 2007;5(1):80-86.
19. Lee SS, Ha HK, Park SH, et al. Usefulness of computed tomography in differentiating transmural infarction from nontransmural ischemia of the small intestine in patients with acute mesenteric venous thrombosis. *J Comput Assist Tomogr.* 2008;32(5):730-737.
20. Amitrano L, Guardascione MA, Scaglione M, et al. Prognostic factors in noncirrhotic patients with splanchnic vein thromboses. *Am J Gastroenterol.* 2007;102(11):2464-2470.
21. Bergqvist D, Svensson PJ. Treatment of mesenteric vein thrombosis. *Semin Vasc Surg.* 2010;23(1):65-68.
22. Di Minno MN, Milone F, Milone M, et al. Endovascular thrombolysis in acute mesenteric vein thrombosis: a 3-year follow-up with the rate of short and long-term sequaelae in 32 patients. *Thromb Res.* 2010;126(4):295-298.
23. Yang S, Fan X, Ding W, et al. Multidisciplinary stepwise management strategy for acute superior mesenteric venous thrombosis: an intestinal stroke center experience. *Thromb Res.* 2015;135(1):36-45.
24. Hollingshead M, Burke CT, Mauro MA, Weeks SM, Dixon RG, Jaques PF. Transcatheter thrombolytic therapy for acute mesenteric and portal vein thrombosis. *J Vasc Interv Radiol.* 2005;16(5):651-661.
25. Morasch MD. Mesenteric venous thrombosis. Current concepts in diagnosis and treatment. In: Pearce WH, Matsumura JS, Yao JST, eds. *Trends in Vascular Surgery.* Chicago: Precept Press; 2002:473.
26. Oderich GS, Bower TC, Sullivan TM, Bjarnason H, Cha S, Gloviczki P. Open and endovascular revascularization for chronic mesenteric ischemia: risk stratification outcomes. *J Vasc Surg.* 2009;4:1472-1479.
27. Jaster A, Choudhery S, Ahn R, et al. Anatomic and radiologic review of chronic mesenteric ischemia and its treatment. *Clin Imaging.* 2016;40(5):961-969.
28. Hansen KJ, Wilson DB, Craven TE, et al. Mesenteric artery disease in the elderly. *J Vasc Surg.* 2004;40(1):45-52.
29. Mitchell EL, Moneta GL. Mesenteric duplex scanning. *Perspect Vasc Surg Endovasc Ther.* 2006;18:175.
30. Moneta GL, Lee RW, Yeager RA, Taylor LM Jr, Porter JM. Mesenteric duplex scanning: a blinded prospective study. *J Vasc Surg.* 1993;17:79.
31. Zwolak RM, Fillinger MF, Walsh DB, et al. Mesenteric and celiac duplex scanning: a validation study. *J Vasc Surg.* 1998;27:1078.
32. Jiminez JG, Huber TS, Ozaki CK, et al. Durability of antegrade synthetic aortomesenteric bypass for chronic mesenteric ischemia. *J Vasc Surg.* 2002;35:1078.
33. Sarac TP, Altinel O, Kashyap V, et al. Endovascular treatment of stenotic and occluded visceral arteries for chronic mesenteric ischemia. *J Vasc Surg.* 2008;47:485.
34. Kougias P, Huynh TT, Lin PH. Clinical outcomes of mesenteric artery stenting versus surgical revascularization in chronic mesenteric ischemia. *Int Angiol.* 2009;28:132.
35. Oderich GS, Panneon JM, Macedo TA, et al. Intraoperative duplex ultrasound of visceral revascularizations: optimizing technical success and outcome. *J Vasc Surg.* 2003;38:684.
36. Gentile AT, Moneta GL, Taylor LM Jr, Park TC, McConnell DB, Porter JM. Isolated bypass to the superior mesenteric artery for intestinal ischemia. *Arch Surg.* 1994;129:926.
37. Wolf YG, Berlatzky Y, Gewertz BL. Sequential configuration for aorto-celiac-mesenteric bypass. *Ann Vasc Surg.* 1997;11:640.
38. Geroulakos G, Tober JC, Anderson L, Smead WL. Antegrade visceral revascularization via a throracoabdominal approach for chronic mesenteric ischemia. *Eur J Vasc Endovasc Surg.* 1999;17:56.
39. Modrall JG, Sadjadi J, Joiner DR, et al. Comparison of superficial femoral and saphenous vein as conduits for mesenteric arterial bypass. *J Vasc Surg.* 2003;37:362.
40. Indes JE, Giocovelli JK, Muhs BE, Sosa JA, Dardik A. Outcomes of endovascular and open treatment for chronic mesenteric ischemia. *J Endovasc Ther.* 2009;16:624.
41. Davies RSM, Wall ML, Silverman SH, et al. Surgical versus endovascular reconstruction for chronic mesenteric ischemia: a contemporary UK series. *Vasc Endovascular Surg.* 2009;43:157.
42. Oderich GS. Open versus endovascular revascularization for chronic mesenteric ischemia: risk-stratified outcomes. *J Vasc Surg.* 2009;49:1472.
43. Stoney RJ, Ehrenfeld WK, Wylie EJ. Revascularization methods in chronic visceral ischemia caused by atherosclerosis. *Ann Surg.* 1977;186:468.

44. Park WM, Cherry KJ, Chua HK, et al. Current results of open revascularization for chronic mesenteric ischemia: a standard for comparison. *J Vasc Surg.* 2002;35:853.

45. Silva JA, White CJ, Collins TJ, et al. Endovascular therapy for chronic mesenteric ischemia. *J Am Coll Cardiol.* 2006;47:944.

46. Aburahma AF, Campbell JE, Stone PA, et al. Perioperative and late clinical outcomes of percutaneous transluminal stentings of the celiac and superior mesenteric arteries over the past decade. *J Vasc Surg.* 2013;57:1052.

47. Aschenbach R, Bergert H, Kerl M, et al. Stenting of stenotic mesenteric arteries for symptomatic chronic mesenteric ischemia. *Vasa.* 2012;41:425.

48. Oderich GS, Erdoes LS, LeSar C, et al. Comparison of covered stents versus bare metal stents for treatment of chronic atherosclerotic mesenteric arterial disease. *J Vasc Surg.* 2013;58:1316-1324.

49. Oderich GS, Gloviczki P, Bower TC. Open surgical treatment for chronic mesenteric ischemia in the endovascular era: when is it necessary and what is the preferred technique? *Semin Vasc Surg.* 2010;23:36.

50. Fenwick JL, Wright IA, Buckenham TM. Endovascular repair of chronic mesenteric occlusive disease: the role of duplex surveillance. *ANZ J Surg.* 2007;77:60.

Aortoenteric Fistula and Visceral Artery Aneurysms

Micah Girotti | Melina R. Kibbe

AORTOENTERIC FISTULAS

Aortoenteric fistulas (AEFs) are rare entities that can quickly lead to sepsis, hemorrhage, and lethal exsanguination if they are not quickly diagnosed and treated. Sir Astley Cooper, an English comparative anatomist and surgeon, was the first to describe AEFs in 1829.[1] An AEF is an abnormal communication between the aorta or branches of the aorta and the gastrointestinal (GI) system. The mortality rate of AEFs ranges from 60% to 100%,[2] and they are fatal if no surgical intervention is undertaken. Two main types of fistulas have been described. Primary AEFs form between the native aorta and the GI tract. Secondary AEFs result from abnormal connections between an aorta that has undergone previous reconstructive surgery and the GI tract and can occur anytime from several weeks to many years after surgery. In the era when aortic aneurysms are primarily repaired with endovascular technology, important types of secondary fistulae are those that form following endovascular aneurysm repair (EVAR) with a stent graft.

INCIDENCE, DEMOGRAPHICS, AND CAUSES OF PRIMARY AORTOENTERIC FISTULAS

An autopsy study of the general population showed that the incidence of primary AEF is 0.04% to 0.07%.[3] Those with an abdominal aortic aneurysm have a higher incidence, from 0.69% to 2.36%.[4,5] The majority of primary AEFs occur in the older population, with a mean age of 64 years, and predominantly in men, with a ratio of 3:1.[6] Fistulas are most often located in the third and fourth portions of the duodenum (54%), followed by the esophagus (28%), small and large bowel (5%), and the stomach (2%). The higher likelihood of a fistula forming between the aorta and duodenum is attributed to their proximity to one another, as the duodenum directly overlies the aorta within the retroperitoneum.

Prior to eradication of infections with modern medical practice and antibiotics, diseases such as tuberculosis, salmonella, syphilis, and mycoses were the most common causes of primary AEFs.[7–9] Currently, the most common causes of primary AEFs are atherosclerotic aortic aneurysms.[10,11] Less common etiologies include radiation,[12] tumors,[12] trauma, and ingestion of foreign material.[13]

INCIDENCE, DEMOGRAPHICS, AND SUBTYPES OF SECONDARY AORTOENTERIC FISTULAS

The incidence of secondary AEFs is higher than primary AEFs, with a reported range of 0.36% to 1.6%.[14–17] Although most secondary AEFs form after an open aortic surgical intervention, a small and increasing number of AEFs have been reported after endovascular aortic repairs.[18] A fistula can form if there is an endoleak with subsequent recurrence of the aortic aneurysm, primary endograft infection, kinking or migration of the graft, or physical breakdown of the graft material.[19–22] There are two main categories of secondary AEFs. Type 1, or graft-enteric fistula, occurs as the result of an erosion of the proximal aortic suture, with or without the presence of a pseudoaneurysm, into the adjacent bowel. There is direct erosion into the aortic lumen with the potential for massive GI hemorrhage if not repaired emergently. Type 2 secondary AEFs, also known as aortoenteric erosions (AEEs), graft enteric erosions, or paraprosthetic erosions, can occur where the aortic graft mechanically erodes into the overlying bowel. In this type of secondary AEF, no fistula is formed with the lumen of an arterial structure. The bleeding ensues from the edges of the eroded bowel and often presents as a chronic GI bleed.

PATHOGENESIS

There are several theories as to the pathogenesis of AEFs and AEEs. In primary AEFs, pressure necrosis may occur where the aorta and bowel come into contact with one another, because of the repetitive mechanical trauma from aortic pulsations, which leads to degradation of the nearby tissue.[17]

Secondary AEFs may form due to suture line breakdown, usually from suture technique that fails to adequately incorporate healthy aortic tissue. Failure to close the aneurysm sac and retroperitoneum will also leave the suture line in direct contact with the duodenum, increasing the odds of erosion of the suture line into the bowel. Another hypothesis involves the presence of chronic infection of the reconstructed aorta, which initiates abscess formation with eventual erosion of the graft into the adjacent bowel (Fig. 88.1).[3] Chronic infection may also originate from the GI tract. Foreign-body ingestion, carcinoma, or infections such as diverticulitis can lead to adhesions that bring the bowel in closer proximity to the aorta. The mechanical pulsations cause thinning of the bowel wall with eventual translocation of enteric organisms into the suture line.[23] If a pseudoaneurysm or aneurysm forms adjacent to the suture line, the weakened blood vessel wall leaves it susceptible to breakdown.

DIAGNOSIS

Symptoms

Timely diagnosis of an AEF is vital because of its high morbidity and mortality. The clinician must harbor a high index of suspicion in patients with known abdominal aneurysms or previous aortic surgery in the setting of GI bleeding. The diagnosis is often delayed because of the rarity of the disease and the wide differential that accompanies the initial mild symptoms. Systemic signs of illness,

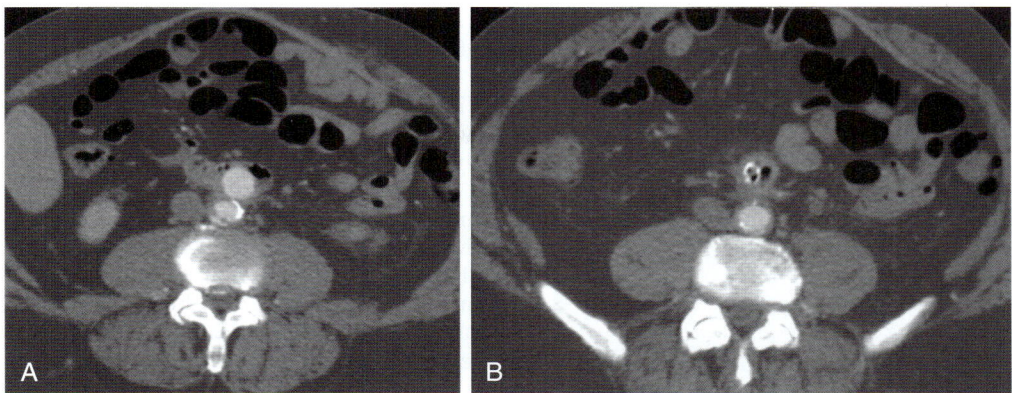

FIGURE 88.1 (A) The aortic portion of an end-to-side aortobifemoral bypass graft has eroded anteriorly and is located directly within the third portion of the duodenum. This is a 66-year-old man who presented with upper gastrointestinal bleeding. (B) Intraluminal air is demonstrated in the iliac limbs of the graft.

such as fever, chills, lethargy, weight loss, anorexia, syncope, and abdominal or back pain, may be present if a patient with a previous aortic reconstruction has an infected graft. AEFs have been described with the classic triad of GI bleeding, pulsating abdominal mass, and abdominal pain. However, this triad is found in only 11% of patients[6] and thus is not a useful diagnostic marker. Intermittent herald bleeds in the form of hematochezia, melena, or hematemesis are common occurrences, being present in 94% of cases.[6] These transient bleeds may recur over a span of hours to weeks and are inexorably followed by a catastrophic GI hemorrhage if not promptly investigated and repair performed. AEEs may present with symptoms consistent with a chronic GI bleed over weeks to months in association with mild abdominal discomfort, fevers, and chills.

Laboratory Studies

Laboratory studies may demonstrate abnormalities, such as an increased white blood cell count and decreased hematocrit. In the presence of fever, aerobic and anaerobic blood cultures should be obtained. Advanced sepsis confirmed by positive preoperative blood cultures is a predictor of poor outcome.[24] Up to 85% of AEFs have blood cultures positive for enteric organisms, with identical organisms found from cultures obtained intraoperatively from the fistula site.[24] Exposure to enteric contents leads to a large number of different organisms that can be implicated in AEFs. The most common organisms isolated from the fistula site include *Staphylococcus aureus* (including methicillin-resistant *S. aureus*), *Staphylococcus epidermidis*, *Escherichia coli*, *Escherichia faecalis*, *Clostridium septicum*, *Lactobacillus*, *Klebsiella*, *Pseudomonas aeruginosa*, *Bacteroides fragilis*, *Salmonella*, *Mycobacterium tuberculosis*, and *Candida*.[6,25,26]

IMAGING

After an AEF or AEE is suspected, a diagnostic work-up should be obtained expediently if the patient is stable. A hemodynamically unstable patient should undergo resuscitation while being prepped for an emergency exploratory laparotomy. Indeed, the exploratory laparotomy is the gold standard, with 100% sensitivity and specificity. If the

patient is stable, further diagnostic tests should be obtained without delay. Currently, computed tomography (CT) and endoscopy are used as first-line diagnostic modalities when an AEF is in the differential.

CT has been endorsed as the preferred diagnostic tool for the evaluation of AEF. CT is a useful tool for evaluating perigraft infections, and its utility in determining the presence of AEFs is also promising. Its advantages are widespread accessibility and rapidity of image acquisition. Intravenous contrast should be routinely used when assessing for an AEF with both arterial and venous or delayed phases; the utility of oral contrast is in debate. Although oral contrast may be useful in distinguishing bowel wall thickening, it may obscure visualization of any arterial extravasation into the GI tract. The overall sensitivity and specificity of CT for AEF are 94% to 100% and 50% to 85%, respectively.[27–29] Among the most specific signs for an AEF are extravasation of contrast from the aorta into the bowel lumen and enteric contrast found in the periaortic space (Fig. 88.2).[29,30] Other signs that may be present on CT scan include periaortic soft tissue edema, periaortic fluid, periaortic stranding, focal bowel wall thickening, pseudoaneurysm formation, and disruption of the aortic wall or aneurysmal wrap.[27,29,31,32] Some of the difficulty in evaluating for AEFs is a result of the overlapping CT findings in AEFs and periaortic graft infections. Periaortic gas, fluid, and soft tissue edema also may be observed with graft infections and are normal findings immediately after the operation. Periaortic gas is abnormal if present 3 to 4 weeks after the operation and may signify a graft infection with or without fistulization or erosion into the GI tract.[29] A perigraft fluid collection that persists beyond 3 months also indicates a possible graft infection and warrants further investigation. The key to determining the relevance of these findings is to correlate the radiologic findings with other clinical signs, such as concurrent GI bleeding.

Endoscopy has also been used as a first-line diagnostic tool in evaluating for AEFs and AEE in the hemodynamically stable patient. A patient exhibiting transient GI bleeding may benefit from an extensive work-up that includes attempts at complete visualization of the GI tract. If there is a high suspicion for an AEF, the endoscopy

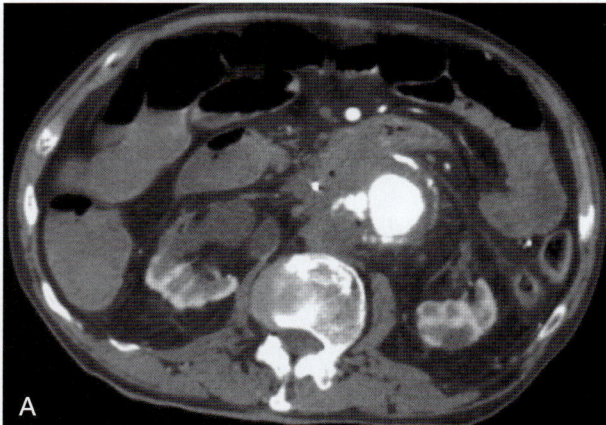

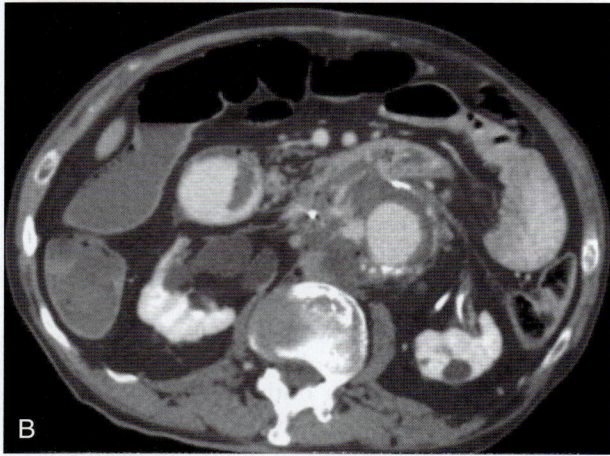

FIGURE 88.2 (A) Patient presented 6 weeks after an open repair of a 5.6-cm abdominal aortic aneurysm with hematemesis and syncope. Computed tomography scan reveals aortoenteric fistula between the aortic graft and the third portion of the duodenum. Air is seen external to the duodenum extending into the aortic graft. (B) Delayed venous-phase views reveal a large amount of contrast in the bowel, confirming active extravasation.

should be performed in the operating room, in the event of a catastrophic hemorrhage. Particular attention should be paid to the third and fourth portions of the duodenum because AEFs and AEEs are most commonly located in these areas. Endoscopy may reveal a portion of the graft protruding into the bowel, active bleeding, ulcerations, petechiae, blood clot, or extrinsic pulsating mass.[17,33] Lack of endoscopic findings does not preclude the possibility of an AEF or AEE, and further investigation may be warranted. In addition, alternative bleeding sites can be uncovered; however, care must be taken not to discount the possibility of an AEF or AEE in conjunction with these findings.[34]

Numerous other diagnostic tools have been used with limited success and are often used in the initial work-up of abdominal complaints or as an adjunct to CT or endoscopy. *Plain abdominal radiographs* may show pneumoperitoneum from the perforated bowel and can be one of the first signs that alert the clinician to the severity of the situation. However, this finding is not common in

the presence of AEF, and there are numerous other causes of free air.

Abdominal ultrasounds are not particularly useful for diagnosing AEFs, and it is currently unclear as to the utility of *magnetic resonance imaging (MRI)* for determining the presence of an AEF. Increased signal intensity in T1- and T2-weighted images indicates localized inflammation, and perigraft fluid seen after the initial postoperative period may signal a graft infection.[31] Although perigraft air also can be detected, it can easily be obscured by motion artifact and can be difficult to distinguish from calcified plaque. In addition, MRI is an expensive imaging technique, not as widely available, and requires more technical proficiency than CT scan.

Indium 111–labeled white blood cell scans or *technetium 99m-hexametazime white blood cell scans* are useful adjuncts to CT and endoscopy in detecting low-grade graft infections. In patients who do not have overt signs of graft infection, radiolabeled white blood cell scans show promising results, with 100% sensitivity and 94% specificity.[35] *Tagged red blood cell scans* are also beneficial in localizing fistulas in patients with active GI bleeding. *Upper GI studies* with barium may demonstrate an AEF with active extravasation of contrast; however, the contrast may be detrimental because it may obscure other diagnostic tests that are more sensitive.

Although rarely used, *aortography* may show aortic contrast extravasation into the bowel lumen, which is pathognomonic for an AEF.[15] Aortography is not often used in diagnosing AEFs because it is difficult to localize the fistula, and its usefulness lies mostly in preoperative planning with visualization of the anatomy. This modality is occasionally therapeutic because it affords the ability to stem temporarily high-volume GI bleeding by placing a stent over the fistula or embolizing a small artery.

TREATMENT

The mainstay of treatment for an AEF is surgery, with almost certain death if intervention is delayed or deferred. A clear distinction should be made between the hemodynamically stable patient and one who is actively bleeding and requires an expedient laparotomy. If the patient is hemodynamically unstable, an arterial line and central line should be placed and rapid resuscitation initiated while preparing the patient for an exploratory laparotomy. The patient should be typed and crossmatched and receive empiric intravenous broad-spectrum antibiotics that cover both gram-positive and enteric organisms. In stable patients, a diagnostic work-up may be initiated with a comprehensive operative plan set in place. Because the treatment for an AEF or AEE is a serious undertaking, if the patient is competent and stable, the surgeon should initiate a conversation regarding the potential complications of the operation and the patient's goals of care. A review of the patient's comorbidities will aid in operative planning because there are several different approaches that are available.

Surgical Technique

The goals of AEF repair are rapid and effective control of hemorrhage, preservation of perfusion to the legs, and treatment and containment of infection. Because good visualization of the surgical field is essential, the initial incision should extend from the xiphoid process to the pubic symphysis. A retroperitoneal approach through a left flank incision can be considered in patients who have had previous abdominal operations or currently have hostile abdomens. Proximal and distal control of the aorta is imperative prior to manipulation of the fistula site to prevent uncontrollable hemorrhage. Systemic heparinization is performed prior to aortic cross-clamping to prevent thromboembolic events. Control is obtained with either aortic clamps or occlusion of the aorta with a Fogarty balloon. The aorta is cautiously exposed and proximal control undertaken either at the subdiaphragmatic level or preferably at the infrarenal level to maintain perfusion to the visceral vessels and renal arteries. The aorta is dissected out and distal control obtained either at the aortic or iliac level.

Repair of the Enteric Fistula or Erosion.
Because a fistula or erosion may be found anywhere along the alimentary tract, the entire GI tract is inspected to determine its location. Again, careful attention should be paid to the third and fourth portions of the duodenum because the majority of AEFs and AEEs occur in this region. Sharp dissection of the bowel is performed away from the aorta with vigilance sustained to minimize the amount of enteric spillage. Contamination of the field provides a nidus of infection and may lead to disastrous postoperative outcomes, such as aortic stump rupture or recurrence of infection at the reconstruction site. After the bowel has been separated from the aorta, inspect the bowel for areas of necrosis or nonviability. Even though most of the enteric defects are small enough to close primarily with a two-layered transverse closure, a resection may be necessary with anastomosis and proximal diversion as the situation dictates. Meticulous débridement of all infected graft material and tissue within the perigraft area is undertaken. Cultures should routinely be obtained from the aorta, periaortic tissue, and any gross purulence in the field to aid in narrowing antibiotic coverage after the reconstruction.

Prior to closure, a thorough washout decreases the likelihood of infection by decreasing the bacterial load. A nasogastric tube should be placed and left for decompression until bowel function has returned. The retroperitoneal region may require placement of a drain if an abscess was present.

Depending on the location of the AEF and other patient factors, several different approaches to aortic reconstruction have been used and are described next.

Extraanatomic Bypass Grafting With Aortic Ligation and Graft Excision.
The traditional and most commonly used surgical approach to AEFs and AEE is the extraanatomic bypass graft. Blaisdell et al. first described the use of an axillobifemoral bypass in 1965 as a treatment for aortic aneurysms.[36] This technique uses a two-team approach to establish an extraanatomic bypass, most often as an axillofemoral bypass, followed by the removal of the infected aortic graft with oversewing of the aorta to create an aortic stump. The aortic stump is closed with two layers of monofilament sutures. Healthy aortic tissue should be incorporated into the stump closure to lessen the risk of aortic rupture. The aortic stump should be protected with omentum, preferably with 360-degree coverage. If omentum

is unavailable, a sartorius or rectus femoris muscle transposition may be used.[37]

A staged procedure involves a short delay between the construction of the extraanatomic bypass and resection of the infected graft. This operative plan may be beneficial in those who have chronic aortic graft infections and should be used only if the patient is hemodynamically stable. After the extraanatomic bypass is established, resection of infected graft is performed, preferably within the next few days, depending on the stability of the patient. One study had a median interoperative interval of 5 days, with a range of 2 to 31 days.[38] Mortality rates for a staged extraanatomic bypass range from 11% to 27%[39,40] and are highly dependent on the patient's preoperative condition, infection load, and hemodynamic status.

One of the most dreaded complications of the extraanatomic bypass in this setting is aortic stump blowout or rupture. It occurs in 5% to 25% of patients[40] and is almost certainly fatal. In addition, pelvic ischemia can occur as a consequence of a lack of perfusion to the internal iliac arteries, and inadequate perfusion to the lower extremities can lead to high amputation rates. The graft itself is subject to both infection and thrombosis, with axillofemoral graft infection rates reported to be between 22% and 40%.[41,42] The primary patency rate of extraanatomic bypass grafts is approximately 43% at 3 years, with the secondary patency rate improved to 65%.[43] With the staged procedure these numbers have improved, with the 5-year primary patency between 64% and 73%,[39,41] and secondary graft patency rate of 92% to 100%.[39,41] Although the extraanatomic bypass grafting technique is the most widely used and has the longest history, it has been criticized for significant mortality and complications. Hence there has been a search for alternative operative methods.

In Situ Graft Replacement.
In situ graft replacement is a surgical option that is particularly attractive for patients who have a number of comorbidities, wherein a long operative time may be detrimental. The infected graft is removed and replaced with an in situ graft. Common conduits include femoral veins, aortic homografts, and prosthetic grafts, which have been soaked in antibiotics, typically rifampin. The advantages to these alternatives are decreased risk of limb loss and pelvic ischemia, lower amputation rates, avoidance of stump blowouts, and better long-term patency.[44,45] The greatest drawbacks to these methods are the possibility of recurrent graft infections, proximal anastomotic rupture, deep vein thrombosis, and chronic limb edema.[37,46,47]

Autogenous reconstruction is a technique that has been used with construction of a neoaortoiliac system. The most commonly used conduits are the femoropopliteal veins because of their high patency and large caliber.[48] Superficial veins have fallen out of favor as a consequence of high stenosis rates and intimal hyperplasia that occlude these conduits.[49] The veins are used reversed or nonreversed with lysed valves and anastomosed if a bifurcated graft is necessary for the aortoiliac junction. The decreased infection risk, circumvention of stump blowout, and lower amputation rates as compared with extraanatomic bypass grafting make this an attractive alternative. The technical complexity of harvesting and lack of appropriate conduits pose obstacles in some cases, and long operative times make this approach not ideal for patients with significant comborbidities. However, a large series from Europe routinely using the neoaortoiliac system reconstruction and tensor fascia lata flap coverage of the proximal anastomosis in 55 patients with AEF over 13 years resulted in a 90% 30-day survival with a minimal number of reinterventions or limb thrombosis.[50]

Cryopreserved arterial homografts are an alternative material for in situ arterial reconstruction. They have been used in the treatment of aortic valve endocarditis by cardiothoracic surgeons, with good success.[51] The cryopreserved arterial homograft is maintained at low temperatures prior to implantation, and may be impregnated with neomycin to heighten its bacterial resistance. Thirty-day mortality rates are approximately 9% to 12%,[52,53] whereas 30-day survival rates range from 67% to 81%.[52,54] Its major benefit arises from the extremely low infection rates as a result of the antibacterial properties of the allograft.[52-54] Complications can include aneurysmal degeneration of the homograft[52] and allograft rejection leading to dilation and rupture. Other disadvantages to the cryopreserved arterial homograft include its lack of availability in all centers and relative expense.

The use of antibiotic-soaked prosthetic grafts is also increasing in popularity, partly because of higher flow rates and the higher patency rates seen in these grafts compared with extraanatomic bypass grafts.[44,45] Grafts may be silver coated, rifampin bonded, or amikacin loaded for greater antibacterial resistance. Rifampin covers a broad spectrum of both gram-positive and gram-negative bacteria, including *S. aureus,* which is why it remains a popular choice. Antibiotic-coated prostheses have been used with moderate success; however, the concern of infection is higher in patients growing methicillin-resistant *S. aureus.*[46] Rifampin has been used in the treatment of methicillin-resistant *S. aureus* but never as a monotherapy because of the rapid emergence of resistance. One approach is to place the graft in a 45- to 60-mg/mL solution of rifampin for 15 minutes at room temperature prior to implantation.[55] The perioperative mortality rate for in situ prosthetic graft replacement ranges from 13% to 21%, with a 30-day mortality rate ranging from 8% to 26%.[37,56]

Endovascular Repair. Endovascular repair has become increasingly popular as an alternative technique in selected situations. In the presence of severe hemorrhage, it can be used to temporize prior to definitive management. This percutaneous technique is less invasive and may be beneficial to those who have significant comorbidities and cannot tolerate significant shifts in their circulatory status, have a limited life expectancy, or have a hostile abdomen from inflammation or previous operations. Placement of a covered aortic stent graft within the surgical graft excludes the AEF from the circulation, leaving the infected graft in place. Endovascular repair is less likely to be helpful in cases of graft erosion because the bleeding originates from the bowel edges rather than an abnormal aortic fistula formation.

Although most of the literature describes the use of endovascular repair as a temporizing measure, there have been cases in which AEFs were managed solely with endovascular repair in high-risk patients. Significant concerns remain because of the high recurrence rate of bleeding and infection. The infected graft remains in place with this repair, and the fistula is not removed, thus providing a continued source of infection. The inability to débride the area of infected tissue leads to a greater risk of long-term infectious complications. Recurrent or new infections or recurrent hemorrhage have been reported to occur in 44% to 60% of patients with an endovascular approach.[57,58] Those with known preoperative signs of infection are more likely to have a poor outcome, and patients with secondary AEFs (compared with those with primary AEFs) tend to have a higher rate of infection, presumably from the retained prosthetic graft.[57]

Numerous adjunctive strategies have been used with endovascular repairs to help to minimize risk of progressive infection. Although there is no clear evidence that lifelong antibiotics prevent sepsis,[57] most vascular surgeons will place their patients on lifelong suppressive antibiotic therapy and maintain close follow-up to monitor for signs of recurrent or progressive infection. Patients have also been treated with CT-guided percutaneous drainage of the aneurysm sac with or without placement of drains within the sac for irrigation with saline or antibiotics.[59,60] A diverting ileostomy may be attempted to prevent further contamination of the graft site.[58] One report of endoscopic injection of fibrin sealant into the fistula tract alleged good success.[60]

Infection of Endografts. In an era when the majority of aortic aneurysms are repaired with endovascular technology, an increasing proportion of AEFs are associated with previously placed endoluminal stent grafts (Fig. 88.3). In a multicenter American review examining more than 200 endovascular aortic graft infections, more than a quarter presented as enteric fistulas.[61] This included aortoesophageal fistulas occurring in a high proportion of infected thoracic endografts (Fig. 88.4A and B). In this

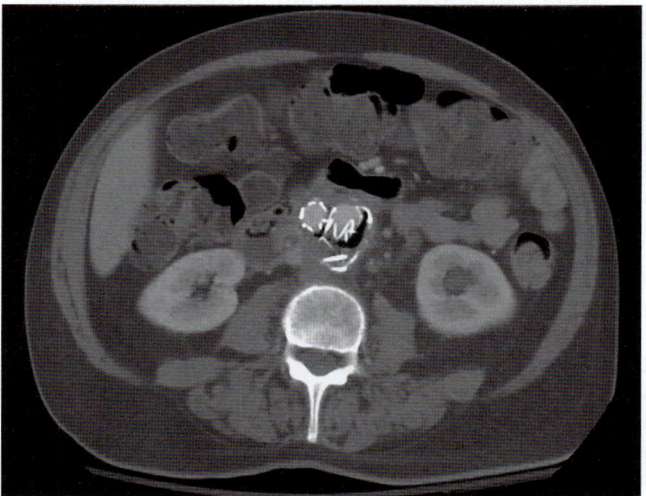

FIGURE 88.3 This 66-year-old male presented 3 years after an endovascular aneurysm repair with 6 weeks of back pain, abdominal pain, and intermittent fevers. Computed tomography scan shows air in the aneurysm sac. On exploration there was a duodenal-aortic erosion with purulence. The endograft was explanted and replaced with rifampin-soaked Dacron and the duodenum repaired primarily.

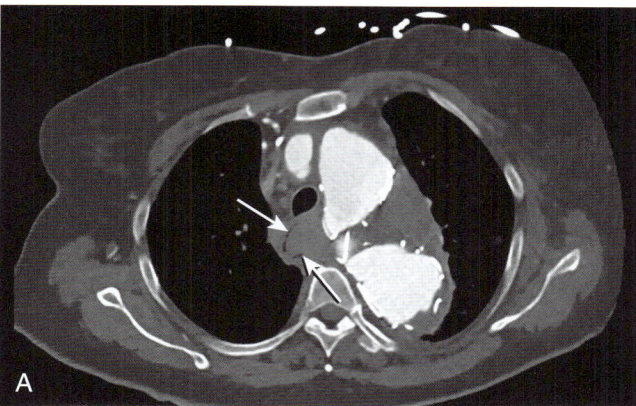
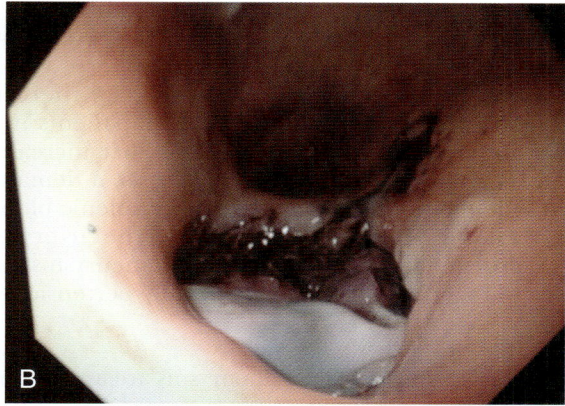

FIGURE 88.4 (A) A 78-year-old female underwent thoracic endovascular aneurysm repair and presented less than 2 years later with a low-volume gastrointestinal bleed. Computed tomography scan revealed a type 1 endoleak, aneurysm sac expansion, and suspicion for esophageal erosion. *Arrows* denote esophageal lumen impinged upon by inflammatory tissue and clot. (B) Upper endoscopy revealed a proximal esophageal ulcer with graft visible in the ulcer. Due to the patient's frailty, she was not a candidate for explant and aortic arch/esophageal reconstructions. She was treated with a carotid-carotid bypass, a midarch thoracic endograft, an esophageal stent, and lifelong antibiotic suppression.

population, aortic fistula in univariate and multivariate analysis was significantly associated with all-cause mortality. In a multicenter Italian study, the incidence of AEF after EVAR in approximately 4000 patients over 16 years was 0.8%.[62] Pseudoaneurysm, as the initial indication for EVAR, and urgent or emergent timing of the initial procedure were significantly associated with later development of AEF.

Management of these patients is parallel to those with prior open aortic reconstruction, with the majority undergoing in-line aortic reconstruction, primarily with antibiotic-soaked prosthetic grafts, although a significant proportion do undergo reconstruction with cryopreserved allograft or autogenous tissue and creation of a neoaortoiliac system.

Infected fenestrated and branched grafts have been reported,[63] and as more centers place these grafts for complex aortic aneurysmal disease, enteric fistulization will mandate creative management solutions.

VISCERAL ANEURYSMS

Although uncommon, visceral aneurysms often prompt urgent surgical consultation. Occasionally, aneurysm rupture may create an acute abdominal emergency with massive intraperitoneal or GI bleeding. Less acute presentations may include abdominal pain, nausea, or a palpable pulsatile mass. More recently, the diagnosis of asymptomatic visceral aneurysms is increasing coincident with cross-sectional imaging performed for other purposes. It is important to be familiar with the variety of presentations, diagnostic tests, and therapeutic options for these potentially lethal visceral aneurysms.

SPLENIC ARTERY ANEURYSMS

Splenic artery aneurysms are the most common visceral aneurysm, accounting for 60% of all visceral aneurysms.[64] They are the third most common intraabdominal aneurysm after aortic and iliac aneurysms. The prevalence in the general population is reported to range between 0.1% and 10.4%.[65,66] Unlike aortic and iliac aneurysms, female

gender predominates, with a female-to-male ratio of 4:1. Patients with splenic artery aneurysms typically present in the fifth decade of life, with the noted exception of those who present during childbearing years. When considering patients with cirrhosis and portal hypertension, the incidence rises and is reported to be between 7% and 17%.[66,67]

Anatomy and Pathology

Splenic artery aneurysms are usually small and saccular. The average size at discovery is 2.1 cm, and it is uncommon for them to be greater than 3 cm.[64] Cirsoid aneurysms of the entire splenic artery have been rarely reported.[67] Typically, a splenic aneurysm is found in the main splenic artery, and 75% are located in the distal third of the artery. The splenic artery provides flow to the greater curvature of the stomach via the short gastrics and left gastroepiploic artery, branches that are relevant to the treatment of distal splenic artery aneurysms.[68] Although the etiology is not fully understood, splenic artery aneurysms can be atherosclerotic and associated with arterial degenerative syndromes. Splenic artery aneurysms are also associated with arterial degeneration from medial fibrodysplasia,[63] autoimmune disorders, and collagen vascular diseases, such as Marfan syndrome and Ehlers-Danlos syndrome.[67,69] However, calcification from atherosclerosis is thought to be a secondary phenomenon and not a primary etiologic event.[64] Histologically, there is usually degeneration or absence of the medial layer and a variable degree of inflammation.[64,66]

Two demographics deserve further consideration in regard to diagnosis and management. The first is multiparous women, and the second is patients with liver failure and portal hypertension. The etiology of splenic aneurysms in pregnancy or the multiparous woman is thought to be secondary to both hemodynamic factors and hormonal influences.[69] The hormonal effects of pregnancy on the arterial wall include internal elastic lamina disruption and medial fibrodysplasia.[69,70] Hormones implicated include estrogen, progesterone, and relaxin.[71]

The resultant mural degeneration combined with increased blood flow can lead to weakening of the vessel wall and aneurysm formation.

In patients with underlying liver disease, there is increased splenic blood flow, but in these patients it is secondary to portal hypertension. As resistance increases in the portal vein with developing cirrhosis, a demand for portosystemic shunts occurs. Increased splenic blood flow and splenic artery size predispose the artery to aneurysmal degeneration. Splenic artery aneurysms are found in up to 17% of those with portal hypertension.[72]

Clinical Presentation

Eighty percent of splenic artery aneurysms are asymptomatic. Splenic aneurysms are increasingly found on abdominal imaging studies performed for other reasons. Of the 20% that are symptomatic, rupture has already occurred in 2% to 10%.[64] Before rupture, there may be a variety of symptoms, including vague or sharp left upper quadrant, epigastric, or flank pain, sometimes radiating to the left shoulder (the Kerr sign). Other symptoms may include nausea, vomiting, dyspepsia, and anorexia.

When rupture occurs, the patient may present with sudden cardiovascular collapse and shock, usually preceded by acute pain; however, a "double rupture phenomenon" can occur. In these patients there is a period of hypotension followed by relative stability as bleeding is tamponaded by the constraints of the lesser sac. Later, when free intraperitoneal extravasation of blood occurs with loss of tamponade, the patient progresses to profound hemorrhagic shock and possible death.[64,68] Clearly there is an opportunity for prompt surgical therapy in patients who do present with a delay in free intraperitoneal rupture. This period allows for intervention in approximately a quarter of patients.[67]

Rupture into the GI tract with subsequent GI bleeding or hemobilia occurs in up to 13% of patients.[64,65] Connections between the aneurysm and the GI tract can occur through erosion into the stomach, colon, or pancreatic duct.

Acute portal hypertension can result if there is erosion into the splenic vein causing an arteriovenous fistula.[64] This has been reported to cause small bowel ischemia from mesenteric steal, although such a steal must be a very rare event.[73,74]

There is a higher incidence of splenic artery rupture following liver transplantation. Increased collagen lysis after laparotomy has been associated with visceral aneurysm rupture in the first week after liver transplantation.[65] Because of this, in patients with cirrhosis approaching the need for liver transplantation, recommendations are for all to have cross-sectional imaging with evaluation for splenic artery aneurysms. If found, the recommendation is to treat these patients during the period of liver transplantation.[65]

Rupture of a splenic artery aneurysm during pregnancy is associated with a high risk of maternal mortality (64% to 75%) and fetal mortality (72.5% to 95%).[69] The risk of rupture increases during the last trimester and can be as high as 25% to 45%.[75] Most ruptured splenic artery aneurysms are in pregnant women, as high as 95%.[64] Rupture often presents as an obstetric catastrophe and can be misdiagnosed as a different obstetric emergency, such as placental abruption, uterine rupture, and amniotic fluid embolism.[69] If a pregnant woman presents with left upper quadrant pain, nausea, and vomiting, consideration must be given to this etiology. Physical examination findings may include tenderness over the uterine fundus, making the diagnosis more challenging.

Diagnosis

A plain radiograph may reveal the calcified splenic artery aneurysm by showing the classic signet ring–shaped calcifications in the left upper quadrant.[64] Ultrasound with pulsed Doppler is advantageous because of its lack of radiation but limited with regard to anatomic detail because of patient factors, such as truncal obesity and bowel gas. It is the preferred modality in pregnancy due to decreased risk to the fetus from ionizing radiation and can be used in any symptomatic patient to detect free fluid in the left upper quadrant.

CT scans provide a detailed three-dimensional image and are the most useful diagnostic modality. However, routine use during pregnancy is limited secondary to radiation. MRI/magnetic resonance angiography can also provide useful three-dimensional imaging. Catheter angiography with selection of the visceral vessels is a valuable diagnostic and potentially therapeutic tool in the armamentarium of the interventionalist or vascular surgeon. However, the use of intravascular contrast media is contraindicated in pregnancy because of the risk to the developing fetus.[69]

Treatment

Current recommendations for treatment of splenic artery aneurysms take into account size, growth characteristics, and clinical setting. Symptomatic splenic arterial aneurysms should be repaired regardless of size. In general, all asymptomatic splenic artery aneurysms should be treated when greater than 2 cm in diameter.[64,76] However, some authors recommend intervention if a smaller aneurysm is found to be growing during surveillance.[64,65,69] It is widely recommended to intervene in pregnant women and multiparous women of childbearing age even if the aneurysm is less than 2 cm because the risk of rupture increases significantly during pregnancy. The timing of intervention for an asymptomatic splenic artery aneurysm discovered during pregnancy is a difficult decision, but surgery during the second trimester is thought to be associated with the least risk to the developing fetus.[69]

There is a wide range of surgical and interventional approaches for splenic artery aneurysms. The choice of treatment may depend on such factors as anatomic location, acuity of symptoms, clinical presentation, and patient and physician preference. Large single-center series reveal the increasing preference to treat these lesions with endovascular techniques. Indeed, a large systematic review of more than 1300 splenic aneurysms treated with either open surgical, endovascular, or conservative therapy revealed endovascular methods to have a much lower incidence of short-term complications and a significantly shorter hospital stay compared with open techniques.[77] These endovascular methods include either coil embolization or exclusion of the lesion with a stent graft. These

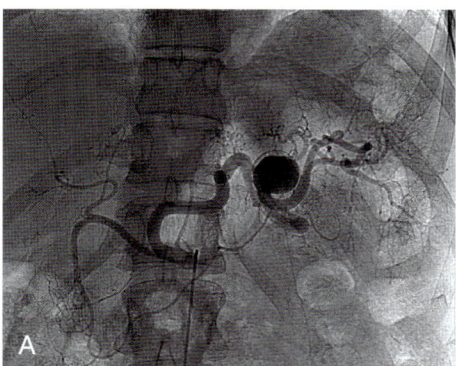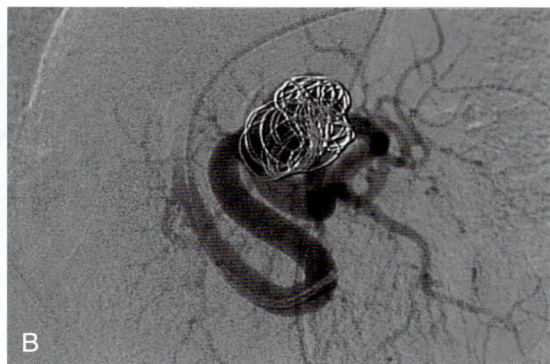

FIGURE 88.5 (A) Selective arteriography of the celiac artery reveals the signet ring opacification of the midsplenic artery aneurysm in this 58-year-old gravida 4 para 2 woman. Calcification of the walls is seen. (B) Coil embolization followed by the introduction of Gelfoam powder–induced arterial stasis and thrombosis of the aneurysm.

techniques were initially more commonly used for elderly or higher-risk patients or for those with concomitant portal hypertension.[70] However, aneurysms of the proximal and midsplenic artery are now preferentially treated with an endovascular approach.[76] Covered stent grafts have been used and have the benefit of maintaining splenic artery patency[78] and allowing for treatment of aneurysms in the middle third of the splenic artery, where the pancreas makes direct surgical exposure more difficult. They are best suited for more proximal aneurysms. Challenges for endovascular stent grafting are a wide neck of the aneurysm and splenic artery tortuosity. Complications include stent graft thrombosis, infection, and access-related complications.[76,79]

Transcatheter embolization can be performed on the main splenic artery (Fig. 88.5). If the hilum is involved, embolization is generally not successful, and splenectomy may be recommended.[64,80] Options for embolization include using coils alone, detachable balloons, vascular plugs, glue, or Gelfoam gelatin.[80–82]

The most common complication of coil embolization is the postembolization syndrome. It can occur in 30% of patients and presents as fever, severe abdominal pain, ileus, and, occasionally, pancreatitis.[65] Other complications include failure of embolization to occlude the aneurysm, splenic infarction, infection or abscess, rupture, and access-related (puncture-site) complications.[64,65,83] Recanalization has also been reported in up to 12.5% of patients.[84]

In terms of open surgical options, for aneurysms located in the distal splenic artery, splenectomy with additional splenic artery resection that includes the aneurysm is curative. In some cases, distal pancreatectomy may also be necessary. Simple ligation of the proximal splenic artery is insufficient for treatment of an aneurysm in the splenic hilum because collateral flow through accessory splenic or gastroepiploic arteries will continue to perfuse the aneurysm. In these cases, subsequent splenectomy is unavoidable.[65,85]

However, proximal splenic artery aneurysms can be treated with ligation with or without interposition grafting or end-to-end reanastomosis. In the midportion of the splenic artery, where there is tortuosity and redundancy, the artery is more amenable to end-to-end reanastomosis.[67] Splenic preservation has been recognized as important

for the immune system and is possible in most cases, except those involving the hilum.[64] For aneurysms in the middle third of the splenic artery, aneurysmectomy alone has been reported leaving the spleen in place and perfused via short gastric collaterals.[79,85]

Surgical techniques also include a laparoscopic approach and the use of robotic assistance.[74] Several series report successful laparoscopic treatment of splenic artery aneurysms. The laparoscopic approach is contraindicated if the patient is hemodynamically unstable or with evidence of rupture. For distal aneurysms, a laparoscopic lateral approach facilitates visualization of the aneurysm, use of the endoscopic stapler, and splenectomy.[64,86]

Combination therapy performed in staged fashion has been used for large aneurysms and in patients at higher risk for surgery. Embolization with subsequent excision has been useful in this group.[65] The mortality rate of elective open surgery is 1.3% to 1.8%, with a morbidity rate of 9%.[65,85] Mortality after emergency surgery for rupture is reported to be as high as 40%.[67]

The surgical approach is either via an anterior or lateral approach.[64] When acute rupture is present, the splenic artery can be controlled quickly via the lesser sac by dividing the gastrohepatic ligament. In addition, supraceliac control of the aorta can temporize bleeding until the splenic artery is controlled.[64]

For pregnant women with splenic artery aneurysm rupture, ligation with or without reanastomosis or splenectomy is recommended. Vigorous fluid resuscitation is vital. Delaying delivery until the splenic artery bleeding is controlled is recommended, but if cardiac arrest has occurred, prompt delivery of the fetus within minutes is crucial.[69] Treatment of splenic artery aneurysms regardless of their size in women contemplating pregnancy should be considered to avoid this catastrophe.

HEPATIC ARTERY ANEURYSMS

Incidence

Hepatic artery aneurysms are the second most common true visceral artery aneurysm, accounting for 20% of this entity. However, pseudoaneurysms are increasingly common, now accounting for nearly half of all reported hepatic artery aneurysms.[64,67] In the past, hepatic artery aneurysms were more frequently extrahepatic (80%), and most were solitary and in either the common or right hepatic arteries.[80] Hepatic artery aneurysms are more common in men.

Anatomy and Pathology

Historically, infection was the most common etiology for hepatic artery aneurysms, classically after intravenous drug abuse or intraabdominal infection. Now, this represents a much less common cause, between 4% and 10%.[80,87,88] The majority are now either degenerative or associated with trauma or interventional biliary and hepatic procedures. Some reports now estimate pseudoaneurysms to approach nearly 50% of all hepatic artery aneurysms.[67,87] Aneurysms associated with liver transplantation now make up an increasing proportion of hepatic artery aneurysms, 17% in some reports.[80,87] Extrahepatic aneurysms are more likely to be degenerative with atherosclerotic changes, whereas intrahepatic aneurysms, representing 20% of hepatic artery aneurysms, are more likely to be pseudoaneurysms, with characteristic saccular appearance.[89] Smaller fusiform aneurysms tend to be extrahepatic (80%).[88] Most patients present with solitary aneurysms, but 20% of patients can have multiple aneurysms.[87]

When associated with liver transplantation, aneurysms are usually extrahepatic and often associated with infection.[87,90] These extrahepatic aneurysms are usually pseudoaneurysms at or near the arterial anastomosis. Intrahepatic aneurysms in liver transplant patients are typically pseudoaneurysms at sites of biopsy or drainage.[90]

In liver transplant recipients, the mean time from transplantation to diagnosis of an aneurysm is reported as averaging between 10 days and 2 months.[90]

Clinical Presentation

Most true hepatic artery aneurysms are asymptomatic and found incidentally during abdominal imaging. Of those patients who present with symptoms, right upper quadrant or epigastric pain is the most common symptom, present in more than 50%.[80] Other symptoms include back pain or biliary colic. Jaundice can also occur without rupture when the bile duct is extrinsically compressed by the aneurysm.[80]

Frank rupture can occur in 10% to 30% of patients and presents with abdominal pain and shock. Of those presenting with rupture, 50% may have rupture into the biliary tree and one-third present with the Quincke triad of abdominal pain, hemobilia, and obstructive jaundice.[67,80,87,89] Fifty percent present with free intraperitoneal rupture. Extrahepatic aneurysms are more likely to rupture intraperitoneally, and intrahepatic aneurysms more typically rupture into the biliary tree and manifest as massive GI bleeding or with the Quincke triad.[87] Ruptured hepatic artery aneurysms are associated with up to a 35% mortality rate.[80,91]

Diagnosis

Most hepatic artery aneurysms are not detectable on physical examination unless large and symptomatic, and presenting with a pulsatile mass. If atherosclerotic changes have occurred, a ring of calcifications may be seen in the right upper quadrant on plain radiograph. Ultrasound

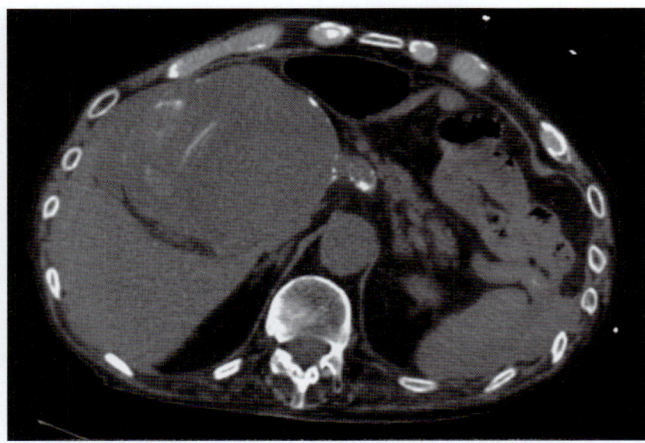

FIGURE 88.6 Noncontrast computed tomography scan of an 86-year-old man presenting with a 1-day history of abdominal pain and coffee-ground emesis. At surgery, a large ruptured hepatic artery aneurysm was identified. Although the duodenum was adherent to the mass, there was no arterial-enteric fistula. The hepatic artery was ligated without reconstruction. He survived and was discharged to home on postoperative day 8.

can detect these, but it does not provide the anatomic detail needed for treatment planning. Ultrasound may also suggest a cystic structure that can be mistaken for a cystic tumor or pseudocyst; thus careful color flow analysis is an important tool to distinguish a solid structure from a vascular structure. CT scanning and arteriography are the mainstay of diagnosis and treatment planning (Fig. 88.6). Angiography provides both information about the aneurysm and can evaluate for other intraabdominal aneurysm, which are present in 20% of patients.[87]

Treatment

The rupture risk as related to size of hepatic artery aneurysms is unknown.[67] Because of this and the known high mortality of rupture, consideration for intervention at any size has been recommended by some authors. However, patients with aneurysms ranging from 1.5 to 5 cm have been safely followed and only intervened upon when symptomatic or with risk factors for rupture.[67,92]

The Mayo Clinic published a large study following patients with true hepatic artery aneurysms. Patients with aneurysms and significant comorbidities were followed, and none ruptured over a mean of 68.4 months.[92] In general, the accepted recommendation is to treat hepatic artery aneurysms when greater than 2 cm if the patient is in good health and has a significant life expectancy.[76,92] The same group published a large series of patients who underwent treatment—males outnumbered females 2:1, the mean size of lesions was 4.5 cm, and nearly half of the patients had associated connective tissue disorders. Nearly all of the patients underwent open surgical treatment. Two of the five patients presenting with frank rupture died.[93]

The preferred modality of treatment largely depends on the location of the aneurysm and the patient's presentation. Extrahepatic aneurysms are typically treated surgically, whereas intrahepatic aneurysms are usually treated with endovascular techniques.[87] Extrahepatic aneurysms can also be treated with endovascular techniques, such as embolization or stent grafting.

Surgical approaches are varied. Extrahepatic aneurysms can occasionally be treated with resection and grafting or aneurysmorrhaphy.[80] Grafts can be autogenous or nonautogenous.[91] Ligation is also an option, regardless of whether or not the aneurysm is proximal to the gastroduodenal artery, because of the extensive collateral circulation to the liver.[89,91] The superior mesenteric artery (SMA) must be evaluated for patency for simple ligation to be an option. Intrahepatic aneurysms may require liver resection if not amenable to endovascular techniques.

Similar to splenic artery aneurysms, endovascular catheter-based therapies are being used more frequently but must face the challenge of maintaining adequate hepatic perfusion. Options again include stent graft coverage and embolization techniques.[80] Aneurysms in the liver transplant population are traditionally treated with surgery, although there are reports of endovascular management.[94]

SUPERIOR MESENTERIC ARTERY ANEURYSMS

Incidence

Aneurysms of the SMA represent the third most common visceral artery aneurysm, occurring in 5.5% of patients with these entities.[80] SMA aneurysms are equally distributed in males and females.[80,95] Mycotic aneurysms typically affect patients younger than age 50 years, whereas degenerative aneurysms are more likely to present in patients age 60 years or older.[95] Aneurysms are most commonly found in the first 5 cm of the SMA.[96]

Anatomy and Pathology

Up to one-third of SMA aneurysms have historically been described as mycotic or septic,[64,80] with septic emboli being a known cause. *Streptococcus* from left-sided cardiac valvular endocarditis has been reported.[67,88] When excluding pseudoaneurysms, infection is currently an etiologic factor in less than 5% of cases,[95] with the primary etiology now being atherosclerotic. Medial degeneration, also seen in splenic and hepatic aneurysms, often with secondary atherosclerosis, accounts for 25% of SMA aneurysms. Other reported causes are inflammatory processes in the abdomen or retroperitoneum (cholecystitis, pancreatitis) and trauma. In one report, nearly 20% of patients had an identifiable collagen vascular disorder.[96]

When secondary to pancreatitis, the etiology is thought to be autodigestive destruction of the arterial wall from activated pancreatic enzymes or mechanical erosion from an adjacent pseudocyst.[96] Arterial dissection also has been a reported cause and, although rare, affects the SMA in this way more than any other visceral artery.[67,88]

Clinical Presentation

Most patients (90%) are symptomatic with abdominal pain and a pulsatile mass.[80] The pulsatile mass may be notably mobile, differentiating it from an abdominal aortic aneurysm.[88] Patients also may present with frank intraperitoneal hemorrhage or symptoms and signs of mesenteric ischemia. Mesenteric ischemia may be secondary to thromboembolism from the aneurysm.[67] Rupture into the duodenum with subsequent massive GI bleeding

has been reported.[97] Overall, 50% of patients present with rupture, and the mortality rate is 30%.[67]

Diagnosis

Diagnosis is not typically incidental, as most patients are symptomatic. CT scanning and angiography are most helpful in diagnosis and treatment planning.[96]

Treatment

Treatment is usually recommended for asymptomatic noninfected aneurysms measuring 2.5 cm or larger and previously has been in open surgical fashion. Ligation without revascularization is an option for elective patients who have adequate collateral arterial supply. Ligation or aneurysm resection with revascularization has been reported to be necessary in 25% of elective procedures.[96] Endovascular stent graft coverage or transcatheter embolization has been reported with success,[96,98] and in a large series from the University of Pittsburgh group, the majority of noninfected SMA aneurysms were treated with endovascular methods, primarily coil embolization.[99] Concern does exist in treating mycotic or infected SMA aneurysms with endovascular methods, and in this setting, open repair is preferred. Bowel resection is often required for emergency cases when rupture or ischemia is present. This is unlikely to be necessary in elective procedures.[96] If catheter procedures are used, careful evaluation and monitoring for the development of bowel ischemia is mandatory.

CELIAC ARTERY ANEURYSMS

Incidence

Celiac artery aneurysms are uncommon, representing only 4% of visceral aneurysms. They occur with equal frequency in men and women, and are usually identified in the fifth decade of life.[88,100]

Anatomy and Physiology

Celiac artery aneurysms are usually secondary to medial degeneration with secondary atherosclerosis.[80,88] However, in the past they were primarily caused by infectious diseases, such as disseminated syphilis, which is now rare. Collagen vascular disorders also account for 17% of these disorders.[88] Pseudoaneurysms are typically caused by trauma, infection, or dissection, and are less common.[80]

Clinical Presentation

Most patients are asymptomatic, as the aneurysm is found incidentally. When symptoms do occur, the most common is epigastric pain. Nausea, vomiting, jaundice, or hematemesis have been reported. Occasionally, a pulsatile mass or bruit may be appreciated.[80]

The rupture risk has been reported as 5% for aneurysms smaller than 2.2 cm and 70% for those larger than 3.2 cm.[101,102] In general, the rupture risk is thought to be 13%,[100] and most often the rupture is into the peritoneal cavity. Presentation with GI bleeding secondary to rupture into the GI tract (stomach) has been reported.

Diagnosis

Plain radiographs have detected celiac aneurysms in a number of cases. The typical finding is that of a curvilinear calcification in the epigastrium.[100] Ultrasound can also lead to the diagnosis. CT and angiography are the most helpful tests in establishing the diagnosis and aiding with treatment planning. Catheter angiography provides the ability to determine the adequacy of collateral flow and helps to establish either catheter-based or surgical options.[103] Attention must be given to other arterial beds because a high proportion of patients with these aneurysms have concomitant aortic, iliac, femoral, or renal aneurysms.

Treatment

Open surgical approaches to celiac artery aneurysms have included ligation alone, reimplantation, aneurysmorrhaphy, and grafting and is recommended at diameters beginning at 2 cm for asymptomatic lesions.[100,103] Aneurysmorrhaphy is sometimes possible if the aneurysm is saccular.[88,103] Ligation alone is the procedure of choice in 35% of procedures and is the recommended choice of treatment in the setting of Ehlers-Danlos syndrome.[88] Although surgical intervention is individualized, consideration should be given to choosing aneurysmectomy and arterial reconstruction with either autogenous vein or prosthetic graft to maintain patency of the artery.[93] For endovascular procedures, both embolization and stent grafting have been described, with good results reported for the latter involving stent graft placement into the celiac axis and down the common hepatic to ensure patency.[104]

Rupture carries with it a mortality risk of 40%.[88] Elective surgery for intact aneurysms has been reported to have a mortality rate of 5%.[100,103,105]

INFERIOR MESENTERIC ARTERY ANEURYSMS

Inferior mesenteric artery (IMA) aneurysms are rare, accounting for 0.5% of visceral artery aneurysms.[93,98] Most are found in the proximal main trunk of the artery.[106]

Although infectious or inflammatory etiologies have been implicated, a unique proposed etiology is concomitant occlusive disease of the celiac and SMA. This increased flow through the IMA, especially if associated with a concomitant IMA origin stenosis, can lead to a poststenotic dilation phenomenon and subsequent aneurysmal degeneration.[106] In these cases, preservation of IMA flow is important because the circulation of the bowel may be dependent on IMA flow.[106]

Rupture with retroperitoneal hemorrhage is the most dramatic mode of presentation. Other manifestations of symptomatic IMA aneurysms include abdominal pain or colonic ischemia. Ligation with aneurysm resection is the most straightforward therapy if bowel viability is not dependent on IMA flow. Resection and reimplantation on the aorta or transposition to the iliac artery have also been reported.[106]

CELIAC ARTERY BRANCH ANEURYSMS: GASTRIC, GASTROEPIPLOIC, AND PANCREATIC ARTERIES

Gastric and gastroepiploic artery aneurysms are the most common of the celiac artery branch aneurysms, representing 4% of visceral aneurysms.[88] Gastroduodenal and pancreaticoduodenal artery aneurysms are less common, accounting for 1.5% to 3% of visceral aneurysms (Fig. 88.7).[80,88]

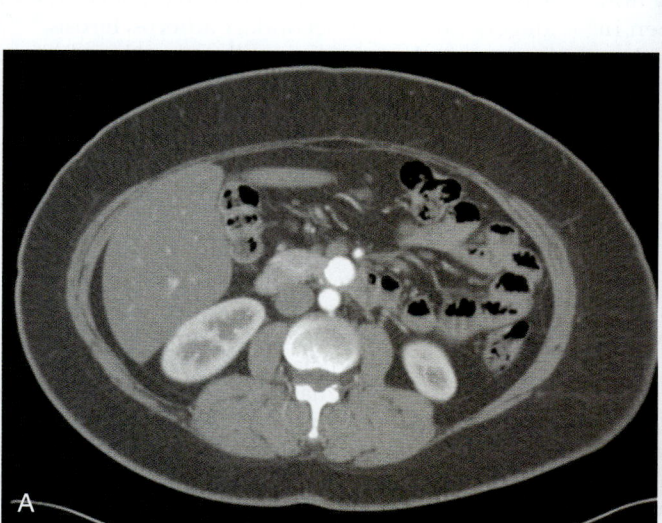
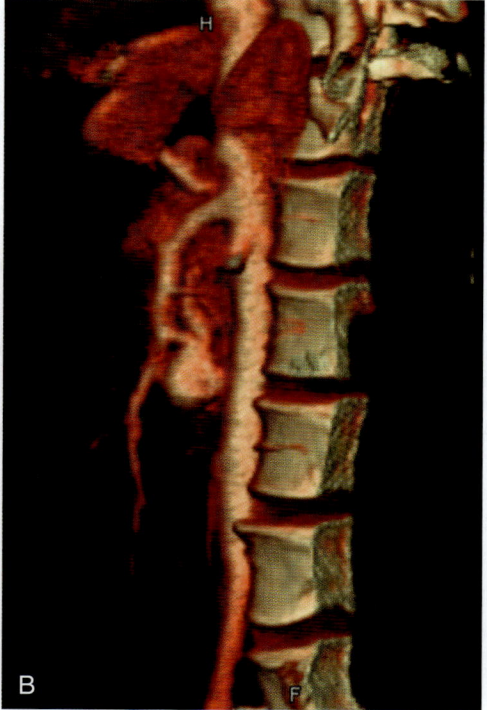

FIGURE 88.7 (A) An abdominal computed tomography scan of the midabdomen with intravenous contrast identifies an aneurysm of the inferior pancreaticoduodenal artery lying between the underlying aorta and the smaller superior mesenteric artery above it. (B) A sagittal three-dimensional reconstruction computed tomography angiogram illustrates the inferior pancreaticoduodenal artery aneurysm arising posterior to the superior mesenteric artery.

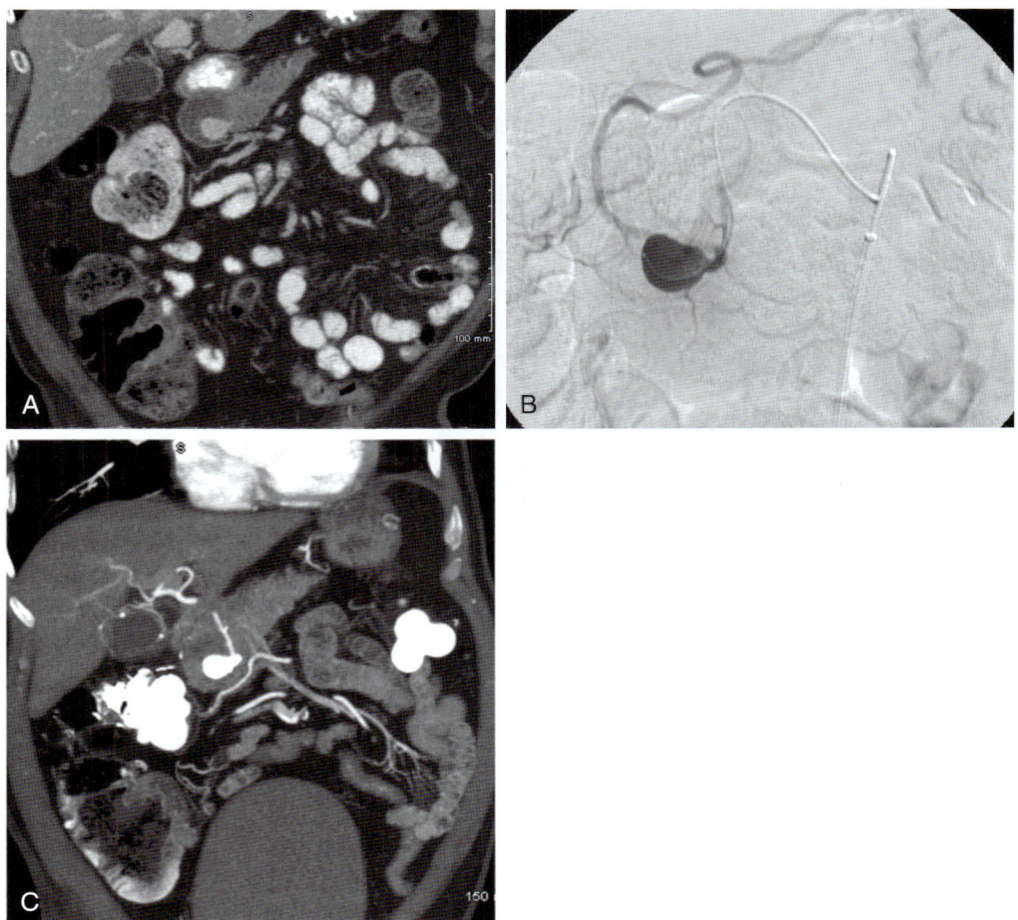

FIGURE 88.8 (A) Coronal computed tomography images reveal a 2-cm aneurysm arising from the distal gastroduodenal artery at the origin of the gastroepiploic artery. This was in a 74-year-old man presenting with abdominal pain. (B) The common hepatic artery had its own origin from the aorta. Initial selective catheterization of the common hepatic artery allowed for selection of the gastroduodenal artery with a microcatheter and embolization with glue. (C) Computed tomography scan 1 day after the embolization procedure reveals complete occlusion of the gastroduodenal aneurysm with glue. There is additional glue present in the gastroepiploic artery, branches to the pancreas, and the gallbladder wall.

When associated with pancreatitis, most arise in men, usually in the fifth decade of life.[80]

Gastroduodenal aneurysms are more common in men than women. They present with rupture in 56% of cases. Abdominal pain and GI hemorrhage or hemobilia are each present in more than half, and jaundice in nearly a third of patients.[99] Associated conditions are pancreatitis in 47% and alcohol abuse in 25%.[107] The majority, 72%, have been treated with ligation, whereas aneurysmectomy has been chosen for 22%.[107]

True pancreaticoduodenal artery aneurysms often occur in the setting of stenosis or occlusion of the celiac axis.[108] Half of true pancreaticoduodenal aneurysms present with rupture, the mortality of which is 26%.[107,108] Most often, this is rupture into the GI tract. Free intraperitoneal rupture may be present in 15% of cases.[60] After pancreaticoduodenectomy, a "herald bleed" from the drain may indicate rupture of a gastroduodenal artery pseudoaneurysm.[67] Most of these aneurysms are thought to be pseudoaneurysms, secondary to necrotizing pancreatitis or infection, where there is erosion into the artery.[67]

Most patients present with epigastric abdominal pain, often radiating to the back. It can be difficult to distinguish from that of pancreatitis.[67,88] Diagnosis is typically with CT and angiography, although ultrasound has been diagnostic. Occasionally, diagnosis is made at laparotomy.[107]

Therapy approaches have included both open surgical and endovascular techniques. Open techniques include ligation, excision of the aneurysm with primary reanastomosis, and aneurysmorrhaphy.[69] Occasionally, pancreatic resection with or without splenectomy has been required for treatment.[80,91] Standard catheter-based techniques, including embolization, have been used successfully (Fig. 88.8).

MESENTERIC BRANCH ANEURYSMS: JEJUNAL, ILEAL, AND COLIC ARTERIES

Jejunal, ileal, and colic artery aneurysms represent less than 3% of visceral aneurysms.[80,88] They occur either in the mesentery or in an intramural location.

Most are usually small, less than 1 cm, solitary, and symptomatic.[80] The etiology includes degenerative

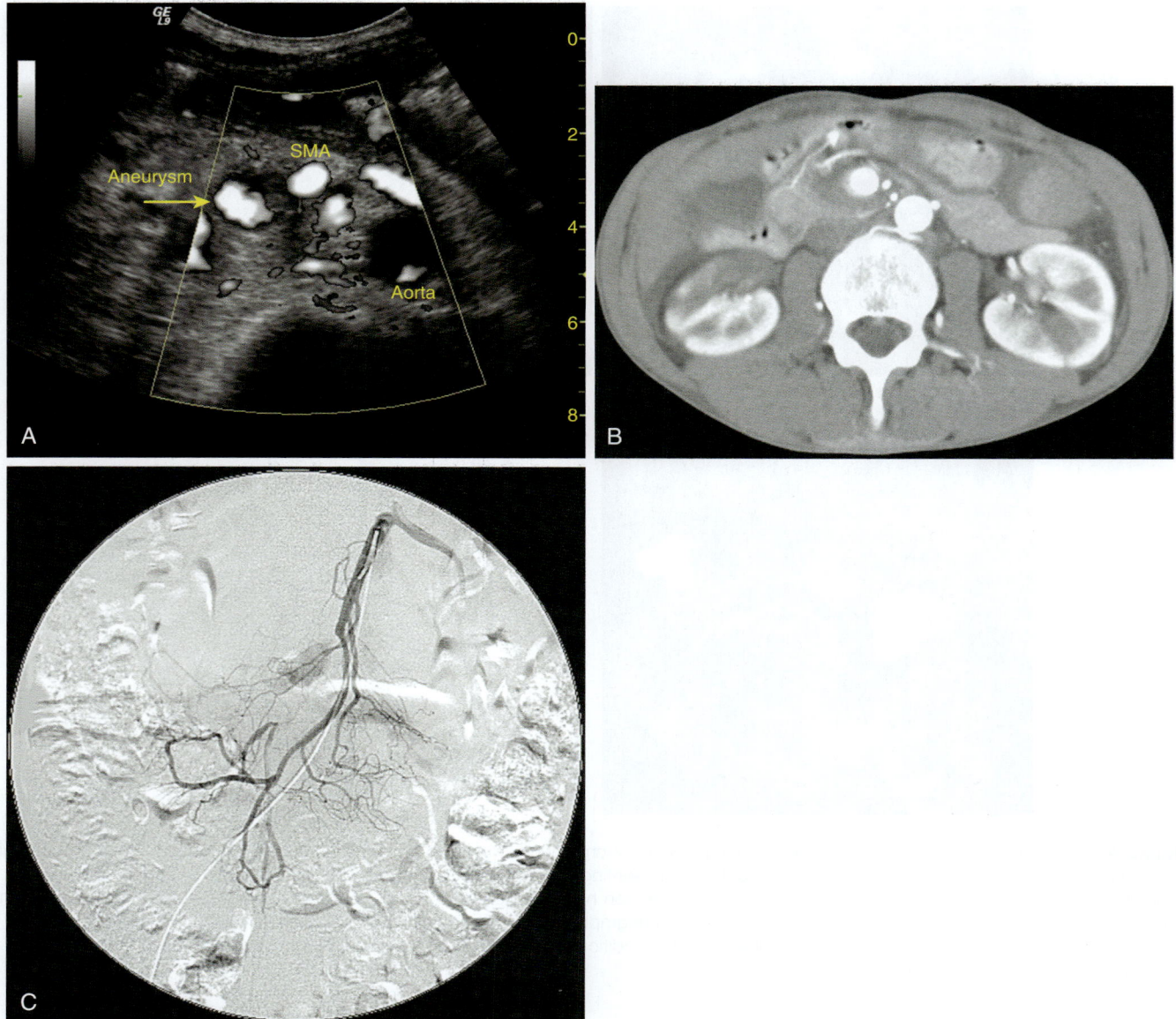

FIGURE 88.9 (A) Transverse lower abdominal power-flow duplex ultrasound showing an ileocolic aneurysm lateral to the superior mesenteric artery (SMA). (B) A computed tomography scan with contrast demonstrates the large size of the ileocolic aneurysm and nonopacified thrombus within it. (C) Selective angiogram of the SMA showing retained contrast within the ileocolic aneurysm, with contrast filling the distal vessel and extrinsic compression and medial displacement of the SMA.

processes, infection, and inflammation. Nearly half present with rupture into either the GI tract or peritoneum. Sometimes large mesenteric hematomas are present and can make locating the aneurysm a challenge at surgery. Surgical ligation with assessment of bowel viability is an option, but intestinal resection is occasionally necessary secondary to inadequate collateral flow.[80] Endovascular embolization can be performed, but evaluation for subsequent bowel viability is mandatory (Fig. 88.9).

RENAL ARTERY ANEURYSMS

Renal artery aneurysms, one of the most uncommon visceral aneurysms, have been reported in autopsy series to occur at rates of 0.01% to 0.1%.[109] In general, these aneurysms are bland and very slow growing, and previous recommendations to repair these aneurysms at 2 cm may be too liberal. Females outnumber males 3:1, and there is a striking association with fibromuscular dysplasia, as well as hypertension. Series document a 70% to 100% incidence of the latter in these patients. Theories for this include associated renal artery occlusive disease, distal embolization to the parenchyma, and turbulent flow within the aneurysm, resulting in decreased parenchymal perfusion. Indeed, many series have shown an improvement in hypertension in patients who undergo repair of their aneurysm.

Open surgical repair options include angioplastic closure with or without branch reimplantation, primary resection with anastomosis, plication of smaller lesions, or bypass from a proximal location, such as the aorta or other splanchnic branches. Endovascular methods have typically consisted of coil embolization of distal lesions and stent graft placement for main branch lesions in the absence of severe tortuosity.

SUMMARY

Aortoenteric fistulas can be a consequence of a primary erosive process in the native aorta but are most commonly associated with previous aortic intervention, either open bypass grafting or placement of endovascular stent grafting. Standards of treatment are resuscitation, assessment of patient comorbidities, resection of the infected graft and associated aorta, débridement of infected tissue, and reconstruction, either with aortic replacement or extraanatomic methods. Morbidity and mortality are high even with the best-risk patients.

Visceral artery aneurysms are uncommon entities when compared with aortic aneurysms, but with the increasing incidence of cross-sectional imaging, more are being detected in the general population. Of these, splenic artery aneurysms are the most common, followed by hepatic artery aneurysms. All of these have a fairly benign natural history and can be repaired on an elective basis, but all can present with rupture and abdominal emergency with hemodynamic instability. Nearly all the visceral artery aneurysms can be repaired with either open surgical or endovascular methods.

ACKNOWLEDGMENT

The authors would like to credit Julie E. Adams, MD and Fuyuki Hirashima, MD as authors on the original chapter.

REFERENCES

1. Cooper A. *The Lectures of Sir Astley Cooper on the Principles and Practice of Surgery with Additional Notes and Cases by F. Tyrrell.* 5th ed. Philadelphia: Haswell. Barrington and Haswell; 1939.
2. Flye MW, Thompson WM. Aortic graft-enteric and paraprosthetic-enteric fistulas. *Am J Surg.* 1983;146:183.
3. Busuttil RW, Reese W, Baker JD, Wilson SE. Pathogenesis of aortoduodenal fistula, experimental and clinical correlates. *Surgery.* 1979;85:1.
4. Hickey NC, Downing R. Hamer JD, Ashton F, Slaney G. Abdominal aortic aneurysm as complicated by spontaneous ileocaval or duodenal fistulae. *J Cardiovasc Surg (Torino).* 1991;32:181.
5. Olcott C 4th, Holcroft JW, Stoney RJ, Wylie EJ. Unusual problems of abdominal aortic aneurysms. *Am J Surg.* 1978;135:426.
6. Saers SJ, Scheltinga MR. Primary aortoenteric fistula. *Br J Surg.* 2005;92:143.
7. Gad A. Aortoduodenal fistula revisited. *Scand J Gastroenterol Suppl.* 1989;167:97.
8. Skourtis G, Gerasimos P, Sotirios M, et al. Primary aortoenteric fistula due to septic aortitis. *Ann Vasc Surg.* 2010;24:e7.
9. Berry SM, Fischer JE. Classification and pathophysiology of enterocutaneous fistulas. *Surg Clin North Am.* 1996;76:1009.
10. Reckless JP, McColl I, Taylor GW. Aorto-enteric fistulae: an uncommon complication of abdominal aortic aneurysms. *Br J Surg.* 1972;59:458.
11. Dossa CD, Pipinos II, Shepard AD, Ernst CB. Primary aortoenteric fistula: Part II. Primary aortoesophageal fistula. *Ann Vasc Surg.* 1994;8:207.
12. Lawlor DK, DeRose G, Harris KA, Forbes TL. Primary aorto/iliac-enteric fistula: report of 6 new cases. *Vasc Endovascular Surg.* 2004;38:281.
13. Kappadath SK, Clarke MJ, Stormer E, Steven L, Jaffray B. Primary aortoenteric fistula due to a swallowed twig in a three-year-old child. *Eur J Vasc Endovasc Surg.* 2010;39:217.
14. O'Hara PJ, Hertzer NR, Beven EG, Krajewski LP. Surgical management of infected abdominal aortic grafts: review of a 25-year experience. *J Vasc Surg.* 1986;3:725.
15. Thompson WM, Jackson DC, Johnsrude IS. Aortoenteric and paraprosthetic-enteric fistulas: radiologic findings. *AJR Am J Roentgenol.* 1976;127:235.
16. Bergqvist D, Alm A, Claes G, et al. Secondary aortoenteric fistulas: an analysis of 42 cases. *Eur J Vasc Surg.* 1987;1:11.
17. Champion MC, Sullivan SN, Coles JC, Goldbach M, Watson WC. Aortoenteric fistula. Incidence, presentation, recognition, and management. *Ann Surg.* 1982;195:314.
18. Ruby BJ, Cogbill TH. Aortoduodenal fistula 5 years after endovascular abdominal aortic aneurysm repair with the Ancure stent graft. *J Vasc Surg.* 2007;45:834.
19. Hausegger KA, Tiesenhausen K, Karaic R, Tauss J, Koch G. Aortoduodenal fistula: a late complication of intraluminal exclusion of an infrarenal aortic aneurysm. *J Vasc Interv Radiol.* 1999;10:747.
20. d'Othée BJ, Soula P, Otal P, et al. Aortoduodenal fistula after endovascular stent-graft of an abdominal aortic aneurysm. *J Vasc Surg.* 2000;31:190.
21. Parry DJ, Waterworth A, Kessel D, Robertson I, Berridge DC, Scott DJ. Endovascular repair of an inflammatory abdominal aortic aneurysm complicated by aortoduodenal fistulation with an unusual presentation. *J Vasc Surg.* 2001;33:874.
22. Norgren L, Jernby B, Engellau L. Aortoenteric fistula caused by a ruptured stent-graft: a case report. *J Endovasc Surg.* 1998;5:269.
23. DeWeese MS, Fry WJ. Small-bowel erosion following aortic resection. *J Am Med Assoc.* 1962;179:882.
24. Rosenthal D, Deterling RA Jr, O'Donnell TF Jr, Callow AD. Positive blood culture as an aid in the diagnosis of secondary aortoenteric fistula. *Arch Surg.* 1979;114:1041.
25. O'Mara CS, Williams GM, Ernst CB. Secondary aortoenteric fistula. A 20-year experience. *Am J Surg.* 1981;142:203.
26. Goldstone J, Cunningham CC. Diagnosis, treatment and prevention of aorto-enteric fistulas. *Acta Chir Scand Suppl.* 1990;555:165.
27. Hughes FM, Kavanagh D, Barry M, Owens A, MacErlaine DP, Malone DE. Aortoenteric fistula: a diagnostic dilemma. *Abdom Imaging.* 2007;32:398.
28. Mark AS, Moss AA, McCarthy S, McCowin M. CT of aortoenteric fistulas. *Invest Radiol.* 1985;20:272.
29. Low RN, Wall SD, Jeffrey RB Jr, Sollitto RA, Reilly LM, Tierney LM Jr. Aortoenteric fistula and perigraft infection: evaluation with CT. *Radiology.* 1990;175:157.
30. Peirce RM, Jenkins RH, Maceneaney P. Paraprosthetic extravasation of enteric contrast: a rare and direct sign of secondary aortoenteric fistula. *AJR Am J Roentgenol.* 2005;184:S73.
31. Orton DF, LeVeen RF, Saigh JA, et al. Aortic prosthetic graft infections: radiologic manifestations and implications for management. *Radiographics.* 2000;20:977.
32. Vu QD, Menias CO, Bhalla S, Peterson C, Wang LL, Balfe DM. Aortoenteric fistulas: CT features and potential mimics. *Radiographics.* 2009;29:197.
33. O'Donnell TF Jr, Scott G, Shepard A, Mackey W, Deterling RA, Callow AD. Improvements in the diagnosis and management of aortoenteric fistula. *Am J Surg.* 1985;149:481.
34. Ihama Y, Miyazaki T, Fuke C, et al. An autopsy case of a primary aortoenteric fistula: a pitfall of the endoscopic diagnosis. *World J Gastroenterol.* 2008;14:4701.
35. Fiorani P, Speziale F, Rizzo L, et al. Detection of aortic graft infection with leukocytes labeled with technetium 99m-hexametazime. *J Vasc Surg.* 1993;17:87; discussion 95.
36. Blaisdell FW, Hall AD, Lim RC Jr, Moore WC. Aorto-iliac arterial substitution utilizing subcutaneous grafts. *Ann Surg.* 1970;172:775.
37. Young RM, Cherry KJ Jr, Davis PM, et al. The results of in situ prosthetic replacement for infected aortic grafts. *Am J Surg.* 1999;179:136.
38. Reilly LM, Stoney RJ, Goldstone J, Ehrenfeld WK. Improved management of aortic graft infection: the influence of operation sequence and staging. *J Vasc Surg.* 1987;5:421.
39. Seeger JM, Pretus HA, Welborn MB, Ozaki CK, Flynn TC, Huber TS. Long-term outcome after treatment of aortic graft infection with staged extra-anatomic bypass grafting and aortic graft removal. *J Vasc Surg.* 2000;32:451; discussion 460.

40. Kuestner LM, Reilly LM, Jicha DL, Ehrenfeld WK, Goldstone J, Stoney RJ. Secondary aortoenteric fistula: contemporary outcome with use of extraanatomic bypass and infected graft excision. *J Vasc Surg.* 1995;21:184.

41. Yeager RA, Moneta GL, Taylor LM Jr, Harris EJ Jr, McConnell DB, Porter JM. Improving survival and limb salvage in patients with aortic graft infection. *Am J Surg.* 1990;159:466.

42. Yashar JJ, Weyman AK, Burnard RJ, Yashar J. Survival and limb salvage in patients with infected arterial prostheses. *Am J Surg.* 1978;135:499.

43. Quiñones-Baldrich WJ, Hernandez JJ, Moore WS. Long-term results following surgical management of aortic graft infection. *Arch Surg.* 1991;126:507.

44. Torsello G, Sandmann W, Gehrt A, Jungblut RM. In situ replacement of infected vascular prostheses with rifampin-soaked vascular grafts: early results. *J Vasc Surg.* 1993;17:768.

45. Torsello G, Sandmann W. Use of antibiotic-bonded grafts in vascular graft infection. *Eur J Vasc Endovasc Surg.* 1997;14:84.

46. Hayes PD, Nasim A, London NJ, et al. In situ replacement of infected aortic grafts with rifampicin-bonded prostheses: the Leicester experience (1992 to 1998). *J Vasc Surg.* 1999;30:92.

47. Oderich GS, Bower TC, Cherry KJ Jr, et al. Evolution from axillofemoral to in situ prosthetic reconstruction for the treatment of aortic graft infections at a single center. *J Vasc Surg.* 2006;43:1166.

48. Clagett GP, Valentine RJ, Hagino RT. Autogenous aortoiliac/femoral reconstruction from superficial femoral-popliteal veins: feasibility and durability. *J Vasc Surg.* 1997;25:255; discussion 267.

49. Clagett GP, Bowers BL, Lopez-Viego MA, et al. Creation of a neo-aortoiliac system from lower extremity deep and superficial veins. *Ann Surg.* 1993;218:239; discussion 248.

50. Heinola I, Kantonen I, Jaroma M, et al. Treatment of aortic prosthesis infections by graft removal and in-situ replacement with autologous femoral veins and fascial strengthening. *Eur J Vasc Endovasc Surg.* 2016;51:232.

51. Zwischenberger JB, Shalaby TZ, Conti VR. Viable cryopreserved aortic homograft for aortic valve endocarditis and annular abscesses. *Ann Thorac Surg.* 1989;48:365; discussion 369.

52. Bisdas T, Bredt M, Pichlmaier M, et al. Eight-year experience with cryopreserved arterial homografts for the in situ reconstruction of abdominal aortic infections. *J Vasc Surg.* 2010;52:323.

53. Kieffer E, Bahnini A, Koskas F, Ruotolo C, Le Blevec D, Plissonnier D. In situ allograft replacement of infected infrarenal aortic prosthetic grafts: results in forty-three patients. *J Vasc Surg.* 1993;17:349; discussion 355.

54. Lesèche G, Castier Y, Petit MD, et al. Long-term results of cryopreserved arterial allograft reconstruction in infected prosthetic grafts and mycotic aneurysms of the abdominal aorta. *J Vasc Surg.* 2001;34:616.

55. Bandyk DF, Novotney ML, Johnson BL, Back MR, Roth SR. Use of rifampin-soaked gelatin-sealed polyester grafts for in situ treatment of primary aortic and vascular prosthetic infections. *J Surg Res.* 2001;95:44.

56. Batt M, Jean-Baptiste E, O'Connor S, et al. In-situ revascularisation for patients with aortic graft infection: a single centre experience with silver coated polyester grafts. *Eur J Vasc Endovasc Surg.* 2008;36:182.

57. Antoniou GA, Koutsias S, Antoniou SA, Georgiakakis A, Lazarides MK, Giannoukas AD. Outcome after endovascular stent graft repair of aortoenteric fistula: a systematic review. *J Vasc Surg.* 2009;49:782.

58. Danneels MI, Verhagen HJ, Teijink JA, Cuypers P, Nevelsteen A, Vermassen FE. Endovascular repair for aorto-enteric fistula: a bridge too far or a bridge to surgery? *Eur J Vasc Endovasc Surg.* 2006;32:27.

59. Burks JA Jr, Faries PL, Gravereaux EC, Hollier LH, Marin ML. Endovascular repair of bleeding aortoenteric fistulas: a 5-year experience. *J Vasc Surg.* 2001;34:1055.

60. Mok VW, Ting AC, Law S, Wong KH, Cheng SW, Wong J. Combined endovascular stent grafting and endoscopic injection of fibrin sealant for aortoenteric fistula complicating esophagectomy. *J Vasc Surg.* 2004;40:1234.

61. Smeds MR, Duncan AA, Harlander-Locke MP, et al. Treatment and outcomes of aortic endograft infection. *J Vasc Surg.* 2016;63:332.

62. Kahlberg A, Rinaldi E, Castelli P, et al. Aorto-enteric fistula following endovascular aortic repair: results from the multicenter study on aorto-enteric fistulization after stent grafting of the abdominal aorta (MAEFISTO) [abstract only]. *Eur J Vasc Endovasc Surg.* 2015; 50:391.

63. Morgan-Rowe L, Simring D, Raja J, Agu O, Richards T, Ivancev K. The use of an endovascular stent graft with 'home-made' fenestrations to treat an infected aortic endograft in an emergency setting: a short report. *Eur J Vasc Endovasc Surg.* 2011;Extra 22:e34.

64. Al-Habbal Y, Christophi C, Muralidharan V. Aneurysms of the splenic artery—a review. *Surgeon.* 2010;8:223.

65. Moon D, Lee S, Hwang S, et al. Characteristics and management of splenic artery aneurysms in adult living donor liver transplant recipients. *Liver Transpl.* 2009;15:1535.

66. Smith EB. Surgical aspects of the visceral arteries. *J Natl Med Assoc.* 1965;57:374.

67. Pasha SF, Gloviczki P, Stanson AW, Kamath PS. Splanchnic artery aneurysms. *Mayo Clin Proc.* 2007;82:472.

68. Valentine RJ, Wind GG. *Anatomic Exposure in Vascular Surgery.* Philadelphia: Lippincott Williams & Wilkins; 2003.

69. Ha JF, Phillips M, Faulkner K. Splenic artery aneurysm rupture in pregnancy. *Eur J Obstet Gynecol Reprod Biol.* 2009;146:133.

70. Mattar S, Lumsden A. The management of splenic artery aneurysms: experience with 23 cases. *Am J Surg.* 1995;169:580.

71. Grotemeyer D, Duran M, Park E, et al. Visceral artery aneurysms—follow-up of 23 patients with 31 aneurysms after surgical or interventional therapy. *Langenbecks Arch Surg.* 2009;394:1093.

72. Sachdev-Ost U. Visceral artery aneurysms: review of current management options. *Mt Sinai J Med.* 2010;77:296.

73. Sendra F, Safran D, McGee G. A rare complication of splenic artery aneurysm. Mesenteric steal syndrome. *Arch Surg.* 1995;130:669.

74. Rao S, Sivina M, Willis I, Sher T, Habibnejad S. Massive lower gastrointestinal tract bleeding due to splenic artery aneurysm: a case report. *Ann Vasc Surg.* 2007;21:388.

75. Lang W, Strobel D, Beinder E, Raab M. Surgery of a splenic artery aneurysm during pregnancy. *Eur J Obstet Gynecol Reprod Biol.* 2002;102:215.

76. Hirsch AT, Haskal ZJ, Hertzer NR, et al. ACC/AHA Guidelines for the management of patients with peripheral arterial disease. *J Am Coll Cardiol.* 2006;47:1239.

77. Hogendoorn W, Lavida A, Hunink MGM, et al. Open repair, endovascular repair, and conservative management of true splenic artery aneurysms. *J Vasc Surg.* 2014;60:1667.

78. Aslam M, Shalev Y. Treatment of splenic artery aneurysm with polytetrafluoroethylene-covered stent. *Catheter Cardiovasc Interv.* 2010;76:229.

79. Osaka S, Maeda H, Umezawa H, et al. Splenic artery aneurysm performed vascular reconstruction: a case report. *Ann Thorac Cardiovasc Surg.* 2009;15:418.

80. Shanley CJ, Weinberger JB. Acute abdominal vascular emergencies. *Med Clin North Am.* 2008;92:627.

81. Mordasini P, Szucs-Farkas Z, Do D, Gralla J, Kettenbach J, Hoppe H. Use of a latest-generation vascular plug for peripheral vascular embolization with use of a diagnostic catheter: preliminary clinical experience. *J Vasc Interv Radiol.* 2010;21:1185.

82. Pietrabissa A, Morelli L, Ferrari M, et al. Mixed reality for robotic treatment of a splenic artery aneurysm. *Surg Endosc.* 2010;24:1204.

83. Pappy R, Sech C, Hennebry T. Giant splenic artery aneurysm: managed in the cardiovascular catheterization laboratory using the modified neck remodeling technique. *Catheter Cardiovasc Interv.* 2010;76:590.

84. Carr SC, Pearce WH, Vogelzang RL, McCarthy WJ, Nemcek AA Jr, Yao JS. Current management of visceral aneurysms. *Surgery.* 1996;120:627.

85. Pulli R, Dorigo W, Troisi N, Pratesi G, Innocenti AA, Pratesi C. Surgical treatment of visceral artery aneurysms: a 25 year experience. *J Vasc Surg.* 2008;48:334.

86. Grover BT, Gundersen SB 3rd, Kothari SN. Laparoscopic distal pancreatectomy and splenectomy for splenic artery aneurysm. *Surg Endosc.* 2010;24:2318.

87. O'Driscoll D, Olliff SP, Ollif JFC. Pictorial review: hepatic artery aneurysm. *Br J Radiol.* 1999;72:1018.

88. Upchurch GR, Zelenock GB, Stanley JC. Splanchnic artery aneurysms. In: Rutherford RB, ed. *Vascular Surgery.* 6th ed. Philadelphia: Elsevier Saunders; 2005:1565.

89. Curran FT, Taylor SA. Hepatic artery aneurysm. *Postgrad Med J.* 1986;62:957.

90. Kim HJ, Kim KW, Kim AY, et al. Hepatic artery pseudoaneurysm in adult living-donor-liver transplantation: efficacy of CT and Doppler sonography. *AJR Am J Roentgenol.* 2005;184:1549.

91. Rogers DM, Thompson JE, Garrett WV, Talkington CM, Patman RD. Mesenteric vascular problems. *Ann Surg.* 1982;195:554.

92. Abbas MA, Fowl RJ, Stone WM, et al. Hepatic artery aneurysm: factors that predict complications. *J Vasc Surg.* 2003;38:41.

93. Erben Y, DeMartino RR, Bjarnason H, et al. Operative management of hepatic artery aneurysms. *J Vasc Surg.* 2015;62:610.

94. Maleux G, Pirenne J, Aerts R, Nevens F. Case report: hepatic artery pseudoaneurysm after liver transplantation: definitive treatment with a stent-graft after failed coil embolisation. *Br J Radiol.* 2005;78:453.

95. Stone WM, Abbas M, Cherry KJ, Fowl RJ, Gloviczki P. Superior mesenteric artery aneurysms: is presence an indication for intervention? *J Vasc Surg.* 2002;36:234.

96. Rocek M, Peregrin JH, Dutka J, Ryska M, Bêlina F, Lastovcková J. Percutaneous treatment of a superior mesenteric artery pseudoaneurysm using a stent-graft. *AJR Am J Roentgenol.* 2002;178:1459.

97. Hall RI, Lavelle MI, Venables CW. Chronic pancreatitis as a cause of gastrointestinal bleeding. *Gut.* 1982;23:250.

98. Tan BS, Reidy JF. Case report: transcatheter embolization of a superior mesenteric artery pseudoaneurysm with interlocking detachable coils. *Clin Radiol.* 1998;53:455.

99. Shukla AJ, Eid R, Fish L, et al. Contemporary outcomes of intact and ruptured visceral artery aneurysms. *J Vasc Surg.* 2015;61:1442.

100. Graham LM, Stanley JC, Whitehouse WM, et al. Celiac artery aneurysms: historic (1745–1949) versus contemporary (1950–1984) differences in etiology and clinical importance. *J Vasc Surg.* 1985;2:757.

101. Carrafiello G, Rivolta N, Fontana F, et al. Combined endovascular repair of a celiac trunk aneurysm using celiac-splenic stent graft and hepatic artery embolization. *Cardiovasc Intervent Radiol.* 2009;33:352.

102. Røkke O, Søndenaa K, Amundsen S, Bjerke-Larssen T, Jensen D. The diagnosis and management of splanchnic artery aneurysms. *Scand J Gastroenterol.* 1996;31:737.

103. Knox R, Steinthorsson G, Sumpio B. Celiac artery aneurysms: a case report and review of the literature. *Int J Angiol.* 2000;9:99.

104. Zhang W, Fu Y, Wei P, E B, Li DC, Xu J. Endovascular repair of celiac artery aneurysm with the use of stent grafts. *J Vasc Interv Radiol.* 2016;27:514.

105. Vasconcelos L, Garcia AC, Silva e Castro J, Albuquerque e Castro J, Mota Capitão L. Celiac artery aneurysms. *Ann Vasc Surg.* 2010;24(554):e17.

106. Sallou C, Cron J, Julia P, Fabiani JN. Aneurysm of the inferior mesenteric artery: case report and review of the literature. *Eur J Vasc Endovasc Surg.* 1997;14:71.

107. Shanley CJ, Shah N, Messina LM. Uncommon splanchnic artery aneurysms: pancreaticoduodenal, gastroduodenal, superior mesenteric, inferior mesenteric, and colic. *Ann Vasc Surg.* 1996;10:506.

108. Katsura M, Gushimiyagi M, Takara H, Mototake H. True aneurysm of the pancreaticoduodenal arteries: a single institution experience. *J Gastrointest Surg.* 2010;14:1409.

109. Coleman DM, Stanley JC. Renal artery aneurysms. *J Vasc Surg.* 2015;62:779.

CHAPTER 89

Mesenteric Arterial Trauma

Eric N. Klein | Orlando C. Kirton

The superior mesenteric artery (SMA) and inferior mesenteric artery are susceptible to injury from both blunt and penetrating trauma. Injuries to the mesenteric arteries compose a small subset of intra-abdominal vascular trauma.[1] A multiinstitutional study involving 34 trauma centers reported only 250 patients with SMA injuries over 10 years.[2] Due to its smaller size, the incidence of injury to the inferior mesenteric artery is even rarer. Mesenteric arterial injuries are associated with high morbidity and mortality and present challenges for even the most experienced trauma surgeon. Patients are susceptible to massive hemorrhage, and those who initially survive remain at risk for early and delayed complications related to visceral ischemia. Proximal injuries to the SMA are rare but highly lethal. Although trauma to the branches of these vessels is more common, it is managed much like injuries to the bowel parenchyma supplied and is not discussed in this chapter. The diagnosis and treatment of injuries to the superior and inferior mesenteric arteries will be covered. The chapter will describe the associated injury pattern between blunt and penetrating trauma to the mesenteric arteries and their intraoperative management.

PENETRATING TRAUMA TO THE MESENTERIC ARTERIES

As with all intraabdominal vessels, the mesenteric arteries are susceptible to injury from penetrating trauma. Due to their deep retroperitoneal location, they are well protected and more likely to be injured from gunshot wounds than stab wounds. Similarly, they are rarely injured in isolation, and, despite varying degrees of selective conservatism in the management of penetrating trauma, most will be diagnosed upon emergent laparotomy for hemorrhage or peritonitis. The intraoperative management algorithm is presented in the section following the diagnosis of blunt mesenteric artery injury.

BLUNT TRAUMA TO THE MESENTERIC ARTERIES

The presentation of mesenteric arterial injury resulting from blunt trauma may vary from a stable patient with an incidental finding of intraperitoneal free fluid, or a mesenteric hematoma on imaging, to a an unstable patient with a major vascular injury causing exsanguinating hemorrhage. The management of these two scenarios is vastly different.

Although blunt mesenteric arterial injury generally causes abdominal pain, some patients may remain asymptomatic. Possible signs of mesenteric arterial injury may include bruising to the abdominal wall (seat belt sign), abdominal tenderness, or other signs of peritonitis. In stable patients, abdominal computed tomography (CT) scans are frequently obtained in a battery of imaging studies. Mesenteric hematomas may be seen in isolation but are frequently associated with other injuries to the gastrointestinal tract or solid organs.[3] With the advent of multidetector CT, the recognition and diagnostic ability of minor mesenteric injury has improved over the past 20 years. Historically, patients with blunt abdominal trauma were evaluated with a diagnostic peritoneal lavage to diagnose solid organ or hollow viscus injury. For hemodynamically stable trauma patients, CT imaging is currently favored in the diagnosis of blunt abdominal trauma. Solid organ injury can readily be identified, but evidence of mesenteric arterial injury remains difficult and signs often overlap with blunt hollow viscus injury.

The newest generation multislice CT scanner has increased sensitivity and specificity in the diagnosis of mesenteric injury. CT findings that may suggest mesenteric injury include free intraperitoneal fluid (Fig. 89.1), mesenteric hematomas that may look triangular or polygonal (Fig. 89.2), fat stranding of the omentum, intramesenteric fluid adjacent to thickening bowel wall (Fig. 89.3), mesenteric vessel beading, abrupt termination of mesenteric vessels, or active extravasation of contrast (Fig. 89.4). Active extravasation has the best positive predictive value. Absence of peritoneal fluid has the best negative predictive value.[4] Oral contrast is not required to detect mesenteric injuries.[5] In children, these radiographic findings are less reliable, and clinical data and physical exam should guide the decision to operate.[6] Although we are now better able to detect a mesenteric hematoma or laceration, predicting the clinical implications of a particular injury remains challenging. Due to variations in collateral supply, some patients can compensate for an injury that would cause bowel ischemia in another patient.

The management of stable patients with mesenteric injury should include close observation with serial abdominal exams and may require repeat CT imaging to evaluate for increase in the size of the hematoma or evidence of bowel ischemia secondary to disruption of the blood supply. If at any point the patient develops worsening abdominal pain, worsening or recurrent metabolic acidosis, worsening or delayed ileus, feeding intolerance, evidence of obstruction, peritonitis, or signs of sepsis, surgical exploration may be required.

A patient with active extravasation on CT imaging may require urgent exploration for control of hemorrhage and evaluation of bowel viability. If there is a question of bowel viability, a planned second-look operation is prudent.

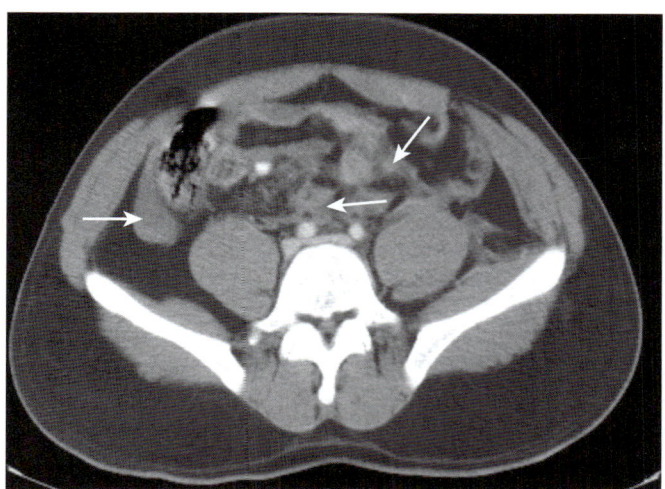

FIGURE 89.1 Mesenteric injury illustrated by associated free intraabdominal fluid (arrows).

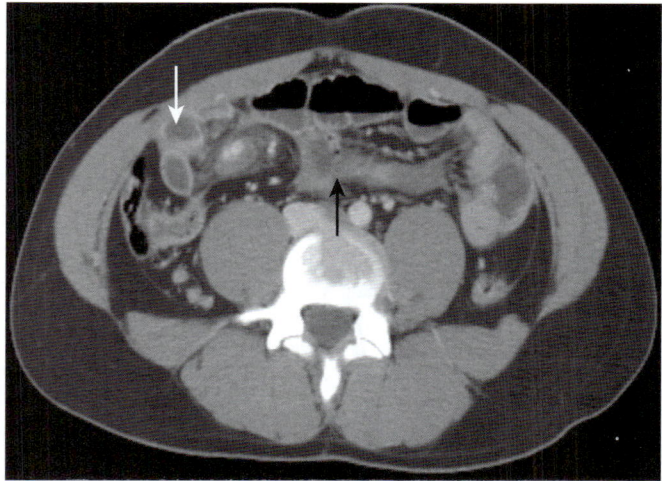

FIGURE 89.3 Mesenteric injury illustrated by intramesenteric fluid (black arrow), as well as thickening of the adjacent small bowel (white arrow).

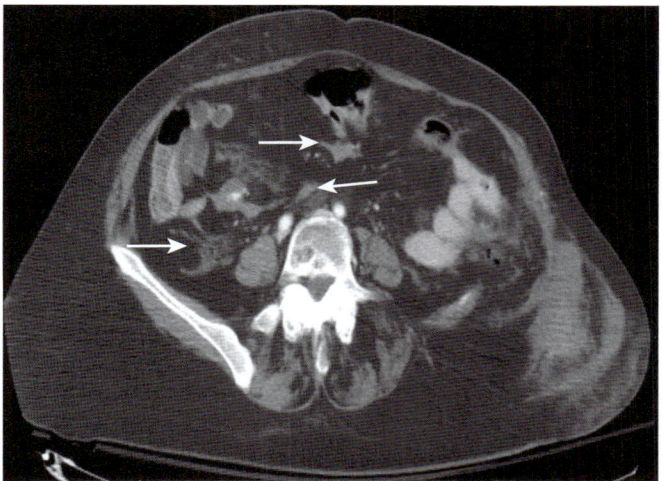

FIGURE 89.2 Mesenteric injury illustrated by associated triangular and polygonal hematomas (arrows).

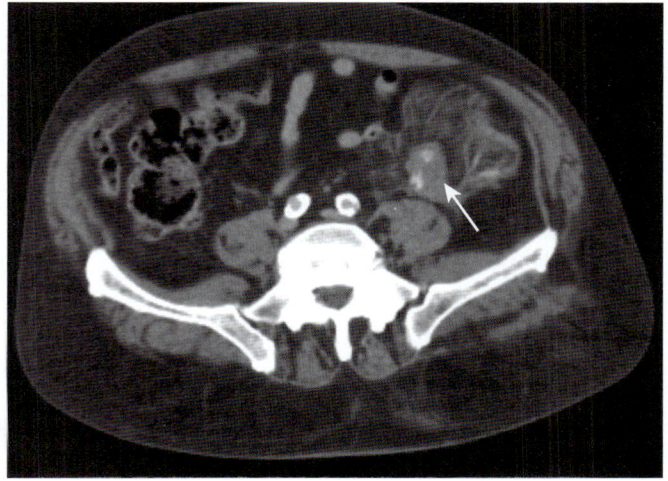

FIGURE 89.4 Mesenteric injury associated with active extravasation of contrast (arrow). Also note the definition of the mesenteric vasculature by this injury.

There are anecdotal case reports of laparoscopic procedures with intracorporeal control of hemorrhage and/or resection, as well as transcatheter arterial embolization of small mesenteric hemorrhage, but these techniques are not currently recommended except in centers with specialized expertise.[7,8]

The long-term consequence of a mesenteric injury is difficult to determine. There are case reports of late small bowel obstruction and mesenteric fibrosis that occurred in patients with a history of blunt abdominal trauma. These late complications are thought to be a result of subclinical bowel perforation or localized gut ischemia caused by injury of the mesenteric vasculature.[9,10] The majority of our discussion refers to injuries of the superior mesenteric arterial system. Injuries to the inferior mesenteric artery are rare and generally can be treated with ligation. An uninjured superior mesenteric system usually prevents ischemic sequelae.

SUPERIOR MESENTERIC ARTERY

ANATOMY AND EXPOSURE

The SMA is the second branch off the abdominal aorta and lies in zone I of the retroperitoneum. Because it is surrounded by critical structures, including the pancreas, duodenum, and portal vein, it is difficult for even the most experienced surgeon to access and control. Fullen et al.[11] eloquently described anatomic zones of the SMA and associated ischemic territories (Fig. 89.5). Zone I is the trunk proximal to the inferior pancreaticoduodenal artery. Zone II is the segment between the inferior pancreaticoduodenal artery and middle colic artery. Zone III is the segment distal to the middle colic artery. Zone IV gives off the segmental branches. The collateral arteries of the SMA are variable, as are their distributions of bowel at risk for ischemia.

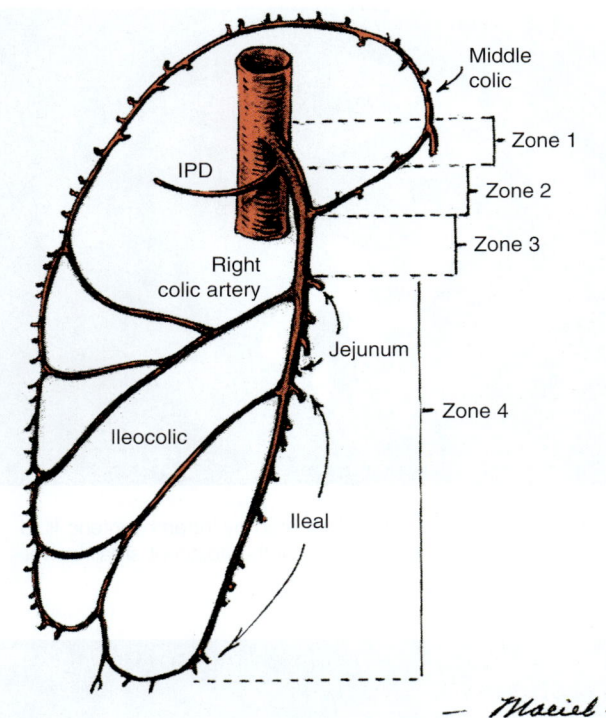

FIGURE 89.5 The Fullen anatomic classification of injuries to the superior mesenteric artery based on the location of the injury in relation to the main arterial branches. *IPD,* Inferior pancreaticoduodenal artery. (From Fullen WD, Hunt J, Altemeier WA. The clinical spectrum of penetrating injury to the superior mesenteric arterial circulation. *J Trauma.* 1972;12:656.)

Exposure of the proximal SMA can be hampered by the dense lymphatics and the adjacent venous plexus, which are often also injured. Dividing the pancreas at its neck or a medial visceral rotation can provide exposure to this difficult area. Mobilizing the left colon, spleen, stomach, tail, and body of the pancreas and the left kidney, commonly known as the Mattox maneuver (Fig. 89.6),[12] provides access to the proximal vessel at its origin from the aorta. To expose injuries in the inframesocolic region, an extended Kocher or Cattell-Braasch maneuver will expose the SMA (Fig. 89.7).[13] The distal SMA and its branches are more accessible and can be approached directly through the mesentery.

INTRAOPERATIVE MANAGEMENT AND REPAIR

Intraoperative techniques are primarily driven by the Fullen zone, American Association for the Surgery of Trauma (AAST)-Organ Injury Scale for abdominal vascular injury, and the patient physiology. Ligation, primary repair, and the use of autogenous vein or prosthetic polytetrafluoroethylene (PTFE) grafts have all been described. It is recommended that zone I and II injuries be repaired, if possible, because of the risk of ischemia. If not completely transected, the artery may be repaired using 5-0 or 6-0 polypropylene suture. In the setting of vasospasm caused by shock and the small size of the vessel, interrupted sutures or a vein patch have been advocated.[14] Ligation of the proximal SMA is usually an act of desperation because of exsanguination but can be effective.[2,14] Reimplantation of the SMA should not be performed at its native location due to its close proximity to the pancreas and risk for pseudoaneurysm. Injuries in the distal zones of the SMA may be ligated, although they may also require a bowel resection.

A damage control approach is advocated when the patient is acidotic, hypothermic, and coagulopathic.

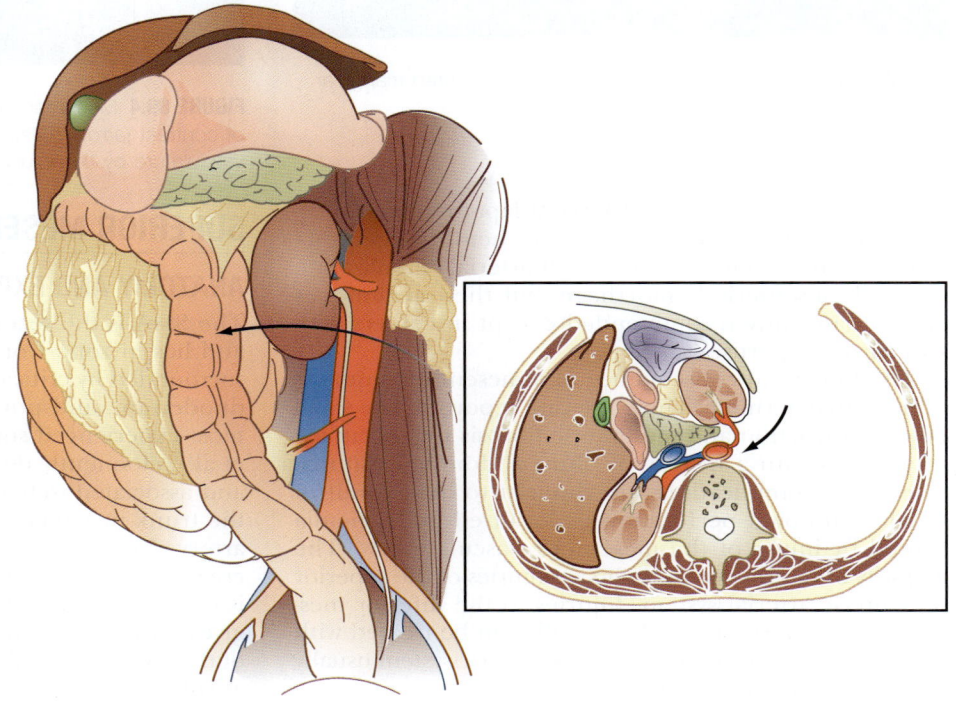

FIGURE 89.6 Left-sided medial visceral rotation (Mattox maneuver). This provides exposure to the proximal trunk of the superior mesenteric artery. (From Hirschberg A, Mattox K. Vascular trauma. In: Townsend CM Jr, Beauchamp RD, Evers BM, et al., eds. *Sabiston Textbook of Surgery.* 18th ed. Philadelphia: Saunders; 2008, Fig. 67.5. Illustration by Jan Redden after Jim Schmidt. Copyright Kenneth L. Mattox, MD.)

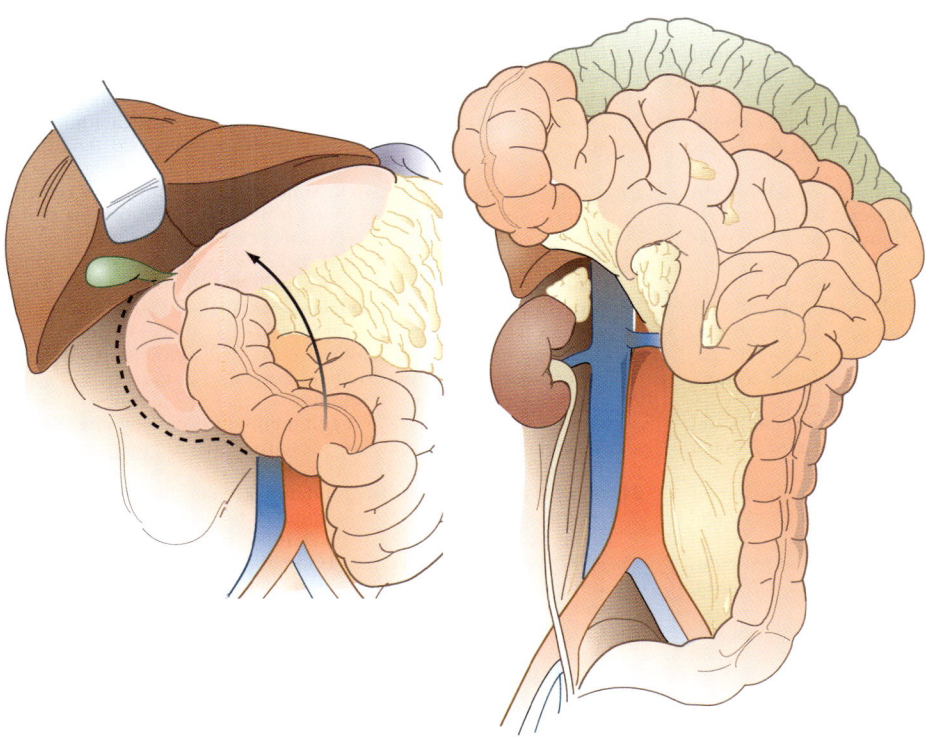

FIGURE 89.7 Extensive retroperitoneal exposure by the Cattell-Braasch maneuver provides access to the root of the mesentery and superior mesenteric artery. (From Hirschberg A, Mattox K. Vascular trauma. In: Townsend CM Jr, Beauchamp RD, Evers BM, et al., eds. *Sabiston Textbook of Surgery*. 18th ed. Philadelphia: Saunders; 2008, Fig. 67.7. Illustration by Jan Redden after Jim Schmidt. Copyright Kenneth L. Mattox, MD.)

Intravascular shunts have been helpful in extremity trauma and may also be an adjunct when dealing with mesenteric arterial injuries. In the damage control setting, systemic anticoagulation is not used. Both the Javid shunt[15] and an 8-French Argyle shunt[16] have been described in the management of SMA injuries. These shunts can be placed in line and secured with rubber vessel loops or silk ties. Patency up to 52 hours in the smaller shunts without anticoagulation has been reported.[17] However, the thrombosis rate of shunts in the SMA is reported to be high.[16] Recent animal data illustrated that SMA shunting was superior to primary anastomosis in the damage control setting.[18] Additional data document 100% patency of SMA shunts for up to 6 hours.[19] This would allow a brief opportunity to reverse physiologic derangements.

OUTCOMES

Injury to the SMA carries a high risk of morbidity and mortality. Overall mortality rates range from 39% to 54%.[1,2,14] Early deaths are a result of exsanguination, whereas late deaths stem from multisystem organ failure and sepsis. Mortality also is increased when concomitant major venous injury is present. Mortality rates can be linked to anatomic Fullen zones. Mortality rates have been demonstrated to be the following: Fullen zone I: 76% to 100%; zone II: 44%; zone III: 25%; and zone IV: 25%.[2,14] Asensio et al. evaluated SMA injuries in isolation and in combination with other intraabdominal vascular injuries. An isolated injury carried a mortality of 47.6%. When in combination with one other abdominal vascular injury, mortality increased to 71.4%. Four or more intraabdominal vascular injuries conferred a mortality of 100%.[1] Other independent predictors of mortality were transfusion of more than 10 units of blood, intraoperative acidosis, dysrhythmias, and multisystem organ failure.[2]

For those patients who survive the initial repair and resuscitation, reperfusion injury to the bowel and ongoing ischemia can present a challenge. A second-look laparotomy is advocated to evaluate the overall perfusion and status of the bowel. Even if the bowel does not appear ischemic, significant reperfusion injury may be present. Experimentally, several agents, including atenolol, L-arginine, simvastatin, intravenous immunoglobulin, and glutamine, help modulate the response in intestinal ischemia–reperfusion models.[20–24] Although none of these are standard yet, they may hold promise.

There are several reports of the development of late pseudoaneurysms and arteriovenous fistulas as a result of both repaired and undiagnosed mesenteric arterial injuries. Fistulas to the superior mesenteric vein[25] and splenic vein[26] have been described. These rare and late sequelae can present as abdominal pain, bruit, or acute heart failure. Gastrointestinal bleeding has also been described secondary to fistulization to the duodenum. The presentation may be 1 week or several years after the original trauma.[26–28] Successful repairs have been reported using both an open approach[28] and endovascular techniques.[25,27–29] Long-term patency after endovascular correction has been reported.[25,30]

REFERENCES

1. Asensio JA, Chahwan S, Hanpeter D, et al. Operative management and outcome of 302 abdominal vascular injuries. *Am J Surg.* 2000;180:528-533; discussion 533–534.
2. Asensio JA, Britt LD, Borzotta A, et al. Multiinstitutional experience with the management of superior mesenteric artery injuries. *J Am Coll Surg.* 2001;193:354-365; discussion 365–366.
3. Yu J, Fulcher AS, Turner MA, Cockrell C, Halvorsen RA. Blunt bowel and mesenteric injury: MDCT diagnosis. *Abdom Imaging.* 2011;36(1):50-61.

4. Atri M, Hanson JM, Grinblat L, Brofman N, Chughtai T, Tomlinson G. Surgically important bowel and/or mesenteric injury in blunt trauma: accuracy of multidetector CT for evaluation. *Radiology.* 2008;249(2):524-533.

5. Stuhlfaut JW, Soto JA, Lucey BC, et al. Blunt abdominal trauma: performance of CT without oral contrast material. *Radiology.* 2004;233(3):689-694.

6. Peters E, LoSasso B, Foley J, Rodarte A, Duthie S, Senac MO Jr. Blunt bowel and mesenteric injuries in children: do nonspecific computed tomography findings reliably identify these injuries? *Pediatr Crit Care Med.* 2006;7(6):551-556.

7. Asayama Y, Matsumoto S, Isoda T, Kunitake N, Nakashima H. A case of traumatic mesenteric bleeding controlled by only transcatheter arterial embolization. *Cardiovasc Intervent Radiol.* 2005;28(2):256-258.

8. Woo K, Margulies DR, Gaon MD, Cunneen SA. Intracorporeal laparoscopic management of mesenteric avulsion in a blunt trauma patient. *J Trauma.* 2009;67(4):E104-E107.

9. Maharaj D, Perry A, Ramdass M, Naraynsingh V. Late small bowel obstruction after blunt abdominal trauma. *Postgrad Med J.* 2003;79(927):57-58.

10. Byard RW, Heath K. Mesenteric fibrosis: a histologic marker of previous blunt abdominal trauma in early childhood. *Int J Legal Med.* 2010;124(1):71-73.

11. Fullen WD, Hunt J, Altemeier WA. The clinical spectrum of penetrating injury to the superior mesenteric arterial circulation. *J Trauma.* 1972;12(8):656-664.

12. Mattox KL, McCollum WB, Beall AC Jr, Jordan GL Jr, Debakey ME. Management of penetrating injuries of the suprarenal aorta. *J Trauma.* 1975;15(9):808-815.

13. Cattell RB, Braasch JW. A technique for the exposure of the third and fourth portions of the duodenum. *Surg Gynecol Obstet.* 1960;111:378-379.

14. Asensio JA, Berne JD, Chahwan S, et al. Traumatic injury to the superior mesenteric artery. *Am J Surg.* 1999;178(3):235-239.

15. Reilly PM, Rotondo MF, Carpenter JP, Sherr SA, Schwab CW. Temporary vascular continuity during damage control: intraluminal shunting for proximal superior mesenteric artery injury. *J Trauma.* 1995;39(4):757-760.

16. Subramanian A, Vercruysse G, Dente C, Wyrzykowski A, King E, Feliciano DV. A decade's experience with temporary intravascular shunts at a civilian level I trauma center. *J Trauma.* 2008;65:316-324; discussion 324–326.

17. Granchi T, Schmittling Z, Vasquez J, Schreiber M, Wall M. Prolonged use of intraluminal arterial shunts without systemic anticoagulation. *Am J Surg.* 2000;180:493-496; discussion 496–497.

18. Ding W, Wu X, Pascual JL, et al. Temporary intravascular shunting improves survival in a hypothermic traumatic shock swine model with superior mesenteric artery injuries. *Surgery.* 2010;147(1):79-88.

19. Ding W, Wu X, Meng Q, et al. Time course study on the use of temporary intravascular shunts as a damage control adjunct in a superior mesenteric artery injury model. *J Trauma.* 2010;68(2):409-414.

20. Taha MO, Miranda-Ferreira R, Simões RS, et al. Intestinal ischemia-reperfusion is attenuated by treatment with atenolol in rabbits. *Transplant Proc.* 2010;42(2):451-453.

21. Taha MO, Miranda-Ferreira R, Paez RP, et al. Role of L-arginine, a substrate of nitric oxide biosynthesis, on intestinal ischemia-reperfusion in rabbits. *Transplant Proc.* 2010;42(2):448-450.

22. Anderson J, Fleming SD, Rehrig S, Tsokos GC, Basta M, Shea-Donohue T. Intravenous immunoglobulin attenuates mesenteric ischemia-reperfusion injury. *Clin Immunol.* 2005;114(2):137-146.

23. Kozar RA, Verner-Cole E, Schultz SG, et al. The immune-enhancing enteral agents arginine and glutamine differentially modulate gut barrier function following mesenteric ischemia/reperfusion. *J Trauma.* 2004;57(6):1150-1156.

24. Slijper N, Sukhotnik I, Chemodanov E, et al. Effect of simvastatin on intestinal recovery following gut ischemia-reperfusion injury in a rat. *Pediatr Surg Int.* 2010;26(1):105-110.

25. Al-Khayat H, Haider HH, Al-Haddad A, Al-Khayat H, Ginzburg E. Endovascular repair of traumatic superior mesenteric artery to splenic vein fistula. *Vasc Endovascular Surg.* 2007;41(6):559-563.

26. Chiriano J, Abou-Zamzam AM Jr, Teruya TH, Ballard JL. Delayed development of a traumatic superior mesenteric arteriovenous fistula following multiple gunshot wounds to the abdomen. *Ann Vasc Surg.* 2005;19(4):470-473.

27. Wu CG, Li YD, Li MH. Post-traumatic superior mesenteric arteriovenous fistula: endovascular treatment with a covered stent. *J Vasc Surg.* 2008;47(3):654-656.

28. Weinstein D, Altshuler A, Belinki A, et al. Superior mesenteric artery to superior mesenteric vein arteriovenous fistula presenting as abdominal pain and gastrointestinal bleeding 3 years after an abdominal gunshot wound: report of a case and review of the literature. *J Trauma.* 2009;66(1):E13-E16.

29. Yeo KK, Dawson DL, Brooks JL, Laird JR. Percutaneous treatment of a large superior mesenteric artery pseudoaneurysm and arteriovenous fistula: a case report. *J Vasc Surg.* 2008;48(3):730-734.

30. Narayanan G, Mohin G, Barbery K, Lamus D, Nanavati K, Yrizarry JM. Endovascular management of superior mesenteric artery pseudoaneurysm and fistula. *Cardiovasc Intervent Radiol.* 2008;31(6):1239-1243.

Index

Page numbers followed by "*f*" indicate figures, "*t*" indicate tables, and "*b*" indicate boxes.

Antimitochondrial antibody (AMA), in primary biliary cholangitis, 1407
Antireflux barrier
lower esophageal sphincter and, 6–7
reestablishment of, in laparoscopic paraesophageal hernia repair, 289
Antireflux mucosectomy, for gastroesophageal reflux disease, 258–259
Antireflux procedures
for GERD, 306
postoperative esophageal imaging in, 73–74, 74f
Antireflux surgery, 48–52
for asthma, 224
barium esophagram before, 51
in Barrett esophagus
decreased risk, 329–330
on metaplasia-dysplasia-neoplasia continuum, 343–344
regression of, 343
subjective and objective outcomes of, 342–343, 342t, 343f
endoscopic evaluation after, 91–92, 92f–93f
endoscopy before, 51–52
gastric emptying studies for, 52
for gastroesophageal reflux disease, 205
impedance manometry before, 51
impedance testing before, 50
laparoscopic Nissen fundoplication in, 234
manometry in, 50–51, 126–127
fundoplication tailoring, 126–127, 127f
pH monitoring before, 48–50, 49f–50f
Anti-*Saccharomyces cerevisiae* antibodies, 866–867
Antisecretory medications, for recurrent ulcer disease, 810
Anti-tumor necrosis factor-α therapies
for Crohn disease, 1903
for ulcerative colitis, 1899–1900
Antral mucosa, 638
Antrectomy
for peptic ulcer disease, 674–675
stomach and duodenum, reoperations on, 810
Antroduodenal manometry, for gastroparesis, 262, 757
Antrum, 446, 755
gastric, 262, 634
Aortic arch, esophageal perforations in, 537t
Aortic bronchus, esophageal perforations in, 537t
Aortobifemoral bypass graft, 1041f
Aortoenteric erosions (AEEs), 1040
Aortoenteric fistulas (AEFs), 903, 1040–1045
causes of, 1040
demographics of, 1040
diagnosis of, 1040–1041
laboratory studies in, 1041
symptoms, 1040–1041
imaging for, 1041–1042, 1042f
incidence of, 1040
pathogenesis of, 1040, 1041f
treatment for, 1042–1045
surgical technique in, 1042–1045
Aortography, for aortoenteric fistulas, 1042
Aortomesenteric endarterectomy, 1037, 1037f
Aperistalsis, 13
Aphthous ulcer, in Crohn disease, 867, 869–870
Appendectomy, 1951

Appendiceal neoplasms, 1956
Appendiceal neuroendocrine tumors, 947
Appendices epiploicae, 1663
Appendicitis
acute, 1951
abdominal exam for, 1951–1952
clinical presentation of, 1951–1952
diagnosis of, 1953
differential diagnosis of, 1953
in infants and toddlers, 1953
interval appendectomy for, 1956
laboratory evaluation for, 1952
laparoscopic appendectomy for, 1953
nonoperative management of, 1954, 1956t
in older adults, 1953
open appendectomy for, 1954, 1955f
pathophysiology of, 1951
pelvic examination for, 1952
during pregnancy, 1953
radiographic evaluation for, 1952, 1952f
signs of, 1951
symptoms of, 1951
treatment of, 1953–1956
gangrenous or perforated, 1954
Appendicular artery, 824f
Appendix, 1665, 1951–1958
Apple peel lesions, 973–974
Appleby procedure, for pancreatic ductal adenocarcinoma, 1202–1203
APR. *see* Abdominoperineal resection
Aquaporins (AQPs), 832, 1677
Arc of Riolan, 1668–1669
ARDS. *see* Acute respiratory distress syndrome
ARE. *see* Acute radiation enteritis
Areolar plane, in laparoscopic paraesophageal hernia repair, 287
Argon plasma coagulation, for Barrett esophagus or dysplasia, 356, 356t
Argyle shunt, for mesenteric arterial trauma, 1058–1059
Arizona-Texas-Oklahoma-Memphis-Arkansas-Consortium (ATOMAC), 1630
ARM. *see* Anorectal manometry
Arterial angiogenesis, in hepatocellular carcinoma, 1543
Arterial cast, of esophageal blood supply, 36f
Arterial circulation, of mesenteric circulation
anatomic variants in, 1018
anatomy of, 1016–1019, 1020f
celiac axis in, 1014, 1016–1018
collateral pathways in, 1018–1019, 1020f
embryology of, 1014, 1015f
hyperemia in, 1021
Arterial emboli, in acute mesenteric ischemia, 1028–1029, 1029f–1031f
Arterial supply
colonic, 1667–1669, 1668f
marginal artery of Drummond (MAoD), 1668
to duodenum, 821f
of extrahepatic biliary tree, anomalies in, 1260
hepatic, 1389–1390
arteries in, 1389–1390
ducts in, 1387f, 1390
Arterial thrombosis, in acute mesenteric ischemia, 1029–1030, 1031f
Arteriovenous fistula, in mesenteric arterial trauma, 1059
Artery, hepatic, anatomy of, 1577, 1577f

Arthritis, in Crohn disease, 866
Artificial anal sphincter, for fecal incontinence, 1729
Artificial liver support system, 1512–1513
As low as reasonably achievable (ALARA) radiation dose, 1627–1628
Ascending colon, 1665, 1666f
Ascites
in Budd-Chiari syndrome, 1520–1521
in hepatocellular carcinoma, 1544
in liver and biliary tract disease, 1412
in portal hypertension, 1580, 1587–1588, 1588f
Asia
Barrett esophagus in people in, 323
prevalence of GERD in, 198–199
Aspartate aminotransferase (AST), 1398
elevated, 1398, 1399t
in pyogenic liver abscess, 1432t
Aspiration
in asthma, 223–224
in chronic cough, 222
in epiphrenic diverticulum, 173
in hepatic cysts, 1420
in polycystic liver disease, 1424
of water-soluble contrast material, 73
Aspirin
for Barrett esophagus, 341
for peptic ulcer disease, 677
AST. *see* Aspartate aminotransferase
Asthma
gastroesophageal reflux disease in, 223–224
in GERD, 47, 47f
Atelectasis, in esophagectomy, 409–410
ATOMAC. *see* Arizona-Texas-Oklahoma-Memphis-Arkansas- Consortium
ATP. *see* Adenosine triphosphate
ATP7B gene, in Wilson disease, 1405
ATP-binding cassette (ABC) transporters, 1261
Atraumatic vascular clamps, 453
Atresia
duodenal, 972–973, 974f–975f
duodenal webs and, 766–767
jejunoileal, 973–978, 975f–977f
Atrial fibrillation, acute mesenteric ischemia and, 1028–1029
Atriocaval shunt, in hepatobiliary trauma, 1452
Attenuation, in ultrasonography, 95
ATZ. *see* Anal transitional zone
Auerbach plexus, 36, 827
Autogenous intestinal reconstruction surgery, for short bowel syndrome, 929
Autoimmune hepatitis, 1404
primary sclerosing cholangitis with, 1380
Autoimmune neutropenia, splenectomy for, 1640
Autoimmune pancreatitis, 1174–1176, 1175f
imaging and radiologic intervention in, 1129–1130
Autoimmune risk factors, associated with chronic pancreatitis, 1087
Autonomic nervous system (ANS)
in control of intestinal motility, 827–828
small intestine and, 823–827
Autosomal dominant polycystic kidney disease (AD-PKD), 1421–1422
Autosomal dominant polycystic liver disease (ADPLD), 1422

F

Factitious hypoglycemia, in insulinoma, 1150
Falciform ligament, 1386–1388
Familial adenomatous polyposis (FAP), 804, 1963–1968
  attenuated, 1968
  chemoprevention for, 1966–1967
  desmoid disease in, 1967–1968, 1967t
  diagnosis of, 1963–1964
  epidemiology and genetics of, 1963, 1964t
  extracolonic manifestations of, 1968
  gastric adenocarcinoma risk and, 712
  initial evaluation and management of, 1964–1965
  MutYH-associated polyposis and, 1968–1969
  NTHL1-associated polyposis and, 1968–1969
  permanent ileostomy in, 991–992
  polymerase proofreading-associated polyposis, 1969
  postoperative surveillance for, 1966
  prophylactic colectomy for, 1965, 1965t
  surgery for, 1965–1966, 1965t–1966t
  upper gastrointestinal tract in, 1968, 1968t
Familial colorectal cancer type X, 1976
Familial GIST syndrome, 957
Family history
  diverticular disease and, 1830
  in increased risk of Barrett esophagus, 328–329
FAP. *see* Familial adenomatous polyposis
Fascia, abdominoperineal resection and, 2036, 2038f
FAST. *see* Focused abdominal sonography for trauma
Fasting motility, 644–645
Fat malabsorption
  in postvagotomy diarrhea, 723
  in radiation enteritis, 915
Fatigue, in Crohn disease, 866
Fats, for short bowel syndrome, 925t
Fat-soluble vitamins, small bowel absorption of, 839, 839t
Fatty acids, 1395
Fatty infiltration, of pancreas, 1127
Fatty liver disease, 1413, 1413b
  liver transplantation in, 1490
Fecal diversion
  for fecal incontinence, 1730
  ileostomy in
    difficult, 995–999, 997f
    diverting loop, 994–995, 996f
    end, 994, 995f
    end-loop, 995, 997f
    laparoscopic loop, 995
  permanent ileostomy in, 992
  preoperative considerations in, 993
  for rectourethral fistula, 1772–1773
Fecal impaction, 1722
Fecal incontinence (FI), 1721–1732
  anal manometry in, 1723–1724
  anorectal physiology testing in, 1723–1725
  biofeedback in, 1726
  causes of, 1721, 1722b
  electromyography in, 1724
  endoanal ultrasound in, 1724, 1725f
  evaluation in, 1721–1725
  fluoroscopic defecography in, 1724
  history of, 1721–1722, 1723f
  magnetic resonance imaging defecography in, 1724

Fecal incontinence (FI) *(Continued)*
  medical therapy for, 1725–1726
  pelvic floor dysfunction and, 1750–1751
  physical examination in, 1722–1723
  pudendal nerve terminal motor latency in, 1724–1725
  surgery for, 1726–1730
    fecal diversion in, 1730
    implantable sphincter in, 1729, 1729f
    injectable biomaterials in, 1727
    rectal prolapse in, 1729
    sacral nerve stimulation in, 1726–1727, 1727f
    sphincter reconstruction in, 1727–1729, 1728f
  treatment of, 1725–1730
    algorithm for, 1730–1731, 1730f
Fecal Incontinence Severity Index (FISI), 1721
Fecal microbiota transplantation, 1900
Fecal stasis, diverticular disease and, 1828
Feeding jejunostomy, in gastric, duodenal, and small intestinal fistulas, 905
FEES. *see* Fiberoptic endoscopic evaluation of swallowing
Feline esophagus, 60, 60f
Felty syndrome, splenectomy for, 1639–1640
Female reproductive health, of ulcerative colitis, 1936
Female sexual function, of ulcerative colitis, 1936
Femoral hernia, 590
  surgical technique in, 603
Fenestration
  laparoscopic, for hepatic cyst, 1421
  for neoplastic cysts, 1426–1427
  for polycystic liver disease, 1424
FENIX magnetic sphincter, 1729, 1729f
Fentanyl, in colonoscopy, 1690
Ferguson closed hemorrhoidectomy, 1853, 1855f
Fetal circulation, congenital diaphragmatic hernia and, 561–562
Fetal endoscopic tracheal occlusion (FETO), 568
Fetal therapy, for congenital diaphragmatic hernia, 568
FETO. *see* Fetal endoscopic tracheal occlusion
α-Fetoprotein (AFP), in hepatocellular carcinoma, 1544
Fever
  in Crohn disease, 866
  open cholecystectomy and, 1352
  in pyogenic liver abscess, 1431, 1432t
2-[^{18}F]-fluoro-2-deoxyglucose-PET/CT (FDG-PET/CT) scans, for esophageal cancer, 374–375, 374f
FI. *see* Fecal incontinence
Fiberoptic endoscopic evaluation of swallowing (FEES), 159
Fiberoptic endoscopic treatment, 167–168
Fiberoptic lighted deep pelvic retractor, 2042
Fibrin glue, 1011
  for anorectal fistulas, 1882
  for rectovaginal fistula, 1765
Fibroblast growth factor, 1067–1068
Fibroma
  esophageal, 108–109
  gallbladder, 1323
Fibromuscular dysplasia, 1033
Fibrosarcoma, hepatic, 1561

Fibrosis
  congenital hepatic, portal hypertension in, 1579
  in radiation enteritis, 914
Fibrovascular polyps, 108, 510–512, 510f–511f
  esophageal, 70, 71f
Fine-needle aspiration
  for acute pancreatitis, 1079
  endoscopic ultrasound-guided, 1314
  for pancreatic cysts, 1316
Fine-needle biopsy, endoscopic ultrasound-guided, 1314
Finney pyloroplasty, for peptic ulcer disease, 680, 680f–681f
Finney strictureplasty, 874–876, 876f
  for Crohn disease, 1943
FIP. *see* Focal intestinal perforation
FISH. *see* Fluorescence in situ hybridization
FISI. *see* Fecal Incontinence Severity Index
Fissurectomy, in anal fissure, 1868–1869
  with Botox, 1867
Fissure-in-ano, 1864–1870
  acute and chronic, 1865f
  algorithm for treatment of, 1869, 1869f
  diagnosis of, 1864–1865, 1865f
  etiology of, 1864, 1865f
  nonsurgical management of, 1866–1867
    Botox for, 1866–1867
    calcium channel blockers for, 1866
    conservative, 1866
    nitroglycerin for, 1866
  surgical therapy for, 1867–1869, 1867f–1868f, 1868t
Fistula plug, for anorectal fistulas, 1882
Fistula Tract-Jejunostomy, 1107–1108, 1109f
Fistula-in-ano, anal
  history of, 1873
  management of, 1880t
Fistulas, 1871
  aortoenteric, 1040–1045
    causes of, 1040
    demographics of, 1040
    diagnosis of, 1040–1041
    imaging for, 1041–1042, 1042f
    incidence of, 1040
    pathogenesis of, 1040, 1041f
    treatment for, 1042–1045
  biliary, after hepatic resection, 2087
  complications in, 1883
  definition of, 1241
  diagnosis of, 1871–1877
  emerging technologies for fistula repair, 1883–1884
  enterocutaneous, in Crohn disease, 880
  etiology of, 1871
  formation, in Crohn disease, 866
  gastric, duodenal, small intestinal and, 886–907
    complications of, 889–890
    control of sepsis (and control of fistula effluent) in, 892–894, 893f–894f
    decision in, 896–898
    definitive operative therapy in, 898–905
    diagnosis of perforations and, 888–889
    enterocutaneous fistula and, 899–901, 900f
    enteroenteric fistula and, 901, 901f
    enterovaginal fistula and, 902–903
    enterovesical fistula and, 901–902, 902f
    etiology of, 888
    gastric and duodenal perforations and fistulas and, 898–899

Liver operation *(Continued)*
　left, with hilar dissection, 1463–1464, 1465*f*
　left lateral sectionectomy in, 1465
　right, with hilar dissection, 1463, 1464*f*
　transecting the hepatic parenchyma in, 1462–1463
Liver resection, for extrahepatic disease, 1568
Liver support systems, 1511–1514, 1511*f*
Liver surgery
　anatomic approach to, 1386, 1389*f*
　Couinaud anatomic approaches to, 1387*f*–1388*f*, 1392–1394
　　left hemiliver (segments II, III, IV) in, 1392
　　left lobe (segments II, III) in, 1392
　　posterior liver (dorsal liver, sector I) in, 1392
　　right hemiliver (segments V, VI, VII, and VIII) in, 1393–1394, 1393*f*
　　right lateral sector (segments VI and VII) in, 1394
　　right paramedian sector (segments V and VIII) in, 1394
　　segment IV in, 1392–1393
　　segment V and VI in, 1394
　　segment VII in, 1394
　　segment VIII in, 1394
　hepatic resections in, Couinaud anatomic approaches to, 1387*f*–1388*f*, 1392–1394
　laparoscopic, 1472, 1473*t*
　　clinical benefits of, 1475–1476
　　economic aspects of, 1477–1478
　　indications for, 1472–1473, 1473*t*
　　left hepatectomy in, 1475
　　oncologic outcomes for, 1476–1477, 1476*t*
　　right hepatectomy in, 1474–1475
　　technical approaches to, 1473–1475, 1473*t*, 1474*f*
Liver transplantation, 1488
　for biliary atresia, 1365
　for Budd-Chiari syndrome, 1521
　for hepatic adenoma, 1538
　hepatic artery thrombosis after, 1518, 1519*f*
　for hepatocellular carcinoma, 1550, 1552*f*
　for intrahepatic cholangiocarcinoma, 1559
　for polycystic liver disease, 1424–1425
　pseudoaneurysm of hepatic artery after, 1517
　splenic artery rupture following, 1046
Living-donor liver transplantation (LDLT), 1499–1500, 1551
Living-donor pancreas transplantation, 1229
Lloyd-Davies position, in abdominoperineal excision, 1988–1989
Lobe of Spieghel, 1392
Localized colon cancer, operative treatment for, 1982–1984
　anastomotic techniques for, 1984
　colectomy in, 1982, 1983*f*
　minimally invasive approaches for, 1982–1984
Localized rectal cancer, operative treatment for, 1984–1990
　abdominoperineal excision for, 1988–1989, 1988*f*–1989*f*
　local excision in, 1990

Localized rectal cancer, operative treatment for *(Continued)*
　minimally invasive approaches for, 1989–1990
　sphincter-saving procedures for, 1986–1988, 1987*f*
　total mesorectal excision for, 1986
Locoregional esophageal cancer, extent of resection of, 405–406, 406*t*
Locoregional recurrence, of recurrent and metastatic colorectal cancer, 2061–2068
Lone Star retractor, 2011
Long segment Barrett esophagus, 87*f*–88*f*, 88, 316
Longitudinal intestinal lengthening and tailoring (LILT), for short bowel syndrome, 930–931, 932*f*–933*f*
Loop end stoma, 2150, 2150*f*
Loop gastrojejunostomy, 715
Loop ileostomy, 2150, 2151*f*
Loop sigmoid colostomy, 2150–2151
Loop stoma, 2150–2152
Loperamide, for decreasing gastrointestinal fistula output, 895
Los Angeles classification
　of esophagitis, 51–52, 51*t*
　of reflux esophagitis, 90–91, 91*f*–92*f*, 91*t*
Low anterior resection, for rectal cancer
　complications of, 2028–2029
　functional outcomes in, 2029–2030
　hand-assisted, 2009–2011
　laparoscopic, 2009–2011, 2009*f*–2010*f*, 2012*t*, 2016*t*, 2018*t*
　oncologic outcomes in, 2029
　open, 2008–2009, 2012*t*
　robotic-assisted, 2011–2020, 2014*f*, 2016*t*, 2018*t*
　single port, 2009–2011
Lower esophageal sphincter (LES), 4–7, 18–22, 19*f*, 159, 206*f*–207*f*, 212*f*
　abdominal esophagus and, 41–42, 41*f*–42*f*
　abdominal segment of, loss of pressure in, 19*f*
　achalasia and, 8–9, 184–185
　antireflux barrier and, 6–7
　botulinum toxin in achalasia and, 123
　damage of
　　GERD in, 15
　　histologic measurement of, 22–27
　　mechanism of, 21–22, 22*t*
　　pathologic test of, 27–28
　　preventing, 29
　　progression of, prediction of, 28
　dynamic failure of, 208
　functional characteristics of, 6–7
　gastroesophageal junction and, 5, 5*f*
　in gastroesophageal reflux disease, 7–8, 253
　gastroesophageal reflux disease and, 248
　hypertensive, 9
　manometry for, 18–21, 19*f*, 20*t*
　permanent failure of, 208–209
　pH electrode placement and, 132
　phase of compensated, 20
　physiologic function and anatomic structure of, 4–6
　process of, 208*f*
　radiofrequency ablation on, 256
　relationship between length and failure, 22
　retroflex endoscopic image of, 214*f*
　schema of components of, 208*f*
　shortening of, 6–7, 7*f*

Lower esophageal sphincter (LES) *(Continued)*
　tone, gastroesophageal reflux disease and, 224
　transient failure of, 209
Lower gastrointestinal bleeding, 1814
　diagnosis of, 1815–1817, 1815*f*
　in diverticulosis, 1814
　etiology of, 1814–1815
　in neoplasia, 1814
　in scant intermittent hematochezia, 1816
　in severe hematochezia, 1816–1817, 1816*f*
　in vascular ectasias, 1814–1815, 1815*b*
Lower thoracic esophagus, 34, 37*f*
　anatomy of, 368
Lower-sphincter relaxing medications, 365
Low-grade dysplasia (LGD)
　in Barrett esophagus, 341*b*, 344–346
　confirmed, 351
　dysplasia and, 332
　intramucosal adenocarcinoma and, 350
　neoplastic progression of Barrett esophagus, 330
　"overdiagnosis" of, 350–351
LPR. *see* Laryngopharyngeal reflux
LS. *see* Laparoscopic splenectomy
Lubricants, for constipation, 1733–1734, 1735*b*
Lugano system, for staging of gastrointestinal lymphomas, 963–964, 963*t*
Lumbar hernia, 606–620
　anatomy and classification of, 606–607, 607*f*–608*f*
　clinical presentation and diagnosis of, 607–609, 608*f*
　treatment of, 609–611, 609*f*–610*f*
Lumbar lymphatic trunks, right and left, 826*f*
Lung
　colorectal cancer metastasis to, 2071
　development of, congenital diaphragmatic hernia and, 561
Lung transplantation
　gastroesophageal reflux disease and, 225–226
　preoperative testing for, 52–53
Lung-to-head ratio (LHR), congenital diaphragmatic hernia and, 563
LVI. *see* Lymphovascular invasion
Lymph, from esophagus, 38, 39*f*
Lymph node
　dissection
　　abdominal, 431–432
　　thoracic, 432
　hepatic, 1255
　metastases, distribution of, 434*f*–435*f*
　tiers, 431, 432*f*
Lymphadenectomy
　for gallbladder cancer, 1326, 1326*f*
　for gastric adenocarcinoma, 715–716, 716*f*, 716*t*
　for gastrointestinal tumors, 507
　implications of, 433–436
　morbidity of, 436
　three-field, 435–436
　total mediastinal, 432
Lymphatic drainage
　of biliary tract, 1255
　of colon, 1669, 1670*f*–1671*f*
　concept of, 39*f*
　of esophageal wall, 38*f*
　of gallbladder, 1324

Patient positioning
  for abdominoperineal resection, 2044, 2044f
  for laparoscopic liver resection, 1473
  for laparoscopic Nissen fundoplication, 236–238, 237f–238f
  for laparoscopic splenectomy, 1598, 1599f
  for reoperative pelvic surgery, 2173–2174, 2174f
  for transanal endoscopic microsurgery for early rectal cancer, 1999
Patient preparation
  for conventional transanal excision for early rectal cancer, 1997
  for reoperative pelvic surgery, 2173
  for transanal endoscopic microsurgery for early rectal cancer, 1997
Patient survival
  in pancreas transplantation, 1231
  in pancreatic islet allotransplantation, 1235–1236
PD. see Pilonidal disease
PDACs. see Pancreatic ductal adenocarcinomas
PDGFRA mutation, in gastrointestinal stromal tumor, 952
Pearson, Griffith, 284
Pectin, for radiation enteritis, 916
Pectineal (Cooper) ligament, in preperitoneal space, 590
Pediatric End-Stage Liver Disease, 1496, 1496t
PEG. see Percutaneous endoscopic gastrostomy
PEH. see Paraesophageal hernia
Peliosis, 1538
  of spleen, 1643
Pelvic arterial blood supply, abdominoperineal resection and, 2036–2037
Pelvic dissection, reoperative, 2174
Pelvic floor dysfunction, 1750–1760
  biofeedback in, 1745t
  evaluations of, 1752–1758
    anorectal manometry (ARM), 1752–1753, 1753f
    defecography, 1755, 1756f
    dynamic magnetic resonance imaging, 1756–1758, 1758f
    endoanal ultrasound, 1754–1755, 1754f–1755f
    magnetic resonance imaging, 1756, 1757f
    neurophysiologic assessment, 1753, 1754f
    pudendal nerve motor terminal latency (PNMTL), 1753–1754
    scintigraphy, 1758
    transit studies, 1758
  history of, 1750–1752, 1751b
  management of, 1758
  physical examination for, 1752, 1752b
Pelvic floor musculature, abdominoperineal resection and, 2036, 2039f
Pelvic floor retraining, in constipation, 1745–1746
Pelvic hernia, 606–620
Pelvic nerves, abdominoperineal resection and, 2037, 2040f
Pelvic organ prolapse, 1858–1860
Pelvic outlet obstruction, 1740–1742, 1741f–1742f
Pelvic plexus, 2006

Pelvic reoperative surgery, 2172–2184
  abdominal entry in, 2174–2175
  adhesiolysis in, 2174–2175
  anatomy in, 2172–2173
  bleeding in, 2176–2177
  drains in, 2177
  equipment for, 2173–2174, 2174f
  identification of pelvic structures in, 2175
  patient positioning for, 2173–2174, 2174f
  pitfalls in, 2172–2173
  preparation for, 2173
  for recurrent rectal cancer, 2181–2183, 2182f–2183f
  in reversal of Hartmann procedure, 2177–2178, 2178f
  surgical technique of, 2173–2175
  timing of, 2173
Pelvic sepsis
  in pouch-specific postoperative complications, 1930
  risk factors for development of, 1931
Pelvis
  reoperative
    anatomy of, 2172–2173
    pitfalls of, 2172–2173
  retrorectal tumor and, 2103
    algorithm for, 2114, 2115f
    anatomy in, 2103, 2104f–2106f
    classification of, 2103, 2107b
    enterogenous cysts, 2108
    epidermoid and dermoid cysts, 2108
    history and physical examination in, 2103–2104
    imaging, 2106
    miscellaneous lesions in, 2112
    neurogenic tumors, 2109, 2110f
    osseous lesions in, 2112
    preoperative biopsy in, 2106–2108, 2107f–2108f
    sacrococcygeal chordomas, 2109–2111
    surgical intervention and approach, 2112–2114
    tailgut cysts, 2108–2109
    teratoma and teratocarcinoma in, 2111–2112, 2111f
PEM. see Phrenoesophageal membrane
Penetrating trauma, to mesenteric arteries, 1056
Penetration-Aspiration Scale, 158
Pentalogy of Cantrell, diaphragmatic hernia and, 562
Pepsinogen, 640–641
Peptic ulcer disease, 649–650
  complicated, 693–698
    bleeding in, 693–695, 694t
    perforation in, 695–698
  drainage procedures for, 679–682, 680f
    Finney pyloroplasty, 680, 681f
    gastrojejunostomy, 681–682
    Heineke-Mikulicz pyloroplasty, 680, 681f
    Jaboulay gastroduodenostomy, 680–681, 682f
  gastric resection procedures for, 682–687, 683f
  pathophysiology of, 675–677
    acid hypersecretory states and, 677
    aspirin and, 677
    classification of gastric and duodenal ulcers, 676b
    Helicobacter pylori and, 676–677
    nonsteroidal antiinflammatory drugs and, 677
    stress ulcer and, 677, 677b

Peptic ulcer disease (Continued)
  recurrent, 690
  surgical treatment of
    history of, 673–675
    indications for, 677–678
  vagotomy for, 678–679
    proximal gastric, 675, 675f, 679
    selective, 675, 675f, 679
    supradiaphragmatic, 679
    truncal, 675f, 678–679
Peptide YY, 828, 832t
Percutaneous balloon dilation, for bile duct injury, 1350
Percutaneous biopsy
  for hemangioma, 1533–1534
  in pancreatic and periampullary cancer, 1140
Percutaneous catheter drainage, for acute pancreatitis, 1080–1081, 1081f
Percutaneous dilation, in bile duct stricture, 1359
Percutaneous drainage
  for hepatobiliary trauma, 1453
  for infected pancreatic necrosis, 1114–1115
  for pseudocysts, 1100–1101
Percutaneous endoscopic gastrostomy (PEG), 160
  in intubation of stomach and small intestine, 667–669, 669f
  perforation and, 887
Percutaneous ethanol injection
  in hepatic neoplasms, 1485
  in hepatocellular carcinoma, 1548
Percutaneous interventions, for echinococcal cysts, 1426
Percutaneous laparoscopic aspiration, in splenic cyst, 1659
Percutaneous liver biopsy, 1456
Percutaneous or transperitoneal biopsy, in PSC, 1383
Percutaneous therapy, for pancreatic pseudocyst, 1115–1117
Percutaneous transarterial catheter embolization, in hepatic artery aneurysm, 1517, 1518f
Percutaneous transcatheter hepatic artery embolization, for polycystic liver disease, 1424
Percutaneous transhepatic biliary drainage, technique of, 1270–1271
Percutaneous transhepatic cholangiography (PTC)
  for bile duct, 1353
  for bile duct injury, 1344–1345, 1345f
  for periampullary cancer, 1139–1140
  for PSC, 1379
  technique of, 1270–1271
Perforating zone, of gastroesophageal junction, 1577, 1577f
Perforation
  of bile ducts, congenital biliary dilatation and, 1371, 1372f
  causing small intestinal fistula formation, 888
  as colonoscopy complication, 1694
  in complicated peptic ulcer disease, 695–698
  in Crohn disease, 879–880
  in duodenal diverticula, 909
  in endoscopic pseudocyst drainage, 1118
  endoscopic ultrasound and, 1318

Z

ZAP classification, for squamocolumnar junction, 88–89

Zenker diverticulum, 81, 82*f*, 162–171
contractility studies in, 164, 164*f*
cricopharyngeal dysfunction and, 157–172
oropharyngeal dysphagia, assessment of, 157–159
treatment of, 160–162, 166*f*
results and discussion, 168–171, 168*t*, 169*f*, 170*t*–171*t*
symptoms and diagnosis of, 164–165, 165*t*, 166*f*

Z-line, of esophagus, 86*f*, 87–88, 88*f*
classification for evaluation of, 88–89

Zollinger-Ellison syndrome, 702–711
anatomy, pathophysiology, and molecular biology of, 702
corticotropin-producing tumor in, 1154–1155
cytotoxic chemotherapy for, 709
diagnosis and medical therapy for, 703–704
gastrointestinal hormones in, 704–705
GRFoma in, 1154
intraoperative imaging of, 706, 707*f*

Zollinger-Ellison syndrome (*Continued*)
metastatic disease in, 708–709
multiple endocrine neoplasia type 1 in, 705, 1152–1153
neuroendocrine tumors, 1571
peptic ulcer disease and, 677
prognosis in, 709
surgical therapy for, 706–708
surveillance in, 709
symptoms and signs of, 703
targeted therapy for, 709
tumor localization in, 705–706, 705*f*–706*f*

Zymogen granule, 1065

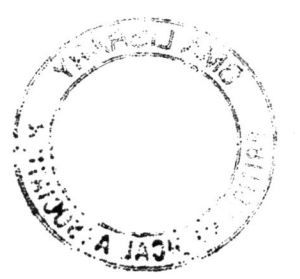

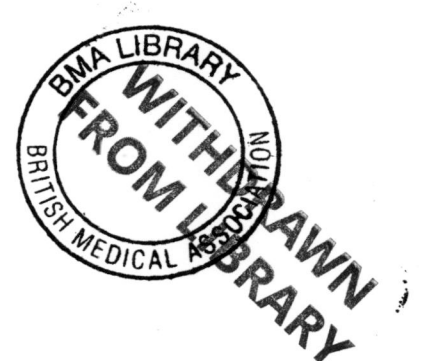

BMA LIBRARY
BRITISH MEDICAL ASSOCIATION

WITHDRAWN
FROM LIBRARY

765954

WITHDRAWN
FROM LIBRARY
BMA LIBRARY
BRITISH MEDICAL ASSOCIATION

WITH
FROM

BRITISH MEDICAL ASSOCIATION

1003511

Y

Shackelford's

SURGERY *of the* ALIMENTARY TRACT

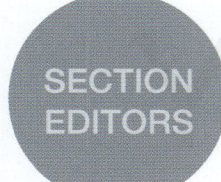

SECTION EDITORS

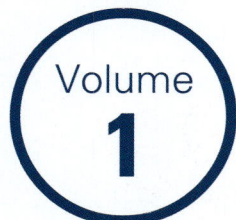

Volume 1

Volume 2

Steven R. DeMeester, MD, FACS

Division of Foregut and Minimally Invasive Surgery
The Oregon Clinic
Portland, Oregon

Section I **Esophagus and Hernia**

David W. McFadden, MD, MBA, FACS

Chairman, Department of Surgery
University of Connecticut
Surgeon-in-Chief
University of Connecticut Health
Farmington, Connecticut

Section II **Stomach and Small Intestine**

Jeffrey B. Matthews, MD, FACS

Dallas B. Phemister Professor and Chairman of Surgery
The University of Chicago
Chicago, Illinois

Section III **Pancreas, Biliary Tract, Liver, and Spleen**

James W. Fleshman, MD, FACS

Seeger Professor and Chairman of Surgery
Baylor University Medical Center
Professor of Surgery
Texas A&M Health Science Center
Dallas, Texas

Section IV **Colon, Rectum, and Anus**

EIGHTH EDITION

Shackelford's SURGERY *of the* ALIMENTARY TRACT

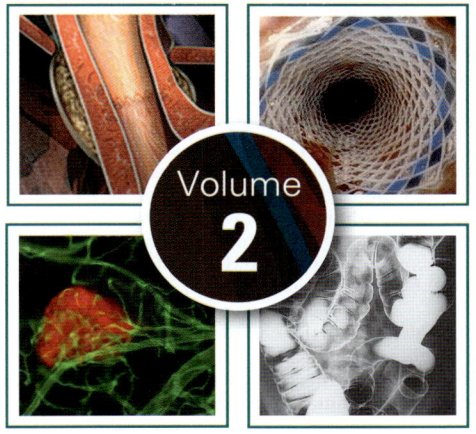

Volume 2

Charles J. Yeo, MD, FACS

Samuel D. Gross Professor and Chair

Department of Surgery

Sidney Kimmel Medical College at Thomas Jefferson University

Philadelphia, Pennsylvania

ELSEVIER

ELSEVIER

1600 John F. Kennedy Blvd.
Ste 1800
Philadelphia, PA 19103-2899

SHACKELFORD'S SURGERY OF THE ALIMENTARY
TRACT, EIGHTH EDITION

ISBN: 978-0-323-40232-3
Volume 1 part number: 9996118169
Volume 2 part number: 9996118223

Copyright © 2019 by Elsevier, Inc. All rights reserved.

No part of this publication may be reproduced or transmitted in any form or by any means, electronic or mechanical, including photocopying, recording, or any information storage and retrieval system, without permission in writing from the publisher. Details on how to seek permission, further information about the Publisher's permissions policies and our arrangements with organizations such as the Copyright Clearance Center and the Copyright Licensing Agency, can be found at our website: www.elsevier.com/permissions.

This book and the individual contributions contained in it are protected under copyright by the Publisher (other than as may be noted herein).

Notices

Knowledge and best practice in this field are constantly changing. As new research and experience broaden our understanding, changes in research methods, professional practices, or medical treatment may become necessary.

Practitioners and researchers must always rely on their own experience and knowledge in evaluating and using any information, methods, compounds, or experiments described herein. In using such information or methods they should be mindful of their own safety and the safety of others, including parties for whom they have a professional responsibility.

With respect to any drug or pharmaceutical products identified, readers are advised to check the most current information provided (i) on procedures featured or (ii) by the manufacturer of each product to be administered, to verify the recommended dose or formula, the method and duration of administration, and contraindications. It is the responsibility of practitioners, relying on their own experience and knowledge of their patients, to make diagnoses, to determine dosages and the best treatment for each individual patient, and to take all appropriate safety precautions.

To the fullest extent of the law, neither the Publisher nor the authors, contributors, or editors, assume any liability for any injury and/or damage to persons or property as a matter of products liability, negligence or otherwise, or from any use or operation of any methods, products, instructions, or ideas contained in the material herein.

Previous editions copyrighted 2013, 2007, 2002, 1996, 1991, 1986, 1983, 1982, 1981, 1978, 1955.
Mayo Foundation retains copyright to their original artwork.

Library of Congress Cataloging-in-Publication Data

Names: Yeo, Charles J., editor.
Title: Shackelford's surgery of the alimentary tract / [edited by] Charles J. Yeo.
Other titles: Surgery of the alimentary tract
Description: Eighth edition. | Philadelphia, PA : Elsevier, [2019] | Includes bibliographical references and index.
Identifiers: LCCN 2017042680 | ISBN 9780323402323 (hardcover : alk. paper)
Subjects: | MESH: Digestive System Surgical Procedures–methods | Digestive System Diseases–surgery
Classification: LCC RD540 | NLM WI 900 | DDC 617.4/3–dc23 LC record available at
https://lccn.loc.gov/2017042680

Executive Content Strategist: Russell Gabbedy
Content Development Specialist: Mary Hegeler
Publishing Services Manager: Patricia Tannian
Senior Project Manager: Amanda Mincher
Design Direction: Patrick Ferguson

Printed in China

Last digit is the print number: 9 8 7 6 5 4 3 2 1

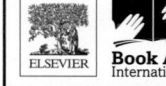 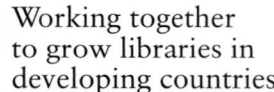

Working together
to grow libraries in
developing countries

www.elsevier.com • www.bookaid.org

To my wife, Theresa, and my children, William and Scott; to my many mentors (some now deceased, many still alive) who have contributed to the science of surgery and to my education; to the many colleagues and friends whose contributions have made this eighth edition possible; and to those young alimentary tract surgeons and other health care professionals who will learn from these pages, move the field forward, and continue to improve our understanding of alimentary tract diseases.

CHARLES J. YEO

To my father, Tom DeMeester, whose passion for understanding the pathophysiology of esophageal and foregut disorders and applying this knowledge to better the lives of patients has been and remains an inspiration for me; to my many mentors who have helped me learn the craft of surgery and encouraged me to constantly strive for perfection; to my colleagues who give up many hours of their evenings, weekends, and vacations to contribute to abstracts, papers, and book chapters; to my fellows and residents who diligently train to be the next generation of expert surgeons; and to my family and friends who support me and graciously accept my long hours away at work caring for people in need of help.

STEVEN R. DeMEESTER

I would like to dedicate this book to all the past residents and fellows with whom I have worked and to thank them for making education such a wonderful part of my life; I hope this will help us to remember the times we've spent together taking care of complex patients and will encourage you to continue to pass on your knowledge to those whom you mentor.

JAMES W. FLESHMAN

To Dr. William Silen and my late grandfather, Dr. Benjamin M. Banks, for their wisdom; to the surgical residents and students, for their thirst for knowledge; and to my wife, Joan, and our boys, Jonathan, David, and Adam, for their love and support.

JEFFREY B. MATTHEWS

To my wife, Nancy, and my children, William, Hunter, and Nora; and to all of my mentors, colleagues, and patients who challenge and inspire me every day.

DAVID W. McFADDEN

Contributors

Abbas E. Abbas, MD, MS, FACS
Professor and Chief, Division of Thoracic Surgery, Department of Thoracic Medicine and Surgery; Director, Thoracic and Foregut Surgery, Temple University School of Medicine, Philadelphia, Pennsylvania

David B. Adams, MD
Professor of Surgery, Medical University of South Carolina, Charleston, South Carolina

Piyush Aggarwal, MBBS
Fellow, Division of Colorectal Surgery, Mayo Clinic, Phoenix, Arizona

Bestoun H. Ahmed, MD, FRCS, FACS, FASMBS
Associate Professor of Surgery, University of Pittsburgh School of Medicine, Pittsburgh, Pennsylvania

Craig Albanese, MD, MBA
Division of Pediatric Surgery, Department of Surgery, Stanford University School of Medicine, Stanford, California

Matthew R. Albert, MD, FACS, FASCRS
Program Director, Florida Hospital Colorectal Fellowship, Department of Colon and Rectal Surgery, Center for Colon and Rectal Surgery, Florida Hospital, Orlando, Florida

Abubaker Ali, MD
Assistant Professor of Surgery, Wayne State University, Detroit, Michigan

Evan Alicuben, MD
General Surgery Resident, Keck School of Medicine of the University of Southern California, Los Angeles, California

Marco E. Allaix, MD, PhD
Department of Surgical Sciences, University of Torino, Torino, Italy

Ashley Altman, MD
Department of Radiology, The University of Chicago Medicine, Chicago, Illinois

Hisami Ando, MD
President, Aichi Prefectural Colony; Emeritus Professor, Department of Pediatric Surgery, Nagoya University Graduate School of Medicine, Nagoya-city, Aichi, Japan

Ciro Andolfi, MD
Department of Surgery, The University of Chicago Pritzker School of Medicine, Chicago, Illinois

Alagappan Annamalai, MD
Surgery, Cedars-Sinai Medical Center, Los Angeles, California

Elliot A. Asare, MD, MS
Chief Resident, General Surgery, Department of Surgery, Medical College of Wisconsin, Milwaukee, Wisconsin

Emanuele Asti, MD, FACS
Assistant Professor, General and Emergency Surgery, IRCCS Policlinico San Donato, University of Milano, Milan, Italy

Hugh G. Auchincloss, MD, MPH
Cardiothoracic Fellow, Massachusetts General Hospital, Boston, Massachusetts

Benjamin Babic, MD
Department of Surgery, Agaplesion Markus Hospital, Frankfurt, Germany

Talia B. Baker, MD
Associate Professor of Surgery, Transplantation Institute, The University of Chicago Medicine, Chicago, Illinois

Chad G. Ball, MD, MSC, FRCSC, FACS
Associate Professor of Surgery, University of Calgary, Foothills Medical Center, Calgary, Alberta, Canada

Arianna Barbetta, MD
Research Fellow, General Surgery Department, Thoracic Surgery Service, Memorial Sloan Kettering Cancer Center, New York, New York

John M. Barlow, MD
Assistant Professor, Department of Radiology, Mayo Clinic College of Medicine, Rochester, Minnesota

Justin Barr, MD, PhD
Department of Surgery, Duke University Medical Center, Durham, North Carolina

Juan Camilo Barreto, MD
Assistant Professor of Surgery, Division of Surgical Oncology, University of Arkansas for Medical Sciences, Little Rock, Arkansas

Linda Barry, MD, FACS
Associate Professor of Surgery, University of Connecticut School of Medicine; Chief Operating Officer, Connecticut Institute for Clinical and Translational Science, Farmington, Connecticut

Eliza W. Beal, MD
Department of Surgery, The Ohio State University Wexner Medical Center, Columbus, Ohio

Kristin Wilson Beard, MD
Baylor Scott and White Medical Center, Round Rock, Texas

David E. Beck, MD, FACS, FASCRS
Professor and Chair, Department of Colon and Rectal Surgery, Ochsner Clinic Foundation, New Orleans, Louisiana; Professor of Surgery, Ochsner Clinical School, University of Queensland, Brisbane, Queensland, Australia

Kevin E. Behrns, MD
Dean, School of Medicine, VP for Medical Affairs, St. Louis University, St. Louis, Missouri

Oliver C. Bellevue, MD
General Surgery Resident, Department of Surgery, Swedish Medical Center, Seattle, Washington

Omar E. Bellorin-Marin, MD
Chief Resident, General Surgery, NewYork-Presbyterian/ Queens, Flushing, New York

Jacques Bergman, MD, PhD
Professor of Gastrointestinal Endoscopy, Department of Gastroenterology and Hepatology, Academic Medical Center, Amsterdam, The Netherlands

James Berry, MD
Department of Surgery, University of Connecticut Health Center, Farmington, Connecticut

Marc G.H. Besselink, MD, MSc, PhD
Department of Surgery, Academic Medical Center, Amsterdam, The Netherlands

Adil E. Bharucha, MBBS, MD
Professor of Medicine, Division of Gastroenterology and Hepatology, Mayo Clinic, Rochester, Minnesota

Anton J. Bilchik, MD, PhD
Professor of Surgery, Chief of Medicine, Chief of Gastrointestinal Research, Gastrointestinal Oncology, John Wayne Cancer Institute at Providence Saint John's Health Center, Santa Monica, California

Nikolai A. Bildzukewicz, MD, FACS
Assistant Professor of Clinical Surgery, Division of Upper GI and General Surgery, Associate Program Director, General Surgery Residency and Advanced GI/MIS Fellowship, Keck School of Medicine of the University of Southern California, Los Angeles, California

Jason Bingham, MD
Department of General Surgery, Madigan Army Medical Center, Tacoma, Washington

Elisa Birnbaum, MD
Professor of Surgery, Section of Colon and Rectal Surgery, Washington University School of Medicine, St. Louis, Missouri

Sylvester M. Black, MD, PhD
Assistant Professor of Surgery, Division of Transplant, The Ohio State University Wexner Medical Center, Columbus, Ohio

Shanda H. Blackmon, MD, MPH
Associate Professor of Surgery, Division of Thoracic Surgery, Mayo Clinic, Rochester, Minnesota

Joshua I.S. Bleier, MD
Associate Professor of Surgery, University of Pennsylvania, Philadelphia, Pennsylvania

Adam S. Bodzin, MD
Assistant Professor, Department of Surgery, Section of Transplantation, The University of Chicago, Chicago, Illinois

C. Richard Boland, MD
Chief, Division of Gastroenterology, Internal Medicine, Baylor Scott and White, La Jolla, California

John Bolton, MD
Chairman Emeritus, Department of Surgery, Ochsner Health Systems, New Orleans, Louisiana

Nathan Bolton, MD
Resident, General Surgery, Ochsner Medical Center, New Orleans, Louisiana

Luigi Bonavina, MD, PhD
Professor and Chief of General Surgery, Department of Biomedical Sciences for Health, IRCCS Policlinico San Donato, University of Milano, Milan, Italy

Morgan Bonds, MD
Surgical Resident, University of Oklahoma Health Science Center, Oklahoma City, Oklahoma

Stefan A.W. Bouwense, MD, PhD
Department of Surgery, Radboud University Medical Center, Nijmegen, The Netherlands

Joshua A. Boys, MD
Thoracic Surgery Research Fellow, Department of Surgery, University of Southern California, Los Angeles, California

Raquel Bravo-Infante, MD
Gastrointestinal Surgery Department, Hospital Clinic of Barcelona, Barcelona, Spain

Ross M. Bremner, MD, PhD
Executive Director, Norton Thoracic Institute, St. Joseph's Hospital and Medical Center, Phoenix, Arizona

Bruce M. Brenner, MD
Associate Professor of Surgery, University of Connecticut, Farmington, Connecticut

Shaun R. Brown, DO, FACS
Clinical Fellow, Department of Colon and Rectal Surgery, Ochsner Medical Center, New Orleans, Louisiana

Mark P. Callery, MD
Professor of Surgery, Harvard Medical School; Chief, Division of General Surgery, Beth Israel Deaconess Medical Center, Boston, Massachusetts

John L. Cameron, MD
Alfred Blalock Distinguished Service Professor of Surgery, Professor of Surgery, The Johns Hopkins Hospital, Baltimore, Maryland

Michael Camilleri, MD
Atherton and Winifred W. Bean Professor, Professor of Medicine, Pharmacology, and Physiology, Consultant, Division of Gastroenterology and Hepatology, Department of Medicine, Mayo Clinic, Rochester, Minnesota

Jacob Campbell, DO, MPH
Department of Surgery, University of Connecticut Health Center, Farmington, Connecticut

Riaz Cassim, MD, FACS, FASCRS
Associate Professor, Department of Surgery, West Virginia University, Morgantown, West Virginia; Chief of Surgery, Louis A. Johnson VA Medical Center, Clarksburg, West Virginia

Manuel Castillo-Angeles, MD, MPH
Research Fellow, Department of Surgery, Beth Israel Deaconess Medical Center, Boston, Massachusetts

Christy Cauley, MD, MPH
Resident, Department of Surgery, Massachusetts General Hospital, Boston, Massachusetts

Keith M. Cavaness, DO, FACS
Surgery, Baylor Scott and White Health, Dallas, Texas

Robert J. Cerfolio, MD, MBA, FACS, FACCP
Professor of Surgery, Chief of Clinical Division Thoracic Surgery, Director of the Lung Cancer Service Line, New York University; Senior Advisor, Robotic Committee, New York, New York

Bradley J. Champagne, MD, FACS, FASCRS
Chairman of Surgery, Fairview Hospital; Director of Services, DDSI West Region; Professor of Surgery, Cleveland Clinic Lerner School of Medicine; Medical Director, Fairview Ambulatory Surgery Center, Cleveland, Ohio

Parakrama Chandrasoma, MD, MRCP
Chief, Surgical and Anatomic Pathology, Los Angeles County + University of Southern California Medical Center; Emeritus Professor of Pathology, Keck School of Medicine of the University of Southern California, Los Angeles, California

Alex L. Chang, MD
Department of General Surgery, University of Cincinnati, Cincinnati, Ohio

Christopher G. Chapman, MD
Assistant Professor of Medicine, Director, Bariatric and Metabolic Endoscopy, Center for Endoscopic Research and Therapeutics, The University of Chicago Medicine and Biological Sciences, Chicago, Illinois

William C. Chapman, MD, FACS
Surgery, Washington University, St. Louis, Missouri

Susannah Cheek, MD
Clinical Instructor in Surgery, University of Pittsburgh, Pittsburgh, Pennsylvania

Harvey S. Chen, MD
Department of Surgery, Mayo Clinic, Rochester, Minnesota

Clifford S. Cho, MD
Department of Surgery, University of Michigan, Ann Arbor, Michigan

Eric T. Choi, MD
Chief, Vascular and Endovascular Surgery, Professor of Surgery, Professor, Center for Metabolic Disease Research, Temple University Lewis Katz School of Medicine, Philadelphia, Pennsylvania

Eugene A. Choi, MD
Associate Professor of Surgery, Baylor College of Medicine, Houston, Texas

Karen A. Chojnacki, MD, FACS
Associate Professor of Surgery, Thomas Jefferson University, Philadelphia, Pennsylvania

Michael A. Choti, MD, MBA
Professor, Department of Surgery, University of Texas Southwestern Medical Center, Dallas, Texas

Ian Christie
Research Assistant, Department of Cardiothoracic Surgery, University of Pittsburgh, Pittsburgh, Pennsylvania

Heidi Chua, MD
Consultant, Department of Colon and Rectal Surgery, Mayo Clinic, Rochester, Minnesota

James M. Church, MBChB, MMedSci, FRACS
Staff Surgeon, Colorectal Surgery, Digestive Disease and Surgery Institute, Cleveland Clinic, Cleveland, Ohio

Jessica L. Cioffi, MD
Assistant Professor of Surgery, University of Florida, Gainesville, Florida

Susannah Clark, MS, MPAS
Boston, Massachusetts

Pierre-Alain Clavien, MD, PhD
Professor and Chairman, Department of Surgery, Division of Visceral and Transplant Surgery, University Hospital Zurich, Zurich, Switzerland

Adam Cloud, MD
Assistant Professor of Surgery, University of Connecticut, Farmington, Connecticut

Paul D. Colavita, MD
Gastrointestinal and Minimally Invasive Surgery, Carolinas Medical Center, Charlotte, North Carolina

Steven D. Colquhoun, MD
Professor of Surgery, Chief, Section of Hepatobiliary Surgery, Director of Liver Transplantation, Department of Surgery, University of California, Davis, Davis, California

William Conway, MD
Surgical Oncology, Ochsner Medical Center, New Orleans, Louisiana

Jonathan Cools-Lartigue, MD, PhD
Assistant Professor of Surgery, McGill University, Montreal, Quebec, Canada

Willy Coosemans, MD, PhD
Professor in Surgery, Clinical Head, Department of Thoracic Surgery, University Hospital Leuven, Leuven, Belgium

Edward E. Cornwell III, MD, FACS, FCCM, FWACS
The LaSalle D. Leffal Jr., Professor and Chairman of Surgery, Howard University Hospital, Washington, D.C.

Mario Costantini, MD
Department of Surgical, Oncological, and Gastroenterological Sciences, University and Azienda Ospedaliera of Padua, Padua, Italy

Yvonne Coyle, MD
Medical Director, Oncology Outpatient Services at the Baylor T. Boone Pickens Cancer Hospital; Texas Oncology and the Baylor Charles A. Sammons Cancer Center at the Baylor University Medical Center; Clinical Associate Professor, Texas A&M Health Science Center, College of Medicine, Dallas, Texas

Daniel A. Craig, MD
Assistant Professor of Radiology, Mayo Clinic, Rochester, Minnesota

Kristopher P. Croome, MD, MS
Assistant Professor of Transplant Surgery, Mayo Clinic, Jacksonville, Florida

Joseph J. Cullen, MD
Professor of Surgery, University of Iowa College of Medicine; Chief Surgical Services, Iowa City VA Medical Center, Iowa City, Iowa

Anthony P. D'Andrea, MD, MPH
Department of Surgery, Division of Colon and Rectal Surgery, Icahn School of Medicine at Mount Sinai, New York, New York

Themistocles Dassopoulos, MD
Adjunct Professor of Medicine, Texas A&M University; Director, Baylor Scott and White Center for Inflammatory Bowel Diseases, Dallas, Texas

Marta L. Davila, MD
Professor, Department of Gastroenterology, Hepatology, and Nutrition, The University of Texas MD Anderson Cancer Center, Houston, Texas

Raquel E. Davila, MD
Associate Professor, Department of Gastroenterology, Hepatology, and Nutrition, The University of Texas MD Anderson Cancer Center, Houston, Texas

Steven R. DeMeester, MD, FACS
Division of Foregut and Minimally Invasive Surgery, The Oregon Clinic, Portland, Oregon

Tom R. DeMeester, MD
Professor and Chairman Emeritus, Department of Surgery, University of Southern California, Los Angeles, California

Daniel T. Dempsey, MD, MBA
Professor of Surgery, University of Pennsylvania; Assistant Director, Perioperative Services, Hospital of the University of Pennsylvania, Philadelphia, Pennsylvania

Gregory dePrisco, MD
Diagnostic Radiologist, Baylor University Medical Center, Dallas, Texas

Lieven Depypere, MD
Joint Clinical Head, Department of Thoracic Surgery, University Hospital Leuven, Leuven, Belgium

David W. Dietz, MD, FACS, FASCRS
Chief, Division of Colorectal Surgery, Vice Chair, Clinical Operations and Quality, Vice President, System Surgery Quality and Experience, University Hospitals, Cleveland, Ohio

Mary E. Dillhoff, MD, MS
Assistant Professor of Surgery, The Ohio State University College of Medicine, Columbus, Ohio

Joseph DiNorcia, MD
Assistant Professor of Surgery, David Geffen School of Medicine, University of California, Los Angeles, Los Angeles, California

Stephen M. Doane, MD
Advanced Gastrointestinal Surgery Fellow, Department of Surgery, Thomas Jefferson University Hospital, Philadelphia, Pennsylvania

Epameinondas Dogeas, MD
Resident, Department of Surgery, University of Texas Southwestern Medical Center, Dallas, Texas

Eric J. Dozois, MD, FACS, FASCRS
Colon and Rectal Surgery, Mayo Clinic, Rochester, Minnesota

Kristoffel Dumon, MD
Associate Professor of Surgery, Hospital of the University of Pennsylvania, Philadelphia, Pennsylvania

Stephen P. Dunn, MD
Chairman, Department of Surgery, Nemours/Alfred I. Dupont Hospital for Children, Wilmington, Delaware; Professor of Surgery, Sidney Kimmel Medical College, Thomas Jefferson University, Philadelphia, Pennsylvania

Christy M. Dunst, MD
Co-Program Director, Advanced GI-Foregut Fellowship, Cancer Center, Providence Portland Medical Center; Foregut Surgeon, Gastrointestinal and Minimally Invasive Surgery, The Oregon Clinic, Portland, Oregon

John N. Dussel, MD
Fellow in Vascular Surgery, University of Connecticut, Farmington, Connecticut

Matthew Dyer, BA
Case Western Reserve University School of Medicine, Cleveland, Ohio

Jonathan Efron, MD
Associate Professor of Surgery and Urology, Johns Hopkins University, Baltimore, Maryland

Yousef El-Gohary, MD
Department of General Surgery, Stony Brook University
School of Medicine, New York, New York

Mustapha El Lakis, MD
Thoraco-Esophageal Postdoctoral Research Fellow, General,
Vascular, and Thoracic Surgery, Virginia Mason Medical
Center, Seattle, Washington

E. Christopher Ellison, MD
Robert M. Zollinger and College of Medicine Distinguished
Professor of Surgery, The Ohio State University College of
Medicine, Columbus, Ohio

James Ellsmere, MD, MSc, FRCSC
Division of General Surgery, Dalhousie University, Halifax,
Nova Scotia, Canada

Rahila Essani, MD, FACS
Department of Surgery, Baylor Scott and White Healthcare,
Texas A&M University College of Medicine, Temple, Texas

Douglas B. Evans, MD
Professor and Chair of Surgery, Medical College of Wisconsin,
Milwaukee, Wisconsin

Sandy H. Fang, MD
Assistant Professor, Department of Surgery, Johns Hopkins
Medical Institutions, Baltimore, Maryland

Geoffrey Fasen, MD, MS
Clinical Instructor in General Surgery, University of Virginia,
Charlottesville, Virginia

Hiran C. Fernando, MBBS, FRCS, FRCSEd
Department of Surgery, Inova Fairfax Medical Campus, Falls
Church, Virginia

Lorenzo Ferri, MD, PhD
Professor of Surgery, McGill University, Montreal, Quebec,
Canada

Alessandro Fichera, MD, FACS, FASCRS
Professor and Section Chief, Gastrointestinal Surgery,
University of Washington Medical Center, Seattle, Washington

Christine Finck, MD
Chief, Division of Pediatric Surgery, Donald Hight Endowed
Chair, Surgery, Connecticut Children's Medical Center,
Hartford, Connecticut; Associate Professor of Pediatrics and
Surgery, University of Connecticut Health Center,
Farmington, Connecticut

Oliver M. Fisher, MD
Gastroesophageal Cancer Program, St. Vincent's Centre for
Applied Medical Research, Department of Surgery, University
of Notre Dame School of Medicine, Sydney, Australia

James W. Fleshman, MD, FACS
Seeger Professor and Chairman of Surgery, Baylor University
Medical Center; Professor of Surgery, Texas A&M Health
Science Center, Dallas, Texas

Yuman Fong, MD
Chairman, Department of Surgery, City of Hope National
Medical Center, Duarte, California

Michael L. Foreman, MS, MD
Chief, Division of Trauma, Critical Care, and Acute Care
Surgery, Department of Surgery, Baylor University Medical
Center; Professor of Surgery, Texas A&M Health Science
Center, College of Medicine, Dallas, Texas

Todd D. Francone, MD, MPH, FACS, FASCRS
Chief, Division of Colon and Rectal Surgery, Newton-
Wellesley Hospital; Director, Robotic Surgery, Newton-
Wellesley Hospital; Associate Chair, Department of Surgery,
Newton-Wellesley Hospital; Staff Surgeon, Massachusetts
General Hospital; Assistant Professor of Surgery, Tufts
Medical School, Boston, Massachusetts

Edward R. Franko, MD, FACS
Assistant Professor of Surgery, Texas A&M University College
of Medicine, Dallas, Texas

Daniel French, MD, MASc, FRCSC
Assistant Professor, Division of Thoracic Surgery, Dalhousie
University, Halifax, Nova Scotia, Canada

Hans Friedrich Fuchs, MD
Department of Surgery, University Hospital Cologne,
Cologne, Germany

Karl Hermann Fuchs, MD
Professor, Department of Surgery, Agaplesion Markus
Hospital, Frankfurt, Germany

Brian Funaki, MD
Professor of Radiology, The University of Chicago Pritzker
School of Medicine; Section Chief, Division of Vascular and
Interventional Radiology, The University of Chicago
Medicine, Chicago, Illinois

Geoffrey A. Funk, MD, FACS
Trauma and General Surgery, Surgical Critical Care, Assistant
Professor of Surgery, Texas A&M University College of
Medicine, Dallas, Texas

Joseph Fusco, MD
Children's Hospital of Pittsburgh, University of Pittsburgh,
Pittsburgh, Pennsylvania

Shrawan G. Gaitonde, MD
Fellow, Surgical Oncology, John Wayne Cancer Institute at
Providence Saint John's Health Center, Santa Monica,
California

Julio Garcia-Aguilar, MD, PhD
Chief, Colorectal Service, Department of Surgery, Benno C.
Schmidt Chair in Surgical Oncology, Memorial Sloan
Kettering Cancer Center; Professor of Surgery, Weill Cornell
Medical College, New York, New York

Susan Gearhart, MD
Associate Professor of Surgery, Johns Hopkins Medical
Institutions, Baltimore, Maryland

David A. Geller, MD, FACS
Richard L. Simmons Professor of Surgery, Chief, Division of Hepatobiliary and Pancreatic Surgery, University of Pittsburgh, Pittsburgh, Pennsylvania

Comeron Ghobadi, MD
Department of Radiology, The University of Chicago Medicine, Chicago, Illinois

Sebastien Gilbert, MD
Associate Professor of Surgery, University of Ottawa; Chief, Division of Thoracic Surgery, Department of Surgery, Clinician Investigator, The Ottawa Hospital Research Institute, The Ottawa Hospital, Ottawa, Ontario, Canada

David Giles, MD
Associate Clinical Professor of Surgery, University of Connecticut School of Medicine, Farmington, Connecticut

Erin Gillaspie, MD
Assistant Professor, Department of Thoracic Surgery, Vanderbilt University Medical Center, Nashville, Tennessee

Micah Girotti, MD
Division of Vascular Surgery, Northwestern University Feinberg School of Medicine, Chicago, Illinois

George K. Gittes, MD
Professor of Surgery, Surgeon-in-Chief, Children's Hospital of Pittsburgh, University of Pittsburgh School of Medicine, Pittsburgh, Pennsylvania

Michael D. Goodman, MD
Assistant Professor of Surgery, University of Cincinnati, Cincinnati, Ohio

Hein G. Gooszen, MD, PhD
Professor, Department of Operating Room/Evidence Based Surgery, Radboud University Medical Center, Nijmegen, The Netherlands

Gregory J. Gores, MD
Executive Dean for Research, Professor of Medicine, Division of Gastroenterology and Hepatology, Mayo Clinic, Rochester, Minnesota

James F. Griffin, MD
Surgical Resident, Department of Surgery, The Johns Hopkins Hospital, Baltimore, Maryland

S. Michael Griffin, OBE, MD, FRCSEd
Professor, Consultant Oesophagogastric Surgeon, Northern Oesophagogastric Cancer Unit, Royal Victoria Infirmary, Newcastle-upon-Tyne, United Kingdom

Leander Grimm Jr., MD, FACS, FASCRS
Assistant Professor of Surgery, Division of Colon and Rectal Surgery, University of South Alabama, Mobile, Alabama

L.F. Grochola, MD, PhD
Department of Visceral and Transplant Surgery, University Hospital Zurich, Zurich, Switzerland

Fahim Habib, MD, MPH, FACS
Esophageal and Lung Institute, Allegheny Health Network, Pittsburgh, Pennsylvania

John B. Hanks, MD
C. Bruce Morton Professor and Chief, Division of General Surgery, Department of Surgery, University of Virginia Health System, Charlottesville, Virginia

James E. Harris Jr., MD
Assistant Professor of Surgery, The Johns Hopkins Hospital, Baltimore, Maryland

Matthew G. Hartwig, MD
Associate Professor of Surgery, Division of Thoracic and Cardiovascular Surgery, Department of Surgery, Duke University Hospital, Durham, North Carolina

Imran Hassan, MD, FACS
Clinical Associate Professor of Surgery, Carver College of Medicine, University of Iowa Health Care, Iowa City, Iowa

Traci L. Hedrick, MD, MS
Associate Professor of Surgery, University of Virginia Health System, Charlottesville, Virginia

Terry C. Hicks, MD, FACS, FASCRS
Colorectal Surgeon, Department of Colon and Rectal Surgery, Ochsner Medical Center, New Orleans, Louisiana

Richard Hodin, MD
Department of Surgery, Massachusetts General Hospital, Boston, Massachusetts

Wayne L. Hofstetter, MD
Professor of Surgery and Deputy Chair, Department of Thoracic and Cardiovascular Surgery, The University of Texas MD Anderson Cancer Center, Houston, Texas

Melissa Hogg, MD, MS
Assistant Professor of Surgery, Division of Surgical Oncology, University of Pittsburgh Medical Center, Pittsburgh, Pennsylvania

Yue-Yung Hu, MD, MPH
Pediatric Surgery Fellow, Connecticut Children's Medical Center, Hartford, Connecticut

Eric S. Hungness, MD
S. David Stulberg, MD Research Professor, Associate Professor in Gastrointestinal and Endocrine Surgery and Medical Education, Northwestern University Feinberg School of Medicine; Attending Surgeon, Northwestern Memorial Hospital, Chicago, Illinois

Steven R. Hunt, MD
Associate Professor of Surgery, Division of General Surgery, Section of Colon and Rectal Surgery, Washington University School of Medicine, St. Louis, Missouri

Khumara Huseynova, MD
Assistant Professor of Vascular and Endovascular Surgery, West Virginia University, Morgantown, West Virginia

Neil H. Hyman, MD
Chief, Section of Colon and Rectal Surgery, Co-Director, Digestive Disease Center, Department of Surgery, The University of Chicago Medicine, Chicago, Illinois

David A. Iannitti, MD
Chief, Division of Hepatobiliary and Pancreatic Surgery, Department of Surgery, Carolinas HealthCare System, Charlotte, North Carolina

Jeffrey Indes, MD
Associate Professor of Surgery, Section of Vascular Surgery, University of Connecticut, Farmington, Connecticut

Megan Jenkins, MD
Department of Surgery, New York University Langone Medical Center, New York, New York

Todd Jensen, MSc
Research Associate, University of Connecticut, Farmington, Connecticut

Paul M. Jeziorczak, MD
Senior Fellow, Division of Pediatric Surgery, St. Louis Children's Hospital, St. Louis, Missouri

Danial Jilani, MD
Department of Radiology, The University of Chicago Medicine, Chicago, Illinois

Marta Jiménez-Toscano, MD, PhD
Gastrointestinal Surgery Department, Hospital Clinic of Barcelona, Barcelona, Spain

Blair A. Jobe, MD, FACS
Director, Esophageal and Lung Institute, Allegheny Health Network; Clinical Professor of Surgery, Temple University School of Medicine, Pittsburgh, Pennsylvania

Lily E. Johnston, MD, MPH
Resident, Department of Surgery, University of Virginia Health System, Charlottesville, Virginia

Peter J. Kahrilas, MD
Gilbert H. Marquardt Professor of Medicine, Northwestern University Feinberg School of Medicine, Chicago, Illinois

Matthew F. Kalady, MD
Professor of Surgery, Colorectal Surgery, Co-Director, Comprehensive Colorectal Cancer Program, Digestive Disease and Surgery Institute, Cleveland Clinic, Cleveland, Ohio

Noor Kassira, MD
Assistant Professor of Surgery, Division of Pediatric Surgery, University of South Florida, Morsani College of Medicine, Tampa, Florida

Namir Katkhouda, MD, FACS
Professor of Surgery, Division of Upper Gastrointestinal and General Surgery, Keck School of Medicine of the University of Southern California, Los Angeles, California

Philip O. Katz, MD, FACG
Director of Motility Laboratories, Jay Monahan Center for Gastrointestinal Health, Weill Cornell Medicine, New York, New York

Deborah S. Keller, MS, MD
Department of Surgery, Baylor University Medical Center, Dallas, Texas

Matthew P. Kelley, MD
General Surgery Resident, Johns Hopkins Medical Institutions, Baltimore, Maryland

Gregory D. Kennedy, MD, PhD
Professor of Surgery, University of Alabama Birmingham, Birmingham, Alabama

Tara Sotsky Kent, MD, MS
Assistant Professor of Surgery, Harvard Medical School, Beth Israel Deaconess Medical Center, Boston, Massachusetts

Leila Kia, MD
Department of Medicine, Northwestern University Feinberg School of Medicine, Chicago, Illinois

Melina R. Kibbe, MD
Chair, Department of Surgery, The University of North Carolina at Chapel Hill, Chapel Hill, North Carolina

John Kim, DO, MPH, FACS
Clinical Assistant Professor of Surgery, Clerkship Director, Surgery, University of Illinois College of Medicine, Champaign-Urbana, Illinois; Attending Surgeon, Acute Care Surgery and Trauma, Carle Foundation Hospital, Urbana, Illinois

Alice King, MD
Junior Fellow, Division of Pediatric Surgery, St. Louis Children's Hospital, St. Louis, Missouri

Ravi P. Kiran, MBBS, MS, FRCS (Eng), FRCS (Glas), FACS, MSc EBM (Oxford)
Kenneth A. Forde Professor of Surgery in Epidemiology, Division Chief and Program Director, Director, Center for Innovation and Outcomes Research, Division of Colorectal Surgery, NewYork-Presbyterian Hospital/Columbia University Medical Center, New York, New York

Orlando C. Kirton, MD, FACS, MCCM, FCCP, MBA
Surgeon-in-Chief, Chairman of Surgery, Abington-Jefferson Health; Professor of Surgery, Sidney Kimmel Medical College of Thomas Jefferson University, Abington, Pennsylvania

Andrew Klein, MD, MBA, FACS
Professor and Vice Chairman, Department of Surgery, Director, Comprehensive Transplant Center, Cedars-Sinai Medical Center, Los Angeles, California

Eric N. Klein, MD
Acute Care Surgeon, North Shore University Hospital, Manhasset, New York

Geoffrey P. Kohn, MBBS(Hons), MSurg, FRACS, FACS
Senior Lecturer, Department of Surgery, Monash University, Melbourne, Australia; Upper Gastrointestinal Surgeon, Melbourne Upper Gastrointestinal Surgical Group, Melbourne, Victoria, Australia

Robert Caleb Kovell, MD
Assistant Professor of Clinical Urology in Surgery, Department of Urology Surgery, Perelman School of Medicine, University of Pennsylvania, Philadelphia, Pennsylvania

Robert Kozol, MD
General Surgery, JFK Medical Center, Atlantis, Florida

Antonio M. Lacy, MD, PhD
Chief, Gastrointestinal Surgery, Hospital Clinic of Barcelona, Barcelona, Spain

Daniela P. Ladner, MD, MPH, FACS
Associate Professor of Transplant Surgery, Division of Organ Transplantation, Feinberg School of Medicine, Northwestern University; Director, Northwestern University Transplant Outcomes Research Collaborative, Northwestern University, Chicago, Illinois

S.M. Lagarde, MD, PhD
Department of Surgery, Erasmus MC–University Medical Center Rotterdam, Rotterdam, The Netherlands

Carrie A. Laituri, MD
Assistant Professor of Surgery, Division of Pediatric Surgery, University of South Florida, Morsani College of Medicine, Tampa, Florida

Alessandra Landmann, MD
Resident Physician, Department of Surgery, University of Oklahoma, Oklahoma City, Oklahoma

Janet T. Lee, MD, MS
Clinical Assistant Professor of Surgery, University of Minnesota, St. Paul, Minnesota

Lawrence L. Lee, MD, PhD, FRCSC
Department of Colon and Rectal Surgery, Center for Colon & Rectal Surgery, Florida Hospital, Orlando, Florida

Jennifer A. Leinicke, MD, MPHS
Department of Surgery, Washington University School of Medicine, St. Louis, Missouri

Toni Lerut, MD, PhD
Emeritus Professor of Surgery, Clinical Head, Department of Thoracic Surgery, University Hospital Leuven, Leuven, Belgium

David M. Levi, MD
Transplant Surgeon, Carolinas Medical Center, Charlotte, North Carolina

Chao Li, MD, MSc, FRCSC
Division of General Surgery, Dalhousie University, Halifax, Nova Scotia, Canada

Yu Liang, MD
Department of Surgery, University of Connecticut Health Center, Farmington, Connecticut

Andrew H. Lichliter, MD
Diagnostic Radiology Resident, Baylor University Medical Center, Dallas, Texas

Warren E. Lichliter, MD
Chief, Colon and Rectal Surgery, Baylor Scott and White Health, Dallas, Texas

Amy L. Lightner, MD
Senior Associate Consultant, Department of Colon and Rectal Surgery, Mayo Clinic, Rochester, Minnesota

Deacon J. Lile, MD
Department of General Surgery, Temple University Hospital, Philadelphia, Pennsylvania

Keith D. Lillemoe, MD, FACS
W. Gerald Austen Professor of Surgery, Harvard Medical School; Surgeon-in-Chief, The Massachusetts General Hospital, Boston, Massachusetts;

Jules Lin, MD, FACS
Associate Professor, Mark B. Orringer Professor, Section of Thoracic Surgery, University of Michigan, Ann Arbor, Michigan

Shu S. Lin, MD, PhD
Associate Professor of Surgery, Pathology, and Immunology, Duke University Medical Center, Durham, North Carolina

John C. Lipham, MD, FACS
Chief, Division of Upper Gastrointestinal and General Surgery, Associate Professor of Surgery, Keck School of Medicine of the University of Southern California, Los Angeles, California

Virginia R. Litle, MD
Professor of Surgery, Division of Thoracic Surgery, Boston University, Boston, Massachusetts

Nayna A. Lodhia, MD
Resident, Department of Internal Medicine, The University of Chicago Medicine, Chicago, Illinois

Walter E. Longo, MD, MBA
Colon and Rectal Surgery, Yale University School of Medicine, New Haven, Connecticut

Reginald V.N. Lord, MBBS, MD, FRACS
Director, Gastroesophageal Cancer Program, St. Vincent's Centre for Applied Medical Research; Professor and Head of Surgery, University of Notre Dame School of Medicine, Sydney, Australia

Brian E. Louie, MD, MPH, MHA
Director, Thoracic Research and Education, Division of Thoracic Surgery, Swedish Cancer Institute and Medical Center, Seattle, Washington

Donald E. Low, MD, FACS, FRCS(C)
Head of Thoracic Surgery and Thoracic Oncology, General, Vascular, and Thoracic Surgery, Virginia Mason Medical Center, Seattle, Washington

Val J. Lowe, MD
Professor of Radiology/Nuclear Medicine, Mayo Clinic, Rochester, Minnesota

Jessica G.Y. Luc, MD
Faculty of Medicine and Dentistry, University of Alberta, Alberta, Canada

James D. Luketich, MD
Henry T. Bahnson Professor and Chairman, Department of Cardiothoracic Surgery, Chief, Division of Thoracic and Foregut Surgery, University of Pittsburgh School of Medicine, Pittsburgh, Pennsylvania

Yanling Ma, MD
Pathologist, Department of Surgical Pathology, Los Angeles County + University of Southern California Medical Center; Associate Professor of Pathology, Keck School of Medicine of the University of Southern California, Los Angeles, Los Angeles, California

Robert L. MacCarty, MD
Professor of Diagnostic Radiology, Emeritus, Mayo Clinic College of Medicine, Rochester, Minnesota

Blair MacDonald, MD, FRCPC
Associate Professor of Medical Imaging, University of Ottawa; Clinical Investigator, The Ottawa Hospital Research Institute; Gastrointestinal Radiologist, The Ottawa Hospital, Ottawa, Ontario, Canada

Robert D. Madoff, MD
Professor of Surgery, University of Minnesota, Minneapolis, Minnesota

Deepa Magge, MD
Fellow in Surgical Oncology, Division of Surgical Oncology, University of Pittsburgh Medical Center, Pittsburgh, Pennsylvania

Anurag Maheshwari, MD
Clinical Assistant Professor of Medicine, Division of Gastroenterology and Hepatology, University of Maryland School of Medicine; Consultant Transplant Hepatologist, Institute for Digestive Health and Liver Diseases, Mercy Medical Center, Baltimore, Maryland

Najjia N. Mahmoud, MD
Professor of Surgery, Division of Colon and Rectal Surgery, University of Pennsylvania, Philadelphia, Pennsylvania

David A. Mahvi, MD
Brigham and Women's Hospital, Boston, Massachusetts

David M. Mahvi, MD
Professor of Surgery, Northwestern University School of Medicine, Chicago, Illinois

Grace Z. Mak, MD
Associate Professor, Section of Pediatric Surgery, Department of Surgery, The University of Chicago Medicine and Biological Sciences, Chicago, Illinois

Sara A. Mansfield, MD, MS
Clinical Housestaff, Department of Surgery, The Ohio State University Wexner Medical Center, Columbus, Ohio

Maricarmen Manzano, MD
Division of Gastroenterology, National Cancer Institute of Mexico, Mexico City, Mexico

David J. Maron, MD, MBA
Vice Chair, Department of Colorectal Surgery, Director, Colorectal Surgery Residency Program, Cleveland Clinic Florida, Weston, Florida

Melvy S. Mathew, MD
Assistant Professor of Radiology, The University of Chicago Pritzker School of Medicine; Division of Body Imaging, The University of Chicago Medicine, Chicago, Illinois

Kellie L. Mathis, MD
Surgery, Mayo Clinic, Rochester, Minnesota

Jeffrey B. Matthews, MD, FACS
Dallas B. Phemister Professor and Chairman of Surgery, The University of Chicago, Chicago, Illinois

David W. McFadden, MD, MBA, FACS
Chairman, Department of Surgery, University of Connecticut; Surgeon-in-Chief, University of Connecticut Health, Farmington, Connecticut

Amit Merchea, MD, FACS, FASCRS
Assistant Professor of Surgery, Colon and Rectal Surgery, Mayo Clinic, Jacksonville, Florida

Evangelos Messaris, MD, PhD
Associate Professor of Surgery, Pennsylvania State University, College of Medicine, Hershey, Pennsylvania

Daniel L. Miller, MD
Clinical Professor of Surgery, Medical College of Georgia, Augusta University, Augusta, Georgia; Chief, General Thoracic Surgery, Program Director, General Surgery Residency Program, Kennestone Regional Medical Center, WellStar Health System/Mayo Clinic Care Network, Marietta, Georgia

Heidi J. Miller, MD, MPH
Assistant Professor of Surgery, University of New Mexico, Sandoval Regional Medical Center, Albuquerque, New Mexico

J. Michael Millis, MD, MBA
Professor of Surgery, Transplant Surgery, The University of Chicago, Chicago, Illinois

Sumeet K. Mittal, MD, FACS, MBA
Surgical Director, Esophageal and Foregut Program, Norton Thoracic Institute, St. Joseph's Hospital and Medical Center, Phoenix, Arizona

Daniela Molena, MD
Surgical Director, Esophageal Cancer Surgery Program, General Surgery Department, Thoracic Surgery Service, Memorial Sloan Kettering Cancer Center, New York, New York

Stephanie C. Montgomery, MD, FACS
Director of Surgery Education, Saint Francis Hospital and
Medical Center; Assistant Professor, University of Connecticut
School of Medicine, Hartford, Connecticut

Ryan Moore, MD
Department of General Surgery, Temple University Hospital,
Philadelphia, Pennsylvania

Katherine A. Morgan, MD, FACS
Professor of Surgery, Chief, Division of Gastrointestinal and
Laparoscopic Surgery, Medical University of South Carolina,
Charleston, South Carolina

Melinda M. Mortenson, MD
Department of Surgery, Permanente Medical Group,
Sacramento, California

Michael W. Mulholland, MD, PhD
Department of Surgery, University of Michigan, Ann Arbor,
Michigan

Michael S. Mulvihill, MD
Resident Surgeon, Department of Surgery, Duke University,
Durham, North Carolina

Matthew Mutch, MD
Chief, Section of Colon and Rectal Surgery, Associate
Professor of Surgery, Washington University, St. Louis,
Missouri

Philippe Robert Nafteux, MD, PhD
Assistant Professor in Surgery, Clinical Head, Department of
Thoracic Surgery, University Hospital Leuven, Leuven,
Belgium

Arun Nagaraju, MD
Department of Radiology, The University of Chicago
Medicine, Chicago, Illinois

David M. Nagorney, MD, FACS
Professor of Surgery, Mayo Clinic, Rochester, Minnesota

Hari Nathan, MD, PhD
Department of Surgery, University of Michigan, Ann Arbor,
Michigan

Karen R. Natoli, MD
Department of Surgery, Community Hospital, Indianapolis,
Indiana

Rakesh Navuluri, MD
Department of Radiology, The University of Chicago
Medicine, Chicago, Illinois

Nicholas N. Nissen, MD
Director, Liver Transplant and Hepatopancreatobiliary
Surgery, Cedars-Sinai Medical Center, Los Angeles, California

Tamar B. Nobel, MD
Department of Surgery, Mount Sinai Hospital, New York, New
York

B.J. Noordman, MD
Department of Surgery, Erasmus MC–University Medical
Center Rotterdam, Rotterdam, The Netherlands

Jeffrey A. Norton, MD
Professor of Surgery, Stanford University School of Medicine,
Stanford, California

Yuri W. Novitsky, MD
Director, Cleveland Comprehensive Hernia Center, University
Hospitals Cleveland Medical Center; Professor of Surgery,
Case Western Reserve School of Medicine, Cleveland, Ohio

Michael S. Nussbaum, MD, FACS
Professor and Chair, Department of Surgery, Virginia Tech
Carilion School of Medicine, Roanoke, Virginia

Scott L. Nyberg, MD, PhD
Professor of Biomedical Engineering and Surgery,
Department of Transplantation Surgery, Mayo Clinic,
Rochester, Minnesota

Brant K. Oelschlager, MD
Byers Endowed Professor of Esophageal Research, Chief,
Division of General Surgery, University of Washington
Medical Center; Vice Chair, Department of Surgery,
University of Washington, Seattle, Washington

Daniel S. Oh, MD
Assistant Professor of Surgery, Thoracic Surgery, University of
Southern California, Los Angeles, California

Ana Otero-Piñeiro, MD
Gastrointestinal Surgery Department, Hospital Clinic of
Barcelona, Barcelona, Spain

Aytekin Oto, MD
Professor of Radiology, The University of Chicago Pritzker
School of Medicine; Section Chief, Division of Body Imaging,
The University of Chicago Medicine, Chicago, Illinois

H. Leon Pachter, MD
Chairman, Department of Surgery, New York University
Langone Medical Center, New York, New York

Charles N. Paidas, MD, MBA
Professor of Surgery and Pediatrics, Chief, Pediatric Surgery,
Vice Dean for Graduate Medical Education, University of
South Florida, Morsani College of Medicine, Tampa, Florida

Francesco Palazzo, MD
Associate Professor of Surgery, Thomas Jefferson University,
Philadelphia, Pennsylvania

Alessandro Paniccia, MD
General Surgery Resident, University of Colorado School of
Medicine, Aurora, Colorado

Harry T. Papaconstantinou, MD, FACS, FACRS
Department of Surgery, Baylor Scott and White Healthcare,
Texas A&M University College of Medicine, Temple, Texas

Theodore N. Pappas, MD, FACS
Distinguished Professor of Surgical Innovation, Chief of Advanced Oncologic and Gastrointestinal Surgery, Duke University School of Medicine, Durham, North Carolina

Emmanouil P. Pappou, MD, PhD
Assistant Professor of Colorectal Surgery, Columbia University Medical Center, New York, New York

Manish Parikh, MD
Associate Professor of Surgery, New York University Langone Medical Center/Bellevue Hospital, New York, New York

Jennifer L. Paruch, MD, MS
Lahey Hospital and Medical Center, Burlington, Massachusetts

Asish D. Patel, MD
Chief Resident, Department of Surgery, University of Nebraska Medical Center, Omaha, Nebraska

Mikin Patel, MD
Department of Radiology, The University of Chicago Medicine, Chicago, Illinois

Marco G. Patti, MD
Center for Esophageal Diseases and Swallowing, University of North Carolina at Chapel Hill, Chapel Hill, North Carolina

Emily Carter Paulson, MD, MSCE
Assistant Professor of Surgery, University of Pennsylvania; Assistant Professor of Surgery, Corporal Michael Crescenz VA Medical Center, Philadelphia, Pennsylvania

Timothy M. Pawlik, MD, MPH, PhD
Professor of Surgery and Oncology, The Urban Meyer III and Shelley Meyer Chair for Cancer Research, Ohio State University; Chair, Department of Surgery, Wexner Medical Center, Columbus, Ohio; Division of Surgical Oncology, Department of Surgery, The Johns Hopkins School of Medicine, Baltimore, Maryland

Isaac Payne, DO
Surgical Resident, University of South Alabama, Mobile, Alabama

John H. Pemberton, MD
Professor of Surgery, College of Medicine, Consultant, Department of Colon and Rectal Surgery, Mayo Clinic, Rochester, Minnesota

Michael Pendola, MD
Staff Colorectal Surgeon, Department of Surgery, Baylor University Medical Center, Dallas, Texas

Alexander Perez, MD, FACS
Chief of Pancreatic Surgery, Duke University Medical Center, Durham, North Carolina; Associate Professor of Surgery, Duke University School of Medicine, Durham, North Carolina

Luise I.M. Pernar, MD
Assistant Professor of Surgery, Boston University School of Medicine; Minimally Invasive and Weight Loss Surgery, Boston Medical Center, Boston, Massachusetts

Walter R. Peters Jr., MD, MBA
Chief, Division of Colon and Rectal Surgery, Baylor University Medical Center, Dallas, Texas

Henrik Petrowsky, MD
Professor of Surgery, Vice Chairman, Department of Visceral and Transplant Surgery, University Hospital Zurich, Zurich, Switzerland

Christian G. Peyre, MD
Division of Thoracic and Foregut Surgery, Department of Surgery, University of Rochester School of Medicine and Dentistry, Rochester, New York

Alexander W. Phillips, MA, FRCSEd, FFSTEd
Consultant Oesophagogastric Surgeon, Northern Oesophagogastric Cancer Unit, Royal Victoria Infirmary, Newcastle-upon-Tyne, United Kingdom

Lashmikumar Pillai, MD
Associate Professor of Vascular and Endovascular Surgery, West Virginia University Medical Center, Morgantown, West Virginia

Joseph M. Plummer, MBBS, DM
Department of Surgery, Radiology, and Intensive Care, University of the West Indies, Mona, Jamaica

David T. Pointer Jr., MD
Surgery, Tulane University School of Medicine, New Orleans, Louisiana

Katherine E. Poruk, MD
Surgical Resident, Department of Surgery, The Johns Hopkins Hospital, Baltimore, Maryland

Mitchell C. Posner, MD, FACS
Thomas D. Jones Professor of Surgery and Vice-Chairman, Chief, Section of General Surgery and Surgical Oncology, Physician-in-Chief, The University of Chicago Medicine Comprehensive Cancer Center, The University of Chicago Medicine, Chicago, Illinois

Russell Postier, MD
Chairman, Department of Surgery, University of Oklahoma, Oklahoma City, Oklahoma

Vivek N. Prachand, MD
Associate Professor, Director of Minimally Invasive Surgery, Chief Quality Officer, Executive Medical Director, Procedural Quality and Safety, Section of General Surgery, Department of Surgery, The University of Chicago Medicine and Biological Sciences, Chicago, Illinois

Timothy A. Pritts, MD, PhD
Professor of Surgery, University of Cincinnati, Cincinnati, Ohio

Gregory Quatrino, MD
Surgical Resident, University of South Alabama, Mobile, Alabama

Sagar Ranka, MD
Resident, Department of Internal Medicine, John H. Stroger Hospital of Cook County, Chicago, Illinois

David W. Rattner, MD
Chief, Division of General and Gastrointestinal Surgery, Massachusetts General Hospital; Professor of Surgery, Harvard Medical School, Boston, Massachusetts

Kevin M. Reavis, MD
Division of Gastrointestinal and Minimally Invasive Surgery, The Oregon Clinic, Portland, Oregon

Vikram B. Reddy, MD, PhD
Colon and Rectal Surgery, Yale University School of Medicine, New Haven, Connecticut

Feza H. Remzi, MD, FACS, FTSS (Hon)
Director, Inflammatory Bowel Disease Center, New York University Langone Medical Center; Professor of Surgery, New York University School of Medicine, New York, New York

Rocco Ricciardi, MD, MPH
Chief, Section of Colon and Rectal Surgery, Massachusetts General Hospital, Boston, Massachusetts

Thomas W. Rice, MD
Professor of Surgery, Cleveland Clinic Lerner College of Medicine; Emeritus Staff, Department of Thoracic Cardiovascular Surgery, Cleveland Clinic, Cleveland, Ohio

Aaron Richman, MD
Department of Surgery, Boston Medical Center, Boston, Massachusetts

Paul Rider, MD, FACS, FASCRS
Associate Professor of Surgery, Division of Colon and Rectal Surgery, University of South Alabama, Mobile, Alabama

John Paul Roberts, MD, FACS
Professor and Chief, Division of Transplant Surgery, University of California, San Francisco, San Francisco, California

Patricia L. Roberts, MD
Chair, Department of Surgery, Senior Staff Surgeon, Division of Colon and Rectal Surgery, Lahey Hospital and Medical Center, Burlington, Massachusetts; Professor of Surgery, Tufts University School of Medicine, Boston, Massachusetts

Kevin K. Roggin, MD
Professor of Surgery and Cancer Research, Program Director, General Surgery Residency Program, Associate Program Director, Surgical Oncology Fellowship, The University of Chicago Medicine, Chicago, Illinois

Garrett Richard Roll, MD, FACS
Assistant Professor of Surgery, Department of Surgery, Division of Transplant, University of California, San Francisco, San Francisco, California

Kais Rona, MD
Chief Resident in General Surgery, Keck School of Medicine of the University of Southern California, Los Angeles, California

Charles B. Rosen, MD
Chair, Division of Transplantation Surgery, Mayo Clinic, Rochester, Minnesota

Samuel Wade Ross, MD, MPH
Chief Resident, Department of Surgery, Carolinas Medical Center, Charlotte, North Carolina

J. Scott Roth, MD
Professor of Surgery, Chief, Gastrointestinal Surgery, Department of Surgery, University of Kentucky, Lexington, Kentucky

Amy P. Rushing, MD, FACS
Assistant Professor, Division of Trauma, Critical Care, and Burn, The Ohio State University Wexner Medical Center, Columbus, Ohio

Bashar Safar, MBBS
Assistant Professor of Surgery, Johns Hopkins Medicine, Baltimore, Maryland

Pierre F. Saldinger, MD
Chairman, Surgery, NewYork-Presbyterian/Queens, Flushing, New York

Kamran Samakar, MD, MA
Assistant Professor of Surgery, Division of Upper Gastrointestinal and General Surgery, Keck School of Medicine of the University of Southern California, Los Angeles, California

Kulmeet K. Sandhu, MD, FACS, MS
Assistant Professor of Clinical Surgery, Division of Upper Gastrointestinal and General Surgery, Keck School of Medicine of the University of Southern California, Los Angeles, California

Lara W. Schaheen, MD
Cardiothoracic Surgery Resident, Department of Cardiothoracic Surgery, University of Pittsburgh, Pittsburgh, Philadelphia

Bruce Schirmer, MD
Stephen H. Watts Professor of Surgery, University of Virginia Health System, Charlottesville, Virginia

Andrew Schneider, MD
General Surgery Resident, The University of Chicago Medicine, Chicago, Illinois

Richard D. Schulick, MD, MBA
Professor and Chair, Department of Surgery, University of Colorado School of Medicine, Aurora, Colorado

Ben Schwab, MD, DC
General Surgery Resident, Northwestern University Feinberg School of Medicine, Chicago, Illinois

Stephanie Scurci, MD
Resident, University of Miami Miller School of Medicine, Palm Beach Regional Campus, Palm Beach, Florida

Anthony Senagore, MD, MS, MBA
Professor, Chief of Gastrointestinal Surgery, Surgery, University of Texas–Medical Branch, Galveston, Texas

Adil A. Shah, MD
Resident, Department of Surgery, Howard University Hospital and College of Medicine, Washington, D.C.

Shimul A. Shah, MD
Director, Liver Transplantation and Hepatobiliary Surgery, Associate Professor of Surgery, University of Cincinnati, Cincinnati, Ohio

Brian Shames, MD
Chief, Division of General Surgery, General Surgery Residency Program Director, University of Connecticut Health Center, Farmington, Connecticut

Skandan Shanmugan, MD
Assistant Professor of Surgery, Division of Colon and Rectal Surgery, University of Pennsylvania, Perelman School of Medicine, Philadelphia, Pennsylvania

David S. Shapiro, MD, FACS, FCCM
Chairman, Department of Surgery, Saint Francis Hospital and Medical Center–Trinity Health New England, Hartford, Connecticut; Assistant Professor of Surgery, University of Connecticut School of Medicine, Farmington, Connecticut

Matthew Silviera, MD
Washington University, St. Louis, Missouri

Douglas P. Slakey, MD, MPH, FACS
Professor, Surgery, Tulane University, New Orleans, Louisiana

Joshua Sloan, DO
Division of Gastroenterology, Einstein Healthcare Network, Philadelphia, Pennsylvania

Nathan Smallwood, MD
Division of Colon and Rectal Surgery, Baylor University Medical Center, Dallas, Texas

Shane P. Smith, MD
General Surgery Resident, Department of Surgery, Swedish Medical Center, Seattle, Washington

B. Mark Smithers, MBBS, FRACS, FRCSEng, FRCSEd
Professor of Surgery, University of Queensland; Director, Upper Gastrointestinal and Soft Tissue Unit, Princess Alexandra Hospital, Brisbane, Queensland, Australia

Rory L. Smoot, MD, FACS
Assistant Professor, Mayo Clinic, Rochester, Minnesota

Kevin C. Soares, MD
Resident, General Surgery, Department of Surgery, Johns Hopkins Medical Institutions, Baltimore, Maryland

Edy Soffer, MD
Professor of Clinical Medicine, Director, GI Motility Program, Keck School of Medicine of the University of Southern California, Los Angeles, California

Julia Solomina, MD
Department of Surgery, The University of Chicago, Chicago, Illinois

Nathaniel J. Soper, MD
Loyal and Edith Davis Professor of Surgery, Northwestern University Feinberg School of Medicine; Chair, Department of Surgery, Northwestern Memorial Hospital, Chicago, Illinois

Stuart Jon Spechler, MD
Chief, Division of Gastroenterology, Co-Director, Center for Esophageal Research, Baylor University Medical Center at Dallas; Co-Director, Center for Esophageal Research, Baylor Scott and White Research Institute, Dallas, Texas

Praveen Sridhar, MD
Department of Surgery, Boston Medical Center, Boston, Massachusetts

Scott R. Steele, MD, FACS, FASCRS
Chairman, Department of Colorectal Surgery, Cleveland Clinic; Professor of Surgery, Case Western Reserve University School of Medicine, Cleveland, Ohio

Joel M. Sternbach, MD, MBA
Bechily-Hodes Fellow in Esophagology, Department of Surgery, Northwestern University Feinberg School of Medicine, Chicago, Illinois

Christina E. Stevenson, MD
Assistant Professor of Surgery, Department of Surgery and Neag Comprehensive Cancer Center, University of Connecticut, Farmington, Connecticut

Scott A. Strong, MD
James R. Hines Professor of Surgery, Northwestern University Feinberg School of Medicine, Chicago, Illinois

Iswanto Sucandy, MD
Clinical Instructor, Department of Surgery, University of Pittsburgh School of Medicine, Pittsburgh, Pennsylvania

Magesh Sundaram, MD, MBA, FACS
Senior Associate Medical Director, Carle Cancer Center, Carle Foundation Hospital, Urbana, Illinois

Sudhir Sundaresan, MD, FRCSC, FACS
Surgeon-in-Chief, The Ottawa Hospital; Wilbert J. Keon Professor and Chairman, Department of Surgery, University of Ottawa, Ottawa, Ontario, Canada

Lee L. Swanstrom, MD
The Institute of Image-Guided Surgery of Strasbourg, University of Strasbourg, Strasbourg, Alsace, France; Director, Division of Gastrointestinal and Minimally Invasive Surgery, The Oregon Clinic, Portland, Oregon

Patricia Sylla, MD
Associate Professor of Surgery, Division of Colorectal Surgery, Icahn School of Medicine at Mount Sinai Hospital, New York, New York

Tadahiro Takada, MD, FACS, FRCSEd
Emeritus Professor, Department of Surgery, Teikyo University School of Medicine, Tokyo, Japan

Ethan Talbot, MD
Resident, General Surgery, Bassett Medical Center, Cooperstown, New York

Vernissia Tam, MD
Resident in General Surgery, University of Pittsburgh Medical Center, Pittsburgh, Pennsylvania

Eric P. Tamm, MD
Professor, Diagnostic Imaging, The University of Texas MD Anderson Cancer Center, Houston, Texas

Talar Tatarian, MD
Department of Surgery, Jefferson Gastroesophageal Center, Sidney Kimmel Medical College at Jefferson University, Philadelphia, Pennsylvania

Ali Tavakkoli, MD, FACS, FRCS
Associate Professor of Surgery, Director, Minimally Invasive and Weight Loss Surgery Fellowship, Co-director, Center for Weight Management and Metabolic Surgery, Brigham and Women's Hospital, Harvard Medical School, Boston, Massachusetts

Helen S. Te, MD
Associate Professor of Medicine, Department of Medicine, Center for Liver Diseases, The University of Chicago Medicine, Chicago, Illinois

Ezra N. Teitelbaum, MD, MEd
Foregut Surgery Fellow, Providence Portland Medical Center, Portland, Oregon

Charles A. Ternent, MD, FACS
Section of Colon and Rectal Surgery, Creighton University School of Medicine, University of Nebraska College of Medicine, Omaha, Nebraska

Jon S. Thompson, MD
Professor of Surgery, University of Nebraska Medical Center, Omaha, Nebraska

Iain Thomson, MBBS, FRACS
Senior Lecturer, University of Queensland; Upper Gastrointestinal and Soft Tissue Unit, Princess Alexandra Hospital, Brisbane, Queensland, Australia

Alan G. Thorson, MD, FACS
Clinical Professor of Surgery, Creighton University School of Medicine, University of Nebraska College of Medicine, Omaha, Nebraska

Chad M. Thorson, MD, MSPH
Pediatric Surgery Fellow, Stanford University, Palo Alto, California

Crystal F. Totten, MD
Department of Surgery, University of Kentucky College of Medicine, Lexington, Kentucky

Mark J. Truty, MD, MsC, FACS
Assistant Professor, Mayo Clinic, Rochester, Minnesota

Susan Tsai, MD, MHS
Associate Professor of Surgical Oncology, Department of Surgery, Medical College of Wisconsin, Milwaukee, Wisconsin

Jennifer Tseng, MD
Surgical Oncology Fellow, The University of Chicago, Chicago, Illinois

Tom Tullius, MD
Department of Radiology, The University of Chicago Medicine, Chicago, Illinois

Andreas G. Tzakis, MD, PhD
Director, Transplant Center, Cleveland Clinic Florida, Weston, Florida

J.J.B. van Lanschot, MD, PhD
Professor, Department of Surgery, Erasmus MC–University Medical Center Rotterdam, Rotterdam, The Netherlands

Hjalmar C. van Santvoort, MD, PhD
Department of Surgery, St. Antonius Hospital, Nieuwegein, The Netherlands

Hans Van Veer, MD
Joint Clinical Head, Department of Thoracic Surgery, University Hospital Leuven, Leuven, Belgium

Jorge A. Vega Jr., MD
Department of Surgery, University of South Florida Morsani College of Medicine, Tampa, Florida

Vic Velanovich, MD
Professor, Department of Surgery, University of South Florida Morsani College of Medicine, Tampa, Florida

Sarah A. Vogler, MD, MBA
Clinical Assistant Professor of Surgery, University of Minnesota, Minneapolis, Minnesota

Huamin Wang, MD, PhD
Professor of Pathology, The University of Texas MD Anderson Cancer Center, Houston, Texas

Mark A. Ward, MD
Minimally Invasive Surgery Fellow, Gastrointestinal and Minimally Invasive Surgery, The Oregon Clinic, Portland, Oregon

Brad W. Warner, MD
Division of Pediatric Surgery, St. Louis Children's Hospital, St. Louis, Missouri

Susanne G. Warner, MD
Assistant Professor of Surgery, City of Hope National Medical Center, Duarte, California

Thomas J. Watson, MD, FACS
Professor of Surgery, Georgetown University School of Medicine; Regional Chief of Surgery, MedStar Washington, Washington, D.C.

Irving Waxman, MD
Sara and Harold Lincoln Thompson Professor of Medicine, Director of the Center for Endoscopic Research and Therapeutics, The University of Chicago Medicine and Biological Sciences, Chicago, Illinois

Carissa Webster-Lake, MD
University of Connecticut, Farmington, Connecticut

Benjamin Wei, MD
Assistant Professor, Division of Cardiothoracic Surgery, University of Alabama-Birmingham Medical Center, Birmingham, Alabama

Martin R. Weiser, MD
Stuart H.Q. Quan Chair in Colorectal Surgery, Department of Surgery, Memorial Sloan Kettering Cancer Center; Professor of Surgery, Weill Cornell Medical College, New York, New York

Dennis Wells, MD
Resident in Thoracic Surgery, Department of Surgery, University of Cincinnati College of Medicine, Cincinnati, Ohio

Katerina Wells, MD, MPH
Director of Colorectal Research, Baylor University Medical Center; Adjunct Assistant Professor, Texas A&M Health Science Center, Dallas, Texas

Mark Lane Welton, MD, MHCM
Chief Medical Officer, Fairview Health Services, Minneapolis, Minnesota

Yuxiang Wen, MD
General Surgery, Cleveland Clinic Florida, Weston, Florida

Mark R. Wendling, MD
Acting Instructor and Senior Fellow, Advanced Minimally Invasive Surgery, CVES, Division of General Surgery, University of Washington, Seattle, Washington

Hadley K.H. Wesson, MD
Assistant Professor of Surgery, The Johns Hopkins Hospital, Baltimore, Maryland

Steven D. Wexner, MD, PhD(Hon)
Director, Digestive Disease Center, Chair, Department of Colorectal Surgery, Cleveland Clinic Florida, Weston, Florida

Rebekah R. White, MD
Associate Professor of Surgery, University of California, San Diego, La Jolla, California

Charles B. Whitlow, MD, FACS, FASCRS
Chairman, Department of Colon and Rectal Surgery, Ochsner Clinic Foundation, New Orleans, Louisiana

B.P.L. Wijnhoven, MD, PhD
Department of Surgery, The Erasmus University Medical Center, Rotterdam, The Netherlands

Justin Wilkes, MD
Department of Surgery, Maine Medical Center, Portland, Maine; Research Fellow, Department of Surgery, University of Iowa, Iowa City, Iowa

Rickesha L. Wilson, MD
General Surgical Resident, Department of Surgery, University of Connecticut, Farmington, Connecticut

Piotr Witkowski, MD, PhD
Associate Professor of Surgery, Department of Surgery, The University of Chicago, Chicago, Illinois

Christopher L. Wolfgang, MD, PhD
Chief, Hepatobiliary and Pancreatic Surgery, Professor of Surgery, Pathology, and Oncology, The Johns Hopkins Hospital, Baltimore, Maryland

Stephanie G. Worrell, MD
Surgery, Keck School of Medicine of the University of Southern California, Los Angeles, California

Jian Yang, MD
Department of Liver Transplantation Center, West China Hospital of Sichuan University, Chengdu, Sichuan Province, China

Charles J. Yeo, MD, FACS
Samuel D. Gross Professor and Chair, Department of Surgery, Sidney Kimmel Medical College at Thomas Jefferson University, Philadelphia, Pennsylvania

Ching Yeung, MD
Thoracic Surgery Fellow, University of Ottawa, The Ottawa Hospital–General Campus, Ottawa, Canada

Evan E. Yung, MD
Fellow in Surgical Pathology, Los Angeles County + University of Southern California Medical Center, Los Angeles, California

Syed Nabeel Zafar, MD MPH
Chief Resident, Department of Surgery, Howard University Hospital, Washington, D.C.

Giovanni Zaninotto, MD
Professor, Department of Surgery and Cancer, Imperial College, London, United Kingdom

Herbert Zeh III, MD
Professor of Surgery, Division of Surgical Oncology, University of Pittsburgh Medical Center, Pittsburgh, Pennsylvania

Joerg Zehetner, MD, MMM, FACS
Adjunct Associate Professor of Surgery, Klinik Beau-Site Hirslanden, Berne, Switzerland

Michael E. Zenilman, MD
Professor of Surgery, Weill Cornell Medicine; Chair, Department of Surgery, NewYork-Presbyterian Brooklyn Methodist Hospital, Brooklyn, New York

Pamela Zimmerman, MD
Associate Professor of Vascular and Endovascular Surgery, West Virginia University, Morgantown, West Virginia

Gregory Zuccaro Jr., MD
Department of Gastroenterology and Hepatology, Cleveland Clinic, Cleveland, Ohio

Preface

The time has come to release the eighth edition of the classic textbook *Shackelford's Surgery of the Alimentary Tract*. This publication has served as an important resource for surgeons, internists, gastroenterologists, residents, medical students, and other medical professionals over the past 61 years. I hope that you will find the eighth edition brimming with new information, beautifully illustrated, up to date, and educationally fulfilling.

BRIEF HISTORY

The first edition of *Surgery of the Alimentary Tract* was written solely by Dr. Richard T. Shackelford, a Baltimore surgeon, and was published in 1955. Following the success of the first edition, the book's publisher, W.B. Saunders Company, urged Dr. Shackelford to produce a second edition. Considerable time passed. A second edition was released, as separate five-volume tomes, between 1978 and 1986, with Dr. Shackelford enlisting the assistance of Dr. George D. Zuidema, the Chairman of the Department of Surgery at Johns Hopkins, as co-editor. It was the second edition that served as my "bible" for alimentary tract diseases during my surgical residency and early faculty appointment.

The third edition, edited by Dr. Zuidema, was published as a five-volume set in 1991 and proved to be a major tour de force. The field of alimentary tract surgery had advanced, new research findings were included in the edition, and emerging techniques were illustrated. For the third edition, Dr. Zuidema enlisted the help of a guest editor for each of the five volumes.

The fourth edition, again headed by Dr. Zuidema, was published in 1996 and remained encyclopedic in scope, breadth, and depth of coverage. The textbook had become a classic reference source for surgeons, internists, gastroenterologists, and other health care professionals involved in the care of patients with alimentary tract diseases.

The fifth edition was published in 2002. At that time, Dr. Zuidema asked me to join him as a co-editor. The fifth edition remained a five-volume set, and it was filled with new operative techniques, advances in molecular biology, and noninvasive therapies. It marked progress in the co-management of patients by open surgical, laparoscopic surgical, and endoscopic techniques.

In 2007, the sixth edition of *Shackelford's Surgery of the Alimentary Tract* was published. The look of the sixth edition was changed. The book went from five volumes to two volumes with the deletion of outdated material, and it included a four-color production scheme, emphasized new procedures, and focused on advances in technology. In 2012, the seventh edition was published.

THE EIGHTH EDITION

The eighth edition maintains the exterior changes and look of the sixth and seventh editions. However, the eighth edition has been carefully planned by me and the four expert section editors to represent the current state of alimentary tract surgery as practiced throughout the world. This edition has been completed with an enormous amount of assistance from my four colleagues, who have served as editors for the four major sections of the book. These section editors have worked tirelessly, planning, organizing, and developing this massive textbook. They have incorporated numerous changes in surgical practice, operative techniques, and noninvasive therapies within the text. Although each area does retain sections on anatomy and physiology, the numerous advances in genomics, proteomics, laparoscopic techniques, and robotics are included. The eighth edition includes the contributions of two new and two retained section editors from the seventh edition, providing both innovation and stability.

Section I, Esophagus and Hernia, is now edited by Dr. Steven R. DeMeester, a Professor of Surgery at the University of Southern California, in Los Angeles. Dr. DeMeester is a nationally and internationally known expert who brings his detailed knowledge of the esophagus and esophageal diseases to the textbook. Dr. DeMeester is the son of Dr. Tom DeMeester, a legendary individual who has made numerous contributions to the field. Steve has enlisted new authors for his chapters and has put together a spectacular section on esophageal diseases, including pathology and ambulatory diagnostics, extensive sections on gastroesophageal reflux disease, esophageal motility disorders, and esophageal neoplasia.

Dr. David W. McFadden remains as the editor for Section II, Stomach and Small Intestine. Dr. McFadden works at the University of Connecticut in Farmington, Connecticut, serving as the Professor and Chairman of the Department of Surgery and the Surgeon in Chief of their health system. Dr. McFadden is an expert in alimentary tract diseases, surgical research, and education. He served for many years as the co-editor-in-chief of the *Journal of Surgical Research*, and he has served as the president of the Society for Surgery of the Alimentary Tract. He has done a superb job of enlisting many new chapter authors so as to present an updated section regarding the luminal structures of the upper gastrointestinal system. Dr. McFadden's section is an outstanding contribution to this area.

For Section III, Pancreas, Biliary Tract, Liver, and Spleen, we have retained our section editor, Dr. Jeffrey B. Matthews, the Dallas B. Phemister Professor and Chairman of the Department of Surgery at the University of Chicago, in Chicago, Illinois. Dr. Matthews' surgical career has focused on diseases of the nonluminal structures of the alimentary tract, and he has done a superb job in enlisting new contributors and reorganizing this section. Dr. Matthews' credentials include serving as the editor-in-chief of the *Journal of Gastrointestinal Surgery*, and he is also a recent past president of the Society for Surgery of the Alimentary Tract. This section serves as an outstanding contribution to the field.

Finally, Section IV, Colon, Rectum, and Anus, has been designed and reorganized by Dr. James W. Fleshman, the Seeger Professor and Chairman of the Department of Surgery at Baylor University Medical Center. Dr. Fleshman is an internationally known figure in his field, and his section has been totally reorganized. Included are various new developments in the field, updates on pelvic floor anatomy and physiology, new therapies for inflammatory bowel disease, increased emphasis on laparoscopic interventions, and new chapters dealing with the topics not previously presented.

ACKNOWLEDGMENTS

The eighth edition would have been impossible to complete without the expertise, dedication, and hard work of each of these four expert section editors. They have been helped immensely by their colleagues, staff, and all the chapter contributors. I would like to thank each of these section editors for their vision, dedication, expertise, and incredible hard work in bringing this project to fruition.

As is often the case with printed works of this size, hundreds of individuals have contributed chapters to this edition. In fact, hundreds of contributors are listed in the contributors section. We understand how difficult it is to produce superb chapters, and I wish to recognize these individuals and thank them for their dedication and commitment. Most of these contributors are nationally and internationally known leaders in their fields. I am deeply indebted to them for sharing their knowledge and enthusiasm about their topic, culminating in an outstanding overall product.

I would also like to thank the publishing team at Elsevier, who again have been instrumental in making this edition a reality. My thanks go out to Michael Houston, Mary Hegeler, Amanda Mincher, and many others who have been involved in overseeing this project. This edition represents an enormous amount of new work, and thousands of hours have been spent on its production. These professionals have made it a labor of love to work on this project.

Finally, I must thank individuals who have helped me during this new edition process over the past three years. Here in my office at Thomas Jefferson University, accolades go out to Claire Reinke, Dominique Vicchairelli, and Laura Mateer who have been outstanding assistants in bringing this work to fruition.

Charles J. Yeo, MD

Contents

PART FIVE

Techniques and Pearls

Pancreas, Biliary Tract, Liver, and Spleen

Anatomy, Physiology, and Embryology of the Pancreas

Joseph Fusco | Yousef El-Gohary | George K. Gittes

The term *pancreas* is derived from Greek meaning "all flesh"[1] and developmental biologists have been intrigued for years with the fascinating embryologic development of the pancreas. It is an endodermally derived organ, consisting of two morphologically distinct tissues, the exocrine and endocrine pancreas (Fig. 90.1). Some have even described it as two organs in one due to the disparate function and organization of these two tissues (exocrine and endocrine) within the pancreas.

Given the importance of a better understanding of the embryologic and molecular biologic mechanisms of pancreatic development, we hope in the future to design strategies to generate therapeutically useful tissue (e.g., pancreas or β cells) from stem cells, and better understand the differentiation pathways that may lead to pancreatic cancer.

The morphologic development of the pancreas is dictated by its two major functions, which are the production of digestive enzymes by the exocrine tissue, and the production of metabolically active hormones by the endocrine tissue. These two tissues exist together within the pancreas despite their contrasting morphology and function. The endocrine pancreas, which comprises only 2% of the adult pancreatic mass, is organized into islets of Langerhans consisting of five cell subtypes, α, β, δ, ε, and PP cells, that secrete glucagon, insulin, somatostatin, ghrelin, and pancreatic polypeptide hormones, respectively. The exocrine tissue on the other hand, which forms nearly 98% of the adult pancreatic mass, is composed of acinar and ductal epithelial cells.[1] This chapter reviews the basic anatomic and embryologic development of the pancreas.

BASIC ANATOMY

The human pancreas is a long, tapered, glandular organ, divided into four anatomic domains, the head, neck, body, and tail, along with one accessory lobe or uncinate process, with the head nestled within the curve of the second part of the duodenum. It is situated in a retroperitoneal position, lying obliquely across and behind the stomach with a firm and lobulated smooth surface, extending transversely toward the hilum of the spleen, measuring between 12 and 15 cm long in adults. The digestive enzymes and bicarbonates are secreted by the exocrine-acinar tissue, which then drain into tiny pancreatic tubular ductal networks, eventually joining to form the main pancreatic ducts (ducts of Wirsung and Santorini) to drain into the duodenum via the major duodenal papilla (ampulla of Vater). The main pancreatic duct (derived from the ventral anlage to become the duct of Wirsung and the distal duct of Santorini) may have a separate accessory pancreatic duct (derived from the proximal duct of Santorini), which drains the uncinate process and lower part of the head of the pancreas into the duodenum via the minor duodenal papilla. Incomplete fusion of the dorsal and ventral pancreatic ducts results in pancreas divisum, but numerous anatomic variations of the pancreatic ductal drainage system exist (Fig. 90.2). The endocrine hormones are produced in the islets of Langerhans (which are scattered throughout the pancreas) and drained by a network of capillaries that invade the islet, and are thus delivered into the bloodstream.[2] The distribution of endocrine cells within the islet is species dependent. In rodents, the core of the islet is occupied by the β cells surrounded in the periphery by a ring of α cells, whereas in humans and monkeys, all the endocrine cell types are intermingled.[3] Nonendocrine cells also exist in the islet, including endothelial cells, neurons, dendritic cells, macrophages, and fibroblasts. Pancreatic surgery requires a good understanding of the anatomic relationships of the pancreas with other structures. The pancreatic head lies in front of the inferior vena cava, right renal artery, both renal veins, and the superior mesenteric vessels, whereas the uncinate process lies posterior to the superior mesenteric vessels. The neck of the pancreas lies directly over the portal vein and vertebral bodies L1 and L2. Because the neck lies over those vertebrae, anterior-posterior blunt trauma can lead to pancreatic trauma with possible ductal injury from a direct blow to the epigastrium. The common bile duct passes in a deep groove on the posterior aspect of the pancreatic head until it joins the main pancreatic duct at the ampulla of Vater in the pancreatic parenchyma. The stomach lies anterior to the body and tail of the

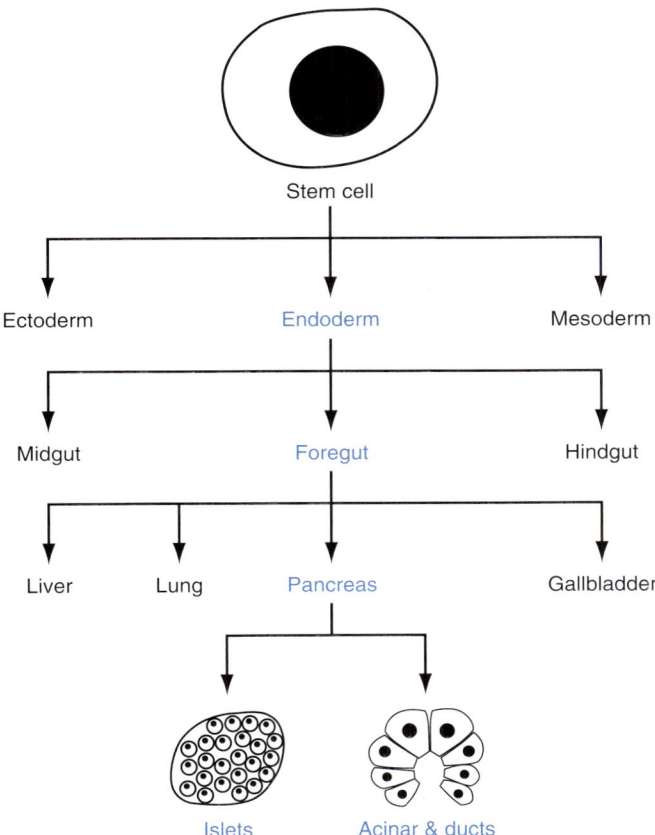

FIGURE 90.1 Cell lineage schematic for pancreatic development from a multipotent progenitor stem cell.

pancreas, whereas the aorta, left adrenal gland, and left kidney lie posterior to the body of the pancreas. The tail lies in the hilum of the spleen with the splenic artery, which is often tortuous, running along the superior border of the pancreas. The major blood supply for the pancreas arises from multiple branches of the celiac trunk and superior mesenteric arteries forming arterial arcades within the body and tail of the pancreas, with the inferior and superior pancreaticoduodenal artery running along the head of the pancreas. Approximately one in every five patients has major variations in the arterial anatomy, such as having the right hepatic artery, which usually originates from the celiac trunk, arising from the superior mesenteric artery (also known as a replaced right hepatic artery) traveling posterior to the pancreatic head toward the liver. Discerning this arterial anomaly is important in preoperative computed tomography (CT) scans to avoid injury (Fig. 90.3).

PHYSIOLOGY

Despite the disparate functions of the endocrine and exocrine parts of the pancreas, the two different components coordinate to regulate and respond to food digestion by secreting different hormones and digestive enzymes, with a regulatory feedback system in place. The pancreas regulates the body's energy metabolism through the

endocrine islet cells of Langerhans, which constitute nearly 2% of the total pancreas. This regulation is delicately balanced through the actions of the hormones insulin and glucagon. Insulin is the hormone of energy storage; it induces an increase in amino acid uptake and facilitates glucose uptake into cells, which increases protein synthesis and decreases lipolysis and glycogenolysis, especially after a meal or in a hyperglycemic state. Glucagon, on the other hand, is viewed as the hormone of energy release; it stimulates higher blood glucose levels by stimulating hepatic gluconeogenesis, glycogenolysis, and lipolysis in the setting of hypoglycemia, and thus counteracts the effects of insulin.

β cells secrete insulin based on blood glucose levels as well as neural and humoral stimuli. The stimulus for insulin release into the bloodstream is far greater when glucose is ingested enterally compared to the parenteral route, indicating that a feed-forward mechanism in the digestive tract is activated, anticipating the rise in blood glucose. This anticipation is mediated by *incretins*. There are two main incretin hormones, glucose-dependent insulinotropic peptide, also known as gastric inhibitory peptide (GIP), and glucagon-like peptide-1 (GLP-1). Both are secreted by endocrine cells located in the small intestinal epithelium when the luminal concentration of glucose increases in the digestive tract, and subsequently they stimulate the β cells to secrete more insulin. Hence, the great interest in the pharmaceutical industry to develop incretin-based therapies to treat diabetes, particularly type 2 diabetes, because of its potent secretagogue effect on β cells. Unlike traditional medications that stimulate β cells to secrete insulin regardless of blood glucose level, incretins augment the β-cell response to blood glucose levels in a glucose-dependent manner, in addition to GLP-1's inhibitory effect on glucagon secretion and the ability to increase food transit time in the stomach.[4,5] Humoral inhibitors for insulin release include somatostatin, amylin, leptin, and pancreastatin. The vagus nerve generally stimulates insulin release, whereas the sympathetic nervous system inhibits it, mediated by various peptidergic molecules secreted from nerve fibers such as substance P, vasoactive intestinal peptide (VIP), and neurotensin.

Exocrine secretion is stimulated by the hormones secretin and cholecystokinin (CCK), and by parasympathetic vagal discharge. The exocrine function is traditionally divided into three phases: (1) the cephalic phase, which is triggered by the sight and smell of food, comprises 10% to 20% of pancreatic excretion; (2) the gastric phase, which is triggered by food entering the stomach and gastric distention, comprises 15% to 20% of enzyme excretion; and (3) the intestinal phase, which is triggered by acidification of the duodenum and proximal jejunum, comprises 60% to 70% of meal-stimulated pancreatic excretion.[6] The exocrine portion of the pancreas is comprised of a ductal tree along with a mass of acinar cells. Acidification and entry of fatty acids along with bile salts in the duodenum stimulate secretin and VIP, in turn leading to the release of a bicarbonate-rich fluid from ductal cells. Vagal stimulation and the entry of either peptides or fatty acids into the duodenum cause release of CCK and acetylcholine, producing the secretion of a digestive enzyme–rich fluid from the acinar cells.

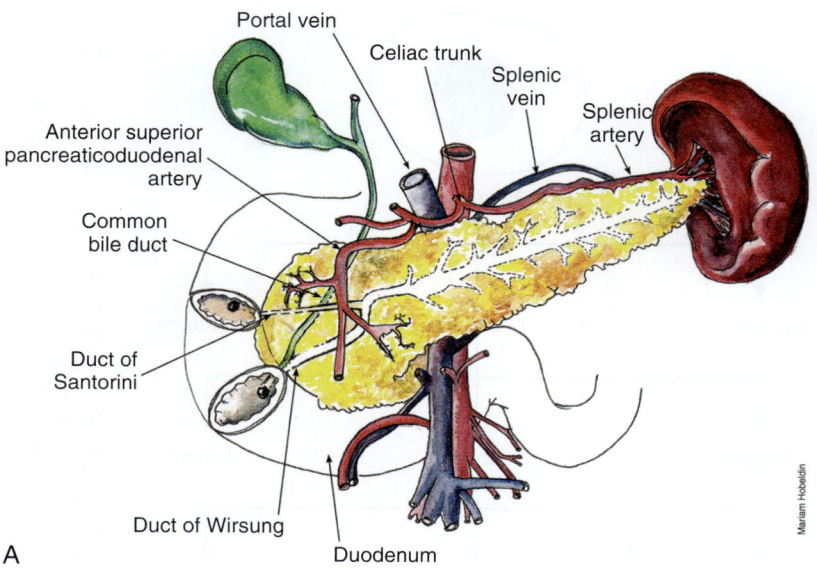

A

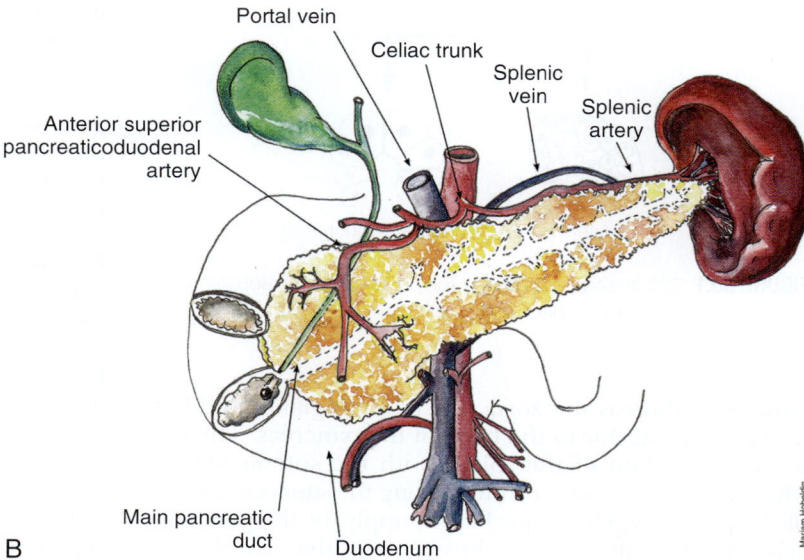

B

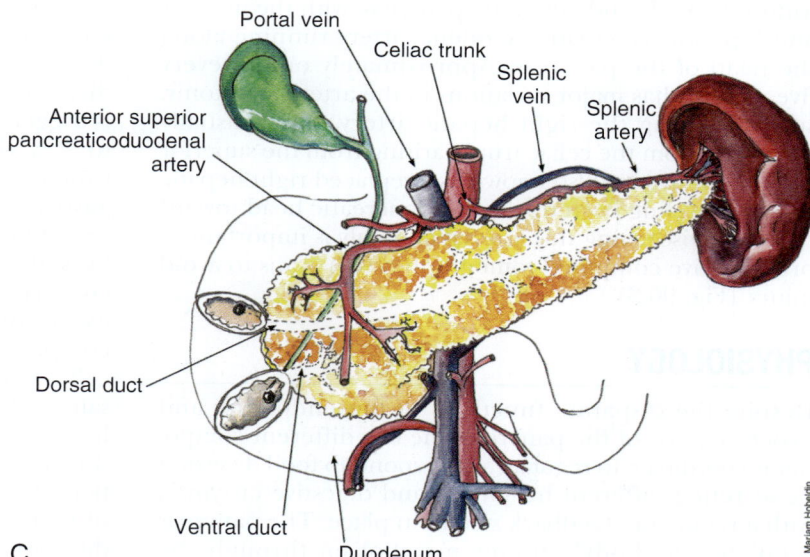

C

FIGURE 90.2 (A–D) Schematic illustration of the anatomic relationship of the pancreas in relation to other anatomic structures.

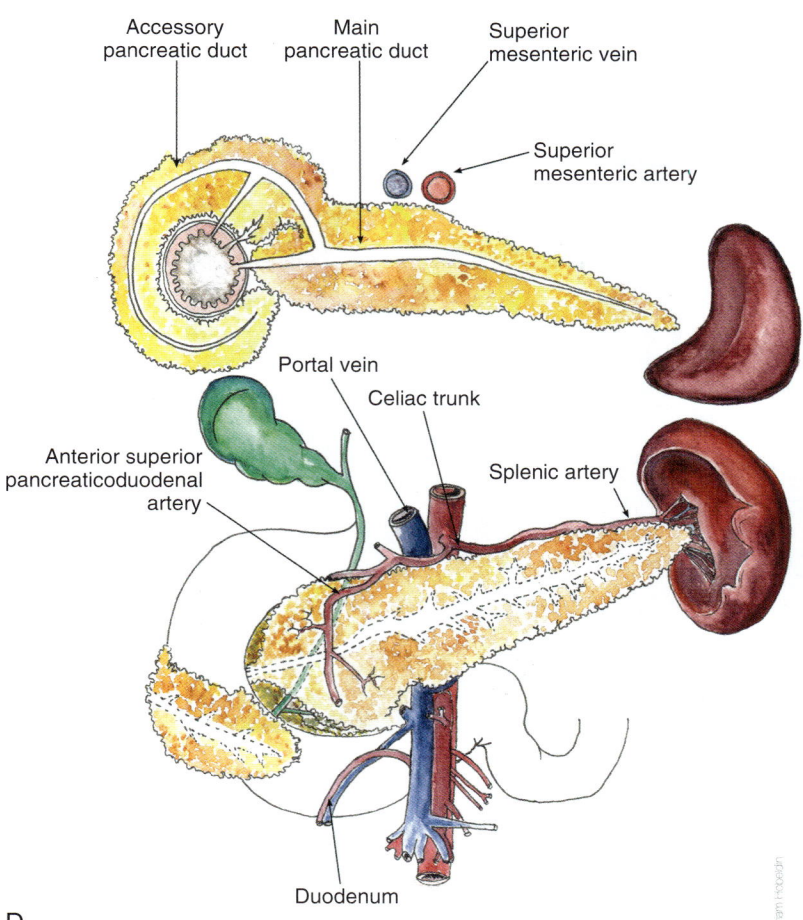

Accessory pancreatic duct

Main pancreatic duct

Superior mesenteric vein

Superior mesenteric artery

Portal vein

Celiac trunk

Anterior superior pancreaticoduodenal artery

Splenic artery

Duodenum

D

FIGURE 90.2, cont'd

Currently, the most widely accepted model of bicarbonate secretion from the ductal cells involves the diffusion of carbon dioxide into the cell from the circulation, where it is hydrated by carbonic anhydrase to form H_2CO_3. H_2CO_3 dissociates into H^+ and HCO_3^-. The bicarbonate is transported into the ductal space by a chloride/bicarbonate exchanger. Secretin binds to receptors on the basolateral membrane, activating adenylate cyclase to produce cyclic adenosine monophosphate (cAMP). cAMP in turn activates the cystic fibrosis transmembrane regulator (CFTR) on the luminal cell surface, allowing for the passage of chloride into the ductal space. The passage of bicarbonate and chloride across the ductal cell membrane generates an ionic and osmotic gradient causing sodium and water to follow.[7] Defects in CFTR lead to both acute and chronic pancreatitis through ductal and glandular obstruction secondary to the inability to hydrate the ductal molecules in the lumen.[8,9] The lack of chloride ions flowing into the lumen prevents the formation of an ionic and osmotic gradient. Therefore, sodium and water do not cross into the lumen, producing a low volume, thickened secretion and subsequent blockage. Pancreatitis is rarely a complication in individuals with mutations of both CFTR alleles because this results in rapid destruction of the pancreas beginning in utero. Patients experience the loss of acinar cells, which are a necessary nidus for pancreatitis, leading to pancreatic insufficiency.[9,10]

Along with bicarbonate secretion, the second arm of pancreatic exocrine function involves the release of digestive enzymes from the acinar cells. Digestive enzymes are synthesized in their inactive form within acinar cells and are packaged into zymogen granules. The granules migrate to the cell surface and fuse to the cell membrane releasing their contents in response to vagal stimulation, peptides, and fatty acids. Some enzymes, including amylase, lipase, RNase, and DNase are synthesized in their active forms, but most (trypsinogen, chymotrypsinongen, procarboxypeptidase, and proelastase) are inactive upon release. The intestinal brush border enzyme, enteropeptidase, cleaves trypsinogen to its active form, trypsin. Trypsin cleaves and activates the remaining digestive enzymes. More than 40 mutations in cationic trypsinogen *(PRSS1),* the gene that encodes trypsin, have been uncovered. The mutations often cause the premature activation of trypsinogen to trypsin, producing a condition characterized by recurrent episodes of pancreatitis ultimately leading to pancreatic insufficiency.[11]

Serum amylase is usually measured to diagnose pancreatitis, which is usually 2.5 times normal within 6 hours after the onset of an acute episode, and then returns to normal within 3 to 7 days. However, the major limitation of serum amylase measurement to diagnose pancreatitis is the lack of specificity because several clinical conditions can result in elevated amylase. In addition, a normal

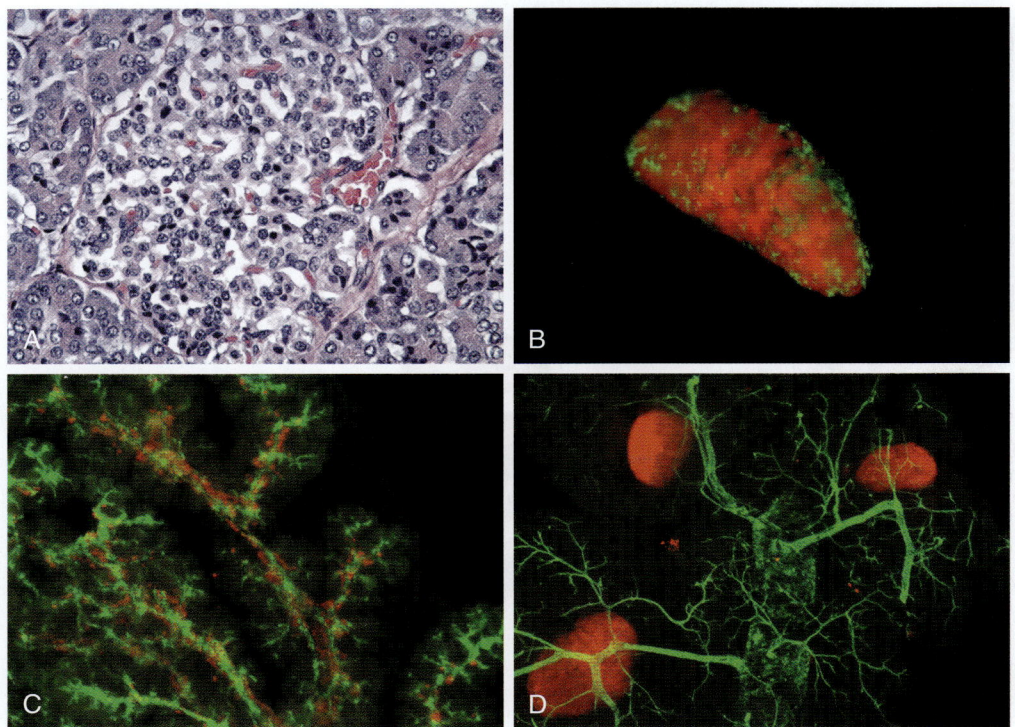

FIGURE 90.3 (A) Standard histologic section of a human pancreas specimen illustrating a small, relatively pale-staining cell known as the islet of Langerhans, which is embedded in darker-stained exocrine tissue. (B) Adult mouse pancreas whole mount image showing an isolated islet stained with insulin, with glucagon in the periphery. (C) Whole mount image of embryonic day 16.5 pancreas illustrating the close relationship between insulin cells and pancreatic ducts. (D) Whole mount image of an adult mouse pancreas stained with insulin and Dolichos biflorus agglutinin for pancreatic ducts.

serum amylase certainly does not exclude pancreatitis. The amylase-to-creatinine ratio (ACR) may help in differentiating acute pancreatitis from other conditions using the following equation:

$$(Urine_{amy}\,U/L \times Serum_{Cr}\,mg/dL)/$$
$$(Serum_{amy}\,U/L/Urine_{Cr}\,mg/dL) \times 100$$

An ACR greater than 5% suggests acute pancreatitis, and ratios less than 1% suggest macroamylasemia. Serum lipase levels, on the other hand, are believed to be more specific in diagnosing pancreatic tissue damage because lipase is only produced in the pancreas. Lipase tends to be higher in alcoholic pancreatitis and the amylase level higher in gallstone pancreatitis, hence the lipase-to-amylase ratio has been suggested as means to distinguish between the two.

BASIC PANCREATIC EMBRYOLOGY

The embryonic pancreas is known to pass through three stages of development.[12] The first is the undifferentiated stage where the endoderm evaginates to initiate pancreatic morphogenesis, with only insulin and glucagon genes being expressed at this stage.[13] The second phase involves epithelial branching morphogenesis with simultaneous formation of primitive ducts. This stage involves the separation of islet progenitors beginning to differentiate and losing their attachments to the basement membrane.[14] The third and final stage begins with the formation of

acinar cells at the apices of the ductal structures, with the development of zymogen granules containing enzymes. Acinar cells usually commence enzyme secretion shortly after birth.[12,15]

During early development, the pancreas initiates by the regional specification of the undifferentiated primitive endodermal foregut tube by these transcription factors: pancreatic and duodenal homeobox 1 (Pdx1), which marks the prepancreatic endoderm, and pancreas-specific transcription factor 1a (PTF1a), where both are expressed in multipotent pancreatic progenitor cells.[16] The pancreas first appears morphologically as a mesenchymal condensation at the level of the duodenal anlagen, distal to the stomach on the dorsal aspect of the foregut tube at embryonic day (E) 9.0 in mice. All cells expressing Pdx1 and PTF1a in the endoderm will eventually give rise to the epithelial cells in the adult pancreas, which includes endocrine, acinar, and duct cells.[1] At around E9.5 gestation in mice and the 26th day of gestation in humans, the dorsal bud begins to evaginate into the overlying mesenchyme while retaining luminal continuity with the gut tube.[17] Approximately 12 hours later in mice, and 6 days after dorsal bud evagination in humans, the ventral bud begins to arise. Gut rotation will bring the ventral lobe dorsally, ultimately fusing with the dorsal pancreatic bud (this event corresponds to around the sixth to seventh week of gestation in humans or E12 to E13 in mice) contributing to the formation of the uncinate process and inferior part of the head of the pancreas, while the rest of the pancreas arises from the dorsal pancreatic bud.

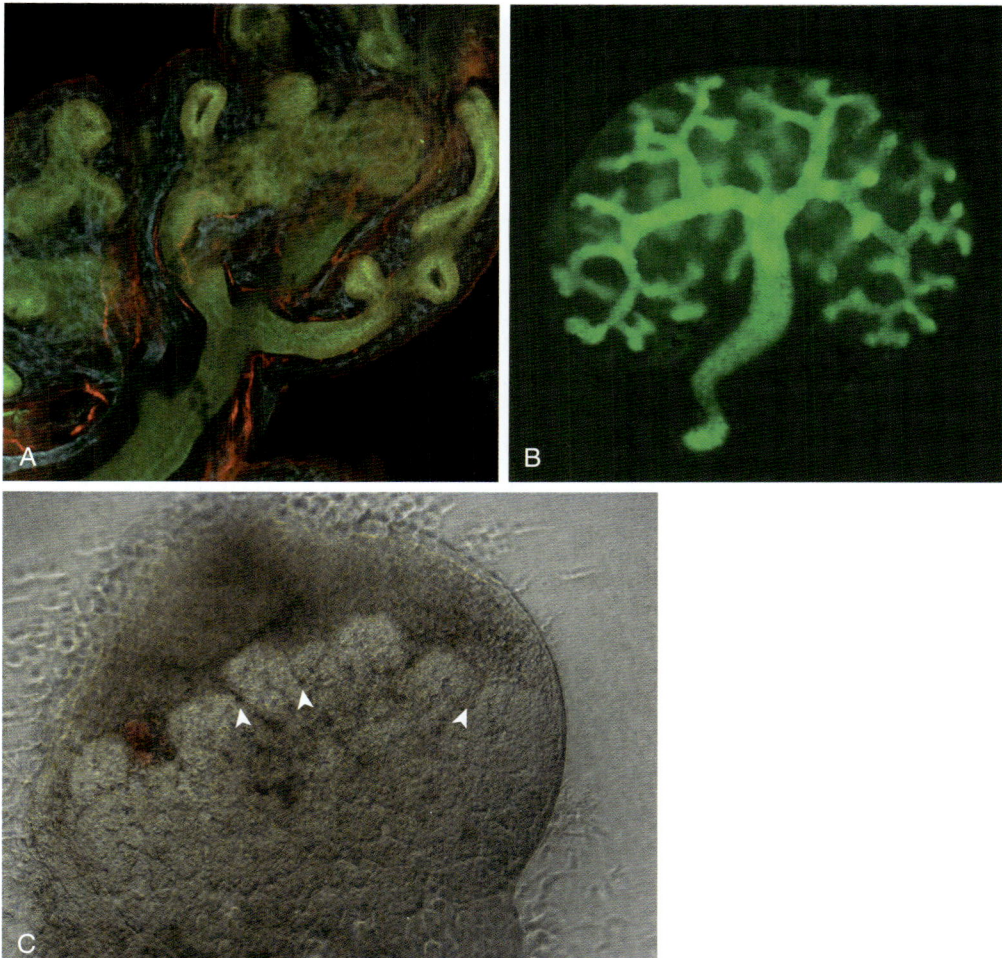

FIGURE 90.4 Pancreatic branching morphogenesis is different from other organ systems such as lung and kidney. (A) Whole mount of E12.5 lung stained for Ecad, PGP9.5 (a neuronal marker), and CD31. (B) E11.5 kidney cultured for 3 days and stained with the epithelial marker Calbindin-D28k, both demonstrating 90-degree branching pattern. (C) E11 whole pancreas from CD-1 cultured for 5 days revealing acute branching pattern mesenchymal exclusion zones *(arrowheads)*. Mesenchyme contains factors that regulate pancreatic growth and differentiation.

The entire ventral pancreatic duct and the distal part of the dorsal pancreatic duct fuse together to form the main pancreatic duct of Wirsung. The remaining proximal part of the dorsal pancreatic duct is either obliterated or persists as a small accessory pancreatic duct of Santorini.[18] This fusion and evagination of the two buds is followed by elongation of the pancreatic bud stalk region (precursor to the main pancreatic duct) and branching morphogenesis of the apical region of the bud. Unlike the usual branching morphogenesis growth patterns seen in the developing kidney, lung, and salivary gland, in which the branching morphogenesis occurs at 90-degree angles, the pancreas grows in an acute-angled branching pattern, which leads to the exclusion or "squeezing out" of mesenchyme from between the closely apposed branches of epithelium (Fig. 90.4). This exclusion of mesenchyme may influence epithelial-mesenchymal interactions and lineage selection. The pancreas then undergoes major amplification of the endocrine cell population through two distinct waves of differentiation within the pancreatic epithelium during embryogenesis, an early primary wave (pre E13.5 in mice),

followed by the secondary wave of differentiation (E13.5 to E16.5 in mice).[1] Over a similar gestational window, the exocrine pancreatic precursors undergo an exponential increase in branching morphogenesis and acinar cell differentiation.

DORSAL AND VENTRAL PANCREATIC BUD DEVELOPMENT

It is important to note that although the morphologic development of the ventral and dorsal pancreatic buds may be similar, they differ markedly at the molecular level, with various lines of evidence suggesting that there are differences in the specification between the pancreatic rudiments, with the notochord playing a key role. Sonic hedgehog (Shh), which is a potent intercellular patterning molecule, is expressed along the entire foregut, but is noticeably suppressed in the prospective pancreatic endoderm. This suppression of Shh appears to be necessary for dorsal pancreatic development, permitting the expression of pancreas-specific genes including Pdx1 and insulin. Deletion of the notochord in chick embryo cultures leads to ectopic Shh being seen in the pancreatic region of the foregut endoderm, with subsequent failure of the pancreas to develop.[19] Activin-βB (a member of the transforming growth factor-β family) and fibroblast growth factor (FGF) 2 both mimic notochord activity in inducing pancreatic genes.[19] In stark contrast to the dorsal bud, developmental gene expression in the ventral pancreatic anlage is not affected when the notochord is removed.[20] The ventral pancreas, on the other hand, develops under the control of signals from the overlying cardiogenic mesenchyme, which also produces prohepatic signals (FGFs) to induce liver formation. Lack of prohepatic FGF signaling in regions of the cardiogenic mesenchyme will lead to the endoderm differentiating into ventral pancreas by default.[21] When ventral foregut endoderm is cultured in the absence of cardiac mesoderm or FGF, it fails to activate liver-specific genes, with Pdx1 being expressed instead. Cardiac mesoderm, through FGF, induces liver formation from the ventral endoderm, and simultaneously inhibits pancreatic development.[21] Further differences between ventral and dorsal pancreas are demonstrated in Hlxb9 mutant mice. The homeobox gene Hlxb9, which is transiently expressed in the endoderm in the region of the dorsal and ventral pancreatic anlage, when inactivated in mice, only dorsal pancreatic development is blocked.[22] Hematopoietically expressed homeobox 1 (Hex1) is an early marker of the anterior endoderm[23] and is expressed at E7.0 in the cells that will subsequently give rise to the ventral pancreas and liver. Hex-null mutant embryos have specific failure of ventral pancreatic bud development, with the dorsal bud developing normally.[24] These examples underscore the significantly different molecular controls governing dorsal and ventral pancreatic bud development.

INITIATION OF THE PANCREAS WITH ENDODERMAL PATTERNING

The signaling molecules that govern the specification of the primitive gut tube into different specialized domains remain yet to be fully elucidated.[25] The pancreas and other endoderm-derived organs develop through a series of reciprocal interactions between the endoderm and the surrounding mesenchyme, which is a critical step in initiating organ specification or *endodermal patterning* along the anterior-posterior axis of the foregut endoderm. Endodermal patterning is manifested by the regional expression of transcription factors in the primitive gut tube; for example, Hex1 and Nkx2.1 (also known as thyroid transcription factor 1) are expressed at E8.5 in defined foregut domains along the anterior-posterior axis of the primitive gut tube, giving rise to liver and lung/thyroid, respectively. Pdx1 and PTF1a are coexpressed in the foregut-midgut endoderm boundary, defining the pancreas and duodenum, whereas Cdx1, and Cdx4 (early markers of posterior endoderm) are expressed in the posterior midgut and hindgut domains that will give rise to the small and large intestines. Thus, various domains of the primitive gut tube are specified (Fig. 90.5).[26,27]

Mesenchyme-induced endodermal patterning is necessary before the initiation of organogenesis. When the pancreatic mesenchyme is removed from the pancreatic epithelium in explant cultures, it results in disrupted pancreatic cell differentiation, with the endocrine lineage being favored over exocrine.[12]

The primitive gut tube is divided into three domains, foregut, midgut, and hindgut regions, each of which will give rise to specialized structures.[16] This subdivision into presumptive gut tube domains is governed by different molecular markers in the gastrula stage endoderm (E7.5).[16,28,29] The endoderm toward the anterior side of the embryo generates the ventral foregut, which will later give rise to the liver, lung, thyroid, and the ventral pancreas. The dorsal region of the definitive endoderm, on the other hand, contributes to the formation of the esophagus, stomach, dorsal pancreas, duodenum, and intestines. The pancreas has been found to form as a result of the actions of some key specific transcription factors and signaling pathways. For example, FGF4 and Wnt signaling from the posterior mesoderm are specifically inhibited in the anterior endoderm to allow foregut development. FGF signaling is required to initially determine, and then to maintain gut tube domains, as demonstrated with cultured mouse endoderm and by in vivo studies in chick embryos. FGF4 is normally expressed in the mesoderm and ectoderm adjacent to the developing midgut-hindgut endoderm, and when isolated mouse endoderm was cultured in the presence of high concentrations of FGF4, a posterior (intestinal) endoderm was induced. On the other hand, lower concentrations of FGF4 induced a more anterior (pancreas-duodenal) cell fate. Similarly, when chick embryos are treated in vivo with FGF4, the Hex1 (anterior endodermal marker) expression domain was reduced, whereas CdxB (posterior endodermal marker) expression expanded anteriorly, inhibiting the development of the foregut.[27,30] Therefore, FGF4 plays a critical role in endodermal patterning by repressing anterior (foregut) fate and promoting posterior (intestinal) endoderm fate. Another molecular pathway that has linked endodermal patterning to the initiation of pancreatic development is Wnt/β-catenin signaling, as demonstrated in frog (*Xenopus*) studies.[31] β-catenin repression in the anterior endoderm is specifically necessary to initiate liver and pancreas development, and to maintain foregut identity. Conversely, forcing high β-catenin activity in the posterior endoderm promotes intestinal development and inhibits foregut development into liver and pancreas. McLin et al.[31] demonstrated that forced β-catenin expression in the anterior endoderm (where β-catenin is usually repressed) led to downregulation of Hhex, as well as other foregut markers for liver (*for1*), pancreas (*pdx1*), lung/thyroid (*nkx2.1*), and intestine (*endocut*),[28] resulting in inhibition of foregut fate, namely liver and pancreas formation. Repressing β-catenin in the posterior endoderm (future hindgut that normally expresses β-catenin) induced ectopic liver and pancreas markers (hhex, Pdx1, elastase, and amylase) with subsequent ectopic liver bud initiation and pancreas development.[31] The homeobox-containing gene Hhex, is a direct target of β-catenin, is one of the earliest foregut markers,[23] and is essential for normal liver and ventral pancreas development in mice.[24,32] *Hex* expression

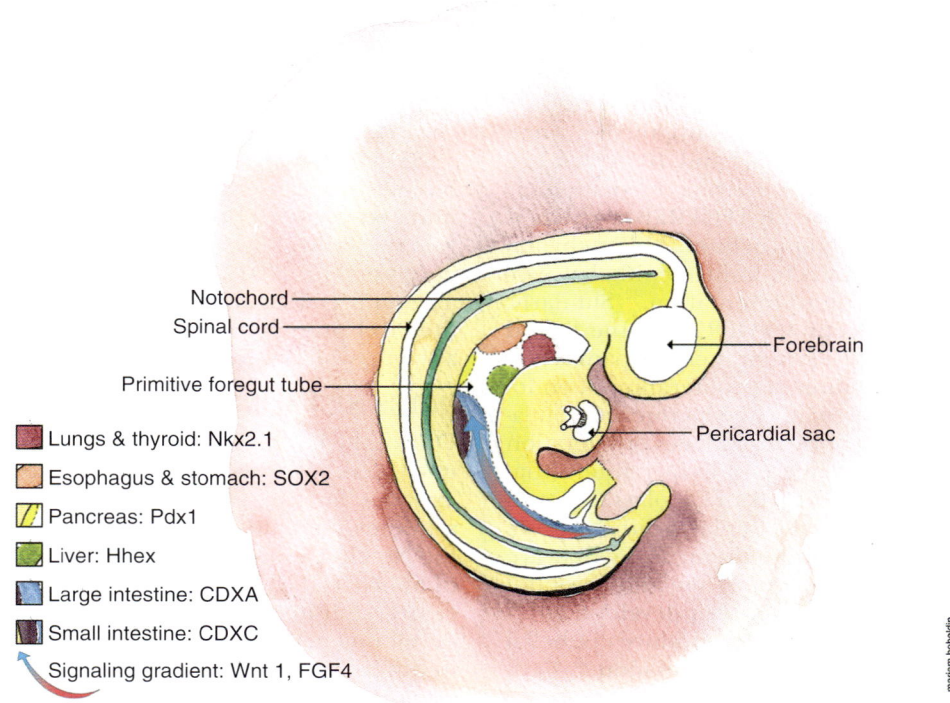

FIGURE 90.5 Schematic representation of the regional specification of the primitive foregut tube (~E8.5) with the various transcription factors. Wnt and FGF4, which are secreted from the posterior mesoderm in a gradient, repress foregut fate and promote hindgut development. Wnt and FGF4 inhibition in the anterior endoderm promotes foregut fate.

was noted to have an important role in the specification and differentiation of the ventral pancreas, where Hex$^{-/-}$ null mutant mouse embryos lacked a ventral pancreas, and lacked liver, thyroid, and parts of the forebrain.[24,33]

Retinoic acid (RA) signaling has been implicated as an important molecule for endodermal patterning in zebrafish. RA signaling is necessary for specification and differentiation of both liver and pancreas.[34] As with RA, bone morphogenetic protein (BMP) signaling has also been shown to have a role in endodermal patterning and in the normal development of the pancreas in zebrafish, but neither RA nor BMP affect the induction of endodermal precursors.[35] Targeted disruption of the Pdx1 gene in mice also prevented pancreatic development.[36] A critical role for Pdx1 in pancreatic initiation and patterning of foregut endoderm in mice was further demonstrated by humans with Pdx1 mutations being apancreatic.[37] Despite our growing knowledge of many molecular signals mediating cross-talk between the pancreatic mesenchyme and the epithelium, most pathways remain poorly understood.

PANCREATIC MESENCHYME

The pancreatic mesenchyme, which envelops the pancreatic epithelium after regional specification, contains important factors that are pivotal for pancreatic morphogenesis. These factors promote growth and differentiation of the developing pancreas, specifically inducing growth of the endocrine cell population and rapid branching

morphogenesis.[1] The pancreatic mesenchyme helps regulate lineage selection by the pancreatic epithelium between the endocrine and exocrine lineages during early stages of pancreatic development.[1,12] This interaction between pancreatic mesenchyme and epithelium is a vital process for pancreatic development. Pure pancreatic epithelium (E11) cultured without its mesenchyme failed to develop at all; however, the epithelium grew into a fully differentiated pancreas (acinar, ductal, and endocrine structures), when cultured with its mesenchyme.[12] The pancreatic mesenchyme has a pro-exocrine effect on the epithelium through cell-cell contact, and also a pro-endocrine effect, mediated by diffusible factors secreted from the mesenchyme.[38] Mesenchymal contact with the epithelium both enhances notch signaling (Hes1), which favors the acinar lineage, and also inhibits neurogenin 3 (Ngn3) expression leading to the suppression of endocrine differentiation.[39] The default differentiation of the pancreatic epithelium in the absence of mesenchyme is endocrine.[12] Interestingly, culturing pure pancreatic epithelium in a basement membrane–rich gel, without its mesenchyme, led to the predominant formation of ductal structures. These results suggest that the basement membrane has factors or components that are conducive to ductal development.[12] To further illustrate the importance of the mesenchyme and mesenchymal signaling in embryonic and organ development, when the normal embryonic separation that occurs between the spleen and the pancreas-associated mesenchyme does not occur in Bapx1-null mutant embryos, the dorsal pancreatic bud becomes intestinalized.[40] Activin

A, which is expressed in the splenic mesenchyme, is a possible mediator for this transdifferentiation because exposing pancreatic buds to activin A in an in vitro culture system also leads to intestinalization.[41]

Some signaling pathways have been implicated in mediating this epithelial-mesenchymal interaction, such as the FGFs. Specifically, FGFs 1, 7, and 10, which are expressed in the pancreatic mesenchyme, mediate their effects through FGF receptor 2B (FGFR2B), which is expressed in the pancreatic epithelium. Mesenchymal FGF signaling has been shown to induce epithelial proliferation, favoring exocrine differentiation.[42] Similarly, null mutations for the receptor FGFR2B or the ligand FGF10 lead to blunting of early branching pancreatic morphogenesis, with inhibition of proliferation of endocrine progenitor cells and premature endocrine differentiation, indicating that FGF10 normally induces proliferation of epithelial cells and prevents endocrine differentiation.[43,44] Despite the positive role that FGF plays in dorsal pancreatic development, it seems to play a different role in ventral pancreatic bud development. FGFs that are secreted from the cardiogenic mesenchyme inhibit ventral pancreatic bud formation and favor liver development.[21] BMP ligands in pancreatic mesenchyme induce epithelial branching and inhibit endocrine differentiation.[45]

KEY SIGNALING MOLECULES

TRANSFORMING GROWTH FACTOR-BETA SIGNALING

Transforming growth factor-beta (TGF-β) superfamily signaling has been implicated in many developmental processes, including pancreatic development. The superfamily consists of three main subfamilies, TGF-β isoforms (numbered 1 to 3 in mammals), BMPs, and activins. In brief, a TGF-β ligand binds to the serine-threonine kinase receptor type 2, which phosphorylates the type 1 receptor. This phosphorylation leads to the phosphorylation of SMADs at a serine region at the C-terminus, which are in turn translocated to the nucleus with SMAD4 to effect transcription. In β cells, this pathway serves to suppress proliferation. Conversely, the proliferative stimulation of β cells comes from factors such as epidermal growth factor (EGF) and hepatocyte growth factor (HGF), which produce phosphorylation in the linker region of the SMAD proteins as opposed to the C-terminus. These signals are terminated through ubiquitination or proteasomal degradation.

TGF-β isoform receptors during the early stages of pancreatic development are distributed throughout the pancreatic epithelium and mesenchyme, but then gradually become restricted to the pancreatic islets and ducts.[46] TGF-β ligands (TGF-β1, -β2, and -β3), on the other hand, are specifically localized to the pancreatic embryonic epithelium as early as E12.5, and then progressively become focused to the acinar cells, where they mediate their actions through TGF-β receptor type II.[46] Blocking TGF-β signaling in the embryonic pancreas, either through in vivo overexpression of a dominant-negative TGF-β type II receptor, or with an in vitro TGF-β-specific pan-neutralizing antibody, leads to a profound increase in the number of proliferating endocrine cells, especially

in the periductal area.[46] Thus overall, TGF-β isoform signaling suppresses the formation of endocrine cells from the ducts in the embryonic pancreas, and TGF-β isoform inhibition promotes pancreatic ductal epithelial cell proliferation and differentiation into endocrine cells.[46]

SMADs have gained interest among developmental biologists because SMAD4 was specifically identified as mutated in 50% of pancreatic cancers.[47] However, a key role for SMAD4 has not been identified yet in pancreatic development.[48] SMAD7 on the other hand, which acts as a general TGF signaling inhibitor, when expressed under the Pdx1 promoter, resulted in a 90% decrease in β cells at birth, which were replaced by glucagon cells.[49]

NOTCH SIGNALING

One of the key decisions that a pancreatic progenitor cell must make is whether to enter the endocrine or the exocrine lineage. Notch signaling has been identified as a master regulator of this fate decision.[50] Activation of the Notch receptor leads to activation of Hairy-Enhancer of Split 1 (HES1) and repression of genes such as Ngn3 (a prerequisite marker for pancreatic endocrine lineage development).[50] Notch also serves to maintain cells in an undifferentiated progenitor-like state. Impairing Notch signaling leads to premature differentiation of pancreatic progenitor cells into endocrine cells. However, the exact mechanism for Notch signaling in pancreatic lineage selection remains elusive, and ambiguity still surrounds the exact role of Notch signaling in pancreatic development.

HEDGEHOG SIGNALING

The mammalian hedgehog family consists of Shh, desert hedgehog (Dhh), and Indian hedgehog (Ihh). Shh signaling is essential for foregut differentiation toward a gastrointestinal fate[51] and its suppression in the prospective pancreatic endoderm is a prerequisite for pancreas formation. However, hedgehog signaling in pancreatic development appears to be complex. Targeted deletion of Shh in the foregut of mice does not lead to an expanded pancreatic field as would be expected.[52,53] Null mutant mice for Ihh develop a small pancreas, indicating a pro-pancreatic role for Ihh.[54] Furthermore, combining an Shh-null mutation with a heterozygous mutation for Ihh results in an annular pancreas.

There appears to be a link between aberrant Hh signaling and pancreatic exocrine neoplasia, with the upregulation of Shh ligand being observed in noninvasive lesions preceding pancreatic adenocarcinoma.[55] In addition, it has been demonstrated that Shh ligand secreted by pancreatic cancer epithelium binds to stromal cells in a paracrine fashion, causing proliferation and *desmoplasia*.[56–58] Clinical trials are in place to neutralize and target Hh molecules in patients with pancreatic adenocarcinoma.[59] Shh was not believed to be expressed in the normal pancreas[19] until recently when Strobel et al.[60] identified expression in a specialized compartment within the proximal ductal system, known as the pancreatic duct glands (PDGs), which are blind-ending outpouches that specifically produce Shh ligand. When exposed to chronic injury, PDGs grow, a condition that is associated with an upregulation of Shh expression (along with gastric mucins and other progenitor markers such as Pdx1 and hes1). This process leads to Shh-mediated mucinous gastrointestinal metaplasia with features of a pancreatic intraepithelial neoplasia (PanIN). PanINs are pancreatic cancer precursor lesions of unclear origin that are known to aberrantly express Shh and gastrointestinal mucins. They are thought to arise from ducts, and thus PDGs may be the missing link between Shh, mucinous metaplasia, and neoplasia.[51]

Wnt SIGNALING

Wnt signaling plays a role in early endodermal specification of pancreas because β-catenin repression in the anterior endoderm is necessary to initiate liver and pancreas development (see earlier in this chapter). However, beyond endodermal patterning, Wnt signaling has multiple pancreatic roles that depend on the time and place of Wnt signaling. Transgenic expression of Wnt1 or Wnt5a in the pancreatic epithelium leads to pancreatic agenesis or severe hypoplasia, respectively, confirming that early Wnt signaling is detrimental to pancreatic development. Others found a role for Wnt signaling in promoting postnatal pancreatic growth,[61] illustrating the complex and multiple roles that Wnt signaling plays in pancreatic development.

ENDOTHELIAL CELLS AND OXYGEN TENSION

It has been shown that cells exposed to low oxygen tension go through adaptive changes such as anaerobic metabolism, increased angiogenesis, and erythropoeisis.[62] In pancreatic development, β-cell differentiation seems to be influenced by oxygen tension. A key mediator for this adaptive response by cells is the hypoxia-inducible factor (HIF).[63] HIF1α is expressed strongly in the rat pancreatic epithelium and mesenchyme at E11.5, then gradually decreases and is virtually undetectable by birth. Hypoxia leads to the stabilization of HIF1α, resulting in absent Ngn3 expression and thus arresting β-cell differentiation. Increasing oxygen tension leads to upregulation of β-cell differentiation with degradation of HIF1α, and restoration of Ngn3. Similarly, inhibiting the degradation of HIF1α resulted in the repression of Ngn3 and arrest of β-cell differentiation, even in normoxia.[63]

ENDOTHELIAL CELLS

Pancreatic islets are highly vascularized, embedded in a capillary network that is 5 to 10 times denser than that of the exocrine pancreas, and allow efficient secretion of islet hormones into the bloodstream[64] (Fig. 90.6). Islet transplantation entails an enzymatic digestion process that also removes some intraislet endothelial cells. This endothelial removal may take away an important vascular niche for the β cells.[65,66] During development, β cells aggregate to form islets, and express high levels of vascular endothelial growth factors (VEGF) to attract endothelial cells.[67] β cells that are deficient in VEGF-A form islets with fewer capillaries, and experimental overexpression of VEGF-A has improved islet graft vascularization.[67,68] Thus, there is an intimate relationship between blood vessels and the pancreatic cells during embryonic development.

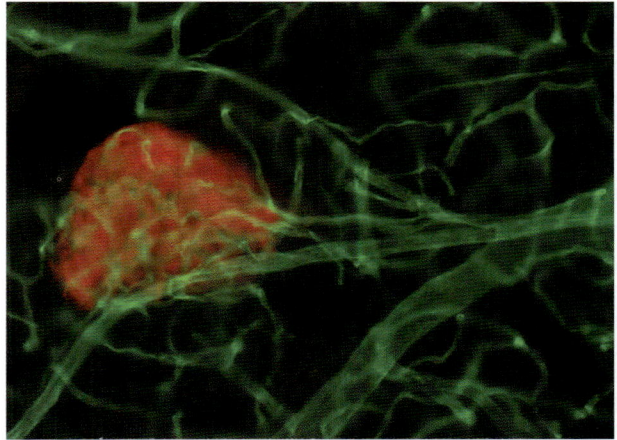

FIGURE 90.6 Whole mount adult mouse pancreas, stained with CD31 and insulin demonstrating the complex microcapillary network within the islet.

As the embryonic pancreas progresses through the different developmental stages, it receives signals from different adjacent structures, including notochord, cardiac mesoderm, and the dorsal aortae. Removal of the dorsal aorta from *Xenopus* embryos led to the absence of pancreatic endocrine development.[69] In addition, aortic endothelial cells can induce dorsal pancreatic bud and β-cell formation in vitro from endoderm. Interestingly, ventral pancreas development seems not to be dependent on the endothelium, despite its close proximity to the vitelline veins.[70] This difference was corroborated in a human with aortic coarctation. The patient lacked the pancreatic body and tail, but not the head of the pancreas, with the latter arising from the ventral bud, which develops independently of the aortae.[71] Here, the prospective pancreatic endoderm presumably lost the inducing signal from the "narrowed" aorta, leading specifically to dorsal pancreatic agenesis.

EXTRACELLULAR MATRIX

The pancreatic epithelium is contained within a continuous sheath of basement membrane, which constitutes the epithelial-mesenchymal interface, and plays an important role in guiding pancreatic development.[72] Basement membrane has also been shown to play an important role in regulating branching morphogenesis in many other organs, with laminin and collagen IV the major protein components of all basement membranes.[73] Laminin-1 was found to induce duct formation in isolated E11 mouse pancreatic epithelium,[12] and to mediate the pro-exocrine inductive effect of the mesenchyme, as well as the pro-β-cell role later in gestation.[38,74] β cells are unable to form their own basement membrane but depend on the endothelial cells to produce a vascular basement membrane. Endothelial cells also produce collagen IV, which interacts with $\alpha_1\beta_1$ integrin to increase insulin secretion.[75] Calcium-dependent adhesion molecules (cadherins), which are critical for cell-cell adhesion, play an essential role in migration and differentiation of pancreatic endocrine progenitor cells. E-cadherin and R-cadherin are initially localized to the ducts, and then become downregulated in endocrine progenitor cells as they move out of the ducts to form islets.[76,77] The neural cell adhesion molecule (NCAM) is expressed in mature α and PP cells[78] and is necessary for aggregation of endocrine cells within the islet.[79]

GLUCAGON

The first detectable endocrine cells during pancreatic development are the glucagon-containing cells at around E9 in the mouse, and recent studies have shown that glucagon signaling is necessary for early differentiation of insulin-expressing cells, which appear at E10 to E13.[17,80] Glucagon is generated from pro-glucagon by the action of pro-hormone convertase 2 (PC2). When PC2 or the glucagon receptor is knocked out, mutant mice lack glucagon and have delayed islet cell differentiation and maturation, but still show the large amplification of insulin-positive cells ("secondary wave") later in gestation.[81] Furthermore, exogenous addition of exendin-4, a GLP-1 analogue, was able to rescue the delay in early insulin differentiation and was shown also to be able to convert rat pancreatic acinar cells (AR42J) and rat pancreatic ductal cells (ARIP) into insulin-expressing cells.[80,82] These studies strongly support the role of glucagon signaling, through its receptor, in initiating early insulin differentiation. Recently it has been demonstrated that α cells can be reprogrammed to form new β cells during regeneration after ablating nearly 99% of the existing β cells.[83]

TRANSCRIPTION FACTORS

PANCREATIC AND DUODENAL HOMEOBOX 1

Transcription factors are key elements for orchestrating the formation of all endocrine and exocrine cell lineages, and their roles have been extensively studied in pancreatic development. The most heavily studied transcription factor is Pdx1, one of the earliest markers of pancreatic progenitors, and is later expressed only in β cells. It is expressed in the pre-pancreatic region of the primitive foregut tube at E8.5, then expands to be expressed in the distal stomach; common bile duct, and duodenum by E10.5 to E11.5.[1] Pdx1 is initially expressed throughout the epithelium; however, its expression becomes suppressed in cells as they commit to the endocrine lineage or ducts. It then reappears as cells differentiate into the insulin-positive β-cell lineage. Pdx1-null mutant mice and humans that lack the Pdx1 gene have pancreatic agenesis.[37] Delayed Pdx1 inhibition using a tetracycline regulatable transgenic knock-in system demonstrated severe blunting of pancreatic development with complete absence of acini and β cells,[84] indicating that Pdx1 continues to have a role in pancreas development beyond early regional specification during endodermal patterning.

PANCREAS-SPECIFIC TRANSCRIPTION FACTOR 1a

PTF1a is an early marker of pancreatic progenitor cells, is expressed slightly later than Pdx1 at around E9.5, and then becomes localized to the acini by E18.5.[85] PTF1a-null mutant mice develop severe pancreatic hypoplasia and absent acini and ducts, an observation that is similar to that seen in Pdx1-null mutant mice; however endocrine cells still develop and, interestingly, the endocrine cells migrate out through the pancreatic mesenchyme to form islets in the spleen.[86] A PTF1a nonfunctioning mutation has been seen in humans, where they are born without a pancreas.[87]

NEUROGENIN 3

Ngn3 is one of the earliest markers specific to the pancreatic endocrine lineage and is required for endocrine lineage development. It is first expressed at E11.0, and then peaks at around E15.5.[88] Ngn3 is believed to be antagonized by Notch signaling through Hes1 in cells with an acinar fate.[89] Ngn3 cells proliferate, giving rise to postmitotic endocrine progenitor cells expressing transcription factors neuroD, nkx6.1, and pax6. Ngn3 shuts off at around E17.5.[88,89] When Ngn3 is deleted from cells, it leads to the absence of the four endocrine cell types (α, β, δ, and PP), which produce glucagon, insulin, somatostatin, and pancreatic polypeptide, respectively.[90] Thus, Ngn3 appears to be a critical and essential factor for pancreatic endocrine differentiation, acting as a pro-endocrine gene. However, how exactly Ngn3 controls the subsequent specification of different endocrine subtypes remains to be fully elucidated. In humans, Ngn3 is not detected between weeks 16 and 38, but reappears scattered throughout the pancreas and the islet.[91] Ngn3 does not colocalize with insulin or Pdx1, which correlates with mouse studies where NGN3 is extinguished when hormone-positive cells appear.[90,92]

Rfx6

Rfx6 is a transcription factor downstream of Ngn3 that has been identified as a key pro-endocrine regulator that directs islet cell differentiation. It is initially expressed broadly in gut endoderm, particularly in Pdx1-positive cells in the prospective pancreatic region, and then becomes restricted to the endocrine lineage in postmitotic islet progenitor cells. Mice that are null-mutant for Rfx6 fail to generate all islet cell types except pancreatic polypeptide cells (insulin, glucagon, somatostatin, and ghrelin). A human syndrome of neonatal diabetes (patients lack pancreatic endocrine cells) with bowel atresia was shown to have mutations in the Rfx6 gene.[93] Thus, Rfx6 is dependent on Ngn3 and is a unique regulator of islet cell development.

Nkx2.2

Nkx2.2 is expressed as early as E9.5, is coexpressed with Pdx1 as a marker of multipotent pancreatic progenitor cells, and eventually becomes restricted to Ngn3-positive cells, persisting in all endocrine lineages except for δ cells.[94] Nkx2.2-null mutant mice develop with no β cells, reduced PP cells, 80% reduction in α cells, but no effect on δ cells. Interestingly, a large number of ghrelin-positive ε cells with no glucagon coexpression were seen, indicating that Nkx2.2 normally induces insulin-positive differentiation and represses ε-cell formation.[94]

MafA/B

There are two distinct waves of amplification of the endocrine cell population, primary (pre-E13.5) and secondary (E13.5 to E16.5) transition periods. MafB is expressed in endocrine cells during both waves. As insulin-positive cells form into mature β cells, MafB turns off and the cells then express MafA.[95] MafA is first expressed only in the secondary wave β cells and in adult β cells. MafA is a critical regulator of the insulin gene, and is viewed as the only transcription factor specific to β cells as well as a marker of a mature β cell. However, it is not absolutely necessary for β-cell formation because mafA-null mutant mice have a normal proportion of insulin-positive cells at birth.[96]

Sox9

Sox9 is a marker for those pancreatic progenitor cells that can give rise to all pancreatic cell types, and is necessary for maintaining those cells in a progenitor state.[97] Postnatally, sox9 expression becomes restricted to the ductal and centroacinar cell compartment.[98] Sox9 mutants display pancreatic hypoplasia as a result of depletion of the pancreatic progenitor pool[98] (Fig. 90.7).

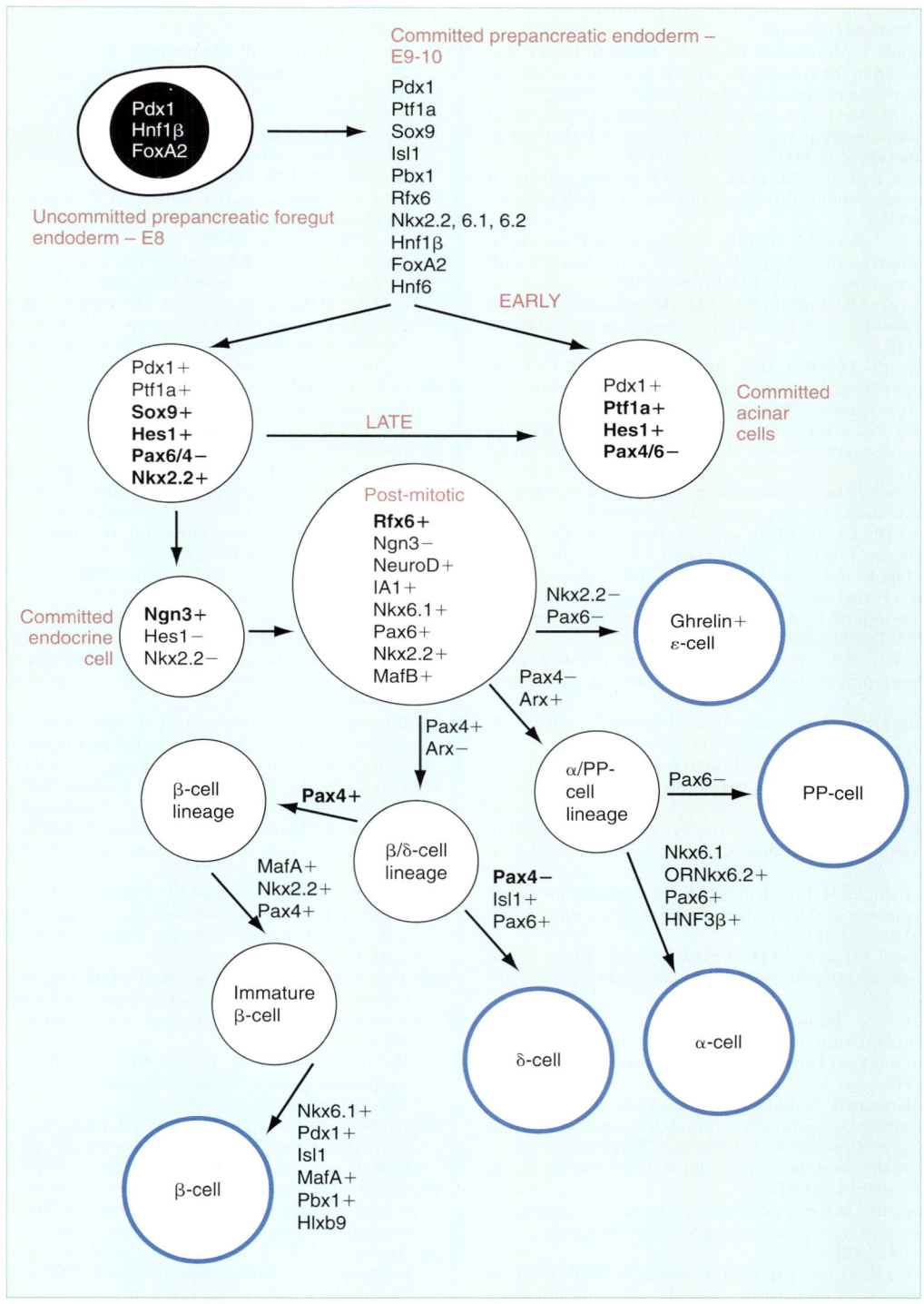

FIGURE 90.7 Overview of the pancreatic endocrine and exocrine cell lineage. *Bold* terms are the key actors in the pathway.

REFERENCES

1. Gittes GK. Developmental biology of the pancreas: a comprehensive review. *Dev Biol.* 2009;326(1):4-35.
2. Gray S, Russo K. *Gray's Anatomy.* Woodstock, IL: Dramatic Publishing; 2008:69.
3. Kim A, Miller K, Jo J, Kilimnik G, Wojcik P, Hara M. Islet architecture: a comparative study. *Islets.* 2009;1(2):129-136.
4. Baggio LL, Drucker DJ. Biology of incretins: GLP-1 and GIP. *Gastroenterology.* 2007;132(6):2131-2157.
5. Scheen AJ, Radermecker RP. Addition of incretin therapy to metformin in type 2 diabetes. *Lancet.* 2010;375(9724):1410-1412.
6. Konturek SJ, Zabielski R, Konturek JW, Czarnecki J. Neuroendocrinology of the pancreas; role of brain-gut axis in pancreatic secretion. *Eur J Pharmacol.* 2003;481(1):1-14.
7. Montero A, Bragado J, Alonso RM, Garcia LJ, Calvo JJ, Lopez MA. Mechanisms involved in the control of exocrine pancreatic secretion in the interdigestive state in the rabbit. *Rev Esp Fisiol.* 1993;49(2):93-99.
8. Ahmed N, Corey M, Forstner G, et al. Molecular consequences of cystic fibrosis transmembrane regulator (CFTR) gene mutations in the exocrine pancreas. *Gut.* 2003;52(8):1159-1164.
9. Kristidis P, Bozon D, Corey M, et al. Genetic determination of exocrine pancreatic function in cystic fibrosis. *Am J Hum Genet.* 1992;50(6):1178-1184.
10. Durno C, Corey M, Zielenski J, Tullis E, Tsui LC, Durie P. Genotype and phenotype correlations in patients with cystic fibrosis and pancreatitis. *Gastroenterology.* 2002;123(6):1857-1864.
11. Whitcomb DC, Gorry MC, Preston RA, et al. Hereditary pancreatitis is caused by a mutation in the cationic trypsinogen gene. *Nat Genet.* 1996;14(2):141-145.
12. Gittes GK, Galante PE, Hanahan D, Rutter WJ, Debase HT. Lineage-specific morphogenesis in the developing pancreas: role of mesenchymal factors. *Development.* 1996;122(2):439-447.
13. Gittes GK, Rutter WJ. Onset of cell-specific gene expression in the developing mouse pancreas. *Proc Natl Acad Sci USA.* 1992;89(3):1128-1132.
14. Argent BE, Githens S, Kalser S, Longnecker DS, Metzgar R, Williams JA. The pancreatic duct cell. *Pancreas.* 1992;7(4):403-419.
15. Kolacek S, Puntis JW, Lloyd DR, Brown GA, Booth IW. Ontogeny of pancreatic exocrine function. *Arch Dis Child.* 1990;65(2):178-181.
16. Moore-Scott BA, Opoka R, Lin SC, Kordich JJ, Wells JM. Identification of molecular markers that are expressed in discrete anterior-posterior domains of the endoderm from the gastrula stage to mid-gestation. *Dev Dyn.* 2007;236(7):1997-2003.
17. Pictet RL, Clark WR, Williams RH, Rutter WJ. An ultrastructural analysis of the developing embryonic pancreas. *Dev Biol.* 1972;29(4):436-467.
18. Sadler TW, Langman J. *Langman's Medical Embryology.* 10th ed. Philadelphia: Lippincott Williams & Wilkins; 2006:xiii-371.
19. Hebrok M, Kim SK, Melton DA. Notochord repression of endodermal Sonic hedgehog permits pancreas development. *Genes Dev.* 1998;12(11):1705-1713.
20. Kim SK, Hebrok M, Melton DA. Notochord to endoderm signaling is required for pancreas development. *Development.* 1997;124(21):4243-4252.
21. Deutsch G, Jung J, Zheng M, Lora J, Zaret KS. A bipotential precursor population for pancreas and liver within the embryonic endoderm. *Development.* 2001;128(6):871-881.
22. Li H, Arber S, Jessell TM, Edlund H. Selective agenesis of the dorsal pancreas in mice lacking homeobox gene Hlxb9. *Nat Genet.* 1999;23(1):67-70.
23. Thomas PQ, Brown A, Beddington RS. Hex: a homeobox gene revealing peri-implantation asymmetry in the mouse embryo and an early transient marker of endothelial cell precursors. *Development.* 1998;125(1):85-94.
24. Bort R, Martinez-Barbera JP, Beddington RS, Zaret KS. Hex homeobox gene-dependent tissue positioning is required for organogenesis of the ventral pancreas. *Development.* 2004;131(4):797-806.
25. Wells JM, Melton DA. Vertebrate endoderm development. *Annu Rev Cell Dev Biol.* 1999;15:393-410.
26. Ehrman LA, Yutzey KE. Anterior expression of the caudal homologue cCdx-B activates a posterior genetic program in avian embryos. *Dev Dyn.* 2001;221(4):412-421.
27. Dessimoz J, Opoka R, Kordich JJ, Grapin-Botton A, Wells JM. FGF signaling is necessary for establishing gut tube domains along the anterior-posterior axis in vivo. *Mech Dev.* 2006;123(1):42-55.
28. Costa RM, Mason J, Lee M, Amaya E, Zorn AM. Novel gene expression domains reveal early patterning of the *Xenopus* endoderm. *Gene Expr Patterns.* 2003;3(4):509-519.
29. Grapin-Botton A. Antero-posterior patterning of the vertebrate digestive tract: 40 years after Nicole Le Douarin's PhD thesis. *Int J Dev Biol.* 2005;49(2-3):335-347.
30. Shamim H, Mason I. Expression of Fgf4 during early development of the chick embryo. *Mech Dev.* 1999;85(1-2):189-192.
31. McLin VA, Rankin SA, Zorn AM. Repression of Wnt/beta-catenin signaling in the anterior endoderm is essential for liver and pancreas development. *Development.* 2007;134(12):2207-2217.
32. Keng VW, Yagi H, Ikawa M, et al. Homeobox gene Hex is essential for onset of mouse embryonic liver development and differentiation of the monocyte lineage. *Biochem Biophys Res Commun.* 2000;276(3):1155-1161.
33. Martinez Barbera JP, Clements M, Thomas P, et al. The homeobox gene Hex is required in definitive endodermal tissues for normal forebrain, liver and thyroid formation. *Development.* 2000;127(11):2433-2445.
34. Stafford D, Hornbruch A, Mueller PR, Prince VE. A conserved role for retinoid signaling in vertebrate pancreas development. *Dev Genes Evol.* 2004;214(9):432-441.
35. Tiso N, Filippi A, Pauls S, Bortolussi M, Argenton F. BMP signalling regulates anteroposterior endoderm patterning in zebrafish. *Mech Dev.* 2002;118(1-2):29-37.
36. Ahlgren U, Jonsson J, Edlund H. The morphogenesis of the pancreatic mesenchyme is uncoupled from that of the pancreatic epithelium in IPF1/PDX1-deficient mice. *Development.* 1996;122(5):1409-1416.
37. Stoffers DA, Zinkin NT, Stanojevic V, Clarke WL, Habener JF. Pancreatic agenesis attributable to a single nucleotide deletion in the human IPF1 gene coding sequence. *Nat Genet.* 1997;15(1):106-110.
38. Li Z, Manna P, Kobayashi H, Spilde T, et al. Multifaceted pancreatic mesenchymal control of epithelial lineage selection. *Dev Biol.* 2004;269(1):252-263.
39. Duvillie B, Attali M, Bounacer A, Ravassard P, Basmaciogullari A, Scharfmann R. The mesenchyme controls the timing of pancreatic beta-cell differentiation. *Diabetes.* 2006;55(3):582-589.
40. Asayesh A, Sharpe J, Watson RP, et al. Spleen versus pancreas: strict control of organ interrelationship revealed by analyses of Bapx1$^{-/-}$ mice. *Genes Dev.* 2006;20(16):2208-2213.
41. van Eyll JM, Pierreux CE, Lemaigre FP, Rousseau GG. Shh-dependent differentiation of intestinal tissue from embryonic pancreas by activin A. *J Cell Sci.* 2004;117(Pt 10):2077-2086.
42. Elghazi L, Cras-Meneur C, Czernichow P, Scharfmann R. Role for FGFR2IIIb-mediated signals in controlling pancreatic endocrine progenitor cell proliferation. *Proc Natl Acad Sci USA.* 2002;99(6):3884-3889.
43. Bhushan A, Itoh N, Kato S, et al. Fgf10 is essential for maintaining the proliferative capacity of epithelial progenitor cells during early pancreatic organogenesis. *Development.* 2001;128(24):5109-5117.
44. Pulkkinen MA, Spencer-Dene B, Dickson C, Otonkoski T. The IIIb isoform of fibroblast growth factor receptor 2 is required for proper growth and branching of pancreatic ductal epithelium but not for differentiation of exocrine or endocrine cells. *Mech Dev.* 2003;120(2):167-175.
45. Ahnfelt-Ronne J, Ravassard P, Pardanaud-Glavieux C, Scharfmann R, Serup P. Mesenchymal bone morphogenetic protein signaling is required for normal pancreas development. *Diabetes.* 2010;59(8):1948-1956.
46. Tulachan SS, Tei E, Hembree M, et al. TGF-beta isoform signaling regulates secondary transition and mesenchymal-induced endocrine development in the embryonic mouse pancreas. *Dev Biol.* 2007;305(2):508-521.
47. Hahn SA, Schutte M, Hoque AT, et al. DPC4, a candidate tumor suppressor gene at human chromosome 18q21.1. *Science.* 1996;271(5247):350-353.
48. Bardeesy N, Cheng KH, Berger JH, et al. Smad4 is dispensable for normal pancreas development yet critical in progression and tumor biology of pancreas cancer. *Genes Dev.* 2006;20(22):3130-3146.
49. Smart NG, Apelqvist AA, Gu X, et al. Conditional expression of Smad7 in pancreatic beta cells disrupts TGF-beta signaling and induces reversible diabetes mellitus. *PLoS Biol.* 2006;4(2):e39.
50. Apelqvist A, Li H, Sommer L, et al. Notch signalling controls pancreatic cell differentiation. *Nature.* 1999;400(6747):877-881.
51. Maitra A. Tracking down the hedgehog's lair in the pancreas. *Gastroenterology.* 2010;138(3):823-825.

52. Litingtung Y, Lei L, Westphal H, Chiang C. Sonic hedgehog is essential to foregut development. *Nat Genet.* 1998;20(1):58-61.

53. Ramalho-Santos M, Melton DA, McMahon AP. Hedgehog signals regulate multiple aspects of gastrointestinal development. *Development.* 2000;127(12):2763-2772.

54. Hebrok M, Kim SK, St Jacques B, McMahon AP, Melton DA. Regulation of pancreas development by hedgehog signaling. *Development.* 2000;127(22):4905-4913.

55. Pasca di Magliano M, Sekine S, Ermilov A, Ferris J, Dlugosz AA, Hebrok M. Hedgehog/Ras interactions regulate early stages of pancreatic cancer. *Genes Dev.* 2006;20(22):3161-3173.

56. Yauch RL, Gould SE, Scales SJ, et al. A paracrine requirement for hedgehog signalling in cancer. *Nature.* 2008;455(7211):406-410.

57. Bailey JM, Swanson BJ, Hamada T, et al. Sonic hedgehog promotes desmoplasia in pancreatic cancer. *Clin Cancer Res.* 2008;14(19):5995-6004.

58. Olive KP, Jacobetz MA, Davidson CJ, et al. Inhibition of Hedgehog signaling enhances delivery of chemotherapy in a mouse model of pancreatic cancer. *Science.* 2009;324(5933):1457-1461.

59. Hidalgo M, Maitra A. The hedgehog pathway and pancreatic cancer. *N Engl J Med.* 2009;361(21):2094-2096.

60. Strobel O, Rosow DE, Rakhlin EY, et al. Pancreatic duct glands are distinct ductal compartments that react to chronic injury and mediate Shh-induced metaplasia. *Gastroenterology.* 2010;138(3):1166-1177.

61. Heiser PW, Lau J, Taketo MM, Herrera PL, Hebrok M. Stabilization of beta-catenin impacts pancreas growth. *Development.* 2006;133(10):2023-2032.

62. Semenza GL. Life with oxygen. *Science.* 2007;318(5847):62-64.

63. Heinis M, Simon MT, Ilc K, et al. Oxygen tension regulates pancreatic beta-cell differentiation through hypoxia-inducible factor 1alpha. *Diabetes.* 2010;59(3):662-669.

64. Eberhard D, Kragl M, Lammert E. 'Giving and taking': endothelial and beta-cells in the islets of Langerhans. *Trends Endocrinol Metab.* 2010;21(8):457-463.

65. Couzin J. Diabetes. Islet transplants face test of time. *Science.* 2004;306(5693):34-37.

66. Konstantinova I, Lammert E. Microvascular development: learning from pancreatic islets. *Bioessays.* 2004;26(10):1069-1075.

67. Lammert E, Gu G, McLaughlin M, et al. Role of VEGF-A in vascularization of pancreatic islets. *Curr Biol.* 2003;13(12):1070-1074.

68. Zhang N, Richter A, Suriawinata J, et al. Elevated vascular endothelial growth factor production in islets improves islet graft vascularization. *Diabetes.* 2004;53(4):963-970.

69. Lammert E, Cleaver O, Melton D. Induction of pancreatic differentiation by signals from blood vessels. *Science.* 2001;294(5542):564-567.

70. Yoshitomi H, Zaret KS. Endothelial cell interactions initiate dorsal pancreas development by selectively inducing the transcription factor Ptf1a. *Development.* 2004;131(4):807-817.

71. Kapa S, Gleeson FC, Vege SS. Dorsal pancreas agenesis and polysplenia/heterotaxy syndrome: a novel association with aortic coarctation and a review of the literature. *JOP.* 2007;8(4):433-437.

72. Hisaoka M, Haratake J, Hashimoto H. Pancreatic morphogenesis and extracellular matrix organization during rat development. *Differentiation.* 1993;53(3):163-172.

73. Hallmann R, Horn N, Selg M, Wendler O, Pausch F, Sorokin LM. Expression and function of laminins in the embryonic and mature vasculature. *Physiol Rev.* 2005;85(3):979-1000.

74. Jiang FX, Georges-Labouesse E, Harrison LC. Regulation of laminin 1-induced pancreatic beta-cell differentiation by alpha6 integrin and alpha-dystroglycan. *Mol Med.* 2001;7(2):107-114.

75. Kaido T, Yebra M, Cirulli V, Montgomery AM. Regulation of human beta-cell adhesion, motility, and insulin secretion by collagen IV and its receptor alpha1beta1. *J Biol Chem.* 2004;279(51):53762-53769.

76. Dahl U, Sjodin A, Semb H. Cadherins regulate aggregation of pancreatic beta-cells in vivo. *Development.* 1996;122(9):2895-2902.

77. Sjodin A, Dahl U, Semb H. Mouse R-cadherin: expression during the organogenesis of pancreas and gastrointestinal tract. *Exp Cell Res.* 1995;221(2):413-425.

78. Cirulli V, Baetens D, Rutishauser U, Halban PA, Orci L, Rouiller DG. Expression of neural cell adhesion molecule (N-CAM) in rat islets and its role in islet cell type segregation. *J Cell Sci.* 1994;107 (Pt 6):1429-1436.

79. Esni F, Taljedal IB, Perl AK, Cremer H, Christofori G, Semb H. Neural cell adhesion molecule (N-CAM) is required for cell type segregation and normal ultrastructure in pancreatic islets. *J Cell Biol.* 1999;144(2):325-337.

80. Prasadan K, Daume E, Preuett B, et al. Glucagon is required for early insulin-positive differentiation in the developing mouse pancreas. *Diabetes.* 2002;51(11):3229-3236.

81. Vincent M, Guz Y, Rozenberg M, et al. Abrogation of protein convertase 2 activity results in delayed islet cell differentiation and maturation, increased alpha-cell proliferation, and islet neogenesis. *Endocrinology.* 2003;144(9):4061-4069.

82. Zhou J, Wang X, Pineyro MA, Egan JM. Glucagon-like peptide 1 and exendin-4 convert pancreatic AR42J cells into glucagon- and insulin-producing cells. *Diabetes.* 1999;48(12):2358-2366.

83. Thorel F, Nepote V, Avril I, et al. Conversion of adult pancreatic alpha-cells to beta-cells after extreme beta-cell loss. *Nature.* 2010;464(7292):1149-1154.

84. Holland AM, Hale MA, Kagami H, Hammer RE, MacDonald RJ. Experimental control of pancreatic development and maintenance. *Proc Natl Acad Sci USA.* 2002;99(19):12236-12241.

85. Cras-Meneur C, Li L, Kopan R, Permutt MA. Presenilins, Notch dose control the fate of pancreatic endocrine progenitors during a narrow developmental window. *Genes Dev.* 2009;23(17):2088-2101.

86. Kawaguchi Y, Cooper B, Gannon M, Ray M, MacDonald RJ, Wright CV. The role of the transcriptional regulator Ptf1a in converting intestinal to pancreatic progenitors. *Nat Genet.* 2002;32(1):128-134.

87. Sellick GS, Barker KT, Stolte-Dijkstra I, et al. Mutations in PTF1A cause pancreatic and cerebellar agenesis. *Nat Genet.* 2004;36(12):1301-1305.

88. Gu G, Dubauskaite J, Melton DA. Direct evidence for the pancreatic lineage: NGN3+ cells are islet progenitors and are distinct from duct progenitors. *Development.* 2002;129(10):2447-2457.

89. Jensen J, Heller RS, Funder-Nielsen T, et al. Independent development of pancreatic alpha- and beta-cells from neurogenin3-expressing precursors: a role for the notch pathway in repression of premature differentiation. *Diabetes.* 2000;49(2):163-176.

90. Gradwohl G, Dierich A, LeMeur M, Guillemot F. Neurogenin3 is required for the development of the four endocrine cell lineages of the pancreas. *Proc Natl Acad Sci USA.* 2000;97(4):1607-1611.

91. Sarkar SA, Kobberup S, Wong R, et al. Global gene expression profiling and histochemical analysis of the developing human fetal pancreas. *Diabetologia.* 2008;51(2):285-297.

92. Schwitzgebel VM, Scheel DW, Conners JR, et al. Expression of neurogenin3 reveals an islet cell precursor population in the pancreas. *Development.* 2000;127(16):3533-3542.

93. Smith SB, Qu HQ, Taleb N, et al. Rfx6 directs islet formation and insulin production in mice and humans. *Nature.* 2010;463(7282):775-780.

94. Sussel L, Kalamaras J, Hartigan-O'Connor DJ, et al. Mice lacking the homeodomain transcription factor Nkx2.2 have diabetes due to arrested differentiation of pancreatic beta cells. *Development.* 1998;125(12):2213-2221.

95. Artner I, Hang Y, Mazur M, et al. MafA and MafB regulate genes critical to beta cells in a unique temporal manner. *Diabetes.* 2010;59:2530-2539.

96. Nishimura W, Bonner-Weir S, Sharma A. Expression of MafA in pancreatic progenitors is detrimental for pancreatic development. *Dev Biol.* 2009;333(1):108-120.

97. Akiyama H, Kim JE, Nakashima K, et al. Osteo-chondroprogenitor cells are derived from Sox9 expressing precursors. *Proc Natl Acad Sci USA.* 2005;102(41):14665-14670.

98. Seymour PA, Freude KK, Tran MN, et al. SOX9 is required for maintenance of the pancreatic progenitor cell pool. *Proc Natl Acad Sci USA.* 2007;104(6):1865-1870.

Acute Pancreatitis

Stefan A.W. Bouwense | Hein G. Gooszen |

Hjalmar C. van Santvoort | Marc G.H. Besselink*

Acute pancreatitis is the most common gastrointestinal disease for which patients are acutely hospitalized and its incidence is rising.[1] Around 80% of patients with acute pancreatitis have a mild disease course where symptoms usually resolve within 1 week.[2,3] Approximately 20% of patients develop severe acute pancreatitis with organ failure and/or necrotizing pancreatitis. Necrotizing pancreatitis is defined by pancreatic parenchymal necrosis and/or peripancreatic fat necrosis.[2,4] Those patients are at risk for a persistent systemic inflammatory response syndrome and/or (multiple) organ failure. Sterile pancreatic necrosis and sterile peripancreatic collections can usually be treated successfully with conservative measures. However, 30% of patients develop secondary infection of necrosis, most often 3 to 4 weeks after the onset of disease. When secondary infection of necrosis occurs, morbidity and mortality increase dramatically.[5,6] Overall mortality in severe pancreatitis is high (15% to 30%) compared with mild pancreatitis (0% to 1%).[7,8]

ETIOLOGY

Gallstones are the most frequent cause of pancreatitis in the Western world, in approximately 50% to 60% of patients, followed by alcohol in 20%. Other infrequent causes of acute pancreatitis are: hypercalcemia, hypertriglyceridemia, medications, hereditary causes, sphincter of Oddi dysfunction, pancreas divisum, and infections.[1,9] Before the final diagnosis of idiopathic pancreatitis is made, it is important to rule out causes that have therapeutic implications; biliary sludge can be ruled out by endoscopic ultrasonography and pancreatic neoplasms can be ruled out by contrast-enhanced computed tomography (CECT).[10]

CLINICAL PRESENTATION AND DIAGNOSIS

The diagnosis of acute pancreatitis requires two of the following three features: (1) abdominal pain consistent with acute pancreatitis (acute onset of a persistent, severe, epigastric pain often radiating to the back); (2) serum lipase activity (or amylase activity) at least three times greater than the upper limit of normal; and (3) characteristic findings of acute pancreatitis on CECT and less commonly, magnetic resonance imaging (MRI) or transabdominal ultrasonography.[2,3]

Usually, the first two criteria are present and CECT is not required for diagnosis. However, CECT may be helpful in patients who have abdominal pain for several days with already normalized amylase and lipase levels. Caution is advised with CECT in the first 72 to 96 hours of disease because CECT often fails to demonstrate pancreatic necrosis and peripancreatic collections in this time period.[11,12]

CLASSIFICATION OF ACUTE PANCREATITIS

The 1992 Atlanta Symposium attempted to offer a global consensus and a universally applicable classification system for acute pancreatitis.[2,13] Due to improvements in diagnostic imaging and therapy, together with a better understanding of the pathophysiology of organ failure and pancreatitis, it was necessary to revise the Atlanta Classification.[2] The aims of the 2012 Revised Atlanta Classification were to clarify terminology and stimulate the use of uniform definitions and standardized reporting in patients with acute pancreatitis. Three categories of acute pancreatitis were defined, based on the absence or presence of local complications and/or organ failure: mild, moderate, and severe (Table 91.1). Based on local complications on diagnostic imaging, acute pancreatitis is divided into interstitial edematous or necrotizing pancreatitis. Four types of local complications can be defined: acute fluid collections, pseudocysts, acute necrotic collections (i.e., sterile or infected), and walled-off necrosis (i.e., sterile or infected) (Table 91.2).

The Revised Atlanta Classification represents a step forward in categorizing patients with acute pancreatitis, but some practical issues with the classification need to be resolved. To distinguish between an acute necrotic collection and walled-off necrosis, a period of 4 weeks is assumed necessary for the development of a wall encapsulating the collection.[14] The rate of encapsulation of collections may differ between patients; therefore, it is best to use the actual presence of encapsulation of a collection instead of time from onset of disease to differentiate between an acute necrotic collection and walled-off necrosis. MRI is particularly helpful in determining whether a collection contains predominantly fluid or solid debris.[14] MRI, however, can be impractical in critically ill patients.[11] CECT has its limitations in defining whether the collection contains mostly fluid or solid material, a distinction that is relevant in clinical decision making. The exact place of CECT and MRI in the diagnosis of acute pancreatitis needs to be addressed in future studies.

PREDICTING SEVERITY

The clinical course of acute pancreatitis is unpredictable and may vary from full recovery within a few days to

---

*For the Dutch Pancreatitis Study Group.

TABLE 91.1 Severity of Acute Pancreatitis as Defined in the 2012 Revised Atlanta Classification

Complications	2012 REVISED ATLANTA CLASSIFICATION		
	Mild	Moderate	Severe
Local complications	No	Yes	Yes
SYSTEMIC COMPLICATIONS			
Transient organ failure	No	Yes	Yes
Persistent organ failure	No	No	Yes
Exacerbation of preexisting comorbidity	No	Yes	Yes

TABLE 91.2 Collections as Defined in the 2012 Revised Atlanta Classification

Definition	Description*
Acute fluid collection (<4 wk after onset and edematous pancreatitis)	• Homogeneous fluid density • Confined by normal peripancreatic fascial planes • No definable wall encapsulating the collection • Adjacent to pancreas (not intrapancreatic)
Pseudocyst (rare, usually >4 wk after onset and edematous pancreatitis)	• Well circumscribed, usually round/oval • Homogeneous fluid density • Well-defined wall and completely encapsulated • Adjacent to pancreas (not intrapancreatic)
Acute necrotic collection (<4 wk after onset and necrotizing pancreatitis)	• Heterogeneous and nonliquid density • No definable wall encapsulating the collection • Location: intrapancreatic and/or extrapancreatic
Walled-off necrosis (usually >4 wk after onset and necrotizing pancreatitis)	• Heterogeneous and nonliquid density • Well-defined wall and completely encapsulated • Location: intrapancreatic and/or extrapancreatic

*Revised Atlanta Classification definitions of morphologic features of acute pancreatitis.

TABLE 91.3 Scoring Systems in Acute Pancreatitis

	Cutoff for Predicted Severe Acute Pancreatitis
APACHE II	≥8 in first 24 h*
BISAP	≥3 in first 24 h
Modified Glasgow (or Imrie)	≥3 in first 48 h
Ranson	≥3 in first 48 h
Urea at admission	>60 mmol/L
C-reactive protein	>150 U/L in first 72 h

*After onset of symptoms.
APACHE, Acute physiology and chronic health evaluation; *BISAP,* bedside index for severity in acute pancreatitis.

own strengths and limitations, and a system with a high negative predictive value and a high positive predictive value is not yet available, as described in a recent systematic review.[15] The most popular scores and their application are listed in Table 91.3.

The presence of (persistent) organ failure is the key determinant for morbidity and mortality in acute pancreatitis, in particular (early) multiorgan failure is associated with high mortality. The International Association of Pancreatology (IAP)/American Pancreatic Association (APA) guidelines recommend using persistent systemic inflammatory response syndrome (SIRS) (>48 hours) as a marker to predict severity of acute pancreatitis.[3] Persistent organ failure is also one of the key determinants of the severity of acute pancreatitis in the Revised Atlanta Classification (see Table 91.2).[2]

MORPHOLOGIC SCORING SYSTEMS

Morphologic abnormalities assessed by CECT can be used in a scoring system such as the Balthazar grade, pancreatic size index, extrapancreatic inflammation on CT score, CT severity index, or the modified CT severity index. Although all these scoring systems have been shown to correlate with morbidity and mortality, it remains difficult, at the time of their admission or early in the course of their hospitalization, to accurately identify individual patients who will develop clinically severe disease.[12,16,17] A study comparing all radiologic scoring systems in the early prediction of severity in acute pancreatitis did not show an advantage of an early CT on admission as an independent predictor as compared to the more easily obtainable clinical scoring systems in terms of accuracy in predicting clinically severe acute pancreatitis and mortality.[12]

PHASES OF ACUTE PANCREATITIS

Traditionally, acute pancreatitis was described as running a biphasic course with two peaks of mortality: early and late.[18,19] The early phase is characterized by a SIRS and lasts about 1 to 2 weeks. The late phase is characterized by a compensatory, antiinflammatory response syndrome (CARS), which can run a protracted course from weeks to months. More recent data suggest that the biphasic course is outdated and that there are not two peaks in the incidence of organ failure and mortality.[5]

Organ failure may already be present at the first presentation to the emergency department; however, in the

multiorgan failure and death within hours after onset of the disease. Predicting the severity of acute pancreatitis in the first days of the disease has been attempted in past decades and many scoring systems have been proposed to provide guidance for clinicians.

PREDICTING DISEASE SEVERITY

Because of large variability in the clinical course of acute pancreatitis, a number of predictive scoring systems have been developed. These scoring systems are based on clinical and biochemical parameters: for example, the Ranson, APACHE-II, Imrie, or modified Glasgow scores. Blood levels of C-reactive protein and blood urea nitrogen are also often used in predicting severity at the time of hospital admission. All these scoring systems have their more severe cases, organ failure is usually diagnosed in the early SIRS phase at a median of 2 days after admission. Overall, approximately one-half of the patients who die in the early phase of acute pancreatitis have no infected necrosis but suffer from multiorgan failure. A recent systematic review of cohort studies demonstrated that the mortality of patients with organ failure in acute pancreatitis is 32%.[6] Patients with both organ failure and infected necrosis had a mortality of 43%.

EARLY PHASE

During the early phase of pancreatic inflammation, cytokine cascades are activated and are the cause of the host systemic response to the local pancreatic disease process. This manifests clinically as SIRS.[7,20] When SIRS persists, organ failure will often develop. As mentioned earlier, the presence and duration of organ failure is important in defining the severity of acute pancreatitis.[2] Transient organ failure is defined as organ failure that resolves within 48 hours. Persistent organ failure lasts more than 48 hours. If organ failure affects more than one organ system, it is defined as multiple organ failure (MOF). A useful scoring system for organ dysfunction is the modified Marshall scoring system.[2] Infections originating from the pulmonary or urogenital tract, not related to local complications of the pancreas, do occur in the early phase of SIRS and may contribute to early organ failure.

Although morphologic abnormalities can be present during the first phase, it may be unreliable to determine the extent and content of the abnormalities, in particular the extent of (peri)pancreatic necrosis. In addition, the severity of acute pancreatitis is not directly proportional to the size of local complications.[2,11,12] Therefore, defining the severity of acute pancreatitis in the early phase depends more on organ failure than on the presence (or extent) of (peri)pancreatic necrosis only.

LATE PHASE

In the late phase, the SIRS of the early phase can be followed by a CARS. Organ failure in the CARS phase is related to local complications and secondary infection such as infected pancreas necrosis. Also in this phase, but more rarely, infection may originate in the pulmonary or urogenital tract. When this is the case, it may be difficult to determine the cause of the CARS reaction (infected necrosis or infection from another organ system) and start the proper treatment.

This was also demonstrated in a large observational cohort study of acute pancreatitis patients where it was demonstrated that these infections were most often diagnosed in the first week of admission.[22]

In the late phase, it is important, with respect to the decision to perform necrosectomy, to adequately characterize the local complications on CECT scan. In clinical practice, this means differentiation between an acute necrotic collection and walled-off necrosis. The combination of adequate characterization of local complications on radiologic imaging and (persistent) organ failure attributable to the local complication remains the basis for performing some form of necrosectomy.

TREATMENT

EARLY SUPPORTIVE MEASURES

Pain Management

In the vast majority of acute pancreatitis patients, intense abdominal pain is the presenting symptom in the emergency department. During the first days of admission, abdominal pain remains one of the most dominant features of the disease. A specific pain treatment regimen for acute pancreatitis is not available, so use of the World Health Organization (WHO) analgesic ladder is recommended.[23] The exact place of pain management and its physiologic and immunologic response is still unknown.[24]

Fluid Therapy

The optimal fluid infusion rate and response measurement for initial fluid resuscitation in acute pancreatitis is still under debate because high-level evidence is still lacking. Intensive care studies in severe sepsis and septic shock have shown that early goal-directed therapy provides a better outcome than standard therapy.[25]

Extensive fluid resuscitation is often needed during the first days of acute pancreatitis to correct or preferably prevent intravascular hypovolemia and maintain microcirculation of the pancreas.[26,27] On the contrary, uncontrolled, aggressive fluid therapy may induce morbidity and even mortality, so careful monitoring of the response to fluid resuscitation is necessary (heart rate, mean arterial pressure, and urinary output 0.5 to 1 mL/kg/h).[3,28,29]

The recent update of the IAP/APA treatment guideline for acute pancreatitis recommends the use of Ringer lactate with an infusion rate of 5 to 10 mL/kg/h until resuscitation goals are reached, monitored by vital parameters and urine production.[3,30]

Prevention of Infection

In acute pancreatitis, early infections (especially bacteremia), and in the later phase secondary infection of pancreas necrosis, often have a significant impact on mortality.[22] Therefore, prophylactic strategies to prevent infection should be initiated as early as possible.

Before the PROPATRIA trial, one study showed that probiotics reduce pancreatic sepsis and the need for surgical intervention[31] and a second study showed that nasojejunal feeding with synbiotics may prevent organ dysfunctions in the late phase of severe acute pancreatitis.[32] Because of the lack of strong evidence in a larger randomized controlled multicenter trial, the PROPATRIA trial compared outcomes after probiotics with placebo in patients with predicted severe pancreatitis. Probiotics were found to have no effect in reducing infectious complications; however an unexpected higher rate of bowel ischemia (9 vs. 0) and mortality (16% vs. 6%) was observed in the probiotics group.[33] The mechanism explaining this adverse effect was unclear but the use of probiotics in acute pancreatitis is not recommended.

An extensively debated issue is the use of prophylactic administration of antibiotics to prevent infection of necrosis in acute pancreatitis. The most recent systematic reviews of randomized trials have shown that prophylactic administration of intravenous antibiotics does not prevent infection of (peri)pancreatic necrosis.[34-36] Antibiotics in acute pancreatitis are therefore only indicated as therapy (not as prophylaxis) for proven infection or strong clinical suspicion of infected necrosis.[3]

Selective decontamination of the intestinal tract reduces mortality in general in intensive care units in a wide variety of diseases.[37] The effects of this approach in acute pancreatitis have been tested with beneficial effects on morbidity, but no impact on mortality.[38] Studies with a proper design and adequate numbers of patients are not available, so the use of selective decontamination should be weighed against the potential for an increase in antibiotic resistance and fungal colonization.[39]

Nutrition

Today much attention is turned to the timing and route of feeding in patients on intensive care units and on surgical wards in general.[40-42] When oral nutrition is not tolerated, enteral or parenteral nutrition should be started. In predicted severe acute pancreatitis, a head-to-head comparison of enteral nutrition through a nasoenteric feeding tube and parenteral nutrition showed that enteral nutrition was superior in terms of reducing organ failure, infected necrosis, and even mortality.[43] The underlying mechanism for the beneficial effect of enteral nutrition could be reduced gut permeability and less bacterial overgrowth with bacterial translocation. This may have a positive influence on intestinal motility and may help to conserve or restore bowel mucosa.[44,45]

In the PYTHON trial, patients with predicted severe pancreatitis were randomized to early nasoenteric tube feeding within 24 hours of presentation to the emergency department, or to an oral diet initiated within the first few days of presentation, with tube feeding only provided if the oral diet was not tolerated after 72 hours.[46] The most important result was that routine early nasoenteral nutrition did not reduce the composite endpoint of infection or mortality. In the on-demand group, most patients (69%) tolerated an oral diet and did not require tube feeding. Therefore, enteral nutrition is only recommended when an oral diet is not tolerated during the first 3 to 5 days of acute pancreatitis.

Role of Endoscopic Retrograde Cholangiography and Papillotomy

An urgent endoscopic retrograde cholangiopancreatography (ERC) with endoscopic sphincterotomy is indicated only for biliary pancreatitis with concurrent cholangitis.[3] In mild biliary pancreatitis and in the absence of symptomatic common bile duct stones and/or cholangitis, there is no evidence that an ERC will beneficially influence the course of acute pancreatitis.[3,47] In predicted severe acute pancreatitis without cholangitis, it was hypothesized that endoscopic sphincterotomy (relieving pressure of the pancreatic duct) may reduce the severity of the course of the disease.[48] However, the evidence on this subject is conflicting and therefore the Dutch Pancreatitis Study Group is currently enrolling patients in the randomized multicenter APEC trial to compare early ERC with endoscopic sphincterotomy in patients with predicted severe pancreatitis without cholangitis (ISRCTN97372133).[3,47,49]

Role of Cholecystectomy

The timing of cholecystectomy in patients with gallstone pancreatitis has been debated for many decades; early cholecystectomy during the same hospital admission is claimed to reduce the risk of recurrent gallstone-related complications, but concern has existed that early cholecystectomy may increase the risk of technical complications.[50,51] Strong evidence was lacking and therefore the PONCHO trial was performed.[52] This trial showed that an early cholecystectomy (just before discharge, when the patient has recovered and severe disease excluded), compared to interval cholecystectomy, effectively reduces the rate of recurrent gallstone-related complications in patients with mild biliary pancreatitis, with a very low added risk of complications.[52] Therefore early cholecystectomy should be performed after mild biliary pancreatitis has resolved.

Evidence on the timing of cholecystectomy in severe pancreatitis is scarce. Cholecystectomy is recommended after all signs of pancreatic necrosis have been resolved or if they persist more than 6 weeks.[3,53]

Management of Infected Necrosis

When the clinical condition of a patient with necrotizing pancreatitis does not improve or worsens over the first 1 to 2 weeks, infected necrosis may have developed. The next step is to perform a CECT in search of acute necrotic collections or walled-off necrosis.[2,3] When gas bubbles are detected in collections, caused by gas-forming bacteria with or without fistulization to the digestive tract, infection of necrosis is considered proven.[11] In the absence of gas bubbles and when there is a persistent suspicion of infection and a need for intervention, fine-needle aspiration (FNA) of the collection can be used as the next diagnostic step.[3] It should be noted that properly designed prospective studies on the clinical importance of FNA are lacking, false-negative FNA results have been reported in 12% to 25% of patients, and there is a risk of introducing infection into the necrotic cavity.[54-56]

Intravenous broad-spectrum antibiotics should be started when infected necrosis is suspected or proven, which can subsequently be narrowed down based on cultures of the infected collection.[3] Some small case series show that treatment with antibiotics alone can be successful in obviating the need for surgical, radiologic, or endoscopic intervention in a small subset (i.e., 5% to 10%) of patients, but in the vast majority of patients, antibiotics should be regarded as supportive care in this phase of the disease, where drainage and/or necrosectomy of (suspected) infected necrotic collections are regarded as the only option for effective treatment.[5]

Traditionally, a primary laparotomy was performed for necrosectomy, even early in the clinical course of necrotizing pancreatitis, but this practice has now largely been abandoned.[57] Today surgical or endoscopic intervention is postponed when clinically feasible until walled-off necrosis (with full encapsulation) is documented on CECT, a process that usually takes 3 to 4 weeks.[11] Waiting for full encapsulation and delaying intervention reduces morbidity and mortality when compared to early intervention in the first 2 weeks, most likely because encapsulation facilitates effective necrosectomy while reducing the risk of complications such as bleeding and perforation.[5,58]

In the acute (early) phase, there is no indication for intervention of sterile collections, because drainage of sterile collections carries a risk of introducing infection, thereby increasing the risk of morbidity and mortality.[3,59] In rare cases of obstruction of the biliary or gastrointestinal tract and persisting pain, sterile collections may need drainage for symptomatic relief, but this is usually performed at least 4 to 6 weeks after the onset of disease.[3]

INVASIVE TREATMENT

The place of primary open surgical necrosectomy by laparotomy has changed in the past few years after the introduction of minimally invasive techniques for necrosectomy.[3,60] Mortality (11% to 39%) and morbidity (up to 95%) with open necrosectomy as performed in past decades were high.[61,62] As a result of improvement in the timing and approach of invasive intervention, combined with improvement in supportive care in the intensive care unit, recent studies have shown that the success rate of necrosectomy has improved significantly (11% to 19%).[55,60]

After the introduction of minimally invasive techniques to first drain and selectively debride pancreatic necrosis (i.e., catheter drainage and video-assisted retroperitoneal debridement [VARD]), the number of laparotomies performed has decreased dramatically.[58,60,63] Still, emergency laparotomy is indicated in acute pancreatitis for patients with abdominal compartment syndrome, bowel ischemia, and bowel perforation.[5,64-66] In these cases, intraabdominal decompression, and not necrosectomy, is the goal of surgical treatment. If early laparotomy is needed for this purpose, it is highly recommended not to explore the retroperitoneum if infected necrosis has not been documented before operation. The international guideline for treatment of an abdominal compartment syndrome proposes a stepwise approach with medication and percutaneous drainage, followed when needed by laparotomy.[67]

MINIMALLY INVASIVE INTERVENTION

Today tertiary referral centers use some form of step-up approach to treat infected necrosis in acute pancreatitis. The first step, which is widely accepted, is to place a percutaneous or endoscopic drain, to decompress the collection.[60,68] When this does not lead to clinical improvement, drains may be added or revised if CECT shows unsuccessful or incomplete decompression. If still unsuccessful, necrosectomy is performed. This stepwise approach, also referred to as the step-up approach, not only reduces surgical trauma (as compared to primary necrosectomy) but also the risk of iatrogenic damage, bowel injury, and hemorrhage requiring surgical or radiologic intervention.[60,68]

Several minimally invasive intervention strategies are available for drainage and/or debridement of infected necrotizing pancreatitis: percutaneous catheter drainage,[69] percutaneous necrosectomy,[70] VARD,[71] laparoscopic necrosectomy,[72] and endoscopic transluminal drainage and necrosectomy.[73]

Percutaneous Catheter Drainage and Video-Assisted Retroperitoneal Debridement

Catheter drainage is the least invasive technique to control sepsis and is the first step in treating infected necrosis. A drain is used to relieve pus that is under pressure in the necrotic collection, prevent further bacteremia, and serve as a bridge to necrosectomy (Fig. 91.1). Distinct advantages of this technique include its simplicity and wide availability. In the PANTER trial, 35% of the patients were solely treated with antibiotics and percutaneous drains; similar results have been shown as well in other studies.[60,74,75]

Most peripancreatic collections can be drained percutaneously through the retroperitoneal or transperitoneal route. The advantage of the route through the retroperitoneum is that it is not very demanding and has a low complication rate (i.e., intestinal perforation and contamination of a compartment).[60,76] When catheter drainage of the collection is clinically unsuccessful, the drain can be used as guidance for minimally invasive retroperitoneal necrosectomy (VARD: Fig. 91.2).

In the PANTER trial, the minimal drain size was 12 French and drains were irrigated three times daily with 250 mL of normal saline to keep them open.[60] When a collection is not optimally drained, drain upsizing or placement of additional drains is advocated.[3,74]

In case of VARD, the next steps need to be taken. The patient is put under general anesthesia in the right lateral position and a subcostal incision of 5 to 7 cm is made close to the drain entrance site. With the most recent CECT scan and drain as guidance, the route to the peripancreatic collection is usually found easily. Visible nonadherent necrosis is removed from the collection with a forceps. Using a 0-degree videoscope, the loosely adherent necrosis

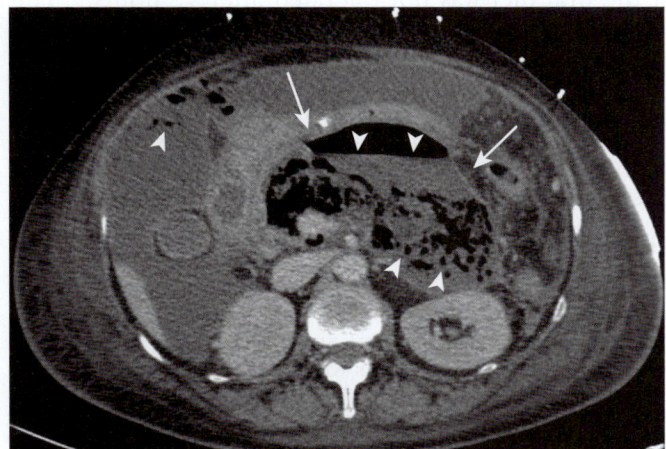

FIGURE 91.1 Imaging of a patient with infected necrotizing pancreatitis. The patient recovered fully after a single large percutaneous drain was placed through the left retroperitoneum, without additional drainage procedures and without necrosectomy. *Arrows* point at the borders of the collection, with *arrowheads* pointing at impacted gas bubbles and at the gas-fluid level. (Reprinted from van Brunschot S, Bakker OJ, Besselink MG, et al. Treatment of necrotizing pancreatitis. Clinical Gastroenterology and Hepatology: The Official Clinical Practice journal of the American Gastroenterological Association. 2012;10:1190–1201, with permission from Elsevier.)

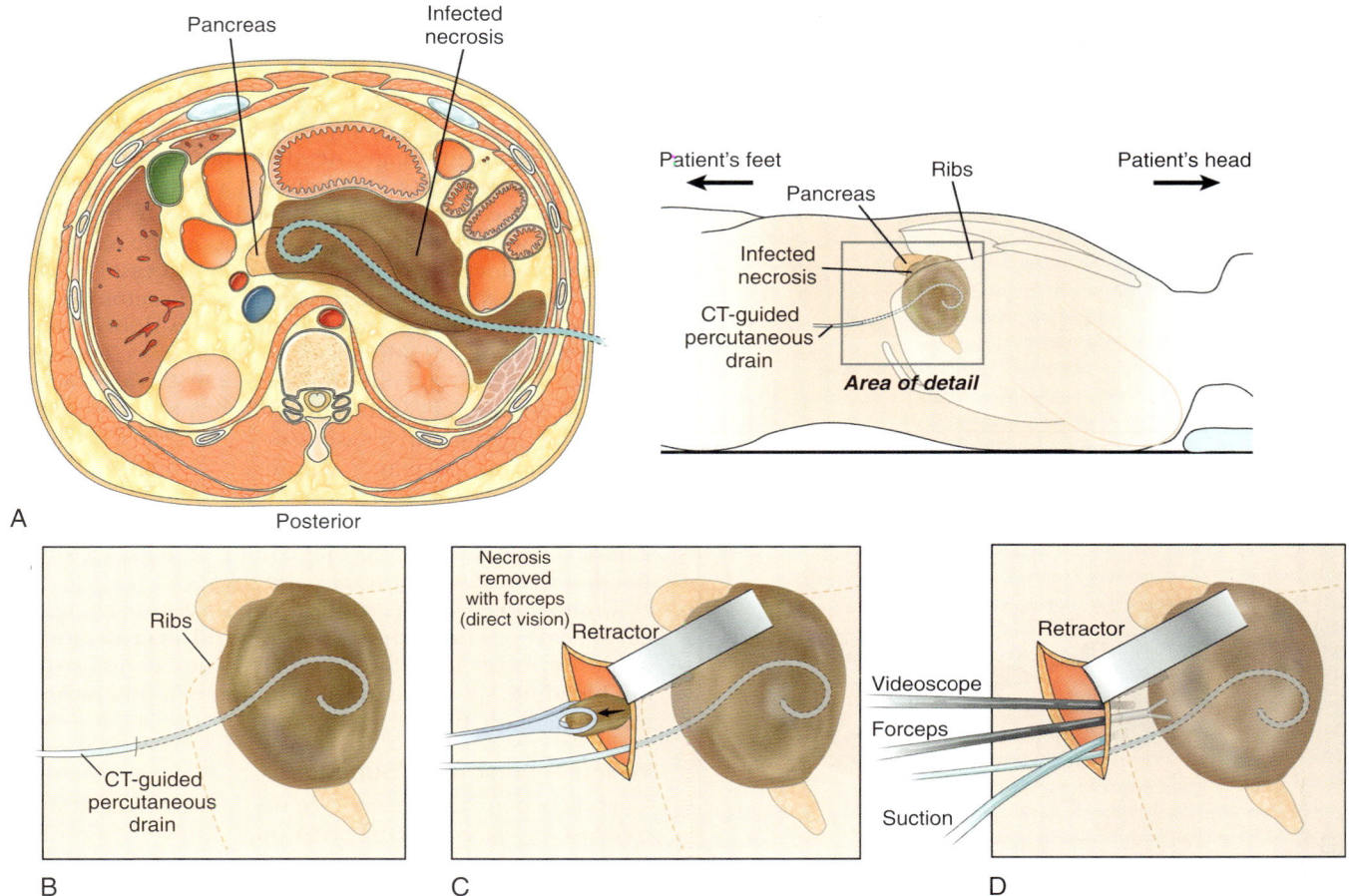

FIGURE 91.2 Percutaneous catheter drainage and video-assisted retroperitoneal debridement. (A) Contrast-enhanced computed tomography image of a patient with necrotizing pancreatitis showing a transverse cross-sectional image. Catheter drainage through the left side of the retroperitoneum is the preferred route. (B) Details on the drained area. (C) Near the puncture site of the percutaneous drain a small subcostal incision is made. The drain is used as a guide to the necrotic collection through the retroperitoneum. All visible necrosis is removed directly. (D) Under vision of a 0-degree videoscope, further debridement is performed with laparoscopic instruments. (Reprinted from van Brunschot S, Bakker OJ, Besselink MG, et al. Treatment of necrotizing pancreatitis. Clinical Gastroenterology and Hepatology: The Official Clinical Practice journal of the American Gastroenterological Association. 2012;10:1190–1201, with permission from Elsevier.)

is removed with a long atraumatic forceps, to reduce the risk of bleeding from viable underlying tissue. For postoperative lavage (up to 10 L per 24 hours) two large catheters are placed and the abdominal wall is closed (see Fig. 91.2). Videos of the VARD procedure can be found on YouTube under the name Dutch Pancreatitis Study Group.

Evidence for the safety and effectiveness of the previously described step-up approach comes from the randomized multicenter PANTER trial. In this study, 88 patients with suspected infected necrotizing pancreatitis were randomized for primary open necrosectomy (by laparotomy) or a surgical step-up approach consisting of percutaneous catheter drainage as the first step, followed after 72 hours by VARD if there is no clinical improvement observed.[60] In the trial, 35% of patients were successfully treated by percutaneous catheter drainage only. This approach was associated with a significantly lower rate of the combined endpoint of mortality and major complications compared to open necrosectomy (40% vs. 69%). Other complications, such as pancreatic fistula formation (28% vs. 38%), incisional hernia (7% vs. 24%),

and new-onset diabetes (16% vs. 38%), were less frequent in the step-up approach group compared to open primary necrosectomy. Complications such as intraabdominal bleeding (16% vs. 22%) and enterocutaneous fistula or perforation of a visceral organ requiring intervention (14% vs. 22%) did not differ significantly between the groups.

The VARD procedure has been followed up by multiple other retroperitoneal approaches, including single-port or multiport procedures and flexible endoscopy.[70,77–79]

Endoscopic Drainage and Necrosectomy

An increasingly popular alternative to the surgical step-up approach is endoscopic internal transluminal catheter drainage of the necrotic collection, followed by endoscopic transluminal necrosectomy if drainage is not completely successful.[73,80,81]

This can be performed through the stomach or through the duodenal wall (Fig. 91.3). If the endoscopic approach is chosen, the following steps are required. The procedure is started with the patient in the left lateral position under deep sedation or general anesthesia. The size, content,

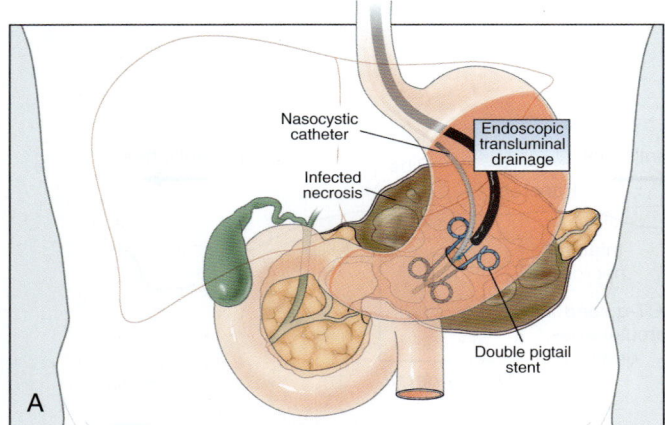

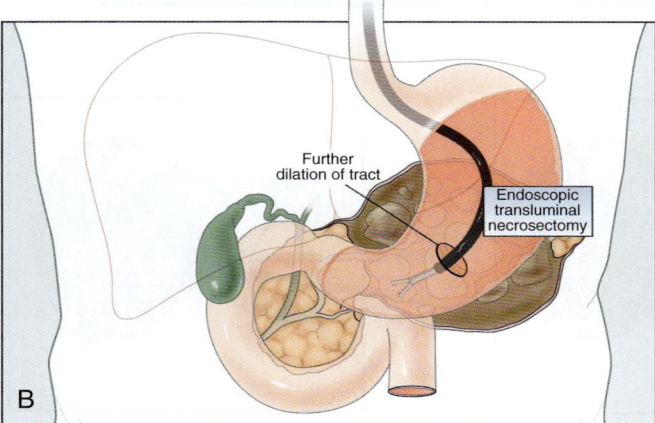

FIGURE 91.3 Endoscopic transluminal drainage and endoscopic transluminal necrosectomy. (A) Through the stomach wall the necrotic collection is punctured and a guidewire is placed in the collection, under guidance of endoscopic ultrasound if needed. Over the guidewire the tract is balloon dilated. Two-pigtail drains and a nasocystic catheter are placed in the collection for continuous lavage. (B) Further dilation of the cystogastrostomy and the collection is performed via endoscope. A necrosectomy can be performed under direct vision. (Reprinted from van Brunschot S, Bakker OJ, Besselink MG, et al. Treatment of necrotizing pancreatitis. Clinical Gastroenterology and Hepatology: The Official Clinical Practice journal of the American Gastroenterological Association. 2012;10:1190–1201, with permission from Elsevier.)

and the relationship of the collection to other structures are explored by endoscopic ultrasound.[82] Drainage not guided by ultrasound is technically feasible, but the success rate is inferior to the ultrasound-guided procedure.[83,84] First, material is collected for bacterial culture. Then a 19-gauge FNA needle and a guidewire are introduced under fluoroscopic guidance and looped in the collection.[85] A fistula tract of 8 to 12 mm is created between the collection and the intestinal lumen using electrocauterization with balloon dilation. A nasocystic catheter and two double pigtails (or metal stents to create a larger and more permanently "supported" opening to the cavity) are placed in the collection, to be used for flushing the contents into the stomach or duodenum (1 L per 24 hours).[86–88] There are reports showing that metal stents may increase the risk of bleeding, and therefore this technique needs

to be validated in randomized trials. Multiple collections can be drained by multiple cystogastrostomies or alternatively by combined percutaneous and endoscopic drainage.[89–91]

Endoscopic necrosectomy, as the next step after technically successful drainage, needs to be performed if no clinical improvement is documented within 72 hours after drainage. The fistula tract is dilated 15 to 18 mm with a forward viewing endoscope and the endoscope is advanced into the collection. With endoscopic accessories (i.e., snares, baskets, nets, and forceps), necrosectomy is performed through this tract, leaving the debris in the stomach. CO_2 insufflation is recommended to reduce the risk of air embolisms, although this is not 100% protective because endoscopes insufflate without pressure control.

Finally, pigtails and a nasocystic catheter are left in the cavity to ensure permanent drainage through the fistula tract.[85,92,93] Endoscopic necrosectomy should be repeated every few days until most necrotic material is removed. There is no data showing that complete necrosectomy is needed to successfully treat patients.

Comparable with the surgical step-up approach, technical success of endoscopic drainage and necrosectomy is achieved in up to 91% of cases.[82] Major complications are bleeding, spontaneous perforation of a hollow organ, and pancreatic fistula.

Which Technique Is Superior?

Currently, convincing evidence on the preferred route of necrosectomy is lacking. Although there is a shift in preference for minimally invasive interventions over necrosectomy, superiority of one of these strategies has not been proven. For example, the Dutch PANTER trial did not compare VARD and open necrosectomy directly, because VARD was always preceded by percutaneous drainage in the step-up approach strategy.[60]

Comparison of VARD and endoscopic transluminal necrosectomy was performed in the PENGUIN trial, a pilot trial in 20 patients with infected necrosis. The primary endpoint, postprocedural proinflammatory response, was significantly lower after endoscopic necrosectomy as compared to VARD (18 patients underwent necrosectomy).[68] A similar effect was shown for the combined endpoint of major complications and death.

The recently completed TENSION trial (ISRCTN-09186711) compares outcomes after an endoscopic and surgical step-up approach (publication expected in 2017). In this trial, the focus is on clinical results (major morbidity and mortality) and cost-effectiveness.[94]

It is clear that patients with necrotizing pancreatitis should be treated by a multidisciplinary team consisting of surgeons, gastroenterologists, radiologists, and intensivists. Most experts recommend a form of step-up approach in patients with infected necrotizing pancreatitis.[95] Treatment is guided by the advice proposed in the Revised Atlanta Classification and the IAP/APA evidence-based guidelines.[2,3]

REFERENCES

1. Peery AF, Dellon ES, Lund J, et al. Burden of gastrointestinal disease in the United States: 2012 update. *Gastroenterology.* 2012;143:1179-1187.e1-e3.

2. Banks PA, Bollen TL, Dervenis C, et al. Classification of acute pancreatitis—2012: revision of the Atlanta classification and definitions by international consensus. *Gut.* 2013;62:102-111.
3. Working Group IAP/AAP. International Association of Pancreatology/American Pancreatic Association evidence-based guidelines for the management of acute pancreatitis. *Pancreatology.* 2013;13:e1-e15.
4. Bakker OJ, van Santvoort H, Besselink MG, et al. Extrapancreatic necrosis without pancreatic parenchymal necrosis: a separate entity in necrotising pancreatitis? *Gut.* 2013;62:1475-1480.
5. van Santvoort HC, Bakker OJ, Bollen TL, et al. A conservative and minimally invasive approach to necrotizing pancreatitis improves outcome. *Gastroenterology.* 2011;141:1254-1263.
6. Petrov MS, Shanbhag S, Chakraborty M, Phillips AR, Windsor JA. Organ failure and infection of pancreatic necrosis as determinants of mortality in patients with acute pancreatitis. *Gastroenterology.* 2010;139:813-820.
7. Johnson CD, Abu-Hilal M. Persistent organ failure during the first week as a marker of fatal outcome in acute pancreatitis. *Gut.* 2004;53:1340-1344.
8. Mofidi R, Duff MD, Wigmore SJ, Madhavan KK, Garden OJ, Parks RW. Association between early systemic inflammatory response, severity of multiorgan dysfunction and death in acute pancreatitis. *Br J Surg.* 2006;93:738-744.
9. Spanier BW, Dijkgraaf MG, Bruno MJ. Epidemiology, aetiology and outcome of acute and chronic pancreatitis: an update. *Best Pract Res Clin Gastroenterol.* 2008;22:45-63.
10. Räty S, Pulkkinen J, Nordback I, et al. Can laparoscopic cholecystectomy prevent recurrent idiopathic acute pancreatitis?: A prospective randomized multicenter trial. *Ann Surg.* 2015;262:736-741.
11. Bollen TL. Imaging of acute pancreatitis: update of the revised Atlanta classification. *Radiol Clin North Am.* 2012;50:429-445.
12. Bollen TL, Singh VK, Maurer R, et al. A comparative evaluation of radiologic and clinical scoring systems in the early prediction of severity in acute pancreatitis. *Am J Gastroenterol.* 2012;107:612-619.
13. Bradley EL III. A clinically based classification system for acute pancreatitis. Summary of the International Symposium on Acute Pancreatitis, Atlanta, Ga, September 11 through 13, 1992. *Arch Surg.* 1993;128:586-590.
14. Bollen TL, Van Santvoort HC, Besselink MG, van Es WH, Gooszen HG, van Leeuwen MS. Update on acute pancreatitis: ultrasound, computed tomography, and magnetic resonance imaging features. *Semin Ultrasound CT MR.* 2007;28:371-383.
15. Gravante G, Garcea G, Ong SL, et al. Prediction of mortality in acute pancreatitis: a systematic review of the published evidence. *Pancreatology.* 2009;9:601-614.
16. Balthazar EJ, Ranson JH, Naidich DP, Megibow AJ, Caccavale R, Cooper MM. Acute pancreatitis: prognostic value of CT. *Radiology.* 1985;156:767-772.
17. Papachristou GI, Whitcomb DC. Predictors of severity and necrosis in acute pancreatitis. *Gastroenterol Clin North Am.* 2004;33:871-890.
18. McKay CJ, Imrie CW. The continuing challenge of early mortality in acute pancreatitis. *Br J Surg.* 2004;91:1243-1244.
19. Blum T, Maisonneuve P, Lowenfels AB, Lankisch PG. Fatal outcome in acute pancreatitis: its occurrence and early prediction. *Pancreatology.* 2001;1:237-241.
20. Buter A, Imrie CW, Carter CR, Evans S, McKay CJ. Dynamic nature of early organ dysfunction determines outcome in acute pancreatitis. *Br J Surg.* 2002;89:298-302.
21. Reference deleted in review.
22. Besselink MG, Van Santvoort HC, Boermeester MA, et al. Timing and impact of infections in acute pancreatitis. *Br J Surg.* 2009;96:267-273.
23. Jadad AR, Browman GP. The WHO analgesic ladder for cancer pain management. Stepping up the quality of its evaluation. *J Am Med Assoc.* 1995;274:1870-1873.
24. Schwartz ES, Christianson JA, Chen X, et al. Synergistic role of TRPV1 and TRPA1 in pancreatic pain and inflammation. *Gastroenterology.* 2011;140:1283-1291.e1-e2.
25. Rivers E, Nguyen B, Havstad S, et al. Early goal-directed therapy in the treatment of severe sepsis and septic shock. *N Engl J Med.* 2001;345:1368-1377.
26. Gardner TB, Vege SS, Chari ST, et al. Faster rate of initial fluid resuscitation in severe acute pancreatitis diminishes in-hospital mortality. *Pancreatology.* 2009;9:770-776.
27. Warndorf MG, Kurtzman JT, Bartel MJ, et al. Early fluid resuscitation reduces morbidity among patients with acute pancreatitis. *Clin Gastroenterol Hepatol.* 2011;9:705-709.
28. Mao EQ, Fei J, Peng YB, Huang J, Tang YQ, Zhang SD. Rapid hemodilution is associated with increased sepsis and mortality among patients with severe acute pancreatitis. *Chin Med J.* 2010;123:1639-1644.
29. Mao EQ, Tang YQ, Fei J, et al. Fluid therapy for severe acute pancreatitis in acute response stage. *Chin Med J.* 2009;122:169-173.
30. Wu BU, Hwang JQ, Gardner TH, et al. Lactated Ringer's solution reduces systemic inflammation compared with saline in patients with acute pancreatitis. *Clin Gastroenterol Hepatol.* 2011;9:710-717.e1.
31. Olah A, Belagyi T, Issekutz A, Gamal ME, Bengmark S. Randomized clinical trial of specific lactobacillus and fibre supplement to early enteral nutrition in patients with acute pancreatitis. *Br J Surg.* 2002;89:1103-1107.
32. Olah A, Belagyi T, Poto L, Romics L Jr, Bengmark S. Synbiotic control of inflammation and infection in severe acute pancreatitis: a prospective, randomized, double blind study. *Hepatogastroenterology.* 2007;54:590-594.
33. Besselink MG, Van Santvoort HC, Buskens E, et al. Probiotic prophylaxis in predicted severe acute pancreatitis: a randomised, double-blind, placebo-controlled trial. *Lancet.* 2008;371:651-659.
34. Villatoro E, Mulla M, Larvin M. Antibiotic therapy for prophylaxis against infection of pancreatic necrosis in acute pancreatitis. *Cochrane Database Syst Rev.* 2010;(5):CD002941.
35. Jiang K, Huang W, Yang XN, Xia Q. Present and future of prophylactic antibiotics for severe acute pancreatitis. *World J Gastroenterol.* 2012;18:279-284.
36. Wittau M, Mayer B, Scheele J, Henne-Bruns D, Dellinger EP, Isenmann R. Systematic review and meta-analysis of antibiotic prophylaxis in severe acute pancreatitis. *Scand J Gastroenterol.* 2011;46:261-270.
37. de Smet AM, Kluytmans JA, Cooper BS, et al. Decontamination of the digestive tract and oropharynx in ICU patients. *N Engl J Med.* 2009;360:20-31.
38. Luiten EJ, Hop WC, Lange JF, Bruining HA. Controlled clinical trial of selective decontamination for the treatment of severe acute pancreatitis. *Ann Surg.* 1995;222:57-65.
39. Daneman N, Sarwar S, Fowler RA, Cuthbertson BH, SuDDICU Canadian Study Group. Effect of selective decontamination on antimicrobial resistance in intensive care units: a systematic review and meta-analysis. *Lancet Infect Dis.* 2013;13:328-341.
40. Bosscha K, Nieuwenhuijs VB, Vos A, Samsom M, Roelofs JM, Akkermans LM. Gastrointestinal motility and gastric tube feeding in mechanically ventilated patients. *Crit Care Med.* 1998;26:1510-1517.
41. Braga M, Gianotti L, Nespoli L, Radaelli G, Di Carlo V. Nutritional approach in malnourished surgical patients: a prospective randomized study. *Arch Surg.* 2002;137:174-180.
42. Preiser JC, Berré J, Carpentier Y, et al. Management of nutrition in European intensive care units: results of a questionnaire. Working group on metabolism and nutrition of the European Society of Intensive Care Medicine. *Intensive Care Med.* 1999;25:95-101.
43. Al-Omran M, Albalawi ZH, Tashkandi MF, Al-Ansary LA. Enteral versus parenteral nutrition for acute pancreatitis. *Cochrane Database Syst Rev.* 2010;(1):CD002837.
44. Rahman SH, Ammori BJ, Holmfield J, Larvin M, McMahon MJ. Intestinal hypoperfusion contributes to gut barrier failure in severe acute pancreatitis. *J Gastrointest Surg.* 2003;7:26-35 [discussion 35–36].
45. Fritz S, Hackert T, Hartwig W, et al. Bacterial translocation and infected pancreatic necrosis in acute necrotizing pancreatitis derives from small bowel rather than from colon. *Am J Surg.* 2010;200:111-117.
46. Bakker OJ, van Brunschot S, van Santvoort HC, et al. Early versus on-demand nasoenteric tube feeding in acute pancreatitis. *N Engl J Med.* 2014;371:1983-1993.
47. Tse F, Yuan Y. Early routine endoscopic retrograde cholangiopancreatography strategy versus early conservative management strategy in acute gallstone pancreatitis. *Cochrane Database Syst Rev.* 2012;(5):CD009779.
48. van Santvoort HC, Besselink MG, de Vries AC, et al. Early endoscopic retrograde cholangiopancreatography in predicted severe acute biliary pancreatitis: a prospective multicenter study. *Ann Surg.* 2009;250:68-75.
49. van Geenen EJ, van Santvoort HC, Besselink MG, et al. Lack of consensus on the role of endoscopic retrograde cholangiography in acute biliary pancreatitis in published meta-analyses and guidelines: a systematic review. *Pancreas.* 2013;42:774-780.
50. van Baal MC, Besselink MG, Bakker OJ, et al. Timing of cholecystectomy after mild biliary pancreatitis: a systematic review. *Ann Surg.* 2012;255(5):860-866.

51. Lankisch PG, Weber-Dany B, Lerch MM. Clinical perspectives in pancreatology: compliance with acute pancreatitis guidelines in Germany. *Pancreatology.* 2005;5:591-593.

52. da Costa DW, Bouwense SA, Schepers NJ, et al. Same-admission versus interval cholecystectomy for mild gallstone pancreatitis (PONCHO): a multicentre randomised controlled trial. *Lancet.* 2015;386:1261-1268.

53. Nealon WH, Bawduniak J, Walser EM. Appropriate timing of cholecystectomy in patients who present with moderate to severe gallstone-associated acute pancreatitis with peripancreatic fluid collections. *Ann Surg.* 2004;239:741-749.

54. van Baal MC, Bollen TL, Bakker OJ, et al. The role of routine fine-needle aspiration in the diagnosis of infected necrotizing pancreatitis. *Surgery.* 2014;155:442-448.

55. Rodriguez JR, Razo AO, Targarona J, et al. Debridement and closed packing for sterile or infected necrotizing pancreatitis: insights into indications and outcomes in 167 patients. *Ann Surg.* 2008;247:294-299.

56. Rau B, Pralle U, Mayer JM, Beger HG. Role of ultrasonographically guided fine-needle aspiration cytology in the diagnosis of infected pancreatic necrosis. *Br J Surg.* 1998;85:179-184.

57. Mier J, Luque-de León E, Castillo A, Robledo F, Blanco R. Early versus late necrosectomy in severe necrotizing pancreatitis. *Am J Surg.* 1997;173:71-75.

58. Besselink MG, Verwer TJ, Schoenmaeckers EJ, et al. Timing of surgical intervention in necrotizing pancreatitis. *Arch Surg.* 2007;142:1194-1201.

59. Besselink MG, van Santvoort HC, Bakker OJ, Bollen TL, Gooszen HG. Draining sterile fluid collections in acute pancreatitis? Primum non nocere! *Surg Endosc.* 2010;25(1):331-332.

60. van Santvoort HC, Besselink MG, Bakker OJ, et al. A step-up approach or open necrosectomy for necrotizing pancreatitis. *N Engl J Med.* 2010;362:1491-1502.

61. Howard TJ, Patel JB, Zyromski N, et al. Declining morbidity and mortality rates in the surgical management of pancreatic necrosis. *J Gastrointest Surg.* 2007;11:43-49.

62. Rau B, Bothe A, Beger HG. Surgical treatment of necrotizing pancreatitis by necrosectomy and closed lavage: changing patient characteristics and outcome in a 19-year, single-center series. *Surgery.* 2005;138:28-39.

63. Hartwig W, Maksan SM, Foitzik T, Schmidt J, Herfarth C, Klar E. Reduction in mortality with delayed surgical therapy of severe pancreatitis. *J Gastrointest Surg.* 2002;6:481-487.

64. De Waele JJ, Hoste E, Blot SI, Decruyenaere J, Colardyn F. Intra-abdominal hypertension in patients with severe acute pancreatitis. *Crit Care.* 2005;9:R452-R457.

65. Mentula P, Hienonen P, Kemppainen E, Puolakkainen P, Leppaniemi A. Surgical decompression for abdominal compartment syndrome in severe acute pancreatitis. *Arch Surg.* 2010;145:764-769.

66. Takahashi Y, Fukushima J, Fukusato T, et al. Prevalence of ischemic enterocolitis in patients with acute pancreatitis. *J Gastroenterol.* 2005;40:827-832.

67. Kirkpatrick AW, Roberts DJ, De Waele J, et al. Intra-abdominal hypertension and the abdominal compartment syndrome: updated consensus definitions and clinical practice guidelines from the World Society of the Abdominal Compartment Syndrome. *Intensive Care Med.* 2013;39:1190-1206.

68. Bakker OJ, van Santvoort HC, van Brunschot S, et al. Endoscopic transgastric vs surgical necrosectomy for infected necrotizing pancreatitis: a randomized trial. *J Am Med Assoc.* 2012;307:1053-1061.

69. Freeny PC, Hauptmann E, Althaus SJ, Traverso LW, Sinanan M. Percutaneous CT-guided catheter drainage of infected acute necrotizing pancreatitis: techniques and results. *AJR Am J Roentgenol.* 1998; 170:969-975.

70. Carter CR, McKay CJ, Imrie CW. Percutaneous necrosectomy and sinus tract endoscopy in the management of infected pancreatic necrosis: an initial experience. *Ann Surg.* 2000;232:175-180.

71. Horvath KD, Kao LS, Wherry KL, Pellegrini CA, Sinanan MN. A technique for laparoscopic-assisted percutaneous drainage of infected pancreatic necrosis and pancreatic abscess. *Surg Endosc.* 2001;15:1221-1225.

72. Gibson SC, Robertson BF, Dickson EJ, McKay CJ, Carter CR. 'Step-port' laparoscopic cystgastrostomy for the management of organized solid predominant post-acute fluid collections after severe acute pancreatitis. *HPB (Oxford).* 2014;16:170-176.

73. Seifert H, Wehrmann T, Schmitt T, Zeuzem S, Caspary WF. Retroperitoneal endoscopic debridement for infected peripancreatic necrosis. *Lancet.* 2000;356:653-655.

74. van Baal MC, van Santvoort HC, Bollen TL, et al. Systematic review of percutaneous catheter drainage as primary treatment for necrotizing pancreatitis. *Br J Surg.* 2011;98:18-27.

75. Mouli VP, Sreenivas V, Garg PK. Efficacy of conservative treatment, without necrosectomy, for infected pancreatic necrosis: a systematic review and meta-analysis. *Gastroenterology.* 2013;144:333-340.e2.

76. Besselink MG, van Santvoort HC, Schaapherder AF, van Ramshorst B, van Goor H, Gooszen HG. Feasibility of minimally invasive approaches in patients with infected necrotizing pancreatitis. *Br J Surg.* 2007;94:604-608.

77. Castellanos G, Pinero A, Doig LA, Serrano A, Fuster M, Bixquert V. Management of infected pancreatic necrosis using retroperitoneal necrosectomy with flexible endoscope: 10 years of experience. *Surg Endosc.* 2013;27:443-453.

78. Sileikis A, Beisa V, Simutis G, Tamosiunas A, Strupas K. Three-port retroperitoneoscopic necrosectomy in management of acute necrotic pancreatitis. *Medicina.* 2010;46:176-179.

79. Tang C, Wang B, Xie B, Liu H, Chen P. Treatment of severe acute pancreatitis through retroperitoneal laparoscopic drainage. *Front Med.* 2011;5:302-305.

80. Working Party of the British Society of Gastroenterology. UK guidelines for the management of acute pancreatitis. *Gut.* 2005;54(suppl 3):iii1-iii9.

81. Isaji S, Takada T, Kawarada Y, et al. JPN Guidelines for the management of acute pancreatitis:surgical management. *J Hepatobiliary Pancreat Surg.* 2006;13:48-55.

82. Fabbri C, Luigiano C, Maimone A, Polifemo AM, Tarantino I, Cennamo V. Endoscopic ultrasound-guided drainage of pancreatic fluid collections. *World J Gastrointest Endosc.* 2012;4:479-488.

83. Park DH, Lee SS, Moon SH, et al. Endoscopic ultrasound-guided versus conventional transmural drainage for pancreatic pseudocysts: a prospective randomized trial. *Endoscopy.* 2009;41:842-848.

84. Varadarajulu S, Christein JD, Tamhane A, Drelichman ER, Wilcox CM. Prospective randomized trial comparing EUS and EGD for transmural drainage of pancreatic pseudocysts (with videos). *Gastrointest Endosc.* 2008;68:1102-1111.

85. Rana SS, Bhasin DK, Rao C, Gupta R, Singh K. Non-fluoroscopic endoscopic ultrasound-guided transmural drainage of symptomatic non-bulging walled-off pancreatic necrosis. *Dig Endosc.* 2013;25:47-52.

86. Yamamoto N, Isayama H, Kawakami H, et al. Preliminary report on a new, fully covered, metal stent designed for the treatment of pancreatic fluid collections. *Gastrointest Endosc.* 2013;77:809-814.

87. Moon JH, Choi HJ, Kim DC, et al. A newly designed fully covered metal stent for lumen apposition in EUS-guided drainage and access: a feasibility study (with videos). *Gastrointest Endosc.* 2014;79:990-995.

88. Sarkaria S, Sethi A, Rondon C, et al. Pancreatic necrosectomy using covered esophageal stents: a novel approach. *J Clin Gastroenterol.* 2014;48:145-152.

89. Bang JY, Wilcox CM, Trevino J, et al. Factors impacting treatment outcomes in the endoscopic management of walled-off pancreatic necrosis. *J Gastroenterol Hepatol.* 2013;28:1725-1732.

90. Ross AS, Irani S, Gan SI, et al. Dual-modality drainage of infected and symptomatic walled-off pancreatic necrosis: long-term clinical outcomes. *Gastrointest Endosc.* 2014;79:929-935.

91. Bang JY, Holt BA, Hawes RH, et al. Outcomes after implementing a tailored endoscopic step-up approach to walled-off necrosis in acute pancreatitis. *Br J Surg.* 2014;101:1729-1738.

92. Freeman ML, Werner J, van Santvoort HC, et al. Interventions for necrotizing pancreatitis: summary of a multidisciplinary consensus conference. *Pancreas.* 2012;41:1176-1194.

93. Gardner TB. Endoscopic management of necrotizing pancreatitis. *Gastrointest Endosc.* 2012;76:1214-1223.

94. van Brunschot S, van Grinsven J, Voermans RP, et al. Transluminal endoscopic step-up approach versus minimally invasive surgical step-up approach in patients with infected necrotising pancreatitis (TENSION trial): design and rationale of a randomised controlled multicenter trial [ISRCTN09186711]. *BMC Gastroenterol.* 2013;13:161.

95. van Grinsven J, van Brunschot S, Bakker OJ, et al. Diagnostic strategy and timing of intervention in infected necrotizing pancreatitis: an international expert survey and case vignette study. *HPB (Oxford).* 2015;doi:10.1111/hpb.12491.

Chronic Pancreatitis

Jennifer Tseng | Eugene A. Choi | Jeffrey B. Matthews

Chronic pancreatitis is a progressive inflammatory disorder that leads to irreversible destruction of the exocrine and endocrine tissue of the pancreas. Fibrotic replacement of the normal pancreas may be associated with persistent abdominal pain, the development of exocrine insufficiency, and ultimately, diabetes mellitus. Inflammation may lead to local complications, including biliary and gastrointestinal obstruction, ascites, mesoportal-splenic thrombosis, pseudocyst formation, hemorrhage, and sepsis. In its advanced stages, chronic pancreatitis is readily apparent clinically, typically associated with pancreatic duct stricture and ductal dilation, stones and diffuse parenchymal calcification, and the digestive and metabolic effects of organ insufficiency. However, recognition of patients with early and mild disease remains a difficult challenge. The absence of a clinically relevant classification system for chronic pancreatitis contributes to inconsistencies in the treatment of the disease. Treatment decisions are better made in the context of individual circumstances such as patient symptoms and anatomic findings rather than classification systems based on etiology or morphologic severity.

DEFINITION

Acute pancreatitis generally refers to a single episode of acute inflammation of the organ, typically associated with histopathologic changes that may include edema, fat necrosis, and hemorrhage. Although often fully reversible, the acute injury may be so severe as to result in permanent parenchymal damage, local or remote complications, or death. Chronic pancreatitis generally refers to an ongoing inflammatory and fibrosing disorder characterized by irreversible morphologic changes, progressive and permanent loss of exocrine and endocrine function, and a clinical pattern of recurrent acute exacerbation or persistent pain. In reality, however, acute and chronic pancreatitis represent more of a spectrum of inflammatory and fibrosing conditions of the pancreas than the two dichotomous terms would otherwise imply. Recurrent episodes (or even a single episode) of acute pancreatitis may lead to chronic changes within the pancreas, although the timing and extent to which such changes merit a change in nomenclature to chronic pancreatitis is somewhat arbitrary. The histopathologic changes of chronic pancreatitis comprise fibrosis, a reduced number of acinar cells and islets of Langerhans, and development of strictures and dilation of pancreatic ducts as well as calcium calculi (pancreatic duct stones). The morphologic/structural changes of chronic pancreatitis can occur years before any clinical symptoms are present. One hypothesis envisions the activation of pancreatic stellate cells, which

induce desmoplasia, as the key pathogenetic "switch" that leads to the transition to chronic pancreatitis.[1]

Efforts to establish consensus for uniform terminology of pancreatitis began with an international conference held in Marseille in 1963, during which participants agreed that chronic pancreatitis was distinguished by irreversible focal, segmental, or diffuse destruction of the exocrine tissue along with dilation or focal strictures of the main pancreatic duct. At a second meeting in Marseille held in 1984,[2,3] chronic pancreatitis was subclassified as chronic pancreatitis with focal or segmental or diffuse fibrosis, and chronic pancreatitis with or without stones, and obstructive chronic pancreatitis was listed as a distinct form. To help define changes associated with clinical risk factors, a 1988 meeting in Rome added the morphologic distinction of chronic calcifying pancreatitis, which is characterized by intraductal calcifications and protein plugs, and chronic inflammatory pancreatitis, which is characterized by dense infiltration of mononuclear inflammatory cells.[4] A consensus conference in Cambridge in 1984 defined the distinction between acute and chronic pancreatitis as the reversibility of the morphologic and functional changes of inflammation.[5] The Cambridge meeting proposed a classification system of chronic pancreatitis based on radiographic findings on endoscopic retrograde cholangiopancreatography (ERCP) (Table 92.1) and ultrasonography (US) or computed tomography (CT). Criteria for chronic pancreatitis from the Japan Pancreas Society focused on findings from an array of diagnostic approaches including US, CT, ERCP, secretin stimulation, and histologic examination of pancreatic tissue. The presence of certain criteria such as pancreatic stones on CT or US is considered definitive evidence of chronic pancreatitis, whereas other criteria such as pancreatic deformity with irregular contour are considered only probable or possible evidence in support of the disease.[6] The shortcoming of all of these consensus approaches has been the inability to establish a definitive diagnosis in the earliest stages of disease. Moreover, no classification system has proven practical applicability in guiding decisions for therapy.

RISK FACTORS

An association between alcohol and acute and chronic pancreatitis has been noted for over half a century. Sarles et al. demonstrated that the relative risk of chronic pancreatitis increases directly with mean daily alcohol consumption.[4] However, even relatively moderate alcohol intake can cause chronic pancreatitis, and the duration of alcohol consumption can be relatively short before the onset of disease. In chronic pancreatitis, alcohol is thought

TABLE 92.1 Cambridge Conference Classification of Chronic Pancreatitis: Endoscopic Retrograde Cholangiopancreatography

Terminology	Main Duct	Abnormal Side Ducts	Additional Features
Normal	Normal	None	—
Equivocal	Normal	<3	—
Mild changes	Normal	≥3	—
Moderate changes	Abnormal	>3	—
Marked changes	Abnormal	>3	1 or more of large cavity, obstruction, filling defects, severe dilation, or irregularity

Modified from Sarner M, Cotton PB. Classification of pancreatitis. *Gut.* 1984;25:756.

TABLE 92.2 Etiologic Risk Factors Associated With Chronic Pancreatitis

Toxic/ metabolic	Alcoholic, tobacco smoking, hypercalcemia (hyperparathyroidism)
	Hyperlipidemia
	Chronic renal failure
	Medications, toxins
Idiopathic	Tropical
Genetic	Cationic trypsinogen *(PRSS1)*
	PRSS2, CTRC
	CFTR, SPINK1
	CSR, CLDN2, CPA1
Autoimmune	Isolated or associated with autoimmune disorders
Recurrent acute and severe	Postnecrotic (severe acute pancreatitis)
	Recurrent acute pancreatitis
	Vascular disease/ischemic
	Postirradiation
Obstructive	Pancreatic divisum
	Sphincter of Oddi disorders
	Duct obstruction (tumor)
	Posttraumatic pancreatic duct scars
	Preampullary duodenal wall cysts

Modified from Etemad B, Whitcomb DC. Chronic pancreatitis: diagnosis, classification, and new genetic developments. *Gastroenterology.* 2001;120:682.

to increase the protein concentration in pancreatic juice, which causes intraductal calcium stone formation, ductal epithelial ulceration, inflammation, and fibrosis. Yet it is only a small percentage (5% to 10%) of alcoholics that develop pancreatic disease, suggesting that alcohol is more of a risk factor than a causative agent for pancreatitis in patients who are susceptible for various unknown or poorly defined reasons. Different disease processes causing similar-appearing injury to the pancreas may follow different clinical courses. Thus, rather than classifying pancreatitis based on the presumed causative agent, Whitcomb et al. proposed a system to classify risk factors that may interact to predispose an individual patient to produce pancreatitis.[7] According to this framework, risk factors are grouped as toxic/metabolic, idiopathic, genetic, autoimmune, recurrent acute, or obstructive (TIGAR-O) (Table 92.2). An additional classification system uses the M-ANNHEIM paradigm: **M**ultiple risk factors of **A**lcohol consumption (excessive >80 g/day, increased 20 to 80 g/day, moderate <20 g/day), **N**icotine consumption, **N**utritional factors (high calorie proportion of fat and protein, hyperlipidemia), **H**ereditary factors, **E**fferent duct factors (pancreas divisum, annular pancreas, tumors, posttraumatic, sphincter of Oddi dysfunction), **I**mmunologic factors and **M**iscellaneous and rare metabolic disorders (hypercalcemia, hyperparathyroidism, chronic renal failure, drugs, toxins).[8]

TOXIC/METABOLIC

Almost 70% of chronic pancreatitis cases are associated with chronic alcoholic intake in Western countries.[9] Tobacco use is associated with the early presentation of alcoholic chronic pancreatitis and is associated with the presentation of calcifications and the development of diabetes. It is unknown if tobacco initiates the disease[10]; however, tobacco is thought to potentiate the progression. In a preclinical model, investigators demonstrated that tobacco exposure increases the risk of pancreatic cancer in chronic pancreatitis patients.[11] Hyperparathyroidism and hypercalcemia are also associated with chronic pancreatitis. Patients with chronic renal failure have a higher risk.

IDIOPATHIC

Historically, no environmental or metabolic risk factor can be identified in approximately 20% of patients who are therefore categorized as having idiopathic acute, recurrent acute, or chronic pancreatitis. Patients with idiopathic disease typically fall into a bimodal age distribution, presenting between the ages of 10 and 20 or after age 50 years. However, many of these patients are increasingly recognized to have underlying genetic mutations and polymorphisms and may be more appropriately recategorized into the genetic subgroup. To better understand the interactions among genetic, environmental, and metabolic factors predisposing to chronic pancreatitis, a consortium (North American Pancreatitis Study 2) has been established to collect patient questionnaires and blood for genomic DNA and biomarker studies.[12]

GENETIC

Although hereditary pancreatitis was recognized as a distinct clinical entity in the 1950s, it was not until 1996 that its genetic basis began to be understood. The inheritance pattern of hereditary chronic pancreatitis is autosomal dominant and has roughly a 78% penetrance rate. Genetic linkage analysis established a locus for hereditary chronic pancreatitis on chromosome 7q, a region that encodes eight different zymogen genes including various trypsins and carboxypeptidase A. Whitcomb et al. performed mutational screening analyses for each of the encoding regions of the cationic and anionic trypsinogen genes and discovered a single G-to-A transition mutation in the cationic trypsinogen gene *(PRSS1)*.[7] This transition mutation resulted in an Arg (CGC)-to-His (CAC) *(R122H)* substitution that did not change the structure or catalytic activity of the enzyme but led to an unusually stable protein. The *R122H* mutation produces a proteolytic-resistant trypsinogen favoring inappropriate activation within the pancreas, leading to autodigestion. Other mutations in *PRSS1* have been identified in various kindreds, although these are less well studied.[13-16] Patients with hereditary pancreatitis, especially those bearing the *R122H* mutation of *PRSS1*, have an estimated 35% lifetime risk of developing pancreatic cancer,[17] a risk that is roughly doubled by smoking.

Variations in a number of other genes have been associated with chronic pancreatitis. Witt et al. studied 96 unrelated children and adolescents with idiopathic chronic pancreatitis and identified frequent mutations in the serine protease inhibitor, Kazal type 1 *(SPINK1)*, a pancreatic trypsin inhibitor.[18] *SPINK1* is colocalized with trypsinogen within zymogen granules and is believed to prevent inappropriate intrapancreatic protease activation. The most frequent mutation associated with chronic pancreatitis is an N34S amino acid substitution in exon 3. Mutations in *SPINK1* or in *PRSS1* lead to an imbalance toward intrapancreatic trypsin activation, thereby leading to autodigestion of the pancreas and inflammation. It is postulated that the *SPINK1* mutations are not directly responsible for pancreatitis but may lower the threshold for the disease from other risk factors.[19]

Chronic pancreatitis is also associated with mutations in the cystic fibrosis transmembrane conductance regulator gene *(CFTR)*. Cystic fibrosis is an autosomal recessive disorder that has been linked to mutation of the *CFTR* gene, which encodes a cyclic adenosine monophosphate–regulated chloride channel located in the apical domain of epithelial cells lining the proximal ducts of the pancreas. More than 1000 mutations have been characterized with a wide range of impact on the characteristics of the channel function. The most common mutation results in a deletion of the single amino acid, phenylalanine, at position 508 *(DF508)*. The clinical manifestations are dependent on the specific mutation and the impact on the functional characteristic of the chloride channel. Sharer et al. found that *CFTR* mutations were more common in patients with idiopathic rather than alcoholic chronic pancreatitis.[20] The *CFTR* mutation is not a direct cause of chronic pancreatitis but may contribute to the disease. Mutation of the *CFTR* may lead to a decrease in bicarbonate secretion, impaired fluid secretion and formation of protein plugs, and pancreatic insufficiency. Alternatively, the *CFTR* mutation may alter vesicular sorting and granule trafficking or cause membrane lipid imbalance. Chronic pancreatitis has also been associated with mutations in the anionic trypsinogen *(PRSS2)* and chymotrypsin C *(CTRC)*. *PRSS2* has a lower incidence of mutations in chronic pancreatitis; a variant of *PRSS2* with a glycine-to-arginine change at codon 191 appears to have a protective effect against chronic pancreatitis.[21] Chymotrypsin C gene mutation may increase the risk and encourage progression of chronic pancreatitis in patients with *CFTR* and *SPINK1* mutations with tobacco and alcohol abuse.[22,23] Calcium-sensing receptor *(CSR)*, X-linked claudin-2 *(CLDN2)*, carboxypeptidase A1 *(CPA1)*, and additional genetic and nongenetic alterations are also associated with chronic pancreatitis.[24-28]

AUTOIMMUNE

Autoimmune pancreatitis, also known as lymphoplasmacytic sclerosing pancreatitis, is a rare cause (1%) of chronic pancreatitis.[29] Gland enlargement, diffuse duct narrowing, and stenosis of the intrapancreatic portion of the bile duct characterize the disease. Histologic examination of the tissue demonstrates pancreas parenchyma infiltrated by both CD4+ and CD8+ lymphocytes and IgG4 plasma cells, with interstitial fibrosis and acinar cell atrophy. Patients with autoimmune pancreatitis have antibodies directed against a peptide that is homologous with the sequence of the plasminogen-binding protein (PBP) of *Helicobacter pylori* and with the ubiquitin-protein ligase E3 component n-recognin 2, which is expressed in the acinar cells of the pancreas.[30] Autoimmune pancreatitis can be associated with other autoimmune diseases including Sjögren syndrome, primary sclerosing cholangitis (PSC), and inflammatory bowel disease. Primary treatment for autoimmune pancreatitis is steroid treatment. Focal inflammation seen with this disease can often mimic a pancreatic mass, which may be difficult to differentiate from a pancreatic malignancy on imaging studies.

RECURRENT ACUTE

Recurrent episodes of acute pancreatitis of any etiology can cause chronic pancreatitis. This mechanism is poorly understood but likely involves the accumulated effects of postinflammatory scarring and necrosis as well as the priming of pancreatic stellate cells to induce fibrosis. In addition, radiation and ischemia may contribute to irreversible histopathologic changes and inflammation characteristic of chronic pancreatitis. However, the term *recurrent acute pancreatitis* (RAP) refers specifically to episodes of acute pancreatitis that do not lead to chronic pancreatitis if the underlying inciting factors are treated.[31]

OBSTRUCTION

Obstructive pancreatitis can be congenital, functional, or acquired. Causes of pancreatic obstruction include pancreatic or ampullary tumors, and postinjury pancreatic duct fibrosis. Elevated basal pressures at the sphincter of Oddi are thought by some to lead to relative outflow obstruction from the proximal duct and thereby contribute to pancreatitis. Patients may also have anatomic variations in the pancreatic ductal system that predispose for obstruction, most notably pancreas divisum. However, the vast majority of patients with pancreas divisum are asymptomatic; thus, the anatomic variation may predispose to pancreatitis in combination with other risk factors.

CLINICAL MANIFESTATIONS

The most common symptom of chronic pancreatitis is abdominal pain (90%), although the pattern of pain is highly variable. In some patients, particularly early in the course of the disease, pain may be a minor feature. The pain may be episodic and minimal or absent between acute exacerbations, but it is often noted to gradually become more constant. In late phases of the disease, pain may disappear ("burnout"), a transition that is often associated with the development of diabetes and exocrine insufficiency. The pain is most frequently localized to the epigastrium, often radiates to the back, and is typically associated with nausea and vomiting. Overall, the course of chronic pancreatitis is highly unpredictable and variable. Lankisch et al. followed 335 patients with chronic pancreatitis, and despite a long-term observation period of more than 10 years, a majority of patients continued to experience pain.[32] Because eating can exacerbate pain, patients may avoid regular meals, leading to weight loss and malnutrition. Between 4% and 30% of patients have significant exocrine insufficiency and report bloating, flatulence, or steatorrhea. Malabsorption leads to weight loss and deficiencies in micronutrients, especially fat-soluble vitamins A, D, and E. Endocrine insufficiency or diabetes mellitus develops later in the course of the disease, typically when 90% of the parenchyma is replaced by fibrosis. Diabetes develops more often in those patients with alcohol-associated chronic calcifying pancreatitis than in hereditary forms of the disease.

EXTRAPANCREATIC COMPLICATIONS OF CHRONIC PANCREATITIS

A subset of patients develops symptoms of gastrointestinal and biliary obstruction. Duodenal, colonic, and bile duct obstruction can occur as a result of significant fibrosis of the head of the pancreas or the development of large pseudocysts (Fig. 92.1). The incidence of biliary obstruction is approximately 3% to 23% among patients diagnosed with chronic pancreatitis, and is even higher (15% to 60%) among patients who require surgery.[33] The incidence of duodenal obstruction/stenosis is 2% in all patients, and again is higher (12%) in patients who require operative therapy. The majority of patients with splenic vein thrombosis are asymptomatic; the incidence of thrombosis varies anywhere from 4% to 45% depending on the population surveyed, but very few patients present with gastric variceal bleeding.[34,35] Additionally, chronic pancreatitis has been

associated with an increased risk of osteoporotic fractures that are likely secondary to a combination of malnutrition and malabsorption.[36]

Epidemiologic and preclinical studies demonstrate that chronic pancreatitis is associated with the development of pancreatic cancer. Lowenfels et al. presented a multi-center historical cohort study of 2015 patients with chronic pancreatitis followed for at least 2 years.[37] The standardized incidence risk ratio for the development of pancreatic cancer was 16.5 and 14.4 at 2- and 5-year follow-up, respectively, for the risk of developing pancreatic cancer. The cumulative incidence of pancreatic cancer in non-hereditary chronic pancreatitis is 2% per decade after initial diagnosis.[36] The incidence of pancreatic cancer in hereditary pancreatitis is 40% by age 70 starting at age 35.[38] The incidence of pancreatic cancer was equally high in patients who presented with pancreatitis associated with chronic alcohol use and those with other risk factors. In a preclinical murine model, Guerrra et al. reported that inflammation associated with chronic pancreatitis is essential for induction of pancreatic cancer by the onco-gene *KRAS* (Figs. 92.2 and 92.3).[39]

MECHANISM OF PAIN IN CHRONIC PANCREATITIS

A number of mechanisms have been proposed to account for the pain of chronic pancreatitis. However, the correlation between the hypothetical cause of the pain and the clinical results of therapies directed at that cause is imperfect at best. Obstruction of the main pancreatic duct in some circumstances is thought to lead to increased ductal pressure leading to pain through stretch-activated neural pathways. Ductal obstruction may also induce missorting and mistargeted basolateral secretion of pancreatic enzymes, triggering protease-activated nociceptive pathways. Relief of main duct obstruction is often effective treatment for pain in these circumstances. Chronic

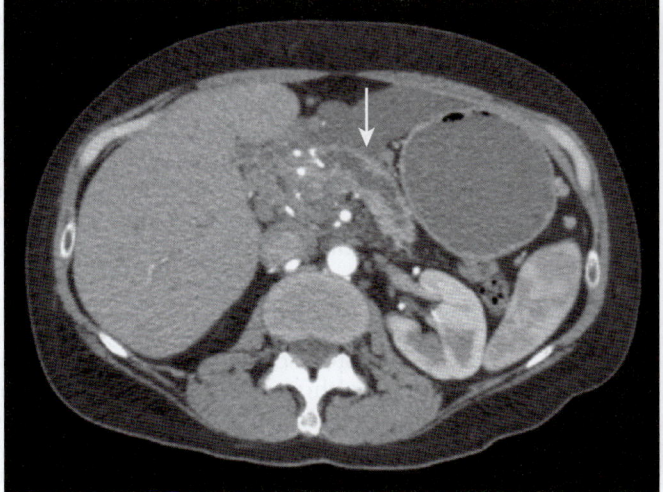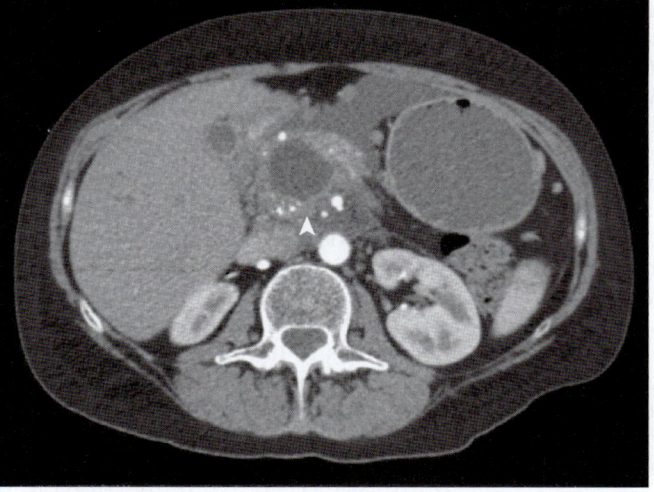

FIGURE 92.1 Chronic pancreatitis in a 48-year-old woman with a history of alcohol use. *(Left)* Axial cross-section abdominal computed tomography demonstrating a dilated pancreatic duct *(arrow)* and *(right)* a pseudocyst in the head of the pancreas communicating with the main duct *(arrowhead)*.

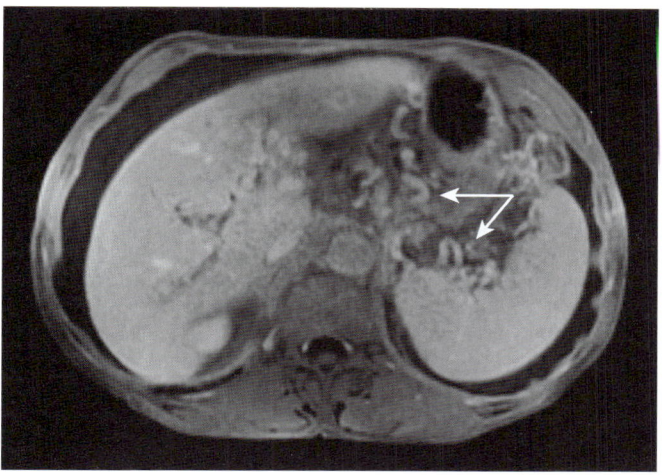

FIGURE 92.2 Chronic pancreatitis in a 50-year-old man with a history of extensive alcohol use. Magnetic resonance imaging demonstrates a thrombosed splenic vein with extensive varices involving the splenic hilum and pancreatic tail *(arrows)*.

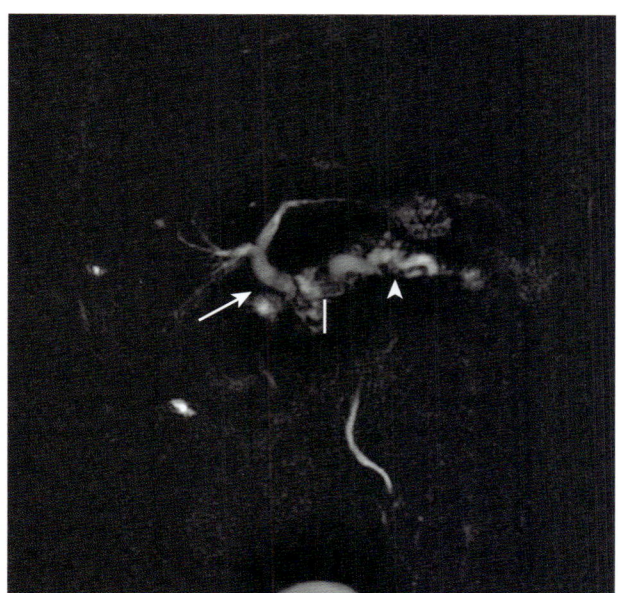

FIGURE 92.3 Chronic pancreatitis in a 52-year-old man with a history of extensive alcohol use. Magnetic resonance cholangiopancreatography demonstrates a dilated common bile duct up to the intrapancreatic portion *(arrow)*, irregularity of and dilation of the pancreatic duct and sides *(arrowhead)*, and intraluminal filling defects at the level of the pancreatic head *(line)*.

inflammation of the pancreas may lead to fibrosis of the peripancreatic capsule and perilobular parenchyma, which has been proposed to impair regional and local blood flow, thereby producing pain through ischemia and consequent tissue acidosis.[40] Parenchymal fibrosis has also been likened to a compartment syndrome, associated with impaired venous drainage.[41] Chronic inflammation associated with chronic pancreatitis may also induce visceral hyperalgesia through neural remodeling of local, spinal, or central nociceptive pathways.[42,43] Superimposed on this background of uncertainty regarding the cellular, organ, and systemic basis of pain is the confounding influence of narcotic addiction that afflicts many affected individuals.

DIAGNOSIS OF CHRONIC PANCREATITIS

The diagnosis of chronic pancreatitis is based on the combination of history and physical examination, blood tests, functional tests, and radiographic studies. The clinician should elicit a clear description of the pain, the recurrent nature of the episodes, and the presence of risk factors for the disease, including alcohol consumption and family history. Because the natural history of pain is highly variable and 20% of patients have painless chronic pancreatitis, it is not unusual that the diagnosis may be delayed. On physical examination, there may be evidence of malnutrition such as temporal wasting and decreased stores of subcutaneous fat. Abdominal fullness may suggest the presence of a pancreatic pseudocyst.

There are no perfect tests for chronic pancreatitis, particularly in its earliest stages. Serum amylase and lipase, as well as fasting serum glucose and glycosylated hemoglobin (Hb_{A1c}) may be helpful. Serum amylase and lipase levels may be elevated during an acute exacerbation of chronic pancreatitis, but with disease progression and pancreatic parenchymal fibrosis, these levels may remain normal even during an episode of acute inflammation. Blood glucose may be elevated in patients with advanced disease as endocrine function deteriorates. Stool samples can be examined for levels of fat. Stool is collected for a 72-hour period and fat content greater than 7 g per day is abnormal. Pancreatic exocrine function can also be assessed by analysis of duodenal bicarbonate concentration before and after stimulation with secretin during an upper endoscopy procedure[44] or by measurement of fecal elastase. However, fecal elastase levels may be insensitive in mild to moderate chronic pancreatitis. A ^{13}C-mixed triglyceride breath test is also in development for the diagnosis of pancreatic exocrine insufficiency due to chronic pancreatitis.[45] For patients with autoimmune pancreatitis, serum IgG4 protein levels, antinuclear antibodies, rheumatoid factor, and erythrocyte sedimentation rate (ESR) may help establish the diagnosis.[46]

Plain radiographs may demonstrate calcifications but are otherwise not helpful and not routinely recommended. Similarly, transabdominal US is usually limited by patient body habitus and is operator dependent. The modality most often used is intravenous contrast-enhanced CT, which is effective in demonstrating late changes of the disease including ductal and parenchymal calcifications, ductal dilation and stricture, and parenchymal atrophy, as well as complications such as pseudocysts, vessel thrombosis, and pseudoaneurysms. ERCP and magnetic resonance cholangiopancreatography (MRCP) can complement CT by better visualizing the pancreatic ductal system. Before the widespread use of magnetic resonance imaging, ERCP was the gold standard to confirm early chronic pancreatitis. ERCP sensitivity and specificity for the diagnosis of chronic pancreatitis has been reported to be 70% to 90%, and 90% to 100%, respectively. Currently, ERCP is not routinely performed purely for diagnostic purposes because it is invasive and can induce acute pancreatitis; its use is largely restricted to situations where endoscopic therapy is contemplated, such as for stone removal. MRCP is noninvasive and avoids the use of nonionizing radiation and contrast media. MRCP with intravenous secretin administration may augment visualization of pancreatic side ducts and provide qualitative and semiquantitative information regarding the exocrine capacity of the pancreas, but it is limited in detecting calcifications. A few studies have demonstrated that endoscopic ultrasound (EUS) may detect early changes/features characteristic of chronic pancreatitis such as ductal wall echogenicity, focal echogenicity, and increased duct branches before changes are seen with CT scan, MRCP, and ERCP.[47] However, the criteria used to make the diagnosis of chronic pancreatitis with endoscopic US are controversial and some of these findings can be identified in individuals without clinical symptoms or known pancreatic disease.

TREATMENT OPTIONS FOR CHRONIC PANCREATITIS

For patients with chronic pancreatitis, treatment begins with lifestyle changes. Patients should cease alcohol intake. Continuous exposure to alcohol may precipitate recurrent episodes of pancreatitis and exacerbate pain. Patients should stop smoking. Patients with pain may need to change their diet and eating patterns. Patients may need to eat six small low-fat meals during the day and increase fluid intake. Oral pancreatic enzyme supplementation with meals may help both with malabsorption and with pain associated with exocrine insufficiency. Scheduled dosing of uncoated enzyme preparations (rather than the more widely available coated preparations) may also reduce pain in chronic pancreatitis according to several small randomized trials, although the efficacy of this approach is controversial. Patients developing type 1 diabetes may require insulin replacement.

One of the greatest challenges in treating patients with chronic pancreatitis is pain control. Patients with persistent pain despite diet modification may require fasting for several days with intravenous fluids, enteral feedings via nasojejunal feeding tubes, or parenteral nutrition via central catheter. A few limited studies suggest that octreotide and antidepressants may help relieve pain and reduce the risk of exacerbation.[48] A recent metaanalysis showed the benefit of antioxidant therapy in pain reduction.[49] Nonsteroidal antiinflammatory drugs, such as ibuprofen, may be used early in the course of the disease. Pregabalin may help prevent central sensitization and hyperalgesia due to chronic pancreatitis.[50] However, a regimen of a combination of long-acting and short-acting narcotics may be needed for refractory pain. For patients who are not candidates for endoscopic or surgical options, a celiac plexus nerve block may be performed percutaneously or endoscopically. The block relieves pain in about half of the patients who undergo the procedures; pain relief typically lasts for 2 months. However, for durable pain relief, patients may require additional treatment 2 to 6 months after the first treatment; however, these are usually

TABLE 92.3 Pain Management Strategy Reflects Presumed Mechanism

Diagnosis	Proposed Treatment
Local inflammation	Pharmacotherapy (pancreatic enzymes, analgesics, narcotics, pregabalin)
Ductal hypertension	Decompression (Puestow, endoscopic stenting)
Organ hypertension	Resection (Whipple, Frey procedures)
Retroperitoneal damage	Neuroablation (celiac block, splanchnicectomy)
Altered nociception	Psychosocial intervention (counseling, detoxification)

ineffective. A variety of agents have been used for the nerve block, including neurolytic agents (alcohol), antiinflammatory agents (steroids), and anesthetics. Alternatively, thoracoscopic denervation of splanchnic nerves has been reported to achieve short-term pain relief. Implantable pumps for intrathecal infusion of narcotics have also been reported (Table 92.3).[51]

ENDOSCOPIC MANAGEMENT

Pancreatic endoscopic therapy may be used for patients with pain and radiographic evidence of duct obstruction by calcified stones.[52] Pancreatic sphincterotomy permits the introduction of endoscopic equipment to dilate pancreatic duct strictures by balloon dilation or coiled wire stent removal device. Endoscopic polyethylene stents, ranging in size from 5.0 to 11.5 French, can be placed across areas of stricture to maintain ductal patency. Opening of strictures allows for the unobstructed flow of pancreatic juice to improve both pain and nutrient absorption. Unfortunately, the patency of the stents is relatively short-lived, usually 2 to 4 months. Stent occlusion and migration can exacerbate pain and lead to suppurative infection. Long-term stenting can paradoxically worsen periductal inflammation, fibrosis, and stricturing. Ductal stents are routinely removed after a period of time (2 to 4 months) and if the pain is improved, patients are observed and given pancreatic enzyme supplementation.

Stones may form within the pancreatic duct, in the duct wall, or in the pancreatic parenchyma, frequently in the segment of the duct proximal to a stricture, exacerbating ductal obstruction and inflammation. Intraductal stones can be removed with Dormia-type baskets. Stones larger than the pancreatic duct orifice can be broken into smaller pieces by mechanical lithotripsy. Extracorporeal shock wave lithotripsy (ESWL) can help remove stones not accessible by basket or mechanical lithotripsy. A metaanalysis and systemic review found ESWL to be effective and safe in patients with a main pancreatic duct stone size greater than 5 mm, in the presence of pancreatic duct strictures, impacted pancreatic duct calculi, or failure of endoscopic methods.[53] Endoscopic therapy can also be used to treat biliary strictures associated with chronic pancreatitis. Duodenal obstruction can be relieved in nonoperative candidates by endoscopic placement of expandable coated metallic stents. In addition, symptomatic pseudocysts can be drained transgastrically or transduodenally in appropriately selected patients to achieve relief of pain.

SURGICAL MANAGEMENT

Surgical management is generally reserved for otherwise unmanageable symptomatic chronic pancreatitis. Indications for surgery include intractable abdominal pain, secondary complications of chronic pancreatitis including biliary stricture, duodenal stenosis, pseudocyst, and suspected pancreatic neoplasm. The goals of surgical management are to relieve pain and address complications, while preserving exocrine and endocrine function as much as possible. The specific choice of procedure is usually determined by anatomic findings, although there may be several reasonable alternatives in any given scenario (Tables 92.4 and 92.5). Useful features in considering surgical options are the presence of so-called large-duct versus small-duct disease as well as the presence and location of an inflammatory mass.

In many patients, inflammation and parenchymal abnormalities appear most prominently within the head of the pancreas. Briggs et al. proposed that the head of the organ was also the prime source of pain in chronic pancreatitis.[54] In view of this notion, and because the three major ductal systems of Wirsung, Santorini, and the uncinate course through the head of the pancreas, it is often said that the head of the pancreas is the "pacemaker" of the disease. Patients may less commonly present with isolated inflammation in the tail of the pancreas, or with only ductal dilation and stricture without focal fibrosis or dominant inflammatory mass.

The optimal timing of surgery is influenced by a global assessment of disease course. Longer disease duration, preoperative opioid usage, and frequent endoscopic procedures have been associated with ongoing pain after surgical management. Patients undergoing surgery within 3 years of symptoms had improved pain relief and delayed loss of endocrine and exocrine function. Long-standing chronic pancreatitis may lead to hyperalgesia as more advanced stages have been correlated with sensitization of central pain pathways.[55,56]

RESECTION

For patients with focal disease largely confined to the head of the pancreas without duct dilation, a Whipple procedure (pancreaticoduodenectomy [PD]) is generally preferred (Fig. 92.4).[57] Removal of the head of the pancreas also addresses bile duct stricture and duodenal obstruction, if present, and improves drainage of the upstream proximal (main) pancreatic duct and its tributaries. The reconstruction includes a two-layered end-to-side pancreaticojejunostomy (Fig. 92.5), an end-to-side hepaticojejunostomy, and a gastrojejunostomy. Pain relief, either complete or partial, is usually achieved in approximately 85% of patients. Following PD, new-onset diabetes is uncommon in patients with otherwise normal glucose tolerance preoperatively, although up to 50% of patients will develop diabetes during the subsequent 10 years.[58] Postoperative exocrine insufficiency requiring enzyme supplementation develops in almost 50% of patients. Mortality associated with the procedure is generally less than 5%, although the overall rate of postoperative complications is typically reported between 30% and 40%. Traverso and Longmire introduced a pylorus-preserving pancreaticoduodenectomy (PPPD), an operation that was intended to improve functional digestive outcomes and quality of life by preserving the physiologic gastric emptying mechanism.[59]

Beger introduced duodenum-preserving pancreatic head resection (DPPHR) as an alternative to PD or PPPD.[60] The procedure includes division of the neck of the pancreas overlying the confluence of the splenic and superior mesenteric veins and removal of the head of

---

TABLE 92.4 Surgical Treatments for Chronic Pancreatitis

Resection	Decompression	Hybrid
Pancreaticoduodenectomy (Kausch-Whipple procedure)	Duval procedure	Frey procedure
Pylorus-preserving pancreaticoduodenectomy (Traverso-Longmire)	Puestow-Gillesby procedure	Hamburg modification
Beger procedure	Partington-Rochelle procedure (Puestow)	Berne modification
Near-total or total pancreatectomy	Izbicki procedure	—

TABLE 92.5 Surgical Treatment Options Based on Pancreas Morphology

	Dilated Pancreatic Duct	Small or Nondilated Duct
No focal mass	1. Decompressive: Partington-Rochelle procedure (Puestow) 2. Hybrid procedure: Frey	1. Observation 2. Resection: pancreaticoduodenectomy, total pancreatectomy 3. Decompressive: Izbicki procedure
Focal mass	1. Resection: pancreaticoduodenectomy, Beger procedure 2. Hybrid procedure: Frey	1. Resection: pancreaticoduodenectomy, Beger procedure

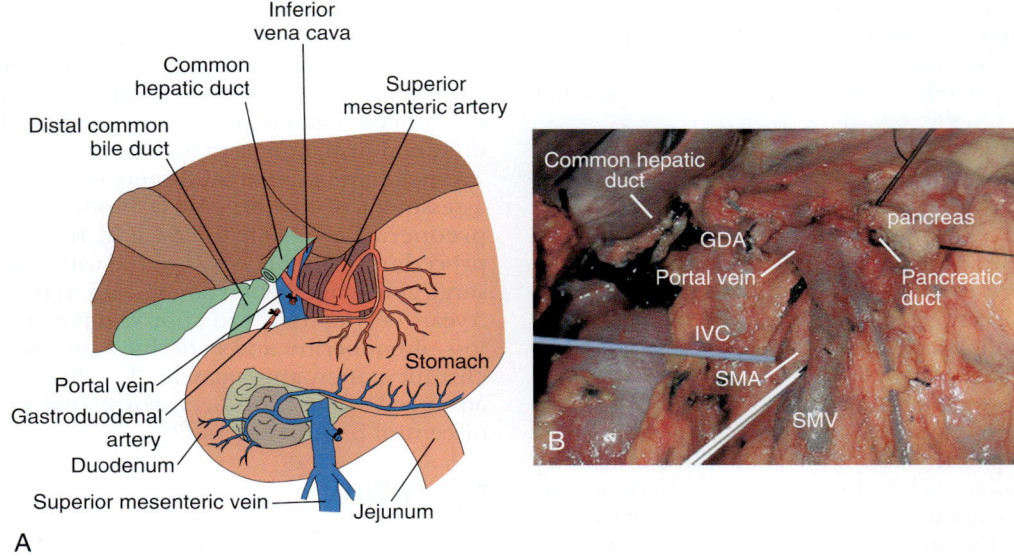

FIGURE 92.4 (A) Pancreaticoduodenectomy (classic Whipple procedure). The procedure involves the resection of the head of the pancreas with the distal common bile duct, distal stomach, duodenum, and proximal jejunum. (B) The features of the retroperitoneum after the Whipple specimen has been removed. *GDA,* Gastroduodenal artery; *IVC,* inferior vena cava; *SMA,* superior mesenteric artery; *SVC,* superior vena cava. (From Ahmad SA, Wray CJ, Rilo HR, et al. Chronic pancreatitis: recent advances and ongoing challenges. *Curr Probl Surg.* 2006;43:184.)

the pancreas, leaving a small rim of pancreatic tissue along the duodenum. The procedure is completed with end-to-end and side-to-side Roux-en-Y pancreaticojejunostomy (Fig. 92.6). DPPHR maintains gastrointestinal and biliary continuity, and achieves similar pain relief[60–62] and improvement in quality of life[63] as PD. Key steps in the procedure include identification and preservation of the posterior branch of the gastroduodenal artery and the intrapancreatic portion of the common bile duct. Gloor et al. described a modification of the DPPHR, known as the Berne procedure, that involves excavation of the central portion of the head without formal division of the neck.[64]

DECOMPRESSION

For patients with large-duct disease and no focal inflammatory mass, duct-enteric drainage is the preferred treatment. In 1954, Duval described drainage of the tail of the pancreas with a Roux-en-Y limb of jejunum as a procedure for chronic pancreatitis. This operation often failed because it did not address disease in the proximal pancreas. Puestow and Gillesby introduced a modified procedure to drain the entire pancreatic duct along the body and tail of the pancreas laterally into a Roux-en-Y limb of jejunum, which was initially described in conjunction with splenectomy and distal pancreatectomy.[65] Partington and Rochelle simplified the Puestow technique by eliminating splenectomy and pancreatic resection.[66] The Puestow procedure, or the lateral pancreaticojejunostomy, involves a retrocolic side-to-side Roux-en-Y pancreaticojejunostomy (Fig. 92.7). Typically, 80% of patients with large-duct disease experience relief of pain, although in long-term studies the durability of relief has been questioned.

HYBRID PROCEDURES

Some patients present with not only large-duct disease but also significant inflammatory disease within the head of the pancreas, and Puestow-type lateral pancreaticojejunostomy may be insufficient to address potential sources of pain within the pancreatic head. Frey introduced a procedure that combines duodenum-sparing resection of the pancreatic head, without formal division of the neck of the pancreas, combined with longitudinal pancreaticojejunostomy of the dorsal duct.[67] The Frey procedure appears to be an acceptable surgical alternative to achieve durable long-term pain relief and decrease opiate dependence in selected patients. In several series, relief of pain and weight gain were achieved in more than 75% of cases after the Frey procedure.[68,69] For patients with an inflammatory head mass but small-duct disease, Izbicki introduced a procedure that combines excavation of the pancreatic head with a V-shaped longitudinal wedge resection, followed by lateral decompressive pancreaticojejunostomy of the pancreatic body and tail.[70]

TOTAL PANCREATECTOMY WITH ISLET AUTOTRANSPLANTATION

Patients with small-duct disease and diffuse parenchymal inflammation or minimal change disease, hereditary syndromes, and failures of prior pancreatic operations present a particular challenge for treatment. Options include near-total or total pancreatectomy for end-stage or refractory disease. The initial attempts at total pancreatectomy were complicated by high postoperative complication rates, most notoriously poor long-term glycemic control and severe exocrine insufficiency.[71] The introduction of long-acting insulin and more effective pancreatic enzyme replacement, as well as advances in islet isolation and preservation, have renewed interest in total pancre-atectomy with islet autotransplantation. Several centers have now reported results with this procedure[72–74] in selected patient populations and typically report complete or near complete pain relief in about 75% of patients, with 60% to 70% achieving narcotic independence.

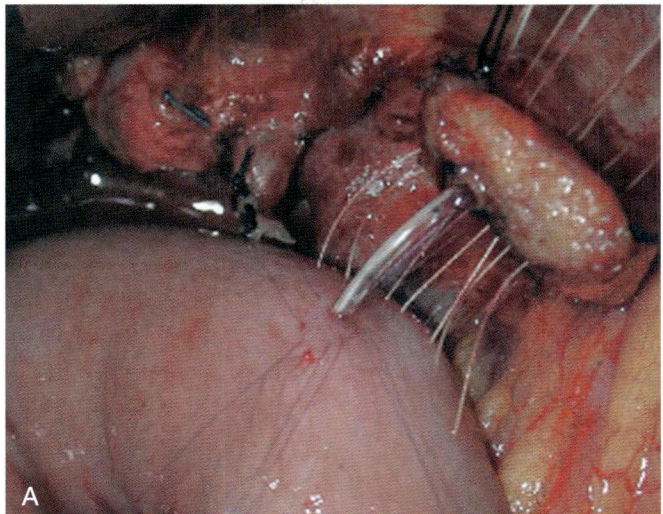

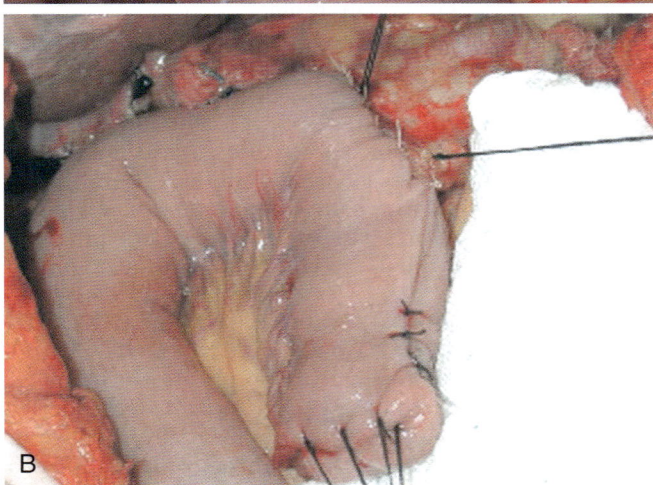

FIGURE 92.5 (A) The reconstruction after resection of a Whipple specimen involves a two-layered end-to-side pancreaticojejunostomy using a 5 French pediatric feeding tube as a pancreatic duct stent. (B) The completed pancreaticojejunostomy anastomosis. (From Ahmad SA, Wray CJ, Rilo HR, et al. Chronic pancreatitis: recent advances and ongoing challenges. *Curr Probl Surg*. 2006;43:185.)

Although a significant minority of patients (40%) is initially insulin-independent after islet autotransplantation, there is a steady drop-off of transplanted islet function over time. However, insulin requirements tend to be small and, overall, postoperative diabetes after islet autotransplantation appears to be facilitated and less vulnerable to wide swings in serum glucose, particularly severe hypoglycemia. The indications and timing for total pancreatectomy with islet autotransplantation is controversial, but potential candidates include those who have failed prior operation, patients with small-duct disease without conventional surgical alternatives, and patients with hereditary pancreatitis syndromes. Early total pancreatectomy with islet autotransplantation may avoid the complications of chronic opioid use and allow a higher islet yield from remaining nonfibrotic pancreatic parenchyma.[75,76]

RESULTS OF SURGICAL AND ENDOSCOPIC PROCEDURES

Interventional therapy should be considered in selected patients who are otherwise refractory to risk modification, dietary modification, analgesic pain medication, and endoscopic treatment. Ammann et al. prospectively followed 245 patients with chronic pancreatitis. Of the patients with alcoholic relapsing pancreatitis, 53% did not require surgery and the number of patients who reported durable pain relief were similar in the operated and nonoperated patient groups.[77] However, numerous retrospective studies suggest that patients who are managed surgically may ultimately require fewer interventions and hospitalizations with an overall better quality of life.[78]

Despite the tendency to consider endoscopic intervention less invasive, there have now been two prospective randomized trials comparing surgery versus endoscopy that indicate a clear superiority of surgical intervention. Díte et al. randomized 72 patients to surgery (resection or drainage) or endoscopic therapy including sphincterotomy, stent placement, and/or stone removal. Surgery provided better long-term pain relief and increase in weight gain.[79] A second study randomized 39 patients with distal obstruction of the pancreatic duct without inflammation to pancreaticojejunostomy or endoscopic duct drainage. After a median follow-up of 24 months, surgical patients had lower pain scores, better physical health summary scores, and durable relief of pain (75% to 32%). Patients randomized to endoscopic therapy required more repeat treatments (Table 92.6).[80] Surgery for patients with large-duct or focal inflammation may be appropriate earlier in the evolution of the disease. The optimal treatment of symptomatic patients with small-duct disease and mild to moderate pain remains controversial.

TABLE 92.6 Randomized Trials Comparing Endoscopic Stenting to Surgical Management

| Author | Year | NO. OF PATIENTS | | % WITH DURABLE RELIEF | | | MEAN NO. OF PROCEDURES | |
		Stenting	Surgery	Stenting	Surgery	P value	Stenting	Surgery
Beger et al.[60]	1999	36	36	61.4	85.9	.002	NA	NA
Izbicki et al.[61]	1994	19	20	32	75	.007	8	3

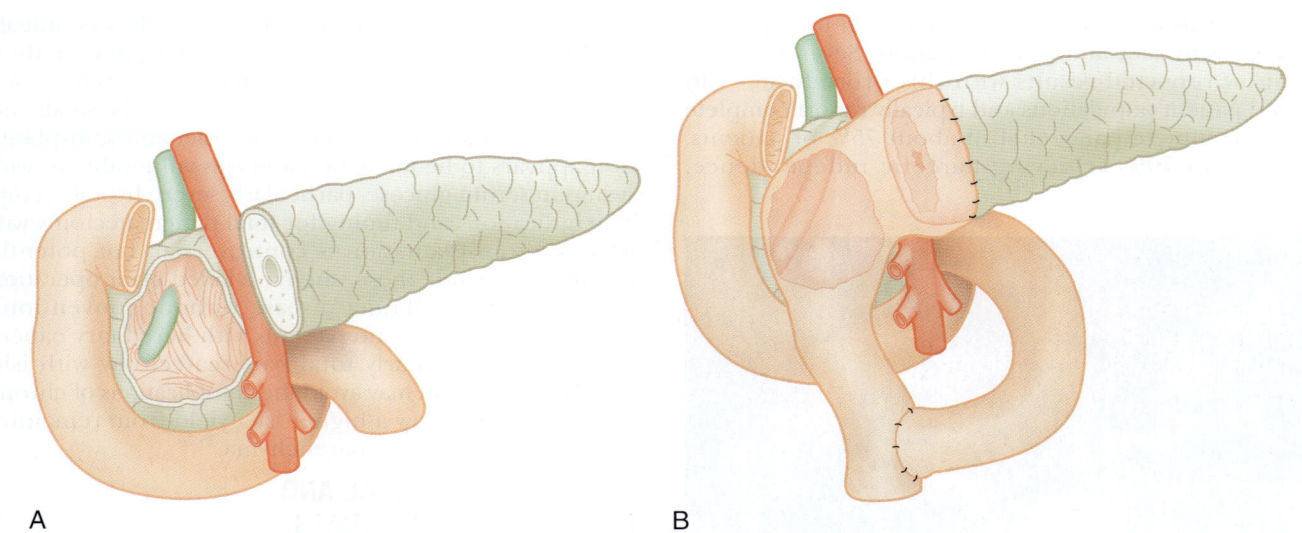

A   B

FIGURE 92.6 The duodenum-preserving pancreatic head resection introduced by Beger. (A) The procedure includes division of the neck of the pancreas, leaving a small rim of pancreatic tissues along the duodenum. (B) The procedure is completed with end-to-end and side-to-side Roux-en-Y pancreaticojejunostomy. (From Beger HG, Buechler M. Duodenum-preserving resection of the head of the pancreas in chronic pancreatitis with inflammatory mass in the head. *World J Surg.* 1990;14:83; and Beger HG, Krauztberger W, Bittner R, et al. Duodenum-preserving resection of the head of the pancreas in patients with severe pancreatitis. *Surgery.* 1985;97:467.)

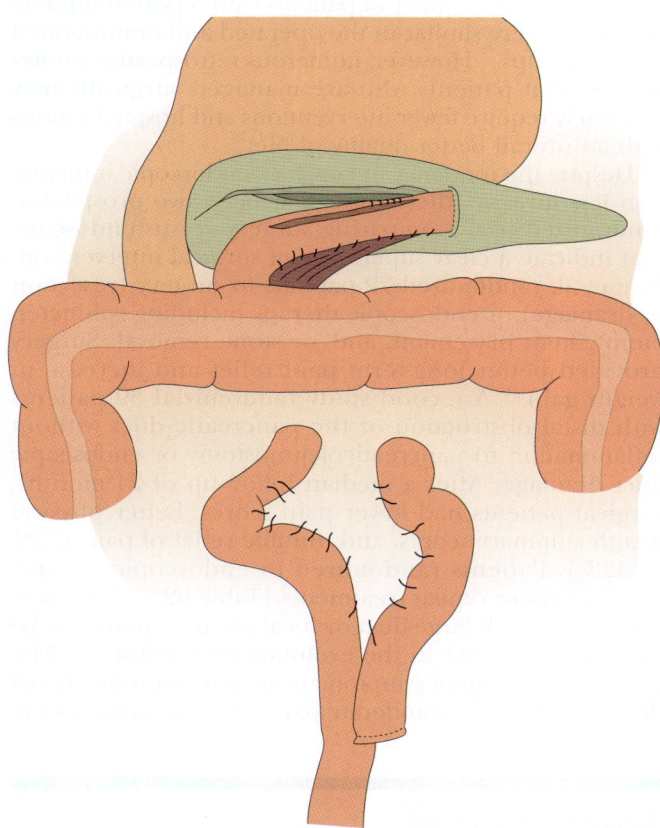

FIGURE 92.7 Lateral pancreaticojejunostomy (Puestow procedure). An illustration of a retrocolic side-to-side Roux-en-Y pancreaticojejunostomy.

Significant long-term pain relief along with weight gain and decreased narcotic dependence are achieved in a majority of patients who undergo operative therapy.[59] The postoperative mortality rate is usually reported to be below 3% and complication rates are typically 10% to 40%. However, the optimal choice of specific surgical alternatives in various settings is less clear. In general, PD and PPPD are associated with higher complication rates than DPPHR and drainage procedures. However, there are no significant differences in pain relief and control of complications to adjacent organs.

Izbicki et al. reported a randomized controlled trial comparing extended drainage with PPPD. The latter procedure had a higher rate of complication (53.3% vs. 19.4%), and the drainage procedure provided a better quality of life. Both procedures were equally effective in terms of pain relief and resolution of complications to adjacent organs.[81] Köninger et al. presented results of a randomized study comparing the Beger procedure with the Berne modification. Sixty-five patients were randomized and followed for 24 months. Operative time and median hospital stay were shorter in patients who underwent the Berne modification. Quality of life was similar in both groups 2 years after the surgery.[82] Strate et al. reported long-term follow-up results of a randomized trial comparing the Beger and Frey procedures and found no differences in late mortality, quality of life, pain score, and exocrine or endocrine insufficiency.[83] The same group reported long-term follow-up of a randomized trial comparing PPPD and the Frey procedure. There were no differences in quality of life and pain control after a median follow-up of 7 years. Müller et al. reported long-term follow-up of a randomized trial comparing the Beger procedure with PPPD.[84] The results demonstrate that both procedures were similar in pain control and exocrine and endocrine pancreatic function.

CONCLUSION

Chronic pancreatitis results in the progressive and irreversible destruction and replacement of the normal pancreatic parenchyma with fibrosis, ultimately leading to exocrine and, later, endocrine insufficiency. There is no simple unifying mechanism of pathogenesis. Rather, it is the interaction among risk factors including environmental exposure, genetic factors, and anatomic anomalies that appears to predispose to the development of chronic pancreatitis. Treatment decisions should be guided by patient presentation but are hampered by the lack of consensus guidelines and by clinician bias. Therapeutic options include risk modification, analgesic therapy, diet, endoscopic therapy, and surgical therapy. Patients may be best treated in high-volume centers with radiologic, endoscopic, and surgical expertise, as well as an ancillary system of social workers, dietitians, and psychologists.

REFERENCES

1. Masamune A, Watanabe T, Kikuta K, Shimosegawa T. Roles of pancreatic stellate cells in pancreatic inflammation and fibrosis. *Clin Gastroenterol Hepatol.* 2009;7(11 suppl):S48-S54.
2. Singer MV, Gyr K, Sarles H. Revised classification of pancreatitis. Report of the Second International Symposium on the Classification of Pancreatitis in Marseille, France, March 28–30, 1984. *Gastroenterology.* 1985;89(3):683-685.
3. Banks PA, Bradley EL 3rd, Dreiling DA, et al. Classification of pancreatitis—Cambridge and Marseille. *Gastroenterology.* 1985;89(4):928-930.
4. Sarles H, Adler G, Dani R, et al. Classifications of pancreatitis and definition of pancreatic diseases. *Digestion.* 1989;43(4):234-236.
5. Sarner M, Cotton PB. Classification of pancreatitis. *Gut.* 1984;25(7):756-759.
6. Homma T, Harada H, Koizumi M. Diagnostic criteria for chronic pancreatitis by the Japan Pancreas Society. *Pancreas.* 1997;15(1):14-15.
7. Whitcomb DC, Gorry MC, Preston RA, et al. Hereditary pancreatitis is caused by a mutation in the cationic trypsinogen gene. *Nat Genet.* 1996;14(2):141-145.
8. Schneider A, Lohr JM, Singer MV. The M-ANNHEIM classification of chronic pancreatitis: introduction of a unifying classification system based on a review of previous classifications of the disease. *J Gastroenterol.* 2007;42(2):101-119.
9. Irving HM, Samokhvalov AV, Rehm J. Alcohol as a risk factor for pancreatitis. A systematic review and meta-analysis. *JOP.* 2009;10(4):387-392.
10. Lin Y, Tamakoshi A, Hayakawa T, Ogawa M, Ohno Y. Cigarette smoking as a risk factor for chronic pancreatitis: a case-control study in Japan. Research Committee on Intractable Pancreatic Diseases. *Pancreas.* 2000;21(2):109-114.
11. Song Z, Bhagat G, Quante M, et al. Potential carcinogenic effects of cigarette smoke and Swedish moist snuff on pancreas: a study using a transgenic mouse model of chronic pancreatitis. *Lab Invest.* 2010;90(3):426-435.
12. Whitcomb DC, Yadav D, Adam S, et al. Multicenter approach to recurrent acute and chronic pancreatitis in the United States: the North American Pancreatitis Study 2 (NAPS2). *Pancreatology.* 2008;8(4-5):520-531.
13. Teich N, Ockenga J, Hoffmeister A, Manns M, Mössner J, Keim V. Chronic pancreatitis associated with an activation peptide mutation that facilitates trypsin activation. *Gastroenterology.* 2000;119(2):461-465.
14. Gorry MC, Gabbaizedeh D, Furey W, et al. Mutations in the cationic trypsinogen gene are associated with recurrent acute and chronic pancreatitis. *Gastroenterology.* 1997;113(4):1063-1068.
15. Witt H, Luck W, Becker M. A signal peptide cleavage site mutation in the cationic trypsinogen gene is strongly associated with chronic pancreatitis. *Gastroenterology.* 1999;117(1):7-10.
16. Nishimori I, Kamakura M, Fujikawa-Adachi K, et al. Mutations in exons 2 and 3 of the cationic trypsinogen gene in Japanese families with hereditary pancreatitis. *Gut.* 1999;44(2):259-263.
17. Felderbauer P, Stricker I, Schnekenburger J, et al. Histopathological features of patients with chronic pancreatitis due to mutations in the PRSS1 gene: evaluation of BRAF and KRAS2 mutations. *Digestion.* 2008;78(1):60-65.
18. Witt H, Luck W, Hennies HC, et al. Mutations in the gene encoding the serine protease inhibitor, Kazal type 1 are associated with chronic pancreatitis. *Nat Genet.* 2000;25(2):213-216.
19. Pfützer RH, Barmada MM, Brunskill AP, et al. SPINK1/PSTI polymorphisms act as disease modifiers in familial and idiopathic chronic pancreatitis. *Gastroenterology.* 2000;119(3):615-623.
20. Sharer N, Schwarz M, Malone G, et al. Mutations of the cystic fibrosis gene in patients with chronic pancreatitis. *N Engl J Med.* 1998;339(10):645-652.
21. Weiss FU, Sahin-Tóth M. Variations in trypsinogen expression may influence the protective effect of the p.G191R PRSS2 variant in chronic pancreatitis. *Gut.* 2009;58:749.
22. Rosendahl J, Witt H, Szmola R, et al. Chymotrypsin C (CTRC) variants that diminish activity or secretion are associated with chronic pancreatitis. *Nat Genet.* 2008;40:78-82.
23. Masson E, Chen JM, Scotet V, Le Maréchal C, Férec C. Association of rare chymotrypsinogen C (CTRC) gene variations in patients with idiopathic chronic pancreatitis. *Hum Genet.* 2008;123(1):83-91.
24. Felderbauer P, Hoffmann P, Einwächter H, et al. A novel mutation of the calcium sensing receptor gene is associated with chronic pancreatitis in a family with heterozygous SPINK1 mutations. *BMC Gastroenterol.* 2003;3:34.
25. Muddana V, Lamb J, Greer JB, et al. Association between calcium sensing receptor gene polymorphisms and chronic pancreatitis in a US population: role of serine protease inhibitor Kazal 1 type and alcohol. *World J Gastroenterol.* 2008;14(28):4486-4491.
26. Whitcomb DC, LaRusch J, Krasinskas AM, et al. Common genetic variants in the CLDN2 and PRSS1-PRSS2 loci alter risk for alcohol-related and sporadic pancreatitis. *Nat Genet.* 2012;44(12):1349-1354.
27. Witt H, Beer S, Rosendahl J, et al. Variants in CPA1 are strongly associated with early onset chronic pancreatitis. *Nat Genet.* 2013;45(10):1216-1220.
28. Xu W, Hui C, Yu SS, et al. MicroRNAs and cystic fibrosis—an epigenetic perspective. *Cell Biol Int.* 2011;35:463-466.
29. Finkelberg DL, Sahani D, Deshpande V, Brugge WR. Autoimmune pancreatitis. *N Engl J Med.* 2006;355(25):2670-2676.
30. Frulloni L, Lunardi C, Simone R, et al. Identification of a novel antibody associated with autoimmune pancreatitis. *N Engl J Med.* 2009;361(22):2135-2142.
31. DiMagno EP, DiMagno MJ. Chronic pancreatitis—landmark papers, management decisions, and future. *Pancreas.* 2016;45:640-650.
32. Lankisch PG, Löhr-Happe A, Otto J, Creutzfeldt W. Natural course in chronic pancreatitis. Pain, exocrine and endocrine pancreatic insufficiency and prognosis of the disease. *Digestion.* 1993;54(3):148-155.
33. Vijungco JD, Prinz RA. Management of biliary and duodenal complications of chronic pancreatitis. *World J Surg.* 2003;27(11):1258-1270.
34. Heider TR, Azeem S, Galanko JA, et al. The natural history of pancreatitis-induced splenic vein thrombosis. *Ann Surg.* 2004;239:876 [discussion 880].
35. Agarwal AK, Raj Kumar K, Agarwal S, Singh S. Significance of splenic vein thrombosis in chronic pancreatitis. *Am J Surg.* 2008;196(2):149-154.
36. Munigala S, Agarwal B, Gelrud A, Conwell DL. Chronic pancreatitis and fracture: a retrospective, population-based Veterans Administration study. *Pancreas.* 2016;45(3):355-361.
37. Lowenfels AB, Maisonneuve P, Cavallini G, et al. Pancreatitis and the risk of pancreatic cancer. International Pancreatitis Study Group. *N Engl J Med.* 1993;328(20):1433-1437.
38. Lowenfels AB, Maisonneuve P, DiMagno EP, et al. Hereditary pancreatitis and the risk of pancreatic cancer. International Hereditary Pancreatitis Study Group. *J Natl Cancer Inst.* 1997;89(6):442-446.
39. Guerra C, Schuhmacher AJ, Cañamero M, et al. Chronic pancreatitis is essential for induction of pancreatic ductal adenocarcinoma by K-Ras oncogenes in adult mice. *Cancer Cell.* 2007;11(3):291-302.
40. Patel AG, Reber PU, Toyama MT, Ashley SW, Reber HA. Effect of pancreaticojejunostomy on fibrosis, pancreatic blood flow, and interstitial pH in chronic pancreatitis: a feline model. *Ann Surg.* 1999;230(5):672-679.
41. Ebbehoj N, Svendsen LB, Madsen P. Pancreatic tissue pressure: techniques and pathophysiological aspects. *Scand J Gastroenterol.* 1984;19(8):1066-1068.
42. Ceyhan GO, Demir IE, Rauch U, et al. Pancreatic neuropathy results in neural remodeling and altered pancreatic innervation in chronic

pancreatitis and pancreatic cancer. *Am J Gastroenterol.* 2009;104(10): 2555-2565.

43. Bockman DE, Buchler M, Malfertheiner P, Beger HG. Analysis of nerves in chronic pancreatitis. *Gastroenterology.* 1988;94(6):1459-1469.

44. Laugier R. Dynamic endoscopic manometry of the response to secretin in patients with chronic pancreatitis. *Endoscopy.* 1994;26(2): 222-227.

45. Domínguez-Muñoz JE, Nieto L, Vilariño M, Lourido MV, Iglesias-García J. Development and diagnostic accuracy of a breath test for pancreatic exocrine insufficiency in chronic pancreatitis. *Pancreas.* 2016;45:241-247.

46. Okazaki K, Uchida K, Ohana M, et al. Autoimmune-related pancreatitis is associated with autoantibodies and a Th1/Th2-type cellular immune response. *Gastroenterology.* 2000;118(3):573-581.

47. Wiersema MJ, Hawes RH, Lehman GA, Kochman ML, Sherman S, Kopecky KK. Prospective evaluation of endoscopic ultrasonography and endoscopic retrograde cholangiopancreatography in patients with chronic abdominal pain of suspected pancreatic origin. *Endoscopy.* 1993;25(9):555-564.

48. Bhardwaj P, Garg PK, Maulik SK, Saraya A, Tandon RK, Acharya SK. A randomized controlled trial of antioxidant supplementation for pain relief in patients with chronic pancreatitis. *Gastroenterology.* 2009;136:149 [e2].

49. Shalimar S, Midha S, Hasan A, Dhingra R, Garg PK. Long-term pain relief with optimized medical including antioxidants and step-up interventional therapy in patients with chronic pancreatitis. *J Gastroenterol Hepatol.* 2016;doi:10.1111/jgh.13410.

50. Olesen SS, Graversen C, Bouwense SA, Wilder-Smith OH, van Goor H, Drewes AM. Is timing of medical therapy related to outcome in painful chronic pancreatitis? *Pancreas.* 2016;45(3):381-387.

51. Kongkam P, Wagner DL, Sherman S, et al. Intrathecal narcotic infusion pumps for intractable pain of chronic pancreatitis: a pilot series. *Am J Gastroenterol.* 2009;104(5):1249-1255.

52. Rösch T, Daniel S, Scholz M, et al. European Society of Gastrointestinal Endoscopy Research Group. Endoscopic treatment of chronic pancreatitis: a multicenter study of 1000 patients with long-term follow-up. *Endoscopy.* 2002;34:765.

53. Moole H, Jaeger A, Bechtold ML, Forcione D, Taneja D, Puli SR. Success of extracorporeal shock wave lithotripsy in chronic calcific pancreatitis management: a meta-analysis and systematic review. *Pancreas.* 2016;45(5):651-658.

54. Briggs JD, Jordan PH Jr, Longmire WP Jr. Experience with resection of the pancreas in the treatment of chronic relapsing pancreatitis. *Ann Surg.* 1956;144:681.

55. Ahmed Ali U, Nieuwenhuijs VB, van Eijck CH, et al. Clinical outcome in relation to timing of surgery in chronic pancreatitis: a nomogram to predict pain relief. *Arch Surg.* 2012;147(10):925-932.

56. Bouwense SA, Olesen SS, Drewes AM, Frøkjær JB, van Goor H, Wilder-Smith OH. Is altered central pain processing related to disease stage in chronic pancreatitis patients with pain? An exploratory study. *PLoS One.* 2013;8(2):e55460.

57. Whipple AO. Radical surgery for certain cases of pancreatic fibrosis associated with calcareous deposits. *Ann Surg.* 1946;124:991.

58. Sakorafas GH, Farnell MB, Nagorney DM, Sarr MG, Rowland CM. Pancreatoduodenectomy for chronic pancreatitis: long-term results in 105 patients. *Arch Surg.* 2000;135(5):517-523 [discussion 523–524].

59. Traverso LW, Tompkins RK, Urrea PT, Longmire WP Jr. Surgical treatment of chronic pancreatitis. Twenty-two years' experience. *Ann Surg.* 1979;190(3):312-319.

60. Beger HG, Schlosser W, Friess HM, Büchler MW. Duodenum-preserving head resection in chronic pancreatitis changes the natural course of the disease: a single-center 26-year experience. *Ann Surg.* 1999;230(4):512-519 [discussion 519–523].

61. Izbicki JR, Bloechle C, Knoefel WT, et al. Complications of adjacent organs in chronic pancreatitis managed by duodenum-preserving resection of the head of the pancreas. *Br J Surg.* 1994;81(9):1351-1355.

62. Prinz RA, Kaufman BH, Folk FA, Greenlee HB. Pancreaticojejunostomy for chronic pancreatitis. Two- to 21-year follow-up. *Arch Surg.* 1978;113(4):520-525.

63. Bloechle C, Izbicki JR, Knoefel WT, Kuechler T, Broelsch CE. Quality of life in chronic pancreatitis—results after duodenum-preserving resection of the head of the pancreas. *Pancreas.* 1995;11(1):77-85.

64. Gloor B, Friess H, Uhl W, Büchler MW. A modified technique of the Beger and Frey procedure in patients with chronic pancreatitis. *Dig Surg.* 2001;18(1):21-25.

65. Puestow CB, Gillesby WJ. Retrograde surgical drainage of pancreas for chronic relapsing pancreatitis. *AMA Arch Surg.* 1958;76(6):898-907.

66. Partington PF, Rochelle RE. Modified Puestow procedure for retrograde drainage of the pancreatic duct. *Ann Surg.* 1960;152:1037-1043.

67. Frey CF, Smith GJ. Description and rationale of a new operation for chronic pancreatitis. *Pancreas.* 1987;2(6):701-707.

68. Frey CF, Amikura K. Local resection of the head of the pancreas combined with longitudinal pancreaticojejunostomy in the management of patients with chronic pancreatitis. *Ann Surg.* 1994;220:492 [discussion 504].

69. Negi S, Singh A, Chaudhary A. Pain relief after Frey's procedure for chronic pancreatitis. *Br J Surg.* 2010;97(7):1087-1095.

70. Izbicki JR, Bloechle C, Broering DC, Kuechler T, Broelsch CE, Longitudinal V. shaped excision of the ventral pancreas for small duct disease in severe chronic pancreatitis: prospective evaluation of a new surgical procedure. *Ann Surg.* 1998;227(2):213-219.

71. Braasch JW, Vito L, Nugent FW. Total pancreatectomy of end-stage chronic pancreatitis. *Ann Surg.* 1978;188(3):317-322.

72. Sutton JM, Schmulewitz N, Sussman JJ, et al. Total pancreatectomy and islet cell autotransplantation as a means of treating patients with genetically linked pancreatitis. *Surgery.* 2010;148:676 [discussion 685].

73. Garcea G, Weaver J, Phillips J, et al. Total pancreatectomy with and without islet cell transplantation for chronic pancreatitis: a series of 85 consecutive patients. *Pancreas.* 2009;38(1):1-7.

74. Ahmad SA, Lowy AM, Wray CJ, et al. Factors associated with insulin and narcotic independence after islet autotransplantation in patients with severe chronic pancreatitis. *J Am Coll Surg.* 2005;201(5):680-687.

75. Bramis K, Gordon-Weeks AN, Friend PJ, et al. Systematic review of total pancreatectomy and islet autotransplantation for chronic pancreatitis. *Br J Surg.* 2012;99(6):761-766.

76. Sutherland DE, Gruessner AC, Carlson AM, et al. Islet autotransplant outcomes after total pancreatectomy: a contrast to islet allograft outcomes. *Transplantation.* 2008;86(12):1799-1802.

77. Ammann RW, Akovbiantz A, Largiader F, et al. Course and outcome of chronic pancreatitis. Longitudinal study of a mixed medical-surgical series of 245 patients. *Gastroenterology.* 1984;86:820.

78. Rutter K, Ferlitsch A, Sautner T, et al. Hospitalization, frequency of interventions, and quality of life after endoscopic, surgical, or conservative treatment in patients with chronic pancreatitis. *World J Surg.* 2010;34:2642.

79. Díte P, Ruzicka M, Zboril V, Novotný I. A prospective, randomized trial comparing endoscopic and surgical therapy for chronic pancreatitis. *Endoscopy.* 2003;35(7):553-558.

80. Cahen DL, Gouma DJ, Nio Y, et al. Endoscopic versus surgical drainage of the pancreatic duct in chronic pancreatitis. *N Engl J Med.* 2007;356(7):676-684.

81. Izbicki JR, Bloechle C, Broering DC, Knoefel WT, Kuechler T, Broelsch CE. Extended drainage versus resection in surgery for chronic pancreatitis: a prospective randomized trial comparing the longitudinal pancreaticojejunostomy combined with local pancreatic head excision with the pylorus-preserving pancreatoduodenectomy. *Ann Surg.* 1998;228(6):771-779.

82. Köninger J, Friess H, Müller M, et al. Duodenum-preserving pancreatic head resection—a randomized controlled trial comparing the original Beger procedure with the Berne modification (ISRCTN No. 50638764). *Surgery.* 2008;143:490.

83. Strate T, Taherpour Z, Bloechle C, et al. Long-term follow-up of a randomized trial comparing the Beger and Frey procedures for patients suffering from chronic pancreatitis. *Ann Surg.* 2005;241(4): 591-598.

84. Müller MW, Friess H, Martin DJ, Hinz U, Dahmen R, Büchler MW. Long-term follow-up of a randomized clinical trial comparing Beger with pylorus-preserving Whipple procedure for chronic pancreatitis. *Br J Surg.* 2008;95(3):350-356.

Pseudocysts and Other Complications of Pancreatitis

Stephen M. Doane | Charles J. Yeo

PANCREATIC AND PERIPANCREATIC FLUID COLLECTIONS

Pancreatitis often results in sequelae of pseudocyst formation or other complications. The consensus guidelines of the revised Atlanta classification of pancreatitis describe various features of acute pancreatitis, distinguishing between interstitial edematous pancreatitis and the more aggressive necrotizing pancreatitis (Table 93.1).[1] Acute peripancreatic fluid collections are defined specifically as fluid lacking the presence of tissue necrosis. A pancreatic pseudocyst is defined as a fluid collection within or adjacent to the pancreas that becomes completely encapsulated with a mature, nonepithelialized, fibrous, inflammatory wall. This process of acute pseudocyst formation requires at least 4 weeks by definition. Pancreatic pseudocysts are typically homogeneous with minimal or no necrosis present and without a significant solid component on contrast-enhanced computed tomography (CT) imaging (Fig. 93.1). Acute necrotic collections often form in the setting of necrotizing pancreatitis and are defined as collections with variable amounts of fluid and necrosis, without a discrete encapsulating wall. If such a collection becomes completely encapsulated with a mature inflammatory wall, it is defined as walled-off pancreatic necrosis, a more specific term replacing the previous concept of pancreatic abscess (Fig. 93.2). Management of walled-off pancreatic necrosis is discussed in Chapter 94, though many of the same principles apply regarding stabilization of acute pancreatitis, pancreatic ductal evaluation, and minimally invasive techniques.

Pancreatic fluid collections and pseudocysts occur in 40% and 5% to 15% of patients, respectively, as a consequence of acute pancreatitis.[2-4] Etiologies of pancreatitis vary by region, but alcohol abuse is most commonly associated with pseudocyst formation (50% to 70% of cases) in most case series. Any other etiologies of pancreatitis, such as gallstones, trauma, and postprocedural issues, can also result in pseudocysts. Biliary causes of pancreatitis more often lead to pseudocysts after acute pancreatitis, whereas alcohol is typically the cause of pseudocysts in patients with chronic pancreatitis. Release of inflammatory cytokines as part of the immunologic response of pancreatitis can lead to profound reactive fluid accumulation around the pancreatic parenchyma. These fluid collections are typically sterile and disappear with resolution of the pancreatitis. Microcirculatory injury and intraacinar activation of digestive enzymes can damage the parenchyma itself. Disruption or occlusion of the pancreatic ductal system can also lead to fluid collections within and surrounding the pancreas due to extravasation of amylase-rich secretions. Factors affecting the responsiveness of fluid collections to treatment include infection and the presence of significant necrotic debris, as well as ongoing communication with the main pancreatic ductal system.

PANCREATIC PSEUDOCYSTS

CLINICAL PRESENTATION

Pseudocysts are located most commonly in the lesser sac adjacent to the pancreas because the inflammatory response associated with pancreatitis prevents fluid from adequate reabsorption. Less often, pseudocysts will form within the pancreatic parenchyma or extend to other intraperitoneal or retroperitoneal locations. Symptoms of pancreatic pseudocysts commonly include abdominal pain and early satiety. Less frequent symptoms include infection of the pseudocyst, jaundice, or intestinal obstruction from their space-occupying nature, intracystic hemorrhage, and peritonitis from pseudocyst rupture. If the pseudocyst is sizable enough, an abdominal mass corresponding to the pseudocyst can be palpated on physical exam. Most pseudocysts are noticed on abdominal imaging after acute pancreatitis, and pseudocysts account for most pancreatic cystic lesions in patients with a history of pancreatitis. Additionally, chronic pancreatitis can lead to development of a pseudocyst in up to 40% of cases.[3] Neoplastic, congenital, and infectious etiologies of cystic lesions must also be considered in the differential diagnosis and are listed in Table 93.2.[5] In patients without a history of pancreatitis or pancreatic symptoms, pseudocysts are rarely the cause of an incidentally found pancreatic cyst.[6,7]

IMAGING

Contrast-enhanced CT imaging is highly sensitive (close to 100%) for the presence of pancreatic cystic lesions but does not reliably exclude the possibility of a cystic neoplasm. Cystic neoplasms may sometimes show a macrocystic phenotype and mural nodularity is not always present. A known history of pancreatitis strongly suggests the diagnosis of a pseudocyst, but cystic neoplasms can also cause ductal obstruction leading to pancreatitis in 5% to 10% of patients. Radiologic findings of chronic pancreatitis such as glandular calcifications, pancreatolithiasis, and pancreatic atrophy should be noted. The presence of nonenhancing internal dependent debris on T2-weighted magnetic resonance imaging (MRI) sequences was a highly specific finding for pseudocysts in a recent review of pancreatic cystic lesions, and may be helpful in excluding neoplasm.[8] Endoscopic retrograde cholangiopancreatography (ERCP) in the past was considered to be the gold standard for

TABLE 93.1 Definitions of Pancreatic and Peripancreatic Fluid Collections by Time From Onset of Disease

Phases of Acute Pancreatitis	Interstitial Edematous Pancreatitis	Necrotizing Pancreatitis
Early phase (0–4 weeks)	Acute peripancreatic fluid collection	Acute necrotic collection
Late phase (>4 weeks)	Pancreatic pseudocyst	Walled-off pancreatic necrosis

Modified from the revised Atlanta classification of Acute Pancreatitis, 2012.

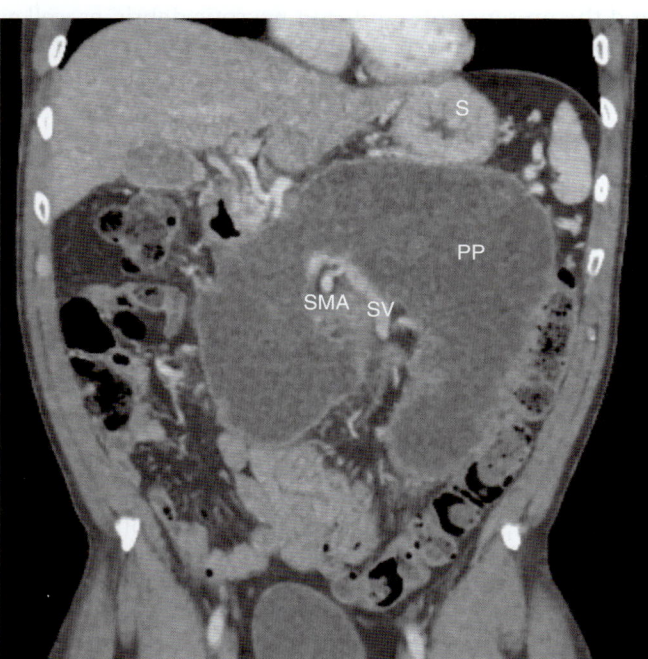

FIGURE 93.1 Computed tomography scan showing a large horseshoe-shaped pancreatic pseudocyst *(PP)* after acute gallstone pancreatitis. *S,* Stomach; *SMA,* superior mesenteric artery; *SV,* splenic vein.

TABLE 93.2 Cystic Lesions of the Pancreas and Peripancreatic Region

Inflammatory fluid collections	Acute peripancreatic fluid collection
	Pancreatic pseudocyst
	Acute necrotic collection
	Walled-off pancreatic necrosis
Cystic neoplasms of the pancreas	Serous cystadenoma
	Mucinous cystadenoma/cystadenocarcinoma
	Intraductal papillary mucinous neoplasm
	Cystic islet cell tumor
	Cystic adenocarcinoma
	Acinar cell cystadenocarcinoma
	Cystic choriocarcinoma
	Cystic teratoma
Parasitic cysts	Echinococcal cyst
	Taenia solium cyst
Dermoid cyst	—
Lymphoepithelial cyst	—
Congenital simple cyst	—
Polycystic disease	Isolated to the pancreas
	Associated with polycystic kidney disease
	Associated with von Hippel-Lindau disease
	Associated with cystic fibrosis
Extrapancreatic cysts	Duplication cyst
	Mesenteric cyst
	Splenic cyst
	Adrenal cyst

Modified from Yeo CJ, Sarr MG. Cystic and pseudocystic diseases of the pancreas. *Curr Probl Surg.* 1994;31:165.

diagnosing pancreatic ductal disruption or stricture, and can usually visualize a pseudocyst if there is communication between it and the pancreatic ductal system. However, ERCP is an invasive procedure carrying its own risk of procedure-related complications, including the risk of contaminating a previously sterile pancreatic fluid collection. Magnetic resonance cholangiopancreatography (MRCP) has demonstrated greater than 90% accuracy in identifying pancreatic duct leakage when compared with ERCP and may be a reliable indicator of the need for early intervention in patients with pancreatitis (Fig. 93.3).[9] Therefore, ERCP is rarely required for diagnosis in the current era.

CYST FLUID ANALYSIS

In the absence of diagnostic certainty of a pseudocyst, endoscopic ultrasound is indicated to better characterize the cystic lesion and to aspirate a sample of cyst fluid for analysis. The measurement of cyst fluid carcinoembryonic antigen (CEA) and amylase levels, and the presence or

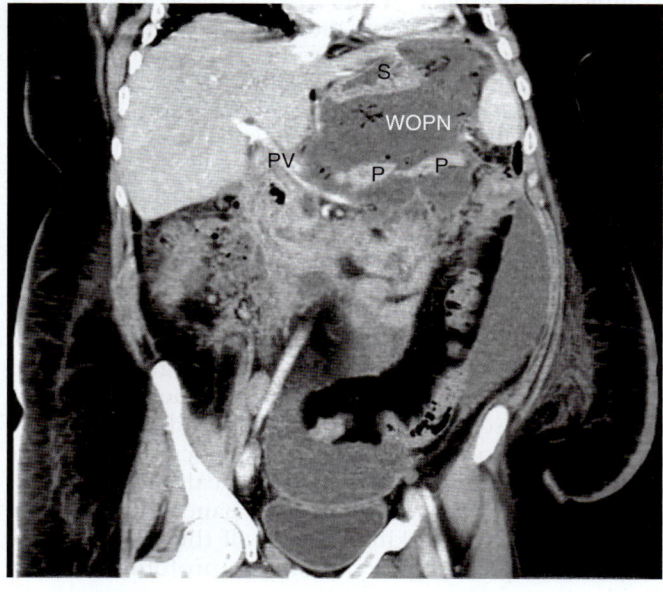

FIGURE 93.2 Computed tomography scan showing walled-off pancreatic necrosis *(WOPN)*. *P,* Pancreas; *PV,* portal vein; *S,* stomach.)

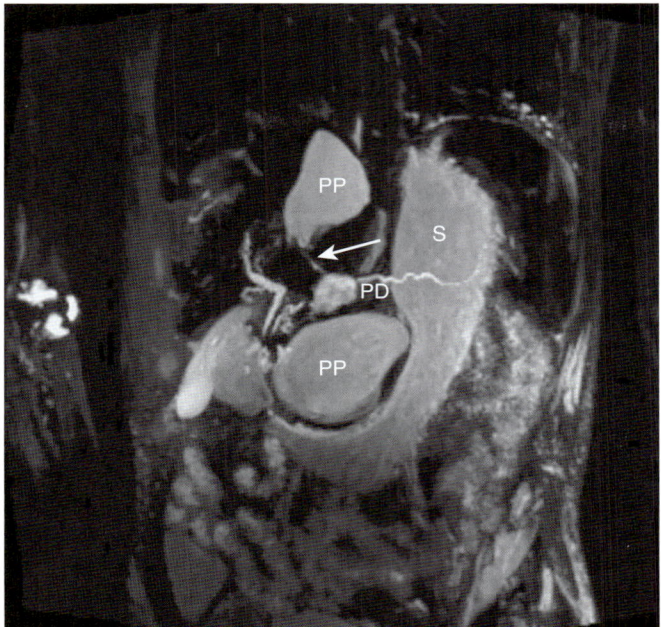

FIGURE 93.3 Magnetic resonance cholangiopancreatography of pancreatic duct *(PD)* disruption with pseudocyst. Thick slab, heavily T2-weighted magnetic resonance cholangiopancreatography image of a patient with smoldering pancreatic symptoms 3 weeks after an acute pancreatitis event with suspected pancreatic duct fistula based on fluid collections on a computed tomography scan. A small communication between the disrupted main pancreatic duct and the pseudocyst is demonstrated *(arrow)*. *PP,* Pancreatic pseudocyst; *S,* stomach. (Modified from Drake LM, Anis M, Lawrence C. Accuracy of magnetic resonance cholangiopancreatography in identifying pancreatic duct disruption. *J Clin Gastroenterol.* 2012;46[8]:696–699.)

TABLE 93.3 Cyst Fluid Concentrations for Commonly Aspirated Cystic Pancreatic Lesions

Cyst Fluid Element	Pancreatic Pseudocyst	Serous Cystadenoma	Mucinous Cystic Neoplasm	Intraductal Papillary Mucinous Neoplasm
CEA	Low	Low	High	Low to high
Amylase	High	Low	Low	High
Mucin	Absent	Absent	Present usually	Present usually

CEA, Carcinoembryonic antigen.
Data from Brugge WR, Lauwers GY, Sahani D, Fernandez-del Castillo C, Warshaw AL. Cystic neoplasms of the pancreas. *N Engl J Med.* 2004;351(12):1218–1226.

absence of mucin, are together accurate at distinguishing between the possibility of a malignant/premalignant cystic neoplasm and a pseudocyst.[10] The most commonly sampled cystic lesions and their respective cyst fluid values are shown in Table 93.3. In addition, other cystic tumors such as cystic endocrine neoplasms, cystadenocarcinomas, or solid pseudopapillary neoplasms with a cystic component can occasionally be confused with pseudocysts. Cytology from fine-needle aspiration can often identify epithelial

cells that exclude pseudocyst, but such findings lack reliable sensitivity.[11]

CLASSIFICATION

Due to imprecise definitions of pseudocyst and small case series, older data on management of pseudocyst can seem contradictory or difficult to interpret. D'Egidio and Schein introduced a classification scheme that has been widely referenced. This scheme divides pseudocysts into three types: type 1, a postnecrotic pseudocyst after acute pancreatitis, rarely involving ductal disruption; type 2, a postnecrotic pseudocyst after an acute exacerbation of chronic pancreatitis, sometimes showing ductal disruption; and type 3, a retention pseudocyst always related to obstruction and dilation of the pancreatic duct.[12] Despite the heterogeneity of patients in this observational series, important conclusions were shown including the low recurrence rate of pseudocyst after percutaneous drainage in the absence of ductal stricture, a high success rate of internal drainage in patients with chronic pancreatitis, and the necessity of ductal decompression (with endoscopic stent placement or surgery) in patients with ductal stricture because pseudocyst drainage alone in the presence of a stricture was found to be associated with recurrence. Nealon et al. further clarified important anatomic relationships related to the prognosis and management of pancreatic pseudocysts, categorizing pseudocysts into types I to IV by the appearance of the main pancreatic duct and the presence or absence of pseudocyst-duct communication (Fig. 93.4).[13]

NONOPERATIVE MANAGEMENT

Older data suggested that nonoperative management of pseudocysts would lead to a significant rate of complications. Those reports may have been influenced by a low sensitivity of abdominal imaging at that time for detection of pseudocysts, causing a selection bias for those patients with large pseudocysts more likely not to resolve without intervention and drainage. Two observational studies of pseudocysts published in the early 1990s helped to change this paradigm. Yeo et al.[14] reported on 75 consecutive patients with pseudocysts identified on CT imaging, of whom 48% were asymptomatic and were managed nonoperatively. Of those asymptomatic pseudocyst patients, 60% had complete resolution of their pseudocysts after 1-year follow-up. The lesions of the other 40% of patients remained stable or decreased in size and there was only one patient with a complication (intracystic hemorrhage), which was self-limited and did not require surgery. Although larger pseudocysts were more likely to require surgery, even 27% of those patients with pseudocysts greater than 10 cm in diameter were successfully managed nonoperatively. Vitas and Sarr[15] similarly reported on 68 patients with minimal or no symptoms from a pseudocyst who were initially managed with a nonoperative approach. Almost two-thirds of these patients were successfully managed without intervention after a median follow-up of 51 months, with initial pseudocyst diameter ranging from 2 to 11 cm. Among nonoperative patients with follow-up imaging, 54% of the pseudocysts completely resolved. Only 7% of patients required an emergent operation for a complication related to the pseudocyst,

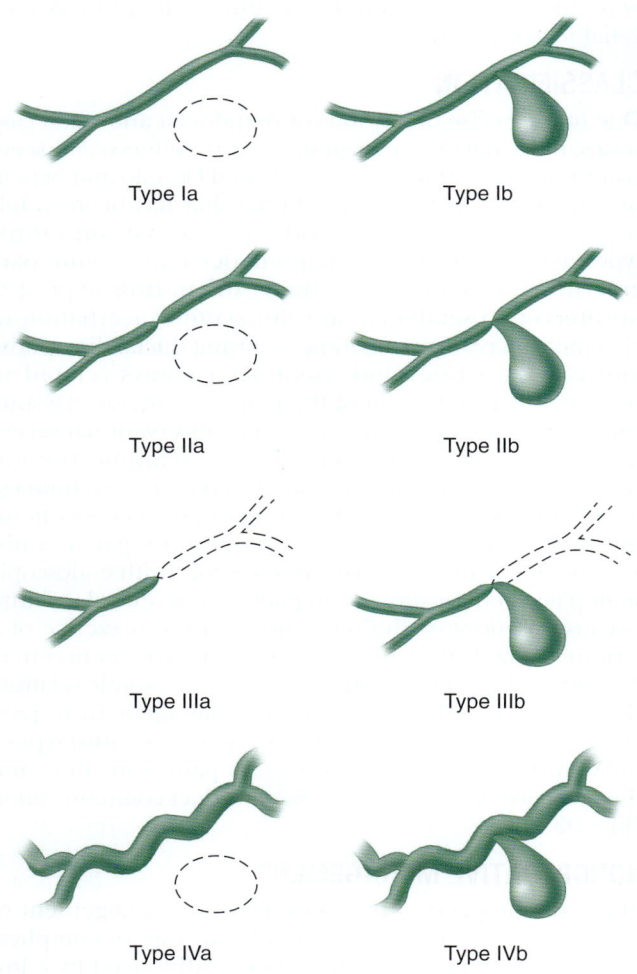

FIGURE 93.4 Nealon classification of pancreatic ductal disruption and pseudocyst formation. Type I is a normal main pancreatic duct. Type II is a pancreatic duct stricture. Type III is pancreatic duct occlusion (disconnected pancreatic duct syndrome). Type IV depicts chronic pancreatitis. Subtypes *a* represent no radiographically demonstrable communication between the pancreatic duct and the pseudocyst. Subtypes *b* represent communication between the pancreatic duct and the pseudocyst. (Modified from Nealon WH, Bhutani M, Riall TS, Raju G, Ozkan O, Neilan R. A unifying concept: pancreatic ductal anatomy predicts and determines the major complications resulting from pancreatitis. *J Am Coll Surg.* 2009;208:790–799.)

emphasizing nonetheless the need for close initial follow-up when pursuing a nonoperative approach to look for signs of pseudoaneurysm formation or impending vascular erosion. More recently, Cui et al. published a prospective study of pseudocysts after acute pancreatitis (median diameter 9.7 cm) demonstrating resolution or decrease in size of the pseudocyst in 84% of patients.[2] In Nealon's large series of 563 pseudocyst patients, 25% resolved spontaneously and there was equivalent likelihood of resolution between pseudocysts with diameter less than 5 cm or greater than 5 cm.[13] Although underpowered, the series reported by Soliani et al. had similar recurrence rates between pseudocysts with diameter less than 10 cm

> **BOX 93.1** **Management Options for Pancreatic Pseudocysts**
>
> Observation
> Percutaneous catheter drainage
> Endoscopic internal drainage
>   Cystogastrostomy
>   Cystoduodenostomy
>   Transpapillary pancreatic duct stenting/pseudocyst
>   drainage
> Surgical interventions (open or laparoscopic)
>   Cystogastrostomy
>   Roux-en-Y cystojejunostomy
>   Cystoduodenostomy
>   Longitudinal pancreaticojejunostomy
>   Partial pancreatic resection
>   External catheter drainage

and greater than 10 cm.[16] Symptoms may be more common in patients developing a pseudocyst after an episode of acute pancreatitis rather than chronic pancreatitis, and in alcoholic-related pancreatitis, which tends to have a more persistent inflammatory process. Normal pancreatic ductal anatomy in the Nealon classification was a significant predictor of spontaneous resolution, with 87% resolution of type I pseudocysts and infrequent resolution of pseudocysts associated with any other ductal anatomy. Nealon type II, III, and IV pseudocysts were typically symptomatic and required intervention.

TREATMENT OPTIONS

When a patient's symptoms are significant enough to affect their quality of life or a pseudocyst continues to increase in size on surveillance imaging, elective decompression is indicated (Box 93.1). Open surgical cystoenterostomy has traditionally been the gold standard for internal drainage, with pseudocyst recurrence rates less than 5%.[17] Newer endoscopic and laparoscopic techniques have demonstrated similar efficacy in pseudocyst resolution along with the benefits of a minimally invasive approach, including decreased morbidity and hospital length of stay.[18,19] These techniques are discussed further in Chapter 94. In the most favorable large study to date, endoscopic drainage has been shown to have a greater than 90% pseudocyst resolution rate at an experienced center.[20] However, a recent series comparing endoscopic and surgical drainage reported a higher primary success rate for laparoscopic or open surgical procedures, suggesting that the efficacy of endoscopic drainage varies widely and remains significantly operator-dependent.[21] When varices or other large vessels are visualized by endoscopic ultrasound (or CT or MRI) between the stomach and the pseudocyst at a proposed cystogastrostomy site, endoscopic drainage is contraindicated and surgery should be performed.

When compared with operative internal drainage, percutaneous drainage of pseudocysts has been shown to result in an increased requirement for repeat interventions[22] and increased mortality,[23] although the latter may result from a selection bias relating to its use in a sicker population of acute pancreatitis patients. When percutaneous drainage fails, there is usually an associated persistent pancreatic fistula and a high rate of sepsis.[24] At hospitals with adequate surgical and endoscopic expertise, percutaneous catheter drainage may be best reserved for patients who are severely malnourished or medically unfit for a more extensive procedure. Percutaneous drainage is helpful for emergent treatment of an infected pseudocyst with sepsis. For stable patients with suspected infection of a pseudocyst, surgical or endoscopic drainage may still be an efficient treatment option.[25]

SURGERY FOR INTERNAL DRAINAGE

Operations for internal drainage follow the same basic principles, whether open or laparoscopic. The wall of the pseudocyst must be mature and thick enough to hold suture for anastomosis, which is typically true more than 6 weeks after the initial appearance of the pseudocyst. In chronic pancreatitis, surgery for a pseudocyst may proceed as soon as any acute inflammation has subsided. Given the usual significant inflammation from the antecedent pancreatitis, dissection around the pseudocyst should be minimized whenever possible. If there is any concern about the possibility of a cystic neoplasm, a full-thickness biopsy of the cyst wall can be excised where the anastomosis will be performed and sent for immediate frozen section evaluation. Residual debris or necrotic material within the pseudocyst cavity should also be gently suctioned or debrided prior to anastomosis. Cystogastrostomy, Roux-en-Y cystojejunostomy, or cystoduodenostomy are options for internal drainage depending on the anatomic location of the pseudocyst. Especially in cases of giant pseudocysts, the anastomosis should be located to optimize dependent drainage of the pseudocyst.[26] Longitudinal pancreaticojejunostomy for duct drainage alone may be adequate for treatment of an associated pseudocyst in chronic pancreatitis. In other more complex cases, pancreatic resection may be necessary. External drainage can result in a prolonged pancreaticocutaneous fistula, but may be necessary in emergent septic situations when a more definitive or extensive intervention is not prudent.

Cystogastrostomy

When the anterior pseudocyst wall is seen to be directly opposed to the posterior stomach wall from its location in the lesser sac, generally cystogastrostomy is the internal drainage procedure of choice. Because there can be significant scarring of tissue planes in the lesser sac, an anterior approach to cystogastrostomy has been described most often (Fig. 93.5). This technique involves a longitudinal gastrotomy at the level of the anterior wall of the stomach, typically in the body. The bulge of a large pseudocyst can be visualized by pressing into the posterior stomach wall, or an aspirating needle can be used to localize a smaller lesion. Ultrasound can also be used if necessary to localize the pseudocyst. The pseudocyst is entered by incision (or excisional biopsy) of the posterior stomach wall at least 3 cm long and the pseudocyst contents are suctioned out. Traditionally, a cystogastrostomy anastomosis is fashioned with a running, locking, absorbable 2-0 or 3-0 suture such as polydioxanone (PDS) or polyglycolic acid, which ensures adequate hemostasis. Surgical gastrointestinal anastomosis (GIA) staplers with a thick cartridge can also be used if the pseudocyst wall is not

thick enough (>5 mm) to risk staple line dehiscence. The anterior gastrotomy is then closed with sutures or a surgical stapler.

Cystojejunostomy

Cystojejunostomy is performed in a Roux-en-Y configuration (as compared to a loop configuration), thus yielding the advantage of keeping the flow of enteric contents away from the pseudocyst lumen. The Roux limb is versatile and can be brought to any pseudocyst location within the abdomen, although most often it is anastomosed to the pseudocyst through a window in the right or left side of the transverse mesocolon. The same Roux limb can be used to drain multiple pseudocysts in disparate locations, or to decompress a dilated common bile duct in the presence of a concomitant biliary stricture. The proximal jejunum is divided about 30 cm from the ligament of Treitz and a jejunojejunostomy is made, creating a Roux limb approximately 40 to 60 cm long. Closure of the mesenteric defect is routine. The cystojejunostomy anastomosis is formed with sutures or a surgical stapler according to surgeon preference. A two-layer anastomosis using silk for the outer layer and continuous absorbable suture for the inner layer is shown for a pseudocyst whose wall was pushing into the transverse mesocolon (Fig. 93.6).

Cystoduodenostomy

Cystoduodenostomy is rarely necessary, except when the pseudocyst is located at the pancreatic head and immediately abutting the duodenal wall. A longitudinal duodenotomy should be used to expose the medial wall of the duodenum. An aspirating needle can be used to identify the area of nearest apposition of the pseudocyst to the duodenal wall. When creating the 2- to 3-cm-long cystoduodenostomy, caution must be taken to avoid injury to the gastroduodenal artery, as well as the common bile duct or the main pancreatic duct. If those structures impede clear access to the pseudocyst from the medial duodenal wall, a cystojejunostomy may be preferable. Interrupted hemostatic sutures can be placed along the cystoduodenostomy if there is any bleeding from intervening pancreatic parenchyma. The lateral duodenotomy is then closed in one or two layers and a closed-suction drain may be placed per surgeon preference. Historically, a lateral side-to-side cystoduodenostomy has a high rate of morbidity and mortality related to anastomotic dehiscence and abscess formation, and therefore it should rarely (if ever) be performed.[27]

Pancreatic Ductal Drainage

For patients with chronic pancreatitis, the primary factor in the persistence of a pseudocyst is believed to be a stricture or obstruction of the main pancreatic duct. Pseudocyst patients initially believed to have acute pancreatitis may also have findings consistent with chronic pancreatitis on MRCP or ERCP. Nealon and Walser studied 103 patients with pseudocyst and chronic pancreatitis with a main pancreatic duct diameter of greater than 7 mm who received longitudinal pancreaticojejunostomy (Puestow procedure) alone for duct drainage or surgical cystojejunostomy combined with duct drainage.[28] Outcomes were similar except that the patients with duct drainage

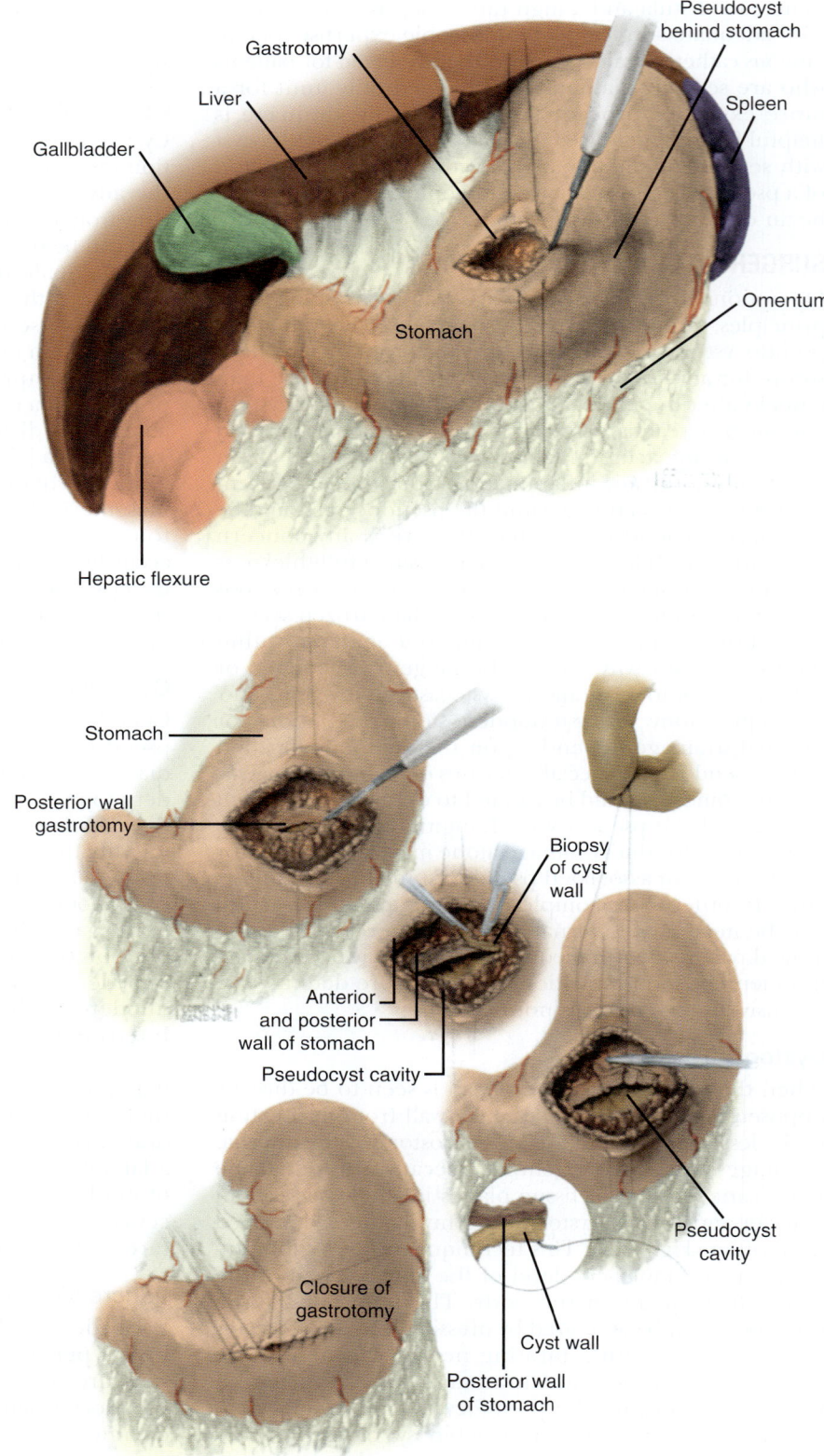

FIGURE 93.5 Anterior technique of cystogastrostomy for pancreatic pseudocyst, as described in the text.

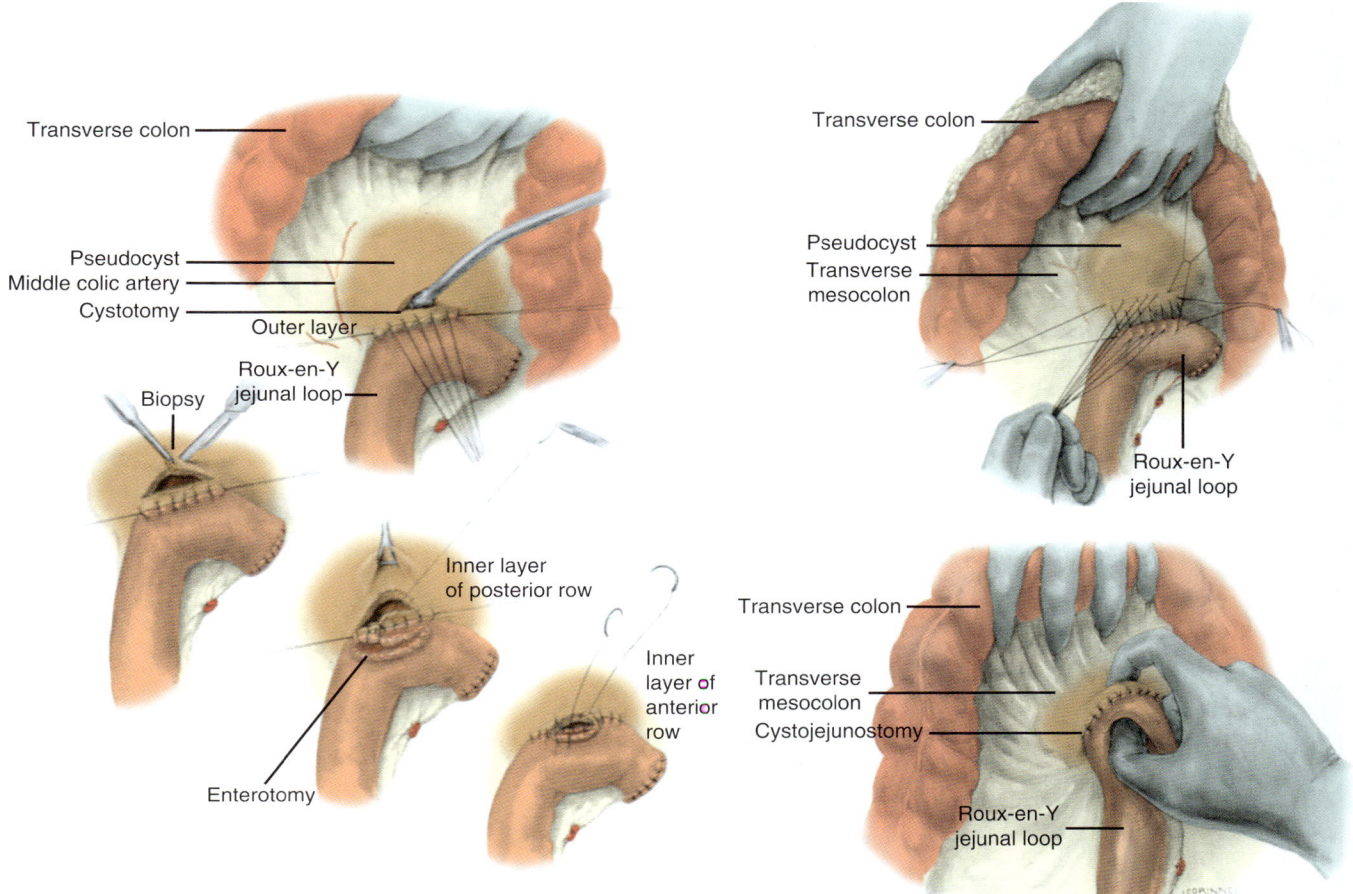

FIGURE 93.6 Roux-en-Y cystojejunostomy for pancreatic pseudocyst, focusing on the actual anastomosis between the pseudocyst and the Roux-en-Y limb.

alone had a shorter operative time and slightly fewer postoperative complications. There were no pseudocyst recurrences in the cohort with duct drainage alone over a mean follow-up of more than 5 years, and 89% of patients had complete resolution of their preoperative pain symptoms. Toward the end of this study, the index pseudocyst was addressed by a single intraoperative aspiration during the ductal drainage procedure. There are data that suggest surgical intervention in chronic pancreatitis may be more efficient and effective for pain relief than endoscopic interventions.[29] Although endoscopic transpapillary pancreatic stent placement can be a successful method of pseudocyst decompression, patients with pseudocyst and a chronically diseased main pancreatic duct may represent a subset that is better treated with early surgical intervention.

Pancreatic Resection

Partial pancreatic resection is generally not considered the first option in the treatment of pseudocysts because of the resultant decrease in pancreatic endocrine and exocrine function and the more extensive surgical dissection required in an area of chronic inflammation and fibrosis. However, even in a study by Murage et al. of an operative strategy favoring internal drainage over resection, the subgroup of patients with pseudocyst and disconnected

pancreatic duct syndrome received a resection 60% of the time.[30] Disconnected pancreatic duct syndrome (Nealon type IIIa and IIIb) occurs when a viable left pancreatic remnant cannot drain its secretions into the duodenum through an intact main pancreatic duct. This scenario can manifest concurrently with acute necrotizing pancreatitis, present in a delayed fashion after damage to the duct from ischemia or prior debridement, or occur as a retention pseudocyst due to occlusion or stricture of the proximal duct related to chronic pancreatitis (Fig. 93.7). Patients with a small pancreatic remnant less than 6 cm long and the presence of splenic vein thrombosis were most likely to have distal pancreatectomy and splenectomy. Other patients treated via resection of the left pancreatic remnant had a small pancreatic duct unsuitable for anastomosis. Pseudocysts in the pancreatic head of patients receiving surgery for symptoms of chronic pancreatitis may be removed along with a duodenum-preserving pancreatic head resection or Whipple procedure, to ensure postoperative pain relief. Fischer et al. managed all of their delayed disconnected pancreatic duct syndrome patients with distal pancreatectomy and splenectomy, due to doubts about pseudocyst accessibility to endoscopy and the long-term patency of endoscopic drainage in the setting of complete pancreatic duct disruption. Splenic artery embolization was performed preoperatively 80%

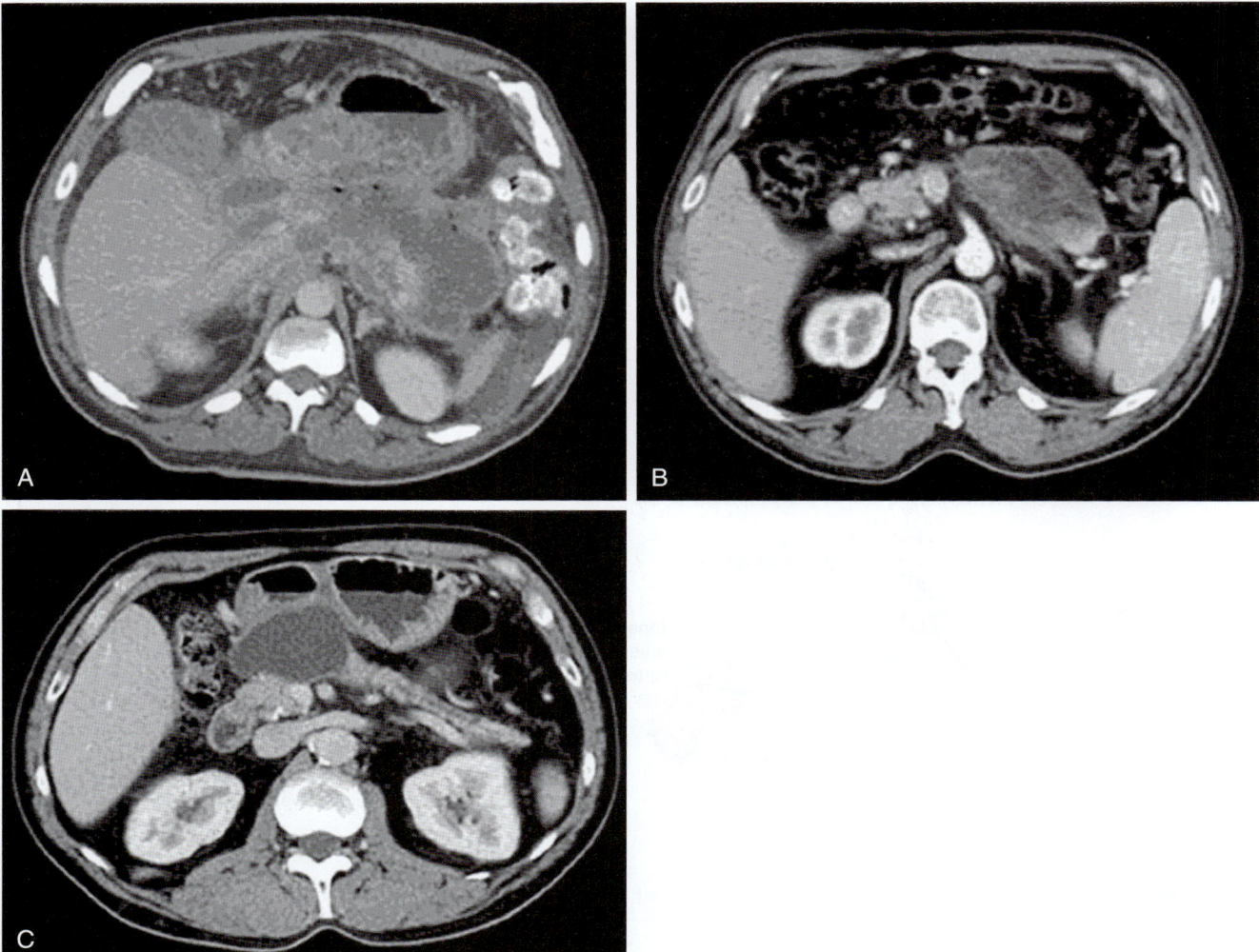

FIGURE 93.7 Computed tomography images of disconnected pancreatic duct syndrome (DPDS). Typical presentations for (A) concurrent DPDS with walled-off pancreatic necrosis, (B) delayed DPDS with loculated pseudocyst, and (C) chronic pancreatitis-associated DPDS with pseudocyst and atrophy of the parenchyma of the body and tail. (Modified rom Fischer TD, Gutman DS, Hughes SJ, Trevino JG, Behrns KE. Disconnected pancreatic duct syndrome: disease classification and management strategies. *J Am Coll Surg.* 2014;219:704–712.)

of the time in an effort to decrease the operative blood loss.[31] Heider and Behrns reviewed a large series of pseudocyst patients and found that 6% had splenic parenchymal involvement by the pseudocyst.[32] The majority of these patients required distal pancreatectomy and splenectomy. As discussed earlier, if preoperative imaging and sampling of cyst fluid from a pancreatic lesion cannot exclude a cystic neoplasm and confirm the diagnosis of pseudocyst, then resection may be necessary.

External Drainage

Open external drainage of a pseudocyst often creates a controlled pancreaticocutaneous fistula and is associated with delayed closure of the fistula, depending on the degree of communication with the underlying pancreatic duct. When emergent surgery is undertaken to control hemorrhage or peritonitis from pseudocyst rupture, external drainage may be the most expedient temporizing action. Definitive endoscopic or surgical treatment can

be deferred until the patient's condition stabilizes. If the pseudocyst wall is unexpectedly too thin and immature for anastomosis, external drainage can be performed. In operations when a planned internal drainage procedure is anatomically unachievable due to adhesions, then external drainage of the pseudocyst is a reasonable "bailout" option. If an infected pseudocyst is encountered at the time of necrosectomy for an acute necrotic collection, external drainage of the pseudocyst is also warranted.

SURGICAL OUTCOMES

Surgical decompression for pseudocysts is a durable intervention with a high initial success rate. Once adequately drained, the pseudocyst cavity obliterates and fuses to the wall of the organ to which it was anastomosed. A review of 451 cystoenterostomy patients from 1960 to 1966 found only a 3.5% pseudocyst recurrence rate and a 5.3% mortality rate.[33] A review of 321 patients receiving surgical cystoenterostomy from 1975 to 2001 showed only a 10% pseudocyst recurrence rate and a 2.5% mortality rate.[34] A more recent review of 118 laparoscopic procedures for pseudocyst (mostly cystogastrostomy) showed only a 2.5% recurrence rate, 0% mortality, and 4.2% complication rate.[35] Likewise, Nealon et al. reported a 2% pseudocyst recurrence rate and 0% mortality in 367 patients receiving an open surgical intervention for pseudocyst.[13] In that study, 25% of patients with pseudocysts experienced spontaneous resolution of the pseudocyst, and surgery was required in 87% of the remaining patients, some of whom had failed endoscopic or percutaneous drainage. These modern series demonstrate the continued importance of surgical treatment for pancreatic pseudocysts. A summary management algorithm for pseudocysts is proposed (Fig. 93.8).

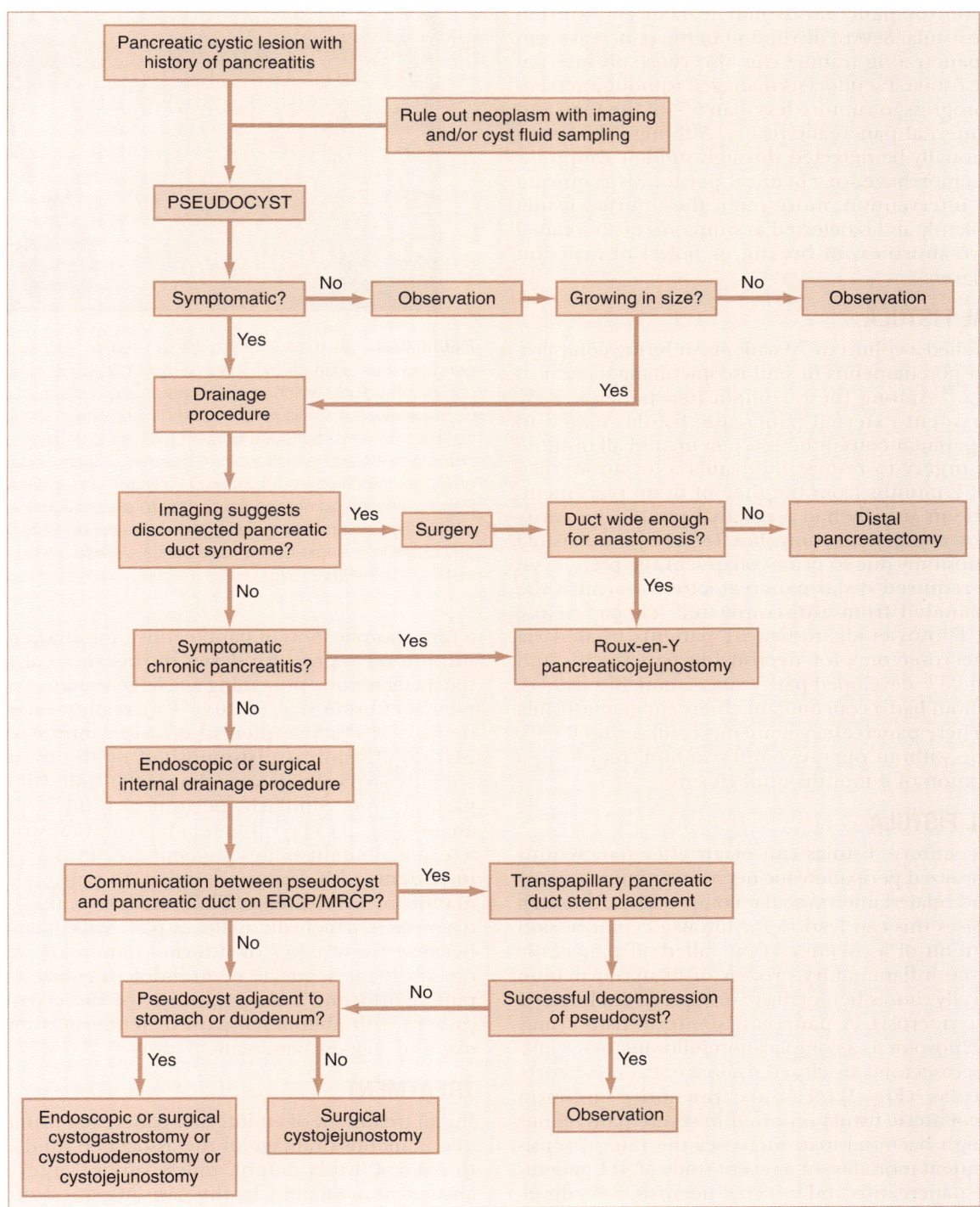

FIGURE 93.8 Algorithm for elective management of pancreatic pseudocysts. *ERCP*, Endoscopic retrograde cholangiopancreatography; *MRCP*, magnetic resonance cholangiopancreatography.

PANCREATIC FISTULAS

DUCTAL DISRUPTION

Pancreatic duct disruption, if uncontained as a pseudocyst, may cause development of an internal pancreatic fistula, variously manifesting as pancreatic ascites, pancreatico-pleural fistula, or pancreaticoenteric fistula. Additionally, prior catheter drainage from a percutaneous or surgical intervention for pancreatitis may lead to an external pancreatic fistula. Severe disruption of the pancreas from blunt or penetrating trauma can also cause an internal pancreatic fistula. Pseudocysts managed without interven-tion can progress to rupture less than 5% of the time and form an internal pancreatic fistula. Although this event can occasionally be detected through sudden symptoms of pain, hemorrhage, or chemical peritonitis requiring emergent intervention, more often the internal fistula develops silently and is detected as symptoms of abdominal discomfort, shortness of breath, or bowel obstruction slowly progress.

EXTERNAL FISTULA

Nealon studied a cohort of 79 patients suffering complica-tions from percutaneous or endoscopic management of pseudocyst.[24] Among these complicated patients, 84% had a persistent external pancreatic fistula related to failure of percutaneous drain placement, and all of those required surgery to resolve the fistula after an average interval of 2 months from the time of drain placement. These patients usually had a residual pseudocyst cavity suitable for cystojejunostomy, but 18% required fistula tract–jejunostomy due to prior collapse of the pseudocyst and 11% required distal pancreatectomy because the fistula emanated from a disconnected left pancreatic remnant. Tsiotos et al. studied 61 patients treated via surgical necrosectomy for necrotizing pancreatitis and found that 23% developed pancreaticocutaneous fistulas, some of whom had a concomitant enterocutaneous fistula as well.[36] These pancreaticocutaneous fistulas closed 64% of the time without operative intervention, requiring a mean duration of 4 months until closure.

INTERNAL FISTULA

Pancreaticoenteric fistulas can occur after pancreatitis due to a localized peripancreatic necrotizing inflammatory process and related microvascular compromise. Although in some cases this can lead to fortuitous decompression and resolution of a pseudocyst or walled-off pancreatic necrosis, the inflammatory process of fistula formation more typically causes hemorrhage or sepsis from infected pancreatic necrosis. A pancreaticoenteric fistula may develop de novo or as a complication following manipula-tion by necrosectomy or closed drainage. Pancreaticoco-lonic fistulas (Fig. 93.9)[37] are the most common pancreaticoenteric fistula reported in severe pancreatitis and the high bacterial load increases the rate of sepsis and subsequent mortality. In a recent study of 311 patients with acute pancreatitis and infected necrosis, 38% devel-oped pancreaticoenteric fistulas and 61% of fistulas involved the colon.[38] Pancreaticobiliary fistula can result in cholangitis or cholestasis. Pancreaticopleural fistula is

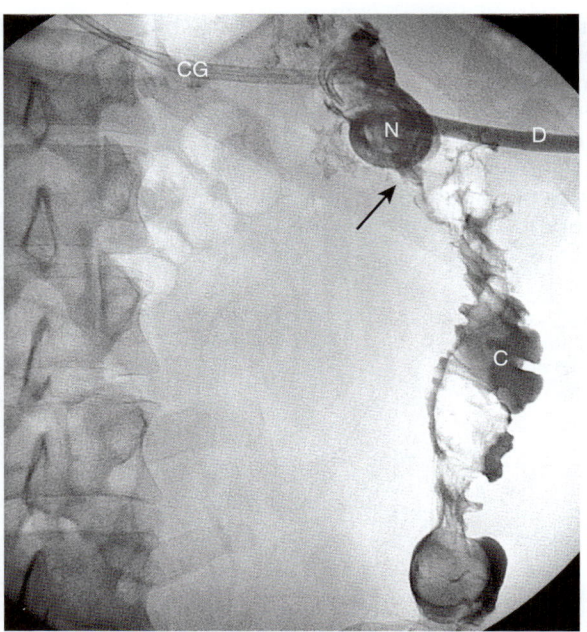

FIGURE 93.9 Pancreaticocolonic fistula seen on fluoroscopic percutaneous drain study. The external drain *(D)* is injected with contrast medium, which opacifies an area of walled-off pancreatic necrosis *(N)*, the fistula *(arrow)*, and descending colon *(C)*. Two cystgastrostomy stents are present *(CG)* for combined percutaneous and endoscopic transenteric ("dual-modality") drainage. (Modified from Heeter ZR, Hauptmann E, Crane R, et al. Pancreaticocolonic fistulas secondary to severe acute pancreatitis treated by percutaneous drainage: successful nonsurgical outcomes in a single-center case series. *J Vasc Interv Radiol.* 2013;24:122–129.)

a rare complication of pancreatitis caused when negative intrathoracic pressure draws retroperitoneal fluid into the mediastinum, presenting as a large-volume symptomatic pleural effusion (Fig. 93.10).[39] Pancreatitis can sometimes provoke a reactive pleural effusion, but a pancreatic pleural effusion is distinguished by the high amylase content (typically greater than 1000 units/liter) of the pleural fluid. Similarly, peritoneal fluid in pancreatic ascites (Fig. 93.11) will have a high amylase content and a serum albumin-ascites gradient greater than 1.1 unlike in patients with ascites secondary to peritoneal inflam-mation or liver disease. Fluid analysis is the key to the diagnosis of pancreatic ascites or pancreaticopleural fistula, because these types of internal pancreatic fistula are classically the sequelae of an indolent course of chronic pancreatitis and only a minority of these patients will present with abdominal pain or tenderness on physical exam to suggest pancreatic pathology.[40]

TREATMENT

Initial treatment of an internal pancreatic fistula involves percutaneous drainage of the associated fluid collection to control fistula output, unless surgical intervention is chosen immediately. In the case of pancreaticopleural fistula, tube thoracostomy is usually adequate treatment, although in some patients lung entrapment from empyema may require eventual decortication to restore normal

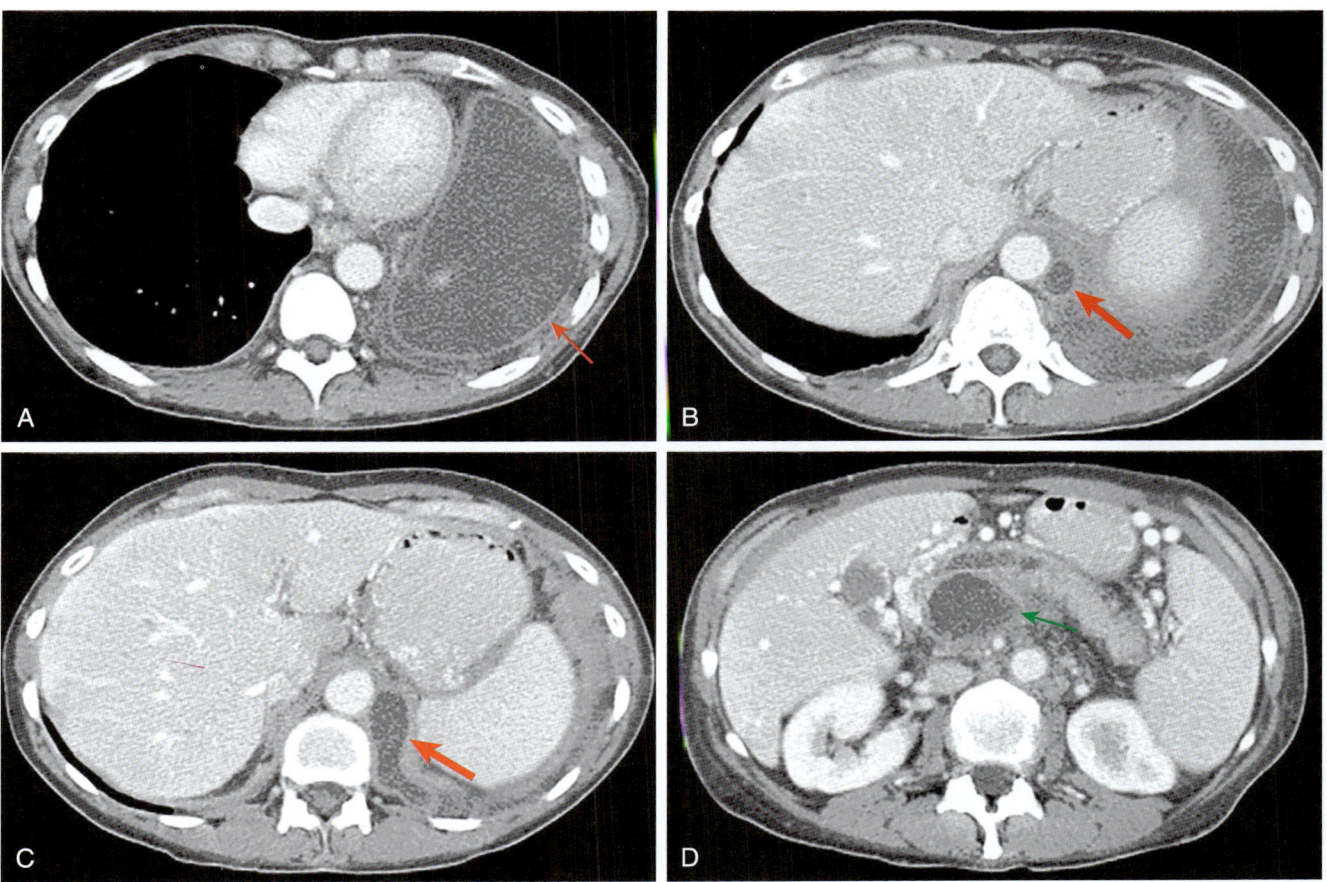

FIGURE 93.10 Computed tomography images of pancreaticopleural fistula. (A–D) Representative sections of preoperative CT scan of chest and abdomen. Note the large left pleural effusion with enhancing rim (*thin red arrow* in [A]), periaortic fistulous tract extending from abdomen into mediastinum (*bold red arrows* in [B] and [C]), and pancreatic pseudocyst deep to the dilated main pancreatic duct (*green arrow* in [D]). (Modified from King JC, Reber HA, Shiraga S, Hines OJ. Pancreatic-pleural fistula is best managed by early operative intervention. *Surgery.* 2010;147:154–159.)

pulmonary function. Diet restriction and parenteral nutrition are often employed to reduce fistula output, although nasojejunal feeding that minimizes pancreatic stimulation may be preferable as long as it does not increase fistula output. Octreotide and other antisecretory medications may decrease the volume of fistula output, but they have not shown a consistent benefit in shortening the time to fistula closure.[41] Endoscopic transpapillary pancreatic duct stent placement has been shown to facilitate fistula closure when the stent is able to traverse a significant ductal stricture.[42] Nasopapillary drainage can also be used for ductal decompression, with the advantage of allowing repeated imaging to check for fistula closure without additional endoscopic procedures. King et al. reviewed published case series of pancreaticopleural fistula and showed that patients who received early operative treatment experienced faster time to fistula closure and a decreased rate of complications as compared to patients who started with medical management.[39] Schweigert et al. also found that prolonged nonoperative management was associated with a significantly higher risk of pleural empyema.[43] MRCP should be obtained early in the evaluation of patients with internal pancreatic fistula because the

anatomy of the pancreatic duct disruption can direct the most efficient therapy. Wronski et al. suggest an MRCP-based algorithm for management of pancreaticopleural fistula that is relevant for all types of internal pancreatic fistula resulting from pancreatitis.[44] When the MRCP shows a pancreatic duct that is normal or mildly dilated, or when there is a ductal stenosis proximal to the ductal disruption, a transpapillary pancreatic duct stent can be placed by ERCP and resolution of the fistula should be expected. If stent placement by ERCP fails to result in fistula healing, or if the MRCP shows a complete blockage of the pancreatic duct with distal disruption, surgical treatment such as a ductal drainage procedure or distal pancreatectomy should be performed.

Fistula Tract–Jejunostomy

Roux-en-Y fistula tract–jejunostomy is recommended for treatment of recalcitrant nonhealing external pancreatic fistulas when pancreatic resection can be avoided, due to its associated decrease in morbidity and mortality (compared to resection). The percutaneous drainage catheter is followed as close as desired to the origin of the pancreatic fistula, but dissection within the inflamed retroperitoneum

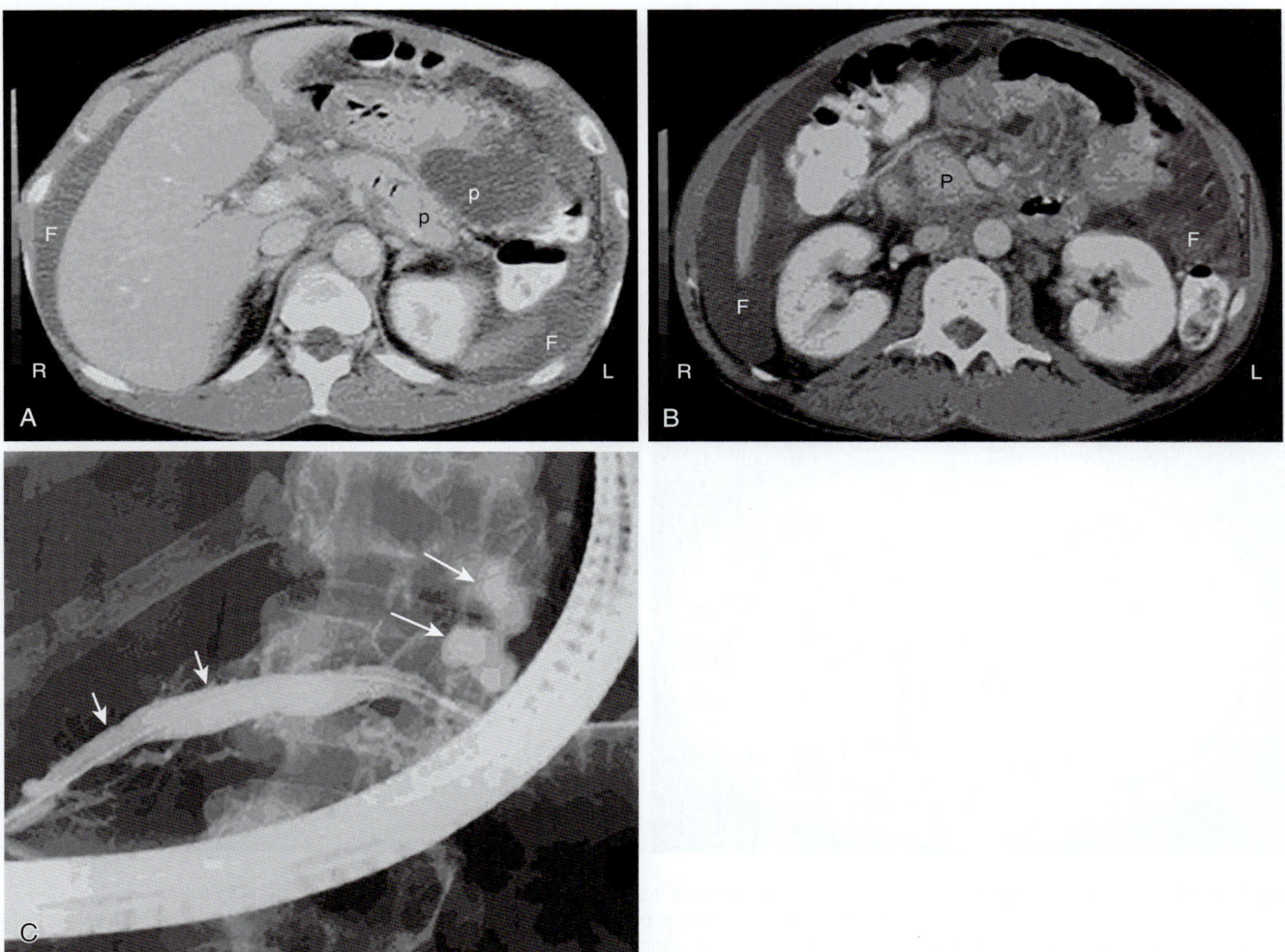

FIGURE 93.11 Pancreatic ascites in a patient with a long history of pancreatitis. (A–B) Computed tomography shows a pancreas with dilation of the main pancreatic duct and a partially loculated fluid collection anterior to the tail of the pancreas consistent with a ruptured pseudocyst. A large amount of retroperitoneal and intraperitoneal fluid is also present. Peritoneal tap showed an amylase level of 20,000 U/L, consistent with pancreatic ascites. (C) Endoscopic retrograde pancreatography examination demonstrates a dilated pancreatic duct *(two small arrows)* and extravasation of contrast material from the tail of the pancreas into the pseudocyst *(two large arrows)*. *F,* Fluid; *p,* pancreas; *P,* pseudocysts. (Modified from Balthazar EJ. Complications of acute pancreatitis: clinical and CT evaluation. *Radiol Clin North Am.* 2002;40:1211–1227.)

is not necessary. The fibrotic fistula tract is cut and its distal end is usually excised. The proximal tract is secured to the Roux limb with interrupted absorbable 4-0 monofilament sutures (Fig. 93.12)[45] and a peritoneal drain is placed near the anastomosis. Although many authors report waiting at least 6 months prior to fistula tract–jejunostomy, Bassi et al. demonstrated 100% success of fistula resolution via internal drainage in 17 patients operated an average of 2 months after fistula onset.[46] They advocate that a 6- to 12-week period after fistula onset is sufficient for the presence of a mature fistula tract.

Distal Pancreatectomy

For internal pancreatic fistulas, as with other cases of disconnected pancreatic duct syndrome, distal pancreatectomy can be performed if the pancreatic fistula originates close to the tail of the pancreas. Roux-en-Y cystojejunostomy is suitable if the fistula involves a mature pseudocyst. Roux-en-Y pancreaticojejunostomy is indicated if the proximal pancreatic duct requires decompression or if the fistula tract is too thin to support an anastomosis. After necrotizing pancreatitis, once a pancreaticoenteric fistula is controlled with external drainage, it may warrant a longer period of nonoperative and endoscopic management prior to surgery. One exception to this rule is a pancreaticocolonic fistula, in which case a temporary proximal stoma for fecal diversion or a segmental colon resection is often necessary to sufficiently control the fistula output and mitigate the development of worsening sepsis.

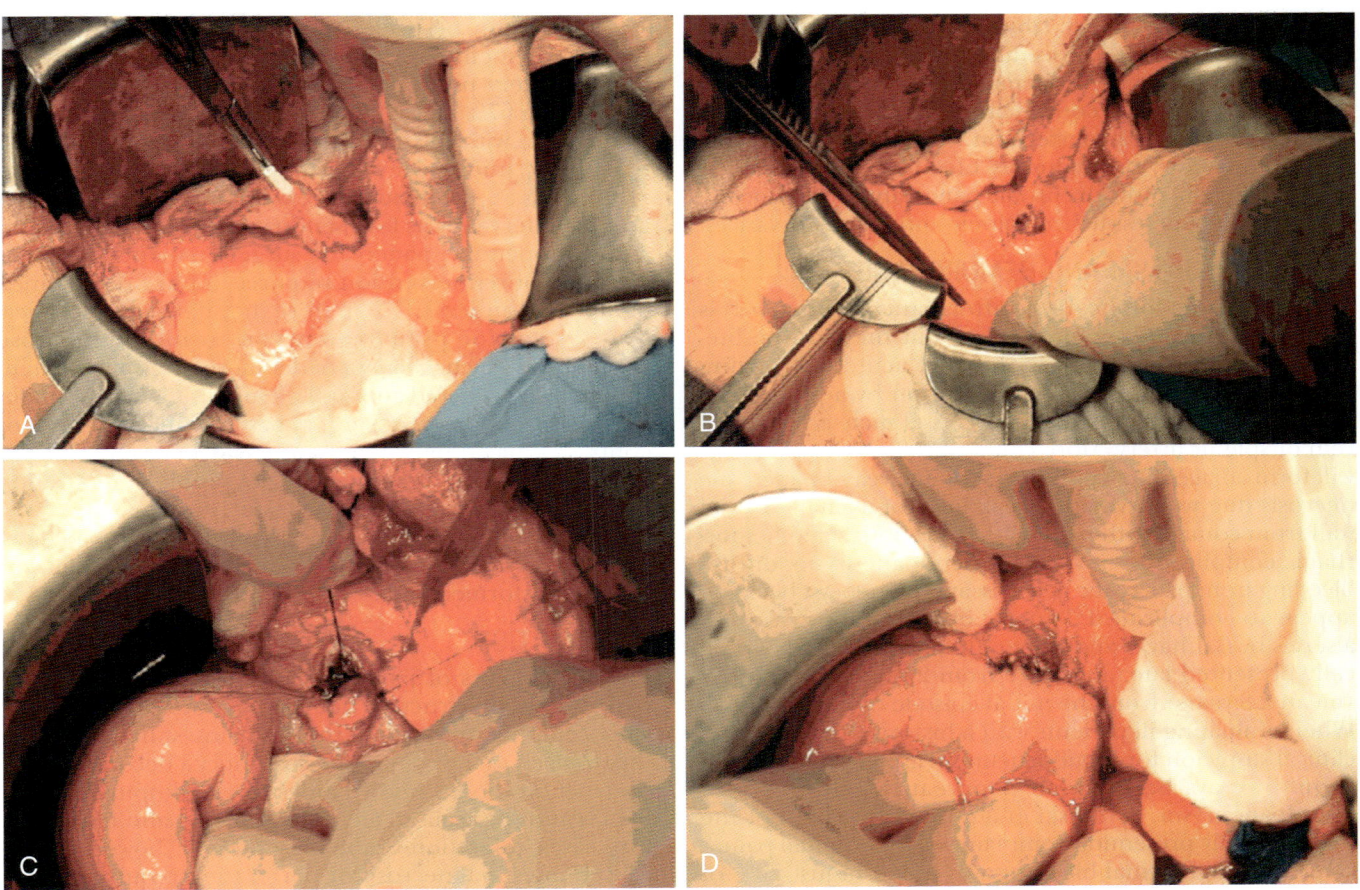

FIGURE 93.12 Roux-en-Y pancreatic fistula tract–jejunostomy for disconnected pancreatic duct syndrome. (A) Dissection of a pancreatic fistula associated with an external pancreatic drainage catheter left through the root of the transverse mesocolon at the time of the initial pancreatic necrosectomy. (B) Opening of a fistula tract and the placement of stay suture. (C) Construction of a Roux-en-Y pancreatic fistula tract–jejunostomy. (D) Completed anastomosis between the fistula tract and the jejunum. (Modified from Pearson EG, Scaife CL, Mulvihill SJ, Glasgow RE. Roux-en-Y drainage of a pancreatic fistula for disconnected pancreatic duct syndrome after acute necrotizing pancreatitis. *HPB [Oxford].* 2012;14:26–31.)

EXTRAPANCREATIC COMPLICATIONS OF PANCREATITIS

SPLENIC VEIN THROMBOSIS

Pancreatitis can often result in splenic vein thrombosis, due to the location of the splenic vein immediately posterior to the pancreas, which is susceptible to peripancreatic fibrosis. Pseudocysts are often present in patients with chronic pancreatitis and splenic vein thrombosis, as seen in 89% of patients in a single-institution review of the natural history of pancreatitis-induced splenic vein thrombosis.[47] According to a metaanalysis of 805 patients, pancreatitis-induced splenic vein thrombosis occurs in approximately 14% of patients with pancreatitis, although that may be an overestimation related to reporting bias.[48] The incidence of gastrointestinal bleeding in those patients was only 12%, considerably less than the rate of bleeding in patients with portal hypertension and a high hepatic venous pressure gradient. Only 53% of splenic vein thrombosis patients had gastric or esophageal varices present and only 52% went on to manifest splenomegaly.

Within this meta-analysis, four out of seven studies published since 1997 showed a 0% rate of spontaneous bleeding. Thus it seems that splenic vein thrombosis in the context of pancreatitis is less consequential than in patients with cirrhosis or cancer. Splenic vein thrombosis is usually an incidental finding on abdominal imaging for patients with chronic pancreatitis, and neither routine anticoagulation nor prophylactic splenectomy is recommended. If esophagogastric variceal bleeding from left-sided portal hypertension occurs, splenectomy is the definitive treatment. Splenic artery embolization is another option for symptomatic patients medically unfit for surgery. Some authors have argued that splenic vein thrombosis patients with asymptomatic gastric varices undergoing pancreatic surgery for another indication (chronic pain, pseudocyst, etc.) should receive splenectomy during the same procedure to prevent future variceal bleeding[49]; we do advocate this approach selectively, but it remains controversial. Nevertheless, splenic vein thrombosis is an important finding to note on preoperative imaging because these patients will have enlarged perigastric and omental venous collaterals that can cause troublesome bleeding during pancreatic surgery. Izbicki et al. compared patients receiving a resectional procedure for chronic pancreatitis and found higher rates of hemorrhage, wound infection, and overall hospital complications in the group with extrahepatic portal hypertension.[50] Distinct from splenic vein thrombosis, spontaneous bleeding has also been reported in patients with chronic pancreatitis from uncommon variceal sources such as colonic and duodenal varices.

PSEUDOANEURYSM AND HEMORRHAGE

Hemorrhagic complications after pancreatitis are less frequent than venous thrombosis, but they can be life-threatening. Rarely in the setting of acute necrotizing pancreatitis there will be direct erosion by a pseudocyst or necrotic collection into a major vessel such as the portal vein or splenic artery. More commonly, pseudoaneurysms will form adjacent to a pseudocyst or an area of pancreatic necrosis due to enzymatic breakdown of a small arterial wall from contact with pancreatic secretions. Late hemorrhagic complications including pseudoaneurysm, diffuse bleeding from pancreatic necrosis, and pseudocyst bleeding appear to complicate 1% to 4% of pancreatitis cases. In a series by Balthazar and Fisher, these complications typically presented late, anywhere from 2 months to 8 years (mean 2.3 years) from the initial episode of pancreatitis.[51] When evaluating ill patients with a history of pancreatitis, clinical suspicion for pseudoaneurysm and occult bleeding should always be high. In pancreatitis patients with pseudoaneurysm, Zyromski et al. noted that 62% of the time, the only presenting complaint was abdominal pain.[52] Overt gastrointestinal bleeding was noted in just 29% of those patients. Angiographic embolization has become first-line therapy for pseudoaneurysm in pancreatitis (Fig. 93.13). Coil embolization is the usual technique, but stent placement can be used if the target artery cannot be sacrificed, such as with a common hepatic or proper hepatic artery pseudoaneurysm. Reported success rates range from 67% to 100% of cases. Pseudoaneurysm communication with the gastrointestinal tract or exposure to pancreatic juice over time may lead to infection and rebleeding. A systematic review by Pang et al. of angiographic interventions for pseudoaneurysm in pancreatitis and postoperative pancreatic surgery patients showed a 20% rate of reintervention required (either repeat angiography or surgery).[53] Therefore they devised a classification system for pseudoaneurysm to highlight those situations in which a benefit of definitive surgical treatment should be considered after using embolization as a stabilizing measure. Emergent surgery has an important role for control of bleeding when a patient is hemodynamically unstable or when attempted angiographic embolization of the bleeding vessel is unsuccessful. Proximal and distal ligation of the bleeding vessel is usually the most expedient procedure, although limited pancreatic resection may also be performed.

OBSTRUCTION

Varying degrees of paralytic ileus are very common in pancreatitis. Obstruction due to pseudocyst compression can occur anywhere along the gastrointestinal tract from the stomach to the colon. After pseudocyst decompression, obstruction should resolve unless the pathophysiology of pancreatitis has caused adjacent ischemia and fibrosis. In rare cases, infarction of the mesentery or bowel wall has caused intestinal necrosis or perforation requiring emergent resection and proximal stoma. Focal ischemic strictures requiring resection or bypass have been reported in the duodenum, jejunum, colon, and common bile

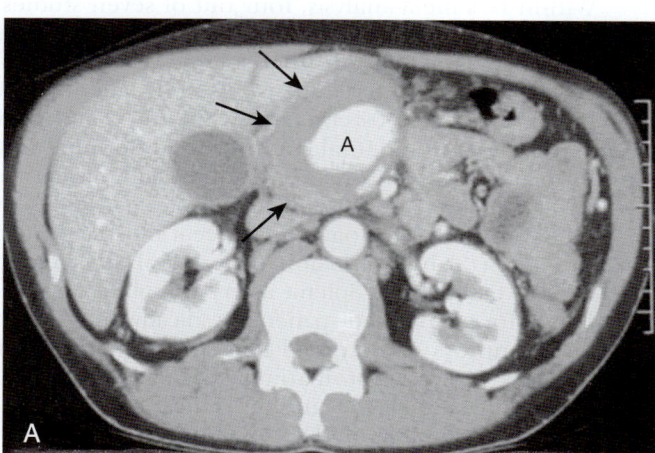
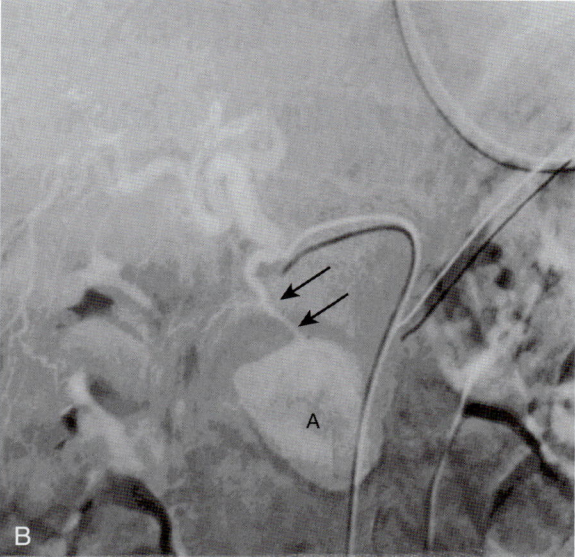

FIGURE 93.13 Pseudoaneurysm within a pseudocyst in a patient with a history of pancreatitis. (A) Computed tomography image showing a large, oval, intravenous contrast–filled structure consistent with pseudoaneurysm *(A)* located in a pseudocyst *(arrows)*. (B) Selective angiogram of the gastroduodenal artery showing the pseudoaneurysm *(A)* arising from the superior pancreaticoduodenal branch *(arrows)*. Pseudoaneurysm was successfully embolized. (Modified from Balthazar EJ. Complications of acute pancreatitis: clinical and CT evaluation. *Radiol Clin North Am.* 2002;40:1211–1227.)

duct.[54,55] Frey et al. reported that 5% to 10% of patients with chronic pancreatitis will require operative decompression of an obstructed common bile duct and that previous pancreaticojejunostomy does not protect against bile duct stricture.[56] Large pseudocysts can obstruct the ureters or the inferior vena cava, which necessitates prompt decompression to avoid chronic sequelae from hydronephrosis or lower extremity edema, respectively.

CONCLUSION

Pseudocysts and pancreatic fistulas are frequent complications after acute or chronic pancreatitis. It is important to have a multidisciplinary approach to treatment including surgeons, endoscopists, radiologists, and interventional radiologists. Understanding the status of the main pancreatic duct is essential for selecting the optimal therapies. There are many scenarios in which surgery remains the most efficient and effective treatment strategy.

REFERENCES

1. Banks PA, Bollen TL, Dervenis C, et al. Classification of acute pancreatitis—2012: revision of the Atlanta classification and definitions by international consensus. *Gut.* 2013;62(1):102-111.
2. Cui ML, Kim KH, Kim HG, et al. Incidence, risk factors and clinical course of pancreatic fluid collections in acute pancreatitis. *Dig Dis Sci.* 2014;59(5):1055-1062.
3. Kourtesis G, Wilson SE, Williams RA. The clinical significance of fluid collections in acute pancreatitis. *Am Surg.* 1990;56(12):796-799.
4. Kim KO, Kim TN. Acute pancreatic pseudocyst: incidence, risk factors, and clinical outcomes. *Pancreas.* 2012;41(4):577-581.
5. Yeo CJ, Sarr MG. Cystic and pseudocystic diseases of the pancreas. *Curr Probl Surg.* 1994;31(3):165-243.
6. Fernández-del Castillo C, Targarona J, Thayer SP, Rattner DW, Brugge WR, Warshaw AL. Incidental pancreatic cysts: clinicopathologic characteristics and comparison with symptomatic patients. *Arch Surg.* 2003;138(4):427-433, [discussion 433–434].
7. Moris M, Bridges MD, Pooley RA, et al. Association between advances in high-resolution cross-section imaging technologies and increase in prevalence of pancreatic cysts from 2005 to 2014. *Clin Gastroenterol Hepatol.* 2016;14(4):585-593.e3.
8. Macari M, Finn ME, Bennett GL, et al. Differentiating pancreatic cystic neoplasms from pancreatic pseudocysts at MR imaging: value of perceived internal debris. *Radiology.* 2009;251(1):77-84.
9. Drake LM, Anis M, Lawrence C. Accuracy of magnetic resonance cholangiopancreatography in identifying pancreatic duct disruption. *J Clin Gastroenterol.* 2012;46(8):696-699.
10. Brugge WR, Lauwers GY, Sahani D, Fernandez-del Castillo C, Warshaw AL. Cystic neoplasms of the pancreas. *N Engl J Med.* 2004;351(12):1218-1226.
11. Maker AV, Lee LS, Raut CP, Clancy TE, Swanson RS. Cytology from pancreatic cysts has marginal utility in surgical decision-making. *Ann Surg Oncol.* 2008;15(11):3187-3192.
12. D'Egidio A, Schein M. Pancreatic pseudocysts: a proposed classification and its management implications. *Br J Surg.* 1991;78(8):981-984.
13. Nealon WH, Bhutani M, Riall TS, Raju G, Ozkan O, Neilan R. A unifying concept: pancreatic ductal anatomy both predicts and determines the major complications resulting from pancreatitis. *J Am Coll Surg.* 2009;208(5):790-799, [discussion 799–801].
14. Yeo CJ, Bastidas JA, Lynch-Nyhan A, Fishman EK, Zinner MJ, Cameron JL. The natural history of pancreatic pseudocysts documented by computed tomography. *Surg Gynecol Obstet.* 1990;170(5):411-417.
15. Vitas GJ, Sarr MG. Selected management of pancreatic pseudocysts: operative versus expectant management. *Surgery.* 1992;111(2):123-130.
16. Soliani P, Franzini C, Ziegler S, et al. Pancreatic pseudocysts following acute pancreatitis: risk factors influencing therapeutic outcomes. *J Pancreas.* 2004;5(5):338-347.
17. Parks RW, Tzovaras G, Diamond T, Rowlands BJ. Management of pancreatic pseudocysts. *Ann R Coll Surg Engl.* 2000;82(6):383-387.
18. Johnson MD, Walsh RM, Henderson JM, et al. Surgical versus nonsurgical management of pancreatic pseudocysts. *J Clin Gastroenterol.* 2009;43(6):586-590.
19. Varadarajulu S, Bang JY, Sutton BS, Trevino JM, Christein JD, Wilcox CM. Equal efficacy of endoscopic and surgical cystogastrostomy for pancreatic pseudocyst drainage in a randomized trial. *Gastroenterology.* 2013;145(3):583-590.e1.
20. Varadarajulu S, Bang JY, Phadnis MA, Christein JD, Wilcox CM. Endoscopic transmural drainage of peripancreatic fluid collections: outcomes and predictors of treatment success in 211 consecutive patients. *J Gastrointest Surg.* 2011;15(11):2080-2088.
21. Melman L, Azar R, Beddow K, et al. Primary and overall success rates for clinical outcomes after laparoscopic, endoscopic, and open pancreatic cystgastrostomy for pancreatic pseudocysts. *Surg Endosc.* 2009;23(2):267-271.
22. Heider R, Meyer AA, Galanko JA, Behrns KE. Percutaneous drainage of pancreatic pseudocysts is associated with a higher failure rate than surgical treatment in unselected patients. *Ann Surg.* 1999;229(6):781-787, [discussion 787–789].
23. Morton JM, Brown A, Galanko JA, Norton JA, Grimm IS, Behrns KE. A national comparison of surgical versus percutaneous drainage of pancreatic pseudocysts: 1997–2001. *J Gastrointest Surg.* 2005;9(1):15-20, [discussion 20–21].
24. Nealon WH, Walser E. Surgical management of complications associated with percutaneous and/or endoscopic management of pseudocyst of the pancreas. *Ann Surg.* 2005;241(6):948-957.
25. Boerma D, van Gulik TM, Obertop H, Gouma DJ. Internal drainage of infected pancreatic pseudocysts: safe or sorry? *Dig Surg.* 1999;16(6):501-505.
26. Johnson LB, Rattner DW, Warshaw AL. The effect of size of giant pancreatic pseudocysts on the outcome of internal drainage procedures. *Surg Gynecol Obstet.* 1991;173(3):171-174.
27. Bradley EL 3rd. Cystoduodenostomy. New perspectives. *Ann Surg.* 1984;200(6):698-701.
28. Nealon WH, Walser E. Duct drainage alone is sufficient in the operative management of pancreatic pseudocyst in patients with chronic pancreatitis. *Ann Surg.* 2003;237(5):614-620, [discussion 620–622].
29. Cahen DL, Gouma DJ, Nio Y, et al. Endoscopic versus surgical drainage of the pancreatic duct in chronic pancreatitis. *N Engl J Med.* 2007;356(7):676-684.
30. Murage KP, Ball CG, Zyromski NJ, et al. Clinical framework to guide operative decision making in disconnected left pancreatic remnant (DLPR) following acute or chronic pancreatitis. *Surgery.* 2010;148(4):847-856.
31. Fischer TD, Gutman DS, Hughes SJ, Trevino JG, Behrns KE. Disconnected pancreatic duct syndrome: disease classification and management strategies. *J Am Coll Surg.* 2014;219(4):704-712.
32. Heider R, Behrns KE. Pancreatic pseudocysts complicated by splenic parenchymal involvement: results of operative and percutaneous management. *Pancreas.* 2001;23(1):20-25.
33. Becker WF, Pratt HS, Ganji H. Pseudocysts of the pancreas. *Surg Gynecol Obstet.* 1968;127(4):744-747.
34. Rosso E, Alexakis N, Ghaneh P, et al. Pancreatic pseudocyst in chronic pancreatitis: endoscopic and surgical treatment. *Dig Surg.* 2003;20(5):397-406.
35. Aljarabah M, Ammori BJ. Laparoscopic and endoscopic approaches for drainage of pancreatic pseudocysts: a systematic review of published series. *Surg Endosc.* 2007;21(11):1936-1944.
36. Tsiotos GG, Smith CD, Sarr MG. Incidence and management of pancreatic and enteric fistulas after surgical management of severe necrotizing pancreatitis. *Arch Surg.* 1995;130(1):48-52.
37. Heeter ZR, Hauptmann E, Crane R, et al. Pancreaticocolonic fistulas secondary to severe acute pancreatitis treated by percutaneous drainage: successful nonsurgical outcomes in a single-center case series. *J Vasc Interv Radiol.* 2013;24(1):122-129.
38. Jiang W, Tong Z, Yang D, et al. Gastrointestinal fistulas in acute pancreatitis with infected pancreatic or peripancreatic necrosis: a 4-year single-center experience. *Medicine (Baltimore).* 2016;95(14):e3318.
39. King JC, Reber HA, Shiraga S, Hines OJ. Pancreatic-pleural fistula is best managed by early operative intervention. *Surgery.* 2010;147(1):154-159.
40. Cameron JL, Kieffer RS, Anderson WJ, Zuidema GD. Internal pancreatic fistulas: pancreatic ascites and pleural effusions. *Ann Surg.* 1976;184(5):587-593.

41. Gans SL, van Westreenen HL, Kiewiet JJ, Rauws EA, Gouma DJ, Boermeester MA. Systematic review and meta-analysis of somatostatin analogues for the treatment of pancreatic fistula. *Br J Surg*. 2012;99(6):754-760.

42. Boerma D, Rauws EA, van Gulik TM, Huibregtse K, Obertop H, Gouma DJ. Endoscopic stent placement for pancreaticocutaneous fistula after surgical drainage of the pancreas. *Br J Surg*. 2000; 87(11):1506-1509.

43. Schweigert M, Solymosi N, Dubecz A, Ofner D, Stein HJ. Length of nonoperative treatment and risk of pleural empyema in the management of pancreatitis-induced pancreaticopleural fistula. *Am Surg*. 2013;79(6):614-619.

44. Wronski M, Slodkowski M, Cebulski W, Moronczyk D, Krasnodebski IW. Optimizing management of pancreaticopleural fistulas. *World J Gastroenterol*. 2011;17(42):4696-4703.

45. Pearson EG, Scaife CL, Mulvihill SJ, Glasgow RE. Roux-en-Y drainage of a pancreatic fistula for disconnected pancreatic duct syndrome after acute necrotizing pancreatitis. *HPB (Oxford)*. 2012;14(1):26-31.

46. Bassi C, Butturini G, Salvia R, et al. A single-institution experience with fistulojejunostomy for external pancreatic fistulas. *Am J Surg*. 2000;179(3):203-206.

47. Heider TR, Azeem S, Galanko JA, Behrns KE. The natural history of pancreatitis-induced splenic vein thrombosis. *Ann Surg*. 2004;239(6):876-880, [discussion 880–882].

48. Butler JR, Eckert GJ, Zyromski NJ, Leonardi MJ, Lillemoe KD, Howard TJ. Natural history of pancreatitis-induced splenic vein thrombosis: a systematic review and meta-analysis of its incidence and rate of gastrointestinal bleeding. *HPB (Oxford)*. 2011;13(12):839-845.

49. Sakorafas GH, Sarr MG, Farley DR, Farnell MB. The significance of sinistral portal hypertension complicating chronic pancreatitis. *Am J Surg*. 2000;179(2):129-133.

50. Izbicki JR, Yekebas EF, Strate T, et al. Extrahepatic portal hypertension in chronic pancreatitis: an old problem revisited. *Ann Surg*. 2002;236(1):82-89.

51. Balthazar EJ, Fisher LA. Hemorrhagic complications of pancreatitis: radiologic evaluation with emphasis on CT imaging. *Pancreatology*. 2001;1(4):306-313.

52. Zyromski NJ, Vieira C, Stecker M, et al. Improved outcomes in postoperative and pancreatitis-related visceral pseudoaneurysms. *J Gastrointest Surg*. 2007;11(1):50-55.

53. Pang TC, Maher R, Gananadha S, Hugh TJ, Samra JS. Peripancreatic pseudoaneurysms: a management-based classification system. *Surg Endosc*. 2014;28(7):2027-2038.

54. Vijungco JD, Prinz RA. Management of biliary and duodenal complications of chronic pancreatitis. *World J Surg*. 2003;27(11):1258-1270.

55. Negro P, D'Amore L, Saputelli A, et al. Colonic lesions in pancreatitis. *Ann Ital Chir*. 1995;66(2):223-231.

56. Frey CF, Suzuki M, Isaji S. Treatment of chronic pancreatitis complicated by obstruction of the common bile duct or duodenum. *World J Surg*. 1990;14(1):59-69.

Endoscopic and Minimally Invasive Therapy for Complications of Pancreatitis

Christopher G. Chapman | Irving Waxman | Vivek N. Prachand

Acute pancreatitis (AP) and chronic pancreatitis (CP) are dynamic inflammatory conditions that can result in local complications necessitating invasive treatment. Although AP and CP were previously considered and managed as distinct clinical entities, advances in experimental pancreatitis models, improved clinical characterization, and discovery of genetic mutations have resulted in a better understanding of the natural history and pathophysiology of what is now recognized as a clinical continuum. Local and systemic complications of AP and CP develop from the intrapancreatic activation of zymogens resulting in an inflammatory cascade, tissue ischemia, and pancreatic fluid leak. AP is differentiated from CP by the resolution of symptoms, histologic improvement, and generally the maintenance of pancreatic endocrine and exocrine function. However, in a subset of patients with persistent pancreatic enzyme activation or recurrent AP, there can be progression to inflammation-induced, permanent structural damage that is diagnostic of CP.

Early medical management of acute exacerbations of AP and CP are generally supportive in nature, focusing on assessment of disease severity, aggressive hydration, and pain control. When complications such as inflammatory pancreatic fluid collections develop, however, interventional therapies are often required. In 2012, the revised Atlanta classifications (Table 94.1) for inflammatory pancreatic and peripancreatic fluid collections were released to provide standardized definitions to differentiate these lesions.[1] Inflammatory pancreatic fluid collections were divided into four types including acute pancreatic fluid collections (APFC), acute necrotic collections (ANC), pancreatic pseudocysts, and walled-off necrosis (WON). The new definitions and classifications of inflammatory pancreatic fluid collections as distinct entities are important to recognize as the natural history, risk of subsequent morbidity and mortality, and outcomes of minimally invasive therapies are varied. Furthermore, the majority of antecedent literature reporting the outcomes of management is based upon heterogeneous combinations of these inflammatory fluid collections.[2] In addition to inflammatory pancreatic fluid collections and their risk of infection, local complications of AP include biliary/gastric/duodenal obstruction, splenic and portal vein thrombosis, gastrointestinal bleeding/pseudoaneurysm, and internal/external fistulization. Patients with CP remain at risk for similar complications, such as pseudocysts and biliary obstruction, in addition to chronic pain with pancreaticolithiasis or ductal strictures.

The endoscopic, minimally invasive surgical and radiologic procedures available to practitioners managing the complications of AP and CP have rapidly expanded and provide an alternative to traditional open surgical management strategies. In concert with the medical technology expansion, the revised Atlanta definitions for inflammatory pancreatic fluid collections have provided more homogeneous data on outcomes and clinical management strategies. Given the heterogeneity of pancreatic fluid collections, local technical expertise, and anatomic variation, management decisions should be individualized within the context of a multidisciplinary team composed of surgeons, radiologists, and gastroenterologists.

LOCAL COMPLICATIONS OF ACUTE PANCREATITIS

AP is a common inflammatory condition accounting for over 200,000 hospital admissions annually in the United States and over $2 billion in annual health care costs.[3] Mortality from acute interstitial edematous pancreatitis is 3% to 5%[4]; however when associated with sterile pancreatic necrosis, the mortality rate increases to 15% and with infected pancreatic necrosis (IPN) to 30% to 40%.[5] The mortality from AP occurs in two phases—an early phase, usually secondary to a severe systemic inflammatory response with multiorgan failure to the primary insult and a second, late phase, secondary to local complications including infected pancreatic and peripancreatic necrosis.[6] Despite these concerning statistics, the vast majority of patients with acute interstitial pancreatitis and preserved perfusion will resolve without complications. Approximately 15% to 20% of patients develop pancreatic and peripancreatic necrosis,[1] but in these cases, ductal disruption is invariable and complications are more frequent and illness is protracted.[4,7]

ACUTE PANCREATIC FLUID AND ACUTE NECROTIC COLLECTIONS

According to the revised Atlanta classification, acute pancreatic collections include APFC and ANC and are diagnosed less than 4 weeks from the presentation of AP. APFCs are predominantly fluid-filled collections that occur subsequent to an episode of acute interstitial pancreatitis with no radiologic evidence of parenchymal or peripancreatic necrosis. ANCs contain a mixture of fluid and solid necrotic debris and tissue secondary to documented pancreatic or peripancreatic necrosis. These collections often do not require any therapeutic intervention as they are generally sterile, lack a well-defined, mature wall, and self-resolve after a few weeks. However, if they become infected or symptomatic, therapy may need to be considered.

TABLE 94.1 2012 Revised Atlanta Classification Definitions and Morphologic Features of Acute Pancreatitis–Associated Inflammatory Pancreatic Fluid Collections

Pancreatic Fluid Collection	Type of Pancreatitis	Time	Well-Defined Wall	Contains Solid Necrotic Debris	Radiographic Features*
Acute pancreatic fluid collection	Interstitial edematous	<4 weeks	No	No	Homogeneous collection with fluid density Confined by normal peripancreatic fascial planes No definable wall encapsulating the collection Adjacent to pancreas (no intrapancreatic extension)
Acute necrotic collection	Necrotizing	<4 weeks	No	Yes	Heterogeneous and nonliquid density of varying degrees in different locations (some appear homogeneous if early) No definable wall encapsulating the collection Intrapancreatic and/or extrapancreatic
Pseudocyst	Interstitial edematous	>4 weeks	Yes	No	Well circumscribed, usually round or oval Homogeneous fluid density No nonliquid component Well-defined wall, completely encapsulated
Walled-off necrosis	Necrotizing	>4 weeks	Yes	Yes	Heterogeneous with liquid and nonliquid density with varying degrees of loculations (some may appear homogeneous) Well-defined wall, completely encapsulated Intrapancreatic and/or extrapancreatic

*Contrast-enhanced CT features.
Modified from Banks PA, Bollen TL, Dervenis C, et al. Classification of acute pancreatitis—2012: revision of the Atlanta classification and definitions by international consensus. *Gut*. 2013;62:102–111.

A better understanding of the natural history of these collections reveals that although APFCs may occur in approximately 40% to 60% of patients with acute interstitial pancreatitis, the vast majority, approximated to be 85% to 90%, undergo spontaneous, self-resolution within 7 to 10 days.[8,9] The residual 10% to 15% that persist beyond 4 weeks progress to pancreatic pseudocysts and are at risk for complications, including intracystic hemorrhage, rupture, or infection. APFCs that are large (> 6 cm), persist more than 6 weeks,[6] are associated with CP,[10,11] contain multiple cystic lesions (~10% of patients),[11,12] are located in the tail,[13] or have a wall greater than 1 cm in size[14] have been reported to have a decreased likelihood of spontaneous resolution and need to be monitored serially to assess the need for intervention.

Patients with ANCs often present with a heightened systemic inflammatory response, multiorgan failure, and admission to the intensive care unit (ICU), which can be confounding when assessing for infection. In the initial 2-week time period, ANCs are typically sterile and should be treated with aggressive medical management. Surgical débridement of ANCs in the early stages should be avoided unless infection is confirmed and until the necrotic material has liquefied as prior data on urgent open surgical débridement was associated with excessive morbidity and mortality. If the patient develops recurrent systemic symptoms, such as fever, new or worsening abdominal pain, rising leukocytosis, an infected ANC should be suspected. In these cases, antibiotics with adequate pancreatic penetration should be initiated in an attempt to allow time for the transition from ANC to WON defined by the development of a mature, well-defined wall. With this transition, the WON can undergo minimally invasive débridement with reduced risk of complications.

INFECTED PANCREATIC NECROSIS

The cornerstone of management of severe AP is supportive care, typically in the ICU, with more invasive treatments, such as surgical, percutaneous, or endoscopic débridement reserved for patients with IPN, which develops in 40% to 70% of patients with pancreatic necrosis.[5] WON was defined by the 2012 revised Atlanta classification as "a mature, encapsulated collection of pancreatic and/or peripancreatic necrosis that has developed a well defined inflammatory wall." WON typically develops as an evolution of an ANC 4 weeks after an episode of severe acute necrotizing pancreatitis. In 2014, Sarathi Patra et al. reported the natural history of fluid collections in severe AP and found that 41% of patients with ANCs have spontaneous resolution, whereas 49% progress to WON.[15] If sterile, treatment for WON is usually conservative; however if IPN is suspected by the presence of gas in a pancreatic or peripancreatic fluid collection on computed tomography (CT) or failure to respond to maximal ICU support and confirmed by aspiration or drainage and culture of the collection, antibiotics and invasive therapy are warranted. If left untreated, IPN has a mortality rate that approaches 100%.

The historical standard approach for the treatment of IPN has been surgical débridement with the goal of removal of all infected tissues. The significant mortality (11% to 39%) and complication rates (34% to 95%) associated with open necrostectomy,[16,17] including the development of pancreaticocutaneous and enterocutaneous fistulas, incisional hernias, and exocrine and endocrine pancreatic insufficiency, led to the development and implementation of less invasive techniques, such as endoscopic necrosectomy and percutaneous drainage.

Standard of therapy for IPN has been a multimodality "step up approach," consisting of percutaneous catheter drainage followed by surgical necrosectomy; however, advances in endoscopic techniques have resulted in an evolving paradigm shift. As a result, clinical guidelines, including the International Association of Pancreatology and the American Pancreatic Association evidence-based guidelines, endorse percutaneous catheter or endoscopic transmural drainage as the first step in the treatment, followed by either endoscopic or minimally invasive surgical necrosectomy.[18] Management strategies can be difficult and therefore require a multidisciplinary assessment. Regardless of approach, because demarcation and organization of necrotic tissues require several weeks and surgical mortality is greater following early intervention, it is preferable to defer débridement of IPN for at least 4 weeks following the onset of severe necrotizing AP.[18]

ENDOSCOPIC NECROSECTOMY

For patients with an organized WON located within close proximity (~1 cm) to the gastric or duodenal wall, endoscopic necrosectomy has emerged as a therapeutic alternative to surgery. The technique for endoscopic necrosectomy involves initial guidewire access to the necroma either via direct puncture (in the case of a luminal bulge) or through the use of endoscopic ultrasound (EUS)-guided needle puncture and subsequent wire guided access. Once access is secured, the tract is dilated using a graduated dilating catheter, needle knife sphincterotome, or cystotome, and subsequent dilation to 15 to 20 mm is performed using a balloon dilator to allow passage of an upper endoscope into the necroma. Débridement is then performed using a combination of endoscopic accessories. Preservation of the tract is achieved by the placement of stents into the cavity across the gastric or duodenal wall. A variety of stenting options are available, including two or more pigtail stents, biliary or esophageal fully covered self-expanding metal stents (FCSEMS) and as of 2013, a FCSEMS with double-walled flanges, known as the lumen-apposing metal stent (LAMS), which can be noncautery enhanced (non-CE) or cautery enhanced (CE) to allow for one-step puncture and stent deployment (Fig. 94.1). LAMS foreshorten on deployment and have the benefit of keeping the necroma wall and luminal wall in close apposition, theoretically reducing the risk of migration, and being large enough diameter to allow upper endoscope passage. Tract maintenance allows for repeated access and débridement following the initial necrosectomy. Placement of a nasocystic drain may be required for continuous lavage; irrigation with hydrogen peroxide and multiport access, known as the multiple transluminal gateway technique, may be beneficial in select cases.

Endoscopic necrosectomy/treatment of WON with plastic double-pigtail stents was evaluated in two multicenter retrospective trials with reported clinical success rates of 80% and 91% after necrosectomy, and procedure-related morbidity rates of 26% and 14% respectively.[19,20] There has been one randomized, comparator trial by the Dutch Pancreatitis Group (PENGUIN study) in which 20 patients were randomized to endoscopic transgastric necrosectomy with plastic stents and surgical necrosectomy via either minimally invasive video-assisted retroperitoneal

débridement (VARD) or, if not feasible, open surgery.[21] In patients with infected necrotizing pancreatitis, endoscopic necrosectomy reduced the inflammatory response, had a lower rate of complications, and prevented new-onset multiple organ failure.

In 2016, a retrospective, multicenter study was published that involved 17 United States institutions that used a fully covered LAMS for the endoscopic management of WON.[22] In this largest series to date of 124 patients, technical success was 100% with LAMS and clinical success was achieved in 86.3% after 3 months of follow-up. The median number of endoscopic interventions was two, the overall stent migration rate was 5.6%, and the overall rate of stent patency was 94%. Early adverse events (<30 days) occurred in 14% of patients and late adverse events occurred in 7.2%. There was no procedure-related mortality, which was an initial concern after the original two endoscopic necrosectomy multicenter retrospective trials had patient deaths attributed directly to the procedure. This difference is multifactorial but likely related to the improved understanding of the importance of a well-formed wall, the development of LAMS, and the use of carbon dioxide insufflation as a standard of care. The results of a large, multicenter (13 European institutions) study using CE-LAMS for inflammatory pancreatic collections, including 52 cases of WON, was published in 2015.[23] Technical success was achieved in 98.9% of patients, and clinical success was achieved in 92.5%. Adverse events were reported in 5.6% of patients. Further prospective, randomized studies are needed to confirm the safety and efficacy of non-CE and CE-LAMS in WON; however, initial data are promising with high clinical success rates and minimal adverse events.

PERCUTANEOUS THERAPY

Another method for drainage of IPN includes placement of a large-caliber percutaneous drainage into the necroma, guided by CT or ultrasound with fluoroscopy. Drains are preferably placed through the retroperitoneum to avoid enteric leaks and leakage of infected contents into the peritoneum. Drains are irrigated 3 to 4 times per day and are progressively upsized to a maximum of 30 French (Fr) to allow drainage and modest débridement of predominantly liquefied necrotic tissue. This approach is occasionally necessary when safe and appropriate endoscopic access to the area of IPN is not anatomically available. Aside from the need for frequent radiographic tube checks and drain changes and relatively ineffective débridement of particulate necrotic tissues, a major drawback to this technique is the high rate of associated chronic pancreaticocutaneous fistula formation.

"STEP-UP" THERAPY AND MINIMAL ACCESS PANCREATIC NECROSECTOMY

Minimal access pancreatic necrosectomy is an approach that has been demonstrated to improve outcomes relative to open surgery. Multiple approaches have been reported, including trans- or intraperitoneal laparoscopic necrosectomy and retroperitoneal necrosectomy via VARD or sinus tract endoscopy. The literature on laparoscopic approaches is limited due to significant heterogeneity of technique and

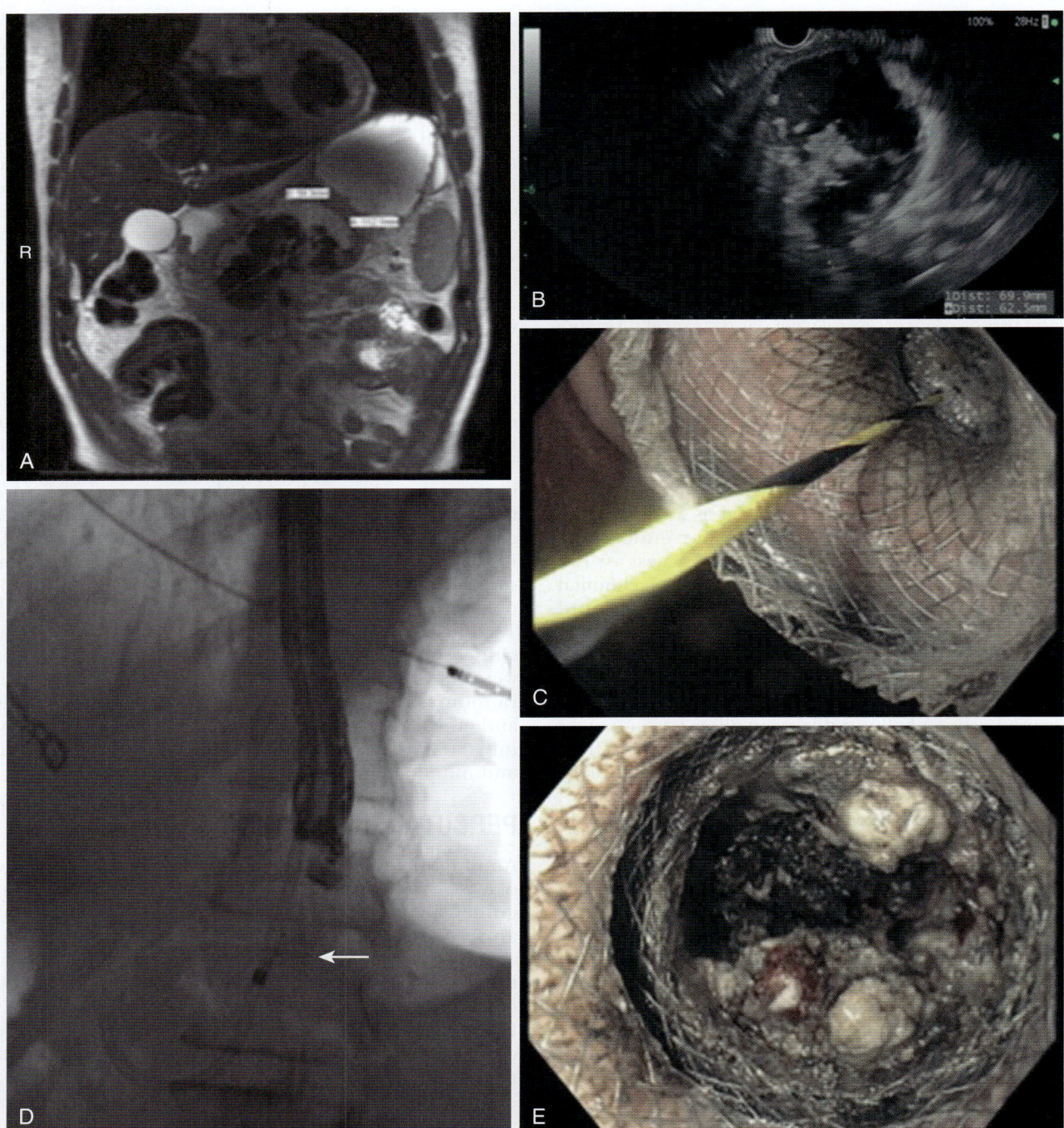

FIGURE 94.1 Endoscopic walled-off pancreatic necrosis drainage. (A) Magnetic resonance imaging scan demonstrating walled-off infected pancreatic necrosis. Note the internal debris present in the collection. (B) Endoscopic ultrasound image demonstrating a transgastric view into the necroma with evidence of internal debris/necrosis. (C) Placement of a lumen-apposing metal stent (LAMS) to provide access to the necroma. (D) Fluoroscopic image of a plastic stent (*arrow*) being placed through the LAMS. (E) Necrotic tissue visualized through an endoscopically dilated LAMS.

timing, but the published data to date have demonstrated a need for repeat surgery in up to 20% of cases and nearly universal need for external drainage, increasing the likelihood for pancreaticocutaneous fistula. As a result, laparoscopic approaches are used less frequently given the advancement in minimally invasive retroperitoneal necrosectomy and endoscopic necrosectomy, and generally reserved for when the latter options are unavailable, technically not feasible, or clinically unsuccessful. Sinus tract endoscopy requires the intraoperative dilation of the drainage tract followed by the lavage and débridement of the necroma with a nephroscope, laparoscope, or other flexible endoscope. For VARD, a 14- to 20-Fr percutaneous catheter is placed into the necroma, typically via CT guidance through a left-retroperitoneal window.[24,25] A small, 5-cm subcostal flank incision is made, and using the retroperitoneal drain as a guide, blunt dissection is completed to allow placement of a port for videoscope insertion. Loose adherent debris is then removed under video guidance. Upon procedure completion, two large-bore drains are inserted (into the deepest point of the cavity and near the incision site) and continuous lavage is completed.

In 2010, a multicenter randomized prospective trial (PANTER) of 88 Dutch patients comparing open débridement with a "step-up" approach to IPN treatment was completed.[26] In this trial, minimal access retroperitoneal pancreatic necrosectomy was performed if two consecutive percutaneous drainage procedures failed to achieve clinical or radiographic improvement, with a primary outcome endpoint that included new organ system failure, perforation, enterocutaneous fistula, and death. The step-up approach was associated with reduced incidence of the primary endpoint (40% vs. 69%), ICU admission (16% vs. 40%), incisional hernia (7% vs. 24%), new-onset diabetes (16% vs. 38%), and use of pancreatic enzyme supplements (7% vs. 33%). Interestingly, 35% of the step-up approach patients responded to percutaneous drainage alone and did not require minimal access retroperitoneal necrosectomy. There was no difference in mortality (17% vs. 16%), and the total costs were $16,000 less per patient in the step-up group. As such, the step-up approach has significant advantages over open necrosectomy.

Endoscopic necrosectomy can also be completed in a step-up approach, consisting of endoscopic transmural drainage followed by endoscopic transmural necrosectomy, if necessary. A systematic review[27] and the aforementioned, randomized controlled PENGUIN study[21] have suggested that an endoscopic approach is safe, feasible, and associated with complications similar to surgical approaches. At this time, multidisciplinary consensus statements recommend that when interventions are indicated, a step-up approach with percutaneous catheter or endoscopic transmural drainage be the first step in the treatment, followed by endoscopic or minimally invasive surgical necrosectomy when necessary. If the WON is endoscopically accessible, transmural drainage is recommended; however for necromas with deep extension, locations not adjacent to the stomach or duodenum, or failure after endoscopic treatment, VARD should be considered.

PANCREATIC PSEUDOCYSTS

Pancreatic pseudocysts are encapsulated fluid collections in the peripancreatic or pancreatic parenchyma with a well-defined nonepithelialized inflammatory wall, high concentration of pancreatic enzymes, and no or minimal solid necrotic component that can develop in both AP and CP.[1] In AP, pseudocysts develop as a maturation of an APFC, generally 4 weeks after the onset of an episode of acute interstitial edematous pancreatitis with associated ductal disruption and leakage of pancreatic enzymes into the peripancreatic or retroperitoneal tissue (occasionally intrapancreatic). Although high-resolution contrast-enhanced CT scans of the abdomen are often the initial diagnostic modality most commonly used at the time of pancreatic fluid collection diagnosis, magnetic resonance imaging (MRI) and EUS have an increased ability to assess for pancreartic duct (PD) integrity and the presence of necrotic debris within the cystic lesion.[2] The importance of differentiating a walled-off pancreatic fluid collection as a pseudocyst versus WON is evident in that successful endoscopic treatment occurs in 86% to 100% of pseudocysts compared with 63% to 81% of patients with WON.[2]

Intervention is reserved for the pancreatic pseudocysts that are symptomatic, infected, or progressively enlarging. Symptoms attributed to pseudocysts that warrant consideration of drainage develop after the patient has recovered from the acute phase of pancreatitis. As a result, new or worsening abdominal, flank, or back pain, intolerance of oral intake and weight loss, mechanical obstruction (gastric, duodenal, or biliary), evidence of infection (gas in a non-intervened-on lesion), or concerns for PD leakage (fistula) should prompt concerns for symptomatic pseudocyst development. Although size alone is generally not considered an indication for drainage in isolation, rapidly growing or larger lesions are more likely to be symptomatic, less likely to spontaneously resolve, and may be at higher risk for complications.[28] Prior to pursuing drainage, an adequate, mature pseudocyst wall is required, which generally requires 4 to 6 weeks. Lesions smaller than 3 cm are considered by some experienced endoscopists not to be amenable to transmural stenting.[2]

Pseudocysts can be drained via surgical (open and laparoscopic), endoscopic, and image-guided percutaneous drainage methods. In centers with technical expertise and appropriate surgical backup, endoscopic methods for pseudocyst drainage have emerged as the first-line therapeutic option with a randomized clinical trial[29] and several single-center retrospective reviews[30,31] demonstrating similar efficacy, shorter length of stay, and greater cost effectiveness as compared with open surgical cystogastrostomy.

In 2008, Varadarajulu et al. completed an initial retrospective case-controlled study comparing EUS-guided drainage and open surgical cystogastrostomy and found no difference in outcomes and increased cost savings and decreased length of stay in the EUS group.[31] In 2013, these results were confirmed by the same author in a follow-up single-center, open-label, randomized trial. None of the patients in the endoscopy group had pseudocyst recurrence during a 24-month follow-up period and the endoscopic group had significantly shorter length of stays (median, 2 days, vs. 6 days in the surgery group; $P < .001$), better physical and mental health, and lower cost ($7,011 vs. $15,052; $P = .003$).[29]

A retrospective review comparing pseudocyst drainage via EUS, laparoscopic, and open cystogastrostomy was reported by Melman et al. in 2009 and remains the only published literature to include laparoscopic surgical techniques as a comparator group.[30] In this study, primary success, defined as the resolution of symptoms or pseudocyst after the initial intervention, was significantly higher in the laparoscopic and open surgical groups compared with EUS (87.5%, 81.2%, and 51.1%, respectively; $P < .01$) with no significant difference in complication rates

(25%, 22.7%, and 15.6%, respectively; $P = .64$). The success rate for the EUS cohort is unexpectedly low with a higher than expected complication rate of 15.6%, which included three patients needing urgent laparotomy and two gastric perforations. These findings are likely due, in part, to early technical experience and the utilization of nonstandardized, pre-2012 revised Atlanta classification definitions of "pseudocysts" and inclusion of pancreatic debris/necrosis-containing collections.

Endoscopic drainage of pseudocysts can be completed using a transmural technique with EUS guidance, without EUS (commonly referred to as conventional transmural drainage [CTD]) or transpapillary technique via endoscopic retrograde cholangiopancreatography (ERCP). CTD is safe and effective in patients with bulging lesions (luminal compression) without obvious portal hypertension[32]; however luminal bulging is seen in only an estimated 42% to 48% of inflammatory pancreatic fluid collections and less likely to be found in pancreatic tail collections.[2,33] Two prospective, randomized trials compared the EUS-guided technique with CTD. In both the Korean[34] and American trials,[35] there were significantly higher technical success rates with EUS guidance versus CTD (94% vs. 72%; $P = .039$ and 100% vs. 33.3%; $P < .001$, respectively). In both trials, 100% of patients with failed CTD had successful drainage on a crossover to EUS. In the Korean study, there were no differences between the groups; however in the American study, the CTD cohort had two instances of major procedure bleeding including one death 4 hours post procedure secondary to massive intracystic bleeding.[35,36] A subsequent meta-analysis identified similar findings concluding that the EUS-guided approach has a higher technical success rate and safety profile than CTD and is the preferred method in nonbulging pseudocysts, portal hypertension, or coagulopathy.[37] As a result, many expert endoscopists believe the EUS-guided technique to be the preferable approach because it can identify cystic debris/necrosis, other cystic lesions, and large intervening vessels.[33,36]

With transmural drainage approaches for pseudocysts, multiple stents are available including plastic pigtail stents, FCSEMS, and CE- and non-CE LAMS. Current literature supports the placement of at least two double-pigtail plastic stents as the standard of care; however this is a rapidly evolving landscape. Although the FCSEMS offers the advantage of ease of placement and larger luminal diameter, allowing for improved drainage and decreased occlusion risk, plastic stents are significantly less expensive and likely safer for long-term drainage due to the concern for stent migration or erosion. An initial prospective study in 2012 of 20 patients with symptomatic pseudocysts drained with a FCSEMS anchored with a double-pigtail plastic stent revealed a 100% technical success rate, 70% pseudocyst resolution rate without recurrence, 15% adverse event rate, and 15% stent migration rate.[38] This was followed by a multicenter retrospective review in 2015 in which 230 patients with pseudocysts drained by double-pigtail plastic stents were compared with FCSEMS.[39] Complete resolution was significantly higher when treated with a FCSEMS versus double-pigtail plastic stents (98% vs. 89%; $P = .01$). Further, double-pigtail plastic stents were associated with a 2.9 times higher risk of adverse events.

Itoi et al. first reported a retrospective review of the LAMS for symptomatic pancreatic pseudocyst drainage in 2012.[40] In all 15 patients, the LAMS was successfully deployed with only one stent migration reported. In 1 year of follow-up, all patients had complete resolution of their collections following the initial procedure without recurrence. Subsequent multicenter, prospective studies in mixed inflammatory pancreatic fluid collections reported similar findings of technical success in 91% to 98% of patients, and resolution of the pancreatic fluid collection in 93% of patients—with one study reporting a rate of resolution of 93% in pseudocysts specifically and 81% in WON.[41,42] Further multicenter, randomized, prospective studies are necessary to determine if the safety and efficacy of LAMS are superior to double-pigtail plastic stents for pseudocyst drainage.

Often in clinical practice, after creation of the cystogastrostomy or cystoduodenostomy, repeat imaging with a CT or magnetic resonance cholangiopancreatography (MRCP) is completed in 4 to 6 weeks to assess the PD integrity and size of the collection. In patients in whom there is no communication between the pseudocyst and the main PD, transmural stents can likely be removed 4 to 6 weeks after the pseudocyst has been completely drained.

The major complications associated with endoscopic pseudocyst drainage—infection, bleeding, stent migration/obstruction, perforation—have been reported to be between 2.5% and 37%.[2,43] Infection is a common complication, and as such, periprocedural antibiotics are typically administered. Infection typically occurs as a result of incomplete evacuation of the cyst cavity, particularly when stents become obstructed or migrate, or because of inadvertent drainage of an organized pancreatic necrosis. The former can typically be avoided through the placement of at least two double-pigtail plastic stents into the cyst cavity and assurance of simultaneous drainage of multiple, communicating pseudocysts. Bleeding associated with pseudocyst drainage is usually a result of puncture of blood vessels during the drainage procedure. Patients at high risk are those with pancreatic tail collections (adjacent to splenic vessels), concomitant portal hypertension, and gastric varices in which the use of EUS with color Doppler can theoretically reduce the risk of inadvertent puncture of adjacent blood vessels. In most cases, however, bleeding is mild and can be treated using endoscopic techniques such as injection with epinephrine, heater probe application, hemoclip placement, dilating balloon tamponade, or placement of an FCSEMS. Other complications of endoscopic therapy, such as free abdominal perforation and stent migration, are rare. Free perforation is usually seen when the pseudocyst is located more than 1 cm away from the gastric or duodenal wall.

Laparoscopic approaches to pseudocyst drainage have been well described and are identical to those of open surgery, in that drainage can be achieved via anterior (intraluminal) and posterior (extraluminal) pseudocyst gastrostomy, Roux-en-Y cystojejunostomy, or cystoduodenostomy, according to the anatomic topography of the cyst. Although more invasive than endoscopic therapies, laparoscopic (and open) procedures allow for concomitant débridement of any necrosis, improved assessment and control of bleeding from the enteric or pseudocyst

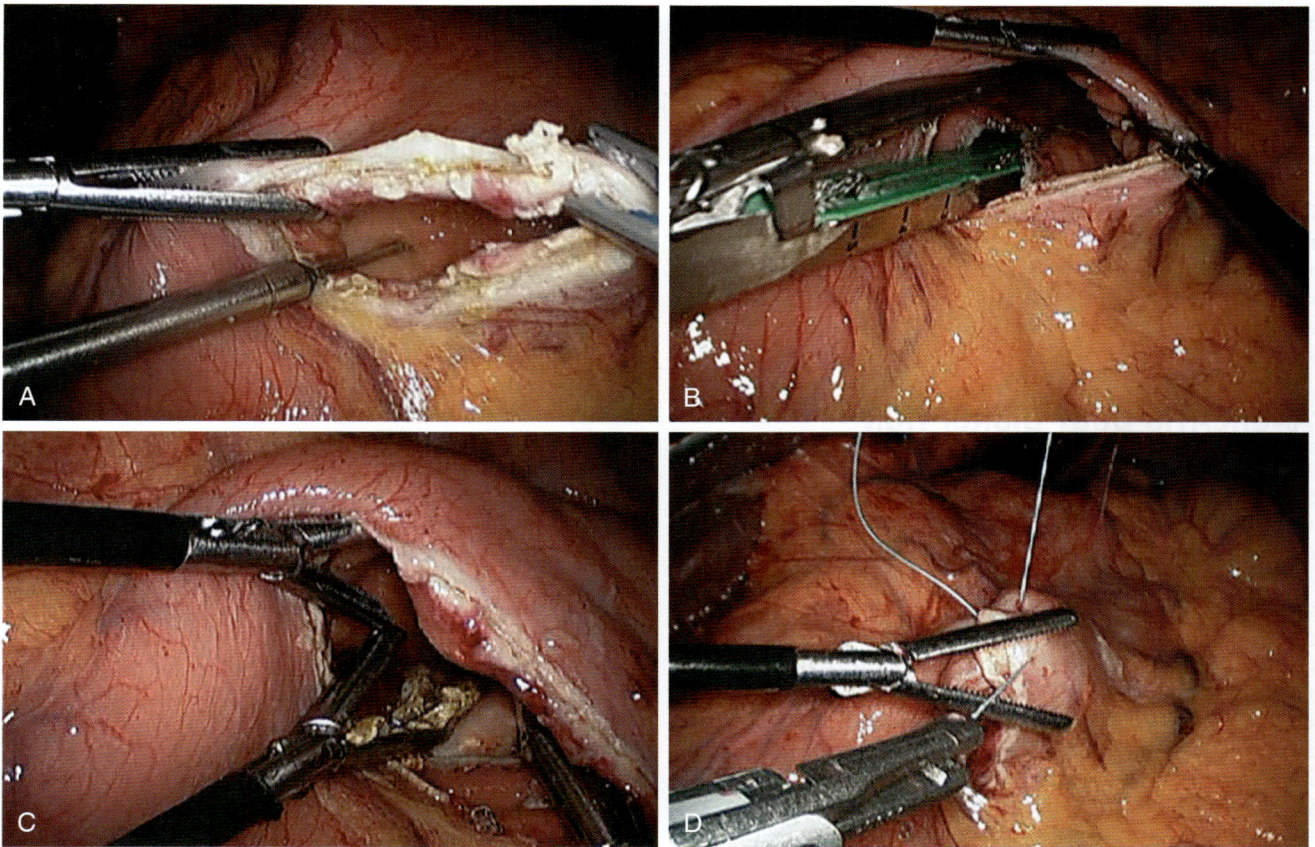

FIGURE 94.2 Laparoscopic cystogastrostomy. (A) Needle aspiration of a pseudocyst through the posterior gastric wall via anterior gastrotomy. (B) Thick-tissue stapler used to create common opening between posterior stomach and cyst wall. (C) Débridement of residual necrotic pancreatic debris within cyst cavity. (D) Sutured closure of anterior gastrotomy.

wall, an opportunity to obtain adequate biopsy of the pseudocyst wall to rule out malignancy, and positioning of the common opening to facilitate dependent drainage. The simplest laparoscopic technique for a lesser sac pseudocyst is cystogastrostomy via an anterior approach (Fig. 94.2). After making a 2- to 3-cm anterior gastrostomy, the pseudocyst can usually be seen bulging against the posterior wall of the stomach, confirmed by inserting a gallbladder aspiration needle through the posterior gastric wall into the pseudocyst cavity. If it is not readily apparent, laparoscopic ultrasound can be used to localize the pseudocyst. The opening into the pseudocyst is widened with monopolar, bipolar, or ultrasonic energy source to accommodate passage of a laparoscopic stapling device, with a portion of the wall excised and sent to pathology to rule out malignancy. The choice of stapler height requires surgical judgment based on the thickness of the common wall of the stomach and pseudocyst to achieve appropriate tissue compression for hemostasis without excessive tissue necrosis. If the tissue thickness exceeds the capacity for stapling, the opening is extended and a running, slowly absorbable monofilament suture is used to approximate the edges of the opening. The pseudocyst cavity is explored, and if any necrotic tissue is present, it is gently débrided. The anterior gastrostomy is closed, and the patient can typically be started on liquids later

that evening. Cystogastrostomy can also be performed via a lesser sac approach, which may be advantageous in allowing better dependent drainage as compared with the anterior approach, after opening the gastrocolic omentum, although the space can be obliterated because of prior pancreatitis episode(s).

Laparoscopic Roux-en-Y cystojejunostomy may be preferable to cystogastrostomy when a large pseudocyst extends inferior to the stomach. In this setting, the pseudocyst can be seen bulging through the transverse mesocolon when viewed from the infracolic perspective. A window is made through the mesocolon to the pseudocyst wall, avoiding injury to the middle colic vessels and inferior mesenteric vein, and following transection of the proximal jejunum 40 cm distal to the ligament of Treitz, the Roux limb is approximated to the pseudocyst wall using interrupted nonabsorbable or slowly absorbable suture with the stapled edge of the bowel and mesentery facing toward the patient's left side, and a stapled or sutured cystojejunostomy is performed as described earlier. The jejunojejunostomy is then performed at least 50 to 60 cm distally to reduce enteric reflux into the cavity.

Outcomes from laparoscopic approaches have primarily consisted of retrospective case series.[44–49] In these studies, treatment success ranged from 83% to 100% with complications occurring in 0% to 27%. Recurrent rates ranged from 0% to 20% and additional surgical or other procedural management strategies were also required in 0% to 20% of patients. Palanivelu et al. published the largest case series to date, a 12-year, single-center retrospective review that evaluated 106 patients undergoing laparoscopic therapy.[49] Treatment success was 100%, complications occurred in 6.6%, and recurrence was identified in 0.9% of patients after a mean follow-up of 54 months. Laparoscopic cystogastrostomy was completed in the majority of cases, accounting for 83.4% of all surgical procedures, compared with laparoscopic cystojejunostomy in 7.4%, open cystogastrostomy in 1.8%, and laparoscopic external drainage in 7.4%.

PANCREATIC DUCT DISRUPTION

Disruption of the main PD or its side branches can be seen in both AP and CP. Virtually every case of AP involves some form of duct leak, which may or may not persist. Persistent leaks in the setting of AP can lead to pseudocyst development, external pancreatic fistula, and internal pancreatic fistula formation leading to pancreatic ascites (if anterior) and high amylase pleural effusions (if posterior) as well as disconnected duct syndrome. Internal pancreatic fistulas can also communicate with other organs including the biliary system, bronchus, small bowel, stomach, or colon. In patients with CP, leaks are invariably associated with a downstream calculus or stricture. Endoscopy plays a significant role in the management of duct leaks in each of these clinical scenarios and includes transmural drainage for pancreatic pseudocysts, transpapillary drainage by placing a stent into the PD via the major or minor papilla, and more recently described, EUS-guided pancreatic duct drainage (EUS-PDD) via pancreaticoduodenostomy or pancreaticogastrostomy to reconnect a completely disconnected PD to the bowel lumen.

Conservative medical therapy for internal pancreatic fistulas that result in pancreatic ascites or pleural effusions includes taking nothing by mouth (NPO), parenteral nutrition, somatostatin or its analogues, and large-volume paracentesis as needed. However, this approach is unsuccessful in a significant proportion of patients.[50,51] There are now several published series reporting transpapillary stents for ductal disruptions in the setting of pancreatic ascites and high amylase pleural effusions in which more than 90% of patients resolve their fluid collection without complication or recurrence. Patients may require simultaneous large-volume paracentesis or concomitant pseudocyst drainage. It is likely that transpapillary stenting works less by leak occlusion and more by bypassing potential areas of downstream obstruction and the pancreatic sphincter, thereby converting the duodenum to the path of least resistance to flow of pancreatic juice. In these cases, transpapillary stenting appears to be most effective if a partial PD disruption is identified and can be successfully bridged. Pancreaticobiliary fistulas almost invariably respond to concomitant pancreaticobiliary stenting[52] for 4 to 6 weeks, assuming that the fistula does not arise from the upstream portion of a disconnected gland.

In the setting of severe necrotizing AP and CP-induced isolation of a viable portion of upstream pancreas, known as disconnected pancreatic duct syndrome (DPDS), the majority (>80% of cases) have a disruption at the head or neck/body of the pancreas.[53] Suspicion for DPDS should arise in the setting of nonresolving or recurrent inflammatory pancreatic fluid collection, and in such cases, pancreatography, either endoscopic or magnetic resonance (with intravenous secretin), may provide a definitive diagnosis. Surgery remains the standard of therapy for DPDS depending on the location of injury and amount of functional pancreatic tissue isolated. In cases with a significant amount of functional pancreatic tissue, laparoscopic or open pancreaticojejunostomy is preferred, whereas if only a small segment is isolated, a distal pancreatectomy-splenectomy may be required. In cases of DPDS-associated pancreatic fluid collections, transmural drainage can be completed endoscopically as previously discussed; however when DPDS has been diagnosed, there have been a few reports of leaving transmural stents permanently as opposed to the typical 4- to 8-week period.[54,55] Although indefinite stent placement allows for long-term drainage of the PD into the bowel lumen, there are risks of stent migration and occlusion. It also is now feasible to drain the disconnected segment into the stomach or duodenum using EUS-PDD with reports of this technique being successful in cases of CP with complete rupture of the main PD and in cases of PD leaks.[56]

PANCREATIC DUCT STRICTURE

Strictures arising within the main PD are typically the result of chronic pancreatic inflammation or relapsing bouts of AP. Pancreatic malignancy is also a part of the differential diagnosis of PD strictures in the appropriate clinical setting. More than one stricture may be present at any given time with varying levels of symptomatology. In patients with CP, strictures may be associated with a ductal calculus. Once a malignancy has been excluded by one or more methods (cross-sectional imaging, biopsy, EUS, cytology, or pancreatoscopy), a variety of therapeutic interventions can be employed in an attempt to alleviate the symptoms (pain and steatorrhea) associated with chronic ductal strictures.

Endotherapy is most effective for single strictures in the pancreatic head, whereas patients with isolated strictures in the tail or multiple strictures may not be amenable to endoscopic treatment. The endoscopic approach to managing PD strictures begins with guidewire access into the PD following a pancreatic sphincterotomy. There are a variety of methods for stricture dilation, including graduated dilating catheters and controlled radial expansion polyethylene balloons. Balloons are used most frequently; the size of balloon selected should approximate that of the PD downstream from the stenosis so as to avoid rupture of the more normal portion of the duct. Dilation is performed to waist effacement.

In strictures that are acutely angulated or impassable by graduated dilating catheters or balloon dilators, the use of a Soehendra stent extractor may be initially required to "drill through" the stricture prior to dilation. This is often the case with large PD calculi. Following dilation, most endoscopists attempt to place a 5- to 10-Fr polyethylene stent approximating the downstream diameter of the duct. In patients who are symptomatically improved, prostheses are retrieved in 2 to 3 months, followed by repeat dilation and upsizing of the stent, if possible. This process is repeated several times over the course of a year, and if there is no stricture or symptom resolution and the patient becomes stent dependent, surgical therapy should be considered.

A single-center randomized prospective study comparing open surgical pancreaticojejunostomy with transampullary endoscopic therapy of 39 patients with symptomatic main duct strictures with a dilated (>5 mm) proximal duct suggested improved pain scores and better physical health summary scores in the surgically treated group, with 75% complete or partial pain relief versus 32% in the endoscopically treated group. Complication rates, length of stay, and changes in pancreatic function were similar between the two groups, although the endoscopically treated group required more procedures than the surgery group (median of eight vs. three). The trial was stopped early because of these findings.[57] In this study, a single 10-Fr stent without side holes was used. In contrast, it has been our practice to place multiple, parallel 5- to 7-Fr prostheses into the PD following stricture dilation. The recent introduction of the FCSEMS into clinical endoscopic practice has raised the possibility of using these larger-caliber devices as a removable endoprosthesis for benign strictures of the pancreas. Three prospective studies using an FCSEMS for CP-related main PD strictures have been published with no relapse of pain in 86% of patients with 5 months of follow-up and 100% stent removal after 2 to 3 months of therapy.[58–60] However, stent migration rates occurred in up to 31% of cases in one report and de novo strictures occurred in 16% in another. Additional study is required prior to advocating the routine use of these significantly more costly devices for benign PD strictures.

Several published series now exist that demonstrate a 60% to 80% reduction in attacks of relapsing pancreatitis following endotherapy for PD strictures.[61–67] Although a decrease in or resolution of chronic pain has also been suggested (immediately, 65% to 95% of patients, and in the long term, 32% to 68%),[68] PD stenting is not without its own risk of iatrogenic complications. Side-branch occlusion, parenchymal atrophy, and glandular fibrosis are all possibilities when stents are placed into relatively normal ducts.[69,70] Moreover, inflammation or "ductitis" induced by a stent side flap or pressure from the internal stent tip can lead to further fibrosis and ductal stenoses.

The existing literature shows at best a 50% rate of resolution when PD strictures are endoscopically treated for 1 year, with most series suggesting rates closer to 20% to 30%.[61,62,65–67] It is important to recognize, however, that the presence of a stricture does not imply symptoms, and indeed, 60% to 80% of patients become asymptomatic following endoscopic therapy, even in the presence of residual stenosis.

ENDOSCOPIC ULTRASOUND-GUIDED PANCREATIC DUCT DRAINAGE

In some patients, the PD cannot be accessed through either the major or minor papilla with conventional transpapillary endoscopic retrograde pancreatography (ERP) because of a severe stenosis, calculus in the head of the pancreas, disconnected PDs, inaccessible ampullas, or postsurgical altered anatomy. The two EUS-guided approaches for PD access and drainage are the EUS-guided "rendezvous" and direct drainage or "antegrade" procedures.[71] In both techniques, a 19-gauge EUS fine-needle aspiration (FNA) needle punctures the main PD upstream to the narrowing and a stiff, hydrophilic 0.025- or 0.035-inch angled or straight wire is passed into the duodenum or looped in the PD.

In the "rendezvous" procedure, after passing the wire in an antegrade fashion into the duodenum, the echoendoscope is removed and a duodenoscope is advanced to the major papilla. The intraluminal guidewire is captured with a snare or forceps. The wire is pulled through the endoscope and brought out the accessory channel of the duodenoscope, over which therapeutic accessories can subsequently be passed. This technique can also be used in patients with altered anatomy who require pancreatic intervention. One such group of patients is those who have undergone pancreaticoduodenectomy and developed a pancreticojejunostomy anastomotic stricture. In the "antegrade" approach, a stent is deployed directly through the bowel lumen into the PD either terminating across the papilla (transpapillary) or within the PD (transmural). For the antegrade technique, tract dilation with a needle knife, cystotome, graduated dilating catheter, or Soehendra stent extractor is obligatory to allow passage of the stent through the gastrointestinal tract wall into the PD. Transpapillary stent placement is preferable; however, bypassing the narrowing with the guidewire may not always be successful, in which case, the distal portion of the stent can remain inside the PD with the proximal portion in the stomach (transmural).

In 2014, Fujii-Lau et al. summarized the current literature on EUS-guided PD drainage, reviewing the cumulative published experience of 222 patients.[72] Including both antegrade and rendezvous techniques, technical success was achieved in 170 patients (76.6%) while complications occurred in 42 patients (18.9%). The most frequent complication was abdominal pain occurring in 17 patients (7.7%) followed by pancreatitis in 7 patients (3.2%). Additional, less frequently reported complications included four patients with bleeding, two patients each with perforation, peripancreatic abscess, or shearing of the guidewire. A single patient was reported to develop fever, pneumoperitoneum, pseudocyst, aneurysm, or perigastric fluid collection. A similar review by Itoi et al. in 2013 reported a technical success rate of greater than 70% in 75 patients using the antegrade technique and a range of success rates from 25% to 100% in 52 patients with the rendezvous technique.[73] The largest experience in the rendezvous cohort was 20 patients with a lower reported technical success rate of 48%.

Although EUS-PDD is emerging as a minimally invasive technique, both EUS-guided rendezvous and antegrade PD access procedures are in their infancy using accessories not specifically designed for the technique. As such, EUS-PDD is arguably one of the most technically challenging therapeutic EUS procedures and should be performed in the hands of adequately trained and experienced endoscopists who have adequate surgical backup, and its use should be limited to appropriately selected patients.

CHRONIC PANCREATITIS–ASSOCIATED BILIARY STRICTURES

Biliary strictures may develop in 3% to 23% of patients with advanced CP secondary to fibrosis, pseudocyst compression, and malignancy, and can result in symptoms such as chronic cholestasis, jaundice, acute and recurrent cholangitis, and secondary biliary cirrhosis.[74] As therapeutic endotherapy for benign biliary strictures typically occurs over a period of 12 months, it is critical to rule out malignancy through EUS-FNA or brushing of the stricture for cytologic analysis prior to pursuing endoscopic treatment. Clinical guidelines published by the European Society of Gastrointestinal Endoscopy (ESGE) for the endoscopic treatment of CP recommend that the choice between endoscopic and surgical treatment should rely upon local expertise, local or systemic patient comorbidities (e.g., cirrhosis, splenic vein thrombosis, varices), and expected patient compliance with endoscopic procedures (Fig. 94.3).[68] If endoscopic therapy is selected, the current gold standard of treatment is the placement of multiple, side-by-side plastic biliary stents, increasing in number or size with exchanges approximately every 3 months primarily due to concerns for stent occlusion.

Temporary, multiple plastic stent placement is technically successful in greater than 90% of patients; long-term success rates have been reported to be 62% in patients with simultaneous, multiple plastic stents compared with 32% in patients with single plastic stents.[68] A single, nonrandomized prospective trial compared multiple versus single plastic stents and found a significant clinical success difference of 92% versus 24%, in favor of multiple stents.[75] Despite this success rate, plastic stents are limited not only by their occlusion rate and subsequent risk of cholangitis if not exchanged, but also the requirement of an average of five ERCP procedures for successful treatment. As a result, FCSEMS have increasingly been used for benign biliary strictures, because they have larger diameters and are less prone to occlusion. A large prospective, nonrandomized, multinational trial of 13 centers evaluated the use of FCSEMS in 187 patients with benign biliary strictures (including 127 patients with CP).[76] Stents were removed a median 11 months after placement with stricture resolution in 76% of patients (79.7% in CP patients), with a stricture recurrence rate of 15% over 20 months of follow-up. The FCSEMS were removed successfully in 80.5% of patients with CP and stent- or removal-related serious adverse events, mostly cholangitis, occurred in 27.3%. These results are similar to another study with FCSEMS for CP strictures whereby a resolution rate of 83.9% was reported in 44 patients after 3 months of insertion.[77] These studies are encouraging and support the consideration and further investigation of FCSEMS for benign biliary strictures, but currently their use is not endorsed by consensus guidelines.

PANCREATIC DUCT STONES

As opposed to their biliary counterparts, PD calculi represent a more vexing clinical problem. Several factors contribute to this, including a significantly harder composition than bile duct stones as a consequence of the predominance of calcium carbonate, in addition to commonly being located upstream from a PD stricture. Indeed, less than half of patients with PD calculi have stones that are amenable to endoscopic extraction alone; the other 50% require lithotripsy to facilitate removal. Finally, the PD distal to impacted calculi can be markedly dilated; the resultant intraductal hypertension can lead to ductal disruption and the development of pancreatic pseudocysts, ascites, and pleural effusions.

The management of PD calculi begins with obtaining high-quality cross-sectional imaging in the form of a CT or MRI/MRCP. This allows for preprocedural planning and estimation of stone size, as well as the identification of sequelae of ductal disruption. Small stones can be removed by standard extraction techniques using an extraction balloon or basket passed alongside or over a hydrophilic guidewire. Dilation of ductal strictures, using a graduated dilation catheter or hydrostatic balloon, is required when stones are impacted distal to a stenosis. In the case of severe stenosis that will not allow passage of a catheter or balloon dilator, the stricture and stone can be "drilled" through using a Soehendra stent extractor. In the majority of cases, endoscopic sphincterotomy is performed to facilitate stone extraction. In some cases of obstructive CP, a "pseudodivisum" may be present in which the ventral PD is obstructed by a large stone or severe stricture. In such cases, access and drainage are typically achieved through the minor papilla.

PANCREATIC LITHOTRIPSY

A majority of patients will require some form of lithotripsy to facilitate stone extraction. Mechanical lithotripsy can be difficult with PD stones, especially in the presence of a PD stricture, because the basket must be passed distal to the calculus to allow for full deployment and stone capture. Probe-based lithotripsy—either electrohydraulic or laser—can be performed at the time of pancreatoscopy;

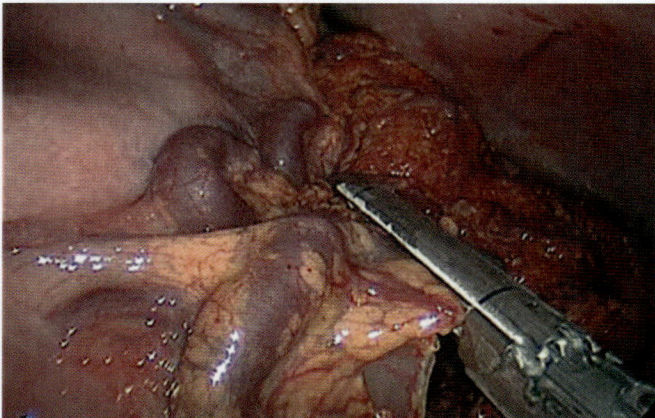

FIGURE 94.3 Perigastric varices caused by splenic vein thrombosis in chronic pancreatitis. Vascular stapler cartridges are used to divide the gastrosplenic ligament in preparation for laparoscopic distal pancreatectomy with splenectomy in a patient with hypersplenism and symptomatic chronic pancreatitis localized to the pancreatic tail.

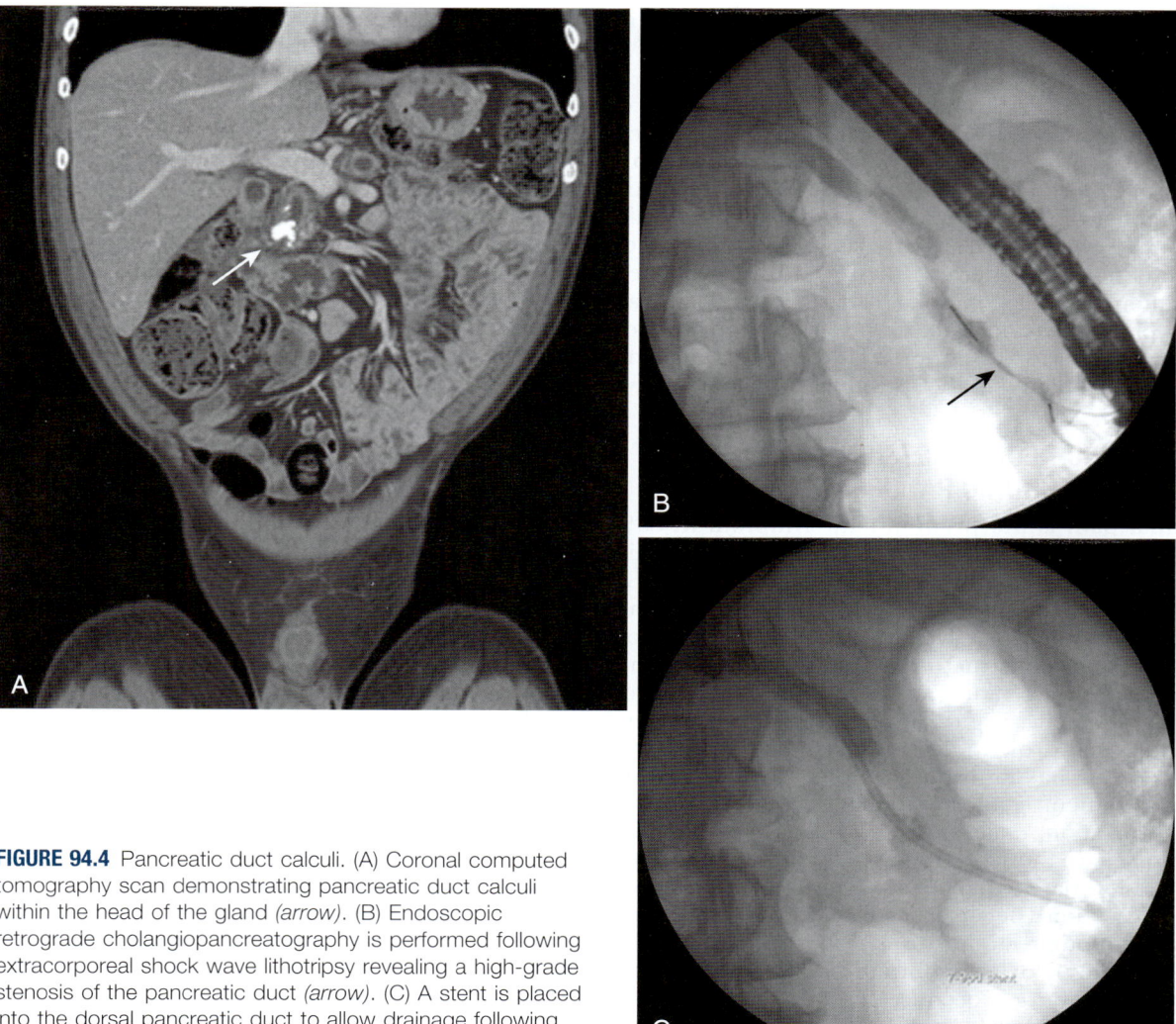

FIGURE 94.4 Pancreatic duct calculi. (A) Coronal computed tomography scan demonstrating pancreatic duct calculi within the head of the gland *(arrow)*. (B) Endoscopic retrograde cholangiopancreatography is performed following extracorporeal shock wave lithotripsy revealing a high-grade stenosis of the pancreatic duct *(arrow)*. (C) A stent is placed into the dorsal pancreatic duct to allow drainage following stone extraction.

however the need to pass a pancreatoscope into a strictured PD to access the stone can be challenging.

Because of the difficulties associated with both mechanical and probe-based lithotripsy, most patients with large PD stones initially undergo extracorporeal shock wave lithotripsy (ESWL) for fragmentation prior to endoscopic extraction. Stone localization and assessment of abdominal vascular calcifications are required prior to ESWL. It is our practice to perform ERCP immediately following ESWL, at which time a PD sphincterotomy and stone extraction are performed. Both saline lavage at the time of post-ESWL ERCP and nasopancreatic drain placement at the time of ERCP seem to facilitate stone fragment passage and may preclude the need for multiple ERCPs. Regardless of whether ESWL was performed, placement of one or more endoprostheses into the PD is performed at the time of ERCP to allow for passage of additional stone fragments and allow for ductal decompression and prevention of pancreatitis secondary to edema from the performance of pancreatic endoscopic sphincterotomy (Fig. 94.4).

Although there are data to suggest that endoscopic stone extraction leads to clinical improvement,[78,79] not all patients with chronic calcific pancreatitis should undergo attempted stone extraction. Poor candidates include those with a major burden of small stones within the pancreatic head (pseudotumor); patients without a dilated PD distal to the calculus; stones in side branches or the distal tail; ductal calculi within the setting of a disconnected duct; and concomitant presence of an inflammatory mass in the pancreatic head. Such individuals should be considered for surgical treatment[80] or managed medically.

Most recent series suggest that approximately two-thirds of patients who have successful stone removal from the PD will have significant improvement in chronic pain and a decrease or elimination of attack of relapsing pancreatitis.[78,79] There have been two recent large retrospective series reporting the long-term outcomes of ESWL in patients with obstructing PD stones in 636 patients and 120 patients, respectively.[81,82] In the larger study published by Tandan et al., 272 patients had more than 5 years of follow-up and 164 patients (60.3%) had no pain, 97 patients (35.7%) had mild or moderate episodes of pain, whereas 11 patients (4.04%) had episodic severe pain.[82] In the smaller study published by Seven et al., with a mean follow-up of 4.3 years, partial pain relief was achieved in 85%, complete pain relief with no narcotic use in 50%, and avoidance of surgery in 84% of patients.[81]

Despite this success and that of others, the requirement for careful patient selection cannot be emphasized enough. Those who are poor candidates for endoscopic therapy, and those in whom repeated ERCP is required over a number of years to manage complications, should be strongly considered for surgery. Even in an era of effective endoscopic therapy for CP and its associated complications, there are reasonable data to conclude that, in the appropriate candidate, surgical decompression or resection is superior to endotherapy in the long-term management of pain in patients with chronic obstructive pancreatitis.[83]

LAPAROSCOPIC DECOMPRESSION AND RESECTION IN CHRONIC PANCREATITIS

Abdominal pain is the predominant symptom in 85% to 90% of CP patients, and despite the advances in endoscopic interventions for the complications of CP (strictures, stones, pseudocysts), nearly half of CP patients continue to have progressively worsening pain, develop strictures of adjacent structures (bile duct, duodenum), or are noted to have radiographic lesions suspicious for neoplasia. As such, surgical intervention continues to play an important role in disease management. Because the pain in CP has multiple etiologies (ductal/tissue hypertension, neurogenic inflammation, visceral/central nerve sensitization, tissue ischemia),[84] surgical therapies for pain relief are thought to achieve their effects through decompression (lateral pancreaticojejunostomy, cystenterostomy), resection (Beger procedure, Berne procedure, pancreaticoduodenectomy, distal pancreatectomy, total pancreatectomy), or a combination of the two (Frey procedure, Hamburg procedure). Details of these procedures and their outcomes are described elsewhere in this textbook. Procedure selection is based on the presence or absence of an inflammatory mass in the pancreatic head, extent of PD dilation (diameter >7 mm is considered to be a "large duct"), extent of gland involvement, suspicion for cancer, and previous pancreatic procedures. Surgical therapy is not curative, but should achieve pain relief, address complications of adjacent structures if present, improve quality of life, and preserve endocrine and exocrine pancreatic function in a safe and durable manner. Minimally invasive surgical treatment of CP has been shown to be technically feasible with good short-term results: laparoscopic lateral pancreaticojejunostomy,[85–87] distal pancreatectomy,[88,89] pancreaticoduodenectomy,[90–92] and the Frey procedure have all been described. Two recent randomized controlled trials with long-term follow-up data comparing duodenum-preserving procedures (e.g., Frey operation) and pancreaticoduodenectomy for CP were published in 2012 and 2013.[93,94] Keck et al. found that after a median of 5 years of follow-up, pylorus-preserving and duodenum-preserving pancreatic head resections were equally effective in pain relief and eventual quality of life without differences in endocrine or exocrine function.[94] Bachmann et al. published the results of 64 patients randomized to pancreaticoduodenectomy or Frey procedure with 15 years of follow-up.[93] Similarly, both pancreaticoduodenectomy and Frey procedure resulted in good and permanent pain relief and improvement of the quality of life in long-term follow-up. However, better short-term results and longer survival were found with the Frey procedure, leading the authors to suggest the duodenum-sparing operation may be more favorable.

Laparoscopic pancreatic surgery has the potential to substantially reduce the morbidity associated with the midline or bilateral subcostal incision used to perform the procedures listed previously. Given that most surgical candidates already have pain that is difficult to manage medically, reduced incisional pain following laparoscopy may be distinctly advantageous. Furthermore, the relative malnutrition of these patients may increase the risk of wound infection and incisional hernia, both of which are substantially reduced with laparoscopy. On the other hand, the inflammation, edema, and dense scar found in CP substantially increase the degree of difficulty of the procedures, whether performed open or laparoscopically, and should be taken into consideration. Additionally, for most of the procedures described, the trauma caused by surgical access to the abdomen (i.e., laparotomy) is substantially outweighed by the trauma of the surgical procedure itself; indeed, the term *minimally invasive pancreaticoduodenectomy* is a significant semantic paradox.

From a technical standpoint, the Beger procedure appears to be the least amenable to laparoscopy, given the need to perform two pancreaticojejunostomies, dissect the portosplenic confluence in the setting of CP, and palpate the head of the pancreas to assess the depth of resection. Laparoscopic intraoperative ultrasound may be useful for the latter, and is a mandatory skill, in addition to facility with intracorporeal suturing using fine suture and needles, in performing any of the procedures laparoscopically. The latter skills can be facilitated using robotic-assisted approaches. In contrast to the Beger procedure, lateral pancreaticojejunostomy, cystenterostomy, and distal pancreatectomy are more readily performed laparoscopically, as they generally avoid the potentially hazardous major vascular dissection in the setting of CP and the required anastomoses are less technically challenging. The Frey and Berne procedures represent an intermediate level of laparoscopic technical difficulty given the resection of the pancreatic head, although its resection is somewhat less extensive than that of the Beger procedure. The Hamburg procedure replicates the pancreatic head resection of the Beger procedure, increasing the laparoscopic degree of difficulty, although its lateral pancreaticojejunostomy is more amenable to a laparoscopic suturing than the Beger procedure.

There are currently only a handful of pancreatic surgeons who have and regularly use the advanced laparoscopic skills necessary to effectively perform procedures for CP that require pancreaticoenteric reconstruction. There are correspondingly very few advanced laparoscopists who have adequate familiarity with the clinical management of CP and who regularly operate in the anatomic region of the duodenum and pancreatic head and neck. As such, collaboration and bilateral education between these two groups of surgeons will be necessary to bridge this gap so that patients may safely and maximally benefit from the available minimally invasive surgical therapies for CP.

Similarly, given the need for individualized management of CP, a cooperative, multidisciplinary team of surgeons, gastroenterologists, radiologists, pain specialists, and dietitians is necessary for the optimal treatment of this challenging disease.

REFERENCES

1. Banks PA, Bollen TL, Dervenis C, et al. Classification of acute pancreatitis—2012: revision of the Atlanta classification and definitions by international consensus. *Gut.* 2013;62:102-111.
2. Holt BA, Varadarajulu S. The endoscopic management of pancreatic pseudocysts (with videos). *Gastrointest Endosc.* 2015;81:804-812.
3. Peery AF, Dellon ES, Lund J, et al. Burden of gastrointestinal disease in the United States: 2012 update. *Gastroenterology.* 2012;143:1179-1187. e1–e3.
4. Singh VK, Bollen TL, Wu BU, et al. An assessment of the severity of interstitial pancreatitis. *Clin Gastroenterol Hepatol.* 2011;9:1098-1103.
5. Trikudanathan G, Attam R, Arain MA, Mallery S, Freeman ML. Endoscopic interventions for necrotizing pancreatitis. *Am J Gastroenterol.* 2014;109:969-981, [quiz 982].
6. Zerem E. Treatment of severe acute pancreatitis and its complications. *World J Gastroenterol.* 2014;20:13879-13892.
7. Bollen TL, Singh VK, Maurer R, et al. A comparative evaluation of radiologic and clinical scoring systems in the early prediction of severity in acute pancreatitis. *Am J Gastroenterol.* 2012;107:612-619.
8. Bradley EL 3rd. The natural and unnatural history of pancreatic fluid collections associated with acute pancreatitis. *Dig Dis Sci.* 2014;59:908-910.
9. Cui ML, Kim KH, Kim HG, et al. Incidence, risk factors and clinical course of pancreatic fluid collections in acute pancreatitis. *Dig Dis Sci.* 2014;59:1055-1062.
10. Bourliere M, Sarles H. Pancreatic cysts and pseudocysts associated with acute and chronic pancreatitis. *Dig Dis Sci.* 1989;34:343-348.
11. Lerch MM, Stier A, Wahnschaffe U, Mayerle J. Pancreatic pseudocysts: observation, endoscopic drainage, or resection? *Dtsch Arztebl Int.* 2009;106:614-621.
12. Aranha GV, Prinz RA, Esguerra AC, Greenlee HB. The nature and course of cystic pancreatic lesions diagnosed by ultrasound. *Arch Surg.* 1983;118:486-488.
13. Maringhini A, Uomo G, Patti R, et al. Pseudocysts in acute nonalcoholic pancreatitis: incidence and natural history. *Dig Dis Sci.* 1999;44:1669-1673.
14. Warshaw AL, Rattner DW. Timing of surgical drainage for pancreatic pseudocyst. Clinical and chemical criteria. *Ann Surg.* 1985;202:720-724.
15. Sarathi Patra P, Das K, Bhattacharyya A, et al. Natural resolution or intervention for fluid collections in acute severe pancreatitis. *Br J Surg.* 2014;101:1721-1728.
16. Connor S, Alexakis N, Raraty MG, et al. Early and late complications after pancreatic necrosectomy. *Surgery.* 2005;137:499-505.
17. Rau B, Bothe A, Beger HG. Surgical treatment of necrotizing pancreatitis by necrosectomy and closed lavage: changing patient characteristics and outcome in a 19-year, single-center series. *Surgery.* 2005;138:28-39.
18. Working Group IAP/APA Evidence-Based Guidelines. IAP/APA evidence-based guidelines for the management of acute pancreatitis. *Pancreatology.* 2013;13:e1-e15.
19. Gardner TB, Coelho-Prabhu N, Gordon SR, et al. Direct endoscopic necrosectomy for the treatment of walled-off pancreatic necrosis: results from a multicenter U.S. series. *Gastrointest Endosc.* 2011;73:718-726.
20. Seifert H, Biermer M, Schmitt W, et al. Transluminal endoscopic necrosectomy after acute pancreatitis: a multicentre study with long-term follow-up (the GEPARD Study). *Gut.* 2009;58:1260-1266.
21. Bakker OJ, van Santvoort HC, van Brunschot S, et al. Endoscopic transgastric vs surgical necrosectomy for infected necrotizing pancreatitis: a randomized trial. *JAMA.* 2012;307:1053-1061.
22. Sharaiha RZ, Tyberg A, Khashab MA, et al. Endoscopic therapy with lumen-apposing metal stents is safe and effective for patients with pancreatic walled-off necrosis. *Clin Gastroenterol Hepatol.* 2016;14(12):1797-1803.
23. Rinninella E, Kunda R, Dollhopf M, et al. EUS-guided drainage of pancreatic fluid collections using a novel lumen-apposing metal stent on an electrocautery-enhanced delivery system: a large retrospective study (with video). *Gastrointest Endosc.* 2015;82:1039-1046.
24. Horvath KD, Kao LS, Wherry KL, Pellegrini CA, Sinanan MN. A technique for laparoscopic-assisted percutaneous drainage of infected pancreatic necrosis and pancreatic abscess. *Surg Endosc.* 2001;15:1221-1225.
25. van Santvoort HC, Besselink MG, Horvath KD, et al. Videoscopic assisted retroperitoneal debridement in infected necrotizing pancreatitis. *HPB (Oxford).* 2007;9:156-159.
26. van Santvoort HC, Besselink MG, Bakker OJ, et al. A step-up approach or open necrosectomy for necrotizing pancreatitis. *N Engl J Med.* 2010;362:1491-1502.
27. Haghshenasskashani A, Laurence JM, Kwan V, et al. Endoscopic necrosectomy of pancreatic necrosis: a systematic review. *Surg Endosc.* 2011;25:3724-3730.
28. Samuelson AL, Shah RJ. Endoscopic management of pancreatic pseudocysts. *Gastroenterol Clin North Am.* 2012;41:47-62.
29. Varadarajulu S, Bang JY, Sutton BS, Trevino JM, Christein JD, Wilcox CM. Equal efficacy of endoscopic and surgical cystogastrostomy for pancreatic pseudocyst drainage in a randomized trial. *Gastroenterology.* 2013;145:583-590.e1.
30. Melman L, Azar R, Beddow K, et al. Primary and overall success rates for clinical outcomes after laparoscopic, endoscopic, and open pancreatic cystgastrostomy for pancreatic pseudocysts. *Surg Endosc.* 2009;23:267-271.
31. Varadarajulu S, Lopes TL, Wilcox CM, Drelichman ER, Kilgore ML, Christein JD. EUS versus surgical cyst-gastrostomy for management of pancreatic pseudocysts. *Gastrointest Endosc.* 2008;68:649-655.
32. Kahaleh M, Shami VM, Conaway MR, et al. Endoscopic ultrasound drainage of pancreatic pseudocyst: a prospective comparison with conventional endoscopic drainage. *Endoscopy.* 2006;38:355-359.
33. Tyberg A, Karia K, Gabr M, et al. Management of pancreatic fluid collections: a comprehensive review of the literature. *World J Gastroenterol.* 2016;22:2256-2270.
34. Park DH, Lee SS, Moon SH, et al. Endoscopic ultrasound-guided versus conventional transmural drainage for pancreatic pseudocysts: a prospective randomized trial. *Endoscopy.* 2009;41:842-848.
35. Varadarajulu S, Christein JD, Tamhane A, Drelichman ER, Wilcox CM. Prospective randomized trial comparing EUS and EGD for transmural drainage of pancreatic pseudocysts (with videos). *Gastrointest Endosc.* 2008;68:1102-1111.
36. Teoh AY, Dhir V, Jin ZD, Kida M, Seo DW, Ho KY. Systematic review comparing endoscopic, percutaneous and surgical pancreatic pseudocyst drainage. *World J Gastrointest Endosc.* 2016;8:310-318.
37. Panamonta N, Ngamruengphong S, Kijsiricharoenchai K, Nugent K, Rakvit A. Endoscopic ultrasound-guided versus conventional transmural techniques have comparable treatment outcomes in draining pancreatic pseudocysts. *Eur J Gastroenterol Hepatol.* 2012;24:1355-1362.
38. Penn DE, Draganov PV, Wagh MS, Forsmark CE, Gupte AR, Chauhan SS. Prospective evaluation of the use of fully covered self-expanding metal stents for EUS-guided transmural drainage of pancreatic pseudocysts. *Gastrointest Endosc.* 2012;76:679-684.
39. Sharaiha RZ, DeFilippis EM, Kedia P, et al. Metal versus plastic for pancreatic pseudocyst drainage: clinical outcomes and success. *Gastrointest Endosc.* 2015;82:822-827.
40. Itoi T, Binmoeller KF, Shah J, et al. Clinical evaluation of a novel lumen-apposing metal stent for endosonography-guided pancreatic pseudocyst and gallbladder drainage (with videos). *Gastrointest Endosc.* 2012;75:870-876.
41. Shah RJ, Shah JN, Waxman I, et al. Safety and efficacy of endoscopic ultrasound-guided drainage of pancreatic fluid collections with lumen-apposing covered self-expanding metal stents. *Clin Gastroenterol Hepatol.* 2015;13:747-752.
42. Walter D, Will U, Sanchez-Yague A, et al. A novel lumen-apposing metal stent for endoscopic ultrasound-guided drainage of pancreatic fluid collections: a prospective cohort study. *Endoscopy.* 2015;47:63-67.
43. Ge PS, Weizmann M, Watson RR. Pancreatic pseudocysts: advances in endoscopic management. *Gastroenterol Clin North Am.* 2016;45:9-27.
44. Barragan B, Love L, Wachtel M, Griswold JA, Frezza EE. A comparison of anterior and posterior approaches for the surgical treatment of pancreatic pseudocyst using laparoscopic cystogastrostomy. *J Laparoendosc Adv Surg Tech A.* 2005;15:596-600.
45. Davila-Cervantes A, Gomez F, Chan C, et al. Laparoscopic drainage of pancreatic pseudocysts. *Surg Endosc.* 2004;18:1420-1426.
46. Hauters P, Weerts J, Navez B, et al. Laparoscopic treatment of pancreatic pseudocysts. *Surg Endosc.* 2004;18:1645-1648.
47. Hindmarsh A, Lewis MP, Rhodes M. Stapled laparoscopic cystgastrostomy: a series with 15 cases. *Surg Endosc.* 2005;19:143-147.

48. Oida T, Mimatsu K, Kawasaki A, et al. Long-term outcome of laparoscopic cystogastrostomy performed using a posterior approach with a stapling device. *Dig Surg.* 2009;26:110-114.

49. Palanivelu C, Senthilkumar K, Madhankumar MV, et al. Management of pancreatic pseudocyst in the era of laparoscopic surgery—experience from a tertiary centre. *Surg Endosc.* 2007;21:2262-2267.

50. Gomez-Cerezo J, Barbado Cano A, Suarez I, Soto A, Ríos JJ, Vázquez JJ. Pancreatic ascites: study of therapeutic options by analysis of case reports and case series between the years 1975 and 2000. *Am J Gastroenterol.* 2003;98:568-577.

51. Kaman L, Behera A, Singh R, Katariya RN. Internal pancreatic fistulas with pancreatic ascites and pancreatic pleural effusions: recognition and management. *ANZ J Surg.* 2001;71:221-225.

52. Kozarek RA, Jiranek GC, Traverso LW. Endoscopic treatment of pancreatic ascites. *Am J Surg.* 1994;168:223-226.

53. Varadarajulu S, Rana SS, Bhasin DK. Endoscopic therapy for pancreatic duct leaks and disruptions. *Gastrointest Endosc Clin N Am.* 2013;23:863-892.

54. Arvanitakis M, Delhaye M, Bali MA, et al. Pancreatic-fluid collections: a randomized controlled trial regarding stent removal after endoscopic transmural drainage. *Gastrointest Endosc.* 2007;65:609-619.

55. Varadarajulu S, Wilcox CM. Endoscopic placement of permanent indwelling transmural stents in disconnected pancreatic duct syndrome: does benefit outweigh the risks? *Gastrointest Endosc.* 2011;74:1408-1412.

56. Tessier G, Bories E, Arvanitakis M, et al. EUS-guided pancreatogastrostomy and pancreatobulbostomy for the treatment of pain in patients with pancreatic ductal dilatation inaccessible for transpapillary endoscopic therapy. *Gastrointest Endosc.* 2007;65:233-241.

57. Cahen DL, Gouma DJ, Nio Y, et al. Endoscopic versus surgical drainage of the pancreatic duct in chronic pancreatitis. *N Engl J Med.* 2007;356:676-684.

58. Moon SH, Kim MH, Park DH, et al. Modified fully covered self-expandable metal stents with antimigration features for benign pancreatic-duct strictures in advanced chronic pancreatitis, with a focus on the safety profile and reducing migration. *Gastrointest Endosc.* 2010;72:86-91.

59. Park DH, Kim MH, Moon SH, Lee SS, Seo DW, Lee SK. Feasibility and safety of placement of a newly designed, fully covered self-expandable metal stent for refractory benign pancreatic ductal strictures: a pilot study (with video). *Gastrointest Endosc.* 2008;68:1182-1189.

60. Sauer B, Talreja J, Ellen K, Ku J, Shami VM, Kahaleh M. Temporary placement of a fully covered self-expandable metal stent in the pancreatic duct for management of symptomatic refractory chronic pancreatitis: preliminary data (with videos). *Gastrointest Endosc.* 2008;68:1173-1178.

61. Binmoeller KF, Rathod VD, Soehendra N. Endoscopic therapy of pancreatic strictures. *Gastrointest Endosc Clin N Am.* 1998;8:125-142.

62. Boerma D, Huibregtse K, Gulik TM, Rauws EA, Obertop H, Gouma DJ. Long-term outcome of endoscopic stent placement for chronic pancreatitis associated with pancreas divisum. *Endoscopy.* 2000;32:452-456.

63. Cremer M, Deviere J, Delhaye M, Balze M, Vandermeeren A. Stenting in severe chronic pancreatitis: results of medium-term follow-up in seventy-six patients. *Endoscopy.* 1991;23:171-176.

64. Delhaye M, Arvanitakis M, Verset G, Cremer M, Devière J. Long-term clinical outcome after endoscopic pancreatic ductal drainage for patients with painful chronic pancreatitis. *Clin Gastroenterol Hepatol.* 2004;2:1096-1106.

65. Ponchon T, Bory RM, Hedelius F, et al. Endoscopic stenting for pain relief in chronic pancreatitis: results of a standardized protocol. *Gastrointest Endosc.* 1995;42:452-456.

66. Rosch T, Daniel S, Scholz M, et al. Endoscopic treatment of chronic pancreatitis: a multicenter study of 1000 patients with long-term follow-up. *Endoscopy.* 2002;34:765-771.

67. Topazian M, Aslanian H, Andersen D. Outcome following endoscopic stenting of pancreatic duct strictures in chronic pancreatitis. *J Clin Gastroenterol.* 2005;39:908-911.

68. Dumonceau JM, Delhaye M, Tringali A, et al. Endoscopic treatment of chronic pancreatitis: European Society of Gastrointestinal Endoscopy (ESGE) Clinical Guideline. *Endoscopy.* 2012;44:784-800.

69. Kozarek RA. Pancreatic stents can induce ductal changes consistent with chronic pancreatitis. *Gastrointest Endosc.* 1990;36:93-95.

70. Smith MT, Sherman S, Ikenberry SO, Hawes RH, Lehman GA. Alterations in pancreatic ductal morphology following polyethylene pancreatic stent therapy. *Gastrointest Endosc.* 1996;44:268-275.

71. Chapman CG, Waxman I, Siddiqui UD. Endoscopic ultrasound (EUS)-guided pancreatic duct drainage: the basics of when and how to perform EUS-guided pancreatic duct interventions. *Clin Endosc.* 2016;49:161-167.

72. Fujii-Lau LL, Levy MJ. Endoscopic ultrasound-guided pancreatic duct drainage. *J Hepatobiliary Pancreat Sci.* 2015;22:51-57.

73. Itoi T, Kasuya K, Sofuni A, et al. Endoscopic ultrasonography-guided pancreatic duct access: techniques and literature review of pancreatography, transmural drainage and rendezvous techniques. *Dig Endosc.* 2013;25:241-252.

74. Abdallah AA, Krige JE, Bornman PC. Biliary tract obstruction in chronic pancreatitis. *HPB (Oxford).* 2007;9:421-428.

75. Catalano MF, Linder JD, George S, Alcocer E, Geenen JE. Treatment of symptomatic distal common bile duct stenosis secondary to chronic pancreatitis: comparison of single vs. multiple simultaneous stents. *Gastrointest Endosc.* 2004;60:945-952.

76. Deviere J, Nageshwar Reddy D, Puspok A, et al. Successful management of benign biliary strictures with fully covered self-expanding metal stents. *Gastroenterology.* 2014;147:385-395, quiz e15.

77. Kahaleh M, Brijbassie A, Sethi A, et al. Multicenter trial evaluating the use of covered self-expanding metal stents in benign biliary strictures: time to revisit our therapeutic options? *J Clin Gastroenterol.* 2013;47:695-699.

78. Brand B, Kahl M, Sidhu S, et al. Prospective evaluation of morphology, function, and quality of life after extracorporeal shockwave lithotripsy and endoscopic treatment of chronic calcific pancreatitis. *Am J Gastroenterol.* 2000;95:3428-3438.

79. Smits ME, Rauws EA, Tytgat GN, Huibregtse K. Endoscopic treatment of pancreatic stones in patients with chronic pancreatitis. *Gastrointest Endosc.* 1996;43:556-560.

80. Kozarek RA. Endoscopic treatment of chronic pancreatitis. *Indian J Gastroenterol.* 2002;21:67-73.

81. Seven G, Schreiner MA, Ross AS, et al. Long-term outcomes associated with pancreatic extracorporeal shock wave lithotripsy for chronic calcific pancreatitis. *Gastrointest Endosc.* 2012;75:997-1004.e1.

82. Tandan M, Reddy DN, Talukdar R, et al. Long-term clinical outcomes of extracorporeal shockwave lithotripsy in painful chronic calcific pancreatitis. *Gastrointest Endosc.* 2013;78:726-733.

83. Deviere J, Bell RH Jr, Beger HG, Traverso LW. Treatment of chronic pancreatitis with endotherapy or surgery: critical review of randomized control trials. *J Gastrointest Surg.* 2008;12:640-644.

84. Demir IE, Tieftrunk E, Maak M, Friess H, Ceyhan GO. Pain mechanisms in chronic pancreatitis: of a master and his fire. *Langenbecks Arch Surg.* 2011;396:151-160.

85. Khaled YS, Ammori MB, Ammori BJ. Laparoscopic lateral pancreaticojejunostomy for chronic pancreatitis: a case report and review of the literature. *Surg Laparosc Endosc Percutan Tech.* 2011;21:e36-e40.

86. Kurian MS, Gagner M. Laparoscopic side-to-side pancreaticojejunostomy (Partington-Rochelle) for chronic pancreatitis. *J Hepatobiliary Pancreat Surg.* 1999;6:382-386.

87. Tantia O, Jindal MK, Khanna S, Sen B. Laparoscopic lateral pancreaticojejunostomy: our experience of 17 cases. *Surg Endosc.* 2004;18:1054-1057.

88. Cuschieri A. Laparoscopic surgery of the pancreas. *J R Coll Surg Edinb.* 1994;39:178-184.

89. Patterson EJ, Gagner M, Salky B, et al. Laparoscopic pancreatic resection: single-institution experience of 19 patients. *J Am Coll Surg.* 2001;193:281-287.

90. Gagner M, Pomp A. Laparoscopic pylorus-preserving pancreatoduodenectomy. *Surg Endosc.* 1994;8:408-410.

91. Kendrick ML, Cusati D. Total laparoscopic pancreaticoduodenectomy: feasibility and outcome in an early experience. *Arch Surg.* 2010;145:19-23.

92. Palanivelu C, Jani K, Senthilnathan P, Parthasarathi R, Rajapandian S, Madhankumar MV. Laparoscopic pancreaticoduodenectomy: technique and outcomes. *J Am Coll Surg.* 2007;205:222-230.

93. Bachmann K, Tomkoetter L, Kutup A, et al. Is the Whipple procedure harmful for long-term outcome in treatment of chronic pancreatitis? 15-years follow-up comparing the outcome after pylorus-preserving pancreatoduodenectomy and Frey procedure in chronic pancreatitis. *Ann Surg.* 2013;258:815-820, discussion 820–821.

94. Keck T, Adam U, Makowiec F, et al. Short- and long-term results of duodenum preservation versus resection for the management of chronic pancreatitis: a prospective, randomized study. *Surgery.* 2012;152:S95-S102.

Imaging and Radiologic Intervention in the Pancreas

Melvy S. Mathew | Brian Funaki | Aytekin Oto

Cross-sectional imaging modalities such as computed tomography (CT), magnetic resonance imaging (MRI), and ultrasonography are commonly used for diagnosis of pancreatic diseases. CT has been the most commonly used technique because it can provide high-resolution images of the pancreas and depict even small lesions and calcifications. With the advent of multidetector computed tomography (MDCT) technology, acquisition speed and image quality have significantly improved. The development of 64-, 128-, 256-, and 320-slice scanners provides images with isotropic voxels on different phases of enhancement. MRI combined with magnetic resonance cholangiopancreatography (MRCP) has a growing role in imaging of the pancreas and biliary ducts. MRCP allows evaluation of the pancreatic parenchyma, biliary and pancreatic ducts, and vessels during the course of a single examination. The lack of ionizing radiation is an important advantage of MRI, making it an excellent choice for serial imaging. Transabdominal ultrasonography is often the primary diagnostic imaging modality in patients with suspected pancreatic/biliary disease. Contrast-enhanced ultrasonography may improve accuracy in detecting pancreatic diseases but is not widely used in the United States. Even with the use of contrast agents, ultrasonography has inherent limitations. Visualization of the entire pancreas is often not possible because of overlying gas or due to patient obesity, and the quality of the examination is dependent on the experience of the operator. This chapter reviews the MDCT, MRI, and ultrasound imaging features of congenital, inflammatory, and neoplastic diseases of the pancreas, and the role of interventional radiologic procedures in their management. There is also ongoing research regarding the utility of dual-energy CT (with its reduced radiation dosage to imaged patients) in the detection of focal pancreatic lesions.

CONGENITAL DISEASE

PANCREAS DIVISUM

Pancreas divisum is the most frequent congenital pancreatic abnormality. This entity may be asymptomatic; however, it is frequently associated with acute or chronic pancreatitis.[1] It is very difficult to diagnose pancreas divisum on CT because the pancreatic duct is difficult to visualize in its entirety, especially when it is normal in size.

On the other hand, MRCP highlights the ducts and allows visualization of the separate entries of the dorsal and ventral pancreatic ducts into the duodenum in patients with pancreas divisum. Because pancreas divisum is a key consideration in individuals with pancreatitis of unknown etiology, MRI plays an important role in the imaging evaluation of these patients. Occasionally, the pancreatic duct is not visualized as a result of its small size or secondary to edema of the pancreas. In these cases, MRCP following secretin administration can improve delineation of the pancreatic ductal anatomy (Fig. 95.1).[2,3]

ANOMALOUS PANCREATICOBILIARY DUCTAL JUNCTION

In anomalous pancreaticobiliary ductal junction, the main pancreatic and common bile ducts join within the duodenal wall and form a common channel (usually measuring more than 15 mm) proximal to the sphincter of Oddi.[4,5] Because anomalous pancreaticobiliary ductal junction is associated with pancreatitis and biliary carcinogenesis, its recognition is critical. Although endoscopic retrograde cholangiopancreatography is the most reliable method for evaluation, endoscopic sonography and MRCP are also useful for diagnosis. MRCP noninvasively detects the anomalous union between the common bile duct and the pancreatic duct. MRCP can also reveal associated choledochal cysts, biliary dilation, pancreatitis, or biliary malignancy (e.g., common bile duct or gallbladder carcinoma).[6]

FATTY INFILTRATION

The distribution of fatty infiltration of the pancreas is generally diffuse but may also be focal and mimic a hypoattenuating mass on CT.[7,8] In these cases, MRI can provide the correct diagnosis via employment of the chemical shift technique,[7,8] which unambiguously demonstrates fatty infiltration of the parenchyma.

On CT, diffuse fatty infiltration appears as separation or replacement of lobules of parenchymal tissue by intermixed, low-attenuating areas. Fatty focal infiltration is seen as hypoattenuating, nonenhancing fat interdigitating between normal pancreatic tissues. The focal sparing of fatty infiltration appears as a hyperdense, platelike, or triangular area,[8] compared to the fat-infiltrated areas of the pancreas. On MRI, areas of focal fatty infiltration demonstrate loss of signal intensity on opposed-phase gradient-echo T1-weighted images compared to in-phase T1-weighted images; this is caused by the presence of intracellular lipids in these focal areas. Unlike pancreatic adenocarcinoma, focal fatty infiltration does not cause upstream pancreatic parenchymal atrophy, ductal dilation, or displacement of adjacent vessels.

CONTOUR ABNORMALITIES

Annular pancreas is a rare congenital abnormality that may require surgical treatment, depending on the degree of duodenal obstruction.[9,10] CT and MRI demonstrate the normal pancreatic tissue encircling and encasing the second portion of the duodenum. Immediate postcontrast images can be helpful in differentiating pancreatic tissue

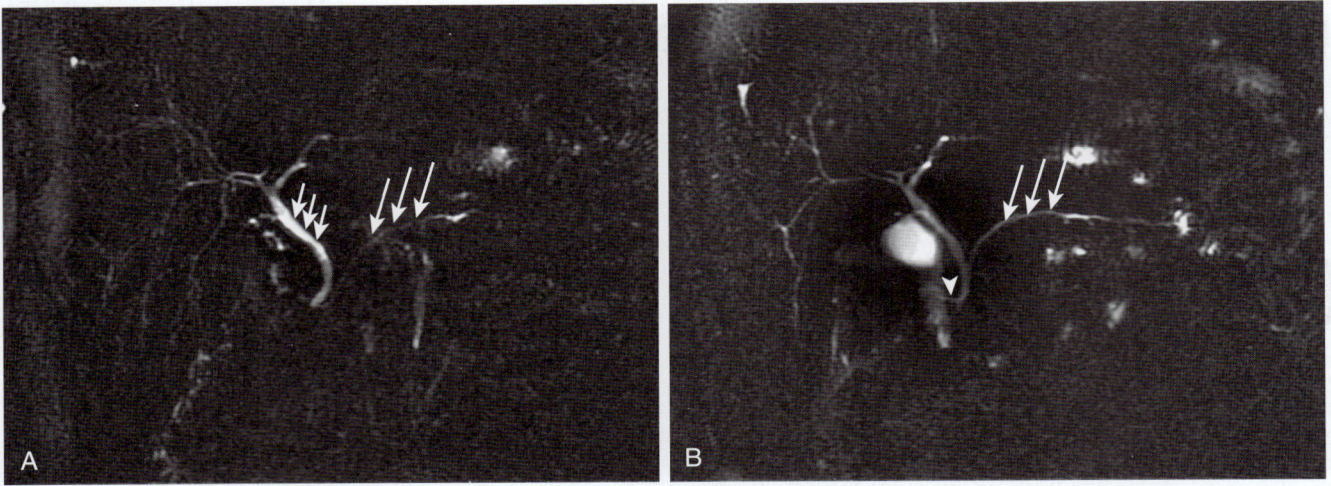

FIGURE 95.1 Pancreas divisum. (A) Thick-slab magnetic resonance cholangiopancreatography image before secretin administration demonstrates the pancreatic duct *(long arrows)*. *Short arrows* indicate the common bile duct. (B) Following secretin administration, the pancreatic duct *(long arrows)* becomes much better defined as a result of distention and its separate opening to the duodenum *(arrowhead)* via the minor papilla and becomes more prominent.

from the duodenum because of its relatively early and avid enhancement and to better demonstrate corresponding circumferential thickening of the duodenal wall. In addition, MRCP is able to depict the course and drainage of the pancreaticobiliary duct system.[9,10] Contour abnormalities are particularly common in the uncinate process and tail of the pancreas, but can also involve the body. Visualization of a normal duct crossing the area of contour abnormality is a very helpful imaging sign to exclude inflammation or neoplasm.

ACUTE PANCREATITIS

Acute pancreatitis is defined as an acute inflammatory process of the pancreas with involvement of adjacent organs and classified into interstitial edematous (70% to 80%) or necrotizing acute pancreatitis (20% to 30%).[11] The initial diagnosis is based on clinical features, but imaging may play a vital role in confirming the diagnosis, determining the severity, and detecting the complications of acute pancreatitis.[12] Ultrasound is frequently the first imaging modality and may identify underlying factors such as gallstones and biliary dilation. However, visualization of the pancreas is usually limited on ultrasonography. Contrast-enhanced CT is a fast and readily available imaging technique for the diagnosis of pancreatitis.[13,14] MRI should be considered for assessment, especially in younger patients, in patients with risk factors for iodinated contrast agents, and for follow-up purposes. MRCP allows evaluation of the entire biliary and pancreatic ductal system and can be helpful in determining the etiology of acute pancreatitis.

The pancreas may appear normal on CT or MRI in mild cases of pancreatitis. Imaging features of the pancreas in acute pancreatitis include diffuse or focal enlargement of the organ with border indistinctness, heterogeneous decreased signal on CT and T1-weighted images, and diminished postcontrast enhancement secondary to edema. Peripancreatic inflammatory changes include stranding

of surrounding fat and peripancreatic fluid (Fig. 95.2). As the severity of the pancreatitis worsens, nonenhancing areas in the pancreas indicative of necrosis may be seen.[12,13] On MRI, peripancreatic fluid is best demonstrated on T2-weighed images with fat saturation as high-signal-intensity collections.[11] Diffusion-weighted MRI may be superior to CT in detecting subtle changes of mild pancreatitis.[15]

Based on the revised Atlanta classification, complications of pancreatitis include acute peripancreatic fluid collections and, if necrosis is present, acute necrotic collections when imaging is being performed less than 4 weeks from the onset of symptoms; beyond this point visualized collections are referred to as pseudocysts or, in the setting of necrosis, walled-off necroses (WONs; Fig. 95.3A and B).[11,12] Infected necrosis is a serious development often associated with complications and may require open surgical treatment or, increasingly, percutaneous drainage. The presence of gas within hypoenhancing or necrotic areas of pancreatic tissue suggests infected necrosis. Pseudocysts occur at least 4 weeks after the acute onset of pancreatitis. These structures are usually round or oval in configuration and demonstrate rim enhancement, corresponding to a fibrous wall. Most pseudocysts are asymptomatic and remain stable or show spontaneous resolution. If pseudocysts are complicated by infection or hemorrhage, percutaneous drainage may be pursued. On MRI, pseudocysts appear hypointense on T1-weighted images, hyperintense on T2-weighted images, and show progressive wall enhancement over time. WONs also persist beyond 4 weeks from the start of acute pancreatitis and are seen in the setting of necrosis. Of note, WONs may appear identical to pseudocysts on CT. MRI is extremely useful in differentiating the two entities and this distinction has important ramifications in treatment planning, as alluded to in the following text.

Interventional radiology plays an increasingly important role in the management of acute pancreatitis. Ultrasound- or CT-guided percutaneous drainage or aspiration of fluid

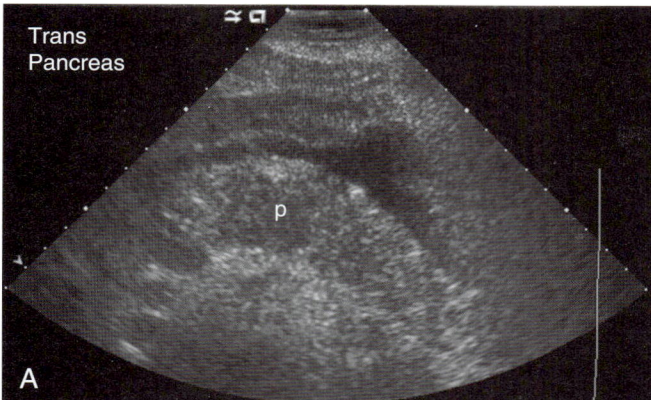

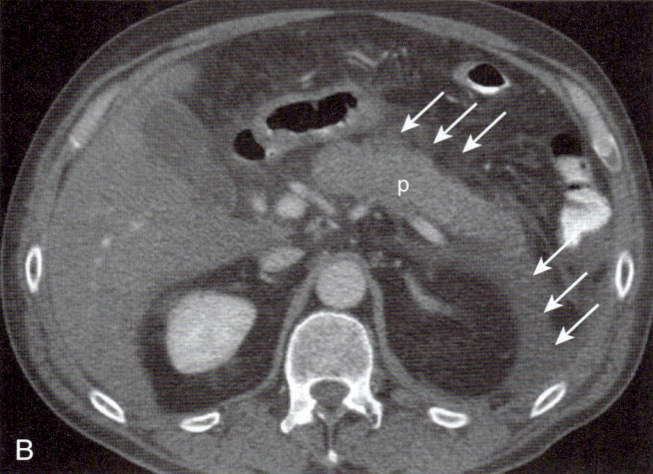

FIGURE 95.2 Acute pancreatitis. (A) On ultrasound, the pancreas *(p)* is enlarged and hypoechoic, compatible with acute pancreatitis. A small amount of peripancreatic fluid is also noted. (B) Contrast-enhanced computed tomography image demonstrates an edematous, enlarged pancreas *(p)* with peripancreatic fluid and inflammatory changes *(arrows)* consistent with acute pancreatitis.

collections is performed to exclude or confirm the diagnosis of infection or for definitive treatment.[12,16] Preprocedural differentiation of a pseudocyst from a WON is useful because more aggressive interventional or surgical approaches may be required in the case of a WON, where a good deal of nonliquefied contents may be present. The diagnosis of a WON on imaging is best achieved using MRI, where fat-saturated T2-weighted imaging can be used to determine whether a hypoattenuating fluid collection seen on CT truly contains fluid or whether it is, in actuality, mostly nonliquefied, necrotizing material. Common access routes include a retroperitoneal approach through the lateral flank or an anterior approach through the peritoneum (see Fig. 95.3C).[16] Often, multiple large-bore drainage catheters (at least 12 or 14 French) with multiple side holes are necessary to drain viscous fluid collections. After placement of a drainage catheter, follow-up CT scans are required. Minimally invasive necrosectomy may be performed by placing a flexible endoscope in the necrotic tissue cavity using an endoscopic

or percutaneous approach, and the necrotic material may then be removed using irrigation, snares, and/or baskets. Emergency angiography and embolization may be required in patients with vascular complications such as hemorrhage or pseudoaneurysms.

CHRONIC PANCREATITIS

MRI in combination with MRCP is the most helpful noninvasive test for the diagnosis of chronic pancreatitis. MRI enables evaluation of both pancreatic parenchymal changes (including alterations in signal and atrophy) and pancreatic ductal changes. CT, on the other hand, is excellent for the demonstration of characteristic pancreatic calcifications (Fig. 95.4).

Among early findings of chronic inflammation is abnormal pancreatic tissue signal, for example, a decrease in the intrinsic T1 signal on precontrast T1-weighted fat-saturated imaging. Late findings include dilation and stenosis of the pancreatic and biliary ducts, intraductal calcifications, and parenchymal atrophy or enlargement.[17] In patients with chronic pancreatitis, the pancreas demonstrates decreased postcontrast enhancement compared to normal pancreatic tissue.

Focal pancreatic enlargement as a result of acute-to-subacute pancreatitis may be difficult to distinguish from cancer. Helpful distinguishing imaging features include the "duct-penetrating sign" (i.e., visualization of the normal or nonobstructed duct in the focally abnormal pancreatic segment) and the presence of calcifications. On the other hand, evidence of vascular invasion is *not* typical of chronic pancreatitis and is, instead, highly indicative of malignancy.

Complications of chronic pancreatitis include gastrointestinal obstruction caused by pseudocyst formation, superimposed infection, and vascular complications (e.g., portal vein or splenic vein thrombosis and arterial pseudoaneurysm), which may require radiologic interventions. MRCP with secretin stimulation allows for the evaluation of the exocrine function of the pancreas and ductal compliance. Negative oral contrast agents should be administered prior to secretin-stimulated MRCP for accurate evaluation of pancreatic function.

AUTOIMMUNE PANCREATITIS

The diagnosis of autoimmune pancreatitis requires a multidisciplinary approach. Imaging modalities, especially CT and MRI, can confirm clinical suspicion and are helpful in monitoring response to treatment.

In autoimmune pancreatitis, pancreatic parenchymal changes and abnormalities of the biliary and pancreatic ducts may be observed. Autoimmune pancreatitis leads to a diffuse "sausage-shaped" or, more rarely, a focal "mass-like" enlargement of the pancreas. The pancreas appears hypointense on T1-weighted images and hyperintense on T2-weighted images. Following intravenous contrast administration, delayed pancreatic parenchymal enhancement or peripancreatic rim enhancement may be appreciated. Irregular narrowing, strictures, and dilations of the main pancreatic duct and of the branch ducts may be best seen on MRCP. Other possible findings include

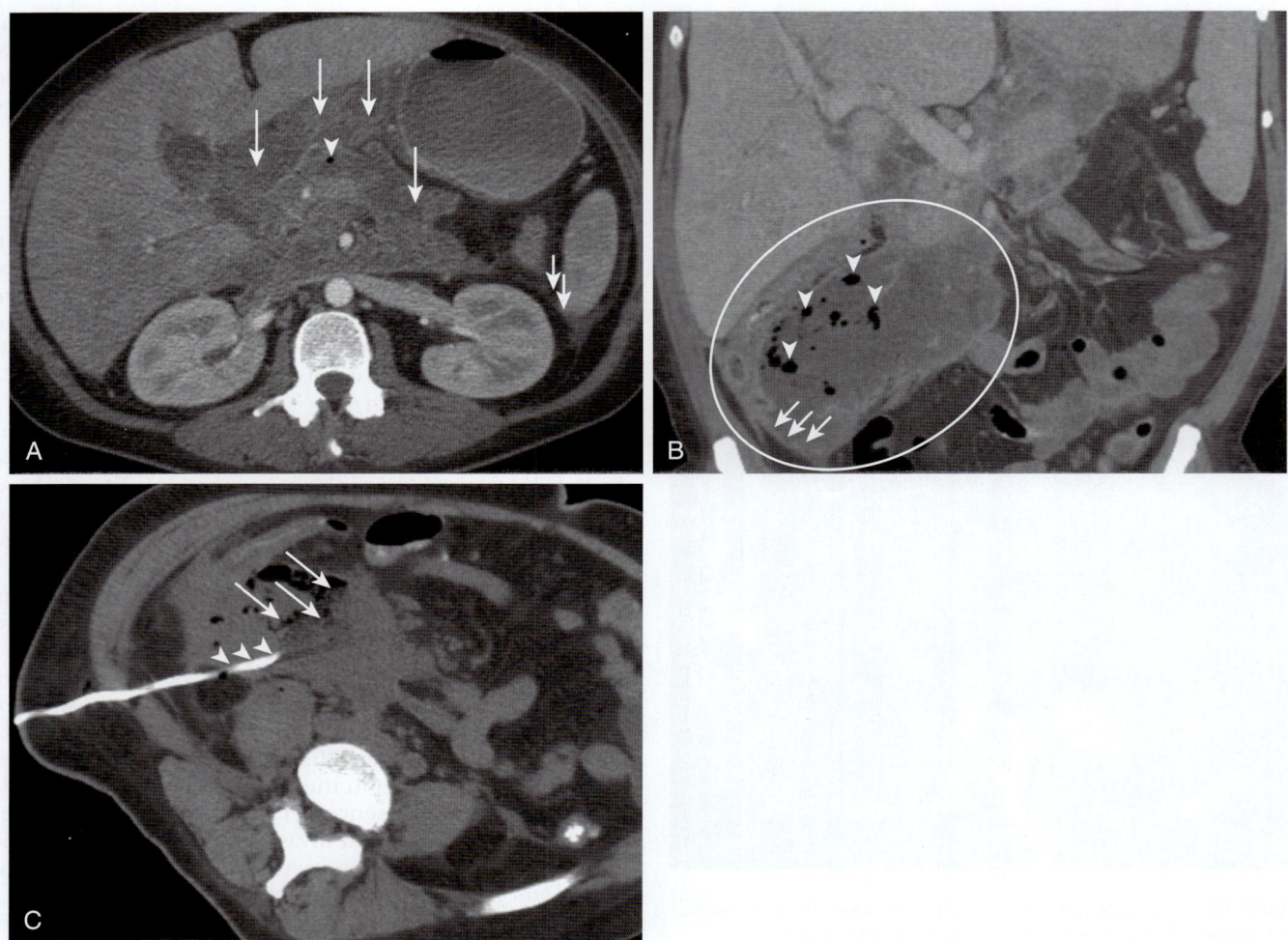

FIGURE 95.3 Necrotizing pancreatitis. (A) Axial contrast-enhanced computed tomography (CT) image demonstrates a nonenhancing pancreas and peripancreatic fluid collections extending into the left upper quadrant *(long arrows)* with foci of air *(arrowhead)*. Free fluid is shown in the left anterior pararenal space *(short arrows)*. (B) Coronal contrast-enhanced CT image demonstrates an infected collection extending inferiorly into the right paracolic gutter *(circle)* with multiple foci of air *(arrowheads)* and wall enhancement *(short arrows)*. Based on CT imaging findings alone, it is difficult to optimally assess the contents of the fluid collection; the appearance is suspicious for a walled-off necrosis. (C) CT-guided drainage of the infected collection. Under CT guidance, a pigtail catheter *(arrowheads)* was placed into the fluid collection and the collection *(arrows)* was drained.

biliary strictures, retroperitoneal adenopathy, and bilateral multiple, small hypodense/hypointense renal lesions.

Focal involvement of the pancreatic head by autoimmune pancreatitis must be distinguished from pancreatic cancer. Differentiation is extremely challenging but of paramount importance. In some cases, differentiation may be very difficult or impossible based on imaging findings alone. Identification of a normal pancreatic duct within the suspicious-appearing focal portion of the pancreas is an important imaging finding suggestive of a benign etiology and should be actively sought after, especially on MRCP. Irregular but gradual tapering obstruction of the main pancreatic duct within the apparent lesion, a normal upstream duct size, and normalization of the pancreatic gland following steroid therapy all suggest the diagnosis of autoimmune pancreatitis.[18,19] Endoscopic ultrasound-guided tissue sampling may also aid in the diagnosis of autoimmune pancreatitis and in the exclusion of underlying neoplasm.

TRAUMA

Management of pancreatic injury is greatly influenced by the grade of the injury, especially the integrity of the main pancreatic duct and the presence of concomitant abdominal injuries.[20,21] CT is the modality of choice with sensitivity and specificity for pancreatic injuries greater than 85%.[22] Other imaging modalities are not as sensitive or specific and/or the examination (as in the case of MRI) may take too long or may not be available in emergency settings.

On CT, imaging features include parenchymal laceration (i.e., areas of intrapancreatic low attenuation), fracture of the pancreas with or without separation of the fracture

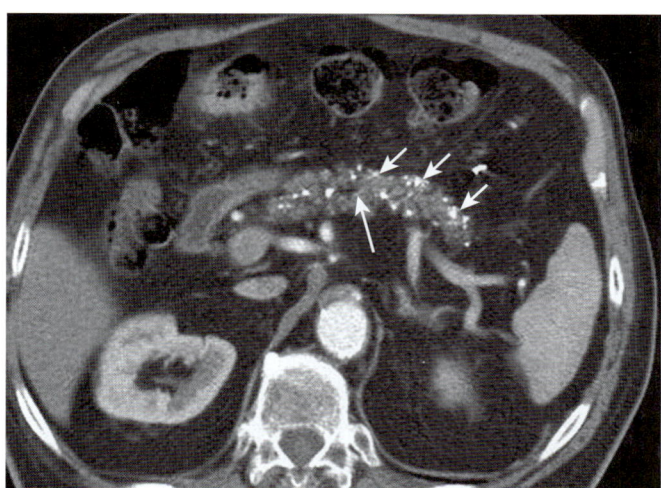

FIGURE 95.4 Chronic pancreatitis. Axial postcontrast computed tomography image demonstrates an atrophic pancreas with multiple calcifications *(short arrows)* and a dilated main pancreatic duct *(long arrow)* consistent with chronic pancreatitis.

segments, hemorrhage, fluid collections, thickening of the anterior renal fascia, and associated injuries involving left upper quadrant structures.[20,21] Follow-up scans are often required to exclude or to monitor complications such as pancreatitis or the formation of a pancreatic fistula or pseudocyst, which may require intervention.

On abdominal radiographs taken of a trauma patient, an altered psoas shadow, mass effect indicating hematoma, or free air are significant findings; however, these occur in only 18% to 20% of patients with pancreatic injury.[23] Ultrasound is very limited in the evaluation of pancreatic injuries. MRI provides not only visualization of the entire pancreas, but also evaluation of the pancreatic duct. This may be useful if a severed pancreatic duct cannot be excluded by CT scan. On T1-weighted images, the compromised pancreatic tissue will show variable decreased signal intensity and will enhance heterogeneously after gadolinium contrast administration.[20,21] Fluid collections are best seen on T2-weighted fat-suppressed images as areas of hyperintensity.

NEOPLASM

ADENOCARCINOMA

Pancreatic ductal adenocarcinoma is characterized by its relatively rapid growth, early invasion of surrounding tissue, and early hepatic and lymphatic metastases. Criteria for unresectability include invasion of the celiac trunk, superior mesentery artery, or common hepatic artery, or distant metastases.

CT is traditionally the most commonly utilized method for diagnosing and staging pancreatic malignancy. MRI combined with MRCP and magnetic resonance angiography also allow detection and characterization of pancreatic lesions.[24] Ultrasonography is very limited in the detection of a focal pancreatic lesion and in the differentiation of cancer from chronic pancreatitis.

With respect to both CT and MRI, imaging in the pancreatic phase (i.e., approximately 45 seconds after contrast administration) and in the portal venous phase (i.e., approximately 70 seconds after contrast administration) is critical for detection of pancreatic adenocarcinoma, which tends to be hypodense/hypointense to the background pancreas on these modalities following intravenous contrast administration (Fig. 95.5A). Mass effect exerted by a tumor located in the head of the pancreas causes upstream pancreatic and biliary ductal dilation (the "double-duct sign") (see Fig. 95.5B). Grading systems for diagnosing and assessing vascular invasion include the extent of contiguity with the vessels, morphologic deformation of vessels (see Fig. 95.5C), dilation of peripancreatic veins, and the "teardrop sign," which refers to the deformed shape of the superior mesenteric vein as a result of tumoral involvement.[25,26] MRI is one of the most sensitive imaging modalities for detection and characterization of liver lesions, in this case, metastases.[27] Liver metastases are hypovascular, hypointense on T1-weighted images, minimally hyperintense on T2-weighted images, and show irregular rim enhancement on postgadolinium images.[24] The presence of malignant lymphadenopathy is often assessed by using size criteria, with a cutoff nodal diameter of 10 mm in maximum short axis dimension.[25] Ascites, abnormal peritoneal enhancement, or nodularity and omental thickening are highly concerning for peritoneal metastatic disease. Recently, diffusion-weighted MRI has been shown to improve detection of liver and peritoneal metastatic lesions.[28]

PANCREATIC NEUROENDOCRINE TUMORS

The role of imaging in functioning pancreatic endocrine tumors is primarily for the detection and verification of the number and location of lesions. Intraoperative ultrasound may play a particularly important role in procuring this information, which is vital for future surgical planning. CT and MRI are also useful in monitoring and follow-up of patients with malignant neuroendocrine tumors. Insulinoma and gastrinoma are the two most common functioning endocrine neoplasms of the pancreas. Insulinomas are typically small (<2 cm) when diagnosed, richly vascularized, and appear as well-defined, round lesions. On unenhanced images, insulinomas generally demonstrate low attenuation on CT and low signal on T1-weighted MR images and increased signal on T2-weighted images. After contrast administration, insulinomas tend to enhance avidly in the arterial phase and remain hyperdense/hyperintense on delayed-phase imaging (Fig. 95.6). Associated liver metastases are also hypervascular and may show a peripheral rim of enhancement or may enhance homogeneously, particularly when the lesions are small.[29]

Gastrinomas are relatively large (with a mean size of 4 cm) when diagnosed.[29] They occur most frequently in the gastrinoma triangle, which is defined as the neck and body of the pancreas medially, the confluence of the cystic and common bile ducts superiorly, and the second and third portion of the duodenum inferiorly. Comparatively speaking, gastrinomas are not as hypervascular as insulinomas. Gastrinomas may manifest on imaging as an isodense mass on unenhanced CT and show diminished signal on T1-weighted fat-suppressed MR images and

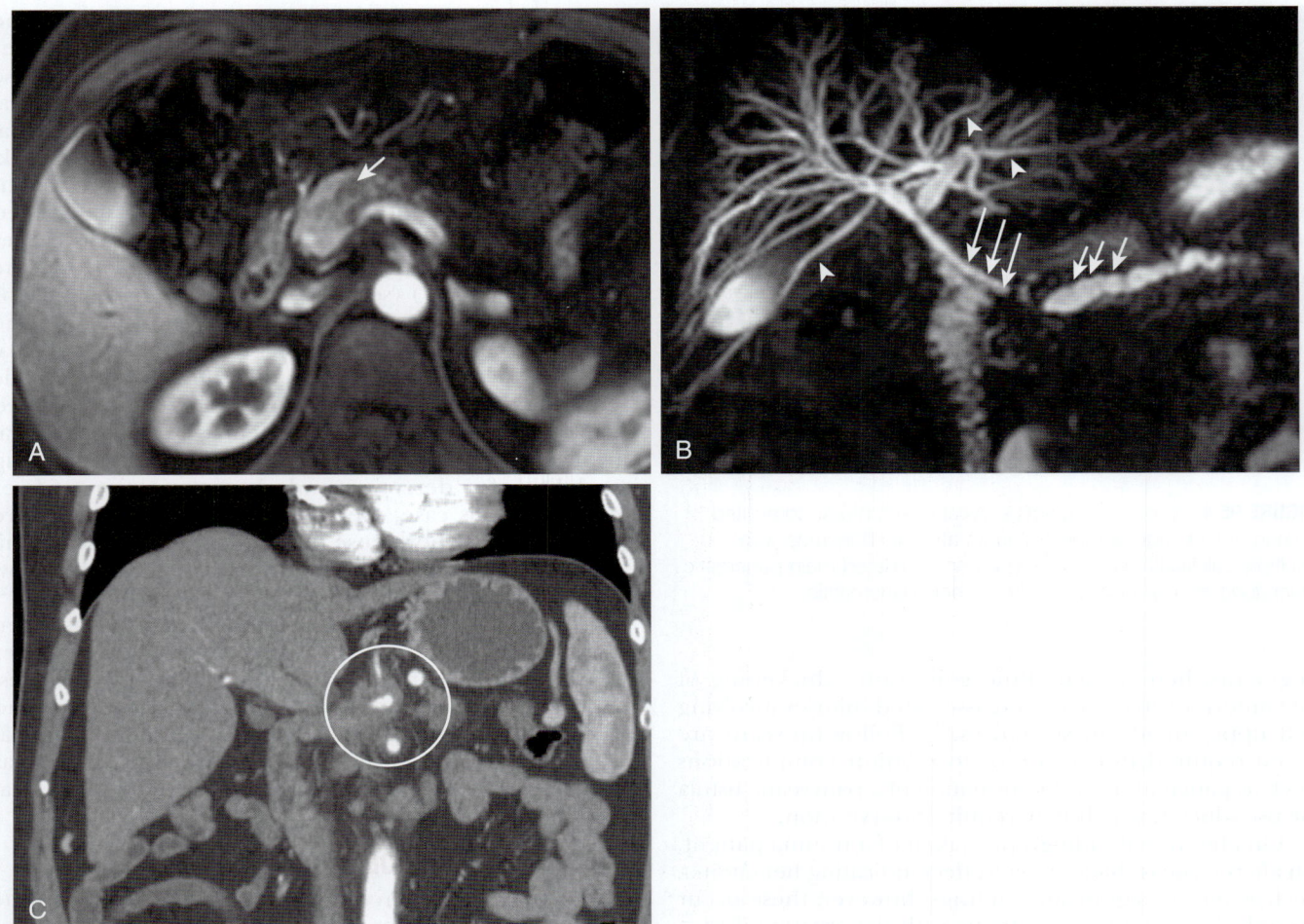

FIGURE 95.5 Adenocarcinoma of the pancreas. (A) On contrast-enhanced T1-weighted imaging, a hypointense, ill-defined lesion within the pancreatic head *(short arrow)* consistent with adenocarcinoma of the pancreas is seen. (B) Coronal maximum-intensity projection magnetic resonance cholangiopancreatography image demonstrates the "double-duct sign" caused by mass effect of the tumor involving the head of the pancreas: Prestenotic dilation of the pancreatic *(short arrows)* and common bile duct *(long arrows)* and dilation of the intrahepatic biliary duct system *(arrowheads)*. (C) Coronal contrast-enhanced computed tomography image in the arterial phase demonstrates encasement of the celiac trunk and the superior mesentery artery *(circle)* by pancreatic adenocarcinoma.

increased signal on T2-weighted images. After contrast media administration, gastrinomas may show mild enhancement with hypoenhancing areas within, reflecting intralesional necrosis.[30] Liver metastases are hyperintense on T2-weighted fat-suppressed images and have well-defined margins. The majority of gastrinomas are malignant and assessing for locoregional infiltration and distant metastases is critical for patient management.

Nonfunctioning pancreatic endocrine tumors are generally large at presentation. Consequently, the main role of imaging is not only for detection but also for more definitive characterization, in particular, differentiation from pancreatic adenocarcinoma.[31] Given that nonfunctioning pancreatic endocrine tumors are often malignant and that patients generally present initially with liver metastases, accurate staging and follow-up are essential. Nonfunctioning pancreatic endocrine tumors are mostly solid and hypervascular. They typically have sharp margins and a capsule, and they may harbor cystic or necrotic areas. The presence of hemorrhagic content and central

calcifications mostly depends on tumor size,[32] and results in complex echogenicity on ultrasound and inhomogeneous enhancement after contrast application on CT and MRI.

CYSTIC NEOPLASMS OF THE PANCREAS

Most cystic pancreatic neoplasms consist of intraductal papillary mucinous neoplasms (IPMNs), serous cystadenomas, or mucinous cystic neoplasms. Cystic neoplasms of the pancreas are being diagnosed with increasing frequency as a result of technologic advances in cross-sectional imaging. In addition to detection and follow-up of these lesions, imaging is also done to differentiate malignant and nonmalignant cystic lesions, which can be challenging due to the overlapping features of each. The following imaging features are important in the differentiation of benign and malignant cystic lesions: The uni- or multilocular nature of the lesion, communication with the pancreatic duct, the size of the tumor and the degree of pancreatic duct dilation, the presence of thick septations

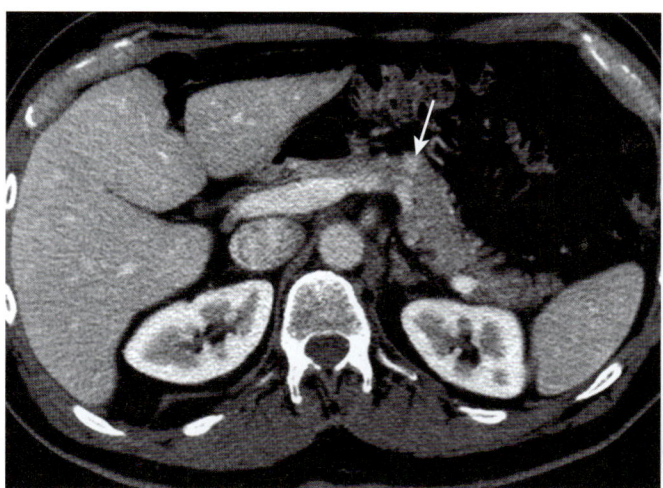

FIGURE 95.6 Insulinoma. Axial contrast-enhanced computed tomography image of the pancreas shows a small, well-defined, round lesion in the pancreatic body *(arrow)*. The lesion is hyperdense compared to the normal pancreas, a typical computed tomography finding for pancreatic neuroendocrine tumors.

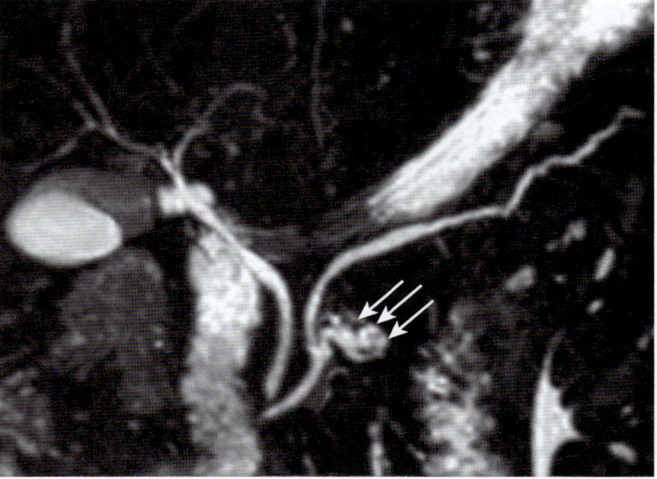

FIGURE 95.7 Branch duct-intraductal papillary mucinous neoplasm. Coronal maximum-intensity projection magnetic resonance cholangiopancreatography demonstrates an oval-shaped cystic mass with lobulated borders located in the uncinate process of the pancreas *(arrows)* that communicates with the main pancreatic duct.

or mural nodules, and the signal of the tumor on T1-weighted images. A history of pancreatitis and a lack of an epithelial lining favor a pseudocyst, whereas the presence of central calcifications, septations, and solid components is more indicative of a cystic neoplasm.[33] CT is advantageous in its ability to detect central calcifications, whereas MRI provides better soft tissue contrast resolution and better delineation of the tumor with respect to the pancreatic duct. MRCP images can be of further use in the anatomic evaluation of the pancreatic duct system and its relationship to the cystic lesion. MRI is also an ideal modality for follow-up imaging because of its lack of ionizing radiation.

Intraductal Papillary Mucinous Neoplasm

IPMNs are divided into three groups: main duct type, branch duct type (BD-IPMN), and mixed type.[34,35] The risk for malignancy depends on the type of IPMN. In 58% to 92% of main duct IPMNs, malignancy has been reported,[34] whereas the risk for malignancy in BD-IPMNs is much lower, with rates ranging from 6% to 46%. Thus an important challenge for diagnostic imaging is the differentiation between the types of IPMNs and the detection of imaging features worrisome for malignancy. IPMNs can be detected on MDCT; however, three-dimensional high-resolution contrast-enhanced MRI with high-resolution MRCP may be more accurate in demonstrating communication with the main pancreatic duct and in identifying small BD-IPMNs.[36,37]

BD-IPMNs can be seen in any segment of the pancreas but are most commonly located in the uncinate process. They appear as oval-shaped cystic masses communicating with the branch ducts of the pancreas (Fig. 95.7). Especially when small, these lesions can mimic cystic changes in the setting of chronic pancreatitis. Imaging features of a combined-type IPMN include the presence of BD-IPMNs as well as dilation of the main pancreatic duct greater

than 6 mm. The main-duct type IPMN may have the appearance of segmental or diffuse dilation of the main pancreatic duct.

Imaging features associated with malignancy include mural nodules, a dilated main pancreatic duct (greater than 8 to 10 mm), thick septae, intraluminal calcifications (best seen on CT scan), ductal filling defects on MRCP, a bulging papilla, local invasion, and/or signs of invasive cancer, such as dilation of the common bile duct.[37]

Serous Cystadenoma

One percent to 2% of all pancreatic tumors and 25% of all cystic pancreatic neoplasms are serous tumors. They are distributed evenly throughout the pancreas.[34] Serous cystadenomas are benign and can generally speaking be classified as microcystic, macrocystic (also known as oligocystic), or mixed; a solid type also exists.[38,39] Typically, they appear as a pancreatic mass with numerous, mostly small fluid-filled or solid-appearing grapelike cysts. The lesions may have a central stellate scar and sunburst pattern of calcifications.[38,39] Serous tumors never communicate with the main pancreatic duct. Small discrete calcifications can be best visualized on CT, whereas MRI provides superior visualization of the small grapelike cysts and their contents. After injection of contrast media, enhancement of thin-walled septae may be seen, producing the characteristic "honeycomb" appearance. In addition, MRI and CT images may reveal a late-enhancing central scar.

Mucinous Cystadenoma/Cystadenocarcinoma

Mucinous cystic neoplasms of the pancreas represent 2% of all pancreatic neoplasms.[34] Mucinous cystadenomas are described pathologically as having borderline malignant potential and as such need to be differentiated from serous cystadenomas. Most mucinous cystic neoplasms are localized to the pancreatic body or tail and their sizes range

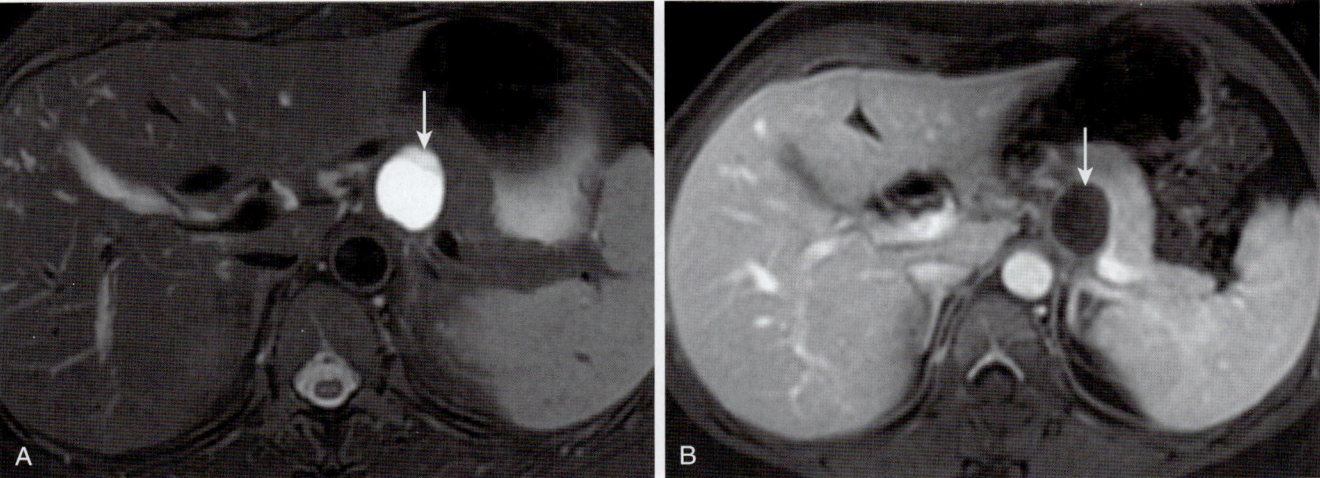

FIGURE 95.8 Mucinous cystadenoma. (A) T2-weighted image with fat saturation demonstrates a large, unilocular cystic lesion *(arrow)*, which does not communicate with the pancreatic duct. (B) After contrast administration, wall enhancement *(arrow)* of the mucinous cystadenoma is shown on T1-weighted imaging.

up to 35 cm.[34] They are characterized by the formation of large unilocular or multilocular cysts with enhancing septations (Fig. 95.8).[35] Mucin production typically results in high signal intensity within these tumors and is also seen with respect to associated liver metastases (in cases of mucinous cystadenocarcinoma) on T1- and T2-weighted MR images.[29] Hemorrhagic content is a strong predictor of mucinous cystic neoplasm and shows high attenuation and high signal on CT and MRI, respectively. Mucinous cystadenomas are well circumscribed and encapsulated; in contrast, mucinous cystadenocarcinomas may be seen infiltrating adjacent organs or structures. The appearance of solid nodules, irregularity or thickening of the cyst wall, a tumor size larger than 6 cm, and the presence of metastatic lesions and/or peripheral eggshell calcifications are additional criteria that are concerning for malignancy.

REFERENCES

1. Fulcher AS, Turner MA. MR pancreatography: a useful tool for evaluating pancreatic disorders. *Radiographics*. 1999;19:5.
2. Motosugi U, Ichikawa T, Araki T, et al. Secretin-stimulating MRCP in patients with pancreatobiliary maljunction and occult pancreatobiliary reflux: direct demonstration of pancreatobiliary reflux. *Eur Radiol*. 2007;17:2262.
3. Sandrasegeran K, Lin C, Akisik FM, Tann M. State-of-the-art pancreatic MRI. *AJR Am J Roentgenol*. 2010;195:42.
4. Yu Z, Zhang L, Fu J, Li J, Zhang QY, Chen FL. Anomalous pancreaticobiliary junction: image analysis and treatment principles. *Hepatobiliary Pancreat Dis Int*. 2004;3:136.
5. Funabiki T, Matsubara T, Miyakwa S, Ishihara S. Pancreaticobiliary maljunction and carcinogenesis to biliary and pancreatic malignancy. *Langenbecks Arch Surg*. 2009;394:159.
6. Kamisawa T, Tu Y, Egawa N, Tsuruta K, Okamoto A, Kamata N. MRCP of congenital pancreaticobiliary malformation. *Abdom Imaging*. 2007;32:129.
7. Isserow JA, Siegelman ES, Mammone J. Focal fatty infiltration of the pancreas: MR characterization with chemical shift imaging. *AJR Am J Roentgenol*. 1999;173:1263.
8. Kawamoto S, Siegelman SS, Bluemke DA, Hruban RH, Fishman EK. Focal fatty infiltration of the head of the pancreas: evaluation

9. Sandrasegaran K, Patel A, Fogel EL, Zyromski NJ, Pitt HA. Annular pancreas in adults. *AJR Am J Roentgenol*. 2009;193:455.
10. Jadvar H, Mindelzun RE. Annular pancreas in adults: imaging features in seven patients. *Abdom Imaging*. 1999;24:174.
11. Balci NC, Bieneman BK, Bilgin M, Akduman IE, Fattahi R, Burton FR. Magnetic resonance imaging in pancreatitis. *Top Magn Reson Imaging*. 2009;20:25.
12. Thoeni RF. The revised Atlanta classification of acute pancreatitis: its importance for the radiologist and its effect on treatment. *Radiology*. 2012;262:751.
13. Vijayaraghavan G, Kurup D, Singh A. Imaging of acute abdomen and pelvis: common acute pathologies. *Semin Roentgenol*. 2009;44:221.
14. Stevens T, Parsi MA, Walsh RM. Acute pancreatitis: problems in adherence to guidelines. *Cleve Clin J Med*. 2009;76:697.
15. Thomas S, Kayhan A, Lakadamyali H, Oto A. Diffusion MRI of acute pancreatitis and comparison with normal individuals using ADC values. *Emerg Radiol*. 2012;19:5.
16. Segal D, Mortele KJ, Banks PA, Silverman SG. Acute necrotizing pancreatitis: role of CT-guided percutaneous catheter drainage. *Abdom Imaging*. 2007;32:351.
17. Miller FH, Keppke AL, Wadhwa A, Ly JN, Dalal K, Kamler VA. MRI of pancreatitis and its complications: part 2, chronic pancreatitis. *AJR Am J Roentgenol*. 2004;183:1645.
18. Carbognin G, Girardi V, Biasiutti C, et al. Autoimmune pancreatitis: imaging findings on contrast-enhanced MR, MRCP and dynamic secretin-enhanced MRCP. *Radiol Med*. 2009;114:1214.
19. Manfredi R, Graziani R, Cicero C, et al. Autoimmune pancreatitis: CT patterns and their chances after steroid treatment. *Radiology*. 2008;247:435.
20. Chrysos E, Athanasakis E, Xynos E. Pancreatic trauma in the adult: current knowledge in diagnosis and management. *Pancreatology*. 2002;2:365.
21. Tkacz JN, Anderson SA, Soto J. MR imaging in gastrointestinal emergencies. *Radiographics*. 2009;29:1767.
22. Ahmed N, Vernick JJ. Pancreatic injury. *South Med J*. 2009;102:1253.
23. Balasegaram M. Surgical management of pancreatic trauma. *Curr Probl Surg*. 1979;16:1.
24. Vachiranubhap B, Kim YH, Balci NC, et al. Magnetic resonance imaging of adenocarcinoma of the pancreas. *Top Magn Reson Imaging*. 2009;20:3.
25. Grenacher L, Klauss M. Computed tomography of pancreatic tumors. *Radiologe*. 2009;49:107.
26. Kinney T. Evidence-based imaging of pancreatic malignancies. *Surg Clin North Am*. 2010;90:235.

27. Ba-Ssalamah A, Uffmann M, Saini S, Bastati N, Herold C, Schima W. Clinical value of liver-specific contrast agents: a tailored examination for a confident non-invasive diagnosis of focal liver lesions. *Eur Radiol.* 2009;19:342.

28. Low RN. MR imaging of the peritoneal spread of malignancy. *Abdom Imaging.* 2007;32:267.

29. Ku YM, Shin SS, Lee CH, Semelka RC. Magnetic resonance imaging of cystic and endocrine pancreatic neoplasm. *Top Magn Reson Imaging.* 2009;20:11.

30. Horton K, Hruban RH, Yeo C, Fishman EK. Multi-detector-row CT of pancreatic islet cell tumors. *Radiographics.* 2006;26:453.

31. Graziani R, Brandalise A, Bellotti M, et al. Imaging of neuroendocrine gastroenteropancreatic tumors. *Radiol Med.* 2010;115:1047.

32. Dörffel Y, Wermke W. Contrast medium sonography of neuroendocrine tumors of the gastroenteropancreatic system. *Radiologe.* 2009;49:206.

33. Sand J, Nordback I. The differentiation between pancreatic neoplastic cysts and pancreatic pseudocyst. *Scand J Surg.* 2005;94:161.

34. Verbesey JE, Munson JL. Pancreatic cystic neoplasms. *Surg Clin North Am.* 2010;90:411.

35. Brambs HJ, Jucherns M. Cystic tumors of the pancreas. *Radiologe.* 2008;48:740.

36. Baiocchi GL, Portolani N, Missale G, et al. Intraductal papillary mucinous neoplasm of the pancreas (IPMN): clinico-pathological correlations and surgical indications. *World J Surg Oncol.* 2010;8:25.

37. Augustin T, VanderMeer TJ. Intraductal papillary mucinous neoplasm: a clinicopathologic review. *Surg Clin North Am.* 2010;9:377.

38. Liu QY, Zhou J, Zeng YR, Lin XF, Min J. Giant serous cystadenoma of the pancreas (>10 cm): the clinical features and CT findings. *Gastroenterol Res Pract.* 2016;2016:8454823.

39. Yasuda A, Sawai H, Ochi N, Matsuo Y, Okada Y, Takeyama H. Solid variant of serous cystadenoma of the pancreas. *Arch Med Sci.* 2011;7(2):353-355.

Pancreatic and Periampullary Cancer

Katherine E. Poruk | James F. Griffin | Christopher L. Wolfgang |

John L. Cameron

Pancreatic and periampullary tumors include a diverse group of malignant neoplasms that arise in the pancreas or at or near the ampulla of Vater. These neoplasms commonly include adenocarcinomas of the pancreas (pancreatic ductal adenocarcinomas [PDACs]), duodenum, distant common bile duct, or ampulla of Vater in addition to pancreatic neuroendocrine tumors (PNETs). Other neoplasms located in this region include intraductal papillary mucinous neoplasms (IPMNs), acinar cell cancer, mucinous cystic neoplasms (MCNs), and solid pseudopapillary neoplasms (SPNs). Presentation of these tumors is often similar given their common location of origin with symptoms including abdominal discomfort, obstructive jaundice and pruritus for lesions located in the head of the pancreas or periampullary region, and pain or abdominal discomfort for pancreatic tail lesions. The surgical management of these neoplasms is often similar given their shared location, but differences in underlying biology can dictate subtle differences in care requiring the need for accurate diagnosis and differentiation of these neoplasms.

INCIDENCE

The most common periampullary malignancy is PDAC, followed by ampullary adenocarcinoma, distal cholangiocarcinoma, and duodenal adenocarcinoma. Other, less common lesions can also be found in this region, including PNETs, acinar cell cancer, IPMNs, sarcomas, gastrointestinal (GI) stromal tumors, MCNs, SPNs, and metastases from other cancers. Although periampullary cancers are generally less common compared to other malignancies including colorectal, breast, and lung, they remain a major cause of mortality often related to their difficulty to diagnose early. An estimated 53,000 cases of pancreatic adenocarcinoma are estimated for 2016, making it the ninth most common cancer in the United States. However, approximately 42,000 deaths due to PDAC are expected for the same time period, making it the fourth leading cause of cancer death with a 5-year overall survival of only 7%.[1] The number of new cases of pancreatic cancer in the United States is approximately 10 to 12 per 100,000 men and women per year, which has remained relatively steady over the past several decades.[2] A similar, stable incidence has been seen in European nations over the past several decades. A dramatic increase has been seen in pancreatic cancer rates in Japan over the past 3 decades, although the overall incidence of PDAC in Japan, the Middle East, and Asia remains lower than in Western nations.

Cholangiocarcinoma is a tumor of the bile ducts found along the biliary tree and occurs less frequently than pancreatic adenocarcinoma. Distal bile duct carcinoma comprises 20% to 40% of all cholangiocarcinomas. The exact incidence and death rate is difficult to ascertain because distal cholangiocarcinomas are usually combined with other cholangiocarcinomas (hilar and intrahepatic) and gallbladder cancer cases when the annual incidence is reported. The overall incidence of extrahepatic cholangiocarcinoma has been suggested at 1 case per 100,000 individuals in the United States, with a higher incidence in Western countries compared with Asian and Eastern countries.

Ampullary adenocarcinoma is a rare tumor arising from the ampulla of Vater that accounts for 6% to 19% of periampullary cancers. Although uncommon, its incidence is estimated at 6 cases per 1 million individuals and has been slowly rising over the past 3 decades. In addition, compared to other periampullary malignancies, ampullary cancers tend to become symptomatic at an earlier stage and thus as many as 80% of these tumors are resectable. Duodenal adenocarcinoma of the periampullary region is the least common of the main periampullary cancers.[3] It is often difficult to estimate the exact incidence of these tumors because duodenal cancers are combined with other malignancies of the small bowel when reporting overall statistics.

PATHOLOGY

Pathologic examination of the surgical specimen after pancreaticoduodenectomy (PD) reveals a disease breakdown with a pattern similar to the overall incidence. The majority (40% to 60%) of resections are for pancreatic adenocarcinoma, 10% to 20% for ampullary adenocarcinoma, 10% for distal cholangiocarcinoma, 5% to 10% for duodenal adenocarcinoma, and 10% to 20% for benign disease. However, it is important to note that this breakdown only involves resectable tumors. Only a minority of patients who present with pancreatic adenocarcinoma are found to have a resectable tumor without distant metastases, and as such it is likely that the incidence of pancreatic adenocarcinoma making up periampullary tumors is much higher than reported.

Most pancreatic adenocarcinomas arise from the head, neck, or uncinate process and are the predominant tumor pathology seen in this region. In addition, rare tumor variants exist for pancreatic adenocarcinoma, including tubular adenocarcinoma, adenosquamous carcinoma, colloid carcinoma (mucinous noncystic), and medullary carcinoma. Each variant has distinct pathologic findings different from the traditional pancreatic adenocarcinoma, often leading to differences in survival following resection. Other less common tumor types in the pancreas include acinar cell cancer, PNETs, MCNs, and SPNs.

Cystic neoplasms of the pancreas have been more frequently identified in recent years, likely due to the increasing use of cross-sectional imaging. The majority of these lesions are benign with little malignant potential, such as serous cystadenomas, whereas others such as IPMNs are of keen interest given their identification as precursors to the development of invasive ductal adenocarcinoma. Noninvasive IPMNs are classified based on their degree of dysplasia into three groups—low grade, intermediate grade, or high grade—although recent discussion has suggested simply categorizing all noninvasive IPMNs as either low/intermediate grade or high grade. In addition, histologic subtypes of IPMNs exist including pancreatobiliary type, gastric type, intestinal type, and oncocytic type, with slightly differing natural histories based on each type.[4] Institutional studies of IPMNs have demonstrated a rate of associated invasive cancer at the time of resection between 30% and 38%.[5,6] Data are equivocal, however, as to whether invasive adenocarcinoma derived from an IPMN possesses improved overall survival when compared to traditional PDAC.[6,7]

Similar precursors of the biliary tree known as intraductal papillary neoplasms of the biliary tract (IPNBs) have also been identified in recent years.[8–10] Analogous to IPMNs, these are also characterized by different histologic subtypes (pancreaticobiliary, intestinal, gastric, and oncocytic), identified based upon histopathologic analysis of cells present and by immunologic staining by cytokeratins and mucin markers.[9] IPNBs are believed to be precursor lesions to the development of cholangiocarcinoma, much like the progression of an IPMN to PDAC. One series of 343 patients found that 11% ($n = 39$) of patients had IPNB by histology after resection of a bile duct tumor, with 29 of 39 patients (74%) having an invasive carcinoma component in association with the IPNB.[9]

Rare causes of periampullary tumors include metastatic disease from the kidney, lung, melanoma, breast, colon, stomach, or tumors from other primary sites of disease. Sarcomas, including gastrointestinal stromal tumors (GISTs), leiomyosarcoma, histiocytomas, and fibrosarcomas, may also arise in the periampullary region. Differentiation among these different sarcoma types is important in terms of management, as GISTs are highly responsive to targeted immunotherapies such as imatinib mesylate (Gleevec). Lymphomas have also been seen in the periampullary region given the presence of large areas of lymphatic tissue around the pancreas and porta hepatis.

RISK FACTORS

PANCREATIC ADENOCARCINOMA

The risk factors for pancreatic adenocarcinoma are the best documented of all the periampullary tumors, although our understanding of them remains incomplete. These risk factors include advanced age, diabetes mellitus, obesity, African American race, a current or prior history of tobacco use, chronic pancreatitis, and family history/genetics.[11] Most cases of PDAC occur in adults older than 50 years, with pancreatic cancer rarely seen under the age of 40 years. Smoking confers an increased risk of developing PDAC compared to nonsmokers (odds ratio [OR] 1.71),

and former smokers who had quit for less than 5 years were also shown to have a higher risk of developing PDAC (OR 1.78).[12] A family history of pancreatic cancer, especially when two or more first-degree relatives are affected, is considered a strong predictor of developing PDAC. Other factors such as alcohol consumption, coffee consumption, prior cholecystectomy, physical inactivity, and a dietary intake of meat and sugar have been suggested to confer an increased risk of PDAC, but these are unlikely to be true risk factors.[13]

Several genetic syndromes and risk factors have been associated with an increased risk of developing pancreatic cancer. However, familial clustering accounts for only 5% to 10% of pancreatic cancer cases.[14] Large population studies have shown an overall risk of 1.8 to 2.3 for the development of PDAC in individuals with an affected first-degree relative.[13,15,16] This risk increases to 6.4-fold with two first-degree affected relatives, and three first-degree relatives with PDAC confers a 32-fold increased risk of an individual developing pancreatic cancer.[13] Individuals with BRCA1 and BRCA2 mutations are at a higher risk of developing pancreatic tumors, with a risk of 3.5- to 10-fold in BRCA2 mutation carriers.[17,18] Germline BRCA2 mutations are also associated with an increased risk of breast, prostate, and ovarian cancer. Peutz-Jeghers syndrome, defined by STK11/LKB1 mutations, is a rare autosomal dominant disorder marked by the development of benign hamartomatous polyps in the GI tract and small, dark-colored macules in and around the mouth. Individuals with this disorder carry a 132-fold increased risk of developing PDAC.[17,19] Familial atypical multiple mole melanoma (FAMMM syndrome) involving mutations in CDKN2A leads to the development of multiple atypical nevi and an increased risk of melanoma, and can confer an almost 22-fold increased risk of pancreatic cancer.[20] Other genetic risk factors include familial adenomatous polyposis (FAP) (APC mutations) with a 4.5-fold increased risk, Lynch syndrome (MSH2, MLH1/HNPCC mutations) with an 8.6-fold increased risk of PDAC, and hereditary pancreatitis (PRSS1 mutations) with a 53-fold increased risk of pancreatic cancer for affected individuals.[17,21]

SOMATIC GENETIC ALTERATIONS AND PANCREATIC CANCER

A high level of detail regarding the global genetic landscape (i.e., cancer genome) is known for pancreatic cancer as the result of several recent publications on this subject. A comprehensive analysis of pancreatic tumors from 24 individuals identified a core set of 12 signaling pathways that were genetically altered in 67% to 100% of the tumors studied.[22] These mutations allow the cancer to evade apoptosis, grow unconstrained, and metastasize to distant organs. All tumors studied were found to have mutations in the KRAS, Wnt/Notch, TGF-β, and hedgehog (Hh) signaling genes, whereas most cancers sampled have mutations in processes that regulate invasion or involve DNA damage control (p53). Overall, an average of 63 mutations were found per individual tumor indicating heterogeneity among most pancreatic tumors despite a core of common mutations. In addition, a comparison of mutations in key pathways such as KRAS, SMAD4, and p53 found a similar rate of mutations in these genes among both familial and sporadic pancreatic cancer cases.

A larger analysis of 100 pancreatic tumors by whole-genome sequencing recently confirmed the presence of many common mutational pathways (KRAS, SMAD4, TP53, CDKN2A, and MAP2K4) while further demonstrating that tumors could be categorized into four subtypes based on the mutations observed: stable, scattered, unstable, and locally rearranged.[23] The stable subtype (20%) contained less than 50 structural variation events, suggesting defects in the cell cycle and mitosis with similar point mutations seen for *KRAS* and *SMAD4*. The locally rearranged subtype (30%) involved a significant focal event on one or two chromosomes, either involving focal regions of copy number gain or complex genomic rearrangements. The scattered subtype (36%) involved tumors with a moderate range of nonrandom chromosomal damage. The least common type of tumor seen was the unstable subtype (14%), which involved tumors with a large number of structural variation events suggesting defects in DNA maintenance. This work suggested that the different subtypes could aid in the understanding of the underlying tumor and offer potential stratification methods for therapeutic intervention.

Genomic data have also suggested a large window of time in which these mutations accumulate and lead to the development of a clinically evident pancreatic tumor. Sequencing of cancer cells from primary and metastatic pancreatic tumors involving data on the accumulation of mutations estimates an average of 11.7 years from tumor initiation to the development of a clinically visible primary pancreatic tumor, with an additional 6.8 years to the development of metastatic disease.[24] This suggests that a large window of time is needed for mutations to occur and tumors to develop, and offers a potentially long window for future screening programs.

OTHER PERIAMPULLARY TUMORS

Risk factors for the remaining periampullary tumors (duodenal, ampullary, and distal cholangiocarcinoma) are often related to genetic or environmental factors, but these are less well understood than pancreatic tumors. Similar to pancreatic adenocarcinoma, most periampullary cancers are seen in patients of advanced age with the tumors rarely occurring before the age of 50 years.[25,26] A higher risk of developing cholangiocarcinoma has been seen in association with primary sclerosing cholangitis (PSC), choledochal cysts, choledocholithiasis, inflammatory bowel disease, and infections including liver flukes (*Clonorchis sinensis*, 4.8-fold risk), hepatitis B (OR 2.6), and hepatitis C (OR 1.8).[27,28] Ampullary carcinoma is increasingly seen in patients with hereditary polyposis syndromes including hereditary nonpolyposis colorectal cancer (HNPCC), Peutz-Jegher syndrome, and FAP.

DIAGNOSIS

CLINICAL FINDINGS

Pancreatic and periampullary malignancies are often difficult to diagnose early given a paucity of specific clinical findings. Many patients, especially those with small tumors and early-stage disease, will be asymptomatic. Furthermore, exact symptoms are vague and depend on the location of the lesion. The most common presenting symptom for periampullary tumors is jaundice caused by biliary outflow obstruction, classically referred to as "painless jaundice." Often, biliary obstruction will be associated with dark urine, pruritus, scleral icterus, and light-colored stools. Additional symptoms of weight loss, fatigue, and mild epigastric pain or discomfort radiating to the back may be present, and nausea and vomiting may be seen in those with duodenal obstruction. Conversely, patients with tumors of the body or tail of the pancreas more commonly present with weight loss, nausea, early satiety, and epigastric pain. Patients with extensive disease burden or tumor invasion into the celiac nerve plexus may present with severe abdominal pain, although this is not common. Rare symptoms of periampullary and pancreatic neoplasms include acute pancreatitis, upper GI bleeding, and cholangitis.

A complete history and physical should be performed for any patient presenting with concern for a pancreatic or periampullary neoplasm, with special focus on any potential risk factors or a family history of malignancy. Physical examination is often nonspecific but may include jaundice, scleral icterus, abdominal discomfort, hepatomegaly, or a palpable gallbladder (Courvoisier sign). Palpation of a periumbilical nodule (Sister Mary Joseph nodule), left supraclavicular node (Virchow node), or pelvic nodules felt on rectal examination (Blumer shelf nodule) may be present in patients with advanced periampullary tumors.

Laboratory findings may be subtle in patients with periampullary tumors. Mildly elevated transaminases, alkaline phosphatase, and bilirubin levels may be seen, and can become severely elevated in those patients with obstructive jaundice. Coagulopathy may be seen in association with biliary obstruction due to vitamin K deficiency, whereas the combination of malnutrition and weight loss can lead to anemia and hypoalbuminemia. New-onset diabetes with an elevated fasting glucose precedes the diagnosis of periampullary tumors in some with pancreatic cancer. Tumor markers should be sent including carcinoembryonic antigen (CEA) and carbohydrate antigen 19-9 (CA 19-9). Although CA 19-9 levels are elevated in most patients with pancreatic and periampullary cancers, it has limited diagnostic capabilities given similar elevations seen in patients with benign pancreas and biliary diseases. However, baseline CA 19-9 levels are important to obtain and trend to allow monitoring for tumor recurrence or evaluating therapy response.

IMAGING STUDIES

Pancreatic and periampullary tumors are most frequently diagnosed through a combination of imaging modalities including right upper quadrant ultrasound (RUQ US), computed tomography (CT) scans, magnetic resonance imaging (MRI), magnetic resonance cholangiopancreatography (MRCP), endoscopic ultrasound (EUS), endoscopic retrograde cholangiopancreatography (ERCP), and percutaneous transhepatic cholangiography (PTC). An RUQ US may be the first imaging obtained to work up a patient with abdominal pain or biliary symptoms,

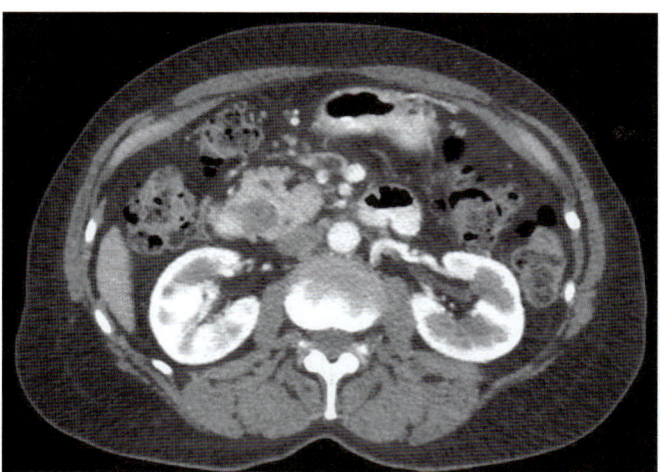

FIGURE 96.1 Computed tomography scan demonstrating a hypodense lesion in the head of the pancreas, confirmed to be pancreatic adenocarcinoma.

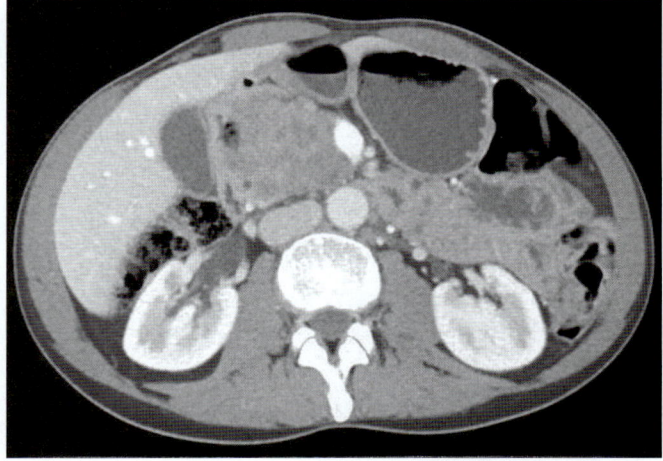

FIGURE 96.2 Computed tomography scan of a large heterogeneous pancreatic head mass with invasion into the duodenum.

and may show a dilated biliary tree, gallstones, or gallbladder distention. Hepatic metastases and ascites suggestive of advanced disease may also be seen by ultrasound. However, this modality is not sensitive for demonstrating a pancreatic or periampullary mass, and additional imaging is needed to sufficiently rule out a tumor in this region.

High-quality cross-sectional imaging is imperative for the detection of a periampullary tumor, assessment of resectability, and the evaluation of metastatic disease. In the majority of patients, periampullary tumors are first identified by CT scan obtained due to vague abdominal complaints or identified incidentally when the patient undergoes imaging for an unrelated etiology. Multidetector computed tomography (MDCT) scans remain the most useful initial imaging modality and provide a highly sensitive way to identify periampullary tumors and their relationship to nearby structures (Fig. 96.1). Three-dimensional reconstruction of the vasculature aids in determining the relationship between the mass and important blood vessels, namely the superior mesenteric artery, celiac artery axis, superior mesenteric vein, and portal vein. MDCT has a sensitivity as high as 90% for evaluating vascular involvement of pancreatic tumors and distal cholangiocarcinoma. Furthermore, MDCT has the capability to detect liver metastases with a relatively high sensitivity, although this is dependent on the size of the lesion. Together, MDCT can aid in the diagnosis of periampullary tumors, assessing for resectability, and determining alternative treatment methods in patients with vascular invasion, local advancement, or distant disease (Fig. 96.2).

MRI is rarely the first imaging modality used for the diagnosis of periampullary tumors, but is often obtained in conjunction with an MDCT scan to better delineate periampullary tumors. This is typically the case when distal biliary obstruction is present or suspected but no discrete mass can be seen on CT scan. MRI and MRCP are especially useful in the detection of distal bile duct tumors, allowing for easier identification of a tumor's extent and visualization of the bile and pancreatic ducts (Fig. 96.3A and B). Often, a tumor of the bile ducts will be identified on MRI

or MRCP by thickening or irregularity of the bile duct wall with proximal dilatation of the biliary tree. MRCP, especially, is a noninvasive method to assess the bile ducts without the risk of invasive cholangiopancreatography but has been shown to be equivalent to ERCP in the diagnosis of cholangiocarcinoma. However, if an intervention such as stent placement or tissue diagnosis is required, ERCP is still necessary.

EUS and ERCP provide useful adjuncts to cross-sectional imaging for the diagnosis of periampullary tumors. These methods provide a method to diagnose a suspected pancreatic or periampullary tumor while also obtaining tissue for pathologic diagnosis. EUS provides direct visualization of ampullary and duodenal cancers with a relatively easy way to obtain tissue for pathologic diagnosis. EUS can also provide information on the location and size of a pancreatic lesion in addition to nodal staging and information on vascular invasion. Fine-needle aspiration can be added to EUS to provide tissue diagnosis prior to surgical resection or neoadjuvant therapies in situations where a definitive diagnosis is unclear. On ERCP, pancreatic cancers will classically demonstrate a long, irregular stricture in the pancreatic duct with distal dilation of both the pancreatic and distal bile ducts (Fig. 96.4). Furthermore, ERCP can be utilized to decompress an obstructive biliary tree with stent placement while obtaining bile duct brushings, thus alleviating jaundice and obtaining a tissue diagnosis. However, routine ERCP and stenting is not advised on all patients with pancreatic or periampullary tumors given the potential increase in wound infections after surgery and associated complications such as post-ERCP pancreatitis.

PTC is an additional method used to define the biliary anatomy. However, given its invasive nature, it is usually reserved for instances when endoscopic decompression is not possible. Tissue biopsies can be performed at the time of cholangiography, and a drainage catheter can be inserted to allow for decompression of the biliary tree when ERCP has failed. PTC has been shown to have a similar sensitivity and specificity when compared to ERCP

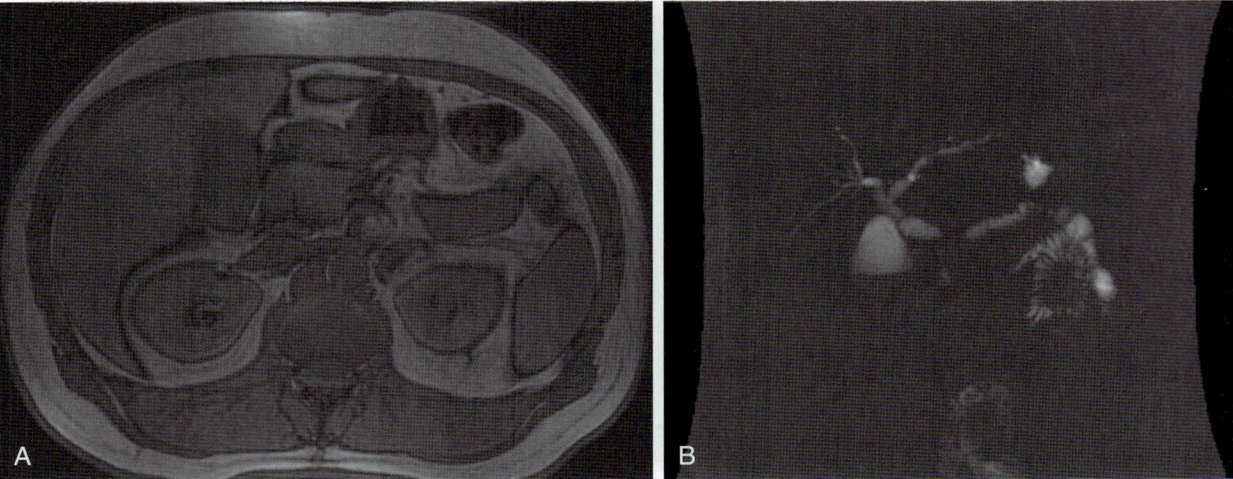

FIGURE 96.3 (A) T2-weighted magnetic resonance image demonstrating a hypodense mass in the head of the pancreas, with (B) associated coronal magnetic resonance cholangiopancreatography demonstrating dilation of the common bile duct and pancreatic duct due to the mass.

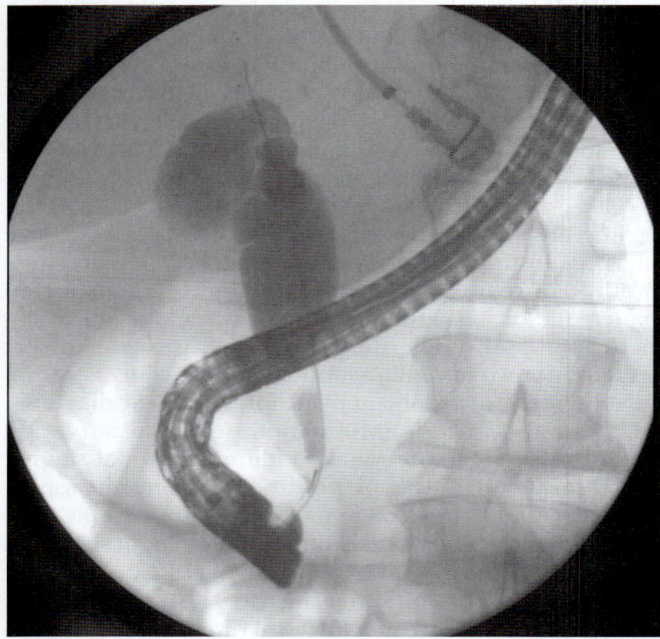

FIGURE 96.4 Endoscopic retrograde cholangiopancreatography showing dilation of the proximal common bile duct due to a distal common bile duct mass.

for obtaining a tissue diagnosis for cholangiocarcinoma. However, PTC is associated with more severe complications such as hemobilia when compared to EUS or ERCP, often due to its more invasive nature.

TISSUE DIAGNOSIS

Surgery is often performed for resectable pancreatic tissues on the basis of imaging findings and clinical presentation alone without confirmation of a tissue diagnosis. However, percutaneous (ultrasound or CT guided) or EUS-guided biopsy can be used to obtain tissue confirmation of the diagnosis for a pancreatic tumor.

Percutaneous biopsy is most often used to assess suspicious liver lesions, whereas EUS is best for biopsy of the primary lesion. Biopsy is highly recommended for patients with unresectable disease to help guide therapy, patients under consideration for neoadjuvant therapy to confirm diagnosis, and patients being considered for palliative therapy. In addition, patients with suspicion for metastatic disease from another site to the pancreas or patients with lymphoma should undergo biopsy, especially if the disease can be best managed without resection.

Tissue diagnosis of distal bile duct cancers can be performed by taking tumor brushings by ERCP or PTC, often performed at the same time a stent is placed to relieve obstruction. Both ERCP and PTC have been shown to have a similar sensitivity and specificity for the ability to obtain a tissue diagnosis.[29,30] However, as with pancreatic tumors, a negative biopsy does not rule out cholangiocarcinoma. Ampullary and duodenal cancers can be biopsied by upper endoscopy.

PREOPERATIVE STAGING

Tumors are staged based on the tumor, nodes, metastases (TNM) staging system set forth by the American Joint Committee on Cancer (AJCC) and the National Comprehensive Cancer Network, with AJCC guidelines present for pancreatic tumors, extrahepatic bile duct tumors, ampulla of Vater tumors, and small intestine tumors. These criteria take into account the size and extent of the primary tumor (T stage), the involvement of lymph nodes (N stage), and the presence of distant metastases (M stage), incorporating all three into an overall stage for each individual. This overall stage can then be used to help guide treatment and provide information on prognosis. Information regarding each aspect of the TNM stage can offer an assessment of tumor resectability. This is predominantly true for pancreatic adenocarcinoma, in which the presence of nodal metastases beyond the field of resection, invasion of the aorta, or tumors with encasement greater than 180 degrees of the superior mesenteric artery or celiac artery is a contraindication to resection of the primary tumor.[31] Currently, there are no formal criteria for determining resectability for nonpancreatic periampullary tumors, and thus the PDAC criteria is usually used in these situations. Additionally, the presence of distant metastases is a contraindication to resection for all the main periampullary tumors.

Preoperative staging is performed prior to treatment for all periampullary tumors, often using the same imaging techniques that are used for diagnosis. MDCT with intravenous contrast is performed in both the venous and arterial phases, and provides information about the resectability of a tumor with respect to nearby vasculature. Three-dimensional reconstruction of CT scans has the added ability to predict resectability of periampullary tumors, with an accuracy of more than 90% according to studies.[32] In addition, three-dimensional CT is highly accurate in determining tumor invasion of the superior mesenteric vessels as well as tumor burden and the ability to obtain a margin negative resection. In addition, MDCT scans are highly effective in detecting the presence of liver metastases, particularly those greater than 1 cm in diameter.[33] Imaging of the chest is also recommended for preoperative workup by CT of the thoracic cavity or chest radiograph, although it is uncommon to have isolated lung metastases without peritoneal metastases.[31]

Staging laparoscopy is a controversial topic and is center dependent with regard to the preoperative staging and management of periampullary tumors. Some surgeons will use staging laparoscopy in all patients prior to surgical resection. Other surgeons will not routinely perform staging laparoscopy, citing improvements in cross-sectional imaging that has substantially decreased the number of tumors found to be unresectable at the time of surgery. Finally, others will use it selectively in those patients with suspicious lesions outside the resection bed. In general, the yield of staging laparoscopy depends on the quality of imaging with higher yields as the quality of the image decreases. Regardless of the institution's practice, staging laparoscopy is only used to identify occult metastases and not to determine local tumor relationships to vessels. This is best accomplished with high-quality imaging.

RESECTION OF PANCREATIC AND PERIAMPULLARY CANCER

PANCREATICODUODENECTOMY

The first successful operation for periampullary cancer was performed at the Johns Hopkins Hospital by William S. Halsted in 1898. This operation involved the local resection of a wedge-shaped portion of the periampullary duodenum with end-to-end closure of the duodenum and reimplantation of the bile and pancreatic ducts for a patient with obstructive jaundice.[34] The patient survived for 7 months after surgery before eventually dying from complications due to local tumor recurrence. The first en bloc resection of the head of the pancreas and duodenum was performed by the Italian surgeon Alessandro Codvilla that same year, but the patient succumbed to complications in the early postoperative period. Walther Kausch performed the first successful two-stage PD in 1909, and in 1914 Hirschel reported the first one-stage

PD with survival of the patient 1-year out from surgery.[35,36] It was not until 1935 with Allen O. Whipple's refinements to the procedure that the operation became a viable, mainstream operation in the United States for the treatment of periampullary tumors.[37] However, the operation was rarely performed over the next several decades given a high morbidity and mortality rate, and in the 1960s and 1970s some surgeons even advocated abandoning the procedure altogether. Beginning in the 1980s, John L. Cameron at the Johns Hopkins Hospital led the charge of refining several aspects of the operation and postoperative care, greatly reducing the mortality of the PD to its current level of 1% to 3% in high-volume academic settings.

PD is the current mainstay of surgical treatment for periampullary cancers. The surgery involves three basic steps: exploration and assessment for occult metastatic disease, resection of the tumor, and reconstruction of the GI tract. A vertical midline incision from the xiphoid process to below the umbilicus is performed to obtain exposure for the operation. Alternatively, a bilateral subcostal incision may be used. A self-retaining retractor is then placed to improve exposure in the operative field. Upon entry, the abdominal cavity is surveyed for evidence of metastases and the tumor is assessed for resectability. The entire liver is inspected and palpated for the presence of metastases, as is the omentum, parietal and visceral peritoneal surfaces, pelvis, and small and large intestine. Any suspicious lesions found during exploration should be sent for intraoperative pathologic analysis because evidence of distant metastasis is a contraindication to resection. Some surgeons advocate starting with staging laparoscopy as stated earlier to perform this portion of the operation.

The viscera are now mobilized. First the right colon is mobilized and the transverse mesocolon is dissected free from the head of the pancreas. The superior mesenteric vein caudal to the neck of the pancreas can be identified running anterior to the third portion of the duodenum. The superior mesenteric vein is identified by dissecting the fatty tissue at the base of the transverse mesocolon and below the neck of the pancreas. Division of the branches emptying into the anterior surface of the superior mesenteric vein—the right gastroepiploic and middle colic may be necessary for safe continued cephalad dissection. Often, a vein retractor to lift the inferior edge of the neck of the pancreas is useful for visualization. The plane anterior to the superior mesenteric vein is developed under direct vision.

A Kocher maneuver is performed by elevating the duodenum and head of the pancreas out of the retroperitoneum. The hepatoduodenal ligament is then divided exposing the portal triad. The gallbladder is mobilized out of the gallbladder fossa and the cystic duct and artery are divided. The portal structures should be assessed during these maneuvers to determine if a replaced right hepatic artery originating from the superior mesenteric artery is present. If found, this vessel should be dissected and protected from injury. The common hepatic duct is encircled and divided close to the level of the cyst duct entry site early in the operation. The gastroduodenal artery is divided following a test clamp to confirm flow through the proper hepatic artery. The bile duct is retracted caudally, and a dissection plane is opened on the anterior surface of the portal vein. After the plane anterior to the portal vein and superior mesenteric vein is complete, a Penrose drain can be looped under the neck of the pancreas.

A classic PD involves the resection of 30% to 40% of the distal stomach and a pylorus-performing PD is performed by dividing the proximal portion of the duodenum 2 to 3 cm distal to the pylorus with a linear stapling device. The GI tract is divided distally at a point of mobile jejunum, in most cases approximately 20 to 30 cm distal to the ligament of Treitz. The mesenteric vasculature to the third and fourth portions of the duodenum and divided jejunum is carefully divided. Once the distal duodenum and proximal jejunum are separated from their mesentery, it can be delivered dorsal beneath the superior mesenteric vessels from the left to the right side.

Stay sutures are placed superiorly and inferiorly on the pancreatic remnant to reduce bleeding from the segmental pancreatic arteries. The pancreatic neck is then divided with a scalpel or with electrocautery. The Penrose drain placed previously under the neck of the pancreas is used to elevate the pancreatic tissue during division, thus protecting the underlying major veins. The main pancreatic duct should be identified so that it can be incorporated into the subsequent reconstruction. The portal vein and superior mesenteric veins are then rolled out of the vascular groove. The specimen is then removed by dividing the uncinate process of the pancreas from the superior mesenteric artery. This is accomplished by serially clamping, dividing, and tying the smaller vascular branches of the superior mesenteric artery and should result in skeletonization of the superior mesenteric artery for at least 180 degrees. The specimen can then be removed. The pancreatic neck margin, uncinate margin, and common hepatic duct margins are marked for pathologic examination.

Focus can now be turned to reconstruction. There are multiple options for reconstruction, with the most common involving creation of a pancreaticojejunostomy to the divided jejunum, followed by hepaticojejunostomy and then gastrojejunostomy. For pylorus-sparing PD, the gastrojejunostomy is replaced by a duodenojejunostomy. The pancreaticojejunostomy is the most problematic anastomosis of the three and is the most common cause of the procedure's morbidity. Controversy exists regarding the best type of pancreaticojejunostomy, the use of pancreatic duct stents, and the use of adjuncts such as fibrin glue or somatostatin analogues. The pancreatic anastomosis can be performed with an invagination technique or a duct-to-mucosa anastomosis. With either technique, the proximal jejunal stump is brought through a defect in the mesocolon to the right of the middle colic artery. The duct-to-mucosa anastomosis is constructed in an end-to-side fashion in which the outer row consists of interrupted 3-0 silk sutures that incorporate the capsule of the transected pancreas and seromuscular bites of the jejunum. A small defect is then made in the jejunum to which a duct-to-mucosa anastomosis is performed that incorporates the pancreatic duct and the full thickness of the jejunum with interrupted 5-0 absorbable monofilament suture. Some

surgeons prefer to stent this anastomosis with a 6-cm pediatric feeding tube. Three centimeters of the stent is placed in the pancreatic duct, and the other half is placed in the jejunum. This stent typically passes through the intestinal tract and into the stool within a couple of weeks.

The invagination technique is performed with an end-to-end or end-to-side pancreaticojejunostomy. The pancreatic remnant is circumferentially cleared and mobilized for 2 to 3 cm to allow for an optimal anastomosis. The pancreaticojejunostomy is performed in two layers, with the outer layer consisting of interrupted 3-0 silk sutures that incorporate the capsule of the pancreas and the seromuscular layers of the jejunum. The inner layer consists of running 3-0 absorbable suture that incorporates the capsule and a portion of the cut edge of the pancreas and the full thickness of the jejunum. An attempt should be made to incorporate the pancreatic duct into the inner layer for several bites to splay it open. When completed, this anastomosis invaginates the cut surface of the pancreatic neck into the jejunal lumen for several centimeters. The stomach can also be used to reconnect the pancreas with an invagination method similar to the one described for the jejunum. However, the pancreaticojejunostomy is more commonly performed.

The biliary anastomosis is performed next with an end-to-side hepaticojejunostomy approximately 5 to 10 cm distal to the pancreaticojejunostomy. This anastomosis is performed with a single layer of interrupted absorbable suture. Finally, the last anastomosis, either a duodenojejunostomy or gastrojejunostomy, is performed depending on whether the pylorus has been preserved. This anastomosis can be performed 10 to 15 cm distal to the hepaticojejunostomy, proximal to the portion of jejunum traversing the defect in the mesocolon. Alternatively, it can be performed in antecolic fashion more distally on the jejunal limb, distal to where it traverses the mesocolic defect.

At the end of the operation, closed suction drains are left in place near the pancreatic and biliary anastomoses. Some groups prefer not to drain and accept that if a fluid collection becomes clinically evident postoperatively, percutaneous drainage by interventional radiology may be required. Postoperative management after PD consists of ensuring that the patient has nothing by mouth for 1 or 2 days and slowly advancing the diet to liquids and then solids as tolerated. The stomach is decompressed overnight after the day of surgery with a nasogastric tube (NGT), which is usually removed the next morning unless the output is high. The drains around the pancreatic anastomosis are typically removed once the patient has been on a regular diet without any significant output of amylase-rich or bilious fluid.

LAPAROSCOPIC PANCREATICODUODENECTOMY

In recent years, a minimally invasive approach involving laparoscopic or robotic PD has been used in selected cases. However, given the technical demands of this operation, it is primarily limited to high-volume centers. Large operative series have shown no difference in morbidity or mortality after laparoscopic PD when compared to open pancreatic resection, when performed by a surgeon facile in the approach.[38–40] In addition, no differences in overall survival have been documented between patients undergoing the laparoscopic or open approach for PD.[41]

At our institution, the laparoscopic operation begins with the placement of six ports in a semicircle around the pancreas from the left upper quadrant to the right upper quadrant. These 10-mm ports are placed evenly to give access from all directions. As with the open approach, the abdomen is first evaluated for metastatic disease. Standing on the patient's right side, the lesser sac is entered and the first portion of the duodenum and antrum is then lifted with a retractor. The hepatic artery is identified and dissected with the hook cautery to find the takeoff of the gastroduodenal artery, which is a landmark for the portal vein below. The gastroduodenal artery is dissected and ligated. At this point, the inferior portion of the pancreas is dissected looking for the superior mesenteric vein. Earlier identification of the portal vein helps with superior mesenteric vein identification. Once found, the tunnel is created under the neck of the pancreas with gentle blunt dissection and encircled with an umbilical tape.

Once the tunnel under the pancreas neck is created, the gallbladder is mobilized and used to find the common bile duct, which is encircled with a vessel loop prior to transection. The common bile duct can be used as an anchor to identify the portal vein below. Following the resection of the common bile duct, the Kocher maneuver can be started by mobilizing the duodenum staying close to the bowel. After the extended kocherization is complete, the distal jejunum is identified 30 to 40 cm distal to the ligament of Treitz and transected with a stapler. The stapled ends of the jejunum are sewn to each other with a 25-cm silk stitch with a large gap to facilitate pulling the distal jejunum through the ligament of Treitz for future anastomosis. Next, the colon is lifted and the ligament of Treitz is freed with a hook cautery and the antrum is divided with a stapler.

The final point of transection is the pancreas. The neck is transected with an energy device. The portal vein and superior mesenteric vein (SMV) are rolled out of the vascular groove and the uncinate, which is taken off the superior mesenteric artery with an energy device. Larger vascular branches may require ligation with clips or suture. As the specimen is pulled to the right upper quadrant, the previously sewn jejunal limb will be pulled through the ligament of Treitz defect into proper place for pancreatic and biliary anastomosis. The jejunal suture can be cut at this point to remove the specimen.

Reconstruction of the three anastomoses can now be done with the jejunum already in proper position. These anastomoses are done similar to the open technique requiring intracorporeal stitches. The pancreatic anastomosis can be done from the duct to the mucosa or using the invagination technique. The hepaticojejunostomy is done with interrupted suture with the assistant holding the bowel up to facilitate this step. The final gastroduodenojejunal anastomosis can be done in a two-layered intracorporeal sewn fashion or stapled. At the end of the operation, drains are placed around the anastomosis. Ports are removed and port sites are closed. The postoperative course is similar for patients after laparoscopic PD as for the open approach.

DISTAL PANCREATECTOMY

A distal pancreatectomy is used for tumors located in the body and tail of the pancreas. Staging laparoscopy is advocated for patients with distal pancreatic cancer because carcinomatosis is a more common finding in patients with cancers of the body and tail. Exposure is provided by a vertical midline incision from the xiphoid process to several centimeters below the umbilicus. A bilateral subcostal incision can also be used. Exposure is greatly enhanced with the use of a mechanical retracting device. The lesser sac is entered by elevating the greater omentum off the transverse colon. The splenic artery is controlled with a vessel loop. The splenic flexure of the colon is then mobilized caudally and away from the spleen by dividing the splenocolic ligament. Splenectomy is usually performed with distal pancreatectomy in patients suspected of having carcinoma to obtain better margins, and to remove the lymph nodes at the tip of the pancreas and the hilum of the spleen. However, for some limited benign pancreatic diseases, the spleen can be preserved. The spleen is mobilized toward the midline by dividing the splenorenal ligament with the electrocautery device. The short gastric vessels in the splenogastric ligament are isolated and ligated. A plane is then developed behind the pancreatic tail and body to also mobilize and control the splenic vein. This dissection is continued until an adequate margin is reached beyond the tumor. The splenic artery and vein are isolated at this level and suture ligated. The electrocautery device is next used to transect the pancreatic parenchyma distal to this suture line. A row of overlapping "U" stitches of absorbable suture should then be placed to control the transected remnant. If the main pancreatic duct can be identified, it should be suture ligated with an absorbable monofilament suture. Alternatively, the pancreas can be transected with a stapling device. A frozen section should be performed on the pancreatic margin to confirm clearance of the lesion prior to completion of the operation.

Postoperative management of patients after distal pancreatectomy has a similar, if not higher, risk of pancreatic fistula than PD. Patients are advanced to a solid diet as tolerated. If an operative drain is left in place, it is monitored for signs of a pancreatic leak. Removing the spleen does place the patient theoretically at increased risk for postsplenectomy sepsis, and vaccines are given preoperatively or after recovery for pneumococcus, *Neisseria meningitidis*, and *Haemophilus influenzae*.

In recent years, the laparoscopic approach has become a standard method to perform a distal pancreatectomy with or without splenectomy. Laparoscopic distal pancreatectomy has been demonstrated to have similar outcomes without any increase in morbidity or mortality when compared to the open approach.[42–46] In addition, long-term survival is equivalent for laparoscopic and open distal pancreatectomy.

OPERATIVE COMPLICATIONS

Remarkable advancements have been made over the past several decades with regards to pancreatic surgery, drastically decreasing the operative morbidity and mortality related to the procedure. Currently at high-volume centers, the mortality rate after PD is only 2% to 3%. However, several postoperative complications continue to be frequent after pancreatic resection. The most common complications are delayed gastric emptying (DGE) and pancreatic fistula; postoperative hemorrhage is much less common but has the potential to be lethal.

DELAYED GASTRIC EMPTYING

DGE is the failure of the stomach to empty properly in the absence of an obstruction. More specifically, DGE is defined by the International Study Group of Pancreatic Surgery (ISGPS) as the inability of a patient to return to a standard diet by the end of the first postoperative week, often necessitating the use of prolonged nasogastric intubation of the patient.[47] Studies have placed the rate of DGE as high as 45% after PD, although most large series have estimated the rate to be between 12% and 15%.[48,49] The ISGPS categorizes DGE into three grades (A, B, and C) based upon the patient's symptoms and postoperative management. Patients with grade A DGE are unable to tolerate oral intake by day 7 and require an NGT on postoperative days (PODs) 4 to 7 or replaced after day 3. Vomiting in this grade is uncommon. Patients with DGE grade B cannot tolerate oral intake by POD 14, with an NGT required on PODs 8 to 14 or reinserted after day 7. In grade C DGE, the most severe form, the patient cannot tolerate oral intake after POD 21, and an NGT cannot be discontinued or is required beyond POD 14. Nausea and vomiting are commonly seen in DGE grades B and C. Diagnosis is often made by symptoms or through delayed gastric transit imaged on an upper GI series. Early research suggested that a pylorus-sparing PD may reduce the rate of DGE, but large series comparing the classic and pylorus-sparing PD have been equivocal. Treatment of DGE depends on the individual grade and the severity of symptoms, often starting with the administration of prokinetic drugs (such as erythromycin) and dietary changes, to prolonged treatment with parenteral nutritional support. With these interventions, symptoms will typically resolve and the majority of patients are able to tolerate an oral diet.

PANCREATIC FISTULA

Pancreatic fistula is an abnormal connection between the pancreatic ductal epithelium and another epithelial surface, allowing for the leakage of pancreatic enzyme-rich fluid. According to the International Study Group on Pancreatic Fistula (ISGPF), a postoperative pancreatic fistula is a result of the failure of the pancreatic-enteric anastomosis to heal or a parenchymal leak not related to the anastomosis.[50] A pancreatic fistula is typically diagnosed by measuring the amylase content of fluid from the peripancreatic drain; a drain amylase content greater than three times the serum amylase on or after POD 3 is pathognomonic for a fistula. Rates of pancreatic fistula remain similar for both PD and distal pancreatectomy, ranging from 3% to 28% for both operations. Three different grades (A, B, and C) of pancreatic fistula have been defined based on the patient's appearance, need for parenteral nutrition and/or drainage, and potential for reoperation. Patients with a mild, or grade A, pancreatic

fistula often appear well and require no intervention. Grade B pancreatic fistulas occur in patients who generally appear well, but may require parenteral nutrition or fistula drainage for the fistula to heal. The most severe form are grade C fistulas, in which patients appear ill and require parenteral nutrition, interventional drainage, and potentially even reoperation for treatment.[50] The development of a pancreatic fistula is associated with longer hospital stays, but most patients can be treated effectively without the need for additional surgery.

POSTOPERATIVE HEMORRHAGE

A rare but life-threatening complication is delayed postoperative hemorrhage, with a higher incidence seen after PD than distal pancreatectomy given the location and extent of resection. The ISGPS defines and categorizes postpancreatectomy hemorrhage based on onset, location, and severity.[51] Mild hemorrhage is defined by a drop in hemoglobin concentration of less than 3 g/dL. Conversely, severe hemorrhage involves large-volume blood loss evidenced by a hemoglobin drop of greater than 3 g/dL and requires urgent intervention to treat. Early hemorrhage occurs within 24 hours of surgery, whereas late hemorrhage is defined as occurring on or beyond 5 days after surgery. Late bleeding is usually caused by a pseudoaneurysm formed by a pancreatic fistula or nearby infection, leading to erosion of the vasculature by amylase-rich fluid. Postoperative bleeding can occur intraluminally into the GI tract or extraluminally into the abdominal cavity. As a result, patients may present with signs of an upper GI bleed, hemodynamic instability, or be asymptomatic except for a drop in hemoglobin. Postoperative hemorrhage is preferentially treated by arterial embolization. Surgical exploration and control is reserved for instances in which the patient is too unstable for interventional radiology or in whom embolization is unsuccessful. Mortality is high if this complication occurs.

SURVIVAL AFTER RESECTION OF PERIAMPULLARY CANCER

A study of 5-year survivors undergoing resection of periampullary adenocarcinoma found the 5-year tumor-specific survival rates after resection to be 15% for pancreatic adenocarcinoma, 27% for distal bile duct cancer, 39% for ampullary adenocarcinoma, and 59% for duodenal adenocarcinoma.[52] Thus, despite a common location and surgical resection, survival is impacted by the underlying tumor biology. In addition, improved 5-year survival is seen for patients with well-differentiated tumors, negative lymph nodes, and negative (or R0) resection margins despite the tumor type. Median and overall survival at 5 years is higher for patients with right-sided lesions in the pancreatic head when compared to left-sided pancreatic cancers.[52] Other factors associated with improved survival include small tumor size, negative lymph nodes, well or moderate tumor differentiation, and negative resection margin. Survival is also improved for early-stage tumors. For pancreatic adenocarcinoma, 5-year survival for localized disease is 27% compared to 11% for regional spread to the lymph nodes and only 2% for patients with metastatic disease at diagnosis.[1] Similar survival differences based on stage are also seen for bile duct tumors, ampullary adenocarcinoma, and duodenal adenocarcinoma.

PALLIATIVE MANAGEMENT OF UNRESECTABLE DISEASE

Management of periampullary cancers with a curative intent is often prevented by the late stage in which many patients present. It is estimated that as many as 80% of patients with pancreatic malignancies will present with unresectable or metastatic disease. As a result, a combination of operative and nonoperative management is usually required for symptom management. In the majority of patients, nonoperative palliation is the first choice in treatment, with surgery reserved for patients unable to be adequately managed by these methods. The three main symptoms necessitating palliation are obstructive jaundice, gastric outlet obstruction, and pain.

BILIARY DECOMPRESSION

The majority of patients with periampullary cancers will present with biliary obstruction due to the location of the tumor. Often, this obstruction will lead to symptoms such as jaundice, abdominal discomfort, pruritus, and nausea. Many patients will require endoscopic or surgical decompression of the biliary tract to relieve obstruction, mitigate symptoms, and improve quality of life. This is accomplished by surgical resection of the primary tumor in patients with early stage, resectable disease. However, for patients with metastatic or unresectable periampullary tumors, this requires biliary stenting or surgical bypass.

Biliary decompression can be accomplished by endoscopic or surgical means. Endoscopic stenting involves the placement of a metallic or plastic stent into the biliary tree to provide passage of bile through the area of obstruction. Plastic stents were historically used but required periodic replacement and were more prone to occlusion and migration. As a result, self-expanding metallic stents have been more commonly used in recent years. These have a larger diameter when compared to plastic stents and are less likely to occlude. However, these can fail due to tumor ingrowth, presenting a problem because they are not readily changeable and cannot be removed after placement.[53] PTC drain placement also offers a mechanism for biliary obstruction when endoscopic means fail, and creates a higher risk of complications including hemobilia and bile leakage.

Alternatively, surgical bypass by hepaticojejunostomy, cholecystojejunostomy, or choledochojejunostomy can be performed providing a direct communication between the biliary tree and the small bowel to bypass the obstruction. The most effective operation is hepaticojejunostomy, which is performed by removing the gallbladder and circumferentially dissecting the common hepatic duct near the bifurcation.[54] The common bile duct is divided, and the anastomosis is performed between the duct and a loop of jejunum (requiring a Braun jejunojejunostomy between afferent and efferent limbs) or to a Roux-en-Y limb. Hepaticojejunostomy has a lower rate of failure compared to other surgical methods. Cholecystojejunostomy

has a higher chance of recurrent biliary obstruction and obstructive jaundice given that the insertion site of the cystic duct into the common bile duct is often close to the site of the original obstruction. However, surgical bypass tends to be reserved for patients who are fit for surgery and have failed endoscopic means to relieve obstruction.[54,55]

Comparisons of endoscopic and surgical biliary decompression have demonstrated no clearly superior method, although each has associated benefits and risks. Most studies are retrospective and include only a small number of patients, although a limited number of early randomized controlled trials were performed to compare the two methods. These randomized trials of endoscopic biliary drainage and surgical bypass have demonstrated no differences in morbidity or overall survival between the two methods.[56–59] In general, endoscopic stenting is associated with a shorter hospital length of stay but has a higher incidence of long-term complications. Conversely, surgical bypass is associated with a longer hospital stay and increased early complications but with fewer long-term complications. Thus, the decision between endoscopic and surgical bypass to manage biliary obstruction involves the consideration of several patient factors to determine the best course of treatment for each individual patient. However, at highly specialized centers, endoscopic therapies are traditionally the first line of treatment with surgery reserved for patients who fail these methods.

GASTRIC DECOMPRESSION

Periampullary tumors can often lead to symptoms of gastric outlet obstruction, including persistent nausea and vomiting, pain, an inability to eat, and decreased quality of life.[60] These symptoms are the result of compression of a tumor on the duodenum or dysmotility due to infiltration of the celiac nerve plexus by the tumor.[61] Patients who are unable to undergo surgical resection of their tumor will require an alternative mechanism to provide symptom relief. In most, this can be achieved by duodenal stenting or percutaneous gastrostomy tube with a jejunal extension.

Patients who undergo exploratory laparotomy and are found to be unresectable can undergo a bypass of the duodenum with a gastrojejunostomy, often in conjunction with operative biliary decompression. Early studies comparing hepaticojejunostomy with or without gastric bypass found a benefit to the double bypass given a significant decrease in the incidence of postoperative gastric outlet obstruction when gastrojejunostomy was performed.[62] One study showed that 19% of patients who underwent hepaticojejunostomy alone went on to develop gastric outlet obstruction, compared to none of the patients undergoing palliative gastrojejunostomy.[63] In addition, there was no difference seen in postoperative hospital stay, morbidity, operative mortality, or overall survival between patients undergoing hepaticojejunostomy with or without gastrojejunostomy. Thus, the majority of patients undergoing palliative bypass will undergo a combination operation involving gastrojejunostomy and hepaticojejunostomy, although controversy still remains.

In patients who are not surgical candidates, duodenal stenting is a potential method for the treatment of gastric outlet obstruction. Upper endoscopy is performed and a self-expandable metal stent is placed in the duodenum, with a success rate between 90% and 100%.[64–66] In addition, a very low complication rate is seen with stent placement. It remains to be seen whether endoscopic stent placement is superior to surgical bypass. Studies have suggested that endoscopic duodenal stent placement has comparable outcomes to surgical bypass without differences in hospital costs, morbidity, or mortality.[67] In addition, endoscopic stenting is associated with a shorter hospital stay and faster return to oral intake. However, few randomized controlled trials exist comparing the two methods, with most studies involving a small number of patients and retrospective analysis. Thus, although both mechanisms are likely to be effective, the decision between endoscopic and surgical bypass should be made based on the individual and the patient's fitness to undergo either procedure. As with biliary decompression, endoscopic means are traditionally preferred as first-line treatment with surgery reserved for patients who fail these methods or are unable to be adequately treated with stenting.

PAIN CONTROL

Adequate pain control remains an important aspect of treatment for patients with resectable or unresectable periampullary tumors. Periampullary tumors, especially those increasing in size, can lead to significant abdominal and back pain, severely reducing the patient's quality of life. Standard management of pain for these tumors involves narcotic and nonnarcotic pain medications, such as nonsteroidal antiinflammatory agents. In addition, percutaneous or open celiac plexus block procedures can be used to alleviate pain and reduce the need for narcotic pain medication. Celiac plexus block involves the destruction of the celiac ganglia and/or splanchnic nerves with alcohol or other neurolytic solutions by fluoroscopic guidance, EUS, or CT.[68,69] This can also be performed intraoperatively during a palliative bypass, although this is less commonly performed given advances in noninvasive techniques. Patients who undergo celiac plexus block have been shown to have lower pain scores after 4 and 8 weeks and also require less narcotic medications to achieve adequate pain control.[68] Other studies have shown that pain relief by celiac plexus block can last for months and even years.[70] Adverse effects after celiac plexus block are minimal and transient, and include local pain, hypotension, and diarrhea.

CHEMOTHERAPY

NEOADJUVANT THERAPY

The timing of chemotherapy and radiation is an important consideration for periampullary tumors, especially in resectable patients, and as such there are several potential benefits to neoadjuvant chemotherapy. Many oncologists and surgeons favor the administration of neoadjuvant chemotherapy to assess the biology of the tumor. Some patients have been found to be resectable only to develop metastases weeks to months after resection.[71] The administration of neoadjuvant chemotherapy would theoretically allow time for the aggressive tumor biology to be evident, thus sparing a patient the morbidity and mortality of

surgery. In addition, with the advent of more efficacious regimens neoadjuvant therapy may be a benefit in getting early systemic control. Moreover, studies have suggested that overall survival is similar whether patients undergo neoadjuvant or adjuvant chemotherapy.[72] However, postoperative complications have been shown to delay or prevent the administration of adjuvant chemotherapy, potentially leading to worse outcomes.[73] Thus, the administration of neoadjuvant chemotherapy also ensures that a patient undergoes a full course of chemotherapy, in case other circumstances prevent the administration of adjuvant therapies.

ADJUVANT THERAPY

The administration of adjuvant chemotherapy after surgical resection of periampullary tumors has been shown to confer a survival benefit. Early studies included all periampullary cancers, but recent trials have appropriately focused on each individual tumor type, giving a better understanding of their biology. The best studied is pancreatic adenocarcinoma, with several trials assessing adjuvant therapies after resection of pancreatic adenocarcinoma. The first large trial was the Gastrointestinal Tumor Study Group (GITSG) trial in 1985. The GITSG trial demonstrated that patients undergoing combined adjuvant radiation and chemotherapy with fluorouracil had better overall survival compared to those who did not undergo additional therapy, including three patients in the treatment group who survived more than 5 years after surgery.[74] This trial was followed in recent years by a series of multiinstitutional European trials further assessing adjuvant therapies for pancreatic cancer after resection. The Charité Onkologie 001 (CONKO-001) trial aimed to assess whether improvements in disease-free survival with adjuvant chemotherapy translated into improved overall survival.[75] Patients were randomized to receive adjuvant gemcitabine therapy for 6 months compared to observation alone. The CONKO-001 study demonstrated both significantly improved disease-free and overall survival in the treatment group compared to the observation group, even as far out as 5 years after surgery.

The European Study Group for Pancreatic Cancer (ESPAC-1) trial randomized patients with pancreatic cancer who underwent surgical resection to four treatment groups: chemoradiotherapy alone (20 Gy over 2 weeks plus fluorouracil), chemotherapy alone (fluorouracil), both chemoradiotherapy and chemotherapy, or observation alone.[76] This study demonstrated a survival benefit for patients who received chemotherapy compared to those that did not. Interestingly, however, this study demonstrated that fluorouracil-based chemotherapy alone offered a significant survival benefit compared to chemoradiation therapy, which was actually shown to have a deleterious effect. This finding has been controversial, given several smaller studies suggesting a potential benefit of chemoradiotherapy, particularly in the prevention of local recurrence. The ESPAC-2 and ESPAC-3 trials further assessed the survival benefit of different chemotherapeutic agents after resection, based on the conclusions of ESPAC-1 that chemoradiotherapy was inferior to chemotherapy alone. ESPAC-3 randomized patients to receive fluorouracil or gemcitabine for 6 months, and found no significant difference in progression-free or overall survival between the two cohorts.[77] Overall, these studies confirm a survival benefit for adjuvant chemotherapy after resection in all patients with pancreatic adenocarcinoma.

The role of adjuvant chemotherapy and radiation after resection of distal bile duct cancer, ampullary cancer, and duodenal cancer is less well understood given the rarity of these diseases and a correlating lack of randomized controlled trials assessing adjuvant therapies. Retrospective reviews and small institutional studies have suggested prolonged overall survival in patients with cholangiocarcinoma who received adjuvant chemotherapy after surgical resection compared to surgery alone.[78,79] However, these studies often include patients with different malignancies of the biliary tract, including gallbladder cancer, limiting their applicability to distal bile duct tumors.

CONCLUSION

Periampullary tumors represent a biologically diverse collection of tumors with a common location and presentation. Although these tumors often present with similar symptoms, prognosis and treatment depend on the specific type of cancer. Pancreatic adenocarcinoma is the most common periampullary tumor and as such remains the best studied, despite having the worst prognosis of the four main tumor types. Surgical resection remains the only opportunity for cure in the majority of these patients, and should be attempted when appropriate. However, it is clear that no single modality can effectively treat these patients; as such, chemotherapy and radiation therapy are used in addition to surgery to prolong survival. As new advancements are made both in the diagnosis and resection of these tumors, the future is promising for the treatment of periampullary tumors.

REFERENCES

1. Siegel RL, Miller KD, Jemal A, et al. Cancer treatment and survivorship statistics, 2016. *CA Cancer J Clin.* 2016;66(1):7-30.
2. Howlader N, Noone A, Krapcho M, et al., eds. *SEER Cancer Statistics Review, 1975–2013*. Bethesda, MD: National Cancer Institute; 2016.
3. He J, Ahuja N, Makary MA, et al. 2564 resected periampullary adenocarcinomas at a single institution: trends over three decades. *HPB (Oxford).* 2014;16(1):83-90.
4. Distler M, Kersting S, Niedergethmann M, et al. Pathohistological subtype predicts survival in patients with intraductal papillary mucinous neoplasm (IPMN) of the pancreas. *Ann Surg.* 2013;258(2):324-330.
5. Sohn TA, Yeo CJ, Cameron JL, et al. Intraductal papillary mucinous neoplasms of the pancreas: an updated experience. *Ann Surg.* 2004;239(6):788-797 [discussion 97–99].
6. Schnelldorfer T, Sarr MG, Nagorney DM, et al. Experience with 208 resections for intraductal papillary mucinous neoplasm of the pancreas. *Arch Surg.* 2008;143(7):639-646 [discussion 646].
7. Yamaguchi K, Kanemitsu S, Hatori T, et al. Pancreatic ductal adenocarcinoma derived from IPMN and pancreatic ductal adenocarcinoma concomitant with IPMN. *Pancreas.* 2011;40(4):571-580.
8. Zen Y, Fujii T, Itatsu K, et al. Biliary papillary tumors share pathological features with intraductal papillary mucinous neoplasm of the pancreas. *Hepatology.* 2006;44(5):1333-1343.
9. Rocha FG, Lee H, Katabi N, et al. Intraductal papillary neoplasm of the bile duct: a biliary equivalent to intraductal papillary mucinous neoplasm of the pancreas? *Hepatology.* 2012;56(4):1352-1360.
10. Schmuck RB, de Carvalho-Fischer CV, Neumann C, Pratschke J, Bahra M. Distal bile duct carcinomas and pancreatic ductal

adenocarcinomas: postulating a common tumor entity. *Cancer Med.* 2016;5(1):88-99.
11. Poruk KE, Firpo MA, Adler DG, Mulvihill SJ. Screening for pancreatic cancer: why, how, and who? *Ann Surg.* 2013;257(1):17-26.
12. Vrieling A, Bueno-de-Mesquita HB, Boshuizen HC, et al. Cigarette smoking, environmental tobacco smoke exposure and pancreatic cancer risk in the European Prospective Investigation into Cancer and Nutrition. *Int J Cancer.* 2010;126(10):2394-2403.
13. Gold EB, Goldin SB. Epidemiology of and risk factors for pancreatic cancer. *Surg Oncol Clin N Am.* 1998;7(1):67-91.
14. Michaud DS. Epidemiology of pancreatic cancer. *Minerva Chir.* 2004;59(2):99-111.
15. Permuth-Wey J, Egan KM. Family history is a significant risk factor for pancreatic cancer: results from a systematic review and meta-analysis. *Fam Cancer.* 2009;8(2):109-117.
16. Jacobs EJ, Chanock SJ, Fuchs CS, et al. Family history of cancer and risk of pancreatic cancer: a pooled analysis from the Pancreatic Cancer Cohort Consortium (PanScan). *Int J Cancer.* 2010;127(6):1421-1428.
17. Shi C, Hruban RH, Klein AP. Familial pancreatic cancer. *Arch Pathol Lab Med.* 2009;133(3):365-374.
18. Howe JR, Klimstra DS, Moccia RD, Conlon KC, Brennan MF. Factors predictive of survival in ampullary carcinoma. *Ann Surg.* 1998;228(1):87-94.
19. Korsse SE, Harinck F, van Lier MG, et al. Pancreatic cancer risk in Peutz-Jeghers syndrome patients: a large cohort study and implications for surveillance. *J Med Genet.* 2013;50(1):59-64.
20. Goldstein AM, Fraser MC, Struewing JP, et al. Increased risk of pancreatic cancer in melanoma-prone kindreds with p16INK4 mutations. *N Engl J Med.* 1995;333(15):970-974.
21. Kastrinos F, Mukherjee B, Tayob N, et al. Risk of pancreatic cancer in families with Lynch syndrome. *J Am Med Assoc.* 2009;302(16):1790-1795.
22. Jones S, Zhang X, Parsons DW, et al. Core signaling pathways in human pancreatic cancers revealed by global genomic analyses. *Science.* 2008;321(5897):1801-1806.
23. Waddell N, Pajic M, Patch AM, et al. Whole genomes redefine the mutational landscape of pancreatic cancer. *Nature.* 2015;518(7540):495-501.
24. Yachida S, Jones S, Bozic I, et al. Distant metastasis occurs late during the genetic evolution of pancreatic cancer. *Nature.* 2010;467(7319):1114-1117.
25. DeOliveira ML, Cunningham SC, Cameron JL, et al. Cholangiocarcinoma: thirty-one-year experience with 564 patients at a single institution. *Ann Surg.* 2007;245(5):755-762.
26. Albores-Saavedra J, Schwartz AM, Batich K, Henson DE. Cancers of the ampulla of Vater: demographics, morphology, and survival based on 5,625 cases from the SEER program. *J Surg Oncol.* 2009;100(7):598-605.
27. Khan SA, Toledano MB, Taylor-Robinson SD. Epidemiology, risk factors, and pathogenesis of cholangiocarcinoma. *HPB (Oxford).* 2008;10(2):77-82.
28. Shin HR, Oh JK, Masuyer E, et al. Epidemiology of cholangiocarcinoma: an update focusing on risk factors. *Cancer Sci.* 2010;101(3):579-585.
29. Silva MA, Tekin K, Aytekin F, Bramhall SR, Buckels JA, Mirza DF. Surgery for hilar cholangiocarcinoma; a 10 year experience of a tertiary referral centre in the UK. *Eur J Surg Oncol.* 2005;31(5):533-539.
30. Park MS, Kim TK, Kim KW, et al. Differentiation of extrahepatic bile duct cholangiocarcinoma from benign stricture: findings at MRCP versus ERCP. *Radiology.* 2004;233(1):234-240.
31. Tempero MA, Malafa MP, Behrman SW, et al. Pancreatic adenocarcinoma, version 2.2014: featured updates to the NCCN guidelines. *J Natl Compr Canc Netw.* 2014;12(8):1083-1093.
32. Gambhir SS, Czernin J, Schwimmer J, Silverman DH, Coleman RE, Phelps ME. A tabulated summary of the FDG PET literature. *J Nucl Med.* 2001;42(5 suppl):1S-93S.
33. Tummala P, Junaidi O, Agarwal B. Imaging of pancreatic cancer: an overview. *J Gastrointest Oncol.* 2011;2(3):168-174.
34. Halsted WS. Contributions to the surgery of the bile passages, especially of the common bile duct. *Boston Med Surg J.* 1899;141:645.
35. Kausch W. Das Carcinoma der Papilla Duodeni und seine radikale entfeinung. *Beitr Z Clin Chir.* 1912;78:439.
36. Hirschel G. Die Resection des Duodenums mit der papille wegen karzinoma. *Munchen Med Worchenschr.* 1914;61:1728.

37. Whipple AO, Parsons WB, Mullins CR. Treatment of carcinoma of the ampulla of Vater. *Ann Surg.* 1935;102(4):763-779.

38. Asbun HJ, Stauffer JA. Laparoscopic vs open pancreaticoduodenectomy: overall outcomes and severity of complications using the Accordion Severity Grading System. *J Am Coll Surg.* 2012;215(6):810-819.

39. Lei P, Wei B, Guo W, Wei H. Minimally invasive surgical approach compared with open pancreaticoduodenectomy: a systematic review and meta-analysis on the feasibility and safety. *Surg Laparosc Endosc Percutan Tech.* 2014;24(4):296-305.

40. Palanivelu C, Rajan PS, Rangarajan M, et al. Evolution in techniques of laparoscopic pancreaticoduodenectomy: a decade long experience from a tertiary center. *J Hepatobiliary Pancreat Surg.* 2009;16(6):731-740.

41. Croome KP, Farnell MB, Que FG, et al. Total laparoscopic pancreaticoduodenectomy for pancreatic ductal adenocarcinoma: oncologic advantages over open approaches? *Ann Surg.* 2014;260(4):633-638 [discussion 8–40].

42. Venkat R, Edil BH, Schulick RD, Lidor AO, Makary MA, Wolfgang CL. Laparoscopic distal pancreatectomy is associated with significantly less overall morbidity compared to the open technique: a systematic review and meta-analysis. *Ann Surg.* 2012;255(6):1048-1059.

43. Vijan SS, Ahmed KA, Harmsen WS, et al. Laparoscopic vs open distal pancreatectomy: a single-institution comparative study. *Arch Surg.* 2010;145(7):616-621.

44. Shin SH, Kim SC, Song KB, et al. A comparative study of laparoscopic vs open distal pancreatectomy for left-sided ductal adenocarcinoma: a propensity score-matched analysis. *J Am Coll Surg.* 2014;260(4):633-638.

45. Kooby DA, Hawkins WG, Schmidt CM, et al. A multicenter analysis of distal pancreatectomy for adenocarcinoma: is laparoscopic resection appropriate? *J Am Coll Surg.* 2010;210(5):779-785, 786-787.

46. Fernandez-Cruz L, Saenz A, Astudillo E, et al. Outcome of laparoscopic pancreatic surgery: endocrine and nonendocrine tumors. *World J Surg.* 2002;26(8):1057-1065.

47. Wente MN, Bassi C, Dervenis C, et al. Delayed gastric emptying (DGE) after pancreatic surgery: a suggested definition by the International Study Group of Pancreatic Surgery (ISGPS). *Surgery.* 2007;142(5):761-768.

48. Welsch T, Borm M, Degrate L, Hinz U, Buchler MW, Wente MN. Evaluation of the International Study Group of Pancreatic Surgery definition of delayed gastric emptying after pancreatoduodenectomy in a high-volume centre. *Br J Surg.* 2010;97(7):1043-1050.

49. DeOliveira ML, Winter JM, Schafer M, et al. Assessment of complications after pancreatic surgery: a novel grading system applied to 633 patients undergoing pancreaticoduodenectomy. *Ann Surg.* 2006;244(6):931-937 [discussion 7–9].

50. Bassi C, Dervenis C, Butturini G, et al. Postoperative pancreatic fistula: an international study group (ISGPF) definition. *Surgery.* 2005;138(1):8-13.

51. Wente MN, Veit JA, Bassi C, et al. Postpancreatectomy hemorrhage (PPH): an International Study Group of Pancreatic Surgery (ISGPS) definition. *Surgery.* 2007;142(1):20-25.

52. Sohn TA, Yeo CJ, Cameron JL, et al. Resected adenocarcinoma of the pancreas-616 patients: results, outcomes, and prognostic indicators. *J Gastrointest Surg.* 2000;4(6):567-579.

53. Kaassis M, Boyer J, Dumas R, et al. Plastic or metal stents for malignant stricture of the common bile duct? Results of a randomized prospective study. *Gastrointest Endosc.* 2003;57(2):178-182.

54. Sohn TA, Lillemoe KD, Cameron JL, Huang JJ, Pitt HA, Yeo CJ. Surgical palliation of unresectable periampullary adenocarcinoma in the 1990s. *J Am Coll Surg.* 1999;188(6):658-666 [discussion 66–69].

55. Di Fronzo LA, Cymerman J, Egrari S, O'Connell TX. Unresectable pancreatic carcinoma: correlating length of survival with choice of palliative bypass. *Am Surg.* 1999;65(10):955-958.

56. Smith AC, Dowsett JF, Russell RC, Hatfield AR, Cotton PB. Randomised trial of endoscopic stenting versus surgical bypass in malignant low bile duct obstruction. *Lancet.* 1994;344(8938):1655-1660.

57. Shepherd HA, Royle G, Ross AP, Diba A, Arthur M, Colin-Jones D. Endoscopic biliary endoprosthesis in the palliation of malignant obstruction of the distal common bile duct: a randomized trial. *Br J Surg.* 1988;75(12):1166-1168.

58. Andersen JR, Sørensen SM, Kruse A, Rokkjaer M, Matzen P. Randomised trial of endoscopic endoprosthesis versus operative bypass in malignant obstructive jaundice. *Gut.* 1989;30(8):1132-1135.

59. Maosheng D, Ohtsuka T, Ohuchida J, et al. Surgical bypass versus metallic stent for unresectable pancreatic cancer. *J Hepatobiliary Pancreat Surg.* 2001;8(4):367-373.

60. DiMagno EP, Reber HA, Tempero MA. AGA technical review on the epidemiology, diagnosis, and treatment of pancreatic ductal adenocarcinoma. American Gastroenterological Association. *Gastroenterology.* 1999;117(6):1464-1484.

61. Thor PJ, Popiela T, Sobocki J, Herman RM, Matyja A, Huszno B. Pancreatic carcinoma-induced changes in gastric myoelectric activity and emptying. *Hepatogastroenterology.* 2002;49(43):268-270.

62. Van Heek NT, De Castro SM, van Eijck CH, et al. The need for a prophylactic gastrojejunostomy for unresectable periampullary cancer: a prospective randomized multicenter trial with special focus on assessment of quality of life. *Ann Surg.* 2003;238(6):894-902 [discussion 902–905].

63. Lillemoe KD, Cameron JL, Hardacre JM, et al. Is prophylactic gastrojejunostomy indicated for unresectable periampullary cancer? A prospective randomized trial. *Ann Surg.* 1999;230(3):322-328 [discussion 8–30].

64. Maire F, Hammel P, Ponsot P, et al. Long-term outcome of biliary and duodenal stents in palliative treatment of patients with unresectable adenocarcinoma of the head of pancreas. *Am J Gastroenterol.* 2006;101(4):735-742.

65. Nassif T, Prat F, Meduri B, et al. Endoscopic palliation of malignant gastric outlet obstruction using self-expandable metallic stents: results of a multicenter study. *Endoscopy.* 2003;35(6):483-489.

66. Adler DG, Baron TH. Endoscopic palliation of malignant gastric outlet obstruction using self-expanding metal stents: experience in 36 patients. *Am J Gastroenterol.* 2002;97(1):72-78.

67. Nagaraja V, Eslick GD, Cox MR. Endoscopic stenting versus operative gastrojejunostomy for malignant gastric outlet obstruction—a systematic review and meta-analysis of randomized and non-randomized trials. *J Gastrointest Oncol.* 2014;5(2):92-98.

68. Arcidiacono PG, Calori G, Carrara S, McNicol ED, Testoni PA. Celiac plexus block for pancreatic cancer pain in adults. *Cochrane Database Syst Rev.* 2011;(3):CD007519.

69. Si-Jie H, Wei-Jia X, Yang D, et al. How to improve the efficacy of endoscopic ultrasound-guided celiac plexus neurolysis in pain management in patients with pancreatic cancer: analysis in a single center. *Surg Laparosc Endosc Percutan Tech.* 2014;24(1):31-35.

70. Eisenberg E, Carr DB, Chalmers TC. Neurolytic celiac plexus block for treatment of cancer pain: a meta-analysis. *Anesth Analg.* 1995;80(2):290-295.

71. Fischer R, Breidert M, Keck T, Makowiec F, Lohrmann C, Harder J. Early recurrence of pancreatic cancer after resection and during adjuvant chemotherapy. *Saudi J Gastroenterol.* 2012;18(2):118-121.

72. Spitz FR, Abbruzzese JL, Lee JE, et al. Preoperative and postoperative chemoradiation strategies in patients treated with pancreaticoduodenectomy for adenocarcinoma of the pancreas. *J Clin Oncol.* 1997;15(3):928-937.

73. Wu W, He J, Cameron JL, et al. The impact of postoperative complications on the administration of adjuvant therapy following pancreaticoduodenectomy for adenocarcinoma. *Ann Surg Oncol.* 2014;21(9):2873-2881.

74. Kalser MH, Ellenberg SS. Pancreatic cancer. Adjuvant combined radiation and chemotherapy following curative resection. *Arch Surg.* 1985;120(8):899-903.

75. Oettle H, Neuhaus P, Hochhaus A, et al. Adjuvant chemotherapy with gemcitabine and long-term outcomes among patients with resected pancreatic cancer: the CONKO-001 randomized trial. *J Am Med Assoc.* 2013;310(14):1473-1481.

76. Neoptolemos JP, Stocken DD, Friess H, et al. A randomized trial of chemoradiotherapy and chemotherapy after resection of pancreatic cancer. *N Engl J Med.* 2004;350(12):1200-1210.

77. Neoptolemos JP, Stocken DD, Bassi C, et al. Adjuvant chemotherapy with fluorouracil plus folinic acid vs gemcitabine following pancreatic cancer resection: a randomized controlled trial. *J Am Med Assoc.* 2010;304(10):1073-1081.

78. Todoroki T. Chemotherapy for bile duct carcinoma in the light of adjuvant chemotherapy to surgery. *Hepatogastroenterology.* 2000;47(33):644-649.

79. Patt YZ, Jones DV Jr, Hoque A, et al. Phase II trial of intravenous flourouracil and subcutaneous interferon alfa-2b for biliary tract cancer. *J Clin Oncol.* 1996;14(8):2311-2315.

Neuroendocrine Tumors of the Pancreas

Daniela P. Ladner | Jeffrey A. Norton

The overall prevalence and incidence of pancreatic neuroendocrine tumors (PNETs) is low, approximately 1 to 6 per million population,[1] but it is increasing.[2] Gastrinoma and insulinoma are the two most common functional NETs. Most PNETs are malignant, except insulinomas, which are generally benign. The diagnosis of malignancy may be based on Ki67, which is a marker of cellular proliferation. Malignancy is difficult to diagnose based on histology, but it is often diagnosed with metastases. The presence of metastases proves that a PNET is cancerous.

Beyond insulinoma, other PNETs include somatostatinoma, glucagonoma, pancreatic peptide–producing tumor (PPoma), vasoactive intestinal peptide–producing tumor (VIPoma), growth hormone–releasing factor–producing tumors (GRFomas), adrenocorticotropic hormone–producing tumors (ACTHomas), parathyroid hormone–related protein–producing tumors (PTHrpomas), neurotensinomas, and nonfunctional neuroendocrine tumors. Nonfunctional tumors are the most common. All PNETs produce chromogranin A, which can be used as a tumor marker.[3] Higher levels correlate with greater tumor burdens. Pancreatic endocrine tumors may produce more than one hormone.[3–5] These findings suggest that pancreatic endocrine tumors originate from dedifferentiation of an immature pancreatic stem cell.[5] A recent study identified a pancreatic NET stem cell and that c-MET expression was a predictor of malignant growth.[6]

Microscopically, pancreatic endocrine tumors are composed of sheets of small, round cells with uniform nuclei and cytoplasm (Fig. 97.1). Mitotic figures are rare (Ki67: 1% to 2%), and the precise determination of malignancy cannot be made by histologic appearance.[7]

Some studies suggest that PNETs can be grouped according to aggressive or nonaggressive behaviors. The aggressive forms include glucagonoma, VIPoma, somatostatinoma, and most nonfunctional tumors. Aggressive tumors are characterized by short disease duration, large size, liver metastases, and a reduced long-term survival rate. Studies have shown a number of clinical and tumoral factors that are predictors of aggressive growth. These include liver metastases, lymph node metastasis, local invasion, large (>2 cm) primary tumor size, nonfunctional tumor, and incomplete tumor resection. PNETs are usually highly vascular in nature and appear bright during the arterial phase of a pancreatic protocol computed tomography (CT). However, some tumors do not appear bright, and this appears to correlate with a more aggressive behavior.[8]

The molecular pathogenesis of PNETs is just beginning to be elucidated. Recent studies demonstrate that alterations in the tumor suppressor gene DPC4 located on 18q21 may be involved in tumorigenesis. The specific role for the MEN1 tumor suppressor gene product menin is unknown, although its diverse interactions suggest possible pivotal roles in transcriptional regulation, DNA processing and repair, and cytoskeletal integrity. As mentioned, c-MET gene expression suggests a more aggressive behavior of a PNET.[6]

Pancreatic endocrine tumors occur in various familial conditions, the most common of which is multiple endocrine neoplasia type 1 (MEN-1). PNETs are found in a higher frequency in patients with von Recklinghausen disease, von Hippel-Lindau disease, and tuberous sclerosis. In patients with von Recklinghausen disease, duodenal somatostatinoma and gastrinomas have been reported. Of patients with von Hippel-Lindau disease, 17% had pancreatic endocrine tumors, including both adenomas and carcinomas. Patients with tuberous sclerosis may have a higher incidence of insulinoma and nonfunctional PNETs.

INSULINOMA

Insulinoma is a tumor of pancreatic beta cells that secrete insulin, leading to hypoglycemia. Insulinomas occur approximately in 1 per million people per year.[9] Unlike other neuroendocrine tumors of the pancreas, these tumors are generally benign (90%) and are only occasionally malignant (10%). They are found uniformly distributed throughout the entire pancreas. Patients present as sporadic cases (80%) or as part of a familial syndrome (MEN-1). In the sporadic form the tumors are solitary and small (<2 cm in diameter), making localization difficult.[9] Tumors in the familial form are typically larger (>3 cm) and often multiple.

SYMPTOMS AND DIAGNOSIS

Diagnosis of insulinoma is suggested by the presence of Whipple triad: neuroglycopenic symptoms, low blood glucose levels (<45 mg/dL), and relief of symptoms with glucose administration. Acute neuroglycopenic symptoms include anxiety, dizziness, obtundation, confusion, unconsciousness, personality changes, and seizures. Symptoms are typically worse following exercise or fasting. Eighty percent of patients gain weight. The majority (60% to 75%) of patients are female, and many have undergone extensive psychiatric evaluation. Many have been diagnosed with a neurologic condition such as seizure disorder, cerebrovascular accident, or transient ischemic attack. In a review of 59 patients with insulinoma, the interval from the onset of symptoms to the time of diagnosis ranged from 1 month to 30 years, with the median time to diagnosis being 2 years. Approximately 5% to 10% of

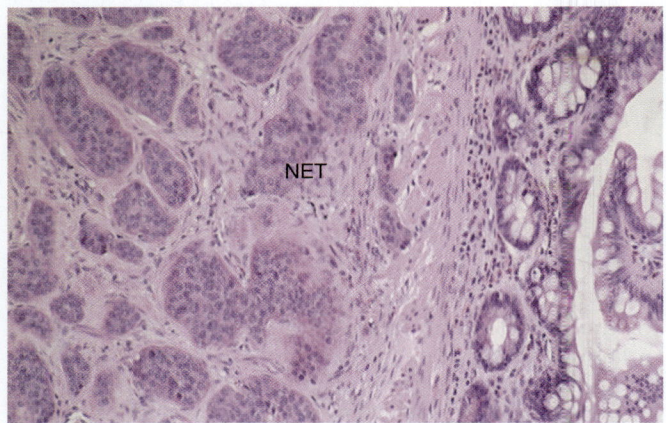

FIGURE 97.1 Neuroendocrine tumor (NET) within the wall of duodenum. This tumor was found to be a somatostatinoma.

patients with insulinoma also have MEN-1, which should be excluded or included based on history, symptoms, physical examination, and biochemical findings.

Patients with a suspicion of having insulinoma should undergo a 72-hour diagnostic fast. Factitious hypoglycemia, in which exogenous insulin or oral hypoglycemic drugs are administered clandestinely, may present with exactly the same symptoms as an insulinoma and must be excluded. Factitious hypoglycemia is seen more commonly in women and may be suspected in individuals with access to insulin or oral hypoglycemic drugs. Urinary sulfonylurea concentration should be measured by gas chromatography–mass spectroscopy to detect abuse of oral hypoglycemic drugs. Antiinsulin antibodies should not be detectable in patients with insulinoma. An increased serum concentration of proinsulin or C-peptide during hypoglycemia effectively excludes the diagnosis of factitious hypoglycemia because exogenously administered insulin does not contain these proteins and actually suppresses their endogenous production. The diagnosis of insulinoma is difficult in patients with chronic renal failure because hypoglycemia may develop for other reasons.

Any patient with a history of neuroglycopenic symptoms and hypoglycemia should undergo a diagnostic 72-hour fast in the inpatient hospital setting under close supervision. During the fast, the patient may drink only water or noncaloric beverages. The study is designed to induce symptoms of hypoglycemia in a controlled setting so that serum levels of glucose and insulin can be measured during symptoms. Blood is tested for serum glucose and immunoreactive insulin concentration every 6 hours and when symptoms develop. If the patient develops neuroglycopenic symptoms, such as confusion, altered mental status, dizziness, or seizure, serum levels of glucose, insulin, C-peptide, and proinsulin are drawn and the fast is terminated. At termination, dextrose is administered intravenously to relieve the symptoms of hypoglycemia.

The diagnosis of insulinoma is made if the patient develops neuroglycopenic symptoms, the serum glucose level is lower than 45 mg/dL, and the concomitant serum level of insulin is higher than 5 µU/L. The symptoms should be ameliorated with the administration of glucose.

Elevated serum levels of C-peptide (>0.7 ng/mL) and proinsulin are confirmatory and exclude factitious hypoglycemia. Sixty percent of patients with insulinoma develop symptoms within 24 hours after fasting, and almost all patients develop symptoms within 72 hours.[10]

PREOPERATIVE LOCALIZATION

Sporadic nonfamilial insulinomas may be difficult to localize precisely preoperatively. For this reason the diagnosis must be unequivocal before contemplating an operation. Ultrasonography is an initial study to try to localize the insulinoma. The tumor appears sonolucent compared with the more echo-dense pancreas. However, ultrasound images only approximately 20% of insulinomas. It is especially limited by overlying bowel gas and obesity.

Thin-cut pancreatic protocol CT with intravenous contrast and serial sections at small intervals through the pancreas (Fig. 97.2) is the noninvasive study of choice. Tumors are hypervascular compared with the surrounding pancreatic parenchyma. CT can demonstrate at least 80% of insulinomas and may be useful for demonstrating liver metastases. Magnetic resonance imaging (MRI) is a newer but similarly sensitive modality for imaging insulinomas. Insulinomas appear bright on T2-weighted images. The sensitivity of MR is equivalent to that of CT and increases with tumor size.

Somatostatin receptor scintigraphy (SRS) or Octreoscan has become an important imaging modality for neuroendocrine tumors of the pancreas. It images tumors based on the density of type 2 somatostatin receptors. Radiolabeled octreotide binds to tumors with somatostatin receptors, causing the tumor to appear as a "hot spot" on whole-body gamma camera scintigraphy. Although SRS correctly identifies 90% of NETs and carcinoid tumors, small insulinomas often are not visible on SRS, although combined with endoscopic ultrasound (EUS) the sensitivity for the diagnosis of insulinoma is reported to be higher than 90%. DOTA scan is a newer type of SRS. It is able to image PNETs better than Octreoscan and has replaced it as the preoperative imaging study of choice.[11]

INVASIVE LOCALIZATION STUDIES

Approximately 50% of patients have small (<2 cm) insulinomas that are not detected by noninvasive imaging tests. EUS (Fig. 97.3) is an important study that can identify tumors as small as 2 to 3 mm. PNETs can be biopsied by fine-needle aspiration for an unequivocal diagnosis and localization.[12] Sensitivity for EUS ranges from 70% to 90%, and specificity is near 100%. It is more accurate in the head of the pancreas than in the body and the tail. Despite the tremendous potential, there are some limitations, including false-positive findings, such as accessory spleens and intrapancreatic lymph nodes. CT is a useful adjunct to EUS to image the liver and rule out disseminated malignancy.

A small number of insulinomas remain occult despite extensive preoperative imaging studies. When the diagnosis is certain based on the result of the 72-hour fast, surgical exploration with careful inspection, palpation, and intraoperative ultrasound (IOUS) is indicated.[13] Studies have shown that the combination of surgical exploration with IOUS identifies nearly all insulinomas.

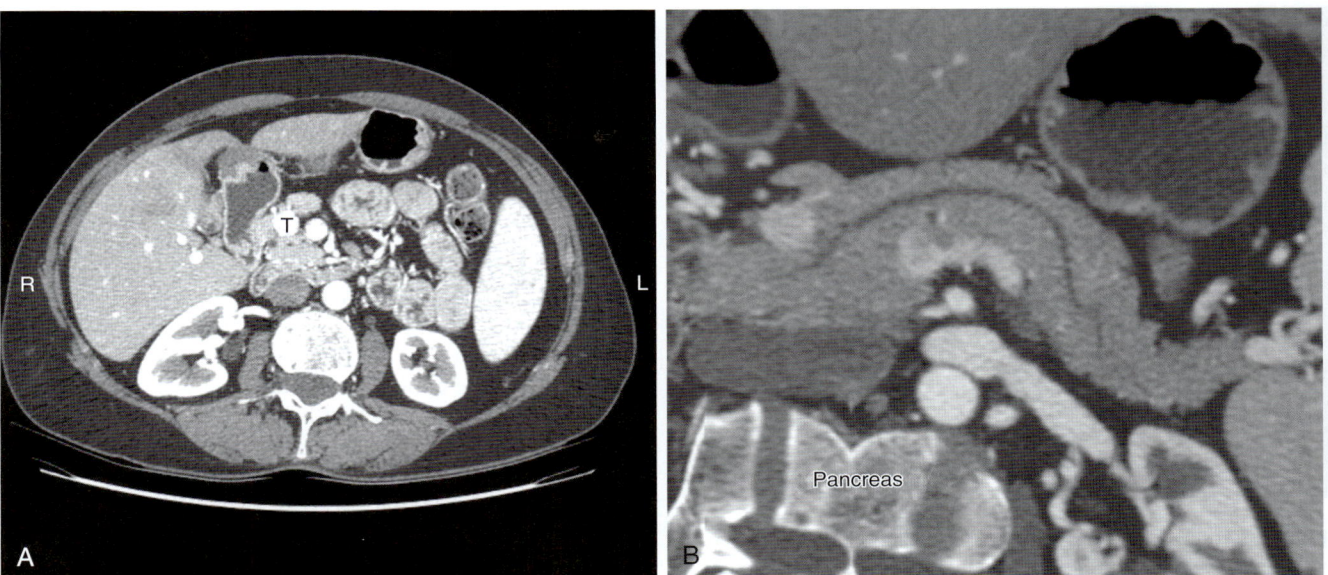

FIGURE 97.2 (A) Computed tomography scan of a small insulinoma *(T)* within the head of the pancreas. (B) Three-dimensional reconstruction of the same computed tomography, which shows the small hypervascular insulinoma within the head of the pancreas.

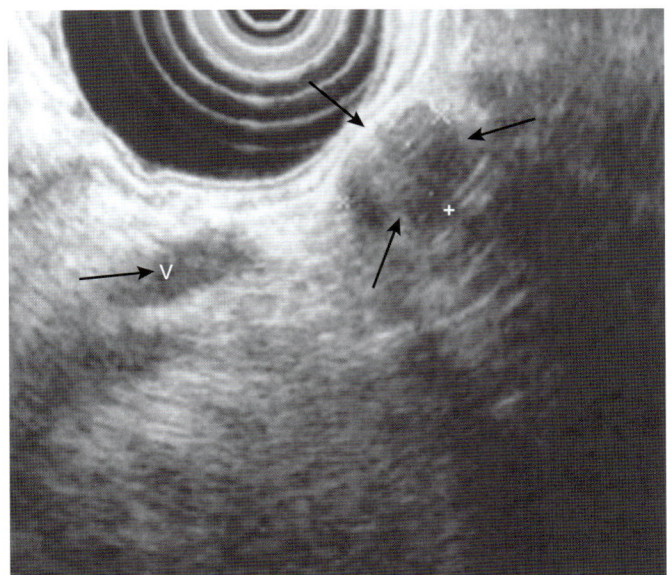

FIGURE 97.3 Endoscopic ultrasound with the transducer in the stomach demonstrating a small hypodense mass (insulinoma) within the tail of the pancreas *(arrows)*. The relationship to the splenic vein *(V)* is also seen.

THERAPY

Medical treatment should prevent hypoglycemia. Acute hypoglycemia is initially treated with intravenous glucose infusion. Hypoglycemia can be prevented while establishing the diagnosis and tumor localization by giving frequent feeds of high-carbohydrate diet, including a night meal. Cornstarch added to the diet may prolong and slow down absorption of glucose. For patients who continue to become hypoglycemic between feedings, diazoxide may be added to the treatment regimen at a dose of 400 to 600 mg orally each day. Diazoxide inhibits insulin release in approximately 50% of patients with insulinoma. In some patients, calcium channel blockers or phenytoin may suppress insulin production. Octreotide binds to and activates somatostatin receptors on cells expressing them. However, its usefulness to inhibit insulin release has been disappointing and unpredictable.

Long-term medical management of hypoglycemia in patients with insulinomas is generally reserved for the few patients (<5%) with unlocalized, unresected tumors after thorough preoperative testing and exploratory laparotomy and for patients with metastatic, unresectable malignant insulinoma. Patients with malignant insulinomas and refractory hypoglycemia may even require the placement of implantable glucose pumps for continuous glucose infusion.

Surgery is the only curative therapy for insulinoma. Because most insulinomas are benign and small, the goal of surgery is to precisely localize the tumor and remove it with minimal morbidity. The major breakthrough in surgery for insulinoma is IOUS.[13] It is the single best intraoperative method to localize insulinomas, although in most cases the tumor is localized by other techniques preoperatively or is visualized or palpated by the surgeon.

Midline or bilateral subcostal incisions allow for good exposure. Because virtually all insulinomas are located within the pancreas, an extended Kocher maneuver is performed and the lesser sac is opened, such that the entire pancreas can be examined. The tumor feels like a firm, nodular, and discrete mass. It may appear brownish-red purple, like a cherry. IOUS should be performed with a high-resolution near-field transducer (10 to 15 MHz).[13] The neuroendocrine tumor is sonolucent compared with the more echodense pancreas (Fig. 97.4). The tumor should be imaged in two directions to identify it as a real

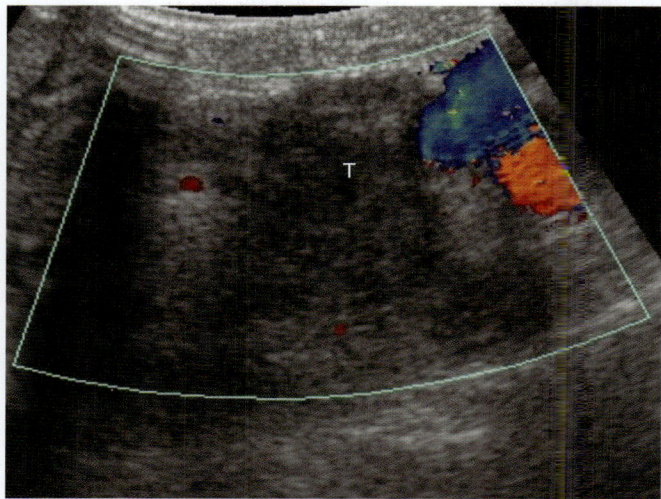

FIGURE 97.4 Intraoperative ultrasound that demonstrates a small, hypodense sonolucent tumor *(T)* within the head of the pancreas to the right of the superior mesenteric vein *(blue)* and artery *(red)*. This tumor was an insulinoma and intraoperative ultrasound facilitated the enucleation.

structure. A recent study of 37 consecutive patients showed that IOUS identified tumors in 35 (95%), and the 2 that were missed were in the pancreatic tail. The liver is examined, and suspicious lesions are biopsied or excised.

Patients who have clear-cut preoperative localization including CT may be candidates for laparoscopic resection. This has been done with good results in these patients using laparoscopic ultrasound to image the tumor and guide the resection. Patients who undergo laparoscopic resection of insulinomas have less postoperative pain, shorter hospitalization, and faster return to work. Insulinomas presenting during pregnancy have been reported and are usually managed medically until the fetus can be delivered or the pregnancy is terminated.

MULTIPLE ENDOCRINE NEOPLASIA TYPE 1

MEN-1 is an inherited autosomal dominant disease in which tumors develop in multiple endocrine organs. Patients classically have primary hyperparathyroidism secondary to four-gland clonal parathyroid adenomas (94%), pituitary adenoma (35%) (most commonly prolactinoma), and multiple PNETs that may be malignant (75%). Gastrinoma and insulinoma are the most common functional neuroendocrine pancreatic tumors in MEN-1 patients, accounting for approximately 50% and 20% of the neuroendocrine tumor syndromes, respectively. Nonfunctional pancreatic endocrine tumor and PPomas are the most common PNETs in MEN-1 patients because these tumors are almost always identified on careful histologic studies of the pancreas. Patients may also have lipomas, thyroid adenomas, adrenal cortical adenomas or carcinomas, and carcinoid tumors of the entire neuroendocrine system.

Of the rare PNETs, MEN-1 is present in approximately 3% of patients with glucagonoma, 1% of patients with VIPoma, 33% of patients with tumors that secrete growth hormone–releasing factor (GRF) (GRFomas), and 5% of patients with somatostatinoma.

The genetic defect in patients with MEN-1 has been localized to the long arm of chromosome 11 and linked to the skeletal muscle glycogen phosphorylase gene. Evidence from these studies suggests that the development of endocrine tumors in MEN-1 patients conforms to the Knudson two-hit model of neoplasm formation, with an inherited mutation in one chromosome unmasked by a somatic deletion or mutation of the other normal chromosome, thereby removing the suppressor effects of the normal gene. In contrast, in sporadic patients with PNETs, tumors do not appear to develop by homozygous inactivation of the same gene. Growth factors have been identified in the plasma of patients with MEN-1. A circulating blood factor that was mitogenic for parathyroid cells in tissue culture has been identified, and a subsequent study demonstrated that the factor was similar to fibroblast growth factor. However, most recent evidence suggests that the parathyroid glands have a clonal abnormality that is similar, and thus they represent the same tumor.[14]

DIAGNOSIS

The possibility of MEN-1 should be considered during the evaluation of all patients presenting with pancreatic NET. A careful family history of first-degree relatives should be taken, and suspicious comorbidities, such as kidney stones, hyperparathyroidism, hypoglycemia, peptic ulcer disease, diarrhea, Cushing syndrome, and prolactinoma should be queried. All patients younger than age 40 years presenting with primary hyperparathyroidism due to multiple gland disease should be screened for pancreatic endocrine tumors even if their family history is negative for MEN-1 syndrome. Physical examination should be done to exclude lipomas that may be present in MEN-1. Screening of other family members is indicated, if suspicion for MEN-1 exists. Evaluation should include serum levels of calcium, gastrin, glucose, PP, chromogranin A, and prolactin.

Each patient with biochemical evidence of a neuroendocrine tumor should undergo complete radiologic assessment of disease to determine the feasibility of surgery. During the radiologic evaluation, medical management should be used to ameliorate symptoms secondary to excessive hormone secretion. It is clear that in some patients with neuroendocrine tumors (e.g., VIPoma) advances in medical control of the hormone production have improved the surgical outcome and reduced the operative complication rate.

THERAPY

In MEN-1 patients with primary hyperparathyroidism and Zollinger-Ellison syndrome, surgery to correct the primary hyperparathyroidism (three and one-half gland parathyroidectomy) should be performed prior to pancreatic surgery because correction of the hypercalcemia will greatly ameliorate the signs and symptoms of Zollinger-Ellison syndrome. If MEN-1 is present, the pathologist will identify multiple neuroendocrine tumors within the pancreas, so patients are seldom cured by surgery, but most experts recommend that patients with neuroendocrine tumors greater than 2 cm undergo surgery because these tumors have a higher probability of developing liver metastases. Medical management can only control the signs and symptoms, and tumor resection is the only potentially curative treatment for malignant PNET. Resection is better in MEN-1 patients because of multiple tumors. Therefore, in patients with localized, potentially resectable, imageable (2 cm or larger) tumors, pancreatic resection by either a Whipple procedure (for pancreatic head tumors) or distal pancreatectomy (for pancreatic body and tail tumors) is indicated.

PROGNOSIS

Many variables associated with an individual patient have an impact on the surgical outcome. These include the extent of disease on preoperative imaging studies, whether the primary tumor is within the pancreas or duodenum, the exact area of the pancreas involved (head, body, or tail), the presence of liver or other distant metastases and whether they are resectable, the occurrence of the neuroendocrine tumor in a familial or a sporadic setting, and the simultaneous occurrence of other medical conditions that may limit the ability of a patient to undergo major surgery. The definition of success need not be equated with cure because decreased medication requirement, decreased symptoms, and increased length of survival may be of considerable clinical value. In each patient, it is clear that neuroendocrine tumors may be malignant, that surgery is an effective way of accurately staging the true extent of disease, and that surgery may be curative, even in the patients with metastatic neuroendocrine tumor.

Genetic counseling and screening should be provided to families at high risk of developing MEN-1. These patients should enter a clinical screening program, which can enable earlier detection and treatment of MEN-1–associated tumors and prompt treatment of hyperparathyroidism.

SOMATOSTATINOMA

Somatostatinoma is a rare endocrine tumor of the pancreatic islet D cells or duodenum that secretes excessive amounts of somatostatin. Somatostatin excess causes a syndrome characterized by steatorrhea, mild diabetes, and cholelithiasis. Somatostatin is an inhibitory hormone originally discovered in the hypothalamus. It was discovered by its ability to inhibit growth hormone and thus was called somatotropin release–inhibiting hormone. The somatostatinoma syndrome included diabetes, cholelithiasis, weight loss, and anemia. Subsequently, diarrhea, steatorrhea, and hypochlorhydria have been added. Somatostatin inhibits the release of most other gastrointestinal hormones. It decreases many gastrointestinal functions, including acid secretion, pancreatic enzyme secretion, and intestinal absorption. It reduces gut motility and transit time. Contrary to their duodenal counterparts, pancreatic somatostatinomas are not associated with von Recklinghausen syndrome.

PRESENTATION

Patients with pancreatic or intestinal somatostatinoma are typically in the sixth decade of life, with an equal proportion of men and women. Initial symptoms are diabetes, cholelithiasis, and steatorrhea. Diabetes mellitus

and glucose intolerance are reported to occur in 60% of patients with pancreatic somatostatinomas; gallstones occur in 70%; diarrhea and steatorrhea are reported in 30% to 68%; and hypochlorhydria presents in 86%. The weight loss may be secondary to diarrhea and malabsorption.

DIAGNOSIS

In most instances, somatostatinomas are found incidentally at the time of cholecystectomy or during routine imaging studies. In 75% of cases, they are metastatic and larger than 5 cm at the time of diagnosis. Most somatostatinomas are located in the pancreas. Despite equal distribution of islet D cells throughout the pancreas, two-thirds of the tumors are located in the head of the pancreas, with the remainder found in the duodenum, at the ampulla, or small intestine.

Diagnosis of somatostatinoma requires the demonstration of elevated tissue concentration of somatostatin or by the documentation of increased fasting plasma somatostatin levels. A level greater than 14 pmol/L is suggestive of the diagnosis of somatostatinoma. CT is a sensitive imaging study, given that the tumor is usually large at the time of diagnosis. Alternatively, MRI and EUS with biopsy and cytology or somatostatin receptor scintigraphy can be helpful in obtaining the diagnosis. The early diagnosis of somatostatinoma may be possible with greater awareness of its existence and reliable assays for the determination of somatostatin in the blood.

THERAPY

Most somatostatinomas are solitary and located within the pancreatic head or duodenum. A high proportion of these tumors are malignant. If the tumor is localized and not widely metastatic, surgical resection is the treatment of choice and the only chance for cure. In some, the severity of diarrhea and steatorrhea correlates with the size and degree of metastatic spread of the tumor, and it improves with tumor resection. Therefore surgical debulking of metastatic disease has been advocated, but patients are few and clear benefits have not been demonstrated. Five-year survival rates of patients with duodenal and pancreatic somatostatinomas are 30% and 15%, respectively.

VASOACTIVE INTESTINAL PEPTIDE–PRODUCING TUMOR

VIPomas are generally located within the pancreas. Most VIPomas have been found in the body and the tail of the pancreas. The initial characterization of what was later recognized to be VIPoma was called the *Verner-Morrison syndrome* and consisted of large-volume diarrhea, severe hypokalemia with muscle weakness, hypercalcemia, and hypochlorhydria. VIPoma typically occurs in adults. Approximately half the VIPomas are benign.

PRESENTATION

The diarrhea is typically large in volume (>5 L/day), and it occurs in 70% of patients. It is a secretory diarrhea and thus persists during a fast. Hypokalemia is present in nearly every patient and is caused by excessive potassium losses in the diarrheal fluid, leading to severe muscle weakness and debilitation. Hypochlorhydria is found in 75% of patients with VIPoma and is due to inhibition of gastric acid secretion by VIP. The vasodilatory action of VIP leads to flushing in a minority of patients. Hyperglycemia occurs in 25% to 50% of patients and is caused by the glycogenolytic action of VIP. Hypercalcemia is present in a significant proportion of patients.

DIAGNOSIS

In patients with secretory diarrhea and hypokalemia suspected of having a VIPoma, a fasting plasma VIP level should be measured. Given that symptomatic tumors are usually larger than 1 cm, CT is a sensitive imaging study. MRI and ultrasound may also be helpful. SRS may also be useful for tumor localization.

TREATMENT

The first step in treating VIPoma includes the correction of the metabolic imbalance. Electrolyte losses from long-standing diarrhea should be aggressively corrected. Long-acting somatostatin analogues can decrease the diarrhea and help to correct hypokalemia and the other metabolic derangements. Surgical resection is the only chance for cure. IOUS may be considered for intraoperative identification. If complete surgical resection cannot be achieved, surgical debulking may be helpful, and postoperative medical treatment of the residual disease with octreotide is recommended.

GLUCAGONOMA

Glucagonoma is an endocrine tumor of the pancreas that secretes excessive amounts of glucagon. This results in a characteristic syndrome that includes a rash called necrolytic migratory erythema (NME), type 2 diabetes mellitus, weight loss, anemia, stomatitis, glossitis, pulmonary and venous thromboembolism, and other gastrointestinal and neuropsychiatric symptoms. Liver disease and zinc deficiency may also add to the symptomatology. Unlike other islet cell tumors, glucagonomas are almost always malignant and usually not resectable for cure. Tumor-related deaths occur in most patients after approximately 5 years of follow-up. Surgery is the only option for cure. Surgical resection leads to complete resolution of all signs and symptoms in many patients.

Patients with glucagonoma typically present between 50 and 60 years of age. The rash is migratory, red, and scaling and is associated with intense pruritus. It commonly occurs in the intertriginous areas, including the groin and lower extremities. NME is pathognomonic for the tumor. The rash is related to markedly decreased plasma levels of amino acids, and can be completely reversed with total parenteral nutrition. Others have also reported that infusion of peripheral amino acids did resolve the rash but it did not reverse hypoaminoacidemia. Diabetes mellitus and glucose intolerance are among the most frequent findings in patients. However, approximately 20% of patients do not present with hyperglycemia.

Weight loss and cachexia are common and may be profound. Thromboembolic symptoms occur more commonly in patients with glucagonoma. Both deep venous thrombosis and pulmonary emboli may ultimately cause death.

DIAGNOSIS

Diagnosis is established by the measurement of elevated plasma levels of glucagon. In all patients with glucagonoma, plasma glucagon concentration is elevated (>150 pg/mL). Plasma levels greater than 1000 pg/mL are diagnostic of glucagonoma. CT identifies the location of the tumor, which is usually larger than 4 cm (Fig. 97.5A). Glucagonomas are almost always found within the body and tail of the pancreas and only rarely in the head. Seventy percent of patients present with liver metastasis at the time of the diagnosis.

THERAPY

Preoperative preparation involves control of diabetes, treatment of complications (such as venous thrombosis), and nutritional support. Resection of the primary tumor usually requires subtotal pancreatectomy with splenectomy. If the primary lesion is not fully resectable, debulking and resection of liver metastases may improve symptoms. Metastatic disease tends to progress slowly (see Fig. 97.5B). Other options include hepatic artery embolization, chemotherapy with bevacizumab (Avastin), 5-fluorouracil, and oxaliplatin or everolimus, long-term octreotide (Sandostatin LAR) for symptoms, and transplantation of the liver and pancreas.

GROWTH HORMONE–RELEASING FACTOR–PRODUCING TUMOR

The GRFoma is a neuroendocrine tumor that secretes excessive amounts of GRF. GRFomas occur most frequently in the lung (bronchus), followed by pancreas, jejunum, adrenal glands, and retroperitoneum. Pancreatic GRFomas are typically large (>6 cm). One-third will have metastasized at the time of diagnosis. Approximately 50% of patients with GRFomas also have Zollinger-Ellison syndrome and 33% have MEN-1. Patients present with acromegaly and a pancreatic mass. If liver metastasis or peptic ulcer disease is present, the diagnosis of GRFoma should also be considered. The diagnosis of GRFoma is established using a plasma assay for GRF. Given that the tumor is usually large at the time of diagnosis, CT scan is a sensitive modality for localization. Surgical resection should be attempted in these patients because complete resection may be curative, and debulking may decrease symptoms and prolong survival. Octreotide therapy can relieve the symptoms of acromegaly.

CORTICOTROPIN-PRODUCING TUMOR

Malignant NETs commonly secrete more than one peptide. When they produce ACTH (corticotropin), patients present with Cushing syndrome. Excessive production of corticotropin by a pituitary tumor may occur in patients with MEN-1 but is usually mild and clinically insignificant. In 5% of patients with Zollinger-Ellison syndrome, Cushing syndrome has been reported. In contrast, these patients

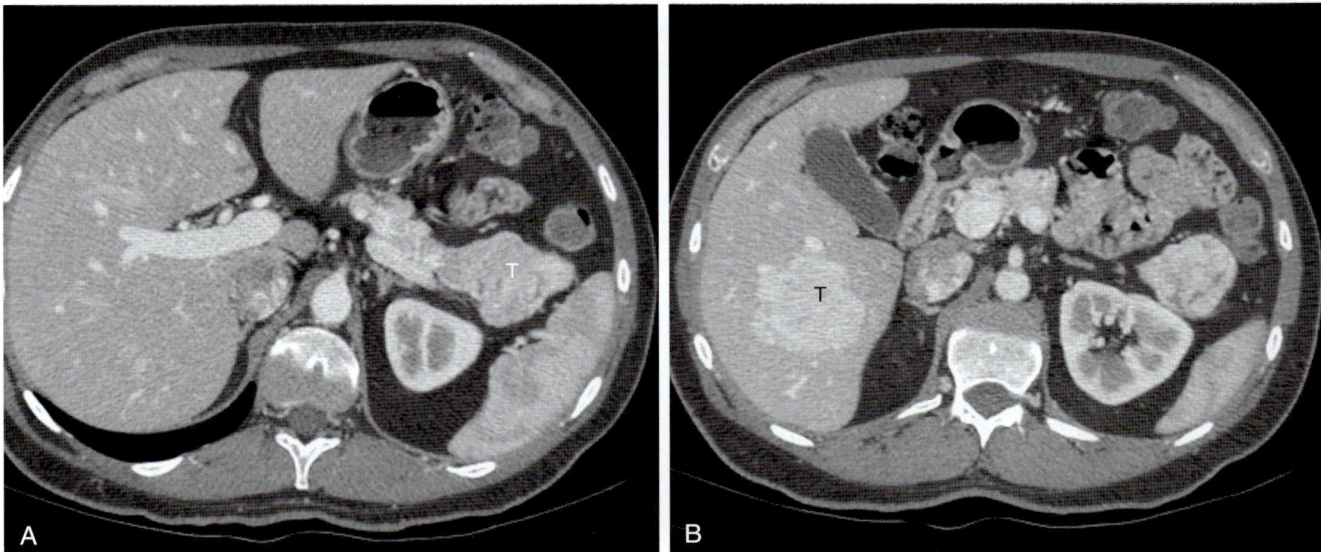

FIGURE 97.5 (A) Glucagonoma *(T)* in the tail of the pancreas is demonstrated on computed tomography scan. The patient presented with a rash known as necrolytic migratory erythema. (B) The patient also had a large metastasis in the right lobe of the liver *(T)*. He underwent a subtotal pancreatectomy/splenectomy and concomitant right hepatic lobectomy and recovered well. The rash resolved, and he has remained without imageable tumor for 2 years.

have severe Cushing syndrome because of ectopic production of corticotropin by the neuroendocrine tumor. Elevated blood levels of cortisol are diagnostic, and CT is used for localization. Corticotropin-producing PNETs are usually not resectable. Therefore either debulking or bilateral adrenalectomy may be indicated to control the severe signs and symptoms of hypercortisolism, given that medical management of the hypercortisolism in these patients is usually inadequate.

TUMOR RELEASING PARATHYROID HORMONE–RELATED PROTEIN

Severe hypercalcemia has been reported to be due to a PNET-releasing parathyroid hormone–related protein (PTHrP). Hypercalcemia associated with PNETs has also been reported to be due to the release of other substances such as VIP. In most cases the pancreatic tumor is malignant and has spread to the liver by the time of diagnosis.

NEUROTENSINOMA

There have been reports of neuroendocrine tumors that secrete neurotensin. Neurotensin is a peptide that is found in the brain and the gastrointestinal tract. It can cause hypotension, tachycardia, cyanosis, pancreatic secretion, intestinal motility, and small intestinal secretion. Patients with neurotensinomas present with diarrhea and hypokalemia, weight loss, diabetes, cyanosis, hypotension, and flushing. Patients may be cured by resection of the tumor; others have responded to chemotherapy. Some have questioned whether a separate neurotensinoma exists. Patients with VIPoma and gastrinoma have been found to have elevated plasma levels of neurotensin. At present, it is unclear whether a separate syndrome exists.

GHRELINOMA

Ghrelin is a novel gastrointestinal hormone that exerts a wide range of metabolic functions. It promotes growth hormone release and is an important regulator of energy balance. It has been demonstrated to increase appetite and food intake and modulate insulin secretion. It has significant homology with motilin, and it stimulates gastric contractility and acid secretion. A study suggested that a patient had a neuroendocrine tumor of the pancreas excreting the hormone ghrelin, a so-called ghrelinoma. This hormone had not been found in any other neuroendocrine tumor of the pancreas.

PANCREATIC PEPTIDE–PRODUCING TUMOR AND NONFUNCTIONING NEUROENDOCRINE TUMOR

Neuroendocrine tumors that are not associated with a syndrome related to hormonal hypersecretion are referred to as nonfunctional. For example, PPomas secrete PP, but this hormone does not appear to cause symptoms; therefore this tumor is considered nonfunctional. It is estimated that 10% to 25% of all neuroendocrine pancreatic tumors are nonfunctional. They are therefore estimated to be among the most frequent neuroendocrine tumors of the pancreas.

PRESENTATION

Typically these tumors are large when diagnosed (>5 cm), and almost all (80%) are malignant and metastatic (Fig. 97.6). The incidence of malignancy is clearly higher than among the functioning PNETs. Symptoms occur secondary to mass effect. Cachexia, abdominal pain, intestinal bleeding, blockage, or hepatomegaly are common symptoms.

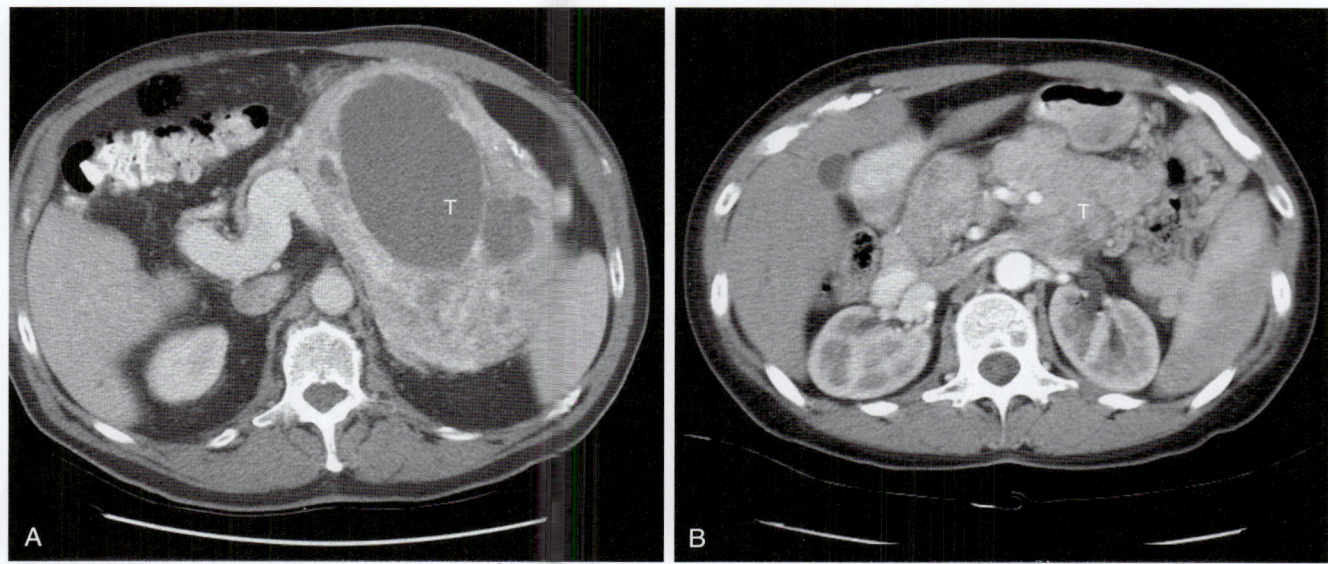

FIGURE 97.6 (A) Large nonfunctional neuroendocrine tumor within the tail of the pancreas (T). This patient presented with stomach bleeding because the tumor had eroded into the posterior wall of the stomach. (B) This patient presented with back pain. She was found to have a localized large nonfunctional neuroendocrine tumor within the body of the pancreas (T). Removal of this tumor required a total pancreatectomy/splenectomy. She has done well except that she developed small liver metastases at the 5-year follow-up.

Some patients present with pancreatitis. Some patients present with small incidentally discovered PNETs found on a CT done for another reason, such as trauma or kidney stones. These incidental PNETs are usually less than 2 cm and may not be malignant or functionally important. Certainly, hormonal secretion must be excluded by careful questioning and blood measurement. In these individuals it is questionable whether or not surgery should be performed. In our opinion, surgical excision should be done in a young, otherwise healthy individual. This should be done in the safest, most pancreatic parenchyma-preserving manner. Enucleation is a possibility as is resection if a fistula could be a complication because of proximity to the pancreatic duct. However, in older patients with more comorbidity and shorter life expectancy, simple MRI follow-up may be a better option reserving surgery for those with progressive and/or metastatic PNETs.

DIAGNOSIS

Tumors are often found incidentally during surgery. Given that these tumors are usually large by the time the patient is symptomatic, CT and MRI are good diagnostic imaging studies. PP and chromogranin A are presently the best serum markers to identify PPomas. Nonfunctioning pancreatic endocrine tumors are differentiated from PPomas on the basis of results of the serum PP assay. Adenocarcinoma of the pancreas can be distinguished from neuroendocrine tumors by immunohistochemical staining with chromogranin A and by DOTA scan (Fig. 97.7).

THERAPY

Therapy includes resection of the tumor and chemotherapy. Most nonfunctioning islet cell tumors are in the head of the pancreas and require a Whipple

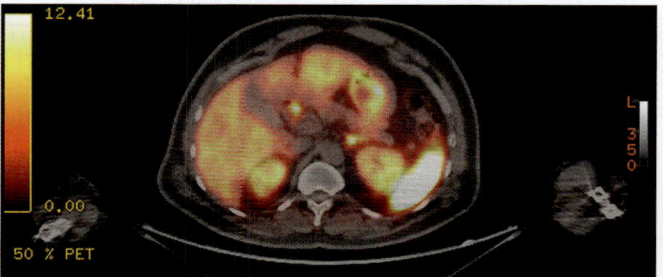

FIGURE 97.7 Positron emission tomography fused axial image of DOTATOC scan of a small neuroendocrine tumor in the head of the pancreas with a second unexpected tumor in the left adrenal. The patient presented with a computed tomography scan that showed a possible neuroendocrine tumor in the head of the pancreas. Subsequent DOTA scan was performed to ascertain if the computed tomography finding was indeed a pancreatic neuroendocrine tumor. DOTA scan was positive for a pancreatic neuroendocrine tumor in the head of the pancreas. It also showed a small tumor in the left adrenal that was subsequently found to be a 1-cm pheochromocytoma.

pancreaticoduodenectomy. Debulking of hepatic tumor mass can be replaced by hepatic embolization. Dopamine agonists have been shown to decrease circulating levels of PP and chromogranin A in patients with large unresectable islet cell tumors. PPomas and nonfunctioning neuroendocrine tumors of the pancreas do not seem to differ in their biologic behavior; however, PP and chromogranin levels may be used to monitor the result of therapy. Everolimus and other chemotherapy regimens have been useful in some tumors. Furthermore, therapy based on tagging somatostatin receptor analogues (peptide related radiation therapy [PRRT]) have been able to induce some partial, but not complete, responses and are useful in some patients. Liver transplantation has also been used in some patients with extensive disease localized to the liver, with reasonable outcomes.[15]

PROGNOSIS

The 5-year survival of nonfunctioning PNETs is typically less than functional neuroendocrine pancreatic tumors.[15] Results may vary due to the small numbers of patients with this disease. Most likely there is no significant difference in behavior between functioning and nonfunctioning tumors. Ki67 rate is the most important predictor of outcome and survival and should be assessed pathologically in all cases.

REFERENCES

1. Phan AT, Oberg K, Choi J, et al. NANETS consensus guideline for the diagnosis and management of neuroendocrine tumors: well differentiated neuroendocrine tumors of the thorax (includes lung and thymus). *Pancreas*. 2010;39:784-798.
2. Yao JC, Hassan M, Phan A, et al. One hundred years after "carcinoid": epidemiology of and prognostic factors for neuroendocrine tumors in 35,825 cases in the United States. *J Clin Oncol*. 2008;26:3063-3072.
3. Kloppel G, Heitz PU. Pancreatic endocrine tumors. *Pathol Res Pract*. 1988;183:155-168.
4. Heitz PU, Kasper M, Polak JM, Klöppel G. Pancreatic endocrine tumors: immunocytochemical analysis of 125 tumors. *Hum Pathol*. 1982;13:263-271.
5. Creutzfeldt W, Arnold R, Creutzfeld C. Pathomorphologic, biochemical, and diagnostic aspects of gastrinomas (Zollinger-Ellison syndrome). *Hum Pathol*. 1975;6:47-76.
6. Krampitz GW, George BM, Willingham SB, et al. Identification of tumorigenic cells and therapeutic targets in pancreatic neuroendocrine tumors. *Proc Natl Acad Sci USA*. 2016;113(16):4464-4469.
7. Tamburrino D, Spoletini G, Partelli S, et al. Surgical management of neuroendocrine tumors. *Best Pract Res Clin Endocrinol Metab*. 2016;30(1):93-102.
8. Worhunsky DJ, Krampitz GW, Poullos PD, et al. Pancreatic neuroendocrine tumours: hypoenhancement on arterial phase computed tomography predicts biological aggressiveness. *HPB (Oxford)*. 2014;16(4):304-311.
9. Norton JA. Neuroendocrine tumors of the pancreas and duodenum. *Curr Probl Surg*. 1994;31:77-156.
10. Doherty GM, Doppman JL, Shawker TH, et al. Results of a prospective strategy to diagnose, localize, and resect insulinomas. *Surgery*. 1999;110:989-996.
11. Ambrosini V, Campana D, Polverari G, et al. Prognostic value of ^{68}Ga-DOTANOC PET/CT SUVmax in patients with neuroendocrine tumors of the pancreas. *J Nucl Med*. 2015;56(12):1843-1848.
12. Rosch T, Lightdale CJ, Botet JF, et al. Localization of pancreatic endocrine tumors by endoscopic ultrasonography. *N Engl J Med*. 1992;326:1721-1726.
13. Weinstein S, Morgan T, Poder L, et al. Value of intraoperative sonography in pancreatic surgery. *J Ultrasound Med*. 2015;34(7):1307-1318.
14. Arnold A, Staunton CE, Kim HG, Gaz RD, Kronenberg HM. Monoclonality and abnormal parathyroid hormone genes in parathyroid adenomas. *N Engl J Med*. 1988;318(11):658-662.
15. Yao JC, Evans DB. Pancreatic neuroendocrine tumors. In: DeVita VT, Lawrence TS, Rosenberg SA, eds. *DeVita, Hellman, and Rosenberg's Cancer: Principles and Practice of Oncolgy*. Wolters Kluwer; 2015:1205-1217.

Primary Pancreatic Cystic Neoplasms

Andrew Schneider   Kevin K. Roggin

Over the past century, clinicians have been challenged by the more frequent identification of primary pancreatic cystic neoplasms (PCNs). Increased use of cross-sectional imaging studies, such as computed tomography and magnetic resonance imaging (MRI), have led to a sustained increased "incidence" of these lesions. Management decisions are extremely difficult due to the uncertain biologic behavior of these lesions and the lack of prognostic biomarkers to assist with counseling patients on treatment. Reports of cystic neoplasms in the pancreas are documented in the literature as early as 1908. However, the distinction between serous and mucinous cysts was not made until 1978 by Compagno and Oertel.[1] This proved to be an important differentiation due to the risk of malignant transformation associated with mucinous cysts. Only a few years later, in 1982 Ohashi et al.[2] published the first report of a mucinous secreting cancer of the pancreas, which was later redefined as an intraductal papillary mucinous neoplasm (IPMN) in 1996.[3] Despite histopathologic advancements in diagnosis, PCNs remain a diagnostic dilemma for even the most experienced clinician to accurately predict the malignant potential of these lesions. This chapter will focus on the classifications and characteristics of PCNs, the diagnostic modalities, the therapies, and future ways of treating this disease.

INCIDENCE AND EPIDEMIOLOGY

Most pancreatic cysts are nonneoplastic, originating from injury, inflammation, or congenital abnormalities of the pancreas. A much smaller percentage of cysts are neoplastic. In spite of previously being defined as a rare entity, PCNs have increased in diagnostic prevalence due to increased use of cross-sectional imaging. Based on a retrospective review in 2010, the overall prevalence of incidental pancreatic cysts discovered by MRI is 13.5% and increases with age.[4] An autopsy study identified PCNs in 378 of 1374 cases (27.5%) with an increased prevalence correlated with age.[5] Thus, as imaging techniques continue to improve, more incidental PCNs will inevitably become discovered.

The three most common types of PCNs are serous cystic neoplasms (SCNs), mucinous cystic neoplasms (MCNs), and IPMNs, representing approximately 90% of all PCNs.[6] MCNs and IPMNs are the most common and more importantly have the highest potential for malignant transformation. SCNs occur much less frequently and are almost always benign.[7]

SEROUS CYSTIC NEOPLASMS

SCNs are most commonly observed in women (3:1 female-to-male ratio), with an average age of diagnosis of 62 years.[8] There are four subtypes of SCNs: serous microcytic

adenoma, serous macrocytic (oligocystic) adenoma, von Hippel-Lindau (VHL)-associated pancreatic cysts, and serous cystadenocarcinoma.

SCNs are characterized by serous fluid–filled cysts lined by a single layer of cuboidal epithelial cells with uniform, round, darkly stained nuclei and a glycogen-rich cytoplasm.[9] Notably, there is a lack of atypia, necrosis, and mitotic features in SCNs. On gross examination, microcystic SCNs have a characteristic honeycomb appearance with multiple thin-walled cysts around a central scar (Fig. 98.1). Commonly, calcifications can be found in the proximity of the central scar. The cystic spaces do not communicate with the pancreatic ductal system. The surrounding stroma usually contains nerves, islets, lymphoid aggregates, and vascular channels.[9]

Serous macrocytic or oligocystic adenomas are rare and usually have larger and fewer cystic structures. The oligocystic variant does not have the central scar that is seen with the microcystic subtype. These cysts are found equally in men and women and usually occur earlier in life, with an average age of 50 years.[10] They are predominately found in the pancreatic head, which can lead to symptoms related to biliary duct obstruction.[9] Microscopically the cellular architecture of macrocystic and microcystic serous adenomas are similar.[10]

Von Hippel-Lindau–Associated Pancreatic Cysts

VHL disease is an autosomal dominant mutation of chromosome 3p25.3 causing multiorgan pathology. VHL-associated pancreatic cysts show a loss of heterozygosity on chromosome 3p25 and mutations in the VHL gene. A 2012 systemic review of the literature by Charlesworth identified 252 out of 420 (60%) patients with VHL and a pancreatic lesion.[11] These lesions are indistinguishable from sporadic serous cystadenomas. In contrast, VHL patients tend to have multifocal disease rather than a single lesion. These lesions behave similarly to non-VHL serous cystadenomas with minimal malignant potential.[11]

Serous Cystadenocarcinoma

Malignant SCNs are exceedingly rare, with a few case reports in the literature. George et al.[12] first described a patient with a serous cystadenocarcinoma in 1989, and since that time, fewer than 40 cases have been published. These malignant cysts are nearly identical to benign serous cystadenomas and are distinguished only by the presence of metastases. Literature suggests the possibility that serous cystadenocarcinomas are misdiagnosed as a malignancy due to the presence of vascular impingement on imaging. Histologic review of these reported serous cystadenocarcinoma specimens failed to demonstrate any malignant attributes.[13]

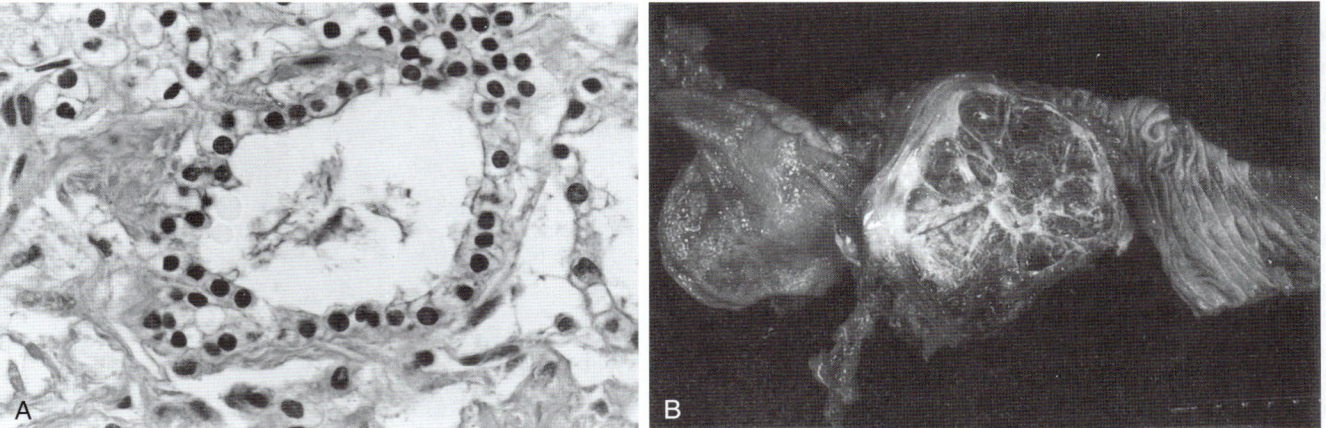

FIGURE 98.1 Serous cystadenoma of the pancreas (serous cystic neoplasm). (A) Simple serous cuboidal cells without dysplasia. (B) Gross appearance with multiple small cysts. (Reproduced with permission from Pyke CM, van Heerden JA, Colby TV, et al. The spectrum of serous cystadenoma of the pancreas: clinical, pathological, and surgical aspects. *Ann Surg*. 1992;215:132.)

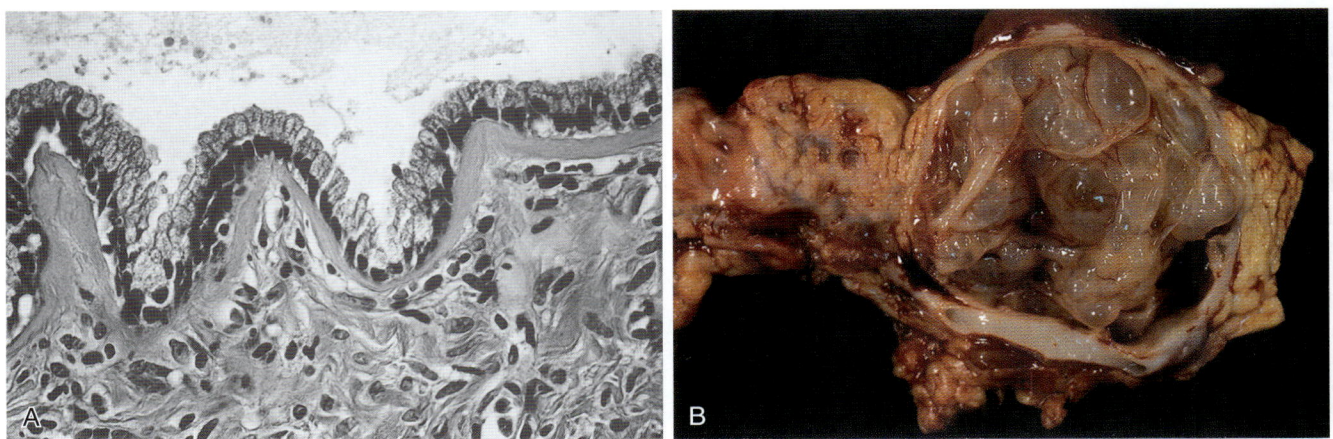

FIGURE 98.2 Mucinous cystic neoplasm of the pancreas. (A) Columnar mucinous cells line the cyst wall. (B) Gross appearance of macrocysts with thin walls and mucinous cystic fluid. (Reproduced with permission from Sarr MG, Carpenter HA, Prabhakar LP, et al. Clinical and pathologic correlation of 84 mucinous cystic neoplasms of the pancreas: can one reliably differentiate benign from malignant [or premalignant] neoplasms? *Ann Surg*. 2000;231:205.)

MUCINOUS CYSTIC NEOPLASMS

MCNs are cystic tumors of the pancreas that have a lower incidence than serous cysts or IPMNs. The average age range of presentation is 40 to 50 years old, and they are found predominantly in perimenopausal women (20:1 female-to-male ratio).[14]

The vast majority of MCNs are found in the body and tail of the pancreas. Most MCNs are approximately 6 to 10 cm at the time of diagnosis but range from 1.5 to 35 cm in diameter.[15] On gross examination, they are spherical and infrequently encapsulated by a calcified fibrous wall (approximately 15%). Almost all MCNs are multiloculated. The cyst can be filled with mucin, blood, or a watery fluid. This fluid tends to be thicker and more viscous than in SCN, due to the presence of mucus. MCNs do not communicate with the pancreatic ductal system except when there is erosion into the duct or the formation of a fistula. Any evidence of solid mural nodules should be thoroughly investigated to rule out stromal invasion.[14]

MCNs are lined by tall mucin-producing columnar cells (Fig. 98.2). These epithelial cells that line the cyst may be papillary or flat and can show a tendency toward gastric or intestinal differentiation. The stroma resembles an ovarian corpora albicantia due to luteinized cells and foci of hyalinization. The ovarian-like stroma that underlies that epithelium is pathognomonic of MCN and thus is required for diagnosis. In difficult to diagnose cases the presence of the ovarian-like stroma can help to differentiate between MCN and IPMN. Areas of denudation in the epithelial lining can occasionally be seen.[14]

The epithelium of MCN demonstrates immunoreactivity for cytokeratins 7, 8, 18, and 19, epithelial membrane antigen, carcinoembryonic antigen (CEA), MUC5AC, and carbohydrate antigen (CA) 19-9. The stroma cells stain for estrogen (25% to 63%), progesterone (50% to 80%), and alpha-inhibin (50% to 70%).[14]

Malignant Potential

In 2010 the World Health Organization (WHO) classification divided noninvasive MCNs into three distinct categories based on the degree of cellular atypia: low-, intermediate-, and high-grade.[16] The classification is based on the greatest degree, and not the average, of the epithelial dysplasia (Fig. 98.3). Less than 20% of MCNs are associated with invasive carcinoma and thus should be considered a potential precursor to pancreatic cancer. In these cases the invasive component is histologically consistent with the classic pancreatic ductal adenocarcinoma, although colloid carcinoma, undifferentiated carcinoma, osteoclast-like giant cells, adenosquamous carcinoma, and sarcomas may infrequently occur. Extensive sampling of the cyst is recommended, given the relatively small volume of the invasive component. It appears that the incidence of malignant transformation is directly correlated to the overall size of the cyst and the complexity of the cyst.[14]

Symptoms

The majority of patients with an MCN present with nonspecific symptoms, including weight loss, nausea, vomiting, diarrhea, and abdominal pain. Approximately 30% of patients with an MCN have a palpable abdominal mass.[14]

INTRADUCTAL PAPILLARY MUCINOUS NEOPLASMS

IPMNs were first recognized in 1982 by Ohashi, but the term IPMN was not officially used until 1993.[2] IPMNs are defined in the WHO Classification of Tumors of the Digestive System as an intraductal, grossly visible epithelial neoplasm of mucin-producing cells.[16] Using imaging and histology, IPMNs can be classified into three types based on duct involvement[17]:

1. *Main-duct IPMN* (approximately 25% of IPMNs): Segmental or diffuse dilation of the main pancreatic duct (>5 mm) in the absence of other causes of ductal obstruction.
2. *Branch-duct IPMN* (approximately 57% of IPMNs): Pancreatic cysts (>5 mm) that communicate with the main pancreatic duct.
3. *Mixed type IPMN* (approximately 18% of IPMNs): Meets criteria for both main and branch duct.

Due to the asymptomatic nature of the disease, the overall incidence of IPMNs is difficult to define but is thought to account for approximately 3% to 5% of all pancreatic tumors.[6] Most IPMNs are discovered as incidental lesions from the workup of an unrelated process by imaging or endoscopy. IPMNs are slightly more prevalent in males than in females, with a peak incidence of 60 to 70 years of age.[18] Branch-duct IPMNs tend to occur in a slightly younger population and are less associated with malignancy compared with main-duct or mixed variants.[17]

In the main-duct variant of IPMN the main pancreatic duct is usually dilated (≥5 mm), mucin filled, and tortuous.[19,20] The ampulla of Vater on endoscopy tends to have a characteristic "fish-mouth" appearance.[21] These tumors are generally found near the head of the pancreas and grow along the main duct.[22] In patients, when the major or minor papilla is involved, evidence of mucin in the

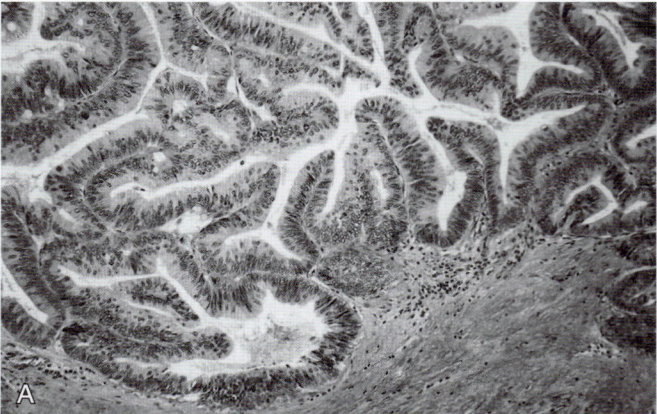
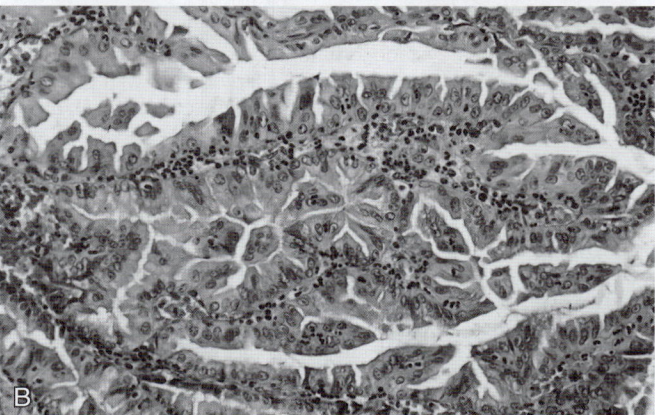
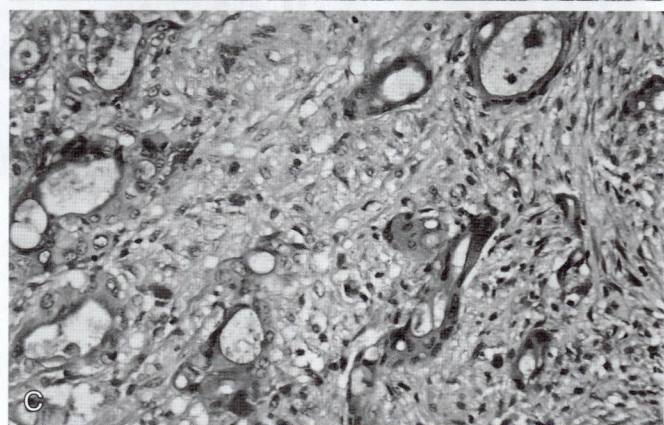

FIGURE 98.3 Spectrum of mucinous cystic neoplasm of the pancreas. (A) Proliferative changes in epithelium with papillary fronds and low-grade dysplasia. (B) High-grade dysplasia with papillary polypoid intracystic growth. (C) Mucinous cystadenocarcinoma with tissue invasion and desmoplastic response. (Reproduced with permission from Sarr MG, Carpenter HA, Prabhakar LP, et al. Clinical and pathologic correlation of 84 mucinous cystic neoplasms of the pancreas: can one reliably differentiate benign from malignant [or premalignant] neoplasms? *Ann Surg.* 2000;231:205.)

duodenum can be visualized when performing endoscopy.[21] Adjacent pancreas can be fibrotic and firm due to chronic pancreatitis.[15,20] Branch-duct IPMNs are most frequently found in the uncinate process.[22] On gross examination, branch-duct IPMNs are grapelike structures that are

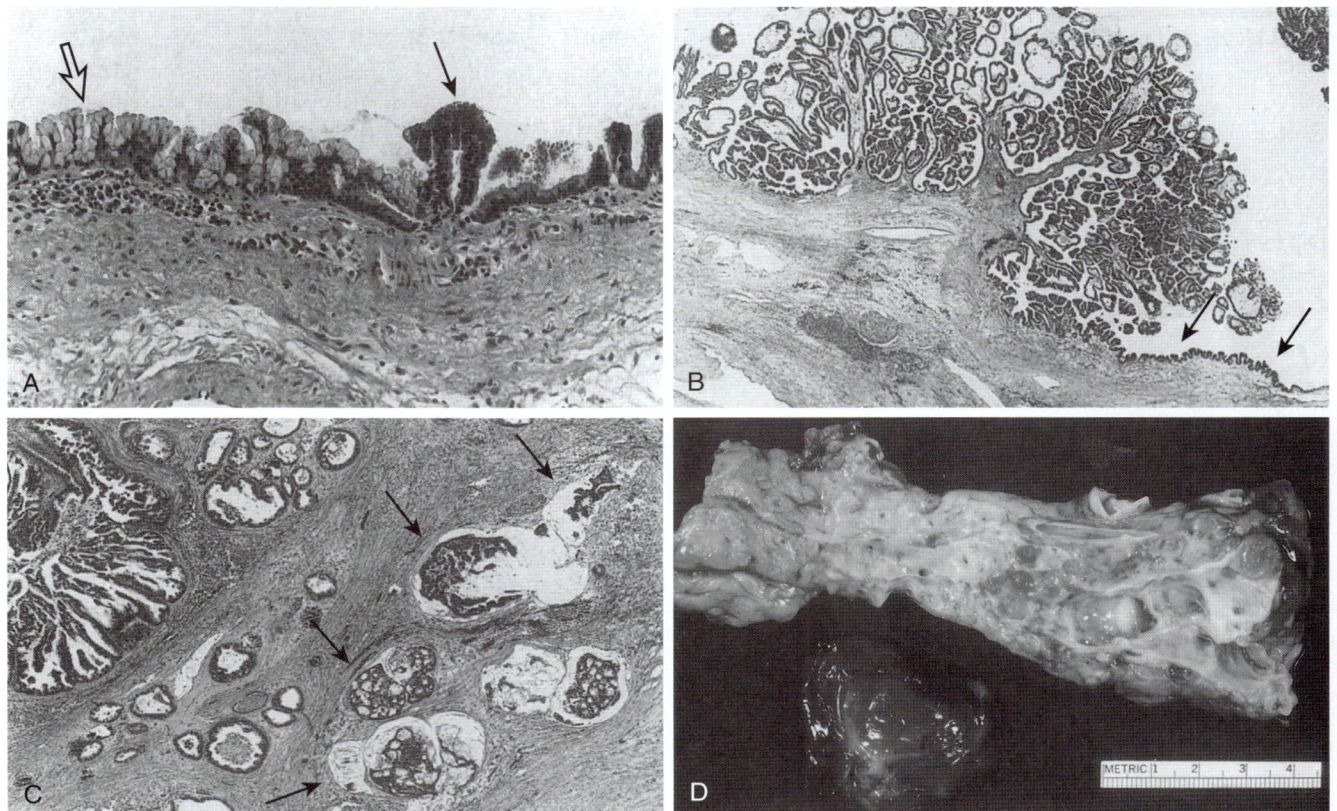

FIGURE 98.4 Intraductal papillary mucinous neoplasm. (A) Ductal epithelium containing nondysplastic, micropapillary mucinous hyperplasia *(open arrow)* and micropapillary dysplasia *(solid arrow)*. (B) Gross papillomatous changes with changes of flat micropapillary dysplasia *(arrows)*. (C) Invasive adenocarcinoma *(arrows)*. (D) Gross findings; main pancreatic duct dilation with copious intraductal mucin and ductal adenomas. (Reproduced with permission from Loftus EV Jr, Olivares-Pakzad BA, Batts KP, et al. Intraductal papillary-mucinous tumors of the pancreas: clinicopathologic features, outcome, and nomenclature. Members of the Pancreas Clinic and Pancreatic Surgeons of Mayo Clinic. *Gastroenterology*. 1996;110:1909.)

multicystic, containing mucin-filled ducts.[23] The adjacent pancreas is usually normal due to noninvolvement of the main pancreatic duct.[15]

Studies have categorized IPMNs based on their epithelial lining of the papillary component (Fig. 98.4).[17] These include gastric, intestinal, pancreatobiliary, and oncocytic.[24] Furthermore, IPMNs contain highly glycosylated proteins called mucins (MUC) that have different gene expression patterns and can help to distinguish between the histopathologic IPMN subtypes.[25] The gastric-subtype IPMNs contain basal small nuclei with apical cytoplasmic mucin, similar in appearance to gastric epithelium. These lesions are almost always low-grade and express MUC5AC and MUC6. The majority of branch-duct IPMNs are of the gastric variant.[17] The intestinal-type IPMNs contain finger-like projections lined by mucin-containing cells with large cigar-like nuclei. These tumors, which express MUCH5AC, MUC2, and CDX2, are strongly associated with colloid carcinomas. A large proportion of main-duct IPMNs are of the intestinal type.[17] Pancreatobiliary-type IPMNs contain cuboidal cells with atypical nuclei and prominent nucleoli. These lesions tend to be a higher grade and are associated with invasive carcinomas that tend to be tubular and aggressive. Their expression pattern includes MUC1 and MUC5A. Finally, the oncocytic subtype contains cells with abundant eosinophilic cytoplasm secondary to large amounts of intracellular mitochondria. This type tends to be complex with arborizing papillae, cribriform formations, and solid nests growing into a dilated duct.[17,24] Most of these lesions are classified as high grade with expression of MUC1 and MUC6.[24]

Because a majority of IPMNs are discovered incidentally, most are asymptomatic. When symptoms do occur, they tend to be nonspecific and include unexplained weight loss, anorexia, abdominal pain, and back pain. Jaundice can occur with mucin obstructing the ampulla or with an underlying invasive carcinoma. The obstruction of the pancreatic duct can also lead to pancreatitis.[26]

IPMNs may represent genomic instability of the entire pancreas. This concept, known as a "field defect," has been described as a theoretical risk of developing a recurrent IPMN or pancreatic adenocarcinoma at a site remote from the original IPMN.[27]

See Table 98.1 for cystic variants of other pancreatic neoplasms.

CLINICAL PRESENTATION

Most primary pancreatic cysts are discovered incidentally by imaging during the evaluation of an unrelated process.[4]

TABLE 98.1 Cystic Variants of Other Pancreatic Neoplasms

Cystic endocrine tumors	Cyst usually contains clear fluid lined by neoplastic endocrine cells Radiographically tumor appears solid with small cystic changes[40]
Cystic acinar cell tumors	Includes: *Acinar cell cystadenoma* (benign proliferation of acinar cells without atypia)[97] *Acinar cell cystadenocarcinoma* (rare, large neoplasm, average >20 cm, with neoplastic acinar cells lining the cyst)[98]
Other pancreatic neoplasms with cystic changes	Includes: ductal adenocarcinoma, adenosquamous carcinoma, undifferentiated carcinoma with osteoclast-like giant cells, and squamous cell carcinoma

Approximately 47% of patients with SCNs are asymptomatic, with the cyst identified only incidentally.[8] The nonspecific symptoms associated with SCNs include abdominal pain (25%), palpable mass (10%), and jaundice (7%).[8] The size of the cyst plays a large role in the manifestation of symptoms with cysts greater than 4 cm compared with less than 4 cm (72% vs. 22%).[8] MCNs and IPMNs are generally more symptomatic (approximately 75%) than SCNs due to their larger size. These lesions are more likely to cause acute pancreatitis due to mass effect on the pancreatic duct (9.2%). IPMNs can also cause acute pancreatitis from mucin production leading to duct obstruction. Other symptoms include abdominal pain (60%), fatigue (10%), and palpable mass (12%).[28] Smaller-size branch-duct IPMNs are more likely to be asymptomatic and diagnosed incidentally.[29]

DIAGNOSTIC EVALUATION

Each of the PCNs has varying degrees of malignant potential and requires an accurate diagnosis to ensure adequate therapeutic decision making. Clinical presentation is variable due to nonspecific or lack of symptoms in patients. To aid in the diagnosis of PCNs, physicians rely on different imaging techniques. The three modalities that will be discussed in this section include multidetector-row computed tomography (MDCT), MRI, and positron emission tomography–computed tomography (PET–CT).

RADIOGRAPHIC CHARACTERIZATION (NONINVASIVE)

Multidetector-Row Computed Tomography

Cross-sectional imaging including MDCT and MRI have become the preferred modalities to assess pancreatic lesions. The initial choice of imaging should include a comprehensive evaluation of the thorax, abdomen, and pelvis with careful attention to the liver and lungs for potential metastatic disease. Each of the different types of PCNs has distinguishing features identified on cross-sectional imaging.

Serous Cystic Neoplasm

SCNs are benign cysts that traditionally contain multiple small thin-walled cysts. Three different imaging patterns exist for SCNs: polycystic, honeycomb, and oligocystic. The polycystic variant is the most common and is identified by the appearance of multiple small cysts, which individually are less than 2 cm. The presence of a central fibrous scar with radial calcifications appearing as a starburst can be found in up to 30% of SCN.[9,30] The less common honeycomb variant is identified by numerous subcentimeter cysts that may appear as a solid mass due to the small cyst on CT imaging. The honeycomb appearance is produced by septal wall enhancement from contrast administration due to the presence of multiple cysts (Fig. 98.5). Finally, the oligocystic pattern, representing less than 2%, is characterized by small cystic areas with stromal hypervascularity.[9] Differentiating unilocular SCNs from MCNs by imaging remains difficult. A 2003 retrospective study identified radiographic criteria that had a specificity of 100% for identifying SCNs when at least three out of four of the criteria were present: (1) location in the pancreatic head, (2) lobulated contour, (3) lack of wall enhancement, and (4) wall thickness equal to or less than 2 mm.[31]

Mucinous Cystic Neoplasm

Normally, MCNs are macrocystic and unilocular (80%) but can also be multilocular (20%). MCNs may lead to pancreatic ductal dilatation due to extrinsic pressure on the duct, but they do not communicate with the ductal system. The walls of the cyst are thick and irregular with papillary excrescences that extend into the cyst (Fig. 98.6). This complex architecture allows differentiation between mucinous and SCNs. The pancreatic parenchyma surrounding the cyst is usually normal compared with the inflammatory parenchyma seen with pseudocysts. Calcifications are rare but when present are typically located in the periphery of the cyst in an eggshell pattern and are associated with malignancy.[9] Radiographic findings of an invasive mucinous cystadenocarcinoma include calcifications, multiple papillary invaginations, intracystic mural nodules, septal enhancement, pericystic mass or reaction, invasion into vascular structures, extrahepatic biliary obstruction, and ascites. Moreover, there is a direct correlation between the size of intracystic mural nodules and the risk of malignant degeneration.[32]

Intraductal Papillary Mucinous Neoplasm

Classically, IPMNs demonstrate cystic dilatation of the main pancreatic duct (main-duct IPMN) or a side branch of the main duct (branch-duct IPMN) located in the uncinate process (Fig. 98.7).[22] Filling defects on cross-sectional imaging represent either mucinous globules or areas of malignant degeneration. Full appreciation of the extent of the IPMN is enhanced by serial sectioning of the pancreas with three-dimensional (3D) reconstructions. Furthermore, imaging can quantify the degree of pancreatic duct dilation and help to differentiate IPMNs from other causes of duct dilation (chronic pancreatitis or other neoplastic processes). Diagnosing mixed-type IPMNs remains elusive. A mixed-type IPMN should be suspected

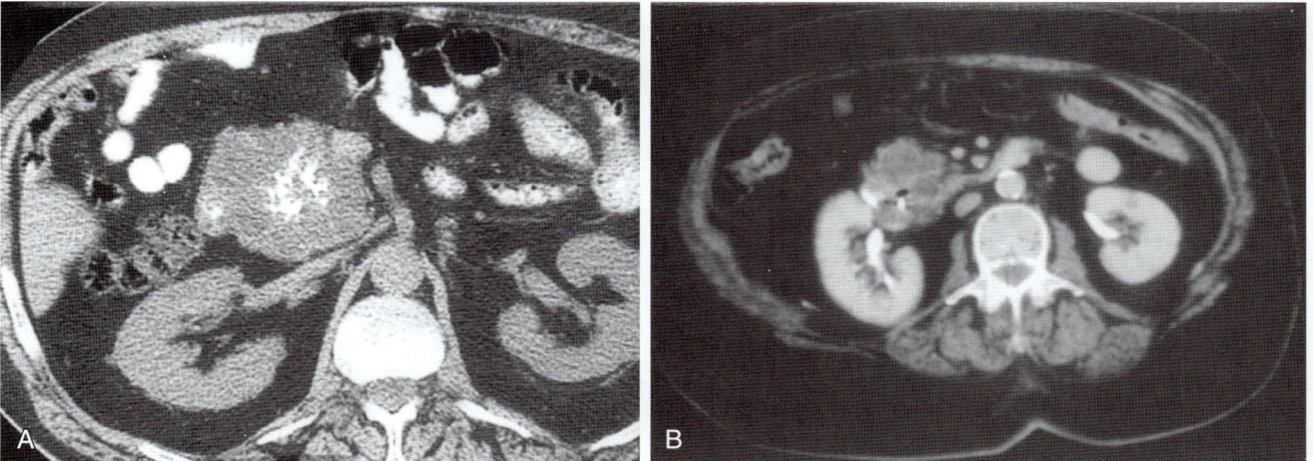

FIGURE 98.5 Computed tomography scan of serous cystic neoplasm. (A) Solid-appearing lesion with central starburst calcification. (B) "Microcystic" mass in head of pancreas. ([A], Reproduced with permission from Pyke CM, van Heerden JA, Colby TV, Sarr MG, Weaver AL. The spectrum of serous cystadenoma of the pancreas: clinical, pathological, and surgical aspects. *Ann Surg.* 1992;215:132; [B], reproduced with permission from Sarr MG, Murr M, Smyrk TC, et al. Primary cystic neoplasms of the pancreas: neoplastic disorders of emerging importance—current state-of-the-art and unanswered questions. *J Gastrointest Surg.* 2003;7:417.)

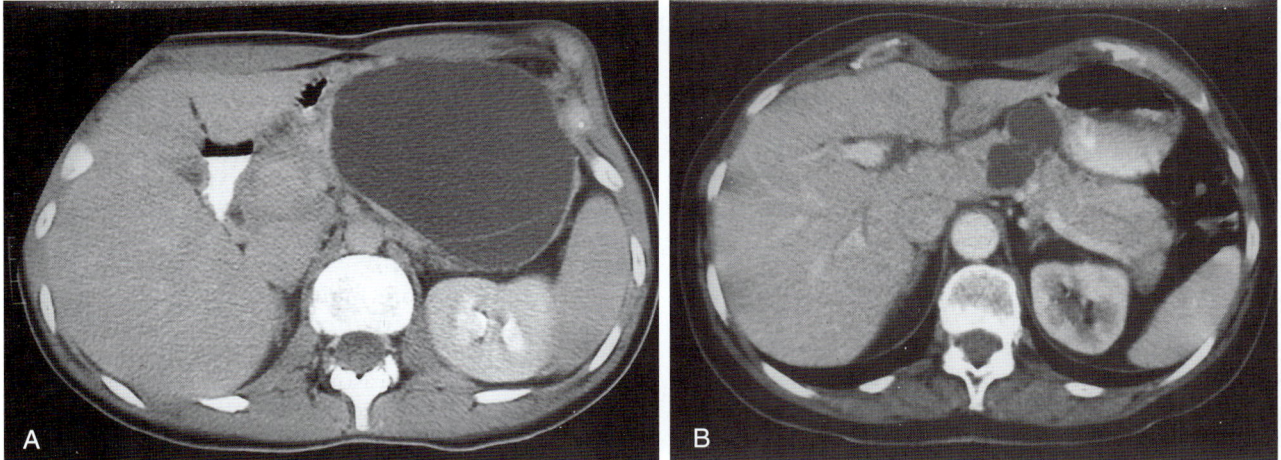

FIGURE 98.6 Computed tomography characteristics of primary mucinous cystic neoplasms of the pancreas. (A) Macrocystic form: note septum and lack of surrounding inflammatory reaction. (B) Several macrocystic areas (>2 cm) in midbody of pancreas. (Reproduced with permission from Yeo CJ, Sarr MG. Cystic and pseudocystic diseases of the pancreas. *Curr Probl Surg.* 1994;31:165.)

in the presence of main pancreatic duct dilation greater than 5 mm with a branch-duct IPMN.[33] Imaging findings with a higher probability of malignancy include main-duct IPMN, presence of mural nodules, and dilation of the biliary tree.[9,30] However, differentiation of benign versus malignant IPMNs by imaging is technically difficult and diagnosis can only be confirmed with adequate tissue sampling. A major limitation of MDCT is the exposure of patients to ionizing radiation, and judicious use of this modality should be practiced.[34]

Magnetic Resonance Cholangiopancreatography

Technologic advances in MRI have led to increased ability to visualize pancreatic lesions. The lack of ionizing radiation exposure compared with CT imaging is a substantial benefit. Moreover, new resonance sequences that allow for fast breath-holding imaging has led to fewer motion artifacts with enhanced imaging during multiple phases of contrast administration. All of these advances have allowed MRI to become the preferred modality for pancreatic imaging of the parenchyma, ductal system, and vasculature.[35] Magnetic resonance cholangiopancreatography (MRCP) is a noninvasive diagnostic method that uses MRI to specifically assess the pancreas and ductal system. This imaging modality has little risk when compared with invasive procedures, such as endoscopic retrograde cholangiopancreatography (ERCP). In addition, MRCP may be more sensitive than ERCP when assessing

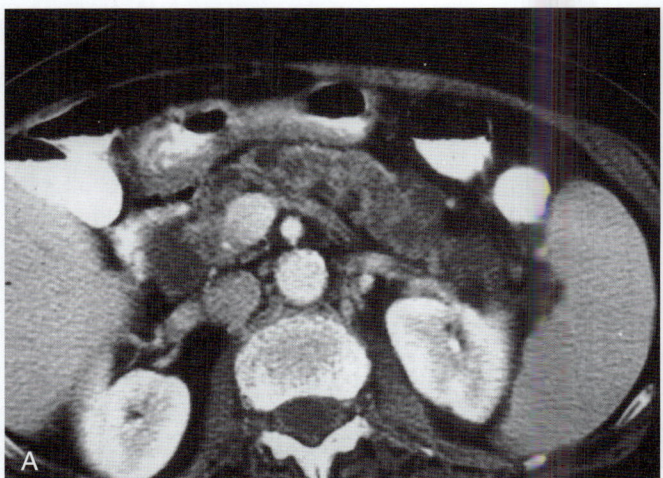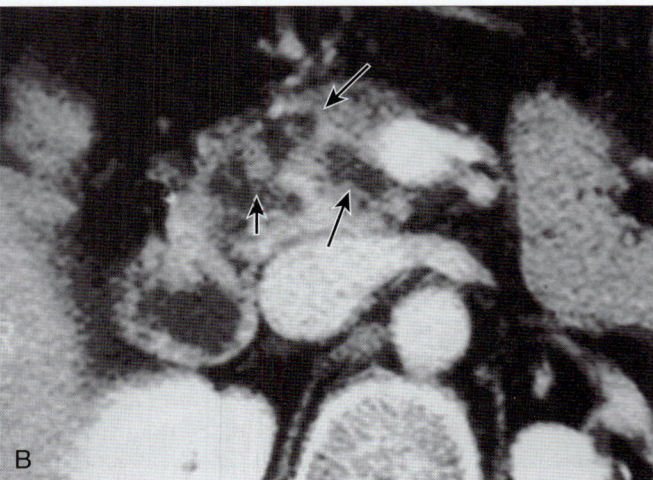

FIGURE 98.7 Computed tomography findings of intraductal papillary mucinous neoplasms of the pancreas. (A) Main-duct disease. Note dilation of main pancreatic duct and atrophy of the parenchyma. (B) Branch-duct intraductal papillary mucinous neoplasm dilation of secondary branches of the ductal system *(arrows)*. ([A], Reproduced with permission from Loftus EV Jr, Olivares-Pakzad BA, Batts KP, et al. Intraductal papillary-mucinous tumors of the pancreas: clinicopathologic features, outcome, and nomenclature. Members of the Pancreas Clinic and Pancreatic Surgeons of Mayo Clinic. *Gastroenterology*. 1996;110:1909; [B], reproduced with permission from Sarr MG, Murr M, Smyrk TC, et al. Primary cystic neoplasms of the pancreas: neoplastic disorders of emerging importance—current state-of-the-art and unanswered questions. *J Gastrointest Surg.* 2003;7:417.)

obscured ductal anatomy due to side-branch filling by mucin.[36,37] MRCP can also assess cysts that do not communicate with the main ductal system.[38] Similar to other imaging techniques, mural nodules, main-duct IPMN, and common bile duct dilation suggest underlying malignancy.[36] Classically, MRCP has been very useful in diagnosing branch-duct IPMNs due to their appearance as a cluster of grapes.[17]

Serous Cystic Neoplasms

SCNs on MRI appear as a "cluster of grapes" on T2-weighted images with multiple small cysts and enhanced septations. MRI is able to detect very small cysts due to superior soft tissue contrast resolution compared with CT. The presence of bright T1-weighted cystic fluid suggests hemorrhagic fluid content. The main disadvantage of MRI is the inability to detect central calcifications commonly seen with SCNs.[39,40]

Mucinous Cystic Neoplasms

MCNs on MRI appear as well-defined, uniloculated or multiloculated cystic lesion(s) with enhanced septations and occasionally solid components. MRI is able to better identify the contents of the cyst compared with CT imaging. High signal intensity on T1- and T2-weighted imaging can result from mucin within the cyst. The proximity of the cyst to the ductal system is better assessed with MRI and can help to differentiate MCNs from pseudocysts and IPMNs. Similar to SCNs, calcifications are not appreciated on MRI.[39,40]

Intraductal Papillary Mucinous Neoplasm

The technologic advances with MRI including 3D high-resolution post-contrast with MRCP have made it possible to perform a detailed evaluation of the pancreatic ductal system and potential IPMNs. The high resolution of the imaging has allowed MRI to diagnose IPMNs without the need of ERCP. Lastly, MRI can be used as the imaging modality of choice to follow patients with pancreatic lesions over time due to the lack of ionizing radiation.[40]

There are certain limitations to performing an MRI to assess for pancreatic disease. Smaller-size IPMNs (<10 mm) are not readily seen with traditional imaging and endoscopic ultrasound (EUS) should be used for full assessment.[35] In addition, patients with pacemakers or implantable defibrillators were previously an absolute contraindication to undergo an MRI due to the risk of severe complications or even death. Nowadays, advances in cardiac implantable devices have allowed certain patients to no longer be contraindicated for MRI, but extreme caution should still be exercised to prevent injury to the patient.[41] Finally, a relative contraindication for MRI is claustrophobia due to the narrow space required to perform the scan.

Positron Emission Tomography–Computed Tomography

PET-CT is an imaging method that identifies tissue metabolism and perfusion using a radiotracer, most commonly ^{18}F-fluorodeoxyglucose (FDG).[42] PET-CT has been proposed as a useful modality to aid in the differentiation of benign versus malignant cystic lesions. A case series has demonstrated a sensitivity and specificity of 92% and 95%, respectively.[43] In 2013 a metaanalysis demonstrated similar results with a pooled sensitivity of 88%.[42] A limitation to PET-CT is the increased uptake that occurs with pseudocysts and inflammatory conditions (e.g.,

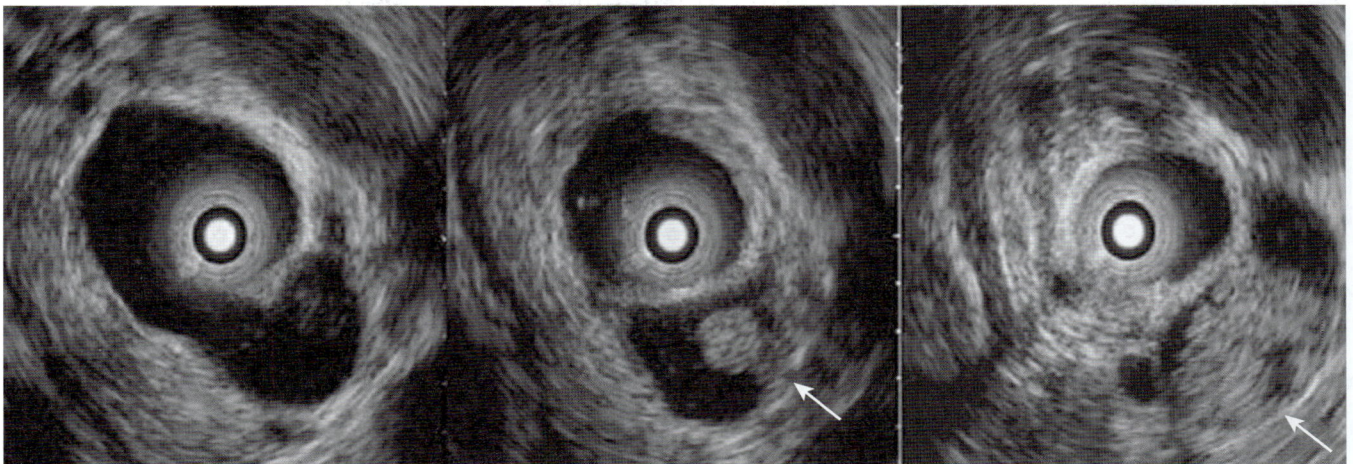

FIGURE 98.8 Intraductal ultrasonography of an intraductal papillary mucinous neoplasm with mural nodules *(arrows)* in the pancreatic head. (Reprinted with permission from Tanaka M, Chari S, Volkan Adsay N, et al. Management of intraductal papillary mucinous neoplasms and mucinous cystic neoplasms of the pancreas. *Pancreatology*. 2006;6:20 [Fig. 6].)

acute pancreatitis). The lack of FDG uptake associated with certain mucinous tumors does not preclude resection. Although this modality may have future applications, it currently does not add sufficient diagnostic value and is not generally recommended outside of experimental studies.

ENDOSCOPIC EVALUATION (INVASIVE)

Advanced Endoscopic Evaluation of Pancreatic Cystic Neoplasms

Despite a thorough history and physical and high-resolution imaging techniques, differentiating the histopathologic subtypes of pancreatic cysts remains elusive. As seen previously, discerning between benign and malignant PCNs is essential for clinical management. The use of EUS with fine-needle aspiration (FNA) by a skilled operator can provide anatomic detail, locoregional staging, and sampling of cystic fluid. Although EUS is considered an invasive procedure, major complications are rare when performed by experienced endoscopists. One prospective study identified an overall complication rate of 1.1% in 540 patients.[44] The use of EUS provides cyst size, morphology, and proximity to vascular and other visceral structures (Fig. 98.8).[45] SCNs typically appear as microcystic compartments with the absence of fluid. The presence of the microcystic appearance usually does not warrant FNA due to the benign nature of disease.[46] Some SCNs have macrocystic components that can resemble MCNs. However, the low mucin concentration and low viscosity provides an easy way to differentiate the two.

MCNs are typically unilocular with high viscous fluid during aspiration.[46] The viscosity of the fluid can make it challenging to obtain an adequate sample.[47] There is great difficulty involved when trying to differentiate MCNs from IPMNs on EUS. Most IPMNs demonstrate a "grape-like" architecture and communication with the pancreatic duct, which is noticeably absent in MCNs.[46]

The diagnosis of IPMNs can be aided by ERCP because it can demonstrate ductal dilatation, filling defects secondary to mucin obstruction, and cystic dilatations of side branches (Fig. 98.9).[46] The major papilla can also have the dilated, fish-mouth appearance in main or mixed-type IPMN with free flow of mucinous fluid into the duodenum.[21] The incidence of morbidity from ERCP and the continual advancements in MRCP imaging technology may have contributed to decreased use of ERCP for diagnosis in PCN. As mentioned earlier, MRCP has a higher sensitivity for detecting branch-duct IPMNs compared with endoscopic equivalents.[48] The one advantage of endoscopic procedures is the ability to perform a sphincterotomy with stent placement for biliary decompression when a neoplastic cyst causes obstructive jaundice.[49] This serves as a temporizing measure until a definitive operative intervention is performed. The main limitation of EUS is the low availability of EUS-trained endoscopists in nontertiary medical centers.

Fine-Needle Aspiration

Examination of the cystic fluid obtained during either percutaneous or endoscopic approach has been shown to have clinical utility.[50] The preferred method to acquire the cystic fluid is endoscopically due to the small risk of potential complications. These complications include bleeding (<1%), intracystic hemorrhage (6%), pancreatitis (1% to 2%), infection (<1%), and potential seeding of malignant cells along the needle tract.[51,52] Antibiotics are usually administered perioperatively to theoretically decrease the risk of infection, and most endoscopists remove as much fluid as possible in an attempt to decrease bacterial inoculation of the cyst fluid.[53]

Fluid Cytology

Cystic fluid cytology can help to differentiate between benign and high-risk/malignant PCNs.[54]

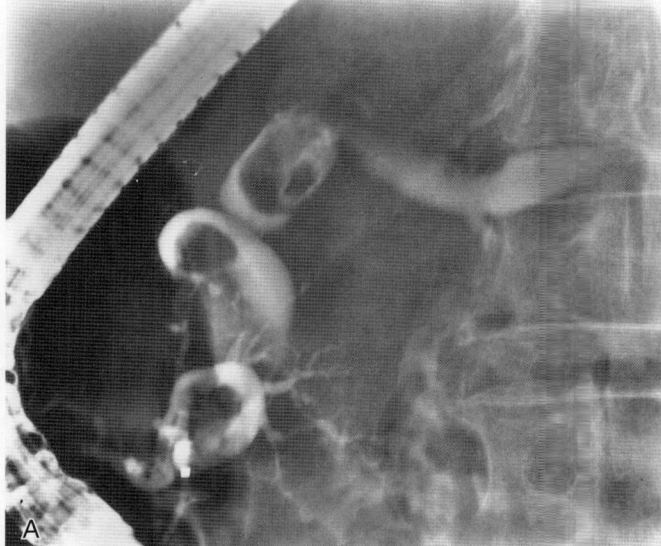

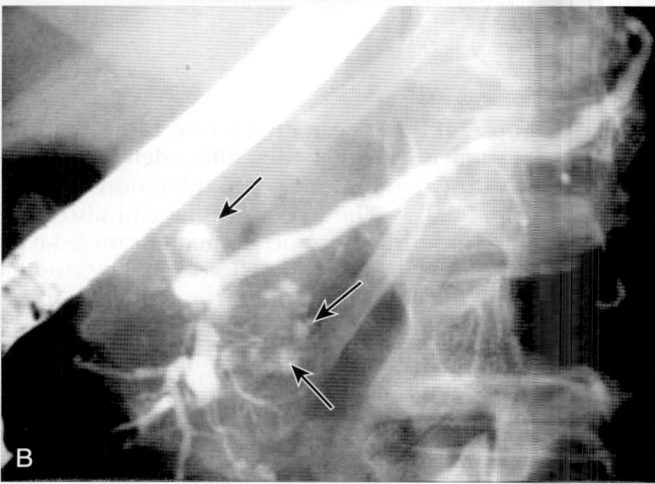

FIGURE 98.9 Endoscopic retrograde pancreatography in intraductal papillary mucinous neoplasms. (A) Main-duct disease. (B) Branch-duct disease. ([A], Reproduced with permission from Loftus EV Jr, Olivares-Pakzad BA, Batts KP, et al. Intraductal papillary-mucinous tumors of the pancreas: clinicopathologic features, outcome, and nomenclature. Members of the Pancreas Clinic and Pancreatic Surgeons of Mayo Clinic. *Gastroenterology*. 1996;110:1909; [B], reproduced with permission from Ear MG, Murr M, Smyrk TC, et al. Primary cystic neoplasms of the pancreas: neoplastic disorders of emerging importance—current state-of-the-art and unanswered questions. *J Gastrointest Surg*. 2003;7:417.)

The cytology of SCNs includes bland cuboidal cells containing glycogen, clear cytoplasm without cellular atypia or necrosis.[13,55] However, it is common for the aspirate to be devoid of any cellular material limiting adequate diagnosis and should be treated as a nondiagnostic result.[56] Low-grade MCN aspirates contain honeycomb sheets and clusters of columnar cells containing mucin. The presence of mucin can help to differentiate between SCNs and MCNs.[57] The heterogeneity of MCNs may lead to differing cytologic and histologic diagnosis, and thus the cytology should only be used to differentiate between serous and mucinous neoplasms. Cytology from IPMNs typically shows the presence of papillary clusters lined by columnar cells containing mucin with varying degrees of atypia.[22] The degree of atypia has been shown to correlate with the risk of malignancy.[58] The cellular aspirate of the inflammatory pancreatic pseudocyst usually contains cellular debris with macrophages, proteinaceous precipitate, and other inflammatory cells.[59]

The main limitation of FNA is the nondiagnostic result due to a lack of adequate cellular material, causing a potential false-negative to occur. A single-center study of 141 cysts found that cytology was diagnostic in only 58% of cysts.[56] The ability to sample solid components of the cyst via endoscopic methods can aid in diagnosis.[50] However, frequent "contamination" of parenchyma in the proximity may further complicate diagnosis.[50]

Cystic Fluid Analysis

Recent research has focused on the biochemical analysis of cystic fluid in hopes to simplify the diagnosis of pancreatic cysts prior to surgical intervention. The analysis typically includes measurement of mucin, CEA, and amylase.[50]

1. Mucin: As mentioned earlier, with adequate sampling, SCNs do not contain any mucin. The presence of mucin is highly specific for MCNs and IPMNs, which can be visualized grossly during endoscopy when smears are prepared after sampling.[50]
2. CEA: Most mucinous neoplasms of the pancreas contain higher concentrations of CEA compared with their SCN counterparts. There is no standardized cutoff value to differentiate between the two, but most centers use 192 ng/mL (established by Brugge et al.[60]), with a sensitivity of 73% and specificity of 84%. Moreover, no other combination of serologic markers provided greater accuracy in diagnosing mucinous lesions than CEA level alone. When CEA levels are less than 5 ng/mL, mucinous neoplasms can essentially be excluded.[61]
3. Amylase: There are very few publications that find amylase to have any diagnostic value.[50] In these reports a value greater than five times serum amylase highly suggests the presence of a pseudocyst. However, cystic fluid amylase concentration from IPMNs may be high due to communication with the pancreatic ductal system.[62]

The value of cyst fluid CA 19-9 remains controversial with uncertain value.[50]

Recent research has focused on analyzing the MUC expression patterns from pancreatic cystic fluid. A prospective study from Memorial Sloan Kettering Cancer Center[25] collected cystic fluid from 40 patients who underwent pancreatic resection. The pancreatic specimens were grouped into low-risk (low-grade or moderate dysplasia) and high-risk groups (high-grade dysplasia or carcinoma). Higher concentrations of MUC2 and MUC4 in the cystic fluid were correlated with high-risk groups.[25] These expression patterns may assist surgeons in selecting patients for resection.

Molecular Diagnostics

The increased availability of molecular testing has given rise to improved understanding of genetic mutations associated with PCNs. These mutations include *KRAS*, *p53*, *p16*, and *SMAD4*.[63] A multiinstitutional prospective analysis from 2009 showed high levels of specificity (96%) associated with these mutations but a lack of sensitivity (50%).[64] To account for the low sensitivity, another gene, *GNAS*, was proposed as the source of mutation when IPMNs lacked *KRAS* mutations.[50] Combining *GNAS* and *KRAS* achieved a 98% specificity and 84% sensitivity when assessing pancreatic cystic fluid from IPMNs.[65]

Although the individual use of molecular markers in cystic fluid has limited utility, studies have started to analyze a panel of markers to aid in diagnosis of cysts from cystic fluid. A study from 2015 included 130 resected pancreatic specimens, and the cystic fluid was analyzed by a panel that included mutations in genes, loss of heterozygosity, and aneuploidy. The combination of molecular markers and clinical features achieved a 90% to 100% sensitivity and a 92% to 98% specificity. Furthermore, the panel identified 67 out of 74 patients that did not require surgery and thus could have reduced the number of unnecessary operations by 91%.[66] Additional studies are necessary to assess applicability to cystic fluid obtained preoperatively and to simplify the molecular marker panels for more efficiency.

OPERATIVE MANAGEMENT

The varying levels of malignant potential among the PCNs dictate separate treatment algorithms for each of the PCNs.

SEROUS CYSTIC NEOPLASM

As previously discussed, nearly all SCNs are benign. Due to the high risks of undergoing resection for a benign process, the general principle has been to observe SCNs.[7] With decreasing perioperative morbidity and mortality associated with pancreatic surgery, there is a trend toward resection of SCNs. Proper risk stratification of each patient is essential prior to surgery. In older or frail patients, conservative approaches continue to be the best ideology. Resection of SCNs should be selected based on patient risk factors, extent of surgery required, and cyst biology. The main indication for operative management of an SCN is the presence of symptoms. Other indications include cyst size greater than 4 cm and uncertainty of diagnosis despite appropriate radiologic assessment.[37] The type of surgical resection that is performed is based on the position of the cyst within the pancreas. These include anatomic pancreatectomy (pancreaticoduodenectomy, distal pancreatectomy) or tissue-preserving procedures (segmental central pancreatectomy). There are limited reports in the literature discussing enucleation of the cyst. This approach is associated with high morbidity (approximately 40%) due to the development of a pancreatic fistula.[67] The size of operative SCNs does not allow for enucleation to be performed. However, small peripheral SCNs can be amendable to enucleation, but this is not common practice. There is no role for lymphadenectomy or extended resections due to the inherent benign nature of SCNs.

The rare instance of serous cystadenocarcinoma remains a therapeutic challenge. The volume of cases published in the literature regarding this malignant process is extremely limited. The preferred method at this time is treating the cystadenocarcinomas as a malignant tumor and following standard operative procedures for pancreatic malignancies.

MUCINOUS CYSTIC NEOPLASM

The varying degrees of metaplasia, dysplasia, carcinoma in situ, and tissue invasion prognosticates the potential malignant degeneration associated with MCNs.[68] The general principle for all mucinous neoplasms is surgical resection irrespective of location in the pancreas or size.[7] Patients with an MCN located in the head of the pancreas should undergo a pancreaticoduodenectomy. However, a majority of MCNs originate in the body and tail of the pancreas, and thus the surgical technique of choice is a distal pancreatectomy.[7] There are controversial data supporting or against a concurrent splenectomy. If there is no evidence of malignancy, spleen preservation can be considered. If there is invasion on frozen section, a completion splenectomy with splenic vessels and regional lymph node dissection should be performed.[69,70] Increasingly, laparoscopic approaches have been used for small and medium MCNs located in the body and tail of the pancreas. Care should be taken to not rupture the cyst intraoperatively, causing seeding of the peritoneal cavity and loss of vital histologic margins for proper pathologic diagnosis.[69] Nonanatomic resections (enucleation, duodenal preserving) have been performed previously but are considered suboptimal due to limitations with intraoperative diagnosis of malignancy.[71] Lymph node excision should be limited to the immediate proximity of the pancreatic lesion due to the small incidence of lymph node metastases even with malignant MCNs.[72] Occasionally, adjacent structures or organs may require resection due to involvement with the MCN. Compared with pancreatic adenocarcinoma, MCNs tend to "push" rather than "invade."[73]

Obtaining frozen sections during the operation is usually not required when resecting MCNs because the borders of the cysts are normally discernable from the pancreatic parenchyma. Intraoperative frozen section should be used when attempting to exclude invasive carcinoma or a palpable firmness is within a close proximity to resection margin. In the event that the pathologist reports an invasive carcinoma on frozen section, the operation should proceed as if treating any other carcinoma of the pancreas.[74]

Some surgeons have taken the nonoperative approach for certain low-risk MCNs. These low-risk factors include asymptomatic MCNs, smaller than 3 cm, absence of mural nodules, absence of pancreatic and biliary duct dilatation, and absence of lymphadenopathy.[72] This observance approach depends on regular surveillance imaging to monitor for signs of increasing cyst size and presence of mural nodules. Unfortunately, long-term data associated with observation are currently unknown. No prospective studies have identified the frequency or modality of imaging for surveillance. Nonoperative management warrants a thorough discussion with patients and their surgeon to discuss the risks of waiting to treat a potential malignant neoplasm. Guidelines at this time recommend resection for MCNs greater than 3 cm or with high-risk features and some recommend resection of all MCNs irrespective of size.[17,75]

INTRADUCTAL PAPILLARY MUCINOUS NEOPLASM

The three different types of IPMNs, main duct, branch duct, and mixed duct, dictate different treatment algorithms. Main-duct IPMNs should be resected in all patients unless the risks of existing comorbidities outweigh the benefits of resection. The goal of operative management of IPMNs is to remove all adenomatous or potentially malignant epithelium to minimize recurrence in the pancreas remnant. There are two theories on the pathophysiologic basis of IPMNs. The first groups IPMNs into a similar category as an adenocarcinoma, a localized process involving only a particular segment of the pancreas. The thought is that removal of the IPMN is the only treatment necessary. In contrast, some believe IPMNs to represent a field defect of the pancreas. All of the ductal epithelium remains at risk of malignant degeneration despite removal of the cyst. Ideally, a total pancreatectomy would eliminate all risk, but this is a radical procedure that is associated with metabolic derangements and exocrine insufficiency.[76] Total pancreatectomy should be limited to the most fit patients, with a thorough preoperative assessment and proper risk stratification prior to undertaking this surgery.[77]

Localized branch-duct IPMN can be treated with a formal anatomic pancreatectomy, pancreaticoduodenectomy, or distal pancreatectomy, depending on the location of the lesion. However, guidelines were established that allow for nonoperative management with certain branch-type IPMN characteristics. These include asymptomatic patients with a cyst size less than 3 cm and lack of mural nodules.[74] The data to support this demonstrate a very low incidence of malignancy (approximately 2%) in this patient group. Which nearly matches the anticipated mortality of undergoing a formal anatomic resection.[17,78] In approximately 20% to 30% of patients with branch-duct IPMNs, there is evidence of multifocality.[79] The additional IPMNs can be visualized on high-resolution CT or MRI imaging. Ideally, patients with multifocal branch-duct IPMNs should undergo a total pancreatectomy. However, as previously mentioned, the increased morbidity and lifestyle alterations associated with a total pancreatectomy allows for a more conservative approach. This would include removing the most suspicious or dominant of the lesions in an anatomic resection and follow-up imaging surveillance of the remaining pancreas remnant.[17] If subsequent imaging demonstrates malignant characteristics, a completion pancreatectomy is usually indicated.[74]

There is less uncertainty with treatment of main-duct IPMNs. The high incidence of underlying malignancy associated with the IPMNs warrants surgical resection. IPMNs localized to the body and tail (approximately 33%) can undergo a distal pancreatectomy with splenectomy.[24] At the time of surgery, a frozen section of the proximal margin should be interpreted by a pathologist to rule out

high-grade dysplasia. A prospective study identified a concordance rate of 94% between frozen section and final pathologic examination.[80] If the margin is positive (high-grade dysplasia, invasion) additional margins may be resected from the pancreas until no evidence of disease is present. However, most surgeons will proceed to a total pancreatectomy after two subsequent margins demonstrate malignant changes.[17] This more extensive procedure should be discussed with the patient prior to surgery, and the patient should be properly consented regarding the risks of a total pancreatectomy. IPMNs localized to the head or uncinate process of the pancreas should undergo a pancreaticoduodenectomy. A frozen section of the distal margin should be analyzed by pathology for evidence of disease. As mentioned before, after two additional margins reveal malignant changes, a total pancreatectomy is usually indicated (approximately 5%).[17,81] The absence of abnormal changes in frozen sections does not equate to negative disease throughout the pancreas remnant. Rather, skip lesions involving the remainder of the pancreas can exist and thus patients ultimately still require imaging surveillance after successful resection.[17,81]

A prophylactic total pancreatectomy is rarely performed because the subsequent pancreatic endocrine (diabetes mellitus) and exocrine deficits (malnutrition) carry an increased morbidity.[79,82]

Recent studies have focused on performing endoscopic cyst ablation using ethanol and occasionally in combination with paclitaxel.[61,83] Ablation serves as an alternative to operative intervention for smaller cysts and for patients with serious comorbidities that would preclude surgery. Endoscopic ablation with ethanol is contraindicated with main-duct IPMNs due to the interaction of the ethanol with the activation of zymogens resulting in acute pancreatitis.[84] Long-term outcomes regarding recurrence and survival remain unclear, and ablation is currently not recommended for patients with neoplastic cysts.[61]

ADJUVANT AND NEOADJUVANT THERAPY

Historically, adjuvant therapy has been reserved for patients with evidence of invasive disease on final pathology even in the absence of positive margins. This management has merely been extrapolated from the treatment of pancreatic adenocarcinoma because no randomized clinical trials exist evaluating adjuvant therapy.[35] Similar to pancreatic adenocarcinoma, the preferred drug of choice is gemcitabine-based chemotherapy with radiotherapy.[85] One study from Johns Hopkins[86] showed a 57% decrease in the relative risk of mortality when 70 patients with IPMNs received chemoradiotherapy with 5-fluorouracil. Individuals with the largest decrease in mortality included those with evidence of lymph node metastases. A retrospective analysis performed at Duke[87] identified 972 patients who underwent surgery for IPMNs, of which 309 (31.8%) received adjuvant radiotherapy. There was no difference in overall survival between the adjuvant and surgery-only groups. However, subgroup analysis demonstrated improved survival for invasive IPMNs, T3/T4 tumors, and lymph node involvement. No generalized recommendation for adjuvant radiotherapy can currently be made. Individuals with high-risk tumors, including lymph node disease and invasion, should have a discussion with their physician regarding the risks and benefits of radiotherapy.[35]

Neoadjuvant therapy should be reserved with patients with unresectable disease. Some of these patients may subsequently become resectable after treatment, but without clinical trials demonstrating this benefit, no formal recommendation can be made.

OUTCOMES

SURVIVAL

Operative resection of SCNs and noninvasive MCNs is curative if the cyst is removed with negative margins.

For MCNs with invasion, previous studies cited 5-year survival rates approaching 70%, but retrospective analysis of these specimens have revealed an incorrect classification of branch-duct IPMNs and mucinous cysts with proliferative epithelium lacking invasion. Newer studies have demonstrated a much lower 5-year survival (26%) when resecting an MCN with invasion.[88] For unresectable invasive MCNs, the prognosis is similar to unresectable pancreatic adenocarcinomas.[77]

A retrospective analysis of the Surveillance, Epidemiology and End Results (SEER) registry analyzed the differences in overall survival between invasive MCNs and IPMNs. Patients with invasive MCNs localized within the pancreas and without nodal disease (stage IA) had significantly better survival than similarly staged IPMNs (74.6% vs. 43.4% at 5 years). However, this survival benefit disappeared in the presence of nodal disease or with extrapancreatic extension.[89]

Recurrence rates with IPMNs are variable. An anatomic resection of a branch-duct IPMN with negative margins has been shown to be curative. The recurrence of a main-duct IPMN in the remnant gland is anywhere from 0% to 10% if the margins are negative and there is no evidence of invasion.[26,77,90] Most case series cite a 5-year survival rate of at least 70% after resection of noninvasive IPMNs.[91] In contrast, evidence of invasive disease, despite negative margins, decreases 5-year survival to 30% to 50%.[91,92] The recurrence rate in either the pancreatic remnant or distant sites approaches 50% to 90% in these patients.[26] Histopathologic subtype of the IPMN is correlated with survival. The aggressive tubular subtype has a 5-year survival ranging from 37% to 55% following surgical resection, whereas the colloid subtype has 5-year survival ranging from 61% to 87% post resection.[93] Factors associated with decreased survival include tubular subtype, lymph node metastases, vascular invasion, and positive margins.[81,94] IPMNs with evidence of invasion should be treated similar to pancreatic adenocarcinomas. Studies show that IPMNs tend to have better survival than pancreatic adenocarcinoma.[94] This survival benefit may be secondary to the less aggressive tumor biology or the earlier diagnosis of IPMNs.

SURVEILLANCE

SCNs and noninvasive MCNs tend to be isolated in the pancreas, and the likelihood of local or distant recurrence is minimal.[95] Regular follow-up with imaging of the abdomen is unnecessary for these types of cysts.[74]

TABLE 98.2 Guidelines for Follow-Up Imaging of Pancreatic Cysts After Resection[17]

Noninvasive MCN	No surveillance imaging necessary
Invasive MCN	Surveillance imaging similar to pancreatic ductal adenocarcinoma (cross-sectional imaging every 6 months for 2 years)
Noninvasive IPMN with negative margins	Surveillance imaging at approximately 2 and 5 years after resection
Noninvasive IPMN with dysplastic margins	Surveillance imaging every 6 months
Invasive IPMN	Surveillance imaging similar to pancreatic ductal adenocarcinoma (cross-sectional imaging every 3–6 months for 2 years)

IPMN, Intraductal papillary mucinous neoplasm; *MCN,* mucinous cystic neoplasm.

The recommended follow-up for MCNs with invasion is surveillance imaging every 3 to 6 months for the first 2 years to monitor for local or distant recurrence.[17,74] The modality of choice remains MRI due to the lack of ionizing radiation. The downside to MRI surveillance remains the cost.

All patients who have a resected IPMN should undergo imaging surveillance. There is continual survival benefit with further resection if an IPMN does recur.[90] International Consensus Guidelines published in 2012[17] offer recommendations for the frequency and modality of imaging surveillance after resection (see Table 98.2). Routine serum measurement of CEA and CA 19-9 has a limited role for detection of an IPMN recurrence. Of note, a new pancreatic lesion discovered on imaging after resection could represent a postoperative pseudocyst, a recurrence of the IPMN from inadequate resection, a new IPMN, or an unrelated new neoplastic process.

IPMNs may also be associated with extrapancreatic neoplasms (stomach, colon, rectum, lung, breast) and pancreatic ductal adenocarcinoma.[17,24,96] It is unclear if this represents a true genetic syndrome. However, patients with IPMNs should have a discussion about the implications of their disease with their physician and are encouraged to undergo colonoscopy to exclude a synchronous neoplastic process.[96]

The incidence of PCNs will continue to increase as imaging technology improves. EUS, cytology, and molecular panels have made differentiating the type of PCN less problematic. The importance of an accurate preoperative diagnosis ensures that operative management is selectively offered to those with high-risk lesions. Management beyond surgery, including adjuvant therapy and surveillance, continue to be active areas of research.

ACKNOWLEDGMENTS

Special thanks to Roberta Carden for proofreading and editing.

Special thanks to George H. Sakorafas, Thomas Schnelldorfer, and Michael G. Sarr for their contributions in the previous edition.

REFERENCES

1. Compagno J, Oertel JE. Mucinous cystic neoplasms of the pancreas with overt and latent malignancy (cystadenocarcinoma and cystadenoma). A clinicopathologic study of 41 cases. *Am J Clin Pathol*. 1978;69(6):573-580.

2. Ohashi K, Murakami Y, Maruyama M. Four cases of mucous-secreting pancreatic cancer. *Prog Dig Endosc*. 1982;20:348-351.

3. Kloppel G, Solica E, Longnecker DS, Capella C, Sobin LH. *Histological Typing of Tumours of the Exocrine Pancreas*. Berlin: Springer 1996:2.

4. Lee KS, Sekhar A, Rofsky NM, Pedrosa I. Prevalence of incidental pancreatic cysts in the adult population on MR imaging. *Am J Gastroenterol*. 2010;105(9):2079-2084.

5. Kimura W. How many millimeters do atypical epithelia of the pancreas spread intraductally before beginning to infiltrate? *Hepatogastroenterology*. 2003;50(54):2218-2224.

6. Kosmahl M, Pauser U, Peters K, et al. Cystic neoplasms of the pancreas and tumor-like lesions with cystic features: a review of 418 cases and a classification proposal. *Virchows Arch*. 2004;445(2):168-178.

7. Chandwani R, Allen PJ. Cystic neoplasms of the pancreas. *Annu Rev Med*. 2016;67:45-57.

8. Zhang XP, Yu ZX, Zhao YP, Dai MH. Current perspectives on pancreatic serous cystic neoplasms: diagnosis, management and beyond. *World J Gastrointest Surg*. 2016;8(3):202-211.

9. Tran Cao HS, Kellogg B, Lowy AM, Bouvet M. Cystic neoplasms of the pancreas. *Surg Oncol Clin N Am*. 2010;19(2):267-295.

10. Chatelain D, Hammel P, O'Toole D, et al. Macrocystic form of serous pancreatic cystadenoma. *Am J Gastroenterol*. 2002;97(10):2566-2571.

11. Charlesworth M, Verbeke CS, Falk GA, Walsh M, Smith AM, Morris-Stiff G. Pancreatic lesions in von Hippel-Lindau disease? A systematic review and meta-synthesis of the literature. *J Gastrointest Surg*. 2012;16(7):1422-1428.

12. George DH, Murphy F, Michalski R, Ulmer BG. Serous cystadenocarcinoma of the pancreas: a new entity? *Am J Surg Pathol*. 1989;13(1):61-66.

13. Reid MD, Choi HJ, Memis B, et al. Serous neoplasms of the pancreas: a clinicopathologic analysis of 193 cases and literature review with new insights on macrocystic and solid variants and critical reappraisal of so-called "serous cystadenocarcinoma". *Am J Surg Pathol*. 2015;39(12):1597-1610.

14. Cooper CL, O'Toole SA, Kench JG. Classification, morphology and molecular pathology of premalignant lesions of the pancreas. *Pathology*. 2013;45(3):286-304.

15. Basturk O, Coban I, Adsay NV. Pancreatic cysts: pathologic classification, differential diagnosis, and clinical implications. *Arch Pathol Lab Med*. 2009;133(3):423-438.

16. The International Agency for Research on Cancer. WHO classification of tumours of the digestive system. In: Bosman FT, Carneiro F, Hruban RH, Theise ND, eds. *World Health Organization Classification of Tumours*. 4th ed. Lyon, France: IARC Press; 2010:417.

17. Tanaka M, Fernández-del Castillo C, Adsay V, et al. International consensus guidelines 2012 for the management of IPMN and MCN of the pancreas. *Pancreatology*. 2012;12(3):183-197.

18. Brugge WR, Lauwers GY, Sahani D, Fernandez-del Castillo C, Warshaw AL. Cystic neoplasms of the pancreas. *N Engl J Med*. 2004;351(12):1218-1226.

19. Spence RA, Dasari B, Love M, Kelly B, Taylor M. Overview of the investigation and management of cystic neoplasms of the pancreas. *Dig Surg*. 2011;28(5-6):386-397.

20. Xiao SY. Intraductal papillary mucinous neoplasm of the pancreas: an update. *Scientifica (Cairo)*. 2012;2012:893632.

21. Beintaris I, Polymeros D, Krivan S, Triantafyllou K. Fish-mouth appearance of the ampulla of Vater. *Ann Gastroenterol*. 2013;26(1):73.

22. Castellano-Megías VM, Andrés CI, López-Alonso G, Colina-Ruizdelgado F. Pathological features and diagnosis of intraductal papillary mucinous neoplasm of the pancreas. *World J Gastrointest Oncol*. 2014;6(9):311-324.

23. Barresi L, Tarantino I, Granata A, Curcio G, Traina M. Pancreatic cystic lesions: how endoscopic ultrasound morphology and endoscopic ultrasound fine needle aspiration help unlock the diagnostic puzzle. *World J Gastrointest Endosc*. 2012;4(6):247-259.

24. Shi C, Hruban RH. Intraductal papillary mucinous neoplasm. *Hum Pathol*. 2012;43(1):1-16.

25. Maker AV, Katabi N, Gonen M, et al. Pancreatic cyst fluid and serum mucin levels predict dysplasia in intraductal papillary mucinous neoplasms of the pancreas. *Ann Surg Oncol*. 2011;18(1):199-206.

26. Raut CP, Cleary KR, Staerkel GA, et al. Intraductal papillary mucinous neoplasms of the pancreas: effect of invasion and pancreatic margin status on recurrence and survival. *Ann Surg Oncol*. 2006;13(4):582-594.

27. Lafemina J, Katabi N, Klimstra D, et al. Malignant progression in IPMN: a cohort analysis of patients initially selected for resection or observation. *Ann Surg Oncol*. 2013;20(2):440-447.

28. Crippa S, Salvia R, Warshaw AL, et al. Mucinous cystic neoplasm of the pancreas is not an aggressive entity: lessons from 163 resected patients. *Ann Surg*. 2008;247(4):571-579.

29. Crippa S, Fernández-Del Castillo C, Salvia R, et al. Mucin-producing neoplasms of the pancreas: an analysis of distinguishing clinical and epidemiologic characteristics. *Clin Gastroenterol Hepatol*. 2010;8(2):213-219.

30. Jani N, Bani Hani M, Schulick RD, Hruban RH, Cunningham SC. Diagnosis and management of cystic lesions of the pancreas. *Diagn Ther Endosc*. 2011;2011:478913.

31. Cohen-Scali F, Vilgrain V, Brancatelli G, et al. Discrimination of unilocular macrocystic serous cystadenoma from pancreatic pseudocyst and mucinous cystadenoma with CT: initial observations. *Radiology*. 2003;228(3):727-733.

32. Ng DZ, Goh BK, Tham EH, Young SM, Ooi LL. Cystic neoplasms of the pancreas: current diagnostic modalities and management. *Ann Acad Med Singapore*. 2009;38(3):251-259.

33. Tan L, Zhao YE, Wang DB, et al. Imaging features of intraductal papillary mucinous neoplasms of the pancreas in multi-detector row computed tomography. *World J Gastroenterol*. 2009;15(32):4037-4043.

34. Sodickson A, Baeyens PF, Andriole KP, et al. Recurrent CT, cumulative radiation exposure, and associated radiation-induced cancer risks from CT of adults. *Radiology*. 2009;251(1):175-184.

35. Fong ZV, Ferrone CR, Lillemoe KD, Fernández-Del Castillo C. Intraductal papillary mucinous neoplasm of the pancreas: current state of the art and ongoing controversies. *Ann Surg*. 2016;263(5):908-917.

36. Machado NO, al Qadhi H, al Wahibi K. Intraductal papillary mucinous neoplasm of pancreas. *N Am J Med Sci*. 2015;7(5):160-175.

37. Barreto G, Shukla PJ, Ramadwar M, Arya S, Shrikhande SV. Cystic tumours of the pancreas. *HPB (Oxford)*. 2007;9(4):259-266.

38. Guarise A, Faccioli N, Ferrari M, et al. Evaluation of serial changes of pancreatic branch duct intraductal papillary mucinous neoplasms by follow-up with magnetic resonance imaging. *Cancer Imaging*. 2008;8:220-228.

39. Buerke B, Domagk D, Heindel W, Wessling J. Diagnostic and radiological management of cystic pancreatic lesions: important features for radiologists. *Clin Radiol*. 2012;67(8):727-737.

40. Dewhurst CE, Mortele KJ. Cystic tumors of the pancreas: imaging and management. *Radiol Clin North Am*. 2012;50(3):467-486.

41. Nordbeck P, Ertl G, Ritter O. Magnetic resonance imaging safety in pacemaker and implantable cardioverter defibrillator patients: how far have we come? *Eur Heart J*. 2015;36(24):1505-1511.

42. Bertagna F, Treglia G, Baiocchi GL, Giubbini R. F18-FDG-PET/CT for evaluation of intraductal papillary mucinous neoplasms (IPMN): a review of the literature. *Jpn J Radiol*. 2013;31(4):229-236.

43. Sperti C, Bissoli S, Pasquali C, et al. 18-Fluorodeoxyglucose positron emission tomography enhances computed tomography diagnosis of malignant intraductal papillary mucinous neoplasms of the pancreas. *Ann Surg*. 2007;246(6):932-937; discussion 937–939.

44. Eloubeidi MA, Tamhane A. Prospective assessment of diagnostic utility and complications of endoscopic ultrasound-guided fine needle aspiration. Results from a newly developed academic endoscopic ultrasound program. *Dig Dis*. 2008;26(4):356-363.

45. Rafique A, Freeman S, Carroll N. A clinical algorithm for the assessment of pancreatic lesions: utilization of 16- and 64-section multidetector CT and endoscopic ultrasound. *Clin Radiol*. 2007;62(12):1142-1153.

46. Khalid A, Brugge W. ACG practice guidelines for the diagnosis and management of neoplastic pancreatic cysts. *Am J Gastroenterol*. 2007;102(10):2339-2349.

47. Alkaade S, Chahla E, Levy M. Role of endoscopic ultrasound-guided fine-needle aspiration cytology, viscosity, and carcinoembryonic antigen in pancreatic cyst fluid. *Endosc Ultrasound*. 2015;4(4):299-303.

48. Doi R, Fujimoto K, Wada M, Imamura M. Surgical management of intraductal papillary mucinous tumor of the pancreas. *Surgery*. 2002;132(1):80-85.

49. Brugge WR. Advances in the endoscopic management of patients with pancreatic and biliary malignancies. *South Med J*. 2006;99(12):1358-1366.

50. Rockacy M, Khalid A. Update on pancreatic cyst fluid analysis. *Ann Gastroenterol.* 2013;26(2):122-127.

51. Matthaei H, Feldmann G, Lingohr P, Kalff JC. Molecular diagnostics of pancreatic cysts. *Langenbecks Arch Surg.* 2013;398(8):1021-1027.

52. Yoon WJ, Brugge WR. The safety of endoscopic ultrasound-guided fine-needle aspiration of pancreatic cystic lesions. *Endosc Ultrasound.* 2015;4(4):289-292.

53. Levy MJ, Clain JE. Evaluation and management of cystic pancreatic tumors: emphasis on the role of EUS FNA. *Clin Gastroenterol Hepatol.* 2004;2(8):639-653.

54. Moparty B, Logroño R, Nealon WH, et al. The role of endoscopic ultrasound and endoscopic ultrasound-guided fine-needle aspiration in distinguishing pancreatic cystic lesions. *Diagn Cytopathol.* 2007;35(1):18-25.

55. Karoumpalis I, Christodoulou DK. Cystic lesions of the pancreas. *Ann Gastroenterol.* 2016;29(2):155-161.

56. Cizginer S, Turner BG, Bilge AR, Karaca C, Pitman MB, Brugge WR. Cyst fluid carcinoembryonic antigen is an accurate diagnostic marker of pancreatic mucinous cysts. *Pancreas.* 2011;40:1024-1028.

57. Recine M, Kaw M, Evans DB, Krishnamurthy S. Fine-needle aspiration cytology of mucinous tumors of the pancreas. *Cancer.* 2004;102(2):92-99.

58. Pitman MB, Genevay M, Yaeger K, et al. High-grade atypical epithelial cells in pancreatic mucinous cysts are a more accurate predictor of malignancy than "positive" cytology. *Cancer Cytopathol.* 2010;118(6):434-440.

59. Stelow EB, Bardales RH, Stanley MW. Pitfalls in endoscopic ultrasound-guided fine-needle aspiration and how to avoid them. *Adv Anat Pathol.* 2005;12(2):62-73.

60. Brugge WR, Lewandrowski K, Lee-Lewandrowski E, et al. Diagnosis of pancreatic cystic neoplasms: a report of the cooperative pancreatic cyst study. *Gastroenterology.* 2004;126(5):1330-1336.

61. Brugge WR. Management and outcomes of pancreatic cystic lesions. *Dig Liver Dis.* 2008;40(11):854-859.

62. van der Waaij LA, van Dullemen HM, Porte RJ. Cyst fluid analysis in the differential diagnosis of pancreatic cystic lesions: a pooled analysis. *Gastrointest Endosc.* 2005;62(3):383-389.

63. Izeradjene K, Combs C, Best M, et al. Kras(G12D) and Smad4/Dpc4 haploinsufficiency cooperate to induce mucinous cystic neoplasms and invasive adenocarcinoma of the pancreas. *Cancer Cell.* 2007;11(3):229-243.

64. Khalid A, Zahid M, Finkelstein SD, et al. Pancreatic cyst fluid DNA analysis in evaluating pancreatic cysts: a report of the PANDA study. *Gastrointest Endosc.* 2009;69(6):1095-1102.

65. Singhi AD, Nikiforova MN, Fasanella KE, et al. Preoperative GNAS and KRAS testing in the diagnosis of pancreatic mucinous cysts. *Clin Cancer Res.* 2014;20(16):4381-4389.

66. Springer S, Wang Y, Dal Molin M, et al. A combination of molecular markers and clinical features improve the classification of pancreatic cysts. *Gastroenterology.* 2015;149:1501-1510.

67. Beger HG, Siech M, Poch B, Mayer B, Schoenberg MH. Limited surgery for benign tumours of the pancreas: a systematic review. *World J Surg.* 2015;39(6):1557-1566.

68. Zhai J, Sarkar R, Ylagan L. Pancreatic mucinous lesions: a retrospective analysis with cytohistological correlation. *Diagn Cytopathol.* 2006;34(11):724-730.

69. Fernandez-del Castillo C. Mucinous cystic neoplasms. *J Gastrointest Surg.* 2008;12(3):411-413.

70. Ohtsuka T, Takahata S, Takanami H, et al. Laparoscopic surgery is applicable for larger mucinous cystic neoplasms of the pancreas. *J Hepatobiliary Pancreat Sci.* 2014;21(5):343-348.

71. Ohigashi S, Shimada S, Suzuki A, Onodera H. Pancreas-sparing tumor enucleation for pancreatic mucinous cystic neoplasms: experience with two patients. *J Hepatobiliary Pancreat Surg.* 2007;14(2):167-170.

72. Testini M, Gurrado A, Lissidini G, Venezia P, Greco L, Piccinni G. Management of mucinous cystic neoplasms of the pancreas. *World J Gastroenterol.* 2010;16(45):5682-5692.

73. Le Borgne J, de Calan L, Partensky C. Cystadenomas and cystadenocarcinomas of the pancreas: a multiinstitutional retrospective study of 398 cases. French Surgical Association. *Ann Surg.* 1999;230(2):152-161.

74. Tanaka M, Chari S, Adsay V, et al. International consensus guidelines for management of intraductal papillary mucinous neoplasms and mucinous cystic neoplasms of the pancreas. *Pancreatology.* 2006;6(1-2):17-32.

75. Stark A, Donahue TR, Reber HA, Hines OJ. Pancreatic cyst disease: a review. *J Am Med Assoc.* 2016;315(17):1882-1893.

76. Stauffer JA, Nguyen JH, Heckman MG, et al. Patient outcomes after total pancreatectomy: a single centre contemporary experience. *HPB (Oxford).* 2009;11(6):483-492.

77. Sarr MG, Murr M, Smyrk TC, et al. Primary cystic neoplasms of the pancreas. Neoplastic disorders of emerging importance—current state-of-the-art and unanswered questions. *J Gastrointest Surg.* 2003;7(3):417-428.

78. Woo SM, Ryu JK, Lee SH, Yoon WJ, Kim YT, Yoon YB. Branch duct IPMNs in a retrospective series of 190 patients. *Br J Surg.* 2009;96:405.

79. Garcea G, Ong SL, Rajesh A, et al. Cystic lesions of the pancreas. A diagnostic and management dilemma. *Pancreatology.* 2008;8(3):236-251.

80. Couvelard A, Sauvanet A, Kianmanesh R, et al. Frozen sectioning of the pancreatic cut surface during resection of intraductal papillary mucinous neoplasms of the pancreas is useful and reliable: a prospective evaluation. *Ann Surg.* 2005;242(6):774-778; discussion 778–780.

81. Schnelldorfer T, Sarr MG, Nagorney DM, et al. Experience with 208 resections for intraductal papillary mucinous neoplasm of the pancreas. *Arch Surg.* 2008;143(7):639-646; discussion 646.

82. Barbier L, Jamal W, Dokmak S, et al. Impact of total pancreatectomy: short- and long-term assessment. *HPB (Oxford).* 2013;15(11):882-892.

83. Kim J. Endoscopic ultrasound-guided treatment of pancreatic cystic and solid masses. *Clin Endosc.* 2015;48(4):308-311.

84. DiMaio CJ, DeWitt JM, Brugge WR. Ablation of pancreatic cystic lesions: the use of multiple endoscopic ultrasound-guided ethanol lavage sessions. *Pancreas.* 2011;40(5):664-668.

85. Caponi S, Vasile E, Funel N, et al. Adjuvant chemotherapy seems beneficial for invasive intraductal papillary mucinous neoplasms. *Eur J Surg Oncol.* 2013;39(4):396-403.

86. Swartz MJ, Hsu CC, Pawlik TM, et al. Adjuvant chemoradiotherapy after pancreatic resection for invasive carcinoma associated with intraductal papillary mucinous neoplasm of the pancreas. *Int J Radiat Oncol Biol Phys.* 2010;76(3):839-844.

87. Worni M, Akushevich I, Gloor B, et al. Adjuvant radiotherapy in the treatment of invasive intraductal papillary mucinous neoplasm of the pancreas: an analysis of the Surveillance, Epidemiology, and End Results registry. *Ann Surg Oncol.* 2012;19(4):1316-1323.

88. Jang KT, Park SM, Basturk O, et al. Clinicopathologic characteristics of 29 invasive carcinomas arising in 178 pancreatic mucinous cystic neoplasms with ovarian-type stroma: implications for management and prognosis. *Am J Surg Pathol.* 2015;39(2):179-187.

89. Kargozaran H, Vu V, Ray P, et al. Invasive IPMN and MCN: same organ, different outcomes? *Ann Surg Oncol.* 2011;18(2):345-351.

90. Marchegiani G, Mino-Kenudson M, Ferrone CR, et al. Patterns of recurrence after resection of IPMN: who, when, and how? *Ann Surg.* 2015;262(6):1108-1114.

91. Bhardwaj N, Dennison AR, Maddern GJ, Garcea G. Management implications of resection margin histology in patients undergoing resection for IPMN: a meta-analysis. *Pancreatology.* 2016;16(3):309-317.

92. Koh YX, Chok AY, Zheng HL, Tan CS, Goh BK. Systematic review and meta-analysis comparing the surgical outcomes of invasive intraductal papillary mucinous neoplasms and conventional pancreatic ductal adenocarcinoma. *Ann Surg Oncol.* 2014;21(8):2782-2800.

93. Fong ZV, Castillo CF. Intraductal papillary mucinous adenocarcinoma of the pancreas: clinical outcomes, prognostic factors, and the role of adjuvant therapy. *Viszeralmedizin.* 2015;31(1):43-46.

94. Winter JM, Jiang W, Basturk O, et al. Recurrence and survival after resection of small intraductal papillary mucinous neoplasm-associated carcinomas (≤20-mm invasive component): a multi-institutional analysis. *Ann Surg.* 2016;263(4):793-801.

95. Tien YW, Hu RH, Hung JS, Wang HP, Lee PH. Noninvasive pancreatic cystic neoplasms can be safely and effectively treated by limited pancreatectomy. *Ann Surg Oncol.* 2008;15(1):193-198.

96. Reid-Lombardo KM, Mathis KL, Wood CM, Harmsen WS, Sarr MG. Frequency of extrapancreatic neoplasms in intraductal papillary mucinous neoplasm of the pancreas: implications for management. *Ann Surg.* 2010;251(1):64-69.

97. Tanaka H, Hatsuno T, Kinoshita M, et al. A resected case of symptomatic acinar cell cystadenoma of the pancreas displacing the main pancreatic duct. *Surg Case Rep.* 2016;2(1):39.

98. Colombo P, Arizzi C, Roncalli M. Acinar cell cystadenocarcinoma of the pancreas: report of rare case and review of the literature. *Hum Pathol.* 2004;35(12):1568-1571.

Unusual Pancreatic Tumors

Elliot A. Asare | Huamin Wang | Eric P. Tamm |

Melinda M. Mortenson | Douglas B. Evans | Susan Tsai

Although pancreatic ductal adenocarcinomas account for approximately 85% of all pancreatic tumors, epithelial tumors of the pancreas are increasingly being identified due to the frequent and improved quality of abdominal imaging modalities, such as computed tomography (CT). Solid pancreatic masses with atypical clinical presentations or unusual imaging characteristics may be diagnostically challenging, and familiarity with less common pancreatic conditions is necessary to develop a comprehensive differential diagnosis and help to avoid a delay in diagnosis. This chapter will focus on unusual solid tumors of the pancreas and discuss optimal diagnostic and therapeutic approaches for management.

ACINAR CELL CARCINOMA

Acinar cell carcinomas (ACCs) account for less than 1% of pancreatic cancers. In contrast to pancreatic ductal adenocarcinoma, ACCs arise from the acinar elements of the exocrine pancreas, not ductal epithelium. As a result, ACCs often retain the exocrine characteristics of normal pancreatic acini and can produce digestive enzymes such as trypsin, chymotrypsin, and lipase. These tumors are more common among men (male to female ratio of 2:1) and usually occur in the sixth and seventh decades of life. Approximately 50% of patients are asymptomatic at initial presentation; however, some patients may present with abdominal pain (45%) or weight loss (35%).[1,2] Approximately 10% of patients with ACC may present with a paraneoplastic syndrome caused by excessive pancreatic enzyme production, which is characterized by the presence of subcutaneous fat necrosis, bony infarcts, arthritis, and eosinophilia. Although no specific serum or plasma tests exist that are diagnostic for ACC, serum lipase levels may be elevated in up to 25% of patients.[1,3] Serum tumor markers such as carbohydrate antigen 19-9 (CA 19-9), α-fetoprotein (AFP), and carcinoembryonic antigen (CEA) are variably expressed.[3] In some patients, the combination of serum lipase and AFP can be quite helpful in assessing tumor burden in response to therapy.

IMAGING

ACCs tend to be large (7 to 10 cm) solitary tumors at presentation. The lesions can be entirely solid when small, but larger tumors often outgrow their blood supply and develop central areas of necrosis. The location of ACC within the pancreas has been reported as head (47%), tail (47%), neck (3%), and uncinate process (3%).[4] Characteristic cross-sectional imaging findings include the presence of a large, exophytic, well-circumscribed mass with capsular enhancement but central hypodensity

(Fig. 99.1). There may also be internal foci of calcifications, although calcifications are not a distinguishing feature.[3,4] Similar to pancreatic adenocarcinoma, ACCs are often metastatic at presentation, with the liver being the most common site of metastasis.[4] Unlike pancreatic ductal adenocarcinomas, ACCs are less likely to cause biliopancreatic ductal dilatation because they originate from the acinus.[5] The radiographic differential diagnosis of ACCs includes pancreatic ductal adenocarcinoma, pancreatic neuroendocrine tumor, solid pseudopapillary tumors (SPTs), pancreatoblastoma, and mucinous cystic neoplasms.

PATHOLOGY

On histopathologic examination, pure ACCs have two predominant cellular patterns of growth: an acinar pattern consisting of cells growing in well-formed acini and a solid pattern characterized by sheets of cells that lack the prominent stromal component seen in pancreatic ductal adenocarcinoma.[6,7] The tumor cells have a uniform appearance with large, centrally located nucleoli with cytoplasm that is typically eosinophilic (Fig. 99.2). Classically, the majority of ACCs will have coarse granular apical cytoplasmic staining for trypsin or chymotrypsin.[8] In contrast to the staining pattern of pancreatic ductal adenocarcinoma, ACCs generally stain negative for CEA and mucicarmine. Although fine-needle aspiration (FNA) biopsy can usually differentiate a pancreatic ductal adenocarcinoma from an ACC, the greater diagnostic dilemma is distinguishing between ACC and a well-differentiated pancreatic neuroendocrine neoplasm and pancreatoblastoma. The diagnosis of ACC can be challenging, owing to the morphologic and immunophenotypical overlap that ACCs have with pancreatic neuroendocrine tumors. ACCs can have scattered neuroendocrine cells present in up to 40% of cells.[6] To distinguish the neuroendocrine cells, additional immunohistochemistry for synaptophysin and chromogranin A may be informative. When neuroendocrine cells comprise greater than 35% of the tumor, it qualifies as a mixed acinar-neuroendocrine carcinoma.[9]

Recently, 21 ACCs were characterized by whole-exome sequencing. On average the tumors had 64 somatic mutations, and no common gene was mutated in more than 30% of cancers.[10] The number of nonsynonymous mutations found in ACC is greater than that observed in such tumors as pancreatic ductal adenocarcinoma or prostate and hepatocellular carcinoma but less than that noted in melanoma and lung cancer. Several genes, including ATM, BRCA2, and PALB2, which have been associated with pancreatic ductal adenocarcinoma, were also identified as mutated in ACCs.[11] However, key driver mutations

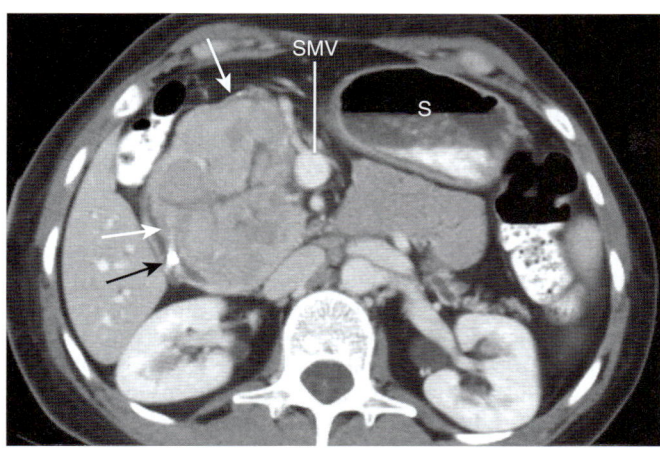

FIGURE 99.1 Axial image of a contrast-enhanced computed tomography scan from a patient with a large acinar cell carcinoma demonstrating local compression of the duodenum (white arrows) causing gastric distention (S) and biliary obstruction that required endobiliary stenting (black arrow). SMV, Superior mesenteric vein.

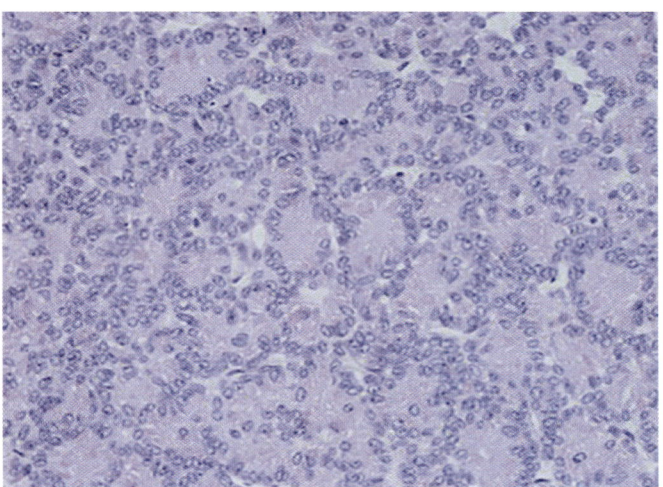

FIGURE 99.2 Histologic appearance of acinar cell carcinoma with periodic acid–Schiff positivity. Note the solid, trabecular, and glandular growth pattern. Nuclei are round to oval with minimal pleomorphism and a single prominent nucleoli.

present in pancreatic adenocarcinoma, including *KRAS*, *TP53*, *CDKN2A*, and *SMAD4*, were found to be infrequently mutated in ACCs. Interestingly, the genetic mutations associated with the major types of pancreatic cancer are now known to be relatively distinct: pancreatic ductal adenocarcinomas are characterized by mutations in *SMAD4*, *TP53*, *KRAS*, and *CDKN2A*; neuroendocrine tumors by mutations in *MEN1*, *DAXX*, *ATRX*, and the mTOR pathway; mucinous cystic neoplasms by mutations in *RNF43*; and intraductal papillary mucinous neoplasms by mutations in *GNAS* and *RNF43*. ACCs have been found to express BCL10, which is absent in pancreatic ductal adenocarcinomas and neuroendocrine tumors.[12] Although ACCs are microsatellite stable, they exhibit a high degree of chromosomal imbalances, which may help to distinguish them from pancreatic ductal adenocarcinoma and

neuroendocrine tumors.[13,14] In a murine model of cells that express *neurogenin-3*, deletion of the *Tsc1* gene leads to activation of mTOR signaling, resulting in the development of ACC.[15] The different molecular alterations found in pancreatic tumors make it possible to use DNA sequencing in those rare situations where the primary tumor or a metastatic biopsy is difficult to classify solely by histopathologic criteria.

TREATMENT

Patients who have localized disease should undergo surgical resection. Although ACCs are generally large, they tend to be well circumscribed and are often amenable to complete surgical resection. In a review of the National Cancer Database, the 5-year survival rate of 865 patients who underwent surgical resection for ACC was 36.2%.[16] Survival durations from single-institution series are even more favorable, with median survivals reported as high as 57 months for patients with localized disease who underwent complete surgical resection.[2,17] ACCs have a high rate of recurrence, with 57% of recurrences occurring at a median follow-up of 15 months and 100% of recurrences occurring at a median of 31.4 months.[1,18] Distant recurrence is most common, and, similar to pancreatic adenocarcinoma, liver and lung predominate. Adjuvant gemcitabine is often administered after complete resection, but ACCs have been reported to be less responsive to systemic chemotherapies as compared with pancreatic ductal adenocarcinoma. However, with the adoption of combination chemotherapy regimens, including chemotherapeutic regimens that use oxaliplatin and irinotecan, partial response rates in patients with metastatic disease have been reported in up to 30% of patients.[16] Anecdotally, we have seen liver and lung recurrence after a long disease-free interval (greater than 4 years) in rare patients with ACC. In such situations, resection of a unifocal metastasis may be considered in an otherwise healthy patient. This also allows for histologic confirmation of the diagnosis and molecular profiling as a guide to further systemic therapy.

SOLID PSEUDOPAPILLARY TUMORS

Solid pseudopapillary tumors (SPTs) of the pancreas are rare neoplasms with low malignant potential. SPTs have been associated with several other names, including Frantz tumors, Hamoudi tumors, and papillary cystic neoplasm. It is estimated that SPTs represent up to 3% of all pancreatic tumors and 6% to 12% of pancreatic cystic neoplasms.[19] SPTs are notable for their high prevalence among women, most commonly occurring in the third decade of life and earlier (mean age, 22 years; range, 2 to 85 years).[20–22] The most common presenting symptoms are abdominal pain (45%) and/or an abdominal mass (34%).[22] In the asymptomatic patient, tumors may be discovered as a palpable mass on routine physical examination, as a mass seen on casual view of the abdomen, or as an incidental finding on imaging for an unrelated complaint. Serologic tests are often of little value with CA 19-9 elevated in 4.3%, amylase in 22.6%, and lipase in 29.3%.

IMAGING

On CT imaging, SPTs are characteristically large, heterogeneously enhancing lesions with solid and cystic

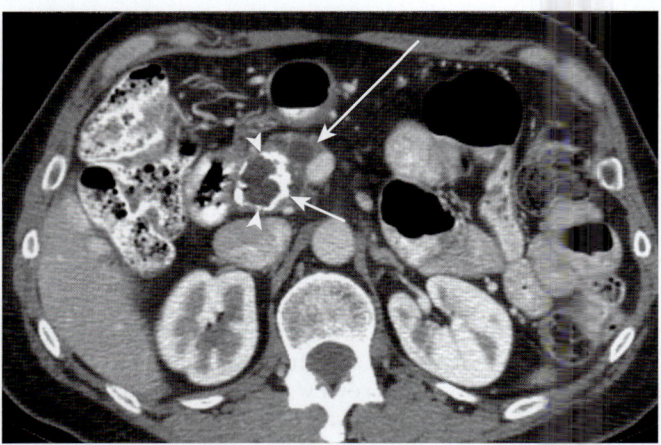

FIGURE 99.3 Axial image of a contrast-enhanced computed tomography scan from a patient with a solid pseudopapillary tumor of the pancreas with solid and cystic characteristics (*long arrow*) and central calcification (*short arrow* and *arrowheads*).

components, and they frequently demonstrate peripheral enhancement and central calcification (Fig. 99.3). On magnetic resonance imaging (MRI), SPTs have a low signal intensity on T1-weighted images and a high signal intensity on T2-weighted images.[23] Ultrasound shows a hypoechoic or isoechoic lesion. These lesions can range from being completely cystic to completely solid.[54] The cystic portion of SPTs is not a true cyst, but rather has a cystic appearance that is secondary to necrotic degeneration of the primary tumor. As the solid papillary-vascular stalks within the tumor slough and hemorrhage, central necrosis can occur, resulting in cystic degeneration. Although SPTs can occur throughout the pancreas, they are perhaps slightly more common in the pancreatic tail and, when discovered, are generally large in size (mean diameter, 5.4 cm).[24] The radiographic differential diagnosis of an SPT should include other cystic neoplasms, including mucinous neoplasms or serous cystadenomas, and intraductal papillary mucinous neoplasms, as well as cystic degeneration of a typically solid neoplasm, such as a pancreatic neuroendocrine tumor or ACC. However, age is important; in a young woman under the age of 30, SPT and pancreatic neuroendocrine tumor would be most likely. In a young woman under the age of 20, SPT would clearly be the most likely diagnosis (even an affected member of a family with multiple endocrine neoplasia type 1 (MEN1) is unlikely to have a large pancreatic neuroendocrine tumor if under the age of 20). FNA biopsy may be useful when routine imaging is inconclusive and diagnostic uncertainty exists. However, because of the tumor's largely necrotic composition, FNA biopsy can frequently be nondiagnostic.

PATHOLOGY

Some defining histologic features of SPTs include the presence of solid cellular hypervascular regions without gland formation, and the presence of branching papillary fronds with sheets and degenerative pseudopapillae.[25] Cells have eosinophilic granules within the nuclei, which are typically grooved. The immunophenotype stains

positively for neuron-specific enolase, CD10, and has atypical nuclear staining for β-catenin, which is generally a cytoplasmic protein.[25,26] Keratins, chromogranin, synaptophysin, and endocrine pancreatic enzymes are generally not expressed. SPTs often stain positive for progesterone receptors, whereas estrogen receptor positivity is more variable.[27] SPTs have also been reported to positively stain for α-methylacyl coenzyme A racemase (AMACR) in contrast to ACC and neuroendocrine tumors of the pancreas, which do not.[28] Aggressive histologic features, such as angioinvasion, perineural invasion, or extension into the surrounding pancreatic parenchyma, that were previously thought to portend worse clinical behavior have not been found to be associated with recurrence or disease-specific survival.[23,29,30] Therefore there is no consensus on factors that are prognostic for patients with SPTs.

The genetic profile associated with SPT is different from adenocarcinoma, most notably for an absence of *KRAS*, *GNAS*, and *SMAD4* mutations. Almost all SPTs harbor alterations in the APC/β-catenin pathway due to a mutation involving *CTNNB1* (exon 3).[31] Nuclear accumulation of β-catenin has been described in 95% of SPTs, and 74% of tumors overexpress cyclin D1, a downstream effector of β-catenin.[32] Interestingly, *BCL9L,* a β-catenin stabilizing gene, is significantly decreased in SPTs, which may help to attenuate the protumorigenic effects of overactivation of the Wnt/β-catenin pathway.[33] In addition, downregulation of miR-194 and SOX 9 (compared with pancreatic ductal adenocarcinomas and nonneoplastic pancreatic tissue) has been reported in SPTs.[34] In addition, genes involved in the hedgehog and androgen receptor signaling pathways, as well as genes involved in epithelial mesenchymal transition, have been shown to be activated in SPTs.[35]

TREATMENT

Given the unpredictable but real metastatic potential of these tumors, surgical resection is recommended for all patients with localized SPT. Although these tumors may be extremely large and can invade critical vasculature, most lesions are usually amenable to complete resection. Pancreaticoduodenectomy or distal pancreatectomy can be performed with en bloc resection of involved adjacent organs when indicated. In a single institution study of 37 patients with SPTs, only 1 patient (3%) had a recurrence, at median follow-up of 4.8 years.[36] A final study reported 26 patients; 2 (8%) recurrences were reported at 6 and 7 years after treatment without any disease-specific mortalities at 73 months of follow-up.[29] Although recurrence rates are low, long-term surveillance is important.

Given the excellent survival rates after surgical resection alone, adjuvant systemic therapy is not routinely used. If metastatic disease occurs, the most common sites include liver, mesentery, and peritoneum. Several series have reported long-term survival after metastasectomy.[37] For unresectable metastatic disease, anecdotal case reports have suggested that gemcitabine-based chemotherapy may be successful in some patients.[38,39]

AUTOIMMUNE PANCREATITIS

Autoimmune pancreatitis (AIP) is a form of pancreatitis characterized by obstructive jaundice with or without a pancreatic mass, lymphoplasmacytic infiltration and fibrosis of the pancreas, and a therapeutic response to corticosteroids.[40] The true incidence of AIP is unknown; however, it is reported to be the diagnosis in 2% to 3% of patients who undergo pancreatic resection for pancreatic cancer.[41,42] Patients with AIP often present with painless obstructive jaundice, which can mimic pancreatic ductal adenocarcinoma. Jaundice has been reported in up to 70% to 80% of patients and is likely due to inflammation and narrowing or stricture of the distal common bile duct.[43] In addition, other common symptoms of AIP include weight loss and abdominal pain; however, other symptoms consistent with pancreatic ductal adenocarcinoma, such as cachexia, inability to eat, and pain requiring narcotic medications, are rarely observed. Up to 60% of patients with AIP are diabetic, the majority of whom have type 2 diabetes with impaired glucose tolerance. Elevation of pancreatic enzymes may also occur.

AIP is currently classified into two subtypes. Patients with type 1 AIP are typically older men, who often have associated elevation in serum immunoglobulin G4 (IgG4) levels and radiographic evidence of extrapancreatic involvement, such as Sjögren syndrome, rheumatoid arthritis, primary sclerosing cholangitis, orbital pseudotumor, and inflammatory bowel disease.[44] Extrapancreatic organ involvement can occur prior to, synchronous with, or after the diagnosis of AIP, with the exception of swelling of salivary and lacrimal glands, which tends to precede the onset of AIP.[44] Biopsy of extrapancreatic sites can be helpful in making the diagnosis because the affected organs often demonstrate the characteristic lymphoplasmacytic infiltrate rich in IgG4-positive cells. In contrast, type 2 AIP is seen with equal frequency in younger patients of both genders, often in the absence of elevated IgG4 levels, and associated autoimmune disease is limited to inflammatory bowel disease, which is found in approximately 30% of patients.[43,45]

Serum IgG4 is the single best serologic marker of AIP, with a sensitivity of 80% in patients with type 1 AIP but only 17% in those with type 2 AIP.[46] IgG4 elevation greater than twice the upper limit of normal is strongly suggestive of AIP in the setting of obstructive jaundice. However, serum IgG4 elevation alone is not sufficient to make a diagnosis of AIP in the absence of typical radiographic findings.

IMAGING

The classic radiographic features of AIP include a diffusely enlarged, sausage-shaped pancreas with homogeneous attenuation and moderate enhancement. In contrast to alcohol-induced pancreatitis, AIP often lacks the radiographic features of ductal dilation, calculi, and pseudocyst formation. Importantly, although AIP may involve a stricture of the pancreatic duct, the upstream dilation characteristic of pancreatic ductal adenocarcinoma is rarely observed.[47] Sometimes, AIP may also present as a focal mass-forming lesion in the pancreas that can be easily confused with pancreatic ductal adenocarcinoma.[48] Recently, international consensus diagnostic criteria were developed for type 1 and type 2 AIP that incorporate the findings from radiographic imaging (including ductal imaging with magnetic resonance cholangiography or

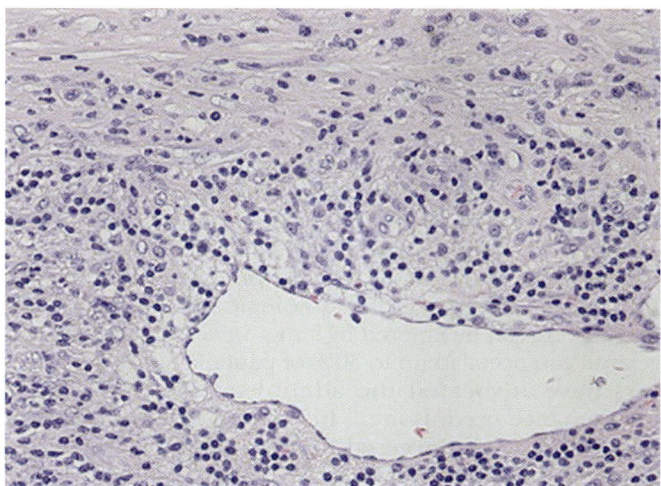

FIGURE 99.4 Histologic changes associated with type 1 autoimmune pancreatitis including periductal lymphoplasmacytic infiltrates.

endoscopic retrograde cholangiopancreatography), as well as serologic and histopathologic data.[40]

PATHOLOGY

Type 1 AIP may not require a histologic diagnosis when the typical clinical, radiographic, and laboratory criteria are present, but because type 2 AIP is often seronegative and lacks other organ involvement, definitive diagnosis requires a pathologic biopsy specimen. A consensus conference of experts from Japan, Korea, Europe, and the United States was convened in Honolulu in 2009 to establish histologic criteria for AIP. Type 1 AIP has three essential features: (1) lymphoplasmacytic infiltrate surrounding small-sized interlobular pancreatic ducts that spare the pancreatic ductal epithelium (Fig. 99.4); (2) fibrosis centered around the ducts and veins affecting predominantly the peripancreatic adipose tissue; and (3) obliterative phlebitis affecting the pancreatic veins. Immunostaining often demonstrates abundant (>10 cells/high-power field) IgG4-positive cells. Type 2 AIP differs from type 1 by less prominent fibrosis, phlebitis, and the lack of IgG4 positivity.[49] In type 2 AIP, lymphoplasmacytic infiltrates may result in obliteration of the pancreatic duct lumen, in contrast to type 1 AIP, in which the ductal epithelium is generally spared. The diagnosis of AIP (especially type 2) can be clinically challenging, and no single diagnostic test is sufficient. Diagnostic criteria rely on a combination of histology, cross-sectional and endoscopic imaging, serologic findings, and a detailed clinical history. In general, the diagnosis of AIP requires a multidisciplinary team consisting of a radiologist, pathologist, and gastroenterologist with expertise in the disease.

TREATMENT

AIP is highly responsive to corticosteroid therapy, and the lack of response should prompt consideration of an alternate diagnosis. Although AIP can resolve spontaneously, treatment with corticosteroids has been associated with an increased remission of AIP when compared with no treatment (98% vs. 75%; $P < .001$).[50] Reversal of jaundice, diabetes, and exocrine dysfunction can be expected (often within weeks, especially with respect to the biliary obstruction) after treatment. The International Consensus Diagnostic Criteria for Autoimmune Pancreatitis recommends a trial of 0.6 mg/kg of prednisone for a period of 2 weeks followed by reimaging and interval assessment of CA 19-9 levels.[40] If the diagnosis of AIP is correct, such radiographic abnormalities as biliary stricture and gland enlargement should improve with steroid therapy. With clinical and radiologic improvement, the prednisone can be tapered by 5 mg/week. Because clinical relapse can occur in up to 30% of patients, some investigators have advocated the administration of low-dose maintenance prednisone.[51] In Japan, prednisone (2.5 to 5 mg/day) is administered for up to 3 years, which has demonstrated lower relapse rates (23% vs. 34%; $P < .05$) in a retrospective analysis of more than 500 patients managed with this approach.[50] Disease relapse is common in type 1 but not in type 2 AIP.[46] Proximal bile-duct involvement and diffuse swelling of the pancreas were factors predictive of disease relapse in type 1 AIP.[1] In addition, IgG4 elevation and evidence of other organ involvement may also be predictive of relapse.[52] AIP patients who demonstrate rapid decline in serum IgG4 levels in response to initial steroid therapy have been reported to have low rates of relapse.[53] In addition, patients who experience a rapid decrease in serum IgG4 levels between pretreatment levels and first posttreatment level (measured within 2 months of steroid therapy) have a low probability of relapse.[53] A repeat challenge of corticosteroids may be effective in disease relapse, and other immunologic therapies, including rituximab and azathioprine, have also been reported.[54,55] A small number of patients with relapsing AIP on corticosteroid therapy have been treated with rituximab with subsequent reduction in IgG4 serum levels and a successful tapering of steroids in less than 2 months.[55]

PRIMARY PANCREATIC LYMPHOMA

Lymphomas involving the pancreas can occur (1) exclusively in the pancreas (primary pancreatic lymphoma [PPL]), (2) via direct extension from adjacent peripancreatic lymphadenopathy and involve the pancreas (secondary pancreatic lymphoma), or (3) originate from lymph nodes distant from the pancreas. PPL is defined by the World Health Organization as "an extranodal lymphoma arising in the pancreas with the bulk of the disease localized to this site; contiguous lymph node involvement and distant spread may be seen but the primary clinical presentation is in the pancreas with treatment directed to this site."[56] PPL is predominantly non-Hodgkin lymphoma of B-cell phenotype, and diffuse large B-cell lymphoma is the most common histologic subtype.[57,58] PPL accounts for less than 0.5% of all pancreatic tumors and less than 2% of extranodal lymphomas. Currently, no specific biochemical markers aid in the diagnosis of PPL. An elevated serum lactate dehydrogenase (LDH) and β2-microglobulin in the setting of normal CA 19-9 levels may have some diagnostic and prognostic value.[59,60] In a review of 523 patients from the SEER database, the most common histologic subtype of PPL was diffuse, large cell lymphoma (56%), follicular lymphoma (12.4%), and other B-cell lymphomas (31%).[61] PPLs predominantly occur in men (7 : 1) and usually present in the fifth to sixth decade of life. Common presenting symptoms include abdominal pain (67% to 73%), B symptoms such as fever, night sweats, chills, weight loss (38% to 58%), jaundice (33% to 42%), and gastric or duodenal outlet obstruction (2% to 26%).[57,58]

IMAGING

Radiographic findings characteristic of PPL include either the presence of a large mass that focally involves the head of the pancreas or occasionally a more diffuse form that is infiltrative and can mimic the appearance of acute pancreatitis (Fig. 99.5). In addition, patients with PPL often present with significant lymphadenopathy involving the peripancreatic nodes and most notably the retroperitoneal lymph nodes below the renal vein. The involved lymph nodes lack central necrosis or calcifications, and the pancreatic duct is rarely dilated despite what appears to be a large pancreatic tumor.[59,62,63] In addition, vascular invasion or occlusion is rarely present in most patients despite the bulky tumor size.[57,64] Similar to pancreatic ductal adenocarcinoma, PPLs are low attenuation and have minimal enhancement on CT scan. On T1-weighted gradient echo (GRE) MRI, PPLs appear as a homogeneous, hypodense mass and have variable signal intensity on T2.[57] PPLs are avid on fluorodeoxyglucose positron emission tomography (FDG-PET) scans, with uptake patterns that may be focal nodular, diffuse, or segmental.[57,65]

PATHOLOGY

Pathologic examination is essential in the diagnosis of PPL. Cytopathologic features include large malignant lymphocytic nuclei, prominent nucleoli, abundant karyorrhexis, and a background of necrosis. In addition, the cells are positive for leukocyte common antigen (LCA) and CD20 and negative for CD34 and CD68.[62] Key

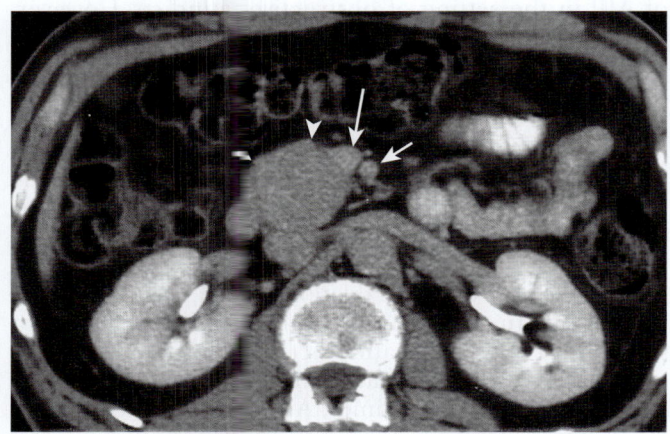

FIGURE 99.5 Primary pancreatic lymphoma involving the head of pancreas. Note the hypodense appearance of the mass *(arrowheads)* and the adjacent abutment of the superior mesenteric vein *(long arrow)* and proximity to the superior mesenteric artery *(short arrow)*.

immunohistochemical stains that are positive in pancreatic endocrine neoplasms, such as synaptophysin, are generally negative in PPL.[62] The addition of flow cytometry has also been reported to have high (84%) sensitivity for the diagnosis of non-Hodgkin lymphoma.[66] However, the use of flow cytometry is limited by the cellularity of fine-needle aspirate specimens; therefore core needle biopsy is recommended when the diagnosis of PPL is suspected.

TREATMENT

The standard of care in the management of PPL is chemotherapy alone, which provides excellent control of symptoms, including jaundice, as well as long-term remission.[67,68] PPL is most commonly treated with a multidrug regimen, such as cyclophosphamide, doxorubicin, vincristine, and prednisone (CHOP). Complete remission can be expected with multidrug therapy in 63% to 77% of patients with large B-cell lymphoma.[67] However, recurrence is common in patients older than 60 years. The use of an anti-CD20 antibody, rituximab, in addition to CHOP has been associated with improved response rates of up to 85% in diffuse large B-cell lymphoma.[68] Other regimens include cyclophosphamide, vincristine, and prednisone (CVP) and methotrexate, Adriamycin, cyclophosphamide, vincristine, prednisone, and bleomycin (MACOP-B).[57] Although surgical resection was previously considered a primary treatment option for PPL, laparotomy should now be reserved for patients in whom the diagnosis is uncertain (inconclusive percutaneous or endoscopic biopsy results often in the setting of biliary obstruction/endoscopic stenting) or therapeutic purposes (palliative surgery) in the setting of gastrointestinal hemorrhage or gastric outlet obstruction.[63]

METASTATIC RENAL CELL CARCINOMA

Metastatic lesions to the pancreas are very rare and represent only 2% (or less) of all pancreatic neoplasms. Although most cancers rarely metastasize to the pancreas, renal cell carcinoma (RCC) accounts for 40% or more of metastatic lesions. Synchronous metastases can occur in up to 25% to 30% of patients with RCC, and metachronous metastases may occur in up to 40% of all patients with a history of RCC.[69,70] RCC metastases to the pancreas usually present after an extended disease-free interval from nephrectomy, with 91% of RCC metastases diagnosed at a mean of 11.2 years after nephrectomy.[71] This emphasizes the importance of long-term follow-up for patients with RCC after initial nephrectomy. Men and women are equally affected, and there are no differences in the laterality of the primary tumor and the location of the metastases within the pancreas. The majority of patients have solitary metastases, which are usually asymptomatic (>50%) and identified incidentally or during follow-up surveillance. Among those who are symptomatic, abdominal pain, weight loss, jaundice, or gastrointestinal hemorrhage may be the presenting complaint. Up to 34% of patients can have extrapancreatic metastases, and therefore a thorough staging evaluation should be performed in patients with suspected or biopsy-proven metastatic RCC to the pancreas.[72]

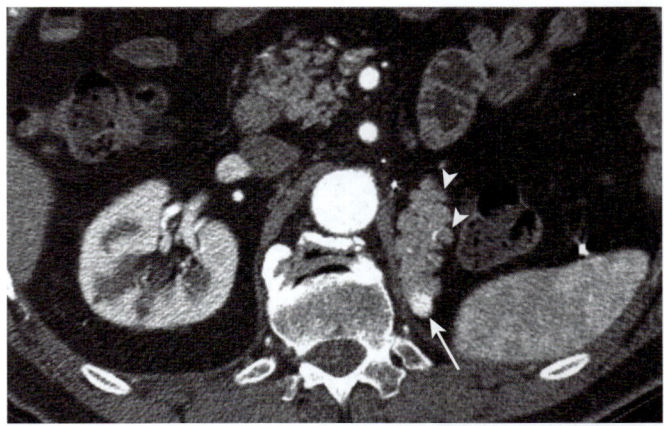

FIGURE 99.6 Axial image of a contrast-enhanced computed tomography scan from a patient who underwent a left nephrectomy for renal cell carcinoma and then developed a metachronous metastasis to the pancreatic tail. Note the characteristic enhancement of the metastatic lesion *(arrow)* on arterial phase imaging, as well as the posterior displacement of the pancreas *(arrowheads)* due to the absence of the left kidney.

IMAGING

CT is the best test for the evaluation of presumed RCC metastases to the pancreas, and findings are usually classic: well-defined hypervascular lesion(s) that demonstrate a central area of low attenuation on the arterial phase (Fig. 99.6). The imaging characteristics can be similar to pancreatic neuroendocrine neoplasms, and these lesions should be included in the differential diagnosis. In contrast, the hypervascularity of the tumor is inconsistent with pancreatic ductal adenocarcinoma.

PATHOLOGY

In the majority of patients with a history of RCC, the CT findings are diagnostic and there is no need for a preoperative biopsy. However, a tissue biopsy may be helpful if there is diagnostic concern for a pancreatic neuroendocrine neoplasm or if there is disease outside of the pancreas suggesting multiple sites of recurrence. The cytomorphic features of RCC can vary depending on the subtype. Histologically, RCC forms solid sheets of tumor cells that are separated into solid acini by vascular septae, which can be distinguished from pancreatic endocrine neoplasms (Fig. 99.7). Metastatic RCC may appear histologically different from the primary RCC because of alterations in differentiation and expression proteins. Positive immunohistochemical staining for CD10 and PAX8 can be used to distinguish between metastatic RCC and other tumors, such as clear cell carcinoma of the pancreas, clear cell pancreatic endocrine tumor, and the solid variant of serous adenoma.[73] Importantly, the tumor-type–specific profiles for primary RCC are usually found in the metastases, but changes in staining intensity have also been reported.[74] Furthermore, depending on the histology of the primary, several stains have 100% positivity (e.g., CD10 for clear cell RCC and AMACR for papillary RCC).[75]

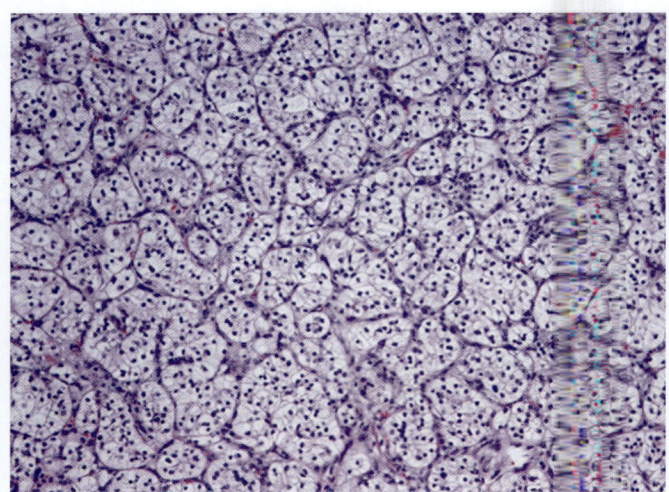

FIGURE 99.7 Histologic appearance of a clear cell renal cell carcinoma metastatic to the pancreas. Note the solid sheets of tumor cells that are separated into acini by vascular septae.

TREATMENT

In general, for all patients with metastatic RCC, long-term survival is poor, with an estimated 5-year survival rate of less than 50%.[76] However, patients with isolated RCC metastases to the pancreas who undergo surgical resection experience much longer survivals. In a systematic review that identified 321 patients with resected pancreatic RCC metastases, the disease-free survival and overall survival were 57% and 73% at 5 years, respectively.[77] A series from the Johns Hopkins pancreas program reported similar results, with an overall survival of 51% at 5 years and the median survival after resection being 5.5 years. Perioperative mortality rates (for pancreatic surgery in patients with RCC) in multiple series ranged between 1.5% and 2.3%, similar to mortality rates associated with pancreatic surgery for primary pancreatic neoplasms at high-volume centers.[72,77] A retrospective review of 276 patients with inoperable metastatic RCC from 11 European centers reported a median overall survival of 56 months (95% confidence interval [CI], 46 to 67 months) and a 5-year overall survival of 48.7% for patients treated with targeted therapies. With improvements in systemic therapy, a more recent study demonstrated that patients who received local pancreatic treatment (surgery or radiotherapy for pancreas-only metastases) had a median overall survival of 106 months (95% CI, 78 to 204 months) and a 5-year overall survival of 75%.[78] Given the relatively favorable prognosis of patients with pancreatic metastases from RCC, aggressive treatment with surgical resection should be considered. In addition, antiangiogenic agents, such as bevacizumab, sunitinib, and sorafenib, have shown promising results in metastatic RCC, necessitating the need for a multidisciplinary approach to the management of these patients.[72]

CONCLUSION

Although the majority of pancreatic neoplasms are pancreatic ductal adenocarcinoma, a thorough understanding of rare and unusual pancreatic neoplasms is important to develop the correct treatment plan for all patients. An accurate pretreatment diagnosis is of obvious importance. This is best achieved by a coordinated approach involving a multidisciplinary team of physicians, with particular attention to radiographic and pathologic analysis. Surgery is the cornerstone of therapy for SPT, ACC, and isolated RCC metastases; however, medical therapy is more appropriate for AIP and PPL.

REFERENCES

1. Holen KD, Klimstra DS, Hummer A, et al. Clinical characteristics and outcomes from an institutional series of acinar cell carcinoma of the pancreas and related tumors. *J Clin Oncol.* 2002;20(24):4673-4678.
2. Seth AK, Argani P, Campbell KA, et al. Acinar cell carcinoma of the pancreas: an institutional series of resected patients and review of the current literature. *J Gastrointest Surg.* 2008;12(6):1061-1067.
3. Chiou YY, Chiang JH, Hwang JI, Yen CH, Tsay SH, Chang CY. Acinar cell carcinoma of the pancreas: clinical and computed tomography manifestations. *J Comput Assist Tomogr.* 2004;28(2):180-186.
4. Bhosale P, Balachandran A, Wang H, et al. CT imaging features of acinar cell carcinoma and its hepatic metastases. *Abdom Imaging.* 2013;38(6):1383-1390.
5. Tian L, Lv XF, Dong J, et al. Clinical features and CT/MRI findings of pancreatic acinar cell carcinoma. *Int J Clin Exp Med.* 2015;8(9):14846-14854.
6. Klimstra DS, Heffes CS, Oertel JE, Rosai J. Acinar cell carcinoma of the pancreas. A clinicopathologic study of 28 cases. *Am J Surg Pathol.* 1992;16(9):815-837.
7. Klimstra DS, Adsay V. Acinar neoplasms of the pancreas—a summary of 25 years of research. *Semin Diagn Pathol.* 2016;33(5):307-318.
8. Sigel CS, Klimstra DS. Cytomorphologic and immunophenotypical features of acinar cell neoplasms of the pancreas. *Cancer Cytopathol.* 2013;121(8):459-470.
9. Klimstra DS, Rosai J, Heffess CS. Mixed acinar-endocrine carcinomas of the pancreas. *Am J Surg Pathol.* 1994;18(8):765-778.
10. Jiao Y, Yonescu R, Offerhaus GJ, et al. Whole-exome sequencing of pancreatic neoplasms with acinar differentiation. *J Pathol.* 2014;232(4):428-435.
11. Furukawa T, Sakamoto H, Takeuchi S, et al. Whole exome sequencing reveals recurrent mutations in BRCA2 and FAT genes in acinar cell carcinomas of the pancreas. *Sci Rep.* 2015;5:8829.
12. Hosoda W, Sasaki E, Murakami Y, Yamao K, Shimizu Y, Yatabe Y. BCL10 as a useful marker for pancreatic acinar cell carcinoma, especially using endoscopic ultrasound cytology specimens. *Pathol Int.* 2013;63(3):176-182.
13. Bergmann F, Aulmann S, Sipos B, et al. Acinar cell carcinomas of the pancreas: a molecular analysis in a series of 57 cases. *Virchows Arch.* 2014;465(6):661-672.
14. Furlan D, Sahnane N, Bernasconi B, et al. APC alterations are frequently involved in the pathogenesis of acinar cell carcinoma of the pancreas, mainly through gene loss and promoter hypermethylation. *Virchows Arch.* 2014;464(5):553-564.
15. Ding L, Han L, Li Y, Zhao J, He P, Zhang W. Neurogenin 3-directed cre deletion of Tsc1 gene causes pancreatic acinar carcinoma. *Neoplasia.* 2014;16(11):909-917.
16. Schmidt CM, Matos JM, Bentrem DJ, Talamonti MS, Lillemoe KD, Bilimoria KY. Acinar cell carcinoma of the pancreas in the United States: prognostic factors and comparison to ductal adenocarcinoma. *J Gastrointest Surg.* 2008;12(12):2078-2086.
17. Lowery MA, Klimstra DS, Shia J, et al. Acinar cell carcinoma of the pancreas: new genetic and treatment insights into a rare malignancy. *Oncologist.* 2011;16(12):1714-1720.
18. Butturini G, Pisano M, Scarpa A, D'Onofrio M, Auriemma A, Bassi C. Aggressive approach to acinar cell carcinoma of the pancreas: a single-institution experience and a literature review. *Langenbeck's Arch Surg/Dtsch Ges Chir.* 2011;396(3):363-369.
19. Casadei R, Santini D, Calculli L, Pezzilli R, Zanini N, Minni F. Pancreatic solid-cystic papillary tumor: clinical features, imaging findings and operative management. *JOP J Pancreas.* 2006;7(1):137-144.

20. Speer AL, Barthel ER, Patel MM, Grikscheit TC. Solid pseudopapillary tumor of the pancreas: a single-institution 20-year series of pediatric patients. *J Pediatr Surg.* 2012;47(6):1217-1222.

21. Patil TB, Shrikhande SV, Kanhere HA, Saoji RR, Ramadwar MR, Shukla PJ. Solid pseudopapillary neoplasm of the pancreas: a single institution experience of 14 cases. *HPB.* 2006;8(2):148-150.

22. Papavramidis T, Papavramidis S. Solid pseudopapillary tumors of the pancreas: review of 718 patients reported in English literature. *J Am Coll Surg.* 2005;200(6):965-972.

23. Tsukamoto M, Hashimoto D, Chikamoto A, Abe S, Ohmuraya M, Baba H. Clinical features and management of pancreatic solid pseudopapillary tumor. *Am Surg.* 2014;80(12):1212-1215.

24. Raman SP, Kawamoto S, Law JK, et al. Institutional experience with solid pseudopapillary neoplasms: focus on computed tomography, magnetic resonance imaging, conventional ultrasound, endoscopic ultrasound, and predictors of aggressive histology. *J Comput Assist Tomogr.* 2013;37(5):824-833.

25. Klimstra DS, Wenig BM, Heffess CS. Solid-pseudopapillary tumor of the pancreas: a typically cystic carcinoma of low malignant potential. *Semin Diagn Pathol.* 2000;17(1):66-80.

26. Suzuki S, Hatori T, Furukawa T, Shiratori K, Yamamoto M. Clinical and pathological features of solid pseudopapillary neoplasms of the pancreas at a single institution. *Dig Surg.* 2014;31(2):143-150.

27. Santini D, Poli F, Lega S. Solid-papillary tumors of the pancreas: histopathology. *JOP J Pancreas.* 2006;7(1):131-136.

28. Shen Y, Wang Z, Zhu J, Chen Y, Gu W, Liu Q. Alpha-methylacyl-CoA racemase (P504S) is a useful marker for the differential diagnosis of solid pseudopapillary neoplasm of the pancreas. *Ann Diagn Pathol.* 2014;18(3):146-150.

29. Zhang H, Wang W, Yu S, Xiao Y, Chen J. The prognosis and clinical characteristics of advanced (malignant) solid pseudopapillary neoplasm of the pancreas. *Tumour Biol.* 2016;37(4):5347-5353.

30. Irtan S, Galmiche-Rolland L, Elie C, et al. Recurrence of solid pseudopapillary neoplasms of the pancreas: results of a nationwide study of risk factors and treatment modalities. *Pediatr Blood Cancer.* 2016;63(9):1515-1521.

31. Springer S, Wang Y, Dal Molin M, et al. A combination of molecular markers and clinical features improve the classification of pancreatic cysts. *Gastroenterology.* 2015;149(5):1501-1510.

32. Abraham SC, Klimstra DS, Wilentz RE, et al. Solid-pseudopapillary tumors of the pancreas are genetically distinct from pancreatic ductal adenocarcinomas and almost always harbor beta-catenin mutations. *Am J Pathol.* 2002;160(4):1361-1369.

33. Hallas C, Phillipp J, Domanowsky L Kah B, Tiemann K. BCL9L expression in pancreatic neoplasia with a focus on SPN: a possible explanation for the enigma of the benign neoplasia. *BMC Cancer.* 2016;16:648.

34. Li P, Hu Y, Yi J, Li J, Yang J, Wang J. Identification of potential biomarkers to differentially diagnose solid pseudopapillary tumors and pancreatic malignancies via a gene regulatory network. *J Translat Med.* 2015;13:361.

35. Park M, Kim M, Hwang D, et al. Characterization of gene expression and activated signaling pathways in solid-pseudopapillary neoplasm of pancreas. *Mod Pathol.* 2014;27(4):580-593.

36. Reddy S, Cameron JL, Scudiere J, et al. Surgical management of solid-pseudopapillary neoplasms of the pancreas (Franz or Hamoudi tumors): a large single-institutional series. *J Am Coll Surg.* 2009;208(5):950-957; discussion 957–959.

37. Martin RC, Klimstra DS, Brennan MF, Conlon KC. Solid-pseudopapillary tumor of the pancreas: a surgical enigma? *Ann Surg Oncol.* 2002;9(1):35-40.

38. Strauss JF, Hirsch VJ, Rubey CN, Pollock M. Resection of a solid and papillary epithelial neoplasm of the pancreas following treatment with cis-platinum and 5-fluorouracil: a case report. *Med Pediatr Oncol.* 1993;21(5):365-367.

39. Maffuz A, Bustamante Fde T, Silva JA, Torres-Vargas S. Preoperative gemcitabine for unresectable, solid pseudopapillary tumour of the pancreas. *Lancet Oncol.* 2005;6(3):185-186.

40. Shimosegawa T, Chari ST, Frulloni L, et al. International Consensus Diagnostic Criteria for Autoimmune Pancreatitis: guidelines of the International Association of Pancreatology. *Pancreas.* 2011;40(3):352-358.

41. de Castro SM, de Nes LC, Nio CY, et al. Incidence and characteristics of chronic and lymphoplasmacytic sclerosing pancreatitis in patients scheduled to undergo a pancreatoduodenectomy. *HPB.* 2010;12(1):15-21.

42. Hardacre JM, Iacobuzio-Donahue CA, Sohn TA, et al. Results of pancreaticoduodenectomy for lymphoplasmacytic sclerosing pancreatitis. *Ann Surg.* 2003;237(6):853-858; discussion 858–859.

43. Okazaki K, Uchida K, Chiba T. Recent concept of autoimmune-related pancreatitis. *J Gastroenterol.* 2001;36(5):293-302.

44. Takuma K, Kamisawa T, Anjiki H, Egawa N, Igarashi Y. Metachronous extrapancreatic lesions in autoimmune pancreatitis. *Int Med.* 2010;49(6):529-533.

45. Chari ST, Longnecker DS, Kloppel G. The diagnosis of autoimmune pancreatitis: a Western perspective. *Pancreas.* 2009;38(8):846-848.

46. Sah RP, Chari ST, Pannala R, et al. Differences in clinical profile and relapse rate of type 1 versus type 2 autoimmune pancreatitis. *Gastroenterology.* 2010;139(1):140-148; quiz e112–e143.

47. Kamisawa T, Imai M, Yui Chen P, et al. Strategy for differentiating autoimmune pancreatitis from pancreatic cancer. *Pancreas.* 2008;37(3):e62-e67.

48. Frulloni L, Scattolini C, Falconi M, et al. Autoimmune pancreatitis: differences between the focal and diffuse forms in 87 patients. *Am J Gastroenterol.* 2009;104(9):2288-2294.

49. Chari ST, Kloeppel G, Zhang L, et al. Histopathologic and clinical subtypes of autoimmune pancreatitis: the Honolulu consensus document. *Pancreas.* 2010;39(5):549-554.

50. Kamisawa T, Shimosegawa T, Okazaki K, et al. Standard steroid treatment for autoimmune pancreatitis. *Gut.* 2009;58(11):1504-1507.

51. Gardner TB, Chari ST. Autoimmune pancreatitis. *Gastroenterol Clin North Am.* 2008;37(2):439-460, vii.

52. Naitoh I, Nakazawa T, Ohara H, et al. Clinical significance of extrapancreatic lesions in autoimmune pancreatitis. *Pancreas.* 2010;39(1):e1-e5.

53. Shimizu K, Tahara J, Takayama Y, et al. Assessment of the rate of decrease in serum IgG4 level of autoimmune pancreatitis patients in response to initial steroid therapy as a predictor of subsequent relapse. *Pancreas.* 2016;45(9):1341-1346.

54. Chatterjee S, Oppong KW, Scott JS, et al. Autoimmune pancreatitis—diagnosis, management and longterm follow-up. *J Gastrointest Liver Dis.* 2014;23(2):179-185.

55. Khosroshahi A, Bloch DB, Deshpande V, Stone JH. Rituximab therapy leads to rapid decline of serum IgG4 levels and prompt clinical improvement in IgG4-related systemic disease. *Arthr Rheum.* 2010;62(6):1755-1762.

56. Hamilton SR, Aaltonen AL, eds. *World Health Organization Classification of Tumours. Pathology and Genetics of Tumours of the Digestive System.* Lyon: IARC Press; 2000.

57. Anand D, Lall C, Bhosale P, Ganeshan D, Qayyum A. Current update on primary pancreatic lymphoma. *Abdom Radiol (NY).* 2016;41(2):347-355.

58. Sadot E, Yahalom J, Do RK, et al. Clinical features and outcome of primary pancreatic lymphoma. *Ann Surg Oncol.* 2015;22(4):1176-1184.

59. Baylor SM, Berg JW. Cross-classification and survival characteristics of 5,000 cases of cancer of the pancreas. *J Surg Oncol.* 1973;5(4):335-358.

60. Grimison PS, Chin MT, Harrison ML, Goldstein D. Primary pancreatic lymphoma—pancreatic tumours that are potentially curable without resection, a retrospective review of four cases. *BMC Cancer.* 2006;6:117.

61. Mishra MV, Keith SW, Shen X, Bar Ad V, Champ CE, Biswas T. Primary pancreatic lymphoma: a population-based analysis using the SEER program. *Am J Clin Oncol.* 2013;36(1):38-43.

62. Naito Y, Okabe Y, Kawahara A, et al. Guide to diagnosing primary pancreatic lymphoma, B-cell type: immunocytochemistry improves the diagnostic accuracy of endoscopic ultrasonography-guided fine needle aspiration cytology. *Diagn Cytopathol.* 2012;40(8):732-736.

63. Sadot E, Yahalom J, Do RK, et al. Clinical features and outcome of primary pancreatic lymphoma. *Ann Surg Oncol.* 2015;22(4):1176-1184.

64. Behrns KE, Sarr MG, Strickler JG. Pancreatic lymphoma: is it a surgical disease? *Pancreas.* 1994;9(5):662-667.

65. Dong A, Cui Y, Gao L, Wang Y, Zuo C, Yang J. Patterns of FDG uptake in pancreatic non-Hodgkin's lymphoma lesions. *Abdom Imaging.* 2014;39(1):175-186.

66. Khashab M, Mokadem M, DeWitt J, et al. Endoscopic ultrasound-guided fine-needle aspiration with or without flow cytometry for the diagnosis of primary pancreatic lymphoma—a case series. *Endoscopy.* 2010;42(3):228-231.

67. Webb TH, Lillemoe KD, Pitt HA, Jones RJ, Cameron JL. Pancreatic lymphoma. Is surgery mandatory for diagnosis or treatment? *Ann Surg.* 1989;209(1):25-30.

68. Coiffier B. Monoclonal antibody as therapy for malignant lymphomas. *Comptes Rendus Biol.* 2006;329(4):241-254.

69. Zweizig SL. Cancer of the kidney. *Clin Obstet Gynecol*. 2002;45(4):884-891.

70. Motzer RJ, Bander NH, Nanus DM. Renal-cell carcinoma. *New Engl J Med*. 1996;335(12):865-875.

71. Tosoian JJ, Cameron JL, Allaf ME, et al. Resection of isolated renal cell carcinoma metastases of the pancreas: outcomes from the Johns Hopkins Hospital. *J Gastrointest Surg*. 2014;18(3):542-548.

72. Sperti C, Moletta L, Patane G. Metastatic tumors to the pancreas: the role of surgery. *World J Gastrointest Oncol*. 2014;6(10):381-392.

73. Cheng SK, Chuah KL. Metastatic renal cell carcinoma to the pancreas: a review. *Arch Pathol Labor Med*. 2016;140(6):598-602.

74. Lew M, Foo WC, Roh MH. Diagnosis of metastatic renal cell carcinoma on fine-needle aspiration cytology. *Arch Pathol Lab Med*. 2014;138(10):1278-1285.

75. Truong LD, Shen SS. Immunohistochemical diagnosis of renal neoplasms. *Arch Pathol Lab Med*. 2011;135(1):92-109.

76. Krabbe LM, Haddad AQ, Westerman ME, Margulis V. Surgical management of metastatic renal cell carcinoma in the era of targeted therapies. *World J Urol*. 2014;32(3):615-622.

77. Tanis PJ, van der Gaag NA, Busch OR, van Gulik TM, Gouma DJ. Systematic review of pancreatic surgery for metastatic renal cell carcinoma. *Br J Surg*. 2009;96(6):579-592.

78. Grassi P, Doucet L, Giglione P, et al. Clinical impact of pancreatic metastases from renal cell carcinoma: a multicenter retrospective analysis. *PLoS One*. 2016;11(4):e0151662.

Techniques of Pancreatic Resection for Cancer

Kevin C. Soares | Timothy M. Pawlik

Pancreatic resection and reconstruction remain a therapeutic challenge to surgeons treating neoplastic disease of the pancreas, distal common bile duct, ampulla of Vater, and proximal duodenum. Despite appreciable improvements in perioperative, postoperative, and intraoperative techniques, morbidity for these procedures remains high. The majority of this morbidity is attributed to pancreatic reconstruction and subsequent anastomotic and pancreatic leaks.

HISTORICAL BACKGROUND

The first reported resection of a pancreatic tumor was a distal pancreatectomy for a spindle cell sarcoma performed by Friedrich Trendelenburg in 1882.[1] Despite a postoperative course complicated by wound infection and malnutrition, the patient was discharged home upon his own insistence only to die a few weeks later secondary to acute respiratory failure.[2] Halsted described the first successful resection of a periampullary tumor in 1898 when he performed a local resection along with an anastomosis of the pancreatic duct and bile duct to the duodenum for a patient with obstructive jaundice.[3] Indeed, most early reports of periampullary tumor resection were performed via a transduodenal approach. That same year, Alessandro Codivilla performed the first pancreaticoduodenectomy in a 46-year-old male with a pancreatic head mass; however, the patient died on postoperative day 18.[4] Walther Kausch[5] performed the first successful two-stage pancreaticoduodenectomy in 1909, followed by Hirschel[6] in 1914, who reported the first successful one-stage pancreaticoduodenectomy. By 1910, 20 pancreatic resections were reported in the literature with a 45% in-hospital mortality rate.[2]

General acceptance for the pancreaticoduodenectomy was not seen until Whipple reported his successful two-stage pancreaticoduodenectomies in 1935.[7] Five years later he performed the first anatomic one-stage pancreaticoduodenectomy for a tumor of the head of the pancreas, where he performed an antrectomy and complete removal of the duodenum.[2,8] The first one-stage pancreaticoduodenectomy in the United States was performed by Trimble in 1941.

Despite numerous technical advances over the next 40 years, morbidity and mortality remained high, 40% to 60% and 20% to 40%, respectively. However, the combination of centralization of pancreatic surgery, as well as the technical advancements led by John Cameron after 1980, resulted in improved outcomes, particularly with mortality, and subsequent widespread acceptance of the procedure.[9]

PREOPERATIVE EVALUATION

One of the most important elements in the preoperative evaluation of a patient with pancreatic cancer is determining resectability. This involves evaluation of both clinical and anatomic parameters, ranging from patient performance status to local tumor relationships relative to major vascular structures. Clinical evaluation involves a thorough history and physical examination. History should focus specifically on a personal and family history of pancreatitis or malignancies, such as pancreatic, colon, or breast cancer. Physical examination should look for evidence of advanced disease, such as palpable metastatic disease in the supraclavicular fossa (Virchow node), palpable periumbilical node (Sister Mary Joseph node), palpable perirectal mass (Blumer shelf), ascites, weight loss, and cachexia. Hepatomegaly and a palpable gallbladder (Courvoisier sign) may signify chronic biliary obstruction. Routine laboratory screening (including complete blood count, electrolyte panel, liver function tests, coagulation panel, and albumin) alerts the clinician to anemia, hyperbilirubinemia, and evidence of new-onset diabetes, pancreatitis, and malnutrition. Pertinent serum tumor markers include carbohydrate antigen 19-9 (CA 19-9) and carcinoembryonic antigen (CEA). Of note, CA 19-9 levels are often elevated in setting of biliary inflammation or obstruction, even among patients with benign disease. Accordingly, its low sensitivity (80%) and specificity (60% to 70%) for pancreatic ductal adenocarcinoma make it unsuitable for use as a screening tool but can be useful when trends are assessed, particularly in determining response to therapy.

Appropriate preoperative imaging is essential to assess resectability of pancreatic tumors. Specifically, identification of distant metastases and locally advanced pancreatic tumors involving major vascular structures is paramount. Multiple preoperative imaging modalities are used; however, in most centers, contrast-enhanced pancreas protocol spiral computed tomography (CT) is the preferred modality (Fig. 100.1). Liver lesions greater than 1 cm in size are easily identified. The role of positron emission tomography–CT (PET-CT) in pancreatic cancer remains poorly defined but may be useful in ruling out distant metastatic disease in patients with suspicious lesions. Tumor encasement of the celiac axis or superior mesenteric artery or occlusion/unreconstructible portal vein (PV) and superior mesenteric vein (SMV) tumor involvement is considered locally advanced disease, and nonsurgical options, such as chemotherapy and chemoradiation, are preferred in these instances. Three-dimensional (3D) reconstruction of the mesenteric vessels both in the arterial

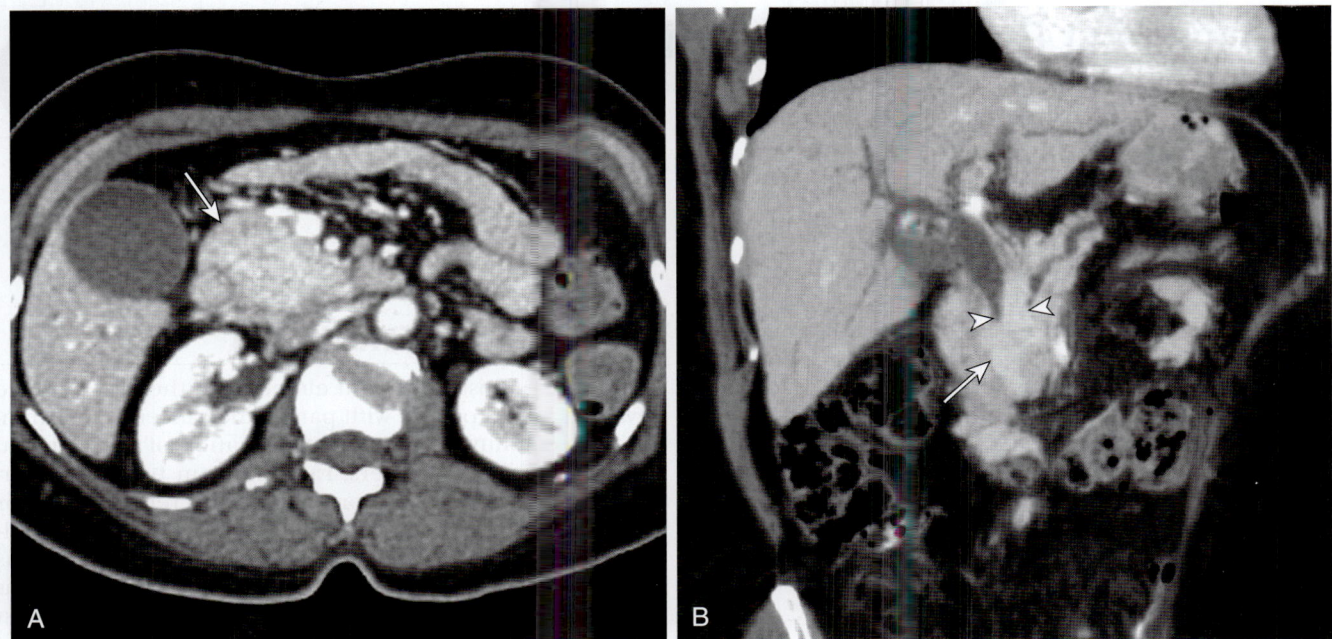

FIGURE 100.1 A 57-year-old female with history of pancreatic adenocarcinoma. (A) Axial computed tomography image of the abdomen obtained in the venous phase demonstrates a large mass in the region of the head of the pancreas *(arrow)*. (B) Minimum intensity projection in the coronal plane better demonstrates the pancreatic mass *(arrow)*, resulting in a "double duct" sign *(arrowheads)*. (Courtesy Ihab Kamel, MD, and Mounes Ghasebeh, MD, Department of Radiology, The Johns Hopkins University School of Medicine.)

and venous phases can preoperatively aid in demonstrating critical anatomic relationships. In addition, 3D CT helps identify surgically relevant aberrant anatomy, such as a replaced right hepatic artery.

The use of endoscopic ultrasound (EUS) for preoperative evaluation is center dependent. The ability of EUS to predict vascular involvement remains controversial. Moreover, the procedure is operator dependent and not particularly useful in the determination of distant metastatic disease. Its main utility is in obtaining a tissue sample via fine-needle aspiration, particularly in patients with locally advanced/unresectable disease prior to beginning chemotherapy. Biopsy is associated with a low incidence of complications, and it is generally reserved for unresectable lesions or patients who may benefit from neoadjuvant therapy prior to resection. Preoperative biliary decompression is associated with increased wound infections and prolonged hospital stay but may be beneficial for malnourished patients or those presenting with jaundice/cholangitis in whom surgery may be delayed.[3–12]

TECHNIQUES OF RESECTION

PANCREATICODUODENECTOMY

Resection

Endotracheal intubation is necessary. Central venous catheters and invasive arterial monitoring lines are inserted as needed, with peripheral venous access typically being sufficient. A nasogastric tube is placed and preoperative antibiotic prophylaxis, as well as deep venous thrombosis prophylaxis, is administered. The patient is positioned in the supine position.

The first step of the procedure is to determine resectability and rule out distant disease. Routine use of staging laparoscopy remains controversial. Some surgeons use it routinely, whereas others prefer to use staging laparoscopy only in select cases when there is a higher probability of metastatic disease, such as adenocarcinoma of body and tail of the pancreas or in the setting of high CA 19-9 levels.[13–15] With the increased sensitivity of modern imaging techniques, many surgeons argue that staging laparoscopy has a low yield, making it less necessary.

Many surgeons prefer an upper abdominal midline incision; however, a bilateral subcostal incision may also be used. The abdomen is explored for evidence of metastatic disease. This exploration includes the liver, peritoneum, omentum, transverse mesocolon, and all serosal surfaces. Involvement of periportal and celiac axis lymph nodes or involvement of the base of the transverse mesocolon is not necessarily a contraindication to resection. The base of the transverse mesocolon may be taken with the specimen, including a segment of the middle colic artery when necessary, given that the marginal artery generally maintains blood supply to the transverse colon.

A wide Kocher maneuver is performed to evaluate local major vascular relationships. Of note, preoperative cross-sectional imaging offers the most accurate assessment of the relationship of the tumor to the vessels, especially the superior mesenteric artery. With mobilization of the duodenum, one can assess whether there is a component of uncinate process involvement with the superior mesenteric artery. In addition, this maneuver allows the surgeon to evaluate for tumor extension into the inferior vena cava and aorta. Next, the common hepatic artery and proper hepatic artery are assessed to confirm resectability. The PV SMV confluence is also assessed for tumor involvement. The hepatoduodenal ligament is incised. The common hepatic duct is identified and divided close to the level of the cystic duct. A more proximal margin on the hepatic duct is sometimes needed for superior pancreatic tumors arising from the head of pancreas. Assessment for a replaced right hepatic artery, typically located lateral and posterior to the common bile duct, is imperative, and the artery should be protected when identified. A replaced hepatic artery should also be readily visible with state-of-the-art preoperative imaging. When an accessory right hepatic artery is present (i.e., a right hepatic artery traveling lateral and posterior to the common bile duct in the presence of a native right hepatic artery), the accessory replaced right hepatic artery can often be ligated with impunity. Rarely, a completely replaced common hepatic artery may be seen originating from the superior mesenteric artery (type IX anatomy); recognition, preservation, or reconstruction of this vessel is critical.

After defining the arterial anatomy, the gastroduodenal artery (GDA) is identified and test clamped to ensure adequate flow in the proper hepatic artery. In instances in which the celiac axis is partially or completely occluded, the hepatic artery flow may be dependent on the GDA. If a weak pulse is noted in the hepatic artery at test clamping, division of the median arcuate ligament is a feasible option to diminish stenosis or occlusion of the celiac axis. After confirming an adequate pulse in the proper hepatic artery, the GDA is ligated and divided. The anterior PV can now be dissected free from the posterior surface of the neck of the pancreas. For a classic Whipple, a distal gastrectomy is performed, which includes ligation of the right gastric artery. For pylorus-preserving pancreaticoduodenectomies (PPPDs) the first portion of the duodenum is divided 3 cm distal to the pylorus. Numerous studies comparing classic Whipple and PPPD have reported no major differences in morbidity or survival. However, other studies have noted decreased delayed gastric emptying (DGE) with classic Whipple compared with less operative time, operative blood loss, and red blood cell transfusion for patients undergoing PPPD.[16,17]

Attention is then turned to the third and fourth portions of the duodenum. This portion of the duodenum is adequately mobilized, allowing for the anterior surface of the SMV to be dissected free. The right gastroepiploic vein and artery are identified and ligated. Cephalad dissection off the anterior surface of the SMV avoids venous branches and ultimately clears a plane anterior to the PV and SMV, posterior to the neck of the pancreas (Fig. 100.2). The transverse pancreatic arterial arcade is controlled with four 3-0 silk stay sutures placed superiorly and inferiorly. The pancreatic neck is slowly transected using electrocautery. The duct is identified and transected with a scalpel when possible. The jejunum is divided distally, approximately 15 to 20 cm distal to the ligament of Treitz. The mesentery is carefully divided, and the proximal jejunum and fourth portion of the duodenum are passed posterior to the mesenteric vessels to the right of the operative field.

The specimen now remains attached by the remaining attachments of the head and uncinate process, which are

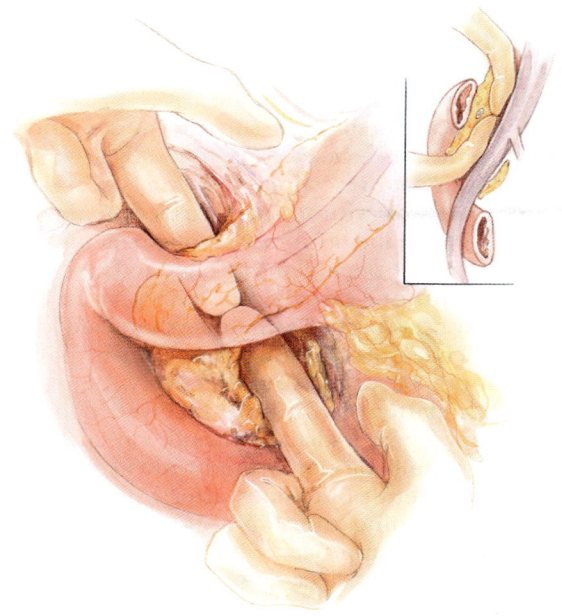

FIGURE 100.2 Creation of the tunnel behind the neck of the pancreas with cephalad dissection off the anterior surface of the superior mesenteric vein avoids venous branches and ultimately clears a plane anterior to the portal vein and superior mesenteric vein, posterior to the neck of the pancreas. (Image drawn by Corinne Sandone, MA, CMI. From Cameron JL, Sandone C. *Atlas of Gastrointestinal Surgery.* Vol 1. 2nd ed. Shelton, CT: People's Medical Publishing House; 2014:290. Used with permission from PMPH-USA, LTD, Shelton, CT.)

subsequently separated from the SMV and SMA through sharp dissection, and serial division of retroperitoneal tissue along the superior mesenteric artery with an electronic dissector (e.g., harmonic scalpel, LigaSure device). The dissection should remain flush with the mesenteric vessels to ensure pancreatic tissue and lymph nodes are excised in their entirety. The specimen consists of the distal stomach or first portion of the duodenum, neck, head, and uncinate process of the pancreas, gallbladder, distal biliary tree, and approximately 10 cm of the jejunum. The pancreatic neck, bile duct, and retroperitoneal margins are marked for intraoperative frozen section. Alternatively, the common hepatic duct and pancreatic neck margins can be sent for examination earlier in the procedure while the main specimen is removed.

Vascular Resection

En bloc resection to include the PV or SMV in pancreatic cancer was first proposed by Fortner in 1973.[18] With the increasing use of neoadjuvant therapies, PV and SMV resection in borderline resectable pancreatic tumors is increasingly being performed. State-of-the-art cross-sectional imaging is very accurate in identifying vascular involvement; as such, the surgeon should rarely be caught off guard and should be prepared for the possibility of vascular reconstruction. Adequate proximal and distal control is obtained by mobilization of the PV and SMV. Primary anastomosis is generally possible for short segment resections (<3 to 4 cm) after adequate mobilization of the portal and SMV (and sometimes the liver itself). For long segment reconstruction, interposition grafts are used, including cadaveric vein or autologous vein, such as the internal jugular or left renal vein.

Arterial encasement of the superior mesenteric artery, hepatic arteries, or celiac axis is generally accepted as a contraindication to resection. However, visceral arterial resections with or without vein resections have been reported.[19] Unlike the outcomes among patients undergoing PV, which have been demonstrated to be comparable to Whipple without vascular resection, visceral artery resection may be associated with worse short- and long-term outcomes. Therefore vascular resection in pancreatic cancer should be used very selectively, being largely restricted to patients who have received neoadjuvant chemotherapy/chemoradiation. In addition, such complex operations should be performed only at experienced centers. In general, outcomes after arterial resection remain disappointing and should therefore not be considered a standard approach, although arterial resection may be beneficial in select cases.

Reconstruction

After closing the defect at the previous ligament of Treitz, reconstruction begins with delivering the jejunum through a rent in the bare area of the transverse mesocolon to the right of the middle colic vessels. The pancreatoenteric reconstruction is responsible for the majority of morbidity associated with the Whipple procedure. Numerous variations of this anastomosis exist. We prefer a duct-to-mucosa anastomosis beginning with a back row of 3-0 silk sutures incorporating the pancreatic capsule and a seromuscular bite of the jejunum. A small jejunostomy in similar dimension to the pancreatic duct is created. A duct-to-mucosa anastomosis with interrupted 5-0 PDS sutures is performed incorporating the pancreatic duct and the full thickness of the jejunum. A 3.5- to 5-mm pediatric feeding tube (depending on the size of the duct) can be used as a pancreatic stent and left in place. Upon completion of the duct-to-mucosa anastomosis, an anterior row of interrupted 3-0 silk Lembert sutures completes the two-layer anastomosis.

Another method of pancreatoenteric reconstruction is the invagination technique, which can be accomplished in an end-to-side or end-to-end fashion. When an invagination technique is used, we prefer the end-to-side technique. Initially, the pancreatic remnant is mobilized for 2 to 3 cm. A back row of interrupted 3-0 silk sutures is placed, followed by a jejunostomy along the length of the pancreatic neck (Fig. 100.3A). The inner posterior layer is made using running 3-0 absorbable sutures, incorporating the pancreatic capsule, cut portion of pancreas, and

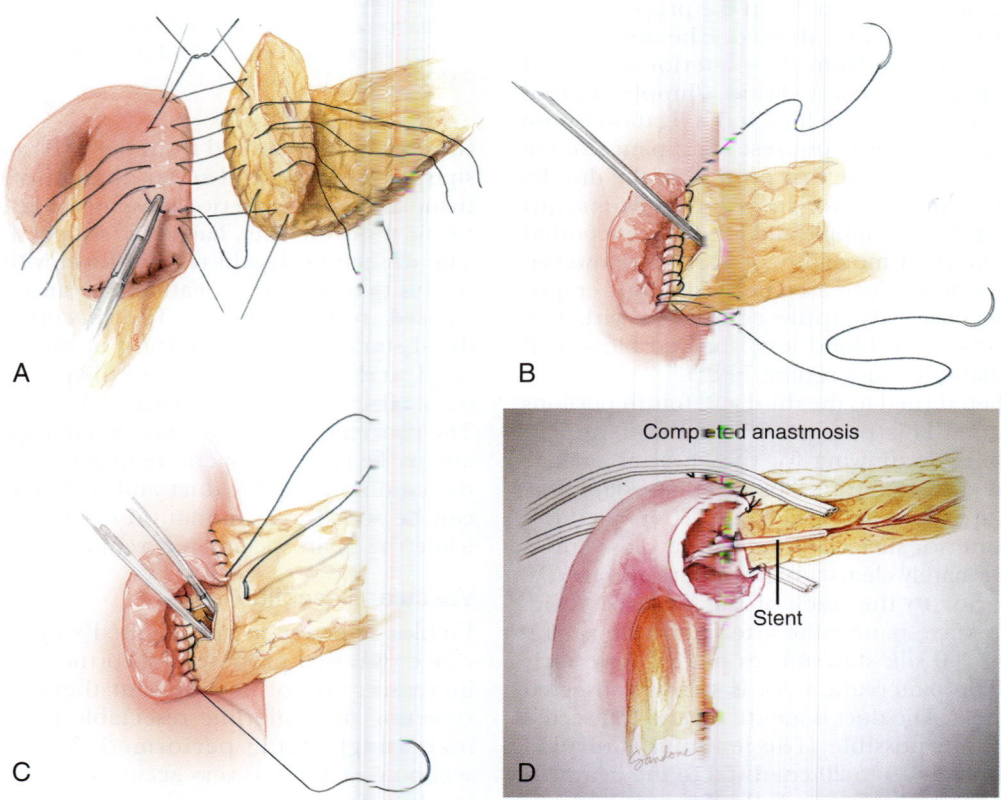

FIGURE 100.3 (A–D) Pancreaticojejunostomy technique beginning with (A) the outer layer of the posterior row followed by (B) inner layer of posterior row and (C) the inner layer of anterior row. (D) Final reconstruction of pancreaticojejunostomy with drains in place. ([A–C], Images drawn by Corinne Sandone, MA, CMI. For Cameron JL, Sandone C. *Atlas of Gastrointestinal Surgery*. Vol 1. 2nd ed. Shelton, CT: People's Medical Publishing House; 2014:294–295. Used with permission from PMPH-USA, LTD, Shelton, CT; [D], From Cameron JL, He J. Two thousand consecutive pancreaticoduodenectomies. *J Am Coll Surg*. 2015;220:530–536.)

full thickness of the jejunum (Fig. 100.3B). When possible, the pancreatic duct should be included in several throws of the running stitch to create a duct-to-mucosa anastomosis. The anterior layer of the inner row is performed in a similar fashion, being sure to include the pancreatic duct when possible, with careful attention to not inadvertently occlude the duct (Fig. 100.3C). Finally, an anterior row of interrupted 3-0 silk Lembert sutures is placed, bringing the jejunum over to cover the anastomosis (Fig. 100.3D).

Pancreatogastrostomy is performed in a similar fashion with the pancreas invaginated into the posterior wall of the stomach. Menahem et al. performed a meta-analysis of randomized controlled clinical trials comparing pancreaticogastrostomy with pancreaticojejunostomy.[20] These authors reported a lower incidence of pancreatic and biliary fistulas with pancreaticogastrostomies; however, other randomized controlled trials and metaanalyses have failed to demonstrate superior outcomes for using pancreaticogastrostomy. Heterogeneity in surgical techniques and definition of pancreatic fistula and complications complicate such analyses.[21,22] Both approaches are acceptable and depend on surgeon experience and preference.

The approach to the biliary anastomosis is less variable. We prefer a single layer of interrupted 4-0, 5-0, or 6-0 PDS sutures (depending on the duct size), located 5 to 10 cm distal to the pancreaticojejunostomy. The posterior row is performed by placing the sutures inside out on the jejunum and outside in on the hepatic duct, leaving the knot inside the anastomosis. The posterior row sutures are secured with clamps until all posterior row sutures are placed. These sutures are then knotted and the anterior row is placed outside in on the jejunum and inside out on the hepatic duct. Previously placed biliary stents may be included in the anastomosis.

Reconstruction of gastrointestinal continuity involves either a gastrojejunostomy or duodenojejunostomy depending on whether a classic or pylorus preserving Whipple is performed. This anastomosis is made approximately 15 cm distal to the hepaticojejunostomy. An end-to-side duodenojejunostomy is performed in two layers; an interrupted layer of 3-0 silk for the outer layers with typically an inner running layer of 3-0 synthetic absorbable suture (Fig. 100.4). For a classic Whipple, a gastrojejunostomy is performed in a similar fashion. Retrocolic versus antecolic reconstruction remains controversial. Retrocolic reconstruction is performed with a proximal portion of jejunum without traversing the mesocolon, while an antecolic anastomosis is performed with a more distal portion of the jejunum "over" the transverse mesocolon. Some groups prefer antecolic reconstruction arguing that venous congestion and bowel edema are increased with a retrocolic technique, thereby leading to increased complications, such as DGE. Others argue that antecolic reconstruction lends itself to increased angulation of the stomach and higher rates of DGE. In addition, some argue that an antecolic anastomosis is less likely to obstruct in the event of a locoregional recurrence. However, multiple randomized controlled trials and metaanalyses have failed to demonstrate a significant difference in postoperative outcomes between a retrocolic versus antecolic reconstruction.[23–27]

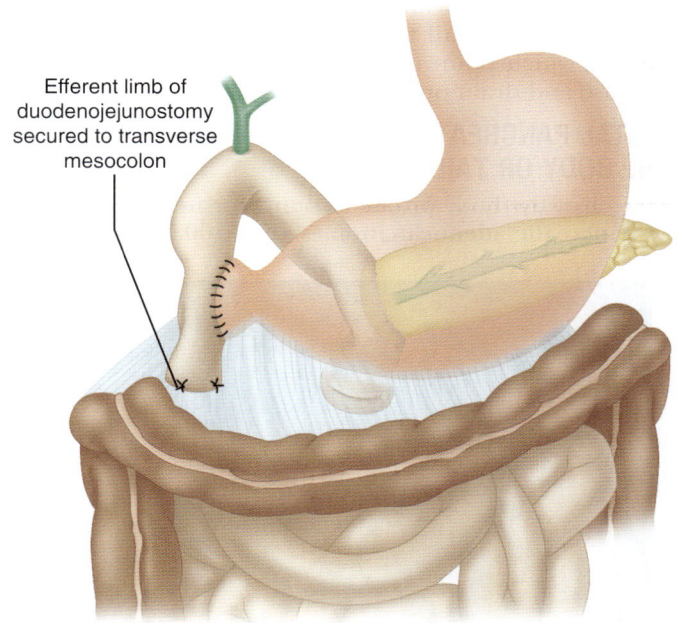

Efferent limb of duodenojejunostomy secured to transverse mesocolon

FIGURE 100.4 Final anatomy after pylorus-preserving pancreaticoduodenectomy. Notice the efferent limb of the duodenojejunostomy secured to the transverse mesocolon. (From Kennedy EP, Brumbaugh J, Yeo CJ. Reconstruction following the pylorus preserving Whipple resection: PJ, HJ, and DJ. *J Gastrointest Surg.* 2010;14:408–415.)

The use of drains after pancreaticoduodenectomy has been extensively studied.[28–31] Some groups prefer to abstain from drains at the time of operation and use interventional radiology to drain any postoperative fluid collections that are clinically relevant. Based on data from a multiinstitutional randomized controlled trial, van Buren et al. reported that the avoidance of drains at the time of a Whipple procedure was associated with an increased frequency and severity of complications.[29] Patients without routine drainage were more likely to have a higher average complication severity, longer length of hospital stay, and increased mortality rates. In fact, the study was stopped early by the Data Safety Monitoring Board. We typically place two closed suction drains by the pancreatic and biliary anastomosis with special attention made to prevent the drains from coming into direct contact with the hepatico- and pancreaticojejunostomy.

Postoperative Care

Routine prolonged nasogastric decompression appears unnecessary.[32,33] As such, the nasogastric tube is removed the next morning. The patient has nothing by mouth except "sips and chips" for the first 1 to 2 postoperative days, and then the diet is advanced daily. With regard to drain management, a prospectively validated study from the Massachusetts General Hospital identified a less than 1% risk of pancreatic fistula if postoperative day (POD) 1 drain amylase levels are lower than 600 U/L and recommend early drain removal in these patients.[34] In instances of high POD 1 drain amylase levels, we prefer to maintain drains in place until the patient is tolerating a regular diet, at which point the drains are removed when low amylase and drain output are low (<20 mL/day).

DISTAL PANCREATECTOMY FOR CANCERS OF THE BODY OR TAIL

Cancer of the body or tail accounts for nearly one-third of pancreatic adenocarcinomas (Fig. 100.5). Symptoms

typically manifest late in the course of the disease and therefore are more likely to present with advanced disease. Accordingly, staging laparoscopy is commonly used for these lesions. In the absence of metastases, distal pancreatectomy is the procedure of choice for these tumors. A "bump" may be placed underneath the patient's left upper back to further elevate the left upper quadrant. A vertical midline incision is typically used, although a bilateral subcostal incision is also acceptable.

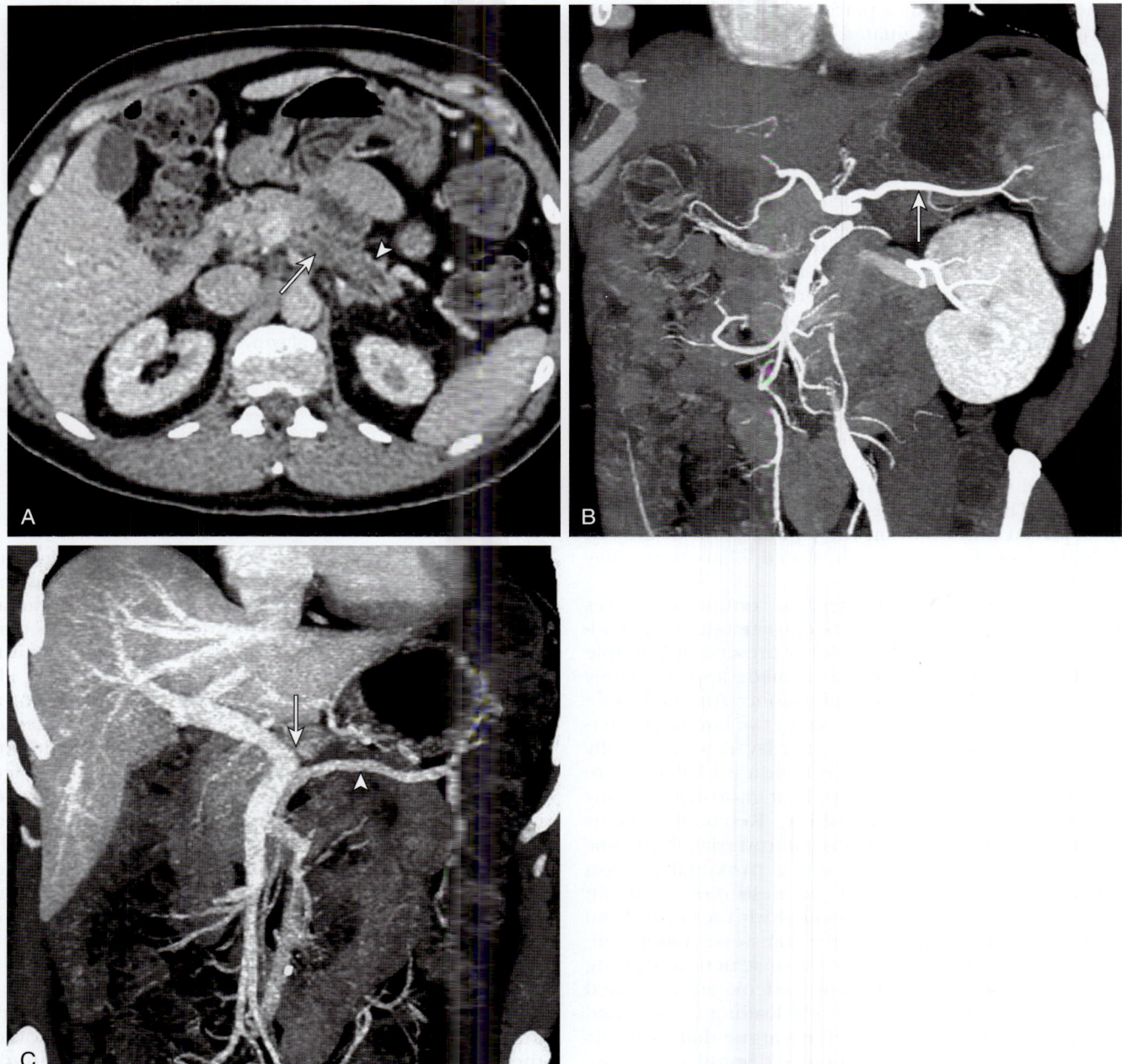

FIGURE 100.5 A 58-year-old male with history of adenocarcinoma in the tail of the pancreas. (A) Axial computed tomography image of the abdomen obtained in the venous phase reveals a subtle mass in the tail of the pancreas *(arrow)*, resulting in atrophy of the pancreatic tail and upstream dilatation of the pancreatic duct *(arrowhead)*. B) Coronal maximum intensity projection image in the arterial phase reveals patent splenic artery *(arrow)*. (C) Coronal maximum intensity projection image in the venous phase reveals complete occlusion of the splenic vein at the confluence *(arrow)*. The splenic artery *(arrowhead)* is not invaded or encased. (Courtesy Ihab Kamel, MD, and Mounes Ghasebeh, MD, Department of Radiology, The Johns Hopkins University School of Medicine.)

The procedure begins with entering the lesser sac by elevating the greater omentum off the transverse colon. The splenic flexure of the colon is mobilized and reflected inferiorly by dividing the splenocolic ligament. The short gastrics are subsequently divided using an electronic sealing device or serial clamp and ties. The spleen is mobilized laterally to medially out of the retroperitoneum by dividing the splenorenal ligament, thereby mobilizing the pancreas out of the retroperitoneum as well. Isolation of the splenic artery and vein may be performed by developing a tunnel behind the pancreatic body and tail. The splenic vein is located posterior to the pancreas often within the pancreatic parenchyma as it courses toward to the spleen; the splenic artery courses along the superior border of the pancreas. The splenic artery should be test clamped and flow in the common hepatic artery confirmed prior to ligating the splenic artery. The splenic artery and vein can be suture ligated or stapled using a vascular load on a linear stapler.

Postoperative pancreatic fistula is the most common complication after distal pancreatectomy. Numerous methods of pancreatic transection and management of the pancreatic remnant have been reported, including using linear stapling devices across the pancreas, direct duct ligation, fibrin glue application, and enteric drainage.[35] No specific method has been demonstrated to be superior. Prior to dividing the pancreas, four stay sutures may be placed along the inferior and superior border of the pancreatic transection line. We prefer to divide the pancreas with electrocautery (Fig. 100.6). The neck of the pancreas is oversewn with overlapping "U"

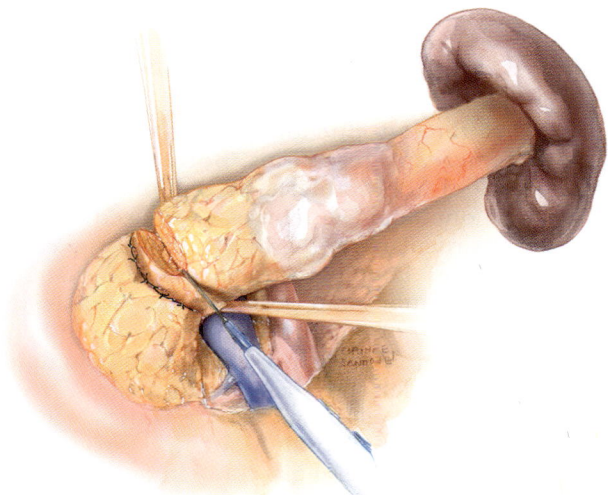

FIGURE 100.6 Transection of pancreatic neck during distal pancreatectomy. A Penrose drain has been placed across the underside of the pancreatic neck, anterior to the portal vein–superior mesenteric vein confluence to aid in elevating the pancreatic neck during transection. (Image drawn by Corinne Sandone, MA, CMI. From Cameron JL, Sandone C. *Atlas of Gastrointestinal Surgery*. Vol 1. 2nd ed. Shelton, CT: People's Medical Publishing House; 2014:315. Used with permission from PMPH-USA, LTD, Shelton, CT.)

stitches, and the duct is directly ligated when it can be identified. One or two 19-French drains are placed in the left upper quadrant and along the edge of the pancreatic remnant.

Postoperative management is relatively straightforward. Diets are advanced as tolerated. The drain output is monitored for evidence of pancreatic leak, and drain amylase levels are measured as indicated. Postsplenectomy vaccines for *Neisseria meningitidis*, *Streptococcus pneumoniae*, and *Haemophilus influenzae* are given preoperatively or on the day of discharge.

Splenic Preservation

Mallet-Guy and Vachon first described a spleen-preserving distal pancreatectomy in 1943.[36,37] Classically, however, splenic preservation is contraindicated in cases where malignancy is suspected given the close proximity of the splenic blood supply to the pancreas and the potential to negatively impact oncologic resection. Some reports demonstrate fewer postoperative complications and improved survival with spleen-preserving distal pancreatectomy compared with distal pancreatectomy and splenectomy.[36,38] In cases of pancreatic adenocarcinoma in the body or tail of the pancreas, we typically prefer resection of the distal pancreas and spleen en bloc. Splenic preservation is more appropriate in cases of benign disease or tumors with low malignant potential.

Splenic preservation can be performed by either preserving the splenic vessels or the Warshaw technique,[39] in which the splenic vessels are ligated but the short gastric are preserved. Outcomes appear similar with both approaches; however, splenic infarcts and secondary splenectomies occur more frequently with the Warshaw technique.[36] In cases of splenic preservation we prefer to preserve the splenic vessels whenever possible. This requires mobilizing the pancreatic tail and careful dissection of the various pancreatic branches from the splenic artery and vein from proximal to distal on the pancreas. The spleen is not mobilized medially to avoid inadvertent injury.

Appleby Procedure

The Appleby procedure was first described in 1953 and includes en bloc resection of the celiac axis, distal pancreatectomy with splenectomy, and total gastrectomy.[40] It was originally intended for locally advanced gastric cancer; however, in 1976 Nimura reported the first Appleby for locally advanced pancreatic adenocarcinoma of the body and tail.[41] With improvements in neoadjuvant pancreatic cancer chemoradiotherapy, an increasing number of patients are presenting with local tumor progression without evidence of metastatic disease. The Appleby procedure has been slow to gain popularity; however, there are an increasing number of series in the literature reporting either the Appleby or modified Appleby procedure for locally advanced pancreatic adenocarcinoma. The modified Appleby includes distal pancreatectomy, splenectomy, combined with celiac axis resection with resection of the common hepatic artery proximal to the GDA without gastrectomy.[42] The arterial blood supply to the liver is subsequently dependent on the pancreatico-duodenal branches from the superior mesenteric artery supplying the GDA. In select cases, arterial reconstruction, most often common hepatic artery to aorta, may be used.[42]

Outcomes of the modified Appleby for locally advanced pancreatic adenocarcinoma have not been clearly defined.[42–44] In a multicenter series derived from the American College of Surgeons National Surgical Quality Improvement Program (NSQIP) Pancreatectomy Demonstration Project that compared standard distal pancreatectomy versus distal pancreatectomy and concurrent celiac axis resection, patients who underwent celiac axis resection had a longer operative time, higher postoperative acute kidney injury, and a 10% operative mortality.[45] Although the modified Appleby procedure may be indicated in certain locally advanced body and tail tumors of the pancreas, these patients are most likely at increased risk of postoperative complications and death; as such, prudent and appropriate patient selection is critical.

TOTAL PANCREATECTOMY

Given the poor overall survival associated with pancreatic cancer, total pancreatectomy was proposed as a more radical approach in the 1960s and 1970s. A more radical resection was thought to potentially improve outcomes by completely removing all of the gland at risk, as well as decreasing morbidity and mortality due to the lack of a pancreaticoenteric anastomosis. Outcomes following total pancreatectomy were initially poor with increased postoperative morbidity and no improvement in long-term disease-free or overall survival. More recently, with improved operative technique and better perioperative care, outcomes following total pancreatectomies have improved and the number of total pancreatectomies for pancreatic cancer has increased.[46] Total pancreatectomy leaves the patient with difficult to manage brittle diabetes and persistent diarrhea and steatorrhea secondary to the loss of exocrine function. However, modern day, long-acting insulin analogues and pancreatic enzyme supplementation have improved the management of these problems. In fact, modern-day surgical series report acceptable long-term quality of life.[47–49] Morbidity and mortality associated with total pancreatectomy has decreased dramatically over time, although perioperative morbidity and mortality rates remain higher among patients undergoing total pancreatectomy versus pancreaticoduodenectomy, particularly when combined with vascular resections.[46,47,50] Despite this, long-term survival is equivalent in most modern series when comparing total pancreatectomy and pancreaticoduodenectomy.[46,47,51,52] As such, total pancreatectomy should be considered when required to achieve a margin-negative resection. Typically, the head or tail has been mobilized, and a total pancreatectomy becomes necessary due to a persistently positive margin. The technique for total pancreatectomy in pancreatic cancer therefore consists of mobilization of the remnant pancreas. In cases in which the pancreatic head has been resected, the remnant pancreas should then be excised along with the spleen. The short gastric vessels are ligated and divided. The splenic artery is taken at its origin, while the splenic vein is divided at the PV/SMV confluence. The remnant pancreas and spleen are then mobilized in a medial to lateral fashion.

MULTIVISCERAL RESECTION

The benefits of extended resections in pancreatic cancer have been debated and extensively studied. One indication for multivisceral resection in pancreatic cancer is an advanced tumor invading the hepatic flexure or transverse colon requiring a hemicolectomy.[53,54] Retrospective series comparing standard pancreatic resections versus resections that include an additional visceral resection demonstrate increased morbidity and mortality in the latter group.[54–56] In an NSQIP database analysis, perioperative mortality and morbidity rate with multivisceral resection at the time of pancreaticoduodenectomy was 8.8% and 56.8%, respectively, versus 2.9% and 30.8% for a standard pancreatoduodenectomy.[54] In multivariate analysis, multivisceral resection was an independent predictor of increased perioperative mortality and morbidity.

The benefit of multivisceral resection in pancreatic cancer is to obtain a curative resection with negative margins. Patients requiring multivisceral resection generally present with larger, more locally advanced tumors needing extended resection for contiguous organ involvment.[57] Despite this, retrospective series analyzing long-term outcomes of pancreatic cancer patients who undergo a multivisceral resection have a comparable 3-year and 5-year overall survival versus a standard pancreatic resection.[56–59] More importantly, overall survival in pancreatic cancer patients with multivisceral resection is significantly improved compared with patients who have unresected pancreatic cancer.[59] As such, multivisceral resections in pancreatic cancer should be attempted when a curative R0 resection can be achieved. Appropriate patient selection and performance by an experienced surgeon in specialized pancreatic cancer centers are important.

MINIMALLY INVASIVE PANCREATIC SURGERY

Further advancements in the field of pancreatic surgery have led to the introduction of both laparoscopic and robotic pancreatic resections. Both techniques have demonstrated acceptable early outcomes and likely equivalent oncologic outcomes compared with open resection, particularly in the hands of experienced pancreatic surgeons. Potential advantages include decreased wound complications and postoperative pain, as well as shortened length of stay. Most of the perceived benefits are derived from retrospective series because no randomized controlled trials have been performed.

More recently, robotic pancreatic resections have increased in popularity. Early results with regard to complications and oncologic outcomes are similar for both distal pancreatectomies and pancreatoduodenectomies; however, there are no randomized control trials that compare robotic resection with traditional open or laparoscopic approaches.[60–63] Ultimately, outcomes appear similar with either minimally invasive approach, and the optimal technique depends mainly on surgeon comfort (see Chapter 101 for a more detailed discussion of this topic).

Laparoscopic Distal Pancreatectomy

Distal pancreatectomy was one of the first pancreatic procedures to be attempted using a minimal invasive approach. Laparoscopic distal pancreatectomy has gained widespread acceptance in the treatment of benign pancreatic disease. More recently, numerous series have reported on the use of laparoscopic distal pancreatectomy for pancreatic ductal adenocarcinoma and noted equivalent oncologic outcomes, fewer complications, and shorter length of stay compared with open distal pancreatectomy.[64-69] For example, in a series of 2753 pancreatectomies, the French Pancreatectomy Study Group demonstrated largely comparable outcomes for laparoscopic distal pancreatectomy versus open distal pancreatectomy, with lower postoperative morbidity and shorter length of stay in the laparoscopic group.[64]

Laparoscopic distal pancreatectomy begins with insertion of an infraumbilical port and establishment of pneumoperitoneum via either Veress needle or Hassan cutdown technique. Three more ports are typically used, one in the left lower quadrant and two additional ports along the upper midline. The dissection begins with taking down the gastrocolic ligament and short gastric vessels using an electronic dissector. The splenic flexure of the colon is mobilized and taken down. The pancreas is mobilized by incising the peritoneum overlying its inferior border, and dissection continues until the splenic vessels are visualized. The pancreatic tail can be suspended by an instrument to allow better visualization of the splenic vessels. The splenic artery is confirmed by tracing it proximally to the celiac axis if necessary. Both the splenic artery and vein are ligated using a linear stapler with a vascular (white) load. The pancreas is divided with an Endo GIA stapler. The spleen is then mobilized from its retroperitoneal attachments, and the specimen is delivered via an Endo Catch bag. The pancreatic neck margin is sent for frozen-section analysis.

Laparoscopic Pancreaticoduodenectomy

The first laparoscopic pancreaticoduodenectomy was reported by Gagner and Pomp in 1994.[70] Since then, the use of minimally invasive pancreaticoduodenectomy (MIPD) has been slowly growing as a result of improved technology and more experience among pancreatic surgeons. As such, laparoscopic pancreaticoduodenectomies are currently performed in centers throughout the world. The data comparing MIPDs are variable, given that minimally invasive Whipple procedures include both laparoscopic and robotic approaches. Zhang et al.[71] performed a systematic review comparing MIPD versus the open approach. They included 1018 MIPDs compared with 5102 open pancreaticoduodenectomies. Despite longer operative times, MIPD Whipple procedures were associated with less blood loss, lower wound infections, and a 3.5-day shorter length of stay.[71] Although outcomes following MIPD appear comparable with open resections for pancreatic cancer, well-designed randomized controlled trials with extensive follow-up are lacking.[62,72,73]

Although a more detailed explanation can be found in the chapter on minimally invasive pancreatic surgery, in brief, six 10-mm ports are positioned in a semicircle around the umbilicus extending from the left upper quadrant to the right upper quadrant.[72] The hepatic artery is identified, and the GDA is then confirmed and ligated. The antrum is retracted, and the first portion of the

duodenum is divided. The inferior border of the pancreas is dissected to identify the SMV. A tunnel underneath the neck of the pancreas is created, and an umbilical tape is placed around the pancreas for retraction. The gallbladder is mobilized, and the common bile duct is encircled and subsequently divided. A wide Kocher maneuver is performed, and the jejunum is divided with a stapler 10 cm from the ligament of Treitz. Finally, the pancreatic neck is transected using an energy device, and the uncinate is then taken off of the superior mesenteric artery in a similar fashion. Of note, the pancreaticoduodenal branches will need to be divided between clips.

The jejunum is brought into the right upper quadrant through the ligament of Treitz defect. Reconstruction is performed in a similar fashion to the open technique, consisting of an end-to-side, duct to mucosa, 1- or 2-layer pancreaticojejunostomy, a single layer end-to-side hepaticojejunostomy, and an end-to-side, antecolic duodenojejunostomy. This final anastomosis is generally stapled, although a sewn 2-layer anastomosis is acceptable.

COMPLICATIONS AFTER PANCREATIC RESECTION

Although the mortality incidence in high-volume pancreatic surgery centers is only 2% to 3%, morbidity remains high, ranging from 30% to 50%.[74] The most common complications after pancreaticoduodenectomy includes DGE (7% to 21%), pancreatic fistula (7% to 15%), and wound infections (8% to 14%) (Table 100.1).[9,74] Older patients (>80 years old) and patients with increased comorbidities are more likely to die during their hospitalization.[9] Distal pancreatectomy for pancreatic adenocarcinoma has a similar mortality (1%) and morbidity (30%).[69] Pancreatic fistula and wound infections are the most common complications.

DGE is generally self-limited and non–life-threatening but may lead to a prolonged length of stay and increased hospital costs.[75] Treatment involves nasogastric decompression and sometimes parenteral nutrition support when the patient has a prolonged DGE course. In severe cases a gastrostomy tube may even be necessary; however, this is rare. The management of a postoperative pancreatic fistula varies from no interventions to the need for reoperation. Pancreatic fistula accounts for a significant proportion of early postoperative deaths after pancreatectomy

TABLE 100.1 Morbidity After Pancreaticoduodenectomy

Complication	n	%
Delayed gastric emptying	410	21
Postoperative pancreatic fistula	295	15
Wound infection	222	11
Cardiac event	69	3
Pneumonia	38	2
Delayed bleeding	32	2
Chyle leak	28	1
Any complication	894	45

From Cameron JL, He J. Two thousand consecutive pancreaticoduodenectomies. *J Am Coll Surg*. 2015;220:530–536.

secondary to sepsis/multisystem organ failure and bleeding secondary to pseuodoaneurysms. If intraoperative drains are in place, amylase levels may be checked to confirm a pancreatic leak. When cross-sectional imaging demonstrates an intraabdominal abscess, percutaneous drainage via interventional radiology techniques is appropriate. If the patient is otherwise well with no evidence of infection, tolerating a regular diet with a seemingly well-controlled leak, conservative management with outpatient drain management is appropriate.

Despite numerous clinical trials, the use of octreotide has not been shown to be effective in preventing postoperative pancreatic fistulas or associated complications. More recently, a single-center, randomized double blind trial examined 300 patients undergoing either pancreaticoduodenectomy or distal pancreatectomy who received either 900 µg subcutaneous pasireotide or placebo.[76] Of these patients, 15% reached the primary end point, which was grade 3 or higher postoperative pancreatic fistula, leak, or abscess. The pasireotide group demonstrated a significantly decreased risk of postoperative pancreatic fistula compared with the placebo group (9% vs. 21%; P = .006). The beneficial effect of pasireotide was noted in both the pancreaticoduodenectomy and distal pancreatectomy cohorts.

Delayed bleeding is one of the most severe postoperative complications after a pancreatectomy. The International Study Group of Pancreatic Surgery developed a consensus definition in 2007 that defined criteria for postpancreatectomy hemorrhage based on clinical factors assessing the severity of bleeding.[77] Fortunately, postpancreatectomy hemorrhage is rare, with an incidence of 1.5%; however, the mortality can be as high as 30% to 40%.[9,78] Postpancreatectomy hemorrhage is most often secondary to a pseudoaneurysm in the presence of a pancreaticojejunostomy leak, although gastrojejunostomy/duodenojejunostomy anastomotic bleeding can also occur. Management preferably consists of interventional radiology techniques to embolize the false aneurysm/gastroduodenal stump. When embolization of the gastroduodenal stump is not feasible, a covered stent across the common/proper hepatic artery that excludes the false aneurysm should be considered. When bleeding is secondary to an intraluminal/enteric anastomotic source, endoscopic techniques can be used. In instances of hemodynamic instability, immediate reexploration is warranted.

CONCLUSION

Surgery remains the only chance of long-term survival for patients with pancreas adenocarcinoma. Although mortality from pancreatic resections has decreased significantly, morbidity remains high. More aggressive surgical approaches, including vascular resection and multivisceral resection, have demonstrated acceptable outcomes and have allowed for an increased number of patients to be considered for surgery. However, proper patient selection, a multidisciplinary approach, and referral to high-volume centers are required to ensure optimal outcomes. Although technical excellence is critical, pancreatic surgeons need to play a role in identifying more effective adjuvant therapy

for this disease if we are to optimize outcomes for our patients.

REFERENCES

1. Witzel O. Beitrage zur Chirurgie der Bauchorgane. *Dtsch Zeitschr Chir.* 1886;24:325-354.
2. Schnelldorfer T, Adams DB, Warshaw AL, Lillemoe KD, Sarr MG. Forgotten pioneers of pancreatic surgery: beyond the favorite few. *Ann Surg.* 2008;247:191-202.
3. Halsted WS. Contributions to the surgery of the bile passages, especially of the common bile-duct. *Boston Med Surg J.* 1899;141:645-654.
4. Sauve L. Des pancréatectomies et specialement de la pancréatectomie céphalique. *Rev Chir.* 1908;37:113-152, 335–385.
5. Kausch W. Das Carcinom der Paiplla duodeni und seine radikale Entfernung. *Beitr Klin Chir.* 1912;78:439-486.
6. Hirschel G. Die Resektion des Duodenums mit der Papille wegen Karzinoms. *Munchen Med Wochenschr.* 1914;61:1728-1729.
7. Whipple AO, Parsons WB, Mullins CR. Treatment of carcinoma of the ampulla of Vater. *Ann Surg.* 1935;102:763-779.
8. Whipple AO. Pancreaticoduodenectomy for islet carcinoma: a five-year follow-up. *Ann Surg.* 1945;121:847-852.
9. Cameron JL, He J. Two thousand consecutive pancreaticoduodenectomies. *J Am Coll Surg.* 2015;220:530-536.
10. Sohn TA, Yeo CJ, Cameron JL, Pitt HA, Lillemoe KD. Do preoperative biliary stents increase postpancreaticoduodenectomy complications? *J Gastrointes Surg* 2000;24:258-267 [discussion 267–258].
11. Povoski SP, Karpeh MS Jr, Conlon KC, Blumgart LH, Brennan MF. Association of preoperative biliary drainage with postoperative outcome following pancreaticoduodenectomy. *Ann Surg.* 1999;230:131-142.
12. Alamo JM, Marin LM, Suarez G, et al. Improving outcomes in pancreatic cancer: key points in perioperative management. *World J Gastroenterol.* 2014;20:14237-14245.
13. Conlon KC, Dougherty E, Klimstra DS, Coit DG, Turnbull AD, Brennan MF. The value of minimal access surgery in the staging of patients with potentially resectable peripancreatic malignancy. *Ann Surg.* 1996;223:134-140.
14. Vollmer CM, Drebin JA, Middleton WD, et al. Utility of staging laparoscopy in subsets of peripancreatic and biliary malignancies. *Ann Surg.* 2002;235:1-7.
15. Allen VB, Gurusamy KS, Takwoingi Y, Kalia A, Davidson BR. Diagnostic accuracy of laparoscopy following computed tomography (CT) scanning for assessing the resectability with curative intent in pancreatic and periampullary cancer. *Cochrane Database Syst Rev.* 2013;(11):CD009323.
16. Hüttner FJ, Fitzmaurice C, Schwarzer G, et al. Pylorus-preserving pancreaticoduodenectomy (pp Whipple) versus pancreaticoduodenectomy (class Whipple) for surgical treatment of periampullary and pancreatic carcinoma. *Cochrane Database Syst Rev.* 2016;(2):CD006053.
17. Wu W, Hong X, Fu L, et al. The effect of pylorus removal on delayed gastric emptying after pancreaticoduodenectomy: a meta-analysis of 2,599 patients. *PLoS One.* 2014;9:e108380.
18. Fortner JG. Regional resection of cancer of the pancreas: a new surgical approach. *Surgery.* 1973;73:307-320.
19. Christians KK, Pilgrim CH, Tsai S, et al. Arterial resection at the time of pancreatectomy for cancer. *Surgery.* 2014;155:919-926.
20. Menahem B, Guittet L, Mulliri A, Alves A, Lubrano J. Pancreaticogastrostomy is superior to pancreaticojejunostomy for prevention of pancreatic fistula after pancreaticoduodenectomy: an updated meta-analysis of randomized controlled trials. *Ann Surg.* 2015;261:882-887.
21. Wellner UF, Sick O, Olschewski M, Adam U, Hopt UT, Keck T. Randomized controlled single-center trial comparing pancreatogastrostomy versus pancreaticojejunostomy after partial pancreatoduodenectomy. *J Gastrointest Surg.* 2012;16:1686-1695.
22. Crippa S, Cirocchi R, Randolph J, et al. Pancreaticojejunostomy is comparable to pancreaticogastrostomy after pancreaticoduodenectomy: an updated meta-analysis of randomized controlled trials. *Langenbecks Arch Surg.* 2016;401:427-437.
23. Joliat GR, Labgaa I, Demartines N, Schäfer M, Allemann P. Effect of antecolic versus retrocolic gastroenteric reconstruction after pancreaticoduodenectomy on delayed gastric emptying: a meta-analysis of six randomized controlled trials. *Dig Surg.* 2016;33:15-25.

24. Gangavatiker R, Pal S, Javed A, Dash NR, Sahni P, Chattopadhyay TK. Effect of antecolic or retrocolic reconstruction of the gastro/duodenojejunostomy on delayed gastric emptying after pancreaticoduodenectomy: a randomized controlled trial. *J Gastrointest Surg.* 2011;15:843-852.

25. Eshuis WJ, van Eijck CH, Gerhards MF, et al. Antecolic versus retrocolic route of the gastroenteric anastomosis after pancreatoduodenectomy: a randomized controlled trial. *Ann Surg.* 2014;259:45-51.

26. Bell R, Pandanaboyana S, Shah N, Bartlett A, Windsor JA, Smith AM. Meta-analysis of antecolic versus retrocolic gastric reconstruction after a pylorus-preserving pancreatoduodenectomy. *HPB (Oxford).* 2015;17:202-208.

27. Tamandl D, Sahora K, Prucker J, et al. Impact of the reconstruction method on delayed gastric emptying after pylorus-preserving pancreaticoduodenectomy: a prospective randomized study. *World J Surg.* 2014;38:465-475.

28. McMillan MT, Malleo G, Bassi C, et al. Drain management after pancreatoduodenectomy: reappraisal of a prospective randomized trial using risk stratification. *J Am Coll Surg.* 2015;221:798-809.

29. Van Buren G 2nd, Bloomston M, Hughes SJ, et al. A randomized prospective multicenter trial of pancreaticoduodenectomy with and without routine intraperitoneal drainage. *Ann Surg.* 2014;259:605-612.

30. Correa-Gallego C, Brennan MF, D'Angelica M, et al. Operative drainage following pancreatic resection: analysis of 1122 patients resected over 5 years at a single institution. *Ann Surg.* 2013;258:1051-1058.

31. Conlon KC, Labow D, Leung D, et al. Prospective randomized clinical trial of the value of intraperitoneal drainage after pancreatic resection. *Ann Surg.* 2001;234:487-493 [discussion 493–484].

32. Kunstman JW, Klemen ND, Fonseca AL, Araya DL, Salem RR. Nasogastric drainage may be unnecessary after pancreaticoduodenectomy: a comparison of routine vs selective decompression. *J Am Coll Surg.* 2013;217:481-488.

33. Fisher WE, Hodges SE, Cruz G, et al. Routine nasogastric suction may be unnecessary after a pancreatic resection. *HPB (Oxford).* 2011;13:792-796.

34. Ven Fong Z, Correa-Gallego C, Ferrone CR, et al. Early drain removal—the middle ground between the drain versus no drain debate in patients undergoing pancreaticoduodenectomy: a prospective validation study. *Ann Surg.* 2015;262:378-383.

35. Diener MK, Seiler CM, Rossion I, et al. Efficacy of stapler versus hand-sewn closure after distal pancreatectomy (DISPACT): a randomised, controlled multicentre trial. *Lancet.* 2011;377:1514-1522.

36. Shi N, Liu SL, Li YT, You L, Dai MH, Zhao YP. Splenic preservation versus splenectomy during distal pancreatectomy: a systematic review and meta-analysis. *Ann Surg Oncol.* 2016;23:365-374.

37. Mallet-Guy P, Vachon A. *Pancreatites Chroniques Gauches.* Paris: Masson & Cie; 1943.

38. Schwarz RE, Harrison LE, Conlon KC, Klimstra DS, Brennan MF. The impact of splenectomy on outcomes after resection of pancreatic adenocarcinoma. *J Am Coll Surg.* 1999;188:516-521.

39. Warshaw AL. Conservation of the spleen with distal pancreatectomy. *Arch Surg.* 1988;123:550-553.

40. Appleby LH. The coeliac axis in the expansion of the operation for gastric carcinoma. *Cancer.* 1953;6:704-707.

41. Nimura Y, Hattori T, Miura K, et al. Resection of advanced pancreatic body-tail carcinoma by Appleby's operation. *Shujutu.* 1976;30:885-889.

42. Latona JA, Lamb KM, Pucci MJ, Maley WR, Yeo CJ. Modified Appleby procedure with arterial reconstruction for locally advanced pancreatic adenocarcinoma: a literature review and report of three unusual cases. *J Gastrointest Surg.* 2016;20:300-306.

43. Wu X, Tao R, Lei R, et al. Distal pancreatectomy combined with celiac axis resection in treatment of carcinoma of the body/tail of the pancreas: a single-center experience. *Ann Surg Oncol.* 2010;17:1359-1366.

44. Jing W, Zhu G, Hu X, et al. Distal pancreatectomy with en bloc celiac axis resection for the treatment of locally advanced pancreatic body and tail cancer. *Hepatogastroenterology.* 2013;60:187-190.

45. Beane JD, House MG, Pitt SC, et al. Distal pancreatectomy with celiac axis resection: what are the added risks? *HPB (Oxford).* 2015;17:777-784.

46. Reddy S, Wolfgang CL, Cameron JL, et al. Total pancreatectomy for pancreatic adenocarcinoma: evaluation of morbidity and long-term survival. *Ann Surg.* 2009;250:282-287.

47. Hartwig W, Gluth A, Hinz U, et al. Total pancreatectomy for primary pancreatic neoplasms: renaissance of an unpopular operation. *Ann Surg.* 2015;261:537-546.

48. Muller MW, Friess H, Kleeff J, et al. Is there still a role for total pancreatectomy? *Ann Surg.* 2007;246:966-974 [discussion 974-965].

49. Belyaev O, Herzog T, Chromik AM, Meurer K, Uhl W. Early and late postoperative changes in the quality of life after pancreatic surgery. *Langenbecks Arch Surg.* 2013;398:547-555.

50. Bhayani NH, Miller JL, Ortenzi G, et al. Perioperative outcomes of pancreaticoduodenectomy compared to total pancreatectomy for neoplasia. *J Gastrointest Surg.* 2014;18:549-554.

51. Johnston WC, Hoen HM, Cassera MA, et al. Total pancreatectomy for pancreatic ductal adenocarcinoma: review of the National Cancer Data Base. *HPB (Oxford).* 2016;18:21-28.

52. Satoi S, Murakami Y, Motoi F, et al. Reappraisal of total pancreatectomy in 45 patients with pancreatic ductal adenocarcinoma in the modern era using matched-pairs analysis: Multicenter Study Group of Pancreatobiliary Surgery in Japan. *Pancreas.* 2016;45:1003-1009.

53. Nikfarjam M, Sehmbey M, Kimchi ET, et al. Additional organ resection combined with pancreaticoduodenectomy does not increase postoperative morbidity and mortality. *J Gastrointest Surg.* 2009;13:915-921.

54. Bhayani NH, Enomoto LM, James BC, et al. Multivisceral and extended resections during pancreatoduodenectomy increase morbidity and mortality. *Surgery.* 2014;155:567-574.

55. Kleeff J, Diener MK, Z'Graggen K, et al. Distal pancreatectomy: risk factors for surgical failure in 302 consecutive cases. *Ann Surg.* 2007;245:573-582.

56. Kulemann B, Hoeppner J, Wittel U, et al. Perioperative and long-term outcome after standard pancreaticoduodenectomy, additional portal vein and multivisceral resection for pancreatic head cancer. *J Gastrointest Surg.* 2015;19:438-444.

57. Hartwig W, Hackert T, Hinz U, et al. Multivisceral resection for pancreatic malignancies: risk-analysis and long-term outcome. *Ann Surg.* 2009;250:81-87.

58. Sasson AR, Hoffman JP, Ross EA, et al. En bloc resection for locally advanced cancer of the pancreas: is it worthwhile? *J Gastrointest Surg.* 2002;6:147-157 [discussion 157–148].

59. Burdelski CM, Reeh M, Bogoevski D, et al. Multivisceral resections in pancreatic cancer: identification of risk factors. *World J Surg.* 2011;35:2756-2763.

60. Huang B, Feng L, Zhao J. Systematic review and meta-analysis of robotic versus laparoscopic distal pancreatectomy for benign and malignant pancreatic lesions. *Surg Endosc.* 2016;30:4078-4085.

61. Lai EC, Yang GP, Tang CN. Robot-assisted laparoscopic pancreaticoduodenectomy versus open pancreaticoduodenectomy—a comparative study. *Int J Surg.* 2012;10:475-479.

62. Zureikat AH, Breaux JA, Steel JL, Hughes SJ. Can laparoscopic pancreaticoduodenectomy be safely implemented? *J Gastrointest Surg.* 2011;15:1151-1157.

63. Sharpe SM, Talamonti MS, Wang CE, et al. Early national experience with laparoscopic pancreaticoduodenectomy for ductal adenocarcinoma: a comparison of laparoscopic pancreaticoduodenectomy and open pancreaticoduodenectomy from the National Cancer Data Base. *J Am Coll Surg.* 2015;221:175-184.

64. Sulpice L, Farges O, Goutte N, et al. Laparoscopic distal pancreatectomy for pancreatic ductal adenocarcinoma: time for a randomized controlled trial? Results of an All-inclusive National Observational Study. *Ann Surg.* 2015;262:868-873 [discussion 873–864].

65. Kooby DA, Hawkins WG, Schmidt CM, et al. A multicenter analysis of distal pancreatectomy for adenocarcinoma: is laparoscopic resection appropriate? *J Am Coll Surg.* 2010;210:779-785, 786–787.

66. DiNorcia J, Schrope BA, Lee MK, et al. Laparoscopic distal pancreatectomy offers shorter hospital stays with fewer complications. *J Gastrointest Surg.* 2010;14:1804-1812.

67. Sharpe SM, Talamonti MS, Wang E, et al. The laparoscopic approach to distal pancreatectomy for ductal adenocarcinoma results in shorter lengths of stay without compromising oncologic outcomes. *Am J Surg.* 2015;209:557-563.

68. Stauffer JA, Rosales-Velderrain A, Goldberg RF, Bowers SP, Asbun HJ. Comparison of open with laparoscopic distal pancreatectomy: a single institution's transition over a 7-year period. *HPB (Oxford).* 2013;15:149-155.

69. Riviere D, Gurusamy KS, Kooby DA, et al. Laparoscopic versus open distal pancreatectomy for pancreatic cancer. *Cochrane Database Syst Rev.* 2016;(4):CD011391.

70. Gagner M, Pomp A. Laparoscopic pylorus-preserving pancreato-duodenectomy. *Surg Endosc.* 1994;8:408-410.

71. Zhang H, Wu X, Zhu F, et al. Systematic review and meta-analysis of minimally invasive versus open approach for pancreaticoduodenectomy. *Surg Endosc.* 2016;[Epub ahead of print].

72. Tee MC, Kendrick ML, Farnell MB. Laparoscopic pancreaticoduodenectomy: is it an effective procedure for pancreatic ductal adenocarcinoma? *Adv Surg.* 2015;49:143-156.

73. Asbun HJ, Stauffer JA. Laparoscopic vs open pancreaticoduodenectomy: overall outcomes and severity of complication using the Accordion Severity Grading System. *J Am Coll Surg.* 2012;215:810-819.

74. He J, Ahuja N, Makary MA, et al. 2564 resected periampullary adenocarcinomas at a single institution: trends over three decades. *HPB (Oxford).* 2014;16:83-90.

75. Eisenberg JD, Rosato EL, Lavu H, Yeo CJ, Winter JM. Delayed gastric emptying after pancreaticoduodenectomy: an analysis of risk factors and cost. *J Gastrointest Surg.* 2015;19:1572-1580.

76. Allen PJ, Gönen M, Brennan MF, et al. Pasireotide for postoperative pancreatic fistula. *N Engl J Med.* 2014;370:2014-2022.

77. Wente MN, Veit JA, Bassi C, et al. Postpancreatectomy hemorrhage (PPH): an International Study Group of Pancreatic Surgery (ISGPS) definition. *Surgery.* 2007;142:20-25.

78. Grützmann R, Rückert F, Hippe-Davies N, Distler M, Saeger HD. Evaluation of the International Study Group of Pancreatic Surgery definition of postpancreatectomy hemorrhage in a high-volume center. *Surgery.* 2012;151:612-620.

Minimally Invasive Pancreas Surgery

Vernissia Tam | Deepa Magge | Herbert Zeh III | Melissa Hogg

The introduction of laparoscopy in the 1980s has revolutionized the field of complex abdominal surgery. Once highly morbid procedures requiring open exposure and prolonged recovery are now accomplished through minimally invasive techniques with comparable outcomes. In 1994 Gagner and Pomp described the first laparoscopic pylorus-sparing pancreaticoduodenectomy (PD) in a 30-year-old female with chronic pancreatitis (CP).[1] The operative time was 10 hours, and her postoperative course was complicated by delayed gastric emptying, necessitating a 30-day hospital stay. Due to concerns of excessive morbidity, the introduction of laparoscopic pancreas surgery was challenged. However, since 2010, there has been growing momentum in laparoscopic surgery and it is now well integrated into routine pancreatic resections and reconstructions at high-volume centers, with equivalent rates of mortality compared with open procedures. Traditional operations for almost all pancreatic resections and reconstructions have been described and replicated through a laparoscopic approach.

Laparoscopic surgery can be generally described as pure laparoscopic, robotic assisted, or a combination. Conventional laparoscopic surgery permits smaller incisions and improved postoperative pain control. Patients benefit from expedited functional recovery and shorter hospital stays. Technically, improved visualization through a magnified view allows meticulous dissection and greater control of intraoperative bleeding. With the advent of robotic assistance, surgeons benefit from binocular three-dimensional vision, scaling, stabilization of tremor, reduced operator fatigue and improved ergonomics from the console-surgeon interface. This chapter will focus on the robotic approach, summarizing the data on the safety, efficacy, and technique of robotic approaches to minimally invasive pancreas surgery for both benign and malignant indications, showcasing the diversity of the platform for complex pancreatic operations.

BENIGN CONDITIONS

ACUTE PANCREATITIS

Complications of acute pancreatitis, including infected pancreatic necrosis, were historically managed with laparotomy and open pancreatic necrosectomy, which were associated with high rates of mortality and morbidity at 56% and 78%, respectively. This has prompted less invasive techniques, such as percutaneous and endoscopic drainage. For infected necrotizing pancreatitis, the step-up approach as described by van Santvoort et al. in the PANTER (PAncreatitis, Necrosectomy versus sTEp up appRoach) trial[2] recommends beginning with percutaneous or endoscopic drainage for sepsis control. After 72 hours, if

there is no clinical improvement or a new collection forms that is inadequately drained, a second drain is recommended. If there is no clinical improvement after another 72 hours, a video-assisted retroperitoneal débridement (VARD) is recommended. This technique in stepwise escalation of invasive intervention was found to have equal rates of mortality compared with traditional necrosectomy. Furthermore, more than one-third of patients were successfully managed with drains alone and had fewer long-term complications of new-onset diabetes, incisional hernias, and pancreatic insufficiency.

The decision to pursue a minimally invasive approach for walled-off pancreatic necrosis (WOPN) depends on timing of presentation, anatomy of collection, and patient history. For patients with WOPN, we would recommend delaying surgical intervention for a minimum of 6 to 12 weeks following presentation, which allows the wall of the collection to mature and its contents to liquefy. Collections that consist of homogenous fluid may successfully be treated by endoscopic or percutaneous drainage, whereas those containing heterogeneous debris usually necessitate mechanical débridement. Patients who present with biliary pancreatitis will need a cholecystectomy, and a laparoscopic or robotic-assisted approach will permit a concurrent opportunity.

Minimally Invasive Cyst-Gastrostomy

A minimally invasive cyst-gastrostomy (CG) allows en bloc débridement of infected necrotic pancreatic tissue and continued drainage via a connection with the stomach. Collections that are likely to be successfully treated by a CG are greater than 15 cm in size, possess a defined capsule, are medially located within the pancreas, and adherent to the posterior wall of the stomach.

Comparing laparoscopic with open CG, Khaled et al. found the laparoscopic approach to have shorter operative times, lower risk of postoperative morbidity, and shorter hospital stay.[3] Although endoscopy and minimally invasive CG have been shown to have similar rates of complications, endoscopically managed patients typically require repeat interventions. Khreiss et al. compared 20 patients who underwent minimally invasive CG with 20 patients who underwent endoscopic drainage and found that 45% of endoscopic patients required repeat drainage for residual WOPN, compared with 15% of patients who received an operation.[4] Similarly, Worhunsky et al. reported 90% of 21 patients with sterile pancreatic necrosis who underwent transgastric necrosectomy were successfully débrided without additional interventions.[5]

Technique. The robotic transgastric CG as described by Khreiss et al.[4] begins with six robotic ports: one 12-mm camera port, three 8-mm robotic arm ports, and two bedside assistant ports (12 mm and 5 mm) as depicted

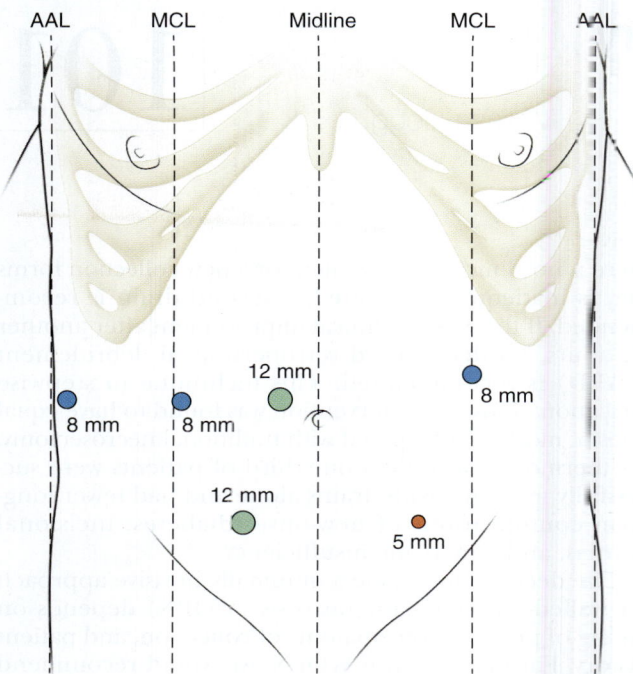

FIGURE 101.1 Robotic cyst-gastrostomy—port placement. Periumbilical 12-mm camera port; three upper 8-mm robotic arms; right lower quadrant 12-mm laparoscopic port; left lower quadrant 5-mm laparoscopic assistant port. *AAL,* Anterior axillary line; *MCL,* midclavicular line.

in Fig. 101.1. Intraoperative ultrasound is used to localize the WOPN and plan the optimal location for CG. A 5-cm anterior gastrostomy is created using monopolar scissors, a minimum of 2 cm away from, and parallel to, the greater gastric curve. A 1-cm posterior gastrostomy is then made to reach the anterior wall of the collection. A suction irrigator is used until the effluent is dry. The CG is fashioned using either a linear cutting stapler or plication of posterior stomach wall to the anterior capsule using running suture. Under direct visualization, the necrotic material is removed through the CG, ideally as a large en bloc necroma. After cavity irrigation, the anterior gastrostomy is closed in 2 layers with a linear stapler or running absorbable suture followed by a second layer of silk sutures (Fig. 101.2). At this point, such adjunct procedures as a cholecystectomy or jejunostomy feeding tube may be performed.

Video-Assisted Retroperitoneal Débridement

The VARD procedure allows pancreatic débridement under direct visualization through a retroperitoneal route. It is indicated for patients who have had a retroperitoneal drain in place. It may be ideal for patients with a significant abdominal surgical history by avoiding a transabdominal route or for patients who are septic and not expected to do well following a laparotomy.

Horvath et al. conducted the largest review of VARD procedures in 25 patients with necrotizing pancreatitis across six tertiary care centers.[6] There were four (16%) primary complications, including bleeding and enteric fistula, and nine (36%) secondary complications, including

pneumonia, deep vein thrombosis, renal failure, and pancreatic fistula. There were no 30-day mortalities and 1 mortality at 3- to 6-month follow-up. Although their rates of morbidity and mortality compare favorably with open débridement, 19% required a second VARD for additional débridement. Garcia-Urena describes seven consecutive patients who underwent VARD for a variety of indications and reported similar results: four (57%) complications, the most common of which being pancreatic fistula, with no mortalities.[7] A second VARD was required in two (29%) of seven patients.

Technique. The technique involves using the percutaneous drain as a guide to enter the pancreatic collection. One method is using the Seldinger technique, in which a flexible guidewire is inserted through the drain followed by an introducer sheath, and a 5-mm laparoscopic port through the introducer. Alternatively, direct cutdown can also be used. Under videoscopic guidance, irrigation, suction, and manual débridement is used to judiciously excavate the purulent necrotic material. A large sump drain is left in the cavity to allow scheduled lavages postoperatively until the effluent becomes clear.

CHRONIC PANCREATITIS

The decision to pursue a minimally invasive approach for CP depends on patient factors, including underlying pathophysiology, age, comorbidities, and history of prior pancreatic interventions. The specific operation of choice for CP depends on anatomic considerations, including the presence of a pancreatic head mass, a dilated pancreatic duct, and peripancreatic fluid collections. Outcomes of the published literature are summarized in Table 101.1.

The majority of surgical interventions for CP are typically executed through an open approach. Therefore data on outcomes following minimally invasive procedures are rare. However, open techniques of pancreatic resection, drainage, and combination procedures have been replicated through conventional laparoscopic and robotic-assisted techniques and have been shown to be safe and feasible. Given the infrequent indication for surgical interventions for CP, they are best delivered at high-volume tertiary centers by multidisciplinary teams. Therefore approach for surgical treatment will largely be dictated by the local expertise.

Minimally Invasive Total Pancreatectomy With Auto Islet Transplantation

Resection procedures for CP include total pancreatectomy, with or without auto islet transplantation (TP ± AIT), PD, distal pancreatectomy (DP), and the Puestow, Frey, and Beger procedures. TP ± AIT is a rarely performed procedure with few reports of a minimally invasive approach. It is indicated for patients with small-duct disease without diabetes. The largest published case series includes 10 patients who underwent a robotic-assisted TP, one of whom received AIT.[8] There were no mortalities at 90 days, and two Clavien-Dindo grade III complications, including one that required reoperation. Galvani et al. retrospectively reviewed a single-institutional series of six patients with CP who underwent a fully robotic-assisted TP + AIT.[9] There were no major complications or mortalities, and all patients were in the process of weaning off chronic

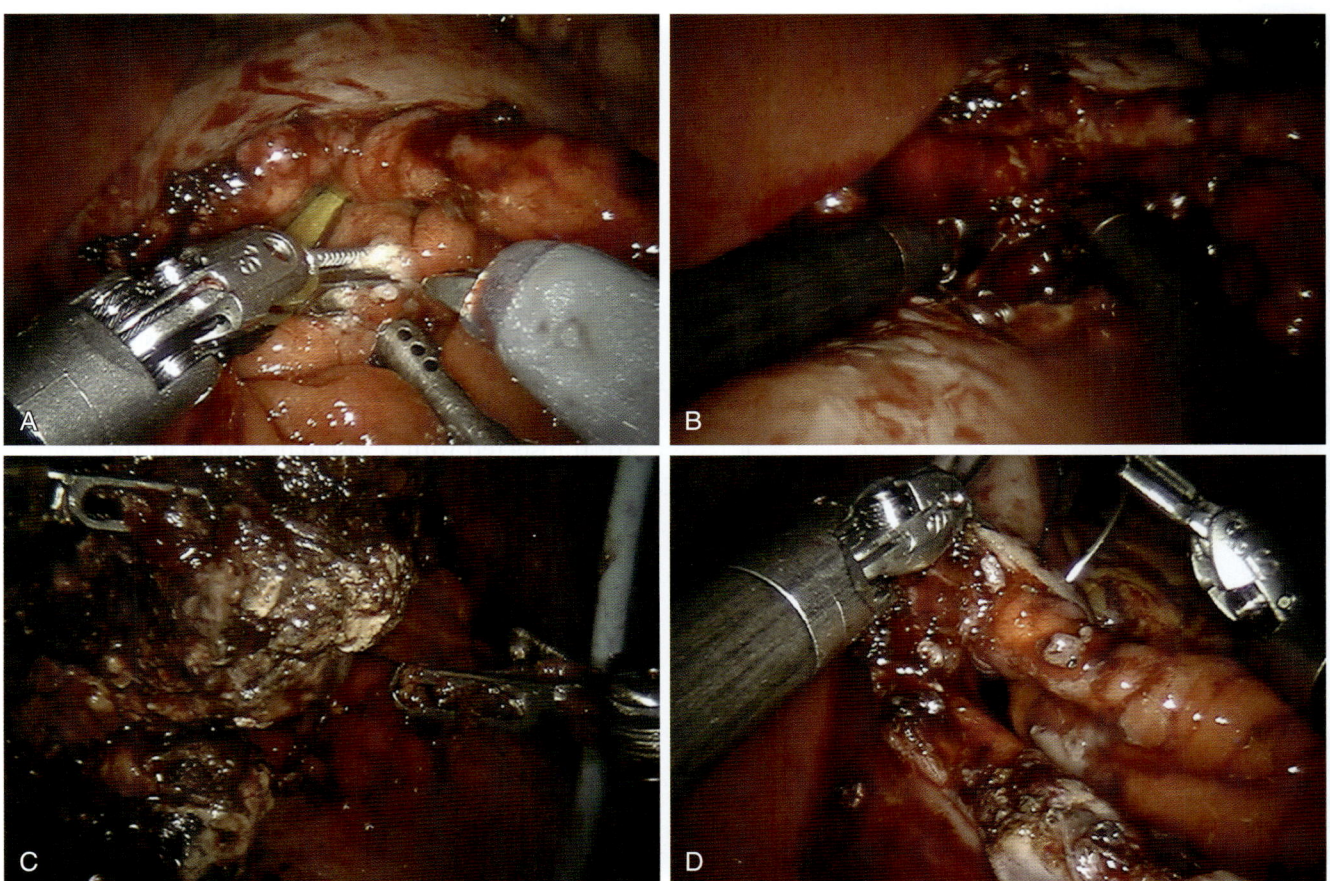

FIGURE 101.2 Robotic cyst-gastrostomy—technique. (A) Anterior gastrostomy. (B) Posterior gastrostomy and entrance to walled-off pancreatic necrosis. (C) En bloc débridement of walled-off pancreatic necrosis. (D) Closure of anterior cyst gastrostomy with running suture.

TABLE 101.1 Clinical Outcomes Following Minimally Invasive Treatment for Pancreatitis

Author	Procedure	Approach	Patients	OR Time (min)	EBL (mL)	Complications	Mortality	LOS (Days)	Symptom Improvement (%)
Galvani et al. (2014)	TP + AIT	Robotic (1 with AIT)	6	712	630	2 (33%)	0	12.6	100
Zureikat et al. (2015)	TP + AIT	Robotic	10	560	650	2 (20%)	0	10	NR
Cuschieri et al. (1996)	DP	Lap	5	240–360	400	1 (20%)	0	6	100
Fernandez-Cruz et al. (2002)	DP	Lap	5	240	450	1 (20%)	0	4.5	100
Khaled et al. (2011)	LPJ	Lap	37	218	NR	5 (13.5%)	0%	5.5	89
Meehan et al. (2011)	LPJ	Robot	1	390	NR	NR	0	8	100
Khaled et al. (2014)	LPJ	Lap	5	278	150	1 (25%)	0	5	80
Khaled et al. (2014)	CG	Lap	30	62	NR	3 (10%)	0	6.2	97 resolution
Worhunsky et al. (2014)	CG	Lap	21	170	50	12 (57%)	1 (5%)	5	NR
Khreiss et al. (2015)	CG	14 Robot 6 Lap	20	167	30	4 (20%)	0 (0%)	7	NR
Horvath et al. (2010)	VARD	Lap	25	135	NR	9 (36%)	0	48	NR
Garcia-Urena et al. (2013)	VARD	Lap	7	63	NR	4 (57%)	0 (0%)	50	NR
Cooper et al. (2014)	Frey	Lap	1	NR	NR	0	0	6	100
Tan et al. (2015)	Frey	Lap	9	323	57	1 (14%)	0	7	100
Khaled et al. (2014)	Beger	Lap	1	285	NR	0	0	5	100

CG, Cyst-gastrostomy; *DP,* distal pancreatectomy; *EBL,* estimated blood loss; *Lap,* conventional laparoscopy; *LOS,* length of stay, median days; *LPJ,* lateral pancreaticojejunostomy (Puestow); *NR,* not reported; *OR time,* operating room time, median minutes; *Robot,* robotic approach; *TP + AIT,* total pancreactectomy and auto islet transplantation; *VARD,* video-assisted retroperitoneal débridement.

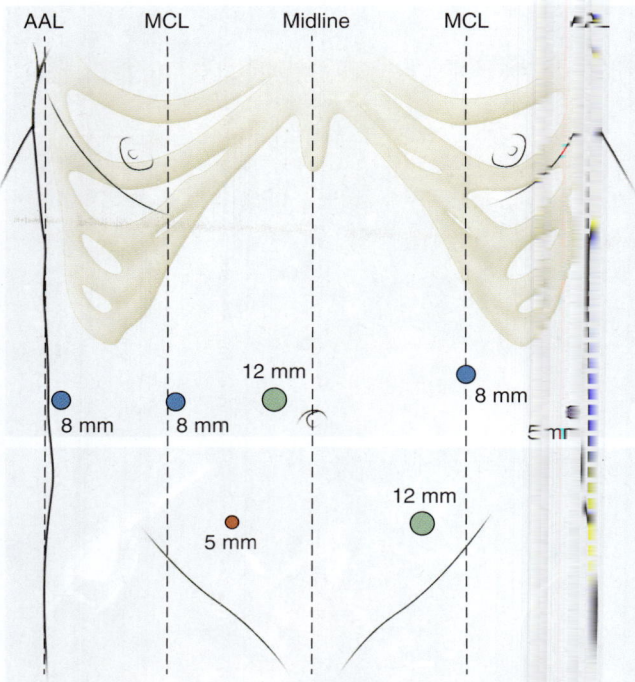

FIGURE 101.3 Robotic total pancreatectomy with auto islet transplantation—port placement. Periumbilical 12-mm camera port; three upper 8-mm robotic arms; left 5-mm self-retaining retractor *(purple)*; left lower quadrant 12-mm laparoscopic port and specimen extraction site; right lower quadrant 5-mm laparoscopic port *(red)*. *AAL,* Anterior axillary line; *MCL,* midclavicular line.

narcotics at 1-month follow-up. These outcomes are comparable with a series of 12 patients who underwent open TP + AIT.

Technique. The robotic approach as described by Zureikat et al.[8] first places seven laparoscopic ports as depicted in Fig. 101.3, composing one 12-mm camera port, three 8-mm robotic ports, two assistant ports (12 mm and 5 mm), and one 5-mm port for a self-retaining liver retractor. The lesser sac is entered, and the posterior stomach is freed from the surface of the pancreas. A medial visceral rotation is performed by mobilizing the right colon, and a Kocher maneuver is used to mobilize the duodenum. The jejunum is transected with a linear cutting stapler approximately 10 cm from the ligament of Treitz and is sutured to the stomach by a single stitch to mark the future gastrojejunostomy, approximately 50 cm downstream. The distal stomach is transected with a linear cutting stapler. The robot is then docked directly over the head of the table.

Dissection of the porta hepatis is performed using robotic hook cautery with isolation of the gastroduodenal artery (GDA), portal vein (PV), and common bile duct (CBD). In a TP the GDA is transected with a vascular linear stapler with enforcement of the stump with a 10-mm clip (Fig. 101.4). With a planned AIT, the GDA transection is delayed until just prior to pancreatic extraction to reduce the warm ischemia time. The CBD is then transected with a linear stapler. The division of the pancreas is delayed to preserve islet cell yield but can be transected

in a TP alone for ease of dissection. Similarly the splenic vein (SV) and artery are transected with vascular staplers but preserved until specimen extraction in the case of an AIT. The retroperitoneum is incised laterally, and the retropancreatic space is developed to include the SV, splenic artery (SA), and pancreatic body and tail. The entire pancreaticosplenic unit is mobilized by dividing the splenic flexure, splenorenal and splenocolic attachments. The pancreas is dissected from the superior mesenteric vein (SMV) and PV to expose the superior mesenteric artery (SMA) posteriorly. This requires dividing the inferior and superior pancreaticoduodenal vessels.

To perform the AIT, the pancreas is elevated from the retroperitoneum, only attached by the GDA, SA, and SV. Heparin is administered (50 IU/kg), and all three vessels are transected with a vascular stapler in the following order: SA, GDA, SV. A generous SV stump facilitates the introduction of a 14-gauge catheter for islet cell infusion. The specimen is then retrieved with an endoscopic bag. An end-to-side hepaticojejunostomy is fashioned in a "neo-duodenal" fashion using a running suture. An antecolic end-to-side gastrojejunostomy is handsewn in two layers. Lastly, a 14-gauge angiocatheter is inserted into the SV stump, and islet cells are infused by gravity, followed by a restapled closure of the SV stump.

Minimally Invasive Pancreaticoduodenectomy

Despite an abundance of literature on single-institution experience with minimally invasive PD and DP, many studies do not stratify between benign and malignant conditions. Therefore the efficacy of minimally invasive approaches for CP cannot be generalized and warrants further study. However, it can be inferred from large studies that minimally invasive PD and DP are safe and feasible in high-volume centers.[10] For example, the largest single-institution review of 132 robotic PDs, including 8% with benign indications, found outcomes similar to the open Whipple. Overall mortality at 30-days was 1.5%, with 21% Clavien-Dindo grade III or IV complications.[11]

Minimally Invasive Distal Pancreatectomy

Cruz et al. compared a series of five patients with CP who underwent laparoscopic DP with 41 patients who received an open DP.[12] The laparoscopic group had 1 (20%) complication (duodenal perforation) versus 20 patients with complications in the open group (48%). There were no mortalities in either group. At 13-month follow-up, all five laparoscopic patients were pain free versus 80% in the open group. There are also data to suggest that robotic DP is associated with higher rates of splenic preservation and lower rates of open conversion when compared with conventional laparoscopy.[13,14]

Technique. The techniques of robotic-assisted PD and DP are similar for benign or malignant conditions. Description of the approach is summarized later for pancreatic adenocarcinoma.

Minimally Invasive Lateral Pancreaticojejunostomy (Puestow)

The lateral pancreaticojejunostomy (LPJ) or "modified Puestow" procedure permits drainage of the pancreatic duct and is commonly indicated for patients with an

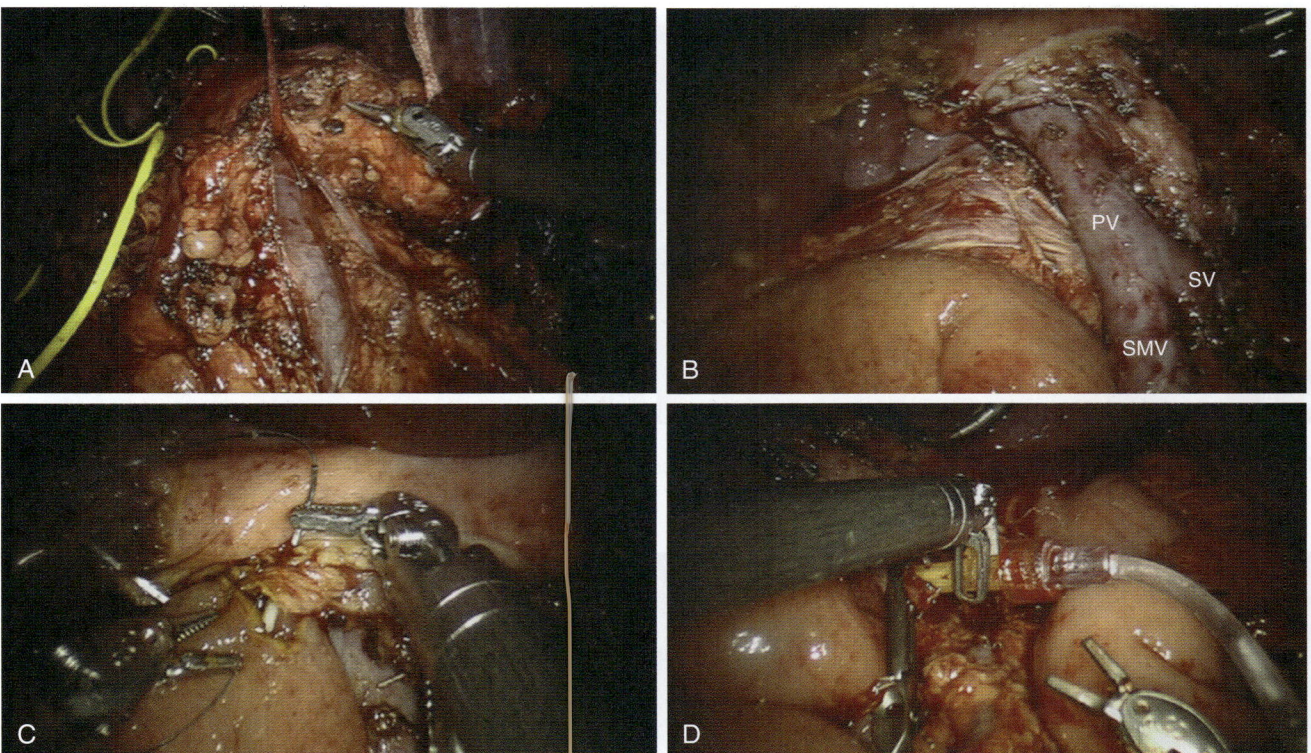

FIGURE 101.4 Robotic total pancreatectomy with auto islet transplantation—technique. (A) Pancreatic neck is freed from the superior mesenteric vein *(SMV)*, splenic vein *(SV)*, and portal vein *(PV)*. (B) Resection of entire pancreas from the retroperitoenum. (C) Creation of hepaticojejunostomy over a stent. (D) Angiocatheter introduced through the SV stump for islet cell infusion.

obstructed or dilated pancreatic duct. It offers the advantage of preserving the head of the pancreas along with exocrine and endocrine function.

In limited case reports of minimally invasive approaches, the laparoscopic approach appears to be safe, feasible, and effective.[15] In a review of five patients with CP who underwent laparoscopic LPJ, there were no reported mortalities, one complication of pancreatic bleeding requiring reoperation (20%), and ultimately four out of five (80%) patients pain free at a median 15-month follow-up. In a single case report of a robotic LPJ, there was no mortality or morbidity, and the patient remained asymptomatic at 2 years postoperatively.[16]

Technique. The robotic approach as described by Meehan and Sawin[16] begins with five ports: one 12-mm camera port, two robotic arm ports, and two assistant ports. The lesser sac is entered using the robotic hook cautery, and the endoscopic ultrasound is used to localize the dilated pancreatic duct. The pancreatic duct is opened longitudinally along the entire length of the pancreas using the hook cautery. To create the Roux limb, the bowel is divided approximately 20 cm beyond the ligament of Treitz using the endoscopic stapler. The Roux limb is aligned along the pancreatic duct, and the distal bowel anastomosis is created on the antimesenteric surface of the bowel, using the endoscopic stapler. The Roux limb is brought up in a retrocolic fashion, and the mesenteric defect is closed. The LPJ is robotically sewn using absorbable 3-0 suture (Fig. 101.5).

Minimally Invasive Frey Procedure

The Frey procedure combines the tenets of resection and drainage and is suited for patients with severe pancreatic head inflammation and/or a mass, as well as an obstructed or dilated pancreatic duct. A minimum pancreatic duct width greater than 8 mm has been recommended for successful laparoscopic intervention.[17]

There are limited data on outcomes following laparoscopic Frey procedure for CP. A single case is reported from the United States of a laparoscopic Frey procedure for a 42-year-old woman with recurrent idiopathic CP.[18] She had no postoperative complications and was discharged home on day 6 without narcotic pain medication. A single institution review in China compared 9 laparoscopic to 37 open Frey procedures.[17] Of seven successful laparoscopic procedures, there was one (22%) complication of postpancreatectomy hemorrhage, no mortality, and seven out of seven patients with improved pain scores at 3-month follow-up. Results were similar to their open cohort.

Technique. The technique of the robotic Frey procedure is similar to that described earlier for the Puestow procedure, with the addition of the pancreatic head enucleation. The pancreatic duct is similarly longitudinally opened, and any pancreatic duct stones are removed (Fig. 101.6). The head of the pancreas is excavated. It has been suggested to extend the excavation to the depth of the posterior wall of the Wirsung duct, preserving a 0.5-cm margin from the duodenum to prevent damage to the

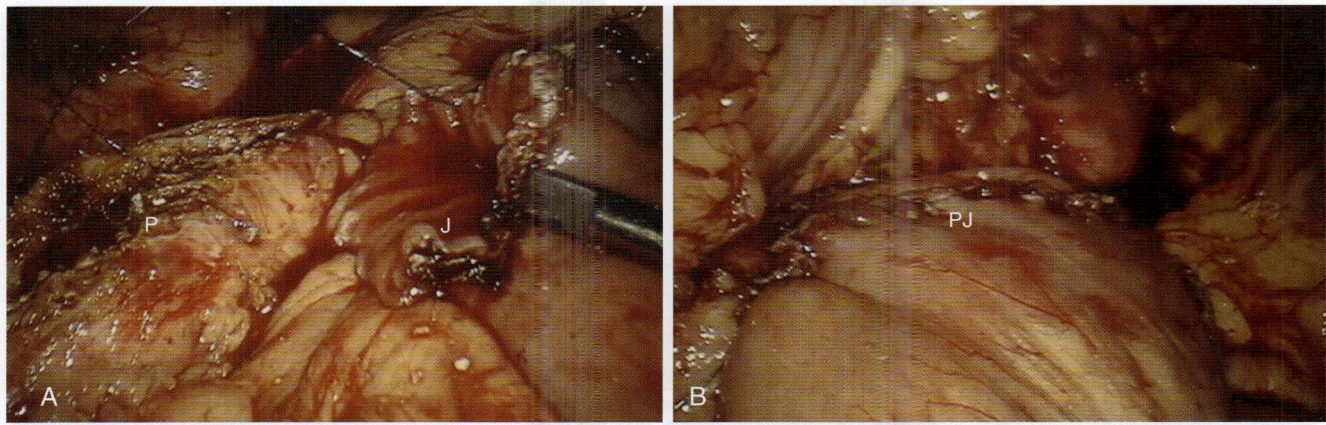

FIGURE 101.5 Robotic lateral pancreaticojejunostomy (Puestow procedure). (A) Pancreatic duct (P) and jejunostomy (J) in preparation for anastomosis. (B) Completed pancreaticojejunostomy anastomosis (PJ).

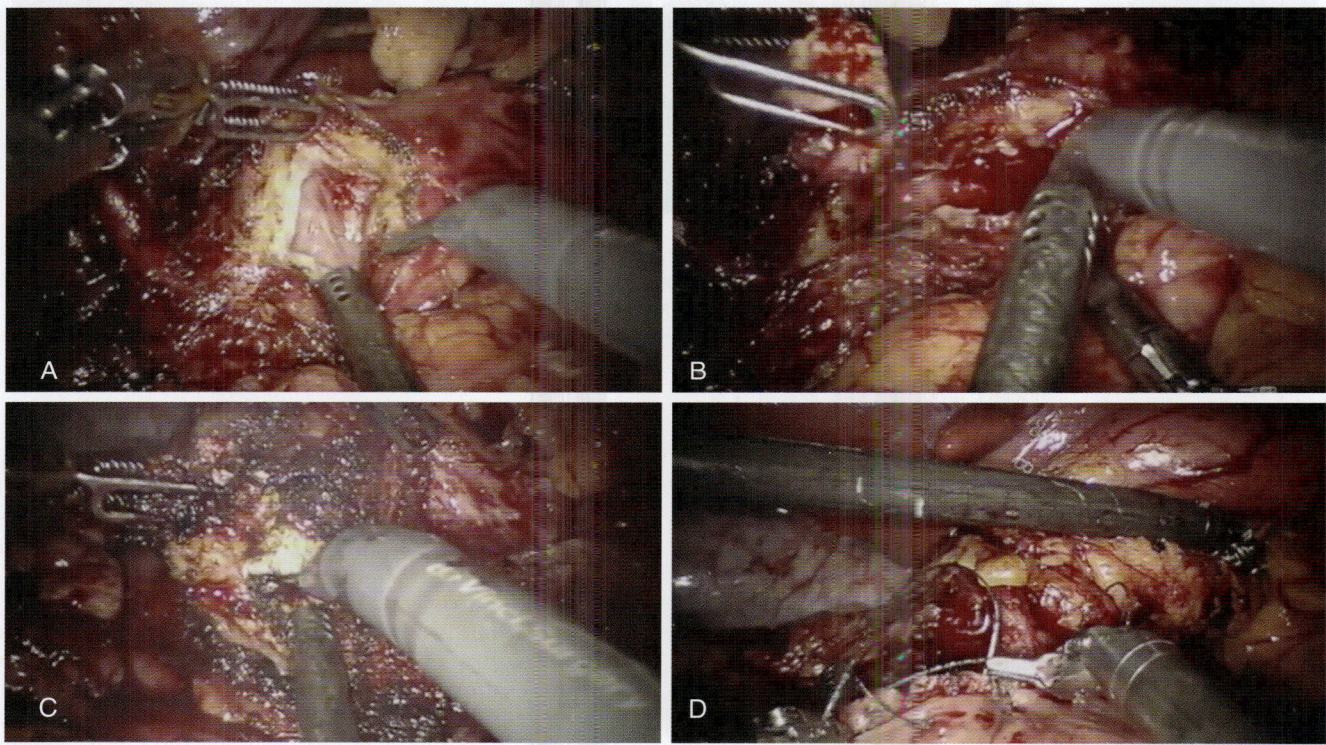

FIGURE 101.6 Robotic Frey procedure. (A) Opening of pancreatic duct. (B) Removal of pancreatic duct stones. (C) Enucleation of pancreatic head. (D) Lateral pancreaticojejunostomy.

biliary duct.[17] The LPJ is created in a similar fashion to the Puestow procedure.

Minimally Invasive Beger Procedure

The Beger procedure combines a duodenum-preserving pancreatic head resection with drainage for patients without pancreatic duct dilatation or pancreatic head enlargement.

Published studies on the laparoscopic approach to the Beger procedure are rare. A single case report from the United Kingdom by Khaled et al. reports laparoscopic Beger procedure with Berne modification in a patient with an inflammatory head mass causing an intrapancreatic CBD stricture.[15] There was no morbidity or mortality, and at 16-month follow-up, the patient had mild pain controlled on a multiopioid oral regimen at one-third of his preoperative dose.

Technique. There are no reports of a robotic-assisted Beger procedure, and this has never been performed at our institution. The laparoscopic Beger technique with Berne modification as described by Khaled et al.[15] uses multiple 3-0 sutures encircling the border of the enlarged pancreatic head mass to assist with hemostasis during excavation. The mass is then cored out using an ultrasonic scalpel (Ethicon, Cincinnati, Ohio), leaving a thin rim of parenchyma until the pancreatic duct is opened. The bile duct is then opened, and the choledochotomy is extended within the limits of the cored cavity. The jejunum is divided 75 cm distal to the ligament of Treitz, and a side-to-side jejunojejunostomy is constructed 60 cm downstream. The Roux loop is brought up in a retrocolic fashion through the transverse mesocolon, and an end-to-side LPJ is created in a single layer. This simplified modification avoids a second anastomosis between the residual pancreatic head remnant and jejunal limb.

PANCREATIC CYSTIC NEOPLASMS

The prevalence of pancreatic cysts has increased over the past several decades, largely due to widespread use and technologic advancement in cross-sectional imaging. Because many of these are discovered in asymptomatic individuals, an accurate diagnosis based on radiologic imaging, endoscopic ultrasound, and cyst fluid analysis helps to differentiate premalignant lesions that necessitate resection from those that can be closely monitored. Many criteria exist to judge surveillance and surgery in mucinous cysts. To date, the most recent are the American Gastroenterological Association Guidelines, which have not been well received.[19] The initial Sendai criteria were published in 2006, with widespread adoption and classification.[20] These have been modified in 2012 with the Fukuoka criteria, with many additional studies now determining the merit of this revision versus the original consensus guidelines.[21]

Mucinous pancreatic cystic neoplasms (MPCNs) have potential for malignant degeneration, and nearly 50% are associated with malignant or premalignant lesions.[22,23] Thus their early detection and treatment are imperative. Based on international consensus guidelines, surgical resection of all MPCNs is recommended in patients who are symptomatic and deemed low surgical risk.[21] These MPCNs are classified as intraductal papillary mucinous neoplasms (IPMNs) and mucinous cystic neoplasms (MCNs). IPMNs are broken into three anatomic classifications: (1) main duct, (2) side branch, or (3) mixed (main and side branch) duct. Molecular cyst fluid analysis, carcinoembryonic antigen (CEA), and amylase can be helpful for classification of these cysts.[24,25] IPMNs can have KRAS mutations, GNAS mutations, elevated CEA, and elevated amylase, whereas MCNs can have KRAS mutations and can have elevated CEA but they do not have GNAS mutations or elevated amylase levels in cyst fluid.

There is a lack of focused reports for outcomes following robotic surgery for MPCNs. However, in the largest review of 250 robotic pancreatic resections by Zureikat et al.,[11] 21% were for premalignant conditions including IPMN and MCN, including 20 PDs and 17 DPs. Overall, there was a 0.8% 30-day mortality and 3.8% 90-day mortality, which compares favorably with published open and laparoscopic series.

Intraductal Papillary Mucinous Neoplasms

IPMNs account for 21% to 33% of pancreatic cystic neoplasms[26,27] and are typically located in the pancreatic head.[28] They are categorized by their ductal involvement, phenotype (which is beyond the scope of this chapter), and highest grade of dysplasia. High-grade dysplasia is found in 20% of IPMNs and invasive carcinoma in up to 45%. Involvement of the main pancreatic duct, dilation of the main pancreatic duct or side branch, mural nodules, an associated mass, advanced age, and presence of symptoms are risk factors for underlying malignancy.[21,29]

Main-duct IPMNs (MD-IPMNs) have the highest likelihood of progression to cancer, with up to 60% of high-grade dysplasia and invasion. Therefore pancreatic resection is recommended for all surgically fit patients.[21] In branch-duct IPMNs (BD-IPMNs), high-grade dysplasia is present in approximately 26%, with invasive cancer found in approximately 18%. Therefore revised guidelines recommend watchful waiting for asymptomatic, simple lesions without a solid component/mural nodule. Size in the new Fukuoka guidelines is not an absolute criterion, whereas the Sendai criteria proposed a size threshold less than 3 cm without worrisome features or "high-risk stigmata" as acceptable for observation without immediate resection.[21]

Technique. Due to frequent localization of IPMNs in the head of the pancreas, a PD is indicated, with the robotic approach described later. Because IPMNs typically grow along the ductal system, analyzing the distal pancreatic margin with frozen section is imperative to confirm complete tumor resection and the absence of high-grade dysplasia.[30] For the minority of patients with distal lesions, DP with splenectomy, described later, with frozen section of the proximal pancreatic margin is indicated.[31] If any high-grade dysplasia or invasive carcinoma is found at the margin, additional resection is required. If clear margins are not achieved after a total of three frozen sections, a TP is generally advised,[32] and in fact 19% of patients with IPMN ultimately receive a TP.[21,33]

Mucinous Cystic Neoplasms

MCNs are found in 14% to 23% of resected pancreatic cystic neoplasms[22,34] and are almost exclusively found in the body and tail of the pancreas. According to the World Health Organization (WHO) classification, MCN sits in the borderline category between benign (mucinous cystadenoma) and malignant (mucinous cystadenocarcinoma) lesions.[35] MCNs that are larger, associated with symptoms, and in older patients harbor a higher risk of malignancy,[36–38] and indeed invasive carcinoma is found in up to 20% of all MCNs.[31]

Due to variable cellular atypia and biologic behavior, surgical resection is advised in all patients of reasonable surgical risk, regardless of size or symptoms.[21] However, observation and surveillance are also reasonable approaches for high-risk patients.[26] Second-line treatments, such as intracystic injection of ethanol and other ablative agents, have also been described for nonsurgical candidates[39] but are not practiced at our institution.

Technique. The robotic approach to the DP and splenectomy are described later for carcinoma. For MCN with low suspicion of underlying malignancy, a spleen-preserving DP is reasonable,[40] as well as central pancreatectomy and enucleation, also described later, although these may be associated with higher morbidity.[41–43] However, any evidence of high-grade dysplasia or invasive carcinoma mandates a traditional pancreatectomy with lymphadenopathy. The use of intraoperative frozen section is not routinely recommended because these cysts typically manifest as solitary, well-defined lesions. With that said, regardless of surgical procedure, care must be taken to avoid cyst rupture and spillage of contents to prevent intraperitoneal contamination.

MALIGNANT CONDITIONS

PANCREATIC DUCTAL ADENOCARCINOMA

Minimally Invasive Pancreaticoduodenectomy

Despite the laparoscopic approach to the Whipple being met with skepticism in the 1990s, the first robotic Whipple was completed in 2007 and is now increasingly used to treat pancreatic malignancy (Fig. 101.7).[44] The minimally invasive approach is now recognized as being safe and

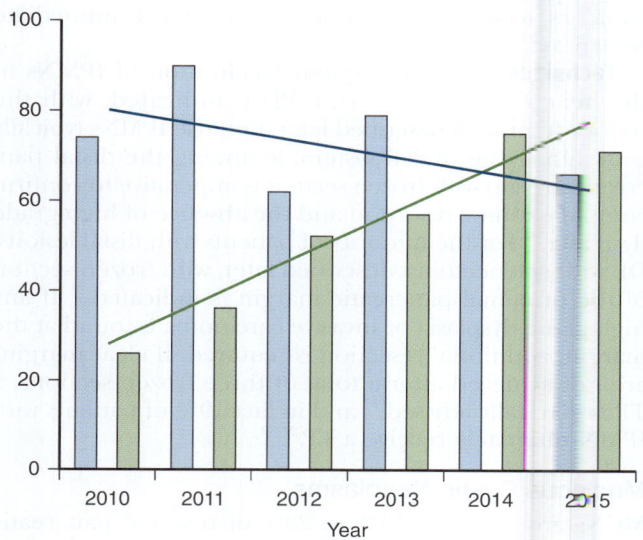

FIGURE 101.7 Open *(blue)* versus robotic *(green)* approaches to the pancreaticoduodenectomy at the University of Pittsburgh Medical Center, Pittsburgh, Pennsylvania, between 2010 and 2015.

feasible when performed at high-volume specialty centers (Table 101.2).[45]

Resectability of pancreatic adenocarcinoma depends largely on the presence of metastatic disease and involvement of the mesenteric vessels.[46] Triphasic computed tomography scanning and EUS are imperative in preoperative planning to determine resectability,[47] especially because manual palpation intraoperatively is not feasible in a minimally invasive approach.

Our institution has performed more than 170 robotic PDs for pancreatic ductal adenocarcinoma, totaling more than 380 robotic procedures for all indications. We have shown that these are safe and feasible procedures, with grade 3 and 4 complication rates of 10.6% and 12%, respectively, which are comparable to the open approach. Studies have shown that the robotic PD is associated with reduced blood loss and length of hospital stay; however, there is no evidence that demonstrates a consistent improvement in overall morbidity, mortality, operative time, or fistula rate. In regard to oncologic outcomes, most studies show an equivalent lymph node harvest, with excellent rates of R0 resection with the robotic approach.[1,48-55]

Technique (Fig. 101.8). The robotic approach to the PD as described by Seh et al.[56] begins with gaining access to the abdomen through a 5-mm left subcostal port and laparoscopically evaluating the abdomen for metastatic disease. After gross metastatic disease is ruled out, one camera port, three robotic ports, and two assistant ports are inserted as illustrated in Fig. 101.3 and the robot is immediately docked. The gastrocolic omentum is divided and a near Cattel-Braasch maneuver is used to expose the SMV at the base of the small bowel mesentery. The ligament of Treitz is divided, and an extended Kocher maneuver is used to pull the jejunum into the right upper quadrant. The jejunum is divided with a linear stapler 10 cm distal to the ligament of Treitz. The posterior stomach is dissected free from the anterior surface of the pancreas, with ligation of the right gastric artery and right gastroepiploic artery. The stomach is then divided with a linear stapler.

TABLE 101.2 Clinical Outcomes Following Robotic Pancreatic Resection for Carcinoma

Author	Procedure	No. of Patients/% Cancer	OR Time (min)	EBL (mL)	POPF (%), Morbidity (%)	30-day Mortality (%)	LOS (Days)	R0, No. of Lymph Nodes
Buchs et al. (2011)	Robotic PD	44/75	444	387	18.2, 35.4	4.5	13	90.9, 16.8
Chalikonda et al. (2012)	Robotic PD	30/47	476	485	6.7, 30	3.3	9.8	100, 13.2
Lai et al. (2012)	Robotic PD	20/75	492	247	35, 50	NR	14	73.3, 10
Boggi et al. (2013)	Robotic PD	34/65	597	220	38.2, 58	0	23	100, 32
Zureikat et al. (2013)	Robotic PD	132/80	527	300	17, 62.3	1.5	10	87.7, 19
Bao et al. (2014)	Robotic PD	28/68	431	100	29, NR	7*	7.4	63, 15
Chen et al. (2015)	Robotic PD	60/63	410	400	13.3, 35	1.7	20	97.8, 13.6
Baker et al. (2015)	Robotic PD	22/77	454	425	4.6, 40.9	0	7	77.8, NR
Kang et al. (2011)	Robotic DP	20/90	348	372	NR, 17	0	7.1	NR, NR
Zureikat et al. (2013)	Robotic DP	83/72	256	150	43, 72	0	6	97, 16
Daouadi (2013)	Robotic DP	30/73	293	212	46, 67	0	6.1	100, 18.6

*90-day mortality.

DP, Distal pancreactectomy; *EBL,* estimated blood loss; *LOS,* length of stay, median days; *NR,* not recorded; *OR time,* median operating room time; *PD,* pancreaticoduodenectomy; *POPF,* postoperative pancreatic fistula; *R0,* curative resection.

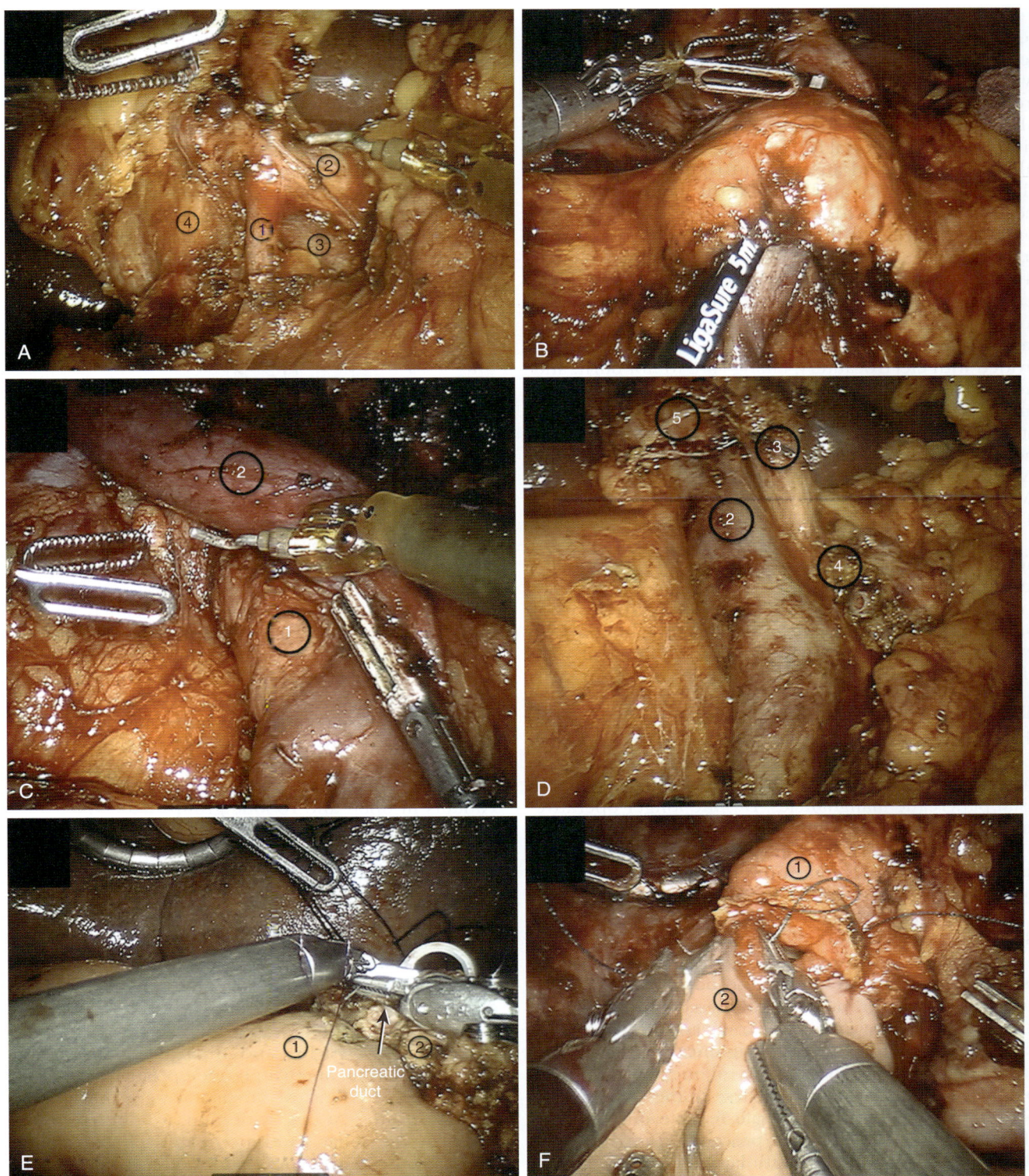

FIGURE 101.8 Robotic pancreaticoduodenectomy—technique. (A) Portal dissection including *(1)* the gastroduodenal artery, *(2)* common hepatic artery, *(3)* portal vein, and *(4)* common bile duct. (B) Dissection along the inferior and superior border of the pancreatic neck to create a retro-pancreatic tunnel above the mesenteric vessels. (C) The resection bed following removal of all tissue along the plane of Leriche, exposing *(1)* the superior mesenteric artery, and *(2)* portal vein. (D) Prior to reconstruction: *(2)* the dissected portal vein, *(3)* gastroduodenal artery stump, *(4)* transected edge of pancreas with visible pancreatic duct, and *(5)* transected common bile duct. (E) Approximation of *(1)* the jejunum and *(2)* pancreatic parenchyma to create the pancreaticojejunostomy using a modified Blumgart technique over a pancreatic stent *(arrow)*. (F) Creation of choledochojejunostomy between *(1)* the common hepatic duct and *(2)* jejunum.

To dissect the porta hepatis, the hepatic artery lymph node is first removed to help to expose the common hepatic artery (CHA), GDA, and PV. The GDA is temporarily occluded with a vessel loop while color flow and Doppler are used to assess flow in the CHA. Once confirmed, the GDA is ligated with a vascular stapler load and reinforced with a clip. A periportal lymphadenectomy is conducted, taking care to avoid an aberrant right hepatic artery. This exposes the PV and CBD. At this point a cholecystectomy may be performed or delayed after specimen removal. The CBD is then dissected and divided with a vascular stapler. The right gastroepiploic vein is followed proximally to locate the SMV, and the right gastroepiploic artery is divided. The SMV is dissected from the inferior border of the pancreas to create a tunnel between the pancreas and the PV. The neck of the pancreas is then divided with electrocautery, taking care to not burn, and intentionally leaving a small extension on the pancreatic duct. The pancreas is then mobilized, starting at the lateral border of the SMV/PV, identifying and preserving the first jejunal branch of the SMV as it crosses over the SMA. The SMV/PV is retracted medially to expose the SMA, which is dissected circumferentially along the plane of Leriche.

The pancreaticojejunostomy is reconstructed in a modified Blumgart fashion with a two-layer end-to-side duct-to-mucosa anastomosis. The choledochojejunostomy is created with a running suture. Finally, a gastrojejunostomy is fashioned using endoscopic staplers, followed by sewing of the common enterotomy in two layers or with a hybrid stapled technique.

Minimally Invasive Distal Pancreatectomy

The minimally invasive approach to the DP has been well accepted by the surgical oncology community and is embraced by many as the preferred method for resecting distal pancreatic malignancies. Despite longer operative times, studies have shown that the laparoscopic approach is associated with reduced blood loss, shorter hospital stays, higher rates of splenic preservation, and decreased complications rates.[13,57–60]

Our institution has analyzed our series of DP, comparing 94 laparoscopic cases with 30 robotic cases, 43% of which in the robotic group were for ductal adenocarcinoma. Using propensity matching, the robotic approach was found to be superior for greater R0 resection rate, lymph node yield, and lower rate of conversion to open. In addition, there was a statistically significant difference in margin-positivity rate favoring the robotic approach (0% robotic vs. 35% laparoscopic). These studies support the robotic approach to the DP as a safe, feasible, oncologically efficient, and possibly superior procedure for pancreatic adenocarcinoma compared with laparoscopy.

Technique. The robotic approach begins with accessing the peritoneum with an optical separator through a 5-mm left subcostal port, which is later exchanged for an 8-mm robotic port, followed by the following ports: a 12-mm right supraumbilical, 8-mm right paraxiphoid, 8-mm left anterior axillary line, 5-mm right subcostal for the liver retractor, 5-mm right lower quadrant, and 12-mm left lower quadrant. The gastrocolic ligament is divided to enter the lesser sac, and the splenic flexure of the left

colon is mobilized inferiorly. A liver retractor is placed to reflect the stomach and tent up the left gastric pedicle, allowing for delineation of the celiac trunk anatomy. The splenic artery is isolated proximally near the celiac trunk and divided with a vascular stapler using the left gastric vein as a landmark and test-clamping to ensure good hepatic blood flow prior to transection. Once the vessels have been mobilized, the pancreatic parenchyma is divided using a linear stapler. A celiac lymphadenectomy is performed beginning from the left side of the SMA and working laterally including the posterior pancreatic fascia en bloc. The spleen is mobilized by dividing its suspending ligaments, and the pancreas-spleen unit is removed through an extension of the left lower quadrant 12-mm port incision.

Minimally Invasive Appleby Procedure

The standard resection for tumors of the body and tail of the pancreas is a DP with concomitant splenectomy; however, tumor involvement of the CHA and/or celiac trunk was previously considered one of the main reasons precluding radical resection. However, DP with en bloc resection of the celiac trunk (DPCAR) has broadened the operative spectrum in pancreatic surgery. Initially described by Appleby in 1953 to achieve complete nodal clearance around the celiac trunk for advanced gastric cancer, Mayum and Kimura et al. adopted this approach for locally advanced adenocarcinoma of pancreatic body.[47] More recent reports from expert centers clearly showed that vascular resection did not increase morbidity and mortality and can offer these patients the possibility of radical surgery.

Comparable outcomes between the open and minimally invasive approach to the DPCAR have been demonstrated. Our institution performed a comparative analysis of 11 robot-assisted DPCARs to 19 open Appleby patients.[60a] Patients in open and robotic groups had similar demographics, including age, tumor size, and neoadjuvant chemotherapy; however, patients in the robotic group had shorter operative times (315 minutes robotic vs. 476 minutes open) estimated blood loss (EBL) (392 mL robotic vs. 1735 mL open), and need for blood transfusion (0 units robotic vs. 7 units open). Outcomes, including 90-day mortality, overall complication rate, hospital length of stay, and hospital readmission rate, were not significantly different between the two groups. The robotic group had a significantly higher lymph node acquisition than the open group (32 vs. 18), and other oncologic outcomes, including R0 rate and lymph node positivity rate, as well as recurrence-free and overall survival, were similar between the two groups. At our institution, we do not routinely embolize the celiac trunk preoperatively but have had two gastric ischemia complications postoperatively requiring total parenteral nutrition.

Technique. Port placement for the robotic DPCAR is identical to the DP. Entry into the lesser sac with careful preservation of the gastroepiploic artery and mobilization of the splenic flexure is similar to that performed in the standard DP, which has been previously described. However, the important technical issue of the Appleby procedure is to preserve the blood flow from the SMA via the pancreaticoduodenal arcades to the GDA to enable adequate retrograde blood flow to the liver following resection of the CHA and stomach via the right gastric artery. Adequate blood flow to the liver has to be well evaluated during the operation by clamping the CHA and detecting changes in the liver parenchyma color as well as ultrasonic Doppler flow. After this is established, vascular control of the CHA is obtained, followed by its stapled transection. The SV and SA are then controlled and transected using a stapled approach. The vein is taken at the confluence; however, because the splenic artery is encased with tumor at the celiac trunk, the inflow is often transected near the tail of the pancreas prior to SV transection to prevent engorgement and back bleeding. Robot-assisted intraoperative ultrasound is then performed to demonstrate the junction of the aorta, celiac trunk, and proximity of the superior mesenteric artery. The SMA is traced superiorly and the aorta from the right crus inferiorly to locate the celiac trunk. The celiac trunk is then transected with a vascular staple load. The specimen is then removed en bloc with the transected vasculature.

NEUROENDOCRINE TUMORS

Central Pancreatectomy and Enucleation

Central pancreatectomy, also referred to as the medial pancreatectomy, is a technique for low-grade malignant neoplasms located to the left of the GDA and close to the splenomesenteric confluence.[61] Open central pancreatectomy remains a high-risk procedure due to the meticulous dissection around the splenic vessels and the magnified risk of fistulas due to pancreatic transection at two sites. A major benefit of central pancreatectomy is preservation of pancreatic parenchyma, thereby decreasing the risk of diabetes and exocrine insufficiency, which would improve postoperative morbidity and patient quality of life. Pancreatic enucleations similarly spare as much unaffected parenchyma as possible and have been reported for small neuroendocrine tumors and premalignant lesions, such as IPMNs.

Abood et al. and Zhan et al. performed the largest single institution series of the central pancreatectomy performed robotically, with 9 and 10 cases, respectively.[14,62] They showed that robotic central pancreatectomy can be performed safely with similar oncologic outcomes to open procedures. In Abood's series the pancreatic fistula rate was 78% (seven of nine patients); however, only 22% (two patients) were clinically significant, with a grade B or C leak, both of which resolved with conservative measures. This mirrors pancreatic fistula rates published in other minimally invasive and open central pancreatectomy reports.[62] In Zhan's study the pancreatic fistula rate was 70%, the majority of which were grade A fistulas that were managed nonoperatively.[14] Overall, the robotic approach did not show inferiority to the open approach in regard to outcomes. However, operative times for robotic (median 219 to 425 minutes) were longer than open approaches in patients whose reconstruction was via a Roux-en-Y pancreaticojejunostomy versus a pancreaticogastrostomy.[14,62]

In Abood's series, no euglycemic patients required insulin upon discharge or at the 30-day postoperative visit, and none of the three preoperatively known noninsulin-dependent diabetic patients required escalation of their oral hyperglycemic medications at discharge or at the 30-day visit.[62] In addition, none of the patients presented with clinical criteria for exocrine insufficiency, consistent with reports of exocrine insufficiency following central pancreatectomy ranging from 0% to 8%. From these studies, central pancreatectomy can be safely performed robotically with similar outcomes to the open technique with the added long-term benefits of avoiding surgically induced diabetes and exocrine insufficiency through a minimally invasive approach.

Technique. At our institution the robotic central pancreatectomy is carried out as a hybrid of our PD and DP approach. The initial dissection is carried out laparoscopically where the lesser sac is entered and the anterior surface of the gland is cleared from the GDA to the lesion.[61] After this is completed, the robot is docked and a tunnel is created over the mesenteric vein confluence. The lesion is resected with an endoscopic stapler on the proximal margin, similar to a DP. To avoid injury to the bile duct, the transection is done at or medial to the GDA. Electrocautery is used on the distal margin with care to avoid thermal injury to the duct. Finally, the reconstruction is created via a pancreaticogastrostomy or pancreaticojejunostomy using a modified Blumgart technique.[61]

Robotic enucleation requires similar exposure to that needed for the more complex procedures, depending on lesion location, but requires intraoperative ultrasound to confirm location of the lesion and its proximity to the pancreatic duct.[11,52] For head lesions, we place a preoperative pancreatic duct stent endoscopically for assistance in surgery and drainage postoperatively as leak rates approach 100%. For smaller lesions and those not involving the pancreatic duct, the high resolution and dexterity afforded by the robotic platform enables the surgeon to carefully dissect around major vasculature to enucleate small pancreatic lesions, thus sparing pancreatic parenchyma. The added benefit of being able to identify the pancreatic duct by real-time ultrasound while performing the enucleation likely helps to reduce pancreatic duct leak. We have not previously reported our series, but currently 38 patients have undergone robotic enucleation between 2009 and 2016.

PERIAMPULLARY TUMORS

Periampullary tumors present anatomic challenges due to their relationship to the major and minor papillae and gastric outlet. Endoscopic resection, including mucosal resection or papillectomy, has been firmly demonstrated to be safe and feasible.[63] However, large lesions in the periampullary region may require multiple endoscopic interventions, are associated with higher risk of bleeding, perforation, incomplete resection, and require frequent endoscopic surveillance following resection.[63] According to the American Society of Gastrointestinal Endoscopy, lesions extending greater than one-third the circumference of the duodenum should be referred for surgical resection.[64]

A multiinstitutional review of 26 robotic resections for benign and low-grade tumors of the duodenum and periampullary region was reported by Downs-Canner et al. and found the robotic approach to be safe and feasible.[63] At 90-day follow-up, there were nine (35%) minor complications (Clavien-Dindo grades 1 to 2) and four (15%)

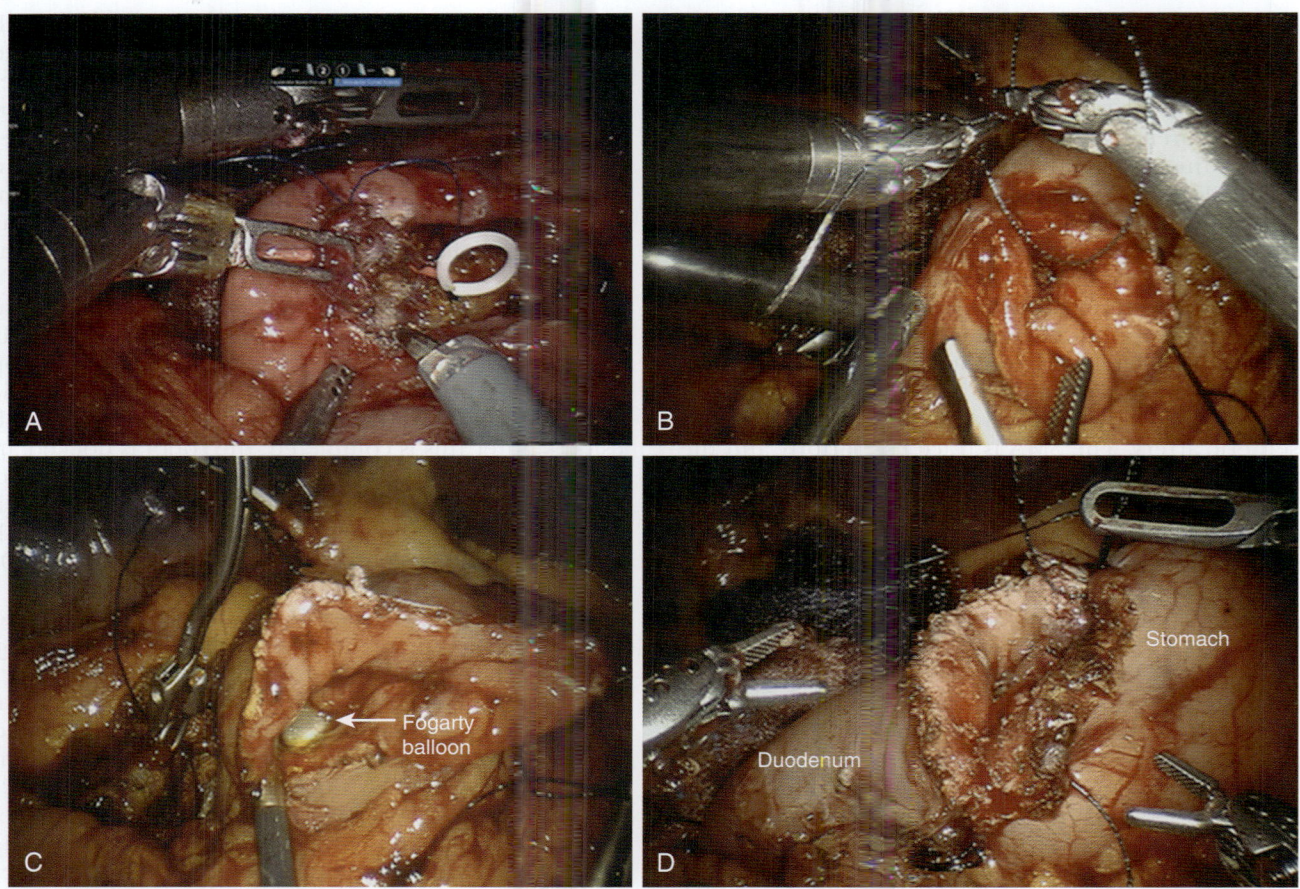

FIGURE 101.9 Robotic transduodenal ampullectomy—technique. (A) Catheters visible in both common bile duct and pancreatic duct during ampullary reconstruction. (B) Following ampullectomy, duodenotomy repaired transversely in two layers. (C) Fogarty catheter used to locate the ampulla. (D) Following duodenal sleeve resection, a duodenoduodenostomy (depicted) or duodenojejunostomy is performed.

major complications (Clavien-Dindo grades 3 to 4), which is comparable to a series of 28 open transduodenal ampullectomies reporting a complication rate of 48%.[35]

Transduodenal Ampullectomy

Robotic trocar placement mimics the configuration for the PD, described earlier, with similar methods of exposure up to the mobilization of the duodenum from the ligament of Treitz. The ampulla is identified by intraoperative ultrasound with the assistance of a preoperatively placed stent or a biliary catheter through the cystic duct following cholecystectomy. A longitudinal duodenectomy is created with electrocautery scissors, and a transfixing suture is placed through the ampulla and stent to maximize exposure of the ampulla (Fig. 101.9). The mucosa around the lesion is incised 0.5 to 1 cm circumferentially and then dissected in the submucosal plane until the bile duct is encountered. After the pancreatic duct is identified following incision of the bile duct, a stent is placed in the pancreatic duct to facilitate reconstruction. The dissection is continued circumferentially in the submucosal plane to remove the specimen. The duodenal mucosa is reapproximated to the bile duct in a clockwise direction beginning at the 12 o'clock position. The duodenum is then closed transversely in two layers.

Segmental Duodenal Resection

For segmental duodenal resection, or sleeve resection, the ampulla is identified, as described earlier, with the assistance of intraoperative endoscopy or ultrasound. The duodenum is divided distal and proximal to the lesion using a stapling device, and the duodenal mesentery and small perforating branches are divided from the head of the pancreas using an energy sealing device. The duodenum is resected using a stapling device, and frozen section is sent to verify complete excision. A side-to-side duodenojejunostomy is fashioned in two layers.

METASTATIC PANCREATIC TUMORS

Metastatic tumors to the pancreas are rare and when present are most frequently from renal cell carcinoma (RCC), melanoma, breast, lung, and colon cancer.[66] The incidence of solitary metastases that are potentially resectable are even less frequent.[67] Time interval between primary tumor and pancreatic metastases diagnosis is typically within 36 months but can be as prolonged as 10 years; many patients are also asymptomatic at the time of metastases diagnosis. This prolonged disease-free survival is especially prevalent in patients with metastatic RCC.[66,68]

Sparse literature is limited to small case series.[66,67] Crippa et al. reviewed 13 patients with histologically proven metastatic tumor of the pancreas from a variety of primary diagnoses who underwent either pylorus-preserving PD, PD, or DP with splenectomy.[66] Of 13 patients, 12 had solitary tumors, and the most common primary diagnosis was renal carcinoma. The median survival following radical pancreatic resection was 26 months, and the 5-year overall survival was 48% in these well-selected patients.

There is a lack of consensus on the surgical treatment of metastatic tumors to the pancreas. There are reports of PD, with or without pylorus preservation, DP, TP, and central pancreatectomy. Some authors recommend surgery for patients with metastases from RCC, breast, colon, and sarcomas, in whom there is some literature to suggest an improved survival. Meanwhile, metastases from melanoma and lung cancer are best managed nonoperatively, due to projected worse outcomes.[66,67,69]

ROBOTIC VERSUS LAPAROSCOPIC APPROACH

Robotic platforms provide the advantages of open surgical technique for complex anastomotic reconstruction while also addressing the limitations of traditional laparoscopy. It has been suggested that the magnified view offered by a laparoscope permits the reconstruction of small pancreatic ducts. Complex pancreatic resections and reconstructions using the robotic platform have been shown to be safe and feasible, with perioperative outcomes comparable to those of open surgery, including postoperative pancreatic fistula (POPF).[70,71]

Outcomes-based recommendations on robotic versus laparoscopic approaches are indeterminate. A systematic review of 25 studies comparing robotic PD ($n = 234$) to laparoscopic PD ($n = 386$), including 17.5% for benign indications, found that conventional laparoscopy had shorter operative times, reduced blood loss, and lower rates of pancreatic fistula.[10] Meanwhile, a systematic review of 9 studies including 1167 patients comparing robotic ($n = 238$) with laparoscopic ($n = 929$) DPs, for benign and malignant indications, showed no difference in operative time, open conversion, spleen preservation rate, transfusion requirements, length of hospital stay, or incidence of pancreatic fistulas.[72] It appears that robotic approaches are safe and feasible among specialized centers, with clinical outcomes equivalent to that of the open approach, although its advantages over conventional laparoscopy are inconclusive.

Data from the American College of Surgeons National Surgical Quality Improvement Program participant user file from 2014 shows that 3137 PDs and 1582 DPs were performed in participating institutions. Only 7% of 201 PDs (133 laparoscopic [56.2%] and 88 robotic [43.8%]) were performed in minimally invasive fashion, whereas 47% of 741 DPs (571 laparoscopic [77.1%] and 170 robotic [22.9%]) were performed minimally invasively (unpublished data). The adoption of minimally invasive DP shifted prior to PD so it would stand to reason the national pendulum toward this would occur prior to PD.

COST

Generalizable studies on the cost efficiency of laparoscopic pancreas surgery with attention to cost per quality-adjusted life year is lacking. The total cost of a laparoscopic Whipple appears to be comparable to that of an open approach. It appears that the benefits of shorter hospital stays afforded by laparoscopy is offset by increased operative time.[73] However, for DP, reduced length of stay has almost consistently been shown to be reduced following laparoscopic surgery, whereas operation time is minimally increased.[73] Therefore, after adjusting for quality-life years gained, laparoscopic DP has been shown to be cost effective.

A robotic console costs $1.2 million, with up to $150,000 per year in maintenance costs. Compared with an open DP, robotic-assisted resection incurs increased costs of approximately $1500 to $6000 USD per procedure; however, postoperative complications and their associated costs have not been comprehensively analyzed through conclusive cost effectiveness studies.[73] For nonpancreatic resections, robotic surgery has been demonstrated to be profitable to hospital systems.[74,75] In summary, the cost-benefit of robotic approaches to pancreas surgery compared with conventional laparoscopy remains to be determined.

LEARNING CURVE

The widespread implementation of laparoscopic pancreas surgery is hindered by a long learning curve.[70] For laparoscopic PD, proficiency is estimated to be obtained after 10 to 20 cases. It is reported that after performing 11 full Whipples laparoscopically, rates of POPF halve from 36% to 18%.

The robotic approach necessitates a second significant learning curve. It has been reported that 20 robotic-assisted laparoscopic Whipples are required to reduce blood loss (600 mL to 250 mL) and open conversion (35% to 3%), 40 cases necessary to reduce POPF rates (28% to 14%), and 80 procedures to reduce operative times (581 minutes to 417 minutes).[70] For robotic-assisted DPs, shorter operative times and lower readmission rates are observed after completing 40 cases.[73]

A "hybrid" approach has been advocated as a bridging strategy in which the resection portion is completed laparoscopically followed by the anastomotic portion through a small laparotomy. Improved operative results have been reported after 50 of such hybrid procedures.[76]

In summary, complex pancreatic resections and reconstructions via conventional laparoscopic or robotic techniques should be performed in specialized, high-volume centers with expertise in minimally invasive hepatobiliary surgery and multidisciplinary teams.

This learning curve is translated into patient outcomes; centers that performed less than 10 laparoscopic Whipple procedures per year had 30-day mortality rates twice as high as open procedures. However, in centers performing more than 10 laparoscopic Whipples, mortality rates did not differ.[73] The concept of a learning curve is not a concept isolated to minimally invasive surgery. The open PD specifically has been shown to have a learning curve greater than 60 cases,[77–79] and the procedure itself took half a century to evolve.[80] Unfortunately, national database studies are not equipped to answer these questions. One National Cancer Database study from 2010–2011[81] called into question an increased mortality of minimally invasive PD; however, most centers had only performed one and the conversion rate was 30%. The analysis failed to account for an increase in high-risk pathology, such as neuroendocrine tumors, and an increase in performance at low-volume hospitals. These are well established as having increased risk in open cohorts.[82,83] The same group looked only at pancreatic ductal cancers from 2010–2012[84] from the same database, and this mortality difference was no longer present after controlling for this significant variable. The true challenge to the dissemination of this technology is not the feasibility of the procedures, but the training of surgeons to incorporate the technology safely

CONCLUSION

A variety of pancreatic surgeries, historically achieved through large open incisions with associated high rates of morbidity and morality, have been replicated through a minimally invasive approach. At high-volume specialized centers, these procedures are safe, feasible, and efficacious; however, the dissemination process is still in an early adopter phase. The robotic interface offers many technical advantages that overcome the limitations of laparoscopic techniques while maintaining the tenets of an open approach to permit meticulous dissection and reconstruction. However, when adopting any new technology, robotic surgery imposes a significant cost and learning curve. As the field of robotics matures, further comparative studies on cost effectiveness and efficacy for improving patient-centered outcomes, such as symptomatic relief and quality of life, are needed.

REFERENCES

1. Gagner M, Pomp A. Laparoscopic pylorus-preserving pancreato-duodenectomy. *Surg Endosc.* 1994;8(5):408-410.
2. van Santvoort HC, Besselink MG, Bakker OJ, et al. A step-up approach or open necrosectomy for necrotizing pancreatitis. *N Engl J Med.* 2010;362(16):1491-1502.
3. Khaled YS, Malde DJ, Packer J, et al. Laparoscopic versus open cystgastrostomy for pancreatic pseudocysts: a case-matched comparative study. *J Hepatobiliary Pancreat Sci.* 2014;21(11):818-823.
4. Khreiss M, Zenati M, Clifford A, et al. Cyst gastrostomy and necrosectomy for the management of sterile walled-off pancreatic necrosis: a comparison of minimally invasive surgical and endoscopic outcomes at a high-volume pancreatic center. *J Gastrointest Surg.* 2015;19 8):1441-1448.
5. Worhunsky DJ, Qadan M, Dua MM, et al. Laparoscopic transgastric necrosectomy for the management of pancreatic necrosis. *J Am Coll Surg.* 2014;219(4):735-743.
6. Horvath K, Freeny P, Escallon J, et al. Safety and efficacy of video-assisted retroperitoneal debridement for infected pancreatic collections: a multicenter, prospective, single-arm phase 2 study. *Arch Surg.* 2010;145(9):817-825.
7. Garcia-Urena MA, Lopez-Monclus J, Melero-Montes D, et al. Video-assisted laparoscopic debridement for retroperitoneal pancreatic collections: a reliable step-up approach. *Am Surg.* 2013;79(4):429-433.
8. Zureikat AH, Nguyen T, Boone BA, et al. Robotic total pancreatectomy with or without autologous islet cell transplantation: replication of an open technique through a minimal access approach. *Surg Endosc.* 2015;29(1):176-183.
9. Galvani CA, Rodriguez Rilo H, Samame J, Porubsky M, Rana A, Gruessner RW. Fully robotic-assisted technique for total pancreatectomy with an autologous islet transplant in chronic pancreatitis patients: results of a first series. *J Am Coll Surg.* 2014;218 3):e73-e78.
10. Boggi U, Amorese G, Vistoli F, et al. Laparoscopic pancreaticoduodenectomy: a systematic literature review. *Surg Endosc.* 2015;29(1):9-23.
11. Zureikat AH, Moser AJ, Boone BA, Bartlett DL, Zenati M, Zeh HJ 3rd. 250 Robotic pancreatic resections: safety and feasibility. *Ann Surg.* 2013;258(4):554-559; discussion 559–562.
12. Fernandez-Cruz L, Saenz A, Astudillo E, Pantoja JP, Uzcategui E, Navarro S. Laparoscopic pancreatic surgery in patients with chronic pancreatitis. *Surg Endosc.* 2002;16(6):996-1003.
13. Chen S, Zhan Q, Chen JZ, et al. Robotic approach improves spleen-preserving rate and shortens postoperative hospital stay of laparoscopic distal pancreatectomy: a matched cohort study. *Surg Endosc.* 2015;29(12):3577-3518.
14. Zhan Q, Deng XX, Han B, et al. Robotic-assisted pancreatic resection: a report of 47 cases. *Int J Med Robot.* 2013;9(1):44-51.
15. Khaled YS, Ammori BJ. Laparoscopic lateral pancreaticojejunostomy and laparoscopic Berne modification of Beger procedure for the treatment of chronic pancreatitis: the first UK experience. *Surg Laparosc Endosc Percutan Tech.* 2014;24(5):e178-e182.
16. Meehan JJ, Sanvin R. Robotic lateral pancreaticojejunostomy (Puestow). *J Pediatr Surg.* 2011;46(6):e5-e8.
17. Tan CL, Zhang H, Li KZ. Single center experience in selecting the laparoscopic Frey procedure for chronic pancreatitis. *World J Gastroenterol.* 2015;21(44):12644-12652.
18. Cooper MA, Data TS, Makary MA. Laparoscopic Frey procedure for chronic pancreatitis. *Surg Laparosc Endosc Percutan Tech.* 2014; 24(1):e16-e20.
19. Singhi AD, Zeh HJ, Brand RE, et al. American Gastroenterological Association guidelines are inaccurate in detecting pancreatic cysts with advanced neoplasia: a clinicopathologic study of 225 patients with supporting molecular data. *Gastrointest Endosc.* 2016;83(6): 1107-1117, e112.
20. Tanaka M, Chari S, Adsay V, et al. International consensus guidelines for management of intraductal papillary mucinous neoplasms and mucinous cystic neoplasms of the pancreas. *Pancreatology.* 2006;6(1-2):17-32.
21. Tanaka M, Fernandez-del Castillo C, Adsay V, et al. International consensus guidelines 2012 for the management of IPMN and MCN of the pancreas. *Pancreatology.* 2012;12(3):183-197.
22. Goh BK, Tan YM, Cheow PC, et al. Cystic lesions of the pancreas: an appraisal of an aggressive resectional policy adopted at a single institution over 15 years. *Am J Surg.* 2006;192(2):148-154.
23. Kimura W, Nagai H, Kuroda A, Muto T, Esaki Y. Analysis of small cystic lesions of the pancreas. *Int J Pancreatol.* 1995;18(3):197-206.
24. Nikiforova MN, Khalid A, Fasanella KE, et al. Integration of KRAS testing in the diagnosis of pancreatic cystic lesions: a clinical experience of 618 pancreatic cysts. *Mod Pathol.* 2013;26(11):1478-1487.
25. Singhi AD, Nikiforova MN, Fasanella KE, et al. Preoperative GNAS and KRAS testing in the diagnosis of pancreatic mucinous cysts. *Clin Cancer Res.* 2014;20(16):4381-4389.
26. Adsay NV, Klimstra DS, Compton CC. Cystic lesions of the pancreas. Introduction. *Semin Diagn Pathol.* 2000;17(1):1-6.
27. Fernandez-del Castillo C, Targarona J, Thayer SP, Rattner DW, Brugge WR, Warshaw AL. Incidental pancreatic cysts: clinicopathologic characteristics and comparison with symptomatic patients. *Arch Surg.* 2003;138(4):427-433; discussion 433–434.
28. Schnelldorfer T, Sarr MG, Nagorney DM, et al. Experience with 208 resections for intraductal papillary mucinous neoplasm of the pancreas. *Arch Surg.* 2008;143(7):639-646; discussion 646.
29. Sakorafas GH, Smyrniotis V, Reid-Lombardo KM, Sarr MG. Primary pancreatic cystic neoplasms revisited. Part III. Intraductal papillary mucinous neoplasms. *Surg Oncol.* 2011;20(2):e109-e118.
30. Couvelard A, Sauvanet A, Kianmanesh R, et al. Frozen sectioning of the pancreatic cut surface during resection of intraductal papillary mucinous neoplasms of the pancreas is useful and reliable: a prospective evaluation. *Ann Surg.* 2005;242(6):774-778; discussion 778–780.
31. Sarr MG, Murr M, Smyrk TC, et al. Primary cystic neoplasms of the pancreas. Neoplastic disorders of emerging importance—current state-of-the-art and unanswered questions. *J Gastrointest Surg.* 2003;7(3):417-428.
32. Farnell MB. Surgical management of intraductal papillary mucinous neoplasm (IPMN) of the pancreas. *J Gastrointest Surg.* 2008;12(3):414-416.
33. Garcea G, Ong SL, Rajesh A, et al. Cystic lesions of the pancreas. A diagnostic and management dilemma. *Pancreatology.* 2008;8(3):236-251.
34. Valsangkar NP, Morales-Oyarvide V, Thayer SP, et al. 851 Resected cystic tumors of the pancreas: a 33-year experience at the Massachusetts General Hospital. *Surgery.* 2012;152(3 suppl 1):S4-S12.
35. Zamboni G, Scarpa A, Bogina G, et al. Mucinous cystic tumors of the pancreas: clinicopathological features, prognosis, and relationship to other mucinous cystic tumors. *Am J Surg Pathol.* 1999;23(4):410-422.

36. Ceppa EP, De la Fuente SG, Reddy SK, et al. Defining criteria for selective operative management of pancreatic cystic lesions: does size really matter? *J Gastrointest Surg.* 2010;14(2):236-244.

37. Crippa S, Salvia R, Warshaw AL, et al. Mucinous cystic neoplasm of the pancreas is not an aggressive entity: lessons from 163 resected patients. *Ann Surg.* 2008;247(4):571-579.

38. Scott J, Martin I, Redhead D, Hammond P, Garden OJ. Mucinous cystic neoplasms of the pancreas: imaging features and diagnostic difficulties. *Clin Radiol.* 2000;55(3):187-192.

39. Gan SI, Thompson CC, Lauwers GY, Bounds BC, Brugge WR. Ethanol lavage of pancreatic cystic lesions: initial pilot study. *Gastrointest Endosc.* 2005;61(6):746-752.

40. Rodriguez JR, Madanat MG, Healy BC, Thayer SP, Warshaw AL, Fernandez-del Castillo C. Distal pancreatectomy with splenic preservation revisited. *Surgery.* 2007;141(5):619-625.

41. Crippa S, Partelli S, Falconi M. Extent of surgical resections for intraductal papillary mucinous neoplasms. *World J Gastrointest Surg.* 2010;2(10):347-351.

42. Madura JA, Yum MN, Lehman GA, Sherman S, Schmidt CM. Mucin secreting cystic lesions of the pancreas: treatment by enucleation. *Am Surg.* 2004;70(2):106-112; discussion 413.

43. Sperti C, Pasquali C, Ferronato A, Pedrazzoli S. Median pancreatectomy for tumors of the neck and body of the pancreas. *J Am Coll Surg.* 2000;190(6):711-716.

44. Cadiere GB, Himpens J, Germay O, et al. Feasibility of robotic laparoscopic surgery: 146 cases. *World J Surg.* 2001;25(11):1467-1477.

45. Bilimoria KY, Bentrem DJ, Ko CY, Stewart AK, Winchester DP, Talamonti MS. National failure to operate on early stage pancreatic cancer. *Ann Surg.* 2007;246(2):173-180.

46. Callery MP, Chang KJ, Fishman EK, Talamonti MS, Traverso L, Linehan DC. Pretreatment assessment of resectable and borderline resectable pancreatic cancer: expert consensus statement. *Ann Surg Oncol.* 2009;16(7):1727-1733.

47. Kondo S, Katoh H, Hirano S, et al. Results of radical distal pancreatectomy with en bloc resection of the celiac artery for locally advanced cancer of the pancreatic body. *Langenbecks Arch Surg.* 2003;388(2):101-106.

48. Baker EH, Ross SW, Seshadri R, et al. Robotic pancreaticoduodenectomy: comparison of complications and cost to the open approach. *Int J Med Robot.* 2016;12(3):554-560.

49. Bao PQ, Mazirka PO, Watkins KT. Retrospective comparison of robot-assisted minimally invasive versus open pancreaticoduodenectomy for periampullary neoplasms. *J Gastrointest Surg.* 2014;18(4):682-689.

50. Buchs NC, Addeo P, Bianco FM, Ayloo S, Benedetti E, Giulianotti PC. Robotic versus open pancreaticoduodenectomy: a comparative study at a single institution. *World J Surg.* 2011;35(12):2739-2746.

51. Chen S, Chen JZ, Zhan Q, et al. Robot-assisted laparoscopic versus open pancreaticoduodenectomy: a prospective, matched, mid-term follow-up study. *Surg Endosc.* 2015;29(12):3698-3711.

52. Giulianotti PC, Sbrana F, Bianco FM, et al. Robot-assisted laparoscopic pancreatic surgery: single-surgeon experience. *Surg Endosc.* 2010;24(7):1646-1657.

53. Lai EC, Yang GP, Tang CN. Robot-assisted laparoscopic pancreaticoduodenectomy versus open pancreaticoduodenectomy—a comparative study. *Int J Surg.* 2012;10(9):475-479.

54. Nguyen KT, Zureikat AH, Chalikonda S, Bartlett DL, Moser AJ, Zeh HJ. Technical aspects of robotic-assisted pancreaticoduodenectomy (RAPD). *J Gastrointest Surg.* 2011;15(5):870-875.

55. Zhou NX, Chen JZ, Liu Q, et al. Outcomes of pancreatoduodenectomy with robotic surgery versus open surgery. *Int J Med Robot.* 2011;7(2):131-137.

56. Zeh HJ 3rd, Bartlett DL, Moser AJ. Robotic-assisted major pancreatic resection. *Adv Surg.* 2011;45:323-340.

57. Daouadi M, Zureikat AH, Zenati MS, et al. Robot-assisted minimally invasive distal pancreatectomy is superior to the laparoscopic technique. *Ann Surg.* 2013;257(1):128-132.

58. Kooby DA, Hawkins WG, Schmidt CM, et al. A multicenter analysis of distal pancreatectomy for adenocarcinoma: is laparoscopic resection appropriate? *J Am Coll Surg.* 2010;210(5):779-785, 786–787.

59. Magge D, Gooding W, Choudry H, et al. Comparative effectiveness of minimally invasive and open distal pancreatectomy for ductal adenocarcinoma. *JAMA Surg.* 2013;148(6):525-531.

60. Napoli N, Kauffmann EF, Perrone VG, Miccoli M, Brozzetti S, Boggi U. The learning curve in robotic distal pancreatectomy. *Updates Surg.* 2015;67(3):257-264.

60a. Ocuin LM, Miller-Ocuin JL, Novak SM, et al. Robotic and open distal pancreatectomy with celiac axis resection for locally advanced pancreatic body tumors: a single institutional assessment of perioperative outcomes and survival. *HPB (Oxford).* 2016;18(10):835-842.

61. Sauvanet A, Partensky C, Sastre B, et al. Medial pancreatectomy: a multi-institutional retrospective study of 53 patients by the French Pancreas Club. *Surgery.* 2002;132(5):836-843.

62. Abood GJ, Can MF, Daouadi M, et al. Robotic-assisted minimally invasive central pancreatectomy: technique and outcomes. *J Gastrointest Surg.* 2013;17(5):1002-1008.

63. Downs-Canner S, Van der Vliet WJ, Thoolen SJ, et al. Robotic surgery for benign duodenal tumors. *J Gastrointest Surg.* 2015;19(2):306-312.

64. Standards of Practice Committee, Adler DG, Qureshi W, et al. The role of endoscopy in ampullary and duodenal adenomas. *Gastrointest Endosc.* 2006;64(6):849-854.

65. Posner S, Colletti L, Knol J, Mulholland M, Eckhauser F. Safety and long-term efficacy of transduodenal excision for tumors of the ampulla of Vater. *Surgery.* 2000;128(4):694-701.

66. Crippa S, Angelini C, Mussi C, et al. Surgical treatment of metastatic tumors to the pancreas: a single center experience and review of the literature. *World J Surg.* 2006;30(8):1536-1542.

67. Sperti C, Moletta L, Patane G. Metastatic tumors to the pancreas: the role of surgery. *World J Gastrointest Oncol.* 2014;6(10):381-392.

68. Sperti C, Pasquali C, Liessi G, Pinciroli L, Decet G, Pedrazzoli S. Pancreatic resection for metastatic tumors to the pancreas. *J Surg Oncol.* 2003;83(3):161-166; discussion 166.

69. Minni F, Casadei R, Perenze B, et al. Pancreatic metastases: observations of three cases and review of the literature. *Pancreatology.* 2004;4(6):509-520.

70. Boone BA, Zenati M, Hogg ME, et al. Assessment of quality outcomes for robotic pancreaticoduodenectomy: identification of the learning curve. *JAMA Surg.* 2015;150(5):416-422.

71. Zureikat AH, Nguyen KT, Bartlett DL, Zeh HJ, Moser AJ. Robotic-assisted major pancreatic resection and reconstruction. *Arch Surg.* 2011;146(3):256-261.

72. Huang B, Feng L, Zhao J. Systematic review and meta-analysis of robotic versus laparoscopic distal pancreatectomy for benign and malignant pancreatic lesions. *Surg Endosc.* 2016;30(9):4078-4085.

73. de Rooij T, Klompmaker S, Hilal MA, Kendrick ML, Busch OR, Besselink MG. Laparoscopic pancreatic surgery for benign and malignant disease. *Nat Rev Gastroenterol Hepatol.* 2016;13:227-238.

74. Geller EJ, Matthews CA. Impact of robotic operative efficiency on profitability. *Am J Obstet Gynecol.* 2013;209(1):20 e21-20 e25.

75. Waters JA, Canal DF, Wiebke EA, et al. Robotic distal pancreatectomy: cost effective? *Surgery.* 2010;148(4):814-823.

76. Speicher PJ, Nussbaum DP, White RR, et al. Defining the learning curve for team-based laparoscopic pancreaticoduodenectomy. *Ann Surg Oncol.* 2014;21(12):4014-4019.

77. Fisher WE, Hodges SE, Wu MF, Hilsenbeck SG, Brunicardi FC. Assessment of the learning curve for pancreaticoduodenectomy. *Am J Surg.* 2012;203(6):684-690.

78. Schmidt CM, Turrini O, Parikh P, et al. Effect of hospital volume, surgeon experience, and surgeon volume on patient outcomes after pancreaticoduodenectomy: a single-institution experience. *Arch Surg.* 2010;145(7):634-640.

79. Tseng JF, Pisters PW, Lee JE, et al. The learning curve in pancreatic surgery. *Surgery.* 2007;141(5):694-701.

80. Are C, Dhir M, Ravipati L. History of pancreaticoduodenectomy: early misconceptions, initial milestones and the pioneers. *HPB (Oxford).* 2011;13(6):377-384.

81. Adam MA, Choudhury K, Dinan MA, et al. Minimally invasive versus open pancreaticoduodenectomy for cancer: practice patterns and short-term outcomes among 7061 patients. *Ann Surg.* 2015;262(2):372-377.

82. Birkmeyer JD, Finlayson SR, Tosteson AN, Sharp SM, Warshaw AL, Fisher ES. Effect of hospital volume on in-hospital mortality with pancreaticoduodenectomy. *Surgery.* 1999;125(3):250-256.

83. Birkmeyer JD, Warshaw AL, Finlayson SR, Grove MR, Tosteson AN. Relationship between hospital volume and late survival after pancreaticoduodenectomy. *Surgery.* 1999;126(2):178-183.

84. Nussbaum DP, Adam MA, Youngwirth LM, et al. Minimally invasive pancreaticoduodenectomy does not improve use or time to initiation of adjuvant chemotherapy for patients with pancreatic adenocarcinoma. *Ann Surg Oncol.* 2016;23(3):1026-1033.

Pancreatic Trauma

Syed Nabeel Zafar | Edward E. Cornwell III | Adil A. Shah

Pancreatic injuries, despite their relative infrequency, are regarded with great respect among experienced trauma surgeons because of their significant associated mortality and morbidity. Pancreatic injuries occur in up to 3% of patients with significant blunt abdominal trauma and a slightly higher percentage of those sustaining abdominal gunshot and stab wounds.[1] Penetrating trauma accounts for more than 70% of pancreatic injuries, and, given its anatomic location, associated injuries are the rule. The mortality rate for pancreatic injuries ranges from 10% to 25%, with the majority of deaths occurring in the first 48 hours from massive bleeding and its complications. The systemic inflammatory response syndrome, sepsis, and multisystem organ failure account for the vast majority of delayed deaths. Among patients with pancreatic injury surviving the initial hemorrhage, nearly half will have a complication of their pancreatic wound, such as abscess, fistula, pseudocyst, false aneurysm, or anastomotic leak.[2,3]

Patients with penetrating trauma to the pancreas experience injuries with equal frequency along the head, body, and tail of the organ. In victims of blunt trauma, the deceleration and direct compression mechanism of injury explain why the neck of the pancreas in the prevertebral segment of the gland is the most commonly injured region. The surgical management of pancreatic injury is complicated by the gland's complex anatomic relationship with the duodenum, biliary tract, splanchnic vessels, liver, spleen, vena cava, and aorta. Operative decisions are challenging because of the unforgiving nature of the gland, relative unfamiliarity with the techniques, controversy regarding the technical details, and the judgment required to decide on the extent of surgery. The overall management is challenging, given its often delayed clinical presentation and lack of specific diagnostic modalities. The use of computed tomographic (CT) scans and endoscopic retrograde cholangiopancreatography (ERCP) has fostered the nonoperative management of pancreatic trauma, yet there remains a role for definitive operative therapy in the setting of hemorrhage and main pancreatic duct disruption.

This chapter will outline the clinical presentation of pancreatic injuries, address critical points regarding technical surgical approaches, and review the common complications related to these difficult injuries.

DIAGNOSIS

Patients with torso trauma who manifest early indications of intraabdominal bleeding or peritonitis require immediate operative intervention, at which time direct evaluation of the pancreas should be carried out. For patients who are hemodynamically stable, a thorough diagnostic evaluation is warranted. The stable patient with blunt abdominal trauma is the person in whom timely diagnosis of pancreatic injury is most challenging.

Physical examination and evaluation of hemodynamic status remain the key factors in the diagnostic algorithm of abdominal trauma. A hypotensive patient with abdominal trauma should proceed to the operating room without delay. For the clinically stable patient, selective management can be successful as long as careful attention is given to clinical progress or deterioration. Even patients with abdominal gunshot wounds, once uniformly accepted as a clear indication for exploratory laparotomy, are now managed selectively at some large trauma centers under the appropriate circumstances. The initial clinical examination (vital signs, physical examination of the abdomen) becomes the main determinant of whether the patient is triaged immediately to the operating room, to other diagnostic testing, or to an observation site where physical examinations and monitoring can be undertaken. Important prerequisites for considering selective management of abdominal gunshot wounds rather than mandatory exploration include (1) experienced in-house surgeons who are available to take the patient to the operating room in the event of change of the initial benign clinical examination; (2) a predetermined site in the hospital that facilitates observation and serial examination (i.e., monitoring the vital signs, urine output, hematocrit, and repeated abdominal examinations); and (3) priority status that allows patients with deteriorating clinical examinations to be triaged immediately to the operating room. Serial physical examination is more universally accepted as a mainstay in the selective management of stab wounds to the anterior abdomen.

A full laboratory panel should be collected including serum amylase and lipase levels. Serum amylase is elevated in 80% of patients with blunt pancreatic injury. This figure is much lower for penetrating wounds, but in either case an elevated amylase level mandates a directed evaluation of the pancreas. Studies show that amylase levels upon admission are not very sensitive. The diagnostic yield of amylase is time sensitive, and a value obtained 3 to 6 hours after presentation has a much higher accuracy in predicting pancreatic trauma.[4,5] An elevated amylase level can be a result of bowel perforation, salivary gland trauma, or nondisruptive pancreatic injury because it is not a very specific test. Serum lipase may be used if there is confusion because it is not elevated when hyperamylasemia is of salivary origin. Pancreatic isoenzyme fractionation can identify salivary amylase but is often not available. It is often useful to repeat the serum amylase in patients being observed for abdominal trauma because first blood specimens may be drawn so close to the time of wounding that a misleading normal value may result.

Additional diagnostic studies are indicated if there is suspicion of pancreatic injury An example should be patients with amylase elevation and upper abdominal tenderness and distention. Plain or contrast radiographs offer little assistance. The focused abdominal sonogram for trauma (FAST) rapidly identifies fluid in the hepatorenal recess of Morrison. As a modality that provides prompt assessment of patients with blunt trauma in the emergency department, it has essentially supplanted the diagnostic peritoneal lavage. Following the initial physical examination, the hemodynamically stable patient should undergo a CT scan of the abdomen and pelvis (with intravenous contrast) to elucidate the presence of any visceral injuries. A pancreatic injury can be challenging to assess, given that some injuries may not be obvious without significant inflammatory changes. Such findings may not be apparent in the initial 24 hours post injury. In 2009 the American Association for the Surgery of Trauma (AAST) published a multicenter study examining the use of CT scan in the evaluation of pancreatic injuries. They enrolled 206 patients with confirmed pancreatic injuries on operative exploration and determined the following radiographic characteristics were "hard signs" of a pancreatic injury:

- Active bleeding
- Pancreatic hematoma or laceration
- Diffuse enlargement or edema of pancreas
- Low pancreatic attenuation

The study also suggested that lacerations greater than 50% of the gland thickness on CT scan should raise concern for a pancreatic ductal injury.[6]

In cases in which the clinical findings leading to the CT scan are persistent and the CT scan is equivocal or even negative, ERCP will delineate the pancreatic ductal anatomy (Fig. 102.1). Magnetic resonance cholangiopancreatography (MRCP) has not been evaluated specifically in large numbers of trauma patients, but its use has been extrapolated from its use in nontraumatic scenarios. Its potential benefits include its noninvasive nature, and the fact it can be performed even after anatomy-altering surgery has made ERCP impossible (i.e., pyloric exclusion or gastric bypass procedures). However, it does have a potential drawback, specifically the need to send an acutely injured patient to a remote location. Although the situation occurs infrequently, ERCP can identify major ductal disruption well before clinical signs lead to laparotomy. Early identification and treatment of pancreatic injury can reduce morbidity.

NONOPERATIVE MANAGEMENT

As stressed previously, to attempt nonoperative management for abdominal trauma, the patient must be hemodynamically stable in a facility where there is an experienced in-house surgeon and facilities available for intensive monitoring, serial examinations, and the option to be in the operating room at a moment's notice in the event that the patient's condition deteriorates. Nonoperative management of pancreatic trauma diagnosed on CT scanning is generally reserved for grade I and II injuries.[7]

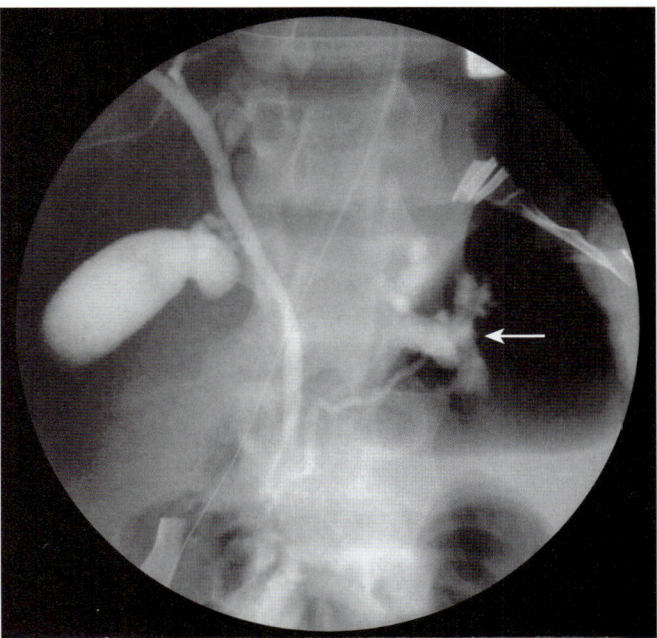

FIGURE 102.1 Endoscopic retrograde cholangiopancreatography performed after original damage control surgery for gunshot wound to abdomen and before reexploration. *Arrow* shows extravasation of contrast from pancreatic duct.

Velmahos et al. conducted a multiinstitutional review of blunt abdominal trauma and studied 230 patients with blunt pancreatoduodenal injury.[8] Ninety-seven (42%) of these were selected for nonoperative management and with a success rate of 90%. A study from the Nationwide Inpatient Sample shows that over a 10-year period from 1998 to 2009 the number of pancreatoduodenal injuries increased by 8.3%; however, the proportion of patients receiving operative intervention declined from 21.7% to 19.8% without affecting morbidity.[9] ERCP can be a very useful adjunct in the diagnosis and management of low-grade pancreatic injuries.[10]

INTRAOPERATIVE EVALUATION

After hemorrhage is controlled in the management of pancreatic trauma, delayed complications, such as pancreatic fistulae and pseudocysts, intraabdominal abscesses, and multisystem organ dysfunction, correlate in frequency with the severity of the pancreatic injury. Therefore the most extensive surgical procedures in the management of pancreatic trauma are reserved for patients with combined pancreaticoduodenal injuries. The overall goals of these surgical procedures are to (1) maintain pancreatic-enteric and biliary-enteric flow, (2) provide wide drainage for all pancreatic and duodenal injuries and anastomoses, and (3) divert the gastrointestinal stream so as to minimize stimulation of the pancreaticobiliary secretions.

In most patients with pancreatic injury, the diagnosis is confirmed intraoperatively. Evaluation of pancreatic trauma requires several surgical maneuvers. A Kocher maneuver entails incising the lateral peritoneal attachments

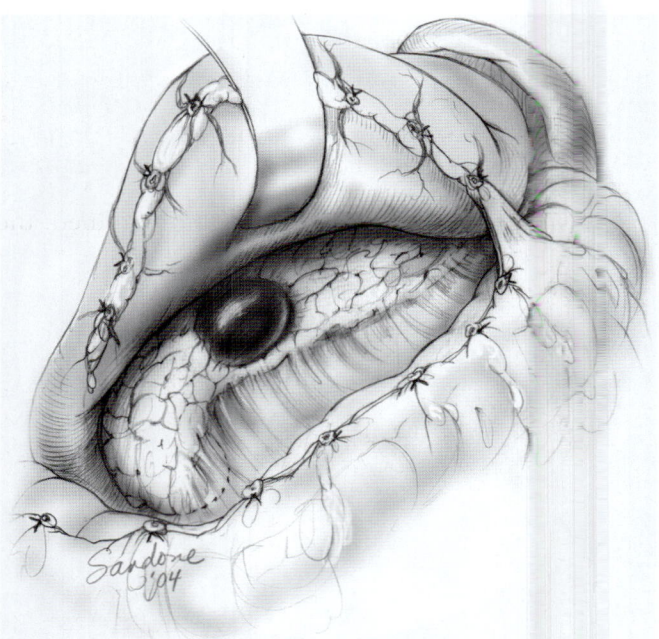

FIGURE 102.2 Any hematomas overlying the gland must be unroofed.

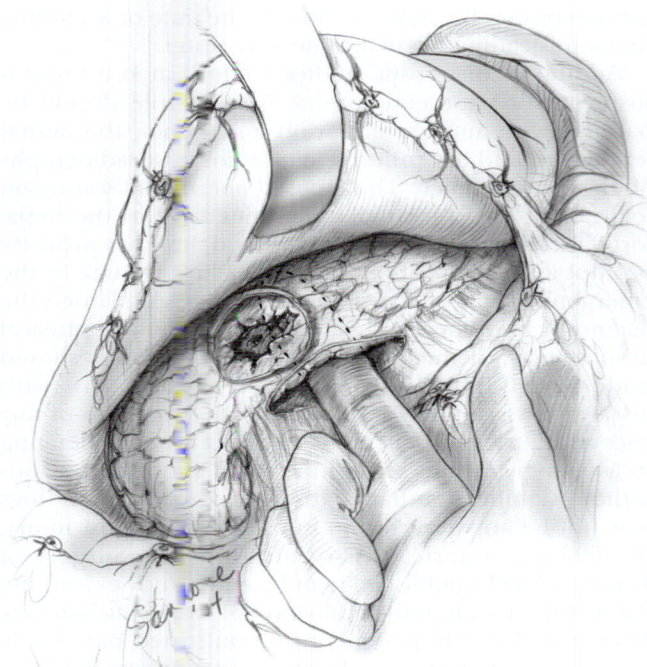

FIGURE 102.3 With the peritoneum along the inferior border of the pancreas divided, the surgeon's finger is slipped behind the gland to evaluate for palpable parenchymal defects.

to the second and third portion of the duodenum and mobilizing the duodenum and the head of the pancreas to the patient's left. This proceeds along the avascular plane to the superior mesenteric vein. A replaced right hepatic artery is occasionally encountered as a branch of the superior mesenteric artery (SMA), and care must be taken because it can be injured during the dissection. This facilitates inspection of the posterior aspect of the head of the gland, as well as the posterior wall of the duodenum, and provides a view of the suprarenal inferior vena cava.

The anterior aspect of the entire gland may be evaluated by entering the lesser sac through the gastrocolic omentum. With a wide incision through the omentum and retraction of the stomach superiorly and the transverse colon inferiorly, a thorough evaluation of the gland becomes possible. Any hematomas overlying the gland must be evacuated and thoroughly explored because they frequently mask underlying severe pancreatic parenchymal or ductal injury (Fig. 102.2). A patient may occasionally present with severe injury to the posterior aspect of the pancreas, with the anterior capsule intact. This is seen most commonly in patients with blunt mechanisms of injury. When hematoma or contusion raises an index of suspicion for injuries that may involve the posterior aspect of the gland, an incision should be made in the peritoneum and areolar tissue along the inferior aspect of the pancreas. Most of these injuries will reside in the prevertebral region of the pancreas. After division of the peritoneum along the inferior border of the pancreas, the surgeon's finger is slipped behind the gland to evaluate for parenchymal defects by palpation and direct visualization (Fig. 102.3).

Full evaluation of the tail of the pancreas can be facilitated by the Aird maneuver.[11] Originally described in 1955

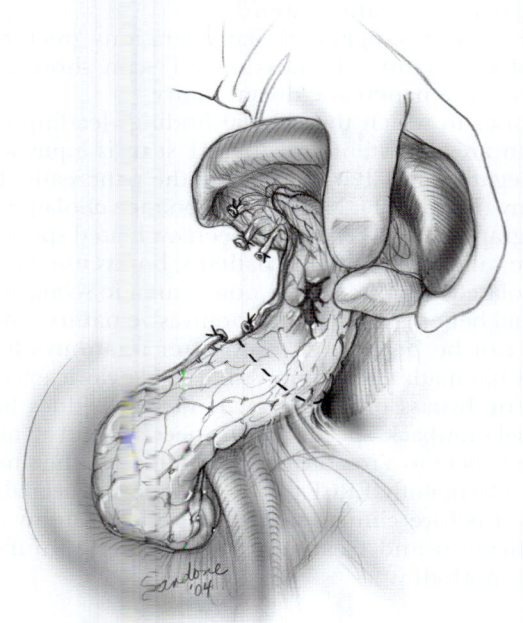

FIGURE 102.4 Aird maneuver is used to mobilize the spleen and tail of the pancreas.

to facilitate adrenalectomy, this procedure entails division of the avascular splenic ligaments (i.e., splenorenal, splenocolic and splenophrenic) and mobilization of the spleen and the tail of the pancreas from the patient's left to right (Fig 102.4).

OPERATIVE TREATMENT

AAST pancreatic organ injury scale grades injuries from I through V (Table 102.1).[12] The use of a combination of the injury grade, injury location, and other concomitant injuries (especially to the duodenum) helps to determine the surgical treatment for the pancreatic injury. Patients with lower-grade pancreatic injuries are significantly easier to manage. Observation and drainage along with débridement and meticulous hemostasis may be all that is necessary for grade I (minor contusion or superficial laceration) or grade II injuries (major contusion or laceration).

Major disruption of the pancreatic tissue requires a decision regarding the likelihood of major ductal injury. Even in major trauma centers, the gold standard ERCP is not available intraoperatively in the middle of the night. Suspicion of ductal involvement is raised by the anatomic location of the injury and the amount of local pancreatic tissue disruption. Pancreatic juice can occasionally be seen leaking at the open ends of a duct. When major ductal injury is suspected, it should, in most instances, prompt definitive therapy. Under some circumstances, such as cardiovascular instability, drainage alone should be performed, after which the patient almost always has a pancreatic fistula.

The popular concept of a continuum of resuscitative care in the operating room/surgical intensive care unit, the acceptance of distal pancreatectomy for wounds to the left of the SMA, and the availability of postoperative ERCP in patients with more severe injuries who have been adequately drained, all render intraoperative pancreatography rarely indicated.

In the rare instance when the duodenum is open already from the traumatic injury, then it is reasonable to perform fluoroscopic pancreatography by cannulating the ampulla to inject contrast. If there is no associated duodenal wound, the duodenum should not be opened for the sole reason of performing a pancreatogram. Another technique for performing a pancreatogram is a cystic duct cholangiogram by passing the catheter into the common bile duct and refluxing contrast into the main pancreatic duct. Such adjuncts as secretin or intravenous opiates may enhance the ability to perform a pancreatogram in this fashion.

After the pancreatic injury has been identified, the location of the injury will determine the appropriate treatment. The pancreatic duct injury can be divided into proximal (at the head or neck, to the right side of the superior mesenteric vessels) and distal injuries (at the distal body and tail to the left side of the mesenteric vessels). Grade III pancreatic injury with a distal transection or parenchymal injury is most easily treated by distal pancreatectomy. In the case of active ongoing hemorrhage, the most expeditious way to perform this is in combination with a splenectomy. The spleen and pancreatic tail will have already been mobilized, leaving only the division of the pancreas itself, the short gastric arteries, splenic artery, and splenic vein. As with all other operations on the pancreas for trauma, the area should be widely drained with closed-suction drains to manage possible postoperative pancreatic leak.

Many options (including staples, sutures, or electrocautery) are acceptable for transecting the pancreas and controlling the transected end of the gland; their use is based on surgeon preference. Ideally the transected pancreatic duct should be identified and closed directly, often with either U stitch or a figure-of-eight suture. Other options include omental patch or fibrin glue for helping control the distal pancreatic stump. The possibility of a distal pancreatectomy without splenectomy (spleen-preserving distal pancreatectomy) can be considered in certain patient populations based on clinical stability and isolated injuries. The small benefit of helping to prevent overriding postsplenectomy sepsis by leaving the spleen in is often outweighed by the significant time that it takes to perform this tedious operation (Fig. 102.5).

An extended distal pancreatectomy can be performed if the laceration resides to the right of the superior mesenteric vessels and may be an option that potentially avoids a Whipple procedure. Another alternative is a central pancreatectomy, which can be considered in the setting of a proximal ductal transection with otherwise normal distal pancreatic parenchyma. The procedure involves resecting the central portion of the gland and débriding back to viable tissue to properly close the end of the proximal duct. The distal pancreatic remnant is then drained by creating a Roux-en-Y pancreaticojejunostomy. Again, wide drainage should be performed to control a postoperative fistula.

Surgical management of severe injuries to the pancreaticoduodenal complex are some of the most complex that a trauma surgeon deals with. These grades IV and V injuries involve proximal ductal injury or massive destruction of the pancreatic head to the right of the superior mesenteric vein and are often in close association with the C-loop of the duodenum. The scope of procedure performed varies with the severity of the injury, reserving the most aggressive surgical treatments for the most severe of these combined pancreaticoduodenal injuries.

TABLE 102.1 American Association for the Surgery of Trauma Organ Injury Scaling: Pancreas

	Type of Injury
GRADE I	
Hematoma	Minor contusion without duct injury
Laceration	Superficial laceration without duct injury
GRADE II	
Hematoma	Major contusion without duct injury or tissue loss
Laceration	Major laceration without duct injury or tissue loss
GRADE III	
Hematoma	Distal transection or parenchymal injury with duct injury
GRADE IV	
Laceration	Proximal transection or parenchymal injury involving ampulla
GRADE V	
Laceration	Massive disruption of pancreatic head

From Moore EE, Cogbill TH, Malangoni MA, et al. Organ injury scaling, II: pancreas, duodenum, small bowel, colon, and rectum. *J Trauma.* 1990;30(11):1427–1429.

There are three main goals in any surgical procedure for severe pancreatic injury. The first is to maintain enteric flow from the pancreas to the biliary tree. The second is to divert any gastrointestinal secretions to minimize stimulation of the pancreatic exocrine function. The third is to widely drain in anticipation of postoperative leaks or fistulas. The main surgical dictum for treatment of the injuries should be to perform the minimal surgical intervention necessary to adequately treat the injury and accomplish these objectives. Significant injuries to the head and neck that do not injure the major pancreatic duct are most appropriately treated with simple débridement and drainage. This approach can be used in the hemodynamically unstable patient undergoing damage control surgery as a temporizing measure, allowing further investigation, such as ERCP or MRCP, after the initial operation. In the patient who is hemodynamically stable or at the second-stage operation after initial damage control, there are multiple options for dealing with injuries to the pancreaticoduodenal complex.

If at the initial operation the pancreas is widely drained and the abdomen is closed, postoperative ERCP is performed to place a pancreatic stent (Fig. 102.6). This can give the main pancreatic duct injury time to heal without performing a major pancreatic resection.

When pancreatic injuries are associated with major duodenal injuries, drainage or resection of pancreas can be combined with suturing or stapling of the pylorus (pyloric exclusion procedure) to divert gastric flow from the duodenum. Gastrointestinal continuity is then accomplished by gastrojejunostomy (Fig. 102.7). It is quite

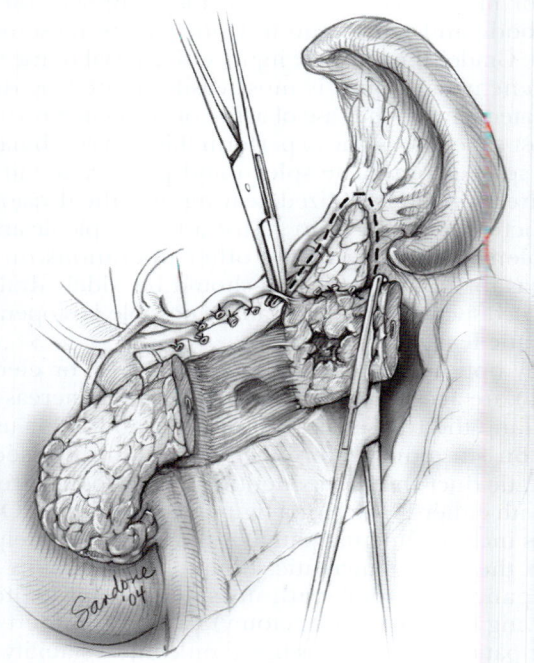

FIGURE 102.5 Distal pancreatectomy with splenic preservation.

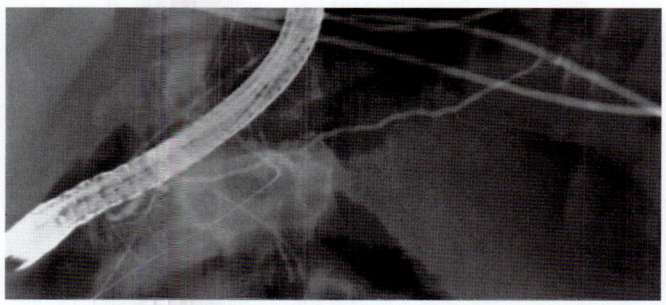

FIGURE 102.6 The same patient as Fig. 102.1 following placement of a pancreatic stent.

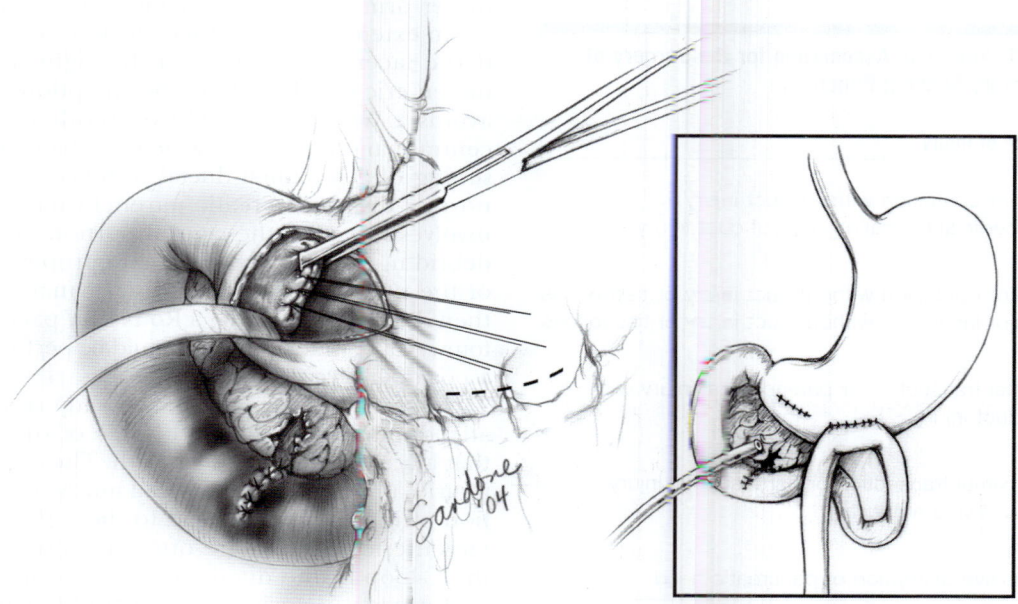

FIGURE 102.7 The pyloric exclusion procedure.

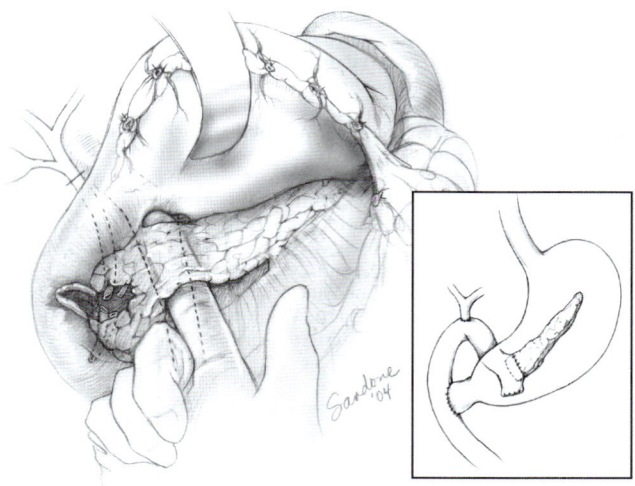

FIGURE 102.8 The Whipple procedure mobilizing the head of the gland.

remarkable that gastroduodenal continuity is reestablished by 4 to 6 weeks after pyloric exclusion even when heavy nonabsorbable sutures or staples are used. The pyloric exclusion procedure has largely replaced the duodenal diverticulization procedure, which entails antrectomy and gastrojejunostomy, as well as drainage and decompression of the duodenal injury and drainage of the pancreatic injury.

When pancreaticoduodenal trauma is so severe that hemorrhage control or extensive destruction of the tissue necessitates resection of the second portion of the duodenum or the head of the pancreas, a pancreaticoduodenectomy (Whipple procedure) is indicated. The avascular plane between the neck of the pancreas and the superior mesenteric vein allows for safe mobilization of the gland for resection (Fig. 102.8). A staged Whipple may be the safest option for the patient after hemorrhage and enteric contamination are controlled because peripancreatic packing and drainage are safe and effective temporary measures until the patient's physiology is restored.[13]

POSTOPERATIVE CONSIDERATIONS

When drainage is performed for major pancreatic injuries, the guideline for removing the drain is tolerance of regular tube feedings and the absence of high-volume or high-amylase content in the drainage fluid. A feeding jejunostomy is an important adjunct to major pancreatic injuries requiring pancreatic resection, pyloric exclusion, or the Whipple procedure because accumulated evidence shows the importance of early enteric feeding in maintaining the immune function of the gut in critically injured patients.

Up to one-third of patients with major pancreatic injuries develop a pancreatic fistula. Most of these resolve spontaneously with adequate drainage. The evidence of a beneficial effect of somatostatin following pancreatic resection for trauma fails to justify the expense associated with its routine use.[14] There is more support for the

concept that somatostatin may reduce the volume of output (and promote closure) after a pancreatic fistula has developed. Rarely, late management of the pancreatic fistula that shows no sign of closure after many weeks of nonoperative management or the patient who forms a pseudocyst after drain removal requires internal drainage via a Roux-en-Y jejunal limb. Postoperative pancreatic abscess usually demands open débridement and wide drainage. However, single uniloculated collections in the absence of much pancreatic necrosis (as determined by dynamic CT scanning) may respond to percutaneous CT-guided drainage with large catheters. Pulmonary and infectious complications also remain high at 20% and 13%, respectively, and need to be identified and managed appropriately.[9] Literature shows that the risk factors for postoperative complications include age, injury location, injury grade, associated vascular injuries, and delay to surgery and are predictors of morbidity.[9,15,16]

SUMMARY

Pancreatic trauma continues to carry a significant risk of mortality and morbidity. Therefore treating other injuries to stabilize the patient may be necessary before definitive operative management of the pancreatic injury can occur. Prompt diagnosis, appropriate resuscitation, and careful surgical technique are paramount in the proper treatment of pancreatic trauma. The grade of the injury, and particularly the presence and location of a pancreatic ductal injury, determines the most appropriate operation (hemostasis, debridement, drainage versus resection, pyloric exclusion, or rarely pancreaticoduodenectomy). Finally, complications are likely to occur, so close observation and early interventions are essential to the recovery of patients with pancreatic trauma.

ACKNOWLEDGMENTS

This chapter is an update from the prior chapters on pancreatic trauma by Edward E. Cornwell III, Elliot R. Haut, and David Kuwayama from the 6th edition of Shackelford's Surgery of the Alimentary Tract *and by Amy Rushing, Edward E. Cornwell III, and Elliott R. Haut from the 7th edition of* Shackelford's Surgery of the Alimentary Tract.

REFERENCES

1. Subramanian A, Dente CJ, Feliciano DV. The management of pancreatic trauma in the modern era. *Surg Clin North Am.* 2007;87(6):1515-1532.
2. Ivatury R, Nallathambi M, Rao P, Stahl W. Penetrating pancreatic injuries. Analysis of 103 consecutive cases. *Am Surg.* 1990;56(2):90-95.
3. Young PR Jr, Meredith JW, Baker CC, Thomason MH. Pancreatic injuries resulting from penetrating trauma: a multi-institution review/discussion. *Am Surg.* 1998;64(9):838.
4. Mahajan A, Kadavigere R, Sripathi S, Rodrigues GS, Rao VR, Koteshwar P. Utility of serum pancreatic enzyme levels in diagnosing blunt trauma to the pancreas: a prospective study with systematic review. *Injury.* 2014;45(9):1384-1393.
5. Takishima T, Sugimoto K, Hirata M, Asari Y, Ohwada T, Kakita A. Serum amylase level on admission in the diagnosis of blunt injury to the pancreas: its significance and limitations. *Ann Surg.* 1997;226(1):70-76.
6. Phelan HA, Velmahos GC, Jurkovich GJ, et al. An evaluation of multidetector computed tomography in detecting pancreatic injury:

results of a multicenter AAST study. *J Trauma.* 2009;67(3):641-646; discussion 646-647.

7. Bokhari F, Phelan H, Holevar M, et al. *EAST Guidelines for the Diagnosis and Management of Pancreatic Trauma.* Chicago: Eastern Association for the Surgery of Trauma (EAST); 2009.

8. Velmahos GC, Tabbara M, Gross R, et al. Blunt pancreatoduodenal injury: a multicenter study of the Research Consortium of New England Centers for Trauma (ReCONECT). *Arch Surg.* 2009;144(5):413-419; discussion 419-420.

9. Ragulin-Coyne E, Witkowski ER, Chau Z, et al. National trends in pancreaticoduodenal trauma: interventions and outcomes. *HPB (Oxford).* 2014;16(3):275-281.

10. Rogers SJ, Cello JP, Schecter WP. Endoscopic retrograde cholangio-pancreatography in patients with pancreatic trauma. *J Trauma.* 2010;68(3):538-544.

11. Aird I, Helman F. Bilateral anterior transabdominal adrenalectomy. *Br Med J.* 1955;2(4941):708-709.

12. Moore EE, Cogbill TH, Malangoni MA, et al. Organ injury scaling, II: pancreas, duodenum, small bowel, colon, and rectum. *J Trauma.* 1990;30(11):1427-1429.

13. Seamon MJ, Kim PK, Stawicki SP, et al. Pancreatic injury in damage control laparotomies: is pancreatic resection safe during the initial laparotomy? *Injury.* 2009;40(1):61-65.

14. Nwariaku FE, Terracina A, Mileski WJ, Minei JP, Carrico CJ. Is octreotide beneficial following pancreatic injury? *Am J Surg.* 1995; 170(6):582-585.

15. Recinos G, DuBose JJ, Teixeira PG, Inaba K, Demetriades D. Local complications following pancreatic trauma. *Injury.* 2009;40(5):516-520.

16. Lin BC, Chen RJ, Fang JF, Hsu YP, Kao YC, Kao JL. Management of blunt major pancreatic injury. *J Trauma.* 2004;56(4):774-778.

Pancreatic Problems in Infants and Children

Noor Kassira | Carrie A. Laituri | Charles N. Paidas

There is much about the pediatric pancreas that can be informative to the adult surgical specialist. Problems that are commonly seen in infants and children, such as annular pancreas, may remain occult until adulthood. Pediatric management strategies, such as the nonoperative management of pancreatic trauma, have been found to be effective in this patient population, and the adult clinician must make an informed decision whether to extend these approaches to adult patients.

This chapter discusses surgical pancreatic conditions commonly seen in infancy, childhood, and adolescence. We review annular pancreas and its relation to duodenal atresia; congenital hyperinsulinism (CHI) of infancy; pancreas divisum; and the pediatric surgical strategies for chronic pancreatitis, tumors, and trauma. The safety and efficacy of endoscopic retrograde cholangiopancreatography (ERCP) in children are also discussed.

ANNULAR PANCREAS

In the fetus the caudal portion of the developing foregut develops into the proximal duodenum, as well as the dorsal and ventral pancreatic buds. At 5 weeks of gestation, rightward rotation begins to bring the ventral pancreatic bud to the right of the duodenum, where it comes to join the dorsal pancreatic bud to give rise to the head of the pancreas (Fig. 103.1). The lumen of the duodenum becomes transiently obliterated with proliferation of the lining cells during the same period of development. By the eighth week of gestation, rotation of the pancreas is complete and recanalization of the duodenum has occurred.[1] Thus it is easy to understand that any perturbation influencing the rotation of pancreatic tissue may also impact recanalization of the duodenum. Therefore annular pancreas is occasionally associated with various degrees of intrinsic duodenal stenosis and atresia. However, in most cases, annular pancreas is associated with external compression of the duodenum resulting in partial or complete obstruction.

Annular pancreas generally presents in the newborn period, with 75% of cases presenting in the first week of life, but it has been reported in an 11-year-old and may be encountered incidentally in adults.[2,3] It has been suggested that a large percentage of patients with annular pancreas remain asymptomatic; however, it is impossible to know because the denominator is unknown.[4] Prenatal ultrasound may detect polyhydramnios or may diagnose duodenal obstruction directly in 30% of patients (Fig. 103.2).[3] At birth, infants have a scaphoid abdomen. Radiographs showing the "double bubble" sign, classically attributed to duodenal atresia, may be seen in more than 88% of patients (Fig. 103.3).[3,5] Emesis may be bilious (up to 50%) or more commonly nonbilious (>90%), depending on whether the obstruction is above or below the ampulla of Vater.[2,3,6]

Associated congenital anomalies occur in approximately 70% of patients (32% chromosomal and 38% other malformations) and should be looked for prior to, and during, operation for annular pancreas.[7] These may include nonsurgical anomalies, such as Down syndrome, and operative conditions, including esophageal atresia, malrotation, Meckel diverticulum, and imperforate anus. In addition, 4% of patients with annular pancreas may have a second duodenal obstruction related to stenosis or web usually noticed intraoperatively as a dilated duodenum distal to the annular pancreas.[8] Congenital cardiac defects must be assessed with preoperative echocardiogram.

At operation, a transverse right upper quadrant skin incision is used. In the newborn the proximal, obstructed, duodenal bulb may be markedly dilated, with the rim of annular pancreas visible just caudal to it. Repair is by duodenoduodenostomy, done in diamond-shaped fashion by making a transverse incision in the proximal duodenum and a perpendicular longitudinal incision in the distal duodenum (Fig. 103.4). The two ends may then be "fish mouthed" or "diamond shaped" together using a single layer of interrupted, absorbable, monofilament suture. If duodenoduodenostomy is precluded by excess tension or a poorly developed distal duodenum, then duodenojejunostomy should be performed. Advances in minimally invasive surgery techniques have allowed attempts at laparoscopic duodenal repair. Laparoscopic duodenoduodenostomy has proven safe with excellent short-term outcomes when completed by pediatric surgeons with advanced laparoscopic skills, with complication rates similar to open duodenoduodenostomy.[9] Thus annular pancreas, which Merrill and Raffensperger in 1976 deemed an "eminently curable lesion," is cured without ever touching the pancreas itself.

Occasionally after correction for annular pancreas, a patient may experience recurrent abdominal pain that may be related to biliary anomalies, such as pancreatic divisum or pancreaticobiliary maljunction.[10] These anomalies can be detected by ERCP or magnetic resonance cholangiopancreatography (MRCP) and may require surgical intervention for recurrent or chronic pancreatitis.

CONGENITAL HYPERINSULINISM

CHI is characterized by dysregulated insulin secretion that results in persistent mild to severe hypoglycemia. The various forms of CHI represent a group of clinically, genetically, and morphologically heterogeneous disorders.[11,12] CHI occurs at a frequency of 1 in 30,000 to 50,000 live births.[6] There has been significant ambiguity surrounding the pathophysiology of CHI. Early recognition of CHI

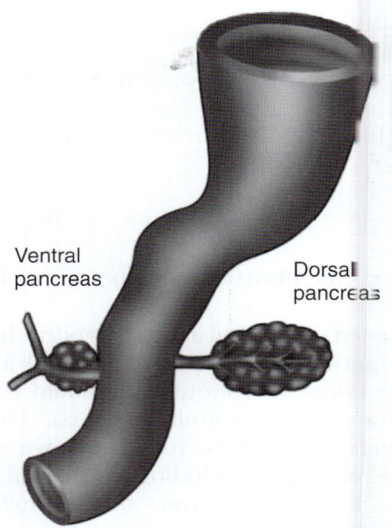
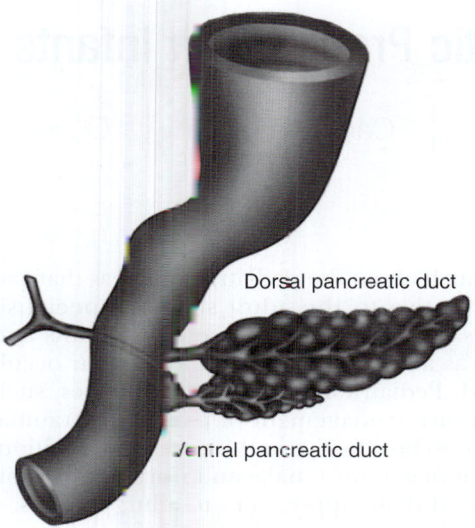

FIGURE 103.1 Embryology of the pancreas at 5 weeks' gestational age. The caudal portion of the foregut gives rise to a ventral and dorsal pancreatic bud. Rotation of the ventral bud to the right allows fusion with the dorsal component. The ventral portion gives rise to the head of the pancreas, and the body and tail are formed from the dorsal bud. (From Godin S. The pancreas. In: Lawrence PF, Bell RM, Dayton MT, eds. *Essentials of General Surgery*. 5th ed. Philadelphia: Lippincott Williams & Wilkins; 2011.)

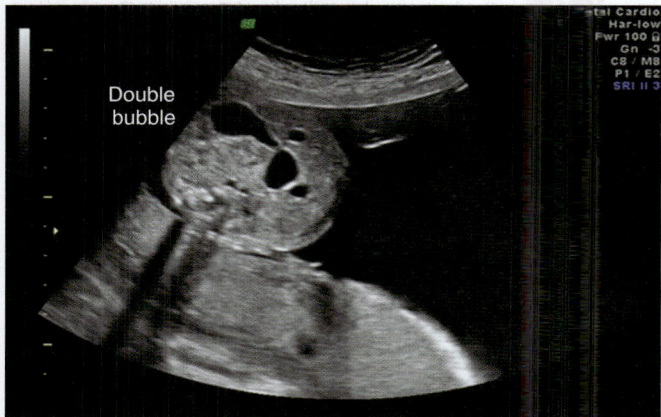

FIGURE 103.2 Antenatal ultrasound showing a double bubble and polyhydramnios indicative of duodenal obstruction or atresia. The double bubble consists of dilated stomach and proximal duodenal obstruction. Polyhydramnios is the result of an inability for the fetus to pass meconium beyond the duodenal obstruction. (Courtesy Victoria Belogolvkin, MD, Assistant Professor, Division of Maternal Fetal Medicine, Department of Obstetrics and Gynecology, University of South Florida College of Medicine, Tampa, Florida.)

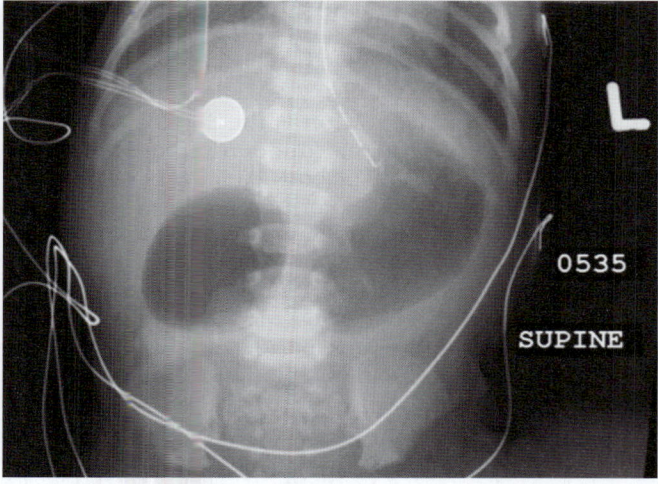

FIGURE 103.3 Postpartum plain abdominal film showing the classic double bubble.

is critical because, if untreated, profound hypoglycemia may lead to brain damage. The clinical manifestations of CHI include babies who are jittery, floppy, or lethargic; seizures are common, and near-death events may occur.[13,14] Diagnosis requires the presence of inappropriately elevated insulin in the setting of hypoglycemia (<2.5 mmol/L, 45 mg/dL), along with the need for continuous glucose infusion (>15 mg/kg/min) to maintain normoglycemia. The presence of low ketone bodies, low free fatty acid, and

an increase in blood glucose after glucagon administration may additionally be used as diagnostic criteria.[13,15]

Mutations in six genes have been associated with CHI: the sulfonylurea receptor 1 (SUR-1; encoded by *ABCC8*)[16]; potassium inward rectifying channel (Kir6.2; encoded by *KCNJ11*)[17]; glucokinase (GK; encoded by *GCK*)[18]; glutamate dehydrogenase (GDH; encoded by *GLUD1*)[19]; short-chain 3-hydroxyacyl-CoA dehydrogenase (SCHAD; encoded by *HADH*),[20] and ectopic expression on β-cell plasma membrane of *SLC16A1* (encodes monocarboxylate transporter 1 [MCT1]).[21] Genetic testing is available through commercial laboratories for four of the six genes known to be associated with CHI (*ABCC8, KCNJ11, GCK, GLUD1*).

SUR-1 and Kir6.2 combine to form the β-cell plasma membrane K$_{ATP}$ channel. Inactivating mutations in the

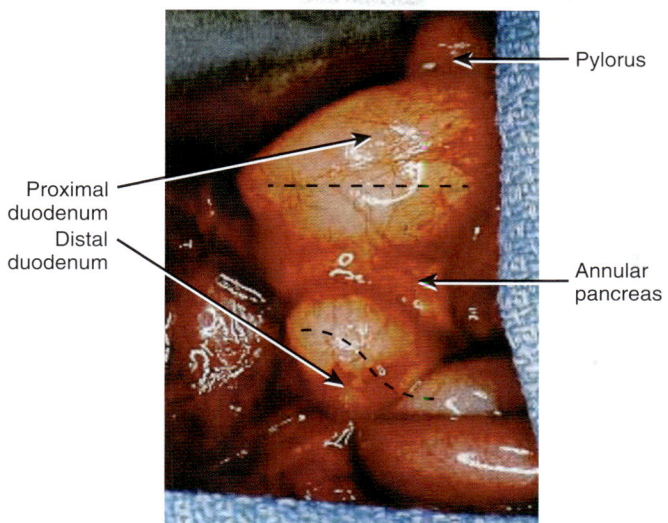

Pylorus

Proximal duodenum

Distal duodenum

Annular pancreas

FIGURE 103.4 Reconstruction of annular pancreas. The absence of ventral and dorsal bud fusion results in an obstructing ring or anulus around the duodenum. Shown in the operative photo is pylorus, annular pancreas, and proximal and distal duodenum. The *dotted lines* represent duodenal incisions for fish-mouth or diamond-shaped duodenoduodenal anastomosis. (Modified from Eckholdt-Wolke F, Hesse A, Krishnaswami S. Duodenal atresia and stenosis. In: Ameh E, Bickler S, Lakhoo K, et al, eds. *Pediatric Surgery: A Comprehensive Text for Africa.* Global HELP; 2011 [Chapter 62]. Available at <www.global-help.org/publications/books/help_pedsurgeryafricavolume02.pdf>.)

K_{ATP} channel result in membrane depolarization and calcium influx into the β cell, resulting in constitutive insulin secretion. This is the most common and severe form of CHI. There are three subtypes of K_{ATP}-CHI, recessively inherited K_{ATP}-CHI, dominantly inherited K_{ATP}-CHI, and focal K_{ATP}-CHI.

GDH CHI is the second most common form of CHI. It is also known as the hyperinsulinism and hyperammonemia (HI/HA) syndrome. GDH-CHI presents with recurrent episodes of hypoglycemia that are less severe than in K_{ATP}-CHI and can be precipitated by a protein-rich meal.[22] These patients do not typically present with hypoglycemia at birth but are frequently diagnosed after several months of age. The hypoglycemia in patients with GDH-CHI is easily controlled with diazoxide.

CHI can also occur in the setting of perinatal stress, resulting in prolonged neonatal hypoglycemia. Transient CHI is seen in the infants of diabetic mothers that develops after birth and resolves spontaneously within the first 3 to 4 weeks of life, but perinatal stress–induced CHI can persist up to a year.[15,23] The mechanism is unknown; however, transient CHI has been associated with shorter gestational age and low birth weight. Transient CHI is believed to be caused by mainly nongenetic factors, whereas persistent CHI likely has genetic etiology. These infants usually respond well to diazoxide; however, via comprehensive analysis, the responsible genes can be identified in only 53% of diazoxide-responsive CHI patients.[15] Mimickers of CHI include neonatal panhypopituitarism,

drug-induced hypoglycemia, insulinoma, antiinsulin and insulin-receptor stimulating antibodies, Beckwith-Wiedemann syndrome, Sotos syndrome, Kabuki syndrome, Costello syndrome, Usher-CHI syndrome, mosaic Turner syndrome, and congenital disorders of glycosylation.

The ability to distinguish focal and diffuse CHI is of paramount importance, in that focal CHI is curable by partial pancreatectomy. Interventional radiology studies, such as transhepatic portal venous insulin sampling[24] and selective pancreatic arterial calcium stimulation,[25] have been used to localize focal lesions. More recently, positron emission tomography (PET) scans with ^{18}F-dihydroxyphenylalanine (DOPA) have been shown to accurately discriminate focal CHI from diffuse CHI.[26–28] PET-CT may offer even better localization because the ^{18}F-DOPA PET scan detects focal lesions as small as 5 mm.[15,29] Supplemental imaging modalities, such as computed tomography (CT), ultrasound, and intraoperative ultrasound, have not yet been validated in the literature for this problem in infancy; however, PET-MRI appears promising.[30] In diffuse CHI, β cells throughout the pancreas are functionally abnormal and have characteristic enlarged nuclei in approximately 2% to 5% of cells (Fig. 103.5). Focal CHI lesions are usually less than 1 cm in diameter and are characterized by the presence of a confluent proliferation of islet cell clusters (focal adenomatosis).[13]

The goal of treatment in infants with CHI is to prevent brain damage from hypoglycemia by maintaining plasma glucose levels greater than 700 mg/L (70 mg/dL). First-line pharmacologic therapy in patients with CHI is diazoxide, a K_{ATP} channel agonist. Because a functional K_{ATP} channel is required for diazoxide to exert an effect, patients with recessive focal or diffuse K_{ATP}-CHI do not respond to therapy with diazoxide. Patients with GDH-CHI, SCHAD-CHI, and perinatal stress–induced hyperinsulinism typically respond well to diazoxide. Second-line medical therapy for infants unresponsive to diazoxide is octreotide. Patients with K_{ATP} channel CHI can be maintained on long-term treatment until spontaneous remission at 2 to 5 years of age.[15]

The decision to operate is based on a laboratory evaluation consistent with CHI, medical responsiveness, genetic testing, and imaging. Operation is necessary in more than two-thirds of cases.[30] The decision to operate should hinge on the demonstration of focality or, in the case of diffuse disease, on the failure of medical management. Treatment of the focal form of CHI is by partial pancreatectomy. Cretolle et al. have reported cure in 44 of 45 patients undergoing partial pancreatectomy following localization, and most, although not all, were found to appropriately correlate with preoperative venous localization. The authors approached lesions of the midportion of the pancreas by means of middle pancreatectomy with preservation of the head, along with Roux-en-Y jejunal loop to the transected portion of the pancreatic tail. Forty-four patients in the series had normal postoperative glucose and glucose tolerance tests, as well as hemoglobin A1c, and all patients were without exocrine dysfunction, with a reported mean follow-up of 3.7 years.[21] Curative laparoscopic enucleation of focal lesions has been reported by others.[31]

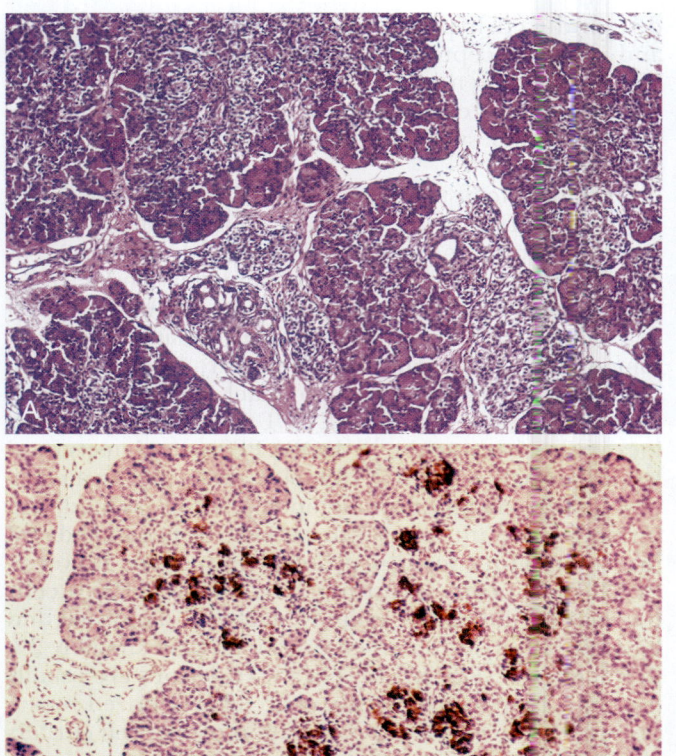

FIGURE 103.5 Diffuse hyperinsulinism from a 95% pancreatectomy specimen of a 1-month-old infant. (A) In the diffuse form of hyperinsulinism, islet cell tissue is increased both at the center of the pancreatic acinus and in connective tissue between the lobules. (B) Pancreas stained by immunocytochemistry using antiinsulin antibody. Numerous small packets of islets scattered throughout the parenchyma and multiple larger islets consistent with the diffuse form of hyperinsulinism. (From Gilbert-Barness E, ed. *Potter's Pathology of the Fetus, Infant and Child*. 2nd ed. New York: Elsevier; 2007 [chapter 25].)

Infants with diffuse disease will normally require a near-total pancreatectomy (95% to 98%) to control the CHI and might require additional therapy with diazoxide, octreotide, and/or frequent feedings to maintain euglycemia. In the diffuse form of CHI, there is diffuse hyperfunction of pancreatic β cells with enlargement of their nuclei, but neither the β-cell proliferation rate nor the overall β-cell mass is increased.[16,17] Diagnosis may also be made by pancreatic venous sampling or by the observation on frozen section of diffuse enlargement of nuclei seen in all specimens. In this case, near-total pancreatectomy is required. Classic anatomic benchmarks, such as removing all pancreatic tissue up to the superior mesenteric vein, should be taken with caution in light of a pediatric autopsy study by Reyes et al., who demonstrated that distal pancreatectomy taken past the mesenteric vessels, up to the left border of the pancreaticoduodenal vessels in the head of the pancreas, accounted for removal of only an average of 71% of the pancreas by weight, with a highly variable range of 43% to 96%.[32] The approach of Fékété et al. is to perform near-total pancreatectomy, leaving only a "small lump of pancreatic tissue in the concavity of the duodenal genu superius, with choledochal dissection."[30] Long-term complications reported following near-total pancreatectomy have included growth disturbance, glucose intolerance or overt diabetes, and variceal bleeding due to splenic vein thrombosis, the latter presenting as late as 15 years postoperatively.[33–35] Reports of long-term pancreatic exocrine deficiency are hard to find. Regeneration of the pancreas following near-total pancreatectomy in infancy has been documented.[13,14] Patients with CHI requiring surgical therapy have a higher incidence of neurodevelopmental problems compared with patients responsive to medical therapy.[36] The risk of developing diabetes has been attributed to pancreatectomy[37]; however, it has also been observed in patients who did not have surgery. In a series of 114 patients with CHI, the incidence of diabetes was as high as 27% after pancreatectomy, and 71% in patients requiring multiple surgical resections.[38]

PANCREAS DIVISUM

Pancreas divisum is a congenital anomaly, but it may or may not manifest itself at any time during life. During fetal development, as the pancreas forms from the rotation and fusion of the ventral pancreatic anlage and the dorsal pancreatic anlage, the ventral duct of Wirsung and the dorsal duct of Santorini ordinarily join. Failure of fusion of the two ducts results in a spectrum of anomalies known as pancreas divisum (Fig. 103.6). In the most common variant the duct of Wirsung drains the uncinate process and variable amounts of the head of the pancreas through the major papilla, while the smaller duct of Santorini drains the majority of the pancreas through a more cephalad accessory papilla. Stenosis of one or both ducts may contribute to the development of pancreatitis.

Pancreas divisum is associated with 25% of patients with recurrent pancreatitis.[39] In contrast, a group of patients with primary biliary disease who had ERCP manifested a 3.5% incidence of pancreas divisum. Necropsy series show a 5% to 10% incidence in the general population. A more recent pediatric study corroborates that of 52 children with relapsing or chronic pancreatitis, 10 had variants of pancreas divisum.[22] The association with chronic or recurrent pancreatitis is unproven but suspected, and, if true, likely is multifactorial in mechanism.

Surgical treatment of recurrent pancreatitis in the setting of pancreas divisum with ductal stenosis includes transduodenal sphincteroplasty of the minor papilla draining the stenotic accessory duct of Santorini, as well as sphincteroplasty of the major papilla.[22,40,41] The sphincteroplasties are done by insinuating a probe into the papilla and sharply dividing anterior to the probe, in gradual fashion. During the course of this sharp division, which serves to splay open the sphincter, interrupted 6-0 or 7-0 synthetic, monofilament, absorbable sutures are sequentially placed from ductal mucosa to surrounding duodenal mucosa. No stent is left. The duodenotomy, opened longitudinally, is closed transversely. Secretin (1 U/kg) given during the operation may assist in the localization of the papilla.

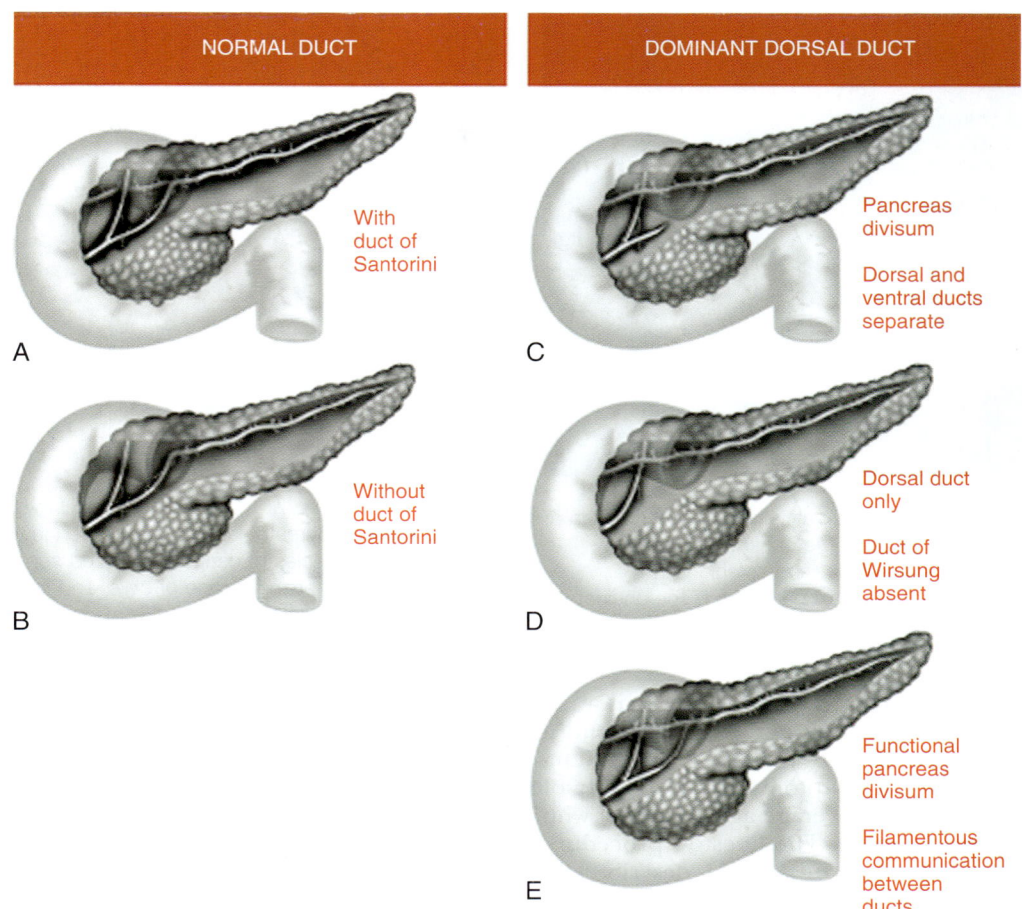

NORMAL DUCT	DOMINANT DORSAL DUCT

A — With duct of Santorini

B — Without duct of Santorini

C — Pancreas divisum / Dorsal and ventral ducts separate

D — Dorsal duct only / Duct of Wirsung absent

E — Functional pancreas divisum / Filamentous communication between ducts

FIGURE 103.6 The spectrum of pancreas divisum. The most common variant is shown in (C). In this case the duct of Wirsung drains the uncinate process and head of the pancreas into the major papilla. Through a more cephalad accessory papilla, the duct of Santorini drains the majority of the head of the pancreas. (From Goldin S. The pancreas. In: Lawrence PF, Bell RM, Dayton MT, eds. *Essentials of General Surgery*. 5th ed. Philadelphia: Lippincott Williams & Wilkins; 2011.)

However, this treatment does not ensure resolution of the patient's symptoms. In one study of six patients, all patients had preoperative evidence of pancreas divisum with ductal obstruction by ERCP.[22] Of the six, only one had a long-term excellent result. Another required ERCP and stenting 3 years later. Two of the six patients continued to have attacks of abdominal pain. Two others went on to have Puestow procedures, with achievement of long-term improvement. Clearly, for some patients with recurrent or chronic pancreatitis and pancreas divisum, sphincteroplasty alone may not address the whole problem, and pancreaticoenteric anastomosis may be required.

ACUTE AND CHRONIC PANCREATITIS

The most common pathologic entity affecting the pancreas in children is acute pancreatitis.[42] Approximately a third of pancreatitis episodes are recurrent. In stark contrast with cases of pancreatitis in adults, where the most frequent causes are alcohol and gallstones, in children the etiology is much more diverse and includes biliary stones, familial, drug ingestion, hypercalcemia, trauma, hypertriglyceridemia, and pancreatic anomalies such as divisum.[42,43] Multi-institutional and single-center studies have indicated an increase in the incidence of acute pancreatitis in children over a 26 year period from 1993–2009.[44–48] The increase is noted to be multifactorial, with one of the most likely culprits being the obesity epidemic, which is a significant independent risk factor for acute biliary pancreatitis.[49–51] There are approximately 3.6 to 13.2 cases of acute pancreatitis per 100,000 pediatric individuals, which approaches the incidence in adults.[46,47] There is also substantial morbidity associated with pancreatitis, with one-quarter developing a severe complication, such as necrotizing pancreatitis, portal vein thrombosis, and diabetes, with mortality rates reaching 4% to 10% (Fig. 103.7).[52]

Medical management of chronic pancreatitis revolves around the use of total parenteral nutrition (TPN), somatostatin, pain management, pancreatic enzyme replacement, and endoscopic sphincterotomy and stenting. When these fail, surgical therapy is indicated. There are three pancreaticoenteric procedures described for the surgical management of chronic pancreatitis in children: the Frey, Puestow, and Duval procedures.

The Frey procedure involves opening the main pancreatic duct throughout its length in the neck, body, and tail of the gland, after which the head is "cored out" in

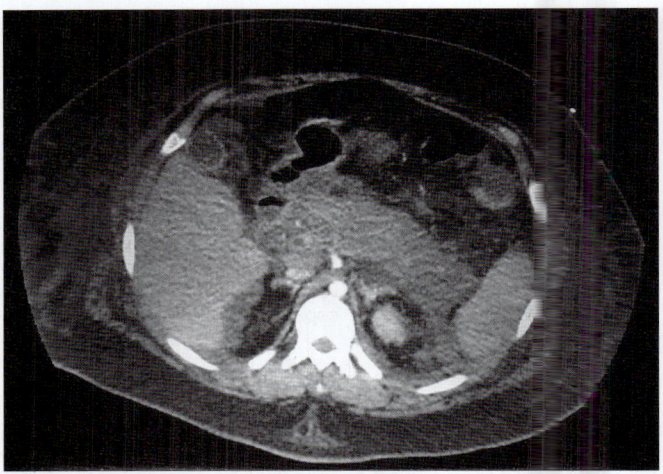

FIGURE 103.7 Acute necrotizing pancreatitis due to gallstones in a 15-year-old morbidly obese female. The patient subsequently developed portal, superior mesenteric, and splenic vein thrombosis. The only remnant of viable pancreas is the uncinate, resulting in the development of diabetes.

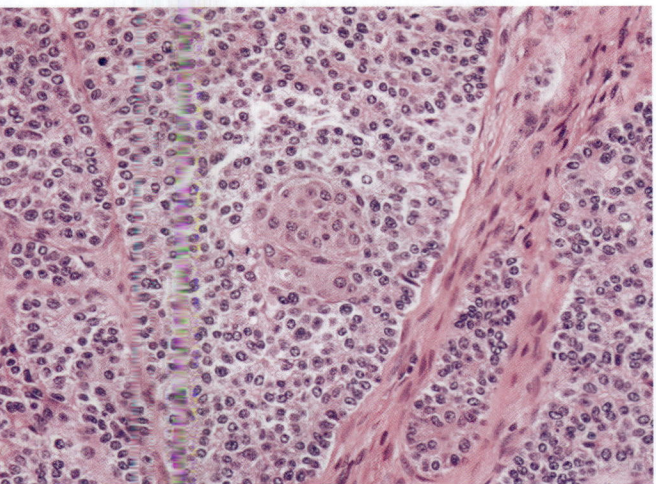

FIGURE 103.8 Pancreatoblastoma. This adenocarcinoma of infancy consists of corpuscles of centrally localized squamous cells, an intermediate dark-staining zone of cells, and finally a peripheral rim of ductlike tubular structures. (From Gilbert-Barness E, ed: *Potter's Pathology of the Fetus, Infant and Child*. 2nd ed. New York: Elsevier 2007 [chapter 25].)

continuity with the opened duct.[53] A longitudinal anastomosis is then constructed between the gland and a Roux-en-Y limb of intestine. A retrospective study demonstrated improvements in symptoms and in quality of life in seven of nine patients (average age: 13 years) who underwent the Frey procedure. The Puestow procedure may also be used in children. DuBay et al. described 12 cases of hereditary pancreatitis treated by modified Puestow.[54] The patients ranged from 2 to 16 years of age, and all had dilated ducts. They used a two-layer side-to-side anastomosis between the opened pancreatic duct and a retrocolic, Roux-en-Y jejunal limb. These authors found significantly decreased rates of hospitalizations after 1 and 3 years and a significant gain in percentage of ideal body weight after 3 years. All but 1 of the 12 patients rated their own outcome as good or excellent. Crombleholme et al. also reported favorable results using the Puestow (with splenectomy) or modified Puestow (without splenectomy) procedure in a group of 10 children with chronic pancreatitis of varying etiologies.[55] The authors found improvement or resolution of pain in all patients, with a mean follow-up of 4 years (range: 7 months to 20 years). The Duval procedure (distal pancreatectomy with Roux-en-Y pancreaticojejunostomy) may also be indicated in some patients.[56] Weber and Keller reviewed 16 patients who had this procedure as the primary operation, and an additional 2 patients who were converted to Duvals following failure of prior Puestow procedures. Half had familial pancreatitis. Of the 18 patients, 13 were weaned entirely off pain medications and required no further hospitalizations, with a mean follow-up of 7.5 years. No claim can be made as to the relative superiority of one operative approach over the other.

TUMORS

Pancreatic tumors are very rare in children and have better outcomes as compared with adult pancreatic tumors.

As a general principle, pancreatic tumors in children are well demarcated rather than infiltrative. Several pancreatic tumors are unique to pediatric patients. Patients are usually asymptomatic; however, presenting signs and symptoms in pediatric patients may include a mass, pain, weight loss, or hypoglycemia, but jaundice is a much less common presentation than is experienced with adults. Surgery figures prominently in the treatment of each of these conditions.

Pediatric pancreatic tumors include pancreatoblastoma, solid pseudopapillary tumors, and primitive neuroectodermal tumors (PNETs). Lymphoid malignancies and metastatic disease may also affect the pancreas. Other pancreatic masses and cysts such as neuroendocrine tumors, serous cystadenomas, and hydatid cysts can occur in children, and their management parallels that of the same conditions in adults.[57–59]

PANCREATOBLASTOMA

Pancreatoblastoma usually presents in the first decade of life. Originally termed *infantile pancreatic carcinoma*, these tumors comprise both epithelial and stromal components. Pathologists look for characteristic squamoid corpuscles, which are nests of squamous-appearing spindle cells that may have keratinization (Fig. 103.8). Tumors are distributed similarly between males and females. There is no predilection for the head versus the tail of the pancreas; however, it has been noted in one study that four of six patients with tumors in the head of the pancreas died, whereas five of five with tumors in the body or tail survived.[60]

Wide local excision carries an important role in pancreatoblastoma, so the surgeon must be prepared for whatever resection is required, whether distal pancreatectomy or pancreaticoduodenectomy, even if in an infant.[61] Involvement of adjacent organs, regional nodes, and vessels is common; many patients present with metastases. Neoadjuvant and adjuvant therapy have been used with variable success. Initial diagnosis may be made by fine-needle aspiration.[38] Recurrences are common and therefore long-term follow-up is critical.[62]

PRIMITIVE NEUROECTODERMAL TUMOR

PNETs are members of the Ewing sarcoma family of tumors. Primary pancreatic PNETs, of which only 15 cases have been reported in the literature,[63–69] are aggressive tumors that typically affect patients in the second or third decades of life. The overwhelming preponderance has occurred in the head of the pancreas, which may explain why patients with pancreatic PNET, unlike those with the other pediatric histologies described here, frequently present with jaundice.

Histologically, PNETs are small round cell tumors. They share the characteristic t(19;37)(q24;q12) chromosomal translocation of Ewing sarcoma, and this results in the *EWS-FLI1* fusion gene. Histologic diagnosis may not be straightforward, and thus obtaining enough tissue to perform molecular diagnostic studies may be critical.

All reported patients have undergone either biopsy or resection. Infiltration into surrounding organs and lymph nodes has been described. Given the similarities with Ewing sarcoma and PNETs at other locations, chemotherapy is indicated; the only survivors reported in the literature have been those who have complied with this. Radiation therapy has also been used.

SOLID PSEUDOPAPILLARY TUMOR

In the past, solid pseudopapillary tumors have also been termed *papillary cystic neoplasm, Hamoudi tumor,* or *Frantz tumor.* It is an epithelial tumor of low-grade malignant potential, occurring more frequently in females of reproductive age that usually presents as an asymptomatic large mass or with pain.[70–72] Radiographically and grossly, solid pseudopapillary tumors have cystic and solid elements (Fig. 103.9). Diagnosis may be made by fine-needle aspirate, which may be accomplished at the time of endoscopic ultrasound in an adolescent patient.[73]

Solid pseudopapillary tumors occur in all regions of the pancreas with equal frequency. They do not tend to invade adjacent organs. Depending on location, pancreaticoduodenectomy, central pancreatectomy with anastomosis of the distal portion to a Roux-en-Y jejunal loop, and distal pancreatectomy have each been applied.[71,73–76] Treatment is by complete excision and, if completely excised, has an excellent prognosis. However, based on recent case reports with follow-up, select cases can be treated by a minimally invasive approach and tissue-sparing resection.[77] There is no established role for chemotherapy or radiation therapy.

OTHER TUMORS

Lymphomas may arise in the pancreas. The pancreas also may be the site of metastatic spread of other pediatric malignancies, such as neuroblastoma (Fig. 103.10).

TRAUMA

Pancreatic trauma is uncommon and is frequently missed during initial evaluation. Blunt injury to the pancreas in children typically occurs in the setting of three characteristic mechanisms. These include handlebar injuries, blows to the abdomen, or motor vehicle crashes. Ordinarily, mechanism, symptoms, or a "seat belt" sign will lead to the performance of a CT scan. The administration of intravenous contrast is essential to suitably visualize solid organ injury, but the utility of oral or intragastric contrast is debatable. Most patients will have grade 3 or 4 injuries usually in the body of the pancreas (Fig. 103.11).[77,78] The accuracy of CT to detect pancreatic injury increases from 70% at time of injury to 90% after 3 days. Hemodynamic instability after volume resuscitation of 40 mL/kg (20 mL/kg × 2) of crystalloid should prompt celiotomy, but this scenario is unusual.

Nonoperative management of pancreatic injuries has been reported in multiple case series since the 1990s. In 1994 a Johns Hopkins group found that of 2900 children admitted for blunt trauma to a pediatric trauma center,

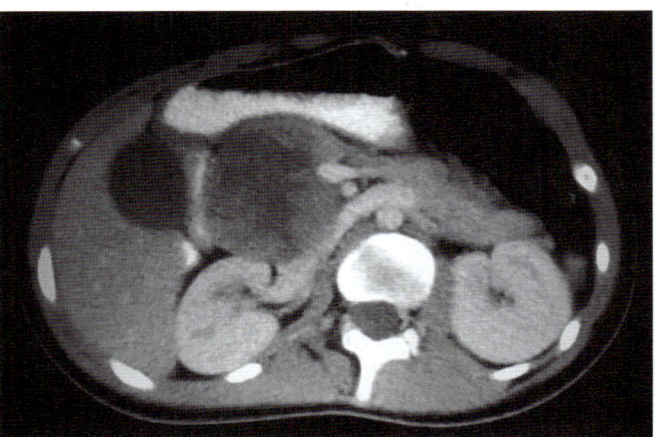

FIGURE 103.9 Solid cystic tumor of the head of the pancreas in a 14-year-old patient consistent with a solid pseudopapillary neoplasm.

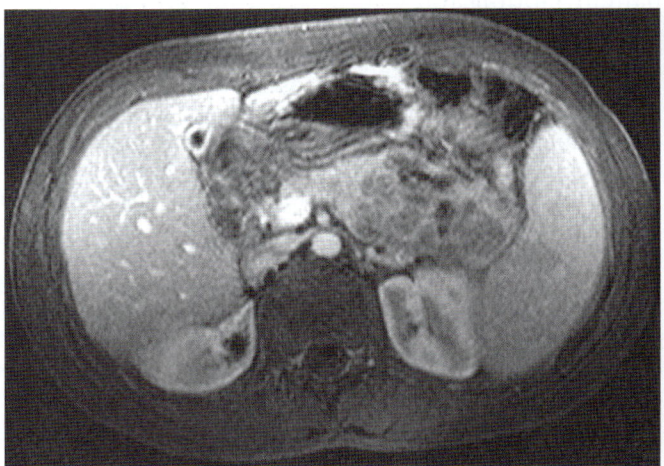

FIGURE 103.10 Magnetic resonance imaging showing neuroblastoma metastatic to the tail of the pancreas in a 16-year-old girl, appearing as a heterogeneous, multilobulated mass.

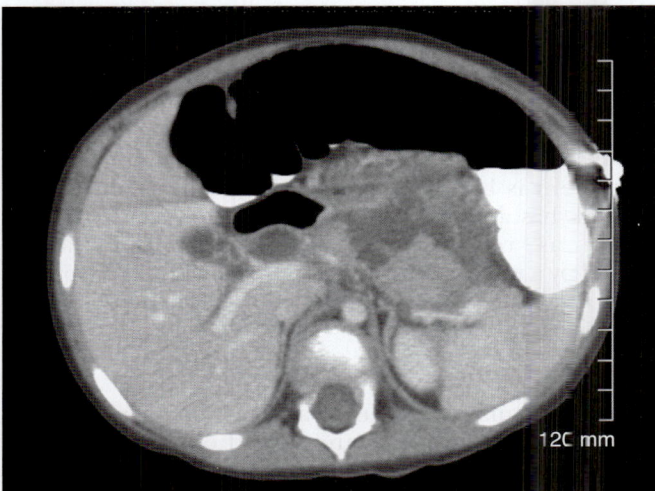

FIGURE 103.11 Midbody pancreas injury following blunt trauma to abdomen in a 5-year-old girl. Note incidental finding of choledochal cyst.

seven had CT-proven lacerations of the pancreas. Four of these seven patients recovered without intervention. The remaining three required partial resection or operative treatment of a pseudocyst.[79] A subsequent review of the National Pediatric Trauma Registry stratified 154 pediatric pancreatic injuries by severity and found that 79% of the children without major ductal injury and 48% of the children with major ductal injury avoided celiotomy.[80] Although encouraging, these data must be counterbalanced by a consideration of the morbidity associated with nonoperative management. Nonoperative management carries complication rates up to 78%.[77,78] However even with the higher complication rate for nonoperative therapy, when compared with operative treatment, the patients had similar lengths of stay and rates of readmission.[81,82] In another review of 19 Japanese children reported in a 1999 series, nonoperative management had complications, including two pseudocyst ruptures secondary to patient motion and one death from TPN-associated complications.[25]

The data on nonoperative management highlight the observation that in some cases, even after complete transection, the pancreatic duct may seal. The resiliency of the duct is illustrated by a case of an 8-year-old patient who sustained a complete, ERCP-proven transection of the proximal duct. Surgical débridement and placement of two Jackson-Pratt drains—but no pancreatic resection or enteric anastomosis—were performed, and in 3 months' time complete reconstitution of the duct was demonstrated.[83] Similarly, a review of nine children with complete pancreatic transection who were treated nonoperatively showed that percutaneous pseudocyst drainage was later required in three of the nine patients. Atrophy of the body and tail were observed in some cases. However, two patients reconstituted completely normal glands.[84] In contrast, other investigators have suggested that given the high complication rate in patients with a transected duct, those are the patients best treated with operative resection.[81] This study also suggested that ERCP was the

tool best used to determine which patients had ductal injury and would require resection. A recent review of the National Trauma Database found that nonoperative management of blunt pancreatic trauma in children is a feasible option with equivalent or better outcomes in regard to death length of stay, Intensive Care Unit length of stay, Intensive Care Unit use, and overall complications.[85]

PROXIMAL VERSUS DISTAL DUCT INJURIES

The decision to render operative or nonoperative treatment to a child with a ductal injury depends, in part, on whether the injury is in the proximal duct or distal duct. The distal duct presents more straightforward surgical options because a distal pancreatectomy may be accomplished by standard suture or staple closure of the pancreatic remnant without the requirement for an enteric anastomosis. Distal resection can be performed laparoscopically.[86] Therefore several groups now advocate early operation for distal duct transections, citing earlier return to health and obviation of the need for TPN.[24,26]

However, proximal duct injuries have prompted wide-ranging solutions, including Whipple procedure[24] and onlay of a Roux limb of jejunum.[27] The track record of nonoperative management makes observation a more attractive alternative than complex operation for proximal ductal transection. All that may be required is interval drainage of the potentially resulting pseudocyst.[28,87]

Alternatively, Canty and Weinman treated their patients with ductal injury by ERCP and transampullary stenting of the pancreatic duct.[88] In this study, both patients healed without pseudocyst formation. Ductal disruption occurred in the midbody in one and in the distal duct in the other, and in one case the stent did not even traverse the injury. Thus the healing of the ductal injury is attributed to decompression of the pancreatic duct as a whole. The investigators pointed out that these cases involved ductal extravasation but not full-scale ductal transection.

OPTIONS FOR PSEUDOCYST DRAINAGE

If a pseudocyst develops (Fig. 103.12), it may be dealt with by standard cystogastrostomy or cystojejunostomy. Percutaneous drainage and internal, endoscopic drainage using a double-pigtail stent into the stomach have also been reported in children as young as 2 years old (Fig. 103.13). Like open operative techniques, these methods rely on the development of a rind around the pseudocyst cavity.[89,90]

ENDOSCOPIC RETROGRADE CHOLANGIOPANCREATOGRAPHY IN CHILDREN

The assumption that ERCP is more dangerous in children than in adults has not been substantiated. Some concerns center on a 2011 study from Montreal Children's Hospital, delineating ERCP procedures performed in children (mean age: 11.5 years; range: 4 to 17 years). Although the success rate was greater than 90%, the authors reported a high complication rate of 33%. Pancreatitis occurred in four patients who underwent sphincterotomy, in one who had a safety diagnostic ERCP, and in one in whom

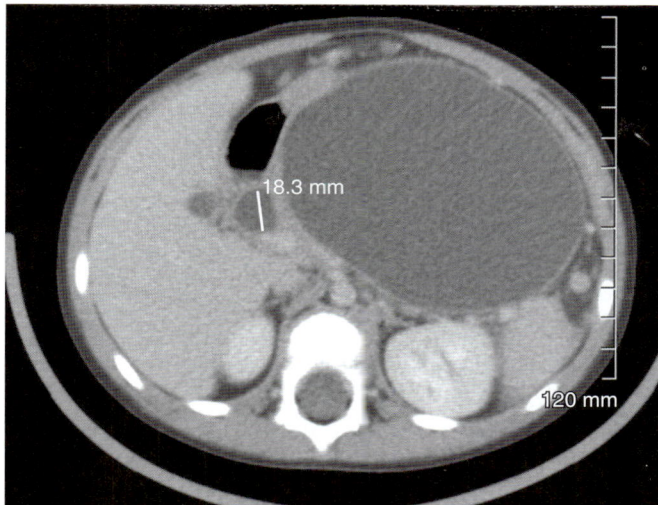

FIGURE 103.12 Posttraumatic pseudocyst in a 4-year-old girl following blunt injury to the abdomen. Extrinsic compression of the common bile duct (18.3 mm).

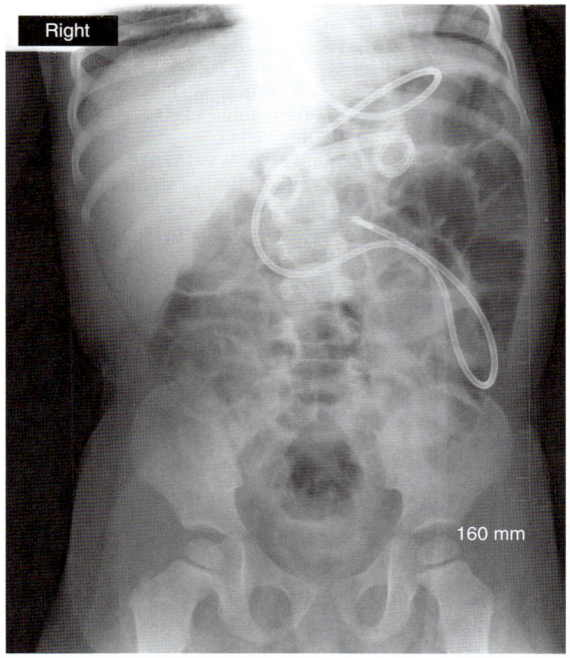

FIGURE 103.13 Pigtail catheter in place following endoscopic cyst gastrostomy for management of posttraumatic pseudocyst in 4-year-old patient shown in Fig. 103.12. Nasoduodenal feeding tube remains in place.

the ampulla could not be cannulated at all. Another patient had bleeding following sphincterotomy, requiring transfusion.[91]

However, these findings are counterbalanced by data from other centers. Allendorph et al. reported four complications among 39 diagnostic and/or therapeutic ERCPs in children (mean age: 12.5 years; range: 6 months to 18 years); all four complications were mild cases of pancreatitis.[92] Guelrud has reported 95% cannulation

success in a series of 155 neonates and infants and 98% success among 125 children older than 1 year, with major complications (cholangitis and pancreatitis) occurring in only two patients.[36] Therapeutic ERCP may be useful for children with chronic pancreatitis, enabling papillotomy, stone extraction, and stenting with an acceptable short-term complication rate.[37]

However, for patients requiring purely diagnostic studies, the use of MRCP to study the pancreatic ducts has been retrospectively validated in a small pediatric series by Arcement et al., who compared findings with those of ERCPs performed on the same children.[38] Given that the only complications of MRCP seem to be those of general anesthesia, MRCP is beginning to supplant ERCP when a diagnostic, not therapeutic, study is needed. For premature infants or children with respiratory concerns, overnight observation in the hospital may still be needed after anesthesia for MRCP.

ACKNOWLEDGMENT

The authors acknowledge David A. Rodeberg, MD for his contributions to previous chapter editions.

REFERENCES

1. Moore KM. *The Developing Human: Clinically Oriented Embryology.* 4th ed. Philadelphia: WB Saunders; 1988.
2. Merrill JR, Raffensperger JG. Pediatric annular pancreas: twenty years' experience. *J Pediatr Surg.* 1976;11:921.
3. Jimenez JC, Emil S, Podnos Y, Nguyen N. Annular pancreas in children: a recent decade's experience. *J Pediatr Surg.* 2004;39:1654.
4. Lainakis N, Antypas S, Panagidis A, et al. Annular pancreas in two consecutive siblings: an extremely rare case. *Eur J Pediatr Surg.* 2005;15:364.
5. Sencan A, Mir E, Gunsar C, Akcora B. Symptomatic annular pancreas in newborns. *Med Sci Monit.* 2002;8:CR434.
6. Lin Y-T, Chang M-H, Hsu H-Y, Lai HS, Chen CC. A follow-up study of annular pancreas in infants and children. *Zhongua Min Guo Xiao Er Ke Yi Xue Hui Za Zhi.* 1998;39:89.
7. Scheida N, Wales PW, Krishnamurthy G, Chait PG, Amaral JG. Ectopic drainage of the common bile duct into the lesser curvature of the gastric antrum in a newborn with pyloric atresia, annular pancreas and congenital short bowel syndrome. *Pediatr Radiol.* 2009;39:66.
8. Papandreou E, Baltogiannia N, Cigliano B, Savanelli A, Settimi A, Keramidas D. Annular pancreas combined with distal stenosis. A report of four cases and review of the literature. *Pediatr Med Chir.* 2004;26:256.
9. Hill S, Koontz CS, Langness SM, Wulkan ML. Laparoscopic versus open repair of congenital duodenal obstruction in infants. *J Laparoendosc Adv Surg Tech A.* 2011;21(10):961-963.
10. Urushihara N, Fukumoto K, Fukuzawa H, et al. Recurrent pancreatitis caused by pancreatobiliary anomalies in children with annular pancreas. *J Pediatr Surg.* 2010;45:741.
11. Palladino A, Bennett MJ, Santley CA. Hyperinsulinism in infancy and childhood: when an insulin level is not always enough. *Clin Chem.* 2008;4:256.
12. Darendeliler F, Bas F. Hyperinsulinism in infancy—genetic aspects. *Pediatr Endocrinal Rev.* 2006;3:521.
13. Aynsley-Green A, Polak JM, Bloom SR, et al. Nesidioblastosis of the pancreas: definition of the syndrome and the management of the severe neonatal hyperinsulinaemic hypoglycaemia. *Arch Dis Child.* 1981;56:496.
14. Schonau E, Deeg KH, Huemmer HP, Akcetin YZ, Böhles HJ. Pancreatic growth and function following surgical treatment of nesidioblastosis in infancy. *Eur J Pediatr.* 1991;150:550.
15. Yorifuji T. Congenital Hyperinsulinism: current status and future perspectives. *Ann Pediatr Endocrinol Metab.* 2014;19(2):57-68.

16. Sempoux C, Poggi F, Brunelle F, Saudubray JM, Fekete C Rahieret J. Nesidioblastosis and persistent neonatal hyperinsulinism. *Diabete Metab (Paris)*. 1995;21:402.

17. Rahier J, Guiot Y, Sempoux C. Persistent hyperinsulinemic hypoglycemia of infancy: a heterogeneous syndrome unrelated to nesidioblastosis. *Arch Dis Child Fetal Neonatal Ed.* 2000;82:F108.

18. Verkarre V, Fournet J-C, de Lonlay P, et al. Paternal mutation of the sulfonylurea receptor (*SUR1*) gene and maternal loss of 11p15 imprinted genes lead to persistent hyperinsulinism in focal adenomatous hyperplasia. *J Clin Invest.* 1998;102:1286.

19. Dubois J, Brunelle F, Touati G, et al. Hyperinsulinism in children: diagnostic value of pancreatic venous sampling correlated with clinical, pathological, and surgical outcome in 25 cases. *Pediatr Radiol.* 1995;25:512.

20. Brunelle F, Negre V, Barth MO, et al. Pancreatic venous samplings in infants and children with primary hyperinsulinism. *Pediatr Radiol.* 1989;19:100.

21. Cretolle C, Fékété CN, Jan D, et al. Partial elective pancreatectomy is curative in focal form of permanent hyperinsulinemic hypoglycemia in infancy: a report of 45 cases from 1983 to 2000. *J Pediatr Surg.* 2002;37:155.

22. Neblett WW, O'Neill JA. Surgical management of recurrent pancreatitis in children with pancreas divisum. *Ann Surg.* 2000;231:899.

23. Silverman JF, Holbrook CT, Pories WJ, Kodroff MB, Joshi VV. Fine-needle aspiration cytology of pancreatoblastoma with immunocytochemical and ultrastructural studies. *Acta Cytol.* 1990;34:632.

24. Jobst MA, Canty TG, Lynch FP. Management of pancreatic injury in pediatric blunt abdominal trauma. *J Pediatr Surg.* 1999;34:818.

25. Kouchi K, Tanabe M, Yoshida H, et al. Nonoperative management of blunt pancreatic injury in childhood. *J Pediatr Surg.* 1999;34:1736.

26. Meier DE, Coln CD, Hicks BA, Guzzetta PC. Early operation in children with pancreas transection. *J Pediatr Surg.* 2001;36:341.

27. Mboyo A, Flurin V, Allamand P, et al. Internal drainage into an onlay-Roux-en-Y jejunal loop in isolated pancreatic injury with ductal transection: short-term and long-term follow-up in two pediatric cases. *Eur J Pediatr Surg.* 2000;10:398.

28. Ohno Y, Ohgami H, Nagasaki A, Hirose R. Complete disruption of the main pancreatic duct: a case successfully managed by percutaneous drainage. *J Pediatr Surg.* 1995;30:1741.

29. Cherubini V, Bagalini LS, Ianilli A, et al. Rapid genetic analysis, imaging with ^{18}F-DOPA-PET/CT scan and laparoscopic surgery in congenital hyperinsulinism. *J Pediatr Endocrinol Metab.* 2010;23:171.

30. Fékété CN, de Lonlay P, Jaubert F, Rahier J, Brunelle F, Saudubray JM. The surgical management of congenital hyperinsulinemic hypoglycaemia in infancy. *J Pediatr Surg.* 2004;39:267.

31. De Vroede M, Bax NMA, Brusgaard K, et al. Laparoscopic diagnosis and cure of hyperinsulinism in two cases of focal adenomatous hyperplasia in infancy. *Pediatrics.* 2004;114:e520.

32. Reyes GA, Fowler CL, Pokorny WJ. Pancreatic anatomy in children: emphasis on its importance to pancreatectomy. *J Pediatr Surg.* 1993;28:712.

33. Soliman AT, Alsalmi I, Darwish A, Asfour MG. Growth and endocrine function after near total pancreatectomy for hyperinsulinaemic hypoglycaemia. *Arch Dis Child.* 1996;74:379.

34. Chevalier SG. Long-term complication following subtotal pancreatectomy for nesidioblastosis: a case report. *Conn Med.* 1996;60:335.

35. Maier JP, Weiss WM. Variceal hemorrhage 18 years after pancreatectomy for nesidioblastosis: a case report and discussion. *J Pediatr Surg.* 2003;38:1102.

36. Guelrud M. Endoscopic retrograde cholangiopancreatography in children. *Gastroenterologist.* 1996;4:81.

37. Kozarek RA, Christie D, Barclay G. Endoscopic therapy of pancreatitis in the pediatric population. *Gastrointest Endosc.* 1993;39:665.

38. Arcement CM, Meza MP, Arumanla S, Towbin RB. MRCP in the evaluation of pancreaticobiliary disease in children. *Pediatr Radiol.* 2001;31:92.

39. Cotton PB. Congenital anomaly of pancreas divisum as cause of obstructive pain and pancreatitis. *Gut.* 1980;21:105.

40. Adzick NS, Shamberger RC, Winter HS, Hendren WH. Surgical treatment of pancreas divisum causing pancreatitis in children. *J Pediatr Surg.* 1989;24:54.

41. O'Rourke RW, Harrison MR. Pancreas divisum and stenosis of the major and minor papillae in an eight-year-old girl: treatment by dual sphincteroplasty. *J Pediatr Surg.* 1998;33:789.

42. Sanchez-Ramirez CA, Larosa-Haro A, Flores-Martinez S, Sánchez-Corona J, Villa-Gómez A, Macías-Rosales R. Acute and recurrent pancreatitis in children: etiological factors. *Acta Paeditr.* 2007;96:534.

43. Stringer MD, Davison DM, McClean P, et al. Multidisciplinary management of surgical disorders of the pancreas in childhood. *J Pediatr Gastroenterol Nutr.* 2005;40:363.

44. Kandula L, Lowe ME. Etiology and outcome of acute pancreatitis in infants and toddlers. *J Pediatr.* 2008;152:106-110.

45. Lopez MJ. The changing incidence of acute pancreatitis in children: a single-institution perspective. *J Pediatr.* 2002;140:622-624.

46. Morinville VD, Barmada MM, Lowe ME. Increasing incidence of acute pancreatitis at an American pediatric tertiary care center: is greater awareness among physicians responsible? *Pancreas.* 2010;39:5-8.

47. Nydegger A, Heine RG, Ranuh R, Gegati-Levy R, Crameri J, Oliver MR. Changing incidence of acute pancreatitis: 10-year experience at the Royal Children's Hospital, Melbourne. *J Gastroenterol Hepatol.* 2007;22:1313-1316.

48. Pant C, Deshpande A, Olyaee M, et al. Epidemiology of acute pancreatitis in hospitalized children in the United States from 2000–2009. *PLoS One.* 2014;9:e95552.

49. Ma MH, Bai HX, Park AJ, et al. Risk factors associated with biliary pancreatitis in children. *J Pediatr Gastroenterol Nutr.* 2012;54:651-656.

50. Poffenberger CM, Gausche-Hill M, Ngai S, Myers A, Renslo R. Cholelithiasis and its complications in children and adolescents: update and case discussion. *Pediatr Emerg Care.* 2012;28:68-76.

51. Svensson J, Makin E. Gallstone disease in children. *Semin Pediatr Surg.* 2012;21:255-265.

52. Benifla M, Weizman Z. Acute pancreatitis in childhood: analysis of literature data. *J Clin Gastroenterol.* 2003;37:169-172.

53. Rollins MD, Meyers RL. Frey procedure for surgical management of chronic pancreatitis in children. *J Pediatr Surg.* 2004;39:817.

54. DuBay D, Sandler A, Kimura K, Bishop W, Eimen M, Soper R. The modified Puestow procedure for complicated hereditary pancreatitis in children. *J Pediatr Surg.* 2000;35:343.

55. Crombleholme TM, deLorimier AA, Way LW, Adzick NS, Longaker MT, Harrison MR. The modified Puestow procedure for chronic relapsing pancreatitis in children. *J Pediatr Surg.* 1990;25:749.

56. Weber TR, Keller MS. Operative management of chronic pancreatitis in children. *Arch Surg.* 2001;136:550.

57. Beccaria L, Bosio L, Burgio G, Paesano PL, Del Maschio A, Chiumello G. Multiple insulinomas of the pancreas: a patient report. *J Pediatr Endocrinol Metab.* 1997;10:309.

58. Montero M, Vazques JL, Rihuete MA, et al. Serous cystadenoma of the pancreas in a child. *J Pediatr Surg.* 2003;38:E36.

59. Arikan A, Sarac A, Erikci VS. Hydatid cyst of the pancreas: a case report with five years' follow-up. *Pediatr Surg Int.* 1999;15:579.

60. Klimstra DS, Wenig BM, Adair CF, Heffess CS. Pancreatoblastoma: a clinicopathologic study and review of the literature. *Am J Surg Pathol.* 1995;19:1371.

61. Jaksic T, Yaman M, Thorner P, Wesson DK, Filler RM, Shandling B. A twenty-year review of pediatric pancreatic tumors. *J Pediatr Surg.* 1992;27:1315.

62. Lee YJ, Hah JO. Long-term survival of pancreatoblastoma in children. *J Pediatr Hematol Oncol.* 2007;29:845.

63. Danner DB, Hruban RH, Pitt HA, Hayashi R, Griffin CA, Perlman EJ. Primitive neuroectodermal tumor arising in the pancreas. *Mod Pathol.* 1994;7:200.

64. Luttges J, Pierre E, Zamboni G, et al. Maligne nichtepthliale tumoren des pancreas. *Pathologe.* 1997;18:233.

65. Bulchmann G, Schuster T, Haas RJ, Joppich I. Primitive neuroectodermal tumor of the pancreas: an extremely rare tumor. *Klin Padiatr.* 2000;212:185.

66. Movahedi-Lankarani S, Hruban RH, Westra WH, Klimstra DS. Primitive neuroectodermal tumors of the pancreas: a report of seven cases of a rare neoplasm. *Am J Surg Pathol.* 2002;26:1040.

67. Shorter NA, Glick RD, Klimstra DS, Brennan MF, LaQuaglia MP. Malignant pancreatic tumors in childhood and adolescence: the Memorial Sloan-Kettering experience, 1967 to present. *J Pediatr Surg.* 2002;37:887.

68. Perek S, Perek A, Sarman K, Tuzun H, Buyukunal E. Primitive neuroectodermal tumor of the pancreas: a case report of an extremely rare tumor. *Pancreatology.* 2003;3:352.

69. Changal KH, Mir MH, Azaz SA, Qadri SK, Lone AR. Primitive neuroectodermal tumour of pancreas; second case from Asia. *Malays J Med Sci.* 2014;21(6):65-69.

70. Martin RCG, Klimstra DS, Brennan MF, Conlon KC. Solid-pseudopapillary tumor of the pancreas: a surgical enigma? *Ann Surg Oncol.* 2002;9:35.

71. Raffel A, Cupisti K, Krausch M, et al. Therapeutic strategy of papillary cystic and solid neoplasm (PCSN): a rare non-endocrine tumor of the pancreas in children. *Surg Oncol.* 2004;13:1.

72. Lee YJ, Jang JY, Hwang DW, Park KW, Kim SW. Clinical features and outcome of solid pseudopapillary neoplasm. *Arch Surg.* 2008;143:218.

73. Nadler EP, Novikov A, Landzberg BR, et al. The use of endoscopic ultrasound in the diagnosis of solid pseudopapillary tumors of the pancreas in children. *J Pediatr Surg.* 2002;37:1370.

74. Wunsch LP, Flemming P, Werner U, Gluer S, Bürger D. Diagnosis and treatment of papillary cystic tumor of the pancreas in children. *Eur J Pediatr Surg.* 1997;7:45.

75. Ward HC, Leake J, Spitz L. Papillary cystic cancer of the pancreas: diagnostic difficulties. *J Pediatr Surg.* 1993;28:89.

76. Casanova M, Collini P, Ferrari A, Cecchetto G, Dall'Igna P, Mazzaferro V. Solid-pseudopapillary tumor of the pancreas (Frantz tumor) in children. *Med Pediatr Oncol.* 2003;41:74.

77. Sacco Casamassima MG, Gause CD, Goldstein SD, et al. Pancreatic surgery for tumors in children and adolescents. *Pediatr Surg Int.* 2016;32(8):779-788.

78. Thomas H, Madanur M, Bartlett A, Marangoni G, Heaton N, Rela M. Pancreatic trauma: 12-year experience from a tertiary center. *Pancreas.* 2009;38:113.

79. Haller JA, Papa P, Drugas G, Colombani P. Nonoperative management of solid organ injuries in children: is it safe? *Ann Surg.* 1994;219:625.

80. Keller MS, Stafford PW, Vane DW. Conservative management of pancreatic trauma in children. *J Trauma.* 1997;42:1097.

81. Wood JH, Partrick DA, Bruny JL, Sauaia A, Moulton SL. Operative vs nonoperative management of blunt pancreatic trauma in children. *J Pediatr Surg.* 2010;45:401.

82. de Blaauw I, Winkelhorst JT, Rieu PN, et al. Pancreatic injury in children: good outcome of nonoperative treatment. *J Pediatr Surg.* 2008;43:1640.

83. Arkovitz MS, Garcia VF. Spontaneous recanalization of the pancreatic duct: case report and review. *J Trauma.* 1996;40:1014.

84. Wales PW, Shuckett B, Kim PCW. Long-term outcome after nonoperative management of complete traumatic pancreatic transection in children. *J Pediatr Surg.* 2001;36:823.

85. Mora MC, Wong K, Friderici J, et al. Operative vs nonoperative management of pediatric blunt pancreatic trauma: evaluation of the National Trauma Data Bank. *J Am Coll Surg.* 2016;222(6):977-982.

86. Yoder SM, Rothenberg S, Tsao K, et al. Laparoscopic treatment of pancreatic pseudocysts in children. *J Laparoendosc Adv Surg Tech A.* 2009;19:S37.

87. Canty TG, Weinman D. Management of major pancreatic duct injuries in children. *J Trauma.* 2001;50:1001.

88. Canty TG, Weinman D. Treatment of pancreatic duct disruption in children by an endoscopically placed stent. *J Pediatr Surg.* 2001;36:345.

89. Kimble RM, Cohen R, Williams S. Successful endoscopic drainage of a posttraumatic pancreatic pseudocyst in a child. *J Pediatr Surg.* 1999;34:1518.

90. Patty I, Kalaoui M, Al-Shamali M, Al-Hassan F, Al-Naqeeb B. Endoscopic drainage for pancreatic pseudocyst in children. *J Pediatr Surg.* 2001;36:503.

91. Prasil P, Laberge J-M, Barkun A, Flageole H. Endoscopic retrograde cholangiopancreatography in children: a surgeon's perspective. *J Pediatr Surg.* 2001;36:733.

92. Allendorph M, Werlin SL, Geenen JE, et al. Endoscopic retrograde cholangiopancreatography in children. *J Pediatr.* 1987;110:206.

Pancreas and Islet Allotransplantation

Piotr Witkowski | Julia Solomina | J. Michael Millis

In 1993 the Diabetes Control and Complications Trial Research Group reported that patients with insulin-dependent diabetes mellitus (IDDM) treated with intensive insulin therapy showed a reduced risk of developing retinopathy, albuminuria or microalbuminuria, and clinical neuropathy, when compared with patients who received conventional insulin therapy.[1] In this trial the intensive therapy group was shown to have achieved sustained lowered blood glucose concentrations over time, as reflected by significantly lower hemoglobin (Hb)A_{1c} values compared with those of the conventional insulin therapy group. Although the intensive therapy group benefited from reduced long-term complications, the risk of severe hypoglycemia, which compromised life quality associated with tight glycemic control, was three times greater than in the conventional therapy group. Successful β-cell replacement therapy in the form of pancreas or islet transplantation offers the advantages of attaining normal or near-normal blood glucose control without the risks of severe hypoglycemia associated with intensive insulin therapy. Thus the goal of pancreas and islet transplantation is to restore normal glycemic control and thereby reduce the complications of IDDM by providing sufficient β-cell mass.[2] Although pancreas transplantation remains the gold standard as β-cell replacement therapy, an alternative approach (i.e., pancreatic islet transplantation), is a developing procedure, and results from studies in 2012 indicate it may be as effective as solitary pancreas transplantation.[3,4] Over the last decade, islet cell allotransplantation has become an approved funded procedure in Canada, Europe, and Australia in selected patients. In the United States it should achieve the same status in a few years because results of the National Institutes of Health (NIH)-sponsored multicenter trial have just been published.[5] Individual islet centers can currently apply to the US Food and Drug Administration (FDA) for a biological product license for the clinical islet cell processing after they can demonstrate safety and effectiveness of islet cell manufacturing and clinical outcome. Such a license is necessary for the center to offer islet allotransplantation as a standard of care procedure and to approach insurance for a reimbursement. All together, as pancreatic islet allotransplantation has become a clinical reality and an alternative β-cell replacement therapy option, we have elected to present it together with pancreas transplantation.

HISTORY OF PANCREAS TRANSPLANTATION

The first pancreas transplants were performed in combination with a kidney in uremic type 1 diabetic patients in 1966 at the University of Minnesota. It was proved that pancreas transplantation could obtain a euglycemic state without the need for exogenous insulin.[6] However, early procedures were complicated by a high rate of morbidity, early graft failure, and poor patient survival, so few transplants were performed.[6] Improvements in transplantation techniques, immunosuppressive therapies, and posttransplantation monitoring of graft function and rejection have resulted in a dramatic improvement in patient morbidity and graft survival. According to the International Pancreas Transplant Registry (IPTR), from 1966 to 2014 more than 48,000 pancreases were transplanted worldwide (over 29,000 in the United States and 19,000 in Europe).[7,5] Up until 2004 the number of pancreas transplants was growing and peaked at level of 1400 performed annually in the United States in 2000–2004, but since then there has been a steady decline in numbers of these procedures.[7,8] Between 2004 and 2011 the number of simultaneous pancreas-kidney transplants (SPKs) dropped by 10% for pancreas transplant alone (PTA) by 34%, but for pancreas after kidney transplantation (PAK) dropped the most—by 55%; the same trend continued over the next few years (data available until 2014).[7,8] Paradoxically, this drop-off occurred in the setting of improvements in graft and patient survival and transplanting higher risk patients. The drop in number of pancreas transplants was attributed to lack of a primary referral source, lack of acceptance by the diabetes care community, improvements in diabetes care and management, changing donor and recipient considerations, inadequate training opportunities, and increasing risk aversion because of regulatory scrutiny.[7] However, at the same time, outside the United States, the number of pancreas transplants has been trending up, reaching 1400 annually in the past few years (Fig. 104.1).[8] Between 2004 and 2014, SPK transplantation has accounted for 74% of pancreas transplants and has been offered to uremic diabetic patients. PAK transplantation accounts for 17% of pancreas transplant procedures and is offered most commonly to those uremic diabetics, who received a living donor kidney transplant previously (80%).[8] PTA is offered to labile diabetics with good renal function and accounts for 9% in the United States.[8] Pancreas retransplantation accounts for 7% of pancreas transplant procedures; among those PAK was the most common one (68%) and performed in patients with stable function of the kidney graft.[8]

HISTORY OF PANCREATIC ISLET TRANSPLANTATION

In 1965 Moskalewski first isolated pancreatic islets from the guinea pig and in 1967 Lacy's group described a novel collagenase-based method to isolate rat islets, thus paving the way for islet transplantation.[9,10] Subsequent studies showed that transplanted islets could reverse diabetes not

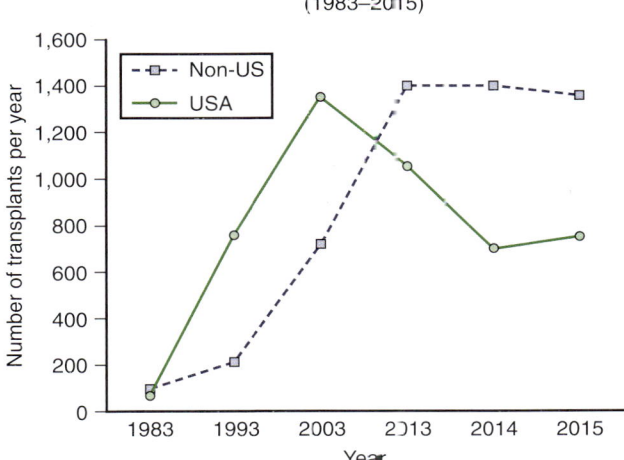

FIGURE 104.1 Annual number of US and non-US pancreas transplants (1983–2015). Number of pancreas transplantations has been recently declining in the United States, whereas the number continues to rise outside the United States. (Modified from Gruessner AC, Gruessner RW. Pancreas transplantation of US and non-US cases from 2005 to 2014 as reported to the United Network for Organ Sharing [UNOS] and the International Pancreas Transplant Registry [IPTR]. *Rev Diabet Stud.* 2016;13:35–58.)

only in rodents but also in nonhuman primates.[11] However, early efforts to treat type 1 diabetics with pancreatic islet transplantation were mostly unsuccessful. Although the first human pancreatic islet allografts were performed in 1977,[12] it was not until 1990 that a pancreatic islet transplant recipient achieved sustained euglycemia off insulin (for 1 year).[13] The same authors reported the first successful series of human islet allografts when transplanted together with the liver from the same donor. Although they did not address the added issue of autoimmunity in type 1 diabetes (none of their patients were type 1 diabetics), this study provided the first evidence of long-term reversal of diabetes after islet allotransplantation, with more than 50% of recipients having sustained insulin independence, lasting in one case up to 5 years.

EDMONTON PROTOCOL

Of the patients receiving islet transplants in the 1990s, only 7% of patients remained insulin free 1 year after islet transplantation. In 2000 the Edmonton group reported seven consecutive islet transplant recipients, all of whom achieved insulin independence at the end of 1 year without major complications.[14] All recipients received islets from at least two donors and were maintained on a glucocorticoid-free immunosuppression protocol using rapamycin and low-dose tacrolimus.[14] The success of the Edmonton program has led to a general acceptance that islet transplantation is a clinically feasible therapy, which may be considered for the treatment of patients with labile type 1 diabetes experiencing hypoglycemia unawareness with severe hypoglycemic episodes (SHEs). Since the report

of success from Edmonton, interest has grown in islet transplantation, and more than 46 centers worldwide have performed this procedure. According to the Collaborative Islet Transplant Registry (CITR), from 1999 to 2012, a total of 1679 allogeneic islet transplantations in 828 recipients were reported.[15]

CANDIDATES FOR PANCREAS OR ISLET ALLOTRANSPLANTATION

Neither pancreas nor islet transplantation is a life-saving intervention. The aim for both procedures is to prevent secondary diabetic complications and improve quality of life. Therefore patient selection criteria are stricter than for other organ transplantation in order to protect patient safety and properly identify candidates who can benefit from the procedures.

Guidelines of the American Diabetes Association for indications for pancreas transplantation include patients with IDDM, with undetected C-peptide who suffer from end-stage renal disease or symptoms of hypoglycemic unawareness with progressive secondary diabetic complications, such as (1) history of frequent, acute, and severe metabolic complications (hypoglycemia, hyperglycemia, ketoacidosis) requiring medical attention; (2) clinical and emotional problems with exogenous insulin therapy that are so severe as to be incapacitating; or (3) consistent failure of insulin-based management to prevent acute complications.[16]

Currently, general indications for islet allotransplantation in most of the clinical studies are the same as described earlier for pancreas transplantation. For example, the NIH-funded, FDA-regulated, multicenter Clinical Islet Transplantation trial targets patients who failed intensive insulin treatment defined as intensive insulin therapy with target HbA$_{1c}$ levels of less than 6.5%, as suggested by the American Association of Clinical Endocrinologists/American College of Endocrinology (AACE/ACE) consensus panel statement on type 1 diabetes mellitus and glycemic control. Following a period of longer than 4 months on this therapy, only patients who evidence continued inadequate glucose control characterized by either HbA$_{1c}$ level higher than 7.5% or HbA$_{1c}$ level less than 7.5% but with SHEs are included.[5]

Currently, one limitation of islet allotransplantation is the insufficient number of islets isolated from a single organ to restore normoglycemia in each type 1 diabetic patient. Even with two or three sequential infusions, success cannot be achieved in patients with high insulin demand. Most studies limit recipients to body mass index (BMI) less than 30 kg/m^2, body weight less than 90 to 100 kg, and daily insulin requirements below 1 unit/kg.[5]

As results of pancreas transplantation have been improving, the percentage of patients older than 50 years who received a pancreas transplant has been increasing, reaching 35% in 2009.[17] Mortality of the uremic patient older than 50 years on the waiting list is extremely high and much higher than after SPK, so this group of patients has actually much more to gain than younger population.[17] Immunologic risk of rejection is also lower in older than younger patients, so those patients should be considered for transplant as long as there is no contraindication for surgery.[17]

It is worth emphasizing that 6% of pancreas transplants (mostly SPK) are performed in selected type 2 diabetic patients (age <55 with low surgical risk).[6,18] United Network for Organ Sharing (UNOS) policy allows for accruing waiting time for SPK when serum C-peptide ≤2 ng/mL, or if higher, then BMI needs to be below maximum allowed (approximately 28).[19] Overall, number of type 2 diabetic patients receiving SPK has increased in recent years and accounted for 9% of those procedures.[8] In addition, 7% of pancreas allografts are implanted in nondiabetic patients after extended intraabdominal resection as part of multiorgan transplantation (including liver, intestine, and/or kidney transplants).[8] Islet transplantation is also an option in such cases with good results, in cases in which the patient is not suitable for whole pancreas transplantation.[13]

In general, the waiting time for pancreas transplantation varies widely, depending on the country and region of the United States. For the United States the shortest waiting time is for PTA, at 4.9 months, and the longest is 10.5 months for PAK.[8]

DONOR CHARACTERISTICS

Most pancreas allografts (95%) come from deceased heart-beating donors. The remainder are from highly selected non–heart-beating donors or from living donors.[2] To improve results, optimal parameters of donors are as follows: age 14 to 45 years; BMI less than 28 kg/m^2; head trauma as the preferred cause of death; and organ procured by a local organ procurement organization to minimize cold ischemic time, preferably less than 12 hours. Pancreas donors are excluded based on presence of diabetes, pancreatitis, sepsis, malignancy, and positive markers for viral infection, such as hepatitis B or C, human immunodeficiency virus (HIV), or human T-lymphocyte virus. Undesired conditions include BMI greater than 30 kg/m^2, Centers for Disease Control and Prevention (CDC) high risk, downtime, disseminated intravascular coagulopathy (DIC), need for pressors, and pancreas injury, fibrosis, or steatosis. Hyperglycemia or need for insulin therapy in the donor at the time of organ procurement is not a contraindication, but it is a minor risk factor for long-term graft loss.[2] Hyperamylasemia can be of salivary origin, and it is not itself a contraindication for donation. Some centers have exclusion criteria for the pancreas based on age (younger than 8 years), body weight (<30 kg), or diameter of the splenic artery (<2 mm).[16] Donors with a BMI greater than 35 kg/m^2 or who are older than 55 years are used very rarely; only 6% of donors are younger than 14 years of age, and 6% are older than 45 years of age.[2]

Exclusion donor criteria for the purpose of islet transplantation are the same as for pancreas transplantation to prevent transmission of disease to the recipient. However, donor and organ quality criteria are much less restrictive. Desired age is older than 18 years without an upper limit, and BMI is unrestricted as long as the patient is not diabetic (HbA_{1c} ≤6%). The main limiting factor regarding

the effectiveness of the islet isolation is cold ischemia time (≤12 hours) but preferably less than 8 hours. In the United States and United Kingdom, preferential pancreas allocation to islet transplant recipients was established for donors older than 50 years or with a BMI greater than 30 kg/m^2.[2] The goal is to limit cold ischemia time and enhance availability of the organ and improve isolation results. Otherwise, the current organ allocation system promotes pancreas transplantation over islet transplantation. Therefore, other than in the United Kingdom, each pancreas is offered first to potential whole-organ recipients, and then if rejected, is considered for islet transplant patients. In this way, mostly lower-quality organs are used for islet isolation. This allocation schema may be changed in the future, after islet transplantation achieves the same effectiveness and status as whole-organ pancreas transplantation, such as currently in the United Kingdom, where there is only one waiting list for islet/pancreas transplant. The next available organ is allocated for pancreas or islet transplantation, depending on the patient on the top of the common list.

Due to more extensive reperfusion injury and increased risk for thrombosis, donation after cardiac death (DCD) of the pancreas for whole-organ transplant is not very popular in the United States, whereas it is well developed in the United Kingdom and Japan.[8] For the same reason of tissue ischemic injury and poor islet isolation yield, DCD donors have not been used broadly. However, the Edmonton group has reported comparable outcomes of islet isolation and transplantation, when pancreas was retrieved from DCD and brain-dead donors.[20]

PANCREAS PROCUREMENT TECHNIQUES

PANCREAS PROCUREMENT FOR WHOLE-ORGAN TRANSPLANTATION

Cadaveric-donor pancreatectomy is performed as part of a multiorgan procurement through a midline incision. The gastrocolic ligament is divided to enter the lesser sac and expose the anterior aspect of the pancreas. At this point the pancreas is evaluated for signs of fat infiltration, edema, injury, hematoma, calcification, and tumor. If the organ is still suitable, a Kocher maneuver is performed to expose the inferior vena cava and aorta. The gastroduodenal artery is ligated and divided. If a replaced (accessory) right hepatic artery is present, it may be divided at its origin. If liver is procured at the same time, usually the liver surgeon decides whether to include the superior mesenteric artery (SMA) with the right replaced hepatic artery, allowing for easier arterial reconstruction of pancreas vasculature and transplantation. Next, the spleen and tail of the pancreas are mobilized to allow for placement of the ice-slush posterior to the gland during perfusion. After the thoracic aorta is cross-clamped, cold preservation solution (most commonly University of Wisconsin or histidine-tryptophan-ketoglutarate) is introduced through cannulas in the inferior mesenteric vein and distal aorta. On completion of organ perfusion, the splenic artery is divided from the celiac trunk; the aorta is divided above and below the origin of the celiac trunk, and the portal vein is divided usually 2.5 cm above the superior border of the pancreas. The SMA is harvested with an aortic Carrel patch and distal to the origin of interior pancreaticoduodenal artery. The duodenum is divided by gastrointestinal anastomosis (GIA) stapler at the level of pylorus and ligament of Treitz after flushing the lumen with an antiseptic solution. The spleen remains attached to the pancreas to protect the tail during the procurement. Iliac venous and arterial grafts are obtained from the donor for the reconstruction of the pancreas vasculature.[16] When the small bowel is procured for transplantation at the same time, it is essential to ensure that the inferior pancreaticoduodenal artery is not divided during dissection of the root of the small bowel. Next the pancreas with spleen and duodenum in continuity are placed in a container with preservation solution and placed on ice during transportation.

PANCREAS PROCUREMENT FOR THE ISLET ALLOTRANSPLANTATION

Basically the pancreas for the islet isolation is procured in the same way. However, different elements of the procurements are more crucial. First, the pancreas for islet procurement is more sensitive to warm injury; therefore, the organ should be well flushed with the preservation solution to eliminate blood. Then the organ should be kept constantly surrounded by ice, even during dissection. Next, because no blood vessels are necessary for the isolation, the presence of a right hepatic artery does not preclude pancreas procurement. Instead, it is extremely important during the dissection not to cut or open the pancreas capsule because it compromises enzyme distention, organ digestion, and eventually the yield of the isolation. Because results of the islet isolation depend strongly on proper pancreas preservation, it is hard to overemphasize the importance of the pancreas procurement technique for the success of the islet isolation and then transplantation. In multivariable analyses the procuring team from the islet isolation center is the strongest independent factor (odds ratio [OR] = 10.9) regarding the success of the isolation.[21]

BACK-TABLE PREPARATION FOR WHOLE PANCREAS TRANSPLANTATION

Before implantation, the pancreas needs to be prepared for transplantation while still on ice at the back table. During this important procedure the pancreas vasculature is restored; excess surrounding fat, connective tissue, and the spleen are removed, followed by meticulous ligation of the surrounding blood vessels. This is all done to minimize unnecessary ischemic or bleeding injury, improving the results of pancreas transplantation. Because the celiac trunk and hepatic artery are allotted to the liver, the splenic artery and SMA are maintained with the pancreas. To make a single arterial pedicle, the donor iliac artery is used as a "Y" graft to suture onto the donor SMA and splenic artery. The portal vein is available for anastomosis and usually does not require elongation. The standard pancreas graft includes the entire pancreas and the second portion of the duodenum. Some authors recommend reconstruction of the gastroduodenal artery as well with an arterial conduit, to improve blood supply to the head and duodenum and decrease risk for

complications; however, the advantage of such a maneuver has not been confirmed in comparative studies.[22]

LIVING-DONOR PANCREAS TRANSPLANTATION

Since 1978, when for the first time a living-donor pancreas transplantation was performed at the University of Minnesota, there have been 160 of those procedures reported to the IPTR, and only three American centers were involved.[23,24] Improved graft survival was the main goal of the procedure when azathioprine and cyclosporine were the main immunosuppressive agents, despite the magnitude and potential complications of the donor operation. However, with the introduction of tacrolimus, mycophenolate mofetil (MMF), and clinical antibodies used for induction therapy, and better donor selection excluding donor-specific antibodies, graft survival improved dramatically for cadaveric-donor pancreas transplants. As a result, the immunologic advantage of pancreas transplantation with living-donor transplants in the recent era is no longer as critical as it was before. Moreover, cadaver donors for pancreas transplantation are more available than for other organ transplants, and there is a substantial risk for donors developing diabetes after donation (26%).[25] Thus living donors for solitary pancreas transplants are only considered in order to limit long waiting times in highly sensitized recipients or if the donor is a nondiabetic identical twin or a six-antigen matched sibling.[2] Of note, living-donor pancreas transplantation has been offered with good results not only as solitary organ but also in setting of SPK with kidney from the same donor or deceased donor.[24,26]

In the living-donor pancreas recovery procedure, the short gastric artery arcade should be preserved so that the spleen can be safely left in place. The splenic artery is divided just distal to its origin, and the splenic vein is divided proximal to its confluence with the superior mesenteric vein. The splenic arterial anastomosis is to the recipient common iliac artery, whereas venous drainage is to the common iliac vein. The pancreatic drainage is accomplished by pancreaticojejunostomy or pancreaticocystostomy.[2]

PANCREAS TRANSPLANTATION

The pancreas may be transplanted as the only organ in PTA or as PAK transplantation. However, most commonly, it is transplanted from the same donor with the kidney as SPK transplantation. In this situation, during the same procedure, the pancreas may be transplanted first because it has a shorter "shelf life" (optimal cold storage time is <12 hours vs. 24 to 48 hours for kidney), so as to reduce preservation injury and the risk of complication.[2] Alternatively, the kidney may be grafted first to reduce the incidence of acute tubular necrosis and to avoid pancreas manipulation during kidney transplantation. The pancreas is usually placed in the right pelvis, as in kidney transplantation, with the arterial anastomosis performed on the recipient common iliac artery. Venous drainage can be connected to the lower vena cava or the common iliac vein (systemic drainage) or superior mesenteric vein (portal drainage). The standard pancreas graft includes the entire pancreas and a portion of the duodenum. The donor duodenum is anastomosed to the recipient's small bowel or urinary bladder allowing drainage of the exocrine pancreas secretions. Each alternative procedure has its own pros and cons.

PORTAL VERSUS SYSTEMIC VENOUS DRAINAGE

Portal venous drainage directs the insulin released by the pancreas transplant initially to the liver, in a fashion similar to normal physiologic conditions, allowing for 50% first-pass metabolism. It also lowers the concentration of low-density lipoprotein and apolipoprotein B, and free cholesterol, as well as very-low-density lipoprotein. It was postulated based on experimental models that portal venous drainage decreases immunologic response to the graft; however, this was not confirmed clinically.[22] On the other hand, systemic drainage omitting first passage through the liver leads to hyperinsulinemia and increased level of low-density lipoprotein. However, clinically the advantages of the portal over systemic drainage in maintaining normal glucose homeostasis or lipid metabolism have never been shown.[22] Similarly, carbohydrate metabolism does not differ in recipients having SPK transplantation compared with nondiabetic recipients after kidney transplantation only, when similar immunosuppression is used.[2] Therefore portal drainage is currently used in only 20% of patients because it is more challenging, requires more experience, and has a somewhat higher risk of graft thrombosis.[27]

ENTERIC DRAINAGE VERSUS BLADDER DRAINAGE

Historically, restoration of pancreatic exocrine secretion drainage was challenging. After the failure of attempts at pancreatic duct ligation and obliteration, the urinary bladder with pancreas-duodenum anastomosis was developed. The advantage of this approach is that amylase concentration in urine allows for monitoring of graft function, enabling early detection of rejection. It is especially useful in PTA and PAK transplantation. However, the major disadvantage is metabolic acidosis because of loss of bicarbonate with the relatively large amount of pancreas juice, frequent reflux pancreatitis (50%), cystitis, urinary tract infection, and perineal irritation.[16] Therefore, after more potent immunosuppression was introduced, including induction therapy, and the need for pancreas monitoring was diminished, enteric drainage was more widely adopted, improving postoperative course and patient satisfaction. In addition, pancreas rejection is usually associated with kidney graft dysfunction in SPK transplantation, which allows additional monitoring of the pancreas graft state. Therefore 90% of patients currently undergo enteric drainage for all three categories of pancreas transplantation.[8] There are many different methods for enteric drainage in use: The duodenum may be connected with a loop of jejunum, ileum, or even recipient duodenum. It is usually a side-to-side configuration with the loop (most common) or Roux-en-Y limb of the bowel (15% to 20%), either a handsewn double layer or a stapled anastomosis.[8] However, in the latter approach, there is a higher risk of postoperative mucosal bleeding. It seems that enteric drainage has a slightly higher incidence of graft thrombosis than bladder anastomosis: 5.5% to 11.6% versus 5% to 7.2%, respectively.[2] Postoperative

enteric leak usually requires reoperation for repair with Roux-en-Y conversion of the bowel loop. In cases of a leak from a bladder anastomosis, drainage with a Foley urinary catheter is usually sufficient.[22] Based on considerable data from both registries and various retrospective and prospective trials, neither of those two drainage techniques has a clear advantage with regard to overall patient or pancreas graft survival.[2]

COMPLICATIONS

The hypoxic injury inherent in cadaveric organ procurement accounts for some of the complications related to the pancreatic allograft. During the 1980s 25% of all pancreata were lost because of surgical technical failure. According to the IPTR, from 2004 through 2008, the incidence was reduced to an 8% average in all three categories (SPK, PTA, and PAK recipients).[7] Nonetheless, surgical complications such as pancreas graft thrombosis, leakage, graft pancreatitis, and bleeding, remain high concerns because the rate of the relaparotomy is as high as 35%.[28]

Pancreas Graft Thrombosis

Pancreas graft thrombosis remains, by far, the most frequent and serious surgical complication (incidence ranges from 3% to 10%).[28] With rare exceptions, it results in graft loss and the need for transplant pancreatectomy. Anticoagulation is often used, and tight postoperative management and monitoring with ultrasound, contrast-enhanced computed tomography (CT), or magnetic resonance imaging (MRI) is required.[29] Ultrasound is less useful in patients with enteric drainage, where bowel gas obscures the window. Recipient obesity carries 50% higher risk of graft thrombosis.[8]

Leakage

Leakage remains a clinically significant entity because it typically causes intraabdominal infection. In the case of enteric drainage, intestinal contents leak and cause peritonitis and sepsis. This complication usually requires graft duodenal diversion with a Roux-en-Y limb. From this perspective bladder drainage has a lower incidence of leakage but also if it occurs, can be managed conservatively.

Graft Pancreatitis

Although only the endocrine part of the pancreas is needed to control normoglycemia, whole pancreas grafts have both islets and exocrine tissue. Postoperative graft pancreatitis occurs more frequently in PAK and PTA recipients with bladder drainage (1.7% and 2.0%, respectively). Postoperative pancreatitis may be treated conservatively, but severe cases may require relaparotomy with débridement or occasionally graft pancreatectomy. In addition, repetitive episodes of reflux pancreatitis in bladder-drained recipients are an indication for conversion from bladder to enteric drainage.

Hemorrhage

Significant intraabdominal bleeding after pancreas transplantation frequently requires relaparotomy; however, less than 2% of all pancreas grafts are currently lost because of bleeding. Gastrointestinal (GI) bleeding may occur in the early postoperative period, most often from mucosal bleeding at the duodenoenteric anastomosis, and especially when the stapler was applied. Furthermore, late GI bleeding may be a sign of chronic graft rejection.[2]

Rejection and Immunosuppression

Pancreas transplantation is associated with graft loss by rejection as a result of alloimmunity or autoimmune recurrence. Even transplants between identical twins need immunosuppression to prevent autoimmune recurrence.[2] Although the introduction of cyclosporine improved overall results of organ transplantation, the pancreas graft rejection rate was still as high as 73% (for PTA), with up to a third of patients experiencing recurrent rejections. Currently, tacrolimus and MMF with low-dose steroids in combination with different induction therapies are most commonly used as the maintenance immunosuppressive regimen. Such combinations lead to rejection rates at the level of 5% to 25%.[2] Anti-T-cell antibody induction with a combination of maintenance treatment is used in 80% of all pancreas transplant recipients.[8,27] Antihuman thymocyte antibody (thymoglobulin), anti-interleukin-2 (IL-2) receptor antibody (basiliximab), or anti-CD52 antibody (alemtuzumab) are most commonly used for induction.

Because acute rejection is a strong predictor of chronic rejection (relative risk [RR]: 4.1), which is the second most common cause of graft loss (after technical failure), there is a hope that reduction of the number and severity of acute graft rejection episodes will improve long-term results.[16] However, so far clinically, it has not been proved that reduced graft rejection rate (diagnosed with biopsy) prolongs pancreas graft or patient survival.[2] Side effects of the immunosuppression compromise overall health and function of the other organs; for example, steroids lead to insulin resistance, dyslipidemia, bone loss, and impaired wound healing, and tacrolimus causes nephrotoxicity. Large trials tested a steroid-free regimen or minimization of calcineurin inhibitors, showing a slightly increased rejection rate of 20% to 30% without the hoped-for improvement in long-term results.[2] Steroid-free protocols seem to compromise kidney graft function in SPK without affecting pancreas graft survival.[8]

OUTCOME OF PANCREAS TRANSPLANTATION

Although pancreas transplantation is not a life-saving procedure but aims to improve quality of life and prevent secondary complications, the benefits of the pancreas transplantation may be considered only in patients with functioning grafts; therefore we primarily assess both graft and patient survival.

Patient Survival

According to the IPTR, the patient survival rate for primary deceased-donor pancreas transplants has constantly improved over the past several years. The 1-year survival rate increased from 67% in 1980 to more than 95% in 2005–2009 and to greater than 97% currently.[2,5,6,8] The 3- and 5-year survival rates recently reached 95% and 89%, respectively, in all three transplantation categories.[27] Fifteen-year actuarial patient survival is 56% in SPK transplants, 42% for PAK transplants, and 59% after PTA.[2]

Interestingly, there was a substantial increase in survival in age-matched diabetics 10 years after SPK transplantation, compared with deceased-donor kidney transplantation.[30] Reddy et al. found similar benefits 5 and 8 years after the procedures.[31] SPK recipients have a 10-year longer expected survival time than do kidney transplantation alone (KTA) recipients (23 vs. 13 years); however, the difference is not obvious for patients older than 50 years before transplantation.[32] The presence of a functioning kidney graft increases survival by almost 20% in SPK patients at 7-year follow-up.[8]

Despite that, there has been a debate whether the benefits of pancreas transplantation translate into patient survival. It turned out that overall patient survival was similar in SPK recipients when compared with living-donor kidney transplantation (LDKT) recipients.[30–32] The adjusted survival rate was 67% for SPK recipients, 65% for LDKT, and 46% for deceased-donor kidney transplantation.[32] In addition, it was also reported that patients with preserved renal function after receiving solitary pancreas transplantation had worse survival rates than those diabetics who were treated with conventional therapy (insulin) while waiting to be transplanted.[33] The RR of dying was 2.7 (confidence interval [CI]: 0.84 to 6.13) for PTA and 2.89 (CI: 1.67 to 5.00) for PAK transplantation within 90 days after the procedure. For SPK transplantation, the risk was lower (RR: 1.7; 95% CI: 0.97 to 2.98), but reversed as late as 4 years after transplantation. However, other authors reanalyzed the same United Network for Organ Sharing data and found several factors that could bias the previous results. Several patients were listed for many procedures at the same time, and the mortality rate of the patients on the waiting list was underestimated.[34] The current conclusion is that the benefit in patient survival starts 3 months after surgery for SPK patients and 1 year after PTA and PAK transplantation, compared with patients on the waiting list.[34] Overall mortality after pancreas transplantation is not higher than mortality on the waiting list and for SPK transplantation is even decreased (hazard ratio [HR]: 0.29; CI: 0.27 to 0.33). At least 40% of patients die within the first 4 years waiting for SPK transplants, whereas only 10% die after the transplantation.[34] For PTA and PAK transplantation, 4-year survival is comparable to survival on the waiting list. For PTA and PAK, the most important factor for long-term patient survival is preservation of the pancreas graft (RR approximately 6 and 5 [for mortality]). However for SPK and PAK patients, kidney graft failure has a much stronger influence on mortality than pancreas graft loss (RR: 18 vs. 3 and 8 vs. 3, respectively).[8]

The benefit of patient survival after pancreas transplantation was confirmed also in an analysis of UNOS 25-year data: median patient survival was 14 years after SPK and solitary transplant, whereas only 3.7 and 7 years on waiting list, respectively.[35] The main causes of death after pancreas transplantation remain cardiac or cerebrovascular incidents (31%) and infection (24%). Infection peaks between 3 and 12 months after the transplantation.[8,36]

Graft Function (Graft Survival)

According to recent UNOS criteria, a patient is considered to have a graft failure when he or she is relisted, has a pancreas graft removed, has died, or needs more than

0.5 unit of insulin/kg body weight/day for 90 days.[8] Previously, transplant outcomes were assessed based on graft survival only in insulin-independent patients. Currently, we determine a presence of the *pancreas graft function* in those patients, who do not meet graft failure criteria (defined previously). In this way, those patients who require small amount of insulin support (often due to insulin resistance) are also included in the group of patients with present graft function.[8] Compared with the period of 2005–2009, in more recent years, pancreas 1-year graft function rate improved from 83% to 91% for SPK, and 81% to 86% for PAK and PTA.[8] Improvement was also observed in the 3-year follow-up and long-term results; half-life for SPK reached 15.5 years, for PAK 8 years, and nearly 7 years for PTA (Fig. 104.2).[8] To date, most recent 5-, 10-, and 20-year graft function were 80%, 68%, and 45% for SPK; 62%, 46%, and 16% for PAK; and 59%, 39%, and 12% for PTA, respectively.[37] Improvement in outcomes was attributed to better donor selection (lower pancreas donor risk index—primarily young trauma victims) and shorter cold ischemia time, as well as tendency to transplanting older recipients (especially for solitary pancreas transplant), and those with lower immunologic risk for rejection.[8] Improved outcomes are observed despite 48% of all SPK procedures being performed in low-volume centers (<5 pancreas transplants per year).[8]

Early technical failure rates (up to 90 days after transplant) related to portal vein thrombosis, bowel leak, bleeding, or infection are similar for all types of pancreas transplantation and approach 8%.[8] Primary graft nonfunction accounts for 4%.[8] Differences in long-term graft survival between SPK and PTA/PAK recipients are mainly caused by immunologic graft loss (acute or chronic rejection). One-year immunologic graft loss rate is 1.8% for SPK, 3.7% for PAK, and 6% for PTA.[38] The second leading cause of graft failure in SPK patients is death with a functioning graft. Loss because of chronic rejection increases with time and dominates in PTA and PAK.[8] In multifactorial analyses of registry data, deceased-donor factors and preservation time impacted outcomes the most. Grafts from younger trauma victims, with shorter preservation time, recipients on tacrolimus and MMF immunosuppression, and those operated on in high-volume centers had better graft survival. Interestingly, young recipients (<30 years old) had worse outcomes than older patients (RR: 1.25 to 2).[36] Bladder versus enteric drainage had no influence on graft survival.[36]

In case of pancreas transplant failure, pancreas retransplantations remain a viable option as long as the patient can tolerate another big surgery. It is more often the case after early graft loss that extensive vascular disease and heart conditions may preclude that option. Islet transplantation after failed pancreas transplantation after failed pancreas may be still a very beneficial procedure with minimal risk and great benefit of restoring improved glucose control in long term.[39]

Impact on the Health Status and Quality of Life of Patients

The effect of pancreas transplantation on diabetic complications and quality of life is often difficult to assess because complications are often too advanced to reverse.

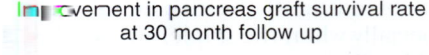

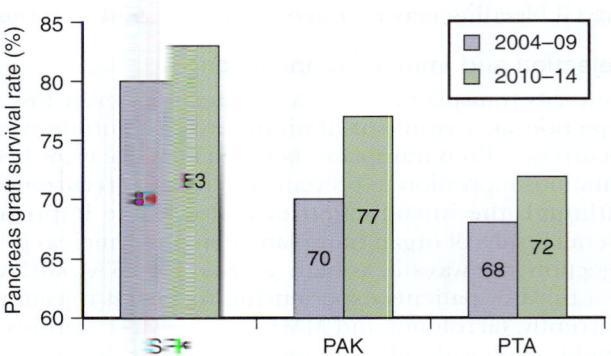

FIGURE 104.2 Improvement in primary deceased donor pancreas graft function in recent era (2010–2014) compared with previous one (2004–2009). Improvement was noticed in all 3 pancreas transplant categories: SKP, PTA, but the most for PAK (8%). *PAK,* Pancreas after kidney; *PTA,* pancreas transplant alone; *SPK,* simultaneous pancreas-kidney (Modified from Gruessner AC, Gruessner RW. Pancreas transplantation of US and non-US cases from 2005 to 2014 as reported to the United Network for Organ Sharing [UNOS] and the International Pancreas Transplant Registry [IPTR]. *Rev Diabet Stud.* 2016;13:35–58.)

In addition, SPK patients are usually younger and in better general health than PTA recipients. Furthermore, conclusions are not drawn from the 5% of SPK patients who die within the first year.[2] There are clear data that the quality of life improves when the patient has an uncomplicated postoperative course and good pancreas graft function. Cessation of insulin injections, removal of dietary constraints, and most importantly the fear about hypoglycemic episodes improve the quality of life in SPK patients and, to less degree, in PTA recipients. However, diabetic patients have also improved quality of life after they have a kidney transplant working, irrespective if they also received a pancreas graft. Nevertheless, successful PTA recipients also report improved quality of life despite surgery and the side effects of immunosuppression.[34] These improvements disappear after the patient develops a pancreas graft failure, serious complication, or serious side effects of immunosuppression.[40]

Glycemic Control

Successful pancreas transplantation restores a normoglycemic state in the majority of the patients immediately after pancreas implantation. Delayed onset of normoglycemia may occur because of organ injury caused by the donor's condition, preservation, extended preservation time, in transplants of a small pancreas into a large adult, or with insulin resistance. Abnormal glucose control may be caused also by complications (arterial or venous thrombosis of the graft, pancreatitis or rejection). Therefore blood glucose levels and insulin requirements should be closely observed in the postoperative period. After the pancreas recovers from perioperative stress, patients typically experience normal fasting and postprandial blood glucose concentrations. Results after glucose challenge are also similar to those who are nondiabetic.[41] However, the most important and long-term benefit is that pancreas transplantations fully protect the patient from disabling and life-threatening severe hypoglycemia unawareness episodes so that the patients can fearlessly resume normal life activities.

Retinopathy

Retinopathy can deteriorate in 10% to 35% of patients with unstable eye disease immediately after pancreas transplantation.[2] However, such complications are preventable if proper pretransplantation screening and treatment is applied. Most of the patients have already developed advanced retinopathy or blindness at the time of transplantation. The long-term effects of pancreas transplantation on diabetic retinopathy have been conflicting. Many early reports showed clear improvement, some found progression of retinal lesions,[42] others reported slower progression of vascular proliferation, improvement of retinal arterial flow velocities, and less need for laser therapy in SPK and PTA recipients.[43] In addition, post–pancreas grafting cataracts may develop or worsen because of calcineurin inhibitors and steroids.[2]

Nephropathy

In general, normoglycemia can stop the progression of diabetic nephropathy in kidneys and even partially reverse histologic changes secondary to diabetes in native kidneys, but the effect is only observed after a long time.[44] The time frame for this improvement is 5 to 10 years after pancreas engraftment, and many patients may never reach that time point and obtain this benefit.[45] Whether native renal function benefits from PTA is uncertain because the nephrotoxic effect of calcineurin inhibitor–based immunosuppression therapy must be considered. Despite the morphologic improvement and reduced urinary protein excretion, creatinine clearance usually gradually deteriorates. Although, according to IPTR data, 2% to 8% of PTA recipients develop end-stage renal failure (6% in 5 years after the transplant), a significant decrease in additional kidney transplant is noted, as well as improved function of previously transplanted kidney in PAK patients.[8,27,46]

Neuropathy

Polyneuropathy is a common complication of both IDDM and end-stage renal failure, and advanced motor, sensory, and autonomic neuropathies are frequently seen in patients undergoing whole pancreas transplantation. Early reports demonstrated that the motor and sensory nerve conduction indices increased significantly at all intervals after pancreas transplantation; however, the clinical examination and autonomic tests improved only slightly.[45] The impact of restored normoglycemia probably depends on the degree of degeneration before transplantation. In more advanced neuropathy, prevention from progression is observed. In those with mild neuropathy before transplantation, some degree of improvement may be observed.

Vascular Disease

Macrovascular disease naturally progresses with age, and it is difficult to observe any beneficial influence following pancreas transplantation. However, coronary atherosclerosis

can regress in nearly 40% of patients with functioning pancreas grafts.[47] Diastolic dysfunction can return to normal after 4 years.[48]

Stabilization and improvement of cardiac autonomic function have also been noted. Peripheral vascular disease is usually too advanced to see substantive improvement after pancreas transplant.

ISLET ALLOTRANSPLANTATION

After the pancreas is procured, it should be immediately shipped to the islet isolation laboratory (good manufacture practice [GMP] facility) to limit cold ischemia time and improve outcome.

ISLET ISOLATION

The pancreas is trimmed from surrounding tissue and blood vessels and then distended with cold enzyme (collagenase) through the pancreatic duct. An intact capsule of the pancreas allows for full distention of the organ and effective digestion in the next step. During enzymatic digestion, the pancreas dissociates into acinar (exocrine tissue) and islets. In the next step the enzymes are washed out of the collected tissue. The digested tissue is then purified to separate islets from acinar tissue. The final product, purified islets, are tested for bacterial contamination, level of endotoxin, and mycoplasma. Quality tests include purity (>40%), viability (intracellular staining assessed under microscope instantly), and stimulation index (an in vitro functional test assessing the response of the islets to high and low glucose concentration). The final criterion is a sufficient amount of islets after the isolation, so as to benefit the patient. The minimal amount based on previous experience is 5000 islet equivalents (IEQ)/kg body mass.[14] Islets may be infused fresh (just after the isolation) or after in vitro culture, usually up to 72 hours.

ISLET INFUSION INTO LIVER

Pancreatic islet allotransplantation, in contrast to whole-organ pancreas transplantation, is a minor procedure usually performed under local anesthesia in a radiology suite. The interventional radiologist first inserts a small (7-French) catheter under ultrasound and fluoroscopy guidance into the main portal vein through a percutaneous, transhepatic approach. Islets (usually 2 to 5 mL; up to 10-mL tissue pellet) are suspended in 200 to 400 mL solution (transplant media) with heparin and human albumin contained in a plastic infusion bag. The procedure starts with portal pressure measurements to ensure absence of portal hypertension. Next, islets are dripped slowly through the intravenous line connecting the harvested islet bag with the portal catheter. Portal pressure is measured at the midpoint and the conclusion of the infusion. Typically, the infusion, performed slowly, takes 30 to 45 minutes. Alternatively, it can be done under general anesthesia and in the operating room during a mini-laparotomy with infusion through the mesocolonic vein if percutaneous access via the portal vein fails. Postoperatively, subcutaneous heparin and insulin are administered for at least 2 weeks to promote islet engraftment.

COLLABORATIVE ISLETS TRANSPLANT REGISTRY

CITR was established by NIH in 2001 to collect, record, analyze, and report data about islet transplantation. To maintain integrity of the data, it is collected only from accredited centers, which meet all requirements and pass CITR audit. Currently, 32 centers in the United States report their own data to the CITR, as well as three centers from Europe, and another three from Australia. Yearly reports summarize the updated results.[15]

INFUSION-RELATED COMPLICATIONS

Infusion of islets into the portal vein usually causes transient transaminase elevation (2 to 5 times), but native liver or liver graft (in the case of simultaneous liver and islet transplantation) long-term dysfunction has not been reported.[15] Postinfusion portal vein thrombosis has been reported based on routine Doppler screening without clinical symptoms in 4% of cases. However, it has always resolved without any treatment.[49] Because the process of purification has been optimized, less tissue is infused, and currently, the risk for thrombosis is even lower. Intraabdominal bleeding was reported initially in 10% of patients.[5,49] However, when the access technique was optimized (smaller catheters, obliteration of the puncture tract), the risk for such a complication has been much decreased (3%).[15] In Edmonton—the most active single islet center in the world (more than 150 patients and more than 300 procedures), intraportal access and sealing off the tract was optimized, reducing risk of bleeding from 13% to close zero.[50,51] It allowed for more aggressive heparin use, which in combination with limited tissue pellet volume (below 5 mL) led to reduced risk of portal vein thrombosis close to zero as well (0 in last 101 procedures). Partial portal vein thrombosis is also very rare—3.7%, based on routine Doppler study on day 1 and 7.[51,52]

Immunosuppression

Since 2000, when the Edmonton group reported success of the corticosteroid-free immunosuppressive regimen, more than 90% of islet programs have followed the same protocol.[14] It consists of rapamycin-based therapy, with low doses of tacrolimus and anti-IL-2 receptor antibody (daclizumab) as induction therapy. Because islets were used in "brittle" type 1 diabetics with preserved kidney function, the main rationale was to improve islet survival and function (thus a steroid-free approach) and protect kidney function (calcineurin inhibitors were minimized). After 5 years of disappointing experience with this approach, many different protocols were developed. The most successful were those involving stronger immunosuppression, involving T-cell depletion induction therapy in the form of thymoglobulin, anti-CD52 antibody (alemtuzumab), or anti-CD3 humanized antibody. Another adjustment in immunosuppression has been a trend to move away from sirolimus (due to side affects profile) to use tacrolimus and MMF to improve outcomes tolerability and patient compliance.[50] Because the immunosuppression for islet transplant currently does not differ from that routinely used for other organ grafts, the side effects are also the same and not unexpected.

Allosensitization

Because pancreatic islet allotransplantation usually requires two or three islet infusions from the same number of different donors there is theoretically an increased risk for allosensitization. Clinical observation confirmed that when patients stop immunosuppression because of islet graft failure or side effects, as many as 70% of them develop donor-specific antibody and high panel-reactive antibody (PRA) (>50%).[53–55] However, reports show that as long as patients remain on adequate immunosuppression, the risk for donor-specific antibody and high PRA is small even after their fourth and fifth islet infusion.[54,56] In addition, data from islet registry showed that despite increased number of human leukocyte antigen (HLA) class I mismatches with each infusion, risk of sensitization remained the same as after one transplant.[57] Moreover, exposure to repeat HLA class I mismatch in second and third islet infusion resulted in less frequent development of de novo HLA class I antibodies compared with new class I mismatch. PRA greater than 20% increases risk for donor-specific antibodies and is associated with poor islet graft outcome.[57]

OUTCOME OF PANCREATIC ISLET ALLOTRANSPLANTATION

Graft Function and Insulin Dependence

Islet allotransplantation is an attractive alternative for pancreas transplantation as β-cell replacement therapy because it is a mini-invasive procedure and does not deal with the exocrine part of the pancreas and vascular anastomosis, limiting the risk for complications.

With the current technology, we are able to retrieve only 30% to 50% of original islet mass, even from the best cadaveric pancreas. It is also estimated that an additional 50% of islets are being destroyed by the native immunity instant blood-mediated inflammatory response.[58–61] Therefore first islet transplantation leads to lower insulin requirements in 40% to 60%, but it is much more important that it allows for instant improvement in glucose control, prevention of SHEs and hyperglycemia, and in the long term hypoglycemia unawareness which were main indications for transplant in those highly selected type 1 diabetic patients.[62] Quality of life is improved instantly, removing fear of the hypoglycemic coma, seizure, and sudden death from SHEs.[20] Therefore the primary endpoint for all islet transplant studies has been prevention of SHEs with improved glucose control of HbA1c at less than 6.5 to 7.[5,63] Partial islet function (which strongly correlates with detectable serum C-peptide) is sufficient to achieve such metabolic outcome. After 1 to 2 months, after islet engraftment is accomplished, the patient is offered subsequent transplant with a chance of additional benefit—insulin independence (secondary endpoint). If required later, patient may be offered supplemental islet infusions to maintain insulin independence. Of course, the ultimate goal of the current islet studies is to improve islet isolation and transplantation procedure to achieve insulin independence with only one infusion from a single donor routinely (currently 15% rate in Edmonton).[64] Because the number of patients is still limited in each study, cumulative results are reported by the CITR, which helps to analyze the data.[15] The most recent CITR report to date included data for 1999–2012 from 30 international islet centers (much less currently active) on 864 allogeneic islet transplant recipients (686 islet transplant alone, ITA, and 178 islet after or simultaneous with kidney, islet after kidney transplantation/simultaneous islet and kidney transplantation [IAK/SIK]), who received 1679 infusions from 2146 donors.[15,59] The North American sites contributed 60% and European and Australian sites 40% of the recipients. Combining the ITA and IAK/SIK recipients, 28% received a single islet infusion, 49% received two, 20% received three, and 3% received four to six infusions.[15]

Because islet transplantation still has status of experimental procedure in the United States, all CITR data come from different phase 1, 2 and 3 clinical studies sponsored by NIH, Juvenile Diabetes Research Foundation, or supported own islet center funding. Results from the more recent phase 3 NIH-sponsored trial involving eight North American centers have been published.[5] The primary endpoint (HbA$_{1c}$ <7 and freedom from SHEs) was achieved in 87.5% of patients at 1-year and 71% at 2-year follow-up, with median HbA$_{1c}$ of 5.6. Islet graft function (C-peptide positive) was preserved in 94% of patients with insulin independence rate of 51% at 1-year follow-up.[5] The insulin independence rate reported in the trial, as well as in CITR, is the average outcome of all participating centers, mixture of those more and much less experienced. As expected for a new and sophisticated procedure, there have been varied results among centers; therefore the average insulin independence rate might be seen as low. Those few, most experienced centers have reported much higher insulin independence rates, as high as 40% to 50% at 5-year follow-up.[50,65–69] Overall, approximately 70% to 90% of all islet recipients are estimated to have achieved insulin independence at some point. The median time to achievement of insulin independence was 6 to 7 months after the first transplant.[4]

Over the past 15 years, the protocols of the islet transplant studies have been changing, implementing novel approaches so that overall outcomes have been improving with time.[4] Safety was enhanced, toxicity of immunosuppression was reduced, and long-term graft function improved: 3-year insulin independence increased from 27% (1999–2002) to 44% (2007–2010) based on the islet registry.[4,50] In addition, durability of the islet transplant measured as serum C-peptide greater than 0.3 ng/mL (partial islet function) improved from 60% to greater than 90% 5 years after transplantation.[4] This result correlated with prevention of SHEs in those patients. The first-year islet reinfusion rate decreased from 66% to 48%.[4] Improved results are attributed to increasing experience of the centers, optimization of the donor selection and donor pancreas preservation, islet isolation technique, and introduction of islet culture prior to the infusion, as well as use of more potent immunosuppression based on T-cell depletion agents rather than IL-2 receptor antibody. Adding anti–tumor necrosis factor-alpha (anti–TNF-α) agents to T cell–depleting induction therapy allowed for an improved 3- to 5-year insulin independence rate to 50% to 62%, which was comparable with results for PTA (Fig. 104.3).[3,4] Interestingly, the beneficial effect of T cell–depleting properties of thymoglobulin was observed only when anti-TNF-α agent was applied simultaneously.[3] The results indicate a positive trend that islet transplantation may be as effective as whole pancreas grafts, with the advantage of harboring less risk of complications. Results from the Edmonton group confirm this observation, and they also have data indicating that supplemental fourth and fifth islet infusions performed a few years after the initial ones may be an effective option for patients, without carrying an additional risk of portal vein thrombosis or appearance of PRA.[56] Long-term observations also confirm that selected patients may have preserved islet function for more than 10 years, protecting them from SHEs without serious adverse effects of immunosuppression.[63,69] In addition, for those patients who failed islet transplantation, subsequent SPK or solitary pancreas transplantation remains a viable option. Analysis of IPTR/UNOS data revealed that pancreas after islet (PAI) is a safe procedure, comparable with primary pancreas transplantation with low recipient mortality and high graft function rates in both short- and long-term and excellent kidney function.[39,70]

Patient Survival

There have been 25 reports of death to the CITR for islet allograft recipients, for 2.4% crude mortality over a mean of 6.7 years elapsed follow-up per patient (including

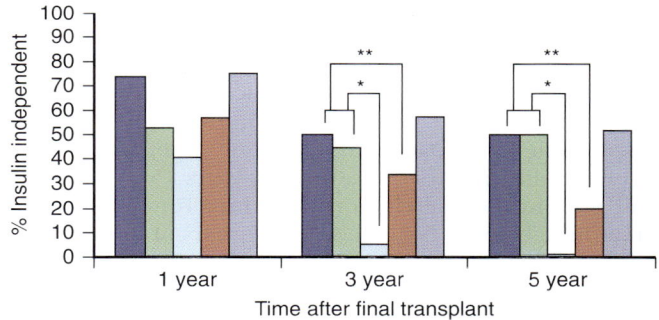

Ns	1 year	3 year	5 year
Group 1 (UMN)	27	22	20
Group 2 (TCDAb+TNF-α)	17	11	4
Group 3 (TCDAb−TNF-α)	34	17	7
Group 4 (IL2RAb)	171	146	105

FIGURE 104.3 Observed insulin independence of recipients of pancreas transplant alone and in islet transplant alone, based on induction immunosuppression administered. Islet transplant groups are indicated as follows: group 1 (University of Minnesota [UMN] recipients; *dark purple*), group 2 (Collaborative Islet Transplant Registry [CITR] recipients receiving T cell depleting antibody [TCDAb] + TNF-α; *green*), group 3 (CITR recipients receiving TCDAb without TNF-α; *light blue*), group 4 (CITR recipients receiving IL-2RAb; *maroon*), group 5 (pancreas transplant alone recipients; *light purple*). Insulin independence was superior in groups 1 and 2 compared with groups 3 and 4 at 3 and 5 years post transplant; groups 1 and 2 did not differ statistically from pancreas transplant alone (group 5).*P < .01; **P ≤ .05. *IL*, Interleukin; *TNF*, tumor necrosis factor. (From Bellin MD, Barton FB, Heitman A, et al. Potent induction immunotherapy promotes long-term insulin independence after islet transplantation in type I diabetes. *Am J Transplant*. 2012;12:1576–1583.)

periods after complete graft failure and loss to observed follow-up). Causes of death were (number of cases): cardiovascular (5), hemorrhage (3), pneumonia (2), diabetic ketoacidosis (1), infection (1), respiratory arrest (1), acute toxicity (1), pneumopathy (1), multiorgan failure of unknown etiology (1), viral meningitis (1), and lung cancer (1). The remaining seven deaths did not have a cause specified.[15]

Kidney Function

Although initial Edmonton protocol implemented sirolimus to avoid nephrotoxicity, subsequently this agent-related heavy proteinuria compromised kidney function. Even low-dose tacrolimus compromised renal function especially in patients with preexisting renal impairment.[50] Three out of 138 (2%) islet transplant patients in Edmonton end up requiring dialysis within 12 years.[50] However, a crossover study from Vancouver showed that renal dysfunction progresses more rapidly despite optimal insulin treatment in labile type 1 diabetic patients on a waiting list for islet transplant than in patients after islet transplant on full dosages of tacrolimus as maintenance immunosuppression therapy.[71,72] Among patients with more than 3 years of follow-up, the decline in glomerular filtration rate (GFR) was 3.55 mL/min per year in the medically treated group, whereas it was 1.4 mL/min per year in the islet transplant group ($P < .0001$).[72] The average HbA$_{1c}$ in those patients was 6.7 versus 7.8 in islet versus medical group, respectively. Of note, most studies report some degree of kidney dysfunction without distinction of the islet graft function and long-term glucose control, implicating that only toxic effects of immunosuppression are responsible for impairment. Our four patients, who have been insulin free for more than 5 years (5 to 11 years) still present completely normal kidney function (serum creatinine below 1 mg/mL) despite years of immunosuppression including tacrolimus or rapamycin.[6]

Retinopathy

In the same crossover study in Vancouver, none of the patients after islet transplant had progression of retinopathy or required eye surgery, whereas in the medical group, there was substantial progression of the eye disease and need for surgery.[71,72] Similar observation with stabilization of the retinal disease and occasional improvement can be found in other reports.[15,50,69,72–74]

Neuropathy

Improved glycemic control after islet transplantation leads to improvement or stabilization of neuropathy in more than 50% of patients.[73] These observations are exciting because they were made after only a 2-year follow-up. Similar observations were reported in Edmonton, Vancouver, and Chicago.[69,75,76]

PATIENT SELECTION

Results of pancreas, as well as islet, transplantation constantly evolve, so algorithms for β-cell replacement therapy should be constantly updated. Nevertheless, medical indications for pancreas and islet transplantation remain the same.

Pancreas transplant candidates must be in good medical condition to safely survive major surgery. There is no age limit for pancreas transplantation. Younger patients have higher rates of rejection, but those older than 50 years of age have higher postoperative complication rates.

The most appropriate type of pancreas transplant depends on patient comorbidity, renal function, and availability of living or cadaveric donor. Patients with hypoglycemic unawareness and stable kidney function (GFR, 80 to 100 mL/min per 1.73 m²) may be candidates for PTA or ITA depending on whether the patient can tolerate major surgery. However, 3% to 30% of those patients will require a kidney transplant in 9 to 10 years because of calcineurin-inhibitor nephrotoxicity, which is an independent risk factor for progression of kidney failure.[2] The rate range is wide because timing and risk of progression strongly depends on kidney function prior to transplant (baseline) and pancreas/islet graft function afterward, indicating how well the glucose was controlled. Patients with a GFR of less than 50 to 60 mL/min per 1.73 m² prior to transplant will likely need a kidney graft before, with, or soon after the pancreas. Of course, preemptive LDKT would be the best option for these patients. If a patient has a GFR less than 80 mL/min per 1.73 m², then they should be prepared to need a kidney graft in the future.

SPK transplantation would be the best option for uremic type 1 diabetics because long-term results are the best for combined kidney and pancreas grafts. However, because of the shortage of deceased-donor organs, instead of waiting long on dialysis for proper organs and developing complications, a better option is to have a preemptive LDKT followed by deceased-donor pancreas transplant. Immediate results of PAK transplantation in such situations are good because the patient has never been uremic. Patient survival for LDKT and SPK transplantation are comparable.[2]

SUMMARY

Both pancreas and islet transplantation offers the advantage of improved glucose control, preventing, reversing, or halting progression of secondary diabetic complications, as well as improved quality of life in properly selected patients with justified lifelong immunosuppression.[46] Both procedures are complementary and use distinct deceased-donor group population, expanding the donor pool and availability of β-cell replacement therapy. Islet transplantation provides an advantage of being a minimally invasive procedure, especially to patients with contraindication for major surgery, whereas pancreas transplantation delivers instant and more durable endocrine effects.[77] To extend benefits of β-cell replacement therapy, islet transplantation can be an effective treatment option for patients who failed previous pancreas transplants; in addition, pancreas transplantation can successfully restore insulin independence in those who failed islet transplants.[46]

REFERENCES

1. The Diabetes Control and Complications Trial Research Group. The effect of intensive treatment of diabetes on the development and progression of long-term complications in insulin-dependent diabetes mellitus. *N Engl J Med.* 1993;329:977.

2. White SA, Shaw JA, Sutherland DE. Pancreas transplantation. *Lancet.* 2009;373:1808.
3. Bellin MD, Barton FB, Heitman A, et al. Potent induction immunotherapy promotes long-term insulin independence after islet transplantation in type I diabetes. *Am J Transplant.* 2012;12(6):1576-1583.
4. Barton FB, Rickels MR, Alejandro R, et al. Improvement in outcomes of clinical islet transplantation: 1999-2010. *Diabetes Care.* 2012;35(7):1436-1445.
5. Hering BJ, Clarke WR, Bridge ND, et al. Phase 3 trial of transplantation of human islets in type 1 diabetes complicated by severe hypoglycemia. *Diabetes Care.* 2016;39(7):1230-1240.
6. Kelly WD, Lillehei RC, Merkel FK, Idezuki Y, Goetz FC. Allotransplantation of the pancreas and duodenum along with the kidney in diabetic nephropathy. *Surgery.* 1967;61:827.
7. Stratta RJ, Fridell AJ, Gruessner AC, Odorico JS, Gruessner RW. Pancreas transplantation: a decade of decline. *Curr Opin Organ Transplant.* 2016;21(4):386-392.
8. Gruessner AC, Gruessner RW. Pancreas transplantation of US and non-US cases from 2005 to 2014 as reported to the United Network for Organ Sharing (UNOS) and the International Pancreas Transplant Registry (IPTR). *Rev Diabet Stud.* 2016;13(1):35-58.
9. Moskalewski S. Isolation and culture of the islets of Langerhans of the guinea pig. *Gen Comp Endocrinol.* 1965;44:342.
10. Lacy PE, Kostianovsky M. Method for the isolation of intact islets of Langerhans from the rat pancreas. *Diabetes.* 1967;16:35.
11. Scharp DW, Murphy JJ, Newton WT, Ballinger WF, Lacy PE. Transplantation of islets of Langerhans in diabetic rhesus monkeys. *Surgery.* 1975;77:100.
12. Najarian JS, Sutherland DE, Matas AJ, Steffes MW, Simmons RL, Goetz FC. Human islet transplantation: a preliminary report. *Transplant Proc.* 1977;9:233.
13. Tzakis AG, Ricordi C, Alejandro R, et al. Pancreatic islet transplantation after upper abdominal exenteration and liver replacement. *Lancet.* 1990;336:402.
14. Shapiro AM, Lakey JR, Ryan EA, et al. Islet transplantation in seven patients with type 1 diabetes mellitus using a glucocorticoid-free immunosuppressive regimen. *N Engl J Med.* 2000;343:230.
15. Collaborative Islet Transplant Registry (CITR). http://www.citregistry.org/.
16. Leeser DB, Bartlett ST. Pancreas transplantation. In: Yeo CJ, Dempsey DT, Klein AS, et al., eds. *Shackelford's Surgery of the Alimentary Tract.* 6th ed. Philadelphia Saunders; 2005:113.
17. Gruessner AC, Sutherland DE. Access to pancreas transplantation should not be restricted because of age: invited commentary on Schenker et al. *Transpl Int.* 2011;24(2):134-135.
18. Weems P, Cooper M. Pancreas transplantation in type II diabetes mellitus. *World J Transplant.* 2014;4(4):216-221.
19. OPTN/UNOS Policy. https://optn.transplant.hrsa.gov/media/1200/optn_policies.pdf#nameddest=Policy_11.
20. Anders A, Kin T, O'Gorman D, et al. Clinical islet isolation and transplantation outcomes with deceased cardiac death donors are similar to neurological determination of death donors. *Transpl Int.* 2016;29(1):34-40.
21. O'Gorman D, Kin T, Murdoch T, et al. The standardization of pancreatic donors for islet isolations. *Transplantation.* 2005;80:801.
22. Boggi U, Amorese G, Marchetti P. Surgical techniques for pancreas transplantation. *Curr Opin Organ Transplant.* 2010;15:102.
23. Sutherland DE, Goetz FC, Najarian JS. Living-related donor segmental pancreatectomy for transplantation. *Transplant Proc.* 1980;12:19.
24. Sutherland DE, Radosevich D, Gruessner R, Gruessner A, Kandaswamy R. Pushing the envelope: living donor pancreas transplantation. *Curr Opin Organ Transplant.* 2012;17(1):106-115.
25. Kirchner VA, Finger EB, Bellin MD, et al. Long-term outcomes for Living Pancreas donors in the modern era. *Transplantation.* 2016;100(6):1322-1328.
26. Kobayashi T, Gruessner AC, Wakai T, Sutherland DE. Three types of simultaneous pancreas and kidney transplantation. *Transplant Proc.* 2014;46(3):948-953.
27. University of Minnesota: International Pancreas Transplant Registry (IPTR). http://www.iptr.umn.edu/.
28. Troppmann C. Complications after pancreas transplantation. *Curr Opin Organ Transplant.* 2010;15:112.
29. Chandra J, Phillips RR, Boardman P, Gleeson FV, Anderson EM. Pancreas transplants. *Clin Radiol.* 2009;54:714.
30. Tyden G, Bolinder J, Solders G, Brattström C, Tibell A, Groth CG. Improved survival in patients with insulin-dependent diabetes mellitus and end-stage diabetic nephropathy 10 years after combined pancreas and kidney transplantation. *Transplantation.* 1999;67:645.
31. Reddy KS, Stablein D, Taranto S, et al. Long-term survival following simultaneous kidney-pancreas transplantation versus kidney transplantation alone in patients with type 1 diabetes mellitus and renal failure. *Am J Kidney Dis.* 2003;41:464.
32. Ojo AO, Meier-Kriesche HU, Hanson JA, et al. The impact of simultaneous pancreas-kidney transplantation on long-term patient survival. *Transplantation.* 2001;71:82.
33. Venstrom JM, McBride MA, Rother KI, Hirshberg B, Orchard TJ, Harlan DM. Survival after pancreas transplantation in patients with diabetes and preserved kidney function. *J Am Med Assoc.* 2003;290:2817.
34. Gruessner RW, Sutherland DE, Gruessner AC. Mortality assessment for pancreas transplants. *Am J Transplant.* 2004;4:2018.
35. Rana A, Gruessner A, Agopian VG, et al. Survival benefit of solid-organ transplant in the United States. *JAMA Surg.* 2015;150(3):252-259.
36. Gruessner AC, Sutherland DE, Gruessner RW. Pancreas transplantation in the United States: a review. *Curr Opin Organ Transplant.* 2010;15:93.
37. Gruessner AC, Sutherland DE, Gruessner RW. Long-term outcome after pancreas transplantation. *Curr Opin Organ Transplant.* 2012;17(1):100-105.
38. Gruessner A. 2011 update on pancreas transplantation: comprehensive trend analysis of 25,000 cases followed up over the course of twenty-four years at the International Pancreas Transplant Registry (IPTR). *Rev Diabet Stud.* 2011;8(1):6-16.
39. Anders A, Livingstone S, Kin T, et al. Islet-after-failed-pancreas and pancreas-after-failed-islet transplantation: two complementary rescue strategies to control diabetes. *Islets.* 2015;7(6):e1126036.
40. Sutherland DE, Gruessner RW, Dunn DL, et al. Lessons learned from more than 1,000 pancreas transplants at a single institution. *Ann Surg.* 2001;233:463.
41. Larsen JL. Pancreas transplantation: indications and consequences. *Endocr Rev.* 2004;25:919.
42. Ramsay RC, Goetz FC, Sutherland DE, et al. Progression of diabetic retinopathy after pancreas transplantation for insulin-dependent diabetes mellitus. *N Engl J Med.* 1988;318:208.
43. Dean PG, Kudva YC, Stegall MD. Long-term benefits of pancreas transplantation. *Curr Opin Organ Transplant.* 2008;13:85.
44. Fioretto P, Steffes MW, Sutherland DE, Goetz FC, Mauer M. Reversal of lesions of diabetic nephropathy after pancreas transplantation. *N Engl J Med.* 1998;339:69.
45. Navarro X, Sutherland DE, Kennedy WR. Long-term effects of pancreatic transplantation on diabetic neuropathy. *Ann Neurol.* 1997;42:727.
46. Gruessner RW, Gruessner AC. Pancreas transplantation alone: a procedure coming of age. *Diabetes Care.* 2013;36(8):2440-2447.
47. Stratta RJ. Mortality after vascularized pancreas transplantation. *Surgery.* 1998;124:823.
48. La Rocca E, Fiorina P, di Carlo V, et al. Cardiovascular outcomes after kidney-pancreas and kidney-alone transplantation. *Kidney Int.* 2001;60:1964.
49. Ryan EA, Paty BW, Senior PA, et al. Five-year follow-up after clinical islet transplantation. *Diabetes.* 2005;54:2060.
50. Senior PA, Kin T, Shapiro J, Koh A. Islet transplantation at the university of Alberta: status update and review of progress over the last decade. *Can J Diabetes.* 2012;36:32-37.
51. Villiger P, Ryan EA, Owen R, et al. Prevention of bleeding after islet transplantation: lessons learned from a multivariate analysis of 132 cases at a single institution. *Am J Transplant.* 2005;5(12):2992-2998.
52. Kawahara T, Kin T, Kashkoush S, et al. Portal vein thrombosis is a potentially preventable complication in clinical islet transplantation. *Am J Transplant.* 2011;11(12):2700-2707.
53. Rickels MR, Kearns J, Markmann E, et al. HLA sensitization in islet transplantation. *Clin Transpl.* 2006;413.
54. Cardani R, Pileggi A, Ricordi C, et al. Allosensitization of islet allograft recipients. *Transplantation.* 2007;84:1413.
55. Campbell PM, Senior PA, Salam A, et al. High risk of sensitization after failed islet transplantation. *Am J Transplant.* 2007;7:2311.
56. Koh A, Imes S, Kin T, et al. Supplemental islet infusions restore insulin independence after graft dysfunction in islet transplant recipients. *Transplantation.* 2010;89:361.

57. Naziruddin B, Wease S, Stablein D, et al. HLA class I sensitization in islet transplant recipients: report from the Collaborative Islet Transplant Registry. *Cell Transplant.* 2012;21(5):901-908.

58. Otsuki K, Ito T, Kenmochi T, et al. Positron emission tomography and autoradiography of (18)F-Fluorodeoxyglucose labeled islet with or without warm ischemic stress in portal transplanted rats. *Transplant Proc.* 2016;48(1):229-233.

59. Pepper AR, Gala-Lopez B, Ziff O, Shapiro AJ. Current status of clinical islet transplantation. *World J Transplant.* 2013;3(4):48-53.

60. Eich T, Eriksson O, Lundgren T, Nordic Network for Clinical Islet Transplantation. Visualization of early engraftment in clinical islet transplantation by positron-emission tomography. *N Engl J Med.* 2007;356(26):2754-2755.

61. Korsgren O, Lundgren T, Felldin M, et al. Optimizing islet engraftment is critical for successful clinical islet transplantation. *Diabetologia.* 2008;51(2):227-232.

62. Rickels MR, Fuller C, Dalton-Baker C, et al. Restoration of glucose counterregulation by islet transplantation in long-standing type I diabetes. *Diabetes.* 2015;64(5):1713-1718.

63. Brennan DC, Kopetskie HA, Sayre PH, et al. Long-term follow-up of the Edmonton protocol of islet transplantation in the United States. *Am J Transplant.* 2016;16(2):509-517.

64. Koh A, Senior P, Salam A, et al. Insulin-heparin infusions peritransplant substantially improve single-donor clinical islet transplant success. *Transplantation.* 2010;89(4):465-471.

65. Shapiro AM. Islet transplantation in type 1 diabetes: ongoing challenges, refined procedures, and long-term outcome. *Rev Diabet Stud.* 2012;9(4):385-406.

66. Bellin MD, Kandaswamy R, Parkey J, et al. Prolonged insulin independence after islet allotransplants in recipient with type 1 diabetes. *Am J Transplant.* 2008;8(11):2463-2470.

67. Posselt AM, Szot GL, Frassetto LA, et al. Islet transplantation in type 1 diabetic patients using calcineurin inhibitor-free immunosuppressive protocols based on T-cell adhesion or costimulation blockade. *Transplantation.* 2010;90(12):1595-1601.

68. Gangemi A, Salehi P, Hatipoglu B, et al. Islet transplantation for brittle type 1 diabetes the UIC protocol. *Am J Transplant.* 2008;8(6):1250-1261.

69. Tekin Z, Garfinkel MR, Chon WJ, et al. Outcomes of pancreatic islet allotransplantation using the Edmonton protocol at the university of Chicago. *Transplant Direct.* 2016;2(10):e105.

70. Gruessner RW, Grusnner AC. Pancreas after islets transplantation: a first report of the International Pancreas Transplant Registry. *Am J Transplan.* 2016;16(2):688-693.

71. Warnock GL, Thompson DM, Meloche RM, et al. A multi-year analysis of islet transplantation compared with intensive medical therapy on progression of complications in type 1 diabetes. *Transplantation.* 2008;86:1762.

72. Thompson DM, Meloche M, Ao Z, et al. Reduced progression of diabetic microvascular complications with islet cell transplantation compared with intensive medical therapy. *Transplantation.* 2011;91(3):373-378.

73. Lee TC, Barshes NR, O'Mahony CA, et al. The effect of pancreatic islet transplantation on progression of diabetic retinopathy and neuropathy. *Transplant Proc.* 2005;37:2263.

74. Koh A, Rudnisky C, Tennant M. Positive effects of clinical islet transplantation on diabetic retinopathy over 5 years. *Diabetes.* 2011;60(1):A205.

75. Albaker W, Koh A, Ryan EA, et al. Diabetic peripheral neuropathy is stabilized after clinical islet transplantation: 7 year follow-up study. *J Clin Endocrinol Metab.* 2008;93(S1):OR26-2.

76. Fenson B, Al Mehthel M, Ao Z, Thompson SE, Warnock GL, Thompson DM. Islet cell transplantation improves diabetic neuropathy compared with intensive medical therapy. *Diabetes.* 2014;63:A22-A22.

77. Gruessner RW, Gruessner AC. What defines success in pancreas and islet transplantation—insulin independence or prevention of hypoglycemia? A review. *Transplant Proc.* 2014;46(6):1898-1899.

Prevention and Management of Complications of Pancreatic Surgery

Mark P. Callery | Manuel Castillo-Angeles | Tara Sotsky Kent

Mortality after pancreatic resection has greatly decreased in comparison with historical series, from 33% following Whipple's initial reports to currently less than 2% in most high-volume centers,[1] resulting in the recognition that assessment of surgical quality for these high-acuity patients warrants further refinement.[1] Birkmeyer et al. have demonstrated the impact of hospital volume on actual operative mortality for pancreatic cancer resections, among other high-acuity operations,[2] but these two measures accounted for only half of the hospital-level variation in mortality. Moreover, van der Geest et al. found that the volume-outcome relationship persists in the highest-volume centers (≥40 procedures annually),[3] yet overall morbidity remains high for pancreatic resections, in the range of 35% to 55%.[1,4] Previously published outcomes after pancreatic resection in a high-volume institution are demonstrated in Table 105.1; the three most common complications were delayed gastric emptying (DGE) in 14%, wound infection in 7%, and pancreatic fistula in 5%.[5] This chapter will also discuss postpancreatectomy hemorrhage (PPH).

Initial efforts to better understand perioperative mortality after pancreatic resection demonstrated the impact of hospital volume on outcome, with a threefold to fourfold greater operative mortality at low-volume hospitals versus high-volume hospitals.[6–8] Fong et al. also demonstrate an ongoing survival benefit (6% at 2 years) for patients undergoing pancreatic cancer resection at a high-volume institution.[8] A recent single-institution study reports that higher surgeon volume is associated with shorter operative time, less intraoperative blood loss, and higher lymph node harvest (for cancer cases).[9] However, surgeon experience mitigated these differences, with experienced surgeons (>50 pancreaticoduodenectomies [PDs]) having significantly lower morbidity compared with less experienced surgeons and, in particular, less blood loss, shorter operative time, and a lower postoperative pancreatic fistula (POPF) rate.[9] Twenty PDs were required to equalize the experienced and inexperienced surgeons. However, adequacy of oncologic resection did not differ based on experience.

This chapter will focus on technical and clinical means of preventing and managing pancreatic surgical complications, but the import of surgeon and hospital volume, as well as experience, on complication and overall outcome after pancreatic resection should not be lost on the reader. Schmidt et al. also emphasize the importance of the institution's systems support for the diagnosis and management of postoperative complications (i.e., interventional radiology and gastroenterology, intensive care, and surgical team members).[9]

POSTPANCREATECTOMY HEMORRHAGE

Hemorrhage associated with pancreatic resection (PPH) occurs in up to 8% of cases but may account for 11% to 38% of mortality.[10–13] Because of the potential consequences of this problem, a consensus definition was developed by the International Study Group of Pancreatic Surgery (ISGPS) in 2007[14] and is seen in Table 105.2. This definition was validated and has been found to correlate well with duration of hospital stay, morbidity, and mortality.[13] It may occur intraoperatively, early in the postoperative period, or late (more than 24 hours postoperatively). Intraoperative hemorrhage may be more likely to occur in the event of aberrant vasculature particularly when not preoperatively identified.[15] Fig. 105.1 demonstrates normal peripancreatic vasculature, as seen on computed tomography (CT) angiography.[15] The common variations include a replaced right hepatic artery (11% to 21%), replaced left hepatic artery (4% to 10%), accessory right or left hepatic artery (<1% to 8%), and celiac artery stenosis (2% to 8%).[15]

Intraoperative vascular complications are known to adversely affect ultimate outcome,[16] including in-hospital mortality and survival rate; thus efforts to delineate vasculature preoperatively by means of a pancreatic protocol CT including arterial, venous, and portal venous phases[15] should allow the surgeon to be better prepared intraoperatively and limit the occurrence of intraoperative hemorrhage related to an unexpected encounter with abnormal vascular anatomy. These efforts should continue intraoperatively by inspection and palpation of the operative field to further define the vascular anatomy. For example, a replaced right hepatic artery may be appreciated by palpation of a pulse posterior and lateral to the bile duct and portal vein. Intraoperative hemorrhage may also occur in the setting of tumor infiltration that involves the relevant vasculature.

To obtain intraoperative control of hemorrhage, direct pressure should be applied initially to allow for mobilization of appropriate anesthetic and surgical resources, such as blood products, vascular sutures, and clamps, and appropriate surgical assistance. Aberrant vasculature, such as a replaced right hepatic artery, may need to be reconstructed or anastomosed to an alternate vessel to preserve hepatic arterial blood flow. Doppler ultrasonography may be useful to determine whether there is already alternate arterial flow. Venous injuries may be able to be addressed with venorrhaphy or with patch venoplasty. In exsanguinating, uncontrolled hemorrhage, portal vein ligation has been described, with a potential for survival, when accompanied by a "second-look" laparotomy in 24 hours

TABLE 105.1 Mortality and Morbidity After Pancreaticoduodenectomy and Distal Pancreatectomy in 616 Patients

	Overall (N = 616)	Pancreaticoduodenectomy/Total Pancreatectomy (n = 564)	Distal Pancreatectomy (n = 52)	P Value
Perioperative mortality	2.3%	2.3%	1.9%	NS
Overall complications	30%	31%	25%	NS
SPECIFIC COMPLICATIONS				
Reoperation	3%	3%	4%	NS
Delayed gastric emptying	—	14%	—	—
Cholangitis	—	3%	—	—
Bile leak	—	2%	—	—
Wound infection	7%	7%	5%	NS
Pancreatic fistula	5%	5%	8%	NS
Intraabdominal abscess	3%	3%	4%	NS
Pneumonia	1%	1%	0%	NS
Pancreatitis	1%	1%	0%	NS
POSTOPERATIVE LENGTH OF STAY				
Mean ± SE	13.7 ± 0.4 days	14.0 ± 0.4 days	11.5 ± 2.2 days	.08
Median	11 days	11 days	7 days	—

NS, Not significant.
From Sohn TA, Yeo CJ, Cameron JL, et al. Resected adenocarcinoma of the pancreas—616 patients: results, outcomes, and prognostic indicators. *J Gastrointest Surg.* 2000;4:567.

TABLE 105.2 Classification of PPH: Clinical Condition and Diagnostic and Therapeutic Consequences

Grade	Time of Onset, Location, Severity and Clinical Impact of Bleeding		Clinical Condition	Diagnostic Consequence	Therapeutic Consequence
A	Early, intraluminal or extraluminal, mild	—	Well	Observation, blood count, ultrasonography and, if necessary, computed tomography	No
B	Early, intraluminal or extraluminal, severe	Late, intraluminal or extraluminal, mild*	Often well/ intermediate, very rarely life-threatening	Observation, blood count, ultrasonography, computed tomography, angiography, endoscopy	Transfusion of fluid/blood, intermediate care unit (or ICU), therapeutic endoscopy,[†] embolization, relaparotomy for early PPH
C		Late, intraluminal or extraluminal, severe	Severely impaired, life-threatening	Angiography, computed tomography, endoscopy[†]	Localization of bleeding, angiography and embolization (endoscopy[†]), *or* relaparotomy, ICU

*Late, intraluminal or extraluminal, mild bleeding may not be immediately life-threatening to patient but may be a warning sign for later severe hemorrhage ("sentinel bleed") and is therefore grade B.
[†]Endoscopy should be performed when signs of intraluminal bleeding are present (melena, hematemesis, or blood loss via nasogastric tube).
ICU, Intensive care unit; *PPH,* postpancreatectomy hemorrhage.
From Wente MN, Veit JA, Bassi C, et al. Postpancreatectomy hemorrhage (PPH)—an International Study Group of Pancreatic Surgery definition. *Surgery.* 2007;142:20.

to evaluate for signs of ischemia.[17] A more recent paper reports on a small series of patients undergoing damage control laparotomy (DCL) for pancreatic surgery,[18] primarily for portal vein injury, with the goal of allowing intensive care unit (ICU) resuscitation to reverse the accompanying hypothermia, acidosis, and coagulopathy. They describe initial venous compression to allow for identification/visualization of the site of injury, as well as for preparation of the surgical and anesthetic teams. Useful maneuvers for compression included the Kocher maneuver and sponge sticks. The pancreas was then divided and the specimen quickly extirpated when possible. Other

techniques used to shorten operating time included external drainage, packing, stapled bowel closure, and rapid abdominal closure.[18] The authors emphasize that there was significant resource use but no mortality. Other risk factors for PPH have been identified including age, pancreatic fistula, pancreatoduodenectomy, and the nutritional risk index (NRI).[16]

Management of early and late PPH is addressed by the ISGPS classification schema.[13,14] Early PPH is most often a result of technical failure to achieve appropriate hemostasis at the index operation or else secondary to underlying coagulopathy. When significant and thought to be technical

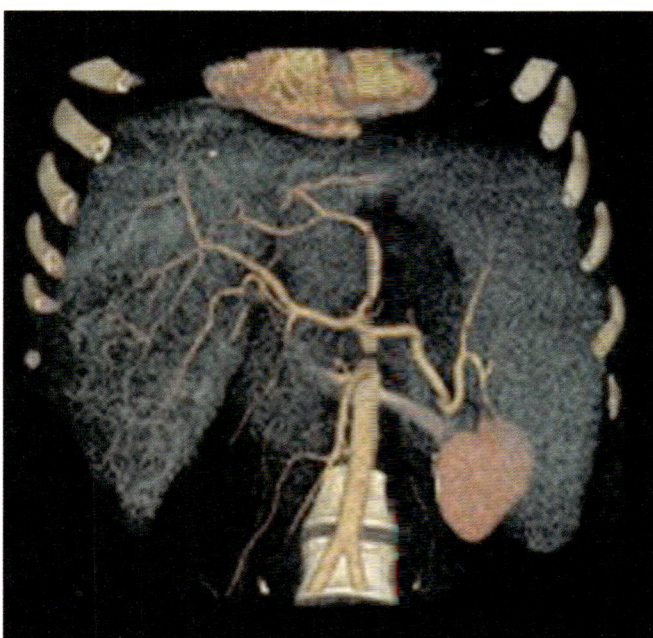

FIGURE 105.1 Computed tomography angiography of normal peripancreatic arterial anatomy. (From Shukla PJ, Barreto SG, Kulkarni A, Nagarajan G, Fingerhut A. Vascular anomalies encountered during pancreatoduodenectomy: do they influence outcomes? *Ann Surg Oncol*. 2010;17 133.)

failure, prompt relaparotomy is mandated.[19] PPH occurring later than the first postoperative day and up to several weeks postoperatively is often a result of other postoperative complications, such as fistula, anastomotic ulceration, or pseudoaneurysm.[11,14,20] PPH may represent bleeding from intraluminal or extraluminal sources: unsecured vessels, vessels with pseudoaneurysm, anastomotic suture lines or ulceration, resection cut surfaces, or hemobilia. Named vascular structures that may be the source of bleeding are the gastroduodenal, hepatic, or splenic artery, branches of the superior mesenteric artery, or the splenic vein stump.[13,14] The classification system for PPH is described in Table 105.2.

After PPH becomes apparent, evaluation must occur in a timely fashion and may include a variety of modalities depending on the hemodynamic status of the patient and apparent location of the bleeding (intraluminal or extraluminal): endoscopy, angiography, CT scan, or reoperation.[14] Early extraluminal PPH requires reexploration. Intraluminal bleeding may manifest as extraluminal if there is associated anastomotic breakdown,[13] and this may be amenable to angiographic intervention when involving the pancreaticojejunostomy. Bleeding from the gastrojejunostomy or duodenojejunostomy may first be excluded by endoscopy. Over time, conservative management has become more successful for late PPH but surgical intervention has continued to be the mainstay of treatment. Mortality in patients with late PPH is much higher than for the routine pancreatic resection with rates of 16% to 27%,[13–21] but is strongly associated with a bleed in the setting of a septic complication, such as pancreatic fistula. Patients present with septic complications and/or a sentinel

bleed. Radiographic embolization has become a more successful modality, with up to 80% success,[13] but is limited by the initially intermittent nature of the bleeding.[20] Furthermore, key factors are the recognition of the sentinel bleed, the presence of pancreatic fistula, and a long gastroduodenal artery stump with radiopaque marker for an effective embolization.[21] Reexploration is indicated when angiographic intervention is not technically feasible or successful or when the site is not visualized on angiography and the patient is hemodynamically unstable.[13]

PANCREATIC FISTULA

POPF continues to be the nemesis of pancreatic resection. Occurring in up to 33% of cases, even in the setting of vast improvements in the safety and efficacy of pancreatic surgery overall as mentioned earlier, fistula rates have failed to decrease significantly.[22–24] One must first recall the definition of *fistula* as "an abnormal communication from one epithelialized surface to another" compared with that of *leakage*, referring to "an abnormal escape of fluid through an orifice or opening."[23]

In addition, POPF occurs with the leakage of amylase-rich fluid from the transection margin of the gland and/or from the pancreatic-enteric anastomosis. Although many literature reports have been devoted to studying the diagnosis, management, and effect of POPF on patient outcome, comparison of these studies has been difficult because there was previously no uniform definition available. To better understand POPF, the ISGPF developed a classification scheme that is presented in Table 105.3.[25] POPF was defined as inclusive of all peripancreatic fluid collections, abscesses, leaks, or fistulas and diagnosed by virtue of drain amylase, output, imaging, and clinical picture (well versus septic).[25] According to the classification scheme, grade A fistulas are biochemical only and not clinically relevant, whereas grades B and C fistulas are clinically relevant, requiring further evaluation and management, such as antibiotics, nutritional support, octreotide, and percutaneous drainage (grade B) or surgical exploration (grade C) in the setting of sepsis.[25] Subsequent efforts to validate this classification scheme demonstrate that grade A fistulas comprise nearly half of all POPF yet have no apparent significant effect on outcome. However, grade B/C fistulas occur less often (40% and 11%, respectively) but are associated with higher resource use (ICU stay, nursing services post discharge, readmission), longer hospital stay, more complications, and, accordingly, increase in cost, grade for grade.[22,24]

RISK STRATIFICATION

Prevention of POPF relates to appropriate risk stratification[26] according to endogenous, perioperative, and operative risk factors.[22] A soft gland or diagnoses of ampullary, duodenal, cystic, or islet cell pathologies increases the risk of POPF development by up to 10-fold.[26,27] Pancreatic duct size is also crucial, with small ducts up to 3 mm in diameter conferring increased risk of POPF,[26,28] with an odds ratio greater than 3. The Fistula Risk Score has been developed and validated as a predictive tool for surgeons, taking the above factors into account.[29,30] As for other endogenous risk factors, conflicting information

TABLE 105.3 Criteria for Grading Pancreatic Fistula (International Study Group of Pancreatic Surgery Classification Scheme)

Criteria	No Fistula	Grade A Fistula	Grade B Fistula	Grade C Fistula
Drain amylase	<3 times normal serum amylase	>3 times normal serum amylase	>3 times normal serum amylase	>3 times normal serum amylase
Clinical conditions	Well	Well	Often well	Ill appearing/bad
Specific treatment	No	No	Yes/No	Yes
Ultrasonography/Computed tomography (if obtained)	Negative	Negative	Negative/positive	Positive
Persistent drainage (>3 weeks)	No	No	Usually yes	Yes
Signs of infection	No	No	Yes	Yes
Readmission	No	No	Yes/No	Yes/No
Sepsis	No	No	No	Yes
Reoperation	No	No	No	Yes
Death related to fistula	No	No	No	Yes

Note: Signs of infection include elevated body temperature >38°C, leukocytosis, and localized erythema, induration, or purulent drainage. Readmission is any hospital admission within 30 days following hospital discharge from the initial operation. Sepsis is the presence of localized infection and positive culture with evidence of bacteremia (i.e., chills, rigors, elevated white blood cell count) requiring intravenous antibiotic treatment, or hemodynamic compromise as demonstrated by high cardiac output and low systemic vascular resistance within 24 hour of body temperature >38°C.
Modified from Bassi C, Dervenis C, Butturini G, et al. Postoperative pancreatic fistula: an international study group definition. *Surgery*. 2005;138:8.

TABLE 105.4 The Impact of Increasing Number of Risk Factors for Pancreatic Fistulas

Outcomes	No Risk Factors (n = 63)	1 Risk Factor (n = 88)	2 Risk Factors (n = 66)	3 Risk Factors (n = 13)	4 Risk Factors (n = 3)	P value
Clinically relevant fistulas (%)	1 (2)	7 (8)	16 (24)	4 (31)	3 (100)	<.001
Nonfistulous complications (%)	22 (35)	38 (43)	38 (53)	6 (42)	2 (67)	.113
Hospital duration (median, days)	8	8	8	9	19	.001
Total hospital costs (median)	$16,969	$17,797	$22,179	$26,776	$40,517	.002
Total cost increase (beyond no risk factors)	—	$828	$5210	$9807	$23,548	—

Risk factors for pancreatic fistulas consist of (1) small pancreatic duct size (<3 mm); (2) pancreatic parenchyma of soft texture; (3) ampullary, duodenal, cystic, or islet cell pathology; and (4) increased intraoperative blood loss (>1000 mL).
Modified from Pratt WB, Callery MP, Vollmer CM Jr. Risk prediction for development of pancreatic fistula using the International Study Group of Pancreatic Surgery classification scheme. *World J Surg*. 2007;31:419.

exists in the literature. Some investigators have identified older age, male gender, coronary artery disease, diabetes mellitus, jaundice, and low creatinine clearance as predictors of POPF.[22,27,31,32] However, even though studies have found a correlation between male gender and POPF, these results are weakened by the design of these studies.[22,28] Moreover, explanations for the impact of gender are still lacking.[22] Interestingly, as a perioperative factor, neoadjuvant therapy appears to reduce the risk of fistula.[22,33] Operative risk factors for POPF include blood loss higher than 1000 mL, the anastomotic technique, routine drain placement, transanastomotic stents, and longer operative time.[22,26,28,31] Importantly, there appears to be an additive effect of these risk factors, whereby the percentage of patients developing a POPF increases sequentially as the number of risk factors increases,[26] as seen in Table 105.4, and is associated with increased cost and hospital stay.

Although the incidence of POPF seems to be similar after distal and central pancreatectomy versus proximal pancreatectomy, the clinical course in the setting of a distal resection is milder.[34] However, risk factors particular to distal resections remain poorly understood. Again, a soft gland is predictive of POPF, as well as primary pancreatic pathology and splenic preservation.[35] Division of

the pancreas at the body rather than the neck and failure to ligate the main pancreatic duct were also identified as predictors of POPF after distal pancreatectomy.[36] Furthermore, there was no difference in fistula rate for stump closure with suture versus stapler, nor for any demographic measures.[35]

PREVENTIVE MEASURES

Many technical variations have been studied with the hope of decreasing the incidence of POPF. For PD, both the type of anastomosis and the technique used have been evaluated. The pancreatic-enteric anastomosis may be to the jejunum or to the stomach. For the more typical pancreaticojejunal anastomosis, a duct-to-mucosa or invagination technique may be used, as demonstrated in Figs. 105.2 and 105.3, respectively.[37] Most groups have found the duct-to-mucosa technique to be superior in terms of fistula rates, according to a large meta-analysis by Poon et al. published in 2002 and reflecting the studies of the 1990s.[7] Additional variations include the use of a single- or double-layer anastomosis, as well as the choice between continuous and interrupted suture. The binding pancreaticojejunostomy, in which invagination is used with ablation of the overlapping jejunal mucosa, has been

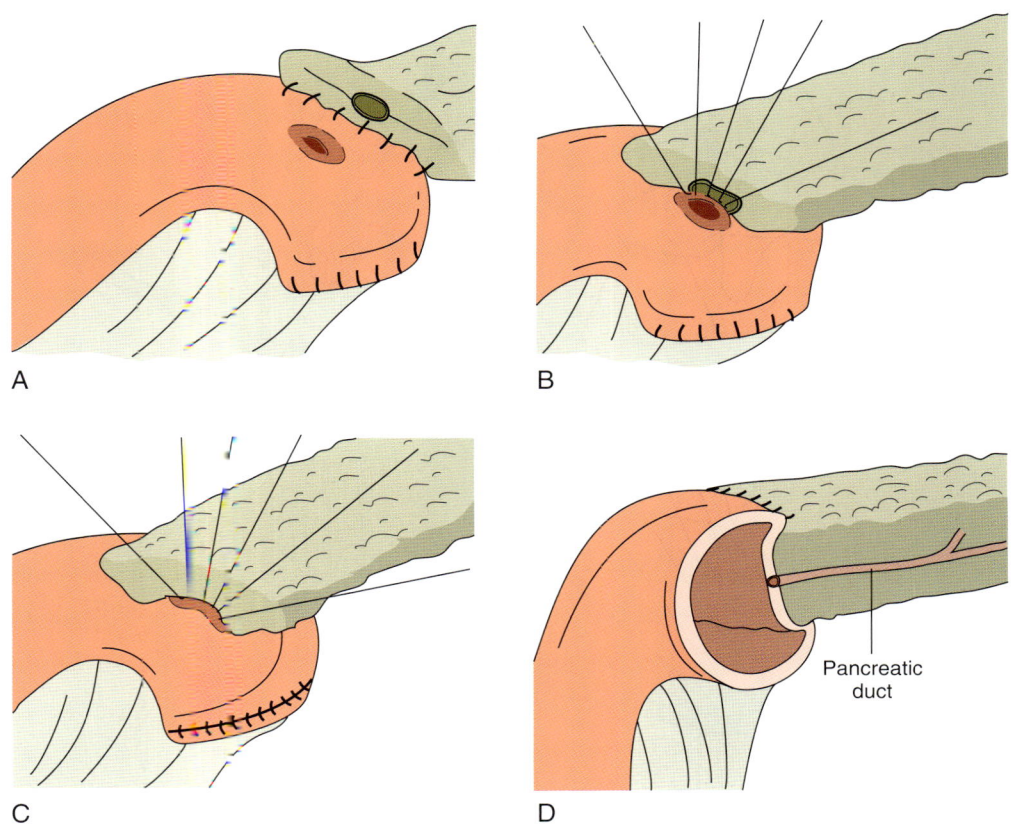

FIGURE 105.2 Duct-to-mucosa pancreaticojejunostomy. (A) Posterior outer row of interrupted silk sutures. (B) Posterior inner layer of duct-to-mucosa sutures. (C) Anterior inner layer of duct to mucosa interrupted sutures have been placed and tied. (D) Side view of completed anastomosis. Note in this trial, indwelling stents were not used. (Modified from Cameron JL, Sandone C. *Atlas of Gastrointestinal Surgery*. Vol. 1. 2nd ed. Hamilton, Ontario: Decker; 2007:296 [Figs. 26, 27, 30, and 31].)

shown to have equivalent fistula rates versus duct-to-mucosa but increased incidence of PPH.[2] There is one recent report of superiority of the invagination technique over the duct-to-mucosa technique in terms of fistula rate,[39] but the usual practice of the surgeons involved is taken into account; thus the results are difficult to interpret, and, at this point, duct-to-mucosa continues to be the preferred technique.

Pancreaticogastrostomy has been postulated to be advantageous with respect to POPF occurrence, because of the thickness and blood supply of the gastric wall, its proximity to the pancreas, and incomplete activation of pancreatic enzymes in the presence of gastric acid.[23,34] Yeo et al.[40] completed a prospective randomized trial comparing pancreaticojejunostomy to pancreaticogastrostomy (Fig. 105.4), which failed to demonstrate any benefit to either technique because the fistula rate was approximately 12% in both groups, which were similar in terms of gland texture and operative characteristics. Of note, surgeon volume did affect fistula rate.[39] There have been several nonrandomized similar studies and two meta-analyses that have concluded that pancreaticogastrostomy does indeed have a lower fistula rate when compared with pancreaticojejunostomy.[22,41] Furthermore, long-term patency and functional results may be problematic with this variation, as described in smaller case series.[38] Thus pancreaticojejunostomy

continues as the mainstay of the reconstruction, although there may be some merit to performing the invagination technique or pancreaticogastrostomy when the duct is very small and/or difficult to delineate, and other high-risk factors are present, or when the surgeon is more practiced with those techniques.

In summary and at a most fundamental level, a successful pancreaticoenteric anastomosis requires a tension-free anastomosis with properly placed and tied sutures, preserved blood supply to the pancreatic remnant and jejunum, and unobstructed flow from the pancreas into the gastrointestinal tract, whatever the chosen technique may be.

Neither internal stenting nor creation of an isolated Roux loop has been found to positively affect fistula rate.[22] However, there is one randomized trial that demonstrates a significantly lower rate of POPF formation with external stenting compared with no stent (6% vs. 22%, respectively).[42] In theory, such external drainage might be advantageous because it should completely divert the pancreatic secretions away from the anastomosis.[42] Moreover, a meta-analysis also concluded that there was a benefit when stents are used; however, further studies need to be performed before asserting this benefit.[43]

After distal pancreatectomy, fistula rates have been studied to compare stapled versus sutured pancreatic

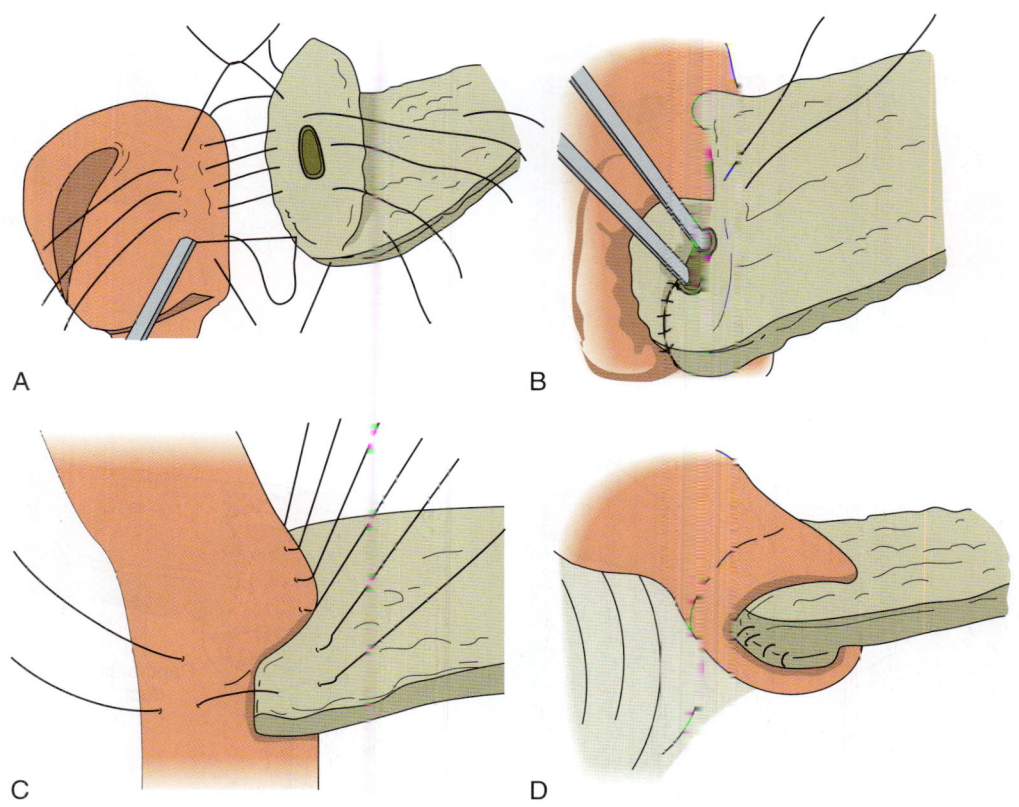

FIGURE 105.3 Invagination pancreaticojejunostomy. (A) Posterior outer row of silk interrupted sutures. (B) Inner continuous suture. (C) Outer layer of interrupted silk sutures. (D) Completed anastomosis demonstrating the "dunking" of the pancreatic remnant. (Modified from Cameron JL, Sandone C. *Atlas of Gastrointestinal Surgery.* Vol. 1. 2nd ed. Hamilton, Ontario: Decker; 2007:294 [Figs. 21, 23, 24, and 25].)

remnant[35] without clear demonstration of benefit with one technique over another found in evaluating the various papers in the literature[35,36]; thus either approach is acceptable. Investigation of the success of fibrin glue for preventing POPF has been marred by bias, and thus no conclusion has been reached as regards its utility.[23]

Octreotide, a long-lasting analogue of somatostatin, inactivates gastric and pancreatic exocrine secretion and may thus support a fragile pancreaticojejunostomy[23] or soft remnant after distal pancreatectomy. Studies of the utility of octreotide for decreasing POPF have been conflicting.[23,35,36] Some authors have found octreotide to be effective for distal[35] or local resection but not helpful in PD.[38] However, the benefit is clearer for high-risk glands[38] after PD. Prophylactic octreotide was efficacious and cost efficient when given to patients at high risk for POPF, with the criteria as listed previously,[26] and thus may be used selectively for those patients. No benefit was found for low-risk patients. On the other hand, a Cochrane review found no benefit in reducing fistula rates.[22] Furthermore, McMillan et al. found that octreotide was associated with higher rates of clinically relevant POPF, specifically in the presence of risk factors, including soft pancreatic parenchyma, high-risk pathologies, small duct diameter (≤4 mm), and elevated intraoperative blood loss.[44] However, a randomized trial found that pasireotide, a longer-acting somatostatin analogue, reduced the rates of clinically relevant POPF.[45]

MANAGEMENT

Management of clinically relevant pancreatic fistulas hinges on timely diagnosis. Especially because latent leaks or fistulas may develop and the patient may be home already, with the operative drain out, it is critical to acknowledge and respond to patient reports of worsening abdominal pain, fever, failure to thrive, or inability to tolerate a diet. According to the ISGPF classification, diagnosis requires drain amylase measurement, as well as clinical and imaging data. Furthermore, a sinister character of drain effluent, or output greater than 200 mL/day after postoperative day 5 may be associated with clinically relevant POPF.[23] Grade A fistulas are not of clinical consequence.[24] Patients having had a proximal or central pancreatectomy are more likely to require aggressive resuscitation and/or intervention than are patients after distal pancreatectomy.[34]

Much of the treatment of clinically relevant POPF is empiric. Initial management often includes hydration, being "nil per os" (NPO), supplemental nutrition, and antibiotics when patients present with signs and symptoms of infection (i.e., fever, leukocytosis). Octreotide may be given for high-output fistulas. Patients with amenable collections may undergo radiology-guided drainage, particularly if the operative drain has already been removed or if it is not adequately draining the site of the collection.

Reexploration is rarely required but may be necessary in the setting of clinical decline, undrainable fistula/abscess, or for the suspicion of pancreaticojejunal anastomotic dehiscence (Fig. 105.5). Options include wide drainage, anastomotic revision or conversion to alternate pancreatic duct drainage site, completion pancreatectomy, or use of a bridge-stent technique,[46] as depicted in Fig. 105.6. Pancreaticojejunal anastomotic dehiscence following PD is a rare but difficult problem to manage. The previously mentioned traditional surgical options are associated with significant morbidity and mortality. With a patient who is already compromised physiologically, the goal is a safe, efficient reoperation. The bridge-stent technique allowed a small group of patients to recover to hospital discharge with limited long-term sequelae[46] and is another option in the armamentarium to deal with this complex problem. However, specifically for patients with grade C POPF, a significant burden is incurred for patients, and aggressive clinical management, including reoperation when indicated (approximately 72% reported in this series), did not impact 90-day mortality.[47]

Patients with clinically relevant POPF are known to have longer hospital stays, more additional complications, ICU requirements, transfusion requirements, and need for services or rehabilitation placement on discharge.[24] Accordingly, total costs increase significantly as the grade of fistula increases.[24]

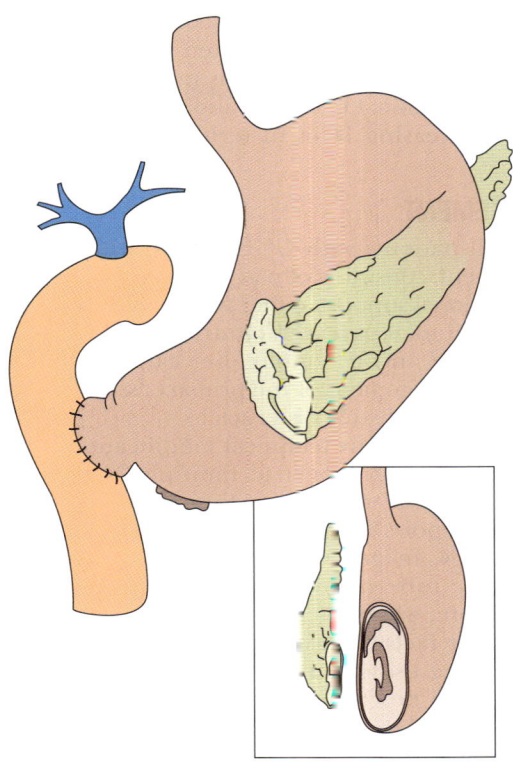

FIGURE 105.4 Pancreaticogastrostomy illustration, with anastomosis of the pancreas to the posterior gastric wall. (From Yeo CJ, Cameron JL, Maher MA, et al. A prospective randomized trial of pancreaticogastrostomy versus pancreaticojejunostomy after pancreaticoduodenectomy. *Ann Surg*. 1995;222:580.)

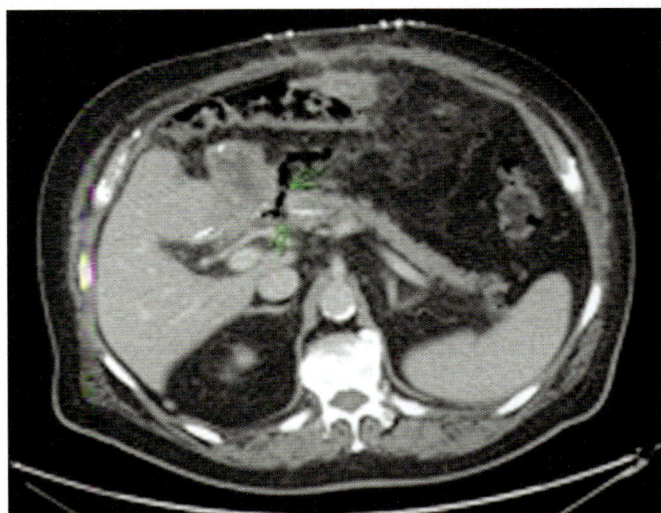

FIGURE 105.5 *Arrows* demonstrate gap between the pancreas and the jejunum, with associated peripancreatic gas. (From Kent TS, Callery MP, Vollmer CM. The bridge-stent technique for salvage of pancreatico-jejunal anastomotic dehiscence. *HPB [Oxford]*. 2010;12:577.)

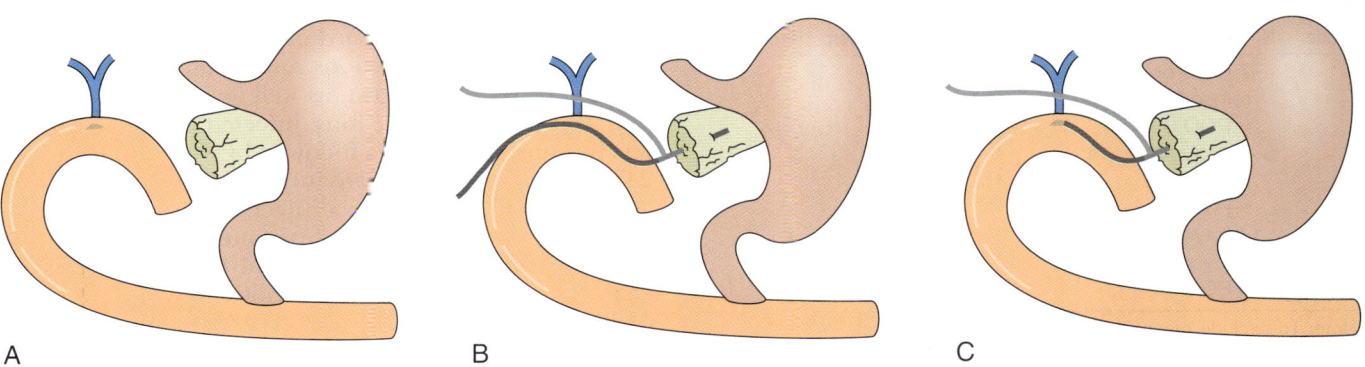

A   B   C

FIGURE 105.6 (A) Dehiscence of the pancreaticojejunal anastomosis is illustrated with a gap between the pancreatic remnant and jejunum. (B) Bridge-stent technique with externalized stent plus external drain. (C) Bridge-stent technique with internal stent and external drain adjacent to gap. (From Kent TS, Callery MP, Vollmer CM. The bridge-stent technique for salvage of pancreatico-jejunal anastomotic dehiscence. *HPB [Oxford]*. 2010;12:577.)

DELAYED GASTRIC EMPTYING

Although DGE is rarely life-threatening and typically is self-limited, it can increase the length of hospital stay, likelihood of readmission, other complications, and ultimately cost.[48,49] Until 2007 there was no standard definition of DGE, and thus it was difficult to compare the multitude of literature reports on the topic, which described an incidence after PD of 6% to more than 50%.[5,48-51] The ISGPS has now created a definition (Table 105.5) of DGE, dividing it into grades of severity. Similar to the consensus definitions for PPH and POPF, this effort resulted in a standardized classification scheme based on duration of NGT decompression required, time until solid food is tolerated, the presence of vomiting or gastric distention, and the use of prokinetics.[47,51]

PREVENTIVE MEASURES

DGE is likely multifactorial but may be related to the decrease in plasma motilin that occurs following duodenal resection, vagal innervation to the pylorus and antrum with gastric atony, and/or relative devascularization of the pylorus.[48] Thus attempts to prevent DGE have centered on technical modifications to modulate the previously mentioned factors.

Some groups have found a decreased rate of DGE with pylorus-preserving versus classic PD, but more recent studies have found the opposite, leaving no clearly better technique at this point in time.[48-52] Still other surgeons advocate pylorus-preserving PD with the addition of a pyloric dilation or pyloromyotomy to decrease the incidence of DGE.[4,48,53] These studies have been difficult to interpret in light of variable DGE definitions and variation in the diagnoses of included cases, and recent reviews conclude equivalency.[54,55] Another decision point is the location (retrocolic or antecolic) of the gastrojejunostomy or duodenojejunostomy. Nikfarjam et al. found a significant decrease in the rate of DGE when they switched from retrocolic to antecolic gastrojejunostomy or duodenojejunostomy.[56] This finding was supported by a meta-analysis in which the incidence of DGE in antecolic duodenojejunostomy was lower when compared with the retrocolic approach (risk ratio: 0.260).[57]

Promotility agents have also been evaluated as to their efficacy at decreasing the incidence of DGE after pancreatic resection. A prospective study in 1993 found that erythromycin, a motilin agonist, was associated with a 37% reduction in the incidence of DGE, and with a significant reduction in the percentage liquid retention in gastric emptying studies.[58] Another similar study supported this finding.[59] Metoclopramide is often used instead of, or in addition to erythromycin, but is not well studied in this patient population. Octreotide also may have an adjunctive role in decreasing DGE in terms of its ability to limit POPF.

MANAGEMENT

Nearly all patients with DGE resolve with conservative management consisting of nasogastric tube decompression and nutritional support, either with a feeding jejunostomy tube or with total parenteral nutrition (TPN) until symptoms resolve and a regular diet can be tolerated. In addition, management of the primary associated problem (i.e., pancreatic fistula) is crucial.

In summary, many technical modifications have been investigated with respect to limiting DGE. Again, the ability to draw meaningful conclusions from most of these published reports is limited by the lack of uniform definition and by, in general, longer time to remove the nasogastric tube or initiate diet in the older studies. Furthermore, when one technical aspect was compared, many other factors varied, again limiting comparison. However, the use of an antecolic duodenojejunostomy does seem to be consistently associated with decreased DGE rates.[55] Most important in the prevention of DGE is the avoidance of other complications, namely POPF, as discussed earlier, because such complications are clearly associated with a secondary DGE.[48,49]

INFECTIOUS COMPLICATIONS

Infectious complications occur frequently following pancreatectomy. In a review of our own data, infections occurred in nearly one-third of patients, including both proximal and distal resections, and accounted for a nearly 40% increase in total cost, as well as one extra hospital day. Among major infections, infected pancreatic fistula was responsible for 28%, followed by wound infection at 24%. Other major infections included pneumonia (17%), abscess (15%), urinary tract infection (10%), and sepsis (6%). Many patients with at least one infection incurred multiple infections. A study found that patient-related characteristics including intraoperative blood transfusion, diabetes, and use of steroids were risk factors for surgical site infections following gastrointestinal surgery.[60] Thus infectious complications, of both minor and major significance, occur frequently following pancreatic resections and are most commonly wound infections and infected pancreatic fistulas. These are responsible for a significant burden to patients, practitioners, and systems alike. Their

TABLE 105.5 Consensus Definition of DGE After Pancreatic Surgery

DGE Grade	NGT Required	Unable to Tolerate Solid Oral Intake by POD	Vomiting/ Gastric Distention	Use of Prokinetics
A	4–7 days or reinsertion > POD 3	7	±	±
B	8–14 days or reinsertion > POD 7	14	+	+
C	>14 days or reinsertion > POD 14	21	+	+

Note: To exclude mechanical causes of abnormal gastric emptying, the patency of either the gastrojejunostomy or the duodenojejunostomy should be confirmed by endoscopy or upper gastrointestinal gastrograph in series. *DGE,* Delayed gastric emptying; *NGT,* nasogastric tube; *POD,* postoperative day.
From Wente MN, Bassi C, Dervenis C, et al. Delayed gastric emptying after pancreatic surgery: a suggested definition by the International Study Group of Pancreatic Surgery. *Surgery.* 2007;142:761.

common occurrence in the setting of excellent adherence to infection control regulations emphasizes the need to discover better process improvements to decrease the incidence of infectious complications, including reevaluating the effectiveness of chosen antimicrobial prophylaxis regimens and adjusting the regimens according to various risk profiles. Fong et al. found discordance between antimicrobial prophylaxis and wound infection cultures in a multicenter study.[61] They suggest that bile cultures should be obtained in patients who undergo preoperative endoscopic retrograde cholangiopancreatography because the identified microorganisms matched the ones found on wound cultures.[61]

SUMMARY

Pancreatic resection remains a high-acuity operation that can be safely performed by appropriately trained and experienced surgeons, in adequately equipped facilities. Although mortality has declined, morbidity remains high. Major potential complications as discussed here include POPF, PPH, and DGE. Other, more generic, complications remain prevalent as well, particularly wound infections, which have been reported at 7% to 15%, and in association with fistulas.[5,40,56]

Aside from efforts to prevent and appropriately manage individual complications, the system of care delivery for pancreatic surgical patients plays a crucial role in improving outcomes overall. Adequate system-wide support for the diagnosis and management of complications must be sufficient to provide the appropriate level of care.[9] For example, services available should include ICU level of care, adequate blood bank, interventional radiology and gastroenterology, nurses accustomed to managing complex postoperative care and drains, and case management. Standardized care plans have been developed to care for postpancreatectomy patients. "Critical" or "clinical" pathways, presently known as enhanced recovery after surgery (ERAS) protocols, have been defined as "structured multidisciplinary care plans that detail essential steps (process measures) in the care of patients with specific problems."[62] Such structured plans have been shown to positively impact outcomes without compromising morbidity and mortality for these patients.[5,64] Multiple studies have confirmed the decreased resource use, readmission, and cost and increased bed/operation theater availability[64,65] and also demonstrated fewer deviations from the expected postoperative course after initiation of the clinical pathway.[23,66] As a result of these data, it has been suggested that development and maintenance of such pathways or protocols should be a requirement for institutions to serve as referral centers.[64,65]

REFERENCES

1. Bliss LA, Witkowski ER, Yang CJ. Tseng JF. Outcomes in operative management of pancreatic cancer. *J Surg Oncol.* 2014;110:592.
2. Birkmeyer JD, Dimick JB, Staiger DO. Operative mortality and procedure volume as predictors of subsequent hospital performance. *Ann Surg.* 2006;243:411.
3. van der Geest LG, van Rijssen LB, Molenaar IQ, et al. Volume-outcome relationships in pancreatoduodenectomy for cancer. *HPB (Oxford).* 2016;18:317.
4. Bassi C, Falconi M, Salvia R, Mascetta G, Molinari E, Pederzoli P. Management of complications after pancreaticoduodenectomy in a high-volume center: results on 150 consecutive patients. *Dig Surg.* 2001;18:453.
5. Sohn TA, Yeo CJ, Cameron JL, et al. Resected adenocarcinoma of the pancreas—616 patients: results, outcomes, and prognostic indicators. *J Gastrointest Surg.* 2000;4:567.
6. Birkmeyer JD, Finlayson SR, Tosteson AN, Sharp SM, Warshaw AL, Fisher ES. Effect of hospital volume on in-hospital mortality with pancreaticoduodenectomy. *Surgery.* 1999;125:250 [Comment in *Surgery* 1999;127:238].
7. Finlayson EV, Goodney PP, Birkmeyer JD. Hospital volume and operative mortality in cancer surgery. *Arch Surg.* 2003;138:721.
8. Fong Y, Gonen M, Rubin D, Radzyner M, Brennan MF. Long-term survival is superior after resection for cancer in high-volume centers. *Ann Surg.* 2005;242:540 [discussion 544].
9. Schmidt CM, Turrini O, Parikh P, et al. Effect of hospital volume, surgeon experience, and surgeon volume on patient outcomes after pancreaticoduodenectomy: a single-institution experience. *Arch Surg.* 2010;145:634.
10. van Berge Henegouwen MI, Allema JH, van Gulik TM, Verbeek PC, Obertop H, Gouma DJ. Delayed massive haemorrhage after pancreatic and biliary surgery. *Br J Surg.* 1995;82:1527.
11. Tien YW, Lee PH, Yang CY, Ho MC, Chiu YF. Risk factors of massive bleeding related to pancreatic leak after pancreaticoduodenectomy. *J Am Coll Surg.* 2005;201:554.
12. Trede M, Schwall G. The complications of pancreatectomy. *Ann Surg.* 1988;207:39.
13. Grutzmann R, Ruckert F, Hippe-Davies N, Distler M, Saeger HD. Evaluation of the International Study Group of Pancreatic Surgery definition of post-pancreatectomy hemorrhage in a high volume center. *Surgery.* 2012;151:612.
14. Wente MN, Veit JA, Bassi C, et al. Postpancreatectomy hemorrhage (PPH)—an International Study Group of Pancreatic Surgery (ISGPS) definition. *Surgery.* 2007;142:20.
15. Shukla PJ, Barreto SG, Kulkarni A, Nagarajan G, Fingerhut A. Vascular anomalies encountered during pancreatoduodenectomy: do they influence outcomes? *Ann Surg Oncol.* 2010;17:186.
16. Darnis B, Lebeau R, Chopin-Laly X, Adham M. Postpancreatectomy hemorrhage (PPH): predictors and management from a prospective database. *Langenbecks Arch Surg.* 2013;398:441.
17. Pachter HL, Drager S, Godfrey N, LeFleur R. Traumatic injuries of the portal vein. *Ann Surg.* 1979;189:383.
18. Morgan K, Mansker D, Adams DB. Not just for trauma patients: damage control laparotomy in pancreatic surgery. *J Gastrointest Surg.* 2010;14:768.
19. Standop J, Glowka T, Schmiltz V, et al. Operative re-intervention following pancreatic head resection: indications and outcome. *J Gastrointest Surg.* 2009;13:1503.
20. De Castro SM, Kuhlmann KF, Busch OR, et al. Delayed massive hemorrhage after pancreatic and biliary surgery. *Ann Surg.* 2005; 241:85.
21. Khalsa BS, Imagawa DK, Chen JI, Dermirjian AN, Yim DB, Findeiss LK. Evolution in the treatment of delayed postpancreatectomy hemorrhage: surgery to interventional radiology. *Pancreas.* 2015;44: 953.
22. McMillan MT, Vollmer CM Jr. Predictive factors for pancreatic fistula following pancreatectomy. *Langenbecks Arch Surg.* 2014;399:811.
23. Callery MP, Pratt WB, Vollmer CM. Prevention and management of pancreatic fistula. *J Gastrointest Surg.* 2009;13:163.
24. Pratt WB, Maithel SK, Vanounou T, Huang ZS, Callery MP, Vollmer CM Jr. Clinical and economic validation of the International Study Group of Pancreatic Fistula (ISGPF) classification scheme. *Ann Surg.* 2007;245:443.
25. Bassi C, Dervenis C, Butturini G, et al. Postoperative pancreatic fistula: an international study group (ISGPF) definition. *Surgery.* 2005;138:8.
26. Pratt WB, Callery MP, Vollmer CM. Risk prediction for development of pancreatic fistula utilizing the ISGPF classification scheme. *World J Surg.* 2007;32:419.
27. Lin JW, Cameron JL, Yeo CJ, Riall TS, Lillemoe KD. Risk factors and outcomes in postpancreaticoduodenectomy pancreaticocutaneous fistula. *J Gastrointest Surg.* 2004;8:951.
28. de Castro SM, Busch OR, van Gulik TM, Obertop H, Gouma DJ. Incidence and management of pancreatic leakage after pancreatoduodenectomy. *Br J Surg.* 2005;92:1117.

29. Callery MP, Pratt WB, Kent TS, Chaikof EL, Vollmer CM Jr. A prospectively validated clinical risk score accurately predicts pancreatic fistula after pancreatoduodenectomy. *J Am Coll Surg.* 2013;216:1.

30. Miller BC, Christein JD, Behrman SW, et al. A multi-institutional external validation of the fistula risk score for pancreatoduodenectomy. *J Gastrointest Surg.* 2014;18:172.

31. Yeh TS, Jan YY, Jeng LB, et al. Pancreaticojejunal anastomotic leak after pancreaticoduodenectomy—multivariate analysis of perioperative risk factors. *J Surg Res.* 1997;67:119.

32. Matsusue S, Takeda H, Nakamura Y, Nishimura S, Koizumi S. A prospective analysis of the factors influencing pancreaticojejunostomy performed using a single method, in 100 consecutive pancreaticoduodenectomies. *Surg Today.* 1998;28:719.

33. Cheng TY, Sheth K, White RR, et al. Effect of neoadjuvant chemoradiation on operative mortality and morbidity for pancreaticoduodenectomy. *Ann Surg Oncol.* 2006;13:66.

34. Pratt W, Maithel SK, Vanounou T, Callery MP, Vollmer CM Jr. Postoperative pancreatic fistulas are not equivalent after proximal, distal, and central pancreatectomy. *J Gastrointest Surg.* 2006;10:1264.

35. Ridolfini MP, Alfieri S, Gourguitis S, et al. Risk factors associated with pancreatic fistula after distal pancreatectomy: which technique of pancreatic stump closure is more beneficial? *World J Gastroenterol.* 2007;13:5096.

36. Pannegeon V, Pessaux P, Sauvanet A, Vullierme MP, Kianmanesh R, Belghiti J. Pancreatic fistula after distal pancreatectomy: predictive risk factors and value of conservative treatment. *Arch Surg.* 2006;141:1071.

37. Cameron JL, Sandone C. *Atlas of Gastrointestinal Surgery.* Vol. 1. 2nd ed. Hamilton, Ontario: Decker; 2007:294.

38. Poon RT, Lo SH, Fong D, Fan ST, Wong J. Prevention of pancreatic anastomotic leakage after pancreaticoduodenectomy. *Am J Surg.* 2002;183:42.

39. Berger AC, Howard TJ, Kennedy EP, et al. Does type of pancreaticojejunostomy after pancreaticoduodenectomy decrease rate of pancreatic fistula? A randomized, prospective, dual-institution trial. *J Am Coll Surg.* 2009;208:738.

40. Yeo CJ, Cameron JL, Maher MA, et al. A prospective randomized trial of pancreaticogastrostomy versus pancreaticojejunostomy after pancreaticoduodenectomy. *Ann Surg.* 1995;222:580.

41. Hallet J, Zih FS, Deobald RG, et al. The impact of pancreaticojejunostomy versus pancreaticogastrostomy reconstruction on pancreatic fistula after pancreatoduodenectomy: meta-analysis of randomized controlled trials. *HPB (Oxford).* 2015;17:113.

42. Motoi F, Egawa S, Rikiyama T, Katayose Y, Unno M. Randomized clinical trial of external stent drainage of the pancreatic duct to reduce postoperative pancreatic fistula after pancreatojejunostomy. *Br J Surg.* 2012;99:524.

43. Markar SR, Vyas S, Karthikesalingam A, Imber C, Malago M. The impact of pancreatic duct drainage following pancreaticojejunostomy on clinical outcome. *J Gastrointest Surg.* 2012;16:1610.

44. McMillan MT, Christein JD, Callery MP, et al. Prophylactic octreotide for pancreaticoduodenectomy: more harm than good? *HPB (Oxford).* 2014;16:954.

45. Allen PJ, Gonen M, Brennan MF, et al. Pasireotide for postoperative fistula. *N Engl J Med.* 2014;370:2014.

46. Kent TS, Callery MP, Vollmer CM. The bridge-stent technique for salvage of pancreatico-jejunal anastomotic dehiscence. *HPB (Oxford).* 2010;12:577.

47. McMillan MT, Vollmer CM Jr, Asbun HJ, et al. The characterization and prediction of ISGPF grade C fistulas following pancreatoduodenectomy. *J Gastrointest Surg.* 2016;20:262.

48. Wente MN, Bassi C, Dervenis C, et al. Delayed gastric emptying (DGE) after pancreatic surgery: a suggested definition by the International Study Group of Pancreatic Surgery (ISGPS). *Surgery.* 2007;142:761.

49. Huttner FJ, Fitzmaurice C, Schwarzer G, et al. Pylorus-preserving pancreaticoduodenectomy (pp Whipple) versus pancreaticoduodenectomy (classic Whipple) for surgical treatment of periampullary and pancreatic carcinoma. *Cochrane Database Syst Rev.* 2016;2:CD006053.

50. Richter A, Niedergethmann M, Sturm JW, Lorenz D, Post S, Trede M. Long-term results of partial pancreaticoduodenectomy for ductal adenocarcinoma of the pancreatic head: 25-year experience. *World J Surg.* 2003;27:324.

51. Welsch T, Borm M, Degrate L, Hinz U, Büchler MW, Wente MN. Evaluation of the International Study Group of Pancreatic Surgery definition of delayed gastric emptying after pancreaticoduodenectomy in a high-volume centre. *Br J Surg.* 2010;97:1043.

52. Witzigmann H, Max D, Uhlmann D, et al. Outcome after duodenum-preserving pancreatic head resection is improved compared with classic Whipple procedure in the treatment of chronic pancreatitis. *Surgery.* 2003;134:53.

53. Kim DK, Hirzenburg AA, Sharma SK, et al. Is pylorospasm a cause of delayed gastric emptying after pylorus-preserving pancreaticoduodenectomy? *Ann Surg Oncol.* 2005;12:222.

54. Lytras D, Paraskevas KI, Avgerinos C, et al. Therapeutic strategies for the management of delayed gastric emptying after pancreatic resection. *Langenbecks Arch Surg.* 2007;392:1.

55. Paraskevas K, Avgerinos C, Manes C, Lytras D, Dervenis C. Delayed gastric emptying is associated with pylorus-preserving but not classical Whipple pancreaticoduodenectomy: a review of the literature and critical reappraisal of the implicated pathomechanism. *World J Gastroenterol.* 2006;12:5951.

56. Nikfarjam M, Kimchi ET, Gusani NJ, et al. A reduction in delayed gastric emptying by classic pancreaticoduodenectomy with an antecolic gastrojejunal anastomosis and a retrogastric omental patch. *J Gastrointest Surg.* 2009;13:1674.

57. Hanna MM, Gadde R, Allen CJ, et al. Delayed gastric emptying after pancreaticoduodenectomy. *J Surg Res.* 2016;202:380.

58. Yeo CJ, Barry MK, Sauter PK, et al. Erythromycin accelerates gastric emptying following pancreaticoduodenectomy: a prospective, randomized placebo controlled trial. *Ann Surg.* 1993;218:229.

59. Ohwada S, Satoh Y, Kawate S, et al. Low-dose erythromycin reduces delayed gastric emptying and improves gastric motility after Billroth I pylorus-preserving pancreaticoduodenectomy. *Ann Surg.* 2001;234:66.

60. Fukuda H. Patient-related risk factors for surgical site infection following eight types of gastrointestinal surgery. *J Hosp Infect.* 2016;93(4):347-354.

61. Fong ZV, McMillan MT, Marchegiani G, et al. Discordance between perioperative antibiotic prophylaxis and wound infection cultures in patients undergoing pancreaticoduodenectomy. *JAMA Surg.* 2016;151:432.

62. Riall TS, Nealon WH, Goodwin JS, Townsend CM Jr, Freeman JL. Outcomes following pancreatic resection: variability among high-volume providers. *Surgery.* 2008;144:133.

63. Kagedan DJ, Ahmed M, Devitt KS, Wei A. Enhanced recovery after pancreatic surgery: a systematic review of the evidence. *HPB (Oxford).* 2015;17:11.

64. Kennedy EP, Rosato EL, Sauter PK, et al. Initiation of a critical pathway for pancreaticoduodenectomy at an academic institution—the first step in multidisciplinary team building. *J Am Coll Surg.* 2007;204:917.

65. Kennedy EP, Grenda TR, Sauter PK, et al. Implementation of a critical pathway for distal pancreatectomy at an academic institution. *J Gastrointest Surg.* 2009;13:938.

66. Vanounou T, Pratt W, Fischer JE, Vollmer CM Jr, Callery MP. Deviation-based cost modeling: a novel model to evaluate the clinical and economic impact of clinical pathways. *J Am Coll Surg.* 2007;204:570.

CHAPTER
106

Anatomy, Embryology, Anomalies, and Physiology of the Biliary Tract

Pierre F. Saldinger | Omar E. Bellorin-Marin

Cholelithiasis represents a significant problem for the health system in both developed and developing societies, affecting 10% to 15% of the adult population, corresponding to 20 to 25 million Americans who have or will have cholelithiasis.[1] Laparoscopic cholecystectomy is the most common surgery performed in the United States, with a considerably low complication rate. Knowledge of the anatomy, embryology, and anomalies of the biliary tract is crucial and will have a positive impact in the decision-making progress of the biliary surgeon.

The anatomy and embryology of the biliary tract is intimately associated with both the liver and the pancreas. Thus, for a complete picture of the anatomy, embryology, and physiology of the biliary tract, the reader is referred to corresponding chapters in the sections on the liver and pancreas.

ANATOMY AND EMBRYOLOGY

The first step in understanding the anatomy of the biliary tract is a review of the embryology of the liver, biliary tract, and pancreas. At the fourth week in the development of the human embryo, a projection appears in the ventral wall of the primitive midgut at the level of the primitive duodenum. At this 3-mm stage, three buds can be recognized. The cranial bud develops into two lobes of the liver, whereas the caudal bud becomes the gallbladder and extrahepatic biliary tree (Fig. 106.1). Part of this caudal bud will become the cystic diverticulum by day 26, which will form the cystic duct (CD) and gallbladder by the end of the fourth week. The gallbladder and CD develop from histologically distinct populations of duodenal cells. The ventral pancreas, which eventually becomes the pancreatic head and uncinate process, also develops from the caudal bud. The third primitive bud develops from the dorsal surface of the midgut to become the anlage of the remainder of the pancreatic head, as well as the neck, body, and tail of the pancreas.[2] At the 5-mm stage, the primitive gallbladder and common bile duct (CBD) have appeared.

At the 7-mm stage (see Fig. 106.1), the liver and hepatic ducts have formed, and the gallbladder, CD, and ventral pancreas have arisen from the common duct. At this stage, the stomach has begun to form, and the ventral pancreas has developed from the dorsal mesogastrium. By the 12-mm stage, the ventral pancreatic bud has rotated 180 degrees clockwise around the duodenum. This rotation causes fusion of the ventral and dorsal buds to form the complete pancreas by the sixth or seventh week of gestation. When this rotation occurs in different directions, the result is a ringlike formation around the second portion of the duodenum called annular pancreas. When the ventral and dorsal buds fuse correctly, their ductal systems also become interconnected. The duct from the dorsal bud usually degenerates leaving the ventral pancreatic duct to be the main pancreatic duct. Within another week, a completely open lumen has formed in the gallbladder, bile ducts, and pancreatic ducts. By the 12th week of fetal life, the liver begins to secrete bile and the pancreas secretes fluid that flows through the extrahepatic biliary tree and pancreatic ducts, respectively, into the duodenum.

INTRAHEPATIC DUCTS

The anatomy of the biliary tract can be divided into various segments, including the intrahepatic ducts, extrahepatic ducts, gallbladder and CD, and sphincter of Oddi. The anatomy of the intrahepatic ducts is intimately associated with the anatomy of the liver. The lobar and segmental anatomy of the liver is determined by the sequential branching of the portal vein, hepatic artery, and biliary tree as they enter the parenchyma at the hilum. All three of these structures follow approximately parallel courses and bifurcate just before entering the liver. This major bifurcation divides the liver into left and right lobes. According to the Couinaud classification, the caudate lobe is segment I; segments II to IV are on the left; and segments V to VIII are on the right (Fig. 106.2).

The biliary drainage of the right and left liver is into the right and left hepatic ducts, respectively. The left hepatic duct is formed within the umbilical fissure from the union of the three segmental ducts draining the left side of the liver (segments II through IV). The left hepatic duct crosses the base of segment IV (medial segment of

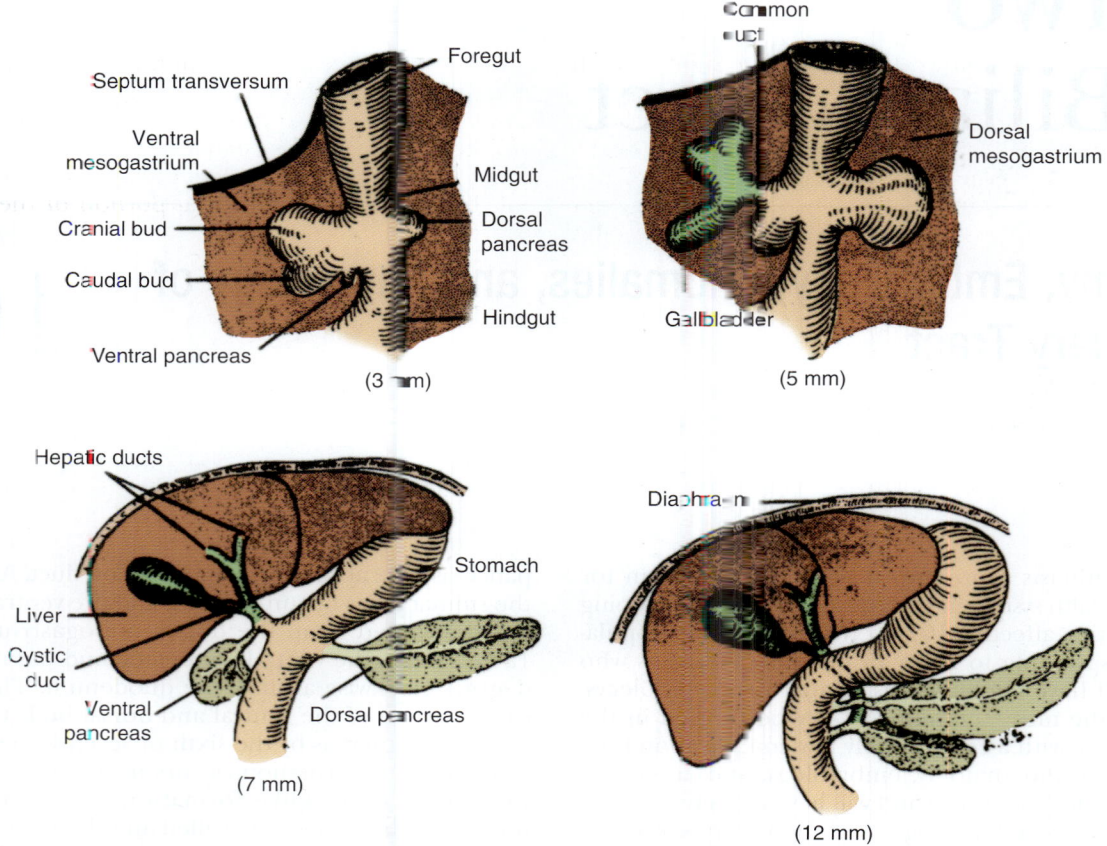

FIGURE 106.1 Embryonic development of the extrahepatic biliary tract and pancreas. (From Linder HH. Embryology and anatomy of the biliary tree. In: Way LW, Pellegrini CA, eds. *Surgery of the Gallbladder and Bile Ducts*. Philadelphia: Saunders; 1987:4.)

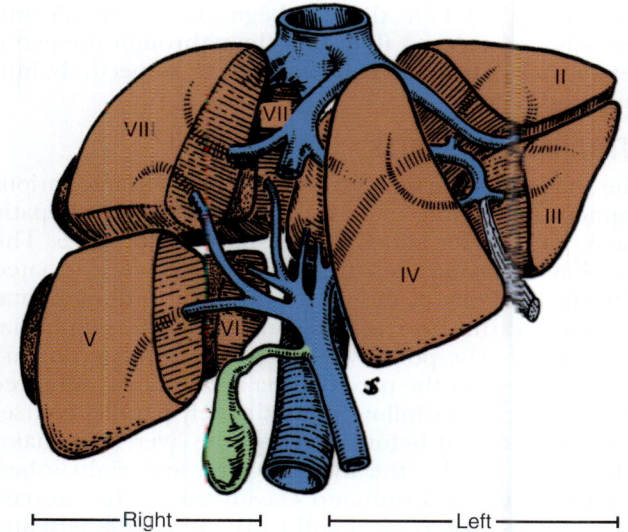

FIGURE 106.2 Segmental biliary drainage of the liver. (From Smadja C, Blumgart LH. The biliary tract and the anatomy of biliary exposure. In: Blumgart LH, ed. *Surgery of the Liver and Biliary Tract*. Edinburgh: Churchill Livingstone; 1988:11.)

the left lobe in a horizontal direction to join the right hepatic duct and form the common hepatic duct (CHD). The right hepatic duct drains segments V through VIII and is formed from the union of the right posterior and right anterior segmental ducts. The right posterior segmental duct is formed by the confluence of ducts draining segments VI and VII. The posterior segmental duct initially courses in a nearly horizontal direction before descending in a more vertical direction to join the anterior segmental duct. The right anterior segmental duct is formed by the union of the ducts draining segments V and VIII. In approximately 15% to 20% of cases, the right posterior duct drains into the left hepatic duct.[3] The posterior right duct usually passes superior to the right anterior portal vein (80%). The ducts from segments II and III join to the left of the intrahepatic left portal vein, and the segment IV duct joins to the right of the umbilical fissure and forms the main left duct. The main left (horizontal) and right hepatic ducts (vertical) join at the hilum to form the CHD in 56% of the cases. The biliary drainage of the caudate lobe (segment I) is variable.[4] In approximately 80% of the individuals, the caudate lobe drains into both the right and left hepatic ducts. In 15% of cases the caudate lobe drains only into the left hepatic duct, and in the remaining 5% of cases the caudate is drained exclusively by the right hepatic duct.[5]

EXTRAHEPATIC DUCTS

Most patients have a bifurcation where the right and left hepatic ducts join to form the CHD. This junction may occur as a wide or an acute angle, or the two hepatic ducts may run parallel to each other before joining. In some patients, three hepatic ducts join to form the CHD. Usually, the hepatic ducts meet just outside of the liver parenchyma, with the CD entering 2 to 3 cm distally. Occasionally, the two hepatic ducts do not unite until after the CD has joined the right hepatic duct. The CHD extends for a variable length from the junction of the right and left hepatic ducts to the entrance of the CD into the gallbladder (Fig. 106.3)

The CBD is formed by the union of the cystic and CHDs. The CBD is approximately 8 cm in length, but, like the hepatic duct, it varies in length according to the point of union of the CD and the CHD. The normal diameter of the CBD ranges from 4 to 9 mm. The CBD is considered enlarged if the duct diameter exceeds 10 mm. The upper third, or supraduodenal portion, of the CBD courses downward in the free edge of the lesser omentum, anterior to the portal vein and to the right of the proper hepatic artery. The middle third, or retroduodenal portion, of the CBD passes behind the first portion of the duodenum, lateral to the portal vein and anterior to the inferior vena cava. The lower third, or intrapancreatic portion, of the CBD traverses the posterior aspect of the pancreas in a tunnel or groove to enter the second portion of the duodenum, where it is usually joined by the pancreatic duct. The intramural or intraduodenal portion of the CBD passes obliquely through the duodenal wall to enter the duodenum at the papilla of Vater.

The relationship between the lower CBD and pancreatic duct is variable: (1) the two structures may rarely unite outside the duodenal wall to form a long common channel; (2) the bile duct and pancreatic duct usually join within the duodenal wall to form a short common channel; or (3) the two structures may rarely enter the duodenum independently through separate orifices. The lower portion of the CBD and the terminal portion of the pancreatic duct are enveloped and regulated by a complex sphincter, the sphincter of Oddi. In 5% to 10% of patients who have pancreas divisum, the dorsal pancreatic duct enters the duodenum through an accessory sphincter, whereas the ventral pancreatic duct joins the CBD at the sphincter of Oddi.

The extrahepatic bile ducts contain a columnar mucosa surrounded by a connective tissue layer. The surface is relatively flat, with basal nuclei and an absent or small nucleolus. The lamina propria consists of collagen, elastic fibers, and vessels. Occasional lymphocytes are found, and pancreatic acini and ducts may be seen in the wall of the intrapancreatic portion of the distal CBD. Muscle fibers in the bile duct are sparse and discontinuous. The muscle fibers that are present are usually longitudinal, although occasional circular fibers are observed. The distal CBD begins to develop a more substantial muscle layer in the intrapancreatic portion of the duct, which becomes prominent at the sphincter of Oddi, where distinct bundles of longitudinal and circular fibers are clearly identified.

GALLBLADDER AND CYSTIC DUCT

The gallbladder is a pear-shaped organ that lies on the inferior surface of the liver at the junction of the left and

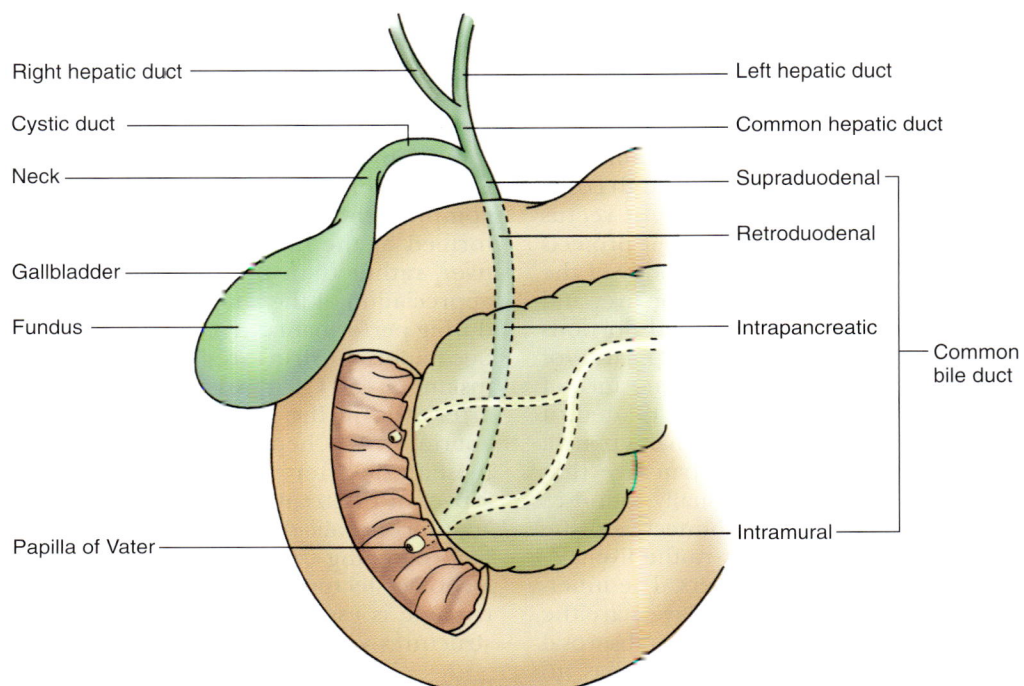

FIGURE 106.3 Anatomic divisions of the gallbladder and extrahepatic biliary tree. (From Gadacz TR. Biliary anatomy and physiology. In: Greenfield LJ, Mulholland MW, Oldham KT, eds. *Surgery: Scientific Principles and Practice*. Philadelphia: Lippincott; 1993:931.)

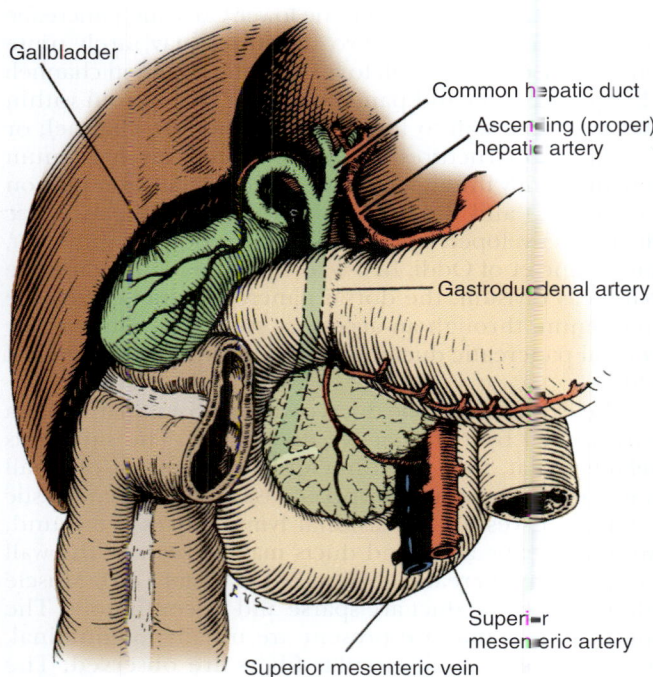

FIGURE 106.4 Anatomic relationships of the gallbladder. (From Linder HH. Embryology and anatomy of the biliary tree. In: Way LW, Pellegrini CA, eds. *Surgery of the Gallbladder and Bile Ducts.* Philadelphia: Saunders; 1987:8.)

right hepatic lobes between Couinaud segments IV and V (Fig. 106.4).[6] The gallbladder varies from 7 to 10 cm in length and from 2.5 to 3.5 cm in width. The gallbladder's volume varies considerably, being large during fasting states and small after eating. A moderately distended gallbladder has a capacity of 50 to 60 mL of bile but may become much larger with certain pathologic states and can get markedly distended containing up to 300 mL. The gallbladder has been divided into four areas: the fundus, body, infundibulum, and neck. The gallbladder fundus is commonly located at the level of the ninth costal cartilage and the external border of the right rectus muscle. It is covered by peritoneum because it projects beyond the inferior border of the liver. The body of the gallbladder occupies the gallbladder fossa of the liver and has intimate contact with the first and second portions of the duodenum. The infundibulum is the portion of the body between the neck and the point of entrance of the cystic artery (CA); when this portion is dilated, it becomes an asymmetric bulge called the Hartmann pouch. The neck curves forming an S-shaped structure that ultimately becomes the CD. The CA is usually found in this region coursing parallel within the connective tissue that attaches the neck of the gallbladder to the liver.

The gallbladder wall consists of five layers. The innermost layer is the epithelium, and the other layers are the lamina propria, smooth muscle, perimuscular subserosal connective tissue, and serosa. The gallbladder has no muscularis mucosae or submucosa. Most cells in the mucosa are columnar cells, and their main function is absorption, but they also are capable of active secretion.[7]

These cells are aligned in a single row, with slightly eosinophilic cytoplasm, apical vacuoles, and basal or central nuclei.

The lamina propria contains nerve fibers, vessels, lymphatics, elastic fibers, loose connective tissue, and occasional mast cells and macrophages. The muscle layer is a loose arrangement of circular, longitudinal, and oblique fibers without well-developed layers. Ganglia are found between smooth muscle bundles. The subserosa is composed of a loose arrangement of fibroblasts, elastic and collagen fibers, vessels, nerves, lymphatics, and adipocytes.

Rokitansky-Aschoff sinuses are invaginations of epithelium into the lamina propria, muscle, and subserosal connective tissue. These sinuses are present in approximately 40% of normal gallbladders and are present in abundance in almost all inflamed gallbladders. The ducts of Luschka are tiny bile ducts found around the muscle layer on the hepatic side of the gallbladder. They are found in approximately 10% of normal gallbladders and have no relation to the Rokitansky-Aschoff sinuses or to cholecystitis.

The CD arises from the gallbladder and joins the CHD to form the CBD (see Fig. 106.3). The length of the CD is variable averaging between 2 and 4 cm. The CD usually courses downward in the hepatoduodenal ligament to join the lateral aspect of the supraduodenal portion of the CHD at an acute angle.[3] Occasionally the CD may join the right hepatic duct, or it may extend downward to join the retroduodenal duct. In addition, the CD may join the CHD at a right angle, may run parallel to the CHD, or may enter the CHD dorsally, on its left side, behind the duodenum, or, rarely, may enter the duodenum directly. The CD contains a variable number of mucosal folds, similar to those found in the neck of the gallbladder. Although referred to as valves of Heister, these spiral folds do not have a valvular function. Variations in the length and course of the CD and its point of union with the CHD are common.

In 1891 Calot described a triangular anatomic region formed by the CHD medially, the CD laterally, and the CA superiorly.[8] Calot triangle is considered by most to comprise the triangular area with an upper boundary formed by the inferior margin of the right lobe of the liver, rather than the CA (Fig. 106.5).[9,10] A thorough appreciation of the anatomy of Calot triangle is essential during performance of a cholecystectomy because numerous important structures pass through this area. In most instances the CA arises as a branch of the right hepatic artery within the hepatocystic triangle. A replaced or aberrant right hepatic artery arising from the superior mesenteric artery usually courses through the medial aspect of the triangle, posterior to the CD. Aberrant or accessory hepatic ducts also may pass through Calot triangle before joining the CD or CHD. During performance of a cholecystectomy, clear visualization of the hepatocystic triangle is essential with accurate identification of all structures within this triangle.

SPHINCTER OF ODDI

The entire sphincteric system of the distal bile duct and the pancreatic duct is commonly referred to as the *sphincter of Oddi*. It regulates the bile and pancreatic juice flow towards the duodenum, preventing the regurgitation of duodenal content into the biliary tree and also diverts bile into the gallbladder leading to its distention. This term is imprecise because the sphincter is subdivided into several sections and contains both circular and longitudinal fibers. The sphincter mechanism functions independently from the surrounding duodenal musculature and has

separate sphincters for the distal bile duct, the pancreatic duct, and the ampulla (Fig. 106.6). In more than 90% of the population, the common channel, where the biliary and pancreatic ducts join, is less than 1.0 cm in length and lies within the ampulla. In the rare situation in which the common channel is longer than 1.0 cm or the biliary and pancreatic ducts open separately into the duodenum, pathologic biliary or pancreatic problems are likely to develop. The entire sphincter mechanism is actually composed of four sphincters containing both circular and longitudinal smooth muscle fibers (Fig. 106.7). The four sphincters are the superior and inferior sphincter choledochus, the sphincter pancreaticus, and the sphincter of the ampulla.[11]

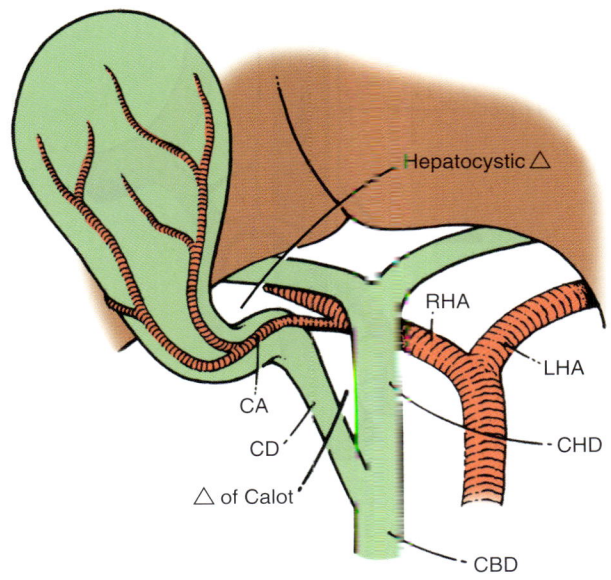

FIGURE 106.5 The triangle *(Δ)* of Calot and the hepatocystic triangle. The two triangles differ in their upper boundaries. The upper boundary of Calot triangle is the cystic artery (CA), whereas that of the hepatocystic triangle is the inferior margin of the liver. *CBD,* Common bile duct; *CD,* cystic duct; *CHD,* common hepatic duct; *LHA,* left hepatic artery; *RHA,* right hepatic artery. (From Skandalakis JE, Gray SW, Rowe JS Jr. Biliary tract. In: Skandalakis JE, Gray SW, eds. *Anatomical Complications in General Surgery*. New York: McGraw-Hill; 1983:31.)

VASCULAR

The hepatic artery represents the 25% of the blood supply to the liver; the rest is provided by the portal vein. The hepatic artery is derived from the celiac trunk in 55% of the cases. The common hepatic and the right or left hepatic arteries may arise from vessels other than the celiac trunk.[12]

The blood supply to the right and left hepatic ducts and upper portion of the CHD is from the CA and the right and left hepatic arteries. The supraduodenal bile duct is supplied by arterial branches from the right hepatic, cystic, posterior superior pancreaticoduodenal, and retroduodenal arteries. The axial blood supply of the supraduodenal bile duct has been emphasized by Terblanche et al. (Fig. 106.8).[13] The most important arteries to the supraduodenal bile duct run parallel to the duct at the 3 and 9 o'clock positions. Approximately 60% of the blood supply to the supraduodenal bile duct originates inferiorly from the pancreaticoduodenal and retroduodenal arteries, whereas 38% of the blood supply originates superiorly from the right hepatic artery and CD artery. Injury to this important axial blood supply may result in the formation of an ischemic ductal stricture. This configuration dictates surgical management when the CBD is injured or is opened purposefully when attempting

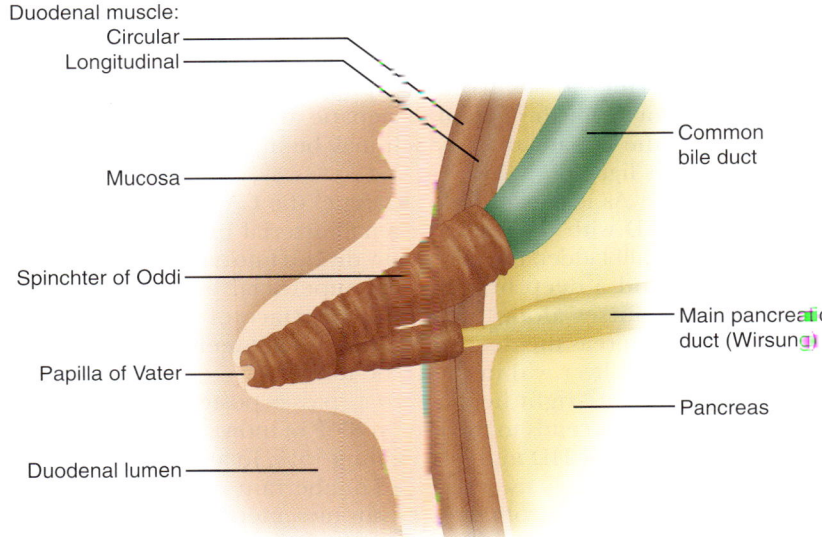

FIGURE 106.6 The junction of the pancreatic and common bile ducts, surrounded by the sphincter of Oddi. (From Hatzaras I, Pawlik T. Gallbladder and biliary tree: anatomy and physiology. In: Stanley WA, ed. *Scientific American Surgery*. Hamilton, Ontario, and Philadelphia: Decker Intellectual Properties; 2016:44.)

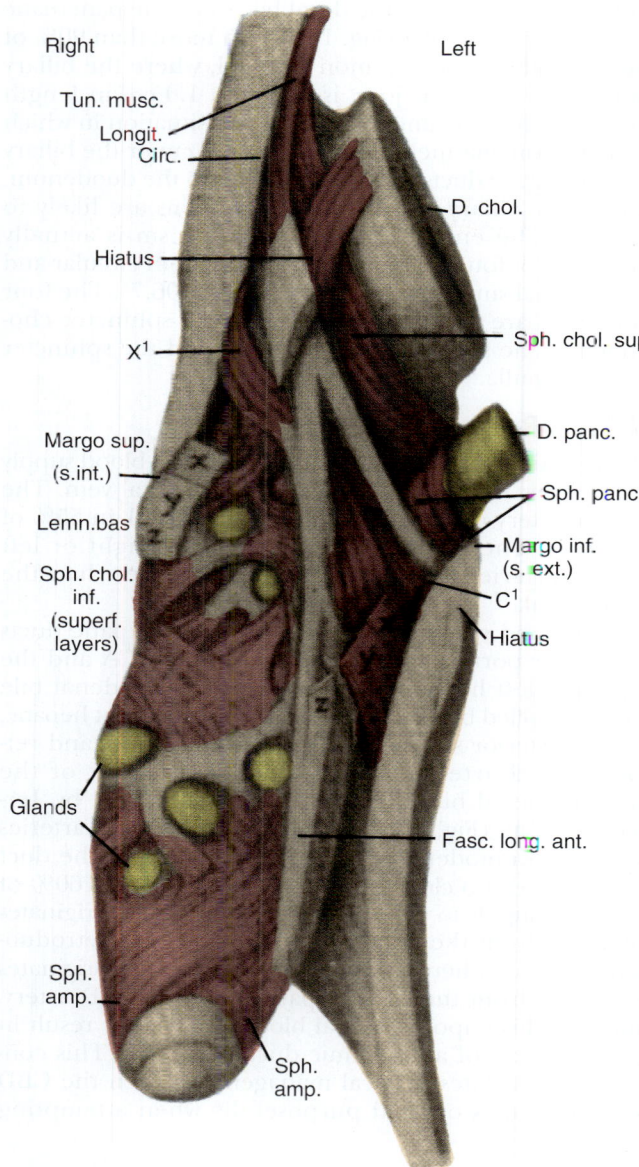

Right   Left

Tun. musc.
Longit.
Circ.

D. chol.

Hiatus

X¹

Sph. chol. sup.

Margo sup.
(s.int.)

D. panc.

Sph. panc.

Lemn.bas

Margo inf.
(s. ext.)

Sph. chol.
inf.
(superf.
layers)

C¹

Hiatus

Glands

Fasc. long. ant.

Sph.
amp.

Sph.
amp.

FIGURE 106.7 Human choledochoduodenal junction at the terminal portion of the common bile duct and pancreatic ducts. (From Boyden EA. The anatomy of the choledochoduodenal junction in man. *Surg Gynecol Obstet.* 1957;104:646.)

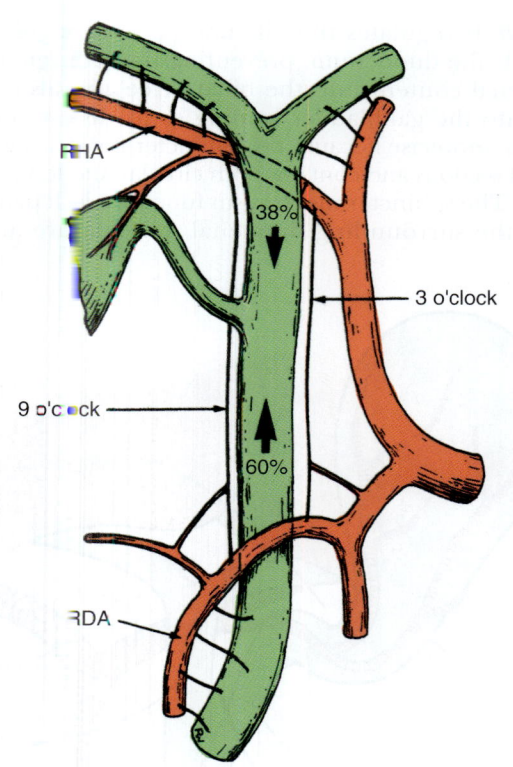

RHA

38%

3 o'clock

9 o'clock

60%

RDA

FIGURE 106.8 Arterial blood supply of the extrahepatic biliary tree. The proximal or hilar ducts and the retropancreatic bile duct receive a rich blood supply. The supraduodenal bile duct supply is axial and tenuous, with 60% from below and 38% from above. The small axial vessels (arteries at the 3 and 9 o'clock positions) are vulnerable and easily damaged. *RDA,* Retroduodenal artery; *RHA,* right hepatic artery. (From Terblanche J, Allison HF, Northover JMA. An ischemic basis for biliary strictures. *Surgery.* 1983;94:56.)

exploration. Most surgeons would suggest that if more than 50% of the diameter of the CBD is transected it will lead unequivocally to stricture if primarily closed, rendering jejunal limb reconstruction necessary in this situation. Only 2% of the arterial blood supply to the supraduodenal bile duct is segmental (nonaxial). These small segmental arterial branches arise directly from the proper hepatic artery as it ascends in the hepatoduodenal ligament, adjacent to the CBD. The blood supply to the retroduodenal and intrapancreatic bile duct is from the retroduodenal and pancreaticoduodenal arteries.

The CA usually arises as a single branch from the right hepatic artery within Calot triangle (Fig. 106.9).[14,15]

Infrequently, the CA may arise from the left hepatic, common hepatic, gastroduodenal, or superior mesenteric artery.[15] When the CA arises from the right hepatic artery, it usually courses parallel, adjacent, and medial to the CD. However, this relation is far from constant; if the artery arises from the proximal right hepatic artery or from the common hepatic artery, it may lie close to the hepatic duct, which may be injured when the artery is ligated.

As it crosses Calot triangle, the CA often supplies the CD with one or more small arterial branches. Near the gallbladder, the CA usually divides into a superficial branch and a deep branch. The superficial branch of the CA courses along the anterior surface of the gallbladder, whereas the deep branch passes between the gallbladder and liver within the cystic fossa.

The right hepatic artery passes posterior to the CHD as it ascends to the liver in 85% of individuals and anterior to the CHD in the remaining 15%. In approximately 15% of individuals, a replaced or aberrant right hepatic artery originates from the superior mesenteric artery and courses through the medial aspect of Calot triangle, posterior to the CD.

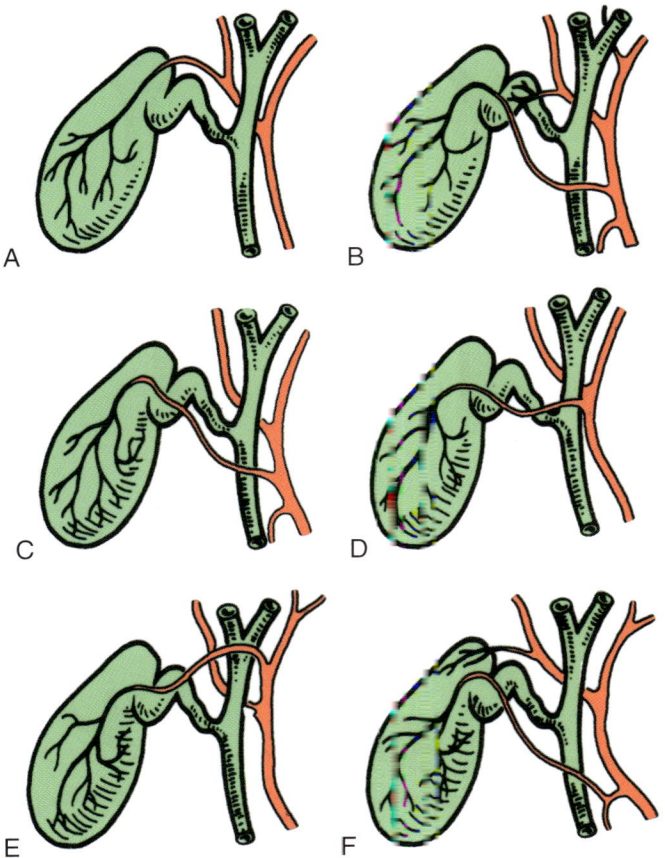

FIGURE 106.9 Cystic artery (CA) and its variations. (A) Usual origin and course of the CA. (B) Double CA. (C) CA crossing anterior to main bile duct. (D) CA originating from the right branch of the hepatic artery and crossing the common hepatic duct anteriorly. (E) CA originating from the left branch of the hepatic artery. (F) CA originating from the gastroduodenal artery. (From Smadja C, Blumgart LH. The biliary tract and the anatomy of biliary exposure. In: Blumgart LH, ed. *Surgery of the Liver and Biliary Tract.* Edinburgh: Churchill Livingstone; 1988:6.)

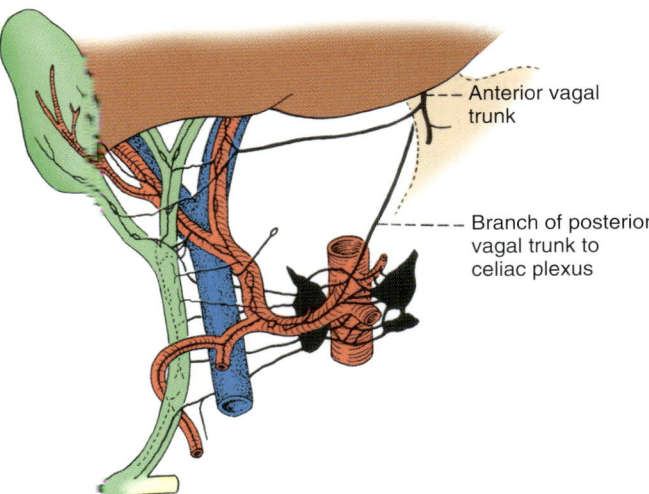

FIGURE 106.10 Nerve supply to the extrahepatic bile tree. (From Linder HH. Embryology and anatomy of the biliary tree. In: Way LW, Pellegrini CA, ed. *Surgery of the Gallbladder and Bile Ducts.* Philadelphia: Saunders; 1987:21.)

The venous drainage from the hepatic ducts and hepatic surface of the gallbladder is through small vessels that empty into branches of the hepatic veins within the liver. A small venous trunk ascending parallel to the portal vein receives veins draining the gallbladder and bile duct before entering the liver, separate from the portal vein.[5] Venous drainage of the lower portion of the bile duct is directly into the portal vein.

LYMPHATIC DRAINAGE

Lymphatic vessels from the hepatic ducts and upper CBD drain into the hepatic lymph nodes, a chain of lymph nodes that follows the course of the hepatic artery to drain into the celiac lymph nodes. Lymph from the lower bile duct drains into the lower hepatic nodes and the upper pancreatic lymph nodes. Lymphatic vessels from the gallbladder and CD drain primarily into the hepatic nodes. Two main trunks descending along the lateral

borders of the gallbladder join together by an oblique trunk, forming a large "N" on the surface. The trunks located to the left of the gallbladder drain into the cystic node, a constant lymph node located at the junction of the CD and CHD. The right trunks do not enter the node but continue down, joining the bile duct lymphatics. Lymphatic vessels from the hepatic surface of the gallbladder may also communicate with lymphatic vessels within the liver.

NEURAL INNERVATION

The gallbladder and biliary tree receive sympathetic and parasympathetic nerve fibers that are derived from the celiac plexus and course along the hepatic artery (Fig. 106.10). The left (anterior) vagal trunk branches into hepatic and gastric components. The hepatic branch supplies fibers to the gallbladder, bile duct, and liver. Sympathetic fibers originating from the fifth to the ninth thoracic segments pass through the greater splanchnic nerves to the celiac ganglion. Postganglionic sympathetic fibers travel along the hepatic artery to innervate the gallbladder, bile duct, and liver. Visceral afferent nerve fibers from the liver, gallbladder, and bile duct travel with sympathetic afferent fibers through the greater splanchnic nerves to enter the dorsal roots of the fifth through ninth thoracic segments. Sensory fibers from the right phrenic nerve also innervate the gallbladder, presumably through the communications between the phrenic plexus and the celiac plexus. This innervation may explain the phenomenon of referred shoulder pain in patients with gallbladder disease.

Burnett et al.[17] described three nerve plexuses within the gallbladder wall: mucosal, muscular, and subserous. There is a decrease in number of ganglion cells from subserous to mucosal plexus. The subserous plexus ganglia are large and spaced farther apart, unlike the myenteric plexus of the gut.

ANOMALIES

BILIARY DUCTS

The anatomy of the extrahepatic biliary tree is highly variable. A thorough knowledge of this variable anatomy is important because failure to recognize the frequent anatomic variations may result in significant ductal injury. Anomalies of the extrahepatic biliary tree may involve the hepatic ducts, CBD, or CD.

Hepatic Ducts

In 57% to 68% of patients, the right anterior and right posterior intrahepatic ducts join and the right hepatic duct unites with the left hepatic duct to form the CHD (Fig. 106.11) [4,18,19] Three other common variations are recognized. In 12% to 18% of patients, the right anterior, right posterior, and left hepatic ducts unite to form the CHD. In 3% to 20% of patients, the right posterior and left hepatic ducts join to form the CHD and the right anterior duct joins below the union. In 4% to 7% of patients, the right posterior duct joins the CHD below the union of the right anterior and the left hepatic ducts. In 1.5% to 3% of patients, the CD joins at the union of all the ducts or with one of the right hepatic ducts.

Accessory hepatic ducts may emerge from the liver to join the right hepatic duct, CHD, CD, CBD, or gallbladder (Fig. 106.12). These ducts are present in approximately 10% of individuals. Although accessory hepatic ducts may approach the size of a normal CD, they are often delicate, thin structures that may easily be overlooked. Accessory hepatic ducts often course through Calot triangle and may be injured during dissection in this area. Cholecystohepatic ducts are small biliary ducts that emerge from the liver to enter the hepatic surface of the gallbladder directly.[20] If a cholecystohepatic duct is discovered during dissection of the gallbladder from the cystic fossa, it should be ligated to avoid a postoperative bile leak.

Common Bile Duct

Malpositions or duplications of the CBD are rare anomalies. However, recognition of their presence is extremely important to prevent serious injury to the CBD during operations on the biliary tract or stomach. Several variations of CBD malposition and duplication have been described: (1) a single duct opening into the pylorus or antrum; (2) a single duct opening into the gastric fundus (3) a single duct entering the duodenum independently of the pancreatic duct; (4) two separate ducts entering the duodenum; (5) a bifurcating duct, with one branch entering the duodenum and the other branch entering the stomach; (6) a bifurcating duct with both branches entering the duodenum; and (7) a septate CBD, with two openings of the single duct into the duodenum. The mere presence of these anomalies does not produce symptoms, and their clinical importance rests solely on their recognition and on the avoidance of injury during an operation.

Cystic Duct

In 1976 Benson and Page described five ductal anomalies of clinical significance to the surgeon during performance of a cholecystectomy.[14] Of these five anomalies, three

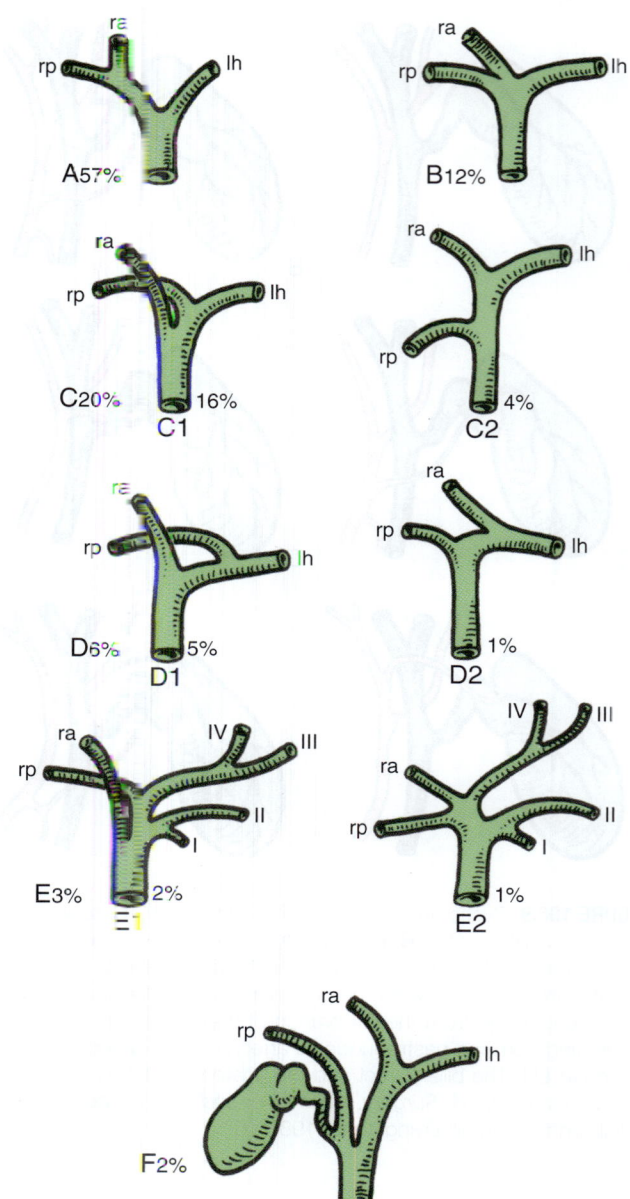

FIGURE 106.11 (A to F) Variations in hepatic ducts and hepatic duct bifurcation. *lh,* Left hepatic duct; *ra,* right anterior segmental duct; *rp,* right posterior segmental duct. The Roman numerals *I* to *IV* refer to hepatic segmental ducts. (From Smadja C, Blumgart LH. The biliary tract and the anatomy of biliary exposure. In: Blumgart LH, ed. *Surgery of the Liver and Biliary Tract.* Edinburgh: Churchill Livingstone; 1988:17.)

involve abnormalities in the length, course, or insertion of the CD into the CHD (see Fig. 106.12). The CD may run parallel to the CHD for a variable distance, or it may spiral anterior or posterior to the CHD to form a left-sided union. Parallel CDs occur in 15% of individuals, whereas spiral CDs are found in approximately 8%. The parallel or spiral CD may be normal in length or may course downward in the hepatoduodenal ligament for a considerable distance before forming a low union with the CHD.

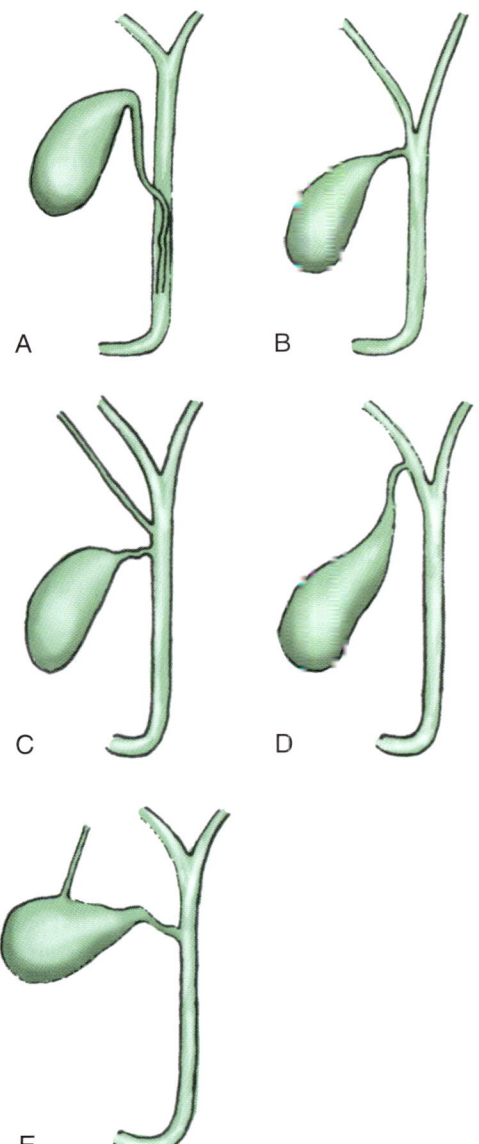

FIGURE 106.12 Duct anomalies. (A) Long cystic duct with low fusion with common hepatic duct. (B) Abnormally high fusion of cystic duct with common hepatic duct (trifurcation). (C) Accessory hepatic duct. (D) Cystic duct entering right hepatic duct. (E) Cholecystohepatic duct. (From Benson EA, Page RE. A practical reappraisal of the anatomy of the extrahepatic bile ducts and arteries. *Br J Surg.* 1976;63:854.)

In both situations, the CD is usually closely adhered to the CHD by a sheath of connective tissue.

The CD may join the right hepatic duct or a right segmental duct. Less often, the CD, right hepatic duct, and left hepatic duct may join at the same level to form a trifurcation. In these situations the right hepatic duct may easily be mistaken for the CD and may be inadvertently ligated and divided. Occasionally, the gallbladder may join the CHD with a short or virtually nonexistent CD. During ligation of a short CD, care must be taken not to compromise the lumen of the CBD.

BOX 106.1 Anomalies of the Gallbladder

FORMATION
Phrygian cap
Bilobed gallbladder
Hourglass gallbladder
Diverticulum of the gallbladder
Rudimentary gallbladder

NUMBER
Absence of the gallbladder (agenesis)
Duplication of the gallbladder

POSITION
Floating gallbladder
Intrahepatic gallbladder
Left-sided gallbladder
Transverse gallbladder
Retrodisplaced gallbladder

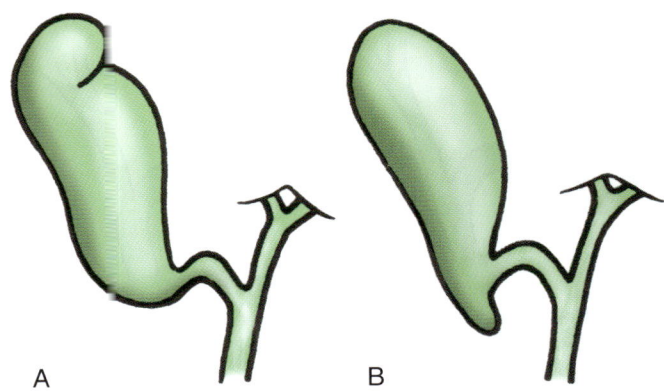

FIGURE 106.13 Deformations of the gallbladder. (A) Phrygian cap deformity. (B) Hartmann pouch of the infundibulum. (From Gray SW, Skandalakis JE. *Embryology for Surgeons*. Philadelphia: Saunders; 1972:254.)

GALLBLADDER

Some apparent anomalies are acquired but most result from arrested or abnormal development at some stage of embryonic growth. These anomalies vary in their clinical significance: Some are only medical curiosities and require no attempt at correction, whereas others require surgical intervention. The gallbladder anomalies may be divided into three groups based on formation, number, and position (Box 106.1).

Phrygian Cap

This anomaly of formation is the most common of the gallbladder (Fig. 106.13A). Phrygian cap occurs in individuals of all ages and more commonly in women. Boyden found that this anomaly was present as confirmed by oral cholecystography in 18% of patients with a functioning gallbladder.[21] The phrygian cap deformity is created by an infolding of a septum between the body and the fundus. The gallbladder functions normally, and this anomaly is not an indication for cholecystectomy.

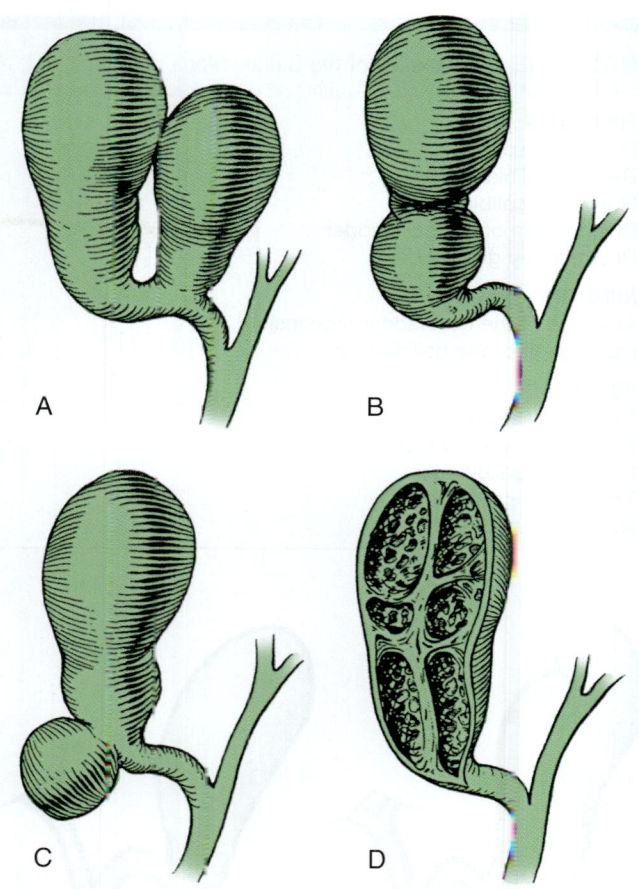

FIGURE 106·14 Anomalies of the gallbladder. (A) Bilobed gallbladder. (B) Hourglass gallbladder. (C) Congenital diverticulum of the infundibulum. (D) Septate gallbladder. (From Linder HH. Embryology and anatomy of the biliary tree. In: Way LW, Pellegrini CA, eds. *Surgery of the Gallbladder and Bile Ducts*. Philadelphia: Saunders; 1987:5.)

Bilobed Gallbladder

This rare anomaly of formation consists of a completely divided gallbladder drained by a common CD (Fig. 106.14A). Bilobed gallbladder occurs in two forms: (1) a type that has the outward appearance of a single gallbladder but is divided internally by a longitudinal fibrous septum; and (2) a type that has the outward appearance of two separate gallbladders that are fused at the neck. A bilobed gallbladder has no clinical significance and does not require excision unless it becomes symptomatic.

Hourglass Gallbladder

Alterations in the contour of the gallbladder may result in a dumbbell or hourglass form (see Fig. 106.14B). These anomalies are not rare and can be congenital or acquired. In children, this anomaly is congenital and does not require removal. In adults, this abnormality usually results from chronic cholecystitis and should be removed in patients with appropriate biliary symptoms.

Diverticulum of the Gallbladder

Congenital diverticula of the gallbladder are rare, being found in only 25 of 29,701 gallbladders removed surgically

at the Mayo Clinic (see Fig. 106.14C).[22] Diverticula may occur in any part of the gallbladder and may vary greatly in size from 0.5 to 9 cm in diameter. These diverticula are clinically insignificant unless they become the site of disease, in which case they may contain stones, become acutely inflamed, or even perforate. Hartmann pouch is an acquired diverticulum of the infundibulum or neck of the gallbladder (see Fig. 106.13B). This pouch projects from the convexity of the gallbladder neck and may adhere to the CBD. Hartmann pouch is associated with pathologic conditions of the gallbladder, especially those involving prolonged obstruction to gallbladder emptying.[23]

Rudimentary Gallbladder

This condition consists of a small nubbin at the end of the CD. When found in infants and children, a rudimentary gallbladder is believed to be caused by congenital hypoplasia and usually requires no treatment. In an older adult, this situation may be the result of fibrosis from cholecystitis and may require removal if causing biliary symptoms.

Absence of the Gallbladder (Agenesis)

More than 300 cases of absence of the gallbladder have been reported. Most cases are associated with other biliary abnormalities, and most of the patients died before 6 months of age. One publication reviewed 185 cases of gallbladder agenesis. In this series, 70 (38%) were completely absent, 60 (32%) were rudimentary, and 55 (30%) were a fibrous structure.[24]

The absence of the gallbladder must not be confused with an intrahepatic gallbladder or a left-sided gallbladder, conditions that can mimic this particular situation. A history of gallbladder disease with subsequent cholecystectomy is not in itself enough to establish absence of the organ. There have been cases where two gallbladders were present in a single patient and only one removed leaving the second behind.[25]

Duplication

The first description of a double gallbladder was made by Blasius in 1674 found at autopsy of a human body,[26] and the first such anomaly to be recorded from observation of a living patient was made by Sherren in 1911.[27] This anomaly occurs in approximately 1 in 4000 persons. A true duplicated gallbladder has two separate cavities, each drained by its own CD and sometimes supplied by its own CA (Fig. 106.15). Duplication occurs as one of two varieties: (1) the more common ductular type, in which each gallbladder has its own CD that empties independently into the same or different parts of the extrahepatic biliary tree; and (2) a type in which the two ducts gradually merge into a common CD before emptying into the CBD. The gallbladder itself may be seen as two distinct organs at variable distances apart or may outwardly have the appearance of a single organ. Each cavity may function normally or become diseased independently of the other. Duplication of the gallbladder is clinically unimportant and generally requires no treatment.

Rarely a gallbladder may be found in an abnormal location. This type of gallbladder requires no treatment

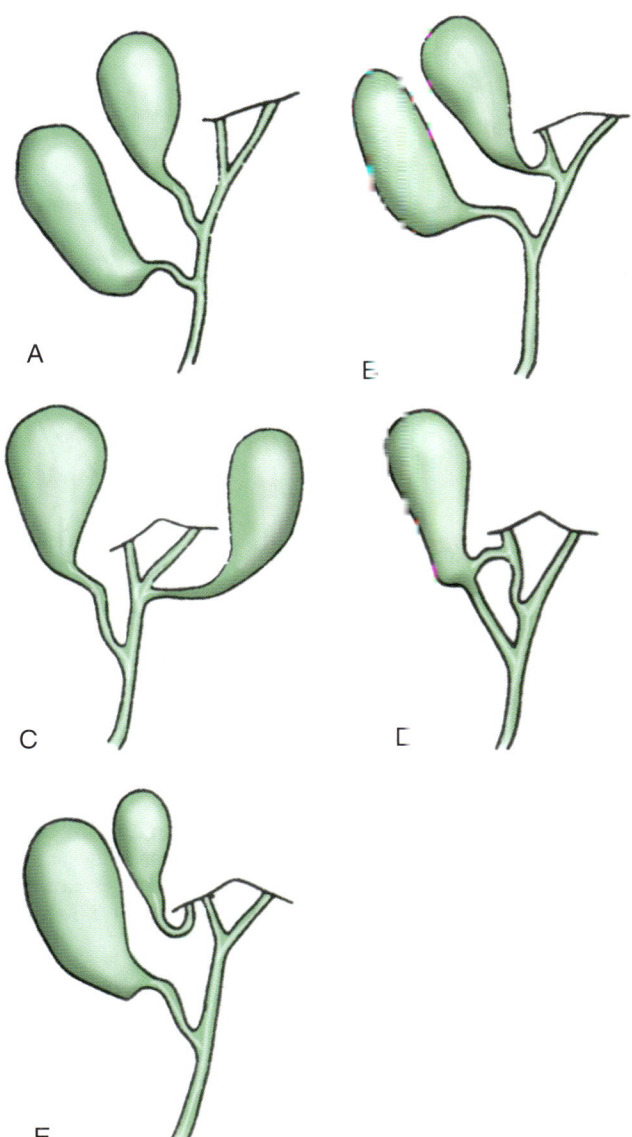

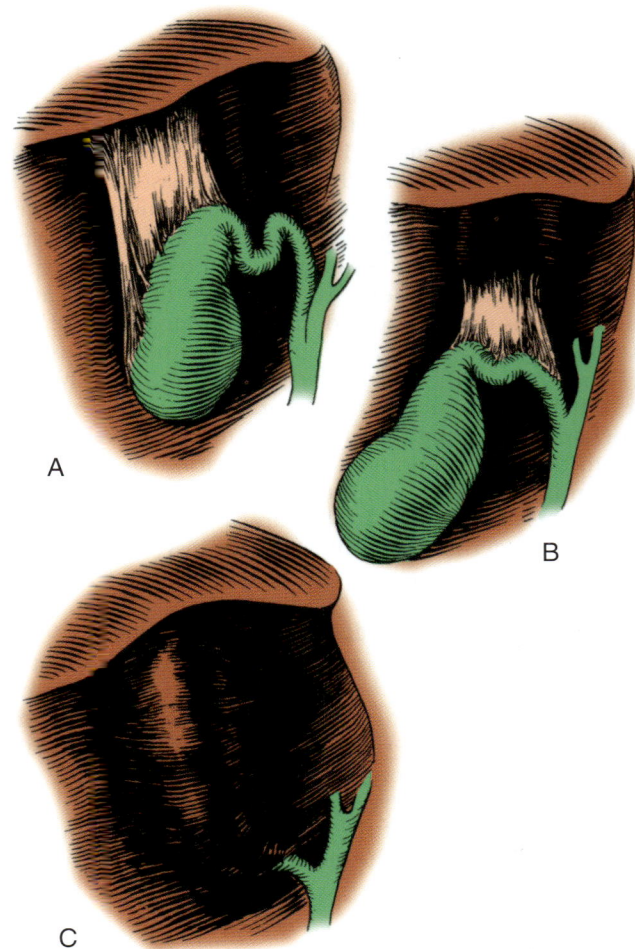

FIGURE 106.16 Anomalies of gallbladder position. (A) Floating gallbladder with mesentery. (B) Cystic duct with mesentery. (C) Intrahepatic gallbladder. (From Linder HH. Embryology and anatomy of the biliary tree. In: Way LW, Pellegrini CA, eds. *Surgery of the Gallbladder and Bile Ducts*. Philadelphia: Saunders; 1987:5.)

FIGURE 106.15 (A to E) Duplication of the gallbladder. (From Glassman JA: A short practical review of surgical anatomy of the biliary tract. In: Glassman JA, ed. *Biliary Tract Surgery: Tactics and Techniques*. New York: Macmillan; 1989:18.)

unless it causes symptoms. Five different conditions are recognized: floating, intrahepatic, left sided, transverse, and retrodisplaced.

Floating Gallbladder. A floating gallbladder has been reported to occur in approximately 5% of persons. In this condition the gallbladder is completely surrounded by peritoneum and is attached to the undersurface of the cystic fossa by the peritoneal reflection from the liver. This attachment may extend the entire length of the gallbladder, or it may include only the CD, thus leaving the gallbladder unsupported and ptosed (Fig. 106.16A and B). This condition usually occurs in women older than 60 years. Such a gallbladder not only is subject to the same pathologic changes as a normally placed gallbladder but also may undergo torsion around its pedicle.

Torsion of the gallbladder usually occurs in persons 60 to 80 years of age, but it also has been reported to occur in young children. When torsion of the gallbladder occurs, an abrupt onset of symptoms may include acute right upper quadrant abdominal pain, nausea, and vomiting. Torsion of the gallbladder requires operative detorsion and removal of the gallbladder, which may be infarcted as a result of occlusion of its blood vessels.

Intrahepatic Gallbladder. The gallbladder is usually intrahepatic during its embryologic period and becomes extrahepatic later in its development. An intrahepatic gallbladder is one that is partially or completely embedded within the substance of the liver (see Fig. 106.16C). The condition may be suspected if the cholecystogram or ultrasound reveals a gallbladder in an unusually high location. In adults, approximately 60% of intrahepatic gallbladders are associated with gallstones. Most intrahepatic gallbladders are only partially embedded within the hepatic parenchyma, and they can usually be easily identified at the time of cholecystectomy. Those that are completely buried within the liver may be a challenge to remove. A completely embedded gallbladder is best approached by first identifying the CD where it joins the CHD and then following the CD back to the gallbladder.

Left-Sided Gallbladder. The two types of left-sided gall-bladders are (1) left-sided gallbladder associated with situs inversus, in which the heart and abdominal viscera are transposed from their usual position; and (2) the type in which the gallbladder alone is transposed. Both types of left-sided gallbladders are rare. The malpositioned gallbladder is usually located on the undersurface of the left lobe of the liver. In most instances, the CD joins the CHD in the usual location, but it may occasionally join the left hepatic duct. Usually there is no malfunction associated with this anomaly. Ultrasonography should be able to detect this anomaly, and the radiologist must be alert and aware of this finding.

Transverse Gallbladder. In this rare anomaly the gallblad-der is positioned horizontally in the transverse fissure of the liver. In these cases the gallbladder is usually deeply embedded within the liver parenchyma.

Retrodisplaced Gallbladder. Retrodisplacement of the gallbladder is a condition in which the organ is not situated in the gallbladder fossa but is bound to another portion of the liver or freely suspended from the liver with the fundus extending posteriorly. The retrodisplaced gallblad-der may be partially or completely located within the retroperitoneum. This type of gallbladder may be difficult to expose and excise. If the gallbladder is located retro-peritoneally, dividing the peritoneum overlying it will facilitate its removal.

VASCULAR

Variations in the arterial supply of the extrahepatic biliary tree are more common than variations in the ductal anatomy. Anatomic variations of the hepatic and CAs are present in approximately 50% of individuals.[5,14,28] Based on their anatomic dissections, Benson and Page described three surgically important variations in the arterial anatomy (Fig. 106.17).[14] An accessory or double CA occurs in approximately 15% to 20% of individuals.[14,29] These arteries usually arise from the right hepatic artery within Calot triangle. Triple CAs are unusual and occur in less than 1% of individuals. During dissection of Calot triangle, care should be taken to exclude the presence of an accessory CA.

In 5% to 15% of individuals, the right hepatic artery courses through Calot triangle in close proximity to the CD before turning upward to enter the hilum of the liver.[14,28] In this location, the CA arises from the convex aspect of the angled or humped portion of the hepatic artery. This "caterpillar hump" right hepatic artery may easily be mistaken for the CA and may be inadvertently ligated during performance of a cholecystectomy. The CA that arises from the caterpillar hump is typically short and may easily be avulsed from the hepatic artery if exces-sive traction is applied to the gallbladder.[14]

The CA may occasionally pass anterior to the CBD or CHD.[15] In this location, the CA, rather than the CD, is usually the first structure encountered during dissection of the lower border of Calot triangle.[29,30] These arteries

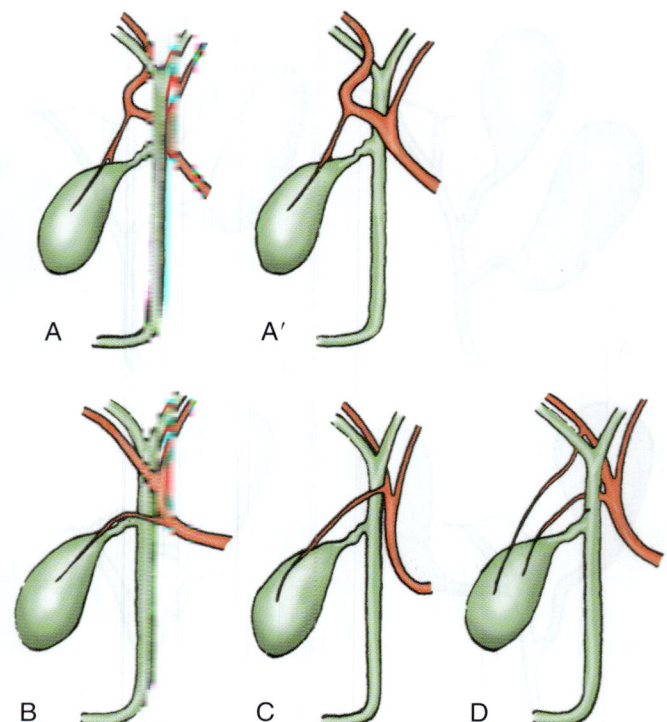

FIGURE 106.17 Vascular anomalies. (A and A') "Caterpillar hump" right hepatic artery. (B) Right hepatic artery anterior to common hepatic (or common bile) duct. (C) Cystic artery anterior to common hepatic (or common bile) duct. (D) Accessory cystic artery. (From Benson EA, Page RE. A practical reappraisal of the anatomy of the extrahepatic bile ducts and arteries. *Br J Surg.* 1976;63:854.)

usually require ligation and division early in the dissection during a cholecystectomy, to provide adequate exposure of the CD.

PHYSIOLOGY

BILE PRODUCTION

Bile Formation and Composition

The formation of bile by the hepatocyte serves two pur-poses. Bile represents the route of excretion for certain organic solutes such as bilirubin and cholesterol, and it facilitates intestinal absorption of lipids and fat-soluble vitamins. Bile secretion results from the active transport of solutes into the canaliculus followed by the passive flow of water. Water constitutes approximately 85% of the volume of bile.

Phospholipids, bile salts, and cholesterol constitute approximately 90% of the solids in bile; the remainder consists of bilirubin, fatty acids, and inorganic salts. Bili-rubin, the breakdown product of spent red blood cells, is conjugated with glucuronic acid by the hepatic enzyme glucuronyl transferase and is excreted actively into the adjacent canaliculus. Normally, a large reserve exists to handle excess bilirubin production, which might exist in hemolytic states. Approximately 250 to 300 mg of bilirubin

TABLE 106.1 Composition of Hepatic and Gallbladder Bile

Characteristics*	Hepatic Bile	Gallbladder Bile
Na	160	270
K	5	10
Cl	90	15
HCO₃	45	10
Ca	4	25
Mg	2	4
Bilirubin	1 5	15
Protein	150	200
Bile acids	50	150
Phospholipids	8	40
Cholesterol	4	18
Total solids	—	125
pH	7.8	7.2

*All determinations are milliequivalents per liter; except for pH. Significant ranges of all elements may occur.

is excreted each day in the bile, 75% of it from break-down of red cells in the reticuloendothelial system and 25% from turnover of hepatic heme and hemoproteins. Bile salts are steroid molecules synthesized by the hepatocyte. The primary bile salts in humans, cholic and chenodeoxycholic acid, account for more than 80% of those produced. The primary bile salts which are then conjugated with either taurine or glycine, can undergo bacterial alteration in the intestine to form the secondary bile salts, deoxycholate and lithocholate. The purpose of bile salts is to solubilize lipids and facilitate their absorption. Phospholipids are synthesized in the liver in conjunction with bile salt synthesis. Lecithin is the primary phospholipid in human bile, constituting more than 95% of its total. The final major solute of bile is cholesterol, which also is produced primarily by the liver with little contribution from dietary sources.

The normal volume of bile secreted daily by the liver is 750 to 1000 mL. Three main factors contribute to bile flow: hepatic secretion, gallbladder contraction, and sphincteric resistance. In the fasting state, the pressure in the CBD is 5 to 10 cm H₂O, and the bile produced is diverted to the gallbladder, storing up to 50 to 60 mL. After a meal, the gallbladder contracts and the sphincter relaxes as response of vagal and cholecystokinin stimulus. As a result the bile is forced to the duodenum as ductal pressure exceeds sphincteric resistance. The pressure within the gallbladder can reach up to 25 cm H₂O, and the CBD pressure may reach up to 30 cm H₂O, favoring a gradient toward the duodenum. Bile is usually concentrated 5- to 10-fold by the absorption of water and electrolytes, leading to a marked change or bile composition (Table 106.1).[31,32] Active sodium chloride transport by the gallbladder epithelium is the driving force for the concentration of bile. Water is passively absorbed in response to the osmotic force generated by solute absorption.

Bile Salt Secretion

Bile is secreted from the hepatocyte into canaliculi that drain their contents into small bile ducts. Secretion of bile salts is the major osmotic force for the generation of bile flow. Bile acids are formed at a rate of 500 to 600 mg per day. The majority of the bile salt pool is maintained in the gallbladder, followed by the liver, the small intestine, and the extrahepatic bile ducts. Bile acids are synthesized from cholesterol via (1) a classic pathway that leads to the formation of cholic acid and (2) an alternate pathway that results in the synthesis of chenodeoxycholic acid, which occurs less commonly in human bile.[33]

In plasma, bile acids circulate in a bound state either to albumin or to lipoproteins. In the space of Disse in the liver, bile salt uptake into the hepatocytes is very efficient. This process is mediated by sodium-dependent and sodium-independent mechanisms. The sodium-dependent pathway accounts for more than 80% of taurocholate uptake but less than 50% of cholate uptake.[34] A number of transport proteins have been identified that play a key role in this process. The bile salt transporter, sodium-taurocholate cotransporting polypeptide (NTCP), is exclusively expressed in the liver and is located in the basolateral membrane of the hepatocyte. Sodium-independent hepatic uptake of bile acids is mediated primarily by a family of transporters termed the *organic anion–transporting polypeptides* (OATPs). In contrast to NTCP, these transporters have a broader substrate affinity and transport a variety of organic anions, including the bile salts. OATP-C is the major sodium-independent bile salt uptake system. OATP-A also uptakes bile acids, and OATP8 mediates taurocholate uptake.

Intracellular bile acid transport occurs within a matter of seconds. Two mechanisms may be responsible for bile acid transcellular movement. One involves transfer of bile acids from the basolateral membrane to the canalicular membrane via bile acid–binding proteins.[35] The other proposed mechanism for intracellular bile salt movement is through vesicular transport. In contrast, the transport of bile salts across the canalicular membrane of hepatocytes represents the rate-limiting step in the overall secretion of bile salts from the blood into bile.

Bile salt concentrations are 1000-fold greater within the canaliculi than in the hepatocyte. This gradient necessitates an active transport mechanism, which is an adenosine triphosphate (ATP)-dependent process. This bile salt export pump (BSEP) is closely related to the proteins encoded by the multidrug resistance (MDR) gene family of ATP-binding cassette (ABC) transporters.[33] The ABC transporters mediate the transport of metabolites, peptides, fatty acids, cholesterol, and lipids in the liver, intestine, pancreas, lungs, kidneys, brain, and macrophages. Although BSEP is the major transporter for monovalent bile salts into the canaliculus, multidrug resistance-associated protein 2 (MRP2), a member of the MDR protein family, also transports sulfated and glucuronidated bile salts into the canaliculus. MRP2 also mediates the export of multiple other organic anions, including conjugated bilirubin, leukotrienes, glutathione disulfide, chemotherapeutic agents, uricosurics, antibiotics, toxins, and heavy metals.[36]

Enterohepatic Circulation

The main functions of the bile salts are to bind calcium ions in bile, to induce the bile flow, and more importantly to facilitate lipid transport. Bile salts are synthesized and conjugated in the liver, secreted into bile, stored temporarily

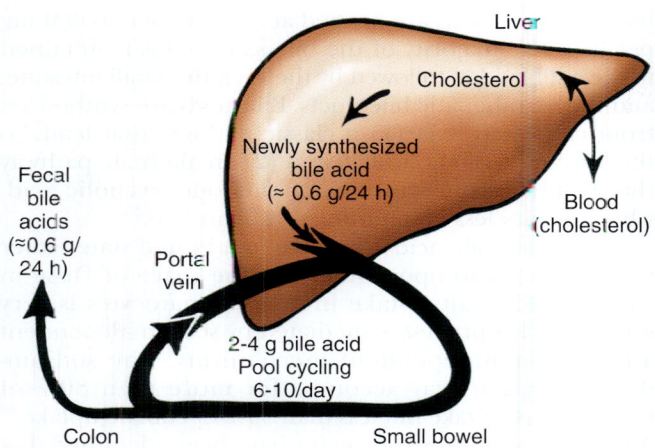

FIGURE 106.18 Enterohepatic circulation of bile salts. Cholesterol is taken up from plasma by the liver. Bile acids are synthesized at a rate of 0.6 g/24 h and are excreted through the biliary system into the small bowel. Most of the bile salts are reabsorbed in the terminal ileum and are returned to the liver to be extracted and reextracted. (Modified from Dietschy JM. The biology of bile acids. *Arch Intern Med.* 1972;130:472.)

in the gallbladder, passed from the gallbladder into the duodenum, absorbed throughout the small intestine but especially in the terminal ileum by an active transport system, and returned to the liver via the portal vein. This cycling of bile acids between the liver and the intestine is referred to as the *enterohepatic circulation* (Fig. 106.18). The total amount of bile acids in the enterohepatic circulation is defined as the circulating bile pool. In this highly efficient system, nearly 95% of bile salts are reabsorbed. Thus, of the total bile salt pool of 2 to 4 g that recycles through the enterohepatic cycle 6 to 10 times daily, only approximately 600 mg of bile salt is actually excreted into the colon. Bacterial action in the colon on the two primary bile salts, cholate and chenodeoxycholate, results in the formation of the secondary bile salts, deoxycholate and lithocholate. Although some deoxycholate is reabsorbed passively by the colon, the remainder is lost in fecal waste.

The enterohepatic circulation provides an important negative feedback system on bile salt synthesis. Should the recirculation be interrupted by resection of the terminal ileum, or by primary ileal disease, abnormally large losses of bile salts can occur. This situation increases bile salt production to maintain a normal bile salt pool. Similarly, if bile salts are lost by an external biliary fistula, increased bile salt synthesis is necessary. However, except for those unusual circumstances in which excessive losses occur, bile salt synthesis matches losses, maintaining a constant bile salt pool size. During fasting, approximately 90% of the bile acid pool is sequestered in the gallbladder.

Cholesterol Saturation

Cholesterol is highly nonpolar and insoluble in water; thus it is insoluble in bile. The key to maintaining cholesterol in solution is the formation of micelles, a bile salt–phospholipid-cholesterol complex. Bile salts are amphipathic compounds containing both a hydrophilic

and hydrophobic portion. In aqueous solutions, bile salts are oriented with the hydrophilic portion outward. Phospholipids are incorporated into the micellar structure, allowing cholesterol to be added to the hydrophobic central portion of the micelle. In this way, cholesterol can be maintained in solution in an aqueous medium. The concept of mixed micelles as the only cholesterol carrier has been challenged by the demonstration that much of the biliary cholesterol exists in a vesicular form. Structurally, these vesicles are made up of lipid bilayers of cholesterol and phospholipids. In their simplest and smallest form, the vesicles are unilamellar, but an aggregation may take place, leading to multilamellar vesicles. Present theory suggests that in states of excess cholesterol production, these large vesicles may also exceed their capability to transport cholesterol, and crystal precipitation may occur (Fig. 106.19).

Cholesterol solubility depends on the relative concentration of cholesterol, bile salts, and phospholipids.[37] By plotting the percentages of each component on triangular coordinates, the micellar zone in which cholesterol is completely soluble can be demonstrated (Fig. 106.20). In a solution composed of 10% solutes similar to bile, the area under the curve represents the concentration at which cholesterol is maintained in solution. In the area above the curve, bile is supersaturated with cholesterol, and precipitation of cholesterol crystals can occur.

A mathematical model of cholesterol solubility has been developed and is influenced by the relative concentrations of lipid components and the total lipid composition.[38] A numerical value, known as the *cholesterol saturation* (or *lithogenic*) *index,* is derived that expresses the relative degrees of cholesterol saturation. When the cholesterol saturation index is greater than 1.0, the solution is supersaturated with cholesterol. Changes in the relative concentrations of bile salts, cholesterol, or phospholipids alter the capacity of micelles, thus changing the solution's cholesterol saturation index.

Gallstone Formation. Gallstones form as a result of the imbalance in concentration of solutes within the bile (bilirubin, bile salts, phospholipids, and cholesterol). After the bile is saturated, it precipitates into a more solid component: gallstones. Gallstones can be differentiated according to their composition into cholesterol and pigment stones. Pigment stones can be further classified as black or brown. Cholesterol stones are usually multiple, of variable size, and irregular with color range from clear yellow to green and black. Most of cholesterol stones are radiolucent, and less than 10% are radiopaque. Pigment stones are dark due to the presence of calcium bilirubinate and only 20% of cholesterol. Black pigment stones are small and black, often formed as a consequence of hemolytic diseases such as hereditary spherocytosis and sickle cell disease. Cholesterol stones are more prevalent in Western countries (>85%), mostly due to obesity. Brown-pigmented stones are predominant in Asia primarily as a result of bacterial infections, biliary parasites, and stasis from partial biliary obstruction.[1]

Bilirubin Metabolism

Heme, released at the time of degradation of senescent erythrocytes by the reticuloendothelial system, is the

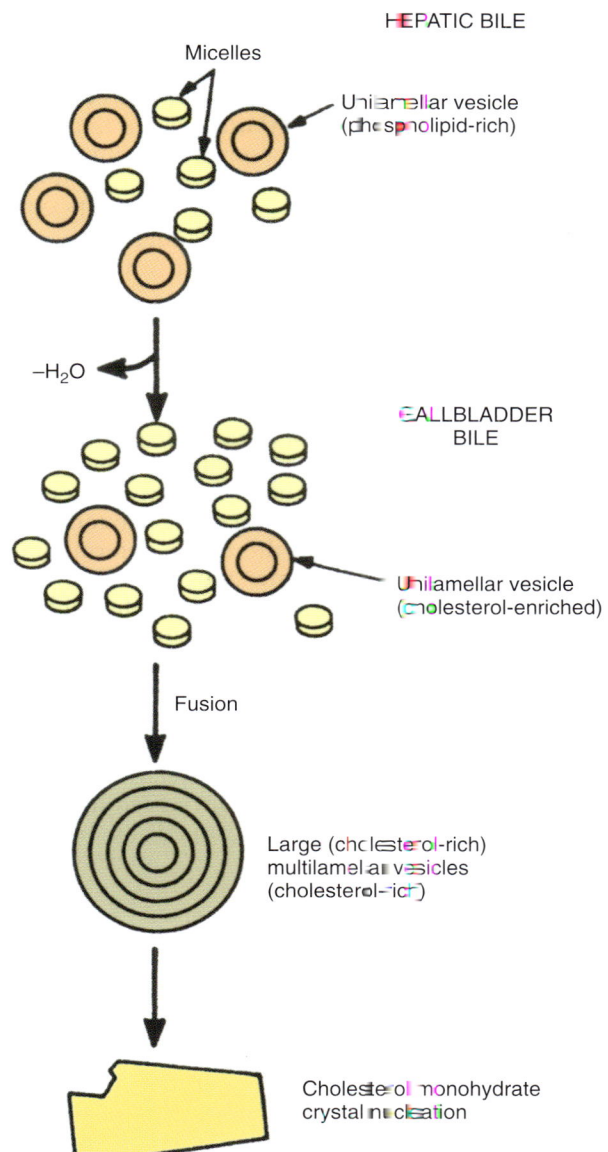

FIGURE 106.19 Concentration of bile leads to net transfer of phospholipids and cholesterol from vesicles to micelles. Phospholipids are transferred more efficiently than cholesterol, leading to cholesterol enrichment of the remaining (remodeled) vesicles. Aggregation of these cholesterol-rich vesicles forms multilamellar liquid crystals of cholesterol monohydrate. (From Vessey DA: Metabolism of drugs and toxins by the human liver. In: Zakin D, Boyer TD, eds. *Hepatology A Textbook of Liver Disease.* 2nd ed. Philadelphia: Saunders; 1990:1492.)

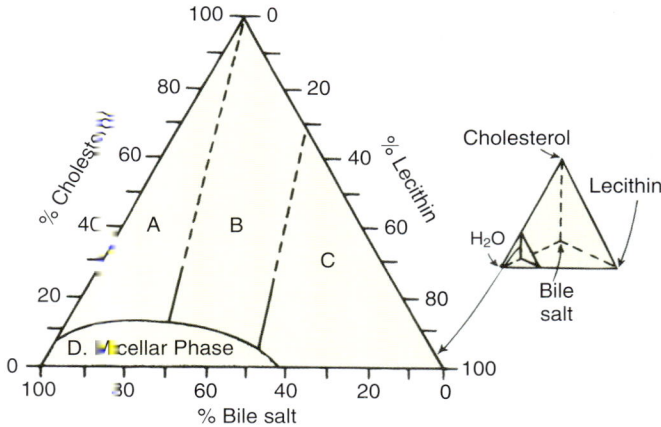

FIGURE 106.20 Interrelationships of bile salts, lecithin, and cholesterol. The graph is a plan taken from a tetrahedron at 90% water concentration. The tetrahedral plot is used to record the relationships of the four major constituents of bile: water, bile salts, lecithin, and cholesterol. The triangular coordinates can be divided into four zones, representing the physical state of the solutes in bile: crystals of cholesterol plus liquid (A); cholesterol crystals plus cholesterol liquid crystals plus liquid (B); liquid crystals plus liquid (C); and the micellar zone in which cholesterol is in water solution through the formation of cholesterol-lecithin-bile salt micelles (D). The solid line is the 10% solute line. (From Admirand WH, Small DM. The physicochemical basis of cholesterol gallstone formation in man. *J Clin Invest.* 1968;47:1043.)

source of approximately 80% to 85% of the bilirubin produced daily. The remaining 15% to 20% is derived largely from the breakdown of hepatic hemoproteins.[39] Both enzymatic and nonenzymatic pathways for the formation of bilirubin have been proposed. Although both may be important physiologically, the microsomal enzyme heme oxygenase, found in high concentration throughout the liver, spleen, and bone marrow, plays a major role in the initial conversion of heme to biliverdin. Biliverdin is then reduced to bilirubin by the cytosolic enzyme biliverdin reductase in a nicotinamide adenine dinucleotide (NADH)-dependent reaction before being released into the circulation. In this unconjugated form, bilirubin has a very low solubility. Bilirubin is bound avidly to plasma proteins, primarily albumin, before uptake and further processing by the liver. The liver is the sole organ capable of removing the albumin-bilirubin complex from the circulation and esterifying the potentially toxic bilirubin to water-soluble, nontoxic monoconjugated and deconjugated derivatives. After being extracted by the hepatocytes, bilirubin is conjugated with glucuronic acid to form bilirubin diglucuronide (conjugated bilirubin). The enzyme responsible for this reaction is glucoronil transferase present in the endoplasmic reticulum of the hepatocyte. Bilirubin is then transported within the hepatocyte by cytosolic binding proteins delivering the molecule to the canalicular membrane for active secretion into bile. Conjugated bilirubin is then excreted into the duodenum in association with mixed lipid micelles. Once in the intestine, bilirubin is converted to urobilinogens by intestinal bacteria, which are then further oxidized to pigmented urobilins. These pigments are responsible for the brown color of stool.

GALLBLADDER FUNCTION

The main function of the gallbladder is to concentrate and store hepatic bile during the fasting state, thus allowing for its coordinated release in response to a meal. To serve this overall function, the gallbladder has absorptive, secretory, and motor capabilities. Absorption of water results from an active process via the sodium-hydrogen exchanger. As a result the gallbladder stores concentrated bile that reenters the distal bile duct and is secreted into the duodenum in response to a meal. In addition to absorption and concentration, the gallbladder's mucosa actively secretes glycoproteins and hydrogen ions. Secretion of mucus glycoproteins occurs primarily from the glands of the gallbladder neck and CD. The resultant mucin gel is believed to constitute an important part of the unstirred layer (diffusion-resistant barrier) that separates the gallbladder cell membrane from the luminal bile.[40,41] This mucus barrier may be very important in protecting the gallbladder epithelium from the strong detergent effect of the highly concentrated bile salts found in the gallbladder. However, considerable evidence also suggests that mucin glycoproteins play a role as pronucleating agents for cholesterol crystallization.[42] The transport of hydrogen ions by the gallbladder epithelium leads to a decrease in gallbladder bile pH through a sodium-exchange mechanism. Acidification of bile promotes calcium solubility, thereby preventing its precipitation as calcium salts. The gallbladder's normal acidification process lowers the pH of entering hepatic bile from 7.5 to 7.8 down to 7.1 to 7.3.[31,32]

Absorption

The gallbladder mucosa has the greatest absorptive capacity per unit of any structure in the body. Bile is usually concentrated fivefold by the absorption of water and electrolytes. Active Na-Cl transport by the gallbladder epithelium is the driving force for the concentration of bile (Fig. 106.21). Water is passively absorbed in response to the osmotic force generated by solute absorption. The concentration of bile may affect both calcium and cholesterol solubilities. The concentration of calcium in gallbladder bile, which is an important factor in gallstone pathogenesis, is influenced by serum calcium, hepatic bile calcium, gallbladder water absorption, and the concentration of organic substances, such as bile salts in gallbladder bile.[43] Although the gallbladder mucosa does absorb calcium, this process is not nearly as efficient as for sodium or water.

As the gallbladder bile becomes concentrated, several changes occur in the bile's capacity to solubilize cholesterol. The solubility in the micellar fraction is increased, but the stability of phospholipid-cholesterol vesicles is greatly decreased. Because cholesterol crystal precipitation occurs preferentially by vesicular rather than micellar mechanisms, the net effect of concentrating bile is an increased tendency to nucleate cholesterol.[42] Absorption of organic compounds also occurs; lipid solubility is the major determinant of movement across the gallbladder mucosa. However, the absorption of bilirubin, cholesterol, phospholipids, and bile salts is minimal compared with that of water. Thus these organic compounds are significantly concentrated by the normal absorptive process that occurs in the gallbladder. Unconjugated bile salts are absorbed more readily than conjugated bile salts and may actually damage the gallbladder's mucosa, causing a nonselective increase in absorption of other solutes. Thus increased absorption of unconjugated bile salts, caused by bacterial

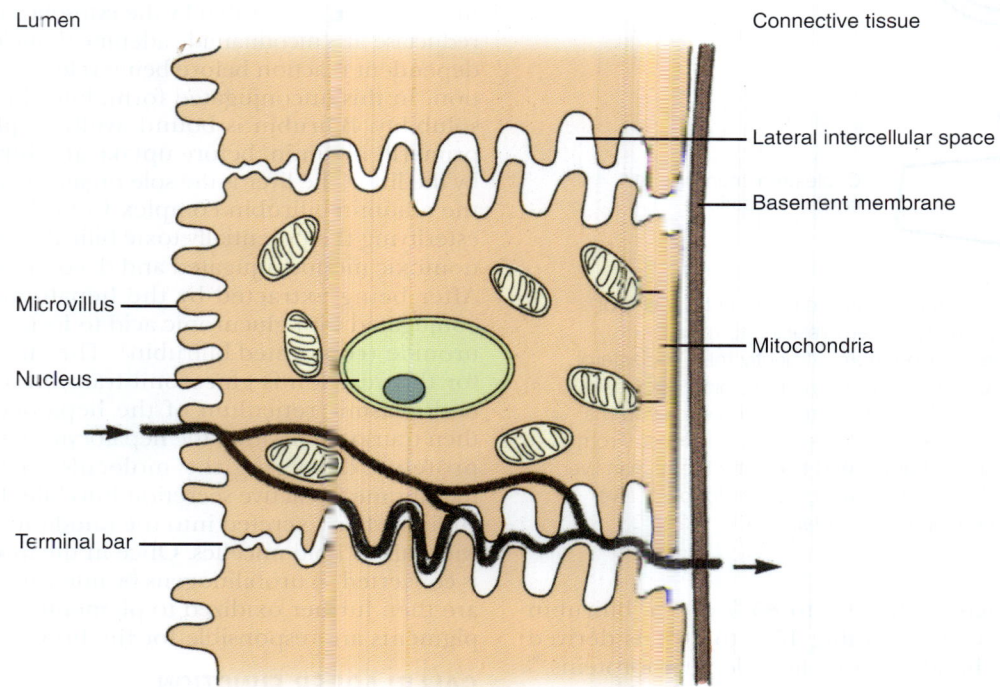

Lumen

Connective tissue

Lateral intercellular space

Basement membrane

Microvillus

Mitochondria

Nucleus

Terminal bar

FIGURE 106.21 Cellular mechanisms of gallbladder mucosal absorption. The *arrows* indicate the route of water flow across the cell membrane and into the intercellular spaces. Sodium chloride is pumped into the intercellular space, and the result is a hypertonic environment. As water is transported into the space, the space distends, and an isotonic solution enters the connective tissue space. (From Gadacz TR. Biliary anatomy and physiology. In: Greenfield LJ, Mulholland MW, Oldham KT, eds. *Surgery: Scientific Principles and Practice*. Philadelphia: Lippincott; 1993:935.)

deconjugation or mucosal inflammation, may impair cholesterol solubility and therefore promote cholesterol gallstone formation.

Secretion

The gallbladder's epithelial cells secrete at least two important products into its lumen: glycoproteins and hydrogen ions. Prostaglandins play an important role as stimulants of gallbladder mucin secretion. Furthermore, mucin glycoproteins are key pronucleating agents for cholesterol crystallization.

The acidification of bile occurs by the transport of hydrogen ions by the gallbladder epithelium, through a sodium-exchange mechanism. Acidification of bile promotes calcium solubility, thereby preventing its precipitation as calcium salts. The gallbladder's normal acidification process lowers the pH of gallbladder bile, which normally varies from approximately 7.1 to 7.3. Compared with gallbladder bile, the bile secreted by the liver is slightly alkaline, pH 7.5 to 7.8, so that excess losses of hepatic bile may cause metabolic acidosis.

Motility

Gallbladder filling is facilitated by tonic contraction of the ampullary sphincter, which maintains a constant pressure in the CBD (10 to 15 mm Hg). However, the gallbladder does not simply fill passively and continuously during fasting. Rather, periods of filling are punctuated by brief periods of partial emptying (10% to 15% of its volume) of concentrated gallbladder bile, which are coordinated with each passage through the duodenum of phase III of the migrating myoelectric complex. This process is mediated, at least in part, by the hormone motilin.[44-46] After a meal, the release of stored bile from the gallbladder requires a coordinated motor response of gallbladder contraction and sphincter of Oddi relaxation. When stimulated by eating, the gallbladder empties 50% to 70% of its contents within 30 to 40 minutes. Gallbladder refilling then occurs gradually over the next 60 to 90 minutes. Many other hormonal and neural pathways are also necessary for the coordinated action of the gallbladder and sphincter of Oddi. Defects in gallbladder motility, which increase the residence time of bile in the gallbladder, play a central role in the pathogenesis of gallstones.[31]

SPHINCTER OF ODDI

The human sphincter of Oddi is a complex structure that is functionally independent from the duodenal musculature. Endoscopic manometric studies have demonstrated that the human sphincter of Oddi creates a high-pressure zone between the bile duct and the duodenum (Fig. 106.22). The sphincter regulates the flow of bile and pancreatic juice into the duodenum and also prevents the regurgitation of duodenal contents into the biliary tract. These functions are achieved by keeping pressure within the bile and pancreatic ducts higher than duodenal pressure.[47] The sphincter of Oddi also has high-pressure phasic contractions, which may play a role in preventing the regurgitation of duodenal contents into the biliary tract.

Both neural and hormonal factors influence the sphincter of Oddi. In humans, sphincter of Oddi pressure

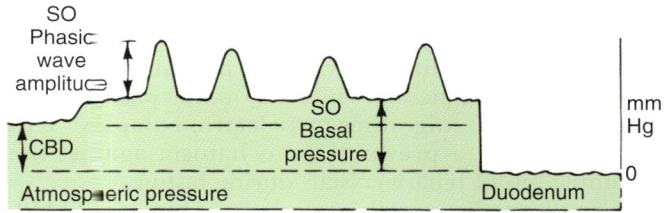

FIGURE 106.22 Sphincter of Oddi (SO) manometric pressure profile obtained by catheter pull-through from the common bile duct (CBD) into the duodenum. The CBD pressure and SO basal pressure are both referenced to duodenal pressure. SO phasic wave amplitude was measured from basal SO pressure. The CBD-to-duodenal pressure gradient is indicated by the *parallel broken lines*. (From Geenen JE, Toouli J, Hogan WJ, et al. Endoscopic sphincterotomy: follow-up evaluation of effects on the sphincter of Oddi. *Gastroenterology*. 1984;87:754.)

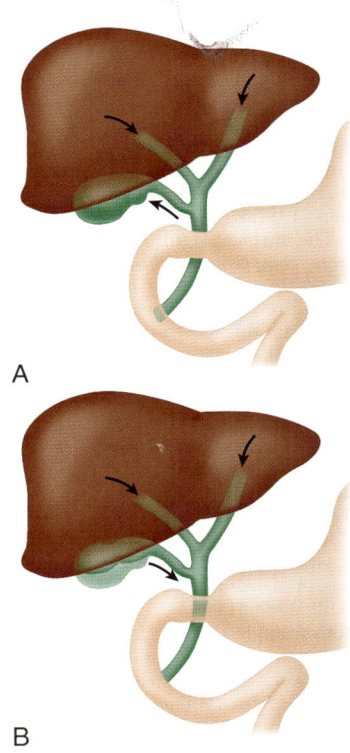

FIGURE 106.23 The effect of cholecystokinin on the gallbladder and sphincter of Oddi. (A) During fasting, with the sphincter contracted and the gallbladder filling. (B) In response to a meal, the sphincter is relaxed and the gallbladder emptying. (From Pham TH, Hunter J. Gallbladder and the extrahepatic biliary system. In Brunicardi F, Andersen D, Billiar T, et al., eds. *Schwartz's Principles of Surgery*. 10th ed. New York: McGraw-Hill; 2015: 314.)

and phasic wave activity diminish in response to cholecystokinin (Fig. 106.23). Thus sphincter pressure relaxes after a meal, allowing the passive flow of bile into the duodenum. During fasting, high-pressure phasic contractions of the sphincter of Oddi persist through all phases of the migrating myoelectric complex. However, recent animal studies suggest that sphincter of Oddi phasic waves do vary to some degree in concert with the migrating myoelectric complex. Thus sphincter of Oddi activity is undoubtedly coordinated with the partial gallbladder emptying and the increases in bile flow that occur during phase III of the migrating myoelectric complex. This activity may be a preventive mechanism against the accumulation of biliary crystals during fasting.[31]

Neurally mediated reflexes link the sphincter of Oddi with the gallbladder and stomach to coordinate the flow of bile and pancreatic juice into the duodenum. The cholecysto–sphincter of Oddi reflex allows the human sphincter to relax as the gallbladder contracts.[48] Similarly, antral distention causes both gallbladder contraction and sphincter relaxation.[49]

ACKNOWLEDGMENT

The authors thank the previous authors, Henri A. Pitt and Thomas R. Gadacz, for their contributions.

REFERENCES

1. Stinton LM, Shaffer EA. Epidemiology of gallbladder disease: cholelithiasis and cancer. *Gut Liver*. 2012;6:172-187.
2. Linder HH. Embryology and anatomy of the biliary tree. In: Way LW, Pellegrini CA, eds. *Surgery of the Gallbladder and Bile Ducts*. Philadelphia: Saunders; 1987:3.
3. Moorman DA. The surgical significance of six anomalies of the biliary duct system. *Surg Gynecol Obstet*. 1970;131:665.
4. Healey JE, Schroy PC. Anatomy of the biliary ducts within the human liver: analysis of the prevailing pattern of branchings and the major variations of the biliary ducts. *Arch Surg*. 1953;66:599.
5. Johnson EV, Anson BJ. Variations in the formation and vascular relationships of the bile ducts. *Surg Gynecol Obstet*. 1952;94:669.
6. Frierson H Jr. The gross anatomy and histology of the gallbladder, extrahepatic bile ducts, vaterian system, and minor papilla. *Am J Surg Pathol*. 1989;13:146.
7. Swartz-Basile DA, Lu D, Basile DP, et al. Leptin regulates gallbladder genes related to absorption and secretion. *Am J Physiol*. 2007;293:84.
8. Rock J, Swan KG, Diego J. Calot's triangle revisited. *Surg Gynecol Obstet*. 1981;153:410.
9. Skandalakis JE, Gray SW, Rowe JS Jr. Biliary tract. In: Skandalakis JE, Gray SW, eds. *Anatomical Complications in General Surgery*. New York: McGraw-Hill; 1983:31.
10. Specht MJ. Calot's triangle [letter]. *J Am Med Assoc*. 1967;200:1186.
11. Boyden EA. The anatomy of the choledochoduodenal junction in man. *Surg Gynecol Obstet*. 1957;104:646.
12. Michels NA. *Blood Supply and Anatomy of the Upper Abdominal Organs*. Philadelphia: Lippincott; 1955.
13. Terblanche J, Allison HF, Northover JMA. An ischemic basis for biliary strictures. *Surgery*. 1983;94:52.
14. Benson E, Page RE. A practical reappraisal of the anatomy of the extrahepatic bile ducts and arteries. *Br J Surg*. 1976;63:853.
15. Michels NA. The hepatic, cystic, and retroduodenal arteries and their relations to the biliary ducts with samples of the entire celiacal blood supply. *Ann Surg*. 1951;133:503.
16. Daseler EH, Anson BJ, Hambley WD, Riemann AF. The cystic artery and constituents of the hepatic pedicle: a study of 500 specimens. *Surg Gynecol Obstet*. 1947;85:47.
17. Burnett W, Cairns FW, Bacsich P. Innervation of the extrahepatic biliary system. *Ann Surg*. 1964;159:8.
18. Couinaud C. Cited in Smadja C, Blumgart LH. The biliary tract and the anatomy of biliary exposure. In: Blumgart LH, ed. *Surgery of the Liver and Biliary Tract*. Edinburgh: Churchill Livingstone; 1988:16.
19. Yoshida J, Chijiiwa K, Yamaguchi K, Yokohata K, Tanaka M. Practical classification of the branching types of the biliary tree: an analysis of 1094 consecutive direct cholangiograms. *J Am Coll Surg*. 1996;182:37.
20. Bockman DE, Freeny PC. Anatomy and anomalies of the biliary tree. *Laparosc Surg Endosc*. 1992;1:92.
21. Boyden E. "Phrygian cap" in cholecystography: a congenital anomaly of the gallbladder. *AJR Am J Roentgenol*. 1935;33:589.
22. Weisel W, Waters W. Diverticulosis of the gallbladder: report of a case. *Proc Staff Meet Mayo Clin*. 1941;16:753.
23. Davies F, Harding HE. The pouch of Hartmann. *Lancet*. 1942;1:193.
24. Stokline C. Congenital abnormalities of gallbladder and extrahepatic ducts. *Br J Child Dis*. 1939;36:115.
25. Suzuki M, Akaishi S, Rikiyama T, Naitoh T, Rahman MM, Matsuno S. Laparoscopic cholecystectomy, Calot's triangle, and variation in cystic arterial supply. *Surg Endosc*. 2000;14:141-144.
26. Blasius G. *Observata Anatomica in Homine, Simia, Equo*. Amsterdam: Gaasbeek; 1674.
27. Sherren J. A double gallbladder removed by operation. *Ann Surg*. 1911;54:10.
28. Browne EZ. Variations in origin and course of the hepatic artery and its branches: importance from a surgical viewpoint. *Surgery*. 1940;8:424.
29. Hugh TB, Kelly TB. Laparoscopic anatomy of the cystic artery. *Am J Surg*. 1992;163:593.
30. Scott-Conner CEH, Hall T. Variant arterial anatomy in laparoscopic cholecystectomy. *Am J Surg*. 1992;163:590.
31. Klein A, Lillemoe K, Yeo C, Pitt HA. Liver, biliary tract, and pancreas. In: O'Leary J, ed. *Physiologic Basis of Surgery*. Baltimore: Wilkins & Wilkins; 1996:441.
32. Gadacz TR. Biliary anatomy and physiology. In: Greenfield LJ, Mulholland MW, Oldham KT, eds. *Surgery: Scientific Principles and Practice*. Philadelphia: Lippincott; 1993:925.
33. Kullak-Ublick GA, Stieger B, Meier PJ, et al. Enterohepatic bile salt transporters in normal physiology and liver disease. *Gastroenterology*. 2004;126:322.
34. Meier PJ, Stieger B. Bile salt transporters. *Annu Rev Physiol*. 2002;64:635.
35. Crawford JM. Role of vesicle-mediated transport pathways in hepatocellular bile secretion. *Semin Liver Dis*. 1996;16:169.
36. Gerk PM, Vore M. Regulation of expression of the multidrug resistance-associated protein 2 (MRP2) and its role in drug disposition. *J Pharmacol Exp Ther*. 2002;302:407.
37. Admirand WH, Small DM. The physicochemical basis of cholesterol gallstone formation in man. *J Clin Invest*. 1968;47:1043.
38. Carey MC. Critical tables for calculating the cholesterol saturation of native bile. *J Lipid Res*. 1978;19:945.
39. Blanckaert N, Schmid R. Physiology and pathophysiology of bilirubin metabolism. In: Zakmin D, Boyer TD, eds. *Hepatology: A Textbook of Liver Disease*. 2nd ed. Philadelphia: Saunders; 1990:246.
40. Smithson KW, Miller DB, Jacobs LR, Gray GM. Intestinal diffusion barrier: unstirred water layer or membrane surface mucous coat? *Science*. 1981;214:1241.
41. Glickerman DJ, Kim MH, Malik R, Lee SP. The gallbladder also secretes. *Dig Dis Sci*. 1997;42:489.
42. Holzbach RT. Recent progress in understanding cholesterol crystal nucleation as a precursor to human gallstone formation. *Hepatology*. 1986;6:405.
43. Moore EW. Biliary calcium and gallstone formation. *Hepatology*. 1990;12:206S.
44. Itoh A, Takahasi I. Periodic contractions of the canine gallbladder during interdigestive state. *Am J Physiol*. 1981;240:G183.
45. Niebergall-Roth E, Teyssen S, Singer MV. Neurohormonal control of gallbladder motility. *Scand J Gastroenterol*. 1997;32:737.
46. Svenberg T, Christofides ND, Fitzpatrick ML, Areola-Ortiz F, Bloom SR, Welbourn RB. Interdigestive biliary output in man: relationship to fluctuations in plasma motilin and effect of atropine. *Gut*. 1982;23:1024.
47. Geenen JE, Hoagan WJ, Dodds WJ, Stewart ET, Arndorfer RC. Intraluminal pressure recording from the human sphincter of Oddi. *Gastroenterology*. 1980;78:317.
48. Muller EL, Lewinski MA, Pitt HA. The cholecysto-sphincter of Oddi reflex. *J Surg Res*. 1984;36:377.
49. Webb TH, Lillemoe KD, Pitt HA. The gastro-sphincter of Oddi reflex. *Am J Surg*. 1988;155:193.

Imaging and Radiologic Intervention in the Biliary Tract

Rakesh Navuluri | Brian Funaki | Danial Jilani | Tom Tullius

Mikin Patel | Ashley Altman | Comeron Ghobadi | Arun Nagaraju

This chapter includes a review of both imaging and percutaneous intervention of the biliary system. A thorough evaluation of a patient with obstructive jaundice includes detailed medical and surgical history, physical examination, laboratory data, and evaluation of pertinent imaging. A multidisciplinary approach including the primary care physician, surgeon, gastroenterologist, and interventional radiologist provides comprehensive management options. Noninvasive imaging studies provide the foundation for treatment planning, including surgical and/or percutaneous intervention. Percutaneous biliary interventions may be the primary diagnostic and therapeutic treatment option or serve as a conduit for later surgical intervention. The principal objectives of the chapter include (1) reviewing the role of noninvasive imaging modalities commonly used in the patient presenting with biliary obstruction and (2) examining the role of minimally invasive percutaneous interventions available for the patient with either benign or malignant biliary disease.

This chapter begins with an overview of the role of ultrasound (US), computed tomography (CT), magnetic resonance imaging (MRI), and nuclear medicine in the evaluation of patients with biliary disease.

The goals of imaging are to not only confirm the presence of obstructive jaundice but also to define the biliary anatomy. Identification of the degree and point of the obstruction using such techniques as magnetic resonance cholangiopancreatography (MRCP) can guide therapeutic management. In the case of a malignant etiology, imaging can also stage the extent of disease.

After the anatomic structure is defined, percutaneous interventions including percutaneous transhepatic cholangiography (PTC) and percutaneous transhepatic biliary drainage (PTBD) can be used. These techniques, as well as other interventions, including percutaneous biopsy, drainage catheter management, percutaneous biliary stricture dilatation, and biliary endoprostheses, are reviewed. The appropriate selection for each approach, as will be discussed, depends on the clinical scenario and etiology of the stricture, whether it be benign, malignant, or iatrogenic. Finally, a brief overview of innovative practices to treat unresectable biliary malignancies will be presented, including radiofrequency ablation (RFA) and yttrium-90 (Y-90) therapy.

The goal of the chapter is to provide readers with a basic understanding of the role of imaging and image-guided intervention for the patient with complex biliary conditions.

DIAGNOSTIC IMAGING

ULTRASOUND

US often serves as an initial imaging modality to evaluate the biliary system. In the hands of a trained operator, US can provide physicians with valuable information to help to manage patients with suspected hepatobiliary disease. It may be used in the evaluation of bile ducts for obstruction (Fig. 107.1A), masses, or stones. US is noninvasive, inexpensive, and does not involve ionizing radiation, which is particularly important in the setting of pediatric and pregnant patients.

The normal gallbladder is an ovoid, anechoic, fluid-filled structure adjacent to the interlobar fissure, which separates the right and left hepatic lobes. The gallbladder wall should be smooth, and the thickness should not exceed 3 mm.[1] When the gallbladder is contracted, as is often seen in nonfasting patients, the wall may appear falsely thickened. Primary causes of wall thickening include cholecystitis (Fig. 107.2), adenomyomatosis, and cancer. Secondary causes of wall thickening include acquired immune deficiency syndrome (AIDS) cholangiopathy, sclerosing cholangitis, hepatitis, pancreatitis, heart failure, hypoalbuminemia, cirrhosis, portal hypertension, and lymphatic obstruction.[2]

The extrahepatic bile ducts are divided into the common bile duct and common hepatic duct. On US the common hepatic duct is the most easily visualized portion of the extrahepatic biliary system. The cystic duct is normally located posterior to and may join with the common hepatic duct at variable distances, forming the common bile duct. In 10% of the population the cystic duct runs parallel to the common hepatic duct for a long segment, where it is joined by a fibrous sheath, which may cause the common hepatic duct to be misinterpreted as the cystic duct.[3] In the majority of patients the common hepatic duct is anterior and lateral to the portal vein and to the right of the hepatic artery. The hepatic artery separates the common hepatic duct from the portal vein within the hepatoduodenal ligament. However, in 10% to 15% of the patients, the hepatic artery is located anterior to the common hepatic duct. The common bile duct travels toward the second portion of the duodenum as it adopts a more posterior position.[1,4] The normal diameter of the extrahepatic bile ducts can range from 4 to 8 mm.[5] The size of the common bile duct may increase with age, after cholecystectomy, and after endoscopic manipulation of the duct. The maximum upper limit of normal in the

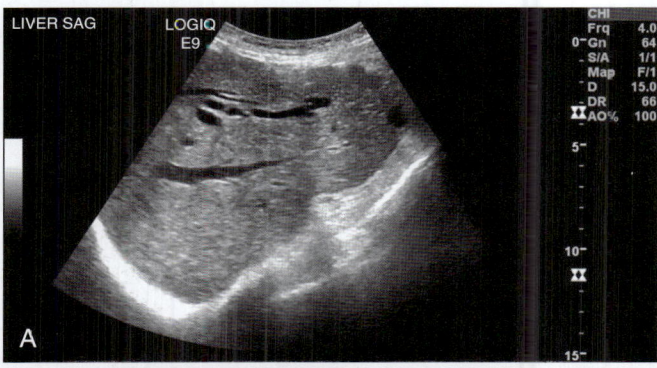

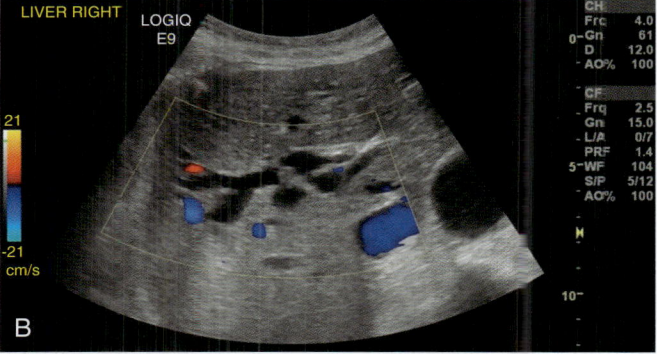

FIGURE 107.1 Gray scale (A) and color Doppler (B) transabdominal sagittal right upper quadrant ultrasound images showing intrahepatic biliary ductal dilatation. The color Doppler scan (B) helps to differentiate dilated ducts from hepatic vessels.

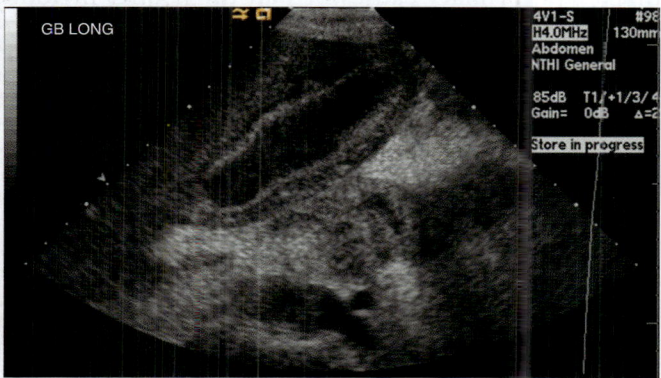

FIGURE 107.2 Transabdominal sagittal right upper quadrant ultrasound image showing marked gallbladder wall thickening in a septic patient with acalculous cholecystitis.

extrahepatic biliary tree after cholecystectomy is 10 mm. However, it is generally accepted that a duct that measures 6 mm or greater in symptomatic patients warrants further investigation.[6]

The intrahepatic bile ducts normally measure less than 2 mm in diameter or less than 40% of the diameter of the accompanying portal vein.[4] Intrahepatic biliary dilation is detected by the parallel channel sign, which is formed by dilated ducts running parallel to the portal vein tributaries.[7] Large intrahepatic biliary ducts located centrally near

the porta hepatis should not be confused with pathologic dilatation. Color Doppler US can be used to differentiate dilated intrahepatic ducts from hepatic vessels (see Fig. 107.1B).[8]

Causes of biliary obstruction include benign etiologies (e.g., stones, infectious, congenital), neoplastic etiologies, and extrinsic compression (e.g., Mirizzi syndrome, pancreatitis, adenopathy).[4] US is able to accurately predict the level of obstruction in 92% of cases and identifies the correct cause in 71% of cases.[9] Further evaluation by CT or MRCP is often needed to help to identify the cause of obstruction or to identify the extent of disease in the case of malignancy prior to therapeutic intervention.[1]

COMPUTED TOMOGRAPHY

Multidetector CT has allowed for improved imaging of the biliary system. Rapid acquisition of volumetric data and the ability to perform multiplanar reconstructions (MPRs) provides more detailed evaluation of both intrahepatic and extrahepatic ducts. Unlike US, CT allows for visualization of the entire common bile duct and better detects etiologies of biliary obstruction. CT is reported to have a sensitivity of 72% to 88% in detecting choledocholithiasis.[10–12] Disadvantages of CT include exposure to ionizing radiation and use of intravenous (IV) contrast, which may be contraindicated in patients with renal impairment or contrast allergy.

The CT technique for evaluation of the biliary system includes obtaining an unenhanced scan through the liver, gallbladder, common bile duct, and pancreas. Unenhanced scans provide a baseline to determine lesion enhancement and to better detect stones, which can be obscured by contrast material. A portal venous scan is obtained 70 to 80 seconds after IV contrast administration. When there is concern for malignancy, a late arterial phase may be obtained at 45 to 50 seconds. In addition to assessing vascularity within a tumor, a late arterial phase allows for detection of vascular involvement surrounding the tumor, which may alter or preclude surgical management (e.g., pancreatic head lesion with nearby vascular encasement). A 10-minute delayed scan should be added when there is suspicion for cholangiocarcinoma because these tumors often demonstrate delayed enhancement relative to the remainder of the hepatic parenchyma. A thin section technique (1 mm or less) allows for higher quality multiplanar reformats (e.g., coronal, sagittal), which are helpful in the assessment of bile ducts.[13]

Normal intrahepatic bile ducts are faintly visualized on an enhanced CT and are often readily differentiated from dilated ducts, which measure greater than 2 mm (Fig. 107.3). The common hepatic duct and common bile ducts appear as tubular water density structures with near imperceptible walls. The distal common bile duct takes on a round or oval configuration at the level of the pancreatic head.[1,13]

Procedural guidance with CT-fluoroscopy serves as an effective tool for percutaneous interventional procedures of the chest, spine, abdomen, and pelvis. CT-fluoroscopy provides near real-time image acquisition similar to that of US, allowing for increased procedural efficiency. In the setting of biliary system pathology, CT-fluoroscopy is particularly helpful when undergoing a challenging biopsy

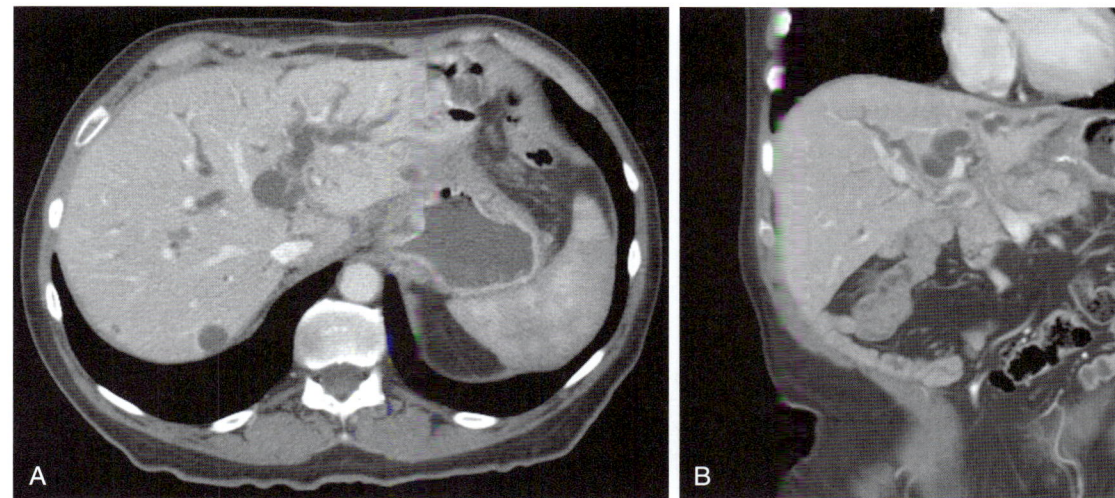

FIGURE 107.3 Axial (A) and reconstructed coronal (B) contrast-enhanced computed tomography scans through the liver and biliary tree demonstrating diffuse intrahepatic biliary ductal dilatation. The patient was found to have a mass at the head of the pancreas causing common bile duct obstruction.

(e.g., hepatic lesion adjacent to bile ducts) or a difficult catheter drainage (e.g., biloma near the aorta).[14]

MAGNETIC RESONANCE IMAGING

US and CT have some advantages over MRI, including cost, availability, speed, and real-time imaging. However, MRI has increasingly played a vital role in biliary imaging. It is considered a highly sensitive and specific noninvasive imaging modality in the evaluation of biliary tract pathology. Indeed, it has become favored over ERCP and percutaneous cholangiogram in most institutions for diagnostic purposes. It is also useful in patients who cannot undergo or have failed ERCP. MRCP may visualize stones as small as 2 mm[15] with sensitivity greatly increasing as stone size increases. Furthermore it is equally useful in visualizing strictures, biliary leaks (Fig. 107.4), and other pathologies.

MRCP uses T2-weighted imaging to visualize the biliary system. These images are then reformatted into multiple planes using MPR and maximal intensity projections (MIPs), allowing for visualization of much of the biliary tract at once. Three-dimensional imaging or two-dimensional imaging in any other plane may also be obtained. Advances in technique, along with growing experience of MRI technicians, allow high-resolution imaging and decreased imaging time. This allows high-quality diagnostic imaging in severely ill patients who may not be able to be positioned properly for extended periods of time or comply with breathing commands.[16-19] These advances, along with inherent benefits of MRI, make MRCP a valuable tool both in diagnostic imaging and presurgical planning.

NUCLEAR MEDICINE

Hepatobiliary scintigraphy is a noninvasive technique that uses derivatives of iminodiacetic acid tagged with radiotracer (technetium) for the evaluation of the biliary system.

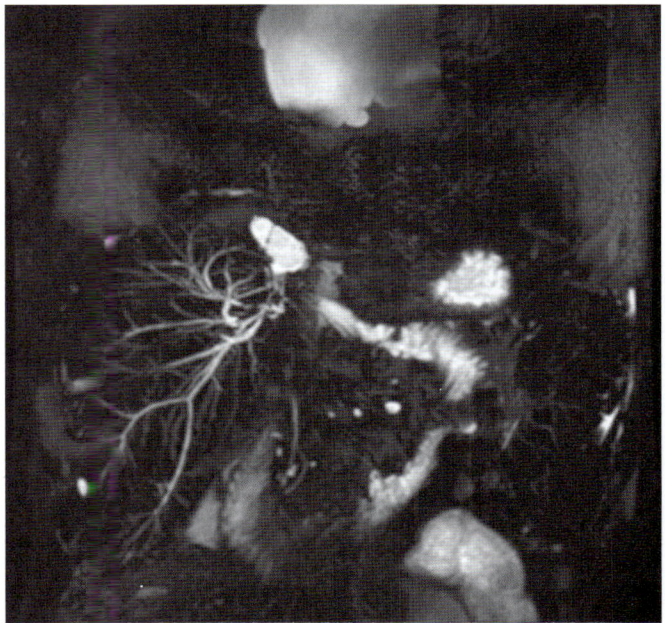

FIGURE 107.4 A biliary leak resulting in large biloma is noted by a region of high T2 signal on this coronal image.

It is commonly referred to as hepatobiliary iminodiacetic acid (HIDA) scan, although paraisopropyl iminodiacetic acid (PIPIDA) is now the more prevalent tracer. Cholescintigraphy is particularly useful in the evaluation for biliary leak, where it is highly sensitive[20] (Fig. 107.5). However, a negative scan in a patient with high clinical suspicion should be followed with ERCP.[21,22] Cholescintigraphy is also an extremely sensitive examination for other biliary pathology, including obstruction and cholecystitis.

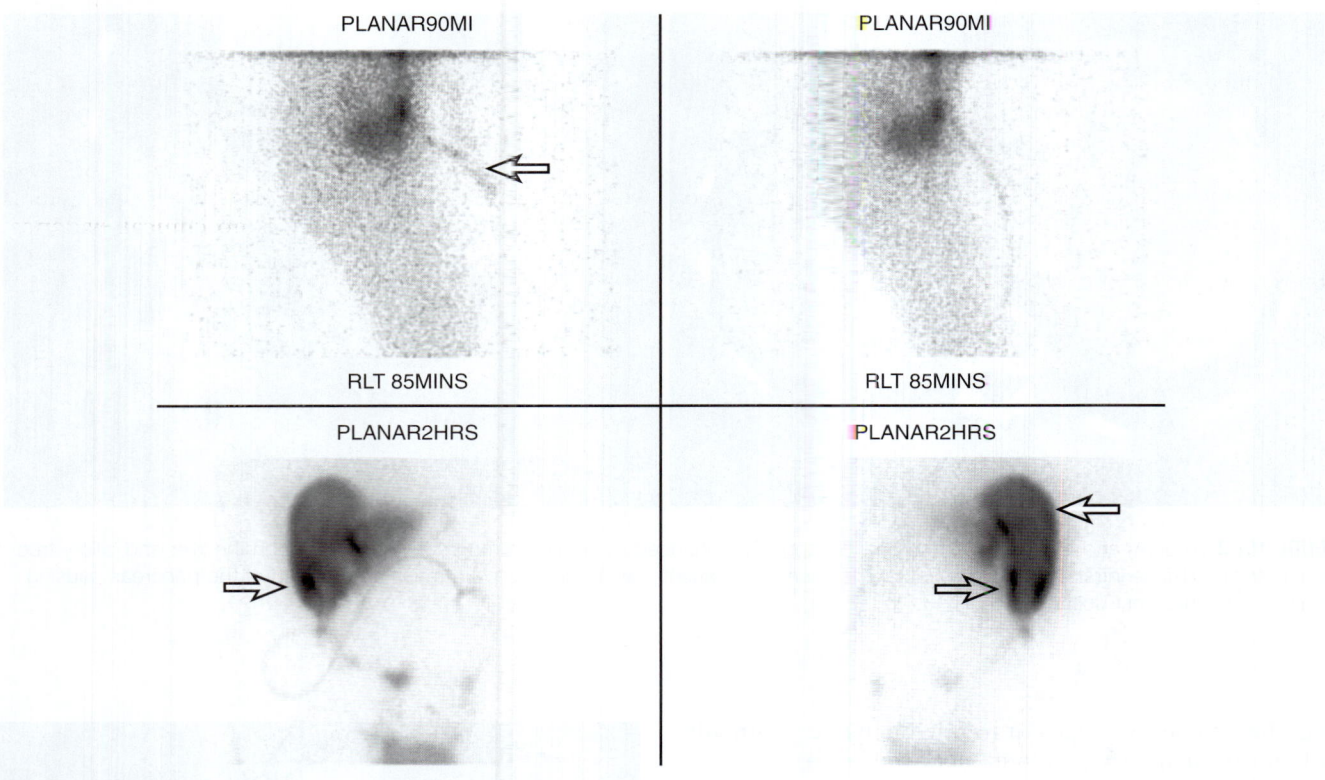

PLANAR90MI PLANAR90MI

RLT 85MINS RLT 85MINS

PLANAR2HRS PLANAR2HRS

FIGURE 107.5 Nuclear medicine scintigraphy 90-minute– and 2-hour–delayed (diisopropyl-iminodiacetic acid [DISIDA] scan) showing extravasation of radiotracer into the inferior percutaneous drain and surrounding the right surface of the liver, extending superiorly consistent with a bile leak *(arrows)*. This patient was status post cholecystectomy and was found to have fusiform dilation of the common bile duct, consistent with a type I choledochal cyst.

BILIARY INTERVENTIONS

PTC as a diagnostic tool has been largely replaced by the cross-sectional imaging techniques already described. In addition, with the development and widespread availability of ERCP, along with advances in endoscopic interventions, the need for percutaneous interventions has declined. In many institutions, after initial clinical, laboratory, and imaging evaluations, ERCP is generally the first minimally invasive procedure performed in patients with known biliary disease—particularly in nondilated systems. However, percutaneous transhepatic interventions remain a valuable tool in the multidisciplinary management of biliary pathology. Interventional radiology is often called on to perform PTBD in patients with known biliary-enteric surgical reconstruction and obstructing tumors at the biliary confluence. Percutaneous interventions are also valuable when ERCP has failed. Not uncommonly, endoscopic stents are unable to reach peripheral biliary obstructions. In addition, patients with high-grade obstruction and subsequent unsuccessful endoscopic bile duct manipulation may require emergent percutaneous transhepatic drainage because of sepsis. Percutaneous techniques are also well suited for patients with biliary bifurcation (i.e., hilar) or intrahepatic lesions and in those patients with prior surgical failures (e.g., anastomotic strictures at the site of a prior biliary-enteric surgical reconstruction).

TECHNIQUE OF PERCUTANEOUS TRANSHEPATIC CHOLANGIOGRAPHY, PERCUTANEOUS TRANSHEPATIC BILIARY DRAINAGE, AND DILATATION OF BILIARY STRICTURE

PTC is an invasive procedure that requires informed consent, moderate sedation, and preprocedural intravenous antibiotics directed against enteric pathogens. Access into the biliary tree via a percutaneous transhepatic route can be accomplished by two main approaches: low right midaxillary and left anterior subxiphoid. Although both fluoroscopy and CT can be used for guidance, fluoroscopy is widely preferred due to its speed and real-time image acquisition. US is often used during the initial puncture to target a specific intrahepatic duct or when the upstream ducts are only minimally dilated. The right midaxillary approach is more commonly used in clinical practice due to a larger volume of hepatic parenchyma and decreased radiation exposure to the operator's hands. The primary risk of the right-sided approach is crossing the pleural space. If US is not used to target a particular duct, a 22-gauge coaxial Chiba needle (Cook Inc., Bloomington, Indiana) is directed toward the 11th intercostal space from the right midaxillary line or three fingerbreadths below the xiphoid in a left-sided approach.[22] The stilette is then removed, and dilute water-soluble contrast is injected into the needle under fluoroscopic guidance as the needle is slowly withdrawn. Often in the setting of benign strictures the peripheral ducts are only minimally dilated, making access more difficult. In this case a second Chiba needle will be inserted into a central duct, through which a cholangiogram will be used as a map for fluoroscopic puncture of a peripheral duct. After an appropriate peripheral duct is selected, the needle is exchanged over an 0.018-inch guidewire and upsized to a 0.035-guidewire, using a coaxial system and sequentially larger diameter sheaths.[23] A cholangiogram may be performed again at this step to define the patient's anatomy and to identify strictures. If no strictures are visualized, an 8- or 10-Fr internal-external biliary drain is placed with the distal end within the proximal small bowel and the multiple side holes spanning the biliary system. Alternatively, a simple external biliary pigtail drain may be placed for temporary decompression, depending on the clinical circumstances and cause of obstruction or leak.

If a benign stricture is identified, the decision must be made whether to cross the stricture with a guidewire with the aim of dilating the narrowed segment and/or placing a drainage catheter beyond the stricture. In general, in the setting of sepsis, cholangitis, or difficult cannulation an external biliary drain will be placed temporarily and the patient will be brought back to the angiography suite for conversion to an internal-external drain after the acute infection has resolved.[24]

After the stricture has been crossed, the interventionalist may either place an internal-external biliary drain, dilate the strictured segment with a balloon, or perform both sequentially. Balloon dilation is a reasonable approach for most benign strictures except in the setting of recent surgical anastomosis (<1 month), in which case narrowing is often due to postoperative edema, which may resolve spontaneously. Furthermore, balloon dilation of a new biliary anastomosis may be dangerous in the early postoperative period and can result in perforation or leak. In such cases it is reasonable to insert an internal-external drain and repeat the cholangiogram in several weeks.[24] Balloon dilation of short-segment strictures has shown greater success than long-segment strictures, with a short-term patency rate of 50% to 90% and long-term patency rate of 56% to 74% for short-segment strictures.[25-29]

Most benign biliary strictures are amenable to balloon dilation. The size of the balloon depends on the caliber of the bile duct proximal and distal to the stricture. In general, balloons that are 8 to 10 mm wide and 2 to 4 cm long are sufficient to dilate a common bile duct (CBD) or common hepatic duct (CHD) stricture, although balloons up to 14 mm in size can be safely used in adults. Smaller 6- to 8-mm diameter balloons are used for peripheral strictures. Larger balloons up to 20 mm may be used at biliary-enteric anastomoses. The balloon is inflated slowly for at least 1 minute and should be repeated multiple times per session. Following dilation, an internal-external biliary catheter is then inserted over a guidewire. In many cases, sequential upsizing of the drainage catheter up to 16 French is performed over multiple sessions. The dilation schedule depends on the institution, but patients usually return every 3 to 6 weeks for sheath cholangiogram, repeat balloon dilatation, and catheter upsizing. Larger balloons may be used at subsequent appointments if the stricture is persistent. Cutting balloons have been used

with some success; however, data on safety and efficacy are still limited.[30]

Successful dilation of the stricture will reveal a patent bile duct with rapid drainage on follow-up cholangiogram. An external pigtail drain is then left in place and capped externally for a trial of several weeks. The drain may be removed if repeat cholangiogram shows no significant residual stenosis and if there is no clinical evidence of obstruction or infection (leakage around the catheter, jaundice, fever, or cholangitis). Successful drain removal was achieved in 87% of patients who completed a full treatment period of 6 to 12 months of sequential upsizing and dilation with a stricture patency rate of 84% at 1 year, 74% at 5 years, and 67% at 10 years.[31] In the setting of treatment failure, the patient may require permanent indwelling internal-external catheter drainage with catheter replacement at 3-month intervals to prevent clogging. In some cases, surgical revision may ultimately be necessary.

Bare metal stents generally have no role in the management of benign biliary strictures. These devices are permanent and irretrievable because they induce intimal hyperplasia and become embedded within the biliary epithelium. Bare metal stents also have a high rate of occlusion and are thus only used for palliation in malignant disease. Fully covered self-expandable metallic stents (FCSEMSs) have shown promising results, with an increasing volume of data supporting efficacy and long-term patency with endoscopic ERCP deployment. These devices are covered in a material that delays intimal hyperplasia and allows for easy removal. A recent study of 68 patients who were treated percutaneously with covered stents showed a clinical success rate of 87% in patients with both primary and refractory strictures and a patency rate of 91% at 1 year.[32] Finally, it is important to recognize that in the endoscopic realm, dilation is rarely performed alone and is usually accompanied by deployment of multiple plastic stents or FCSEMSs.[33]

PERCUTANEOUS MANAGEMENT OF BILIARY STONES

Up to one-fifth of patients undergoing cholecystectomy have common biliary duct stones that can be treated with surgical exploration or endoscopic retrograde cholangiopancreatography (ERCP). Sphincterotomy or (less commonly) sphincteroplasty is performed with cholecystectomy to clear the common bile duct.

When an endoscopic approach fails due to anatomic anomalies, alternative treatment for common bile duct stones can be pursued through either the postoperative drain (T-tube or transcystic) placed during cholecystectomy or via a transhepatic approach. Success rates are reported at greater than 95%, with the most common complication, cholangitis, occurring in less than 3% of cases.[34,35] Anterograde wire access is gained into the duodenum followed by percutaneous balloon dilation of the ampulla of Vater (Fig. 107.6). The balloon catheter is then deflated, reinflated proximal to the stone, and then used to push the stones into the duodenum. For stones larger than 15 mm, basket lithotripsy can be used prior to dilation of the ampulla (Fig. 107.7).

For patients with intrahepatic lithiasis or stones for which direct visualization is desired but not feasible via

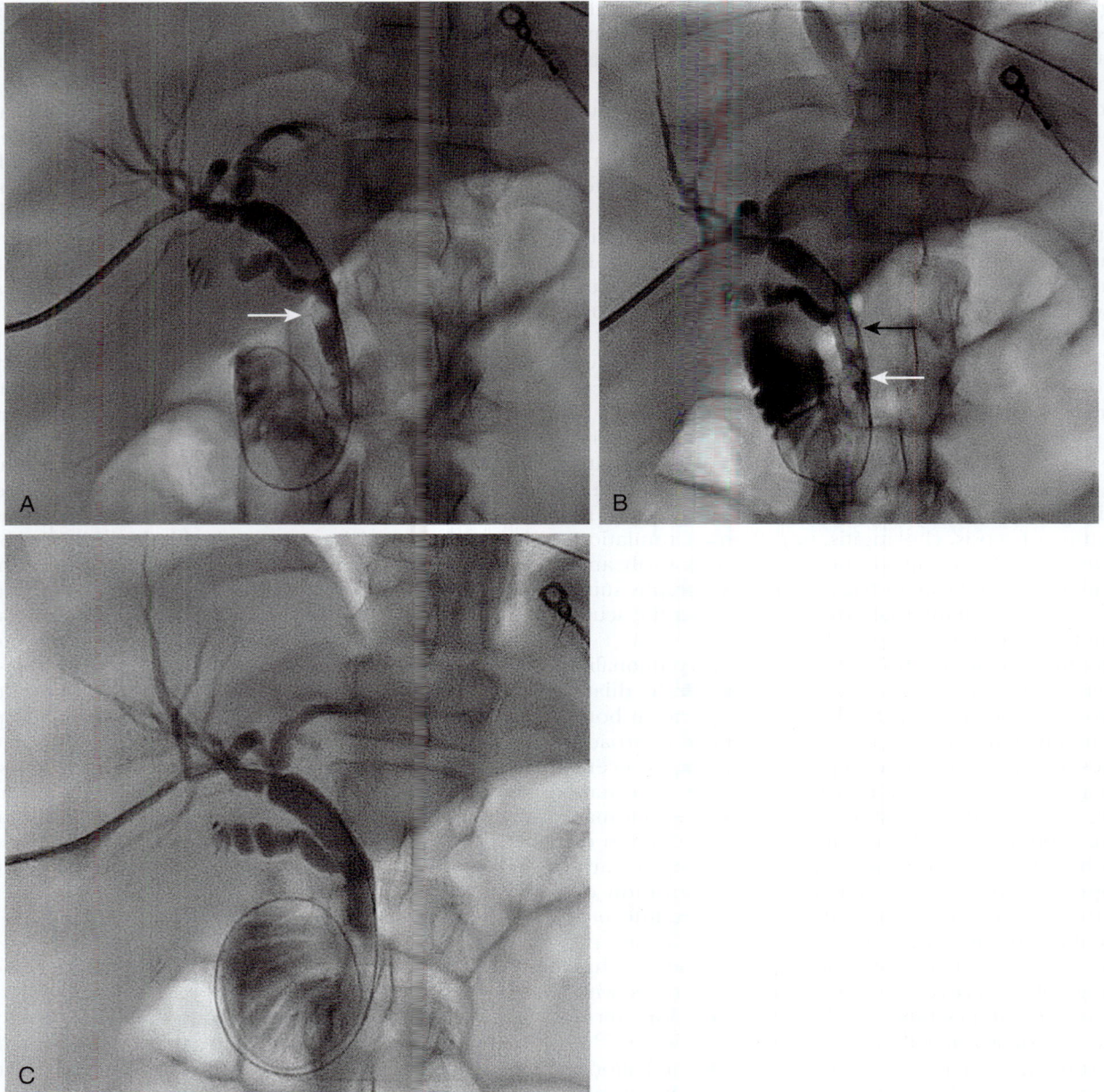

FIGURE 107.6 A 27-year-old woman with history of cholecystectomy and duodenal switch, now with pain and jaundice. (A) Percutaneous transhepatic cholangiogram shows a filling defect within the common bile duct *(white arrow)* compatible with a stone. (B) Following balloon dilation of the ampulla, the balloon *(black arrow)* is inflated proximal to the stone *(white arrow)* and pushed into the duodenum. (C) Completion cholangiogram shows patent common bile duct without stone. Internal-external biliary drain was subsequently placed.

ERCP, transhepatic cholangioscopy can be used.[36] For larger ductal stones, cholangioscopy can be combined with percutaneous intracorporeal lithotripsy to remove the stones.[37]

In patients with high surgical risk unable to undergo cholecystectomy, percutaneous cholecystolithotomy can be considered as a minimally invasive alternative. Success rates are reported as high as 97%, with the major complications, bile leak after tube removal, occurring in less than 10% of patients.[38] The major disadvantage of percutaneous cholecystolithotomy is that gallstones often recur.

PERCUTANEOUS IMAGE-GUIDED THERAPY OF MALIGNANT BILIARY TRACT DISEASE

Bile duct obstruction is commonly caused by malignant neoplasms, such as cholangiocarcinoma, gallbladder cancer, and pancreatic neoplasms, which are often unresectable at the time of presentation. Palliative relief of pruritus and management of cholangitis can be obtained through placement of percutaneous biliary drainage catheters, endoscopic or percutaneous biliary stenting, and surgical bypass.

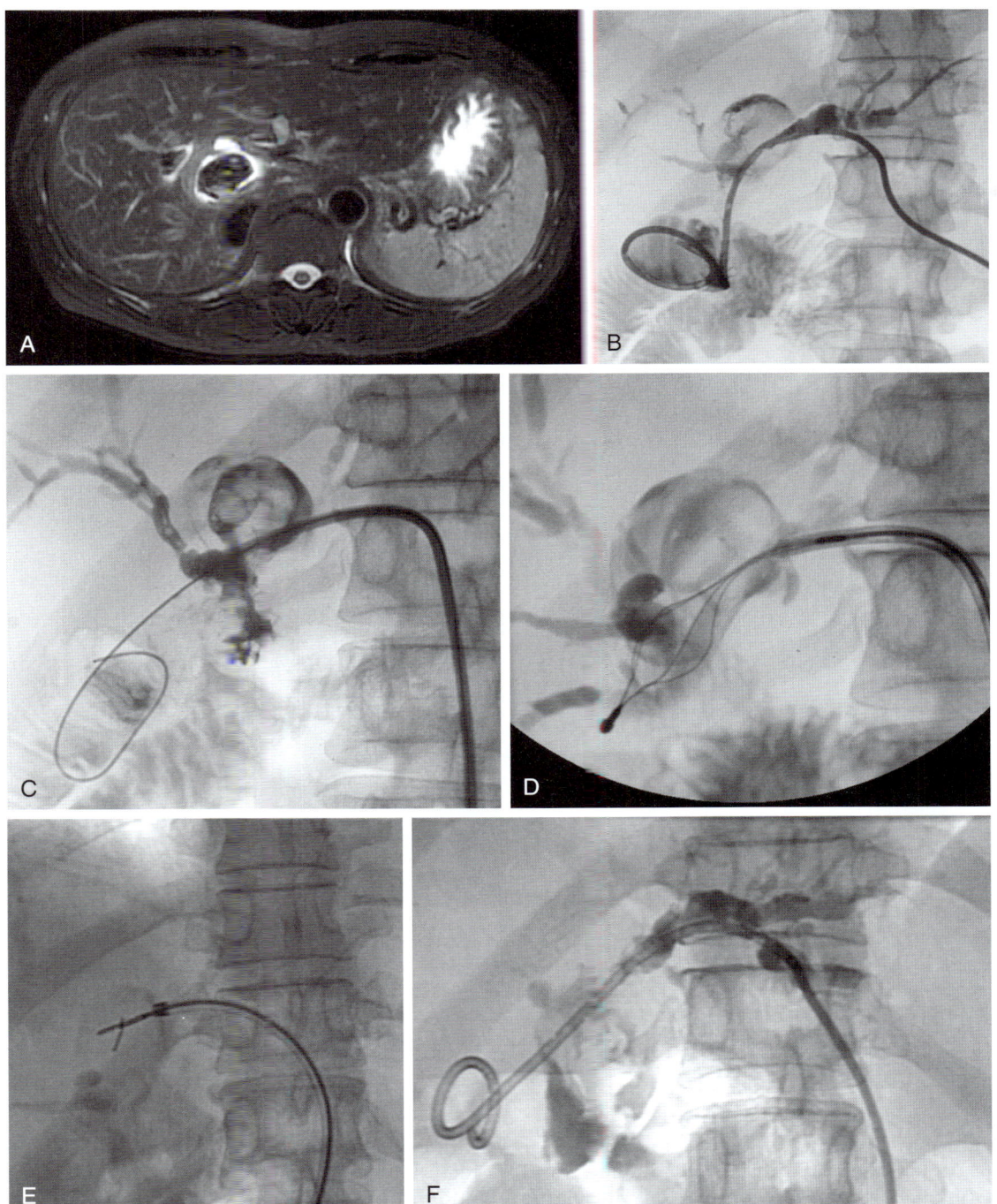

FIGURE 107.7 (A) A 51-year-old woman status post Whipple procedure for pancreatic cancer presented with a left hepatic lobe choledochal cyst containing a large 3 × 2 cm stone and associated with mild biliary ductal dilatation. (B) After left-sided percutaneous transhepatic biliary drainage placement. (C) stone fragmentation and extraction was performed over multiple visits to infrared using a combination of a (D) stone fragmentation basket and (E) biliary forceps. (F) Completion cholangiogram.

PTBD is achieved as described previously by either placing a pigtail catheter into the biliary system for drainage (external) or placement of a multiple side-hole catheter into the duodenum (internal to external). PTBD is efficacious for both distal and proximal malignant bile duct obstructions and large studies have reported technical success rates of greater than 90% and clinical success rates of greater than 75%.[39]

Internalization of drainage for malignant biliary strictures removes the external catheter, thus eliminating the need for daily care of the catheter and frequent exchanges and providing enhanced quality of life to the patient.

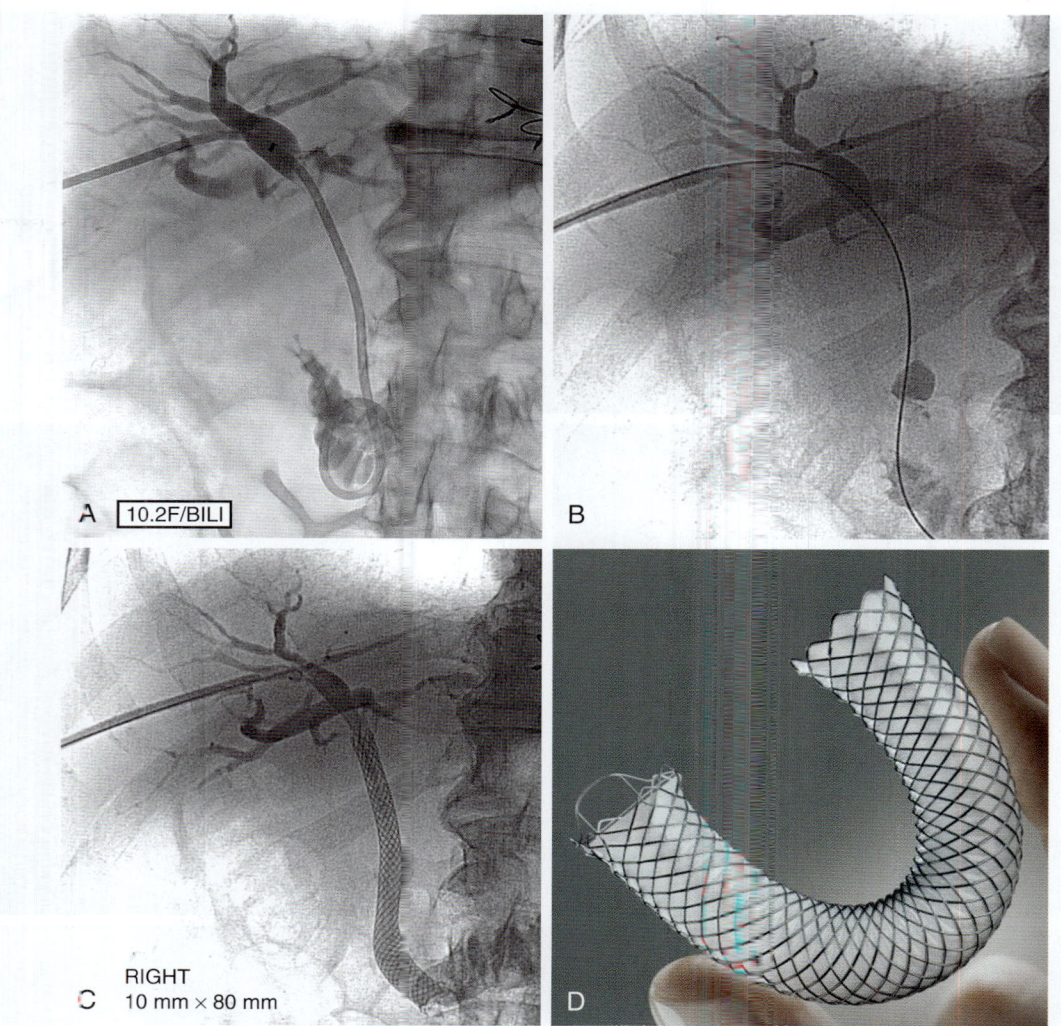

FIGURE 107.8 (A) A 79-year-old man admitted with worsening jaundice due to biliary obstruction secondary to metastatic gastric cancer. Internal-external drain was placed in the acute setting to allow decompression of the biliary system. (B) Two weeks later the patient returned for placement of a fully covered self-expandable metallic stent. A cholangiogram was performed over a guidewire in preparation for stent deployment. (C) Successful stent deployment with brisk drainage of contrast from the intrahepatic biliary ductal system into the small bowel. (D) Photograph of a self-expanding covered biliary endoprosthesis (WallFlex) similar to the one that was used in the case. ([D] Courtesy Boston Scientific Corporation, Natick, Massachusetts.)

Internalization may be achieved using either plastic or metal stents. Metallic stents are of larger diameter and have better long-term patency in comparison with plastic stents; however, they are more expensive. Metal stents are typically preferred in patients who have life expectancies of greater than 3 to 6 months, whereas plastic stents are appropriate for patients with shorter life expectancies. Metal stents may become obstructed by bile debris, or tumor ingrowth. To counteract tumor ingrowth and prevent recurrent jaundice, covered metal stents were developed (Fig. 107.8). Covered biliary stents exhibit improved patency compared with noncovered metallic stents, although the rate of stent migration and acute cholecystitis is increased.[40–43]

Primary stenting involves placing the stent percutaneously in the same session as the initial biliary system access. Primary stenting has been found to be more effective with fewer complications compared with secondary stenting, which is a staged procedure. In a study of 61 patients undergoing PTBD with stent placement for malignant biliary duct obstruction, the major complication rate was 23% and 54% in the primarily and secondarily stented groups, respectively.[44] Primary stenting resulted in a shorter hospital stay, making it more cost effective with reduced morbidity.[45,46]

Endoscopic placement of stents for biliary obstruction was long preferred over percutaneous means due to higher technical success rates, lower complication rates, and the absence of an external catheter.[47] Studies using advances in technique and improved catheter technology have showed that percutaneous stent placement is associated with improved technical success and fewer complications than endoscopic procedures. Cholangitis, a major procedural complication, occurred up to five times more commonly in the endoscopic group compared with the percutaneous group.[48–50]

The Bismuth classification is a commonly used system for grading bile obstruction due to a hilar mass. The grading system can be useful for both the determination of tumor resectability and planning for the drainage procedure. Preprocedural planning using imaging, including US, CT, or MRCP, is crucial, especially in the setting of hilar obstruction.[51] Radiographic evaluation of the exact level of obstruction facilitates the selection of the point of access and the most appropriate liver segment for drainage. Multiple studies have evaluated the effect of the optimal location and number of stents necessary to adequately drain an obstructed biliary system. Drainage and stenting of a single complete lobe is typically adequate; however, draining several segments in one lobe is typically not sufficient and may result in increased complication rates.[52] Evaluating which lobe constitutes greater than 70% of the liver volume, demonstrates less tumor burden, and is supplied by a patent lobar portal vein branch are vital.[53] The main predictive indicator for clinical success in patients with hilar tumors is adequate drainage of a liver volume of more than 50%, which may require bilateral stent placement.[54] Draining of an atrophic lobe should be avoided because it is ineffective and only indicated when cholangitis is suspected in this lobe.

BENIGN BILIARY DISEASE: IATROGENIC OR TRAUMATIC INJURIES OF THE BILIARY SYSTEM

Iatrogenic bile duct injuries (IBDIs) cause a significant amount of morbidity and mortality each year, as well as contribute to rising health care cost. The most frequent cause of IBDI remains laparoscopic cholecystectomies—one of the most common procedures in the world. It is essential to recognize IBDI early to prevent severe complications. Percutaneous interventions play a crucial role in management of IBDI, most often as a temporizing measure prior to definitive surgical management. Bilomas and biliary leaks are the most common types of IBDI requiring intervention.[55] The interventional radiologist plays a critical role in delineating biliary anatomy and providing biliary diversion. Imaging is essential for the diagnosis and planning of bile duct injuries, with each modality contributing different advantages and limitations. The most helpful modalities for diagnosis and management include cholescintigraphy, MRCP, ERCP, and PTC.[55] CT is useful in detecting fluid collections and assessing for arterial injuries.Bilomas may lead to serious complications, such as an abscess formation, cholangitis, and sepsis. Fluid collections that are suspected to contain bile should be drained urgently. Single or bilateral percutaneous biliary drains may be required in bile duct injuries. U tube placement may be considered in patients requiring both biliary diversion and biliary drainage. A U tube is a simple straight drain with multiple side holes and two percutaneous exits.[55] A Roux-en-Y hepaticojejunostomy is the surgery of choice for major bile duct injuries unable to be resolved through percutaneous or endoscopic interventions. Blunt abdominal trauma is commonly associated with injuries of the gallbladder, common bile duct, and the intrahepatic ducts. These can include contusions, lacerations, perforations, and avulsions. Most traumatic biliary injuries are treated with surgery.[56]

COMPLICATIONS OF BILIARY INTERVENTIONS

Serious complications related to percutaneous biliary drainage occur in 6.7% of cases, with fatal outcomes in 1.7%.[57] Overall, the complication rate of percutaneous biliary drainage is comparable to the rates associated with endoscopic techniques, although the types of complications differ. Bile leakage is more typically seen after PTBD, whereas ERCP is more likely to be complicated by pancreatitis. Major complications related to percutaneous biliary interventions include arterial bleeding, pseudoaneurysm formation, and biliary sepsis. Incidence of serious complications after PTBD is increased in patients with coagulopathies, cholangitis, biliary stones, malignant obstruction, or more proximal biliary obstruction.[57]

Due to the close relationship between the intrahepatic bile duct and the branches of the hepatic arteries and portal vein, needle punctures from percutaneous interventions can easily cause fistulous communications leading to hemobilia. Avoidance of major vessels during needle placement may be facilitated by US guidance of PTC/PTBD, although subsegmental branches can be difficult to avoid for even the most experienced operators. The rate of vascular complications after PTBD is relatively low—reported at 2.3% in one series.[58] Another series found the incidence of hemobilia from PTBD to be higher (2.2%) than the rate from PTC alone (0.7%), suggesting that the process of tract dilatation and drain placement can cause inadvertent enlargement of an iatrogenic vascular-biliary tract fistula.[59] Delayed bleeding that occurs weeks after drain placement can be caused by a combination of pressure from a relatively stiff biliary drainage catheter and local inflammation. Together, these may lead to erosion of the blood vessel wall, resulting in pseudoaneurysm formation and eventually hemobilia upon rupture into an adjacent bile duct.[60] Hemorrhage into the biliary tree is predominantly arterial in origin due to the high-pressure differential between the hepatic artery and bile ducts. On the other hand, biliary-venous communications are more likely to stop spontaneously, owing to the low-pressure gradient, although venous hemobilia can still occur, particularly in the setting of portal hypertension.[61]

Minor hemobilia typically presents as blood-tinged output from a biliary drainage catheter. Bleeding is most commonly caused by injury to a vein during PTBD. Treatment is generally conservative in these cases and should begin with correcting any underlying coagulopathies. A trial of capping of the drain may also facilitate hemostasis by eliminating an outlet for hemorrhage. However, it is important to recognize that if an internal-external type biliary drain has been placed, bleeding may continue into the upper gastrointestinal (GI) tract through the transpapillary route. If bloody output persists, the patient should be brought to interventional radiology (IR) for fluoroscopic interrogation of the drain and the biliary system. It is important to first check that the most proximal (i.e., peripheral) side hole is not outside the biliary system because it can allow for egress of blood along the drain tract. Other maneuvers to manage minor hemobilia include slightly retracting or advancing the drain so that side

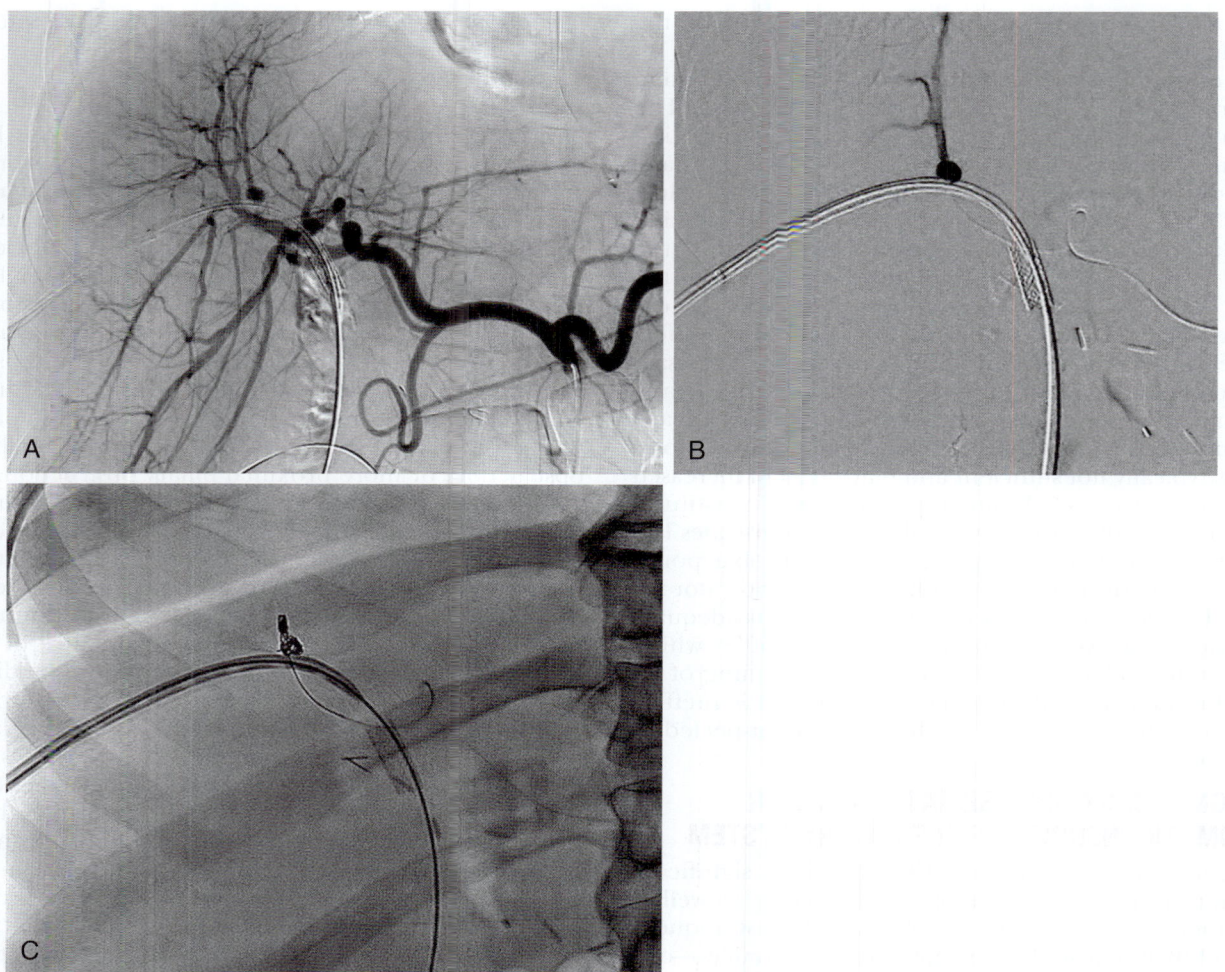

FIGURE 107.9 A 50-year-old woman with history of cholangiocarcinoma status post right percutaneous transhepatic biliary drainage placed 2 weeks prior presented with blood output from the drain. (A) Celiac arteriogram demonstrated a 4-mm pseudoaneurysm adjacent to the percutaneous transhepatic biliary drainage tract. (B) Superselective angiography of the segmental right hepatic artery supplying the (C) pseudoaneurysm treated with coil embolization across the neck of the aneurysm from distal to proximal to prevent recurrent bleeding from collateral hepatic arterial blood flow.

holes do not engage the injured vessel or upsizing drain to create a tamponade effect.[62]

Major hemobilia is characterized by rapid accumulation of blood in an external biliary drainage bag or GI bleeding. Cholangiography in these cases rarely reveals a vascular communication because the direction of bleeding is into the bile duct. Instead, patients should undergo prompt angiography by interventional radiology (Fig. 107.9). The existing biliary drains should be removed over a guidewire prior to angiography to relieve the relative tamponade effect of the drain and to allow for better visualization of the vasculature. Superselection of the right and left hepatic arteries, or of any vessels along the path of the biliary drain, should be performed if no active bleeding or lesion is seen on celiac arteriography. Superior mesenteric arteriography is also recommended to exclude accessory right hepatic arterial sources of hemobilia. Just as with other causes of upper GI bleeding, hemobilia can be intermittent in nature and consequently missed on angiography. After the site of the bleeding is identified,

superselective catheterization with a microcatheter and microcoil embolization is performed. Pseudoaneurysms should be embolized across the neck of the aneurysm from distal to proximal to avoid back bleeding from collateral arterial supply. Because they lack a true wall, pseudoaneurysms may continue to expand if they are simply packed. Other embolic agents, such as glue (n-butyl cyanoacrylate) can be useful in select cases, although they require greater operator experience. Placement of a covered stent across the site of vascular injury is an alternative option to embolization. This allows preservation of distal flow, which can be particularly beneficial in liver transplant patients. Percutaneous thrombin injection is an option for cases of hemobilia secondary to hepatic artery pseudoaneurysm. There are numerous case reports of percutaneous thrombin injection treatment of hepatic artery pseudoaneurysms, and it has been proven to be a safe and effective treatment.[63]

Even with appropriate preprocedure antibiotic prophylaxis, inadvertent puncture of blood vessels in patients with cholangitis can result in bacteremia and potentially frank sepsis. The risk of infection is increased during cholangiography because injected contrast can increase pressure within the biliary tract, particularly in an obstructed system, and cause bacteremia. Sepsis occurs in up to 2.5% of patients after interventional biliary procedures.[57] The risk of infection is greater in patients with malignant rather than benign biliary obstruction.[64] Bacteremia presents as fever, chills, and tachycardia and typically occurs shortly after the procedure as the patient is recovering from anesthesia. Prompt administration of a broad-spectrum antibiotic can forestall acute sepsis, but should it occur, the patient should be managed immediately with vasopressors, inotropic agents, and transfer to an intensive care setting. Percutaneous biliary drainage catheters should be left to bag drainage after intervention to allow clearance of infected blood or bile.

Inadvertent puncture of nontarget structures, such as lung, can occur in up to 0.5% of cases.[57] This complication, typically associated with right-sided PTBD placement, is best avoided by proper preprocedural planning and technique because the pleural reflection is difficult to detect by ultrasonography performed at the time of needle puncture. Because of the negative pressure within the pleural space, percutaneous biliary drains that traverse the pleura can result in bilothorax.[58] Transpleural catheters should be managed by placement of a pleural drain.

Pericatheter leakage can result in subcapsular or perihepatic bile collections. This commonly occurs when the drainage catheter side holes are positioned within the liver parenchyma or in the peritoneum. Bile leakage along PTBD drain occurs as a late complication in 18.8% to 21.7% of patients.[66] Large bilomas should be treated with percutaneous drainage, along with repositioning and/or upsizing of the biliary drain. Leakage of ascites along a PTBD tract can also occur and is more challenging to manage. These patients often require serial paracenteses or placement of a tunneled peritoneal drainage catheter.

INTERVENTIONAL ONCOLOGY

Malignant hepatobiliary disease may present with a variety of clinical presentations. Traditional palliative approaches, such as biliary decompression and intraductal stenting, are still widely used and discussed in prior sections. Newer alternatives, such as transarterial chemoembolization (TACE), radioembolization (Y-90), and RFA, are being used with increasing frequency and successful outcomes.

TRANSARTERIAL CHEMOEMBOLIZATION

Malignant hepatic disease is the most widespread application of TACE. By interrupting the tumoral blood supply, chemoembolization induces ischemic tumoral necrosis through embolization after delivering targeted high-dose intraarterial chemotherapy, sparing systemic exposure.[67] Although hepatocellular carcinoma and colonic metastases remain the most common indications for a TACE, it is increasingly used in patients with intrahepatic cholangiocarcinoma who present with unresectable disease. Data suggest response rates and survival times increase with intraarterial therapy in the setting of inoperable disease.[68]

Evaluating the hepatic arterial anatomy is crucial to the success of the procedure and to prevent nontarget embolization.[67] The procedure entails obtaining arterial access, most commonly by puncturing the common femoral artery, and eventually accessing the common hepatic and proper hepatic arteries, then ultimately branches which supply the tumor. After being selected, the vessels feeding the tumor are injected with both embolic material and a chemotherapeutic agent. Injected agents include Lipiodol, gelatin sponge, and microspheres. Doxorubicin is the most common chemotherapy drug currently used.

RADIOEMBOLIZATION (Y-90)

Radioembolization, also known as selective internal radiation therapy or radiation microsphere therapy, is an effective and increasingly popular treatment alternative for both primary and metastatic malignant hepatobiliary disease. It is a minimally invasive, multiphasic procedure halting blood flow through embolization and providing radiation through the radioactive isotope Y-90. It plays a critical role in inoperable patients.[69] Radioembolization allows targeted radiation therapy allowing sparing of radiosensitive normal hepatocytes, lowering the risk of hepatocellular dysfunction from whole liver radiation.[69]

Research has demonstrated both antitumoral responses and survival benefit in patients with intrahepatic cholangiocarcinoma. The treatment is particularly promising in patients with solitary tumors, with tumors regressing to the point of curative resection. There have also been reported cases of intraductal brachytherapy.[70]

RADIOFREQUENCY ABLATION

Another alternative to surgical resection is percutaneous thermal ablation. Numerous thermal and nonthermal ablation modalities are used, including RFA, microwave ablation, cryoablation, high-intensity focused ultrasonography, and laser ablation. Each modality has its advantages and disadvantages. Heat is generally preferred over cryoablation in the liver due to the increased bleeding risk and the possibility of a diffuse intravascular coagulation–like reaction with cryoablation. RFA induces thermal coagulation necrosis through the delivery of high-frequency alternating current through a needle electrode.[71] Studies are currently investigating RFA in conjunction with locally administered chemotherapy, such as TACE, with the belief that the chemotherapy-containing liposomes are heat-sensitive and ultimately trigger release of the chemotherapeutic agent. RFA has been shown to increase survival rate and local tumor control in patients with primary intrahepatic cholangiocarcinoma. Patients with untreated unresectable cholangiocarcinoma have a median survival of 3.9 months. A study reported a median overall survival period of 38.5 months in patients with unresectable primary intrahepatic cholangiocarcinoma treated with RFA.[72]

CONCLUSION AND SUMMARY

Patients with biliary disease present with complex issues, which often require a multidisciplinary approach. The role of the radiologist is to detect benign and life-threatening diseases, as well as assess for any potential interventions that may be offered. Imaging modalities continue to evolve, with each modality offering certain advantages and disadvantages. Imaging has widespread applications in biliary disease, particularly in identifying obstruction, delineating biliary anatomy, staging malignant disease, and guiding percutaneous and nonsurgical management. The interventional radiologist offers minimally invasive, image-guided therapeutic procedures in patients with biliary disease. This includes obtaining percutaneous access to define biliary anatomy, providing biliary decompression and diversion, and obtaining tissue for pathologic diagnosis. In addition, interventional radiologists provide percutaneous management of biliary strictures, stones, and leaks, as well as newer techniques in interventional oncology.

REFERENCES

1. Levy AD. Noninvasive imaging approach to patients with suspected hepatobiliary disease. *Tech Vasc Interv Radiol.* 2001;4:132.
2. van Breda Vriesman AC, Engelbrecht MR, Smithuis RH, Puylaert JB. Diffuse gallbladder wall thickening: differential diagnosis. *AJR Am J Roentgenol.* 2007;188:495.
3. Catalano OA, Singh AH, Uppot RN, Hahn PF, Ferrone CR, Sahani DV. Vascular and biliary variants in the liver: implications for liver surgery. *Radiographics.* 2008;28:374.
4. Khalili K, Wilson SR. The biliary tree and gallbladder. In: Rumack CM, Wilson SR, Charboneau JW, Levine D, eds. *Diagnostic Ultrasound.* Vol. 1. 4th ed. Philadelphia: Mosby; 2011:172.
5. Niederau C, Müller J, Sonnenberg A, et al. Extrahepatic bile ducts in healthy subjects, in patients with cholelithiasis, and in post-cholecystectomy patients: a prospective ultrasonic study. *J Clin Ultrasound.* 1983;11:23.
6. Graham MF, Cooperberg PL, Cohen MM, Burhenne HJ. The size of the normal common hepatic duct following cholecystectomy: an ultrasonographic study. *Radiology.* 1980;135:137.
7. Conrad MR. Sonographic "parallel channel" sign in obstructive jaundice. *AJR Am J Roentgenol.* 1986;146:645.
8. Berland LL, Lawson TL, Foley WP. Porta hepatis sonographic discrimination of bile ducts from arteries with pulsed Doppler with new anatomic criteria. *AJR Am J Roentgenol.* 1982;138:833.
9. Laing FC, Jeffrey RB Jr, Wing VW, Nyberg DA. Biliary dilatation: defining the level and cause by real-time US. *Radiology.* 1986;160:39.
10. Anderson SW, Lucey BC, Varghese JC, Soto JA. Accuracy of MDCT in the diagnosis of choledocholithiasis. *AJR Am J Roentgenol.* 2006;187:179.
11. Neitlich JD, Topazian M, Smith RC, Gupta A, Burrell MI, Rosenfield AT. Detection of choledocholithiasis: comparison of unenhanced helical CT and endoscopic retrograde cholangiopancreatography. *Radiology.* 1997;203:753-757.
12. Anderson SW, Rho E, Soto JA. Detection of biliary duct narrowing and choledocholithiasis: accuracy of portal venous phase multidetector CT. *Radiology.* 2008;247:418-427.
13. Yeh BM, Liu PS, Soto JA, Corvera CA, Hussain HK. MR imaging and CT of the biliary tract. *Radiographics.* 2009;29:6.
14. Paulson EK, Douglas SH, Enterline DS, McAdams HP, Yoshizumi TT. CT fluoroscopy-guided interventional procedures: techniques and radiation dose to radiologists. *Radiology.* 2001;220:161.
15. Patel HT, Shah AJ, Khandelwal SR, Patel HF, Patel MD. MR cholangiopancreatography at 3.0 T. *Radiographics.* 2009;29(6):1689-1706.
16. Sodickson A, Mortele K, Barish M, Zou KH, Thibodeau S, Tempany CM. Three-dimensional fast-recovery fast spin-echo MRCP: comparison with two-dimensional single-shot fast spin-echo techniques. *Radiology.* 2006;238:549.
17. Glockner JF, Saranathan M, Bayram E, Lee CU. Breath-held MR cholangiopancreatography (MRCP) using a 3D Dixon fat-water separated balanced steady state free precession sequence. *Magn Reson Imaging.* 2013;31(8):1263-1270.
18. Glockner JF, Lee CU. Balanced steady state-free precession (b-SSFP) imaging for MRCP: techniques and applications. *Abdom Imaging.* 2014;39(6):1309-1322.
19. Yokoyama E, Takaura T, Iyama Y, et al. Usefulness of 3D hybrid profile order technique with 3T magnetic resonance cholangiography: comparison of image quality and acquisition time. *J Magn Reson Imaging.* 2014;4(5):1346-1353.
20. Banzo I, Blanco I, Gutiérrez-Mendiguchía C, Gómez-Barquín R, Quirce R, Carril JM. Hepatobiliary scintigraphy for the diagnosis of bile leaks produced after T-tube removal in orthotopic liver transplant. *Nucl Med Commun.* 1998;19(3):229-236.
21. Tripathi M, Chandrashekar N, Kumar R, et al. Hepatobiliary scintigraphy. An effective tool in the management of bile leak following laparoscopic cholecystectomy. *Clin Imaging.* 2004;28(1):40-43.
22. Venbrux A, Sherman F. Malignant obstruction of the hepatobiliary system. In: Baum S, Pentecost MS, eds. *Abrams' Angiography.* New York: Little, Brown; 1997:472-482.
23. Covey AM, Brown KT. Percutaneous transhepatic biliary drainage. *Tech Vasc Interv Radiol.* 2008;11(1):14-20.
24. Fidelman N. Benign biliary strictures: diagnostic evaluation and approaches to percutaneous treatment. *Tech Vasc Interv Radiol.* 2015;18(3):210-217.
25. Köcher M, Cerná M, Havlík R, Král V, Gryga A, Duda M. Percutaneous treatment of benign bile duct strictures. *Eur J Radiol.* 2007;62(2):170-174.
26. Cantwell CP, Pena CS, Gervais DA, Hahn PF, Dawson SL, Mueller PR. Thirty years' experience with balloon dilation of benign postoperative biliary strictures: long-term outcomes. *Radiology.* 2008;249(3):1050-1057.
27. Zajko AB, Sheng R, Zetti GM, Madariaga JR, Bron KM. Transhepatic balloon dilation of biliary strictures in liver transplant patients: a 10-year experience. *J Vasc Interv Radiol.* 1995;6(1):79-83.
28. Weber A, Rosca B, Neu B, et al. Long-term follow-up of percutaneous transhepatic biliary drainage (PTBD) in patients with benign bilioenterostomy stricture. *Endoscopy.* 2009;41(4):323-328.
29. Ramos-de la Medina A, Misra S, Leroy AJ, Sarr MG. Management of benign biliary strictures by percutaneous interventional radiologic techniques (PIRT). *HPB (Oxford).* 2008;10(6):428-432.
30. Saad WE, Davies MG, Saad NE, et al. Transhepatic dilation of anastomotic biliary strictures in liver transplant recipients with use of a combined cutting and conventional balloon protocol: technical safety and efficacy. *J Vasc Interv Radiol.* 2006;17(5):837-843.
31. Depietro DM, Shlansky-Goldberg RD, Soulen MC, et al. Long-term outcomes of a benign biliary stricture protocol. *J Vasc Interv Radiol.* 2015;26(7):1032-1039.
32. Gwon DI, Lee IS, Ko HK, Yoon HK, Sung KB. Percutaneous transhepatic treatment using retrievable covered stents in patients with benign biliary strictures: mid-term outcomes in 68 patients. *Dig Dis Sci.* 2013;58(11):3270-3279.
33. Ferreira R, Loureiro R, Nunes N, et al. Role of endoscopic retrograde cholangiopancreatography in the management of benign biliary strictures: what's new? *World J Gastrointest Endosc.* 2016;8(4):220-231.
34. Ozcan N, Kahriman G, Mavili E. Percutaneous transhepatic removal of bile duct stones: results of 261 patients. *Cardiovasc Intervent Radiol.* 2012;35:890-897.
35. Hatzidakis A, Krokidis M, Gourtsoyiannis N. Percutaneous removal of biliary calculi. *Cardiovasc Intervent Radiol.* 2009;32:1130-1138.
36. Hatzidakis A, Alexandrakis G, Kouroumalis H, Gourtsoyiannis NC. Percutaneous cholangioscopy in the management of biliary disease: experience in 25 patients. *Cardiovasc Intervent Radiol.* 2000;23:431-440.
37. Picus D, Hicks M, Darcy M, et al. Percutaneous cholecystolithotomy: analysis of results and complications in 58 consecutive patients. *Radiology.* 1992;183:779-784.
38. Kim YH, Lim YJ, Shin TB. Fluoroscopy-guided percutaneous gallstone removal using a 12-Fr sheath in high-risk surgical patients with acute cholecystitis. *Korean J Radiol.* 2011;12:210-215.
39. van Delden OM, Laméris JS. Percutaneous drainage and stenting for palliation of malignant bile duct obstruction. *Eur Radiol.* 2008;18:448-456.
40. Bezzi M, Zolovkins A, Cantisani V, et al. New ePTFE/FEP-covered stent in the palliative treatment of malignant biliary obstruction. *J Vasc Interv Radiol.* 2002;13:581-589.
41. Schoder M, Rossi P, Uflacker R, et al. Malignant biliary obstruction: treatment with ePTFE-FEP-covered endoprostheses initial technical and clinical experiences in a multicenter trial. *Radiology.* 2002;225:35-42.
42. Hausegger KA, Thurnher S, Bodendörfer G, et al. Treatment of malignant biliary obstruction with polyurethane-covered Wallstents. *AJR Am J Roentgenol.* 1998;170:403-408.

43. Miyayama S, Matsui O, Akakura Y, et al. Efficacy of covered metallic stents in the treatment of unresectable malignant biliary obstruction. *Cardiovasc Intervent Radiol.* 2004;27:349-354.

44. Chatzis N, Pfiffner R, Glenck M, Stolzmann P, Pfammatter T, Sharma P. Comparing percutaneous primary and secondary biliary stenting for malignant biliary obstruction: a retrospective clinical analysis. *Indian J Radiol Imaging.* 2013;23:38-45.

45. Inal M, Aksungur E, Akgül E, Oguz M, Seydaoglu G. Percutaneous placement of metallic stents in malignant biliary obstruction: one-stage or two-stage procedure? Pre-dilate or not? *Cardiovasc Intervent Radiol.* 2003;26:40-45.

46. Yoshida H, Mamada Y, Taniai N, et al. One-step palliative treatment method for obstructive jaundice caused by unresectable malignancies by percutaneous transhepatic insertion of an expandable metallic stent. *World J Gastroenterol.* 2006;12:2423-2426.

47. Speer AG, Cotton PB, Russell RC, et al. Randomized trial of endoscopic versus percutaneous stent insertion in malignant obstructive jaundice. *Lancet.* 1987;2:57-62.

48. Saluja SS, Gulati M, Garg PK, et al. Endoscopic or percutaneous biliary drainage for gallbladder cancer: a randomized trial and quality of life assessment. *Clin Gastroenterol Hepatol.* 2008;6:944-950, e3.

49. Kloek JJ, van der Gaag NA, Aziz Y, et al. Endoscopic and percutaneous preoperative biliary drainage in patients with suspected hilar cholangiocarcinoma. *J Gastrointest Surg.* 2010;14:119-125.

50. Walter T, Ho CS, Horgan AM, et al. Endoscopic or percutaneous biliary drainage for Klatskin tumors? *J Vasc Interv Radiol.* 2013;24:113-121.

51. Freeman ML, Overby C. Selective MRCP and CT-targeted drainage of malignant hilar biliary obstruction with self-expanding metallic stents. *Gastrointest Endosc.* 2003;58:41-49.

52. Inal M, Akgül E, Aksungur E, et al. Percutaneous self-expandable uncovered metallic stents in malignant biliary obstruction. Complications, follow-up and reintervention in 154 patients. *Acta Radiol.* 2003;44:139-146.

53. Veal DR, Lee AY, Kerlan RK Jr, Gordon RL, Fidelman N. Outcomes of metallic biliary stent insertion in patients with malignant bilobar obstruction. *J Vasc Interv Radiol.* 2013;24:1003-1010.

54. Vienne A, Hobeika E, Gouya H, et al. Prediction of drainage effectiveness during endoscopic stenting of malignant hilar strictures: the role of liver volume assessment. *Gastrointest Endosc.* 2010;72:728-735.

55. Thompson CM, Saad NE, Quazi RR, et al. Management of iatrogenic bile duct injuries: role of the interventional radiologist. *Radiographics.* 2013;33(1):117-134.

56. Gupta A, Stuhlfaut JW, Fleming KW, Lucey BC, Soto JA. Blunt trauma of the pancreas and biliary tract: a multimodality imaging approach to diagnosis. *Radiographics.* 2004;24(5):1381-1395.

57. Saad WE, Wallace MJ, Wojak JC, Kundu S, Cardella JF. Quality improvement guidelines for percutaneous transhepatic cholangiography, biliary drainage, and percutaneous cholecystostomy. *J Vasc Interv Radiol.* 2010;21(6):789-795.

58. Rivera-Sanfeliz GM, Assar OS, Laberge JM, et al. Incidence of important hemobilia following transhepatic biliary drainage: left-sided versus right-sided approaches. *Cardiovasc Intervent Radiol.* 2004;27:13-139.

59. Fidelman N, Bloom AI, Kerlan RK Jr, et al. Hepatic arterial injuries after percutaneous biliary interventions in the era of laparoscopic surgery and liver transplantation: experience with 930 patients. *Radiology.* 2008;247(3):880-886.

60. Gandhi V, Doctor N, Marar S, Nagral A, Nagral S. Major hemobilia—experience from a specialist unit in a developing country. *Trop Gastroenterol.* 2011;32(3):214-218.

61. Mutignani M, Shah SK, Bruni A, Perri V, Costamagna G. Endoscopic treatment of extrahepatic bile duct strictures in patients with portal biliopathy carries high risk of haemobilia: report of 3 cases. *Dig Liver Dis.* 2002;34(8):587-591.

62. Srivastava DN, Sharma S, Pal S, et al. Transcatheter arterial embolization in the management of hemobilia. *Abdom Imaging.* 2006;31:439-448.

63. Krueger K, Zaehringer M, Strohe D, Stuetzer H, Boecker J, Lackner K. Postcatheterization pseudoaneurysm: results of US-guided percutaneous thrombin injection in 240 patients. *Radiology.* 2005;236:1104-110.

64. Cohan RH, Illescas FF, Saeed M, et al. Infectious complications of percutaneous biliary drainage. *Invest Radiol.* 1986;21:705-709.

65. Saro A, Yotsumoto T. Bilothorax as a complication of percutaneous transhepatic biliary drainage. *Asian Cardiovasc Thorac Ann.* 2016;24(1):101-103.

66. Garcarek J, Kurcz J, Guziński M, Janczak D, Sasiadek M. Ten years single center experience in percutaneous transhepatic decompression of biliary tree in patients with malignant obstructive jaundice. *Adv Clin Exp Med.* 2012;21:621-635.

67. Lee KH, Sung KB, Lee DY, Park SJ, Kim KW, Yu JS. Transcatheter arterial chemoembolization for hepatocellular carcinoma: anatomic and hemodynamic considerations in the hepatic artery and portal vein. *Radiographics.* 2002;22(5):1077-1091.

68. Zeccanski JJ, Rilling WS. Transarterial therapies for the treatment of intrahepatic cholangiocarcinoma. *Semin Intervent Radiol.* 2013;30(1):21-27.

69. Murthy R, Nunez R, Szklaruk J, et al. Yttrium-90 microsphere therapy for hepatic malignancy: devices, indications, technical considerations, and potential complications. *Radiographics.* 2005;25:S41-S55.

70. Mouli S, Memon K, Baker T, et al. Yttrium-90 radioembolization for intrahepatic cholangiocarcinoma: safety, response, and survival analysis. *J Vasc Interv Radiol.* 2013;8:1227-1234.

71. Hinshaw JL, Lubner MG, Ziemlewicz TJ, Lee FT Jr, Brace CL. Percutaneous tumor ablation tools: microwave, radiofrequency, or cryoablation—what should you use and why? *Radiographics.* 2014;34(5):1344-1362.

72. Kim KH, Won HJ, Shin YM, Kim KA, Kim PN. Radiofrequency ablation for the treatment of primary intrahepatic cholangiocarcinoma. *AJR Am J Roentgenol.* 2011;196(2):W205-W209.

Operative Management of Cholecystitis and Cholelithiasis

Alexander Perez | Theodore N. Pappas

With an annual rate of greater than a quarter of a million hospital admissions and an associated cost of greater than two billion dollars, cholelithiasis and cholecystitis have a tremendous impact on the health care system. Their diagnosis and associated symptoms are one of the most common reasons for clinic visits and the second most common reason for gastrointestinal-related hospital admissions in the United States.[1] Minimally invasive surgery has revolutionized the way these patients are managed. This technique provides a safe and effective therapy that also results in reduced wound-related complications compared with open cholecystectomy. This enhanced recovery has made the laparoscopic cholecystectomy one of the most commonly performed abdominal surgeries in the Unites States, with more than 500,000 performed each year.[2]

CHOLELITHIASIS

The incidence of cholelithiasis varies greatly (10% to 70%) and is influenced by ethnicity, gender, age, genetic predisposition, obesity, and the presence of certain diseases, such as hemolytic anemia and cirrhosis.[3] The vast majority of gallstones (90%) result from the crystallization and precipitation of excess biliary cholesterol from endogenous and dietary lipids.[4] Most patients diagnosed with gallstones present without symptoms or with mild symptoms, and the majority resolve spontaneously. Expectant management is recommended for these patients because the majority will remain without clinically significant symptoms (78%).[5] Patients with symptomatic cholelithiasis who are surgical candidates should undergo cholecystectomy due to its safe and definitive resolution of symptoms and prevention of future gallstone-related complications. A select group of patients (15%) who are either unable or unwilling to undergo a surgical intervention may be managed nonoperatively with oral gallstone lytic therapy (hydrophilic ursodeoxycholic acid), as long as they present with mild symptoms and small, noncalcified cholesterol gallstones in a functioning gallbladder with a patent cystic duct.[4]

The main symptom of uncomplicated cholelithiasis is biliary colic, which is characterized by sporadic pain localized in the epigastrium or right upper abdomen. This is caused by the intermittent obstruction of the cystic duct by a gallstone. It is usually preceded by a fatty meal, which stimulates gallbladder contraction. This pain may radiate to the back and may be accompanied by nausea and vomiting. Ultrasonography (US) detects cholelithiasis in most patients (98%).[6] These patients benefit from an elective laparoscopic cholecystectomy because their symptoms are likely to persist and surgery will avoid future bouts of cholecystitis and gallstone-related complications, such as pancreatitis, cholangitis, and gallstone ileus.

Pancreatitis that progresses into infected pancreatic necrosis may require pancreatic débridement. Simultaneous cholecystectomy at the time of pancreatic débridement should be considered because gallstones are the most common etiology in these patients (41%), and patients who undergo the combined procedure do not incur an increased incidence of intraoperative biliary ductal injury or postoperative morbidity or mortality. One-third of patients who do not undergo simultaneous cholecystectomy develop biliary-associated complications within a year of the necrosectomy.[7]

Cholangitis may develop in the setting of biliary obstruction secondary to stone impaction within the common bile duct (CBD). Stones in this location are amenable to extraction via endoscopic retrograde cholangiopancreatography (ERCP) and sphincterotomy. Gallstones may also cause major biliary obstruction from impaction within the gallbladder or cystic duct by external compression or "Mirizzi syndrome." This requires cholecystectomy with possible reconstruction or bypass of the extrahepatic biliary tract. Although few patients undergoing cholecystectomy present with this entity (0.18%), most of these patients present with abdominal pain and jaundice. Preoperative ERCP is used to define the biliary anatomy. Most favor an open approach due to the high rate of conversion associated with a laparoscopic approach (67%). There is a significant postoperative morbidity (31%) and a prolonged length of hospitalization associated with this entity.[8] Preoperative biliary stenting and the enhanced dexterity provided by robotic assistance may reduce conversion rate. This technique provides the advantage of minimally invasive surgery such as shorter length of hospitalization but comes at the expense of a longer operative time.[9]

Gallstones may also erode through the gallbladder into the duodenum and then lodge themselves in the distal small bowel. This creates a mechanical bowel obstruction or "gallstone ileus" requiring an emergent laparotomy. This rare condition is associated with a significant morbidity (35%) and mortality rate (6%). The obstruction is typically addressed via stone extraction alone, whereas bowel resection is less often required. Simultaneous cholecystectomy is associated with increased operative time and increased length of postoperative stay, but because there is no significant increase in major postoperative morbidity this option may be considered in select patients.[10]

CHOLECYSTITIS

The inflammation in cholecystitis is for the most part (90%) due to cystic duct obstruction secondary to prolonged gallstone impaction. As this inflammatory process progresses, secondary infection may develop and result in emphysematous cholecystitis and even gangrenous cholecystitis and perforation. These advanced stages of cholecystitis are associated with a significant increase in morbidity and mortality compared with earlier stages of cholecystitis.[11]

Acute cholecystitis usually presents as biliary colic that persists and localizes in the right upper quadrant. Physical findings reflect this level of local inflammation, and patients demonstrate "Murphy's sign" with cessation of inspiration with palpation of the right upper abdomen.[6] Diagnosis is confirmed radiologically by US, which has been proven to be safe, widely available, and highly sensitive for the diagnosis of acute cholecystitis. Findings on US include gallstones, gallbladder wall thickening ($\geq$5 mm), and pericholecystic fluid. When the diagnosis is in doubt, a hepatoimino diacetic acid (HIDA) scan can aid in the diagnosis by identifying cystic duct obstruction with the absence of gallbladder filling within 60 minutes after the radiotracer administration. HIDA has a significantly higher sensitivity and specificity than US in the setting of acute cholecystitis.[12]

There are cases of severe inflammation during cholecystitis in which no obstruction from stone impaction is found (acalculous cholecystitis) and is thought to be related to bile stasis and/or systemic hypoperfusion, as seen in critically ill patients.[3] Patients who develop acalculous cholecystitis may require a percutaneous cholecystostomy tube for immediate decompression with or without an interval cholecystectomy depending on their overall status. Subsequent cholecystectomy in this patient cohort is associated with a significantly increased operative time, open conversion rate, biliary-related complications, surgical site infections (both superficial and deep), and total length of hospitalization compared with those who undergo cholecystectomy without the need for preoperative tube placement.[14]

SPECIAL CONSIDERATIONS

Diabetes is present in some patients (9%) undergoing cholecystectomy for symptomatic gallstones. This comorbidity has been shown to be associated with a higher conversion rate of laparoscopic to open procedure. However, patients with diabetes whose cholecystectomy is completed laparoscopically benefit with a significant reduction in length of hospital stay, morbidity and mortality compared with the open group with diabetes.[15]

Although the vast majority of gallstones are cholesterol based, there are also pigment-based stones, which are more prevalent in certain metabolic conditions, such as hemolytic anemia and cirrhosis. Advanced stage and decompensated cirrhosis is associated with poor outcomes after elective cholecystectomy. The Model for End-Stage Liver Disease (MELD) score has been shown to better predict outcome (sensitivity: 86%; specificity: 61%) than Child-Pugh classification in patients with cirrhosis undergoing cholecystectomy. A MELD score greater than 13 was associated with a higher postoperative morbidity rate and longer hospitalization.[16]

Symptomatic cholelithiasis is common during pregnancy. Timing of the cholecystectomy must take into consideration the burden of gallbladder-related symptoms, complications on the pregnancy, and the safety profile of cholecystectomy. The majority of cholecystectomies were performed within a 3-month period after the delivery. Prior to surgery, most patients present with recurrent biliary symptoms that commonly result in repeat hospitalizations.[17] Cholecystectomies performed during pregnancy usually take place during the second trimester, are associated with a low rate of complications, and can be completed laparoscopically without need for conversion.[18]

Increased age (>85 years) and the Charlson Comorbidity Index were significantly associated with a decreased probability of undergoing surgery within 1 year after the initial visit and an increased probability of undergoing nonsurgical therapies, such as cholecystostomy tube placement and ERCP.[19] Older patients who did not receive cholecystectomy had a higher gallstone-related readmission rate and worse survival compared with patients undergoing cholecystectomy.[20] Older age is an independent predictor for worse outcome after cholecystectomy because it is associated with an increased conversion rate, longer hospital stay, and higher mortality rate.[21]

Infants with cholelithiasis usually have a known underlying risk factor for gallstone development. These children may develop gallstone-related complications, including choledocholithiasis, cholecystitis, and pancreatitis. Most of these patients undergo a laparoscopic cholecystectomy, whereas those managed nonoperatively occasionally have resolution of gallstones. Because infants less than 1 year of age have higher anesthetic and surgical risks, a nonsurgical approach may be considered.[22]

CHOLECYSTECTOMY

The timing of cholecystectomy impacts outcomes in the setting of acute cholecystitis. Cholecystectomy performed within 24 to 48 hours of admission is favored because it is associated with a lower conversion rate, lower incidence of major bile duct injury, less morbidity, lower reoperation rates, shorter total hospital length of stay, shorter postoperative stay, and lower overall cost compared with cholecystectomy performed at later time points.[23–25]

Cholecystectomy in the setting of mild biliary pancreatitis (Ranson score $\leq$3) should be performed during the index admission because it is associated with fewer readmissions, fewer recurrent biliary events, and a similar rate of intraoperative complications and conversion rate compared with interval cholecystectomy.[26] Performing the cholecystectomy in this cohort of patients within 48 hours of admission regardless of the resolution of abdominal pain or laboratory abnormalities results in a shorter length of hospital stay without increasing rates of conversion or perioperative complications.[27]

OPERATIVE TECHNIQUE

Significant changes in the surgical approach to gallbladder disease due to widespread adoption of minimally invasive techniques and education within the residency training programs have resulted in significantly fewer open cholecystectomies performed, lower conversion rate, and more cholecystostomy tubes being placed. Patients undergoing a laparoscopic cholecystectomy have better

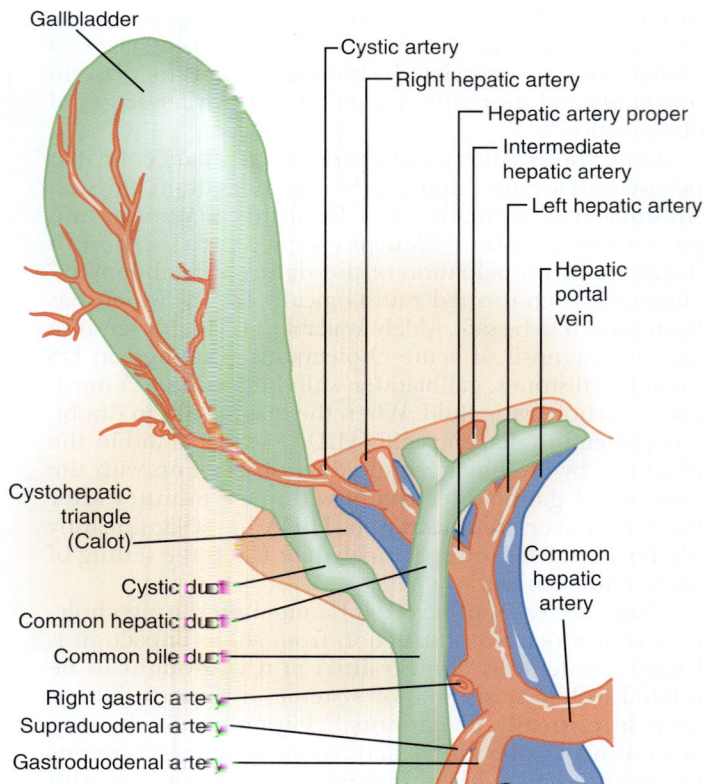

FIGURE 108.1 Gallbladder anatomy.

Labels in figure:
Gallbladder
Cystic artery
Right hepatic artery
Hepatic artery proper
Intermediate hepatic artery
Left hepatic artery
Hepatic portal vein
Cystohepatic triangle (Calot)
Common hepatic artery
Cystic duct
Common hepatic duct
Common bile duct
Right gastric artery
Supraduodenal artery
Gastroduodenal artery

outcomes, including shorter postsurgical stay and fewer complications compared with open cholecystectomy and cholecystostomy tube placement.[28]

Contraindications to a laparoscopic approach include lack of surgeon experience, patient intolerance to pneumoinsufflation, and the inability to safely dissect and identify the pertinent anatomic structures. The patient should be placed in the supine position while in reverse Trendelenburg and rotated with the patient's right side up. The patient's arm should be out and the surgeon stands on the patient's left side. All access approaches are equally safe and should be determined based on surgeon preference and adjusted to each individual situation. In general, patients with morbid obesity and previous surgery involving the umbilicus can be approached with the Veress needle or with the assistance of a transparent optical trocar away from the area with possible intraabdominal adhesions. This allows for direct visualization with the laparoscope while dissecting through the abdominal wall.

Safe dissection and mobilization of the gallbladder away from its attachments require identification of the relevant anatomy (Fig. 108.1). Whether the dissection is performed via a subcostal incision or via a minimally invasive approach, the dissection should be adjusted to the level of inflammation and the ability to adequately and safely identify the gallbladder and adjacent structures. In most cases the fundus of the gallbladder is retracted cephalad to provide adequate retraction of the overlying liver and expose the infundibulum. After being exposed, this is retracted laterally and away from the liver to place adequate tension on the cystic duct without overly retracting the CBD into the dissection field. Depending on the

body habitus, the CBD may be clearly identified and aid with confirmation of the cystic duct; however, it is not recommended to attempt exposure of the CBD to avoid inadvertent injury. The peritoneum is scored at the level of the infundibulum, and dissection is carried out alongside of the gallbladder where it meets the liver both medially and laterally. Exposure for this is provided by lateral retraction of the infundibulum and cephalad traction on the fundus. Various tools can be used to facilitate the dissection, including electrocautery, suction-irrigation, and blunt and sharp dissectors. Careful hemostasis ensures optimal visualization, but excessive thermal use may result in delayed injury. The goal is to provide a circumferential dissection of the gallbladder away from the liver so that only two structures are left tethering it—the cystic duct and the cystic artery. After this is achieved, the cystic duct and artery are dissected close to the gallbladder. This level of dissection achieves the "Critical View of Safety" and allows these structures to be safely controlled and transected (Fig. 108.2).[29] Due to the highly variable nature of anatomic variations in this area, the surgeon should always take all the necessary precautions to ensure a safe dissection.

The early phase of the learning curve for the laparoscopic cholecystectomy (1990s) was associated with an increased rate of bile duct injury (2.2%) in the first 13 patients of the series compared with the rate (0.1%) for all the patients thereafter, which is comparable to the rate of injury in the open control from the same time period.[30] A contemporary series demonstrates a lower rate of the incidence of bile duct injury (0.08%) associated with laparoscopic cholecystectomy.[31] This improvement is likely

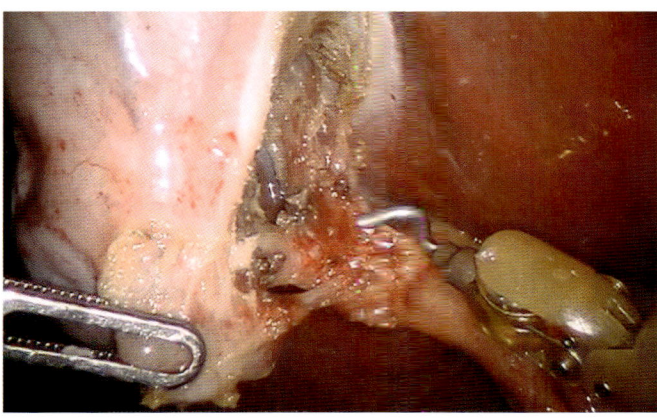

FIGURE 108.2 Critical View of Safety.

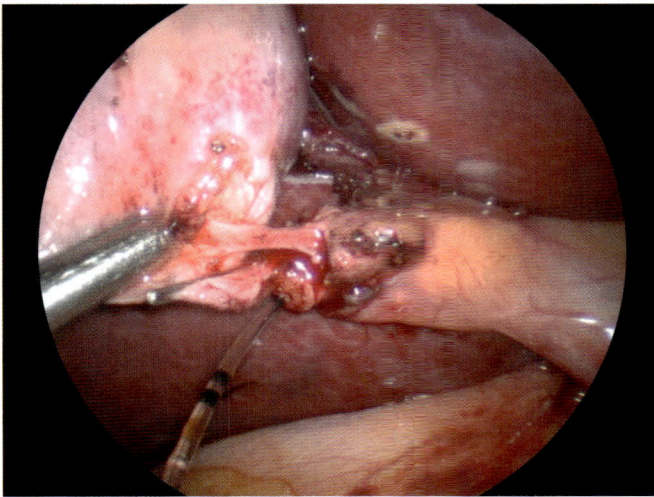

FIGURE 108.3 Intraoperative cholangiogram.

a result of increased experience, improved instrumentation with enhanced dexterity and visualization, and widespread teaching of advanced minimally invasive techniques in residency training programs.

Intraoperative cholangiography typically uses contrast dye injected directly into the suspected cystic duct or gallbladder infundibulum, along with real-time fluoroscopy to aid in identifying biliary ductal structures (Fig. 108.3). When correctly interpreted, this may decrease the risk or severity of injury and improve biliary ductal injury recognition. In experienced hands, intraoperative laparoscopic ultrasound may also help to delineate relevant anatomy and thus decrease the risk of injury. An analysis of eight randomized trials with 1715 patients failed to demonstrate a significant advantage to routine over selective use of intraoperative cholangiography to reduce the rate of bile duct injuries (0.1%) but did demonstrate a longer operative time. This study also concludes that due to its low incidence, any future study would require greater than 15,000 patients to demonstrate a significant difference in bile duct injury prevention.[33]

Other methods for identifying ductal anatomy without the need for accessing the biliary tract directly include preoperative intravenous indocyanine green administration and intraoperative near-infrared fluorescence cholangiography with a specialized camera system to visualize the biliary tract. This method has been shown to be able to identify the cystic duct sooner than with a conventional imaging system.[34]

Repairs to biliary ductal injuries done by nonhepatobiliary surgeons are associated with higher rates of restricturing, recurrent cholangitis, need for dilations, redo reconstructions, and overall morbidity compared with repairs done by hepatobiliary surgeons. The timing of these repairs also impacts outcome because early repairs (≤21 days) have been shown to result in lower rates of restricturing, less need for dilations, and less overall morbidity compared with late repairs.[35]

Uncomplicated bile leaks are for the most part successfully managed by endoscopic measures alone (96%) without the need for surgical intervention. More complex biliary ductal injuries are best managed with surgical management (88%) and most require biliary stenting for a prolonged period of time (>6 months). Outcomes for the surgical repair of these complex biliary injuries have improved over recent years.[36] Even though the rate of laparoscopic cholecystectomies continues to rise, it has been without an increase in the rate of complex biliary injuries requiring surgical biliary reconstruction and a significant decrease in annual mortality.[37]

OTHER TECHNICAL APPROACHES

Partial cholecystectomy is a procedure that removes only a portion of the gallbladder when the gallbladder cannot be safely removed in its entirety. A meta-analysis of 30 studies including 1231 patients showed that most of these procedures are performed laparoscopically and mostly for case of severe acute cholecystitis, cirrhosis and portal hypertension, or gallbladder perforation. Rates of bile duct injury were lower, whereas the rate of postoperative bile leak was higher than historical controls for the standard cholecystectomy. The laparoscopic group had fewer wound infections but a higher rate of bile leaks compared with the open group. Lack of closure of the cystic duct or Hartmann pouch was associated with a higher rate of bile leaks and subhepatic collections than those who had undergone closure of these structures.[38] Patients are routinely managed by leaving a drain in the resection bed and using ERCP as needed for stenting in the postoperative setting.

Cholecystostomy or gallbladder drainage via a percutaneously placed drain in nonsurgical candidates with cholecystitis has proven to be safe and effective. Early drainage via percutaneous cholecystostomy tube placement (within 2 days of admission) results in lower conversion rate during subsequent laparoscopic cholecystectomy compared with a drainage procedure performed at a later time frame. Those who required conversion to an open procedure had a longer hospital stay than those who had their procedure completed laparoscopically.[39] Patients with acute cholecystitis who undergo a drainage procedure with a cholecystostomy tube are typically sicker, older, and have more comorbidities, including cardiovascular disease and diabetes, than those who undergo a cholecystectomy. These patients also have a longer length of hospitalization and a higher mortality rate compared with patients who underwent cholecystectomy.[40,41] Over the years, mortality rates after percutaneous cholecystostomy tube placement have significantly decreased (36% to 12%).[42]

Single incision laparoscopic surgery (SILS) was developed with the goal of improving such outcomes as postoperative pain reduction and improved patient-perceived cosmesis by reducing the number of skin incisions to one through which multiple instruments can be introduced. This technique has required a new learning curve and the development of articulating instrumentation to facilitate the dissection. Concern has been expressed due to the increased rate of bile duct injuries (0.72%) compared with historical rates. This is apparent even though these procedures have been performed for the most part in the absence of acute cholecystitis (91%), thus with less inflammation and theoretically better conditions for proper identification of anatomic structures.[43] Other studies have shown consistently longer operative times without significant improvements in other intraoperative or postoperative outcomes compared with standard laparoscopic cholecystectomy.[44,45] Increased body mass index is associated with a higher rate of conversion from SILS to standard laparoscopy.[46]

Natural orifice transluminal endoscopic surgery was also developed with a similar goal to improve postoperative pain and cosmesis outcomes by eliminating the incisions associated with laparoscopy and performing the surgical resection and extraction via natural orifices, such as the mouth, vagina, and anus. This approach has resulted in longer operative times without significant improvements in other intraoperative or postoperative outcomes compared with standard laparoscopy.[47,48]

The use of robotic assistance in the area of cholecystectomy has resulted in increased costs but has not significantly decreased the complication rates or length of postoperative hospital stay.[49] The lack of haptic feedback has been noted as a disadvantage of this system while potential advantages may include its utility as an educational platform for teaching and mentoring in addition to stimulating interest in the field of surgery.[50] These important aspects will continue to be evaluated and play an important role in the future of surgery as the technology itself evolves and access to these platforms becomes more widespread and cost effective.

REFERENCES

1. Peery AF, Dellon ES, Lund J, et al. Burden of gastrointestinal disease in the United States: 2012 update. *Gastroenterology.* 2012;143:1179.
2. Cullen KA, Hall MJ, Golosinskiy A. Ambulatory surgery in the United States, 2006. *Natl Health Stat Report.* 2009;28:1.
3. Stinton LM, Myers RP, Shaffer EA. Epidemiology of gallstones. *Gastroenterol Clin N Am.* 2010;39:157.
4. Portincasa P, Moschetta A, Palasciano G. Cholesterol gallstone disease. *Lancet.* 2006;368:230.
5. Festi D, Reggiani ML, Attili AF, et al. Natural history of gallstone disease: expectant management or active treatment? Results from a population-based cohort study. *J Gastroenterol Hepatol.* 2010;25:719.
6. Strasberg SM. Clinical practice. Acute calculous cholecystitis. *N Engl J Med.* 2008;358:2804.
7. Fong ZV, Peev M, Warshaw AL, et al. Single-stage cholecystectomy at the time of pancreatic necrosectomy is safe and prevents future biliary complications: a 20-year single institutional experience with 217 consecutive patients. *J Gastrointest Surg.* 2015;19:32.
8. Erben Y, Benavente-Chenhalls LA, Donohue JM, et al. Diagnosis and treatment of Mirizzi syndrome: 23-year Mayo Clinic experience. *J Am Coll Surg.* 2011;213:114.
9. Lee KF, Chong CN, Ma KW, et al. A minimally invasive strategy for Mirizzi syndrome: the combined endoscopic and robotic approach. *Surg Endosc.* 2014;28:2690.
10. Mallipeddi MK, Pappas TN, Shapiro ML, Scarborough JE. Gallstone ileus: revisiting surgical outcomes using National Surgical Quality Improvement Program data. *J Surg Res.* 2013;184:84.
11. Ganapathi AM, Speicher PJ, Englum BR, Perez A, Tyler DS, Zani S. Gangrenous cholecystitis: a contemporary review. *J Surg Res.* 2015;197:18.
12. Kaoutzanis C, Davies E, Leichtle SW, et al. Is hepato-imino diacetic acid scan a better imaging modality than abdominal ultrasound for diagnosing acute cholecystitis? *Am J Surg.* 2015;210:473.
13. Huffman JL, Schenker S. Acute acalculous cholecystitis: a review. *Clin Gastroenterol Hepatol.* 2010;8:15.
14. Mizrahi I, Mazeh H, Yuval JB, et al. Perioperative outcomes of delayed laparoscopic cholecystectomy for acute calculous cholecystitis with and without percutaneous cholecystostomy. *Surgery.* 2015;158:728.
15. Paajanen H, Suuronen S, Nordstrom P, Miettinen P, Niskanen L. Laparoscopic versus open cholecystectomy in diabetic patients and postoperative outcome. *Surg Endosc.* 2011;25:764.
16. Delis S, Bakoyiannis A, Madariaga J, Bramis J, Tassopoulos N, Dervenis C. Laparoscopic cholecystectomy in cirrhotic patients: the value of MELD score and Child-Pugh classification in predicting outcome. *Surg Endosc.* 2010;24:407.
17. Jorge AM, Keswani RN, Veerappan A, Soper NJ, Gawron AJ. Non-operative management of symptomatic cholelithiasis in pregnancy is associated with frequent hospitalizations. *J Gastrointest Surg.* 2015;19:598.
18. Dhupar R, Smaldone GM, Hamad GG. Is there a benefit to delaying cholecystectomy for symptomatic gallbladder disease during pregnancy? *Surg Endosc.* 2010;24:108.
19. Bergman S, Sourial N, Vedel I, et al. Gallstone disease in the elderly: are older patients managed differently? *Surg Endosc.* 2011;25:55.
20. Riall TS, Zhang D, Townsend CM Jr, Kuo YF, Goodwin JS. Failure to perform cholecystectomy for acute cholecystitis in elderly patients is associated with increased morbidity, mortality, and cost. *J Am Coll Surg.* 2010;210:668.
21. Nielsen LB, Harboe KM, Bardram L. Cholecystectomy for the elderly: no hesitation for otherwise healthy patients. *Surg Endosc.* 2014;28:171.
22. Jeanty C, Derderian SC, Courtier J, Hirose S. Clinical management of infantile cholelithiasis. *J Pediatr Surg.* 2015;50:1289.
23. Banz V, Gsponer T, Candinas D, Güller U. Population-based analysis of 4113 patients with acute cholecystitis: defining the optimal time-point for laparoscopic cholecystectomy. *Ann Surg.* 2011;254:964.
24. de Mestral C, Rotstein OD, Laupacis A, et al. Comparative operative outcomes of early and delayed cholecystectomy for acute cholecystitis: a population-based propensity score analysis. *Ann Surg.* 2014;259:10.
25. Gutt CN, Encke J, Köninger J, et al. Acute cholecystitis: early versus delayed cholecystectomy: a multicenter randomized trial (ACDC study, NCT00447304). *Ann Surg.* 2013;258:385.
26. van Baal MC, Besselink MG, Bakker OJ, et al. Timing of cholecystectomy after mild biliary pancreatitis: a systematic review. *Ann Surg.* 2012;255:860.
27. Aboulian A, Chan T, Yaghoubian A, et al. Early cholecystectomy safely decreases hospital stay in patients with mild gallstone pancreatitis: a randomized prospective study. *Ann Surg.* 2010;251:615.
28. Wiseman JT, Sharuk MN, Singla A, et al. Surgical management of acute cholecystitis at a tertiary care center in the modern era. *Arch Surg.* 2010;145:439.
29. Strasberg SM, Brunt LM. Rationale and use of the critical view of safety in laparoscopic cholecystectomy. *J Am Coll Surg.* 2010;211:132.
30. Meyers WC, Branum GD, Farouk M, et al. A prospective analysis of 1518 laparoscopic cholecystectomies. The Southern Surgeons Club. *N Engl J Med.* 1991;324:1073.
31. Halbert C, Pagkratis S, Yang J, et al. Beyond the learning curve: incidence of bile duct injuries following laparoscopic cholecystectomy normalize to open in the modern era. *Surg Endosc.* 2016;30(6):2239-2243.

32. Overby DW, Apelgren KN, Richardson W, Fanelli R. Society of American Gastrointestinal and Endoscopic Surgeons. SAGES guidelines for the clinical application of laparoscopic biliary tract surgery. *Surg Endosc.* 2010;24:2368.

33. Ford JA, Soop M, Du J, Loveday BP, Rogers M. Systematic review of intraoperative cholangiography in cholecystectomy. *Br J Surg.* 2012;99:160.

34. van Dam DA, Ankersmit M, van de Ven P, van Rijswijk AS, Tuynman JB, Meijerink WJ. Comparing near-infrared imaging with indocyanine green to conventional imaging during laparoscopic cholecystectomy: a prospective crossover study. *J Laparoendosc Adv Surg Tech A.* 2015;25:486.

35. Perera MT, Silva MA, Hegab B, et al. Specialist early and immediate repair of post-laparoscopic cholecystectomy bile duct injuries is associated with an improved long-term outcome. *Ann Surg.* 2011;253:553.

36. Pitt HA, Sherman S, Johnson MS, et al. Improved outcomes of bile duct injuries in the 21st century. *Ann Surg.* 2013;258:490.

37. Worth PJ, Kaur T, Diggs BS, Sheppard BC, Hunter JG, Dolan JP. Major bile duct injury requiring operative reconstruction after laparoscopic cholecystectomy: a follow-on study. *Surg Endosc.* 2016;30:1839.

38. Elshaer M, Gravante G, Thomas K, Sorge R, Al-Hamali S, Ebdewi H. Subtotal cholecystectomy for "difficult gallbladders": systematic review and meta-analysis. *JAMA Surg.* 2015;150:159.

39. Bickel A, Hoffman RS, Loberant N, Weiss M, Eitan A. Timing of percutaneous cholecystostomy affects conversion rate of delayed laparoscopic cholecystectomy for severe acute cholecystitis. *Surg Endosc.* 2015;30:1028.

40. Anderson JE, Chang DC, Talamini MA. A nationwide examination of outcomes of percutaneous cholecystostomy compared with cholecystectomy for acute cholecystitis 1998-2010. *Surg Endosc.* 2013;27:3406.

41. Jang WS, Lim JU, Joo KR, Cha JM, Shin HP, Joo SH. Outcome of conservative percutaneous cholecystostomy in high-risk patients with acute cholecystitis and risk factors leading to surgery. *Surg Endosc.* 2015;29:2359.

42. Smith TJ, Manske JG, Mathiason MA, Kallies KJ, Kothari SN. Changing trends and outcomes in the use of percutaneous cholecystostomy tubes for acute cholecystitis. *Ann Surg.* 2013;257:1112.

43. Joseph M, Phillips MR, Farrell TM, Rupp CC. Single incision laparoscopic cholecystectomy is associated with a higher bile duct injury rate: a review and a word of caution. *Ann Surg.* 2012;256:1.

44. Ma J, Cassera MA, Spaun GO, Hammill CW, Hansen PD, Aliabadi-Wahle S. Randomized controlled trial comparing single-port laparoscopic cholecystectomy and four-port laparoscopic cholecystectomy. *Ann Surg.* 2011;254:22.

45. Chang SK, Wang YL, Shen L, Iyer SG, Madhavan K. A randomized controlled trial comparing post-operative pain in single-incision laparoscopic cholecystectomy versus conventional laparoscopic cholecystectomy. *World J Surg.* 2015;39:897.

46. Han HJ, Choi SB, Kim WB, Choi SY. Single-incision multiport laparoscopic cholecystectomy: things to overcome. *Arch Surg.* 2011;146:68.

47. Sodergren MH, Markar S, Pucher PH, Badran IA, Jiao LR, Darzi A. Safety of transvaginal hybrid NOTES cholecystectomy: a systematic review and meta-analysis. *Surg Endosc.* 2015;29:2077.

48. Borchert DH, Federlein M, Fritze-Büttner F, et al. Postoperative pain after transvaginal cholecystectomy: single-center, double-blind, randomized controlled trial. *Surg Endosc.* 2014;28:1886.

49. Kaminski JP, Bueltmann KW, Rudnicki M. Robotic versus laparoscopic cholecystectomy inpatient analysis: does the end justify the means? *J Gastrointest Surg.* 2014;18:2116.

50. Perez A, Zinner MJ, Ashley SW, Brooks DC, Whang EE. What is the value of telerobotic technology in gastrointestinal surgery? *Surg Endosc.* 2003;17:811.

Management of Common Bile Duct Stones

Ben Schwab | Eric S. Hungness | Nathaniel J. Soper

Choledocholithiasis is a common condition that often requires a procedural intervention in order to treat. There are a number of different treatment strategies used when managing patients who present with common bile duct (CBD) stones. As such, the debate about the optimal management of patients with choledocholithiasis has persisted for many years. The currently available options include surgical intervention, most commonly with laparoscopic common bile duct exploration (LCBDE), endoscopic retrograde cholangiography (ERC) with or without endoscopic sphincterotomy (ES), and percutaneous transhepatic cholangiography. The choice of which option to pursue is dependent both on patient-level considerations, including the presence of comorbidities that make the risk of surgical intervention prohibitive, in addition to the timing of diagnosis of CBD stones (preoperatively, postoperatively, or intraoperatively). In addition, the level of support present in the health care facility to which the patient presents often dictates treatment options, given that the use of nonsurgical options requires the presence of endoscopic and/or interventional radiology capability. In this chapter, we review the various techniques available to clear the CBD of stones, with a focus on the use of LCBDE, including a discussion of the overall use of surgical approaches to the management of choledocholithiasis. In addition, we propose an updated algorithm that assumes an advanced laparoscopic surgeon with excellent endoscopic and radiologic support (Fig. 109.1) and that takes into account the ability to clear the CBD in the safest and most cost-effective manner.

DETECTION OF COMMON DUCT STONES

The most common clinical presentations for patients with choledocholithiasis are cholecystitis, pancreatitis, biliary colic, cholangitis, and jaundice. Cholangitis is most predictive, with some studies showing 100% specificity.[1] However, none of the other more common clinical presentations are predictive. Tranter and Thompson demonstrated a 14% incidence of choledocholithiasis in 1000 consecutive laparoscopic cholecystectomies (LCs) during which routine intraoperative cholangiogram was performed. Patients presenting with cholecystitis, biliary colic, pancreatitis, and jaundice were found to have common duct stones 7%, 16%, 20%, and 45% of the time, respectively.[1]

Transabdominal ultrasonography is the most common imaging modality used in the initial evaluation of patients who present with biliary symptoms. However, compared with its high accuracy in diagnosing cholelithiasis and cholecystitis, transabdominal ultrasound has only 50% to 80% sensitivity in detecting common duct stones, depending mostly on the presence of CBD dilation.[2,3] Some studies have shown that if sonographic CBD dilation is combined with age older than 55 years and abnormal liver enzymes, choledocholithiasis can be predicted up to 95% of the time.[4]

For these patients in whom choledocholithiasis is suspected, more definite preoperative tests may be performed. ERC is highly specific in diagnosing common duct stones and may be therapeutic with sphincterotomy and duct clearance. However, this procedure is invasive and associated with significant morbidity, including post-ERC pancreatitis, bleeding, sepsis, and perforation. A prospective study of 1177 consecutive ERCs demonstrated a 30-day morbidity rate of 15.9%, with a procedure-related mortality of .7%.[5] The morbidity of the ERC procedure is thought to be caused by two primary mechanisms: mechanical injury from repeated instrumentation of the sphincter of Oddi and the biliary and pancreatic ducts, in addition to hydrostatic injury incurred during injection of the contrast under pressure. In addition, up to 60% of patients undergoing ERC prior to LC will be found not to have common duct stones and will therefore have undergone an unnecessary and invasive test.[6,7]

Endoscopic ultrasound (EUS) and magnetic resonance technology have been used to diagnose choledocholithiasis. To decrease unnecessary ERC/ES, some centers now routinely perform EUS before ERC. The sensitivity and specificity of EUS have been reported as high as 98% and 99%, respectively.[8] In light of these findings and the decreased risk of pancreatitis when compared with ERC, two clinical guidelines advocate EUS in symptomatic patients with indeterminate risk of choledocholithiasis.[9,10] In addition, magnetic resonance imaging has shown promise as an alternative means to diagnose choledocholithiasis, with a study showing a positive predictive value of 95%.[11] In patients with indeterminate risk for choledocholithiasis, magnetic resonance cholangiopancreatography (MRCP) is a valuable, noninvasive option that does not incur the same morbidity risks as ERC and, to less degree, EUS. MRCP is also useful in patients who have had a prior Billroth II or Roux-en-Y gastrojejunostomy, particularly in patients having undergone a gastric bypass operation for the treatment of morbid obesity. However, MRCP is quite expensive and does not have the therapeutic possibilities of ERC.

PREOPERATIVE ENDOSCOPIC THERAPY

ERC plays an important role in the treatment of common duct stones for older adults or debilitated patients and in patients who present with jaundice, cholangitis, or severe pancreatitis. For patients who may not tolerate an operation, performing ERC/ES and leaving the gallbladder in situ is a good alternative to cholecystectomy, because up to 85% of patients remain symptom free with up to

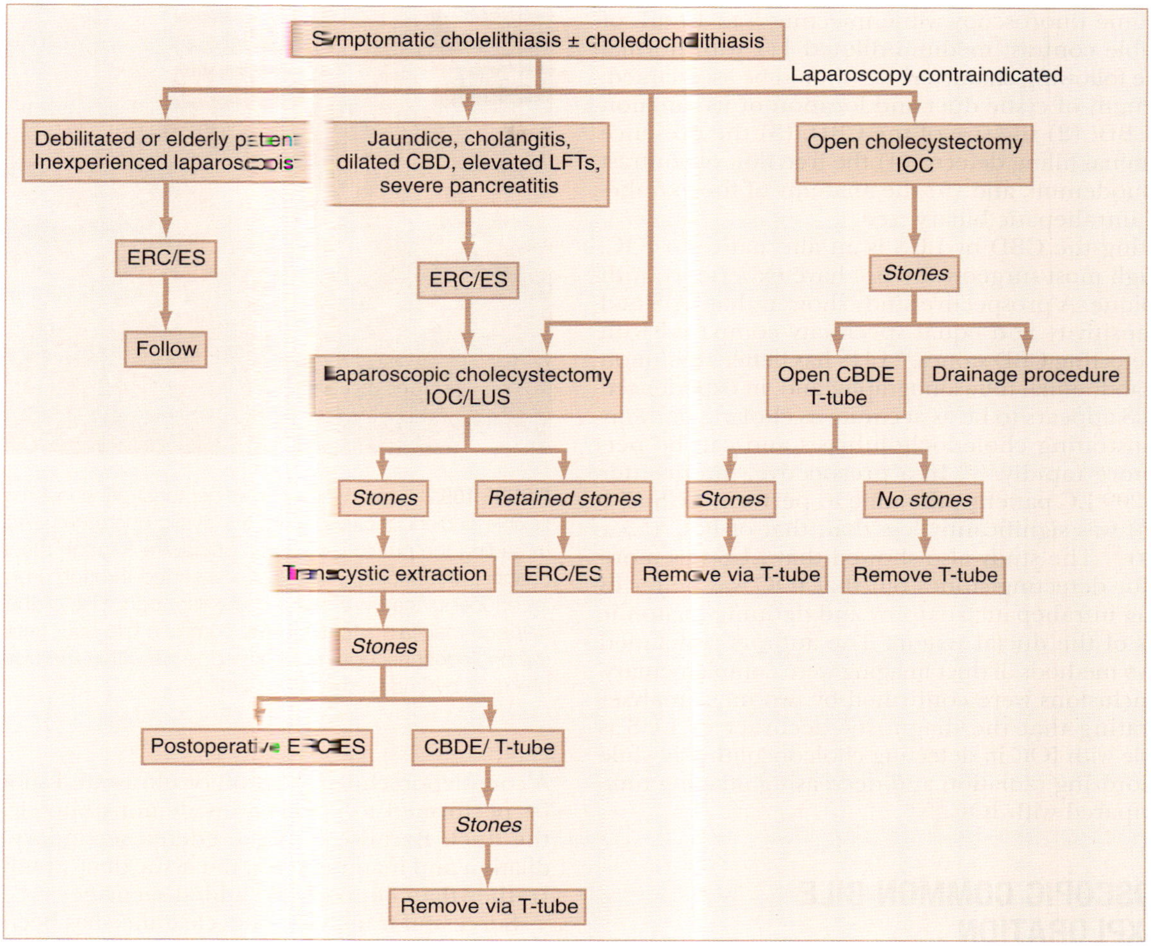

FIGURE 109.1 Management algorithm for treatment of common bile duct stones. This approach assumes that the laparoscopist is experienced in transcystic techniques and that endoscopic retrograde cholangiography and endoscopic sphincterotomy are at least 90% successful at CBD stone clearance. *CBD,* Common bile duct; *CBDE,* common bile duct exploration; *ERC,* endoscopic retrograde cholangiography; *ES,* endoscopic sphincterotomy; *LFT,* liver function test; *IOC,* intraoperative cholangiography; *LUS,* laparoscopic ultrasonography. (From Jones DB, Soper NJ. The current management of common bile duct stones. *Adv Surg.* 1996;29:271.)

70-month follow-up.[12,13] Other studies have demonstrated a decreased mortality for patients undergoing ERC versus surgical drainage for cholangitis and severe pancreatitis.[14–16] If a patient with choledocholithiasis does undergo successful preoperative ERC, early LC could be considered because a randomized trial showed 36% recurrent biliary events within 6 to 8 weeks.[17] In addition, two prospective randomized trials and a systematic review comparing two-stage versus single-stage management demonstrate equivalent success rates for LCBDE versus preoperative ERC/ES followed by LC.[18–20] One-stage LCBDE has also been shown to significantly reduce hospital stays and hospital costs.[19,21] Tai et al showed that LCBDE had a 100% success rate in salvaging failed preoperative ERC/ES.[22]

Much of the morbidity associated with ERC/ES is associated with the sphincterotomy. Endoscopic papillary dilation has been suggested as an alternative; a multicenter randomized study demonstrated that endoscopic balloon dilation resulted in a higher rate of pancreatitis when compared with sphincterotomy and recommended that it should be avoided in routine practice.[23] However, in patients with coagulopathy, dilation should be the preferred method for endoscopic removal of common duct stones.[24]

INTRAOPERATIVE DIAGNOSIS OF COMMON BILE DUCT STONES

For patients undergoing LC, the CBD should be imaged intraoperatively if choledocholithiasis is suspected (past or present elevation of liver function tests, gallstone pancreatitis, CBD dilation, or choledocholithiasis on preoperative ultrasound) or if the biliary anatomy is unclear.[25] This can be achieved by intraoperative cholangiography (IOC) or laparoscopic ultrasonography (LUS). Before either procedure, a clip is applied high on the cystic duct at its junction with the gallbladder to prevent stones migrating down the duct. To perform IOC, the cystic duct is partially transected and "milked," moving stones away from the CBD and out the ductotomy. A cholangiography catheter is inserted into the cystic duct and secured in place with a clip, grasping jaws, or balloon fixation. Cholangiography is preferentially performed with real-time fluoroscopy while injecting 5 to 10 mL of water-soluble contrast medium diluted 1:1 with normal saline. The following characteristics should be ascertained: (1) the length of cystic duct and location of its junction with the CBD, (2) the size of the CBD, (3) the presence of intraluminal filling defects, (4) the free flow of contrast into the duodenum, and (5) the anatomy of the extrahepatic and intrahepatic biliary tree.

Evaluating the CBD by LUS is an alternative to IOC, even though most surgeons do not have experience with this technique. A prospective study showed that LUS had greater sensitivity and equal specificity compared with IOC for detecting CBD stones.[26] LUS has better resolution than transabdominal ultrasonography, and, in experienced hands, LUS appears to be as accurate as cholangiography for demonstrating choledocholithiasis and can be performed more rapidly.[27,28] In a prospective, multicenter trial with 209 LC patients, the time to perform LUS (7 ± 3 minutes) was significantly less than that of IOC (13 ± 6 minutes).[27] The study also showed that LUS was more sensitive for detecting stones but that IOC was better in delineating intrahepatic anatomy and defining anatomic anomalies of the ductal system. The authors concluded that the two methods of duct imaging were complementary. These conclusions were confirmed by two meta-analyses demonstrating that the diagnostic accuracy of LUS is comparable with IOC in detecting choledocholithiasis while avoiding ionizing radiation and decreasing imaging time when compared with IOC.[29,30]

LAPAROSCOPIC COMMON BILE DUCT EXPLORATION

When CBD stones are found, laparoscopic CBD exploration can take place through the cystic duct (transcystic technique) or by directly incising and opening the CBD with stone retrieval (laparoscopic choledochotomy). In the transcystic duct approach, small stones (<2 to 3 mm) can often be flushed through the ampulla into the duodenum. Intravenous glucagon (1 to 2 mg) may be used to relax the sphincter of Oddi, followed by vigorous flushing of 100 to 200 mL of saline. When these methods fail, a helical stone basket can be passed over a guidewire through the cystic duct and into the CBD to extract stones under fluoroscopic guidance. If attempts at transcystic basket extraction fail, a choledochoscope (≤10 French) should be tried next to remove the stones under direct vision. If the CBD stone is larger than the lumen of the cystic duct, the cystic duct should first be balloon dilated to a maximum of 8 mm diameter but never larger than the internal diameter of the CBD.[31] The choledochoscope is then passed into the peritoneal cavity through the midaxillary port, using a sheath to prevent damage to the scope by the port's valve. The choledochoscope is then inserted through the cystic ductotomy into the CBD under direct vision (Fig. 109.2). Continuously infusing saline through the biopsy channel helps to dilate the lumen of the duct facilitating visualization. The tip of a Segura-type stone basket is advanced through the working channel of the scope beyond the stone and opened. As the basket is pulled backward and rotated, the stone is ensnared (Fig. 109.3).[32]

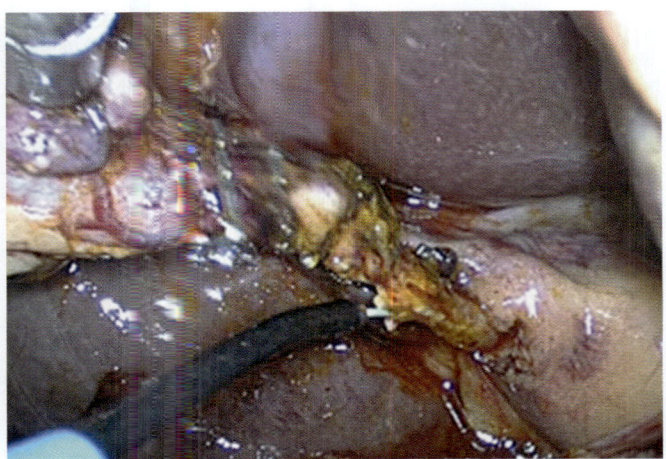

FIGURE 109.2 Laparoscopic view demonstrating insertion of flexible choledochoscope into the cystic ductotomy. After threading the previously placed guidewire through the working channel, the choledochoscope is inserted through a protective introducer placed within the midaxillary port. Use of the guidewire helps to maintain access to the common bile duct until the tip of the choledochoscope is confirmed to be within the distal common bile duct by endoscopic visualization

A completion cholangiogram or ultrasound should always be performed to conclusively demonstrate clearance of the duct. Because of tissue edema secondary to ductal dilation and manipulation, the cystic duct stump is ligated (rather than clipped) for added security.

Successful transcystic duct clearance has been reported in 80% to 98% of patients in recent series.[18,33,34] Complications, such as infection and pancreatitis, have been reported in 5% to 10% of patients, with a mortality rate of 0% to 2%. The duration of hospitalization following an uncomplicated transcystic duct stone extraction is the same as that for LC alone, averaging 1 to 2 days. The main advantage of the transcystic approach is that it avoids choledochotomy. Poor candidates for transcystic extraction techniques are those with large or multiple CBD stones, those with stones in the proximal ductal system, and those with small or tortuous cystic ducts.[35]

Other novel transcystic approaches include balloon dilation of the sphincter of Oddi and antegrade sphincterotomy. Carroll et al. reported successful clearance of CBD stones in 17 (85%) of 20 patients by balloon dilation; however, even in this small series, three patients (15%) experienced mild postoperative pancreatitis.[36] This method should be avoided in patients with preexisting pancreatitis, biliary dyskinesia, or anatomic sphincter anomalies. A sphincterotome may be inserted through the cystic duct and its tip placed just through the ampulla of Vater into the duodenum. A duodenoscope is passed transorally and used to allow proper positioning of the sphincterotome before applying current to perform a sphincterotomy. DePaula et al. have reported the performance of transcystic antegrade sphincterotomy at the time of LC in 22 patients, and all had successful stone clearance without complications; the procedure added only 17 minutes to the operation.[37]

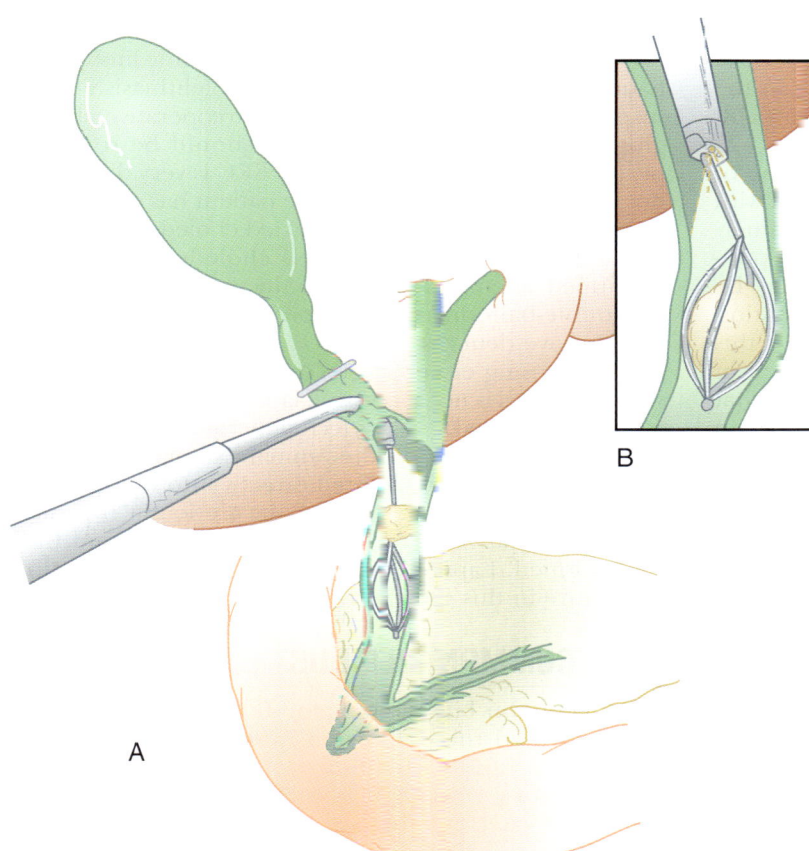

B

A

FIGURE 109.3 Transcystic choledochoscopy. (A) The flexible choledochoscope is passed into the common bile duct through the cystic duct. Under direct vision the basket is advanced distal to the stone and opened. (B) As the basket is withdrawn through the working channel of the choledochoscope, the stone is ensnared. The basket, stone, and choledochoscope are then removed as a unit. (From Jones DB, Soper NJ. The current management of common bile duct stones. *Adv Surg.* 1996;29:271.)

If the transcystic approach fails, there are two primary options for management. For surgeons comfortable with intracorporeal suturing technique, a laparoscopic choledochotomy can be performed. Alternatively, the surgeon can choose to complete the cholecystectomy and refer the patient for postoperative ERC to obtain clearance of the CBD stones. The indications for performance of a laparoscopic choledochotomy are multiple or large stones or those positioned within the proximal bile ducts in patients with a CBD diameter larger than 8 to 10 mm.[38,39] Stay sutures are usually placed on either side of the midline of the anterior CBD wall to allow anterior traction on the duct. A longitudinal choledochotomy is made on the distal CBD, of adequate length to allow easy placement of a choledochoscope and removal of the largest stone.

After the stones are removed under endoscopic visualization, the ductotomy is closed either primarily or over an appropriately sized T tube. Some centers have used transcystic tubes (C tubes) or antegrade stenting with choledochorrhaphy for CBD drainage.[40,41] Common duct closure is accomplished with fine absorbable sutures using intracorporeal suturing techniques and if a T tube or C tube is used, it is exteriorized through the lateral port site. Following transcholedochal stone extraction, an active drain is placed in the subhepatic space. Studies have demonstrated comparable results regardless of the technique of duct closure.[42] Others have shown decreased complications with primary closure compared with T tube use, as well as decreased operative time and hospital stay.[40,43–45] The patient is generally discharged 2 to 4 days

postoperatively. If a T tube is used, a final cholangiogram is performed 14 to 21 days postoperatively with removal of the tube if no abnormalities are noted. Retained stones demonstrated by T tube cholangiography may be effectively removed percutaneously after allowing maturation of the T tube tract. Percutaneous extraction is successful in more than 95% of patients with retained stones[46]; otherwise postoperative ERC will be required.

Overall, laparoscopic choledochotomy is successful in 84% to 94% of patients, with a minor morbidity rate of 4% to 16% and a mortality rate of 0% to 2%.[18,33,34] Potential complications of this technique include CBD laceration, bile leak, sewn-in T tubes, and stricture formation.[38] Many surgeons have not mastered laparoscopic suturing and feel uncomfortable closing the choledochotomy for fear of a resultant stricture; however, no biliary strictures have been identified in three recently published studies that looked at the long-term outcomes of more than 640 patients undergoing LCBDE with a mean follow-up of more than 3 years.[47–49] Similarly, there was no increased risk of recurrent CBD stones for patients who underwent primary choledochorrhaphy compared with T tube closure.[4,50]

Some centers have used intraoperative ERC as an alternative to CBD exploration. Enochsson et al. reported that the technique was safe, with 93.5% duct clearance; however it added 1 hour of operative time compared with LC alone.[51] In another study, intraoperative ERC was as effective as LCBDE in duct clearance (approximately 90%), but morbidity was doubled, and hospital costs were significantly increased.[52] Intraoperative ERC also relies on preoperative coordination with a skilled endoscopist if the surgeon is not trained in ERC. Positioning in the operating room also makes the technique more difficult than in the endoscopy suite.

The possibility of finding CBD stones at the time of LC and potential treatment plans must be discussed with the patient before the operation. Many surgeons routinely leave CBD stones in place during LC for planned postoperative endoscopic removal. This strategy may be appropriate in centers with expert interventional endoscopists with demonstrated high cannulation rates. If this expertise is not available, intraoperative management of the CBD is warranted. A prospective study reported that more than 50% of clinically silent CBD stones passed spontaneously within 6 weeks.[53] Neither the number of stones nor stone size was predictive of spontaneous stone passage. The authors suggested a short-term expectant management approach for patients with clinically silent choledocholithiasis.

POSTOPERATIVE ENDOSCOPIC THERAPY

Postoperative ERC/ES should be considered when (1) LCBDE fails to clear the duct, (2) the surgeon is inexperienced in LCBDE, (3) retained stones are discovered postoperatively, (4) a patient's comorbidities make a prolonged operation risky, and (5) the CBD is small and prone to postoperative stricture. Multiple studies have shown that the clinical incidence of retained CBD stones after LC is approximately 2.5%.[48,54] Regardless of the reason, postoperative ERC/ES maintains the goals of minimally invasive treatment with a rapid return to full activity. However, relying on postoperative ERC/ES subjects the patient to an additional procedure with its associated morbidity and possibly a second operation if endoscopic stone extraction fails. In a study by Rhodes et al., 80 patients discovered to have choledocholithiasis at the time of LC were randomized to have LCBDE versus postoperative ERCP.[55] Clearance of the duct was 100% for LCBDE and 93% for ERC, with a significantly decreased hospital stay for patients undergoing LCBDE. Other studies have shown that even in experienced hands, ES has an overall failure rate for stone clearance of 4% to 18%.[56] Because of the uncertainty of postoperative ERC, it may be reasonable to insert a catheter through the cystic duct into the CBD at the time of LC when CBD stones cannot be removed laparoscopically. Leaving a transcystic catheter in the CBD may facilitate spontaneous passage of retained CBD stones or may increase postoperative ERC success by allowing a guidewire to be passed into the duodenum, thereby ensuring cannulation of the duct.[57,58]

PATIENTS WITH Roux-en-Y GASTROJEJUNOSTOMY

Patients who have had a prior Roux-en-Y gastrojejunostomy, most commonly performed now during gastric bypass operation for the treatment of obesity, and who present with choledocholithiasis pose certain challenges that must be considered (Fig. 109.4). The typical anatomy consists of a small gastric pouch connected to a 75- to 150-cm Roux limb and a 40- to 50-cm biliopancreatic limb. If the patient presents with symptomatic cholelithiasis and/or suspected choledocholithiasis, an intraoperative cholangiogram with or without LCBDE should be routinely performed because postoperative ERC is very difficult, if not impossible to perform. If the patient has already had a cholecystectomy and has suspected choledocholithiasis, MRCP should be performed. If choledocholithiasis is confirmed, attempts at ERC with the assistance of a single- or double-balloon enteroscope can be made. Recent studies have demonstrated 60% to 80% successful CBD clearance using either single- or double-balloon enteroscopes.[59] If this is not successful, laparoscopic-assisted ERC has been described.[60] In this technique, after a laparoscopic gastrotomy is created in the remnant stomach, a 15-mm laparoscopic trocar is inserted directly into the stomach. The endoscope is then passed into the previously "bypassed" gastrointestinal (GI) tract through this trocar, and ERC is performed. Laparoscopic choledochotomy is another alternative in this group of challenging patients.

OPEN COMMON BILE DUCT EXPLORATION

Open common bile duct exploration (OCBDE) should be considered the default position, not a "failure," if LCBDE and/or ERC are unsuccessful. The most common reason to convert to OCBDE is an impacted stone at the ampulla of Vater, and these cases require a transduodenal exploration. This entails performing either a choledochoenterostomy or a sphincterotomy ("-plasty"). Studies have shown overall similar results with either of the two operations. Therefore surgeon experience should dictate which procedure is performed.[61] However, some authors have suggested choledochoenterostomy for CBD greater than 2 cm in diameter to create a large opening between the bile duct and intestine.

SPHINCTEROTOMY AND SPHINCTEROPLASTY

Sphincterotomy consists of incising the distal part of the sphincter musculature for a distance of approximately 1 cm. This incision should not extend beyond the outer wall of the duodenum. A sphincteroplasty requires complete division of the sphincter muscle. This creates a patulous, wide opening that is followed by suture approximation of the wall of the duodenum to the wall of the CBD.

After a choledochotomy is made as described earlier, a catheter or dilator is passed distally and left in place to serve as a guide. A generous Kocher maneuver is then performed, after which a longitudinal anterior duodenotomy is made at the level of the ampulla, which can be palpated. The dilator is then used to bring the ampulla into the operative field being careful not to perforate the duct. For sphincterotomy, the ampulla is then incised sufficiently along the anterosuperior side (opposite the pancreatic duct orifice) to permit removal of the impacted calculus.

For sphincteroplasty, the ampulla and distal CBD are divided for a distance of 1.5 to 2 cm directed anteromedially. The sphincter is usually divided sequentially between small clamps with sequential suture approximation of the duodenal and bile duct mucosa. This is done using fine interrupted absorbable suture. The duodenum is

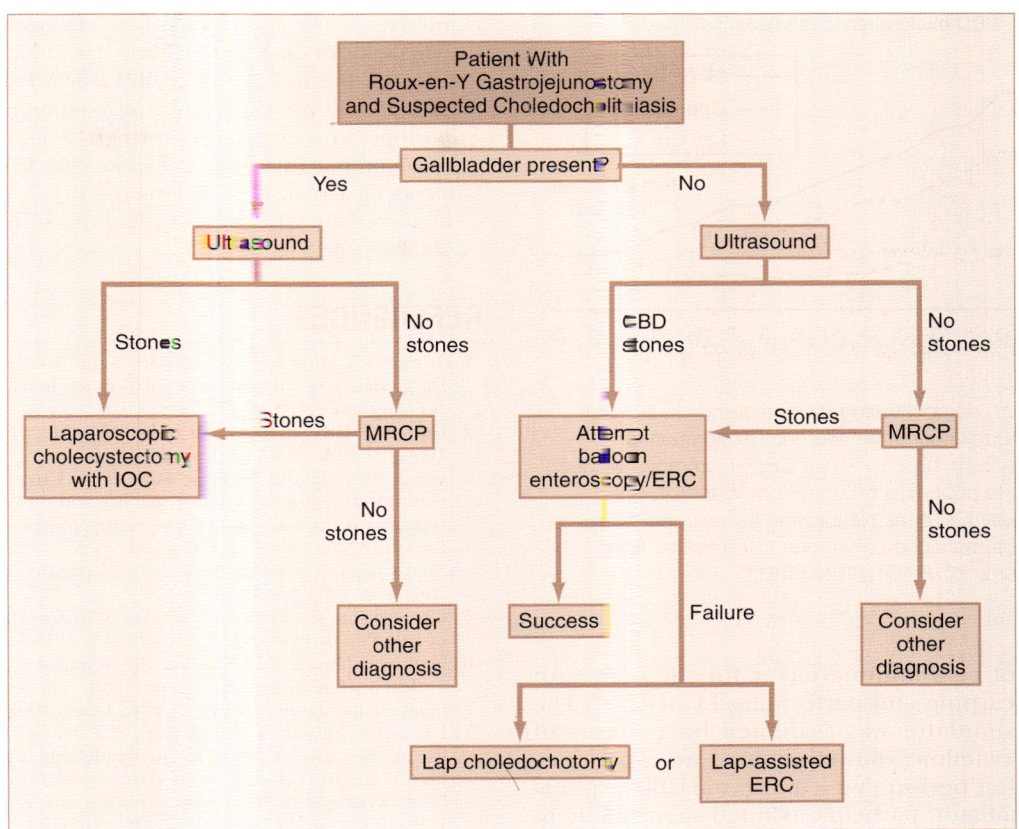

FIGURE 109.4 Treatment algorithm for patients with suspected choledocholithiasis and Roux-en-Y gastrojejunostomy. *CBD,* Common bile duct; *ERC,* endoscopic retrograde cholangiography; *IOC,* intraoperative cholangiography; *MRCP,* magnetic resonance cholangiopancreatography.

closed transversely, and the choledochotomy is managed as described earlier.

CHOLEDOCHOENTEROSTOMIES

The most common choledochoenterostomy is the side-to-side choledochoduodenostomy, usually in the setting of a dilated CBD with multiple stones. A generous Kocher maneuver is performed, and the distal CBD is exposed. A 2- to 3-cm longitudinal choledochotomy is made close to the lateral border of the duodenum along with a similar-sized longitudinal duodenotomy at the corresponding location. A "diamond-shaped" anastomosis is made with interrupted absorbable sutures. One potential postoperative complication from this is the "sump syndrome" caused by food or other debris becoming lodged and impacted in the distal CBD. This complication is rare (approximately 1%) and can be managed with ERC/ES.[62,63] Other authors have suggested end-to-side choledochoduodenostomy and choledochojejunostomy as alternatives,[64] although endoscopic biliary access following these operations is technically challenging.

FUTURE OF SURGICAL COMMON BILE DUCT EXPLORATION

Surgical management of CBD stones has been proven in numerous studies to be an efficacious, safe, and cost-effective strategy for managing patients with choledocholithiasis. Despite this, the utilization rate of ERC for patients with CBD stones far surpasses that of the surgical options, including both LCBDE and OCBDE. In a national analysis looking at selected in-hospital management strategies for patients admitted with CBD stones, Poulose et al. found that ERC was selected 93% of the time compared with 7% of cases managed by surgical exploration. The same study demonstrated that hospital length of stay (LOS) and total hospital costs were reduced for patients who underwent CBDE compared with those who underwent endoscopic management.[65] Wandling et al. demonstrated that there has been an ongoing decline in the nationwide use of surgical CBDE for patients admitted with CBD stones, down from 40% in 1998 to 8.5% in 2013, while the rate of ERC increased from 53% to over 85% over the same time period (Fig. 109.5). The same study again demonstrated a decreased LOS for patients who underwent a surgical approach for managing their CBD stones.[66]

One of the commonly cited reasons for the decline in use of CBDE is surgeon unfamiliarity with the technical aspects of the procedure. In an effort to increase use of LCBDE, a simulator was developed, evaluated, and incorporated into a standardized LCBDE curriculum for general surgery residents. All participants attained the mastery standard after a short period of targeted practice. These results suggest that perceived lack of technical

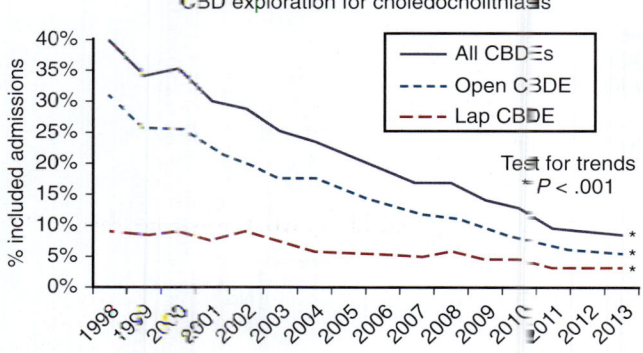

FIGURE 109.5 Graph demonstrating national trends in surgical (open and laparoscopic) common bile duct exploration for choledocholithiasis from 1998 to 2013. *CBD,* Common bile duct; *CBDE,* common bile duct exploration. (From Wandling MW, Hungness ES, Pavey ES, et al. Nationwide assessment of trends in choledocolithiasis management in the United States from 1998 to 2013. *JAMA Surg.* 2016;151:1125-1130.)

skills should not be a limiting factor for surgeons with an interest in learning and performing LCBDE.[67,68] The same LCBDE simulator was evaluated by a cohort of pediatric surgery fellows with minimal to no experience with LCBDE. After performing a transcystic CBD exploration on the simulator, participants rated their ability to perform the individual tasks of LCBDE highly. Again, this result suggests that even novice surgeons are comfortable with the necessary techniques needed to safely perform an LCBDE when given the opportunity to practice on a targeted simulator.[69] The use of such simulation-based curricula is one potential way to stem the decline in the use of CBDE. Available data suggest strongly that a single-stage strategy for treatment of patients with CBD stones is more cost effective and less morbid than relying on an ERC-based strategy.

CONCLUSION

Many treatment alternatives exist for patients who present with choledocholithiasis. The authors feel that the single-stage approach to managing choledocolithiasis should be the primary approach for patients who are deemed to be good operative candidates, with the understanding that ERC still plays a valuable role in the overall management of these patients. The algorithm proposed is only a guideline, and ultimate treatment will depend on physician experience and available resources.

SUGGESTED READINGS

Collins C, Maguire D, Ireland A, Fitzgerald E, O Sullivan GC. A prospective study of common bile duct calculi in patients undergoing laparoscopic cholecystectomy: natural history of choledocholithiasis. *Ann Surg.* 2004;239:28.

Cuschieri A, Lezoche E, Morino M, et al. E.A.E.S. multicenter prospective randomized trial comparing two-stage versus single-stage management of patients with gallstone disease and ductal calculi. *Surg Endosc.* 1999;13:952.

Hunter JG, Soper NJ. Laparoscopic management of common bile duct stones. *Surg Clin North Am.* 1992;72:1077.

Rhodes M, Sussman L, Cohen L, Lewis MP. Randomised trial of laparoscopic exploration of common bile duct versus postoperative endoscopic retrograde cholangiography for common bile duct stones. *Lancet.* 1998;351:159.

Williams EJ, Green J, Beckingham I, et al. Guidelines on the management of common bile duct stones (CBDS). *Gut.* 2008;57:1004.

REFERENCES

1. Tranter SE, Thompson MH. Spontaneous passage of bile duct stones: frequency of occurrence and relation to clinical presentation. *Ann R Coll Surg Engl.* 2003;85:174.
2. Cronan JJ. US diagnosis of choledocholithiasis: a reappraisal. *Radiology.* 1986;161:133.
3. Gross BH, Harter LP, Gore RM, et al. Ultrasonic evaluation of common bile duct stones: prospective comparison with endoscopic retrograde cholangiopancreatography. *Radiology.* 1983;146:471.
4. Barkun AN, Barkun JS, Fried GM, et al. Useful predictors of bile duct stones in patients undergoing laparoscopic cholecystectomy. *Ann Surg.* 1994;220:32.
5. Christensen M, Matzen P, Schulze S, Rosenberg J. Complications of ERCP: a prospective study. *Gastrointest Endosc.* 2004;60:721.
6. Nataly Y, Merrie AE, Stewart ID. Selective use of preoperative endoscopic retrograde cholangiopancreatography in the era of laparoscopic cholecystectomy. *ANZ J Surg.* 2002;72:186.
7. Lakatos L, Mester G, Reti G, Nagy A, Lakatos PL. Selection criteria for preoperative endoscopic retrograde cholangiopancreatography before laparoscopic cholecystectomy and endoscopic treatment of bile duct stones: results of a retrospective, single-center study between 1996-2002. *World J Gastroenterol.* 2004;10:3495.
8. Buscarini E, Tansini P, Vallisa D, Zambelli A, Buscarini L. EUS for suspected choledocholithiasis: do benefits outweigh costs? A prospective, controlled study. *Gastrointest Endosc.* 2003;57:510.
9. Williams EJ, Green J, Beckingham I, et al. Guidelines on the management of common bile duct stones (CBDS). *Gut.* 2008;57:1004.
10. The Standards of Practice Committee. The role of endoscopy in the evaluation of suspected choledocholithiasis. *Gastrointest Endosc.* 2010;71:1.
11. Kejriwal R, Liang J, Anderson G, Hill A. Magnetic resonance imaging of the common bile duct to exclude choledocholithiasis. *ANZ J Surg.* 2004;74:619.
12. Vazquez-Iglesias JL, Gonzalez-Conde B, Lopez-Roses L, et al. Endoscopic sphincterotomy for prevention of the recurrence of acute biliary pancreatitis in patients with gallbladder in situ. *Surg Endosc.* 2004;18:1442.
13. Schreurs WH, Vles WJ, Stuifbergen WH, Oostvogel HJ. Endoscopic management of common bile duct stones leaving the gallbladder in situ: a cohort study with long-term follow-up. *Dig Surg.* 2004;21:60.
14. Lai EC, Mok FP, Tan ES, et al. Endoscopic biliary drainage for severe acute cholangitis. *N Engl J Med.* 1992;326:1582.
15. Neoptolemos JP, Carr-Locke DL, London NJ, Bailey IA, James D, Fossard DP. Controlled trial of urgent ERCP versus conservative treatment for acute pancreatitis due to gallstones. *Lancet.* 1988; 2:979.
16. Fan S, Lai EC, Mok FP, Lo CM, Zheng SS, Wong J. Early treatment of acute biliary pancreatitis by endoscopic papillotomy. *N Engl J Med.* 1993;328:228.
17. Reinders JK, Goud A, Timmer R, et al. Early laparoscopic cholecystectomy improves outcomes after endoscopic sphincterotomy for choledochocystolithiasis. *Gastroenterology.* 2010;138:2315.
18. Cuschieri A, Lezoche E, Morino M, et al. E.A.E.S. multicenter prospective randomized trial comparing two-stage versus single-stage management of patients with gallstone disease and ductal calculi. *Surg Endosc.* 1999;13:952.
19. Rogers S, Cello JP, Horn JK, et al. Prospective randomized trial of LC + LCBDE vs ERCP/S + LC for common bile duct stone disease. *Arch Surg.* 2010;145:28.
20. Dasari BV, Tan CJ, Gurusamy KS, et al. Surgical versus endoscopic treatment of bile duct stones. *Cochrane Database Syst Rev.* 2013;(9):CD003327.

21. Topol B, Vromman K, Aerts R, Vertruyen C, Van Steenbergen W, Penninckx F. Hospital cost categories of one-stage versus two-stage management of common bile duct stones. *Surg Endosc.* 2010; 24:413.

22. Tai CK, Tang CN, Ha JP, Chau CH, Siu WT, Li MK. Laparoscopic exploration of common bile duct in difficult choledocholithiasis. *Surg Endosc.* 2004;18:910.

23. Disario JA, Freeman ML, Bjorkman DJ, et al. Endoscopic balloon dilation compared with sphincterotomy for extraction of bile duct stones. *Gastroenterology.* 2004;127:1291.

24. Baron TH, Harewood GC. Endoscopic balloon dilation of the biliary sphincter compared to endoscopic biliary sphincterotomy for removal of common duct stones during ERCP: a meta-analysis of randomized, controlled trials. *Am J Gastroenterol.* 2004;99:1455.

25. Horwood J, Akbar F, Davis K, Morgan R. Prospective evaluation of a selective approach to cholangiography for suspected common bile duct stones. *Ann R Coll Surg Engl.* 2010;92:206.

26. Tranter SE, Thompson MH. A prospective single-blinded controlled study comparing laparoscopic ultrasound of the common bile duct with operative cholangiogram. *Surg Endosc.* 2003;17:216.

27. Stiegmann GV, McIntyre RC, Pearlman NW. Laparoscopic intracorporeal ultrasound: an alternative to cholangiography? *Surg Endosc.* 1994;8:167.

28. Halpin VJ, Dunnegan D, Soper NJ. Laparoscopic intracorporeal ultrasound versus intraoperative cholangiography: after the learning curve. *Surg Endosc.* 2002;16:336.

29. Jamal KN, Smith H, Ratnasingham K, et al. Meta-analysis of the diagnostic accuracy of laparoscopic ultrasonography and intraoperative cholangiography in detection of common bile duct stones. *Ann R Coll Surg Engl.* 2016;98:244.

30. Aziz O, Ashrafian H, Jones C, et al. Ultrasonography versus intraoperative cholangiogram for the detection of common bile duct stones during laparoscopic cholecystectomy: a meta-analysis of diagnostic accuracy. *Int J Surg.* 2014;12:712.

31. Hunter JG, Soper NJ. Laparoscopic management of common bile duct stones. *Surg Clin North Am.* 1992;72:1077.

32. Jones DB, Soper NJ. The current management of common bile duct stones. *Adv Surg.* 1996;29:271.

33. Rojas-Ortega S, Arizpe-Bravo D, Marin Lopez ER, Cesin-Sánchez R, Roman GR, Gómez C. Transcystic common bile duct exploration in the management of patients with choledocholithiasis. *J Gastrointest Surg.* 2003;7:492.

34. Thompson MH, Tranter SE. All-comers policy for laparoscopic exploration of the common bile duct. *Br J Surg.* 2002;89:1608.

35. Strömberg C, Nilsson M, Leijonmarck CE. Stone clearance and risk factors for failure in laparoscopic transcystic exploration of the common bile duct. *Surg Endosc.* 2008;22:1194.

36. Carroll BJ, Phillips EH, Chandra M, Fallas M. Laparoscopic transcystic duct balloon dilatation of the sphincter of Oddi. *Surg Endosc.* 1993;7:514.

37. DePaula AL, Hashiba K, Bafutto M, Zago R, Machado M. Laparoscopic antegrade sphincterotomy. *Semin Laparosc Surg.* 1997;4:42.

38. Dion YM, Ratelle R, Morin J, Grave D. Common bile duct exploration: the place of laparoscopic choledochotomy. *Surg Laparosc Endosc.* 1994;4:419.

39. Phillips EH. Laparoscopic transcystic duct common bile duct exploration. *Surg Endosc.* 1998;12:365.

40. Isla AM, Griniatsos J, Karvounis E, Arbuckle JD. Advantages of laparoscopic stented choledochorrhaphy over T-tube placement. *Br J Surg.* 2004;91:862.

41. Hotta T, Taniguchi K, Kobayashi Y, et al. Biliary drainage tube evaluation after common bile duct exploration for choledocholithiasis. *Hepatogastroenterology.* 2003;50:315.

42. Petelin JB. Laparoscopic common bile duct exploration. *Surg Endosc.* 2003;17:1705.

43. Zhu QD, Tao CL, Zhou MT, Yu ZP, Shi HQ, Zhang QY. Primary closure versus T-tube drainage after common bile duct exploration for choledocholithiasis. *Langenbecks Arch Surg.* 2011;396:53.

44. El-Geidie AA. Is the use of T-tube necessary after laparoscopic choledochotomy? *J Gastrointest Surg.* 2010;14:844.

45. Gurusamy KS, Koti R, Davidson BR. T-tube drainage versus primary closure after laparoscopic common bile duct exploration. *Cochrane Database Syst Rev.* 2013;(6):CD005641.

46. Burhenne HJ. Garland lecture. Percutaneous extraction of retained biliary tract stones: 661 patients. *AJR Am J Roentgenol.* 1980;134:889.

47. Waage A, Strömberg C, Leijonmarck CE, Arvidsson D. Long-term results from laparoscopic common bile duct exploration. *Surg Endosc.* 2003;17:1185.

48. Riciardi R, Islam S, Canete JJ, Arcand PL, Stoker ME. Effectiveness and long-term results of laparoscopic common bile duct exploration. *Surg Endosc.* 2003;17:19.

49. Yi HJ, Hong G, Min SK, Lee HK. Long-term outcome of primary closure after laparoscopic common bile duct exploration combined with choledochoscopy. *Surg Laparosc Endosc Percutan Tech.* 2015;25:250.

50. Zhang HW, Chen YJ, Wu CH, Li WD. Laparoscopic common bile duct exploration with primary closure for management of choledocholithiasis: a retrospective analysis and comparison with conventional T-tube drainage. *Am Surg.* 2014;80:178.

51. Enochsson L, Lindberg B, Swahn F, Arnelo U. Intraoperative endoscopic retrograde cholangiopancreatography (ERCP) to remove common bile duct stones during routine laparoscopic cholecystectomy does not prolong hospitalization: a two-year experience. *Surg Endosc.* 2004;18:367.

52. Wei Q, Wang JG, Li LB, Li JD. Management of choledocholithiasis: comparison between laparoscopic common bile duct exploration and intraoperative endoscopic sphincterotomy. *World J Gastroenterol.* 2003;9:2856.

53. Collins C, Maguire D, Ireland A, et al. A prospective study of common bile duct calculi in patients undergoing laparoscopic cholecystectomy: natural history of choledocholithiasis. *Ann Surg.* 2004;239:28.

54. Anwer S, Rahim R, Agwunobi A, Bancewicz J. The role of ERCP in management of retained bile duct stones after laparoscopic cholecystectomy. *N Z Med J.* 2004;117:U1102.

55. Rhodes M, Sussman L, Cohen L, Lewis MP. Randomised trial of laparoscopic exploration of common bile duct versus postoperative endoscopic retrograde cholangiography for common bile duct stones. *Lancet.* 1998;351:159.

56. Tranter SE, Thompson MH. Comparison of endoscopic sphincterotomy and laparoscopic exploration of the common bile duct. *Br J Surg.* 2002;89:1495.

57. Deslandres E, Gagner M, Pomp A. Intraoperative endoscopic sphincterotomy for common bile duct stones during laparoscopic cholecystectomy. *Gastrointest Endosc.* 1993;39:54.

58. Khabbuli B, Velanovich V. Management of preoperatively suspected choledocholithiasis: a decision analysis. *J Gastrointest Surg.* 2008;12:1973.

59. Saleem A, Baron TH, Gostout CJ, et al. Endoscopic retrograde cholangiopancreatography using a single-balloon enteroscope in patients with altered Roux-en-Y anatomy. *Endoscopy.* 2010;42:656.

60. Lopes TL, Clements RH, Wilcox CM. Laparoscopic-assisted ERCP: experience of a high-volume bariatric surgery center (with video). *Gastrointest Endosc.* 2009;70:1254.

61. Baker AR, Neoptolemos JP, Leese T, James DC, Fossard DP. Long-term follow-up of patients with side-to-side choledochoduodenostomy and transduodenal sphincteroplasty. *Ann R Coll Surg Engl.* 1987;68:253.

62. Escudero-Fabre A, Escallon A Jr, Sack J, Halpern NB, Aldrete JS. Choledochoduodenostomy: analysis of 71 cases followed for 5 to 15 years. *Ann Surg.* 1991;213:635.

63. Cardi-Josc FX, Demarquay JF, Peten EP, et al. Endoscopic management of sump syndrome after choledochoduodenostomy: retrospective analysis of 30 cases. *Gastrointest Endosc.* 2000;51:180.

64. Cuschieri A. Common bile duct exploration. In: Zinner MJ, Schwartz SI, Ellis H, eds. *Maingot's Abdominal Operations.* Norwalk, CT: Appleton & Lange; 1997:1875.

65. Poulose BK, Arbogast PG, Holzman MD. National analysis of in-hospital resource utilization in choledocholithiasis management using propensity scores. *Surg Endosc.* 2006;20:186.

66. Wandling MW, Hungness ES, Pavey ES, et al. Nationwide assessment of trends in choledocholithiasis management in the United States from 1998 to 2013. *JAMA Surg.* 2016;151:1125-1130.

67. Santos BF, Reif TJ, Soper NJ, Nagle AP, Rooney DM, Hungness ES. Development and evaluation of a laparoscopic common bile duct exploration simulator and procedural rating scale. *Surg Endosc.* 2012;26:2403.

68. Teitelbaum EN, Soper NJ, Santos BF, et al. A simulator-based resident curriculum for laparoscopic common bile duct exploration. *Surgery.* 2014;156:880.

69. Schwab B, Rooney DM, Hungness ES, Barsness KA. Preliminary evaluation of a laparoscopic common bile duct simulator for pediatric surgical education. *J Laparoendosc Adv Surg Tech A.* 2016;26:831-835.

Biliary Dyskinesia and Sphincter of Oddi Dysfunction

Katherine A. Morgan | David B. Adams

Biliary dyskinesia and sphincter of Oddi dysfunction (SOD) are functional disorders of the pancreas and biliary tract that challenge the practicing surgeon. Both disease entities are characterized by pancreatobiliary pain syndromes and are fraught with controversy over their definition, diagnosis, and management. In addition, both disorders have been the subject of recent important study, potentially affecting management.

BILIARY DYSKINESIA

Acalculous gallbladder disease has been recognized by surgeons for almost a century. In 1924 Alfred Blalock described a series of greater than 100 patients who underwent cholecystectomy in the absence of gallstones with excellent results in pain relief (83% were improved).[1] In 1926 Allen Oldfather Whipple reported on 36 of 47 patients (76%) who were improved with cholecystectomy for acalculous biliary disease.[2]

Biliary dyskinesia is a disease process characterized by right upper quadrant biliary-type pain in the absence of gallstones.[3] Biliary dyskinesia is also referred to as *chronic acalculous cholecystitis, acalculous biliary pain, and functional gallbladder disorder*. Biliary dyskinesia is presumed to represent pain secondary to the abnormal motile function of the gallbladder. The frequency of acalculous biliary pain may be as high as 8% in men and 21% in women.

PHYSIOLOGY

The purpose of the gallbladder is to store and concentrate bile after production by the liver. Gallbladder emptying is achieved by contraction of the smooth muscle of the gallbladder wall, which occurs in coordination with sphincter of Oddi relaxation. In the fasting state the gallbladder empties partially cyclically in conjunction with the migrating motor complex. In response to meal intake, contraction of the gallbladder occurs because of neural reflex stimuli, as well as enterohormonal cues from the foregut, most notably cholecystokinin (CCK).

The pathophysiology of biliary dyskinesia is incompletely understood. In some cases the cystic duct is implicated as problematic, with narrowing, possibly because of inflammation or fibrosis, and a resultant obstruction to gallbladder emptying. In other cases an intrinsic functional motility disorder of the smooth muscle of the gallbladder wall or the cystic duct seems to be causative. Biliary dyskinesia has been associated with other gastrointestinal motility disorders, including irritable bowel syndrome, colonic inertia, and gastroparesis. Alterations in bile composition, as well as inflammatory mediators (prostaglandin E_2), have also been implicated in biliary dyskinesia. Interestingly,

up to 43% of gallbladders on final pathology after cholecystectomy for presumed biliary dyskinesia show no histologic abnormalities.

Likely, biliary dyskinesia encompasses a diverse group of patients with variable factors contributing to poor gallbladder emptying.

CLINICAL PRESENTATION

Patients with biliary dyskinesia present with typical pancreatobiliary-type pain, as outlined by the Rome IV diagnostic criteria, in the absence of gallstones (Box 110.1).[4] The pain is located in the right upper quadrant or epigastrium, is colicky in nature, occurs postprandially, and is typically associated with nausea or bloating. The patient may have associated emesis or diarrhea. In addition, the patient may report anorexia and weight loss.

DIAGNOSIS

The essential component of the diagnostic evaluation of the patient with suspected biliary dyskinesia is a typical pain history. The physical examination may be remarkable for abdominal tenderness, particularly in the right upper quadrant, but often the abdominal examination is entirely benign. Liver biochemistries and pancreatic enzymes are within normal limits. A transabdominal ultrasound of the right upper quadrant should exclude the presence of gallstones (sensitivity >95%).

The differential diagnosis of upper abdominal pain in patients with an intact gallbladder but without gallstones is broad, including peptic ulcer disease, SOD, microlithiasis, chronic pancreatitis, and generalized functional gut motility disorders. In addition, there is often overlap with these disorders making diagnosis and management decisions challenging. In fact, some authors have reported residual or recurrent abdominal pain in patients treated with cholecystectomy for symptomatic cholelithiasis. Accordingly, these alternative or additional diagnoses should be sought with appropriate diagnostic studies where indicated by the clinical picture, including upper endoscopy.

CCK-stimulated hepatoiminodiacetic acid (CCK-HIDA) nuclear scintigraphy is considered the cornerstone diagnostic test for biliary dyskinesia, despite controversy over testing methodology and variable evidence correlating abnormal studies to treatment outcomes. CCK-HIDA is used to quantify gallbladder ejection fraction (EF) as a marker for abnormal motility. Most physicians define an abnormal gallbladder EF as less than 35% to 40%, based on the original descriptive study by Krishnamurthy et al. in 1982. This group evaluated seven subjects with a fast (1 to 3 minutes) technique of CCK injection and defined an abnormal study as two standard deviations below the mean

---

BOX 110.1 Rome IV Diagnostic Criteria for Functional Gallbladder and Sphincter of Oddi Disorders

BILIARY PAIN

Pain located in the epigastrium and/or right upper quadrant and all of the following:

1. Builds up to steady level and lasting 30 minutes or longer
2. Occurring at different intervals (not daily)
3. Severe enough to interrupt daily activities or lead to an emergency room visit
4. Not significantly (<20%) related to bowel movements
5. Not significantly (<20%) relieved by postural change or acid suppression

Supportive Criteria

The pain may be associated with:

1. Nausea and vomiting
2. Radiation to the back and/or right infrascapular region
3. Waking from sleep

FUNCTIONAL GALLBLADDER DISORDER

1. Biliary pain
2. Absence of gallstones or other structural pathology

Supportive Criteria

1. Low ejection fraction on gallbladder scintigraphy
2. Normal liver enzymes, conjugated bilirubin, amylase/lipase

FUNCTIONAL BILIARY SPHINCTER DISORDER

1. Biliary pain
2. Elevated liver enzymes or dilated bile duct, but not both
3. Absence of bile duct stones or other structural abnormalities

Supportive Criteria

1. Normal amylase/lipase
2. Abnormal sphincter of Oddi manometry
3. Hepatobiliary scintigraphy

PANCREATIC SPHINCTER OF ODDI DISORDER

1. Documented recurrent episodes of pancreatitis (typical pain with amylase or lipase >3 times normal and/or imaging evidence of acute pancreatitis)
2. Other etiologies of pancreatitis excluded
3. Negative endoscopic ultrasound
4. Abnormal sphincter manometry

From Cotton PB, Elta GH, Carter CR, Pasricha PJ, Corazziari ES. Gallbladder and sphincter of Oddi disorders. *Gastroenterology* 2016;150:1420–1429.

---

of normal subjects.[5] The current technique advocated by the Society of Nuclear Medicine entails a slow infusion (over 60 minutes) of a weight-based (0.02 µg/kg) dose of CCK, with abnormal EF defined as 38%.[6] In addition, some have advocated that reproduction of pain symptoms with infusion of CCK is confirmatory of disease presence, although evidence supporting this assertion is lacking and the effects of CCK on small bowel and gastric motility in addition to the biliary tree are certainly confounding.

Study is being undertaken of alternative methods of diagnosis using functional magnetic resonance cholangiopancreatography and dynamic computed tomography (CT) scanning, with results that appear comparable to cholescintigraphy.

TREATMENT

Cholecystectomy is the primary treatment undertaken for biliary dyskinesia. With the introduction of laparoscopic technology in the late 1980s, the number of patients undergoing cholecystectomy for this indication has at least tripled. Biliary dyskinesia is now reported to feature 10% to 20% of cases in adults and up to 50% in children in the United States.[7,8] Interestingly, cholecystectomy for this indication is much less commonly reported in other developed countries.

Outcomes after cholecystectomy for biliary dyskinesia have not been well defined.[8–10] In the hallmark prospective study, Yap et al. in 1991 evaluated 40 patients with biliary-type pain with CCK-HIDA. Twenty-one patients with a CCK-HIDA–determined EF less than 40% were randomized to cholecystectomy (11 patients) or observation (10 patients). Of 11 undergoing surgery, 10 experienced complete symptom resolution and one improvement. Of the 10 in the observation group, all remained symptomatic, and two subsequently underwent surgery and experienced pain relief. Of the patients with pain but a normal CCK-HIDA, treatment was undertaken at the discretion of the surgeon, and those undergoing surgery fared no better than those who did not. The authors concluded from this small study that cholecystectomy is effective in the management of biliary dyskinesia as directed by an abnormal CCK-HIDA scan, and this conclusion has driven common practice for the management of biliary dyskinesia.[11] More recently, in 2016 Richmond and colleagues randomized 30 patients with abnormal CCK-HIDA (<38%) to cholecystectomy or medical management (low-dose tricyclic antidepressant). They measured preoperative and postoperative quality of life (Short Form-8) scores as their primary end point. Fourteen of the 15 patients randomized to medical management opted to cross over to surgery at a median of 3.5 days. Of 26 patients who underwent surgery, all reported pain relief and significant improvement in physical and mental health quality-of-life scores.[2] Although this study is limited in size and allowed immediate crossover essentially eliminating the control group, it lends credence to cholecystectomy as a valid treatment for biliary dyskinesia. Larger studies, including ideally a randomized controlled trial, are clearly needed.[10]

SPHINCTER OF ODDI DYSFUNCTION

Francis Glisson described circular muscle fibers surrounding the distal common bile duct in 1654. As a young medical student in 1887, Ruggero Oddi elucidated the sphincter of the hepatopancreatic ampulla. He went on to become an acclaimed academician in Genoa, but his career was thwarted by a series of professional and financial indiscretions; he was therefore obligated to practice clinical medicine to make a living. Perhaps fittingly, since its description by this controversial man, the sphincter of Oddi, along with its associated disorders, has been viewed with skepticism. Patients with SOD are often challenging in their factious presentation, difficult diagnosis, and laborious management.

SOD classically is believed to represent a benign, noncalculous obstruction to the flow of biliary or pancreatic secretions through the pancreaticobiliary junction. SOD is known by many names, including ampullary stenosis, papillary stenosis, papillitis, and postcholecystectomy syndrome. It is a disorder of the contractile function of the ampullary sphincter. It is a heterogeneous disorder, consisting of a fixed obstruction because of a stenotic ampulla in some patients and a functional obstruction due to abnormal motility in others. Alternative theories of pathophysiology not related to obstruction have recently emerged. Interruption of the cholecystosphincteric reflex with cholecystectomy may affect sphincter behavior. Alternatively, inflammation during cholecystitis may be an inciting painful stimulus which leads to nociceptive sensitization and ultimately allodynia during physiologic bile duct or duodenal distention.

SOD is an uncommon disorder, affecting most often middle-aged women. Approximately 10% of patients develop pain post cholecystectomy, and 10% of those will have SOD. Depending on the group studied, 15% to 76% of cases of idiopathic recurrent pancreatitis are attributed to SOD.

ANATOMY AND PHYSIOLOGY

The sphincter of Oddi is located at the terminal portions of the common bile duct and main pancreatic duct as they enter into the second portion of the duodenum. The sphincter consists of a common muscular complex, also known as the ampullary zone, as well as an intrapancreatic and an intrabiliary sphincteric mechanism.

The sphincter of Oddi exhibits a baseline zone of elevated pressure, with superimposed phasic contractions. It demonstrates a cyclical change in motor activity that is closely associated with the migrating motor complex. There is some neural influence on the sphincter through the parasympathetic and sympathetic systems. However, hormonal factors seem to play a significant role in the motility pattern. CCK is a potent inhibitor of the ampullary sphincter. Secretin acts to inhibit the pancreatic portion of the sphincter of Oddi.

SOD is marked by aberrations in the function of the sphincteric mechanism. It is most commonly defined by elevated intraductal pressures on manometric evaluation.

CLINICAL PRESENTATION

Patients with SOD are marked clinically by classic pancreatobiliary-type pain, similar to the pain of biliary dyskinesia. This pain, as defined by the Rome IV criteria (see Box 110.1),[2] is episodic upper abdominal pain, typically postprandial in nature and associated with nausea. The physical examination is generally unremarkable. Patients

may have transient elevation of their liver or pancreatic serum biochemical markers, or they may present with recurrent idiopathic pancreatitis.

Of important historical note, Hogan and Geenen in Milwaukee developed a classification system for patients presenting with presumed SOD (Table 110.1).[13] This system was valuable in that it served to predict diagnosis as well as management options and outcomes (Table 110.2).[14] Type I patients had typical pancreatobiliary pain, elevated liver or pancreatic biochemistries, and a dilated biliary or pancreatic duct. Type II patients had typical pain, along with one other objective finding, and type III patients had pain alone. This classification system has been mostly abandoned in the modern era, given more recent clinical outcomes studies. Patients previously designated as type I often have organic stenosis and are treated with sphincterotomy. Type III patients (with pain only and no objective findings) have been shown in the recent EPISOD (Evaluating Predictors and Interventions in Sphincter of Oddi Dysfunction) trial to not respond to sphincterotomy any better than sham treatment and are no longer considered for intervention.[15] Prior type II patients (pain and one objective finding) are considered for further evaluation and for sphincterotomy.

DIAGNOSIS

The most important component of the diagnostic evaluation for SOD is a consistent history of pancreatobiliary-type pain. Other more common etiologies of abdominal pain

TABLE 110.1 Milwaukee Classification System

Type	Criteria
I	Pancreatobiliary pain **and** Elevated liver or pancreatic biochemistries* **and** Dilated bile or pancreatic duct† **and** Delayed drainage of contrast on ERCP]‡
II	Pancreatobiliary pain **and** Elevated liver or pancreatic biochemistries* **or** Dilated bile or pancreatic duct† **or** Delayed drainage of contrast on ERCP]‡
III	Pancreatobiliary pain **only**

*Aspartate aminotransferase, alkaline phosphatase or amylase, lipase greater than twice normal on two occasions.
†Common bile duct greater than 12 mm or pancreatic duct greater than 5 mm.
‡Not generally included in the modern criteria.
ERCP, Endoscopic retrograde cholangiopancreatography.
From Hogan WJ, Geenen JE. Biliary dyskinesia. *Endoscopy.* 1988;20:179.

TABLE 110.2 Milwaukee Classification System and Response to Therapy

SOD Type	Probability of Abnormal Manometry	Response to Treatment if Manometry Abnormal	Response to Treatment if Manometry Normal	Manometry Recommended?
I	75–95%	90–95%	90–95%	No
II	55–65%	85%	35%	Yes
III	25–60%	55–65%	<10%	Yes

SOD, Sphincter of Oddi dysfunction.
Modified from Sherman S, Lehman G. Sphincter of Oddi dysfunction: diagnosis and treatment. *JOP.* 2001;2:382.

should be excluded with appropriate tests, including CT, esophagogastroduodenoscopy, and colonoscopy.

Historically, many elaborate tests of the elusive sphincter of Oddi have been described. In the Nardi test (morphine-prostigmine provocation test), the patient is administered morphine and neostigmine, and then evaluated for pain or elevated liver or pancreatic serum biochemistries. Biliary scintigraphy can evaluate for delayed hepatic hilum to duodenum transit time of the nuclear medicine tracer, correlating with ampullary obstruction. Ultrasound stimulation tests (transabdominal, endoscopic) have been used to evaluate the biliary or pancreatic duct diameter after administration of CCK or secretin, respectively. Sustained ductal enlargement from baseline suggests a relative obstruction caused by SOD. Similarly, secretin-stimulated magnetic resonance cholangiopancreatography (ssMRCP) can show a persistent increase in the pancreatic duct diameter after secretin administration. In general, these tests are of variable accuracy because of operator inconsistencies.

The most standard test used for evaluation of SOD is endoscopic retrograde cholangiopancreatography (ERCP) with endoscopic sphincter of Oddi manometry (ESOM) (Fig. 110.1). ESOM allows for the direct measurement of ductal pressures to assess for sphincteric hypertension. A small-caliber (typically 5 French) multilumen perfusion

catheter with an aspiration port is used for pressure monitoring. Sustained ductal pressures greater than 35 to 40 mm Hg above baseline are indicative of SOD. Abnormal pressures can be localized to the pancreatic duct, the bile duct, or may be present in both. ERCP with ESOM does carry some risk for morbidity, with pancreatitis reported in 4% to 31% of patients. A small percentage of these will be clinically significant. Pancreatitis is minimized by use of an aspiration port and by limiting perfusion time and pressure. In cases with equivocal manometry or where manometry is not available, alternative endoscopic interventions have been used. Endoscopic transpapillary stenting has been undertaken but is generally avoided due to high risk of pancreatitis. Endoscopic intrasphincteric injection of botulinum toxin has been shown to be potentially predictive of response to endoscopic sphincterotomy (ES) therapy.

TREATMENT

The indications for intervention in patients with SOD are debilitating pain episodes or episodes of recurrent pancreatitis.

The medical approach to SOD has shown limited success, but because of the risks and uncertainties involved in invasive approaches, it is considered frontline management. Smooth muscle–relaxing agents such as nifedipine, phosphodiesterase inhibitors, trimebutine, hyoscine butylbromide, and nitric oxide have been used, although without data to show long-term improvement. Alternative strategies of pain management, including amitriptyline and duloxetine as well as electroacupuncture, biofeedback, and use of transcutaneous electrical nerve stimulation have also been described.

ENDOSCOPY

The current standard for management of types I and II SOD (typical pain with objective findings) is ES. Successful pain relief is achieved in 55% to 95% of patients after this intervention, depending on patient selection. Three randomized, controlled trials have demonstrated the efficacy of ES in properly selected patients (Table 110.3).[16-18] ES does carry a significant risk for postprocedure pancreatitis, 10% to 15%, even in expert hands and with the use of prophylactic endoscopic stenting and/or rectal nonsteroidal antiinflammatory drugs. Restenosis rates of 15% to 33% are reported after intervention.

A recent prospective trial (the EPISOD trial) randomized 214 patients with type III SOD (typical pain but no objective findings) to either ERCP with ES or ERCP with no intervention (sham). The authors found that sphincterotomy was not better than sham in decreasing disability due to pain in these patients.[15] Therefore ES is not routinely recommended in this challenging group of patients with pancreatobiliary pain but no supporting objective findings.

SURGERY

Historically, before the modern endoscopic era, operative transduodenal sphincteroplasty with pancreatic septoplasty was the treatment of choice for patients with SOD, with good outcomes reported. However, with the success of endoscopic therapies, the surgical approach to SOD

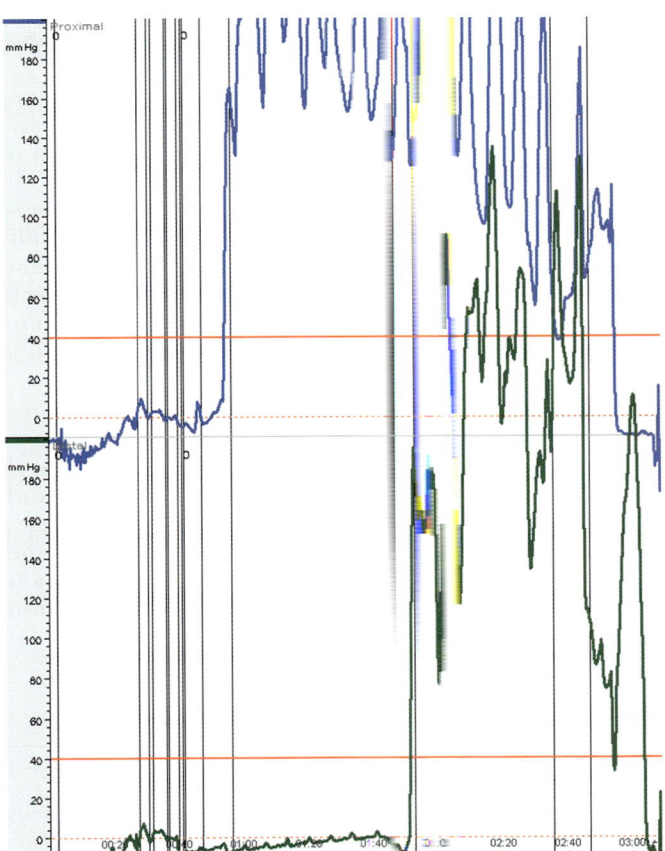

FIGURE 110.1 Endoscopic sphincter of Oddi manometry tracing shows abnormally high pressures (>40 mm Hg) measured in both the proximal and distal channels of the catheter.

TABLE 110.3 Randomized Controlled Trials of Endoscopic Sphincterotomy for Sphincter of Oddi Dysfunction

Study	N	Follow-Up (years)	Design	Response
Geenen et al.[16]	47	4	ES vs. Sham All SOM	+SOM ES, 90% +SOM Sham, 30% −SOM ES, 35% −SOM Sham, 35%
Sherman et al.[17]	23	3	ES vs. SSpx vs. ESham	ES, 83% SSpx, 80% ESham, 29%
Toouli et al.[18]	58	2	ES vs. Sham	+SOM ES, 85% +SOM Sham, 38% −SOM ES = Sham

ES, Endoscopic sphincterotomy; *Esham,* endoscopy without sphincterotomy; *Sham,* endoscopy without sphincterotomy; *SOM,* sphincter of Oddi manometry (+ abnormal; − normal); *SSpx,* surgical sphincteroplasty. From Geenen JE, Hogan WJ, Dodds WJ, Toouli J, Venu RP. The efficacy of endoscopic sphincterotomy after cholecystectomy in patients with sphincter-of-Oddi dysfunction. *N Engl J Med.* 1989;320:82; Sherman S, Lehman GA, Jamidar P, et al. Efficacy of endoscopic sphincterotomy and surgical sphincteroplasty for patients with sphincter of Oddi dysfunction: randomized, controlled study. *Gastrointest Endosc.* 1994;40:A125; and Toouli J, Roberts-Thomson IC, Kellow J, et al. Manometry based randomised trial of endoscopic sphincterotomy for sphincter of Oddi dysfunction. *Gut.* 2000;46:98.

is relevant to two groups of patients currently: those patients who have failed prior endoscopic intervention (generally because of restenosis) and those patients who have undergone previous gastric surgery, particularly gastric bypass with Roux-en-Y reconstruction, in which endoscopic access to the ampulla is difficult except with advanced techniques.[19,20]

Transduodenal sphincteroplasty is undertaken through a midline laparotomy. A generous Kocher maneuver is used to fully mobilize the duodenum and bring it up into the operative field. The duodenum and head of pancreas are assessed, noting signs of chronic pancreatitis, which may portend a poor prognosis for postoperative relief of symptoms. A fibrotic ampulla may be palpable through the duodenal wall and can help to guide the location of the duodenotomy. An oblique duodenotomy is made overlying the estimated location of the ampulla using electrocautery. The ampulla is sought within the duodenum, with care taken not to traumatize the duodenal mucosa. A lacrimal duct probe is used to cannulate the distal common bile duct. The needle-tipped cautery is used to make a generous sphincterotomy, dividing the duodenal mucosa and sphincter on top of the lacrimal duct probe. The sphincterotomy is continued until there is easy flow of bile into the operative field.

The pancreatic duct is then sought and cannulated with a separate lacrimal duct probe. The septum between the bile duct and pancreatic duct is divided using electrocautery. The septotomy is continued until there is good flow of pancreatic secretions. Interrupted fine absorbable monofilament suture (such as 5-0 polydioxanone) is used to approximate duodenal mucosa to bile duct mucosa and bile duct mucosa to pancreatic duct mucosa to complete

the biliary sphincteroplasty and pancreatic septoplasty. The duodenotomy is closed obliquely with a running 3-0 absorbable monofilament suture.

In the modern era, pain relief rates in excess of 60% can be expected on long-term follow-up after operative transduodenal sphincteroplasty with pancreatic septoplasty. Younger patients and patients with chronic pancreatitis have poorer outcomes.

POSTGASTRIC SURGERY PATIENTS

In patients who have undergone prior gastric surgery, and are therefore not easily amenable to ESOM, the diagnosis of SOD can be difficult. In these patients the most important component of the evaluation is a proper history. Laboratory evidence with abnormal biliary or pancreatic serum biochemistries, particularly during a pain exacerbation episode, is sought. Other more common diagnoses, such as ulcer disease, anastomotic stricture, internal hernia, or adhesions, are excluded with proper tests, including upper endoscopy and abdominal CT. ssMRCP can be used to evaluate for biliary or pancreatic ductal dilation at baseline or a persistently dilated pancreatic duct after secretin administration, both suggestive of SOD. ssMRCP seems to be specific but not very sensitive in the diagnosis of SOD. ssMRCP can help to exclude other pathology such as stones or neoplasm. Importantly, ssMRCP can also help to evaluate for chronic pancreatitis, as patients who have chronic pancreatitis tend to have a poor response to sphincteroplasty and may do better with an alternative procedure such as total pancreatectomy with islet autotransplantation.

These patients are well treated with operative transduodenal sphincteroplasty with pancreatic septoplasty. With proper patient selection, long-term pain relief is expected in 85% of patients.[20]

Alternatively, in the patient who is post–gastric bypass, the excluded stomach can be accessed by radiographic or operative means. This site can then be used to allow endoscopic access for ERCP, ESOM, and ES. This approach has been favored by some authors. However, it does require multiple procedures and carries morbidity.

SUMMARY

Biliary dyskinesia and SOD, the functional disorders of the biliary tract and pancreas, are vexing in diagnosis and management. They are becoming increasingly recognized, and more objective means of evaluation have become available over the past two decades. However, significant controversy still remains regarding their ideal evaluation and therapy.

REFERENCES

1. Blalock A. A statistical study of eight hundred and eighty-eight cases of biliary tract disease. *Johns Hopkins Hosp Bull.* 1926;35:391.
2. Whipple AO. Surgical criteria for cholecystectomy. *Am J Surg.* 1926;40:129.
3. Behar J, Corazziari E, Guelred M, Hogan W, Sherman S, Toouli J. Functional gallbladder and sphincter of Oddi disorders. *Gastroenterology.* 2006;130:1498-1509.
4. Cotton PB, Elta GH, Carter CR, Pasricha PJ, Corazziari ES. Gallbladder and sphincter of Oddi disorders. *Gastroenterology.* 2016;150:1420-1429.

5. Krishnamurthy GT, Bobba VR, Kingston E, Turner F. Measurement of gallbladder emptying sequentially using a single dose of 99mTc-labeled hepatobiliary agent. *Gastroenterology*. 1982;83:773.

6. Tulchinsky M, Ciak B, Debelke D, et al. SNM practice guidelines for hepatobiliary scintigraphy 4.0. *J Nuc Med Technol*. 2010;38:210-218.

7. Bielefeldt K, Saligram S, Zickmund SL, Dudekula A, Olyaee M, Yadav D. Cholecystectomy for biliary dyskinesia: how did we get there? *Dig Dis Sci*. 2014;59:2850-2865.

8. Adams DB. Biliary dyskinesia: does it exist? If so how do we diagnose it? Is laparoscopic cholecystectomy effective or a sham operation? *J Gastrointest Surg*. 2013;17(9):1550-1552.

9. Ponsky TA, Desagun R, Brody F. Surgical therapy for biliary dyskinesia: a metaanalysis and review of the literature. *J Laparoendosc Adv Surg Tech*. 2005;15:439-442.

10. Gurusamy KS, Junnarkar S, Farouk M, Davidson BR. Cholecystectomy for suspected gallbladder dyskinesia. *Cochrane Database Syst Rev*. 2009;(1):CD007086.

11. Yap L, Wycherly AG, Morphett AD, Toouli J. Acalculous biliary pain: cholecystectomy alleviates symptoms in patients with abnormal cholescintigraphy. *Gastroenterology*. 1991;101:786.

12. Richmond BK, Grodman C, Walker J, et al. Pilot randomized controlled trial of laparoscopic cholecystectomy vs active non-operative therapy for the treatment of biliary dyskinesia. *J Am Coll Surg*. 2016;222(6):1156-1163.

13. Hogan WJ, Geenen JE. Biliary dyskinesia. *Endoscopy*. 1988;20:179.

14. Sherman S, Lehman G. Sphincter of Oddi dysfunction: diagnosis and treatment. *JOP*. 2001;2:382.

15. Cotton PB, Durkalski V, Romagnuolo J, et al. A multicenter, randomized trial of endoscopic sphincterotomy for suspected sphincter of Oddi dysfunction in patients with pain after cholecystectomy—the EPISOD trial. *JAMA*. 2014;311:2101-2109.

16. Geenen JE, Hogan WJ, Dodds WJ, Toouli J, Venu RP. The efficacy of endoscopic sphincterotomy after cholecystectomy in patients with sphincter-of-Oddi dysfunction. *N Engl J Med*. 1989;320:82.

17. Sherman S, Lehman GA, Jamidar P, et al. Efficacy of endoscopic sphincterotomy and surgical sphincteroplasty for patients with sphincter of Oddi dysfunction: randomized, controlled study. *Gastrointest Endosc*. 1994;40:A125.

18. Toouli J, Roberts-Thomson IC, Kellow J, et al. Manometry based randomised trial of endoscopic sphincterotomy for sphincter of Oddi dysfunction. *Gut*. 2000;46:98.

19. Morgan KA, Romagnuolo J, Adams DB. Transduodenal sphincteroplasty in the management of sphincter of Oddi dysfunction and pancreas divisum in the modern era. *J Am Coll Surg*. 2008;206:908.

20. Morgan KA, Glenn JB, Byrne TK, Adams DB. Sphincter of Oddi dysfunction after Roux-en-Y gastric bypass. *Surg Obes Relat Dis*. 2009;5:571.

Endoscopic Evaluation and Management of Pancreaticobiliary Disease

Christopher G. Chapman | Nayna A. Lodhia |

Maricarmen Manzano | Irving Waxman

Since the first endoscopic visualization and cannulation of the major papilla with cholangiopancreatogram was completed in 1968, rapid advances in the field of endoscopy have increased the capabilities of physicians to detect, classify, and more recently, provide therapy to disease involving the pancreaticobiliary system. The development of side-viewing endoscopes and introduction of endoscopic sphincterotomy (ES) permitted less invasive diagnostic and therapeutic maneuvers in the pancreatic and bile ducts that were previously limited to open surgical and percutaneous techniques. In recent years, advances in cross-sectional radiologic imaging techniques, namely magnetic resonance cholangiopancreatography (MRCP), have transitioned the role of endoscopic retrograde cholangiopancreatography (ERCP) to a modality primarily for pancreatobiliary therapeutics. However, technologic advances, including intraductal ultrasound, direct cholangioscopy, and pancreatoscopy, have been built on the scaffold of ERCP and have anchored ERCP as a widely applied method of choice for many clinical problems involving the pancreatic duct and the hepatobiliary system.

Endoscopic ultrasound (EUS) burgeoned into the field of pancreaticobiliary disease beginning in the 1980s for the diagnosis and staging of pancreatic cancers and has rapidly progressed to allow minimally invasive tissue acquisition and an increasing breadth of interventional and therapeutic management strategies. New tools, accessories, and stents continue to develop providing access to various intraabdominal fluid collections or gastrointestinal tract and organs. In pancreaticobiliary cases where tissue acquisition may be limited, enhanced endoscopic-based imaging modalities such as confocal laser endomicroscopy, contrast-enhanced ultrasonography, and elastography may aid in diagnosis and, in certain cases, be accepted as surrogates for histologic diagnosis.

ENDOSCOPIC RETROGRADE CHOLANGIOPANCREATOGRAPHY

INDICATIONS

The role for diagnostic ERCP alone has diminished as other less invasive/noninvasive imaging techniques (e.g., EUS and MRCP) have become increasingly prevalent. ERCP is indicated in clinical settings in which there are significant suspicions of obstructing, inflammatory, or neoplastic pancreaticobiliary lesions that, if detected or ruled out, would alter clinical management. A list of appropriate indications for ERCP and ES is reported in Box 111.1. ERCP is generally not indicated for the evaluation of abdominal pain of unclear etiology in the absence of objective findings supporting hepatobiliary or pancreatic disease in other laboratory or imaging studies, in suspected gallbladder disease without evidence of bile duct disease, or for further evaluation of proven pancreatic malignancy if management will not change.[1,2]

BENIGN BILIARY TRACT DISEASE

CHOLEDOCHOLITHIASIS

Choledocholithiasis develops in 5% to 10% of patients with symptomatic cholelithiasis undergoing laparoscopic cholecystectomy.[3] The introduction of ES by Classen and Kawai in 1974 initiated a change in the management of common bile duct (CBD) stones. Before that time, laparotomy with open CBD exploration was the main therapeutic recourse for patients with choledocholithiasis. While laparoscopic cholecystectomy has since become the standard, accepted, and preferred technique for the treatment of gallbladder stones (due to less postoperative pain, reduced hospitalization time, shorter convalescence, and better cosmetic results than open cholecystectomy), laparoscopic management of common duct stones is significantly more complex. Advanced surgical skills and sophisticated instrumentation are required, and neither widely available. As a result, ERCP plays an integral role in the treatment of common duct stones in the laparoscopic cholecystectomy era.

The timing and need for ERCP in relation to laparoscopic cholecystectomy are dependent on the likelihood of stones being present (low, medium, and high), the skill of the endoscopist, and the ability of the laparoscopist to perform common duct exploration. There is little value of routine ERCP before laparoscopic cholecystectomy in patients with a low likelihood of having bile duct stones. When comparing the low yield of detecting clinically important anatomic variants and unsuspected bile duct stones with the generally accepted 3% to 7% ERCP complication rate, the routine use of ERCP before cholecystectomy cannot be justified. In patients with symptomatic cholelithiasis, a completely normal liver biochemical panel has a significant clinical utility in excluding the presence of CBD stones with a negative predictive value of more than 97%. Conversely, there is no one clinical variable that can reliably identify the subset of patients with concomitant choledocholithiasis with good positive predictive value. The most reliable

BOX 111.1 Indications for Endoscopic Retrograde Cholangiopancreatography

SUSPECTED BILIARY DUCTAL DISORDER
Jaundice or cholestasis of suspected obstructive origin
Acute cholangitis
Gallstone pancreatitis
Clarification of biliary lesion seen on one imaging tests
Biliary fistula

SUSPECTED PANCREATIC DUCTAL DISORDER
Pancreatic cancer
Mucinous or cystic neoplasm
Unexplained recurrent pancreatitis
Chronic pancreatitis with unrelenting pain
Clarification of pancreatic lesion detected on other imaging
  tests
Ascites or pleural effusion of suspected pancreatic origin
Pancreatic pseudocyst or fistula

TO DIRECT ENDOSCOPIC THERAPY
Sphincterotomy
Biliary drainage
Pancreatic drainage

TO DIRECT ENDOSCOPIC TISSUE/FLUID SAMPLING
Biopsy, brush, fine-needle aspiration
Bile/pancreatic juice collection

PREOPERATIVE DUCTAL MAPPING
Malignant tumors
Benign strictures
Chronic pancreatitis
Pancreatic pseudocysts and ductal disruptions
Mucinous or cystic tumors of the pancreas

TO PERFORM MANOMETRY
Sphincter of Oddi
Ductal

---

predictors include a stone visualized within the CBD on ultrasound; however, the sensitivity of transabdominal ultrasound for detecting a stone is low (22% to 50%). Ascending cholangitis, bilirubin level greater than 1.7 mg/dL, and a dilated CBD on ultrasound are additional high risk/strong likelihood features. Using multiple modality abnormalities, patients can be determined to be low (<10% risk of choledocholithiasis), medium (10% to 50%), or high risk (>50%).[3]

Patients judged to have a high likelihood of harboring duct stones are likely to benefit from preoperative ERCP and stone extraction (if stones are present). Patients in the medium-risk group create a diagnostic and therapeutic dilemma because a failure to identify and remove choledocholithiasis can result in serious complications including recurrent symptoms, cholangitis, and acute gallstone pancreatitis. To lower this risk, additional biliary imaging is warranted, and patients should undergo preoperative EUS or MRCP or intraoperative laparoscopic intraoperative cholangiogram (IOC) or ultrasound; however, these imaging modalities are operator dependent and not universally available (Fig. 111.1). When intraoperative laparoscopic IOC is positive, the patient should undergo a postoperative ERCP or laparoscopic duct exploration.

METHODS OF STONE EXTRACTION

Standard (Basket and Balloon Catheters)

After identification of a common duct stone, an ES is typically performed. Balloon catheters are most useful for extracting one or more relatively small or fragmented stones (≤10 mm) in a nondilated duct (Fig. 111.2). They are not as effective for extracting larger stones or small stones in a markedly dilated bile duct because the balloon will often slide past the stone. Stone retrieval wire baskets with different configurations, length/width, types of wire, and number of wires are commercially available. Settings in which a basket may be preferred over a balloon include larger stones (>10 mm), intrahepatic stones, smaller stones in a dilated duct, and stones that are larger than the downstream duct (e.g., stone proximal to a stricture). A risk with a wire basket stone retrieval is the possibility of the wires getting impacted within the stone in the CBD. The basket and stone apparatus are then anchored within the CBD and cannot be easily retrieved. The emergency mechanical lithotripsy may allow a rescue of the impacted basket; however, surgery may be required to remove the basket.

In experienced centers, common duct stones can be successfully removed in 80% to 90% of patients after sphincterotomy with standard baskets and balloon catheters. Difficulty clearing or failure to clear the common duct of stones may occur for a variety of reasons. In most cases, stone size is the major determinant of success. Stones greater than 15 mm are generally considered large; equally important, however, are stone factors (such as number, consistency, shape, and location) and ductal factors (such as contour, diameter at the level of and distal to the stone, and the presence of coexisting pathology such as a stricture or tumor).

Lithotripsy Techniques

A variety of lithotripsy techniques (mechanical, electrohydraulic, laser, and extracorporeal shock wave lithotripsy [ESWL]) have been used to facilitate the retrieval of stones not removable by standard methods.[4] The simplest endoscopic adjunct for the management of common duct stones that have failed to be removed by conventional baskets and balloons is the mechanical lithotripter or crushing basket. There are through-the-scope mechanical lithotripters and lithotriptor devices that require endoscope removal. Mechanical lithotripsy is a safe, effective, low-cost procedure that can be performed at the time of the initial ERCP. In experienced centers, mechanical lithotripsy allows for the removal of more than 85% to 90% of difficult bile duct stones that are refractory to standard extraction techniques. However, up to 30% of patients may require more than one ERCP. Failure of mechanical lithotripsy is typically due to an inability to engage the stone within the basket and rarely to insufficient shearing power to fragment the stone.

Since being used for the first time in 1985 to treat gallstones,[5] ESWL has had decreasing use in biliary disease, given the frequent difficulty visualizing stones for targeting shock wave therapy and the frequent recurrence and incomplete clearance of therapy. ESWL is currently relegated mostly for use in chronic pancreatitis–associated

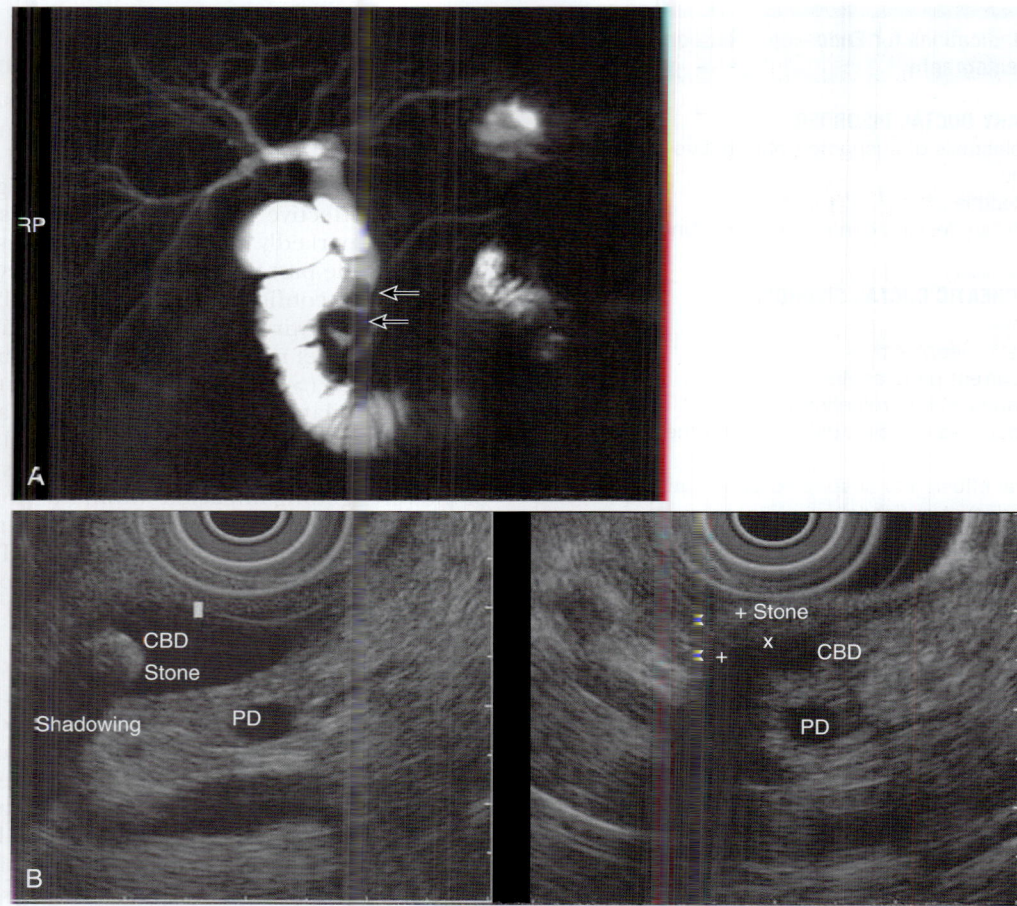

FIGURE 111.1 (A) Magnetic resonance cholangiopancreatography demonstrating bile duct stones *(arrows)*. (B) Endoscopic ultrasound showing bile duct stones with acoustic shadowing. *CBD*, Common bile duct; *PD*, pancreatic duct.

lithiasis, which is discussed further in another chapter. In contrast to ESWL, intraductal (laser or electrohydraulic) modalities have become standard adjuncts to traditional endoscopic management when attempting bile duct clearance.

The choice between these methods or surgery largely depends on availability because they are usually concentrated in tertiary centers. Intraductal lithotripsy can be achieved by producing a shock wave directly on the surface of the stone with either a flexible electrohydraulic probe or a flexible quartz fiber to deliver light from a laser. Both of these techniques are most frequently performed under direct endoscopic control via a cholangioscope (i.e., mother–baby endoscope system, single operator cholangioscopes or ultrathin gastroscopes).

Biliary Stents

When stone extraction is incomplete or has failed, biliary drainage should be established to prevent stone impaction and cholangitis. In most situations, this therapy serves as a temporizing measure that allows for improvement in the patient's clinical condition pending repeat attempts at stone removal. The stent is placed so that one limb is above the stone and the other is in the duodenum (Fig. 111.3). Most authorities recommend double-pigtail stents,

although favorable experience is reported with straight 10-French (Fr) stents.[6] Biliary stenting not only serves to drain the bile duct but may also aid in mechanically fragmenting the stone and thereby facilitating subsequent attempts at endoscopic removal. The addition of oral dissolution therapy may also soften and reduce the size of the stone and thus aid endoscopic removal.

ACUTE GALLSTONE PANCREATITIS

In Western countries, gallstone disease is a leading cause of acute pancreatitis and accounts for 34% to 54% of cases. Most patients with acute gallstone pancreatitis (AGP) have a mild attack and can be treated conservatively. However, the case fatality rate in severe pancreatitis remains unacceptably high, approaching 10%. In the open cholecystectomy era, urgent surgical intervention for severe AGP did not gain general acceptance because of the increased morbidity and mortality associated with this approach. Coincident with these surgical reports were uncontrolled endoscopic series reporting the efficacy and safety of ERCP and ES in the setting of AGP. Although the results were encouraging, the studies varied in their criteria for patient selection and timing of ES in relation to the acute attack (many were performed in the recovery phase, when surgery is also safe). These early series prompted the three randomized

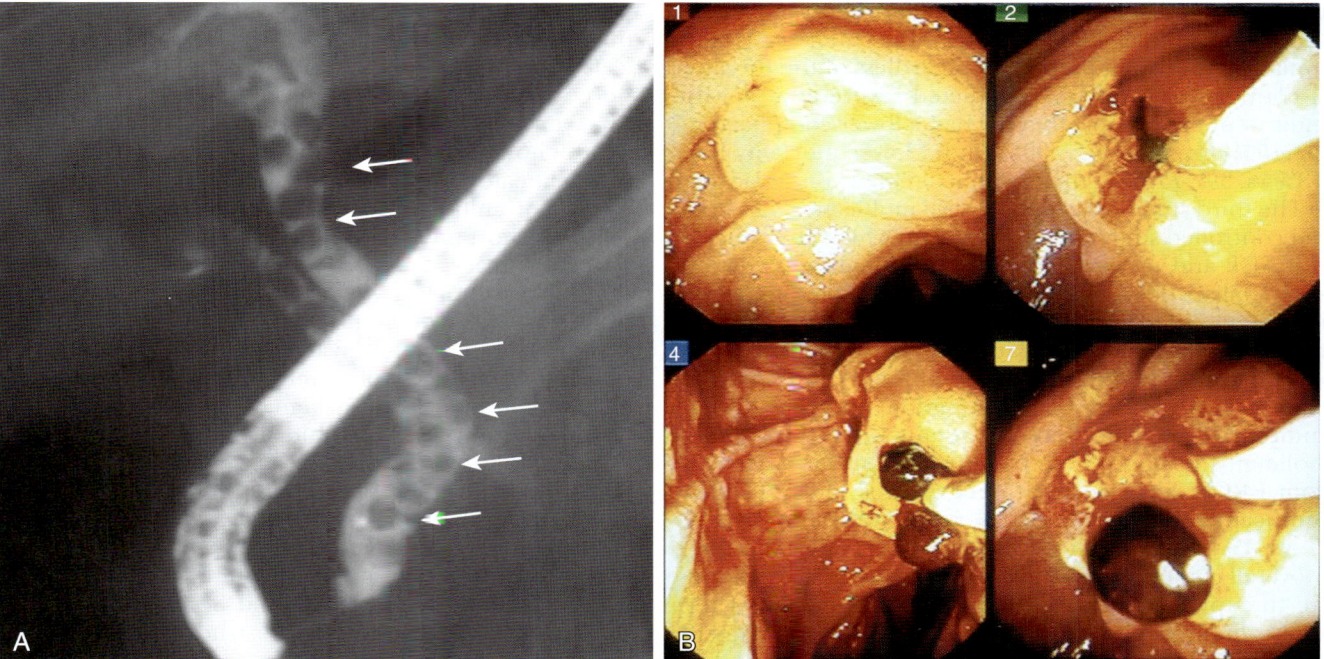

FIGURE 111.2 (A) Numerous bile duct stones present in the entire common duct *(arrows)*. Note stones also in the cystic duct. (B) Stones removed after biliary sphincterotomy. *Top left,* Normal papilla. *Top right,* Completed biliary sphincterotomy. *Bottom left* and *bottom right,* Stones being removed with a stone retrieval balloon.

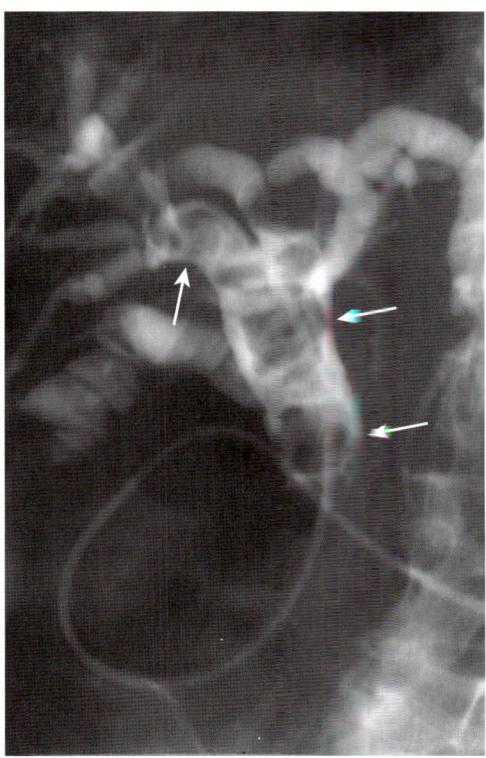

FIGURE 111.3 A nasobiliary tube has been placed to provide temporary biliary drainage in this patient with multiple large bile duct stones *(arrows)*.

controlled trials[7–9] that now serve as the basis for the endoscopic treatment of AGP. The therapeutic principle for ES in AGP is simply removal of the obstructing calculus and reestablishment of bile and pancreatic juice flow.

In a randomized prospective controlled trial from the United Kingdom, 121 patients with AGP either received conventional therapy (i.e., gut rest, analgesics, intravenous fluids, and antibiotics) or underwent urgent (within 72 hours after admission) ERCP with ES and stone extraction (if stones were present in the CBD at the time of ERCP).[7] Patients were stratified by the predicted severity of their attacks with the modified Glasgow system. Choledocholithiasis was found in 25% of patients with predicted mild attacks and 63% with predicted severe attacks. The four important findings were that (1) ERCP could be safely performed in the setting of gallstone pancreatitis, (2) there was a significant reduction in major complications in patients who underwent urgent ERCP and ES, (3) the reduction in morbidity was apparent only in patients with predicted severe attacks (61% vs. 24%; $P = .007$), and (4) there was a significant reduction in hospital stay for those with severe attacks treated by urgent ERCP and ES (median of 9.5 vs. 17 days; $P = .03$). The mortality rate was improved, but the difference was not statistically significant.

A second randomized controlled study was performed by the department of surgery at the University of Hong Kong.[8] One hundred ninety-five patients with acute pancreatitis were randomized to early ERCP (within 24 hours of admission) or conservative therapy. Although the methodology, patient selection, and assessment of the severity of the acute pancreatitis used in this study differed from that in the United Kingdom study, the results in the subgroup of patients with gallstone pancreatitis ($n = 127$) were quite similar. Patients with mild pancreatitis had similar morbidity and mortality regardless of the therapy. In contrast, patients with predicted severe attacks who underwent endoscopic therapy had a lower complication rate (54% vs. 13%; $P = .003$) and a lower mortality rate (18% vs. 3% $P = .07$) than patients treated conservatively.

The third study[9] was a prospective multicenter randomized controlled study from Germany in which 238 patients with AGP and no evidence of severe biliary obstruction (severe biliary obstruction defined as a bilirubin concentration >5 mg/dL) were randomized to ERCP with ES and stone extraction or conservative therapy within 72 hours of symptom onset. This study attempted to address the major criticism of the United Kingdom and Hong Kong studies: the need to exclude patients with concomitant cholangitis because these patients are known to benefit from ERCP. The two treatment groups did not differ significantly in mortality (11% vs. 6% overall mortality, 8% vs. 4% AGP mortality, ERCP vs. conservative therapy) or overall complications (46% vs. 51%, ERCP vs. conservative therapy) regardless of the predicted severity of the pancreatitis. However, respiratory failure was more frequent in the ERCP group (12% vs. 5%; $P = .03$), and jaundice was more frequent in patients who received conservative treatment (11% vs. 1%; $P = .02$).

Although all three studies concluded that there was no difference in outcomes for patients with mild pancreatitis treated conservatively or by ERCP, only the study from Germany suggested that early ERCP was of no benefit in patients with severe gallstone pancreatitis. Even though ERCP is clearly indicated in patients with AGP complicated by cholangitis or biliary obstruction, its role in the setting of severe AGP alone warrants further investigation. A meta-analysis[9] of these three published studies revealed a statistically significant reduction in morbidity from 38% to 25% and mortality from 9% to 5% in the ERCP/ES group versus the conservatively treated group. A subgroup analysis based on the severity of pancreatitis was not reported in this meta-analysis.

ACUTE CHOLANGITIS

Cholangitis is a potentially life-threatening disease that results from bacterial infection of obstructed bile. Systemic toxicity occurs when intraductal pressure is sufficiently elevated to cause reflux of bacteria or endotoxin into blood. Thus obstruction plays a key role by both increasing intraductal pressure and promoting bacterial overgrowth as a result of bile stasis. The most common cause of acute cholangitis is choledocholithiasis, which occurs in approximately 80% to 90% of unselected cases. Therapy for cholangitis must be individualized because of the spectrum of severity of illness. Antibiotic therapy should be initiated promptly. Analysis of bile and stone cultures indicates that *Escherichia coli*, *Klebsiella* spp., *Enterobacter* spp., *Enterococcus* spp., and *Streptococcus* spp. are the most commonly isolated bacteria. The antibiotic selected should preferably penetrate an obstructed biliary tree. The majority of patients will respond to conservative management, thereby allowing for a more elective approach to biliary decompression.[10] Urgent decompression is indicated if improvement is not seen within a few hours of initial resuscitation. The latter group will invariably have a fatal outcome if conservative treatment is continued.

Options for bile duct decompression include surgical, percutaneous, and endoscopic methods. Endoscopic intervention is now accepted as definitive therapy for acute cholangitis. The advantages of ERCP are that it can delineate the cause of obstruction, facilitate sampling of bile for culture, and decompress the biliary tree in a relatively short time with low morbidity. Biliary decompression is the goal of therapy and can be complete (e.g., stone removal) or temporary (e.g., placement of a stent without stone removal), pending more definitive management (to allow stabilization of an unstable patient). The endoscopic procedure consists of sphincterotomy with stone extraction or biliary drainage with a stent.

Ideally the patient should be stabilized or made as stable as possible before performing ERCP. Patients with respiratory compromise can have their ERCP performed while on ventilatory assistance. Because intrabiliary pressure is increased in acute cholangitis, contrast injection should be limited to reduce further systemic seeding of bacteria. Enough contrast should be injected to define the anatomy and the cause of obstruction. Aspirated bile should be cultured. In a stable patient, definitive therapy can be performed. In an unstable patient, the length of the procedure should be limited. In such cases a stent should be placed, and once the patient is stabilized, more definitive therapy can be performed.

The high morbidity and mortality associated with surgical and percutaneous therapy for acute cholangitis prompted evaluation of the safety and utility of endoscopic management. In a retrospective analysis, Leese et al.[11] reported on 71 patients with stone-related cholangitis treated by early decompression either surgically ($n = 28$) or by ES ($n = 43$). Early surgery was associated with significantly higher 30-day mortality (21% vs. 5%) and morbidity (57% vs. 8%) than sphincterotomy. The endoscopic group was significantly older than the surgical group and had more medical risk factors, but there were no significant differences in the severity of cholangitis. Leung et al.[10] reported their experience in a retrospective analysis of 105 patients with acute calculous cholangitis who did not respond to conservative management and underwent urgent endoscopic decompression at a mean of 1.5 days after admission. Of these patients, 39% had coexisting medical problems, 85% had Charcot triad, and 40% were in shock at the time of admission. Endoscopic drainage was successful in 102 patients (97%). Ninety-seven percent of patients responded with striking improvement in abdominal pain, and 93% had resolution of fever within 3 days. The overall 30-day mortality was 5%. Among those in shock, 2 of 4 who had been drained after 72 hours died, as compared with 3 of 38 who had been drained before 72 hours. There were no deaths in the group without shock, irrespective of the timing of drainage. The mortality of 5% compares favorably with that of urgent surgical intervention in which mortality has been reported to be greater than 40% in some series. The ERCP complication rate was 5% and was limited to five postsphincterotomy bleeding episodes managed by endoscopic techniques. The safety and efficacy of endoscopic therapy were corroborated in a large retrospective study of 947 patients with cholangitis secondary to stones ($n = 898$) or stricture ($n = 49$).[12] In a randomized prospective study, Lai et al. compared the safety and efficacy of biliary decompression by surgical and endoscopic techniques in 82 patients with severe cholangitis as a result of stones.[1] Patients treated with laparotomy and CBD exploration had significantly higher morbidity (64% vs. 34%) and mortality (32% vs. 10%) than those treated with endoscopic therapy. These and other studies clearly demonstrate the efficacy and safety of biliary decompression either as definitive therapy or as a temporizing measure, pending more definitive intervention once the patient is stabilized.

BENIGN BILIARY STRICTURES

Endoscopic therapy for the management of benign biliary strictures has emerged as an effective and safe treatment with significantly less morbidity and mortality than the traditional surgical and percutaneous management strategies. Benign biliary strictures amenable to endoscopic intervention develop most frequently secondary to inflammatory conditions, such as chronic pancreatitis or as postoperative complications. Additional less frequent causes are primary sclerosing cholangitis, infection, ischemia (e.g., portal biliopathy), papillary stenosis, autoimmune pancreatitis/cholangiopathy, trauma, and bile duct stones. Regardless of etiology, benign biliary strictures necessitate therapeutic intervention in the presence of jaundice, chronic cholestasis, or cholangitis, to reduce the risk of developing secondary biliary cirrhosis.

Endoscopic Management of Benign Biliary Strictures

Irrespective of the site or pathogenesis of the stricture, the primary aim of endoscopy is to pass a guidewire through the stricture to permit passage of dilators (balloon or catheter) and stents. In 2012, the European Society for Gastrointestinal Endoscopy (ESGE) published guidelines for endoscopic biliary drainage and recommended the use of temporary placement of multiple plastic stents for benign strictures of the CBD as standard of care.[14] The sequential placement of multiple plastic stents is technically feasible in more than 90% of patients and provides the highest long-term biliary patency rate (90% for postoperative biliary strictures and 65% for those complicating chronic pancreatitis). The limitation to this approach is the requirement of multiple endoscopic procedures over a 1-year period with stent exchange, upsizing, redilation every 3 months, and subsequent increased costs, procedure risks, and potential decreased patient compliance. The use of dilating balloons in isolation or temporary placement of single plastic stents is associated with high recurrence. The goals of treatment are to render the patient free of symptoms and to achieve sustained normalization of liver test results after the stents are permanently removed.

Placement of self-expanding metal stents (SEMSs) with a streamlined delivery system offers the benefit of increased patency and larger diameter, with single stent providing prompt dilation to an estimated radial dilation force equivalent to approximately three side-by-side plastic stents.[15] Recently there have been two large studies evaluating the use of fully covered SEMSs (FCSEMSs) in benign biliary strictures. In 2014, Deviere et al.[16] reported

their results of a large, prospective multinational study designed to evaluate removability, stricture resolution, safety, and early stricture recurrence. In cases of chronic pancreatitis or cholecystectomy, FCSEMS removal was scheduled at 10 to 12 months and for patients with liver transplant at 4 to 6 months. In 177 patients, removal success was accomplished in 74.6% (95% confidence interval [CI], 67.5% to 80.8%). Removal success was more frequent in the chronic pancreatitis group (80.5%) than in the liver transplantation (63.4%) or cholecystectomy (61.1%) groups ($P = .017$). FCSEMSs were removed by endoscopy from all patients in whom this procedure was attempted. Stricture resolution without restenting upon FCSEMS removal occurred in 76.3% of patients (95% CI, 69.3% to 82.3%). Over a median follow-up period of 20.3 months (interquartile range, 12.9 to 24.3 months), the rate of stricture recurrence was 14.8% (95% CI, 8.2% to 20.9%). Stent- or removal-related serious adverse events, most often cholangitis, occurred in 27.3% of patients. This was followed in 2016 by an American open-label, multicenter, randomized clinical trial[15] to test the hypothesis that FCSEMS would be noninferior to multiple plastic stents as first-line endoscopic treatment of benign bile duct strictures. Over a 3-year period, 112 patients with treatment-naive benign biliary strictures due to orthotopic liver transplant ($n = 73$), chronic pancreatitis ($n = 35$), or postoperative injury ($n = 4$) were randomized to receive multiple plastic stents or a single FCSEMS. Fifty-five patients were randomized to the plastic stent group and 57 patients to the FCSEMS group. Compared with plastic stents (41/48, 85.4%) the FCSEMS resolution rate was 50 of 54 patients (92.6%, with a rate difference of 7.2% (1-sided 95% CI, −3.0% to >; $P < .001$). Among patients with benign biliary strictures and a bile duct diameter greater than 6 mm, FCSEMSs were not inferior to multiple plastic stents after 12 months in achieving stricture resolution. Collectively, these data support the use of endoscopic therapy, and there is increasing data to support the use of FCSEMS for benign biliary strictures. Surgically fit patients who fail initial endoscopic therapy or have recurrent strictures are best managed by a bilioenteric bypass.

Postoperative Biliary Strictures

Postoperative strictures can occur within the extrahepatic bile duct after cholecystectomy or orthotopic liver transplantation (OLT) or at the biliary-enteric anastomosis after pancreaticoduodenectomy, OLT, liver resection, and Roux-en-Y hepaticojejunostomy. Iatrogenic injury to the bile duct during cholecystectomy, either open or more commonly laparoscopic, can result in the development of an extrahepatic biliary stricture. The advent and recent predominance of laparoscopic techniques has been associated with an increased incidence of bile duct injury, with reported incidence of postlaparoscopic cholecystectomy bile duct stricture of 0.2% to 0.7% (Fig. 111.4). In one of the largest series to date, the group from Amsterdam published their 10-year data in 74 patients with postcholecystectomy bile duct stenosis.[17] Two 10-Fr stents were inserted for a maximum of 12 months with stent exchange every 3 months to avoid cholangitis caused by loss of patency. Stent insertion was successful in 80% of patients, and in the 44 patients who completed 12 months of stent therapy, recurrent

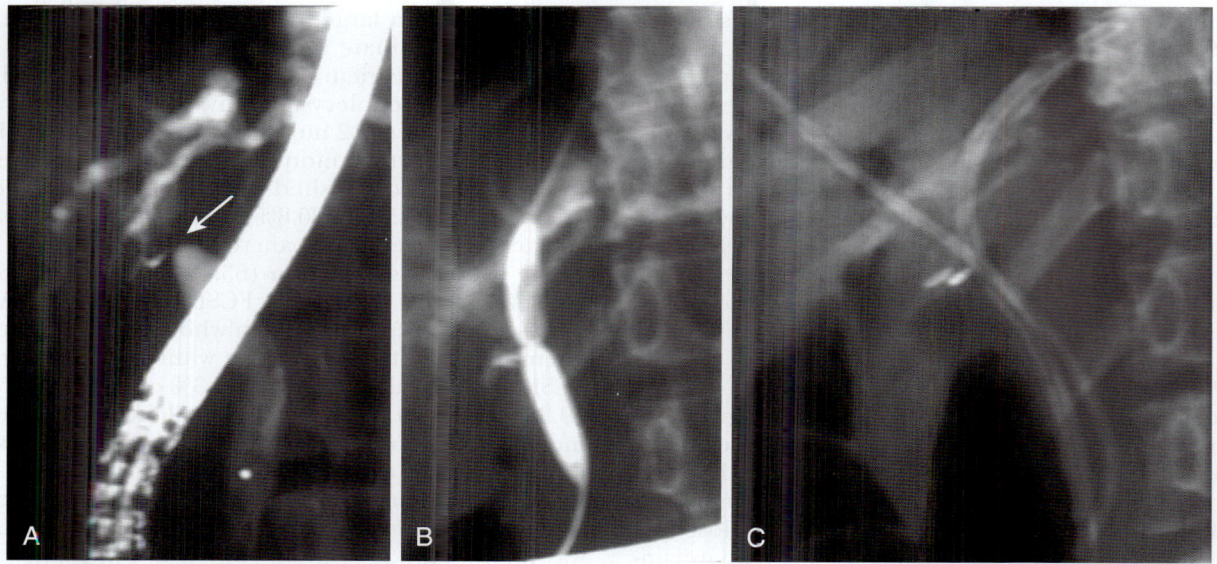

FIGURE 111.4 This patient was evaluated for obstructive jaundice 2 months after laparoscopic cholecystectomy. (A) The cholangiogram shows a common duct stricture *(arrow)*. Note the clips in the region of the common duct. (B) The stricture was then dilated with a balloon-dilating catheter. (C) Two biliary stents were placed to bridge the stricture.

stenosis occurred in 20% after a median follow-up of 9.1 years—with the majority within the first 6 months and all cases within 2 years of stent removal. This was followed by the 10-year experience from the group in Rome in which 55 patients (35 postcholecystectomy) with postoperative biliary stenoses were treated endoscopically. Costamagna et al.[18] undertook a more aggressive endoscopic approach than the group in Amsterdam. Each patient received as many large-diameter stents as necessary (based on stricture tightness and bile duct diameter) to eliminate the stricture. Stents were exchanged electively at 3-month intervals and were removed after complete resolution of the stricture. By intention-to-treat analysis, the success rate was 89% of patients. Early complications developed in 9% of patients (three cholangitis, one pancreatitis) and stent occlusion that required early exchange occurred in 18% of patients. There was one death caused by a stroke 2 months after a stent exchange. Among the patients with long-term follow-up (76% of patients), there was no recurrence of symptoms caused by relapsing biliary stricture at a mean follow-up of 48.8 months. In summary, the majority of retrospective data for postoperative (predominantly cholecystectomy) reports an approximate 74% to 90% resolution of strictures with endoscopic therapy.[19] Complete transection of the bile duct is significantly more difficult to treat endoscopically, and although case reports have been reported, surgical intervention is frequently required.

Biliary strictures are one of the more frequent complications of both living donor and deceased donor liver transplant and can be classified as anastomotic or nonanastomotic (ischemic, e.g., hepatic artery thrombosis). Anastomotic strictures are more common, single, present earlier (<1 month), and short, and tend to be more responsive to endoscopic therapy than strictures occurring at nonanastomotic sites, which are longer, less

common, present later (>1 month), and often multifocal. Anastomotic strictures can account for up to 80% of post-OLT biliary strictures. Endoscopic therapy with balloon dilation and sequential plastic stent placement achieves a long-term patency rate in the range of 75% to 90%. Contrarily, nonanastomotic strictures are associated with a lower long-term treatment response rate of 50% to 75% and frequently require more endoscopic procedures.[19] There is increasing experience with FCSEMS in the post-OLT population, and in the large, prospective multinational study from Europe, the stricture resolution rate was 68.3% in OLT patients after 4 to 6 months of therapy.[16] Previous FCSEMS anastomotic stricture resolution rates have ranged from 61.3% to 95.5%.

Distal Common Bile Duct Strictures Secondary to Chronic Pancreatitis

Intrapancreatic CBD strictures have been reported to occur in 3% to 46% of patients with chronic pancreatitis (Fig. 111.5). When these strictures are complicated by cholestasis, jaundice, and cholangitis, they can be treated with plastic and fully covered SEMS. The long-term outcome after endoscopic biliary stenting of postoperative biliary strictures has previously been shown to be superior to that after stenting of biliary strictures in the setting of chronic pancreatitis; however, in the recent Deviere et al.[16] publication for FCSEMS in benign biliary strictures, the stricture resolution rate was 79.7% for chronic pancreatitis patients, 68.3% for OLT, and 72.2% for cholecystectomy patients. Chronic pancreatitis accounted for two-thirds of the population, and both favorable short-term resolution rates and low recurrence rates (10.5%) were identified. The authors theorize that the diameter of the FCSEMS and the duration of indwell may have contributed to the unexpectedly high observed resolution rate and low recurrence rate in the chronic pancreatitis group.

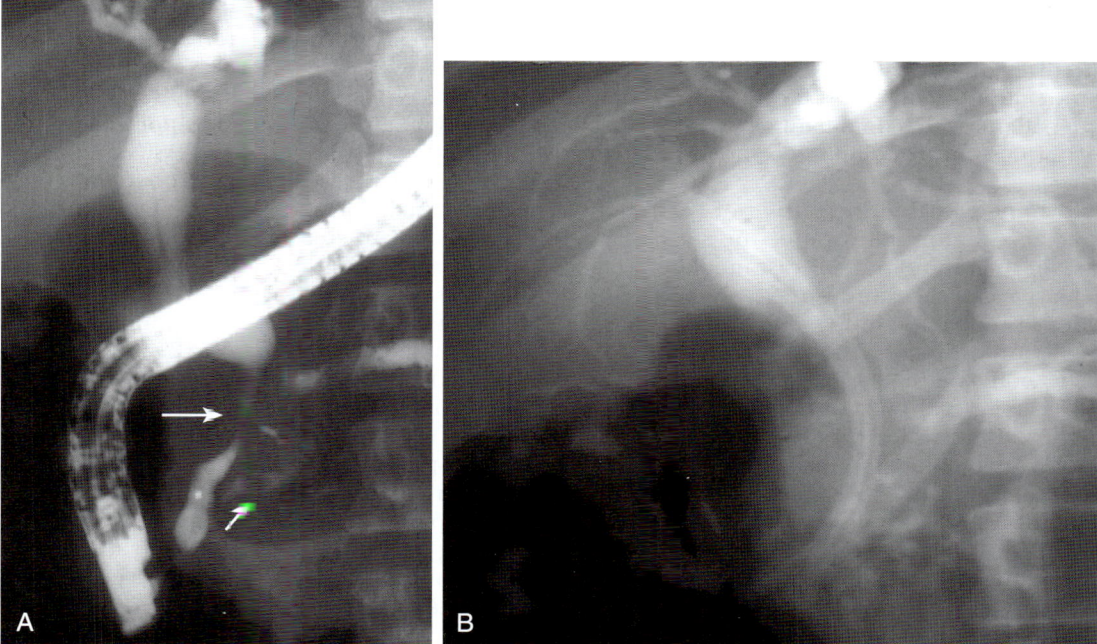

FIGURE 111.5 Chronic pancreatitis-induced common bile duct (CBD) stricture. A The cholangiogram shows a 2-cm CBD stricture *(large arrow)* with proximal dilation. Note the pancreatic duct stone *(small arrow)* and pancreatic stricture. (B) Two biliary stents were placed.

This endoscopic treatment of chronic pancreatitis is discussed further in another chapter in this book on the endoscopic management of complications of acute and chronic pancreatitis.

PRIMARY SCLEROSING CHOLANGITIS

Cholangiographic imaging is the gold standard for diagnosing primary sclerosing cholangitis (PSC), although conditions that mimic PSC must be excluded. Although both percutaneous transhepatic cholangiography (PTC) and ERCP can be used to show the characteristic changes associated with PSC, given the possible complications with these procedures, MRCP has become the ESGE/European Association for the Study of the Liver (EASL) recommended first-line noninvasive imaging test for suspected PSC.[20] A meta-analysis using ERCP as the standard reference measure found MRCP to have a high sensitivity and specificity of 86% and 94%, respectively, for the diagnosis of PSC.[21] ERCP still has a diagnostic role in patients with equivocal MRCP images with negative liver biopsies or in patients with contraindications for MRCP. The classic cholangiographic features in PSC are diffuse multifocal strictures of the intrahepatic and extrahepatic bile ducts (Fig. 111.6). These strictures are usually short, with intervening normal or dilated segments giving a beaded appearance. Other frequent findings on cholangiography include pseudodiverticula, mural irregularities, and biliary stones and sludge.

The rationale for endoscopic intervention is based on the hypothesis that progressive liver disease and deterioration of liver function may be aggravated or accelerated by backpressure from dominant strictures and stones or debris when present. It is further hypothesized that relief of obstruction may halt, delay, or even reverse progression to

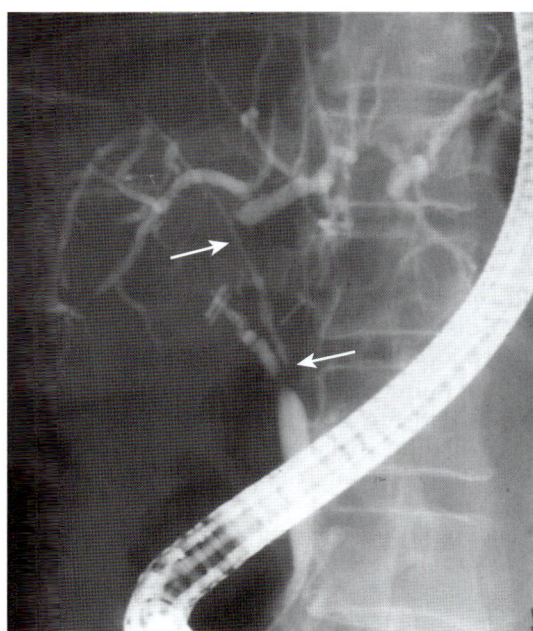

FIGURE 111.6 This patient has primary sclerosing cholangitis involving the extrahepatic and intrahepatic ducts. There is a long, high-grade stricture involving the common hepatic duct *(arrows)* and the right and left hepatic ducts, as well as narrowings/irregularities of the intrahepatic ducts.

cirrhosis and liver failure. Because no medical therapy has definitively proved effective for PSC, a trial of endoscopic therapy in symptomatic patients is reasonable. Indications for considering endoscopic management of PSC are treatment of jaundice or pruritus and symptomatic cholangitis, deteriorating serum hepatic chemical profile, and when concern for bile duct cancer is high with new dominant strictures or progression of existing dominant strictures, tissue sampling. The most favorable candidates for therapy are patients with a dominant extrahepatic stricture with or without stones and limited or no intrahepatic involvement.

When performing ERCP in the setting of PSC, therapeutic skills are mandatory because of the serious risk for infection. Not uncommonly, contrast media will take the path of least resistance and enter the cystic duct and gallbladder; intrahepatic filling is therefore limited. Preferably, a balloon catheter is then manipulated above the cystic duct takeoff, and higher-pressure injection of the intrahepatic radicles is performed with the balloon inflated. Moreover, because the risk for post-ERCP cholangitis in patients with PSC may be as high as 20% to 30% after diagnostic and therapeutic procedures (particularly in those in whom obstructed segments are not decompressed), antibiotic prophylaxis is mandatory.

All therapeutic procedures aim at improving bile flow. Endoscopic techniques that may be used to achieve this goal are ES, stone/sludge removal, stricture dilation with balloons and catheters, placement of stents, and combinations of therapy. Endoscopic stricture dilation and stenting have been reported in PSC patients since the early 1980s. The techniques have been standardized. The goals of endoscopic intervention in patients with PSC are to relieve jaundice and pruritus, treat cholangitis, and theoretically delay the onset of biliary cirrhosis and thus buy time before liver transplantation. In reviewing the efficacy of endoscopic interventions in PSC it must be acknowledged that the majority of studies are of retrospective design, prone to selection bias, and report nonuniform treatments, including dilation with and without stenting of dominant strictures as well as, in some cases, treatment with ursodeoxycholic acid.

Balloon Dilation With or Without Stenting in Primary Sclerosing Cholangitis

Johnson and associates[22] reported their results of endoscopic dilation in 35 symptomatic PSC patients (29 with cholangitis and 6 with jaundice alone). Patients were treated by dilation (balloon or catheter) with or without biliary stenting. During a mean follow-up period of 24 months, there was a significant reduction in the frequency of hospitalization for cholangitis, bilirubin, and stricture score. Cholangitis occurred shortly after treatment in six patients; five of the six had a biliary stent placed. As a result, these authors recommended avoiding biliary stents in patients with PSC.

Lee and associates[23] retrospectively reviewed the records of 85 PSC patients who underwent 175 ERCP procedures (75 diagnostic and 100 therapeutic). Endoscopic therapy was associated with a 15% major complication rate (7% pancreatitis and 8% cholangitis). Clinical follow-up (median of 31 months) was obtained in 50 of 53 patients who underwent 85 therapeutic procedures. Twenty-eight patients improved clinically, whereas 21 felt the same and 1 felt worse. Serum liver chemistry results obtained within 3 months of the endoscopic intervention were significantly improved in comparison to pretreatment values. Overall,

41 of 53 patients (77%) had improvement in their clinical symptoms, liver function test results, or cholangiograms.

Stenting in Primary Sclerosing Cholangitis

Van Milligen de Wit et al.[24] reported the results of stent therapy in 25 patients with PSC and dominant extrahepatic strictures. Stents were exchanged or removed electively at 2- to 3-month intervals or because of symptoms attributable to stent clogging. Endoscopic therapy was technically successful in 21 patients (84%). In these 21 patients, the results of all serum biochemical liver tests improved significantly within 6 months of stent therapy. During a median follow-up of 29 months (range, 2 to 120 months) after stent removal, 12 patients (57%) remained asymptomatic with stable biochemical liver test results and 4 (19%) had clinical and biochemical relapse of disease that responded favorably to repeat endoscopic therapy. Early procedure-related complications occurred in 14% of the procedures. The value of short-term endoscopic stenting (mean 11 days; range, 1 to 23 days) for 32 patients with dominant strictures was reported by Ponsioen et al.[25] Cholestatic symptoms improved in 83%, and there were statistically significant reductions in abdominal pain, fatigue, and pruritus. Serum liver chemistry results were significantly improved. Eighty percent of patients were free of reinterventions at 1 year and 60% at 3 years. Procedure-related complications occurred in 15%, but there were no episodes of cholangitis. The authors advocated this technique because it was efficacious and overcame the complications associated with stent occlusion.

Balloon Dilation Versus Dilation With Stenting

Kaya et al.[26] reported in a retrospective review of 71 patients with dominant PSC strictures, comparing balloon dilation alone versus balloon dilation with stenting. Stenting after balloon dilation (median stenting interval of about 4.5 months) of dominant strictures provided no additional benefit and was associated with more complications, including increased number of procedures and bile duct perforations. Recently the European multicenter randomized DILSTENT trial comparing single-balloon dilatation and short-term stenting was prematurely discontinued, with preliminary results showing no differences in outcome but a significantly higher serious adverse event rate in the stent group.[20]

The 2017 ESGE guidelines for the role of endoscopy in PSC recommend that if stenting is going to be completed, the endoscopist should use a single 10-Fr plastic stent for dominant stricture in the extrahepatic ducts or two 7-Fr stents for hilar strictures extending into the left or right hepatic duct and that the stents should be removed in 1 to 2 weeks following insertion.[20]

Primary Sclerosing Cholangitis–Associated Cholangiocarcinoma

Cholangiocarcinoma is a dreaded complication of PSC that occurs in 9% to 15% of patients with a 400-fold relative increase in risk compared with the general population. The risk appears to be greatest in patients with long-standing ulcerative colitis and cirrhosis. Sudden worsening of jaundice, weight loss, and raised serum CA19-9 should raise the possibility of the development of cholangiocarcinoma. Cholangiographic findings that suggest malignant transformation include markedly dilated ducts of the ductal segments proximal to a stricture, the presence of a polypoid mass, and progressive stricture formation. Comparison with previous ERCP results is essential to signal the presence of complicating cholangiocarcinoma because with PSC uncomplicated by malignancy, the cholangiographic appearance frequently remains static for years. Unfortunately, early diagnosis of cancer is difficult because of the absence of a sensitive, specific serologic marker and the relative insensitivity of bile duct tissue sampling. However, tissue sampling of any suspicious lesion at ERCP is indicated.

BILIARY LEAKS/FISTULAS

Biliary fistulas most commonly occur as a complication of cholecystectomy, CBD exploration or inadvertent operative injury of the bile duct or as a consequence of a local infection. Rarely, biliary fistulas result from long-standing untreated biliary tract disease. With more widespread use of laparoscopic cholecystectomy, the incidence of bile duct injury, including biliary fistula, has increased. Bile leakage from the cystic duct remnant is among the most common injuries reported as a complication of laparoscopic cholecystectomy. The most common cause of cystic duct leaks involves imprecise application of clips on the duct or their subsequent dislodgment during the procedure. Biliary fistulas may also arise from the intrahepatic ducts and common duct. A duct of Luschka in the gallbladder bed, if present, is quite vulnerable to transection during cholecystectomy. Distal obstruction from a stone, stricture, or papillary stenosis increases ductal pressure proximally and may promote and maintain the biliary fistula.

Postoperative bile duct leaks are usually manifested within a week after surgery.[27] In a series of 62 patients with postcholecystectomy leaks, initial symptoms included abdominal pain in 89%, abdominal tenderness in 81%, fever in 74%, nausea and vomiting in 45%, and jaundice in 43%.[27] Only 2% had a clinically detectable mass or ascites. Biochemical testing is usually nonspecific with variable elevations in serum hepatic chemistry values and the white blood cell count.

A high index of suspicion for bile duct injuries after laparoscopic cholecystectomy should be maintained in any patient who fails to follow a smooth, uneventful postoperative course. Patients with suspected biliary fistulas often undergo abdominal ultrasonography or computed tomography (CT) to look for evidence of a biloma, as well as a hepatobiliary iminodiacetic acid (HIDA) scan to diagnose the leak. However, direct cholangiography (most often by ERCP) is the most sensitive test to detect a biliary fistula.[27]

Treatment options for biliary leaks include percutaneously or endoscopically placed biliary drains or stents and surgical drainage and repair of the leak. Patients with large bilomas should undergo percutaneous drainage of the fluid collection (unless surgery is performed). Endoscopic therapy has been shown to be definitive therapy in this setting, with low morbidity. Patients with leaks from the cystic duct, duct of Luschka, and T-tube tract are optimal candidates for endoscopic treatment. However, patients

with injuries of the CBD, common hepatic duct, and intrahepatic ducts can also be managed by endoscopic techniques.

The primary goal of endoscopic therapy is to decrease the pressure gradient between the bile duct and duodenum and thereby allow drainage of bile along the path of least resistance and away from the site of leakage (to permit the defect to seal). This objective can be accomplished with biliary sphincterotomy alone, stenting alone, an NBT alone, or any combination thereof.[27-31] Kaffes et al.[30] performed ES alone (n = 18), bile duct stenting alone (n = 40), or ES plus stenting (n = 31) in 89 patients, with leaks arising in 80 from the cystic duct stump (n = 48), duct of Luschka (n = 15), T-tube tract (n = 7), common duct (n = 5), an intrahepatic duct (n = 4), and an uncertain site (n = 1). The biliary fistula closure rate was 95%, and significantly more patients in the sphincterotomy-alone group required surgery to control leaks than in the other groups (22% vs. 0%; P = .001). Sandha et al.[31] recommended a systematic approach to bile duct fistulas based on their experience in 207 patients. Low-grade leaks (leak identified only after intrahepatic opacification) resolved in 91% with sphincterotomy alone (along with bile duct stone removal when present), and 100% of high-grade leaks (leak observed before intrahepatic opacification) resolved with stenting with or without ES (and stone extraction when present). Patients with clinically evident leaks not identified on cholangiography usually have a disconnected duct. Kalacyi et al.[32] showed that MRCP may be helpful in identifying the upstream disconnected bile duct and the site of injury. This occurs most frequently when there is low insertion of a right posterior sectoral duct, which is clipped along with the cystic duct.

Biliary stents are a very effective therapy for resolving biliary leaks. The observation from several uncontrolled studies that patients treated with stents alone experience equally good outcomes as patients treated with a combination of stents and sphincterotomy suggests that sphincterotomy can be avoided in patients with otherwise unobstructed ducts. Therapeutic efficacy of 7-Fr stents has been high. However, Foutch et al.[29] reported a 22% failure rate with 7-Fr stents; these fistulas resolved by upsizing the stent to 10 Fr. Larger caliber stents are certainly preferred when a concomitant stricture is present. In most reported series, stents were inserted with the proximal end positioned above the leak site. It is assumed that the stent can partially mechanically occlude the leak site, thus favoring more rapid closure. However, Bjorkman et al.[28] reported a 100% fistula closure rate in 15 patients after placing one short (2 to 3 cm) 10-Fr stent with the stent tip distal to the leak site. The results of this study confirm the importance of eliminating the transpapillary pressure gradient. Most studies that monitor drain output or reassess the fistula by repeat cholangiography report rapid closure of the fistula in most cases with cessation of bile extravasation in 1 to 7 days. The precise time when the fistula site is permanently closed is difficult to determine from reported series, however.

The available data suggest that biliary fistulas are likely to heal regardless of the therapy used to decrease the pressure gradient in the direction of the duodenum. Biliary fistulas associated with bile duct strictures will

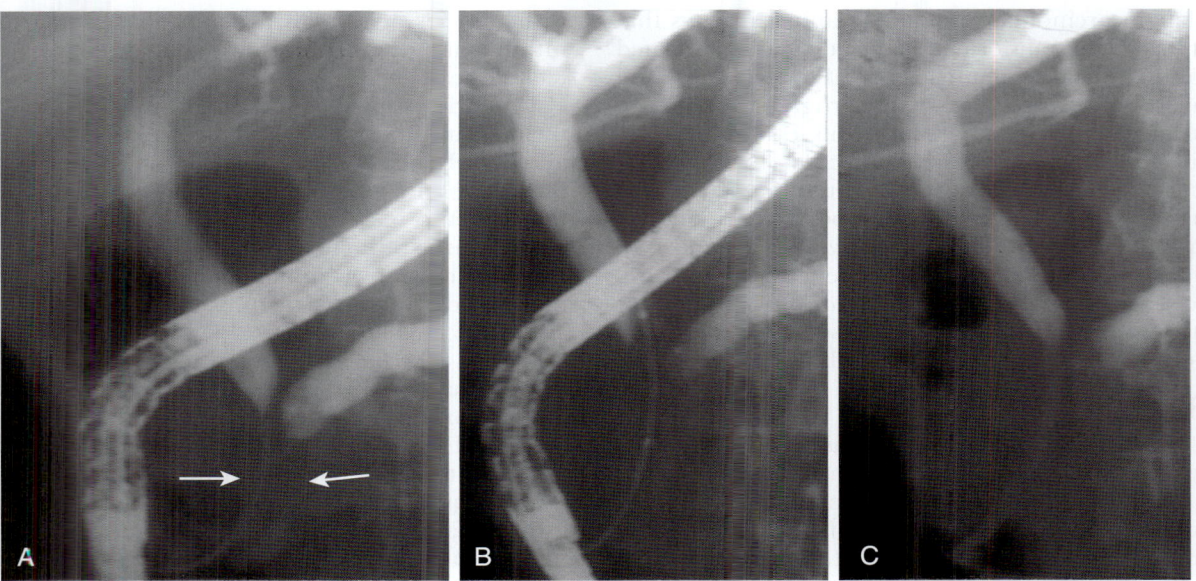

FIGURE 111.7 This patient has pancreas cancer. (A) Endoscopic retrograde cholangiopancreatography demonstrates a classic double-duct sign with strictures of both the common bile duct *(left arrow)* and the pancreatic duct *(right arrow)* in the pancreas head with upstream ductal dilation. (B) The stricture was then dilated and (C) a biliary stent was placed.

require long-term stenting, preferably with large-bore plastic stents or FCSEMSs.

MALIGNANT BILE DUCT OBSTRUCTION

Malignant biliary obstruction can occur as a consequence of pancreatic head cancer, cholangiocarcinoma, periampullary cancer, or external compression secondary to lymph node metastases. A variety of palliative options can be offered to a patient with malignant obstructive jaundice, including surgical, percutaneous, endoscopic, and medical therapy (chemotherapy and radiation therapy). Certainly a surgically fit patient with a resectable tumor after staging should be offered the option of surgical resection for cure.

Palliative Management of Malignant Biliary Obstruction

In a high-risk patient or one with an unresectable tumor, endoscopic placement of plastic or SEMS has become a widely accepted method of management (Fig. 111.7). Soehendra and Reyinders-Frederix[33] first described endoscopic biliary stenting in 1980. Since then, many advances in stent technology have been made. With plastic stents, stent patency remains a major problem, with 10-Fr stents frequently becoming occluded after 3 to 6 months. The success rate of plastic stent insertion is about 90%, and it is higher with distal than with proximal tumors. One of the major advances in stent technology was development of the SEMS. Expandable metal stents may offer improved biliary drainage with prolonged patency rates because of their large diameter and small surface area. Several types of expandable metal stents are available that are characterized by different insertion devices, methods of deployment, radial forces, covered/uncovered, and metal composition. Five prospective, randomized trials (four endoscopic and one percutaneous)[34-37] have shown that a metal expandable biliary stent occludes less frequently

and less rapidly than conventional 10- and 11.5-Fr plastic stents. Further, a 2015 meta-analysis of 19 studies involving 1989 patients (1045 SEMSs and 944 plastic stents) to compare SEMSs and plastic stents for occlusion rate and 30-day mortality rate revealed SEMS are associated with a statistically significantly lower occlusion rate, less therapeutic failure, less need for reintervention, and lower cholangitis incidence.[38] This translates into a reduction in hospitalization requirements (for cholangitis and stent change) and an overall cost savings for the metal stents. Based on data, we typically recommend that patients with a life expectancy of more than 3 months be potential candidates for the use of a SEMS. An additional indication for the use of metal stents is in the small group of patients who suffer rapid and repeated obstruction of plastic stents.

The optimal palliative management of unresectable hilar obstructing lesions remains without definitive consensus. There is considerable debate about whether patients with strictures involving the confluence require ductal decompression of both the right and left intrahepatic systems. Advocates of a single stent argue that ductal decompression of one lobe improves symptoms of cholestasis and allows jaundice to resolve. Proponents of decompressing both sides of the liver point to the 30% to 40% incidence of cholangitis, increased mortality, and death from sepsis when only one lobe is drained. De Palma et al.[39] randomized 157 consecutive patients with malignant hilar obstruction to undergo unilateral or bilateral hepatic duct drainage. In the intention-to-treat analysis, unilateral drainage was associated with significantly higher rates of successful drainage and lower early complication rates (primarily because of lower rates of cholangitis). Thirty-day mortality, late complications, and median survival were similar for the two groups. MRCP can help in selecting the liver lobe to be drained, thus avoiding injection of contrast medium into the contralateral lobe. Sawas et al.[38] recently reviewed seven studies that compared unilateral with bilateral (metal and plastic) stenting involving 634 patients (346 unilateral and 268 bilateral). SEMSs had a lower 30-day occlusion rate and lower long-term occlusion rate than plastic stents in both hilar malignant obstruction (OR 0.16; 95% CI, 0.04 to 0.62 and OR 0.28; 95% CI, 0.19 to 0.39), respectively. Bilateral stenting for hilar obstruction was not associated with a lower obstruction rate than unilateral stenting (OR 1.49; 95% CI, 0.77 to 2.89) or a lower 30-day mortality rate (OR 0.73; 95% CI, 0.29 to 1.79).

When palliation is the goal of therapy for patients with malignant bile duct obstruction, endoscopic decompression compared with percutaneous and surgical procedures[40] was associated with more frequent successful drainage (81% vs. 61%; $P < .05$), a lower complication rate (19% vs. 67%; $P < .05$), and lower 30-day mortality (15% vs. 33%; $P < .05$). Median survival was similar for the two groups (23 vs. 16 weeks). Three prospective, randomized trials[41–43] have compared endoscopic and surgical drainage for malignant distal biliary obstruction. Endoscopic stenting and surgery were equally effective palliative treatments, with endoscopic treatment having a lower early complication rate and mortality, but a higher risk for late complications such as stent blockage and gastric outlet obstruction. None of these studies demonstrated a difference in survival rates between treatment groups.

Preoperative Malignant Biliary Obstruction

Preoperative biliary drainage for malignant bile duct obstruction has been debated and still remains controversial. Studies to date have reported differing outcomes, and some have suggested that morbidity and mortality are greater in patients undergoing drainage than in those proceeding directly to surgery. In 2010 a multicenter, randomized trial compared preoperative biliary drainage with surgery alone for patients with cancer of the pancreatic head.[44] In 202 patients, 96 were assigned to undergo early surgery (within 1 week of randomization) and 106 were assigned to undergo preoperative biliary drainage. Although surgery-related complications and mortality did not differ between the two groups, the rates of serious complications were 39% (37 patients) in the early-surgery group and 74% (75 patients) in the biliary-drainage group (relative risk in the early-surgery group, 0.54; 95% CI, 0.41 to 0.71; $P < .001$). A follow-up study in 2016 using SEMS for preoperative biliary drainage similarly showed that patients in an early-surgery group had significantly less serious complications.[45] Based on available evidence, preoperative biliary drainage is unnecessary, except for patients with cholangitis or poor hepatic function, before pancreatoduodenectomy or less invasive surgery. However, neoadjuvant therapy is increasingly being used in borderline resectable and locally advanced tumors, which could delay surgery by 3 to 4 months. In these clinical situations, preoperative biliary drainage may be beneficial.

Tissue Sampling at Endoscopic Retrograde Cholangiopancreatography.
ERCP frequently provides the first opportunity to obtain a histologic or cytologic specimen from an unexplained biliary or pancreatic stricture. A variety of tissue-sampling techniques are available to the endoscopist at the time of ERCP, including bile and pancreatic juice cytology, brush cytology, intraductal forceps biopsy, intraductal fine-needle aspiration (FNA), stent cytology, and juice and tissue evaluation for aneuploidy, tumor markers (e.g., carcinoembryonic antigen [CEA], CA 19-9), p53 immunoreactivity, and K-ras oncogene mutations.

Brush cytology is the most commonly applied method of tissue sampling and the most extensively studied. Although the technical success rate is high (90% to 95%), most studies demonstrate cancer detection rates in the 20% to 60% range.[46] The sensitivity of bile duct brush cytology is higher for cholangiocarcinoma than for pancreatic cancer. Although prior research has shown that brushing the pancreatic duct may increase the diagnostic yield of brush cytology (vs. brushing the bile duct) in pancreatic cancer. EUS has emerged as the principal endoscopic method to obtain diagnostic tissue for suspected pancreatic cancer.

Endobiliary forceps biopsy allows examination of tissue specimens below the bile duct epithelium. The results of six selected studies have shown improved cancer detection rates in comparison to cytologic techniques, with a cancer detection rate of 56% in 502 patients.[47] Although it would be preferable to have one technique that would have a cancer detection rate similar to that seen with biopsy of upper gastrointestinal and colonic neoplasms, this goal has not been reached in the pancreaticobiliary tree. Investigators have therefore evaluated the added sensitivity of combining a number of tissue sampling techniques. Jailwala et al.[46] reported their results of the cumulative sensitivity of triple tissue sampling at one ERCP session with brush cytology, FNA, and forceps biopsy in 104 patients with malignant bile duct obstruction. Tissue sampling sensitivity varied according to the type of cancer; the highest yield was seen in patients with ampullary cancer. The combination of techniques was superior to individual methods, with the addition of a second or third technique increasing cancer sensitivity rates in most instances.

It is clear that the cancer detection sensitivity of these standard techniques individually is suboptimal. Methods to improve this sensitivity are therefore being evaluated. Preliminary studies suggest that the yield may be increased by using direct cholangioscopy, evaluating aspirated fluid, and tissue for aneuploidy and tumor markers such as CEA and CA 19-9. Recent investigation has suggested that evaluation of tissue or fluid for K-ras mutations is more accurate than cytology in the diagnosis of pancreatic cancer. However, some authors have identified K-ras mutations in patients with chronic pancreatitis, thus reducing the specificity of this test. Further study is warranted to determine the role of these new techniques in the assessment of pancreatic and biliary strictures.

Other ancillary cytologic tests such as digital image analysis (DIA) and fluorescence in situ hybridization (FISH) have been also developed to improve the sensitivity of routine cytology. DIA and FISH use cells obtained from ERCP brushing specimens. DIA is used to assess for aneuploidy by determining the DNA content of cells. FISH is a technique that uses fluorescently labeled DNA probes to examine cells for chromosomal abnormalities. The detection of nondiploid (DIA) or chromosomally abnormal (FISH) cells generally correlates with the presence of tumor. Recent studies showed that FISH and DIA may enhance the accuracy of standard techniques in evaluation of indeterminate pancreatobiliary strictures.[48]

CHOLEDOCHAL CYSTS AND ANOMALOUS PANCREATICOBILIARY UNION

Choledochal cysts are uncommon anomalies of the biliary tree that are manifested as cystic dilation of the intrahepatic or extrahepatic ducts (or both). These cysts are most often classified by the scheme proposed by Todani et al. Type I cysts, which involve only the extrahepatic biliary tree, are the most common form and account for 80% to 90% of all choledochal cysts. In this form of the anomaly, the cystic duct generally enters the choledochal cyst, and the right and left hepatic ducts and the intrahepatic ducts are normal in size. Type II cysts are extrapancreatic bile duct diverticula and make up 2% of reported cases. Type III cysts, which account for 1.4% to 5% of cases, are choledochoceles and most often involve only the intraduodenal part of the CBD, but occasionally the intrapancreatic portion. Type IV cysts are subdivided into type IV A, or multiple intrahepatic and extrahepatic cysts, and type IV B, or multiple extrahepatic cysts. Type IV A cysts account for approximately 19% of reported cases, whereas type IV B cysts are much less common. Finally, a type V cyst, or Caroli disease, consists of either single or multiple solely intrahepatic cysts. This form of cystic disease within the liver communicates with the biliary system, as opposed to fibrocystic disease, in which cysts filled with bile do not.

An anomalous pancreaticobiliary union is an anomaly frequently combined with choledochal cyst that is more common in the Asian population. However, anomalous pancreaticobiliary union is not associated with choledochal cyst in 22% to 37%.[49] An anomalous pancreaticobiliary union is considered to be present when the common channel is longer than 15 mm. In this situation, the pancreatic duct and bile duct junction is outside the duodenal wall and proximal to the sphincter of Oddi, thus promoting reflux of pancreatic juice into the biliary tree. Japanese criteria emphasize the junction of the ducts outside the duodenal wall.[49] Reflux of pancreatic juice has been postulated to be involved in the pathogenesis of carcinoma, which occurs in 2.5% to 17% of patients with choledochal cysts.

Surgery is the recommended treatment for most patients with choledochal cysts (most notably types I and II). Cholangiography is the gold standard for diagnosing choledochal cysts. Because ERCP and PTC are inherently invasive, MRCP should be used to assess the cyst anatomy, site of biliary origin, extent of intrahepatic and extrahepatic disease, associated biliary tract anomalies, and complications (e.g., bile duct strictures, stones); in addition, they shed light on possible therapeutic intervention, either definitive or temporizing pending surgery.

ERCP has become the procedure of choice to evaluate and treat most patients with type III choledochal cysts.[50] Patients with choledochoceles will commonly have biliary symptoms (biliary colic, cholestatic jaundice, jaundice) or unexplained pancreatitis prompting evaluation by ERCP. The endoscopic features of a choledochocele include the following: the intramural segment of the CBD protrudes into the duodenum in continuity with an enlarged papilla, the papilla is soft and smooth, ballooning of the papilla is noted with contrast injection, on contrast injection a cyst-filled structure is apparent on fluoroscopy and in continuity with the CBD, and no impacted stone is present. Several small series have reported the utility of endoscopic cyst unroofing and sphincterotomy for both pancreatic and biliary indications.[50,51] Ladas et al.[50] identified 15 symptomatic choledochocele patients among 1019 (1.5%) referred for ERCP. Twelve patients were treated by endoscopic therapy. During long-term follow-up (mean, 26 months; range, 4 to 56 months), 10 of 12 patients were asymptomatic with normal liver test results. One patient had a mild episode of cholangitis, and carcinoma developed in the choledochocele in another. This unusually high frequency of choledochoceles may represent overdiagnosis because several of these patients appeared to have only bile duct and ampulla of Vater dilation associated with ductal stones (not true choledochoceles). Although the risk for cancer in these patients is uncertain, it appears appropriate to recommend long-term follow-up in patients treated by endoscopic therapy alone. How this follow-up should be pursued remains to be clarified. Elton et al.[51] described a variant of a choledochocele that they called a dilated common channel syndrome. These patients have enlarged common pancreaticobiliary channels that were thought to have developed because of papillary stenosis. Among 77 patients treated by unroofing and sphincterotomy, 77% had complete and long-lasting resolution of symptoms.

Management of anomalous pancreaticobiliary union in the absence of a choledochal cyst is unclear. Because of the high risk for gallbladder cancer, prophylactic cholecystectomy has been recommended by some.[49] In one series of 15 patients with an anomalous pancreaticobiliary union (7 had choledochal cysts) and recurrent pancreatitis or abdominal pain (or both) treated by ES, 13 had resolution or a reduction in the frequency of pancreatitis and pain.[52] Ng et al.[53] similarly reported resolution of pain and pancreatitis in 5 of 6 patients with a long common channel after endoscopic therapy. Whether patients with anomalous junctions without choledochal cysts treated by sphincterotomy need surveillance for cancer remains unclear.

PANCREAS DIVISUM

Pancreas divisum, the most common congenital variant of pancreatic ductal anatomy, occurs when the ductal systems of the dorsal and ventral pancreatic ducts fail to fuse during the second month of gestation. With nonunion of the ducts, the major portion of pancreatic exocrine juice drains into the duodenum via the dorsal duct and minor papilla. It has been proposed that a relative obstruction to pancreatic exocrine juice flow through the minor papilla could result in pancreatic pain or acute pancreatitis (or both) in a subpopulation of patients with pancreas divisum. Endoscopic attempts to decompress the dorsal duct in symptomatic patients with pancreas divisum have been performed primarily by dilation, stent insertion, minor papilla sphincterotomy, or any combination of these

TABLE 111.1 Approximate Frequencies of Complications After Endoscopic Retrograde Cholangiopancreatography (ERCP) and Sphincterotomy (%)

Complication	AVERAGE-RISK PATIENTS		HIGH-RISK PATIENTS*	
	ERCP	Sphincterotomy	ERCP	Sphincterotomy
Pancreatitis	3	5	8	12
Bleeding	0.2	5	0.4	3.5
Perforation	0.1	8	0.3	1.5
Infection	0.1	5	2	2
Sedation reaction or cardiopulmonary	0.5	5	2	2
Total[†]	3.9[‡]	3[‡]	12.7[‡]	21[‡]

*Certain patient characteristics and technical aspects of the procedure increase the risk for complications, including suspected sphincter of Oddi dysfunction, recurrent pancreatitis, difficult cannulation, precut sphincterotomy, coagulopathy, renal dialysis, cirrhosis, and advanced cardiopulmonary disease.
[†]Some patients have more than one complication.
[‡]Approximate severity of complications: mild, 70%; moderate, 20%; and severe, 10%.

techniques.[54–56] Lans et al.[54] reported their results of a randomized controlled trial of long-term (12 months) stenting of the minor papilla in patients with recurrent pancreatitis (n = 19). Follow-up continued for at least 12 months after stent removal. Stented patients had fewer hospitalizations and episodes of pancreatitis (P < .05) and were more frequently judged to be improved (90% vs. 11% for controls; P < .05). Although the symptomatic improvement after this therapy has been encouraging, multiple stent changes are generally required, and the risk for stent-related complications is considerable. Ertan[55] reported that stent-induced ductal changes developed in 21 of 25 patients (84%) with pancreas divisum after stenting periods of 6 to 9 months.

A more permanent enlargement of the minor papilla orifice is possible with sphincterotomy. Lehman et al.[56] attempted to evaluate the efficacy of minor papilla ES for patients with pancreas divisum (n = 52) and disabling pancreatic-type pain (n = 24), idiopathic acute recurrent pancreatitis (n = 17), or chronic pancreatitis (n = 11). A short 4- to 7-Fr stent was placed in the minor papilla and a 3- to 6-mm sphincterotomy was performed over the stent, with the stent used as a guide for cutting and a bridge to prevent edema–induced closure of the cut. The stent was then removed in approximately 2 weeks. The mean duration of preintervention symptoms was 5.1 years, and follow-up averaged 1.7 years, with all patients being observed for at least 6 months after therapy. Although 76.5% of the acute recurrent pancreatitis group improved after therapy, only 26% of the chronic pain group (P = .002) and 27% of the chronic pancreatitis group (P = .01) benefited. Similarly, when compared with the chronic pain and chronic pancreatitis groups, the acute recurrent pancreatitis group had a significant reduction in mean pain score and number of hospital days per month required for severe pain or pancreatitis (or both). These discordant results in responsiveness to therapy for the acute recurrent pancreatitis group versus the chronic pancreatitis and chronic pain groups were noted in several surgical series evaluating dorsal duct decompression and other endoscopic series. Pancreatitis complicating therapy occurred in 15% but in general was mild and managed conservatively. Stent-induced dorsal duct changes occurred in 50%. Heyries et al.[57] reported

that 22 of 24 patients (92%) had no further episodes of pancreatitis during a median follow-up period of 39 months (range, 24 to 105 months) after minor papilla sphincterotomy in eight patients and dorsal duct stenting for a mean time of 8 months in 16 patients. When summarizing eight published studies that evaluated the efficacy of minor papilla therapy in 127 patients, no further attacks occurred in 81% monitored for a mean of 27 months after the intervention.[58] The results of these studies suggest that patients with pancreas divisum and acute recurrent pancreatitis are good candidates for endoscopic therapy, whereas patients with chronic pancreatitis or chronic pain alone (or both) do not appear to do as well.

ADVERSE EVENTS OF ENDOSCOPIC RETROGRADE CHOLANGIOPANCREATOGRAPHY

Complications of ERCP and ES are undesirable outcomes related to some portion of the procedure or sedation required for the procedure. Unsuccessful cannulation, stent placement, or stone removal and making an incorrect diagnosis are failures of the procedure but are not generally included as complications. Table 111.1 lists the more common complications of diagnostic and therapeutic ERCP.

ENDOSCOPIC ULTRASOUND

BACKGROUND

Ultrasound is widely used in modern medicine for diagnostic and therapeutic purposes, given its ability to provide rapid, real-time images without radiation exposure; however, the equipment used to collect and process this information varies among medical specialties. Knowledge of the basic principles of ultrasound and how they are applied to EUS is essential to understanding the utility of EUS in hepatobiliary and pancreatic disease.

Sound is a form of energy that is propagated through mediums such as air, water, or tissue as vibrations. At low frequencies (20 to 20,000 Hz) sound is audible to the human ear. Ultrasound is defined as sound vibrations that are propagated at frequencies higher than the audible range (≥20,000 Hz). This high-frequency mechanical energy disrupts and displaces molecules from their average position, which may propagate the oscillatory wave in a three-dimensional manner.

The acoustic velocity, or how the ultrasound is propagated through a specific medium, is dependent on the density, compressibility, and bulk modulus of the medium through which the wave is traveling. Density is defined as the mass per unit volume of medium, whereas compressibility is the decrease in volume as pressure is applied to the medium. Bulk modulus represents the stiffness of the medium and is defined as the negative ratio of the pressure applied to the fractional change in volume of the medium. Bulk modulus and compressibility most affect the acoustic velocity because they change at a faster rate than density does.

When ultrasound waves and tissue interface, the waves may reflect, refract, scatter, or be absorbed. The energy that is reflected creates a feedback signal received by a transducer. Transducers convert electrical signals into mechanical ultrasound signals, which are propagated onto a medium. The mechanical energy that is reflected back to the transducer is processed into electrical energy thereby providing the image of the tissue.

In EUS, the transducer on the tip of the endoscope assists in providing real-time images of the intramural gastrointestinal tract and organs and adjacent structures that otherwise would not be visible. Given the relative anatomic proximity of the pancreaticobiliary organs relative to the stomach and duodenum, the liver, pancreas, lymph nodes, and bile ducts/gallbladder can easily be examined. Echoendoscopes may be classified as radial or linear ("curved linear array" [CLA]). Radial echoendoscopes provide a 360-degree view in a plane perpendicular to the long axis of the echoendoscope, while the linear EUS provides images longitudinal to the long axis of the echoendoscope. Radial echoendoscopes are appropriate for diagnosis only; however, the CLA echoendoscopes, which contain an elevator and therapeutic channel, allow for the passage of aspiration/biopsy needles, guidewires, and stents under direct endosonographic visualization and are suitable for diagnostic and therapeutic purposes.

The development of CLA echoendoscopes has led to the development of EUS-guided tissue acquisition techniques, including FNA and more recently fine-needle biopsy (FNB) enabling histologic sampling. The goal of EUS-FNA and EUS-FNB is to provide the largest sample size, while minimizing adverse events. EUS-FNA needles are currently available in 19-gauge, 20-gauge, 22-gauge, and 25-gauge sizes with adjustable sheaths that can be advanced between 1 and 8 cm. To aid in obtaining an adequate sample, specific techniques can be used including fanning or use of negative-pressure suction, although this may result in increased blood contamination. Needle selection is often dependent on the target lesion—for example, in pancreatic cysts, a larger bore 19-gauge needle may be required to aspirate thick, mucinous cystic fluid.

INDICATIONS

EUS may be used for number of diagnostic and therapeutic purposes. Gastrointestinal subepithelial lesions, suspected bile duct stones, and pancreatic cysts, including main duct and side branch duct intraductal papillary mucinous neoplasias, may be detected using EUS. Diagnostic yield

is increased by use of EUS-FNA, which provides histologic and cytologic samples of gastrointestinal tissue, nongastrointestinal masses, and lymph nodes. The application of EUS-FNA to obtain tissue has been found to be up to 90% accurate in the diagnosis and staging of luminal and pancreaticobiliary disease,[59] and the ability to obtain tissue for preoperative diagnosis has been demonstrated to lower the likelihood of surgery for benign indications.[60–62]

Therapeutic indications of EUS include aspiration of fluid from pancreatic cysts, injection of solutions (alcohol, steroids, anesthetics), accessing adjacent luminal and nonluminal structures for diagnostic and therapeutic purposes. The EUS-guided pancreaticobiliary therapeutic interventions include pancreatitis-associated inflammatory pancreatic fluid collection drainage, pancreaticobiliary duct access/drainage, gallbladder drainage, celiac plexus neurolysis/block, gastroenterostomy creation, and ablative therapies. Ablative therapies include EUS–fine-needle injection (FNI) of local chemotherapeutics in malignancy. Most recently, the development of new imaging technologies such as needle-based confocal laser endomicroscopy, contrast-enhanced ultrasonography, and elastography have increased the diagnostic capabilities of EUS.

PANCREATIC DISEASE

EUS examination of the pancreas is technically challenging and requires examination from multiple positions for a complete evaluation of the entire pancreas; however, when mastered, it allows for the most sensitive nonoperative imaging for identification of benign or malignant pancreatic lesions.

Endoscopic Ultrasound in Inflammatory Diseases of Pancreas

Inflammation of the pancreas begins in the microscopic exocrine glands of the pancreas and progresses to macroscopic changes such as enlarged or atrophic pancreas, ductal abnormalities, cysts, and later calcifications, which indicates chronic pancreas inflammation. Traditional methods of imaging the pancreas in its inflammatory state such as CT or magnetic resonance imaging (MRI) may assist in the diagnosis of late-stage pancreatitis by detecting things such as duct size, cysts, and calcification.[63] EUS, however, may be more sensitive in disease detection because it can visualize small parenchymal changes.

The Rosemont criteria were developed as a consensus of major and minor EUS imaging findings for the diagnosis of acute and chronic pancreatic inflammation. However, these criteria have not been found to improve interobserver variability, and have not been validated against the conventional diagnostic criteria.[64–66] Both systems comment on hyperechoic foci, lobules and strands, cysts, irregular duct contour, side branches, and dilated ducts as criteria for the diagnosis of inflammation of the pancreas. It is widely accepted that calcifications are diagnostic for chronic pancreatitis regardless of the other criteria that may or may not be met.

Endoscopic Ultrasound in Pancreatic Tumors (Adenocarcinoma, Pancreatic Neuroendocrine Tumors)

Current literature demonstrates that EUS is more sensitive in the diagnosis of pancreatic tumors than traditional

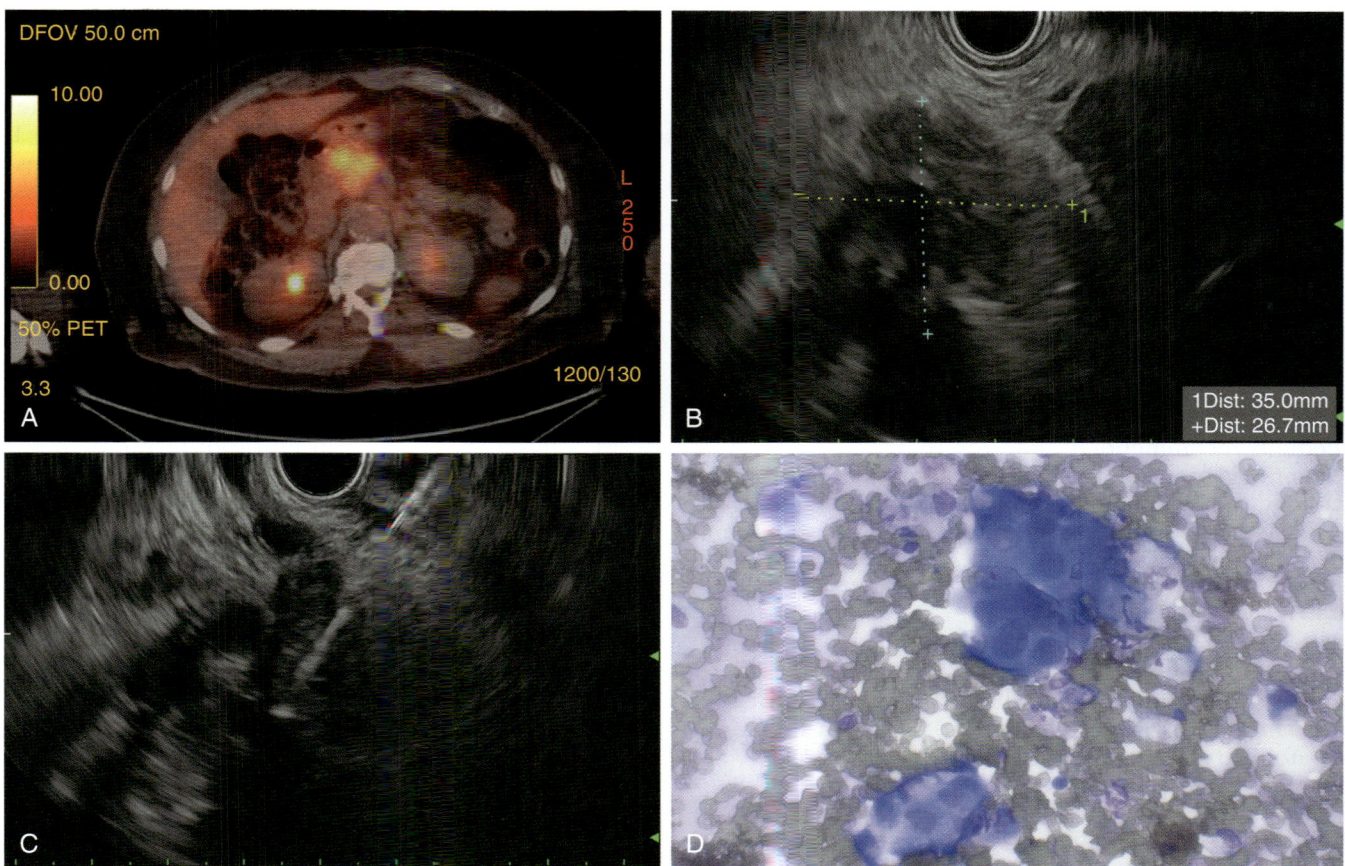

FIGURE 111.8 (A) Positron emission tomography (*PET*) computed tomography of the abdomen and pelvis, demonstrating an ill-defined hypermetabolic mass in region of pancreas head/neck measuring up to 4.7 × 4.5 cm. (B) Endoscopic ultrasound (EUS) confirmed a large 4-cm, hypoechoic irregular mass in the pancreatic neck with vascular involvement, including encasement of the splenic vein and splenic artery and superior mesenteric vein abutment. (C) EUS-guided fine-needle aspiration is performed with a 25-gauge needle. (D) Preliminary, on-site cytology reveals adenocarcinoma. (Images courtesy Uzma D. Siddiqui, MD.)

imaging modalities, such as CT and MRI (Fig. 111.8). A summary of published literature assessing EUS for the detection of a pancreatic mass has found a sensitivity of 95% (range, 85% to 100%). However, it is important to note that some of the studies included in this summary may have favored EUS because they included benign pancreatic disease and ampullary tumors. Subset analyses in this summary found that EUS (98%) is more sensitive than CT (77%), MRI (88%), transabdominal ultrasound (76%), positron emission tomography (87%), and ERCP (90%).[29] EUS has also been reported to have higher sensitivity (90% to 100%) for small pancreatic tumors (<20 mm) when compared with both CT (40% to 67%) and MRI (33%).[67,68] Despite these promising statistics, EUS is less successful in identifying patients with pancreatic cancer in patients with comorbid chronic pancreatitis, diffuse infiltration of carcinoma, recent episode of acute pancreatitis, or prominent ventral/dorsal split. Therefore a follow-up imaging study is recommended in patients with equivocal results owing to their pancreatic inflammation.

Given its high sensitivity in detecting masses, EUS is often also used tool in the staging of pancreatic tumors using the American Joint Committee on Cancer (AJCC)

TNM classification system (tumor extension, lymph node, and distant metastases). However, wide ranges have been reported for the accuracy of EUS in T staging (63% to 94%) and N staging (41% to 86%). In pancreatic cancer, EUS alone is 28% to 92% sensitive in detecting metastatic adenopathy and 42% to 91% sensitive in detecting malignant vascular invasion. EUS is limited in assessing nonnodal metastatic disease due to the constraints of anatomic visualization. Currently, determination of resectability should be completed with multimodality assessment, including radiologic (CT or MRI) in conjunction with EUS.[69,70] EUS-FNA increases the sensitivity and specificity of EUS to 85% to 89% and 98% to 99%, respectively.[71,72] Because there is no clear consensus on what imaging studies provided the highest diagnostic yield, institutional factors, such as equipment and expertise available, should be taken into account when determining the best method of diagnosis.

Endoscopic Ultrasound in Pancreatic Cysts

Pancreatic cysts may represent benign, premalignant, or malignant neoplasms, and EUS alone is insufficient in this diagnosis. A multimodality approach combining EUS, fluid cytology, carcinoembryonic level, and mucin staining is used to differentiate the etiology of pancreatic cysts. After a pancreatic cyst is identified in EUS, the size, location (including adjacent vessels and organs), locoregional or distant metastases, wall thickness, septations, and echo-dense mucus/debris should be noted. If the cyst has a thick wall, a nearby solid mass, or a mural nodule, or if it causes focal dilation of the main pancreatic duct (5 to 9 mm) or another large pancreatic duct (>10 mm), there is an increased likelihood of malignant transformation.

EUS-FNA provides additional data to assist in the diagnosis of pancreatic cysts. Complete aspiration of the cystic contents is recommended to increase sample size and to theoretically decrease the chances of infection. If there is concern for a vascular component, a smaller gauge needle is recommended; however, there are no specific recommended needle sizes. Cyst fluid may be analyzed for cytology, tumor markers (e.g., carcinoembryonic antigen or CA 19-9), or molecular markers (e.g., K-ras mutation, *VHL, RNF43, CTNNB1*, or *GNAS*).

HEPATOBILIARY DISEASE

EUS examination of the entire hepatobiliary system may be challenging depending on the patient's anatomy; however, extrahepatic bile ducts and portions of the liver should be visible to diagnose and treat common hepatobiliary diseases.

Endoscopic Ultrasound in Bile Duct, Gallbladder, and Ampullary Lesions

ERCP is considered gold standard in the diagnosis and removal of CBD stones. However, it carries significant risks of complications and death (4% to 6.85% and 0.1% to 0.33%, respectively), even when performed by experienced endoscopists.[73-76] Furthermore, patients often have an endoscopic sphincterotomy with the ERCP, which carries higher complication and mortality rates (5% to 10% and <1%, respectively). In patients with low to moderate probability of CBD stones, this risk of complications or mortality is unacceptable.

The most accurate diagnostic tools for CBD stones are EUS and MRCP.[77-79] While MRCP is also a noninvasive and radiation-free imaging technique in the diagnosis of choledocholithiasis, its limited availability due to cost and expertise, limited spatial resolution, and ability to diagnose CBD stones in the periampullary region make it less advantageous overall than EUS in the diagnosis of CBD.[80] EUS is superior in its spatial resolution (0.1 vs. 1 to 1.5 mm) and in its sensitivity for detecting stones less than 10 mm when compared to MRCP.[81-83] When EUS was compared with MRCP in the detection of CBD stones, it trended toward a higher sensitivity (93% vs. 33% to 85%) and specificity (38% to 96% vs. 89% to 93%).[84,85]

The use of noninvasive imaging such as EUS to guide the decision for an ERCP has decreased the number of inappropriate bile duct instrumentation in 67.1% of patients and has reduced the relative risk of complications to 0.35.[86] Therefore it is generally agreed upon that ERCP may be a first-line therapy in patients at a high risk for CBD stones but should be preceded by noninvasive imaging in moderate-risk patients.[87-89] Ideally EUS and ERCP, if indicated, would be performed in one session.

Transabdominal ultrasound (TUS) is an inexpensive method of detecting gallstones with an excellent sensitivity and specificity (97% and 95%, respectively).[90] However, its sensitivity decreases in obese patients, given their thick abdominal walls or in small stones (<3 mm). In cases where TUS results are equivocal but there remains a high clinical suspicion for gallstones, bile crystal analysis has been used for diagnosis. EUS has been found to be as accurate as biliary crystal analysis for the diagnosis of microlithiasis.[91] This is particularly useful in the diagnosis of idiopathic pancreatitis, which is often caused by biliary sludge or microlithiasis. In studies of patients with idiopathic pancreatitis, EUS diagnosed gallbladder sludge or microlithiasis in 40% of patients, and detected a cause for the acute pancreatitis in 80% of patients.[92]

EUS has also become a useful tool in the diagnosis of biliary obstruction, such as bile duct strictures and neoplasia, and in small gallbladder polyps (5 to 10 mm). EUS alone has 78% sensitivity and 84% specificity in the diagnosis of malignant biliary structures, but when combined with EUS-FNA, the sensitivity increases to 80% to 88% and specificity to 97% to 100%.[93-95] The diagnosis of proximal strictures, such as Klatskin tumors, is less sensitive given its distance from the EUS probe. In the detection of polyps, EUS was better than TUS at diagnosing polyps smaller than 2 cm in size (87% vs. 52%, respectively).[96] Overall, EUS is better at characterizing gallbladder polyps than TUS and should be used in the diagnosis of small gallbladder polyps.

EUS is also helpful in the diagnosis of ampullary tumors, which originate from the pancreaticobiliary-duodenal junction proximal to the sphincter of Oddi. Diagnosis of ampullary tumors is limited because many tumors extend intramurally, and the pathologic difference between inflammatory changes and biopsies may be an inadequate sample or be difficult for a pathologist to differentiate, especially in the case of inflammatory cells versus low-grade dysplasia. EUS has been studied in the diagnosis of ampullary tumors, and while it has high sensitivity (92%), its specificity (75%) is low.[97] Given its low specificity, EUS should be used as a follow-up in patients who are suspected to have an ampullary tumor by endoscopy but have inconclusive biopsies secondary to intramural spread; EUS-FNA may be safely used.[98] After diagnosis, EUS is the most reliable method for preoperative staging of ampullary lesions.[99,100] EUS is the most accurate method to determine the primary tumor stage (T) of ampullary carcinoma, which determines the choice of treatment.[101] In its early stage when the primary tumor is in situ or only limited to the ampulla of Vater or sphincter of Oddi, without duodenal mucosa invasion, the primary tumor may be endoscopically resected. The tumor must be surgically resected at higher stages.

Endoscopic Ultrasound-Guided Biliary/Gallbladder and Pancreatic Duct Drainage

EUS-guided gallbladder drainage (EUS-GBD) is an emerging treatment for acute cholecystitis in high-risk patients. This approach was first described in 2007, and since then several case reports have described the utility and complications of EUS-GBD.[102] The largest study to date has published a series of 30 patients who had a technical and clinical success rate of 97% and 100%, respectively, with two cases complicated by pneumoperitoneum.[103] Other complications that have been reported include bile leak, bile peritonitis, stent migration, hematoma, and abdominal pain.[104] EUS-GBD is technically limited in cases where the gallbladder wall is thickened and its lumen is not distended, and when the gallbladder is located more than 2 cm farther from the gastrointestinal lumen.

In patients with severe pancreatic duct stenosis, calculus in the head of the pancreas, disconnected pancreatic ducts, inaccessible ampullae, or postsurgical altered anatomy, the pancreatic duct may not be easily accessed through conventional transpapillary endoscopic retrograde pancreatography. In these cases, two separate EUS-guided pancreatic duct drainage (EUS-PDL) approaches (direct "anterograde" and "rendezvous") have been described that can provide access and drainage of the pancreatic duct. Further discussion on these procedures is found in a subsequent chapter of this textbook.

Endoscopic Ultrasound-Guided Ablation and Celiac Plexus Neurolysis

The utility of EUS has progressed from diagnostic imaging to tissue diagnosis and recently to provide endoscopic therapies. Radiofrequency ablation (RFA) and celiac plexus neurolysis are two such newer therapies in the treatment of pancreatic diseases. RFA uses thermal injury of the target tissue to induce necrosis. This is accomplished by using EUS to introduce a needle into the target tissue, inducing necrosis in the tissue 1 to 3 cm surrounding the needle catheter. In initial case studies in humans, EUS-RFA has been shown to decrease the size in two out of five pancreatic ductal adenocarcinomas and two out of two patients with neuroendocrine tumors and a complete resolution of six out of six pancreatic cystic neoplasms.

Pancreatic neoplasms or chronic pancreatitis is thought to cause severe pain in some patients because the efferent nerves from the pancreas travel within the celiac plexus. The celiac plexus is in the retrogastric space, which gives it an ideal location for targeted injection therapies in the treatment of this pain. It was first described with promising results in 1996 in the treatment of pain from pancreatic cancer.[105] Nearly 80% of patients had improvement in their pain scores after neurolysis of the celiac plexus, and the effect was sustained for 24 weeks. However, this effect is not appreciated in the treatment of pain associated with chronic pancreatitis. In patients with chronic pancreatitis, only 50% achieve some pain relief with results lasting on average 1 month.[106,107]

NOVEL TECHNIQUES

Elastography

Benign and malignant tumors may be differentiated by differences in the elasticity, or hardness, of the tumors. Malignant tumors are oftentimes stiffer when compared with benign tumors. Elastography is a method to assess the elasticity of tumors in real-time to potentially diagnose tumors as benign or malignant. Real-time sonoelastography refers to a method by which small compressions of the transducer or surrounding vessel movements is used to estimate tissue strain. The strain is calculated by the relative change in tissue with each compression through a complex algorithm and converted into a hue color scale transposed over the grayscale ultrasound image.[108] The hue color scale is a numerical representation of the elasticity and may be averaged over a specified area for quantified comparisons.

EUS elastography has been found to be sensitive and specific in the differential diagnosis of focal pancreatic masses (92.3% and 80.0%) and in the differential diagnosis of lymph nodes (91.8% and 82.5%).[109] Given its high sensitivity, specificity, and interobserver variability with kappa coefficient (κ) 0.785 and κ 0.657 for pancreatic masses and lymph nodes, respectively, EUS elastography is superior to conventional grayscale EUS. It has been suggested as a tool for patients with pancreatic masses and negative EUS-FNA to increase the yield of FNA by differentiating benign and malignant lymph nodes.[99,110]

Contrast-Enhanced Endoscopic Ultrasound

Contrast-enhanced (CE) EUS is showing promise in detecting microvasculature within lesions and may also help characterize autoimmune pancreatitis. In this technique, microbubbles are injected into a peripheral vein and circulate through the pancreas and highlight the vasculature of target organs. These features of contrast-enhanced EUS may help direct FNA or core needle biopsy of lesions because malignant tumors have a different vascular pattern than normal tissue. For example, pancreatic adenocarcinomas are known to have hypovascular patterns in 90% of cases based on contrast-enhanced CT or angiography. CE EUS may be used to identify and biopsy the lesion immediately with EUS-FNA to obtain multiple diagnostics in one study. Through this method, CE EUS has a sensitivity of 92% and specificity of 100% in the diagnosis of pancreatic tumors.[111] Furthermore, CE EUS has been used to identify 94% of mural nodules, with 75% of these correctly identified as high-grade dysplasia or invasive carcinoma.[112]

Endoscopic Ultrasound-Guided Gastroenterostomy

Both benign pancreatic disease including advanced chronic pancreatitis and malignancy can result in duodenal or gastric outlet obstruction and result in an inability to tolerate oral food intake. Typically this is treated surgically with a gastrojejunostomy or endoscopically with balloon dilation or a placement of SEMS. In 2013, a novel EUS-guided gastrojejunostomy technique was reported using lumen-opposing metal stent (LAMS).[113] It is a technique that involves using a specially created double-balloon enteric tube (Tokyo Medical University type; Create Medic, Yokohama, Japan) to help stabilize the small bowel adjacent to the stomach in the area of the puncture and LAMS placement. In animal studies, different types of LAMS (e.g., cautery-enhanced LAMS) were used to create the gastrojejunostomy, there were no signs of infection, and the animals maintained normal eating habits for 1 month post procedure. At the 1-month follow-up endoscopy, the LAMS was patent, and once removed, a mature stoma was noted that allowed for easy scope passage from the stomach into the jejunum.[113] In the first prospective human study, EUS-guided double-balloon occluded gastrojejunostomy bypass using LAMS was performed in 20 patients in 2015. The technical success rate was 90%; however, in the two failed cases, there was misdeployment of the distal flange, resulting in pneumoperitoneum and perforation.[114] EUS-guided gastroenterostomy is a promising technique; however, prospective, multicenter trials as well as equipment designed specifically for this application are needed.

Needle-Based Confocal Laser Endomicroscopy

Using a low-power laser for tissue illumination with subsequent detection of the fluorescence of light reflected from the tissue through a pinhole, confocal laser endomicroscopy (CLE) provides real-time cellular imaging and evaluation of tissue architecture during endoscopy through the use of topical and/or intravenous fluorescence contrast agents to generate images with a resolution similar to that of traditional histologic examination. Needle-based confocal endomicroscopy (nCLE) uses the AQ-Flex 19 probe and can be passed through a 19-gauge EUS-FNA needle. A preliminary study by Konda et al.[115] in pancreatic cystic lesions identified the highly specific finding of papillary (finger-like projections for intraductal papillary mucinous neoplasms (IPMNs). However, due to variations in the location of the probe within a cyst and the epithelium of IPMNs themselves, nCLE was associated with a low sensitivity of 59%. In 2015, Napoleon et al.[116] identified a new imaging criterion for diagnosing serous cystadenomas: superficial vascular network (SVN). Although nCLE again had a low sensitivity of 69%, if the SVN was visualized, it was 100% specific for serous cystadenomas, with a 100% positive predictive value. nCLE is a promising technique that needs further investigation to confirm ease of learning, diagnostic accuracy, reproducibility by independent investigators and cost-benefit analysis.

ADVERSE EVENTS

Adverse events in EUS are minimized by its few absolute contraindications to intervention, including high-risk sedation, coagulopathy (INR >1.5), thrombocytopenia (platelets <50,000), or anatomic structures that do not allow for a biopsy.[1–120] Relative contraindications include new diagnosis of cancer that has not been worked up, altered anatomy that makes accessing anatomic sites difficult, and mild coagulopathy or thrombocytopenia.[121,122]

The most common risks of performing diagnostic and therapeutic EUS on patients who do not have any contraindications to the procedure include perforation, bleeding, infection, pancreatitis, and the known medical risks of all procedures under sedation (e.g., deep vein thrombosis, cardiovascular events). The incidence of perforation secondary to EUS is higher than the incidence of patients undergoing upper endoscopy (0% to 0.4% vs. 0.03% to 0.11%).[123–127] This is likely because moving the rigid EUS tip makes it more difficult to navigate around

complex anatomy (e.g., stenosis, diverticula). While some luminal bleeding is expected in EUS-FNA, EUS-FNB, and EUS-FNI, the incidence of clinically extraluminal bleeding has been reported to be 1.3%.[128] The incidence of bacteremia in patients undergoing EUS and EUS-FNA was 2% and 4%, respectively.[129] The introduction of prophylactic periprocedural antibiotics has greatly diminished the rate of infections in the EUS-FNA of cysts.[129–131] EUS-FNA of solid lesions carries a 0.3% to 0.6% incidence of pancreatitis, and the risk increases in cystic lesions to 1% to 2%.[132,133]

DIRECT PANCREATOSCOPY AND CHOLANGIOSCOPY

CHOLANGIOSCOPY

Cholangioscopy or choledoscopy is another tool frequently used to evaluate and treat difficult bile duct stones or indeterminate biliary strictures. This endoscopic technique carries the advantage of direct vision therapy. The traditional "mother and baby" cholangioscope model needed two endoscopists to manage it and consumes more time. The only available single-operator cholangioscope is the SpyGlass System by Boston Scientific Corp (Natick, Massachusetts). Although it also has a "mother and baby" conformation, it can be used by one endoscopist. One of the therapeutic indications of the cholangioscope is intracorporeal electrohydraulic or laser lithotripsy for choledocholithiasis (Fig. 111.9). Intracorporeal lithotripsy is very useful in difficult-extraction biliary stones by ERCP for any reason (large size, location in the intrahepatic biliary ducts, hard consistency, impacted, piston shape, small bile duct, sigmoid bile duct shape).[134] When compared with ESWL, stone clearance of the bile duct was superior with intracorporeal laser lithotripsy (97% vs. 73%; $P < .05$), with fewer number of sessions and reduced time of treatment.[135] However, it does carry a 7% complication rate and is not widely available at all centers, which limits its utility.[15]

PANCREATOSCOPY

Pancreatoscopes provide direct visualization of the pancreatic ducts at the time of ERCP for the diagnosis and treatment of pancreatic duct stones, with or without lithotripsy. Furthermore, pancreatoscopes may assist in evaluating pancreatic duct strictures through direct visualization and by biopsies. While its use has been limited to tertiary referral centers, advances in instrumentation and ease of use are promising for more widespread use in the future. Pancreatoscopy by visual inspection alone has a sensitivity of 87% and specificity of 86% in the detection of pancreatic duct neoplasia; however, it increases to 91% and 95%, respectively, when combined with pancreatoscopy-guided tissue sampling.[137] Complication rates have been reported to range from 7% to 12%.[137,138]

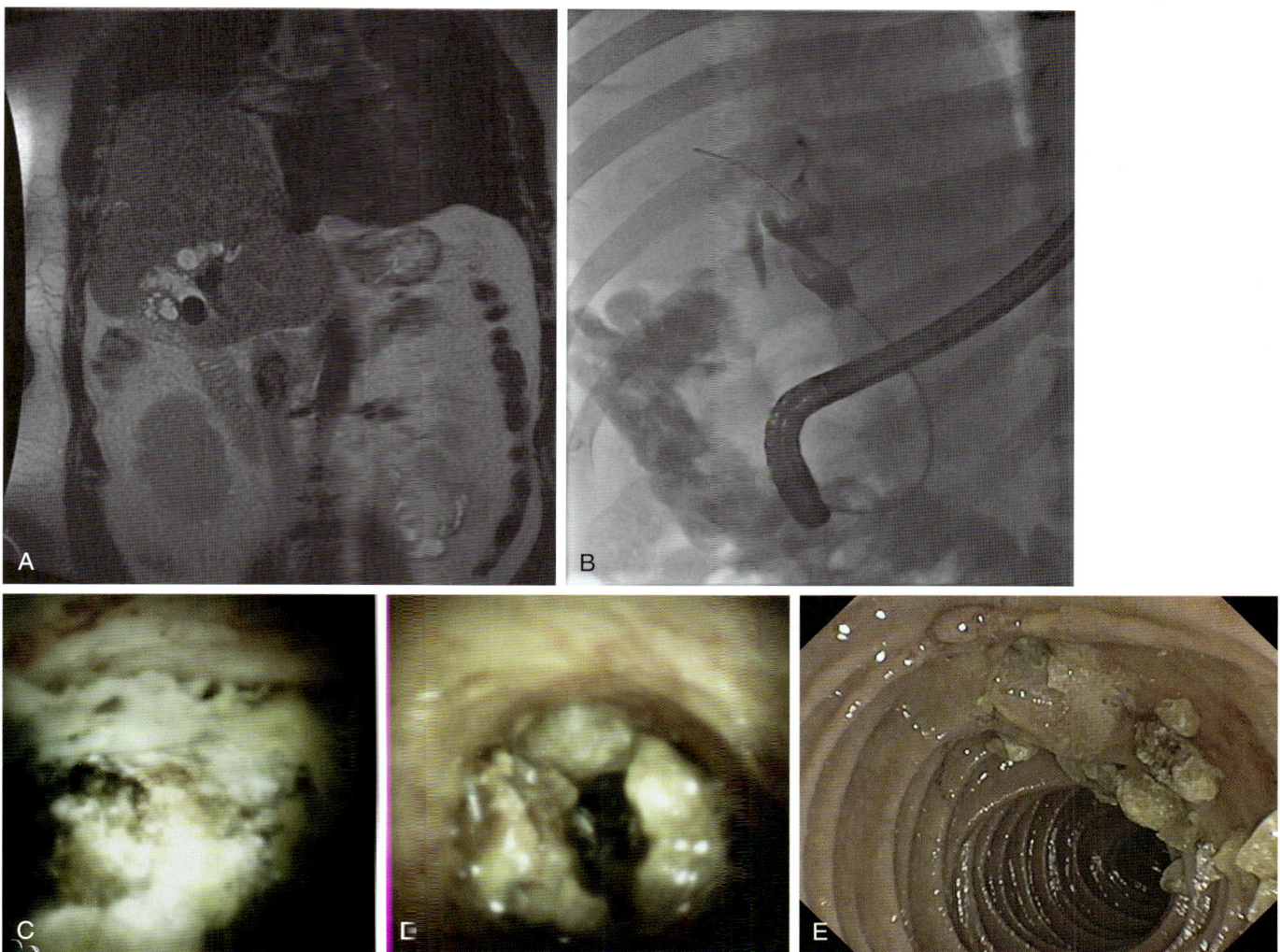

FIGURE 111.9 (A) Magnetic resonance imaging-magnetic resonance cholangiopancreatography demonstrating a large stone at the level of the Klatskin point measuring 2 cm causing significant intra- and extrahepatic biliary dilatation in the liver. (B) Endoscopic retrograde cholangiopancreatography cholangiogram confirming the presence of a large stone. (C) Direct cholangioscopy visualizes the large stone to allow for directed intracorporeal electrohydraulic lithotripsy (EHL). (D) After EHL the stone is partially fragmented. (E) Stone fragments were then successfully removed from the common bile duct using a mechanical lithotripsy basket and 15-mm balloon. (Images courtesy Uzma D. Siddiqui, MD.)

REFERENCES

1. Committee ASop, Early DS, Ben-Menachem T, et al. Appropriate use of GI endoscopy. *Gastrointest Endosc.* 2012;75:1127-1131.
2. Adler DG, Lieb JG 2nd, Cohen J, et al. Quality indicators for ERCP. *Gastrointest Endosc.* 2015;81:54-66.
3. Committee ASop, Maple JT, Ben-Menachem T, et al. The role of endoscopy in the evaluation of suspected choledocholithiasis. *Gastrointest Endosc.* 2010;71:1-9.
4. Yoo KS, Lehman GA. Endoscopic management of biliary ductal stones. *Gastroenterol Clin North Am.* 2010;39:209-227, viii.
5. Sauerbruch T, Delius M, Paumgartner G, et al. Fragmentation of gallstones by extracorporeal shock waves. *N Engl J Med.* 1986;314:818-822.
6. Bergman JJ, Rauws EA, Tijssen JG, Tytgat GN, Huibregtse K. Biliary endoprostheses in elderly patients with endoscopically irretrievable common bile duct stones: report on 117 patients. *Gastrointest Endosc.* 1995;42:195-201.
7. Neoptolemos JP, Carr-Locke DL, London NJ, Bailey IA, James D, Fossard DP. Controlled trial of urgent endoscopic retrograde cholangiopancreatography and endoscopic sphincterotomy versus conservative treatment for acute pancreatitis due to gallstones. *Lancet.* 1988;2:979-983.
8. Fan ST, Lai EC, Mok FP, Lo CM, Zheng SS, Wong J. Early treatment of acute biliary pancreatitis by endoscopic papillotomy. *N Engl J Med.* 1993;328:228-232.
9. Sharma VK, Howden CW. Metaanalysis of randomized controlled trials of endoscopic retrograde cholangiography and endoscopic sphincterotomy for the treatment of acute biliary pancreatitis. *Am J Gastroenterol.* 1999;94:3211-3214.
10. Leung JW, Chung SC, Sung JJ, Banez VP, Li AK. Urgent endoscopic drainage for acute suppurative cholangitis. *Lancet.* 1989;1:1307-1309.
11. Leese T, Neoptolemos JP, Baker AR, Carr-Locke DL. Management of acute cholangitis and the impact of endoscopic sphincterotomy. *Br J Surg.* 1986;73:988-992.
12. Siegel JH, Rodriquez R, Cohen SA, Kasmin FE, Cooperman AM. Endoscopic management of cholangitis: critical review of an alternative technique and report of a large series. *Am J Gastroenterol.* 1994;89:1142-1146.
13. Lai EC, Mok FP, Tan ES, et al. Endoscopic biliary drainage for severe acute cholangitis. *N Engl J Med.* 1992;326:1582-1586.

14. Dumonceau JM, Tringali A, Blero D, et al. Biliary stenting: indications, choice of stents and results: European Society of Gastrointestinal Endoscopy (ESGE) clinical guideline. *Endoscopy*. 2012;44:277-298.

15. Cote GA, Slivka A, Tarnasky P, et al. Effect of covered metallic stents compared with plastic stents on benign biliary stricture resolution: a randomized clinical trial. *JAMA*. 2016;315:1250-1257.

16. Deviere J, Nageshwar Reddy D, Puspok A, et al. Successful management of benign biliary strictures with fully covered self-expanding metal stents. *Gastroenterology*. 2014;147:385-395, quiz e15.

17. Bergman JJ, Burgemeister L, Bruno MJ, et al. Long-term follow-up after biliary stent placement for postoperative bile duct stenosis. *Gastrointest Endosc*. 2001;54:154-161.

18. Costamagna G, Pandolfi M, Mutignani M, Spada C, Perri V. Long-term results of endoscopic management of postoperative bile duct strictures with increasing numbers of stents. *Gastrointest Endosc*. 2001;54:162-168.

19. Zepeda-Gomez S, Baron TH. Benign biliary strictures: current endoscopic management. *Nat Rev Gastroenterol Hepatol*. 2011;8:573-581.

20. Aabakken L, Karlsen TH, Albert J, et al. Role of endoscopy in primary sclerosing cholangitis: European Society of Gastrointestinal Endoscopy (ESGE) and European Association for the Study of the Liver (EASL) Clinical Guideline. *Endoscopy*. 2017;49(6):588-608.

21. Dave M, Elmunzer BJ, Dwamena BA, Higgins PD. Primary sclerosing cholangitis: meta-analysis of diagnostic performance of MR cholangiopancreatography. *Radiology*. 2010;256:387-396.

22. Johnson GK, Geenen JE, Venu RP, Schmalz MJ, Hogan WJ. Endoscopic treatment of biliary tract strictures in sclerosing cholangitis: a larger series and recommendations for treatment. *Gastrointest Endosc*. 1991;37:38-43.

23. Lee JG, Schutz SM, England RE, Leung JW, Cotton PB. Endoscopic therapy of sclerosing cholangitis. *Hepatology*. 1995;21:661-667.

24. van Milligen de Wit AW, van Bracht J, Rauws EA, Jones EA, Tytgat GN, Huibregtse K. Endoscopic stent therapy for dominant extrahepatic bile duct strictures in primary sclerosing cholangitis. *Gastrointest Endosc*. 1996;44:293-299.

25. Ponsioen CY, Lam K, van Milligen de Wit AW, Huibregtse K, Tytgat GN. Four years experience with short term stenting in primary sclerosing cholangitis. *Am J Gastroenterol*. 1999;94:2403-2407.

26. Kaya M, Petersen BT, Angulo P, et al. Balloon dilation compared to stenting of dominant strictures in primary sclerosing cholangitis. *Am J Gastroenterol*. 2001;96:1059-1066.

27. Barkun AN, Rezieg M, Mehta SN, et al. Postcholecystectomy biliary leaks in the laparoscopic era: risk factors, presentation, and management. McGill Gallstone Treatment Group. *Gastrointest Endosc*. 1997;45:277-282.

28. Bjorkman DJ, Carr-Locke DL, Lichtenstein DR, et al. Postsurgical bile leaks: endoscopic obliteration of the transpapillary pressure gradient is enough. *Am J Gastroenterol*. 1995;90:2128-2133.

29. Foutch PG, Harlan JR, Hoefer M. Endoscopic therapy for patients with a post-operative biliary leak. *Gastrointest Endosc*. 1993;39:416-421.

30. Kaffes AJ, Hourigan L, De Luca N, Byth K, Williams SJ, Bourke MJ. Impact of endoscopic intervention in 100 patients with suspected postcholecystectomy bile leak. *Gastrointest Endosc*. 2005;61:269-275.

31. Sandha GS, Bourke MJ, Haber GB, Kortan PP. Endoscopic therapy for bile leak based on a new classification: results in 207 patients. *Gastrointest Endosc*. 2004;60:567-574.

32. Kalayci C, Aisen A, Canal D, et al. Magnetic resonance cholangiopancreatography documents bile leak site after cholecystectomy in patients with aberrant right hepatic duct where ERCP fails. *Gastrointest Endosc*. 2000;52:277-281.

33. Soehendra N, Reynders-Frederix V. Palliative bile duct drainage—a new endoscopic method of introducing a transpapillary drain. *Endoscopy*. 1980;12:8-11.

34. Davids PH, Groen AK, Rauws EA, Tytgat GN, Huibregtse K. Randomised trial of self-expanding metal stents versus polyethylene stents for distal malignant biliary obstruction. *Lancet*. 1992;340:1488-1492.

35. Knyrim K, Wagner HJ, Pausch J, Vakil N. A prospective, randomized, controlled trial of metal stents for malignant obstruction of the common bile duct. *Endoscopy*. 1993;25:207-212.

36. Wagner HJ, Knyrim K, Vakil N, Klose KJ. Plastic endoprostheses versus metal stents in the palliative treatment of malignant hilar biliary obstruction. A prospective and randomized trial. *Endoscopy*. 1993;25:213-218.

37. Kaassis M, Boyer J, Dumas R, et al. Plastic or metal stents for malignant stricture of the common bile duct? Results of a randomized prospective study. *Gastrointest Endosc*. 2003;57:178-182.

38. Sawas T, Al Halabi S, Parsi MA, Vargo JJ. Self-expandable metal stents versus plastic stents for malignant biliary obstruction: a meta-analysis. *Gastrointest Endosc*. 2015;82:256-267.e7.

39. De Palma GD, Galloro G, Siciliano S, Iovino P, Catanzano C. Unilateral versus bilateral endoscopic hepatic duct drainage in patients with malignant hilar biliary obstruction: results of a prospective, randomized, and controlled study. *Gastrointest Endosc*. 2001;53:547-553.

40. Speer AG, Cotton PB, Russell RC, et al. Randomised trial of endoscopic versus percutaneous stent insertion in malignant obstructive jaundice. *Lancet*. 1987;2:57-62.

41. Andersen JR, Sorensen SM, Kruse A, Rokkjaer M, Matzen P. Randomised trial of endoscopic endoprosthesis versus operative bypass in malignant obstructive jaundice. *Gut*. 1989;30:1132-1135.

42. Smith AC, Dowsett JF, Russell RC, Hatfield AR, Cotton PB. Randomised trial of endoscopic stenting versus surgical bypass in malignant low bile duct obstruction. *Lancet*. 1994;344:1655-1660.

43. Shepherd HA, Royle G, Ross AP, Diba A, Arthur M, Colin-Jones D. Endoscopic biliary endoprosthesis in the palliation of malignant obstruction of the distal common bile duct: a randomized trial. *Br J Surg*. 1988;75:1166-1168.

44. van der Gaag NA, Rauws EA, van Eijck CH, et al. Preoperative biliary drainage for cancer of the head of the pancreas. *N Engl J Med*. 2010;362:129-137.

45. Tol JA, van Hooft JE, Timmer R, et al. Metal or plastic stents for preoperative biliary drainage in resectable pancreatic cancer. *Gut*. 2016;65:1981-1987.

46. Jailwala J, Fogel EL, Sherman S, et al. Triple-tissue sampling at ERCP in malignant biliary obstruction. *Gastrointest Endosc*. 2000;51:383-390.

47. de Bellis M, Sherman S, Fogel EL, et al. Tissue sampling at ERCP in suspected malignant biliary strictures (Part 2). *Gastrointest Endosc*. 2002;56:720-730.

48. Fritcher EG, Kipp BR, Halling KC, et al. A multivariable model using advanced cytologic methods for the evaluation of indeterminate pancreatobiliary strictures. *Gastroenterology*. 2009;136:2180-2186.

49. Funabiki T, Matsubara T, Miyakawa S, Ishihara S. Pancreaticobiliary maljunction and carcinogenesis to biliary and pancreatic malignancy. *Langenbecks Arch Surg*. 2009;394:159-169.

50. Ladas SD, Katsogridakis I, Tassios P, Tastemiroglou T, Vrachliotis T, Raptis SA. Choledochocele, an overlooked diagnosis: report of 15 cases and review of 56 published reports from 1984 to 1992. *Endoscopy*. 1995;27:233-239.

51. Elton E, Hanson BL, Biber BP, Howell DA. Dilated common channel syndrome: endoscopic diagnosis, treatment, and relationship to choledochocele formation. *Gastrointest Endosc*. 1998;47:471-478.

52. Samavedy R, Sherman S, Lehman GA. Endoscopic therapy in anomalous pancreatobiliary duct junction. *Gastrointest Endosc*. 1999;50:623-627.

53. Ng WD, Liu K, Wong MK, et al. Endoscopic sphincterotomy in young patients with choledochal dilatation and a long common channel: a preliminary report. *Br J Surg*. 1992;79:550-552.

54. Lans JL, Geenen JE, Johanson JF, Hogan WJ. Endoscopic therapy in patients with pancreas divisum and acute pancreatitis: a prospective, randomized, controlled clinical trial. *Gastrointest Endosc*. 1992;38:430-434.

55. Ertan A. Long-term results after endoscopic pancreatic stent placement without pancreatic papillotomy in acute recurrent pancreatitis due to pancreas divisum. *Gastrointest Endosc*. 2000;52:9-14.

56. Lehman GA, Sherman S, Nisi R, Hawes RH. Pancreas divisum: results of minor papilla sphincterotomy. *Gastrointest Endosc*. 1993;39:1-8.

57. Heyries L, Barthet M, Delvasto C, Zamora C, Bernard JP, Sahel J. Long-term results of endoscopic management of pancreas divisum with recurrent acute pancreatitis. *Gastrointest Endosc*. 2002;55:376-381.

58. Klein SD, Affronti JP. Pancreas divisum, an evidence-based review. Part II: patient selection and treatment. *Gastrointest Endosc*. 2004;60:585-589.

59. Dye C, Waxman I. Interventional endoscopy in the diagnosis and staging of upper gastrointestinal malignancy. *Surg Oncol Clin N Am*. 2002;11:305-320.

60. Kallimanis GE, Gupta PK, al-Kawas FH, et al. Endoscopic ultrasound for staging esophageal cancer, with or without dilation, is clinically important and safe. *Gastrointest Endosc*. 1995;41:540-546.

61. Van Dam J, Rice TW, Catalano MF, Kirby T, Sivak MV Jr. High-grade malignant stricture is predictive of esophageal tumor stage. Risks of endosonographic evaluation. Cancer 1993;71:2910-2917.

62. Wallace MB, Hawes RH, Sahai AV, Van Velse A, Hoffman BJ. Dilation of malignant esophageal stenosis to allow EUS guided fine-needle aspiration: safety and effect on patient management. Gastrointest Endosc. 2000;51:309-313.

63. Dimastromatteo J, Brentnall T, Kelly KA. Imaging in pancreatic disease. Nat Rev Gastroenterol Hepatol. 2017;14:97-109.

64. Catalano MF, Sahai A, Levy M, et al. EUS-based criteria for the diagnosis of chronic pancreatitis: the Rosemont classification. Gastrointest Endosc. 2009;69:1251-1261.

65. Stevens T, Lopez R, Adler DG, et al. Multicenter comparison of the interobserver agreement of standard EUS scoring and Rosemont classification scoring for diagnosis of chronic pancreatitis. Gastrointest Endosc. 2010;71:519-526.

66. Kalmin B, Hoffman B, Hawes R, Romagnuolo J. Conventional versus Rosemont endoscopic ultrasound criteria for chronic pancreatitis: comparing interobserver reliability and intertest agreement. Can J Gastroenterol. 2011;25:261-264.

67. Legmann P, Vignaux O, Dousset B, et al. Pancreatic tumors: comparison of dual-phase helical CT and endoscopic sonography. AJR Am J Roentgenol. 1998;170:1315-1322.

68. Muller MF, Meyenberger C, Bertschinger P, Schaer R, Marincek B. Pancreatic tumors: evaluation with endoscopic US, CT, and MR imaging. Radiology. 1994;190:745-751.

69. Soriano A, Castells A, Ayuso C, et al. Preoperative staging and tumor resectability assessment of pancreatic cancer: prospective study comparing endoscopic ultrasonography, helical computed tomography, magnetic resonance imaging and angiography. Am J Gastroenterol. 2004;99:492-501.

70. Tierney WM, Francis IR, Eckhauser F, Elta G, Nostrant TT, Scheiman JM. The accuracy of EUS and helical CT in the assessment of vascular invasion by peripapillary malignancy. Gastrointest Endosc. 2001;53:182-188.

71. Hewitt MJ, McPhail MJ, Possamai L, Dhar A, Vlavianos P, Monahan KJ. EUS-guided FNA for diagnosis of solid pancreatic neoplasms: a meta-analysis. Gastrointest Endosc. 2012;75:319-331.

72. Hebert-Magee S, Bae S, Varadarajulu S, et al. The presence of a cytopathologist increases the diagnostic accuracy of endoscopic ultrasound-guided fine needle aspiration cytology for pancreatic adenocarcinoma: a meta-analysis. Cytopathology. 2013;24:159-171.

73. Andriulli A, Loperfido S, Napolitano G, et al. Incidence rates of post-ERCP complications: a systematic survey of prospective studies. Am J Gastroenterol. 2007;102:1781-1788.

74. Davis WZ, Cotton PB, Arias R, Williams D, Onken JE. ERCP and sphincterotomy in the context of laparoscopic cholecystectomy: academic and community practice patterns and results. Am J Gastroenterol. 1997;92:597-601.

75. Loperfido S, Angelini G, Benedetti G, et al. Major early complications from diagnostic and therapeutic ERCP: a prospective multicenter study. Gastrointest Endosc. 1998;48:1-10.

76. Cotton PB, Garrow DA, Gallagher J, Romagnuolo J. Risk factors for complications after ERCP: a multivariate analysis of 11,497 procedures over 12 years. Gastrointest Endosc. 2009;70:80-88.

77. Anderson SW, Rho E, Soto JA. Detection of biliary duct narrowing and choledocholithiasis: accuracy of portal venous phase multidetector CT. Radiology. 2008;247:418-427.

78. Okada M, Fukada J, Toya K, Ito R, Ohashi T, Yorozu A. The value of drip infusion cholangiography using multidetector-row helical CT in patients with choledocholithiasis. Eur Radiol. 2005;15:2140-2145.

79. Kondo S, Isayama H, Akahane M, et al. Detection of common bile duct stones: comparison between endoscopic ultrasonography, magnetic resonance cholangiography, and helical-computed-tomographic cholangiography. Eur J Radiol. 2005;54:271-275.

80. MacEneaney P, Mitchell MT, McDermott R. Update on magnetic resonance cholangiopancreatography. Gastroenterol Clin North Am. 2002;31:731-746.

81. Savides TJ. EUS-guided ERCP for patients with intermediate probability for choledocholithiasis: is it time for all of us to start doing this? Gastrointest Endosc. 2008;67:669-672.

82. Mendler MH, Bouillet P, Sautereau D, et al. Value of MR cholangiography in the diagnosis of obstructive diseases of the biliary tree: a study of 58 cases. Am J Gastroenterol. 1998;93:2482-2490.

83. Zidi SH, Prat F, Le Guen O, et al. Use of magnetic resonance cholangiography in the diagnosis of choledocholithiasis: prospective comparison with a reference imaging method. Gut. 1999;44:118-122.

84. Verma D, Kapadia A, Eisen GM, Adler DG. EUS vs MRCP for detection of choledocholithiasis. Gastrointest Endosc. 2006;64:248-254.

85. De Castro Cano D. Suspected choledocholithiasis: endoscopic ultrasound or magnetic resonance cholangio-pancreatography? A systematic review. Eur J Gastroenterol Hepatol. 2007;19:1007-1011.

86. Petrov MS, Savides TJ. Systematic review of endoscopic ultrasonography versus endoscopic retrograde cholangiopancreatography for suspected choledocholithiasis. Br J Surg. 2009;96:967-974.

87. Napoleon B, Dumortier J, Keriven-Souquet O, Pujol B, Ponchon T, Souquet JC. Do normal findings at biliary endoscopic ultrasonography obviate the need for endoscopic retrograde cholangiography in patients with suspicion of common bile duct stone? A prospective follow-up study of 238 patients. Endoscopy. 2003;35:411-415.

88. Canto MI, Chak A, Stellato T, Sivak MV Jr. Endoscopic ultrasonography versus cholangiography for the diagnosis of choledocholithiasis. Gastrointest Endosc. 1998;47:439-448.

89. Palazzo L, Girollet PP, Salmeron M, et al. Value of endoscopic ultrasonography in the diagnosis of common bile duct stones: comparison with surgical exploration and ERCP. Gastrointest Endosc. 1995;42:225-231.

90. Shea JA, Berlin JA, Escarce JJ, et al. Revised estimates of diagnostic test sensitivity and specificity in suspected biliary tract disease. Arch Intern Med. 1994;154:2573-2581.

91. Dill JE, Hill S, Callis J, et al. Combined endoscopic ultrasound and stimulated biliary drainage in cholecystitis and microlithiasis—diagnoses and outcomes. Endoscopy. 1995;27:424-427.

92. Frossard JL, Sosa-Valencia L, Amouyal G, Marty O, Hadengue A, Amouyal P. Usefulness of endoscopic ultrasonography in patients with "idiopathic" acute pancreatitis. Am J Med. 2000;109:196-200.

93. Garrow D, Miller S, Sinha D, et al. Endoscopic ultrasound: a meta-analysis of test performance in suspected biliary obstruction. Clin Gastroenterol Hepatol. 2007;5:616-623.

94. Lee JH, Salem R, Aslanian H, Chacho M, Topazian M. Endoscopic ultrasound and fine-needle aspiration of unexplained bile duct strictures. Am J Gastroenterol. 2004;99:1069-1073.

95. Navaneethan A, Mohamadnejad M, Islami F, et al. Diagnostic yield of EUS-guided FNA for malignant biliary stricture: a systematic review and meta-analysis. Gastrointest Endosc. 2016;83:290-298.e1.

96. Azuma T, Yoshikawa T, Araida T, Takasaki K. Differential diagnosis of polypoid lesions of the gallbladder by endoscopic ultrasonography. Am J Surg. 2001;181:65-70.

97. Will U, Bosseckert H, Meyer F. Correlation of endoscopic ultrasonography (EUS) for differential diagnostics between inflammatory and neoplastic lesions of the papilla of Vater and the peripapillary region with results of histologic investigation. Ultraschall Med. 2008;29:275-280.

98. Defrain C, Chang CY, Srikureja W, Nguyen PT, Gu M. Cytologic features and diagnostic pitfalls of primary ampullary tumors by endoscopic ultrasound-guided fine-needle aspiration biopsy. Cancer. 2005;105:289-297.

99. Rosch T, Braig C, Gain T, et al. Staging of pancreatic and ampullary carcinoma by endoscopic ultrasonography. Comparison with conventional sonography, computed tomography, and angiography. Gastroenterology. 1992;102:188-199.

100. Artifon EL, Couto D Jr, Sakai P, da Silveira EB. Prospective evaluation of EUS versus CT scan for staging of ampullary cancer. Gastrointest Endosc. 2009;70:290-296.

101. Cannon ME, Carpenter SL, Elta GH, et al. EUS compared with CT, magnetic resonance imaging, and angiography and the influence of biliary stenting on staging accuracy of ampullary neoplasms. Gastrointest Endosc. 1999;50:27-33.

102. Baron TH, Topazian MD. Endoscopic transduodenal drainage of the gallbladder: implications for endoluminal treatment of gallbladder disease. Gastrointest Endosc. 2007;65:735-737.

103. Jang JW, Lee SS, Song TJ, et al. Endoscopic ultrasound-guided transmural and percutaneous transhepatic gallbladder drainage are comparable for acute cholecystitis. Gastroenterology. 2012;142:805-811.

104. Itoi T, Itokawa F, Kurihara T. Endoscopic ultrasonography-guided gallbladder drainage: actual technical presentations and review of the literature (with videos). J Hepatobiliary Pancreat Sci. 2011;18:282-286.

105. Wiersema MJ, Wiersema LM. Endosonography-guided celiac plexus neurolysis. Gastrointest Endosc. 1996;44:656-662.

106. Puli SR, Reilly JB, Bechtold ML, Antillon MR, Brugge WR. EUS-guided celiac plexus neurolysis for pain due to chronic pancreatitis or pancreatic cancer pain: a meta-analysis and systematic review. *Dig Dis Sci.* 2009;54:2330-2337.

107. LeBlanc JK, DeWitt J, Johnson C, et al. A prospective randomized trial of 1 versus 2 injections during EUS-guided celiac plexus block for chronic pancreatitis pain. *Gastrointest Endosc.* 2009;69:835-842.

108. Saftoiu A, Vilmann P, Hassan H, Gorunescu F. Analysis of endoscopic ultrasound elastography used for characterisation and differentiation of benign and malignant lymph nodes. *Ultraschall Med.* 2006;27:535-542.

109. Giovannini M, Thomas B, Erwan B, et al. Endoscopic ultrasound elastography for evaluation of lymph nodes and pancreatic masses: a multicenter study. *World J Gastroenterol.* 2009;15:1587-1593.

110. Xu W, Shi J, Zeng X, et al. EUS elastography for the differentiation of benign and malignant lymph nodes: a meta-analysis. *Gastrointest Endosc.* 2011;74:1001-1009, quiz 1115 e1-4.

111. Dietrich CF, Ignee A, Braden B, Barreiros AP, Ott M, Hocke M. Improved differentiation of pancreatic tumors using contrast-enhanced endoscopic ultrasound. *Clin Gastroenterol Hepatol.* 2008;6:590-597.e1.

112. Wang KX, Ben QW, Jin ZD, et al. Assessment of morbidity and mortality associated with EUS-guided FNA: a systematic review. *Gastrointest Endosc.* 2011;73:283-290.

113. Itoi T, Itokawa F, Uraoka T, et al. Novel EUS-guided gastrojejunostomy technique using a new double-balloon enteric tube and lumen-apposing metal stent (with videos). *Gastrointest Endosc.* 2013;78:934-939.

114. Itoi T, Ishii K, Ikeuchi N, et al. Prospective evaluation of endoscopic ultrasonography-guided double-balloon-occluded gastrojejunostomy bypass (EPASS) for malignant gastric outlet obstruction. *Gut.* 2016;65:193-195.

115. Konda VJ, Meining A, Jamil LH, et al. A pilot study of in vivo identification of pancreatic cystic neoplasms with needle-based confocal laser endomicroscopy under endosonographic guidance. *Endoscopy.* 2013;45:1006-1013.

116. Napoleon B, Lemaistre AI, Pujol B, et al. A novel approach to the diagnosis of pancreatic serous cystadenoma: needle-based confocal laser endomicroscopy. *Endoscopy.* 2015;47:26-32.

117. Baron TH, Kamath PS, McBane RD. Management of antithrombotic therapy in patients undergoing invasive procedures. *N Engl J Med.* 2013;368:2113-2124.

118. Eisen GM, Baron TH, Dominitz JA, et al. Guideline on the management of anticoagulation and antiplatelet therapy for endoscopic procedures. *Gastrointest Endosc.* 2002;55:775-779.

119. Kearon C, Hirsh J. Management of anticoagulation before and after elective surgery. *N Engl J Med.* 1997;336:1506-1511.

120. Kwok A, Faigel DO. Management of anticoagulation before and after gastrointestinal endoscopy. *Am J Gastroenterol.* 2009;104:3085-3097, quiz 3098.

121. Bissonnette J, Paquin S, Sahai A, Pomier-Layrargues G. Usefulness of endoscopic ultrasonography in hepatology. *Can J Gastroenterol.* 2011;25:621-625.

122. Wang AJ, Li BM, Zheng XL, Shu X, Zhu X. Utility of endoscopic ultrasound in the diagnosis and management of esophagogastric varices. *Endosc Ultrasound.* 2016;5:218-224.

123. Chirica M, Champault A, Dray X, et al. Esophageal perforations. *J Visc Surg.* 2010;147:e117-e128.

124. Cotton PB, Eisen GM, Aabakken L, et al. A lexicon for endoscopic adverse events: report of an ASGE workshop. *Gastrointest Endosc.* 2010;71:446-454.

125. Eloubeidi MA, Tamhane A, Lopes TL, Morgan DE, Cerfolio RJ. Cervical esophageal perforations at the time of endoscopic ultrasound: a prospective evaluation of frequency, outcomes, and patient management. *Am J Gastroenterol.* 2009;104:53-56.

126. O'Toole D, Palazzo L, Arotcarena R, et al. Assessment of complications of EUS-guided fine-needle aspiration. *Gastrointest Endosc.* 2001;53:470-474.

127. Wiersema MJ, Vilmann P, Giovannini M, Chang KJ, Wiersema LM. Endosonography-guided fine-needle aspiration biopsy: diagnostic accuracy and complication assessment. *Gastroenterology.* 1997;112:1087-1095.

128. Affi A, Vazquez-Sequeiros E, Norton ID, Clain JE, Wiersema MJ. Acute extraluminal hemorrhage associated with EUS-guided fine needle aspiration: frequency and clinical significance. *Gastrointest Endosc.* 2001;53:221-225.

129. Fujii LL, Levy MJ. Basic techniques in endoscopic ultrasound-guided fine needle aspiration for solid lesions: adverse events and avoiding them. *Endosc Ultrasound.* 2014;3:35-45.

130. Fabbri C, Luigiano C, Cennamo V, et al. Complications of endoscopic ultrasonography. *Minerva Gastroenterol Dietol.* 2011;57:159-166.

131. Ryan AG, Zamvar V, Roberts SA. Iatrogenic candidal infection of a mediastinal foregut cyst following endoscopic ultrasound-guided fine-needle aspiration. *Endoscopy.* 2002;34:838-839.

132. Eloubeidi MA, Gress FG, Savides TJ, et al. Acute pancreatitis after EUS-guided FNA of solid pancreatic masses: a pooled analysis from EUS centers in the United States. *Gastrointest Endosc.* 2004;60:385-389.

133. Eloubeidi MA, Tamhane A, Varadarajulu S, Wilcox CM. Frequency of major complications after EUS-guided FNA of solid pancreatic masses: a prospective evaluation. *Gastrointest Endosc.* 2006;63:622-629.

134. Williamson JB, Draganov PV. The usefulness of SpyGlass choledochoscopy in the diagnosis and treatment of biliary disorders. *Curr Gastroenterol Rep.* 2012;14:534-541.

135. Neuhaus H, Zillinger C, Born P, et al. Randomized study of intracorporeal laser lithotripsy versus extracorporeal shock-wave lithotripsy for difficult bile duct stones. *Gastrointest Endosc.* 1998;47:327-334.

136. Sethi A, Chen YK, Austin GL, et al. ERCP with cholangiopancreatoscopy may be associated with higher rates of complications than ERCP alone: a single-center experience. *Gastrointest Endosc.* 2011;73:251-256.

137. El H II, Brauer BC, Wani S, Fukami N, Attwell AR, Shah RJ. Role of per-oral pancreatoscopy in the evaluation of suspected pancreatic duct neoplasia: a 13-year US single-center experience. *Gastrointest Endosc.* 2017;85:737-745.

138. Parbhu SK, Siddiqui AA, Murphy M, et al. Efficacy, safety, and outcomes of endoscopic retrograde cholangiopancreatography with per-oral pancreatoscopy: a multicenter experience. *J Clin Gastroenterol.* 2017; Jan 5 [Epub ahead of print].

Biliary Tract Tumors

Susanne G. Warner | Clifford S. Cho | Yuman Fong

BENIGN GALLBLADDER TUMORS

Benign tumors of the gallbladder are relatively common, with up to 5% of patients undergoing abdominal ultrasonography being found to harbor gallbladder polyps.[1] Benign gallbladder tumors can be broadly categorized as epithelial (adenomas), mesenchymal (fibromas, lipomas, hemangiomas), or as pseudotumors (cholesterol polyps, inflammatory polyps, and adenomyomas). Cholesterol polyps are the most common of the benign tumors, accounting for approximately 60% of all gallbladder polyps. Adenomyomas account for approximately 25% of gallbladder polyps. They can appear polypoid or infiltrative in morphology and can be associated with biliary colic–like symptoms.[2] Adenomas make up approximately 4% of polyps and are thought by some to be neoplastic.[3,4] That being said, most gallbladder cancers do not arise from precursor adenomas, and K-ras mutations are not typically found in gallbladder cancers arising from adenomas.[5]

Clinical presentation of gallbladder polyps varies widely. One large retrospective series showed that of polyps diagnosed on ultrasound, 64% were found during work-up of unrelated problems, 23% had abdominal symptoms, and 13% had liver function test abnormalities.[6] The likelihood of malignancy in gallbladder polyps increases with increasing polyp size and decreasing polyp number. A classic review of 182 cases of resected gallbladder polyps identified only 13 cases of malignancy; likelihood of malignancy in this series was associated with patient age more than 50 years and solitary polyps greater than 1 cm in size.[7] Most studies recommend resection for polyp size greater than or equal to 1 cm in diameter. Of note, even in two more modern series, between 27% and 32% of patients thought to have polyps on ultrasound were found to have no polypoid lesion on final pathology.[6,8]

The management of gallbladder polyps is dictated by the presence of symptoms and their likelihood of harboring occult malignancy. Risk factors include primary sclerosing cholangitis, congenital polyposis syndromes, and chronic hepatitis B.[9–11] Any patient with symptoms referable to gallbladder polyps should undergo cholecystectomy. In addition, patients with suspicious polyps (size >10 mm, number <3, sessile lesions, or sonographic evidence of mucosal invasion) should undergo cholecystectomy. Cholecystectomy for patients with suspicious polyps can be performed laparoscopically, but great pains should be taken to minimize the likelihood of tumor spillage. Furthermore, for a high level of suspicion, intraoperative frozen-section analysis of the resected gallbladder specimen should be undertaken because confirmation of malignancy could mandate an extended oncologic resection. This can also be done minimally invasively and should be discussed with the patient in advance. Patients who do not undergo surgical therapy for borderline polyps deserve close radiographic follow-up, with serial sonograms performed at 6- to 12-month intervals to identify any rapid interval size progression that may indicate the presence of malignancy.

GALLBLADDER CANCER

Cancer of the gallbladder is the most common biliary malignancy, and it is the fifth most common gastrointestinal cancer. Because of its aggressive nature (manifested by its propensity toward nodal metastases, direct hepatic invasion, and seeding of peritoneal surfaces), it is usually diagnosed at an advanced stage, resulting in an overall median survival of less than 6 months.[12] However, advances in our understanding of its tumor biology accompanied by progress in diagnostic and surgical extirpative techniques have motivated a fresh approach to this once universally fatal disease; indeed, the possibility of cure is real for a subset of patients presenting with gallbladder cancer.

EPIDEMIOLOGY

The prevalence of gallbladder cancer appears to be highest in South America, intermediate in Europe, and lower in the United States and United Kingdom. In the United States the incidence is 1 to 2 per 100,000, but incidence rates are as high as 22 per 100,000 in women in Delhi, India.[13] Epidemiologic analysis suggests that processes promoting chronic gallbladder irritation and inflammation are also risk factors: history of biliary disease, Mirizzi syndrome, age, female gender, obesity, high carbohydrate diet, ethanol abuse, and tobacco abuse (all of which are associated with calculous biliary disease) have been associated with a higher risk of gallbladder cancer.[14–17] Moreover, 69% to 86% of patients with gallbladder cancer have a personal history of gallstone disease.[14,18] The presence of an abnormal pancreaticobiliary duct junction, thought to promote chronic biliary inflammation, has been associated with both choledochal cyst disease and gallbladder cancer.[19] The incidence of gallbladder cancer in the so-called porcelain gallbladder, presumably resulting from chronic inflammation and calcification of the gallbladder wall, was once estimated to be as high as 61%; however, more contemporary analyses suggest that the correct figure is more likely between 7% and 25%.[20,21]

The exact nature of the relationship between chronic inflammation and gallbladder tumorigenesis is unclear. It has been estimated that only 0.3% to 3% of patients with gallstones will develop gallbladder cancer, eliminating any theoretical benefit for prophylactic cholecystectomy (with the exception of porcelain gallbladder).

ANATOMY

The anatomic relationships of the gallbladder to surrounding structures dictate the surgical strategies that must be used in its treatment. The gallbladder fossa, against which the fundus and body of the gallbladder lie, is found beneath the junction of hepatic segments IVB and V. As a result, the likelihood of direct hepatic invasion of gallbladder cancer typically mandates resection of these segments. The infundibulum of the gallbladder lies adjacent to the right portal pedicle within the porta hepatis; as a result, tumors arising in the infundibulum commonly invade the right portal pedicle and require a right trisectionectomy for complete surgical extirpation.

The thin gallbladder wall is composed of an inner mucosa, a thin lamina propria, and a single muscularis layer (unlike the two muscle layers that line most hollow viscera). The serosa of the gallbladder is typically opened during a standard cholecystectomy, with the avascular subserosal layer being used as the surgical plane of dissection; the ability of mucosally based tumors to microscopically invade across the serosa explains the high prevalence of positive resection margins after standard cholecystectomy for gallbladder cancer.

The lymphatic drainage of the gallbladder has been well characterized. The pattern of lymphatic flow appears to be directed initially toward the cystic and pericholedochal lymph nodes, then to the posterior pancreaticoduodenal, periportal, and common hepatic artery nodes within the hepatoduodenal ligament, and eventually to the celiac, aortocaval, and superior mesenteric artery nodes.[22] There appears to be no ascending lymphatic drainage into the hilum of the liver. For this reason, meticulous lymphadenectomy within the hepatoduodenal ligament is a critical component of surgical strategy in the management of gallbladder cancer. Unfortunately, the potential for direct drainage from the pericholedochal nodes into the aortocaval nodes explains the difficulty of completely encompassing the extent of lymphatic involvement after surgical resection.

PATHOLOGY

Approximately 60% of gallbladder cancers arise in the fundus, with 30% arising from the body and 10% from the neck.[23] Although it is likely that gallbladder cancer may follow the pathogenic sequence of mucosal dysplasia to carcinoma in situ to invasive cancer, it is unlikely that most gallbladder cancers arise from precursor adenomata.

Gallbladder cancers have been categorized as infiltrative, nodular, combined nodular-infiltrative, papillary, and combined papillary-infiltrative. Infiltrative tumors, which are the most common variety, initially appear as indurated areas of gallbladder wall thickening that spread into the subserosal plane, which is typically violated during routine cholecystectomy. Nodular tumors invade into adjacent pericholecystic structures early, but unlike infiltrative cancers, induce sharply defined borders that can facilitate curative resection. Papillary tumors tend to grow in a polypoid fashion, often filling into the lumen of the gallbladder with minimal wall invasion; as such, this variety

of tumors tends to be associated with more favorable prognoses.

Microscopically, adenocarcinoma is the most common histologic subtype seen with gallbladder malignancies. Other histologic subtypes that have been reported include adenosquamous carcinoma, oat cell carcinoma, sarcoma, carcinoid, lymphoma, and melanoma. Histologic grading for gallbladder cancer, which has been recognized as a significant prognostic variable, is categorized from G1 (well differentiated) to G4 (undifferentiated); patients most commonly present with G3 (poorly differentiated) tumors.

The propensity of gallbladder cancer to penetrate beyond the single muscle layer of the gallbladder wall results in a high likelihood of tumor penetration into the liver, peritoneal cavity, and lymphovascular spaces at the time of diagnosis. Review of the literature suggests that only 10% of cases are confined to the gallbladder wall at the time of diagnosis; 59% exhibit direct invasion into hepatic parenchyma, 45% demonstrate lymph node metastases, and 20% present with distant extrahepatic metastases.[24] Indeed, a high level of suspicion for occult intraperitoneal metastases should be maintained throughout the diagnostic process for patients with gallbladder cancer. The most common site of extraabdominal spread is the lungs although pulmonary metastases are rare in the absence of extensive intraperitoneal disease.

MUTATIONS AND TARGETED THERAPIES

In the coming years, relevant evidence for this section should grow dramatically. Traditionally, biliary and gallbladder cancers have been poorly researched and thereby mechanisms of carcinogenesis remain poorly understood. Earlier studies posited that gallbladder carcinoma develops via distinct pathways, either occurring de novo with predominant *p53* alteration with low percentage of K-ras mutation, or via adenoma-carcinoma sequence in the absence of p53, K-ras, or adenomatous polyposis coli (APC) gene mutations.[25] Although targeted therapies have yielded promising results in other more uniformly developed malignancies, it appears that a variety of heterogeneous pathways can result in gallbladder cancer development.[26] This may explain lack of success in targeted agents against biliary tract cancers thus far because few have examined targeted therapies in relationship to mutations carried. Mutations identified thus far include BRAF mutations in 7 of 21 (33%) resected specimens, and interestingly K-ras and BRAF mutations were not identified in the same specimens.[27] There is much left to learn, but targeted therapies do represent a promising avenue for future adjuvant therapies.

DIAGNOSIS

Patients with gallbladder cancer may experience complaints that mimic those of benign biliary colic. Symptoms of persistent pain, weight loss, anorexia, jaundice, and a palpable right upper quadrant mass are typically indicative of advanced disease that is not amenable to surgical resection. A review of the Memorial Sloan Kettering Cancer Center (MSKCC) experience highlighted the observation that 95% of patients presenting with jaundice were ultimately noted to harbor unresectable disease.[28]

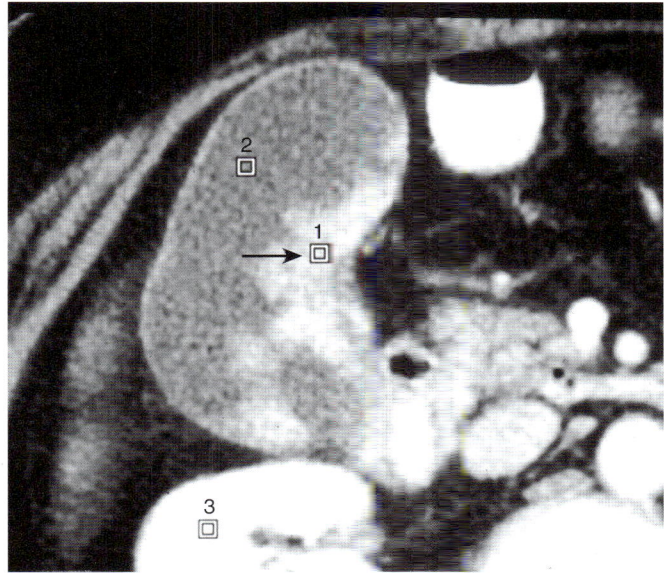

FIGURE 112.1 Appearance of gallbladder cancer on computed tomography; *arrow* notes extensive sessile polypoid lesion within lumen of gallbladder wall.

TABLE 112.1 American Joint Committee on Cancer System for Gallbladder Cancer

T1a	Tumor invades lamina propria of gallbladder wall
T1b	Tumor invades muscular layer of gallbladder wall
T2	Tumor invades perimuscular connective tissue but not across serosa
T3	Tumor invades across serosa of gallbladder wall and/or invades liver and/or one adjacent structure or organ
T4	Tumor invades main portal vein or hepatic artery or two or more extrahepatic structures or organs
N0	No lymph node involvement
N1	Lymph node involvement within hepatoduodenal ligament
N2	Lymph node involvement beyond hepatoduodenal ligament
M0	No distant metastases
M1	Distant metastases
Stage I	T1 N0 M0
Stage II	T2 N0 M0
Stage IIIA	T3 N0 M0
Stage IIIB	T1-3 N1 M0
Stage IVA	T4 N0-1 M0
Stage IVB	T1-4 N2 M0
	T1-4 N0-2 M1

Tumor markers provide limited assistance with diagnosis. In the presence of appropriate symptomatology, carcinoembryonic antigen (CEA) elevations greater than 4 ng/mL have been shown to predict gallbladder cancer with 50% sensitivity and 93% specificity.[29] Similarly, elevations of carbohydrate antigen (CA) 19-9 greater than 20 U/mL are 79.4% sensitive and 79.2% specific.[30] Radiographic findings on ultrasonography include the presence of a polypoid gallbladder mass (seen in 27% of gallbladder cancer cases) or an invasive gallbladder-based lesion (seen in 50% of cases); other sonographic findings consistent with gallbladder cancer include discontinuous gallbladder mucosa, echogenic mucosa, or submucosal echolucency.[31] Computed tomographic (CT) findings seen in patients with gallbladder cancer include a mass filling the gallbladder lumen in 42% of cases, a polypoid mass in 26%, a mass in the region of the gallbladder fossa without a distinctly recognizable gallbladder in 26%, and diffuse wall thickening in 6% (Fig. 112.1).[32] Magnetic resonance imaging (MRI) and magnetic resonance cholangiopancreatography (MRCP) are especially accurate means of identifying small hepatic metastases and involvement of the common bile duct.

Despite the high frequency of nodal involvement, definitive preoperative identification of lymph node metastases is challenging. Enlarged benign inflammatory lymph nodes are commonly encountered at the time of laparotomy. Although the CT finding of ringlike or heterogeneous enhancement of a more than 10-mm large lymph node has been found to identify lymph node metastases with 89% accuracy, only 38% of nodal metastases are preoperatively identified by CT.[3] Endoscopic ultrasonography may be useful for assessing peripancreatic and periportal adenopathy. Fluorodeoxyglucose positron emission tomography (PET) is used for identifying distant metastases that may contraindicate surgical intervention, but PET efficacy for nodal metastases is limited.[34]

The striking ability of disseminated gallbladder cancer cells to implant within needle tracts limits the utility of percutaneous core biopsy for diagnosis. Percutaneous fine-needle aspiration appears to have a lower incidence of needle tract seeding while providing satisfactory diagnostic accuracy, and it can be used in cases of surgically unresectable disease in which a definitive tissue diagnosis may direct nonoperative therapy.[35] Cytologic analysis of bile samples collected either percutaneously or endoscopically is not often helpful for diagnosing gallbladder cancer, with suboptimal sensitivities of approximately 50%.[35]

STAGING

The most accurate predictor of outcome is tumor stage. With changes and improvements in surgical therapy, the impact of various staging criteria has evolved. For example, previous iterations of the American Joint Committee on Cancer (AJCC) staging system categorized patients with tumors extending into the liver as having unresectable stage IV disease.[36] With the increased implementation of modern hepatic resection techniques, curative resection is now possible for this subset of patients with gallbladder cancer. The current AJCC system (Table 112.1) now categorizes patients with disease invasive into the liver within stage III. In addition, nodal metastases found outside of the hepatoduodenal ligament (N2) have been shown to carry the same ominous prognostic weight as distant nonnodal metastases (M1)[37]; for this reason, the current AJCC system categorizes any patients with N2 disease within stage IV.

This emphasizes the importance of thorough lymphadenectomy. To reiterate, the cystic duct, common bile duct, hepatic artery, and periportal lymph nodes are considered N disease in the 7th edition of AJCC staging manual, whereas the paraaortic, paracaval, superior mesenteric artery, and celiac lymph nodes are N2 nodes.[36] Standard lymphadenectomy for regional clearance is thus limited to the hepatoduodenal ligament. If N disease is suspected, most surgeons will sample nodes in the N2 distribution for staging purposes but will not completely clear these nodal basins in the interest of sparing the patient added morbidity. Imaging plays a critical role when considering surgical re-resection after incidentally found gallbladder cancer, or when planning surgery for suspected gallbladder cancer. Most authors advocate for some combination of CT, MRI, and PET.[38–40]

Stage I Gallbladder Cancer

The setting in which a surgeon is most apt to encounter stage I gallbladder cancer occurs after routine cholecystectomy for presumed benign stone disease, when pathologic analysis of the resected gallbladder unexpectedly identifies cancer within the muscular layer of the gallbladder wall. As stated earlier, the plane of dissection used during a typical cholecystectomy is along the subserosal plane, which should not violate a T1 tumor. The likelihood of N1 disease is low for patients with T1a tumors, and, for this reason, simple cholecystectomy should be curative.[41–43] A notable exception to this is the situation in which the cystic duct margin remains positive, in which case re-resection to negative margins is imperative. On occasion, this may necessitate common bile duct excision with reestablishment of biliary-enteric continuity. Additional debate surrounds the management of T1b disease, with studies suggesting that T1b disease can present with lymph node metastases in up to 20% of patients and many authors advocating for radical resection.[44,45]

Stage II Gallbladder Cancer

The subserosal plane of dissection used in the standard cholecystectomy is likely to violate T2 tumors; indeed, patients with T2 tumors resected by simple cholecystectomy have a 40% to 50% likelihood of margin positivity.[37,41] Furthermore, approximately one-half of patients with T2 tumors harbor nodal metastases. For these reasons, extended cholecystectomy with portal lymphadenectomy is the procedure of choice for patients with stage II disease. The importance of performing an extended cholecystectomy with negative margins is underscored by the observation that 5-year survival rates are 70% to 90% for patients with stage II disease treated with extended cholecystectomy, as compared with 20% to 40% after simple cholecystectomy alone (with no 5-year survivors among those with positive margins).[42,43]

Stage III Gallbladder Cancer

Performance of an extended cholecystectomy for patients with stage III disease has been associated with 5-year survival estimates of 33% to 67%.[37,46] Occasionally, tumors localized to the infundibulum of the gallbladder can present unique surgical challenges because extensive tumor within the region of the adjacent right portal pedicle may necessitate removal of the right hemiliver, in addition to resection of segment IVA; this is undertaken in the form of an extended right hepatectomy or right trisectionectomy.

Stage IV Gallbladder Cancer

Unfortunately, no long-term survival has been observed among patients with stage IV disease. Involvement of N2 nodes outside of the hepatoduodenal ligament and distant metastases are indicative of more aggressive tumor biology than that seen in bulky tumors extending into the hepatic parenchyma or in those with nodal disease confined to the hepatoduodenal ligament.

SURGICAL MANAGEMENT

The standard template on which all gallbladder cancer operations should be based is the so-called radical or extended cholecystectomy. This consists of cholecystectomy with en bloc resection of a rim of segments IVB and V and lymphadenectomy of the cystic, pericholedochal, periportal, and posterior pancreaticoduodenal lymph nodes residing in the hepatoduodenal ligament and local aortocaval lymph nodes (Fig. 112.2). Knowledge of a patient's tumor stage and familiarity with the general biologic proclivities of gallbladder cancer allow the surgeon to tailor surgical therapy to the individual oncologic needs of each patient. For example, lymphadenectomy can often be performed by simply skeletonizing the porta hepatis. However, in cases of prior dissection in which cicatricial changes in the porta hepatis might blur any distinction between tumor and postoperative changes, in patients with infundibular tumors extending into the region of the common bile duct or in very obese patients, resection of the extrahepatic biliary system with Roux-en-Y hepaticojejunostomy reconstruction may be necessary to accomplish a margin-negative resection and adequate lymphadenectomy.

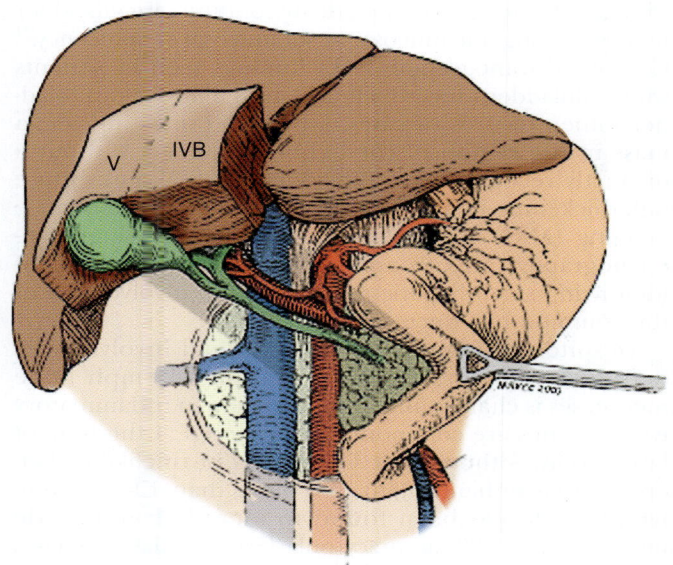

FIGURE 112.2 Portal lymphadenectomy and radical cholecystectomy with en bloc segment IVB/V hepatic resection for gallbladder cancer. (From Bartlett DL, Fong Y. Gallbladder cancer. In: Blumgart LH, et al, eds. *Hepatobiliary Cancer*. Hamilton, ON: BC Decker; 2001:216.)

In practice, the surgeon is often confronted with gallbladder cancer diagnosed incidentally on final pathology after a routine simple cholecystectomy. In the scenario in which the diagnosis of gallbladder cancer is unexpectedly made at the time of laparoscopy, the operating surgeon should discuss the situation with the patient's family and either convert to an open exploration for possible extended cholecystectomy with portal lymphadenectomy, or abort the procedure with subsequent reexploration or referral. The only exception to this is if the patient is at a specialty center where surgeons are well-versed in minimally invasive techniques and are capable of safely performing resection and lymphadenectomy laparoscopically or robotically.

In a more recent series, 66% of those presenting after incidental discovery were eligible for reexploration, and, of those, 17% had no evidence of residual disease.[47] Ultimately, 62% of those reexplored underwent R0 or curative resections, but this represents only 41% of those presenting following incidental disease discovery.[47] Still more discouraging, evidence suggests that the presence of residual disease identified on liver resection following cholecystectomy with incidentally discovered gallbladder cancer confers similar survival to patients with stage IV disease.[39] This makes the case for prudent preoperative investigation prior to index operations and likely reflects the invariable violation of the subserosal plane during laparoscopic cholecystectomy that can result in inadvertent peritoneal seeding. This also underscores the importance of staging laparoscopy, which remains an effective means of identifying patients with unresectable gallbladder cancer.

ADJUVANT THERAPY

In MSKCC data, among those patients undergoing curative resection, a median survival of 26 months and a 5-year actuarial survival of 38% were observed. Factors predictive of poor survival were advanced T stage and N stage.[48] Gallbladder cancer is unfortunately highly resistant to chemotherapy, and its proclivity toward diffuse peritoneal spread limits the applicability of radiation therapy. Uncontrolled studies investigating the use of adjuvant chemotherapy and radiation have provided mixed outcomes with no consistent benefit. One phase III trial examining the efficacy of 5-fluorouracil (5-FU)/mitomycin as adjuvant therapy for various pancreaticobiliary malignancies demonstrated a measurable but modest improvement in 5-year overall survival (26% vs. 15%) and 5-year disease-free survival (20% vs. 11%) for patients with gallbladder cancer treated with adjuvant chemotherapy versus those treated with surgical resection alone.[48] Notably, no such survival benefit was observed among patients with pancreatic cancer, cholangiocarcinoma or ampullary carcinoma in this series.[49] Meta-analysis of studies using palliative and adjuvant radiation therapy for patients with gallbladder cancer suggests a small benefit in survival for those treated with radiotherapy.[49] One report observed a 5-year survival of 64% among a cohort of 21 gallbladder cancer patients treated with concurrent 5-FU and 54-Gy external beam radiation treatment (EBRT) after resection, suggesting that the use of adjuvant chemoradiation may potentiate the therapeutic benefit of surgical treatment.[50] Unfortunately, there have been no large randomized trials from which recommendations regarding the routine use of adjuvant chemotherapy and/or radiotherapy for gallbladder cancer can be made. However, in practice, patients with positive resection margins or nodal metastases are often offered adjuvant therapy without definitive proof of demonstrable efficacy.

PALLIATION

Because of the very high likelihood of surgical unresectability, comprehensive care for patients with gallbladder cancer must also include an armamentarium of palliative procedures. Unfortunately, the median survival of patients with unresectable gallbladder cancer is typically only 2 to 4 months (with a 1-year survival <5%). Therefore, effective palliation should be accompanied by minimal risk of morbidity. Surgical palliation in the form of a segment III biliary bypass provides a relatively simple means of durable biliary decompression because of its distance from the gallbladder and hepatic hilum.[51] However, in very advanced disease, percutaneous biliary drainage usually provides a more reasonable method of palliation when the expected duration of survival is brief. When feasible, resection of port site recurrences after prior laparoscopic cholecystectomy can help to prevent the pain and local cutaneous complications associated with necrotic abdominal wall wounds. Palliative chemotherapy and radiation therapy have not been shown to provide consistent benefit.[52]

SURGICAL TECHNIQUE FOR GALLBLADDER CANCER

As discussed earlier, surgical therapy is reserved for the subset of patients who demonstrate resectability on preoperative imaging. With the exception of those patients who have undergone cholecystectomy with a pathologically confirmed T1a tumor not extending past the lamina propria, patients are offered an extended cholecystectomy with portal lymphadenectomy and partial hepatectomy.

The operative strategy begins with exploratory laparoscopy. If no evidence of peritoneal or unsuspected hepatic spread is noted, the surgeons proceed with open deliberate abdominal exploration through a bilateral subcostal or right transverse incision with a vertical extension to the xiphoid process. If no evidence of technically unresectable disease, distant disease, or N2 nodal metastases is identified, the lymphadenectomy is begun by mobilizing the duodenal sweep with an extensive Kocher maneuver. The retroduodenal lymphatic tissue is harvested with care taken to include aortocaval and superior mesenteric nodes. The portal lymphatic tissue may be skeletonized off of the extrahepatic biliary system, but in cases of prior hilar dissection, tumor extension into the bile duct, or extreme obesity, comprehensive portal lymphadenectomy may require excision of the extrahepatic bile ducts. In this scenario the supraduodenal bile duct is divided and elevated, and its surrounding lymphatic tissue is swept off of the underlying portal vein and hepatic artery as dissection proceeds toward the hepatic hilus.

At the hilus, the hilar plate is lowered by incising Glisson capsule along the base of segment IVB. A determination is made at this point regarding the extent of hepatic resection that will be necessary for complete tumor extirpation. For patients with extensive invasion into the porta hepatis, an extended right hemihepatectomy or right trisectionectomy may be necessary. If the bile duct has been divided, a right hemihepatectomy or trisectionectomy will require division of the left hepatic duct; if the bile duct has been divided and resection of segments IVB and V is sufficient for tumor clearance, the common hepatic duct is typically divided below the confluence of the right and left hepatic ducts.

In the absence of significant tumor extension into the porta hepatis, resection of segments IVB and V is performed. Prior to hepatectomy, care is taken to maintain a low central venous pressure, and the patient is placed into a moderate Trendelenburg position to minimize the risk of air embolism. Inflow control to segment IVB can be obtained by dissection in the region of the umbilical fissure, where the vessels to IVB can be identified and ligated to minimize intraoperative hemorrhage. Control of the segment V vessels is usually achieved after parenchymal transection has commenced; care must be exercised to avoid inadvertent injury to the adjacent right anterior sectoral branches or to the segment VIII vessels. Importantly, the middle hepatic vein draining segments IVB and V runs between segments IVA and VIII and enters the portion of liver to be resected; care must be taken to avoid injury to this vessel, which is divided during parenchymal transection. Inflow and outflow control and accurate segmental resection are facilitated by the use of intraoperative ultrasonography, which can identify the anatomy and course of the relevant vessels. In cases in which extrahepatic biliary resection has been performed, a retrocolic Roux-en-Y hepaticojejunostomy is constructed to reestablish biliary-enteric continuity. Finally, for patients who have previously undergone laparoscopic cholecystectomy, the surrounding skin and fascia of the laparoscopic port sites can be excised and submitted for pathologic analysis for staging, based upon surgeon preference.

BENIGN BILIARY TUMORS

Benign tumors of the biliary tract are exceedingly rare but can cause symptoms not dissimilar from those resulting from malignant causes. The most common benign biliary tumors are papillomas and adenomas. Less common benign tumors include granular cell myoblastomas, neural tumors, endocrine tumors, and leiomyomas. Because they are found most frequently in the region of the ampulla of Vater or along the common bile duct, benign biliary tumors typically present with jaundice that is slowly progressive or intermittent in nature. Optimal treatment includes local excision with removal of a portion of the duct wall from which they originate because local recurrences have been reported after subtotal resection.

Bile duct adenomas are benign intrahepatic tumors that are typically found incidentally at the time of laparoscopy or laparotomy. They often appear as well-demarcated white subcapsular lesions ranging from several millimeters to 1 or 2 cm in size. Histologically, they are characterized by numerous well-differentiated bile duct–like structures surrounded by a fibrous stroma. They are generally asymptomatic and have not been proven to be precancerous in nature.

Biliary cystadenomas are unusual benign tumors often characterized by a multiloculated cystic appearance. Most cystadenomas are mucinous in nature; such mucinous cystadenomas may be associated with pancreatic mucinous cystic neoplasms and are histologically also associated with an ovarian-like stroma in females. Far less common are the serous cystadenomas. The occasional presence of dysplasia suggests the possibility that these tumors may harbor a potential for malignant transformation into biliary cystadenocarcinomas.

Several noteworthy benign conditions must be considered in the differential diagnosis of obstructing biliary tract lesions. Primary sclerosing cholangitis is an idiopathic, premalignant disorder characterized by progressive biliary tract fibrosis whose cholangiographic appearance can mimic that of malignant biliary disease. Untreated, it can ultimately progress to cholestatic liver failure and cholangiocarcinoma. Mirizzi syndrome is an unusual benign condition resulting from a chronically impacted stone in the neck of the gallbladder that itself compresses the common bile duct or that over time induces sufficient pericholecystic inflammation to obstruct the adjacent common hepatic duct or common bile duct. Finally, another unusual benign process that can produce biliary tract obstruction is benign idiopathic focal stenosis, or the so-called malignant masquerade. Because of its propensity to involve the confluence of the hepatic ducts, this benign fibroproliferative disorder is often indistinguishable from cholangiocarcinoma without extensive surgical intervention.[53]

CHOLANGIOCARCINOMA

Cholangiocarcinoma is an uncommon cancer, accounting for only 2% of all reported malignancies. Its incidence in the United States has been estimated at 1 to 2 per 100,000. It may arise anywhere along the entire length of the biliary system; 40% to 60% develop in the hilum (hereafter referred to as hilar cholangiocarcinomas), 20% to 30% in the distal lower biliary tract (distal cholangiocarcinomas), 10% arise intrahepatically (the so-called peripheral or intrahepatic cholangiocarcinomas), and less than 10% develop in a diffuse or multifocal manner. Because of their anatomic differences, these subtypes are associated with distinct patterns of clinical presentation and require distinct strategies for surgical resection. As is the case with gallbladder cancer, the majority of patients with cholangiocarcinoma present with advanced disease that is not amenable to surgical resection; as a result, most patients die within 6 to 12 months of diagnosis from hepatic insufficiency or cholangitis. However, also like gallbladder cancer, improvements in diagnosis and surgical technique have given rise to new optimism in their management.

EPIDEMIOLOGY

In the United States, cholangiocarcinoma is more common among Native Americans and Japanese Americans. Most patients are diagnosed after the age of 65, with a peak incidence occurring during the eighth decade of life. Unlike gallbladder cancer, men appear to have intrahepatic cholangiocarcinoma slightly more frequently than do women. Incidence is similar between the sexes for extrahepatic cholangiocarcinoma.[54,55] Known risk factors include primary sclerosing cholangitis, choledochal cyst disease, chronic viral hepatitis, cirrhosis, prior operative transduodenal sphincteroplasty, chronic biliary parasitic infestation, and numerous teratogens, including thorotrast, asbestos, dioxin, and nitrosamines.[56,57] In Thailand, many cases of cholangiocarcinoma are attributed to the liver fluke *Opisthorchis viverrini*, which has been classified as a type 1 carcinogen as a result.[58] Coordinated public health efforts have dramatically decreased the incidence of *O. viverrini* infestation in Thailand.[59,60] Officials are hopeful that this will decrease the incidence of cholangiocarcinoma; however, it will take 20 to 30 years to see this decrease reflected in the population. Moreover, there remain somewhere between 6 and 8 million people infected with *O. viverrini*; thus public health efforts in Thailand are heavily focused on designing effective screening programs.[61]

PATHOLOGY

Intrahepatic Cholangiocarcinoma

On gross examination, intrahepatic cholangiocarcinomas appear as scirrhous primary hepatic lesions with a non-encapsulated infiltrative pattern of growth that produces poorly defined tumor margins. The most common histologic type is poorly differentiated adenocarcinoma; as a result, they are often misdiagnosed as metastatic adenocarcinomas. Indeed, it is quite likely that many hepatic tumors classified as metastatic adenocarcinoma of unknown primary in the past were truly intrahepatic cholangiocarcinomas. Variants with focal areas of papillary carcinoma, signet ring cells, squamous cells, mucoepidermoid cells, and spindle cells have been described.[62]

Hilar and Extrahepatic Cholangiocarcinoma

Extrahepatic hilar and distal cholangiocarcinomas are categorized into three macroscopic subtypes: sclerosing (70%, usually hilar in location, characterized by circumferential ductal thickening with residual fibrosis and inflammation), nodular (20% firm tumors extending irregularly into the duct lumen, occasionally growing in a nodular-sclerosing pattern), and papillary (5% to 10%, soft and friable tumors typically projecting into the duct lumen in a pedunculated fashion, usually distal in location, and associated with higher resectability and more favorable outcomes).[63,64] Their pattern of growth is insidiously longitudinal, with tumor cells often extending both proximally and distally beneath normal ductal epithelium. This pattern of growth mandates careful microscopic attention to margins at the time of surgical extirpation to ensure complete tumor resection. Another pathologic feature of cholangiocarcinoma is the exuberant desmoplastic reaction that often accompanies these tumors. Histologic analysis of these tumors occasionally identifies only small foci of malignant cells within densely fibrotic stroma. This characteristic can render the analysis of needle biopsy specimens challenging and highly susceptible to sampling error. Pathologic evaluation can be aided by fluorescence in situ hybridization (FISH) in patients with chronic inflammatory states such as primary sclerosing cholangitis. However, although FISH is specific (93%), it has limited sensitivity (51%).[65]

The tendency of extrahepatic cholangiocarcinoma to occlude biliary ducts and to invade portal venous branches often results in hepatic atrophy. Gradually progressive segmental or lobar atrophy in the setting of cholangiocarcinoma is indicative of chronic biliary obstruction; comparatively rapid parenchymal atrophy is typically the result of portal obstruction.[66] Distant metastases are not uncommon, perineural and lymphovascular spread are often observed, and up to one-third of patients present with nodal metastases.

PRESENTATION

Symptoms associated with intrahepatic cholangiocarcinomas are nonspecific, including malaise and abdominal pain. Unlike hilar and distal cholangiocarcinomas, a minority of patients develop jaundice. Hilar and distal cholangiocarcinomas can present with nonspecific symptoms of pain, anorexia, and weight loss. Distal cholangiocarcinoma can be clinically indistinguishable from other periampullary neoplasms. Pruritis is a common symptom for patients with extrahepatic cholangiocarcinoma, and it typically precedes clinically apparent jaundice. It is jaundice or the presence of abnormal liver enzymes that usually prompts medical attention. However, it is helpful to note that, although most patients with hilar and distal cholangiocarcinoma ultimately develop jaundice, segmental or incomplete lobar obstruction can produce considerable hepatic atrophy without frank jaundice.

Some of the more nonspecific presenting symptoms of cholangiocarcinoma can closely resemble those associated with benign gallstone disease, and malignant biliary disease can often coexist with benign calculous disease. The level of hyperbilirubinemia can be informative in distinguishing benign from malignant biliary obstruction; benign causes of obstructive jaundice typically produce bilirubin levels ranging from 2 to 4 mg/dL (rarely exceeding 5 mg/dL), whereas biliary obstruction from cholangiocarcinoma usually results in serum bilirubin levels greater than 10 mg/dL (with a mean level of approximately 18 mg/dL).[67] On occasion, intraluminal growth of papillary cholangiocarcinomas (more common among distal tumors) can induce a physiologic ball-valve effect that produces intermittent episodes of obstructive jaundice.

Although a 30% rate of bactibilia has been observed among patients with extrahepatic cholangiocarcinoma, clinically evident cholangitis is unusual as a presenting symptom.[68] The noteworthy variance from this observation comes from patients who undergo biliary instrumentation (either percutaneously or endoscopically), because these patients uniformly develop bactibilia and not uncommonly develop manifestations of cholangitis.

DIAGNOSIS

The finding of an intrahepatic mass prompts an extensive diagnostic work-up that can, in large part, be directed by relevant findings from the patient's history and physical examination. For example, a history of colon cancer or hepatitis might direct the diagnostic evaluation toward hepatic colorectal metastases or hepatocellular carcinoma, respectively. Otherwise, evaluation begins with measurement of tumor markers, including CEA, alpha fetoprotein, and CA 19-9, as well as hepatitis B and C viral serologies.

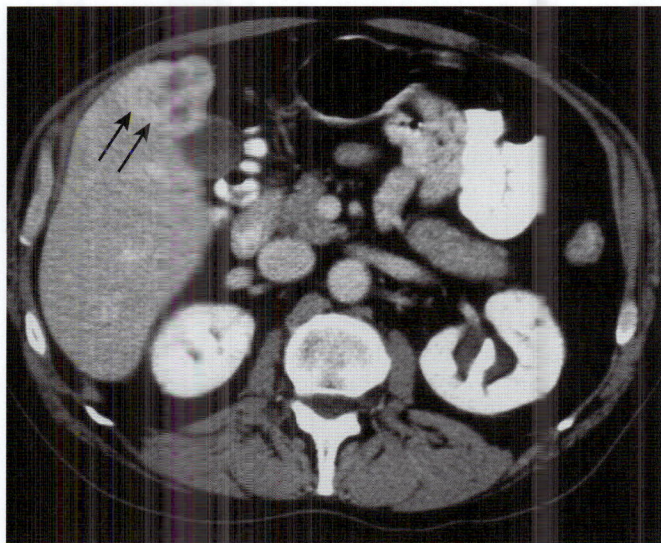

FIGURE 112.3 Computed tomographic appearance of large intrahepatic cholangiocarcinoma. (From Koea J, Fong Y. Primary hepatic malignancies. In: Blumgart LH, et al, eds. *Hepatobiliary Cancer.* Hamilton, ON: EC Decker; 2001:59.)

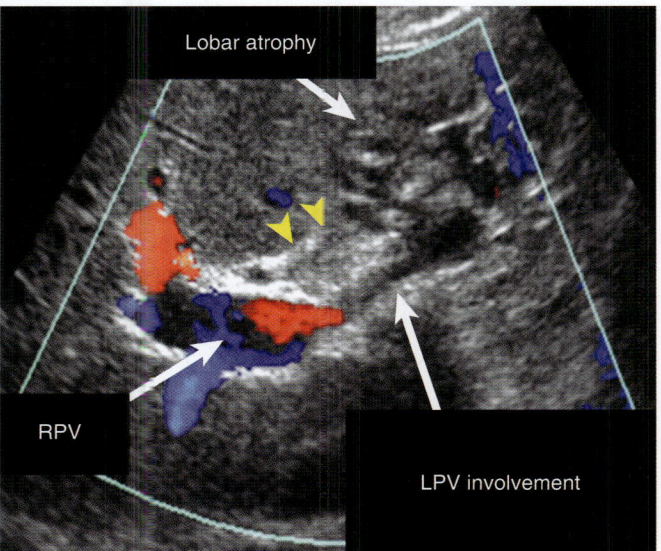

FIGURE 112.4 Ultrasonographic duplex image of hilar cholangiocarcinoma with lobar atrophy. *Yellow arrowheads* indicate tumor compression at hilus. *LPV,* Left portal vein; *RPV,* right portal vein.

Colonoscopic evaluation can be used to identify primary colorectal adenocarcinoma if pathology is equivocal. In general, cholangiocarcinomas are often accompanied by elevations in CA 19-9. Levels of CA 19-9 greater than 100 U/mL have been shown to correspond with the presence of cholangiocarcinoma with a sensitivity of 89% and a specificity of 86%.[69] Of course, one must bear in mind that biliary obstruction results in falsely elevated CA 19-9. Thus baseline measurements should be regarded as correct only after adequate biliary decompression is achieved. In addition, 10% of patients may be Lewis antigen nonproducers, in which case CA 19-9 measurement is unhelpful.[70] Typical imaging modalities include ultrasonography followed by high-quality cross-sectional imaging, which is best performed prior to biliary instrumentation to prevent inflammatory and instrumentation artifacts.[71] Thin section (minimum 2.5 mm reconstructed at 1.25 mm), high-resolution CT performed with rapid intravenous contrast bolus in arterial and portovenous phases can accurately determine resectability in the majority of cases. MRI with MRCP can better delineate intrahepatic tumor extension and precise biliary radicle involvement but has limited vascular accuracy and is therefore less helpful in determining resectability. If both modalities are used, resectability should be predicted more than 75% of the time.[71]

Intrahepatic cholangiocarcinomas often appear as hypovascular masses on standard imaging techniques and can appear similar to other primary and metastatic hepatic malignancies (Fig. 112.3). In general, intrahepatic cholangiocarcinoma appears hypodense with irregular margins in the unenhanced phase, with peripheral rim enhancement in the arterial phase, and progressive hyperattenuation on venous and delayed phases.[72] Hilar cholangiocarcinoma often requires the full gamut of radiologic and endoscopic examinations to achieve a

diagnosis. In experienced hands, duplex ultrasonography can provide data regarding extent of biliary ductal, periductal, and vascular involvement with a sensitivity and specificity matching or exceeding that of CT angiography (Fig. 112.4).[73,74] MRCP provides an accurate assessment of biliary ductal anatomy and can evaluate distal or proximal ductal systems that are excluded by the tumor and therefore not imaged by percutaneous or endoscopic cholangiography. MRCP also avoids the biliary instrumentation (and potential infectious complications) associated with invasive cholangiography. The finding of hepatic parenchymal atrophy is indicative of biliary and/or portal venous obstruction from tumor. It is also an indication that partial hepatectomy of the atrophic segment or lobe is likely to be necessary for complete extirpation of disease (Fig. 112.5). Because of its proximity to the duodenum, the radiographic evaluation of distal cholangiocarcinoma more commonly uses endoscopic retrograde cholangiopancreatography (ERCP) and endoscopic ultrasound. Although the primary lesions are often too small to be visible on cross-sectional imaging, CT is useful for evaluating the extent of metastatic disease. Endoscopic brushings and biliary cytology are associated with very low diagnostic sensitivity; this, combined with their typical inaccessibility to percutaneous biopsy techniques, often requires that therapeutic intervention be undertaken for extrahepatic cholangiocarcinoma in the absence of a definitive tissue diagnosis. It should be noted that in patients without suspicion for benign biliary obstruction etiology, preoperative pathologic confirmation is not required to proceed with resection.[71] More importantly, percutaneous and laparoscopic biopsies should be avoided in patients who might be candidates for transplantation. However, if systemic or locoregional therapies are pursued, then tissue diagnosis is necessary. In the case of intrahepatic cholangiocarcinoma, if biopsy demonstrates adenocarcinoma,

ta

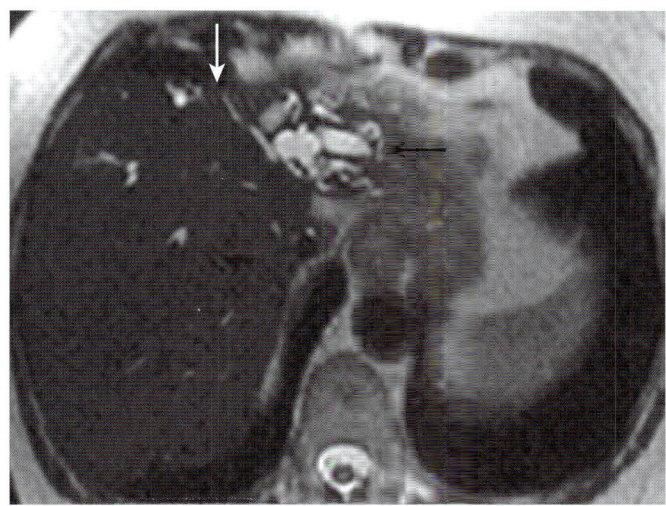

FIGURE 112.5 Magnetic resonance imaging appearance of hilar cholangiocarcinoma with lobar atrophy. Note crowded, dilated ducts *(white arrow)* denoting presence of small, hypoperfused left hepatic lobe *(black arrow).*

immunostains are required to detect other possible metastatic lesions and to differentiate from mixed hepatocellular tumors.[75] Unless immunostains are clearly consistent with intrahepatic cholangiocarcinoma, thorough work-up for occult primary tumor should be undertaken.[75] Although PET can be helpful in identifying distant disease, findings rarely change treatment course if thorough cross-sectional imaging has been used. Thus PET is not routinely recommended.[71,75]

STAGING

The two major conventional staging systems for cholangiocarcinoma are the Bismuth-Corlette system and the AJCC tumor, node, metastasis staging system (Table 112.2).[36,76] The Bismuth-Corlette system is an anatomically based, surgically oriented system that is not very predictive of patient outcome. Previous iterations of the AJCC system were pathology-driven constructs that correlated poorly with surgical resectability and patient outcome. The current AJCC system appropriately differentiates hilar and intrahepatic and distal cholangiocarcinoma. Staging criteria for intrahepatic cholangiocarcinoma resemble those used for other primary hepatic tumors, and staging criteria for distal cholangiocarcinoma resemble those used for other periampullary carcinomas. Moreover, as with gallbladder cancer, the new staging systems for cholangiocarcinoma incorporate determinants of surgical resectability and outcome.

In the absence of effective chemotherapy or radiation therapy, surgical resection remains the mainstay of curative treatment for cholangiocarcinoma. Within this context, the ability to affect a margin-negative R0 complete resection is critical. Other factors influencing long-term survival after potentially curative surgery include number of tumors, vascular invasion, and lymph node metastases.[77–80] Nodal status is also of great import. Some authors have shown that intrahepatic cholangiocarcinoma patients with lymph node metastases and R0 resections fare the same as those

BOX 112.1 Criteria for Unresectability for Cholangiocarcinoma

Medical contraindication to surgical intervention
Advanced cirrhosis or portal hypertension
  Inadequate size of future liver remnant
Bilateral second-order biliary radicle involvement
  Bilateral hepatic artery and/or portal venous branch involvement
  Involvement of unilateral hepatic artery with contralateral ductal spread
Main portal vein involvement or encasement
Lobar atrophy with contralateral second-order biliary radicle involvement
Lobar atrophy with contralateral portal vein involvement
Nodal involvement
Distant metastases

with R1 resections.[78] Nevertheless, the role of routine lymphadenectomy remains controversial.

The criteria for surgical unresectability for hilar cholangiocarcinoma are listed in Box 112.1.[81] As discussed previously, the presence of hepatic segmental or hemiliver atrophy is indicative of biliary and/or portal venous obstruction, and resection of the atrophic segment or hemiliver is generally required for complete tumor removal. Therefore the observation of portal venous or biliary obstruction contralateral to an atrophic lobe is suggestive of bilobar tumor involvement that would not be amenable to surgical resection. Importantly, these criteria have been shown to correlate strongly with surgical resectability (Table 112.3).[81] The current iteration of the AJCC staging system for hilar cholangiocarcinoma appropriately incorporates these criteria for resectability. That being said, some investigators advocate that T-stage classification should measure the depth of invasion of a tumor rather than structures invaded and locations thereof.[80]

SURGERY

The goal of surgical therapy for cholangiocarcinoma is complete R0 resection.

Intrahepatic Cholangiocarcinoma

Techniques of anatomic hepatic resection for intrahepatic cholangiocarcinoma follow those used for other hepatic malignancies. With appropriate patient selection, 5-year overall survival rates following attempted curative resection can range from 30% to 40%.[79,80,82] In the historical MSK experience, patients with disease amenable to surgical resection exhibited a median survival of 37 months and a 3-year actuarial survival of 55%; predictors of poor survival were vascular invasion, positive resection margins, and multiple tumors.[75,83] A more recent series builds on these data and reports 82 patients undergoing potentially curative resections, with a median disease-specific survival of 36 months.[77] Recurrence was found in 62% of patients with a median follow-up of 26 months. The liver remnant was the most frequent site of recurrence. Independent predictors of poor disease-specific survival include multiple tumors, regional nodal involvement, and large tumor size (>5 cm).[77]

TABLE 112.2 American Joint Committee on Cancer Staging System for Cholangiocarcinoma

A. HILAR CHOLANGIOCARCINOMA

T1	Tumor confined to bile duct
T2a	Tumor invades beyond bile duct wall into surrounding adipose tissue
T2b	Tumor invades beyond bile duct wall into adjacent hepatic parenchyma
T3	Tumor invades unilateral portal vein or hepatic artery
T4	Tumor invades bilateral portal veins or hepatic arteries or;
	Tumor invades second-order biliary radicles bilaterally or;
	Tumor invades second-order biliary radicles unilaterally and contralateral portal vein or hepatic artery
N0	No lymph node involvement
N1	Lymph node involvement within hepatoduodenal ligament
N2	Lymph node involvement beyond hepatoduodenal ligament
M0	No distant metastases
M1	Distant metastases
Stage I	T1 N0 M0
Stage II	T2 N0 M0
Stage IIIA	T3 N0 M0
Stage IIIB	T1-3 N1 M0
Stage IVA	T4 N0-1 M0
Stage IVB	T1-4 N2 M0
	T1-4 N0-2 M1

B. INTRAHEPATIC CHOLANGIOCARCINOMA

T1	Solitary tumor without vascular invasion
T2a	Solitary tumor with vascular invasion
T2b	Multiple tumors with or without vascular invasion
T3	Tumor directly invades local extrahepatic structures
T4	Tumor invades periductal tissues
N0	No lymph node involvement
N1	Lymph node involvement
M0	No distant metastases
M1	Distant metastases
Stage I	T1 N0 M0
Stage II	T2 N0 M0
Stage III	T3 N0 M0
Stage IVA	T4 N0 M0
	T1-4 N1 M0
Stage IVB	T1-4 N0-1 M1

C. DISTAL CHOLANGIOCARCINOMA

T1	Tumor confined to bile duct
T2	Tumor invades beyond bile duct
T3	Tumor invades the gallbladder, pancreas, duodenum, or adjacent organs without involvement of the celiac axis or superior mesenteric artery
T4	Tumor invades the celiac axis or superior mesenteric artery
N0	No lymph node involvement
N1	Lymph node involvement
M0	No distant metastases
M1	Distant metastases
Stage I	T1 N0 M0
Stage IB	T2 N0 M0
Stage IIA	T3 N0 M0
Stage IIB	T1-3 N1 M0
Stage III	T4 N0-1 M0
Stage IV	T1-4 N0-1 M1

Hilar Cholangiocarcinoma

As outlined in Table 112.3, surgical resectability is determined by the extent of portal venous involvement, biliary radicle involvement, and lobar atrophy. Those patients who are found to harbor resectable disease should undergo operative exploration; complete extirpation will require extrahepatic biliary excision with partial hepatectomy and hepaticojejunostomy. Laparoscopy can also be of assistance prior to attempted curative resection, especially in the setting of equivocal preoperative imaging studies. A prospective evaluation of the ability of staging laparoscopy to identify patients with unresectable disease demonstrated

TABLE 112.3 Correlation of Tumor Extent and Resectability

Biliary Involvement	Ipsilateral Lobar Atrophy	Ipsilateral Portal Vein Involvement	Main Portal Vein Involvement	Resectability (%)
Hilus and/or unilateral bile duct	No	No	No	48
Hilus and/or unilateral bile duct	Yes	No	No	43
Hilus and/or unilateral bile duct	Yes/No	Yes	No	25
Bilateral second-order radicles	Yes/No	Yes/No	Yes	0

From Burke EC, Jarnagin WR, Hochwald SN, Pisters PW, Fong Y, Blumgart LH. Hilar cholangiocarcinoma: patterns of spread, the importance of hepatic resection for curative operation, and a presurgical clinical staging system. *Ann Surg*. 1998;228:385.

that 14 of 56 patients with hilar cholangiocarcinoma undergoing exploratory laparoscopy at MSKCC were found to have laparoscopic evidence of unresectable disease; of the remaining 42 patients who then underwent laparotomy with curative intent, an additional 19 patients were found to have unresectable tumors for reasons not appreciated laparoscopically.[75]

Because of its propensity for longitudinal ductal spread, partial hepatectomy is often necessary in addition to extrahepatic biliary excision for complete resection of extrahepatic cholangiocarcinoma. Generally speaking, the rate of negative-margin resection closely approximates the frequency with which partial hepatectomy is performed. The proximity of the caudate lobe to the hepatic hilus often mandates concomitant caudate lobectomy for hilar tumors; this is particularly evident for left-sided hilar tumors because the major caudate lobe ducts drain into the left hepatic duct. Classically, up to 50% of those presenting for resection have evidence of unresectable disease.[84] Rates of attempted margin-negative resections are expected to diminish as sensitivity of modern imaging continues to improve.[71] In more recent series, 75% to 80% of patients undertaking potentially curative resections are able to achieve margin-negative resection.[84-86] Five-year overall survival following resection ranges in the literature from 25% to 50%.[84,87] In a classic series from Memorial Sloan Kettering, patients undergoing resection exhibited an overall median survival of 59 months; predictors of improved survival were well-differentiated tumors, negative resection margin, and the performance of a concomitant hepatic resection. The importance of obtaining negative resection margins is underscored by the observation that patients with histologically positive margins of resection demonstrated survival outcomes indistinguishable from those with locally advanced tumors undergoing operative exploration without attempted resection. It appears that the performance of partial hepatectomy at the time of resection of hilar cholangiocarcinoma is critical for optimizing outcome. Indeed, the 5-year actuarial survival among those patients undergoing partial hepatectomy was 37%, compared with 0% for those treated with bile duct excision alone. Interestingly, even within the cohort of patients who underwent complete R0 resection, the performance of partial hepatectomy conferred a statistically significant survival advantage on multivariate analysis.[84] The correlation between concomitant partial hepatectomy and improved disease-free and disease-specific survival outcomes has also been confirmed in other centers.[88]

Distal Cholangiocarcinoma

Most distal cholangiocarcinomas will require pancreaticoduodenectomy for complete resection. A review of the MSKCC experience with distal cholangiocarcinomas demonstrated that only 13% of these tumors could be removed with bile duct excision alone.[89] As mentioned previously, distal cholangiocarcinomas are often clinically indistinguishable from other periampullary neoplasms, including pancreatic adenocarcinoma. However, possibly because of the inherent likelihood of earlier presentation with biliary symptoms, they are associated with less frequent lymphovascular invasion, lower margin positivity, and higher resectability and therefore were classically thought to have better survival compared with pancreatic ductal adenocarcinoma.[89,90] Newer studies have shown no significant difference between survival from distal cholangiocarcinoma and pancreatic ductal adenocarcinoma.[91] When compared between equivalent stages and resections, there do not appear to be any meaningful survival differences between hilar and distal cholangiocarcinomas.[92]

Orthotopic Liver Transplant

Orthotopic liver transplant for hilar cholangiocarcinoma, often done for patients with underlying primary sclerosing cholangitis, has traditionally been associated with suboptimal survival outcomes. However, the Mayo Clinic has demonstrated promising results among a select cohort of patients undergoing neoadjuvant chemoradiation followed by cadaveric or living donor liver transplant. In this protocol, eligibility is reserved for patients with confirmed cholangiocarcinoma who have technically unresectable disease above the cystic duct and no evidence of intrahepatic or extrahepatic metastases. Patients must have a radial tumor diameter of less than or equal to 3 cm and be a good candidate for liver transplantation.[93] For those entering the protocol, neoadjuvant therapy begins with an initial period of EBRT with intravenous fluorouracil, followed by transcatheter iridium-based brachytherapy, then subsequent maintenance therapy with oral capecitabine. After completion of their neoadjuvant radiotherapy, all patients undergo a staging laparotomy to confirm absence of extrahepatic disease. In their most recent report of their experience, 184 patients have begun neoadjuvant therapy. Of those, 120 patients had favorable findings at the staging operation and have successfully undergone transplant, yielding a 5-year overall survival of 73%.[94] Interestingly, 5-year survival is better for those patients with underlying primary sclerosing cholangitis (79%) versus those with de novo cholangiocarcinoma (63%). A recurrence rate of 18% is noted. These novel observations suggest that a highly selective subset of patients with unresectable but nonmetastatic hilar cholangiocarcinoma may experience considerable survival benefit after orthotopic liver transplant.

ADJUVANT THERAPY

Systemic Therapy

As is the case with gallbladder cancer, there have not been sufficiently large or controlled trials rigorously examining the efficacy of adjuvant chemotherapy or radiotherapy for patients undergoing resection of cholangiocarcinoma to dictate general treatment guidelines. Moreover, because of the relative rarity of cholangiocarcinomas, the subtypes of distal, intrahepatic, and hilar are frequently lumped together, which may confound available data. For instance, an earlier phase III trial examining the effect of 5-FU and mitomycin-C on 508 patients with pancreatobiliary malignancies (139 of which were cholangiocarcinomas) demonstrated an observable but not statistically significant survival benefit of R0 resection plus adjuvant treatment over surgical resection alone for cholangiocarcinoma.[49,84] Much of current adjuvant practice is extrapolated from trials studying chemotherapy in patients with locally advanced or metastatic biliary tract cancers. In 2010, the ABC-02 trial published results of 410 patients with intrahepatic or extrahepatic cholangiocarcinoma, gallbladder cancer, or ampullary cancer. Patients received either cisplatin with gemcitabine for eight 3-week cycles or gemcitabine alone in six 4-week cycles.[95] A median survival benefit was noted in the gemcitabine-cisplatin group (11.7 months vs. 8.1 months) and this treatment arm also experienced improved progression-free survival and locoregional control.[95]

Locoregional Therapy

Unlike gallbladder cancer, initial recurrence sites following resection are more likely to be locoregional in patients with hilar cholangiocarcinoma (59%) when compared with gallbladder cancer (15%).[96] This provides the basis for locoregional adjuvant strategies in the treatment of hilar lesions following resection, and accordingly several authors have demonstrated survival benefit of postoperative chemoradiotherapy on multivariate analyses.[97,98] Postoperative chemoradiotherapy administered to patients with risk factors for recurrence, such as positive margins or positive nodes, has been shown to yield similar locoregional recurrence rates (38% vs. 37%) and similar overall 5-year survival as those patients without the high-risk features who did not receive radiation therapy.[99] Todoroki et al. demonstrated the benefits of radiation therapy (in the form of either intraoperative and/or external beam therapy), showing substantially improved locoregional control in those patients receiving radiation compared with those receiving surgery alone.[100] However, 90% of the patients in that series had a positive resection margin, which hinders the efficacy of these results in margin-negative cases. An older but oft cited study demonstrated no survival benefit for radiation in perihilar cholangiocarcinoma.[101] Thus a

clear role for radiation therapy has yet to be defined in the literature.

Molecular Therapy

A number of different molecular markers have been identified as major players in biliary tract carcinogenesis and cancer progression.[102] Whole-genome analysis of cholangiocarcinoma has identified two genomic classes of disease occurrence: those activated via inflammatory pathways and those activated via proliferative oncogene pathways.[108] The latter portends a worse prognosis.[103] Regarding specific markers, a comprehensive genomic profile of 104 surgically resected cholangiocarcinomas yielded a subgroup of patients with poor overall survival and early recurrence that were characterized by the presence of K-ras mutations and multiple aberrations in cellular regulation, including activated human epidermal growth factor receptor 2 (HER2) and epidermal growth factor receptor (EGFR) signaling.[104] Interestingly, although BRAF mutations have been noted in gallbladder cancer patients, only one of 59 patients analyzed in the aforementioned study demonstrated BRAF V600E mutations, again indicating varied tumor biology among biliary tract cancers.[104]

Several studies have attempted to establish synergy of molecular targeting therapies with more traditional regimens with little success thus far. For instance, the ABC-03 trial studied the addition of cediranib (a vascular endothelial growth factor inhibitor with additional activity against platelet derived growth factor receptors and c-KIT) to cisplatin and gemcitabine in patients with advanced biliary tract cancers and showed no improvement in progression-free survival.[105] In another instance the French Biliary Cancers group put on the BINGO trial which randomized 101 patients with intrahepatic or extrahepatic cholangiocarcinoma, gallbladder cancer, or ampullary cancer to receive gemcitabine and oxaliplatin with or without cetuximab (an EGFR inhibitor). Unfortunately no added benefit was noted for these patients.[106] However, many would argue that molecular targeting in the absence of molecular profiling is a significant waste of resources. A publication by Churi et al. details the MD Anderson experience with mutation profiling and resultant targeted therapies and demonstrated radiologic and clinically significant responses following use of EGFR, fibroblast growth factor receptor (FGFR), C-met, BRAF, and MEK inhibitors.[107] Among patients with intrahepatic cholangiocarcinoma, this study noted a worse prognosis with KRAS, TP53, and MAPK/mTOR genetic aberrations, whereas those patients with FGFR aberrations had a more indolent course.[107]

PALLIATION

Palliation in the setting of unresectable cholangiocarcinoma is usually directed toward the control of refractory malignant jaundice. Palliation of jaundice is generally indicated for cases of cholangitis or intractable pruritus or for patients requiring optimization of hepatic function before initiation of chemotherapy. Several important principles guide the manner in which biliary decompression should be undertaken. First, jaundice is typically not relieved until more than one-third of functional liver mass is effectively decompressed. Because of the propensity of advanced cholangiocarcinoma obstruct and isolate multiple hepatic segments or lobes that may necessitate separate drainage of more than one biliary ductal system. Second, decompression of an atrophic segment or hemiliver will not control jaundice. Third, it is possible for jaundice to develop in the absence of biliary obstruction. Portal venous obstruction or thrombosis from cholangiocarcinoma can produce rapid hepatic atrophy and dysfunction; jaundice in such patients will not be relieved by biliary decompression.

Selection of the optimal method of biliary decompression requires a careful balance between the expected duration of treatment benefit and the anticipated length of patient survival, as well as between the potential for treatment-related morbidity and patient quality of life. Operative bypass options, which include hepaticojejunostomy for hilar cholangiocarcinoma or choledochoenterostomy for distal cholangiocarcinoma, are generally associated with high durability and patency but at the cost of high potential morbidity, mortality, and recovery time. As such, operative biliary bypass is generally reserved for patients in whom unresectability and present or impending biliary obstruction are recognized at the time of attempted surgical resection or for patients whose expected survival exceeds 6 months. Operative bypass to the segment III ducts is particularly appealing in the setting of unresectable hilar cholangiocarcinoma because of their distance from the hepatic hilus and demonstrates an 80% patency rate at 1 year; bypass to the right anterior or posterior sectional duct can also be performed.[108] For others, percutaneously or endoscopically placed self-expanding metallic biliary stents may be preferable. Percutaneous biliary drainage can help patients with hilar cholangiocarcinoma, whose tumors can be difficult to traverse with endoscopically placed stents. Bile duct occlusion from distal cholangiocarcinoma is ideally treated with endobiliary stenting, which can demonstrate 1-year patency rates of up to 89%.[109] The total duration of patency for permanent metallic stents (3 to 10 months) doubles that of temporary plastic endobiliary stents (4 to 5 months).[110] There is some evidence that intraluminal brachytherapy with iridium-based radiation may prolong patency by delaying in-growth of tumor into the lumen of the stent. However, the palliative use of intraluminal radiotherapy, even when used in conjunction with EBRT, has not consistently shown a measurable survival benefit over that seen with biliary decompression alone.[111]

SURGICAL TECHNIQUE FOR CHOLANGIOCARCINOMA

The technique of resection for intrahepatic cholangiocarcinoma follows standard procedure of hepatic resection (Fig. 112.6). Similarly, surgical extirpation of distal cholangiocarcinoma is performed by pancreaticoduodenectomy. In this section, we will review the basic technique of surgical management of hilar cholangiocarcinoma.

If preoperative imaging demonstrates no clear evidence of unresectability, operative intervention is undertaken. In selected cases, this may begin with an initial laparoscopic inspection. Alternatively, abdominal exploration through a bilateral subcostal or right transverse incision with a midline extension to the xiphoid process is commenced. Careful visual and manual inspection is performed to

identify evidence of distant or N2 nodal metastases that would preclude resection. The ligamentum teres is ligated, divided and elevated to permit careful inspection of the liver for previously unidentified intrahepatic lesions. The lesser omentum is opened to permit careful inspection of hepatic segment I (the caudate lobe), and a Kocher maneuver is performed to inspect the retroduodenal lymph nodes. Should evidence of unresectable disease be encountered at this point, the surgical strategy turns to one of palliation of biliary obstruction by operative biliary-enteric bypass or nonoperative drainage.

If tumor resectability is confirmed, preparations are begun for possible partial hepatectomy. Low central venous pressure is maintained to minimize blood loss during hepatic parenchymal transection, and the patient is placed in a moderate Trendelenburg position for prevention of air embolism. The supraduodenal bile duct is divided, and a cholecystectomy is performed to begin mobilization and inspection of the extrahepatic biliary system. The bile duct is dissected free from the underlying portal vein and hepatic artery in an ascending fashion toward the hepatic hilus; direct tumor invasion into the portal vein may preclude resection unless a segmental portal vein resection and reconstruction can be performed with restoration of sufficient portal venous blood flow to the liver. The course of the left hepatic duct is exposed by dividing the bridge of hepatic tissue that typically joins the bases of segments IVB and III, and the hilar plate is lowered by incising Glisson capsule along the base of segment IVB. By exposing the hepatic hilus in this fashion, the need for partial hepatectomy may be determined. If evidence of unilateral second-order biliary radicle involvement or ipsilateral portal vein involvement is detected, partial hepatectomy of the involved lobe is mandated to maximize the likelihood of a complete R0 resection. In the limited number of cases in which second-order biliary radicles are not involved and vascular involvement is absent, segmental extrahepatic bile duct excision may be sufficient.

When segmental bile duct excision can be performed, the right and left bile ducts are divided well above the proximal extent of visible tumor. In certain cases this may require division of the bile ducts above the level of a sectoral confluence, resulting in more than two duct orifices. Biliary-enteric continuity is then reestablished by construction of a retrocolic Roux-en-Y hepaticojejunostomy. Whenever possible, separated ipsilateral sectoral ducts are first sutured close to one another so that they may be used as a single functional duct when constructing the hepaticojejunostomy. Alternatively, separated sectoral ducts can be sequentially anastomosed into a single enterotomy site. To accomplish this, a row of anterior sutures is first placed along the separated ducts. Retraction of the anterior row of sutures facilitates exposure to the posterior wall of the duct. A posterior row of sutures is then placed along the ducts and the jejunotomy and serially tied to bring the back wall of the separated ducts into direct apposition against the back wall of the jejunum. The preplaced anterior row of sutures can then be placed along the anterior wall of the jejunum.

In the more common situation in which partial hepatectomy is deemed to be necessary for complete resection, the liver is mobilized by dividing its peritoneal and

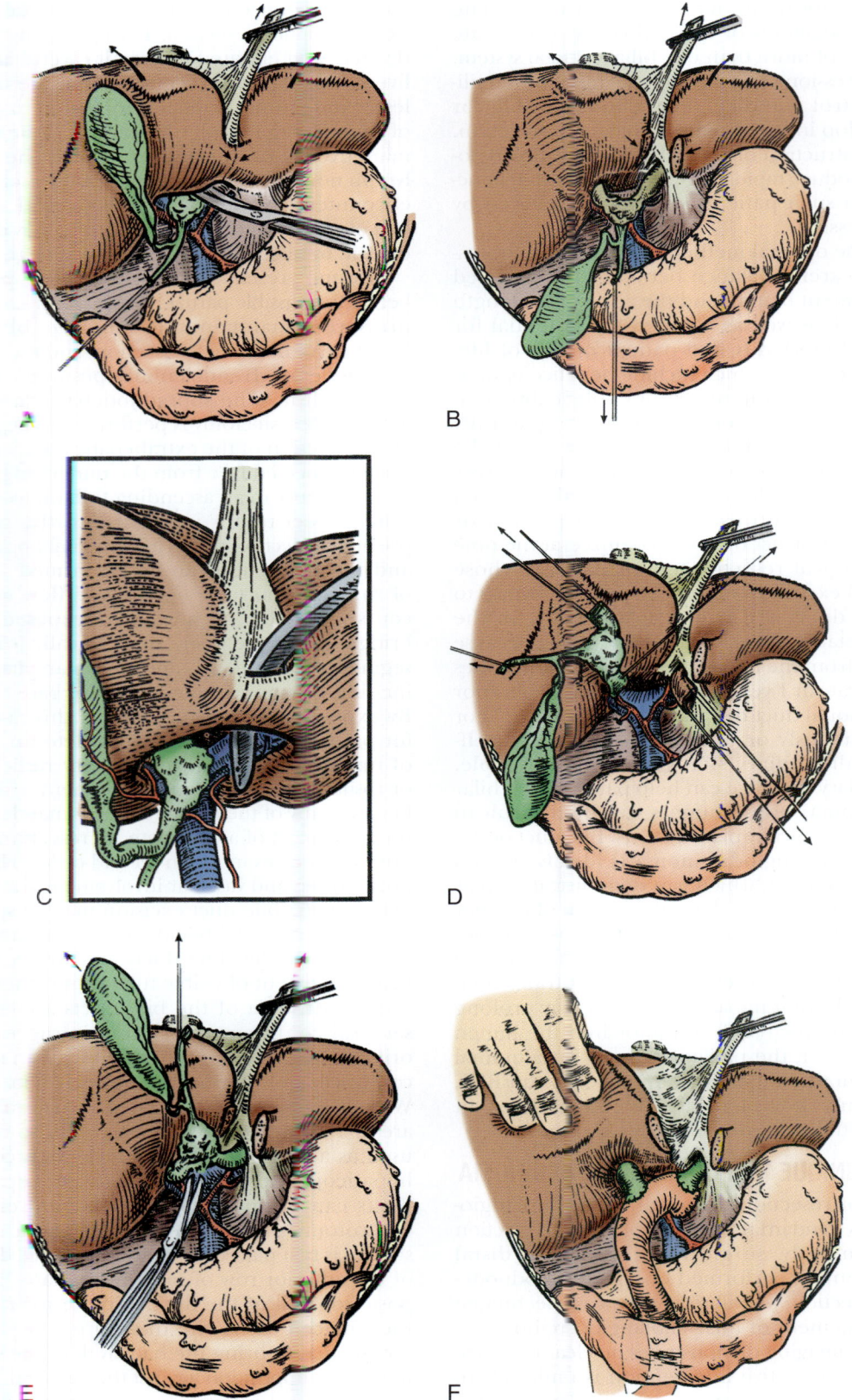

FIGURE 112.6 Resection of hilar cholangiocarcinoma with partial hepatectomy. (From Jarnagin WR, et al: Hilar cholangiocarcinoma. In: Blumgart LH, Fong Y, eds. *Surgery of the Liver and Biliary Tract*. London: Saunders, 2000:1033.)

diaphragmatic attachments. For patients with left-sided tumors, careful inspection of the caudate lobe is necessary because involvement of the usual left-sided caudate ducts usually requires en bloc segment I (caudate lobectomy). The hepatic artery and portal vein to the involved lobe or segment are divided, as is the draining hepatic vein. Hepatic parenchymal transection is performed to complete the resection, and construction of a Roux-en-Y hepaticojejunostomy to the contralateral duct or ducts is performed. External drains are routinely placed close to the biliary-enteric anastomoses.

In a select group of patients with hilar or intrahepatic cholangiocarcinoma, a central mesohepatectomy can be performed. This involves resection of segments IVA, IVB, V, and VIII. This is most helpful in patients whose liver function, future liver remnant volume, or tumor location will not allow for an extended left or extended right hepatectomy. Patient selection is critical because risks of morbidity and mortality are as high as 55% and 6%, respectively.[112] However, with judicious use of partial or total inflow occlusion (and outflow occlusion when necessary), margin negative resection can be achieved that may not otherwise be possible.

OTHER MALIGNANT BILIARY TUMORS

MIXED HEPATOCELLULAR AND CHOLANGIOCARCINOMA

Limited experience exists with the management of this distinct primary hepatic malignancy. These intrahepatic tumors possess histologic features of both hepatocellular carcinoma and cholangiocarcinoma. Demographics of patients with these mixed tumors appear to be more similar to those with pure intrahepatic cholangiocarcinoma than hepatocellular carcinoma. Furthermore, the survival outcomes of patients undergoing surgical resection of these mixed tumors appear to more closely parallel those of patients treated for cholangiocarcinoma.[83] This favors resection rather than transplantation treatment strategies in these patients because their poor prognosis obviates judicious organ use.[113]

BILIARY CYSTADENOCARCINOMA

Biliary cystadenocarcinomas are rare malignancies that are typically intrahepatic in location. The presence of an associated ovarian-like stroma in female patients appears to signify a favorable prognosis and these lesions may arise from preexisting biliary cystadenomas. In a large multiinstitutional analysis, 248 patients were identified over 30 years, and, of these, 10% were biliary cystadeoncarcinomas. In that study, no reliable preoperative indicators could be established to enhance preoperative detection of malignancy.[114]

REFERENCES

1. Boulton RA, Adams DH. Gallbladder polyps: when to wait and when to act. *Lancet.* 1997;349(9055):817.
2. Persley K. Acalculous cholecystitis, cholesterolosis, adenomyomatosis, and polyps of the gallbladder. *Gastrointest Liver Disease.* 2006;1:1443-1459.
3. Kozuka S, Tsubone N, Yasui A, Hachisuka K. Relation of adenoma to carcinoma in the gallbladder. *Cancer.* 1982;50(10):2226-2234.
4. Harrison J, Reynolds JV, Sheahan K, Gibney RG, Hyland JM. Evidence for the polyp-cancer sequence in gallbladder cancer. *Irish Med J.* 1997;90(3):98.
5. Goldin RD, Roa JC. Gallbladder cancer: a morphological and molecular update. *Histopathology.* 2009;55(2):218-229.
6. Hann LE, D'Angelica M, et al. Polypoid lesions of the gallbladder: diagnosis and followup. *J Am Coll Surg.* 2009;208(4):570-575.
7. Yang HL, Sun YG, Wang Z. Polypoid lesions of the gallbladder: diagnosis and indications for surgery. *Br J Surg.* 1992;79(3):227-229.
8. Zielinski MD, Atwell TD, Davis PW, Kendrick ML, Que FG. Comparison of surgically resected polypoid lesions of the gallbladder to their pre-operative ultrasound characteristics. *J Gastrointest Surg.* 2009;13(1):19-25.
9. Komorowski RA, Tresp MG, Wilson SD. Pancreaticobiliary involvement in familial polyposis coli/Gardner's syndrome. *Dis Colon Rectum.* 1986;29(1):55-58.
10. Wada K, Tanaka M, Yamaguchi K, Wada K. Carcinoma and polyps of the gallbladder associated with Peutz-Jeghers syndrome. *Dig Dis Sci.* 1987;32(8):943-946.
11. Gallahan WC, Conway JD. Diagnosis and management of gallbladder polyps. *Gastroenterol Clin North Am.* 2010;39(2):359-367, x.
12. Henley SJ, Weir HK, Jim MA, Watson M, Richardson LC. Gallbladder cancer incidence and mortality, United States 1999–2011. *Cancer Epidemiol Biomarkers Prev.* 2015;24(9):1319-1326.
13. Randi G, Franceschi S, La Vecchia C. Gallbladder cancer worldwide: geographical distribution and risk factors. *Int J Cancer.* 2006;118(7):1591-1602.
14. Hsing AW, Gao YT, Han TQ, et al. Gallstones and the risk of biliary tract cancer: a population-based study in China. *Br J Cancer.* 2007;97(11):1577-1582.
15. Maringhini A, Moreau JA, Melton LJ 3rd, Hench VS, Zinsmeister AR, DiMagno EP. Gallstones, gallbladder cancer, and other gastrointestinal malignancies. An epidemiologic study in Rochester, Minnesota. *Ann Intern Med.* 1987;107(1):30-35.
16. Larsson SC, Wolk A. Obesity and the risk of gallbladder cancer: a meta-analysis. *Br J Cancer.* 2007;96(9):1457-1461.
17. Tazuma S, Kajiyama G. Carcinogenesis of malignant lesions of the gall bladder. The impact of chronic inflammation and gallstones. *Langenbeck's Arch Surg.* 2001;386(3):224-229.
18. Panagevopoulos JA, Dennison A, Ross B, Johnson AG. Primary carcinoma of the gallbladder: a 10-year experience. *Ann R Coll Surg Engl.* 1992;74(3):222.
19. Herman CJ, Lagerwaard FJ, Bueno de Mesquita HB, van Dalen A, van Leeuwen MS, Schrover PA. Gallstone size and the risk of gallbladder cancer. *Scand J Gastroenterol.* 1993;28(6):482-486.
20. Berk RN, Armbuster TG, Saltzstein SL. Carcinoma in the porcelain gallbladder. *Radiology.* 1973;106(1):29-31.
21. Stephen AE, Berger DL. Carcinoma in the porcelain gallbladder: a relationship revisited. *Surgery.* 2001;129(6):699-703.
22. Ito M, Yasui K, Morimoto T, et al. Visualization of routes of lymphatic drainage of the gallbladder with a carbon particle suspension. *J Am Coll Surg.* 1996;183(4):345-350.
23. Shaffer EA. Gallbladder cancer: the basics. *Gastroenterol Hepatol.* 2008;4(10):737-741.
24. Bosma EJ. Towards an oncological resection of gall bladder cancer. *Eur J Surg Oncol.* 1994;20(5):537-544.
25. Itoi T, Watanabe H, Ajioka Y, et al. APC, K-ras codon 12 mutations and p53 gene expression in carcinoma and adenoma of the gall-bladder suggest two genetic pathways in gall-bladder carcinogenesis. *Pathol Int.* 1996;46(5):333-340.
26. Chen E, Berlin J. Biliary tract cancers: understudied and poorly understood. *J Clin Oncol.* 2015;33(16):1845-1848.
27. Saetta AA, Papanastasiou P, Michalopoulos NV, et al. Mutational analysis of BRAF in gallbladder carcinomas in association with K-ras and p53 mutations and microsatellite instability. *Virchows Arch.* 2004;445(2):179-182.
28. Hawkins WG, DeMatteo RP, Jarnagin WR, Ben-Porat L, Blumgart LH, Fong Y. Jaundice predicts advanced disease and early mortality in patients with gallbladder cancer. *Ann Surg Oncol.* 2004;11(3):310-315.
29. Strom BL, Maislin G, West SL, et al. Serum CEA and CA 19-9: potential future diagnostic or screening tests for gallbladder cancer? *Int J Cancer.* 1990;45(5):821-824.

30. Ritts RE Jr, Nagorney DM, Jacobsen DJ, Talbot RW, Zurawski VR Jr. Comparison of preoperative serum CA19-9 levels with results of diagnostic imaging modalities in patients undergoing laparotomy for suspected pancreatic or gallbladder disease. *Pancreas*. 1994;9(6):707-716.

31. Wibbenmeyer LA, Sharafuddin MJ, Wolverson MK, Heiberg EV, Wade TP, Shields JJ. Sonographic diagnosis of unsuspected gallbladder cancer: imaging findings in comparison with benign gallbladder conditions. *AJR J Roentgenol*. 1995;165(5):1169-1174.

32. Kumar A, Aggarwal S. Carcinoma of the gallbladder: CT findings in 50 cases. *Abdom Imag*. 1994;19(4):304-308.

33. Ohtani T, Shirai T, Tsukada K, Hatakeyama K, Muto T. Carcinoma of the gallbladder: CT evaluation of lymphatic spread. *Radiology*. 1993;189(3):875-880.

34. Petrowsky H, Wildbrett P, Husarik DB, et al. Impact of integrated positron emission tomography and computed tomography on staging and management of gallbladder cancer and cholangiocarcinoma. *J Hepatol*. 2006;45(1):43-50.

35. Akosa AB, Barker F, Desa L, Benjamin I, Krausz T. Cytologic diagnosis in the management of gallbladder carcinoma. *Acta Cytol*. 1995;39(3):494-498.

36. Edge SB, Compton CC. The American Joint Committee on Cancer: the 7th edition of the AJCC cancer staging manual and the future of TNM. *Ann Surg Oncol*. 2010;17(6):1471-1474.

37. Bartlett DL, Fong Y, Fortner JG, Brennan MF, Blumgart LH. Long-term results after resection for gallbladder cancer. Implications for staging and management. *Ann Surg*. 1996;224(5):639-646.

38. Rodriguez-Fernandez A, Gomez-Rio M, Medina-Benitez A, et al. Application of modern imaging methods in diagnosis of gallbladder cancer. *J Surg Oncol*. 2006;93(8):650-664.

39. Butte JM, Kingham TP, Gonen M, et al. Residual disease predicts outcomes after definitive resection for incidental gallbladder cancer. *J Am Coll Surg*. 2014;219(3):416-429.

40. Furlan A, Ferri JV, Hosseinzadeh K, Borhani AA. Gallbladder carcinoma update: multimodality imaging evaluation, staging, and treatment options. *AJR Am J Roentgenol*. 2008;191(5):1440-1447.

41. Tsukada K, Kurosaki I, Uchida K, et al. Lymph node spread from carcinoma of the gallbladder. *Cancer*. 1997;80(4):661-667.

42. Shirai Y, Yoshida K, Tsukada K, Muto T. Inapparent carcinoma of the gallbladder. An appraisal of a radical second operation after simple cholecystectomy. *Ann Surg*. 1992;215(4):326-331.

43. de Aretxabala XA, Roa IS, Burgos LA, Araya JC, Villaseca MA, Silva JA. Curative resection in potentially resectable tumours of the gallbladder. *Eur J Surg*. 1997;163(6):419-426.

44. Fetzner UK, Hölscher AH, Stippel DL. Regional lymphadenectomy strongly recommended in T1b gallbladder cancer. *World J Gastroenterol*. 2011;17(39):4347-4348.

45. Abramson MA, Pandharipande P, Ruan D, Gold JS, Whang EE. Radical resection for T1b gallbladder cancer: a decision analysis. *HPB*. 2009;11(8):656-663.

46. Chijiiwa K, Tanaka M. Carcinoma of the gallbladder: an appraisal of surgical resection. *Surgery*. 1994;115(6):751-756.

47. Duffy A, Capanu M, Abou-Alfa GK, et al. Gallbladder cancer (GBC): 10-year experience at Memorial Sloan-Kettering Cancer Centre (MSKCC). *J Surg Oncol*. 2008;98(7):485-489.

48. Fong Y, Jarnagin W, Blumgart LH. Gallbladder cancer: comparison of patients presenting initially for definitive operation with those presenting after prior noncurative intervention. *Ann Surg*. 2000;232(4):557-569.

49. Takada T, Amano H, Yasuda H, et al. Is postoperative adjuvant chemotherapy useful for gallbladder carcinoma? A phase III multicenter prospective randomized controlled trial in patients with resected pancreaticobiliary carcinoma. *Cancer*. 2002;95(8):1685-1695.

50. Kresl JJ, Schild SE, Henning GT, et al. Adjuvant external beam radiation therapy with concurrent chemotherapy in the management of gallbladder carcinoma. *Int J Radiat Oncol Biol Phys*. 2002;52(1):167-175.

51. Kapoor VK, Pradeep R, Haribhakti SP, et al. Intrahepatic segment III cholangiojejunostomy in advanced carcinoma of the gallbladder. *Br J Surg*. 1996;83(12):1709-1711.

52. Taal BG, Audisio RA, Bleiberg H, et al. Phase II trial of mitomycin C (MMC) in advanced gallbladder and biliary tree carcinoma. An ECRTC Gastrointestinal Tract Cancer Cooperative Group Study. *Ann Oncol*. 1993;4(7):607-609.

53. Hadjis NS, Collins NA, Blumgart LH. Malignant masquerade at the hilum of the liver. *Br J Surg*. 1985;72(8):659-66

54. McLean L, Patel T. Racial and ethnic variations in the epidemiology of intrahepatic cholangiocarcinoma in the United States. *Liver Int*. 2006;26(9):1047-1053.

55. Siegel RL, Miller KD, Jemal A. Cancer statistics, 2016. *CA Cancer J Clin*. 2016;66(1):7-30.

56. Braconi C, Patel T. Cholangiocarcinoma: new insights into disease pathogenesis and biology. *Infect Dis Clin North Am*. 2010;24(4):871-884, vii.

57. Patel T. New insights into the molecular pathogenesis of intrahepatic cholangiocarcinoma. *J Gastroenterol*. 2014;49(2):165-172.

58. Bouvard V, Baan R, Straif K, et al. A review of human carcinogens—part B: biological agents. *Lancet Oncol*. 2009;10(4):321-322.

59. Khampitak T, Knowles J, Yongvanit P, et al. Thiamine deficiency and parasitic infection in rural Thai children. *Southeast Asian J Trop Med Public Health*. 2006;37(3):441-445.

60. Jongsuksuntigul P, Imsomboon T. Opisthorchiasis control in Thailand. *Acta Trop*. 2003;88(3):229-232.

61. Sripa B, Bethony JM, Sithithaworn P, et al. Opisthorchiasis and *Opisthorchis*-associated cholangiocarcinoma in Thailand and Laos. *Acta Trop*. 2011;120(suppl 1):S158-S168.

62. Sempoux C, Jibara G, Ward SC, et al. Intrahepatic cholangiocarcinoma: new insights in pathology. *Semin Liver Dis*. 2011;31(1):49-60.

63. Vauthey JN, Blumgart LH. Recent advances in the management of cholangiocarcinomas. *Semin Liver Dis*. 1994;14(2):109-114.

64. de Groen PC, Gores GJ, LaRusso NF, Gunderson LL, Nagorney DM. Biliary tract cancers. *N Engl J Med*. 1999;341(18):1368-1378.

65. Navaneethan U, Njei B, Venkatesh PG, Vargo JJ, Parsi MA. Fluorescence in situ hybridization for diagnosis of cholangiocarcinoma in primary sclerosing cholangitis: a systematic review and meta-analysis. *Gastrointest Endosc*. 2014;79(6):943-950, e943.

66. Hadjis NS, Blumgart LH. Role of liver atrophy, hepatic resection and hepatocyte hyperplasia in the development of portal hypertension in biliary disease. *Gut*. 1987;28(8):1022-1028.

67. Way L, Dunphy J. Biliary tract. *Curr Surg Diagn Treat*. 1994;537-566.

68. Blechacz BR, Gores GJ. Cholangiocarcinoma. *Clin Liver Dis*. 2008;12(1):131-150, ix.

69. Nichols JC, Gores GJ, LaRusso NF, Wiesner RH, Nagorney DM, Ritts RE Jr. Diagnostic role of serum CA 19-9 for cholangiocarcinoma in patients with primary sclerosing cholangitis. *Mayo Clin Proc*. 1993;68(9):874-879.

70. Patel AH, Harnois DM, Klee GG, LaRusso NF, Gores GJ. The utility of CA 19-9 in the diagnoses of cholangiocarcinoma in patients without primary sclerosing cholangitis. *Am J Gastroenterol*. 2000;95(1):204-207.

71. Mansour JC, Aloia TA, Crane CH, Heimbach JK, Nagino M, Vauthey JN. Hilar cholangiocarcinoma: expert consensus statement. *HPB*. 2015;17(8):691-699.

72. Valls C, Guma A, Puig I, et al. Intrahepatic peripheral cholangiocarcinoma: CT evaluation. *Abdominal Imag*. 2000;25(5):490-496.

73. Hann LE, Greatrex KV, Bach AM, Fong Y, Blumgart LH. Cholangiocarcinoma at the hepatic hilus: sonographic findings. *AJR Am J Roentgenol*. 1997;168(4):985-989.

74. Bach AM, Hann LE, Brown KT, et al. Portal vein evaluation with US: comparison to angiography combined with CT arterial portography. *Radiology*. 1996;201(1):149-154.

75. Weber SM, DeMatteo RP, Fong Y, Blumgart LH, Jarnagin WR. Staging laparoscopy in patients with extrahepatic biliary carcinoma. Analysis of 100 patients. *Ann Surg*. 2002;235(3):392-399.

76. Bismuth H, Nakache R, Diamond T. Management strategies in resection for hilar cholangiocarcinoma. *Ann Surg*. 1992;215(1):31-38.

77. Endo I, Gonen M, Yopp AC, et al. Intrahepatic cholangiocarcinoma: rising frequency, improved survival, and determinants of outcome after resection. *Ann Surg*. 2008;248(1):84-96.

78. Luo X, Yuan L, Wang Y, Ge R, Sun Y, Wei G. Survival outcomes and prognostic factors of surgical therapy for all potentially resectable intrahepatic cholangiocarcinoma: a large single-center cohort study. *J Gastrointest Surg*. 2014;18(3):562-572.

79. Ribero D, Pinna AD, Guglielmi A, et al. Surgical approach for long-term survival of patients with intrahepatic cholangiocarcinoma: a multi-institutional analysis of 434 patients. *Arch Surg*. 2012;147(12):1107-1113.

80. de Jong MC, Nathan H, Sotiropoulos GC, et al. Intrahepatic cholangiocarcinoma: an international multi-institutional analysis of prognostic factors and lymph node assessment. *J Clin Oncol*. 2011;29(23):3140-3145.

81. Burke EC, Jarnagin WR, Hochwald SN, Leer PW, Fong Y, Blumgart LH. Hilar Cholangiocarcinoma: pattern of spread, the importance of hepatic resection for curative operation, and a presurgical clinical staging system. *Ann Surg*. 1998;228:385-394.

82. Lang H, Sotiropoulos GC, Sgourakis G, et al. Operations for intrahepatic cholangiocarcinoma: single-institution experience of 158 patients. *J Am Coll Surg*. 2009;208(2):218-228.

83. Weber SM, Jarnagin WR, Klimstra D, DeMatteo RP, Fong Y, Blumgart LH. Intrahepatic cholangiocarcinoma: resectability, recurrence pattern, and outcomes. *J Am Coll Surg*. 2001;193(4):384-391.

84. Jarnagin WR, Fong Y, DeMatteo RE, et al. Staging, resectability, and outcome in 225 patients with hilar cholangiocarcinoma. *Ann Surg*. 2001;234(4):507-517; discussion 517-519.

85. Rocha FG, Matsuo K, Blumgart LH, Jarnagin WR. Hilar cholangiocarcinoma: the Memorial Sloan-Kettering Cancer Center experience. *J Hepatobiliary Pancreat Sci*. 2010;17(4):490-496.

86. Nagino M, Ebata T, Yokoyama Y, et al. Evolution of surgical treatment for perihilar cholangiocarcinoma: a single-center 34-year review of 574 consecutive resections. *Ann Surg*. 2013;258(1):129-140.

87. Kobayashi A, Miwa S, Nakata T, Miyagawa S. Disease recurrence patterns after R0 resection of hilar cholangiocarcinoma. *Br J Surg*. 2010;97(1):56-64.

88. Ito F, Agni R, Rettammel RJ, et al. Resection of hilar cholangiocarcinoma: concomitant liver resection decreases hepatic recurrence. *Ann Surg*. 2008;248(2):273-279.

89. Fong Y, Blumgart LH, Lin E, Fortner JL, Brennan MF. Outcome of treatment for distal bile duct cancer. *Br J Surg*. 1996;83(12):1712-1715.

90. Yeo CJ, Sohn TA, Cameron JL, Hruban RH, Lillemoe KD, Pitt HA. Periampullary adenocarcinoma: analysis of 5-year survivors. *Ann Surg*. 1998;227(6):821-831.

91. Courtin-Tanguy L, Rayar M, Bergeat D, et al. The true prognosis of resected distal cholangiocarcinoma. *J Surg Oncol*. 2016;113(5):575-580.

92. Nagorney DM, Donohue JH, Farnell MB, Schleck CD, Ilstrup DM. Outcomes after curative resections of cholangiocarcinoma. *Arch Surg*. 1993;128(8):871-877; discussion 877-879.

93. Gores GJ, Darwish Murad S, Heimbach JK, Rosen CB. Liver transplantation for perihilar cholangiocarcinoma. *Dig Dis*. 2013;31(1):126-129.

94. Rosen CB, Heimbach JK, Gores CJ. Liver transplantation for cholangiocarcinoma. *Transpl Int*. 2010;23(7):692-697.

95. Valle J, Wasan H, Palmer DH, et al. Cisplatin plus gemcitabine versus gemcitabine for biliary tract cancer. *N Engl J Med*. 2010;362(14):1273-1281.

96. Jarnagin WR, Ruo L, Little SA, et al. Patterns of initial disease recurrence after resection of gallbladder carcinoma and hilar cholangiocarcinoma: implications for adjuvant therapeutic strategies. *Cancer*. 2003;98(8):1689-1700.

97. Kim TH, Han SS, Park SJ, et al. Role of adjuvant chemoradiotherapy for resected extrahepatic biliary tract cancer. *Int J Radiat Oncol Biol Physics*. 2011;81(5):e853-e859.

98. Nakeeb A, Tran KQ, Black MJ, et al. Improved survival in resected biliary malignancies. *Surgery*. 2002;132(4):555-563; discussion 563-554.

99. Borghero Y, Crane CH, Szklaruk J, et al. Extrahepatic bile duct adenocarcinoma: patients at high-risk for local recurrence treated with surgery and adjuvant chemoradiation have an equivalent overall survival to patients with standard-risk treated with surgery alone. *Ann Surg Oncol*. 2008;15(11):3147-3156.

100. Todoroki T, Ohara K, Kawamoto T, et al. Benefits of adjuvant radiotherapy after radical resection of locally advanced main hepatic duct carcinoma. *Int J Radiat Oncol Biol Phys*. 2000;46(3):581-587.

101. Pitt HA, Nakeeb A, Abrams RA, et al. Perihilar cholangiocarcinoma. Postoperative radiotherapy does not improve survival. *Ann Surg*. 1995;221(6):788-797; discussion 797-788.

102. Ghafoori E, Iyer R. Biliary cancer: current management and emerging targeted therapies. *Targeted Oncology* 2015.

103. Sia D, Hoshida Y, Villanueva A, et al. Integrative molecular analysis of intrahepatic cholangiocarcinoma reveals 2 classes that have different outcomes. *Gastroenterology*. 2013;144(4):829-840.

104. Andersen JB, Spee B, Blechacz BR, et al. Genomic and genetic characterization of cholangiocarcinoma identifies therapeutic targets for tyrosine kinase inhibitors. *Gastroenterology*. 2012;142(4):1021-1031, e1015.

105. Valle JW, Wasan H, Lopes A, et al. Cediranib or placebo in combination with cisplatin and gemcitabine chemotherapy for patients with advanced biliary tract cancer (ABC-03): a randomised phase 2 trial. *Lancet Oncol*. 2015;16(8):967-978.

106. Malka D, Cervera P, Foulon S, et al. Gemcitabine and oxaliplatin with or without cetuximab in advanced biliary-tract cancer (BINGO): a randomised, open-label, non-comparative phase 2 trial. *Lancet Oncol*. 2014;15(8):819-828.

107. Churi CR, Shroff R, Wang Y, et al. Mutation profiling in cholangiocarcinoma: prognostic and therapeutic implications. *PLoS One*. 2014;9(12):e115383.

108. Jarnagin WR, Burke E, Powers C, Fong Y, Blumgart LH. Intrahepatic biliary enteric bypass provides effective palliation in selected patients with malignant obstruction at the hepatic duct confluence. *Am J Surg*. 1998;175(6):453-460.

109. Becker CD, Glattli A, Maibach R, Baer HU. Percutaneous palliation of malignant obstructive jaundice with the Wallstent endoprosthesis: follow-up and reintervention in patients with hilar and non-hilar obstruction. *J Vasc Interv Radiol*. 1993;4(5):597-604.

110. Davids PH, Groen AK, Rauws EA, Tytgat GN, Huibregtse K. Randomised trial of self-expanding metal stents versus polyethylene stents for distal malignant biliary obstruction. *Lancet*. 1992;340(8834-8835):1488-1492.

111. Kuvshinoff BW, Armstrong JG, Fong Y, et al. Palliation of irresectable hilar cholangiocarcinoma with biliary drainage and radiotherapy. *Br J Surg*. 1995;82(11):1522-1525.

112. Miyazo M, Frilling A, Li J, Lang H, Broelsch CE. Cholangiocellular carcinoma—the role of caudate lobe resection and mesohepatectomy. *HPB* 2008;10(3):179-182.

113. Vilchez V, Shah MB, Daily MF, et al. Long-term outcome of patients undergoing liver transplantation for mixed hepatocellular carcinoma and cholangiocarcinoma: an analysis of the UNOS database. *HPB*. 2016;18(1):29-34.

114. Anagnostakis DJ, Kim Y, Pulitano C, et al. Management of biliary cyst tumors: a multi-institutional analysis of a rare liver tumor. *Ann Surg*. 2015;261(2):361-367.

Prevention and Management of Bile Duct Injury

Chad G. Ball | Keith D. Lillemoe

Bile duct injuries most commonly occur after primary operations on the gallbladder or biliary tree. Biliary injuries themselves are also among the most difficult challenges that a surgeon will face. Although numerous technologic developments have facilitated diagnosis and management, bile duct injuries remain a significant clinical problem. If they go unrecognized or are managed improperly life-threatening early complications such as sepsis and multisystem organ failure or late complications of biliary cirrhosis, portal hypertension, and cholangitis can develop. To avoid these complications, virtually every patient with a bile duct stricture should undergo evaluation and treatment with the goal of relieving the obstruction to bile flow and its associated hepatic injury. Finally, the occurrence of a major bile duct injury during an elective cholecystectomy remains one of the most common indications of medical malpractice claims within the United States.

EPIDEMIOLOGY OF BILE DUCT INJURIES

Most benign bile duct strictures result from operations in or near the right upper quadrant. More than 80% of strictures occur after injury to the bile ducts during cholecystectomy (Fig. 113.1). The exact incidence of bile duct injury is unknown because many cases go unreported in the literature. Data suggest that the incidence of bile duct injury during the "open cholecystectomy era" was 1 in 500 to 1000 cases. The incidence of bile duct injury during laparoscopic cholecystectomy is clearly higher. Although a wide range in the incidence of injury can be found in reported series, the most accurate data are derived from surveys encompassing thousands of patients. These reports reflect the results from a large number of surgeons in both community and teaching hospitals. These series suggest an incidence of bile duct injury during laparoscopic cholecystectomy ranging from 0.3% to 0.7%.[1] Fortunately now over 25 years after its introduction in the United States, the incidence of bile duct injury associated with laparoscopic cholecystectomy may be starting to trend downward in recent reports. The increase in incidence of biliary injuries when compared with the open technique is likely inherent within the laparoscopic approach and certainly no longer the function of a learning curve. Furthermore, the introduction of new techniques such as single-port laparoscopic cholecystectomy and robotic cholecystectomy to raise some concerns that injuries could become more common. Finally, as experience in open cholecystectomy in surgical training programs has decreased, there are also concerns for a potential increase in the incidence (and severity) of injuries during difficult laparoscopic cases that are converted to open procedures.

GENERAL PREVENTION OF BILE DUCT INJURIES

A number of factors are associated with bile duct injury during either open or laparoscopic cholecystectomy, including acute or chronic inflammation, inadequate exposure, patient obesity, and failure to identify structures before clamping, ligating, or dividing them. Bleeding from the cystic or hepatic arteries can lead to bile duct injury during attempts to achieve hemostasis. The generous application of Ligaclips at either open or laparoscopic cholecystectomy to hilar areas not well visualized can result in placing a clip on or across a bile duct, with resultant injury. Failure to recognize congenital anatomic anomalies of the bile ducts, such as the low insertion of the right hepatic duct or even into the cystic duct, or a long common wall between the cystic duct and the common bile duct, can also lead to injury. There have been many discussions concerning the risks of bile duct injury during cases of severe acute cholecystitis, as well as how these risks are affected by timing of cholecystectomy. Although 30-day postoperative morbidity and mortality rates may remain independent of timing, it is clear that patients who undergo laparoscopic cholecystectomy beyond 24 hours are more likely to require an open procedure and sustain significantly longer postoperative and overall lengths of hospital admission (and therefore cost).[2]

Numerous technical factors that are associated with laparoscopic cholecystectomy can also increase the risk of bile duct injury compared with the open procedure. These factors include the use of an end-viewing laparoscope, which alters the surgeon's perspective of the operative field. The issue of visual alignment and perspective has become ever more topical with the proliferation of single-incision laparoscopic cholecystectomy that is known to be associated with a higher rate of common bile duct injury than the traditional four-incision laparoscopic technique using an angled scope.[3] Excessive cephalad retraction of the gallbladder fundus can cause the cystic duct and common bile duct to become aligned in the same plane. This distortion often results in the classic laparoscopic injury, in which the common bile duct is mistaken for the cystic duct and clipped and divided.[4]

The role of intraoperative cholangiography (IOC) in preventing bile duct injury during laparoscopic cholecystectomy remains controversial. Individual series have failed to demonstrate that either performing routine or selective IOC affects the incidence of bile duct injury. Although an initial retrospective nationwide cohort analysis of Medicare patients undergoing laparoscopic cholecystectomy between 1992 and 1999 demonstrated that common bile duct

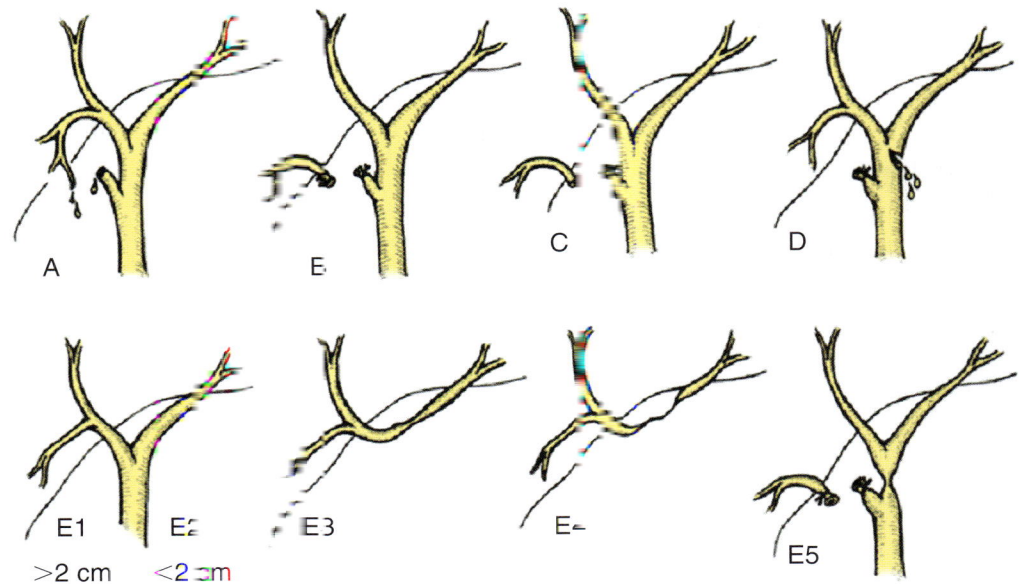

FIGURE 113.1 Strasberg bile duct injury classification scheme. (From Strasberg SM, Hertl M, Soper NJ. An analysis of the problem of biliary injury during laparoscopic cholecystectomy. *J Am Coll Surg.* 1995;180:101.)

injuries occurred in 0.39% of patients in which IOC was performed versus 0.58% in patients not undergoing IOC (unadjusted relative risk, 1.49; 95% confidence interval, 1.42 to 1.57),[5] a more recent Medicare-based study (2000–2009), analyzing over 92,000 patients undergoing cholecystectomy identified no statistically significant association between IOC and common bile duct injury. The authors therefore concluded that IOC is not effective as a preventive strategy against common duct injury during cholecystectomy.[6] Despite this controversy, the proper interpretation of IOC can minimize the extent of injury. Nevertheless, only 27% of surgeons in the United States perform IOC routinely (see Fig. 113.1).[7] Finally, ample evidence exists to support the conclusion that the experience of the surgeon in performing laparoscopic cholecystectomy can be correlated with the risk of bile duct injury.

COGNITIVE FACTORS RELATED TO THE PREVENTION OF BILE DUCT INJURIES

In recent years, there has been a growing understanding of surgeon cognitive factors associated with bile duct injury during laparoscopic cholecystectomy. An analysis examining 252 biliary injuries during laparoscopic cholecystectomy using human error factor and cognitive science techniques found that 97% of injuries were caused by visual-perceptual illusion or inadequate visualization. Further work from the same group has determined a range of explanation for the surgeon's frequent inability to recognize bile duct injury. These bile duct injuries appear to be associated with confirmation bias, which is a process by to seek cues to confirm a belief and to discount cues that might discount the belief. Although cognitive factors are important for the understanding of the psychological issues associated with bile duct injuries, surgeons must continue to have the

appropriate corrective mechanisms in place to minimize the chance of these injuries, including knowledge of anatomy, typical mechanisms of injury, and a true sense of suspicion and logic. An example of such a corrective mechanism occurs within the operative technique of laparoscopic cholecystectomy, which defines the "critical view of safety," and therefore helps prevent misidentification and injury of the major bile ducts (Fig. 113.2).[9] This concept mandates that the fundus of the gallbladder be retracted superiorly while the infundibulum is retracted laterally. This exposure generally allows the surgeon to carefully dissect out the triangle of Calot, leaving only two structures connected to the lower end of the gallbladder: the cystic artery and cystic duct. The critical view of safety has also been enhanced to now describe both anterior and posterior views.

While this maneuver is the single most effective means of preventing a bile duct injury, the reality is substantially more complex. In scenarios of a short or nonexistent cystic duct, or a small common bile duct (common in acute cholecystitis), these structures can be confused for each other. Furthermore, inappropriate or overzealous traction then makes these associations even more challenging. Similarly, inflammation closes the space between the gallbladder and the bile duct. In extreme cases, they may even be fused and move as a single unit (Mirizzi type A). This not uncommon reality makes identification of associated regional anatomy even more important for the surgeon in an attempt to orient the critical structures of interest and proceed with a safe procedure. These spatial-regional issues can be further challenged by a loss of perspective given the tendency of many camera operators to move ever closer to the operative dissection itself.

In all laparoscopic cholecystectomies for acute cholecystitis, the surgeon should perform a "bile duct time out" to evaluate their understanding of targeted anatomy

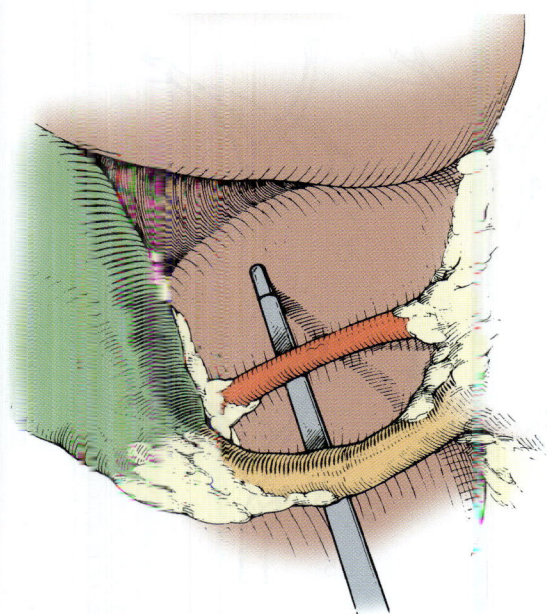

FIGURE 13.2 The critical view needed to avoid bile duct injury. Here, the triangle of Calot has been dissected free of all tissue except the cystic duct and cystic artery. A laparoscopic instrument is shown dorsal to the cystic duct and artery. (From Strasberg SM, Hertl M, Soper NJ. An analysis of the problem of biliary injury during laparoscopic cholecystectomy. *J Am Coll Surg.* 1995;180:101.)

BOX 113.1 Bile Duct "Time Out" (B.E. S.A.F.E.)

B—Bile duct
E—Enteric (duodenum) position
S—Sulcus of Rouvier
A—Artery (hepatic artery)
F—Fissure (umbilical fissure)
E—Environment (back the camera out for improved perspective)

---

based on regional structures (Box 113.1). After a wide laparoscopic view of the subhepatic space is obtained, the surgeon should lift the liver off the porta hepatis and identify a checklist of landmarks around the gallbladder, including duodenum, sulcus of Rouvier, umbilical fissure, pulsations of the common hepatic artery, and the bile duct itself. Once these landmarks are identified, a careful dissection of the triangle of Calot can be accomplished with minimal cautery. A specific search for a sectoral duct should also be completed. Then with a cleared triangle and the true gallbladder cystic duct angle identified, the correct "cognitive map" of the biliary tree can be superimposed on the patient's specific anatomy in the correct location. In cases of severe acute cholecystitis, it may be unclear if the operator can safely even obtain this anatomic viewpoint (and therefore the ability to safely proceed with a laparoscopic technique). In most scenarios, however, if the surgeon can still obtain a clear dissection of the junction between the cystic duct and the

gallbladder on the lateral edge, then it is safe to continue. Initial dissection in the lateral tissues for cases of a severely inflamed field is also safest from a bile duct injury point of view. If it is unsafe to proceed with further dissection medial to the gallbladder, however, a subtotal cholecystectomy may represent the best option. The gallbladder should be opened, all stones and debris extracted, and then closed using the surgeon's preferred minimally invasive modality (Endoloops, suturing, thick stapler) as low as is safe given the regional inflammation.

During the entire operation, a surgeon must maintain a vigilant attitude, and when ambiguity arises, must slow down and back out the camera to widen the view of all landmarks (complete another "bile duct time out"). The surgeon must avoid both physical and mental "tunnel vision." Inability to accurately place the cognitive map is a stop signal. If this cannot be resolved, conversion to open surgery with top down dissection will improve safety. For patients with inflammatory obliteration of the triangle of Calot, near-total cholecystectomy or cholecystostomy can prevent injury. Furthermore, any dissection on the left side of the bile duct should be considered a "near miss." Surgeons must also have several "cognitive maps" in their minds—normal, caudal sectoral duct, and short cystic duct. The maps must be somewhat "plastic" as size and distances vary with each patient.

VASCULOBILIARY INJURIES

The importance of ischemia of the bile duct in the formation of postoperative strictures is significant. Injury to the hepatic artery at the time of biliary injury during laparoscopic cholecystectomy has been recognized at an increased incidence, as high as 50%, when investigated at the time of presentation.[10] The true impact of an arterial injury, however, remains debated. It is clear that the most common site of vasculobiliary injury is the right hepatic artery (Fig. 113.3).[11] Damage to this vessel may lead to a higher injury level on the bile duct than the initial grossly observed mechanical trauma. As a result, concurrent injury to the right hepatic artery may prompt the surgeon to delay biliary reconstruction for a later date to allow the level of the final injury to become more apparent upon exploration. Similarly, trauma to the right hepatic artery is also a significantly larger problem in the context of higher biliary injuries. More specifically, disruption of the crossing arterial plexus at the hilar bifurcation remains a more challenging reconstruction issue worthy of thoughtful consideration. Vasculobiliary injuries may also have specific effects on the arteries (pseudoaneurysm with delayed hemorrhage), bile ducts (necrosis, stenosis, cholangitis), and/or liver (necrosis, atrophy) over variable lengths of time.[11] Concurrent hepatic artery and portal vein injuries can have catastrophic effects on the liver, including rapid necrosis, potentially requiring urgent liver transplant. Finally, a clinically important and a more common cause of bile duct ischemia is excessive dissection around the bile duct during bile duct anastomosis for repair of an injury, which can divide or injure the major arteries of the bile duct that run in the 3-o'clock and 9-o'clock positions.[12,13]

Another important factor contributing to the formation of biliary strictures is the intense connective tissue

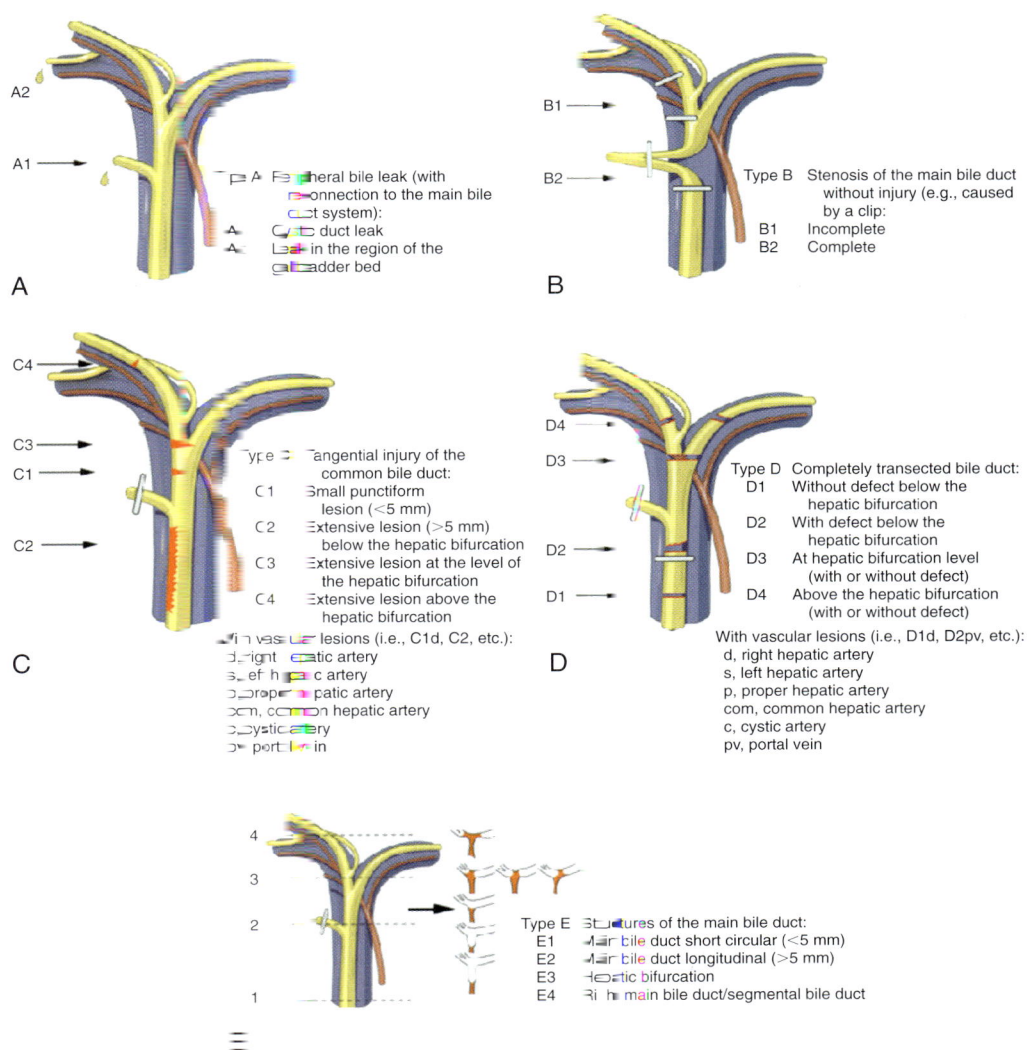

FIGURE 113.3 Hannover bile duct injury classification scheme. (A) Type A, peripheral bile leak. (B) Type B, bile duct obstruction. (C) Type C, tangential bile duct injury. (D) Type D, transected bile duct. (E) Type E, late bile duct stenosis. Vascular injury modifiers include right hepatic artery (d), left hepatic artery (s), proper hepatic artery (p), common hepatic artery (com), cystic artery (c), and portal vein (pv). (From Bektas H, Schrem H, Winny M, et al. Surgical treatment and outcome of iatrogenic bile duct lesions after cholecystectomy and the impact of different clinical classification systems. Br J Surg. 2007;94:1119.)

response with fibrosis and scarring that can occur after bile duct injury. Experimental studies of bile duct ligation in a canine model have demonstrated immediate and sustained elevation of bile duct pressure and progressive increase in bile duct diameter. Histologic changes at 1 month after ligation have shown that the bile duct wall is thickened, with a reduction of mucosal folds and loss of surface microvilli, associated with a well-defined epithelial degeneration. Biochemical analysis of connective tissue response to ligation showed that collagen synthesis and proline hydroxylase activity are increased within 2 weeks in the obstructed bile duct and are sustained throughout the period of observation. Finally, a marked local inflammatory response can develop in the adjacent tissue in association with bile leakage, which occurs with many bile duct injuries. This inflammation can be further intensified in the face of infection. This inflammation results in fibrosis and scarring in the periductal tissue, further contributing to stricture

formation. These factors can be of *major* importance in bile duct injuries during laparoscopic cholecystectomy, which are frequently associated with bile leaks.[12,13]

After cholecystectomy and common bile duct exploration, the two most common operations associated with bile duct injury are gastrectomy and hepatic resection. The typical situation resulting in bile duct injury during gastrectomy involves dissection of the pyloric region and the first portion of the duodenum. The injury occurs during mobilization of the duodenum either for creation of a Billroth I gastroduodenostomy or for closure of the duodenal stump. Biliary injury during liver resection is most likely to occur during dissection of the hepatic hilum.

Unfortunately, the recurrence of bile duct strictures after an initial attempt at repair is not uncommon and can also account for a number of anastomotic strictures. A number of factors have been evaluated in patients who have a recurrent bile duct stricture, including the location of the stricture, the length of follow-up, the influence of previous operations, the type of operation performed, the type of sutures used, and the use and duration of postoperative stenting.[8] Previous attempts at repair, performance of a procedure other than choledochojejunostomy or hepaticojejunostomy, and stricture location higher in the biliary tree appear to be associated with a higher incidence of recurrent stricture. Finally, long-term follow-up of a bile duct anastomosis is important because strictures can develop years after the original anastomosis.

CLINICAL PRESENTATION OF PATIENTS WITH BILE DUCT INJURIES

Most patients with biliary injuries present early after their initial operation. After open cholecystectomy, only approximately 10% of postoperative strictures are actually suspected within the first week, but nearly 70% are diagnosed within the first 6 months, and more than 80% are diagnosed within 1 year of surgery. In series reporting bile duct injuries during laparoscopic cholecystectomy, the injury is usually recognized either during the procedure (25% to 30%) or, more commonly, in the early postoperative period.

Patients suspected of having a postoperative bile duct injury within days to weeks of initial operation usually present in one of two ways. One presentation is the progressive elevation of liver function test results, particularly total bilirubin and alkaline phosphatase levels. These changes can often be seen as early as the second or third postoperative day. The second mode of early presentation is with leakage of bile from the injured bile duct. This presentation appears to occur most often in patients presenting with bile duct injuries after laparoscopic cholecystectomy. Bilious drainage from operatively placed drains or through the wound after cholecystectomy is abnormal and represents some form of biliary injury. In patients without drains (including patients in whom the drains have been removed), the bile can leak freely into the peritoneal cavity or it can loculate as a collection. Free accumulation of bile into the peritoneal cavity results in either biliary ascites or bile peritonitis. Similarly, a loculated bile collection can result in sterile biloma or in an infected subhepatic or subdiaphragmatic abscess.

Patients with postoperative bile duct strictures who present months to years after the initial operation frequently have evidence of cholangitis. The episodes of cholangitis are often mild and respond to antibiotic therapy. Repetitive episodes usually occur before the definitive diagnosis. Less commonly, patients may present with painless jaundice and no evidence of sepsis. Finally, patients with markedly delayed diagnoses may present with advanced biliary cirrhosis and its complications.

DIAGNOSTIC RECOGNITION AND EVALUATION—LABORATORY TESTS

Liver function tests usually show evidence of cholestasis. In patients with bile leakage, the bilirubin can be normal or minimally elevated because of absorption from the peritoneal cavity. When elevated, serum bilirubin usually ranges from 2 to 6 mg/dL, although it can rise higher in the context of delayed recognition. Serum alkaline phosphatase is also usually elevated. Serum aminotransferase levels can be normal or minimally elevated except during episodes of cholangitis. If advanced liver disease exists, hepatic synthetic function can be impaired, with lowered serum albumin and a prolongation of prothrombin time. Serum electrolytes and complete blood count are typically normal unless there is associated biliary sepsis.

DIAGNOSTIC RECOGNITION AND EVALUATION—RADIOLOGY

The imaging techniques of abdominal ultrasound and computed tomography (CT) play an important initial role in the evaluation of patients with benign postoperative biliary strictures. In patients who present in the early postoperative period with evidence of a bile leak or biliary sepsis, these studies are useful to rule out the presence of intraabdominal collections that might require drainage. CT and ultrasound are also important in the initial evaluation of the patient presenting with a bile duct stricture months to years after initial operation. Both studies can confirm biliary obstruction by demonstrating a dilated biliary tree. CT is especially useful in identifying the level of obstruction of the extrahepatic bile duct. It is also essential to ensure an arterial phase to the CT if a hepatic artery (typically right) injury is suspected.

In patients suspected of having early postoperative bile duct injury, a radionucleotide biliary scan can confirm bile leakage. In patients with postoperative external bile fistula, injection of water-soluble contrast media through the drainage tract/drain (sinography) can often define the site of leakage and the anatomy of the biliary tree.

The "gold standard" for evaluation of patients with bile duct strictures remains cholangiography (Fig. 113.4). Percutaneous transhepatic cholangiography (PTC) is usually more valuable than endoscopic retrograde cholangiography (ERC) in patients with major bile duct injuries following laparoscopic cholecystectomy. PTC is more useful in that it defines the anatomy of the proximal biliary tree that is to be used in the surgical reconstruction. Furthermore, PTC can be followed by placement of percutaneous transhepatic catheters, which can be useful in decompressing the biliary system to either treat or prevent cholangitis and to control an ongoing bile leak. These catheters can also be of assistance in surgical reconstruction and provide access to the biliary tree for nonoperative dilation. ERC is less useful than PTC in major bile duct transections during laparoscopic cholecystectomy because the discontinuity of the extrahepatic bile duct usually prevents adequate filling of the proximal biliary tree. Often, ERC can demonstrate a normal-size distal bile duct up to the site of the stricture without visualization of the proximal biliary system. This finding is frequently the case in patients with injury during laparoscopic cholecystectomy, when the distal bile duct is often clipped and divided. ERC is extremely valuable for identifying and treating cystic duct leaks, as well as partial injuries appropriate for biliary stenting. The development of magnetic resonance cholangiopancreatography (MRCP)

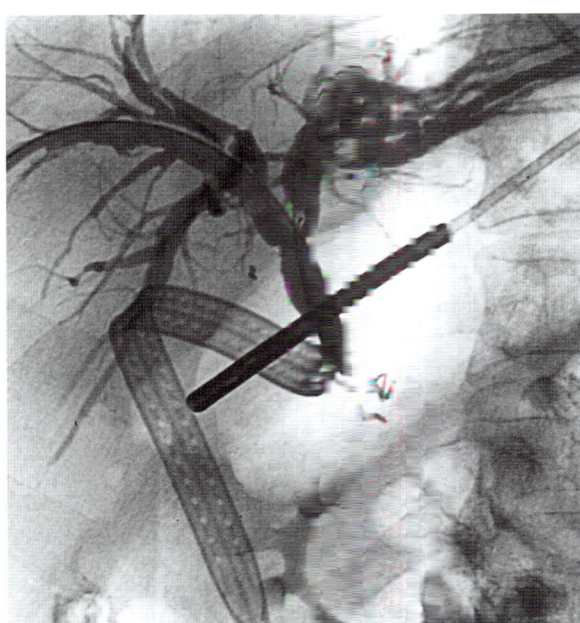

FIGURE 113.4 A percutaneous transhepatic cholangiogram from a patient with a complete transection of the common hepatic duct, which ends close to several surgical clips. A surgical drain is in place, as well as a duodenal feeding tube (which crosses obliquely over the common hepatic duct).

has provided a noninvasive technique that provides excellent delineation of the biliary anatomy. The quality of these images has led some surgeons to advocate this technique as the initial step in the evaluation of patients with suspected bile duct injuries and may eliminate the need for a diagnostic ERC in many patients. MRCP is especially worth considering if the referral surgeon has a low pretest probability of using transhepatic stents for subsequent reconstructive purposes.

MANAGEMENT OF BILE DUCT INJURY

The preoperative management of a patient with a postoperative bile duct injury depends primarily on the timing of the presentation. Optimally if a bile duct injury is recognized at the time of cholecystectomy, either immediate reconstruction or "damage control" steps can be employed. Unfortunately, recognition of bile duct injuries at the time of laparoscopic cholecystectomy occurs in less than half of all cases. Patients presenting in the early postoperative period can be septic with either cholangitis or intraabdominal bile collections. Sepsis must be controlled first with broad-spectrum parenteral antibiotics, percutaneous biliary drainage, and percutaneous or operative drainage of biliary leaks. Once sepsis and the ongoing bile leak are controlled, there is no rush to proceed with surgical reconstruction of the bile duct injury. The combination of proximal biliary decompression and external drainage allows most biliary fistulas to be controlled or even to close. The patient can then be discharged home to allow several weeks to elapse for resolution of the inflammation in the periportal region and recovery of overall health.

The management of a suspected bile duct injury after laparoscopic cholecystectomy presenting with a bile leak deserves special mention. Often, when bile leakage is suspected, the surgeon believes that urgent surgical exploration is necessary. Unfortunately, at laparotomy, the marked inflammation associated with bile spillage and the small decompressed biliary tree that appears retracted high into the porta hepatis make recognition of the injury and repair virtually impossible. In such cases, every attempt should be made to define the biliary anatomy by preoperative cholangiography (PTC or MRCP) and to control the bile leak with percutaneous biliary drainage. In many cases, early operative intervention is not required because the bile collections or ascites can either be drained percutaneously or simply are absorbed from the peritoneal cavity. Delayed reconstruction, aided by percutaneous biliary catheters, then allows optimal surgical results.[14]

In patients who present with a biliary stricture remote from the initial operation, symptoms of cholangitis can necessitate urgent cholangiography and biliary decompression. Biliary drainage is best accomplished by the transhepatic method, although successful endoscopic stent placement can also be accomplished. Parenteral antibiotics and biliary drainage should be continued until sepsis is controlled. In patients who present with jaundice but without cholangitis, cholangiography should be performed to define the anatomy. Preoperative biliary decompression in patients without cholangitis has not been demonstrated to improve outcome.

SURGICAL MANAGEMENT OF BILE DUCT INJURY

The goal of operative management of bile duct stricture is the establishment of bile flow into the proximal gastrointestinal tract in a manner that prevents cholangitis, sludge or stone formation, restricture, and biliary cirrhosis. This goal is best accomplished with a tension-free anastomosis between healthy tissues. A number of surgical alternatives exist for primary repair of bile duct strictures, including end-to-end repair, Roux-en-Y hepaticojejunostomy or choledochojejunostomy, or choledochoduodenostomy. The choice of repair depends on a number of factors, including the extent and location of the strictures, the experience of the surgeon, and the timing of the repair.

IMMEDIATE REPAIR OF INTRAOPERATIVE BILE DUCT INJURY

In many cases, initial proper management of bile duct injury recognized at the time of cholecystectomy can avoid the development of a bile duct stricture. This includes but is not limited to minimizing the extent of the injury, avoiding complications, and performing a satisfactory repair using all of the advanced principles discussed here. Unfortunately, recognition of a bile duct injury is uncommon during either open or laparoscopic cholecystectomy. If bile leakage is observed or atypical anatomy is encountered during laparoscopic cholecystectomy, early conversion

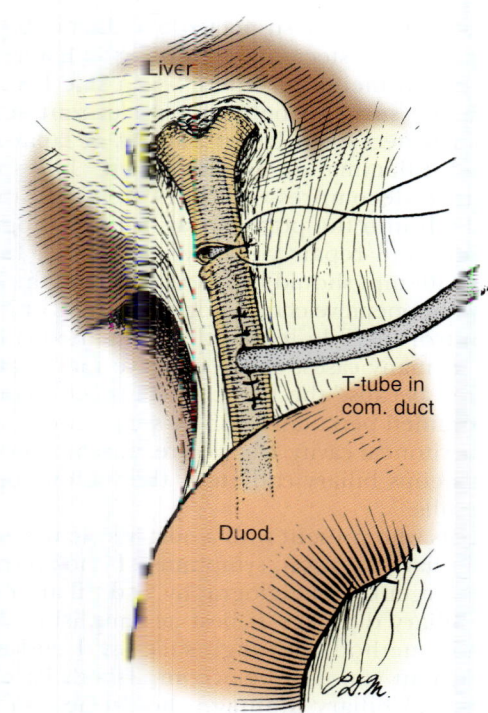

FIGURE 113.5 Primary end-to-end repair of a bile duct injury over a T-tube. In general, this technique is used for partial transections of the bile duct when there has been no associated loss of ductal length. Note that the T-tube does not exit at the site of injury.

to an open technique and prompt cholangiography are imperative. If a segmental or accessory duct less than 3 mm has been injured and cholangiography demonstrates segmental or subsegmental drainage of the injured ductal system, simple ligation of the injured duct is adequate. If the injured duct is 4 mm or larger, however, it is likely to drain multiple hepatic segments or the entire right or left lobe and thus requires operative repair.

If the injury involves the common hepatic duct or the common bile duct, repair should also be performed at the time of injury. The aims of any repair should be to maintain ductal length and not to sacrifice tissue as well as to affect a repair that will not result in postoperative bile leakage. To accomplish these goals, all repairs at the time of initial operation should involve some sort of external drainage. If the injured segment of the bile duct is short (<1 cm) and the two ends can be opposed without tension, an end-to-end anastomosis can be performed with placement of a T-tube through a separate choledochotomy either above or below the anastomosis (Fig. 113.5). Generous mobilization of the duodenum out of the retroperitoneum (Kocher maneuver) can be useful to help approximate the injured ends of the bile duct. An end-to-end repair, however, should be avoided if the ductal injury is near the hepatic duct bifurcation. Although seemingly an attractive option, end-to-end repair is often associated with postoperative stricture. Fortunately, such strictures can often be successfully managed with endoscopic dilation and stenting.

For proximal injuries or if the injured segment of the bile duct is greater than 1 cm in length, an end-to-end bile duct anastomosis should be avoided because of the excessive tension that usually exists in these situations. In these circumstances, the distal bile duct should be oversewn, and the proximal bile duct should be débrided of injured tissue and anastomosed in an end-to-side fashion to a Roux-en-Y jejunal limb. The use of a Roux-en-Y jejunal limb is preferable to anastomosis to the duodenum because, in the latter case, an anastomotic leak results in a duodenal fistula. A transanastomotic Silastic stent can be placed retrograde through the transected duct and exiting the hepatic parenchyma to allow for postoperative external drainage.

Unfortunately, most bile duct injuries during laparoscopic cholecystectomy occur in the hands of surgeons who are not experienced in performing complex biliary reconstruction. In such settings, the surgeon should consider *not* repairing the injury and not risk further worsening the situation. If the biliary tree has been transected, a retrograde catheter can be placed into the duct system to facilitate cholangiography at a later date. The bile duct should not be ligated, as ligation of the proximal bile duct most often leads to stump necrosis, subsequent bile leakage, and a more challenging reconstruction due to proximal migration of the injury itself.[15] The subhepatic space should be well drained to control the biliary leak. Furthermore, if the cholecystectomy has not yet been completed at the time of recognition, the procedure can be aborted to prevent further extending the injury proximally. Prompt transfer to a tertiary hepatobiliary center should then be made. The long-term results of immediate repair of common bile duct injuries are uncertain. Most injuries occur away from major centers; therefore even the successes are unlikely to be reported in the literature. In a Swedish report, early primary repair with end-to-end anastomosis resulted in good outcomes in only 22% of patients. Anastomotic leak requiring reoperation occurred in 32% of patients, and late stricture occurred in another 37% of patients. In patients undergoing immediate repair with a biliary-enteric anastomosis, good results were seen in 54% of patients, with strictures occurring in only 12% of patients. Similar poor late results were observed in another series in which 29 of 36 patients with primary end-to-end repair had postoperative strictures within 4 years.

DELAYED REPAIR OF BILE DUCT INJURIES

Several principles are associated with successful repair of a biliary injury or stricture: exposure of healthy proximal bile ducts that provide drainage of the entire liver; preparation of a suitable segment of intestine that can be brought to the area of the stricture without tension, most frequently a Roux-en-Y jejunal limb; and creation of a direct biliary-enteric mucosal-to-mucosal anastomosis (Fig. 113.6). A number of alternatives for elective repair of bile duct strictures exist. The choice of procedure is dictated by the location of the stricture, the history of previous unsuccessful attempts at repair, and the surgeon's personal preference. Simple excision of a bile duct stricture and end-to-end bile duct anastomosis or repair of the damaged duct can rarely be accomplished because of the invariable

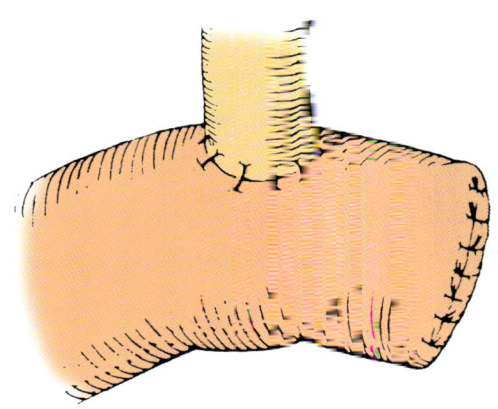

FIGURE 113.6 A completed Roux-en-Y hepaticojejunostomy. The anastomosis is typically performed with interrupted sutures in a single layer. The Roux limb is usually 40 to 60 cm long.

loss of duct length as a result of fibrosis associated with the injury. Similarly, anastomosis of the proximal bile duct to the duodenum as a choledochoduodenostomy is not suitable for most postcholecystectomy strictures because an adequate length of bile duct to create a tension-free anastomosis to the duodenum usually cannot be obtained. Thus, in almost all cases, hepaticojejunostomy constructed to a Roux-en-Y limb of jejunum is the preferred procedure.

Many surgeons believe that the use of an anastomotic stent is helpful in the majority of cases (Fig. 113.7). In the early postoperative period, a stent is used to decompress the biliary tree and provide access for cholangiography. If the injury involves the common bile duct or the common hepatic duct at least 2 cm distal to the hepatic duct bifurcation and adequate proximal bile duct mucosa can be defined, the use of long-term biliary stents is not necessary. In these situations, the preoperatively placed percutaneous transhepatic catheter is used to decompress the biliary-enteric anastomosis for 4 to 6 weeks after surgery. When adequate proximal bile duct is not available for a good mucosa-to-mucosa anastomosis, a longer period of stenting of the biliary-enteric anastomosis with a Silastic transhepatic stent is recommended. For strictures involving the hepatic duct bifurcation, both the right and left main hepatic ducts should be individually stented.

An operative technique for biliary reconstruction with transhepatic stents using the preoperatively placed percutaneous transhepatic catheters begins with dissection of the porta hepatis, which usually involves separating adhesions of the duodenum and hepatic flexure of the colon to the Glisson capsule and gallbladder fossa.[6] Identification of the proximal biliary segment can be difficult and can be aided by the presence of the preoperatively placed transhepatic biliary catheter. This is particularly true for bile duct transections that will retract high into the porta. If a primary duct stricture exists, the bile duct is then divided at the lowest extent of the stricture and dissected proximally. A segment of the strictured duct should be resected and submitted for pathologic examination. The distal duct is then oversewn, and the bile duct proximal to the stricture is carefully dissected circumferentially in a cephalad direction for a distance not to exceed 5 mm.

Excess in dissection should be avoided to prevent vascular compromise of this segment of duct, which will be used for the anastomosis. After mobilization and division of the bile duct, the biliary catheters protrude through the proximal end. A radiologic guidewire is then placed through these catheters. The preoperatively placed catheter can then be exchanged over the wire for a properly sized Silastic stent. These stents are 70 cm long and range from 12 French to 22 French. Multiple side holes are present along 40% of the length of the stent. These side holes are left to reside within the intrahepatic biliary tree and the portion of the Roux-en-Y jejunal limb used for the biliary anastomosis. The end of the stent without the side holes exits through the hepatic parenchyma and is brought out through a stab wound in the upper anterior abdomen. After stent placement, a Roux-en-Y jejunal limb is prepared, and the anastomosis is then performed as an end-to-side hepaticojejunostomy.

The importance of the hilar (epicholedochal) arterial plexus in cases of proximal bile duct injuries is also worth mentioning. More specifically, performing a "high" hepaticojejunostomy reconstruction to an intact proximal hilar bridge between the right and left hepatic ducts uses robust crossing arterial anatomy and is believed by many surgeons to minimize the risk of subsequent biliary stenosis. In patients with an injury to the right hepatic artery during cholecystectomy, this arterial plexus is particularly important to maintain healthy well-vascularized right hepatic duct for reconstruction.

An alternative technique has been described for management of bile duct strictures involving the bifurcation and one or both of the hepatic ducts in which a side-to-side anastomosis of the left hepatic duct to the Roux-en-Y limb is constructed. A long opening along the anterior surface of the left hepatic duct is anastomosed to the side of the Roux-en-Y limb. Because it is possible to dissect the anterior surface of the left hepatic duct high up into the hepatic parenchyma, this procedure permits anastomosis to normal mucosa even though there can be fibrosis and stricture at the bifurcation of the ducts and in the distal portion of the hepatic duct. This technique can avoid the need for postoperative stenting.

SURGICAL OUTCOMES

POSTOPERATIVE MORBIDITY AND MORTALITY

Repair of bile duct strictures are performed primarily in major medical centers by experienced surgeons; however, these operations are still associated with significant morbidity and mortality. In 1982, a review of 38 series published since 1900 that included more than 7643 procedures performed on 5586 patients reported an overall operative mortality rate of 8.3%.[17] More recently the incidence of operative mortality has decreased markedly with improved technology and a multidisciplinary approach as well as improved surgical experience. A series of 200 consecutive patients managed at the Johns Hopkins Hospital reported three deaths in patients who did not undergo an attempt at repair who were referred with sepsis secondary to an uncontrolled biliary leak for a mortality rate of 1.5%. Definitive surgical reconstruction was performed in 175

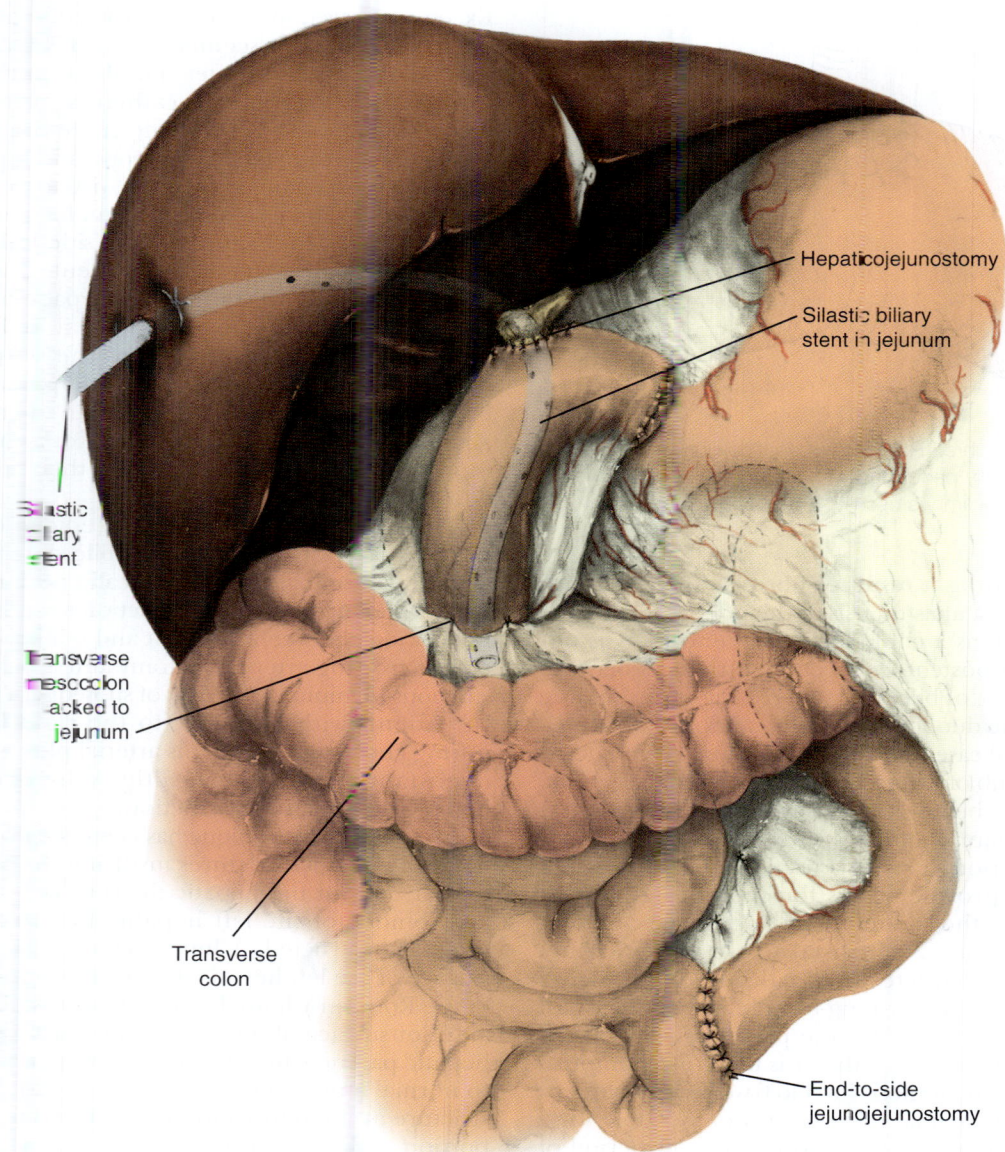

Hepaticojejunostomy

Silastic biliary
stent in jejunum

Silastic
biliary
stent

Transverse
mesocolon
tacked to
jejunum

Transverse
colon

End-to-side
jejunojejunostomy

FIGURE 113.7 Completed repair showing the Silastic biliary stent traversing the liver and the hepaticojejunostomy. The Roux-en-Y jejunal limb has been brought to the hepatic hilum in retrocolic position. (From Cameron JL. *Atlas of Surgery*. Vol 1. Toronto: BC Decker; 1990:57.)

patients with a perioperative mortality of 1.7%.[18] In this series, the timing of repair, the mode of presentation, previous attempts of repair, and the level of injury did not influence outcome. Chronic liver disease can be an important factor for operative mortality and morbidity with advanced biliary cirrhosis and portal hypertension leading to mortality rates approaching 30%. Fortunately in the modern era, such advanced disease is uncommon. In most series, postoperative morbidity rates are in the range of 20% to 40%. In the Johns Hopkins series, complications occurred in 41% of patients. Most of the complications are minor and could be managed with either interventional radiology techniques or conservative management. No patient required reoperation for postoperative complications, and the median length of stay in this series was 8 days.

LONG-TERM RESULTS AND QUALITY OF LIFE

Historically, excellent long-term results were achieved in 70% to 90% of patients who underwent repair of bile duct strictures. The definition of satisfactory results in most series requires that patients have no symptoms, jaundice, or cholangitis. Length of follow-up is important in analyzing final results, because recurrent strictures can occur up to 20 years after the initial procedure.[12,13] Approximately, two-thirds of restrictures are evident within 2 years, and 90% are seen within 7 years. The percentage of patients with good results is inversely related to the number of previous repairs. Other factors that favor a good outcome include young age at the time of stricture repair, use of a Roux-en-Y biliary-enteric anastomosis, absence of infection and hepatic fibrosis, and use of transhepatic stents.

As illustrated earlier, in the era before laparoscopic cholecystectomy, excellent long-term results were obtainable in tertiary care centers specializing in the management of these problems. Questions were raised as to whether the excellent results of bile duct strictures after open cholecystectomy could be directly transferred to patients sustaining laparoscopic bile duct injuries. Some researchers had suggested that the mechanism of bile duct injury during laparoscopic cholecystectomy, the complex nature of many of these injuries, and the frequent association of significant inflammation and fibrosis secondary to sustained, unrecognized bile leakage might result in poor long-term results. Furthermore, the high percentage of these patients who have undergone unsuccessful operations, often performed by the primary laparoscopic surgeon, might also lead to a poor long-term outcome. Evidence for the latter hypothesis was provided by a review of the records of 85 patients who underwent a total of 112 biliary repairs.[9] Four factors determined the success or failure of treatment in this series. These factors included performance of preoperative cholangiography, the choice of surgical repair, details of the operative repair, and experience of the surgeon performing the repair. The importance of preoperative delineation of anatomy was clear, in that 96% of procedures in which cholangiograms were not obtained before repair were unsuccessful, and 69% of repairs were not successful when the cholangiographic data were incomplete. When cholangiographic data were complete, the initial repair was successful in 84% of patients. The type of repair was also of significance in influencing outcome. A primary end-to-end ductal repair over a T-tube was unsuccessful in all patients in whom a complete transection of the bile duct had taken place, whereas 63% of Roux-en-Y hepaticojejunostomies were successful. Attempts at repair by the primary surgeon were successful only in 17% of cases, and in no case was a secondary repair by the primary surgeon successful. In those cases in which the first repair was performed by a tertiary care biliary surgeon, a 94% success rate was obtained.

To better define the optimal outcome of the repair of bile duct injuries at tertiary care centers in the laparoscopic era, a series of 142 patients with major bile duct injuries treated during the 1990s has been reported.[20] Laparoscopic cholecystectomy was the initial operation in 75% of these patients, and 41% had undergone a previous attempt or attempts at surgical repair before referral. In this series with a median follow-up of 58 months (range, 11 to 119 months), a successful outcome was obtained in 91% of patients. In this series the level of initial clinical presentation, history of prior repair, and length of biliary stenting did not influence outcome. Comparable results have been reported from other high-volume hepatobiliary centers.[21,22] These results suggest that surgical reconstruction of major bile duct injuries after laparoscopic cholecystectomy can still result in excellent long-term results.

Despite the overall success of biliary reconstruction, there is a small subset of patients with major bile duct injuries in whom standard repair techniques appear to be inadequate. Factors such as delayed diagnosis, complex injuries above the hepatic confluence, associated vasculobiliary injuries, and liver atrophy can all negatively affect

the outcomes of standard reconstruction. In this select population, excellent results have been observed with major hepatectomy.[23] A classic example of this scenario would be a patient who has sustained a right posterior sectoral bile duct injury, and subsequent hepatic atrophy with associated recurrent cholangitis. These patients typically benefit most from a right posterior hepatic sectionectomy, as opposed to an attempt at a challenging hepaticojejunostomy reconstruction to a small duct within an abnormal liver. Finally, in rare cases with failure of all standard surgical techniques of reconstruction with resultant end-stage liver disease, liver transplantation may offer the opportunity for survival.[24] Interestingly, many of these extreme injuries are caused during open cholecystectomy and therefore trauma caused by migration from the cystic plate into the hilar plate itself.[11]

Although large series from tertiary referral centers have reported excellent long-term results, the overall impact of bile duct injuries on society is significant in terms of health care costs, disability, and even mortality. In an analysis of patients undergoing laparoscopic cholecystectomy from the US Medicare database, Flum et al. demonstrated that the adjusted hazard ratio for death during the follow-up period was significantly higher (2.79; 95% confidence level, 2.71 to 2.85) for patients with a bile duct injury than in those patients without a bile duct injury.[25] The hazard increased with advancing age and comorbidities and decreased with the experience of the repairing surgeon. The adjusted hazard of death during follow-up was 11% greater if the repairing surgeon was the same as the injuring surgeon. These data certainly further support the referral of most patients with bile duct injuries to centers with greater experience in the management of the injuries.

Finally, although the overall success of the surgical management of laparoscopic bile duct injuries associated with laparoscopic cholecystectomy is excellent, there is an impression that patients may have an impaired quality of life even after successful repair of their bile duct injury. Quality-of-life assessments after laparoscopic cholecystectomy bile duct injury have been addressed in several recent reports.[26,27] These results have generally reported either comparable or mildly diminished quality of life compared with matched controls. Interestingly, in one study, patients who reported pursuing a lawsuit following their injury had significantly worse quality-of-life scores in all domains when compared with those who did not entertain legal action.[26] The most recent study, which spanned a 23-year period (169 month median follow-up), evaluated 62 patients who had generally undergone a Roux-en-Y hepaticojejunostomy (86%) reconstruction, confirmed that mental health concerns were more common-place than physical or general health issues following bile duct injuries. While most patients displayed an eventual return to their physical baseline, psychological quality of life was much more difficult to correct over time.[28]

NONOPERATIVE MANAGEMENT STRATEGIES

Operative management of bile duct strictures is technically difficult and continues to be associated with significant postoperative morbidity and mortality. Moreover, in all series recurrent strictures develop in a proportion of patients. These factors, in addition to technical advances in the fields of therapeutic radiology and endoscopy, have led to the development of nonoperative techniques for management of bile duct strictures. The optimal method for management using these techniques is dependent on the presence and anatomy of biliary-enteric continuity.

PERCUTANEOUS BALLOON DILATION

The management of benign bile duct strictures using the percutaneous transhepatic route is indicated primarily in patients with a failed prior biliary-enteric anastomosis to a jejunal limb. The procedure in many cases can be performed with a combination of local anesthesia and intravenous sedation. In this technique, access to the proximal biliary tree is gained and the stricture is traversed with a guidewire under fluoroscopic guidance. At this point the stricture is dilated using angioplasty-type balloon catheters, chosen based on the location of the stricture and the diameter of the normal duct. After the procedure, a transhepatic stent is left in place across the stricture to allow access to the biliary tree for follow-up cholangiography, repeat dilation, and maintenance of a lumen during the healing process. In most series, numerous dilations are required.

The results from a number of series have been encouraging. In a multicenter review of bile duct strictures treated in the open cholecystectomy era, 3-year follow-up showed a 67% patency rate for anastomotic and a 76% patency rate for iatrogenic primary bile duct strictures, yielding an overall 70% success rate.[29] A report of 51 patients with bile duct strictures after laparoscopic cholecystectomy managed with percutaneous dilation showed a success rate of 58% with a mean follow-up of 76 months.[30]

Complications of balloon dilation are frequent. Cholangitis, hemobilia, and bile leaks can occur in up to 20% of patients. Bleeding, usually from the hepatic parenchyma, has been reported, with transfusions often necessary. Sepsis due to cholangitis can occur despite antibiotic prophylaxis. Sepsis and significant bleeding seldom occur in patients dilated by a T-tube tract, suggesting that much of the morbidity is the result of traversing the hepatic parenchyma by the large percutaneously placed catheters.

ENDOSCOPIC BALLOON DILATION

Endoscopic balloon dilation is often considered technically possible only in patients with primary bile duct strictures or with strictures at a prior primary end-to-end repair or choledochoduodenal anastomosis. With the advent of double-balloon enteroscopy, however, more patients are now able to undergo endoscopic retrograde cholangiopancreatography following preceding hepaticojejunostomies as well as myriad gastric or bariatric procedures. This technique begins with ERC and endoscopic sphincterotomy. The stricture is traversed retrograde with an atraumatic guidewire, and sequential balloon dilation is used. Reevaluation with cholangiography is performed every 3 to 6 months, and redilation is performed as necessary. In most cases, an endoprosthesis is left in place after dilation for at least 12 months.

There are now large reported experiences with endoscopic dilation of benign bile duct strictures. The largest experience comes from the group in The Netherlands who recently reported their experience in 110 patients.[31] The mean number of stents placed was two, the mean duration of stenting was 11 months, and stent-related complications occurred in 33% of patients with one death. Twenty percent of patients were eventually referred for surgery. The overall reported success rate was 74% with a mean follow-up of 7.6 years. A similar experience was reported in the United States.[32,33] In this series, 18 of 25 strictures were postoperative. Strictures were located at the cystic duct junction in 17 patients and in the distal bile duct in the remaining 8 patients. Of 25 patients, 22 (88%) had significant clinical benefit from the therapy. Only two complications occurred in this series—one case each of pancreatitis and cholangitis.

In a large comparative study, the group from The Netherlands compared endoscopic versus surgical treatment of benign bile duct strictures.[34] Thirty-five patients were treated surgically, and 66 were treated by endoscopic stenting. Patient characteristics, initial injury, previous repairs, and the level of obstruction were comparable in both groups. Surgical therapy consisted of Roux-en-Y hepaticojejunostomy, and endoscopic therapy consisted of placement of an endoprosthesis with trimonthly elective exchange for 1 year. Successful stent placement was accomplished in 94% of patients managed endoscopically. Six of the 66 endoscopic patients, however, underwent surgical reconstruction either for failed stent placement or for other reasons. Early complications occurred more frequently in the surgically treated group (26% vs. 8%; $P <$ .03). However, the only procedure-related death occurred in a patient in whom severe pancreatitis developed after endoscopic stent placement. Late complications, which included primarily episodes of cholangitis, occurred only in the endoscopic group (27%). The overall complication rates, therefore, were similar at 26% for surgical patients and 35% for endoscopic patients. The mean follow-up and definition of success were similar to those in the aforementioned study. After surgery, excellent results were observed in 83% of patients with a recurrent stricture developing in six patients at a mean of 40 months after the initial operation. After endoscopic stenting, excellent results were observed in 72% of patients, with restricture developing in 18% of patients at a mean of 3 months after stent removal. The investigators concluded that endoscopic stenting should be considered for the initial attempt at definitive management in suitable patients in the hope of avoiding reoperation.

The final and most recent comparative study describing 528 patients over 18 years has confirmed a number of interesting observations.[35] More specifically, patients with all types of bile duct injuries were most commonly treated by endoscopists (40%), followed by surgeons (36%) and interventional radiologists (24%). Success rates, however, were higher for surgery (88%) compared with either endoscopy (76%) or interventional radiology (50%). This observation was accomplished with an overall morbidity among the surgical cohort of 24% with no 90-day mortality. Not surprisingly, outcomes also improved dramatically over time among all approaches. Although the reason for this progress is clearly multifactorial, issues such as improved selection of patients for each approach, increased experience in reconstruction at the surgeon level (and therefore fewer surgeons performing repairs overall), and perhaps pursuit of more proximal biliary-enteric anastomoses and/or more selective use of transhepatic stents may each play a role. Overall, the modern analysis of bile duct injuries confirms the importance of ensuring significant clinician experience with this complication; a multidisciplinary team composed of hepatopancreatobiliary surgeons, interventional endoscopists, and interventional radiologists; and thoughtful selection of a given patient for the appropriate therapeutic option with the highest chance of long-term success.

CONCLUSION

Iatrogenic bile duct injuries remain extremely challenging to the individual surgeon, as well as the health care system and most importantly the patient. Preoperative planning, surgeon vigilance, achieving the critical view of safety, and completing the bile duct time out can reduce the risk of creating a bile duct injury. In cases of suspected bile duct injury, an expedient diagnostic work-up, control of sepsis, and referral to a surgeon experienced in the reconstruction of these injuries is essential. If mistakes and misadventures are avoided the long-term outcome and quality of life in the vast majority of patients should be excellent.

REFERENCES

1. Hall JG, Pappas TN. Current management of biliary strictures. *J Gastrointest Surg*. 2004;8:1098.
2. Brooks KR, Scarborough JE, Vaslef SN, Shapiro ML. No need to wait: an analysis of the timing of cholecystectomy during admission for acute cholecystitis using the American College of Surgeons National Surgical Quality Improvement Program database. *J Trauma Acute Care Surg*. 2012;74:167.
3. Joseph M, Phillips MR, Farrell TM, Rupp CC. Single incision laparoscopic cholecystectomy is associated with a higher bile duct injury rate: a review and word of caution. *Ann Surg*. 2012;256:1.
4. Branum G, Schmitt C, Baillie J, et al. Management of major biliary complications after laparoscopic cholecystectomy. *Ann Surg*. 1993;17:532.
5. Flum DR, Dellinger EP, Cheadle A, Chan L, Koepsell T. Intraoperative cholangiography and risk of common bile duct injury during laparoscopic cholecystectomy. *JAMA*. 2003;289:1639.
6. Sheffield KM, Riall TS, Kuo YF, Kuo Y, Townsend CM Jr, Goodwin JS. Association between cholecystectomy with vs without intraoperative cholangiography and risk of common duct injury. *JAMA*. 2013;310:812.
7. Massaruch NN, Devlin A, Elrod JAB, Symons RG, Flum DR. Surgeon knowledge, behavior and opinions regarding intraoperative cholangiography. *J Am Coll Surg*. 2008;207:2.
8. Way LW, Stewart L, Gantert W, et al. Causes and prevention of laparoscopic bile duct injuries: analysis of 252 cases from a human factors and cognitive psychology perspective. *Ann Surg*. 2003;273:460.
9. Strasberg SM, Hertl M, Soper NJ. An analysis of the problem of biliary injury during laparoscopic cholecystectomy. *J Am Coll Surg*. 1995;180:101.
10. Alves A, Farges O, Nicolet J, Watrin T, Sauvanet A, Belghiti J. Incidence and consequence of an hepatic artery injury in patients with postcholecystectomy bile duct strictures. *Ann Surg*. 2003;230:93.
11. Strasberg SM, Helton WS. An analytical review of vasculobiliary injury in laparoscopic and open cholecystectomy. *HPB*. 2011;13:1.
12. Pitt HA, Miyamoto T, Parapatis SK, Tompkins RK, Longmire WP Jr. Factors influencing outcome in patients with postoperative biliary strictures. *Am J Surg*. 1982;144:14.
13. Pellegrini CA, Thomas MJ, Way LW. Recurrent biliary stricture: patterns of recurrent and outcome of surgical therapy. *Am J Surg*. 1984;147:175.
14. Lillemoe KD, Martin SA, Cameron JL, et al. Major bile duct injuries during laparoscopic cholecystectomy: follow-up after combined surgical and radiologic management. *Ann Surg*. 1977;225:459.
15. Mercado MA, Chan C, Jacinto JC, Sanchez N, Barajas A. Voluntary and involuntary ligature of the bile duct in iatrogenic injuries: a nonadvisable approach. *J Gastrointest Surg*. 2008;12:1029.
16. Lillemoe KD. Treatment of laparoscopic bile duct injuries. *Curr Tech Gen Surg*. 1997;6:1.
17. Warren KW, Christophi C, Armendari ZR. The evolution and current perspectives of the treatment of benign bile duct strictures: a review. *Surg Gastroenterol*. 1982;1:141.
18. Sicklick JK, Camp MS, Lillemoe KD, et al. Surgical management of bile duct injuries sustained during laparoscopic cholecystectomy: perioperative results in 200 patients. *Ann Surg*. 2005;241:786.
19. Stewart L, Way LW. Bile duct injuries during laparoscopic cholecystectomy. *Arch Surg*. 1995;130:1123.
20. Lillemoe KD, Melton GB, Cameron JL, et al. Postoperative bile duct strictures: management and outcome in the 1990s. *Ann Surg*. 2000;232:430.
21. Murr MM, Gigot JI, Nagorney DM, Harmsen WS, Ilstrup DM, Farnell FB. Long-term results of biliary reconstruction after laparoscopic bile duct injuries. *Arch Surg*. 1999;134:604.
22. Walsh RM, Henderson JM, Vogt DP, Brown N. Long-term outcome of biliary reconstruction for bile duct injuries from laparoscopic cholecystectomies. *Surgery*. 2007;142:450.
23. Laurent A, Sanvanet A, Farges O, Watrin T, Rivkine E, Belghiti J. Major hepatectomy for the treatment of complex bile duct injury. *Ann Surg*. 2008;248:77.
24. de Santibanes E, Ardilles V, Gadano A, Palavecino M, Pekolj J, Ciardullo M. Liver transplantation: the last measure in the treatment of bile duct injuries. *World J Surg*. 2008;32:1714.
25. Flum DR, Cheadle A, Prela C, Dellinger EP, Chan L. Bild duct injury during cholecystectomy and survival in Medicare beneficiaries. *JAMA*. 2003;290:2168.
26. Melton GB, Lillemoe KD, Cameron JL, Sauter PA, Coleman J, Yeo CJ. Major bile duct injuries associated with laparoscopic cholecystectomy: effect on quality of life. *Ann Surg*. 2002;235:888.
27. Morgan AM, Hoti E, Winter DC, et al. Quality of life after iatrogenic bile duct injury: a case control study. *Ann Surg*. 2009;249:292.
28. Lazo A, Spolverato G, Kim Y, et al. Long-term health-related quality of life after iatrogenic bile duct injury repair. *J Am Coll Surg*. 2014;219:923.
29. Mueller PR, van Sonnenberg E, Ferrucci JT Jr, et al. Biliary stricture classification: multicenter review of clinical management in 73 patients. *Radiology*. 1986;160:17.
30. Misra S, Melton GB, Geschwind JF, Venbrux AC, Cameron JL, Lillemoe KD. Percutaneous management of bile duct strictures and injuries associated with laparoscopic cholecystectomy: a decade of experience. *J Am Coll Surg*. 2004;198:218.
31. de Reuver P, Rauws EA, Vermeulen M, Dijkgraaf MGW, Gouma DJ, Bruno MJ. Endoscopic treatment of post-surgical bile duct injuries: long term outcomes and predictors of success. *Gut*. 2007;56:1599.
32. Geenen DJ, Geenen JE, Hogan WJ, et al. Endoscopic therapy for benign bile duct strictures. *Gastrointest Endosc*. 1989;35:367.
33. Pitt HA, Kaufman SL, Coleman J, White RI, Cameron JL. Benign postoperative biliary strictures: operate or dilate? *Ann Surg*. 1989;210:417.
34. Davids PHP, Tanka AKF, Rauws EAJ, et al. Benign biliary strictures: surgery or endoscopy? *Ann Surg*. 1993;217:237.
35. Pitt HA, Sherman S, Johnson MS, et al. Improved outcomes of bile duct injuries in the 21st century. *Ann Surg*. 2013;258:490.

Operative Management of Bile Duct Strictures

Karen A. Chojnacki | Charles J. Yeo

Bile duct strictures can result from a myriad of conditions, both benign and malignant. These strictures represent a significant clinical problem and if not managed correctly can result in major morbidity, both short and long term, and possible mortality. Complications of untreated or improperly treated strictures include cholangitis, biliary cirrhosis, portal hypertension, and end-stage liver disease. The goal of treatment is to reestablish unobstructed biliary flow into the intestinal tract.

PATHOGENESIS

The most common cause of bile duct stricture is surgery of the gallbladder or biliary tree. In the era of open surgery the incidence of bile duct injury following cholecystectomy was 0.2% to 0.3%.[2] Since the introduction of laparoscopic cholecystectomy, the rate of bile duct injury has doubled. Several studies have published an injury rate of 0.4% to 0.6%.[2-4] This rate of injury has remained essentially stable.[5] Less than 30% of bile duct injuries are recognized intraoperatively.[6] Therefore most patients will go on to develop a leak or stricture. The classification of these injuries and strictures has been defined by Strasberg and Bismuth and is shown in Figs. 114.1 and 114.2.[2]

Not all bile duct strictures caused by a previous surgery result from laparoscopic cholecystectomy. Endoscopic, percutaneous, and operative procedures on the bile duct may result in stricture. Injury may also occur during gastric and duodenal procedures, liver resection and transplantation, and pancreatic procedures. These injuries typically involve a failure to recognize the extrahepatic biliary tree at the time of antral or duodenal dissection/division. The anatomy in this region may be distorted by inflammation or a neoplastic process. The intrapancreatic bile duct may be injured during surgery of the pancreatic head or ampulla of Vater. Inflammatory or congenital conditions may also cause strictures of the bile duct (Box 114.1). Benign and malignant neoplasms of the biliary tree and surrounding organs are additional causes of biliary stricture (Box 114.2).

CLINICAL PRESENTATION

Patients with postoperative bile duct injuries typically present early after the procedure. In a study of patients with bile duct injury following open cholecystectomy, 69% of patients were diagnosed within the first 6 months and 82% were diagnosed within the first year following surgery.[7] Patients with early postoperative complications have three types of injury: bile leak, obstruction, or a combination of leak and obstruction. Patients with a leak often complain of vague symptoms such as abdominal fullness, abdominal pain, nausea, vomiting, fever, and/or chills. Their pain is often similar to the biliary colic that brought them to surgery. These patients may have bile leaking from their incisions or operatively placed drains, or the leak may be contained within the abdomen. Any patient who is not improving daily following a cholecystectomy should be suspected of harboring a bile duct injury. Liver function tests can be normal or show only mild elevations of bilirubin. Bilirubin elevation is typically a result of peritoneal absorption. Serum alkaline phosphatase is often elevated as the biliary epithelium is damaged. Levels of alanine aminotransferase and aspartate aminotransferase are usually normal. Patients with obstruction will have evidence of jaundice, scleral icterus, abdominal pain, and/or anorexia. If cholangitis is present, patients will also have fever, chills, and malaise, and these patients will also have abnormalities in their liver function tests. Hyperbilirubinemia is present. Cholangitis will cause leukocytosis. If the obstruction is long-standing with progression to biliary cirrhosis, there will be evidence of decreased hepatic synthetic function (i.e., hypoalbuminemia and prolonged prothrombin time).

Patients undergoing uncomplicated laparoscopic cholecystectomy should recover quickly with minimal discomfort. Most patients have little to no pain in the first postoperative days. There is little requirement for analgesics. Most are back to normal activities within the first week. Any patient with persistent pain, nausea, vomiting, abdominal distention, or declining activity level should be evaluated for a suspected bile duct injury.

RADIOLOGIC WORK-UP

Initial radiologic evaluation includes abdominal ultrasound and/or computed tomography (CT). Both can identify intraabdominal fluid collections and dilated intrahepatic or extrahepatic bile ducts. Small fluid collections are found in the gallbladder fossa in 10% to 14% of patients after cholecystectomy, and these typically resolve without intervention.[8,9] Large fluid collections, fluid collections outside of the gallbladder fossa, or ascites are findings worrisome for bile leak. CT and ultrasound cannot distinguish between seroma, lymphocele, hematoma, or biloma. Aspiration, drainage, and/or catheter placement into a fluid collection may be necessary to define the fluid collection. CT and ultrasound can both be used to evaluate for signs of unsuspected malignancy, such as mass or adenopathy.

Hepatobiliary iminodiacetic acid (HIDA) scanning can be used to assess for bile leak or biliary obstruction. However, the exact location of a leak or extent of injury cannot be uniformly assessed with HIDA scan. If a drain was placed at the time of cholecystectomy, water-soluble contrast can be injected through the catheter (sinography)

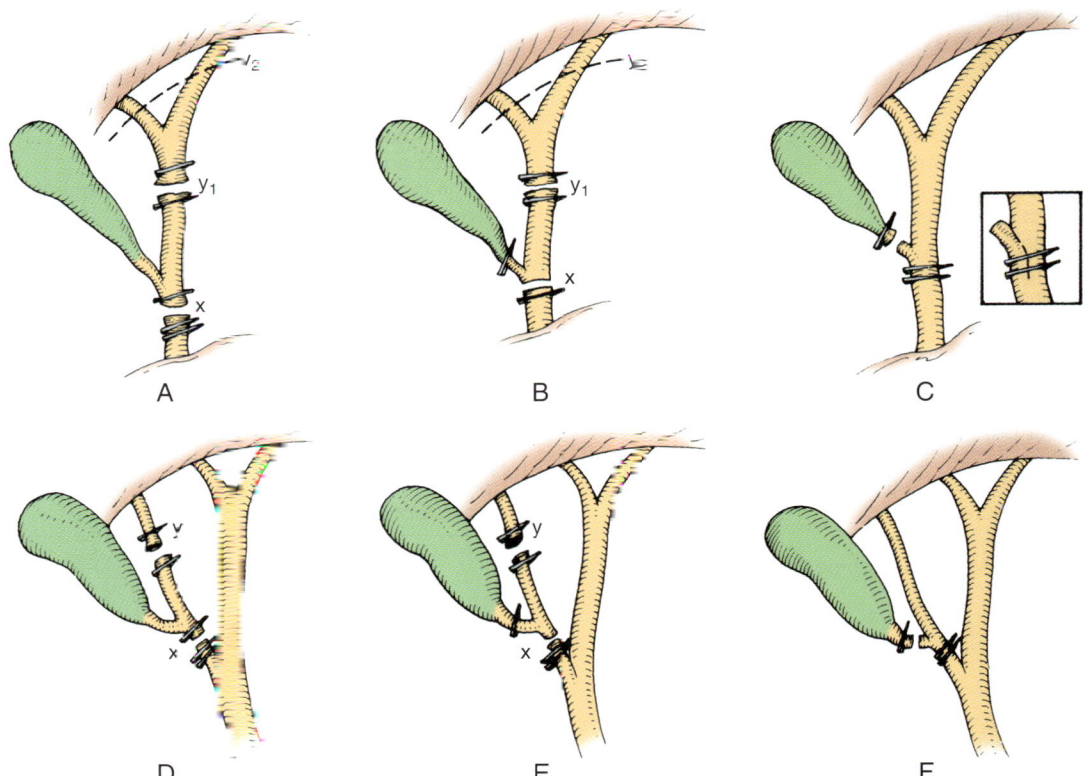

FIGURE 114.1 Various patterns of biliary duct injury. (A) Classic injury. (B and C) Variants of the classic injury. (D to F) Different injuries resulting from the cystic duct originating from an aberrant right hepatic duct. (From Strasberg SM, Hertl M, Soper NJ. An analysis of the problem of biliary injury during laparoscopic cholecystectomy. *J Am Coll Surg* 1995;180:101.)

to define the leak or injury. Alternatively, if a percutaneous drainage catheter has been placed, a sinogram can be obtained via this catheter, to confine the leak site and the relevant biliary anatomy.

In most cases, cholangiography will be necessary for accurate evaluation of the biliary tree. Three techniques exist for imaging the bile ducts: percutaneous transhepatic cholangiography (PTC), endoscopic retrograde cholangiography (ERC), and magnetic resonance cholangiopancreatography (MRC). PTC has the ability to detect the exact location of leak, injury, or obstruction (Fig. 114.3A). It is particularly useful in the management of cystic stump leaks and partial injuries to the extrahepatic biliary tree. If a leak or partial injury is detected at ERC, an endoprosthesis can be placed. An endoprosthesis can serve two purposes. As a stent across a leak, the endoprosthesis decreases the pressure gradient between the biliary system and the duodenum by traversing the sphincter of Oddi. This creates a path of least resistance allowing the bile to flow away from the leak. An endoprosthesis can also bridge and occlude a defect, allowing it to heal and minimize stricture formation.[10] However, ERC is less valuable in cases of complete common bile duct transection or occlusion. In these cases the proximal biliary tree cannot be evaluated by ERC (see Fig. 114.3B). Of note, ERC provides no information about concomitant vascular injuries.

PTC is useful for evaluating the proximal extrahepatic and intrahepatic biliary tree (Fig. 114.3). Information gained from this study is essential for planning future

reconstruction. First the intrahepatic biliary tree is visualized with a Chiba needle, and then using the Seldinger technique, a wire is passed into the biliary tree. This is followed by the placement of a percutaneous transhepatic catheter. This allows for therapeutic procedures, such as drainage, dilation, and control of a bile leak. This is an invasive procedure with a complication rate as high as 6.9%. Complications include bleeding, hemobilia, bile duct injury, and cholangitis. Although challenging, even nondilated intrahepatic ducts can be cannulated safely.[11] At the time of the biliary reconstruction, it is helpful to wedge the catheter at the caudal-most extent of the transected, obstructed extrahepatic biliary tree or advance the catheter for a few centimeters in the subhepatic space in the case of an open proximal biliary tree. This greatly facilitates identification of the injured duct.

MRC is a noninvasive technique for imaging of the biliary tree. Besides evaluating the bile ducts proximal and distal to an injury, MRCP can also assess for other intraabdominal injuries, fluid collections, vascular injury, and hepatic ischemia or necrosis. These high-quality images have led some to suggest that MRCP is superior to PTC or ERC and should become the initial step in evaluating patients with suspected bile duct strictures.[12,13] Information gained from MRCP can determine which patients will have therapeutic benefit from an invasive study (e.g., cystic duct leak requiring biliary endoprosthesis). It can also guide which invasive procedure will most benefit a patient (e.g., ERC for complete common bile duct transection).

BOX 114.1 Causes of Benign Biliary Strictures

IATROGENIC
Postoperative strictures following biliary procedures
Laparoscopic cholecystectomy
Open cholecystectomy
Common bile duct exploration
Prior stricture repair
Endoscopic retrograde cholangiopancreatography
Endoscopic sphincterotomy
Percutaneous biliary manipulation
Postoperative strictures following other operative
  procedures
Gastrectomy
  Duodenal ulcer procedures
Hepatic resection
   Hepatic transplantation
   Pancreatic procedures
   Portacaval shunt
   Stricture at biliary-enteric anastomosis

TRAUMATIC
Blunt injury
Penetrating injury

INFLAMMATORY
Chronic pancreatitis
Cholelithiasis and choledocholithiasis
Mirizzi syndrome
Primary sclerosing cholangitis
Duodenal ulcer
Duodenal diverticulum
Crohn disease
Sphincter of Oddi stenosis
Viral infections
Toxic drugs
Radiation fibrosis
Subhepatic abscess
Parasitic infections

CONGENITAL
Choledochal cyst
Caroli disease
Congenital stricture webs
Biliary atresia

BOX 114.2 Neoplastic Causes of Biliary Stricture

BENIGN
Bile duct hamartoma
Bile duct adenoma
Benign inflammatory tumors (benign inflammatory
  pseudotumors)

MALIGNANT—INTRINSIC
Cholangiocarcinoma

MALIGNANT—EXTRINSIC
Pancreatic carcinoma
Ampullary carcinoma
Duodenal carcinoma
Gallbladder carcinoma
Lymphoma
Lymphadenopathy from gastric carcinoma, colorectal
  carcinoma

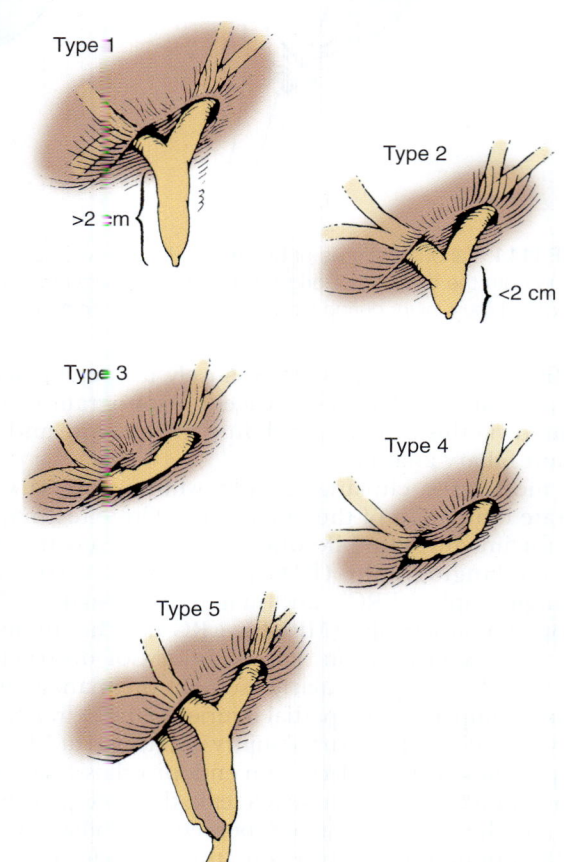

FIGURE 114.2 Classification of bile duct strictures based on the level of the stricture in relation to the confluence of the hepatic ducts. Types 3, 4, and 5 are typically considered complex injuries. (From Bismuth H. Postoperative strictures of the bile ducts. In: Blumgart LH, ed. *The Biliary Tract. Clinical Surgery International Series*, Vol 5. Edinburgh: Churchill Livingstone; 1983:209.)

The importance of accurate understanding of the biliary anatomy in patients with bile duct stricture cannot be overstated. The success of reconstruction depends on clear delineation of the site of the stricture and the biliary anatomy. In one study, 96% of bile duct reconstructions were unsuccessful when preoperative cholangiography was not obtained, and 69% of repairs were unsuccessful if the cholangiographic data were incomplete. When cholangiographic data were complete, 84% of initial repairs were successful.[14]

SURGICAL MANAGEMENT OF BILE DUCT STRICTURES

After the anatomy of a bile duct stricture has been defined, decisions must be made regarding the timing of repair and

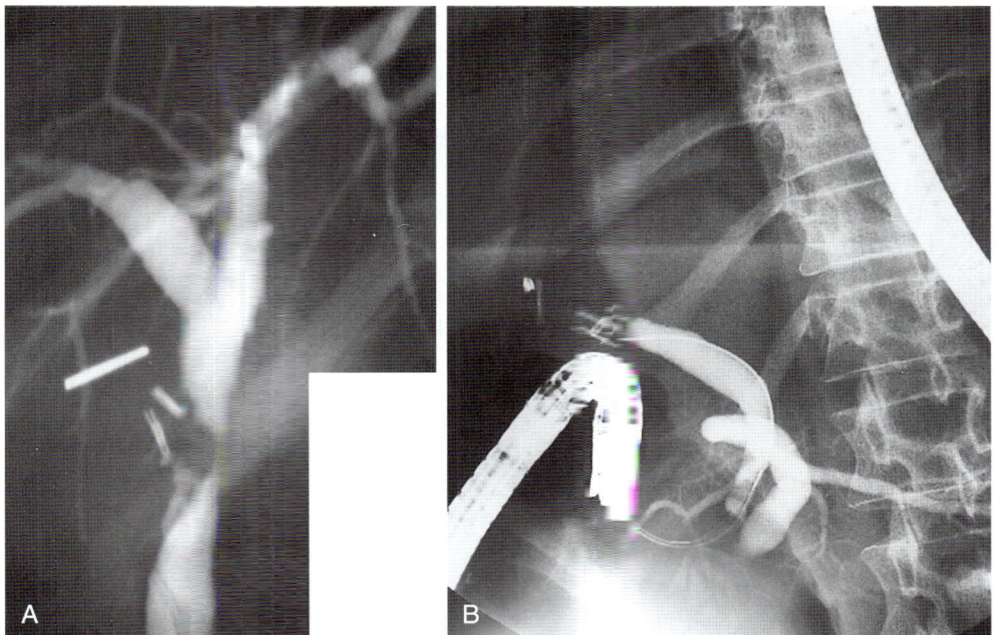

FIGURE 114.3 (A) An endoscopic retrograde cholangiopancreatogram from a patient with elevated liver function tests 4 years after open cholecystectomy. Note the extensive narrowing of the bile duct below the bifurcation and the surgical clips close to the strictured area. (B) A cholangiopancreatogram from a patient with a total transection of the common bile duct during laparoscopic cholecystectomy. Note the multiple clips across the common bile duct and the abrupt termination of the column of contrast medium at the site of the clips.

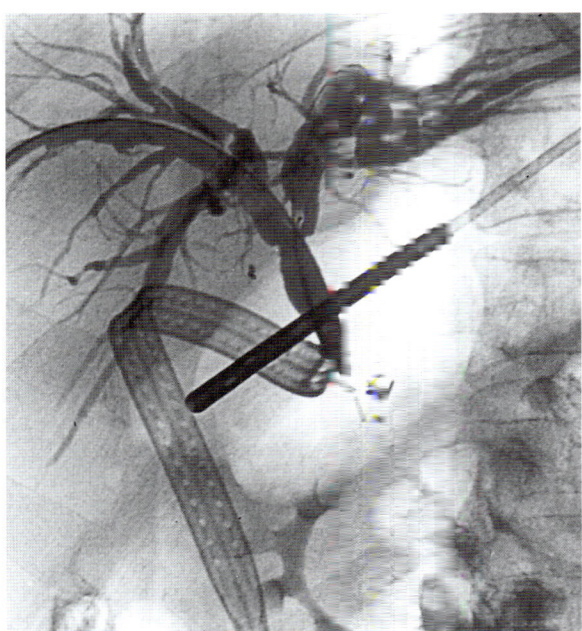

FIGURE 114.4 A percutaneous transhepatic cholangiogram from a patient with a complete transection of the common hepatic duct, which ends close to several surgical clips. A surgical drain is in place, as well as a duodenal feeding tube, which crosses obliquely over the common hepatic duct.

the type of repair. *There are no randomized controlled trials studying early versus late repair of bile duct injury. Therefore optimal timing of repair has not been conclusively determined. Successful results, with little clinical differences, have been obtained in both early and late repair. Early repair of bile duct injury has been shown to be most cost effective.*[15]

EARLY REPAIR

Patients who present early after surgery and show no signs of sepsis, intraabdominal collections, or vascular injury should be considered for early repair within 72 hours. These patients tend to have simpler injuries. The type of injury guides the appropriate intervention. Strasberg type A injuries, cystic duct leaks, can be managed with endoscopic sphincterotomy and stenting, via the placement of a biliary endoprosthesis (typically 8- to 10-French plastic stent). Leaks from a duct of Luschka can be managed in a similar manner.

Strasberg type D injuries can also be approached in the early postoperative period. These injuries are also amenable to endoscopic sphincterotomy and stenting. Of note, if a partial transection of the common bile duct is recognized at the time of initial surgery, it can be repaired primarily over a T tube. Fine, monofilament, absorbable sutures should be used for the repair. The T tube should be brought out of the common bile duct at a distant site away from the repair site (Fig. 114.5). If the injury is secondary to the use of cautery or results in complete transection of the duct, results of primary repair are poor. One study reported a restricture rate of nearly 100% for end-to-end repairs of the common bile duct.[14]

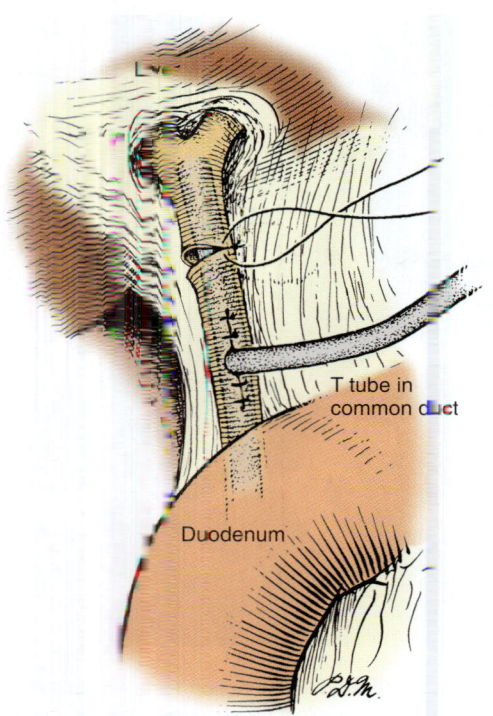

FIGURE 114.5 Primary end-to-end repair of a bile duct injury over a T tube. In general, this technique is used for partial transections of the bile duct, when there has been no associated loss of ductal length. Note that the T tube does not exit at the site of injury.

These patients are best managed with a biliary-enteric anastomosis as later described.

DELAYED MANAGEMENT OF BILIARY STRICTURE

If operative repair cannot be completed within 72 hours of injury because of patient condition or inability to complete radiographic work-up, delay of repair *for 6 weeks* is often advocated.[15,17] This will allow time for inflammation to subside and infection and sepsis to resolve. Others argue that this approach results in dense adhesions, making definitive repair more difficult.[18] Regardless of timing of repair intraabdominal sepsis and patient condition must be stabilized before repair of complex injuries. *Sepsis control prior to repair has been shown to be a significant protective factor of postoperative complications and anastomotic failure (stenosis and cholangitis). Delay in the timing of repair is especially important in patients undergoing a second attempt at repair. These patients benefit from better operative planning, control of sepsis, improved nutritional status, and decreased inflammation.*

Patients with a delayed presentation will typically be suffering from an ongoing bile leak or biliary obstruction. Patients with a leak require drainage of intraabdominal collections, volume and electrolyte replacement/correction, correction of anemia, and nutritional assessment. Infection and sepsis will require antibiotic treatment. Patients with obstruction may have signs and symptoms of cholangitis. These patients will require antibiotic therapy and drainage

of the biliary tree by percutaneous transhepatic biliary drainage. All patients will require adequate radiologic assessment of the biliary tree. This is most often achieved by PTC. Percutaneous drainage catheters, left in place above the stricture or through the injured, leaking duct, are often useful during reconstruction for identification of the injured/strictured duct.

Successful bile duct–enteric reconstruction is dependent on several factors:

1. Adequate preoperative assessment of biliary anatomy
2. Exposure of proximal, healthy bile ducts with adequate blood supply
3. The repair must include all injured/strictured ducts to ensure adequate drainage of the entire liver, and control of bile leakage
4. Use of a healthy segment of intestine that can be brought to the anastomosis without tension (most often a Roux-en-Y jejunal limb)
5. Creation of a tension-free biliary mucosa-to-bowel mucosa anastomosis

Operative intervention is most often done through a midline incision. Careful dissection of the porta hepatis is required. There may be dense adhesions in this area; therefore the duodenum and hepatic flexure of the colon must be carefully mobilized. Identification of the strictured or injured bile duct can be difficult. Dissection in this area must proceed with caution to avoid injury to the portal vein, proper hepatic artery, or proximal bile duct. Identification of the injured duct can be aided by the presence of a previously placed percutaneous biliary catheter or catheters. If the injured duct(s) is transected, the duct should be dissected circumferentially for a distance of 5 mm. An end-to-side hepaticojejunostomy to the newly created, defunctionalized 50- to 60-cm-long Roux-en-Y jejunal limb is then performed (Fig. 114.6). The distal bile duct, if it remains open, is oversewn with absorbable, running suture. Most often, the distal bile duct has been closed with clips at the time of cholecystectomy. If this is the case the clips are left undisturbed. If the injured duct is strictured or inflamed, the duct proximal to the stricture is cleared anteriorly for 1 to 2 cm. The biliary-enteric anastomosis is accomplished with absorbable monofilament suture in one layer, typically 4-0, 5-0, or 6-0 polydioxanone. If multiple ducts are injured, then more than one anastomosis may be required. Proximal injuries may require the anastomosis to be positioned at the extrahepatic portion of the left hepatic duct after it is lowered by dividing the hepatic plate, the Hepp-Couinaud approach.[20] Continuity of the left and right ducts is required for this approach to work. This technique works well for Bismuth type 2 and 3 strictures. At completion of the anastomosis, a closed suction drain is left in the right upper quadrant to drain any residual collection or small bile leak in the early postoperative period.

The duodenum can also be used for restoration of biliary continuity to the gastrointestinal tract. A duodenal anastomosis is most often done end to side. Full mobilization of the duodenum by a generous Kocher maneuver with release of the right hepatic colonic flexure enables the duodenum to reach the hepatic confluence without tension. "Sump syndrome" is not reported with this approach because the end-to-side anastomosis avoids the

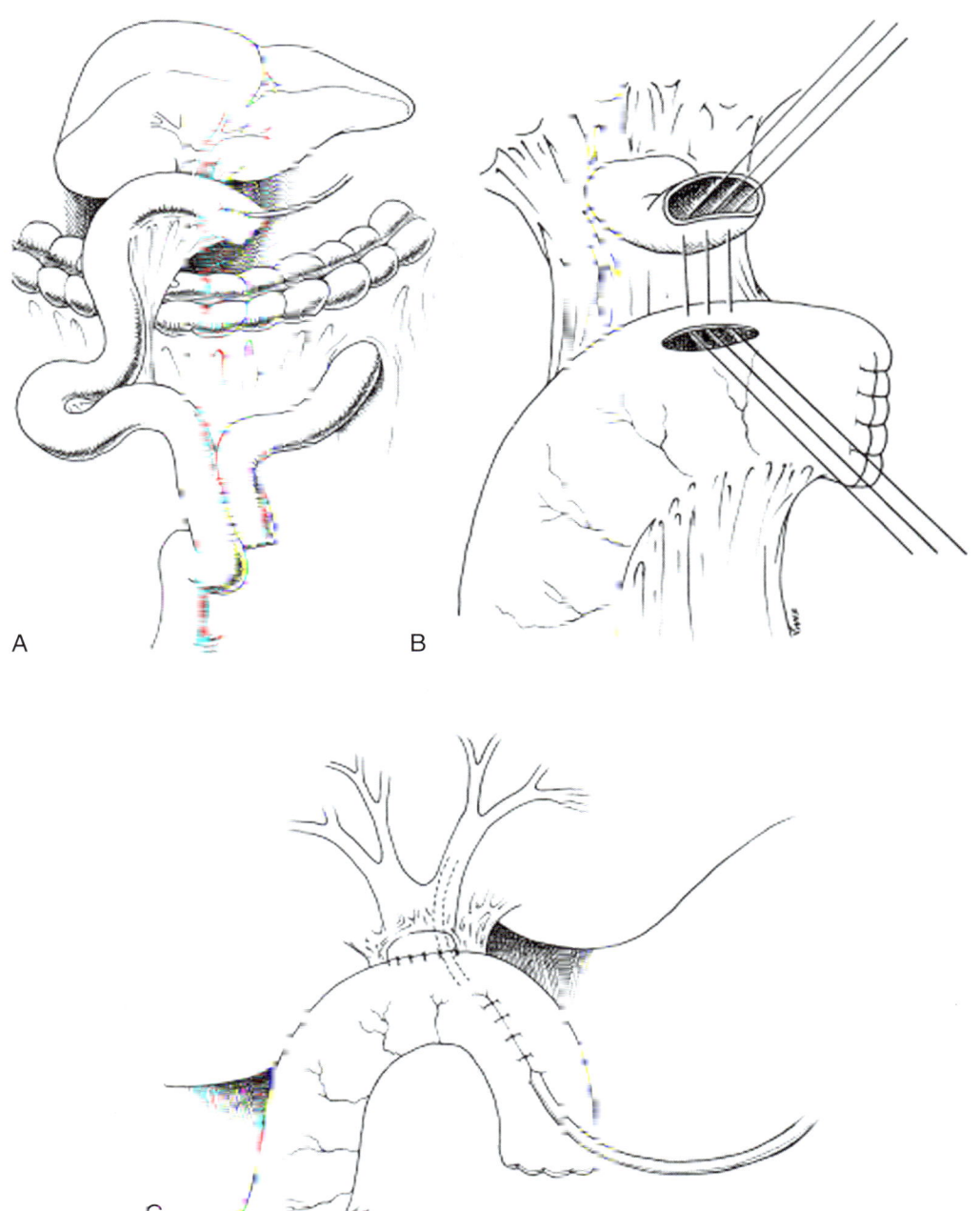

FIGURE 114.6 (A) Completed Roux-en-Y hepaticojejunostomy with 5-French pediatric feeding tube as biliary stent. (B) Close-up view of hepaticojejunostomy using interrupted 5-0 PDS absorbable suture. Note back-wall knots on inside of anastomosis. (C) Biliary stent secured with Witzel tunnel and used for imaging postoperatively. Omission of stent is acceptable. (From McPartland KJ, Pomposelli JJ. Iatrogenic biliary injuries: classification, identification, and management. *Surg Clin N Am*. 2008;88:1329, figure 3, p 1339.)

creation of the blind distal pouch seen in the side-to-side anastomosis. Stricture rates of 35% have been reported for this approach.[21]

If the left and right ducts are not in communication (e.g., in Bismuth type 4 and 5 injuries), sufficient exposure of both the right and left ducts or the injured aberrant right duct is required for adequate repair. Because the extrahepatic length of the right duct is often quite short, exposure of this duct can be difficult. Dissection along the left duct provides a guide to the coronal plane in which the right ducts will be found. Along this plane,

liver tissue can be removed to better expose the right ducts. Exposure can be further improved by dividing the bridge of tissue between liver segments 3 and 4 by fully opening the gallbladder fossa. Partial resection of segments 4b and 5 will open the upper porta hepatic tissue, further exposing the right duct to allow for a standard biliary-enteric anastomosis.

The use of stents across the biliary reconstruction is controversial. Good results have been reported by groups who routinely stent and also by those who do not. Advocates of stenting argue that a transanastomotic stent decompresses the biliary tree and anastomosis, provides a scaffold for scarring of the biliary anastomosis, and maintains patency of the anastomosis.[22] Intraoperatively, transhepatic stents facilitate identification of the bile duct. Postoperatively, stents allow for easy radiologic assessment and intervention at the point of repair. Those arguing against the use of stents note their increased risk of infecting the biliary tree and the increased incidence of hemobilia related to the transhepatic stent. Contaminated bile increases the risk of postoperative infectious complications.[23] Transanastomotic stents may also cause pressure necrosis of the duct. Arteriobiliary and biliary pleural fistula formation have also been reported.[20] Some experts advocate selective use of transanastomotic stents for small ducts (<4 mm), more than one anastomosis, a scarred and/or inflamed duct, and a proximal anastomosis.[24] If the decision is made to use a transanastomotic stent, the percutaneously placed transhepatic stent can be used or a new Silastic stent can be placed. The stent is typically left in place for a minimum of 6 to 8 weeks, occasionally longer. A cholangiogram should be obtained prior to removing the stent. This is best done as an over-the-wire cholangiogram, pulling the transhepatic stent back so that it does not transverse the repair at the time of cholangiography.

In those rare instances in which a biliary anastomosis cannot be achieved, hepatectomy/resection of the affected liver segments may be required so as to remove the hepatic parenchyma without continuity to the biliary tree.

POSTOPERATIVE COMPLICATIONS

Complications for bile duct stricture repair range from 20% to 40% in the literature.[25,26] In one large series, the postoperative complication rate was 42.9% with many complications being minor, including wound infection, cholangitis, anastomotic leak, intraabdominal abscess/biloma, and stent-related complications.[24] Nonsurgical complications typically include cardiopulmonary complications, ileus, and short-term diarrhea. Reported mortality rates ranged from 1.7% to 2.7%.[27,28]

SURGICAL RESULTS

Excellent long-term results of bile duct stricture repair have been reported. Success rates of 80% to 90% for all types of benign strictures have been achieved (Table 114.1). Studies of repair following laparoscopic cholecystectomy have reported similar success rates (Table 114.2). Success is defined by the absence of symptoms, jaundice, and

cholangitis. Postoperative stricture formation can occur in the early or late postoperative period. With long-term follow-up, recurrent stricture rates of 10% to 14% have been reported.[16,29] Eighty percent of recurrent strictures occur within 5 years of repair. Five percent of strictures occur more than 12 years after repair.[7] The factor most associated with recurrent stricture is the initial injury or stricture level. One-third of injuries proximal to the bile duct bifurcation will develop stricture.[30] A small minority of patients may also develop chronic liver disease following repair of a bile duct stricture. Rates of chronic liver disease have been reported between 6% and 22%.[31,32] Risk factors for the development of chronic liver disease include a prolonged interval between injury diagnosis and referral to a tertiary care center, cholangitis, and preexisting liver disease. Patients should be followed closely postoperatively for the development of chronic liver disease and recurrent stricture. Most cases of recurrent stricture can be managed with endoscopic or percutaneous dilation. Rarely, patients with liver failure will require transplantation. In several studies, the long-term quality of life for patients undergoing repair of bile duct injuries approaches the quality of life of the general population.[33]

NONOPERATIVE MANAGEMENT OF BILE DUCT STRICTURES

Endoscopic or percutaneous transhepatic stenting or dilation can be used for simple bile duct injuries or strictures, such as cystic stump leaks, duct of Luschka leaks, small

TABLE 114.1 Selected Results of Surgical Repair of Bile Duct Strictures

Authors, Year	No. of Patients	Success Rate (%)	Follow-up (months)	Reference
Pellegrini et al., 1984	60	78	102	41
Genest et al., 1986	105	82	60	42
Innes et al., 1988	22	95	72	43
Pitt et al., 1989	25	88	57	44
David et al., 1993	35	83	50	36
Chapman et al., 1995	104	76	86	45
McDonald et al., 1995	72	87	<60	46
Tocchi et al., 1996	84	83	108	47
Lillemoe et al., 2000	156	91	58	27
Dominguez-Rosado et al., 2016	614	78.5	40.5	19

TABLE 114.2 Studies of Repair Following Laparoscopic Cholecystectomy

Authors, Year	No. of Patients	Recognized at Laparoscopic Cholecystectomy (%)	Bismuth Types 3–5 (%)	Success Rate (%)	Reference
Stilling et al., 2015	139	42	25	70	48
Walsh et al., 2007	84	43	61	91	31
Bauer et al., 1998	32	31	24	83	37
Lillemoe et al., 1997	52	8	53	92	38
Mirza et al., 1997	27	22	33	81	39
Neason et al., 1996	23	70	26	100	40

partial common bile duct transection, and focal strictures less than 1 cm in length.[34] The success of nonoperative management for more extensive injuries or strictures is less than that of operative repair

For patients who develop a bile duct stricture following repair, nonoperative therapies may provide relief of the stricture. These patients have developed a stricture after biliary-enteric anastomosis. In one report, 58% of 51 patients with biliary stricture were successfully managed by percutaneous dilation.[35] Another report compared 35 patients managed with surgery with 35 patients treated with endoscopic stenting.[36] The surgical patients were managed with a Roux-en-Y hepaticojejunostomy. Endoscopic therapy involved the placement of an endoprosthesis that was exchanged every 3 months. Excellent results were achieved in 83% of the surgical patients with a recurrent stricture rate of 17% at 40 months. After endoscopic stenting, 72% of patients achieved excellent results. Eighteen percent of these patients developed recurrent strictures at a mean of 3 months after stent removal. In cases of stricture following repair, endoscopic stenting should be considered.

SUMMARY

Bile duct injuries and strictures are complex problems requiring a multidisciplinary approach involving surgeons, radiologists, and gastroenterologists. Failure to properly diagnose and/or manage these problems can result in chronic liver disease and/or chronic disabilities. Complete and accurate preoperative imaging is essential to successful outcomes. Appropriate surgical management with careful attention to detail and technique is also imperative. Excellent outcomes can be achieved by following these principles.

REFERENCES

1. Roslyn JJ, Pinns GS, Hughes EF, Saunders-Kirkwood K, Zinner MJ, Cates JA. Open cholecystectomy: a contemporary analysis of 42,474 patients. *Ann Surg*. 1993;218:129.
2. Strasberg SM, Hertl M, Soper NJ. An analysis of the problem of biliary injury during laparoscopic cholecystectomy. *J Am Coll Surg*. 1995;180:101.
3. Fletcher DR, Hobbs MST, Tan P, et al. Complications of cholecystectomy: risks of the laparoscopic approach and protective effects of cholangiography—a population-based study. *Ann Surg*. 1999;229:449.
4. Deziel DJ, Millikan KW, Economou SG, Doolas A, Ko ST, Airan MC. Complications of laparoscopic cholecystectomy: a national survey of 4,292 hospitals and an analysis of 77,604 cases. *Am J Surg*. 1993;165:9.
5. Wherry DC, Marohn MR, Malanoski MP, Hetz SP, Rich NM. An external audit of laparoscopic cholecystectomy in the steady state performed in medical treatment facilities of the Department of Defense. *Ann Surg*. 1996;224:145.
6. Carroll BJ, Birth M, Phillip EH. Common bile duct injuries during laparoscopic cholecystectomy that result in litigation. *Surg Endosc*. 1998;12:310.
7. Pitt HA, Miyamoto T, Parapatis SK, Tompkins RK, Longmire WP Jr. Factors influencing outcome in patients with postoperative biliary strictures. *Am J Surg*. 1982;114:14
8. McAlister VC. Abdominal fluid collection after laparoscopic cholecystectomy. *Br J Surg*. 2000;87:1126.
9. Moran J, Del Grosso E, Wills J, Hagy JA, Baker R. Laparoscopic cholecystectomy: imaging of complications and normal postoperative CT appearance. *Abdom Imaging*. 1994;19:143
10. Weber A, Feussner H, Winkelmann F, Siewert JR, Schmid RM, Prinz C. Long term outcome of endoscopic therapy in patients with bile duct injury after cholecystectomy. *J Gastroenterol Hepatol*. 2009;24:762.
11. Oh HC, Lee SK, Lee TY, et al. Analysis of percutaneous transhepatic cholangioscopy-related complications and the risk factors for those complications. *Endoscopy*. 2007;39:731.
12. Yeh TS, Jan YY, Tseng JH, Hwang TL, Jeng LB, Chen MF. Value of magnetic resonance cholangiopancreatography in demonstrating major bile duct injuries following laparoscopic cholecystectomy. *Br J Surg*. 1999;86:181.
13. Bujanda L, Calvo MM, Cabriada JL, Orive V, Capelastegui A. MRCP in the diagnosis of iatrogenic bile duct injury. *NMR Biomed*. 2003;16:475.
14. Stewart L, Way LW. Bile duct injuries during laparoscopic cholecystectomy. *Arch Surg*. 1995;130:1123.
15. Dageforde LA, Landman MP, Feurer ID, Poulose B, Pinson CW, Moore DE. A cost effectiveness analysis of early vs. late reconstruction of iatrogenic bile duct injuries. *J Am Coll Surg*. 2012;214:6.
16. Lillemoe KD. Current management of bile duct injury. *Br J Surg*. 2008;95:403.
17. Sahajpal AK, Chow SC, Dixon E, Greig PD, Gallinger S, Wei AC. Bile duct injuries associated with laparoscopic cholecystectomy: timing of repair and long term outcomes. *Arch Surg*. 2010;145:757.
18. McPartland KJ, Pomposelli JJ. Iatrogenic biliary injuries: classification, identification, and management. *Surg Clin North Am*. 2008;88:1329.
19. Dominguez-Rosado I, Sanford DE, Liu JL, Hawkins WG, Mercado MA. Timing of surgical repair after bile duct injury impacts postoperative complications but not anastomotic patency. *Ann Surg*. 2016;264:544.
20. Hepp J, Couinaud C. [Approach to and use of the left hepatic duct in reparation of the common bile duct]. *Presse Med*. 1956;64:947. [in French].
21. Rose JB, Bilderback P, Raphaeli T, et al. Use the duodenum, it's right there: a retrospective cohort study comparing biliary reconstruction using either the jejunum or the duodenum. *JAMA Surg*. 2013;148:9.
22. Mercado AM, Chan C, Orozco H, et al. To stent or not to stent bilioenteric anastomosis after iatrogenic injury. *Arch Surg*. 2002;137:60.
23. Hochwald SN, Burke EC, Jarnagin WR, Fong Y, Blumgart LH. Association of preoperative biliary stenting with increased postoperative infectious complications in proximal cholangiocarcinoma. *Arch Surg*. 1999;134:261.
24. Wu V, Linehan DC. Bile duct injuries in the era of laparoscopic cholecystectomies. *Surg Clin North Am*. 2010;90:787.
25. Robinson TN, Stiegmann GV, Durham JD, et al. Management of major bile duct injury associated with laparoscopic cholecystectomy. *Surg Endosc*. 2001;15:1381.
26. Sicklick JK, Camp MS, Lillemoe KD, et al. Surgical management of bile duct injuries sustained during laparoscopic cholecystectomy: perioperative results in 200 patients. *Ann Surg*. 2005;241:786.
27. Lillemoe KD, Melto GB, Cameron JL, et al. Postoperative bile duct strictures: management and outcome in the 1990's. *Ann Surg*. 2000;232:430.
28. Flum DL, Cheadle A, Prela C, Dellinger EP, Chan L. Bile duct injury during cholecystectomy and survival in Medicare beneficiaries. *JAMA*. 2003;290:2168.
29. Murr MM, Gigo JF, Nagorney DM, Harmsen WS, Ilstrup DM, Farnell MB. Long-term results of biliary reconstruction after laparoscopic bile duct injuries. *Arch Surg*. 1999;134:604.
30. Mercado MA, Chan C, Orozco H, et al. Prognostic implication of preserved bile duct confluence after iatrogenic injury. *Hepatogastroenterology*. 2005;52:40.
31. Walsh RM, Henderson JM, Voight DP, Brown N. Long term outcome of biliary reconstruction for bile duct injuries from laparoscopic cholecystectomy. *Surgery*. 2007;142:450.
32. Nordin A, Holme L, Makisalos H, Isoniemi H, Höckerstedt K. Management and outcome of major bile duct injury after laparoscopic cholecystectomy: from therapeutic endoscopy to liver transplantation. *Liver Transpl*. 2002;8:1036.
33. Melton GB, Lillemoe KD, Cameron JL, Sauter PA, Coleman J, Yeo CJ. Major bile duct injuries associated with laparoscopic cholecystectomy: effect on quality of life. *Ann Surg*. 2002;235:888.
34. Winslow ER, Fialkowski EA, Linehan DC, Hawkins WG, Picus DD, Strasberg SM. Sideways: results of repair of biliary injuries using a policy of side to side hepatico-jejunostomy. *Ann Surg*. 2009;94:1119.
35. Misra S, Melton GB, Beschwind JF, Venbrux AC, Cameron JL, Lillemoe KD. Percutaneous management of bile duct strictures and injuries associated with laparoscopic cholecystectomy: a decade of experience. *J Am Coll Surg*. 2004;198:218.
36. Davids PHP, Tanka AKF, Rauws EAJ, et al. Benign biliary strictures. Surgery or endoscopy? *Ann Surg*. 1993;217:237.

37. Bauer TW, Morris JB, Lowenstein A, Wolferth C, Rosato FE, Rosato EE. The consequences of a major bile duct injury during laparoscopic cholecystectomy. *J Gastrointest Surg.* 1998;2:61.

38. Lillemoe KD, Martin SA, Cameron JL, et al. Major bile duct injuries during laparoscopic cholecystectomy: follow-up after combined radiological and surgical management. *Ann Surg.* 1997;225:459, discussion 468.

39. Mirza DF, Narsimhan KL, Ferrazneto BH, Mayer AD, McMaster P, Buckels JAC. Bile duct injury following laparoscopic cholecystectomy: referral pattern and management. *Br J Surg.* 1997;34:786.

40. Nealon WH, Urrutia F. Long term follow up after bilioenteric anastomosis for benign bile duct stricture. *Ann Surg.* 1996;223:639.

41. Pellegrini CA, Thomas JM, Way IW. Recurrent biliary stricture. Pattern of recurrence and outcome of surgical therapy. *Am J Surg.* 1984;147:175.

42. Genest JF, Nanos E, Grundfest-Broniatowski S, Vogt D, Hermann RE. Benign biliary strictures: an analytic review (1970 to 1984). *Surgery.* 1986;90:409.

43. Innes JT, Ferara JJ, Kairey LC. Biliary reconstruction without transanastomotic stent. *Am Surg.* 1988;54:27.

44. Pitt HA, Kaufman HS, Coleman J, White RI, Cameron JL. Benign postoperative biliary strictures: operate or dilate? *Ann Surg.* 1989;210:417.

45. Chapman WC, Halevy A, Blumgart LH, Benjamin IS. Postcholecystectomy bile duct strictures: management and outcome in 130 patients. *Arch Surg.* 1995;130:597.

46. McDonald ML, Farnell MB, Nagorney DM, Ilstrup DM, Kutch JM. Benign biliary strictures: repair and outcome with a contemporary approach. *Surgery.* 1995;118:582.

47. Tocchi A, Costa G, Lepre L, Liotta G, Mazzoni G, Sita A. The long-term outcome of hepaticojejunostomy in the treatment of benign bile duct stricutres. *Ann Surg.* 1996;224:162.

48. Stilling NM, Fristrup C, Wettergren A. Long-term outcome after early repair of iatrogenic bile duct injury. A national Danish multicenter study. *HPB (Oxford).* 2015;17:394.

Biliary Atresia and Biliary Hypoplasia

Stephen P. Dunn

Biliary atresia is a disease characterized by progressive obliterative destruction of intrahepatic and extrahepatic biliary structures.[1] It is the most common cause of direct hyperbilirubinemia in infancy and must be quickly and effectively differentiated from the numerous other causes of jaundice.[2] Early surgical intervention and appropriate postoperative medical management are necessary to prolong native liver function.[3] Ultimately liver transplantation is required in most cases. However, the combination of early surgical intervention and hepatic transplantation has transformed the prognosis in this disease characterized as fatal in the 1950s to one in which the great majority survive with an excellent quality of life.[4,5] *Biliary hypoplasia* is the liver biopsy finding of a reduced number of small bile ducts and is most common as a component of Alagille syndrome.[6] Many of these patients may have serious cardiac anomalies as well as growth deficiency and decreased renal function. Progressive biliary cirrhosis may occur in the syndromic and nonsyndromic varieties, requiring hepatic transplantation.

DIAGNOSIS

Jaundice is common in newborns and is secondary to immature hepatic enzyme activity resulting in indirect hyperbilirubinemia. Jaundice persisting beyond the age of 2 weeks should be evaluated by fractionated bilirubin determination. Diagnostic evaluation should be initiated promptly if the direct bilirubin fraction is greater than 20% of the total.[8] Infection, especially when caused by gram-negative bacteria, may cause jaundice. Serologic testing for congenital infection, testing for α_1-antitrypsin deficiency, sweat testing or genetic studies for cystic fibrosis, tests to exclude galactosemia and tests for defects of oxidative enzyme and amino acid metabolism are included in this evaluation.[1,2] Ultrasound examination of the abdomen should be obtained early in the evaluation.[9] In biliary atresia, the gallbladder is normally shrunken, and no common bile duct is visible. A "triangle cord sign" found on ultrasound has a predictive accuracy of 95%.[10] Hepatobiliary scintigraphy with technetium-99m disofenin (hepatic iminodiacetic acid [HIDA]) with 3 to 5 days of preimaging phenobarbital administration demonstrates no intestinal excretion initially or at 24 hours.[11] Percutaneous liver biopsy is helpful and can yield approximately 90% accuracy in experienced hands.[12] Typical histology demonstrates intracanalicular cholestasis with proliferation of bile ducts. Findings compatible with neonatal hepatitis, periportal fibrosis, and giant cell formation also may be present. Biopsy cannot differentiate biliary atresia from other diseases including α_1-antitrypsin deficiency or parenteral nutrition associated liver disease. The most common findings in biliary atresia published in the recent Biliary Atresia Research Consortium experience were bile duct proliferation, portal fibrosis, and absence of sinusoidal fibrosis.[13]

In the absence of a definitive diagnosis excluding biliary atresia, operative cholangiography must be performed and, if possible, before the age of 60 days. The patient must be prepared for definitive hepatoportoenterostomy at the time of operative cholangiography.

Biliary hypoplasia is diagnosed by the findings on liver biopsy and operative cholangiography. A diminished number of interlobular bile ducts and the cholangiography findings of small intrahepatic and extrahepatic biliary structures with the presence of bile in the gallbladder at exploration are typical. The syndromic form of this disease described by Alagille includes several other important findings. These include characteristic facies, butterfly-like vertebral arch defects, the ophthalmologic finding of posterior embryotoxon, and cardiac anomalies, of which the most common is branch pulmonary artery stenosis. Renal tubular abnormalities may also be present on ultrasound. Recent work has identified the abnormal gene *JAG*.[6] Testing for this gene is available.

ETIOLOGY

The cause of biliary atresia remains enigmatic. Although approximately 15% of cases occur in the context of other associated anomalies suggesting a genetic basis, most occur randomly or sporadically, which is consistent with a toxic or infectious cause.[14,15] Animal models of biliary injury have been developed with reovirus and rotavirus as the infectious agent.[1,14] These agents have not been definitively implicated in biliary atresia in humans. It is suggested that exposure of antigen on biliary epithelium secondary to the consequences of infection leads to an autoimmune-type process. This hypothesis is speculative but is supported by the investigations of the inflammatory process found in biliary atresia.[14] Of particular interest in the sporadic cases is the not-uncommon history that an affected newborn had pigmented stools initially. This history suggests the progressive nature of the biliary injury and is one of the intriguing aspects of this disease.

The most common presentation of the syndromic variety of biliary atresia is in association with splenic and vascular malformations. This grouping of biliary atresia, biliary atresia splenic malformation syndrome, is frequently abbreviated BASM syndrome. In these cases, the associated anomalies may include polysplenia; malrotation; situs inversus; interrupted inferior vena cava with azygous continuation; and preduodenal portal vein, hepatic arterial anomalies and cardiac anomalies, including heterotaxia or more severe lesions.[14,16,17]

The genetic abnormality underlying Alagille syndrome has been discovered during the past decade. Studies of *JAG1* expression patterns have shown that the associated

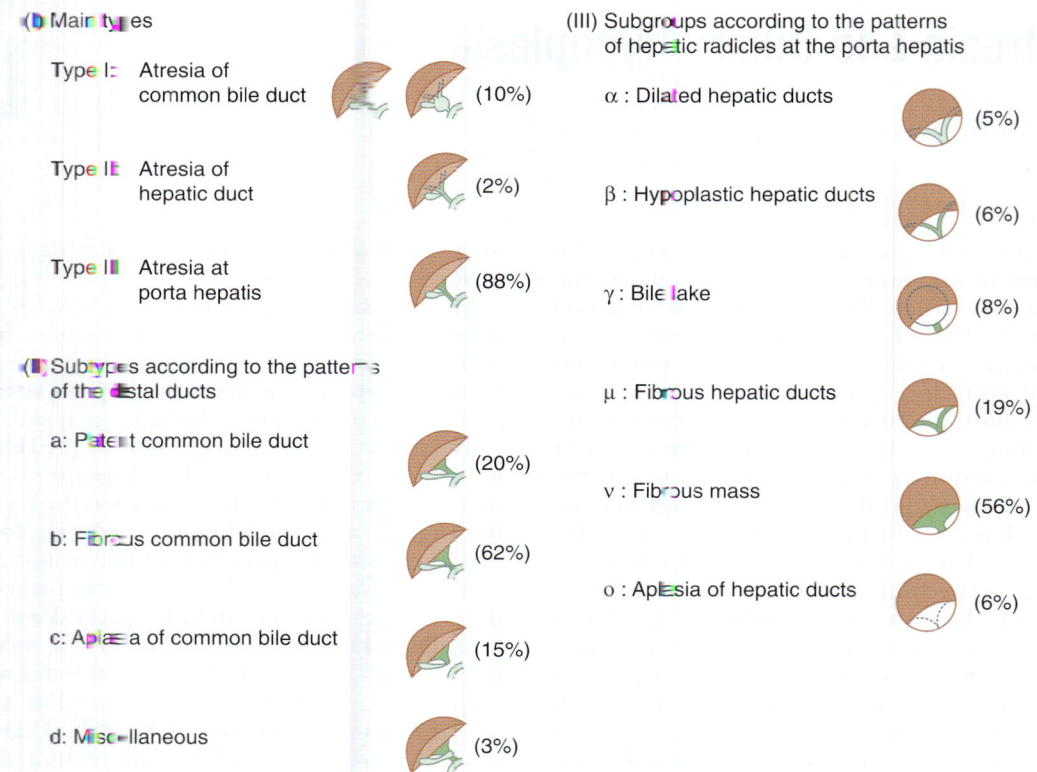

(I) Main types

Type I: Atresia of common bile duct (10%)

Type II: Atresia of hepatic duct (2%)

Type III: Atresia at porta hepatis (88%)

(II) Subtypes according to the patterns of the distal ducts

a: Patent common bile duct (20%)

b: Fibrous common bile duct (62%)

c: Aplasia of common bile duct (15%)

d: Miscellaneous (3%)

(III) Subgroups according to the patterns of hepatic radicles at the porta hepatis

α : Dilated hepatic ducts (5%)

β : Hypoplastic hepatic ducts (6%)

γ : Bile lake (8%)

μ : Fibrous hepatic ducts (19%)

ν : Fibrous mass (56%)

o : Aplasia of hepatic ducts (6%)

FIGURE 115-1 Morphologic classification of biliary atresia based on macroscopic and cholangiographic findings. (From Ohi R, Nio M. The jaundiced infant: biliary atresia and other obstructions. In: O'Neill JA, Rowe MI, Grosfeld JA, et al, eds. *Pediatric Surgery*. 5th ed. St. Louis: Mosby; 1998:1466.)

abnormalities of Alagille syndrome are not coincidental but related to abnormalities of this gene, which codes for a ligand of NOTCH 1.

CLASSIFICATION

Ohi et al.[17] created an effective classification scheme for the biliary abnormalities found in biliary atresia (Fig. 115.1). This scheme allows each case to be designated by the operative findings. One of the important findings of the Childhood Liver Disease Research and Education Network study of 244 infants undergoing the Kasai procedure is that Ohi types II and III including subtypes b, c, and d have a worse prognosis than type I and subtype a. In addition, the BASM category had a worse prognosis than type I.[18] This is important for outcome comparison between centers as well as for individual patient prognosis.

The most common findings at operation are atresia at the porta hepatis (type III) with a fibrous common bile duct (subtype b) and a fibrous mass at the hepatic radicles (subgroup ν). When biliary atresia was first classified, terms such as *correctable* and *noncorrectable* were used. These terms are misleading, as Kasai and Suzuki described their surgical procedure for the noncorrectable form of the disease.[19] Most patients have the uncorrectable form of the disease and are still excellent candidates for surgical therapy with a high expectation of benefit if surgery is performed before 60 to 75 days of age.[17,18] Nevertheless, as many as 10% of all patients never achieve bile drainage because

of damage incurred to the intrahepatic biliary tree, and these cases are correctly identified as uncorrectable. At present, we have no way to identify these cases for whom hepatoportoenterostomy will have no merit. However, the biopsy finding of increased periportal fibrosis is highly correlated with poor response to hepatoportoenterostomy.[20]

The work of Bezerra et al. has identified mechanistic explanations for the progression of the atretic process. This appears to be immune in nature and highly correlated with the age of onset of the inflammatory process. Pathologic findings document both from histology and heat maps of genetic markers a progression from inflammation to fibrosis.[14] This progression suggests possibilities for intervention based on the inflammatory process at the time of the Kasai. However, current data are not yet available that would confirm the benefit of this approach.

OPERATIVE MANAGEMENT

BILIARY ATRESIA

The operation for biliary atresia begins as a diagnostic procedure with a small incision to inspect the gallbladder and biliary tree. In the presence of a small, shrunken, or scarred gallbladder that may contain a small amount of clear fluid, further investigation is not needed. The incision is lengthened to facilitate portal dissection. If the gallbladder is of reasonable caliber, cholangiography is performed through the dome of the gallbladder. Flow into the duodenum may be encountered necessitating external pressure to the distal common bile duct to facilitate flow into the proximal ductal structures. If these structures cannot be seen, dissection of the porta is required. Presence of a fibrous extrahepatic biliary tree and, in some cases, its disruption or absence is consistent with biliary atresia. Portal dissection is facilitated by division of the fibrous remnant of the extrahepatic biliary tree near the duodenum. The fibrous remnant is then lifted from the portal vein and separated from the hepatic artery branches. Care must be taken not to injure these vessels. The target of the dissection is the fibrous cone of tissue just anterior to the bifurcation of the right and left branches of the portal vein. Removal of the fibrous remnant between the point of entry of the portal vein branches into the hepatic parenchyma is the goal and is the highest safe point for dissection. Gentle traction on the portal vein branches has been advocated to facilitate this dissection. Small vessels from the main porta vein to the biliary plate need to be carefully ligated with fine suture to achieve an adequate dissection (Fig. 115-5).

Reconstruction of bile drainage is through a hepaticojejunostomy. A Roux-en-Y limb of jejunum is formed by dividing the proximal jejunum approximately 10 cm from the ligament of Treitz. The distal end is passed through the transverse mesocolon to the area of the porta hepatis. The anastomosis of the proximal jejunum is to the side of the distal jejunum approximately 30 cm from the initial point of jejunal division. The portal reconstruction is performed using an anastomosis of the antimesenteric side of the Roux limb of the jejunum close to the blind end to the tissue surrounding the biliary plate. This is usually performed with fine absorbable sutures. Especially on the inside row a single layer of suture creates the inside back wall of the anastomosis. A running technique for this suture is a useful alternative and avoids the placement of intraluminal knots. The anastomosis should incorporate the entire biliary plate resulting in an area of the biliary plate covered by the Roux that is roughly the shape of an hourglass that is lying on its side.

At the completion of the hepaticojejunostomy, the retrocolic tunnel and the mesenteric defects are repaired. A single, closed-suction drain is placed posterior to the anastomosis, exiting through the side of the infant. A needle biopsy of the liver is always obtained at the time of operation to document the degree of hepatic inflammation and fibrosis. Analysis of this issue may become very helpful in determining the postoperative medical management. Biliary diversion or formation of one-way valves in the Roux limb has not measurably altered the progression of this disease to biliary cirrhosis, although the incidence of cholangitis may be decreased. The presence of BASM may complicate the operative procedure. Placement of the initial incision should be guided by ultrasound location of the porta or palpation of the liver under general anesthesia. Malrotation may also be found associated with the syndrome and may make retrocolic placement of the Roux limb impossible. Abnormalities of hepatic arterial supply and the presence of a preduodenal portal vein should be anticipated and recognized during portal dissection. Placement of the hepaticojejunostomy is guided by identification of the portal vein bifurcation.

Report of a laparoscopic approach to hepatoportoenterostomy are found in the literature with initial favorable results.[21] However, other authors have not found this approach to be of subsequent benefit in reducing intraoperative blood loss or dissection time at liver transplantation.[22] It is also noted that there is a general moratorium on this approach in Japan.[18] Technical accuracy is paramount and large outcome studies of a laparoscopic approach are not available.[23]

Repeat Kasai has been attempted in the setting of once established bile flow with acute cessation. This clinical situation is usually precipitated by cholangitis with subsequent damage to bile ducts and decreased bile flow due to that damage and the effect of infection on bile production. Most surgeons do not advocate second or even more than two attempts to reopen the hepatoportoenterostomy. That procedure is very challenging and may lead to vascular injury to the portal vein or hepatic artery. Subsequently, the effect of repeated Kasai procedures is deleterious for liver transplantation.[24]

BILIARY HYPOPLASIA

Biliary hypoplasia can be indistinguishable from biliary atresia leading to the need for operative cholangiography. That procedure is undertaken just as it would be for an infant who may have biliary atresia. The gallbladder is visualized through a small incision. This may be facilitated by intraoperative ultrasound localization. The gallbladder is usually normal or small in caliber and often contains bile, although it may be dilute. Once a catheter is secured in the cone of the gallbladder, injection of the contrast is performed with fluoroscopic visualization of the contrast injection. Contrast is usually seen flowing into the duodenum, but the extrahepatic biliary structures and the intrahepatic ducts are quite small. A liver biopsy is obtained for permanent section. No further operative treatment is performed, and the incision is closed without a drain after suture closure of the gallbladder with absorbable sutures.

POSTOPERATIVE MANAGEMENT

BILIARY ATRESIA

Bile flow is achieved in most infants who receive surgery before 60 days of life. Bile flow may be slow at first and not reach normal proportions for several months. A medical regimen of corticosteroids, ursodeoxycholic acid and prophylactic antibiotics to prevent cholangitis appears to enhance and sustain bile flow. However, no standard regimen to improve outcomes is recognized. Wide variation is found in choice and length of treatment with antibiotics, steroids, and ursodeoxycholic acid.[25] Enhanced bile flow is not associated with long-term avoidance of liver transplantation. The recently completed prospective randomized trial of steroids post hepatoportoentereostomy (the START trial) did not show improvement in bile flow rate.[18]

An earlier study did show improvement in clearance of jaundice but not in avoidance of liver transplantation.[26] Recurrence of jaundice implies cholangitis but other causes should be investigated. Liver biopsy may be helpful in diagnosis, although presumptive treatment is standard

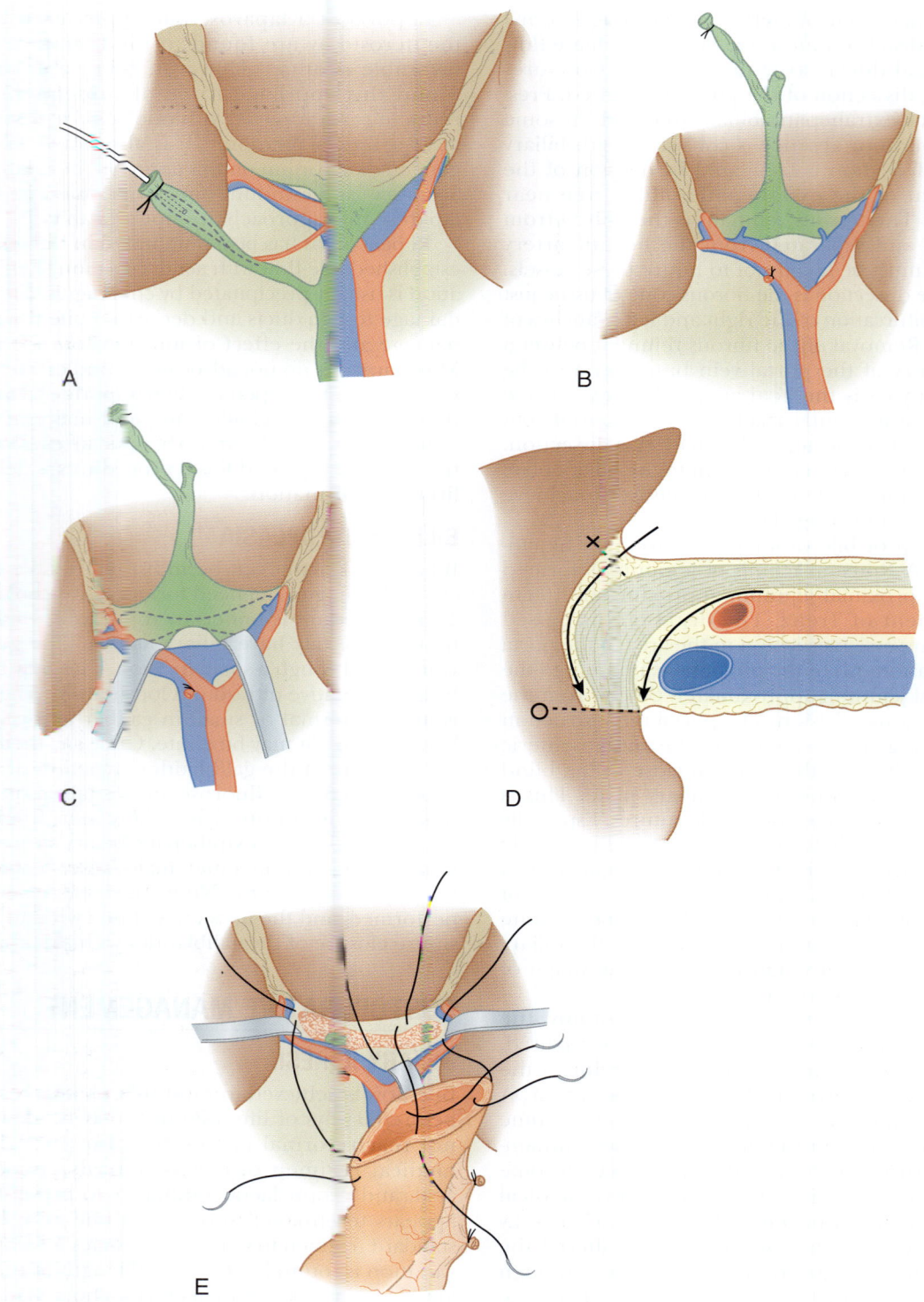

FIGURE 115.2 Sequential depiction of the dissection and reconstruction of the porta hepatis during operation for hepatoportoenterostomy: (A) Usual findings at exploration with fibrosis of the extrahepatic biliary tree. (B) Dissection of the fibrous duct from the portal vein and hepatic artery. (C and D) Level of transection of the fibrous remnant of the bile duct. (E) Reconstruction of the porta in progress. (From Ohi R, Nio M. The jaundiced infant: biliary atresia and other obstructions. In: O'Neill JA, Rowe MI, Grosfeld JA, et al, eds. *Pediatric Surgery*. 5th ed. St Louis: Mosby; 1998:1470.)

practice. Systemic antibiotics and increased corticosteroids may result in improved bile flow; at one time, repeat operation was advocated for infants who had drained bile initially and subsequently became jaundiced. This treatment is no longer advocated because it has not had a high rate of success. Infants whose jaundice does not clear or those with recurrent jaundice should be referred for early evaluation for liver transplantation. The average length of survival in those infants whose total bilirubin did not decrease below 5 mg/dL after hepatoportoenterostomy was 18 months.[27] Prevention of malnutrition secondary to fat and fat-soluble vitamin malabsorption avoids unnecessary liver dysfunction, poor growth, bone disease, and coagulopathy. Nutritional requirements for all biliary atresia patients are greater than normal and especially so for those who remain jaundiced. Aggressive support of nutritional needs improves outcomes.

BILIARY HYPOPLASIA

The postoperative course of biliary hypoplasia is one of rapid recovery and the need to identify if the patient has the syndromatic or nonsyndromatic condition. Genetic consultation will identify children with Alagille syndrome. In the syndromatic condition, the search for associated anomalies includes consultation with ophthalmology, cardiology, nephrology, and gastroenterology. The child will require long-term follow-up to assess their progression of liver disease. Some require liver transplantation for progressive cholestatic liver disease.

OUTCOMES

BILIARY ATRESIA

The perioperative mortality rate is approximately 1.5% after hepatoportoenterostomy.[19] Most infants clear their jaundice if operated on before age 60 days. A recent systematic review of native liver survival without transplantation at 10 years ranged between 24% and 52.8%.[5] Of importance, survival with native liver was highest in centers with larger volumes of hepatoportoenterostomy cases (>5 cases per year).[25] Clearance of jaundice (defined as total bilirubin less than 2 mg/dL at 3 months after surgery) is favorable but progression of liver disease to frank cirrhosis may occur over a number of years. Recurrent bouts of cholangitis accelerate the progression of liver disease. Almost one-third of patients have only modest or no improvement in the jaundice after hepatoportoenterostomy. Liver disease progression in these infants is rapid. Liver transplantation is the next line of therapy for the jaundiced child and for those with the sequelae of progressive liver disease.[28]

LIVER TRANSPLANTATION

Biliary atresia is the most common indication for liver transplantation in children.[5] Most children with biliary atresia require transplantation at some time in their lives because of the progression of liver disease. Transplantation may be required in infancy because of the inability to obtain bile drainage with hepatoportoenterostomy or at the time of initial diagnosis if end-stage liver disease is present. Indications for transplantation are persistent

cholangitis, gastrointestinal bleeding from esophageal varices, uncontrolled ascites, and declining synthetic function. Most challenging for the child facing liver transplantation is the inadequacy of the donor organ pool. Segmental transplantation from cadaveric or live donors can meet this need but is neither universally practiced nor possible without the cooperation of adult transplant surgeons. Sadly, the majority of adult donor organs are not split (i.e., separated) into two useable donor grafts suitable for both a child and an adult. Deaths while on the waiting list may be as high as 10% in the youngest age group. Liver transplantation, whether prior to or after hepatoportoenterostomy, is straightforward, although technically challenging. Biliary drainage is by choledochojejunostomy to a Roux-en-Y limb of jejunum. Hepatic artery and portal vein anastomoses are facilitated by operating loupes or microscope. Patient and graft survival rates are excellent; more than 90% of children are alive at 1 year, and of those, most are alive at 10 years.[29]

REFERENCES

1. Kobayashi H, Stringer MD. Biliary atresia. *Semin Neonatol.* 2003;8:383.
2. Sokol RJ. Clinical problems with developmental anomalies of the biliary tract. *Semin Gastrointest Dis.* 2003;14:156.
3. Chin R. Surgery for biliary atresia. *Liver.* 2001;21:175.
4. Chin JB, deVille DE, de Goyet J, et al. Sequential treatment of biliary atresia with Kasai portoenterotomy and liver transplantation: a review. *Hepatology.* 1994;20:41.
5. Ryckman FC, Alonso MH, Bucuvalas JC, Balistreri WF. Biliary atresia: surgical management and treatment options as they relate to outcome. *Liver Transpl Surg.* 1998;4(5 suppl 1):S24.
6. Hadchouel M. Alagille syndrome. *Indian J Pediatr.* 2002;69:815.
7. Alagille D, Estrada A, Hadchouel M, Gautier M, Odièvre M, Dommergues JP. Syndromatic paucity of interlobal bile ducts (Alagille syndrome or arteriohepatic hypoplasia): review of 80 cases. *J Pediatr.* 1987;110:195.
8. Balistreri WF. Neonatal cholestasis. *J Pediatr.* 1985;106:171.
9. Cubernick JA, Rosenberg HK, Ilaslan H, Kessler A. US approach to jaundice in infants and children. *Radiographics.* 2000;20:173.
10. Park WH, Choi SO, Lee HJ. Technical innovation for noninvasive and early diagnosis of biliary atresia: the ultrasonographic "triangular cord" sign. *J Hepatobiliary Pancreat Surg.* 2001;8:337.
11. Chin R, Klingensmith WC III, Lilly JR. Diagnosis of hepatobiliary disease in infants and children with Tc-99m-diethyl-IDA imaging. *Clin Nucl Med.* 1981;6:297.
12. McKiernan PJ. Neonatal cholestasis. *Semin Neonatal.* 2002;7:153-165.
13. Russo P, Magee JC, Boitnott J, et al. Design and validation of the biliary atresia research consortium histologic assessment for cholestasis in infancy. *Clin Gastroenterol Hepatol.* 2011;9:357-362.
14. Bessho K, Bezerra J. Biliary atresia: will blocking inflammation tame the disease? *Annu Rev Med.* 2011;62:171-185.
15. Sokol RJ, Mack C. Etiopathogenesis of biliary atresia. *Semin Liver Dis.* 2001;21:517.
16. Chandra RS. Biliary atresia and other structural anomalies in congenital polysplenia syndrome. *J Pediatr.* 1974;85:649.
17. Oh R, Nio M. The jaundiced infant: biliary atresia and other obstructions. In: O'Neill JA, Rowe MI, Grosfeld JL, et al., eds. *Pediatric Surgery.* 5th ed. St. Louis: Mosby; 1998:1465.
18. Superina R, Magee J, Brandt M, et al. The anatomic pattern of biliary atresia at time of Kasai hepatoportoenterostomy and early postoperative clearance of jaundice are significant predictors of transplant-free survival. *Ann Surg.* 2011;254:577-585.
19. Kasai M, Suzuki S. A new operation for "non-correctable" biliary atresia: hepatic portoenterostomy. *Shujyutsu.* 1959;13:733.
20. Pape L, Olsson K, Peterson C, von Wasilewski R, Melter M. Prognostic value of computerized quantification of liver fibrosis in children with biliary atresia. *Liver Transpl.* 2009;15:876.
21. Liu S, Li L, Cheng W, et al. Laparoscopic hepatojejunostomy for biliary atresia. *J Laparoendosc Adv Surg Tech A.* 2009;19(suppl):S31-S35.

22. Oetzmann von Sochaczewski C, Peterson C, Ure BM, et al. Laparoscopic versus conventional Kasai portoenterostomy doesn't facilitate subsequent liver transplantation in infants with biliary atresia. *J Lap Adv Surg*. 2012;22:408-411.

23. Wong KK, Chung PH, Chan KL, Fan ST, Tam PK. Should open Kasai portoenterostomy be performed for biliary atresia in the era of laparoscopy? *Pediatr Surg Int*. 2008;24:931.

24. Ibrasku T, Hara Y, Sanada Y, et al. Effect of repeat Kasai hepatic portoenterostomy on pediatric live-donor liver graft for biliary atresia. *Exp Clin Transpl*. 2013;3:259-263.

25. Jimenez-Rivera C, Jolin-Dahel K, Fortinsky K, Benchimol EI, Gozdyra P. International incidence and outcomes of biliary atresia. *J Pediatr Gastroenterol Nutr*. 2013;56:344-354.

26. Davenport M, Stringer MD, Tizzard SA, McClean P, Mieli-Vergani G, Hadzic N. Randomized, double-blind, placebo-controlled trial of corticosteroids after Kasai portoenterostomy for biliary atresia. *Hepatology*. 2007;46:1821.

27. Kasai M, Mochizuki I, Ohkohchi N, Chiba T, Ohi R. Surgical limitation for biliary atresia: indication for liver transplantation. *J Pediatr Surg*. 1989;24:851.

28. Ohi R. Biliary atresia: a surgical perspective. *Clin Liver Dis*. 2000;4:779.

29. Colombani P, Dunn S, Harmon W, Magee JC, McDiarmid SV. Sprayf TL. SRTR report on the state of transplantation. Pediatric transplantation. *Am J Transpl*. 2003;3(suppl 4):53.

Cystic Disorders of the Bile Ducts

Hisami Ando | Tadahiro Takada

CLASSIFICATION OF CYSTIC DISORDERS OF THE BILE DUCTS

In 1959 Alonso-Lej[1] first classified extrahepatic bile duct cystic dilatation into the following three types: type I is congenital cystic dilatation of the common bile duct in which the intrahepatic tree is usually normal; type II is congenital diverticulum of the common bile duct and is extremely rare; type III is choledochocele—cystic dilatation of the distal segment of the common bile duct protruding into the duodenal lumen. However, Alonso-Lej's classification did not include intrahepatic bile duct dilatation or pancreaticobiliary maljunction, the abnormal union between the pancreatic and biliary ducts. Todani et al.[2,3] refined the classification of bile duct cystic disorders into five types and included the concept of pancreaticobiliary maljunction (Fig. 116.1). Type IV-A is congenital biliary dilatation associated with intrahepatic duct dilatation. Type V is multiple intrahepatic bile-duct dilatations. Todani type I (except for type Ib) and type IV-A are both accompanied by pancreaticobiliary maljunction in almost all cases, whereas this condition rarely arises in types Ib, II, III, IV-B, or V.[4] The frequencies of the types of bile duct cystic disorders are as follows: type I, 73.5%; type II, 0.4%; type III, 1.1%; type IV-A, 24%; and type V, 1.1% of patients.[5]

CONGENITAL BILIARY DILATATION (TYPES Ia, Ic, AND IV-A)

GENERAL DESCRIPTION

Term

Congenital biliary dilatation used to be known as "congenital choledochal cyst" or "choledochal cyst" in Western countries. The dilated lesion of biliary dilatation used to be called a "cyst." However, because there are patients who do not present cystic dilatation, it has been referred to as the "dilated part of the bile duct" and the Japanese Study Group on Pancreaticobiliary Maljunction has recommended the term "congenital biliary dilatation" (Fig. 116.2).[4,6] Congenital biliary dilatation is subdivided into cystic, cylindrical, or fusiform dilatation. However, there is no difference in symptoms, signs, complications, or surgical care among the types.

History

Congenital biliary dilatation is characterized by localized dilatation of the choledochus and is associated with pancreaticobiliary maljunction. The first description of a fusiform dilatation of the common bile duct was published by Vater in 1723, and the first authentic case of congenital biliary dilatation was reported by Douglas[7] in

1852. On the other hand, pancreaticobiliary maljunction, which was first noted by Kozumi and Kodama[8] in an autopsy case with congenital biliary dilatation in 1916, is a congenital anomaly defined as an abnormal union of the pancreatic and biliary ducts. This initial observation did not attract attention for many years, but the concept has been accepted widely since Babbitt[9] reported the anomaly in 1969.

Incidence

Congenital biliary dilatation has generally been considered a rarity, but recently the number of cases reported in the literature has steadily increased. The incidence of congenital biliary dilatation in Western countries is 1 in 100,000 to 190,000 live births,[10,11] whereas it is not uncommon in Asia and a marked increase has been seen in the Japanese population with an incidence of 1 in 1000.[12] The preponderance of female patients is well known, with the female-to-male ratio being 3 or 4 to 1.[12,13] Congenital biliary dilatation may be found at any age, but more than two-thirds of cases are diagnosed in children younger than 10 years of age, and some cases are diagnosed prenatally by ultrasound examinations as early as the 15th week of gestation.[14]

Embryology

Many theories have been proposed to explain the origin of bile duct dilatation and can be divided into two groups: (1) that due to an obstructive factor localized at the junction of the choledochus with the duodenum as an abnormal angularity or congenital stenosis of the terminal common bile duct and (2) that due to a weakness originating in the common bile duct proper. In 1936 Yotuyanagi[15] suggested that inequality in the proliferation of epithelial cells of the upper portion and the lower portion of the common bile duct in the primitive stage might produce an abnormally dilated structure following recanalization. However, the mechanism of bile duct dilatation remains uncertain.

On the other hand, pancreaticobiliary maljunction is thought to develop as a misarrangement of the embryonic connections in the pancreaticobiliary ductal system, with the terminal bile duct joined to the second branch of the ventral pancreas.[16] During the development of the bile duct, abnormal fusion may occur between the bile duct and branches of the right ventral pancreatic duct. The site in the bile duct where a branch of the pancreatic duct joins it is likely to develop atresia due to a disturbance of the recanalization process.[17] However, the embryogenesis of pancreaticobiliary maljunction remains obscure because observation of the fetal development of this anomaly is extremely difficult, and there is also a lack of suitable animal models.

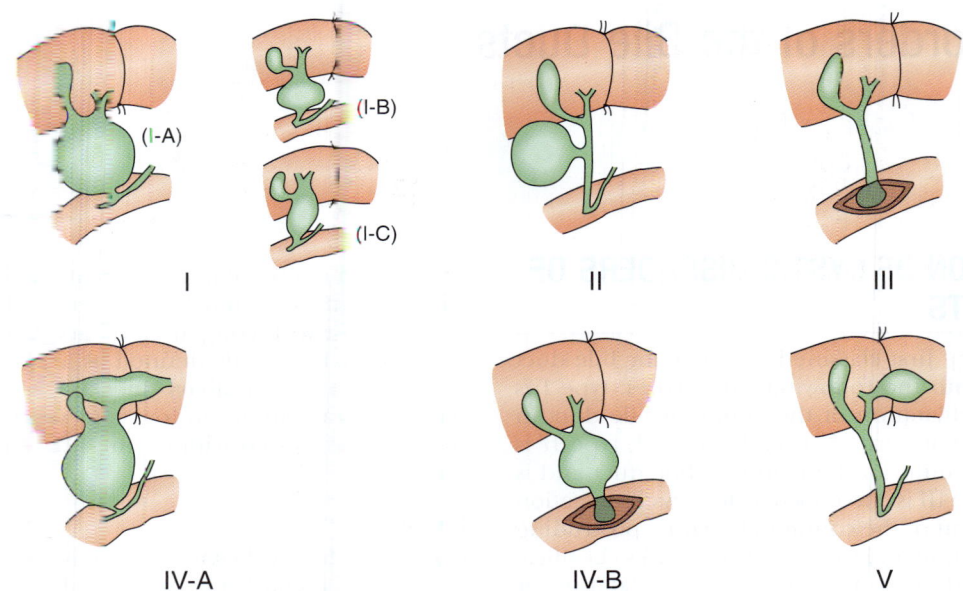

FIGURE 116.1 Classification of cystic disorders of the bile ducts. (From Todani T. Congenital choledochal dilatation: classification, clinical features, and long-term results. *J Hepatobiliary Pancreat Surg.* 1997;4:276–282.)

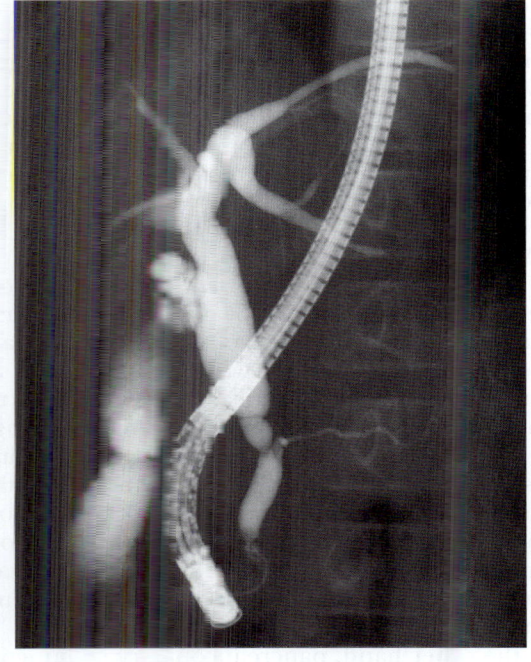

FIGURE 116.2 Endoscopic retrograde cholangiopancreatography shows congenital biliary dilatation without cystic dilatation of the extrahepatic bile duct.

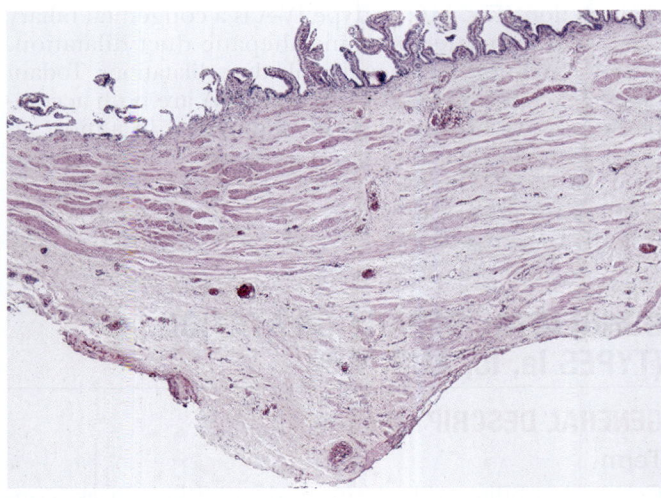

FIGURE 116.3 Hematoxylin and eosin–stained section shows numerous smooth muscle bundles in the lower part of the common bile duct wall.

Pathophysiology

The dilated bile duct wall is usually 1 to 2 mm thick and composed mainly of a fibromuscular layer. This layer is made up of dense connective tissue that is fibrocollagenous and sometimes contains smooth muscles and elastic elements (Fig. 116.3). The epithelium is sometimes lacking, but columnar epithelium is identified by gently manipulating the bile duct during surgery. On rare occasion,

ectopic pancreatic tissue may be found in the bile duct wall.[18]

The pancreaticobiliary junction is located outside the duodenal wall, where the normal sphincter does not work (Fig. 116.4). This permits reflux of pancreatic juice into the biliary tract and destruction of the bile duct wall. Bile containing regurgitated pancreatic juice has been reported to produce substances hazardous to the biliary epithelium, including activated pancreatic enzymes, lysolecithin, secondary or unconjugated bile acids, and a mutagen.[19] These agents may injure the epithelium of the biliary tract and induce metaplasia and may be a key factor in the pathogenesis of malignant changes in congenital biliary dilatation.[20]

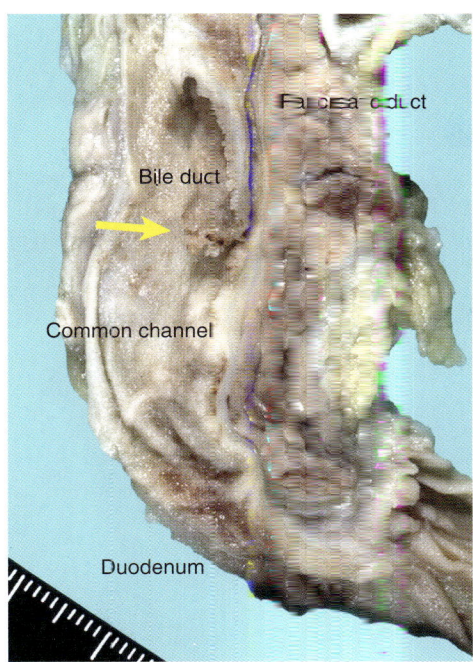

FIGURE 116.4 Gross dissection shows the long common channel and pancreaticobiliary junction complicated with biliary cancer (arrow).

SYMPTOMS AND SIGNS

Patients with congenital biliary dilatation, including type IV-A, most often present with nonspecific symptoms, and half of the patients appear asymptomatic, particularly adults. In children, the major clinical symptoms are recurrent abdominal pain (82%) that may occur repeatedly for several days, nausea and vomiting (36%), mild jaundice (44%), an abdominal mass (29%) and fever (29%). The classical triad of abdominal pain, jaundice, and abdominal mass was originally described as one of the key features of congenital biliary dilatation, but now it is only present in fewer than 20% of patients.[2] The simultaneous occurrence of symptoms may be explained by the disturbance in bile and pancreatic secretory flow caused by a protein plug, which resolves spontaneously, in the common channel.[22]

DIAGNOSIS AND DEFINITION

Patients with congenital biliary dilatation sometimes temporarily show abnormal values for serum bilirubin levels, serum amylase, and serum hepatic transaminases. However, abnormalities in blood examination tests are transient, and they are only evident during the symptomatic phase.[4] In addition, age must be considered when evaluating the biliary amylase levels, because the serum amylase levels are low in neonates and infants.[3]

For a diagnosis of congenital biliary dilatation, both abnormal dilatation of the bile duct and pancreaticobiliary maljunction must be evidenced by radiographic or anatomic abnormalities.[6] Characteristic images include localized bile duct dilatation involving the common bile duct, stenosis at the lower portion of the dilated bile duct, abnormal junction of the pancreatic and bile duct away

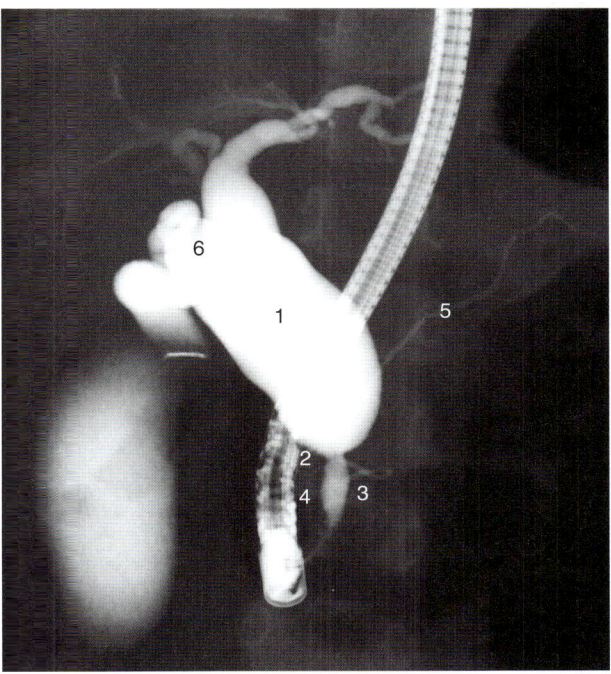

FIGURE 116.5 Endoscopic retrograde cholangiopancreatography provides characteristic images of congenital biliary dilatation: (1) localized bile duct dilatation involving the common bile duct, (2) stenosis at the lower portion of the dilated bile duct, (3) abnormal junction of the pancreatic and bile ducts away from the papilla, (4) dilated common channel, (5) normal dorsal pancreatic duct, and (6) dilated cystic duct.

from the papilla, dilated common channel, normal dorsal pancreatic duct, dilated cystic duct, and stenoses at the hepatic ducts (Fig. 116.5).[24] On the other hand, diagnostic criteria for pancreaticobiliary maljunction by radiography are that (1) the pancreatic duct and the bile duct connect with an obviously long common channel (usually ≥15 mm) or (2) the ducts unite in an apparently anomalous form.[24,25]

The noninvasiveness and accuracy of ultrasonography support its use as the initial investigative procedure. Because the standard diameter of the bile duct on ultrasonography significantly correlates with age, diagnosis of bile duct dilatation should be considered based on the upper limit of the bile duct diameter for each patient.[26,27] Biliary sludge or stones within the dilated bile duct also can be identified in some cases. Focal thickening of the bile duct wall raises the suspicion of carcinoma.

Endoscopic retrograde cholangiopancreatography (ERCP) gives an excellent visualization of the bile ducts, duct anatomy, and pancreaticobiliary maljunction (see Figs. 116.2 and 116.5).[28] This examination is important to avoid intraoperative injury of the pancreatic duct and to recognize protein plugs within the common channel. However, ERCP is invasive and associated with a small risk of complications, such as pancreatitis, and must be performed under general anesthesia in children.

Magnetic resonance cholangiopancreatography (MRCP) can play an important role as a noninvasive examination without radiation exposure and should be considered a

FIGURE 116.6 (A) Magnetic resonance cholangiopancreatography provides images of congenital biliary dilatation characterized by dilated bile ducts and pancreaticobiliary maljunction. (B) Multiplanar reconstruction image shows the pancreaticobiliary junction outside the duodenal wall.

first-choice imaging technique for evaluation of congenital biliary dilatation as an attractive alternative to ERCP (Fig. 116.6A).[29,30] The detection rate of pancreaticobiliary maljunction by MRCP is reported to be 82% to 100% in adults and 40% to 80% in children.[31,32] However, MRCP can be hindered by the technical difficulty of children holding their breath, and motion artifacts can affect image quality, and it can sometimes be difficult in patients with a short common channel.[4,33]

The great advantage of computed tomography (CT) is its ability to produce high-quality images without respiratory artifacts and to provide more anatomic detail of the biliary tract.[3] High-resolution multidetector CT (MD-CT), which provides multiplanar reconstruction (MPR) images, and three-dimensional CT (3D-CT) have become available, and by combining them with drip-infusion cholangiography (DIC-CT), clear 3D images (3D-DIC-CT) of the intrahepatic and extrahepatic ducts or postoperative evaluation of bilioenteric anastomosis can be obtained (see Figs. 116.6B and 116.7).[3] However, in cases with a relatively short common channel, it is necessary to confirm that the effect of the papillary sphincter does not extend to the junction by direct cholangiography. An additional disadvantage in children is the exposure to radiation.

COMPLICATIONS

Biliary Stones

Biliary stones are the most frequent complication associated with congenital biliary dilatation. The prevalence of biliary stones ranges from 9.0% in children to 24.1% in adults, with the stone site being cholecystolithiasis in 12.7%, choledocholithiasis in 65.8%, and hepatolithiasis in 21.5% of cases.

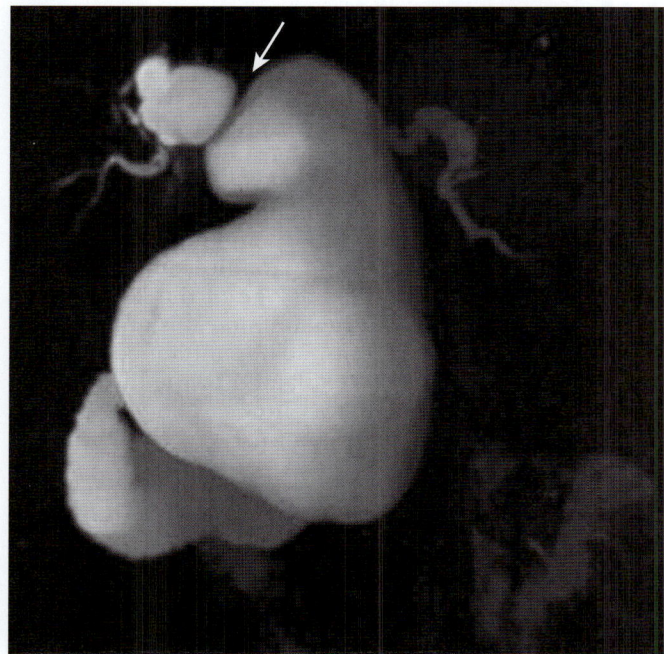

FIGURE 116.7 Computed tomography with drip-infusion cholangiography shows clear images of the intrahepatic and extrahepatic ducts and membranous stenosis of the right hepatic duct (arrow).

Pancreatitis

The association of pancreatitis with congenital biliary dilatation is well recognized. A history of clinical pancreatitis is present in nearly 30% of patients.[13] The pattern

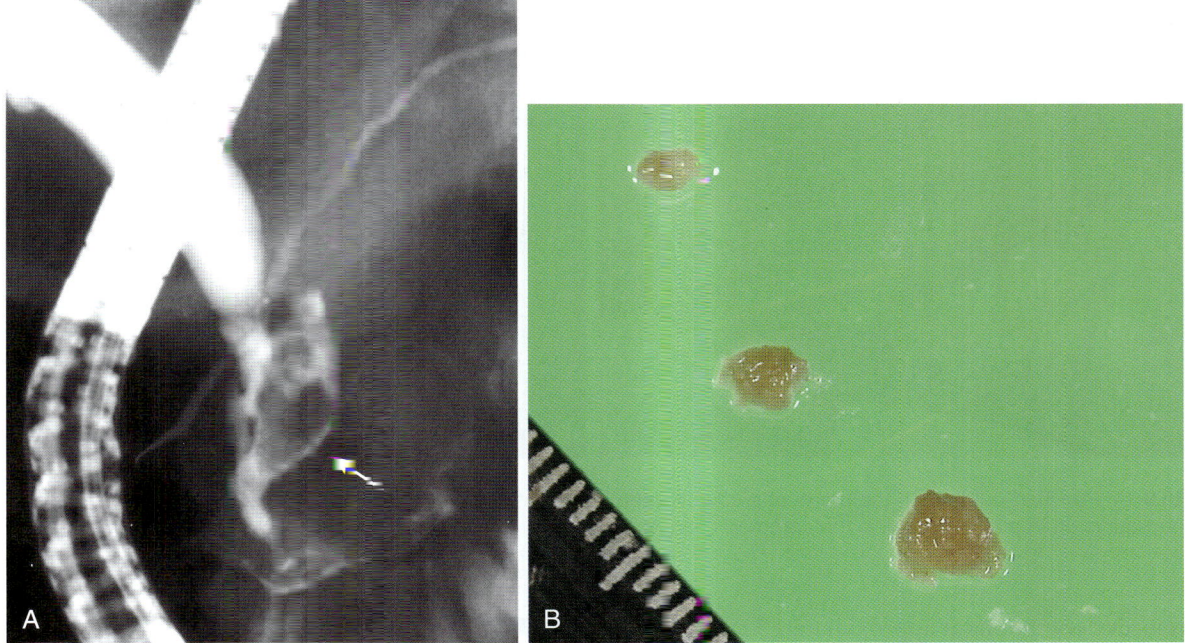

FIGURE 116.8 (A) Protein plugs present at the common channel (arrow). (B) The plugs consist mainly of protein, and most are soluble.

of pancreatitis is often characterized by a clinically transient or a clinically mild, but recurrent clinical course and may be caused by protein plug impaction within the common channel or bile duct, where the plug acts like a ball valve, producing a transient and abrupt elevation in the intraluminal pressure in both the bile and pancreatic ducts (Fig. 116.8A).[22] Most protein plugs are fragile and disappear spontaneously because they consist of more than 98% protein, which explains the self-limiting nature of the symptoms (see Fig. 116.8B).[5]

Spontaneous Perforation of the Bile Duct

Dijkstra[36] reported the first case of spontaneous perforation of the bile duct in 1932. Lilly et al.[37] in 1974 described a series of 53 cases collected from the world literature and Yamaguchi[38] reported a collective of 26 Japanese cases in 1433 patients of congenital biliary dilatation. Most patients are children, with 60% being younger than 1 year of age. An abdominal ultrasound, biliary radionuclide scan, or MRCP can facilitate diagnosis.[39] Perforation of the bile duct occurs as a small, punched-out hole and, although found mainly in the anterior aspect, can be found in any part of the bile duct (Fig. 116.9A).

Carcinoma

The association of bile duct carcinoma with congenital biliary dilatation was first reported by Irwin and Morison[40] in 1944. Tumors may develop anywhere within the intrahepatic and extrahepatic bile ducts, but more than one-half occur within the dilated part of the bile duct itself. The incidence of hepatobiliary malignancies associated with congenital biliary dilatation ranges from 3.2% to 39.4%.[12,40,41] Malignant degeneration according to age at initial operation has also been reported, and it has

been estimated that the risk of cancer in patients who had congenital biliary dilatation diagnosed in the first decade is 0.7%, whereas in those who had congenital biliary dilatation diagnosed at 11 to 20 years of age and at more than 20 years of age it is 6.8% and 14.3%, respectively.[42] The youngest reported patient with primary adenocarcinoma associated with a congenital biliary dilatation was a 3-year-old boy.[43]

SURGICAL MANAGEMENT

General Description Before Surgery

Internal drainage by choledochoenterostomy has fallen out of favor due to increased frequency of cholangitis, biliary stones, and the risk of malignant degeneration in the retained bile duct or gallbladder.[44,45] The mean age of the affected patients was approximately a decade less than the mean age of patients who developed malignancy in unoperated patients.[44] In 1970 Kasai et al.[46] and Ishida et al.[47] reported that the dilated extrahepatic bile duct should be removed to reduce postoperative morbidity and prevent cancer. Currently the definitive treatment of congenital biliary dilatation is to excise the whole extrahepatic bile duct and perform Roux-en-Y hepaticojejunostomy to separate the bile and pancreatic ducts to prevent free reflux of pancreatic juice into the bile duct.

There are no clear evidence-based recommendations as to when patients with congenital biliary dilatation should undergo surgery. However, because pancreaticobiliary maljunction enhances the chances of developing biliary carcinoma and because cancer can develop in juvenile patients, immediate surgery is recommended after a definitive diagnosis is established. Symptomatic neonates and infants should be operated on as soon as possible,

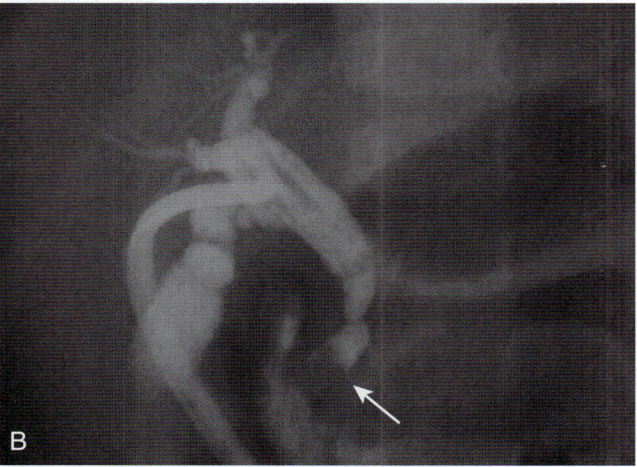

FIGURE 116.9 (A) Punched-out hole of the bile duct *(arrow)* is seen in the anterior aspect. (B) A T tube is inserted to the bile duct through the punched-out hole. The plug is seen in the common channel *(arrow).*

whereas elective operations at approximately 3 to 6 months of age may be considered for asymptomatic patients while their main organ functions, such as that of the liver, are monitored carefully.[21]

In patients with spontaneous perforation of the bile duct, emergency treatment is designed to improve the patient's condition and treat the biliary peritonitis, usually by means of T-tube drainage, followed by delayed surgery after the inflammation has subsided and after the anomalous anatomy has been clarified.[48] In many cases, cholangiography reveals the presence of protein plugs (see Fig. 116.9B).

Operative Technique

First, the gallbladder is mobilized. Intraoperative choledochoscopy via the cystic duct may be useful to exclude retained ductal stones and to biopsy the abnormal epithelium to exclude malignancy. A cholangiocatheter can be advanced through the cystic duct for bile aspiration and intraoperative cholangiography, which can be used to confirm the orientation of the pancreatic duct and check for protein plugs in the common channel or stenoses of the intrahepatic bile ducts. Dissection of the intrapancreatic bile duct proceeds on the outer plane of the epicholedochal plexus, where only loose fibrous tissue exists, so as to leave the plexus with the bile duct wall.[49] Further dissection should reveal that the narrow distal segment connecting the bile duct and the main pancreatic duct is located not at the bottom of the choledochus but almost always to the right and ventral to the dilated bile duct (Fig. 116.10). Attention must be directed to the main pancreatic duct just ventral to the dilated bile duct. The distal narrow segment is ligated carefully with absorbable suture to prevent narrowing of the pancreatic duct. For patients with protein plugs stuck in the common channel, irrigation with saline solution through a thin tube placed in the common channel or removal using a blunt spoon through the narrow segment is recommended.[50] In Lilly's and Okada's method,[51,52] the dilated bile duct is accomplished using a plane of dissection between the inner and

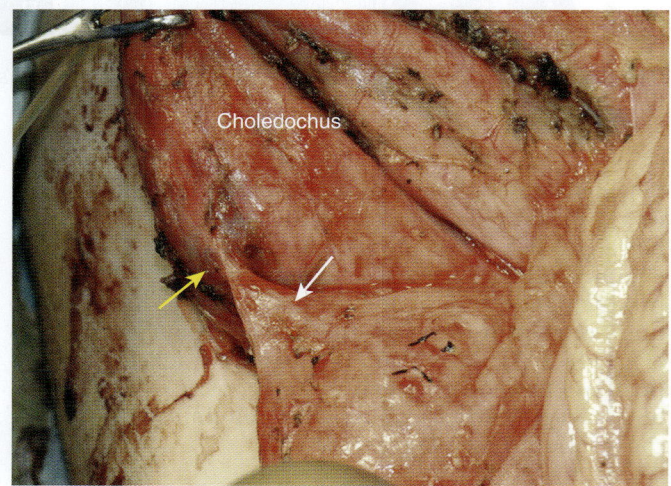

FIGURE 116.10 Operation for congenital biliary dilatation shows the narrow segment *(yellow arrow)* connecting the choledochus and the main pancreatic duct *(white arrow),* which is located not at the bottom of the dilated bile duct but almost always to the right and ventral to the dilated bile duct.

outer layers of the bile duct. However, this approach causes massive bleeding because there are many vessels in this layer and the distal narrow segment may become unclear. Because incomplete excision of the choledochus causes protein plug formation and may permit malignant change, whole extrahepatic bile duct excision should be performed.[53,54]

Next, the choledochus is elevated ventrally off the portal vein and mobilized proximally to the common hepatic duct. The hepatic duct near the confluence is transversely incised for assessment of possible stenoses at the orifice of the left and right hepatic ducts. If no stenosis is present at the bile ducts, the proximal bile duct is transected and the dilated choledochus removed. However, in patients with Todani type IV-A, stenoses are frequently found at

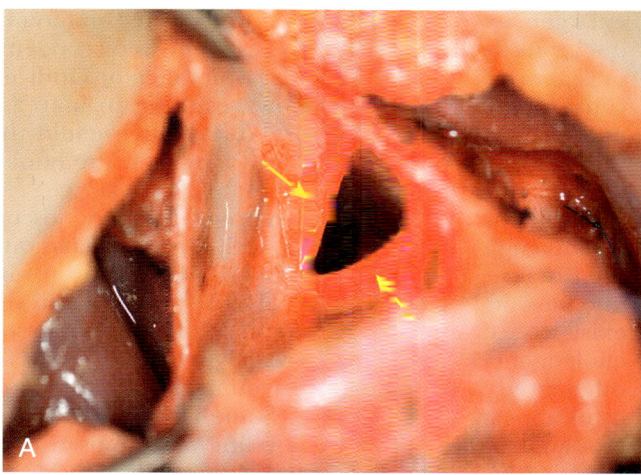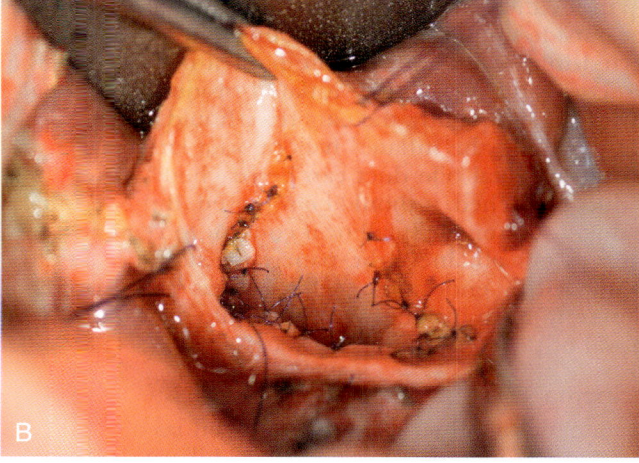

FIGURE 116.11 (A) The membranous stenosis at the right hepatic duct is characterized by the presence of a thin wall *(arrows)*. (B) The right hepatic duct can be dilated by resection of the membrane from the divided end of the common hepatic duct.

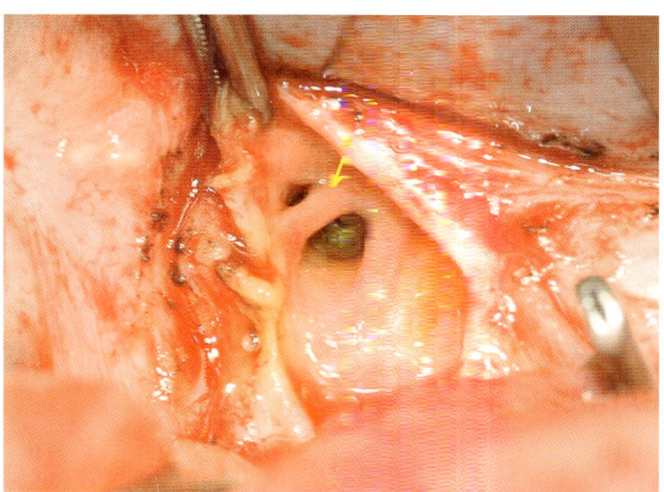

FIGURE 116.12 The septal stenosis *(arrow)* is characterized by a slender column of tissue.

the orifice of the left and right hepatic ducts. There are two different types of stenosis: membranous and septal (Figs. 116.11A and 116.12).[5] Because these stenoses near the hepatic hilum associated with upstream biliary dilatation can trigger postoperative cholangitis, hepatolithiasis, and possibly carcinogenesis, these stenoses should be treated by incising the hepatic ducts laterally to obtain a large anastomosis or they can be dilated by resection from the divided end of the common hepatic duct (see Fig. 116.11B).[56,57] Biliary reconstruction is accomplished by a 45-cm retrocolic Roux-en-Y hepaticojejunostomy.

POSTOPERATIVE COMPLICATIONS

Early complications can include anastomotic leakage, postoperative bleeding, acute pancreatitis, ileus, gastrointestinal bleeding, and pancreatic fistula. The prognosis

for congenital biliary dilatation is satisfactory; however, considerable numbers of articles have been published about the development of postoperative long-term complications.[58]

Cholangitis and Hepatolithiasis

Recurrent cholangitis from anastomotic strictures occurs in 10% to 25% of patients.[3,59] The incidence of hepatolithiasis, usually occurring in Todani type IV-A, has been reported in as many as 2.7% to 10.7% of cases after long-term follow-up.[56,59,60] Although some cases do have a stricture of the anastomosis, in many other cases, especially type IV-A, calculi occur by residual stenoses near the confluence of the left and right hepatic duct.[57,59]

In patients in whom hepatolithiasis develops postoperatively, it is important not only to remove the stone(s) but also to relieve the stenoses. When the stenotic site is dilated with an instrument inserted percutaneously, such as a balloon, the success rate is reported to be 70% to 90%.[61] However, there is a risk of stenosis recurring despite obtaining a favorable short-term outcome, and the approaches noted above are not generally effective for septal stenosis. It is important to ensure that smooth biliary flow is resumed by resecting the lithogenic membranous and/or septal stenosis. Hepatectomy is also a useful method to resect the stenotic site, although in pediatric patients it should be limited to cases in which the stenosis cannot be dealt with from the hepatic hilum, or when the stenosis is limited to either the right or the left lobe of the liver.[4]

Pancreatic Stones

Because protein plugs may form in the remnant bile duct, incomplete removal of the intrapancreatic bile duct might cause persistent pancreatitis or stone formation. The treatment for such stone(s) is complete extraction of the residual bile duct. When the residual bile duct can be localized from outside the pancreas, the bile duct should be extracted by a procedure similar to that performed in the initial operation. If the residual bile duct is buried deep inside the pancreas such that it is difficult to identify from outside the pancreas, a balloon catheter should be inserted intraoperatively via the papilla of Vater, using endoscopy, and the balloon inflated inside the residual bile duct. Subsequently, the pancreas should be cut open while palpating the inflated balloon as a landmark and until the residual bile duct can be reached.[65] After the bile duct is reached, it should be removed. If the residual bile duct is extremely small or if consent to remove it by surgery is not obtained, the pancreatic stone(s) should be removed by endoscopy.[53] However, as protein plugs continue to form inside the residual bile duct, repeated removal of the stone(s) will be necessary.

Carcinoma

Extrahepatic bile duct excision has been recognized as the definitive operation for congenital biliary dilatation; however, reports of bile duct cancer after bile duct excision are gradually increasing. Thistlethwaite and Horwitz[63] reported that cholangiocarcinoma occurred on the anastomotic portion 4 years after extrahepatic bile duct excision. Moreover, Gallagher et al.[64] reported that cholangiocarcinoma developed in the intrahepatic bile ducts, although the extrahepatic bile duct had been excised 7 years previously. Watanabe et al.[65] reported 23 patients with bile duct cancer developing after extrahepatic bile duct excision. Index malignant changes may occur before bile duct excision or choledochoenterostomy and may advance after bile duct excision. Long-term follow-up is important, even after excision of the dilated bile duct, because the entire residual biliary tree is believed to be at increased risk for cholangiocarcinoma.[66–69] Therefore careful follow-up for the rest of their lives is strongly recommended.

DIVERTICULUM (TYPE II)

A type II diverticulum arises laterally from the wall of the common bile duct. However, because of its rarity, experience with this type is limited.[70] In this type the weakness factor is limited to one small area of the side of the wall. The treatment of choice is simple cyst excision, a procedure that can be performed open or laparoscopically. Type II diverticulum is not usually associated with pancreaticobiliary maljunction.

CHOLEDOCHOCELE (TYPE III)

Choledochocele is an uncommon abnormality of cystic or diverticular dilatation of the terminal intramural portion of the common bile duct, first described by Wheeler[71] in 1940. The term choledochocele was introduced by Wheeler, who saw the analogy with congenital ureterocele. The first classification of choledochocele was proposed by Scholz et al. in 1976 and has been classified by various authors according to this scheme. There are two different types of the internal cyst wall component. One is lined by duodenal mucosa and the other lined by bile duct mucosa. The former type suggests that the choledochocele is a congenital duodenal duplication arising near the main duodenal papilla, which communicates with the common bile duct. The latter type suggests a diverticular enlargement of the terminal portion of the common bile duct.[72] In the latter type, papillary stenosis or congenital or acquired dysfunction of the sphincter of Oddi may cause obstruction of bile flow, resulting in increased pressure within the distal bile duct, which could then evaginate into the duodenum.[74] However, the etiology remains unclear in many cases.

Choledochocele can be diagnosed by duodenoscopic or cholangiographic findings, with a cystic dilatation of the distal segment of the common bile duct protruding into the duodenal lumen (Fig. 116.13).[75] Some controversy exists concerning the size cutoff for the diagnosis of a choledochocele. Despite the widely recognized view that other biliary cysts are truly congenital, some choledochoceles appear to be acquired. Some authors have stated that an arbitrary 1-cm dividing line may be used to differentiate between a choledochocele and a dilated common channel or normal variants.[76,77] Choledochocele usually shows a normal pancreaticobiliary junction but is associated with pancreaticobiliary maljunction in rare cases. Patient age may range from 1 to 89 years (median: 40 years), and there appears to be no gender predominance.[73] Patients with choledochocele clinically present with intermittent episodes of upper abdominal pain accompanied by nausea and vomiting, obstructive jaundice, cholangitis, or recurrent acute pancreatitis.[72,73,77] Associated stone disease occurs in approximately 20% of cases, but the risk of malignant changes is extremely low.[73]

Although surgical excision of the duodenal luminal portion of the cyst wall has been performed, endoscopic papillotomy has been increasingly chosen as the preferred treatment for this type. Asymptomatic choledochoceles, incidentally identified during ERCP examinations, are best left alone and observed.[73]

CAROLI DISEASE (TYPE V)

In 1958 Caroli described a disease entity characterized by (1) segmental cystic dilatation of the intrahepatic ducts; (2) increased incidence of biliary lithiasis, cholangitis, and abscesses; (3) absence of cirrhosis and portal hypertension; and (4) association of renal tubular ectasia or similar renal cystic disease. Still later, Caroli[78] recognized two entities: a simple type and a periportal fibrosis type. The so-called simple or pure type, originally described in 1958, is a very rare congenital abnormality, whereas the more common type is associated with congenital hepatic fibrosis, which is present in childhood.[79] As a term, Caroli disease has been applied broadly to describe patients with segmentally ectatic appearance of the intrahepatic bile ducts, identical to that seen in intrahepatic involvement of the congenital biliary dilatation. However, Caroli disease and congenital biliary dilatation are separate diseases. Caroli disease is not accompanied by pancreaticobiliary maljunction or localized common bile duct dilatation.

Caroli disease is generally considered autosomal recessive, but there are some cases of autosomal dominant inheritance.[80] The male-to-female ratio is 3:2, and the age at diagnosis ranges between 1 and 60 years (median: 25 years).[80] The dilated hepatic ducts connect with the common hepatic duct and are liable to become infected and contain stones. Biliary infection and stones account

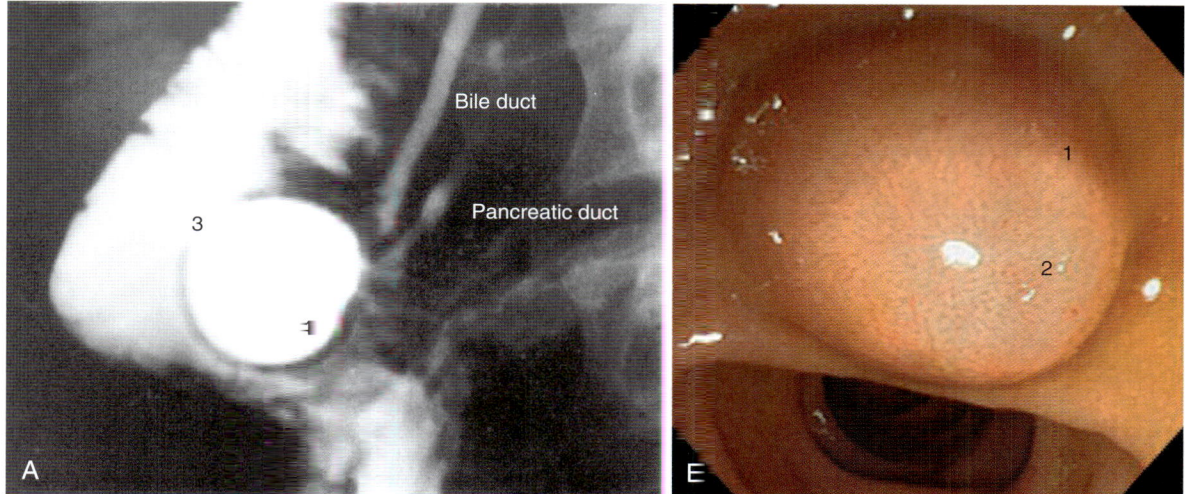

FIGURE 116.13 Endoscopic retrograde cholangiopancreatography (A) and endoscopy (B) show characteristic images of a type III choledochocele: *(1)* an intramural segment of the common bile duct protruding into the duodenum in continuation with an enlarged papilla with a spherical shape; *(2)* soft overlying mucosa with a smooth appearance; *(3)* ballooning of the papilla during contrast injection; and *(4)* a rather spherical, cystlike, contrast-filled structure in continuity with the terminal common bile duct.

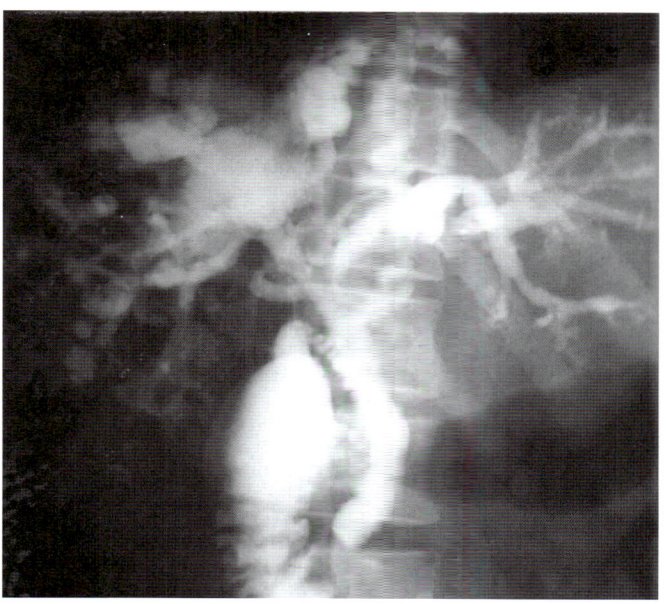

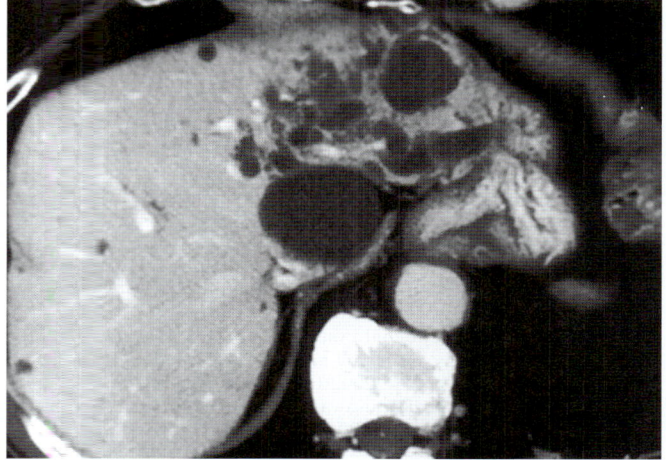

FIGURE 6.15 Computed tomography shows saccular dilatation of the intrahepatic bile ducts. The sacculi are large and distributed within the left lobe.

FIGURE 116.14 Endoscopic retrograde cholangiopancreatography shows Caroli disease, with multiple communicating sacculi of the intrahepatic biliary tree. The sacculi are large and are distributed within the right lobe.

for the symptoms of fever and abdominal pain. The clinical onset of Caroli disease usually occurs during childhood and symptoms include cholangitis (46%), portal hypertension (22%), and abdominal pain in the right upper quadrant (18%).[80,81]

Caroli disease can be diagnosed by the cholangiographic finding of a multiple saccular appearance of intrahepatic bile ducts (Fig. 116.14).[82] Ultrasound, MRCP, and CT have been shown to be useful in detecting saccular dilatation of the intrahepatic bile ducts (Figs. 116.15 and 116.16).

The sacculi may vary greatly in size and distribution within the liver.[79] CT scans of the liver show tiny dots with strong contrast enhancement within the dilated intrahepatic bile ducts or the *central dot sign*, which corresponds to intraluminal portal radicles surrounded by the dilated intrahepatic bile ducts.[79,83] Liver involvement may be limited to a single lobe or segment.

The long-term prognosis for patients with Caroli disease is quite poor, with a marked predisposition to septicemia, liver abscess, resultant hepatic failure, portal hypertension, or cholangiocarcinoma.[81] Cholangiocarcinoma has been reported in approximately 7% of patients.[81,82] The therapeutic management of Caroli disease is difficult, whether using conservative medical management or surgical interventions. Liver transplantation should be considered if the patient's condition deteriorates.[84,85]

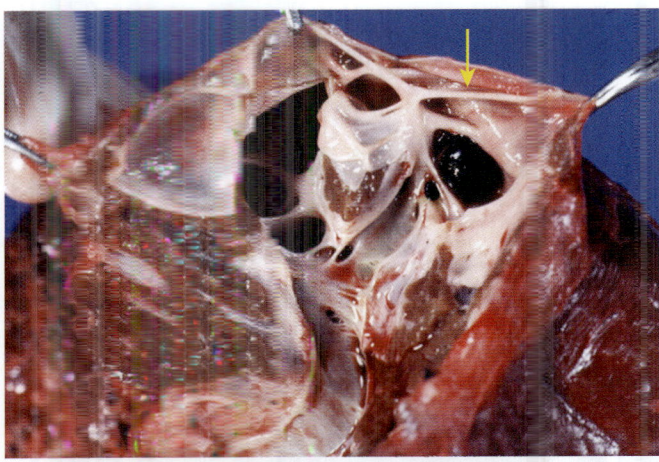

FIGURE 116.16 Gross pathology sections of the liver in Caroli disease show multiple saccular dilatations of the intrahepatic bile ducts and black-pigmented calcium bilirubinate stones. Septum-like fibrovascular bundles *(arrow)* are seen on the wall of the cut sacculi.

REFERENCES

1. Alonso-Lej E, Ferrer WB, Pessagno DJ. Congenital choledochal cysts, with a report of 2, and an analysis of 94, cases. *Int Abstr Surg.* 1959;108: 1-30.
2. Todani T, Watanabe Y, Narusue M, Tabuchi K, Okajima K. Congenital bile duct cysts: classifications, operative procedures, and review of 37 cases including cancer arising from choledochal cyst. *Am J Surg.* 1977;134:263-269.
3. Todani T. Congenital choledochal dilatation: classification, clinical features, and long-term results. *J Hepatobiliary Pancreat Surg.* 1997; 4:276-282.
4. Kamisawa T, Ando H, Suyama M, et al. Japanese clinical practice guidelines for pancreaticobiliary maljunction. *J Gastroenterol.* 2012; 47:731-759.
5. Stringer MD. Choledochal cysts. In: Howard ED, Stringer MD, Colombani PM, eds. *Surgery of the Liver, Bile Ducts and Pancreas in Children.* London: Arnold; 2002:149-168.
6. Hamada Y, Ando H, Kamisawa T, et al. Diagnostic criteria for congenital biliary dilatation 2015. *J Hepatobiliary Pancreat Sci.* 2016; 23:342-346.
7. Douglas AH. Case of dilatation of the common bile duct. *Month J Med Sci.* 1852;2:497-501.
8. Kozumi I, Kodama T. A case report and the etiology of choledochal cystic dilatation. *Tokyo Med Assoc.* 1916;30:1413-1423. [in Japanese].
9. Babbitt DP. Congenital choledochal cysts: new etiological concept based on anomalous relationships of common bile duct and pancreatic bulb. *Ann Radiol (Paris).* 1969;12:231-240.
10. Lenriot JP, Gigot JF, Segol P. Bile duct cysts in adults: a multi-institutional retrospective study. French Association for Surgical Research. *Ann Surg.* 1998;228:159-166.
11. Benhamou JS. Biliary cystic disease: the risk of cancer. *J Hepatobiliary Pancreat Surg.* 2003;10:335-339.
12. Miyano T, Yamataka A. Choledochal cysts. *Curr Opin Pediatr.* 1997;9:283-288.
13. Nagorney DM. Choledochal cysts in adults. In: Blumgart LH, Fong Y, eds. *Surgery of the Liver and Biliary Tract.* 3rd ed. London: Saunders; 2000:1229-1244.
14. Lugo-Vicente HL. Prenatally diagnosed choledochal cyst: obstruction or early surgery? *J Pediatr Surg.* 1995;30:1288-1290.
15. Yotuyanagi S. Contributions to the aetiology and pathogeny of idiopathic cystodilatation of the common bile-duct with report of three cases: a new aetiological theory based on supposed unequal epithelial proliferation at the stage of the physiological epithelial occlusion of the primitive choledochus. *Gann.* 1936;30:601-652.
16. Matsumoto Y, Fujii H, Itakura J, et al. Pancreaticobiliary maljunction: pathophysiological and clinical aspects and the impact on biliary carcinogenesis. *Langenbecks Arch Surg.* 2003;388:122-131.
17. Ando H, Kaneko K, Ito F, Seo T, Harada T, Watanabe Y. Embryogenesis of pancreaticobiliary maljunction inferred from development of duodenal atresia. *J Hepatobiliary Pancreat Surg.* 1999;6:50-54.
18. Kattepura S, Nanjegowda NB, Babu MK, Das K. Macroscopic pancreatic heterotopia on a congenital biliary dilatation. *Pediatr Surg Int.* 2010;26:847-849.
19. Funabiki T, Sugiue K, Matsubara T, Amano H, Ochiai M. Bile acids and biliary carcinoma in pancreaticobiliary maljunction. *Keio J Med.* 1991;40:118-122.
20. Kato T, Hebiguchi T, Matsuda K, Yoshino H. Action of pancreatic juice on the bile duct: pathogenesis of congenital choledochal cyst. *J Pediatr Surg.* 1981;16:146-151.
21. Lipsett PA, Pitt HA. Surgical treatment of choledochal cysts. *J Hepatobiliary Pancreat Surg.* 2003;10:352-359.
22. Kaneko K, Ando H, Ito T, et al. Protein plugs cause symptoms in patients with choledochal cysts. *Am J Gastroenterol.* 1997;92:1018-1021.
23. Todani T, Urushihara N, Morotomi Y, et al. Characteristics of choledochal cysts in neonates and early infants. *Eur J Pediatr Surg.* 1995;5:143-145.
24. Kamisawa T, Ando H, Hamada Y, et al. Diagnostic criteria for pancreaticobiliary maljunction 2013. *J Hepatobiliary Pancreat Sci.* 2014;21:159-161.
25. Itokawa F, Kamisawa T, Nakano T, et al. Exploring the length of the common channel of pancreaticobiliary maljunction on MRCP. *J Hepatobiliary Pancreat Sci.* 2015;22:68-73.
26. Itoi T, Kamisawa T, Fujii H, et al. Extrahepatic bile duct measurement by using transabdominal ultrasound in Japanese adults: multi-center prospective study. *J Gastroenterol.* 2013;48:1045-1050.
27. Kamisawa T, Ando H, Shimada M, et al. Recent advances and problems in the management of pancreaticobiliary maljunction: feedback from the guidelines committee. *J Hepatobiliary Pancreat Sci.* 2014;21:87-92.
28. Hiramatsu T, Itoh A, Kawashima H, et al. Usefulness and safety of endoscopic retrograde cholangiopancreatography in children with pancreaticobiliary maljunction. *J Pediatr Surg.* 2015;50:377-381.
29. Kim MJ, Han SJ, Yoon CS, et al. Using MR cholangiopancreatography to reveal anomalous pancreaticobiliary ductal union in infants and children with choledochal cysts. *AJR Am J Roentgenol.* 2002;179:209-214.
30. Sacher VY, Davis JS, Sleeman D, Casillas J. Role of magnetic resonance cholangiopancreatography in diagnosing choledochal cysts: case series and review. *World J Radiol.* 2013;5:304-312.
31. Irie H, Honda H, Jimi M, et al. Value of MR cholangiopancreatography in evaluating choledochal cysts. *AJR Am J Roentgenol.* 1998; 171:1381-1385.
32. Matos C, Nicaise N, Devière J, et al. Choledochal cysts: comparison of findings at MR cholangiopancreatography and endoscopic retrograde cholangiopancreatography in eight patients. *Radiology.* 1998;209:443-448.
33. Lam WW, Lam TP, Saing H, Chan FL, Chan KL. MR cholangiography and CT cholangiography of pediatric patients with choledochal cysts. *AJR Am J Roentgenol.* 1999;173:401-405.
34. Hamada Y, Sato M, Sanada T, Tsuji M, Kogata M, Hioki K. Spiral computed tomography for biliary dilatation. *J Pediatr Surg.* 1995;30: 694-696.
35. Kaneko K, Ando H, Seo T, Ono Y, Tainaka T, Sumida W. Proteomic analysis of protein plugs: causative agent of symptoms in patients with choledochal cyst. *Dig Dis Sci.* 2007;52:1979-1986.
36. Dijkstra OH. Jaundice from rupture of choledochus in nurseling; cause unknown. *Maandschr Kindergeneeskd.* 1932;1:409-414.
37. Lilly JR, Weintraub WH, Altman RP. Spontaneous perforation of the extrahepatic bile ducts and bile peritonitis in infancy. *Surgery.* 1974;75:664-673.
38. Yamaguchi M. Congenital choledochal cyst. Analysis of 1,433 patients in the Japanese literature. *Am J Surg.* 1980;140:653-657.
39. Lee MJ, Kim MJ, Yoon CS. MR cholangiopancreatography findings in children with spontaneous bile duct perforation. *Pediatr Radiol.* 2010;40:687-692.
40. Irwin ST, Morison JE. Congenital cyst of the common bile duct containing stones and undergoing cancerous change. *Br J Surg.* 1944;32:319-321.
41. Hasumi A, Matsui H, Sugioka A, et al. Precancerous conditions of biliary tract cancer in patients with pancreaticobiliary maljunction:

reappraisal of nationwide survey in Japan. *J Hepatobiliary Pancreat Surg.* 2000;7:551-555.

42. Voyles CR, Smadja C, Shands WC, Blumgart LH. Carcinoma in choledochal cysts. Age-related incidence. *Arch Surg.* 1983;118:986-988.

43. Saikusa N, Naito S, Iinuma Y, Ohtani T, Toyama N, Nitta K. Invasive cholangiocarcinoma identified in congenital biliary dilatation in a 3-year-old boy. *J Pediatr Surg.* 2009;44:2202-2205.

44. Todani T, Watanabe Y, Toki A, Urushihara N. Carcinoma related to choledochal cysts with internal drainage operations. *Surg Gynecol Obstet.* 1987;164:51-64.

45. Tocchi A, Mazzoni G, Liotta G, Lepre L, Cassini D, Miccini M. Late development of bile duct cancer in patients who had biliary-enteric drainage for benign diseases: a follow-up study of more than 1,000 patients. *Ann Surg.* 2001;234:210-214.

46. Kasai M, Asakura Y, Taira Y. Surgical treatment of choledochal cyst. *Ann Surg.* 1970;172:844-851.

47. Ishida M, Tsuchida Y, Saito S, Hori T. Primary excision of choledochal cysts. *Surgery.* 1970;68:884-888.

48. Ando H, Ito T, Watanabe Y, Seo T, Lane GJ, Nagaya M. Spontaneous perforation of choledochal cyst. *J Am Coll Surg.* 1995;181:125-128.

49. Ando H, Kaneko K, Ito T, et al. Complete excision of the intrahepatic portion of choledochal cysts. *J Am Coll Surg.* 1996;183:317-321.

50. Ando H, Kaneko K, Ito F, et al. Surgical removal of protein plugs complicating choledochal cysts: primary repair after adequate opening of the pancreatic duct. *J Pediatr Surg.* 1998;33:1265-1267.

51. Lilly JR. Total excision of choledochal cyst. *Surg Gynecol Obstet.* 1978;146:254-256.

52. Okada A, Nakamura T, Okumura K, Iguchi K, Kamata S. Surgical treatment of congenital dilatation of bile duct (choledochal cyst) with technical considerations. *Surgery.* 1987;101:238-243.

53. Chiba K, Kamisawa T, Egawa N. Relapsing acute pancreatitis caused by protein plugs in a remnant choledochal cyst. *J Hepatobiliary Pancreat Sci.* 2010;17:729-730.

54. Millar A, Cywes S. Choledochal cyst: is complete excision of the intrapancreatic cyst necessary? *HPB Surg.* 1997;11:61-70.

55. Ando H, Ito T, Kaneko K, Seo T. Congenital stenosis of the intrahepatic bile duct associated with choledochal cyst. *J Am Coll Surg.* 1995;181:426-430.

56. Todani T, Watanabe Y, Urushihara N, Noda T, Morotomi Y. Biliary complications after excision procedure for choledochal cyst. *J Pediatr Surg.* 1995;30:478-481.

57. Ando H, Kaneko K, Ito F, Seo T, et al. Operative treatment of congenital stenoses of the intrahepatic bile ducts in patients with choledochal cyst. *Am J Surg.* 1997;173:491-494.

58. Saing H, Han H, Chan KL, et al. Early and late results of excision of choledochal cysts. *J Pediatr Surg.* 1997;32:1563-1566.

59. Uno K, Tsuchida Y, Kawarasaki H, Ohmiya H, Honna T. Development of intrahepatic cholelithiasis long after primary excision of choledochal cyst. *J Am Coll Surg.* 1996;183:583-588.

60. Chijiiwa K, Komura M, Kameoka N. Postoperative follow-up of patients with type IV-A choledochal cyst after excision of extrahepatic cyst. *J Am Coll Surg.* 1994;179:641-645.

61. Vos PM, van Beek EJ, Smits NJ, Rauws EA, Gouma DJ, Reeders JW. Percutaneous balloon dilatation for benign hepaticojejunostomy strictures. *Abdom Imaging.* 2000;25:134-138.

62. Koshinaga T, Hoshino M, Inoue M, et al. Pancreatitis complicated with dilated choledochal remnant after congenital choledochal cyst excision. *Pediatr Surg Int.* 2005;21:936-938.

63. Thistlethwaite JR, Horwitz A. Choledochal cyst followed by carcinoma of the hepatic duct. *South Med J.* 1967;60:1872-1874.

64. Gallagher PJ, Millis R, Mitchinson MJ. Congenital dilatation of the intrahepatic bile ducts with cholangiocarcinoma. *J Clin Pathol.* 1972;25:804-808.

65. Watanabe Y, Toki A, Todani T. Bile duct cancer developed after cyst excision for choledochal cyst. *J Hepatobiliary Pancreat Surg.* 1999;6:207-212.

66. Goto N, Yoshida K, Shirai Y, et al. A case of carcinoma arising in the intrapancreatic terminal choledochus 12 years after primary excision of a giant choledochal cyst. *Am J Gastroenterol.* 1986;81:378-384.

67. Ishibashi T, Kasahara K, Yasuda Y, Nagai H, Makino S, Kanazawa K. Malignant change in the biliary tract after excision of choledochal cyst. *Br J Surg.* 1997;84:1687-1689.

68. Kobayashi S, Asano T, Yamasaki M, Kenmochi T, Nakagohri T, Ochiai T. Risk of bile duct carcinogenesis after excision of extrahepatic bile ducts in pancreaticobiliary maljunction. *Surgery.* 1999;126:939-944.

69. Goto N, Yasuda I, Uematsu T, et al. Intrahepatic cholangiocarcinoma arising 10 years after the excision of congenital extrahepatic biliary dilatation. *J Gastroenterol.* 2001;36:856-862.

70. Hewitt PM, Kringe JEJ, Bornman PC, Terblanche J. Choledochal cysts in adults. *Br J Surg.* 1995;82:382-385.

71. Whitler WIC. An unusual case of obstruction to the common bile duct (choledochocele?). *Br J Surg.* 1940;27:446-448.

72. Scholz FJ, Carrera GF, Larsen CR. The choledochocele: correlation of radiological, clinical and pathological findings. *Radiology.* 1976;118:25-28.

73. Masetti R, Antinori A, Coppola R, et al. Choledochocele: changing trends in diagnosis and management. *Surg Today.* 1996;26:281-285.

74. Stampfl G, Sauer H, Goriupp U, Becker H. Choledochocele: importance of histological evaluation. *J Pediatr Surg.* 1993;28:1562-1565.

75. Ladas SD, Katsogridakis I, Tassios P, Tastemiroglou T, Vrachliotis T, Raptis SA. Choledochocele, an overlooked diagnosis: report of 15 cases and review of 56 published reports from 1984 to 1992. *Endoscopy.* 1995;27:233-239.

76. Savader SJ, Benenati JF, Venbrux AC, et al. Choledochal cysts: classification and cholangiographic appearance. *AJR Am J Roentgenol.* 1991;156:327-331.

77. Elton E, Hanson BL, Biber BP, Howell DA. Dilated common channel syndrome: endoscopic diagnosis, treatment, and relationship to choledochocele formation. *Gastrointest Endosc.* 1998;47:471-478.

78. Desmet J. Disease of the intrahepatic biliary tree. *Clin Gastroenterol.* 1983;12:147-161.

79. Miller WJ, Sechtin AG, Campbell WL, Pieters PC. Imaging findings in Caroli's disease. *AJR Am J Roentgenol.* 1995;165:333-337.

80. Tsuchida Y, Sato T, Sanjo K, et al. Evaluation of long-term results of Caroli's disease: 21 years' observation of a family with autosomal "dominant" inheritance, and review of the literature. *Hepatogastroenterology.* 1995;42:175-181.

81. Dayton MT, Longmire WP, Tompkins RK. Caroli's disease: a premalignant condition? *Am J Surg.* 1983;145:41-48.

82. Sherlock S, Dooley J. Cysts and congenital biliary abnormalities. In: Sherlock S, Dooley J, eds. *Diseases of the Liver and Biliary System.* 10th ed. Oxford: Blackwell; 1997:579-591.

83. Choi BI, Yeon KM, Kim SH, Han MC. Caroli disease: central dot sign in CT. *Radiology.* 1990;174:161-163.

84. Ibrahim M, Umemoto S, Inimata Y, et al. Living-donor liver transplantation for Caroli's disease with intrahepatic adenocarcinoma. *J Hepatobiliary Pancreat Surg.* 2001;8:284-286.

85. Millwala C, Deutscher J, Müller S, et al. Successful liver transplantation in a child with Caroli's disease. *Pediatr Transplant.* 2008;12:483-486.

Surgical Treatment of Primary Sclerosing Cholangitis

Kristopher P. Croome | Gregory J. Gores | Charles B. Rosen

Primary sclerosing cholangitis (PSC) is a chronic, cholestatic liver disease of unknown cause characterized by diffuse inflammation and fibrosis of intrahepatic and/or extrahepatic bile ducts and is strongly associated with inflammatory bowel disease (IBD).[1] PSC is ultimately progressive, leading to obliteration of the biliary tree and subsequently to biliary cirrhosis.[1] To date, the etiology of PSC remains unknown and effective medical therapy is not currently available. Patients with PSC have shortened life expectancy. Orthotopic liver transplantation (OLT) extends the life of patients with advanced-stage PSC. Development of colon cancer, gallbladder cancer, cholangiocarcinoma (CCA), and hepatocellular carcinoma are known complications of the disease.

EPIDEMIOLOGY

PSC usually affects more young males than females.[1] The mean age of diagnosis is the late 30s. In the United States, population-based studies have estimated an age-adjusted incidence for PSC to be 1.25 and 0.54 per 100,000 in men and women, respectively.[2] Moreover, the calculated prevalence of PSC was 20.9 and 6.3 per 100,000 in men and women, respectively.[2] Approximately 75% to 80% of northern European origin patients with PSC suffer from IBD, with chronic ulcerative colitis (CUC) being more common (approximately 90%) than Crohn disease.

PSC is associated with a lack of smoking. In one study the incidence of current smoking was 19% in patients with PSC compared with 38% of controls.[3] In another study, 1.9% of PSC patients were reported to smoke compared with 26.1% of controls. The odds of having PSC in current smokers or former and current smokers compared with never-smokers were 0.13 and 0.41, respectively, regardless of the presence or absence of IBD.[4] Studies have also reported that prior appendectomy may delay the onset of PSC but does not affect either the prevalence or severity of the latter.[5]

CLINICAL PRESENTATION

The clinical presentation of PSC is heterogeneous and varies widely depending on the disease stage at the time of diagnosis. Asymptomatic individuals typically come to medical attention because of abnormal liver biochemistry detected during routine screening. Symptomatic patients present with symptoms/signs of cholestasis and complications of chronic cholestatic liver disease. The symptoms may include fatigue, pruritus, right upper quadrant pain, weight loss, and manifestations related to portal hypertension (i.e., ascites, gastrointestinal bleed from esophageal/

gastric varices). Symptoms of bacterial cholangitis are less common, except if the patient has dominant biliary strictures and/or biliary stones. The physical examination of symptomatic patients may reveal jaundice, hepatomegaly, splenomegaly, skin excoriations, ascites, and peripheral edema.

A frequent clinical scenario is a patient with CUC who presents with a cholestatic pattern of liver enzymes. PSC can affect any age group, including children. Children may present with an overlap syndrome of PSC and autoimmune hepatitis (AIH), which can be as high as 35% according to a recent study.[6]

DIAGNOSIS

The criteria used to diagnose PSC are based on the clinical presentation, biochemical abnormalities, histologic features, and the characteristic cholangiographic changes that affect the intrahepatic and extrahepatic bile ducts. In addition, secondary biliary cirrhosis needs to be excluded. The most frequent clinical presentation currently is an asymptomatic patient with persistently increased levels of alkaline phosphatase noted on routine serum biochemical testing.

Liver biopsy is recommended, but it is not always required to make the diagnosis. In a study of 79 patients with a PSC diagnosis established by cholangiography, liver biopsy performed following diagnosis did not affect the management in the vast majority of patients.[7] The role of liver biopsy in PSC is to (1) exclude other causes of cholestatic liver disease; (2) diagnose or exclude small-duct PSC; and (3) define the PSC stage, which may have prognostic value. Small-duct PSC is a variant of PSC that accounts for approximately 5% of histologically proven cases.[8] Small-duct PSC presents with a cholestatic pattern of liver enzymes and normal cholangiography, but liver biopsy reveals evidence of PSC. Small-duct PSC has a better long-term prognosis compared with classic PSC. However, a portion of patients with small-duct PSC progress to classic PSC over time.[8]

In most patients the history, clinical presentation, serum biochemical profile, and cholangiography distinguish PSC from other causes of chronic cholestatic liver disease.

PATHOLOGY

The pathologic findings in PSC depend on the duration and extent of the disease. Early on in the disease the liver may appear grossly normal, whereas in established PSC, biliary cirrhosis may be present with associated portal hypertension, ascites, and splenomegaly. The bifurcation of the hepatic duct is macroscopically involved in most cases. Enlarged lymph nodes are often present in the porta hepatis and along the proper and common hepatic arteries and the hepatic and common bile duct.

Liver biopsy is recommended for staging liver disease to determine the prognosis. PSC is staged histologically (1 to 4) according to the following system': stage 1 (portal stage), there is edema, inflammation, and ductal proliferation; stage 2 (periportal stage), periportal fibrosis and inflammation are noted; stage 3 (septal stage) is defined by septal fibrosis or bridging necrosis; stage 4 (cirrhotic stage) is characterized by biliary cirrhosis. Unfortunately, histologic changes can be markedly varied from segment to segment of the liver at any given point in time.

IMAGING STUDIES

Cholangiography is required to diagnose a patient with PSC. Endoscopic retrograde cholangiopancreatography (ERCP) is the standard approach to evaluate the bile ducts. Magnetic resonance cholangiography (MRC) may suffice, and percutaneous transhepatic cholangiography (PTC) is sometimes necessary when ERCP is not possible. The classic cholangiographic findings of PSC include multifocal stricturing and beading throughout the biliary tree (Fig. 117.1). Strictures are often diffusely distributed with intervening segments of dilated ducts (i.e., ectasia). The cholangiographic findings usually involve both the intrahepatic and extrahepatic bile ducts. Strictures can vary from 1 or 2 mm to several centimeters in length, and 30% to 40% of PSC patients may have mural irregularities, producing a shaggy appearance. These lesions may vary from a "fine brush border" to "frank nodularity." Pseudodiverticula (i.e., tiny diverticulum-like outpouchings) of the extrahepatic bile ducts are nearly pathognomonic

for PSC. In approximately 20% of PSC patients, only the intrahepatic and perihilar extrahepatic bile ducts are involved, and as many as 15% of PSC patients have involvement of the gallbladder and cystic duct. Moreover, approximately 5% of patients have small-duct PSC (i.e., normal cholangiogram but liver disease detectable on biochemical testing and histology).[8]

MRC is a noninvasive substitute for ERCP for the diagnosis of PSC. In a study of 73 patients with clinically suspected biliary disease, the sensitivity and specificity of MRC for diagnosing PSC were 82% and 98%, respectively.[10] These authors reported that MRC had comparable diagnostic accuracy to ERCP, leading to reduced cost when used as the initial approach to diagnose PSC. In PSC patients, MRC could be used as a noninvasive imaging method for the detection of CCA. Indeed, some clinicians now prefer MRC over ERCP for the diagnosis of PSC.

PTC is used less frequently to image the bile ducts in patients with suspected PSC. PTC is an alternative approach to access the biliary tree when ERCP is not technically possible. Abdominal ultrasonography is valuable to evaluate the bile ducts for dilation and/or stones, and liver parenchyma for cirrhosis. Computed tomography (CT) can reveal morphologic features of liver cirrhosis. Atrophy of the left lateral segments and hypertrophy of the caudate lobe may differentiate cirrhosis associated with PSC from that seen in other causes of chronic liver disease.[11] CT can also complement cholangiography in evaluating for malignancy, given its ability to detect peripheral, intrahepatic CCA and metastatic spread within the hepatic parenchyma or the abdomen.[12] It is important to note that perihilar lymphadenopathy is common in PSC, and this finding alone cannot be taken as evidence of malignancy or metastasis.

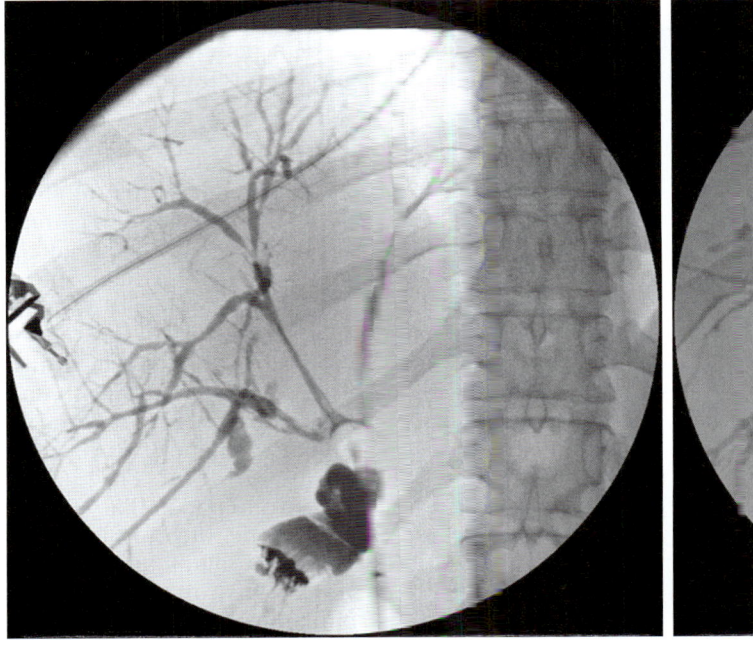
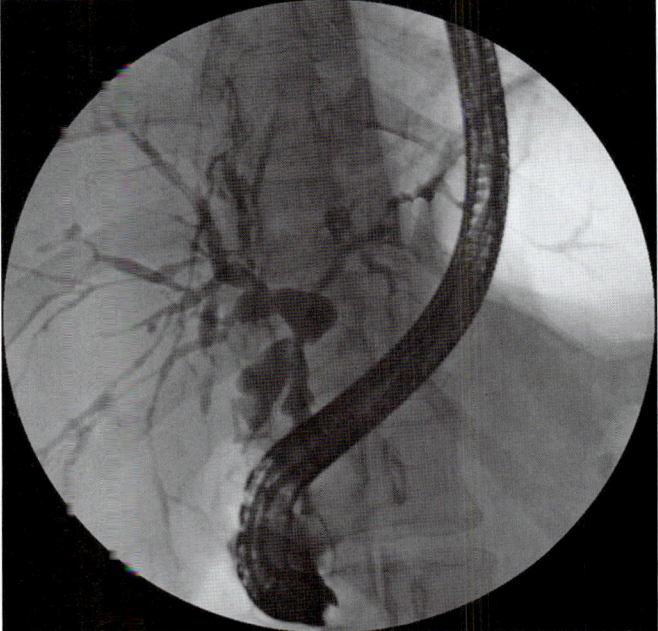

FIGURE 117.1 Endoscopic retrograde cholangiopancreatographic images depicting typical cholangiographic findings of primary sclerosing cholangitis.

ASSOCIATED INFLAMMATORY BOWEL DISEASE

IBD is seen in approximately 70% to 80% of patients with PSC and ulcerative colitis accounts for approximately 85% to 90% of these patients.[13] Usually, the diagnosis of IBD is established approximately 8 to 10 years before the diagnosis of PSC, although cases of IBD occurring years after the diagnosis of PSC have also been reported.[13] Conventional treatment of IBD does not alter the course of PSC, and severity of the former does not affect the disease seriousness of the latter. Proctocolectomy, the most aggressive treatment for CUC, has had no effect on PSC natural history. PSC patients with CUC have increased risk of colorectal dysplasia and neoplasia after OLT.[15] The increased neoplastic potential is of concern in PSC patients following OLT particularly because of the life-long immunosuppression that is required. Thus, in PSC patients who undergo OLT, annual colonoscopy with surveillance biopsies is recommended.

OVERLAP WITH AUTOIMMUNE HEPATITIS

PSC can coexist with AIH.[1] These patients typically fulfill definitive criteria for both diseases and have elevated serum alkaline phosphatase and aminotransferases, increased IgG, and antinuclear and/or anti–smooth muscle antibodies. Liver biopsy shows moderate to severe interface hepatitis with or without biliary destruction. Aminotransferase levels are higher than what one would expect for classic PSC. Patients with overlap syndrome may show improvement of AIH with immunosuppressive therapy. Indeed, patients who present with AIH and do not respond entirely to immunosuppressant therapy should be suspected of having concurrent PSC.

NONMALIGNANT COMPLICATIONS AND MANAGEMENT

CHOLELITHIASIS AND CHOLEDOCHOLITHIASIS

Twenty-five percent to 30% of PSC patients have or will develop calculi in the gallbladder or bile ducts during the course of the disease. In a study of 121 patients with PSC, 32 (26%) patients had gallstones, half of which were pigment stones, and 13 (15%) patients had PSC involving the gallbladder.[16]

Intrahepatic calculi are present in approximately 3% of PSC patients.[17] Biliary calculi can serve as a nidus for the development of bacterial cholangitis in these patients, although the latter is less common in the absence of dominant biliary strictures or prior bile duct surgery. Following diagnosis of bacterial cholangitis, ERCP is required to remove possible bile duct calculi, and/or to dilate biliary strictures allowing satisfactory bile drainage. Nevertheless, bacterial cholangitis can occur in PSC patients after ERCP. To prevent this complication, we suggest prophylactic coverage with intravenous antibiotics before and oral ciprofloxacin for 10 days after ERCP.

GALLBLADDER POLYPS

The risk of malignancy in PSC patients with gallbladder polyps is much higher than that for the general population. A study by Buckles et al. investigating 102 patients with PSC who underwent a cholecystectomy at the Mayo Clinic found that 13.7% of gallbladders contained polyps and 57% of those were malignant. In addition, they found presence of dysplasia in both adenomatous and malignant lesions, supporting the adenoma-carcinoma sequence. Most importantly, their study found no statistical difference between the size of benign and malignant lesions.[18] Based on studies such as this one in patients with PSC and the presence of a gallbladder polyp, cholecystectomy is indicated regardless of size.

PRURITUS

Patients with advanced-stage PSC frequently complain of intense pruritus. This distressing symptom can improve using various medical therapies.[19] Cholestyramine is a nonabsorbable resin that decreases the intestinal absorption of bile acids and alleviates pruritus; it is the standard of care. Phenobarbital has rarely been used in conjunction with cholestyramine to treat PSC patients with nocturnal pruritus. Ursodeoxycholic acid (UDCA) (i.e., ursodiol), a hydrophilic bile acid that likely replaces hydrophobic, toxic bile acids from the bile pool, may also improve pruritus in PSC patients. Antihistamines, such as hydroxyzine and diphenhydramine, have been used as supplements to cholestyramine or UDCA but are seldom effective because of their sedative properties. Rifampin may also improve pruritus, although its potential side effects (i.e., drug-induced hepatitis) make rifampin a second-line agent following cholestyramine for this upsetting symptom. In patients with PSC, opiate antagonists, such as naloxone, nalmefene, and naltrexone, have been used to alleviate pruritus but are fraught with psychiatric-type side effects. Molecular adsorbent recirculating system (MARS) (albumin liver dialysis) has been used in patients with acute and chronic liver failure and has been reported to abate cholestatic itch.[20]

DOMINANT BILIARY STRICTURES

Dominant biliary strictures are present in 20% to 45% of patients with PSC and cause an increased rate of jaundice, pruritus, right upper quadrant pain, and bacterial cholangitis. ERCP is required to assess the bile ducts, rule out the possibility of CCA, and allow therapeutic dilation with or without biliary stenting to relieve cholestasis. In the modern era, nontransplant surgical intervention for dominant strictures has largely been replaced with endoscopic management. The largest published nontransplant surgical experience in the management of patients with PSC investigated 146 patients with PSC. Fifty patients underwent resection of the extrahepatic biliary tract; 40 of these patients were noncirrhotic. Mean follow-up was 62 months. All patients had symptomatic biliary obstruction, and the primary indications for treatment were persistent jaundice and cholangitis. Operative mortality in patients with and without cirrhosis was 20% and 2.5%, respectively. Postoperative complications developed in 32% of patients, the most common being cholangitis.

The overall 1-, 3-, and 5-year survival rates after bile duct resection were 86%, 84%, and 76%, respectively; survival rates that are now surpassed by liver transplantation.[21]

Multiple studies have shown excellent results with endoscopic management of biliary strictures. A prospective study of 12 symptomatic PSC patients with major ductal strictures treated with repeated balloon dilation and nasobiliary catheter perfusion showed sustained improvement in eight patients following an average of three treatment sessions (mean follow-up, 23 months).[22] A retrospective study of 25 PSC patients with symptomatic dominant strictures reported that endoscopic stenting was technically successful in 21 (84%) patients and was associated with significant improvement of liver function tests. Moreover, 12 (57%) of the 21 PSC patients remained asymptomatic with stable liver biochemistries, whereas 4 (19%) patients had clinical and biochemical relapse over a median follow-up of 29 months. All four patients with relapse responded to additional endoscopic therapy.[23] The same authors reported 16 symptomatic PSC patients treated with short-term biliary stent placement (median duration only 9 days); 13 (81%) patients remained symptom-free and without biochemical evidence of cholestasis after a median follow-up of 19 months.[24] In spite of these studies, it is uncertain if dominant biliary strictures are directly accountable for cholestasis in PSC patients. The authors of a retrospective study of 125 patients with PSC reported that 56 (45%) patients had dominant biliary strictures defined by stenosis of the common bile duct to less than 1.5 mm in diameter and/or stenosis of the right or left hepatic duct to less than 1.0 mm. Of interest, between the 56 patients with and the 69 patients without dominant strictures, alkaline phosphatase and bilirubin levels were not significantly different up to 2 and 12 months after cholangiography.[25]

Endoscopic management should be the initial approach to patients with PSC and dominant strictures. When endoscopy fails, surgical interventions, such as extrahepatic biliary resection with transhepatic stenting, can be considered for noncirrhotic patients in centers with appropriate expertise.[21] In patients with end-stage PSC and advanced liver disease, liver transplantation should be considered the treatment of choice. However, all patients should be carefully assessed for CCA prior to transplantation.

DECOMPENSATED CIRRHOSIS AND PORTAL HYPERTENSION

Complications of decompensated cirrhosis and portal hypertension should be managed expectantly as in other end-stage liver diseases. As PSC progresses, the complications of end-stage liver disease become intractable and liver transplantation becomes the only effective cure.

ORTHOTOPIC LIVER TRANSPLANTATION

OLT remains the most effective treatment for PSC. At Mayo Clinic Rochester, 1- and 5-year survival rates for PSC patients following OLT are 95% and 86%, respectively. These rates compare favorably with results of OLT for other chronic liver diseases. Risk factors that adversely affect outcomes of patients who underwent OLT for PSC are divided into those that influence the general OLT outcome and those

specific for PSC.[26] The former include stay in the intensive care unit (ICU) or being on life support prior to OLT, age greater than 65 years old, poor nutritional status, Child-Pugh class C cirrhosis, and renal failure requiring dialysis prior to or after OLT. These factors are also predictive of increased operative blood loss, prolonged ICU stay, and major postoperative complications. Risk factors specific for PSC include disease severity, previous biliary or shunt surgery, coexistent CCA, and presence of IBD. Using the Mayo PSC natural history model as a measure of disease severity, survival following transplantation was higher than non-transplantation therapy for all stages of disease.[27] Thus earlier OLT has been advised for patients with PSC to improve both patient outcome and resource use.

Controversy exists on the impact of prior biliary surgery on OLT for PSC. There is little doubt that prior biliary surgery increases the technical difficulty of OLT, but it is unknown if this increased difficulty actually affects survival. In a combined series of 216 patients from the University of Pittsburgh and the Mayo Clinic, prior biliary tract and/or portal hypertensive surgery was associated with less favorable survival after OLT, but the difference in survival did not reach statistical significance.[27] In a study from the University of California at San Francisco, increased operative time and blood loss, but not mortality, were found in PSC patients with a history of prior colectomy or biliary surgery.[28] These reports suggest that prior biliary tract surgery increases the technical difficulty of OLT for PSC and is associated with a trend toward slightly increased mortality even when performed at large transplant centers.

Patients develop complications unique to PSC after liver transplantation. PSC patients have increased rates of biliary strictures occur due to PSC recurrence. However, not all biliary strictures represent PSC recurrence; other factors may cause biliary strictures, including ischemia related to chronic rejection or chronic bacterial cholangitis resulting from the Roux-en-Y anastomosis. The University of Pittsburgh found a significantly increased incidence of biliary strictures in allografts of patients transplanted for PSC versus patients who underwent OLT with choledocho-jejunostomy for non-PSC causes of end-stage liver disease.[29] Because cholangiographic, clinical, and biochemical criteria for recurrent disease have not been widely accepted, there is no consensus regarding the incidence of recurrent PSC in liver allografts. Nevertheless, careful analysis of a registry of transplanted PSC patients at our institution concluded that 20% of patients developed recurrent disease based on characteristic cholangiographic and histologic features.[30] Several transplant centers have reported increased incidence and severity of rejection in patients transplanted for PSC.[28] In a study of 100 consecutive PSC patients who underwent transplantation at Baylor University Medical Center, chronic rejection and disease recurrence occurred in 13% and 16% of patients, respectively, following OLT. These events adversely affected both graft and patient survival.[31] Five-year graft survival rates were 38% and 65% for patients with chronic rejection and disease recurrence, respectively, compared with 76% for patients free of chronic rejection or recurrence.

Because many patients with PSC have concurrent CUC, life-long immunosuppression after OLT may increase the risk and disease progression of colorectal carcinoma. In a study of 108 patients with PSC and concomitant IBD who underwent OLT, Loftus et al. reported a fourfold increase in colon carcinoma in the group that did not have a prior colectomy compared with the expected colon cancer rate in a group with comparable (pre-OLT) duration of IBD.[32] However this finding was not statistically significant and did not affect patient survival. Gos et al. also reported that posttransplant colectomy for dysplasia-carcinoma or symptomatic colitis does not affect PSC patient survival.[33] Given the lack of impact on patient survival, we do not recommend prophylactic proctocolectomy in PSC patients with IBD who undergo OLT. Nonetheless, the high risk of colonic neoplasia in transplanted PSC patients warrants annual surveillance colonoscopy with biopsies, and colectomy in cases in which low-grade dysplasia is detected.

Biliary reconstruction remains controversial for patients with PSC undergoing OLT. Two popular options are Roux-en-Y cauded-chojejunostomy and choledochocholedochostomy (a duct-to-duct anastomosis). Initial publications reported that Roux-en-Y reconstruction may reduce the incidence of postoperative stricture formation and improve patient and graft survival when compared with duct-to-duct anastomosis.[34] A more recent meta-analysis demonstrated no difference in 1-year recipient survival rates (odds ratio [OR], 1.02; 95% confidence interval [CI], 0.65 to 1.60; *P* = .95), 1-year graft survival rates (OR, 1.11; CI, 0.72 to 1.71; *P* = .64), risk of biliary leaks (OR, 1.25; CI, 0.59 to 2.59 *P* = .33), risk of biliary strictures (OR, 1.99; CI, 0.93 to 4.06; *P* = .06), or rate of recurrence of PSC (OR, 1.94 CI, 0.19 to 4.78; *P* = .94).[35] This study suggests that selected recipients with a disease-free common bile duct do quite well with a duct-to-duct anastomosis. Another option is choledochoduodenostomy. This anastomosis is more problematic if there were to be a leak after transplantation, but the advantages are that it avoids use of a potentially diseased common bile duct and does not require a bowel anastomosis (which is also subject to leaking or bleeding). We have reported excellent results in a limited number of PSC patients, and this anastomosis is now our preferred method for biliary reconstruction for PSC patients.[5]

SURGICAL MANAGEMENT OF ULCERATIVE COLITIS IN THE PRESENCE OF PRIMARY SCLEROSING CHOLANGITIS

The presence of PSC can influence the management of ulcerative colitis. The current indications for surgical intervention in this population are the same as for patients without PSC—medical failure to control severe symptoms or presence of colon dysplasia or neoplasia. Complications associated with surgical management of ulcerative colitis are highly affected by the degree of liver disease present at the time of surgery. The decision to perform Brooke ileostomy versus ileal pouch–anal anastomosis (IPAA) is greatly influenced by the presence of PSC. In a retrospective study of 72 patients with PSC and CUC treated with either Brooke ileostomy (*n* = 32) or IPAA (*n* = 40), 8 of 32 (25%) patients who underwent ileostomy developed peristomal varices and subsequent bleeding; however,

none of the 40 patients who underwent IPAA developed perianastomotic varices or perineal bleeding.[37] Of interest, the cumulative risk of pouchitis at 10 years after IPAA was 61% for patients with PSC and CUC, as compared with 36% for patients with CUC alone.[38] Therefore patients with PSC have increased risk of pouchitis if treated for CUC with IPAA. In our practice, we prefer IPAA and not Brooke ileostomy, because treating pouchitis is simpler than managing bleeding peristomal varices and has less of an impact on subsequent OLT.

MALIGNANT COMPLICATIONS AND MANAGEMENT

HILAR CHOLANGIOCARCINOMA

Patients with PSC have a 10% to 15% lifetime risk of developing CCA. The Mayo Clinic developed a novel therapeutic protocol combining neoadjuvant chemoradiation and OLT in 1993 to treat patients with unresectable hilar CCA or CCA arising in the setting of PSC. Initial publications following this protocol demonstrated 5-year survival rates of 82%.[39] Since that time, other centers have replicated these results, making this an established standard of care at select centers.[40]

Liver transplantation for patients with CCA arising in the setting of PSC fare significantly better than patients with de novo CCA, both for survival after initiation of neoadjuvant therapy and survival after OLT.[41] PSC patients have underlying liver disease, multiple strictures, and often undergo endoscopic cholangiography for evaluation of jaundice or treatment of cholangitis. Therefore the PSC patients are more likely to have detection of CCA earlier in the course of the malignancy than patients with de novo CCA. Underlying liver disease and the potential for tumor multicentricity often preclude liver resection in patients with PSC and hilar CCA; these patients are best treated with neoadjuvant therapy and OLT. Patients with PSC meeting the entry criteria for the Mayo protocol should undergo liver transplantation.

As of March 2016 Mayo Clinic Rochester had entered 283 patients with hilar CCA into their neoadjuvant therapy protocol. Five-year survival following initiation of neoadjuvant therapy was 60% ± 4% for 171 patients with underlying PSC and 37% ± 5% for 112 patients with CCA arising de novo; 181 patients ultimately underwent liver transplantation (PSC, *n* = 113; de novo, *n* = 68). Patient survival at 5 years for patients with underlying PSC was 77% ± 4% and 56% ± 7% with CCA arising de novo.

BRUSH CYTOLOGY FOR HILAR STRICTURES SUSPICIOUS FOR CHOLANGIOCARCINOMA

Brush cytology of strictures, obtained at ERCP, has a specificity approaching 97% to 100% in most studies (with the exception of one[42]), but sensitivity varies. Repeated brushings can improve the sensitivity[43] and are highly recommended when the obtained material proves suspect or negative in the presence of high clinical suspicion. Fluorescence in situ hybridization (FISH) assay is a technique that uses four fluorescently labeled DNA probes, hybridized to the centromere of chromosomes 3, 7, and 17 and to the p16 gene on chromosome 9 (9p21), to detect chromosomal aberrations in the brushed cholangiocytes. The sensitivity of FISH for the detection of malignant strictures was significantly higher (34%) compared with that of cytology (15%; $P < .01$), but the diagnostic specificity of FISH and cytology was comparable, at 97% and 98%, respectively.

Percutaneous or transperitoneal biopsy of the tumor mass is an absolute contraindication for transplantation due to a high rate of seeding and recurrence after transplantation.[45] Thus endoscopic ultrasound or percutaneous biopsy of the primary tumor should not be done unless transplantation has been ruled out as a treatment option. Patients with suspected CCA arising in PSC should be referred to a transplant center with experience in the diagnosis and treatment—including transplantation—for this disease.

INTRAHEPATIC CHOLANGIOCARCINOMA

The annualized cumulative risk of CCA is 1.5% per year.[46] Intrahepatic cholangiocarcinoma (ICC) often develops two to three decades earlier in patients with PSC than in those with sporadic tumors.[47] Liver resection for ICC is often limited by amount of underlying liver disease secondary to PSC. An R0 resection must be performed to achieve a survival benefit. Although there are no size criteria for what constitutes resectable disease, a clear 1-cm margin with a well-vascularized remnant and adequate venous and biliary drainage is required for success. Resection may be considered in the setting of regional lymph node metastases, but stability of disease with neoadjuvant therapy should be considered due to the poor prognosis associated with nodal metastases. Liver resection is usually limited to patients with Child A liver disease. Multifocal intrahepatic tumors and metastatic disease to distant sites are generally considered contraindications to resection.

Incidental CCA in explanted livers following transplantation for PSC has been reported to be as high as 8%.[33] In addition, small intrahepatic CCA can masquerade as hepatocellular carcinoma (HCC) in patients with cirrhosis, including patients with PSC. Transplantation for ICC less than 2 cm has been associated with survival comparable to that achieved for patients with small HCC. A Spanish multicenter study followed eight patients with "very early" ICC, including four incidental tumors, who experienced excellent 5-year survival, at 73% without tumor recurrence.[48] In another study, 10 patients with small incidental ICC less than 1 cm in diameter did not experience tumor recurrence and had a 5-year survival rate of 83%.[33]

Larger intrahepatic CCA is considered to be an absolute contraindication to transplantation outside of established research protocols. A single-center experience examining OLT for known ICC as part of a research protocol in 25 patients has previously been published. In this study the 5-year disease-free patient survival was 47%.[49] Despite this being shown to be superior to surgical resection, it is substantially lower than the 70% 5-year threshold needed to justify the usage of scarce deceased donor livers.

HEPATOCELLULAR CARCINOMA

PSC patients with end-stage disease are at risk of developing HCC. Although the true incidence of HCC for PSC cirrhotics has not been well studied, a previous study based

on liver explant pathology showed an increased incidence for HCC in patients with PSC.[50] HCC was identified in 3 (2% of 134 PSC patients who underwent transplantation.[50] PSC patients with cirrhosis and HCC should be referred for liver transplantation according to established transplant criteria, such as the Milan criteria, which are widely adopted in North America and Europe (a single lesion ≤5 cm or up to three lesions, none larger than 3 cm).[51]

MIXED HEPATOCELLULAR CARCINOMA AND CHOLANGIOCARCINOMA

Combined HCC and cholangiocarcinoma (cHCC-CCA) is an uncommon form of primary liver cancer containing components of both HCC and IHC. The traditional classification includes double tumor, combined type, and mixed type.[52] The reported prognosis after resection for cHCC-CCA tumors was similar to that of IHC and poorer than that of HCC.[53] Surgical resection for cHCC-CCA should follow similar principles to resection in the setting of ICC.

The presence of a mixed HCC-CCA tumor is a contraindication to liver transplantation; however, on occasion, misdiagnosis may lead to its identification on explanted livers. Review of the United Network for Organ Sharing database identified 2% of patients having mixed HCC-CCA had a diagnosis of PSC.[54]

GALLBLADDER MALIGNANCY

The prevalence of gallbladder carcinoma (GBC) in patients with PSC is estimated at 3% to 14%. PSC patients are predisposed to gallbladder abnormalities, including gallstones, inflammation, and malignancies.[16,18] Males represent greater than 60% of those with GBC among PSC patients.[55] Patients with PSC and GBC tend to be younger than GBC patients without PSC; 70% of PSC/GBC patients are less than 60 years of age, with a median age at diagnosis of 58 versus median age of 70 years in the general population.[56] In a study of 121 PSC patients, 41% had one or more abnormal gallbladder findings—gallstones in 26%, probable PSC involving the gallbladder in 15%, and benign or malignant neoplasms in 4%.[16] Another study of 286 PSC patients reported similar findings.[57] Of note, 56% (10 of 18) of the mass lesions proved to be a gallbladder carcinoma. In gallbladders from 102 PSC patients, a high prevalence (8 of 14; 57%) of carcinomas in polyps was also found.[18] The risk of malignant transformation of the gallbladder epithelium in PSC may be related to a neoplastic "field effect" along the entire biliary tree. Based on this high risk of malignancies in gallbladder polyps in PSC, it has been recommended that patients are followed with regular ultrasound of the gallbladder and that cholecystectomy is carried out for all polyps, even if a mass lesion is less than 1 cm in diameter.[57,58]

LIVER RESECTION IN PATIENTS WITH UNDERLYING LIVER DISEASE SECONDARY TO PRIMARY SCLEROSING CHOLANGITIS

Underlying liver disease secondary to PSC can present major obstacles to liver resection. Major resection is generally limited to patients with no more than Child-Turcotte-Pugh (CTP) Class A liver disease. Limited resection of small superficial tumors can sometimes be considered in Child class B, whereas Child class C is generally a contraindication to resection. Previous authors have shown that in patients with cirrhosis undergoing resection, Model for End-Stage Liver Disease (MELD) score less than or equal to 8 was associated with no perioperative mortality versus 29% for patients with a MELD score greater than or equal to 9 ($P < .01$).[59]

Assessment of the volume of the liver remnant is important in patients with underlying liver disease secondary to PSC. In general, a remnant liver volume of 40% to 50% of the total liver volume is a minimum for considering resection.[60] Such techniques as portal vein embolization can be used prior to surgery to achieve contralateral liver hypertrophy. Although the associating liver partition and portal vein ligation for staged hepatectomy (ALPPS) procedure has gained significant interest in future liver remnant growth, high rates of morbidity secondary to sepsis in the setting of biliary pathology make it a poor choice for patients undergoing resection in the setting of PSC.[61]

Postoperative biliary fistula is also a major concern in patients with intrahepatic or extrahepatic biliary strictures. Unlike biliary fistula in the non-PSC setting, these fistulas often persist indefinitely due to distal obstruction.

REFERENCES

1. Chapman R, Fevery J, Kalloo A, et al. Diagnosis and management of primary sclerosing cholangitis. *Hepatology*. 2010;51:660.
2. Bambha K, Kim WR, Talwalkar J, et al. Incidence, clinical spectrum, and outcomes of primary sclerosing cholangitis in a United States community. *Gastroenterology*. 2003;125:1364.
3. van Erpecum KJ, Smits SJ, van de Meeberg PC, et al. Risk of primary sclerosing cholangitis is associated with nonsmoking behavior. *Gastroenterology*. 1996;110:1503.
4. Loftus EV Jr, Sandborn WJ, Tremaine WJ, et al. Primary sclerosing cholangitis is associated with nonsmoking: a case-control study. *Gastroenterology*. 1996;110:1496.
5. Florin TH, Pandeya N, Radford-Smith GL. Epidemiology of appendicectomy in primary sclerosing cholangitis and ulcerative colitis: its influence on the clinical behaviour of these diseases. *Gut*. 2004;53:973.
6. Feldstein AE, Perrault J, El-Youssif M, Lindor KD, Freese DK, Angulo P. Primary sclerosing cholangitis in children: a long-term follow-up study. *Hepatology*. 2003;38:210.
7. Burak KW, Angulo P, Lindor KD. Is there a role for liver biopsy in primary sclerosing cholangitis? *Am J Gastroenterol*. 2003;98:1155.
8. Bjornsson E, Olsson R, Bergquist A, et al. The natural history of small-duct primary sclerosing cholangitis. *Gastroenterology*. 2008;134:975.
9. Ludwig J, Dickson ER, McDonald GS. Staging of chronic nonsuppurative destructive cholangitis (syndrome of primary biliary cirrhosis). *Virchows Arch A Pathol Anat Histol*. 1978;379:103-112.
10. Talwalkar JA, Angulo P, Johnson CD, Petersen BT, Lindor KD. Cost-minimization analysis of MRC versus ERCP for the diagnosis of primary sclerosing cholangitis. *Hepatology*. 2004;40:39.
11. Caldwell SH, Hespenheide EE, Harris D, de Lange EE. Imaging and clinical characteristics of focal atrophy of segments 2 and 3 in primary sclerosing cholangitis. *J Gastroenterol Hepatol*. 2001;16:220.
12. Campbell WL, Peterson MS, Federle MP, et al. Using CT and cholangiography to diagnose biliary tract carcinoma complicating primary sclerosing cholangitis. *AJR Am J Roentgenol*. 2001;177:1095.
13. Loftus EV Jr, Sandborn WJ, Lindor KD, Larusso NF. Interactions between chronic liver disease and inflammatory bowel disease. *Inflamm Bowel Dis*. 1997;3(4):288-302.
14. Cangemi JR, Wiesner RH, Beaver SJ, et al. Effect of proctocolectomy for chronic ulcerative colitis on the natural history of primary sclerosing cholangitis. *Gastroenterology*. 1989;96:790.
15. Bleday R, Lee E, Jessurun J, Heine J, Wong WD. Increased risk of early colorectal neoplasms after hepatic transplant in patients with inflammatory bowel disease. *Dis Colon Rectum*. 1993;36:908.
16. Brandt DJ, MacCarty RL, Charboneau JW, LaRusso NF, Wiesner RH, Ludwig J. Gallbladder disease in patients with primary sclerosing cholangitis. *AJR Am J Roentgenol*. 1988;150:571-574.
17. Dodd GD 3rd, Niedzwiecki GA, Campbell WL, Baron RL. Bile duct calculi in patients with primary sclerosing cholangitis. *Radiology*. 1997;203:443.
18. Buckles DC, Lindor KD, Larusso NF, Petrovic LM, Gores GJ. In primary sclerosing cholangitis, gallbladder polyps are frequently malignant. *Am J Gastroenterol*. 2002;97(5):1138-1142.
19. Bergasa NV. An approach to the management of the pruritus of cholestasis. *Clin Liver Dis*. 2004;8:55.
20. Steiner C, Mitzner S. Experiences with MARS liver support therapy in liver failure: analysis of 176 patients of the International MARS Registry. *Liver*. 2002;22(suppl 2):20-25.
21. Ahrendt SA. Surgical approaches to strictures in primary sclerosing cholangitis. *J Gastrointest Surg*. 2008;12:423-425.
22. Wagner S, Gebel M, Meier P, et al. Endoscopic management of biliary tract strictures in primary sclerosing cholangitis. *Endoscopy*. 1996;28:546.
23. van Milligen de Wit AW, van Bracht J, Rauws EA, Jones EA, Tytgat GN, Huibregtse K. Endoscopic stent therapy for dominant extrahepatic bile duct strictures in primary sclerosing cholangitis. *Gastrointest Endosc*. 1996;44:293.
24. Marc van Milligen de Wit AW, van Bracht J, Rauws EAJ, et al. Lack of complications following short-term stent therapy for extrahepatic bile duct strictures in primary sclerosing cholangitis. *Gastrointest Endosc*. 1997;46:344.
25. Bjornsson E, Lindqvist-Ottosson J, Asztely M, Olsson R. Dominant strictures in patients with primary sclerosing cholangitis. *Am J Gastroenterol*. 2004;99:502.
26. Wiesner RH, Porayko MK, Hay JE, et al. Liver transplantation for primary sclerosing cholangitis: impact of risk factors on outcome. *Liver Transpl Surg*. 1996;2:99.
27. Abu-Elmagd KM, Malinchoc M, Dickson ER, et al. Efficacy of hepatic transplantation in patients with primary sclerosing cholangitis. *Surg Gynecol Obstet*. 1993;177:335.
28. Narumi S, Roberts JP, Emond JC, Lake J, Ascher NL. Liver transplantation for sclerosing cholangitis. *Hepatology*. 1995;22:451.
29. Sheng R, Zajko AB, Campbell WL, Abu-Elmagd K. Biliary strictures in hepatic transplants: prevalence and types in patients with primary sclerosing cholangitis vs those with other liver diseases. *AJR Am J Roentgenol*. 1993;161:297.
30. Graziadei IW, Wiesner RH, Marotta PJ, et al. Long-term results of patients undergoing liver transplantation for primary sclerosing cholangitis. *Hepatology*. 1999;30:1121.
31. Jeyarajah DR, Netto GJ, Lee SP, et al. Recurrent primary sclerosing cholangitis after orthotopic liver transplantation: is chronic rejection part of the disease process? *Transplantation*. 1998;66:1300.
32. Loftus EV Jr, Aguilar HI, Sandborn WJ, et al. Risk of colorectal neoplasia in patients with primary sclerosing cholangitis and ulcerative colitis following orthotopic liver transplantation. *Hepatology*. 1998;27:685.
33. Goss JA, Shackleton CR, Farmer DG, et al. Orthotopic liver transplantation for primary sclerosing cholangitis. A 12-year single center experience. *Ann Surg*. 1997;225:472; discussion 481.
34. Welsh FK, Wigmore SJ. Roux-en-Y choledochojejunostomy is the method of choice for biliary reconstruction in liver transplantation for primary sclerosing cholangitis. *Transplantation*. 2004;77(4):502-604.
35. Wells MM, Croome KP, Boyce E, Chandok N. Roux-en-Y choledochojejunostomy versus duct-to-duct biliary anastomosis in liver transplantation for primary sclerosing cholangitis: a meta-analysis. *Transplant Proc*. 2013;45(6):2263-2271.
36. Peacock J, Heimbach J, Nyberg S, Rosen C. Choledochoduodenostomy is an excellent alternative to Roux Y choledochojejunostomy. *HPB (Oxford)*. 2012;14(suppl 2):187.
37. Kartheuser AH, Dozois RR, LaRusso NF, Wiesner RH, Ilstrup DM, Schleck CD. Comparison of surgical treatment of ulcerative colitis associated with primary sclerosing cholangitis: ileal pouch-anal anastomosis versus Brooke ileostomy. *Mayo Clin Proc*. 1996;71:748.
38. Penna C, Dozois R, Tremaine W, et al. Pouchitis after ileal pouch-anal anastomosis for ulcerative colitis occurs with increased frequency in patients with associated primary sclerosing cholangitis. *Gut*. 1996;38:234.

39. Rea DJ, Heimbach JK, Rosen CB, et al. Liver transplantation with neoadjuvant chemoradiation is more effective than resection for hilar cholangiocarcinoma. *Ann Surg* 2005;242(3):451-458; discussion 458-461.

40. Darwish Murad S, Kim WR, Harnois DM, et al. Efficacy of neoadjuvant chemoradiation, followed by liver transplantation, for perihilar cholangiocarcinoma at 12 US centers. *Gastroenterology*. 2012;143(1): 88-98.e3; quiz e14.

41. Croome KP, Rosen CB, Heimbach JK, Nagorney DM. Is liver transplantation appropriate for patients with potentially resectable de novo hilar cholangiocarcinoma? *J Am Coll Surg*. 2015;221(1):130-139.

42. Ponsioen CY, Vrouenraets SM, van Milligen de Wit AW, et al. Value of brush cytology for dominant strictures in primary sclerosing cholangitis. *Endoscopy*. 1999;31:305-309.

43. Rabinovitz M, Zajko AB, Hassanein T, et al. Diagnostic value of brush cytology in the diagnosis of bile duct carcinoma: a study in 65 patients with bile duct strictures. *Hepatology*. 1990;12:747-752.

44. Kipp BR, Stadheim LM, Halling SA, et al. A comparison of routine cytology and fluorescence in situ hybridization for the detection of malignant bile duct strictures. *Am J Gastroenterol*. 2004;99:1675-1681.

45. Heimbach JK, Sanchez W, Rosen CB, Gores GJ. Trans-peritoneal fine needle aspiration biopsy of hilar cholangiocarcinoma is associated with disease dissemination. *HPB (Oxford)*. 2011;13(5):356-360. doi: 10.1111/j.1477-2574.2011.00298.x.

46. Farrant JM, Hayllar KM, Wilkinson ML, et al. Natural history and prognostic variables in primary sclerosing cholangitis. *Gastroenterology*. 1991;100(6):1710-1717.

47. Bergquist A, Said K, Broomé U. Changes over a 20-year period in the clinical presentation of primary sclerosing cholangitis in Sweden. *Scand J Gastroenterol*. 2007;42:88-93.

48. Sapisochin G, Rodríguez de Lope C, Gastaca M, et al. "Very early" intrahepatic cholangiocarcinoma in cirrhotic patients: should liver transplantation be reconsidered in these patients? *Am J Transplant*. 2014;14:660-667.

49. Hong JC, Jones CM, Duffy JP, et al. Comparative analysis of resection and liver transplantation for intrahepatic and hilar cholangiocarcinoma: a 24-year experience in a single center. *Arch Surg*. 2011;146: 683-689.

50. Harnois DM, Gores GJ, Ludwig J, Steers JL, LaRusso NF, Wiesner RH. Are patients with cirrhotic stage primary sclerosing cholangitis at risk for the development of hepatocellular cancer? *J Hepatol*. 1997;27:512-516.

51. Mazzaferro V, Regalia E, Doci R, et al. Liver transplantation for the treatment of small hepatocellular carcinomas in patients with cirrhosis. *N Engl J Med*. 1996;334(11):693-699.

52. Allen RA, Lisa JR. Combined liver cell and bile duct carcinoma. *Am J Pathol*. 1949;25:647-655.

53. Chu KJ, Lu CD, Dong H, Fu XH, Zhang HW, Yao XP. Hepatitis B virus-related combined hepatocellular-cholangiocarcinoma: clinicopathological and prognostic analysis of 390 cases. *Eur J Gastroenterol Hepatol*. 2014;26:192-199.

54. Vilchez V, Shah MB, Daily MF, et al. Long-term outcome of patients undergoing liver transplantation for mixed hepatocellular carcinoma and cholangiocarcinoma: an analysis of the UNOS database. *HPB (Oxford)*. 2016;18(1):29-34.

55. Lazcano-Ponce EC, Miquel JF, Muñoz N, et al. Review epidemiology and molecular pathology of gallbladder cancer. *CA Cancer J Clin*. 2001;51(6):349-364.

56. Malik IA. Gallbladder cancer: current status. *Expert Opin Pharmacother*. 2004;5(6):1271-1277.

57. Said K, Glaumann H, Bergquist A. Gallbladder disease in patients with primary sclerosing cholangitis. *J Hepatol*. 2008;48(4):598-605. doi:10.1016/j.jhep.2007.11.019.

58. Lewis JT, Talwalkar JA, Rosen CB, Smyrk TC, Abraham SC. Prevalence and risk factors for gallbladder neoplasia in patients with primary sclerosing cholangitis: evidence for a metaplasia–dysplasia–carcinoma sequence. *Am J Surg Pathol*. 2007;31:907-913.

59. Teh SH, Christein J, Donohue J, et al. Hepatic resection of hepatocellular carcinoma in patients with cirrhosis: Model of End-Stage Liver Disease (MELD) score predicts perioperative mortality. *J Gastrointest Surg*. 2005;9(9):1207-1215; discussion 1215.

60. Azoulay D, Castaing D, Krissat J, et al. Percutaneous portal vein embolization increases the feasibility and safety of major liver resection for hepatocellular carcinoma in injured liver. *Ann Surg*. 2000;232(5):665-672.

61. Schadde E, Ardiles V, Slankamenac K, et al. ALPPS offers a better chance of complete resection in patients with primarily unresectable liver tumors compared with conventional-staged hepatectomies: results of a multicenter analysis. *World J Surg*. 2014;38(6):1510-1519.

CHAPTER

118

Anatomy and Physiology of the Liver

Adam S. Bodzin | Talia B. Baker

Our understanding of functional surgical hepatic anatomy evolved significantly through technical advances in repair of hepatobiliary injury, liver transplantation, hepatic resection, and radiologically guided intervention. This evolution was essential to the development of live-donor and deceased-donor segmental liver transplantation.[1-3] Molmenti described this reconception of hepatic anatomy as derived from an anatomic-physiologic inside-out approach, as opposed to the purely topographic outside-in view of the past (Fig. 118.1).[2]

Human anatomy may be classified and is classifiable, but variation is the rule. This chapter reviews basic concepts of hepatic anatomy, with the important caveat that these simple concepts will not always hold true in all circumstances. There are now tools that allow the individual anatomy of the subject to be outlined preoperatively and intraoperatively in cases such as hepatic resection or live liver donation.

MODERN ANATOMIC APPROACH TO LIVER SURGERY

The liver is a single organ that can be functionally regarded as two hemilivers. The parenchyma can be further subdivided into several regions sharing common arterial, portal, and biliary supply and venous drainage. The portal and venous systems define these regions that are named sectors and segments, respectively (Figs. 118.2–118.5).[2-5] The liver has a rather constant anatomic pattern, the knowledge of which allows for a safe surgical approach. Nevertheless, there are some anatomic irregularities, and in particular instances, exact knowledge of the anatomy specific to the individual patient being examined or operated on is necessary (live donors, left extended or central hepatectomies, caudate lobe masses). In these cases a computed three-dimensional reconstruction of each anatomic detail is possible following an accurate computed tomographic or magnetic resonance imaging contrast scan. Several software packages are currently available that allow for the mapping of the individual anatomy, as well as for the calculation of volumes corresponding to the whole liver, liver sectors, and segments (Hepavision, DeVis-Germany Hitachi-Japan, Hepavis-Slovenia, Université de Strasbourg-France). The reliability of virtual three-dimensional reconstructions based on standard anatomic landmarks for both surgical planning and graft volume calculations has been demonstrated (Fig. 118.6).[7] For standard liver surgery, the operating surgeon should be familiar with the basic anatomic pattern of the liver and the most frequent variations that have been described.

EMBRYOLOGY OF THE LIVER

The liver primordium, also known as *diverticulum hepatis* or *liver bud*, arises from endoderm in weeks 3 through 4 of embryologic development and invades the septum transversum, vitelline (omphalomesenteric) veins, and umbilical veins. Its connection to the embryologic duodenum (foregut) will eventually become the bile duct.[8,9] Embryologically the liver receives blood from both portal and umbilical veins, themselves connected by the left portal vein.[10,11] Although the primitive portal veins arise from the caudal part of the vitelline veins, the primitive hepatic veins arise from the cranial part of the vitelline veins.[8,12] In humans and many other mammals the inferior vena cava (IVC), ductus venosus, and umbilical vein are initially surrounded by liver parenchyma and become extrahepatic only in later stages of embryologic development.[11] The arteries develop in conjunction with the bile ducts at a later period than the veins. On the right side, arteries and bile ducts follow the trajectory of the portal venous branches. On the left side, although arterial and biliary branching follows a symmetric pattern similar to that of the right side, the portal vein branches do not.[12] During early stages of development, there are three hepatic arteries: (1) a left hepatic artery arising from the left gastric artery, (2) a middle hepatic artery arising from the celiac trunk, and (3) a right hepatic artery arising from the superior mesenteric artery. Although in most cases the middle artery is the only one that persists, variations in regression and origin of these three early arteries account for the so-called accessory and replaced variants.[11] A complete ductal system is present by the 10th week of intrauterine life.[9,11] The mesoderm of the septum between liver and abdominal wall develops into the *falciform ligament*. The surface of the developing liver in contact with the diaphragm is devoid of peritoneum, and the so-called bare area is a reminder of such association.[8,9] By week 10 of development, the liver is involved in hematopoietic

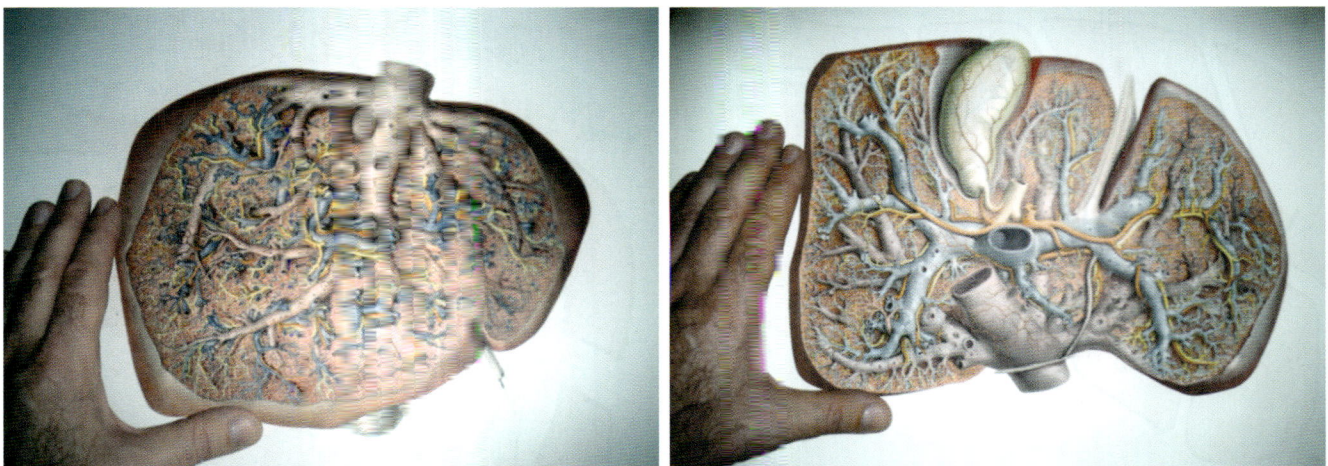

FIGURE 118.1 Classic depictions of the liver anatomy. (From Bourgery JM, Jacob NH. Traité Complet de L'anatomie de L'homme. In: Delaunay CA, ed. *Tome Cinquième*. Paris: CA Delaunay (Éditeur); 1839. [Private collection of Ernesto P. Molmenti, MD, PhD, MBA.])

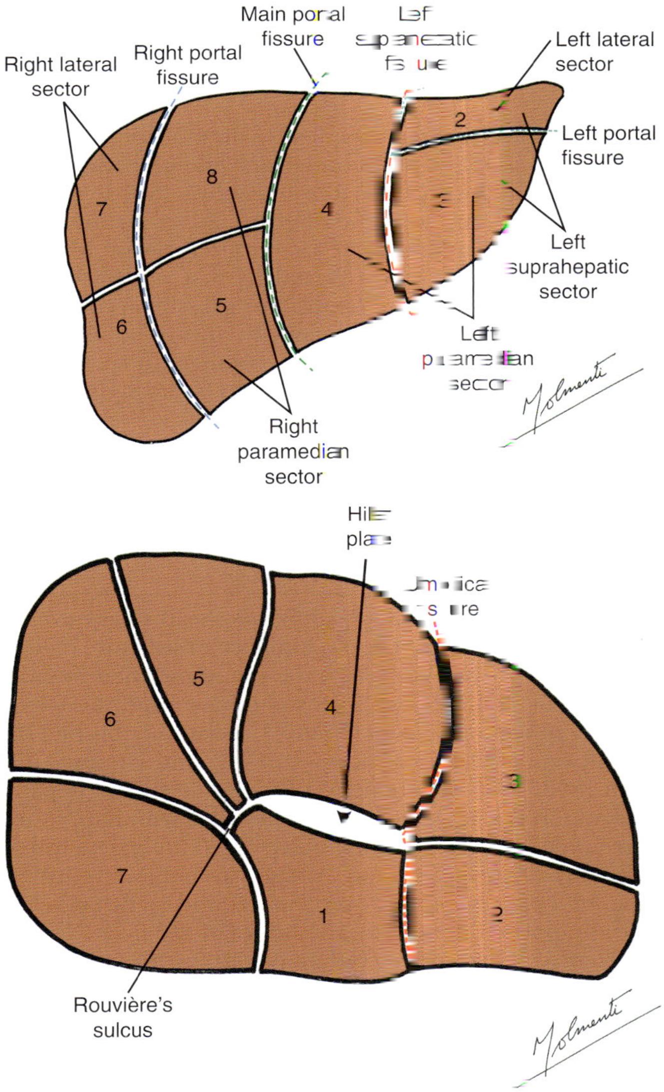

FIGURE 118.2 Schematic representation of the liver anatomy. The hepatic segments have been numbered and the major structures have been labeled.

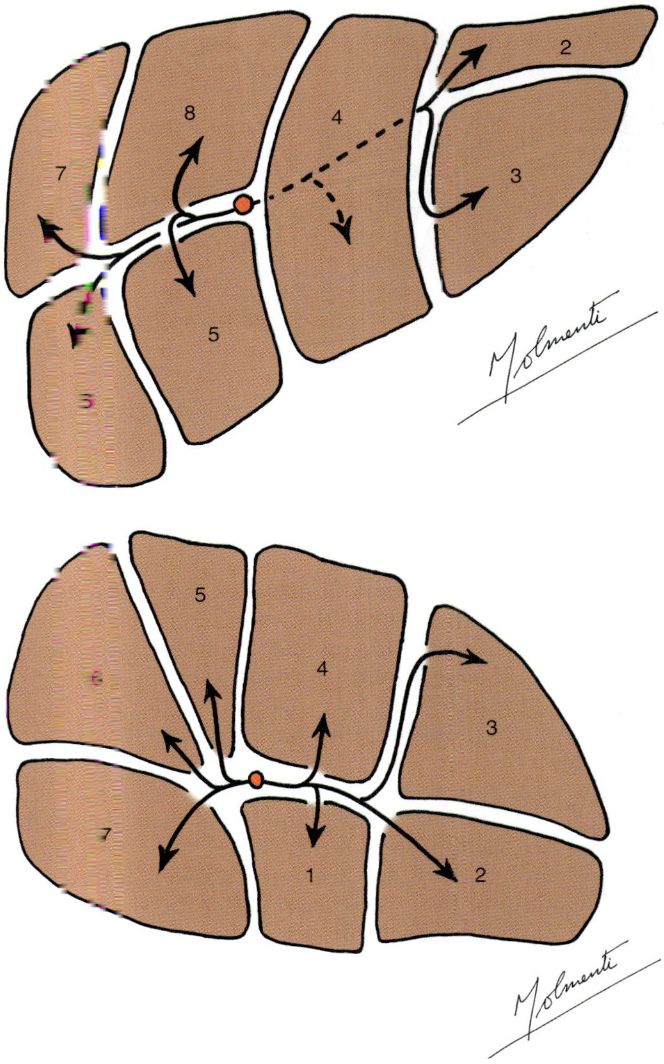

FIGURE 118.3 Schematic representation of the arteriobiliary liver anatomy.

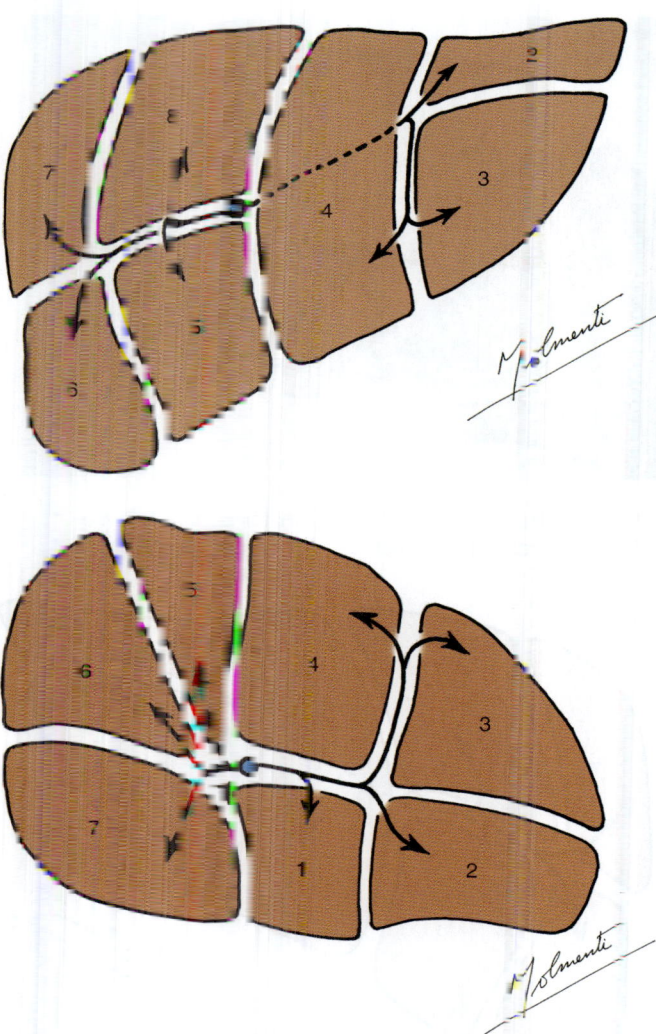

FIGURE 118.4 Schematic representation of the portal venous liver anatomy.

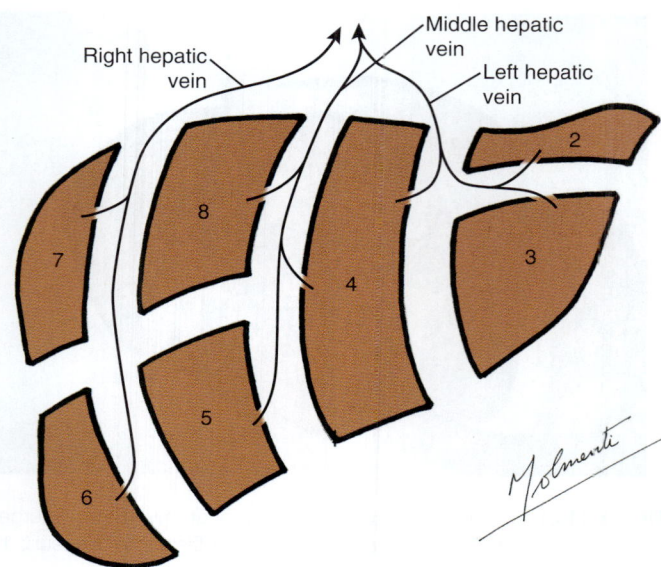

FIGURE 118.5 Schematic representation of the hepatic venous liver anatomy.

function, an activity that diminishes markedly during gestational months 8 and 9.[8] By week 12 of development, the liver is already producing bile.[8] However, hepatocytes only attain single-cell plate configuration by the age of 5 years.[12] Several events take place at birth. The *ductus venosus*, which optimized venous return from the placenta to the fetus by connecting the left umbilical and common hepatic vein crosses and becomes the *ligamentum venosus*. Also at birth, the *extrahepatic* umbilical vein closes and becomes the *ligamentum teres*.[12]

True anomalies of the liver are relatively infrequent. Prolongations of liver tissue from either the right (Riedel lobe) or left lobe usually present as incidental abdominal masses. In other instances, hepatic tissue connected by an isthmus to the liver is found in the chest. Small accessory collections of tissue attached to the liver by a pedicle are also occasionally encountered.[9]

HEPATIC DIVISIONS

Several nomenclatures and topographic divisions have been proposed. According to Couinaud, the right

and left hemilivers are supplied by first-order branches. Sectors are supplied by second-order branches. Segments are supplied by third-order branches. Subsegments are supplied by fourth-order or other branches.[11] Segments are numbered in a counterclockwise fashion, from I to VIII.[11] A main portal fissure, a right portal fissure, and a left portal fissure are grossly or conceptually defined because they may not always be anatomically present.[11,12] Left and right paramedian sectors are adjacent to the main portal fissure. Left and right lateral sectors are located on the outer side of the corresponding paramedian ones (see Figs. 118.2–118.5).[2–5,11] During our discussion, we follow this nomenclature with some modifications.[11,12]

VASCULOBILIARY SHEATHS

Couinaud referred to the vasculobiliary sheaths that envelop the portal elements as "the most important structure of liver anatomy."[11,14] They seem to have been described initially by Walaeus in 1640, and thus some have used the terms *walaean pedicles* or *walaean sheaths*.[11,15] Glisson published his description of the liver "tunic" in 1642, and Laennec did so in 1803.[11,16,17] The elements of the *portal pedicle* (hepatic artery, portal vein, bile ducts, nerves, and lymphatics) are surrounded throughout their trajectory to the parenchymal plates by connective tissue. Not so the hepatic veins.[11,18] The *hilar plate* is located over the left and right pedicles, and the portal division, on the hilum of the liver.[11,18] The *umbilical plate* is found in continuity with the hilar plate and the round ligament, covering the left paramedian pedicle in its upper surface.[11] According to Couinaud and others, dissection of the hilar plate allows for the detachment of the hilar contents.[1,2,11,18] Exposure of the umbilical plate is the gateway to the segmental and sectoral pedicles of the left liver. Because dissection at the level of the plates can lead to complications, an approach to the sheaths is recommended.[11] This strategy has been applied by

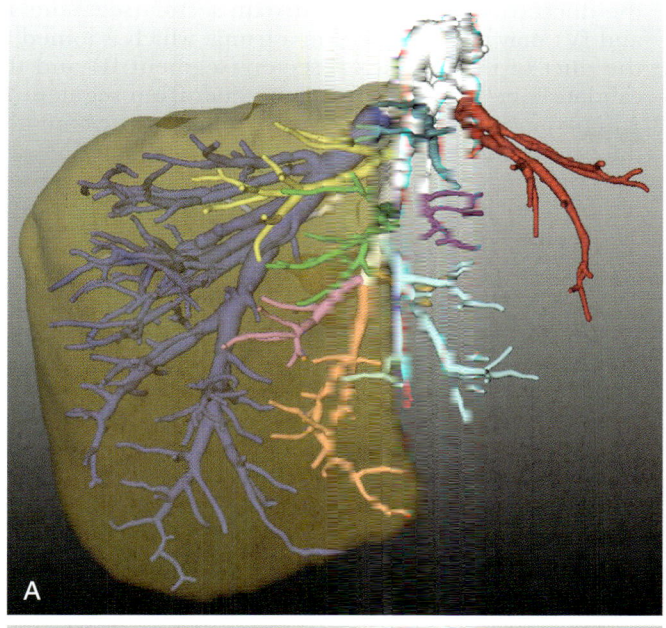

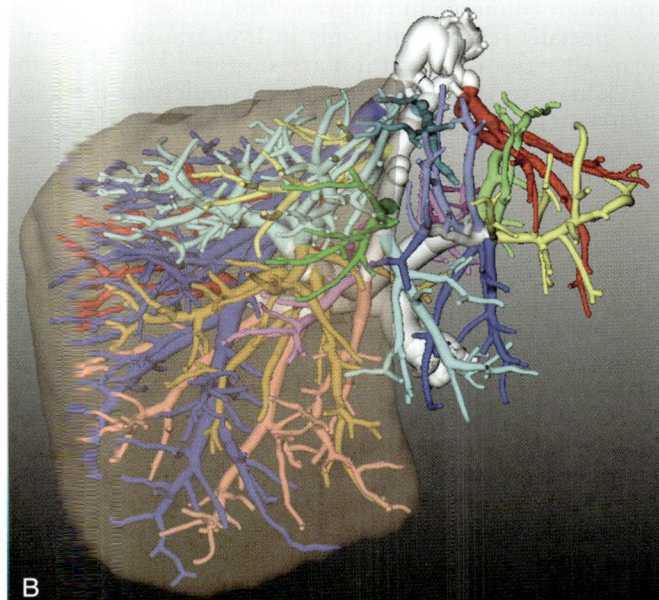

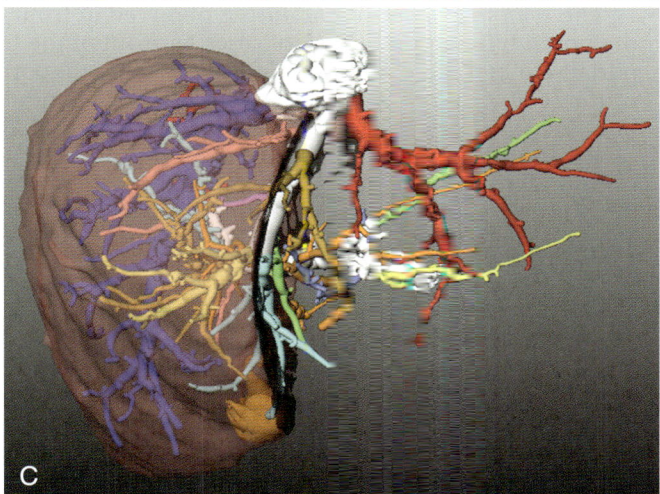

FIGURE 118.6 Virtual three-dimensional reconstruction of the liver anatomy by means of Hepavision, MeVis-Germany software. The right lobe has been reconstructed in a virtual fashion, together with the hepatic veins (A), hepatic veins and portal veins (B), and hepatic veins and biliary system (C).

Lazorthes et al. in the so-called suprahilar approach for anatomic hepatectomies and segmentectomies.[19] Sheaths originate at the right edge of the hilum, at the umbilical plate, and at the posterior margin of the hilar plate. From these sites they will reach the right over the left liver, and the caudate area, respectively.[11] In cases of narrow hila or hila of difficult access, consideration should be given to dividing the anterior portion of the main portal fissure. This maneuver does not damage any structures of significance and allows better exposure of the hilar elements.[11]

Couinaud recognized the following three types of approaches to a portal pedicle:

1. Intrafascial—dissection within the sheath, where the elements are identified
2. Extrafascial—dissection around the pedicle sheath
3. Extrafascial and transfissural—dissection of the sheaths at their origin from the hilar and umbilical plates (considered the safest approach, especially for second- and third-order branches)

ARTERIAL AND BILIARY SYSTEMS

According to Couinaud and Houssin, the most frequent arterial and biliary configurations, accounting for almost 90% of cases in their series, are the following[20]:

- A unique artery and bile duct on right and left (24%)
- Two right bile ducts (17%)
- Two left arteries (26%)
- Two right ducts and two left arteries (22%)

Bile ducts are usually located above the portal branches and arteries below the corresponding veins.[18] The bile ducts derive their blood supply predominantly from arterial branches.[11,13] However, preliminary results from our observations in live-donor liver transplantation would point to some differences in the classically accepted (see Fig. 118.5) anatomic similarities among arteries and bile ducts.

HEPATIC ARTERIES

Mongeretti et al. noted that "the occurrence of (arterial) variants that differ from the usual pattern is both surprisingly common and unpredictable."[21] Such findings are especially relevant not only in liver transplantation but in all types of hepatobiliary surgery.[1,2,21,22] When addressing arterial polymorphism and nomenclature, it is essential to keep in mind the embryologic reality that the liver has a tripartite arterial supply during developmental life. Although all these structures may not be patent in adulthood vestigial remnants such as fibrous bands will always be encountered by the hand and sight of gifted surgeons.

The *common hepatic artery* originates from the celiac trunk in more than 80% of cases. In 5% of instances, there is a *replaced common hepatic artery*, most frequently arising from the superior mesenteric artery. In approximately 10% of cases, there is an *absent common hepatic artery*. In such instances the right and left hepatic arteries originate independently.[21]

The *right hepatic artery* originates from the proper hepatic artery in more than 80% of cases. In approximately 15% to 20% of cases, there is a *replaced right hepatic artery* that arises in most instances from the superior mesenteric artery. In slightly more than 5% of individuals, there is an *accessory right hepatic artery* that may arise from the superior mesenteric artery. The right hepatic artery crosses underneath the common hepatic duct in 65% of cases, anterior to it in approximately 10% of cases, and underneath the common bile duct in approximately 10% of cases.[21,5]

The *left hepatic artery* arises from the hepatic artery proper in more than 80% of instances. In approximately 15% to 20% of cases, there is a *replaced left hepatic artery* that most frequently may arise from the left gastric artery, celiac axis, or replaced common hepatic artery. An *accessory left hepatic artery* may be seen in up to 35% of individuals.[21] Finding such vessels is of help during surgical interventions. Replaced and accessory left hepatic arteries can usually be detected by palpation of the gastrohepatic ligament. Replaced and accessory right hepatic arteries can be identified by palpating the posterior right portion of the hepatoduodenal ligament, with one finger inserted into the foramen of Winslow. The most frequent left-sided arterial distribution is a common trunk formed by the arteries of segments II and IV, which is joined by the artery of segment III. When the latter enters the former near the left-right bifurcation, the left hepatic artery is short. When the entrance occurs at the bifurcation or at the hepatic artery proper, there is a duplication of the left hepatic artery.[21] The hepatic artery is rarely involved by severe atherosclerotic changes, even in elderly individuals.[6]

HEPATIC DUCTS

The *left hepatic duct* drains segments II to IV. It is formed by the junction of ducts from segments II and III into a common trunk that is subsequently joined by the duct from segment IV (see Fig. 118.3). Duct IV usually joins at the umbilical fissure or somewhat to its right. In most cases the left hepatic duct lies in the most superior location of the left portal pedicle. The most frequent left biliary distribution is a common trunk from segments II and III that is joined by that of segment IV. In cases in which duct IV joins late, it may form the upper edge of the left portal pedicle.[11,18,19] In a very small number of cases

the ducts from the left paramedian sector (segments III and IV) may themselves form a trunk, which is joined by the duct of the left lateral sector (segment II) and the caudate lobe (segment I), or the duct from segment IV enters the confluence of the other ducts or the common duct itself. Such variations may lead to the finding of a short left hepatic duct (approximately 17% of cases) or a double left hepatic duct (approximately 12% of cases).[11] The left duct has a classic configuration in almost 70% of cases.[18] Biliary drainage may be achieved by performing a bilioenteric anastomosis to the left hepatic duct at the hilum or to ducts III or IV by accessing them at the umbilical fissure (Hepp-Couinaud operation).[23] Variations in anatomic patterns should be kept in mind.[11,18]

The *right hepatic duct* is present in slightly more than 50% of cases (see Fig. 118.3). It is harder to reach than its left counterpart, is usually short, and may even be missing in cases of an early second-degree bi-trifurcation (or division). It drains segments V to VIII. The duct draining segments VI and VII has a horizontal trajectory. The duct draining segments V and VIII has a vertical course.[11,18]

The caudate lobe has its own bile drainage.[18]

The *confluence of the hepatic ducts* is observed in front of the portal bifurcation in 57% of cases, in front of the left portal vein in 37% of cases, and in front of the right portal vein in 6% of cases. Isolated segmental or subsegmental bile ducts, usually arising from segments I, IV, and V,[11] can lead to biliary fistulas after interventions in the hilar region. The confluence of the right and left hepatic ducts is described as following a normal configuration in approximately 70% of cases. Other possible configurations and their approximate incidences include trifurcation with left, paramedian and lateral right ducts (10%), right sectoral duct merging into the common bile duct (20%), and right sectoral duct joining the left duct (5%).[18]

PORTAL VEIN AND PORTAL VEIN ANOMALIES

The left portal, left paramedian, left lateral, and right paramedian veins are constant structures within the liver architecture.[11] The absence of the bifurcation of the portal vein can be an extremely dangerous situation. In such cases the portal vein follows a curvilinear trajectory within the liver, arching from right to left, and giving off collateral branches along the way until it reaches the caudate lobe. Ligation of the presumed right portal vein branch leads to complete interruption of portal blood into the liver.[11,24,25] The classically accepted portal venous branching is illustrated in Fig. 118.4.

HILUM, PLATES, FISSURES, AND OTHER STRUCTURES

Couinaud reminded us that "*hilum* meant in Latin a tiny black point seen in beans" and that anatomists in antiquity referred to that region as *porta hepatis*, or gateway of the liver.[11] It contains the bifurcation of the portal elements, with the short right and the long left branches. In approximately 23% of cases the right portal vein is not present but rather is replaced by several branches. In 47% of cases the right hepatic duct is not present as such.[11]

The location of the *main portal fissure* described by Rex, may vary (see Fig. 118.2). It is identified by the posterior extremity of the cystic plate and, in cases of normal right portal vein anatomy, tends to be located to the right of the portal vein, less frequently at the site of the bifurcation of the portal vein or even less frequently to its left. In cases of right portal vein variants the fissure is almost always at the level of the bifurcation or at the left portal vein. Its topographic location on the liver is not outlined by superficial markings in Humans and can be traced from the gallbladder fossa to the left anterior surface of the IVC. Furthermore, it has been noted that when the main portal fissure lies on the left, the biliary confluence is located in more than 70% of cases in front of the left portal vein.[11,26,27]

The *hilar plate* (see Fig. 118.2) is detached from the liver parenchyma by dissecting in between the left portal pedicle and liver tissue. The left hepatic duct is the structure located in the superior aspect of the portal elements. No major vessels or biliary ducts are encountered in this pathway. Only in the posterior region are there branches to the caudate lobe.[2,11,18,23,28]

The *umbilical fissure and plate* (see Fig. 118.2) is the site of origin of segmental and sectoral pedicles to the left liver. Its anatomic landmarks are the falciform ligament and the left longitudinal sulcus. The left paramedian pedicle and the umbilical plate can be identified by following the round ligament in continuity with the left portal vein. No walaean pedicles cross the umbilical fissure.[1] This structure divides the left lobe from the rest of the liver and is a landmark point for the evaluation and performance of left lobectomies and trisectorectomies (trisegmentectomies in the classic diction).[29]

The *sulcus of Rouvière* is an irregular fissure in continuity with the right hilum (see Fig. 118.2). It represents the extrahepatic anatomic landmark of the right fissure, usually buried in liver parenchyma. Following this structure leads to the pedicles of segments V and VI and further deeply and posteriorly to the pedicles of segments VII and VIII. The maneuver of isolating these structures is advantageous in the difficult procedures of right sectorectomy (segments VI to VII resection) or left sectorectomy (trisegmentectomy) (segments I-II-III-IV-VIII resection).

The right paramedian portal pedicle is according to Couinaud, "one of the most constant vessels of the liver."[11]

The *parabiliary venous system* of Couinaud is an accessory venous system with collateral branches to the duodenum, pancreas, and stomach, located within the hilar plate. It is associated with liver parenchyma, especially in the caudate and quadrate lobes, as well as with cystic veins. It may act as a collateral pathway in cases of portal hypertension and may serve as a connection between the right and left livers.[11]

The *cystic vein(s)* usually drain into the right portal vein but may also drain into the right liver, the left liver, and/or enter the parabiliary venous system.[1-3]

In 20% to 50% of cases, *small ducts* that are not part of a portal pedicle and do not communicate with the gallbladder are encountered in the cystic fossa. These ducts, described by Luschka, represent part of the "vasa

aberrantia." They are different from the *cystohepatic ducts*, which are true biliary ducts that traverse from liver tissue to the gallbladder.[11,30]

HEPATIC, SUPRARENAL, AND PHRENIC VEINS

There are three main hepatic veins that drain into the IVC (see Fig. 118.5): the right hepatic vein (RHV), middle hepatic vein (MHV), and left hepatic vein (LHV). Accessory inferior, right inferior, right middle, or dorsal hepatic veins also drain directly into the IVC.[31] The MHV and LHV show a relative lack of anatomic diversity, whereas the RHV exhibits multiple variants.[32]

RIGHT HEPATIC VEIN

In most cases the RHV is single; rarely, it is double. In more than 50% of cases, it has no tributaries within 1 cm of its entrance into the IVC. In such cases, it is possible to ligate it before parenchymal transections. In the other variants, attempts to ligate it may lead to profuse bleeding and potentially air emboli in cases where injuries occur.[18,31]

MIDDLE HEPATIC VEIN

The MHV travels in the liver parenchyma along the main portal fissure (Cantlie line). In approximately 85% of cases the MHV and LHV join in a common trunk before their entrance into the IVC. There are five most frequent venous confluence patterns when a length of approximately 1 cm from the IVC is considered (percentiles are approximate numbers)[31]:

- No venous branches (10% of cases)
- Bifurcation (40% of cases)
- Trifurcation (25% of cases)
- Quadrifurcation (5% of cases)
- Independent MHV and LHV (15% of cases)

LEFT HEPATIC VEIN

The LHV has two main tributaries, which usually converge more than 2 cm away from the common trunk's entrance (MHV and LHV) into the IVC.[31] The confluence of the LHV and the MHV represents the posterior part of the sulcus venosus. A posterior vein usually follows the posterior margin of the left lobe.[11] The LHV has a wide variety of branching patterns. However, all principal branches are within the territory limited by the left portal fissure (fissure that separates segments II and III).[11]

INFERIOR HEPATIC VEINS

There are multiple inferior hepatic veins (IHVs) that drain directly into the IVC. According to their location, they can be classified as posterior, posterolateral, posteroinferior, and caudate. Posteroinferior veins were observed in 95% of cases. The veins of the caudate lobe usually range in number from 1 to 4.[31]

RIGHT SUPRARENAL VEIN

There are four frequent suprarenal venous configurations, as follows:

- Single vein flows directly into the IVC, on the right side (75% of cases)

- Single vein merges together with a dorsal hepatic vein before entering the IVC (22% of cases)
- Single vein flows into the confluence of the right renal vein and the IVC (1% of cases)
- Two veins (2% of cases)

PHRENIC VEINS

There are one to five phrenic veins observed. Their confluence into the IVC or hepatic veins was observed with the following frequency patterns (approximate percentages)[31]:

- Supradiaphragmatic IVC, right anterior wall (25% of cases)
- Infradiaphragmatic IVC, right anterior wall (90% of cases)
- Retrohepatic IVC, right posterior wall (50% of cases)
- Supradiaphragmatic IVC, left anterior wall (5% of cases)
- Infradiaphragmatic IVC, left anterior wall (35% of cases)
- Common trunk of MHV and LHV (30% of cases)

ANATOMIC APPROACHES TO HEPATIC RESECTIONS (ACCORDING TO COUINAUD)

See Figs. 118.3 through 118.5.

POSTERIOR LIVER (DORSAL LIVER, SECTOR I)

Couinaud[1] proposed a posterior or dorsal liver that he designated as *sector I*. This area encompasses right and left dorsal segments. The left dorsal segment is known as segment I, while segment I is the liver parenchyma also known as caudate lobe, spigelian lobe (or lobe of Spiegel). The right dorsal segment, also called *segment Ir* is the remainder of the liver parenchyma ventral to the IVC, inferior to the right superior and MHVs, and posterior to the right pedicle.[11] Others view the caudate lobe as "embracing" the IVC and contacting segment VI in approximately half of all cases.[18] Its pathologic involvement may be associated with invasion of the IVC.[4]

Portal vein branches originate from the left portal vein, from the portal bifurcation, from the right portal vein, and from the parabiliary system. There is an artery and bile duct accompanying each vein within the walaean sheaths. Efferent veins drain into the retrohepatic IVC, and hepatic veins.[1]

When attempting to resect part or all of the posterior liver, the sector can be divided into three. The area in front of the IVC, in between the left and MHVs, can be reached anteriorly by removing segment IV. The area in between the middle and right superior hepatic veins can be reached anteriorly by removing segment VII (a difficult task). The area below the right superior hepatic vein can be reached anterolaterally by resecting segment VI.[11] Alternatively, a completely posterior approach to the dorsal or paracaval liver can be used after detachment of the liver from the IVC. Caution should be paid to the posterior aspect of the hilum.

LEFT HEMILIVER (SEGMENTS II, III, IV)

Segment II makes up the left posterior angle, whereas segment III constitutes the left anterior angle of the liver. The left lateral sector encompasses segment II and III, whereas the left paramedian sector is made up of segment IV.[2]

Removal of the left liver along the main portal fissure entails ligation and transection of the left portal pedicle, LHV, and left-sided tributaries of the MHV. The caudate lobe is usually not included when performing a left hepatectomy. The left posterior dissection, dividing the left liver from segment I, is limited by the sulcus of Arantius. Approximately 40% of the functional liver mass is represented by the left hemiliver.[4,11,18,33] Preoperative imaging studies provide a road map, especially useful when anatomic variations are present. The hilar plate is identified and dissected, ligating and transecting any branches to segment IV. The left portal pedicle is encircled and tied, providing a vascular demarcation of the territory to be resected along the main portal fissure. The left hemiliver is mobilized by transecting its ligaments. As dissection is carried out through the liver parenchyma toward the LHV, collaterals are tied or clipped. A venous branch from segment IV may be encountered posteriorly. The LHV is identified, tied, and transected.[4,11,18]

Potential complications based on liver anatomy include walaean sheaths, variations in hepatic vein topography, portal branches that supply the right liver but arise in the left portal vein or traverse close to it, bile ducts that drain the right liver but end in the left hepatic duct or traverse close to it, and vice versa.[11]

LEFT LOBE (SEGMENTS II, III)

Access to and knowledge of the *umbilical plate* provides the gateway to left liver surgery. As outlined by Couinaud the *left portal fissure* separates segments II and III and constitutes the plane where all the main branches of the LHV lie. This fissure should not be confused with the *umbilical (left suprahepatic) fissure*, which runs on the lateral edge of segment IV.[11] Second-order portal branches supply segment II, whereas third-order ones supply segment III. A large posterior branch of the LHV follows the posterior edge of segment II. Resection of segments II or III individually entails dissection by careful identification of pedicles, preservation of veins, and guidance by means of color demarcation.[4,11] The ligamentum teres (round ligament) joins the terminal part of the left portal vein. In this region the bile duct lies above whereas the artery lies anterior and below the left portal vein. The surgical approach always entails the identification of the artery, followed by dissection and division of the most posterior segment III branches of the portal vein, and finally by the identification of the bile duct. In cases in which biliary obstruction must be resolved, the bile duct of segment III can be accessed on the left of the ligamentum teres and a biliary–enteric anastomosis constructed.[2,18,23]

SEGMENT IV

Segment IV can be resected without altering the integrity of the remaining liver mass.[4] Third-order portal branches supply this segment. Resection entails in all cases access to the umbilical fissure, with subsequent ligation and transection of all sheaths arising from the left portal branch and entering segment IV. The liver is divided along the left border of the MHV, allowing for its preservation.

However, when necessary it can also be resected.[4,11] If specific cases in which pathologic findings demand it, segment IV can be removed in continuity with segments II, III, V, VIII ± I.

RIGHT HEMILIVER (SEGMENTS V, VI, VII, AND VIII)

Segment V constitutes the right border of the gallbladder bed. Segment VI makes the right anterior angle of the liver and is occasionally delimited by the sulcus of Rouvière to the right, whereas segment VII configures the right posterior angle. Segment VII is not visible from the inferior surface of the liver.[5] Anatomic variations in portal and hepatic venous configurations are much more frequent in the right than in the left liver.[1] In 1888 Rex described the main portal and the right portal fissures. The *main portal fissure* extends from the anterior-left surface of the IVC to the cystic fossa. The MHV runs within it. In cases in which the fissure is at the level of the right portal vein, there is a very low incidence of right portal vein anatomic variants. When the portal vein anatomy shows no variants, the convergence of the right and left hepatic ducts is usually located in front of the bifurcation of the portal vein. In cases of absent right portal vein, the convergence is in front of the left portal vein. The *right portal fissure* has a posterior edge at the RHV but is otherwise devoid of topographic anatomic landmarks. The right superior hepatic vein runs within it.[1,26]

There are several intraoperative ways to outline hepatic territories. Such maneuvers are especially useful in cases of anatomic distortions caused by tumors. Isolating the right (Fig. 118.7) or left branches of the portal vein and hepatic artery and clamping them temporarily (*right* or *left Pringle maneuver*) leads to a color demarcation of the right or left hemilivers, respectively. In the *Halagó maneuver* the territory of the right hemiliver drained by the MHV is delineated. This maneuver entails the temporary clamping of the right branch of the portal vein, the right branch of the hepatic artery, and subsequently the RHV. Temporary nonperfusion of the area of the liver supplied by the right portal system is achieved and is physically demarcated by a darkened color of the liver parenchyma. When the clamp on the right hepatic artery is released, the arterial perfusion will revascularize the right lobe of the liver. However, by maintaining the RHV clamped, its territory will remain demarcated, and only the parenchyma of the right liver drained by the MHV will regain its color. The Halagó maneuver is especially useful in right liver resections in live-donor liver transplantation.

Segmental pedicles on the right, as opposed to what is encountered on the left liver, arise within the liver parenchyma. As such, the gateway to right liver surgery is the right hilar extremity. The right pedicle is short (see Fig. 118.7), and sometimes the division of the portal pedicle is so early that it replaces the pedicle itself. The right portal vein is estimated to be missing in slightly more than 3% of cases.[11] Anatomically, the right paramedian portal sheath has an oblique configuration, entering the liver parenchyma from the right area of the hilum. The right paramedian portal vein is a constant structure. The right lateral portal sheath can be found parallel to the inferior surface of the liver.[11,18]

The right hepatic duct is believed to be absent in almost 50% of cases, with variations of trifurcation or right segmental biliary drainage emptying into the left-sided biliary ducts in the majority of the remaining cases.[11,34]

Drainage of the right liver (see Fig. 118.5) is by means of the right and MHVs. The MHV drains segment V on its left side by means of the anterior branches and segment VIII by means of its posterior branches. Couinaud made a distinction between superior, middle, and inferior RHVs and noted their high anatomic variability. Small drainage veins originating in segments VII and VIII can be found to enter the IVC independently.[11] Couinaud related that "the facility and safety of right hepatectomy depends on the length of the right portal pedicle." Broelsch stated that "control of the afferent and efferent vessels is of vital importance." Ease of access to the right pedicle may be encountered by accessing the sulcus of Rouvière, which prolongs the right edge of the hilum, or by addressing its lateral and paramedian pedicles.[4,11,35,36] Small branches that

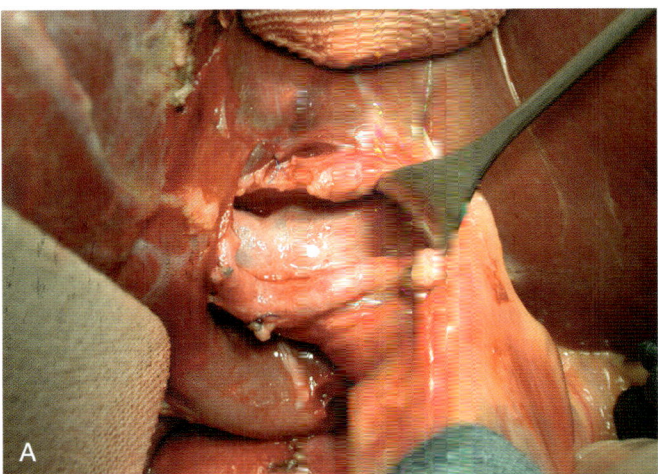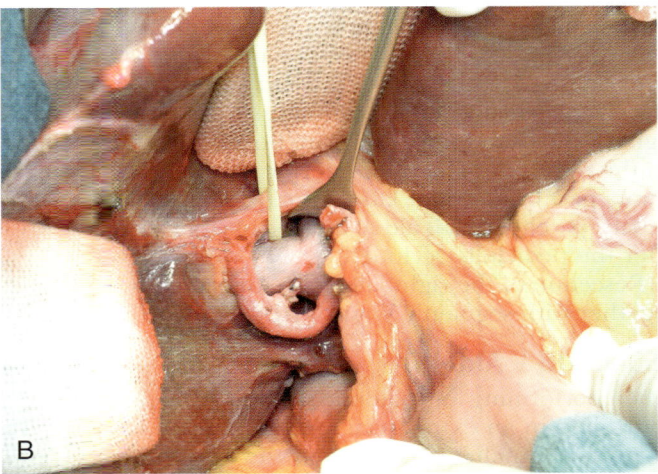

FIGURE 118.7 Surgical dissection of the right portal pedicle. (A) The right hepatic artery and right portal vein have been dissected. (B) The right hepatic duct was subsequently selected and circled with a rubber band.

originate from the right portal vein may go toward the precaval parenchyma, segment VII, or the caudate process.[11] Mobilization of the right lobe is of vital importance. Hepatic veins can be approached by rotating the right lobe medially or from the transected parenchyma at the main portal fissure. Approximately 60% of the functional liver mass is represented by the right hemiliver.[4,11]

RIGHT PARAMEDIAN SECTOR (SEGMENTS V AND VIII)

The right paramedian sector is of variable extent. It is limited by the main portal fissure, the right portal fissure, and the dorsal liver. In approximately 75% of cases, interruption of its pedicle has no associated anatomic complications. In the remainder of cases, variants that may lead to surgical challenges include the origin of branches to segments VI or VII, duplication of its usual branches, and absence of the portal vein bifurcation. In most cases in which the main portal fissure is to the right of the portal vein at the level of the hilum, there are no anatomic variants. As suggested by Couinaud, control of the paramedian portal pedicle should be preferably attained through an extrafascial approach at the level of the hilum as it ascends into the liver parenchyma. Variations in branching of the portal distribution manifest as changes in the pattern of color demarcation after occlusion of inflow. When resecting this sector, the RHV (if not atrophic) should be preserved.[11] The right paramedian sector can be resected in continuity with segments IV, V, and VII.[11]

RIGHT LATERAL SECTOR (SEGMENTS VI AND VII)

The right lateral sector is located lateral to the right portal fissure. On gross inspection the right margin of the liver is part of the right lateral sector. The plane of the right portal fissure is along the RHV. However, the RHV may be unusually small in approximately 25% of cases. Couinaud described the fissure as a "very large" fissure, with an oblique orientation, that encompasses "the whole width of the right liver." When performing a resection of the right lateral sector, the portal pedicle can be identified on the right edge of the hilum, usually 2 cm to the right of the main portal fissure. The right lateral pedicle follows a course parallel to the liver surface. Anatomic variations that can be encountered include branches to the right lateral sector originating from the right paramedian sector and duplication of the pedicle of the latter. In more than 80% of cases in which the main portal fissure is located to the right of the portal vein, there are no anatomic variations on the right side. The right inferior and middle veins are always part of the right lateral sector. Transection of the hepatic parenchyma is along the line of color demarcation after the pedicle is occluded.[11,18]

Resection of the right lateral sector can be performed together with segments V and VIII.[11]

SEGMENTS V AND VI

When performing anatomic resection, the pedicles are controlled in an extrafascial way. Segment V is supplied by portal branches arising from the anterior aspect of the right paramedian bundle. Branches to segment VI arise from the anterior aspect of the right lateral pedicle. Occasionally, there is a single pedicle for segment VI.

Venous drainage of segment V is into the MHV, whereas that of segment VI is into the RHV. Resection is guided by the coloration changes associated with vascular occlusion.[11]

SEGMENT VII

The border between segments VII and VIII is the right portal fissure. Segment VII has the peculiarity of being supplied by a single portal pedicle, known as *Rex's ramus arcuatus*. This pedicle originates from the right lateral portal bundle, distal and posterior to the branches for segment VI. Occasionally, such as in cases of right portal trifurcation, it may arise on its own. Venous drainage is usually into the RHV. When resecting this segment, it is recommended to expose the IVC and RHV.[11]

SEGMENT VIII

Segment VIII is supplied by posterior branches of the right paramedian portal bundle. Its venous drainage is mostly through the MHV.[11]

LYMPHATICS

The lymphatic system of the liver is not yet fully understood. Lymphatic channels are encountered in the portal tract and collect lymph that may originate in the spaces of Disse. Lymphatics travel together with other elements of the portal bundle to the hilum of the liver, eventually reaching the aortic lymph nodes and the thoracic duct. Lymphatic vessels also travel with the hepatic veins, along the IVC, and subsequently into the thoracic region. There are also superficial lymphatics within the capsule of the liver.[13,37]

NERVES

The liver receives both sympathetic and parasympathetic innervation. Sympathetic supply is through the celiac plexus. Stimulation leads to increases in glucose and lactate. Parasympathetic innervation is through the vagus nerve. Stimulation leads to glycogen synthesis, decreased glucose release, and gallbladder contraction.[13,37,38]

MICROSCOPIC STRUCTURE

Given the surgical nature of our chapter, we describe here only the basic aspects of the hepatic microscopic structure. The hexagonal lobule, portal lobule, and acinus have been described as hepatic functional units by Kiernan, Mall, and Rapaport, respectively.[37] This anatomic-physiologic configuration is associated with topographic variations in hepatocyte metabolic activity, exposure to toxic substances, and oxygen concentrations.[13] It is estimated that the liver has approximately 100 billion hepatocytes that make up 80% of hepatic cells. Hepatocytes are polyhedral in shape and arranged in one-cell-thick plates lining the sinusoids. Hepatocytes have a basolateral (sinusoidal, vascular) domain, canalicular (apical, biliary) domain, and lateral domain.[37] The basolateral (vascular, sinusoidal) domain is located toward the sinusoids and space of Disse. The corresponding hepatocytic membrane is lined with microvilli and is a zone of active transport between blood and the hepatocyte. It is responsible in part for maintaining the liver pH around 7.2.[37] The canalicular membrane contains active transport systems and is also responsible in part for maintaining the liver pH around 7.2. This domain contains multiple enzymes with active sites directed toward the exterior of the cell. Bile canaliculi, 1 to 2 μm in diameter, located in between the canalicular domains of hepatocytes, merge into canal of Hering, which in turn drain into bile ductules lined by cholangiocytes. These in turn lead to ducts of larger size and eventually form the common bile duct.[37] The lateral domain separates the former two domains and contains junctional complexes.[37] The perisinusoidal space of Disse is a site where fluids can move freely given the absence of basement membranes in both hepatocytes and sinusoid–lining cells. There are four types of cells in the sinusoids: hepatic sinusoidal endothelial cells, Kupffer cells, lymphocytes, and stellate (Ito) cells. The latter store vitamin A and would contribute to the pathogenesis of cirrhosis.[13,37]

Large and septal bile ducts express blood group antigens.[13] Chronic rejection, toxin reactions, graft-versus-host disease, and other afflictions involve mostly ducts smaller than 0.1 mm.[13]

HEPATIC BLOOD FLOW AND METABOLISM

The liver weighs approximately 1800 g in men and 1400 g in women. It receives approximately 1500 mL of blood per minute, 30% from the hepatic artery and the remaining 70% from the portal vein. There are 25 to 30 mL of blood per 100 g of liver under normal conditions, but that volume may reach up to 60 mL/100 g in cases of congestion. Blood flow also varies as a result of other physiologic conditions, such as ingestion of a meal. Portal blood flow is most sensitive to protein meals. Carbohydrate intake has a moderate effect on increases in portal flow. The influence of lipids is thought to be of minimal importance.[13,37]

The liver is the main site of protein and amino acid metabolism. More than 90% of circulating plasma proteins come from the liver. The liver receives dietary amino acids through the portal circulation. Their availability is limited by hepatocyte membrane transport activity. Hepatocytes are also able to internalize large proteins and other macromolecules by endocytosis. Nonessential amino acids are synthesized in the liver from pathways based on pyruvate, α-ketoglutarate, and oxaloacetate (from the Krebs cycle). Amino acid catabolism occurs mostly in the liver. Those that are not destined to become hepatocytic or plasma proteins are degraded into pyruvate, acetyl coenzyme A (CoA), or members of the tricarboxylic acid cycle intermediaries. The nitrogen from the amino groups is excreted as urea in the urine after being processed by the urea cycle.[37,39]

The liver produces fatty acids from excess sugar. Fatty acids are stored intracellularly mainly as triglycerides. Oxidation of fatty acids in the liver produces ketone bodies.[37] The liver is intimately involved in lipoprotein physiology. It is the site of production of very-low-density lipoprotein (VLDL) and a great part of plasma high-density lipoprotein.[40] Austin Flint was the first to describe hypercholesterolemia in liver disease. Incidentally, he is also credited by some as being the first to report the hepatorenal syndrome.[40,41]

The liver must provide for its own physiologic needs as well as for those of other organs. This is best exemplified when addressing hepatic physiology during fed, postabsorptive, and fasting states.[42] In the *prandial state,* most of the glucose during fed states is converted in the liver to glycogen through three-carbon fragments. The liver can store up to a maximum of 65 g of glycogen for each kilogram of liver tissue. Excess glucose can be directed in a variety of ways. An important such way is the synthesis of fatty acids. Fatty acids are esterified and transported as VLDL to adipocytes.[42] In the *postprandial state,* hepatic glycogen is broken down into glucose mainly at the brain and red blood cells. Adipocytes release fatty acids that act as an energy source for most tissues.[42] In the *fasting state,* glycogen depletion is encountered within 48 hours. Glucose for the brain and red blood cells is produced by means of gluconeogenesis. Gluconeogenesis reaches its peak rate at 24 to 48 hours. In the liver, glycerol, rather than fatty acids, provides the carbon source for gluconeogenesis. During prolonged starvation, glucose use by the brain decreases, and ketone bodies generated by the liver become the major source of energy.[42]

LIVER REGENERATION

The regenerative nature of the liver was initially unearthed by Prometheus in an ancient myth, involving his liver being consumed repeatedly by an eagle only to grow back night after night. This was in retaliation for stealing fire from the gods.[43] This myth has proven true in modern times with the regenerative nature of the liver allowing modern medicine to take advantage of this phenomenon with the likes of extensive liver resection and live-donor liver transplantation. The capacity of the liver to regenerate has provided patients and surgeons with multitude of treatment options that have evolved over decades.

The regenerative ability is usually incited by an insult such as resection or ischemia/reperfusion injury that is inherent in donor livers with regard to liver transplantation, including both live and deceased donors (Fig. 118.8). This capability begins at the molecular level and was initially described in the 1960s in a partial hepatectomy animal model. To recover after injury, hepatocytes must maintain function while replicating at high frequency to maintain physiologic needs of patients. This ability is affected by external as well as internal factors, which include ischemia, preservation injury, steatosis of liver, and age. The fully differentiated hepatocytes are the means by which rapid liver regeneration occurs after a partial hepatectomy. Tumor necrosis factor-α (TNF-α) and interleukin-6 (IL-6) have been implicated in the initial cytokine response within hours of insult initiating cascades that in turn give rise to regeneration. IL-6 and TNF-α released from Kupffer cells, function as primers in the first hours after liver injury along with transforming growth factor (TGF)-α, hepatocyte growth factor (HGF), and heparin binding–epidermal growth factor, which then help hepatocytes enter cell cycles to begin rapid proliferation.[44] Phosphorus levels after liver resection as well as transplantation are often followed closely as levels may drop precipitously. The reason for this is often glossed over as just "a part of regeneration of the liver";

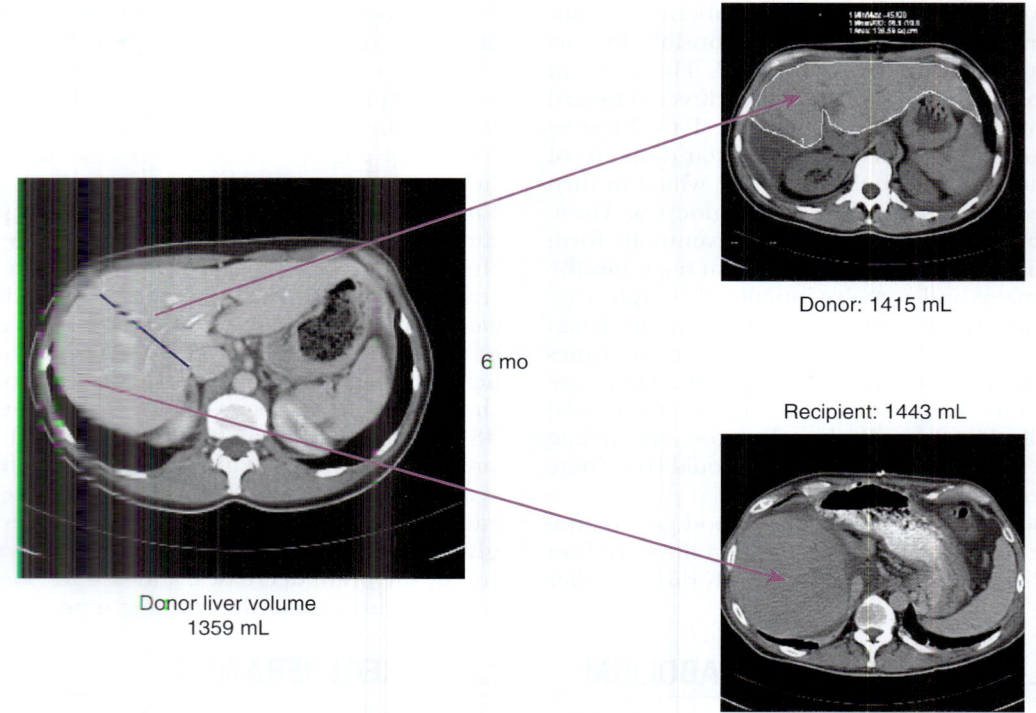

Donor: 1415 mL

Recipient: 1443 mL

6 mo

Donor liver volume
1359 mL

FIGURE 118.8 Computed tomography imaging of a live liver donor before resection *(left)* and the subsequent regrowth of remnant and allograft hemilivers in donor and recipient, respectively *(right)*.

however, this mechanism is important to understand. Phosphorylation of HGF as early as 30 minutes after partial hepatectomy has been shown in animal models and is thought of as an initiator of liver regeneration." Activation of growth factors such as HGF will often explain postresection hypophosphatemia.[45]

IL-6 and TNF-α are also charged with activation of transcription factors, including nuclear factor kappa B and signal transductor and activator of transcription 3, as well as extracellular signal–regulated kinase and c-jun N terminal kinase.[4] The transcription of these genes fosters cell cycle progression and ultimately contributes to the repair and regeneration after either liver resection or ischemic injury within the realm of transplantation. It is important to reiterate the ability to repair and regenerate is affected by degree of injury, condition of underlying liver, as well as the patient's physiologic reserve.

BILE FORMATION

Bile consists of an aqueous solution of salts, electrolytes, amino acids, proteins, lipids, vitamins, steroids, toxins, drugs, and heavy metals." It is formed based on an osmotic filtration and the transport of substances that lead to the development of such osmotic gradient. Its function involves absorption and digestion of dietary substances, cholesterol excretion, and the elimination of toxic substances.[46]

ACKNOWLEDGMENTS

We acknowledge the prior authors of this chapter whose work was extremely detailed and accurate, accompanied with exceptional authorship. (Ernesto P. Molmenti, George C. Sotiropoulos, Arnold Radtke, Jeffrey M. Nicastro, Gene F. Coppa, Eduardo de Santibañes, and Massimo Malagó.)

REFERENCES

1. Molmenti EP, Klintmalm GB. *Atlas of Liver Transplantation*. Philadelphia: Saunders; 2002.
2. Lasala AJ, Molmenti LA. Reoperaciones en vias biliares por lesiones quirurgicas. Buenos Aires: Lopez Libreros Editores; 1966.
3. Malagó M, Testa G, Frilling A, et al. Right living donor liver transplantation—an option for adult patients: single-institution experience with 74 patients. *Ann Surg*. 2003;238:853 [discussion 862].
4. Broelsch CE. *Atlas of Liver Surgery*. New York: Churchill-Livingstone; 1993.
5. Lang H, Malagó M, Broelsch CE. Liver transplantation in children and segmental transplantation. In: Blumgart LH, Fong Y, eds. *Surgery of the Liver and Biliary Tract*. 3rd ed. Philadelphia: Saunders; 2000:2107.
6. Starzl TE, Putnam CW. *Experience in Hepatic Transplantation*. Philadelphia: Saunders; 1969.
7. Radtke A, Schroeder T, Molmenti EP, et al. Anatomical and physiological comparison of liver volumes among three frequent types of parenchyma transection in live-donor liver transplantation. *Hepatogastroenterology*. 2005;52:333.
8. Sadler TW. *Langman's Medical Embryology*. 11th ed. Philadelphia: Lippincott Williams & Wilkins; 2010.
9. Skandalakis JE, et al. The liver. In: Skandalakis JE, Gray SW, eds. *Embryology for Surgeons: The Embryological Basis of the Treatment of Congenital Anomalies*. 2nd ed. Baltimore: Williams & Wilkins; 1994:283.
10. Sappey C. Traité d'anatomie descriptive. Paris: Lecrosnier er Babe; 1889.
11. Couinaud C, ed. *Surgical Anatomy of the Liver Revisited*. Paris: C. Couinaud; 1989.
12. Strasberg SM. Terminology of liver anatomy and liver resection: coming to grips with hepatic Babel. *J Am Coll Surg*. 1997;184:413.

13. Wanless IR. Physioanatomic considerations. In: Schiff ER, Sorrell MF, Maddrey WC, eds. *Schiff's Diseases of the Liver*. 10th ed. Philadelphia: Lippincott Williams & Wilkins; 2007.

14. Couinaud C. Les envelopes vasculo-biliaire de fcie ou capsule de Glisson: Leur intérêt dans la chirurgie vésiculaire, les resections hépatiques et l'abord du hile du foie. *Lyon Chir*. 954;49:589.

15. Johannis Walaei epistolae duae e motu chili et sanguinis ad Thomam Bartholeum. In: *Thomas Bartholes Anatomica auges*. Lataviae (Leyden): Franciscus Hackius; 1640.

16. Glisson F. *Anatomia Hepatis*. London: O Pulein; 642.

17. Laennec RTH. Sur les tuniques qui enveloppent certains viscéres, et fournissent des gaines membaneuses à leurs vasseaux. J De Méd Chir et Pharm Vendémiaire an XI:539, et Germinal an XI:73; 1803.

18. Blumgart LH, Hann LE. Surgical and radologic anatomy of the liver and biliary tract. In: Blumgart LH, ed. *Surgery of the Liver, Biliary Tract and Pancreas*. 4th ed. Philadelphia: Saunders; 2006:3.

19. Lazorthes F, Chiotasso P, Chevreau P, Materre JP, Roques J. Hepatectomy with initial suprahilar control of intrahepatic portal pedicles. *Surgery*. 1993;113:103.

20. Couinaud C, Houssin D. *Partition Regle du Foie pour Transplantation: Contraites Anatomiques*. Paris: Couinaud Editeur; 1991.

21. Molmenti EP, Pinto PA, Klein J, Klein AS. Normal and variant arterial supply of the liver and gallbladder. *Pediatr Transplant*. 2003;7:80.

22. Molmenti EP, Klein AS, Henry ML. Procurement of liver and pancreas allografts in donors with replaced/accessory right hepatic arteries. *Transplantation*. 2004;78:770.

23. Hepp J, Couinaud C. L'abord et l'utilisation du canal hépatique gauche dans la reparation de l voie biliaire principale. *Presse Méd*. 1956;64:947.

24. Couinaud C. Etude sur la veine porte intra-hepatique. *Presse Méd*. 1953;61:1434.

25. Agossou-Veyeme AK. La segmentation hépatique en tomodensito-métrie, Paris: Thése, 3e Cycle; 1982.

26. Rex H. Beitrage zur Morphologie der Säuretheber. *Morph Jb*. 1888;14:517.

27. Reynaud B, Coucouravas G, Amoros P et al. Clampage direct du pedicle glissonien lateral droit. *J Chir*. 1982;11:523.

28. Couinaud C. Recherches sur la chirurgie du confluent biliaire supérieur et des canaux hépatiques. *Presse Méc*. 1955;63:669.

29. http://www.ihpba.org/. Accessed 5 October 2012.

30. Luschka H. Die Anatomie des Menschen. B II. Die Secretionszelle und der Gallenleitende Apparat. Tübingen laupp und Siebeckl; 1863.

31. Nakamura S, Tsuzuki T. Surgical anatomy of the hepatic veins and the inferior vena cava. *Surg Gynecol Obstet*. 1981;152:43.

32. Radtke A, Schroeder T, Sotiropoulos GC, et al. Anatomical and physiological classification of hepatic veir dominance applied to liver transplantation. *Eur J Med Res*. 2005;10:187.

33. Couinaud C. A simplified method for controlled left hepatectomy. *Surgery*. 1985;105:385.

34. Tanaka K, Inomata Y, Kaihara S, Daigaku K. *Living-Donor Liver Transplantation: Surgical Techniques and Innovations*. Barcelona, Spain: Arcus Science; 2003.

35. Rouvière H. Sur la configuration et la signification du sillon du processus caudé. *Bull Soc Anat Paris*. 1924;60:355.

36. Couinaud C. Bases anatomiques des hépatectomies droite et gauche: techniques qui en découlent. *J Chir*. 1954;70:933.

37. Saxena R, Zucker SD, Crawford JM. Anatomy and physiology of the liver. In: Zakim D, Boyer TD, eds. *Hepatology. A Textbook of Liver Disease*. 4th ed. Philadelphia: Saunders; 2003:3.

38. Bourgery JM, Jacob NH. Traité complet de l'anatomie de l'homme: Tome cinquième. Paris: CA Delaunay (Éditeur); 1839.

39. Cooper AJL. Amino acid metabolism and synthesis of urea. In: Zakim D, Boyer TD, eds. *Hepatology: A Textbook of Liver Disease*. 4th ed. Philadelphia: Saunders; 2003:81.

40. Mike JP. Liver disease, alcohol, and lipoprotein metabolism. In: Zakim D, Boyer TD, eds. *Hepatology: A Textbook of Liver Disease*. 4th ed. Philadelphia: Saunders; 2003:127.

41. Kim A. Experimental researches into a new excretory function of the liver: consisting in the removal of cholesterine from the blood, and its discharge from the body in the form of stercorine. *Am J Med Sci*. 1862;44:305.

42. Zakim D. Metabolism of glucose and fatty acids by the liver. In: Zakim D, Boyer TD, eds. *Hepatology: A Textbook of Liver Disease*. 4th ed. Philadelphia: Saunders; 2003:49.

43. Fausto R. Liver regeneration: from myth to mechanism. *Nat Rev Mol Cell Biol*. 2004;5(10):836-847.

44. Olthoff KM. Hepatic regeneration in living donor liver transplantation. *Liver Transpl*. 2003;9(10 suppl 2):S35-S41.

45. Michalopoulos GK. Liver regeneration. *J Cell Physiol*. 2007;213(2):286-300.

46. Wolkoff AW, Berk PD. Bilirubin metabolism and jaundice. In: Schiff ER, Sorrell MF, Maddrey WC, eds. *Schiff's Diseases of the Liver*. 10th ed. Philadelphia: Lippincott Williams & Wilkins; 2007.

Laboratory Measurement of Hepatic Function

Helen S. Te

Liver function tests or a *hepatic function panel* consists of serum biochemical tests that include serum albumin, bilirubin, alkaline phosphatase, aspartate aminotransferase (AST), and alanine aminotransferase (ALT). These terms, however, are misleading because only the serum albumin truly measures the liver's synthetic function. Hence this group of tests is better named as *liver chemistry tests*.

Elevations in liver chemistry tests usually reflect pathology in the liver, but normal liver chemistry tests do not necessarily exclude liver disease. Certainly, chronic hepatitis B or C may exist with normal serum AST and ALT, particularly when there is little or no inflammation in the liver. In addition, burnt-out cirrhosis from any etiology may also be accompanied by normal serum AST and ALT, along with a normal serum albumin and bilirubin when the liver remains well compensated. Conversely, liver disease is not identified in a minority of patients with mildly elevated serum aminotransferases despite a thorough evaluation that includes a liver biopsy. Such patients may never truly develop liver disease, but approximately 20% of them eventually evolve to have a specific liver-related diagnosis during long-term follow-up.[1] Hence both elevated and normal liver chemistry tests need to be interpreted in the context of the clinical setting, keeping in mind that when risk factors for a particular liver disease exist for a patient, and/or when evidence of liver disease is suggested by the history, physical examination, or radiologic studies, a full evaluation for liver disease may be warranted.

The interpretation of abnormal liver chemistry tests should be guided by the pattern and acuity of the elevations, which can narrow the differential diagnoses to some degree. Elevations that consist predominantly of serum AST and ALT more than the alkaline phosphatase suggest a disease process that involves hepatocellular injury or necrosis. On the other hand, a predominant elevation of serum alkaline phosphatase with or without increased bilirubin suggests a disease process that interferes with bile flow into and through the bile ducts. An isolated hyperbilirubinemia may represent an increase in bilirubin production, or disorders in its conjugation or canalicular transport. In cases in which a mixed pattern of AST and ALT elevation as well as alkaline phosphatase and/or bilirubin elevation are present, the differential diagnosis will have to remain broad. The duration of elevation is also another important consideration because the differential diagnosis for an acute, shorter process can be different from a chronic, longer-lasting disease (Table 119.1).

LIVER CHEMISTRY TESTS

MARKERS OF CELLULAR INJURY

The serum aminotransferases AST and ALT catalyze the reversible transfer of the α-amino group of the amino acids aspartic acid and alanine, respectively, to the α-keto group of α-ketoglutaric acids, forming oxaloacetic acid and pyruvic acid, respectively.[2] These enzymes are present in the serum at low levels in the blood (usually up to 35 to 60 IU/L, depending on the laboratory reference values) and are released into the blood whenever hepatocyte plasma membrane damage occurs. ALT is found primarily in the cytoplasm of liver cells and is relatively a more specific indicator of liver damage than the AST, which can be found in the mitochondria of the skeletal and cardiac muscles, kidney, pancreas, red blood cells, and brain. Small rises of ALT can occasionally also be seen in muscle injury.

Although serum levels of aminotransferases are elevated to some degree in almost all liver diseases, the highest levels are seen with acute viral hepatitis, toxin-induced hepatic necrosis, and ischemic liver injury. Mild cases of viral hepatitis are accompanied by elevations in the few hundreds, and values greater than 1000 IU/mL are usually seen only in patients who develop jaundice from acute viral hepatitis. Values greater than 3000 IU/mL are more typical of acetaminophen-induced toxic injury or severe cases of ischemic hepatitis. The degree of elevation has little prognostic significance because it does not reflect the integrity of the remaining viable hepatocytes and the ability of the liver to recover. The remaining synthetic function of the liver is more accurately measured by the prothrombin time, which serves as the best tool for predicting hepatic outcome.[3]

In cases of mild to moderate aminotransferase elevations up to 300 IU/mL, a ratio of AST to ALT of greater than 2 is suggestive of alcoholic liver disease (ALD). Cases of nonalcoholic fatty liver disease (NAFLD) or viral hepatitis typically have a higher serum ALT level than the AST, whereas hypoxic or toxic injury has a higher AST than ALT. The serum AST has a shorter mean plasma half-life (17 hours) as compared with the ALT (47 hours),[2] so it declines more rapidly than the serum ALT, allowing the serum ALT to become higher than the serum AST in the recovery phase of the illness. If the serum AST is significantly elevated out of proportion to a normal or minimally elevated serum ALT, extrahepatic sources of the serum AST should be considered, such as myocardial infarction, rhabdomyolysis, strenuous exercise, or hemolysis.

TABLE 119.1 Common Differential Diagnosis of Elevated Liver Chemistry Tests by Pattern and Acuity of Elevation

Hepatocellular	Cholestatic
ACUTE	
Ischemic hepatitis	Bile duct obstruction
Drug- or toxin-induced liver injury	Drug-induced cholestasis
	Sepsis-induced cholestasis
Acute viral hepatitis	Parenteral nutrition–related
Choledocholithiasis	cholestasis
Autoimmune hepatitis	Critical illness–related
Wilson disease	cholestasis
CHRONIC	
Chronic viral hepatitis	Primary biliary cholangitis
Alcoholic liver disease	Hepatic sarcoidosis
Nonalcoholic fatty liver disease	Primary sclerosing cholangitis
Autoimmune hepatitis	Immunoglobulin G4–
Hereditary hemochromatosis	associated cholangitis
Wilson disease	Drug-induced cholestasis
Alpha1-antitrypsin deficiency	Chronic bile-duct obstruction
Drug-induced liver injury	

An acute elevation of the serum aminotransferases may represent a recent onset of injury from ischemia, drug or toxins, acute viral infection, or in some cases, choledocholithiasis, whereas a chronic elevation of 6 months or longer may represent chronic viral hepatitis, autoimmune hepatitis (AIH), or metabolic diseases of the liver.

MARKERS OF BILE SECRETION AND FLOW

Alkaline phosphatase is a group of zinc metalloenzymes that hydrolyze organic phosphate esters. It is found in the canalicular membrane of hepatocytes, as well as in a variety of other tissues, including bone, intestine, placenta, kidney, and leukocytes.[2] Normal serum levels are highly dependent on age, with high levels in childhood and puberty correlating with active bone growth and a second elevation during older age correlating with bone resorption.[4] In liver disease the enzyme apparently increases by virtue of new protein synthesis, probably induced by certain bile acids. Although modest elevations are seen in many forms of hepatocellular disease, values that are threefold or more above normal range are indicative of bile duct obstruction or intrahepatic cholestasis.[3]

Another enzyme used to evaluate cholestasis, γ-glutamyl transpeptidase (GGT), is present in the liver and in other organs, such as the small intestine, kidney, testes, pancreas, spleen, heart, and brain. This enzyme catalyzes the transfer of γ-glutamyl groups from glutathione and other peptides to other amino acids. Serum GGT is a sensitive, but nonspecific, test for detecting biliary tract disease. It is highly inducible by alcohol and drugs and may be elevated in certain medical conditions such as diabetes mellitus, renal failure, myocardial infarction, and chronic obstructive pulmonary disease. Its main value in the clinical setting is in determining if an elevated alkaline phosphatase level is due to liver disease or not and perhaps in monitoring

alcohol abstinence in a patient with normal serum AST and ALT.[3]

Acute cholestasis may be due to an acute obstruction in the bile duct, which may result from the passage of a gallstone into the common bile duct or from a rapidly growing malignancy. It may also result from hepatotoxicity from certain drugs, such as macrolide antibiotics and azole class of antifungal agents, or as a consequence of sepsis, parenteral nutrition (PN), or other complications of critical illness. Drug-induced cholestasis may linger to become chronic, but other causes of chronic cholestasis include chronic bile duct obstruction from a benign biliary stricture or a slower growing malignancy, primary biliary cholangitis (PBC), primary sclerosing cholangitis (PSC), immunoglobulin G4 (IgG4)-associated cholangitis (IAC), and hepatic sarcoidosis. Infiltrative diseases of the liver often also lead to an increase in serum alkaline phosphatase levels

MARKERS OF BILIRUBIN METABOLISM

Unconjugated bilirubin is the by-product of hemoglobin degradation in the spleen. It binds to serum albumin and is brought to the liver, where it is taken up by the hepatocyte to undergo conjugation, and conjugated bilirubin is excreted in bile. Serum unconjugated bilirubin levels increase in disorders that result in overproduction of unconjugated bilirubin or in disorders of the conjugation process. Serum conjugated bilirubin is commonly elevated in most liver diseases, including conditions in which there is hepatocellular injury, bilirubin transport disorders, or bile duct diseases. In the evaluation of hyperbilirubinemia, it is important to attempt to identify the type of bilirubin that is elevated to allow for the identification of the pathologic step in bilirubin metabolism.[3]

MEASURES OF SYNTHETIC FUNCTION

Albumin is the most abundant serum plasma protein synthesized by the liver. It has a half-life of approximately 20 days, which limits its utility as a synthetic marker during acute liver disease. It is also insensitive to mild degrees of hepatic injury, but a significant decline signals a prolonged, and usually major, insult to the liver. Other factors that may affect the serum albumin levels include nutrition and losses through the gastrointestinal and renal systems. In patients with edema and ascites, the volume of distribution for albumin may be expanded, leading to a reduction in the measured serum levels.[3]

The liver synthesizes six coagulation factors: factor I (fibrinogen), II (prothrombin), V, VII, IX, and X. The prothrombin time measures the rate of conversion of prothrombin to thrombin in the test serum with added thromboplastin and calcium and indirectly assesses for the availability of the coagulation factors.[3] Prolongation of the prothrombin time may be due to inadequate factor synthesis by the liver in cases of severe liver dysfunction, but dietary vitamin K deficiency, antibiotic administration, vitamin K malabsorption, disseminated intravascular coagulation, and drugs (such as warfarin) are other causes. Administration of parenteral vitamin K may aid in differentiation of vitamin K deficiency from synthetic dysfunction of the liver.

COMMON HEPATOBILIARY DISEASES IN THE PRESURGICAL AND POSTSURGICAL PATIENT

ISCHEMIC HEPATITIS

Ischemic hepatitis, also called shock liver or hypoxic liver injury, results from ischemia to the hepatocytes from either hypoperfusion or systemic hypoxemia, resulting in extensive hepatocyte necrosis. It is characterized by a transient but massive rise in serum aminotransferases that is typically followed by a rapid decline, after oxygen supply to the hepatocytes is restored. The diagnosis is typically made in the setting of either known hypotension or hypoxemia in critically ill or postoperative patients, and the absence of such risk factors should prompt a search for other etiologies, such as viral hepatitis and drug injury.

In a recent meta-analysis, the pooled incidence of ischemic hepatitis in patients admitted to an intensive care unit (ICU) was 2.5 of every 100 admissions. However, only approximately half of the patients had detected hypotension. The majority of cases (79%) had a predisposing acute cardiac event, and sepsis was present in 23%.[5] Passive congestion of the liver seems to predispose patients to ischemic hepatitis, wherein the elevated right-sided pressures increase the sinusoidal pressure and impedes forward flow from the portal vein. In one large study of 32,209 ICU patients, patients with ischemic hepatitis were found to have elevated mean pulmonary capillary wedge pressure at 19.4 mm Hg and systemic vascular resistance at 1375 dynes-s/cm⁻⁵. Another study of 1066 ICU patients reported an elevated wedge pressure in all patients without underlying trauma or hemorrhage, with sepsis patients having a median wedge pressure of 17 mm Hg.[7] Hence, patients who develop ischemic hepatitis without obvious compromise in blood pressure may have incurred acute cardiac injury such as myocardial stunning.[5] Finally, sepsis may also reduce oxygen extraction and increase oxygen consumption at the hepatocellular level, which may lead to some amount of ischemia to the hepatocytes.[8]

Management of ischemic hepatitis is focused on improving splanchnic perfusion and oxygenation, either by restoration of adequate blood pressure by expansion of intravascular volume and/or with inotropic support, as indicated, to allow for improved hepatic perfusion.

DRUG-INDUCED LIVER INJURY

As the core center for drug uptake, metabolism, and excretion, the liver is predisposed to injury from toxic effects of drugs or their metabolites. Drug-induced liver injury (DILI) may be intrinsic or idiosyncratic in nature. Intrinsic hepatotoxins include agents that cause liver injury by direct physiochemical effects on the hepatocytes (e.g., carbon tetrachloride, phosphorus) and those whose metabolites interfere with metabolic pathways that in turn disrupt the structural process of the hepatocytes (e.g., *Amanita phalloides*, ethanol, acetaminophen, or tetracycline). Toxic hepatitis caused by intrinsic hepatotoxins is dose dependent and is generally predictable in individuals exposed to the offending agent. Acetaminophen is the most common cause of DILI, occurring in the setting of an overdose or at therapeutic doses when taken in combination with a cytochrome P-450 inducer, such as alcohol.[9]

Idiosyncratic hepatotoxicity is less common and affects only susceptible individuals. Hypersensitivity reactions resulting in hepatic injury develop within 1 to 5 weeks of exposure to the offending agent, recur promptly on readministration of the agent (after one or two doses), and are usually accompanied by fever, rash, arthralgia, and eosinophilia. Drugs that may cause hypersensitivity reactions include halothane, chlorpromazine, methyldopa, sulfonamides, phenytoin, and dapsone. Metabolically mediated hepatic injury results from an aberrant metabolic pathway for the drug in a susceptible patient, which leads to the production of hepatotoxic metabolites. Drugs that may cause this type of injury include isoniazid, valproic acid, methyldopa, and perhexiline maleate.[9]

The diagnosis of DILI requires careful history-taking for possible drug offenders and meticulous exclusion of other possible etiologies of the liver dysfunction. DILI events usually occur within 6 months of starting a new drug, although some drugs may still cause DILI after a longer latency period (e.g., nitrofurantoin, minocycline, and statins). Antibiotics and antiepileptics account for greater than 60% of all cases of DILI, and herbal drug supplements should be considered as possible offenders. The diagnostic approach to DILI can be tailored according to the pattern of liver injury at presentation, using the R-value, which is defined as the ratio of ALT to its upper limit of normal (ULN) divided by the ratio of serum alkaline phosphatase to its ULN. An $R \geq 5$ is considered as hepatocellular DILI, an $R < 2$ is considered as cholestatic DILI, and $R = 2$ to 4.9 is considered as mixed pattern DILI.[10]

Hepatocellular DILI may present with serum AST and ALT in the few hundreds to several thousands, as seen with acetaminophen hepatotoxicity. Acute liver failure can occur but is rare and may require liver transplantation or lead to death. Competing causes, such as acute viral hepatitis (including Epstein-Barr virus [EBV], cytomegalovirus [CMV], and herpes simplex virus [HSV] infection), undiagnosed Wilson disease (WD) in individuals younger than 40 years, and acute Budd-Chiari syndrome, must be excluded. AIH should also be considered in the differential diagnosis, although this is complicated by some idiosyncratic hepatotoxins causing DILI with features that mimic AIH (e.g., minocycline and nitrofurantoin). A liver biopsy can help to confirm a clinical suspicion of DILI, although it is often difficult to pinpoint the exact drug that is responsible for the injury, based on the liver biopsy alone, except for the few drugs that are known to have specific histologic patterns of injury, such as azathioprine or valproic acid. The prediction of serious DILI is best estimated with Hy's law, which predicts serious hepatotoxicity if, (1) the serum aminotransferases are greater than or equal to 3 times the ULN, (2) the total bilirubin is greater than 2 times the ULN with little or no alkaline phosphatase elevation, and (3) there is no other good explanation for the hepatocellular injury. Cases that fulfill all these criteria have a 1 out of 10 chance of developing acute liver failure with a 10% to 50% mortality rate.[11] Thus 90% of patients do recover from hepatocellular DILI. Withdrawal of the offending drug is the hallmark of management, and reexposure to the drug is strongly discouraged, particularly if the initial DILI episode was associated with significant serum aminotransferase elevation or jaundice.

Drug-induced cholestasis is characterized by an elevation in serum alkaline phosphatase level in the presence of a drug currently or recently administered and exclusion of other causes of cholestasis.[12] Risk factors for drug-induced cholestasis include older age (>50 years) and specific genetic determinants for an increased risk with certain drugs. Drugs that are absorbed in the portal circulation are taken up by the transporters at the basolateral membrane of the hepatocytes for detoxification in the hepatocyte, before extrusion into the canaliculi by the canalicular transporters of the multidrug-resistant protein (MDRP) family to be excreted with bile. Drugs and metabolites that affect these canalicular efflux transporters are particularly involved in cholestatic DILI. Most drugs implicated in cholestatic injury are believed to inhibit bile salt export pump (BSEP), and most patients with mutations in multidrug resistance 3 (MDR3) or BSEP have 3 times increased risk for cholestatic DILI.[13]

Many other drugs cause cholestasis by causing bile duct injury or portal inflammation with varying amounts of hepatocyte injury and necrosis. Antimicrobials are the most common drug class associated with cholestatic DILI, with amoxicillin-clavulanate being the most common offender. Sulfonamides, macrolides, fluoroquinolones, tetracyclines, antifungal agents, and antiretroviral agents are also commonly associated with drug-induced cholestasis, along with antiinflammatory agents and some psychotropes. A few drugs, such as oral contraceptives and anabolic steroids, cause bland cholestasis (i.e., pure canalicular cholestasis with no inflammatory component) (Table 119.2). Chronic cholestatic DILI lasting more than 6 months from the initial insult may take the form of vanishing bile duct syndrome or ductopenia (e.g., from trimethoprim-sulfamethoxazole, quinolones, or sclerosing cholangitis (e.g., from floxuridine). Vanishing bile duct syndrome, diagnosed by liver biopsy, has a protracted course of chronic bile duct injury that eventually leads to bile duct loss. Sclerosing cholangitis results from injury to the hepatic arterioles that supply the biliary radicles, inducing ischemic cholangiopathy that manifests as biliary strictures.[13]

Most cases of drug-induced cholestasis will resolve with withdrawal of the offending medication. However, persistent cholestasis can lead to biliary cirrhosis and eventual hepatic decompensation. Mortality rate for cholestatic DILI is at 5% to 14% and for mixed DILI at 2% to 5%.[13] Although the use of ursodeoxycholic acid in cholestatic DILI is common in practice, its true efficacy in this condition has not been established.[14]

VIRAL HEPATITIS

Hepatitis A, B, C, D, and E can cause acute hepatitis, although acute hepatitis C is usually mild and undetected. Acute viral hepatitis may be subclinical but those who develop symptoms typically also have elevated serum AST and ALT in the hundreds, with the serum ALT being much higher than the AST. Severe cases accompanied by jaundice may have serum aminotransferase levels of up to 2000 IU/mL. Hepatitis A infections are self-limited, whereas the other hepatitides may evolve to chronic infections, although chronic hepatitis E occurs only in immunocompromised or immunosuppressed individuals.

However, when the hepatocellular injury and necrosis are severe, the liver may develop acute liver failure, and some cases may require liver transplantation or lead to death. Pregnant women are particularly at higher risk for mortality in the setting of acute liver failure from hepatitis E.[15]

Hepatitis A and E are transmitted by oral-fecal route and are commonly encountered in a traveler returning from an endemic area. However, outbreaks of acute hepatitis A have occurred in the United States from contaminated produce or raw oysters.[16] Acute hepatitis A is diagnosed by the detection of hepatitis A IgM antibody in the serum. This later converts to hepatitis A IgG after recovery which confers lifelong immunity. Similarly, acute hepatitis E can be diagnosed by the detection of hepatitis E IgM antibody in the serum. Chronic hepatitis E has been documented in immunocompromised or immunosuppressed individuals, and the diagnosis of such sometimes requires hepatitis E RNA detection when the suspicion is high but initial serologies are negative.[17]

Hepatitis B is a highly infectious virus, with a risk of transmission far exceeding that of human immunodeficiency virus (HIV). Adolescents or adults usually acquire acute hepatitis B by sexual or parenteral means and may become symptomatic, whereas infants and young children tend to acquire it perinatally or horizontally and have a subclinical course. Risk factors for acquiring the infection include exposure to infected individuals at birth, sexually or within the household, having a history of blood transfusion or parenteral drug use, working in the health care sector, being on hemodialysis, or being institutionalized, such as in a prison or mental institution. The diagnosis of acute hepatitis B is based on the detection of hepatitis B surface antigen (HBsAg) and hepatitis B core (HBc) IgM antibody (Table 119.3). The HBc IgM eventually converts to IgG after 4 to 6 months. When one recovers fully from acute hepatitis B, HBsAg converts to the hepatitis B surface antibody, confering immunity. The risk of progression from acute hepatitis B to a chronic infection is inversely proportional to the age at infection, with the risk as high as 70% to 90% in infected infants.[18,19]

When HBsAg persists for 6 months or longer following the diagnosis of acute hepatitis B, the infection has become chronic. Chronic hepatitis B may be marked with normal or mild to moderate elevations in the serum aminotransferases up to a few hundreds. Serologic markers detected in chronic hepatitis B infection include the total HBc antibody (a marker of exposure to hepatitis B), hepatitis B e (HBe) antigen (HBeAg) (a marker of active viral replication and high infectivity), or hepatitis B e antibody (anti-HBe) (indicates decreasing viral replication when the HBe antigen was previously positive). However, there are viral mutant strains that have limited or no capability to produce HBe antigen; patients infected with such viruses would have a negative HBe antigen, a positive anti-HBe and a high hepatitis B DNA level.[18,19] Chronic hepatitis B cases characterized by active viral replication in large amounts and elevated serum ALT are at increased risk for progressive liver disease, cirrhosis, and hepatocellular carcinoma. Such patients should be considered for therapy with pegylated interferon or nucleoside/nucleotide analogues, which are effective in suppressing the virus, although a complete cure still remains elusive.[18]

TABLE 119.2 Common Drugs Involved in Drug-Induced Cholestasis

Drug Classes	Drugs
BLAND CHOLESTASIS	
Hormones	Anabolic steroids, some antiandrogens, oral contraceptives
Others	Azathioprine, cetirizine, cyclosporine, glimepiride, infliximab, metolazone, nevirapine, prochlorperazine, thiabendazole, tamoxifen, warfarin
INFLAMMATORY CHOLESTASIS	
Penicillins	Amoxicillin, amoxicillin-clavulanate, carbenicillin, cloxacillin, dicloxacillin, flucloxacillin, oxacillin, penicillin, ticarcillin
Sulfonamides	Sulfasalazine, trimethoprim-sulfamethoxazole
Macrolides	Azithromycin, clarithromycin, erythromycin, telithromycin
Fluoroquinolones	Ciprofloxacin, levofloxacin, moxifloxacin, temafloxacin, trovafloxacin
Tetracyclines	Doxycycline, minocycline, tetracycline
Cephalosporins	Ceftriaxone, cephalexin
Antifungal agents	Griseofulvin, itraconazole, ketoconazole, terbinafine
Antiretroviral agents	Didanosine, nevirapine, stavudine
Antimycobacterial agents	Isoniazid, rifabutin, rifampin
Antiinflammatory agents	Allopurinol, celecoxib, diclofenac, gold salts, ibuprofen, penicillamine, phenylbutazone, piroxicam, sulindac, tenoxicam
Tricyclic antidepressants	Imipramine, desipramine, amitriptyline
Antipsychotics	Risperidone, quetiapine, duloxetine
Benzodiazepines	Chlordiazepoxide, diazepam
Other psychotropes	Chlorpromazine, fluphenazine, thioridazine
Chemotherapeutic agents	Carmustine, cytosine arabinoside, gemcitabine
Antidiabetic agents	Metformin, repaglinide
Lipid-lowering agents	Fenofibrate, atorvastatin
Immunomodulators	Azathioprine, cyclosporine
Others	Barbiturates, captopril, carbamazepine, chlorambucil, chlorpropamide, dextromethorphan, dextropropoxyphene, fenofibrate, gabapentin, glibenclamide, hydralazine, hydrochlorthiazide, methimazole, methyldopa, orlistat, phenytoin, propafenone, propylthiourea, ticlopidine, tolbutamide
VANISHING BILE DUCT SYNDROME	
Psychotropes	Amineptine, amitriptyline, acepromethazine, barbiturates, carbamazepine, chlorpromazine, cyamemazine, cyproheptadine, diazepam, haloperidol, imipramine, phenytoin, trifluoperazine
Antibiotics	Amoxicillin, amoxicillin-clavulanate, ampicillin, flucloxacillin, clindamycin, quinolones, trimethoprim-sulfamethoxazole, macrolides, tetracycline
Nonsteroidal antiinflammatory agents	Diclofenac, ibuprofen
Others	Amiodarone, ajmaline, azathioprine, carbutamide, cimetidine, chlorothiazide, cromolyn sodium, cyclohexyl propionate, D-penicillamine, estradiol, glyburide, glycyrrhizin, methyltestosterone, norandrostenolone, phenylbutazone, terbinafine, thiabendazole, tolbutamide, tiopronin, xenalamine, zonisamide
SCLEROSING CHOLANGITIS	
Chemotherapy	Floxuridine
Intralesional agents	Absolute alcohol, formaldehyde, hypertonic saline, iodine solution, silver nitrate

TABLE 119.3 Interpretation of Hepatitis B Serologic Markers

HBsAg	Anti-HBs	ANTI-HBc		HBeAg	Anti-HBe	HBV DNA (IU/mL)	Stage of Infection
		IgG	IgM				
+	−	+	+++	+/−	−	+/+++	Acute hepatitis B
+	−	++	−	−	+	<10⁴	Inactive HBsAg carrier
+	−	++	−	+	−	>10⁴	Chronic hepatitis B, eAg+ strain
+	−	++	−	−	+/−	>10⁴	Chronic hepatitis B, eAg− strain
−	+	++	−	−	−	−	Distant (>6 mo) HBV infection, resolved
−	+	−	−	−	−	−	HBV vaccinated person

Anti-HBc, Hepatitis B core antibody; *Anti-HBe,* hepatitis B e antibody; *Anti-HBs,* hepatitis B surface antibody; *HBsAg,* Hepatitis B surface antigen; *HBV,* hepatitis B virus; *Ig,* immunoglobulin.

Patients are managed with dietary modification and phlebotomy, but in individuals who cannot tolerate phlebotomy, chelating agents (such as deferoxamine or deferasirox) may be needed. First-degree relatives should be screened for genetic hemochromatosis with fasting transferrin saturation levels

WD is an autosomal recessive disease of copper deposition that has an average prevalence of approximately 30 per million population worldwide. The gene, ATP7B, is located on chromosome 13 and encodes a metal-transporting P-type ATPase, which functions in the transmembrane transport of copper in the hepatocyte. Any one of the more than 200 different mutations in the gene causes absent or reduced function of the ATP7B protein, which leads to decreased hepatocellular excretion of copper into bile and inability to incorporate copper into ceruloplasmin. These result in hepatic copper accumulation and injury to the hepatocyte. Eventually, copper is released from the liver and is deposited in various other organs, including the brain, kidneys, and cornea.[30]

The disease can present with no symptoms or with liver dysfunction, progressive neurologic disorder, or psychiatric illness between ages 5 and 35 years of age. Some patients may have a brief clinical illness that resembles viral hepatitis or AIH, whereas others may present with clinical signs of cirrhosis. Acute liver failure may also occur, with an associated Coombs-negative hemolytic anemia and acute renal failure. Neurologic manifestation of WD typically present later than the liver disease and usually consist of extrapyramidal symptoms (i.e., tremor, motor incoordination, drooling, dysarthria, dystonia, and spasticity. Psychiatric manifestations may include depression, anxiety, and even psychosis.

In the setting of elevated serum aminotransaminases, the diagnosis of WD is suggested by a low serum ceruloplasmin level of less than 20 mg/dL. Kayser-Fleischer rings detected by slit lamp examination are considered to be diagnostic in the presence of neurologic symptoms. However, ceruloplasmin may be falsely elevated in settings of acute inflammation and hyperestrogenemia and falsely low in conditions with marked renal or enteral protein loss or severe end-stage liver disease of any etiology. The serum uric acid may also be low due to associated renal tubular dysfunction (Fanconi syndrome). In cases of acute liver failure, the serum alkaline phosphatase may be low and a ratio of alkaline phosphatase to total bilirubin of less than 2 may be seen. Urinary copper reflects the amount of free copper in the circulation, and a level greater than 40 µg over 24 hours in the absence of other cholestatic liver diseases, is suggestive of WD. Urinary copper excretion greater than 1600 µg/24 hours with D-penicillamine challenge is a useful diagnostic tool in the pediatric population. Hepatic copper content greater than or equal to 250 µg/g dry weight is the best histologic evidence for WD, although the distribution of copper within the liver becomes heterogeneous in later stages of WD. An MRI of the brain may demonstrate structural abnormalities in the basal ganglia in patients with WD who have neurologic manifestations.[30]

Treatment of WD involves chelation of the copper with penicillamine or trientene to allow for renal excretion, and/or use of zinc to compete with copper absorption in the gut. First-degree relatives should be screened for WD.

AATD is a common genetic disorder in individuals of Scandinavian and Northern European descent, affecting approximately 1 in 1600 to 1800 live births. It is characterized by a mutation in the SERPINA1 gene that codes for the alpha1-antitrypsin protein. A homozygous mutation leads to the production of the Z protein, which takes an abnormal configuration that prevents its secretion from the hepatocyte, leading to a concomitant deficiency of the protein in the lung. While emphysema results from uninhibited proteolytic destruction of the connective tissue backbone of the lung, the retained mutant Z protein in the endoplasmic reticulum of the hepatocyte activates a cascade of cell injury that leads to apoptosis, fibrosis, and, in some individuals, cirrhosis.

Clinical manifestation and disease course are highly variable, even among protease inhibitor (Pi) ZZ homozygote individuals, suggesting contributions from other genetic and environmental influences in the phenotypic penetrance of the disease. Clinical signs and symptoms may be detected early in infancy but AATD may not be diagnosed until later in childhood or adulthood when patients present with asymptomatic hepatomegaly or elevated transaminases, or with jaundice during the course of an untreated illness. A minority of patients will present with evidence of portal hypertension and synthetic dysfunction, and a few may present with cholestasis.[31] The diagnosis of AATD is established by obtaining an AAT protein phenotype where M is the most common normal allelic variant and S and Z proteins are the aberrant proteins. Liver disease is associated with the homozygous PiZZ phenotype as well as with the compound heterozygous PiSZ phenotype. Heterozygous MZ phenotype is not associated with liver disease by itself.[32] A low circulating serum AAT protein level is expected, but such level may be falsely elevated to normal or near-normal ranges by a concomitant inflammatory host response and may also be falsely low in patients with advanced cirrhosis. The histologic feature of periodic acid-Schiff–positive, diastase-resistant globules in the endoplasmic reticulum of hepatocytes confirms the diagnosis.

Current treatment for liver disease from AATD consists mostly of supportive care and liver transplantation if indicated, but new and promising therapeutic approaches that include gene therapy, stem cell transplantation, and stimulation of autophagy are currently under investigation.

SEPSIS-INDUCED AND PARENTERAL NUTRITION–ASSOCIATED CHOLESTASIS

Cholestasis in the critically ill or postoperative patient is typically multifactorial in etiology, resulting from any combination of sepsis, PN, positive end-expiratory pressure levels, multiple blood transfusions, renal insufficiency, and drugs. The underlying mechanism involves either hepatocellular injury that leads to decreased bilirubin uptake, decreased intrahepatic processing, decreased canalicular transport, decreased clearance of conjugated bilirubin and/or decreased flow through the bile ducts.[8]

Sepsis is the most common cause of cholestasis in critically ill patients and presents with increased bilirubin and alkaline phosphatase levels up to 2 to 3 times normal, and only mild elevations of aminotransferases. Although the primary site of infection is most often intraabdominal, infections at other sites have also been associated with this condition. The mechanism of cholestasis involves decreased basolateral and canalicular transport of bile acids resulting from endotoxemia and its consequent cytokine release.[33] Management of sepsis-induced cholestasis revolves around treatment of the underlying infection, as well as optimizing supportive care and avoidance of additional hepatic insults. Although ursodeoxycholic acid has potential to improve bile flow, data on its benefit in sepsis-induced cholestasis are lacking.

PN is a life-saving therapy in patients with intestinal failure, but PN administration may cause liver dysfunction in as many as 65% of patients.[34] Within the first 2 weeks of administration, mild to moderate elevations in serum aminotransferases may be observed; these may not be associated with significant histologic changes and levels eventually plateau, but it may progress to a more cholestatic pattern of liver test abnormalities in some patients. In adults, PN-associated liver disease may start early as steatosis, which can evolve to steatohepatitis and cholestasis of varying severity with continuing administration of the PN. The pathophysiology of PN-associated liver disease is multifactorial, but excess calories in the PN solution and lipids administered greater than 1 g/kg are believed to predispose to this complication.[35] Phytosterol content in the lipid emulsion, particularly, has been implicated.[36] Sepsis is another major risk factor, and other conditions, such as nutrient deficiencies, nutrient toxicities, and the lack of enteral stimulation, may also play a role in the pathogenesis of liver disease. Diagnosis of PN-associated cholestasis is made by exclusion of biliary obstruction and other possible etiologies of cholestasis, such as drugs. Earlier stages of PN-associated liver disease would typically show steatosis or steatohepatitis with or without fibrosis on liver biopsy, but PN-associated cholestasis is marked by the presence of mild to moderate intrahepatic cholestasis with minimal inflammation, with or without portal fibrosis, and some cases may eventually progress to cirrhosis.[35]

Nonpharmacologic management strategies for PN-related liver disease include enteral stimulation, optimizing PN composition, and avoidance of excess carbohydrate and lipid calories. Pharmacologic therapy with ursodeoxycholic acid has had some success, and antibiotic therapy, such as metronidazole, to reduce the risk of bacterial translocation, has also been used. Liver and intestinal transplantation may be necessary in those patients with permanent intestinal failure who develop persistent, severe liver disease from PN.[37]

BILE DUCT OBSTRUCTION

Bile duct obstruction may result acutely from a gallstone that travels down the cystic duct into the common hepatic duct, causing transient elevations in either serum aminotransferases or alkaline phosphatase levels. It may also result from a rapidly growing mass lesion that encroaches upon the common bile duct or the right or left hepatic duct. A slower, more insidious obstruction of the bile ducts may result from benign biliary or ampullary stricture or a slow-growing malignancy. Elevations in serum bilirubin

(predominantly conjugated) and alkaline phosphatase are typical in both situations. Patients with gallstone disease have a smaller increase in bilirubin (usually less than 20 mg/dL) than those with extrahepatic malignant biliary obstruction (who may have serum bilirubin as high as 35 to 40 mg/dL). Serum aminotransferases may also rise initially until obstruction is relieved. The serum alkaline phosphatase may be as high as 10 times normal in the setting of normal serum aminotransferases in cases of obstruction due to malignancy. Tumor markers (e.g., carbohydrate antigen [CA] 19-9, carcinoembryonic antigen [CEA], CA 125) may be elevated in benign or malignant biliary obstruction.[38]

Ultrasound is a good initial screening tool due to its noninvasive nature, low cost, and wide availability. In equivocal cases a cholescintigraphy (diisopropyl-iminodiacetic acid [DISIDA], hepatobiliary iminodiacetic acid [HIDA]) may be obtained to evaluate the patency of the cystic duct. A CT scan may demonstrate a mass lesion that is causing obstruction of the common bile duct, but an MRI with magnetic resonance cholangiography (MRC) can provide additional details on the biliary tree. However, when intervention is needed, it requires an endoscopic retrograde cholangiopancreatography (ERCP) or a percutaneous biliary cholangiogram. Endoscopic ultrasound (EUS) is gaining traction in detecting choledocholithiasis in patients with acute pancreatitis. It is also more sensitive in detecting small pancreatic and ampullary tumors than cross-sectional radiologic images. Fine-needle aspiration performed during the EUS is useful for the diagnosis of malignancy. More specialized tests, such as intraductal ultrasound and cholangioscopy, may provide additional details in characterizing indeterminate biliary strictures, and intraductal ultrasound may also be useful in detecting pancreatic carcinoma in situ, but these are expensive and technically demanding with very limited availability.[38]

PRIMARY BILIARY CHOLANGITIS AND HEPATIC SARCOIDOSIS

PBC, formerly known as primary biliary cirrhosis, is a chronic cholestatic liver disease characterized by intrahepatic interlobular and septal bile duct destruction. It is predominantly seen in middle-aged women and is associated with other autoimmune disorders, such as thyroiditis, sicca syndrome, Raynaud phenomenon, CREST (calcinosis, Raynaud phenomenon, esophageal dysmotility, sclerodactyly, and telangiectasia) syndrome/scleroderma, ulcerative colitis, celiac disease, and rheumatoid arthritis.

PBC is believed to be an immune-mediated disease that develops in genetically predisposed individuals, and bacterial infection has been proposed as the inciting factor. Some bacteria have been found to possess similar nucleotide sequences as the lipoyl domain of the pyruvate dehydrogenase complex E2 (PDC-E2) on the inner mitochondrial membrane of the biliary epithelial cell. Exposure to such organisms may lead to the development of an immune response with M2 antimitochondrial antibody (AMA), which also targets the PDC-E2 antigens in the biliary epithelial cell, a process called "molecular mimicry."[39,40]

The most common symptom reported by patients with PBC is fatigue (40% to 80% of patients), followed by generalized pruritus. Approximately 25% of patients may be asymptomatic at the time of diagnosis, presenting only with mildly cholestatic liver tests. Jaundice usually occurs later in the disease. On examination, patients may have hepatosplenomegaly, xanthelasmas or xanthomas. Evidence of portal hypertension may be present, and those who have developed cirrhosis may have symptoms of liver failure.

The hallmarks for diagnosis of PBC are the detection of AMA in 95% and a chronically elevated alkaline phosphatase in a middle-aged woman presenting with fatigue or pruritus. The 5% of patients with PBC who are negative for the AMA, also known as autoimmune cholangitis, are diagnosed by a liver biopsy that demonstrates the presence of a florid duct lesion (i.e., a nonsuppurative granulomatous destruction of the interlobular and septal bile ducts) and eosinophilic infiltrates. Patients with PBC may also have hypergammaglobulinemia and elevated ANA titers.

PBC usually progresses over time, and cirrhosis with its complications typically develops within 15 to 20 years of diagnosis. Although asymptomatic patients appear to have similar survival as healthy patients, those who develop symptoms will have a diminished survival. Patients with PBC are at risk for developing osteoporosis. Many patients have elevations in cholesterol levels, mostly of the high-density lipoprotein (HDL) component in the earlier stages of the disease and converting to the low-density lipoprotein (LDL) component in later stages. Because of the involvement of portal tracts in this disease, portal hypertension may develop even in the absence of cirrhosis. With chronic cholestasis, malabsorption of dietary fatty acids and fat-soluble vitamins may also develop.[39]

Ursodeoxycholic acid at lower doses of 12 to 15 mg/kg per day can improve or normalize serum alkaline phosphatase in 70% of patients and improve transplant-free survival.[41] In patients who are intolerant or unresponsive to ursodeoxycholic acid, obeticholic acid is an alternative treatment that improves serum alkaline phosphatase levels, but its effect on survival is not yet known.[42]

Sarcoidosis is a systemic granulomatous inflammatory disease that affects 36 per 100,000 African Americans and 11 per 100,000 white individuals in the United States. Immunologic, genetic, environmental, and oxidative stress factors are hypothesized to contribute to the development of the disease. The lungs are involved in 90% of cases, but the liver may be involved in up to 80%. Hepatic sarcoidosis is usually asymptomatic, presenting with hepatomegaly, cholestatic liver chemistry tests, or nodular abnormalities in the liver on radiographic imaging. Those who have symptoms may complain of right upper quadrant abdominal pain, nausea, emesis, weight loss, and fevers. The diagnosis of hepatic sarcoidosis is based on clinical and radiographic findings with compatible histologic findings in a biopsy obtained from the liver or any other organ involved with sarcoidosis, after excluding other causes of hepatic granulomas.[3] Mild cases of hepatic sarcoidosis may have spontaneous remission and do not need therapy, but more severe cases or those with complications warrant consideration of corticosteroid therapy,

which may improve clinical symptoms, serum liver chemistry tests, and hepatomegaly, but has no proven histologic benefit. Corticosteroids particularly benefit patients who have portal lymphadenopathy that causes biliary obstruction, as resolution of the jaundice has been observed. Similarly, treatment with ursodeoxycholic acid has also led to clinical and biochemical improvement with unknown histologic benefit.[44]

PRIMARY SCLEROSING CHOLANGITIS AND IMMUNOGLOBULIN G4-ASSOCIATED CHOLANGITIS

PSC is a chronic progressive, immune-mediated disease characterized by patchy inflammation of the biliary tree leading to obliterative fibrosis. The exact cause of PSC is still unknown, although both genetic and environmental factors seem to be at play. Two-thirds of affected individuals are males, and the mean age at diagnosis is 40 years.[45] PSC is strongly associated with inflammatory bowel disease, with ulcerative colitis being diagnosed in up to 82% and Crohn disease in up to 13% of patients with PSC. From another vantage, PSC is present in approximately 2.4% to 7.5% of patients with ulcerative colitis.[46] PSC may be asymptomatic in up to 55% of affected individuals but when symptoms are present, they consist of fatigue, pruritus and bouts of bacterial cholangitis accompanied by transient jaundice. Signs of portal hypertension and liver failure may eventually develop.

The diagnosis of PSC is made on the presence of segmental or diffuse irregularity, stricturing, or pruning of the bile ducts on ERCP or magnetic resonance cholangiopancreatography (MRCP) images, in the setting of compatible clinical findings and chronically elevated serum alkaline phosphatase levels, although rare patients may have normal serum alkaline phosphatase levels. Biliary strictures are typically short and annular, alternating with normal or minimally dilated segments to produce a characteristic "beaded" appearance. Histologic findings may be nonspecific due to the segmental nature of the disease and the larger size of the ducts involved, but if the characteristic lesion is captured on the biopsy, it appears as "onion-skinning" or extensive periductular fibrosis with obliteration of the bile ducts (fibroobliterative lesion).[4] Serologic testing for specific autoimmune antibodies does not contribute to the diagnosis of this disease.

Management of PSC includes endoscopic or percutaneous balloon dilation and stenting if a dominant stricture involving the larger extrahepatic biliary ducts is present. Hepaticojejunostomy may be considered for noncirrhotic patients who have severe cholestasis or recurrent bacterial cholangitis attributed to a dominant extrahepatic or hilar stricture that is not amenable to endoscopic or percutaneous dilation and drainage. Liver transplantation is resorted to in patients with cirrhosis; recurrent bacterial cholangitis despite intensive endoscopic or percutaneous and medical therapy; severe extrahepatic biliary obstruction that precludes operative intervention; uncontrolled peristomal variceal bleeding; or intractable pruritus. Unfortunately, no effective medication for PSC exists,[45] although ursodeoxycholic acid in doses up to 15 mg/kg per day is often used to promote bile flow in patients with recurrent bacterial cholangitis. High doses of ursodeoxycholic acid

(28 to 30 mg/kg per day) have been found to lead to detrimental outcomes in PSC.[48]

IgG4-associated cholangitis (IAC) is an immune-mediated systemic disorder that has a predilection for the pancreas and the liver, causing autoimmune pancreatitis and IAC. It also causes cholecystitis, sialadenitis, other gastrointestinal organ involvement, retroperitoneal fibrosis, lymphadenopathy, pulmonary or renal involvement, prostatitis, aortitis, and thyroid gland or bone marrow infiltration.[49] The most common presentation of IAC is obstructive jaundice, sometimes with radiologic images demonstrating lesions that mimic cholangiocarcinoma or pancreatic cancer, leading to unnecessary surgical resections of the liver or pancreas. The diagnosis is based on increased serum levels of total IgG in 42% to 70% and IgG4 in 73% to 90% of patients[50] and the presence of intrahepatic and extrahepatic biliary strictures on cholangiographic imaging, which may also be accompanied by a diffusely enlarged pancreas and narrowing of the main pancreatic duct in up to 90% of cases. However, IAC cases with normal IgG4 have also been documented, and it should be noted that some patients with PSC or pancreatic cancer also have elevated IgG4 levels. Histologically, infiltration of IgG4-positive lymphoplasmacytic cells in the biliary duct wall and the pancreas are the hallmarks of this disease, as opposed to the fibroobliterative lesion and bile duct paucity that are seen in PSC. Immunosuppression, typically with a course of steroids, is highly effective clinically,[51] although a few cases may need maintenance immunosuppression with azathioprine or mycophenolate mofetil.

ISOLATED UNCONJUGATED AND CONJUGATED HYPERBILIRUBINEMIA

Disorders of bilirubin metabolism may occur at any of the several steps in the pathway. Unconjugated hyperbilirubinemia may result from bilirubin overproduction, reduced hepatic uptake, or defective bilirubin conjugation. Conjugated hyperbilirubinemia results from bile canalicular transporter defects or impairment of bile flow through the intrahepatic and extrahepatic bile ducts. These isolated cases of hyperbilirubinemia are typically accompanied by normal serum AST, ALT, and alkaline phosphatase as well as normal liver histology.

Unconjugated hyperbilirubinemia may be due to overproduction of bilirubin, as may occur in hemolysis. The serum total bilirubin rarely increases to greater than 5 mg/dL, and the conjugated value is less than 15% of the total value. The serum conjugated bilirubin also increases because of saturation of the excretory mechanisms with regurgitation of conjugated bilirubin into plasma. Unconjugated hyperbilirubinemia may also result from decreased bilirubin uptake into the hepatocyte due to competition for a carrier-mediated binding site on the hepatocyte plasma membrane by drugs, such as rifampicin and oral cholecystographic drugs.

Unconjugated hyperbilirubinemia due to inadequate intrahepatic bilirubin binding and conjugation is seen in Gilbert syndrome. Gilbert syndrome results from decreased uridine-diphosphoryl-glucuronosyltransferase (UDP-GT) activity that afflicts up to 7% of the general population. Serum unconjugated bilirubin levels tend to increase during fasting, stress, or illness but rarely increase to greater than 5 mg/dL. This is a benign condition that is inherited via a variable pattern and does not affect long-term survival, although it may affect the risk for certain drug toxicity when UDP-GT is involved in the drug detoxification process.[52] A rare autosomal recessive disease, Crigler-Najjar syndrome, is caused by a deficiency in UDP-GT activity. In type I Crigler-Najjar syndrome, there is complete absence of enzyme activity, resulting in severe hyperbilirubinemia (serum total bilirubin >30 mg/dL) and usually, death. In type II, there is partial transferase activity, and this may present with mild to moderate hyperbilirubinemia (5 to 30 mg/dL). This condition may be compatible with life, and medical treatment with phenobarbital can induce expression of UDP-GT to lower the serum unconjugated bilirubin levels.[52]

Conjugated hyperbilirubinemia results from inherited disorders in canalicular transport of conjugated bilirubin, such as Dubin-Johnson syndrome and Rotor syndrome. Dubin-Johnson syndrome is an autosomal recessive disorder characterized by intermittent mild jaundice, caused predominantly by a conjugated hyperbilirubinemia (bilirubin 2 to 5 mg/dL). This is thought to be mediated by an inherited defect in the canalicular transport of conjugated bilirubin, due to a mutation of the MRP2 gene that results in defective expression of the MRP2 transporter. Dark pigment accumulates in the hepatic lysosomes. Rotor syndrome is similar to the Dubin-Johnson syndrome, but there is no dark pigment accumulation in the lysosomes.[52] However, the exact pathogenesis is not clear. Most patients are asymptomatic and can lead normal lives.

SUMMARY

Liver chemistry tests are useful in providing a window into the health of the liver. However, normal liver chemistry tests may accompany significant liver disease, and liver disease may not be identified in a few patients who have persistent elevations. Both elevated and normal liver chemistry tests need to be interpreted in the context of the clinical setting. The interpretation of abnormal liver chemistry tests should be guided by the pattern and acuity of the elevations, which can narrow the differential diagnoses to some degree and allow for a more efficient and tailored evaluation to achieve the diagnosis.

REFERENCES

1. Strasser M, Stadlmayr A, Haufe H, et al. Natural course of subjects with elevated liver tests and normal liver histology. *Liver Int.* 2016; 36:119-125.
2. Woreta TA, Alqahtani SA. Evaluation of abnormal liver tests. *Med Clin North Am.* 2014;98:1-16.
3. Herlong HF. MMCJ: laboratory tests. In: Schiff E, Maddrey WC, Sorrell MF, eds. *Schiff's Diseases of the Liver.* 11th ed. Chichester, West Sussex, UK: John Wiley & Sons; 2012:17-43.
4. Schiele F, Henny J, Hitz J, Petitclerc C, Gueguen R, Siest G. Total bone and liver alkaline phosphatases in plasma: biological variations and reference limits. *Clin Chem.* 1983;29:634-641.
5. Tapper EB, Sengupta N, Bonder A. The incidence and outcomes of ischemic hepatitis: a systematic review with meta-analysis. *Am J Med.* 2015;128:1314-1321.
6. Birrer R, Takuda Y, Takara T. Hypoxic hepatopathy: pathophysiology and prognosis. *Intern Med.* 2007;46:1063-1070.

7. Fuhrmann V, Kneidinger N, Herkner H, et al. Impact of hypoxic hepatitis on mortality in the intensive care unit. *Intensive Care Med.* 2011;37:1302-1310.

8. Horvatits T, Trauner M, Fuhrmann V. Hypoxic liver injury and cholestasis in critically ill patients. *Curr Opin Crit Care.* 2013;19:128-132.

9. Chitturi S, Farrell GC. Drug-induced liver disease. In: Schiff ER, Maddrey WC, Sorrell MF, eds. *Schiff's Diseases of the Liver.* Chichester, West Sussex, UK: John Wiley & Sons; 2012:703-783.

10. Chalasani NP, Hayashi PH, Bonkovsky HL, et al. ACG Clinical Guideline: the diagnosis and management of idiosyncratic drug-induced liver injury. *Am J Gastroenterol.* 2014;109:950-966; quiz 967.

11. Temple R. Hy's law: predicting serious hepatotoxicity. *Pharmacoepidemiol Drug Saf.* 2006;15:241-243.

12. Tajiri K, Shimizu Y. Practical guidelines for diagnosis and early management of drug-induced liver injury. *World J Gastroenterol.* 2008;14:6774-6785.

13. Bhamidimarri KR, Schiff E. Drug-induced cholestasis. *Clin Liver Dis.* 2013;17:519-531, vii.

14. Chalasani N, Fontana RJ, Bonkovsky HL, et al. Causes, clinical features, and outcomes from a prospective study of drug-induced liver injury in the United States. *Gastroenterology.* 2008;135:1924-1934, 1934.e1921-1934.e1924.

15. Watson J, Sjogren M. Hepatitis A and E. In: Schiff E, Maddrey WC, Sorrell MF, eds. *Schiff's Diseases of the Liver.* 11th ed. Chichester, West Sussex, UK: John Wiley & Sons; 2012:521-535.

16. Foodborne Hepatitis A Outbreaks in the U.S. Are Well-documented; Vaccine Provides Lifetime Protection. http://www.immunize.org/catg.d/p2104.pdf. Accessed 22 May 2016.

17. Te HS, Drobeniuc J, Kamili S, Dong C, Hart J, Sharapov UM. Hepatitis E virus infection in a liver transplant recipient in the United States: a case report. *Transplant Proc.* 2013;45:810-813.

18. Lok ASF, Negro F. Hepatitis B and D. In: Schiff ER, Maddrey WC, Sorrell MF, eds. *Schiff's Diseases of the Liver.* 11th ed. Chichester, West Sussex, UK: John Wiley & Sons; 2012:537-581.

19. Te HS. Diagnostic approach to hepatitis B virus (HBV) infection. *N Am J Med Sci.* 2011;4:27-34.

20. Darling JM, Lemon SM, Fried MW. Hepatitis C. In: Schiff ER, Maddrey WC, Sorrell MF, eds. *Schiff's Diseases of the Liver.* 11th ed. Chichester, West Sussex, UK: John Wiley & Sons; 2012:582-652.

21. Thursz MR, Richardson P, Allison M, et al. Prednisolone or pentoxifylline for alcoholic hepatitis. *N Engl J Med.* 2015;372:1619-1628.

22. Lazo M, Hernaez R, Eberhardt MS, et al. Prevalence of nonalcoholic fatty liver disease in the United States: the Third National Health and Nutrition Examination Survey, 1988-1994. *Am J Epidemiol.* 2013; 178:38-45.

23. Browning JD, Szczepaniak LS, Dobbins R, et al. Prevalence of hepatic steatosis in an urban population in the United States: impact of ethnicity. *Hepatology.* 2004;40:1387-1395.

24. Williams CD, Stengel J, Asike MI, et al. Prevalence of nonalcoholic fatty liver disease and nonalcoholic steatohepatitis among a largely middle-aged population utilizing ultrasound and liver biopsy: a prospective study. *Gastroenterology.* 2011;140:124-131.

25. Ahmed M. Non-alcoholic fatty liver disease in 2015. *World J Hepatol.* 2015;7:1450-1459.

26. Sanyal AJ, Chalasani N, Kowdley KV, et al. Pioglitazone, vitamin E, or placebo for nonalcoholic steatohepatitis. *N Engl J Med.* 2010;362:1675-1685.

27. Liberal R, Vergani D, Mieli-Vergani G. Update on autoimmune hepatitis. *J Clin Transl Hepatol.* 2015;3:42-52.

28. Pietrangelo A. Genetics, genetic testing, and management of hemochromatosis: 15 years since hepcidin. *Gastroenterology.* 2015;149:1240-1251.e1244.

29. Salgia RJ, Brown K. Diagnosis and management of hereditary hemochromatosis. *Clin Liver Dis.* 2015;19:187-198.

30. Roberts EA, Schilsky ML, American Association for Study of Liver D. Diagnosis and treatment of Wilson disease: an update. *Hepatology.* 2008;47:2089-2111.

31. Perlmutter DH. Alpha-1-antitrypsin deficiency: diagnosis and treatment. *Clin Liver Dis.* 2004;8:839-859, viii-ix.

32. Nelson DR, Teckman J, Di Bisceglie AM, Brenner DA. Diagnosis and management of patients with alpha1-antitrypsin (A1AT) deficiency. *Clin Gastroenterol Hepatol.* 2012;10:575-580.

33. Chand N, Sanyal AJ. Sepsis-induced cholestasis. *Hepatology.* 2007;45:230-241.

34. Cavicchi M, Beau P, Crenn P, Degott C, Messing B. Prevalence of liver disease and contributing factors in patients receiving home parenteral nutrition for permanent intestinal failure. *Ann Intern Med.* 2000;132:525-532.

35. Raman M, Allard JP. Parenteral nutrition related hepato-biliary disease in adults. *Appl Physiol Nutr Metab.* 2007;32:646-654.

36. Zaloga GP. Phytosterols, lipid administration, and liver disease during parenteral nutrition. *JPEN J Parenter Enteral Nutr.* 2015;39:39S-60S.

37. Guglielmi FW, Regano N, Mazzuoli S, et al. Cholestasis induced by total parenteral nutrition. *Clin Liver Dis.* 2008;12:97-110, viii.

38. Adley JL, Mitchell RM. Advances in the investigation of obstructive jaundice. *Curr Gastroenterol Rep.* 2012;14:511-519.

39. Bhandari BM, Bayat H, Rothstein KD. Primary biliary cirrhosis. *Gastroenterol Clin North Am.* 2011;40:373-386, viii.

40. Poupon R. Primary biliary cirrhosis: a 2010 update. *J Hepatol.* 2010;52:745-758.

41. Poupon RE, Lindor KD, Cauch-Dudek K, Dickson ER, Poupon R, Heathcote EJ. Combined analysis of randomized controlled trials of ursodeoxycholic acid in primary biliary cirrhosis. *Gastroenterology.* 1997;113:884-890.

42. Hirschfield GM, Mason A, Luketic V, et al. Efficacy of obeticholic acid in patients with primary biliary cirrhosis and inadequate response to ursodeoxycholic acid. *Gastroenterology.* 2015;148:751-761.e758.

43. Cremers J, Drent M, Driessen A, et al. Liver-test abnormalities in sarcoidosis. *Eur J Gastroenterol Hepatol.* 2012;24:17-24.

44. Cremers JP, Drent M, Baughman RP, Wijnen PA, Koek GH. Therapeutic approach of hepatic sarcoidosis. *Curr Opin Pulm Med.* 2012;18:472-482.

45. Silveira MG, Lindor KD. Primary sclerosing cholangitis. *Can J Gastroenterol.* 2008;22:689-698.

46. Fausa O, Schrumpf E, Elgjo K. Relationship of inflammatory bowel disease and primary sclerosing cholangitis. *Semin Liver Dis.* 1991;11:31-39.

47. MacCarty RL, LaRusso NF, Wiesner RH, Ludwig J. Primary sclerosing cholangitis: findings on cholangiography and pancreatography. *Radiology.* 1983;149:39-44.

48. Lindor KD, Kowdley KV, Luketic VA, et al. High-dose ursodeoxycholic acid for the treatment of primary sclerosing cholangitis. *Hepatology.* 2009;50:808-814.

49. Alderliste YA, van den Elzen BD, Rauws EA, Beuers U. Immunoglobulin G4-associated cholangitis: one variant of immunoglobulin G4-related systemic disease. *Digestion.* 2009;79:220-228.

50. Nishimori I, Otsuki M. Autoimmune pancreatitis and IgG4-associated sclerosing cholangitis. *Best Pract Res Clin Gastroenterol.* 2009;23: 11-23.

51. Deshpande V. IgG4-related disease of the gastrointestinal tract: a 21st century chameleon. *Arch Pathol Lab Med.* 2015;139:742-749.

52. Fabris L, Cadamuro M, Okolicsanyi L. The patient presenting with isolated hyperbilirubinemia. *Dig Liver Dis.* 2009;41:375-381.

Perioperative Management and Nutritional Support in Patients With Liver and Biliary Tract Disease

Joseph DiNorcia | Steven D. Colquhoun

Even the most straightforward surgical procedure can become exceptionally challenging when performed on a patient with an underlying hepatobiliary disorder. Hepatic dysfunction, as manifest by portal hypertension, synthetic impairment, and cholestasis may be present to varying degrees, and can have a profound influence on the physiology of other organ systems. Depending on the severity of the underlying dysfunction and the nature of the operation, even seemingly minor procedures can precipitate a cascade of events resulting in hemodynamic instability, bleeding, and hepatic decompensation. To avoid such complications, the surgeon must anticipate and appropriately assess in advance any patient who falls along the spectrum of hepatobiliary disease. This chapter focuses on the perioperative issues related to patients with varying degrees of dysfunction caused by primary liver disease and/or the consequences of biliary obstruction. A review of the pathophysiology of hepatobiliary disease first allows a context for understanding the importance of perioperative care in this patient population. A detailed examination of the preoperative, intraoperative, and postoperative considerations for surgical candidates with hepatobiliary dysfunction then follows.

PATHOPHYSIOLOGY OF CIRRHOSIS AND OBSTRUCTIVE JAUNDICE

As evidenced by the suffering of Prometheus in classical Greek mythology, the unique regenerative capacity of the liver has long been appreciated. In the clinical setting, regeneration of a healthy liver usually restores normal hepatic function. However, repeated cycles of regeneration due to chronic inflammation lead to significant alterations to the normal parenchymal architecture. This results in fibrosis, and ultimately cirrhosis, with progressive liver dysfunction.[1,2] The dual arterial and portal venous perfusion of the hepatic sinusoids also changes as fibrosis progresses. The resultant regenerative nodules have only hepatic arterial inflow, as portal venous flow cannot penetrate the fibrotic collagen deposits. Impairment in the first-pass metabolism of substances absorbed from the gastrointestinal tract then becomes one of the first clinically relevant aspects of managing such patients.

In addition to mechanical resistance, a decrease in the secretion of vasodilators and an increase in the secretion of vasoconstrictors in the sinusoids contribute to an increased resistance to portal venous flow *within* the liver.[3,4] *Outside* the liver, there is a further release of vasodilators in the splanchnic circulation to compensate for the increased resistance to portal venous flow. Portal hypertension thus develops as a result of both resistance to blood flow through the liver and overall increased inflow in the splanchnic bed. The increased pressure gradient between the portal and systemic circulations gives rise to the shunting of blood to the spleen and the development of collateral pathways of portal venous flow around the liver. These portosystemic collaterals typically form gastroesophageal, retroperitoneal, periumbilical, and rectal varices, which can lead to gastrointestinal bleeding in the perioperative period and major hemorrhage intraoperatively. Splenomegaly, hypersplenism, and spontaneous splenorenal shunts are other direct consequences of portal hypertension that have clinical implications. Patients with cirrhosis and portal hypertension display multiple interacting physiologic changes that greatly complicate perioperative care (Fig. 120.1).

HEMODYNAMIC CONSIDERATIONS

Cirrhosis leads to profound hemodynamic changes that are part of a complex pathophysiology based primarily on vasodilation. Portal hypertension leads to a release of vasodilators, such as nitric oxide in the splanchnic vasculature to augment blood flow through the cirrhotic liver.[5] These vasodilators are not metabolized normally by the dysfunctional liver and so accumulate, causing further splanchnic, and ultimately systemic, vasodilation. Vasodilation causes low systemic vascular resistance and decreased effective circulatory volume. This leads to activation of both neural and hormonal changes that move to restore effective circulatory volume through vasoconstriction and sodium and water retention.[6] This compensatory vasoconstriction can cause renal ischemia, and the resultant sodium and water retention can contribute to worsening hyponatremia, ascites, and edema. Because of these changes, patients with cirrhosis usually display a baseline tachycardia, relative hypotension, and elevated cardiac output, all reflective of a significant hyperdynamic state.

A variety of interventions may improve overall hemodynamics in patients with cirrhosis.[7] Judicious administration of intravenous colloid can help to temporarily restore intravascular volume. However, excess fluid administration can exacerbate ascites and peripheral edema and lead to volume overload. Splanchnic vasoconstrictor therapy may improve hemodynamics, particularly when renal dysfunction is present. In later stages of cirrhosis, patients may require vasopressors to support blood pressure. Pulmonary artery catheterization, or other assessments of central pressure, may be helpful in some cases to guide fluid resuscitation and vasopressor management. Hypotension despite adequate filling pressures indicates advanced

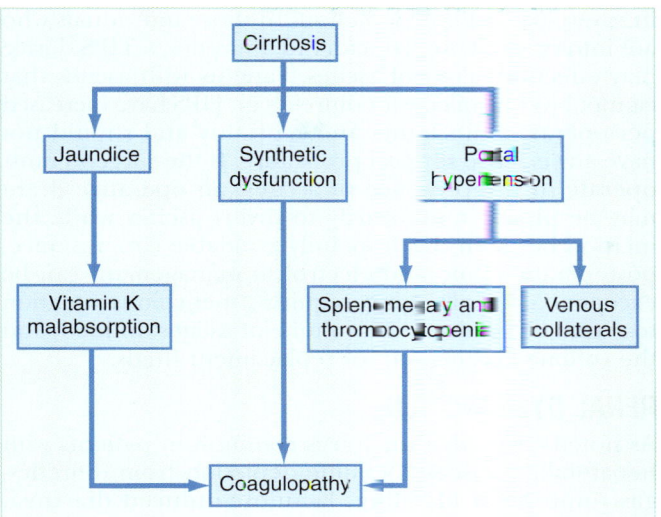

FIGURE 120.1 Schematic showing the interrelationship of multiple physiologic disturbances occurring in patients with cirrhosis and portal hypertension.

hepatobiliary dysfunction and should give the surgeon pause to reassess the indications for the proposed surgical intervention.

CARDIOPULMONARY ISSUES

Cardiopulmonary disease often is present in patients with cirrhosis. The persistence of chronic volume overload and a high cardiac output state can lead to valvular dysfunction and progressive heart failure, with portal hypertension itself contributing to overall cardiac impairment.[8] Patients with alcoholic liver disease or hemochromatosis are particularly predisposed to cardiomyopathy and arrhythmia. Many cirrhotic patients are also at risk for coronary artery disease from long-standing associations such as those related to cigarette smoking or diabetes mellitus.

Liver disease can also significantly impact the lungs. Patients with cirrhosis and ascites are at risk for developing hepatic hydrothorax, hepatopulmonary syndrome, and portopulmonary hypertension.[9] Hepatic hydrothorax (HH) is most commonly found in the right chest and is usually a transudative pleural effusion that results from passage of ascites across the diaphragm. This can often be appreciated on a preoperative physical exam or on a simple chest radiography.[10] Patients with HH are at risk for spontaneous bacterial empyema. Consideration should be given to treating HH perioperatively depending on size and symptoms. When significant, it can impair mechanical ventilation during or after surgery. It can also cause pressure on the right hemidiaphragm sufficient to limit exposure and mobilization of the liver for the surgeon. Similar to ascites, HH is managed with dietary salt restriction, diuretics, thoracentesis, transjugular intrahepatic portosystemic shunt (TIPS) and ultimately liver transplantation.

Both the hepatopulmonary syndrome (HPS) and portopulmonary hypertension (PPH) result when various vasoactive substances bypass the diseased liver and accumulate in a manner that alters the pulmonary vasculature.[11]

HPS is defined by pulmonary vascular dilation causing ventilation-perfusion mismatch and chronic hypoxemia ($Pao_2 <$) mm Hg) in the setting of chronic liver disease.[12,13] Transthoracic echocardiography with bubble contrast can identify intrapulmonary shunts to confirm the diagnosis. Supplemental oxygen and oral garlic supplementation can temporize HPS, but liver transplantation is the only definitive treatment. PPH is defined by pulmonary vascular constriction causing pulmonary hypertension (mean pulmonary artery pressure >25 mm Hg) in the setting of portal hypertension.[14-16] Echocardiography can suggest the diagnosis when estimated pulmonary artery systolic pressures are 40 to 50 mm Hg, but pulmonary artery catheterization is necessary for confirmation. Temporizing treatment of PPH consists of pulmonary vasodilators such as prostaglandin analogues, phosphodiesterase inhibitors, nitric oxide, and endothelin receptor antagonists. Again, liver transplantation is the only definitive cure.

Finally, it should be appreciated that some underlying liver diseases, such a primary biliary cirrhosis or sarcoidosis also have associated intrinsic pulmonary disease.

CHOLESTASIS

Cholestasis is defined as the impaired flow of bile from the liver into the gastrointestinal tract, and pathology at any point between the hepatocyte and the duodenum can be its cause. This can range from mechanical obstruction, for instance gallstones or a malignancy, to metabolic abnormalities such as sepsis or even genetic defects. Cholestasis per se can lead to hepatocellular injury that, in turn, can result in parenchymal changes and impaired liver function similar to that seen with early cirrhosis. Indeed chronic biliary obstruction can lead to secondary biliary cirrhosis.

Cholestasis does not immediately reverse with correction of metabolic abnormalities or relief of biliary obstruction, and the systemic accumulation of those substances normally excreted in the bile can impact and injure biological membranes and cause cellular dysfunction throughout the body. Cholestasis can thus profoundly affect many organs, including the nervous, cardiovascular, gastrointestinal, renal, hematologic, and immune systems. Patients with jaundice often develop impaired cardiac function, nutritional deficiencies, acute renal failure, and infectious complications. One critically important consideration in the perioperative period is the association between cholestasis and coagulopathy (as further discussed in subsequent text).

In patients with obstructive jaundice, preoperative decompression of the biliary tree has been used theoretically to improve liver function and decrease morbidity. However, biliary decompression does not always expeditiously normalize the serum bilirubin level, particularly in the setting of long-standing obstruction and consequent hepatocellular dysfunction. Mounting evidence of greater rates of serious complications argues against routine use of preoperative biliary decompression in patients undergoing surgery for obstructive jaundice.[7] Instrumentation of the biliary tree is also associated with increased infectious complications, and stent placement itself can delay or complicate the planned operation.[18] Percutaneous or endoscopic decompression of the biliary tree is appropriate in patients unfit for surgery and in limited cases where preoperative decompression and nutritional supplementation may be beneficial.

COAGULOPATHY

Perioperative hemorrhage due to coagulopathy is of particular concern when contemplating any surgical intervention on a patient with liver disease. Most proteins involved in hemostasis and fibrinolysis are synthesized exclusively by the liver, including vitamin K-dependent factors II, VII, IX, X, protein C, and protein S; factors V and XIII; fibrinogen, antithrombin, α_2-plasmin inhibitor, and plasminogen. Prolonged prothrombin time (PT) and international normalized ratio (INR) result from the liver's reduced synthesis of these coagulation factors. Whether from intrinsic hepatocyte dysfunction or extrahepatic biliary obstruction, cholestasis further contributes to coagulopathy by inhibiting the absorption of vitamin K and the function of all those requiring this cofactor. Thrombocytopenia results from the reduced synthesis of thrombopoietin and sequestration of platelets due to portal-hypertensive hypersplenism, further potentiating bleeding in the perioperative period.

Treatment of coagulopathy in patients with hepatobiliary disease is based on the underlying pathology. Parenteral administration of vitamin K can correct the coagulopathy related to chronic biliary obstruction or malnutrition, but is less effective for the coagulopathy related to severe hepatic parenchymal disease. Transfusion of fresh-frozen plasma (FFP) and platelets can correct coagulopathy and thrombocytopenia prior to invasive procedures or in patients with active bleeding.[19] Hypofibrinogenemia may require transfusion of cryoprecipitate, and acute bleeding due to fibrinolysis may require aminocaproic or tranexamic acid infusion. The prophylactic uses of recombinant factor VIIa for severe coagulopathy or thrombopoietin for severe thrombocytopenia remain under investigation.[20]

ASCITES

Ascites can be a transudate (low protein, low lactate dehydrogenase [LDH], high pH, normal glucose, and few white blood cells) or exudate (high protein, high LDH, low pH, low glucose, and numerous white blood cells). In hepatobiliary disease, ascites most often is a transudate as a result of the portal hypertension and hypoalbuminemia of chronic liver disease, which cause increased capillary hydrostatic pressure and decreased capillary oncotic pressure in the splanchnic bed. Exudative ascites suggests malignancy and should prompt concern for metastatic peritoneal disease. The serum ascites albumin gradient (SAAG) is a useful calculation to differentiate transudate versus exudate, with a high SAAG greater than 1.1 g/dL suggesting transudative ascites caused by portal hypertension.

The perioperative control of ascites is essential, since ascites predisposes patients to bacterial peritonitis, impairs ventilation, and delays wound healing. Management of ascites includes a dietary salt restriction, diuretics, and paracentesis, with the goal of an ascites-free peritoneal cavity prior to abdominal operation. However, the use of both diuresis and paracentesis should be measured, as these can contribute to acute kidney injury (AKI) due to intravascular volume depletion. In those individuals who are intolerant of, or refractory to, diuretics, a TIPS device may effectively control ascites. Patients with ascites that cannot be controlled with diuretics or TIPS have increased perioperative morbidity and mortality and should not have any elective surgical procedure. If the surgeon must operate in the presence of ascites, an operative drain may be placed temporarily to divert ascites while the incision heals. In this hopefully avoidable circumstance, postoperative fluid and electrolyte management can be exceptionally challenging, requiring meticulous attention to serum electrolytes, the volume of ascites drained, and the volume and content of replacement fluids.

RENAL DYSFUNCTION

As noted, renal dysfunction is common in patients with hepatobiliary disease. Volume depletion from diuretics, gastrointestinal bleeding, lactulose-induced diarrhea, or large-volume paracentesis or thoracentesis can precipitate AKI. Contrast-, infection-, or medication-related nephropathies are other common causes of AKI in the perioperative period. In the absence of a definable cause, AKI in patients with cirrhosis can be attributed to hepatorenal syndrome (HRS).[21] Ultimately, HRS is caused by severe renal vasoconstriction related to the hemodynamic changes discussed earlier.[22] HRS is defined as an increase in serum creatinine to greater than 1.5 mg/dL that does not improve after withdrawal of diuretics and 48 hours of fluid resuscitation. Two types of HRS are differentiated based on time course. Type 1 HRS is defined as the doubling of the initial serum creatinine to a level greater than 2.5 mg/dL in less than 14 days. Type 2 HRS is characterized by diuretic-resistant ascites with slowly progressive, moderate renal dysfunction. The development of HRS portends a poor prognosis with a median survival of 2 weeks in type 1 and 6 months in type 2 HRS.

Renal dysfunction can lead to electrolyte abnormalities, metabolic derangements, and volume overload. Common electrolyte abnormalities include hyperkalemia and hyponatremia, and common metabolic derangements include acidosis and uremia. Treatment of renal dysfunction in the perioperative period depends on the underlying cause. Whereas prerenal AKI requires fluid resuscitation, HRS usually is treated with midodrine, an oral α-adrenergic, and octreotide, a somatostatin analogue.[23] Finally, severe AKI and HRS often require renal replacement therapy for control of electrolytes, acid-base balance, and volume.

HEPATIC ENCEPHALOPATHY

Portosystemic hepatic encephalopathy (PSE) is yet another manifestation of portal hypertension. It may manifest anywhere on a continuum from subtle personality changes and sleep disturbances to frank coma. In the preoperative evaluation, careful questioning of the patient or family can suggest the diagnosis. When present, PSE should be a major warning to the surgeon regarding the extent of underlying liver disease and the extreme potential for postoperative exacerbation of this daunting problem. The pathophysiology of hepatic encephalopathy remains incompletely understood but does appear to be related to the action substances normally metabolized by the liver gaining access to the systemic circulation through shunting and hepatic dysfunction. One example is that of ammonia from the gastrointestinal tract, which can accumulate and lead to changes in neuro-function. Other factors that may contribute to PSE include the production of false neurotransmitters, activation of γ-aminobutyric acid receptors, altered cerebral metabolism, and disturbed sodium-potassium adenosine triphosphatase activity.[24] Electrolyte abnormalities such as hyponatremia and uremia can further alter cerebral function. Dehydration, a large gastrointestinal protein load from either diet or gastrointestinal bleeding, and infection can acutely exacerbate encephalopathy. Proper management of the underlying causes usually can reverse even the most severe cases of encephalopathy. Encephalopathy that does not respond to treatment may indicate the presence of a large portosystemic shunt.

Lactulose, a nonabsorbable disaccharide, is considered first-line treatment. It is metabolized by bacteria in the intestine, lowering the intraluminal pH and rendering the environment unfavorable for the growth of ammonia-producing bacteria. The result is lower serum levels of ammonia. Lactulose is a powerful laxative that can cause volume depletion, which may require resuscitation in the perioperative period. Rifaximin, a poorly absorbed oral antibiotic, is another option that has proven efficacy in both the prevention and treatment of encephalopathy with less risk of dehydration.[24,25]

INFECTIOUS CONSIDERATIONS

Patients with hepatobiliary disease have a systemic immune dysfunction from a number of different factors and therefore are at increased risk for serious infections.[26] The liver contains the majority of the reticuloendothelial system cells (e.g., Kupffer cells, sinusoidal endothelial cells) that are central to clearing cytokines, endotoxin, and bacteria from the circulation. A diseased liver consequently has an impaired immune clearance. Portosystemic shunting of blood around the liver further impairs this hepatic clearance, and the hypersplenism of portal hypertension contributes to neutropenia. Moreover, hepatobiliary disease affects chemotaxis, phagocytosis, and overall immune cell function. The malnutrition often present in these patients further compounds this immunodeficiency.

Liver disease contributes to intestinal motility slowing and an increased permeability of the intestinal mucosa. This can lead to bacterial overgrowth and bacterial translocation, respectively.[27-29] Coupled with the impaired systemic immune function, these factors can certainly predispose to infection. Due to the nature of ascites, patients so afflicted are at further risk of spontaneous bacterial peritonitis. Equally ominous, biliary obstruction puts an individual at risk of cholangitis which is, by definition, a life-threatening condition. Both conditions require immediate recognition, diagnosis, and treatment with broad-spectrum antibiotics.

PREOPERATIVE CONSIDERATIONS

An understanding of these complex pathophysiologic changes associated with hepatobiliary dysfunction guides the preoperative evaluation. An adequate preoperative assessment must include a focus not only on those parameters specific to hepatobiliary function, but also broadly on the functional status of the individual. Those subtle cues that are found through interviewing the patient and family and seen on a thorough physical exam are paramount.

PATIENT

The history and physical exam should focus on the known signs and symptoms of hepatobiliary disease. A thorough history cannot be discounted. One should elucidate any personal or family account of liver disease (Table 120.1) and note risk factors for relevant entities such as fatty liver disease (Box 120.1) or hepatitis. Even a distant history of activities such as intravenous drug use, tattoos, or blood transfusions can be relevant. Remote or vague accounts of jaundice or hepatitis should also raise concern. Recent weight loss (or weight gain in cases of worsening ascites, edema, and anasarca), progressive malaise and confusion, easy bruising, gastrointestinal bleeding, or delayed wound healing may suggest underlying hepatobiliary dysfunction.

In addition to the standard physical examination, the surgeon should look for signs of chronic liver disease, such as asterixis, temporal wasting, scleral icterus, gynecomastia,

TABLE 120.1 Potential Etiologies of Occult Hepatic Disease

Category	Entity	Action/Associations
Infectious	HBV ± delta	History and serology
	HCV	
Metabolic	NAFLD	(See Box 120.1)
	Iron overload	History/specific testing
	Others	
Toxic	Alcohol	History/screen
	Drugs	Amiodarone,
	Environmental	chemotherapy
		Aflatoxin
Structural	Cholestasis	Stone or neoplasm
	Hepatic venous outflow	Budd-Chiari syndrome
		Heart failure
		Pericardial disease
Immune-mediated	PSC	IBD/colorectal tumor
	PBC	Cholangiocarcinoma
	Autoimmune	
Others	Granulomatous disease	
	Cryptogenic	

HBV, Hepatitis B virus; *HCV*, hepatitis C virus; *IBD*, inflammatory bowel disease; *NAFLD*, nonalcoholic fatty liver disease; *PBC*, primary biliary cirrhosis; *PSC*, primary sclerosing cholangitis.

BOX 120.1 Fatty Liver Disease Associations

Obesity
Steroid use
Diabetes
Alcohol
Chemotherapy
Rheumatoid arthritis
Others

TABLE 120.2 Physical Exam Findings of Hepatobiliary Disease

SKIN	Jaundice
	Spider angiomas
	Dupuytren contracture
HEAD	Temporal wasting
	Scleral icterus
	Fetor hepaticus
CHEST	Gynecomastia
LUNGS	Right effusion
ABDOMEN	Caput medusae
	Fluid wave
	Palpable spleen
	Shrunken liver
	Enlarged liver
	Venous hum
EXTREMITIES	Edema
	Anasarca
	Sarcopenia
NEUROLOGIC	Asterixis

TABLE 120.3 Common Laboratory Tests and Interpretations

METABOLIC PANEL	Sodium	Hyponatremia
	BUN/creatinine	AKI
		HRS
	AST/ALT	Ongoing cellular injury
		ETOH: increased ratio
	Alkaline phosphatase	Biliary mass or obstruction
	GGT	Acute ETOH-associated
	Total/direct bilirubin	Nature of cholestasis
COAGULATION	INR	Synthetic dysfunction
		Vitamin K deficiency
	Fibrinogen	Fibrinolysis
BLOOD COUNT	Hemoglobin	Anemia
	MCV/MCHC	Nature of anemia
	Platelets	Portal hypertension

AKI, Acute kidney injury; *ALT,* alanine aminotransferase; *AST,* aspartate aminotransferase; *BUN,* blood urea nitrogen; *ETOH,* ethanol; *GGT,* γ-glutamyltransferase; *HRS,* hepatorenal syndrome; *INR,* international normalized ratio; *MCHC,* mean corpuscular hemoglobin concentration; *MCV,* mean corpuscular volume.

spider angiomas, jaundice, palmar erythema, splenomegaly, prominent superficial abdominal veins, distended abdomen with fluid wave, or peripheral edema and anasarca (Table 120.2). Patients with portosystemic shunting may have high serum ammonia and ketone levels, which are noticeable on exam by a sickly sweet smell known as fetor hepaticus. A unique, albeit rare, clinical sign of portal hypertension is the Cruveilhier-Baumgarten bruit, a venous hum that can be auscultated over the paraumbilical veins.

Laboratory tests should include a complete blood count, coagulation profile, and comprehensive metabolic panel. Interpretation of the results can help characterize the nature and severity of the underlying hepatobiliary disease (Table 120.3). The degree of anemia indicated by the hemoglobin and hematocrit is important for perioperative planning. Patients with normal hemoglobin may be candidates for acute normovolemic hemodilution (ANH),[30] whereas patients with significant anemia more likely will need transfusion intraoperatively. Details such as the mean corpuscular volume can help characterize the anemia and potentially reveal associated behaviors or diseases. For example, a megaloblastic anemia may indicate chronic alcohol use, whereas a microcytic anemia may indicate occult gastrointestinal bleeding. Arguably, the most useful value in the complete blood count is the platelet count. Thrombocytopenia correlates well with hepatocellular dysfunction and portal hypertension.[31] Thrombocytopenia results from decreased hepatic synthesis of thrombopoietin and increased sequestration of platelets in the spleen. Thus thrombocytopenia is a surrogate for the degree of underlying liver dysfunction, and any surgery should be reconsidered in a patient with a platelet count less than 100,000 per cubic millimeter.

Testing of coagulation should include a PT, INR, and partial thromboplastin time (PTT). Additional assessment of fibrinolytic activity requires measuring fibrin degradation products and fibrinogen. Coagulation abnormalities can reveal bleeding risk and guide perioperative transfusion strategies. There is growing evidence that evaluation of total clotting capacity by thromboelastography (TEG) or thromboelastometry (TEM) can more accurately guide transfusion management.[32-35] These dynamic tests provide a composite picture that more closely reflects the in vivo interaction of plasma, platelets, and blood cells than the static conventional blood tests.

The comprehensive metabolic panel can reveal abnormalities in electrolytes and renal function, which are common in patients with hepatobiliary disease. Hyponatremia is usually dilutional and a result of increased levels of aldosterone and antidiuretic hormone that favor sodium and water retention to augment effective circulatory volume. The kidney ultimately retains free water more than the total body needs, exacerbating hyponatremia, ascites, and anasarca. Hyponatremia should be corrected with free water restriction to sodium levels of 130 mEq/L prior to surgery. In certain circumstances, this may require renal replacement therapy. Increased urinary excretion of potassium, particularly in patients on diuretics, may cause hypokalemia, whereas progressive renal dysfunction may result in hyperkalemia. Serum potassium levels should be corrected preoperatively to reduce the risk of cardiac dysrhythmia. Serum blood urea nitrogen and creatinine indicate renal dysfunction, although creatinine may underestimate the degree of dysfunction in patients with sarcopenia. Urine electrolytes and 24-hour creatinine clearance can help clarify both the severity and etiology of renal dysfunction. HRS is diagnosed only after all other causes of renal dysfunction are excluded, and is a major risk to any surgical procedure. Uremia can compound hepatic encephalopathy and platelet dysfunction and may need correction with renal replacement therapy. Uremic bleeding may require desmopressin administration or platelet and cryoprecipitate transfusion perioperatively.

Finally, a thorough assessment of cardiopulmonary function is imperative. Preoperative evaluation should include electrocardiography and transthoracic echocardiography at a minimum, with a low threshold to perform stress echocardiography or cardiac catheterization in elderly patients with significant risk factors for cardiac disease. Formal pulmonary function testing should be performed based on the history and clinical findings. An arterial blood gas on room air in patients with significant pulmonary risk factors such as smoking, chronic cough, or shortness of breath can help rule out HPS or PPH.

The comprehensive preoperative evaluation of the patient thus pays special attention to the organ systems commonly affected by hepatobiliary disease. After completing the evaluation, the surgeon should have an opinion of the patient's suitability for surgery. While there is no substitute for the impression of an experienced surgeon, the Karnofsky score or Eastern Cooperative Oncology Group (ECOG) score can help aggregate and stratify overall patient functional status to guide perioperative decision making.[36] One cannot discount the overall gestalt appearance of the patient versus the magnitude of the proposed surgery: the surgeon's "eyeball" test should be freely invoked in this patient population.

HEPATOBILIARY FUNCTION

The functional status of the patient may belie the functional status of the patient's liver, and specific evaluation of hepatic reserve is crucial.[37] For patients undergoing a general surgical procedure, as before, the patient's hepatic function and overall condition should be weighed against the necessity and magnitude of the proposed procedure. For those requiring hepatic or biliary resection, even more consideration should be given. While there is little concern in patients with normal liver function who undergo small hepatic resections, there should be major concern in patients with underlying liver disease who undergo any hepatic or biliary resection. An insufficient functional hepatic remnant will lead to liver failure, a primary cause of morbidity and mortality after hepatobiliary surgery. Postoperative liver function largely depends on the volume and quality of the future liver remnant (FLR) which, in turn, depends on extent of resection and the degree of underlying cholestasis, steatosis, or cirrhosis.

Currently, computed tomography or magnetic resonance imaging volumetry is the standard method to determine the quantity of the FLR and the safety and feasibility of liver resection.[38–40] In patients with normal liver parenchyma, the surgeon can safely resect to an FLR larger than 25% to 30% of the total liver volume. In patients with underlying liver disease, a 40% margin is added to ensure an FLR larger than 65% to 70% of the total liver volume. Preoperative embolization of the portal vein with a several-week delay may allow for an increase in the size of the FLR to allow liver resection in select patients with significant disease.[41–43]

Liver volume alone, however, does not reflect function, and while no single test exists, several methods can be used in combination to assess overall liver function. Biochemical liver function tests include serum levels of bilirubin, albumin, and coagulation factors. Bilirubin levels reflect the uptake, conjugation, and excretion function

of the liver; levels of albumin and the proteins involved in coagulation reflect liver synthetic function.

Clinical scoring systems exist to combine biochemical tests and clinical symptoms to estimate overall liver function. The Child-Turcotte-Pugh (CTP) score, for example, assigns points for encephalopathy, ascites, bilirubin, albumin, and PT/INR, and classifies patients as class A, B, or C, with Child A patients having good, Child B moderate, and Child C poor operative risk. In general, Child A patients are eligible for surgery while most Child B and C patients should be evaluated for liver transplantation. The CTP score is particularly useful in selecting patients with cirrhosis and hepatocellular carcinoma for liver resection versus transplantation. The Model for End-Stage Liver Disease (MELD) calculates a score with serum total bilirubin, creatinine, and INR. Used initially to predict mortality after TIPS, the MELD score is used currently to assess the severity of liver dysfunction and prioritize patients awaiting liver transplantation. The MELD score correlates with an increased risk of mortality in patients with cirrhosis who undergo abdominal surgery, and evidence suggests that it may predict mortality after liver resection.[44]

Dynamic quantitative liver function tests, such as indocyanine green (ICG) clearance and galactose elimination capacity, can assess overall liver function by measuring the elimination of substances cleared exclusively by the liver. Their clinical applications are limited, and they do not assess function of the FLR. New nuclear imaging tests, such as 99mTc-galactosyl serum albumin scintigraphy and 99mTc-mebrofenin hepatobiliary scintigraphy, can assess overall liver function as well as FLR function and show promise in identifying patients at risk of liver failure after liver resection.[45]

NUTRITION

Malnutrition is common in patients suffering from hepatobiliary disease and is an important prognostic factor associated with suboptimal surgical outcomes. Perioperative treatment of malnutrition may improve liver function and ultimately surgical morbidity and mortality. The European Society for Clinical Nutrition and Metabolism (ESPEN) provides useful nutrition evaluation and treatment guidelines for patients with hepatobiliary disease that are beyond the scope of the chapter.[46,47]

The liver integrates several physiologic processes that are essential for a well-nourished state.[48–50] The metabolism of carbohydrates, fat, proteins, and vitamins, as well as the excretion of bile and transport of lipids, are important for the catabolic-anabolic balance of healing and recovery. Already at a disadvantage because of underlying disease, the hepatobiliary patient's nutritional status can worsen rapidly during the postoperative period due to preoperative malnutrition, surgical stress, complications, and repeated fasting, highlighting the importance of perioperative nutritional assessment and optimization.[51,52]

Traditional methods of nutritional assessment often are not accurate in patients with hepatobiliary disease because of the effects of liver dysfunction on protein synthesis, fluid status, and metabolism. The history and physical examination remain most important. Comparison of the patient's current state to the premorbid state is essential, as an individual with apparent normal weight or musculature may have started from baseline obesity or greater muscle mass. Subtle exam findings such as temporal and thenar wasting may precede overt cachexia, and profound loss of skeletal muscle mass (i.e., sarcopenia), portends significant risk of organ dysfunction, impaired immunity, and poor wound healing.

Objective measurements of nutritional status include: serum albumin, prealbumin, and transferrin; total lymphocyte count; body mass index (BMI), mid-arm muscle circumference, and triceps or subcapsular skin fold thickness; indirect calorimetry; and more recently, body cell mass (BCM) calculation and bioelectrical imped-ance analysis (BIA).[53] Characteristics of patients with malnutrition who have greater perioperative risk include serum albumin less than 3 g/dL, serum transferrin less than 200 mg/dL, weight loss of 10% to 15% over a 3- to 4-month period, impaired performance of ordinary tasks, and inability to perform functional tests such as hand dynamometry. Whereas serum albumin alone may be the best predictor of morbidity after a range of abdominal operations, none of the tests is uniformly reliable in patients with hepatobiliary disease, particularly when ascites, peripheral edema, and anasarca are present.[54–56] Moreover, the latter tests are cumbersome, costly and not widely available, with no proven superiority over the judgment of an experienced clinician. A simplified subjective global assessment that combines a thorough history and physical to rate patients as "well-nourished," "moderately nourished," or "severely malnourished" may be the best guide to treatment.[57]

Nutritional supplementation has long been used to improve surgical outcomes, and adequate nutritional support for hepatobiliary patients is essential in all phases of the perioperative period.[58,59] The enteral route is pre-ferred, even if it requires placement of a nasogastric or nasojejunal tube for feeding. Early enteral nutrition in both trauma and burn patients attenuates the inevitable hypercatabolic response,[60] and studies have shown that enteral nutrition prevents small bowel atrophy and sub-sequent bacterial translocation, sepsis, and multisystem organ failure,[61,62] which is particularly important in patients with hepatobiliary disease and impaired portal clearance of bacteria.[63,64]

Total parenteral nutrition (TPN) should only be used when enteral feeding is contraindicated, as it increases perioperative morbidity.[65] Usually a minimum of 2 weeks of TPN is required to obtain sufficient nutritional enhance-ment to improve outcomes in severely malnourished patients. Despite best intentions, patients with hepatobiliary disease only rarely make significant improvement in pre-operative nutritional status after a course of supplementa-tion. Decompression of the biliary tree in patients with obstructive jaundice can stimulate appetite and caloric intake, but the effect is usually insufficient to improve surgical outcome.

With rising obesity rates, it is important to note the presence of nonalcoholic fatty liver disease (NAFLD) in the perioperative nutritional evaluation. Steatosis and steatohepatitis greatly increase the morbidity and mortality of liver resection.[66–69] Several studies have shown that weight loss after bariatric surgery can improve and even cure steatosis, steatohepatitis, and fibrosis.[70] Furthermore, short-term calorie restriction before liver resection can sig-nificantly reduce both hepatic steatosis and steatohepatitis, allowing for safer liver resection.[71] Preoperative dietary modification and bariatric surgery should be considered in select patients with significant obesity and NAFLD.

INTRAOPERATIVE CONSIDERATIONS

Management of the complex physiology associated with hepatobiliary disease and minimization of blood loss are the major considerations during the intraoperative period. Here we examine the commonly used anesthetic and surgical techniques.

ANESTHESIA

The anesthesiologist must manage all the systemic effects of hepatobiliary disease, including the hemodynamic changes of portal hypertension, electrolyte and acid-base derangements, and coagulation abnormalities. In addition, the hepatic metabolism of many routinely used drugs poses a challenge for intraoperative medication administration. The half-life of drugs cleared by the liver can be significantly prolonged, altering dosage, dura-tion of action, and lipid solubility. The ascites or edema present in cirrhotic patients can increase the volume of distribution, whereas the increased capacity for enzymatic metabolism in chronic alcoholics can result in larger drug requirements. Finally, hypoalbuminemia can increase the plasma concentrations of normally protein-bound drugs, leading to an exaggerated response.

Inhalational agents such as isoflurane and desflurane have been studied extensively and found to be safe in patients with liver disease. Both agents undergo negligible hepatic metabolism,[72] and isoflurane preserves hepatic blood flow and the hepatic artery buffer response better than other volatile anesthetics.[73] In contrast, halothane and other halogenated hydrocarbons must be avoided due to the risk of hepatitis and fulminant hepatic failure, which is most likely mediated by immunologic mechanisms.[74] The use of local anesthesia should be encouraged, especially for minor procedures. Amide-linked local anesthetics, such as lidocaine and bupivacaine, undergo hepatic metabolism and should be used in smaller doses. Regional anesthesia is an excellent adjunct, and placement of a continuous epidural catheter can enhance pain control in the intraoperative and postoperative period. However, significant coagulopathy or thrombocytopenia may con-traindicate a spinal or epidural puncture.

The anesthesiologist aims to minimize the potential for blood loss by reducing hepatic venous congestion through optimum fluid management, judicious use of vasoactive drugs, and correction of coagulopathy.[75] Excessive blood loss clearly is associated with increased adverse outcomes after hepatobiliary surgery.[76] The combination of ANH and careful control of the central venous pressure (CVP) during hepatic resection can reduce intraoperative blood loss.[77–80] Limiting intravenous fluid and pharmacologic or epidural-based vasodilation help control the CVP. The routine avoidance of high positive end-expiratory pressure (PEEP) is common in hepatobiliary surgery, although the actual effect on CVP may be minimal.[75] The low CVP technique can lead to cardiovascular instability, hypovolemia, and reduced renal and splanchnic blood flow and may require vasopressors to maintain organ perfusion. Although a low intraoperative urine volume may result, this is not necessarily associated with an increased incidence of postoperative renal failure.[81] A rapid infusion system should be readily available to provide emergency fluid and blood product infusion. Effective communication between the surgeon and anesthesiologist cannot be overemphasized.

SURGERY

Beyond the basic tenets of surgery, special intraoperative factors must be considered in hepatobiliary surgery. Adequate exposure is critical, and proper consideration must be given to the type and extent of the incision. Extension of the incision should be performed whenever safety requires. In addition, a dependable self-retaining retractor system is essential.

Resting total hepatic blood flow represents about 25% of cardiac output or 1200 to 1400 mL/min, so transection of the liver parenchyma risks major blood loss. A variety of methods can be used to limit intraoperative blood loss. The most commonly used method is either intermittent or continuous clamping of the portal triad known as the Pringle maneuver. The Pringle maneuver is limited by the degree of underlying parenchymal disease. Whereas 60 minutes of total clamp time is considered safe in normal livers, only 30 minutes is considered safe in cirrhotic livers.[82] Prolonged clamping increases the risk of ischemia-reperfusion injury to the remnant liver. The intermittent Pringle maneuver involves 15 to 20 minutes of clamping followed by 5 minutes of reperfusion. Evidence suggests that diseased livers tolerate intermittent better than continuous clamping, perhaps because of ischemic preconditioning.[83,84] Total vascular isolation of the liver involves clamping of the supra- and infrahepatic vena cava as well as the Pringle maneuver. Its use during major liver resection is feasible but carries significant risk of perioperative morbidity and should be discussed in advance with the anesthesiologist. Venovenous bypass may be a useful adjunct in select circumstances, such as in patients with large tumors involving the vena cava.

Several methods of liver parenchymal transection are available and surgeon-dependent. Multiple hemostatic agents also are available and very effective. The use of drains after hepatobiliary surgery is largely idiosyncratic. Evidence suggests against the routine use of drains, although drains may be helpful in cases of biliary reconstruction.[85] Consideration of the placement of feeding tubes for postoperative nutritional supplementation should be given to patients with severe malnutrition. Wound closure can be performed by any standard method, but special consideration should be given to patients with ascites or sarcopenia.

POSTOPERATIVE CONSIDERATIONS

Collaborative advances in anesthesia, surgery, and critical care have lowered the morbidity and mortality of major hepatobiliary surgery to acceptable levels.[75] In general, patients are cared for in a surgical intensive care unit

immediately postoperatively, where management involves not only recovery from anesthesia and pain control, but also close assessment of hepatic function. Hemodynamic monitoring is performed with an arterial catheter for continuous blood pressure measurements and a central venous catheter for fluid administration and CVP measurements. Pulmonary artery catheters are not used routinely, but they may be helpful in select patients with cardiopulmonary comorbidities. Intravenous fluids are given to maintain adequate organ perfusion as measured by blood pressure and urine output. Bolus fluids in the form of crystalloids, colloids, or blood products may be given as necessary depending on laboratory values, with a goal of maintaining relatively low CVP to avoid bleeding from any cut liver surface or the vena cava. Nasogastric tubes are not required after hepatobiliary surgery,[86] but they may be useful in cases that involve bilioenteric anastomoses or significant manipulation of the stomach. Patients should be allowed to eat as soon as clinically acceptable, because early oral intake allows for discontinuation of intravenous fluids and accelerates recovery.[75]

Several issues specific to hepatic resection require attention in the postoperative period. Liver resection may alter anesthetic clearance and drug metabolism, requiring careful selection and dosing of medications. Coagulation parameters should be followed closely; a rapidly rising INR in the first 48 to 72 hours may indicate impending hepatic failure. To avoid postoperative hemorrhage, FFP can be administered for rapid correction of coagulopathy; vitamin K also can be given in cases of suspected deficiency related to preoperative biliary obstruction. Despite elevated serum coagulation parameters, patients who undergo hepatobiliary surgery are still at risk of venous thromboembolism because of postoperative hypercoagulability.[87-89] In general, early mobilization and pharmacologic venous thromboembolism prophylaxis are recommended unless there is a contraindication.[90]

Hepatobiliary surgery may incite hepatic decompensation or exacerbate preexisting liver dysfunction as manifest by encephalopathy, jaundice, coagulopathic bleeding, or ascites. Treatment of hepatic decompensation is largely supportive until the remnant liver regenerates and should be guided by the best standards of surgical critical care. Liver regeneration involves an adenosine triphosphate-dependent process of hepatocyte division that can deplete phosphorus stores and lead to life-threatening hypophosphatemia (phosphorus <1.0 g/dL).[91,92] Serum phosphorus levels must be monitored and replaced diligently to avoid postoperative complications such as cardiac dysfunction, hypoventilation, and impaired immunity. There is conflicting data on the use of N-acetylcysteine (NAC) infusion in patients with postoperative liver dysfunction.[93-95] Vigilant monitoring in the postoperative period thus aims to recognize and treat problems promptly to avoid perioperative complications.

CONCLUSION

A thorough understanding of the pathophysiology of the liver and biliary tree is the foundation for the appropriate care of the patient with hepatobiliary dysfunction. Advances in perioperative management have allowed surgeons to perform complex operations on high acuity patients with low morbidity and mortality. The combination of comprehensive preoperative evaluation, meticulous intraoperative technique, and diligent postoperative care has greatly improved the overall success of surgery for patients with hepatobiliary disease.

REFERENCES

1. Popper H. Pathologic aspects of cirrhosis. A review. *Am J Pathol.* 1977;87(1):228-264.
2. Schuppan D, Afdhal NH. Liver cirrhosis. *Lancet.* 2008;371(9615):838-851.
3. Bosch J, Garcia-Pagan JC. Complications of cirrhosis. I. Portal hypertension. *J Hepatol.* 2000;32(1 suppl):141-156.
4. Sanyal AJ, Bosch J, Blei A, Arroyo V. Portal hypertension and its complications. *Gastroenterology.* 2008;134(6):1715-1728.
5. Gatta A, Bolognesi M, Merkel C. Vasoactive factors and hemodynamic mechanisms in the pathophysiology of portal hypertension in cirrhosis. *Mol Aspects Med.* 2008;29(1-2):119-129.
6. John S, Thuluvath PJ. Hyponatremia in cirrhosis: pathophysiology and management. *World J Gastroenterol.* 2015;21(11):3197-3205.
7. Nadim MK, Durand F, Kellum JA, et al. Management of the critically ill patient with cirrhosis: a multidisciplinary perspective. *J Hepatol.* 2016;64(3):717-735.
8. De BK, Majumdar D, Das D, et al. Cardiac dysfunction in portal hypertension among patients with cirrhosis and non-cirrhotic portal fibrosis. *J Hepatol.* 2003;39(3):315-319.
9. Surani SR, Mendez Y, Anjum H, Varon J. Pulmonary complications of hepatic diseases. *World J Gastroenterol.* 2016;22(26):6008-6015.
10. Roussos A, Philippou N, Mantzaris GJ, Gourgouliannis KI. Hepatic hydrothorax: pathophysiology, diagnosis and management. *J Gastroenterol Hepatol.* 2007;22(9):1388-1393.
11. Hoeper MM, Krowka MJ, Strassburg CP. Portopulmonary hypertension and hepatopulmonary syndrome. *Lancet.* 2004;363(9419):1461-1468.
12. Rodriguez-Roisin R, Krowka MJ. Hepatopulmonary syndrome—a liver-induced lung vascular disorder. *N Engl J Med.* 2008;358(22):2378-2387.
13. Lv Y, Fan D. Hepatopulmonary syndrome. *Dig Dis Sci.* 2015;60(7):1914-1923.
14. Krowka MJ. Hepatopulmonary syndrome versus portopulmonary hypertension: distinctions and dilemmas. *Hepatology.* 1997;25(5):1282-1284.
15. Kuo PC, Plotkin JS, Johnson LB, et al. Distinctive clinical features of portopulmonary hypertension. *Chest.* 1997;112(4):980-986.
16. Halank M, Ewert R, Seyfarth HJ, Hoeffken G. Portopulmonary hypertension. *J Gastroenterol.* 2006;41(9):837-847.
17. Fang Y, Gurusamy KS, Wang Q, et al. Pre-operative biliary drainage for obstructive jaundice. *Cochrane Database Syst Rev.* 2012;(9):CD005444.
18. van der Gaag NA, Rauws EA, van Eijck CH, et al. Preoperative biliary drainage for cancer of the head of the pancreas. *N Engl J Med.* 2010;362(2):129-137.
19. Youssef WI, Salazar F, Dasarathy S, Beddow T, Mullen KD. Role of fresh frozen plasma infusion in correction of coagulopathy of chronic liver disease: a dual phase study. *Am J Gastroenterol.* 2003;98(6):1391-1394.
20. Chavez-Tapia NC, Alfaro-Lara R, Tellez-Avila F, et al. Prophylactic activated recombinant factor VII in liver resection and liver transplantation: systematic review and meta-analysis. *PLoS One.* 2011;6(7):e22581.
21. Baraldi O, Valentini C, Donati G, et al. Hepatorenal syndrome: update on diagnosis and treatment. *World J Nephrol.* 2015;4(5):511-520.
22. Durand F, Graupera I, Gines P, Olson JC, Nadim MK. Pathogenesis of hepatorenal syndrome: implications for therapy. *Am J Kidney Dis.* 2016;67(2):318-328.
23. Esrailian E, Pantangco ER, Kyulo NL, Hu KQ, Runyon BA. Octreotide/Midodrine therapy significantly improves renal function and 30-day survival in patients with type 1 hepatorenal syndrome. *Dig Dis Sci.* 2007;52(3):742-748.
24. Riordan SM, Williams R. Treatment of hepatic encephalopathy. *N Engl J Med.* 1997;337(7):473-479.
25. Bass NM, Mullen KD, Sanyal A, et al. Rifaximin treatment in hepatic encephalopathy. *N Engl J Med.* 2010;362(12):1071-1081.
26. Bonnel AR, Bunchorntavakul C, Reddy KR. Immune dysfunction and infections in patients with cirrhosis. *Clin Gastroenterol Hepatol.* 2011;9(9):727-738.
27. Chang CS, Chen GH, Lien HC, Yeh HZ. Small intestine dysmotility and bacterial overgrowth in cirrhotic patients with spontaneous bacterial peritonitis. *Hepatology.* 1998;28(5):1187-1190.
28. Chesta J, Defilippi C, Defilippi C. Abnormalities in proximal small bowel motility in patients with cirrhosis. *Hepatology.* 1993;17(5):828-832.
29. Wiest R, Garcia-Tsao G. Bacterial translocation (BT) in cirrhosis. *Hepatology.* 2005;41(3):422-433.
30. Jarnagin WR, Gonen M, Maithel SK, et al. A prospective randomized trial of acute normovolemic hemodilution compared to standard intraoperative management in patients undergoing major hepatic resection. *Ann Surg.* 2008;248(3):360-369.
31. Plura A, Gutkowski K, Hartleb M. Coagulopathy in liver diseases. *Adv Med Sci.* 2010;55(1):16-21.
32. Mallett SV, Chowdary P, Burroughs AK. Clinical utility of viscoelastic tests of coagulation in patients with liver disease. *Liver Int.* 2013;33(7):961-974.
33. Afshari A, Wikkelso A, Brok J, Moller AM, Wetterslev J. Thromboelastography (TEG) or thromboelastometry (ROTEM) to monitor haemotherapy versus usual care in patients with massive transfusion. *Cochrane Database Syst Rev.* 2011 (3):CD007871.
34. Krzanicki D, Sugavanam A, Mallett S. Intraoperative hypercoagulability during liver transplantation as demonstrated by thromboelastography. *Liver Transpl.* 2013;19(8):852-861.
35. Stravitz RT. Potential applications of thromboelastography in patients with acute and chronic liver disease. *Gastroenterol Hepatol.* 2012;8(8):513-520.
36. Oken MM, Creech RH, Tormey DC, et al. Toxicity and response criteria of the Eastern Cooperative Oncology Group. *Am J Clin Oncol.* 1982;5(6):649-655.
37. Clavien PA, Petrowsky H, DeOliveira ML, Graf R. Strategies for safer liver surgery and partial liver transplantation. *N Engl J Med.* 2007;356(15):1545-1559.
38. Shoup M, Gonen M, D'Angelica M, et al. Volumetric analysis predicts hepatic dysfunction in patients undergoing major liver resection. *J Gastrointest Surg.* 2003;7(3):325-330.
39. Vauthey JN, Chaoui A, Do KA, et al. Standardized measurement of the future liver remnant prior to extended liver resection: methodology and clinical associations. *Surgery.* 2000;127(5):512-519.
40. Clavien PA, Emond J, Vauthey JN, Belghiti J, Chari RS, Strasberg SM. Protection of the liver during hepatic surgery. *J Gastrointest Surg.* 2004;8(3):313-327.
41. Farges O, Belghiti J, Kianmanesh R, et al. Portal vein embolization before right hepatectomy: prospective clinical trial. *Ann Surg.* 2003;237(2):208-217.
42. Ribero D, Abdalla EK, Madoff DC, Donadon M, Loyer EM, Vauthey JN. Portal vein embolization before major hepatectomy and its effects on regeneration, resectability and outcome. *Br J Surg.* 2007;94(11):1386-1394.
43. Abulkhir A, Limongelli P, Healey AJ, et al. Preoperative portal vein embolization for major liver resection: a meta-analysis. *Ann Surg.* 2008;247(1):49-57.
44. Ross SW, Seshadri R, Walters AL, et al. Mortality in hepatectomy: Model for End-Stage Liver Disease as a predictor of death using the National Surgical Quality Improvement Program database. *Surgery.* 2016;159(3):777-792.
45. Hoekstra LT, de Graaf W, Nibourg GA, et al. Physiological and biochemical basis of clinical liver function tests: a review. *Ann Surg.* 2013;257(1):27-36.
46. Plauth M, Cabre E, Riggio O, et al. ESPEN guidelines on enteral nutrition: liver disease. *Clin Nutr.* 2006;25(2):285-294.
47. Plauth M, Cabre E, Campillo B, et al. ESPEN Guidelines on Parenteral Nutrition: Hepatology. *Clin Nutr.* 2009;28(4):436-444.
48. Dudrick SJ, Kavic SM. Hepatobiliary nutrition: history and future. *J Hepatobiliary Pancreat Surg.* 2002;9(4):459-468.
49. Cabre E, Gassull MA. Nutrition in liver disease. *Curr Opin Clin Nutr Metab Care.* 2005;8(5):545-551.
50. O'Brien A, Williams R. Nutrition in end-stage liver disease: principles and practice. *Gastroenterology.* 2008;134(6):1729-1740.
51. Kaido T, Mori A, Ogura Y, et al. Pre- and perioperative factors affecting infection after living donor liver transplantation. *Nutrition.* 2012;28(11-12):1104-1108.
52. Iida T, Kaido T, Yagi S, et al. Posttransplant bacteremia in adult living donor liver transplant recipients. *Liver Transpl.* 2010;16(12):1379-1385.
53. Hammad A, Kaido T, Uemoto S. Perioperative nutritional therapy in liver transplantation. *Surg Today.* 2015;45(3):271-283.

54. The Veterans Affairs Total Parenteral Nutrition Cooperative Study Group. Perioperative total parenteral nutrition in surgical patients. *N Engl J Med*. 1991;325(8):525-532.

55. Kudsk KA, Tolley EA, DeWitt RC, et al. Preoperative albumin and surgical site identify surgical risk for major postoperative complications. *JPEN J Parenter Enteral Nutr*. 2003;27(1):1-9.

56. Detsky AS, McLaughlin JR, Baker JP, et al. What is subjective global assessment of nutritional status? *JPEN J Parenter Enteral Nutr*. 1987;11(1):8-13.

57. Stephenson GR, Moretti EW, El-Moalem H, Clavien PA, Tuttle-Newhall JE. Malnutrition in liver transplant patients: preoperative subjective global assessment is predictive of outcome after liver transplantation. *Transplantation*. 2001;72(4):666-670.

58. Sax HC, Souba WW. Enteral and parenteral feedings. Guidelines and recommendations. *Med Clin North Am*. 1993;77(4):863-880.

59. Moore EE, Jones TN. Benefits of immediate jejunostomy feeding after major abdominal trauma—a prospective, randomized study. *J Trauma*. 1986;26(10):874-881.

60. Mochizuki H, Trocki O, Dominioni L, Brackett KA, Joffe SN, Alexander JW. Mechanism of prevention of postburn hypermetabolism and catabolism by early enteral feeding. *Ann Surg*. 1984;200(3):297-310.

61. Qiu JG, Delany HM, Teh EL, et al. Contrasting effects of identical nutrients given parenterally or enterally after 70% hepatectomy: bacterial translocation. *Nutrition*. 1997;13(5):431-437.

62. Alverdy J, Holbrook C, Rocha F, et al. Gut-derived sepsis occurs when the right pathogen with the right virulence genes meets the right host: evidence for in vivo virulence expression in *Pseudomonas aeruginosa*. *Ann Surg*. 2000;232(4):480-489.

63. Zulfikaroglu B, Zulfikaroglu E, Ozmen MM, et al. The effect of immunonutrition on bacterial translocation, and intestinal villus atrophy in experimental obstructive jaundice. *Clin Nutr*. 2003;22(3):277-281.

64. Chuang JH, Shieh CS, Chang NK, Chen WJ, Lin JN. Role of parenteral nutrition in preventing malnutrition and decreasing bacterial translocation to liver in obstructive jaundice. *World J Surg*. 1993;17(5):580-585, discussion 586.

65. Archer SB, Burnett RJ, Fischer JE. Current uses and abuses of total parenteral nutrition. *Adv Surg*. 1996;29:165-189

66. Gomez D, Malik HZ, Bonney GK, et al. Steatosis predicts postoperative morbidity following hepatic resection for colorectal metastasis. *Br J Surg*. 2007;94(11):1395-1402.

67. Vauthey JN, Pawlik TM, Ribero D, et al. Chemotherapy regimen predicts steatohepatitis and an increase in 90-day mortality after surgery for hepatic colorectal metastases. *J Clin Oncol*. 2006;24(13):2065-2072.

68. McCormack L, Petrowsky H, Jochum W, Furrer K, Clavien PA. Hepatic steatosis is a risk factor for postoperative complications after major hepatectomy: a matched case-control study. *Ann Surg*. 2007;245(6):923-930.

69. Kooby DA, Fong Y, Suriawinata A, et al. Impact of steatosis on perioperative outcome following hepatic resection. *J Gastrointest Surg*. 2003;7(8):1034-1044.

70. Clanton J, Subichin M. The effects of metabolic surgery on fatty liver disease and nonalcoholic steatohepatitis. *Surg Clin North Am*. 2016;96(4):703-715.

71. Reeves JG, Suriawinata AA, Ng DP, Holubar SD, Mills JB, Barth RJ Jr. Short-term preoperative diet modification reduces steatosis and blood loss in patients undergoing liver resection. *Surgery*. 2013;154(5):1031-1037.

72. Elliott RH, Strunin L. Hepatotoxicity of volatile anaesthetics. *Br J Anaesth*. 1993;70(3):339-348.

73. Berendes E, Lippert G, Loick HM, Brussel T. Effects of enflurane and isoflurane on splanchnic oxygenation in humans. *J Clin Anesth*. 1996;8(6):456-468.

74. Trey C, Lipworth L, Chalmers TC, et al. Fulminant hepatic failure. Presumable contribution to halothane. *N Engl J Med*. 1968;279(15):798-801.

75. Snowden C, Prentis J. Anesthesia for hepatobiliary surgery. *Anesthesiol Clin*. 2015;33(1):125-141.

76. Jarnagin WR, Gonen M, Fong Y, et al. Improvement in perioperative outcome after hepatic resection: analysis of 1,803 consecutive cases over the past decade. *Ann Surg*. 2002;236(4):397-406, discussion 406-407.

77. Jones RM, Moulton CE, Hardy KJ. Central venous pressure and its effect on blood loss during liver resection. *Br J Surg*. 1998;85(8):1058-1060.

78. Moggia E, Rouse B, Simillis C, et al. Methods to decrease blood loss during liver resection: a network meta-analysis. *Cochrane Database Syst Rev*. 2016;(10):CD010683.

79. Chen H, Merchant NB, Didolkar MS. Hepatic resection using intermittent vascular inflow occlusion and low central venous pressure anesthesia improves morbidity and mortality. *J Gastrointest Surg*. 2000;4(2):162-167.

80. Li Z, Sun YM, Wu FX, Yang LQ, Lu Z, Yu WF. Controlled low central venous pressure reduces blood loss and transfusion requirements in hepatectomy. *World J Gastroenterol*. 2014;20(1):303-309.

81. Melendez JA, Arslan V, Fischer ME, et al. Perioperative outcomes of major hepatic resections under low central venous pressure anesthesia: blood loss, blood transfusion, and the risk of postoperative renal dysfunction. *J Am Coll Surg*. 1998;187(6):620-625.

82. Smyrniotis VE, Kostopanagiotou GG, Contis JC, et al. Selective hepatic vascular exclusion versus Pringle maneuver in major liver resections: prospective study. *World J Surg*. 2003;27(7):765-769.

83. Petrowsky H, McCormack L, Trujillo M, Selzner M, Jochum W, Clavien PA. A prospective, randomized, controlled trial comparing intermittent portal triad clamping versus ischemic preconditioning with continuous clamping for major liver resection. *Ann Surg*. 2006;244(6):921-928, discussion 928-930.

84. Gomez D, Homer-Vanniasinkam S, Graham AM, Prasad KR. Role of ischaemic preconditioning in liver regeneration following major liver resection and transplantation. *World J Gastroenterol*. 2007;13(5):657-670.

85. Gurusamy KS, Samraj K, Davidson BR. Routine abdominal drainage for uncomplicated liver resection. *Cochrane Database Syst Rev*. 2007;(3):CD006232.

86. Pessaux P, Regimbeau JM, Dondero F, Plasse M, Mantz J, Belghiti J. Randomized clinical trial evaluating the need for routine nasogastric decompression after elective hepatic resection. *Br J Surg*. 2007;94(3):297-303.

87. Senzolo M, Sartori MT, Lisman T. Should we give thromboprophylaxis to patients with liver cirrhosis and coagulopathy? *HPB (Oxford)*. 2009;11(6):459-464.

88. Lesmana CR, Inggriani S, Cahyadinata L, Lesmana LA. Deep vein thrombosis in patients with advanced liver cirrhosis: a rare condition? *Hepatol Int*. 2010;4(1):433-438.

89. Cerutti E, Stratta C, Romagnoli R, et al. Thromboelastogram monitoring in the perioperative period of hepatectomy for adult living liver donation. *Liver Transpl*. 2004;10(2):289-294.

90. Reddy SK, Turley RS, Barbas AS, et al. Post-operative pharmacologic thromboprophylaxis after major hepatectomy: does peripheral venous thromboembolism prevention outweigh bleeding risks? *J Gastrointest Surg*. 2011;15(9):1602-1610.

91. Pomposelli JJ, Pomfret EA, Burns DL, et al. Life-threatening hypophosphatemia after right hepatic lobectomy for live donor adult liver transplantation. *Liver Transpl*. 2001;7(7):637-642.

92. Pomposelli JJ, Burns DL. Hypophosphatemia and the live liver donor. *Transplantation*. 2004;78(2):305.

93. Harrison PM, Wendon JA, Gimson AE, Alexander GJ, Williams R. Improvement by acetylcysteine of hemodynamics and oxygen transport in fulminant hepatic failure. *N Engl J Med*. 1991;324(26):1852-1857.

94. Walsh TS, Hopton P, Philips BJ, Mackenzie SJ, Lee A. The effect of N-acetylcysteine on oxygen transport and uptake in patients with fulminant hepatic failure. *Hepatology*. 1998;27(5):1332-1340.

95. Robinson SM, Saif R, Sen G, et al. N-acetylcysteine administration does not improve patient outcome after liver resection. *HPB (Oxford)*. 2013;15(6):457-462.

Hepatic Cysts

Hari Nathan | Michael W. Mulholland

Hepatic cysts are a diverse group of lesions, ranging from developmental to infectious to neoplastic in etiology. The clinical implications of these lesions also vary widely. The increased use and sensitivity of abdominal imaging have led to the increasingly common incidental diagnosis of cystic lesions of the liver. The majority of these are simple cysts, usually of little clinical consequence. In contrast, echinococcal cysts remain a major public health problem worldwide, and hepatic cystadenocarcinomas are aggressive malignancies. The task of differentiating cystic lesions of the liver that need intervention from those that do not often falls to the surgeon.

SIMPLE HEPATIC CYSTS

Simple hepatic cysts are presumed to originate from the biliary tree, likely from microhamartomas or peribiliary glands that become isolated from the bile ducts. They are lined with a simple cuboidal epithelium and surrounded by a fibrous, hypocellular stroma. Cyst contents are typically serous, but proteinaceous material from previous hemorrhage may be present. The presence of mucinous or solid contents should prompt consideration of an infectious or neoplastic process.

Hepatic cysts have long been recognized as an incidental finding at laparotomy, during autopsy, or on imaging studies. Estimates of the prevalence of liver cysts range from 11% to 18%, depending on the imaging modality used.[1,2] Hepatic cysts become more common with increasing patient age; more than 92% of cysts occur in those older than 40 years.[1,3] Some studies have shown a higher incidence of cysts in female patients.[1,2]

Although the majority of simple hepatic cysts are asymptomatic and discovered incidentally, some patients will experience abdominal pain or distention. Symptoms may be related to stretch of the liver capsule causing pain or mass effect on surrounding structures. Symptoms are more common in older patients with larger cysts. Progressive cyst enlargement may lead to early satiety, nausea, and vomiting. A palpable mass on physical examination may be infrequently noted.

Simple cysts do not generally result in abnormalities of liver function tests. Echinococcal serology should be obtained if there is appropriate clinical suspicion or characteristic imaging findings. Liver abscesses are usually accompanied by other signs of infection. For most patients, the main challenge is to differentiate neoplastic from nonneoplastic cysts, which depends on imaging.

Hepatic ultrasound is the preferred initial study because it is inexpensive, noninvasive, and highly informative. It reliably distinguishes between cystic and solid hepatic lesions and can suggest the diagnosis of a cystic neoplasm.

Simple hepatic cysts appear sonographically as anechoic masses with smooth margins and imperceptibly thin walls (Fig. 121.1). The differential reflection of ultrasound waves by the cyst wall and cyst fluid leads to back-wall enhancement. Septations or nodularity should prompt suspicion of a neoplastic cyst. Lack of septations is highly predictive of a simple hepatic cyst.[4] However, it is important to remember that simple cysts are common, whereas neoplastic cysts are rare. Therefore, even if septations or other complex features are found in a liver cyst, it is still more likely than not to be nonneoplastic.

Cross-sectional imaging with either computed tomography (CT) or magnetic resonance imaging (MRI) can be very useful in further characterizing a cyst and assessing its anatomic relationships. CT scans should be performed with intravenous contrast timed to delineate arterial, portal venous, and hepatic venous structures. On CT, simple cysts should appear as nonenhancing lesions of water density (0 to 10 Hounsfield units) with smooth, imperceptible walls (Figs. 121.2 and 121.3).[5] Wall thickening or irregularity, papillary mural projections or nodules, internal septations, and intracystic debris should prompt consideration of a neoplastic etiology. CT scans are widely available and well tolerated by patients, but they may fail to adequately characterize smaller lesions. MRI is particularly useful for evaluating smaller lesions[6] and is our imaging modality of choice for patients with newly discovered liver lesions.

On MRI, simple hepatic cysts have homogeneous, very low signal intensity relative to surrounding liver parenchyma on T1-weighted images but very high signal intensity on T2-weighted images. They do not enhance with administration of gadolinium chelates (Fig. 121.4).[5,7] Cysts with internal hemorrhage will appear hyperintense on both T1- and T2-weighted images and often demonstrate a fluid-fluid level (Fig. 121.5).[7] MRI provides detailed information about internal cystic structure, including septations, papillary nodules, and debris. In addition, small lesions that are indeterminate on CT scan can often be accurately characterized by MRI (Fig. 121.6). Diffusion-weighted MRI is particularly useful in distinguishing small hepatic cysts from other benign and malignant liver lesions.[8]

Intervention is indicated in patients with symptoms attributable to a hepatic cyst or uncertainty regarding a neoplastic etiology. Image-guided aspiration is ineffective, with a recurrence rate of 100%.[5] However, aspiration can provide fluid for biochemical and cytologic analyses. Aspiration may also help to assess whether symptoms are related to the cyst because it should provide temporary improvement of symptoms.

Aspiration with the addition of a sclerosant, such as ethanol, hypertonic saline, or tetracycline, has resulted

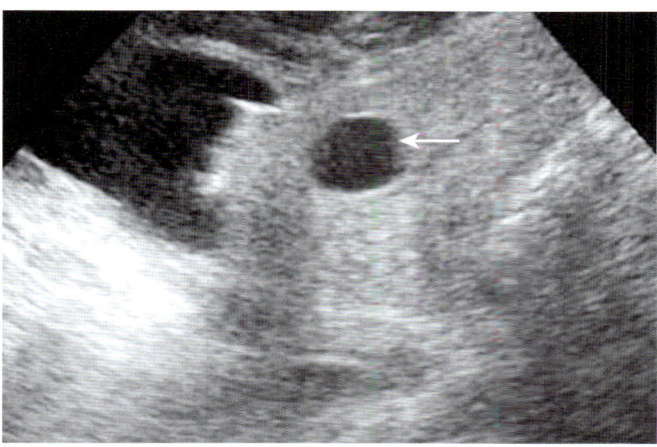

FIGURE 121.1 Simple hepatic cyst. Transverse ultrasound image of the left lobe shows an anechoic cyst *(arrow)* with smooth imperceptible walls and increased through transmission.

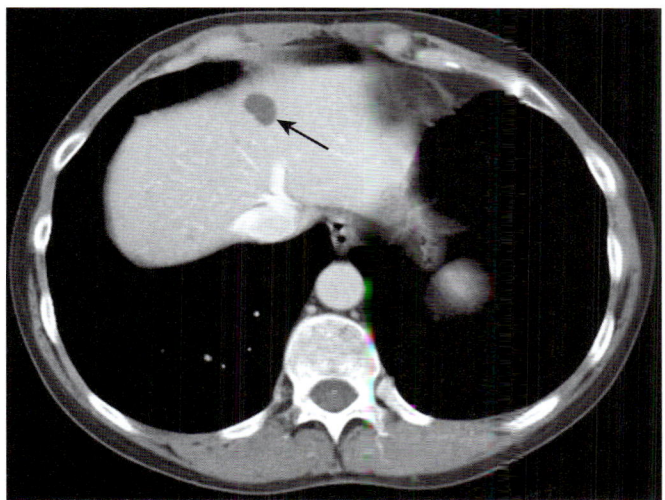

FIGURE 121.2 Simple hepatic cyst. Contrast-enhanced computed tomography image shows a simple cyst *(arrow)* in the left lobe of the liver. The cyst has water attenuation, an imperceptible wall, and little to no enhancement with intravenous contrast.

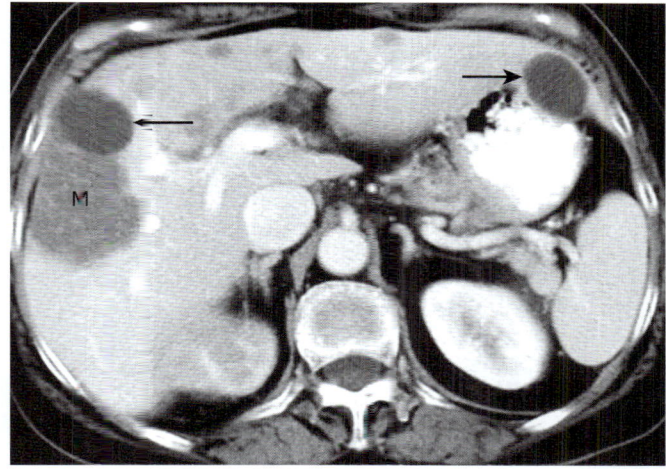

FIGURE 121.3 Two simple hepatic cysts and a liver metastasis. Contrast-enhanced computed tomography image shows two simple hepatic cysts *(arrows)* with water attenuation in the right and left lobes of the liver. The cysts are unenhanced and have imperceptible walls. Compare with the enhancing metastasis *(M)* adjacent to the cyst in the right lobe. Note several other small metastatic lesions in the liver.

in improved recurrence rates. Communication with the biliary tree must be ruled out before a sclerosant is used. In one prospective study of percutaneous aspiration and ethanol injection, 80% of patients demonstrated recurrent cysts; however, the majority of these regressed and did not require retreatment.[10] Other small series have reported recurrence in as few as 17% of patients.[1] The majority of cysts treated with percutaneous aspiration and sclerosant injection decrease in size, with a mean volume reduction of 92% to 98% at a 30-month follow-up.[12,13]

Surgical cyst fenestration or resection remains the mainstay of treatment for symptomatic simple hepatic cysts. Cysts that are deep in the parenchyma may not be suitable for fenestration, but only a portion of the wall needs to be removed to achieve symptomatic relief and rule out neoplasm. Therefore cyst fenestration is a reasonable first step in any medically fit patient with even a

portion of the cyst that is superficial and accessible. Cyst fenestration or resection may be carried out via a laparoscopic or an open approach.

Regardless of the surgical treatment selected, the operation begins with visual inspection. Intraoperative ultrasound can identify and define the cyst's relationship to the biliary tree and vasculature. The cyst should then be aspirated, with fluid sent for cytology. A large portion of the cyst wall (as much as can be removed without a liver resection) should be resected. Nodules or papillary projections in the remaining cyst wall may be separately biopsied. Bilious cyst fluid should prompt careful examination for a connection to the biliary tree, and bile leaks should be oversewn. If there is sufficient preoperative concern for a neoplastic process, a formal resection or enucleation may be carried out rather than fenestration.

For patients who undergo cyst fenestration, whether laparoscopic or open, recurrence rates are less than 10%.[15,16] Morbidity is also less than 10%.[15,17-19] For patients treated with hepatic resection, recurrence is extremely rare but morbidity and mortality rates exceed those associated with fenestration. A prospective nonrandomized study of 40 patients with simple hepatic cysts demonstrated increased length of stay, operative blood loss, and complication rates in patients treated with resection compared with open fenestration. Laparoscopic fenestration carried the lowest morbidity, with no significant difference in recurrence rates among the different surgical procedures.[20] Therefore laparoscopic fenestration should be considered the procedure of choice for symptomatic simple hepatic cysts with low suspicion for neoplasm.

POLYCYSTIC LIVER DISEASE

Polycystic liver disease (PLD) is a benign condition that usually occurs in patients with autosomal dominant

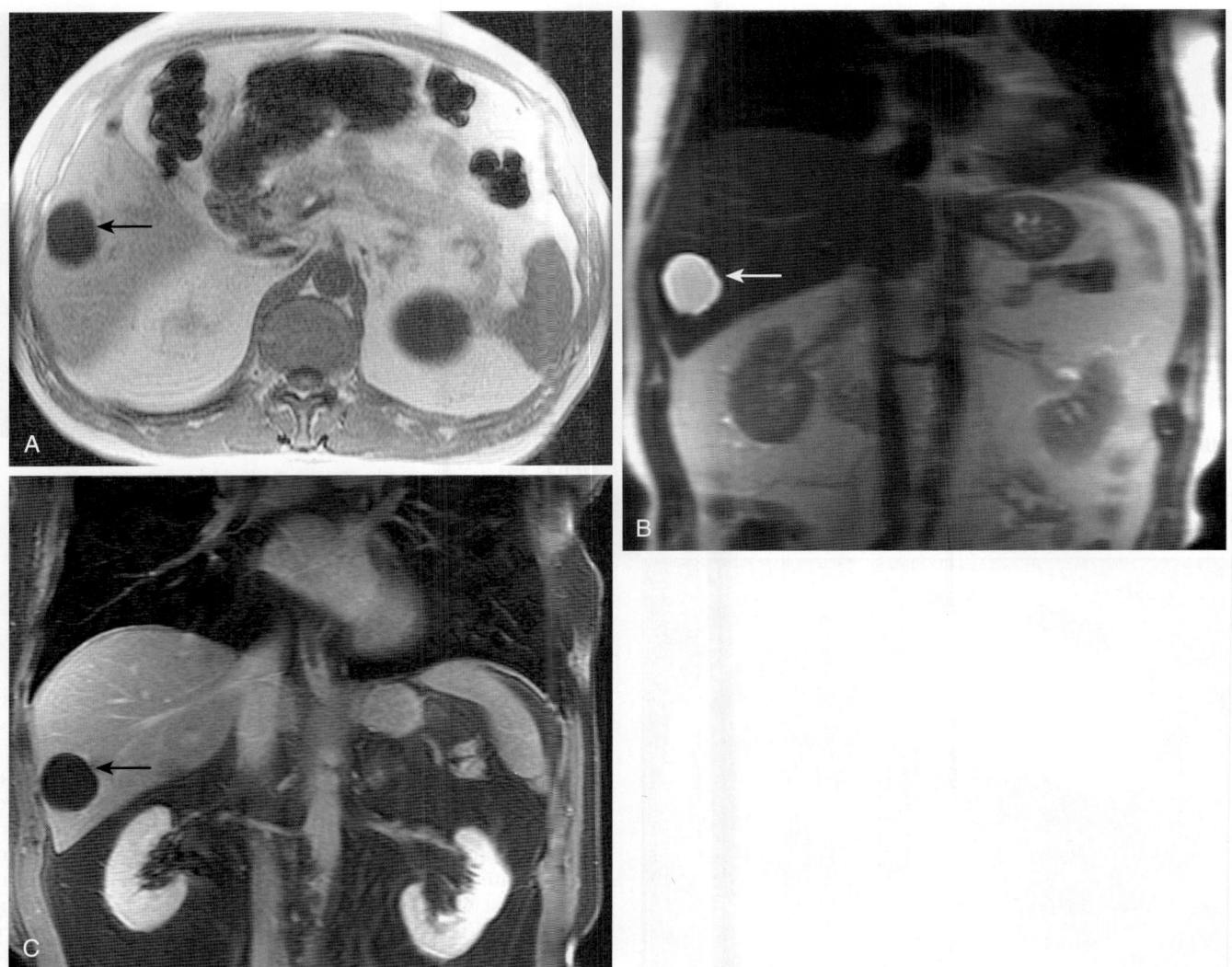

FIGURE 121.4 Simple hepatic cyst *(arrows)* on magnetic resonance imaging. Axial T1-weighted (A) and coronal T2-weighted (B) images of the liver show a well-defined mass with low signal intensity on T1-weighted and very high signal intensity on T2-weighted imaging. The mass does not enhance on the coronal postgadolinium image (C).

polycystic kidney disease (ADPKD). Patients develop a multitude of cysts that closely resemble their solitary counterparts, and the involvement of other organs, such as the kidneys or brain, may be the only way to distinguish multiple simple liver cysts from PLD. In ADPKD, hepatic cysts become increasingly prevalent with age, occurring in 10% of patients younger than 30 years and greater than 50% in those older than 60 years, based on ultrasound studies.[21–23] Studies using MRI suggest a prevalence of greater than 80%.[24] PLD is more common in women, and greater numbers of cysts develop in those having experienced pregnancy or received exogenous hormones. In one study, exposure of patients with ADPKD to conjugated estrogens corresponded to a 7% increase in liver cyst size over 1 year relative to untreated controls.[25]

ADPKD is caused by defects in two genes, *PKD1* and *PKD2*.[26] The extent of disease in the kidney and the liver is poorly correlated, and the ADPKD genotype predicts

the severity and growth rate of renal cysts but not of liver cysts.[27,28] This observation, coupled with the age-dependence of hepatic cyst formation, suggests that additional disease-modifying factors beyond the germline disease-conferring mutation significantly influence the progression of liver cysts in ADPKD. Autosomal dominant polycystic liver disease (ADPLD) is a much less common disorder that is not associated with renal cysts or cerebral aneurysms. ADPLD may be caused by mutations in PRKCSH or SEC63, both of which encode protein products important to the function of the endoplasmic reticulum.[29]

PLD is asymptomatic in most patients, and liver dysfunction is rare. Hepatic enlargement does cause symptoms in a minority of patients. Abdominal pain and distention, early satiety, vomiting, respiratory compromise, and lower extremity edema may occur. Although such problems are not usually life-threatening, they may result in a poor quality of life. Complications attributable to PLD are rare, occurring in fewer than 5% of affected individuals. Cyst

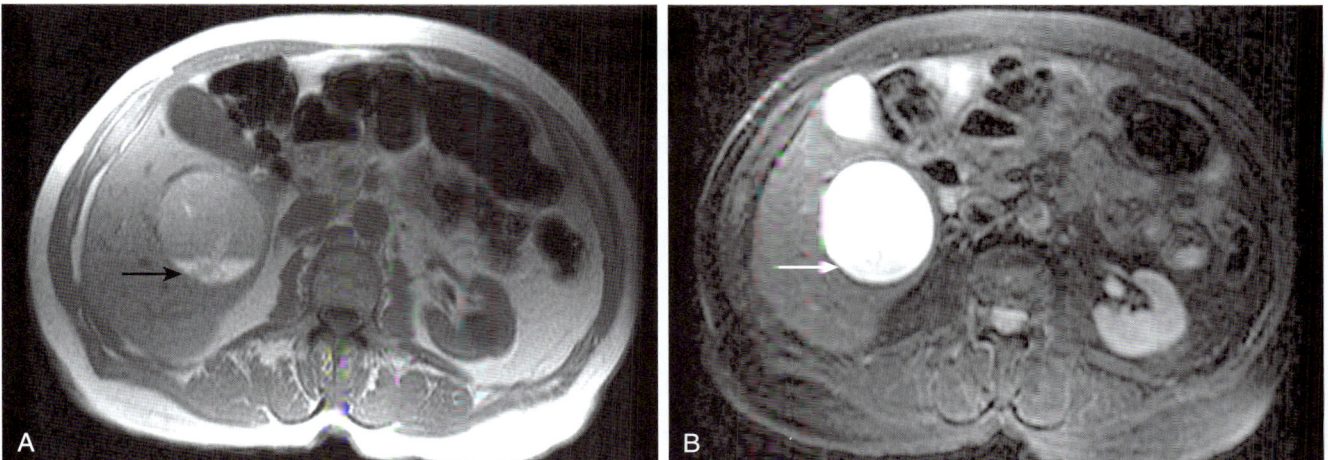

FIGURE 121.5 Hemorrhage within a simple cyst. T1-weighted (A) and T2-weighted (B) magnetic resonance imaging images show a cyst with layering high-T1 and low-T2 signal intensity material *(arrows)* in the dependent portion of the cyst indicating the presence of hemorrhagic products (methemoglobin).

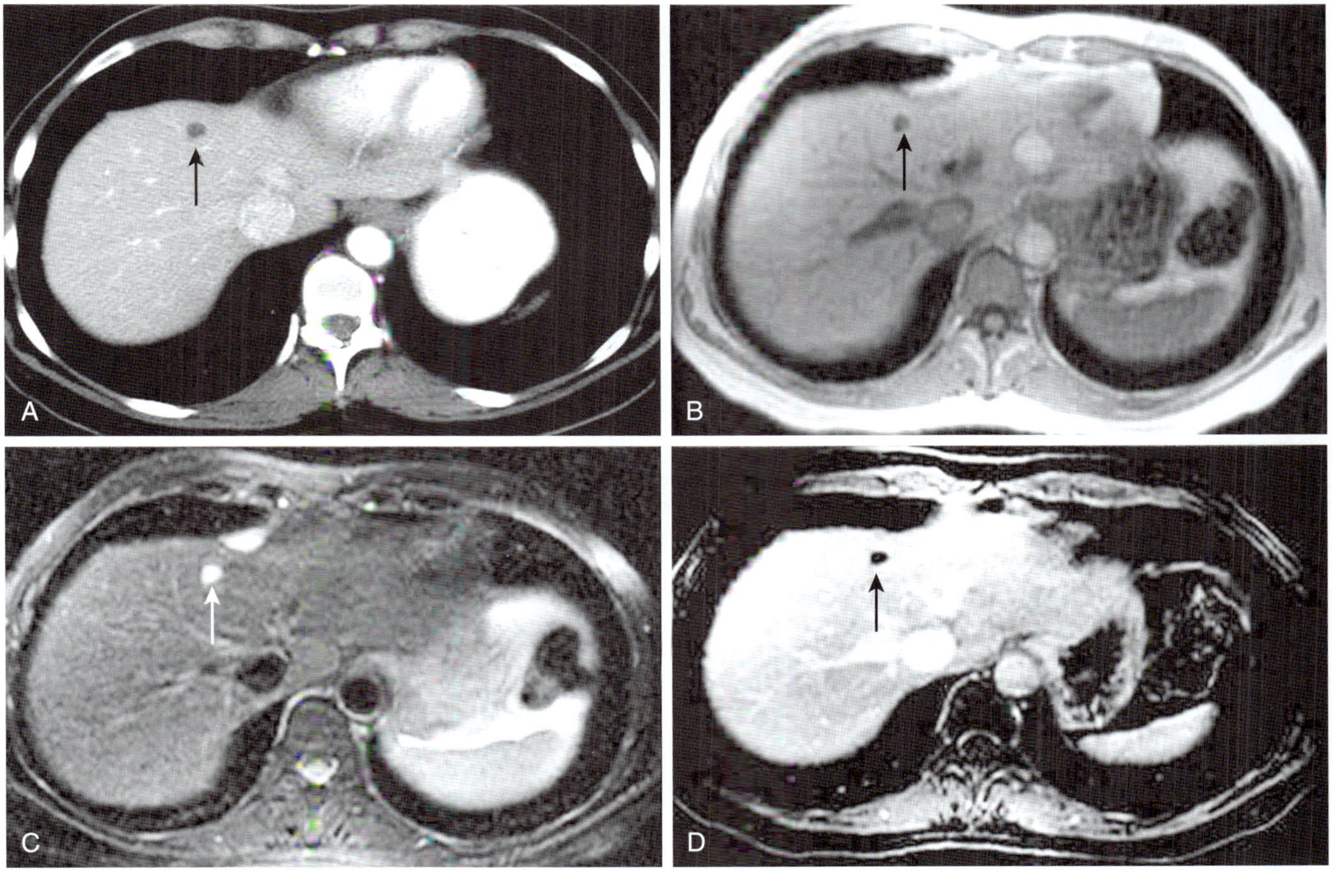

FIGURE 121.6 A small incidentally detected simple cyst on computed tomography (CT) and magnetic resonance imaging (MRI) in a patient with no history of malignancy or chronic liver disease. (A) Contrast-enhanced CT image shows a 1-cm hypocense mass in the medial segment of the left lobe *(arrow)*. The mass is too small to be accurately characterized. T1-weighted (B) and T2-weighted MR (C) images of the liver show the mass *(arrows)* to be hypointense relative to liver on T1-weighted imaging and markedly hyperintense on T2-weighted imaging. The mass does not enhance on the gadolinium-enhanced image (D).

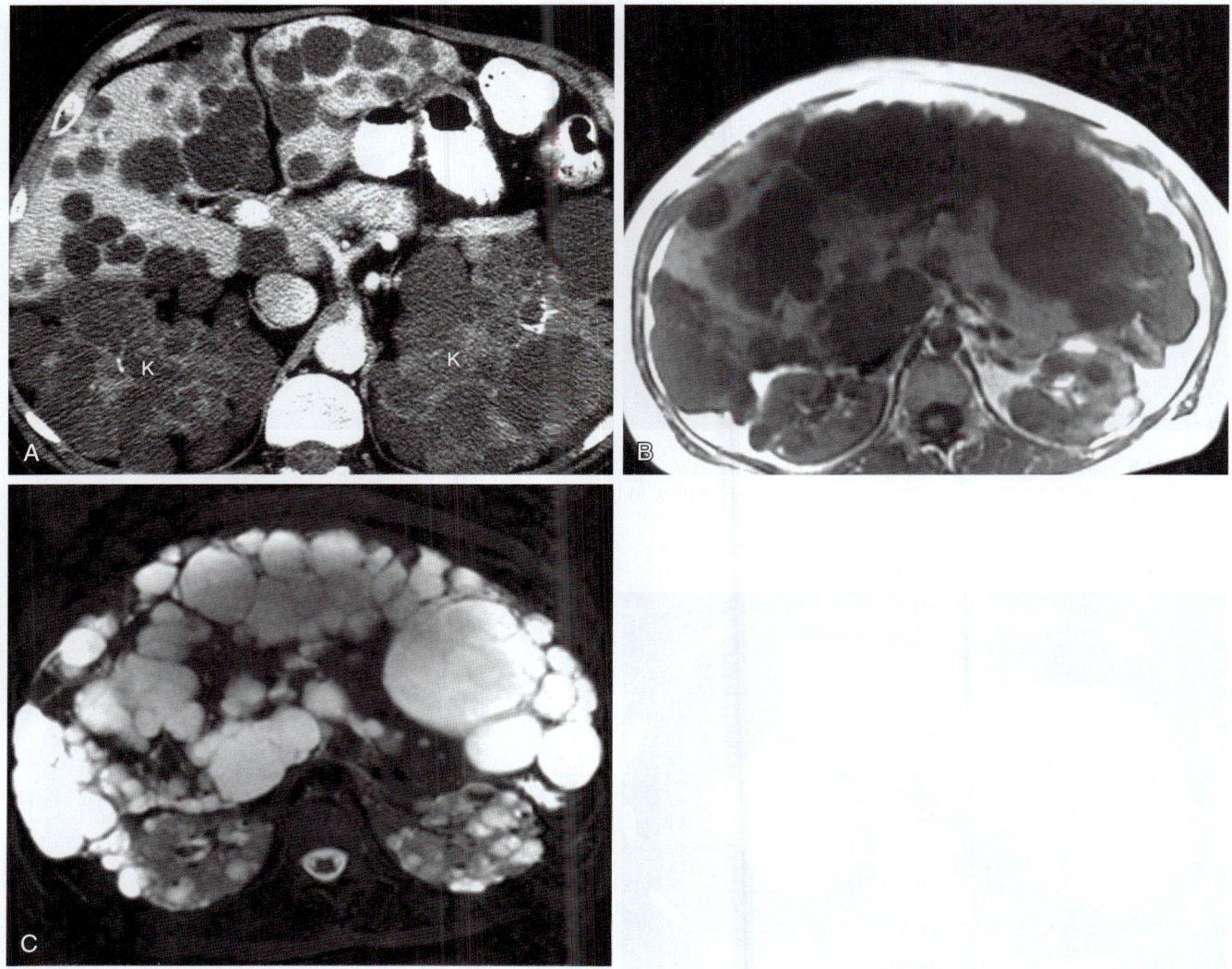

FIGURE 121.7 Hepatic cysts in two patients with autosomal dominant polycystic kidney disease. Contrast-enhanced computed tomography image (A) shows numerous nonenhancing cysts in the liver and kidneys (K). T1-weighted (B) and T2-weighted (C) images of the liver showing numerous simple hepatic and renal cysts with homogeneous low-T1 and high-T2 signal intensity.

infection or rupture, portal hypertension with ascites or variceal bleeding, and hepatic venous outflow obstruction secondary to cyst compression occur infrequently.

A classification of liver cysts proposed by Gigot et al. is useful in classifying patients and comparing treatments.[30]

- Type 1: 10 or fewer large cysts (>10 cm) with large areas of noninvolved liver parenchyma on CT scan.
- Type 2: Diffuse involvement of liver parenchyma by medium-sized cysts but with large areas of noncystic parenchyma on CT scan.
- Type 3: Massive and diffuse involvement of liver parenchyma with only a few areas of normal substance between cysts (Fig. 121.7).

Intervention for PLD should be considered only if it can both significantly reduce cyst-associated hepatomegaly and provide long-term relief of symptoms. Medical therapy with somatostatin analogues and even the immunosuppressive agent sirolimus[31] has been reported to palliate symptoms and reduce liver size. Several surgical options also exist.

Cyst aspiration followed by instillation of a sclerosing agent has been proposed when a small number of dominant cysts are believed to cause symptoms. This approach is limited by the ability to treat only a small number of cysts per session and by the potential for sclerosant extravasation. Experience is limited, and recurrence rates are high (30%–100%).[32,33]

Cyst fenestration, as described previously, is most applicable to patients with type 1 PLD. In properly selected patients with type 1 PLD, a recurrence rate of 11% at 30 months has been reported.[34,35] For patients with type 2 or 3 disease, recurrence rates exceed 70%. The most common postoperative complication is ascites formation, occurring when cyst fluid secretion exceeds the absorptive capacity of the peritoneum. Resection may be undertaken if fenestration is not feasible. Percutaneous transcatheter hepatic artery embolization may be used in patients who are poor surgical candidates.[36]

Liver transplantation for PLD was first reported in the 1990s.[37] Combined liver-kidney transplants have also been performed. The most appropriate candidates for liver transplantation are those with type 3 disease who have failed other palliative measures and those who are also candidates for renal transplantation. Although no survival advantage has been demonstrated for PLD patients undergoing transplantation, long-term survival does exceed that of patients requiring transplantation for other indications.[35] In addition, improved quality of life has been reported in more than 90% of survivors.[5-8]

ECHINOCOCCAL CYSTS

Hepatic infection with *Echinococcus granulosus* is a major public health problem worldwide and a common cause of cystic liver lesions in endemic areas. Transcontinental travel and immigration make recognition of echinococcal liver cysts important also in Western countries. Human infection occurs following oral intake of cestode eggs. Within the upper gastrointestinal tract, the oncospheres are released. They then penetrate the intestinal wall and enter the portal venous system. Hematogenous dissemination occurs primarily to the liver, although other organs may also be infected, including the lungs, brain, and bone. Following tissue lodgement, cestode proliferation occurs in the form of a slowly enlarging cyst. In 80% of affected individuals the only manifestation of echinococcal disease is a solitary cyst in a single organ

Cyst expansion is slow, typically less than 1 cm of diameter per year,[39] and symptoms are unusual until cysts reach 10 cm in size. With time, multiple daughter cysts may form within a single larger cyst. The slow cyst growth causes compression atrophy of the adjacent liver. Host reaction incites the formation of a fibrous surrounding capsule, termed a *pericyst*.

Symptoms of hydatid disease may be caused by compression, obstruction, or displacement of adjacent organs or structures. Symptoms are often vague and nonspecific. Malaise, weight loss, and chronic wasting are common. Mass effect from the cyst can cause abdominal pain, early satiety, or obstructive jaundice. Untreated, erosion into surrounding structures or organs may result in hematogenous dissemination or cystbiliary fistula. Spontaneous rupture with release of infected material into the peritoneum is rare but can cause anaphylaxis. Cyst rupture may also be precipitated by minor blunt abdominal trauma.[40]

The diagnosis of echinococcal infection is confirmed by serologic demonstration of an antibody response. Sensitivity and specificity both approximate 90%.[41] Children, in particular, may have a low antibody response. False-positive reactions may occur in individuals infected with other helminthic organisms.

Ultrasonography is an appropriate first-line diagnostic test for patients with echinococcal disease. Hydatid cysts can be distinguished from simple cysts by the presence of daughter cysts. Although some echinococcal cysts are anechoic, these are often characterized by a thickened cyst wall that is not present in simple cysts.[42] In Western countries, sonography has a specificity of 90%.[43]

If surgical therapy is planned, cross-sectional imaging with CT or MRI should be considered. Both can demonstrate the size and depth of cysts, the presence of daughter cysts, and extrahepatic involvement (Fig. 121.8).[44] Both

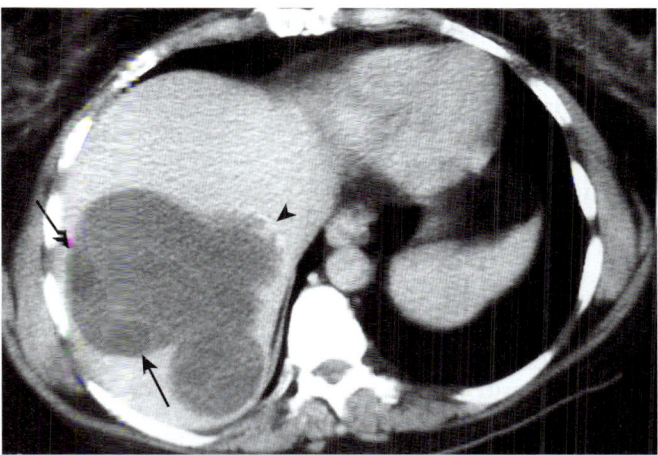

FIGURE 121.8 Hydatid cyst. Nonenhanced computed tomography image shows a cystic mass containing several daughter cysts (arrows) and peripheral calcification (arrowhead).

can also define the surrounding anatomy and relationship to biliary and vascular structures, but MRI with magnetic resonance cholangiopancreatography (MRCP) offers the added benefit of possible preoperative diagnosis of cyst-biliary fistula. In one series, sensitivity and specificity were reported as 78% and 100%, respectively, for diagnosis of cyst-biliary communication in patients with high pretest probability based on symptoms.[45]

Diagnosis of hydatid disease should prompt therapy to alleviate symptoms, halt progression of infection, and prevent complications. Both operative and percutaneous options are available. The goals of hydatid surgery are fourfold: (1) inactivate infectious cyst contents (scolices and the germinative membrane); (2) prevent spillage of cyst contents; (3) evacuate all viable elements; and (4) manage the residual cavity. Although these principal goals are widely accepted, debate continues regarding the extent of surgery and optimal management of the cyst cavity. Cysts may be resected, with or without adjacent liver. More conservative procedures seek to sterilize and then evacuate cyst contents, leaving the pericyst intact. Formal resection has at least a theoretical benefit of lower recurrence and risk of spillage. The only randomized controlled trial to date evaluated 32 patients with cystic echinococcus randomized to resection or fenestration. The conservative therapy group had significantly higher rates of recurrence and morbidity, with no difference in operative time, blood loss, or length of hospital stay.[46] Recurrent helminthic infection occurs in 2% to 10% of patients.[47]

Surgery begins by isolating the area immediately adjacent to the cyst with disinfectant-soaked pads to reduce the risk of contamination. A scolicidal agent is then instilled into the cyst. Ethanol (70%–95%), hypertonic saline (15%–20%), and cetrimide solution (5%) have been widely used at acceptably low risk. In cases of spillage of scolices, postoperative treatment with albendazole or mebendazole may be indicated to reduce the risk of subsequent intraperitoneal recurrence.[39] The residual cavity may be left open to the peritoneum, leaving the pericyst intact. The cyst edges may be sutured to prevent bleeding. An omental flap may also be used to fill the cyst cavity. Laparoscopic approaches are now used in many centers with good results.[48,49]

Percutaneous interventions offer an alternative to operative therapy for hydatid cysts. The most extensively evaluated technique is puncture-aspiration-injection-reaspiration (PAIR). Cyst contents are aspirated percutaneously under CT or sonographic guidance. A scolicidal agent such as hypertonic saline is injected, then reaspirated after a delay of hours to days. This procedure may also be followed by the use of a sclerosing agent, such as ethanol. Before percutaneous intervention, cyst-biliary communication should be excluded with cholangiography. Reported cure, recurrence, and complication rates vary widely, and a Cochrane review found insufficient evidence to make a recommendation.[50] Univesicular cysts may be particularly well suited to this approach.[51–53]

NEOPLASTIC CYSTS

Neoplastic cysts of the liver are much less common than nonneoplastic cysts. They include both metastatic lesions with cystic degeneration and primary cystic tumors of the liver. Cystic metastases usually result from central necrosis of solid metastases. These may arise from any primary cancer, but most common are ovarian, pancreatic, colorectal, renal, and neuroendocrine cancers.

Primary neoplastic cysts of the liver include cystadenomas (alternately referred to as hepatic mucinous cystic neoplasms) and cystadenocarcinomas and comprise less than 5% of intrahepatic cysts. Published data on these rare tumors are limited to small case series.[54–59] More than 90% of cystadenomas occur in women.[60] In contrast, cystadenocarcinomas may be more equally distributed between male and female patients.[54] Both neoplasms are most commonly identified in middle-aged patients, but cystadenocarcinomas have been reported in patients in their thirties.[54]

These lesions are believed to arise from, and may communicate with, the biliary tree. Histologically, cystadenomas

are lined by a simple columnar epithelium resembling bile duct epithelium. In most cases the stroma underlying the epithelium is distinctive, resembling ovarian stroma or primitive biliary mesenchyme.[61] They may express estrogen and progesterone receptors within their stroma, suggesting an embryologic origin from ectopic rests of ovarian tissue similar to those that putatively give rise to mucinous cystic neoplasms of the pancreas. Cystadenomas without ovarian stroma occur much more commonly in men.

Patients may present with a history of abdominal pain or mass, but usually the diagnosis is made incidentally due to the increasing use of cross-sectional imaging. Differentiating cystadenoma or cystadenocarcinoma from a simple liver cyst is a major clinical challenge. The diagnosis may be suggested by ultrasonography, CT, or MRI. Internal septations (Fig. 121.9), papillary projections from the cyst wall, or mural nodules strongly suggest a neoplastic cyst.[62–64] The cyst contents may have variable signal intensity on MRI T1- and T2-weighted imaging, depending on the presence of hemorrhage, protein content, or solid components (Fig. 121.10). Invasion of surrounding structures indicates malignancy, but this finding is rare. Cystadenomas and cystadenocarcinomas are usually large. The presence of other simple cysts in the liver may help to distinguish a dominant large simple cyst from a neoplastic cyst. Serum and cyst fluid levels of the tumor markers carcinoembryonic antigen (CEA) and carbohydrate antigen 19-9 (CA 19-9) may be elevated but are not reliable.[59,62,64,65] Moreover, percutaneous cyst wall biopsy or aspiration risks biopsy tract or peritoneal dissemination of a possible malignancy.[61,66]

Because there are no imaging findings that reliably distinguish cystadenomas from simple cysts, the distinction is often made based on a surgical specimen. Because of the difficulty of making the diagnosis preoperatively, some centers perform cyst fenestration to obtain a large portion of the cyst wall.[67] If the cyst is confirmed to be neoplastic, either based on intraoperative frozen section or final pathology, complete excision can be carried out. Although this approach carries the theoretical risk of allowing

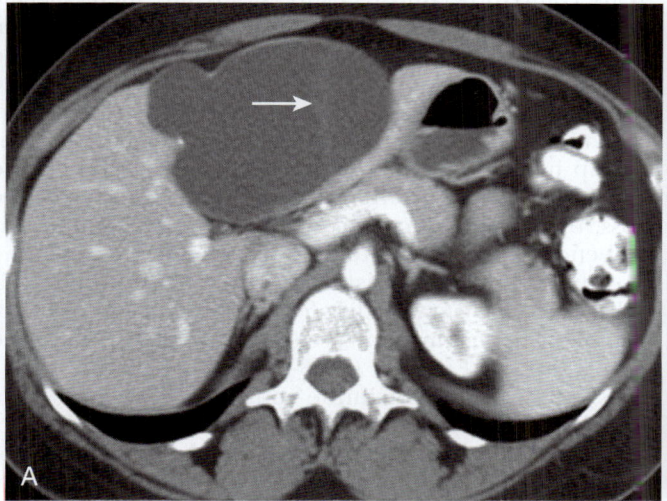 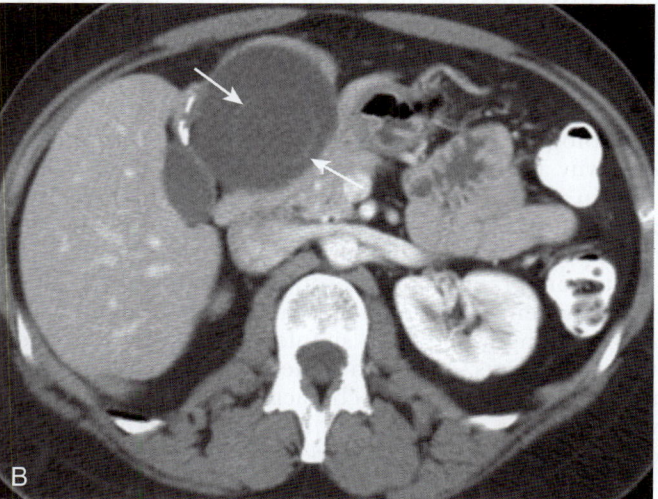

FIGURE 121.9 Hepatic cystadenoma. (A and B) Contrast-enhanced computed tomography images show a cystic mass in the left lobe containing thin enhancing septae *(arrows)*. Identification of septae such as these raises suspicion for a cystic neoplasm.

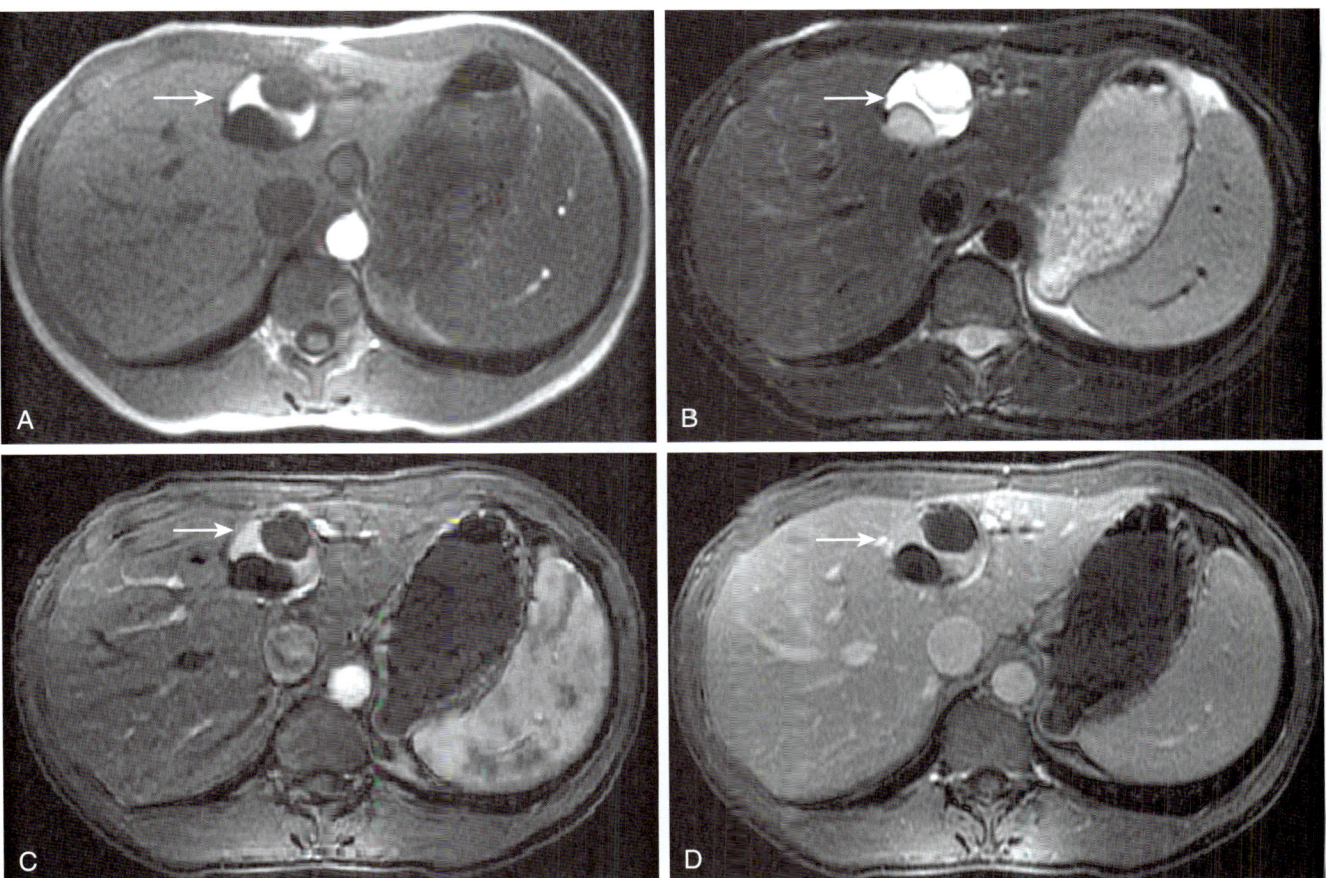

FIGURE 121.10 Hepatic cystadenoma *(arrows)* with ovarian stroma. T1-weighted (A) and T2-weighted (B) images of the liver show a complex multilocular mass in the left lobe. The mucinous content of the mass has mixed high and low signal intensity on T1-weighted imaging and high and intermediate signal intensity on T2-weighted imaging. The mass does not enhance on early (C) or delayed (D) postgadolinium imaging.

dissemination of cancer cells in a patient with cystadenocarcinoma, it should be noted that cystadenocarcinoma remains exceedingly rare. Therefore routine resection of all complex cysts without confirmation of a neoplastic etiology is likely to inflict significant morbidity on many patients but benefit only the very rare patient with a malignant cystadenocarcinoma. Formal hepatic resection is the only adequate procedure for cystadenocarcinoma; cystadenomas may be treated with either resection or enucleation.

Intraductal papillary mucinous neoplasms of the bile duct (IPMNs-B) are recently characterized cystic neoplasms that are similar in appearance and behavior to intraductal papillary mucinous neoplasms (IPMNs) of the pancreas.[68-70] These lesions demonstrate numerous papillary infoldings in the lumen of the bile duct that produce mucin, which uncommonly may result in biliary obstruction. They may present as diffusely dilated bile ducts (bile duct ectatic type) or a large cystic mass (cystic type). Cases are equally distributed between men and women. Invasive cancer is found in up to 60% of resected specimens. As with IPMNs of the pancreas, IPMN-B appears to have a better prognosis than other bile duct cancers, with a 5-year survival of 60%–80%.[71]

ACKNOWLEDGMENT

The authors acknowledge the contributions of Danielle M. Fritze and Hero K. Hussain to the previous edition of this chapter.

REFERENCES

1. Larsen TB, Rørvik J, Hoff SR, Horn A, Rosendahl K. The occurrence of asymptomatic and symptomatic simple hepatic cysts. A prospective, hospital-based study. *Clin Radiol.* 2005;60(9):1026-1029.
2. Carrim ZI, Murchison JT. The prevalence of simple renal and hepatic cysts detected by spiral computed tomography. *Clin Radiol.* 2003;58(8):626-629.
3. Caremani M, Vincenti A, Benci A, Sassoli S, Tacconi D. Ecographic epidemiology of non-parasitic hepatic cysts. *J Clin Ultrasound.* 1993;21(3):115-118.
4. Hansman MF, Ryan JA Jr, Holmes JH 4th, et al. Management and long-term follow-up of hepatic cysts. *Am J Surg.* 2001;181(5):404-410.
5. Horton KM, Bluemke DA, Hruban RH, Soyer P, Fishman EK. CT and MR imaging of benign hepatic and biliary tumors. *Radiographics.* 1999;19(2):431-451.
6. Mueller GC, Hussain HK, Carlos RC, Nghiem HV, Francis IR. Effectiveness of MR imaging in characterizing small hepatic lesions: routine versus expert interpretation. *AJR Am J Roentgenol.* 2003;180(3):673-680.
7. Mortelé KJ, Ros PR. Cystic focal liver lesions in the adult: differential CT and MR imaging features. *Radiographics.* 2001;21(4):895-910.

8. Miller FH, Hammond N, Siddiqi AJ, et al. Utility of diffusion-weighted MRI in distinguishing benign and malignant hepatic lesions. *J Magn Reson Imaging*. 2010;32(1):138-147.

9. Saini S, Mueller PR, Ferrucci JT Jr, Simeone JF, Wittenberg J, Butch RJ. Percutaneous aspiration of hepatic cysts does not provide definitive therapy. *Am J Roentgenol*. 1983;141(3):559-560.

10. Hahn ST, Han SY, Yun EH, et al. Recurrence after percutaneous ethanol ablation of simple hepatic, renal, and splenic cysts: is it true recurrence requiring an additional treatment? *Acta Radiol*. 2008;49(9):982-986.

11. Simonetti G, Profili S, Sergiacomi GL, Meloni GB, Orlacchio A. Percutaneous treatment of hepatic cysts by aspiration and sclerotherapy. *Cardiovasc Intervent Radiol*. 1993;16(2):81-84.

12. Larssen TB, Rosendahl K, Horn A, Jensen DK, Rørvik J. Single-session alcohol sclerotherapy in symptomatic benign hepatic cysts performed with a time of exposure to alcohol of 10 min: initial results. *Eur Radiol*. 2003;13(12):2627-2632.

13. Yang CF, Liang HL, Pan HB, et al. Single-session prolonged alcohol-retention sclerotherapy for large hepatic cysts. *AJR Am J Roentgenol*. 2006;187(4):940-943.

14. Zerem E, Imamović G, Omerović S. Percutaneous treatment of symptomatic non-parasitic benign liver cysts: single-session alcohol sclerotherapy versus prolonged catheter drainage with negative pressure. *Eur Radiol*. 2008;18(2):400-406.

15. Palanivelu C, Jani K, Malladi V. Laparoscopic management of benign nonparasitic hepatic cysts: a prospective nonrandomized study. *South Med J*. 2006;99(10):1063-1067.

16. Katkhouda N, Mavor E. Laparoscopic management of benign liver disease. *Surg Clin North Am*. 2000;80(4):1203-1211.

17. Cowles RA, Mulholland MW. Solitary hepatic cysts. *J Am Coll Surg*. 2000;191(3):311-321.

18. Mazza OM, Fernandez DL, Pekolj J, et al. Management of nonparasitic hepatic cysts. *J Am Coll Surg*. 2009;209(6):733-739.

19. Szabó LS, Takács I, Arkosy P, Sápy P, Szentkereszty Z. Laparoscopic treatment of nonparasitic hepatic cysts. *Surg Endosc*. 2006;20(4):595-597.

20. Tan YM, Chung A, Mack P, Chow P, Khin LW, Ooi LL. Role of fenestration and resection for symptomatic solitary liver cysts. *ANZ J Surg*. 2005;75(7):577-580.

21. Chauveau D, Fakhouri F, Grünfeld JP. Liver involvement in autosomal-dominant polycystic kidney disease: therapeutic dilemma. *J Am Soc Nephrol*. 2000;11(9):1767-1775.

22. Everson GT. Hepatic cysts in autosomal dominant polycystic kidney disease. *Am J Kidney Dis*. 1993;22(4):520-525.

23. Gabow PA, Johnson AM, Kaehny WD, Manco-Johnson ML, Duley IT, Everson GT. Risk factors for the development of hepatic cysts in autosomal dominant polycystic kidney disease. *Hepatology*. 1990;11(6):1033-1037.

24. Bae KT, Zhu F, Chapman AB, et al. Magnetic resonance imaging evaluation of hepatic cysts in early autosomal-dominant polycystic kidney disease: the Consortium for Radiologic Imaging Studies of Polycystic Kidney Disease cohort. *Clin J Am Soc Nephrol*. 2006;1(1):64-69.

25. Sherstha R, McKinley C, Russ P, et al. Postmenopausal estrogen therapy selectively stimulates hepatic enlargement in women with autosomal dominant polycystic kidney disease. *Hepatology*. 1997;26(5):1282-1286.

26. Mochizuki T, Wu G, Hayashi T, et al. PKD2, a gene for polycystic kidney disease that encodes an integral membrane protein. *Science*. 1996;272(5266):1339-1342.

27. Chebib FT, Jung Y, Heyer CM, et al. Effect of genotype on the severity and volume progression of polycystic liver disease in autosomal dominant polycystic kidney disease. *Nephrol Dial Transplant*. 2016;31(6):952-960.

28. Torres VE, Chapman AB, Perrone RD, et al. Analysis of baseline parameters in the HALT polycystic kidney disease trials. *Kidney Int*. 2012;81(6):577-585.

29. Fedeles SV, Tian X, Gallagher AR, et al. A genetic interaction network of five genes for human polycystic kidney and liver diseases defines polycystin-1 as the central determinant of cyst formation. *Nat Genet*. 2011;43(7):639-647.

30. Gigot JF, Jadoul P, Que F, et al. Adult polycystic liver disease: is fenestration the most adequate operation for long-term management? *Ann Surg*. 1997;225(3):286-294.

31. Qian Q, Du H, King BF, et al. Sirolimus reduces polycystic liver volume in ADPKD patients. *J Am Soc Nephrol*. 2008;19(3):631-638.

32. Bistritz L, Tamboli C, Bigam D, Bain VG. Polycystic liver disease: experience at a teaching hospital. *Am J Gastroenterol*. 2005;100(10):2212-2217.

33. Tikkakoski T, Mäkelä JT, Leinonen S, et al. Treatment of symptomatic congenital hepatic cysts with single-session percutaneous drainage and ethanol sclerosis: technique and outcome. *J Vasc Interv Radiol*. 1996;7(2):235-239.

34. Katkhouda N, Hurwitz M, Gugenheim J, et al. Laparoscopic management of benign solid and cystic lesions of the liver. *Ann Surg*. 1999;229(4):460-466.

35. Russell RT, Pinson CW. Surgical management of polycystic liver disease. *World J Gastroenterol*. 2007;13(38):5052-5059.

36. Takei R, Ubara Y, Hoshino J, et al. Percutaneous transcatheter hepatic artery embolization for liver cysts in autosomal dominant polycystic kidney disease. *Am J Kidney Dis*. 2007;49(6):744-752.

37. Lang H, von Woellwarth J, Oldhafer KJ, et al. Liver transplantation in patients with polycystic liver disease. *Transplant Proc*. 1997;29(7):2832-2833.

38. Kirchner GI, Rifai K, Cantz T, et al. Outcome and quality of life in patients with polycystic liver disease after liver or combined liver-kidney transplantation. *Liver Transpl*. 2006;12(8):1268-1277.

39. Pakala T, Molina M, Wu GY. Hepatic echinococcal cysts: a review. *J Clin Transl Hepatol*. 2016;4(1):39-46.

40. Kurt N, Oncel M, Gulmez S, Ozkan Z, Uzun H. Spontaneous and traumatic intra-peritoneal perforations of hepatic hydatid cysts: a case series. *J Gastrointest Surg*. 2003;7(5):635-641.

41. Sbihi Y, Rmiqui A, Rodriguez-Cabezas MN, Orduña A, Rodriguez-Torres A, Osuna A. Comparative sensitivity of six serological tests and diagnostic value of ELISA using purified antigen in hydatidosis. *J Clin Lab Anal*. 2001;15(1):14-18.

42. Caremani M, Lapini L, Caremani D, Occhini U. Sonographic diagnosis of hydatidosis: the sign of the cyst wall. *Eur J Ultrasound*. 2003;16(3):217-223.

43. Sayek I, Onat D. Diagnosis and treatment of uncomplicated hydatid cyst of the liver. *World J Surg*. 2001;25(1):21-27.

44. Polat P, Kantarci M, Alper F, et al. Hydatid disease from head to toe. *Radiographics*. 2003;23(2):475-494.

45. Hosch W, Stojkovic M, Jänisch T, et al. MR imaging for diagnosing cysto-biliary fistulas in cystic echinococcosis. *Eur J Radiol*. 2008;66(2):262-267.

46. Yüksel O, Akyürek N, Şahin T, et al. Efficacy of radical surgery in preventing early local recurrence and cavity-related complications in hydatic liver disease. *J Gastrointest Surg*. 2007;12(3):483-489.

47. Buttenschoen K, Carli Buttenschoen D. *Echinococcus granulosus* infection: the challenge of surgical treatment. *Langenbecks Arch Surg*. 2003;388(4):218-230.

48. Chen W, Xusheng L. Laparoscopic surgical techniques in patients with hepatic hydatid cyst. *Am J Surg*. 2007;194(2):243-247.

49. Palanivelu C, Senthilkumar R, Jani K, et al. Palanivelu hydatid system for safe and efficacious laparoscopic management of hepatic hydatid disease. *Surg Endosc*. 2006;20(12):1909-1913.

50. Nasseri-Moghaddam S, Abrishami A. Percutaneous needle aspiration, injection, and reaspiration with or without benzimidazole coverage for uncomplicated hepatic hydatid cysts. *Cochrane Database Syst Rev*. 2006;(2):CD003623.

51. Giorgio A, Di Sarno A, de Stefano G, Malekzadeh R. Sonography and clinical outcome of viable hydatid liver cysts treated with double percutaneous aspiration and ethanol injection as first-line therapy: efficacy and long-term follow-up. *AJR Am J Roentgenol*. 2009;193(3):W186-W192.

52. Kabaalioğlu A, Ceken K, Alimoglu E, Apaydin A. Percutaneous imaging-guided treatment of hydatid liver cysts: do long-term results make it a first choice? *Eur J Radiol*. 2006;59(1):65-73.

53. Zerem E, Jusufovic R. Percutaneous treatment of univesicular versus multivesicular hepatic hydatid cysts. *Surg Endosc*. 2006;20(10):1543-1547.

54. Ishak KG, Willis GW, Cummins SD, Bullock AA. Biliary cystadenoma and cystadenocarcinoma: report of 14 cases and review of the literature. *Cancer*. 1977;39(1):322-338.

55. Devaney K, Goodman ZD, Ishak KG. Hepatobiliary cystadenoma and cystadenocarcinoma. A light microscopic and immunohistochemical study of 70 patients. *Am J Surg Pathol*. 1994;18(11):1078-1091.

56. Regev A, Reddy KR, Berho M, et al. Large cystic lesions of the liver in adults: a 15-year experience in a tertiary center. *J Am Coll Surg*. 2001;193(1):36-45.

57. Wheeler DA, Edmondson HA. Cystadenoma with mesenchymal stroma (CMS) in the liver and bile ducts. A clinicopathologic study of 17 cases, 4 with malignant change. *Cancer.* 1985;56(6):1434-1445.

58. Soares KC, Arnaoutakis DJ, Kamel I, et al. Cystic neoplasms of the liver: biliary cystadenoma and cystadenocarcinoma. *J Am Coll Surg.* 2014;218(1):119-128.

59. Arnaoutakis DJ, Kim Y, Pulitano C, et al. Management of biliary cystic tumors: a multi-institutional analysis of a rare liver tumor. *Ann Surg.* 2015;261(2):361-367.

60. Daniels JA, Coad JE, Payne WD, Kosari K, Sielaff TD. Biliary cyst-adenomas: hormone receptor expression and clinical management. *Dig Dis Sci.* 2006;51(3):623-628.

61. Manouras A, Markogiannakis H, Lagoudianakis E, Katergiannakis V. Biliary cystadenoma with mesenchymal stroma: report of a case and review of the literature. *World J Gastroenterol.* 2006;12(37):6062-6069.

62. Choi HK, Lee JK, Lee KH, et al. Differential diagnosis for intrahepatic biliary cystadenoma and hepatic simple cyst: significance of cystic fluid analysis and radiologic findings. *J Clin Gastroenterol.* 2010; 44(4):289-293.

63. Korobkin M, Stephens DH. Lee JK, et al. Biliary cystadenoma and cystadenocarcinoma: CT and sonographic findings. *AJR Am J Roentgenol.* 1989;153(3):507-511.

64. Seo JK, Kim SH, Lee SH, et al. Appropriate diagnosis of biliary cystic tumors: comparison with atypical hepatic simple cysts. *Eur J Gastro-enterol Hepatol.* 2010;22(8):989-996.

65. Koffron A, Rao S, Ferrario M, Abecassis M. Intrahepatic biliary cys adenoma: role of cyst fluid analysis and surgical management in the laparoscopic era. *Surgery.* 2004;136(4):926-936.

66. Hai S, Hirohashi K, Uenishi T, et al. Surgical management of cystic hepatic neoplasms. *J Gastroenterol.* 2003;38(8):759-764.

67. Doussot A, Gluskin J, Groot-Koerkamp B, et al. The accuracy of preoperative imaging in the management of hepatic cysts. *HPB (Oxford).* 2015;17(10):889-895.

68. Budzynska A, Hartleb M, Nowakowska-Dulawa E. Krol R, Remiszewski P, Mazuriewicz M. Simultaneous liver mucinous cystic and intraductal papillary mucinous neoplasms of the bile duct a case report. *World J Gastroenterol.* 2014;20(14):4102-4105.

69. Shibahara H, Tamada S, Goto M, et al. Pathologic features of mucin-producing bile duct tumors: two histopathologic categories as counterparts of pancreatic intraductal papillary-mucinous neoplasms. *Am J Surg Pathol.* 2004;28(3):327-338

70. Zen Y, Fedica F, Patcha VR, et al. Mucinous cystic neoplasms of the liver: a clinicopathological study and comparison with intraductal papillary neoplasms of the bile duct. *Mod Pathol.* 2011;24(8):1079-1089.

71. Takanami K, Yamada T, Tsuda M, et al. Intraductal papillary mucininous neoplasm of the bile duct: multimodality assessment with pathologic correlation. *Abdom Imaging.* 2011;36(4):447-456.

CHAPTER 122

Liver Abscess

Eliza W. Beal | Sylvester M. Black

Liver abscess is an uncommon entity that over the past 100 years has seen fairly dramatic changes in demographics, etiology, diagnosis, and treatment. Although the mortality from liver abscess has decreased significantly since the early 20th century, the incidence appears to be increasing.[1-3] Traditionally, it has been useful to think of hepatic abscesses in two broad categories: those of bacterial origin, otherwise known as pyogenic liver abscess (PLA) or those of parasitic origin primarily caused by *Entamoeba histolytica* leading to amebic liver abscess (ALA). With the increase in the number of patients with various forms of immunosuppression, including but not limited to neutropenia secondary to cancer treatment and transplant immunosuppression, the reports of other unusual types of liver abscess, such as mycobacterial abscess and fungal abscess, also appear to be increasing. Improvements in mortality and morbidity appear to be associated with early diagnosis, refinements in diagnostic imaging in the form of ultrasound and computed tomography (CT) scan, as well as the evolution of minimally invasive percutaneous and endoscopic aspiration and drainage techniques. General improvements in antibiotic usage and the development of critical care medicine have likely also contributed to further reductions in mortality from these diseases.

PYOGENIC LIVER ABSCESSES

Ochsner in 1938 demonstrated that surgical drainage combined with antibiotic therapy could considerably improve survival in patients with PLA. Patients undergoing surgical drainage in addition to antibiotic therapy had a 62% survival rate compared with nearly a 100% mortality in those who did not receive this treatment.[4] The standard of care until the 1950s was surgical drainage combined with antibiotic therapy. The mortality rate from PLA continued to remain high although significantly improved when compared with the results at the turn of the 21st century. Improvement in patient survival with PLA remained elusive, and likely contributing factors included the relatively late presentation of patients and inaccuracy of localization, which was primarily by manual palpation and detection of induration and/or fluctuance during surgery. Thus further advancement in the treatment of PLA would depend on refinement in diagnostic imaging, localization, and minimally invasive techniques. In 1953 McFadzean reported 14 patients who survived with percutaneous drainage for PLA.[5] However, percutaneous drainage would not be widely advocated until the 1980s, when several reports of percutaneous drainage combined with antibiotics showed improved survival in patients with PLA.[6,7]

Early detection and localization secondary to advancements in CT and ultrasonography (US) advanced the treatment of PLA considerably. Nowadays, percutaneous treatment of PLA, whether single or multiple abscesses are present, has become the standard of care. In addition, endoscopic and laparoscopic options for drainage in patients who are not responsive to antibiotic treatment have been explored with good outcomes.[8-14] Open operation is reserved primarily for cases of failure of nonoperative treatment, presence of fungal growth on culture, or communication of the abscess cavity with an obstructed biliary tree that cannot be managed nonoperatively, or with endoscopic or laparoscopic techniques.[15,16] The mortality associated with open operation under these circumstances is high.

INCIDENCE AND DEMOGRAPHICS

PLA is associated with significant morbidity, mortality, and health care costs. Reported incidence varies from 1.1 to 3.6 per 100,000 population in the Western literature to 17.6 per 100,000 population in the Eastern literature, and it appears that incidence of PLA is increasing.[1,3,17,18] The recently reported incidence of PLA in the United States is 3.6 per 100,000, with an increase in PLA-based hospitalizations between 1994 and 2005 from 2.7 to 4.1 per 100,000 population.[1] In Canada the reported incidence is 2.3 per 100,000 population.[19] In Taiwan, where PLA has been described as an emerging endemic disease, the reported incidence has increased from 11.2 per 100,000 population in 1996 to 17.6 per 100,000 in 2004.[17] The mortality from PLA has decreased significantly from Ochsner's early series in which mortality from PLA was reported to be approximately 72% (Table 122.1).[4] Currently, mortality from PLA in most North American and European series ranges from 5.6% to 10%, whereas mortality worldwide ranges from 3% to 30%. Importantly, although incidence of PLA appears to be increasing, mortality has remained stable and the demographics of the patient with PLA have changed significantly.[1] At the turn of the century, the patient with PLA was typically a 20- to 30-year-old male with pylephlebitis secondary to appendicitis, diverticulitis, or other intraabdominal infection. With improved management of the underlying cause of the intraabdominal infection in the form of early diagnosis and improvements in antibiotic therapy, the demographics of PLA have shifted considerably. Now the typical patient with PLA is predominately a male in his 60s with an actively treated advanced hepatobiliary malignancy or benign biliary tract pathology as the underlying cause of PLA.[1,4,15,16]

Reported risk factors associated with development of PLA include diabetes (odds ratio [OR] = 3.6; 95% confidence interval [CI], 2.9 to 4.5).[2] This may relate to patients with diabetes' increased risk for severe gram-negative infections and bacteremia.[20] Patients with cirrhosis

TABLE 122.1 Selected Series of Pyogenic Hepatic Abscesses

Author	Location	No. of Cases	Time Period	Age (yr)	Male-to-Female Ratio	Incidence	Mortality Rate (%)
Ochsner et al.[4]	New Orleans	47	1928–1937	30–39 (mean)	2.35 : 1.0	47/540,776 admissions	72.3
Pitt and Zuidema[71]	Baltimore	80	1952–1972	60	1.0 : 1.0	13/100,000	65
Branum et al.[7]	Durham	73	1970–1986	53 (median)	1.1 : 1.0	1970–1978: 11.5/100,000 1979–1986: 22/100,000	19
Seeto and Rockey[22]	San Francisco	142	1979–1994	51 (median)	1.3 : 1.0	22/100,000 admissions	11
Chu et al.[24]	Hong Kong	83	1984–1995	60.2 (mean)	1.3 : 1.0	NR	18
Huang et al.[25]	Baltimore	153	1973–1993	55.5 (mean)	1.3 : 1.0	20/100,000 admissions	31
Alvarez et al.[28]	Spain	133	1985–1997	58.1–64.9 (mean)	1.6 : 1.0	NR	14
Mohsen et al.[30]	United Kingdom	65	1988–1999	64 (median)	1.3 : 1.0	18.5/100,000	12.3
Wong et al.[72]	Hong Kong	80	1991–2001	63.4 (mean)	1.67 : 1.0	NR	6

NR, Not reported.

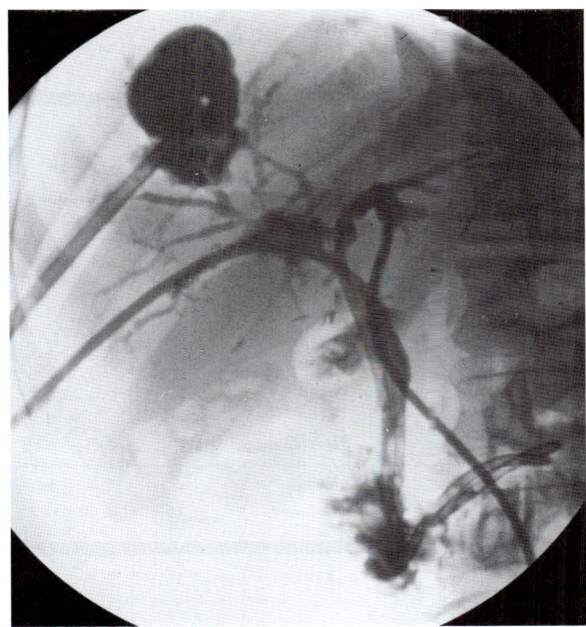

FIGURE 122.1 Cholangiogram demonstrating a perihilar cholangiocarcinoma and an abscess near the dome of the right lobe of the liver.

are also at increased risk for PLA with standardized incidence ratio of 15.4 (95% CI, 9.2 to 23.6) versus 1.0 in the background population.[21]

ETIOLOGY AND PATHOGENESIS

Although there are multiple etiologies of PLA, ascending infection of the biliary tree associated with obstruction is currently the most commonly identified cause.[15,16,22] Geographic differences account for observed differences in etiology of obstruction leading to ascending infection and subsequent PLA. In many Asian countries, hepatolithiasis with associated biliary stricture accounts for most of the cases of PLA,[23,24] whereas in Western countries obstruction secondary to underlying malignancy, such as an obstructing cholangiocarcinoma (Fig. 122.1) with associated ascending cholangitis, is a very common

scenario.[5,16,25] Furthermore, the widespread use of bile duct stents and biliary tract manipulation in these situations has also greatly increased the risk of cholangitis and subsequent PLA.

Other causes of PLA include hematogenous spread from sources other than the gastrointestinal (GI) tract, such as bacterial endocarditis, intravenous drug use, and other infectious processes that can produce bacteremia. Locoregional tumor therapies, including radiofrequency ablation and transarterial chemoembolization (TACE), can also lead to liver necrosis, which may then become secondarily infected, leading to PLA. Traumatic liver injury that results in necrosis may predispose a patient to development of PLA. Prior biliary reconstructive procedures may lead to biliary stricture and subsequent biliary tract infection, predisposing the patient to the development of PLA. Trauma is an additional rare cause of PLA; in a series of 2143 blunt and penetrating abdominal trauma patients, 11 (0.5%) were found to have liver abscesses. Eight of these had penetrating gunshot wounds and the remainder had blunt abdominal trauma.[26]

When no identifiable cause of PLA is found, the abscess is described as cryptogenic. Cryptogenic PLA is currently reported to represent approximately 25% of all liver abscesses in some series (Table 122.2).

CLINICAL PRESENTATION

The clinical presentation of PLA can be quite variable, and the early presentation of symptoms is nonspecific or vague. Prodromal symptoms, such as weight loss, fever, fatigue, malaise, anorexia, and myalgia, may occur many weeks before more specific symptoms, which may localize the process, such as right upper quadrant pain, hepatomegaly, or jaundice. The classic triad of right upper quadrant pain, fever or chills, and generalized malaise is not universally seen. Fever is the most common presenting sign and is present in at least two-thirds of patients. Right upper quadrant pain is also frequently present (Table 122.3). Other signs or symptoms are variable. PLA most often occurs in the setting of other intraabdominal pathology, such as hepatobiliary malignancy or ascending biliary tract infection with obstruction, in which the underlying disease process influences the severity and duration of the symptoms.

TABLE 122.2 Etiology of Pyogenic Hepatic Abscess

Author	No. of Cases	Cryptogenic (%)	Hepatobiliary (%)	Portal (%)	Hepatic Artery (%)	Other (%)
Ochsner et al.[4]	47	60	6	19	N/A	15
Pitt and Zuidema[71]	80	20	51	15	1	<10*
Branum et al.[7]	73	27	31.4	18.2	10	14†
Seeto and Rockey[22]	153	16	60	<10	10	<10*
Chu et al.[24]	83	45	52	1	N/A	2‡
Huang et al.[25]	142	40	37	11	N/A	12§
Alvarez et al.[28]	133	26	25‖	13	2	33¶
Mohsen et al.[30]	65	24 (18 uninvestigated)	28	48	N/A	N/A
Wong et al.[72]	80	N/A	61	N/A	1.25	N/A

*Trauma.
†Trauma, other solid tumors, direct extension, Crohn disease.
‡Hematogenous spread.
§Includes direct extension, abdominal trauma, and chronic granulomatous disease.
‖Includes seven patients with recent hepatic surgery.
¶Trauma, direct extension.
N/A, Not available.

TABLE 122.3 Presenting Symptoms and Signs in Pyogenic Hepatic Abscess

Author	No. of Cases	Fever (%)	Abdominal Pain (%)	Nausea/ Vomiting (%)	Weight Loss (%)	Diarrhea (%)	Jaundice (%)	Hepatomegaly (%)
Pitt and Zuidema[71]	80	92	74	N/A	51	23	54	48
Branum et al.[7]	73	75	55	27	29	8	23	38
Seeto and Rockey[22]	153	89	55	N/A	43	10	50	35
Chu et al.[24]	83	67	89	N/A	13	N/A	24	7
Huang et al.[25]	142	79	55	30/37	28	20	22	28
Alvarez et al.[28]	133	92	69	29	42	N/A	21	24
Mohsen et al.[30]	65	67	67	41	35	23	14	30
Wong et al.[72]	80	99	35	N/A	10	N/A	14	18

N/A, Not available.

TABLE 122.4 Laboratory Findings in Pyogenic Hepatic Abscesses

Author	Leukocytosis (%)	Elevated Alkaline Phosphatase Level (%)	Hypoalbuminemia (%)	Hyperbilirubinemia (%)	ALT (%)	AST (%)	Anemia (%)
Pitt and Zuidema[71]	69	90	62	68	82	90	N/A
Branum et al.[7]	68	78	N/A	36	N/A	57	67
Seeto and Rockey[22]	77	70	71	49	67	64	N/A
Chu et al.[24]	89	92	67	22	N/A	N/A	13
Huang et al.[25]	64	80	>67	N/A*	69†	57†	75
Alvarez et al.[28]	65	56	50	23	N/A	41	56
Mohsen et al.[30]	88	64	N/A	36	67	49	*Male:* 74
							Female: 47
Pitt and Zuidema[72]	84	73	94	48	50–63	N/A	76

*Exact numbers not provided, but was present in most patients with biliary tract disease and hepatic abscess.
†Specific to patients with biliary tract and hepatic abscess.
ALT, Alanine aminotransferase; *AST*, aspartate aminotransferase; *N/A*, not available.

DIAGNOSIS

Laboratory investigations are nonspecific. Many patients present with an elevated white blood cell count. Hypoalbuminemia is also frequently present, likely reflecting disease chronicity (Table 122.4). Transaminases and alkaline phosphatase are also frequently elevated. An elevation of serum bilirubin may suggest underlying biliary obstruction as an etiologic factor.

Chest radiographic examination in 50% of the cases may show an elevated right hemidiaphragm, subdiaphragmatic

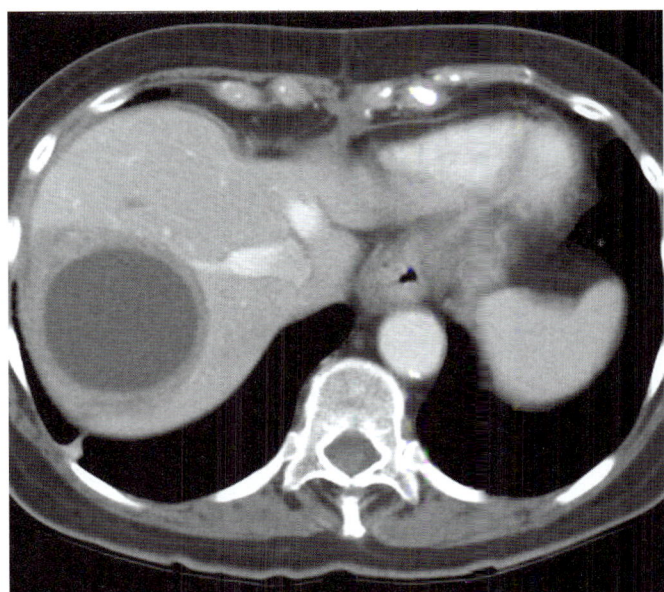

FIGURE 122.2 Contrast-enhanced computed tomography through the liver reveals a unilocular low-density mass near the dome, representing a pyogenic abscess. Note the peripheral enhancing rim, which is relatively narrow.

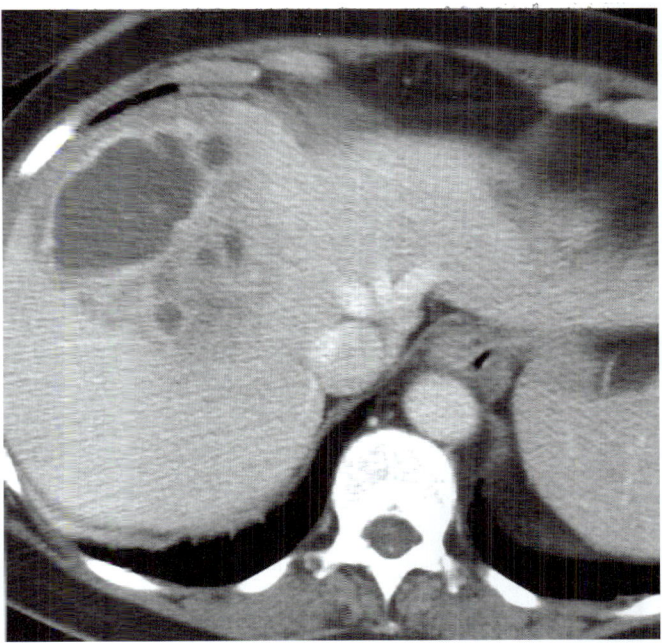

FIGURE 122.3 Contrast-enhanced computed tomography through the liver reveals the "cluster" appearance of a pyogenic hepatic abscess with several smaller peripheral abscesses that have coalesced.

air-fluid levels if gas-forming organisms are present, pleural effusions, and atelectasis.[22] US is usually the initial study of choice for imaging of the liver and biliary tree due to its low cost, the lack of exposure to ionizing radiation, and the high sensitivity.[27] US has a reported sensitivity of 83% to 95%.[25,28] US can also characterize the degree of maturation of liver abscess. Early in the formation of a PLA, the abscess is hyperechoic and not distinct. However, as the abscess matures with the formation of pus, a distinct wall forms and the abscess becomes hypoechoic. Another advantage of US is the ability to characterize underlying biliary pathology such as dilated bile ducts, hepatolithiasis, and choledocholithiasis.

CT scanning is highly sensitive to distinguish PLA from other intrahepatic lesions. The reported sensitivity for detection of PLA is between 93% and 100%.[22,27] In addition to high sensitivity for detection of PLA, CT scanning is also efficient at detecting small PLAs with a diameter of less than 2 cm, so-called microabscesses. CT scanning can detect abscesses within the liver parenchyma as small as 0.5 cm. Based on size, PLAs are classified as either microabscesses (<2 cm) or macroabscesses (>2 cm). Microabscesses will appear as small, multiple, hypodense lesions with distribution throughout the liver parenchyma. During CT scan and especially during the portal venous phase with intravenous contrast, PLAs will often exhibit peripheral rim enhancement, whereby the PLA will appear as a hypodense cystic lesion demonstrating segmental wall enhancement with surrounding low-density edema (Fig. 122.2). There is often a transition zone between the low-density center of the abscess and the peripheral rim. This transition zone is typically narrow, which is a feature that can help to differentiate PLA from necrotic metastasis.[27,29]

Classically, microabscesses have been described as having two distinct appearances on CT scan. First, microabscesses may appear as multiple, widely scattered, miliary-type lesions or they may appear as adjacent "daughter" abscesses clustering around central large abscesses. The clustering phenomenon may represent coalescence of multiple smaller abscesses and has been postulated to represent an early stage in the evolution of the PLA cavity.[29] Many of these multifocal clustered abscesses tend to form intercommunicating cavities, essentially forming larger multiseptate abscesses (Fig. 122.3).

Magnetic resonance (MR) imaging does not appear to offer any significant advantage in the detection of PLA when compared with US and CT, given their high sensitivity. However, if there is diagnostic uncertainty, MR imaging may be able to better characterize intrahepatic lesions and delineate differences between PLA and cystic or necrotic lesions. PLA tends to be hypointense on T1-weighted MR images and hyperintense on T2-weighted MR images (Fig. 122.4). Magnetic resonance cholangiopancreatography (MRCP) may be beneficial if biliary obstruction is suggested clinically. MRCP may help to identify the level of obstruction, allowing for more precise preoperative planning.

MICROBIOLOGY

Bacteria are more likely to be isolated from the abscess cavity than from blood culture.[1,21] Reports in the literature describe varying rates of monomicrobial versus polymicrobial isolates in PLA, with 33% to 55% of hepatic abscess cultures being polymicrobial, compared with a lower rate of polymicrobial blood culture isolates.[22,30–32] There have been many series of PLA in the literature, which have

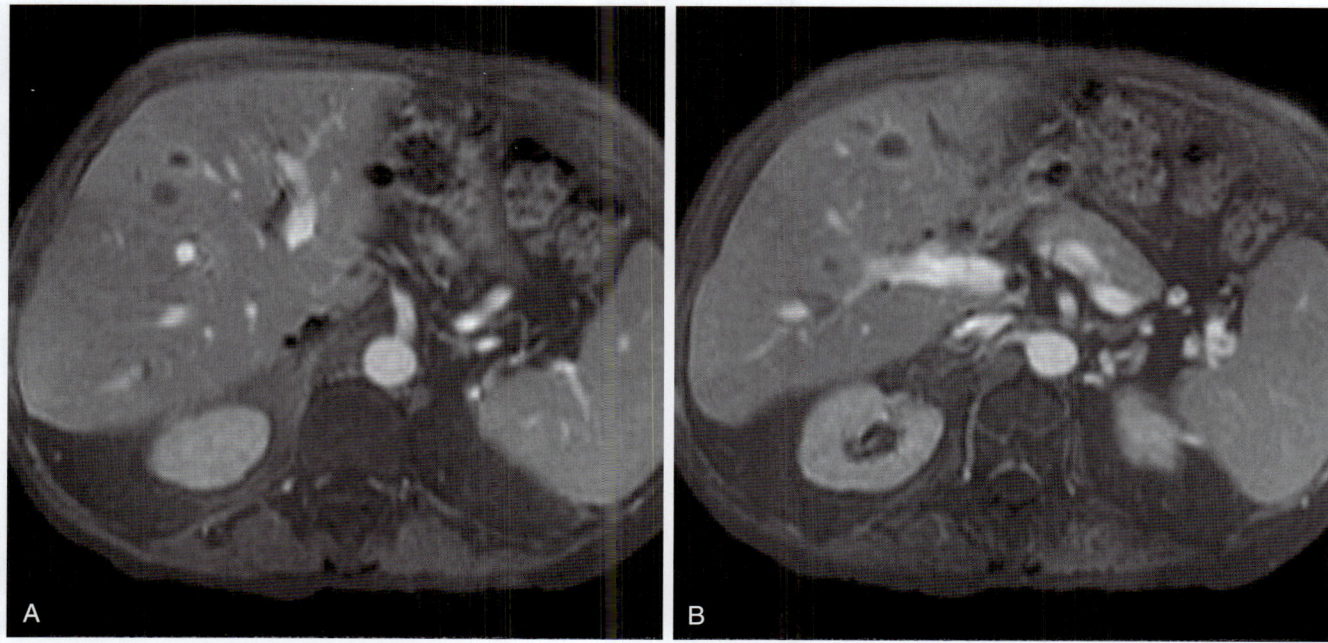

FIGURE 122.4 Gadolinium-enhanced T1-weighted magnetic resonance imaging through the liver reveals multiple low-signal lesions with a thin peripheral ring of enhancement in this patient with multiple pyogenic microabscesses.

BOX 122.1 **Microbiology of Pyogenic Liver Abscess**

Gram-Positive Organisms
  Streptococcus
  Staphylococcus
  Pneumococcus
  Enterococcus mycobacterium
Gram-Negative Organisms
  Escherichia
  Klebsiella
  Pseudomonas
  Proteus
  Haemophilus
  Serratia
Anaerobic Organisms
  Bacteroides
  Fusobacterium
  Pasteurella
  Polymicrobial
  Yeast

---

identified multiple species of bacterial flora presumed to be etiologic agents most commonly responsible for hepatic abscesses (Box 122.1). *Escherichia coli*, *Streptococcus*, *Enterococcus*, and *Klebsiella* are often cultured in patients with PLA, with *E. coli* and *Streptococcus* being the most frequently isolated bacterial flora in most series in the Western literature.[31] PLA with *Clostridium perfringens* has also been reported.[33]

Klebsiella pneumoniae is especially prevalent in Asia compared with Western populations.[23,34,35] A separate syndrome, invasive *K. pneumoniae* liver abscess syndrome

associated with synchronous metastatic *Klebsiella* infection has been described,[36,37] most commonly reported in individuals of Asian descent with diabetes. Metastatic sites of infection may include the lungs, central nervous system (CNS), and eyes. *K. pneumoniae* involved in this syndrome appears to possess additional virulence factors, including capsular type K1 or K2 antigen, the mucoviscosity associated gene (*magA*), *rmpA*, which aids in capsule synthesis, and aerobactin, a type of siderophore.[37] In a single-center study of this syndrome, mortality was 17% in comparison with simple *Klebsiella* PLA with mortality of 0%.[36] A single-center comparison of patients with *E. coli* versus *K. pneumoniae* PLA concluded that, although patients with *Klebsiella* were older, more commonly had ischemic heart disease, and had PLA more commonly associated with underlying biliary disease, outcomes were similar between the groups.[35]

Evolution and refinement of culture technique have led to the increasing identification of anaerobic and microaerophilic organisms in PLA. Sabbaj et al. in 1972 demonstrated that when using strict anaerobic culture techniques, 45% of cultures obtained from hepatic abscesses were in fact anaerobic, a finding that was much higher than prior studies.[38] Huang et al. demonstrated a significant increase in anaerobic isolates over a period of 42 years from 1952 to 1993 at Johns Hopkins.[25] Similarly, Chemaly et al. identified *Streptococcus milleri*, a microaerophilic or anaerobic collection of streptococcal bacteria, and anaerobic gram-negative bacilli as the most common bacterial isolates from culture.[39] In recent studies, *Bacteroides* species are the most commonly isolated anaerobes.[40] Improvement in culture technique suggests that abscesses previously thought to be "sterile" or cryptogenic may actually be caused by anaerobic organisms that were not previously identified secondary to inadequate technique.

PLA due to hematogenous spread not associated with a GI source is often monomicrobial. These PLAs are often the result of infection with *Staphylococcus aureus* or *Streptococcus* species and tend to be solitary abscesses. In contrast, infections that are from enteric or biliary sources tend to be polymicrobial and associated with aerobic gram-negative bacteria and anaerobes.[22,30,3] The clinician should be mindful that, as with many infections, bacteria associated with PLA have developed increased resistance to many antimicrobial agents. This antimicrobial resistance is likely the result of increasing use of indwelling biliary stents and biliary tract manipulation with recurrent episodes of cholangitis treated with antibiotics. PLA may contain multiple species of bacteria, and antibiotic choices should initially have broad coverage to reflect this fact until definitive culture results can be obtained. Abscess cavity culture is not usually immediately available. However, Gram stain of liver abscess aspirates in addition to blood culture provides useful information for the initiation of therapy for PLA. Gram stain of liver abscess aspirates is reported to have sensitivity of 90% with a specificity of 100% for gram-positive cocci. The reported sensitivity and specificity for gram-negative bacilli is 52% and 94%, respectively.[39]

TREATMENT

The principles of treatment of PLA are to drain the abscess cavity, identify the pathogen, initiate appropriate antibiotic therapy, and treat the underlying disease process associated with the abscess.

ANTIBIOTIC THERAPY

After the diagnosis of PLA is suspected, blood cultures should be immediately obtained. Diagnostic imaging in the form of US and/or CT scanning is helpful in localizing the process and in identifying any associated intraabdominal pathology. If a hepatic abscess is identified by diagnostic imaging, *E. histolytica* serology should be obtained to assist in differentiating between the two major types of hepatic abscess because amebic abscesses usually do not require drainage. Percutaneous aspiration or drainage with Gram stain and culture of abscess cavity contents is helpful to guide initial antibiotic management. Therapy should not be delayed while waiting for blood or abscess culture results, and broad-based empiric antibiotic coverage should be started immediately. Biliary disorders commonly yield gram-negative bacteria, whereas abscesses as a result of pylephlebitis often yield gram-negative and anaerobic bacteria. Antimicrobials, such as the extended-spectrum penicillins (piperacillin-tazobactam, ticarcillin-clavulanate, ampicillin-sulbactam), carbapenems (imipenem, meropenem, ertapenem), or second-generation cephalosporins with or without metronidazole depending on antimicrobial anaerobic coverage, are good initial antibiotic choices for the treatment of PLA. Modifications of the antibiotic regimen can be made after the speciation and sensitivities are obtained from blood cultures or abscess cavity aspirate cultures. Antimicrobial therapy is usually initiated parenterally for a duration of 2 to 3 weeks, with conversion to oral antibiotics to complete a 4- to 6-week course.[41] *K. pneumoniae* abscesses should be treated with third-generation cephalosporins, especially in the setting of meningitis or

endophthalmitis.[37] It is important to individualize the antimicrobial therapeutic regimen, with consideration given to such factors as the number of abscesses, likely underlying pathology, toxicity of the antibiotic regimen, and clinical response. In situations in which there are multiple PLAs that are very small and widespread in distribution, and therefore impossible to percutaneously drain, antimicrobial therapy may be the only treatment option available. In this instance, duration of therapy is likely to be longer and the mortality rate has been reported to be as high as 29%.[23]

DRAINAGE PROCEDURES

Percutaneous aspiration and/or catheter-based drainage along with antibiotic therapy are the mainstay of treatment for PLA. Morbidity from percutaneous aspiration and catheter-based drainage is very low, and the effectiveness in treating PLA is well established.[5,7,15,16,42] The vast majority of PLA can be treated with percutaneous procedures, either by aspiration or percutaneous catheter-based drain placement. Both treatment strategies are efficacious, so consideration of which technique to use depends on a multitude of factors, such as abscess size, location, number, and viscosity of abscess cavity contents. Previously, multiple abscesses were an indication to use surgical drainage; however, placement of multiple percutaneous drains or multiple aspirations has been shown to be quite effective.[42] It is important to consider underlying disorders, especially biliary obstruction, which has been associated with a high rate of failure for percutaneous drainage.[16] Underlying biliary obstruction requires treatment either by endoscopic, percutaneous, or surgical means in addition to abscess drainage for resolution of the PLA.

PERCUTANEOUS ASPIRATION AND PERCUTANEOUS CATHETER DRAINAGE

Percutaneous intervention has become the first-line treatment of PLA with diminished need for open surgical drainage. There has been some debate concerning whether catheter-based drain placement is superior to aspiration. Arguments for the advantages of needle aspiration include procedure simplicity, patient comfort, and price.[42] Yu et al. demonstrated that intermittent needle aspiration of PLA was equivalent to percutaneous catheter-based drainage. This study included 64 PLA patients over a period of 5 years treated with intravenous antibiotics and randomized to either percutaneous catheter drain placement or percutaneous needle aspiration. The percutaneous aspiration group trended toward a higher success rate, a shorter duration of hospital stay, and a lower mortality rate, although these findings did not reach statistical significance.[42] O'Farrell et al. reported that in 61 patients, 82% were successfully treated with percutaneous intervention for PLA, with 15% managed medically and 1 patient requiring operative intervention. In this series, there were no mortalities and the average hospital stay was 23 days.[15]

Particularly difficult patients are those with hepatobiliary malignancies, which have traditionally been associated with high failure rates for percutaneous drainage and high mortality rates in general. However, when the often-associated underlying biliary communication or obstruction is treated, percutaneous drainage becomes an effective and safe therapeutic option. Mezhir et al. reported that in 51 patients with a history of actively treated pancreatic cancer, cholangiocarcinoma, or colon or gallbladder cancer, 66% of the time percutaneous drainage was successful. In the 26% of the patients who died with their drainage catheters in place, more than 60% had cancer progression and had no clinical evidence of sepsis. In this series, 9% of the patients required operative intervention and 3% died postoperatively of sepsis.[16] Predictors of failure with percutaneous drainage included abscess culture isolates containing yeast and communication of the abscess cavity with the biliary tree.[16] Lai et al. reported on 44 patients with history of actively treated cholangiocarcinoma, hepatocellular carcinoma, pancreatic carcinoma, carcinoma of the ampulla of Vater, and gallbladder cancer; 66% of the time percutaneous drainage was successful. Of the 15 patients with failure of percutaneous drainage, 12 required surgical intervention and three died with drain in place prior to resolution of their abscess. Of the 12 who required surgical intervention, 7 had abscess drains in place, 3 died of uncontrolled sepsis, and 2 died of liver failure versus progression of malignancy. The authors identified that multiloculated abscesses and lesions with biliary communication were associated with failure on multivariate analysis.[43] Although percutaneous methods are safe and effective, attention must be paid to patients worsening clinically or failing to improve, in which case surgical drainage and/or hepatic resection may be the most effective option.

ENDOSCOPIC MANAGEMENT

Endoscopic ultrasound (EUS)-guided needle drainage accompanied in some cases by transgastric or transduodenal placement of a stent is an emerging technique for drainage of liver abscesses in the left and caudate lobes. There are several case reports and small series reporting successful cases of EUS-guided drainage via transgastric or transduodenal approach with placement of plastic or metal stents, or catheters.[8,44–46] Seewald et al. reported transgastric EUS-guided drainage using a modified Seldinger approach and nasoabscess Teflon catheter irrigation.[9]

Endoscopic management has also been used to manage liver abscesses with communication with the intrahepatic bile ducts. Sharma et al. reported on 38 patients with biliary fistulas who were treated with endoscopic sphincterotomy and 7-French nasobiliary drains or biliary stents. Closure of the fistula was confirmed with cessation of bile leakage and cholangiography. Stents were removed after 4 to 6 weeks. The median time to fistula closure was 6 days (range, 4 to 40 days) after endoscopic treatment.[47]

LAPAROSCOPIC MANAGEMENT OF PYOGENIC LIVER ABSCESSES AND ASSOCIATED PATHOLOGY

Laparoscopic PLA drainage is a viable option for patients requiring surgical therapy. Indications for laparoscopic drainage of PLA are similar to those for open drainage. Wang et al. define indications for laparoscopic drainage as follows: failure of medical management and percutaneous drainage, or contraindications to percutaneous drainage; septic shock on presentation requiring emergency

surgical intervention; a surgically accessible liver abscess with minimal risk of injury to major vessels and the biliary tree; no previous major surgery in the right upper quadrant; no concomitant conditions requiring additional surgery.[11]

Some authors use laparoscopic drainage in patients requiring other procedures. In a comparison of 31 patients undergoing laparoscopic (13 patients) and open (18 patients) operation for treatment of PLA with biliary pathology, Tu et al. report that there were no differences in operation time, intraoperative blood loss and transfusion, postoperative complication rate, and abscess recurrence rate. Coexisting biliary pathology in these patients included cholelithiasis with acute cholecystitis, choledocholithiasis with cholangitis, hepatolithiasis, and intrahepatic biliary stricture, and these pathologies were well distributed between the two groups. There was shorter time to oral intake and length of postoperative hospital stay in the laparoscopic group ($P < .05$).[12]

In a literature review identifying 51 PLAs and 2 ALAs treated with laparoscopy, there was a 90.5% mean success rate and 0% conversion to an open procedure.[13] Tay et al. reported on 20 liver abscesses drained laparoscopically and concluded that the procedure is a safe alternative to open surgery in patients who have failed medical and/or percutaneous treatment.[14]

Purported advantages of laparoscopic hepatic abscess drainage are those attributed to laparoscopic surgery for other indications as well, including shorter length of hospital stay, faster recovery, reduced immunosuppression, and better cosmesis. Operative time and time to oral intake have been reported to be shorter in patients with laparoscopically drained PLA.[11,12]

Barriers to the use of laparoscopic approaches to liver abscess treatment include lack of tactile sensation in palpating the abscess and in breaking down septations and perihepatic adhesions, although this can be partially resolved with the use of intraoperative laparoscopic sonography to aid in localization of the abscesses.[11] The possibility of air embolism if there were injury to the hepatic vein is also a concern.

Additional novel procedures have been reported in the literature. Klink et al. report video-assisted hepatic abscess drainage was performed in 10 patients between 2010 and 2014 at two institutions. Patients were selected on the basis of at least one previous failed percutaneous drainage. This procedure involved preoperative placement of a CT-guided percutaneous drain as posterior as possible on the flank. The patient is then placed under general anesthesia, and a spindle-shaped incision is made at the drain site. Video-assisted retroperitoneal débridement of the liver abscess is then performed using a 10-mm 0 degree scope, and purulent material is aspirated from the abscess cavity using a laparoscopic suction device.[48]

SURGICAL DRAINAGE AND HEPATIC RESECTION

The role of surgical therapy for the treatment of PLA has changed dramatically since the early part of the 20th century. In Ochsner's original series,[4] surgery was the primary treatment modality; however, currently, open operation is primarily indicated for failure of medical management, failure of percutaneous drainage, and complications secondary to percutaneous treatments, such as bleeding or spillage of pus into the peritoneal cavity. Primary surgical treatment may be required to treat abdominal pathology responsible for the PLA, such as diverticulitis, appendicitis, and PLA rupture into the peritoneal cavity with subsequent peritonitis or an obstructed biliary tree, which cannot be treated by endoscopic or interventional means.

Traditionally the open surgical approach to hepatic abscess is through a midline laparotomy or an extended subcostal incision. Exploration of the abdomen with control of any associated intraabdominal pathology is then performed. Localization of all hepatic abscesses with palpation of the liver and intraoperative ultrasound is performed next. At this point, it is often useful to perform needle aspiration to confirm location of the abscess and obtain material for culture and Gram stain. The area of the liver containing the abscess is then isolated from the rest of the abdomen with laparotomy sponges. The abscess cavity is then entered with electrocautery in an area that will allow it to drain in a dependent fashion. A suction catheter is then inserted into the abscess cavity to evacuate the pus and gently break up any loculations. Biopsies of the abscess wall should be obtained at this time to rule out a neoplasm as the etiology for the PLA. Drainage catheters are then placed into the abscess cavity in as dependent a position as possible to ensure adequate drainage. These catheters are brought through the abdominal wall with separate incisions. These drains can be used for drainage, irrigation, or radiologic contrast studies to ensure collapse of the abscess cavity. Omentum may also be placed in the abscess cavity as an adjunct to drain placement.

There are circumstances in which single or multiple PLA is associated with severe hepatic destruction, and in these instances partial hepatectomy may be the best therapeutic option. Chou et al. have advocated hepatic resection in these circumstances and have reported a low mortality rate in patients undergoing partial hepatectomy.[23] Likely outcomes in these particular cases are largely dependent on the underlying cause of the PLA and the general condition of the patient. Patients with underlying malignancies who require hepatectomy for liver destruction secondary to PLA generally have poor outcomes.

OUTCOMES

Mortality rates vary from series to series and typically range in North American and European series from 5% to 10% and worldwide from 3% to 30%. The difference is likely reflective of differences in patient populations and underlying disease processes responsible for PLA. When considering the change in demographics from a younger to an older patient and the change in etiology to a patient with actively treated malignancy or biliary tract disease, it is not surprising that a population-based study noted increased incidence of PLA without a decrease in mortality from 1994 to 2005.[1] In this study, mortality was increased in older adult patients and those with multiple medical comorbidities, including cirrhosis, renal failure, sepsis, and malignancy. Interestingly, patients who were culture positive for bacteria had a negative association with mortality, suggesting the importance of early culture

and speciation in guiding antimicrobial therapy. Patients who underwent percutaneous aspiration or drainage for PLA had half the mortality of patients who did not undergo drainage. In this study, surgical drainage was not associated negatively or positively with mortality.[1]

In an epidemiologic study conducted using the United States Nationwide Inpatient Sample database for years 1994 to 2005, diabetes in patients with PLA was shown to be negatively associated with death with an OR of 0.78 (95% CI, 0.65 to 0.93),[1] although other studies have failed to show positive or negative association with death.[2,49] The authors speculate that the negative association with death may relate to clinicians' inclination to treat diabetic patients earlier with broad-spectrum antibiotics on an empiric basis.[1] Patients with cirrhosis and PLA have a fourfold increased risk of death after adjustment for age, gender, and comorbidity in comparison with other patients with PLA.[2]

PYOGENIC LIVER ABSCESS AND CANCER RISK

In two population-based studies conducted using Taiwan's National Health Insurance Research Database, the incidence of GI cancers was found to be significantly higher in patients with PLA. The first study identified 1257 patients with PLA without prior cancers and followed them for the appearance of cancer. They determined that PLA patients were at increased risk for liver cancer, biliary tract cancer and colorectal cancer and that this risk was highest in the 90 days of follow-up after PLA. The authors concluded that PLA may herald hepatobiliary or colorectal cancer and that such patients should undergo enhanced screening to increase early detection of these cancers.[50] The second of these examined 14,690 patients with PLA in comparison with 58,760 controls over a 7-year period. They determined that the incidence of GI cancer was 4.3 times higher in patients with PLA compared with controls and that patients with PLA had highest incidence of colorectal cancer, followed by cancers of the biliary tract, pancreas and small intestine.[51]

AMEBIC LIVER ABSCESSES

Amebiasis is a parasitic infection caused by *E. histolytica*, the third leading parasitic cause of death worldwide, affecting approximately 50 million people and resulting in approximately 100,000 deaths per year. In some countries *E. histolytica* antibody prevalence rate exceeds 50%; in the United States the seroprevalence is estimated at only 4%. The majority of those who are infected (90%) remain relatively asymptomatic. The liver is the most common site of extraintestinal amebiasis. The incidence of hepatic abscess in amebiasis is 3% to 9%. The long-touted concept that 10% of the world's population is infected with *E. histolytica* is now thought to be incorrect. Another species, *Entamoeba dispar*, is morphologically indistinguishable from *E. histolytica* and more common in humans in many parts of the world. Similarly *Entamoeba moshkovskii*, which was long considered to be a free-living ameba, is also morphologically identical to *E. histolytica* and *E. dispar* and is highly prevalent in some *E. histolytica*–endemic countries. However, the only species to cause invasive amebiasis and clinical disease in humans is

E. histolytica. Many older epidemiologic data on *E. histolytica* are unusable because the techniques used do not differentiate between these three *Entamoeba* species. Molecular tools are now available not only to diagnose these species accurately but also to study intraspecies genetic diversity.[52]

DEMOGRAPHICS

The highest prevalence of amebiasis is found in developing countries, particularly in Mexico, India, Central and South America, and tropical areas of Asia and Africa. The incidence is increased in areas with high poverty and is a reflection of poor sanitation and hygiene. Risk factors for infection include travel or residence in endemic areas. In industrialized countries, risk groups include male homosexuals, travelers and recent immigrants, and institutionalized populations. There is a 7 to 12 times higher incidence in males than females despite an equal gender distribution of noninvasive colonic amebic disease among adults. Possible reasons include heavy alcohol consumption in men, hormonal effects in premenopausal women, and a possible protective effect of iron-deficiency anemia in menstruating women. Individuals in their fourth and fifth decades of life are most commonly affected. The prevalence of infection is higher than 5% to 10% in endemic areas. In a 4-year observational study of 289 preschool children in an urban slum in Bangladesh *E. histolytica* infection was detected at least once in 80%, and repeat infection in 53%, after 4 years of observation.[53]

The impact of the acquired immunodeficiency syndrome (AIDS) pandemic on the prevalence of invasive amebiasis remains controversial. Although the incidence of invasive amebiasis in human immunodeficiency virus (HIV) is rare, reports suggest that ALA is an emerging parasitic infection in individuals with HIV infection in disease-endemic areas.[54] Despite immunosuppression, ALAs and colitis responded favorably to medical treatment.[55]

ETIOLOGY AND PATHOGENESIS

Infection by *E. histolytica* occurs by ingestion of mature quadrinucleate cysts in fecally contaminated food, water, or hands (Fig. 122.5). The cysts are resistant to the acidic pH of the stomach. Excystation occurs in the alkaline pH of the small intestine and trophozoites are released, which migrate to the large intestine. The trophozoites multiply by binary fission and produce cysts (Fig. 122.6). Both stages are passed in the feces, and the cysts can survive days to weeks in the external environment. However, trophozoites passed in the stool are rapidly destroyed after being outside the body, and if ingested would not survive exposure to the gastric environment. In many cases the trophozoites remain confined to the intestinal lumen of individuals who are asymptomatic carriers, passing cysts in their stool. Depending on the genetic and immunoenzymatic profile, and the parasite's ability to produce proteolytic enzymes and resist complement-mediated lysis, the trophozoite becomes virulent and starts its invasion of the intestinal mucosa. Spread is usually through the portal venous radicles to the liver. The hepatic lesion is usually solitary and most frequently located in the right lobe. In some cases, it may occupy more than 80% of the whole liver surface. This may be explained by the larger volume of the right lobe, which receives most of the venous drainage from the right colon, a segment of the bowel frequently affected by intestinal amebiasis. Lesions of the left lobe are less common, and multiple abscesses may occasionally occur in advanced cases.

Amebic-induced lysis of neutrophils at the edge of the lesion releases cytotoxic mediators leading to hepatocyte death, extending the damage to distant hepatic cells and thereby increasing the number of small lesions that coalesce to develop a larger ALA. The content of its central cavity is a thick, viscous exudate. This is generally homogeneous and varies in color, ranging from creamy white to dirty brown and pink. This classic sign is often described as "anchovy paste" (Fig. 122.7). This material is almost always sterile, except when a secondary infection has occurred, allowing differential diagnosis from a pyogenic abscess. The amebae can be found at the edge of the lesion but are rarely detected in the pus or within the abscess cavity itself.

IMMUNOPATHOLOGY

During the establishment of infection, *E. histolytica* confronts a series of innate host defenses, such as the intestinal epithelial barrier, leukocytes, and the complement system.[56] Although the host cells elaborate diverse mechanisms of defense, amebae have also developed complex strategies to evade host defenses and facilitate their own survival.[57]

The early stage of the ALA lesion is characterized by a dominant infiltration of polymorphonuclear leukocytes surrounding the trophozoites. In later stages, usually occurring after 3 days, lymphocytes, macrophages, and epithelioid cells are recruited to the developing lesion, which leads to the formation of a granuloma. This process contributes to the confinement of invading trophozoites.

CLINICAL PRESENTATION

Most patients with amebiasis are asymptomatic and clear their infection without any sign of disease. Clinical amebiasis usually has a subacute presentation, which occurs over 1 to 3 weeks. Symptoms can range from mild diarrhea to severe dysentery with abdominal pain. High-grade fever and right upper quadrant abdominal pain are the main presenting symptoms in ALA, and a history of gastroenteritis is often noted. Pleuritic and right scapular pain are present if the diaphragmatic surface of the liver is involved with or is close to the abscess. It is important to distinguish ALA from PLA because their treatment and prognosis differ. In a retrospective review of 577 adults with liver abscesses, 82% of whom had amebic abscesses, patients with amebic abscess were more likely to be young males with a tender, solitary, right-lobe abscess.[58] This is frequently accompanied by a history of diarrhea and abdominal pain/tenderness, and amebic serology titers greater than 1:256 IU.[58]

Jaundice is relatively uncommon in ALA and if present is a marker of abscess erosion into the biliary tract, although varying incidence has been reported. The most commonly accepted pathogenic mechanism is obstruction of the biliary system by the abscess. Multiple, large abscesses, especially on the inferior surface of the liver, have also been directly linked to elevation of serum

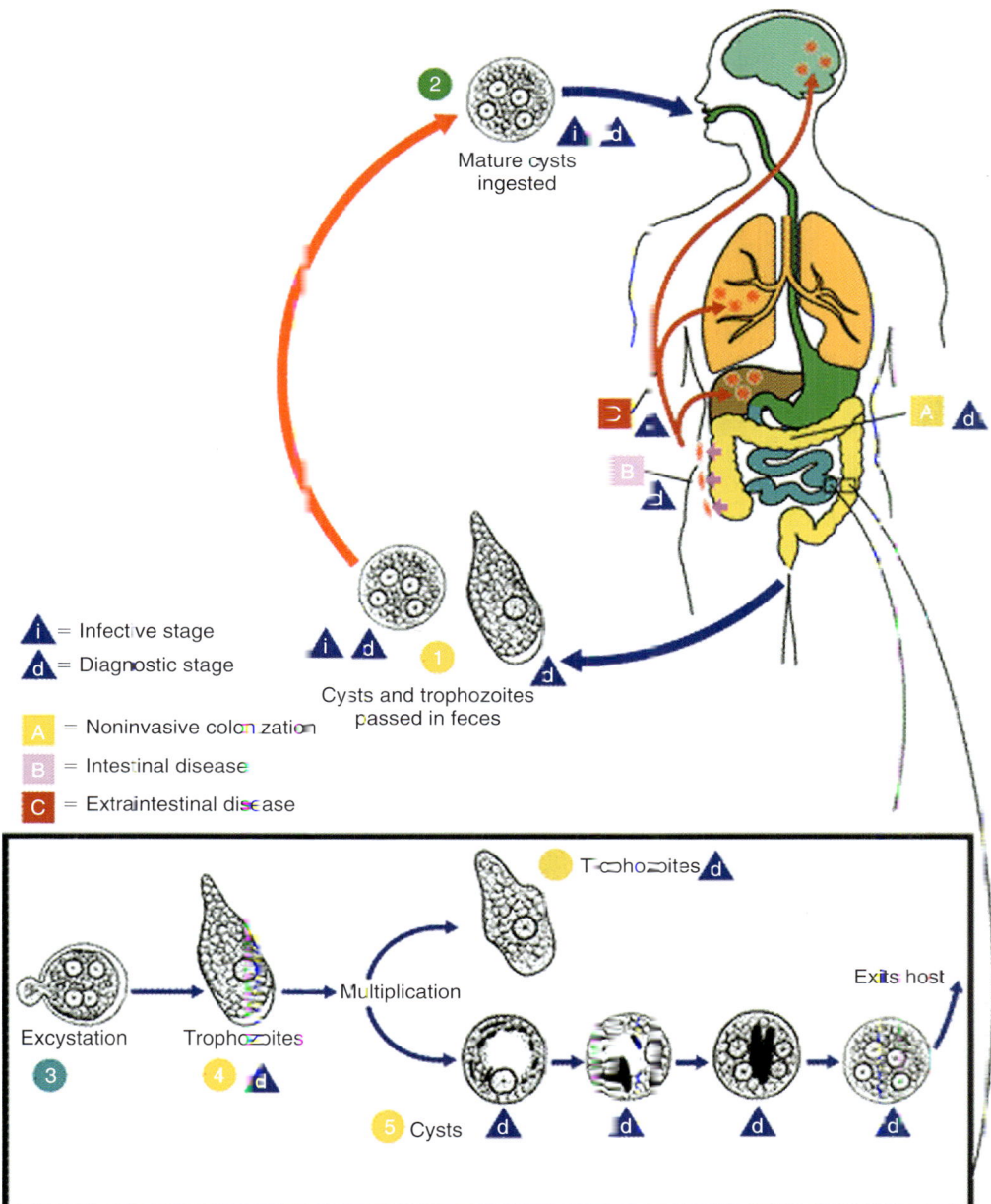

FIGURE 122.5 Life cycle of *Entamoeba histolytica*. (From US Centers for Disease Control and Prevention. http://www.dpd.cdc.gov/dpdx/HTML/Amebiasis.htm.)

bilirubin levels. The prolonged duration and poor response to drug therapy allow the abscess to enlarge; compress biliary radicles, producing jaundice; and finally penetrate the tough fibrous vasculobiliary sheath that surrounds the portal triad structures, with resultant biliary communication.

LABORATORY FINDINGS

Light microscopic examination of fecal specimens is often the first step in diagnosis.[59] In the stages of dysentery/amebic colitis, trophozoites are readily detected in submucosal tissue or fecal samples by permanent stains. Submission of three stool specimens on different days over a period of 10 days is recommended. Because *E.*

histolytica invades the colonic mucosa, feces are almost universally positive for occult blood. The presence of Charcot-Leyden crystals and blood is the most common finding in the acute stage. In addition to the red blood cells, macrophages and polymorphonuclear cells can also be seen on microscopy in cases of amebic dysentery. Microscopy alone cannot differentiate *E. histolytica* from *E. dispar* and *E. moshkovskii*, and additional tests are required for definitive speciation. Identification methods include biopsy, serology, antigen detection, and molecular assays.

Diagnosis of liver abscess is confirmed by a positive serologic test because amebic serology is highly sensitive (>94%) and highly specific (>95%). A false-negative

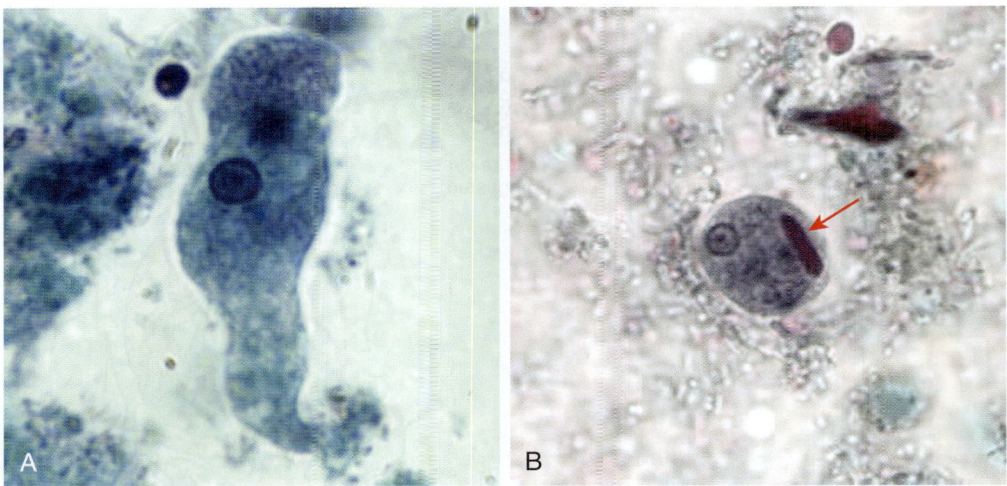

FIGURE 122.6 (A) *Entamoeba histolytica/Entamoeba dispar* trophozoites have a single nucleus, which has a centrally placed karyosome and uniformly distributed peripheral chromatin. (B) Mature *E. histolytica/E. dispar* cysts have four nuclei that characteristically have centrally located karyosomes and fine, uniformly distributed peripheral chromatin. Cysts usually measure 12 to 15 μm. The *red arrow* signifies a chromatid body with blunt ends. (From US Center for Disease Control and Prevention. http://www.dpd.cdc.gov/dpdx/HTML/ImageLibrary/Amebiasis_il.htm.)

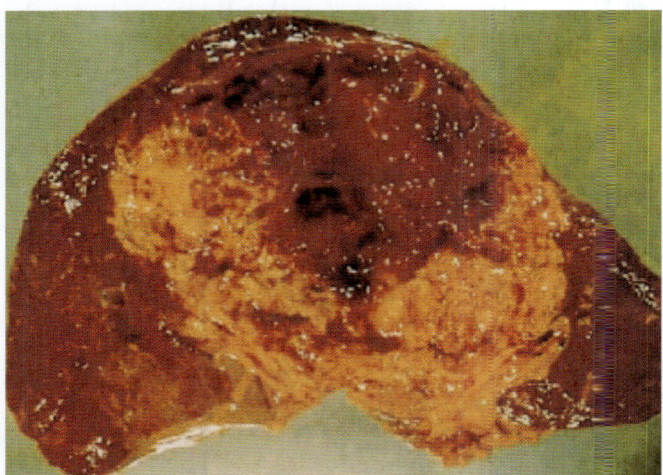

FIGURE 122.7 Amebic abscess. Photograph of a gross liver specimen shows an amebic abscess filled with a chocolate-colored, pasty material (anchovy paste). (From Mortele KJ, Segatto E, Ros PR. The infected liver: radiologic-pathologic correlation. *Radiographics*. 2004;24:937.)

serologic test can be obtained early during infection (within the first 7 to 10 days), but a repeat test is usually positive. Many different assays have been developed for the detection of antibodies, including indirect hemagglutination assay (IHA), latex agglutination, immunoelectrophoresis, counterimmunoelectrophoresis (CIE), the amebic gel diffusion test, immunodiffusion, complement fixation, indirect immunofluorescence assay (IFA), and enzyme-linked immunosorbent assay (ELISA). Of these, ELISA is the most popular assay throughout the world and has been used to study the epidemiology of asymptomatic disease. Serum immunoglobulin G (IgG) antibodies persist for years after *E. histolytica* infection.

In nonendemic areas, a positive amebic serology almost always reflects acute infection and, in the setting of hepatic abscess, is essentially diagnostic of an amebic etiology. However, in regions where amebiasis is very prevalent, positive serology does not carry the same diagnostic yield. Serologic IHA titers usually become negative within 1 year of acute infection but may remain elevated for 5 to 6 years after cure in some patients. Serologic titers less than 1:256 IU were predictive of pyogenic abscess in both univariate and multivariate analyses.[58] Although there was no difference between the white blood cell count in patients with amebic or pyogenic abscesses, hypoalbuminemia was more severe in those with bacterial abscess. Lodhi et al. found serum liver enzymes to be of no value in distinguishing between amebic and pyogenic abscess, although bacterial abscesses may be more frequently associated with greater elevations of serum alanine transferase and alkaline phosphatase.[58]

Polymerase chain reaction (PCR)-based approaches are the method of choice for clinical and epidemiologic studies in the developed countries and are endorsed by the World Health Organization (WHO).[59] *E. histolytica* can be identified in a variety of clinical specimens, including feces, tissues, and liver abscess aspirate. They offer the highest sensitivity and specificity and can also differentiate between the various *Entamoeba* species.

IMAGING

Chest radiographic examination is abnormal in 50% of cases showing elevated right hemidiaphragm, subdiaphragmatic air-fluid levels, pleural effusions, and consolidating infiltrates. US reveals hypoechoic and well-defined lesions with rounded edges and has a diagnostic accuracy of 90%.[60] CT is more sensitive in detecting hepatic abscesses and contiguous organ extension and is the imaging study of choice (Fig. 122.8). CT and MRI also allow for better detection of smaller lesions. All three techniques may facilitate guided needle biopsy and drainage if indicated.

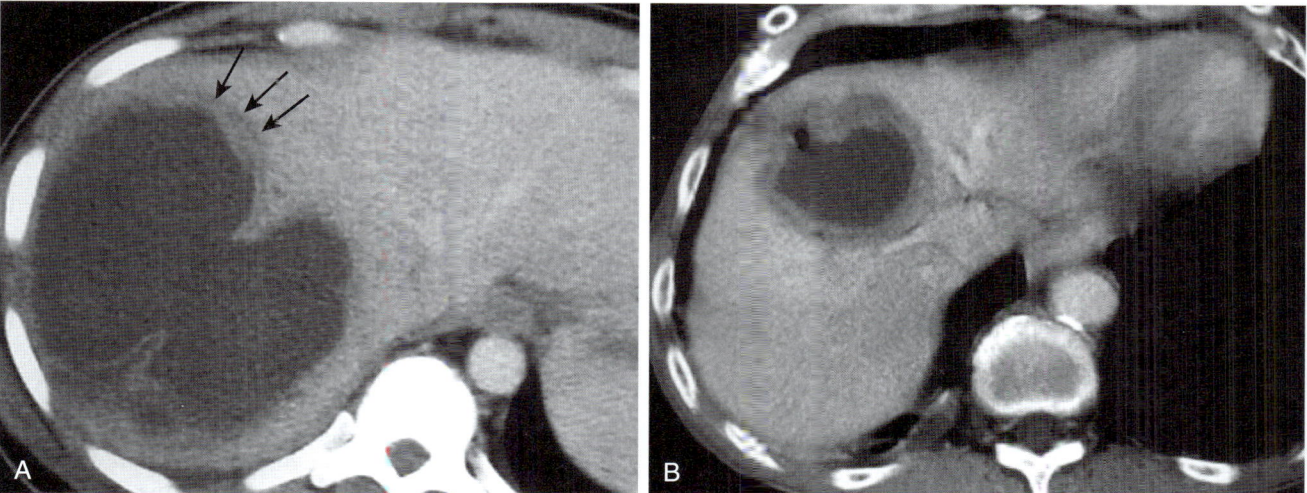

FIGURE 122.8 Amebic abscess. (A) Contrast-enhanced computed tomography scan demonstrates a large, lobulated, well-defined cystic mass in the right hepatic lobe. Note the enhanced, thickened wall of the lesion (*arrows*). (B) Contrast-enhanced computed tomography scan obtained in a different patient shows a rounded, well-defined low-attenuation lesion in the right hepatic lobe with a small focus of air and mild hyperemia of the adjacent liver parenchyma. (From Mortele KJ, Segatto E, Ros PR. The infected liver: radiologic-pathologic correlation. *Radiographics.* 2004;24:937.)

An abscess can usually be distinguished from solid lesions and biliary tract disease, but the differentiation between bacterial and amebic abscesses is less clear. Imaging studies cannot always distinguish between liver abscess and other hepatic lesions and in this case aspiration of purulent drainage with subsequent culture can confirm the diagnosis.

The average time to radiologic resolution is 3 to 9 months and can take years in some patients. Studies have shown that more than 90% of the visible lesions demonstrate disappearance on imaging, but a small percentage of patients are left with a clinically irrelevant residual lesion.[61]

SITES OF AMEBIC ABSCESSES

The liver is the most common site of extraintestinal amebiasis. *E. histolytica* also has been reported to cause brain abscesses from hematogenous spread. Cerebral amebiasis has an abrupt onset and rapid progression to death in 12 to 72 hours. Presentation is with altered consciousness and focal neurologic signs. CT scanning reveals irregular lesions without a surrounding capsule or enhancement. A tissue biopsy sample reveals the trophozoites. Amebomas are localized masses of infected granulation tissue in the intestine whose appearance can mimic colon cancers, and these masses can extend to involve the perianal skin. Cases of ameboma causing GI bleeding, and rectovaginal fistula have been reported. Rare presentation of amebiasis as acute appendicitis has also been reported.

AMEBIC LIVER ABSCESS IN CHILDREN

Pyogenic abscesses constitute the majority of hepatic abscesses in children. Studies suggest that amebic abscesses are rare in children. The treatment of ALA in children is by amebicides. Metronidazole is currently the amebicide of choice. All uncomplicated ALAs can be managed

medically and do not require aspiration. Rupture of an ALA is relatively rare in children. Surgical drainage is necessary when the abscess has ruptured. Porras-Ramirez et al. conducted a study that determined criteria for percutaneous aspiration, which included the following: no clinical improvement, the abscess is 6 cm or more in diameter, and the patient is septic, or there is imminent risk of rupture.[62] In regard to both pyogenic and ALAs in children, Sharma et al. suggest percutaneous drainage when (1) volume of abscess is large and there is risk of spontaneous rupture, (2) when actual rupture has occurred and in this case the abscess and any extraneous collection are drained, (3) when there is a lack of response to medical therapy, and (4) when there is evidence of liver failure. In addition, they suggest surgical drainage for (1) children who have failed percutaneous drainage, (2) those who require management for an underlying abdominal problem, (3) selected patients with multiple macroscopic abscesses, (4) those on steroids, and (5) patients with ascites.

TREATMENT

The mainstays of treatment for uncomplicated amebic hepatic abscesses are amebicidal drugs (Table 122.5). The discovery of systemic amebicides, mainly in the nitroimidazole group with high tissue diffusion and enhanced capability to cross the wall and reach the interior of the abscess at a very high concentration (four times the minimum inhibitory concentration [MIC] for *E. histolytica*) has been responsible for a dramatic change in the treatment of invasive amebiasis, reducing complications and therefore mortality. The drugs of choice for amebic colitis and ALAs include nitroimidazole derivatives (metronidazole, tinidazole, and ornidazole), of which only metronidazole is available in the United States. It is given in doses of 750 mg three times a day by mouth or intravenously for 5 to 10 days. It is activated in anaerobic organisms by

TABLE 122.5 Treatment of Amebic Liver Abscess

Drug treatment	Uncomplicated amebic hepatic abscess
	Both amebic colitis and liver abscess— nitroimidazole derivatives (e.g., metronidazole)
	Amebic colitis—luminal agents such as paromomycin, diloxanide furoate, iodoquinol
Percutaneous drainage	Deterioration in clinical condition despite adequate treatment
	Bacterial superinfection
	Abscess with high risk of rupture
Surgery	Ruptured abscess
	Impending rupture
	Inadequate catheter drainage

reduction, and when activated damages DNA. The main side effects include metallic aftertaste, nausea, vomiting, and diarrhea. Dehydroemetine is an additional drug that inhibits protein synthesis and is mainly used in fulminant colitis or patients with ruptured ALA when administered in combination with metronidazole, but controlled trials are lacking. The drugs for amebic colitis include luminal agents, such as paromomycin, which is the drug of choice; diloxanide furoate; and iodoquinol. The conventional indications for percutaneous drainage include deterioration in clinical condition on adequate treatment, bacterial superinfection, and an abscess having a high risk of rupture, whereas surgery is reserved for patients with ruptured abscess, impending rupture, or inadequate drainage through a catheter.

In a retrospective analysis of 966 patients, 68% of whom had ALAs, the predictive factors for a patient requiring aspiration of their liver abscess included age 55 years or older, size 5 cm or more, involvement of both lobes of the liver, and duration of symptoms of at least 7 days. Hospital stay in the aspiration group was longer than that in the nonaspiration group, and no statistically significant difference in mortality was observed between the two groups.[64]

A meta-analysis of seven low-quality randomized trials was performed.[65] Pooled analysis of three homogeneous trials showed that needle aspiration did not significantly increase the proportion of patients with fever resolution. Reduction in the number of days to resolution of pain, number of days to resolution of abdominal tenderness, and duration of hospitalization were observed in the needle aspiration group only. However, the value of therapeutic aspiration in addition to metronidazole to hasten clinical or radiologic resolution of uncomplicated ALAs could not be supported or refuted by the current evidence. A prospective study of 200 patients with confirmed ALA comparing ultrasound-guided needle aspiration and medications to drug treatment alone showed the initial response (after 15 days) being better in the aspirated group, but resolution of abscess after 6 months was similar. This rapid clinical response was particularly noted in those with larger (>6 cm) abscesses, and there were no complications.[66]

One of the reasons for nonresolution of amebic abscesses seems to be the presence of communication with the biliary tree. In a study of 13 patients who underwent catheter drainage of ALA with persistent drainage after the procedure probably due to abscess-biliary communication, therapeutic endoscopic retrograde cholangiopancreatography was done with sphincterotomy followed by placement of either a pigtail biliary stent or a nasobiliary drain. The procedure resulted in decreased drainage in 48 hours, and in 11 of 13 patients the drainage catheter was removed by 1 week and after 10 days in the remaining two patients. Clinical improvement and significant decrease was noted in the volume of the abscess cavity, and no recurrence of abscess was noted after 9 to 25 months of follow-up.[67]

Patients with abscesses communicating with the biliary tree presented more frequently with jaundice (67% vs. 0%; $P < .005$), with a longer duration of illness (median, 20 vs. 12 days; $P < .001$), had larger lesions, and required catheter drainage for longer periods (median, 17 vs. 6.5 days; $P < .001$).[68]

COMPLICATIONS

The failure of medical therapy for ALA may be heralded by abscess perforation, a complication associated with high mortality. Rupture into the thorax or abdomen are the most common. Factors used to predict rupture include diameter 5 to 10 cm, progressive increase in size, and left lobe location. Rupture into the peritoneal cavity occurs in 18% to 70% of cases. Amebic pericarditis accounts for 4% of all extraintestinal amebiasis, with a mortality rate of approximately 30%. Other rare complications of ALA include hepatic vein and inferior vena cava thrombosis. Bacterial superinfection, anemia, acute respiratory distress syndrome (ARDS), and sepsis also can develop in severe cases.

OUTCOMES

The mortality rate for all patients with ALA is approximately 5% and does not appear to be affected by the addition of aspiration to metronidazole therapy or chronicity of symptoms. For ruptured abscess, the mortality rate is reported to be from 6% to as high as 50%. Factors independently associated with poor outcome are elevated serum bilirubin (>3.5 mg/dL), encephalopathy, hypoalbuminemia (<2.0 g/dL), multiple abscess cavities, abscess volume greater than 500 mL, anemia, and diabetes.[69] Follow-up imaging should be used to monitor response to therapy; continue treatment until CT scan shows complete or near-complete resolution of cavity. Using PCR-based method of genotyping, Ali et al. found that parasite genome might play a role in determining the outcome of infection with *E. histolytica*.[70]

In summary, amebiasis is a disease of high prevalence and morbidity in developing countries. In industrialized nations, risk groups include male homosexuals, travelers and recent immigrants, and institutionalized populations. ALA is the commonest manifestation of extraintestinal amebiasis. Presentation of ALA varies from PLA in that patients with ALA are more likely to be young males with tender, solitary right-lobe abscess. Presence of jaundice is more common in PLA and if present in ALA is indicative of biliary tract obstruction or abscess erosion into the

TABLE 122.6 Selected Signs and Symptoms in Series Comparing Pyogenic and Amebic Hepatic Abscesses*

	CONTER ET AL.[73] (UNIVERSITY OF CALIFORNIA, LOS ANGELES): DATA PERIOD 1968–1983		BARNES ET AL.[74] (UNIVERSITY OF SOUTHERN CALIFORNIA, LOS ANGELES): DATA PERIOD 1979–1985		LODHI ET AL.[58] (KARACHI, PAKISTAN): DATA PERIOD 1988–1998	
	Pyogenic Abscess	Amebic Abscess	Pyogenic Abscess	Amebic Abscess	Pyogenic Abscess	Amebic Abscess
STUDY DESCRIPTORS						
No. of cases	42	40	48	96	106	471
Age (years, mean)	46.5	37.6	—	28	51	40
Male-to-female ratio	2.5:1.0	3.4:1.0	1.4:1.0	18.2:1.0	2.9:1.0	6.1:1.0
SYMPTOMS						
Fever (%)	88	93	—	87	43	67
Abdominal pain (%)	64	93	65	90 (P < .001)	N/A	N/A
Diarrhea (%)	12	60 (P < .005)	25	35	22	30
Symptom duration (%)	N/A	N/A	63, <14 days	86, <14 days	N/A	N/A
—	—	—	37, >14 days	14, >14 days	—	—
Nausea/vomiting (%)	31	50	62/43	85/32	N/A	N/A
SIGNS						
Abdominal tenderness (%)	50	75	48	67	77	87
Jaundice (%)	36	5	25	10	43	32
Shock/sepsis (%)	26	0	N/A	N/A	N/A	N/A
Hepatomegaly (%)	26	53	18	25	67	74

*Listed P value indicates significant difference between pyogenic and amebic abscesses in that specific study.
N/A, Not available.

TABLE 122.7 Selected Laboratory Parameters in Series Comparing Pyogenic and Amebic Hepatic Abscesses*

Laboratory Parameter	CONTER ET AL.[73] (UNIVERSITY OF CALIFORNIA, LOS ANGELES): DATA PERIOD 1968–1983		BARNES ET AL.[74] (UNIVERSITY OF SOUTHERN CALIFORNIA, LOS ANGELES): DATA PERIOD 1979–1985		LODHI ET AL.[58] (KARACHI, PAKISTAN): DATA PERIOD 1988–1998	
	Pyogenic Abscess	Amebic Abscess	Pyogenic Abscess	Amebic Abscess	Pyogenic Abscess	Amebic Abscess
Amebic serology (% positive)	0	95	4	94	33	72
Mean alkaline phosphatase or % with elevation	319 IU	198 IU	52%, >220 U/L	35%, >220 U/L	236 U	211 IU
Mean total bilirubin or % elevated	4.1 mg/dL	0.9 mg/dL	13%	2% (P < .005)	2.4 mg/dL	1.9 mg/dL
Albumin level or % with hypoalbuminemia	2.7 g/dL	2.9 g/dL	51%	16%	2.1 g/dL	2.4 g/dL
WBC × 10³/mm³ or % elevation > 10³/mm³	13.4	13.5	9%	92%	18.9	19.1

*Listed P value indicates difference between pyogenic and amebic hepatic abscesses.
WBC, White blood cell.

biliary tract. Patients are also more likely to have a history of fever, right upper quadrant abdominal pain, and diarrhea. Tender hepatomegaly is twice as common in ALA compared with PLA, and amebic serology titers greater than 1:256 IU are diagnostic (Tables 122.6 and 122.7). Amebic serology is highly sensitive and specific as a diagnostic tool. Ultrasonographic and CT scans have good diagnostic accuracy and also facilitate needle biopsy and drainage if needed. PCR-based studies can also differentiate between various *Entamoeba* species. Most patients with uncomplicated ALA can be treated with medical management alone. Drainage procedures for amebic abscess should be reserved for those patients who do not respond to medical therapy, whose abscess appears to have a high likelihood of rupture, or those whose diagnosis is in question. Surgical procedures are used for patients who fail these management approaches or experience complications of the abscess, such as peritoneal rupture or empyema. Prevention efforts would include improvement of sanitation and hygiene and use of safe sexual practices. Vaccination strategies especially with recombinant antigens are being studied as well.

ACKNOWLEDGMENTS

We would like to acknowledge former authors of this chapter, Sangeetha Prabhakaran and Selwyn M. Vickers.

REFERENCES

1. Meddings L, Myers RP, Hubbard J, et al. A population-based study of pyogenic liver abscesses in the United States: incidence, mortality, and temporal trends. *Am J Gastroenterol.* 2010;105(1):117-124.
2. Thomsen RW, Jepsen P, Sørensen HT. Diabetes mellitus and pyogenic liver abscess: risk and prognosis. *Clin Infect Dis.* 2007;44(9):1194-1201.
3. Jepsen P, Vilstrup H, Schønheyder HC, Sørensen HT. A nationwide study of the incidence and 30-day mortality rate of pyogenic liver abscess in Denmark, 1977–2002. *Aliment Pharmacol Ther.* 2005; 21(10):1185-1188.
4. Ochsner A, DeBakey M, Murray S. Pyogenic abscess of the liver: II. An analysis of forty-seven cases with review of the literature. *Am J Surg.* 1938;40:292-319.
5. Mcfadzean AJ, Chang KP, Wong CC. Solitary pyogenic abscess of the liver treated by closed aspiration and antibiotics: a report of 14 consecutive cases with recovery. *Br J Surg.* 1953;41(166):141-152.
6. Bertel CK, van Heerden JA, Sheedy PF. Treatment of pyogenic hepatic abscesses. Surgical vs percutaneous drainage. *Arch Surg.* 1986;121(5):554-558.
7. Branum GD, Tyson GS, Branum MA, Meyers WC. Hepatic abscess. Changes in etiology, diagnosis, and management. *Ann Surg.* 1990; 212(6):655-662.
8. Noh SH, Park DH, Kim YR, et al. EUS-guided drainage of hepatic abscesses not accessible to percutaneous drainage (with videos). *Gastrointest Endosc.* 2010;71(7):1314-1319.
9. Seewald S, Imazu H, Omar S, et al. EUS-guided drainage of hepatic abscess. *Gastrointest Endosc.* 2005;61(3):495-498.
10. Sharma BC, Garg V, Reddy R. Endoscopic management of liver abscess with biliary communication. *Dig Dis Sci.* 2012;57(2):524-527.
11. Wang W, Lee WJ, Wei PL, Chen TC, Huang MT. Laparoscopic drainage of pyogenic liver abscesses. *Surg Today.* 2004;34(4):323-325.
12. Tu JF, Huang XF, Hu RY, You HY, Zheng XF, Jiang FZ. Comparison of laparoscopic and open surgery for pyogenic liver abscess with biliary pathology. *World J Gastroenterol.* 2011;17(38):4339-4343.
13. Aydin C, Piskin T, Sumer F, Barut B, Kayaalp C. Laparoscopic drainage of pyogenic liver abscess. *JSLS.* 2010;14(3):418-420.
14. Tay KH, Ravintharan T, Hoe MN, See AC, Chng HC. Laparoscopic drainage of liver abscesses. *Br J Surg.* 1998;85(3):330-332.
15. O'Farrell N, Collins CG, McEntee GP. Pyogenic liver abscesses: diminished role for operative treatment. *Surgeon.* 2010;8(4):192-196.
16. Mezhir JJ, Fong Y, Jacks LM, et al. Current management of pyogenic liver abscess: surgery is now second-line treatment. *J Am Coll Surg.* 2010;210(6):975-983.
17. Tsai FC, Huang YT, Chang LY, Wang JT. Pyogenic liver abscess as endemic disease, Taiwan. *Emerg Infect Dis.* 2008;14(10):1592-1600.
18. Chen YC, Lin CH, Chang SN, Shi ZY. Epidemiology and clinical outcome of pyogenic liver abscess: an analysis from the National Health Insurance Research Database of Taiwan, 2000–2011. *J Microbiol Immunol Infect.* 2016;49(5):646-653.
19. Kaplan GG, Gregson DB, Laupland KB. Population-based study of the epidemiology of and the risk factors for pyogenic liver abscess. *Clin Gastroenterol Hepatol.* 2004;2(11):1032-1038.
20. Thomsen RW, Hundborg HH, Lervang HH, Schønheyder HC, Sørensen HT. Diabetes mellitus as a risk and prognostic factor for community-acquired bacteremia due to enterobacteria: a 10-year, population-based study among adults. *Clin Infect Dis.* 2005; 40(4):628-631.
21. Mølle I, Thulstrup AM, Vilstrup H, Sørensen HT. Increased risk and case fatality rate of pyogenic liver abscess in patients with liver cirrhosis: a nationwide study in Denmark. *Gut.* 2001;48(2):260-263.
22. Seeto RK, Rockey DC. Pyogenic liver abscess. Changes in etiology, management, and outcome. *Medicine (Baltimore).* 1996;75(2):99-113.
23. Chou FF, Sheen-Chen SM, Chen YS, Chen MC. Single and multiple pyogenic liver abscesses: clinical course, etiology, and results of treatment. *World J Surg.* 1997;21(4):384-388; discussion 388–389.
24. Chu KM, Fan ST, Lai EC, Lo CM, Wong J. Pyogenic liver abscess. An audit of experience over the past decade. *Arch Surg.* 1996;131(2): 148-152.
25. Huang CJ, Pitt HA, Lipsett PA, et al. Pyogenic hepatic abscess. Changing trends over 42 years. *Ann Surg.* 1996;223(5):600-607; discussion 607–609.
26. Danlin O, Valle EJ, Pimentha G, et al. Pyogenic liver abscess after gunshot injury: 10 years' experience at a single level 1 trauma center. *Ir J Med Sci.* 2016;185(4):797-804.
27. Saini S. Imaging of the hepatobiliary tract. *N Engl J Med.* 1997; 336(25):1889-1894.
28. Alvarez JA, González JJ, Baldonedo RF, Sanz L, Carreño G, Jorge JI. Single and multiple pyogenic liver abscesses: etiology, clinical course, and outcome. *Dig Surg.* 2001;18(4):283-288.
29. Benedetti NJ, Desser TS, Jeffrey RB. Imaging of hepatic infections. *Ultrasound Q.* 2008;24(4):267-278.
30. Mohsen AH, Green ST, Read RC, McKendrick MW. Liver abscess in adults: ten years experience in a UK centre. *QJM.* 2002;95(12): 797-802.
31. Alvarez Pérez JA, González JJ, Baldonedo RF, et al. Clinical course, treatment, and multivariate analysis of risk factors for pyogenic liver abscess. *Am J Surg.* 2001;181(2):177-186.
32. Rahimian J, Wilson T, Oram V, Holzman RS. Pyogenic liver abscess: recent trends in etiology and mortality. *Clin Infect Dis.* 2004;39(11): 1654-1659.
33. Rives C, Chaudhari D, Swenson J, Reddy C, Young M. *Clostridium perfringens* liver abscess complicated by bacteremia. *Endoscopy.* 2015;47(suppl 1 UCTN):E457.
34. Wang JH, Liu YC, Lee SS, et al. Primary liver abscess due to *Klebsiella pneumoniae* in Taiwan. *Clin Infect Dis.* 1998;26(6):1434-1438.
35. Sheat VG, Chia CL, Yeo CS, Qiao W, Woon W, Junnarkar SP. Pyogenic liver abscess: does *Escherichia coli* cause more adverse outcomes than *Klebsiella pneumoniae?* *World J Surg.* 2015;39(10):2535-2542.
36. Shin SU, Park CM, Lee Y, Kim EC, Kim SJ, Goo JM. Clinical and radiological features of invasive *Klebsiella pneumoniae* liver abscess syndrome. *Acta Radiol.* 2013;54(5):557-563.
37. Siu LK, Yeh KM, Lin JC, Fung CP, Chang FY. *Klebsiella pneumoniae* liver abscess: a new invasive syndrome. *Lancet Infect Dis.* 2012; 12(11):881-887.
38. Sabbaj J, Sutter VL, Finegold SM. Anaerobic pyogenic liver abscess. *Ann Intern Med.* 1972;77(4):627-638.
39. Chemaly RF, Hall GS, Keys TF, Procop GW. Microbiology of liver abscesses and the predictive value of abscess Gram stain and associated blood cultures. *Diagn Microbiol Infect Dis.* 2003;46(4):245-248.
40. Johannsen EC, Sifri CD, Madoff LC. Pyogenic liver abscesses. *Infect Dis Clin North Am.* 2000;14(3):547-563, vii.
41. Ng FH, Wong WM, Wong BC, et al. Sequential intravenous/oral antibiotic vs. continuous intravenous antibiotic in the treatment of pyogenic liver abscess. *Aliment Pharmacol Ther.* 2002;16(6):1083-1090.
42. Yu SC, Ho SS, Lau WY, et al. Treatment of pyogenic liver abscess: prospective randomized comparison of catheter drainage and needle aspiration. *Hepatology.* 2004;39(4):932-938.
43. Lai KC, Cheng KS, Jeng LB, et al. Factors associated with treatment failure of percutaneous catheter drainage for pyogenic liver abscess in patients with hepatobiliary-pancreatic cancer. *Am J Surg.* 2013; 205(1):52-57.
44. Ogura T, Takagi W, Onda S, et al. Endoscopic ultrasound-guided drainage of a right liver abscess with a self-expandable metallic stent. *Endoscopy.* 2015;47(suppl 1 UCTN):E397-E398.
45. Ogura T, Higuchi K. Video of the month: endoscopic ultrasound-guided drainage for liver abscess using a fully covered metallic stent. *Am J Gastroenterol.* 2015;110(3):379.
46. Kawakami H, Kawakubo K, Kuwatani M, et al. Endoscopic ultrasonography-guided liver abscess drainage using a dedicated, wide, fully covered self-expandable metallic stent with flared-ends. *Endoscopy.* 2014;46(suppl 1 UCTN):E982-E983.
47. Sharma BC, Agarwal N, Garg S, Kumar R, Sarin SK. Endoscopic management of liver abscesses and cysts that communicate with intrahepatic bile ducts. *Endoscopy.* 2006;38(3):249-253.
48. Klink CD, Binnebösel M, Schmeding M, et al. Video-assisted hepatic abscess debridement. *HPB (Oxford).* 2015;17(8):732-735.
49. Foo NP, Chen KT, Lin HJ, et al. Characteristics of pyogenic liver abscess patients with and without diabetes mellitus. *Am J Gastroenterol.* 2010;105(2):328-335.
50. Kao WY, Hwang CY, Chang YT, et al. Cancer risk in patients with pyogenic liver abscess: a nationwide cohort study. *Aliment Pharmacol Ther.* 2012;36(5):467-476.
51. Lai HC, Lin CC, Cheng KS, et al. Increased incidence of gastrointestinal cancers among patients with pyogenic liver abscess: a

population-based cohort study. *Gastroenterology.* 2014;146(1):129-137. e121.

52. Ali IK, Clark CG, Petri WA. Molecular epidemiology of amebiasis. *Infect Genet Evol.* 2008;8(5):698-707.

53. Haque R, Mondal D, Duggal P, et al. *Entamoeba histolytica* infection in children and protection from subsequent amebiasis. *Infect Immun.* 2006;74(2):904-909.

54. Hung CC, Chen PJ, Hsieh SM, et al. Invasive amoebiasis: an emerging parasitic disease in patients infected with HIV in an area endemic for amoebic infection. *AIDS.* 1999;13(17):2421-2428.

55. Hung CC, Ji DD, Sun HY, et al. Increased risk for *Entamoeba histolytica* infection and invasive amebiasis in HIV seropositive men who have sex with men in Taiwan. *PLoS Negl Trop Dis.* 2008;2(2):e175.

56. Guo X, Houpt E, Petri WA. Crosstalk at the initial encounter: interplay between host defense and amebia survival strategies. *Curr Opin Immunol.* 2007;19(4):376-384.

57. Santi-Rocca J, Rigothier MC, Guillén N. Host-microbe interactions and defense mechanisms in the development of amoebic liver abscesses. *Clin Microbiol Rev.* 2009;22(1):65-75.

58. Lodhi S, Sarwari AR, Muzammil M, Salam A, Smego RA. Features distinguishing amoebic from pyogenic liver abscess: a review of 577 adult cases. *Trop Med Int Health.* 2004;9(6):718-723.

59. Fotedar R, Stark D, Beebe N, Marriot D, Ellis J, Harkness J. Laboratory diagnostic techniques for *Entamoeba* species. *Clin Microbiol Rev.* 2007;20(3):511-532.

60. Reid-Lombardo KM, Khan S, Sclabas G. Hepatic cysts and liver abscess. *Surg Clin North Am.* 2010;90(4):679-697.

61. Blessmann J, Khoa ND, Van An L, Tannich E. Ultrasound patterns and frequency of focal liver lesions after successful treatment of amoebic liver abscess. *Trop Med Int Health.* 2006;11(4):504-508.

62. Porras-Ramírez G, Hernández-Herrera MH, Porras-Hernández JD. Amebic hepatic abscess in children. *J Pediatr Surg.* 1995;30(5):662-664.

63. Sharma MP, Kumar A. Liver abscess in children. *Indian J Pediatr.* 2006;73(9):813-817.

64. Khan R, Hamid S, Abid S, et al. Predictive factors for early aspiration in liver abscess. *World J Gastroenterol.* 2008;14(13):2089-2093.

65. Chavez-Tapia NC, Hernandez-Calleros J, Tellez-Avila FI, Torre A, Uribe M. Image-guided percutaneous procedure plus metronidazole versus metronidazole alone for uncomplicated amoebic liver abscess. *Cochrane Database Syst Rev.* 2009;(1):CD004886.

66. Ramani A, Ramani R, Kumar MS, Lakhkar BN, Kundaje GN. Ultrasound-guided needle aspiration of amoebic liver abscess. *Postgrad Med J.* 1993;69(811):381-383.

67. Sandeep SM, Banait VS, Thakur SK, et al. Endoscopic biliary drainage in patients with amebic liver abscess and biliary communication. *Indian J Gastroenterol.* 2006;25(3):125-127.

68. Agarwal DK, Baijal SS, Roy S, Mittal BR, Gupta R, Choudhuri G. Percutaneous catheter drainage of amebic liver abscesses with and without intrahepatic biliary communication: a comparative study. *Eur J Radiol.* 1995;20(1):61-64.

69. Hughes MA, Petri WA. Amebic liver abscess. *Infect Dis Clin North Am.* 2000;14(3):565-582, viii.

70. Ali IK, Mondal U, Roy S, Haque R, Petri WA Jr, Clark CG. Evidence for a link between parasite genotype and outcome of infection with *Entamoeba histolytica. J Clin Microbiol.* 2007;45(2):285-289.

71. Pitt HA, Zuidema GD. Factors influencing mortality in the treatment of pyogenic hepatic abscess. *Surg Gynecol Obstet.* 1975;140(2):228-234.

72. Wong WM, Wong BC, Hui CK, et al. Pyogenic liver abscess: retrospective analysis of 80 cases over a 10-year period. *J Gastroenterol Hepatol.* 2002;17(9):1001-1007.

73. Conter RL, Pitt HA, Tompkins RK, Longmire WP Jr. Differentiation of pyogenic from amebic hepatic abscesses. *Surg Gynecol Obstet.* 1986;162(2):114-120.

74. Barnes PF, De Cock KM, Reynolds TN, Ralls PW. A comparison of amebic and pyogenic abscess of the liver. *Medicine (Baltimore).* 1987;66(6):472-483.

Management of Hepatobiliary Trauma

Michael D. Goodman | Timothy A. Pritts

Despite improvements in motor vehicle safety and altered patterns in trauma epidemiology over the past 20 years, the liver remains the most commonly injured intraabdominal organ. While the treatment of hepatic injuries has evolved over the past 100 years, areas of controversy remain.[1] Improved resuscitation strategies, critical care, and abdominal imaging modalities have placed the primary focus of the surgeon on selection of appropriate patients for operative as compared with nonoperative treatment, with operative options reserved for failure of nonoperative strategies. The operative techniques for treatment of hepatic injuries have generally remained standard.

HISTORICAL PERSPECTIVE

As there is significant historical literature describing hepatobiliary injuries, understanding the historical approaches to the care of these patients is informative in appreciating recent evolutions in care. Some of the first descriptions of liver injuries and their treatment can be traced back to Greek and Arabic medical literature near the turn of the first millennium. The first successful treatment of a liver injury is attributed to Hildanus in the early 17th century, who described the care of a young man stabbed in the abdomen with resultant severe hemorrhage.[2] A large piece of liver that eviscerated through the wound was removed and cauterized, and the patient subsequently recovered. Otis painstakingly reviewed Civil War injuries in which he documented 37 individuals who recovered after gunshot wounds (GSWs) to the liver.[3] Twenty-three of these cases were complicated by injury of other viscera in the abdomen, foreshadowing the challenge of caring for patients with multiple intraabdominal injuries. In 1905, Tilton reported on a series of 189 injuries to the liver, emphasizing that hepatic wounds are very frequently associated with concomitant injuries to other visceral organs.[4] In one of his most important observations, he noted that "there are many mild cases of laceration of the liver to go onto recovery without complications and with very few symptoms. The number of these cases is, I think, larger than is generally supposed." Tilton's review of the literature at that time showed that injury of the liver was associated with a 78.1% mortality if the wound was caused by blunt forces, 39% if caused by GSWs, and 37.5% if caused by stab wounds. In addition, he reviewed all of the New York hospitals with large accident services over a 10-year period and found that there were 25 liver injuries: 12 were caused by blunt injuries, 9 by GSWs, and 4 by stab wounds, with an overall mortality of 44%. Twenty of the 25 patients were operated on, with a mortality of 40%. In his paper, he discussed current therapy of the day and acknowledged that some surgeons recommended nonoperative management. Tilton stated, "This seems a wrong principle to work on. Many cases might recover without interference but others will prove fatal from oversight, an intestinal perforation or foreign body or from insufficient drainage of the wound in the liver." He also made the point that the surgeon "has no choice" but to operate on those patients with aggressive symptoms of internal hemorrhage. His recommended method of hemorrhage control was to use sutures or gauze packing. He stated that "the thermal cautery is of very little value in arresting hemorrhage from the liver." His opinion on the treatment of these injuries would shape the management of hepatobiliary injuries for the next 75 years.[4]

Despite these early advances, hepatobiliary trauma during the first half of the 20th century was marked by high morbidity and mortality, with reported mortality for patients with liver injuries during World War I being as high as 66%. Packing of liver wounds was frequently practiced and often resulted in perihepatic infection and abscess. However, during World War II, major advances in resuscitation, anesthetic techniques, early operation, hemorrhage control, establishment of liver drainage, and use of antibiotics reduced the mortality rate. In their book *Trauma to the Liver*, which referenced their World War II experience, Madding and Kennedy stated that "before the war, house surgeons advocated expectant or conservative treatment, or no treatment at all for the majority of wounds of the liver....Peritonitis, hepatitis, fistulas and numerous other complications often followed this form of treatment."[5] In an 18-month period during the latter part of World War II, they cared for 829 wounds of the liver in 3154 patients with abdominal and thoracoabdominal wounds. Overall mortality was reduced to 27%, a significant improvement that they felt was due to the use of drainage and "aggressive resectional débridement" as needed. They further stated that "use of packing either with gauze or absorbable hemostatic agents should be avoided, except for temporary purposes." The lessons that were advocated for the next four decades could be summarized as follows: (1) most patients with liver wounds require operation, (2) all wounds should be drained, (3) hepatic tissue should be judiciously débrided, and (4) liver packing should not be performed.[5]

After World War II, the mortality from hepatic injuries decreased greatly,[6,7] likely due to a decline in death from infection. Contributing factors included earlier transport, better resuscitation, advances in antibiotic therapy, and improved supportive care. A 36-year view of liver injury mortality from the Ben Taub Hospital in Houston, Texas, noted that the mortality declined from 20.6% in 1939 to 9.2% by the early 1970s.[8] However, as highway speeds increased and civilian GSWs became more prevalent, deaths from infection were supplanted by deaths from hemorrhage, leading to increased aggressiveness in operative treatment for these injuries during the 1960 to 1990 time period, including major formal hepatic resections including hepatic lobectomy, hepatic artery ligation for hemorrhage control, atriocaval shunting, and tractotomy to expose deep bleeding.[9-12] Although each of these techniques continues to be used in the treatment of major hepatic injuries, these methods are reserved for difficult cases rather than routine practice.

Over the past 20 years, it has become recognized that aggressive operative strategies often failed to prevent deaths from hemorrhage and that, even if operative treatment was prompt and efficient, the vascularity of the liver and overall physiologic state of the patient was such that ongoing bleeding not amenable to control by standard maneuvers often occurred, leading to mortality from ongoing bleeding and coagulopathy.[5] Recent advances in management include updated imaging, improved resuscitation strategies, damage control operative strategies, better hemostatic agents, and the use of percutaneous techniques for angiography, embolization, and drainage. Together, these advances allow a customized approach to the care of these complex patients.

CLASSIFICATION OF LIVER INJURIES

Although the Couinaud and Bismuth anatomic classifications of hepatic segmental anatomy have proven useful in planning elective operations and therapy, most liver injuries are nonanatomic in nature or cross multiple anatomic segments. To characterize these injuries and allow development of treatment strategies as well as ongoing research, the American Association for the Surgery of Trauma developed and validated a liver injury scoring system (Table 123.1).[13-15] This scoring system was originally based on operative findings so that the severity of injuries and mortality increases with higher grade. One known concern with this system is that, while it is valuable as a general guide, it is not precise enough to predict which patients will require intervention and which will not, as some patients will present with low-grade lesions that bleed significantly and many will present with high-grade lesions that do not require operative intervention.

INITIAL EVALUATION

The initial assessment and resuscitation of trauma patients undergoing evaluation for hepatobiliary injury is no different than for any other injured patient. General principles of the Advanced Trauma Life Support Program as taught by the American College of Surgeons should be followed, including initial evaluation of airway, breathing, and circulation; evaluation for additional injuries; and monitoring the response to resuscitation.[16] Special attention is paid to the patient's abdominal examination, vital signs, and physiologic and hemostatic response to treatment. The specific goals of the initial evaluation in all trauma patients is to efficiently determine the presence of potentially life-threatening injuries, assess the hemodynamic stability of the patient, and initiate a therapeutic plan that is based on the initial response to resuscitation and findings on the initial surgeon-performed ultrasound, diagnostic

TABLE 123.1 American Association for the Surgery of Trauma Liver Injury Scale

Grade I	*Hematoma:* Subcapsular, <10% surface area *Laceration:* Capsular tear, <1 cm parenchymal depth
Grade II	*Hematoma:* Subcapsular: 10%–15% surface area; intraparenchymal: <10 cm depth *Laceration:* Capsular tear 1–3 parenchymal depth, <10 cm in length
Grade III	*Hematoma:* Subcapsular, >50% surface area of ruptured subcapsular or parenchymal hematoma; Intraparenchymal hematoma >10 cm or expanding *Laceration:* >3 cm parenchymal depth
Grade IV	*Laceration:* Parenchymal disruption involving 25%–75% hepatic lobe or 1–3 Couinaud segments
Grade V	*Laceration:* Parenchymal disruption involving >75% of hepatic lobe or >3 Couinaud segments within a single lobe *Vascular:* Juxtahepatic venous injuries (i.e., retrohepatic vena cava/central major hepatic veins)
Grade VI	*Vascular:* Hepatic avulsion

Modified from Tinkoff G, et al. American Association for the Surgery of Trauma Organ Injury Scale I: spleen, liver, and kidney, validation based on the National Trauma Data Bank. *J Am Coll Surg.* 2008;207(5):646–655.

peritoneal lavage, or abdominal computed tomography (CT) scan. The response to resuscitation serves as an early decision point in the treatment of patients with hepatobiliary injuries.

Further evaluation of the patient will be dependent on the mechanism of injury, hemodynamic instability, and the ongoing response to resuscitation. In general, patients who are hemodynamically unstable due to hemorrhage from abdominal trauma should be treated with exploratory laparotomy in the operating room. In a similar fashion, urgent operation should be considered for most patients with penetrating injuries. In a patient with blunt trauma who is hemodynamically stable and responsive to resuscitation, the nature of the injury can be more thoroughly evaluated with a complete physical exam and imaging.

In most trauma centers, the initial diagnostic modality of choice is the focused assessment with sonography for trauma (FAST exam). FAST is an effective and accurate technique for rapid imaging in hemodynamically stable or unstable patients with possible hepatic injuries.[17] FAST involves four views of the abdomen, including cardiac (to evaluate for pericardial effusion), right and left upper quadrants, and suprapubic (to evaluate for the presence of fluid). With training and practice, the sensitivity and specificity for detection of fluid in these views is 83% and 99.7%, respectively. Of note, when using FAST for patients with blunt abdominal trauma who are hypotensive, the sensitivity and specificity may increase to 100%.[18] FAST has proven extremely useful as a decision making tool for hypotensive blunt trauma patients. In our practice, an unstable patient with a positive FAST is taken for laparotomy. If the patient is hemodynamically unstable

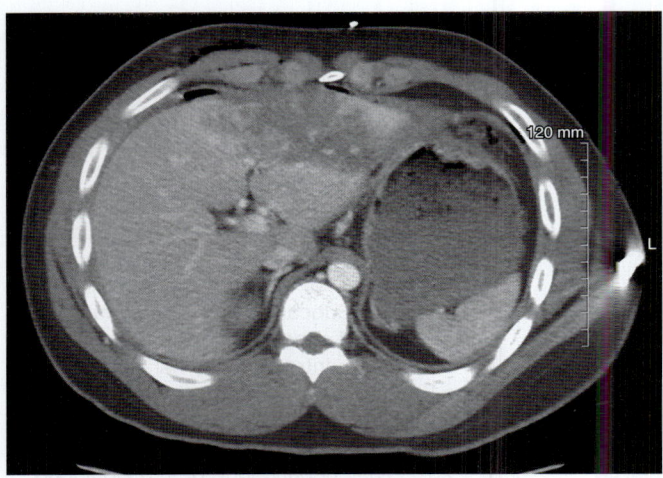

FIGURE 123.1 Computed tomography scan reveals a large liver laceration with active extravasation of contrast.

and has a negative FAST, a search for extraabdominal injuries contributing to shock should be undertaken. If extraabdominal sources of shock are not present or if hemoperitoneum remains a concern in an unstable patient with a negative FAST, the FAST may be repeated or diagnostic peritoneal lavage may be performed. If concern for hemoperitoneum persists, the patient may require an exploratory laparotomy as a diagnostic and potentially therapeutic modality.

If a patient is hemodynamically stable, the patient then undergoes CT scanning of the abdomen and pelvis to document the presence and magnitude of injuries to the liver and other intraabdominal organs. CT of the abdomen and pelvis in the hemodynamically stable patient performed after the intravenous injection of contrast remains the most sensitive and specific imaging modality for the evaluation of hepatobiliary trauma. In our institution, we do not use oral contrast for CT scans in trauma patients. CT findings of interest to the surgeon include the presence and magnitude of the hepatic parenchymal injury, the presence and magnitude of intraperitoneal blood, and the presence and magnitude of associated intraperitoneal and retroperitoneal visceral, mesenteric, and vascular injuries. Hepatic injuries typically noted on a CT study include parenchymal lacerations, intrahepatic hematoma, or subcapsular hematoma with or without active extravasation of intravenous contrast (Fig. 123.1). In addition, CT studies worrisome for active IV contrast extravasation can be quickly repeated to survey for ongoing active bleeding on venous phase imaging.

MANAGEMENT

Similar to the evaluation phase, management of patients with hepatic trauma is driven by hemodynamic status, mechanism of injury, and associated injuries. Guidelines generated by the Western Trauma Association, the Eastern Association for the Surgery of Trauma, and, more recently, the World Society of Emergency Surgery each provide important direction in the care of these patients.[19–21]

Nonoperative management of stab wounds or GSWs to the liver has been shown to be safe,[22–24] but there is a high incidence of concomitant intraabdominal injuries, and these patients must be carefully and thoughtfully selected.[25] Potential candidates for nonoperative management of penetrating injuries to the liver should undergo CT scans.[26] In one series, 15% of patients (and 80% of those presenting with isolated liver injury) were managed nonoperatively.[26] In our practice, patients with penetrating abdominal trauma undergo laparotomy under most circumstances, with the exception of those in whom a reliable abdominal exam is present, additional injuries can be reliably excluded, and serial abdominal exams and physiologic status can be monitored.

Nonoperative management is more common in patients with injuries from blunt trauma. A study of patients from the National Trauma Data Bank examined the role of nonoperative management in patients with high grade (Abbreviated Injury Scale of 4 or higher) liver injuries.[27] Of these, 73% were managed nonoperatively with a 7% failure rate. Of note, failed nonoperative management was independently associated with higher mortality. Predictors of need for conversion to operative management included older age, female gender, higher injury severity score, and hypotension.[27] Previous series have examined the relationship between solid organ injuries and hollow viscus injuries and, perhaps unsurprisingly, noted a positive relationship between the two injury patterns.[28,29] Thus, in the presence of liver injuries, hollow viscus injuries must be strongly considered, even in the absence of supporting CT scan findings.

In our practice, patients who are hemodynamically unstable, fail to respond to resuscitation, have hollow viscus injuries, or have evidence of peritonitis on exam are taken for laparotomy. All other patients are considered for nonoperative management. Patients with American Association for the Surgery of Trauma (AAST) grade I, II, and III injuries as determined by CT scan are admitted to the surgical floor for observation with hemoglobin assessment every 8 hours for 24 hours. These patients are considered for discharge after 24 hours of stable hemoglobin measurements if they are tolerating a diet. If they become unstable or require a blood transfusion, they are transferred to the intensive care unit with consideration for additional imaging and operation. Patients with AAST grade IV and V injuries are admitted to the surgical intensive care unit and undergo hemoglobin measurement every 6 hours for 24 hours. Need for blood transfusion or the occurrence of hemodynamic instability prompts thorough reassessment and consideration of angiography or operation. If initial nonoperative management is successful, these patients undergo interval CT scan prior to discharge to evaluate for interval development of hepatic artery pseudoaneurysm or bile collections.

If the initial CT scan reveals evidence of contrast blush with suspected hemorrhage or the formation of hepatic artery pseudoaneurysm, consideration is made for immediate selective angiography with embolization. In a hemodynamically unstable patient with no additional injuries, we pursue selective angioembolization primarily rather than proceeding to laparotomy. These situations are challenging in that they may require transporting a critically ill and unstable patient to the angiography suite. Our practice is to "bring the surgical intensive care unit to the patient" and continue active resuscitation with the intensive care unit and trauma team regardless of physical location. The advent of advanced hybrid operating rooms, with the capability for open operative intervention and high quality fluoroscopy, may alleviate this challenge, but these are not yet in widespread use.

PRINCIPLES OF OPERATIVE TREATMENT

With rare exception, operations for trauma should use a midline incision to permit rapid exploration of the entire abdomen as well as extension as needed to gain needed exposure.[30] Transverse incisions, which are commonly used in elective hepatic procedures, may not permit a thorough abdominal evaluation and are not the standard incision for trauma patients. The use of an upper abdominal retraction system greatly facilitates exposure of the liver. If further exposure is required, the incision may be extended laterally in a subcostal direction or cephalad either partially or completely through the sternum. Although a median sternotomy may be required to control life-threatening bleeding, opening the sternum for a bicavitary procedure increases evaporative heat loss and may worsen coagulopathy. Therefore this should be done only if it confers a major advantage in exposure. The conduct of the operation will be determined to a considerable degree by the extent of hemoperitoneum encountered and the site of the presumed source of bleeding. If a large volume of free blood is encountered, packs should be placed in the four quadrants of the abdomen in an attempt to determine the primary site of bleeding. If liver bleeding can be controlled with packs initially, these can be left in place while other potential injuries are evaluated and addressed. A seriously injured spleen should be removed promptly and any concomitant gastrointestinal injuries rapidly evaluated and managed.

When addressing hemorrhage from the liver, a series of operative maneuvers may be employed to obtain hemostasis. A very useful algorithm to provide guidance on the approach to liver hemorrhage has been developed by the Western Trauma Association (Fig. 123.2).[19] Minor bleeding from hepatic trauma may be encountered in association with other intraabdominal injuries and is often due to low-grade (AAST I and II) liver injuries. These injuries can usually be managed by compression and temporary packing alone or with electrocautery, argon beam coagulation, with adjunct use of topical hemostatic agents. Packing with temporary abdominal closure will rarely be required for isolated low-grade injuries.

Severe hepatic injuries (AAST grace III to V) require a rapid but logical approach to hemorrhage control. In our practice, we typically initially perform manual compression and perihepatic packing then allow resuscitation of the patient and transfusion of blood products as needed. Once the patient's resuscitation is underway, we proceed with obtaining further hemostasis. Compression and packing often lead to temporary hemorrhage control and allow definitive hemorrhage control. If hemorrhage is not amenable to temporary packing, bimanual compression is held, resuscitation is performed by the anesthesia team, and

---

BOX 123.1 **Operative Techniques for Control of Liver Injury**

Cautery
   Argon beam coagulation
   Hemostatic adjuncts
Individual vessel ligation
Parenchyma reapproximation with large mattress sutures
Selective hepatic artery ligation
Resectional débridement
Hepatic lobectomy (or major resection)
Omental packing
Packing and planned reoperation

---

the operation progresses immediately to definitive control. If significant bleeding is encountered, the institution's massive transfusion protocol should be activated. We typically transfuse in a balanced ratio of packed red blood cells, plasma and platelets (1:1:1) with minimal infusion of crystalloid, as this strategy has been demonstrated to reduce mortality and morbidity from hemorrhage in trauma patients.[31-33]

A number of operative tactics are available to control hepatic bleeding (summarized in Box 123.1). The technique employed will depend on the geometry and depth of the wound as well as the nature of the injured vessels.[34,35] Bleeding hepatic parenchyma responds well to cautery, argon beam coagulation, and hemostatic agents. Bleeding parenchymal injuries are best managed by vessel ligation if feasible. In general, direct suture ligation of vessels is preferable to control with surgical clips due to the susceptibility of the latter to dislodge with manipulation of the liver. As needed, use of the finger fracture technique can be used to expose and allow ligation of deeper vessels. We also find the use of stapling devices useful in the event that removal of devitalized tissue is needed or to control hemorrhage with a limited hepatic resection. These are used in a similar fashion as in elective hepatic surgery. We also find that reapproximation of hepatic parenchyma with adjunct use of hemostatic agents will lead to cessation of bleeding in many injuries.

In the event of major bleeding that is not controlled by parenchymal compression, our next maneuver is to obtain control of the porta hepatis and perform a Pringle maneuver followed by additional hemorrhage control. Gentle dissection to encircle the hepatoduodenal ligament is performed and the resident structures are compressed between a thumb and forefinger. This can then be exchanged for a gentle, noncrushing fine vascular clamp or umbilical tape with a Rumel tourniquet to obtain more secure control. The duration of safe occlusion of the porta hepatis in the setting of traumatic injury with concomitant hypotension and shock is unknown.

If arterial bleeding from deep within the parenchyma is present and this is not amenable to direct control, additional strategies must be employed. If the bleeding slows or ceases with portal triad compression, selective hepatic artery ligation (SHAL) may be performed. Although used frequently in the past,[9,10] SHAL is rarely performed in our current practice. We frequently perform a damage control operation with the control of venous hemorrhage and

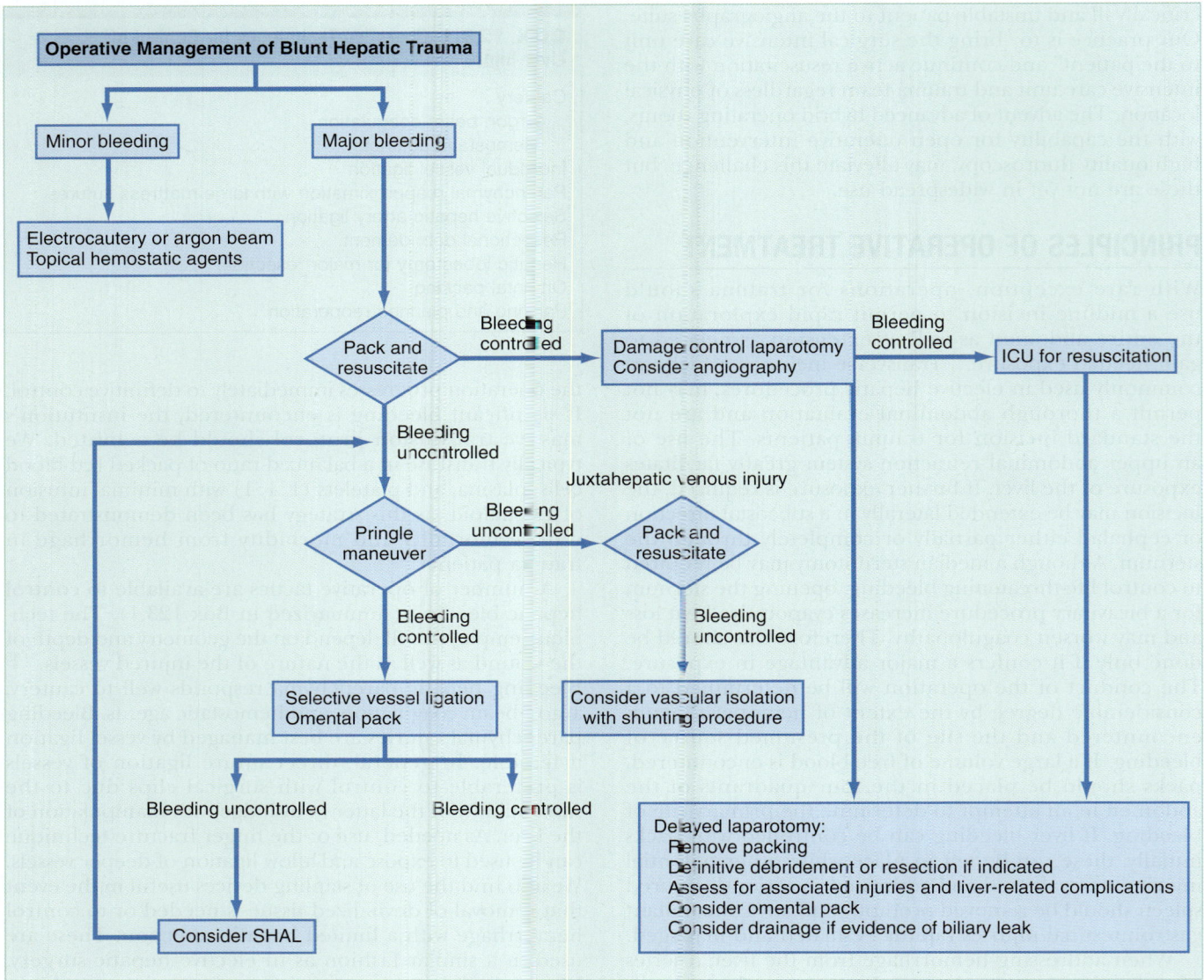

FIGURE 123.2 The Western Trauma Association algorithm for management of blunt liver injuries requiring operation. *SHAL,* Selective hepatic artery ligation. (From Kozar RA, Moore FA, Moore E, et al. Western Trauma Association critical decision in trauma: non-operative management of blunt hepatic trauma. *J Trauma.* 2009;67:1144.)

placement of perihepatic packing and then transport the patient to the angiography suite for selective angiography and embolization.[37–41] If the Pringle maneuver fails to even temporarily control arterial bleeding, one may consider an aberrant left hepatic artery in the lesser omentum as the bleeding source. In the event of penetrating trauma to the liver with uncontrolled hemorrhage, balloon occlusion of the wound may be lifesaving.[42,43] To perform this, a red rubber catheter is placed inside a tied-off Penrose drain. This is passed through the path of the projectile and then inflated until hemorrhage control is achieved. In most cases, the patient undergoes resuscitation and hepatic packing, followed by selective angioembolization. The balloon is removed at subsequent laparotomy. There are also reports of the use of extensive tractotomy for exposure of deep arterial bleeding. In our present practice, we prefer to pursue angioembolization in these patients.

Hepatorrhaphy or reapproximation of the liver parenchyma may be useful for control of venous bleeding or bile leakage. The technique usually involves the placement of large absorbable sutures, often in horizontal mattress fashion, for the reapproximation of the liver (Fig. 123.3). Critics of the procedure argue that the use of large sutures may cause necrosis of hepatic tissue, which can be minimized with control of tension on the sutures. Attempting to control oozing from nonviable liver is an inappropriate use of hepatorrhaphy, as this tissue should be débrided. However, small bleeding cracks can often be closed with the arrest of hemorrhage by this technique without causing tissue necrosis or unnecessarily extending the wound by tractotomy or finger fracture. We have also encountered large injuries with significant lacerations in the liver with little bleeding from the exposed surfaces. After the major vessels and ducts have been controlled by

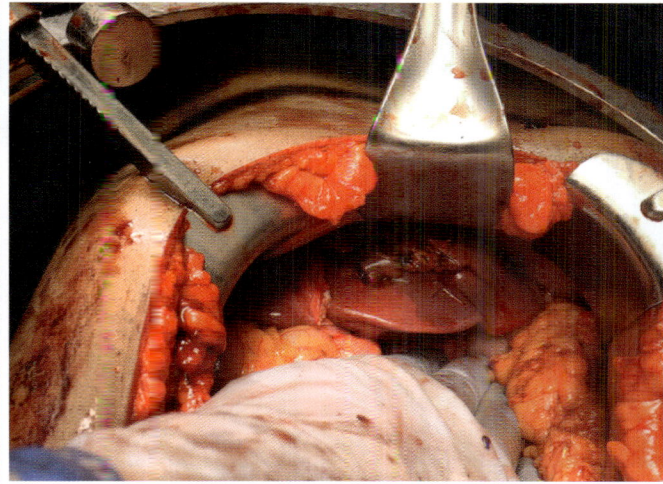

FIGURE 123.3 Sutured hepatorrhaphy. Multiple gunshot wounds to the abdomen result in complex liver laceration *(left)*. After compression and control of larger vessels, hepatorrhaphy is performed with absorbable suture on a large blunt needle *(right)*.

suture techniques, gentle reapproximation of the divided portions may decrease oozing from the raw surfaces. This technique may be augmented by an omental flap, packing with topical hemostatic agents, or both. If used appropriately, hepatorrhaphy can be a useful tool, but it will not control major arterial bleeding.

Omental pedicle flaps can be very useful for prevention of diffuse oozing from raw surfaces of the liver.[44] This was commonly used, but in the era of primarily operative management, the need for this maneuver has diminished considerably. The omental flap is created in a standard fashion and is used in our practice to cover large exposed liver surfaces. Indications for its use vary but might include the aforementioned crevasses in hepatic tissues, coverage of the remaining surface following resection or débridement of hepatic tissue, and for any larger area where there is no liver capsule. In the unusual instance where a subcapsular hematoma has ruptured or been surgically entered, diffuse bleeding from the exposed liver surface usually ensues. The use of an omental flap in this circumstance may be extremely useful.

Formal anatomic resection of the liver is not commonly indicated for trauma. However, there are several instances where a major hepatic resection is indicated: devitalizing injuries along anatomic planes, completion lobectomy when the injury has transected the liver along lobar anatomy, and for exposure of major venous bleeding associated with a major hepatic parenchymal injury. The use of hepatic artery embolization has occasionally resulted in lobar hepatic necrosis that requires a formal lobectomy for resolution.[40,41] Unlike a planned lobar resection for hepatic tumors, major resections for injury must often be performed under an emergent, less-than-optimal situation in a patient who is at grave risk for exsanguination. In this circumstance, operative speed is imperative. The use of techniques employed by elective hepatic surgeons such as vascular and hepatic staplers is a useful adjunct in such cases. Formal resection may also be performed in delayed fashion at a second look operation to delineate

and débride necrotic hepatic tissue following the initial packing and correction of coagulopathy.

MAJOR VENOUS BLEEDING

Although major arterial hemorrhage must be controlled by surgical or radiologic means and is not amenable to cessation by packing, major venous bleeding is a great impediment to patient survival as well.[11,45–47] Major venous bleeding may result from injury to one of the main hepatic veins, from a major injury associated with the vena cava, or from a retrohepatic vena cava wound itself. Isolated vena cava lacerations without involvement of a hepatic vein branch are unusual in blunt trauma but may occur with a GSW. Major hepatic venous injuries confined to the liver parenchyma can generally be successfully managed by suture ligation. If the injury is not readily apparent and blood is welling up from a deep crevasse, it may be necessary to expose the venous injury more clearly with finger fracture or tractotomy. Suture ligation can generally be used to control hemorrhage. Once major bleeding has been lessened, packing may be used to control the remaining bleeding.

Avulsion of one or more of the hepatic veins from the vena cava is a very serious and potentially lethal event (Fig. 123.4). On occasion, this problem can be solved by packing the area of injury and allowing the low-pressure venous system to tamponade. However, the packing may not succeed in hemorrhage control and if the packs are placed too aggressively, the venous return from the lower body may be completely occluded, with resultant unsustainably low cardiac output. Using inflow occlusion, the bleeding may be decreased enough to allow suture control but inflow occlusion of the portal triad does not prevent back-bleeding from the vena cava. The direct application of fine vascular clamps to reapproximate the anterior wall of the vena cava and the major hepatic veins has been reported with good success.[48] The clamps can be allowed to remain in place with the abdomen packed in a damage control strategy. There have also been reports of

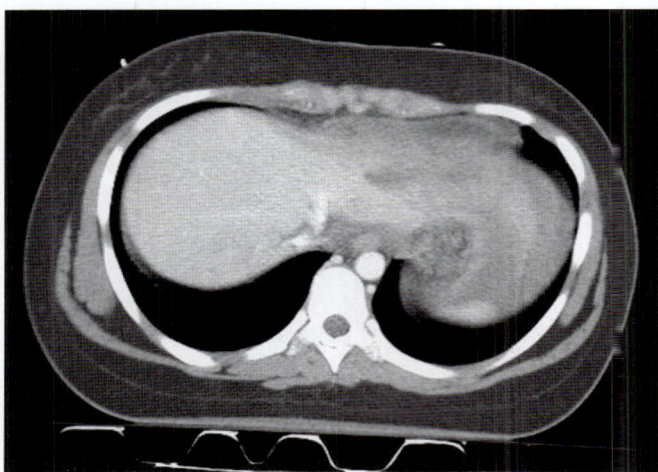

FIGURE 123.4 Complex retrohepatic cava injury. Computed tomography image from a young woman who presented after a motor vehicle crash. She suffered laceration of the left lobe of the liver with avulsion of the left hepatic vein from the inferior vena cava.

successful management by using fenestrated endovascular stent grafts.[49] This method usually involves a contained injury in which extravasation was demonstrated on a CT scan.

One technique for the isolation of the retrohepatic and suprahepatic inferior vena cava involves total hepatic vascular exclusion. This procedure involves the control of all hepatic inflow and outflow from an abdominal approach. Direct hepatic inflow can be controlled with a Pringle maneuver, and additional minimization of inflow can be achieved with supraceliac aortic control to minimize portal blood flow and intestinal venous congestion. The pericardium and diaphragm are then separated to preserve pericardial integrity. The diaphragm is then incised longitudinally to expose the suprahepatic and intrathoracic vena cava, which is then encircled with umbilical tape.[50] Additional infrahepatic vena cava control can be accomplished with an umbilical tape encircling the suprarenal, infrahepatic vena cava. This maneuver will allow for hepatic vascular repairs in a bloodless field with the advantage of a single open cavity.

Historically, the method of choice for management of juxtahepatic major venous injuries has involved the use of an atriocaval shunt.[11,45] This involves the placement of a tube (usually either a modified thoracostomy or endotracheal tube) through the right atrium into the inferior vena cava. Snares are used around the vena cava above and below the liver in an attempt to divert flow through the tube and away from the area of injury, permitting a bloodless field and, theoretically, a more controlled repair. This operation requires an incredible amount of skill and good fortune to be successful. It requires opening a second body cavity (the thorax), which worsens hypothermia and bleeding, and many wounds are difficult to repair even if the shunt is functioning. The best reported results are from San Francisco in the 1980s in which 45% of 27 patients survived. A review of the world's literature revealed 412 cases with 88% mortality.[1] Based on the

---

BOX 123.2 **Principles of Hepatic Packing**

Choose the appropriate patient
  Control arterial bleeding surgically or with
    angioembolization
  Packing is ideal for lesser venous bleeding, coagulopathy
Use packing before excess bleeding and coagulopathy
  develops
  Beware of the patient with acute traumatic coagulopathy
Pack to compress liver in superior to inferior plane
  Anteroposterior packing tends to compress the vena cava
Count sponges
  When feasible as this facilitates later removal
Consider use of nonadherent material over liver
Temporary abdominal closure must avoid tension and
  secondary abdominal compartment syndrome

---

high complexity of the injury as well as high mortality, juxtahepatic venous injuries remain an unsolved problem in hepatic trauma. No single technique is successful and no algorithm for management can be constructed with a reasonable likelihood of patient survival.

PERIHEPATIC PACKING AND DAMAGE CONTROL STRATEGIES

In the early 1980s, several reports presenting a reappraisal of perihepatic packing occurred, which demonstrated a major survival advantage in patients who would have likely died with conventional surgical treatment.[51–53] The term *damage control surgery*, in which packing was an integral part of that strategy, became a recognized and accepted concept.[54] The tenets of liver packing begin with the choice of an appropriate patient as arterial hemorrhage will likely require control by suture or embolization. Good judgment is required to not forego appropriate attempts at technical control of bleeding without delaying for an inappropriate time, which might prevent patient survival.[55] Other technical features we have found useful are outlined in Box 123.2. Secondary effects of abdominal compartment syndrome can generally be ameliorated by avoiding fascial closure, often accompanied by some method of temporary closure usually involving a dressing or vacuum pack technique.[56] Some advocate return to the operating suite for pack removal when the patient is rewarmed and coagulopathy corrected. These goals may be accomplished within 6 hours. However, we prefer to leave packs for at least 24 hours to allow for coagulation of exposed vessels that may rebleed with early pack removal. Issues regarding abdominal compartment syndrome and management of the open abdomen may complicate the decision for perihepatic packing, but they are outside the scope of this discussion.[57]

REQUIREMENTS OF ADJUNCTIVE INVASIVE TREATMENT

The use of nonoperative management (NOM) does not imply that other types of interventions may not be required to treat the patients. Therefore the mindset for NOM should not be to avoid needed therapeutic interventions but instead to allow the patient to recover as rapidly as possible. Angiography has been previously discussed and may be very useful for patients with an arterial blush on CT or evidence of arterial extravasation on angiography. Delayed bleeding from hemobilia may require angiographic treatment as well. Patients with prolonged bile leaks may improve with endoscopic retrograde cholangiography, and sphincterotomy, and biliary stent placement.[39,58,59]

Patients with small perihepatic fluid collections may benefit from percutaneous drainage. When large accumulations of blood and bile are present they may cause bile peritonitis, a systemic inflammatory response syndrome (SIRS), or an abdominal compartment syndrome. To prevent and/or treat these problems, laparoscopy may be performed for evacuation of major accumulations of blood and bile and placement of intraperitoneal drains.[12] If available, a gasless system should be used to prevent the theoretical problem of gas embolism. Laparoscopy permits the evacuation of virtually all of the fluid from the abdominal quadrants and the pelvis itself. We do not attempt to remove organized clot from around the liver and generally place a perihepatic drain to monitor subsequent bile output. This approach to laparoscopic abdominal washout can ameliorate the systemic inflammatory response with a low risk of complications.[60]

SPECIAL PROBLEMS

SUBCAPSULAR HEMATOMAS

Subcapsular hematomas occur in about 2% to 3% of major blunt liver injuries. The natural history of subcapsular hematomas is not clearly defined, but unlike a similar injury to the spleen, which has a real risk of delayed rupture, subsequent bleeding seems to be much less in common hepatic hematomas. In the previous era of uniform operation for suspected liver injury, it was advised to leave these lesions intact if they were encountered. If subcapsular hematomas are encountered, indications for further operative intervention include continued expansion of the hematoma and management of its rupture. Arteriography and embolization may be useful for expanding lesions. If a suspected subcapsular hematoma is detected on CT scan, no therapy is recommended unless it is associated with an arterial blush, suggesting the possibility of continued bleeding. In such instances, angiographic embolization is recommended. If the capsule is ruptured, then operation may be required to control the diffuse bleeding from the exposed surface of the liver. Temporary packing will usually control such bleeding and an omental flap may be useful to prevent rebleeding

HEMOBILIA

Hemobilia is defined as bleeding from the liver which is expressed from the biliary tree. Typically, bleeding occurs several days to a few weeks after the injury and may be manifested by several clinical presentations. These patients most commonly present with melena. Brisk upper gastrointestinal bleeding is less common. Jaundice or subclinical elevation of bilirubin is frequently present. Hemobilia should be suspected in those who sustained recent liver injury with gastrointestinal bleeding and/or jaundice.

The diagnostic modality of choice is arteriography, which commonly shows an abnormality within the liver parenchyma. Selective embolization of the vascular abnormality is nearly always effective in treating this problem and operation is rarely required. Operative treatment is indicated for failure of angiographic treatment, for débridement of associated necrotic liver, or for intrahepatic sepsis.

BILHEMIA

In contradistinction to hemobilia where bleeding occurs through the biliary system, bilhemia is an abnormal communication between an intrahepatic bile duct and a vein. The bile flows into the venous system and may result in profound jaundice. There are few reports of bilhemia in the literature. Care of these patients often requires a two-pronged approach aimed at obliterating the offending vessel through angiographic techniques and decompression of the biliary system through endoscopic retrograde cholangiography and stenting.[61]

AVULSION OF THE LIVER

Grade VI injuries consist of total avulsion of the liver. Although most of these injuries are rapidly fatal, an occasional patient survives his or her operative treatment. There are several reports of successful venovenous bypass with the patient in an anhepatic state followed by emergency liver autotransplantation. These cases require a mindset of preparedness and ingenuity to salvage an otherwise fatal situation.

MORTALITY FROM HEPATIC INJURIES

Mortality from liver injuries has declined considerably in the past several decades. In World War II, the fatality rate was 66%; by the Vietnam War, it had declined to 15% to 20%. As large civilian experiences with liver injuries were reported after midcentury, the mortality was often reported as 8% to 15%. The concept of "liver-related mortality" was introduced in an attempt to define those deaths likely due to the liver injury itself versus those related to associated trauma such as head injury. A comprehensive review of major series published since 1900 shows the downward trend in mortality (Fig. 123.5).[1] Within the past decade with improvement in resuscitation, overall mortality in patients with hepatic injuries has been reported at less than 5%.[6]

GALLBLADDER INJURY

Injuries to the gallbladder may result from either blunt or penetrating trauma. Regardless of mechanism, isolated gallbladder injuries are relatively uncommon. Although there are anecdotal reports of cholecystorrhaphy, the treatment of choice should be cholecystectomy. Attempts to repair even minor gallbladder injuries should generally be avoided because of the propensity for bile leakage and the risk of gallstone formation engendered by the inflammation around the suture used for repair.[63]

Acalculous cholecystitis may also follow treatment modalities that interrupt the gallbladder's blood supply. Both SHAE and angiographic embolization of the hepatic artery may lead to acalculous cholecystitis or gallbladder necrosis.[4]

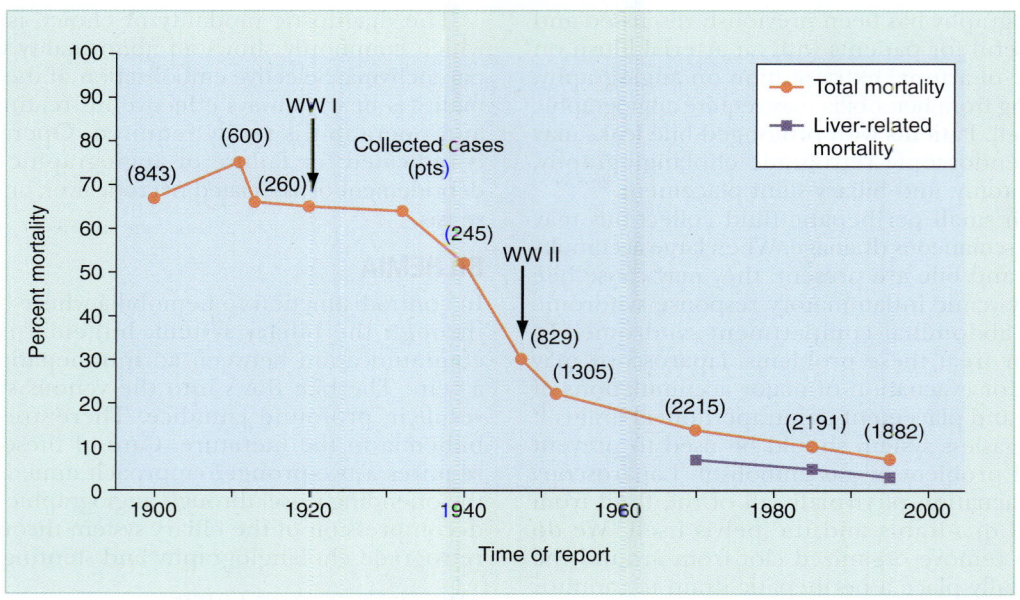

FIGURE 123.5 A review of several thousand cases of liver injury demonstrates a progressively downward trend. Mortality related to liver injury itself is in the 2% to 4% range at present.

INJURIES OF THE EXTRAHEPATIC BILE DUCTS

Injuries of the extrahepatic bile ducts may follow both blunt and penetrating injuries and, as in the case of gallbladder injuries, rarely occur in isolation.[64] When the extrahepatic ductal system is injured by penetrating injuries, other structures are invariably injured, and given the close approximation of the bile ducts to major vessels, massive hemorrhage often accompanies such injuries. We do not recommend repair of these injuries at the initial operation but undertake hemorrhage control, drainage, and damage control. When the patient is resuscitated, we recommend defining the injury, then a planned return to the operating room with the company of an experienced hepatobiliary surgeon for reconstruction.

ACKNOWLEDGMENTS

We recognize the significant contributions of Jason Smith, MD, PhD, FACS and J David Richardson, MD, FACS which are carried over from the previous edition of this chapter.

REFERENCES

1. Richardson JD. Changes in the management of injuries to the liver and spleen. *J Am Coll Surg.* 2005;200(5):648-669.
2. Hardy KJ. Liver surgery: the past 2000 years. *Aust N Z J Surg.* 1990;60(10):811-817.
3. Otis G. Medical and surgical history of the rebellion. 1877;2:129.
4. Tilton BT II. Some considerations regarding wounds of the liver. *Ann Surg.* 1905;41(1):20-30.
5. Madding GF, Kennedy PA. *Trauma to The Liver.* Philadelphia/London: WB Saunders Company; 1965.
6. Peitzman AB, Richardson JD. Surgical treatment of injuries to the solid abdominal organs: a 50-year perspective from the Journal of Trauma. *J Trauma.* 2010;69(5):1011-1021.
7. Trunkey DD, Shires GT, Mc Clelland R. Management of liver trauma in 811 consecutive patients. *Ann Surg.* 1974;179(5):722-728.
8. Defore WW Jr, Mattox KL, Jordan GL Jr, Beall AC Jr. Management of 1,590 consecutive cases of liver trauma. *Arch Surg.* 1976;111(4):493-497.
9. Mays ET, Conti S, Fallahzadeh H, Rosenblatt M. Hepatic artery ligation. *Surgery.* 1979;86(4):536-543.
10. Flint LM Jr, Polk HC Jr. Selective hepatic artery ligation: limitations and failures. *J Trauma.* 1979;19(5):319-323.
11. Schrock T, Blaisdell FW, Mathewson C Jr. Management of blunt trauma to the liver and hepatic veins. *Arch Surg.* 1968;96(5):698-704.
12. Carrillo EH, Richardson JD. The current management of hepatic trauma. *Adv Surg.* 2001;35:39-59.
13. Tinkoff G, Esposito TJ, Reed J, et al. American Association for the Surgery of Trauma organ injury scale I: spleen, liver, and kidney, validation based on the National Trauma Data Bank. *J Am Coll Surg.* 2008;207(5):646-655.
14. Moore EE, Cogbill TH, Jurkovich GJ, Shackford SR, Malangoni MA, Champion HR. Organ injury scaling: spleen and liver (1994 revision). *J Trauma.* 1995;38(3):323-324.
15. Moore EE, Shackford SR, Pachter HL, et al. Organ injury scaling: spleen, liver, and kidney. *J Trauma.* 1989;29(12):1664-1666.
16. ATLS Subcommittee; American College of Surgeons Committee on Trauma. *Advanced Trauma Life Support.* 9th ed. Chicago: American College of Surgeons; 2013.
17. Rozycki GS, Ochsner MG, Feliciano DV, et al. Early detection of hemoperitoneum by ultrasound examination of the right upper quadrant: a multicenter study. *J Trauma.* 1998;45(5):878-883.
18. Rozycki GS, Ballard RB, Feliciano DV, Schmidt JA, Pennington SD. Surgeon-performed ultrasound for the assessment of truncal injuries: lessons learned from 1540 patients. *Ann Surg.* 1998;228(4):557-567.
19. Kozar RA, Feliciano DV, Moore EE, et al. Western Trauma Association/critical decisions in trauma: operative management of adult blunt hepatic trauma. *J Trauma.* 2011;71(1):1-5.
20. Stassen NA, Bhullar I, Cheng JD, et al. Nonoperative management of blunt hepatic injury: an Eastern Association for the Surgery of Trauma practice management guideline. *J Trauma Acute Care Surg.* 2012;73(5 suppl 4):S288-S293.
21. Coccolini F, Catena F, Moore EE, et al. WSES classification and guidelines for liver trauma. *World J Emerg Surg.* 2016;11:50.
22. MacGoey P, Navarro A, Beckingham IJ, Cameron IC, Brooks AJ. Selective non-operative management of penetrating liver injuries at a UK tertiary referral centre. *Ann R Coll Surg Engl.* 2014;96(6):423-426.
23. Demetriades D, Gomez H, Chahwan S, et al. Gunshot injuries to the liver: the role of selective nonoperative management. *J Am Coll Surg.* 1999;188(4):343-348.
24. Demetriades D, Hadjizacharia P, Constantinou C, et al. Selective nonoperative management of penetrating abdominal solid organ injuries. *Ann Surg.* 2006;244(4):620-628.

25. Berg RJ, Karamanos E, Inaba K, Okoye O, Teixeira PG, Demetriades D. The persistent diagnostic challenge of thoracoabdominal stab wounds. *J Trauma Acute Care Surg.* 2014;76(2):418-423.

26. Schnuriger B, Talving P, Barbarino R, Barmparas G, Inaba K, Demetriades D. Current practice and the role of the CT in the management of penetrating liver injuries at a Level I trauma center. *J Emerg Trauma Shock.* 2011;4(1):53-57.

27. Polanco PM, Brown JB, Puyana JC, Billiar TR, Peitzman AB, Sperry JL. The swinging pendulum: a national perspective of nonoperative management in severe blunt liver injury. *J Trauma Acute Care Surg.* 2013;75(4):590-595.

28. Swaid F, Peleg K, Alfici R, et al. Concomitant hollow viscus injuries in patients with blunt hepatic and splenic injuries: an analysis of a National Trauma Registry database. *Injury.* 2014;45(9):1409-1412.

29. Nance ML, Peden GW, Shapiro ML, Kauder DR, Rotondo MF, Schwab CW. Solid viscus injury predicts major hollow viscus injury in blunt abdominal trauma. *J Trauma.* 1997;43(4):618-622, discussion 622-623.

30. Carrillo EH, Wohltmann C, Richardson JD, Polk HC Jr. Evolution in the treatment of complex blunt liver injuries. *Curr Probl Surg.* 2001;38(1):1-60.

31. Ball CG, Dente CJ, Shaz B, et al. The impact of a massive transfusion protocol (1:1:1) on major hepatic injuries: does it increase abdominal wall closure rates? *Can J Surg.* 2013;56(5):E128-E134.

32. Holcomb JB, Tilley BC, Baraniuk S, et al. Transfusion of plasma, platelets, and red blood cells in a 1:1:1 vs a 1:1:2 ratio and mortality in patients with severe trauma: the PROPPR randomized clinical trial. *JAMA.* 2015;313(5):471-482.

33. Campion EM, Pritts TA, Dorlac WC, et al. Implementation of a military-derived damage-control resuscitation strategy in a civilian trauma center decreases acute hypoxia in massively transfused patients. *J Trauma Acute Care Surg.* 2013;75(2 suppl 2):S221-S227.

34. Peitzman AB, Marsh JW. Advanced operative techniques in the management of complex liver injury. *J Trauma Acute Care Surg.* 2012;73(3):765-770.

35. Uranus S, Mischinger HJ, Pfeifer J, et al. Hemostatic methods for the management of spleen and liver injuries. *World J Surg.* 1996;20(8):1107-1111, discussion 1111-1112.

36. Pringle JH. V. Notes on the arrest of hepatic hemorrhage due to trauma. *Ann Surg.* 1908;48(4):541-549.

37. Ciraulo DL, Luk S, Palter M, et al. Selective hepatic arterial embolization of grade IV and V blunt hepatic injuries: an extension of resuscitation in the nonoperative management of traumatic hepatic injuries. *J Trauma.* 1998;45(2):353-358, discussion 358-359.

38. Wahl WL, Ahrns KS, Brandt MM, Franklin GA, Taheri PA. The need for early angiographic embolization in blunt liver injuries. *J Trauma.* 2002;52(6):1097-1101.

39. Carrillo EH, Spain DA, Wohltmann CD, et al. Interventional techniques are useful adjuncts in nonoperative management of hepatic injuries. *J Trauma.* 1999;46(4):619-622, discussion 622-624.

40. Green CS, Bulger EM, Kwan SW. Outcomes and complications of angioembolization for hepatic trauma: a systematic review of the literature. *J Trauma Acute Care Surg.* 2016;80(3):529-537.

41. Letoublon C, Morra I, Chen Y, Monnin V, Voirin D, Arvieux C. Hepatic arterial embolization in the management of blunt hepatic trauma: indications and complications. *J Trauma.* 2011;70(5):1032-1036, discussion 1036-1037.

42. Poggetti RS, Moore EE, Moore FA, Mitchell ME, Read RA. Balloon tamponade for bilobar transfixing hepatic gunshot wounds. *J Trauma.* 1992;33(5):694-697.

43. Ball CG, Wyrzykowski AD, Nickolas JM, Rozycki GS, Feliciano DV. A decade's experience with balloon catheter tamponade for the emergency control of hemorrhage. *J Trauma.* 2011;70(2):330-333.

44. Stone HH, Lamb JM. Use of pedicled omentum as an autogenous pack for control of hemorrhage in major injuries of the liver. *Surg Gynecol Obstet.* 1975;141(1):92-94.

45. Ciresi KF, Lim RC Jr. Hepatic vein and retrohepatic vena caval injury. *World J Surg.* 1990;14(4):472-477.

46. Cogbill TH, Moore EE, Jurkovich GJ, Feliciano DV, Morris JA, Mucha P. S vere hepatic trauma: a multi-center experience with 1,335 liver injuries. *J Trauma.* 1988;28(10):1433-1438.

47. David Richardson J, Franklin GA, Lukan JK, et al. Evolution in the management of hepatic trauma: a 25-year perspective. *Ann Surg.* 2000;232(3):324-330.

48. Carrillo EH, Spain DA, Miller FB, Richardson JD. Intrahepatic vascular clamping in complex hepatic vein injuries. *J Trauma.* 1997;43(1):131-133.

49. Briggs CS, Morcos OC, Moriera CC, Gupta N. Endovascular treatment of iatrogenic injury to the retrohepatic inferior vena cava. *Ann Vasc Surg.* 2014;28(7):1794.e13-1794.e15.

50. Mizuno S, Yagihara M, Tanemura A, et al. An approach to the intra-thoracic inferior vena cava through the abdominal cavity preparing for total hepatic vascular exclusion by sagittal diaphragmotomy. *Hepatogastroenterology.* 2013;60(126):1409-1412.

51. Carmona RH, Peck DZ, Lim RC Jr. The role of packing and planned reoperation in severe hepatic trauma. *J Trauma.* 1984;24(9):779-784.

52. Cue JI, Cryer HG, Miller FB, Richardson JD, Polk HC Jr. Packing and planned reexploration for hepatic and retroperitoneal hemorrhage: critical refinements of a useful technique. *J Trauma.* 1990;30(8):1007-1011, discussion 1011-1013.

53. Feliciano DV, Mattox KL, Jordan GL Jr. Intra-abdominal packing for control of hepatic hemorrhage: a reappraisal. *J Trauma.* 1981;21(4):285-290.

54. Rotondo MF, Schwab CW, McGonigal MD, et al. 'Damage control': an approach for improved survival in exsanguinating penetrating abdominal injury. *J Trauma.* 1993;35(3):375-382, discussion 382-383.

55. Garrison JR, Richardson JD, Hilakos AS, et al. Predicting the need to pack early for severe intra-abdominal hemorrhage. *J Trauma.* 1996;40(6):923-927, discussion 927-929.

56. Barker DE, Kaufman HJ, Smith LA, Ciraulo DL, Richart CL, Burns RP. Vacuum pack technique of temporary abdominal closure: a 7-year experience with 112 patients. *J Trauma.* 2000;48(2):201-206, discussion 206-207.

57. Open Abdomen Advisory P, Campbell A, Chang M, et al. Management of the open abdomen: from initial operation to definitive closure. *Am Surg.* 2009;75(11 suppl):S1-S22.

58. Goldman R, Zilkoski M, Mullins R, Mayberry J, Deveney C, Trunkey D. Delayed celiotomy for the treatment of bile leak, compartment syndrome, and other hazards of nonoperative management of blunt liver injury. *Am J Surg.* 2003;185(5):492-497.

59. Carrillo EH, Richardson JD. Delayed surgery and interventional procedures in complex liver injuries. *J Trauma.* 1999;46(5):978.

60. Franklin GA, Richardson JD, Brown AL, et al. Prevention of bile peritonitis by laparoscopic evacuation and lavage after nonoperative treatment of liver injuries. *Am Surg.* 2007;73(6):611-616, discussion 616-617.

61. Glaser K, Wetscher G, Pointner R, et al. Traumatic bilhemia. *Surgery.* 1994;116(1):24-27.

62. Snell K, Skandarajah AR, Knowles B, Judson R, Thomson BN. Changes in the management of liver trauma leading to reduced mortality: 15-year experience in a major trauma centre. *ANZ J Surg.* 2016;86(11):894-899.

63. Jaggard MK, Johal NS, Choudhry M. Blunt abdominal trauma resulting in gallbladder injury: a review with emphasis on pediatrics. *J Trauma.* 2011;70(4):1005-1010.

64. Feliciano DV, Bitondo CG, Burch JM, Mattox KL, Beall AC Jr, Jordan GL Jr. Management of traumatic injuries to the extrahepatic biliary duct. *Am J Surg.* 1985;150(6):705-709.

Diagnostic Operation of the Liver and Techniques of Hepatic Resection

Alessandro Paniccia | Richard D. Schulick

LIVER BIOPSY

PERCUTANEOUS AND TRANSJUGULAR LIVER BIOPSY

Liver biopsy was originally described by Ehrlich in 1883 to determine glycogen stores in patients with diabetes.[1] A variety of approaches and techniques have been described for performing liver biopsy, including percutaneous, transjugular, laparoscopic, and open techniques.

For focal lesions, percutaneous liver biopsies are often conducted under image guidance either with the use of ultrasound, computed tomography (CT), or magnetic resonance imaging (MRI). The goal of percutaneous biopsy is to obtain a core of tissue with good preservation of the underlying hepatic architecture.

The presence of significant ascites or underlying coagulopathy is a relative contraindication to percutaneous biopsy. In this scenario a transjugular biopsy may be necessary. However, transjugular biopsies are best used for large and easily targetable lesions and are of limited use for small focal lesions because of the inability to accurately place the needle. Furthermore, the amount of tissue obtained is often smaller and more fragmented compared with percutaneous core needle biopsies, making pathologic assessment more difficult.

If multiple percutaneous attempts have failed to obtain adequate material, if there is suspicion that a liver lesion is highly vascularized and prone to bleeding, if there is a need to obtain tissue from multiple sites, or if it is otherwise preferable to biopsy the liver under direct vision, then either laparoscopic or open liver biopsy may be used.

LAPAROSCOPY AND BIOPSY

Laparoscopy examination of the liver consists of visual inspection, palpation (using standard laparoscopic instruments is possible to appreciate any parenchymal nodularity or change in tissue consistency), and tissue biopsy. Superficial lesions can be biopsied under direct visualization using cupped biopsy forceps, whereas deeper lesions might require laparoscopic ultrasound guidance and the use of percutaneous core needle biopsy devices. The authors recommend performing core needle biopsy rather than fine-needle aspiration (FNA) because the former allows for the identification of the architectural structure of the underlying liver parenchyma and often delivers more reliable results compared with FNA. In addition, the direct laparoscopic visualization of the liver parenchyma allows for quick identification and treatment of any potential bleeding complications caused by a large needle biopsy.

Preoperative laparoscopy, as a diagnostic tool in hepatobiliary malignancies, has been discussed extensively during the past two decades. Although no definitive consensus has been achieved, with the improvement of modern radiographic imaging modalities its role appears to be limited to select cases. A particular case is represented by gallbladder and hilar cholangiocarcinoma where the yield of staging laparoscopy and ultrasonography is relatively high and the value of surgical palliation is relatively low, thus arguing in favor of laparoscopic staging in order to prevent an unnecessary laparotomy.

OPEN LIVER BIOPSY AND EXAMINATION

An open liver biopsy can be performed through a limited right subcostal incision. The incision should be placed over the inferior edge of the liver but should be at least 3 cm below the costal margin to allow for adequate fascial closure. The liver can be examined both visually and by palpation, but care should be taken to not disturb any portosystemic collateral vessels. If these friable vessels are disrupted, or if the hepatic capsule is ruptured during examination, a major abdominal operation may be required to gain control. Visual inspection for gross evidence of cirrhosis, nodularity, abnormal color or texture, or neoplasm may be revealing. A laparoscopic ultrasound probe can be used through a small incision, or, if the incision is large enough, the regular probe may be used. A wedge biopsy can be obtained using a No. 15 scalpel and removing a specimen measuring 1 cm at its base. A core needle biopsy can be obtained through the same site, directed deeper into the liver parenchyma but away from the porta hepatis. If significant bleeding is expected, hemostatic 2-0 chromic catgut or Vicryl mattress sutures can be placed in an interlock V shape outside the biopsy site prior to biopsy. After the biopsies are taken, the base of the biopsy site is treated with the argon beam coagulator for hemostasis. The fascia should be closed with running permanent suture if ascites is anticipated. Similarly, the skin should be closed with a running long-lasting suture if ascites is anticipated.

INCISION FOR LIVER OPERATIONS

SUBCOSTAL APPROACH

Most hepatectomies can be accomplished via a right subcostal incision made 3 to 4 cm below the right costal margin with an upper midline extension in a supine patient. The right rectus abdominis muscle is completely divided, as are the medial portions of the external oblique, internal oblique, and transversus abdominis muscles.

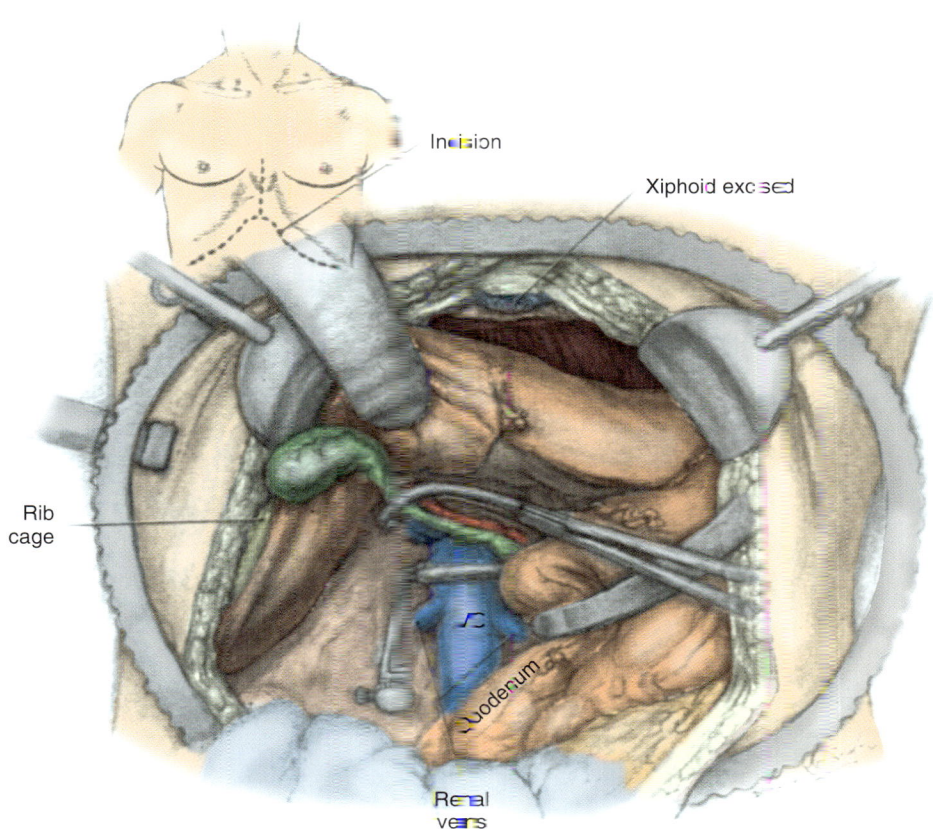

Incision

Xiphoid excised

Rib cage

Duodenum

Renal veins

FIGURE 124.1 Bilateral subcostal incision with a short midline extension. This is a versatile incision appropriate for most major hepatic resections and portosystemic shunts. *VC,* Vena cava.

Depending on the exposure required, the incision can be made up to and beyond the midaxillary line between the costal margin and the iliac bone. This incision exposes the anterior and inferior surfaces of the right and left liver and provides good access to the porta hepatis. For exposure of the dome of the liver, a midline extension over and above the xiphoid is performed and the xiphoid removed. For even more exposure, the incision can be extended under the left subcosta area (Figs. 124.1 and 124.2). With this full incision, the surgeon has excellent exposure to the entire upper abdomen, including the liver as well as the retrohepatic and suprahepatic inferior vena cava (IVC). Because of the appearance when closed, this incision is often referred to as the *Mercedes incision.*

In extreme circumstances, a median sternotomy or right thoracotomy through the costal margin can even further increase access and exposure.

MIDLINE APPROACH

The midline incision can be used in thin patients, especially when a pelvic procedure, such as a low anterior resection, is being performed at the same time, or if the hepatic resection will be limited to the left half of the liver. The patient is positioned supine. This approach does not generally allow good access to the retrohepatic vena cava, the right hepatic vein, or the right posterior sector of the liver until the liver is completely mobilized off the diaphragm and retroperitoneum. It is commonly used in exploration for trauma where hepatic injury may be found.

If greater exposure is required, a median sternotomy or right thoracotomy through the costal margin can be performed.

RIGHT THORACOABDOMINAL APPROACH

The thoracoabdominal incision is sometimes used in patients with large bulky lesions involving the right dome or right posterior section of the liver. It gives the best access to the suprahepatic and retrohepatic vena cava, as well as the right hepatic vein. In addition, it is sometimes used in instances of significant right diaphragmatic involvement. The patient is positioned on a bean bag with the chest in a lateral position but the hips at 45 degrees. The incision is made from the umbilicus to the right costal margin, and, depending on the location of the lesion, the seventh, eight, or even ninth rib interspace is opened. If keeping the right lung unventilated will help, then a double-lumen endotracheal tube should be used. The diaphragm should be incised circumferentially to avoid the neurovascular bundle supplying it. Care should be taken to leave 3 to 4 cm of diaphragm on the rib cage to allow for later closure.

MORPHOLOGIC AND FUNCTIONAL ANATOMY

The morphologic and functional anatomy of the liver has been discussed and revised for more than a century, and it is paramount that the surgeon performing any hepatic resection is intimately familiar with the most current anatomic understanding and most recent nomenclature.[2–5]

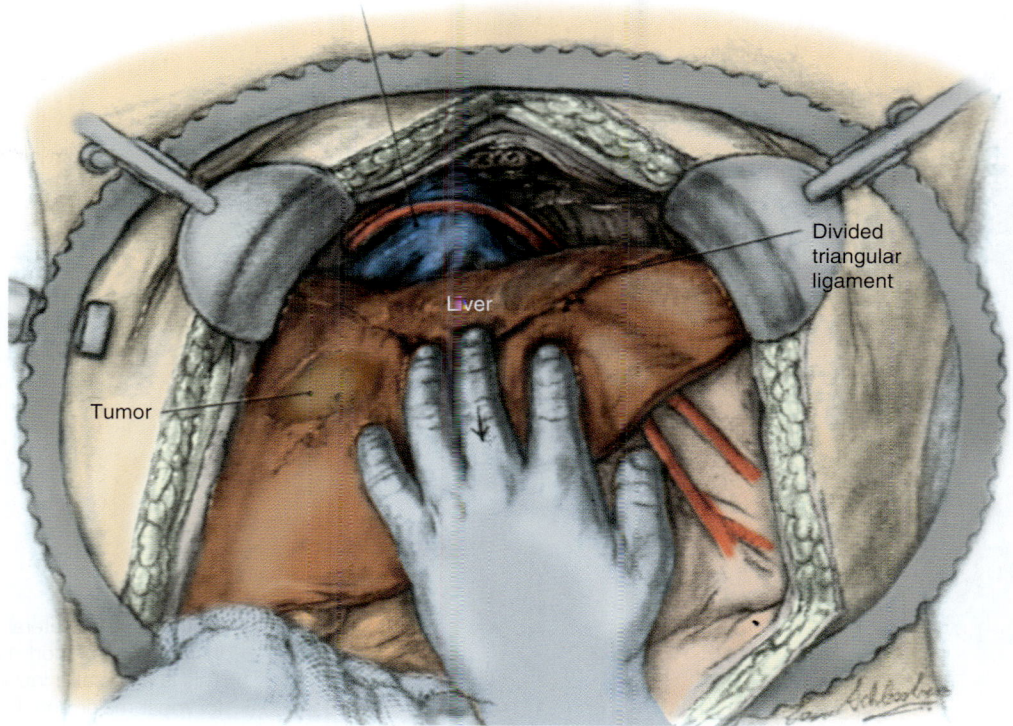

Suprahepatic inferior vena cava and right, middle, and left hepatic veins

Liver

Divided triangular ligament

Tumor

FIGURE 124.2 Mercedes sign incision. Excision of the xiphoid process and downward traction on the liver provide excellent exposure of the hepatic veins and suprahepatic inferior vena cava.

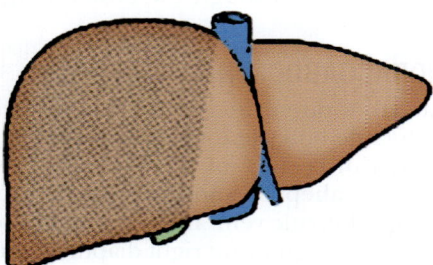

FIGURE 124.3 The liver can be divided into right and left halves by forming a plane through the gallbladder fossa (Cantlie line) and inferior vena cava. (From Blumgart LH, Fong Y. *Surgery of the Liver and Biliary Tract: Selected Operative Procedures.* CD-ROM, 3rd ed. London: Harcourt; 2000.)

Historically, the liver anatomy has been defined by morphologic landmarks visible on the liver surface. As such, the liver can be divided into right and left halves by forming a plane through the gallbladder fossa (Cantlie line) and the IVC (specifically at its junction with the middle hepatic vein, when visible) (Fig. 124.3).[6] Furthermore, the left half of the liver can be further subdivided into a left medial section and left lateral section, based on the location of the umbilical fissure and the falciform ligament. In addition, the caudate of the liver is identified as lying posterior to the gastrohepatic ligament and

emanating from a process of liver situated posterior to the main portal pedicle and anterior to the IVC.

The need for an understanding of the liver's functional anatomy has led to the acceptance of division of the liver anatomy based on the vascular watershed area rather than purely based on liver surface landmarks. As such, the most widely accepted nomenclature of liver anatomy is based on Couinaud's description of eight discrete anatomic segments of the liver (Fig. 124.4). Therefore, in addition to surface anatomy (i.e., Cantlie line, umbilical fissure, and falciform ligament), the eight segments of the liver are determined using the location of the three main hepatic veins and the location of the portal pedicle bifurcation. The right and left halves of the liver are delineated by a plane through the middle hepatic vein and IVC. Segment II, III, and IV lie to the left of this plane and form the left half of the liver. Segments V, VI, VII, and VIII lie to the right of this plane and form the right half of the liver. Segment I, or the caudate, is morphologically distinct from the two halves of the liver and emanates from a process of liver lying posterior to the portal pedicle and anterior to the IVC. The right and left halves of the liver derive blood supply from the corresponding right and left portal veins and hepatic arteries, respectively, whereas segment I derives blood from both. In addition, the right half of the liver has venous drainage mostly through the right and middle hepatic vein, and the left half of the liver has drainage mostly through the left and

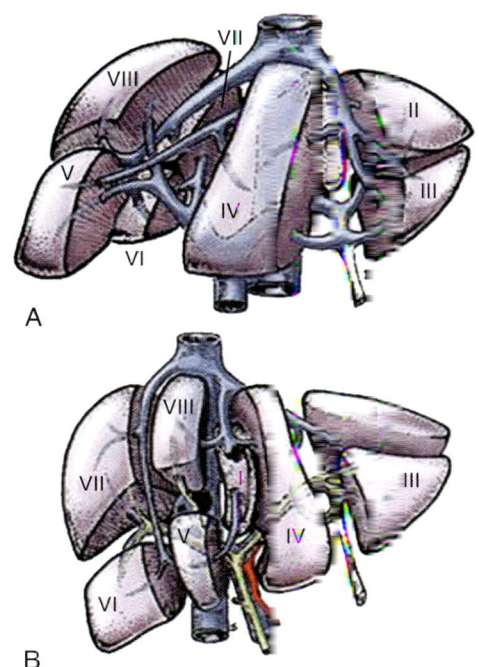

FIGURE 124.4 Couinaud's eight anatomic segments of the liver: anterior (A) and posterior (B) views. *From Blumgart LH, Fong Y. Surgery of the Liver and Biliary Tract Selected Operative Procedures.* CD-ROM, 3rd ed. London: Harcourt 2000.)

middle hepatic veins. However segment I drains directly via small branches into the IVC.

The right half of the liver can be further subdivided using a plane through the right hepatic vein and the IVC. The liver anterior to this plane forms the right anterior sector of the liver, and liver posterior to this plane forms the right posterior sector. The right anterior sector of the liver comprises segment V (caudal to the bifurcation) and segment VIII (cephalad to the portal bifurcation). The right posterior sector of the liver comprises segment VI (caudal to the portal bifurcation) and segment VII (cephalad to the portal bifurcation).

The left half of the liver can be further subdivided using a plane through the umbilical fissure and falciform ligament. Liver medial to this plane forms the left medial section of the liver or segment IV, and liver lateral to this plane forms the left lateral section of the liver. The left lateral section of the liver is further subdivided into segment II (closer to segment I) and segment III (closer to segment IV), which are supplied by separate portal pedicles from the umbilical fissure.

PREOPERATIVE EVALUATION OF HEPATIC RESERVE

A functional liver remnant (FLR) must be ensured at the end of every liver resection; as such, fundamental principles of liver resection require ensuring appropriate hepatic arterial and portal venous inflow, adequate venous outflow, and biliary drainage in continuity with the small bowel.

TABLE 124.1 Child-Pugh Classification*

Parameter	Score 1	2	3
Bilirubin (mg/dL)	<2	2–3	>3
Albumin (g/dL)	>3.5	2.8–3.5	<2.8
Ascites	Absent	Moderate	Severe
Encephalopathy	Absent	Moderate	Severe
PROTHROMBIN TIME			
Seconds prolonged	<4	4–6	>6
INR	<1.7	1.7–2.3	>2.3

*The Child-Pugh classification: grade A = 5–6 points; grade B = 7–9 points; grade C = 10–15 points.
INR, International normalized ratio.

Therefore, when proper hepatic inflow and outflow are secured, up to 70% to 75% of hepatic volume can be resected in patients with relatively normal hepatic parenchyma (without active hepatitis, cirrhosis, or metabolic derangements). Several different strategies have been described to predict hepatic reserve; however, many hepatobiliary centers in the United States commonly rely on the two following strategies:

- Child-Pugh score that assesses hepatic synthetic ability (albumin, prothrombin time, and ascites), bile excretory function (total bilirubin), and metabolic function (changes in mental status from ammonia retention) (Table 124.1).[7]
- Volumetric measurements of the liver and predicted liver remnant after resection based on three-dimensional reconstruction from CT scan and MRI.[8]

When the predicted FLR is inadequate, a technique of portal vein embolization to the right or left half of the liver can be used to generate a compensatory hypertrophy of the future liver remnant prior to resection. However, following embolization, the liver requires approximately 4 to 6 weeks to reach an adequate hypertrophic response.[9-11]

Another available strategy is associating liver partition and portal vein ligation for staged hepatectomy (ALPPS) because this technique produces a rapid increase of the FLR, usually within 7 to 14 days. A key aspect is that the liver partition results in ligation of the bridging veins between the two hemilivers and therefore truly isolates the future specimen from the liver remnant.[12-14] However, the ALPPS technique remains at the center of a heated debate due to its associated complications, between 7% and 36%, among which the most common are sepsis and bile leak.[15-16] The indications for ALPPS are still being debated; however, its best outcomes are seen in patients with colorectal liver metastasis and in patients ≤60 years of age.[5] Nevertheless, portal vein embolization is still the preferred method to obtain hypertrophy of the FLR, and additional studies are needed to properly delineate the role of ALPPS. Particular attention should be given to patient undergoing preoperative chemotherapy, such as in the setting of metastatic colorectal cancer. In fact, modern chemotherapeutic agents are associated with considerable liver toxicity. Two of the most common chemotherapeutic agents including oxaliplatin and irinotecan are associated with sinusoidal congestion and

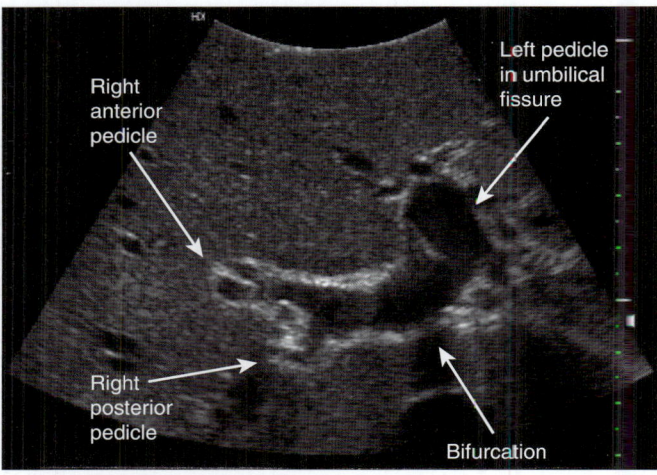

FIGURE 124.5 Intraoperative ultrasound image of bifurcation of the main portal pedicle into the right and left branches.

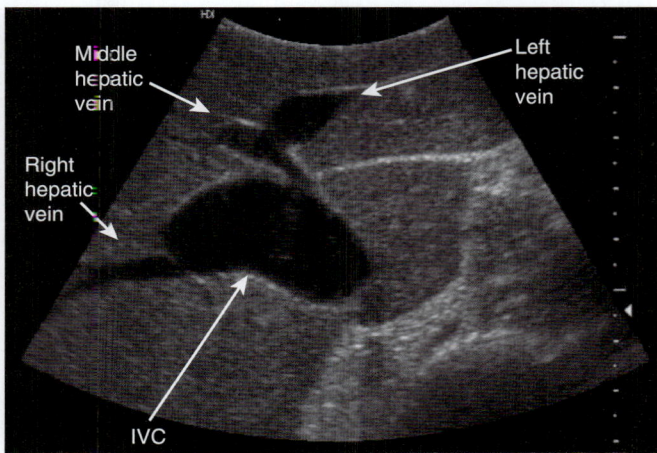

FIGURE 124.6 Intraoperative ultrasound image of the three main hepatic veins. The left and middle hepatic veins often join together before emptying into the inferior vena cava *(IVC)*.

steatohepatitis, respectively.[18] Therefore thorough understanding of the underlying metabolic status of the liver parenchyma is of primary importance to appropriately define the extent of hepatic resection that will guarantee an adequate FLR. A common rule of thumb is to consider adequate an FLR of greater than or equal to 25% of total liver volume in patients with healthy liver. However, patients with chronic liver disease but without cirrhosis require an FLR of at least greater than or equal to 30%, whereas patients with cirrhosis but without portal hypertension require an FLR of at least 40%.[19,20]

INTRAOPERATIVE ASSESSMENT

Intraoperative assessment of the liver allows the surgeon to identify unrecognized lesions missed by preoperative imaging, to delineate the plane of resection and proximity to the index lesions, and to identify any aberrant anatomy. Intraoperative ultrasonography is of incommensurable value and each hepatobiliary surgeon should be intimately familiar with its application.

Mobilization of the liver is often required if the surgeon's intent is to perform a thorough bimanual examination or a diagnostic intraoperative ultrasonography evaluation.

Ultrasonography evaluation begins with the identification of the main portal pedicle within the hepatoduodenal ligament. This is followed cephalad to the portal bifurcation to the main right and left pedicles. It is key to understand that the portal pedicles are invested with the Glisson capsule and have a very echogenic covering, which is in contrast to hepatic vein branches. The main portal pedicle is followed toward the right, where it gives off an anterior and posterior branch (Fig. 124.5). The right anterior branch gives off separate pedicles to segment V (caudal) and to segment VIII (cephalad). The right posterior branch gives off separate pedicles to segment VI (caudal) and to segment VII (cephalad). The main left pedicle is usually much longer and courses intact to the base of the umbilical fissure before branching into various segmental pedicles. At the base of the umbilical fissure, the main left pedicle courses anteriorly toward the round ligament

and gives off a pedicle to segment IV medially and pedicle to segments II and III laterally. Next, if the bare areas around the junction of the hepatic veins and IVC have been well mobilized, the hepatic veins can easily be visualized using intraoperative ultrasonography (Fig. 124.6). As described previously, usually a larger right hepatic vein can be delineated, and smaller left and middle hepatic veins joining into a common trunk before emptying into the IVC are seen. Commonly, an umbilical hepatic vein branch can be identified coursing between the middle and left hepatic veins and running under the falciform ligament. Not uncommonly, significant accessory right hepatic veins can be seen emptying from the posterior surface of the right liver directly into the IVC as it courses posterior to the liver. The identification of these accessory right hepatic veins is quite important for both vascular control and preservation of outflow from the liver. Finally, the hepatic parenchyma is systematically scanned to identify lesions within the liver.

GENERAL MANEUVERS FOR HEPATECTOMY

The porta hepatis can be dissected to identify the main bifurcation of the hepatic artery, bile duct, and portal vein and to allow individual ligation of these structures. Ligation of the hepatic artery and portal vein to one side causes the liver parenchyma to demarcate between the right and left liver. Greater exposure of the cephalad aspect of the hepatic hilum and exposure of a high or intraparenchymal bifurcation of the portal triad structures may be aided by lowering the hilar plate (Fig. 124.7) and dividing the Glisson capsule at the most inferior border of segment IV. Control of the inflow hepatic artery and portal vein branches to a specific anatomic section of the liver may also be obtained by pedicle ligation in which small hepatotomies are made around the main right pedicle, main left pedicle, right anterior pedicle, or right posterior pedicle after identification with ultrasound (Fig. 124.8).[21] The pedicle of interest can be dissected out bluntly with a right angle or by finger fracture. The pedicle should be test clamped atraumatically to confirm that it does indeed

Segment IV

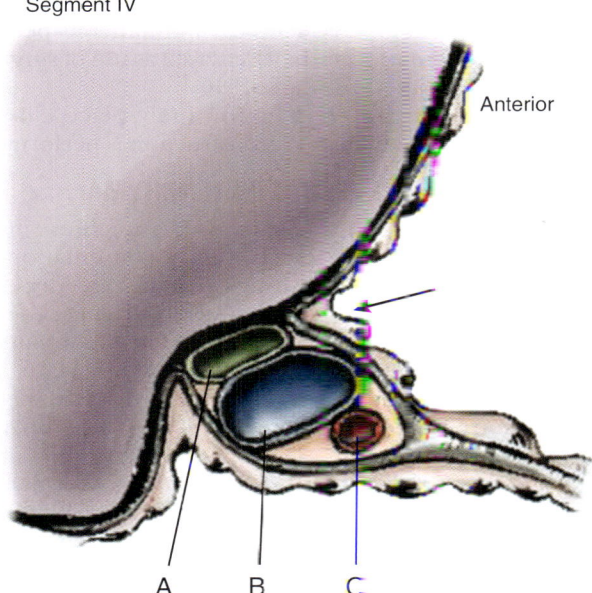

Anterior

FIGURE 124.7 The hilar plate of the liver can be "lowered" by dividing the Glisson capsule at the lowest edge of segment IV. This maneuver gains access to the most cephalad portion of the bifurcation of the porta hepatis. (A) Left hepatic duct. (B) Portal vein. (C) Hepatic artery. (Modified from Blumgart LH, Fong Y. *Surgery of the Liver and Biliary Tract: Selected Operative Procedures*. CD-ROM, 3rd ed. London: Harcourt; 2000.)

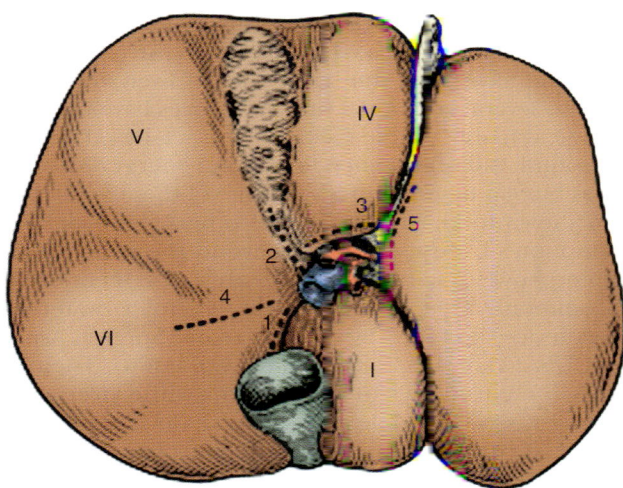

FIGURE 124.8 Sites for intraparenchymal portal pedicle ligation. Incisions at *1* and *2* allow isolation of the main right pedicle. Incisions at *1* and *4* allow isolation of the right posterior pedicle. Incisions at *2* and *4* allow isolation of the right anterior pedicle. Incisions at *3* and *5* allow isolation of the left pedicle. (From Fong Y, Blumgart LH. Useful stapling techniques in liver surgery. *J Am Coll Surg.* 1997;185:93.)

supply the area of liver of interest. If the proper pedicle is clamped, the appropriate portion of the liver (i.e., right half, left half, right anterior section, right posterior section) should demarcate. Once confirmed, it can be divided. Alternatively, the specific inflow pedicles can be divided

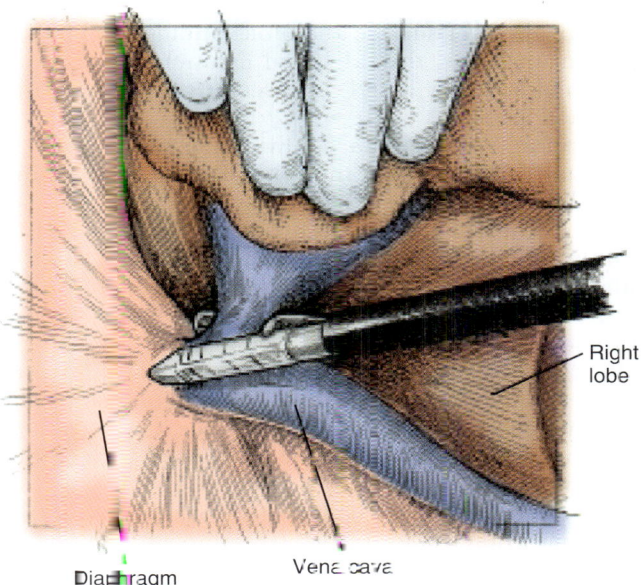

Right lobe

Diaphragm   Vena cava

FIGURE 124.9 The right hepatic vein can be divided with the aid of an endoscopic stapling device with a vascular load. (From Fong Y, Blumgart LH. Useful stapling techniques in liver surgery. *J Am Coll Surg.* 1997;185:93.)

as they are encountered during parenchymal transection. With this technique, hemorrhage can be minimized by intermittent portal inflow occlusion accomplished by atraumatically clamping the main portal triad within the hepatoduodenal ligament (Pringle maneuver).

Outflow control of the hepatic veins can be obtained at different time points, depending on the situation. If there is a sufficient length of extraparenchymal hepatic vein often it is easier to divide the hepatic vein early and prior to parenchymal transection (but after inflow control). If the extraparenchymal portion of the hepatic vein is short (or absent), it may be easier and safer to divide the hepatic vein or veins within the hepatic parenchyma after most of the parenchymal transection has been performed. The use of endoscopic vascular stapling devices has made the ligation of the hepatic veins whether extraparenchymally or intraparenchymally much quicker and safer (Fig. 124.9).[21] Another technique used to minimize blood loss is a low central venous pressure technique in which the central venous pressure of the patient is kept low (<5 mm Hg) until after parenchymal transection.[22] After the parenchymal transection is completed and the bleeding is controlled, the patient is made euvolemic. This minimizes the bleeding coming from hepatic vein branches.

MAJOR HEPATECTOMIES

To understand the different types of hepatectomies, one must be familiar with the hepatic anatomy and nomenclature. A great effort was made by the International Hepato-Pancreato-Biliary Association in the Brisbane 2000 Nomenclature of Hepatic Anatomy and Resections to unify and standardize the terminology in the field of hepatic surgery.[23]

This new terminology transitions from a nomenclature driven by the liver surface anatomic landmarks (i.e., the ligamentum teres, the falciform ligament) to a more functional anatomy based on vascular distribution and watershed areas.

Therefore the liver can be divided in two hemilivers (right and left) based on the vertical plane intersecting the gallbladder fossa and the IVC.

The Couinaud classification remains largely used to identify the different segments of the liver (i.e., I to VIII) and a major liver resection is still defined as the resection of three or more contiguous segments based on the aforementioned classification.

Right hepatectomy or right hemihepatectomy involves the resection of segment V through VIII; left hepatectomy or left hemihepatectomy involves the resection of segment II through IV. Segment I may or may not be included in either of these resections.

Extended right hepatectomy (also known as right trisectionectomy) involves the resection of segment IV through VIII; extended left hepatectomy (also known as left trisectionectomy) involves the resection of segment II through V plus VIII. Again either of these extended resections may or may not include resection of segment I.

Right anterior sectionectomy includes segment V and VIII. Right posterior sectionectomy includes segment VI and VII. Left medial sectionectomy removes segment IV. Left lateral sectionectomy includes segments II and III. A segmentectomy involves the resection of a single segment, and a bisegmentectomy involves the resection of two contiguous segments.

In general, there are four key steps involved in major hepatectomies; these consist of optimal exposure, vascular inflow control, vascular outflow control, and parenchymal transection.

Vascular inflow control may be obtained by directly ligating the main right or left branches of the hepatic artery and portal vein in the hilum and/or by intermittent 10- to 20-minute intervals of a Pringle maneuver with 3 minutes in between to reestablish blood flow. The authors prefer to encircle the hepatoduodenal ligament twice with a $\frac{1}{4}$-inch Penrose drain that is tightened and clamped for a Pringle maneuver. Alternatively, pedicle ligation can be performed as described previously, or the pedicle can be controlled as they are encountered during parenchymal transection. The authors prefer to obtain vascular inflow control by ligating the appropriate vessels in the hilum or by pedicle ligations and to supplement this with intermittent Pringle maneuvers as necessary during parenchymal transection for hemihepatectomies. Vascular outflow to the right or left liver can be obtained by exposing and ligating the hepatic veins as previously described or by ligating the vessels intraparenchymally during transection of the tissue.

The routine use of closed-suction drains after a major hepatectomy remains controversial because no definitive decrease in postoperative intervention has been consistently shown.[24,25] Furthermore, a series from the Memorial Sloan Kettering Cancer Center reviewed 2173 hepatectomies and found that symptomatic perihepatic collections (SPHCs) developed in only 200 cases (9% of patients), and in one-third were nonbilious and noninfected. On multivariate analysis, major hepatic resections, greater than median blood loss (>360 mL), simultaneous performance of colorectal procedure use, as well as use of surgical drains were associated with an SPHC.[26]

The authors of this chapter routinely place closed-suction drainage when biliary reconstruction is performed.

TRANSECTING THE HEPATIC PARENCHYMA

Several different techniques are used to achieve liver parenchymal transection; most often a combination of different techniques is used during the same case, depending on the surgeon's preference and experience, tumor location within the liver parenchyma, and need for margin clearance. Regardless of the method used, certain key principles must be adhered to. These include safety, speed, minimization of blood loss, and avoidance of significant liver injury.

It is good practice to identify the plane of liver parenchymal transection and to demarcate the area of interest by incising the liver capsule with the use of electrocautery. This will not only facilitate parenchymal transection but will also provide an easily visible reference on the liver surface to orient the surgeon along the resection boundaries.

The most classic approach to liver parenchyma transection consists of digitoclasy (also known as finger fracture technique) or clamp crushing technique; both these techniques allow for fracture of the liver parenchyma while sparing vessels and bile ducts encountered along the transection plane. These tubular structures are then controlled with a variety of approaches, including suture ligation metal clips placement, energy device, or stapling device application, according to vessel size and to surgeon's preference. Although the digitoclasy and the clamp crush technique have been the backbones of liver surgery for decades, several additional surgical devices have currently become available. These include water jet–based devices, ultrasound, radiofrequency, microwave energy devices, as well as bipolar devices; however, none of these devices has been shown to be superior to the others.[27–31] A detailed description of these devices is beyond the scope of this chapter; however, a few key points are worth mentioning.

Commonly used devices are the Hydrojet (water jet–based device) and the Cavitron Ultrasonic Surgical Aspirator (CUSA; Valleylab, Inc., Boulder, Colorado). Their use allows for parenchymal destruction while preserving crossing vessels and bile ducts. These devices allow for greater accuracy compared with the clamp-crushing technique and may increase the speed of dissection; however, they have poor to no hemostatic capacity.

Radiofrequency-based devices, including the TissueLink, Aquamantys, and Habib 4X, are considered hemostatic devices and can facilitate liver parenchymal transection, as they are able to rapidly coagulate the cut edge of the liver surface, requiring ligation of only larger vessels. Other devices able to achieve parenchymal coagulation include bipolar (i.e., LigaSure) and ultrasonic vessel-sealing device (i.e., Harmonic Scalpel); both devices are able to seal vessels up to 7 to 8 mm in diameter. In addition, the argon beam coagulator can be used to control diffuse blood oozing from the cut edge of the liver parenchyma.

An important transection technique is the use of stapling devices, especially in the setting of laparoscopic liver resection.[32] Stapling devices can be used to control large vessels crossing through the transection plane or alternatively can be used as the primary means of liver parenchymal transection.[38] In the latter scenario, a track along the liver parenchyma is usually created with the application of a large clamp and the parenchyma is then transected with serial application of the stapling device.

The operating surgeon should be mindful of the effect that the various available transection techniques have on the resection margins width and on the interpretation of margin positivity in the setting of oncologic resection. In fact, the use of nonablating techniques (digitoclasy, clamp crush technique), as opposed to ablative techniques such as the CUSA, Harmonic Scalpel Ligasure and Aquamantys, has been shown to have an impact on the importance of margin width and on the interpretation of margin positivity.[34-37] Hammond et al. conducted an experimental study comparing different surgical devices commonly used to accomplish liver parenchyma transection and concluded that the use of the CUSA was associated with a parenchymal ablation of approximately 7 mm at the edge of the transection that was greater than all the other tested devices.[38]

RIGHT HEPATECTOMY WITH HILAR DISSECTION

A right hepatectomy can usually be accomplished through a right subcostal incision with upper midline extension and involves resection of segments V, VI, VII, and VIII. If greater exposure of the left is required, a trifurcated incision can be used. The hepatic flexure of the colon is mobilized caudad. The round ligament and falciform ligament are divided. The right bare area of the liver is exposed by dividing the right triangular ligament. The right inferior liver edge is mobilized out of the retroperitoneum. This dissection reveals the upper pole of the right kidney, right adrenal gland, and suprahepatic IVC. The liver is then rotated to the left and the subhepatic IVC is dissected by controlling the small venous branches draining directly from the liver. Care must be given to the IVC ligament; this structure is often present and extends from the right liver and around the right side of the IVC just caudad to the right hepatic vein and occasionally contains liver parenchyma or a vein. This can be often controlled with an endoscopic stapler with a vascular load after it is dissected out. At this point the right hepatic vein can be identified and dissected out, whereupon a vessel loop can be placed around it. If dissection of the right hepatic vein is not safe at this time, it can be controlled later after parenchymal transection.

A cholecystectomy is then performed. The hepatic artery bifurcation is localized. The right hepatic artery is ligated. The common hepatic duct is then dissected and mobilized anteriorly and to the left to expose the portal vein (Fig. 124.10). Dissection is then continued into the hilum of the liver to expose the bifurcation of the portal vein. The right portal vein is circumferentially dissected (Fig. 124.11). Care should be taken to make sure that the left portal vein takeoff is clear of the dissection and that small branches draining the caudate are sufficiently controlled and divided. The right portal vein can be divided with ties using a reinforcing suture ligature on

the stump or with an endoscopic stapler with a vascular load. Hilar dissection is then completed by identifying and isolating the right hepatic duct, which is next ligated and divided.

The liver is then rotated to the left and the previously isolated right hepatic vein is divided between vascular clamps or an endoscopic stapler with a vascular load. If vascular clamps are used, the caval stump is closed with a running 4-0 Prolene suture and the specimen side simply suture ligated. Several minutes after the right hepatic artery and portal vein are ligated, the right liver should become devascularized and turn dusky. The Glisson capsule is then scored with an electrocautery device, starting at the level of the divided right hepatic vein to the gallbladder fossa on the anterior surface. If preservation of the middle hepatic vein is intended, then the line of transection should be moved slightly lateral. If the intention is to take the middle hepatic vein, then the line of transection should be moved medially. Intraoperative ultrasound should be used to carefully map this out. On the posterior surface of the liver, the liver is scored along the right lateral border of the IVC, toward the portal bifurcation. Parenchymal transection is then performed by any of the previously-described techniques. Intermittent portal inflow clamping as described previously, can be used to help decrease blood loss if this is a problem during parenchymal transection. During parenchymal transection vascular and biliary structures are controlled by the appropriate combination of clips, suture ligatures, and stapling devices. After the parenchyma is transected, the specimen can be removed.

LEFT HEPATECTOMY WITH HILAR DISSECTION

A left hepatectomy can also be accomplished through a right subcostal incision with an upper midline extension and involves resection of segments II, III, and IV. For large bulky tumors on the left or if the liver extends significantly laterally, a left subcostal component may be needed to trifurcate the incision. Alternatively, a midline incision can be used, but this may limit exposure to the right liver should unexpected findings be encountered during exploration. The round ligament and falciform ligament are divided. The left bare area is next exposed by dissection of the left triangular ligament. Usually the left hepatic vein and middle hepatic vein join together within the parenchyma of the liver before emptying into the IVC, which precludes extrahepatic dissection of these vessels without taking the middle hepatic vein. If it is separate and dissectible, a vessel loop is encircled around it. A cholecystectomy is performed. The lesser omentum is divided to fully expose the margins of the hepatoduodenal ligament. Care should be taken to note a replaced or accessory left hepatic artery running in this location. The proper hepatic artery is identified and dissected above the bifurcation of the right and left branches. The left hepatic artery is then divided.

The common hepatic duct is next exposed, and the left hepatic duct is then divided above the bifurcation. The left portal vein can then be identified at the base of segment IV and traced to the hilus of the liver. It is circumferentially dissected and can be ligated or controlled with an endoscopic stapler with a vascular load. The left

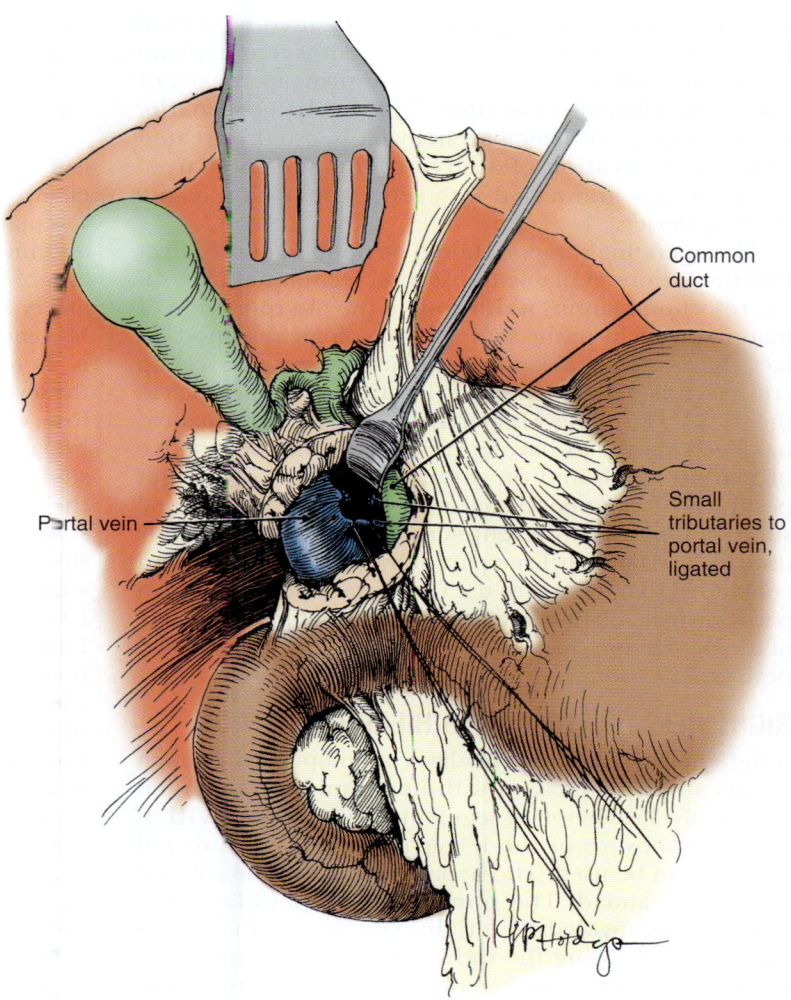

FIGURE 124.10 Right hepatectomy. Initial exposure of the portal vein before hilar ligation of its right branch is shown. The area to be dissected, closer to the hilus of the liver than shown, has no branches. (From Nora PE. *Operative Surgery: Principles and Techniques*. Philadelphia: Lea and Febiger; 1980:647.)

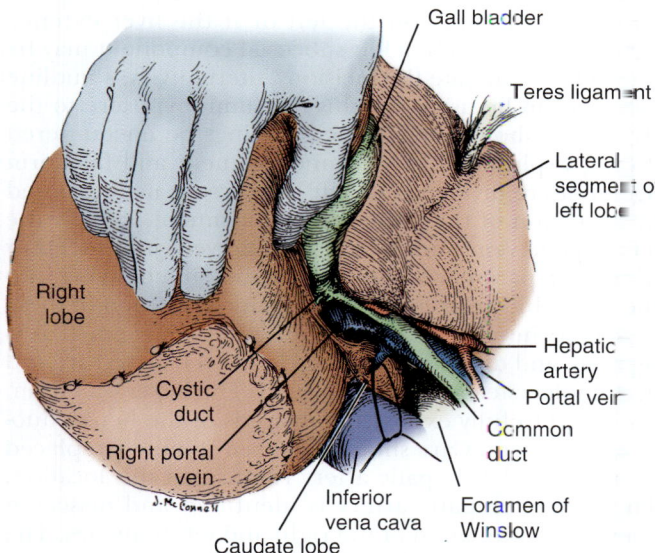

FIGURE 124.11 Right hepatectomy: Exposure of the right branch of the portal vein from the posterior approach. The liver has been retracted anteriorly and to the left. The looped ligature is around a branch to the caudate lobe. (From Starzl TE, Bell RH, Baert RV. Hepatic trisegmentectomy and other liver resections. *Surg Gynecol Obstet*. 1975;141:429.)

liver should become devascularized and become dusky. If the left hepatic vein was previously successfully dissected, then it can be divided with either ligatures or an endoscopic stapler with a vascular load. The anterior surface of the liver is then scored with the electrocautery device from the left hepatic vein (or stump) to the top of the gallbladder fossa. The posterior surface of the liver is then scored with the electrocautery device from the top of the gallbladder fossa to the portal bifurcation. If preservation of the middle hepatic vein is intended, then the line of transection should be moved slightly to the left; if the intention is to take the middle hepatic vein, then the line of transection should be moved to the right. Intraoperative ultrasound can be used to carefully map this out. Parenchymal transection is then performed by any of the previously described techniques. Intermittent portal inflow clamping as described previously can be used to help decrease blood loss if this is a problem during parenchymal transection. During parenchymal transection, vascular and biliary structures are controlled by the appropriate combination of clips, sutures, suture ligatures, and stapling devices. After the parenchyma is transected, the specimen can be removed (Fig. 124.12). If the caudate must also be removed to provide adequate tumor clearance, it can be mobilized off the IVC by sequentially dividing the short veins that directly drain into the IVC.

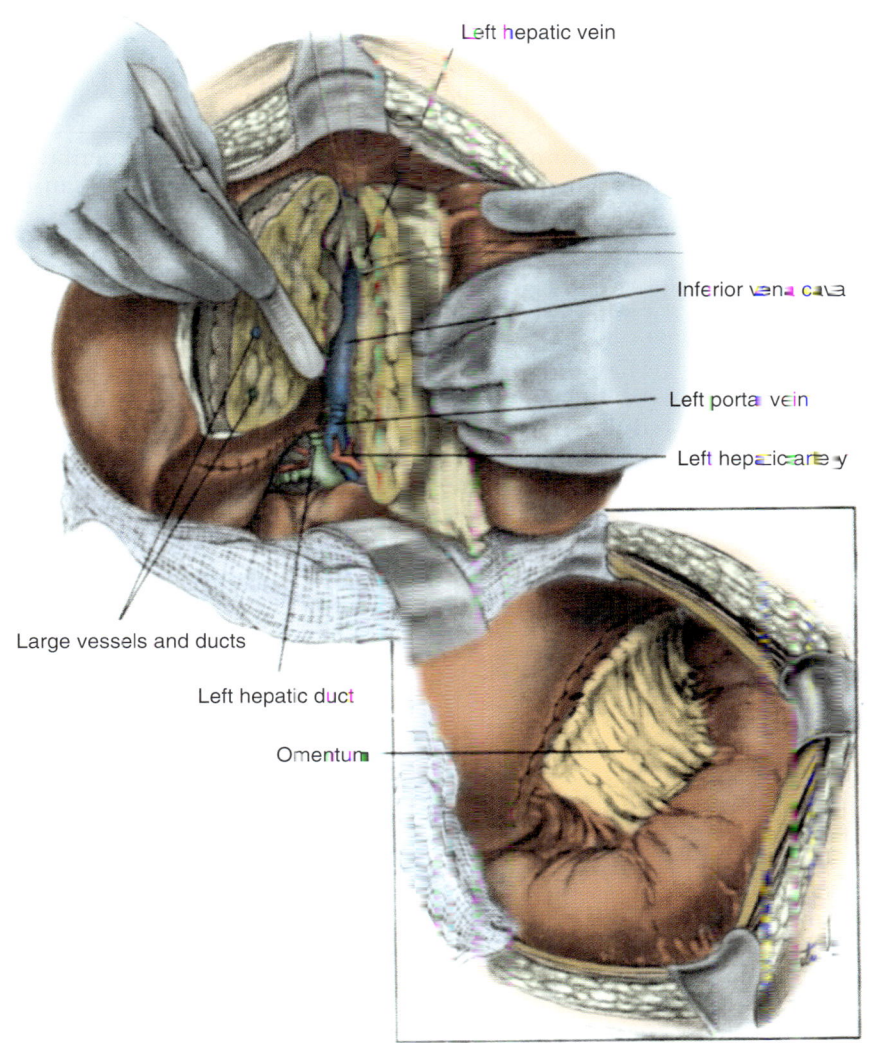

Left hepatic vein

Inferior vena cava

Left portal vein

Left hepatic artery

Large vessels and ducts

Left hepatic duct

Omentum

FIGURE 124.12 Left hepatectomy. The hilar structures have been dissected and ligated, and the parenchymal transection is complete. In this case, the left hepatic vein has been left for last. This also depicts a resection that includes the caudate lobe. (From Schwartz SI. *Surgical Diseases of the Liver*. New York: McGraw-Hill; 1964:254.)

LEFT LATERAL SECTIONECTOMY

Left lateral sectionectomy can usually be performed through an upper midline incision and involves resection of segments II and III of the liver. However, if unexpected findings in the right liver are discovered during exploration, a midline incision may be limiting. Alternatively, a bilateral subcostal incision can be used. The bridge of liver parenchyma between segment III and IV over the round ligament is divided either with electrocautery or with an endoscopic stapler with a vascular load. The left bare area is next exposed by dissecting the left triangular ligament.

For resection of tumor, the surface of the liver is then scored 1 cm to the left of the falciform ligament and to the left of the umbilical fissure (provided that the margin is adequate). This preserves the blood supply and biliary drainage to segment IV of the remnant liver. For donor hepatectomy, the anterior surface of the liver is scored 1 cm to the right of the falciform ligament and to the right of the umbilical fissure. This preserves the blood supply and biliary drainage to segments II and III of the

donor liver. Parenchymal transection is then performed by any of the previously described techniques. Intermittent portal inflow clamping is usually not required for left lateral sectionectomy. As the main portal pedicles to the segments are encountered within the parenchyma, they are controlled with clamps, divided, and ligated or stapled with an endoscopic stapler with a vascular load. The left hepatic vein can then be finally controlled within the hepatic parenchyma either with ligatures or a stapler.

EXTENDED RIGHT AND LEFT HEPATECTOMIES

Extended right and left hepatectomies are perhaps the most difficult and complicated types of liver resections and are covered in classic manuscripts.[39,40] The initial maneuvers for the extended right hepatectomy are similar to right hepatectomy. The cystic artery and duct are ligated and divided, but the gallbladder can be left attached to the specimen because segment IV, V, VI, VII, and VIII are to be resected in continuity. The portal structures are dissected and divided as before. The right hepatic vein is controlled and divided, if possible as before. Because the line of parenchymal transection is just to the right of the umbilical fissure and falciform ligament, the feedback structure to segment IV must be controlled. The bridge of liver parenchyma between segment III and IV is divided. The liver parenchyma is scored with the electrocautery device along the plane of transection. Parenchymal transection is then performed by any of the previously described techniques. As the main portal pedicles to segment IV are encountered within the parenchyma, they are controlled with clamps, divided, and ligated or stapled with an endoscopic stapler with a vascular load. This dissection is carried to the base of the umbilical fissure (Fig. 124.13). Parenchymal transection is continued posteriorly ligating the middle hepatic vein and/or its branches. Great care is taken to preserve the left hepatic vein (Fig. 124.14). Intermittent portal inflow clamping as described previously can be used to help decrease blood loss if this is a problem during parenchymal transection. The caudate is either preserved or resected with the specimen. Because of the risk of torsion of the liver remnant, it should be attached back to the falciform ligament.

The initial maneuvers for an extended left hepatectomy are similar to left hepatectomy. The cystic artery and duct are ligated and divided, but the gallbladder can be left attached to the specimen as segments II, III, IV, V, and VIII are to be resected in continuity. The right triangular ligament, in addition to the left, is also divided. The portal structures are dissected and divided as before. The left hepatic vein (with the middle hepatic veins) is controlled and divided, if possible, as before. The difficulty with extended left hepatectomy is performing the parenchymal transection to preserve the right posterior pedicle and the right hepatic vein while taking the right anterior section of the liver (segments V and VIII). Intraoperative ultrasound is useful in locating and protecting these structures. Intermittent portal inflow clamping as described previously is usually required because of the magnitude of parenchymal transection and difficulty in early control

of the right anterior pedicle. Parenchymal transection is then performed by any of the previously described techniques (Figs. 124.15 and 124.16).

SEGMENTAL RESECTIONS

To maximize functional reserve, (multi)segmental or subsegmental (or nonanatomic) hepatectomies can be

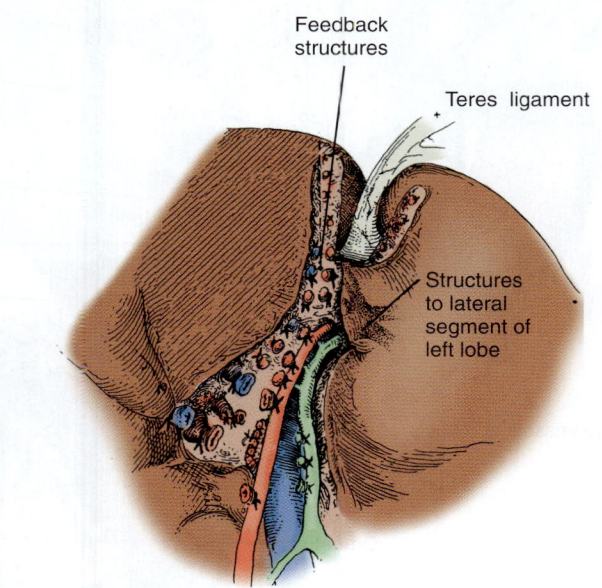

FIGURE 124.13 Right extended hepatectomy. Control of the feedback vessels to segment IV. Blunt dissection in liver substance just to the right of the umbilical fissure exposes these vessels. Each vascular and biliary structure is ligated individually to complete devascularization of segment IV. (From Starzl TE, Bell RH, Baert RW. Hepatic trisegmentectomy and other liver resections. *Surg Gynecol Obstet.* 1975;141:429.)

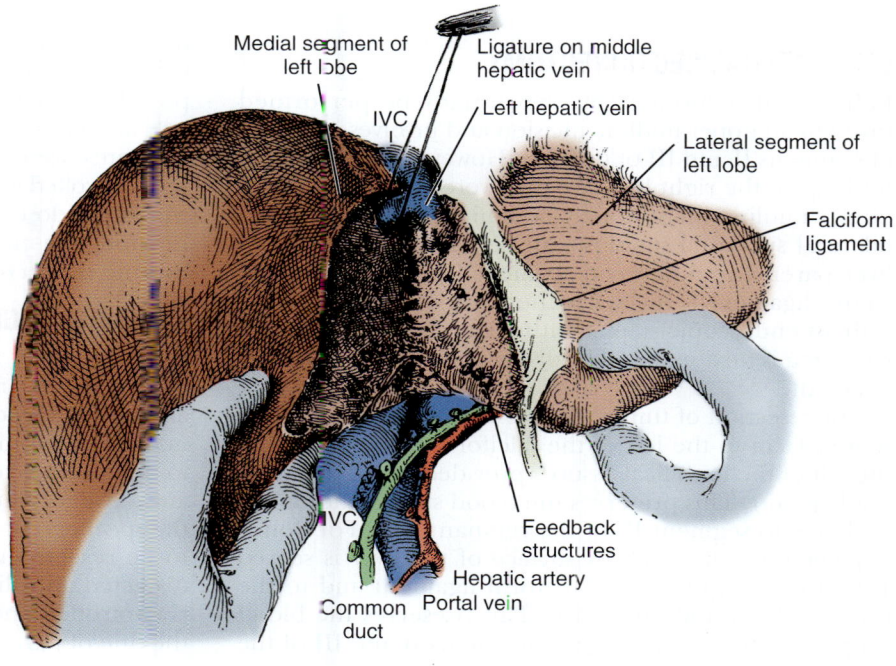

FIGURE 124.14 Right extended hepatectomy. Parenchymal transection is nearly complete. The main trunk of the middle hepatic vein is exposed, with a ligature around it. At this juncture, the caudate still may be left in situ. *IVC,* Inferior vena cava. (From Starzl TE, Bell RH, Baert RW. Hepatic trisegmentectomy and other liver resections. *Surg Gynecol Obstet.* 1975;141:429.)

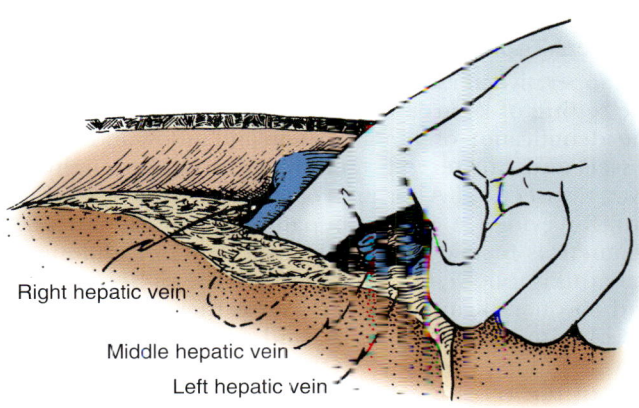

FIGURE 124.15 Left extended hepatectomy: superior-to-inferior dissection between the right anterior section and the right posterior section. The dissecting finger is kept anterior to the right hepatic vein. The left and middle hepatic veins have been ligated or sutured. (From Starzl TE, Iwatsuki S, Shaw BW Jr, et al. Left hepatic trisegmentectomy. *Surg Gynecol Obstet*. 1982;155:25.)

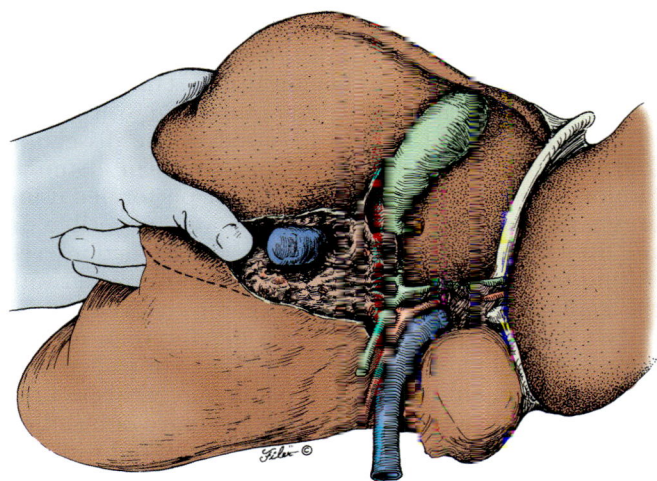

FIGURE 124.16 Left extended hepatectomy. Further development of the plane between the anterior and posterior sections of the right liver. (From Starzl TE, Iwatsuki S, Shaw BW Jr, et al. Left hepatic trisegmentectomy. *Surg Gynecol Obstet*. 1982;155:25.)

performed. For example, left lateral sectionectomy (segments II and III), central hepatectomy to remove the right anterior section (segments V and VIII) and left medial section (segment IV), right posterior sectionectomy (segments VI and VII), or caudate resection (segment I) are examples in which one, two, or three contiguous segments are removed to eradicate tumors within those regions of the liver. These resections are often done with intermittent Pringle maneuvers until the specific pedicles supplying these areas are controlled.

WEDGE RESECTIONS

When a simple wedge resection of the liver is appropriate, the area to be resected is isolated between two interlocking mattress sutures of heavy absorbable material (Fig. 124.17).

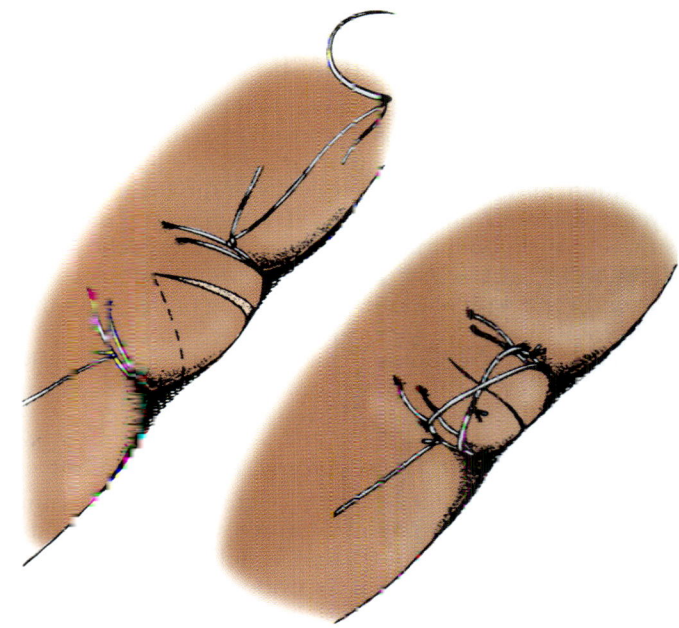

FIGURE 124.17 Wedge biopsy of the free margin of the liver. The two mattress sutures of heavy absorbable material actually should be placed as a V shape and should intersect at the apex, not run parallel as shown. (From Grewe HE, Kremer K. *Atlas of Surgical Operations* vol. 2. Philadelphia: Saunders; 1980:321.)

The two mattress sutures are placed in the form of a V intersecting at the apex. After the wedge resection is performed, the mattress sutures can be tied to each other to approximate the two opposing raw liver surfaces.

LAPAROSCOPIC LIVER RESECTION

Since the first laparoscopic liver resection, performed by Reich in 1991, minimally invasive approaches to liver resection have been popularized, ranging from minor procedures such as wedge resections, to more extensive segmentectomies, sectionectomies, and even hemihepatectomies.[41,42] Several minimally invasive techniques have been reported, such as pure laparoscopy, hand-assisted laparoscopy, and a hybrid technique in which both laparoscopic and open approaches are used during the procedure. The Second International Consensus Conference on Laparoscopic Liver Resection (Japan 2014) issued a recommendation statement, based mainly on observational studies, suggesting that laparoscopic liver resection is associated with decreased wound complications, postoperative pain, and length of stay.[43] Furthermore, laparoscopic liver resection is neither associated with increased mortality nor increased rate of positive margin in the setting of neoplastic diseases, making it an attractive approach in liver surgery. However, in interpreting the available literature, one must be cautious because no randomized clinical trials exist comparing open versus laparoscopic liver resection, and the available data consist mainly of small cohort studies with short follow-up and significant selection bias. Proper patient selection appears to be of critical importance for a safe and successful outcome of the minimally invasive approach.

PORT PLACEMENT AND PATIENT POSITIONING FOR THE LAPAROSCOPIC APPROACH

Proper visualization and easy access to the surgical resection bed is mandatory, especially considering the limitations added by the laparoscopic approach, such as loss of tactile sensation, and increased complexity of the maneuvers of liver mobilization and retraction. The patient is positioned supine on the operating table; care should be taken to elevate the right side of the patient, which can be easily accomplished with placement of padding underneath the right flank.

Four to five laparoscopic ports are used, and the port position varies slightly based on the type of procedure performed (i.e., left vs. right liver resection).

Laparoscopic Right Hepatectomy, Port Placement

Access to the abdominal cavity is obtained with a 10-mm port placed approximately 2 cm above the umbilicus through which CO_2 insufflation is delivered. First, the peritoneal cavity is explored for evidence of extrahepatic disease; this can be promptly accomplished with the use of a 30-degree laparoscope. A 12-mm port is placed along the right midclavicular line; this port will be used for the insertion of stapling devices and energy-based devices. Two 5-mm ports are positioned laterally, along the right subcostal margin. These two ports are of the utmost importance because they will be used to achieve optimal retraction. In addition, a 5-mm port can be inserted in the epigastrium/subxiphoid region to facilitate visualization and mobilization of the liver dome (Fig. 124.18). If a hybrid approach is used, the supraumbilcal port access site can be extended to allow for the placement of a hand port.

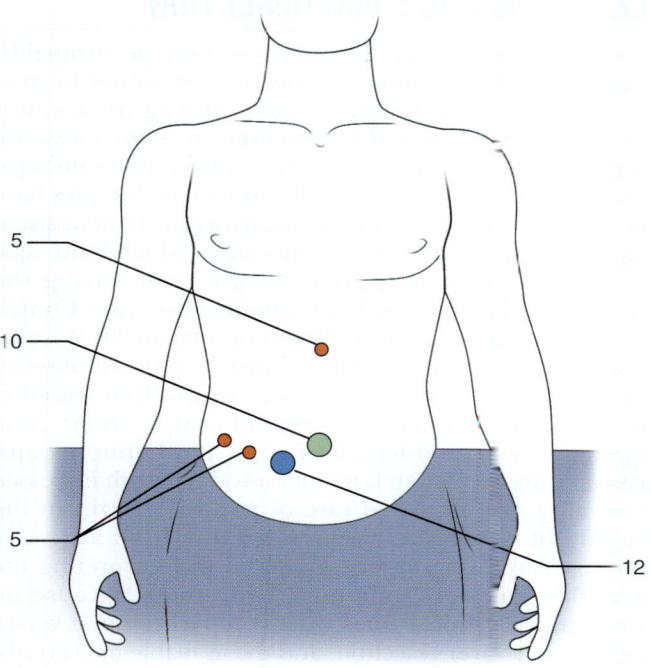

FIGURE 124.18 Optimal port placement for laparoscopic right hepatectomy. For hand-assist access, the supraumbilical port can be extended.

Laparoscopic Right Hepatectomy Surgical Technique

Intraoperative ultrasound provides significant assistance in the setting of laparoscopic liver resection and allows for the identification of tumor location and inflow and outflow vessels and can serve as guidance during parenchymal liver transection. After appropriate peritoneal exploration for evidence of extrahepatic disease, the falciform ligament is first separated from the anterior abdominal wall; this is followed by transection of the right triangular and coronary ligaments. The liver is then freed from its retroperitoneal attachments, and the right hemiliver is elevated to expose the IVC; this allows for the identification of the retrohepatic vessels (draining directly into the IVC), which are carefully ligated with surgical clips proceeding from the inferior liver edge cranially toward the right hepatic vein. Visualization of the liver hilum can be facilitated by cranial retraction of the round ligament, this is accomplished using a transcutaneously placed Endoloop (loaded on a Carter-Thomason needle suture passer) around the round ligament. The gallbladder is then dissected from the gallbladder fossa (proceeding from the fundus to the level of the hilum) with attachment to the cystic duct maintained; this can be used as a handle to facilitate liver retraction and exposure of the hilar structures. The right hepatic artery is dissected free from the surrounding tissues and transected with the use of a stapling device. This is followed by the dissection and transection of the right hepatic vein in a similar fashion. Parenchymal transection can be performed using an energy device along the demarcation line visible on the liver surface. The small hepatic vessels encountered during parenchymal transection can be controlled with the application of an energy device; alternatively, larger vessels (i.e., branches of the right hepatic vein, middle hepatic vein, and the right bile duct) are controlled with the use of a stapling device. It is paramount to inspect the cut edge of the liver surface for any evidence of bleeding or bile leakage. These can often be controlled with the use of additional clips or with the application of the argon beam coagulator, as needed. The liver specimen can be positioned in a laparoscopic extraction bag and retrieved through the supraumbilical incision; this incision can be extended as needed to allow safe retrieval of the specimen. The authors routinely reattach the falciform ligament to the anterior abdominal wall to minimize the risk of liver torsion; this can be easily accomplished with the use of an endoscopic suture device.

Of note, control of the liver hilum is occasionally necessary; therefore a vascular loop or an umbilical tape should be positioned around the portal triad to allow for a prompt Pringle maneuver as needed. This maneuver can easily be accomplished by tightening the umbilical tape or the vessel loop and securing it with the use of a bulldog clamp.

Laparoscopic Left Hepatectomy, Port Placement and Surgical Technique

Access to the abdominal cavity is obtained with a 10-mm port placed approximately 2 cm above the umbilicus through which CO_2 insufflation is delivered. First, the peritoneal cavity is explored for evidence of extrahepatic

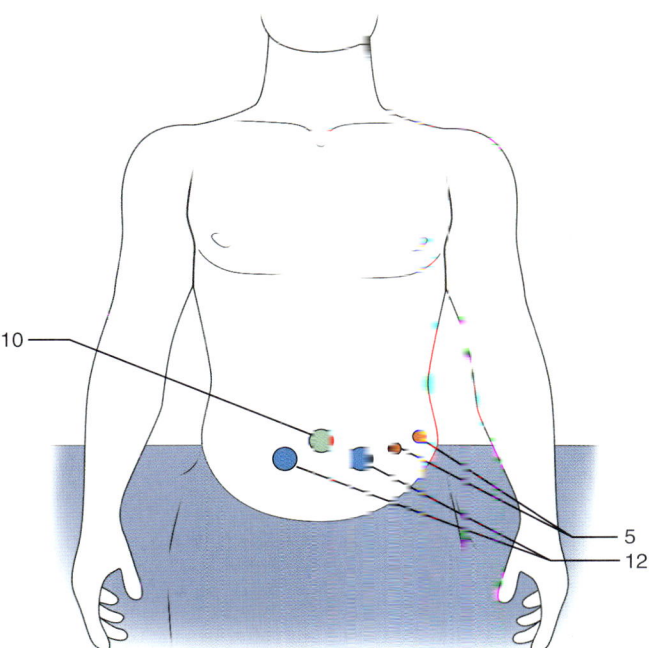

FIGURE 124.19 Optimal port placement for laparoscopic left hepatectomy. For hand-assist access the supraumbilical port can be extended.

disease; this can be promptly accomplished with the use of a 30-degree laparoscope. A 12-mm port is placed along the left midclavicular line; this one will be used for the insertion of stapling devices and energy-based devices, and a second 12-mm port is placed along the right midclavicular line. Two 5-mm ports are positioned laterally, along the left subcostal margin. Once again, if a hybrid approach is used, the supraumbilical port access site can be extended to allow for the placement of a hand port (Fig. 124.19). Attention is first turned to the identification of the left hepatic artery and left portal vein, which are usually ligated at the level of the umbilical fissure. Parenchymal transection can proceed in a similar fashion to the one described during a laparoscopic right hepatectomy (see earlier). The left hepatic vein as well as branches from the middle hepatic vein and the left bile duct, can be controlled with a stapling device as they are encountered during the parenchymal transection. The liver specimen is retrieved as described previously and the falciform ligament is secured to the abdominal wall.

POSTOPERATIVE MANAGEMENT

Liver resection has evolved into a safe and reproducible procedure with an estimated perioperative mortality of less than 5% when performed for metastatic disease and less than 10% for primary hepatocellular carcinoma.[44] However, metabolic derangements can still occur, especially when large portions of liver parenchyma are resected, and this must be expected and anticipated.

Characteristic of the initial perioperative phase is a transient hyperbilirubinemia (occasionally manifested as frank jaundice), a transient elevation of serum transaminase (aspartate transaminase/alanine transaminase), hypophosphatemia, and prolonged international normalized ratio (INR).

The serum bilirubin level usually peaks around the third or fourth postoperative day and quickly resolves as the liver remnant recovers and regenerates. This phenomenon is not uncommon and is usually driven by loss of hepatic parenchyma and sporadically by blood transfusion when used.

Serum transaminases elevations are expected and usually plateau at less than 1000 units/L, and are not usually ominous in the absence of severe prolongation in INR, decreased fibrinogen, hepatic encephalopathy, acidosis, and elevated serum ammonia level. Hypophosphatemia is to be expected and is a sign of liver regeneration; phosphate is consumed during hepatocyte DNA regeneration and serum phosphate level should be monitored closely. In addition, hypokalemia, hypoglycemia, and hypoalbuminemia commonly occur, and again careful monitoring should be implemented and appropriate replacement instituted. Particular attention should be given to any evidence of coagulopathy, often characterized by a prolonged INR; this can arise as a result of a combination of intraoperative blood loss, dilution of clotting factors, blood product transfusion, or as an ominous sign of inadequate liver function.

POSTOPERATIVE COMPLICATIONS

The rate and specific type of complications that can be expected following liver resection is highly influenced by the type of operation performed (i.e., open vs. laparoscopic; major vs. minor resection; with or without biliary duct reconstruction), by the status of the liver parenchyma (cirrhotic vs. not cirrhotic), and by the quality of the FLR. Intraabdominal fluid collections are not uncommon and are often seen along the transected edge of the liver. The significance of these collections can vary; if symptomatic (i.e., pain compression of the hilar structures) or in the setting of clinical signs of infection, they often need to be percutaneously drained; however, if asymptomatic, they can be left alone.[26] In case of persistent biliary leakage, an endoscopic retrograde cholangiopancreatogram can be both diagnostic and therapeutic as it might allow for the identification of the site of leakage and for decompression of the biliary duct via sphincterotomy.

Perhaps one of the most severe complications following hepatectomy is the development of progressive and refractory postoperative hepatic failure (POHF). This complication has been described in the literature to occur in approximately 1.2% to 32% of cases and has an associated mortality estimated between 1.6% and 2.8% of cases.[45,46] It is important to note that POHF can manifest as early as a few days to many weeks after the initial liver resection, and its presentation can range from acute fulminant liver failure to a progressive insidious deterioration over weeks to months.

SUMMARY

The indications for liver resection are a myriad and cover both primary and secondary conditions of the liver.

Nonetheless, the hepatobiliary surgeon needs to adhere to a few surgical principles to ensure a successful outcome: first, intimate knowledge of the conventional liver anatomy and its common variants; second, development of an appropriate operative plan based on the understanding of the preoperative functional status of the liver parenchyma. The ultimate goal is to obtain appropriate parenchymal transection while maintaining an adequate liver remnant with good vascular inflow, vascular outflow, and biliary drainage in continuity with the enteric tract.

The third principle is knowledge and anticipation of the most common complications known to arise after hepatic resections and familiarity with the available treatment strategies.

ACKNOWLEDGMENT

This chapter is a combination and update of a previous chapter on diagnostic operation of the liver and techniques of hepatic resection. The authors acknowledge Aram N. Demirjian, MD, for his contribution to the previous chapter on which this update is based.

REFERENCES

1. von Frerichs FT. *Uber den Diabetes*. Berlin: Hirschweld; 1884.
2. Healey JE, Schroy PC. Anatomy of the biliary ducts within the human liver: analysis of the prevailing pattern of branchings and the major variations of the biliary ducts. *AMA Arch Surg.* 1953;66:599.
3. Goldsmith NA, Woodburne RT. The surgical anatomy pertaining to liver resection. *Surg Gynecol Obstet.* 1957;105(3):310-318.
4. Bismuth H, Houssin D, Castaing D. Major and minor segmentectomies "réglées" in liver surgery. *World J Surg.* 1982;6(1):10-24.
5. Strasberg SM. Nomenclature of hepatic anatomy and resections: a review of the Brisbane 2000 system. *J Hepatobiliary Pancreat Surg.* 2005;12(5):351-355.
6. Couinaud C. *Le Foi: Etudes Anatomiques et Chirurgicales*. Paris: Masson; 1957.
7. Pugh R, Lyon IM, Dawson JL. Transection of the oesophagus for bleeding oesophageal varices. *Br J Surg.* 1973;60:646.
8. Shoup M, Gönen M, D'Angelica M, et al. Volumetric analysis predicts hepatic dysfunction in patients undergoing major liver resection. *J Gastrointest Surg.* 2003;7(3):325-330.
9. Makuuchi M, Thai BL, Takayama K, et al. Preoperative portal embolization to increase safety of major hepatectomy for hilar bile duct carcinoma: a preliminary report. *Surgery.* 1990;107(5):521-527.
10. Covey AM, Tuorto S, Brody LA, et al. Safety and efficacy of preoperative portal vein embolization with polyvinyl alcohol in 58 patients with liver metastases. *Am J Roentgenol.* 2005;185(6):1620-1626.
11. Khatri VP, Petrelli NJ, Belghiti J. Extending the frontiers of surgical therapy for hepatic colorectal metastases: is there a limit? *J Clin Oncol.* 2005;23:8490.
12. Schnitzbauer AA, Lang SA, Goessmann H, et al. Right portal vein ligation combined with in situ splitting induces rapid left lateral liver lobe hypertrophy enabling 2-staged extended right hepatic resection in small-for-size settings. *Ann Surg.* 2012;255(3):405-414.
13. Aloia TA, Vauthey J-N. Associating liver partition and portal vein ligation for staged hepatectomy (ALPPS): what is gained and what is lost? *Ann Surg.* 2012;256(3):e9; author reply e16-e19.
14. Andriani OC. Long-term results with associating liver partition and portal vein ligation for staged hepatectomy (ALPPS). *Ann Surg.* 2012;256(3):e5; author reply e16-e19.
15. Hernandez-Alejandro R, Bertens KA, Pineda-Solis K, Croome KP. Can we improve the morbidity and mortality associated with the associating liver partition with portal vein ligation for staged hepatectomy (ALPPS) procedure in the management of colorectal liver metastases? *Surgery.* 2015;157(2):194-201.
16. Chan ACY, Poon RTP, Lo CM. Modified anterior approach for the ALPPS procedure: how we do it. *World J Surg.* 2015;39(11):2831-2835.
17. Cai Y-L, Song P-P, Tang W, Cheng N-S. An updated systematic review of the evolution of ALPPS and evaluation of its advantages and disadvantages in accordance with current evidence. *Medicine (Baltimore).* 2016;95(24):e3941.
18. Qadan M, Garden OJ, Corvera CU, Visser BC. Management of postoperative hepatic failure. *J Am Coll Surg.* 2016;222(2):195-208.
19. Clavien P-A, Petrowsky H, DeOliveira ML, Graf R. Strategies for safer liver surgery and partial liver transplantation. *N Engl J Med.* 2007;356(15):1545-1559.
20. Hou W, Zhu X. Extravascular interventional treatment of liver cancer, present and future. *Drug Discov Ther.* 2015;9(5):335-341.
21. Fong Y, Blumgart LH. Useful stapling techniques in liver surgery. *J Am Coll Surg.* 1997;185:93.
22. Melendez JA, Arslan V, Fischer ME, Wuest D. Perioperative outcomes of major hepatic resections under low central venous pressure anesthesia: blood loss, blood transfusion, and the risk of postoperative renal dysfunction. *J Am Coll Surg.* 1998;187:620.
23. The Terminology Committee of the IHPBA. The Brisbane 2000 terminology of hepatic anatomy and resections. *HPB.* 2000;2:333.
24. Fuster J, Llovet JM, Garcia-Valdecasas JC, et al. Abdominal drainage after liver resection for hepatocellular carcinoma in cirrhotic patients: a randomized controlled study. *Hepatogastroenterology.* 2004;51(56):536-540.
25. Fong Y, Brennan MF, Brown K, Heffernan N, Blumgart LH. Drainage is unnecessary after elective liver resection. *Am J Surg.* 1996;171(1):158-162.
26. Konstantinidis IT, Mastrodomenico P, Sofocleous CT, et al. Symptomatic perihepatic fluid collections after hepatic resection in the modern era. *J Gastrointest Surg.* 2016;20(4):748-756.
27. Pamecha V, Gurusamy KS, Sharma D, Davidson BR. Techniques for liver parenchymal transection: a meta-analysis of randomized controlled trials. *HPB (Oxford).* 2009;11:38.
28. Takayama T, Makuuchi M, Kubota K. Randomized comparison of ultrasonic vs clamp transection of the liver. *Arch Surg.* 2001;136:922.
29. Arita J, Hasegawa K, Kokudo N, Sano K. Randomized clinical trial of the effect of a saline-linked radiofrequency coagulator on blood loss during hepatic resection. *Br J Surg.* 2007;94:287.
30. Lupo L, Gallerani A, Panzera F, Tandoi F. Randomized clinical trial of radiofrequency-assisted versus clamp-crushing liver resection. *Br J Surg.* 2007;94:287.
31. Lesurtel M, Selzner M, Petrowsky H. How should transection of the liver be performed?: a prospective randomized study in 100 consecutive patients: comparing four different transection strategies. *Ann Surg.* 2005;242:814, discussion 22.
32. Buell JF, Gayet B, Han HS, Wakabayashi G, Kim KH. Evaluation of stapler hepatectomy during a laparoscopic liver resection. *HPB (Oxford).* 2013;11:845.
33. Delis SG, Bakoyiannis A, Karakaxas D, Athanassiou K. Hepatic parenchyma resection using stapling devices: peri-operative and long-term outcome. *HPB (Oxford).* 2009;11:38.
34. Paniccia A, Schulick RD. Surgical margin in hepatic resections for colorectal metastasis: should we care? *Curr Colorectal Cancer Rep.* 2016;1–8.
35. Pawlik TM, Scoggins CR, Zorzi D, et al. Effect of surgical margin status on survival and site of recurrence after hepatic resection for colorectal metastases. *Ann Surg.* 2005;241(5):715-724.
36. Figueras J, Burdio F, Ramos E, et al. Effect of subcentimeter nonpositive resection margin on hepatic recurrence in patients undergoing hepatectomy for colorectal liver metastases. Evidences from 663 liver resections. *Ann Oncol.* 2007;18(7):1190-1195.
37. Busquets J, Pelaez N, Alonso S, Grande L. The study of cavitational ultrasonically aspirated material during surgery for colorectal liver metastases as a new concept in resection margin. *Ann Surg.* 2006;244(4):634-635.
38. Hammond JS, Muirhead W, Zaitoun AM, Cameron IC, Lobo DN. Comparison of liver parenchymal ablation and tissue necrosis in a cadaveric bovine model using the Harmonic Scalpel, the LigaSure, the Cavitron Ultrasonic Surgical Aspirator and the Aquamantys devices. *HPB (Oxford).* 2012;14(12):828-832.
39. Starzl TE, Koep LJ, Weil R 3rd, Lilly JR, Putnam CW, Aldrete JA. Right trisegmentectomy for hepatic neoplasms. *Surg Gynecol Obstet.* 1980;150:208.
40. Starzl TE, Iwatsuki S, Shaw BW Jr, et al. Left hepatic trisegmentectomy. *Surg Gynecol Obstet.* 1982;155:21.

41. Cherian PT, Mishra AK, Kumar P, et al. Laparoscopic liver resection: wedge resections to living donor hepatectomy, are we heading in the right direction? *World J Gastroenterol.* 2014;20(37):13369-13381.

42. Soubrane O, Schwarz L, Cauchy F, et al. A conceptual technique for laparoscopic right hepatectomy based on facts and oncologic principles: the caudal approach. *Ann Surg.* 2015;261(6):1226-1231.

43. Wakabayashi G, Cherqui D, Geller DA, et al. Recommendations for laparoscopic liver resection: a report from the second international consensus conference held in Morioka. *Ann Surg.* 2015;261(4):619-629.

44. Belghiti J, Hiramatsu K, Benoist S, Massault P, Sauvanet A, Farges O. Seven hundred forty-seven hepatectomies in the 1990s: an update to evaluate the actual risk of liver resection. *J Am Coll Surg.* 2000;191(1):38-46.

45. Rahbari NN, Garden OJ, Padbury R, et al. Posthepatectomy liver failure: a definition and grading by the International Study Group of Liver Surgery (ISGLS). *Surgery.* 2011;149(5):713-724.

46. Muller T, Ribero D, Reddy SK, et al. Hepatic insufficiency and mortality in 1,059 noncirrhotic patients undergoing major hepatectomy. *J Am Coll Surg.* 2007;204(5):854-862; discussion 862-864.

Minimally Invasive Techniques of Hepatic Resection

Iswanto Sucandy | Susannah Cheek | David A. Geller

The field of hepatobiliary surgery has evolved dramatically in the past few decades, with improved understanding of the anatomic segments of the liver, advancements in modern imaging techniques, better operative instrumentation, and improved anesthesia care, as well as postoperative management. At the same time, minimally invasive surgery has become an integral part of each surgical subspecialty. However, the application of minimally invasive techniques to liver surgery has been slower to develop, and it is still far from being a standard option for most practicing hepatobiliary surgeons. This reluctance stems in part from the complexity of liver surgery, concerns for significant bleeding or gas embolism, and lack of formal training in minimally invasive surgery for the more "senior" hepatobiliary surgeons.

However, a dramatic progress in minimally invasive hepatic surgery has been made in recent years.[1] Since the First International Consensus Conference in Louisville, Kentucky in 2008 the number of laparoscopic liver resections (LLRs) performed worldwide has increased exponentially.[2-4] The recently published International Survey on Technical Aspects of Laparoscopic Liver Resection (INSTALL) study demonstrated an expanding indication for LLR that includes larger tumor size, increased number of tumors, and lesions in difficult locations.[5] LLR is now considered a safe option when performed by experienced surgeons in a major hepatobiliary center. In addition to the laparoscopic approach for liver resection, the current minimally invasive techniques also include robotic liver resections (RLRs).[2,6] Large reviews and series have reported the safety and feasibility of LLR for both benign lesions and malignant tumors,[3-21] including anatomic right hepatectomies,[22-26] left hepatectomies,[1,7,28] and even extended hepatectomies.[29,30] In a world review of 2804 cases of LLR, 50% of the resections were done for malignancy, with the majority being performed for hepatocellular carcinoma (HCC) or colorectal cancer (CRC) metastases.[1] A plan for conducting a randomized clinical trial comparing laparoscopic with open hepatic resection for cancer had initially been discussed at the First International Conference in Louisville.[3] There are currently two randomized clinical trials of laparoscopic versus open liver resection (OLR) being conducted in Europe. They are the ORANGE II PLUS trial in the Netherlands and the OSLO CoMet study in Norway.[31] In the latter trial the primary outcome is 30-day perioperative morbidity. The secondary outcomes include 5-year survival (overall, disease-free, and recurrence-free), resection margins, recurrence pattern, postoperative pain, health-related quality of life, and evaluation of the inflammatory response.

INDICATIONS FOR LAPAROSCOPIC LIVER SURGERY

An important principle of minimally invasive surgery is that the availability of this technique does not alter the indication. Therefore an LLR should be considered only for lesions that would otherwise be treated with open hepatic surgery. Indications and contraindications for laparoscopic liver surgery are shown in Table 125.1. Malignant liver lesions, symptomatic hemangioma or focal nodular hyperplasia (FNH), and hepatic adenomas larger than 4 cm should be resected. Ideally suited lesions are masses that are located in the right anterior segments (V and VI) or left lateral segments (II and III). However, experienced groups have shown that even laparoscopic major hepatectomies can be safely accomplished.[22-25] Although approximately 36% of LLRs are performed in cirrhotic patients, postoperative liver insufficiency has always been an important factor in deciding extent of hepatic resection, whether in open or laparoscopic hepatectomy.[2] In a multiinstitutional Japanese propensity matched study, Takahara et al. reported that the frequency of postoperative liver failure after LLR for HCC is lower than after OLR (0.5% vs. 1.8%).[32] To avoid postoperative liver failure, for minor LLR (≤2 segments), the majority of surgeons set the upper limit of a total bilirubin at 2.0 mg/dL, whereas for major resection (≥3 segments) the threshold is lowered to 1.5 mg/dL or less.[5] The INSTALL study reported that more than 80% of surgeons set the cutoff at 40% volume for future liver remnant when the liver is found to be cirrhotic.[5]

In liver surgery the main differences between benign and malignant lesions are related to achieving adequate margins and avoidance of tumor rupture. Malignant liver tumors, lesions abutting major vasculature, or tumors that are too large to be manipulated laparoscopically should be resected by an open approach. Perihilar cholangiocarcinomas are often challenging even by an open approach, and in general should not be done with a minimally invasive technique. The presence of dense adhesions that prevent safe dissection, unexpected difficulty in manipulating the liver, or failure to make progress are indications for conversion to an open technique. Such a decision is never considered a failure but rather a good judgment call, used to prevent avoidable complications. Another less common indication for LLR is live donor hepatectomy for liver transplantation. Only 5% of LLRs are performed for this indication around the world.[5] Laparoscopic live donor hepatectomy has been described for left lateral sectionectomy (LLS)[33] and adult-to-adult

TABLE 125.1 Indications and Contraindications for Laparoscopic Liver Resection

Indications	Contraindications
Benign liver lesions	Any contraindications to open
Symptomatic	liver resection
hemangioma	Patients who cannot tolerate
Symptomatic focal	pneumoperitoneum
nodular hyperplasia	Dense adhesions that
Adenoma	cannot be lysed
Symptomatic giant	laparoscopically
hepatic cyst	Lesion too close to
Malignant liver lesions	vasculature
Hepatocellular	Lesion too large to be safely
carcinoma	maximized laparoscopically
Colorectal cancer liver	Resection that requires
metastasis	extensive portal
Other malignant lesions	lymphadenectomy
Live donor hepatectomy	—
for liver transplant	
Indeterminate lesions—	—
cannot rule out cancer	

From Nguyen KT, Gamblin TC, Geller DA. World review of laparoscopic liver resection—2804 patients. *Ann Surg*. 2009;250:331.

TABLE 125.2 Types of Laparoscopic Liver Resection in the Published Literature

Total No. of Reported Cases	**2804**
INDICATIONS FOR LAPAROSCOPIC LIVER RESECTION	
Malignant lesions	1395 (49.8%)
Benign lesions	1253 (44.7%)
Live donor hepatectomies for liver transplant	49 (1.7%)
Indeterminate	107 (3.8%)
MINIMALLY INVASIVE APPROACHES TO LIVER RESECTION	
Totally laparoscopic	2105 (75.1%)
Hand-assisted laparoscopic	463 (16.5%)
Laparoscopy-assisted open (hybrid)	60 (2.1%)
Gasless laparoscopic	52 (1.8%)
Thoracoscopic	5 (0.2%)
Robotics-assisted	3 (0.1%)
Converted to open	116 (4.1%)
TYPES OF RESECTIONS PERFORMED LAPAROSCOPICALLY	
Wedge resection/segmentectomy	1253 (44.9%)
Left lateral sectionectomy	570 (20.3%)
Right hepatectomy	253 (9.0%)
Bisegmentectomy	209 (7.4%)
Left hepatectomy	191 (6.8%)
Deroofing/enucleation	142 (5.1%)
Extended right hepatectomy	19 (0.7%)
Caudate lobectomy	18 (0.6%)
Central hepatectomy	8 (0.3%)
Extended left hepatectomy	3 (0.1%)
Other	16 (0.6%)
Not documented	117 (4.2%)

From Nguyen KT, Gamblin TC, Geller DA. World review of laparoscopic liver resection—2804 patients. *Ann Surg*. 2009;250:331.

right hepatectomy.[34–36] Caution is advised in that these operations should only be done by transplant teams with extensive open live donor liver transplant expertise, as well as minimally invasive liver resection experience.

TECHNICAL APPROACHES TO LAPAROSCOPIC LIVER RESECTION

There are two main approaches for performing minimally invasive liver resection—pure laparoscopic and hand assisted. A third option is using the laparoscopic technique for mobilization of the liver before entering the abdomen and completing the resection through a relatively small laparotomy incision (so-called hybrid technique).[37] Some authors use a hand port for all cases whereas others use it selectively and some never use it at all. The benefits of the hand-assisted technique are the relative ease in manipulation of the liver, direct palpation for improved tactile sensation, and the ability for faster control of bleeding in the case of a major vascular injury. Because most specimens mandate a utility incision for intact specimen extraction, the main difference between hand-assisted and pure laparoscopy is the position of the incision. There have been no comparative studies to support benefit or inferiority of the three techniques and the choice is strictly surgeon's preference. The hand-assisted and hybrid methods are claimed by their proponents to be beneficial for larger lesions, posteriorly located lesions, donor hepatectomy, and for training of surgeons in major LLR techniques.[2,35,37,38] In a large review of more than 2800 LLRs,[1] the majority of minimally invasive liver resections were pure laparoscopic (75%). The hand-assisted approach was the next most common (17%), and the "hybrid" technique was used rarely (2%) (Table 125.2).

In the operating room the patient is placed in the supine position with both arms extended. Some authors favor the French lithotomy position. The preparation is similar to that of major liver resection, including line placement, bladder catheterization, and orogastric tube insertion. We use a foot board and strapping that allow for steep rotational manipulations of the table during the operation. In the case of a planned major hepatectomy, we use a hand port and place it at the beginning of the procedure, as a supraumbilical midline incision (Fig. 125.1). In the case of a small patient (e.g., <68 inches in height) the incision can be infraumbilical. The pneumoperitoneum is established via a trocar inserted through the hand port. The hand port incision may be used for a rapid conversion, by extending it to a longer midline.

The most recent development in minimally invasive liver surgery is robotic hepatectomy. The first report of robotic-assisted liver resection was published in 2006 by Ryska et al[39] The known advantages of robotic technology include improved precision, dexterity, degree of movement, and distal magnification, as well as decreased tremor and fatigue. Robotic liver surgery has gained significant popularity because of its potential to overcome limitations of conventional laparoscopy. Over the past 5 years, many case reports and single-institutional case series of RLRs have emerged. In 2014 Tsung et al. reported their experience of robotic versus laparoscopic hepatectomy with a

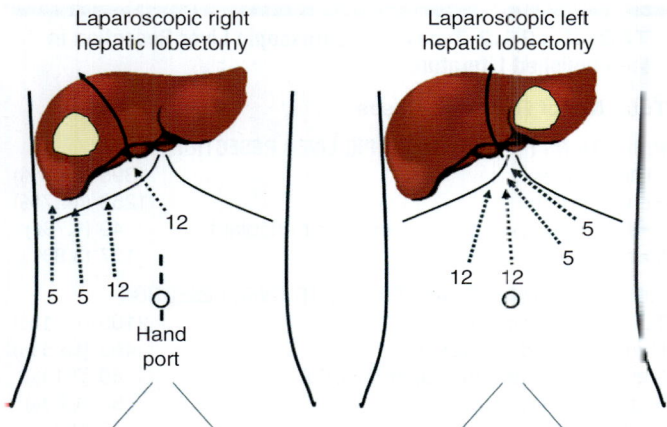

Laparoscopic right
hepatic lobectomy

Laparoscopic left
hepatic lobectomy

FIGURE 125.1 Trocar placement for laparoscopic right and left hepatic lobectomy.

1 : 2 matched analysis.[6] The patients were matched for presence of background liver disease, extent of hepatic resection, diagnosis, body mass index, age, gender, and American Society of Anesthesiologists (ASA) class. With the exception of higher operative time and overall room time in the robotic group, there were no significant differences between perioperative outcomes of robotic and laparoscopic groups. R0 negative margin status was also comparable, which indicates that the oncologic outcome is not compromised by either approach. However the technical advantages associated with robotic approach allows completion of a greater percentage of minor and major hepatectomies using the purely minimally invasive technique. Ninety-three percent of the RLRs were accomplished without the need for hand-assist ports or the hybrid technique, compared with only 49.1% of those performed with the laparoscopic approach.[40] This finding suggests that robotic system may offer technical ease for surgeons in accomplishing purely minimally invasive liver resections. Robotic approach may also facilitate better vascular control during major liver resections compared with its laparoscopic counterpart. Pretransection extrahepatic inflow control is more easily achieved with the robot. Laparoscopic stapling of the portal vein extrahepatically is sometimes difficult to accomplish with the laparoscopic approach due to a poor stapler angle. Increased degree of freedom with the robotic instrumentation mitigates this problem by allowing control of the portal vein extrahepatically using suture ligation. Similar issues apply to the extrahepatic outflow control. During hepatic parenchymal transection, improved three-dimensional magnification provided by the robotic camera may allows surgeon to identify individual vessels more clearly for precise control and ligation. The downside of robotic approach is added costs for the robotic system, in addition to the longer operative time.[41] However the overall perioperative outcomes are comparable between the laparoscopic and RLRs. A future, larger scale, prospective multicenter study is needed to objectively determine the ultimate superiority of robotic over laparoscopic technique. Based on the most recent international consensus in Morioka, Japan, major robotic liver surgery is

still recommended to be done within institutional review board–approved registry.[2]

Despite established advantages of laparoscopy, hemorrhage during LLR remains a major concern. The initial slow development of laparoscopic liver surgery is partly explained by the fear of inability to control bleeding. This important question was discussed among a panel of 34 experts covering five continents during the Second International Conference on Laparoscopic Liver Resection Surgery in Morioka, Iwate, Japan, in October 2014.[2] Several studies have been designed to elucidate potential factors responsible for reduced blood loss during LLR. It is widely accepted that the main reasons for reduced blood loss are the positive pressure of the CO_2 pneumoperitoneum (10 to 14 mm Hg), low central venous pressure (≤ 5 mm Hg), the emergence of new transection devices, and the facilitation of inflow and outflow controls.[42] Experts present in Morioka agreed that low central venous pressure and pneumoperitoneum act in a synergistic manner to reduce bleeding. Image magnification provided by a laparoscope may also allow more precise dissections and facilitates good control of segmental or subsegmental portal pedicles. In cases of severe bleeding, increasing the pneumoperitoneum pressure and decreasing the airway pressure by a brief pause in the artificial ventilation are maneuvers that can be used to decrease back bleeding.[5] Decailliot et al. demonstrated in a nonrandomized study that Pringle maneuver during LLR is as efficient as Pringle maneuver during open liver surgery in decreasing blood loss.[43] Types of instruments by energy sources and technique used in parenchymal transection vary among each surgeon and institution. We recommend that hepatobiliary surgeons should select techniques and instruments based on their familiarity and complete understanding of the system for each specific LLR case. There have been no randomized controlled trials that answer the question of the best technique or device for laparoscopic hepatic parenchymal transection. All studies on this subject have been case-controls, case series, case reports, experimental studies, and reviews.[44] In addition to the use of multiple hemostatic methods, such as bipolar cautery (for vessels ≤ 2 mm), vessel sealing device or clips (for vessels 3 to 7 mm), locked clips or staplers (for vessels ≥ 7 mm), thermofusion, and precoagulation, experts advocate that liver surgeons should master intracorporeal suturing techniques when performing laparoscopic liver surgery. Careful inspection of the transection surface for bleeding and bile leak after decreasing the pneumoperitoneal pressure should be performed routinely prior to ending the operation.

LAPAROSCOPIC RIGHT HEPATECTOMY

After inserting the hand port and establishing the pneumoperitoneum to a pressure limit of 14 mm Hg, four additional trocars are placed, as depicted (see Fig. 125.1). The falciform ligament is divided with endoshears and the round ligament divided using a stapler or with LigaSure or harmonic scalpel. The falciform ligament is left long on the liver side to facilitate retraction. Intraoperative ultrasound is performed to identify the lesion and mark the parenchymal transection line. After taking down the right coronary and triangular ligaments, the right lobe is gradually rotated off the retroperitoneum and lifted from the inferior vena cava (IVC). Short hepatic veins are clipped with 5-mm hemolocks. Small veins can be divided with the LigaSure. At that stage the right hepatic vein is exposed and can be divided with a vascular stapler. If the exposure of the right hepatic vein is not optimal, it can be divided inside the liver at the end of the procedure after the parenchymal transection. The next step is the hilar dissection. It is started with the cholecystectomy and exposure of the right hepatic artery, right portal vein, and bile duct. The right hepatic artery is doubly secured with locking clips. The right portal vein is dissected and encircled. It can be transected with the vascular stapler; however, if the angle precludes stapling, it can be left to the end of the procedure and controlled with a small bulldog clamp inserted through the hand port to allow for an ipsilateral Pringle maneuver. Next, the parenchymal transection is started with an ultrasonic dissector or LigaSure. The deeper parenchyma with crossing middle hepatic vein branches is divided with a vascular stapler. Some surgeons use a bipolar pinching forceps and/or Cavitron ultrasonic surgical aspirator (CUSA) or hydrojet to help divide the parenchyma. During the parenchymal transection, as in an open hepatic resection, the central venous pressure is kept low to minimize blood loss. If not already done, the right portal vein and right hepatic veins are divided as the parenchymal transection is deepened, along with the right hepatic duct inside the liver. If a hand port is used, the hand can provide a laparoscopic hanging maneuver to facilitate exposure and transection. Wakabayashi et al.[45] and Soubrane et al.[46] advocated limited liver mobilization before transection, as a potential technique to decrease bleeding during LLR. The anterior approach provides the advantage of performing LLR without having to mobilize the liver before transection, which is not always easy and safe to accomplish laparoscopically, particularly in case of heavy liver weight or a large-sized tumor. The caudal approach is the main conceptual change in LLR.[2] The caudal approach, which relies on visual magnification, offers improved exposure around the right adrenal gland and the vena cava. This approach also greatly facilitates identification of the Laennec capsule and Glissonian pedicle at the hilar plate. Using this technique the IVC from caudal to cranial can be efficiently exposed, which is then followed by division of the short hepatic veins before parenchymal transection.[46] A meticulous caudal to cranial parenchymal transection with laparoscopic magnification results in better identification of intraparenchymal structure for optimal liver parenchymal division. Placement of patients in reverse Trendelenburg position helps to lower the venous pressure and improve gravitational shifting of visceral structures away from the liver hilum. A recently introduced concept of superior and lateral approaches with or without the use of intercostal and transthoracic ports requires patients to be placed in the left lateral decubitus position or even prone position. This new technical advancement in LLR offers better exposure of the right posterosuperior segments and lifts the right hepatic vein higher than the vena cava to reduce hepatic venous back bleeding.[47,48] Any oozing from the cut edge is controlled with cautery or TissueLink sealing device. Any visible bile leaks are

oversewn with a 4-0 absorbable suture. The specimen is extracted through the hand port, and the abdomen is reinspected for bleeding. A closed-suction drain is left next to the cut surface of the liver and brought out through one of the 5-mm trocar sites.

LAPAROSCOPIC LEFT HEPATECTOMY

The technique of laparoscopic left hepatectomy is similar to that of the right lobe. The position of the trocars is depicted (see Fig. 125.1). Often laparoscopic LLS and left lobectomy can be done with a pure laparoscopic approach with the hand port being reserved for a large tumor or difficult case. Care must be given to avoiding injury to the left phrenic and left hepatic veins when taking down the left triangular ligament. Next, the gastrohepatic ligament is divided (watching for a replaced left hepatic artery), and the left hilum is dissected at the base of the falciform ligament after opening the liver bridge from segment III to IVB. The left hepatic artery is doubly clipped and divided, followed by dissection of the left portal vein. The left portal vein can be controlled/divided in a manner similar to the description of the right portal vein. The left hepatic duct is transected laterally at the base of the umbilical fissure to avoid injury to a not-infrequent right posterior (or right anterior) duct coming off the proximal end of the left hepatic duct. A hepatotomy is made in segment IVB and stapler insinuated to divide the left hepatic duct. Parenchymal transection is done using LigaSure or a harmonic scalpel, followed by vascular staplers to divide the left hepatic vein after the parenchyma is divided.

CLINICAL BENEFITS OF LAPAROSCOPIC LIVER SURGERY

More than 150 publications have shown the safety and efficacy of LLR. In the world review of LLR, conducted by Nguyen et al., in 2804 patients overall mortality was 0.3% (9 of 2804 patients) and morbidity was 10.5%.[1] Two studies reviewed the clinical benefits of laparoscopic versus OLR. The first study is a critical appraisal of 31 publications that directly compared LLR with OLR in 2473 patients.[49] In case-cohort studies of well-matched patients, LLR was associated with less blood loss, less packed red blood cell transfusion, quicker resumption of oral diet, less pain medication requirement, and shorter length of stay, as compared with OLR. Furthermore, seven publications in this analysis reported a lower morbidity (complication rates) in LLR versus OLR, whereas the remaining studies found no difference in complication rates.[32] Other potential advantages include better cosmetic results and, potentially, less of a physiologic stress response, including lower frequency of postoperative liver insufficiency, which was mentioned earlier.[50] This result might be explained by less destruction of the collateral blood/lymphatic flow in LLR during liver mobilization. In those patients undergoing laparoscopic hepatic resection for cancer, there was no difference in 3- or 5-year overall survival when compared with well-matched open hepatic resection cases. The subsequent review is a meta-analysis of 26 articles comparing LLR with OLR from 1998 to 2009.[51] In this study the LLR group had a lower operative blood loss, shorter hospital stay, less intravenous narcotic use, fewer days until oral intake, and lower relative risk of postoperative complications compared with the OLR group. Furthermore, the hazards ratio (HR) for recurrence of malignant tumors was not significantly different between the two groups (HR = 0.79; P = .37).[51] In another study, Martin et al. reported on 90 laparoscopic versus 360 open formal hepatic lobectomies.[52] Patients in the two arms were matched in a 1:4 ratio for age, ASA class, tumor size, histology, and tumor location. Benign tumors were more common in the laparoscopic group. Estimated intraoperative blood loss, Pringle time, total and pulmonary complication rates, and hospital length of stay were significantly lower for the laparoscopic group.

ONCOLOGIC OUTCOMES FOR LAPAROSCOPIC LIVER RESECTION

To date, no randomized clinical trial comparing LLR to OLR for cancer has been performed. Given the large number of cases already performed, as well as multiple case-cohort matched studies reported, it may be challenging to accrue patients to a randomized clinical trial, especially given the large number of patients required and difficulties in managing patient preference of suitable LLR candidates. The patients who are eligible for both approaches may not be willing to be randomized into the OLR group. In liver surgery the two basic surgical techniques commonly used to obtain optimal oncologic

outcome and reduce disease recurrences are anatomic resection for HCC and margin-negative parenchyma-sparing resection for CRC liver metastasis.[2] Anatomic resection refers to parenchyma-preserving resections of portal territories, including sectionectomy, segmentectomy, and subsegmentectomy.

In 2015 Maarschalk et al. reported the first case of port site metastasis involving peritoneum and abdominal wall in a patient who underwent a laparoscopic left lateral segmentectomy for an HCC nearly 3 years earlier.[53] Suffice it to say, however, from the vast body of literature available, there is no evidence for compromise of tumor margins or R0 resection rates, or worse oncologic outcomes using 5-year overall or disease-free survival when comparing LLR with OLR for CRC metastases or HCC (Table 125.3). A brief summary of a few noteworthy studies is provided.

COLORECTAL CANCER METASTASES

In a multicenter international series, Nguyen et al. described 109 patients who underwent minimally invasive liver resection for CRC metastasis, in four American and two French centers.[13] Major liver resections (three or more segments) were performed in 45% of patients. Median operating room time was 234 minutes (range, 60 to 555 minutes) and blood loss was 200 mL (range, 20 to 2500 mL), with 10% receiving a blood transfusion. There were four conversions to open surgery (3.7%), all due to bleeding. Median length of postoperative hospital stay for the entire series was 4 days (range, 1 to 22 days). The median interval from primary colon surgery to liver metastasectomy was 12 months (range, 0 to 60 months).

TABLE 125.3 Overall Survival After Laparoscopic Liver Resection Versus Open Liver Resection for Cancer in Comparative Studies

Reference	Year	Country	Journal	Tumor	OVERALL SURVIVAL			
					LLR	OLR	F/U (Year)	P-Value
Shimada et al.[54]	2001	Japan	Surg Endosc	HCC	50	38	5	NS
Laurent et al.[19]	2003	France	Arch Surgery	HCC	89	70	3	NS
Kaneko et al.[20]	2005	Japan	Am J Surgery	HCC	61	62	5	NS
Lee et al.[55]	2007	Hong Kong	Hong Kong Med J	CRC	81	79	3	NS
Cai et al.[56]	2008	China	Surg Endosc	Mix*	50	51	5	NS
Belli et al.[57]	2009	Italy	Br J Surgery	HCC	67	61	3	NS
Ito et al.[58]	2009	USA	J GI Surgery	CRC	72	56	3	NS
Lai et al.[59]	2009	Hong Kong	Arch Surgery	HCC	60	60	3	NS
Castaing et al.[60]	2009	France	Ann Surgery	CRC	64	56	5	NS
Endo et al.[50]	2009	Japan	Surg Lap Endo Tech	HCC	57	48	5	NS
Sarpel et al.[61]	2009	USA	Ann Surg Oncology	HCC	95	75	5	NS
Tranchart et al.[62]	2010	France	Surg Endosc	HCC	46	37	5	NS
Cannon et al.[63]	2012	USA	Surgery	CRC	36	42	5	NS
Iwahashi et al.[64]	2013	Japan	Surg Endosc	CRC	42	51	5	NS
Montalti et al.[65]	2014	Belgium	Surg Endosc	CRC	60	65	5	NS
Takahara et al.[32]	2015	Japan	J Hepatobiliary Pancreat Sci	HCC	77	71	5	NS
Beppu et al.[66]	2015	Japan	J Hepatobiliary Pancreat Sci	CRC	70	68	5	NS
Allard et al.[67]	2015	France	Ann Surg	CRC	78	75	5	NS
Meguro et al.[68]	2015	Japan	Surgery	HCC	82.1	61.8	5	NS
Komatsu et al.[69]	2016	Japan	Surg Endosc	HCC	69.2	73.4	3	NS
de'Angelis et al.[70]	2015	France	J Laparoendosc Adv Surg Tech A	CRC	73	62	5	NS

*Survival analysis of patients with malignant liver tumors (24 HCC, 2 CRC, 1 breast cancer metastasis, and 4 intrahepatic cholangiocarcinoma).
CRC, Colorectal carcinoma; *F/U*, follow-up; *HCC*, hepatocellular carcinoma; *LLR*, laparoscopic liver resection; *OLR*, open liver resection; *NS*, not significant.

The median tumor size was 3.0 cm, and negative margins were achieved in 94.4% of patients with a median margin of 10 mm. At 1, 3, and 5 years overall survival rates were 88%, 69%, and 50%, respectively, whereas disease-free survival rates were 65%, 43%, and 33%, respectively. Other studies by Sasaki et al.[14] and Kazaryan et al.[7] report similar 5-year overall survival rates of 64% and 51%, respectively, after LLR performed for CRC metastases. The report by Kazaryan et al. reflects a 12-year Norwegian single-center experience in 122 patients. The R0 resection rate was 93.4%, and the median tumor resection margin was 6 mm. These 5-year overall survival rates after LLR of CRC metastases are comparable to 5-year overall survival rates in the range of 37% to 50% reported in modern open hepatic resection series from large liver cancer centers.

In a prospective, head-to-head study, Castaing et al. described the results of two French groups, one performing laparoscopic and the other open hepatectomy, for metastatic CRC.[60] They matched 60 laparoscopic to 60 open cases, based on nine preoperative prognostic criteria predictive of survival: sex, age, primary tumor localization, number, size, and distribution of metastases, presence of extrahepatic disease, initial resectability, and prehepatectomy chemotherapy administration. The mean operative time, 60-day mortality (1.7% in both groups), general and hepatic complication rates, and median postoperative length of stay (10 days for the laparoscopic vs. 11 days for the open group), and mean resection margin were similar between the groups. The transfusion rate was significantly lower in the laparoscopic group (15% vs. 36%; P <.007). At a median follow-up of 34 months, the 5-year overall survival for the laparoscopic group was 64%, versus 56% for the open group (P = .32). The recurrence-free survival at 5 years was 30% for the laparoscopic and 20% for the open group (P = .12).

The most recent large study on long-term outcomes of LLR versus OLR for colorectal liver metastases is a 1:2 propensity score matched multiinstitutional study from 32 Japanese centers between 2005 and 2010.[66] Five-year recurrence-free survival (53.4% vs. 512%), overall survival (70.1% vs. 68%), and disease specific survival (73.2% vs. 69.8%) did not differ significantly between LLR and OLR groups, respectively.[66] Several meta-analyses have also shown comparable oncologic outcomes and survival between OLRs and LLRs.[72-76]

HEPATOCELLULAR CARCINOMA

Many studies have reported 5-year overall survival after LLR performed for HCC in the range of 50% to 75%, and 5-year disease-free survival ranging from 31% to 38%.[1] Kaneko et al. reported the results of 30 LLRs versus 28 OLRs for HCC.[20] The strength of this study is that all patients were offered a laparoscopic approach, but some elected open hepatectomy at the time of informed consent, thereby minimizing surgeon selection bias. The patients were well matched for age, gender, degree of cirrhosis, tumor size, ICG clearance, and extent of surgery. The laparoscopic group had a shorter time to ambulation, initiation of oral intake, and length of hospital stay. There were no significant differences in 5-year overall (61% vs. 62%) or disease-free (31% vs. 29%) survival between the LLR and OLR groups.

Tranchart et al. reported a case-control matched comparison of 42 patients who underwent LLR versus 42 patients undergoing OLR for HCC.[62] The LLR group had significantly less intraoperative blood loss (364 vs. 724 mL; P <.001), postoperative ascites (7.1% vs. 26.1%; P = .03), and shorter length of hospital stay (6.7 vs. 9.6 days; P <.001). There were no differences in transfusion rates or resection margins positivity. With a median follow-up of 30 months, there were no differences in overall survival. Sarpel et al. reported a case-cohort study of 20 LLRs versus 56 OLRs for HCC.[61] The two groups were well matched with no significant difference in age, gender degree of cirrhosis, or tumor size between the groups. There were no significant differences in rates of blood transfusion, operative time, or positive margins between the groups. The LLR group demonstrated a shorter length of stay, and there were no differences in overall or disease-free survival between the groups.

In a large series of 163 LLRs for HCC, Dagher et al. reported the results from three European centers from 1998 to 2008.[77] Seventy-four percent of patients were cirrhotic and the liver resection was anatomic in 107 (65.6%) patients and was a major resection (three or more segments) in 16 (9.8%). A totally laparoscopic approach was used in 155 (95.1%) patients. Median operative time was 180 minutes. Median blood loss was 250 mL, and 16 (9.8%) patients received a blood transfusion. Conversion to open surgery was required in 15 (9.2%) patients. Median tumor size was 3.6 cm, and median surgical margin was 12 mm. Liver-specific and general complications occurred in 19 (11.6%) and 17 (10.4%) patients, respectively. Postoperative hospital length of stay was 7 days. The 5-year overall survival was 64.9%, and 5-year recurrence-free survival was 32.2%. Similar to LLR for CRC metastases, the 5-year overall survival for HCC reported after LLR is comparable to the best data available for OLR for HCC.

Moreover, a study from an experienced hepatobiliary center showed that prior LLR (vs. OLR) for HCC facilitated subsequent salvage liver transplantation with decreased morbidity.[78] Of 24 patients who underwent salvage liver transplant after prior LLR (12 patients) or OLR (12 patients), patients who had previous LLR had shorter explant hepatectomy, decreased total operative time, less blood loss and reduced need for blood transfusions, as compared with the OLR patients.

The latest large multiinstitutional propensity matched study on long-term oncologic and perioperative outcomes of LLR versus OLR for HCC between 2000 and 2010 from 31 centers in Japan was published by Takahara et al.[32] Five-year overall survival (76.8% vs. 70.9%) and disease-free survival (40.7% vs. 39.3%) were comparable between the LLR and OLR groups, respectively.

ECONOMIC ASPECTS OF LAPAROSCOPIC LIVER SURGERY

One of the concerns regarding laparoscopic surgery is related to the cost of the procedure, particularly with the added costs of the laparoscopic instruments in the operating room, many of which are single-use disposables. Koffron et al. showed that the operating room costs for minimally invasive liver resections were higher than OLRs; however, the nonoperating room costs were higher in the open cases, with the primary determinant being greater length of hospital stay, leading to higher costs.[12] Vanounou et al. compared 44 laparoscopic LLSs with 29 open hepatic LLSs at the University of Pittsburgh Medical Center.[79] A deviation-based cost modeling (DBCM) approach was used to compare the economic impact of LLR with OLR approaches. The LLR cases had a shorter length of stay (3 vs. 5 days; $P < .001$) and a weighted average median cost savings of $2939, as compared with the OLR group. Likewise, in a comparative analysis from Dundee, United Kingdom, 25 patients undergoing LLR were compared with 25 well-matched OLR patients between 2005 and 2007.[80] The two groups were homogeneous by age, sex, coexistent morbidity, magnitude of resection, prevalence of liver cirrhosis, and indications. Hospital costs were obtained from the Scottish Health Service Costs Book (ISD Scotland). Overall hospital cost was significantly lower in the laparoscopic group by an average of 2571 pounds sterling (~3312 USD; $P < .04$). The most recent study on the economic comparison between LLR and OLR was reported by Bhojani et al. from Toronto, Canada using a 2:1 matched pair analysis.[81] The median length of stay was lower in the LLR group when compared with the open group. The median overall cost for the LLR was also lower at $11,376 versus $12,523 for the open group ($P = .077$). Therefore LLR appears to be the more fiscally advantageous approach when performed in appropriately selected patients.

During the Second International Consensus Conference on Laparoscopic Liver Resection held in Morioka, jury recommendations and expert technical recommendations were discussed and summarized.[2] Minor LLR was confirmed to be a standard practice because it has been adopted by an increasing proportion of surgeons. Major LLR is considered an innovative procedure, and it should continue to be introduced cautiously. As mentioned previously, major robotic hepatectomy has only limited data available for evaluation at this current time. Laparoscopic donor liver surgery should be performed under institutional ethical approval and reporting registry. General agreement among the liver surgery experts is achieved that experience in both open liver surgery and advanced laparoscopy is mandatory for successful LLRs. Surgeons must also begin with minor laparoscopic resections before embarking on the more complex ones. The hand-assisted and hybrid technique can help overcome certain difficulties associated with the pure LLR and may be useful in minimizing conversions. Conceptual changes include the caudal approach that optimizes hilar dissection and transection of the liver parenchyma for major and/or anterior resections. The lateral approach (left lateral decubitus position) can be used to optimize access to lesions located in posterior segments. Hilar approach includes individual hilar dissection and Glissonian approach. Although individual hilar dissection is considered the standard technique by many surgeons, the Glissonian approach is feasible and can be useful for anatomic liver resection, especially hemihepatectomy,

sectionectomy, or less. Although it can reduce operative time, this approach needs expertise, skills, and thorough knowledge of liver anatomy. Energy devices are efficient and reliable, but they should not replace the acquisition of basic skills of hepatic surgery, such as meticulous dissection, direct visualization, and proper sealing of the vascular structures.

SUMMARY

Laparoscopic liver surgery is an evolving discipline in the field of hepatobiliary surgery. Multiple studies have shown that LLR is safe and effective in the hands of experienced surgeons in selected patients. Clinical benefits to the patients include reduced blood loss, postoperative pain, narcotic use, and earlier discharge, with no overall financial disadvantage. From the oncologic standpoint, LLRs have been shown to yield equivalent cancer outcomes for HCC and CRC metastases with similar rates of negative margins, as well as 5-year overall and disease-free survival.

REFERENCES

1. Nguyen KT, Gamblin TC, Geller DA. World review of laparoscopic liver resection—2,804 patients. *Ann Surg*. 2009;250(5):831-841.
2. Wakabayashi G, Cherqui D, Geller DA, et al. Recommendations for laparoscopic liver resection: a report from the second international consensus conference held in Morioka. *Ann Surg*. 2015;261(4):619-629.
3. Buell JF, Cherqui D, Geller DA, et al. The international position on laparoscopic liver surgery: The Louisville Statement, 2008. *Ann Surg*. 2009;250(5):825-830.
4. Ciria R, Cherqui D, Geller DA, Briceno J, Wakabayashi G. Comparative short-term benefits of laparoscopic liver resection: 9000 cases and climbing. *Ann Surg*. 2016;263:761-767.
5. Hibi T, Cherqui D, Geller DA, Itano O, Kitagawa Y, Wakabayashi G. Expanding indications and regional diversity in laparoscopic liver resection unveiled by the International Survey on Technical Aspects of Laparoscopic Liver Resection (INSTALL) study. *Surg Endosc*. 2016; 30:2975-2983.
6. Tsung A, Geller DA, Sukato DC, et al. Robotic versus laparoscopic hepatectomy: a matched comparison. *Ann Surg*. 2014;259(3):549-555.
7. Viganò L, Tayar C, Laurent A, Cherqui D. Laparoscopic liver resection: a systematic review. *J Hepatobiliary Pancreat Surg*. 2009;16(4):410-421.
8. Pulitanò C, Aldrighetti L. The current role of laparoscopic liver resection for the treatment of liver tumors. *Nat Clin Pract Gastroenterol Hepatol*. 2008;5(11):648-654.
9. Koffron A, Geller D, Gamblin TC, Abecassis M. Laparoscopic liver surgery: shifting the management of liver tumors. *Hepatology*. 2006; 44(6):1694-1700.
10. Cherqui D, Laurent A, Tayar C, et al. Laparoscopic liver resection for peripheral hepatocellular carcinoma in patients with chronic liver disease: midterm results and perspectives. *Ann Surg*. 2006;243(4): 499-506.
11. Buell JF, Thomas MT, Rudich S, et al. Experience with more than 500 minimally invasive hepatic procedures. *Ann Surg*. 2008;248(3): 475-486.
12. Koffron AJ, Auffenberg G, Kung R, Abecassis M. Evaluation of 300 minimally invasive liver resections at a single institution: less is more. *Ann Surg*. 2007;246(3):385-392.
13. Nguyen KT, Laurent A, Dagher I, et al. Minimally invasive liver resection for metastatic colorectal cancer: a multi-institutional, international report of safety, feasibility, and early outcomes. *Ann Surg*. 2009;250(5):842-848.
14. Sasaki A, Nitta H, Otsuka K, Takahara T, Nishizuka S, Wakabayashi G. Ten-year experience of totally laparoscopic liver resection in a single institution. *Br J Surg*. 2009;96(3):274-279.
15. Kazaryan AM, Pavlik Marangos I, Rosseland AR, et al. Laparoscopic liver resection for malignant and benign lesions: ten-year Norwegian single-center experience. *Arch Surg*. 2010;145(1):34-40.
16. Descottes B, Glineur D, Lachachi F, et al. Laparoscopic liver resection of benign liver tumors. *Surg Endosc*. 2003;17(1):23-30.

17. Gamblin TC, Holloway SE, Heckman JT, Geller DA. Laparoscopic resection of benign hepatic cysts: a new standard. *J Am Coll Surg.* 2008;207(5):731-736.

18. Gigot JF, Glineur D, Santiago Azagra J, et al. Laparoscopic liver resection for malignant liver tumors: preliminary results of a multicenter European study. *Ann Surg.* 2002;236(1):90-97.

19. Laurent A, Cherqui D, Lesurtel M, Brunetti F, Tayar C, Fagniez PL. Laparoscopic liver resection for subcapsular hepatocellular carcinoma complicating chronic liver disease. *Arch Surg.* 2003;138(7):763-769.

20. Kaneko H, Takagi S, Otsuka Y, et al. Laparoscopic liver resection of hepatocellular carcinoma. *Am J Surg.* 2005;189(2):190-194.

21. Nguyen KT, Gamblin TC, Geller DA. Laparoscopic liver resection for cancer. *Future Oncol.* 2008;4(5):661-670.

22. Dagher I, O'Rourke N, Geller DA, et al. Laparoscopic major hepatectomy: an evolution in standard of care. *Ann Surg.* 2009;250(5):856-860.

23. O'Rourke N, Fielding G. Laparoscopic right hepatectomy: surgical technique. *J Gastrointest Surg.* 2004;8(2):213-216.

24. Topal B, Aerts R, Penninckx F. Laparoscopic intrahepatic Glissonian approach for right hepatectomy is safe, simple, and reproducible. *Surg Endosc.* 2007;21(11):2111.

25. Gayet B, Cavaliere D, Vibert E, et al. Total laparoscopic right hepatectomy. *Am J Surg.* 2007;194(5):685-689.

26. Dagher I, Di Giuro G, Dubrez J, Lainas P, Smadja C, Franco D. Laparoscopic versus open right hepatectomy: a comparative study. *Am J Surg.* 2009;198(2):173-177

27. Samama G, Chiche L, Bréfort JL, Le Roux Y. Laparoscopic anatomical hepatic resection. Report of four left lobectomies for solid tumors. *Surg Endosc.* 1998;12(1):76-78.

28. Vibert E, Perniceni T, Levard H, Denet C, Shahri NK, Gayet B. Laparoscopic liver resection. *Br J Surg.* 2006;93(1):67-72.

29. Gumbs AA, Bar-Zakai B, Gayet B. Totally laparoscopic extended left hepatectomy. *J Gastrointest Surg.* 2008;12(7):1152.

30. Gumbs AA, Gayet B. Multimedia article. Totally laparoscopic extended right hepatectomy. *Surg Endosc.* 2008;22(9):2076-2077.

31. Fretland ÅA, Kazaryan AM, Bjørnbeth BA, et al. Open versus laparoscopic liver resection for colorectal liver metastases (the Oslo-CoMet Study): study protocol for a randomized controlled trial. *Trials.* 2015;16:73.

32. Takahara T, Wakabayashi G, Beppu T, et al. Long-term and perioperative outcomes of laparoscopic versus open liver resection for hepatocellular carcinoma with propensity score matching: a multiinstitutional Japanese study. *J Hepatobiliary Pancreat Sci.* 2015;22(10):721-727.

33. Soubrane O, Cherqui D, Scatton O, et al. Laparoscopic left lateral sectionectomy in living donors: safety and reproducibility of the technique in a single center. *Ann Surg.* 2006;244(5):815-820.

34. Kurosaki I, Yamamoto S, Kitami C, et al. Video-assisted living donor hemihepatectomy through a 12-cm incision for adult-to-adult liver transplantation. *Surgery.* 2006;139(5):695-703.

35. Koffron AJ, Kung R, Baker T, Fryer J, Clark L, Abecassis M. Laparoscopic-assisted right lobe donor hepatectomy. *Am J Transplant.* 2006;6(10):2522-2525.

36. Soubrane O, de Rougemont O, Kim KH, et al. Laparoscopic living donor left lateral sectionectomy: a new standard practice for donor hepatectomy. *Ann Surg.* 2015;262(5):757-763.

37. Koffron AJ, Kung RD, Auffenberg GB, Abecassis MM. Laparoscopic liver surgery for everyone: the hybrid method. *Surgery.* 2007;142(4):463-468.

38. Cardinal JS, Reddy SK, Tsung A, Marsh JW, Geller DA. Laparoscopic major hepatectomy: pure laparoscopic approach versus hand-assisted technique. *J Hepatobiliary Pancreat Sci.* 2013;20(2):114-119.

39. Ryska M, Fronek J, Rudis J, Jurenka B, Langer D, Pudil J. Manual and robotic laparoscopic liver resection. Two case-reviews. *Rozhl Chir.* 2006;85(10):511-516.

40. Tsung A, Geller DA. Reply to Letter: "Does the robot provide an advantage over laparoscopic liver resection?". *Ann Surg.* 2015;262(2):e70-e71.

41. Packiam V, Bartlett DL, Tohme S, et al. Minimally invasive liver resection: robotic versus laparoscopic left lateral sectionectomy. *J Gastrointest Surg.* 2012;16(12):2233-2238.

42. Tranchart H, O'Rourke N, Van Dam R, et al. Bleeding control during laparoscopic liver resection: a review of literature. *J Hepatobiliary Pancreat Sci.* 2015;22(5):371-378.

43. Decailliot F, Streich B, Heurtematte Y, Duvaldestin P, Cherqui D, Stéphan F. Hemodynamic effects of portal triad clamping with and without pneumoperitoneum: an echocardiographic study. *Anesth Analg.* 2005;100(3):617-622.

44. Otsuka Y, Kaneko H, Cleary SP, Buell JF, Cai X, Wakabayashi G. What is the best technique in parenchymal transection in laparoscopic liver resection? Comprehensive review for the clinical question on the 2nd International Consensus Conference on Laparoscopic Liver Resection. *J Hepatobiliary Pancreat Sci.* 2015;22(5):363-370.

45. Wakabayashi G, Nitta H, Takahara T, Shimazu M, Kitajima M, Sasaki A. Standardization of basic skills for laparoscopic liver surgery towards laparoscopic donor hepatectomy. *J Hepatobiliary Pancreat Surg.* 2009;16(4):439-444.

46. Soubrane O, Schwarz L, Cauchy F, et al. A conceptual technique for laparoscopic right hepatectomy based on facts and oncologic principles: the caudal approach. *Ann Surg.* 2015;261(6):1226-1231.

47. Wakabayashi G, Cherqui D, Geller DA, Han HS, Kaneko H, Buell JF. Laparoscopic hepatectomy is theoretically better than open hepatectomy: preparing for the 2nd International Consensus Conference on Laparoscopic Liver Resection. *J Hepatobiliary Pancreat Sci.* 2014;21(10):723-731.

48. Ikeda T, Mano Y, Morita K, et al. Pure laparoscopic hepatectomy in semiprone position for right hepatic major resection. *J Hepatobiliary Pancreat Sci.* 2013;20(2):145-150

49. Nguyen KT, Marsh JW, Tsung A, Steel JJ, Gamblin TC, Geller DA. Comparative benefits of laparoscopic versus open hepatic resection: a critical appraisal. *Arch Surg.* 2011;146:348

50. Endo Y, Ohta M, Sasaki A, et al. A comparative study of the long-term outcomes after laparoscopy-assisted and open left lateral hepatectomy for hepatocellular carcinoma. *Surg Laparosc Endosc Percutan Tech.* 2009;19:71.

51. Croome KP, Yamashita MH. Laparoscopic vs open hepatic resection for benign and malignant tumors: an updated meta-analysis. *Arch Surg.* 2010;145(11):1109-1118.

52. Martin RC, Scoggins CR, McMasters KM. Laparoscopic hepatic lobectomy: advantages of a minimally invasive approach. *J Am Coll Surg.* 2010;210(5):627.

53. Marschalk J, Robinson SM, White SA. Port site metastases following laparoscopic liver resection for hepatocellular carcinoma. *Ann R Coll Surg Engl.* 2015;97(4):e52-e53.

54. Shimada M, Hashizume M, Maehara S, et al. Laparoscopic hepatectomy for hepatocellular carcinoma. *Surg Endosc.* 2001;15:541.

55. Lee KF, Cheung YS, Chong CN, et al. Laparoscopic versus open hepatectomy for liver tumours: a case control study. *Hong Kong Med J.* 2007;13(6):442-448.

56. Cai XJ, Yang J, Yu H, et al. Clinical study of laparoscopic versus open hepatectomy for malignant liver tumors. *Surg Endosc.* 2008;22(11):2350-2356.

57. Belli G, Limongelli P, Fantini C, et al. Laparoscopic and open treatment of hepatocellular carcinoma in patients with cirrhosis. *Br J Surg.* 2009;96(9):1041-1048.

58. Ito K, Ito H, Are C, et al. Laparoscopic versus open liver resection: a matched-pair case control study. *J Gastrointest Surg.* 2009;3:2276.

59. Lai EC, Tang CN, Ha JP, Li MK. Laparoscopic liver resection for hepatocellular carcinoma: ten-year experience in a single center. *Arch Surg.* 2009;144(2):143-147.

60. Castaing D, Vibert E, Ricca L, Azoulay D, Adam R, Gayet B. Oncologic results of laparoscopic versus open hepatectomy for colorectal liver metastases in two specialized centers. *Ann Surg.* 2009;250(5):849-855.

61. Sarpel U, Hefti MM, Wisnievsky JP, Roayaie S, Schwartz ME, Labow DM. Outcome for patients treated with laparoscopic versus open resection of hepatocellular carcinoma: case-matched analysis. *Ann Surg Oncol.* 2009;16(6):1572-1577

62. Tranchart H, Di Giuro G, Lainas P, et al. Laparoscopic resection for hepatocellular carcinoma: a matched-pair comparative study. *Surg Endosc.* 2010;24(5):1170-1176.

63. Cannon RM, Scoggins CR, Callender GG, McMasters KM, Martin RC 2nd. Laparoscopic versus open resection of hepatic colorectal metastases. *Surgery.* 2012;152(4):567-573; discussion 573-574.

64. Iwahashi S, Shimada M, Utsunomiya T, et al. Laparoscopic hepatic resection for metastatic liver tumor of colorectal cancer: comparative analysis of short- and long-term results. *Surg Endosc.* 2014;28(1):80-84.

65. Montalti R, Tomassini F, Laurent S, et al. Impact of surgical margins on overall and recurrence-free survival in parenchymal-sparing laparoscopic liver resections of colorectal metastases. *Surg Endosc.* 2015;29(9):2736-2747.

66. Beppu T, Wakabayashi G, Hasegawa K, et al. Long-term and perioperative outcomes of laparoscopic versus open liver resection for colorectal

liver metastases with propensity score matching: a multi-institutional Japanese study. *J Hepatobiliary Pancreat Sci.* 2015;22(10):711-720.

67. Allard MA, Cunha AS, Gayet B, et al. Early and long-term oncological outcomes after laparoscopic resection for colorectal liver metastases: a propensity score-based analysis. *Ann Surg.* 2015;262(5):794-802.

68. Meguro M, Mizuguchi T, Kawamoto M, et al. Clinical comparison of laparoscopic and open liver resection after propensity matching selection. *Surgery.* 2015;158(3):573-587.

69. Komatsu S, Brustia R, Goumard C, Perdigao F, Soubrane O, Scatton O. Laparoscopic versus open major hepatectomy for hepatocellular carcinoma: a matched pair analysis. *Surg Endosc.* 2016;30:1965-1974.

70. de'Angelis N, Eshkenazy R, Brunetti F, et al. Laparoscopic versus open resection for colorectal liver metastases: a single-center study with propensity score analysis. *J Laparoendosc Adv Surg Tech A.* 2015; 25(1):12-20.

71. Kazaryan AM, Marangos IP, Røsok BI, et al. Laparoscopic resection of colorectal liver metastases: surgical and long-term oncologic outcome. *Ann Surg.* 2010;252(6):1005-1012.

72. Schiffman SC, Kim KH, Tsung A, Marsh JW, Geller DA. Laparoscopic versus open liver resection for metastatic colorectal cancer: a metaanalysis of 610 patients. *Surgery.* 2015;157(2):211-222.

73. Parks KR, Kuo YH, Davis JM, O' Brien B, Hagopian EJ. Laparoscopic versus open liver resection: a meta-analysis of long-term outcome. *HPB (Oxford).* 2014;16(2):109-118.

74. Wei M, He Y, Wang J, Chen N, Zhou Z, Wang Z. Laparoscopic versus open hepatectomy with or without synchronous colectomy

for colorectal liver metastasis: a meta-analysis. *PLoS One.* 2014;9(1): e87461.

75. Luo LX, Yu ZY, Bai YN. Laparoscopic hepatectomy for liver metastases from colorectal cancer: a meta-analysis. *J Laparoendosc Adv Surg Tech A.* 2014;24(4):213-222.

76. Zhou Y, Xiao Y, Wu L, et al. Laparoscopic liver resection as a safe and efficacious alternative to open resection for colorectal liver metastasis: a meta-analysis. *BMC Surg.* 2013;13:44.

77. Dagher I, Belli G, Fantini C, et al. Laparoscopic hepatectomy for hepatocellular carcinoma: a European experience. *J Am Coll Surg.* 2010;211(1):16-23.

78. Laurent A, Tayar C, Andréoletti M, Lauzet JY, Merle JC, Cherqui D. Laparoscopic liver resection facilitates salvage liver transplantation for hepatocellular carcinoma. *J Hepatobiliary Pancreat Surg.* 2009;16(3): 310-314.

79. Vanounou T, Steel JL, Nguyen KT, et al. Comparing the clinical and economic impact of laparoscopic versus open liver resection. *Ann Surg Oncol.* 2010;17(4):998-1009.

80. Polignano FM, Quyn AJ, de Figueiredo RS, Henderson NA, Kulli C, Tait IS. Laparoscopic versus open liver segmentectomy: prospective, case-matched, intention-to-treat analysis of clinical outcomes and cost effectiveness. *Surg Endosc.* 2008;22(12):2564-2570.

81. Bhojani FD, Fox A, Pitzul K, et al. Clinical and economic comparison of laparoscopic to open liver resections using a 2-to-1 matched pair analysis: an institutional experience. *J Am Coll Surg.* 2012;214(2): 184-195.

Ablative Therapies for Hepatic Neoplasms

David A. Mahvi | David M. Mahvi

The liver is a common site for both primary and metastatic oncologic disease. Primary hepatocellular carcinoma (HCC) has an annual incidence of 6 per 100,000 in the United States.[1] Worldwide HCC is the second leading cause of cancer-related death in men and sixth leading cause in women. Furthermore, the worldwide incidence and number of deaths per year for HCC are nearly identical, highlighting the aggressive nature of the disease.[2]

The liver is also the most common site for gastrointestinal (GI) tumor metastasis. Colorectal cancer is the third leading cancer cause of death in the United States.[3] Approximately 15% to 20% of patients with colorectal cancer present with synchronous liver metastases, and approximately 50% will develop liver metastases at some point.[4] There are limited data suggesting a role for liver-directed therapies in other metastatic GI tumors at this time, although there is some evidence that certain neuroendocrine and GI stromal tumors may also benefit from resection or ablation.

The first-line therapy for both primary and metastatic liver neoplastic disease is resection by partial hepatectomy or, in the case of select HCC total hepatectomy and transplantation. The liver can tolerate extensive resection because of its regenerative capacity, but underlying liver disease and the presence of multiple lesions limit the number of candidates for this potentially curative therapy. Ablative therapies were developed to expand the number of patients amenable to treatment. The widespread use of ablative techniques has been limited by the lack of randomized trials comparing ablation to other therapies. Specifically, ablative techniques have not been directly compared with surgical resection in randomized trials, except in the treatment of small HCC lesions. All non-randomized comparisons are limited by the variation in the definition of "unresectable." Resection studies tend to find fewer unresectable tumors, and ablation studies tend to find more. These caveats make direct comparisons challenging.

This chapter will focus on the multitude of ablative treatment options. The most established is radiofrequency ablation (RFA). Newer strategies include microwave ablation (MWA), high-intensity focused ultrasound, irreversible electroporation (IRL), and percutaneous laser ablation. It will also touch on cryotherapy and percutaneous ethanol injection (PEI), which are used less frequently nowadays.

RADIOFREQUENCY ABLATION

RFA is the most commonly used nonsurgical therapy for liver neoplasms. RFA can be performed open, laparoscopically, or percutaneously. RFA uses a needle electrode to deliver a high-frequency electrical current to generate heat, ultimately resulting in cellular necrosis.[5] Fig. 126.1 shows the characteristic posttreatment appearance on computed tomography (CT) scan.

A major limiting factor for RFA efficacy is the proximity of target lesions to blood vessels, which function as a heat sink, resulting in smaller-diameter treatment areas, and can be a cause of persistent disease. Specifically, proximity to blood vessels larger than 3 mm has been shown to be an independent predictor of incomplete tumor ablation by RFA.[6] The heat sink effect can be partially mitigated with either the Pringle maneuver or percutaneous balloon occlusion of a large hepatic or portal vessel, although the effect may only work in smaller tumors.[7]

Controversy also exists over the best access method, percutaneous versus a surgical approach. Early studies showed lower recurrence rates with an open surgical approach.[8] However, recurrence rates overlap broadly in different studies. The American Society of Clinical Oncology (ASCO) review of RFA concluded that there is insufficient evidence to resolve the issue of optimal approach.[9] It may be advisable to avoid a percutaneous RFA approach if the stomach, duodenum, diaphragm, or transverse colon are in close proximity to one of the target lesions.

RFA is typically well tolerated. The mortality rate is 0% to 2% and the major complication rate was 6% to 9%.[9] Common complications included liver abscess, biliary leakage or stricture, hemorrhage, pleural effusion, pneumothorax, hypoxemia during treatment, and subcapsular hematoma.[10]

Local recurrence rates were analyzed in a meta-analysis and found multiple contributing factors. Namely, tumor size greater than 5 cm, close proximity to a major vessel, subcapsular tumor location, intentional margin less than 1 cm, lack of vascular occlusion, and physician experience were all statistically significant predictors of local recurrence after RFA.[11]

RADIOFREQUENCY ABLATION IN HEPATOCELLULAR CARCINOMA

RFA has been extensively used either alone or combined with other therapies for localized HCC both as primary therapy and as a bridge to hepatic transplantation. The most important predictor of efficacy is size of the tumor(s) being treated. Complete radiographic response is seen in 30% to 90% of tumors less than 3 cm, as compared with 50% to 70% in lesions 3 to 5 cm in size.[12–14] Table 126.1 shows representative series of patients with HCC treated with RFA.[15–24] Five-year overall survival (OS) ranged from 17% to 76%, with complication rates of 1% to 12%.

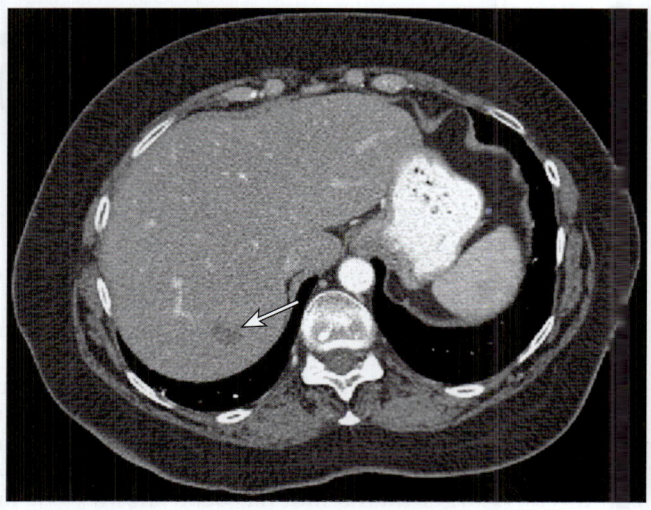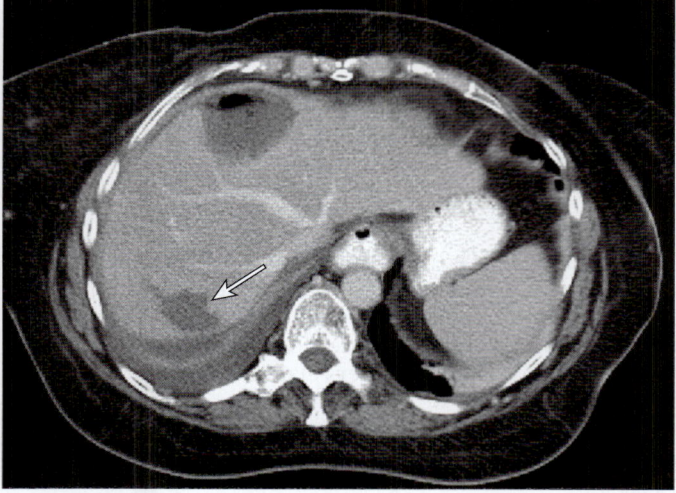

FIGURE 126.1 Computed tomography scan of a liver tumor before *(left; arrow)* and 1 month after *(right; arrow)* radiofrequency ablation. (Courtesy Dr. David J. Bentrem, Department of Surgery, Northwestern University Feinberg School of Medicine, Chicago, Illinois.)

TABLE 126.1 Series of Radiofrequency Ablation in Patients With Hepatocellular Carcinoma

Author	Year	Patients	1-Year Overall Survival (%)	3-Year Overall Survival (%)	5-Year Overall Survival (%)	Complications (%)	Incomplete Ablation (%)	Local Recurrence (%)
Wong*	2013	76	87.3	61	48.6	4.7	17.5	24.7
Wong†	2013	100	92.8	68.7	47.2	4.7	15.4	29.4
Shiina	2012	1170	96.6	80.5	60.2	2.2	0.6	2.9
Rossi	2011	706	—	67	47.1	1	1.4	12.1% at 3 years
Livraghi	2008	218	—	76	55	1.8	1.8	0.90%
Choi	2007	570	95.2	69.5	58	1.9	3.3	11.8% at 3 years
Takahashi	2007	171	98.8	91.1	76.8	—	—	17.7% at 3 years
Chen	2006	71	95.8	71.4	64	4.2	4.2	—
Tateishi	2005	319	94.7	77.7	54.3	—	—	2.4% at 3 years
Lencioni	2005	187	97	71	48	—	—	10% at 3 years
Raut	2005	194	84.5	68.1	55.4	12	2.1	4.6

*Accessed laparoscopically or open.
†Accessed percutaneously.

There have been several trials directly comparing RFA with primary surgical resection for HCC. In one large study of patients with HCC tumors less than 2 cm, OS was similar at 1 and 2 years (98% vs. 99% and 94% vs. 95%, respectively). However, disease-free survival was significantly higher in the surgery group at both 1 and 2 years (91% vs. 84% and 70% vs. 58%, respectively).[25] More recently, a randomized trial between RFA and surgery in HCC tumors less than 4 cm found no statistically significant difference in OS or recurrence-free survival, although there was a trend toward the surgical group faring better.[26] Another randomized trial of 230 patients who met the Milan criteria showed statistically improved overall and recurrence-free survival in the surgery group compared with RFA.[27] At this point in time, patients who are surgical candidates and whose HCC is technically resectable should undergo surgical resection as first-line therapy.

RFA is also a viable option for recurrent HCC. Two representative series of patients with HCC recurrence after a liver resection treated with RFA found 1-year OS of 82% to 91.8% and 5-year OS of 38.2%.[22,28]

RADIOFREQUENCY ABLATION IN COLORECTAL CANCER METASTASES

Patients with isolated liver metastases from colorectal cancer deemed not to be surgical candidates also benefit from RFA.[29] RFA has also been studied both with and in place of chemotherapy in these patients with a significantly improved progression-free survival (PFS)[30] and OS.[31] Table 126.2 shows a select series of larger patient cohorts treated with RFA for colorectal cancer metastases to the liver.[30–36]

There have been no randomized controlled trials comparing surgical resection to RFA for patients with potentially resectable liver metastases. Retrospective series have been done which show improved PFS and OS in

TABLE 126.2 Series of Radiofrequency Ablation in Patients With Metastatic Colorectal Cancer to the Liver

Author	Year	Patients	1-Year Overall Survival (%)	3-Year Overall Survival (%)	5-Year Overall Survival (%)	Complications (%)	Incomplete Ablation (%)	Local Recurrence (%)
Kennedy*	2013	130	93.5	50.1	23.8	8.4	—	9.2
Veltri†	2012	248	93	62	35	7.3	0	—
Solbiati‡	2012	99	93	69.3	47.8	1.3	6.9	11.9
Hammill§	2011	101	87.6	52	33.1	2	—	11.9
Siperstein	2007	234	—	20.2	18.4	—	—	—
Sorensen	2007	102	95	64	44	10.9	—	—
Machi‖	2006	100	90	42	30.5	4.8 (major)	—	6.7

*Access was all laparoscopically.
†Median survival was 41 months if less than 3 cm and 21.7 months if greater than 3 cm.
‡10 years OS 18%. Fifty-four percent of locally aggressive tumors were retreated with RFA and survival significantly improved compared with no retreatment.
§Access was all laparoscopically. Patients with technically resectable disease had significantly longer OS but similar DFS.
‖Median survival was 48 months when RFA used as first-line treatment and 22 months when second-line or salvage therapy after failed chemotherapy.
DFS, Disease-free survival; OS, overall survival; RFA, radiofrequency ablation.

patients in the surgical arm.[37-39] Of note, in these and other similar studies, patients typically underwent RFA only if their disease was unresectable or if they were deemed poor operative candidates. Based on these and similar studies, both ASCO[9] and a Cochrane review[40] concluded that surgical resection should be favored over RFA in patients with potentially resectable liver metastases from colorectal cancer.

One interesting series compared 39 patients who received RFA with 39 who received systemic chemotherapy prospectively after a laparotomy revealed unresectable disease.[41] There was a nonsignificant trend toward improved OS in the RFA group at both 2 years (56% vs. 51%) and 5 years (27% vs. 15%). There was also a significant improvement in quality-adjusted life years in the RFA group, which is an important outcome for oncologic patients.

A randomized trial of 119 patients with nonresectable colorectal cancer liver metastases between chemotherapy (FOLFOX ± bevacizumab) with or without RFA was done. In the 10-year follow-up, patients in the combination group had a significantly longer median survival (45.6 vs. 40.5 months) and 8-year OS (36% vs. 9%).[42] A creative study compared the RFA arm of the above trial to the surgical arm of another prospective randomized trial, which randomized patients with metastatic colorectal cancer to surgery alone or surgery with neoadjuvant and adjuvant FOLFOX4.[43] In comparing the two trials,[44] the group found the local recurrence rate for surgery was 5.5% per lesion compared with 10% per lesion in their RFA group; the rate for RFA local recurrence of lesions smaller than 3 cm was 2.9%. Although this study is limited because the two sets of patients were different and the RFA trial had patients with, on average, more advanced disease, it does provide some preliminary evidence that RFA may provide similar local control for limited liver metastases compared with surgery when combined with systemic chemotherapy.

The benefit of RFA for regional treatment of liver metastases in patients with extrahepatic disease who are undergoing systemic chemotherapy remains uncertain, and this approach is not considered standard of care.[9,40]

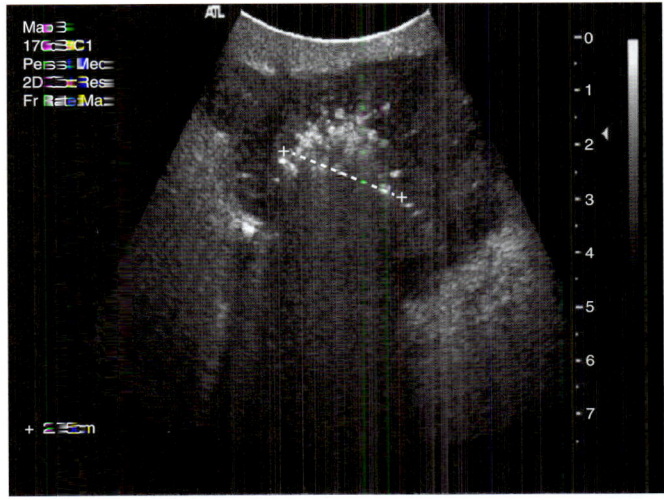

FIGURE 126.2 Intraoperative ultrasound of a liver tumor undergoing microwave ablation.

MICROWAVE ABLATION

MWA is a therapy initially developed for lung cancers that is increasingly being used to treat liver tumors. MWA generates heat using electromagnetic waves to create a zone of energy that causes hyperthermic injury to tumor cells. Ablation zones using third-generation MWA antennas can be up to 6 cm. Fig. 126.2 shows an intraoperative ultrasound of MWA in use. Compared with RFA, MWA has several potential advantages. MWA has shorter treatment times, is less susceptible to the heat sink effect, and produces more predictable ablation zone.[46] In a systematic review the MWA major complication rate was 4.6% and mortality rate of 0.23%. The most common complications were bleeding, bile leak, liver abscess, and portal vein thrombosis.[47] Table 126.3 shows that the range of 1-year OS in representative published series for HCC is 72% to 92% and 5-year OS range is 30% to 72%.[13,48-50]

There have been several studies that compare MWA with RFA in patients with liver tumors. A nonrandomized trial from China evaluated 155 patients with HCC tumors

TABLE 126.3 Series of Microwave Ablation in Patients With Hepatocellular Carcinoma

Author	Year	Patients	1-Year Overall Survival (%)	3-Year Overall Survival (%)	5-Year Overall Survival (%)	Complications (%)	Incomplete Ablation (%)	Local Recurrence (%)
Dong	2003	234	92.7	72.85	56.7	8.9 (all minor)	7.2	7.2
Lu	2005	49	81.6	50.5	—	8.2	6.9	11.8
Yin*	2009	109	75.8	30.9	15.4	9.2	7.4	22
Swan	2013	54	72.3	58.8 (2 year)	—	28.9	5.9	2.9

*HCC tumors in this series were 3 to 7 cm in size.

less than 5 cm treated with either RFA or MWA.[51] Local tumor progression was seen in 10.5% of MWA patients (vs. 11.8% of RFA). For small tumors (<3 cm) and larger tumors (3.1 to 5.0 cm) there was a nonsignificant trend toward improved disease-free survival in the RFA group. In another representative retrospective study, in 197 patients, the disease-free survival in the MWA group at 1, 2, 3, and 4 years was 75.0%, 59.4%, 32.1%, and 16.1%, respectively (compared with 80.3%, 61.8%, 39.5%, and 19.0% in the RFA group; P = .376).[52] A recent meta-analysis between MWA and RFA in HCC found a nonsignificant trend that MWA was superior for larger nodules and also a nonsignificant higher complication rate with MWA; the authors concluded that the two treatments have similar efficacy based on present studies.[53]

MWA is also beginning to be used in metastatic colorectal cancer lesions. In a systematic review of MWA of colorectal liver metastases, the local recurrence rate with MWA was between 5% and 13%, with mean 1-, 3-, and 5-year survival of 73%, 30%, and 16%, respectively.[54] A Cochrane review determined that there was insufficient evidence to recommend treatment of resectable liver metastases with MWA.[55]

HIGH-INTENSITY–FOCUSED ULTRASOUND ABLATION

High-intensity–focused ultrasound ablation (HIFU) is a noninvasive thermal ablation therapy. Acoustic energy from a high-intensity ultrasound beam is delivered to a focal zone, where it is converted into heat and induces coagulative necrosis with minimal damage to surrounding normal structures.[56]

There are no comparative studies of HIFU with either surgical resection or other ablation techniques. Response rates were higher in one series in the left lobe (90.5%) compared with the right (64.1%), likely due to interference of the overlying ribs.[57] There are currently minimal long-term follow-up data for HIFU for liver tumors. One representative study reported 1- and 3-year OS of 87.7% and 62.4%, respectively.[58]

Given the concern of using thermal-based ablation near major vascular structures, an important advantage of HIFU is that it does not rely on thermal energy and can avoid these complications. This was reported in a cohort of 39 patients with HCC treated with HIFU that found no evidence of a major blood vessel injury treating tumors located less than 1 cm from the inferior vena cava, portal vein, or a main hepatic vein.[59]

IRREVERSIBLE ELECTROPORATION

IRE is an ablative technique that uses electrodes to destabilize the cell membrane by creating nanopores in the lipid bilayer.[60] Because IRE is nonthermal, it does minimal damage to surrounding structures outside the ablative zone[61] and is ideal to treat lesions near major vascular or biliary structures in the liver.[62] It also avoids the heat-sink phenomenon seen with RFA and other thermal ablative techniques. IRE requires general anesthesia to perform, and the coordination of multiple parallel probes can be very complex to plan.

As IRE is a relatively new technology, long-term follow-up data are sparse at this time. Small series report a complete ablation rate of 73% to 100%. One series of 28 patients had a 6-month recurrence rate of 5.7%.[63] A series of 44 patients by another group showed a recurrence-free survival rate of 59.5% at 1 year.[64] A systematic review of the safety of IRE reported an overall complication rate of 16% in 129 patients.[65] The most common complications were portal vein thrombosis, pneumothorax, biliary occlusion, and arrhythmias.

IRE is an exciting new ablative technique, given its avoidance of thermal complications. However, long-term outcomes have yet to be reported, and it is still considered investigational at this time.

LASER ABLATION

Percutaneous laser ablation converts light energy into heat energy to induce coagulative necrosis.[66] It is used frequently in Italy. A large representative series included 432 patients with unresectable HCCs with either a single tumor less than 4 cm or two to three nodules all less than 3 cm in size. Median disease-free survival was 26 months. The 3- and 5-year OS rates were 61% and 34%, respectively.[67] Laser ablation has a reported 0.4% mortality rate. The rates of major and minor complications are 1.5% and 6.2%, respectively.[68] A small randomized trial of 30 patients compared laser ablation to RFA.[69] The study found similar complete response rates (87% vs. 93%, respectively). However, patients with tumors greater than 2 cm treated with laser ablation did show a significantly higher recurrence rate at 12 months.

CRYOABLATION

Cryoablation uses a cryoprobe that can rapidly cool hepatic tissue with argon or liquid nitrogen to cause irreversible cell death by intracellular ice crystal formation.[70] In the largest reported series to date, 856 patients with 1197 HCC lesions were treated with cryotherapy. The complete response rate was 96%. Median OS was 57.9 months, with 1-year OS of 98.6% and 5-year OS of 60.3%. Major complications occurred in 2.4% of patients and minor complications in 10.6%.[71]

A randomized controlled trial compared RFA with cryotherapy for HCC smaller than 4 cm in diameter. Local tumor progression was significantly lower in the cryotherapy group at 1, 2, and 3 years (3%, 7%, and 7%, respectively) compared with the RFA group (9%, 11%, and 11%, respectively; $P = .043$). However OS and tumor-free survival were similar between the two groups. Major complication rates were also similar between the two groups.[72]

Many centers stopped performing cryotherapy for liver tumors due to the impression of higher reported complication rates compared with other ablative techniques. Complications include hemorrhage, biliary injury, abscess formation, liver shearing, and "cryoshock." Cryoshock is a unique complication of cryoablation resulting from release of cytokines causing multiorgan failure and a disseminated intravascular coagulation.[6] Notably, cryoablation for tumor ablation seems to be increasing in popularity as newer probes have been introduced.

PERCUTANEOUS ETHANOL INJECTION

Percutaneous chemical ablation can be performed with ethanol, acetic acid, or sodium hydroxide. Of the three, PEI has been the most studied. PEI is performed by injecting concentrated ethanol into the tumor to induce coagulative necrosis.[73] PEI is the lowest cost ablative therapy.

PEI is more efficacious in smaller HCC tumors. Complete response rates can approach 100% in lesions smaller than 2 cm, approximately 70% to 80% in tumors 2 to 3 cm, and only 50% to 60% in tumors larger than 3 cm.[73,74] Survival is also largely dependent on size. In one large series, the 5-year OS was 54% for HCC less than 2 cm compared with 39% in lesions 2 to 5 cm.[75] The degree of cirrhosis also impacts survival; 5-year OS was reported in one series to be 78% among patients with HCC tumors smaller than 2 cm and who were Child-Pugh class A.[74]

PEI is infrequently used currently despite the cost advantage. Multiple randomized controlled trials and meta-analyses demonstrated superiority of RFA over PEI. A Cochrane review included six randomized trials of RFA versus PEI. RFA was found to be significantly superior to PEI in terms of local control (hazard ratio [HR]: 2.44) and OS (HR: 1.64).[76] Results of RFA and PEI seem to be similar in lesions smaller than 2 cm.[77] Following the results of these and similar trials, PEI has largely been supplanted by RFA. However, PEI may be considered in smaller HCCs that are not amenable to RFA (ie, near major vascular structures, the gallbladder, or the liver hilum).[78]

CONCLUSION

Surgery remains the primary treatment modality for both HCC and most liver-only metastatic disease when technically feasible. However, the lack of adequate hepatic reserve and medical comorbidities preclude many patients from surgical resection. Ablation technologies, most notably radiofrequency and MWA, have expanded the patient population amenable to oncologic treatment for liver neoplasms and offer the opportunity for long-term local control and survival. There are no clinical data suggesting that RFA or MWA is superior.

There continues to be debate about the use of ablation for technically resectable liver tumors. A multidisciplinary clinical team should evaluate patients with resectable tumors before a decision is made that the patient is not a surgical candidate. Randomized clinical trials should focus on ablation as an adjunct to systemic therapy in the treatment of unresectable primary and metastatic liver cancers in terms of both OS and quality adjusted life years.

REFERENCES

1. El-Serag HB, Kanwal F. Epidemiology of hepatocellular carcinoma in the United States: where are we? Where do we go? *Hematology.* 2014;60(6):1767-1775.
2. Jemal A, Bray F, Center MM, Ferlay J, Ward E, Forman D. Global cancer statistics. *CA Cancer J Clin.* 2011;61(2):69-90.
3. Ryerson AB, Eheman CR, Altekruse SF, et al. Annual report to the nation on the status of cancer, 1975–2012, featuring the increasing incidence of liver cancer. *Cancer.* 2016;122(9):1312-1337.
4. Adam R. Colorectal cancer with synchronous liver metastases. *Br J Surg.* 2007;94(2):129-131.
5. McGahan J, Brock JM, Tesluk H, Gu WZ, Schneider P, Browning PD. Hepatic ablation with use of radio-frequency electrocautery in the animal model. *J Vasc Interv Radiol.* 1992;3:291-297.
6. Lu DS, Raman SS, Limanond P, et al. Influence of large peritumoral vessels on outcome of radiofrequency ablation of liver tumors. *J Vasc Interv Radiol.* 2003;14:1267-1274.
7. de Baere T, Deschamps F, Briggs P, et al. Hepatic malignancies: percutaneous radiofrequency ablation during percutaneous portal or hepatic vein occlusion. *Radiology.* 2008;248(3):1056-1066.
8. Kuvshinoff BW, Ota DM. Radiofrequency ablation of liver tumors: influence of technique and tumor size. *Surgery.* 2002;132:605-611.
9. Wong SL, Mangu PB, Choti MA, et al. American Society of Clinical Oncology 2009 clinical evidence review on radiofrequency ablation of hepatic metastases from colorectal cancer. *J Clin Oncol.* 2010;28(3): 493-508.
10. de Baere T, Risse O, Kuoch V, et al. Adverse events during radiofrequency treatment of 582 hepatic tumors. *AJR Am J Roentgenol.* 2003;181(3):695-700.
11. Mulier S, Ni Y, Jamart J, Ruers T, Marchal G, Michel L. Local recurrence after hepatic radiofrequency coagulation: multivariate meta-analysis and review of contributing factors. *Ann Surg.* 2005; 242:158-171.
12. Livraghi T, Meloni F, Morabito A, Vettori C. Multimodal image-guided tailored therapy of early and intermediate hepatocellular carcinoma: long-term survival in the experience of a single radiologic referral center. *Liver Transpl.* 2004;10(2):98-106.
13. Yin XY, Xie XY, Lu MD, et al. Percutaneous thermal ablation of medium and large hepatocellular carcinoma: long-term outcome and prognostic factors. *Cancer.* 2009;115(9):1914-1923.
14. Buscarini L, Buscarini E, Di Stasi M, Vallisa D, Quaretti P, Rocca A. Percutaneous radiofrequency ablation of small hepatocellular carcinoma: long-term results. *Eur Radiol.* 2001;11(6):914-921.
15. Wong J, Lee KF, Yu SC, et al. Percutaneous radiofrequency ablation versus surgical radiofrequency ablation for malignant liver tumours: the long-term results. *HPB.* 2013;15(8):595-601.
16. Shiina S, Tateishi R, Arano T, et al. Radiofrequency ablation for hepatocellular carcinoma: 10-year outcome and prognostic factors. *Am J Gastroenterol.* 2012;107(4):569-577.
17. Livraghi T, Meloni F, Di Stasi M. Sustained complete response and complications rates after radiofrequency ablation of very early hepatocellular carcinoma in cirrhosis: is resection still the treatment of choice? *Hepatology.* 2008;47(1):82-89.
18. Rossi S, Ravetta V, Rosa L, et al. Repeated radiofrequency ablation for management of patients with cirrhosis with small hepatocellular carcinomas: a long-term cohort study. *Hepatology.* 2011;53(1):136-147.

19. Choi D, Lim HK, Rhim H, et al. Percutaneous radiofrequency ablation for early-stage hepatocellular carcinoma as a first-line treatment: long-term results and prognostic factors in a large single-institution series. *Eur Radiol.* 2007;17(3):684-692.

20. Takahashi S, Kudo M, Chung H, et al. Initial treatment response is essential to improve survival in patients with hepatocellular carcinoma who underwent curative radiofrequency ablation therapy. *Oncology.* 2007;72:98-103.

21. Chen MS, Li JQ, Zheng Y, et al. A prospective randomized trial comparing percutaneous local ablative therapy and partial hepatectomy for small hepatocellular carcinoma. *Ann Surg.* 2006;243(3):321-328.

22. Tateishi R, Shiina S, Teratani T, et al. Percutaneous radiofrequency ablation for hepatocellular carcinoma: an analysis of 1000 cases. *Cancer.* 2005;103(6):1201-1209.

23. Lencioni R, Cioni D, Crocetti L, et al. Early-stage hepatocellular carcinoma in patients with cirrhosis: long-term results of percutaneous image-guided radiofrequency ablation. *Radiology.* 2005;234(3):961-967.

24. Raut CP, Izzo F, Marra P, et al. Significant long-term survival after radiofrequency ablation of unresectable hepatocellular carcinoma in patients with cirrhosis. *Ann Surg Oncol.* 2005;12(8):616.

25. Takayama T, Makuuchi M, Hasegawa K. Single HCC smaller than 2 cm: surgery or ablation?: surgeon's perspective. *J Hepatobiliary Pancreat Sci.* 2010;17(4):422-424.

26. Feng K, Yan J, Li X, et al. A randomized controlled trial of radiofrequency ablation and surgical resection in the treatment of small hepatocellular carcinoma. *J Hepatol.* 2012;57:794-802.

27. Huang J, Yan L, Cheng Z, et al. A randomized trial comparing radiofrequency ablation and surgical resection for HCC conforming to the Milan criteria. *Ann Surg.* 2010;252:903-912.

28. Choi D, Lim HK, Kim MJ, et al. Recurrent hepatocellular carcinoma: percutaneous radiofrequency ablation after hepatectomy. *Radiology.* 2004;230(1):135-141.

29. Nordlinger B, Guiguet M, Vaillant JC, et al. Surgical resection of colorectal carcinoma metastases to the liver. A prognostic scoring system to improve case selection, based on 1568 patients. Association Française de Chirurgie. *Cancer.* 1996;77(7):1254-1262.

30. Solbiati L, Ahmed M, Cova L, Ierace T, Brioschi M, Goldberg SN. Small liver colorectal metastases treated with percutaneous radiofrequency ablation: local response rate and long-term survival with up to 10-year follow-up. *Radiology.* 2012;265(3):958-968.

31. Machi J, Oishi AJ, Sumida K, et al. Long-term outcome of radiofrequency ablation for unresectable liver metastases from colorectal cancer: evaluation of prognostic factors and effectiveness in first- and second-line management. *Cancer J.* 2006;12(4):318-326.

32. Siperstein AE, Berber E, Ballem N, Parikh RT. Survival after radiofrequency ablation of colorectal liver metastases: 10-year experience. *Ann Surg.* 2007;246(4):559-565.

33. Sorensen SM. Radiofrequency ablation of colorectal liver metastases: long-term survival. *Acta Radiol.* 2007;48(3):253-258.

34. Veltri A, Guarnieri T, Gazzera C, et al. Long-term outcome of radiofrequency thermal ablation (RFA) of liver metastases from colorectal cancer (CRC): size as the leading prognostic factor for survival. *Radiol Med.* 2012;117(7):1139-1151.

35. Kennedy TJ, Cassera MA, Khajanchee YS, Diwan TS, Hammill CW, Hansen PD. Laparoscopic radiofrequency ablation for the management of colorectal liver metastases: 10-year experience. *J Surg Oncol.* 2013;107(4):324-328.

36. Hammill CW, Billingsley KG, Cassera MA, Wolf RF, Ujiki MB, Hansen PD. Outcome after laparoscopic radiofrequency ablation of technically resectable colorectal liver metastases. *Ann Surg Oncol.* 2011;18(7):1947-1954.

37. Abdalla EK, Vauthey JN, Ellis LM, et al. Recurrence and outcomes following hepatic resection, radiofrequency ablation, and combined resection/ablation for colorectal liver metastases. *Ann Surg.* 2004;239(6):818-825.

38. White RR, Avital I, Sofocleous CT, et al. Rates and patterns of recurrence for percutaneous radiofrequency ablation and open wedge resection for solitary colorectal liver metastasis. *J Gastrointest Surg.* 2007;11(3):256-263.

39. Lee WS, Yun SH, Chun HK, et al. Clinical outcomes of hepatic resection and radiofrequency ablation in patients with solitary colorectal liver metastasis. *J Clin Gastroenterol.* 2008;42(8):945-949.

40. Cirocchi R, Trastulli S, Boselli C, et al. Radiofrequency ablation in the treatment of liver metastases from colorectal cancer. *Cochrane Database Syst Rev.* 2012;(6):CD006317.

41. Ruers TJ, Joosten JJ, Wiering B, et al. Comparison between local ablative therapy and chemotherapy for non-resectable colorectal liver metastases: a prospective study. *Ann Surg Oncol.* 2007;14(3):1161-1169.

42. Ruers TJ, Punt CJA, van Coevorden F, et al. Radiofrequency ablation combined with chemotherapy for unresectable colorectal liver metastases: long-term survival results of a randomized phase II study of the EORTC-NCRI CCSG-ALM Intergroup 40004 (CLOCC). 2015 ASCO Annual Meeting. Abstract 3501.

43. Nordlinger B, Sorbye H, Glimelius B, et al. Perioperative FOLFOX4 chemotherapy and surgery versus surgery alone for resectable liver metastases from colorectal cancer (EORTC 40983): long-term results of a randomised, controlled, phase 3 trial. *Lancet Oncol.* 2013;14(12):1208-1215.

44. Tanis E, Nordlinger B, Mauer M, et al. Local recurrence rates after radiofrequency ablation or resection of colorectal liver metastases. Analysis of the European Organisation for Research and Treatment of Cancer #40004 and #40983. *Eur J Cancer.* 2014;50(5):912-919.

45. Kang TW, Rhim H. Recent advances in tumor ablation for hepatocellular carcinoma. *Liver Cancer.* 2015;4:176-187.

46. Poulou LS, Botsa E, Thanou I, Ziakas PD, Thanos L. Percutaneous microwave ablation vs radiofrequency ablation in the treatment of hepatocellular carcinoma. *World J Hepatol.* 2015;7(8):1054-1063.

47. Lahat E, Eshkenazy R, Zendel A, et al. Complications after percutaneous ablation of liver tumors: a systematic review. *Hepatobiliary Surg Nutr.* 2014;3(5):317-323.

48. Dong B, Liang P, Yu X, et al. Percutaneous sonographically guided microwave coagulation therapy for hepatocellular carcinoma: results in 234 patients. *AJR Am J Roentgenol.* 2003;180(6):1547-1555.

49. Lu MD, Xu HX, Xie XY, et al. Percutaneous microwave and radiofrequency ablation for hepatocellular carcinoma: a retrospective comparative study. *J Gastroenterol.* 2005;40(11):1054-1060.

50. Swan RZ, Sindram D, Martinie JB, Iannitti DA. Operative microwave ablation for hepatocellular carcinoma: complications, recurrence, and long-term outcomes. *J Gastrointest Surg.* 2013;17(4):719-729.

51. Zhang L, Wang N, Shen Q, Cheng W, Qian GJ. Therapeutic efficacy of percutaneous radiofrequency ablation versus microwave ablation for hepatocellular carcinoma. *PLoS One.* 2013;8(10):e76119.

52. Ding J, Jing X, Liu J, et al. Comparison of two different thermal techniques for the treatment of hepatocellular carcinoma. *Eur J Radiol.* 2013;82:1379-1384.

53. Facciorusso A, Di Maso M, Muscatiello N. Microwave ablation versus radiofrequency ablation for the treatment of hepatocellular carcinoma: a systematic review and meta-analysis. *Int J Hyperthermia.* 2016;32(3):339-344.

54. Pathak S, Jones R, Tang JM, et al. Ablative therapies for colorectal liver metastases: a systematic review. *Colorectal Dis.* 2011;13(9):252-265.

55. Bala MM, Riemsma RP, Wolff R, Kleijnen J. Microwave coagulation for liver metastases. *Cochrane Database Syst Rev.* 2013;(6):CD009058.

56. Hsiao YH, Kuo SJ, Tsai HD, Chou MC, Yeh GP. Clinical application of high-intensity focused ultrasound in cancer therapy. *J Cancer.* 2016;7(3):225-231.

57. Chen L, Wang K, Chen Z, et al. High intensity focused ultrasound ablation for patients with inoperable liver cancer. *Hepatogastroenterology.* 2015;62:140-143.

58. Ng KK, Poon RT, Chan SC, et al. High-intensity focused ultrasound for hepatocellular carcinoma: a single-center experience. *Ann Surg.* 2011;253(5):981-987.

59. Zhang L, Zhu H, Jin C, et al. High-intensity focused ultrasound (HIFU): effective and safe therapy for hepatocellular carcinoma adjacent to major hepatic veins. *Eur Radiol.* 2009;19(2):437-445.

60. Knavel EM, Brace CL. Tumor ablation: common modalities and general practices. *Tech Vasc Interv Radiol.* 2013;16:192-200.

61. Lee EW, Chen C, Prieto VE, Dry SM, Loh CT, Kee ST. Advanced hepatic ablation technique for creating complete cell death: irreversible electroporation. *Radiology.* 2010;255(2):426-433.

62. Ryan MJ, Willatt J, Majdalany BS, et al. Ablation techniques for primary and metastatic liver tumors. *World J Hepatol.* 2016;8(3):191-199.

63. Kingham TP, Karkar AM, D'Angelica MI, et al. Ablation of perivascular hepatic malignant tumors with irreversible electroporation. *J Am Coll Surg.* 2012;215:379-387.

64. Cannon R, Ellis S, Hayes D, Narayanan G, Martin RC 2nd. Safety and early efficacy of irreversible electroporation for hepatic tumors in proximity to vital structures. *J Surg Oncol.* 2013;107:544-549.

65. Scheffer HJ, Nielsen K, de Jong MC, et al. Irreversible electroporation for nonthermal tumor ablation in the clinical setting: a systematic review of safety and efficacy. *J Vasc Inter Radiol*. 2014;25:997-1011.

66. Goldberg SN, Grassi CJ, Cardella JF, et al. Image-guided tumor ablation: standardization of terminology and reporting criteria. *Radiology*. 2005;235:728-739.

67. Pacella CM, Francica G, Di Lascio FML, et al. Long-term outcome of cirrhotic patients with early hepatocellular carcinoma treated with ultrasound-guided percutaneous laser ablation: a retrospective analysis. *J Clin Oncol*. 2009;27(16):2615-2621.

68. Arienti V, Pretolani S, Pacella CM, et al. Complications of laser ablation for hepatocellular carcinoma: a multicenter study. *Radiology*. 2008;246(3):947-955.

69. Orlacchio A, Bolacchi F, Chegai F, et al. Comparative evaluation of percutaneous laser and radiofrequency ablation in patients with HCC smaller than 4 cm. *Radiol Med*. 2014;119(5):298-308.

70. Bryant G. DSC measurement of cell suspensions during successive freezing runs: implications for the mechanisms of intracellular ice formation. *Cryobiology*. 1995;32(2):114-128.

71. Rong G, Bai W, Dong Z, et al. Long-term outcomes of percutaneous cryoablation for patients with hepatocellular carcinoma within Milan criteria. *PLoS One*. 2015;10(4):1-15.

72. Wang C, Wang H, Yang W, et al. Multicenter randomized controlled trial of percutaneous cryoablation versus radiofrequency ablation in hepatocellular carcinoma. *Hepatology*. 2015;61:1579-1590.

73. Livraghi T, Bolondi L, Lazzaroni S, et al. Percutaneous ethanol injection in the treatment of hepatocellular carcinoma in cirrhosis. A study of 207 patients. *Cancer*. 1992;69:925.

74. Ebara M, Okabe S, Kita K, et al. Percutaneous ethanol injection for small hepatocellular carcinoma: therapeutic efficacy based on 20-year observation. *J Hepatol*. 2005;43(3):458-464.

75. Arii S, Yamaoka Y, Futagawa S, et al. Results of surgical and nonsurgical treatment for small-sized hepatocellular carcinomas: a retrospective and nationwide survey in Japan. The Liver Cancer Study Group of Japan. *Hepatology*. 2000;32(6):1224-1229.

76. Weis S, Franke A, Mössner J, Jakobsen JC, Schoppmeyer K. Radiofrequency (thermal) ablation versus no intervention or other interventions for hepatocellular carcinoma. *Cochrane Database Syst Rev*. 2013;(12):CD003046.

77. Giorgio A, Di Sarno A, De Stefano G, et al. Percutaneous radiofrequency ablation of hepatocellular carcinoma compared to percutaneous ethanol injection in treatment of cirrhotic patients: an Italian randomized controlled trial. *Anticancer Res*. 2011;31(6):2291-2295.

78. Wang XY, Lu MD. Percutaneous ablation for small hepatocellular carcinoma. *Expert Rev Gastroenterol Hepatol*. 2009;3(2):121-130.

Hepatic Transplantation

Nicholas N. Nissen | Alagappan Annamalai | Andrew Klein

Liver transplantation has now been the accepted standard of care for the treatment of end-stage liver disease and related conditions for more than 25 years. Although it was in 1963 that Thomas Starzl and his team performed the first successful human liver transplant, it was not until 1967 that the first 1-year survival was celebrated.[1] Indeed, acceptable and reliable outcomes came significantly later. Starzl and others went on to refine and overcome most of the technical aspects of the procedure, but truly satisfactory results became possible only after 1979. It was in that year that advances in immunosuppression and the efforts of Sir Roy Calne, another pioneer surgeon, made the availability of cyclosporine possible. Ultimately the National Institutes of Health (NIH) convened a consensus development conference in 1984 to evaluate this new clinical option and concluded "that liver transplantation is a therapeutic modality for end-stage liver disease that deserves broader application."[2] With this endorsement, a "broader application" unquestionably occurred as evidenced by the rather swift growth in the United States from a single liver transplant center, to eventually 144 programs nationwide as of December 31, 2015.[3] Most importantly, liver transplantation was firmly established as the standard of care for selected patients with end-stage cirrhosis. Patients who would have succumbed to their disease a few years earlier now completely recovered, and once again enjoyed normal and productive lives.

Ironically, improved results, expanded indications, and wider availability of expertise have all led to undoubtedly the single greatest ongoing challenge facing the field of liver transplantation: the persistent shortage of suitable organs for transplantation. At its worst, in the span of 5 years between 1996 and 2001, the number of patients awaiting liver transplantation increased at a seemingly exponential rate from just more than 7000 to an all-time high of more than 18,000 (Fig. 127.1). In the absence of a commensurate increase in the availability of suitable donor organs, there was a predictable corresponding increase in deaths among potential recipients waiting for organs.

These frustrating facts have led to a number of strategies for increasing the number of available organs, including improved nationwide donor awareness campaigns, dividing deceased donor organs to provide allografts to two recipients, the acceptance of increasingly "marginal" or "extended criteria" deceased donors, the use of "non-heartbeating" donors, and, finally, the general acceptance of adult-to-adult living donor liver transplantation.

In this chapter, many of the clinically relevant details of liver transplantation will be discussed, including the current challenges and opportunities faced by those in the field.

EPIDEMIOLOGY

Chronic end-stage cirrhotic liver disease is the most frequent indication for orthotopic liver transplantation. In the United States, the overall incidence of cirrhosis of any etiology is in the range of 70 to 100,000, with rates higher for men than women (95 vs. 50 to 100,000). Currently in the United States there are estimated to be nearly 6 million individuals with cirrhosis and the most recent National Vital Statistics Reports lists a rate of 9.7 deaths per 100,000.[4] Viral hepatitis, cholestatic liver diseases, and alcoholic and fatty liver diseases are some of the more common causes of end-stage liver failure (Table 127.1).

ETIOLOGIES OF END-STAGE LIVER DISEASE

HEPATITIS C

Estimates vary, but worldwide there are likely more than 200 million individuals infected with the hepatitis C virus (HCV). According to the Centers for Disease Control and Prevention (CDC), the prevalence of hepatitis C in the United States is estimated to be much more than 3 million. In fact, cirrhosis from HCV remains the most common indication for liver transplantation in the United States, accounting for approximately 29% of the activity at most centers.[5] HCV is a parenterally transmitted RNA virus with no DNA intermediates. The HCV genome was elucidated in 1989 and screening of blood products began shortly thereafter. Acute HCV infections are usually subclinical with no icteric phase. The disease becomes chronic in the majority of those infected, with cirrhosis developing between 1 and 2 decades later. The interval to cirrhosis is greatly accelerated by heavy alcohol consumption.[6] In the United States, 1% to 2% of the population is infected with HCV: from blood transfusions prior to 1990, intravenous drug use, or other parenteral routes, such as tattoos. Despite blood product screening and efforts at greater public awareness, and because of the prolonged course of the disease, HCV is predicted to be an increasing problem for at least another decade.

As the leading indication for liver transplantation in the United States, HCV recurrence postorthotopic liver transplant (OLT) is universal. Recurrence is associated with accelerated fibrosis progression and reduced graft and patient survival.[7] With the introduction of the new direct-acting antiviral therapies for HCV in the past several years, studies treating decompensated cirrhotic patients were done with the goals of stabilizing disease, preventing decompensation, and preventing graft infection. Two large clinical trials done in Child B and C decompensated

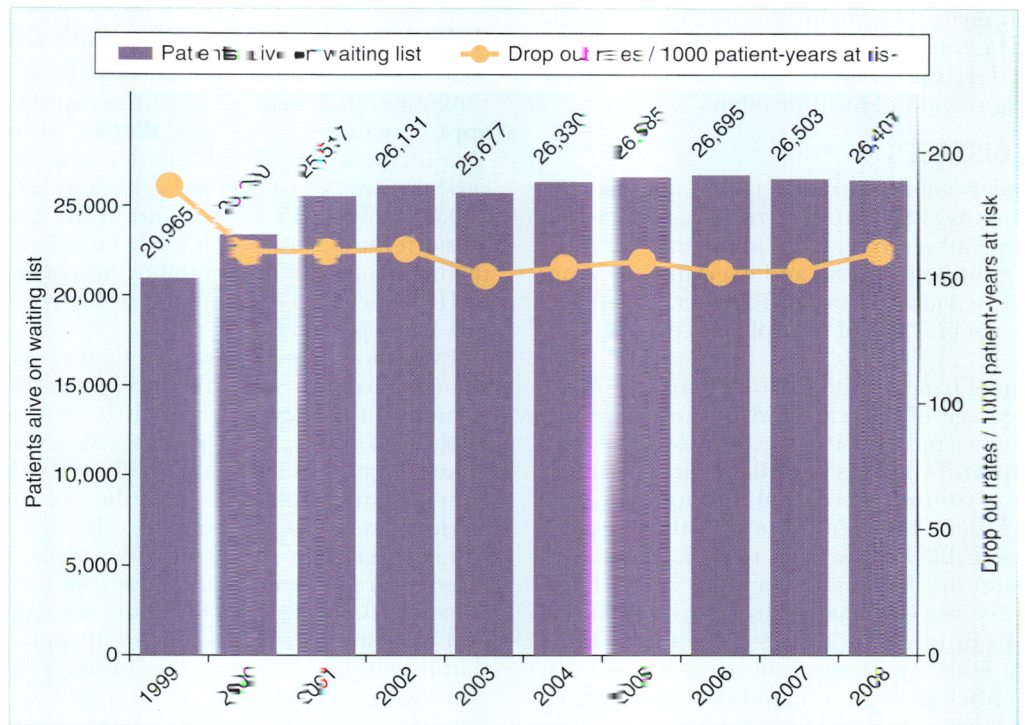

FIGURE 127.1 Patients alive on the waiting list at any time during the year and annual dropout (removal for death or being too sick) rates from the liver waiting list per 1000 patient-years. From Scientific Registry of Transplant Recipients. Data as of May 2009.)

TABLE 127.1 Chronic End-Stage Liver Disease: Etiologies

Category	Disease	Frequency
Hepatitis	(Hepatitis A)	Never chronic
	Hepatitis B	10%–15%
	Hepatitis C	40%
Noncholestatic	Laennec cirrhosis	
	Cryptogenic cirrhosis	
	Autoimmune hepatitis	
Cholestatic	Primary sclerosing cholangitis	
	Primary biliary cirrhosis	
Metabolic	Hemochromatosis	
	Wilson disease	
	α_1-Antitrypsin deficiency	
Malignancies	Hepatocellular carcinoma	Adults
	Hepatoblastoma	Children
	Cholangiocarcinoma	Investigational
	Carcinoid/neuroendocrine	Rare
	Hemangioendothelioma	Rare
	Hemangiosarcoma	
Atresia: children	Biliary atresia	50%
Others	Budd-Chiari	Rare
	Cystic fibrosis	
	Congenital hepatic fibrosis	
	Benign tumors	

cirrhotic patients conducted in North America and Europe using sofosbuvir, ledipasvir, and ribavirin for 12 or 24 weeks yielded sustained virologic response (SVR) rates of 78% to 96%, with lower rates reported in the Child C cohort. Additionally, those treated post-OLT had excellent SVR rates if they were treated early fibrosis (F)0–F3 (96% to 98%). In the Model for End-Stage Liver Disease (MELD) era (see discussion on MELD that follows), determining the appropriate timing of therapy (pre- vs. post-OLT) is essential because in some cases treatment may improve MELD score but may leave the patient in "MELD limbo" as HCV cure may not prevent the need for liver transplant due to other complications (hepatocellular carcinoma [HCC] or portal hypertensive complications). The remarkable progress made in HCV therapies with cure rates of greater than 95%, even in advanced liver disease or post-OLT, will likely reduce the numbers of patients needing liver transplant in the future as other more challenging etiologies are increasing.

HEPATITIS B

Hepatitis B is a DNA virus endemic in many countries, especially those of the Pacific Rim. Although effective vaccines have been available for more than 20 years, it continues to be a major worldwide health problem, due especially to vertical transmission. Hepatitis B virus (HBV)-related liver disease currently accounts for up to 15% of transplant activity at most centers. In the earlier days of liver transplantation, postoperative reinfection was a major issue leading to dismal results and the general acceptance of HBV as a relative contraindication to transplant. A dramatic success story followed the development of improved prophylactic strategies using HBV immune globulin, and the subsequent availability of effective antiviral agents. Hepatic allograft reinfection with HBV is no longer a significant clinical problem.[9]

CHOLESTATIC DISEASES

Collectively, primary biliary cirrhosis (PBC) and primary sclerosing cholangitis (PSC) are referred to as the cholestatic liver diseases. Although both are idiopathic, each has a genetic/autoimmune element, and overlap syndromes with autoimmune hepatitis can occur. Together, on average, they account for roughly 8% of transplant activity at most centers.[5]

Ninety percent of patients with PBC are female, presenting at an average age of 50 years and not uncommonly with familial clustering. Pruritus is the most common presenting symptom, whereas the diagnostic hallmark is the presence of antimitochondrial antibodies, which are present in virtually 100% of those with the disease.[10]

Men are twice as likely as women to be afflicted with PSC, usually presenting between 25 and 45 years of age. Many cases are discovered incidentally on routine blood tests with the finding of an elevated serum alkaline phosphatase. Patients with symptoms are equally likely to present with either pruritus or jaundice. In the proper clinical context, diagnosis is confirmed with endoscopic retrograde cholangiography showing irregular stricturing and beading of the intrahepatic biliary tree. As discussed in some detail later, there is a strong association between PSC and inflammatory bowel disease. A major concern among patients with PSC is the 15% to 30% overall associated risk for the development of cholangiocarcinoma (CCA).[11] Unfortunately there is as yet no reliable method for predicting or detecting this malignancy in its early stages. Ironically, demonstrable disease was, until relatively recently, considered a contraindication for transplantation because of generally dismal outcomes. However, those transplanted and found to have incidental CCA actually fare quite well.[12] As of November 2009, organ allocation policies now facilitate transplantation in highly selected patients with early-stage CCA in the context of aggressive adjuvant therapy.

ALCOHOLIC LIVER DISEASE

Alcoholic liver disease ranks as one of the most common causes of death in the United States and the second most common indication for liver transplantation in adults.[13] Interestingly, only between 10% and 15% of alcoholics develop cirrhosis. Nevertheless, it has been determined that upward of 80 g of alcohol per day for more than 5 years will put most individuals at risk. As already noted, alcohol acts synergistically with HCV or HBV infection. Alcohol-related liver injury can manifest across a spectrum, from acute alcoholic hepatitis to chronic fatty changes and on to cirrhosis and HCC. Most transplant centers maintain strict abstinence guidelines for determining candidacy when alcohol is the cause of liver failure. Most often, a 6-month period of sobriety is required to allow demonstration of insight and compliance. Another very practical reason for a period of abstinence is to avoid transplanting those who will recover from the acute effects of alcohol and no longer meet transplant criteria.

UNRESECTABLE HEPATOCELLULAR CARCINOMA

HCC is one of the most common malignancies worldwide, ranking eighth among all cancers while accounting for approximately 90% of those that are primary to the liver. The incidence of HCC in endemic regions of Asia and sub-Saharan Africa can be as high as 20 to 40 cases per 100,000 Although rates found in the United States and Western Europe are much lower (1 to 5 cases per 100,000) the incidence is rising. In the United States, the incidence of HCC is currently estimated to be from 8500 to 11,500 new cases per year.[14-18]

Even though environmental toxins pose a major risk in some parts of the world, the incidence of HCC is primarily related to the prevalence of cirrhosis from chronic viral hepatitis B and C, with a relative risk several-hundred-fold greater than those who are unaffected. Cirrhosis per se is a premalignant condition, regardless of etiology. Although cirrhosis remains the common denominator, the DNA intermediates in the replicative cycle of HBV may be directly carcinogenic, even in the absence of cirrhosis. The irony of HCC is that such tumors are typically multifocal and almost exclusive to those with underlying cirrhosis that precludes resection. The intuitive appeal of OLT is the elimination of the tumor as well as the underlying liver disease, which creates a fertile environment for developing neoplasms.

FATTY LIVER DISEASE

Nonalcoholic fatty liver disease (NAFLD) is generally considered to be a benign disease and is typically diagnosed incidentally on abdominal imaging confirming steatohepatitis with or without minor elevations in liver function tests. In the United States, the prevalence of NAFLD approaches 30% to 40% in parallel with the obesity epidemic and is associated with type 2 diabetes mellitus, dyslipicemia, and metabolic syndrome, all of which are presumed to occur secondary to a common pathophysiology of insulin resistance.[19] Nonalcoholic steatohepatitis (NASH) is differentiated from NAFLD by evidence of fatty accumulation causing histologic hepatocyte injury with inflammation. NASH has the potential to progress to hepatic fibrosis and cirrhosis and lead to significant morbidity and mortality. Nearly 15% to 20% of patients with NAFLD develop NASH, which is predicted to be the most common reason for OLT in the near future. Unfortunately, there is currently no cure for NASH and most treatment options are targeted toward controlling its underlying associated disease states.[20]

UNUSUAL TUMORS

The early transplant experience in patients with secondary hepatic malignancy was dismal, and consequently metastatic tumors are generally still considered an absolute contraindication. However, a few exceptions do exist. Although largely anecdotal, acceptable outcomes have been described in patients with metastatic midgut carcinoid tumors, whereas patients transplanted for other unresectable neuroendocrine tumors have generally not fared as well. Outcomes for primary hepatic angiosarcoma and biliary cystadenocarcinoma have been disappointing. Hepatic epithelioid hemangioendothelioma has also

TABLE 127.2 Acute Liver Failure: Etiologies

Toxic	Infectious	Metabolic	Cardiovascular
Drugs or chemicals	Viral hepatitis	Wilson disease	Acute Budd-Chiari syndrome
Acetaminophen	Yellow fever	Acute fatty liver of pregnancy	Portal vein thrombosis
Halothane	Q fever	Reye syndrome	"Shock" liver
Isoniazid	Other virus	Other inborn errors	Heat stroke
Valproate			
Amanita phalloides			

been successfully treated using OLT but outcomes are unpredictable.[21] When considering OLT in this setting of secondary tumors, the tradeoff is between the survival advantages offered by traditional therapies for otherwise slowly progressive tumors versus the potential for rapid progression of occult residual disease under the influence of posttransplant immunosuppression. A small number of symptomatic and otherwise unresectable benign tumors, or those with the potential for malignant degeneration, such as adenomas, have also been treated with transplantation.[22]

OTHER ETIOLOGIES

A number of other chronic disorders that can also lead to liver failure and the need for transplantation do exist, but they are beyond the scope of this discussion. Metabolic abnormalities of iron and copper underlie the disorders of hemochromatosis and Wilson disease, respectively. Other entities include autoimmune hepatitis, α_1-antitrypsin deficiency, nonalcoholic fatty liver disease, and the Budd-Chiari syndrome. In addition, there are a host of other disorders that occur in the pediatric population, the most common of which is biliary atresia.

ACUTE LIVER FAILURE

Although the vast majority of patients undergoing liver transplantation suffer from chronic diseases, an estimated 2000 individuals in the United States each year present with conditions leading to acute (or *fulminant*) liver failure (ALF) (Table 127.2). The most common etiologies include toxic drug exposures such as acetaminophen or idiosyncratic reactions to other drugs. Mushroom poisoning (e.g., *Amanita phalloides*) and industrial or environmental toxins have also led to ALF. Other causes include acute hepatitis A, acute or reactivated hepatitis B, and Wilson disease (a hereditary disease of copper metabolism). Other conditions, such as an acute Budd-Chiari syndrome, fatty liver of pregnancy, autoimmune conditions, and even shock can give rise to ALF. In up to 20% of cases, no apparent etiology can be identified. As discussed later, patients presenting with ALF must undergo urgent evaluation and listing for transplantation, as death can occur within hours.[23]

HEPATIC DECOMPENSATION SECONDARY TO CIRRHOSIS

Patients with end-stage liver disease often have significant associated conditions affecting other organ systems. Those that are more common, surprising, or sinister are briefly

mentioned here by organ system. An understanding of these conditions can be critical to the management of a patient's severe cirrhosis and the maintenance of transplant candidacy.

HEMODYNAMICS

Perhaps the most pervasive physiologic changes associated with cirrhosis are those affecting hemodynamics which, in turn can affect each of the organ systems.[24] Cirrhosis leads to a generalized vasodilation and hyperdynamic state. In addition to a reduced systemic vascular resistance, a host of attendant changes can occur, including increased peripheral blood flow, reduced arteriovenous oxygen difference, reduced effective blood volume with reduced cortical renal blood flow, and activation of the renin-angiotensin axis with sodium and water retention contributing to ascites formation. Patients with cirrhosis are generally observed to have an elevated cardiac output, tachycardia, and low blood pressure. As cirrhosis progresses, patients with a history of hypertension no longer require antihypertensive medications. Many of the common physical findings seen in cirrhotic patients, such as palmar erythema and cutaneous spider angiomata, are also explained by these vascular changes.

HEART

Iron overload states, such as that seen with genetic hemochromatosis, can lead to cardiac iron deposition. Although overt abnormalities may be discovered with echocardiography, those afflicted are at risk for conduction abnormalities, severe dysrhythmias, and right heart failure, especially during the significant stress of surgery. Magnetic resonance imaging can detect cardiac iron overload, and cardiac catheterization is usually required to determine transplant candidacy. In some circumstances, patients have been considered for simultaneous dual-organ (heart-liver) transplantation. As a group, those with either primary or secondary iron overload fare worse with transplantation than those without iron overload.[25]

LUNG

Up to one-third of patients with cirrhosis may be found to have reduced arterial oxygen saturation. A number of conditions common to cirrhosis may affect pulmonary function (Box 127.1). Two of the most serious conditions are portopulmonary hypertension and the hepatopulmonary syndrome. Both are likely related to the hyperdynamics of cirrhosis.[26]

Although the etiology of portopulmonary hypertension is unclear and the incidence is low, 2% of patients with

---

BOX 127.1 Pulmonary Issues in Cirrhosis

Hepatopulmonary syndrome
Pulmonary hypertension
Pleural effusions
Raised hemidiaphragm
Basal atelectasis
Ventilation-perfusion mismatch

TABLE 127.3 Stages of Encephalopathy

Stage	Clinical Findings
I	Irritability, altered sleep cycles
II	Disorientation, asterixis
III	Confusion, somnolence
IV	Coma

---

severe liver disease are at risk for developing pulmonary arterial changes indistinguishable from those seen in primary idiopathic pulmonary hypertension. If suspected based on echocardiography, right heart catheterization must be performed. A mean pulmonary arterial pressure (MPAP) greater than 25 mm Hg defines the disease, whereas an MPAP greater than 35 mm Hg (peripheral vascular resistance [PVR] ≥240 dynes/s per·cm^5) is considered the threshold for an increased risk of death. Treatment with prostacyclins, nitric oxide, or similarly active agents can be used in an attempt to lower pressures and facilitate a safe OLT.

Hepatopulmonary syndrome is another uncommon entity defined by the triad of (1) chronic hypoxemia (Pao$_2$ <60 mm Hg), (2) pulmonary vascular dilation as seen on examinations such as angiography or bubble echo, both in the context of (3) severe underlying chronic liver disease. This is a progressive condition that can be reversed following transplantation.

GASTROINTESTINAL

Portal hypertensive bleeding is a well-known complication of cirrhosis and about 90% of such episodes can be successfully treated with endoscopic and/or pharmacologic interventions. When indicated, an experienced interventional radiologist can place transjugular intrahepatic portal systemic shunts (TIPSS).[27] Surgical shunts remain appropriate in the nonacute setting when the most prominent feature of disease is bleeding in an otherwise well-compensated patient. TIPSS may be contraindicated by significant hepatic encephalopathy or bilirubin levels elevated much higher than 3.0 mg/dL, in which case progressive liver failure may ensue without shunt reversal.

Inflammatory bowel disease is strongly associated with PSC.[11] Among patients with PSC, there is a 75% prevalence of ulcerative colitis (UC), whereas the converse is true in only 5%. PSC may also be associated with colonic Crohn disease. In those with PSC and UC, the risk for colonic malignancy may be greater than for those with UC alone and is an indication for vigilant screening colonoscopy, both before and after transplantation.

BONE

Hepatic osteodystrophy can be a complication of end-stage liver disease, especially among those with cholestatic diagnoses. Steroid treatments before or after transplantation can also exacerbate this problem. Consequences include bone pain, fractures, and vertebral collapse.[24] Aggressive calcium replacement and hormonal therapy are usually indicated.

KIDNEY

In the absence of other identifiable pathology, the development of severe renal dysfunction in the presence of end-stage liver failure defines the hepatorenal syndrome.[28] Although the etiology remains uncertain, it is likely related to the hemodynamic changes noted earlier. Because this is largely a functional problem, renal failure can be expected to resolve after liver transplantation. However, in patients with long-standing hepatorenal dysfunction, normalization may be unpredictable. The hepatorenal syndrome has been subdivided into type I and type II based on the pace of functional loss. Patients with type I hepatorenal syndrome experience a rapidly progressive deterioration, with a doubling of the initial serum creatinine in a period of less than 14 days. Such patients have 90% mortality within 90 days. Those with type II syndrome have a less rapid progression and fare better as a group. In either case, patients often require hemodialysis. When renal dysfunction is severe and of a long-standing nature, consideration must be given to combined liver and kidney transplantation. Because one of the parameters for the MELD calculation is serum creatinine, such patients are favored and nationwide there are an increasing number of patients undergoing dialysis at the time of transplantation as well as a growing population of liver transplant recipients receiving simultaneous renal transplants.

BRAIN

Hepatic encephalopathy is a neuropsychiatric condition associated with severe liver disease.[29] It can have manifestations that affect the spectrum of neurologic function from changes in personality and intellect to altered levels of consciousness (Table 127.3). Although it can complicate either chronic liver disease or acute liver failure, there are distinct clinical differences between the two conditions. In chronic disease, symptoms of encephalopathy may wax and wane with dietary indiscretion, poor compliance to medications, gastrointestinal bleeding, or infection. In the worst scenario, stage IV coma may require endotracheal intubation for airway protection. However, with proper management, even in the most severe circumstance, the mental status changes are temporary and reversible. On the other hand, encephalopathy associated with *acute* liver failure may also lead to coma, but unlike its counterpart, it is also associated with cerebral edema and acute brainstem herniation. The optimal management of acute hepatic encephalopathy may require intracranial pressure monitoring, which is not indicated in the chronic setting.

INFECTIOUS DISEASES

Cholangitis can be a significant pre-transplant issue, especially in those patients with biliary strictures, such as those seen with PSC or other rare congenital or acquired conditions. Such patients may require repeated endoscopic balloon dilations or stenting of prominent strictures. Occasionally, the chronic administration of rotating antibiotics may be necessary. Although extrahepatic infection is a contraindication to liver transplantation, it may be impossible to clear cholangitis in a patient with biliary strictures and chronic liver disease until the liver is removed. In the absence of florid sepsis, such patients may still remain candidates for liver transplantation.

SKIN

Intractable pruritus is occasionally seen in patients with cholestatic liver disease. Curiously the symptoms do not correlate well with the level of cholestasis and the exact etiology remains unclear. A variety of treatment options can be used, but none with predictable results. These include ursodeoxycholate, cholestyramine, rifampin, opioid receptor antagonists such as naloxone or serotonin receptor agonists such as ondansetron.[4] Some patients may be driven to the point of considering suicide, and despite the fact that liver transplantation provides definitive relief, additional MELD points are rarely considered appropriate. Patients with chronic HCV cirrhosis may develop small vessel vasculitis and cryoglobulinemia, manifest by palpable cutaneous purpura. In addition to those mentioned here and earlier, a number of other skin changes can be associated with specific liver diseases.

EVALUATION PROCESS

There is unlikely to be another area in the field of medicine in which the word *team* more aptly applies. Organ transplantation in general, and liver transplantation in particular, is so complex as to only be possible through the coordinated efforts of many individuals with special expertise, working in concert. The patient's first encounter through the evaluation process is illustrative. The three goals of evaluation are to (1) confirm the presence of end-stage liver disease and the indication for transplant, (2) exclude contraindications, and (3) initiate patient and family education regarding the transplantation process. To that end, each patient is seen by a core group of individuals composed of a transplant hepatologist, a transplant surgeon, a psychiatrist, a social worker, a certified transplant nursing coordinator, and a nutritionist (Table 127.4). Additional consultations are obtained as indicated in cardiology, pulmonology, nephrology, neurology, anesthesiology, dentistry, and infectious disease. Each of the consultants has acknowledged experience in working with liver failure patients and understands the special concerns and challenges presented by liver disease and transplantation. In the evaluation of healthy volunteer candidates for living donor liver donation, a team composed of a physician, social worker, and nurse coordinator, all independent from the team of individuals caring for the recipient, act as dispassionate advocates for the potential donor. Increasingly, transplant programs are

engaging in regular interactions with hospital ethicists to ensure the appropriateness of details related to living donation and other aspects of transplantation.[30]

TABLE 127.4 Preoperative Assessment

Labs	Tests	Consultations
CMP	CXR	Surgery
CBC	ECG	Hepatology
INR/Protime	PFT w/ABG	Psychiatry
Hepatitis	Axial imaging	Nursing
serology	Doppler ultrasonography	Social work
Iron	PPD/*Candida*/Mumps/	Nutrition
AMA, ANA	Tetanus	Cardiology PRN
CMV	Mammogram >45 years	Pulmonology PRN
EBV	Echocardiogram >45	Nephrology PRN
	years	Infectious disease
TSH, T₃/T₄	CT chest if tumor	PRN
HIV	Bone scan if tumor >	
	stage II	
CEA, AFP		
U/A		
Type & screen		
VDRL		

ABG, Arterial blood gas; *AMA*, antimitochondrial antibody; *ANA*, antinuclear antibody; *CBC*, complete blood count; *CEA/AFP*, carcinoembryonic antigen/α-fetoprotein; *CMP*, comprehensive metabolic panel; *CMV*, cytomegalovirus; *CT*, computed tomography; *CXR*, chest x-ray; *ECG*, electrocardiograph; *EBV*, Epstein-Barr virus; *HIV*, human immunodeficiency virus; *INR*, international normalized ratio; *PFT*, pulmonary function testing; *PPD*, purified protein derivative; *PRN*, as needed; *TSH*, thyroid-stimulating hormone; *U/A*, urinalysis; *VDRL*, Venereal Disease Research Laboratory.

TRANSPLANT CANDIDACY

There are three interrelated aspects of determining transplant candidacy, including criteria defining indications and contraindications, but also the appropriate prioritization of candidates in the context of the limited resource of available organs. There has been an ongoing effort and continuous evolution of policies to better prioritize potential recipients and to maintain the spirit of "sickest first" in organ allocation. Specifically, there has been a determined progression toward more objective and evidence-based criteria.

INDICATIONS FOR TRANSPLANTATION

CHRONIC DISEASE

The basic clinical indications for liver transplant candidacy among patients with chronic disease have remained relatively constant over the past 3 decades and include: (1) progressive hyperbilirubinemia, (2) portal hypertension as evidenced by signs of gastrointestinal bleeding (usually from esophageal or gastric varices), hypersplenism with thrombocytopenia, (3) disabling symptoms of portosystemic or hepatic encephalopathy, and finally (4) synthetic dysfunction as assessed by pro time (PT) or international normalized ratio (INR). More subjective criteria include general wasting or a "failure-to-thrive" condition, which certainly can afflict patients with the constellation of problems associated with end-stage liver disease, as well as poor quality of life (secondary to fatigue, weakness, and intractable pruritus).

ACUTE DISEASE

Patients presenting with ALF have a much more dramatic clinical presentation. In such circumstances, there is a prominent defining role for encephalopathy, which in contrast to the chronic setting, can progress to cerebral edema with herniation. In the acute setting, more than chronic, clinical jaundice parallels the degree of hepatocyte injury. Fundamentally, any previously healthy individual presenting with a rapid decline in liver function associated with coagulopathy and an altered mental status meets the criteria defining ALF.[23] There are two standard definitions for fulminant liver failure and both require the absence of any preexisting chronic liver disease. The first includes a clinical presentation with encephalopathy 8 weeks or less from the onset of symptoms and the second is based on the development of encephalopathy 2 weeks or less from the onset of clinical jaundice (Table 127.5). Acute hepatic decompensation secondary to a diagnosis of Wilson disease of any length is also considered ALF. Interestingly, a longer interval between the development of jaundice and encephalopathy is associated with a poorer clinical prognosis.

CONTRAINDICATIONS

The contraindications to liver transplantation can be relative or absolute, but both lists continue to diminish. Extremes of age, for example, were once limitations that have since broadened dramatically. Human immunodeficiency virus disease was once considered an absolute contraindication, but this too has been reconsidered.[31,32] More so than the other organs, candidacy for liver transplantation weighs equally the medical and the psychosocial considerations. Transplant centers must be compassionate but deliberate and consistent in light of the ongoing shortage of organs, government oversight, and the court of public opinion with a history of misunderstanding regarding issues of substance abuse and mischaracterized celebrity transplants.

In general, the contraindications to OLT are those comorbid conditions that would preclude an operative procedure of its magnitude. The hemodynamic changes that can occur during a liver transplantation may be extreme, stressing any or all of the major organ systems.

Severe cardiac and pulmonary conditions are the most frequently identified medical contraindications. Although advanced age per se is uncommonly cited as a contraindication, it is rare for most programs to consider

candidates aged much beyond the mid-70s. Many centers do adhere to programmatically agreed-on age thresholds. More important than age is the overall condition of a potential recipient. This assessment can be difficult, in that liver failure has dramatic systemic effects that may lead to severe deconditioning. At first glance, the inexperienced clinician might consider many typical transplant candidates to be "too sick." Careful consideration often finds that organ dysfunction is attributable to the liver disease and will reverse with a normally functioning allograft.

The shortage of organs and the methodology of the organ allocation algorithm, which provides priority to the "sickest first," makes it increasingly common that patients undergoing OLT are extremely ill, often hospitalized, or in an intensive care unit setting. For such patients with decompensated chronic disease, or those with fulminant liver failure, other more specific, acute criteria are applicable (Tables 127.6 and 127.7). Patients must display adequate hemodynamics and be maintained on no more than a single pressor agent. Those on a ventilator should have oxygen requirements not greater than an FiO_2 of 50%. As noted earlier, patients with acute liver failure can develop cerebral edema. In such circumstances, if cerebral perfusion pressures have been inadequate, then

TABLE 127.5   Acute Liver Failure: Definitions

Jaundice to Encephalopathy	Days
Hyperacute	≤7
Subacute	8–28
Subacute	29–60

TABLE 127.6   Contraindications: Acute

Organ System	Observation	Contraindication
Cardiac	CAD risks	Recent MI
	Unstable hemodynamics	Inadequate CO
		≥Single pressor required
Pulmonary	Pneumonia	Active/progressive
	ARDS	PEEP ≥10 mm Hg
	Ventilator dependency	FiO₂ ≥50%
Neurologic	Altered mental status	Recent/acute CVA
	Acute encephalopathy/ cerebral edema	Herniation or CPP ≤50
	Seizures	Uncontrolled activity
Infectious disease	Chronic condition	Untreated TB or similar
	Acute infection	Untreated or progressive
Renal	Azotemia	Inadequate renal replacement therapy
	Hyperkalemia	
	Acidosis	
	Hypervolemia	
Psychiatric*	Substance abuse	Inadequate abstinence period
	Suicide attempt(s)	
	Schizophrenia or bipolar (refractory)	Repeated despite therapy
		Jeopardy to follow-up care
Social*	Inadequate support	Jeopardy to follow-up care

*Relative.
ARDS, Acute respiratory distress syndrome; *CAD*, coronary artery disease; *CO*, cardiac output; *CPP*, cerebral perfusion pressure; *CVA*, cerebrovascular accident; *FiO₂*, fraction of inspired oxygen; *MI*, myocardial infarction; *PEEP*, positive end-expiratory pressure; *TB*, tuberculosis.

TABLE 127.7 Contraindications: Severe Chronic

Organ System	Contraindication*
Cardiac	CAD
	Valvular disease
	Cardiomyopathy
Pulmonary	COPD
	Pulmonary HTN
	Hepatopulmonary
	Pulmonary fibrosis
Infectious diseases	HIV
	Untreated TB
	Syphilis
	Other
Psychiatric	Jeopardy to follow-up care
Social	Inadequate transportation
	Inadequate communication
	Homeless
	Inadequate support general

*Relative/evolving.
CAD, Coronary artery disease; COPD, chronic obstructive pulmonary disease; HIV, human immunodeficiency virus; HTN, hypertension; TB, tuberculosis.

TABLE 127.8 Preexisting Malignancy: Risk of Posttransplantation Liver Transplant Recurrence

Low (0%–10%)	Intermediate (11%–22%)	High (≥23%)
Renal cell	Lymphoma	Breast
Uterine	Wilms	Bladder
Testicular	Prostate	Renal cell (large)
Uterine cervix	Colon	Sarcoma
Papillary thyroid	Melanoma	Myeloma

OLT, Orthotopic liver transplant.

an acceptable outcome is unlikely, and the use of an organ is unwarranted. Infectious issues can also present acute contraindications, such as an active pneumonia or other systemic processes. Occasionally, severe psychiatric or extreme social conditions may also present as relative contraindications. In the common circumstance of acetaminophen overdose, for example, multiple prior suicide attempts despite adequate psychiatric therapy would likely contraindicate proceeding to transplant. Similarly, patients with a history of liver failure related to substance abuse but without an adequate period of abstinence, or the patient with no evidence of social support, may also be denied candidacy.

One final, but extremely important, potential contraindication to transplantation is any prior history of extrahepatic malignancy in the candidate. Early in the experience of organ transplantation, it was appreciated that immunosuppression can have profound effects on the growth of a malignancy, including subclinical residual tumor. Many common cancers may recur even years after definitive treatment. Despite modern imaging technology, in many cases only the passage of time can be the determinant of cure. The histologic cell type, the stage and grade of a tumor, as well as the interval between treatment and transplantation are the factors considered in the selection process. Based on the propensity to recur after transplantation, various tumor cell types have been categorized as low (0% to 10%), intermediate (11% to 25%), or high (>25%) risk (Table 127.8). Most programs avoid transplants in patients with a history of histologically aggressive tumors.

A key consideration in evaluating patients with a prior history of extrahepatic malignancy is determining the likelihood of recurrence absent liver transplant. Predicted recurrence rates of less than 5% over the next 2 years are generally required. For the majority of the more commonly occurring malignancies, a 2- to 5-year waiting period is usually imposed.[14] Of those who do recur after transplantation, the majority are evident within 2 years of transplantation.

LIVER ALLOCATION

In the earliest days of organ transplantation, the matching of available donor organs (primarily kidneys) to appropriate recipients and the sharing of these organs between transplant centers relied upon personal relationships and center-to-center phone calls. In the 1960s, the Kidney Disease and Control Agency of the Public Health Service awarded seven contracts to US transplant centers to prove the feasibility of procuring kidneys in one location, preserving, matching, and transporting them to another center. This test of change evolved into two confederations of transplant centers: one in the eastern part of the United States, and one in the west. By the early 1970s, the use of a computerized database to track patient information was implemented in the east within an entity known as the Southeastern Organ Procurement Foundation (SEOPF), which included 18 members spread across six states. With further refinements and the inclusion of non-SEOPF members who desired access to the computerized kidney sharing system, the United Network for Organ Sharing (UNOS) was formed in 1977.

UNOS incorporated in 1984 as a private, nonprofit organization that maintained a nationwide transplant candidate registry for kidney, liver, heart, pancreas, and lung transplantation. That same year, the National Organ Transplant Act created the Organ Procurement and Transplant Network (OPTN), a nonprofit private sector network operated by transplant professionals with oversight by the US government. The mandate of the OPTN was to ensure equitable organ allocation system in the public's interest. UNOS was awarded a federal contract by the Department of Health and Human Services to establish the OPTN in 1986 and has been the administrator of the OPTN ever since.[15]

RECIPIENT CONSIDERATIONS AND EXCEPTIONS FOR ALLOCATION

In an ongoing effort to balance utility with equity and optimize outcomes, the algorithms for allocating livers have been under constant revision. Geography has been used as the dominant variable in liver allocation to minimize ischemia times. Until relatively recently, organs were first allocated locally, followed by regional and then national placement, and time on the waiting list weighed heavily in determining priority. This approach has since been

TABLE 127.9 Child-Turcotte-Pugh Scoring

Points	1 Point	2 Points	3 Points
Encephalopathy	None	Stage 1 or 2	Stage 3 or 4
Bilirubin (noncholestatic disease)	<2	2–3	>3
Bilirubin (cholestatic disease)	<4	4–10	>10
Albumin	>3.5	3.5–2.8	<2.8
Ascites	None	Moderate	Severe

TABLE 127.10 Model for End-Stage Liver Disease: Formula*

MELD score =	$0.957 \times \log$ (creatinine mg/dL)
+	$0.378 \times \log$ (bilirubin mg/dL)
+	$1.120 \times \log$ (INR)
+	0.643

*Multiply score × 10 and round to nearest whole number. Lab test <1.0 is set to 1.0.
MELD, Model for End-Stage Liver Disease.

TABLE 127.11 Pediatric End-Stage Liver Disease: Formula*

PELD score =	$0.480 \times \log$ (bilirubin mg/dL)
+	$1.857 \times \log$ (INR)
+	$0.687 \times \log$ (albumin g/dL)
+	0.436 if patient <1 year of age
+	0.667 if growth failure (≤2 standard deviations)

*Multiply score × 10 and round to nearest whole number. Lab test <1.0 is set to 1.0.
PELD, Pediatric End-Stage Liver Disease.

TABLE 127.12 United Network for Organ Sharing Hepatocellular Tumor, Node, Metastasis/Staging

T1	Single nodule <1.9 cm	Stage I
T2	Single nodule 2.0–5.0 cm or up to three nodules all <3.0 cm	Stage II
T3	Single nodule >5.0 cm or up to three nodules, one >3.0 cm	Stage III
T4a	Four or more nodules	Stage IVA
T4b	Any of the above with portal vein involvement on imaging	Stage IVA2
	Any N1 or M1	Stage IVB

essentially eliminated and replaced by a greater emphasis on the philosophy of "sickest first." Patients with acute conditions are now prioritized above those with chronic disease, and also take precedence regionally over local primacy. Initially, the Child-Turcotte-Pugh (CTP) (Table 127.9) system was used to prioritize patients, but was found to be excessively subjective while also inadequately partitioning patients into only four categories and failing to account for a vast spectrum of disease severity.

Under government pressure to decrease the disparity of waiting times between regions, the MELD system was introduced in February of 2002. MELD scores had the advantage of assessing three objective variables: serum bilirubin, serum creatinine, and INR (International Normalized Ratio for prothrombin time). Despite its development for another purpose, the MELD system was shown to be predictive of death on the waiting list, and allowed improved patient discrimination by severity of disease.[33] The more discrete data offered by the MELD system have also facilitated statistical analyses providing additional insights such as the risk-benefit threshold of transplantation versus medical management of chronic liver disease. The Pediatric End-Stage Liver Disease (PELD) system provides a similar objective system for children aged 11 or younger. The current liver allocation formulas are outlined in Tables 127.10 and 127.11. In summary, patients can be placed on the UNOS transplant waiting list with a minimum MELD score of 6, organs are offered first to patients above the "minimum transplant" MELD score of 15, and the maximum score rests at 40. With exceptions, organs are offered within blood groups only.

Despite the significant improvements offered by the MELD system, allocation remains imperfect.[22] It has been estimated that up to 10% of patients have conditions that are under-appraised. The best example of such a deficiency is the circumstance of HCC. Because cirrhosis of any etiology may predispose to the development of HCC, many patients present with or develop such tumors.

Even in those who are well compensated, only about 15% are amenable to liver resection because of issues of tumor size and location in the context of underlying cirrhosis and portal hypertension. Because allocation schemes have been designed to assess the degree of liver failure, patients with HCC were thus disadvantaged. Importantly, patients with early-stage HCC (stage I–II; see Table 127.12) were shown to have excellent long-term survival and a low incidence of tumor recurrence after liver transplantation.[34] With the introduction of the MELD system, its limited ability to adequately prioritize HCC patients was acknowledged and additional MELD points were granted for patients with stage I to II HCC. HCC patients with more advanced clinical staging have a poorer prognosis following OLT and thus fail the utility criteria on which allocation policy is based. Such patients are not afforded additional MELD points. This policy change was successful in improving access to transplant for patients with early HCC. Following implementation, the percent of transplants performed for HCC increased from 2.4% to 21% and 87% of patients with HCC were transplanted within 3 months of listing. Unfortunately, 39% (260/796) of the liver explants removed from patients transplanted with a primary diagnosis of HCC had no evidence of tumor on pathologic examination.[35] The HCC exception policy has subsequently undergone several revisions to reduce the likelihood that patients who do not have liver cancer are mistakenly classified as having HCC, and to balance timely access to liver transplant for patients with HCC, and fair, equitable distribution to non-HCC patients. Currently, priority is limited to patients with stage II disease, stringent diagnostic and imaging standards must be met, and MELD exception points are only granted 6

TABLE 127.13 Current Exceptions to Model for End-Stage Liver Disease

Hepatocellular carcinoma
Cholangiocarcinoma
Hepatopulmonary syndrome
Portopulmonary hypertension
Familial amyloid polyneuropathy
Primary hyperoxaluria
Cystic fibrosis
Hepatic artery thrombosis (<14 days post-OLT)

OLT, Orthotopic liver transplant.

TABLE 127.14 Deceased Donor Liver Allocation

Priority	Sharing Area	Recipient Classification
1	Region	Acute liver failure (Status 1)
2	Local DSA	MELD/PELD 40
3	Region	MELD/PELD 40
4	Local DSA	MELD/PELD 39
5	Region	MELD/PELD 39
6	Local DSA	MELD/PELD 38
7	Region	MELD/PELD 38
8	Local DSA	MELD/PELD 37
9	Region	MELD/PELD 37
10	Local DSA	MELD/PELD 36
11	Region	MELD/PELD 36
12	Local DSA	MELD/PELD 35
12	Region	MELD/PELD 35
14	Local DSA	MELD/PELD at least 15
15	Region	MELD/PELD at least 15
16	Nation	Acute liver failure (status 1)
17	Nation	MELD/PELD at least 15
18	Local DSA	MELD/PELD <15
19	Region	MELD/PELD <15
20	Nation	MELD/PELD <15

DSA, Donation service area; *MELD*, Model for End-Stage Liver Disease; *PELD*, Pediatric End-Stage Liver Disease.

months after meeting HCC exception criteria, after which time automatic increases in MELD points are given every 3 months to patients who continue to meet HCC criteria.

Additional conditions have been considered for incremental MELD point assignment similar to HCC (Table 127.13). In general, these are also conditions in which the MELD system inadequately captures the magnitude of the patient's need. Recognizing the fact that hyponatremia is a significant risk factor for patients with end-stage liver disease, a second MELD calculation, referred to as the "sodium MELD" (MELD-Na) was introduced in 2016 for patients with an initial MELD (MELD$_{(i)}$) score greater than 11. Sodium MELD can add as many as 11 points to the initial MELD score and is calculated using the following equation[36]:

$$MELD\text{-}Na = MELD_{(i)} + 1.32 \times (137\text{-}Na)$$
$$- [0.033 \times MELD_{(i)} * (137\text{-}Na)]$$

Additional MELD points may be granted to specific patients with special considerations through an appeals process to a "jury of peers" provided by the UNOS Regional Review Board (RRB).

The current liver allocation scheme is outlined in Table 127.14.[36] In summary, organs are offered first to patients with life-threatening acute liver failure (Status 1) listed within the same region as the deceased donor. Next in priority are chronically ill patients with MELD scores between 35 and 40 with preference at each integral value given to recipients listed at a transplant center in the same local donation service area (DSA) as the donor. This is followed by local and then regional recipients with MELD scores between 15 and 34; national Status 1 patients; national patients with MELD scores of at least 15; and finally local, then regional then national patients with MELD scores less than 15.

The benefits of the current liver allocation system are that it is objective, simple, easily understood, and readily verifiable. Unfortunately, the fact that local areas and regions are not uniformly defined has created a system wherein access to transplantation is dramatically different across the country.[37] The median MELD score at the time of transplantation varies by 10 points across regions (35 for Region 5; 25 for Regions 3 and 11).[38] Massie et al. demonstrated that a patient with a MELD score of 38 to 39 has a probability of 14% to 82% of dying on the waiting list, depending on the local DSA in which their transplant center resides.[39] To address this inequity,

computer models have been developed to simulate a variety of re-districting proposals.[40] Discussions regarding such changes are ongoing, but a complete resolution of these issues seems unlikely in the near future.

DONORS AFTER BRAIN DEATH

The report of the Ad Hoc Committee of the Harvard Medical School to Examine the Definition of Brain Death, published in *JAMA* in 1968, begins with the following statement: Our primary purpose is to define irreversible coma as a new criterion for death."[1] These findings served as the basis for the Uniform Brain Death Act of 1978, later clarified by the Uniform Determination of Death Act (UDDA) of 1980, which was subsequently adopted by all 50 states. Under the UDDA, "An individual who has sustained either (1) irreversible cessation of circulatory and respiratory functions, or (2) irreversible cessation of all functions of the entire brain, including the brain stem, is dead. A determination of death must be made in accordance with accepted medical standards."[42]

The criteria for establishing a diagnosis of brain death are summarized in Box 127.2. A patient must have irreversible coma with a known etiology. Medical disorders or conditions that could potentially interfere with neurologic function (electrolyte disturbances, acid-base or hormonal imbalance, encephalopathy, shock, etc.) must be absent. The patient must be free of central nervous system (CNS)-altering drugs, toxins, or infections and must have a core body temperature greater than 32°C.

Although certain tests and imaging techniques may be used as adjunctive techniques, brain death is a clinical diagnosis. A complete neurologic exam by a physician trained to perform brain death determinations forms the basis for determining whether a patient is brain dead.

BOX 127.2 Criteria for Establishing a Diagnosis of Brain Death

1. Prerequisites
   a. Known irreversible cause of coma
   b. Exclusion of potentially reversible conditions (drug intoxication, poisoning, electrolyte or acid-base imbalance, endocrine disturbance)
   c. Core body temperature $\geq 35°C$
   d. Systolic blood pressure ≥ 90 mm Hg
2. No spontaneous movement
3. No response to deep painful stimuli
4. Absent brain stem reflexes
   a. Pupillary reflex
   b. Oculovestibular reflex
   c. Corneal reflex
   d. Pharyngeal (gag) reflex
   e. Tracheal (cough) reflex
   f. Facial sensation and motor response

BOX 127.3 The Apnea Test for Supporting a Diagnosis of Brain Death (N.B. Exact Values and Times Differ by Local Preference)

1. Prerequisites
   a. Core body temperature $\geq 35°C$
   b. Systolic blood pressure ≥ 90 mm Hg
   c. Pco_2 between 35 and 45 mm Hg
   d. Normal electrolytes
   e. Euvolemia
2. Preoxygenation
   a. 100% O_2 for at least 10 min
   b. $Po_2 \geq 200$ mm Hg
3. Disconnect ventilator
4. Observe for respiratory movement
5. Positive test supporting the diagnosis of brain death: Respiratory movements are absent when Pco_2 ≥ 60 mm Hg or Pco_2 increases to ≥ 20 mm Hg above baseline.

BOX 127.4 Risk Factors for Transmission of HIV, Hepatitis B, and Hepatitis C[37]

- People who have had sex with a person known or suspected to have HIV, HBV, or HCV infection in the preceding 12 months
- MSM in the preceding 12 months
- Women who have had sex with a man with a history of MSM behavior in the preceding 12 months
- People who have had sex in exchange for money or drugs in the preceding 12 months
- People who have had sex with a person who had sex in exchange for money or drugs in the preceding 12 months
- People who have had sex with a person who injected drugs by intravenous, intramuscular, or subcutaneous route for nonmedical reasons in the preceding 12 months
- A child who is ≤ 18 months of age and born to a mother known to be infected with, or at increased risk for, HIV, HBV, or HCV infection
- A child who has been breastfed within the preceding 12 months and the mother is known to be infected with, or at increased risk for, HIV infection
- People who have injected drugs by intravenous, intramuscular, or subcutaneous route for nonmedical reasons in the preceding 12 months
- People who have been in lockup, jail, prison, or a juvenile correctional facility for more than 72 consecutive hours in the preceding 12 months
- People who have been newly diagnosed with, or have been treated for, syphilis, gonorrhea, chlamydia, or genital ulcers in the preceding 12 months

HBV, Hepatitis B virus; *HCV,* hepatitis C virus; *HIV,* human immunodeficiency virus; *MSM,* men who have had sex with men.

Generally, this exam, which includes testing of brainstem reflexes, is repeated by a second trained physician after a period of time that varies according to state and institutional policies. If both neurologic assessments demonstrate absent brainstem reflexes, an apnea test is performed (Box 127.3). The absence of respiratory effort when Pco_2 exceeds 60 mm Hg or increases by more than 20 mm Hg over baseline is a positive result that supports the diagnosis of brain death. It is important to note that the presence of brain death does not preclude certain spontaneous body movements. Patients who have absent brain and brainstem function may exhibit twitching of fingers and limbs, arching of the back and shoulders, or other deep tendon or spinal reflexes. The "Lazarus sign" in which a brain dead patient's arms are raised and then folded across their chest is an example of a spinal reflex arc.[43]

DECEASED DONOR ASSESSMENT

Organ procurement organizations (OPOs) are nonprofit entities certified by the Centers for Medicare and Medicaid

Services (CMS) that are responsible for the evaluation and management of deceased organ donors within their DSA. OPOs review the deceased donor's medical record, obtain a medical and behavioral history from one or more individuals familiar with the donor, and complete a physical exam. A key element of the assessment is the identification of transmissible diseases or malignancies that could be transmitted by the donor organ. The OPO is required to perform blood and urine cultures for all deceased donors and to test for the presence of the following infectious diseases: human immunodeficiency virus (HIV), hepatitis B, hepatitis C, cytomegalovirus (CMV), Epstein-Barr virus (EBV), and syphilis. Testing for *Strongyloides*, *Trypanosoma cruzi*, and/or West Nile virus must be performed for donors from an endemic area.

In addition to laboratory testing and clinical assessment, the screening process is designed to elucidate behavioral factors that may increase the risk for transmission of disease from donor to recipient, despite negative results obtained at the time of brain death. The risk factors associated with an increased likelihood of HIV, hepatitis B, or hepatitis C infection have been defined by the Public Health Service (Box 127.4).[44] Transplant centers are required to discuss with potential recipients the use of organs from donors who have any of these behavioral risk factors and document this discussion and informed consent from the recipient in the medical record.

LIVER TRANSPLANT PROCEDURE

DECEASED DONOR LIVER PROCUREMENT

The recovery of hepatic allografts from brain-dead donors is one component of the organ procurement procedure that requires coordination of multiple abdominal and thoracic operative teams. With respect to liver procurement, techniques vary in terms of approaches to and timing of portal dissection (e.g., while the donor's heart is beating or after cessation of cardiac function). Below is a summary of the technique used by the authors.

The heart-beating donor is placed on the operating room table in the supine position. The abdomen and chest are prepared and draped in sterile fashion. A midline incision is made from sternal notch to pubis and the sternum is divided with a saw or Lebsche knife. Sternal and abdominal retractors are placed and an examination of the exposed viscera is conducted to rule out external evidence of tumor, infection, or other condition that would preclude the use of organs for transplantation.

The ligamentum teres is transected and the falciform ligament is transected cephalad to expose the suprahepatic inferior vena cava (IVC). The left triangular ligament is then dissected to free the left lobe of the liver. A small defect is made in the gastrohepatic ligament near the porta hepatis and the ligament is palpated to determine the presence of a replaced left hepatic artery. Care is taken to preserve the replaced left hepatic artery, which may be encountered when the gastrohepatic ligament is transected to expose the caudate lobe. At this point, a Pringle maneuver is performed and the right lateral and posterior porta hepatis is palpated to determine the presence of a replaced right hepatic artery.

Next, the right colon is mobilized to expose the right kidney, IVC, aorta, and the left renal vein. The second portion of the duodenum is also mobilized so that the superior mesenteric artery is exposed. Retroperitoneal attachments of the small bowel are dissected cephalad to the ligament of Treitz to expose the inferior mesenteric vein (IMV). The IMV and aortic bifurcation are skeletonized to facilitate cannulation of the vessels at the time of cross-clamp. The crus of the diaphragm is then transected to expose the supraceliac aorta, which is encircled with an umbilical tape for traction at the time of cross-clamp. Once the thoracic team and abdominal donor teams are ready, 500 units/kg of heparin is administered intravenously. The IMV is encircled with two 2-0 silk ties and ligated distally. The distal aorta is encircled with two umbilical tapes and ligated distally. Perfusion cannulas are then placed in the IMV and the aorta. The gallbladder is also opened and flushed. A large venotomy is made in the IVC just below the heart. The supraceliac aorta is cross-clamped and visceral perfusion is initiated with chilled preservation solution in the portal venous system through the IMV and into the systemic arterial system through the aorta. The peritoneal cavity is filled with saline slush. A total of 3 L of preservation solution is flushed through the aortic cannula and 2 L is flushed through the IMV.

When cold perfusion is completed, the order of organ recovery is generally heart, lungs, liver, pancreas, and finally kidneys. Once the heart and lungs are removed, the diaphragm is transected across the right dome of the liver to the infrahepatic IVC. The cava is transected above the renal vein. The aorta is transected superiorly at the level of the superior mesenteric artery (SMA), taking care not to injure the renal arteries. The portal structures are then transected at the distal common bile duct and the portal vein at the level of the coronary vein. The common hepatic artery is dissected retrograde to the celiac trunk. The distal gastroduodenal artery, the left gastric artery, and the splenic arteries are transected, allowing dissection of the celiac axis to its aortic origin. A cuff of aorta including the celiac axis origin is then dissected free. The remaining retroperitoneal attachments of the liver are carefully divided and the liver is removed from the donor. A back-table flush of the portal vein with one additional liter of preservation solution is commonly performed to ensure adequate perfusion of the portal system. The liver is then sterilely packaged and tagged for transport.

With the increasing number of intestinal and multi-visceral transplants being performed, en bloc abdominal organ recovery is becoming more common. This may minimize injury to other transplantable abdominal organs such as the pancreas, intestines, stomach, and kidneys. In this procedure, described elsewhere, the entire abdominal viscera complex is removed en masse with minimal dissection. Organs are then separated after cold perfusion on the back table.

TOTAL NATIVE HEPATECTOMY

Because of the location of the liver in the right upper quadrant, a number of different incisions have been employed to gain adequate access for the transplant procedure. One of the more commonly used is the bilateral subcostal incision with an upward midline extension to the xiphoid process, euphemistically referred to as the "Mercedes-Benz" incision. Although this incision offers excellent exposure, it carries a significant risk of incisional hernia. A hockey stick incision in the right subcostal and midline area can also provide excellent exposure in many patients and has a lower risk of hernia. Often the xiphoid process is removed, both to increase exposure and to prevent lacerating the graft during manipulation. All ligamentous attachments to the liver are divided with cautery. The hepatoduodenal ligament is opened and the hepatic artery and bile duct are divided close to the liver to leave maximal length with the recipient. The gastrohepatic ligament is divided and the suprahepatic and infrahepatic IVC are isolated. If a standard orthotopic approach is used, the infrahepatic and suprahepatic IVC will be clamped and the intrahepatic portion of the IVC will be resected with the native liver. If a "piggyback" approach is used, the liver is separated from the intrahepatic IVC by dividing all penetrating hepatic veins up to the level of the main hepatic vein orifices and the native IVC is then left in situ.

The decision as to whether to proceed with a piggyback approach must obviously be made during the explant phase, and a number of factors should be considered. In cases in which a tumor is close to the hepatic vein and IVC, a standard approach (removal of the intrahepatic IVC) is favored to allow a better resection margin.

Obesity or other factors that make an end-to-end IVC anastomosis difficult to complete may make the piggyback option attractive because it is essentially a side-to-side anastomosis. Living donor liver transplant (LDLT) must use a piggyback technique, because the donor graft has no caval component. If the piggyback technique can be performed without complete caval occlusion with a side-biting vascular clamp, which thereby leaves some flow through the native IVC, there may also be hemodynamic benefits because of improved venous return during the anhepatic phase. This may in turn allow the physician to avoid the use of venovenous bypass and associated morbidity. In the majority of cases, the decision on which option to use is largely one of surgeon familiarity and personal preference.

BACK-TABLE PREPARATION OF THE DONOR ORGAN

Prior to implantation, the donor organ is prepared in a saline ice slush "back table" basin to minimize rewarming. All extraneous peritoneal and diaphragmatic tissues are excised and phrenic and adrenal veins on the vena cava are ligated. The portal vein and hepatic artery are skeletonized and side branches are ligated to facilitate efficient vascular anastomoses during implantation. When using the piggyback technique, the infrahepatic IVC is ligated because it will not be used during implantation. A small cannula is typically placed in the portal vein to allow perfusion of the organ with cold saline during implantation, which flushes out retained preservative solution before organ reperfusion. Aberrant arterial anatomy is managed by reconstructing the vessels to provide a single inflow to all hepatic arteries.[45] It is paramount that all vessels be preserved to prevent segmental biliary ischemic changes or graft dysfunction.[45] Most aberrant left hepatic arteries do not need reconstruction because the left gastric artery from which they arise is preserved with the donor celiac trunk. Aberrant right hepatic arteries typically require reconstruction because they arise from the superior mesenteric artery off a completely separate trunk from the celiac and common hepatic artery. The standard approach to reconstructing an accessory right hepatic artery is to either attach the aberrant right vessel to the splenic or gastroduodenal artery off the celiac trunk or to put the aortic sides of the celiac and superior mesenteric artery stumps together to create a single inflow through the more distal superior mesenteric artery trunk. Because the superior mesenteric artery trunk is also used during pancreas transplantation, the finding of an aberrant right hepatic vessel during organ recovery may have implications for whether the pancreas can be successfully transplanted. Recovery teams and transplant teams should work jointly during the donor surgery to resolve these issues, but priority and final approval is typically given to the liver procurement.

VENOVENOUS BYPASS

Venovenous bypass is a technique that reroutes blood from the clamped splanchnic and lower extremity venous circulation to the right heart using a nonheparinized centrifugal pump circuit. The decision to use venovenous bypass should be made prior to dividing the portal vein during the total hepatectomy. The use of such bypass is a matter of preference and patient selection. Once considered a major technical advance in liver transplantation, some transplant programs routinely use venovenous bypass, whereas in others it is virtually never used.[46]

Still another approach is to use bypass selectively by performing a test-clamp of the IVC and/or portal vein to determine relative stability during cross-clamp, which will be followed by bypass if instability is demonstrated. Another factor to consider in using bypass is the size of the allograft versus the recipient's abdominal space. Bypass may be required to minimize edematous enlargement of the intestines, thereby facilitating implantation of large allografts. In addition, the presence of excessive portal hypertensive bleeding may be managed by temporary portal decompression through bypass.

If a decision for venovenous bypass is made, an inflow cannula is placed in the saphenous or femoral vein and an outflow cannula is inserted into the jugular, subclavian, or axillary vein to bypass the occluded IVC and to maintain preload during cross-clamp. Bypass cannulas may be placed using a cutdown technique or percutaneous techniques. In the former, the cannulation sites are usually saphenous vein and axillary veins, whereas the latter use the femoral and jugular or cephalic veins. Flow rates of 1.5 L/min can be achieved without difficulties using a simple centrifugal pump. Portal vein inflow is easily added to the inflow circuit using an additional cannula in the portal vein. Portal vein decompression is needed. In cases in which cannulation of the portal vein is difficult or dangerous, such as during retransplantation, portal decompression can be accomplished by cannulation of the IMV. A heat exchanger is often safely added to the circuit to reduce ambient heat loss in the extracorporeal tubing and to warm patients with obligatory heat loss during the procedure.[47] If left untreated, hypothermia can lead to cardiac arrest during reperfusion.[48]

VASCULAR RECONSTRUCTION

Implantation of the donor organ must be accomplished quickly and efficiently to minimize ischemic time. Cold ischemic time is considered the time from cessation of endogenous organ perfusion in the donor (which typically occurs at the time of aortic cross-clamp) to the time that the donor organ is removed from cold storage for implantation in the recipient. The maximal allowable cold ischemic time for any given liver varies with the quality of the graft. In general, low-risk organs can tolerate cold ischemic times of up to 12 hours, whereas higher-risk organs should be implanted within 8 hours or less. Warm ischemic time is considered the time from which the organ is removed from cold storage until the time the organ is reperfused in the recipient.

Vascular reattachment of the donor organ follows a logical sequence with emphasis on both quality and speed. The first anastomosis is created between the suprahepatic cuff of the IVC of the allograft and the recipient IVC (or the hepatic vein confluence if the piggyback technique is used). The second anastomosis is an end-to-end anastomosis between the infrahepatic IVC of the donor and recipient (this is eliminated in the piggyback technique). These anastomoses are usually performed with running nonabsorbable suture. During completion of the IVC anastomosis the donor organ is flushed with cold saline through the portal vein cannula to remove preservative solution. The third step is an end-to-end anastomosis between donor and recipient portal veins. This is also performed with a running suture with care taken to avoid excessive redundancy that could predispose to kinking and thrombosis. A growth factor roughly half the circumference of the portal vein is usually included in the anastomosis to allow maximal dilation and to prevent a purse-string compromise of the vessel caliber. The organ is typically reperfused with portal flow after completion of the portal vein anastomosis, followed by immediate arterial reconstruction and subsequent arterial reperfusion. However, if the hepatic arterial anastomosis can be completed quickly, some prefer to proceed to this anastomosis before portal reperfusion which allows the graft to have complete simultaneous portal and arterial reperfusion. The arterial anastomosis can be performed in a number of different ways but should always adhere to vascular surgery principles of maximizing vessel caliber, minimizing intimal injury, and avoiding vessel kinking. A common approach that can be performed quickly is to create a running end-to-end anastomosis between the celiac trunk of the donor organ and a branch patch of the common hepatic artery at the gastroduodenal artery takeoff of the recipient.

REPERFUSION SYNDROME

With the reintroduction of blood flow to the allograft, significant hypotension and/or cardiac dysrhythmia can occur, which is collectively termed *reperfusion syndrome*.[49] Such changes can occur across a spectrum from very mild and transient bradycardia and peaked T waves, to cardiac failure and asystole. Sudden exposure of the heart to cold, hyperkalemic fluid and the milieu of cytokines released from the transplanted organ are the likely causes. An ominous sign is that of an escalating pulmonary artery pressure associated with a falling systolic blood pressure. This scenario is more common in recipients with preexisting pulmonary hypertension, diastolic dysfunction, or any other condition leading to fixed cardiac output or limited cardiac reserve. Although the best measure is to prevent severe reperfusion syndrome, it may be unavoidable in certain circumstances, especially when combining marginal organs with sick recipients. Remarkably, intraoperative cardiac arrest due to reperfusion syndrome can be survived if the patient has sufficient reserve and the graft failure is not profound.

CONTROL OF BLEEDING

Once the organ has been fully reperfused, attention is turned to obtaining hemostasis in a systematic and safe fashion. The vascular anastomoses are inspected individually, along with the retroperitoneal area along the diaphragmatic attachments and the bare area. Over-aggressive attempts to inspect the retroperitoneum or suprahepatic IVC with a liver rotation maneuver can lead to kinking of the IVC and a sudden drop in blood pressure, and this should always be done with attention of the anesthesia team. Even more problematic is the fragile liver that is firm, fatty, or develops subcapsular blebs because in these cases aggressive rotation can lead

to liver fracture and catastrophic bleeding. This degree of bleeding is rarely amenable to surgical control and is best handled with packing. In rare cases, this degree of bleeding and liver injury may require urgent retransplantation.

BILIARY RECONSTRUCTION

The final phase of the transplant procedure is creation of the biliary anastomosis. The donor gallbladder is removed and the donor and recipient bile ducts are trimmed to appropriate lengths and to the point of demonstrating healthy bleeding from periductal vessels. Most often, an end-to-end anastomosis between donor and recipient ducts is fashioned with interrupted absorbable suture. In the past, T-tubes were used commonly but were associated with a number of biliary complications.[50] Most programs now avoid the use of T-tubes except in unusual circumstances, such as in cases where the risk of bile leak is felt to be high. In the circumstance of an unhealthy or unusable recipient duct, a Roux-en-Y hepaticojejunostomy reconstruction is performed.

INTRAOPERATIVE PROBLEM SOLVING

Portal Vein Thrombosis

Preoperative assessment of recipient portal vein patency is vital to planning the transplant procedure. Patients with preexisting portal vein thrombosis (PVT) can be expected to have higher blood product requirements and more postoperative complications. When preoperative PVT is present, several management options exist. Most acute and chronic thrombi can be removed with eversion atherectomy with restoration of portal venous inflow. If the lumen is obliterated or the occlusion extends substantially into the superior mesenteric vein, this technique may not be sufficient, and consideration should be given to use of an interposition venous graft. Iliac veins from the deceased donor should always be obtained at the time of organ procurement for just this purpose. The inability to identify a vessel with adequate portal flow to reperfuse the allograft is a rare but potentially catastrophic occurrence. In such circumstances, flow from the IVC can be diverted to the allograft with a cava-portal anastomosis. This is termed *portacaval transposition* or *hemi-portacaval transposition*. In these cases, the retrohepatic IVC is constricted or even ligated to increase portal perfusion pressure. Although this technique may allow the patient to survive surgery, they are left with persistent portal hypertension as well as vena caval obstruction and its sequelae.[51]

Hepatic Artery Insufficiency

During preparation of the recipient hepatic artery, the dissection is usually carried back to at least the common hepatic artery to allow for an anastomosis of adequate size. If the inflow at this level is inadequate, then it may be necessary to create alternative hepatic arterial inflow. Donor iliac artery can be used to fashion a conduit from other sources most commonly the infrarenal aorta. Other options include taking a graft off the recipient splenic artery or the supraceliac aorta. Supraceliac aortic cross-clamp carries some risk of paralysis and should be employed with caution. In some cases, hepatic artery flow may be compromised by the recipient arcuate ligament, which is most often identified by noting a significant variation in arterial flow with each ventilator breath. A dramatic improvement can be effected with release of the celiac axis from this ligament at its origin off the aorta.

Graft Function and Primary Nonfunction

The assessment of graft function relies on clinical signs, laboratory analysis, and a certain amount of intuition. In the ideal scenario, the graft shows a healthy perfusion pattern and starts producing bile within 30 minutes of reperfusion. The organ should be soft, and hemostasis and hypothermia should improve rapidly. Over the next 12 to 24 hours, acidosis should resolve, and hemodynamics, mental status, and urine output should improve. INR should correct within 24 to 48 hours and the peak aspartate aminotransferase (AST) elevation should be under 3000 IU/L.

When a transplanted organ shows signs of dysfunction in the first several hours or days after transplant, several factors must be considered. Vascular and other technical complications are discussed later. In the absence of any technical complications, severe graft dysfunction within the first 7 days is termed *primary nonfunction* (PNF).[52] This poorly defined circumstance is a diagnosis of exclusion and can occur across a spectrum from mild to catastrophic. Although most grafts do show at least partial function, the signs and symptoms of a truly nonfunctional graft are easy to recognize. These grafts appear hyperemic, "blebbed," and firm, and may fracture with manipulation. Recipient acidosis, persistent vasodilation, renal failure, coagulopathy, and even cerebral edema may occur. AST levels are usually greater than 5000 IU/mL. In extreme circumstances, if no suitable replacement organ is available and a patient is unstable, removal of the nonfunctional graft and creation of a temporary portacaval shunt may allow the patient to stabilize. This anhepatic state represents a true emergency, and survival without a new liver is typically less than 48 hours. Other manipulations, such as plasmapheresis or utilization of experimental artificial hepatic support devices have been attempted with varying degrees of success.[53] Because of this risk of rapid deterioration and death from PNF, UNOS guidelines allow for patients meeting strict criteria of PNF to be listed for retransplantation at the highest priority level (status 1).

Much more common than the patient with PNF is the patient with delayed graft function, which manifests as failure of INR to correct, persistently climbing bilirubin, albumin, creatinine, and moderate elevations of AST (3000 to 5000 IU/L).[54] Graft dysfunction of this sort is often accompanied by ileus and renal insufficiency, and if a T-tube is present, by poor bile output. Some of these grafts may recover, provided other major complications such as infection do not destabilize the patient. In other cases, graft dysfunction leads to a cascade of events leading to multiorgan dysfunction syndrome and a "failure to thrive," which may ultimately lead to sepsis and death. It is up to the transplant team to weigh the risks of watchful waiting versus that of retransplantation. Although early retransplantation can be technically straightforward, it is not to be taken lightly as it removes another donor organ from the pool and subjects the recipient to a renewed period of intense immunosuppression. Patients

with delayed graft function who do not meet criteria for PNF are typically resisted according to the new MELD score, and as such the wait time for a new liver can be significant.

EARLY COMPLICATIONS

Hepatic Artery Thrombosis

Thrombosis of the hepatic artery occurs in 2% to 10% of liver transplants and usually results in early or delayed graft loss.[55] Because the hepatic artery is the sole blood supply to the biliary tree, hepatic artery thrombosis (HAT) causes biliary ischemia, which has several manifestations depending on the interval since transplant. HAT within the first 1 to 2 weeks after transplant, before anastomotic healing is secure, often leads to breakdown of the biliary anastomosis and bile leak. Occasionally, in a liver heavily reliant on hepatic arterial flow, thrombosis of the hepatic artery will result in a picture of graft failure similar to PNF. HAT occurring more than 30 days after transplant typically presents as mild elevation in liver tests or as biliary stricture with cholangitis or hepatic abscess.

The diagnosis of HAT should be considered in the presence of unexplained changes in liver function tests or if biliary complications are identified. Doppler ultrasound is performed at the first suspicion of HAT at most transplant centers, but is very operator dependent. Definitive diagnosis is often obtained by surgical exploration, angiography, or cross-sectional imaging. If the interval between diagnosis and discovery of HAT is less than 24 hours, there may be value to surgical thrombectomy and attempted hepatic revascularization. Biliary damage occurs quickly, however, and most patients with established HAT are best served with timely retransplantation.[56,57]

The mechanism by which HAT occurs is not always clear. Small donor arteries and the need for revision of the arterial anastomosis are risk factors for HAT, supporting the contention that technical factors play a significant role. Other risk factors suggested by some studies, which are less intuitive, include an HCV-positive recipient, CMV infection, and female donor organ into a male recipient.[55,58] HAT may also be more likely in those with conditions causing postoperative abdominal inflammation such as bacterial peritonitis or pancreatitis.

In the past, UNOS guidelines allowed patients with HAT diagnosed within 7 days of transplant to be listed at the highest priority (status 1). In recent years, it has become increasingly appreciated that HAT is rarely associated with PNF-like organ dysfunction.[59] For this reason, current UNOS guidelines allow for HAT that occurs within 7 days of transplant to receive a MELD score of 40, but not to receive status 1 designation unless PNF criteria are met.

Portal Vein Thrombosis

Fortunately, PVT is exceptionally uncommon after liver transplantation, occurring in only about 1% of cases.[60] Because the portal vein provides the majority of oxygen delivery to the parenchyma, severe parenchymal injury, graft loss, and patient death are common in the face of PVT. Occasionally, thrombectomy may be possible if detected early. The main risk factor for PVT is the need for thrombectomy at the time of the initial transplant.

Biliary Complications

Complications related to the biliary tree occur in up to 15% of deceased donor liver transplant patients, and with a reported incidence often greater than 30% among recipients of living donor transplants.[51,62] Biliary strictures are the most common complication, which usually occur at the site of the biliary anastomosis. Strictures at this level can often be managed with endoscopic or percutaneous interventional radiology techniques, but occasionally surgical revision with hepaticojejunostomy is required. Intrahepatic strictures and those that are remote from the anastomosis generally reflect a more diffusely diseased biliary tree. HAT and recurrent PSC should be excluded. Other factors such as the use of extended-criteria grafts, long ischemic times during transplantation, CMV infection, and primary choledocholithiasis should also be considered. Many grafts with intrahepatic structures can be temporized with aggressive and repeated percutaneous or endoscopic interventions, but some will require repeat transplantation because of recurrent cholangitis or secondary biliary cirrhosis.

Bile leaks typically occur within the first 1 to 2 weeks after transplant and usually reflect either technical error or HAT. If the bile leak is of a large volume or is associated with peritonitis, surgical repair should be attempted promptly. A skilled endoscopist or radiologist can often manage smaller volume leaks by stenting the anastomosis and decompressing the biliary tree.[3]

LATE COMPLICATIONS

Late complications of liver transplantation can be divided into those due to rejection, those due to immunosuppressant medications, and those due to recurrent liver disease.[64]

Rejection

The number of medications available for preventing and treating rejection, as well as knowledge regarding mechanism of action and optimal drug combinations, is growing rapidly.[65] Acute cellular rejection occurs with a reported incidence of 18% in the first 6 months after liver transplant and 29% to 39% by 14 month.[66] Typically, an episode of rejection is asymptomatic and the diagnosis is suspected based on abnormal liver tests. The diagnosis is confirmed by liver biopsy. Treatment options include simply increasing the maintenance immunosuppression in mild cases, and initiating a steroid pulse in cases that are more severe. Although acute rejection itself does not appear to impact long-term graft function, diseases such as hepatitis C have greater risk of recurrence in those requiring treatment of acute rejection. The augmented immunosuppression used to treat rejection is thought to play a role in viral replication and the more aggressive return of viral hepatitis.

Chronic rejection is a poorly understood entity often referred to as "vanishing bile duct syndrome." This condition is characterized by a cholestatic pattern typically occurring several years after transplantation and is diagnosed by paucity of bile ducts on liver biopsy. There is no effective therapy and some of these patients may ultimately require retransplantation.

Complications of Immunosuppressive Medications

Infection. Not surprisingly, the use of medications designed to disrupt immune competence puts individuals at increased risk for infection. The nature of that risk depends on a number of parameters including the interval since transplantation, the intensity of immunosuppression, preexisting exposures to certain infectious agents, the age of the recipient, and the nature and extent of other comorbid conditions (Table 127.15). As with other surgical procedures, the risk for bacterial infections is greatest in the first few weeks after transplant. Fungal infections peak during the first 1 to 2 months posttransplant and are largely related to the patient's nutritional state, the extent of antibiotic use in the perioperative period, and the need for massive transfusions or reoperations at the time of transplant, and the presence of perioperative bacterial infections such as spontaneous bacterial peritonitis.[7]

High-risk donor/recipient CMV exposure history can also predispose to CMV infection or reactivation.[68] Three to 4 months after transplantation, Pneumocystis, CMV, EBV, and varicella-zoster virus (VZV) all become a concern. Because of their impaired cell-mediated immunity, transplant patients remain at higher than normal risk for viral and fungal infections for life. Prophylactic antibiotics are given after transplant, although the exact agent and duration varies among programs. An example of the success of prophylaxis is in the treatment of CMV. This agent was once a common cause of morbidity and death of liver transplant but is now seen with an incidence of less than 5%.

Malignancy. Although the exact mechanisms are still incompletely understood, immunosuppression clearly increases the risk of some types of malignancy. Transplant

---

TABLE 127.15 Immunosuppressant Profiles

Agent	Use	Toxicity	Typical Duration
Corticosteroids	Primary immunosuppressant	Diabetes, hypertension, wound healing	6 months
Cyclosporin A	Primary immunosuppressant	Nephrotoxicity, neurotoxicity, hyperkalemia	Lifelong
Tacrolimus	Primary immunosuppressant	Nephrotoxicity, neurotoxicity, hyperkalemia	Lifelong
Mycophenolate	Used as adjunct to primary agent	Diarrhea, leukopenia	As needed
OKT3	Inductor	Cytokine storm, pulmonary edema	5 days
IL-2 receptor antibodies	Inductor		2 weeks

IL-2, Interleukin-2; OKT3, mouse monoclonal CD3 antibody.

immunosuppression places recipients at a threefold to fourfold increased incidence of cancer compared with age-matched controls. The largest increases are in skin cancers in sun-exposed areas. Although the incidence of other primary neoplasms, such as those of the breast and colon, are not increased in solid organ recipients, they tend to demonstrate a more aggressive behavior in the transplant patient when they do occur. All transplant patients should undergo vigilant screening for breast, prostate, colorectal, gynecologic, and skin cancer.

Cardiovascular Side Effects

Cardiovascular disease has become one of the leading causes of long-term morbidity in liver transplant survivors.[69] Several factors likely contribute to this morbidity, including the increasing frequency of older and obese transplant recipients and medication-related dyslipidemias and diabetes mellitus.

STRATEGIES TO ADDRESS THE ORGAN SHORTAGE

The greatest crisis facing the field of liver transplantation remains the donor organ shortage. Although adult-to-adult LDLT has made some impact, the number of such transplants performed yearly has plateaued in the United States in recent years. Arguments in support of LDLT include a more thorough and accurate assessment of the donor, the opportunity to perform the transplant before the recipient's health deteriorates, and minimization of cold ischemia time. Opponents of LDLT contend that the technical failure rate is higher and that partial liver allografts are inadequate in the setting of severe portal hypertension. The most compelling objection focuses on the morbidity and mortality risk associated with live liver donation. In a survey of 71 transplant programs that performed 11,553 donor hepatectomies, Cheah et al. found that the morbidity rate was 24% and mortality rate was 0.2%.[70] The risk that 1 in every 500 healthy live liver donors will die is unacceptable to many surgeons. A description of the living donor partial hepatectomy and the living donor transplant procedure is beyond the scope of this chapter.

There are ongoing efforts to increase the deceased donor organ pool by several other distinct pathways. The first approach is to increase the number of potential donors by improving intensive care unit and resuscitation protocols for patients with lethal brain injury, so that organ quality is maintained until organ recovery can be coordinated. The second approach is to decrease the number of donors that are lost because of lack of family consent by using a variety of public educational and public health measures. The third approach is to increase the utilization of organs that are not ideal and that might otherwise not be recovered. These marginal, or "extended criteria" donors, include older or less hemodynamically stable donors, non-heartbeating donors, or those with comorbid conditions such as severe hepatic steatosis. Use of these organs, however, may carry an increased risk of graft loss and death. Center-specific transplant outcomes data are available to the public and to third-party payers through the OPTN Internet portal. Although this system of reporting has many benefits, it also serves as a disincentive for the use of marginal grafts, because these

grafts by definition carry an increased risk of graft failure, retransplantation, and death.

Adult-to-Adult Living Donor Transplantation

The first LDLTs were performed from adults to children in the late 1980s, but the evolution to adult-to-adult LDLT in the United States has been much more recent. Only after the shortage of organs reached a critical threshold was consideration given to performing such a procedure, which poses substantial perioperative and perhaps long-term risks to the healthy donor. Many ethical issues continue to be raised including the age, relationship to recipient, and the social circumstances of potential donors.[71] The advantages of this procedure are primarily twofold. First, transplantation can be timed to intervene before a recipient becomes severely decompensated, thereby minimizing the risks of certain complications, avoiding repeated hospitalizations, and even minimizing costs. Second, the quality of the allograft should be optimal with minimal cold ischemia and without the physiologic insults often suffered by deceased donors. On the other hand, the relatively smaller volume and the increased technical anastomotic challenges presented by partial grafts create a new set of potential recipient problems. Add to that the most paramount concern of donor health, and the advantages of living versus deceased donors become less distinct. Indeed, data from the Scientific Registry of Transplant Recipients (SRTR) has shown inferior outcomes for right lobe allografts compared with those from deceased-donor whole organs.[72] The magnitude of this surgery and its potential impact on the donor is evident when viewing an intraoperative photograph (Fig. 127.2).

One of the greatest concerns regarding adult-to-adult LDLT is the adequacy of the liver volume provided by a partial allograft. A pattern of graft failure is now recognized and referred to as the *small-for-size (SFS) syndrome*.[73,74] This can occur when the actual or functional volume of an allograft is inadequate for the recipient. As a general rule, the liver is approximately 2% to 3% of body weight in

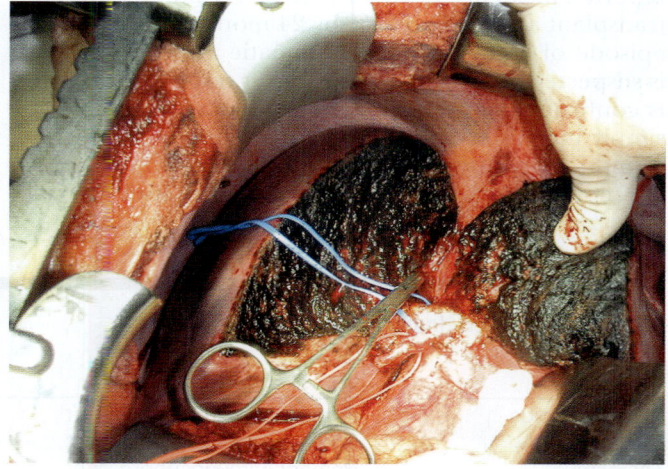

FIGURE 127.2 The magnitude of the living donor procedure is evident in this intraoperative photograph. The blue tape surrounds the vascular pedicle while a vascular clamp has been temporarily placed on a segment VIII hepatic vein.

healthy individuals, but there is considerable individual variability. An SFS graft is now generally accepted to have a graft-to-recipient weight ratio of less than 0.8%, or less than 30% to 50% of the standard estimated liver volume required by the recipient. Factors such as fatty change, the donor's age, duration of ischemia, and the adequacy of venous drainage can all contribute to a functionally diminished graft volume. Severe cholestasis, ongoing coagulopathy, and ascites are all prominent features of the SFS syndrome. Although recovery is possible, outcomes are unpredictable and survival without retransplantation may be uncertain. Sepsis and multiorgan failure can follow, and retransplantation must often be performed within a narrow window of time. Because recipients of living donors have otherwise not drawn from the "pool" of deceased-donor organs, RRBs generally grant additional points when necessary to ensure timely retransplantation in such circumstances.

The Adult-to-Adult Living Donor Liver Transplant Cohort (A2ALL) is a multicenter prospective study, funded by the NIH, undertaken to assess risks and outcomes for this procedure.[75] The most recent results indicate a 1-year graft survival of 81% in which 11.2% of grafts failed within 90 days. Biliary complications were the most common, with 30% early and 11% late. Graft failure was notably greater among transplant programs with less experience.

In the United States, the initial enthusiasm for adult-to-adult LDLT has waned, as indicated by the number of such transplants performed each year and the number of centers actively involved. At this juncture, only a handful of higher-volume programs exist, yet recent donor deaths have been reported in the media. The role for this procedure in the armamentarium for liver transplant surgeons is still in evolution.

Split Grafts

The increasing shortage of deceased donor organs has led to a number of methods to expand the donor organ pool. One such option is that of dividing a healthy donor liver into two portions for use in two recipients. Most often, the liver is split into a left lateral segment (Couinaud segments 2 and 3) for use in a child while the remaining right-trisegmentectomy (Couinaud segments 1, 4 to 8) is used for an appropriately sized adult. On rare occasions, an organ may be of adequate size and quality to split into true right and left lobar grafts if appropriate size-matched recipients are identified. Because a split graft carries the additional risk of a bile leak from the cut edge, a T-tube or internal stent may be useful to maximally decompress the biliary tree.

Perhaps the most important factor when considering split liver transplantation is patient selection. Technical aspects to consider include the possible need for a piggyback technique (depending on which half of the split is being used), the shortened and smaller vessels that may accompany a split graft, and the increased risk of SFS syndrome and bile leak following split liver transplantation. These factors may lead to increased morbidity and mortality in the severely ill recipient, and split grafts should be used sparingly in this group.[76] Patients with high risk of vascular complications, such as those with preexisting portal vein or HAT, may also be at higher risk with split grafts.

DISEASE RECURRENCE

Recurrence of underlying liver disease is a common cause of long-term morbidity and mortality in liver transplant recipients. Because of its prevalence as an indication for transplantation, its propensity to reinfect the new allograft, and our relatively ineffectual ability to treat in the posttransplant setting, recurrence of hepatitis C is a significant problem facing liver transplant physicians.[77] In patients with active replication of hepatitis C, graft reinfection is virtually guaranteed, although for most patients no treatment is needed for several years. An unfortunate unpredictable subgroup will manifest early aggressive recurrence, often leading to graft failure within the first year. The mainstay of treatment at the present is interferon-based viral suppression. Specific guidelines for optimal treatment of recurrent HCV after transplant remain elusive. Clearly, more effective HCV treatment strategies such as protease inhibitors will represent a major advance in the field of liver transplantation.

Although the recurrence of HCV after transplant is the most widely recognized, virtually every condition for which transplant is undertaken can recur after transplant. Hepatitis B activation, once common after transplant, is now rare because of improved antiviral regimens. PBC, PSC, and autoimmune hepatitis can also recur and may even require retransplantation.

LIVER TRANSPLANT OUTCOMES

An important advance in the field of organ transplantation in the United States came with the establishment of the SRTR in 1987. Its purpose is to maintain the data from all solid-organ transplant centers and perform large-scale analyses that are available to professionals and to the general public and transplant candidates. Their reports provide crucial collections of evidence on which the transplant community—including policy makers—makes informed decisions on topics such as procurement and allocation. According to the most recent SRTR data, the survival of a patient undergoing a first-time liver transplant at 1 month, 1 year, and 3 years is 97.2%, 91.8%, and 82.9%. Similarly, graft survival, which is the percentage of grafts still functioning at 1 month, 1 year, and 3 years is 95.5%, 86.7%, and 79.9%, respectively (Fig. 127.3).[78] By tracking results, the SRTR has played an important role in facilitating the progress of liver transplantation.

CONCLUSION

The field of liver transplant has evolved faster than almost any other field of surgery. From an experimental procedure just 35 years ago, this operation is now performed over 6000 times per year in the United States with remarkable outcomes. The last 5 years have seen even more advances, including the near-eradication of the prior nemesis of liver transplant, hepatitis C, and the acceptance of transplantation in HIV-positive patients in many centers. Continued efforts are needed in the areas of donor pool expansion, the treatment of fatty liver disease, management and transplant of the intensive care unit patient, and further refinement of the selection process for high-risk cancer patients.

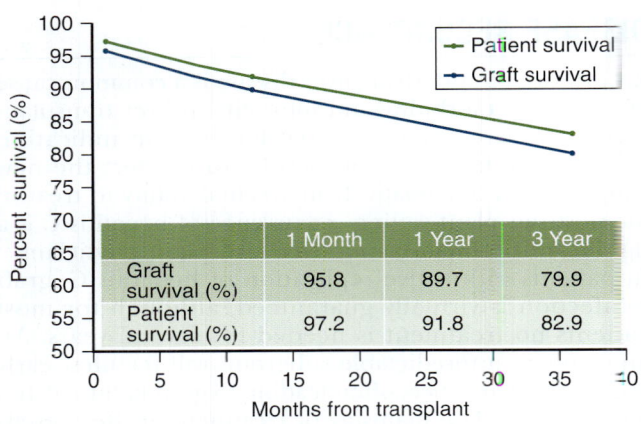

FIGURE 127.3 Patient and graft survival in the United States after deceased donor liver transplantation as of 2016 according to the Scientific Registry of Transplant Recipients (SRTR). Each data point collected from 12 to 13,888 cases. Data only include first-time isolated liver transplants (redo and multiorgan transplants excluded). Based on collection of greater than 12,573 to 13,888 over 3 years. Referenced September 15, 2016. (Data from Scientific Registry of Transplant Recipients. *SRTR Program-Specific Report.* <http://www.srtr.org/csr/current/Centers/201606/pdf/CACSTX1LI201606PNEW.pdf>.)

REFERENCES

1. Starzl TE, Groth CG, Brettschneider L, et al. Orthotopic homotransplantation of the human liver. *Ann Surg.* 1968;168:392.
2. Kolata G. Liver transplants endorsed. An NIH consensus panel recommends more transplants but does not say who will pay. *Science.* 1983;221:139.
3. Scientific Registry of Transplant Recipients (SRTR). US Hospitals With Liver Transplant Centers. http://www.srtr.org/csr/current/Centers/TransplantCenters.aspx?organcode=LI; 2016 Accessed 8 November 2016.
4. Xu J, Kochanek KD, Murphy SL, Tejada-Vera B. Deaths: final data for 2007. *Natl Vital Stat Rep.* 2010;58:1-36.
5. OPTN/SRTR Annual Data Report. http://onlinelibrary.wiley.com/doi/10.1111/ajt.13668/epdf; 2014 Accessed 7 November 2016.
6. Day CP. Heavy drinking greatly increases the risk of cirrhosis in patients with HCV hepatitis. *Gut.* 2001;49:750.
7. Forman LM, Lewis JD, Berlin JA, Feldman HI, Lucey MR. The association between hepatitis C infection and survival after orthotopic liver transplantation. *Gastroenterology.* 2002;122:889-896.
8. Charlton M, Everson GT, Flamm SL, et al. Ledipasvir and sofosbuvir plus ribavirin for treatment of HCV infection in patients with advanced liver disease. *Gastroenterology.* 2015;149:649-659.
9. Colquhoun SD, Belle SH, Samuel D, Pruett TL, Teperman LW. Transplantation in the hepatitis B patient and current therapies to prevent recurrence. *Semin Liver Dis.* 2000;20:7.
10. Neuberger J, Bradwell AR. Anti-mitochondrial antibodies in primary biliary cirrhosis. *J Hepatol.* 2002;37:712.
11. Wiesner RH. Liver transplantation for primary sclerosing cholangitis: timing, outcome, impact of inflammatory bowel disease and recurrence of disease. *Best Pract Res Clin Gastroenterol.* 2001;15:667.
12. Rea DJ, Heimbach JK, Rosen CB, et al. Liver transplantation with neoadjuvant chemoradiation is more effective than resection for hilar cholangiocarcinoma. *Ann Surg.* 2005;242:458.
13. Vong S, Bell BP. Chronic liver disease mortality in the United States, 1990–1998. *Hepatology.* 2004;39:476.
14. Penn I. Evaluation of transplant candidates with pre-existing malignancies. *Ann Transplant.* 1997;2:14.
15. Williams MC, Creger JH, Belton AM, et al. The organ center of the United Network for Organ Sharing and twenty years of organ sharing in the United States. *Transplantation.* 2004;77:641.
16. El-Serag HB, Mason AC. Rising incidence of hepatocellular carcinoma in the United States. *N Engl J Med.* 1999;340:745.
17. El-Serag HB. Hepatocellular carcinoma: recent trends in the United States. *Gastroenterology.* 2004;127:S27.
18. Thomas M, Jaffe D, Choti D. Hepatocellular carcinoma: consensus recommendations of the National Cancer Institute Clinical Trials Planning Meeting. *J Clin Oncol.* 2010;28:3994.
19. Zezos P, Renner EL. Liver transplantation and non-alcoholic fatty liver disease. *World J Gastroenterol.* 2014;29(42):15532-15538.
20. Malhi H, Allen AM, Watt KD. Nonalcoholic fatty liver: optimizing pretransplant selection and posttransplant care to maximize survival. *Curr Opin Organ Transplant.* 2016;2:99-106.
21. Grossman E, Millis JM. Liver transplantation for non-hepatocellular carcinoma malignancy: indications, limitations, and analysis of the current literature. *Liver Transpl.* 2010;16:930.
22. Olthoff KM, Brown RS Jr, Delmonico FL, et al. Summary report of a national conference: evolving concepts in liver allocation in the MELD and PELD era. December 8, 2003, Washington, DC, USA. *Liver Transpl.* 2004;10:A6.
23. American Association for the Study of Liver Diseases. Practice Guidelines. http://www.aasld.org/sites/default/files/guideline_documents/AcuteLiverFailureUpdate201journalformat1.pdf; 2010 Accessed 7 November 2016.
24. Sherlock SAD, Dooley J. *Diseases of the Liver and Biliary System.* 11th ed. Oxford: Blackwell Science; 2002.
25. Kowdley KV, Brandhagen DJ, Gish RG, et al. Survival after liver transplantation in patients with hepatic iron overload: the national hemochromatosis transplant registry. *Gastroenterology.* 2005;129:494.
26. Mandell MS. Hepatopulmonary syndrome and portopulmonary hypertension in the model for end-stage liver disease (MELD) era. *Liver Transpl.* 2004;10:S54.
27. Bass NM, Yao FY. The role of the interventional radiologist. Transjugular procedures. *Gastrointest Endosc Clin N Am.* 2001;11:131.
28. Cardenas A. Hepatorenal syndrome: a dreaded complication of end-stage liver disease. *Am J Gastroenterol.* 2005;100:460.
29. Colquhoun SD, Lipkin C, Connelly CA. The pathophysiology, diagnosis, and management of acute hepatic encephalopathy. *Adv Intern Med.* 2001;46:155.
30. Freeman RB. MELD: the holy grail of organ allocation? *J Hepatol.* 2005;42:16.
31. Coffin CS, Stock PG, Dove LM, et al. Virologic and clinical outcomes of hepatitis B virus infection in HIV-HBV coinfected transplant recipients. *Am J Transplant.* 2010;10:1268.
32. Schreibman I, Gaynor JJ, Jayaweera D, et al. Outcomes after orthotopic liver transplantation in 15 HIV-infected patients. *Transplantation.* 2007;84:697.
33. Wiesner RH, McDiarmid SV, Kamath PS, et al. MELD and PELD: application of survival models to liver allocation. *Liver Transpl.* 2001;7:567.
34. Mazzaferro V, Regalia E, Doci R, et al. Liver transplantation for the treatment of small hepatocellular carcinomas in patients with cirrhosis. *N Engl J Med.* 1996;334(11):693-699.
35. UNOS data courtesy Richard Freeman, MD.
36. U.S. Department of Health and Human Services: Organ Procurement and Transplantation Network. https://optn.transplant.hrsa.gov/governance/policies/; Accessed 2 November 2016.
37. Gentry SE, Massie AB, Cheek SW, et al. Addressing geographic disparities in liver transplantation through redistricting. *Am J Transplant.* 2013;13(8):2052-2058.
38. United Network for Organ Sharing. "Share 35" Liver Policy: Analysis at 1 Year. https://www.transplantpro.org/wp-content/uploads/sites/3/14-Share-35_Edwards.pdf.
39. Massie AB, Caffo B, Gentry SE, et al. MELD exceptions and rates of waiting list outcomes. *Am J Transplant.* 2011;11(11):2362-2371.
40. Gentry S, Chow E, Massie A, Segev D. Gerrymandering for justice: redistricting U.S. liver allocation. *Interfaces.* 2015;45(5):462-480.
41. A definition of irreversible coma: report of the Ad Hoc Committee of the Harvard Medical School to Examine the Definition of Brain Death. *JAMA.* 1968;205(6):337-340.
42. National Conference of Commissioners on Uniform State Laws. Legislative Fact Sheet—determination of Death Act. www.uniformlaws.org/LegislativeFactSheet.aspx?title=DeterminationofDeathAct.
43. Döşemeci L, Cengiz M, Yilmaz M, Ramazanoğlu A. Frequency of spinal reflex movements in brain-dead patients. *Transplant Proc.* 2004;36(1):17-19.
44. Seem DL, Lee I, Umscheid CA, Kuehnert MJ, United States Public Health Service. PHS guideline for reducing human immunodeficiency

virus, hepatitis B virus, and hepatitis C virus transmission through organ transplantation. *Public Health Rep.* 2012;127(4):247-343.

45. Melada E, Maggi U, Rossi G, et al. Back-table arterial reconstructions in liver transplantation: single-center experience. *Transplant Proc.* 2005;37:2587.

46. Griffith BP, Shaw BW Jr, Hardesty RL, Iwatsuki S, Bahnson HT, Starzl TE. Veno-venous bypass without systemic anticoagulation for transplantation of the human liver. *Surg Gynecol Obstet.* 1985;160:270.

47. Neelakanta G, Colquhoun S, Csete M, Koroleff D, Mahajan A, Busuttil RW. Efficacy and safety of heat exchanger added to venovenous bypass circuit during orthotopic liver transplantation. *Liver Transpl Surg.* 1998;4:506.

48. Shi XY, Xu ZD, Xu HT, Jiang JJ, Liu G. Cardiac arrest after graft reperfusion during liver transplantation. *Hepatobiliary Pancreat Dis Int.* 2006;5:185-189.

49. Aggarwal S, Kang Y, Freeman JA, Fortunato FL Jr, Pinsky MR. Postreperfusion syndrome: hypotension after reperfusion of the transplanted liver. *J Crit Care.* 1993;8:154.

50. Shimoda M, Saab S, Morrisey M, et al. A cost-effectiveness analysis of biliary anastomosis with or without T-tube after orthotopic liver transplantation. *Am J Transplant.* 2001;1:157.

51. Tzakis AG, Kirkegaard P, Pinna AD, et al. Liver transplantation with cavoportal hemitransposition in the presence of diffuse portal vein thrombosis. *Transplantation.* 1998;65:619.

52. Nissen NN, Colquhoun S. Graft failure: cause, etiology, recognition and treatment. In: Busuttil RW, Klintmalm GB, eds. *Transplantation of the Liver.* Philadelphia: Saunders; 2005.

53. Mandal AK, King KE, Humphreys SL, Manley VR, Burdick JF, Klein AS. Plasmapheresis: an effective therapy for primary allograft nonfunction after liver transplantation. *Transplantation.* 2000;70:216.

54. Stockmann M, Lock JF, Malinowski M, et al. How to define initial poor graft function after liver transplantation?—a new functional definition by the LiMAx test. *Transpl Int.* 2012;:1023-1032. doi:10.1111/j.1432-2277.2010.01089.

55. Vivarelli M, Cucchetti A, La Barba G, et al. Ischemic arterial complications after liver transplantation in the adult: multivariate analysis of risk factors. *Arch Surg.* 2004;139:1069.

56. Drazan K, Shaked A, Olthoff KM, et al. Etiology and management of symptomatic adult hepatic artery thrombosis after orthotopic liver transplantation (OLT). *Am Surg.* 1996;62:237.

57. Stange B, Glanemann M, Nuessler NC, Settmacher U, Steinmüller T, Neuhaus P. Hepatic artery thrombosis after adult liver transplantation. *Liver Transpl.* 2003;9:612.

58. Madalosso C, Souza NF Jr, Ilstrup DM, Wiesner RH, Krom RA. Cytomegalovirus and its association with hepatic artery thrombosis after liver transplantation. *Transplantation.* 1998;66:294.

59. Wiesner RH. MELD/PELD and the allocation of deceased donor livers for status 1 recipients with acute fulminant hepatic failure, primary nonfunction, hepatic artery thrombosis, and acute Wilson's disease. *Liver Transpl.* 2004;10:S17.

60. Varotti G, Grazi GL, Vetrone G, et al. Causes of early acute graft failure after liver transplantation: analysis of a 17-year single-centre experience. *Clin Transplant.* 2005;19:492.

61. Guichelaar MM, Benson JT, Malinchoc M, Krom RA, Wiesner RH, Charlton MR. Risk factors for and clinical course of non-anastomotic biliary strictures after liver transplantation. *Am J Transplant.* 2003;3:885.

62. Fondevila C, Ghobrial RM, Fuster J, Bombuy E, Garcia-Valdecasas JC, Busuttil RW. Biliary complications after adult living donor liver transplantation. *Transplant Proc.* 2003;35:1902.

63. Thuluvath PJ, Thomson BN, Pleass H, et al. Management of biliary tract complications after orthotopic liver transplantation. *Clin Transplant.* 2004;18:647.

64. Jain A, Reyes J, Kashyap R, et al. Long-term survival after liver transplantation in 4,000 consecutive patients at a single center. *Ann Surg.* 2000;232:490.

65. Fung J, Kelly D, Kadry Z, Patel-Tom K, Eghtesad B. Immunosuppression in liver transplantation: beyond calcineurin inhibitors. *Liver Transpl.* 2005;11:267.

66. Kim WR, Lake JR, Smith JM, et al. OPTN/SRTR 2013 Annual Data Report: liver. *Am J Transplant.* 2015;15(suppl 2):1-28.

67. Winston DJ, Pakrasi A, Busuttil RW. Prophylactic fluconazole in liver transplant recipients. A randomized, double-blind, placebo-controlled trial. *Ann Intern Med.* 1999;131:729.

68. Winston DJ, Busuttil RW. Randomized controlled trial of sequential intravenous and oral ganciclovir versus prolonged intravenous ganciclovir for long-term prophylaxis of cytomegalovirus disease in high-risk cytomegalovirus-seronegative liver transplant recipients with cytomegalovirus-seropositive donors. *Transplantation.* 2004;77:305.

69. Rabkin JM, de la Melena V, Orloff SL, Corless CL, Rosen HR, Olyaei AJ. Late mortality after orthotopic liver transplantation. *Am J Surg.* 2001;181:475.

70. Cheah YL, Simpson MA, Pomposelli JJ, Pomfret EA. Incidence of death and potentially life-threatening near-miss events in living donor hepatic lobectomy: a world-wide survey. *Liver Transpl.* 2013;19(5):499-506.

71. Truog RD. The ethics of organ donation by living donors. *N Engl J Med.* 2005;353:444.

72. Brown RS Jr, Russo MW, Lai M, et al. A survey of liver transplantation from living adult donors in the United States. *N Engl J Med.* 2003;348:818.

73. Emond JC, Renz JF, Ferrell LD, et al. Functional analysis of grafts from living donors. Implications for the treatment of older recipients. *Ann Surg.* 1996;224:544, discussion 552.

74. Kiuchi T, Tanaka K, Ito T, et al. Small-for-size graft in living donor liver transplantation: how far should we go? *Liver Transpl.* 2003;9:S29.

75. Olthoff KM, Merion RM, Ghobrial RM, et al. Outcomes of 385 adult-to-adult living donor liver transplant recipients: a report from the A2ALL Consortium. *Ann Surg.* 2005;242:314, discussion 323.

76. Renz JF, Emond JC, Yersiz H, Ascher NL, Busuttil RW. Split-liver transplantation in the United States: outcomes of a national survey. *Ann Surg.* 2004;239:172.

77. NIH Consensus Statement on Management of Hepatitis C: 2002. *NIH Consens State Sci Statements.* 2002;19:1.

78. Scientific Registry of Transplant Recipients (SRTR). SRTR Program-Specific Report. http://www.srtr.org/csr/current/Centers/201606/pdf/CACTX1LI201606PNEW.pdf; 2016.

Acute Liver Failure and Bioartificial Liver Support

Harvey S. Chen | Jian Yang | Scott L. Nyberg

The failing liver represents a syndrome with profound morbidity and mortality. The morbidity of liver failure is secondary to the tremendous decline in metabolic and synthetic functions inherent to the liver. With the decline in metabolic activity, accumulation of toxic substances occurs. The most notable of these toxins is ammonia. Cerebral edema (the most feared complication) is strongly associated with elevated levels of ammonia.[1] In addition to ammonia accumulation, drugs metabolized by the liver require strict regulation, if they are used at all. One of the leading synthetic functions of the liver is the production of coagulation factors. As the time in failure progresses, the patient will become more coagulopathic. In addition, the liver is home to an abundant source of resident macrophages, Kupffer cells,[2,3] which are believed to produce cytokines leading to systemic inflammation in the setting of the failing liver.[4-6] The systemic inflammatory response syndrome (SIRS) occurs in approximately 60% of patients with a failing liver.[7] The SIRS can lead to failure of other organ systems (kidneys, lungs, etc.), further complicating the course and treatment of patients with failing livers.

The failing liver can be separated into two groups: acute liver failure (ALF) and acute decompensation of a cirrhotic liver (Fig. 128.1). Patients suffering from a failing liver have the possibility of recovering spontaneously. However, for the patients who are not likely to recover spontaneously, the only proven treatment is liver transplantation. Before liver transplantation, the mortality rate of patients with acutely failing livers was greater than 80%.[8] Nowadays this mortality rate has decreased to approximately 30%, thanks to liver transplantation and the high level of intensive care now available.[8] Nonetheless, there are still issues with liver transplantation. For example, these patients are fated to lifetime immunosuppression. More importantly, there is shortage of livers for patients on the transplant waiting list. Thus adding patients in ALF or acute decompensation to this already overextended list only worsens the problem. According to work done by the US ALF Study Group, patients with ALF currently wait a median of 1 day for transplant after listing. However, ALF patients on the transplant list who waited 3 days or longer had a much greater risk of death.[8]

The solution to this shortage is unclear but likely requires multiple advances, including improved knowledge of the etiology, high-quality medical care, and some form of artificial liver support until the supply of donor liver organs can be increased. Over the course of this chapter, the most common etiologies of ALF will be reviewed, current medical protocols will be listed, artificial liver support systems will be described, and potential future directions will be explored.

DEFINITION

The current definition of ALF is acute liver injury associated with coagulopathy (international normalized ratio [INR] of 1.5 or greater) and altered mental status (encephalopathy) for less than 26 weeks and no past history of liver disease.[9] After a patient has been diagnosed with ALF, management ensues based upon the level of encephalopathy and the specific etiology (if identified). The most complete set of guidelines for acutely failing liver management are listed in a position paper[9] on the American Association for the Study of Liver Diseases website (www.aasld.org).

ETIOLOGY OF ACUTE LIVER FAILURE

The incidence of ALF in the United States has been estimated to be approximately 2000 to 3000 per year.[10] However, defining good estimates of the causes of ALF in the United States was difficult due to small sample sizes. In an effort to better define and treat ALF in the United States, the US Food and Drug Administration and the National Institutes of Health (NIH) allotted funding for the development of the US ALF Study Group. Since then, the group has accumulated a robust sampling of ALF patients (2102 patients) between 1998 and 2014 in the United States (Fig. 128.2). This sampling has allowed for a high-quality estimation of the various etiologies of ALF common to the United States.

ACETAMINOPHEN AND DRUG INDUCED

Acetaminophen overdose leads to a buildup of its reactive intermediate N-para-aminoquinonimine (NAPQI). The sulfhydryl groups of glutathione bind to NAPQI and form nontoxic by-products. After glutathione is depleted from hepatocytes, a centrilobular pattern of hepatocyte necrosis ensues.[11,12] Acetaminophen-induced liver failure most commonly occurs at dose greater than 12 g/day.[13] However, ALF after consumption of 3 to 4 g/day has been observed.[13a] Forty-six percent of ALF cases are secondary to acetaminophen overdose. It is the most common cause of ALF in the United States. According to ALF Study Group registry data in 2015, 23% of the patients were listed for transplant, 8% received a liver transplant, 73% recovered spontaneously, and 19% died without receiving a liver transplant.[14] Data showed that patients who recovered spontaneously from acetaminophen had an 89.5% 2-year survival rate, whereas patients who received a liver transplant had a 92.4% 2-year survival rate.[15] For patients who ingested acetaminophen within 4 hours, activated charcoal can be effective in decontamination.[9,16] Besides advances in intensive care, the use of N-acetylcysteine has proven

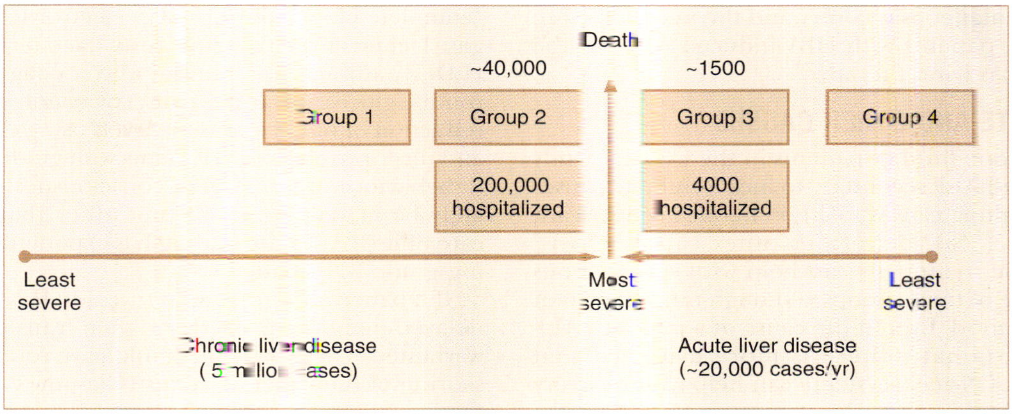

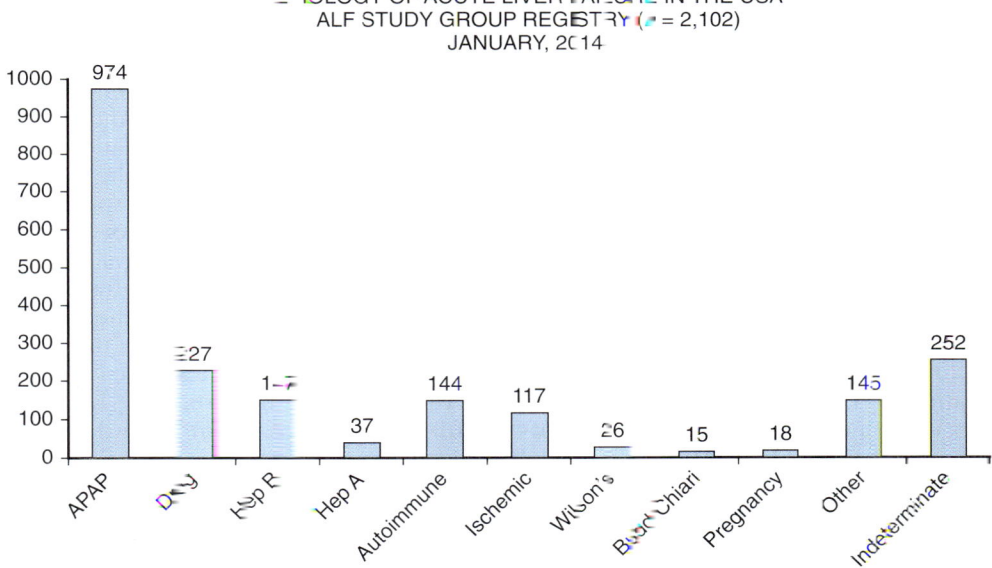

FIGURE 128.1 Liver disease is separated into acute and chronic forms with prevalences of approximately 20,000 and 5 million cases per year, respectively. The cases requiring hospitalization are shown here on a spectrum of severity. Groups 1 and 4 represent those cases that do not lead to hospitalization. However, group 2 (acute decompensation) and group 3 (acute liver failure) are recognized by those that lead to hospitalization. Unfortunately, approximately 35% of the acute liver failure group and 20% of the acutely decompensated group die as a result of their failing liver.

FIGURE 128.2 Etiology of acute liver failure in the United States. A total of 2102 cases were recorded as of January 1, 2014. *ALF*, Acute liver failure; *APAP*, N-acetyl-para-aminophenol *Hep A*, hepatitis A; *Hep B*, hepatitis B. (Data from Acute Liver Failure Study Group Registry. http://www.utsouthwestern.edu/labs/acute-liver/clinical-trials/.)

efficacious and safe in preventing liver injury and has shown promise in improving brain dysfunction (encephalopathy) in animal models.[17,18]

Another 11% of the cases of ALF from the US ALF Study Group were caused by other drug toxicities. More than 60 different drugs, alone or in combination, are thought to induce ALF. Antimicrobials (46% of total cases), especially antituberculosis medications, are the most commonly implicated offenders. The outcome is less favorable than acetaminophen overdose. Only 27.1% of these patients spontaneously recovered (less than half of those who had acetaminophen-induced ALF), and 54.9% of these patients required transplantation. Patients who received liver transplant had a 92.9% 3-week

survival rate. Liver transplant remains the most efficacious treatment.

VIRAL

The two main causes of viral hepatitis leading to ALF are hepatitis A virus (HAV) and hepatitis B virus (HBV). Combined these two viral etiologies account for 10% (HAV—3%, HBV—7%) of the ALF cases seen in the United States. Patients with HAV-induced ALF have a better prognosis both with spontaneous recovery (58% vs. 24%) and overall survival (87% vs. 61%) compared with those with HBV-induced ALF.[8] Treatment for HAV-related ALF remains supportive care because no virus-specific treatment has proven to be effective so far.[9] Because of the lower spontaneous recovery and the need for more transplantation, patients with HBV-induced ALF may be considered for antiviral therapy.[20]

INDETERMINATE AND OTHER CAUSES

The remaining one-third of patients in the US ALF Study Group developed ALF secondary to indeterminate causes (12%), autoimmune causes (7%), ischemic events (6%), Wilson disease (1%), or various other causes (7%).[8] Etiologic-specific treatments can help with spontaneous recovery in some of these groups, although transplantation may still be required. Even if the cause of a patient's ALF may be indeterminate, there is more evidence that administration of N-acetylcysteine can help with recovery or bridge the time to transplant as many of these indeterminate cases may have a combination of causes, which include acetaminophen.[21]

SURGICAL CAUSES OF ACUTE LIVER FAILURE

ALF can occur following massive hepatic resection in otherwise healthy patients or with smaller resections in patients with marginal hepatic function. In a large retrospective study from Memorial Sloan Kettering Cancer Center, the rate of ALF following hepatic resection was 1% (19 out of 1803 patients). This study included consecutive resections ranging from nonanatomic wedge resections to extended hepatectomies (up to six segments). The incidence of failure was not listed for the number of segments resected; however, 583 patients had five or six segments resected.[22] To answer the question of how much liver is safe to resect, a study from MD Anderson Cancer Center looked at outcomes from 301 consecutive extended right hepatectomies. Three groups were identified and compared according to ratio of future liver remnant (FLR) to standardized liver volume (SLV) prior to resection: FLR/SLV ≤ 20%, 20% < FLR/SLV ≤ 30%, FLR/SLV > 30%. Of the 301 patients receiving extended right hepatectomy, 44 patients were determined to have liver insufficiency following resection. The FLR/SLV ≤ 20% group had a significantly higher percentage of patients (34%) with liver insufficiency compared with the 20% < FLR/SLV ≤ 30% group (10%; $P < .001$) and the FLR/SLV > 30% group (15%; $P = .01$).[23] For patients who develop liver failure after resection, supportive therapies may provide time in facilitating remnant hypertrophy and recovery, or bridge the patient to liver transplantation.

MEDICAL THERAPY

Medical therapy for the failing liver has seen improvement over the past decades. Much credit is given to improvement in the quality of intensive care delivered to ALF patients. Effective medical management requires early recognition of a failing liver. After being recognized, coordination is a necessity between primary care and referral centers and medical and surgical disciplines at the referral center. Quality intensive care aims to counteract hemodynamic instability and prevent extrahepatic manifestation of liver failure, including cerebral edema, and potentially allow for recovery or sufficient time for transplant.

Management common to all grades of hepatic encephalopathy (HE) includes baseline and routine lab work (complete blood count [CBC], electrolytes, arterial blood gas, lactate, liver function tests, lactate dehydrogenase [LDH], ammonia, albumin, and a coagulation panel), routine glucose measurements, correction of coagulopathy, reduction of blood ammonia levels using enteral lactulose, and ulcer prophylaxis.[24] Patients with grade I HE (changes in behavior but not level of consciousness) can appropriately be managed in a setting other than the intensive care unit (ICU) if the staffing has experience with monitoring grade I HE patients.[24]

If a patient progresses on to grade II HE (disoriented, delayed mentation, asterixis), then transfer to the ICU is warranted. These patients should have routinely scheduled scoring of their mental status (Glasgow Coma Scale, Full Outline of Unresponsiveness score).[25] In addition to clinical scoring, a head computed tomography (CT) scan should be obtained to rule out other causes of acute mental status change, such as subdural hematoma, before placement of an intracranial pressure (ICP) monitor. However, CT scanning is not routinely used to evaluate cerebral edema because it is a late finding in ALF and transport of patients in advanced ALF to radiology for scanning can be problematic. Nutrition (enteral or parenteral) should be initiated at this juncture to maintain intake of calories, prevent hypoglycemia, stabilize ammonia production, and assist in healing the injured liver.[26] Electrolytes should be monitored closely and derangements corrected promptly.[9] During grades I and II HE, sedation should be avoided to allow for accurate scoring of the patient's mental status; however, short-acting agents, such as propofol, may be effective and safe when for procedures.[27]

With progression of cerebral edema to grade III (in and out of consciousness, confusion), protection of the patient's airway via endotracheal intubation becomes necessary. Grade III HE marks the point at which placement of ICP monitor should be considered.[28,29] However, a retrospective study from the US ALF Study Group in 2014 suggests that ICP monitor does not improve survival in acetaminophen-induced ALF patients, and it may be associated with worse outcomes in patients with nonacetaminophen ALF.[30] Further study, ideally a prospective randomized control trial, is needed to validate this finding. In preparation for ICP monitor placement, the patient's coagulation profile should be corrected to an INR of 1.5 or less to avoid intracranial hemorrhage during ICP catheter placement. INR may be allowed to rise after ICP catheter placement to assess liver synthetic function, but an INR greater than 3.0 should be avoided with the catheter in place. A rising INR is a poor prognostic sign, whereas stabilization or decline in INR is a useful measure of liver recovery from acute injury. With the ICP monitor in place, the goal-directed therapy is now maintaining a cerebral perfusion pressure (CPP) greater than 60 mm Hg. The patient should have the head of the bed elevated to 30 to 45 degrees, minimal stimulation from lighting and noise, and sedation with propofol. In ALF patients with high risk for cerebral edema (serum ammonia >150 μM, grade III/IV HE, acute kidney injury, require vasopressors to maintain mean arterial pressure [MAP]), prophylactic hypertonic saline can be used to maintain serum sodium at 145 to 155 mEq/L.[9,31] If intracranial hypertension is encountered, mannitol bolus of 0.5 to 1.0 g/kg body weight is the first-line treatment.[9] Phenytoin and short-acting benzodiazepines should be used to treat seizures.[9] If the intracranial hypertension is refractory to osmotic agent, hypothermia with goal core body temperature of 34 to 35°C may be started to halt the progression of cerebral edema.[32] However, there is no set standard for the duration of hypothermia. Some centers continue hypothermia for up to 24 hours after transplantation.

ALF patients are high risk for infection. Periodic cultures are recommended with prompt treatment at earliest signs of infection. Although not proven to improve overall outcome, prophylactic antibiotics (antibacterial, antifungal, and antiviral) may be considered due to high infection rates and future possibility of further immunosuppression should transplantation occur.[33]

Given the hemodynamic changes that occur with ALF, vasopressors are initiated to help to increase the MAP to maintain adequate CPP. If renal dysfunction occurs, then continuous venovenous hemodialysis is preferred over intermittent hemodialysis because intermittent hemodialysis can cause hemodynamic changes worsening CPP.[34]

Transplantation is currently the best modality for ALF. So far, no prognostic scoring system satisfactorily predicts outcome and determines liver allocation in patients with ALF.[35,36] Based on United Network for Organ Sharing (UNOS) policy, an ALF patient who (1) is older than 18 years, (2) has less than 7 days life expectancy without liver transplant, (3) has onset of HE within 8 weeks, (4) has no preexisting liver disease, (5) is currently under ICU care, and one of the following: (a) is ventilator dependent, (b) requires renal replacement therapy, or (c) INR greater than 2.0, qualifies for adult status 1A (most urgent) on the waiting list.

LIVER SUPPORT SYSTEMS

The best treatment currently for a liver that will inevitably fail is liver transplantation. However, there is a profound shortage of transplantable donor livers. This shortage leads to approximately 40% of listed patients per year not receiving a liver transplant, with a majority of these patients either dying or becoming too sick to transplant (www.unos.org). One potential solution for decreasing the number of ALF patients requiring liver transplantation is a liver support system that would allow time for recovery and avoid transplantation. The ideal liver support system would detoxify blood to physiologic levels, accomplish all hepatic synthetic functions, attenuate systemic inflammation, and allow for the regenerative capacity of the liver.

The most important identified toxin requiring clearance by the liver is ammonia. Ammonia concentration correlates with the most feared complication of the acutely failing liver, cerebral edema. For ammonia to be effectively detoxified and eliminated by the body, a functioning urea cycle must be present (Fig. 128.3). During the development of a potentially successful liver support system, investigators should take effort in demonstrating urea cycle function not only by measuring levels of urea production and ammonia removal but also by showing effective levels of urea cycle gene expression by hepatocytes in the liver support device.

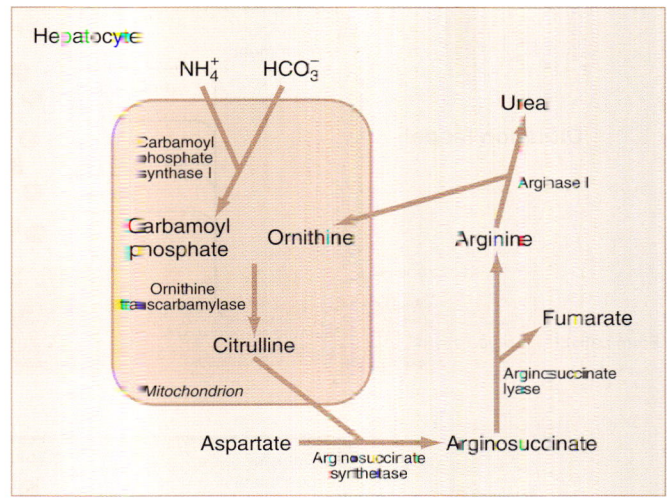

FIGURE 128.3 The urea cycle occurs within hepatocytes. Ammonia (in the form of ammonium, NH₄⁺) enters into the hepatocyte and then is transported into the mitochondria. The first two steps of the urea cycle occur within the mitochondria. The remaining three steps occur in the cytosol of the hepatocyte. After urea and ornithine are produced from arginine, the urea diffuses out of the hepatocyte and ornithine is transported back into the mitochondria to continue the cycle

Two important synthetic functions of the liver are production of albumin and coagulation proteins. Albumin production serves as a useful marker of liver-specific protein production in support systems using hepatocytes. Coagulation pathway restoration is an important part of the ideal liver support system. An effective coagulation pathway profile by a bioartificial liver not only prevents bleeding complications but also reduces the use of transfused blood products, avoids complications of their use, and saves resources for other patient populations.

Important design features of any liver support system include free passage of toxins requiring breakdown, free passage of newly synthesized proteins (bioartificial support system) exclusion of the patient's antibodies/complement components to prevent cytotoxic effects (bioartificial support system), and prevention of cells in the support system entering the patient's circulation (bioartificial support system) (Fig. 128.4). To control the passage or exclusion of various molecules, the permeability of the filter separating the patient's blood from the detoxifying agent compartment (dialyzer or cells), and the flow rate of the patient's blood passing by the detoxifying agent compartment are adjusted for optimal performance. In the setting of a bioartificial liver support system, this concept of controlling the flow rate can be demonstrated in two models (the diffusion model and the convection model). The diffusion model considers the transfer of waste molecules and product molecules across a semipermeable membrane according to concentration gradients of these molecules. In this model the semipermeable membrane separates the patient's blood from the hepatocyte compartment. On the other hand, the convection model considers the transfer of waste molecules and

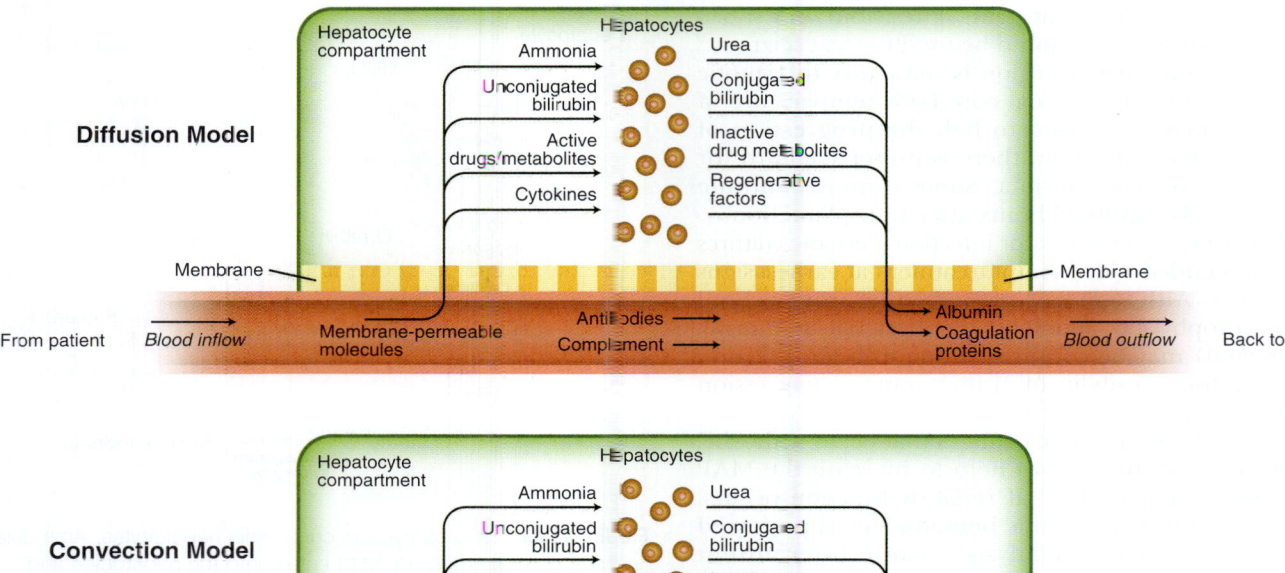

FIGURE 128.4 Two conceptual models are displayed for bioartificial liver support devices. The top model is based upon diffusion—molecules filter from high concentration to low concentration. The bottom model relies on pumps (convection) to allow for increased filtration of larger molecules. Both models contain a semipermeable membrane that allows for passage of nonimmunologic molecules. Toxins from the patient are metabolized, and proteins are synthesized within the hepatocyte compartment and returned back to the patient.

product molecules according to pressure gradients and fluid flow. The convection model incorporates pumps that force flow across the semipermeable membrane and allow for a theoretical advantage of increased passage of larger toxins and liver-synthesized proteins into and out of the hepatocyte compartment.

Work done by Nedredal et al. demonstrated that optimal toxin removal in a bioartificial liver support system (the spheroid reservoir bioartificial liver) occurred with a 400-kDa (kilodalton) membrane incorporating mass transport by both diffusion and high flow rate convection. Under these conditions, ammonia, direct and indirect bilirubin, tumor necrosis factor, and albumin were shown to cross the membrane at high rates. Equally important, immunoglobulin G (IgG) and IgM were shown to cross at negligible levels, thus significantly reducing the risks of cytotoxic effects.[37]

In addition to detoxifying and maintaining synthetic function, the support system should help to attenuate the SIRS associated with the acutely failing liver, as well as promote liver regeneration within the patient. Various

cytokines have been shown to play pivotal roles in both the SIRS of the acutely failing liver and liver regeneration.[4–6] To successfully treat the SIRS of ALF, the liver support device should lower high circulating levels of proinflammatory cytokines, such as interleukin-1β (IL-1β) and tumor necrosis factor-α (TNF-α), while maintaining levels of both proinflammatory and regenerative cytokines, such as IL-6, which favor liver regeneration. Failure to attenuate the SIRS will accentuate the extrahepatic manifestations of liver failure and inflammation and worsen the inability to recover adequate functioning liver mass to maintain homeostasis.

There are two current types of liver support systems, artificial and bioartificial systems. Both systems have been tested in various trials, which will be discussed. However, the ideal liver support system has not yet been developed.

ARTIFICIAL LIVER SUPPORT

Artificial liver support systems are extracorporeal devices intended to assist the failing liver that do not use biologic material, such as cell lines or primary hepatocytes, to remove toxins. Historical examples of artificial liver support include charcoal hemoperfusion and hemodialysis. Both were used in an effort to remove small toxins that cause HE and improve survival. Early devices were successful in reducing HE but did not improve survival in controlled studies in the era before liver transplantation.[38–40] The three most common forms of artificial liver support currently used are plasma exchange, hemodiafiltration, molecular adsorbent recirculating system (MARS), and fractionated plasma separation and absorption (Prometheus). Each of these forms of therapy will be discussed.

Plasma exchange/hemodiafiltration involves a combination of two detoxification methods. The first, plasma exchange, involves the removal of the noncellular components of the patient's blood for detoxification and replacement with an equal volume of fresh frozen plasma containing liver-specific synthetic factors. The second, hemodiafiltration (a combination of hemodialysis and hemofiltration), washes the plasma in high volumes of dialysate and aids in the removal of toxins, such as ammonia. This combined method of artificial liver support is most commonly used in Japan secondary to the low number of cadaveric organ donations performed in that country. In a recent study by Inoue et al., 12 patients (7 with indeterminate etiology and 5 with acute HBV infection) received artificial liver support using plasma exchange/hemodiafiltration. The overall survival was 42% (5 of 12), with seven patients dying from lack of donor livers. All patients had reduction of HE and regained consciousness during treatments.[4]

MARS uses albumin dialysis within a three-circuit system. The extracorporeal blood circuit is separated from the albumin dialysate circuit by a restrictive 70-kDa pore size membrane that allows for selective removal of water-soluble and albumin-bound molecules from the patient's blood. The third circuit then allows for removal of water-soluble toxins from the second albumin circuit.[42] Toxins are also removed from the second albumin circuit by a charcoal filter and resin binding column placed in the second circuit. The majority of the studies testing MARS have been conducted in the setting of acute decompensation of the cirrhotic patient. Multiple randomized studies have demonstrated significant recovery from HE with MARS plus standard medical therapy (SMT) compared with SMT alone.[43–45] For example, the pivotal US trial by Hassanein et al. showed that HE improvement occurred more quickly in the MARS treatment group than SMT alone; the median time to improve two grades in HE occurred 36 hours sooner in the MARS treatment group (72 hours vs. 108 hours).[43] In another study, Heemann et al. showed a statistically significant improvement in survival at 30 days for the MARS plus SMT group (92%, 11 of 12) compared with the SMT-only group (55%, 6 of 11).[44] Interestingly, Sen et al. demonstrated that the improvement in HE in the MARS plus SMT group was independent of changes of ammonia and cytokine levels compared with the SMT-only group.[45] In 2013 Saliba et al. published the first prospective, randomized control trial on MARS in ALF patients (FULMAR study). The study was carried out across 16 liver transplant centers in France. A total of 102

patients were included in the study. Forty-nine patients were assigned to conventional treatment and 53 to MARS treatment. The study showed no statistical significance in 6-month and 1-year overall survival. In subgroup analysis, the paracetamol-related ALF group showed 68.4% survival in the conventional treatment group and 85.0% survival in the MARS group.[46] However, the difference did not reach statistical significance. The RELIEF trial, published by Banares et al. in 2013, is the most recent and largest randomized control trial, to date, studying the effect of MARS in acute-on-chronic liver failure (ACLF) patients. The study did not show any significant survival benefit. However, it showed short-term improvement in bilirubin and creatinine. Improvement in HE from grade II to IV to grade 0-I was also observed, but statistical significance was not reached ($P = .07$). On the other hand, MARS treatment was not associated with increased risk of adverse events.[47]

Prometheus is a second form of albumin dialysis therapy. Prometheus differs from MARS by using a larger porosity membrane (molecular weight cut-off 200 kDa) to fractionate the patient's blood and allow removal of toxins while bound to albumin. The fractionated plasma (containing albumin) is then passed over two adsorption columns, allowing for direct detoxification of the albumin. In contrast, the patient's albumin does not cross the MARS membrane, so toxins must enter the albumin circuit of MARS as free, unbound molecules.[48] Results from a large prospectively randomized trial comparing Prometheus and SMT versus SMT alone in the setting of acute decompensation of cirrhotic patients (HELIOS study) were discussed at the 2010 International Liver Meeting and published in 2012.[49] One-hundred forty-five patients (77 Prometheus + SMT; 68 SMT only) were enrolled. Overall, no survival advantage was demonstrated between the groups at either 28 days or 90 days following initial treatment. However, a predefined subgroup analysis demonstrated a survival advantage for the Prometheus group in patients with a model of end-stage liver disease (MELD) score greater than 30 and patients with hepatorenal syndrome type I (doubling of serum creatinine to >2.5 mg/dL or reduction of creatinine clearance by 50% to >20 mL/min in a period of less than 2 weeks).

BIOARTIFICIAL LIVER SUPPORT

The most important difference between an artificial liver support system and a bioartificial liver (BAL) support system is the use of cells in the latter. The ideal bioartificial liver support system would use human hepatocytes; however, a good-quality source of large numbers of human hepatocytes is currently not available. Most human hepatocytes currently come from unused cadaveric donors (discarded because of poor quality) or from nondiseased partial hepatectomy specimens which are relatively uncommon. Good-quality donor livers are not available because they are in great demand for use in liver transplantation. Novel solutions to expand the availability of human hepatocytes will be discussed later in this chapter. Currently, the two cell sources with the most use in human clinical trials of BAL therapy are the human hepatoblastoma cell line HepG2/C3A and primary hepatocytes from healthy pig livers.

The use of HepG2/C3A cells comprises the foundation of the extracorporeal liver assist device (ELAD). This device allows for hemoperfusion from the patient through columns containing immortalized C3A cells. By use of ultrafiltration, toxins can be detoxified and synthesized proteins can return to the patient. The device contains two acellular membranes to prevent the spread of hepatoblastoma cells back to the patient. Work by Kelly et al. from 1991 to 1993 using the Hepatix ELAD demonstrated the potential safety for patients suffering from ALF. However, this device was composed of a single cartridge containing 100 g of HepG2/C3A cells.[50] Ellis et al. then conducted a small randomized controlled trial using two 100-g Hepatix HepG2/C3A cartridges in a single circuit. A total of 24 patients were enrolled in the study, with 12 treated with ELAD plus SMT and 12 with SMT only. Groups were stratified based upon who met criteria for transplantation and who did not. Overall, the survival was not different between the two groups (ELAD plus SMT 67%, 8 of 12 vs. SMT only 58%, 7 of 12). There was also no difference between the groups when they were further separated based upon meeting or not meeting transplantation criteria.[51] More recently, the use of the HepG2/C3A cell line in the ELAD device has been improved. The latest generation of ELAD uses four HepG2/C3A columns. VTI-208 is the largest randomized control trial to date using ELAD in the United States. It included patients with severe acute alcoholic hepatitis (sAAH) and alcohol-induced liver decompensation (AILD); study results were presented at the 2015 AASLD meeting.[52] Of the 203 patients enrolled, 96 were randomized to the ELAD plus SMT and 107 to the SMT alone. No significant change in overall survival was observed between the treatment group and control group at 28 and 91 days. When stratified, ELAD demonstrated improved outcomes in a subgroup of younger patients (less than 50 years old) with MELD scores lower than 30. A follow-up clinical trial, VTL-308, may be pursued to further study the effects of ELAD in this subgroup of alcoholic patients.

The largest trial to date using HepatAssist device was published by Demetriou et al. in 2004.[53] This BAL device used 70 g of cryopreserved porcine hepatocytes. The trial was conducted at 20 institutions (11 in the United States and 9 in Europe) in which 171 patients were prospectively randomized (85 to BAL plus SMT and 86 to SMT alone). The primary endpoint for this study was the overall 30-day survival. There was no statistically significant difference between the two groups in overall 30-day survival (BAL plus SMT 71%, 60 of 85 vs. SMT alone 62%, 53 of 85). On further analysis, 147 of the 171 patients enrolled suffered from fulminant or subfulminant hepatic failure. The overall survival between these patients favored the BAL plus SMT group (73%, 53 of 73) over the SMT-alone group (59%, 44 of 74); however, this 14% improvement in survival did not reach statistical significance.[53] A further post hoc analysis of 83 patients with known causes of ALF did show significance in survival of BAL therapy over SMT ($P < .009$). The HepatAssist device first performed plasmapheresis before pumping the patient's fractionated plasma into an activated charcoal column for initial detoxification. The charcoal effluent was then oxygenated and passed through the hepatocyte bioreactor before returning back to the patient's circulation.

Despite the promising results from these two methods of BAL therapy for both ALF patients and acutely decompensated cirrhotic patients, concerns exist for both therapies. The biggest concern for the ELAD is the theoretical risk of HepG2/C3A tumor cell migration into the patient's circulation. Another concern of ELAD therapy is the deficiency of HepG2/C3A cells to perform functions specific to primary hepatocytes. Nyberg et al. demonstrated that primary rat hepatocytes had statistically higher ureagenesis and drug metabolism compared with HepG2/C3A in the setting of a gel entrapment BAL device.[54] As for the therapeutic use of porcine hepatocytes, the greatest concern is the possibility of zoonotic infections, such as porcine endogenous retrovirus (PERV) transmission to the patient. During the large trial with the HepatAssist device, there was no detection of PERV transmission to a patient.[53] The other concern with isolated primary hepatocytes is that they have been shown to lose function and undergo apoptosis under ex vivo conditions.[55-57] However, culturing hepatocytes as spheroids (three-dimensional clusters) has been shown to maintain function and prevent apoptosis longer than in monolayer systems.[58,59] Although hepatocyte spheroids have been shown to maintain function longer than isolated hepatocytes, no randomized control trials have been performed to test BAL support devices using this culturing technique.

FUTURE EFFORTS

The ideal therapy for a patient suffering from an acutely failing liver should perform liver-specific detoxification and synthetic functions, attenuate the SIRS often associated with the failing liver, and allow for regeneration of the injured liver. Thus the ideal therapy should either increase the likelihood of spontaneous recovery or effectively serve as a bridge to transplant with the ultimate goal of improved survival. The device that best fulfills these criteria is likely a cell-based support device, such as BAL. Cellular transplantation of 10^7 to 10^{10} allogeneic hepatocytes has also been tested as therapy for human liver failure with modest results.[60] Our discussion of future efforts will focus on those related to improving extracorporeal BAL devices, but these efforts may also have application in the field of hepatocyte transplantation. Efforts to improve BAL therapy continue to improve the microenvironment and architecture of the cells within the device to optimize long-term functionality. The optimal architecture of the hepatocytes will need to prevent cell death and dedifferentiation secondary to the lack of normal cell-to-cell and cell-to-matrix adhesion.

More importantly, the functionality of the cells in the BAL device should resemble that of human hepatocytes as closely as possible. For example, investigators working with the metabolic defect seen in human hereditary tyrosinemia type 1 have shown successful engraftment and rapid expansion of human hepatocytes in the livers of knockout mice with this defect. These mice are deficient of the enzyme fumarylacetoacetate hydrolase (FAH), which provides a selective advantage to normal transplanted human hepatocytes over FAH-deficient mouse hepatocytes in a tyrosine-rich environment.[61] A saline version of this model has been developed.[62] This significant advance can potentially allow for large-scale production of high-quality and readily available human hepatocytes for use in BAL support systems.

Besides using repopulation models, advancements have been made in the field of stem cell research in induced pluripotent stem cells (iPSCs) also has shown promising results in an individualized approach to treating liver disease.[63] iPSCs involve reprogramming normal somatic cells to multipotent stem cells, which can then be differentiated back to cells that closely resemble human hepatocytes in function (hepatocyte-like cells).[64] These new hepatocyte-like cells have the same genetic makeup as the donor, making cellular therapies such as hepatocyte transplantation possible without the need for immunosuppression. These patients could either undergo transplantation using their own hepatocytes or their new hepatocyte-like cells following genetic correction of the inherent deficiency in these cells.

Hepatocyte-like cells can also serve as an autologous cell source for a BAL support system. In 2016 Shi et al. from China developed the first BAL using human fibroblast-derived hepatocyte-like cells (hiHeps).[65] A preclinical trial using a D-galactosamine-induced porcine ALF model showed remarkable survival advantage.[66] Pigs that underwent standard medical treatment ($n = 6$) had 0% 5-day survival, BAL with no cell ($n = 5$) had 17% 5-day survival, and BAL with cells had 83% 5-day survival ($P < .01$). The study also showed attenuated inflammation on liver histology and decreased inflammatory cytokines level.

Currently, no clinically available liver support device has been shown to have definitive survival benefits in ALF. However, continuous improvements have been made to the new-generation liver support devices. Since 2015 a few of these devices have been shown to have survival benefits in preclinical trials using drug-induced porcine ALF models.[66–69]

ACKNOWLEDGMENT

The authors of this chapter acknowledge and greatly appreciate the contribution of previous authors, Drs. James E. Fisher and Joseph B. Lillegard.

REFERENCES

1. Clemmesen JO, Larsen FS, Kondrup J, Hansen BA, Ott P. Cerebral herniation in patients with acute liver failure is correlated with arterial ammonia concentration. *Hepatology*. 1999;29(3): 648-653.
2. Correll PH, Morrison AC, Lutz MA. Receptor tyrosine kinases and the regulation of macrophage activation. *J Leukoc Biol*. 2004;75(5): 731-737.
3. Mackay IR. Hepatoimmunology: a perspective. *Immunol Cell Biol*. 2002;80(1):36-44.
4. Schmidt LE, Larsen FS. Prognostic implications of hyperlactatemia, multiple organ failure, and systemic inflammatory response syndrome in patients with acetaminophen-induced acute liver failure. *Crit Care Med*. 2006;34(2):337-343.
5. Boermeester MA, Houdijk AP, Meyer S, et al. Liver failure induces a systemic inflammatory response. Prevention by recombinant N-terminal bactericidal/permeability-increasing protein. *Am J Pathol*. 1995;147(5):1428-1440.
6. Sekiyama KD, Yoshiba M, Thomson AW. Circulating proinflammatory cytokines (IL-1 beta, TNF-alpha, and IL-6) and IL-1 receptor antagonist (IL-1Ra) in fulminant hepatic failure and acute hepatitis. *Clin Exp Immunol*. 1994;98(1):71-77.
7. Rolando N, Wade J, Davalos M, Wendon J, Philpott-Howard J, Williams R. The systemic inflammatory response syndrome in acute liver failure. *Hepatology*. 2000;32(4 Pt 1):734-739.
8. Lee WM, Squires RH Jr, Nyberg SL, Doo E, Hoofnagle JH. Acute liver failure: summary of a workshop. *Hepatology*. 2008;47(4):1401-1415.
9. Lee WM, Larson AM, Stravitz RT. AASLD position paper: the management of acute liver failure: update 2011. *Hepatology*. 2012;55:965-967.
10. Ostapowicz G, Fontana RJ, Schiodt FV, et al. Results of a prospective study of acute liver failure at 17 tertiary care centers in the United States. *Ann Intern Med*. 2002;137(12):947-954.
11. Mitchell JR, Thorgeirsson SS, Potter WZ, Jollow DJ, Keiser H. Acetaminophen-induced hepatic injury: protective role of glutathione in man and rationale for therapy. *Clin Pharmacol Ther*. 1974;16(4): 676-684.
12. Pumford NR, Hinson JA, Benson RW, Roberts DW. Immunoblot analysis of protein containing 3-(cystein-S-yl)acetaminophen adducts in serum and subcellular liver fractions from acetaminophen-treated mice. *Toxicol Appl Pharmacol*. 1990;104(3):521-532.
13. Makin AJ, Wendon J, Williams R. A 7-year experience of severe acetaminophen-induced hepatotoxicity (1987-1993). *Gastroenterology*. 1995;(6):1907.
13a. Schiodt FV, Rochling FA, Casey DL, Lee WM. Acetaminophen toxicity in an urban county hospital. *N Engl J Med*. 1997;337(16):1112.
14. Speiser J, Lee WM, Karvellas CJ, US Acute Liver Failure Study Group. Predicting outcome on admission and post-admission for acetaminophen-induced acute liver failure using classification and regression tree models. *PLoS One*. 2015;10(4):e0122929.
15. Fontana RJ, Ellerbe C, Durkalski VE, et al. Two-year outcomes in initial survivors with acute liver failure: results from a prospective, multicentre study. *Liver Int*. 2015;35(2):370-380.
16. Sato RL, Wong JJ, Sumida SM, Marn RY, Enoki NR, Yamamoto LG. Efficacy of superactivated charcoal administered late (3 hours) after acetaminophen overdose. *Am J Emerg Med*. 2003;21(3):189-191.
17. Smilkstein MJ, Knapp GL, Kulig KW, Rumack BH. Efficacy of oral N-acetylcysteine in the treatment of acetaminophen overdose. Analysis of the national multicenter study (1976 to 1985). *N Engl J Med*. 1988;319(24):1557-1562.
18. Keays R, Harrison PM, Wendon JA, Forbes A, Gove C, Alexander GJ. A prospective controlled trial of intravenous N-acetylcysteine in paracetamol-induced fulminant hepatic failure. *Br Med J*. 1991;303: 1026-1029.
19. Reuben A, Koch DG, Lee WM, Acute Liver Failure Study Group. Drug-induced acute liver failure: results of a U.S. multicenter, prospective study. *Hepatology*. 2010;52:2065-2076.
20. Jochum C, Gieseler RK, Gawlista I, et al. Hepatitis B-associated acute liver failure: immediate treatment with entecavir inhibits hepatitis B virus replication and potentially its sequelae. *Digestion*. 2009;80(4): 235-240.
21. Lee WM, Hynan LS, Rossaro L, et al. Intravenous N-acetylcysteine improves transplant-free survival in early stage non-acetaminophen acute liver failure. *Gastroenterology*. 2009;137:856-864, 864.e1.
22. Jarnagin WR, Gonen M, Fong Y, et al. Improvement in perioperative outcome after hepatic resection: analysis of 1,803 consecutive cases over the past decade. *Ann Surg*. 2002;236(4):397-406, discussion 406-407.
23. Lisi Y, Abdalla EK, Chun YS, et al. Three hundred and one consecutive extended right hepatectomies: evaluation of outcome based on systematic liver volumetry. *Ann Surg*. 2009;250(4):540-548.
24. Polson J, Lee WM. AASLD position paper: the management of acute liver failure. *Hepatology*. 2005;41(5):1179-1197.
25. Wijdicks EF, Bamlet WR, Maramattom BV, Manno EM, McClelland RL. Validation of a new coma scale: the FOUR score. *Ann Neurol*. 2005;58(4):585-593.
26. Merli M, Riggio O. Dietary and nutritional indications in hepatic encephalopathy. *Metab Brain Dis*. 2009;24(1):211-221.
27. Wijdicks EF, Nyberg S. Propofol to control intracranial pressure in fulminant hepatic failure. *Transplant Proc*. 2002;73:1965-1968.
28. Lidofsky SD, Bass NM, Prager MC, et al. Intracranial pressure monitoring and liver transplantation for fulminant hepatic failure. *Hepatology*. 1992;16(1):1-7.
29. Davis M, Plevak DJ, Wijdicks EF, et al. Acute liver failure: results of a clinical protocol. *Liver Transpl Surg*. 1995;1(4):210-219.

30. Karvellas CJ, Fix OK, Battenhouse H, et al. Outcomes and complications of intracranial pressure monitoring in acute liver failure: a retrospective cohort study. *Crit Care Med.* 2014;42(5):1157-1167.

31. Murphy N, Auzinger G, Bernel W, Wendon J. The effect of hypertonic sodium chloride on intracranial pressure in patients with acute liver failure. *Hepatology.* 2004;39(2):464-470.

32. Jalan R, Olde Damink SW, Deutz NE, Hayes PC, Lee A. Moderate hypothermia in patients with acute liver failure and uncontrolled intracranial hypertension. *Gastroenterology.* 2004;27(5):1338-1346.

33. Vaquero J, Polson J, Chung C, et al. Infection and the progression of hepatic encephalopathy in acute liver failure. *Gastroenterology.* 2003;125(3):755-764.

34. Davenport A, Will EJ, Davidson AM. Improved cardiovascular stability during continuous modes of renal replacement therapy in critically ill patients with acute hepatic and renal failure. *Crit Care Med.* 1993;21(3):328-338.

35. Bailey B, Amre DK, Gaudreault P. Fulminant hepatic failure secondary to acetaminophen poisoning: a systematic review and meta-analysis of prognostic criteria determining the need for liver transplantation. *Crit Care Med.* 2003;31(1):299-305.

36. Shakil AO, Kramer D, Mazariegos GV, Fung JJ, Rakela J. Acute liver failure: clinical features, outcome analysis, and applicability of prognostic criteria. *Liver Transpl.* 2000;6(2):163-169.

37. Nedredal GI, Amiot BP, Nyberg P, et al. Optimization of mass transfer for toxin removal and immunoprotection of hepatocytes in a bioartificial liver. *Biotechnol Bioeng.* 2009;104(5):995-1003.

38. Kiley JE, Pender JC, Welch HF, Welch CS. Ammonia intoxication treated by hemodialysis. *N Engl J Med.* 1958;259(24):1156-1161

39. Merrill JP, Smith S 3rd, Callahan EJ 3rd, Thorn GW. The use of an artificial kidney. II. Clinical experience. *J Clin Invest.* 1950;29(4):425-438.

40. O'Grady JG, Gimson AE, O'Brien CJ, Pucknell A, Hughes RD, Williams R. Controlled trials of charcoal hemoperfusion and prognostic factors in fulminant hepatic failure. *Gastroenterology.* 1988;94(5 Pt 1):1186-1192.

41. Inoue K, Kourin A, Watanabe T, Yamada M, Yoshiba M. Artificial liver support system using large buffer volumes removes significant glutamine and is an ideal bridge to liver transplantation. *Transplant Proc.* 2009;41(1):259-261.

42. Stange J, Mitzner SR, Risler T, et al. Molecular adsorbent recycling system (MARS): clinical results of a new membrane-based blood purification system for bioartificial liver support. *Artif Organs.* 1999;23(4):319-330.

43. Hassanein TI, Tofteng F, Brown RS Jr, et al. Randomized controlled study of extracorporeal albumin dialysis for hepatic encephalopathy in advanced cirrhosis. *Hepatology.* 2007;46(6):1853-1862.

44. Heemann U, Treichel U, Loock J, et al. Albumin dialysis in cirrhosis with superimposed acute liver injury: a prospective, controlled study. *Hepatology.* 2002;36(4 Pt 1):949-958.

45. Sen S, Davies NA, Mookerjee RP, et al. Pathophysiological effects of albumin dialysis in acute-on-chronic liver failure: a randomized controlled study. *Liver Transpl.* 2004;10(9):1109-1119.

46. Saliba F, Camus C, Durand F, et al. Albumin dialysis with a non-cell artificial liver support device in patients with acute liver failure: a randomized, controlled trial. *Ann Intern Med.* 2013;159(8):522-531.

47. Banares R, Nevens F, Larsen FS, et al. Extracorporeal albumin dialysis with the molecular adsorbent recirculating system in acute-on-chronic liver failure: the RELIEF trial. *Hepatology.* 2013;57(3):1153-1162.

48. Rifai K, Ernst T, Kretschmer U, et al. Prometheus—a new extracorporeal system for the treatment of liver failure. *J Hepatol.* 2003;39(6):984-990.

49. Kribben A, Gerken G, Haag S, et al. Effects of fractionated plasma separation and adsorption on survival in patients with acute-on-chronic liver failure. *Gastroenterology.* 2012;142(4):782.e3-789.e3.

50. Kelly JH, Sussman NL. The hepatix extracorporeal liver assist device in the treatment of fulminant hepatic failure. *ASAIO J.* 1994;40(1):83-85.

51. Ellis AJ, Hughes RD, Wendon JA, et al. Pilot-controlled trial of the extracorporeal liver assist device in acute liver failure. *Hepatology.* 1996;24(6):1446-1451.

52. Reich DJ. *The Effect of Extracorporeal C3A Cellular Therapy in Severe Alcoholic Hepatitis—The VTI-208 ELAD Trial.* San Francisco, CA: AASLD; 2015.

53. Demetriou AA, Brown RS Jr, Busuttil RW, et al. Prospective, randomized, multicenter, controlled trial of a bioartificial liver in treating acute liver failure. *Ann Surg.* 2004;239(5):660-667, [discussion 667-670].

54. Nyberg SL, Remmel RP, Mann HJ, Peshwa MV, Hu WS, Cerra FB. Primary hepatocytes outperform Hep G2 cells as the source of biotransformation functions in a bioartificial liver. *Ann Surg.* 1994;220(1):59-67.

55. Frisch SM, Francis H. Disruption of epithelial cell-matrix interactions induces apoptosis. *J Cell Biol.* 1994;124(4):619-626.

56. Grossmann J. Molecular mechanisms of detachment-induced apoptosis—anoikis. *Apoptosis.* 2002;7(3):247-260.

57. Zvibel I, Smets F, Soriano H. Anoikis: roadblock to cell transplantation? *Cell Transplant.* 2002;11(7):621-630.

58. Ambrosino G, Basso SM, Varotto S, Zardi E, Picardi A, D'Amico DF. Isolated hepatocytes versus hepatocyte spheroids: in vitro culture of rat hepatocytes. *Cell Transplant.* 2005;14(6):397-401.

59. Sakai Y, Yamagami S, Nakazawa K. Comparative analysis of gene expression in rat liver tissue and monolayer- and spheroid-cultured hepatocytes. *Cells Tissues Organs (Print).* 2010;191(4):281-288.

60. Fox IJ, Roy-Chowdhury J. Hepatocyte transplantation. *J Hepatol.* 2004;40(6):878-886.

61. Azuma H, Paulk N, Ranade A, et al. Robust expansion of human hepatocytes in Fah$^{-/-}$/Rag2$^{-/-}$/Il2rg$^{-/-}$ mice. *Nat Biotechnol.* 2007;25(8):903-910.

62. Hickey RD, Elgilani F, Mao SA, et al. Autologous hepatocyte transplantation after ex vivo gene therapy in a large animal model of metabolic liver disease. *Hepatology.* 2015;62:Abstract 2.

63. Yu J, Hu K, Smuga-Otto K, et al. Human induced pluripotent stem cells free of vector and transgene sequences. *Science.* 2009;324(5928):797-801.

64. Si-Tayeb K, Noto FK, Nagaoka M, et al. Highly efficient generation of human hepatocyte-like cells from induced pluripotent stem cells. *Hepatology.* 2010;51(1):297-305.

65. Huang P, Zhang L, Gao Y, et al. Direct reprogramming of human fibroblasts to functional and expandable hepatocytes. *Cell Stem Cell.* 2014;14(3):370-384.

66. Shi XL, Gao Y, Yan Y, et al. Improved survival of porcine acute liver failure by a bioartificial liver device implanted with induced human functional hepatocytes. *Cell Res.* 2016;26(2):206-216.

67. Glorioso J, Mao S, Rodysill B, et al. Pivotal preclinical trial of the spheroid reservoir bioartificial liver. *J Hepatol.* 2015;63(2):388-398.

68. Lee EC, Baker LA, Stanzani G, et al. Extracorporeal liver assist device to exchange albumin and remove endotoxin in acute liver failure: results of a pivotal pre-clinical study. *J Hepatol.* 2015;63(3):634-642.

69. Zhou N, Li J, Zhang Y, et al. Efficacy of coupled low-volume plasma exchange with plasma filtration adsorption in treating pigs with acute liver failure: a randomised study. *J Hepatol.* 2015;63(2):378-387.

Vascular Diseases of the Liver

David M. Levi | Andreas G. Tzakis

The topic *vascular diseases of the liver* encompasses an array of disparate clinicopathologic entities, with the common thread that they specifically affect the hepatic vasculature. They can be arbitrarily classified into those that involve the hepatic artery and its branches, those that involve the portal vein, and those that involve the hepatic veins. The topics *portal hypertension* and *portal vein thrombosis* are addressed separately in Chapter 135.

HEPATIC ARTERY DISORDERS

ANEURYSMS OF THE HEPATIC ARTERY

Hepatic artery aneurysms are rare, comprising approximately 20% of all visceral aneurysms. True aneurysms may be a manifestation of systemic diseases, including atherosclerosis or vasculitides such as polyarteritis nodosa[1] and systemic lupus erythematosus.[2] Pseudoaneurysms of the hepatic artery can result from hepatic trauma,[3] iatrogenic, surgical injury to the artery,[4] or rarely as a sequela of acute pancreatitis.[5] Mycotic pseudoaneurysms resulting from bacterial endocarditis[6] or following liver transplantation[7] have also been reported.

Most commonly, hepatic artery aneurysms are solitary, involve the extrahepatic portion of the artery, and are 3 to 4 cm in diameter at the time of presentation.[8,9] The clinical presentation varies considerably. Some are discovered incidentally by noninvasive imaging studies (Fig. 129.1). Patients with mycotic pseudoaneurysms may present with pain, fever, or other signs of infection. Hemobilia following laparoscopic cholecystectomy,[4] liver biopsy, or interventional radiologic procedures can result from rupture of a pseudoaneurysm into the biliary tree. Intraperitoneal or gastrointestinal hemorrhage–related rupture is associated with a high mortality rate.[10]

The diagnosis may be suspected based on the presentation but is confirmed by Doppler ultrasonography, intravenous contrast–enhanced computed tomography (CT), or magnetic resonance (MR) imaging. Angiography can be diagnostic, and with the aid of endovascular techniques, can be therapeutic as well.[11]

The treatment of hepatic artery aneurysms is dictated by their cause, size, location, and patient condition. Although the natural history of these aneurysms is unclear, it seems that size correlates with the risk of rupture. In addition, the ubiquitous use of high-quality imaging techniques has led to an increased detection of small, asymptomatic aneurysms. The concern of eventual complications, especially hemorrhage, warrants the consideration of treating all of these lesions, even those that are asymptomatic or are discovered incidentally.[12] Underlying conditions must be recognized and addressed, and adequate resuscitation is required for patients presenting with intraperitoneal or gastrointestinal hemorrhage.

Aneurysms of the extrahepatic portion of the artery are classically managed surgically. Despite advancements in endovascular technology, open repair remains the mainstay of treatment.[13] Those affecting the common hepatic artery may be ligated proximally and distally if adequate collateral circulation to the liver is afforded by the gastroduodenal artery via the pancreaticoduodenal arcade. Those originating distal to the gastroduodenal artery affecting the proper hepatic artery, can be treated by aneurysmectomy and revascularization of the liver.

A pseudoaneurysm of the hepatic artery following liver transplantation at the site of the arterial anastomosis is a serious complication. The usual treatment is resection of the pseudoaneurysm and revascularization of the liver.[14] In an emergency, ligation of the artery proximally and distally may be the only option but is associated with a high likelihood of graft loss.[5] Urgent retransplantation may be necessary.

Intrahepatic aneurysms can be managed by percutaneous transarterial catheter embolization (Fig. 129.2). This approach is especially useful if the lesions are multiple, as seen in cases of polyarteritis nodosa.[1] The risk of significant hepatic ischemia is minimized if there is adequate portal venous blood flow and the affected artery branch or branches are distal within the liver. Solitary, posttraumatic intrahepatic pseudoaneurysms, confined to a hepatic segment or lobe, may be treated by hepatic resection if an endovascular approach is not possible.[15]

HEPATIC ARTERY INJURY

Traumatic injury of the hepatic artery is uncommon. Penetrating injuries to the portal triad outnumber blunt injuries, and associated injuries are the rule.[17] The diagnosis is usually made at the time of laparotomy or postmortem. Portal triad injuries carry a high mortality rate because of exsanguinating hemorrhage or refractory shock. Successful treatment requires control of bleeding, aggressive resuscitation, and temporization of other injuries. Often concomitant biliary tract and/or portal vein injury must be addressed.[17] Treatment options for the injured artery include ligation or primary repair. Better survival has been reported with hepatic artery ligation as compared with repair.[18] The late sequelae of portal triad injuries, including hepatic ischemia, biliary strictures, portal hypertension, and liver failure, may mandate liver transplantation.[19]

Iatrogenic injury of the hepatic artery is an uncommon but potentially devastating complication of laparoscopic cholecystectomy. Approximately one-fifth of cholecystectomy-related bile duct injuries have an associated hepatic artery injury, usually the right hepatic

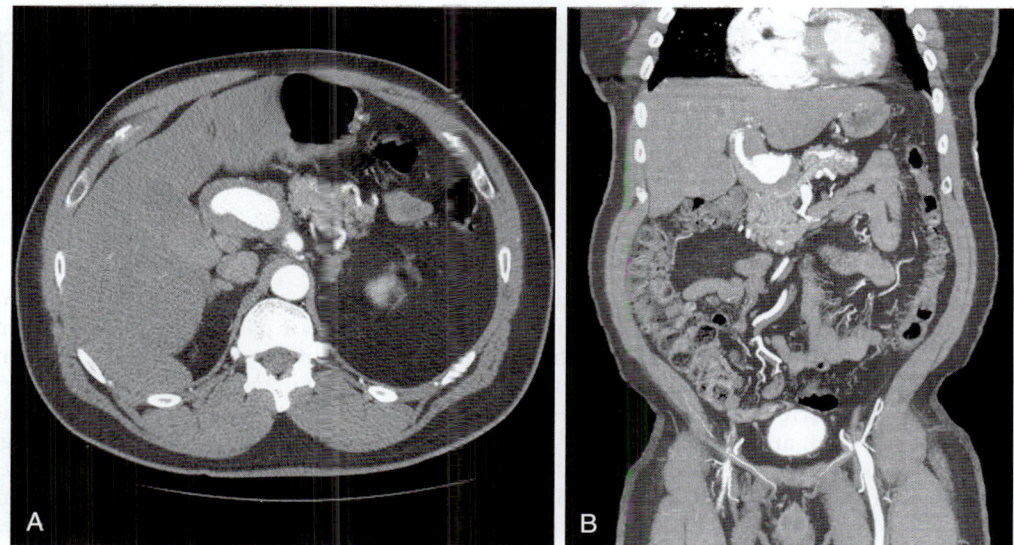

FIGURE 129.1 (A and B) Computed tomography demonstration (axial and coronal image) of a large, solitary hepatic artery aneurysm.

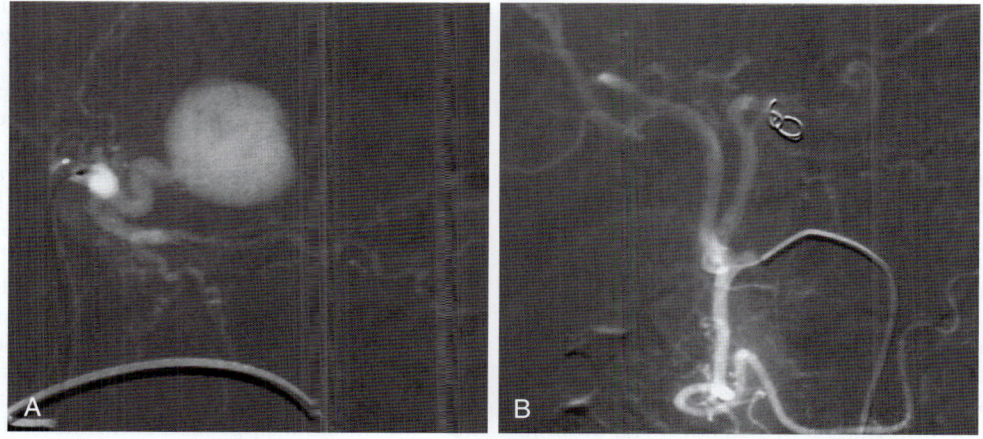

FIGURE 129.2 (A and B) Transarterial catheter embolization of a traumatic pseudoaneurysm of the left hepatic artery. (Courtesy Victor Javier Casillas, MD.)

artery. The addition of an injury to the artery was thought to portend a higher complication rate after biliary reconstruction and a greater risk of mortality.[20] A more recent literature review does not confirm the association between a concomitant arterial injury and failure of biliary repair.[21] The injury is often not recognized at the time of surgery, even if the biliary injury is identified and corrected immediately. In the patient presenting with bile duct strictures after cholecystectomy, the presence of a concomitant arterial injury should be suspected based on the severity of the bile duct injury and the discovery of a report of difficulty gaining hemostasis during the cholecystectomy. The treatment of these injuries is usually directed toward repairing the bile duct endoscopically by primary repair or by Roux-en-Y hepaticojejunostomy. Arterial reconstruction, except when the injury is noted immediately, is seldom indicated or performed. Rarely, an injury to the right hepatic artery results in acute necrosis of the right hepatic lobe or intrahepatic strictures amenable to hepatic resection.[22]

HEPATIC ARTERY THROMBOSIS

Hepatic artery thrombosis is the most dreaded vascular complication following liver transplantation. With an incidence of 2% to 8% of cases, it has a high associated morbidity and mortality. Pediatric recipients[23] and cases requiring aortohepatic conduits[24] are at increased risk for the development of this complication. Advanced donor age increases the risk of liver graft loss from hepatic artery thrombosis.[25] When it occurs early, within the few weeks following transplantation, it usually results in acute graft necrosis necessitating urgent retransplantation (Fig. 129.3).[26] Protocol surveillance of the hepatic artery using Doppler ultrasound may detect early or impending thrombosis allowing for immediate revascularization and potential graft salvage.[27]

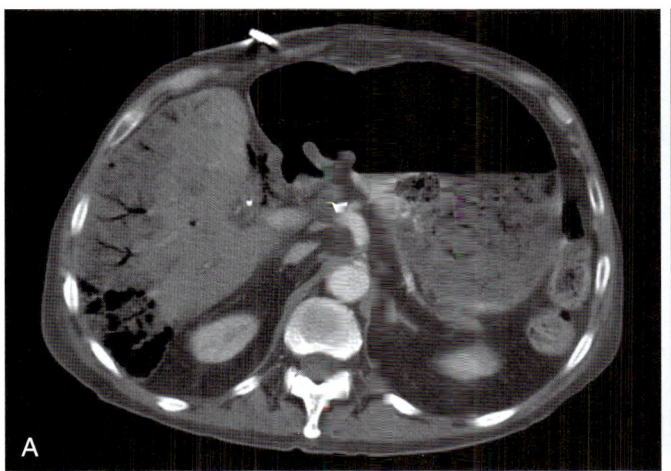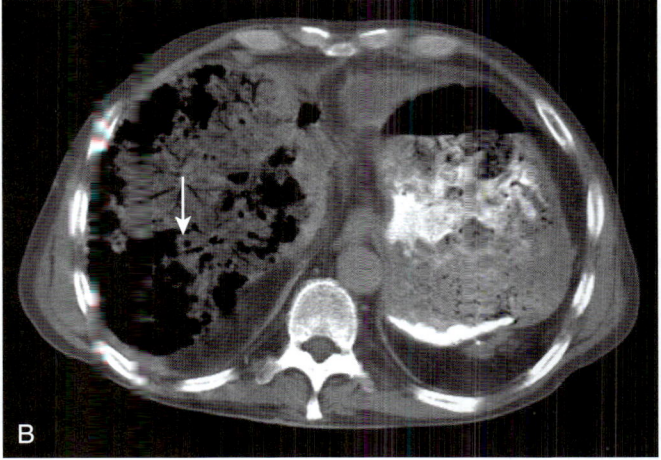

FIGURE 129.3 Computed tomography scan images of hepatic artery thrombosis after liver transplantation. A) The *arrow* marks the thrombus in the hepatic artery. (B) The *arrow* denotes the gangrenous liver allograft. (Courtesy Victor Javier Casillas, MD.)

Late hepatic artery thrombosis is less well understood than early thrombosis and has a wider spectrum of presentation. Some patients are asymptomatic, and the diagnosis is discovered incidentally. For others, the sequelae are biliary tract complications including stricture formation, bile leak, cholangitis, hemobilia, and hepatic biloma/abscess. Cholangitis can be managed by percutaneous or endoscopic catheter decompression of the biliary tree. Infected bilomas are treated by percutaneous drainage and antibiotics. Attempts at biliary reconstruction or hepatic artery revascularization are rarely successful. Although some asymptomatic patients spontaneously develop arterial collaterals and can be treated conservatively, most survivors with late hepatic artery thrombosis will ultimately require retransplantation.[26]

Some cases of late hepatic artery thrombosis follow a period of artery stenosis. When detected, it may be addressed with endovascular techniques, including percutaneous transluminal angioplasty or primary stent placement, avoiding the dire complications of thrombosis.[28]

HEPATIC ARTERIOPORTAL AND ARTERIOVENOUS SHUNTS

Aberrant communication between the hepatic artery and either portal or hepatic venous branches is seen in a variety of diseases and is of variable clinical significance. These shunts can result from iatrogenic injury,[29] penetrating or blunt liver trauma,[30] benign and malignant hepatic neoplasms, or may develop congenitally,[31] such as in patients with hereditary hemorrhagic telangiectasia (Rendu-Osler-Weber disease). Iatrogenic causes include core liver biopsy,[32] hepatic resection, and radiofrequency tumor ablation.[33] Hepatocellular carcinoma can produce a vascular fistula by eroding into a vein branch,[34] and tumors, such as cavernous hemangioma, focal nodular hyperplasia, and infantile hepatic hemangioendothelioma, can develop abnormal shunts. Hereditary hemorrhagic telangiectasia is an autosomal dominant disorder characterized by microscopic and macroscopic arteriovenous

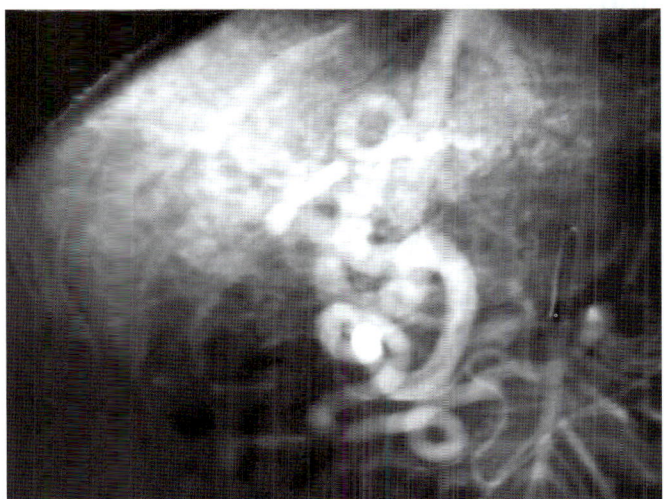

FIGURE 129.4 This angiogram of a patient with hereditary hemorrhagic telangiectasia with liver involvement depicts an enlarged, tortuous hepatic artery with shunting to the hepatic veins. (Courtesy Victor Javier Casillas, MD.)

malformations with rare but well-described liver involvement (Fig. 129.4).[35]

The pathophysiologic and clinical impact of these shunts depends on their type and hemodynamic magnitude. A large shunt from the high-pressure hepatic artery to the low-pressure portal vein can lead to the development of portal hypertension and its consequences, particularly variceal hemorrhage.[31,32] In addition, the increase in portal venous blood flow can cause fibrous tissue proliferation and nodular regeneration within the liver. A large shunt from the hepatic artery to the hepatic venous system can have two main effects. First, this shunt siphons oxygenated blood away from the hepatic parenchyma and biliary tree. Hepatic necrosis and/or ischemic biliary injury can result. Second, the shunt can provoke a hyperdynamic response eventually leading to high-output cardiac failure. This is typically seen in infantile hepatic hemangioendothelioma.[36]

The treatment of intrahepatic arterioportal and arteriovenous shunts is dependent on the size, location, and cause of the shunt. Small, focal, hemodynamically insignificant shunts may be found incidentally on radiologic imaging studies and may not require specific treatment. Shunts that are confined to one lobe or segment of the liver, such as those related to a hepatic tumor, may be amenable to resection. Those shunts resulting from trauma or iatrogenic injury affecting the extrahepatic artery and portal vein may be treated by surgical interruption of the fistula and primary repair of the vessels. As interventional radiologic techniques have improved, more shunts have been treated by percutaneous transarterial catheter embolization.[30,37] Finally, selected patients presenting with multifocal or diffuse intrahepatic arteriovenous shunts, as seen in infantile hemangioendothelioma and hereditary hemorrhagic telangiectasia, may be candidates for liver transplantation.[38,39]

PORTAL VEIN DISORDERS

PORTAL VEIN ANEURYSM

Aneurysmal dilation of the portal vein is an exceedingly rare entity. First described in 1956, there have since been fewer than 200 reported cases.[40] Venous aneurysms are possibly congenital in nature or may develop as a result of trauma to the portal vein. They sometimes develop in the presence of portal hypertension. Some present with epigastric abdominal pain or cause symptoms by compressing adjacent structures, typically the common bile duct, duodenum, or inferior vena cava (IVC).[41] Those patients with portal hypertension may present with variceal hemorrhage. Many are discovered incidentally (Fig. 129.5). Rupture is rare but has been reported, and even spontaneous resolution has been documented. Although their etiology and natural history are not clear, it is reasonable

to suspect that the incidence of compressive symptoms and risk of complications correlate with the size of the aneurysm. There is no consensus regarding the treatment of these lesions but asymptomatic, small (<3 cm) aneurysms of the portal vein can be observed.[42] Larger-diameter, symptomatic aneurysms have been addressed with an array of surgical procedures. The options may be stratified by whether or not the patient has portal hypertension. For those patients without portal hypertension, aneurysmorrhaphy and aneurysmectomy have been performed. For those with concomitant portal hypertension, a variety of shunt procedures with or without splenectomy and even liver transplantation has been reported.[40]

HEPATIC VEIN DISORDERS

BUDD-CHIARI SYNDROME

Budd-Chiari syndrome can result from an array of disorders and has a variable clinical presentation. The common denominator in the pathogenesis of this syndrome is hepatic venous outflow obstruction characterized by the classic clinical triad of abdominal pain, hepatomegaly, and ascites. In most cases the cause is an identifiable, inherited or acquired, hypercoagulable state. Many patients are affected by a myeloproliferative disorder.[43] Other etiologies include tumor invasion of the hepatic outflow tract typically by liver,[44] adrenal,[45] or renal malignancies,[46] iatrogenic outflow obstruction following liver surgery or transplantation, vascular webs, and trauma.

Hepatic vein occlusion results in increased sinusoidal pressure and decreased sinusoidal blood flow. Hepatic congestion can cause liver enlargement and abdominal pain. Diminished sinusoidal blood flow is thought to be important in the pathogenic progression of fibrosis and regenerative nodule formation leading to cirrhosis. Portal hypertension contributes to ascites formation and the development of varices. Concomitant portal vein thrombosis is commonly present in the most severe cases.[43]

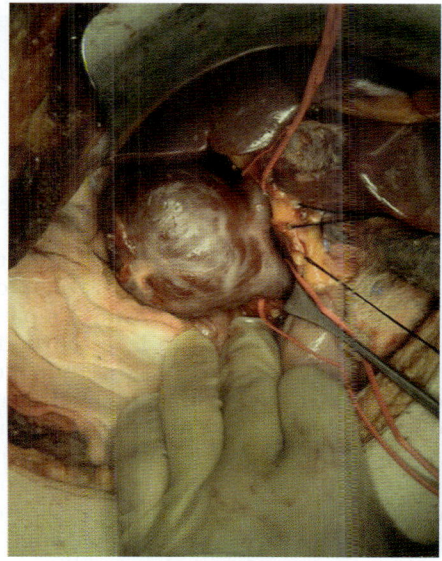
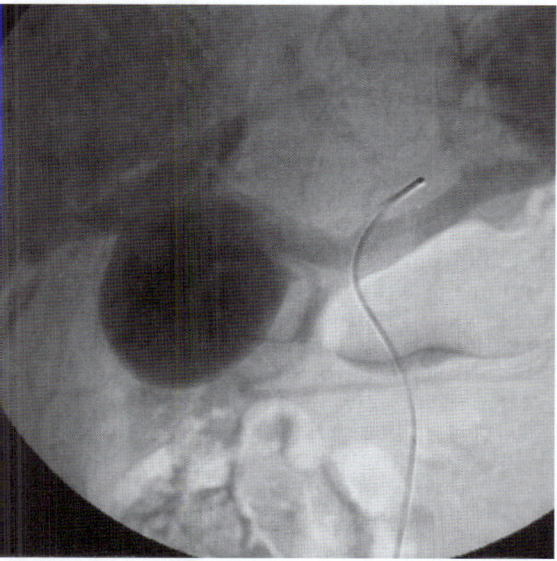

FIGURE 129.5 Images of a symptomatic saccular aneurysm of the portal vein. (Courtesy Victor Javier Casillas, MD.)

Because the venous outflow for the caudate lobe is separate from the major hepatic veins, compensatory hypertrophy of this hepatic segment is common. The enlarged caudate lobe can extrinsically compress the adjacent IVC, producing a pressure gradient across it.

The clinical presentation of patients with Budd-Chiari syndrome varies depending on the extent and acuity of the obstruction to the hepatic venous outflow. Sudden-onset, complete hepatic vein thrombosis may on occasion present as fulminant liver failure. If the onset is gradual and/or the degree of obstruction is incomplete, there is the opportunity for the development of venous collaterals. The degree to which these collaterals decompress the portal venous system impacts the clinical manifestations of the syndrome and determines the preferred treatment. Some patients develop liver enlargement and intractable ascites with relatively preserved hepatic function, whereas others develop cirrhosis with hepatic decompensation.[43]

The diagnosis of Budd-Chiari syndrome should be considered in any patient with hepatomegaly and ascites. Laboratory investigation of liver function may reveal abnormalities, but these tests are nonspecific. Ascitic fluid analysis may reveal a high serum-ascites albumin gradient and an elevated protein level (>3 g/dL).[43] Doppler ultrasonography is excellent for visualizing the hepatic vasculature, revealing the level and extent of the obstruction of the hepatic outflow.[47] It is also useful for evaluating the retrohepatic vena cava and the portal vein. CT and MR imaging may reveal obliterated hepatic veins, heterogeneously perfused hepatic parenchyma and areas of necrosis, hepatomegaly, caudate lobe hypertrophy, narrowing of the retrohepatic vena cava, and ascites (Fig. 129.6). When the underlying cause is tumor invasion of the hepatic veins, these imaging studies are important for determining the local extent of the disease. Hepatic venography is often not needed for establishing a diagnosis but may be useful for direct measurement of a pressure gradient across a narrowed IVC or stenotic hepatic outflow tract. Interventional radiologic techniques including transluminal angioplasty, vein stenting, and transjugular intrahepatic portosystemic shunt (TIPS) placement may be used therapeutically at the time of hepatic venography.[48]

The treatment of Budd-Chiari syndrome must be individualized to the patient and is enhanced by a multidisciplinary team approach.[49] The principles of treatment include addressing the underlying cause, decreasing hepatic sinusoidal pressure and congestion, and preserving liver function. After the diagnosis is established, a liver biopsy may be needed to determine the extent of hepatic fibrosis and cirrhosis. Because the hepatic parenchyma may not be uniformly affected, bilobar biopsies may be useful to avoid sampling error. Liver biopsy is unnecessary in cases in which it is clear that the liver cannot be salvaged, such as some cases with fulminant liver failure or decompensated cirrhosis.

A variety of medical therapies, interventional radiologic techniques, and surgical procedures are available for the patient with Budd-Chiari syndrome. The best therapy or combination of therapies depends on the patient's individual anatomic and physiologic condition as much as the expertise and bias of the team caring for the patient. Medical therapies include anticoagulation, thrombolysis, and pharmacologic treatment of ascites and portal hypertension. Interventional radiologic techniques that have been developed include percutaneous transluminal angioplasty with or without stent placement and TIPS. Surgical procedures include a variety of portosystemic shunts and liver transplantation.

Percutaneous thrombolysis/thrombectomy alone has been attempted for acute hepatic vein thrombosis anecdotally but with limited success.[50] Its best place in therapy may be as a prelude to a more definitive procedure, such as a TIPS or a surgical shunt. Vein angioplasty with or without stent placement also has been tried in selected cases. It is indicated for short-segment stenoses of a hepatic vein or veins, hepatic venous outflow tract stenosis following liver transplantation,[51] or IVC webs. Angioplasty with stenting of the retrohepatic IVC has been performed in conjunction with surgical portosystemic shunting when a pressure gradient exists across this segment of the IVC from caudate lobe compression.[52]

Physiologically a TIPS is a central portosystemic shunt. It is indicated in the patient with Budd-Chiari syndrome and chronic, well-compensated liver disease to relieve portal hypertension and treat intractable ascites. Some patients who have presented with acute liver failure have been treated with TIPS with excellent long-term survival. For patients with fulminant liver failure or decompensated cirrhosis, the procedure has a high incidence of complications. Disadvantages of the TIPS procedure are that its placement may be technically difficult, especially if the ostia of the hepatic veins are occluded, and it often needs revision over time. The introduction of covered stents may yield better results.[53]

Although interventional radiology techniques have evolved and improved, surgical intervention remains the standard for the definitive treatment of Budd-Chiari syndrome. However, there is no consensus as to the best procedure for the disease. The decision between TIPS or

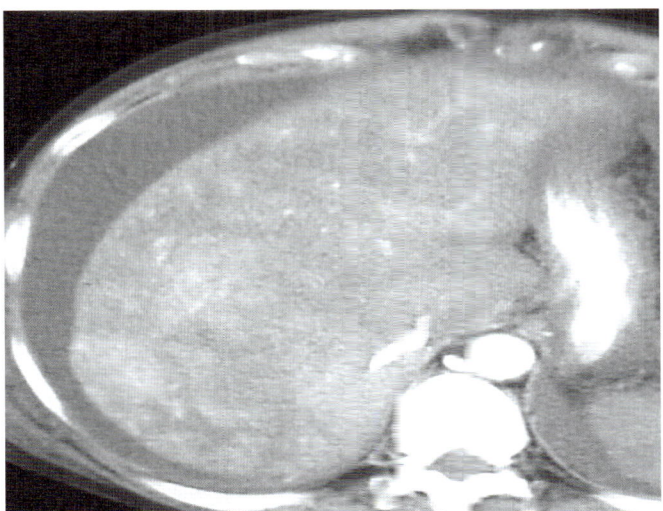

FIGURE 129.6 Computed tomography image of a patient with Budd-Chiari syndrome characterized by heterogeneously appearing hepatic parenchyma, caudate lobe enlargement, ascites, and no visualization of the hepatic veins. (Courtesy Victor Javier Casillas, MD.)

a surgical shunt and which shunt depends largely on the experience of the treatment team. For those patients with chronic, symptomatic Budd-Chiari syndrome, a variety of surgical shunts are available to decompress the portal venous system and preserve liver function. Survival following these procedures is determined primarily by the rate of progression of the liver disease and the long-term patency of the shunt.

If the IVC is widely patent, either a mesocaval shunt, a central splenorenal shunt, or a side-to-side portacaval shunt are the available options. Mesocaval and splenorenal shunts are used most commonly. Mesocaval shunts require an interposition graft of synthetic material or autologous vein between the superior mesenteric vein and the infrahepatic IVC. If the graft thromboses, the superior mesenteric vein will probably not be available should liver transplant eventually become warranted. A direct, side-to-side splenorenal shunt preserves the hepatic hilum and does not require a vein graft. Although side-to-side portacaval shunts have a reported high-patency rate,[54] hypertrophy of the caudate lobe can make direct shunting impossible. In addition, dissection of the hepatic hilum can make subsequent liver transplantation difficult. Finally, portal vein thrombosis is an obvious contraindication for the procedure.

The long-term patency of these surgical shunts depends on the presence of a pressure gradient between a high-pressure portal venous system and a low-pressure infrahepatic IVC. If the retrohepatic vena cava is stenotic or thrombosed, this pressure gradient may be insufficient. In this situation, the retrohepatic vena cava may be stented prior to the surgical shunt.[52] The mesoatrial shunt is a rarely performed option that, in one series, has been replaced completely by combined portacaval shunt and cavoatrial shunt.[54]

Most would agree that liver transplantation is the procedure of choice for the patient with fulminant liver failure or decompensated cirrhosis related to the Budd-Chiari syndrome.[55] The shortage of available organs for transplant and the need for immunosuppression after transplant are the main reasons for reserving this option for those patients with liver failure. Depending on the underlying cause, liver replacement may correct the hypercoagulable state providing a phenotypic cure. For the remaining patients, long-term anticoagulation is essential after transplantation to avoid recurrence of the syndrome. Regardless of the treatment—TIPS, surgical shunt, or liver transplantation—the eventual outcome depends largely on the ability to control the underlying disorder.

ACKNOWLEDGMENT

The authors are grateful to Victor Javier Casillas, MD, for providing us with the radiologic images for this chapter.

REFERENCES

1. Battula N, Tsapralis D, Morgan M, Mirza D. Spontaneous liver haemorrhage and haemobilia as initial presentation of undiagnosed polyarteritis nodosa. *Ann R Coll Surg Engl.* 2012;94(4):e163-e165.
2. Liu C, Tang QB, Zeng H, Yu XH, Xu LB, Li Y. Clinical and pathological analysis of hepatic artery aneurysm in a patient with systemic lupus erythematosus. *Surg Today.* 2011;41(11):1571-1574.
3. Bardes JM, Caranasos TG, Vaughan RA. Hepatic artery pseudoaneurysm: delayed presentation after bicycle accident. *J Trauma.* 2011; 71(3):783.
4. Yao CA, Arnell TD. Hepatic artery pseudoaneurysm following laparoscopic cholecystectomy. *Am J Surg.* 2010;199(1):e10-e11.
5. Yu YH, Sohn JH, Kim TY, et al. Hepatic artery pseudoaneurysm caused by acute idiopathic pancreatitis. *World J Gastroenterol.* 2012; 18(18):2291-2294.
6. Chaudhari D, Saleem A, Patel P, Khan S, Young M, LeSage G. Hepatic artery mycotic aneurysm associated with staphylococcal endocarditis with successful treatment: case report with review of the literature. *Case Reports Hepatol.* 2013;2013:610818.
7. Jones VS, Chennapragada MS, Lord DJ, Stormon M, Shun A. Post-liver transplant mycotic aneurysm of the hepatic artery. *J Pediatr Surg.* 2008;43(3):555-558.
8. Abbas MA, Fowl RJ, Stone WM, et al. Hepatic artery aneurysm: factors that predict complications. *J Vasc Surg.* 2003;38(1):41-45.
9. Lu M, Weiss C, Fishman EK, Johnson PT, Verde F. Review of visceral aneurysms and pseudoaneurysms. *J Comput Assist Tomogr.* 2015; 39(1):1-6.
10. Sebastian JJ, Pena E, Blas JM, Cena G. Fatal upper gastrointestinal bleeding due to hepatic artery pseudoaneurysm diagnosed by endoscopy. *Dig Dis Sci.* 2008;53(4):1152-1153.
11. Kamath V, Gunabushanam V, Hanna A, Siegel D, Sung C, Dolgin SE. Life-threatening postoperative hemorrhage from hepatic artery pseudoaneurysm successfully treated by transcatheter embolization in a 5-year old child. *J Pediatr Surg.* 2012;47(3):585-587.
12. Pulli R, Dorigo W, Troisi N, Pratesi G, Innocenti AA, Pratesi C. Surgical treatment of visceral artery aneurysms: a 25-year experience. *J Vasc Surg.* 2008;48(2):334-342.
13. Erben Y, De Martino RR, Bjarnason H, et al. Operative management of hepatic artery aneurysms. *J Vasc Surg.* 2015;62(3):610-615.
14. Reznichenko AA, Bondoc A, Paterno F, Shah SA. Hepatic artery pseudoaneurysm after liver transplantation. *J Gastrointest Surg.* 2016;20(7):1405-1406.
15. Volpin E, Pessaux P, Sauvanet A, et al. Preservation of the arterial vascularization of the hepatic artery pseudoaneurysm following orthotopic liver transplantation: long-term results. *Ann Transplant.* 2014;19:346-352.
16. Komatsu S, Iwasaki T, Nishioka N, Toyokawa A, Teramura K. Hemobilia associated with a giant thrombosed aneurysm of the hepatic artery requiring hepatectomy. *Ann Vasc Surg.* 2014;28(8):1934.e13-1934. e17.
17. Pearl J, Chao A, Kennedy S, Paul B, Rhee P. Traumatic injuries to the portal vein: case study. *J Trauma.* 2004;56(4):779-782.
18. Croce MA, Fabian TC, Spiers JP, Kudsk KA. Traumatic hepatic artery pseudoaneurysm with hemobilia. *Am J Surg.* 1994;168(3):235-238.
19. Delis SG, Bakoyiannis A, Selvaggi G, Weppler D, Levi D, Tzakis AG. Liver transplantation for severe hepatic trauma: experience from a single center. *World J Gastroenterol.* 2009;15(13):1641-1644.
20. Schmidt SC, Settmacher U, Langrehr JM, Neuhaus P. Management and outcome of patients with combined bile duct and hepatic arterial injuries after laparoscopic cholecystectomy. *Surgery.* 2004; 135(6):613-618.
21. Pulitanò C, Parks RW, Ireland H, Wigmore SJ, Garden OJ. Impact of concomitant arterial injury on the outcome of laparoscopic bile duct injury. *Am J Surg.* 2011;201(2):238-244.
22. Truant S, Boleslawski E, Lebuffe G, Sergent G, Pruvot FR. Hepatic resection for post-cholecystectomy bile duct injuries: a literature review. *HPB (Oxford).* 2010;12(5):334-341.
23. Duffy JP, Hong JC, Farmer DG, et al. Vascular complications of orthotopic liver transplantation: experience in more than 4,200 patients. *J Am Coll Surg.* 2009;208(5):896-903; discussion 903–905.
24. Hibi T, Nishida S, Levi DM, et al. Long-term deleterious effect of aortohepatic conduits in primary liver transplantation: proceed with caution. *Liver Transpl.* 2013;19(8):916-925.
25. Stewart ZA, Locke JE, Segev DL, et al. Increased risk of graft loss from hepatic artery thrombosis after liver transplantation with older donors. *Liver Transpl.* 2009;15(12):1688-1695.
26. Mourad MM, Liossis C, Gunson BK, et al. Etiology and management of hepatic artery thrombosis after adult liver transplantation. *Liver Transpl.* 2014;20(6):713-723.

27. Nishida S, Kato T, Levi D, et al. Effect of protocol Doppler ultrasonography and urgent revascularization on early hepatic artery thrombosis after pediatric liver transplantation. *Arch Surg.* 2002;137(11):1279-1283.

28. Hamby BA, Ramirez DE, Loss GE, et al. Endovascular treatment of hepatic artery stenosis after liver transplantation. *J Vasc Surg.* 2013; 57(4):1067-1072.

29. Zhou HB. Hemobilia and other complications caused by percutaneous ultrasound-guided liver biopsy. *World J Gastroenterol.* 2014;20(13): 3712-3715.

30. O'Hanlon DM, McDonnell CO, Walsh T, Fenlon HM, McEntee GP. Traumatic arteriovenous fistula of the liver. *J Am Coll Surg.* 2001; 193(5):575.

31. Zhang DY, Weng SQ, Dong L, Shen XZ, Qu XD. Portal hypertension induced by congenital hepatic arterioportal fistula: report of four clinical cases and review of the literature. *World J Gastroenterol.* 2015;21(7):2229-2235.

32. Iwaki T, Miyatani H, Yoshida Y, Matsuura K, Eminaga Y. Gastric variceal bleeding caused by an intrahepatic arterioportal fistula that formed after liver biopsy: a case report and a review of the literature. *Clin J Gastroenterol.* 2012;5(2):101-107.

33. Kanogawa N, Chiba T, Ogasawara S, et al. Successful interventional treatment for arterioportal fistula caused by radiofrequency ablation for hepatocellular carcinoma. *Case Rep Oncol.* 2014;7(3):833-839.

34. Ishii H, Sonoyama T, Nakashima S, et al. Surgical treatment of hepatocellular carcinoma with severe intratumoral arterioportal shunt. *World J Gastroenterol.* 2010;16(25):3214-14.

35. Khalid SK, Garcia-Tsao G. Hepatic vascular malformations in hereditary hemorrhagic telangiectasia. *Semin Liver Dis.* 2008;28(3): 247-258.

36. Moon SB, Kwon HJ, Park KW, Yun WJ, Jung SE. Clinical experience with infantile hepatic hemangioendothelioma. *World J Surg.* 2009; 33(3):597-602.

37. Warmann S, Bertram H, Kardorff R, Sasse M, Hausdorf G, Fuchs J. Interventional treatment of infantile hepatic hemangioendothelioma. *J Pediatr Surg.* 2003;38(8):177-181.

38. Bonaccorsi-Riani E, Lerut JP. Liver transplantation and vascular tumors. *Transpl Int.* 2010;23:686.

39. Dupuis-Girod S, Chesnais AL, Ginon I, et al. Long-term outcome of patients with hereditary hemorrhagic telangiectasia and severe hepatic involvement after orthotopic liver transplantation: a single-center study. *Liver Transpl.* 2010;16(3):340-347.

40. Laurenzi A, Ettorre GM, Lionetti R, Meniconi RL, Colasanti M, Vennarecci G. Portal vein aneurysm: what to know. *Dig Liver Dis.* 2015;47(11):918-923.

41. Cho SW, Marsh JW, Fontes PA, et al. Extrahepatic portal vein aneurysm—report of six patients and review of the literature. *J Gastrointest Surg.* 2008;12(1):145-152.

42. Moreno A, Fleming MD, Farnell MB, Gloviczki P. Extrahepatic portal vein aneurysm. *J Vasc Surg.* 2011 54(1):225-226.

43. Plessier A, Valla DC. Budd-Chiari syndrome. *Semin Liver Dis.* 2008;28(3):259-269.

44. Lao WT, Hung HH, Lu HC, et al. Hepatocellular carcinoma with presentation of Budd-Chiari syndrome. *J Chin Med Assoc.* 2010; 73(2):93-96.

45. Eckie S, Ciancio G. Surgical management of large adrenal masses with or without thrombus extending into the inferior vena cava. *J Urol.* 2004;172(6):2340-2343.

46. Cerwinka WH, Ciancio G, Salerno TA, Soloway MS. Renal cell cancer with invasive atrial tumor thrombus excised off-pump. *Urology.* 2005;66(3):1319.

47. Boozari B, Bahr MJ, Kubicka S, Kempnauer J, Manns MP, Gebel M. Ultrasonography in patients with Budd-Chiari syndrome: diagnostic signs and prognostic implications. *J Hepatol.* 2008;49(4):572-580.

48. Cura M, Haskal Z, Lopera J. Diagnostic and interventional radiology for Budd-Chiari syndrome. *Radiographics.* 2009;29(3):669-681.

49. Seijo S, Plessier A, Hoekstra J, et al. Good long-term outcome of Budd-Chiari syndrome with a step-wise management. *Hepatology.* 2013;57(5):1962-1968.

50. Doyle A, Nicoll A, Dowling R. Use of AngioJet percutaneous thrombectomy system for the treatment of acute Budd-Chiari syndrome. *BMJ Case Rep.* 2013;3:2013.

51. Cho JW, Jae HJ, Kim HC, et al. Long-term outcome of endovascular intervention in hepatic venous outflow obstruction following pediatric liver transplantation. *Liver Transpl.* 2015;12 1219-1226.

52. Oldhafer KJ, Frerker M, Prokop M, Lang H, Böker K, Pichlmayr R. Two-step procedure in Budd-Chiari syndrome with severe intrahepatic vena cava stenosis: vena cava stenting and portocaval shunt. *Am J Gastroenterol.* 1998;93(7):1165-1166.

53. Neumann AB, Andersen SD, Nielsen DT, Holland-Fischer P, Vilstrup H, Grønbæk H. Treatment of Budd-Chiari syndrome with a focus on transjugular intrahepatic portosystemic shunt. *World J Hepatol.* 2013;5(1):38-42.

54. Orloff MJ, Isenberg JI, Wheeler HO, Daily PO, Girard B. Budd-Chiari syndrome revisited: 38 years' experience with surgical portal decompression. *J Gastrointest Surg.* 2012;16(2):286-300; discussion 300.

55. Ulrich F, Pratschke J, Neumann U, et al. Eighteen years of liver transplantation experience in patients with advanced Budd-Chiari syndrome. *Liver Transpl.* 2008;14(2):144-150.

Drug-Induced Liver Injury

Anurag Maheshwari | Sagar Ranka

D rug-induced liver injury (DILI) is a frequent cause of liver injury.[1,2] It is the most frequent reason for withdrawal from the market of an approved drug and accounts for one-third to one-half of the cases of acute liver failure in this country.[3] It can mimic both acute and chronic forms of liver disease and often represents an important diagnostic and therapeutic challenge for the treating physician.[4,5] Although more than 1100 drugs, including herbal, vitamin, dietary supplements, and prescription medications, are believed to have the potential to cause DILI,[6] only a handful are associated with acute liver failure and resultant death or liver transplantation.[7]

EPIDEMIOLOGY

DILI is a relatively underreported clinical entity, with a crude incidence ranging from 10 to 20 per 100,000 persons exposed.[8-12] The true incidence remains unknown due to the lack of systemic reporting, controversy regarding the diagnosis in the context of polypharmacy, and the lack of a simple objective test to establish the diagnosis.

The Acute Liver Failure Study Group in the United States has reported the incidence of mortality or liver transplantation as 10% among a large group of 300 cases of DILI. Data from the national liver transplantation network in the United States suggest that DILI accounts for 15% of all cases requiring transplantation in patients who present with acute liver failure.[13]

The low incidence of DILI makes it difficult to ascertain the type and severity of hepatotoxicity of new drugs during phase III clinical trials. Therefore the modified *Hy's rule* is used by the US Food and Drug Administration (FDA) to categorize the severity of hepatotoxicity. Drugs that can cause an alanine aminotransferase (ALT) level 3 or more times the upper limit of normal (ULN) with bilirubin levels 2 or more times ULN are historically associated with greater than 10% mortality[14] and are considered at risk for life-threatening liver damage.

In general, drugs that cause liver injury can be divided into two categories: those that cause dose-dependent toxicity, such as acetaminophen or tetracycline, and the vast majority of others (>90% to 95%) that cause idiosyncratic reactions. For the former group, factors such as dose, blood level, and duration of intake play an important role in determining toxicity. For the latter group, host factors such as age, gender, concomitant diseases, and other drug exposure are important factors (Fig. 130.1).

AGE

Hepatic drug reactions are more common in the elderly (probably due to the presence of polypharmacy)[15] and much less frequent among children. The exceptions include valproic acid, where hepatotoxicity is frequently seen among children younger than 3 years of age.[16] Salicylic acid–induced Reye syndrome is also exclusively seen in children, although now rarely so due to widespread education and awareness.

GENDER

Women seem to be particularly predisposed to drug-induced hepatotoxicity from medications such as minocycline, methyldopa, and nitrofurantoin in which the injury histologically resembles autoimmune hepatitis. Women also seem to be predisposed to the development of severe liver injury, as shown by a female preponderance in most studies of acute liver failure and liver transplantation related to DILI.[17]

CONCOMITANT DRUGS

Recipients of polypharmacy are more likely to experience liver toxicity due to various mechanisms, including enhanced cytochrome P450 metabolism that results in accumulation of the toxic metabolite or delayed biliary excretion.[18] Chronic alcohol ingestion can increase the severity of liver injury from certain agents, such as acetaminophen and isoniazid (INH), due to depletion of glutathione.

CONCOMITANT ILLNESSES

In general, patients with preexisting liver disease, including cirrhosis, are not predisposed to DILI, but they are believed to be at higher risk for complicated courses and outcomes of DILI.[19] Human immunodeficiency virus (HIV) infection increases the risk of sulfonamide toxicity, and renal transplantation is considered a risk factor for azathioprine-induced vascular injury. Most medications metabolized in the liver will demonstrate altered pharmacokinetics with elevated area under the curve (AUC), and clinical judgment should determine the safety of their use in patients with decompensated cirrhosis.

GENETICS

Genetics play an important role in the susceptibility of an individual at multiple phases of the processing of a drug.[20] A major role is played by genes encoding cytochrome P450 (CYP) isoenzymes responsible for drug metabolism. A common example is *slow acetylator* genotype responsible for isoniazid-related liver injury.[21] Genetic mutations affecting the cytokeratin proteins on hepatocytes have also been implicated in the causation of severe DILI. In addition, immune-mediated pathogenesis for DILI has brought to light the susceptible human leukocyte antigen (HLA) haplotypes seen in some cases of DILI.[22] This approach of genetic screening has shown promise in reducing the incidence of idiosyncratic reactions of drugs. A solid example is the HLA-B*5701 genotyping prior to institution

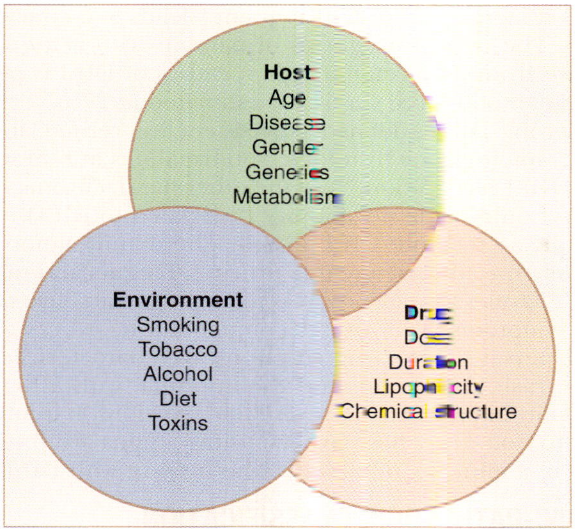

FIGURE 130.1 Venn diagram demonstrating the interaction of various factors affecting the development of drug-induced liver injury.

of abacavir therapy, which has almost eliminated the incidence of a potentially severe hypersensitivity reaction to the drug.

INTRINSIC PROPERTIES OF THE DRUG

The most commonly implicated group of drugs are antimicrobials.[23] The hepatotoxic potential of drugs dosed at more than 50 to 100 mg/day is higher than those dosed at under 20 mg daily.[24-26] In addition, drugs with greater lipophilicity and predominantly hepatic metabolism are more prone to DILI. Interestingly drugs used at higher doses have shorter latency to the onset of DILI.[27]

PATHOPHYSIOLOGY

The liver is the site of first-pass metabolism and is highly exposed to drugs that are absorbed from the gastrointestinal tract. Drugs tend to be lipophilic compounds that are not readily excreted in bile or urine so one of the functions of drug metabolism in the liver is its conversion to a hydrophilic substrate. Drug metabolism in the liver is divided into three series of pathways: Phase 1 metabolism alters the parent molecule, phase 2 produces a conjugate of the drug or its metabolite, and phase 3 metabolism comprises energy-dependent pathways for excretion of the conjugate from the hepatocyte.

PHASE 1

Phase 1 pathways include oxidation, reduction, and hydrolytic reactions. Most reactions are catalyzed by microsomal drug oxidases that act by way of the cytochrome P450 system. Reduced nicotinamide adenine dinucleotide phosphate (NADPH) in the cytosol acts as cofactor. A typical example is the production of N-acetyl-p-benzoquinone imine (NAPQI) from acetaminophen mediated by the CYP2E1 pathway. Enzyme inducers include barbiturates, alcohol, anticonvulsants, rifampin, inhaled anesthetics, and oral hypoglycemic agents. Enzyme induction has

implications for metabolism of other drugs and mechanisms for DILI.

PHASE 2

These reactions involve the conjugation of the parent drug or its metabolite with a small endogenous molecule. The conjugates are highly water soluble and readily excreted in bile or urine. Conjugation is dependent on cofactors, such as glucuronic acid, and can be impaired by their depletion.

PHASE 3

This involves the active excretion of drug and drug metabolites into bile or sinusoids and involves energy-dependent pathways mediated by the adenosine triphosphate (ATP)-binding cassette transport proteins. This system is located at the biliary pole of the hepatocyte and can be saturated, with implications for drug accumulation and cholestatic DILI.

MECHANISMS OF LIVER INJURY

Various mechanisms of drug-induced injury, as follows, have been identified that involve the hepatocyte,[28,29] and the manner in which the intracellular organelles are affected defines the pattern of disease:

1. Disruption of calcium homeostasis can result in actin disruption and loss of ionic gradient, which results in cell swelling and rupture.
2. Covalent binding of drug to the cytochrome P450 system involving high-energy reactions can lead to the formation of nonfunctioning adducts. Such covalent binding may inactivate key enzymes in the cell; the protein-drug adducts may serve as immune targets, inducing the formation of antibodies, or they can evoke a direct cytolytic T-cell response.
3. Oxidative stress in the liver can produce reactive oxygen species that disrupt mitochondrial DNA and microsomal electron transport systems. This results in the disruption of fatty acid metabolism and energy production with ensuing anaerobic metabolism and can result in lactic acidosis and microvesicular steatosis.
4. Drugs that affect transport proteins at the canalicular membrane can interrupt bile flow. Interruption of transport pumps, such as multidrug resistance–associated protein 3 (MRP-3), prevents the excretion of bilirubin, resulting in intracellular cholestasis, causing secondary injury to the hepatocytes.
5. Other cells within the liver may be targets of injury or serve as modulators of injury. Activation of Kupffer cells may release reactive oxygen species and cytokines that amplify the injury to hepatocytes. Injury to hepatic sinusoidal endothelium can result in drug-induced vascular injury and the development of venoocclusive disease. Activation of hepatic stellate cells by methotrexate or vitamin A can result in increased matrix deposition with resultant fibrosis and cirrhosis.

Drugs can be divided into dose-dependent hepatotoxins or dose-independent (idiosyncratic) hepatotoxins. Dose-dependent hepatotoxins require activation to a toxic metabolite and interference with the function of intracellular organelles, such as the mitochondria or canalicular biliary secretion. Liver injury caused by these drugs occurs after a short latent period characterized by zonal necrosis and can be reproduced in other species. In contrast, idiosyncratic reactions cause a wide variety of histologic changes, exhibit a variable latent period to onset of injury, and cannot be reliably reproduced. Idiosyncratic hepatotoxicity is thought to occur by two major mechanisms: metabolic idiosyncrasy or immunoallergy. Metabolic idiosyncrasy is the susceptibility of rare individuals to a drug, which in conventional doses is usually safe. This susceptibility may be the result of genetic or acquired differences in drug metabolism or excretion. Immunoallergy indicates immune-mediated injury in response to the formation of adducts or hapten molecules, which may result from the interaction between the drug metabolite and the cell proteins or cytochrome P450 enzyme.

DIAGNOSIS AND TREATMENT OF DRUG-INDUCED LIVER DISEASE

Almost any drug has the potential for hepatotoxicity and should be suspected when considering the diagnosis. Clinicians must have a high index of suspicion, and the history should include the dose, route, duration, and concomitant administration of all drugs. Particular interest should be paid to the use of alternative and complementary medications because that history is not easily forthcoming. Currently there is no objective test or a marker to ascertain the diagnosis or cause of DILI and thus expert opinion after careful examination of clinical, biochemical, and histologic evidence is essential.[30]

Most presentations of DILI are asymptomatic, but it can also present as acute or chronic liver disease. It may present as a mild asymptomatic rise in liver enzymes or as life-threatening acute liver failure. The usual time to onset of liver injury after drug administration is 5 to 90 days but can occur within 24 to 48 hours if there is prior sensitization, such as by sulfonamide antibiotics. Antibiotics are the most widely implicated drugs and manifest[31] liver injury typically within a week, although exceptions such as minocycline and nitrofurantoin can present as late as 1 year. Polypharmacy and comorbid illnesses predispose to a sixfold increase in the risk of developing DILI.[32]

The symptomatic patients present with malaise, nausea, vomiting, anorexia, jaundice, acholic stools, dark urine, and right-sided abdominal pain. The presentation of DILI can often mimic other liver diseases, so tests for other forms of chronic liver diseases, such as viral hepatitis, autoimmune liver diseases, and genetic causes of liver damage, are an essential part of the evaluation process. Jaundice, although a hallmark of liver diseases, is present only in up to 5% to 10% of the cases.[33] Hepatomegaly may be present on physical examination. Up to 75% of the DILI patients with presence of liver injury at 6 months continue to have liver injury on a prolonged follow-up.[34] Older patients and those with cholestatic injury are more likely to have persistent liver abnormalities at prolonged follow-up.[34] In severe cases, coagulopathy and hepatic encephalopathy may develop, indicative of acute liver failure. These patients typically present with jaundice and altered mental status that frequently leads to a comatose state. The overall prognosis of patients with acute liver failure from nonacetaminophen causes of DILI is poor; transplantation-free survival is estimated at 27%.[35]

Chronic DILI is defined as persistent liver-related laboratory, radiologic, or histologic abnormalities at 6 months after DILI recognition.[36] On the other hand, chronic liver injury could be de novo injury (unrelated to DILI) or as a sequelae to acute DILI as well. The manifestations of chronic liver disease include pruritus, fatigue, and raised liver enzymes. It may progress to cirrhosis and have signs and symptoms of hepatic decompensation.

Hypersensitivity drug reactions are characterized by fever, rash, and peripheral eosinophilia, with a higher mortality in patients with severe skin reactions. It is important to note that these hypersensitivity signs are present only in a minority of patients who present with DILI.[37,38]

CLINIC-PATHOLOGIC CLASSIFICATION

There are many clinical, histopathologic, and pharmacologic classifications of DILI; the one mentioned later is most useful for the clinician. The liver injury is classified into three categories based on the elevation of liver enzymes using the R ratio (ratio of ALT to alkaline phosphatase [ALT/ALP], both expressed as multiples of the ULN range). Hepatocellular injury is defined as an R ratio greater than 5, cholestatic injury has an R ratio less than 2, and "mixed" cholestatic-hepatocellular injury has an R ratio between 2 and 5. This terminology is used regardless of the presence of jaundice (Fig. 130.2).

1. *Hepatocellular injury*: Drug-induced liver disease that resembles acute viral hepatitis and demonstrates prominent hepatocellular pattern of injury. Liver biopsy, if available, usually shows marked liver cell necrosis and inflammation with only mild bile stasis, at least in the early stages. Hepatocellular injury is the most common form on injury[39] and can also be suggested by clinical and laboratory features. If present, symptoms are nonspecific and include fatigue. Serum ALT and AST levels typically are markedly elevated (usually >10-fold), whereas the ALP or gamma-glutamyl transpeptidase (GGT) is only modestly increased. An R ratio greater than 5 is used to define a pattern of hepatocellular injury but may not always be accurate. Agents that typically give a hepatocellular pattern of injury include isoniazid, green tea, nitrofurantoin, and methyldopa.

2. *Cholestatic injury*: A cholestatic picture of DILI resembles a picture of biliary obstruction. The liver biopsy findings are generally of bile stasis, portal inflammation, and proliferation or injury of bile ducts and ductules. Clinically, symptoms of jaundice and itching predominate. Serum ALP and GGT levels are prominently elevated, whereas ALT and AST levels are minimally or modestly increased. An R ratio of less than 2 is used to define a cholestatic pattern of injury but may not always be accurate. Drugs that typically cause a cholestatic liver injury pattern include amoxicillin/clavulanic acid (Augmentin), ciprofloxacin, and the sulfonylureas.

3. *Mixed hepatocellular-cholestatic injury*: A mixture of hepatocellular and cholestatic injury is typical of most drugs, occurring rarely in other forms of acute liver disease. In cases of mixed injury, liver biopsy shows prominent

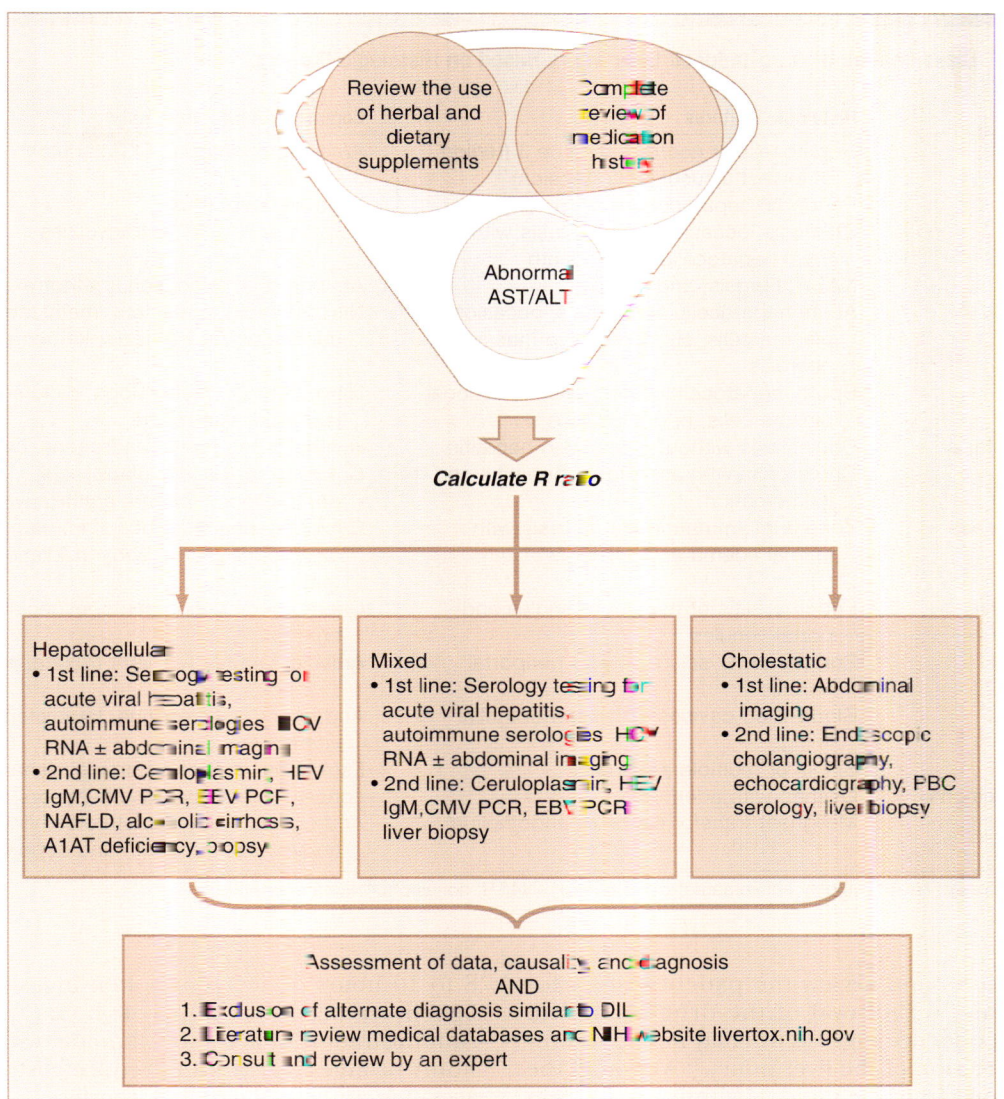

FIGURE 130.2 Algorithm for patient with suspected liver damage secondary to drug. *A1AD,* Alpha1-antitrypsin deficiency; *ALT,* alanine transaminase; *AST,* aspartate transaminase; *CMV PCR,* cytomegalovirus polymerase chain reaction; *DILI,* drug-induced liver damage; *EBV PCR,* Epstein-Barr virus polymerase chain reaction; *HCV RNA,* hepatitis C virus RNA; *HEV IgM,* immunoglobulin M antibody for hepatitis E virus; *NAFLD,* nonalcoholic fatty liver disease; *NIH,* National Institutes of Health Sciences; *PBC,* primary biliary cirrhosis.

hepatocyte necrosis and inflammation accompanied by marked bile stasis. Symptoms may include both fatigue and itching, and laboratory tests show similar elevations in serum ALT and ALP. An *R* ratio between 2 and 5 is used to define a mixed pattern of injury. Drugs that cause a mixed hepatocellular-cholestatic pattern of injury include the sulfonamides, phenytoin, and enalapril.

Role of liver biopsy is to characterize and establish the histologic patterns during ongoing liver injury because different drugs cause different pattern of damage (Table 130.1).

ASSESSMENT OF CAUSALITY AND SEVERITY

It is difficult to implicate a particular drug in the causation of the drug-induced liver disease to prevent reexposure and further harm.[40] The currently used Roussel-Uclaf Causality Assessment Method (RUCAM) scale in clinical practice has a low interobserver reproducibility and reliability compared with expert consensus opinion.[30,41] Clinically, there is lack of an objective scale to ascertain the cause of DILI.[41] The measure of severity of liver damage can be done on criteria mentioned (Table 130.2).

MANAGEMENT OF DRUG-INDUCED LIVER INJURY

The management of DILI has historically been the same, but newer insights into pathogenesis and biomarkers have improved the assessment and treatment of DILI. The primary step is to withdraw the suspected drug,

TABLE 130.1 Classification of Drug-Induced Liver Injury Based on Histologic Damage

Histologic Damage	Histologic Features	Commonly Associated Drugs
Zone 3 necrosis	Hepatocellular necrosis in zone 3 (region of lowest sinusoidal O_2 tension)	*Amanita* mushroom, CCl_4, acetaminophen
Zone 1 necrosis	Periportal hepatocellular necrosis	Yellow phosphorus
Mitochondrial cytopathies	Steatosis, occasional cholestasis with focal hepatocellular cell death	Valproate, HAART, tetracyclines
Steatohepatitis	NASH, fibrosis, and cirrhosis	Amiodarone, tamoxifen, methotrexate, perhexiline
Acute hepatitis	Acute hepatocellular necrosis, occasional plasma cells, submassive to massive necrosis	Nitrofurantoin, phenytoin, methyldopa, disulfiram, sulfonamides, isoniazid, ketoconazole, troglitazone
Chronic hepatitis	Spotty hepatocellular necrosis, occasional plasma cells, bridging fibrosis	Nitrofurantoin, methyldopa, diclofenac, minocycline, isoniazid, dantrolene
Canalicular cholestasis	Cholestasis without associated hepatitis	Synthetic estrogens, androgens, cyclosporine
Hepatocanalicular cholestasis	Cholestasis with associated hepatitis and inflammation	Chlorpromazine, clavulanic acid, dextropropoxyphene, erythromycin
Venoocclusive disease	Zone 3 inflammation and fibrosis with intimal edema and sclerosis	Cyclophosphamide, busulfan, carmustine, etoposide, azathioprine, total body irradiation, Jamaican bush tea, comfrey
Nodular regenerative hyperplasia	Endothelialitis of hepatic arterioles and portal venules	Chemotherapeutic agents, especially alkylating agents
Noncirrhotic portal hypertension	Portal venular sclerosis with periportal fibrosis	Arsenic, vitamin A, methotrexate, vinyl chloride
Peliosis hepatitis	Blood-filled cavities without endothelial lining	Androgens, azathioprine, tamoxifen, estrogens, vitamin A
Hepatic adenoma	Single or multiple adenomas	Estrogens, anabolic steroids, danazol
Hepatocellular carcinoma	Overlap with adenoma	Long-term estrogen use (>8 years)
Angiosarcoma	Malignant transformation of endothelium	Androgenic metabolic steroids, vinyl chloride, arsenic salts, thorium and copper salts

CCl_4, Carbon tetrachloride; *HAART*, highly active antiretroviral therapy; *NASH*, nonalcoholic steatohepatitis.

prevent reexposure, and review the patient history for other causes. Early withdrawal of the drug is advised, although current evidence suggests this may not necessarily impact the progression of the liver injury.[42] Although the serum enzymes may improve rapidly (within 2 to 4 weeks of stopping the medication), sometimes they improve spontaneously (referred to as *adaptation*; e.g., isoniazid).[43] Thus, in a case of asymptomatic liver enzyme elevation, the necessity of drug discontinuation needs to be weighed against its hepatotoxic profile on a case-to-case basis.

Patients with moderate to severe DILI should be hospitalized with frequent monitoring, preferably in the intensive care unit.[7] In patients with acetaminophen overdose, *N*-acetylcysteine (NAC) is the accepted antidote and has been shown to be effective in numerous controlled trials.[44,45] Serum acetaminophen levels are frequently not a reliable marker of the degree of acetaminophen injury despite the availability of a nomogram due to confusion about initial dose and timing of ingestion. Clinical parameters such as markedly elevated aminotransferase levels with a low bilirubin in absence of shock or hypotension has shown to be predictive of spontaneous recovery from acetaminophen liver injury. NAPQI-protein adduct levels may serve as a reliable marker of suspected acetaminophen toxicity up to 12 days after the initial injury.[46] More recently serum micro-RNA levels have also been explored as markers for liver injury in case of acetaminophen poisoning.[47] Early administration of NAC is recommended within 8 to 10 hours of acetaminophen ingestion, but clinical benefit has been shown up to 48 hours after ingestion.[45,48] Administration of activated charcoal within the first few hours of ingestion helps to reduce gastric absorption of acetaminophen and does not interfere with the absorption of NAC.[49,50]

In a randomized controlled trial, NAC appeared to improve spontaneous survival when administered early in the setting of nonacetaminophen acute liver failure in adults, particularly in patients with early-stage encephalopathy.[35,51,52] This effect is partly due to the antiinflammatory, vasodilator, and inotropic benefits of NAC, in addition to the primary benefit of repletion of glutathione stores. Interestingly, in another recent clinical trial, NAC was not found to be useful in children with nonacetaminophen-related liver injury.[52] Other antidotes, such as L-carnitine for valproic acid, silymarin for *Amanita* mushroom poisoning, or cholestyramine in cases of toxicity with leflunomide, should be considered in specific situations.[53]

Glucocorticoids are of unproven benefit for most forms of drug hepatotoxicity but may have a role in patients with hypersensitivity reactions associated with fever, rash, and/or eosinophilia that leads to development of a clinical picture resembling autoimmune hepatitis.[54,55] Symptomatic management of pruritus in the form of bile acid sequestrants (e.g., cholestyramine) should be considered in patients with cholestatic liver disease.

TABLE 130.2 Assessment of Severity of Liver Damage*

Mild	Patient has elevation in ALT and/or alkaline phosphatase levels but total serum bilirubin is <2.5 mg/dL *and* INR is <1.5
Moderate	Patient has elevation in ALT and/or alkaline phosphatase levels *and* serum bilirubin is ≥2.5 mg/dL *or* INR is ≥1.5
Moderate-Severe	Patient has elevation in ALT, alkaline phosphatase, bilirubin, and/or INR levels *and* patient is hospitalized or an ongoing hospitalization is prolonged because of DILI
Severe	Patient has elevation in ALT and/or alkaline phosphatase levels *and* total serum bilirubin is ≥2.5 mg/dL or greater and there is **at least one of the following:** (1) hepatic failure (INR ≥1.5, ascites or encephalopathy); (2) other organ failure believed to be due to DILI event
Fatal	Patient dies or undergoes liver transplantation because of DILI event

*In addition, cases are rated for presence or absence of symptoms (A = asymptomatic; S = symptomatic). Symptoms include fatigue, nausea, vomiting, right upper quadrant pain, itching, skin rash, jaundice, weakness, anorexia, or weight loss, which in the opinion of the investigator are due to DILI. *ALT*, Alanine transaminase; *AST*, aspartate transaminase; *INR*, international normalized ratio; *DILI*, drug-induced liver disease.
From Fontana RJ, Watkins PB, Bonkovsky HL, et al. Drug-Induced Liver Injury Network (DILIN) prospective study: rationale, design and conduct. *Drug Saf.* 2009;32(1):55–68.

PREVENTION

Preventive measures to include patient education and periodic liver test screening should be undertaken to help recognize DILI early. Patients need to be educated regarding the possible drug interactions of concomitant drugs and alcohol.[55] Finally, patients who suffer an episode of DILI should be warned to avoid re-exposure to the implicated drug, and the reaction should be noted in the medical record as an allergy. Periodic screening of liver biochemistries, particularly serum ALT, is recommended for many drugs that have been associated with liver injury. This strategy is not completely effective because liver injury can occur despite monitoring or may resolve on its own with continued administration of the drug.[56,57]

PROGNOSIS

Most mild to moderate cases of DILI usually recover completely with no residual damage. The others may progress to chronic DILI or acute liver failure. The mortality in such severe cases ranges from 30% to 70% without a transplant.[7,45] Many new risk factors have been evaluated affecting the short- and long-term outcomes in patients with drug-induced liver disease. Patients with lung disease, low serum albumin and/or platelet levels, and high levels of total serum bilirubin and/or alanine aminotransferase have a higher risk of death or transplantation.[58]

ALTERNATIVE REMEDIES, RECREATIONAL DRUGS, AND ENVIRONMENTAL AGENTS

Numerous other medicinal and nonmedicinal compounds, including vitamins, herbal remedies, environmental agents, and recreational drugs, can cause various forms of hepatotoxicity. Recreational drugs such as "ecstasy" (MDMA; 3,4-methylenedioxy-methamphetamine) and cocaine have been associated with hepatotoxicity severe enough to require liver transplantation.

HERBAL AND DIETARY SUPPLEMENTS

This umbrella term comprises herbal, natural, mineral, and vitamin products that are commercially available and are used commonly by the lay public (by up to 50% of the adult US population).[59,60] These supplements are now the second most common cause of liver injury,[1] with bodybuilding and weight loss supplements being the most common agents implicated in development of DILI.[61] Factors that predict supplement use are age, availability of health insurance, self-reported good health, endorsement from health care professionals, lower body mass indexes (BMIs), moderate alcohol use, exercise activity, abstinence from smoking, and chronic illness.[62] The increasing popularity of alternative medicines has led to many reports of associated toxicity. In most cases, the hepatotoxin is not readily apparent and many preparations contain more than one ingredient that may be the culprit. Due to lack of FDA oversight of the manufacturing process, these supplements frequently vary in potency and quantity from batch to batch.[16,63–66] They may also contain unlabeled contaminants such as antimicrobials or heavy metals.[67–70] The spectrum of toxicity ranges from acute hepatitis, chronic hepatitis with cirrhosis, cholestasis, to vascular injury. Chinese herbal teas and other mixed preparations can cause a host of toxic reactions, and patient self-reporting may be unreliable to establish temporal relationships. Bodybuilding products such as protein powders can contain anabolic steroids associated with cholestatic hepatitis.[71–73]

Hypervitaminosis A is now more commonly recognized as secondary to self-medication of large doses of vitamin A over prolonged periods. The pathologic spectrum of liver disease due to vitamin A toxicity can range from abnormal liver function tests (LFTs), stellate cell hyperplasia, noncirrhotic portal hypertension, cirrhosis, to rare cases of peliosis hepatis. The prognosis is poorer in cases with established cirrhosis and portal hypertension, and patients with chronic liver diseases should be cautioned against vitamin A supplementation. The list of case reports of DILI associated with alternative and herbal supplements is a rapidly growing area of medical literature.[5,74–79]

Unlike other prescription medications, herbal and dietary supplement–induced liver damage can best be assessed by process of expert referral and opinion. Expert opinion allows assessors to consider all available clinical information, including a qualitative assessment of the published literature and personal experience with any given product. There are multiple products with dissimilar patterns of injury, making it difficult for a clinician to suspect and diagnose the same.[62] Clinicians must query patients about their use of herbal and dietary supplements, realizing that many will not be forthcoming with this history.[80] Voluntary reporting of suspected hepatotoxicity cases associated with supplement use should be encouraged through the FDA MedWatch system.

CONCLUSION

Clinical trials are often inadequate in identifying a drug's potential for liver injury, and this may be evident only after the drug has been approved for public use. Although several drugs cause asymptomatic transient elevations of LFTs, the safety of such a reaction is questionable. LFTs should be monitored 3 to 4 weeks after commencing therapy with any drug that has the potential to cause liver toxicity. Continued administration of the offending drug after development of liver toxicity is the most common cause of poor outcome, necessitating early recognition of the syndrome. The increasing use of complementary medications has raised awareness of their potential for liver toxicity among the medical community, although the lay public must also be cautioned about the dangers of unregulated nonproprietary preparations. Practitioners are encouraged to report suspected drug reactions because underreporting is common and improved reporting may help early recognition of drug toxicity.

REFERENCES

1. Kaplowitz N. Drug-induced liver disorders—implications for drug development and regulation. *Drug Saf.* 2001;24(7):483-490.
2. Watkins PB. Drug safety sciences and the bottleneck in drug development. *Clin Pharmacol Ther.* 2011;89(6):788-790.
3. Navarro VJ, Senior JR. Drug-related hepatotoxicity. *N Engl J Med.* 2006;354(7):731-739.
4. Hayashi PH, Fontana RJ, Chalasani NP, et al. Under-reporting and poor adherence to monitoring guidelines for severe cases of isoniazid hepatotoxicity. *Clin Gastroenterol Hepatol.* 2015;13(9):1676-1682.e1.
5. Agarwal VK, McHutchison JG, Hoofnagle JH. Important elements for the diagnosis of drug-induced liver injury. *Clin Gastroenterol Hepatol.* 2010;8(5):463-470.
6. Larrey D. Epidemiology and individual susceptibility to adverse drug reactions affecting the liver. *Semin Liver Dis.* 2002;22(2):145-155.
7. Ostapowicz G, Fontana RJ, Schiødt FV, et al. Results of a prospective study of acute liver failure at 17 tertiary care centers in the United States. *Ann Intern Med.* 2002;137(12):947-954.
8. Björnsson ES, Bergmann OM, Björnsson HK, Kvaran RB, Olafsson S. Incidence, presentation, and outcomes in patients with drug-induced liver injury in the general population of Iceland. *Gastroenterology.* 2013;144(7):1419-1425.e3.
9. Sgro C, Clinard F, Ouazir K, et al. Incidence of drug-induced hepatic injuries: a French population-based study. *Hepatology.* 2002;36(2):451-455.
10. Shapiro MA, Lewis JH. Causality assessment of drug-induced hepatotoxicity: promises and pitfalls. *Clin Liver Dis.* 2007;11(3):477-505, v.
11. Chalasani N, Fontana RJ, Bonkovsky HL, et al. Causes, clinical features, and outcomes from a prospective study of drug-induced liver injury in the United States. *Gastroenterology.* 2008;135(6):1924-1934, 1934.e1-e4.
12. Bell LN, Chalasani N. Epidemiology of idiosyncratic drug-induced liver injury. *Semin Liver Dis.* 2009;29(4):337-347.
13. Russo MW, Galanko JA, Shrestha R, Fried MW, Watkins P. Liver transplantation for acute liver failure from drug induced liver injury in the United States. *Liver Transpl.* 2004;10(8):1018-1023.
14. Björnsson E. Drug-induced liver injury: Hy's rule revisited. *Clin Pharmacol Ther.* 2006;79(6):521-528.
15. Lucena MI, Andrade RJ, Kaplowitz N, et al. Phenotypic characterization of idiosyncratic drug-induced liver injury: the influence of age and sex. *Hepatology.* 2009;49(6):2001-2009.
16. Benecetti MS, Whomsley R, Canning M. Drug metabolism in the paediatric population and in the elderly. *Drug Discov Today.* 2007;12(15-16):599-610.
17. Chalasani N, Bonkovsky HL, Fontana R, et al. Features and outcomes of 899 patients with drug-induced liver injury: the DILIN prospective study. *Gastroenterology.* 2015;148(7):1340-1352.e7.
18. Kalgutkar AS, Obach RS, Maurer TS. Mechanism-based inactivation of cytochrome P450 enzymes: chemical mechanisms, structure-activity relationships and relationship to clinical drug-drug interactions and idiosyncratic adverse drug reactions. *Curr Drug Metab.* 2007;8(5):407-447.
19. Verbeeck RK. Pharmacokinetics and dosage adjustment in patients with hepatic dysfunction. *Eur J Clin Pharmacol.* 2008;64(12):1147-1161.
20. Zhou SF. Structure, function and regulation of P-glycoprotein and its clinical relevance in drug disposition. *Xenobiotica.* 2008;38(7-8):802-832.
21. Daly AK, Day CP. Genetic association studies in drug-induced liver injury. *Semin Liver Dis.* 2009;29(4):400-411.
22. Andrade RJ, Lucena MI, Alonso A, et al. HLA class II genotype influences the type of liver injury in drug-induced idiosyncratic liver disease. *Hepatology.* 2004;39(6):1603-1612.
23. Reuben A, Koch DG, Lee WM. Drug-induced acute liver failure: results of a U.S. multicenter, prospective study. *Hepatology.* 2010;52(6):2065-2076.
24. Chen M, Borlak J, Tong W. High lipophilicity and high daily dose of oral medications are associated with significant risk for drug-induced liver injury. *Hepatology.* 2013;58(1):388-396.
25. Lammert C, Einarsson S, Saha C, Niklasson A, Bjornsson E, Chalasani N. Relationship between daily dose of oral medications and idiosyncratic drug-induced liver injury: search for signals. *Hepatology.* 2008;47(6):2003-2009.
26. Lammert C, Bjornsson E, Niklasson A, Chalasani N. Oral medications with significant hepatic metabolism at higher risk for hepatic adverse events. *Hepatology.* 2010;51(2):615-620.
27. Vuppalanchi R, Gotur R, Reddy KR, et al. Relationship between characteristics of medications and drug-induced liver disease phenotype and outcome. *Clin Gastroenterol Hepatol.* 2014;12(9):1550-1555.
28. Chun LJ, Tong MJ, Busuttil RW, Hiatt JR. Acetaminophen hepatotoxicity and acute liver failure. *J Clin Gastroenterol.* 2009;43(4):342-349.
29. Tujios S, Fontana RJ. Mechanisms of drug-induced liver injury: from bedside to bench. *Nat Rev Gastroenterol Hepatol.* 2011;8(4):202-211.
30. Rockey DC, Seeff LB, Rochon J, et al. Causality assessment in drug-induced liver injury using a structured expert opinion process: comparison to the Roussel-Uclaf causality assessment method. *Hepatology.* 2010;51(6):2117-2126.
31. Ghabril M, Fontana R, Rockey D, Jiezhun G, Chalasani N. Drug-induced liver injury caused by intravenously administered medications: the Drug-induced Liver Injury Network experience. *J Clin Gastroenterol.* 2013;47(6):553-558.
32. de Abajo FJ, Montero D, Madurga M, García Rodríguez LA. Acute and clinically relevant drug-induced liver injury: a population based case-control study. *Br J Clin Pharmacol.* 2004;58(1):71-80.
33. Bjornsson E, Ismael S, Nejdet S, Kilander A. Severe jaundice in Sweden in the new millennium: causes, investigations, treatment and prognosis. *Scand J Gastroenterol.* 2003;38(1):86-94.
34. Fontana RJ, Hayashi PH, Barnhart H, et al. Persistent liver biochemistry abnormalities are more common in older patients and those with cholestatic drug induced liver injury. *Am J Gastroenterol.* 2015;110(10):1450-1459.
35. Lee WM, Hynan LS, Rossaro L, et al. Intravenous N-acetylcysteine improves transplant-free survival in early stage non-acetaminophen acute liver failure. *Gastroenterology.* 2009;137(3):856-864, 864.e1.
36. Fontana RJ, Watkins PB, Bonkovsky HL, et al. Drug-Induced Liver Injury Network (DILIN) prospective study: rationale, design and conduct. *Drug Saf.* 2009;32(1):55-68.
37. Andrade RJ, Lucena MI, Fernández MC, et al. Drug-induced liver injury: an analysis of 461 incidences submitted to the Spanish registry over a 10-year period. *Gastroenterology.* 2005;129(2):512-521.
38. Ibanez L, Pérez E, Vidal X, Laporte JR; Grup d'Estudi Multicèntric d'Hepatotoxicitat Aguda de Barcelona (GEMHAB). Prospective surveillance of acute serious liver disease unrelated to infectious, obstructive, or metabolic diseases: epidemiological and clinical features, and exposure to drugs. *J Hepatol.* 2002;37(5):592-600.
39. Larrey D. Drug-induced liver diseases. *J Hepatol.* 2000;32(1 suppl):77-88.

40. Hayashi PH, Barnhart HX, Fontana RJ, et al. Reliability of causality assessment for drug, herbal and dietary supplement hepatotoxicity in the Drug-Induced Liver Injury Network (DILIN). *Liver Int.* 2015;35(5):1623-1632.

41. Rochon J, Protiva P, Seeff LB, et al. Reliability of the Roussel Uclaf Causality Assessment Method for assessing causality in drug-induced liver injury. *Hepatology.* 2008;48(4):1175-1183.

42. Lee WM. Drug-induced hepatotoxicity. *N Engl J Med.* 1995;333(17):1118-1127.

43. National Institutes of Health. U.S. Department of Health and Human Services. *Liver Toxicity.* Last updated: 2015-09-10 08:39:12 AM (EST); Available from: <http://livertox.nih.gov/index.html>.

44. Keays R, Harrison PM, Wendon JA, et al. Intravenous acetylcysteine in paracetamol induced fulminant hepatic failure: a prospective controlled trial. *BMJ.* 1991;303(6809):1026-1029.

45. Larson AM, Polson J, Fontana RJ, et al. Acetaminophen-induced acute liver failure: results of a United States multicenter, prospective study. *Hepatology.* 2005;42(6):1364-1372.

46. Bond GR. Acetaminophen protein adducts: a review. *Clin Toxicol (Phila).* 2009;47(1):2-7.

47. Starkey Lewis PJ, Dear J, Platt V, et al. Circulating microRNAs as potential markers of human drug-induced liver injury. *Hepatology.* 2011;54(5):1767-1776.

48. Harrison PM, Keays R, Bray GP, Alexander GJ, Williams R. Improved outcome of paracetamol-induced fulminant hepatic failure by late administration of acetylcysteine. *Lancet.* 1990;335(8705):1572-1573.

49. Green R, Grierson R, Sitar DS, Tenenbein M. How long after drug ingestion is activated charcoal still effective? *J Toxicol Clin Toxicol.* 2001;39(6):601-605.

50. Sato RL, Wong JJ, Sumida SM, Marn RY, Enoki NR, Yamamoto LG. Efficacy of superactivated charcoal administered late (3 hours) after acetaminophen overdose. *Am J Emerg Med.* 2003;21(3):189-191.

51. Polson J, Lee WM, American Association for the Study of Liver Disease. AASLD position paper: the management of acute liver failure. *Hepatology.* 2005;41(5):1179-1197.

52. Squires RH, Dhawan A, Alonso E, et al. Intravenous N-acetylcysteine in pediatric patients with nonacetaminophen acute liver failure: a placebo-controlled clinical trial. *Hepatology.* 2013;57(4):1542-1549.

53. Bohan TP, Helton E, McDonald I, et al. Effect of L-carnitine treatment for valproate-induced hepatotoxicity. *Neurology.* 2001;56(10):1405-1409.

54. Giannattasio A, D'Ambrosi M, Volpicelli M, Iorio R. Steroid therapy for a case of severe drug-induced cholestasis. *Ann Pharmacother.* 2006;40(6):1196-1199.

55. Davern TJ. Drug-induced liver disease. *Clin Liver Dis.* 2012;16(2):231-245.

56. Graham DJ, Green L, Senior JR, Noonan P. Troglitazone-induced liver failure: a case study. *Am J Med.* 2003;114(4):299-306.

57. Watkins PB, Zimmerman HJ, Knapp MJ, Gracon SI, Lewis KW. Hepatotoxic effects of tacrine administration in patients with Alzheimer's disease. *JAMA.* 1994;271(13):992-998.

58. Fontana RJ, Hayashi PH, Gu J, et al. Idiosyncratic drug-induced liver injury is associated with substantial morbidity and mortality within 6 months from onset. *Gastroenterology.* 2014;147(1):96-108.e4.

59. Gahche J, Bailey R, Burt V, et al. Dietary supplement use among U.S. adults has increased since NHANES III (1988–1994). *NCHS Data Brief.* 2011;61:1-8.

60. Bailey RL, Lentino CV, Dwyer JT, et al. Dietary supplement use in the United States, 2003–2006. *J Nutr.* 2011;141(2):261-266.

61. Navarro VJ, Barnhart HX, Bonkovsky HL, et al. The rising burden of herbal and dietary supplement induced hepatotoxicity in the USA. (abstr). *Hepatology.* 2013;58:264A.

62. Bailey RL, Gahche JJ, Miller PE, Thomas PR, Dwyer JT. Why US adults use dietary supplements. *JAMA Intern Med.* 2013;173(5):355-361.

63. Komes D, Belščak-Cvitanović A, Horžić D, Rusak G, Likić S, Berendika M. Phenolic composition and antioxidant properties of some traditionally used medicinal plants affected by the extraction time and hydrolysis. *Phytochem Anal.* 2011;22(2):172-180.

64. Scheepmaker MM, Gower NT. The quality of selected South African and international homoeopathic mother tinctures. *Afr J Tradit Complement Altern Med.* 2011;8(5 suppl):46-52.

65. Sundaresan V, Sahni G, Verma RS, Padalia RC, Mehrotra S, Thul ST. Impact of geographic range on genetic and chemical diversity of Indian valerian (*Valeriana jatamansi*) from northwestern Himalaya. *Biochem Genet.* 2012;50(9-10):797-808.

66. Xiao W, Motley TJ, Unachukwu UJ, et al. Chemical and genetic assessment of variability in commercial Radix Astragali (*Astragalus* sp.) by ion trap LC-MS and nuclear ribosomal DNA barcoding sequence analyses. *J Agric Food Chem.* 2011;59(5):1548-1556.

67. Kneifel W, Czech E, Kopp B. Microbial contamination of medicinal plants—a review. *Planta Med.* 2002;68(1):5-15.

68. Saper RB, Phillips RS, Sehgal A, et al. Lead, mercury, and arsenic in US- and Indian-manufactured ayurvedic medicines sold via the internet. *JAMA.* 2008;300(8):915-923.

69. Ernst E. Heavy metals in traditional Indian remedies. *Eur J Clin Pharmacol.* 2002;57(12):891-896.

70. Stickel F, Droz S, Patsenker E, Bögli-Stuber K, Aebi B, Leib SL. Severe hepatotoxicity following ingestion of Herbalife nutritional supplements contaminated with *Bacillus subtilis. J Hepatol.* 2009;50(1):111-117.

71. Elsharkawy AM, McPherson S, Masson S, Burt AD, Dawson RT, Hudson M. Cholestasis secondary to anabolic steroid use in young men. *BMJ.* 2012;344:e468.

72. Haupt HA, Rovere GD. Anabolic steroids: a review of the literature. *Am J Sports Med.* 1984;12(6):469-484.

73. Ishak KG. Hepatic lesions caused by anabolic and contraceptive steroids. *Semin Liver Dis.* 1981;1(2):116-128.

74. Chojkier M. Hepatic sinusoidal-obstruction syndrome: toxicity of pyrrolizidine alkaloids. *J Hepatol.* 2003;39(3):437-446.

75. Stillman AS, Huxtable R, Consroe P, Kohnen P, Smith S. Hepatic veno-occlusive disease due to pyrrolizidine (Senecio) poisoning in Arizona. *Gastroenterology.* 1977;73(2):349-352.

76. Weston CF, Cooper BT, Davies JD, Levine DF. Veno-occlusive disease of the liver secondary to ingestion of comfrey. *Br Med J (Clin Res Ed).* 1987;295(6591):183.

77. Mohabbat O, Younos MS, Merzad AA, Srivastava RN, Sediq GG, Aram GN. An outbreak of hepatic veno-occlusive disease in north-western Afghanistan. *Lancet.* 1976;2(7980):269-271.

78. Tandon BN, Tandon HD, Tandon RK, Narendranathan M, Joshi YK. An epidemic of veno-occlusive disease of liver in central India. *Lancet.* 1976;2(7980):271-272.

79. Chalasani N, Vuppalanchi R, Navarro V, et al. Acute liver injury due to flavocoxid (Limbrel), a medical food for osteoarthritis: a case series. *Ann Intern Med.* 2012;156(12):857-860, W297–W300.

80. Blendon RJ, DesRoches CM, Benson JM, Brodie M, Altman DE. Americans' views on the use and regulation of dietary supplements. *Arch Intern Med.* 2001;161(6):805-810.

Benign Hepatic Neoplasms

L.F. Grochola | Henrik Petrowsky | Pierre-Alain Clavien

The widespread use and progress in modern imaging modalities have led to an increase in the incidental finding of asymptomatic benign hepatic lesions, including cystic and solid tumors. In contrast to most cystic lesions, the latter group is composed of tumors that often harbor true neoplastic characteristics. The most frequent benign solid lesions are hemangioma and focal nodular hyperplasia (FNH), which only rarely require treatment or long-term follow-up. Less frequent lesions include hepatocellular adenoma and angiomyolipoma, which carry a higher risk for complications, such as bleeding or malignant transformation, and therefore are more likely to necessitate surgical intervention. To account for these marked differences in biology and clinical characteristics between the different tumor types and ensure an accurate diagnosis, as well as an appropriate management of the patients, it is crucial to have a thorough understanding of clinical, biologic, radiologic, and pathologic characteristics of each liver lesion. Indeed, refinements in magnetic resonance imaging (MRI) and contrast-enhanced ultrasonography (ce-US) and computed tomography (ce-CT) allow an accurate diagnosis based only on imaging in a majority of cases and have thus reduced the need for percutaneous biopsy or surgical resection for definitive diagnosis. After the diagnosis has been established, the vast majority of benign hepatic neoplasms do not require surgical resection. However, indications for surgery include diagnostic uncertainty after an extensive diagnostic work-up, symptomatic patients, lesions with a mass effect on gastrointestinal (GI) organs or the biliary tree and tumors that have a potential for complications, as well as malignant transformation. In this chapter, we will cover solid benign hepatic lesions in adults and describe the etiology, clinical presentation, diagnostic work-up, and treatment strategy for each tumor type.

HEMANGIOMA

Hepatic hemangiomas are also termed cavernous hemangiomas and account for approximately 70% off all solid benign liver tumors.[1,2] The prevalence of this most common type of benign neoplasms of the liver is estimated to be in the range from 3% to 20% of the population (Table 131.1).[1,2] Cavernous hemangiomas have a female predilection, with a female-to-male ratio of 5 : 1, and are most frequently detected in middle-aged women.[1,2] They are usually small (<5 cm). Lesions that are larger than 10 cm have been arbitrarily termed giant hemangiomas.[3] Hemangiomas are often solitary, even though multiple lesions may be present in up to 40% of patients.[4] If more than one lesion is present, these are usually located in the same hepatic lobe.[4,5]

Hemangiomas appear as dark purple, soft, and compressible lesions that are well demarcated and frequently surrounded by a thin capsule.[3] They arise from endothelial cells that build multiple vascular channels, supported by fibrous septa, resulting in cavernous vascular spaces lined by endothelium and separated by connective tissue.[6] They obtain their blood supply mainly from the hepatic artery and lack biliary or portal structures.[6] By immunohistochemistry, the endothelium displays vascular as opposed to sinusoidal differentiation.[6] Large tumors may have necrotic areas or dystrophic calcifications, and their lumens are often occluded by thrombi, which are caused by prothrombic conditions in these irregularly shaped vascular structures.[3]

Hemangiomas are typically asymptomatic hepatic lesions that are incidentally discovered at laparotomy, autopsy, or during routine imaging studies for unrelated reasons.[7] If symptoms are present, those are mostly observed in patients with giant hemangiomas and include abdominal pain and discomfort.[8] Very large hemangiomas can cause mass effects due to their size, such as early satiety by gastric compression, biliary stasis, or vascular obstruction.[8,9] Rupture is an extremely rare complication, even in very large hemangiomas or during pregnancy.[10] Rarely, thrombosis of a part of the hemangioma can lead to an inflammatory reaction, which can result in abdominal pain accompanied by slight fever, loss of weight, anemia, thrombocytosis, and increased levels of fibrinogen.[11] The adult Kasabach-Merritt syndrome constitutes a related but even less frequent complication, which mainly occurs in giant hepatic hemangioma but can also be observed in other vascular liver lesions.[12] It is a local consumptive coagulopathy, which is caused by an intravascular coagulation, clotting, and fibrinolysis within the hemangioma.[12] These effects can in turn lead to a secondary increase in systemic fibrinolysis and thrombocytopenia and result in a systemic disseminated intravascular coagulation, which is associated with a high mortality (30% to 40%) as a result of uncontrollable bleeding.[12,13] This complication is reversible by surgical removal of the hemangioma.[12,13]

ETIOLOGY

Hepatic hemangioma is considered to be a vascular malformation or a hamartoma of congenital origin. Enlargement occurs by ectasia rather than hypertrophy or hyperplasia. The observation that hemangiomas have a clear female predilection, are mostly diagnosed in middle-aged women, and show an accelerated growth during puberty and pregnancy and with oral contraceptive use has led to the hypothesis that estrogen has a causative role for growth of hemangiomas.[14] However, these associations have not been consistently found, and the expression of sex hormone receptors could not be clearly linked to

TABLE 131.1 Differential Diagnosis of Benign Hepatic Neoplasms

	Cavernous Hemangioma	Focal Nodular Hyperplasia	Hepatocellular Adenoma
Prevalence	3%–20%	1%	<0.05%
Pathogenesis	Vascular malformation, congenital	Hyperplastic response to vascular malformation, hereditary	Steroid hormones (estrogen, progesterone, androgen), NASH, type I and III glycogen storage disease
Imaging	ce-US, ce-CT, MRI	ce-US, ce-CT, MRI	US, ce-CT, MRI
α-Fetoprotein	Normal	Normal	Normal
Macroscopic features	Dark purple, soft, compressible lesions that are well demarcated and frequently surrounded by a thin capsule; blood-filled "cyst"	Light brown, well-circumscribed lobulated tumor without capsule and a central scar	Well-circumscribed masses with a pseudocapsule of compressed hepatic parenchyma. Areas of inhomogeneous, yellow-brown lipid-rich tissue, as well as hemorrhage, necrosis, and calcifications
Microscopic features	Cavernous vascular spaces lined by endothelium and separated by connective tissue; no biliary or portal structures	Normal hepatocytes arranged in thickened plates, containing Kupffer cells and hepatocyte-derived biliary ductules at the interface between fibrous bands and nodules, no bile ducts	Composed of large lipid and glycogen-containing hepatocytes arranged in plates, separated by dilated sinusoids that are fed by arterial perfusion
Complications	Mass effect, inflammatory reaction, Kasabach-Merritt syndrome	Mass effect, torsion of pedunculated FNH	Mass effect, inflammatory reaction, bleeding, hemorrhagic shock
Malignant transformation	No	No	Yes. Risk factors for malignant transformation include male gender, androgen use, b-HCA subtype and tumor diameter >5 cm
Treatment	Surgical enucleation or resection only if symptomatic; Liver transplantation, embolization and radiation if unresectable	Surgical resection if symptomatic or pedunculated; cessation of hormonal therapy not recommended	Indication for surgical resection depends on size, gender, adenoma subtype. Liver transplantation in exceptional circumstances; discontinue hormonal therapy

b-HCA, β-Catenin–mutated hepatocellular adenoma; *ce-US,* contrast-enhanced ultrasound; *ce-CT,* contrast-enhanced computed tomography; *FNH,* focal nodular hyperplasia; *MRI,* magnetic resonance imaging; *NASH,* nonalcoholic steatohepatitis; *US,* ultrasound.

hemangioma growth, and therefore the estrogen-driven theory has not been proven to date.[14,15]

DIAGNOSIS

Hemangiomas can often be unequivocally identified by imaging studies because of their typical radiographic features. On ultrasonography hemangiomas appear as a well-defined hyperechoic mass with acoustic enhancement and sharp margins.[3,16] However, larger lesions often have an atypical appearance because of calcifications or lumen occlusion by thrombi.[3] In a fatty liver the lesion might actually appear hypoechoic compared with the surrounding parenchyma on ultrasound. When standard ultrasound does not provide an unequivocal diagnosis, contrast-enhanced examinations are necessary to differentiate the hemangioma from other lesions. Typical findings of such contrast-enhanced examinations, which include ce-US, ce-CT, and MRI, are rapid peripheral and nodular enhancement on arterial phases, followed by centripetal filling of the lesion (Fig. 131.1).[16,17] To date, MRI is considered to be the best imaging modality for the detection and characterization of hemangioma.[3] Typical findings are hypointensity on T1-weighted sequences and strong

hyperintensity on T2-weighted sequences. On diffusion-weighted MRI sequences, the signal of hemangioma weakens with increasing b-values, and consequently the apparent diffusion coefficient value is high.[3] However, calcified, hyalinized, sclerotic, cystic or pedunculated hemangiomas, as well as very slow filling lesions or hemangiomas with fluid-fluid level or capsular retraction can have an atypical MRI appearance and require the use of additional imaging modalities.[18] Scintigraphy with technetium 99m pertechnetate–labeled erythrocytes documents gradual accumulation of red blood cells inside the hepatic lesion.[19] Although the specificity is extremely high and can be further improved by using single-photon emission CT (SPECT), the technique is cumbersome and infrequently used. Hepatic angiography is also rarely used for diagnosis; yet it can be helpful in selected cases in which definitive diagnosis cannot be established by noninvasive imaging modalities. Classic angiographic features include the characteristic "cotton wool" appearance that circumscribes a large feeding vessel with displacement and diffuse pooling of intravenous contrast material. Percutaneous biopsy has a low diagnostic yield and carries the risk of severe bleeding complications.[20] Therefore biopsies are

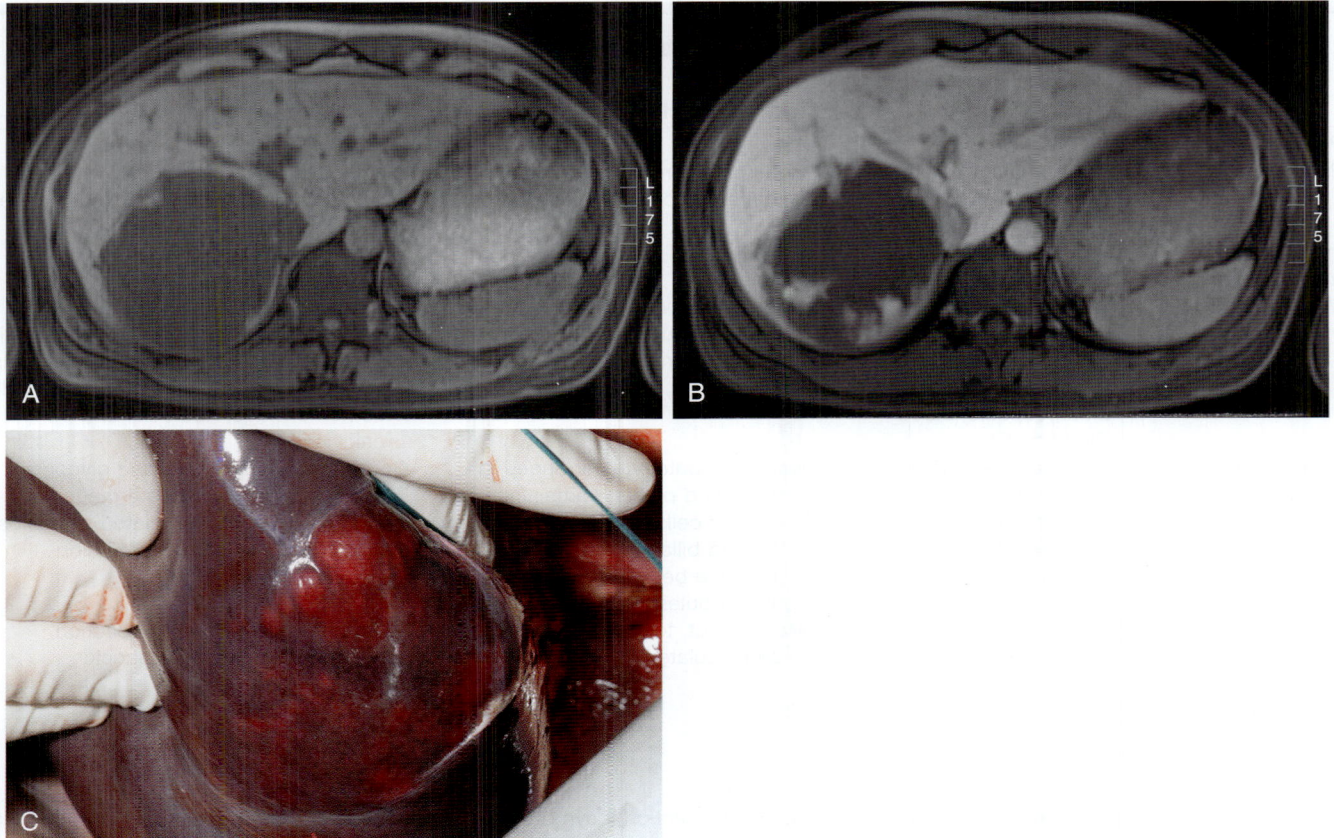

FIGURE 131.1 A typical hemangioma on magnetic resonance imaging. (A) The lesion located in the right liver lobe is hypointense on a precontrast T1 sequence and (B) shows a peripheral and nodular enhancement on a portal venous phase. (C) Intraoperative image of this lesion, which has a typical, well-demarcated, dark purple appearance.

limited to exceptional cases when diagnosis remains uncertain after the use of all available imaging modalities and techniques (Fig. 131.2).

TREATMENT

Most patients with hemangiomas do not have any symptoms or complications and therefore do not require any treatment.[21] One series observed 97% of 249 patients with liver hemangioma for up to 14 years without adverse events or morphologic changes of the lesions.[5] It has been concluded that asymptomatic patients with a firmly established diagnosis do not need to undergo serial imaging studies and a further follow-up is routinely not recommended.[3] Women should neither discontinue oral contraception nor avoid pregnancy, and any specific advice regarding physical activities is also not justified.[3]

Surgical intervention is necessary only in a small subset of patients.[22] Indications for surgery include diagnostic uncertainty, severe symptoms, extrinsic compression of adjacent structures, inflammatory reaction, the Kasabach-Merritt syndrome, and the extremely rare spontaneous rupture.[1,2,5,12] The most important surgical options include formal resection or enucleation using both open and laparoscopic techniques, following the same rules as for all other liver tumors. Enucleation is possible because

of a pseudocapsule of compressed hepatic parenchyma between the hemangioma and the surrounding tissue.[23] This technique offers the presumed advantage of maximal preservation of functional liver tissue and does not involve the transection of biliary structures.[24] However, overall the advantages of enucleation are small, and we prefer standard liver resection for hemangioma. Occasionally, giant hemangiomas can be technically challenging to resect, and special surgical techniques, such as total vascular exclusion, must be used. In the extraordinary case of a technically unresectable, complicated giant hemangioma, liver transplantation can be considered as a feasible treatment option.[25] In patients who do not qualify for surgical resection because of medical or technical reasons, arterial embolization or radiation therapy may be used as therapeutic alternatives.[26,27] In the Kasabach-Merritt syndrome, the gold standard treatment is the removal of the underlying hemangioma, which will correct the consumptive coagulopathy. However, surgical resection of the hemangioma under these circumstances could be hazardous in the presence of uncontrolled coagulopathy secondary to disseminated intravascular coagulation (DIC). Therefore, perioperative administration of fresh-frozen plasma and platelet concentrates may reduce perioperative bleeding.[13]

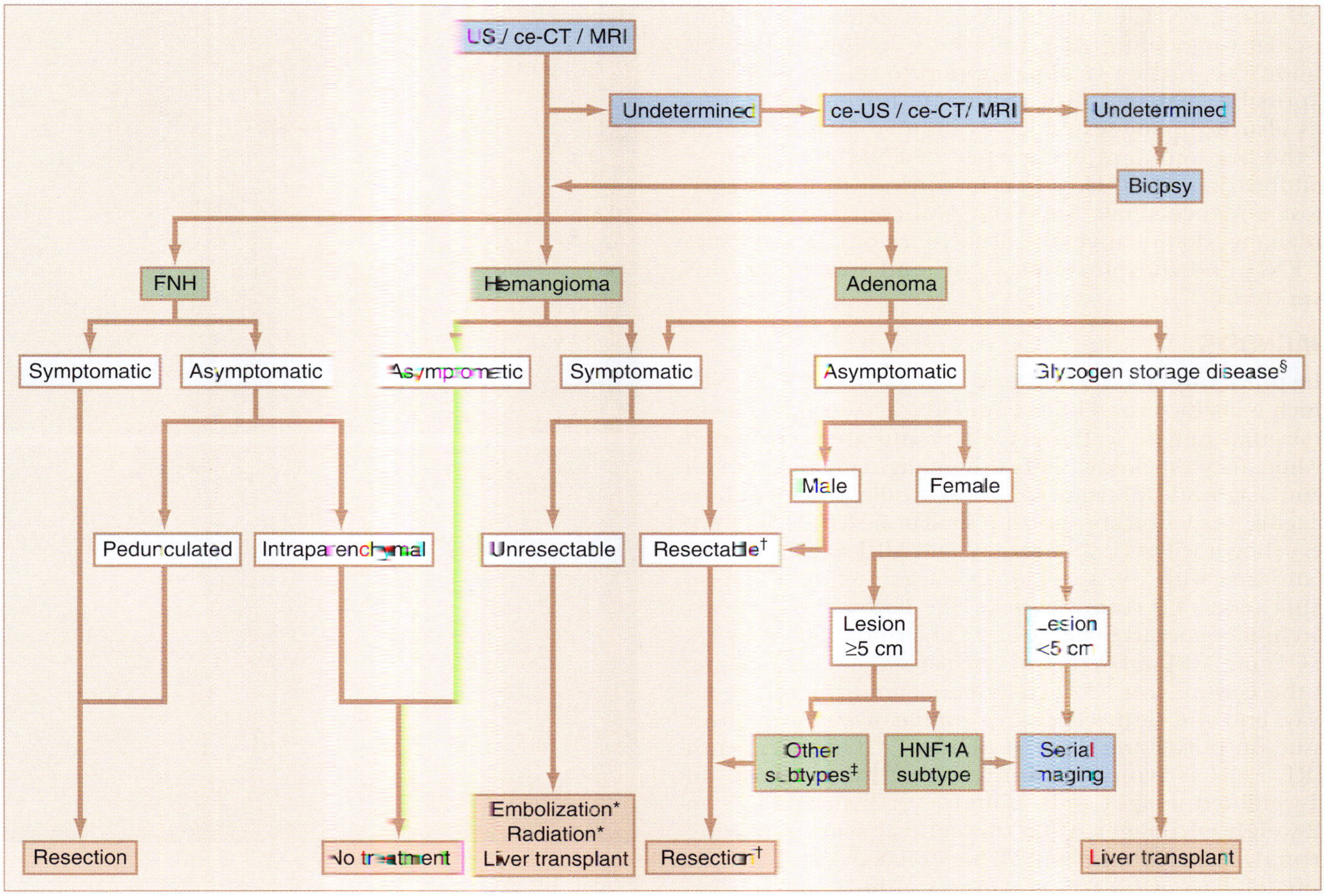

FIGURE 131.2 Flowchart depicting the diagnostic and therapeutic management for suspected focal benign liver lesion (hemangioma, FNH, adenoma) in noncirrhotic patients. *Embolization and radiation are accepted treatment options for hemangioma. †Instead of resection, enucleation of a hemangioma can be performed. ‡IHCA, b-HCA, unclassified subtypes. §Glycogen storage diseases that are indications for liver transplantation include glycogenosis type 1a (defect in G6PC gene), type 4 (GBE1 gene defect) and type 9 (PHKG2 gene defect), whereby type 1a glycogenosis shows the strongest association with adenomatosis.[55] ce-US, Contrast-enhanced ultrasound; ce-CT, contrast-enhanced computed tomography; FNH, focal nodular hyperplasia; MRI, magnetic resonance imaging; IHCA, inflammatory hepatocellular adenoma; b-HCA, β catenin–mutated hepatocellular adenoma; HNF1A, HNF1α-mutated hepatocellular adenoma.

FOCAL NODULAR HYPERPLASIA

FNH is the second most common benign hepatic tumor. Similar to hemangioma, FNH also shows a large predominance in middle-aged women, with a female-to-male ratio of 8:1 (see Table 131.1).[28,29] The lesions are usually less than 5 cm in diameter and solitary in 80% of cases.[28,29] Only 3% are larger than 10 cm, although FNH of up to 19 cm have been reported.[28,29] Macroscopically, FNH appears as a light brown, well-circumscribed lobulated tumor. In contrast to hemangioma, FNH lacks a capsule and has a central scar around a prominent arterial vessel with fibrous septa radiating outward. Histology reveals morphologically normal hepatocytes arranged in thickened plates. FNH contains Kupffer cells and hepatocyte-derived biliary ductules at the interface between fibrous bands and nodules but lacks actual bile ducts. Atypical or nonclassical forms of FNH exist, constituting as much as 20% in series of resected cases; these include telangiectatic FNH, a mixed hyperplastic and adenomatous form, and FNH with cytologic atypia.[29]

Similar to hemangiomas, patients with FNH are usually asymptomatic and the tumors are discovered incidentally.[21] Infrequently, symptoms are reported by patients with large lesions and include abdominal pain and discomfort, which is mostly caused by a mass effect with compression of adjacent GI organs.[3] Other rare symptoms are acute onset of abdominal pain due to the torsion of a pedunculated FNH or a mild elevation of bilirubin, alkaline phosphatase, and liver blood tests owing to extrinsic compression of intrahepatic biliary ducts or vascular structures.[3] Complications such as rupture or bleeding are extremely rare, and malignant transformation of an FNH has not been documented thus far.

ETIOLOGY

FNH develops as a hyperplastic, regenerative response to malformed arterial structures. This theory is supported by the observation that FNH associates with other vascular malformations and hereditary diseases, such as hepatic hemangioma and hereditary hemorrhagic telangiectasia (Osler-Weber-Rendu disease)[30,3] In addition, molecular analyses of FNH lesions suggest that genes involved in vascular remodeling are significantly deregulated in this tumor type, further lending support to this hypothesis.[32] A possible association with female hormonal factors has also been suggested as a causative factor because of the predominant occurrence of FNH in women of childbearing age.[33] However, in contrast to this theory, most evidence shows that both oral contraception and pregnancy do not affect the occurrence or characteristics of FNH and therefore does not lend support to this hypothesis[33,34]

DIAGNOSIS

The previously described histopathologic findings of FNH, which is characterized by a central fibrous scar and fibrous septa that radiate to the periphery and are surrounded by hepatocytes, closely reflect the imaging features of all main diagnostic modalities.[35,36] Specifically, on precontrast imaging, the lesion appears with similar or slightly different US echogenicity, CT attenuation, and MRI signal intensity compared with the surrounding liver tissue.[35,36] Upon application of a contrast agent, the lesion shows strong and homogeneous enhancement on arterial phase ce-US, ce-CT, and MRI with a central vascular supply and a sparing of the central scar.[35,36] This enhancement rapidly fades away, and the signal becomes similar to adjacent liver tissue on portal and delayed phases.[35,36] On precontrast MRI, FNH is typically isointense or hypointense on T1-weighted images and isointense or hyperintense on T2-weighted images, with the central scar appearing strongly hyperintense on T2 sequences[36] (Fig. 131.3). Hepatobiliary MRI contrast agents can be used to underscore the hepatocellular origin of the tumors and distinguish it from hepatic adenomas. In addition, the presence of Kupffer cells in FNH leads to an uptake of superparamagnetic iron oxide (SPIO) contrast agents, which can help to differentiate it from adenoma on MRI. The same effect can be used by scintigraphy with technetium 99m–sulfur colloid. Angiography demonstrates a "spoked wheel" appearance but is usually not indicated for diagnosis. We do not advocate biopsy unless diagnostic uncertainty persists after all available imaging modalities have been exhausted, because of its low diagnostic yield with false-negative diagnosis rates of up to 30%.[37]

TREATMENT

The vast majority of patients with FNH have no symptoms and do not require surgical treatment. In asymptomatic patients with a firmly established diagnosis of FNH, a further follow-up is not recommended, and female patients should not be advised to avoid oral contraceptive use or pregnancy.[3] In the presence of symptomatic FNH, the most frequent indications for operative treatment are mass effect symptoms on digestive organs or the biliary tree. Resection is furthermore indicated in patients with pedunculated lesions due to the risk of pedicle torsion and when diagnosis cannot be established with the available imaging techniques. Due to the presence of large veins, which frequently surround the lesion, liver resection is preferred over enucleation. This can be performed laparoscopically or by traditional open partial hepatectomy.

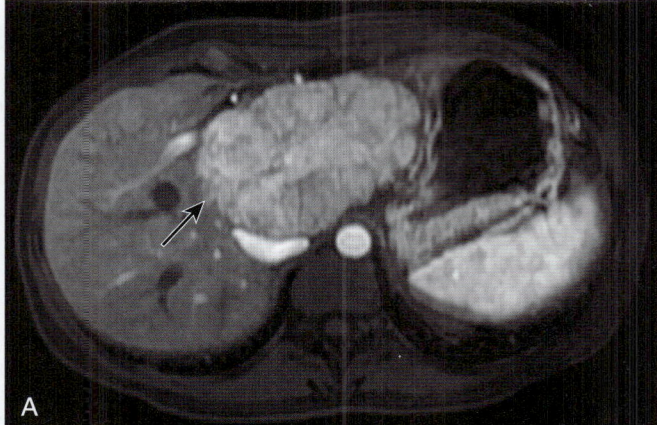

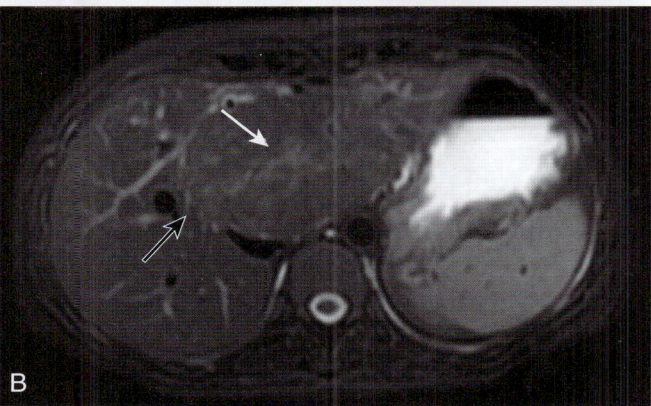

FIGURE 131.3 Dynamic contrast-enhanced magnetic resonance imaging of a focal nodular hyperplasia located in the left liver lobe. (A) The lesion *(black arrow)* shows strong enhancement on the arterial phase and (B) contains a central scar *(white arrow)* that is hyperintense on T2-weighted sequences.

HEPATIC ADENOMA

Hepatic adenoma, or hepatocellular adenoma, is a rare benign hepatic neoplasm that typically affects young women of childbearing age (see Table 131.1).[38] Since the introduction of oral contraceptive pills (OCPs) in the early 1960s, it has become increasingly apparent that long-term use of OCPs is associated with a 30-fold increase in hepatic adenoma incidence, as illustrated by numerous epidemiologic outcome studies.[39] With the advent of newer low-dose estrogen and/or progesterone formulations, the incidence of hepatic adenomas is declining again. Approximately 30% of patients have multiple adenomas, and the presence of multiple such tumors in all liver segments is called adenomatosis.[40] The latter condition represents a distinct disease entity because it is associated with rare genetic syndromes, including glycogen storage diseases (particularly type 1a glycogenosis), and there is no relationship with hormone exposure.[3,40] Hepatic adenoma is thought to be a heterogeneous disease that comprises four main tumor subtypes with distinct clinical and radiologic characteristics.[3,41] This distinction is mainly based on different mutation patterns in those four subtypes and includes the HNF1α-mutated hepatocellular adenoma (HNF1A), inflammatory hepatocellular adenoma (IHCA),

TABLE 131.2 Subtype Classification of Hepatocellular Adenoma

	HNF1α–Mutated	β-Catenin Activated	NONMUTATED	
			Inflammatory	Noninflammatory
Prevalence (relative)	Common	Rare	Rare	Rare
Histologic hallmarks	Marked steatosis	Pseudoglandular formations and cellular atypias; enlarged, irregular, and hyperchromatic nuclei	Clusters of small arteries surrounded by extracellular matrix, inflammatory infiltrates, sinusoidal dilatation or congestion	No specific histologic features
Steatosis	Frequent	Rare	Moderate	Moderate
Cytologic abnormalities	Very rare	Frequent	Moderate	Rare
Inflammatory infiltrates	Very rare	Rare	Yes	None
Pseudoglandular formation	Rare	Frequent	Very rare	Very rare
Specific complications	None	Malignant transformation	Bleeding, inflammatory syndrome	Rarely malignant transformation
Management for tumors <5 cm in females	Follow-up with annual imaging (at least 1 year)	Follow-up with annual imaging (at least 5 years)	Follow-up with biannual imaging (at least 5 years)	Follow-up with annual imaging (at least 5 years)
Management for tumors >5 cm in females	Regular follow-up with imaging	Resection	Resection	Resection
Management for all tumor sizes in males	Resection	Resection	Resection	Resection

β-catenin–mutated hepatocellular adenoma (b-HCA), and unclassified subtypes (Table 131.2)[3,41] Macroscopically, adenomas are well-circumscribed masses with a pseudocapsule of compressed hepatic parenchyma. The cut surface is inhomogeneous, displaying areas of yellow-brown lipid-rich tissue, as well as hemorrhage, necrosis, and calcifications. Histologically, adenomas are composed of large lipid- and glycogen-containing hepatocytes arranged in plates, separated by dilated sinusoids that are fed by arterial perfusion. In contrast to FNH, adenoma contains few or no Kupffer cells and contains no bile ductules.

Similar to hepatic hemangiomas and FNH, the vast majority of patients with hepatocellular adenomas are asymptomatic and the lesions are discovered incidentally during imaging studies for unrelated medical conditions.[21] The most common symptom is abdominal pain, and some patients with IHCA can present with an inflammatory syndrome that includes fever.[42] A frequent complication of hepatic adenoma is bleeding, which can lead to a sudden onset of abdominal pain and even hemorrhagic shock.[43,44] It occurs in approximately 25% of all patients, specifically those with large tumors (≥ cm).[43,44] Other risk factors for hemorrhage include lesional arteries, the IHCA subtype, location of the tumor in the left lateral liver, and exophytic growth.[43–4] Importantly, in contrast to other frequent benign hepatic neoplasms, hepatocellular adenomas harbor the risk of malignant transformation, whereby the overall risk is estimated to be in the range from 4% to 5%.[45] The risk for malignant transformation differs strongly between individuals, whereby the risk factors include male gender (8- to 10-fold increased risk), tumor diameter of greater than 5 cm, androgen use, and b-HCA subtype.[44,45]

ETIOLOGY

Although the underlying molecular mechanisms are not well understood, the association of steroid hormones and OCP use with the development of hepatic adenomas is well established.[39] Specifically, two-thirds of hepatic adenomas express estrogen and progesterone receptors, and enlargement or even rupture has been reported during pregnancy.[46] An increased risk of hepatic adenoma has also been noted with the use of androgen preparations, such as in aplastic anemia, hypogonadism, hypopituitarism, and other endocrine disorders.[47] Furthermore, the illicit use of androgens by bodybuilders has also been reported to promote hepatic adenoma formation.[48] Hepatocellular adenomas have also been increasingly reported in patients with nonalcoholic steatohepatitis (NASH).[49] Other predisposing conditions are type I and III glycogen storage disease, in which adenomas predominantly affect male patients.[50]

DIAGNOSIS

Due to improvements in imaging techniques, the accurate diagnosis of hepatic adenoma can be made without a percutaneous biopsy or surgical resection in the vast majority of patients. Hereby, of all available imaging modalities, to date the highest sensitivity (up to 91%) and specificity (up to 100%) has been shown for MRI imaging, owing in part to the availability of fat-suppressed sequences.[3,51,52] It can help to differentiate the various subtypes of hepatic adenomas. For example, HNF1A adenomas are homogeneous on MRI and have a variable signal on T2 sequences (Fig. 131.4).[51,52] Other features include a slight hyperintensity on non–fat-suppressed

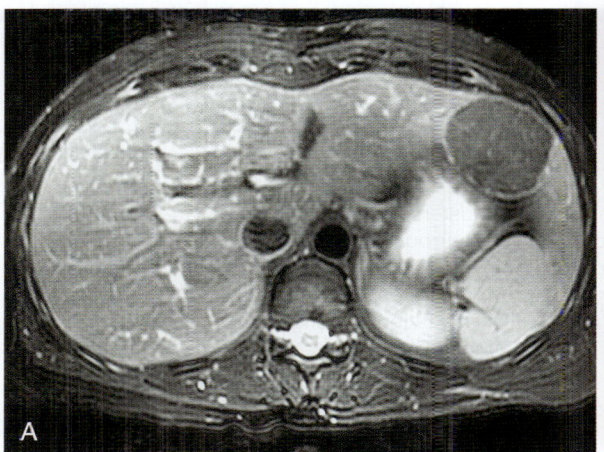
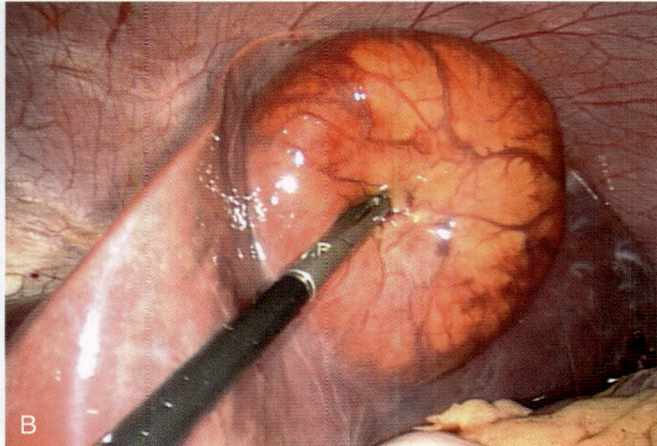

FIGURE 131.4 (A) Hepatic adenoma in the left lateral segment presenting as a T2-weighted hypointense encapsulated lesion. (B) Laparoscopic view of the lesion.

sequences and isointensity or hypointensity on T2-weighted fat-suppressed sequences.[51,52] In addition, they are characterized by a diffuse and homogeneous signal dropout on chemical shift T1-weighted images.[51,52] In contrast to FNH, hepatocellular adenomas usually show only mild to moderate arterial enhancement with significantly higher contrast enhancement ratios on arterial phase images.[53] However, the histologic variation in liver adenomas is known to affect the degree of arterial enhancement whereby inflammatory subtypes can also show strong arterial enhancement similar to that of FNH.[53] Therefore, and despite those marked advances in noninvasive diagnostic techniques, an accurate diagnosis may not be possible in a small subset of patients, and percutaneous biopsy may be necessary to differentiate hepatic adenomas from FNH or identify b-HCA subtypes.[44]

TREATMENT

Treatment recommendations for adenoma are based on the previously described risk factors for complications and malignant transformation, most importantly tumor size, subtype, and gender.[3,33,44] Due to the high risk of malignancy in male patients, hepatic adenomas should be resected independent of the tumor size or subtype of the lesion.[3,33,44] Female patients with tumors smaller than 5 cm in diameter can be closely followed for at least 5 years after cessation of hormonal therapy with annual or biannual MRI surveillance, dependent on the tumor subtype (biannual imaging for the IHCA subtype and annual imaging for non-IHCA lesions).[3,33,44] For female patients with tumors larger than 5 cm, some centers advocate conservative management with regular follow-up for the HNF1A subtype due to its presumed very low risk of complications.[3,33,44] With regard to other adenoma subtypes larger than 5 cm, a resection is always indicated because of the high risk of malignant transformation and complications.[3,33,44] Liver transplantation is reserved for symptomatic unresectable hepatocellular adenoma and patients with liver adenomatosis associated with glycogen storage disease unresponsive to medical treatment.[54,55] Emerging evidence suggests that radiofrequency ablation can be considered as a therapeutic option for adenomas smaller than 4 cm in diameter. However, follow-up data are currently lacking to clearly support routine clinical use.[56,57]

OTHER BENIGN TUMORS

A variety of rare benign tumors that occur in the liver have been described, such as bile duct adenoma, biliary hamartomas (von Meyenburg complexes), solitary fibrous tumors, schwannoma, lipoma, leiomyoma, teratoma, lymphangioma, and peliosis. Among them are also angiomyolipomas, rare mesenchymal tumors derived from perivascular epithelioid cells, which mostly occur in the kidney but sometimes also appear in the liver.[58] They can be associated with tuberous sclerosis and are most commonly diagnosed in women between 30 and 50 years of age.[59] Most lesions are asymptomatic and are found incidentally during routine imaging. The accuracy of diagnosis using imaging techniques is low due to the inconsistent appearance of angiomyolipomas.[3] This inconsistent appearance is caused by the varying content of the components of this lesion, including smooth muscle cells, adipose tissue, and blood vessels, and liver biopsy is often necessary to distinguish it from other solid lesions.[3,60] Surveillance with serial imaging is recommended in patients without symptoms whose lesions are smaller than 5 cm in diameter.[60] Lesions larger than 5 cm should be resected due to a high risk of malignant transformation.[61]

Inflammatory pseudotumor of the liver (IPL) is another rare benign lesion that can mimic cholangiocarcinoma.[62,63] It is a reactive fibroblastic proliferation infiltrated by polymorph inflammatory cells. The lesion is symptomatic in a majority of cases and can cause fever, abdominal pain, weight loss, and jaundice.[63] Diagnosis of IPL is challenging because imaging studies often show diffuse and infiltrative large tumors, and multiple forms of this lesion can be found.[64] The low diagnostic accuracy of imaging techniques results in the frequent need for liver biopsy to rule out other differential diagnoses, such as cholangiocarcinoma, autoimmune cholangiopathy, and primary sclerosing cholangitis.[3] Because IPL constitutes a benign condition without malignant potential, medical treatment by antibiotics, steroids, and observation is justified, which has been shown to result in complete regression rates in more than 90% of patients.[363]

REFERENCES

1. Choi BY, Nguyen MH. The diagnosis and management of benign hepatic tumors. *J Clin Gastroenterol.* 2005;39:401-412.
2. Toro A, Mahfouz AE, Ardiri A, et al. What is changing in indications and treatment of hepatic hemangiomas: a review. *Ann Hepatol.* 2014;13:327-339.
3. Belghiti J, Cauchy F, Paradis V, Vilgrain V. Diagnosis and management of solid benign liver lesions. *Nat Rev Gastroenterol Hepatol.* 2014;11:737-749.
4. Tait N, Richardson AJ, Muguti G, Little JM. Hepatic cavernous haemangioma: a 10 year review. *Aust N Z J Surg.* 1992;62:521-524.
5. Herman P, Costa ML, Machado MA, et al. Management of hepatic hemangiomas: a 14-year experience. *J Gastrointest Surg.* 2005;9:853-859.
6. Duff B, Weigel JA, Bourne P, Weigel PH, McGary CT. Endothelium in hepatic cavernous hemangioma does not express the hyaluronan receptor for endocytosis. *Hum Pathol.* 2002;33:265-269.
7. Trotter JF, Everson GT. Benign focal lesions of the liver. *Clin Liver Dis.* 2001;5:17-42, v.
8. Erdogan D, Busch OR, van Delden OM, et al. Management of liver hemangiomas according to size and symptoms. *J Gastroenterol Hepatol.* 2007;22:1953-1958.
9. Kim DY, Pantelic MV, Yoshida A, Jerius J, Abouljoud MS. Cavernous hemangioma presenting as Budd-Chiari syndrome. *J Am Coll Surg.* 2005;200:470-471.
10. Cobey FC, Salem RR. A review of liver masses in pregnancy and a proposed algorithm for their diagnosis and management. *Am J Surg.* 2004;187:181-191.
11. Bornman PC, Terblanche J, Blumgart RL, Jones EP, Pickard H, Kalvaria I. Giant hepatic hemangiomas: diagnosis and therapeutic dilemmas. *Surgery.* 1987;101:445-449.
12. Concejero AM, Chen CL, Chen TY, Eng HL, Kuo FY. Giant cavernous hemangioma of the liver with coagulopathy: adult Kasabach-Merritt syndrome. *Surgery.* 2009;145:245-247.
13. McCormack L, Petrowsky H, Clavien PA. Image of the month. Kasabach-Merritt syndrome in a giant cavernous liver hemangioma. *Arch Surg.* 2007;142:399-400.
14. Glinkova V, Shevah O, Boaz M, Levin A, Shirin H. Hepatic haemangiomas: possible association with female sex hormones. *Gut.* 2004;53:1352-1355.
15. Gemer O, Moscovici O, Ben-Horin CL, Linov L, Peled R, Segal S. Oral contraceptives and liver hemangioma: a case-control study. *Acta Obstet Gynecol Scand.* 2004;83:1199-1201.
16. von Herbay A, Vogt C, Willers R, Häussinger D. Real-time imaging with the sonographic contrast agent SonoVue: differentiation between benign and malignant hepatic lesions. *J Ultrasound Med.* 2004;23:1557-1568.
17. Quaia E, Bertolotto M, Dalla Palma L. Characterization of liver hemangiomas with pulse inversion harmonic imaging. *Eur Radiol.* 2002;12:537-544.
18. Coumbaras M, Wendum D, Monnier-Cholley L, Dahan H, Tubiana JM, Arrivé L. CT and MR imaging features of pathologically proven atypical giant hemangiomas of the liver. *AJR Am J Roentgenol.* 2002;179:1457-1463.
19. Farlow DC, Chapman PR, Gruenewald SM, Ananda VF, Farrell GC, Little JM. Investigation of focal hepatic lesions: is tomographic red blood cell imaging useful? *World J Surg.* 1990;14:463-467.
20. Yoon SS, Charny CK, Fong Y, et al. Diagnosis, management, and outcomes of 115 patients with hepatic hemangioma. *J Am Coll Surg.* 2003;197:392-402.
21. Charny CK, Jarnagin WR, Schwartz LH, et al. Management of 155 patients with benign liver tumours. *Br J Surg.* 2001;88:808-813.
22. Farges O, Daradkeh S, Bismuth H. Cavernous hemangiomas of the liver: are there any indications for resection? *World J Surg.* 1995;19:19-24.
23. Baer HU, Dennison AR, Mouton W, Stain SC, Zimmermann A, Blumgart LH. Enucleation of giant hemangiomas of the liver.

24. Kuo PC, Lewis WD, Jenkins RL. Treatment of giant hemangiomas of the liver by enucleation. *J Am Coll Surg.* 1994;178:49-53.
25. Ercolani G, Grazi GL, Pinna AD. Liver transplantation for benign hepatic tumors: a systematic review. *Dig Surg.* 2010;27:68-75.
26. Deutsch GS, Yeh KA, Bates WB 3rd, Tannehill WB. Embolization for management of hepatic hemangiomas. *Am Surg.* 2001;67:159-164.
27. Gaspar L, Mascarenhas F, da Costa MS, Dias JS, Afonso JG, Silvestre ME. Radiation therapy in the unresectable cavernous hemangioma of the liver. *Radiother Oncol.* 1993;29:45-50.
28. Wanless IR. Benign liver tumors. *Clin Liver Dis.* 2002;6:513-526, ix.
29. Nguyen BN, Flejou JF, Terris B, Belghiti J, Degott C. Focal nodular hyperplasia of the liver: a comprehensive pathologic study of 305 lesions and recognition of new histologic forms. *Am J Surg Pathol.* 1999;23:1441-1454.
30. Mathieu D, Zafrani ES, Anglade MC, Dhumeaux D. Association of focal nodular hyperplasia and hepatic hemangioma. *Gastroenterology.* 1989;97:154-157.
31. Buscarini E, Danesino C, Plauchu H, et al. High prevalence of hepatic focal nodular hyperplasia in subjects with hereditary hemorrhagic teleangiectasia. *Ultrasound Med Biol.* 2004;30:1089-1097.
32. Paradis V, Bieche I, Dargere D, et al. A quantitative gene expression study suggests a role for angiopoietins in focal nodular hyperplasia. *Gastroenterology.* 2003;124:651-659.
33. Mathieu D, Kobeiter H, Maison P, et al. Oral contraceptive use and focal nodular hyperplasia of the liver. *Gastroenterology.* 2000;118:560-564.
34. Scalori A, Tavani A, Gallus S, La Vecchia C, Colombo M. Oral contraceptives and the risk of focal nodular hyperplasia of the liver: a case-control study. *Am J Obstet Gynecol.* 2002;186:195-197.
35. Hussain SM, Terkivatan T, Zondervan PE, et al. Focal nodular hyperplasia: findings at state-of-the-art MR imaging, US, CT, and pathologic analysis. *Radiographics.* 2004;24:3-17; discussion 18-19.
36. Mortele KJ, Praet M, Van Vlierberghe H, Kunnen M, Ros PR. CT and MR imaging findings in focal nodular hyperplasia of the liver: radiologic-pathologic correlation. *AJR Am J Roentgenol.* 2000;175:687-692.
37. Fabre A, Audet P, Vilgrain V, et al. Histologic scoring of liver biopsy in focal nodular hyperplasia with atypical presentation. *Hepatology.* 2002;35:414-420.
38. Nault JC, Bioulac-Sage P, Zucman-Rossi J. Hepatocellular benign tumors—from molecular classification to personalized clinical care. *Gastroenterology.* 2013;144:888-902.
39. Rooks JB, Ory HW, Ishak KG, et al. Epidemiology of hepatocellular adenoma. The role of oral contraceptive use. *J Am Med Assoc.* 1979;242:644-648.
40. Flejou JF, Barge J, Menu Y, et al. Liver adenomatosis. An entity distinct from liver adenoma? *Gastroenterology.* 1985;89:1132-1138.
41. Zucman-Rossi J, Jeannot E, Nhieu JT, et al. Genotype-phenotype correlation in hepatocellular adenoma: new classification and relationship with HCC. *Hepatology.* 2006;43:515-524.
42. Paradis V, Champault A, Ronot M, et al. Telangiectatic adenoma: an entity associated with increased body mass index and inflammation. *Hepatology.* 2007;46:140-146.
43. Stoot JH, van der Linden E, Terpstra OT, Schaapherder AF. Life-saving therapy for haemorrhaging liver adenomas using selective arterial embolization. *Br J Surg.* 2007;94:1249-1253.
44. Dokmak S, Paradis V, Vilgrain V, et al. A single-center surgical experience of 122 patients with single and multiple hepatocellular adenomas. *Gastroenterology.* 2009;137:1698-1705.
45. Stoot JH, Coelen RJ, De Jong MC, Dejong CH. Malignant transformation of hepatocellular adenomas into hepatocellular carcinomas: a systematic review including more than 1600 adenoma cases. *HPB (Oxford).* 2010;12:509-522.
46. Torbenson M, Lee JH, Choti M, et al. Hepatic adenomas: analysis of sex steroid receptor status and the Wnt signaling pathway. *Mod Pathol.* 2002;15:189-196.
47. Velazquez I, Alter BP. Androgens and liver tumors: Fanconi's anemia and non-Fanconi's conditions. *Am J Hematol.* 2004;77:257-267.
48. Socas L, Zumbado M, Perez-Luzardo O, et al. Hepatocellular adenomas associated with anabolic androgenic steroid abuse in bodybuilders: a report of two cases and a review of the literature. *Br J Sports Med.* 2005;39:e27.
49. Brunt EM, Wolverson MK, Di Bisceglie AM. Benign hepatocellular tumors (adenomatosis) in nonalcoholic steatohepatitis: a case report. *Semin Liver Dis.* 2005;25:230-236.

50. Labrune P, Trioche P, Duvaltier I, Chevalier P, Odièvre M. Hepatocellular adenomas in glycogen storage disease type I and III: a series of 43 patients and review of the literature. *J Pediatr Gastroenterol Nutr.* 1997;24:276-279.

51. Laumonier H, Bioulac-Sage P, Laurent C, Zucman-Rossi J, Balabaud C. Trillaud H. Hepatocellular adenomas: magnetic resonance imaging features as a function of molecular pathological classification. *Hepatology.* 2008;48:808-818.

52. Ronot M, Bahrami S, Calderaro J, et al. Hepatocellular adenomas: accuracy of magnetic resonance imaging and liver biopsy in subtype classification. *Hepatology.* 2011;53:1182-1191.

53. Grazioli L, Bondioni MP, Haradome H, et al. Hepatocellular adenoma and focal nodular hyperplasia: value of gadoxetic acid-enhanced MR imaging in differential diagnosis. *Radiology.* 2012;262:520-529.

54. Lerut JP, Ciccarelli O, Sempoux C, et al. Glycogenosis storage type I diseases and evolutive adenomatosis: an indication for liver transplantation. *Transpl Int.* 2003;16:879-884.

55. Petrowsky H, Brunicardi FC, Leow VM, et al. Liver transplantation for lethal genetic syndromes: a novel model of personalized genomic medicine. *J Am Coll Surg.* 2013;216:534-543; discussion 543–544.

56. Atwell TD, Brandhagen DJ, Charboneau JW, Nagorney DM, Callstrom MR, Farrell MA. Successful treatment of hepatocellular adenoma with percutaneous radiofrequency ablation. *AJR Am J Roentgenol.* 2005;184:828-831.

57. van der Sluis FJ, Bosch JL, Terkivatan T, de Man RA, Ijzermans JN, Hunink MG. Hepatocellular adenoma: cost-effectiveness of different treatment strategies. *Radiology.* 2009;252:737-746.

58. Tsui WM, Colombari R, Portmann BC, et al. Hepatic angiomyolipoma: a clinicopathologic study of 30 cases and delineation of unusual morphologic variants. *Am J Surg Pathol.* 1999;23:34-48.

59. Yang CY, Ho MC, Jeng YM, Hu RH, Wu YM, Lee PH. Management of hepatic angiomyolipoma. *J Gastrointest Surg.* 2007;11:452-457.

60. Sawai H, Manabe T, Yamanaka Y, Kurahashi S, Kamiya A. Angiomyolipoma of the liver: case report and collective review of cases diagnosed from fine needle aspiration biopsy specimens. *J Hepatobiliary Pancreat Surg.* 1998;5:333-338.

61. Flemming P, Lehmann U, Becker T, Klempnauer J, Kreipe H. Common and epithelioid variants of hepatic angiomyolipoma exhibit clonal growth and share a distinctive immunophenotype. *Hepatology.* 2000;32:213-217.

62. Deng FT, Li YX, Ye L, Tong L, Yang XP, Chai XQ. Hilar inflammatory pseudotumor mimicking hilar cholangiocarcinoma. *Hepatobiliary Pancreat Dis Int.* 2010;9:219-221.

63. Park JY, Choi MS, Lim YS, et al. Clinical features, image findings, and prognosis of inflammatory pseudotumor of the liver: a multicenter experience of 45 cases. *Gut Liver.* 2014;8:58-63.

64. Goldsmith PJ, Loganathan A, Jacob M, et al. Inflammatory pseudotumours of the liver: a spectrum of presentation and management options. *Eur J Surg Oncol.* 2009;35:1295-1298.

Hepatocellular Carcinoma

Garrett Richard Roll | John Paul Roberts

EPIDEMIOLOGY AND ETIOLOGY

Hepatocellular carcinoma (HCC) is the sixth most common malignancy in the world and the fastest growing cause of cancer-related death.[1] This is in part due to endemic viral hepatitis in developing countries and the epidemic of obesity in the Western world.[2] Currently, 3–% of patients with HCC live in Asia and Africa but the incidence of HCC in the United States has been steadily increasing since 1975, and HCC is projected to be the third leading cause of cancer death by 2030.[1,3] More common among men, the incidence of HCC in the United States has increased since 1975 to 2000 from 1.4 to more than 5 per 100,000, respectively.[4] Of the 600,000 deaths per annum worldwide, 50% occur in China.

Hepatitis B virus (HBV) and hepatitis C virus (HCV) are both strongly associated with the development of HCC. This association increases significantly with coinfection of both of these viruses. Hepatitis B has a higher prevalence in Asia and Africa, whereas hepatitis C is more prevalent in Japan, Europe, and the United States.[5] The incidence of HCC has actually been decreasing recently in China and Korea, likely demonstrating successful HBV vaccination programs.[6] This is in stark contrast to the increasing incidence in the United States, the Middle East, and Japan, driven by HCV- and obesity-related liver disease.[7–9]

The average age at the time of diagnosis of HCC in the United States is 65 years, with a 75% male predominance.[10] In the United States, hepatitis C and B and alcohol consumption are the commonest causes of HCC. The rise of HCC in Western countries was previously fueled by the increase in the prevalence of hepatitis C. The greatest incidence of hepatitis C infection was during the late 1970s and early 1980s, with a dramatic drop in incidence in the late 1980s (Fig. 132.1). Because of the time necessary for cancer to develop in infected patients and the increased risk in older patients, the number of patients with HCC has risen rapidly as this bolus of patients infected many years ago matures (Fig. 132.2).[11] Current estimate of the prevalence of HCV in the US population is 3.5 million (1.1%).[12] With the advent of direct-acting antiviral medications many patients will be cured of the virus, but the risk of developing HCC is still 5.1% over 10 years after sustained viral response.[13]

STEATOHEPATITIS

With the explosion of obesity in many parts of the world, it is clear that a large proportion of patients suffering from obesity have steatohepatitis, and many will progress to cirrhosis, putting them at risk for HCC. Approximately 20% of adults in the United States have metabolic syndrome, and the incidence of nonalcoholic steatohepatitis

(NASH) is estimated to be 12.2%.[14–16] The yearly incidence of the development of HCC in patients with NASH is similar to patients suffering from HCV (2.6% vs. 4.0% per year), but the worldwide burden of NASH is projected to be much greater than that of HCV.[17] The potential magnitude of the disease burden of NASH can be realized by the fact that 1.1% of the US population has HCV and 25% of liver transplants are done for HCV-related HCC while 12.2% of the population has steatohepatitis and the annual risk of development of HCC in the two populations appears to be similar. The main reason NASH-related liver disease has not reached its zenith is that the epidemic of obesity is a relatively recent event.[18]

OTHER RISK FACTORS

In sub-Saharan Africa, Southeast Asia, and China, aflatoxin, a contaminant in maize and nuts, produced by the fungi *Aspergillus*, is a potent carcinogen. The carcinogenic potential increases 30-fold in the presence of chronic HBV infection (Table 132.1). The estimate of the percentage of HCC related to aflatoxin ranges between 5% and 28%.[19] Programs to reduce exposure to aflatoxins, in combination with HBV vaccination efforts, have been effective.[20]

Pathogenesis

Hepatitis B, a DNA virus, integrates itself into hepatocyte DNA and is thought to increase the rate of oncogene transcription. Hepatitis C, an RNA virus, does not incorporate into DNA of the hepatocytes, and its relationship with HCC is thought to be through chronic inflammation. After cirrhosis develops, HCV continues to replicate, which sustains inflammation and a rapid cell turnover, resulting in mutation and dysplastic changes that lead to neoplastic growth.[21] The pathogenesis in steatohepatitis is poorly understood, although the associated chronic inflammation is thought to contribute to the development of HCC. Termed the *immune-metabolic interface*, the influences of altered insulin signaling and nuclear factor κB are still being elucidated.[2]

Pathophysiology

Understanding the pathophysiology of HCC is critical when considering diagnosis and treatment for this relatively unique malignancy. The three most important clinical aspects of the pathophysiology of HCC are (1) its relationship to cirrhosis and chronic inflammation, (2) arterial angiogenesis, and (3) portal vein invasion.

CIRRHOSIS

Traditionally, more than 90% of patients who developed HCC had liver fibrosis. In patients with hepatitis C, almost all the patients with HCC have cirrhosis, and the risk of developing HCC after cirrhosis is established is

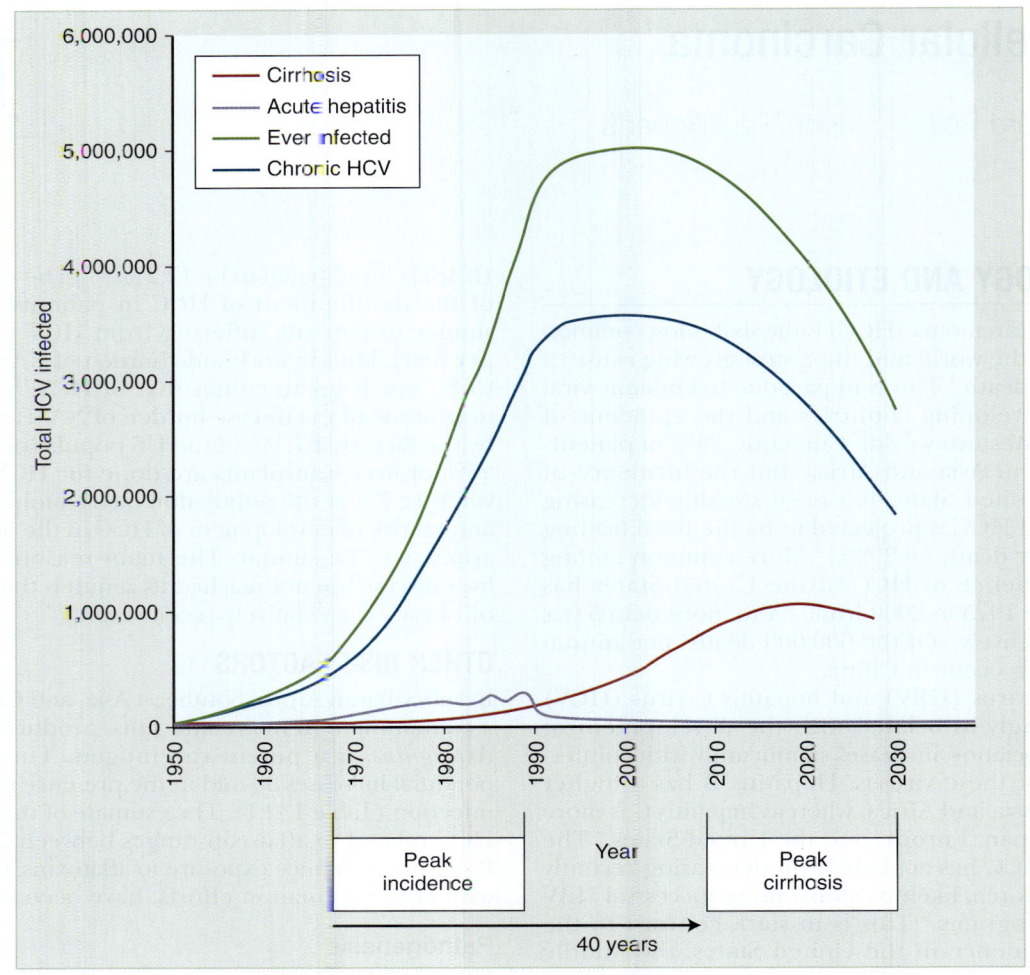

FIGURE 132.1 Estimates by year of prevalent cases ever infected *(green line)*, with chronic hepatitis C *(blue line)*, and cirrhosis *(red line)*. Acute infections *(purple line)* peaked between 1970 and 1990. The peak of chronic hepatitis prevalence was 2001, whereas the highest prevalence of cirrhosis is projected to be between 2010 and 2030, approximately 40 years after the peak of acute infections. (From Davis GL, Alter MJ, El-Serag H, Poynard T, Jennings LW. Aging of hepatitis C virus [HCV]-infected persons in the United States: a multiple cohort model of HCV prevalence and disease progression. *Gastroenterology.* 2010;138:513.)

TABLE 132.1 Major Risk Factors for Hepatocellular Carcinoma

Infection	Hepatitis B
	Hepatitis C
Toxin/drug	Alcoholic cirrhosis
	Aflatoxins
	Anabolic steroids
Genetic	Hemochromatosis
	α_1-Antitrypsin deficiency
Immunologic	Autoimmune chronic active hepatitis
	Primary biliary cirrhosis
Other	Obesity
	Nonalcoholic steatohepatitis
	Cirrhosis (other causes and idiopathic)

approximately 3% to 5% per year. Increasingly, patients without cirrhosis are developing HCC. This shifting trend is not completely understood, but it is clear that most of these patients have a significant amount of chronic inflammation from HBV or NASH.

The cirrhotic liver consists of regenerative nodules surrounded by fibrosis. It appears that because of chronic inflammation, progression from regenerative nodules to dysplasia and finally to HCC occurs. This is a multistep process of a precancerous lesion progressing from a dysplastic foci to a low-grade dysplastic nodule, then high-grade dysplastic nodule, and eventually to HCC.[22] Dysplastic nodules generally range from 1 to 2 cm and contain areas of dysplasia or carcinoma in situ.[23] The risk of liver cancer is not localized to one specific site in the liver but rather is uniform across all the hepatocytes, so the resulting carcinogenic potential is termed a *field defect*. This field defect is responsible for the high rate of recurrence after resection of HCC because the remaining liver contains oncogenic potential. This is why recurrence after

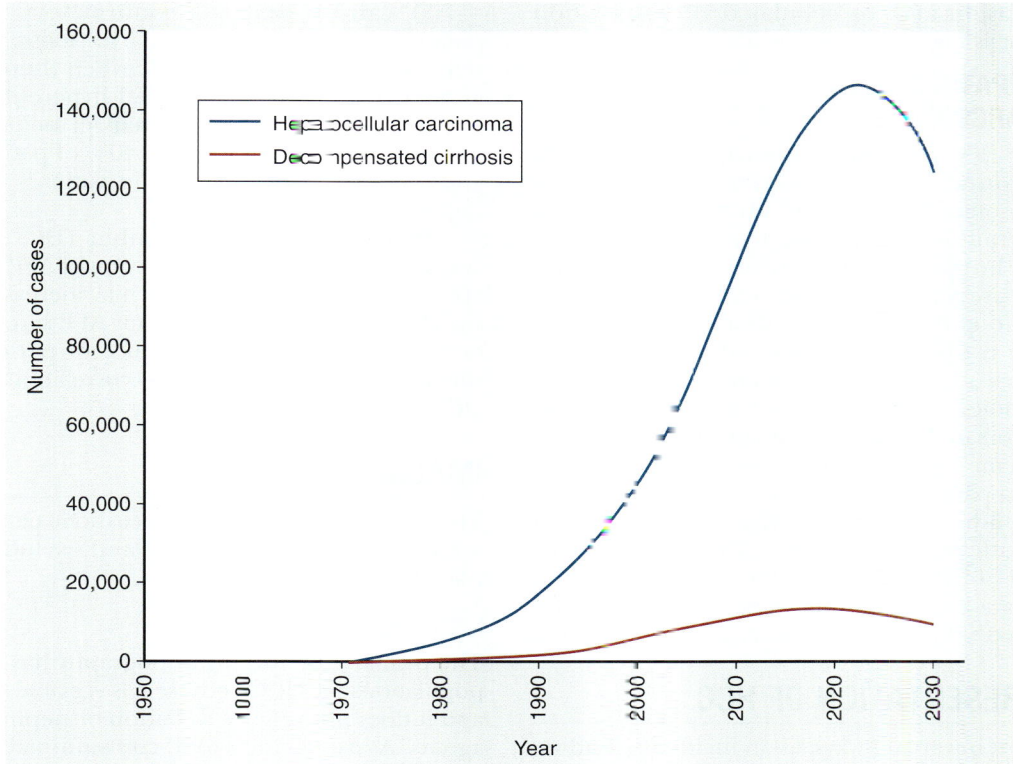

FIGURE 132.2 Projected number of cases by year of decompensated cirrhosis *(red line)* and hepatocellular carcinoma *(blue line)*. The model assumes a first-year mortality of 80% to 85%, so in contrast to the decompensated cirrhosis projection, for the number of cases of hepatocellular carcinoma, the prevalence demonstrated here closely resembles annual incidence of liver cancer. (From Davis GL, Alter MJ, El-Seraq H, Poynard T, Jennings LW. Aging of hepatitis C virus-infected persons in the United States: a multiple cohort model of HCV prevalence and disease progression *Gastroenterology*. 2010;138:513.)

resection most commonly takes the form of a second primary lesion rather than a recurrence of the resected lesion itself.[24] This powerful field defect is why a patient's response to locoregional therapy prior to liver resection does not predict the likelihood of recurrence.[25,26] The field defect is why the greatest risk factor for the development of HCC is a previous HCC, with the risk in the HCV cirrhotic patient increasing from 3% to 5% per year to 20% per year after a diagnosis of HCC.

ARTERIAL ANGIOGENESIS

The normal and cirrhotic liver both are supplied by a unique dual blood flow, dominated by portal venous inflow. Dysplastic nodules are predominantly supplied by the portal vein, but HCC derives its blood supply primarily from the hepatic artery. This clinically useful feature of HCC is due to the dysregulation of angiogenesis and lack of a basement membrane that occurs with malignant tumors.[27] This propensity for HCC to undergo neoangiogenesis and hepatic arterial hyperperfusion allows characterization of lesions and diagnosis of typical appearing lesions as HCC via imaging without requiring a biopsy. On computed tomography (CT) and magnetic resonance imaging (MRI), the HCC lesion will be hyperdense during the arterial phase compared with the surrounding liver parenchyma. HCC will then "washout" during the portal

venous phase, as the predominantly arterial blood supply has already passed through the lesion by the time the portal venous contrast phase is peaking. The arterial blood vessels supplying the tumor have a characteristic appearance of tortuous vessel size and branch density. This abnormal arterial perfusion allows for treatment of HCC via embolization of the predominant artery(ies) supplying the tumor.

PORTAL VEIN INVASION

Another characteristic of HCC is its propensity to invade the portal vein.[28] Tumors measuring more than 2 cm have an increased risk of portal vein invasion, which can be assessed on imaging.[29]

Predictably, the risk of local or remote recurrence of HCC in patients with microscopic or macroscopic portal venous invasion is higher following liver resection or transplantation. Macroscopic portal vein invasion is a contraindication to transplantation and, in many cases, to liver resection as well. It is likely that portal venous invasion is either a mechanism for dissemination of the tumor and/or a marker that the metastatic cells are able to invade and survive in other organs, such as the lung or bone.

It is well recognized that the recurrence of HCC after transplantation is related to the total tumor burden. This finding is likely a reflection of the increased probability of vascular invasion and/or cellular dedifferentiation when the tumor is large or multifocal.

COMBINED HEPATOCELLULAR-CHOLANGIOCARCINOMA

Approximately 1% of liver tumors in patients with cirrhosis are found to be combined hepatocellular-cholangiocarcinoma. These mixed lesions do not seem to follow the traditional multistep sequence of HCC carcinogenesis, but possibly result from malignant transformation of a progenitor cell that retains the ability to differentiate into either cell type.[30] Biopsy of HCC prior to resection or transplant is rarely indicated, so these mixed lesions are frequently presumed to be HCC until the explant pathology is available. The outcome of patients with mixed tumors undergoing transplant is not frequently described, but a multicenter, retrospective matched cohort study found that patients with combined lesions have the same 1-, 3- and 5-year actuarial survival when compared with patients with pure HCC (93%, 78%, and 78% vs. 97%, 86%, and 86%, respectively; $P = .9$).[31] The results, derived from data including only 15 patients with mixed tumors compared with 30 controls, needs to be replicated.

CLINICAL PRESENTATION OF HCC

HCC can present in varying ways: as an incidental finding during ultrasound for right upper quadrant pain, abdominal mass, weight loss, anorexia, or onset of ascites or while screening for patients at risk for HCC, with or without evidence of cirrhosis.

A patient with known cirrhosis who develops any of the symptoms previously mentioned should be suspected of having developed HCC. The finding of small asymptomatic liver lesions during the radiologic evaluation for liver transplantation is another common presentation, particularly in patients with hepatitis C or NASH.

Physical examination is most often dominated by the signs of cirrhosis, such as jaundice, ascites, cachexia, splenomegaly, hepatomegaly, spider angiomata, or palmar erythema. Conversely, the physical exam may be normal in patients with HBV or NASH who can experience HCC prior to the development of cirrhosis.

LABORATORY FINDINGS

Due to the limited success of treatment of advanced HCC, early detection is critical. Blood tests can reveal abnormal liver function and elevated liver enzymes, again, most often driven by the underlying cirrhosis. Viral serologies including hepatitis B surface antigen and hepatitis C antibody tests are also necessary. Patients with cirrhosis may also demonstrate thrombocytopenia, which is a marker of portal hypertension. α-Fetoprotein (AFP) may be elevated in patients with HCC; however, this is neither highly sensitive nor specific. The American Association for the Study of Liver Disease (AASLD) updated their guidelines for screening patients at risk of developing HCC in 2010, recommending liver ultrasound and serum AFP measurement every 6 months.[32] The evidence for screening patients with risk factors other than HBV is somewhat controversial.[33]

AFP can be used as a confirmatory test in cases in patients with cirrhosis and a liver mass. A level greater than 400 ng/mL is diagnostic when there is a liver mass greater than 2 cm with arterial hyperenhancement.[34] It is important to remember that serum AFP can be less than 20 ng/mL in more than 40% of patients with HCC, and the AFP can be elevated in patients with active viral hepatitis without cancer.[35]

The des-carboxyprothrombin (DCP) and the lens culinaris agglutinin-reactive fraction of AFP, termed *AFP-L3*, are candidate biomarkers that may increase the specificity for HCC when used with serum AFP screening.[36] DCP is elevated in approximately 40% of patients with HCC smaller than 2 cm. There is no correlation between serum DCP and AFP levels.[37]

IMAGING

The purpose of imaging in the cirrhotic patient is threefold: screening/diagnosis, staging, and excluding other complications of cirrhosis.

SCREENING

The primary use for ultrasonography has been screening populations for HCC because it is versatile and inexpensive and it does not require radiation or nephrotoxic contrast agents. As a screening tool, conventional ultrasound has a variable sensitivity of 63% to 85% but specificity greater than 90%.[38,39] A prospective randomized controlled trial suggested that surveillance of high-risk individuals with ultrasound and AFP every 6 months reduces HCC-related mortality by close to 40%; however, the screening compliance at that time was only approximately 60%.[40] HCC screening is recommended in patients with non-HBV cirrhosis from HCV, alcohol, genetic hemochromatosis, and primary biliary cirrhosis.[32,33] Data are lacking regarding screening in patients with other non-HBV etiologies of cirrhosis, so screening in these patients is controversial.

In patients with HBV, screening is clearly indicated. Current guidelines suggest patients with the highest risk for HCC, including all patients with HBV cirrhosis, patients with a family history of HCC, males older than 40 years and females older than 50 years (older than 20 years in Africans), and patients with active HBV viral replication and/or active necroinflammatory activity on biopsy, undergo serum AFP and ultrasound screening every 6 months. There is insufficient evidence about screening of young inactive HBV carriers. When screening populations in which the incidence of HCC may be quite high and the picture is complicated by the nodular nature of the cirrhotic liver, such as patients awaiting liver transplantation, ultrasound may be less useful.[41]

Contrast-enhanced ultrasound (CEUS) has been used for more than a decade in other countries, but is only recently approved by the US Food and Drug Administration (FDA).[42] The use of nonnephrotoxic contrast agents containing microbubbles may increase the specificity of ultrasound because these agents will allow demonstration of arterialization.[43] CEUS has a higher sensitivity but is not widely available for screening. CEUS is as sensitive as contrast-enhanced MRI or CT scan and is safe in patients with renal failure. CEUS is not currently in the AASLD guidelines for the diagnosis of HCC because there is concern that CEUS cannot reliably differentiate HCC from intrahepatic cholangiocarcinoma.

LESIONS LESS THAN 2 CENTIMETERS

The regenerating nodules that are commonplace in cirrhosis limit the specificity of ultrasound particularly if the lesion is less than 2 cm in diameter. In a cirrhotic liver a lesion measuring less than 1 cm on imaging carries less than 50% risk of being a malignant transformation. Thus ultrasound surveillance every 3 months is recommended in these patients until lesions increase to a diameter of greater than 1 cm. If the size remains stable for 24 months, the imaging interval can increase, first to every 6 months, then to 1 year.[44]

For lesions between 1 and 2 cm, if on two modalities the image findings, such as arterialization and washout, are characteristic for HCC, then nothing further is needed to make the diagnosis. If one or more of the modalities demonstrate features that are atypical for HCC, then tissue biopsy is recommended.[44,45] Biopsy of small lesions can yield a false-negative result, so ongoing surveillance with contrast-enhanced imaging is recommended for follow-up instead of ultrasound.

LESIONS GREATER THAN 2 CENTIMETERS

Due to advances in imaging the combination of clinical features and image findings provides a positive predictive value of 95% and is thus reliable for diagnosis. Current diagnostic consensus is that with an elevated AFP (>200 ng/mL) with a lesion greater than 2 cm that has classic imaging features (see later), the probability of HCC is so high that biopsy is not required and management can be commenced following staging. However, atypical imaging findings do require tissue biopsy.[30]

COMPUTED TOMOGRAPHY

CT has a relatively high sensitivity and specificity for detecting HCC. The current imaging guidelines for liver and pancreatic disease include precontrast axial images of the upper abdomen. After completion of the unenhanced CT, contrast is then injected intravenously; then scanning at the early arterial phase is performed. This usually occurs at 12 to 30 seconds after injection depending on the patient's hemodynamics. Due to the arterial angiogenesis of the tumor, and its predominantly hepatic arterial blood supply, the arterial phase demonstrates enhancement of the tumor. This is in contrast to the surrounding liver, which is maximally enhanced during the portovenous phase.[46]

Fifteen years ago the sensitivity of identifying HCC on multidetector CT was approximately 86% which dropped to approximately 60% for lesions less than 2 cm in size.[47] However, recently improved imaging acquisition techniques have improved the sensitivity and specificity to as high as 93% and 97%, respectively, confirmed by liver explant and resection pathology.[48]

Intravenous ionized poppyseed oil (Lipiodol) is no longer used for planning and staging. However, Lipiodol is still injected when transarterial embolization therapy is delivered and is used as a marker of treatment on follow-up CT because the lesions can be identified on the noncontrast phase of the CT scan. The Lipiodol is normally cleared by lymphatic vessels and Kupffer cells that the tumor lacks and can be retained by the tumor for months after arterial injection, which can reduce the sensitivity of posttreatment surveillance by sheltering viable tumor. Heterogeneous uptake of Lipiodol after transcatheter arterial embolization (TACE) with residual tumor enhancement is suggestive of presence of viable tumor. CT is also used to assess for complications of embolization therapy, such as hepatic or gallbladder necrosis.[49]

MAGNETIC RESONANCE IMAGING

MRI is becoming the predominant imaging modality for characterizing liver tumors. MRI can be used to assess fat and iron content, as well as acquiring angiographic images and enhancement patterns of multiple contrast phases, similar to CT scan. Classically, HCC has high signal intensity on T2-weighted sequences, with strong early arterial enhancement and delayed washout; however, smaller HCCs can vary in their appearance on MRI.[50] Even with the variation seen in smaller HCC lesions, MRI has the highest sensitivity and specificity for detection of 1- to 2-cm HCC of 90% and 82%, respectively.[51] The capsule surrounding HCC may be of low signal intensity. The lesion may show a "mosaic" appearance because of combined areas of growth and necrosis. Early malignant growth within dysplastic nodules can be identified simply as an area within a nodule that has a different intensity and arterial enhancement in comparison to the remainder of the nodule. This is known as a "nodule within a nodule" appearance.

MRI needs less contrast volume than CT, and injection time is shorter. There is also no ionizing radiation in MRI. Contrast agents used include gadolinium chelates, superparamagnetic iron oxide, and hepatocyte-directed agents (mangafodipir trisodium). Gadolinium is avoided in patients with renal dysfunction, due to the risk of nephrogenic systemic fibrosis.

STAGING

Staging of HCC is important because acquiring information about the degree of spread/metastases can help to plan management and predict prognosis and outcome. The staging system can act as a prognostic tool and is used to direct treatment.

The commonest classifications used are the following:
- *Barcelona Clinic Liver Cancer (BCLC) staging system* provides information on prognosis and aids with planning patients' treatment. It takes into account a variety of factors, including clinically relevant portal hypertension. Stage A (early tumor) is suitable for all treatment modalities; stages B (intermediate) and C (advanced) are more suitable for palliative care and use of new agents and stage D (end stage) should be treated symptomatically only (Fig. 132.3).[52]
- *Tumor, node, metastasis (TNM)*, which assesses only the tumor and not the function of the remaining liver. TNM is difficult to use in the preoperative patient because it relies on histologic assessment of the liver. Currently in the United States, this staging system has

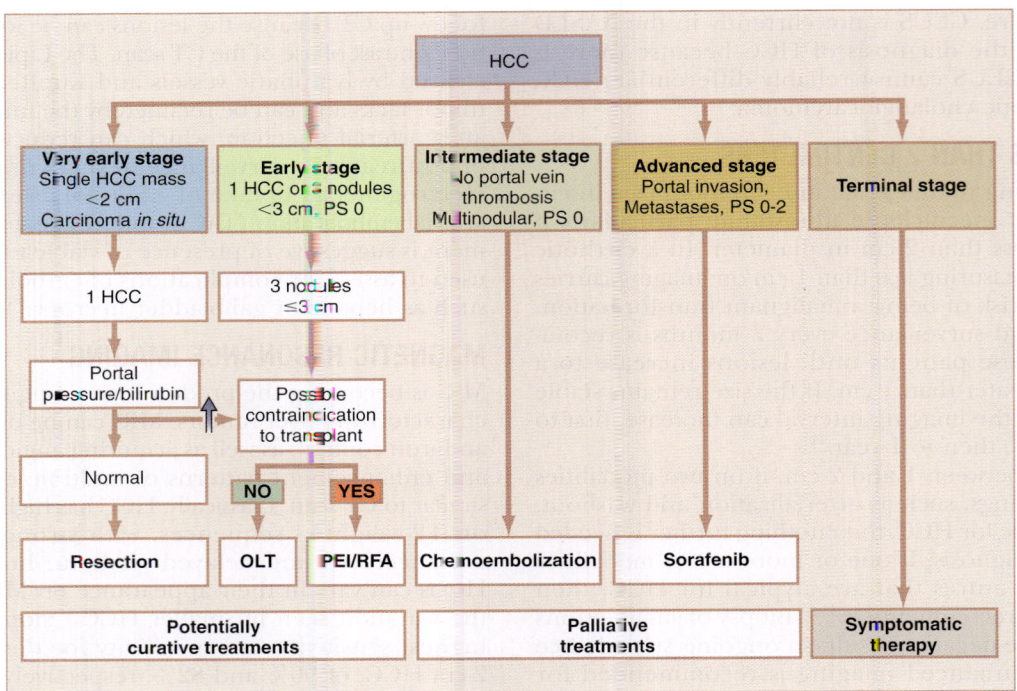

FIGURE 132.3 Management guideline using modified Barcelona Clinic Liver Cancer staging system. *HCC,* Hepatocellular carcinoma; *PEI,* percutaneous ethanol injection; *OLT,* orthotopic liver transplantation; *PS,* performance status; *RFA,* radiofrequency ablation. (From El-Seraq HB, Marrero JA, Rudolph L, Reddy KR. Diagnosis and treatment of hepatocellular carcinoma. *Gastroenterology.* 2008;134: 1752.)

been modified for use to prioritize patients with HCC based on radiologic imaging. This modified staging system is used to allow for prioritization of patients with HCC for transplantation.

- *Okuda classification* assesses both the tumor and the liver. It takes into account the tumor size and liver function tests, such as albumin and bilirubin levels. It does *not* take into account vascular invasion or whether or not the tumor is single or multiple. This is a commonly used staging system (stages I, II, and III).
- *Cancer of the Liver Italian Program (CLIP)* includes the Child-Pugh stage, tumor extension, AFP levels, and portal vein thrombosis. The CLIP staging has been viewed as an easy and acceptable method of staging HCC, which takes into account all the factors needed to allow assessment and management in a patient with the tumor. However, it is poor at staging patients undergoing surgery or transplantation.

The use of staging systems is exemplified by the use of the modified TNM classification in prioritizing patients with HCC for transplantation in the United States. In this classification, patients are stratified by the size and number of the tumor. Patients with a single lesion between 2 and 5 cm in size are given priority for transplantation. If more than one lesion is present, there must be fewer than three lesions with no individual lesion greater than 3 cm in size for the patient to be given priority for transplantation. Patients with single lesions greater than 5 cm, with more than three lesions, with multiple lesions where one lesion is greater than 3 cm, or with radiologic evidence of vascular invasion are not given priority for transplantation.

MANAGEMENT

Treatment decisions in patients with HCC are based on the overall health of the patient, extent and trajectory of tumor burden, and data regarding the results of any particular treatment. In addition to these considerations, it should be remembered that HCC frequently arises in a cirrhotic liver. The risk of liver decompensation due to cancer therapy can limit treatment options. Furthermore, because of the field defect in the liver, patients with HCC are at high risk to develop additional primary lesions, and this risk is significant (Fig. 132.4).[24] The risk of developing a second primary after resection for HCC is approximately 35% at 1 year, 40% to 50% over 3 years, and as high as 70% at 5 years.[53,54] Accounting for this risk of recurrence is fundamental when making treatment decisions in patients with HCC. Also critical is the likelihood of the patient undergoing liver transplantation, and the availability of donor livers in the area.

Much of the future of therapy for this disease will be aimed at reducing the risk of second primary lesions. These therapies may either identify patients at risk for development of a second primary lesion or prevent the ongoing production of new cancers by limiting viral damage, inflammation, or progression of dysplasia to cancer. Unfortunately, many patients present at a stage too advanced for surgical resection or transplantation. These patients may be candidates for locoregional therapy to reduce the tumor burden within transplant criteria, or for systemic chemotherapy.

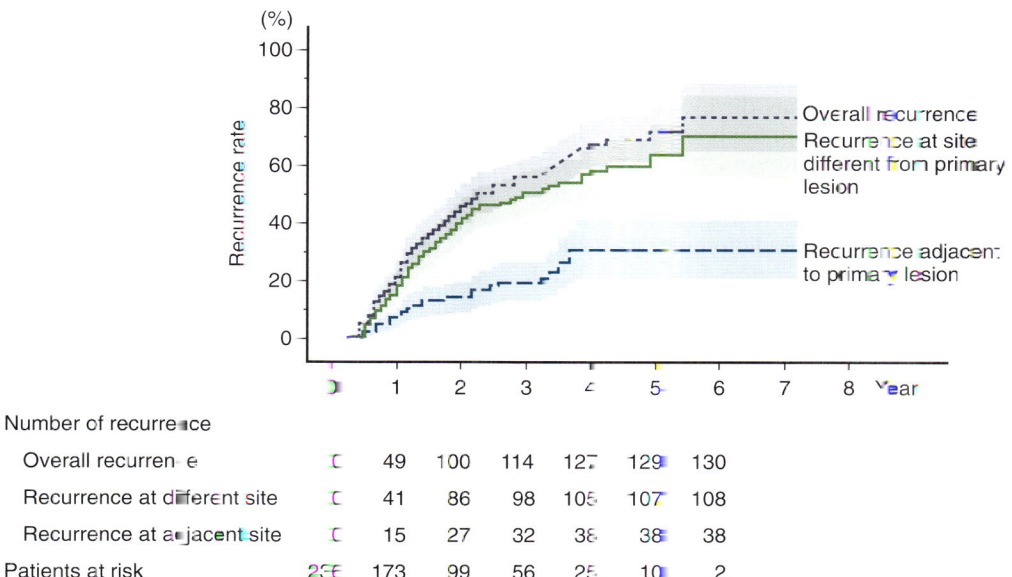

FIGURE 132.4 Risk factors for hepatocellular carcinoma recurrence. (From Koike Y, Shiratori Y, Sato S, et al. Risk factors for recurring hepatocellular carcinoma differ according to infected hepatitis virus—an analysis of 236 consecutive patients with a single lesion. *Hepatology.* 2000;32:1220.)

SYSTEMIC CHEMOTHERAPY

In patients with intermediate or advanced HCC, surgical intervention is often contraindicated, and thus chemotherapy has a potential role. However, cirrhosis often limits the patient's ability to tolerate chemotherapy. This, in combination with the known chemoresistant character of HCC, has previously limited the role of chemotherapy in the management of HCC. In 2007 the FDA approved sorafenib for patients with advanced HCC. This drug is a tyrosine-kinase inhibitor that limits cell proliferation and angiogenesis. Sorafenib has proven benefit in patients with advanced renal cell carcinoma and has been shown to reduce radiologic disease progression in patients with advanced HCC when compared with a placebo group (5.5 vs. 2.8 months, respectively).[55,56] Better survival rates were also demonstrated in the study in comparison with the placebo group, with an increase in the median survival (10.7 vs. 7.9 months). Similar results were seen in an Asian study of sorafenib.[57] No other systemic therapy has generated better results than the modest survival benefit from sorafenib. Subsequent trials failed to demonstrate efficacy of sorafenib as an adjuvant to locoregional therapies.[58] The mammalian target of rapamycin (mTOR) pathway is frequently overactive in patients with HCC, and this led to the use of mTOR inhibitors everolimus and sirolimus. Sirolimus failed to demonstrate a long-term survival benefit in patients after liver transplant, although recurrence-free survival and overall survival up to 3 years was improved in patients whose explant pathology was within the Milan criteria.[59] Another trial showed that the addition of everolimus to sorafenib in patients with unresectable or metastatic HCC increased toxicity but unfortunately did not improve outcomes.[60] Everolimus also did not prolong survival in patients who failed or did not tolerate sorafenib.[61]

ABLATIVE THERAPIES

Locoregional therapy is the use of radiofrequency, microwaves, or toxic substances, such as alcohol, to destroy the lesions. These therapies can be used to destroy a cancer in a cirrhotic liver, with a relatively low risk of decompensation of the remaining liver as compared with resection. These therapies are particularly attractive if they can be done percutaneously, although the positioning of the lesion sometimes requires either a laparoscopic or open approach. These techniques have undergone rapid improvement in the past 10 years.

Radiofrequency Ablation

Radiofrequency ablation (RFA) consists of a high-frequency alternating current that causes agitation and frictional heat up to 120°C, resulting in denaturing of proteins and the tumor cells' bilayer lipid, resulting in tissue destruction and coagulative necrosis. Once temperatures reach 60°C, complete circumferential tissue damage between 0.5 and 3 cm begins, with a further 8-mm rim of partial destruction.[52]

The stainless steel insulated needle is inserted into the tumor site, and the prongs are then deployed to provide heating over a larger area. Repeated applications of the heating can be used to treat larger tumors.[62] When the needles are withdrawn, diathermy is used to prevent tumor seeding.

Advantages of Radiofrequency Ablation. Indications for RFA include reducing tumor bulk in patients with unresectable disease in preparation for surgery or transplantation or in patients who cannot tolerate surgery because of other comorbidities and/or coagulopathies. Multiple studies have demonstrated the role of RFA for small HCC.[53–] There is clearly a role for percutaneous ablation in the management of patients with HCC who have limited access to liver transplantation, especially for tumors smaller than 3 cm, in which local recurrence rates are similar to liver resection. Although center-specific approaches vary slightly, RFA, along with TACE, has developed into the backbone of the multimodal approach to controlling HCC while patients await transplantation, are being down-staged with the eventual goal of transplant, and in the control of disease that falls outside transplant criteria.

Limitations and Disadvantages of Radiofrequency Ablation.

Percutaneous RFA is used with caution for lesions that are close to the diaphragm, heart, gallbladder, duodenum, stomach, or colon. When treating central lesions, RFA can injure the bile duct, resulting in biliary stricture. The use of a laparoscopic or open surgical approach offers the advantage of being able to inspect the surface of the liver and the ability to move extrahepatic structures, such as the colon away from the planned ablation site, as well as simultaneous insertion of multiple electrodes into satellite lesions.

Complete ablation is difficult for larger tumors, due to the large area that must be ablated, and for tumors near large vessels because the flowing liquid draws heat away from the tumor. Occlusion of the portal triad with a Pringle maneuver may decrease the heat sink caused by blood flow, allowing adequate ablation of large central tumors. Patients who undergo RFA or any form of locoregional therapy must be monitored at least every 3 months with CT scans or MRI and serum AFP to detect evidence of residual disease or recurrence.

Percutaneous Ethanol Injection

Ethanol induces coagulative necrosis, cell dehydration, and denaturation. It is relatively inexpensive and has few side effects. Percutaneous injection takes place under ultrasound guidance using 95% alcohol. The tumor is injected, and the needle is left in situ for 1 to 2 minutes and then withdrawn with negative pressure. Because this procedure can be difficult for lesions near the dome of the liver, CT- or MRI-guided injection is preferred. Percutaneous ethanol injection (PEI) frequently achieves complete necrosis of tumors smaller than 3 cm, and 50% necrosis in 3- to 5-cm tumors. Side effects of the procedure include pain, transient hyperthermia, intoxication, portal venous system thrombosis, right pleural effusion, and hemobilia. PEI is reserved for patients who cannot tolerate more aggressive treatment of HCC.

RFA has largely replaced PEI. In tumors of less than 2 cm, the outcome is similar for both treatments; however, RFA has better survival rates and lower local recurrence in tumors larger than 4 cm.[67]

Transcatheter Arterial Chemoembolization

Transcatheter arterial embolization (TAE)/chemoembolization (TACE is another first-line treatment in the management of advanced HCC (Figs. 132.5 and 132.6). The technique involves occlusion of the hepatic artery supplying the tumor, with or without local delivery of chemotherapeutic agent. The vascular occlusion increases the tumor's susceptibility to the chemotherapeutic agent. Selective arterial catheterization is performed under digital subtraction angiography followed by infusion of chemotherapy (e.g., doxorubicin or cisplatin) suspended in Lipiodol

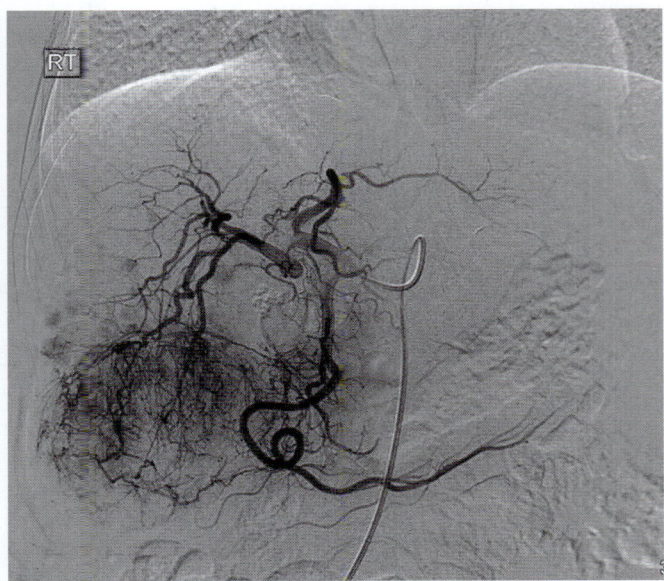

FIGURE 132.5 Digital subtraction angiography demonstrating right hepatic lobe hepatocellular carcinoma with characteristic angiogenesis.

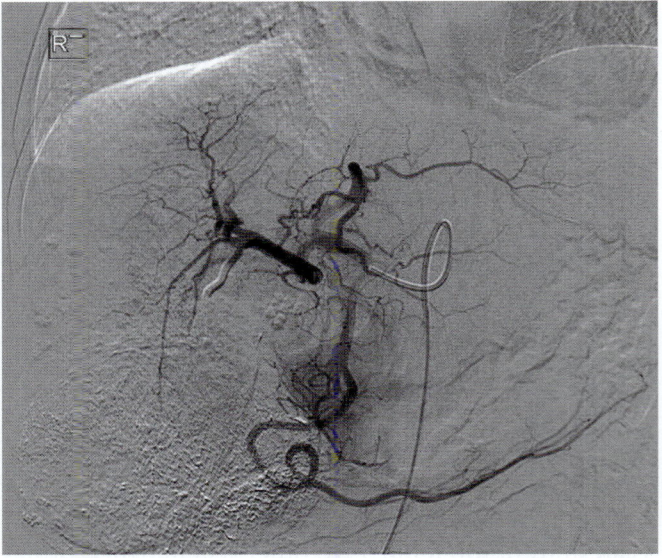

FIGURE 132.6 Posttranscatheter arterial chemoembolization showing complete occlusion of the feeding vessels and hepatocellular carcinoma no longer visualized. The "grainy" appearance shown at the site of the known tumor is residual Lipiodol.

(oily contrast agent) followed by occlusion of the artery using polyvinyl alcohol (PVA) or gelatin sponge.[68] Lipiodol has the tendency to remain in the tumor, and its pattern of distribution is assessed on follow-up imaging. Tissue enhancement within areas of Lipiodol uptake is a sign of persistent viable tumor.

This procedure can be used in patients who are not suitable candidates for anesthesia and/or transplantation. Portal vein thrombosis is a relative contraindication for

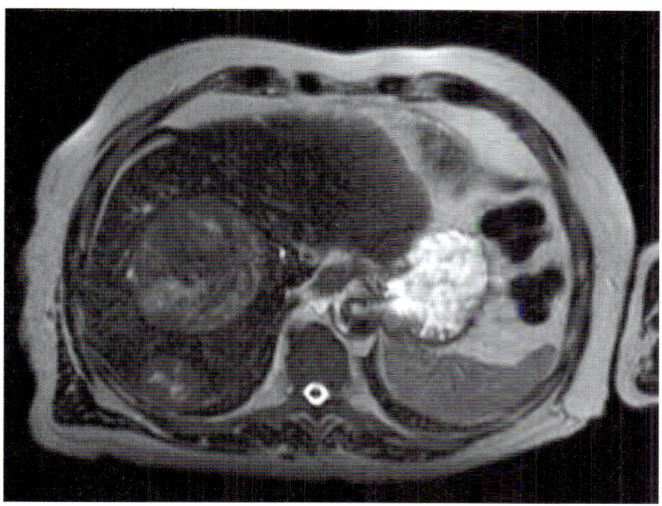

FIGURE 132.7 Magnetic resonance imaging—two hepatocellular carcinoma lesions within the right hepatic lobe.

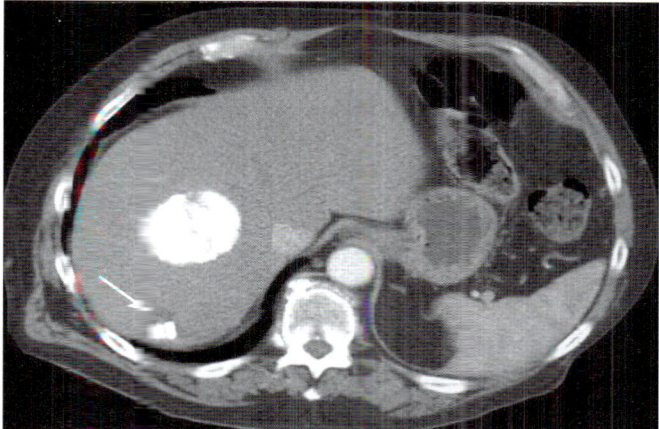

FIGURE 132.8 Contrast-enhanced computed tomography follow-up imaging posttranscatheter arterial chemoembolization. The larger lesions demonstrate Lipiodol within the lesion. Although the smaller lesion, posteriorly, demonstrates a smaller, nonenhanced area *(white arrow)*, the appearances are in keeping with response to treatment. Both lesions show tumor size reduction.

TACE due to the risk of hepatic ischemia and resulting decompensation. Use of highly selective arterial catheterization may decrease the risk of liver failure after TACE. A study by Llovet and Bruix has shown promising survival rates in use of TACE in unresectable HCC at 1, 2, and 3 years at 96%, 77%, and 47%, respectively.[69] The role of TACE as a bridge to transplantation was controversial[70] but has become commonplace in areas where the waiting time for transplant is longer than 1 to 2 months. Because tumor progression can result in patient ineligibility for liver transplantation, patients awaiting a transplant regularly undergo TACE, as well as RFA, to control the burden of disease.

Transcatheter Arterial Chemoembolization/ Radiofrequency Ablation Combination Therapy

Studies suggest that combining the tissue necrosis achieved with RFA with the tissue hypoxia secondary to vessel occlusion during TACE results in better survival.[71,72] One study reported the midterm results of a randomized trial of TACE/RFA compared with RFA alone. There was a trend toward improvement in 3-year survival of the patients treated with TACE plus RFA and the rate of local tumor progression in patients who received the combination therapy than in patients who underwent RFA alone (Figs. 132.7 and 132.8).[73]

Other Treatments

Microwave Therapy. In RFA the electrodes act as an active source of energy. This is in counterdistinction to microwave thermotherapy, during which kinetic energy between molecules is converted into heat by a probe inserted into the tumor. Similar to RFA, microwave therapy can be delivered percutaneously, laparoscopically, or via open surgery. Microwave therapy is thought to penetrate tissue better than radiofrequency therapy, resulting in larger areas of ablation, which, unlike RFA, is not limited by areas of tissue desiccation. Complications include pain, fever, hematoma formation, and bleeding. Several studies have reported the efficacy of microwave ablation. One

study reported 1- and 5-year survival rates of 93% and 51%, respectively.[74]

Resection If the HCC is limited to one lobe and there is no extrahepatic invasion, the remaining liver is functional enough to support life and surgical resection should be considered. The advantages of resection are that the patient does not have to wait for a donor liver to become available for transplant, and wide margins can often be achieved for an optimal local oncologic result. Similar to locoregional therapy, resection does not address the field defect present in the liver remnant. A meta-analysis examined the outcome of patients with small HCC who underwent locoregional therapy versus resection and found no difference in survival at 1 year or 3 years, but the patients who underwent resection had a higher survival at 5 years.[75]

EVALUATING HEPATIC FUNCTION AND RESERVE

Due to the advanced nature of HCC at the time of presentation and/or the concurrent severity of background liver disease, surgical resection is not an option for most patients. For the select group of patients in whom resection is possible, thoughtful patient selection results in perioperative mortality as low as 1% and 5-year survival of 40% to 70% depending on tumor stage.

Several tests assess hepatic function before resection to determine the expected functional liver remnant. Indocyanine green (ICG) clearance is used in patients with normal synthetic function (bilirubin, albumin, and prothrombin time). If hepatic ICG retention is greater than 20% at 15 minutes after injection, no more than one-sixth of the liver should be resected. If ICG retention is greater than 30%, then limited resection or RFA is appropriate.[76] The ICG test is not widely used in the United States.

A commonly accepted guide is that patients with Child-Pugh score A can have up to 50% of their liver resected.

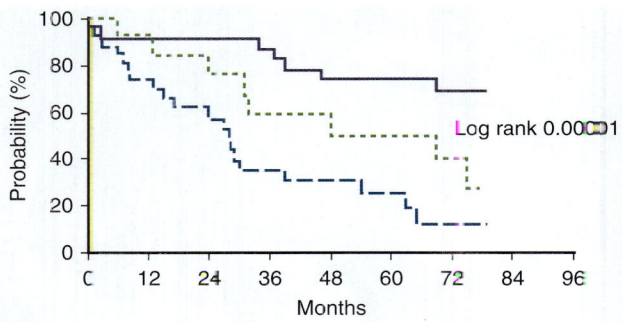

FIGURE 132.9 Actuarial survival for patients with hepatocellular carcinoma treated with resection. (From Llovet J, Fuster J and Bruix J. Intention-to-treat analysis of surgical treatment for early hepatocellular carcinoma: resection versus transplantation. *Hepatology.* 1999;30:1437.)

This value decreases to 25% for Child-Pugh B, and resection is contraindicated in patients with Child-Pugh C.[77] It is not certain that more complex testing has a greater predictive value than this rule of thumb.

The presence of portal hypertension, as measured by the hepatic vein wedge pressure, in the setting of an elevated serum bilirubin appears to be a combined risk factor for postoperative decompensation and may predict patient suitability for resection (Fig. 132.9).[78] It is thought that portal hypertension prevents functional regeneration of the liver.

Since the 1990s portal vein embolization has been used to assess the ability of a patient to tolerate liver resection and minimize the risk of liver failure after resection.[79–81] The portal vein is accessed percutaneously, and the branch of the portal vein that supplies the lobe to be resected is permanently occluded. Portal vein embolization diverts portal blood from the lobe to be resected, and hyperperfusion induces compensatory hypertrophy of the lobe that is to remain after resection. Significant growth of the future liver remnant signifies that the liver is capable of regeneration. The technique may improve postoperative survival in patients with fibrosis or cirrhosis who undergo resection. Portal vein embolization is not efficacious in patients who have clear evidence of portal hypertension.

Intraoperative ultrasonography has been used to ascertain vessel orientation, which, when combined with preoperative knowledge of the tumor and its blood supply, makes accurate resection of the tumor and its associated segments possible. After the tumor and its associated vessels are identified, the surface markings are made on the liver using diathermy. The information gained by this technique may allow for segmental or subsegmental resections that are sufficient from an oncologic standpoint and spare as much liver as possible.

OPERATIVE TECHNIQUES

The appropriate technique depends on the location of the tumor, the degree of cirrhosis, and the experience of the surgeon. The principles are the prevention of blood loss and the preservation of as much functional liver as possible. It does appear that margins greater than 5 to 10 mm are adequate. Anatomic resection does not appear

to decrease recurrence rates when compared with non-anatomic resection.[82]

Several techniques are used to minimize blood loss. These include inflow occlusion, total vascular isolation, and the use of clamps to compress the parenchyma. The intermittent inflow occlusion technique (Pringle maneuver) is used to minimize blood loss during hepatectomies. Fifteen minutes of occlusion followed by 5 minutes of reperfusion is commonly used. Another technique is total vascular isolation of the liver in which occlusion of the infrahepatic and suprahepatic vena cava is combined with occlusion of portal triad inflow. This technique can be helpful when the resection requires dividing parenchyma that is close to a major hepatic vein that cannot be sacrificed.

The expectation is that as instrumentation improves and surgeons gain more experience with laparoscopic resection, it will become routine. Currently both right and left lobes of the liver can be resected laparoscopically. Laparoscopic resection results in less blood loss and shorter hospital stay, although overall survival does not appear to be improved.[83]

Outcome of Resection

HCC recurrence after resection due to the field defect in the liver remnant is common, occurring in 50% and 80% of patients within 5 years, the majority occurring within 2 years. Recurrence may be in the form of residual viable tumor or the development of a second primary lesion. Of these two possibilities, the more common is a second primary lesion. Given the field defect throughout the liver, and the inability of cross-sectional imaging to identify very small HCC, it is not surprising some cancers are missed during preoperative staging. Some additional lesions may be found by the use of intraoperative ultrasound, but the specificity of the technique is limited in a nodular liver.

Transplantation

Solid organ transplantation is not commonly used in the treatment of cancer, but HCC is an exception. Liver transplantation is an effective way to remove both the carcinoma and the remaining cirrhotic liver with its propensity for tumorigenesis. It has taken years to develop insight about which patients with HCC benefit the most from transplant. Overall survival and recurrence-free survival after transplantation are better than resection for selected tumor stages. Criteria first defined by Mazzaferro et al.,[84] referred to as the *Milan criteria* (Fig. 132.10), proposed transplantation for patients with a single tumor smaller than 5 cm or fewer than three tumors, each of which are smaller than 3 cm. Using these criteria yielded an overall 4-year survival rate of 74%, similar to that for patients who received a liver transplant but did not have HCC. The 4-year survival of patients with tumor burden greater than the Milan criteria was only approximately 40%. Because of these poorer results, patients with more tumor burden have been excluded from deceased donor transplantation in the United States.

There has been criticism that the Milan criteria may be too strict, excluding patients from transplantation who would have a significant likelihood of survival. More

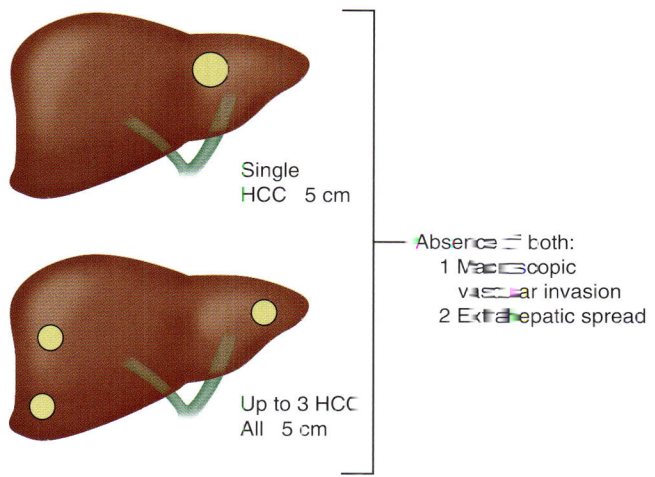

FIGURE 132.10 Milan criteria.

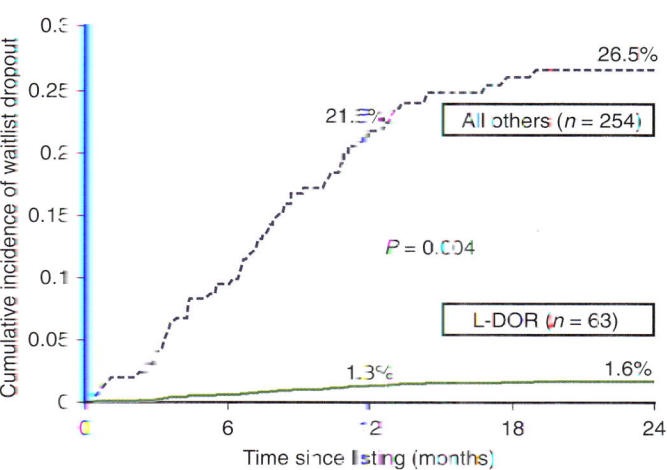

FIGURE 132.11 Cumulative incidence of waitlist dropout due to tumor progression or death by dropout risk groups. (From Mehta N, Dodge JL, Goel A, Roberts JP, Hirose R, Yao FY. Identification of liver transplant candidates with hepatocellular carcinoma and a very low dropout risk: implications for the current organ allocation policy. *Liver Transpl.* 2013;19:1343–1353.)

aggressive criteria, known as the *University of California San Francisco (UCSF) criteria,* were proposed by Yao et al.[85] These criteria offered transplantation to patients with a single tumor less than 6.5 cm or fewer than three tumors, the total diameter of all being less than 8 cm and the largest tumor less than 4.5 cm. The 1- and 5-year survival after transplant were 90% and 75%, respectively. The use of the UCSF criteria was prospectively validated.[86] Patients who present with tumor burden beyond the accepted limit can be treated with locoregional therapy and down-staged within criteria. A study compared 118 patients who presented with tumor beyond Milan criteria with 488 patients who did not. Patients with a serum AFP greater than 1000 ng/mL and Child B (vs. Child A) cirrhosis were more likely to develop progression of tumor resulting in dropout, but if that did not occur, patients who underwent downstaging had similar HCC recurrence rates and 5-year survival compared with patients who did not require downstaging.[87]

In February 2002 the United Network for Organ Sharing (UNOS) modified their criteria, giving priority to patients with HCC. This increased the number of liver transplants among patients with HCC. Patients meeting the Milan criteria gain a priority for transplantation if one of the tumors is greater than 2 cm in diameter. Patients with single lesions less than 2 cm do not receive priority. In October of 2015 UNOS further modified the HCC model of end-stage liver disease (MELD) exception system over concern that patients with HCC had an advantage over patients without cancer. The liver allocation system is clearly becoming more equitable, but wide regional variation in the United States in the number of deceased donors and patients with the need for liver transplant has made this an ongoing, complex discussion. Patients with HCC must now wait 6 months from the time of HCC diagnosis until they can undergo transplant with a deceased donor graft. In addition, the maximum MELD exception score they can be given is 34, when previously that was not capped.

While patients are on the waiting list for a liver transplant, tumor progression or even death can occur. A major obstacle for patients awaiting transplant is the lengthy waiting time during which the tumor may progress beyond

the Milan criteria, causing them to drop off the waiting list. Driven by the shortage of deceased donor organs, control of tumor burden with systematic and aggressive locoregional therapies dominated by TACE and RFA have become commonplace. The dropout rate of some patients with HCC has been reported to be as high as 70%, depending on the tumor burden and the length of time the patient waits for transplantation.[83] There is clearly a group of patients who are at a very low risk of dropout (Fig. 132.11).[89] This has led to the concept of a waiting time "sweet spot" between 6 and 18 months to allow for an understanding of each patient's individual tumor biology. If the HCC does not respond well to locoregional therapy during this window, then the likelihood of recurrence after transplant is restrictively high, and the patient should be removed from the waiting list. Again, regional variation in the number of donors and recipients in the United States make this discussion complex.

Living-donor liver transplantation (LDLT) is another source of organs for transplantation. Originally, LDLT was performed in children, with an organ donated from an adult relative; however, adult-to-adult LDLT is now performed throughout the world. Due to cultural differences leading to drastically different rates of deceased donation, LDLT is much more common in India and Asia compared with Western countries. Some studies suggest similar outcomes in cadaveric and LDLT, whereas other studies have shown an increased risk following LDLT.[90] Decision analyses have shown that LDLT for patients with HCC improves life expectancy and is more cost effective than waiting on the transplant list for more than 7 months.[91] Because the waiting time before transplantation can be quite short, it is possible that LDLT may result in a higher risk of recurrence, but more studies may be needed.[92,93]

LDLT is a relatively safe operation, given its inherent invasiveness. LDLT raises a number of ethical issues that need to be dealt with on an individual basis. These include (1) ascertaining that a donor's decision to donate part

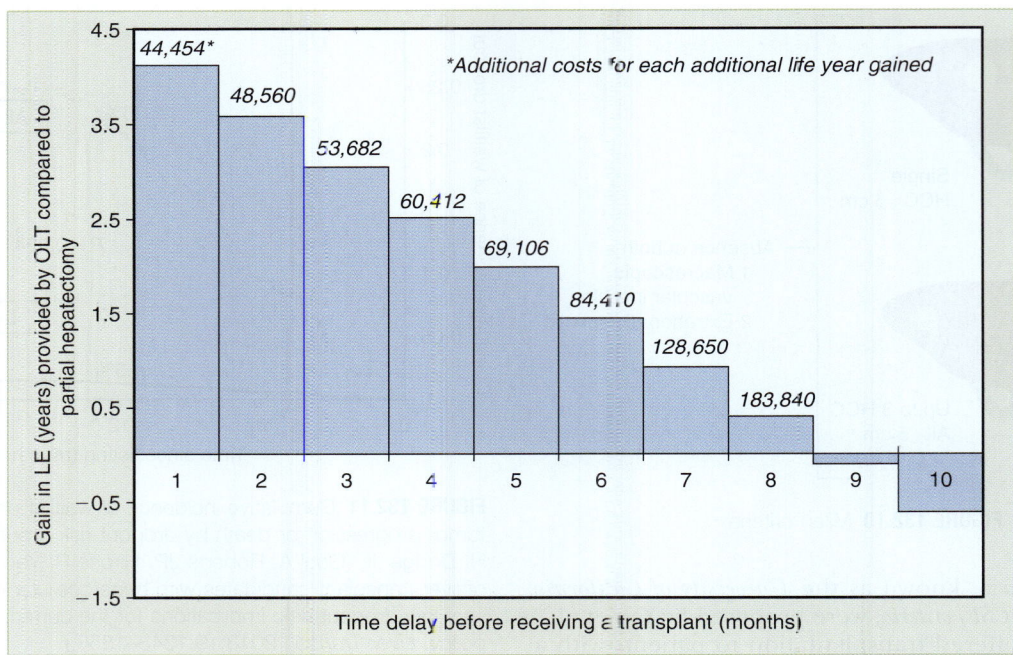

FIGURE 132.12 Tabular demonstration of life expectancy *(LE)* in patients who undergo orthotopic liver transplant versus resection. (From Sarasin FP, Giostra E, Mentha G, Hadengue A. Partial hepatectomy or orthotopic liver transplantation for the treatment of resectable hepatocellular carcinoma? A cost-effectiveness perspective. *Hepatology.* 1998;28:436.)

of their organ is voluntary; (2) ensuring a clear understanding by the donor that the procedure, unlike most operations, is not being done for their own medical problem; (3) noting that donation is associated with complications both intraoperatively and postoperatively; and (4) that there is uncertainty if the donor operation affects long-term survival of donors in any way or has an effect on their quality of life.

Resection Versus Transplantation

In countries with the required resources and infrastructure, controversy continues about whether a patient with HCC should undergo resection or liver transplantation. Although patients with HCC usually have portal hypertension and hepatic decompensation, a small group of patients with small tumors with hepatic reserve are potentially suitable for either resection or transplantation. However, to date, no randomized controlled studies have been published comparing resection and transplantation in such groups of patients. It appears that for tumors that fit the Milan or UCSF criteria, the outcome after transplantation is better than the outcome 5 years after resection. A recent literature review demonstrated that disease-free survival rates after resection at 1, 3, and 5 years were 64%, 38%, and 27%, respectively.[92] The disease-free survival rates following liver transplantation at the same time intervals were 79%, 62.5%, and 54.5%.

However, a major issue is that patients on the transplant waiting list risk tumor progression while awaiting transplantation. As the Milan criteria limit the total tumor burden within which transplantation is indicated, progression risks the suitability for transplantation. In addition, patients with cirrhosis generally have progression of their disease, meaning they are at risk for developing liver decompensation, which could mean they are no longer a candidate for transplantation. One factor that merits consideration in the decision about resection versus liver transplantation is the waiting time to obtain a liver transplant; an immediate resection has a better outcome than waiting a year for a liver transplant, because the immediate resection prevents progression of the disease (Fig. 132.12).[94]

Prior to the HCC MELD exception changes that took place in October 2015, in approximately half of the United States, the waiting time to transplantation was less than 3 months. In that situation, liver transplantation had a better survival at a lower cost per life-year than resection.[95] More time is needed to see how the allocation changes influence survival after transplant now that patients with HCC are required to wait 6 months prior to transplantation. This rule makes the LDLT even more attractive for patients with HCC, because they are not required to wait for 6 months.

Controversy exists about the strategy of initially resecting patients who would be transplant candidates and having transplantation as a means of salvage if the tumor recurs. This strategy takes advantage of the fact that approximately 30% of patients who undergo resection or ablation will be alive and disease free 5 years after resection, meaning they would not require the use of a liver from the deceased donor pool. Currently, there is no way to prospectively select the patients who will survive. This presupposes that transplantation after resection, termed *salvage transplantation,* does not have a different survival rate compared with transplantation without resection, which does not appear to be the case.[96] Furthermore, it appears that many patients who experience recurrence are no longer a candidate for transplant and only approximately 1 in 5 patients will receive a salvage transplantation.[97]

REFERENCES

1. Ferlay J, Shin HR, Bray F, Forman D, Mathers C, Parkin DM. Estimates of worldwide burden of cancer in 2008: GLOBOCAN 2008. *Int J Cancer*. 2010;127:2893-2917.

2. Zoller H, Tilg H. Nonalcoholic fatty liver disease and hepatocellular carcinoma. *Metabolism*. 2016;65(8):1151-1160.

3. Rahib L, Smith BD, Aizenberg R, Rosenzweig AB, Fleshman JM, Matrisian LM. Projecting cancer incidence and deaths to 2030: the unexpected burden of thyroid, liver, and pancreas cancers in the United States. *Cancer Res*. 2014;74:2913-2921.

4. Centers for Disease Control. Hepatocellular carcinoma—United States, 2001–2006. http://www.cdc.gov/mmwr/preview/mmwrhtml/mm5917a3.htm. 2010.

5. Marrero CR, Marrero JA. Viral hepatitis and hepatocellular carcinoma. *Arch Med Res*. 2007;38:612-620.

6. Kao JH, Chen DS. Changing disease burden of hepatocellular carcinoma in the Far East and Southeast Asia. *Liver Int*. 2005;25:696-703.

7. Altekruse SF, McGlynn KA, Reichman ME. Hepatocellular carcinoma incidence, mortality, and survival trends in the United States from 1975 to 2005. *J Clin Oncol*. 2009;27:1485-1491.

8. Younossi ZM, Koenig AB, Abdelatif D, Fazel Y, Henry L, Wymer M. Global epidemiology of non-alcoholic fatty liver disease—meta-analytic assessment of prevalence, incidence and outcomes. *Hepatology*. 2016;64(1):73-84.

9. Makarova-Rusher OV, Altekruse SF, McNeel TS, et al. Population attributable fractions of risk factors for hepatocellular carcinoma in the United States. *Cancer*. 2016;122(11):1757-1765.

10. El-Serag HB. Hepatocellular carcinoma: recent trends in the United States. *Gastroenterology*. 2004;127:S27-S34.

11. Davis GL, Alter MJ, El-Serag H, Poynard T, Jennings LW. Aging of hepatitis C virus (HCV)-infected persons in the United States: a multiple cohort model of HCV prevalence and disease progression. *Gastroenterology*. 2010;138:513-521, 521.e1–521.e6.

12. Centers for Disease Control. Viral hepatitis—hepatitis C information. http://www.cdc.gov/hepatitis/hcv/hcvfaq.htm#a1. 2016.

13. van der Meer AJ, Veldt BJ, Feld JJ, et al. Association between sustained virological response and all-cause mortality among patients with chronic hepatitis C and advanced hepatic fibrosis. *J Am Med Assoc*. 2012;308:2584-2593.

14. Ogden CL, Carroll MD, Kit BK, Flegal KM. Prevalence of childhood and adult obesity in the United States, 2011–2012. *J Am Med Assoc*. 2014;311:806-814.

15. Beltrán-Sánchez H, Harhay MO, Harhay MM, McElligott S. Prevalence and trends of metabolic syndrome in the adult US population, 1999–2010. *J Am Coll Cardiol*. 2013;62:697-703.

16. Williams CD, Stengel J, Asike MI, et al. Prevalence of nonalcoholic fatty liver disease and nonalcoholic steatohepatitis among a largely middle-aged population utilizing ultrasound and liver biopsy: a prospective study. *Gastroenterology*. 2011;140:124-131.

17. Ascha MS, Hanouneh IA, Lopez R, Tamimi TA, Feldstein AF, Zein NN. The incidence and risk factors of hepatocellular carcinoma in patients with nonalcoholic steatohepatitis. *Hepatology*. 2010;51:1972-1978.

18. Centers for Disease Control. Obesity trends. http://www.cdc.gov/obesity/downloads/obesity_trends_2010.ppt. 2010.

19. Liu Y, Wu F. Global burden of aflatoxin-induced hepatocellular carcinoma: a risk assessment. *Environ Health Perspect*. 2010;118:818-824.

20. Chang MH, You SL, Chen CJ, et al. Decreased incidence of hepatocellular carcinoma in hepatitis B vaccinees: a 20-year follow-up study. *J Natl Cancer Inst*. 2009;101:1348-1355.

21. Di Bisceglie AM. Natural history of hepatitis C: its impact on clinical management. *Hepatology*. 2000;31:1014-1018.

22. Niu ZS, Niu XJ, Wang WH, Zhao J. Latest developments in precancerous lesions of hepatocellular carcinoma. *World J Gastroenterol*. 2016;22:3305-3314.

23. Rocken C, Carl-McGrath S. Pathology and pathogenesis of hepatocellular carcinoma. *Dig Dis*. 2001;19:269-278.

24. Koike Y, Shiratori Y, Sato S, et al. Risk factors for recurring hepatocellular carcinoma differ according to infected hepatitis virus—an analysis of 236 consecutive patients with a single lesion. *Hepatology*. 2000;32:1216-1223.

25. Chua TC, Liauw W, Saxena A, et al. Systematic review of neoadjuvant transarterial chemoembolization for resectable hepatocellular carcinoma. *Liver Int*. 2010;30:166-174.

26. Park JY, Kim EK. Pathologic response to preoperative transarterial chemoembolization for resectable hepatocellular carcinoma may not predict recurrence after liver resection. *Hepatobiliary Pancreat Dis Int*. 2016;15:158-164.

27. Semela D, Dufour JF. Angiogenesis and hepatocellular carcinoma. *J Hepatol*. 2004;41:864-880.

28. Esnaola NF, Lauwers GY, Mirza NQ, et al. Predictors of microvascular invasion in patients with hepatocellular carcinoma who are candidates for orthotopic liver transplantation. *J Gastrointest Surg*. 2002;6:224-232; discussion 232.

29. Sakata J, Shirai Y, Wakai T, Kaneko K, Nagahashi M, Hatakeyama K. Preoperative predictors of vascular invasion in hepatocellular carcinoma. *Eur J Surg Oncol*. 2008;34:900-905.

30. Komuta M, Spee B, Vander Borght S, et al. Clinicopathological study on cholangiolocellular carcinoma suggesting hepatic progenitor cell origin. *Hepatology*. 2008;47:1544-1556.

31. Sapisochin G, de Lope CR, Gastaca M, et al. Intrahepatic cholangiocarcinoma or mixed hepatocellular–cholangiocarcinoma in patients undergoing liver transplantation: a Spanish matched cohort multicenter study. *Ann Surg*. 2014;259:944-952.

32. American Association for the Study of Liver Diseases. Guidelines: hepatocellular carcinoma management. http://www.aasld.org/practiceguidelines/Documents/Bookmarked%20Practice%20Guidelines_HCCUpdate2010.pdf. 2010.

33. Atiqin D, Foss D, Kelley M. Acting in the face of uncertainty. *Ann Intern Med*. 2014;161:300-301.

34. Song do S, Bae SH. Changes of guidelines diagnosing hepatocellular carcinoma during the last ten-year period. *Clin Mol Hepatol*. 2012;18:253-257.

35. Ren FY, Piao XX, Jin AL. Efficacy of ultrasonography and alpha-fetoprotein on early detection of hepatocellular carcinoma. *World J Gastroenterol*. 2006;12:4656-4659.

36. Wong RJ, Ahmed A, Gish RG. Elevated alpha-fetoprotein: differential diagnosis—hepatocellular carcinoma and other disorders. *Clin Liver Dis*. 2015;19:309-323.

37. Saton S, Ikeda K, Koida I, et al. Small hepatocellular carcinoma: evaluation of portal blood flow with CT during arterial portography performed with balloon occlusion of the hepatic artery. *Radiology*. 1994;193:67-70.

38. Bolondi L, Sofia S, Siringo S, et al. Surveillance programme of cirrhotic patients for early diagnosis and treatment of hepatocellular carcinoma: a cost effectiveness analysis. *Gut*. 2001;48:251-259.

39. Kim do Y, Han KH. Epidemiology and surveillance of hepatocellular carcinoma. *Liver Cancer*. 2012;1:2-14.

40. Zhang BH, Yang BH, Tang ZY. Randomized controlled trial of screening for hepatocellular carcinoma. *J Cancer Res Clin Oncol*. 2004;130:417-422.

41. Van Thiel DH, Yong S, Li SD, Kennedy M, Brems J. The development of de novo hepatocellular carcinoma in patients on a liver transplant list: frequency, size, and assessment of current screening methods. *Liver Transpl*. 2004;10:631-637.

42. Dietrich CF, Ignee A, Trojan J, Fellbaum C, Schuessler G. Improved characterisation of histologically proven liver tumours by contrast enhanced ultrasonography during the portal venous and specific late phase of SHU 508A. *Gut*. 2004;53:401-405.

43. Liu GJ, Wang W, Lu MD, et al. Contrast-enhanced ultrasound for the characterization of hepatocellular carcinoma and intrahepatic cholangiocarcinoma. *Liver Cancer*. 2015;4:241-252.

44. Bruix J, Sherman M, Practice Guidelines Committee, American Association for the Study of Liver Diseases. Management of hepatocellular carcinoma. *Hepatology*. 2005;42:1208-1236.

45. Llovet JM, Burroughs A, Bruix J. Hepatocellular carcinoma. *Lancet*. 2003;362:1907-1917.

46. Perez-Johnston R, Lenhart DK, Sahani DV. CT angiography of the hepatic and pancreatic circulation. *Radiol Clin North Am*. 2010;48:311-330, viii.

47. Murakami T, Kim T, Takamura M, et al. Hypervascular hepatocellular carcinoma: detection with double arterial phase multi-detector row helical CT. *Radiology*. 2001;218:763-767.

48. Tsurusaki M, Sugimoto K, Fujii M, Fukuda T, Matsumoto S, Sugimura K. Combination of CT during arterial portography and double-phase CT hepatic arteriography with multi-detector row helical CT for evaluation of hypervascular hepatocellular carcinoma. *Clin Radiol*. 2007;62:1189-1197.

49. Schima W, Ba-Ssalamah A, Kurtaran A, Schindl M, Gruenberger T. Post-treatment imaging of liver tumours. *Cancer Imaging*. 2007;7 Spec No A:S28-S36.

50. van den Bos IC, Hussain SM, Dwarkasing RS, et al. MR imaging of hepatocellular carcinoma: relationship between lesion size and imaging findings, including signal intensity and dynamic enhancement patterns. *J Magn Reson Imaging*. 2007;26:1548-1555.

51. Villacastin Ruiz E, Caro-Patón Gómez A, Calero Aguilar H, et al. Review of imaging techniques in the diagnosis of hepatocellular carcinoma in patients who require a liver transplant. *Eur J Gastroenterol Hepatol*. 2016;28:419-424.

52. Weber SM, Lee FT Jr. Expanded treatment of hepatic tumors with radiofrequency ablation and cryoablation. *Oncology (Williston Park)*. 2005;19:27-32.

53. Jaeck D, Bachellier P, Oussoultzoglou E, Weber JC, Wolf P. Surgical resection of hepatocellular carcinoma. Post-operative outcome and long-term results in Europe: an overview. *Liver Transpl*. 2004;10:S58-S63.

54. Minagawa M, Makuuchi M, Takayama T, Kokudo N. Selection criteria for repeat hepatectomy in patients with recurrent hepatocellular carcinoma. *Ann Surg*. 2003;238:703-710.

55. Cha CH, Saif MW, Yamane BH, Weber SM. Hepatocellular carcinoma: current management. *Curr Probl Surg*. 2010;47:10-67.

56. Llovet JM, Ricci S, Mazzaferro V, et al. Sorafenib in advanced hepatocellular carcinoma. *N Engl J Med*. 2008;359:378-390.

57. Cheng AL, Kang YK, Chen Z, et al. Efficacy and safety of sorafenib in patients in the Asia-Pacific region with advanced hepatocellular carcinoma: a phase III randomised, double-blind, placebo-controlled trial. *Lancet Oncol*. 2009;10:25-34.

58. Bruix J, Takayama T, Mazzaferro V, et al. Adjuvant sorafenib for hepatocellular carcinoma after resection or ablation (STORM): a phase 3, randomised, double-blind, placebo-controlled trial. *Lancet Oncol*. 2015;16:1344-1354.

59. Geissler EK, Schnitzbauer AA, Zülke C, et al. Sirolimus use in liver transplant recipients with hepatocellular carcinoma: a randomized, multicenter, open-label phase 3 trial. *Transplantation*. 2016;100:116-125.

60. Koeberle D, Dufour JF, Demeter G, et al. Sorafenib with or without everolimus in patients with advanced hepatocellular carcinoma (HCC): a randomized multicenter, multinational phase II trial (SAKK 77/08 and SASL 29). *Ann Oncol*. 2016;27(5):856-861.

61. Zhu AX, Kudo M, Assenat E, et al. Effect of everolimus on survival in advanced hepatocellular carcinoma after failure of sorafenib: the EVOLVE-1 randomized clinical trial. *J Am Med Assoc*. 2014;312:57-67.

62. Hori T, Nagata K, Hasuike S, et al. Risk factors for the local recurrence of hepatocellular carcinoma after a single session of percutaneous radiofrequency ablation. *J Gastroenterol*. 2003;38:977-981.

63. Chen MS, Li JQ, Zheng Y, et al. A prospective randomized trial comparing percutaneous local ablative therapy and partial hepatectomy for small hepatocellular carcinoma. *Ann Surg*. 2006;243:321-328.

64. Xie X, Dendukuri N, McGregor M. Percutaneous radiofrequency ablation for the treatment of early stage hepatocellular carcinoma: a health technology assessment. *Int J Technol Assess Health Care*. 2010;26:390-397.

65. Seror O, N'Kontchou G, Nault JC, et al. Hepatocellular carcinoma within Milan criteria no-touch multibipolar radiofrequency ablation for treatment—long-term results. *Radiology*. 2016;280(3):150743.

66. Yang W, Yan K, Goldberg SN, et al. Ten-year survival of hepatocellular carcinoma patients undergoing radiofrequency ablation as a first-line treatment. *World J Gastroenterol*. 2016;22:2993-3005.

67. Lin SM, Lin CJ, Lin CC, Hsu CW, Chen YC. Radiofrequency ablation improves prognosis compared with ethanol injection for hepatocellular carcinoma < or = 4 cm. *Gastroenterology*. 2004;127:1714-1723.

68. Vogl TJ, Naguib NN, Nour-Eldin NE, et al. Review on transarterial chemoembolization in hepatocellular carcinoma: palliative, combined, neoadjuvant, bridging, and symptomatic indications. *Eur J Radiol*. 2009;72:505-516.

69. Llovet JM, Bruix J. Systematic review of randomized trials for unresectable hepatocellular carcinoma: chemoembolization improves survival. *Hepatology*. 2003;37:429-442.

70. Ravaioli M, Grazi GL, Ercolani G, et al. Partial necrosis on hepatocellular carcinoma nodules facilitates tumor recurrence after liver transplantation. *Transplantation*. 2004;78:1780-1786.

71. Cheng BQ, Jia CQ, Liu CT, et al. Chemoembolization combined with radiofrequency ablation for patients with hepatocellular carcinoma larger than 3 cm: a randomized controlled trial. *J Am Med Assoc*. 2008;299:1669-1677.

72. Kagawa T, Koizumi J, Kojima S, et al. Transcatheter arterial chemoembolization plus radiofrequency ablation therapy for early stage hepatocellular carcinoma: comparison with surgical resection. *Cancer*. 2010;116:3638-3644.

73. Morimoto M, Numata K, Kondou M, Nozaki A, Morita S, Tanaka K. Midterm outcomes in patients with intermediate-sized hepatocellular carcinoma: a randomized controlled trial for determining the efficacy of radiofrequency ablation combined with transcatheter arterial chemoembolization. *Cancer*. 2010;116:5452-5460.

74. Liang P, Dong B, Yu X, et al. Prognostic factors for survival in patients with hepatocellular carcinoma after percutaneous microwave ablation. *Radiology*. 2005;235:299-307.

75. Dong W, Zhang T, Wang ZG, Liu H. Clinical outcome of small hepatocellular carcinoma after different treatments: a meta-analysis. *World J Gastroenterol*. 2014;20:10174-10182.

76. Makuuchi M, Imamura H, Sugawara Y, Takayama T. Progress in surgical treatment of hepatocellular carcinoma. *Oncology*. 2002;62(suppl 1):74-81.

77. Llovet JM, Schwartz M, Mazzaferro V. Resection and liver transplantation for hepatocellular carcinoma. *Semin Liver Dis*. 2005;25:181-200.

78. Llovet JM, Fuster J, Bruix J. Intention-to-treat analysis of surgical treatment for early hepatocellular carcinoma: resection versus transplantation. *Hepatology*. 1999;30:1434-1440.

79. Farges O, Belghiti J, Kianmanesh R, et al. Portal vein embolization before right hepatectomy: prospective clinical trial. *Ann Surg*. 2003;237:208-217.

80. Makuuchi M, Thai BL, Takayasu K, et al. Preoperative portal embolization to increase safety of major hepatectomy for hilar bile duct carcinoma: a preliminary report. *Surgery*. 1990;107:521-527.

81. Palavecino M, Chun YS, Madoff DC, et al. Major hepatic resection for hepatocellular carcinoma with or without portal vein embolization: perioperative outcome and survival. *Surgery*. 2009;145:399-405.

82. Cho SH, Chun JM, Kwon HJ, Han YS, Kim SG, Hwang YJ. Outcomes and recurrence pattern after non-anatomic liver resection for solitary hepatocellular carcinomas. *Korean J Hepatobiliary Pancreat Surg*. 2016;20:1-7.

83. Leong WQ, Ganpathi IS, Kow AW, Madhavan K, Chang SK. Comparative study and systematic review of laparoscopic liver resection for hepatocellular carcinoma. *World J Hepatol*. 2015;7:2765-2773.

84. Mazzaferro V, Regalia E, Doci R, et al. Liver transplantation for the treatment of small hepatocellular carcinomas in patients with cirrhosis. *N Engl J Med*. 1996;334:693-699.

85. Yao FY, Ferrell L, Bass NM, et al. Liver transplantation for hepatocellular carcinoma: expansion of the tumor size limits does not adversely impact survival. *Hepatology*. 2001;33:1394-1403.

86. Yao FY, Xiao L, Bass NM, Kerlan R, Ascher NL, Roberts JP. Liver transplantation for hepatocellular carcinoma: validation of the UCSF-expanded criteria based on preoperative imaging. *Am J Transplant*. 2007;7:2587-2596.

87. Yao FY, Mehta N, Flemming J, et al. Downstaging of hepatocellular cancer before liver transplant: long-term outcome compared to tumors within Milan criteria. *Hepatology*. 2015;61:1968-1977.

88. Lo CM, Fan ST, Liu CL, Chan SC, Wong J. The role and limitation of living donor liver transplantation for hepatocellular carcinoma. *Liver Transpl*. 2004;10:440-447.

89. Mehta N, Dodge JL, Goel A, Roberts JP, Hirose R, Yao FY. Identification of liver transplant candidates with hepatocellular carcinoma and a very low dropout risk: implications for the current organ allocation policy. *Liver Transpl*. 2013;19:1343-1353.

90. Fisher RA, Kulik LM, Freise CE, et al. Hepatocellular carcinoma recurrence and death following living and deceased donor liver transplantation. *Am J Transplant*. 2007;7:1601-1608.

91. Sarasin FP, Majno PE, Llovet JM, Bruix J, Mentha G, Hadengue A. Living donor liver transplantation for early hepatocellular carcinoma: a life-expectancy and cost-effectiveness perspective. *Hepatology*. 2001;33:1073-1079.

92. Morris-Stiff G, Gomez D, de Liguori Carino N, Prasad KR. Surgical management of hepatocellular carcinoma: is the jury still out? *Surg Oncol*. 2009;18:298-321.

93. Ninomiya M, Shirabe K, Facciuto ME, et al. Comparative study of living and deceased donor liver transplantation as a treatment for hepatocellular carcinoma. *J Am Coll Surg*. 2015;220:297-304, e3.

94. Sarasin FP, Giostra E, Mentha G, Hadengue A. Partial hepatectomy or orthotopic liver transplantation for the treatment of resectable hepatocellular carcinoma? A cost-effectiveness perspective. *Hepatology.* 1998;28:436-442.

95. Majno PE, Sarasin FP, Mentha G, Hadengue A. Primary liver resection and salvage transplantation or primary liver transplantation in patients with single, small hepatocellular carcinoma and preserved liver function: an outcome-oriented decision analysis. *Hepatology.* 2000;31:899-906.

96. Del Gaudio M, Ercolani G, Ravaioli M, et al. Liver transplantation for recurrent hepatocellular carcinoma or cirrhosis after liver resection: University of Bologna experience. *Am J Transplant.* 2008;8: 1177-1185.

97. Botha JF, Campos BD. Salvage transplantation: does saving livers save lives? *Am J Transplant.* 2008;8:1085-1086.

Management of Primary Malignant Hepatic Neoplasms Other Than Hepatocellular Cancer

Epameinondas Dogeas | Michael A. Choti

Primary hepatic malignancies consist of a diverse spectrum of tumors that arise from an equally diverse population of cells that constitute this complex organ. In addition to hepatocytes, the liver is made of cholangiocytes, neuroendocrine cells, hepatic progenitors, myofibroblastic mesenchymal cells, and vascular endothelial cells. Hepatocellular carcinoma (HCC) represents the vast majority (80% to 90%) of primary liver cancers.[1,2] All other primary liver neoplasms, including cholangiocarcinoma, account for 10% to 20%.[3] Table 133.1 outlines the primary hepatic malignancies with their corresponding cellular progenitors. This chapter focuses on nonhepatocellular primary malignancies of the liver. While less common than HCC, these tumor types can be aggressive and are being diagnosed with increasing frequency. The clinician should have a better understanding in the recognition and management of these malignancies

INTRAHEPATIC CHOLANGIOCARCINOMA

Intrahepatic cholangiocarcinoma (ICC) is the second most common primary liver malignancy, accounting for up to 15% of all liver cancers.[4] ICC is defined as cholangiocarcinoma proximal to the second-degree bile ducts and it consists of approximately 10% of all cholangiocarcinomas.[5] The incidence of ICC appears to be increasing, in contrast to the incidence of extrahepatic (hilar and distal) cholangiocarcinoma, which has decreased both in the United States and worldwide.[5] The increasing incidence of ICC could be partially attributed to our ability to more accurately diagnose these tumors, both radiographically and pathologically. In the past, many patients with ICC were erroneously diagnosed with liver metastasis, frequently called *adenocarcinoma of unknown origin*. However, there is epidemiologic evidence that the true incidence of ICC is also rising.[7]

Recently, cirrhosis and hepatitis B and C have been identified as risk factors for the development of ICC.[4,7,8] Much as with HCC, it has been hypothesized that the inflammatory cytokines and cell death associated with the aforementioned conditions promote oncogenesis and the development of ICC. In a recent meta-analysis of epidemiologic studies on ICC risk factors, cirrhosis had an odds ratio (OR) of 22.92 (95% confidence interval [CI], 18.24 to 28.79), hepatitis B: OR, 5.10 (CI, 2.91 to 8.95), and hepatitis C: OR, 4.84 (CI, 2.41 to 9.71).[9] Hepatolithiasis has also been associated with the development of ICC.[8] However, the vast majority of ICC develops de novo without any associated risk factors.

New studies have begun to elucidate the genetic profile of ICC and the mechanics driving tumorigenesis and tumor survival.[10–12] These findings have also begun to identify potential targets for biologic therapies in patients with ICC.[13] Sia et al. performed gene expression and mutation analysis on 149 ICC samples.[14] They identified two classes of ICC, one in which inflammatory signals predominate (38% of ICC in their study) and another one in which proliferation pathways predominate (62%). In the inflammation class, cytokines were overexpressed and signal transducer and activator of transcription 3 (STAT3) was activated. In the proliferation class, the RAS/MAPK/MET signaling pathways were activated and KRAS and BRAF were frequently mutated. In another study, Andersen et al. profiled the transcriptome of 104 ICC and discovered frequent deregulation of the HER2 network and frequent overexpression of epidermal growth factor receptor (EGFR).[15] Jiao et al. sequenced the exome of 32 ICCs and discovered frequent inactivating mutations in chromatin remodeling genes (ARID1A, BAP1, and PBRM1). They also discovered frequent mutations in the IDH1 and IDH2 genes that encode the metabolic enzymes isocitrate dehydrogenase.[16] Mutations of IDH1 and IDH2 in ICC have been identified in several other studies as well.[17–19] IDH1 and IDH2 mutations lead to hypermethylation of DNA and histones, which can result in altered gene expression and carcinogenesis. In addition, novel fibroblast growth factor receptor 2 (FGFR2) gene fusions have also been identified in ICC.[20] Finally, notch signaling has also been studied and implicated in ICC.[21] This pathway has been found to be important for cell differentiation and bile duct formation.[22] In two preclinical models, mature hepatocytes with activated Notch converted into ICC precursors.[23,24] Sia et al. have also demonstrated that the transcriptome of ICC has similarities to HCC.[14] These studies challenge the theory that ICC arises from cholangiocytes and raises the question of which is the true cell of origin of ICC.[25]

Our novel understanding of the genetic heterogeneity of ICC has important clinical implications. Zhu et al. analyzed 200 resected ICCs from seven centers and discovered that most somatic mutations were prevalent in low frequency.[26] In fact, the majority (61.5%) of patients harbored no mutations. In the remaining minority of patients with mutations, only two mutations, KRAS and IDH, were identified with a frequency greater than 5%. These data suggest that applying targeted therapies in ICC is unlikely to benefit all patients. It calls for a personalized approach with sequencing of individual tumors and identification of mutations that would confer sensitivity to biologic therapies. Fortunately, all the commonly altered cancer driver pathways in ICC (IDH, FGFR2, EGFR, mammalian target of rapamycin [mTOR], Notch, chromatin remodelers, and MET) have "actionable" targets.[11,13,27,28]

Histologically, ICC can be classified as mass-forming, periductal-infiltrating, intraductal, superficial spreading, and undefined categories.[29–31] The mass-forming subtype is defined as a mass located in the liver parenchyma, invading through the portal venous system and is the most common form of ICC. The periductal-infiltrating subtype extends longitudinally along the bile duct and can cause peripheral biliary dilation. It often displays lymphatic invasion. The intraductal subtype proliferates into the bile duct, forming an intraductal tumor thrombus.[30] Historically, superficial spreading and intraductal ICC have been associated with better prognosis, while periductal and mass-forming have had worse outcomes.[11] ICC has a distinct immunohistochemistry profile that can help differentiate it from adenocarcinoma liver metastases and HCC. ICC stains strongly positive for CK7 and negative or weakly positive for CK20.[32] In contrast to HCC, ICC does not express hepatocyte paraffin antibody 1 (HepPar-1).[33] Expression of N-cadherin can further differentiate ICC from extrahepatic cholangiocarcinoma, as the combination of CK7 and N-cadherin positivity has a specificity of 98% for ICC.[34]

ICC is most often identified on cross-sectional imaging, computed tomography (CT), or magnetic resonance imaging (MRI) as a mass lesion (Fig. 133.1A). In most cases, ICC has imaging characteristics similar to adenocarcinoma metastases, including peripheral venous enhancement and central necrosis. Less commonly, ICC can appear with arterial enhancement or intravascular thrombus, mimicking radiologic findings of HCC.[32,35] Contrast-enhanced MRI can help differentiate between ICC and other tumor types, including mixed cholangiohepatocellular carcinoma. More commonly, extracellular gadolinium contrast media is used in liver MRI. However, newer contrast agents such as gadoxetic acid (Eovist) and gadobenate dimeglumine

TABLE 133.1 Cellular Phenotype and Primary Hepatic Neoplasms

Cellular Phenotype	Primary Hepatic Tumor
Epithelial	
Hepatocellular	Hepatocellular carcinoma
Hepatic progenitor	Hepatoblastoma
Cholangiocellular	Intrahepatic cholangiocarcinoma
	Hepatic cystadenocarcinoma
Mixed	Mixed cholangiohepatocellular carcinoma
Other	Primary squamous cell carcinoma
Mesenchymal	
Muscular	Leiomyosarcoma
	Rhabdomyosarcoma
Fibroblastic	Fibrosarcoma
Adipose	Liposarcoma
Neural	Schwannoma
Vascular	Angiosarcoma
	Epithelioid hemangioendothelioma

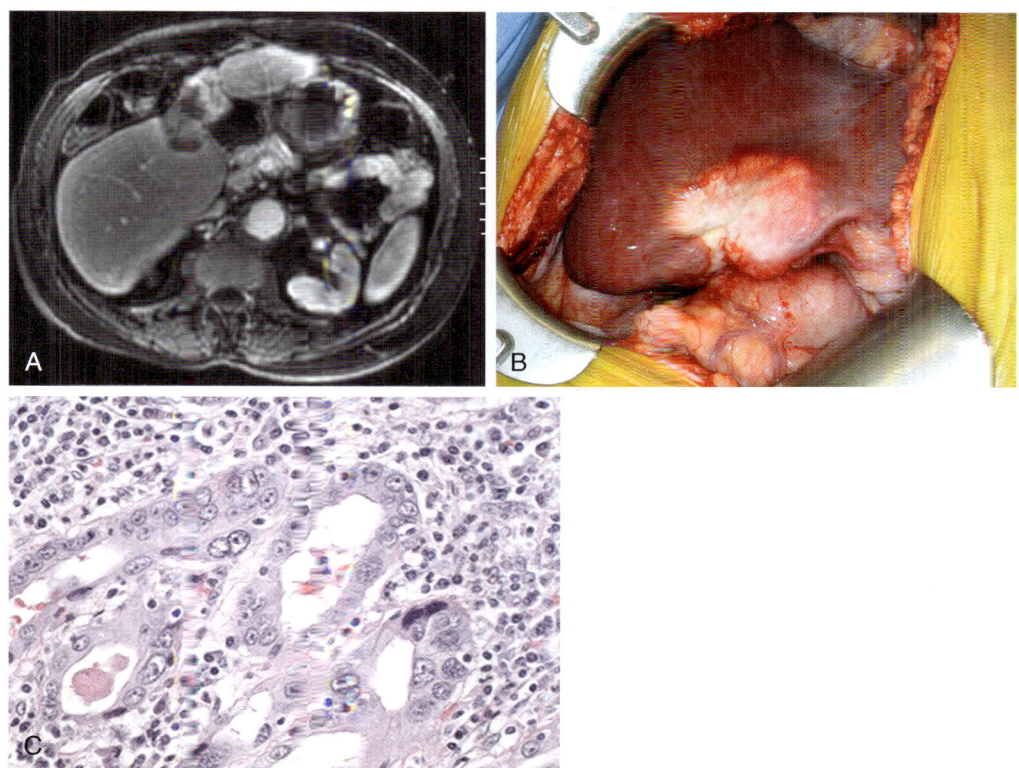

FIGURE 133.1 (A) Magnetic resonance imaging demonstrating a 6-cm intrahepatic cholangiocarcinoma involving the left hemiliver. (B) Intraoperative photograph demonstrating the same tumor prior to planned resection. (C) Photomicrograph of an intrahepatic cholangiocarcinoma. The small glandular structures with nuclei are oval and vesicular. There is also demonstrable mucin production within the ducts. (Courtesy M.S. Torbenson, Department of Pathology, Johns Hopkins Hospital.)

(Multihance) have been shown to have improved ability to characterize ICC.[36] Fluorodeoxyglucose positron emission tomography (FDG-PET) can also be useful as an adjunctive imaging modality. In particular, FDG-PET can be useful to detect nodal involvement or unsuspected distant metastases.[37]

In some cases when a definitive diagnosis needs to be established to plan management, a percutaneous needle biopsy may be indicated. When a biopsy of a suspicious liver tumor reveals adenocarcinoma, it is important not to mistake the diagnosis of ICC from that of a hepatic metastasis from an extrahepatic origin. In such cases, a history of a previous malignancy, identification of other risk factors, and scrutiny of tumor markers are helpful. Moreover, multifocal lesions within the liver increase the likelihood that these are metastases. Staging of the chest and abdomen using CT scanning is useful to help rule out other potential primary tumors as well as metastatic disease. Upper and lower endoscopy should be considered to rule out an intestinal primary malignancy and, in women, mammography and gynecologic screening should be considered.

In ambiguous cases, serum tumor markers such as CA 19-9 can also aid in establishing the diagnosis of ICC. Bergquist et al. using the National Cancer Data Base (NCDB)[38] reported that CA 19-9 was elevated in 66.7% of ICC patients. Additionally, elevated CA 19-9 was an independent predictor of mortality, similar to node positivity and positive resection margins. More recently, other biomarkers have been studied. Ferrone et al. found that tumor staining for albumin RNA using in situ hybridization was highly predictive of primary liver tumor origin rather than metastasis.[39]

ICC is staged based on primary tumor characteristics, lymph nodal involvement, and distant metastasis per the American Joint Commission on Cancer (AJCC) 7th edition Cancer Staging Manual (Table 133.2).[40] This was a departure from previous staging systems that classified ICC with criteria similar to HCC. Notably, tumor size is no longer part of the T classification. Conversely, micro- or major vascular invasion, the number of total lesions, invasion of adjacent structures, and periductal invasion convey important prognostic information. The presence of involved regional lymph nodes (hilar, periduodenal, or peripancreatic) is classified as stage IV disease, as lymph nodal involvement has been shown to negatively affect survival in large multiinstitutional studies.[41] The 7th edition AJCC staging system for ICC has been independently validated and found to distribute patients more equally among stages and to predict survival more accurately than older systems.[42–44]

When possible, surgical resection is the treatment of choice for ICC. The criteria for resectability of ICC are similar to other malignancies. Unlike HCC, where the presence of cirrhosis can impact resectability, ICC is typically associated with normal liver function. Staging laparoscopy prior to laparotomy for ICC is controversial and more commonly only recommended in high-risk circumstances (e.g., multicentric disease, high CA 19-9, radiologic findings suspicious for major vascular invasion or peritoneal disease).[44] In two prospective studies evaluating operations for various hepatobiliary malignancies, staging laparoscopy avoided open exploration in

TABLE 133.2	Staging of Intrahepatic Cholangiocarcinoma		
PRIMARY TUMOR (T)			
Tx	Primary tumor cannot be assessed		
T0	No evidence of primary tumor		
Tis	Carcinoma in situ (Intraductal tumor)		
T1	Solitary tumor without vascular invasion		
T2a	Solitary tumor with vascular invasion		
T2b	Multiple tumors, with or without vascular invasion		
T3	Tumor perforating the visceral peritoneum or with direct invasion of local extrahepatic structures		
T4	Tumor with periductal invasion		
REGIONAL LYMPH NODES (N)			
Nx	Regional lymph nodes cannot be assessed		
N0	No regional lymph node metastasis		
N1	Regional lymph node metastasis present		
DISTANT METASTASIS (M)			
M0	No distant metastasis		
M1	Distant metastasis present		
ANATOMIC STAGE			
Stage 0	Tis	N0	M0
Stage I	T1	N0	M0
Stage II	T2	N0	M0
Stage III	T3	N0	M0
Stage IVa	T4	N0	M0
Stage IVb	Any T	N1	M0
	Any T	Any N	M1

From Edge SB, American Joint Committee on Cancer. *AJCC Cancer Staging Manual.* 7th ed. New York: Springer; 2010.

approximately one third of patients due to the discovery of occult metastatic disease.[45,46] However, neither study specifically examined ICC.

Intraoperatively, ICC can appear much like other hepatic malignancies, often with normal appearing surrounding liver (see Fig. 133.1B). As with most liver surgery, intraoperative ultrasonography is important to determine resectability and rule out occult multifocal disease. The goal of resection is complete extirpation of all gross disease with negative margins while maintaining adequate remnant portal and arterial inflow, hepatic venous outflow, intact biliary drainage, and sufficient uninvolved remnant liver volume. Inclusion of a resection of the extrahepatic biliary tree with reconstruction or inclusion of major vascular (portal vein or inferior vena cava) resection may be required in some circumstances. In one series, 12% of hepatectomies were combined with major vascular resection with no difference in short- and long-term outcomes.[47] In another multiinstitutional Italian series, biliary and major vascular resection were required in 19% and 5% of cases, respectively. With this aggressive surgical approach, negative-margin (R0) resection can be achieved in up to 80% of patients.[48]

Complete resection is associated with improved long-term survival in patients with ICC, with reported 5-year overall survival rates of 30% to 40%.[41,48,49] A meta-analysis of all published series of surgically resected ICC identified the following factors to be associated with worse survival: age, tumor size, multifocal tumors, lymph node metastasis, vascular invasion, and poor tumor differentiation.[50] Hyder et al. studied 514 patients who underwent resection for ICC in United States, Europe, and Asia and used proportional hazards regression modeling to identify factors associated with survival and construct a nomogram.[51] They also identified age at diagnosis, tumor size, multiple tumors, cirrhosis, lymph node metastasis, and macrovascular invasion to negatively impact survival. Fortunately, recent reports suggest improving outcomes in patients undergoing resection for ICC. Endo et al. reported improved disease-free survival when comparing patients resected between 2001 and 2006 compared with those resected between 1990 and 1999.[52] Similarly, Nathan et al. found in a review of ICC outcomes in the United States using the Surveillance Epidemiology and End Results (SEER) database a trend toward better outcome following resection, despite overall poorer outcome in patients with ICC.[42]

ICC can be associated with regional (periportal, periduodenal, or peripancreatic) nodal involvement.[53] Moreover, involved lymph nodes are an important predictor of poor long-term outcome following resection.[12,54] De Jong et al. found a 30% rate of lymph nodal metastasis among patients receiving lymphadenectomy in a multiinstitutional database of 449 patients.[41] However, as node dissection was performed only selectively in this series, this is likely an overestimation of node positivity in resected ICC. In this study, positive nodes were associated with worse survival (median 24 vs. 30 months). Based on these data, some have questioned the value of resection in patients with ICC and lymph node involvement. Uenishi et al. found that while patients with negative nodes had better survival, those with lymph nodes still had favorable outcomes, with a 5-year survival rate of 26%.[55] Similarly, Vitale et al. identified a survival benefit in patients who underwent therapeutic lymphadenectomy (defined as removal of more than three lymph nodes) in a propensity scores analysis using the SEER database.[56] While still controversial, surgical resection can reasonably be offered to patients even with preoperative evidence of nodal involvement, provided all disease can be completely removed. Many experts now recommend routine hilar and periportal lymphadenectomy in all patients undergoing surgical resection for ICC.[44,48,57]

In patients with unresectable disease confined to the liver, a variety of locoregional therapies have the potential of "downstaging" initially unresectable ICC, allowing curative intent resection in selected patients. Intraarterial liver therapies, such as bland transarterial embolization (TAE), transarterial chemoembolization (TACE), hepatic arterial infusion therapy (HAI), and yttrium-90 radioembolization have been reported. Among the arterial therapies, TACE historically has been most often used. A recent meta-analysis on TACE for ICC revealed a pooled partial and complete radiologic response of 22% and 10%.[58] In some selected series, TACE can achieve 40% to 70% response rates and median survival times of 12 to 29 months.[59-61] Continuous HAI therapy with an implanted catheter and pump has been promoted by some groups. While reports are limited to highly selected unresectable ICC

patients, response rates of up to 50% when combined with systemic chemotherapy have been reported.[62,63] More recently, radioembolization with yttrium-90 microspheres is being used with increasing frequency as liver-directed therapy for unresectable ICC. While data are limited, the results appear promising and comparable to other intraarterial therapies, with reported median survival of 9 to 22 months.[64-66] Alternatively, external beam stereotactic body radiotherapy (SBRT) is currently being investigated for unresectable ICC. A phase I/II study of 26 patients with either HCC or ICC treated with SBRT demonstrated a response rate of 42% with a 1-year survival of 45%.[67] Local ablative therapies, radiofrequency ablation (RFA), and microwave ablation (MWA) have been reported in small series of patients with ICC.[68] Because ablation is typically used only in small tumors, it is rarely recommended in unresectable ICC. However, in selected cases, ablation can be used in a patient with a small tumor who is not a candidate for surgery, during surgery as an adjunct to liver resection, or with recurrent disease following prior resection.

Unlike for HCC, the role of liver transplantation for cholangiocarcinoma is limited. Historically, 5-year survival after transplant for cholangiocarcinoma (combining hilar and intrahepatic tumors) was below 20%, leading many centers to consider cholangiocarcinoma as a contraindication for transplantation.[69] More recently, a retrospective cohort multicenter study from Spain showed a 5-year actuarial survival rate of 51% after liver transplantation for ICC.[70] Others have reported encouraging long-term survival in patients with incidentally discovered, early-stage cholangiocarcinomas in the explanted livers of patients with cirrhosis.[71] In addition, some centers such as the Mayo Clinic have found favorable outcomes in patients with cholangiocarcinoma treated with transplant combined with neoadjuvant chemotherapy and chemoradiation.[72,73] However, these patients had hilar cholangiocarcinoma, many with primary biliary cirrhosis, and not ICC. While encouraging, there is no established role for liver transplant in patients with ICC at this time outside of a clinical trial.

Most patients diagnosed with ICC have advanced disease at the time of diagnosis resulting in a median survival of less than 1 year.[74] Randomized, phase III clinical trials examining chemotherapy have been difficult to conduct for ICC due to the small number of patients and the heterogeneous nature of biliary tract malignancies. Historically, 5-fluorouracil was offered as a single agent in unresectable ICC with only a 10% response rate.[75] More recently, combination chemotherapy including platinum-containing regimens have shown increased efficacy. Specifically, Valle et al. reported in a large randomized phase III trial (ABC trial) that patients with advanced cholangiocarcinoma had significantly improved survival with gemcitabine plus cisplatin compared with gemcitabine alone (11.7 vs. 8.1 months).[76] Ongoing trials are examining regimens to improve on these outcomes, including the addition of biologics.[77,78] Advances in genomic sequencing may allow identification of potential actionable targets that can be exploited therapeutically. For example, studies are underway in ICC using targeting of FGFR2 fusions and IDH1/2 mutations.[17,79]

There are currently limited data on the use of chemotherapy in the adjuvant setting for ICC following resection. The presence of high risk factors for recurrence, including lymphovascular and perineural invasion, lymph node metastasis, and positive surgical margins, increases enthusiasm for recommending adjuvant therapy. However, there are no controlled trials demonstrating benefit of adjuvant therapy for ICC. Patients with complete resection (R0) and absence of the above factors should be followed with observation alone. If a decision to administer adjuvant therapy is made, options include fluoropyrimidine chemoradiation, or fluoropyrimidine-based or gemcitabine-based chemotherapy.[80,81] These recommendations are based on phase II trials. Participation in ongoing clinical trials should also be considered.

COMBINED HEPATOCELLULAR CARCINOMA-CHOLANGIOCARCINOMA

Our recently increased understanding of the bipotential nature of hepatic progenitor cells has revealed that they can differentiate between hepatocyte and biliary lineages.[82] Therefore it is not surprising that tumors can develop with heterogeneous cellularity, termed as *combined hepatocellular carcinoma-cholangiocarcinoma (cHCC-CC)*. These tumors are rare, with an estimated incidence of 1.3%. However, their true incidence might be higher, given the significant potential for misdiagnosis.[83] Based upon the concomitant cytokeratin profile consistent with a biliary lineage, albumin expression consistent with a hepatocytic lineage, as well as carcinoembryonic antigen (CEA) and alpha-fetoprotein (AFP) levels, indeed, mixed cholangiohepatocellular carcinomas should be distinguishable from ICC and HCC. Much like HCC, these tumors are commonly associated with chronic viral hepatitis and cirrhosis, suggesting that chronic injury and expansion of hepatic progenitors may be earlier events in tumor progression. Yet, similar to ICC, these mixed tumors may occur sporadically without any risk factors.[85] Histologically, cHCC-CC is defined as a tumor containing intimately mixed elements of both HCC and ICC. The presence of "transition zones," which contain cells with intermediate morphology, is particularly important for the diagnosis. These transition zones distinguish "true" cHCC-CC from "collision tumors," where the HCC and ICC components are clearly separated.[84] Imaging characteristics, such as HCC, typically demonstrate arterial enhancement and heterogeneous necrosis on contrast CT or MRI (Fig. 133.2).

Management of cHCC-CC should include liver resection when possible.[55] Some experts, extrapolating from the data on ICC, have recommended the addition of lymphadenectomy to resection.[86] In cirrhotic patients, liver transplantation can be considered based on similar criteria to that of HCC. However, studies thus far have produced mixed results as to the outcomes of liver transplantation for cHCC-CC.[70,87] Given the infrequency of this tumor type, no reliable histopathologic prognostic factors have been identified.[88] In cases of advanced disease, it remains unclear whether systemic treatment strategies directed toward HCC or ICC are more effective in these tumors.

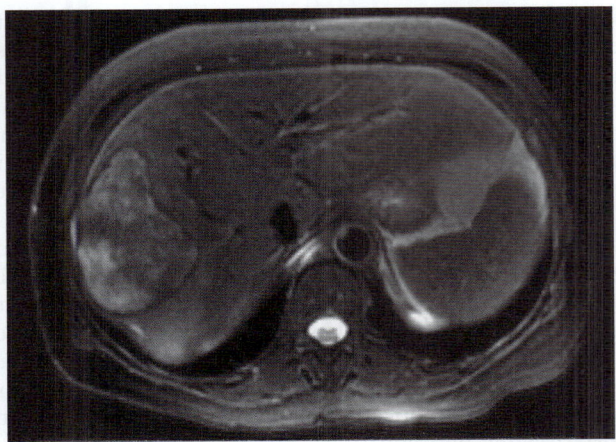

FIGURE 133.2 Abdominal magnetic resonance imaging revealing a large right liver mass. Pathologic analysis following resection demonstrated findings consistent with a mixed cholangiohepatocellular carcinoma.

BILIARY CYSTADENOCARCINOMA

Biliary or hepatic cystadenocarcinoma (BCAC) is an uncommon epithelioid tumor of the liver with less than 250 cases reported in the literature.[89–91] There is controversy whether BCAC arises de novo from the intrahepatic bile ducts or whether benign biliary cystadenomas undergo malignant transformation to form BCAC.[92] Interestingly, while biliary cystadenomas have a clear female predominance, cystadenocarcinoma tends to occur with equal frequency in men and women.[89] It usually presents with nonspecific abdominal symptoms, for example, pain, fullness, early satiety, jaundice.[90] As with other intrahepatic biliary malignancies, this tumor is increasingly found incidentally on CT, MRI, or ultrasound. Thick or irregular wall, peripheral enhancement, associated mass, or papillary tumor projections into a cystic lesion help distinguish BCAC from benign liver cystic lesions. However, CT and MRI frequently fail to make this diagnosis preoperatively.[91] One study reported a positive predictive value of 11% and specificity of 21% when differentiating cystadenocarcinoma versus benign cystadenoma.[90] Analysis of the cyst fluid can occasionally be helpful in establishing the diagnosis of BCAC using needle aspiration, but concerns regarding peritoneal or pleural tumor seeding diminish enthusiasm for its routine use.[93–95] Given the concern for malignant progression of biliary cystadenomas and the difficulties of definitively excluding malignancy preoperatively, most experts recommend surgical resection of hepatic cystic lesions suspicious for these neoplasms. In some cases when a benign disease is suspected, operative biopsy and intraoperative frozen-section analysis can be performed.[96]

When the cystadenocarcinoma is localized and amenable to surgical removal, hepatectomy to clear margins is indicated.[89,95] Survival rates following resection of BCAC have been reported in the range of 25% to 100% at 5 years.[90,91] Positive margins and the presence of spindle cell/ovarian stroma in the tumor are associated with risk of recurrence.[90]

SQUAMOUS CELL CARCINOMA OF THE LIVER

Primary squamous cell carcinoma (SCC) of the liver is extremely rare, with less than 40 cases reported in the literature.[97-99] This histologic diagnosis is often a liver metastasis and should prompt a thorough search for a primary site of SCC, including the skin, oropharynx, and anus. Primary liver SCC is a diagnosis of exclusion when the search for another SCC site is negative. Hepatic teratoma, cyst, and hepatolithiasis have been associated with this rare disease.[98,100] Histologically these tumors are described with keratinized-type cellular features, often with benign appearing metaplastic squamous epithelium. Overall, survival is poor in these patients with median survival of less than 1 year when left untreated or not resected.[97-99] Treatment recommendations are based on limited evidence given the rarity of the disease. Liver resection, when possible, is generally recommended based on several reports of long-term survival following hepatectomy.[97,99]

PRIMARY HEPATIC SARCOMA: LEIOMYOSARCOMA, RHABDOMYOSARCOMA, FIBROSARCOMA, LIPOSARCOMA, UNDIFFERENTIATED EMBRYONAL SARCOMA

Sarcomas of the liver are extremely rare, representing less than 1% of primary liver malignancies.[101-103] Their incidence is higher in the pediatric population, but all subtypes have been described in adults as well. They can arise from a plethora of connective tissue cellular progenitors, including smooth muscle, liver mesenchymal cell, or fatty tissue. Sarcomas are more often hypervascular in appearance on contrast imaging with a lack of venous invasion. These features can help differentiate primary hepatic sarcomas from HCC, especially in noncirrhotic patients.[104,105] Immunohistochemistry with staining for vimentin, a mesenchymal marker, without staining for epithelial markers can confirm the diagnosis. The possibility of sarcoma liver metastasis from another primary site must always be entertained, and a careful evaluation of gastrointestinal, retroperitoneal, gynecologic, and extremity sites should occur before establishing the diagnosis of primary liver sarcoma. As with other hepatic malignancies, resection is generally the treatment of choice when possible. Careful evaluation of the extent of disease both within and outside of the liver is important when evaluating such a patient. In some cases with unresectable liver-dominant disease, intraarterial therapy, either chemoembolization or yttrium-90 radioembolization, can be considered; but evidence of its benefit is limited.

VASCULAR HEPATIC MALIGNANCIES

Vascular malignancies are exceedingly uncommon primary tumors of the liver. Among these, *angiosarcoma* is the most common. Most angiosarcomas are sporadic. However, exposure to thorium dioxide (Thorotrast), arsenicals, and vinyl chloride have been linked to the development of hepatic angiosarcoma.[106,107] There can be significant latency on the order of decades between exposure and development of disease. Insight into the genetics of hepatic angiosarcoma

remains limited with the exception of the recent discovery that the alternative lengthening of telomeres (ALT) phenotype is prevalent.[108] The presenting symptoms are generally similar to other hepatic malignancies with two exceptions. Hepatic angiosarcomas can cause spontaneous tumor hemorrhage or consumptive coagulopathy due to Kasabach-Merritt phenomenon. Angiosarcomas can present as multiple nodules or as a solitary tumor. They appear to have unique characteristics on contrast MRI that can differentiate them from benign vascular liver lesions. They demonstrate heterogeneous signal intensities and septally progressing enhancement.[109,110] When multifocal and unresectable, operative biopsy via an open or laparoscopic approach is recommended for tissue diagnosis due to the high risk of bleeding during percutaneous procedures.

Most patients with angiosarcoma are not resectable, and overall survival rates for these patients are poor, with a median survival of 5 to 6 months and a 2-year survival rate of only 3%.[110,111] Yet, in selected patients with apparently localized disease, surgical therapy should be considered. Liver transplantation for hepatic angiosarcinoma has been associated with very high recurrence rates and is no longer recommended.[112] In unresectable patients, regional or systemic approaches can be offered. Specifically, TAE can control intraabdominal bleeding in case of tumor rupture.

Hepatic epithelioid hemangioendothelioma (HEHE) is another rare vascular hepatic tumor accounting for less than 1% of primary hepatic malignancies. These tumors primarily occur in patients without underlying liver disease and specifically more often in middle-aged women. An association between HEHE and vinyl chloride and oral contraceptives has been reported, but risk factors for HEHE remain largely unknown.[113] HEHE does not have a distinctive clinical presentation and a large percentage of these tumors are diagnosed incidentally. Radiologic evaluation can be helpful in identifying HEHE and distinguishing it from angiosarcoma. CT scan can show irregular hypodense lesions that may have hypervascular enhancement in the periphery following injection of intravenous contrast.[104] Tumor calcification can occasionally also be seen. HEHE also has distinctive features on MRI, including low signal intensity on T1-weighted images and heterogeneous high signal intensity on T2-weighted images.[114] The extent of the tumor can often be difficult to evaluate radiologically, because they tend to be multifocal and widespread within the liver at the time of diagnosis. The final diagnosis is established by histologic examination. When not resectable, operative biopsy via an open or laparoscopic approach is recommended for tissue diagnosis due to the high risk of bleeding during percutaneous procedures. HEHE stains strongly positive for coagulation factor VIII expression. The cells are typically epithelioid with abundant cytoplasm, but a dendritic cell type has also been recognized (Fig. 133.3).

When HEHE is confined to the liver, surgical therapy should be considered. However, the diffuse nature of these tumors often precludes surgical resection; therefore survival rates following liver resection are poor. TACE appears to have comparable outcomes to liver resection.[115] Unlike angiosarcoma, selected patients with HEHE may benefit from liver transplantation.[116,117] Some authors advise watchful waiting after initial diagnosis of HEHE and reserve surgery for those who remain resectable/

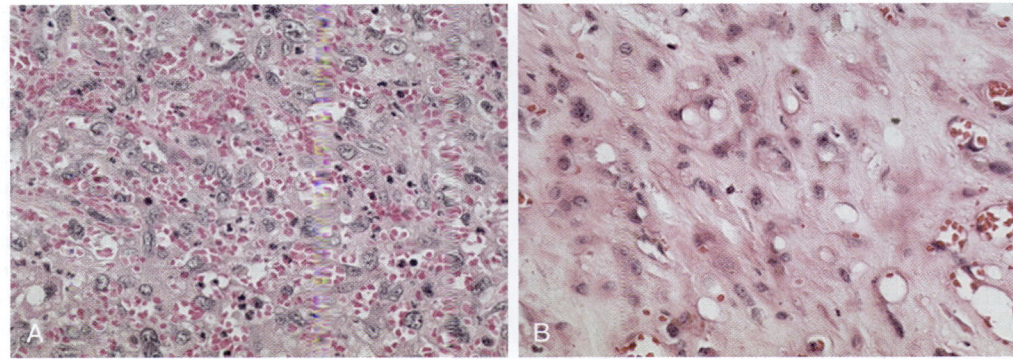

FIGURE 133.3 Comparison of vascular tumors of the liver. (A) Photomicrograph of an angiosarcoma. Note the small, highly aggressive-appearing cells with disruption of the hepatic parenchymal architecture. (B) Photomicrograph of an epithelioid hemangioendothelioma. Note the tumor cells' abundant cytoplasm. Although the tumor cells are often surrounded by sclerotic stroma with diffuse hepatic involvement, the liver architecture is preserved. (Courtesy M.S Torbenson, Department of Pathology, Johns Hopkins Hospital.)

transplantable.[118] There is currently no standardized chemotherapy regimen for patients with advanced disease, although a recent study of mTOR inhibitor sirolimus showed promising results.[119]

SUMMARY

The modern liver surgeon should consider a broad differential diagnosis when approaching primary hepatic malignancies. Although HCC remains the most common primary liver cancer, the incidence of ICC is increasing. While many of the other liver tumors are rare and therapeutic decisions cannot be based on large prospective studies, and hepatic resection with a curative intent should be considered when possible. Careful imaging of the liver and extrahepatic sites should always precede the determination of resectability. The roles of liver transplantation, tumor ablation, regional intraarterial approaches, and systemic chemotherapy with biologic therapies are still being established. As with other diseases, it is prudent when managing these patients to do so with a multidisciplinary team involving hepatic surgeons, medical and radiation oncologists, diagnostic and interventional radiologists, and hepatologists.

REFERENCES

1. Nordenstedt H, White DL, El-Serag HB. The changing pattern of epidemiology in hepatocellular carcinoma. *Dig Liver Dis.* 2010;42(suppl 3):S206-S214.
2. Augustine MM, Fong Y. Epidemiology and risk factors of biliary tract and primary liver tumors. *Surg Oncol Clin N Am.* 2014;23:171-188.
3. Charbel H, Al-Kawas FH. Cholangiocarcinoma: epidemiology, risk factors, pathogenesis, and diagnosis. *Curr Gastroenterol Rep.* 2011;13:182-187.
4. Shaib YH, El-Serag HB, Davila JA, et al. Risk factors of intrahepatic cholangiocarcinoma in the United States: a case-control study. *Gastroenterology.* 2005;128:620-626.
5. DeOliveira ML, Cunningham SC, Cameron JL, et al. Cholangiocarcinoma: thirty-one-year experience with 564 patients at a single institution. *Ann Surg.* 2007;245:755-762.
6. Khan SA, Emadossadaty S, Ladep NG, et al. Rising trends in cholangiocarcinoma: is the ICD classification system misleading us? *J Hepatol.* 2012;56:848-854.

7. Welzel TM, Graubard BI, El-Serag HB, et al. Risk factors for intrahepatic and extrahepatic cholangiocarcinoma in the United States: a population-based case-control study. *Clin Gastroenterol Hepatol.* 2007;5:1221-1228.
8. Donato F, Gelatti U, Tagger A, et al. Intrahepatic cholangiocarcinoma and hepatitis C and B virus infection, alcohol intake, and hepatolithiasis: a case-control study in Italy. *Cancer Causes Control.* 2001;12:959-964.
9. Palmer WC, Patel T. Are common factors involved in the pathogenesis of primary liver cancers? A meta-analysis of risk factors for intrahepatic cholangiocarcinoma. *J Hepatol.* 2012;57:69-76.
10. Zabron A, Edwards RJ, Khan SA. The challenge of cholangiocarcinoma: dissecting the molecular mechanisms of an insidious cancer. *Dis Model Mech.* 2013;6:281-292.
11. Razumilava N, Gores GJ. Cholangiocarcinoma. *Lancet.* 2014;383:2168-2179.
12. Zou S, Li J, Zhou H, et al. Mutational landscape of intrahepatic cholangiocarcinoma. *Nat Commun.* 2014;5:5696.
13. Moeini A, Sia D, Bardeesy N, et al. Molecular pathogenesis and targeted therapies for intrahepatic cholangiocarcinoma. *Clin Cancer Res.* 2016;22:291-300.
14. Sia D, Hoshida Y, Villanueva A, et al. Integrative molecular analysis of intrahepatic cholangiocarcinoma reveals 2 classes that have different outcomes. *Gastroenterology.* 2013;144:829-840.
15. Andersen JB, Spee B, Blechacz BR, et al. Genomic and genetic characterization of cholangiocarcinoma identifies therapeutic targets for tyrosine kinase inhibitors. *Gastroenterology.* 2012;142:1021-1031.e1015.
16. Jiao Y, Pawlik TM, Anders RA, et al. Exome sequencing identifies frequent inactivating mutations in BAP1, ARID1A and PBRM1 in intrahepatic cholangiocarcinomas. *Nat Genet.* 2013;45:1470-1473.
17. Borger DR, Tanabe KK, Fan KC, et al. Frequent mutation of isocitrate dehydrogenase (IDH)1 and IDH2 in cholangiocarcinoma identified through broad-based tumor genotyping. *Oncologist.* 2012;17:72-79.
18. Wang P, Dong Q, Zhang C, et al. Mutations in isocitrate dehydrogenase 1 and 2 occur frequently in intrahepatic cholangiocarcinomas and share hypermethylation targets with glioblastomas. *Oncogene.* 2013;32:3091-3100.
19. Kipp BR, Voss JS, Kerr SE, et al. Isocitrate dehydrogenase 1 and 2 mutations in cholangiocarcinoma. *Hum Pathol.* 2012;43:1552-1558.
20. Wu YM, Su F, Kalyana-Sundaram S, et al. Identification of targetable FGFR gene fusions in diverse cancers. *Cancer Discov.* 2013;3:636-647.
21. Zender S, Nickeleit I, Wuestefeld T, et al. A critical role for notch signaling in the formation of cholangiocellular carcinomas. *Cancer Cell.* 2013;23:784-795.
22. Hofmann JJ, Zovein AC, Koh H, et al. Jagged1 in the portal vein mesenchyme regulates intrahepatic bile duct development: insights into Alagille syndrome. *Development.* 2010;137:4061-4072.
23. Sekiya S, Suzuki A. Intrahepatic cholangiocarcinoma can arise from Notch-mediated conversion of hepatocytes. *J Clin Invest.* 2012;122:3914-3918.

24. Fan B, Malato Y, Calvisi DF, et al. Cholangiocarcinomas can originate from hepatocytes in mice. *J Clin Invest*. 2012;122:2911-2915.

25. Razumilava N, Gores GJ. Notch-driven carcinogenesis: the merging of hepatocellular cancer and cholangiocarcinoma into a common molecular liver cancer subtype. *J Hepatol*. 2013;58:1244-1245.

26. Zhu AX, Borger DR, Kim Y, et al. Genomic profiling of intrahepatic cholangiocarcinoma: refining prognosis and identifying therapeutic targets. *Ann Surg Oncol*. 2014;21:3827-3834.

27. Geynisman DM, Catenacci DV. Toward personalized treatment of advanced biliary tract cancers. *Discov Med*. 2012;14:41-57.

28. Borad MJ, Champion MD, Egan JB, et al. Integrated genomic characterization reveals novel, therapeutically relevant drug targets in FGFR and EGFR pathways in sporadic intrahepatic cholangiocarcinoma. *PLoS Genet*. 2014;10: 1004135.

29. Yamasaki S. Intrahepatic cholangiocarcinoma: macroscopic type and stage classification. *J Hepatobiliary Pancreat Surg*. 2003;10:288-291.

30. Blechacz B, Komuta M, Roskams T, et al. Clinical diagnosis and staging of cholangiocarcinoma. *Nat Rev Gastroenterol Hepatol*. 2011;8:512-522.

31. Razumilava N, Gores GJ. Classification, diagnosis, and management of cholangiocarcinoma. *Clin Gastroenterol Hepatol*. 2013;11:13-21. e11, quiz e13-14.

32. Rullier A, Le Bail B, Fawaz R, et al. Cytokeratin 7 and 20 expression in cholangiocarcinomas varies along the biliary tract but still differs from that in colorectal carcinoma metastasis. *Am J Surg Pathol*. 2000;24:870-876.

33. Lamps LW, Folpe AL. The diagnostic value of hepatocyte paraffin antibody 1 in differentiating hepatocellular neoplasms from nonhepatic tumors: a review. *Adv Anat Pathol*. 2003;10:39-43.

34. Mosnier JF, Kandel C, Cazals-Hatem D, et al. N-cadherin serves as diagnostic biomarker in intrahepatic and perihilar cholangiocarcinomas. *Mod Pathol*. 2009;22 182-190.

35. Kim SA, Lee JM, Lee KB, et al. Intrahepatic mass-forming cholangiocarcinomas: enhancement patterns at multiphasic CT, with special emphasis on arterial enhancement pattern—correlation with clinicopathologic findings. *Radiology*. 2011;260:148-157.

36. Kim R, Lee JM, Shin CI, et al. Differentiation of intrahepatic mass-forming cholangiocarcinoma from hepatocellular carcinoma on gadoxetic acid-enhanced liver MR imaging. *Eur Radiol*. 2016;26:1808-1817.

37. Lee SW, Kim HJ, Park JH, et al. Clinical usefulness of 18F-FDG PET-CT for patients with gallbladder cancer and cholangiocarcinoma. *J Gastroenterol*. 2010;45:560-566.

38. Bergquist JR, Ivanics T, Storlie CB, et al. Implications of CA19-9 elevation for survival, staging, and treatment sequencing in intrahepatic cholangiocarcinoma: a national cohort analysis. *J Surg Oncol*. 2016;114:475-482.

39. Ferrone CR, Ting DT, Shahid M, et al. The ability to diagnose intrahepatic cholangiocarcinoma definitively using novel branched DNA-enhanced albumin RNA in situ hybridization technology. *Ann Surg Oncol*. 2016;23:290-296.

40. Edge SB, American Joint Committee on Cancer. *AJCC Cancer Staging Manual*. 7th ed. New York: Springer; 2010.

41. de Jong MC, Nathan H, Sotiropoulos GC, et al. Intrahepatic cholangiocarcinoma: an international multi-institutional analysis of prognostic factors and lymph node assessment. *J Clin Oncol*. 2011;29:3140-3145.

42. Nathan H, Aloia TA, Vauthey JN, et al. A proposed staging system for intrahepatic cholangiocarcinoma. *Ann Surg Oncol*. 2009;16:14-22.

43. Farges O, Fuks D, Le Treut YP, et al. AJCC 7th edition of TNM staging accurately discriminates outcomes of patients with resectable intrahepatic cholangiocarcinoma: by the AFC-IHCC-2009 study group. *Cancer*. 2011;117:2170-2177.

44. Weber SM, Ribero D, O'Reilly EM, et al. Intrahepatic cholangiocarcinoma: expert consensus statement. *HPB (Oxford)*. 2015;17:669-680.

45. D'Angelica M, Fong Y, Weber S, et al. The role of staging laparoscopy in hepatobiliary malignancy: prospective analysis of 401 cases. *Ann Surg Oncol*. 2003;10:183-189.

46. Goere D, Wagholikar GD, Pessaux P, et al. Utility of staging laparoscopy in subsets of biliary cancers: laparoscopy is a powerful diagnostic tool in patients with intrahepatic and gallbladder carcinoma. *Surg Endosc*. 2006;20:721-725.

47. Ali SM, Clark CJ, Zaydfudim VM, et al. Role of major vascular resection in patients with intrahepatic cholangiocarcinoma. *Ann Surg Oncol*. 2013;20:2023-2028.

48. Ribero D, Pinna AD, Guglielmi A, et al. Surgical approach for long-term survival of patients with intrahepatic cholangiocarcinoma: a multi-institutional analysis of 434 patients. *Arch Surg*. 2012;147:1107-1113.

49. Lang H, Sotiropoulos GC, Sgourakis G, et al. Operations for intrahepatic cholangiocarcinoma: single-institution experience of 158 patients. *J Am Coll Surg*. 2009;208:218-228.

50. Mavros MN, Economopoulos KP, Alexiou VG, et al. Treatment and prognosis for patients with intrahepatic cholangiocarcinoma: systematic review and meta-analysis. *JAMA Surg*. 2014;149:565-574.

51. Hyder O, Marques H, Pulitano C, et al. A nomogram to predict long-term survival after resection for intrahepatic cholangiocarcinoma: an Eastern and Western experience. *JAMA Surg*. 2014;149:432-438.

52. Endo I, Gonen M, Yopp AC, et al. Intrahepatic cholangiocarcinoma: rising frequency, improved survival, and determinants of outcome after resection. *Ann Surg*. 2008;248:84-96.

53. Poultsides GA, Zhu AX, Choti MA, et al. Intrahepatic cholangiocarcinoma. *Surg Clin North Am*. 2010;90:817-837.

54. Guglielmi A, Ruzzenente A, Campagnaro T, et al. Intrahepatic cholangiocarcinoma: prognostic factors after surgical resection. *World J Surg*. 2009;33:1247-1254.

55. Uenishi T, Kubo S, Yamazaki O, et al. Indications for surgical treatment of intrahepatic cholangiocarcinoma with lymph node metastases. *J Hepatobiliary Pancreat Surg*. 2008;15:417-422.

56. Vitale A, Moustafa M, Spolverato G, et al. Defining the possible therapeutic benefit of lymphadenectomy among patients undergoing hepatic resection for intrahepatic cholangiocarcinoma. *J Surg Oncol*. 2016;113:685-691.

57. Abou-Alfa GK, Geschwind JF, Chot M, et al. Consensus conference on intrahepatic cholangiocarcinoma. *HPB (Oxford)*. 2015;17:661-663.

58. Yang L, Shan J, Shan L, et al. Trans-arterial embolisation therapies for unresectable intrahepatic cholangiocarcinoma: a systematic review. *J Gastrointest Oncol*. 2015;6:570-588.

59. Cantore M, Mambrini A, Fiorentini G, et al. Phase II study of hepatic intraarterial epirubicin and cisplatin, with systemic 5-fluorouracil in patients with unresectable biliary tract tumors. *Cancer*. 2005;103:1402-1407.

60. Burger I, Hong K, Schulick R, et al. Transcatheter arterial chemoembolization in unresectable cholangiocarcinoma: initial experience in a single institution. *J Vasc Interv Radiol*. 2005;16:353-361.

61. Gusani N, Balaa FK, Steel JL, et al. Treatment of unresectable cholangiocarcinoma with gemcitabine-based transcatheter arterial chemoembolization (TACE): a single-institution experience. *J Gastrointest Surg*. 2008;12:129-137.

62. Kasai K, Kooka Y, Suzuki Y, et al. Efficacy of hepatic arterial infusion chemotherapy using 5-fluorouracil and systemic pegylated interferon alpha-2b for advanced intrahepatic cholangiocarcinoma. *Ann Surg Oncol*. 2014;21:3638-3645.

63. Konstantinidis IT, Groot Koerkamp B, Do RK, et al. Unresectable intrahepatic cholangiocarcinoma: systemic versus hepatic arterial infusion chemotherapy is associated with longer survival in comparison with systemic chemotherapy alone. *Cancer*. 2016;122:758-765.

64. Mosconi C, Gramenzi A, Ascanio S, et al. Yttrium-90 radioembolization for unresectable/recurrent intrahepatic cholangiocarcinoma: a survival efficacy and safety study. *Br J Cancer*. 2016;115:297-302.

65. Rayar M, Sulpice L, Edeline J, et al. Intra-arterial yttrium-90 radioembolization combined with systemic chemotherapy is a promising method for downstaging unresectable huge intrahepatic cholangiocarcinoma to surgical treatment. *Ann Surg Oncol*. 2015;22:3102-3108.

66. Al-Adra DP, Gill RS, Axford SJ, et al. Treatment of unresectable intrahepatic cholangiocarcinoma with yttrium-90 radioembolization: a systematic review and pooled analysis. *Eur J Surg Oncol*. 2015;41:120-127.

67. Weiner AA, Olsen J, Ma D, et al. Stereotactic body radiotherapy for primary hepatic malignancies—report of a phase I/II institutional study. *Radiother Oncol*. 2016;121 79-85.

68. Han K, Ko HK, Kim KW, et al. Radiofrequency ablation in the treatment of unresectable intrahepatic cholangiocarcinoma: systematic review and meta-analysis. *J Vasc Interv Radiol*. 2015;26:943-948.

69. Meyer CG, Penn I, James L. Liver transplantation for cholangiocarcinoma results in 207 patients. *Transplantation*. 2000;69:1633-1637.

70. Sapisochin G, de Lope CR, Gastaca M, et al. Intrahepatic cholangiocarcinoma or mixed hepatocellular-cholangiocarcinoma in patients undergoing liver transplantation: a Spanish matched cohort multicenter study. *Ann Surg*. 2014;259:944-952.

71. Sapisochin G, Facciuto M, Rubbia-Brandt L, et al. Liver transplantation for "very early" intrahepatic cholangiocarcinoma: international retrospective study supporting a prospective assessment. *Hepatology*. 2016;64:1178-1188.

72. Gores GJ, Darwish Murad S, Heimbach JK, et al. Liver transplantation for perihilar cholangiocarcinoma. *Dig Dis*. 2013;31:126-129.

73. Mantel HT, Westerkamp AC, Adam R, et al. Strict selection alone of patients undergoing liver transplantation for hilar cholangiocarcinoma is associated with improved survival. *PLoS One*. 2016;11:e0156127.

74. Park I, Lee JL, Ryu MH, et al. Prognostic factors and predictive model in patients with advanced biliary tract adenocarcinoma receiving first-line palliative chemotherapy. *Cancer*. 2009;115:4148-4155.

75. Ducreux M, Van Cutsem E, Van Laethem JL, et al. A randomised phase II trial of weekly high-dose 5-fluorouracil with and without folinic acid and cisplatin in patients with advanced biliary tract carcinoma: results of the 40955 EORTC trial. *Eur J Cancer*. 2005;41:398-403.

76. Valle J, Wasan H, Palmer DH, et al. Cisplatin plus gemcitabine versus gemcitabine for biliary tract cancer. *N Engl J Med*. 2010;362:1273-1281.

77. Lee JK, Capanu M, O'Reilly EM, et al. A phase II study of gemcitabine and cisplatin plus sorafenib in patients with advanced biliary adenocarcinomas. *Br J Cancer*. 2013;109:915-919.

78. El-Khoueiry AB, Rankin C, Siegel AB, et al. S0941: a phase 2 SWOG study of sorafenib and erlotinib in patients with advanced gallbladder carcinoma or cholangiocarcinoma. *Br J Cancer*. 2014;110:882-887.

79. Javle MM, Shroff RT, Zhu A, et al. A phase 2 study of BGJ398 in patients (pts) with advanced or metastatic FGFR-altered cholangiocarcinoma (CCA) who failed or are intolerant to platinum-based chemotherapy. *J Clin Oncol*. 2016;34:abstr 335.

80. Horgan AM, Amir E, Walter T, et al. Adjuvant therapy in the treatment of biliary tract cancer: a systematic review and meta-analysis. *J Clin Oncol*. 2012;30:1934-1940.

81. Hezel AF, Zhu AX. Systemic therapy for biliary tract cancers. *Oncologist*. 2008;13:415-423.

82. Alison MR. Liver stem cells: implications for hepatocarcinogenesis. *Stem Cell Rev*. 2005;1:253-260.

83. O'Connor K, Walsh JC, Schaeffer DF. Combined hepatocellular-cholangiocarcinoma (cHCC-CC): a distinct entity. *Ann Hepatol*. 2014;13:317-322.

84. Goodman ZD, Ishak KG, Langloss JM, et al. Combined hepatocellular-cholangiocarcinoma. A histologic and immunohistochemical study. *Cancer*. 1985;55:124-135.

85. Bergquist JR, Groeschl RT, Ivanics T, et al. Mixed hepatocellular and cholangiocarcinoma: a rare tumor with a mix of parent phenotypic characteristics. *HPB (Oxford)*. 2016;18(11):886-892.

86. Kassahun WT, Hauss J. Management of combined hepatocellular and cholangiocarcinoma. *Int J Clin Pract*. 2008;62:1271-1278.

87. Groeschl RT, Turaga KK, Gamblin TC. Transplantation versus resection for patients with combined hepatocellular carcinoma-cholangiocarcinoma. *J Surg Oncol*. 2013;107:608-612.

88. Yoon YI, Hwang S, Lee YJ, et al. Postresection outcomes of combined hepatocellular carcinoma-cholangiocarcinoma, hepatocellular carcinoma and intrahepatic cholangiocarcinoma. *J Gastrointest Surg*. 2016;20:411-420.

89. Vogt DP, Henderson JM, Chmielewski E. Cystadenoma and cystadenocarcinoma of the liver: a single center experience. *J Am Coll Surg*. 2005;200:727-733.

90. Arnaoutakis DJ, Kim Y, Pulitano C, et al. Management of biliary cystic tumors: a multi-institutional analysis of a rare liver tumor. *Ann Surg*. 2015;261:361-367.

91. Soares KC, Arnaoutakis DJ, Kamel I, et al. Cystic neoplasms of the liver: biliary cystadenoma and cystadenocarcinoma. *J Am Coll Surg*. 2014;218:119-128.

92. Wheeler DA, Edmondson HA. Cystadenoma with mesenchymal stroma (CMS) in the liver and bile ducts. A clinicopathologic study of 17 cases, 4 with malignant change. *Cancer*. 1985;56:1434-1445.

93. Sang X, Sun Y, Mao Y, et al. Hepatobiliary cystadenomas and cystadenocarcinomas: a report of 33 cases. *Liver Int*. 2011;31:1337-1344.

94. Seo JK, Kim SH, Lee SH, et al. Appropriate diagnosis of biliary cystic tumors: comparison with atypical hepatic simple cysts. *Eur J Gastroenterol Hepatol*. 2010;22:989-996.

95. Lee JH, Lee KG, Park HK, et al. Biliary cystadenoma and cystadenocarcinoma of the liver: 10 cases of a single center experience. *Hepatogastroenterology*. 2009;56:844-849.

96. Doussot A, Gluskin J, Groot-Koerkamp B, et al. The accuracy of pre-operative imaging in the management of hepatic cysts. *HPB (Oxford)*. 2015;17:889-895.

97. Naik S, Waris W, Carmosino L, et al. Primary squamous cell carcinoma of the liver. *J Gastrointestin Liver Dis*. 2009;18:487-489.

98. Yagi H, Ueda M, Kawachi S, et al. Squamous cell carcinoma of the liver originating from non-parasitic cysts after a 15 year follow-up. *Eur J Gastroenterol Hepatol*. 2004;16:1051-1056.

99. Zhang XF, Du ZQ, Liu XM, et al. Primary squamous cell carcinoma of liver: case series and review of literatures. *Medicine (Baltimore)*. 2015;94:e868.

100. Zhu KL, Li DY, Jiang CB. Primary squamous cell carcinoma of the liver associated with hepatolithiasis: a case report. *World J Gastroenterol*. 2012;18:5830-5832.

101. Weitz J, Klimstra DS, Cymes K, et al. Management of primary liver sarcomas. *Cancer*. 2007;109:1391-1396.

102. Hamed MO, Roberts KJ, Merchant W, et al. Contemporary management and classification of hepatic leiomyosarcoma. *HPB (Oxford)*. 2015;17:362-367.

103. Lin YH, Lin CC, Concejero AM, et al. Surgical experience of adult primary hepatic sarcomas. *World J Surg Oncol*. 2015;13:87.

104. Yu RS, Chen Y, Jiang B, et al. Primary hepatic sarcomas: CT findings. *Eur Radiol*. 2008;18:2196-2205.

105. Harman M, Nart D, Acar T, et al. Primary mesenchymal liver tumors: radiological spectrum, differential diagnosis, and pathologic correlation. *Abdom Imaging*. 2015;40:1316-1330.

106. Lipshutz GS, Brennan TV, Warren RS. Thorotrast-induced liver neoplasia: a collective review. *J Am Coll Surg*. 2002;195:713-718.

107. Sherman M. Vinyl chloride and the liver. *J Hepatol*. 2009;51:1074-1081.

108. Liau JY, Tsai JH, Yang CY, et al. Alternative lengthening of telomeres phenotype in malignant vascular tumors is highly associated with loss of ATRX expression and is frequently observed in hepatic angiosarcomas. *Hum Pathol*. 2015;46:1360-1366.

109. Pickhardt PJ, Kitchin D, Lubner MG, et al. Primary hepatic angiosarcoma: multi-institutional comprehensive cancer centre review of multiphasic CT and MR imaging in 35 patients. *Eur Radiol*. 2015;25:315-322.

110. O'Grady JG. Treatment options for other hepatic malignancies. *Liver Transpl*. 2000;6:S23-S29.

111. Zheng YW, Zhang XW, Zhang JL, et al. Primary hepatic angiosarcoma and potential treatment options. *J Gastroenterol Hepatol*. 2014;29:906-911.

112. Orlando G, Adam R, Mirza D, et al. Hepatic hemangiosarcoma: an absolute contraindication to liver transplantation—the European Liver Transplant Registry experience. *Transplantation*. 2013;95:872-877.

113. Mehrabi A, Kashfi A, Fonouni H, et al. Primary malignant hepatic epithelioid hemangioendothelioma: a comprehensive review of the literature with emphasis on the surgical therapy. *Cancer*. 2006;107:2108-2121.

114. Gan LU, Chang R, Jin H, et al. Typical CT and MRI signs of hepatic epithelioid hemangioendothelioma. *Oncol Lett*. 2016;11:1699-1706.

115. Wang LR, Zhou JM, Zhao YM, et al. Clinical experience with primary hepatic epithelioid hemangioendothelioma: retrospective study of 33 patients. *World J Surg*. 2012;36:2677-2683.

116. Grotz TE, Nagorney D, Donohue J, et al. Hepatic epithelioid haemangioendothelioma: is transplantation the only treatment option? *HPB (Oxford)*. 2010;12:546-553.

117. Mehrabi A, Hoffmann K, Weiss KH, et al. Long term follow up after resection emphasizes the role of surgery in primary hepatic epithelioid hemangioendothelioma. *Ann Med Surg (Lond)*. 2016;11:1-4.

118. Thomas RM, Aloia TA, Truty MJ, et al. Treatment sequencing strategy for hepatic epithelioid haemangioendothelioma. *HPB (Oxford)*. 2014;16:677-685.

119. Stacchiotti S, Provenzano S, Dagrada G, et al. Sirolimus in advanced epithelioid hemangioendothelioma: a retrospective case-series analysis from the Italian rare cancer network database. *Ann Surg Oncol*. 2016;23:2735-2744.

Management of Secondary Hepatic Neoplasms

Juan Camilo Barreto | Mitchell C. Posner

Secondary hepatic neoplasms refer to a heterogeneous collection of tumors that metastasize to the liver. By definition, these cancers develop from other organ sites but share a common metastatic pathway. Tumors that hematogenously disseminate to the liver include carcinomas (e.g., colorectal, pancreatic, gastric, breast, lung), neuroendocrine cancers, and certain types of retroperitoneal sarcomas and gastrointestinal stromal tumors. Systemic chemotherapy may be associated with improved survival compared with untreated patients, but it rarely results in cure. The enhanced efficacy of systemic chemotherapeutic regimens has increased tumor response rates and improved the progression-free and overall survival of patients with these malignancies. The ability to effectively control systemic disease with chemotherapy and reduce either the size of large or the number of diffuse hepatic metastases has expanded the pool of patients eligible to receive curative surgical therapy. Advances in the perioperative management of patients undergoing liver surgery undoubtedly contribute to these improved outcomes. Most importantly, our enhanced collective understanding of the molecular and biologic behavior of these tumors facilitates the appropriate use, combination, and sequencing of cancer-directed treatments. Although much of our knowledge has been drawn from retrospective analyses, several prospective, randomized trials provide an evidence-based rationale for therapy.

As the primary drainage basin of the portal circulatory system, the liver is the most common site of gastrointestinal tract metastases. Colorectal cancer (CRC) is the second leading cause of cancer-specific mortality in the United States and the most frequent tumor type classified as secondary hepatic neoplasm. Up to half of patients with CRC develop hepatic metastases during the course of their disease. Combination treatment with systemic chemotherapy and complete hepatic metastasectomy has been associated with long-term (5-year) survival rates that may approach 50%.[1] A smaller percentage of patients are completely cured of their disease.[2] In neuroendocrine carcinomas with spread to the hepatic parenchyma, complete surgical resection of isolated metastases has been associated with improved survival. Although hepatectomy and locoregional ablative therapies have been used for noncolorectal, nonneuroendocrine (NCNN) metastases, the biology of these tumors is variable, and surgical resection should be reserved for patients with excellent performance status and adequate control of the primary lesion and in select clinical scenarios in which the disease-free interval can be measured in years.

Generally accepted criteria for hepatic metastasectomy include (1) acceptable patient performance status to tolerate the necessary hepatic resection; (2) the liver as the only or predominant site of metastatic disease; (3) the primary tumor (and all other sites of disease) must be completely resectable and not progressing on the most effective systemic chemotherapy regimen; (4) favorable tumor biology, such that rapid progression or widespread micrometastatic disease is unlikely; (5) resection of metastasis will result in either the possibility of a long-term disease-free state or cure. Factors that influence the extent of hepatic resection are the number, size, and location of hepatic lesions, baseline hepatic function, and size of the anticipated postresection liver remnant. Traditionally, the presence of bilobar hepatic metastases and extrahepatic disease (EHD) (in distant nodal basins or lungs) had been considered absolute contraindications to complete hepatic metastasectomy. The combination of effective neoadjuvant chemotherapy, increasingly effective local ablative therapies, and aggressive surgical resection has broadened the indications for surgical resection. The ability to achieve an R0 (negative gross and microscopic margins) resection appears to be a significant factor that is associated with improved disease-free survival rates. Although hepatic recurrence rates have been shown to be higher when the microscopic margins are positive for residual disease, several retrospective reports suggest that this may not influence long-term survival.[2] Positive margins likely reflect poor tumor biology and increased risk of hepatic recurrence. Anatomic resections along the vascular inflow and outflow structures and biliary ducts, are indicated for metastatic disease in which subanatomic or "wedge" resections would lead to a higher probability of positive margins, major blood loss, or a bile leak. The unique capability of the liver parenchyma to regenerate after hepatectomy allows the surgeon to resect up to 80% of the original volume if baseline hepatic function is normal. The oncologic principles regarding CRC, neuroendocrine, and other hepatic metastasis will be discussed here, as a separate chapter will address the surgical and technical details of liver resection more thoroughly.

COLORECTAL CANCER METASTASES

The liver is the most common site of distant metastatic disease in CRC patients. Approximately half of patients with CRC will develop metastases during their course of disease, and up to 25% will have liver metastases at the time of presentation.[4] The historical results of resection, before the development of current-day chemotherapeutic regimens, typically yielded 5-year survival rates between 20% and 40%.[5] Selected patients undergoing modern chemotherapeutic regimens in combination with complete metastasectomy can achieve durable 5-year survival rates exceeding 50%[1,6] and as high as 70% in those with solitary liver metastasis.[7] Approximately 17% to 25% of these patients are cured of their disease.[2] These results have established surgery as the standard of care for patients with resectable liver metastasis. These improved survival trends are likely related to improved patient selection with favorable tumor biology, dramatic improvement in the systemic chemotherapeutic regimens, and the concomitant development of new, targeted therapeutics.

The historical selection criteria used to identify stage IV patients who might benefit from metastasectomy have focused on disease burden: number and size of metastatic lesions, bilateral hepatic disease, lymph node–positive primary tumors, and high carcinoembryonic antigen (CEA) levels. The Fong Clinical Risk Score consolidates these factors into prognostic elements that can be used to select patients for hepatic metastasectomy. Patients who have 0 to 2 of these high-risk factors have 5-year survival rates of 40% to 60%, whereas patients with a score of 3 or higher have less than a 25% chance of surviving beyond the same time interval.[8] Because the data to construct these scoring systems were generated before the advent of modern combination chemotherapy, the clinical usefulness of this model has been debated. Retrospective data suggest that tumor response to induction or "neoadjuvant" therapy as a marker of favorable biology may have more value than the aforementioned variables.[9] Recently, multigene expression profiling of tumor tissue has been demonstrated to be highly predictive of overall survival in patients with resected hepatic colorectal metastases.[10] Improved perioperative therapy, concentrating on minimizing blood loss, maintaining an appropriate and functional remnant liver volume, and maximizing hepatic regeneration and recovery through state-of-the-art surgical intensive care techniques, likely has contributed to the improved results in recent retrospective case series. Patients with normal hepatic and renal function can tolerate up to an 80% hepatectomy without significant perioperative morality. The selective use of portal vein embolization to induce in vivo hepatic regeneration of the anticipated remnant liver is a technique that is predictive of the response to hepatectomy and can help certain patients who could tolerate complete metastasectomy. Portal vein embolization can be combined with neoadjuvant chemotherapy without compromising liver growth.[11] Furthermore, our improved understanding of hepatic anatomy, physiology, and the factors responsible for regeneration has expanded the indications for operation and allowed more patients with stage IV disease to be considered for combination therapy. The ability to achieve a complete resection (i.e., R0 resection) with both gross and microscopically negative margins has been associated with improved recurrence-free survival. It is no longer necessary to perform anatomic or segmental resections on all patients with hepatic metastases to achieve disease control.[3]

ROLE OF SYSTEMIC CHEMOTHERAPY IN RESECTABLE METASTATIC DISEASE

The most effective single agent as first-line therapy for metastatic CRC has historically been the fluoropyrimidine analogue, 5-fluorouracil (5-FU). For more than two decades, the synergistic combination of 5-FU and leucovorin or folinic acid (which inhibits thymidylate synthase) was the standard of care both as an adjuvant treatment for node-positive, resected colon cancers and as treatment for metastatic disease. The addition of oxaliplatin, a platinum-based alkylating agent, to the 5-FU–leucovorin backbone (FOLFOX) has increased the response rates and progression-free survival with lower rates of nephrotoxicity and myelosuppression. In some studies, FOLFOX has resulted in an overall survival benefit in the metastatic setting.[12] Irinotecan is a topoisomerase inhibitor that when combined with 5-FU and leucovorin (FOLFIRI) is superior to 5-FU alone and comparable to FOLFOX.[13] Capecitabine, an oral fluoropyrimidine antimetabolite with similar efficacy to 5-FU, is an equivalent, orally administered substitute for 5-FU in most regimens.[14] Several biologic agents have been added to these combination regimens in an attempt to improve survival in patients with metastatic disease. Bevacizumab, a recombinant monoclonal antibody that blocks the activity of vascular endothelial growth factor A (VEGF-A), has proved of benefit in extending survival in patients with metastatic disease[15] and is frequently added to the FOLFOX and FOLFIRI regimens. Cetuximab and panitumumab are monoclonal antibodies that block the epidermal growth factor receptor (EGFR) pathway. These anti-EGFR agents have efficacy against primary tumors that lack activating mutations in the KRAS gene (wild-type gene variant).[16]

The surgeon treating patients with metastatic CRC must be familiar with safety profiles and potential deleterious effects of these regimens. The extended use of these agents (usually >6 to 12 weeks) may be associated with higher rates of postoperative complications and liver insufficiency. Irinotecan has been associated with both drug-induced steatosis and steatohepatitis, which may lead to increased morbidity and mortality.[17] Oxaliplatin may produce sinusoidal dilatation, which can also increase the risk of postoperative complications.[18] The rare, but potentially lethal side effects of bevacizumab include hypertension, increased risk of arterial thromboembolism, gastrointestinal bleeding, and perforation.[19] Its antiangiogenic effects and long circulating half-life (approximately 6 to 8 weeks) have been associated with delayed wound healing. Most physicians interrupt bevacizumab therapy at least 4 to 6 weeks before surgical metastasectomy.[20] Anti-EGFR agents, in particular cetuximab, have not been associated with the same risk profile or increase in postoperative morbidity or mortality.[21]

Patients with unresectable CRC liver metastases who are treated with modern systemic chemotherapy alone have a median survival of 22 months,[22] compared with the dismal natural history of the disease in untreated patients (median survival of 6 to 12 months). Several randomized controlled, multicenter trials have established the efficacy of the current standards of care for the treatment of metastatic disease.[12,13,15]

The rate of complete pathologic response to chemotherapy has been estimated to be less than 5%.[23] In addition, there is a poor correlation between complete radiologic and pathologic responses; residual disease (documented by pathologic examination of the resected liver) is present in more than 80% of lesions that disappear on high-resolution cross-sectional and metabolic imaging studies.[24] Surgical metastasectomy alone can yield disease-free survival rates in the range of 20% and 5-year survival rates of 25% to 40%.[5] Unfortunately, recurrence after

TABLE 134.1 Survival Outcomes in Patients With Metastatic Colorectal Cancer Treated With Modern Combined Chemotherapy and Resection

Study	No. of Patients	Initially Resectable	Regimen	Disease-Free Survival	Overall Survival
EORTC 40983[25,26] phase III RCT (EPOC)	152	Yes	Surgery	28.1%	47.8%
	151		FOLFOX + Surgery + FOLFOX	36.2%	51.2%
				(3 yr) P = .04	(5 yr) P = NS
Ychou et al.[28] phase III RCT	153	Yes	5-FU + leucovorin	46%	71.6%
	153		FOLFIRI	51%	72.7%
				(2 yr) P = .04	(3 yr) P = .69
Adam et al.[29]	701	No	FOLFOX	NA	34%
					(5 yr)
Wein et al.[30] phase II trial	20	Yes	FOLFOX	52%	80%
				(2 yr)	(2-yr DSS)
Taieb et al[31] phase II trial	47	Yes	FOLFOX followed by FOLFIRI	47%	89%
				(2 yr)	(2 yr)
Barone et al.[32]	40	No	FOLFIRI	NA	63.5%
					(2 yr)
Masi et al.[33]	196	No	FOLFOX/FOLFIRI?	29%	42%
				(5 yr)	(5 yr)
First-BEAT trial[34]	107	No	Bev + 5-FU based	NA	89%
					(2 yr)
N016966 study[34]	34	No	Placebo + XELOX/FOLFOX	NA	82.3%
	44		Bev + XELOX/FOLFOX		90.9%
					(2 yr)
New EPOC[27]	117	Yes	FOLFOX or XELOX	20.5 months	NA
	119		Above regimen + cetuximab	14.1 months	
				(PFS) P = .03	

BEAT, Bevacizumab Expanded Access Trial; *Bev*, bevacizumab; *DSS*, disease-specific survival; *EORTC*, European Organization for Research and Treatment of Cancer; *FOLFIRI*, 5-fluorouracil, leucovorin, and irinotecan; *FOLFOX*, 5-fluorouracil, leucovorin, and oxaliplatin; *5-FU*, 5-fluorouracil; *NA*, not available or not reported; *NS*, not significant; *PFS*, progression-free survival; *RCT*, randomized controlled trial; *XELOX*, capecitabine and oxaliplatin.

resection is common. In approximately 50% of these cases, the recurrence occurs within the liver and it is the only site of disease.[5] Long-term disease-free survival is unlikely without a combination of complete metastasectomy and modern chemotherapy. The proper sequencing of surgery and chemotherapy remains unclear. The European Organization for Research and Treatment of Cancer (EORTC) trial 40983 (EPOC), a randomized, controlled phase III trial of perioperative FOLFOX versus surgery alone in patients with resectable hepatic CRC metastases, showed a significant improvement in progression-free survival from 28% to 36%, with an objective tumor response rate in all treated patients of 43%. Postoperative complications were more frequent in the chemotherapy group, although they were reversible and there was no increase in mortality.[25] The median overall survival was 61 months in the chemotherapy group versus 54 months in the surgery-only group, which was not statistically significant, although the study was likely underpowered to detect a difference and only 63% of patients in the chemotherapy group received treatment post resection.[26] A trial attempting to determine the optimal timing of systemic treatment (NSABP C-11, postoperative chemotherapy vs. preoperative and postoperative chemotherapy) was terminated due to poor accrual. The impact of biologic agents on survival after resection of hepatic metastases is still uncertain. The addition of cetuximab to standard chemotherapy in patients with resectable tumors was shown to be detrimental

to progression-free survival and was an unexpected finding in a randomized trial.[27] A summary of the outcomes of current combined-modality treatment is shown in Table 134.1. Many of these studies included patients who initially had unresectable disease and became resectable after chemotherapy. Along the same lines as the EORTC EPOC trial, there have been two meta-analyses evaluating the role of chemotherapy in patients with resectable liver metastases. Both studies found a benefit in disease-free survival but not for overall survival.[35,36]

There are potential advantages and disadvantages to the neoadjuvant approach. The theoretical advantages include eliminating micrometastatic disease, in vivo cytoreduction to reduce the amount of hepatic parenchyma required for complete resection, the ability to individualize the chemotherapeutic regimen to improve efficacy, and, most importantly, to select patients who may benefit from metastasectomy. The potential disadvantages are biologic or chemotherapy-induced toxicity, inducing a complete radiologic response making the lesion(s) difficult to identify intraoperatively, and missing a window of opportunity to cure patients with resectable lesions that may progress on therapy and become unresectable.

SYNCHRONOUS VERSUS METACHRONOUS DISEASE

Fifteen percent to 25% of CRC patients have synchronous liver metastases at the time of diagnosis.[4] In most cases, metastatic disease is recognized within the first year (or

>6 months) after diagnosis. The biologic importance of synchronous metastatic disease is controversial. One hypothesis is that there may be no significant difference between synchronous and metachronous metastatic disease (i.e., lead-time bias). Several studies suggest that the presence of synchronous disease may be associated with a more adverse prognosis secondary to more aggressive tumor behavior (i.e., higher incidence of bilobar liver and extrahepatic metastases).[37] The optimal treatment of synchronous metastases has been debated. Most patients are treated with a limited period (2 to 3 months) of systemic chemotherapy and are restaged. Surgical resection may be appropriate in the absence of disease progression and if both the primary and all sites of metastatic disease can be resected with acceptable morbidity and mortality.

The concept of staged resection has evolved in response to retrospective data that suggest higher rates of morbidity and mortality with combined resections. There are now multiinstitutional, retrospective data to suggest that simultaneous resections are not only feasible, but may be advantageous in selected cases when performed in high-volume centers. More recent reports have shown that morbidity and mortality are not increased in simultaneous hepatic and colorectal resections, even when major liver resections are performed. Simultaneous resection can translate to decreased total hospital stay, lower costs, and, in some single-institution reports, lower total complication rates. In an international multicenter study, postoperative morbidity was 20% and mortality was 3%, with no increased risk of complications when comparing staged or simultaneous approaches.[38,39] In a separate report with long-term follow-up, the oncologic outcomes were also found to be similar with both approaches.[40] These are retrospective reports, and simultaneous resections were more frequently performed in patients with fewer or smaller metastases, with more proximal tumors, and better prognostic features.[38] When synchronous hepatic metastatic disease is present in the setting of the primary tumor located in the rectum as opposed to the colon, the timing of systemic therapy and local regional therapy (i.e., radiation therapy) may well be the most critical factor in determining the sequencing of hepatic resection and resection of the rectal primary.[41,42] In the absence of evidence-based data, most treatment decisions are individualized based on tumor biology, patient factors (e.g., performance status, liver health), and the location and distribution of metastatic disease.

LIVER RESECTION IN THE PRESENCE OF EXTRAHEPATIC DISEASE

Patients with CRC liver metastases and EHD have traditionally not been considered as candidates for metastasectomy. The improved efficacy of chemotherapy has allowed some to reconsider the role of surgical resection in these individuals. The most prudent approach involves a limited period of neoadjuvant chemotherapy to allow patients with favorable tumor biology to be selected for aggressive surgical intervention.

Five-year survival rates of up to 20% to 30% have been reported in patients with EHD.[43] Two of the largest series of patients undergoing liver resection and extrahepatic

metastasectomy to date reported a 5-year predicted survival of 27%, which is consistent with the previous reports with smaller sample sizes. The majority (84% to 95%) of patients in these series eventually developed recurrence, emphasizing that liver resection in the presence of EHD is very often not curative.[44,45] A systematic review of the outcomes of resection for patients with synchronous liver and EHD reported similar results in terms of survival.[46]

The value of removing metastatic disease in "distant" regional lymphatic basins (e.g., periaortic or hepatic pedicle) remains controversial. It is likely that this clinical situation reflects adverse tumor biology associated with poor long-term survival. Reports of hepatic resection and aggressive portal lymphadenectomy in combination with chemotherapy have been associated with 5-year survival rate approaching 20% when lymph node metastases are limited to the portal basin, with no long-term survivors found among patients with celiac or retroperitoneal metastases.[47]

The evolution of hyperthermic intraperitoneal chemotherapy in combination with cytoreductive surgery offers another possible aggressive treatment for selected patients with peritoneal disease. The value of this treatment in the setting of concomitant solid-organ metastases is unknown.[48]

TREATMENT OF UNRESECTABLE DISEASE: SYSTEMIC THERAPY AND ABLATION TECHNIQUES

Most patients with metastatic CRC are not candidates for surgical resection. Some patients with "unresectable" disease treated with modern chemotherapy have been converted to a resectable state resulting in a durable disease-free interval with the combination of neoadjuvant chemotherapy and aggressive surgical metastasectomy. In a large series of 1439 patients with metastatic CRC and disease limited to the liver, a regimen of FOLFOX or FOLFIRI induced a favorable response in 138 patients, allowing subsequent resection. Although 80% of patients developed eventual recurrence, survival at 5 years was 33%.[49] Defining the criteria for "unresectable" disease in this era remains a challenging proposition. Nonsurgical treatment options for patients who are truly unresectable or have progressed after treatment with either first- or second-line combination systemic therapy include regional chemotherapy (i.e., hepatic arterial infusion [HAI]), percutaneous ablative therapies (i.e., radiofrequency ablation [RFA] or microwave ablation), and experimental therapies. Novel investigational modalities include the use of radiation therapies (including intensity modulated radiation therapy, proton- and gamma-beam irradiation), chemoembolization, and hepatic arterial injection of radioactive materials (e.g., yttrium 90 glass microspheres). The technical aspects of ablative techniques are described in a separate chapter. Table 134.2 summarizes the results of nonsurgical regional therapies. Direct comparison between resection and ablation techniques is difficult because the latter is usually offered to patients who are not optimal surgical candidates. Aside from the selection bias and retrospective nature of the data, most published studies suggest a higher risk of recurrence after ablative techniques, with variable rates across studies.[57] A small, randomized phase II comparative trial compared the

TABLE 134.2 Nonsurgical Regional Therapies for Metastatic Colorectal Cancer to the Liver

Treatment Modality	Limitations	Outcomes	Complications
RFA[50]	Higher recurrence compared with resection	Up to 34% local recurrence rate	Morbidity 5%–30%: abscess, hemorrhage, bile leak
	Lesion proximity to blood vessels	Survival benefit not established	
	Lesion size >5 cm		
Cryoablation[51]	Similar to RFA, but possible higher rate of complications	Local recurrence rate: 10%–60%	Morbidity 15%–30%: hemorrhage, bile leak, cryoshock syndrome, myoglobinuria
HAI[52]	Laparotomy needed to implant infusion device	Response rate >50%	Hepatobiliary toxicity
	Limited centers with experience	No proven survival benefit	Pump complications
			Gastritis/duodenitis
Radioembolization (yttrium 90 microspheres)[53]	Emerging experience	Response rate: 44%	Morbidity: 24%
		Progression-free survival: 16–18 months	Abdominal pain and fever
			Gastritis/duodenitis
		Combined with systemic chemotherapy or HAI	Radiation hepatitis
Conformal/stereotactic radiotherapy[54]	Low liver tolerance to radiation	Median survival: 17 months	Radiation hepatitis: 5%
	Lesion proximity to adjacent organs	Local control rates >60%	Skin erythema
			Chest wall pain
Irreversible electroporation[55,56]	Emerging experience	NA	Abscess, bile leak

HAI, Hepatic artery infusion; *NA*, not available; *RFA*, radiofrequency ablation.

combination of RFA and chemotherapy with systemic therapy alone. Progression-free survival was improved in the group that included RFA (10 months compared with 17 months).[58] Overall survival was not significantly different between both groups, although the survival rates were higher than expected in the systemic treatment alone arm.[59]

HAI has generated interest among some investigators because liver metastases derive most of their blood supply from the hepatic artery. Several randomized trials demonstrated a superior response rate from chemotherapeutic HAI compared with noncontemporary systemic chemotherapy regimens. In the Cancer and Leukemia Group B 9481 trial, systemic chemotherapy using 5-FU and leucovorin was compared with HAI using floxuridine, leucovorin, and dexamethasone in 135 patients. HAI prolonged survival from 20 to 24 months, increased the response rate from 24% to 47%, and was associated with improved physical functioning.[60] Other multiinstitutional clinical trials have attempted to establish the role of adjuvant or neoadjuvant HAI chemotherapy (in combination with 5-FU chemotherapy) plus hepatic resection versus resection alone. Phase III trials have shown an improvement in disease-free, but not overall survival, when compared with resection alone.[61] A more recent retrospective study compared 125 patients who underwent resection of their liver metastases followed by HAI, with 125 patients who underwent resection followed by a modern chemotherapy regimen including oxaliplatin or irinotecan. They found that HAI was associated with improved recurrence-free survival and disease-specific survival.[62] In the era of current-day chemotherapy, which

yields enhanced response rates and improved survival, the role of HAI in the management of CRC hepatic metastases remains unclear in the absence of more contemporary randomized trials, and it has not been embraced by most medical or surgical oncologists.

Irreversible electroporation (IRE) is a novel ablation technique that induces permanent permeabilization of cell membranes and subsequent cell death. It does not involve thermal energy, which allows use in proximity to bile ducts and blood vessels without a heat sink effect. Current available data have shown the relative safety of this approach, and there are several trials underway to assess its efficacy in terms of oncologic outcomes.[55,56]

SURVEILLANCE AFTER LIVER RESECTION FOR COLORECTAL CANCER

The recommended guidelines for surveillance of stage IV CRC patients are based on the results of several clinical trials comparing low- and high-intensity follow-up programs.[63] A history and physical examination should be performed every 3 to 6 months for the first 2 years, and then every 6 months up to 5 years; serum CEA measurements should occur at each of these visits. This only applies to patients with an abnormally elevated baseline CEA level at diagnosis. These evidence-based recommendations also apply to patients who underwent resection of their primary tumor. Because 2% to 5% of patients with CRC will develop metachronous primary lesions, an interval colonoscopy to detect new CRCs and to evaluate for local (anastomotic) recurrence appears reasonable. In the setting of resected metastatic disease, other experts have recommended more intensive imaging surveillance with computed tomography (CT) scans of the chest, abdomen, and pelvis in each of these visits.[64] However, this approach is not supported by data and subjects patients to the harmful and cumulative effects of CT-induced radiation exposure. Magnetic resonance imaging can be used as an effective substitute for CT surveillance without the deleterious effects of radiation exposure. In patients with elevated or rising CEA levels, the use of positron emission tomography scans combined with the anatomic detail of noncontrast-enhanced CT may be helpful to detect the site of recurrent disease.

NEUROENDOCRINE METASTASES

Neuroendocrine tumors (NETs) are malignant gastroenteropancreatic neoplasms of the amine precursor uptake and decarboxylation cells. These heterogeneous collections of tumors include carcinoid tumors, pancreatic endocrine tumors, and all other NETs (e.g., pheochromocytoma, neuroblastoma, medullary thyroid carcinoma). These tumor subtypes are further classified by their location, cell of origin, functionality, and specific production of hormones. Carcinoid tumors are usually slow-growing neuroendocrine tumors that arise from the enterochromaffin cells along the gastrointestinal tract. They typically secrete a range of hormones, but primarily elaborate serotonin (5-hydroxytryptamine [5-HT]). The majority (approximately 70%) of pancreatic endocrine tumors or islet cell tumors of the pancreas secrete specific hormones that may have characteristic physiologic and biologic consequences. Approximately one-third of pancreatic endocrine tumors are completely nonfunctional.

Malignant NETs frequently metastasize to the liver. Their biologic behavior, often indolent in nature, is strikingly different from adenocarcinomas of the colon, rectum, small bowel, and pancreas. The role of metastasectomy or debulking is determined by the distribution of disease, presence of symptoms, and the anticipated impact of resection on long-term disease control or palliation.

Ninety percent of NETs have receptors to somatostatin or its analogue, octreotide. Approximately 60% to 80% of patients have either an objective tumor response or symptomatic improvement with the subcutaneous administration of somatostatin analogues.[65] The duration of response can range from weeks to years, but the vast majority of patients eventually become refractory to its effect.[66] Two phase III randomized trials, CLARINET and PROMID, analyzed their use versus placebo in patients with metastatic neuroendocrine tumors. They demonstrated an improvement in disease-free survival with the use of octreotide or lanreotide in patients with well to moderately differentiated tumors from the gastrointestinal tract or pancreas, with or without carcinoid syndrome. Functionally active or inactive tumors responded similarly to somatostatin analogues. They could not draw conclusions regarding overall survival, in part due to the low number of deaths that occurred during follow-up.[67,68] Several large retrospective reports suggest a progression-free and possible overall survival benefit with the administration of radiolabeled octreotide compared with patients treated with best medical care.[69] Somatostatin analogues have also been used in the form of liver-directed radiation therapy.

In a multicenter study, radiolabeled intravenous edotreotide induced tumor response or stabilization in 74% of patients with carcinoid tumors that were refractory to octreotide, with a reasonable progression-free survival of 16 months.[70] The NETTER-1 phase III randomized trial has been designed to compare ^{177}Lu-DOTA^0-Tyr^3-octreotate versus octreotide in patients with progressive metastatic neuroendocrine tumors. Preliminary data showed improvement in tumor response rates, disease-free survival, and a trend toward improved overall survival.[71] In addition to the available options in patients with unresectable or metastatic tumors, two targeted therapy drugs have been approved based on the results of recent randomized trials. Everolimus, a mammalian target of rapamycin (mTOR) inhibitor, has demonstrated improvement in progression-free survival compared with placebo in metastatic neuroendocrine tumors of intestinal or pancreatic origin, including nonfunctional lesions.[72–74] Sunitinib, a VEGF and EGFR inhibitor, improved progression-free and overall survival in advanced, well differentiated pancreatic neuroendocrine tumors.[75]

In the absence of symptomatic control with somatostatin analogues, a palliative resection may be considered to remove or debulk intrahepatic metastatic disease. Nonoperative ablative techniques (e.g., RFA, ethanol injection), chemoembolization, and systemic chemotherapy have been used in patients who have failed somatostatin therapy and are not candidates for surgical resection.[76] In asymptomatic patients, curative resection should be considered in patients with an excellent performance status and in clinical situations where both the primary and all sites of metastatic disease can be safely extirpated. The goal of surgery (curative vs. palliative) should be established before operative intervention. Unfortunately, most of the evidence that would influence surgical management is based on retrospective data, and therefore most treatment decisions are individualized and generated within the context of multidisciplinary tumor boards.

Medical management of NETs typically results in 5-year survival rates that range from 20% to up to 70%, depending on the histology and grade.[77] When resection is performed with curative intent, durable long-term survival is associated with the complete removal of all disease and reported to be as high as 74% at 5 years and 51% at 10 years.[78] Liver transplantation has been attempted in selected patients with hepatic metastases from NETs. In older reports, actuarial 5-year survival for patients with carcinoid tumors was significantly higher (69%) than for patients with other types of NETs (36%). These outcomes were tempered by the high reported postoperative mortality rate (19% overall; 7% for carcinoid, 31% other NETs).[79] The Milan group has proposed selection guidelines, which include curative resection of the primary lesion, age younger than 55 years, low-grade tumors with a Ki-67 index lower than 10%, primary tumors confined to the portal venous drainage system, and disease involving less than 50% of the liver volume.[80] With stringent selection criteria, these investigators have reported remarkable survival rates, of 97% at 5 years and 88% at 10 years.[81]

The most common NETs that metastasize to the liver are carcinoids and gastrinomas, which are discussed in more detail subsequently.

CARCINOID TUMORS

Carcinoid tumors give rise to two-thirds of NET liver metastases. After the regional lymph nodes, the liver is the most common site of metastasis, although this occurs in only 5% of patients. These enterochromaffin cell tumors most commonly arise from the small bowel and tend to have an indolent nature. There is a correlation between their metastatic potential and their size and location. Rectal carcinoids have the highest risk of metastasis, and appendiceal have the lowest. The clinical course of patients with metastatic liver disease is variable. Patients may remain completely asymptomatic for extended time periods before their disease burden produces hepatic failure, metabolic disturbances, or cachexia. Ninety-percent of symptomatic patients have metastatic disease. A minority (<10%) of patients with metastatic disease to the liver develop the classic "carcinoid syndrome" manifest by flushing, diarrhea, bronchospasm, and/or right-sided heart failure. An elevated serum chromogranin A level has been associated with a worse prognosis.[82]

As with all NETs, treatment options are dictated by the extent of disease, presence of symptoms, and surgical risk for the patient. Prolonged survival can be obtained with complete resection of the primary and metastatic disease.[83] To prevent a life-threatening carcinoid crisis exacerbated by anesthesia, surgery or invasive procedures, intravenous octreotide should be readily available for administration during any of these interventions. In addition, it is recommended that all patients with carcinoid tumors in whom the use of somatostatin analogues is anticipated have their gallbladder removed at the time of surgery because somatostatin analogues increase the risk of developing gallstones.

GASTRINOMAS

Gastrinomas (Zollinger-Ellison syndrome) are foregut NETs that produce excess gastrin, which is a potent stimulator of hydrochloric acid secretion from the parietal cells of the stomach. Peptic ulceration is common, and the disease has both sporadic and inherited forms. Sixty percent to 80% of gastrinomas are malignant, but less than 10% metastasize to the liver. Hepatic metastases are the most important predictor of survival and primary cause of death in the majority of patients.[] As is the case in other NETs, complete resection can result in long-term survival in more than 70% of patients.[85] Unfortunately, less than 15% of patients are candidates for curative resection. In the past, complications of gastrin secretion resulted in significant morbidity and mortality, and palliative surgery was indicated in cases refractory to acid suppression therapy. The use of proton pump inhibitors can control symptomatic disease in many patients by near-complete suppression of gastric acid production.

OTHER NEUROENDOCRINE TUMORS

The remainder of NETs that cause liver metastases are far more uncommon. Insulinomas are the most common islet cell tumor, although only 10% are malignant. Even with widely disseminated disease, aggressive surgical debulking may improve hypoglycemic episodes. Fifty percent of vasoactive intestinal peptide tumors (NET-producing VIPomas)

and the majority of glucagonomas, somatostatinomas, and pancreatic-polypeptide tumors (PPomas) are malignant. Specific data regarding their surgical management in the setting of metastatic liver disease are limited, but the same principles used in patients with all NETs can be extrapolated to these clinical situations.

RESULTS OF LOCAL ABLATIVE THERAPY FOR NEUROENDOCRINE TUMORS

In patients who are not candidates for curative resection or cytoreduction, ablative modalities offer a possibility of palliation of symptoms. Laparoscopic RFA has been reported as a successful technique to ameliorate symptoms in more than 90% of patients, with minimal risk of morbidity and mortality.[86] Hepatic artery embolization has also been described in patients who have failed RFA, because the blood supply to neuroendocrine metastases arises from the hepatic artery. It has been used in combination with cytotoxic chemotherapy or alone to improve pain or hormonal symptoms.[87] A small phase II study of chemoembolization showed a decrease in size of lesions in 33% of patients and symptomatic relief in most, with a median duration of the response of 14 months.[83] Complications with RFA are common and include infection, bleeding, ileus, abdominal pain, fever, elevated liver enzymes, and cholecystitis. Treatment-related mortality ranges from 2% to 5%.[88]

NONCOLORECTAL, NONNEUROENDOCRINE METASTASES

NCNN metastases represent a heterogeneous collection of all other nonprimary hepatic metastases. This group includes metastatic extremity and retroperitoneal sarcomas, renal cell carcinomas, breast cancers, gastrointestinal stromal tumors, melanoma, non-CRC gastrointestinal tumors, and non–small cell lung carcinoma. Although the biologic spectrum of NCNN metastatic disease is variable, centers of experience have attempted to collectively group these tumors en masse to provide retrospective data that may influence medical and surgical therapy. The role of hepatic resection for NCNN metastases is more controversial, and it is generally not considered to be the standard of care. Although reports of actuarial 3-year cancer-specific survival rates over 50% have been reported, these numbers likely cannot be extrapolated to all patients with NCNN.[89] Favorable prognostic factors included a long disease-free interval, the ability to perform a complete metastasectomy, and a primary tumor originating from the reproductive tract or urologic tract.[89,90] In summary, current data suggest that in highly selected patients, resection can be associated with favorable outcomes.

CONCLUSION

The progress in the management of patients with metastatic liver disease has been significant and continues to evolve. Resection is the current standard of care for patients with limited metastatic disease from CRC, and combined treatment has resulted in improved survival rates. There is a role for resection in selected patients with neuroendocrine tumors and in rare patients with NCNN and favorable risk factors. Despite these advances, most patients with liver metastases have incurable disease, and further development of novel therapies is awaited.

ACKNOWLEDGMENT

The authors thank Roberta Carden for proofreading and editing this manuscript.

REFERENCES

1. Adam R, Vibert E, Pitombo M. Induction chemotherapy and surgery of colorectal liver metastases. *Bull Cancer.* 2006;93:S45.
2. Tomlinson JS, Jarnagin WR, DeMatteo RP, et al. Actual 10-year survival after resection of colorectal liver metastases defines cure. *J Clin Oncol.* 2007;25:4575.
3. Pawlik TM, Scoggins CR, Zorzi D, et al. Effect of surgical margin status on survival and site of recurrence after hepatic resection for colorectal metastases. *Ann Surg.* 2005;241:715.
4. Reddy SK, Barbas AS, Clary BM. Synchronous colorectal liver metastases: is it time to reconsider traditional paradigms of management? *Ann Surg Oncol.* 2009;16:2395.
5. Fong Y, Cohen AM, Fortner JG, et al. Liver resection for colorectal metastases. *J Clin Oncol.* 1997;15:938.
6. Choti MA, Sitzmann JV, Tiburi MF, et al. Trends in long-term survival following liver resection for hepatic colorectal metastases. *Ann Surg.* 2002;235:759.
7. Aloia TA, Vauthey JM, Loyer EM, et al. Solitary colorectal liver metastasis. Resection determines outcome. *Arch Surg.* 2006;141:460.
8. Fong Y, Fortner J, Sun RL, Brennan MF, Blumgart LH. Clinical score for predicting recurrence after hepatic resection for metastatic colorectal cancer. Analysis of 1001 consecutive cases. *Ann Surg.* 1999;230:309; discussion 318.
9. Allen PJ, Kemeny N, Jarnagin W, DeMatteo R, Blumgart L, Fong Y. Importance of response to neoadjuvant chemotherapy in patients undergoing resection of synchronous colorectal liver metastases. *J Gastrointest Surg.* 2003;7:109.
10. Ito H, Mo Q, Qin LX, et al. Gene expression profiles accurately predict outcome following liver resection in patients with metastatic colorectal cancer. *PLoS One.* 2013;8:e81680.
11. Covey AM, Brown KT, Jarnagin WR, et al. Combined portal vein embolization and neoadjuvant chemotherapy as a treatment strategy for resectable hepatic colorectal metastases. *Ann Surg.* 2008;247:451.
12. Goldberg RM, Sargent DJ, Morton RF, et al. A randomized controlled trial of fluorouracil plus leucovorin, irinotecan, and oxaliplatin combinations in patients with previously untreated metastatic colorectal cancer. *J Clin Oncol.* 2004;22:23.
13. Douillard JY, Cunningham D, Roth AD, et al. Irinotecan combined with fluorouracil compared with fluorouracil alone as first-line treatment for metastatic colorectal cancer: a multicentre randomized trial. *Lancet.* 2000;355:1041.
14. Twelves C, Wong A, Nowacki MP, et al. Capecitabine as adjuvant treatment for stage III colon cancer. *N Engl J Med.* 2005;352:2696.
15. Hurwitz H, Fehrenbacher L, Novotny W, et al. Bevacizumab plus irinotecan, fluorouracil and leucovorin for metastatic colorectal cancer. *N Engl J Med.* 2004;350:2335.
16. Van Cutsem E, Köhne CE, Hitre E, et al. Cetuximab and chemotherapy as initial treatment for metastatic colorectal cancer. *N Engl J Med.* 2009;360:1408.
17. Vauthey JN, Pawlik TM, Ribero D, et al. Chemotherapy regimen predicts steatohepatitis and an increase in 90-day mortality after surgery for hepatic colorectal metastases. *J Clin Oncol.* 2006;24:2065.
18. Aloia T, Sebagh M, Plasse M, et al. Liver histology and surgical outcomes after preoperative chemotherapy with fluorouracil plus oxaliplatin in colorectal cancer liver metastases. *J Clin Oncol.* 2006; 24:4983.
19. Scappaticci FA, Skillings JR, Holden SN, et al. Arterial thromboembolic events in patients with metastatic carcinoma treated with chemotherapy and bevacizumab. *J Natl Cancer Inst.* 2007;99:1232.
20. Kesmodel SB, Ellis LM, Lin E, et al. Preoperative bevacizumab does not significantly increase postoperative complication rates in patients
21. Adam R, Aloia T, Lévi F, et al. Hepatic resection after rescue cetuximab treatment for colorectal liver metastases previously refractory to conventional systemic therapy. *J Clin Oncol.* 2007;25:4593.
22. Meyerhardt JA, Mayer RJ. Systemic therapy for colorectal cancer. *N Engl J Med.* 2005;352:476.
23. Adam R, Wicherts DA, de Haas RJ, et al. Complete pathologic response after preoperative chemotherapy for colorectal liver metastases: myth or reality? *J Clin Oncol.* 2008;26:1635.
24. Benoist S, Brouquet A, Penna C, et al. Complete response of colorectal liver metastases after chemotherapy: does it mean cure? *J Clin Oncol.* 2006;24:3939.
25. Nordlinger B, Sorbye H, Glimelius B, et al. Perioperative chemotherapy with FOLFOX4 and surgery versus surgery alone for resectable liver metastases from colorectal cancer (EORTC Intergroup trial 40983): a randomised controlled trial. *Lancet.* 2008;371:1007.
26. Nordlinger B, Sorbye H, Glimelius B, et al. Perioperative FOLFOX4 chemotherapy and surgery versus surgery alone for resectable liver metastases from colorectal cancer (EORTC 40983): long-term results of a randomised, controlled, phase 3 trial. *Lancet Oncol.* 2013;14:1208.
27. Primrose J, Falk S, Finch-Jones M, et al. Systemic chemotherapy with or without cetuximab in patients with resectable colorectal liver metastasis: the New EPOC randomised controlled trial. *Lancet Oncol.* 2014;15:601.
28. Ychou M, Hohenberger W, Thezenas S, et al. A randomized phase III study comparing adjuvant 5-fluorouracil/folinic acid with FOLFIRI in patients following complete resection of liver metastases from colorectal cancer. *Ann Oncol.* 2009;20:1964.
29. Adam R, Avisar E, Ariche A, et al. Five-year survival following hepatic resection after neoadjuvant therapy for nonresectable colorectal liver metastases. *Ann Surg Oncol.* 2001;8:347.
30. Wein A, Riedel C, Brückl W, et al. Neoadjuvant treatment with weekly high-dose 5-fluorouracil as 24-hour infusion, folinic acid and oxaliplatin in patients with primary resectable liver metastases of colorectal cancer. *Oncology.* 2003;64:131.
31. Taieb J, Artru P, Paye F, et al. Intensive systemic chemotherapy combined with surgery for metastatic colorectal cancer: results of a phase II study. *J Clin Oncol.* 2005;23:502.
32. Barone C, Nuzzo G, Cassano A, et al. Final analysis of colorectal cancer patients treated with irinotecan and 5-fluorouracil plus folinic acid neoadjuvant chemotherapy for unresectable liver metastases. *Br J Cancer.* 2007;97:1035.
33. Masi G, Loupakis F, Pollina L, et al. Long-term outcome of initially unresectable metastatic colorectal cancer patients treated with 5-fluorouracil/leucovorin, oxaliplatin, and irinotecan (FOLFOXIRI) followed by radical surgery of metastases. *Ann Surg.* 2009;249:420.
34. Okines A, Puerto OD, Cunningham D, et al. Surgery with curative-intent in patients treated with first-line chemotherapy plus bevacizumab for metastatic colorectal cancer. First BEAT and the randomised phase-III N016966 trial. *Br J Cancer.* 2009;101:1033.
35. Ciliberto D, Prati U, Roveda L, et al. Role of systemic chemotherapy in the management of resected or resectable colorectal liver metastases: a systematic review and meta-analysis of randomized controlled trials. *Oncol Rep.* 2012;27:1849.
36. Wang ZM, Chen YY, Chen FF, Wang SY, Xiong B. Peri-operative chemotherapy for patients with resectable colorectal hepatic metastasis: a meta-analysis. *Eur J Surg Oncol.* 2015;41:1197.
37. Tsai MS, Su YH, Ho MC, et al. Clinicopathological features and prognosis in resectable synchronous and metachronous colorectal liver metastases. *Ann Surg Oncol.* 2007;14:786.
38. Martin R, Paty P, Fong YG, et al. Simultaneous liver and colorectal resections are safe for synchronous colorectal liver metastasis. *J Am Coll Surg.* 2003;197:233.
39. Mayo SC, Pulitano C, Marques H, et al. Surgical management of patients with synchronous colorectal liver metastasis: a multicenter international analysis. *J Am Coll Surg.* 2013;216:707.
40. Silberhumer GR, Paty PB, Denton B, et al. Long-term oncologic outcomes for simultaneous resection of synchronous metastatic liver and primary colorectal cancer. *Surgery.* 2016;160(1):67-73. doi:10.1016/j.surg.2016.02.029.
41. Ayez N, Burger JWA, van der Pool AE, et al. Long-term results of the "liver first" approach in patients with locally advanced rectal cancer and synchronous liver metastases. *Dis Colon Rectum.* 2013; 56:281.

42. Gall TMH, Basyouny M, Frampton AE, et al. Neoadjuvant chemotherapy and primary-first approach for rectal cancer with synchronous liver metastases. *Colorectal Dis.* 2013;16:O197.

43. Elias D, Ouellet JF, Bellon N, Pignon JP, Pocard M, Lasser P. Extrahepatic disease does not contraindicate hepatectomy for colorectal liver metastases. *Br J Surg.* 2003;90:567.

44. Carpizo DR, Are C, Jarnagin W, et al. Liver resection for metastatic colorectal cancer in patients with concurrent extrahepatic disease: results in 127 patients treated at a single center. *Ann Surg Oncol.* 2009;16:2138.

45. Pulitano C, Bodingbauer M, Aldrighetti L, et al. Liver resection for colorectal metastases in presence of extrahepatic disease: results from an international multi-institutional analysis. *Ann Surg Oncol.* 2011;18:1380.

46. Chua TC, Saxena A, Liauw W, Chu F, Morris DL. Hepatectomy and resection of concomitant extrahepatic disease for colorectal liver metastases—a systematic review. *Eur J Cancer.* 2012;48:1757.

47. Adam R, de Haas RJ, Wicherts DA, et al. Is hepatic resection justified after chemotherapy in patients with colorectal liver metastases and lymph node involvement? *J Clin Oncol.* 2008;26:3672.

48. Yan TD, Black D, Savady R, Sugarbaker PH. Systematic review on the efficacy of cytoreductive surgery combined with perioperative intraperitoneal chemotherapy for peritoneal carcinomatosis from colorectal carcinoma. *J Clin Oncol.* 2006;24:4011.

49. Adam R, Delvart V, Pascal G, et al. Rescue surgery for unresectable colorectal liver metastases downstaged by chemotherapy. A model to predict long-term survival. *Ann Surg.* 2004;240:644.

50. Abdalla EK, Vauthey JN, Ellis LM, et al. Recurrence and outcomes following hepatic resection, radiofrequency ablation, and combined resection/ablation for colorectal liver metastases. *Ann Surg.* 2004;239:818.

51. Pearson AS, Izzo F, Fleming RY, et al. Intraoperative radiofrequency ablation or cryoablation for hepatic malignancies. *Am J Surg.* 1999;178:592.

52. Lorenz M, Muller HH. Randomized, multicenter trial of fluorouracil plus leucovorin administered either via hepatic artery or intravenous infusion versus fluorodeoxyuridine administered via hepatic artery infusion in patients with nonresectable liver metastases from colorectal carcinoma. *J Clin Oncol.* 2000;18:243.

53. Gulec SA, Fong Y. Yttrium 90 microsphere selective internal radiation treatment of hepatic colorectal metastases. *Arch Surg.* 2007;142:675.

54. Swaminath A, Dawson LA. Emerging role of radiotherapy in the management of liver metastases. *Cancer J.* 2010;16:150.

55. Scheffer HJ, Nielsen K, van Tilborg AAJM, et al. Ablation of colorectal liver metastases by irreversible electroporation: results of the COLDFIRE-I ablate-and-resect study. *Eur Radiol.* 2014;24:2467.

56. Scheffer HJ, Vroomen LGPH, Nielsen K, et al. Colorectal liver metastatic disease: efficacy of irreversible electroporation—a single arm phase II clinical trial (COLDFIRE-2 trial). *BMC Cancer.* 2015;15:772.

57. Abdalla EK, Adam R, Bilchik AJ, Jaeck D, Vauthey JN, Mahvi D. Improving resectability of hepatic colorectal metastases: expert consensus statement. *Ann Surg Oncol.* 2006;13:1271.

58. Ruers T, Punt CJ, van Coevorden L, et al. Final results of the EORTC intergroup randomized study 40004 (CLOCC) evaluating the benefit of radiofrequency ablation combined with chemotherapy for unresectable colorectal liver metastases. *J Clin Oncol.* 2010;28:15s.

59. Ruers T, Punt C, Van Coevorden F, et al. Radiofrequency ablation combined with systemic treatment versus systemic treatment alone in patients with non-resectable colorectal liver metastases: a randomized EORTC Intergroup phase II study (EORTC 40004). *Ann Oncol.* 2012;23:2619.

60. Kemeny NE, Niedzwiecki D, Hollis DR, et al. Hepatic arterial infusion versus systemic therapy for hepatic metastases from colorectal cancer: a randomized trial of efficacy, quality of life, and molecular markers (CALGB 9481). *J Clin Oncol.* 2006;24:1395.

61. Lorenz M, Müller HH, Schramm H, et al. Randomized trial of surgery versus surgery followed by adjuvant hepatic arterial infusion with 5-fluorouracil and folinic acid for liver metastases of colorectal cancer: German Cooperative on Liver Metastases (Arbeitsgruppe Lebermetastasen). *Ann Surg.* 1998;228:756.

62. House MG, Kemeny NE, Gonen M, et al. Comparison of adjuvant systemic chemotherapy with or without hepatic arterial infusional chemotherapy after hepatic resection for metastatic colorectal cancer. *Ann Surg.* 2011;254:851.

63. Desch CE, Benson AB 3rd, Somerfield MR, et al. Colorectal cancer surveillance: 2005 update of an American Society of Clinical Oncology practice guideline. *J Clin Oncol.* 2005;23:8512.

64. Bensor AB 3rd, Venook AP, Bekaii-Saab T, et al. National Comprehensive Cancer Network. Clinical practice guidelines in oncology: colon cancer. NCCN Guidelines, 2016. Available at www.nccn.org.

65. Sarmiento JM, Heywood G, Rubin J, Ilstrup DM, Nagorney DM, Que FG. Surgical treatment of neuroendocrine metastases to the liver: a plea for resection to increase survival. *J Am Coll Surg.* 2003; 197:29.

66. Wynick D, Anderson JV, Williams SJ, Bloom SR. Resistance of metastatic pancreatic endocrine tumours after long-term treatment with the somatostatin analogue octreotide (SMS 201–995). *Clin Endocrinol (Oxf).* 1989;30:385.

67. Caplin ME, Pavel M, Cwikla J, et al. Lanreotide in metastatic enteropancreatic neuroendocrine tumors. *N Engl J Med.* 2014;371: 224.

68. Rinke A, Muller HH, Schade-Brittinger CS, et al. Placebo-controlled, double-blind, prospective, randomized study on the effect of octreotide LAR in the control of tumor growth in patients with metastatic neuroendocrine midgut tumors: a report from the PROMID Study Group. *J Clin Oncol.* 2009;27:4656.

69. Kwekkeboom DJ, de Herder WW, Kam BL, et al. Treatment with the radiolabeled somatostatin analog [^{177}Lu-DOTA0-Tyr^3]octreotate: toxicity, efficacy, and survival. *J Clin Oncol.* 2008;26:2124.

70. Bushnell DL, O'Dorisio TM, O'Dorisio MS, et al. ^{90}Y-Edotreotide for metastatic carcinoid refractory to octreotide. *J Clin Oncol.* 2010;28: 1652.

71. Strosberg JR, Wolin EM, Chasen B, et al. NETTER-1 phase III: progression-free survival, radiographic response, and preliminary overall survival results in patients with midgut neuroendocrine tumors treated with 177-Lu-Dotatate. *J Clin Oncol.* 2016;34(4 suppl):194. [meeting abstracts].

72. Yao JC, Shah MH, Ito T, et al. Everolimus for advanced pancreatic neuroendocrine tumors. *N Engl J Med.* 2011;364:514.

73. Pavel ME, Hainsworth JD, Baudin E, et al. Everolimus plus octreotide long-acting repeatable for the treatment of advanced neuroendocrine tumours associated with carcinoid syndrome (RADIANT-2): a randomised, placebo-controlled, phase 3 study. *Lancet.* 2011;378: 2005.

74. Yao JC, Fazio N, Singh S, et al. Everolimus for the treatment of advanced non-functional neuroendocrine tumours of the lung or gastrointestinal tract (RADIANT-4): a randomised, placebo-controlled, phase 3 study. *Lancet.* 2016;387:968.

75. Raymond E, Dahan L, Raoul JL, et al. Sunitinib malate for the treatment of pancreatic neuroendocrine tumors. *N Engl J Med.* 2011;364:501.

76. Eriksson BK, Larsson EG, Skogseid BM, Lofberg AM, Lorelius LE, Oberg KE. Liver embolizations of patients with malignant neuroendocrine gastrointestinal tumors. *Cancer.* 1998;83:2293.

77. Chamberlain RS, Canes D, Brown KT, et al. Hepatic neuroendocrine metastases: does intervention alter outcomes? *J Am Coll Surg.* 2000;190:432.

78. Mayo SC, de Jong MC, Pulitano C, et al. Surgical management of hepatic neuroendocrine tumor metastasis: results from an international multi-institutional analysis. *Ann Surg Oncol.* 2010;17:3129.

79. Le Treut YP, Delpero JR, Dousset B, et al. Results of liver transplantation in the treatment of metastatic neuroendocrine tumors. A 31-case French multicentric report. *Ann Surg.* 1997;225:355.

80. Mazzaferro V, Pulvirenti A, Coppa J. Neuroendocrine tumors metastatic to the liver: how to select patients for liver transplantation? *J Hepatol.* 2007;47:460.

81. Mazzaferro V, Sposito C, Coppa J, et al. The long-term benefit of liver transplantation for hepatic metastases from neuroendocrine tumors. *Am J Transplant.* 2016;15(10):2892-2902. doi:10.1111/ajt.13831.

82. Janson ET, Holmberg L, Stridsberg M, et al. Carcinoid tumors: analysis of prognostic factors and survival in 301 patients from a referral center. *Ann Oncol.* 1997;3:685.

83. Chen H, Hardacre JM, Uzar A, Cameron JL, Choti MA. Isolated liver metastases from neuroendocrine tumors: does resection prolong survival? *J Am Coll Surg.* 1998;187:88.

84. Yu F, Venzon DJ, Serrano J, et al. Prospective study of the clinical course, prognostic factors and survival in patients with longstanding Zollinger-Ellison syndrome. *J Clin Oncol.* 1999;17:615.

35. Norton JA, Warren RS, Kelly MG, Zuraek MB, Jensen RT. Aggressive surgery for metastatic liver neuroendocrine tumors. *Surgery*. 2003;134:1057.

36. Berber E, Flesher N, Siperstein AE. Laparoscopic radiofrequency ablation of neuroendocrine liver metastases. *World J Surg*. 2002;26:985.

37. Yao KA, Talamonti MS, Nemcek A, et al. Indications and results of liver resection and hepatic chemoembolization for metastatic gastrointestinal neuroendocrine tumors. *Surgery*. 2001;130:677.

88. Ruszniewski P, Rougier P, Roche A, et al. Hepatic arterial chemoembolization in patients with liver metastases of endocrine tumors. A prospective phase II study in 24 patients. *Cancer*. 1993;71:2624.

89. Weitz J, Blumgart LH, Fong Y, et al. Partial hepatectomy for metastases from noncolorectal, nonneuroendocrine carcinoma. *Ann Surg*. 2005;241:269.

90. Adam R, Chiche L, Aloia T, et al. Hepatic resection for noncolorectal nonendocrine liver metastases. Analysis of 1452 patients and development of a prognostic model. *Ann Surg*. 2006;244:524.

Management of Portal Hypertension

Alex L. Chang | Shimul A. Shah

Portal venous hypertension is an entity that is defined by the presence of elevated hydrostatic pressure in the hepatic portal veins greater than 8 mm Hg. In practice it is understood as the constellation of clinical consequences from an abnormally high pressure gradient between hepatic inflow and outflow venous systems. The wide spectrum of clinical manifestations and syndromes, including variceal bleeding, ascites, liver failure, encephalopathy, hepatopulmonary syndrome (HPS), and portopulmonary hypertension, makes the management of these patients complex even for experienced practitioners. As technology advances, there are an ever-increasing number of diagnostic modalities and medical and surgical therapies in the arsenal for portal hypertension. The surgeon's role in the treatment of liver disease and portal hypertension is also evolving. A shift from surgical decompressive shunts toward orthotopic liver transplantation has changed the role of the surgeon in the treatment of portal hypertension. A cunning surgeon must apply an understanding of the pathophysiology of portal hypertension along with a multidisciplinary approach of surgical and nonsurgical therapies, to achieve an optimal result.

HISTORY

In early civilizations, Egyptians, Greeks, and Romans tried to ascribe function to the liver. The Babylonians and Assyrians took note of the fulness of blood in the liver and postulated that this was the "seat of the soul."[1] Writings from Hippocrates reference liver failure by stating "in cases of jaundice it is a bad sign when the liver becomes hard." An understanding of splanchnic and hepatic circulation has existed since empiric evidence of transhepatic blood flow was demonstrated by Francis Glisson in the early 17th century. Despite the long fascination with this organ, a conceptual understanding of its function and dysfunction has only developed over the past one to two centuries. It was not until microscopic examination became possible that the liver lobule with its hexagonal appearance, portal venous and hepatic arterial inflow from the periphery, and hepatic venous drainage from the center could be fully understood.[2]

Clinical consequences of portal hypertension ailed ancient societies, with mention of ascites in ancient Egyptian, Mayan, and Greek texts. Gastroesophageal varices were recognized in the mid-19th century; however, the etiology of portal hypertension was elusive for nearly 100 years. In 1883 Italian physician Guido Banti observed that patients with anemia, leukopenia, and splenomegaly had elevated portal pressures and cirrhosis. From these observations, Banti postulated that splenomegaly and portal hypertension resulted primarily from increased blood flow to the spleen, which in turn damaged the liver. The popularity of Banti's "forward-flow" theory of portal hypertension led to the term hepatosplenopathy to describe these patients disease process. In the 1920s a New Zealand surgeon Archibald McIndoe proposed a "backward-flow" hypothesis which attributes portal hypertension to an obstruction of flow along the portal circulation. Except in rare situations (e.g., arteriovenous fistulas), portal hypertension results from increased resistance and decreased portal flow. The relationship between flow and resistance and their contribution to the development of porta-systemic collaterals remained incompletely understood.[5,3]

Banti's forward-flow hepatosplenopathies led to numerous therapies focused on prehepatic blood flow with splenectomy and omentopexy and other "preobstructive" operations. As this school of thought gave way to the backward-flow hypothesis, treatment shifted toward decompressive operations. The first end-to-side portacaval shunt was performed on dogs by Nicolai Eck in St. Petersburg in the late 19th century. The "Eck fistula" was later used by Ivan Pavlov (better known for his work in gastric physiology and classical conditioning) to shunt all portal flow away from the liver to demonstrate encephalopathy, progressive muscle wasting, and inanition, which he termed "meat intoxication."[4] Early use of portacaval shunts in humans were unsuccessful until the pioneering work of Whipple and his colleagues at Columbia University in New York in the 1930s.[3] Although surgical shunts were able to control bleeding and ascites, subsequent acceleration of liver failure nullified any survival advantage to their patients.

Portal hypertension has evolved over the past 60 years because of the multiple randomized controlled trials performed for all treatment modalities introduced. This was one of the earliest fields of medicine to receive such scrutiny and therefore was early to use level 1 evidence since the 1950s. Initial trials compared surgical shunts with medical therapy in patients prior to the first variceal bleed and showed that mortality was increased with such intervention. Subsequent studies comparing medical therapy and surgical shunts in patients following their initial variceal bleed showed no improvement in overall survival, but rather the mode of death shifted from variceal bleeding to liver failure. These observations stimulated the investigators of that time to look for new treatment modalities.

Selective shunts pioneered by Warren et al.[5] and Inokuchi et al.,[6] who developed distal splenorenal shunts (DSRSs) and left gastric venous-caval shunts. These shunts could achieve variceal decompression while maintaining adequate portal flow to the liver. Partial shunting via portacaval H-grafts was studied and championed by Sarfeh et al.[7] in the 1980s. Preservation of portal flow resulted in lower rates of encephalopathy and liver failure.

Simultaneously, less invasive methods of treated variceal bleeding related to portal hypertension were developed. Chafoord and Frenckner first described esophagoscopic injection sclerotherapy in the treatment of esophageal varices.[8] American surgeon Gregory Stiegmann and colleagues developed endoscopic variceal ligation as an alternative to sclerotherapy in 1989.[9] Relatively recent technologic advances revolutionized portal venous decompression using the method of transjugular intrahepatic portosystemic shunting (TIPS) first described by Rösch et al.[10] Intrahepatic shunting by means of TIPS is now a mainstay of therapy. The evolution of these interventions were combined with an increasingly sophisticated understanding of portal venous pathophysiology.[11] A recognition that portal hypertension can be exacerbated by splanchnic hyperemia and hyperdynamic systemic circulation led to the introduction of noncardioselective β-blockers in 1980 by Lebrec et al.[12] to ameliorate these changes. Since that time, medical therapy to reduce portal pressure and decrease variceal wall tension has become a mainstay of management.

Finally, the history of portal hypertension must recognize the role of liver transplantation introduced by Starzl and Calne in the 1970s[13] and coming of age in the mid-1980s and 1990s. Their perseverance and pioneering work to resolve many of the technical issues of liver transplantation bore fruit. However, it was really the immunologic advances and the introduction of powerful new immunosuppressants that gave life to liver transplantation. The clinical reality is that most interventions address only the complications of late-stage liver disease, and in many patients survival improved only by liver transplantation. For the surgeon, this brings the management of such patients full circle, where the surgeon's role is now largely in the field of liver transplantation as part of the multidisciplinary team taking care of such patients.

ANATOMY

The portal venous system arises from two embryologic sources: (1) the intraembryonic anterior and posterior cardinal venous system, which become the main systemic veins, and (2) the extraembryonic vitelline and umbilical veins, which become the portal venous system.[14] The vitelline veins intercommunicate in the septum transverse where later liver sinusoids develop. The left vitelline vein forms most of the extrahepatic portal venous system draining the primitive intestine and plays a critical role in utero as the ductus venosus, which communicates directly from the rudimentary portovenous system via the vitelloumbilical anastomosis to the hepatic and cardiac channels, bypassing primitive hepatic sinusoids.

The portal vein is formed behind the neck of the pancreas by the joining of the superior mesenteric and splenic veins. It is normally 10 to 20 mm in diameter but in portal hypertension may enlarge. It courses along the free edge of the gastrohepatic ligament to the liver hilus, where it divides into right and left branches (Fig. 135.1). Its feeding tributaries have some variability, with the

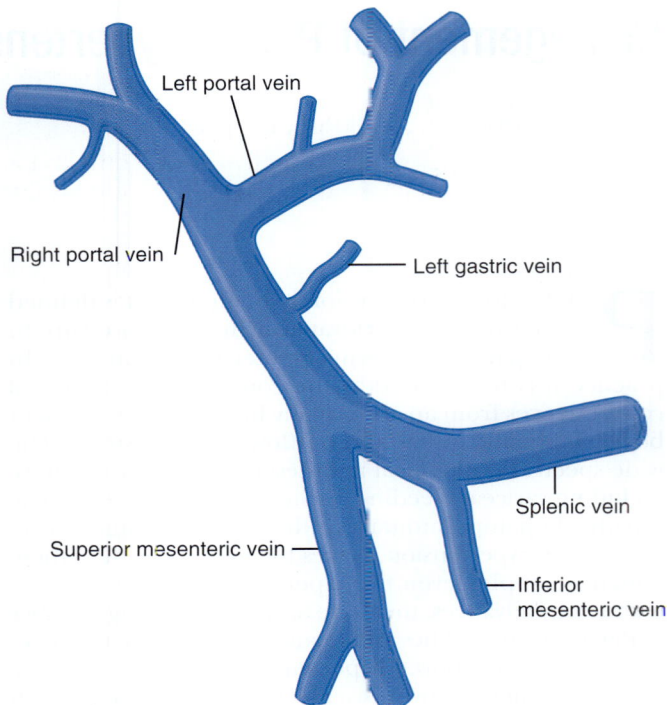

FIGURE 135.1 Portal venous anatomy. The portal vein is formed by the union of the superior mesenteric and splenic veins behind the neck of the pancreas. The inferior mesenteric vein enters the splenic vein in two-thirds of patients and the left gastric vein enters the portal vein in two-thirds of patients.

inferior mesenteric vein entering the splenic vein in approximately two-thirds of persons and superior mesenteric vein in one-third. Similarly the left gastric or coronary vein enters the portal vein in approximately two-thirds and the splenic vein in one-third. The latter may vary considerably in size in portal hypertension and is often one of the major veins feeding into gastroesophageal varices. The umbilical vein is remarkably constant in its communication with the left branch of the portal vein, and in portal hypertension when recanalized this may be quite large. The major changes of clinical significance are around the gastroesophageal junction in portal hypertension. Radiologic studies using corrosion casting and morphometry have clarified the venous pathologic changes at this location in portal hypertension. These are schematically represented in Fig. 135.2, where the following four zones are recognized:

1. The gastric zone extends 2 to 3 cm below the gastroesophageal junction. These veins run longitudinally in the submucosa and lamina propria to the short gastric and left gastric veins.
2. The palisade zone extends 2 to 3 cm superiorly from the gastric zone in the lower esophagus. These parallel palisades run longitudinally and correspond to the esophageal mucosal folds. There are multiple communications between these veins in the lamina propria, but there are no perforating veins in the palisade zone linking the intrinsic and extrinsic venous plexuses.

3. The perforating zone extends approximately 2 cm higher up the esophagus just superior to the palisade zone. In this zone the vessels perforate through the esophageal wall linking the internal and external veins.

4. The truncal zone extends 8 to 10 cm up the esophagus and is characterized by four or five longitudinal veins in the lamina propria. In this zone, there are irregular perforating veins from the submucosa to the external esophageal venous plexuses.

Hepatic arterial anatomy is highly variable, with anomalies being of clinical importance to transplant surgeons, particularly during donor hepatectomy. The normal arterial anatomy is a common hepatic artery arising from the celiac axis that gives rise to a right and left artery just above the gastroduodenal artery. In approximately 20% of persons, there is an anomalous right accessory or replaced hepatic artery arising from the superior mesenteric artery. Similarly, there is an approximately 20% incidence for an accessory or replaced left hepatic artery arising from the left gastric artery. These two anomalies may coexist (Fig. 135.3).

Functional anatomy of the liver can be divided based on their vascular supply. The liver is divided into four sections, which in turn consist of two hepatic segments each. The eight segments of the liver possess their own hepatic artery and portal venous inflow and hepatic venous drainage (Fig. 135.4). Division of these planes allows for functional remnant and donor grafts during liver resection and living-donor liver transplantation. The microarchitecture of the liver parenchyma is also divisible into structural units. The primary modular unit of the liver

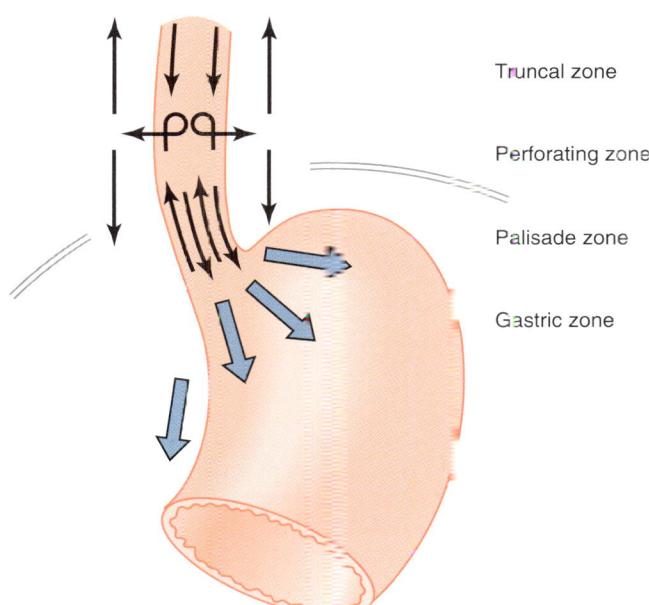

FIGURE 135.2 Diagrammatic representation of the venous zones at the gastroesophageal junction. The perforating zone is the site of highest variceal bleeding risk. Details of the zones are given in the text. (Modified from Vianna A, Hayes PC, Moscoso G, et al. Normal venous circulation of the gastroesophageal junction. A route to understanding varices. *Gastroenterology*. 1987;93:876.)

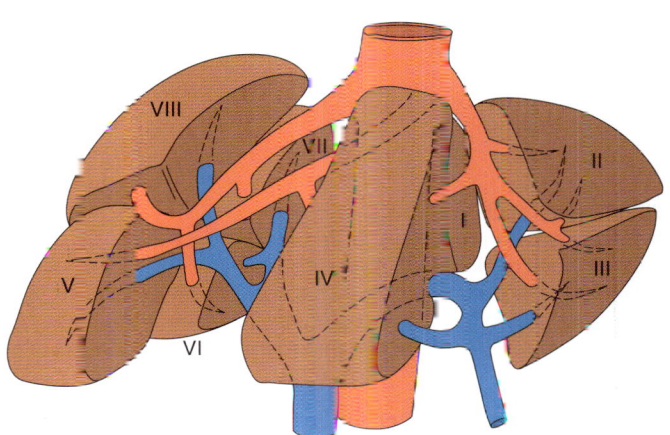

FIGURE 135.4 Liver segmental anatomy is based on portal inflow and hepatic venous outflow. Each of the eight segments is its own functional anatomic unit. (Redrawn from Henderson JM. Atlas of liver surgery. In: Bell RH, Rikkers LF, Mulholland MW, eds. *Digestive Tract Surgery: A Text and Atlas*. Philadelphia: Lippincott-Raven; 1995.)

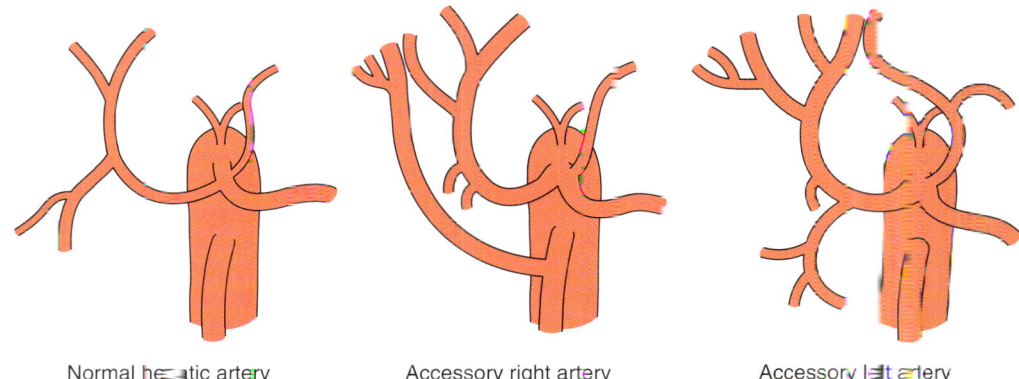

Normal hepatic artery   Accessory right artery   Accessory left artery

FIGURE 135.3 Hepatic arterial anatomy is highly variable. The most common anomalies are accessory—or replaced—right and left hepatic arteries arising from the superior mesenteric and left gastric arteries, respectively. These occur in approximately 20% of the population each; they may coexist. (Redrawn from Henderson JM. Atlas of liver surgery. In: Bell RH, Rikkers LF, Mulholland MW, eds. *Digestive Tract Surgery: A Text and Atlas*. Philadelphia: Lippincott-Raven; 1995.)

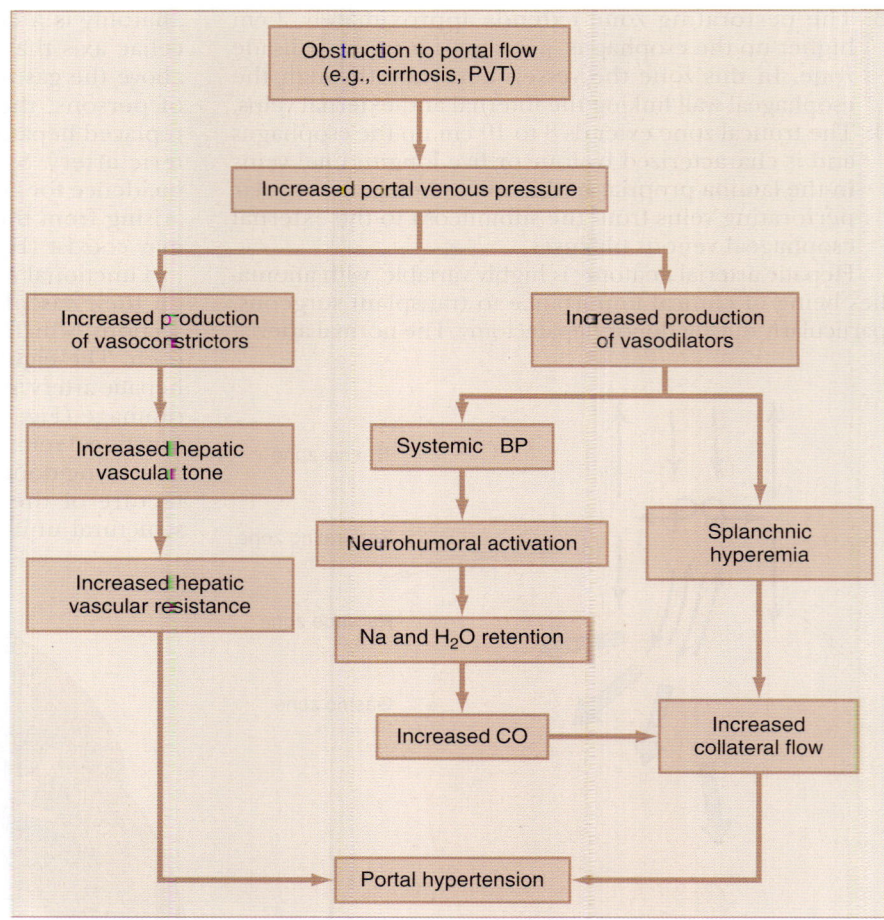

FIGURE 135.5 Pathophysiology of portal hypertension. Complex vascular and neurohumoral responses that affect splanchnic, renal, and peripheral vascular control are shown. *BP*, Blood pressure; *CO*, cardiac output; *PVT*, portal vein thrombosis.

parenchyma are polyhedral structures where the portal venous and hepatic arterial tree terminates. These primary lobules aggregate to form a secondary structure often called the "classical lobule." Blood flow through these structures transverse septum like inflow fronts to pass through sinusoids and eventually drain into central hepatic veins.[15,16]

PATHOPHYSIOLOGY

The hepatic venous pressure gradient (HVPG) is the pressure difference between the portal vein and the vena cava. Portal hypertension is defined by an elevation in the HVPG greater than 6 mm Hg. This gradient can be caused by increased resistance to blood flow in the presinusoidal, sinusoidal, or postsinusoidal portal circulation.[7] As in all venous systems, portal pressure is equivalent to the portal flow × resistance to portal flow. In rare cases, increases in flow in the portal system without concomitant increase in resistance may lead to clinically significant portal hypertension (i.e., splanchnic arteriovenous fistula).

Portal blood flow is determined by vasoconstriction and dilation of the mesenteric and splanchnic arterioles. In healthy individuals, portal flow is responsible for 75% to 80% of the inflow to the liver, with the remainder coming from the hepatic artery. Total flow ranges from 800 to 1200 mL/min, approximately 25% of total cardiac output.[18] Normal portal pressures are in the range of 6

to 10 mm Hg. Regulation of hepatic artery flow can compensate for changes in portal venous flow by intrinsic regulatory system known as the hepatic arterial buffer response.[19]

The changes in portal hypertension occur on this physiologic background. The steps in the development of the pathophysiology of portal hypertension have been carefully elucidated in the past two decades in animal models. Portal hypertension is present when portal pressure exceeds 8 mm Hg, but variceal bleeding rarely occurs until portal pressure exceeds 12 mm Hg. There is a well-defined sequence of events, as follows, that occurs in the pathophysiology of portal hypertension (Fig. 135.5):

- Obstruction to portal venous flow is usually secondary to an intrahepatic block with cirrhosis. However, the inciting event may be one of the other etiologic causes of portal hypertension.
- Functional increase in resistance occurs secondary to activated hepatic stellate cells and myofibroblasts in the fibrous septa of the sinusoid. These represent a potentially reversible component to intrahepatic resistance.
- There is an imbalanced production of vasoconstrictors, such as endothelin, norepinephrine, and angiotensin, with an insufficient release of hepatic vasodilators, such as nitric oxide and prostaglandins.
- Splanchnic vasodilation occurs with increased splanchnic flow aggravating and contributing to the portal

hypertensive syndrome. This is multifactorial, with neurogenic, humoral, and local mediators.

- Portosystemic collaterals develop not only at the gastroesophageal junction but also in the abdominal wall and retroperitoneum.
- There is an increase in plasma volume secondary to the vascular changes.
- A systemic hyperdynamic circulation develops with increased cardiac output, low total systemic vascular resistance, and further aggravation of the splanchnic hyperemia and overall hyperdynamic state.

This sequence of pathophysiologic changes in the hepatic, splanchnic, and finally systemic circulation offers an opportunity for pharmacologic manipulation and management of portal hypertension.

ETIOLOGY OF PORTAL HYPERTENSION

Portal hypertension can be attributed to processes that can be classified as (1) prehepatic, (2) intrahepatic obstruction, and (3) posthepatic venous outflow obstruction. Etiologies found under each category are summarized in Box 135.1.

Prehepatic portal hypertension comprises 5% to 10% of portal hypertension patients in the United States and Europe.[20] In other parts of the world, such as India, this may be the etiology in a higher percentage of portal hypertension patients. Prehepatic portal venous obstruction results from thrombosis, invasion by malignant tumor, or constriction from external surrounding processes. Portal and splenic vein thrombosis is the most common cause of prehepatic portal hypertension. Portal vein thrombosis may be associated with umbilical vein catheterization or other causes of sepsis and dehydration in infancy.[21] In the adult patient the hypercoagulable syndromes should be sought in patients with a newly diagnosed portal or splenic vein thrombosis, with a full hematologic work-up. Other etiologies include pancreatitis and pancreatic tumors, with the later portending a poor prognosis related to the cancer. Prehepatic portal vein thrombosis is typically associated with few downstream signs of liver injury except in preexisting cirrhosis.

Extrinsic pressure on the portal vein from lymph nodes or other tumors can occasionally lead to portal hypertension, but this is unusual because the vein normally passes around surrounding masses. Finally, hepatic artery-to-portal venous fistulas, usually secondary to a liver biopsy, can occur and if large can lead to portal hypertension. Fistulas are diagnosed with radiologic imaging and can usually be managed with endoluminal angiographic techniques for their occlusion.

One important variant of portal hypertension is left-sided (sinistral) portal hypertension with isolated splenic vein thrombosis, a normal portal vein, and no intrahepatic block. The most common causes of this are pancreatitis and carcinoma of the body and tail of the pancreas. This is increasingly recognized on computed tomographic (CT) scan with large collaterals coming from the splenic hilus up to the fundus of the stomach. From a portal hypertension perspective, this is readily handled with splenectomy, but clearly an understanding of the underlying pathology is most important in prognosis.

The intrahepatic causes of portal hypertension account for 90% of the cases in the United States and Europe. Most patients with an intrahepatic block have cirrhosis, which has multiple etiologies. These include alcohol, hepatitis B, hepatitis C, the cholestatic liver diseases (primary sclerosing cholangitis and primary biliary cirrhosis), hemochromatosis, and the other metabolic causes of cirrhosis. Although hepatitis C and alcoholic liver disease account for the majority of cirrhosis in adults, nonalcoholic fatty liver disease is an increasing cause of cirrhosis in the developed world. Portal hypertension due to cirrhosis is thought to be primarily a function of increased hepatic vascular resistance in the hepatic sinusoids due to fibrosis, scarring and distortion of the microvasculature, as well as dysregulation of contractile elements, including hepatic myofibroblasts.[22] In the course of patient evaluation, full definition of the underlying disease is important for management. It is the natural history, activity, and rate of progression of the underlying liver disease that ultimately sets the prognosis.

Schistosomiasis is still an important cause of portal hypertension on a worldwide basis. Still seen in the Middle and Far East and in South America, the pathologic block in schistosomiasis is fibrosis of the terminal portal venules. Although it is an intrahepatic disease process, presinusoidal obstruction of the terminal portal venous branches is balanced by an increase in hepatic arterial inflow. Lobular architecture is preserved and total hepatic inflow is typically normal. Prototypical Symmers clay pipestem fibrosis is present in all patients.[23] In addition, many patients with schistosomiasis may also have hepatitis as a concomitant disease with implications of liver function impairment.

Congenital hepatic fibrosis is a relatively rare cause of an intrahepatic block in the United States and Europe, but it is important to recognize because it is usually associated with preserved liver function. However, more recently there have been reports of progression of congenital hepatic fibrosis to end-stage liver disease requiring liver transplantation. A similar entity is seen in India as noncirrhotic portal fibrosis, which is a cause for portal hypertension in that country.[24] The implication of preserved liver function is that there is a broader range of options for treatment, particularly for variceal bleeding.

BOX 135.1 Etiology of Portal Hypertension

PREHEPATIC
Portal or splenic vein thrombosis
Extrinsic portal vein compression
Arteriovenous fistula

INTRAHEPATIC
Cirrhosis: multiple etiologies
Schistosomiasis
Congenital hepatic fibrosis
Rare causes

POSTHEPATIC
Budd-Chiari syndrome
Constrictive pericarditis

Portal hypertension due to posthepatic venous outflow obstruction is occasionally due to constrictive pericarditis. It is much more commonly attributed to a broad category of Budd-Chiari syndrome[25] and the occasional patient with a constrictive pericarditis. Classic Budd-Chiari syndrome involves thrombosis of the main hepatic veins, but other etiologies, such as inferior vena cava (IVC) webs, may cause this syndrome. The outflow block leads to an increase in sinusoidal pressure, centrilobular hepatocyte injury, and ultimately fibrosis, scarring, and cirrhosis. These are exceedingly rare syndromes, accounting for 1% to 2% of the cases of portal hypertension.

CLINICAL MANIFESTATION OF PORTAL HYPERTENSION

VARICEAL BLEEDING

Esophagogastric varices occur with an incidence of 8% to 11% a year in the cirrhotic patient. Once present, progression of small varices to larger varices and the propensity for those varices to bleed varies widely between studies.[26] Upper gastrointestinal (GI) bleeding from varices is one of the most common and life-threatening complications of portal hypertension. One-third to half of cirrhotic patients will develop varices, and one-third of those patients will develop a clinically significant variceal bleed. Risk of bleeding increases as variceal size increases, and survival is proportional to the severity of underlying liver disease. Despite advances in therapy, mortality from acute variceal hemorrhage is still as high as 15% to 20%.

All patients with documented or suspected cirrhosis should have an upper endoscopy to document whether or not they have varices. Due to the natural history of varices and morbidity of variceal hemorrhage, surveillance of esophageal varices is recommended every 2 to 3 years and every 1 to 2 years in patients with small esophageal varices and compensated liver disease. In the presence of decompensated liver disease, upper endoscopy should be performed annually.[27]

ASCITES

Accumulation of ascites is considered a late sign of portal hypertension, occurring later in the natural history than compared with varices.[28] When unresponsive to simple treatment with diuretics and salt restriction, refractory ascites is a sign of decompensation of the underlying liver disease. Due to its appearance along with advanced liver disease, the presence of ascites is associated with renal dysfunction. In addition, patients developing spontaneous bacterial peritonitis (SBP) portend a poor prognosis, with a 1-year mortality rate between 50% and 70%.[29]

LIVER FAILURE AND ENCEPHALOPATHY

Complications of portal hypertension are commonly caused by progressive underlying liver disease. Recurring encephalopathy due to liver failure, termed hepatic encephalopathy, presents with a spectrum of symptoms ranging from cognitive changes, loss of coordination, and asterixis, to coma. One-year survival following overt signs of hepatic encephalopathy is 43% and has remained largely unchanged in the past several decades. Clinically significant encephalopathy will prompt evaluation for liver transplant as treatment options are limited after this clinical presentation occurs.

HEPATOCELLULAR CARCINOMA

The incidence of hepatocellular carcinoma (HCC) is a clinically significant factor in the manifestation of portal hypertension. This is largely due to the high prevalence of hepatitis C in cirrhosis but can occur in long-standing liver disease of any etiology, with an annual incidence of 3%.[30] HCC in the setting of cirrhosis must be followed with serial imaging and α-fetoprotein measurement. Patients presenting with HCC must be managed with respect to the malignancy, as well as the remaining liver function. Transplantation should be considered for carefully selected patients who are otherwise not candidates for resection, either due to tumor characteristics or underlying liver disease. Liver transplantation remains the best option for long-term survival for patients with HCC.

PORTOPULMONARY SYNDROME

The triad of liver disease, arterial hypoxemia, and intrapulmonary vascular dilation is defined as the HPS. There are two broad groups of patients: (1) those with HPS that is marked by hypoxemia secondary to intrapulmonary shunting in patients with chronic liver disease, in the absence of pulmonary hypertension, and (2) patients with pulmonary hypertension and chronic underlying liver disease who have a more sinister syndrome with a poor prognosis. Medical treatment options have had limited success and transplantation is indicated in these patients, especially in the pediatric population.[31]

WORK-UP

The work-up of patients presenting with portal hypertension requires a multidisciplinary approach. The diagnostic and prognostic priorities will vary for each patient based on the etiology, presentation, and severity of disease. The essential components of such evaluation are summarized in Box 135.2.

Radiologic and endoscopic evaluation are the first-line modalities in most circumstances. Upper GI endoscopy plays a principle role because evaluation of presence and severity of esophagogastric varices is often the most serious complication of portal hypertension. Endoscopy allows for identification of risk factors for variceal bleeding and provides immediate therapy of at-risk variceal columns. Portal gastropathy can also be identified on upper GI endoscopy. Increased variceal diameter and thin variceal wall thickness indicated by a red color sign are predictive of variceal bleeding due to increased wall tension in these vessels. Grading systems for esophageal varices and portal gastropathy are critical to standardizing prognosis and treatment in these patients.[32,33]

Radiologic evaluation of the portal venous system is the next important step. Doppler ultrasonography is used to visualize the size and flow through the portal vein and its tributaries. Patency and wave-flow patterns through hepatic veins can also be assessed.[34] Ultrasound is a useful screening modality for defining liver morphology in the case of cirrhosis or focal lesions.

BOX 135.2 Evaluation of Patients With Portal Hypertension

ENDOSCOPY
Size of varices
Extent of varices
Risk factor, red-color signs
Portal gastropathy

IMAGING
Doppler ultrasound
CT scan
HVPG and imaging
Angiography

LIVER FUNCTION
Clinical: ascites, encephalopathy, jaundice, muscle wasting
Laboratory data
Child score
MELD score

CT, Computed tomography; *HVPG*, hepatic venous pressure gradient; *MELD*, model for end-stage liver disease.

BOX 135.3 Model for End-Stage Liver Disease Score for Liver Disease Severity

$$\text{Score} = 0.957 \times \log_e \text{creatinine (mg/dL)}$$
$$+ 0.378 \times \log_e \text{bilirubin (mg/dL)} + 1.120 \log_e \text{INR}$$

TABLE 135.1 Child-Pugh Grading of Severity of Liver Disease*

Clinical and Laboratory Measurement	PATIENT SCORE FOR INCREASING ABNORMALITY		
	1	2	3
Encephalopathy (grade)	None	1 or 2	3 or 4
Ascites	None	Mild	Moderate
Bilirubin (mg/dL)	1–2	2.1–3	≥3.1
Albumin (g/dL)	≥3.5	2.8–3.5	≤2.7
Prothrombin time (increase, seconds)	1–4	4–6	≥6.1

*Grade A, 5–6 points; grade B, 7–9 points; grade C, 10–15 points.

Axial imaging of the liver by CT or magnetic resonance (MR) imaging is commonly performed. Morphologic assessment of liver parenchyma as well as liver tumors is easily done through both modalities. CT and MR angiography have also become sophisticated enough to evaluate arterial and venous flow to the liver and replace the need for visceral angiography in many settings.

Hepatic venous pressures measured via transhepatic or transvenous catheterization of the hepatic veins is the gold standard of diagnosing portal hypertension. The wedge hepatic venous pressure (WHVP) is measured by use of a balloon catheter, creating a static column of fluid that transmits pressure data from the hepatic sinusoids. In most cases of cirrhotic liver failure intersinusoidal connections are obliterated and sinusoidal pressure equilibrates with portal pressure. Free hepatic venous pressure (FHVP) is subtracted from the WHVP to reveal the HVPG. Increasing emphasis is being placed on the value of this measurement in the era of more sophisticated pharmacologic therapies. A therapeutic response reducing the HVPG to less than 10 mm Hg or less will dramatically reduce the risk of variceal bleeding.

Patients with suspicion of portal hypertension will require an assessment of liver function via clinical and laboratory evaluation. The important parts in clinical assessment of liver function are the detection of ascites, evaluation for encephalopathy, detection of clinical jaundice, and assessment of muscle wasting. All of these clinical signs are indications of advanced liver disease.

Laboratory data that are important are those that directly assess liver status: bilirubin, albumin, prothrombin time, aspartate aminotransferase, alanine transaminase, and alkaline phosphatase. In addition, hematologic parameters (i.e., hemoglobin, platelet count, and white blood cell count) may be affected by portal hypertension. A platelet count less than 100,000 is indicative of significant portal hypertension. A prothrombin time international normalized ratio (INR) of 1.5 indicates poor liver function. All patients should have checks made of specific liver

disease markers, including hepatitis panels, antinuclear antibody, antimitochondrial antibody, and metabolic disease markers for iron, copper, and alpha1-antitrypsin. Finally, hepatoma risk can be assessed with α-fetoprotein.

Calculation of prognostic indices is important when developing a treatment algorithm for patients with portal hypertension. The Child-Pugh score (Table 135.1)[35] and the model for end-stage liver disease (MELD) score (Box 135.3)[36] are used to assess severity of liver dysfunction.

MANAGEMENT OF VARICEAL BLEEDING

PRIMARY PROPHYLAXIS

The past half century has seen a shift in the treatment paradigm of esophageal varices from expectant management to screening, pharmacologic, and endoscopic prophylaxis. All patients with signs of cirrhosis should be screened for esophageal varices at time of diagnosis and every 2 to 3 years thereafter. After small varices develop or liver disease progresses to Child class B or beyond, the screening frequency should be increased to yearly intervals. Efforts to prevent or delay the first episode of variceal hemorrhage are followed by pharmacologic therapy to reduce the rate of rebleeding.

Small varices detected on endoscopic surveillance require no intervention and can be followed up with annual upper endoscopy. Moderate (5 to 10 mm) to large (>10 mm) varices or presence other risk factors (i.e., red-color sign, Child class C cirrhosis), the risk of variceal rupture and hemorrhage requires prophylactic pharmacologic intervention. First-line therapy with nonselective β-blockers (propranolol, nadolol) has decreased the rate of variceal bleeding from 30% to 14%. Nonselective β-blockers reduce portal pressure by β2-receptor antagonism, increasing splanchnic vasoconstriction and decreasing portal blood flow. Carvedilol has been shown to be more effective in reducing HVPG due to additional α1-receptor antagonist activity and can be used in

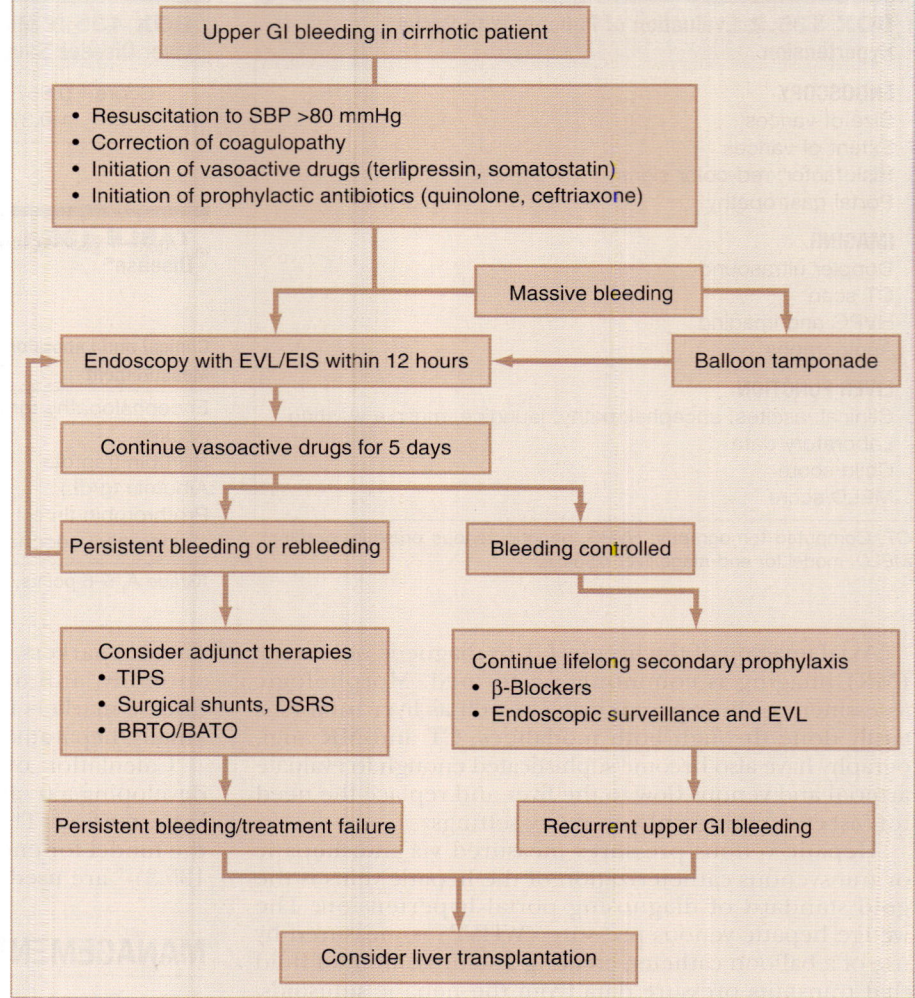

FIGURE 135.6 Algorithm for prevention of recurrent variceal bleeding. Primary therapy for all patients is with β-blockers and banding. Secondary therapy may be variceal decompression for recurrent bleeding or transplant for advanced disease and recurrent bleeding. *BATO*, Balloon-occluded antegrade obliteration; *BRTO*, balloon-occluded retrograde obliteration; *DSRS*, distal splenorenal shunt; *EIS*, endoscopic injection sclerotherapy; *EVL*, endoscopic variceal ligation; *GI*, gastrointestinal; *SBP*, systolic blood pressure; *TIPS*, transjugular intrahepatic portosystemic shunt.

Within the figure:

- Upper GI bleeding in cirrhotic patient
- Resuscitation to SBP >80 mmHg
- Correction of coagulopathy
- Initiation of vasoactive drugs (terlipressin, somatostatin)
- Initiation of prophylactic antibiotics (quinolone, ceftriaxone)
- Massive bleeding
- Endoscopy with EVL/EIS within 12 hours
- Balloon tamponade
- Continue vasoactive drugs for 5 days
- Persistent bleeding or rebleeding
- Bleeding controlled
- Consider adjunct therapies
  - TIPS
  - Surgical shunts, DSRS
  - BRTO/BATO
- Continue lifelong secondary prophylaxis
  - β-Blockers
  - Endoscopic surveillance and EVL
- Persistent bleeding/treatment failure
- Recurrent upper GI bleeding
- Consider liver transplantation

propranolol nonresponders.[37] Endoscopic band ligation should be used as primary prophylaxis of variceal bleeding in nonselective β-blockers (NSBB) nonresponders. NSBB can be used to slow progression of small varices, but the long-term benefits are unclear.[38]

ACUTE VARICEAL BLEEDING

Initial measures in the management of patients once variceal bleeding is suspected include airway protection, hemodynamic stabilization, pharmacologic therapy, and balloon tamponade. Stabilization measures bridge these patients to definitive control of bleeding, usually by means of endoscopic ligation. Efforts are taken to reduce the substantial risk of rebleeding because this recurrent variceal hemorrhage occurs in 50% to 80% of survivors. An overview of the treatment of acute variceal bleeding is diagrammed in Fig. 135.6.

PHARMACOLOGIC INTERVENTION

Initial pharmacologic therapy consists of intravenous infusion of a somatostatin analogue and vasoconstrictive therapy.[38] NSBB should be discontinued when clinically significant bleeding is encountered. Somatostatin and its analogues are effective in variceal hemorrhage due to

their ability to cause splanchnic vasoconstriction and inhibition of glucagon. Octreotide is administered as a bolus of 50 μg followed by a continuous infusion of 50 μg per hour. This infusion is continued for 5 days or longer, although tachyphylaxis may decrease its efficacy in controlling hemorrhage.[27]

Vasoconstrictive agents, including vasopressin and terlipressin, have been studied as an adjunct therapy for acute variceal bleeding. These agents are potent splanchnic vasoconstrictors but are associated with significant side effects, including cardiac arrhythmias, hypertension, and bowel ischemia. In a meta-analysis, the efficacy of octreotide and vasopressin do not reduce the mortality following variceal hemorrhage but did reduce the rate of rebleeding from 32% to 19%.[39]

RESUSCITATION

Severe variceal bleeding frequently requires volume and blood product resuscitation. This is best done in an intensive care setting with continuous hemodynamic monitoring. Data regarding resuscitation strategies during variceal bleeding are limited, and resuscitation is frequently complicated by decompensation of underlying liver disease and inability of these patients to tolerate volume shifts and susceptibility to dilutional coagulopathy. Patients with active variceal bleeding may benefit from conservative volume resuscitation due to increased risk for recurrent bleeding when splanchnic venous volume is overexpanded. A restrictive blood transfusion strategy with hemoglobin thresholds of 8 g/dL or hematocrit of 24% is recommended.[40]

The utility of standard coagulation assays, including prothrombin and partial thromboplastin is limited in the context of significant underlying hepatic dysfunction. Evaluation of coagulation in cirrhotic patients demonstrates a rebalanced hemostasis in some patients despite thrombocytopenia and elevated prothrombin time/INR. Platelet aggregation studies and thromboelastography (TEG) can be used to guide correction of coagulopathy in the face of hemorrhage and chronic liver dysfunction.[41]

BALLOON TAMPONADE

In up to 15% of patients, bleeding continues despite initial maneuvers; balloon tamponade with a Blakemore tube may be necessary to stabilize the patient as a bridge to portal decompression. The high rate of complication mandates a knowledgeable team and careful protocols prior to its use. Patients requiring balloon tamponade should have endotracheal intubation for control of their airway. The tube can be passed either through the nose or the mouth. The position of the gastric balloon in the stomach should be confirmed with a radiograph after inflating it with 25 to 30 mL of air. After the position is confirmed, the gastric balloon is inflated to approximately 200 mL and brought up snugly in the gastric fundus. Occasionally, the esophageal balloon may need to be inflated to 40 mm Hg (monitored through a pressure cuff), but usually this is not required. After being deployed, it is mandatory that measures to decompress varices be undertaken within 24 hours of tamponade.

ENDOSCOPY

Upper endoscopy is the mainstay of diagnosis and treatment in the face of acute variceal bleeding. The technique of endoscopic band ligation was first proposed by Stiegmann[9] in 1988 and has largely replaced endoscopic injection sclerotherapy as the preferred endoscopic intervention. In large studies, variceal ligation has achieved similar degrees of primary hemostasis compared with endoscopic injection sclerotherapy with lower rates of rebleeding. Mortality in Child class A and B patients is decreased with the use of variceal ligation compared with injection sclerotherapy.[8,43] Repeat sessions 7 to 10 days after initial therapy are also recommended with variceal ligation; however, complete variceal obliteration is achieved in fewer sessions with ligation as compared with sclerotherapy. Evidence supports the use of combined endoscopic and pharmacologic therapy to reduce rebleeding rates.[44]

BALLOON-OCCLUDED OBLITERATION OF VARICES

Twenty percent to 30% of variceal bleeding presents with gastric varices, which may not be amenable to endoscopic therapy. Gastric varices related to portal hypertension are often associated with compensatory gastrorenal (Fig. 135.7) or gastrocaval shunts, which are less amenable to

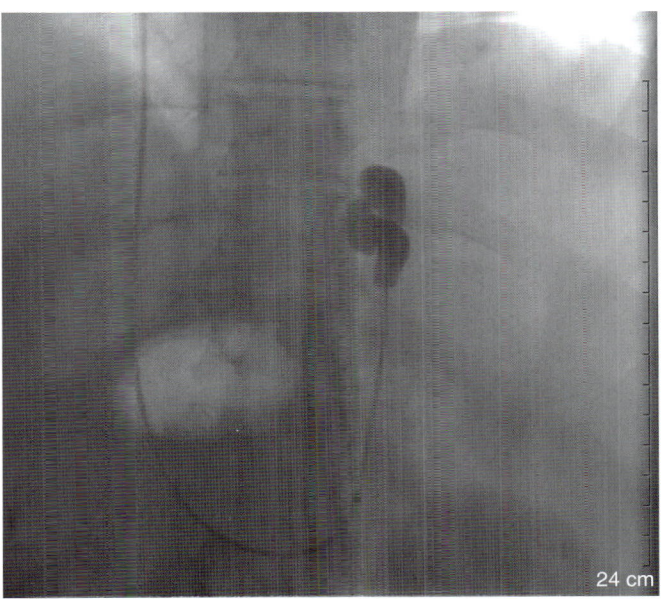

24 cm

FIGURE 35.7 Spontaneous gastrorenal shunt accessed through the left renal vein commonly associated with bleeding gastric varices.

portal decompression (discussed in the next section). Balloon-occluded endovascular techniques, first reported by Kanagawa in 1996, can be a helpful adjunct approach to these varices.

Balloon-occluded retrograde obliteration (BRTO) or balloon-occluded antegrade obliteration (BATO) of varices is dependent on the vascular anatomy in relation to the problematic varices. Balloon catheters are introduced via the femoral or internal jugular approach. Gastrorenal shunts are commonly accessed via the left renal vein; however, the vascular anatomy is highly variable. Technical success rates of BRTO/BATO in appropriately selected patients is 84% to 100%.[45] Full occlusion of the shunt is critical to the delivery of high concentrations of sclerosing agent and obliteration of the varices, and the use of coil embolization in conjunction with sclerosing agents is preferred in some centers (Fig. 135.8). Variceal drainage into one or two distinct shunts is most amenable to successful balloon-occluded endovascular obliteration.

DECOMPRESSION OF VARICES

The current recommendations for variceal decompression are to use either TIPS or a surgical shunt. It is only approximately 10% to 15% of patients with variceal bleeding who will need this level of treatment.

TRANSJUGULAR INTRAHEPATIC PORTOSYSTEMIC SHUNT

Intrahepatic portosystemic shunting has been used for three decades for decompression of portal hypertension in the treatment of variceal bleeding, as well as refractory ascites.[46,47] Early experience showed that new onset or worsening encephalopathy, right heart failure, and

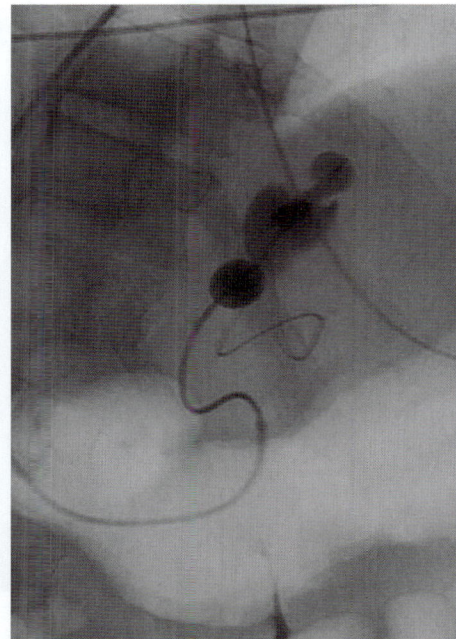
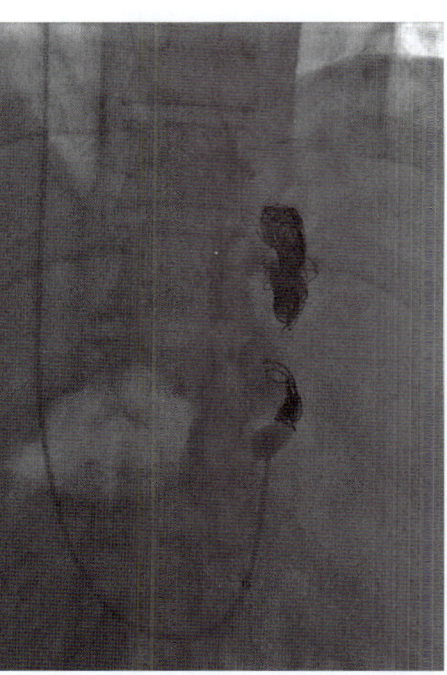

FIGURE 135.8 Gastric varices selected in a retrograde fashion from the left renal vein via a gastro/splenorenal shunt *(left)*. Ablation and coil embolization performed under fluoroscopic guidance *(right)*.

BOX 135.4 Contraindications to Transjugular Intrahepatic Portosystemic Shunting Procedure

ABSOLUTE CONTRAINDICATIONS
Primary prevention of variceal bleeding
Congestive heart failure
Severe pulmonary hypertension
Multiple hepatic cysts
Active infections or sepsis
Unrelieved biliary obstruction

RELATIVE CONTRAINDICATIONS
Single hepatic cyst or central hepatoma
Hepatic vein thrombosis
Portal vein thrombosis
Severe coagulopathy or thrombocytopenia
Moderate pulmonary hypertension

---

restenosis were common. Patients being considered for TIPS must be evaluated for cardiopulmonary function, portal vein patency, and assessment of liver function. Consultation for potential transplantation should be obtained in high-risk patients. A list of absolute and relative contraindications for TIPS is given in Box 135.4.

TRANSJUGULAR INTRAHEPATIC PORTOSYSTEMIC SHUNT: THE PROCEDURE

TIPS is usually placed via a right transjugular route to the right or middle hepatic vein (Fig. 135.9), but any hepatic vein can be used and the choice is dictated by liver morphology. Direct access from the IVC to the portal vein has been used in some cases of Budd-Chiari syndrome. Next, the hepatic parenchyma is traversed with a needle to puncture the portal vein; ultrasound guidance can be used, but experienced interventional radiologists can usually access the portal vein readily. It is important to enter the right or left portal vein within the liver cephalad to the bifurcation that sits outside the liver—puncture and dilation of the tract at the bifurcation can result in a major intraabdominal bleed. A catheter is placed over a guidewire into the portal vein, pressure is measured, and a portogram contrast study performed. The transparenchymal tract is dilated, and the stent(s) placed to keep the tract open. The stent is dilated to reduce the portal-to-right atrial gradient to equal 10 mm Hg. Stent placement is important: not too low into the portal vein and not too high into the suprahepatic IVC, both of which can create technical problems if subsequent transplant is needed. However, the tract must be adequately stented because the most common site for subsequent stenosis is the hepatic vein end of the stent. Covered stents require more fastidious placement to be sure the covered components do not protrude into the portal vein or IVC. Covered stents have a short uncovered segment at the end. A completion study should document patency and appropriate pressure gradient reduction (to ≤10 mm Hg).

Follow-up requires careful monitoring, but recent patency rates are excellent, with 1 year patency around 90%. Doppler ultrasound is adequate for screening and documenting total thrombosis. Covered stents do not transmit the Doppler signal for several days, so initial evaluation should be 3 to 4 days after the procedure. Ultrasound does not always document stenosis, which requires stent recatheterization and pressure measurement and possibly imaging. Gradients greater than 12 mm Hg or stenosis greater than 50% require dilation. Additional stents may be required if the stenosis is refractory to dilation or occurs at either end of the initial stents(s). The necessary frequency of recatheterization is undefined:

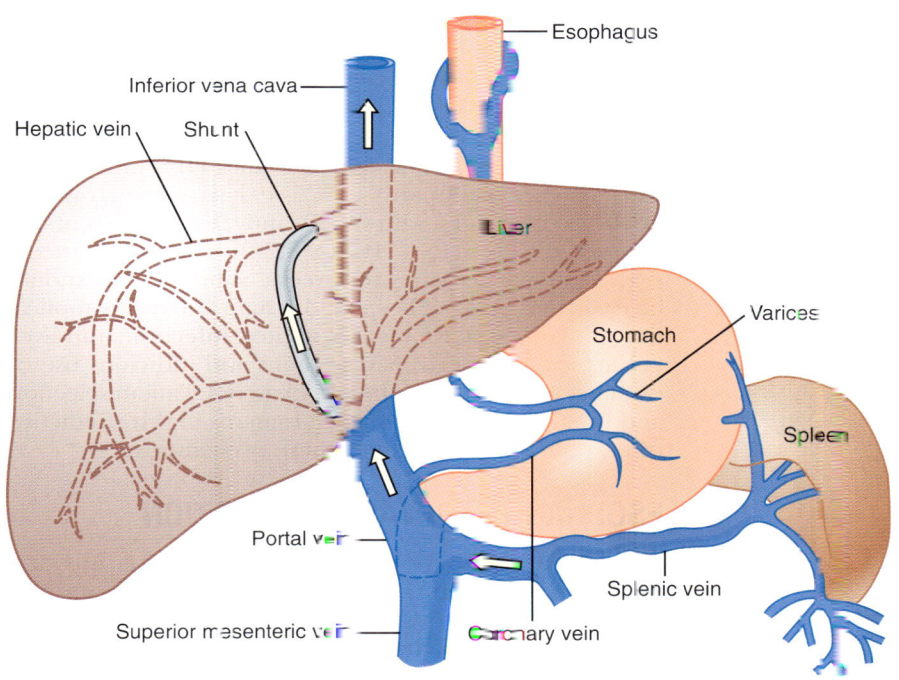

FIGURE 135.9 Transjugular intrahepatic portosystemic shunt is diagrammatically illustrated. The stent is placed between the hepatic vein and the portal vein, dilated to 10 to 12 mm, and the portal-to-right atrial pressure gradient is reduced to less than 10 mm Hg. (From Henderson JM. Portal hypertension. In: Corson JD, Williamson R, eds. *Surgery*. London: Mosby; 2001.)

current indications are when Doppler ultrasound studies change—increased or decreased velocities.

TRANSJUGULAR INTRAHEPATIC PORTOSYSTEMIC SHUNT: OUTCOMES

In large series, complications are as low as 1.4% to 3% and include intraabdominal hemorrhage, right heart failure, and progression of liver disease due to portal diversion. Technical success of TIPS to decrease portal pressure less than 12 mm Hg is achieved in 95% of cases, and clinical resolution of bleeding is achieved in 90% of cases.[48] Results for refractory ascites are less clear. Rebleeding rates following TIPS are in the 11% to 15% range, and long-term restenosis rates have improved as newer covered stents replaced original bare metal stents. One-year survival rates following TIPS procedure vary from 48% to 90%. Improvement in stent patency of as much as 15% following TIPS is seen with the use of covered stents.[49]

SURGICAL SHUNTS

Surgical decompression of portal hypertension in animal models was described by Nikolai Eck in the late 1800s. Eck's early experiments described a large (>15 mm) side-to-side anastomosis of the portal vein to the vena cava, followed by ligation of the distal portal vein before it divides and enters the liver. In 1903 Vidal reported the first Eck fistula in human patients. Central surgical shunts were not popularized until the 1940s when Whipple, Blakemore, and colleagues at the Presbyterian Hospital in New York successfully used central shunts in the treatment of variceal bleeding.[3,50] Although there was much enthusiasm for this mode of therapy, initial success was limited by chronic or recurrent encephalopathy and high rates of hepatic failure.[50] Prophylactic surgical shunts were abandoned for portal hypertension without variceal bleeding but

remained the only effective therapy in the face of active variceal hemorrhage until the introduction of endoscopic interventions. Even nowadays, portosystemic surgical shunts remain a viable option for long-term bridge to transplant in carefully selected patients with preservation of hepatic reserve and for those who fail medical management.[51]

Surgical shunts fall into three broad categories: total, partial, and selective shunts. Complete or near-complete diversion of the portal flow to the vena cava via portacaval, mesocaval, or proximal splenorenal shunts are generally avoided due to the high rates of encephalopathy and liver failure with these total shunts. Partial shunts, including small-diameter shunts, H-shunts, and graft shunts, maintain a portion of portal flow to the liver and have been used successfully by some groups with rebleeding rates in the 5% to 10% range. Because some portal perfusion is preserved, encephalopathy rates are lower with partial shunts than total shunts. Due to the smaller diameter and higher resistance through partial shunts, shunt thrombosis occurs in up to 23% of cases.[52] Selective shunts, accomplished by DSRSs, are currently the most common method of surgical decompression. Selective shunts selectively decompress gastroesophageal varices while maintaining portal pressures in the splanchnic-to-portal axis, thereby maintaining portal flow. Selective shunts remain the most widely used surgical shunts at the present time.

DISTAL SPLENORENAL SHUNT: THE PROCEDURE

DSRS is performed through a long left subcostal incision carried across the midline to the right rectus muscle (Fig. 135.10). Exposure of the splenic and left renal veins is key. Access to the pancreas is obtained through the lesser sac, taking down the gastroepiploic vessels from the pylorus to the short gastric veins—this also serves as part of the portal/azygos disconnection. In addition, the splenic flexure of the colon should be taken down from the

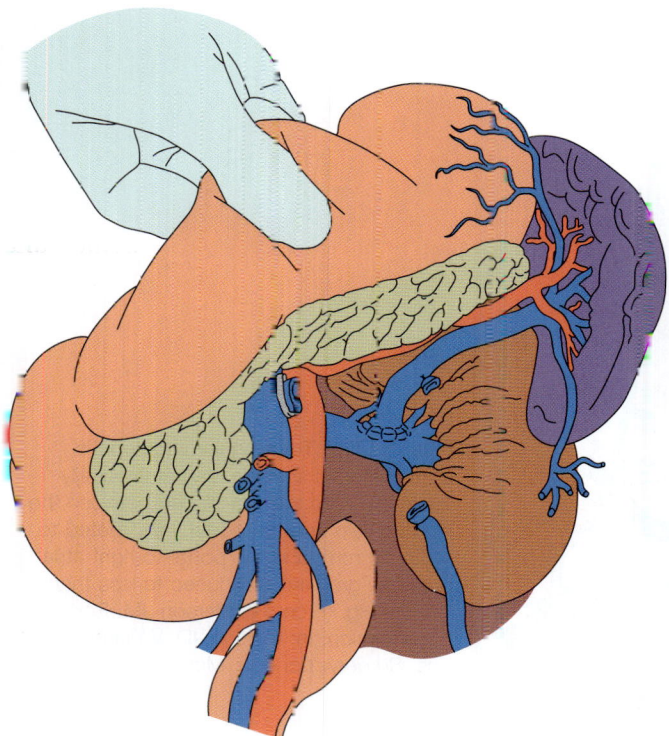

FIGURE 135.10 Distal splenorenal shunt selectively decompresses gastroesophageal varices through the spleen and splenic vein to the left renal vein. Portal hypertension and porta perfusion of the liver are maintained in the superior mesenteric and portal veins.

spleen—this both improves access to the posterior surface of the pancreas and interrupts potential collaterals to the shunt. The pancreas is fully mobilized along its inferior margin from the superior mesenteric vein to the splenic hilus—it is turned cephalad to expose its posterior surface and the splenic vein. Dissection of the splenic vein from the pancreas is done from the superior mesenteric vein over sufficient distance to mobilize enough vein to come down to the left renal vein without kinking. The posteroinferior surface is cleared first, then the small draining tributaries from the pancreas are isolated and ligated. The left renal vein is then identified in the retroperitoneum—a move made easier by preoperative venographic imaging. The left renal vein is mobilized with the left adrenal vein ligated and the gonadal vein left intact. This mobilization must be sufficient to allow the vein to come up into a side-biting clamp. The splenic vein is then divided at the splenic–superior mesenteric–portal junction and brought down for end-to-side anastomosis to the renal vein. We recommend interrupted sutures to the anterior row of the anastomosis to avoid purse-stringing. The shunt is opened, and the spleen can be seen to decompress. The operation is completed with further portal/azygos dissection mainly by interrupting the left gastric vein both at the portal vein and above the pancreas.

DISTAL SPLENORENAL SHUNT: OUTCOMES

Several uncontrolled series of DSRS in the 1990s to early 2000s showed rebleeding rates of 5% to 6%,

encephalopathy rates around 15%, and 1- and 3-year survival rates of 85% and 75%, respectively, in good-risk Child class A and B patients.[51,53,54] Controlled studies of Child class A and B patients with varices refractory to endoscopic and pharmacologic therapy showed similar rebleeding rates following DSRS and TIPS with similar rates of encephalopathy and 5-year survival. However, DSRS was associated with significantly fewer interventions compared with TIPS (11% vs. 82%). Complete variceal regression may require 4 to 8 weeks. Shunt patency should be evaluated prior to hospital discharge. Major complications following DSRS include ascites, infection, and liver failure. Careful fluid management and judicious use of diuretics may minimize the risk of ascites. Patient selection and liver status at presentation remains highly predictive of mortality following all of these procedures.

ESOPHAGEAL DEVASCULARIZATION

Esophageal transection and devascularization was first introduced by Sugiura and Futagawa to control variceal bleeding in 1973.[56] Sugiura originally described extensive paraesophagogastric devascularization with distal esophageal transection, splenectomy, vagotomy and pyloroplasty, often performed in separate thoracic and abdominal stages. Compared with portosystemic shunting procedures, esophageal devascularization successfully controls esophagogastric variceal disease without the increased risk of encephalopathy or reducing flow to the liver.[55]

OPERATIVE TECHNIQUE

The originally described technique included a left lateral thoracotomy, as well as an abdominal incision. The inferior mediastinum is entered through the sixth intercostal space, and the thoracic esophagus is devascularized from the esophageal hiatus to the inferior pulmonary vein. The esophagus is then clamped and the anterior muscular wall, circumferential submucosa, and mucosa are transected, dividing veins in the submucosa. A two-layer anastomosis is performed.

The abdominal portion is performed as a separate operation in high-risk patients. From an upper midline incision, devascularization of the abdominal esophagus is performed and continued through the proximal 7 cm of the lesser curve. A splenectomy, vagotomy, and pyloroplasty are performed. Meticulous disruption of paraesophageal collaterals to the azygous system was emphasized by Sugiura in preventing recurrence and bleeding. Since that time, modifications to the Sugiura procedure included single-incision operations through abdominal, thoracic, or abdominothoracic incisions; preservation of the vagus; use of mechanical staplers; and devascularization without esophageal transection.

ESOPHAGEAL DEVASCULARIZATION: OUTCOMES

Although initial reports from Japan are excellent, these results have not been reproducible in the United States and Europe. Perioperative mortality in emergent settings are in excess of 21% with esophageal transection alone. This increases to 57% to 100% in Child class C cirrhotic patients. In nonemergent settings, operative mortality is 0% to 22%. Relatively poor outcomes in Western nations may be attributed to the high rate of alcoholic cirrhosis compared with schistosomiasis and portal venous thrombosis. Significant complications following esophageal devascularization include bleeding, hepatic failure, anastomotic leak, and esophageal stricture.

Current indications for esophageal devascularization are limited to rescue therapy in patients who are not candidates for selective shunting or TIPS. Patients with end-stage liver disease who do not meet criteria for transplantation may also benefit from devascularization.

ASCITES

Ascites is the most common complication of cirrhosis, with approximately two-thirds of patients with compensated cirrhosis developing ascites within 10 years. After a patient with cirrhosis develops ascites, particularly as it becomes increasingly difficult to manage, there is an approximately 50% mortality over the next 3 years without liver transplantation.

PATHOPHYSIOLOGY

Ascites develops in patients with cirrhosis because of overall hemodynamic changes, vasoconstrictor and sodium-retaining systems being triggered in the kidneys, with the accompanying renal dysfunction. As indicated earlier in this chapter, one of the early vascular responses to portal hypertension is marked arterial vasodilation of the splanchnic circulation. This in turn leads to a hyperdynamic systemic circulation, decreased systemic vascular resistance, and lowered blood pressure. This in turn activates the vasoconstrictor and antinatriuretic systems that affect the kidneys, with sodium and water retention and renal vasoconstriction. The inability of the kidneys to excrete sodium is thus the first event, with water retention subsequently leading to dilutional hyponatremia. This gives the deceptive laboratory picture of low serum sodium yet high total body sodium.

A second pathologic factor in the development of ascites is the hepatic sinusoidal change. Cirrhosis results in high intrasinusoidal pressure and further damage to the already discontinuous endothelium of the sinusoid. This high pressure leads to excess fluid filtration through the sinusoid, and much of the ascitic fluid forms from the liver surface.

DIAGNOSIS

Ascites of as low as 100 mL can be seen on ultrasound and cross-sectional imaging in many cirrhotic patients. A clinical diagnosis of ascites should be made on physical exam, often appearing with unexpected weight gain, peripheral edema, and abdominal distention demonstrable by fluid wave on exam.

A diagnostic paracentesis should be performed on all patients with cirrhosis when they first present with ascites. This is done to characterize the ascites and to exclude the diagnosis of SBP, the most lethal complication of cirrhotic ascites. The fluid (30 to 50 mL) should be sent for cytologic examination, albumin concentration, total protein content, white blood cell counts, and differential and bacterial culture. Ascites total protein level of less than 2.5 g/dL with a serum ascites albumin gradient greater than 1.1 is highly indicative of ascites being of cirrhotic origin. In malignant ascites the total protein content is usually greater than 2.5 g/dL and the serum/ascites albumin gradient is less than 1.1. The white blood cell count is important in differentiating SBP, with a count of $500/mm^3$ being diagnostic and the 250 to $500/mm^3$ range being highly suspicious. Samples for culture should be placed in blood culture bottles with both aerobic and anaerobic media. The minimum amount of ascitic fluid in these bottles should be 10 mL.

MANAGEMENT

The management of ascites in cirrhosis is diagrammed in Fig. 135.11. Initial management of patients with ascites includes dietary modification and diuretics to reduce sodium intake and retention. Low-sodium diets limited to 2 g of sodium daily are recommended. Water restriction is not typically required unless significant hyponatremia results. Hyperaldosteronemia is a major factor in sodium retention, and aldosterone antagonists have proven effective at management of ascites. Spironolactone at an initial dose of 100 mg/day and titrated to a maximum of 400 mg/day is the treatment of choice. Aldosterone antagonists act at the sodium-potassium pumps of the renal distal tubules. Effective antagonism by spironolactone can be confirmed by urinary excretion of sodium greater than urinary excretion of potassium. Some patients develop significant gynecomastia with spironolactone, and in such patients amiloride is an alternative, starting at 5 mg/day and titrating up to 25 mg/day.

A loop diuretic, such as furosemide, may be added to the spironolactone. Furosemide has a quick onset of action (within the first hour of administration) and is given only if the spironolactone is ineffective. Started at 40 mg/day it may be increased up to 160 mg/day. Although spironolactone retains potassium, furosemide will promote potassium loss. A combination of aldosterone antagonist and loop diuretic is optimal, but there is no consensus as to the exact ratio of one to the other.

REFRACTORY ASCITES

Ascites that is not responsive to maximal dietary modification and pharmacologic therapy is termed refractory and requires more aggressive measures. Approximately 10% of patients will be unresponsive to medical management and require additional therapy, including large volume paracentesis, TIPS, or transplantation for refractory ascites.

Removal of 4 to 6 L of ascitic fluid during paracentesis is occasionally necessary. Circulatory dysfunction due to volume shifts can be minimized by concomitant infusion of albumin if necessary. This can be assessed on a case-by-case basis. The major limitation of large-volume paracentesis as a treatment for refractory ascites is the frequency at which ascites will reaccumulate. As frequently as once a month may be required in some patients, although more frequent paracentesis warrants further intervention.

Surgical shunts and TIPS are able to decrease intrahepatic sinusoidal pressure and reduce HVPG to less than 10 mm Hg.[7] Return of hyperdynamic splanchnic blood flow to the systemic circulation can maintain effective blood volume and renal perfusion. Several randomized

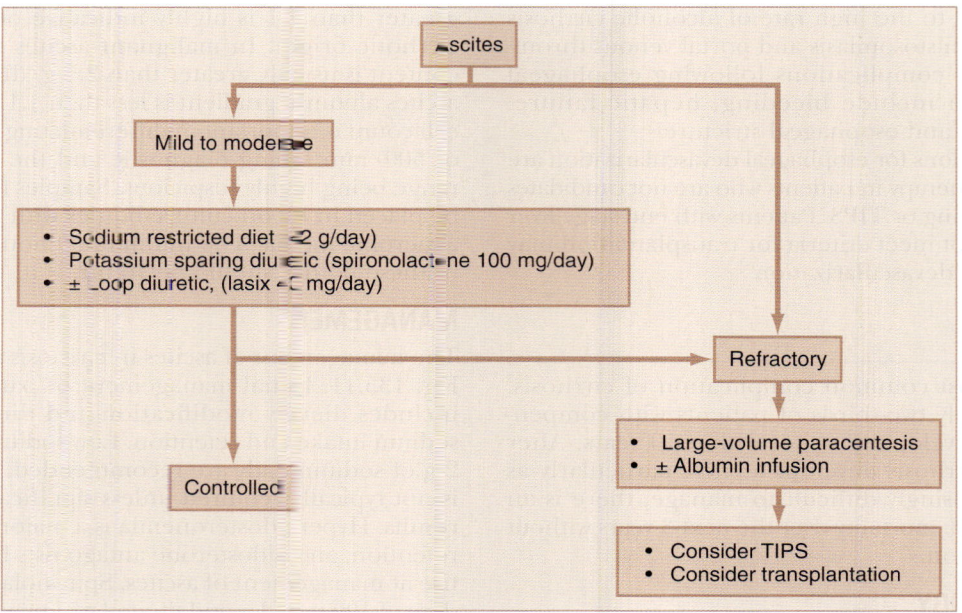

FIGURE 135.11 Treatment of ascites. Most patients are managed with diet and diuretics. Refractory ascites portends a poor prognosis and the need for more aggressive therapy. *TIPS,* Transjugular intrahepatic portosystemic shunt.

trials have shown favorable results with TIPS compared with repeated large volume paracentesis.[58] TIPS is best considered in patients with MELD score less than 18 to avoid hepatic decompensation.

PULMONARY SYNDROMES IN LIVER DISEASE

Some degree of pulmonary abnormality is present in 40% to 70% of patients undergoing evaluation for cirrhosis or portal hypertension. Specific pulmonary vascular disorders related to chronic liver disease and portal hypertension are increasingly well understood. These are currently divided broadly into a vasoconstrictive process leading to pulmonary hypertension termed portopulmonary hypertension or microvascular dilation with associated hypoxemia in HPS.[31,59] The major features of these two syndromes are summarized in Table 135.2

HEPATOPULMONARY SYNDROME

HPS is defined as the presence of liver dysfunction or portal hypertension associated with a widened alveolar-arterial oxygen gradient with intrapulmonary vasodilation. Clinically, HPS presents with concomitant cirrhosis and insidious onset dyspnea, especially while standing. The presence of spider angiomata, digital clubbing, and cyanosis can raise the suspicion for HPS as pulmonary complaints are common. Widened alveolar-arterial oxygen gradient greater than 20 mm Hg is typically present but lacks specificity for HPS. Contrast echocardiography, lung perfusion scanning, and pulmonary angiography have classically been used to diagnose pulmonary vasodilation. Recently, high-resolution CT scanning has been used to correlate gas exchange abnormalities to intrapulmonary vasodilation. A hundred percent oxygen inspiration can measure the degree of

TABLE 135.2 Pulmonary Syndromes in Liver Disease

Variables	Hepatopulmonary Syndrome	Portopulmonary Hypertension
Prevalence	8%–20% of cirrhosis	3%–12% of cirrhosis
Clinical findings	Clubbing, cyanosis, platypnea, systolic flow murmur	Right ventricular heave, systolic flow murmur, lower extremity edema
Pulmonary vascular changes	Vasodilation	Vasoconstriction
Contributing factors	Liver dysfunction, portal hypertension	Portal hypertension
Place of transplant	Curative	Contraindicated

oxygen shunting if PaO_2 fails to rise above 300 mm Hg; however, this is not present in all patients.

Studies indicate that intrapulmonary nitric oxide regulation is implicated in the development of HPS. Reports of HPS in prehepatic portal hypertension without significant liver disease suggest cirrhosis is not a prerequisite for development of HPS. Medical therapies for HPS have little effect, and patients with HPS are supported with supplemental oxygen therapy. Liver transplantation remains the only effective treatment and is effective in reversing HPS in 80% of patients. Patients with PaO_2 of less than 50 mm Hg who are going into liver transplant have poorer survival rates than those with PaO_2 greater than 50 mm Hg. Currently, patients with HPS and PaO_2 less than 60 mm Hg are given priority in the MELD system or organ allocation for liver transplantation.[60]

PORTOPULMONARY HYPERTENSION

In portopulmonary hypertension, flow to the pulmonary arterial bed is obstructed due to vasoconstriction, proliferation of endothelial smooth muscle, and thrombosis. Hypoxemia associated with this syndrome is less pronounced than HPS, but increasing pulmonary arterial pressure and right heart strain leads to right heart failure and death. Clinically, portopulmonary hypertension is less symptomatic than HPS. Decreased single breath diffusing capacity of carbon monoxide on pulmonary function testing and elevated right heart pressure on echocardiography are present in portopulmonary syndrome but lacks specificity for diagnosis. Right heart catheterization with mean pulmonary artery pressure greater than 24 mm Hg and capillary wedge pressure of less than 15 mm Hg is necessary for the diagnosis of these patients.

Mild degrees of pulmonary artery hypertension up to 35 mm Hg do not preclude liver transplantation in otherwise acceptable candidates but pressures greater than 35 mm Hg require aggressive evaluation and treatment. At the present time, pulmonary artery pressures greater than 50 mm Hg are considered an absolute contraindication to liver transplantation because of the high perioperative mortality.[61] Intravenous prostacyclin infusions using epoprostenol have successfully bridged patients to liver transplantation. Oral vasodilatory agents including sildenafil and bosentan have also been reported to dramatically improve pulmonary hemodynamics in some studies; however, a lack of controlled studies makes definitive recommendations difficult.[62]

TRANSPLANTATION

Finally, a discussion of liver transplantation must be included in the management of portal hypertension and its complications. The progression of liver disease heralded by these complications is often best addressed by transplantation. The MELD developed by the United Network for Organ Sharing (UNOS) is used in organ allocation to maximize the utility of available organs by predicting 3-month survival. Serum bilirubin, creatinine, INR for prothrombin time, and etiology of liver disease are used to mathematically calculate MELD scores based on the formula in Box 135.3. Although the individual complications of portal hypertension including SBP, variceal hemorrhage, and refractory ascites, do not significantly add to the predictive power of the MELD score,[63] multidisciplinary evaluation of these patients and comprehensive treatment algorithms must include evaluation for the appropriateness of liver transplantation.

REFERENCES

1. Walker RM. Francis Glisson and his capsule. *Ann R Coll Surg Engl*. 1966;38(2):71-91.
2. Zimmerman HJ. Backward- versus forward flow hypothesis. In: Seeff LB, Leiws JH, eds. *Current Perspectives in Hepatology: Festschrift for Hyman*. 1st ed. Totowa, NJ: Plenum Publishing Company; 1989:114.
3. Whipple AO. The problem of portal hypertension in relation to the hepatosplenopathies. *Ann Surg*. 1945;122(4):449-475.
4. Li JC, Henderson JM. Portal hypertension. In: Holzheimer RG, Mannick JA, eds. *Surgical Treatment: Evidence-based and Problem-oriented*. Munich: Zuckschwedt; 2001.
5. Warren WD, Zeppa R, Fomon JJ. Selective trans-splenic decompression of gastroesophageal varices by distal splenorenal shunt. *Ann Surg*. 1967;160(3):437-455.
6. Inokuchi K, Kobayashi M, Kusaba A, Ogawa Y, Saku M, Shiizaki T. New selective decompression of esophageal varices: by a left gastric venous-caval shunt. *Arch Surg*. 1970;100(2):157-162.
7. Sarfeh IJ, Rypins EB, Mason GR. A systematic appraisal of portacaval H-graft diameters. Clinical and hemodynamic perspectives. *Ann Surg*. 1986;204(4):356-363.
8. Crafoord C, Frenckner P. New surgical treatment of varicous veins of the oesophagus. *Acta Otolaryngol*. 1939;27(4):422-429.
9. Stiegmann GV, Goff JS, Sun JH, Wilborn S. Endoscopic elastic band ligation for active variceal hemorrhage. *Am Surg*. 1989;55(2):124-128.
10. Rosch J, Hanafee WN, Snow H. Transjugular portal venography and radiologic portacaval shunt: an experimental study 1. *Radiology*. 1969;92:1112-1114.
11. Garcia-Tsan JC, Groszmann R, Bosch J. Portal hypertension. In: Weinstein WM, Hawkey JC, Bosch J, eds. *Clinical Gastroenterology and Hepatology, Part 2, Section 4: Diseases of the Gut and Liver*. Philadelphia: Elsevier; 2005:707.
12. Lebrec D, Corbic M, Nouel O, Benhamou J. Propranolol—a medical treatment for portal hypertension? *Lancet*. 1980;316(8187):180-182.
13. Starzl TE, Iwatsuki S, Van Thiel DH, et al. Evolution of liver transplantation. *Hepatology*. 1982;2(5):614-636.
14. Marks C. Developmental basis of the portal venous system. *Am J Surg*. 1969;117(5):671-681.
15. Teutsch HF. The modular microarchitecture of human liver. *Hepatology*. 2005;42(2):317-325.
16. Matsumoto T, Kawakami M. The unit-concept of hepatic parenchyma—a re-examination based on angioarchitectural studies. *Acta Pathol Jpn*. 1982;32(suppl 2):285-314.
17. Roberts LR, Kamath PS. Pathophysiology and treatment of variceal hemorrhage. *Mayo Clin Proc*. 1996;71(10):973-983.
18. Greenway CV, Lautt WW. Hepatic circulation. In: Schultz SG, Wood JL, eds. *Handbook of Physiology. Section 6: The Gastrointestinal System Volume 1: Motility and Circulation*. Oxford: Oxford University Press; 1989:1519-1564.
19. Eipel C, Abshagen K, Vollmar B. Regulation of hepatic blood flow: the hepatic arterial buffer response revisited. *World J Gastroenterol*. 2010;16(48):6046-6057.
20. Valla D, Condat B. Portal vein thrombosis in adults: pathophysiology, pathogenesis and management. *J Hepatol*. 2000;32(5):865-871.
21. Cohen J, Edelman RR, Chopra S. Portal vein thrombosis: a review. *Am J Med*. 1992;92(2):173-182.
22. Bosch J, Pizcueta P, Feu F, Fernandez M, Garcia-Pagan JC. Pathophysiology of portal hypertension. *Portal*. 1992;15:24.
23. Cheever AW, Andrade ZA. Pathological lesions associated with *Schistosoma mansoni* infection in man. *Trans R Soc Trop Med Hyg*. 1976;70(6):626-639.
24. Sarin S, Kapoor D. Non-cirrhotic portal fibrosis: current concepts and management. *J Gastroenterol Hepatol*. 2002;17(5):526-534.
25. Zeitoun G, Escolano S, Hadengue A, et al. Outcome of Budd-Chiari syndrome: a multivariate analysis of factors related to survival including surgical portosystemic shunting. *Hepatology*. 1999;30(1):84-89.
26. Merli M, Nicolini G, Angelon S, et al. Incidence and natural history of small esophageal varices in cirrhotic patients. *J Hepatol*. 2003;38(3):266-272.
27. Garcia-Tsao G, Sanyal AJ, Grace ND, Carey W. Prevention and management of gastroesophageal varices and variceal hemorrhage in cirrhosis. *Hepatology*. 2007;46(3):922-938.
28. Fernandez-Esparrach G, Sánchez-Fueyo A, Ginès P, et al. A prognostic model for predicting survival in cirrhosis with ascites. *J Hepatol*. 2001;34(1):46-52.
29. Evans LT, Kim W, Poterucha JJ, Kamath PS. Spontaneous bacterial peritonitis in asymptomatic outpatients with cirrhotic ascites. *Hepatology*. 2003;37(4):897-901.
30. Mazzaferro V, Regalia E, Doci R, et al. Liver transplantation for the treatment of small hepatocellular carcinomas in patients with cirrhosis. *N Engl J Med*. 1996;334(11):693-700.
31. Krowka MJ. Hepatopulmonary syndromes. *Gut*. 2000;46(1):1-4.
32. Beppu K, Inokuchi K, Koyanagi N, et al. Prediction of variceal hemorrhage by esophageal endoscopy. *Gastrointest Endosc*. 1981;27(4):213-218.
33. Stewart CA, Sanyal AJ. Grading portal gastropathy: validation of a gastropathy scoring system. *Am J Gastroenterol*. 2003;98(8):1758-1765.

34. Bolondi L, Gatta A, Groszmann RJ, et al. Baveno II consensus statements: imaging techniques and hemodynamic measurements in portal hypertension. In: De Franchis R, ed. *Portal Hypertension II: Proceedings of the Second Baveno International Consensus Workshop on Definitions, Methodology and Therapeutic Strategies.* Oxford: Blackwell Science; 1996:67.

35. Angermayr B, Cejna M, Karnel F, et al. Child-Pugh versus MELD score in predicting survival in patients undergoing transjugular intrahepatic portosystemic shunt. *Gut.* 2003;52(6):879-885.

36. Kamath PS, Wiesner RH, Malinchoc M, et al. A model to predict survival in patients with end-stage liver disease. *Hepatology.* 2001; 33(2):464-470.

37. Bañares R, Moitinho E, Matilla A, et al. Randomized comparison of long-term carvedilol and propranolol administration in the treatment of portal hypertension in cirrhosis. *Hepatology.* 2002;36(5): 1367-1373.

38. de Franchis R. Revising consensus in portal hypertension: report of the Baveno V consensus workshop on methodology of diagnosis and therapy in portal hypertension. *J Hepatol.* 2010;53(4):762-768.

39. Corley DA, Cello JP, Adkisson W, Ko W, Kerlikowske K. Octreotide for acute esophageal variceal bleeding: a meta-analysis. *Gastroenterology.* 2001;120(4):946-954.

40. Villanueva C, Colomo A, Bosch A, et al. Transfusion strategies for acute upper gastrointestinal bleeding. *N Engl J Med.* 2013;368(1):11-21.

41. Stravitz RT. Potential applications of thromboelastography in patients with acute and chronic liver disease. *Gastroenterol Hepatol (N Y).* 2012; 8(8):513-520.

42. Gimson A, Ramage J, Panos M, et al. Randomised trial of variceal banding ligation versus injection sclerotherapy for bleeding oesophageal varices. *Lancet.* 1993;342(8868):391-394.

43. Stiegmann GV, Goff JS, Michaletz-Onody PA, et al. Endoscopic sclerotherapy as compared with endoscopic ligation for bleeding esophageal varices. *N Engl J Med.* 1992;326(23):1527-1532.

44. Bañares R, Albillos A, Rincón D, et al. Endoscopic treatment versus endoscopic plus pharmacologic treatment for acute variceal bleeding: a meta-analysis. *Hepatology.* 2002;35(3):609-615.

45. Saad WE, Sabri SS. Balloon-occluded retrograde transvenous obliteration (BRTO): technical results and outcomes. *Semin Intervent Radiol.* 2011;28(3):333-338.

46. Rossle M, Haag K, Ochs A, et al. The transjugular intrahepatic portosystemic stent-shunt procedure for variceal bleeding. *N Engl J Med.* 1994;330(3):165-171.

47. Ochs A, Rössle M, Haag K, et al. The transjugular intrahepatic portosystemic stent-shunt procedure for refractory ascites. *N Engl J Med.* 1995;332(18):1192-1197.

48. Boyer TD, Haskal ZJ. The role of transjugular intrahepatic portosystemic shunt in the management of portal hypertension. *Hepatology.* 2005;41(2):386-400.

49. Bureau C, carlos Garcia-Pagan J, Otal P, et al. Improved clinical outcome using polytetrafluoroethylene-coated stents for TIPS: results of a randomized study. *Gastroenterology.* 2004;126(2):469-475.

50. D'amico G, Pagliaro L, Bosch J. The treatment of portal hypertension: a meta-analytic review. *Hepatology.* 1995;22(1):332-354.

51. Rikkers LF, Jin G, Langnas AN, Shaw BW Jr. Shunt surgery during the era of liver transplantation. *Ann Surg.* 1997;226(1):51-57.

52. Rosemurgy AS, Bloomston M, Clark WC, Thometz DP, Zervos EE. H-graft portacaval shunts versus TIPS: ten-year follow-up of a randomized trial with comparison to predicted survivals. *Ann Surg.* 2005;241(2):238-246.

53. Jenkins RL, Gedaly R, Pomposelli JJ, Pomfret EA, Gordon F, Lewis WD. Distal splenorenal shunt: role, indications, and utility in the era of liver transplantation. *Arch Surg.* 1999;134(4):416-420.

54. Orozco H, Mercado MA, Granados J, et al. Selective shunts for portal hypertension: current role of a 21-year experience. *Liver Transpl Surg.* 1997;3(5):475-480.

55. Dagenais M, Langer B, Taylor BR, Greig PD. Experience with radical esophagogastric devascularization procedures (Sugiura) for variceal bleeding outside Japan. *World J Surg.* 1994;18(2):222-228.

56. Sugiura M, Futagawa S. A new technique for treating esophageal varices. *J Thorac Cardiovasc Surg.* 1973;66(5):677-685.

57. Rössle M, Ochs A, Gülberg V, et al. A comparison of paracentesis and transjugular intrahepatic portosystemic shunting in patients with ascites. *N Engl J Med.* 2000;342(23):1701-1707.

58. Sanyal AJ, Genning C, Reddy KR, et al. The North American study for the treatment of refractory ascites. *Gastroenterology.* 2003;124(3):634-641.

59. Rodríguez-Roisin R, Krowka MJ. Hepatopulmonary syndrome—a liver-induced lung vascular disorder. *N Engl J Med.* 2008;358(22): 2378-2387.

60. Iyer VN. Liver transplantation for hepatopulmonary syndrome. *Clin Liver Dis.* 2014;4(2):38-41.

61. Krowka MJ, Plevak DJ, Findlay JY, Rosen CB, Wiesner RH, Krom RA. Pulmonary hemodynamics and perioperative cardiopulmonary-related mortality in patients with portopulmonary hypertension undergoing liver transplantation. *Liver Transpl.* 2000;6(4):443-450.

62. Swanson K, Wiesner RH, Nyberg S, Rosen C, Krowka MJ. Survival in portopulmonary hypertension: Mayo Clinic experience categorized by treatment subgroups. *Am J Transpl.* 2008;8(11):2445-2453.

63. Kamath PS, Wiesner RH, Malinchoc M, et al. A model to predict survival in patients with end-stage liver disease. *Hepatology.* 2001;53(2): 464-470.

Anatomy and Physiology of the Spleen

Luise I.M. Pernar | Ali Tavakkoli

The spleen has been a source of intrigue and mystery since ancient times, and its anatomy and function have been contemplated by ancient Egyptians and Chinese as far back as 1550 BC. The spleen was variably thought to be associated with emotions, and both ill temper and glee have been thought to arise from the spleen. Across centuries the true significance of the spleen was questioned by a variety of physicians ranging from Galen to Princelsus, and it was not until the turn of the 20th century that the role of the spleen started to be understood.[1-3] Surgery to remove the spleen preceded a good understanding of its function: the first reported splenectomy was performed in 1549 by Zaccarella of Italy, and the first documented splenectomy, performed in 1826, is credited to Quitterbaum of Germany. The first laparoscopic splenectomy was not performed until 1991 by Delaitre and Maignien of France.[4] Although the first splenectomies were performed with little knowledge of the function of the organ, our increased awareness of the role of the spleen as an immunologic organ has changed the preoperative preparation of patients due to undergo an elective splenectomy.

The spleen serves important functions as a secondary lymphoid tissue, contributing through phagocytosis and orchestration of humoral and cellular immunity.[5] The spleen is also associated with multiple nonimmunologic functions, serving as the differentiation site for platelets, reticulocytes, and monocytes; the reservoir for granulocytes and erythrocytes; and the removal site for aged and deformed red blood cells.[5,6] The spleen additionally plays a role in embryogenesis of the pancreas[7] and may serve as a reservoir for islet cell precursors.[8] This function appears to be clinically significant because impaired glucose tolerance after splenectomy has been observed.[9] The spleen also is a source of other stem cell precursors, specifically those expressing HOX11, a protooncogene, and thus may also be involved in oncogenesis of leukemia.[10]

EMBRYOLOGY

The splenic primordium appears during the fifth week of development as a mesodermal proliferation between the two leaves of the dorsal mesogastrium. In the early stages of development the splenic mesenchyme is also adherent to the dorsal pancreatic bud.[11] As the stomach rotates around an anteroposterior axis, with its caudal portion moving upward and to the right and its cephalic portion moving downward and to the left, a portion of the dorsal mesogastrium eventually fuses with the peritoneum of the posterior abdominal wall. The splenic mesenchyme then separates from the pancreas, and the spleen remains intraperitoneal.[11] The splenic primordium is eventually infiltrated by lymphoid cells. Hematopoiesis is prominent in the spleen from the third to the fifth months of embryonic life. By the fourth month, the red pulp structure begins to appear.[5]

ANATOMY

The spleen lies underneath the ninth, tenth, and eleventh ribs on the left, measures 7 to 13 cm in length, and weighs an average of 150 g, although normal weights range from 70 to 250 g and may decrease with age. Splenomegaly is usually considered if splenic weight is greater than 500 g or length greater than 15 cm; massive splenomegaly is defined as splenic weight exceeding 1500 g. The spleen becomes palpable underneath the left costal margin in instances where its size is at least twice normal. The spleen is asymmetric in shape with a smooth convex portion abutting the diaphragm and a concave surface medially (Fig. 136.1).[12,13]

Externally, the spleen is enveloped almost entirely by peritoneum, which is adherent to the splenic capsule and forms several ligaments to surrounding structures. The surgically significant ligaments are the gastrosplenic ligament, containing the short gastric vessels, and the splenocolic and splenorenal ligaments that tether the spleen to the colon and kidney, respectively (Fig. 136.2). The splenic ligaments develop collateral vessels in cases of portal hypertension. Knowledge of these ligaments is critical because they need to be carefully divided when mobilizing the spleen. The gastrosplenic ligament is particularly important because it contains the splenic vessels, which are also often accompanied by the tails of the pancreas. Knowledge of the location of the tail of the pancreas is clinically relevant during a splenectomy to help avoid pancreatic injury. Computed tomography (CT) image analysis has shown that the distance between the pancreatic tail and the splenic hilum averages 3.4 ± 1.5 cm and is typically at least 1 cm. Therefore surgeons

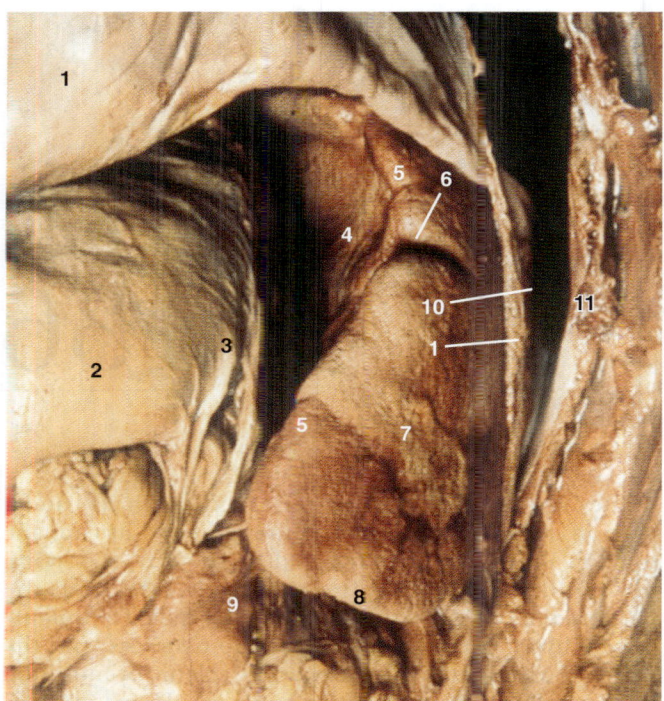

FIGURE 136.1 Gross anatomy photograph of the relationship of the spleen to the diaphragm and other organs. The left upper abdominal and lower anterior thoracic walls have been removed, and part of the diaphragm (1) has been turned upward to show the spleen in its normal position, lying adjacent to the stomach (2) and colon (9), with the lower part against the kidney. The spleen is connected to the stomach by the gastrosplenic ligament (3) and the colon by the splenocolic ligament. The organ's convex shape results from the gastric impression (4) and its position against the thoracic wall (11). When viewed from the front, one can see the spleen's superior border (5), notch (6), diaphragmatic surface (7), and inferior border (8). Also shown here is the costodiaphragmatic recess (10). (From McMinn RMH, Hutchings RT, Pegington J, Abrahams PH. *Color Atlas of Human Anatomy.* 3rd ed. St Louis: Mosby-Year Book; 1993:230–231.)

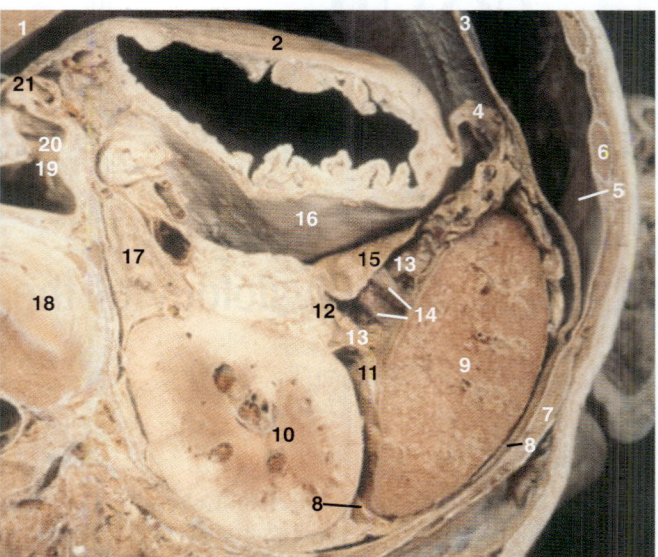

FIGURE 136.2 Gross anatomy photograph of the spleen in transverse section (level of the 12th thoracic and 1st lumbar vertebrae) illustrating the anatomic relationship of the spleen to the stomach, colon, and kidney, and the clinically important splenic ligaments. (1) Left lobe of liver, (2) stomach, (3) diaphragm, (4) gastrosplenic ligament, (5) costodiaphragmatic recess of pleura, (6) ninth rib, (7) tenth rib, (8) peritoneum of greater sac, (9) spleen, (10) left kidney, (11) posterior layer of splenorenal ligament, (12) tail of pancreas, (13) splenic artery, (14) splenic vein, (15) anterior layer of splenorenal ligament, (16) lesser sac, (17) left suprarenal gland, (18) intervertebral disc, (19) abdominal aorta, (20) celiac trunk, and (21) left gastric artery. (From McMinn RMH, Hutchings RT, Pegington J, Abrahams PH. *Color Atlas of Human Anatomy.* 3rd ed. St Louis: Mosby-Year Book; 1993:230–231.)

need to stay within 1 cm of the splenic hilum during a splenectomy to avoid injury to the pancreas.[11,13,14]

Approximately 20% of the population has one or more accessory spleens, usually located within the splenic hilar region. Accessory spleens may also be found in the pancreas, omentum, and even in the pelvis and reproductive glands (Fig. 136.3).[15] A technetium 99m (^{99m}Tc)-labeled red blood cell scan can be used to help localize accessory spleens[16] if complete splenectomy is mandatory, as in surgical management of immune thrombocytopenic purpura (ITP). The incidence of accessory spleens may be as high as 30% in individuals with hematologic pathology.[13]

BLOOD SUPPLY, LYMPHATIC DRAINAGE, AND INNERVATION

The spleen receives approximately 5% of the cardiac output, via the splenic artery, the largest of the three branches of the celiac trunk (Fig. 136.4). However, the spleen also receives some accessory supply from branches of the left gastroepiploic artery. The splenic artery is a tortuous artery that lies posterior to the superior border of the body of the pancreas, forming multiple coils, and eventually divides into two or three main branches that penetrate through the hilum of the spleen. There are two main patterns of splenic artery anatomy, the magistral type, in which a long splenic artery trunk reaches close to the splenic hilum before dividing into branches, and the distributed type, in which there is a short splenic artery trunk with branching far from the splenic hilum. The distributive type is the more common variation.[13,17]

The splenic artery branches in turn divide into segmental arteries that enter along the splenic trabeculae (Fig. 136.5). There is little collateral circulation at this level, and occlusion of one of these arteries usually is associated with infarction of the corresponding region of the spleen, a phenomenon seen in embolic diseases. Segmental arteries give rise to trabecular arteries, which in turn, and by means of perpendicular branches, give origin to central arteries.[12] There is an ongoing debate regarding the paths of blood flow after it enters the spleen. In general, it is thought that the blood takes two paths: a fast (closed) circulation that takes the blood directly from the arterioles to venules and has a predominance referred to as Kehr sign, is observed particularly after splenic rupture.[18]

HISTOLOGY OF THE SPLEEN

The human spleen is composed of red and white pulp, which are separated by a thin marginal zone (Fig. 136.6). The red pulp makes up approximately 75% of the spleen and is predominantly composed of splenic cords, capillaries, and venous sinuses, which express endothelial markers (e.g., clotting factor VIII), within loose reticular tissue. This richly vascular, specialized portion of the spleen enables it to function as a filter of blood.

The white pulp consists of lymphoid follicles (mostly B lymphocytes) and the periarterial lymphoid sheath (PALS) (mostly T lymphocytes). These, along with the lymphoid, nonfiltering red pulp (both B and T lymphocytes), are responsible for the spleen's immunologic function. Although comprising only a minority of the overall mass, this lymphoid compartment plays an important role in the early immunologic response against blood-borne antigens and is the compartment primarily responsible for splenic involvement with lymphoproliferative disorders.[5,6,19] The spleen's lymphoid cells express characteristic cluster designation (CD) and other markers that confer specific immunophenotypes to various regions of the spleen. Table 136.1 shows significant markers of lymphoid tissue. A full discussion is beyond the scope of this chapter, but it suffices to say that studying the immunophenotypes of cells in lymphomas can determine if they are related to the spleen.

FUNCTIONS OF THE SPLEEN

It is helpful to think about the functions of the spleen under the following headings, where we will also review expected changes following a surgical splenectomy.

ERYTHROCYTE QUALITY CONTROL AND REMOVAL OF DEFECTIVE RED CELLS

The red pulp is responsible for "quality control" of erythrocytes. This is achieved through pitting and culling. Pitting refers to the removal of nondeformable intracellular substances from deformable cells. The rigid element is removed while the deformable cytoplasmic mass returns to the general circulation. In the case of red cells, this involves removal of Heinz bodies (denatured intracellular hemoglobin), Howell-Jolly bodies, and hemosiderin granules from red cells. Absence of this function following splenectomy explains the presence of circulating erythrocyte with Howell-Jolly and Pappenheimer bodies (siderotic granules). Indeed, the number of pitted cells is inversely proportional to splenic function. Pits represent vesicles containing hemoglobin, ferritin, and mitochondrial remnants. Under normal circumstances, there are less than 2% pitted cells.[20]

Culling is the term applied to the spleen's ability to remove aged red cells at the end of their 120-day life cycle. As the red cell ages, it loses its membrane integrity and therefore deformability, which result in their phagocytosis by splenic macrophages.[20] However, the spleen is not the only site for red cell destruction and there is no difference

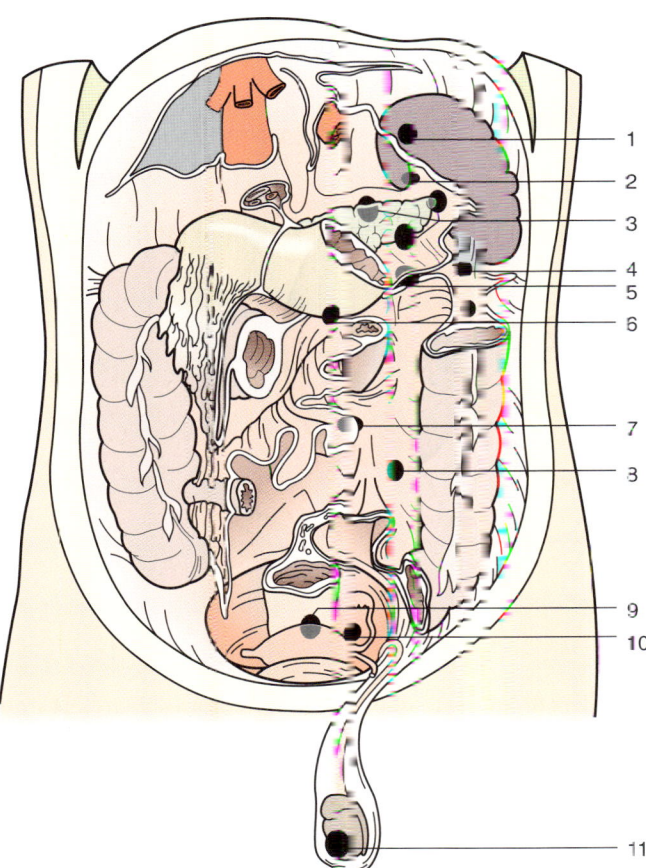

FIGURE 136.3 Schematic of common locations of accessory spleens. *(1)* Gastrosplenic ligament, *(2)* splenic hilum, *(3)* tail of the pancreas, *(4)* splenocolic ligament *(5)* left transverse mesocolon, *(6)* greater omentum along the greater curvature of the stomach, *(7)* mesentery, *(8)* left mesocolon, *(9)* left ovary, *(10)* Douglas pouch, and *(11)* left testis. (From Giroot JF, Lenge B, Gianello P, Etienne J, Claeys N. Present status of laparoscopic splenectomy for hematologic diseases: certitudes and unresolved issues. *Semin Laparosc Surg.* 1998;5:147– 67.)

of plasma, and a slower (open) circulation that takes the blood through the pulp. The majority (90%) of flow is in fact of the slow (open) type, which exposes the circulating cells and erythrocytes to splenic macrophages in the red pulp.

Irrespective of the circulation in the spleen, veins leave the spleen through fibrous bands, or trabeculae, attached to the capsule, and coalesce to form the splenic vein. The splenic vein joins the superior mesenteric vein behind the neck of the pancreas to give origin to the portal vein (see Fig. 136.4).

Lymphatic drainage follows the vasculature. Drainage is into the splenic hilar and celiac nodes via the pancreaticosplenic lymph nodes.[12]

The splenic nervous plexus is formed by branches of the celiac plexus, left celiac ganglion, and right vagus. It runs together with the splenic artery and is composed mainly of sympathetic fibers that reach blood vessels and nonstriated muscle of the capsule and trabeculae. Referred pain from the spleen to the left shoulder, commonly

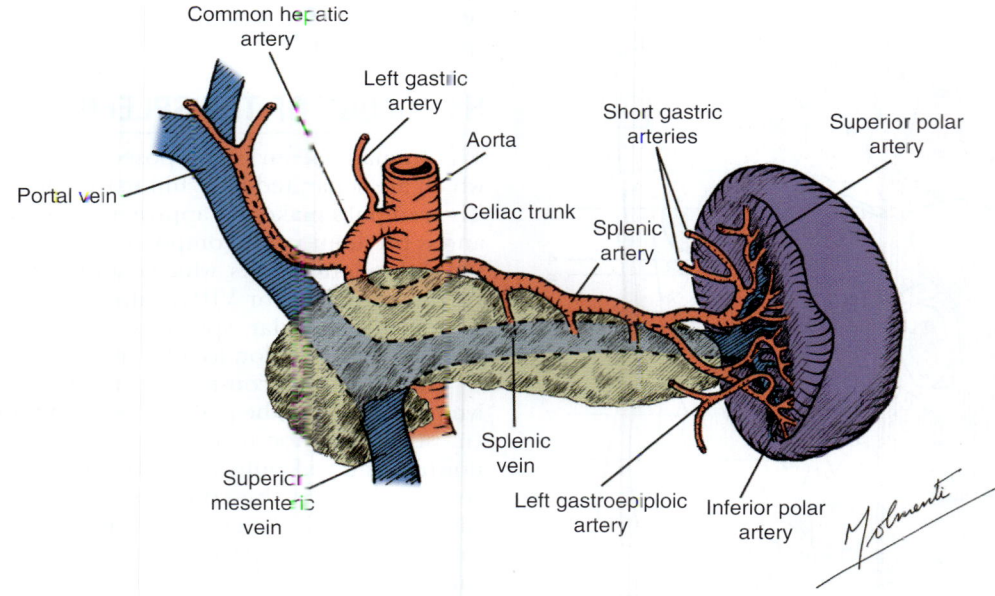

FIGURE 136.4 Arterial and venous supply of the spleen.

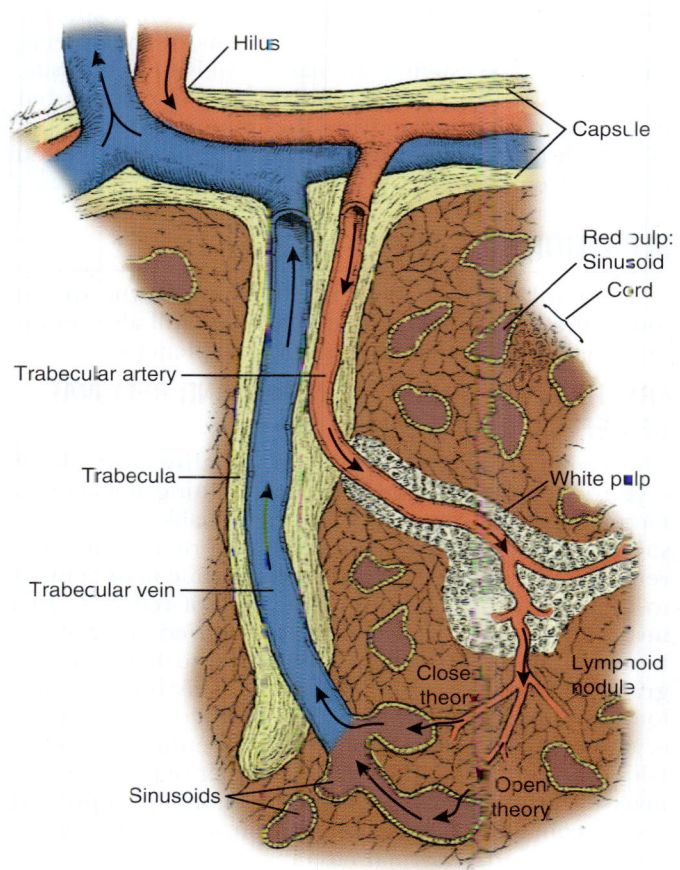

FIGURE 136.5 Details of the splenic structure, highlighting relationship of the white and red pulp to trabecular arteries and closed and open circulation. (From Groom AC. Microcirculatory Society Eugene M. Landis award lecture—microcirculation of the spleen: new concepts, new challenges. *Microvasc Res.* 1987;34:270.)

in red cell survival following splenectomy. Platelets and leukocytes are not predominantly removed by the spleen as they age but rather marginate and die in other tissues.

POOLING

In health, the spleen is not an important reservoir for blood cells but is so for platelets. Approximately one-third of the platelet mass is pooled in the spleen. With splenomegaly, a large proportion of platelets are sequestered in the spleen (up to 80%) and this, along with increased platelet destruction in an enlarged spleen, can result in thrombocytopenia. The role of the spleen in platelet storage also explains the increase in platelet count following a splenectomy.[20]

Neutrophils have a short half-life, and majority either migrate at random into tissues or are destroyed within 24 hours. Hypersplenic states can be associated with neutropenia because of accelerated sequestration of granulocytes or because of enhanced splenic removal of altered granulocytes, as seen in immune neutropenias.

HEMATOPOIESIS

The spleen has an important hematopoietic function in fetal life. Active hematopoiesis can be seen into the third trimester. Late in the second trimester hematopoietic function is transitioned to the bone marrow. In general, splenic hematopoiesis does not occur in healthy adults. Under certain pathologic conditions in which the bone marrow is unable to produce blood cells (e.g., myelofibrosis) or is unable to meet production demands (e.g., chronic hemolytic anemia), extramedullary hematopoiesis in the spleen increases. Typically the resulting cells will be more immature than those produced by the bone marrow.[20]

ANTIBODY SYNTHESIS IN THE WHITE PULP

In addition to the phagocytosis of antibody-coated cells, the immunologic functions of the spleen include antibody synthesis (especially immunoglobulin M). Foreign antigens are filtered in the white pulp and presented to lymphoid

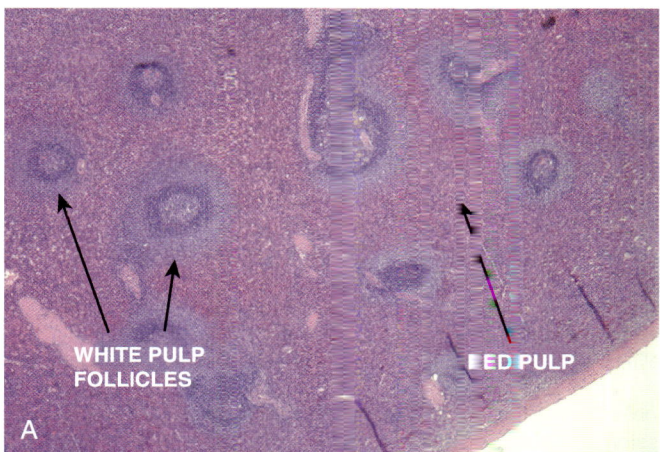

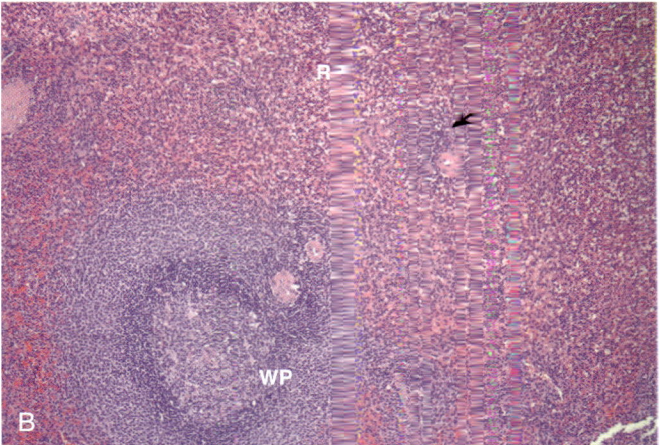

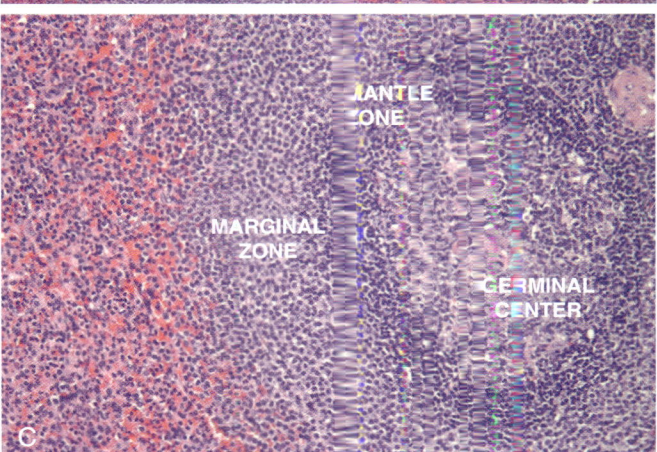

FIGURE 136.6 Normal human spleen on hematoxylin-eosin staining. (A) Low-power photomicrograph showing relationship and relative proportions of red and white pulp. (B) Medium-power photomicrograph (*arrow* indicates periarterial lymphoid sheath). (C) High-power photomicrograph showing detailed secondary follicle architecture. *RP*, Red pulp; *WP*, white pulp secondary follicle).

cells, where an immunoglobulin response is mounted, leading to release of antibodies.

FILTRATION

Macrophages residing in the splenic parenchyma, particularly in the marginal zone, capture cellular and

noncellular material from blood, including encapsulated bacteria, such as pneumococci and meningococci, and destroy them. Splenic macrophages are particularly sensitive to opsonization when compared with macrophages in other sites.[20] This important function explains the increased risk of infections caused by encapsulated organisms that is seen after splenectomy and can lead to the devastating overwhelming postsplenectomy infection (OPSI)

OPSI is a life-threatening complication seen in asplenic individuals that gained significant acceptance in 1953 after an observation by King and Shumacker.[19,21] OPSI is encountered with greatest frequency within 2 years after splenectomy, in the very young, in those with other medical comorbidities, and in those with malignancies. Children, particularly those younger than 2 years of age, are at particularly high risk of OPSI because of their relatively immature immune system. The risk of postsplenectomy sepsis increases according to the specific indications for splenectomy; trauma, hematologic disorders, portal hypertension, Hodgkin disease, sickle cell disease, and thalassemia are associated with increasing cumulative incidence of sepsis.[20] Overall, OPSI is estimated to occur in 0.9% to 5.2% of adults and 3.3% to 4.4% of children; the mortality rate is estimated to be between 0.8% and 1.3% in adults and 1.7% and 2.2% in children.[22,23] OPSI occurs mostly in association with encapsulated organisms that require opsonization for effective phagocytosis. The most frequent of such pathogens are *Neisseria meningitidis*, *Haemophilus influenzae* type b, and *Streptococcus pneumoniae*. There are effective vaccines against all of them, and it is recommended that for adults they be administered ideally 2 weeks before an elective splenectomy to allow for an effective immune response. If this is not achievable because of need for urgent or emergent splenectomy, vaccinations should be administered after the operation. There are multiple guidelines, which vary slightly between countries. The current guidelines from the Centers for Disease Control and Prevention (CDC) are summarized in Table 136.5 and recommend administration of a second dose of vaccine against *N. meningitidis* and *S. pneumoniae* 8 weeks after initial vaccination.[24,25] Daily prophylactic antibiotic use is not clinically proven to be beneficial and generally is not recommended.[26,27] The exception to this rule may be the administration of prophylactic antibiotics in children under 2 years of age to prevent pneumococcal infection.[28] Oral penicillin V or amoxicillin can be used. Other groups for whom prophylaxis might be considered include those high-risk postsplenectomy patients with thalassemias, Hodgkin disease, and immunodeficiencies.[20]

Even with vaccinations and other preventive measures, OPSI can occur, and early recognition is key to reduce morbidity and mortality. Asplenic or hyposplenic patients should be instructed to seek immediate medical attention at the first sign of illness, with some physicians advocating a personal supply of prescribed antibiotics to have on hand. With the onset of fever the patients should take the first dose of antibiotics and then seek immediate medical evaluation. Amoxicillin-clavulanate or levofloxacin are appropriate choices for this purpose.[25]

TABLE 136.1 Significant Cluster Designations (Markers) and Other Antigens: Description of Function and Clarification of Cell Type Typically Expressing the Antigen

Cluster Designation	Function	Physiologic Staining
CD3	Antigen recognition	Thymocytes, peripheral T cells, NK cells
CD4	T-cell activation	Thymocytes, mature T cells (~65%, T-helper subset), macrophages, Langerhans cells, dendritic cells, granulocytes
CD5	Signal transducer	B cells of mantle zone of spleen and lymph nodes, almost all T cells
CD8	Increases avidity of cell–to–cell interactions	Mature T cells (~35% of peripheral T cells, most cytotoxic T cells), NK cells, cortical thymocytes (70%–80%)
CD10	Inactivates bioactive peptides	Pre-B cells, cortical thymocytes; follicular center cells; granulocytes; lymphohematopoietic precursors; neutrophils
CD19	Regulates B-cell development, activation, differentiation	Pre-B cells, B cells, first B-cell antigen after HLA-DR, follicular dendritic cells
CD20	Early activation of B cells	Most B cells (after CD19 and CD10 expression, before CD21/22 expression and surface immunoglobulin expression), retained on mature B cells until plasma cell development, follicular dendritic cells
CD23	Regulates IgE synthesis; B-cell growth factor	Activated mature B cells expressing IgM or IgD, monocytes/macrophages, T-cell subsets, platelets, eosinophils, Langerhans cells, follicular dendritic cells
CD45	T- and B-cell antigen receptor–mediated activation	All hematopoietic cells; stronger in lymphocytes (10% of surface area)
CD79a	Encodes Ig proteins	Early in B-cell differentiation (often positive when mature B-cell markers are negative), plasma cells
BCL2	Induces apoptosis	Mantle zone B cells, germinal center centrocytes
BCL6	Regulates transcription	Germinal center centroblasts and centrocytes

HLA-DR, Human leukocyte antigen D-related; *IgD*, immunoglobulin D; *IgM*, immunoglobulin M; *NK*, natural killer.

TABLE 136.2 Centers for Disease Control and Prevention Recommended Vaccination Schedule for Planned Splenectomy*/Asplenic Patients[†24,25]

	Pneumococcal Vaccination	Meningococcal Vaccination	Haemophilus Influenzae Type B Vaccination
Children	*Immunologically naïve 2–6 years[‡]:* PCV13 followed by PCV13 8 weeks later; PPSV23 8 weeks later; repeat PPSV23 at 5 years *Immunologically naïve 6–18 years[‡]:* PCV13 followed by PSV23 8 weeks later; repeat PPSV23 at 5 years	MenACWY series AND MenB series[§]	Hib once if 15 months or older and previously not vaccinated
Adults (age 19 and older)	*Immunologically naïve[‡]:* PCV13 followed by PPSV23 8 weeks later; repeat PPSV23 every 5 years	MenACWY or MPSV4 2 months apart; repeat MenACWY every 5 years AND MenB series[§] once	Hib once

*First vaccination should be administered at least 2 weeks before splenectomy if elective.
[†]Even with vaccination, oral antibiotic prophylaxis with penicillin V or amoxicillin should be considered for children under 2 years of age, or high-risk postsplenectomy patients.
[‡]For patients who have previously received any PCV or PPSV 23 or a combination of these vaccinations, the recommendations vary and are outlined in the CDC guidelines accessible online.[24,25]
[§]MenB-4C 2 doses 1 month apart or MenB-FHbp 3 doses, 1 each at 0, 2, and 6 months.
Hib, H. influenzae type b; *MenACWY,* Meningococcal 4-valent conjugate; *MPSV4,* Meningococcal 4-valent polysaccharide; *PCV13,* Pneumococcal 13-valent conjugate; *PPSV23,* Pneumococcal 23-valent polysaccharide.

REFERENCES

1. Paraskevas GK, Koutsouflaniotis KN, Nitsa Z, Demesticha T, Skandalakis P. Knowledge of the anatomy and physiology of the spleen throughout Antiquity and the Early Middle Ages. *Anat Sci Int.* 2016; 91(1):43-55.
2. McClusky DA, Skandalakis LJ, Colborn GL, Skandalakis JE. Tribute to a triad: history of splenic anatomy, physiology, and surgery—part 1. *World J Surg.* 1999;23(3):311-325.
3. McClusky DA, Skandalakis LJ, Colborn GL, Skandalakis JE. Tribute to a triad: history of splenic anatomy, physiology, and surgery—part 2. *World J Surg.* 1999;23(5):514-526.
4. Delaitre B, Maignien B. Laparoscopic splenectomy—technical aspects. *Surg Endosc.* 1992;6(6):305-308.
5. Paraskevas F. Lymphocytes and lymphatic organs. In: Greer JP, ed. *Wintrobe's Clinical Hematology.* 13th ed. Philadelphia: Wolters Kluwer Health/Lippincott Wiliams & Wilkins; 2014.
6. Mebius RE, Kraal G. Structure and function of the spleen. *Nat Rev Immunol.* 2005;5(8):606-616.
7. Hörnblad A, Eriksson AU, Sock E, Hill RE, Ahlgren U. Impaired spleen formation perturbs morphogenesis of the gastric lobe of the pancreas. *PLoS One.* 2011;6(6):e21753.
8. Park S, Hong SM, Ahn IS. Can splenocytes enhance pancreatic beta-cell function and mass in 90% pancreatectomized rats fed a high fat diet? *Life Sci.* 2009;84(11-12):358-363.

9. Wu S-C, Fu C-Y, Muo C-H, Chang Y-J. Splenectomy in trauma patients is associated with an increased risk of postoperative type II diabetes: a nationwide population-based study. *Am J Surg.* 2014;208(5):811-816.

10. Dieguez-Acuna FJ, Gygi SP, Davis M, Faustman DL. Splenectomy: a new treatment option for ALL tumors expressing Hox-11 and a means to test the stem cell hypothesis of cancer in humans. *Leukemia.* 2007;21(10):2192-2194.

11. Asayesh A, Sharpe J, Watson RP, et al. Spleen versus pancreas: strict control of organ interrelationship revealed by analyses of Bapx1−/− mice. *Genes Dev.* 2006;20(16):2208-2213.

12. Fraker D. The spleen. In: Greenfield LJ, Mulholland MW, eds. *Greenfield's Surgery: Scientific Principles and Practice* 5th ed. Philadelphia: Wolters Kluwer Health/Lippincott Williams & Wilkins; 2010.

13. Tavakkoli A. The spleen. In: Zinner MJ, Ashley SW, eds. *Maingot's Abdominal Operations.* 12th ed. New York: McGraw Hill Medical; 2013.

14. Saber AA, Helbling B, Khaghany K, Nirmit G, Pimental R, McLeod MK. Safety zone for splenic hilar control during splenectomy: a computed tomography scan mapping of the tail of the pancreas in relation to the splenic hilum. *Am Surg.* 2007;73(9):890-894.

15. Koshenkov VP, Pahuja AK, Németh ZH, Abzin A, Carter MS. Identification of accessory spleens during laparoscopic splenectomy is superior to preoperative computed tomography for detection of accessory spleens. *JSLS.* 2012;16(3):387-391.

16. Bergeron E, Ratte S, Jeannotte S, Recoskie MJ. The use of a handheld gamma probe for identifying two accessory spleens in difficult locations in the same patient. *Ann Nucl Med.* 2008;22(4):331-333.

17. Poulin EC, Thibault C. The anatomical basis for laparoscopic splenectomy. *Can J Surg.* 1993;36(5):484-488.

18. Harpel A. [Does Kehr's sign derive from Hans Kehr? A critical commentary on its documentation]. *Chirurg.* 2004;75(1):80-83.

19. Foreman MR, Doyle M, Chapman WC. Disorders of the spleen. In: Greer JP, ed. *Wintrobe's Clinical Hematology,* 13th ed. Philadelphia: Wolters Kluwer Health/Lippincott Williams & Wilkins; 2014.

20. Connell NT, Shurin SB, Schiffman FJ. The spleen and its disorders. In: Hoffman R, Benz EJ Jr, Silberstein LE, et al., eds. *Hematology: Basic Principles and Practice.* 6th ed. Philadelphia: Elsevier; 2013.

21. Sinwar PD. Overwhelming post splenectomy infection syndrome—review study. *Int J Surg.* 2014;12(12):1314-1316.

22. Holdsworth RJ, Irving AD, Cuschieri A. Postsplenectomy sepsis and its mortality rate: actual versus perceived risks. *Br J Surg.* 1991;78(9):1031-1038.

23. Bisharat N, Omari H, Lavi I, Raz R. Risk of infection and death among post-splenectomy patients. *J Infect.* 2001;43(3):182-186.

24. Birth-18 Years Immunization Schedule. CDC [Internet]. http://www.cdc.gov/vaccines/schedules/hcp/imz/child-adolescent.html; 2016. Accessed 7 November 2016.

25. Adult Immunization Schedule by Medical and Other Indications. CDC [Internet]. http://www.cdc.gov/vaccines/schedules/hcp/adult.htm; 2016. Accessed 21 April 2016.

26. Makris M, Greaves M, Winfield DA, Preston FE, Lilleyman JS. Long-term management after splenectomy. Lifelong penicillin unproved in trials. *BMJ.* 1994;309(6921):131-132.

27. Hari DP, Launoo SS, Mistry P, Nesargikar PN. Immunoprophylaxis in asplenic patients. *Int J Surg.* 2009;7(5):421-423.

28. Prevention of Pneumococcal Disease. Recommendations of the Advisory Committee on Immunization Practices (ACIP) [Internet]. https://www.cdc.gov/mmwr/preview/mmwrhtml/00047135.htm. 2016. Accessed 7 November 2016.

Technique of Splenectomy

Megan Jenkins | Manish Parikh | H. Leon Pachter

Since 1991 when it was first described by Delaitre,[1] the laparoscopic approach has become the standard technique for most cases of elective splenectomy. An increased technical skill among surgeons has extended the application for laparoscopic splenectomy to safely include patients with massive splenomegaly.[2] Some limitations to the laparoscopic approach remain for patients with splenomegaly, splenic trauma, and serious medical conditions.[3]

Hematologic diseases, such as idiopathic thrombocytopenic purpura (ITP) and thrombotic thrombocytopenic purpura (TTP), are the most common indications for elective splenectomy. These patients typically present with normal or moderately enlarged spleens, and, as such, treatment by a minimally invasive technique is highly valuable.[3] Following the procedure, as many as 85% will have long-term normalization of platelet counts with complete remission of disease. Other hematologic conditions, such as hereditary spherocytosis, myeloproliferative disorders (chronic and acute myeloid leukemia), and autoimmune hemolytic anemia, are general indications for splenectomy.[5]

Malignant disease does not preclude the laparoscopic approach. Splenectomy for therapeutic or diagnostic purposes may be necessary in malignancies involving the spleen, such as myelofibrosis, Hodgkin lymphomas, and hairy cell leukemias.[5] In addition, in the case of splenic cysts, spleen-conserving techniques, such as laparoscopic partial splenectomy, unroofing, or fenestration of the cyst, can be safely performed.

For elective splenectomy in patients with splenomegaly, the foremost limitation to a minimally invasive approach is the surgeon's experience.[2] In addition, the laparoscopic approach may be contraindicated in emergent situations due to splenic trauma. The added time required to set up the laparoscopic equipment and position the patient, as well as the inability to effectively explore and pack the patient, may preclude a minimally invasive approach in emergent settings.

PREOPERATIVE EVALUATION AND PREPARATION

The preoperative evaluation is important in elective splenectomy to facilitate operative planning. A combination of abdominal exam and imaging is used to determine the exact size of the spleen. Preoperative abdominal computed tomography (CT) can accurately establish anatomic considerations, such as spleen size and vascular conditions.[3] Moderate splenomegaly (>11 cm) or severe splenomegaly (>20 cm) may change the operative approach to either an anterior, hand-assisted, or open technique as described

later. Preoperative imaging is not reliable in the detection of accessory splenic tissue, and therefore exploration at the onset of surgery is recommended to avoid disease recurrence, particularly in patients with autoimmune hematologic diseases.[3]

The spleen plays a major role in elimination of encapsulated organisms. Overwhelming postsplenectomy infection in the form of life-threatening sepsis is a major risk with a mortality rate of 40% to 50%. Therefore vaccination against *Streptococcus pneumoniae*, *Haemophilus influenzae* type B, and *Neisseria meningitides* should be administered at least 2 weeks prior to elective splenectomy.[5]

Because hematologic conditions are the most common indication for splenectomy, close communication with a hematologist in the perioperative period is important. For autoimmune thrombocytopenia (ITP), when the platelet count is below a certain threshold (generally <20 × 10⁹/L), preoperative steroids, immunoglobulins, and possibly intraoperative platelet transfusion are beneficial. Prednisone (1 mg/kg per day beginning 5 to 7 days before surgery) can be used to increase preoperative platelet counts. In addition, in certain cases, immunoglobulins (2 g/kg divided into two doses) may be given 48 hours prior to surgery. With thrombocytopenia (platelets <50,000), it is important to have platelets on standby for the operating room because it is most beneficial to transfuse platelets after ligation of the splenic artery.[5]

TECHNICAL CONSIDERATIONS

PATIENT POSITIONING

Laparoscopic splenectomy may be performed using a variety of positions, depending on surgeon preference, spleen size, need for concomitant procedures, and patient characteristics. The most widely used position is the lateral approach with the patient placed in left lateral decubitus position. The surgeon and assistant stand on the right side of the patient (Fig. 137.1A).

In this positioning the spleen and viscera fall medially due to gravity. This facilitates the dissection of the ligaments and hilar structures. Positioning devices, such as a bean bag or foam rolls, should be placed under the right flank, and a protective roll should be placed beneath the right axilla. The left arm is extended, and all bony prominences should be padded. It is important when positioning the patient to ensure the ability to hyperextend the left side with table flexion. This allows the surgeon to maximize the working space between the left costal margin and iliac crest. In correct positioning the flank muscles should appear taut. The patient's legs and torso should be secured to the table to allow safe intraoperative manipulation of the operating table.

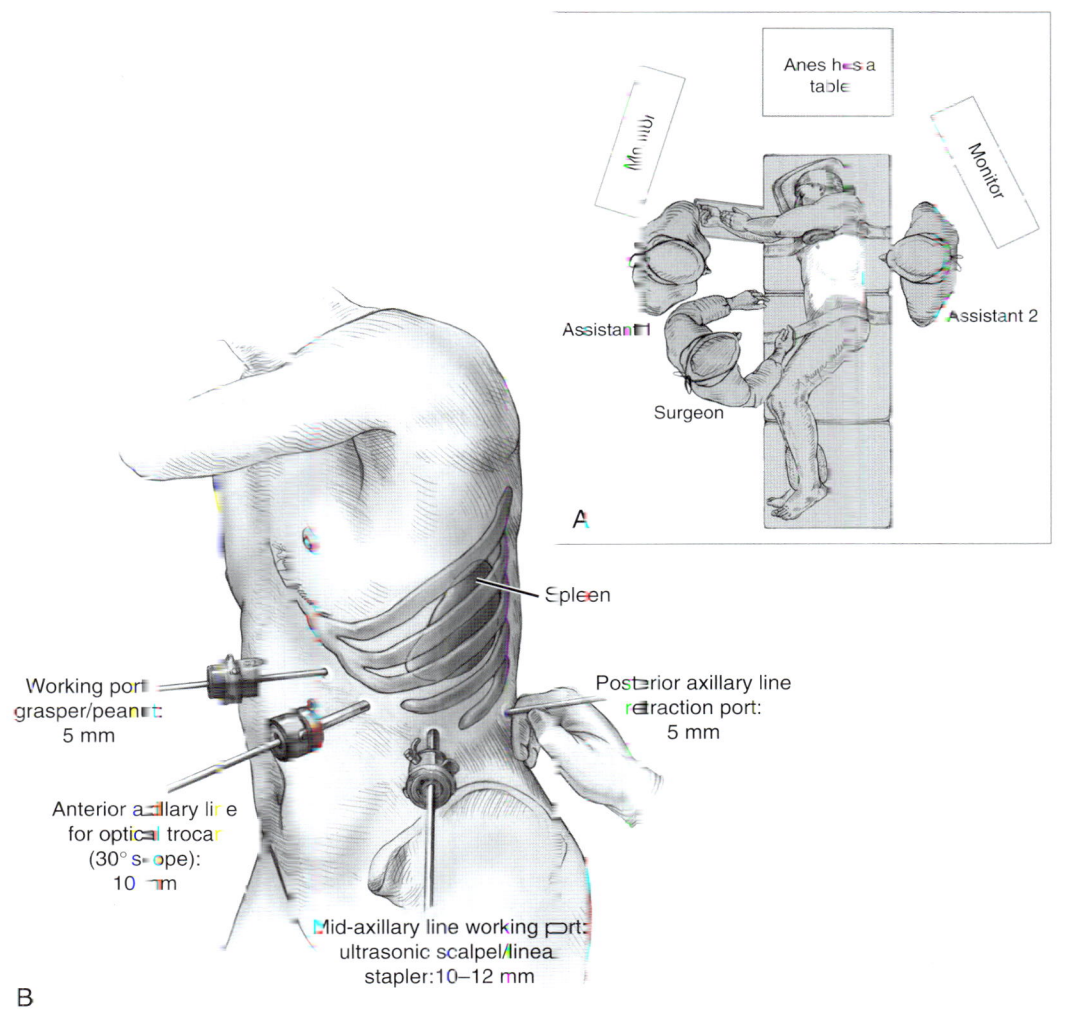

FIGURE 137.1 (A) Patient positioning and (B) trocar placement—lateral decubitus position. (Copyright Jennifer N. Gentry.)

Intravenous (IV) antibiotics (first-generation cephalosporin) are frequently used for operative prophylaxis. The surgical field is prepared with antiseptic solution extending from the nipple to the anterior iliac spine and from the umbilicus to the spine. An orogastric tube is used to decompress the stomach.

TROCAR PLACEMENT

The abdominal cavity is usually entered via the open (Hasson) technique under direct vision just medial to the left anterior axillary line approximately 2 cm below and parallel to the costal margin. After entrance into the peritoneal cavity is confirmed, a 10-mm trocar is placed and carbon dioxide is insufflated to a pressure of 15 mm Hg. A 10-mm, 30-degree angled laparoscope is used to allow improved visualization throughout the procedure. All additional trocars are placed under direct vision to ensure no injury to the viscera. A 10-mm trocar is placed under the 11th rib at the midaxillary line parallel to the costal margin, for the surgeon's right hand. A 5-mm trocar is placed along the midclavicular line lateral to the rectus muscle, medial and anterior to the optical trocar, for the

surgeon's left hand. A fourth 5-mm trocar may be placed dorsally at the costovertebral angle for additional retraction (after mobilization of the splenic flexure) (see Fig. 137.1B).

SURGICAL TECHNIQUE

It is important to perform a routine search for accessory spleens at the beginning of the procedure. The splenic flexure is mobilized inferomedially. This is best performed with a laparoscopic peanut in the surgeon's left hand for retraction and the ultrasonic scalpel in the surgeon's right hand. Alternatively, in patients with ITP, some surgeons prefer entering the lesser sac first and ligating the splenic artery first with 0-silk sutures to allow platelet transfusion prior to hilar dissection (Fig. 137.2).

The splenorenal and splenophrenic ligaments are divided to mobilize the spleen. Next, the lesser sac is entered. A Nathanson liver retractor may occasionally be helpful to retract the left lateral lobe of the liver to better expose the gastroesophageal junction and short gastric vessels. The short gastric vessels are divided with the ultrasonic scalpel. The remainder of the spleen is fully mobilized to the left crus.

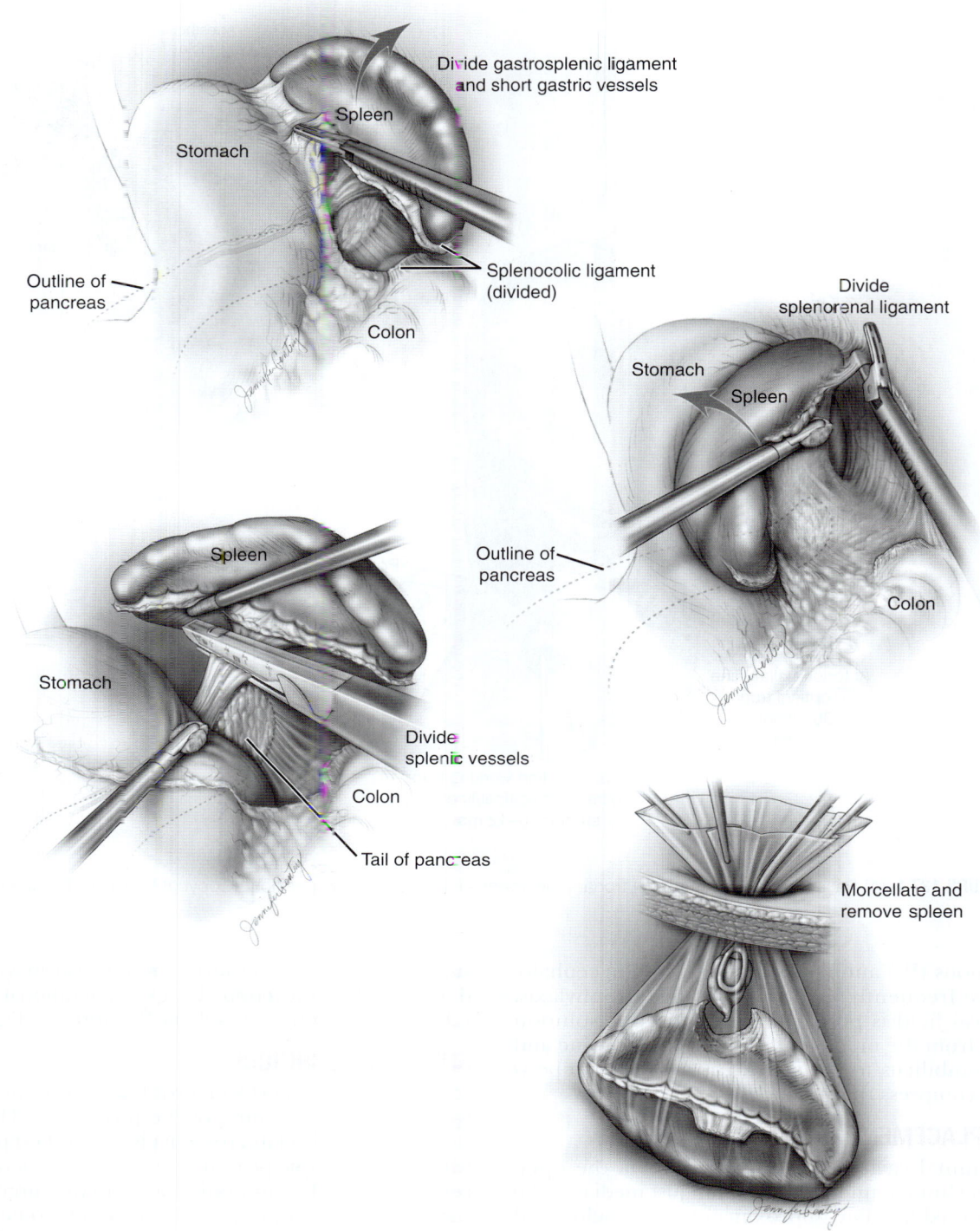

FIGURE 137.2 Surgical technique. (Copyright Jennifer N. Gentry.)

At this point the spleen may be elevated to identify the hilar structures. The most lateral trocar may be helpful to elevate the spleen (using a bowel grasper) to better expose the hilum and tail of pancreas. The peritoneum overlying the hilum is incised with the ultrasonic scalpel. After the hilum is freed from the pancreatic tail, the splenic vein and artery can be dissected. We prefer the 10-mm right angle dissector for dissection of the splenic vein and artery. We avoid clips in this area because they may interfere with appropriate firing of the stapler during transection. When feasible, we individually divide the hilar vessels with vascular load staplers. Alternatively, both the artery and vein can be divided en masse with one vascular load stapler. Some studies have demonstrated safe use of

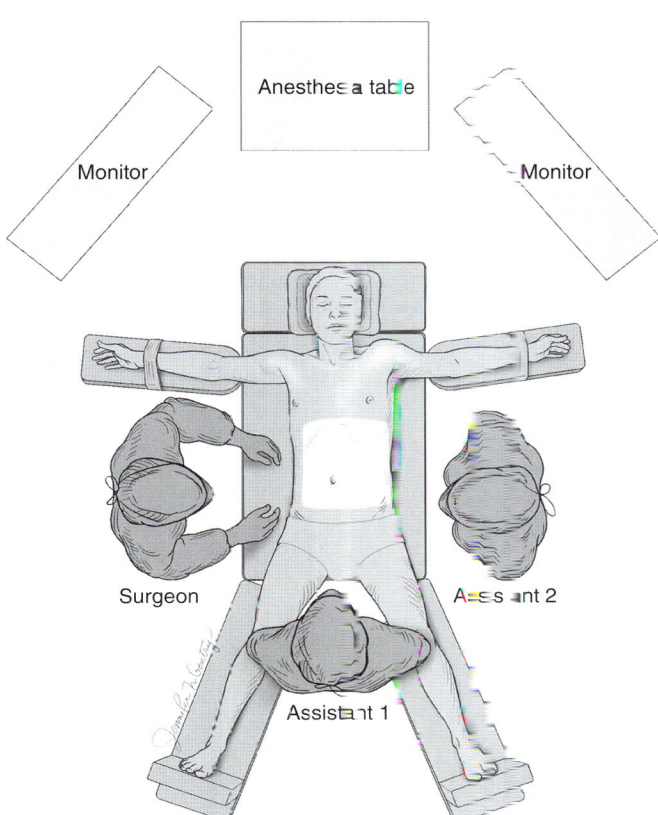

FIGURE 137.3 Alternate anterior approach for splenomegaly—split-leg positioning. (Copyright Jennifer N. Gentry.)

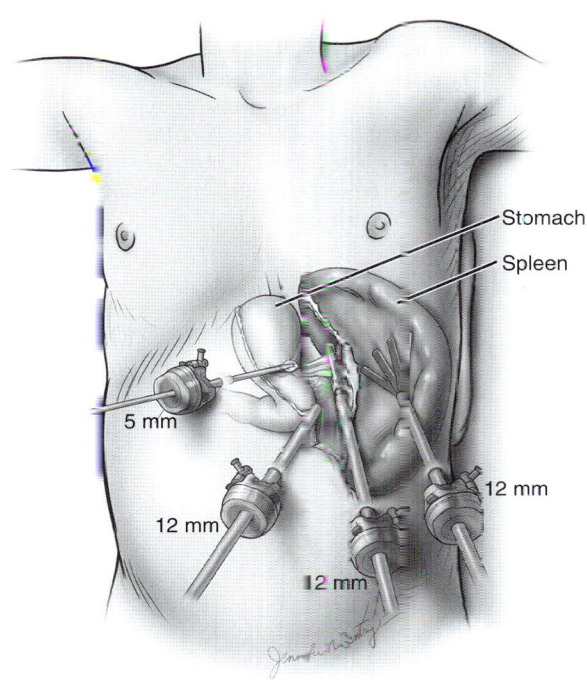

FIGURE 137.4 Trocar placement for splenomegaly. (Copyright Jennifer N. Gentry.)

the LigaSure (Covidien Medtronic, Minnesota) for hilar vessels with a diameter up to 7 mm in normal to moderately enlarged spleens.[5]

An Endo Catch bag (Covidien Medtronic) is used to remove the specimen. The opening of the bag is pulled through the trocar site, and ring forceps are used to morcellate the specimen. It is important to use an adequately durable extraction bag and blunt instruments during morcellation to prevent disruption of the bag and spillage of contents. Drains are not routinely left in the surgical bed. However, if there is concern for pancreatic injury due to extensive dissection of the pancreatic tail at the splenic hilum, a Jackson-Pratt (JP) drain should be placed and its output monitored postoperatively.

OTHER TECHNICAL CONSIDERATIONS INCLUDING SPLENOMEGALY

An alternative approach is to dissect the hilum first and mobilize the spleen after the hilum has been transected ("hanging spleen technique").[7] This takes advantage of the lateral decubitus position and provides exposure of the spleen, which "hangs" from the diaphragm by the peritoneal attachments. The inferior pole splenic vessels, short gastric vessels, and hilar vessels can be transected successively.

In the case of splenomegaly, we prefer the anterior approach (Fig. 137.3). The patient is placed in split-leg position and rotated 45 degrees to the right. The main challenge in massive splenomegaly is adequate retraction

for exposure of the hilum. An additional left lower quadrant trocar may be placed to allow use of the 10-mm fan liver retractor to retract the spleen (Fig. 137.4). If using the fan liver retractor, the utmost care needs to be exerted on the degree of retraction, to avoid injuring the spleen with resultant bleeding that may obscure the operative field.

For splenomegaly due to lymphoma, the hilar dissection may be difficult due to bulky lymphadenopathy. In these cases it may be safest to incise the peritoneum on the inferior border of the pancreas and create a posterior plane behind the tail of the pancreas, just proximal to the lymphadenopathy. Then staple across the most distal tail of the pancreas including the splenic vein with an Endo GIA (Covidien Medtronic, Minnesota) 60 mm blue or purple load buttressed with bioabsorbable Seamguard (Gore, Arizona).[8] In these instances we typically leave a 10-Fr JP drain in the splenic bed.

Specimen extraction for splenomegaly and massive splenomegaly may be challenging. If the 15-mm Endo Catch bag is not large enough, the LapSac (Cook Medical, Bloomington, Indiana) may be used.

Preoperative splenic artery embolization has been described to facilitate a minimally invasive approach in massive splenomegaly. We do not routinely practice this. It is our preference in these cases to preligate the splenic artery prior to hilar dissection.

POSTOPERATIVE CARE

The postoperative care of the patient is largely dependent on the clinical scenario. In general, patients may be started on a clear liquid diet in the evening of postoperative day zero or the following morning. Their diet may be advanced as tolerated. Pain is usually most severe at the specimen extraction site. Oral pain medications are typically sufficient to control postoperative pain. Ketorolac (nonsteroidal antiinflammatory) is a useful adjunct for effective pain control. Patients are frequently discharged home on the first or second postoperative day.

REFERENCES

1. Delaitre B, Maignien B, Icard P. Laparoscopic splenectomy. *Br J Surg*. 1992;79:1334.
2. Bo W, He-Shui W, Guo-Bin W, Kai-Xiong T. Laparoscopic splenectomy for massive splenomegaly. *J Invest Surg*. 2013;26:154-157.
3. Habermalz B, Sauerland S, Decker G, et al. Laparoscopic splenectomy: the clinical practice guidelines of the European Association for Endoscopic Surgery. *Surg Endosc*. 2008;22:821-848.
4. Maurus C, Schäfer M, Müller MK, Clavien PA, Weber M. Laparoscopic versus open splenectomy for nontraumatic diseases. *Would J Surg*. 2008;32:2444-2449.
5. Hammerquist RJ, Messerschmidt KA, Pottenbaum AA, Hellwig TR. Vaccinations in asplenic adults. *Am J Health Syst Pharm*. 2016;73:220-228.
6. Romano F, Caprotti R, Franciosi C, De Fina S, Colombo G, Uggeri F. Laparoscopic splenectomy using Ligasure: preliminary experience. *Surg Endosc*. 2002;16:1608-1611.
7. Delaitre B, Bonnichon P, Barthes T, Dousset B. Laparosopic splenectomy. The hanging spleen technique. *Ann Chir*. 1995;49:471-476.
8. Yamamoto M, Hayashi M, Nguyen N, Nyugen T, McCloud S, Imagawa DK. Use of Seamguard to prevent pancreatic leak following distal pancreatectomy. *Arch Surg*. 2009;144:894-899.

Minimally Invasive Surgical and Image-Guided Interventional Approaches to the Spleen

Ciro Andolfi | Jeffrey B. Matthews

The treatment of spleen disorders in modern surgery requires an extensive knowledge of traditional "open" surgical approaches, minimally invasive surgical procedures, and image-guided interventional techniques that can be tailored to the specific disease. The two sections of this chapter will focus on minimally invasive and image-guided interventional approaches to the spleen.

Minimally invasive approaches to the spleen were crafted upon the rapid expansion of laparoscopic surgery in the early 1990s. Laparoscopic splenectomy (LS) rapidly became the procedure of choice for elective surgery in patients with a normal-sized spleen. Due to its fragility, rich blood supply, and close anatomic relationships with colon, stomach, pancreas, and kidney, the spleen poses special challenges for laparoscopic surgery. However, due to improvements in minimally invasive techniques and instrumentation we are now able to perform more challenging surgeries.

Image-guided percutaneous interventional techniques for spleen disorders are becoming increasingly frequent. This trend started in the early 1970s when Maddison reported the first successful splenic artery embolization in a patient with hepatic cirrhosis and recurrent gastrointestinal bleeding.[1] Today, therapeutic embolization continues to play an important role in managing splenic problems and, for selected patients, it is considered a safe and effective alternative to surgical splenectomy.

MINIMALLY INVASIVE SURGERY FOR THE SPLEEN

LS, first described in 1991 by Delaitre and Maignien, has rapidly gained worldwide acceptance as the first-line treatment for patients requiring elective splenectomy for normal-sized spleens. Conversion to open splenectomy is reported in less than 4% of cases—intraoperative bleeding being the most frequent cause.[2] Improvements in laparoscopic techniques and instrumentation enable us to attempt the laparoscopic approach with more challenging cases, including patients with larger spleen or spleens in complex reoperative settings. The benefits from a minimally invasive approach are those of minimally invasive surgery established for other procedures and include reduced blood loss, better pain control, decreased perioperative morbidity, and shorter hospital length of stay.[3–5]

INDICATIONS

Trauma

Trauma is the most common cause of death in people under the age of 45 years. Moreover, recent data from the Center for Disease Control and Prevention show that nearly 200,000 people die from injury every year. Among these patients, the prevalence of intraabdominal injuries is about 15%, with the spleen being the most injured organ.[6,7] Accordingly trauma is the most common indication for splenectomy, with the vast majority of these being performed via laparotomy. However, over the past 30 years, efforts to preserve functional splenic tissue wherever feasible have been increasingly emphasized. As a consequence of this, the treatment of patients with blunt splenic injury has shifted from operative to nonoperative management. The current literature shows that 60% to 90% of patients are treated nonoperatively, and the accepted criteria for operative management are hemodynamic instability and associated intraabdominal or pelvic injury, which all require surgery.[8] In the management of the injured spleen, the laparoscopic approach appears to have limited indications, and most trauma surgeons view minimally invasive surgery as contraindicated in major abdominal trauma.[9] Only a few studies in literature report the performance of LS in the setting of blunt trauma, without conversion or major morbidity, and it has been suggested that laparoscopy may be reasonable in hemodynamically stable patients with spleen injury grade III (Table 138.1). Instead, there is absolute contraindication in patients with hemodynamic instability and high bleeding rate (>500 mL/h).[10,11] Furthermore, delayed LS may also be safe—especially if combined with adjunctive preoperative embolization, which appears to reduce the risk of continued or delayed hemorrhage. Delayed splenectomy is required in some of these patients because of continued bleeding or infarction with abscess formation. Successful delayed LS in this setting has been reported.[12,13] In addition, laparoscopic techniques can be used to selectively apply electrocautery, fibrin, Gelfoam, suture repair, or to perform a partial splenectomy to control bleeding and preserve splenic tissue.[14–18]

Although some authors have shown that laparoscopy can be a safe tool in the armamentarium for the treatment of splenic injury, additional studies are needed to define the selection criteria for these patients.[11,14,18,19]

Hematologic Disorders

Indications for elective LS are similar to "open" splenectomy, and the most common is hematologic disorders. For a normal-sized spleen, LS has now achieved standard-of-care status. Benign hematologic diseases such as idiopathic thrombocytopenic purpura (ITP), thrombotic thrombopenic purpura, human immunodeficiency virus (HIV)-related thrombocytopenia, hereditary spherocytosis, autoimmune hemolytic anemia, thalassemia intermedia, thalassemia major, sickle cell disease, and Evans syndrome

TABLE 138.1 American Association for the Surgery of Trauma Organ Injury Scale Spleen

Grade	Injury Type	Description of Injury
I	Hematoma	Subcapsular: <10% surface area
	Laceration	Capsular tear: <1 cm parenchymal depth
II	Hematoma	Subcapsular: 10%–50% surface area; intraparenchymal <5 cm in diameter
	Laceration	1–3 cm parenchymal depth that does not involve a trabecular vessel
III	Hematoma	Subcapsular: >50% surface area or expanding; ruptured subcapsular or parenchymal hematoma; intraparenchymal hematoma >5 cm or expanding
	Laceration	>3 cm parenchymal depth or involving trabecular vessels
IV	Laceration	Laceration involving segmental or hilar vessels producing major devascularization (>25% of the spleen)
V	Laceration	Completely shattered spleen
	Vascular	Hilar vascular injury with devascularized spleen

BOX 138.1 Indications for Laparoscopic Splenectomy

PLATELET DISORDERS
Idiopathic thrombocytopenic purpura
Human immunodeficiency virus–related idiopathic thrombocytopenic purpura
Thrombotic thrombocytopenic purpura
Evans syndrome

ANEMIAS/RED BLOOD CELL DISORDERS
Autoimmune hemolytic anemia
Hereditary spherocytosis
Hereditary elliptocytosis
Hereditary pyropoikilocytosis
White blood cell disorders/malignancy
Hodgkin lymphoma
Non-Hodgkin lymphoma
Chronic myeloid leukemia
Chronic lymphocytic leukemia
Hairy cell leukemia
Myelofibrosis
Primary splenic tumors

MISCELLANEOUS
Splenic abscess
Splenic cysts
Splenic trauma
Sarcoidosis
Hypersplenism—Gaucher disease, Felty syndrome, systemic lupus erythematosus, splenic vein thrombosis

are the absolute indications. Relative indications are unresponsiveness to medical therapy, disease relapse, splenomegaly, frequent transfusions, adverse effects, or dependency on steroid therapy.[20–42] Current literature suggests that in patients who come under any of the previously mentioned indications, LS should be offered as the surgical treatment of choice.[21,25,26,36,37] Among hematologic disorders, the most common indication is idiopathic thrombocytopenic purpura.[43–45] Kovaleva et al. reviewed their 20-year experience with more than 1000 ITP patients. First-line treatment for ITP remains medical therapy, usually steroids. Second-line treatment after failure of medical therapy is splenectomy, which achieves 80% remission, with good long-term results (60 months or longer) in 32% of patients.[46]

Box 138.1 summarizes the indications for LS.

Contraindications

Absolute contraindications in the setting of hematologic disorders are uncorrected coagulopathy, severe comorbidities that increase the operative risks, and hematologic malignancies localized outside of the spleen.[23,47,48] A low platelet count (<10×10^9/L) should no longer be considered as an absolute contraindication.[40] Current literature states that the increased surgical experience, as well as advances in laparoscopic techniques and instruments, have made it possible to operate on patients with low platelet counts safely and effectively.[24] Although the European Association for Endoscopic Surgery guidelines consider portal hypertension as an absolute contraindication for LS,[49] several publications reported on the safety of this method in patients with cirrhosis and portal hypertension.[39,50–54] Cai et al., for instance, described 24 successful cases of splenectomy for hypersplenism in cirrhotic patients.[55]

Absolute contraindications in the setting of trauma are splenic injury grade IV and V (see Table 138.1), and acute hemorrhage, with a bleeding rate greater than 500 mL/h on serial ultrasound examinations.

PATIENT SELECTION

Spleen size remains the most important determinant in patient selection for elective open versus LS, as well as in predicting success of the minimally invasive surgical approach. LS should be performed with caution in cases of massive splenomegaly, which is defined as a maximum spleen diameter greater than 25 cm, or as an estimated spleen volume exceeding 1000 mL. Under these circumstances, laparoscopy is correlated with higher conversion rate, and intra- and postoperative complications.[21,25,26,56,37] At a threshold of 500 g for defining a "large" spleen, there are no differences in conversion rates, lengths of stay, or complications.[56] However, at a threshold of 1000 g, conversion rates for large spleens may approach 60%.[57] Few surgeons use 2 kg as an exclusion criteria for LS.[58] Although spleen weight can retrospectively correlate with minimally invasive splenectomy success or failure, it is difficult to assess preoperatively. Spleen size based on computed tomography (CT) or ultrasound imaging measurements provides a more practical preoperative selection criterion. As a guideline, spleen size on ultrasound or CT scan should be less than 20 to 25 cm in the craniocaudal axis.[57–59] Larger spleens have been removed laparoscopically, but the procedure is technically demanding due to the limited abdominal working space, an increased risk of bleeding, and difficulty in retrieving the spleen. If LS is chosen, it can be performed using the same surgical technique, providing that the ports are placed more caudally on the abdominal wall, according to the location of the lower pole of the spleen.[48] For these patients, hand-assisted LS has been proposed as an effective, safe, and feasible alternative.[26,35,60,61] Analyzing the feasibility of LS in cases of massive splenomegaly (spleen weight >2000 g), Al-Mulhim et al.[22] concluded that although LS was feasible in 90% of patients, the condition was significantly associated with prolonged operative time, more blood loss, increased postoperative morbidity, and prolonged postoperative hospital stay. Splenic weight above a cutoff value of 1311.5 g has been proposed to be associated with higher risk of conversion and transfusion, and has also been found to be a significant independent risk factor for portal and splenic vein thrombosis after LS.[38]

Laparoscopic success may be improved by preoperative splenic artery embolization, and a hand-assisted technique. Grahn reported a 10-year retrospective review of LS for 85 patients of whom 25 (29%) had massive or supermassive spleens, with an increasing number of these (40% to 50%) approached laparoscopically during the later years of the study. Despite the increase in giant spleens in the minimally invasive group, conversion rates declined from 33% halfway through the 10-year period to 0% for the final 2 years of the study, with no reoperations for bleeding and no deaths.[44] This study showed that experience remains a key predictor of successful LS.

PREOPERATIVE CONSIDERATIONS

Imaging

Preoperative imaging with ultrasound and/or CT scan is essential for operative planning. Imaging can help assess spleen size and can also delineate useful anatomic relationships that impact the conduct of surgery. The normal spleen measures about 11 cm in length. Moderate splenomegaly, from 11 to 25 cm, should be noted in preoperative planning. Massive splenomegaly, greater than 25 cm length, may change preoperative and intraoperative strategy. Preoperative imaging may also identify accessory spleens, reported in 10% to 20% of patients. In addition, ultrasound is critical in trauma settings because it helps the decision-making process by assessing the bleeding rate.

Although not indicated for a normal-sized spleen, preoperative splenic artery embolization can be useful in patients with massive splenomegaly. Timing is important because patients can develop significant pain from infarcted splenic tissue; it is suggested to perform angioembolization within 24 hours before surgery. Preoperative angioembolization of the splenic artery for LS is safe and reduces the conversion rate.[7]

General Considerations: Antibiotic Prophylaxis, Deep Venous Thrombosis Prophylaxis, Bowel Preparation

A broad-spectrum antibiotic prophylaxis should be administered at the time of induction to anesthesia and continued postoperatively for at least 24 hours.[22,25,2] Patients undergoing splenectomy for a hematologic disorder should undergo the same preparation that they would for open splenectomy, which may include administration of steroids, immune globulin, fresh-frozen plasma, cryoprecipitate, or platelets. Blood products must be available intraoperatively,

especially platelets for patients with severe thrombocytopenia. Prophylactic platelet transfusions are typically given only when the platelet count is below 50,000 and the platelets are administered only after the splenic artery has been ligated.[43]

All patients require deep venous thrombosis (DVT) prophylaxis, including pneumatic sequential compression devices,[25,26] pre- and postoperative low-dose subcutaneous unfractionated heparin prophylaxis, and early postoperative ambulation.[5,28,35] Controversy remains over the length of postoperative DVT prophylaxis. For high-risk patients, DVT prophylaxis should be considered up to and beyond 14 days after surgery.

Bowel preparation before splenectomy is not mandatory. A limited prep the night before surgery may clear the left colon of stool bulk, with the purposes of improving colon mobilization and avoiding postoperative constipation.

Immunization Against Overwhelming Postsplenectomy Infection

Patients who undergo splenectomy are at increased risk of overwhelming postsplenectomy infection (OPSI), with a lifetime risk of 3% to 5%. The annual incidence of OPSI is between 0.23% and 0.42%. Risk is highest in three groups: (1) patients at the extremes of age, (2) immunocompromised patients, and (3) patients with hematologic disorders. Previously healthy patients who require splenectomy due to trauma are the lowest risk groups. When OPSI occurs, it is a true emergency, can be lethal, and requires immediate parenteral antibiotics and intensive care support. Intravenous immunoglobulin may play a beneficial role. OPSI carries a mortality rate of 38% to 69%. In general, OPSI results from decreased antigenic clearance, loss of opsonization, and decreased immunologic response. *Streptococcus pneumoniae* is the most common infective agent isolated in 50% to 90% of patients, followed by *Haemophilus influenzae* type B (Hib), *Streptococcus* group B, *Staphylococcus aureus*, *Escherichia coli*, and other coliforms. Increased susceptibility to parasites and malaria is noted in endemic areas. Increased risk to *Neisseria meningitidis* infection has not been documented but remains a theoretical risk.[62,63] Ideally, immunization against encapsulated organisms should be given 14 days prior to surgery.[25,26] Recommended immunizations include polyvalent pneumococcal, meningococcal, and *Haemophilus* vaccination.[23] Pneumovax provides protection against 73% of OPSI-causing organisms. Data on revaccination remain unclear, but current consensus favors a Pneumovax booster every 5 to 10 years, which may be protective against all OPSI bacteria. Hib/Meningococcal/Influenza vaccine benefit is unconfirmed but recommended. For patients who do not receive recommended OPSI immunizations prior to surgery (such as trauma patients), vaccination is performed just before hospital discharge and is preferred over relying on patient compliance.

OPERATIVE APPROACH

There is wide variation in the technique of LS with respect to approach, patient positioning, port site placement, number of ports, and instrumentation.

Minimally invasive surgery requires a high-technology environment. The surgeon should review with the operative team the equipment as part of the "time out" before the procedure starts to ensure that all instruments are available, including the following: video towers with high-definition cameras, insufflator, high-intensity light source, video-capture device, preferred energy sources (Harmonic scalpel, LigaSure, etc.), angled telescope (preferably a 45-degree telescope), suction irrigator, additional laparoscopic ports (if needed), laparoscopic retractor, retrieval bags, endoscopic staplers, endoclips, morcellator (if needed), and other special tools such as hand-assist devices.

Anatomic Considerations

LS is not a forgiving procedure. Methodical control of the hemostasis is the key for success. The splenic parenchyma is fragile, has a rich blood supply, and is particularly vulnerable to capsular tear and hemorrhage. Understanding the variation of splenic anatomy is essential for a safe intraoperative management.

Michels' 1942 review of 100 spleens suggested that no two spleens have the same anatomy.[64] Michels divided splenic blood supply into two types: distributed and magistral—with the distributed type being present in 70% of patients. Splenic size does not correlate with the number or distribution of splenic arteries, although the number of splenic notches and tubercles does. Splenic hilar anatomy can include numerous branches with various division levels. In addition, six or more short gastric arteries may be found in the gastrosplenic ligament arising from the fundus of the stomach. The lienorenal ligament contains hilar vessels and the tail of the pancreas. In nearly three-quarters of patients, the tail of the pancreas lies within 1 cm from the spleen, and direct contact between pancreas and spleen is found in about one-third of patients.[64]

Technique of Laparoscopic Splenectomy

There are eight steps to LS:
1. Positioning and safe access to establish pneumoperitoneum
2. Diagnostic laparoscopy, including a search for accessory spleens
3. Mobilization of the spleen with dissection of splenic ligaments
4. Division of the splenic vessels, including splenic hilum and short gastric vessels
5. Division of remaining attachments completely detaching the spleen and spleen placement within a specimen bag
6. Extraction of the spleen within the specimen bag from the peritoneal cavity
7. Inspection of the operative field for hemostasis, pancreatic injury, etc.
8. Removal of trocars, abdomen desufflation, and port site closure

Step 1: Positioning and Safe Access for Pneumoperitoneum

Anterior Approach. The anterior approach was the first LS technique to be described. However, after 15 years of experience with LS worldwide, it is seldom used today. The anterior approach may be better suited when the spleen is very large, particularly with prior splenic artery embolization, and when the hand-assist technique is to be employed. The anterior approach may also be preferable if other procedures such as diagnostic laparoscopy

or cholecystectomy are planned, as in patients with spherocytosis.

The operation begins with safe laparoscopic abdominal access. This can be accomplished with an open or closed technique and depends on the skill, experience, and comfort level of the surgeon. Although an open cutdown technique for the direct insertion of the first trocar is sometimes favored, an optical trocar technique with preinsufflation using a Veress needle can be quite useful, especially in patients who are obese. The use of the Veress needle is contraindicated in patients with massive splenomegaly or severe thrombocytopenia and in children because of the limited working space and risk of splenic injury. The laparoscopic insufflator is preset for abdominal pressure at 12 mm Hg or less to minimize the untoward effects of intraabdominal hypertension. Port size is the surgeon's choice. However, it is useful to place at least one 10- to 12-mm port to have immediate access for use of an endoscopic stapler or large endoclips device. Port locations also vary according to individual surgeon preference but generally include three to four additional ports in a V-shaped placement adjacent to the left upper quadrant, with the initial port for the camera at the base of the V. One line of the V extends from the initial port to the xiphoid process; the other line of the V extends from the initial port to the most lateral left subcostal region. Two dissection ports are placed, one near the midline and one along the lateral V line. A 10- to 12-mm port at this location may be preferable because it is the likely port for introduction of an endoscopic stapler or endoclips device. An additional port for retraction is placed further lateral at the anterior axillary line (Fig. 138.1). If a fifth port is necessary for retraction, it is placed in the subxiphoid position. The patient is then placed in reverse Trendelenburg and tilted slightly to the right. The surgeon stands between the legs if the patient is in low lithotomy position, or adjacent to the right hip if the patient lies supine, with the monitor placed at the head of the bed to the patient's left. Surgical assistants and the scrub nurse stand at the patient's sides.[65,66]

Lateral Approach. The lateral approach is useful for normal or moderately enlarged spleens and has several

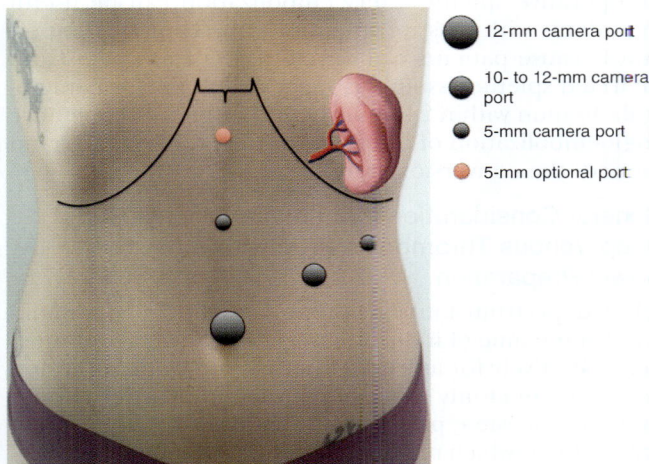

FIGURE 138.1 Laparoscopic splenectomy, anterior approach.

12-mm camera port

10- to 12-mm camera port

5-mm camera port

5-mm optional port

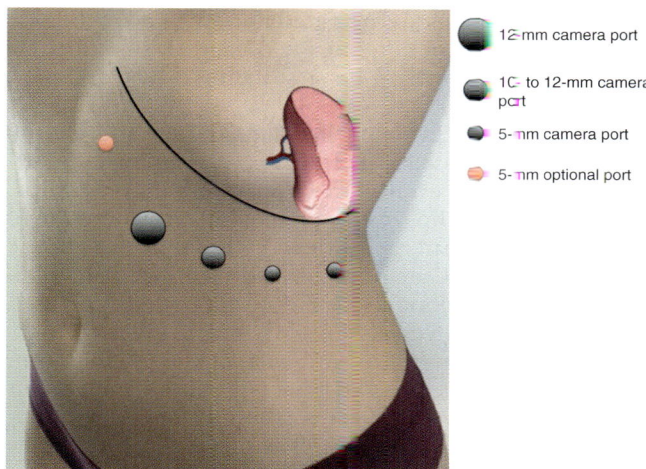

12-mm camera port

10- to 12-mm camera port

5-mm camera port

5-mm optional port

FIGURE 138.2 Laparoscopic splenectomy, lateral approach.

advantages if compared to the anterior approach. It is technically easier, it allows access to the splenic vasculature through the relatively avascular retroperitoneum, and decreases inadvertent trauma to the spleen because gravity helps in retraction along with the instruments. Dissection planes are opened more easily, enhancing identification of key ligaments and dissection planes, and the tail of the pancreas is more accessible and less susceptible to injury.

The position is similar to that used for posterolateral thoracotomy and/or laparoscopic left adrenalectomy. Patients are initially positioned supine on a beanbag. Once general anesthesia is established and the airway is secured, the operative team repositions the patient in lateral decubitus with the right side down. Care is taken to ensure adequate padding, including placing an axillary roll. The beanbag is desufflated, and additional tapes are placed to secure the patient. Security and safety of patient positioning must be tested by moving the operating table. The kidney rest is raised, and the operating table is flexed. The goal is to maximize the working space between the left costal margin and the left anterior superior iliac spine.

As with the anterior approach, an optical trocar technique with preinsufflation through a Veress needle is the preferred method. In the lateral decubitus, however, the umbilicus is avoided, and the first port is positioned approximately one-third the distance from the umbilicus to the splenic hilum. After securing access to the peritoneal cavity, typically three additional ports are placed along the costal margin. Depending on the spleen size and body habitus, it may be necessary to place the trocars inferiorly or medially. A 10- to 12-mm port, capable of accommodating an endostapler or large endoclips device, is typically placed in the left subcostal anterior axillary line. A 5-mm port is placed in the left subcostal region in the midaxillary line. A fourth port, usually 5 mm, is placed in the far left lateral subcostal position. Occasionally an additional port is required for retraction toward the midline near the xiphoid process (Fig. 138.2).

Step 2: Diagnostic Laparoscopy, Including a Search for Accessory Spleens. Diagnostic laparoscopy is performed to survey the abdominal cavity, confirm location of the spleen, assess anatomic relationships of adjacent organs

(colon, stomach, pancreas, etc.), search for accessory spleens, and plan operative strategy.

Up to 20% of people harbor an accessory spleen. The vast majority of patients have only one accessory spleen. However, as many as 20% of patients with accessory spleens have two, and up to 17% have three or more. Accessory spleens range in size from 0.2 cm to 10 cm but typically are less than 1.5 cm in diameter. Approximately two-thirds of them are located at or near the splenic hilum; 20% are close to the tail of the pancreas. The remainder are found in the omentum, along the splenic artery, in the mesentery, or along the left gonadal vessels.[67,68] When the presence of accessory spleens is suspected and a complete splenectomy is necessary to treat the underlying hematologic condition, preoperative imaging with technetium scan may be helpful. This technique can be supplemented by intraoperative localization with laparoscopic gamma probe, after preoperative administration of technetium.

Step 3: Mobilization of the Spleen With Dissection of Splenic Ligaments. Although some surgeons describe a step-by-step approach to the laparoscopic dissection, variable splenic anatomy often forces a "strategy of opportunity." Laparoscopic dissection begins by partially mobilizing the splenic flexure of the left colon, dividing the splenocolic ligament, the distal phrenocolic ligament, and the sustentaculum lienis. This dissection can be accomplished with endoscopic scissors, Harmonic scalpel, or other endosurgical electrocautery devices. This dissection creates access to the gastrosplenic ligament, which is then easily separated from the splenorenal ligament. The lower pole of the spleen is carefully elevated. When dissecting the splenocolic and splenorenal ligament, it is important to leave a remnant of the ligament, which will be used as a handle to avoid grasping the splenic capsule. The dissection continues medially and cranially, with the spleen gradually rolling laterally. This maneuver provides access to the hilum. A cautious, stepwise approach is taken to divide the phrenocolic ligament, enabling the spleen to be rolled laterally away from the tail of the pancreas, exposing the hilum.

Step 4: Division of the Splenic Vessels, Including Splenic Hilum and Short Gastric Vessels. Vascular anatomy can be "distributed" or "magistral." The vascular pattern can usually be recognized by inspecting the inner surface of the spleen during initial laparoscopy. If the vessels appear to cover more than three-quarters of the surface, a distributed pattern is present. If the vessels appear to enter the spleen more uniformly and cover only one-third of the splenic surface, a magistral pattern is present. In the more commonly encountered distributed variant, there is a short splenic vascular trunk and many long branches entering along the medial surface of the spleen. Division of the distributed array of splenic vessels can be performed using sequential applications of an energy source device and endoclips.

The less-common magistral pattern is characterized by a long main splenic artery that divides into short branches close to the hilum.[65,67,69] The optimal approach for this pattern is to isolate the hilum as much as possible, preparing a window to access with an endoscopic linear stapler. The final goal is to identify and isolate the splenic artery and vein and to achieve a separate vascular control, avoiding the risk of bleeding and the theoretical concern of an arteriovenous fistula. One potentially helpful maneuver before staple firing is using an atraumatic bowel grasper to mimic the staple transection. Subsequently, short gastric vessels are divided. Care must be taken with the use of energy devices to avoid gastric necrosis and resultant gastric fistula.

Step 5: Division of Remaining Attachments and Spleen Placement Into a Specimen Bag. The final mobilization of the spleen is completed by dividing the proximal phrenocolic ligament along its entire length to the diaphragm and left crus. Careful dissection ensures complete mobilization of the spleen for safe placement in the specimen bag. Placing the spleen into the bag can be a difficult and frustrating portion of LS. Several different retrieval sacs are available. The surgeon should make sure that these sacs are sturdy enough to prevent rupture and large enough to envelop the entire spleen. Some surgeons prefer leaving the superior-most portion of the phrenosplenic ligament intact. This method leaves the spleen tethered to the diaphragm, and can facilitate its placement into the endoscopic bag. Opening the bag widely and having a handle can greatly facilitate placement of the spleen into the retrieval sac. Some surgeons have used sterilized medium or large, heavy-duty plastic freezer bags as an acceptable alternative.[66,70,71] After the spleen is placed in the bag, it is extracted under direct laparoscopic visualization through a 12-mm trocar site.

Step 6: Extraction of the Spleen From the Peritoneal Cavity. Morcellation or piecemeal extraction of the spleen is then undertaken, unless the spleen must be removed intact for pathologic purpose. The endoscopic bag is usually grasped and extracted through a port site. When the anterior approach is used, the extraction site is the umbilicus. When the lateral approach is used, extraction of the specimen bag is often through one of the lateral left subcostal ports. Typically, the surgeon morcellates the spleen within the bag, allowing extraction of fragments through the small port incision. Caution is needed to avoid crashing the bag, as peritoneal spillage can lead to splenosis (disseminated splenic implantation), a particularly troubling problem after splenectomy for hematologic disorders. Rarely it is necessary to enlarge the incision. For larger spleens, extraction may be preferred through a Pfannenstiel incision, or through a hand port incision, if a hand-assisted laparoscopic surgery (HALS) device has been used.

Step 7: Inspection of the Operative Field. After the spleen has been successfully extracted, the operative field is carefully inspected for hemostasis, previously undetected accessory spleens, or other unexpected damages. No surgical drains are needed, reflecting the established experience from open surgery. The exception to this guideline is the presence of pancreatic tail injury. In this case a closed suction drain along the pancreatic tail is recommended.

Step 8: Removal of Trocars, Pneumoperitoneum Cessation, and Port Site Closure. Once the operative team is satisfied with inspection of the operative field, all ports are removed under direct visualization. The abdomen is desufflated. Fascia at all port sites greater than 5 mm in diameter are closed. Port sites are irrigated and injected with local anesthetic. The skin edges are closed with subcuticular closure, and Steri-Strips or tissue sealant is placed, followed by simple dressings.

Tips Regarding Evolving Instrumentation and Energy Sources. Larger vessels are often challenging for standard endoclip control, even with larger metallic endoclips. Self-locking endoclips are available and provide control of larger vessels. Energy devices such as the Harmonic Scalpel (Ethicon, Cincinnati, Ohio) and LigaSure (Valleyabs, Boulder, Colorado) have evolved; both can be used to divide and seal vessels up to 7 mm in diameter.[72-75] Each device has strengths and weaknesses. The 10-mm LigaSure has a lower risk of adjacent tissue damage, but it is cumbersome to use for a splenic hilar dissection. The 5-mm diameter LigaSure is easier to use but results in higher risks of adjacent tissue damage because of its smaller surface area to absorb the impedance of the device. The 5-mm diameter Harmonic scalpel has a gentle curve to facilitate dissection but it should be used with caution to avoid contact with adjacent tissues, and to ensure that the device is completely across target vessels to seal them. Both Harmonic scalpel and LigaSure technologies are safe, effective, and have shortened operative times.

Minimally Invasive Surgery Approaches to Massive Spleens

Hand-Assisted Laparoscopic Splenectomy. LS is the standard of care for normal to moderately enlarged spleens. However, to successfully manage massive spleens, minimal-access splenectomy employing hybrid technologies such as HALS has proved beneficial in patients with splenomegaly (craniocaudal length >22 cm or width >19 cm).[59,60,61,76] For inexperienced surgeons, HALS may shorten the learning curve; for experienced surgeons, it may facilitate minimally invasive splenectomy for massively enlarged spleens that otherwise would not be amenable to a purely laparoscopic approach.[77,78]

HALS can be used with the anterior or lateral approach because it uses a combination of laparoscopic and open splenectomy techniques. HALS employs a device to enable intraabdominal placement of a hand and forearm, usually the nondominant, through a small incision. The HALS device, while maintaining the pneumoperitoneum, facilitates performing laparoscopic surgery. In addition, HALS improves manipulation of instruments intraabdominally, assists in restoring depth perception and three-dimensional (3D) orientation, and can serve as a bridge to enhance laparoscopic skills.

Optimal placement of the hand port is important. There is a need for "stand-off" distance between the hand port and the target organ so that the surgeon's hand has working room within the abdomen and does not interfere with laparoscopic instruments and visualization. The incision should be 7 to 8 cm (or 1 cm less than the surgeon's glove size) and should be located 2 to 4 cm caudal to the inferior pole of the enlarged spleen. Options for hand port placement include the midline just above the umbilicus, the lower midline, or the left lower quadrant using a muscle-splitting incision. The most common location for the hand port is in the midline, between the xiphoid and the umbilicus. For massive spleens, a Pfannenstiel incision has also been described.[59,69,79] Pneumoperitoneum is established after the hand port is placed.

The biggest technical challenge is to avoid hemorrhage. Small series have reported successful HALS splenectomy for severe splenomegaly, with spleen mean length of 27.9 cm (range, 23 to 32 cm), with acceptable operative times, morbidity, and outcomes.[79] Petrabissa et al. reported a 10-year retrospective registry review of 85 splenectomies comparing 43 patients who underwent HALS to 42 patients who underwent conventional laparoscopy, with spleens weighing more than 700 g in the HALS group. Rates of conversion to open surgery and perioperative mortality were similar. Of note, the incidence of portal venous thrombosis was also similar in both groups. With HALS, a minimally invasive surgical option can also be offered to patients with massive splenomegaly.[61,8]

Emerging Minimally Invasive Options

Single-Port Laparoscopic Splenectomy Single-port access (SPA) is an alternative to traditional multiport laparoscopy, with the goal of exploiting proven benefits of minimally invasive surgery through a single umbilical incision. The use of SPA is controversial, and technical issues such as decreased triangulation and iatrogenic hernia at the port site are still a matter of debate in the surgical community. The evolution to flexible and/or curved instruments and adoption of crossing instrument techniques is helping to address these challenges.

Curcillo et al., a group of SPA pioneers, reported a single-port splenectomy for a patient with normal-sized spleen, using standard instrumentation to lower costs and increase familiarity with the procedure. Outcomes at 18-month follow-up were good and no hernia at the port site was reported.[81] Targarona et al. described a series of eight successful single-incision laparoscopic surgeries (SILS). Six out of eight patients underwent splenectomy.[32] Monclova et al., in a more recent study, compared LS to reduced-port access splenectomy (RPAS) and to single-port access splenectomy (SPAS) for the treatment of patients suffering from benign hematologic disorders. Blood loss and morbidity were similar in the three groups, as were the clinical outcomes in terms of complications, reoperation, and duration of hospital stay. No patients were converted to laparotomy, but three patients in the SPAS group required additional trocars.[31] Successful single-port laparoscopy has also been described for a more challenging procedure, such as partial splenectomy.[83] However, these results are insufficient to establish any evidence of superiority of SPAS over LS, apart from the better postoperative comfort and cosmetic result.

Robot-Assisted Laparoscopic Splenectomy. Robotic surgery restores a three-dimensional view, allows greater degrees of freedom, and improves surgical precision. Limitations are the absence of haptic feedback, the costs, and the unproven benefit for some procedures where laparoscopy is still the gold standard. The robotic approach has been reported by few authors and it has been proposed as a valuable option for complex situations, such as partial splenectomy for patients with splenomegaly.[84,85] However, its role in the treatment of splenic disease still remains unclear.[86] A retrospective review compared six robot-assisted splenectomies to six laparoscopic splenectomies—all for ITP, with patients matched for age, American Society

of Anesthesiologists score, body mass index (BMI), and preoperative platelet levels. There were no conversions. No complications were reported. Mean postoperative stay was 1 day longer, and costs were almost one-third higher in the robotic group. Operative time was approximately 20% longer with the robot. This analysis failed to show any relevant benefit with robot-assisted splenectomy.[87] Another comparative study by Gelmini et al. retrospectively reviewed two well-matched groups of 45 patients, finding no differences in intraoperative blood loss, conversion to laparotomy, return to diet, morbidity, and length of stay.[88]

Natural Orifice Transluminal Endoscopic Surgery for Splenectomy. Natural orifice transluminal endoscopic surgery (NOTES) represents another potential step in the evolution of minimally invasive surgery, with the promise of "no scar." NOTES remains premature in clinical experience and application. Since Reddy and Rau's first video of a NOTES appendectomy in 2004, the evolution of this approach has been very slow. Transvaginal extraction of a laparoscopically dissected spleen was described in the early 1990s but has not been widely adopted.[89-91] Feasibility and benefits of this approach await further studies and instrument development.

MINIMALLY INVASIVE SPLENECTOMY POSTOPERATIVE CARE

Postoperative care following an LS is straightforward, provided that the procedure is uneventful. Orogastric tubes and urinary catheters are removed immediately after the operation. Routine postoperative chest radiograph is not required. Pneumothorax following LS is rare. DVT prophylaxis is continued postoperatively with pneumatic sequential compression devices and heparin or enoxaparin, unless contraindicated. A diet is restarted as tolerated. Typical length of stay following an elective LS is 1 day, although most series report average length of stay of 2 to 3 days.[21-24,27,32,34-37,92]

All patients undergoing splenectomy should be counseled regarding their increased lifetime risk of infections. OPSI is a medical emergency for which only prompt diagnosis and immediate treatment can reduce mortality.[93] The mortality rate is 50% to 70%, and most deaths occur within the first 24 hours.[94] Patients should be advised to seek medical attention immediately if they develop a febrile illness. Asplenic patients in general have poor knowledge about their condition and risks. Information on the Internet for asplenic patients is a resource they are likely to access, and although many websites have incomplete information, almost all discuss the long-term risk of serious infection and need for vaccination.[95]

The use of long-term prophylactic antibiotics after splenectomy remains controversial and there is no evidence-based information. The actual effectiveness of antibiotics is unknown and there is no agreement on how long they should be taken or which subgroups to treat.[96,97] In addition, the major risk of long-term antibiotic therapy is the selection of resistant microbial strains. In adults, guidelines recommend prophylaxis with 250 to 500 mg per day of amoxicillin or 500 mg per day of phenoxymethylpenicillin.[97] Although there is no consensus, long-term treatment is recommended in patients with concomitant hematologic diseases or an impaired immune system.[96] In the pediatric population, hematologists often recommend treatment for 2 years postsplenectomy with a penicillin-based regimen, especially in children with sickle cell disease.

SURGICAL COMPLICATIONS

Intraoperative complications, particularly hemorrhage, can be challenging to manage. Recognition that splenic vascular anatomy is variable and complex, and that the spleen is a fragile solid organ with a delicate capsule underscore preemptive efforts to avoid bleeding. Instruments should be introduced to the operative field under direct visualization, avoiding inadvertent injury to the splenic parenchyma. Dissection should be methodical—identifying, isolating, and controlling vessels sequentially. The lateral approach decreases traction-related splenic capsular tears. Constant intraoperative monitoring for hemostasis is important. Energy sources have limitations, as do clip and linear stapler devices. Improper cautery application can cause injury to adjacent organs. Improper Harmonic scalpel application can result in hemorrhage from a partially sectioned vessel. Improper clip application can result in injury to an adjacent vessel. Blind linear stapler application can result in damage to the tail of the pancreas. The tip of the linear stapler should always be seen before it is fired. Hemorrhage can occur from partial division of a major splenic vessel after release of the stapler.

Postoperative complications for LS are similar to those for the open procedure. Early complications include bleeding, pneumonia, left pleural effusions, atelectasis and, rarely, injury to other organs (colon, small bowel, stomach, liver, and pancreas). Late complications include subphrenic abscess, splenic vein and/or portal vein thrombosis, failure to control the primary disease, recurrent disease due to accessory spleens, and OPSI. A multicenter analysis of LS reported data from 1993 to 2007 including 25 centers and 676 cases. Conversion rate to open splenectomy was 6%, complications were reported in 17% of patients, and perioperative death was 0.4%. Multivariate analysis found that BMI and presence of hematologic malignancy were independent predictors for intraoperative complications and surgical conversion. Spleen longitudinal size and surgical conversion were independent predictors of postoperative complications.[98]

Approximately 6% to 10% of patients undergoing open splenectomy develop splenic or portal vein thrombosis.[69] The incidence of portal vein thrombosis after LS has been reported to be higher at 14%.[99,100] A prospective comparison of open splenectomy and LS using helical CT imaging pre- and postoperatively identified portal venous thrombosis in 19% of patients in the open group and 55% in the laparoscopic group.[99] Most instances of splenoportal venous thrombosis are asymptomatic. When present, symptoms are vague and include fatigue, nausea, vomiting, and nonspecific abdominal pain. The overall risk of *symptomatic* splenic or portal vein thrombosis is about 3%. Risk factors include splenomegaly and hereditary hemolytic anemias, whereas risk may be lower in autoimmune thrombocytopenia and trauma. Treatment of splenic/portal vein thrombosis with heparin and warfarin leads to complete or partial resolution of thrombosis in 80% of cases and persistent occlusion, portal hypertension, or

cavernoma in 20% of patients. Well-designed prospective studies on prophylaxis of visceral venous thrombosis following splenectomy are lacking.[92,102]

Patients with persistent postoperative fever, increased white blood cell count, and abdominal pain should undergo CT of the abdomen. Subphrenic abscesses are treated with drainage and intravenous antibiotics.

IMAGE-GUIDED INTERVENTIONAL THERAPY FOR THE SPLEEN

The spleen possesses a single, accessible feeding artery with a relatively simple branching pattern, making the splenic artery well suited to routine, safe catheter access. Its brisk blood flow and rich vascular parenchyma provides high-quality arteriograms, parenchymal opacification, and portal venous imaging using digital subtraction angiography (DSA). Minimally invasive vascular interventional techniques for the spleen were rapidly popularized in the 1970s and 1980s and play an increasing role in algorithms of contemporary surgical practice, particularly with the shift toward preservation of functioning splenic tissue through nonoperative management. This section reviews techniques and provides updates on clinical applications of image-guided splenic interventions, which include splenic trauma, splenic artery pseudoaneurysm, hypersplenism, drainage of splenic collections, and splenic biopsy, with focus on the complementary role of image-guided interventions for the spleen as adjuncts to minimally invasive surgery—particularly in the management of splenic trauma and giant spleens.

TRANSARTERIAL SPLENIC EMBOLIZATION

Anatomy

Although surgical splenectomy can be performed efficiently and safely, it is now clear that removal of this reticuloendothelial organ is accompanied by significant risks of OPSI. Catheter-directed therapies provide an adjunct to surgery achieving therapeutic goals while preserving adequate functioning splenic tissue for host immunity. In some cases, image-guided splenic intervention, such as splenic embolization, can obviate the need for surgery and support the nonoperative trauma management.[12,103] In other cases, splenic embolization can facilitate LS for the subset of patients failing nonoperative management.[13] The embolization can also be used for patients with giant spleens being prepared for laparoscopic or HALS splenectomy.[45] The splenic artery is usually a large single vessel arising anterolaterally from the celiac axis. Anatomic variations of the splenic artery are uncommon but include a separate origin from the aorta.[104] The artery corkscrews clockwise or anticlockwise while undulating across the posterosuperior aspect of the pancreas body. It gives off sequentially the dorsal pancreatic and pancreatica magna arteries before dividing into extrasplenic polar branches in the region of the pancreatic tail (Fig. 138.3). One should note that the pancreas also receives a blood supply from the pancreaticoduodenal and transverse pancreatic arcades, and the spleen has a rich vascular network from the short gastric and gastroepiploic arteries. This anatomy may be depicted

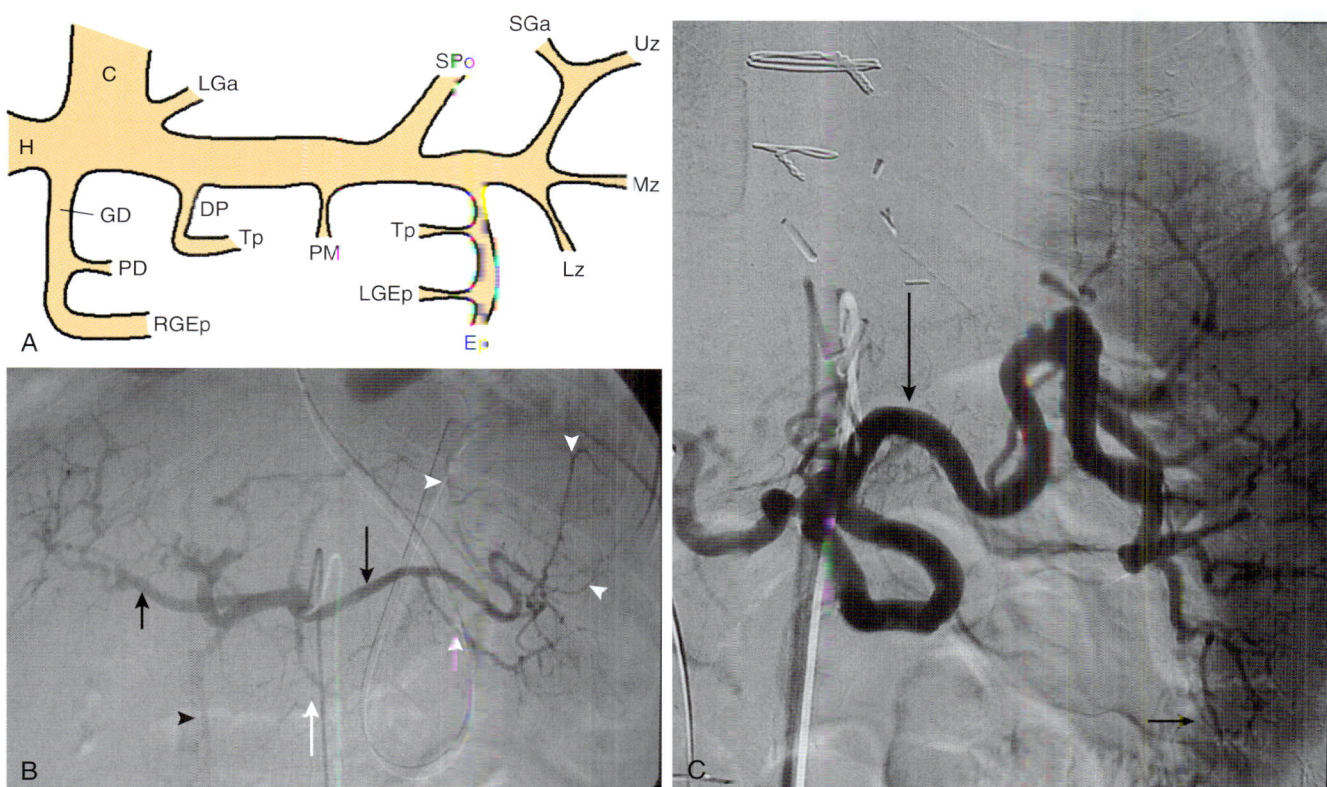

FIGURE 138.3 (A) Schematic illustration of the splenic artery and its branches seen at splenic arteriography. (B) Forty-one-year-old woman with gastrointestinal bleeding. Normal anteroposterior celiac arteriogram demonstrating splenic artery *(long black arrow)*, dorsal pancreatic artery *(long white arrow)*, pancreatica magna *(short white arrow)*, splenic artery hilar branches *(white arrowheads)*, hepatic artery *(short black arrowhead)*, and gastroduodenal artery *(arrowhead)*. (C) Fifty-year-old man with pancreatic carcinoma. Normal anteroposterior celiac arteriogram demonstrates the splenic artery *(long arrow)* and parenchymal phase enhancement of the spleen *(short arrow)*. *C*, Celiac artery; *Ep*, epiploic artery; *GD*, gastroduodenal artery; *H*, hepatic artery; *LGa*, left gastric artery; *LGEp*, left gastroepiploic artery; *Lz*, inferior pole of splenic artery; *Mz*, midzone splenic artery; *PD*, pancreaticoduodenal artery; *PM*, pancreatica magna; *RGEp*, right gastroepiploic artery; *SGa*, short gastric arteries; *SPo*, superior polar artery; *Tp*, transverse pancreatic artery; *Uz*, upper pole splenic artery.

on current 3D multidetector-row CT angiography (CTA) and MR angiography (MRA) with a diagnostic quality comparable to invasive splenic angiography (Fig. 138.4).

Technique

Most splenic interventions can be performed with conscious sedation, though pediatric patients may require general anesthesia. An initial aortogram is performed with a 5-French (5-Fr) flush catheter through a 5-Fr sheath in the femoral artery. This assesses globally for sites of bleeding and depicts the normal and variant anatomy for selective angiography. The celiac axis and splenic artery are selected using a combination of 5-Fr Simmons 1 or Cobra glide catheter and a 0.035 glide wire. With proximal placement of the catheter, a selective splenic angiogram is performed with arterial, parenchymal, and portal venous phase timing of the contrast bolus. Smaller, more distal hilar and branch vessels may be selected with the 5-Fr catheter combined with a 3-Fr microcatheter over a 0.014 to 0.018 microwire. Standard DSA suffices, though newer 3D fluoroscopy units may benefit cases with difficult anatomy (Fig. 138.5).

Embolization is performed from distal to proximal within the artery. Embolic materials available include Gelfoam, particles, and coils. Smaller, more distal arteries and parenchyma may be temporarily embolized with gelatin sponge pledgets or slurry or autologous blood clot. Permanent distal parenchymal vascular occlusion is achieved with 300- to 900-μm particulate polyvinyl alcohol, silicone, or acrylic embolic spheres. The embolic agents may be soaked in antibiotic to decrease the risk of abscess formation. The splenic artery may be permanently embolized with metallic coils from the second-order branches into the main splenic artery. Coils are deployed distal to the dorsal pancreatic and pancreatica magna arteries in an effort to avoid splenic infarction by preserving collateral supply to functioning splenic pulp.[105] Coils must be sized to the target vessel to avoid inadvertent distal embolization of nontarget vessels or proximal migration into the celiac axis or aorta. Depending on the indication, a combination approach of coil and embolic agents may be employed. One must remain cognizant that proximally placed coils may limit future interventions if required.

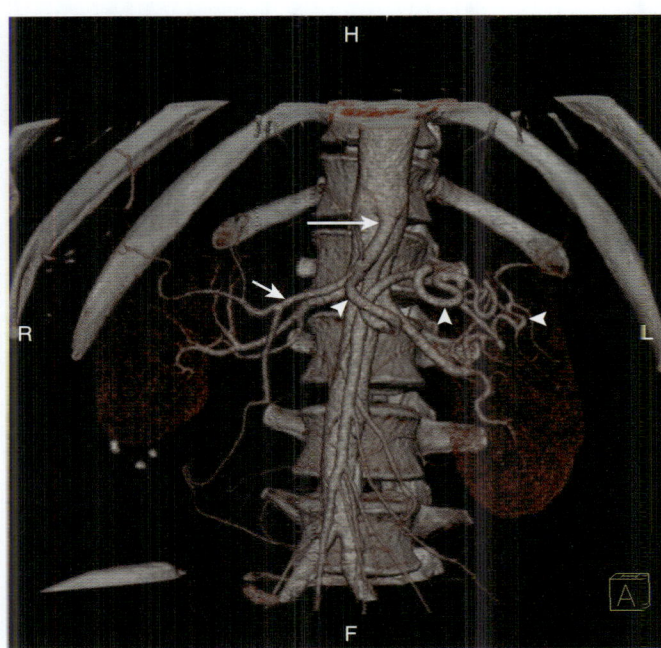

FIGURE 138.4 Thirty-year-old woman being evaluated for renal organ donation. Three-dimensional volume-rendered anteroposterior projection multidetector-row computed tomography of the splenic artery *(arrowheads)*. Celiac axis *(long arrow)* and hepatic artery *(short arrow)*.

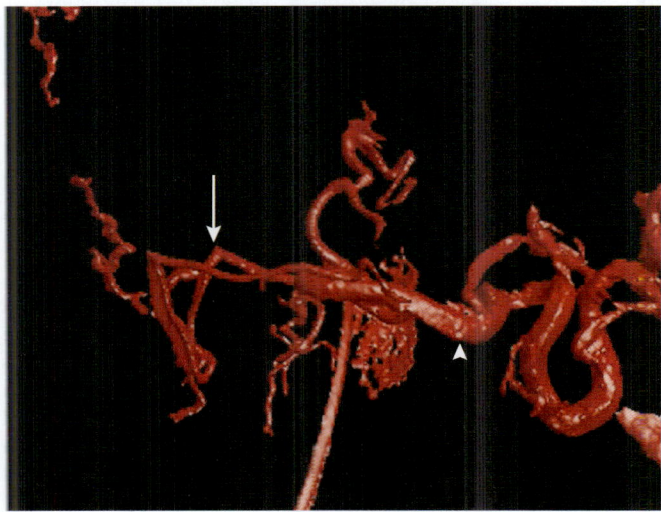

FIGURE 138.5 Forty-year-old woman receiving hepatic chemoembolization. Three-dimensional fluoroscopic digital subtraction angiography that offers infinite planes and projections for interpretation and can unravel complex anatomy. Hepatic artery *(arrow)* and splenic artery *(arrowhead)*.

SPLENIC BLEEDING AND TRANSARTERIAL SPLENIC EMBOLIZATION

The spleen represents the most commonly injured organ from blunt or penetrating trauma. The algorithm for managing the patient with splenic injury is an evolving practice and, in the past decades, the treatment of patients

with blunt splenic injury has shifted from operative to nonoperative management. First described by Sclafani et al. in 1995, transarterial embolization has become commonly available and is well studied.[106] This has led to nonoperative management being the treatment of choice, decreasing splenectomies in adults and children and increasing the number of patients managed by transarterial splenic embolization (TASE). Outcomes are predominantly based on large-volume studies from level 1 trauma centers in the United States, but emerging data suggest good outcomes even from smaller centers.[103] Assignment of patients to operative or nonoperative groups and to interventional or noninterventional groups is best achieved through reconciliation of the clinical picture, imaging findings, and injury scale (American Association for the Surgery of Trauma [AAST] Organ Injury Scale [OIS])[106,107] Grading of the injury is now largely based on CT scan and the most widely accepted indication for TASE is evidence of an arterial lesion.[106–111]

Broadly speaking, most would agree that the hypotensive, unstable patient refractory to resuscitation mandates surgical exploration (usually grade III to V).[107] The majority of injuries present as hemodynamically stable patients with a grade I or II, no signs of continued bleeding, and may be managed conservatively with observation.[112,113] The role of endovascular therapy lies between these broadly defined groups and is still actively debated. Management today largely depends on local expertise and organization of the trauma team, which evaluates each case on its individual merits. Most splenic injuries treated by embolization are grade 2.8 to 3.[107,109,112] TASE has little role in the shattered or devascularized spleen. In centers with rapid access to interventional services as part of trauma triage, there is some evidence to support TASE in patients who respond transiently to minimal resuscitation[114] and in endovascular treatment of higher-grade injuries. Up to 10% of hemodynamically stable patients may have imaging signs of continued bleeding from grade III injuries and are potential candidates for TASE. A retrospective study over 7 years at a level 1 trauma center reviewed 499 patients who suffered blunt splenic trauma; the authors found that 407 (81.6%) patients were successfully treated with nonoperative management and 92 (18.4%) underwent splenectomy within 1 hour of the admission. Splenic embolization was protective against splenectomy for lower-grade injuries.[104] Early experience with splenic embolization for higher-grade splenic trauma is favorable, but requires a vigilant team and algorithm. One group reported 46 patients with splenic trauma of whom 17 were treated surgically, 15 conservatively, and 14 with splenic artery embolization. Hemodynamically stable patients were treated conservatively and 14 patients with grade IV injury were managed with embolization—embolizing proximally the main splenic artery with diffuse organ damage, and embolizing distally selective splenic branches for localized injury. In 13 of the 14 patients (92.9%), embolization was successful and there were no periprocedural complications, with the remaining patient undergoing splenectomy within 24 hours because of recurrent bleeding.[105]

Endovascular therapy for splenic trauma begins with review of the contrast-enhanced CT or magnetic resonance imaging (MRI). The aortogram may demonstrate generalized vasoconstriction and renal retention of contrast in the patient in shock. Splenic angiography findings include abrupt termination of vessels, vasospasm, pseudoaneurysm, and arteriovenous fistula formation. Intrasplenic vessels may be displaced and the extrasplenic artery may be "accordioned" from the hematoma. The parenchymal phase may demonstrate contrast extravasation, avascular segments, abnormal accumulation of contrast within the pulp, and loss of the smooth splenic contour. In the setting of large subcapsular hematoma, the spleen will be displaced anteromedially and the left kidney may be displaced inferiorly. Bleeding may initially be treated with a temporary distal particulate agent but the definitive therapy is permanent coil embolization of the splenic artery. If there are only two to three identifiable bleeding sites, they may be selectively coiled distally. However, if there are multiple sites, a more proximal embolization will be required. Embolization slows arterial inflow and permits distal clot to form.[115] In addition, some authors found no difference in outcomes between proximal and distal embolization.[110,116] After therapy, one may see complete stasis or markedly slowed flow. Absence of extravasation at angiography is a reliable sign of successful therapy,[166] and such patients will not likely need later laparotomy.

The success of TASE and its contribution to nonoperative management is largely from retrospective data. Patients failing nonoperative management (3% to 17%) and requiring splenectomy are decreasing.[109,110] Overall, the success of TASE for controlling splenic bleeding and splenic salvage is more than 80% in adults and children.[106,111,117,118] Haan et al. reviewed 648 patients with blunt splenic injury of whom 132 had embolization with salvage rates of 90%. The presence of an arteriovenous fistula may predict operative failure, but this will depend on how aggressively the fistula is treated. Those who fail an initial TASE may yet be considered for a second therapy if they remain stable, and can account for 2% to 5% of patients treated (Fig. 138.6).[110]

Complications of TASE include delayed recurrent bleeding, due to continued bleeding through the embolization, lysis of the clot at the injured site, pseudoaneurysm rupture, or relaxation of acutely vasospastic vessels.[119,120] Delayed bleeds may occur days to weeks after therapy. Postembolization syndrome presents with abdominal pain and fever and may be associated with CT findings of necrotic, air-containing parenchyma and left-side pleural effusion. This is usually self-limited unless superimposed with infection. Bacterial peritonitis, septicemia, splenic abscesses, and rupture are other possible complications. Hematomata may evolve into calcified splenic hematomata or cysts. Postembolization infarction rates are quoted to be up to 20% but depend on the site of injury and the extent of embolization required.[119-121] Controversy remains regarding proximal versus distal splenic artery embolization. A recent meta-analysis tried to specifically address this issue. Studies evaluating adult trauma patients sustaining blunt splenic injury managed by angioembolization were systematically evaluated for grade of splenic injury, indication, site (proximal vs. distal), and outcomes. Fifteen of 147 studies were included, all retrospective, for a cohort of 479 embolized patients. The overall embolization failure rate was 10% (range, 0.0% to 33.3%). Rebleeding was the most common reason for failure but did not differ between distal and proximal angioembolization techniques. Minor complications occurred more often after distal than proximal embolization, and this is explained by a higher rate of segmental infarctions after distal embolization.[116]

Nonoperative management of splenic trauma assumes that splenic preservation maintains its function. To verify this assumption, immune function was assessed in 43 patients with splenic injury (grades I to IV), analyzing the lymphocyte subpopulation responses and antibody production to *Streptococcus pneumoniae* and *Haemophilus influenzae* vaccinations. Splenectomy patients exhibited significant decrease in CD4$^+$ T lymphocytes, B cells, IgM, and IgD compared to splenic preservation patients, reinforcing the importance of conservative options in splenic trauma.[122]

PSEUDOANEURYSM OF THE SPLENIC ARTERY

The splenic artery is the third most common intraabdominal artery affected by aneurysms and pseudoaneurysms and is second only to aorta and iliac arteries. Although the precise etiology of splenic artery aneurysm remains unknown, it has been associated with systemic hypertension, portal hypertension, cirrhosis, liver transplantation, and pregnancy.[123-125] Less commonly associated conditions include arterial fibrodysplasia, arteritis, collagen deficiency, and inflammatory and infectious disorders.[123] The causes of splenic artery pseudoaneurysm include pancreatitis, trauma and, rarely, peptic ulcer disease.[126-128] It has been suggested that the increased nonoperative management of splenic injuries may lead to a greater prevalence of traumatic pseudoaneurysms that would otherwise have been resected, but there is also an increased incidental detection of splenic aneurysms because of the widespread application of cross-sectional imaging.[127] There is higher prevalence in women and they are more prone to rupture during pregnancy. Splenic aneurysms are typically saccular and situated in the distal third of the splenic artery. Rarely, intrasplenic aneurysms have also been reported.[129] They contain a variable amount of mural thrombus, are frequently calcified, but they do not affect splenic perfusion. CTA is highly accurate for detection and characterization of splenic aneurysms, although 3D reconstruction is required to differentiate from false positives, such as normal vessel tortuosity and atherosclerotic changes. There is some debate on which aneurysm or pseudoaneurysms should be treated. Most agree that larger sizes (above 2 to 2.5 cm) and presence of symptoms should be considered as indication for treatment. In addition, up to 60% of those who bleed will be unstable and the mortality rate of bleeding is quoted as high as 15%.[127] Many also advocate a treatment for smaller aneurysms in women of childbearing age, whereas some argue that lesions less than 2.5 cm and small pediatric splenic aneurysms may be managed conservatively with close follow-up.[127,129,130]

The majority of splenic aneurysms may be treated by TASE, with direct embolization of the aneurysmal sac or its feeding artery. For broad-necked, saccular, or fusiform aneurysms, coils are deployed from a distal to proximal direction, within the splenic artery. In saccular lesions with a narrow neck, one may deploy detachable coils or balloons within the aneurysm sac itself (Fig. 138.7). More

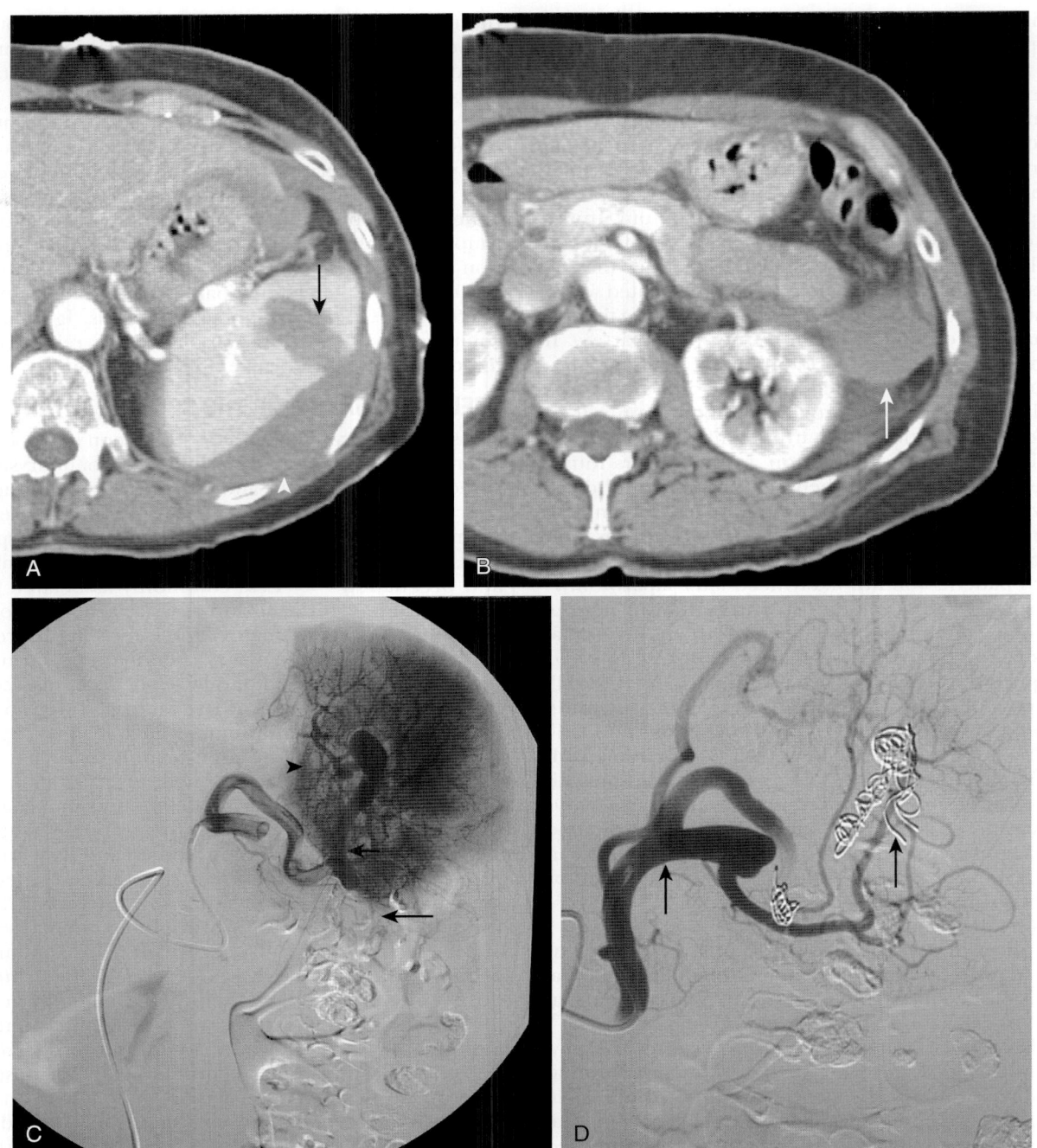

FIGURE 138.6 (A) Axial contrast-enhanced computed tomography (CT) scan in a 32-year-old female who fell from a horse and had active splenic bleeding. Grade IV laceration *(black arrow)* and subcapsular hematoma *(white arrowhead)* of the spleen. (B) Axial contrast-enhanced CT. Moderate retroperitoneal hematoma in the left anterior pararenal space *(arrow)*. (C) Anteroposterior digital subtraction angiography (DSA) of splenic arteriogram demonstrates splenic artery *(short arrow)* supplying remaining upper-pole splenic pulp *(arrowhead)* although there is a sharp cutoff from the avascular lower-pole segment because of the expanding hematoma *(long arrow)*. (D) Treatment with transarterial splenic embolization. Hemostasis was achieved with coil embolization of the splenic artery. Splenic artery DSA demonstrates decreased splenic perfusion and coils in the distal lobar branch of the splenic artery *(black arrows)*.

recently, covered stents placed across the aneurysm neck have been suggested as a form of therapy that will exclude the aneurysm and preserve blood flow and future access.[131] This procedure, however, may be of higher risk in very tortuous arteries and requires careful patient selection.

Percutaneous injection of thrombin has also been reported, but it is an uncommon approach.[132] Localized treatment of pseudoaneurysm preserves splenic function. A recent retrospective review of 38 patients with splenic artery aneurysm (all >2 cm in diameter) included 9 treated with

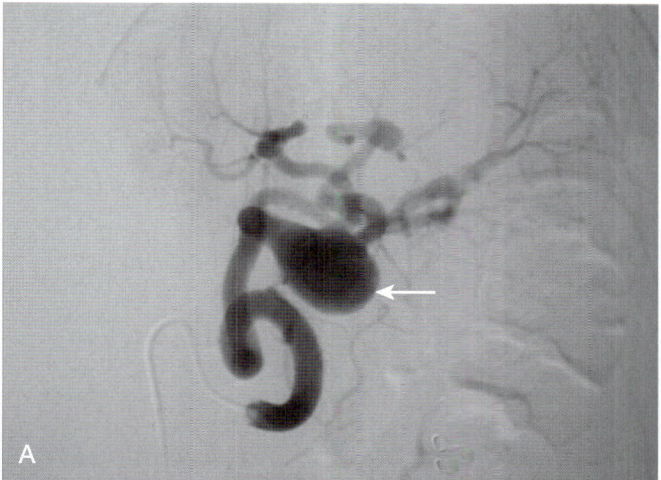
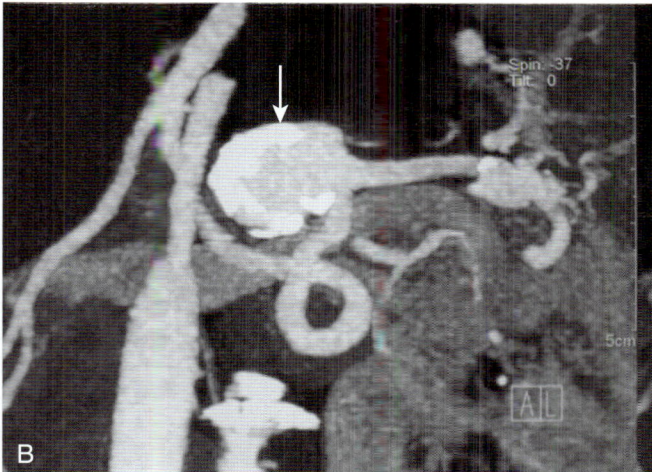
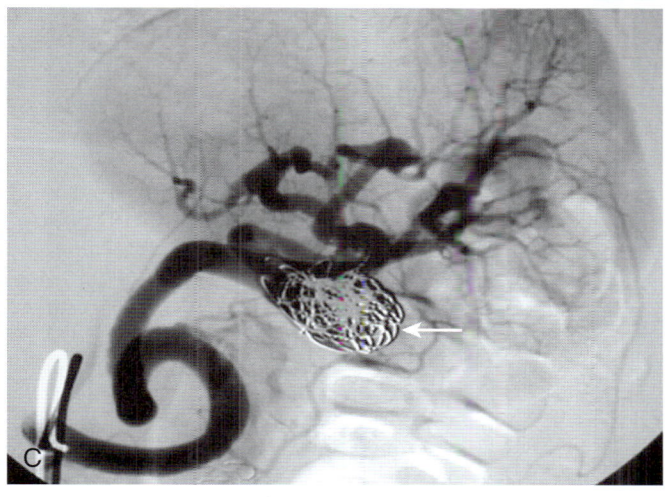

FIGURE 138.7 Pseudoaneurysm of the distal splenic artery. (A) Anteroposterior digital subtraction angiography (DSA) demonstrates a large saccular pseudoaneurysm (*arrow*). (B) Anteroposterior maximum-intensity multidetector-row computed tomography arteriogram demonstrates the saccular pseudoaneurysm (*arrow*). (C) Anteroposterior DSA demonstrates successful coil embolization with detachable coils (*arrow*). (Courtesy Dr. A. Arapally, Johns Hopkins Hospital.)

transcatheter embolization, 8 treated by open repair, and 21 who only required observation. The success rate was 100% in both the transcatheter embolization and open surgical repair groups, with shorter length of stay (8 vs. 16 days) in the angioembolization group, and no recurrence at 45 and 57 months, respectively.[133,134]

The results of endovascular management have improved and it is now recommended for all splenic aneurysms.[153] In cases where surgery is necessary, balloon occlusion catheters may control bleeding intraoperatively.[127]

Splenic artery and vein aneurysm with splenic arteriovenous fistula is rare, but amenable to image-guided intervention. Surgical ligation and percutaneous embolization have been reported to be equally effective. In addition, percutaneous placement of an occlusion device has been reported as yet another emerging alternative.[135]

HYPERSPLENISM AND PARTIAL SPLENIC EMBOLIZATION

Splenic embolization can be used for hypersplenism and pancytopenia with or without massive splenomegaly (e.g., thalassemia, myelofibrosis).[136] In addition to improving hematologic parameters and decreasing splenic size, it may improve liver function and decrease gastric or splenic variceal bleeding.[121,137,138] The combination of antibiotic prophylaxis and partial splenic embolization (PSE) is considered an effective and safer alternative to surgical splenectomy.[139]

Treatment is usually with small (300 to 900 μm) permanent particulate embolic agents (e.g., polyvinyl alcohol, silicone, or acrylic embolic spheres) that seek to deprive peripheral, intraparenchyma segmental regions of the spleen of their blood flow. Coils are not used because it is harder to gauge and stage the percentage of parenchyma treated and they limit access for future treatments. The risk of pancreatitis is reduced by placement of the catheter as distal as possible to avoid particulate agent going to nontarget sites. Selection of individual hilar branches may also be possible, to better distribute the embolic agent throughout the spleen. The percentage of embolization is estimated through the parenchymal phase of the angiography, right after particulate injection. It has been suggested that embolization of less than 50% of the splenic pulp predisposes to relapse,[121,140] but with embolization of more than 70%, greater long-term efficacy may be achieved.[127] Most accomplish this 70% in staged treatments to limit postembolization syndrome and complications. The response in organ size is best appreciated from CT or MRI and is noticed within 2 to 4 months of therapy. The hematologic response may be seen

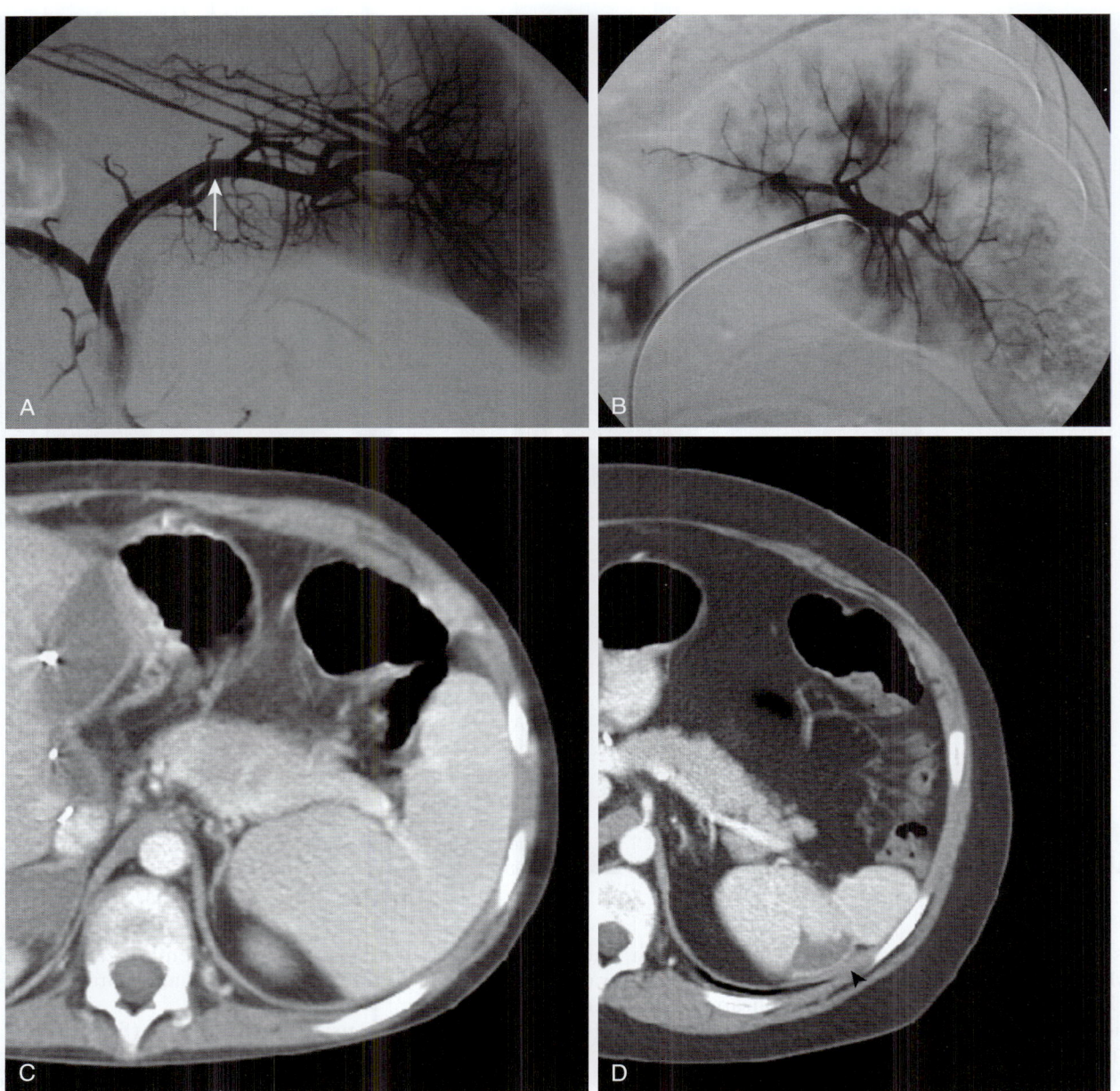

FIGURE 138.8 Fourteen-year-old with hypersplenism and thrombocytopenia after hepatic transplant. (A) Normal splenic arteriogram *(arrow)* with parenchymal phase enhancement. (B) Splenic arteriogram digital subtraction angiography after 70% embolization demonstrating mottled enhancement pattern. (C) Contrast-enhanced computed tomography (CT) before embolization. Note the size of the spleen. (D) Contrast-enhanced CT 3 months after embolization. Note the decreased size of the spleen and small peripheral infarct *(arrowhead)*. ([A] Courtesy Dr. A. Arapally, Johns Hopkins Hospital.)

within weeks,[141] but a prolonged long-term response has also been demonstrated (Fig. 138.8).[142] The success rate is higher for decreased variceal bleeding and improved liver function. Relapse may be related to the rate of splenic regeneration. Reported complications of the procedure include splenoportal venous thrombosis, splenic necrosis, abscess, and septicemia, which are potentially lethal.[121,141]

A similar technique is used for splenic embolization before a splenectomy is performed. In general, the surgical splenectomy has good control of bleeding and limited blood loss (Fig. 138.9). However, it may be more challenging in the patient with massive splenomegaly where access to the hilum is more difficult. Proximal coil embolization may limit blood flow into the hilar vessels. Although the coils may affect placement of surgical clamps and ligatures, they can be easily removed if placed close to the operation.[45] Intraparenchymal particulate Gelfoam slurry embolization may also be used to limit bleeding of an intrasplenic mass (hemangiosarcoma or fibrosarcoma).

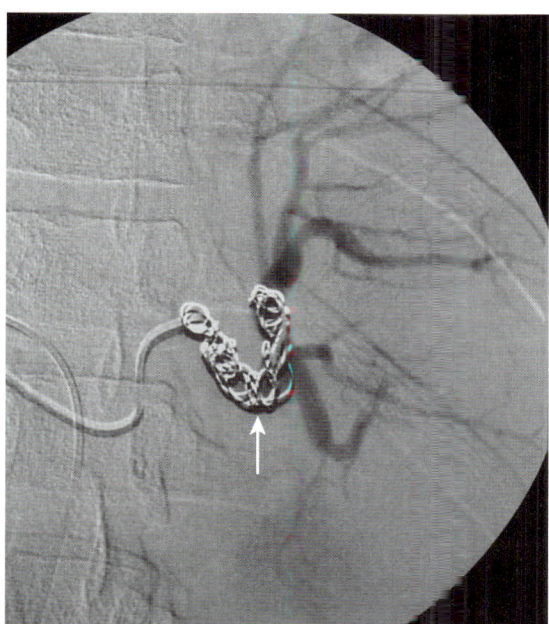

FIGURE 138.9 Sixty-two-year-old man who presented for preoperative embolization before splenectomy for lymphoma and splenomegaly. Note coils in the splenic artery *(arrow)* and decreased blood flow distally.

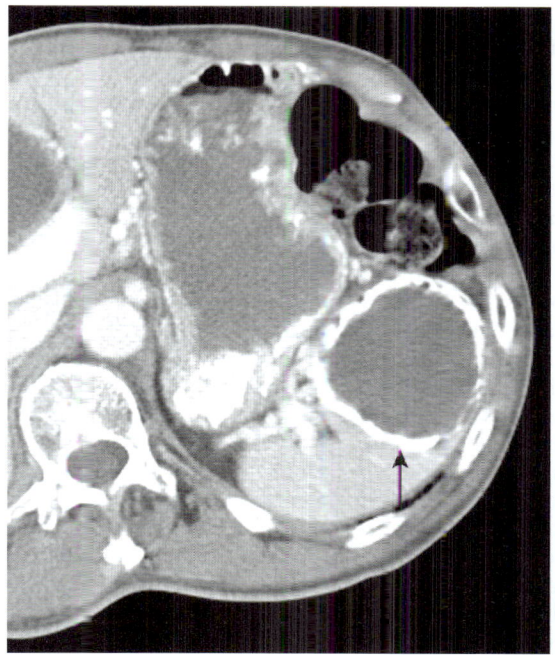

FIGURE 138.10 Axial contrast-enhanced computed tomography demonstrating a calcified splenic hematoma *(arrow)*.

SPLENIC ABSCESS AND PSEUDOCYST

The most common splenic collections are old hematomas, pseudocysts and cysts (Fig. 138.10), and splenic abscesses (Fig. 138.11). Cysts commonly seen on cross-sectional imaging require therapy only when they are large enough to cause early satiety or left shoulder pain. Noninfected splenic cysts may be treated by percutaneous puncture and aspiration with sclerosis. The volume of aspirate is replaced with 100% dehydrated ethanol or doxycycline and the patient is placed in alternate postures for an hour before the fluid is aspirated.[143,144] Repeated therapy may be required. Splenic abscess may be iatrogenic and may be complicated by mycotic pseudoaneurysm. Usually, the access is guided by ultrasound, with a single-wall 18-gauge needle, followed by a 10-Fr drain placed over a 0.035 guidewire. When drainage tapers off and imaging indicates that the cavity has collapsed, the drain can be safely removed.[145,146] Sterile collections that repeatedly accumulate may be sclerosed with tetracycline.[146]

IMAGE-GUIDED BIOPSY OF THE SPLEEN

Percutaneous image-guided biopsy of the spleen is still a controversial topic. Traditionally, the common opinion has always been that the risk of bleeding is too high. However, a meta-analysis by McInnes et al. has shown high diagnostic accuracy, with pooled major complication rate (hemorrhage most frequently, followed by pain) of only 1%, when needles of 18 gauge or smaller were used.[147] Thus, percutaneous image-guided splenic biopsy is considered to be a reasonable option.[148]

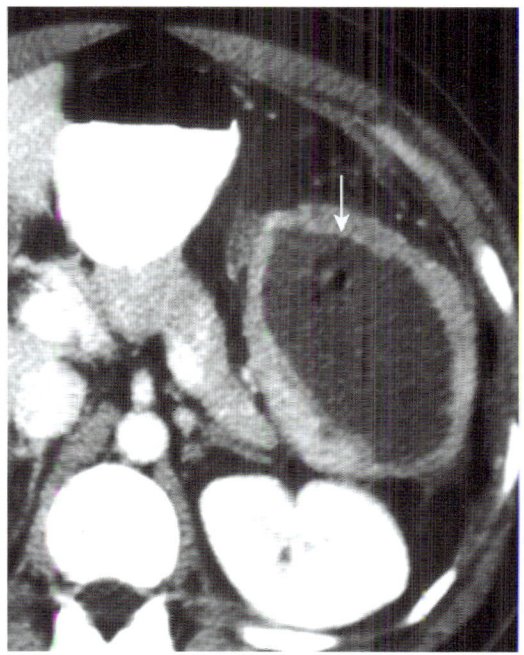

FIGURE 138.11 Axial contrast-enhanced computed tomography demonstrating an air-containing splenic abscess *(arrow)*.

SUMMARY

LS is still the gold standard for most elective cases with normal or slightly enlarged spleen. Surgical innovation, technology, and growing experience have also made the laparoscopic approach doable for medical conditions that once were considered a contraindication. Even though LS still has limited applications in the acute and unstable trauma patient, the increased adoption of nonoperative management and adjunctive treatments, such as embolization, have made delayed LS a valuable option for patients who fail the conservative approach. For elective splenectomy, the minimally invasive approach is applied to increasingly complex splenic disorders, reoperative settings, and massive splenomegaly—often with the application of hand-assisted devices. Single-port, robotic, and NOTES splenectomy require further study for safety and cost-effectiveness.

Diagnostic splenic angiography is shifting from interventional diagnostic techniques to noninvasive 3D CT scan and MRI, which produce studies of similar quality. Therapeutic image-guided percutaneous interventions for the spleen continue to expand. There has been growth in splenic artery embolization for trauma patients, helping to achieve organ preservation. Angioembolization has also enhanced the application of minimally invasive surgery to the giant spleen. Even if further study is needed, image-guided management of splenic artery aneurysm and pseudoaneurysm is emerging as a first-line strategy, as is the application of image-guided splenic biopsy. Collaboration between the surgeon and interventional radiologist is essential in the management of splenic disorders.

ACKNOWLEDGMENT

This is an update of the original chapter by Michael R. Marohn, Kimberly E. Steele, and Leo P. Lawler (Chapter 133 in the previous edition).

REFERENCES

1. Maddison FE. Embolic therapy of hypersplenism. *Invest Radiol.* 1973;8(4):280-281.
2. Moris D, Dimitriou N, Griniatsos J. Laparoscopic splenectomy for benign hematological disorders in adults. A systematic review. *In Vivo.* 2017;31:291-302.
3. Delaitre B, Maignien B. Splenectomy by the laparoscopic approach. Report of a case. *Presse Med.* 1991;20:2263.
4. Park A, Marcaccio M, Sternbach M, Witzke D, Fitzgerald P. Laparoscopic vs open splenectomy. *Arch Surg.* 1999;134:1263.
5. Targarona EM, Espert JJ, Cerdan G, et al. Effect of spleen size on splenectomy outcome. A comparison of open and laparoscopic surgery. *Surg Endosc.* 1999;13:559.
6. Centers for Disease Control and Prevention, National Center for Injury Prevention and Control. Web-based Injury Statistics Query and Reporting System (WISQARS) Fatal Injury Data. 2016.
7. Rhee P, Joseph B, Pandit V, et al. Increasing trauma deaths in the United States. *Ann Surg.* 2014;260(1):13-21.
8. Olthof DC, Sierink JC, Van Delden OM, Luitse JSK, Goslings JC. Time to intervention in patients with splenic injury in a Dutch level 1 trauma center. *Injury.* 2014;45(1):95-100.
9. Smith RS, Fry WR, Morabito DJ, Koehler RH, Organ CH Jr. Therapeutic laparoscopy in trauma. *Am J Surg.* 1995;170:632.
10. Carobbi A, Romagnani F, Antonelli G, Bianchini M. Laparoscopic splenectomy for severe blunt trauma: initial experience of ten consecutive cases with a fast hemostatic technique. *Surg Endosc.* 2010;24:1325.
11. Ermolov AS, Tlibekova MA, Yartsev PA, et al. Laparoscopic splenectomy in patients with spleen injuries. *Surg Laparosc Endosc Percutan Tech.* 2015;25(6):483-486.
12. Ransom KJ, Kavic MS. Laparoscopic splenectomy for blunt trauma: a safe operation following embolization. *Surg Endosc.* 2009;23:352.
13. Davoodi P, Budde C, Minshall CT. Laparoscopic repair of penetrating splenic injury. *J Laparoendosc Adv Surg Tech A.* 2009;19:795.
14. Olthof DC, van der Vlies CH, Goslings JC. Evidence-based management and controversies in blunt splenic trauma. *Curr Trauma Rep.* 2017;3:32-37.
15. Isaev AF, Alimov AN, Safronov EP, Otlygin I, Useinov EB, Muradov IU. Evaluation of status severity in patients with isolated and combined injury of abdomen associated with spleen disruption. *Khirurgiia (Mosk).* 2005;9:31.
16. Shen HB, Lu XM, Zheng QC, Cai XT, Zhou H, Fei KL. Clinical application of laparoscopic spleen-preserving operation in traumatic spleen rupture. *Chin J Traumatol.* 2005;8:293.
17. Mostofa G, Matthews BD, Sing RF, Prickett D, Heniford BT. Elective laparoscopic splenectomy for grade III splenic injury in an athlete. *Surg Laparosc Endosc Percutan Tech.* 2002;12:283.
18. Li H, Wei Y, Peng B, Li B, Liu F. Feasibility and safety of emergency laparoscopic partial splenectomy: a retrospective analysis. *Medicine (Baltimore).* 2017;96(16):e6450.
19. Longo WE, Baker CC, McMillen MA, Modlin IM, Degutis LC, Zucker KA. Nonoperative management of adult blunt splenic trauma: criteria for successful outcome. *Ann Surg.* 1989;210:626.
20. Sotomayor-Ramirez RK. Efficacy and safety of laparoscopic splenectomy: review of 14 adult cases using the lateral approach. *Bol Asoc Med P R.* 2009;101(2):43-49.
21. Vecchio R, Intagliata E, Marchese S, La Corte F, Cacciola RR, Cacciola E. Laparoscopic splenectomy coupled with laparoscopic cholecystectomy. *JSLS.* 2014;18(2):252-257.
22. Al-Mulhim AS. Laparoscopic splenectomy for massive splenomegaly in benign hematological diseases. *Surg Endosc.* 2012;26(11):3186-3189.
23. Bai YN, Jiang H, Prasoon P. A meta-analysis of perioperative outcomes of laparoscopic splenectomy for hematological disorders. *World J Surg.* 2012;36(10):2349-2358.
24. Chen X, Peng B, Cai Y, Zhou J, Wang Y, Wu Z, et al. Laparoscopic splenectomy for patients with immune thrombocytopenia and very low platelet count: is platelet transfusion necessary? *J Surg Res.* 2011;170(2):e225-e232.
25. Corcione F, Pirozzi F, Aragiusto G, Galante F, Sciuto A. Laparoscopic splenectomy: experience of a single center in a series of 300 cases. *Surg Endosc.* 2012;26(10):2870-2876.
26. Fraser SA, Bergman S, Garzon J. Laparoscopic splenectomy: learning curve comparison between benign and malignant disease. *Surg Innov.* 2012;19(1):27-32.
27. Gonzalez-Porras JR, Escalante F, Pardal E, et al. Safety and efficacy of splenectomy in over 65-yrs-old patients with immune thrombocytopenia. *Eur J Haematol.* 2013;91(3):236-241.
28. Li B, Liu J, Shangguan Y, Liu B, Qi Y. Laparoscopy-assisted small incision splenectomy and open splenectomy in the treatment of hematologic diseases: a single-institution comparative experience. *Surg Laparosc Endosc Percutan Tech.* 2013;23(3):309-311.
29. Marte G, Scuderi V, Rocca A, Surfaro G, Migliaccio C, Ceriello A. Laparoscopic splenectomy: a single-center experience. Unusual cases and expanded inclusion criteria for laparoscopic approach. *Updates Surg.* 2013;65(2):115-119.
30. Mohamed SY, Abdel-Nabi I, Inam A, et al. Systemic thromboembolic complications after laparoscopic splenectomy for idiopathic thrombocytopenic purpura in comparison to open surgery in the absence of anticoagulant prophylaxis. *Hematol Oncol Stem Cell Ther.* 2010;3(2):71-77.
31. Monclova JL, Targarona EM, Vidal P, et al. Single incision versus reduced port splenectomy—searching for the best alternative to conventional laparoscopic splenectomy. *Surg Endosc.* 2013;27(3):895-902.
32. Nobili C, Romano F, Ciravegna AL, et al. Consecutive concomitant laparoscopic splenectomy and cholecystectomy: an Italian experience of 30 patients and proposition of a technique. *J Laparoendosc Adv Surg Tech A.* 2011;21(4):313-317.
33. Patel NY, Chilsen AM, Mathiason MA, Kallies KJ, Bottner WA. Outcomes and complications after splenectomy for hematologic disorders. *Am J Surg.* 2012;204(6):1014-1019, discussion 1019-1020.
34. Sasaki A, Nitta H, Otuska K, Kimura Y, Obuchi T, Wakabayashi G. Concomitant laparoscopic splenectomy and cholecystectomy. *Surg Laparosc Endosc Percutan Tech.* 2010;20(2):66-68.
35. Tran T, Demyttenaere SV, Polyhronopoulos G, et al. Recommended timing for surveillance ultrasonography to diagnose portal splenic vein thrombosis after laparoscopic splenectomy. *Surg Endosc.* 2010;24(7):1670-1678.
36. Vecchio R, Cacciola E, Cacciola RR, Marchese S, Intagliata E. Portal vein thrombosis after laparoscopic and open splenectomy. *J Laparoendosc Adv Surg Tech A.* 2011;21(1):71-75.

37. Vecchio R, Marchese S, Sweh E, Intagliata E. Splenic hilum management during laparoscopic splenectomy. *J Laparoendosc Adv Surg Tech A.* 2011;21(8):717-720.

38. Wang M, Zhang M, Li J, Zhou J, Wu Z, Peng B. Risk factors of portal vein thrombosis in patients with beta thalassemia major after splenectomy: laparoscopic versus open procedure. *Hepatogastroenterology.* 2014;61(129):48-54.

39. Wu Z, Zhou J, Li J, Zhu Y, Peng B. The feasibility of laparoscopic splenectomy for ITP patients without preoperative platelet transfusion. *Hepatogastroenterology.* 2012;59(113):81-85.

40. Wu Z, Zhou J, Pankaj P, Peng B. Laparoscopic splenectomy for immune thrombocytopenia (ITP) patients with platelet counts lower than $10 \times 10^9/l$. *Int J Hematol.* 2011;94(6):533-538.

41. Zheng CX, Ji ZQ, Zhang LJ, et al. Proteomics-based identification of haptoglobin as a favorable serum biomarker for predicting long-term response to splenectomy in patients with primary immune thrombocytopenia. *J Transl Med.* 2012;10:208.

42. Zheng CX, Zheng D, Chen LH, Yu JF, Wu ZM. Laparoscopic splenectomy for immune thrombocytopenic purpura at a teaching institution. *Chin Med J.* 2011;12-(8):1175-1180.

43. Cameron JL. Current surgical therapy. In: Park AE, ed. *Laparoscopic Splenectomy.* Philadelphia: Elsevier Mosby; 2004:1-54.

44. Grahn SW, Alvarez J 3rd, Kirkwood K. Trends in laparoscopic splenectomy for massive splenomegaly. *Arch Surg.* 2006;141:755.

45. Reso A, Brar MS, Church N, Mitchell P, Dixon E, Debru E. Outcome of laparoscopic splenectomy with preoperative splenic artery embolization for massive splenomegaly. *Surg Endosc.* 2010;24:2008.

46. Uranues S, Alimoglu O. Laparoscopic surgery of the spleen. *Surg Clin North Am.* 2005;85:75.

47. Heniford BT, Matthews BD, Answini GA, Walsh RM. Laparoscopic splenectomy for malignant diseases. *Semin Laparosc Surg.* 2000;7(2):93-100.

48. Casaccia M, Torelli P, Squarcia S, et al. Laparoscopic splenectomy for hematological diseases: a preliminary analysis performed on the Italian Registry of Laparoscopic Surgery of the Spleen (IRLSS). *Surg Endosc.* 2006;20(8):1214-1220.

49. Habermalz B, Sauerland S, Decker G, et al. Laparoscopic splenectomy: the clinical practice guidelines of the European Association for Endoscopic Surgery (EAES). *Surg Endosc.* 2008;22(4):821-848.

50. Bo W, He-Shui W, Guo-Bin W, Kai-Xiong T. Laparoscopy splenectomy for massive splenomegaly. *J Invest Surg.* 2013;26(3):154-157.

51. Zhan XL, Ji Y, Wang YD. Laparoscopic splenectomy for hypersplenism secondary to liver cirrhosis and portal hypertension. *World J Gastroenterol.* 2014;20(19):5794-5800.

52. Zhu JH, Wang YD, Ye ZY, et al. Laparoscopic versus open splenectomy for hypersplenism secondary to liver cirrhosis. *Surg Laparosc Endosc Percutan Tech.* 2009;19(3):258-262.

53. Kawanaka H, Akahoshi T, Kinjo N, et al. Effect of laparoscopic splenectomy on portal haemodynamics in patients with liver cirrhosis and portal hypertension. *Br J Surg.* 2014;101(12):1585-1593.

54. Zhou J, Wu Z, Pankaj P, Peng B. Long-term postoperative outcomes of hypersplenism: laparoscopic versus open splenectomy secondary to liver cirrhosis. *Surg Endosc.* 2012;26(12):3391-3400.

55. Friedman R, Hiatt J, Korman L, Facklis K, Cymerman J, Phillips EH. Laparoscopic or open splenectomy for hematologic disease: which approach is superior? *J Am Coll Surg.* 1997;185:52.

56. Heniford BT, Park A, Walsh RM, et al. Laparoscopic splenectomy with normal-sized spleens versus splenomegaly: does size matter? *Am Surg.* 2001;67:854.

57. Mahon D, Rhodes M. Laparoscopic splenectomy. Size matters. *Ann R Coll Surg Engl.* 2003;85:248.

58. Terrosu G, Baccarani U, Bresadola V, Sistu MA, Uzzau A, Bresadola F. The impact of splenic weight on laparoscopic splenectomy for splenomegaly. *Surg Endosc.* 2002;16:103.

59. Kercher KW, Matthews BD, Walsh RM, Sing RF, Backus CL, Heniford BT. Laparoscopic splenectomy for massive splenomegaly. *Am J Surg.* 2002;183:192.

60. Barbaros U, Dinccag A, Sume A, et al. Prospective randomized comparison of clinical results between hand-assisted laparoscopic and open splenectomies. *Surg Endosc.* 2010;24(1):25-32.

61. Swanson TW, Meneghetti AT, Sampath S, Connors JM, Panton ON. Hand-assisted laparoscopic splenectomy versus open splenectomy for massive splenomegaly: 20-year experience at a Canadian centre. *Can J Surg.* 2011;54:189.

62. Davidson RN, Wall RA. Prevention and management of infections in patients without a spleen. *Clin Microbiol Infect.* 2001;7:657.

63. Recommendations of the Advisory Committee on Immunization Practices (ACIP): use of vaccines and immune globulins in persons with altered immunocompetence. *MMWR Recomm Rep.* 1993; 42:4.

64. Michels NA. The variational anatomy of the spleen and splenic artery. *Am J Anat.* 1942;70:21.

65. Scott-Conner CE. The SAGES manual—fundamentals of laparoscopy and GI endoscopy. In: Rege RV, ed. *Laparoscopic Splenectomy.* New York: Springer-Verlag; 1999:327.

66. Soper N. Mastery of endoscopic and laparoscopic surgery. In: Poulin EC, ed. *Laparoscopic Splenectomy.* 2nd ed. Philadelphia: Lippincott Williams & Wilkins; 2005:374.

67. Skandalakis JE. Surgical anatomy and technique. In: *Accessory Spleens.* New York: Springer-Verlag; 2000:521.

68. Barawi M, Bekal P, Gress F. Accessory spleen: a potential cause of misdiagnosis at EUS. *Gastrointest Endosc.* 2000;52:769.

69. Souba WW, Fink GJ, Jurkovich LR, et al. ACS surgery principles and practice. In: Poulin EC, Schlachta CM, Mamazza J, eds. *Laparoscopic Splenectomy.* New York: Web MD Professional Publishing; 2005:578.

70. Brodsky A, Brody FJ, Walsh RM, Malm JA, Ponsky JL. Laparoscopic splenectomy. *Surg Endosc.* 2002;16(5):851-854.

71. Glasgow RE, Mulvihill SJ. Laparoscopic splenectomy. *World J Surg.* 1999;23(4):384-388.

72. Misawa T, Yoshida K, Iida T, Sakamoto T, Gocho T, Hirohara S. Minimizing intraoperative bleeding using a vessel-sealing system and splenic hilum hanging maneuver in laparoscopic splenectomy. *J Hepatobiliary Pancreat Surg.* 2009;16(6):786-791.

73. Canda AE, Ozsoy Y, Yuksel S. Laparoscopic splenectomy using LigaSure in benign hematologic diseases. *Surg Laparosc Endosc Percutan Tech.* 2009;19(1):69-71.

74. Romano F, Gelmini R, Caprotti R, Andreotti A, Guaglio M, Franzoni C. Laparoscopic splenectomy: LigaSure versus EndoGIA: a comparative study. *J Laparoendosc Adv Surg Tech A.* 2007;17(6):763-767.

75. Gelmini R, Romano F, Quaranta N, Caprotti R, Tazzioli G, Colombo G. Sutureless and stapleless laparoscopic splenectomy using radiofrequency: Ligasure device. *Surg Endosc.* 2006;20(6):991-994.

76. Wang KX, Hu SY, Zhang GY, Chen B, Zhang HF. Hand-assisted laparoscopic splenectomy for splenomegaly: a comparative study with conventional laparoscopic splenectomy. *Chin Med J.* 2007;120(1):41-45.

77. Rosen M, Brody F, Walsh RM, Ponsky J. Hand-assisted laparoscopic splenectomy vs conventional laparoscopic splenectomy in cases of splenomegaly. *Arch Surg.* 2002;137(12):1348-1352.

78. Kaban GK, Czerniach DR, Cohen R, et al. Hand-assisted laparoscopic splenectomy in the setting of splenomegaly. *Surg Endosc.* 2004;18(9):1340-1343.

79. Borrazzo EC, Daly JM, Morrisey KP, et al. Hand-assisted laparoscopic splenectomy for giant spleens. *Surg Endosc.* 2003;17:918.

80. Pietrabissa A, Moretti L, Peri A, et al. Laparoscopic treatment for splenomegaly: a case for hand assisted laparoscopic surgery. *Arch Surg.* 2011;146:818.

81. Rottman SJ, Podolsky ER, Kim E, et al. Single port access (SPA) splenectomy. *JSLS.* 2010;14:48.

82. Targarona EM, Pallares JL, Balague C, et al. Single incision approach for splenic diseases: a preliminary report on a series of 8 cases. *Surg Endosc.* 2010;24:2236.

83. Hong TH, Lee SK, You YK, et al. Single-port laparoscopic partial splenectomy: a case report. *Surg Laparosc Endosc Percutan Tech.* 2010;20:164.

84. Giulianotti PC, Buchs NC, Coratti A, et al. Robot-assisted treatment of splenic artery aneurysms. *Ann Vasc Surg.* 2011;25:377-383.

85. Pietrabissa A, Morelli L, Ferrari M, et al. Mixed reality for robotic treatment of a splenic artery aneurysm. *Surg Endosc.* 2010;24:1204.

86. Chapman W, Albrecht R, Kim V, et al. Computer-assisted laparoscopic splenectomy with the da Vinci surgical robot. *J Laparoendosc Adv Surg Tech A.* 2002;12:155.

87. Bodner J, Kafka-Ritsch R, Lucciarini P, et al. A critical comparison of robotic versus conventional laparoscopic splenectomies. *World J Surg.* 2005;29:982.

88. Gelmini R, Franzoni C, Spaziani A, et al. Laparoscopic splenectomy: conventional versus robotic approach—a comparative study. *J Laparoendosc Adv Surg Tech A.* 2011;21:393.

89. Zornig C, Emmermann A, Von Waldenfels HA, et al. Colpotomy for specimen removal in laparoscopic surgery. *Chirurg.* 1994;65:883.

90. Vereczkei A, Illenyi L, Arany A, et al. Transvaginal extraction of the laparoscopically removed spleen. *Surg Endosc.* 2003;17:157.

91. Targarona EM, Gomez C, Rovira R, et al. NOTES-assisted transvaginal splenectomy: the next step in the minimally invasive approach to the spleen. *Surg Innov.* 2009;16:218.

92. Wang H, Kopac D, Brisebois R, et al. Randomized controlled trial to investigate the impact of anticoagulation on the incidence of splenic or portal vein thrombosis after laparoscopic splenectomy. *Can J Surg.* 2011;54:227.

93. Brigden ML, Pattullo AL. Prevention and management of overwhelming postsplenectomy infection—an update. *Crit Care Med.* 1999;27(4):836-842.

94. Waghorn DJ. Overwhelming infection in asplenic patients: current best practice preventive measures are not being followed. *J Clin Pathol.* 2001;54(3):214-218.

95. Downing MA, Omar AH, Sabri E, et al. Information on the internet for asplenic patients: a systematic review. *Can J Surg.* 2011;54:5510.

96. Davies JM, Barnes R, Milligan D, British Committee for Standards in Haematology. Working Party of the Haematology/Oncology Task Force. Update of guidelines for the prevention and treatment of infection in patients with an absent or dysfunctional spleen. *Clin Med.* 2002;2(5):440-443.

97. Kaplinsky C, Spirer Z. Post-splenectomy antibiotic prophylaxis—unfinished story: to treat or not to treat? *Pediatr Blood Cancer.* 2006;47(5 suppl):740-741.

98. Casaccia M, Torelli P, Pasa A, et al. Putative predictive parameters for the outcome of laparoscopic splenectomy: a multicenter analysis performed on the Italian Registry of Laparoscopic Surgery of the Spleen. *Ann Surg.* 2010;252:287.

99. Ikeda M, Sekimoto M, Takiguchi S, et al. High incidence of thrombosis of the portal venous system after laparoscopic splenectomy. A prospective study with contrast-enhanced CT scan. *Ann Surg.* 2005;241:208.

100. Harris W, Marcaccio M. Incidence of portal vein thrombosis after laparoscopic splenectomy. *Can J Surg.* 2005;48:352.

101. Deleted in review.

102. Krauth MT, Lechner K, Neugebauer EA, et al. The postoperative splenic/portal vein thrombosis after splenectomy and its prevention—an unresolved issue. *Haematologica.* 2008;93:1227.

103. van der Vlies CH, Hoekstra J, Ponsen KJ, et al. Impact of splenic artery embolization on the success rate of nonoperative management for blunt splenic injury. *Cardiovasc Intervent Radiol.* 2012;35:76.

104. Jeremitsky E, Kao A, Carlton C, et al. Does splenic embolization and grade of splenic injury impact nonoperative management in patients sustaining blunt splenic trauma? *Am Surg.* 2011;77:215.

105. Franco F, Monaco D, Volpi A, et al. The role of arterial embolization in blunt splenic injury. *Radiol Med.* 2011;116:454.

106. Sclafani SJ, Shaftan GW, Scalea TM, et al. Nonoperative salvage of computed tomography-diagnosed splenic injuries: utilization of angiography for triage and embolization for hemostasis. *J Trauma.* 1995;39:818; discussion 826.

107. Moore EE, Cogbill TH, Jurkovich GJ, et al. Organ injury scaling: spleen and liver (1994 revision). *J Trauma.* 1995;38:323.

108. Haan JM, Biffl W, Knudson MM, et al. Splenic embolization revisited: a multicenter review. *J Trauma.* 2004;56:542.

109. Wahl WL, Ahrns KS, Chen S, et al. Blunt splenic injury: operation versus angiographic embolization. *Surgery.* 2004;136:891.

110. Haan JM, Bochicchio GV, Kramer N, et al. Nonoperative management of blunt splenic injury: a 5-year experience. *J Trauma.* 2005;58:492.

111. Sekikawa Z, Takebayashi S, Kurihara H, et al. Factors affecting clinical outcome of patients who undergo transcatheter arterial embolisation in splenic injury. *Br J Radiol.* 2004;77:308.

112. Brasel KJ, DeLisle CM, Olson CJ, et al. Splenic injury: trends in evaluation and management. *J Trauma.* 1998;44:283.

113. Gaunt WT, McCarthy MC, Lambert CS, et al. Traditional criteria for observation of splenic trauma should be challenged. *Am Surg.* 1999;65:689; discussion 691.

114. Peitzman AB, Heil B, Rivera L, et al. Blunt splenic injury in adults: multi-institutional study of the Eastern Association for the Surgery of Trauma. *J Trauma.* 2000;49:177; discussion 187.

115. Lawler LP, Fishman EK. Celiomesenteric anomaly demonstration by multidetector CT and volume rendering. *J Comput Assist Tomogr.* 2001;25:802.

116. Schnuriger B, Inaba K, Konstantinidis A, et al. Outcomes of proximal versus distal splenic artery embolization after trauma: a systematic review and meta-analysis. *J Trauma.* 2011;70:252.

117. Hagiwara A, Murata A, Matsuda T, Matsuda H, Shimazaki S. The usefulness of transcatheter arterial embolization for patients with blunt polytrauma showing transient response to fluid resuscitation. *J Trauma.* 2004;57:271; discussion 276.

118. Liu PP, Lee WC, Cheng YF, et al. Use of splenic artery embolization as an adjunct to nonsurgical management of blunt splenic injury. *J Trauma.* 2004;56:768; discussion 773.

119. Frumiento C, Sartorelli K, Vane D. Complications of splenic injuries: expansion of the nonoperative theorem. *J Pediatr Surg.* 2000;35:788.

120. Cocanour CS, Moore FA, Ware DN, Marvin RG, Clark JM, Duke JH. Delayed complications of nonoperative management of blunt adult splenic trauma. *Arch Surg.* 1998;133:619; discussion 624.

121. Sakai T, Shiraki K, Inoue H, et al. Complications of partial splenic embolization in cirrhotic patients. *Dig Dis Sci.* 2002;47:388.

122. Oller-Sales B, Troya-Diaz J, Martinez-Arconada MJ, et al. Post-traumatic splenic function depending on severity of injury and management. *Transl Res.* 2011;158:118.

123. Abbas MA, Stone WM, Fowl RJ, et al. Splenic artery aneurysms: two decades experience at Mayo Clinic. *Ann Vasc Surg.* 2002;16:442-449.

124. Lee PC, Rhee RY, Gordon RY, Fung JJ, Webster MW. Management of splenic artery aneurysms: the significance of portal and essential hypertension. *J Am Coll Surg.* 1999;189:483-490.

125. Selo-Ojeme DO, Welch CC. Review: spontaneous rupture of splenic artery aneurysm in pregnancy. *Eur J Obstet Gynecol Reprod Biol.* 2003;109:124-127.

126. Goffette PP, Laterre PF. Traumatic injuries: imaging and intervention in post-traumatic complications (delayed intervention). *Eur Radiol.* 2002;12:994.

127. Tessier DJ, Stone WM, Fowl RJ, et al. Clinical features and management of splenic artery pseudoaneurysm: case series and cumulative review of literature. *J Vasc Surg.* 2003;38:969-974.

128. Agrawal GA, Johnson PT, Fishman EK. Splenic artery aneurysms and pseudoaneurysms: clinical distinctions and CT appearances. *AJR Am J Roentgenol.* 2007;188(4):992-999.

129. Gorg C, Colle J, Wied M, et al. Spontaneous non traumatic intrasplenic pseudoaneurysm: causes, sonographic diagnosis, and prognosis. *J Clin Ultrasound.* 2003;31:129.

130. Yardeni D, Polley TZ Jr, Coran AG. Splenic artery embolization for post-traumatic splenic artery pseudoaneurysm in children. *J Trauma.* 2004;57:404.

131. Arepally A, Dagli M, Hofmann LV, et al. Treatment of splenic artery aneurysm with use of a stent-graft. *J Vasc Interv Radiol.* 2002;13:631.

132. Huang IH, Zuckerman DA, Matthews JB. Occlusion of a giant splenic artery pseudoaneurysm with percutaneous thrombin-collagen injection. *J Vasc Surg.* 2004;40:574.

133. Davis KA, Fabian TC, Croce MA, et al. Improved success in nonoperative management of blunt splenic injuries: embolization of splenic artery pseudoaneurysms. *J Trauma.* 1998;44:1008; discussion 1013.

134. Kagaya H, Miyata T, Hoshina K, et al. Long-term results of endovascular treatment for splenic artery aneurysms. *Int Angiol.* 2011;30:359.

135. Moghaddam MB, Kalra M, Bjarnason H, et al. Review: splenic arteriovenous fistula: successful treatment with an Amplatz occlusion device. *Ann Vasc Surg.* 2011;25:556.e17.

136. Mozes MF, Spigos DG, Pollak R, et al. Partial splenic embolization, an alternative to splenectomy—results of a prospective, randomized study. *Surgery.* 1984;96:694.

137. Nio M, Hayashi Y, Sano N, et al. Long-term efficacy of partial splenic embolization in children. *J Pediatr Surg.* 2003;38:1760.

138. Sakata K, Hirai K, Tanikawa K. A long-term investigation of transcatheter splenic arterial embolization for hypersplenism. *Hepatogastroenterology.* 1996;43:309.

139. Kumpe DA, Rumack CM, Pretorius DH, et al. Partial splenic embolization in children with hypersplenism. *Radiology.* 1985;155:357.

140. Sangro B, Bilbao I, Herrero I, et al. Partial splenic embolization for the treatment of hypersplenism in cirrhosis. *Hepatology.* 1993;18:309.

141. N'Kontchou G, Seror O, Bourcier V, et al. Partial splenic embolization in patients with cirrhosis: efficacy, tolerance and long-term outcome in 32 patients. *Eur J Gastroenterol Hepatol.* 2005;17:179.

142. Palsson B, Hallen M, Forsberg AM, et al. Partial splenic embolization: long-term outcome. *Langenbecks Arch Surg.* 2003;387:421.

143. Akhan O, Baykan Z, Oguzkurt L, et al. Percutaneous treatment of a congenital splenic cyst with alcohol: a new therapeutic approach. *Eur Radiol.* 1997;7:1067.
144. Moir C, Guttman F, Jequier S, et al. Splenic cysts: aspiration, sclerosis, or resection. *J Pediatr Surg.* 1989;24:646.
145. Chou YH, Tiu CM, Chiou HJ, et al. Ultrasound-guided interventional procedures in splenic abscesses. *Eur J Radiol.* 1998;28:167.
146. Green BT. Splenic abscess: report of six cases and review of the literature. *Am Surg.* 2001;67:80.

147. McInnes MD, Kielar AZ, Macdonald DB. Percutaneous image-guided biopsy of the spleen: systematic review and meta-analysis of the complication rate and diagnostic accuracy. *Radiology.* 2011;260: 699.
148. Olson MC, Atwell TD, Harmsen WS, et al. Safety and accuracy of percutaneous image-guided core biopsy of the spleen. *AJR Am J Roentgenol.* 2016;206(3):655-652.

Management of Splenic Trauma in Adults

Sara A. Mansfield | Amy P. Rushing

The spleen, an important component of the reticuloendothelial system in normal adults, is a highly vascular solid organ that arises as a mass of differentiated mesenchymal tissue during early embryonic development. The normal adult spleen weighs between 75 and 100 g and receives an average blood flow of 300 mL/min. It functions as the primary filter of the reticuloendothelial system by sequestering and removing antigens, bacteria, and senescent or damaged cellular elements from the circulation. In addition, the spleen has an important role in humoral immunity because it produces immunoglobulin M and opsonins for the complement activation system.[1]

Although the spleen resides under the confines of the left lower rib cage, it is frequently subject to both blunt and penetrating trauma. Isolated splenic injury after blunt trauma is common in children, whereas the adult trauma population will often sustain associated injuries to the thorax, kidneys, extremities, and head.[2] The mechanism of injury in blunt trauma stems from abrupt deceleration resulting in vascular torsion of the splenic hilum, shearing of the short gastric vessels within the gastrosplenic ligament, or capsular tearing at sites of ligamentous fixation. Clinical features that suggest splenic trauma include left upper quadrant or flank ecchymosis and abrasions, as well as left shoulder pain caused by irritation of the left hemidiaphragm by subphrenic blood (Kehr sign). In instances of penetrating trauma, a wound track traversing the left upper quadrant raises the suspicion for splenic injury. Regardless of mechanism, all trauma patients should receive the primary survey, followed by the appropriate secondary evaluation and ancillary studies.

Currently, the accepted standard of care for most splenic trauma is expectant management with close observation. Operative intervention is reserved for the hemodynamically labile patient who shows signs of active hemorrhage and who does not respond appropriately to fluid resuscitation. Although these clinical scenarios seem straightforward, it is often the condition of the patient who falls in between the two ends of the spectrum that can be the most challenging to manage. In the setting of advanced imaging techniques and interventional radiology, the trauma surgeon has more diagnostic information and more treatment options for the patient with splenic trauma.

DIAGNOSIS

Patients who present with evidence of ongoing intraabdominal hemorrhage should undergo immediate operative exploration. For those who present with normal hemodynamics, a thorough diagnostic evaluation should be completed. Following the primary survey, a focused abdominal examination should be performed, looking for signs of significant intraabdominal injuries. Abdominal wall ecchymosis, abrasions, flank pain, and distention should raise suspicion for an injury and prompt further diagnostic work-up. The patient who presents with left-sided rib fractures should also be evaluated for a concomitant splenic laceration.

A laboratory panel should be sent to obtain an index hemoglobin and hematocrit, platelet count, and coagulation profile. While in the emergency department, the focused abdominal sonography for trauma (FAST) exam offers a rapid and noninvasive approach to detecting intraperitoneal blood. The sensitivity of FAST has been reported between 43% and 93%, whereas its specificity ranges in various reports between 90% and 98%.[3,4] The primary limitations of FAST are the heavy operator dependence of the ultrasonographic exam, as well as the technical limitations caused by the patient's body habitus or intestinal gas. Branney et al. demonstrated the technical shortcomings of the technique by infusing volumes of diagnostic peritoneal lavage fluid into the peritoneal cavity and found that only 10% of participants performing FAST could detect fluid volumes of less than 400 mL.[5] In spite of these obstacles, the FAST exam is helpful in the preliminary evaluation of the patient, especially when the patient cannot undergo further imaging because of hemodynamic instability. Given the ranges in sensitivity, it is important to remember a negative FAST without a computed tomography (CT) may result in missed intraabdominal injuries. In addition, in hemodynamically labile patients, the decision of exploratory laparotomy should not be distracted by a negative FAST.[6]

Unlike ultrasonography, CT has dramatically changed the way we characterize splenic injuries. The CT scan is the diagnostic modality of choice for the hemodynamically stable patient in whom a splenic injury is suspected. The sensitivity and specificity of CT imaging approaches 100% and 98%, respectively.[7] Current-generation multislice scanners provide a detailed survey of the splenic architecture and allow the clinician to differentiate simple subcapsular hematomas from more severe parenchymal and vascular injuries. Although exposing patients to increased radiation, the arterial phase of CT image acquisition—in addition to traditionally obtained portal venous and delayed phase images—should be considered to optimize the detection of traumatic splenic injuries.[8]

Several grading systems have been used for classifying splenic injuries, and these have important implications in both the operative and nonoperative management decisions. The Organ Injury Scaling Committee of the American Association for the Surgery of Trauma (OISC-AAST) devised an anatomic grading system that defines the severity of splenic injuries.[9] The system incorporates both CT scan findings and intraoperative assessment of the spleen and consists of five grades (Table 139.1). This grading scale provides universal definitions that all

TABLE 139.1 Organ Injury Scaling Committee of the American Association for the Surgery of Trauma (1994 Revision)

Grade	Injury Description
I	Hematoma—subcapsular, <10% surface area
	Or
	Laceration—capsular tear, <1 cm parenchymal depth
II	Hematoma—subcapsular, 10%–50% surface area, intraparenchymal <5 cm in diameter
	Or
	Laceration 1–3 cm parenchymal depth which does not involve a trabecular vessel
III	Subcapsular, >50% surface area or expanding, ruptured subcapsular or parenchymal hematoma, intraparenchymal hematoma >5 cm or expanding
	Or
	Laceration >3 cm parenchymal depth or involving trabecular vessels
IV	Laceration involving segmental or hilar vessels producing major devascularization (>25% of spleen)
V	Completely shattered spleen
	Or
	Hilar vascular injury which devascularizes spleen

Advance one grade for multiple injuries, up to grade III.
Modified from Moore EE, Cogbill TH, Jurkovich GJ, Shackford SR, Malangoni MA, Champion HR. Organ injury scaling: spleen and liver (1994 revision). *J Trauma*. 1995;38:323.

clinicians can understand, and it becomes particularly useful when a patient requires transfer to a tertiary trauma center from an acute care hospital as the severity of injury is readily appreciated. Although the trauma community recognizes that the primary predictor of operative intervention is hemodynamic instability, the organ injury severity scale can also serve as a predictor of further therapeutic intervention. Haan et al. reported a splenic salvage rate of 94% over a 5-year period; however, they found that the salvage rate decreased with increased splenic injury grade.[16]

NONOPERATIVE MANAGEMENT

The increased availability of high-resolution CT scan and advances in arterial angiography and embolization techniques have contributed to the success of nonoperative management of splenic injuries. The hemodynamically stable patient with blunt splenic trauma can be adequately managed with bed rest, serial abdominal exams, and hemoglobin and hematocrit monitoring. This approach, in combination with occasional angiography, especially for grade III and IV injuries, confers a splenic salvage rate of up to 95%.[11,12] In the setting of expectant management, indications for angiography have been delineated by several studies and include the following CT scan features: contrast extravasation, the presence of a pseudoaneurysm, significant hemoperitoneum, high-grade injury, and evidence of a vascular injury.[13] The goal of angiography is to localize bleeding and embolize the source with coils or a gelatin foam product. Embolization can occur either at the main splenic artery just distal to the dorsal pancreatic portion of the vessel—known as proximal embolization—or selectively at the distal branch of the injured vessel. The goal behind the former technique is to decrease the perfusion pressure to the spleen to encourage hemostasis. The disadvantage to this technique is global splenic ischemia, and many have questioned the spleen's immunocompetence following proximal embolization. Malhotra et al. examined the effects of angioembolization on splenic function by examining serum levels of a particular T-cell line. T-cell proportions between patients who had undergone splenic embolization with asplenic patients and healthy controls were similar suggesting some degree of splenic immunocompetency was maintained.[14] A Norwegian study comparing blood samples from patients who had undergone angioembolization with healthy controls demonstrated that the study samples had similar levels of pneumococcal immunoglobulins and no Howell-Jolly bodies, suggesting normal splenic function.[15] Although these preliminary studies remain encouraging, there is no definitive evidence that splenic immunocompetency is fully maintained following angioembolization.

There is no question that advancements in interventional techniques have contributed to the successful nonoperative management of splenic injuries. This has certainly changed the strategy, but it has not completely replaced operative intervention. The challenge now remains predicting those patients who will ultimately require splenectomy. Many groups have studied potential predictors of nonoperative failure. Earlier studies found that a higher injury grade, increased transfusion requirement and hypotension on initial presentation consistently predicted failure of nonoperative management. More recent literature reflects the use of advanced imaging techniques for predicting which patients will ultimately require splenectomy. Haan looked at the overall outcomes of patients admitted with blunt splenic trauma and reported several radiographic findings that were prevalent among patients requiring splenectomy after angioembolization: contrast extravasation, pseudoaneurysm, significant hemoperitoneum, and arteriovenous fistula. Among these characteristics, an arteriovenous fistula had the highest rate of nonoperative failure at 40%.[10] Nonradiographic features associated with significant risk of nonoperative failure include age greater than 40, injury severity score of 25 or greater or presence of large-volume hemoperitoneum.[16,17]

Aside from radiographic findings, some groups have also examined the mechanism of injury and its association with nonoperative failure. Purad et al. conducted a retrospective review over a 15-year period and found that patients who were victims of blunt assault were more likely to fail nonoperative management: 36% of these patients required splenectomy versus 11.5% of patients from all other mechanisms combined. These findings suggest that regardless of overall injury severity, individuals who sustain a direct transfer of injury to the left torso are more likely to require splenectomy.[18]

OPERATIVE MANAGEMENT

When a patient presents with hemodynamic lability in spite of timed resuscitation, operative intervention remains the most prudent course of treatment. In this situation, standard principles of trauma care are followed: the patient should have reliable intravenous access, appropriate volume resuscitation, preparation of type and cross-matched packed red blood cells, nasogastric decompression, and preoperative intravenous antibiotic administration. It is standard practice to use a vertical midline incision for laparotomy because this affords the quickest access to the peritoneal cavity. If this incision proves to be insufficient, it can be extended cephalad and to the left of the xiphoid process. In addition, the left triangular ligament of the liver may be incised to allow reflection of the liver away from the area of interest. Although it may seem practical, an oblique left upper quadrant incision for a presumed isolated splenic injury is more time-consuming and offers little access to the remainder of the peritoneal cavity should a concomitant injury present itself.

After entering the peritoneal cavity, a standard initial survey should be performed. All four quadrants should be packed and systematically inspected for bleeding or enteric contamination. If other injuries are recognized and require more urgent attention, one can achieve adequate hemostasis of the spleen with proper packing. Multiple laparotomy packs should be placed around the splenic parenchyma in such a manner that a tamponade effect is maintained between the diaphragm, lateral abdominal wall, and retroperitoneum. When it is time to address the injury, mobilization is achieved by placing laparotomy packs posterior to the spleen and lifting it directly into the operative field. Following its inspection, the spleen's ligamentous attachments to the diaphragm, kidney, and colon should be sharply incised. These connections are avascular and can be divided with impunity in most circumstances. The spleen can then be rotated to the midline and further elevated, thus enabling complete access to its anterior and posterior surfaces, as well as to the hilum. Once accomplished, the operator can easily achieve virtually complete hemostasis of any splenic injury by direct manual compression of the splenic parenchyma or by control of the splenic artery and vein at the hilum. At this point, a decision is made regarding splenectomy or splenorrhaphy.

After the spleen has been fully mobilized, one may proceed with splenectomy by first individually ligating and dividing the short gastric vessels. These vessels should be addressed far from the greater curvature of the stomach so that the risk of gastric wall necrosis is minimized. Because the short gastric vessels are divided and the splenic hilum is skeletonized, one must pay attention to the tail of the pancreas. Careless technique can result in disruption of the pancreatic capsule and the development of a pancreatic fistula with subsequent morbidity. Following the division of the short gastric vessels, the splenic artery is then doubly ligated and divided within the splenic hilum. The splenic vein is dealt with in the same manner, and the splenectomy is completed. After removal of the spleen, the splenic bed should be thoroughly irrigated and inspected for hemostasis. These steps are essential to minimize the chances of postoperative splenic bed hematoma, which in turn predisposes to the risk of a subphrenic abscess. Although there are no conclusive data regarding the use of closed-suction drains in the surgical bed, we do not routinely drain the

splenic fossa following splenectomy. Meticulous hemostasis tends to be the best method in avoiding splenic bed complications.

The term *splenorrhaphy* refers to a variety of "spleen-sparing" techniques aimed at controlling hemorrhage so that the patient may retain the immunologic benefits of the spleen. The intraoperative decision to attempt splenorrhaphy should be made only after the spleen has been fully mobilized and inspected.[19,20] As a general rule, splenorrhaphy is most appropriately considered in cases of less severe injury (e.g., grades I and II, and occasionally grade III). Splenorrhaphy should not be attempted to repair extensive or complex injuries of the spleen, nor is it well advised to undertake splenorrhaphy in the face of multiple concomitant injuries or associated hypotension. With the spleen fully mobilized and controlled in the surgeon's hand, splenorrhaphy may consist of mere manual compression of the parenchyma to achieve hemostasis of simple lacerations. In addition, there are a variety of topical hemostatic agents that may be applied directly to the bleeding parenchymal surface. Other options include suture repair of the spleen using a monofilament suture in a mattress technique, where one can also incorporate a piece of omentum or gelatin sponge product into the repair. Alternatively, wrapping the entire spleen in absorbable mesh has been described as a means of effective tamponade and has not been associated with a significant increase in infectious complications.[20] Examining splenic salvage rates over a 9-year period, Feliciano et al. found that the majority of splenorrhaphy cases were accomplished with simple techniques and less than 10% required a mesh wrap. In this series, the incidence of rebleeding was 1.3%.[21]

POSTOPERATIVE CONSIDERATIONS

Overwhelming postsplenectomy sepsis (OPSS), first described by Diamond in 1969, is an infrequent but potentially catastrophic complication of splenectomy resulting from an increased susceptibility to infection by encapsulated microorganisms.[22] The overall standard incidence ratio for hospitalization for sepsis was 5.7, with lower incidences in trauma patients (3.4; 95% confidence interval [CI], 3.0 to 3.8), compared with 18 (95% CI, 16 to 19) for patients with hematologic malignancies.[23] Early reports of OPSS indicated mortality rates of 50% to 70% in spite of the use of intravenous antibiotics and intensive therapeutic intervention. With advances in antibiotic therapy and intensive care, the mortality rate of OPSS can be expected to be approximately 10%, with more than half of all fatalities occurring within 48 hours of presentation.[1,24] Given these findings, it is a widely accepted practice to immunize patients with pneumococcal vaccine shortly after undergoing emergency splenectomy prior to discharge from the hospital.[25] The incidence of OPSS does not appear to have decreased during the vaccine era.[23] In fact, *Streptococcus pneumoniae* remains the causative organism in 42% of cases.[26] The efficacy and clinical importance of *Neisseria meningitidis* and *Haemophilus influenzae* type b vaccination in splenectomized individuals is unknown but should be considered in patients who are deemed more likely to encounter these organisms.[25] We typically administer all three of the vaccines to patients undergoing emergency splenectomy. Although these patients should take all necessary precautions to avoid serious infections, prophylactic antibiotics are not thought to be necessary following splenectomy in adults.[27] Antibody response appears to be preserved following splenic artery embolization, especially in selective embolization, indicating vaccines may not be needed; however, larger studies are needed to confirm this.[28]

REFERENCES

1. Lynch AM, Kapila R. Overwhelming postsplenectomy infection. *Infect Dis Clin North Am*. 1996;10:693.
2. Miller PR, Croce MA, Bee TK, Malhotra AK, Fabian TC. Associated injuries in blunt solid organ trauma: implications for missed injury in nonoperative management. *J Trauma*. 2002;53:238.
3. Rozycki GS, Ballard RB, Feliciano DV, Schmidt JA, Pennington SD. Surgeon-performed ultrasound for the assessment of truncal injuries: lessons learned from 1540 patients. *Ann Surg*. 1998;228:557.
4. Natarajan B, Gupta PK, Cemaj S, Sorensen M, Haroudis GI, Forse RA. FAST scan: is it worth doing in hemodynamically stable blunt trauma patients? *Surgery*. 2010;148:695.
5. Branney SW, Wolfe RE, Moore EE, et al. Quantitative sensitivity of ultrasound in detecting free intraperitoneal fluid. *J Trauma*. 1995;39:375.
6. Carter JW, Falco MH, Chopko MS, Flynn WJ Jr, Wiles Iii CE, Guo WA. Do we really rely on FAST for decision-making in the management of blunt abdominal trauma? *Injury*. 2015;46:817.
7. Wing VW, Federle MP, Morris JA, Jeffrey RB, Bluth R. The clinical impact of CT for blunt abdominal trauma. *AJR Am J Roentgenol*. 1985;145:1191.
8. Uyeda JW, LeBedis CA, Penn DR, Soto JA, Anderson SW. Active hemorrhage and vascular injuries in splenic trauma: utility of the arterial phase in multidetector CT. *Radiology*. 2014;270:99.
9. Moore EE, Cogbill TH, Jurkovich GJ, Shackford SR, Malangoni MA, Champion HR. Organ injury scaling: spleen and liver (1994 revision). *J Trauma*. 1995;38:323.
10. Haan JM, Bochicchio GV, Kramer N, Scalea TM. Nonoperative management of blunt splenic injury: a 5-year experience. *J Trauma*. 2005;58:492.
11. Miller PR, Chang MC, Hoth JJ, et al. Prospective trial of angiography and embolization for all grade III to V blunt splenic injuries: nonoperative management success rate is significantly improved. *J Am Coll Surg*. 2014;218:644.
12. Renzulli P, Gross T, Schnurger B, et al. Management of blunt injuries to the spleen. *Br J Surg*. 2010;97:1696.
13. Haan JM, Biffl W, Knudson MM, et al. Splenic embolization revisited: a multicenter review. *J Trauma*. 2004;56:542.
14. Malhotra AK, Carter RF, Lebman DA, et al. Preservation of splenic immunocompetence after splenic artery angioembolization for blunt splenic injury. *J Trauma*. 2010;69:1126.
15. Skattum J, Titze TL, Dormagen JB, et al. Preserved splenic function after angioembolisation of high grade injury. *Injury*. 2012;43:62.
16. Olthof DC, Joosse P, van der Vlies CH, de Haan RJ, Goslings JC. Prognostic factors for failure of nonoperative management in adults with blunt splenic injury: a systematic review. *J Trauma Acute Care Surg*. 2013;74:546.
17. Bhangu A, Nepogodiev D, Lal N, Bowley DM. Meta-analysis of predictive factors and outcomes for failure of non-operative management of blunt splenic trauma. *Injury*. 2012;43:1337.
18. Plurad DS, Green DJ, Inaba K, et al. Blunt assault is associated with failure of nonoperative management of the spleen independent of organ injury grade and despite lower overall injury severity. *J Trauma*. 2009;66:630.
19. Berry ME, Rosato EF, Williams NN. Dexon mesh splenorrhaphy for intraoperative splenic injuries. *Am Surg*. 2003;69:176.
20. Pachter HL, Hofstetter SR, Spencer FC. Evolving concepts in splenic surgery: splenorrhaphy versus splenectomy and postsplenectomy drainage—experience in 105 patients. *Ann Surg*. 1981;194:262.
21. Feliciano DV, Spjut-Patrinely V, Burch JM, et al. Splenorrhaphy—the alternative. *Ann Surg*. 1990;211:569.
22. Diamond LK. Splenectomy in childhood and the hazard of overwhelming infection. *Pediatrics*. 1969;43:886.
23. Edgren G, Almqvist R, Hartman M, Utter GH. Splenectomy and the risk of sepsis: a population-based cohort study. *Ann Surg*. 2014;260:1081.
24. Brigden ML, Pattullo AL. Prevention and management of overwhelming postsplenectomy infection—an update. *Crit Care Med*. 1999;27:836.
25. Shatz DV. Vaccination practices among North American trauma surgeons in splenectomy for trauma. *J Trauma*. 2002;53:950.
26. Theilacker C, Ludewig K, Serr A, et al. Overwhelming postsplenectomy infection: a prospective multicenter cohort study. *Clin Infect Dis*. 2016;62:871.
27. Working Party of the British Committee for Standards in Haematology Clinical Haematology Task Force. Guidelines for the prevention and treatment of infection in patients with an absent or dysfunctional spleen. *BMJ*. 1996;312:430.
28. Olthof DC, Lammers AJ, van Leeuwen EM, Hoekstra JB, ten Berge IJ, Goslings JC. Antibody response to a T-cell-independent antigen is preserved after splenic artery embolization for trauma. *Clin Vaccine Immunol*. 2014;21:1500.

Splenic Trauma in Children

Grace Z. Mak

Abdominal injury occurs in approximately 10% to 15% of pediatric trauma patients, with the spleen being the most commonly injured intraabdominal organ, accounting for a significant proportion of the management expenses incurred with blunt traumatic injuries.[1-4] Historically the initial management of splenic injury was emergent splenectomy. However, as the immunologic importance of the spleen became evident with the recognition of postsplenectomy sepsis, spleen-preserving strategies were implemented, particularly in children. In 1952 King and Shumacher first reported two deaths among five infants who developed severe sepsis following splenectomy for hereditary spherocytosis.[5] The spleen is now known to play important immune functions, including the eradication of such encapsulated bacteria as *Streptococcus pneumoniae*, *Neisseria meningitidis*, and *Haemophilus influenzae* type B. The rate of postsplenectomy sepsis in children less than 5 years of age is greater than 10%, compared with less than 1% in adults, with a reported life-long risk greater than 85 times that of the normal population and a mortality rate approaching 70%.[4,6,7] Thus, following splenectomy, patients must take penicillin prophylaxis for varying periods of time to decrease the risk of developing postsplenectomy sepsis. In addition, splenectomy increases the risks of short-term hematologic complications and long-term cardiovascular complications.[8] Comparisons of "quality-adjusted life expectancy" after blunt splenic trauma for the treatment options of observation, splenorrhaphy, and splenectomy have shown a decreased life expectancy for patients undergoing splenectomy.[9] Long-term cost savings from splenic preservation could include prescription drug costs both from prophylactic antibiotics and vaccinations, as well as decrease in hospitalizations associated with postsplenectomy infections.[10]

In light of these findings and the observation that bleeding from splenic injuries had often ceased by the time of laparotomy, the treatment of children with blunt splenic injuries evolved from emergent splenectomy to splenic preservation. Upadhyaya and Simpson first described in 1968 selective nonoperative management (NOM) of splenic injuries in children sustaining blunt trauma.[11] Since this initial description, multiple guidelines and protocols have been described, all with success rates greater than 90%. Thus NOM is now the standard of care for blunt splenic injuries in children. Interestingly, the success of NOM in children prompted the application of NOM to blunt splenic injuries in adult trauma patients, although the success rate has been lower.[12]

SPLEEN ANATOMY AND PHYSIOLOGY

The unique segmental blood supply of the spleen readily permits repair and resection of the injured spleen. Vascular anatomy usually consists of superior and inferior segments in 84% compared with superior, middle, and inferior segments in 16% (Fig. 140.1). These segments are separated by avascular planes that pass obliquely to the longitudinal axis of the spleen and often do not traverse the full thickness of the spleen from the parietal to visceral surfaces. Intrasplenic vessels are lobar, segmented, and generally without intersegmental communication. Dixon et al. divided the spleen into three-dimensional zones (hilar, intermediate, and peripheral), with each zone requiring a specific technique for hemostasis. Bleeding from the peripheral zone may be managed with topical agents, whereas ligation is recommended for the trabecular and segmental vessels in the intermediate and hilar zones (Fig. 140.2).[13,14]

Compared with the adult spleen, the splenic capsule in children is relatively thicker and contains abundant myoepithelial cells that favor hemostatic control of hemorrhage.[15] The more efficient contraction and retraction of splenic arterioles, as well as the lack of atherosclerosis, confer greater vascular compliance, further improving contraction leading to more effective hemostasis.[16] Inferior rib fractures are commonly associated with splenic injuries in adults, with the broken rib often penetrating the splenic capsule. In contrast, rib fractures are rarely seen in children because their ribs have greater elasticity, allowing the ribs to recoil rather than fracture, thereby reducing the direct force to the spleen and the risk of penetrating the splenic capsule.[16,17]

EVALUATION OF SPLENIC TRAUMA IN THE CHILD

Evaluation of the pediatric trauma patient proceeds systematically as outlined by Advanced Trauma Life Support (ATLS), prioritizing the assessment and management of the airway, breathing, and circulation.[18] Sequential assessment and maintenance of airway patency, adequacy of gas exchange, and perfusion are the priorities of resuscitation, preventing and/or correcting hypoxemia due to inadequate oxygen delivery.

Many children with abdominal injuries have either equivocal or absent physical findings, with a reported overall accuracy of initial physical examination varying from 16% to 45%. Thus reliance on physical examination alone is an inadequate evaluation of the child with potential abdominal injury. Diagnostic adjuncts in the evaluation of the abdomen include focused assessment sonography in trauma (FAST) and computed tomography (CT). However, if the patient is hemodynamically unstable from an intraabdominal source, the child undergoes immediate surgical exploration. If the patient responds

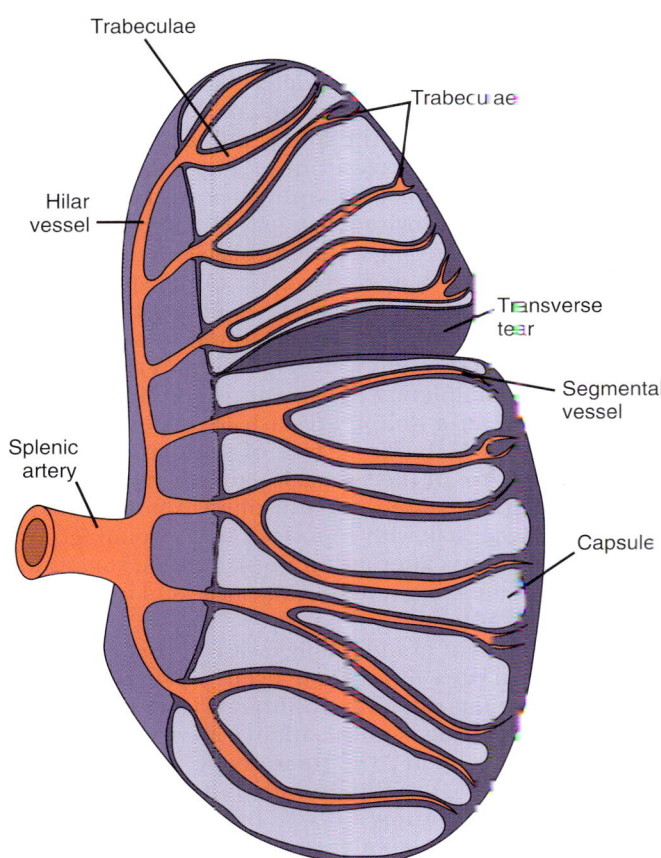

FIGURE 140.1 Diagram of segmental splenic vasculature.

Labels: Trabeculae, Trabeculae, Hilar vessel, Transverse tear, Segmental vessel, Splenic artery, Capsule

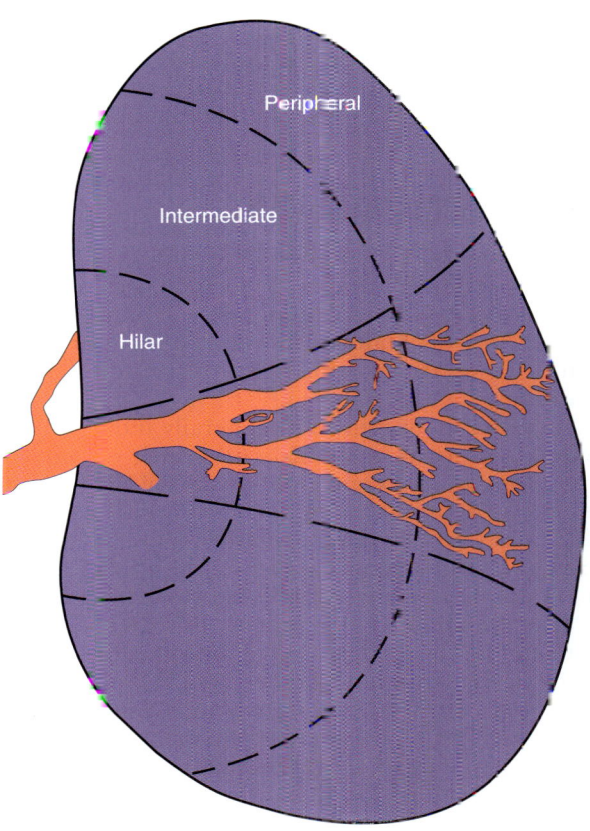

FIGURE 140.2 Diagram of hilar, intermediate and peripheral zones.

Labels: Peripheral, Intermediate, Hilar

to resuscitation, more definitive diagnostic imaging can then be performed.

Ultrasound has many advantages, including portability, immediate availability, lack of ionizing radiation, noninvasiveness, and low cost. During the FAST exam, the operator focuses on identifying free fluid in the subxiphoid region (heart), left flank (spleen), right upper quadrant and Morrison pouch (liver), and pelvis and pouch of Douglas.[19] Although fast, FAST does not reliably identify the injured organ or the quality of the identified free fluid (blood, succus, urine) and can miss solid organ injuries not associated with free fluid. Thus ultrasound may miss intraparenchymal injuries or downgrade injuries.[20] In addition, the quality of the exam is dependent upon the operator in both performing and interpreting the exam. In a systematic review and meta-analysis, abdominal ultrasound was found to have modest sensitivity (66%) in the detection of hemoperitoneum in children sustaining blunt trauma but low specificity. Moreover, a negative ultrasound examination has questionable utility as the sole diagnostic test to rule out intraabdominal injuries in the pediatric trauma patient. Rather, the utility of FAST exam seems to be in the evaluation of the hemodynamically unstable patient to aid in the identification of areas of injury and help to prioritize interventions.[19–21]

CT of the abdomen and pelvis is the current standard of care for the evaluation of the peritoneal cavity and retroperitoneum. Intravenous contrast provides maximal

information regarding organ perfusion, presence of free intraperitoneal fluid, and characteristics of the bowel. Enteral contrast is generally not required in the acute trauma setting and can lead to aspiration.[19] There is a reported correlation between the severity of the solid organ injury and the likelihood and volume of associated free fluid. The most common location of free fluid regardless of the site of injury (spleen or liver) is the pelvis. Free fluid is more common in splenic injury (82%) compared with liver injury (69%).[20]

Due to concern regarding the long-term risk of radiation exposure, the use of any ionizing radiation in children has been particularly scrutinized and limited as much as possible. Although CT is an essential imaging modality, there is an obligatory exposure to ionizing radiation that has been demonstrated to increase the risk of cancer, particularly in children.[22] Compared with adults, the cancer risk from radiation exposure in children is not insignificant and may be more pronounced due to a number of factors. The same amount of radiation exposure results in a relatively higher dose to children due to their smaller cross-sectional area, compared with adults. Tissues and organs that are growing and developing are more sensitive to radiation effects than mature tissue, and the oncologic effect of radiation may have a longer latent period. In addition, an infant or child has a longer life expectancy during which to manifest the potential oncologic effects of radiation compared with the adult. Thus, to decrease radiation exposure radiologists use radiation doses that are as low as reasonably achievable (ALARA), which means that no more radiation should be used than is required to achieve the necessary diagnostic information and to perform these studies only when they are necessary.[23]

OPERATIVE MANAGEMENT

The presence of intraperitoneal blood on CT or FAST does not necessarily mandate exploration because bleeding from solid organ injury is generally self-limited. Overall, less than 10% of children with solid organ injury and less than 15% of those with hemoperitoneum require laparotomy.

Operative management is generally indicated in the hemodynamically unstable child with concomitant intraabdominal injury and in those who fail NOM; however, the precise definition of hemodynamically unstable and NOM failure is elusive. Some define failure as packed red blood cell transfusion exceeding 40 mL/kg, whereas others define it as any blood transfusion requirement. Because no single vital sign, test, or other physiologic parameter has been identified to indicate ongoing bleeding, clinical judgment is the best tool.[24]

The goal of operative management is control of hemorrhage and splenic preservation, if possible. Trauma laparotomy for splenic injury is generally performed through an upper midline incision allowing access to other potentially injured organs as well. Splenic mobilization should be done in a stepwise fashion to allow for adequate inspection of the spleen while minimizing the chance of increased injury. With splenic trauma, hematoma has generally dissected the ligamentous attachments and rapid delivery of the spleen into the wound is facilitated. The lateral attachments of the splenophrenic and splenorenal ligaments are first divided, allowing delivery of the spleen and tail of the pancreas as a unit from lateral to medial. The short gastric vessels are then divided; due to the dual blood supply of the spleen, the short gastric vessels can be ligated without compromising splenic viability. The final step in splenic mobilization is the division of the splenocolic ligament.[25,26]

The spleen is then inspected in its entirety, and a decision is then made regarding splenic preservation (splenorrhaphy) versus splenectomy. The factors in this decision include the presence of ongoing bleeding, degree of splenic injury, the overall condition of the patient, and the presence of associated injuries. Repair should be attempted only if the patient is hemodynamically stable. There are a variety of techniques to repair the injured spleen, depending upon the location and degree of injury. Small lacerations can be managed by compression and topical application of hemostatic agents, such as oxidized regenerated cellulose, absorbable gelatin sponge (plain or saturated with thrombin), or microfibrillar collagen, as well as tissue adhesives, such as fibrin glue and other agents. Hemorrhage from exposed areas of splenic parenchyma can be controlled using electrocautery or the argon beam coagulator. Severe disruptions of the splenic parenchyma with intact capsule can be managed with absorbable sutures that traverse the capsule and incorporate the parenchyma; pledgets may be useful to buttress the repair. Omentum can be further used to reinforce the repair, suturing it over the raw surface of the spleen or packing it into a defect. Partial splenectomy is also possible given the segmental nature of the splenic blood supply. Wrapping the spleen with absorbable mesh is another described technique. The most common complication after splenorrhaphy is persistent bleeding or rebleeding, thereby requiring splenectomy.[25,26]

When splenic bleeding is uncontrollable or other factors mandate expeditious operative procedures, splenectomy should be performed. Following splenic mobilization as previously described, the splenic hilum is isolated to a pedicle of the artery and vein. The hilum is then ligated and divided, completing the splenectomy. Hemostasis is then checked in a deliberate fashion, assessing three major areas: the inferior surface of the diaphragm, the greater curvature of the stomach particularly the region of the short gastric vessels, and the hilum. Autotransplantation is controversial, with reports of overwhelming post-splenectomy sepsis after autotransplantation, suggesting that this technique is not universally successful in restoring immune function.[25,26]

With the advent of minimally invasive surgery, laparoscopic techniques have been used more and more, including in trauma situations, although usually confined to hemodynamically stable patients. In a retrospective review by Feliz et al. in 2006, laparoscopy had a diagnostic accuracy of 100%, avoiding nontherapeutic laparotomy in 40% and laparotomy in 57% of patients. Over the course of the study a greater proportion of patients who required operative intervention underwent laparoscopy.[27] Reported laparoscopic splenic salvage techniques include the use of fibrin glue and collagen fleece–bound sealants.[28,29] Thus emergency laparoscopy has been shown to be a safe diagnostic and therapeutic modality in the management of abdominal injuries in the hemodynamically stable child.

NONOPERATIVE MANAGEMENT

NOM for blunt splenic injuries includes a defined period of bed rest allowing assessment of the degree of ongoing bleeding, serial hematocrit monitoring, initial period of nothing by mouth (NPO), followed by resumption of diet and ambulation, while being monitored prior to discharge. There has been significant controversy regarding the ideal time periods of bed rest, NPO status, and the frequency of serial hematocrits, as well as the need for further imaging and the length of full activity (i.e., contact sports, bicycle riding, etc.) restrictions.

First described by Upadhyaya and Simpson from Toronto in 1968, the use of selective NOM in hemodynamically stable children suffering from blunt splenic injury has gained increasing popularity and universal acceptance both in children and adults from the historic emergent splenectomies. Avoiding postsplenectomy sepsis as well as the concomitant operative morbidity and mortality prompted the initiation of NOM. Initially met with skepticism and fear that it would result in increased transfusion rates and mortality, NOM has proven to be safe and effective with surprisingly decreased transfusion rates and hospital stays.[30–34] Critics of NOM also cite the possibility of missing other intraabdominal injuries as well as the inability to apply NOM in the multiply injured patient. However, studies have not substantiated concerns regarding missed intraabdominal injuries, including the more elusive hollow viscus injuries.[35,36] There are also no absolute contraindications to NOM in the hemodynamically stable child with a concomitant closed head injury or other nonabdominal injuries because NOM has been successful in multiply injured children with other injuries remote from the abdomen, including those with unreliable abdominal examinations and altered mental status.[37,38]

NOM, by a surgical team, has thus become the standard of care for splenic injury in the hemodynamically stable child, with success rates greater than 90%. The great success of NOM in pediatric blunt solid organ injury actually led to the adoption of similar protocols in the adult population, such that NOM for blunt trauma to the liver and spleen are now the standard of care in both children and adults. The rate of NOM success for blunt splenic injury in adults has not been as high as in the pediatric population, which is thought to be due to the more elastic spleen of the child with increased ability of the vessels to contract and retract.[12]

Since its initial description, disparities in practice patterns were noted among physicians caring for children with solid organ injury.[39,40] Thus NOM has undergone significant revisions and refinements to minimize the length of bed rest and hospital stay while maintaining the safest treatment plan for children with blunt splenic injury. In 2000 the American Pediatric Surgical Association (APSA) first published its evidence-based guidelines for the NOM of blunt liver and splenic trauma based on multi-institutional data analysis stratified according to CT grade of injury (Table 140.1).[40,41] These initial guidelines were fairly conservative, with length of bed rest equal to the radiologic grade of injury plus 1 day and restriction from normal activities equal to grade of injury plus 2 weeks. Admission to the intensive care unit (ICU) was reserved for grade IV injuries. No follow-up imaging was recommended.[40] This was followed by prospective validation of its safety from 1998 to 2000 at 16 centers, resulting in 312 children with isolated liver and spleen injuries treated nonoperatively without adverse consequences. This has led to improved conformity in patient management, as well as resource use with significant reductions in imaging and laboratory studies, ICU stay, length of hospital stay, postdischarge imaging, length of activity restrictions, and subsequent reduced costs with no change in outcome, mortality, or hospital readmission rates.[42,43] Of note, they reported no adverse sequelae in 87% of patients with no follow-up imaging.[42] More recent studies have been published showing the safety and efficacy of abbreviated bed rest and activity restriction protocols as well as some using physiologic parameters rather than radiologic grade.

A prospective study by Mehall et al. reported that hemodynamically stable children do not require ICU monitoring or prolonged hospitalization and that management of pediatric solid organ injury should be based on hemodynamic stability rather than CT grade of organ injury.[33] This center further retrospectively reviewed the use of this protocol over a 5-year period and concluded that NOM of children with isolated splenic injuries, based

on physiologic response to resuscitation and hemodynamic status, is not only safe but results in decreased hospital length of stay. They also reported that returning to normal childhood activities, restricting only gym and contact sports, upon discharge is safe and effective.[44] An abbreviated protocol recommended that the number of days of bed rest equal the grade of injury plus 1 (grade I and II) or plus 2 (grades III and IV). It was projected that implementation of this protocol would have affected 65.8% of their patients and would have saved a mean of 2.0 ± 1.5 hospital days per patient.[45]

The Hospital for Sick Children in Toronto, where NOM was first proposed in 1968, summarized their five-decade institutional experience, including 485 patients with blunt splenic injury. The proportion of patients being managed nonoperatively increased to 99% in the most recent era. The mortality rate and use of blood products steadily decreased through the series. The observed decrease in hospital stay was attributed not only to surgeon comfort but also to resource restraints, with a mean length of stay of 5 days. Only a single death (0.33%) was reported in the most recent series from 1992 to 2006, due to delayed bleeding ≤3 days after injury despite following APSA guidelines.[52]

St. Peter et al. reported the application of an abbreviated bed rest protocol in which bed rest consists of overnight for grade I and II injuries and two nights for grade III and IV injuries. Admission to the ICU was based solely on physiologic parameters. Need for blood transfusion restarted the period of bed rest. They did not routinely perform follow-up imaging unless patients were symptomatic and allowed return to normal activity after

TABLE 140.1 Spleen Injury Scale (1994 Revision)

Grade	Injury Type	Description of Injury
I	Hematoma	Subcapsular, <10% surface area
	Laceration	Capsular tear, <1 cm parenchymal depth
II	Hematoma	Subcapsular, 10%–50% surface area; intraparenchymal depth, <5 cm in diameter
	Laceration	Capsular tear, 1–3 cm parenchymal depth that does not involve a trabecular vessel
III	Hematoma	Subcapsular, >50% surface area or expanding; ruptured subcapsular or parenchymal hematoma; intraparenchymal hematoma ≥5 cm or expanding
	Laceration	>3 cm parenchymal depth or involving trabecular vessels
IV	Laceration	Laceration involving segmental or hilar vessels producing major devascularization (>25% of spleen)
V	Laceration	Completely shattered spleen
	Vascular	Hilar vascular injury with devascularized spleen

Modified from Moore EE, Cogbill TH, Jurkovich GJ, Shackford SR, Malangoni MA, Champion HR. Organ injury scaling: spleen and liver (1994 revision). *J Trauma.* 1995;38:323.

discharge with no contact sports for 6 weeks. They reported no increase in delayed bleeding events. Physiologically, they treated bed rest as an observation period rather than a treatment variable, assuming that stable patients were no longer actively bleeding.[46,47] No evidence has been reported suggesting that bed rest prevents rebleeding.[24] They further published in 2014 the largest long-term national evaluation of blunt liver and splenic management in children using national databases from 2000 to 2009 to identify more than 22,000 injured children. They reported decreased length of stay compared with APSA guidelines with an overall decrease in operative trends and improved safety of NOM. In addition, projected application of their abbreviated bed rest protocol would have resulted in significantly decreased length of stay and potentially significant cost savings. These studies support the concept that the physiologic response to resuscitation is more important than the radiologic findings.[1,24]

In 2012 the Arizona-Texas-Oklahoma-Memphis-Arkansas-Consortium (ATOMAC), a pediatric trauma consortium, developed practice management guidelines for blunt liver and splenic injury, with specific parameters defining ICU admission, serial hemoglobin measurements, bed rest, diet, transfusion, and consideration of angioembolization or surgery. Radiologic grade of injury is not part of these guidelines, only physiologic parameters. These guidelines are based in part on findings that more than 50% of injured children with hypotension have severe traumatic brain injury rather than significant intraabdominal bleeding. They also note that greater than 80% of children with blush on CT do not require embolization.[24]

As radiologic techniques have improved, we are able to obtain increasingly more information. However, the best application of this knowledge in treatment algorithms can be controversial. Initial intravenous contrast–enhanced CT scans can often show contrast blush or extravasation, indicating active bleeding from the spleen. Multiple studies have aimed at determining if this radiologic contrast blush on initial CT evaluation is associated with negative outcomes in children with blunt splenic injury, specifically failure of NOM and/or the need for operative intervention. The adult literature has shown the presence of contrast blush to be predictive of NOM failure, further prompting the evaluation of this finding in the pediatric population.[8] Although this may identify a subset of children with blunt splenic injury who require intervention, overemphasis on the predictive value of the contrast blush could also potentially result in unnecessary surgical intervention with splenectomy.[49] Several groups consider the contrast blush an anatomic lesion that predisposed the patient to subsequent deterioration but was not an absolute indication for laparotomy in the absence of significant change in hemodynamic stability.[12,50–52] Davies et al. reported contrast blush in 6.5% of their patients with blunt splenic injury and an association with higher grades of injury and lower initial hemoglobin levels without increased transfusion rate, prolonged hospital stay, mortality, or severity of overall injury. Their institutional rate of successful NOM of pediatric blunt splenic injury was 97%. They concluded that children with contrast blush were not at increased risk of delayed splenic bleeding or need for operative splenic intervention.[32,49]

Angiographic embolization has been shown to be an effective and safe adjunct in NOM of blunt splenic injury in hemodynamically stable children with evidence of ongoing hemorrhage.[53] A systematic review of the literature from 1985 to 2009 assessing the failure rate of NOM both with and without angioembolization in children with blunt liver and/or splenic injury and contrast blush on CT suggested that angioembolization may lead to fewer failures but cited the generally low levels of evidence and the absence of randomized trials.[54]

Another area of controversy in NOM is follow-up imaging, as well as the length and type of activity restriction following hospital discharge. The rationale for follow-up imaging has been to ensure adequate healing of the spleen and to detect and treat long-term complications prior to symptoms. Similarly, postdischarge activity restrictions aim to minimize reinjuring the spleen and avoid delayed splenic bleeding. Pranikoff et al. reported complete healing by CT 6 weeks after injury in 10 of 13 (77%) grade I and grade II injuries but in only 1 of 12 (8%) grade III, IV, or V injuries managed nonoperatively. The 6-week follow-up CT showed disappearance of the majority of splenic fractures and reperfusion of previously nonperfused regions of the spleen. They thus recommended 3 months of restricted activity for all patients without follow-up CT scan or 6 weeks for patients with grade I and II injuries with follow-up CT scan demonstrating injury resolution.[55] Lynch et al. prospectively evaluated the role of serial ultrasounds in assessing splenic healing until complete homogeneity of the splenic tissue was observed without residual defect or fluid. Mean time to ultrasound healing of grade I, II, III, and IV injuries was 3.1, 8.2, 12.1, and 20.7 weeks, respectively. They concluded that the time to radiographic healing was proportional to the severity of the CT-graded splenic injury.[56] However, despite these studies, there have been no studies showing that radiographic evidence of healing correlates with histopathologic healing.[40] Thus current guidelines do not include routine follow-up imaging.[42] Restricting the return to full activities can result in significant decrease in quality-of-life parameters, as well as hidden costs, including loss of work days and wages for caregivers and need for additional caregivers during those missed activities when children are homebound.[44]

Although there are no definite data to suggest a correlation between the initial grade of splenic injury and the incidence of long-term complications, there is significant concern for potentially life-threatening complications, such as splenic pseudoaneurysms and delayed splenic bleeding. However, NOM of pediatric blunt splenic injury is associated with minimal complications. In a series of 228 patients with blunt splenic injury and a mean follow-up of 5 years, there was a 0.44% incidence of long-term complications despite some returning to full activity prior to the recommended APSA guidelines, suggesting that prolonged periods of restricted activity (e.g., 6 months or greater) is not necessary.[57] The reported incidence of delayed complications (e.g., splenic artery pseudoaneurysms, splenic abscesses, and delayed bleeding) ranges from 0% to 7.5%.[58]

Perhaps the most concerning of these are splenic artery pseudoaneurysms, which appear as actively bleeding intraparenchymal hematomas with contrast blush on CT scan and can also be detected by Doppler ultrasound. In adults a significant proportion of these pseudoaneurysms are thought to expand and rupture, resulting in delayed bleeding in 5% to 6% of adults with blunt splenic trauma.[59] In contrast, the incidence of splenic artery pseudoaneurysms in children appears to be lower, with greater likelihood of spontaneous resolution attributed to self-tamponade and thrombosis due to the inherent characteristics of the pediatric spleen. In addition, the severity of the splenic injury does not seem to have predictive value for the development of splenic artery pseudoaneurysms in children. Unfortunately, the natural history of splenic pseudoaneurysms is not known, particularly in children. Although the majority spontaneously resolve, those that persist can gradually increase in size and rupture, resulting in significant bleeding with a reported mortality rate as high as 15%.[12,58-60] Thus appropriate management remains controversial. Treatment options include observation, splenorraphy, partial splenectomy, and splenic artery embolization.[6,50,60,51] Angioembolization in children is also not without its inherent risks and morbidity and thus should not be entered into lightly. The smaller vessel size and increased vasoreactivity in children can make embolization difficult as well as result in the formation of arteriovenous fistulas at the access site. Postembolization complications, although rare, include pain, pleural effusions, arterial puncture site injury or hematoma, acute limb-threatening ischemia, chronic leg ischemia, contrast nephropathy, splenic rupture, splenic abcess, cysts, coil migration, splenic infarction, and overwhelming postsplenectomy infection.[53,54,59,60] In addition, there has been significant debate regarding the preferred location for embolization. Embolization of distal vessels confers the advantage of more targeted embolization although it may cause infarction; proximal embolization can better preserve the reticuloendothelial function of the spleen and also control injuries with multiple bleeding sites. Proximal embolization theoretically allows maintenance of overall perfusion to the spleen from collateral vessels (short gastrics, left gastroepiploic, and branches of left gastric), potentially allowing for better long-term splenic preservation. If the artery is embolized proximal to branches feeding the pancreas, ischemia can result in necrotizing pancreatitis.[53,62] Because many pseudoaneurysms have been shown to spontaneously resolve, there is currently no consensus recommendations for routine imaging or treatment guidelines for pseudoaneurysms. Most recommend obtaining imaging based on clinical symptoms only and then treating accordingly.[24,40,59,60,63]

Delayed splenic bleeding, defined by McIndoe in 1931 as hemorrhage from a ruptured spleen occurring more than 48 hours after trauma, remains a controversial entity because it is difficult to differentiate between true delayed ruptures and delayed presentation of acute injuries.[64] In a retrospective review the incidence of delayed splenic bleeding was 0.33% (1/305). Only 14 cases of delayed splenic bleeding have been reported since 1980 and the advent of NOM. Despite the low incidence, families should be educated about this possible complication and its associated signs and symptoms, including pain, pallor, dizziness, difficulty breathing, vomiting, worsening shoulder

pain, gastrointestinal bleeding or black tarry stools.[24,65] The maximum risk of delayed splenic rupture is estimated to be 0.3%, and thus the use of routine follow-up imaging of children with blunt splenic trauma is not supported.[66]

The management of the traumatized diseased spleen and the management of spontaneous rupture of the diseased spleen remain controversial. Advocates of NOM in the hemodynamically stable patient suggest that the patient with a pathologically enlarged spleen, due to infectious mononucleosis, human immunodeficiency virus (HIV)/acquired immunodeficiency syndrome (AIDS), leukemia, or sickle cell anemia, and spontaneous rupture, may be particularly susceptible to postsplenectomy infection and may benefit from splenic preservation. Successful NOM has been reported in patients with pathologic splenomegaly secondary to infectious mononucleosis and leukemia with spontaneous rupture and in similar patients sustaining blunt splenic injury.[67] Patients with hemophilia and blunt splenic injury do not always require splenectomy; operative splenic salvage with perioperative correction of the coagulopathy has been reported (Fig. 140.3).[68]

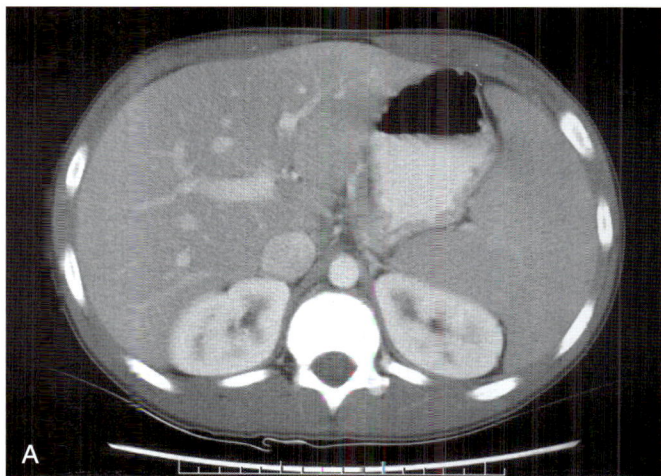

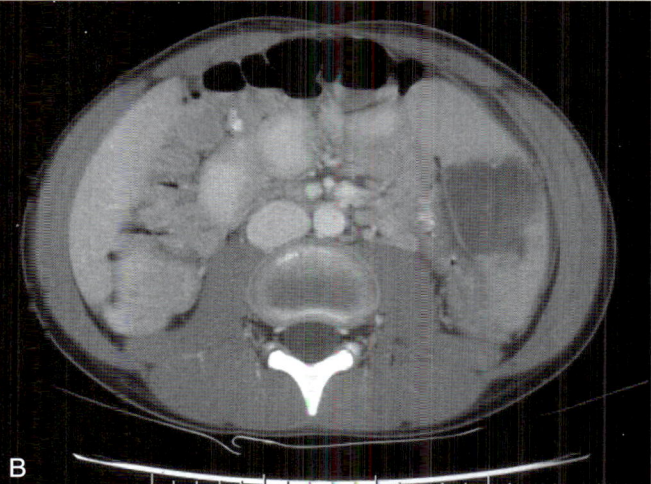

FIGURE 140.3 Abdominal computed tomography scan demonstrating pathologic splenomegaly due to infectious mononucleosis (A), and the traumatic laceration in the same diseased spleen (B).

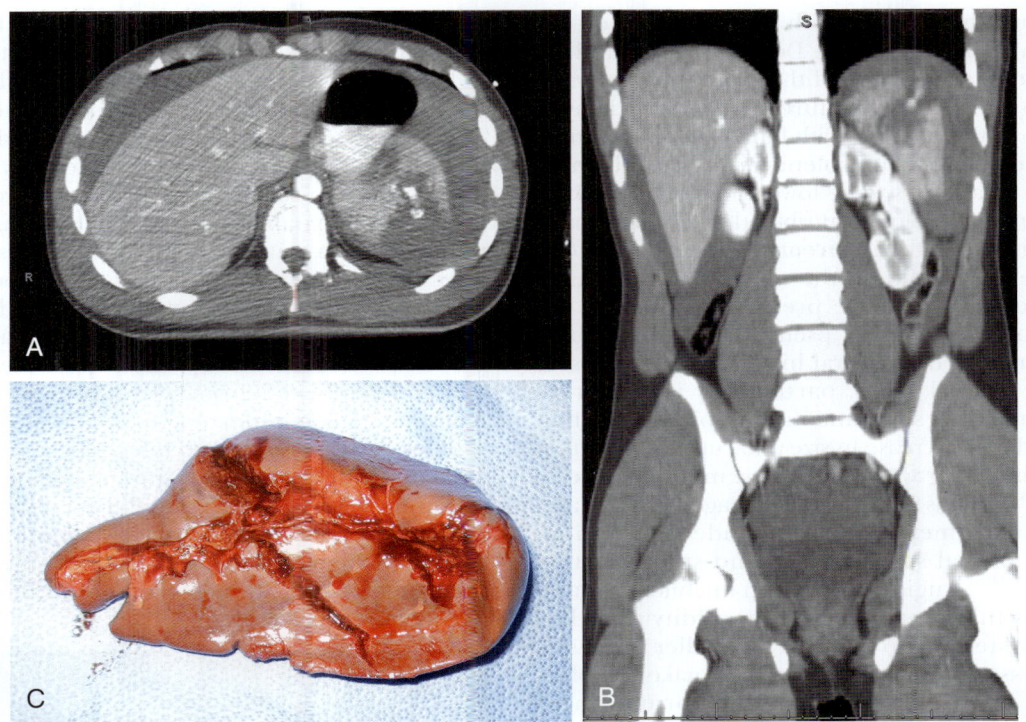

FIGURE 140.4 Abdominal computed tomography scan demonstrating laceration with extravasation of contrast: cross section (A), coronal (B). This patient had an associated closed head injury with two episodes of hypotension and because of his hemodynamic instability underwent splenectomy; operative photo (C).

The threshold for NOM failure has not been clearly defined as most consider it to be hemodynamic instability and the need for persistent blood transfusions. Perhaps the most agreed upon parameter is a transfusion requirement exceeding half the child's blood volume, or 40 mL/kg, during the first 24 hours after injury.[24] In children requiring operation for solid organ injury, the necessity for operative exploration presents itself generally within the first 24 hours. NOM of confirmed abdominal visceral injuries is a surgical decision made by surgeons, as is the decision to operate. The decision to operate continues to be based on abnormal physiologic parameters and the volume of blood lost (Fig. 140.4).

OUTCOMES

NOM of blunt splenic injury has become the standard of care in the hemodynamically stable child, with success rates greater than 90%. Only a small percentage of children will require laparotomy, and studies have attempted to characterize this cohort of children. A retrospective review from Pennsylvania showed that children undergoing splenectomy were older (15 to 16 years of age) and sustained more severe injury overall in motor vehicle or bicycle crashes and sports-related activities. In contrast, children injured by falls, assault, or abuse had significantly lower rates of splenectomy. The independent determinants of splenectomy included Glasgow Coma Scale scores 3 to 8, high grade of spleen injury, and nonspleen abdominal injury.[4] Similar results were noted in a review of pediatric patients with solid organ injury treated at seven level I

pediatric trauma centers over a 6-year period. The majority who fail NOM do so early in their hospital course, with an overall peak failure rate at 4 hours post admission.[69]

Retrospective cohorts from seven level I pediatric trauma centers identified 2944 children who sustained blunt abdominal trauma over a 10-year interval. Two operative groups were characterized: immediate operation and failed NOM (defined as laparotomy more than 3 hours after arrival). The overall rate of operation was low, with 5% requiring laparotomy; 50% of the patients in this group had splenic injuries. The mean age did not differ in the control versus operative groups though patients requiring operation had greater injury severity (higher injury severity scale) and significantly lower median Glasgow Coma Scale scores. Of the 140 patients requiring operative intervention, 81 patients required immediate operation, of whom 54% had splenic injuries and 59 patients failed NOM with 44% having splenic injuries. The most common indication for operation in both groups was hemodynamic instability or bleeding. Their analysis showed no adverse outcomes if NOM was initially attempted but then failed.[70]

Despite the now widespread use of NOM in the treatment of children with blunt splenic injury, there is wide variation in practice based not only on surgeon preference but also on institutions, the most pronounced existing between pediatric and adult surgeons and hospitals. Lee et al. reported in 2012 an increase in operative intervention with decreased use of angiography in rural hospitals, likely due to availability of resources.[71] Mooney et al. examined 2191 children with splenic injuries in 25 states covering

68% of the nation's population for the year 2000. They noted an increased risk of splenectomy with higher grades of splenic injury, increased patient age, and presence of multiple injuries. Three types of pediatric hospitals were recognized: freestanding pediatric, pediatric unit within an adult hospital, and adult hospital. Overall, the rate of splenectomy was 12%; however, the splenectomy rate varied significantly among the pediatric hospital types: 3% at freestanding children's hospitals, 9% at pediatric units within an adult hospital, and 15% at adult hospitals. Teaching hospitals and hospitals with higher patient volume were associated with lower risk for splenectomy.[72] Compared with nontrauma centers, trauma centers have a significantly lower rate of operation for both multiply injured patients and those with isolated injury.[73] Multiple studies report higher rates of operative intervention in nonpediatric hospitals compared to pediatric hospitals.[3,7,8,19,74-78]

Since the great majority of children are not treated at freestanding children's hospitals or by pediatric surgeons, it is incumbent upon pediatric surgeons to better educate adult general and trauma surgeons in the inherent differences between adult and pediatric physiology, as well as the ability of children to spontaneously heal fairly significant injuries, thereby avoiding splenectomy.[72]

ACKNOWLEDGMENTS

I would like to thank Dr. Mindy Statter and the late Dr. Donald Liu for their intellectual contributions in writing the original chapter in the 7th edition.

REFERENCES

1. Dodgion CM, Gosain A, Rogers A, St. Peter SD, Nichol PF, Ostlie DJ. National trends in pediatric blunt spleen and liver injury management and potential benefits of an abbreviated bed rest protocol. *J Pediatr Surg.* 2014;49:1004-1008.
2. Golden J, Mitchell I, Kuzniewski S, et al. Reducing scheduled phlebotomy in stable pediatric patients with blunt liver or spleen injury. *J Pediatr Surg.* 2014;49:759-762.
3. Petrosyan M, Guner YS, Emami CN, Ford HR. Disparities in the delivery of pediatric trauma care. *J Trauma.* 2009;67(2):S114-S119.
4. Potoka DA, Schall LC, Ford HR. Risk factors for splenectomy in children with blunt splenic trauma. *J Pediatr Surg.* 2002;37:294.
5. King H, Shumacher HB. Splenic studies. I. Susceptibility to infection after splenectomy performed in infancy. *Ann Surg.* 1952;136:239.
6. Naess PA, Gaarder C, Dormagen JB. Nonoperative management of pediatric splenic injury with angiographic embolization. *J Pediatr Surg.* 2005;40:E63-E64.
7. Davis DH, Localio AR, Stafford PW, Helfaer MA, Durbin DR. Trends in operative management of pediatric splenic injury in a regional trauma system. *Pediatrics.* 2005;115(1):89-94.
8. Liu S, Bowman SM, Smith TC, Sharar SR. Trends in pediatric spleen management: do hospital type and ownership still matter? *J Trauma Acute Care Surg.* 2015;78(5):935-942.
9. Velanovich V, Tapper D. Decision analysis in children with blunt splenic trauma: the effects of observation, splenorrhaphy, or splenectomy on quality-adjusted life expectancy. *J Pediatr Surg.* 1993;28:179.
10. Bowman SM, Sharar SR, Quan L. Impact of a statewide quality improvement initiative in improving the management of pediatric splenic injuries in Washington state. *J Trauma.* 2008;64(6):1478-1483.
11. Upadhyaya P, Simpson JS. Splenic trauma in children. *Surg Gynecol Obstet.* 1968;126:781.
12. Cloutier DR, Baird TB, Gormley P, McCarten KM, Bussey JG, Luks FI. Pediatric splenic injuries with a contrast blush: successful nonoperative management without angiography and embolization. *J Pediatr Surg.* 2004;39:969.
13. Dixon JA, Miller F, McCloskey D, Siddorway J. Anatomy and techniques in segmental splenectomy. *Surg Gynecol Obstet.* 1980;150:516.
14. Skandalakis JE, Gray SW. *Embryology for Surgeons.* Baltimore: Williams & Wilkins; 1994:334.
15. Rodrigues CJ, Sacchetti JC, Rodrigues AJ. Age-related changes in the elastic fiber network of the human splenic capsule. *Lymphology.* 1999;32:64.
16. Konstantakos AK, Barnoski AL, Plaisier BR, Yowler CJ, Fallon WF, Malangoni MA. Optimizing the management of blunt splenic injury in adults and children. *Surgery.* 1999;126(4):805-813.
17. Hazel MS. Traumatic rupture of spleen, with special reference to its characteristics in young children. *J Pediatr.* 1945;26:82.
18. American College of Surgeons. *Advanced Trauma Life Support.* 8th ed. Chicago: American College of Surgeons; 2008.
19. Stylanos S. Outcomes from pediatric solid organ injury: role of standardized care guidelines. *Curr Opin Pediatr.* 2005;17:402-406.
20. Nance ML, Mahboubi S, Wickstrom M, Prendergast F, Stafford PW. Pattern of abdominal free fluid following isolated blunt spleen and liver injury in the pediatric patient. *J Trauma.* 2002;52:85.
21. Holmes JF, Gladman A, Chang CH. Performance of abdominal ultrasonography in pediatric blunt trauma patients: a meta-analysis. *J Pediatr Surg.* 2007;42:1588.
22. Rice HE, Frush DP, Farmer D, Waldhausen JH, APSA Education Committee. Review of radiation risks from computed tomography: essentials for the pediatric surgeon. *J Pediatr Surg.* 2007;42:603.
23. Brody AS, Frush DP, Huda W, Brent RL, AAP Section on Radiology. Radiation risk to children from computed tomography. *Pediatrics.* 2007;120:677.
24. Notrica DM, Eubanks JW, Tuggle DW, et al. Nonoperative management of blunt liver and spleen injury in children: evaluation of the ATOMAC guideline using GRADE. *J Trauma Acute Care Surg.* 2015;79(4):683-693.
25. Jacoby RC, Wisner DH. Injury to the spleen. In: Feliciano DV, Mattox KL, Moore EE, eds. *Trauma.* 6th ed. New York: McGraw Hill; 2008.
26. Mucha P. Splenic repair and partial splenectomy (preservation of splenic function). In: Baker RJ, Fischer JE, eds. *Mastery of Surgery.* Philadelphia: Lippincott Williams & Wilkins; 2001.
27. Feliz A, Shultz B, McKenna C, Gaines BA. Diagnostic and therapeutic laparoscopy in pediatric abdominal trauma. *J Pediatr Surg.* 2006;41:72.
28. Schmal H, Geiger G. Laparoscopic splenic salvage in delayed rupture by application of fibrin glue in a 11 year old boy. *J Trauma.* 2005;58:528.
29. Carbon RT, Baar S, Waldschmid J, Huemmer HP, Simon SI. Innovative minimally invasive pediatric surgery is of therapeutic value for splenic injury. *J Pediatr Surg.* 2002;37:1146.
30. Schwartz MZ, Kangah R. Splenic injury in children after blunt trauma: blood transfusion requirements and length of hospitalization for laparotomy versus observation. *J Pediatr Surg.* 1994;29:596.
31. Partrick DA, Bensard DD, Moore EE, Karrer FM. Nonoperative management of solid organ injuries in children results in decreased blood transfusion. *J Pediatr Surg.* 1999;34:1695.
32. Davies DA, Pearl RH, Ein SH, Langer JC, Wales PW. Management of blunt splenic injury in children: evolution of the nonoperative approach. *J Pediatr Surg.* 2009;44:1005.
33. Mehall JR, Ennis JS, Saltzman DA, et al. Prospective results of a standardized algorithm based on hemodynamic status for managing pediatric solid organ injury. *J Am Coll Surg.* 2001;193:347.
34. Myers JG, Dent DL, Stewart RM, et al. Blunt splenic injuries: dedicated trauma surgeons can achieve a high rate of nonoperative success in patients of all ages. *J Trauma.* 2000;48(5):801-806.
35. Morse MA, Garcia VF. Selective nonoperative management of pediatric blunt splenic trauma: risk for missed associated injuries. *J Pediatr Surg.* 1994;29:23.
36. Stassen NA, Bhullar I, Cheng JD, et al. Selective nonoperative management of blunt splenic injury: an Eastern Association for the Surgery of Trauma practice management guideline. *J Trauma Acute Care Surg.* 2012;73(5 suppl 4) S294-S300.
37. Coburn MC, Pfeifer J, DeLuca FG. Nonoperative management of splenic and hepatic trauma in the multiply injured pediatric and adolescent patient. *Arch Surg.* 1995;130:332.
38. Keller MS, Sartorelli KH, Vane DW. Associated head injury should not prevent nonoperative management of spleen or liver injury in children. *J Trauma.* 1996;41:471.
39. Falat ME, Casale AJ. Practice patterns of pediatric surgeons caring for stable patients with traumatic solid organ injury. *J Trauma.* 1997;43:820.

40. Stylianos S. APSA Trauma Committee. Evidence-based guidelines for resource utilization in children with isolated spleen or liver injury. *J Pediatr Surg.* 2000;35:164.

41. Moore EE, Cogbill TH, Jurkovich GJ, Shackford SR, Malangoni MA, Champion HR. Organ injury scaling: spleen and liver (1994 revision). *J Trauma.* 1995;38:323.

42. Stylianos S. Compliance with evidence-based guidelines in children with isolated spleen or liver injury: a prospective study. *J Pediatr Surg.* 2002;37:453.

43. Gutierrez IM, Zurakowski D, Chen Q, Mooney DP. Clinical practice guidelines (CPGs) reduce costs in the management of isolated splenic injuries at pediatric trauma centers. *Langenbecks Arch Surg.* 2013;398:313-315.

44. McVay MR, Kokoska ER, Jackson RJ, Smith SD. Throwing out the "grade" book: management of isolated spleen and liver injury based on hemodynamic status. *J Pediatr Surg.* 2008;43:1072.

45. St. Peter SD, Keckler SJ, Spilde TL, Holcomb GW 3rd, Ostlie DJ. Justification for an abbreviated protocol in the management of blunt spleen and liver injury in children. *J Pediatr Surg.* 2008;43:191.

46. St. Peter SD, Sharp SW, Snyder CL, et al. Prospective validation of an abbreviated bedrest protocol in the management of blunt spleen and liver injury in children. *J Pediatr Surg.* 2011;46:173-177.

47. St. Peter SD, Aguayo P, Juang D, et al. Follow up of prospective validation of an abbreviated bedrest protocol in the management of blunt spleen and liver injury in children. *J Pediatr Surg.* 2013;48:2437-2441.

48. Olthof DC, Joosse P, van der Vlies CH, de Haan RJ, Goslings JC. Prognostic factors for failure of nonoperative management in adults with blunt splenic injury: a systematic review. *J Trauma Acute Care Surg.* 2013;74(2):546-557.

49. Davies DA, Ein SH, Pearl R, et al. What is the significance of contrast "blush" in pediatric blunt splenic trauma. *J Pediatr Surg.* 2010;45:916.

50. Cox CC, Geiger JD, Liu DC, Garver K. Pediatric blunt abdominal trauma: role of computed tomography vascular blush. *J Pediatr Surg.* 1997;32:1196.

51. Nwomeh BC, Nadler EP, Meza MP, Bron K, Gaines BA, Ford HR. Contrast extravasation predicts the need for operative intervention in children with blunt splenic trauma. *J Trauma.* 2004;56:537.

52. Lutz N, Mahboubi S, Nance ML, Stafford PW. The significance of contrast blush on computed tomography in children with splenic injuries. *J Pediatr Surg.* 2004;39:491.

53. Kiankhooy A, Sartorelli KH, Vane DM, Bhave AD. Angiographic embolization is safe and effective therapy in blunt abdominal solid organ injury in children. *J Trauma.* 2010;68:526.

54. Van der Vlies CH, Saltzherr TP, Wilde JCH, van Delden OM, de Haan RJ, Goslings JC. The failure rate of nonoperative management in children with splenic or liver injury with contrast blush on computed tomography: a systematic review. *J Pediatr Surg.* 2010;45:1044.

55. Pranikoff T, Hirschl RB, Schlesinger AE, Polley TZ, Coran AG. Resolution of splenic injury after nonoperative management. *J Pediatr Surg.* 1994;29:1366.

56. Lynch JM, Meza MP, Newman B, Gardner MJ, Albanese CT. Computed tomography grade of splenic injury is predictive of the time required for radiographic healing. *J Pediatr Surg.* 1997;32:1093.

57. Kristoffersen KW, Mooney DP. Long-term outcome of non-operative pediatric splenic injury management. *J Pediatr Surg.* 2007;42:1038.

58. Frumiento C, Sartorelli K, Vane D. Complications of splenic injuries: expansion of the nonoperative theorem. *J Pediatr Surg.* 2000;35:788.

59. Martin K, VanHouwelingen L, Butter A. The significance of pseudoaneurysms in the nonoperative management of pediatric blunt splenic trauma. *J Pediatr Surg.* 2011;46:933-937.

60. Yardeni D, Polley TZ Jr, Coran AG. Splenic artery embolization for post-traumatic splenic artery pseudoaneurysm. *J Trauma.* 2004;57:404.

61. Schuster T, Leissner G. Selective angioembolization in blunt solid organ injury in children and adolescents: review of recent literature and own experiences. *Eur J Pediatr Surg.* 2013;23:454-463.

62. Schnuriger B, Inaba K, Konstantinidis A, Lustenberger T, Chan LS, Demetriades D. Outcomes of proximal versus distal splenic artery embolization after trauma: a systematic review and meta-analysis. *J Trauma.* 2011;70(1):252-260.

63. Safavi A, Beaudry P, Jamieson D, Murphy JJ. Traumatic pseudoaneurysms of the liver and spleen in children: is routine screening warranted? *J Pediatr Surg.* 2011;46:938-941.

64. McIndoe AH. Delayed haemorrhage following traumatic rupture of the spleen. *Br J Surg.* 1931;20:249.

65. Davies DA, Fecteau A, Himidan S, Mikrogianakis A, Wales PW. What is the incidence of delayed splenic bleeding in children after blunt trauma? An institutional experience and review of the literature. *J Trauma.* 2009;67:573.

66. Huebner S, Reed MH. Analysis of the value of imaging as part of the follow-up of splenic injury in children. *Pediatr Radiol.* 2001;31:852.

67. Statter MB, Liu DC. Nonoperative management of blunt splenic injury in infectious mononucleosis. *Am Surg.* 2005;71:376.

68. Korer JP, Klein RL, Kavic MS, Krill CE Jr. Management of splenic trauma in the pediatric hemophiliac patient: case series and review of the literature. *J Pediatr Surg.* 2002;37:568.

69. Holmes JH, Wiebe DJ, Tataria M, et al. The failure of nonoperative management in pediatric solid organ injury: a multi-institutional experience. *J Trauma.* 2005;59:1309.

70. Tataria M, Nance ML, Holmes JH, et al. Pediatric blunt abdominal injury: age is irrelevant and delayed operation is not detrimental. *J Trauma.* 2007;63:608.

71. Lee J, Moriarty KP, Tashjian DB. Less is more: management of pediatric splenic injury. *Arch Surg.* 2012;147(5):437-441.

72. Mooney DP, Rothstein DH, Forbes MA. Variation in the management of pediatric splenic injuries in the United States. *J Trauma.* 2006;61:330.

73. Stylianos S, Egorova N, Guice KS, Arons RR, Oldham KT. Variation in treatment of pediatric spleen injury at trauma centers versus nontrauma centers: a call for dissemination of American Pediatric Surgical Association benchmarks and guidelines. *J Am Coll Surg.* 2006;202:247.

74. Li D, Yanchar N. Management of pediatric blunt splenic injuries in Canada—practices and opinions. *J Pediatr Surg.* 2009;44:997-1004.

75. Jen HC, Tillou A, Cryer HG, Shew SB. Disparity in management and long-term outcomes of pediatric splenic injury in California. *Ann Surg.* 2010;251(6):1162-1166.

76. Hsiao M, Sathya C, de Mestral C, Langer JC, Gomez D, Nathens AB. Population-based analysis of blunt splenic injury management in children: operative rate is an informative quality of care indicator. *Injury.* 2014;45:859-863.

77. Lippert SJ, Hartin CW, Ozgediz DE, et al. Splenic conservation: variation between pediatric and adult trauma centers. *J Surg Res.* 2013;182:17-20.

78. Matsushima K, Kulaylat AN, Won EJ, Stokes AL, Schaefer EW, Frankel HL. Variation in the management of adolescent patients with blunt abdominal solid organ injury between adult versus pediatric trauma centers: an analysis of a statewide trauma database. *J Surg Res.* 2013;183:808-813.

Splenectomy for Conditions Other Than Trauma

Rory L. Smoot | Mark J. Truty | David M. Nagorney

Splenectomy for nontraumatic disorders demands careful risk-benefit analysis and surgical planning. Crucial factors considered include the nature of the underlying disease, the severity of symptoms, alternative therapeutic options, the operative risk, and the success rate of splenectomy. During the past decade, the underlying diseases have become better understood; more and effective medical therapies have become available, specifically immunomodulatory/immunosuppressive regimens; laparoscopic techniques have expanded and decreased operative risks; and prophylaxis has minimized the risk of postsplenectomy infections. These advances have challenged some of the traditional concepts regarding splenectomy. This chapter aims to summarize the current indications and contemporary outcomes of splenectomy for nontraumatic conditions encountered by surgeons in consultation. These conditions mainly include hematologic disorders but also splenic mass lesions, splenic vascular disease, iatrogenic injuries, and other rare diseases.

SPLENECTOMY FOR HEMATOLOGIC DISORDERS

The spleen performs important hematologic and immunologic functions. It maintains the circulating blood components by filtering and removing damaged or senescent cells. As the largest aggregate of lymphoid tissue in the reticuloendothelial system, the spleen functions in both antibody production and phagocytosis. Accordingly, cytopenia and splenomegaly are two common manifestations of hematologic disorders involving the spleen. Cytopenia is associated with hypersplenism, the excessive destruction of one or more blood components. Splenomegaly, defined as splenic weight of more than 175 g (normal, 90 to 150 g), can become massive (>1000 to 15,000 g). Mechanical symptoms of splenomegaly include pain and early satiety. When the spleen is the sole site of the disease or a major contributor to the underlying pathophysiology, splenectomy is performed with curative intent. In most conditions, it is performed for effective palliation of symptoms and complications in patients refractory to medical management. In general splenectomy for hematologic disease can be diagnostic, therapeutic, curative, or palliative and is performed for specific clinical indications rather than for specific diagnoses.

DISORDERS CAUSING THROMBOCYTOPENIA

Thrombocytopenia is defined as platelet count less than 150×10^9/L. Patients with platelet counts of 50×10^9/L or greater are usually asymptomatic and are discovered incidentally. Excessive oozing after surgery or bruising after minor trauma usually does not occur until the platelet count is less than 30×10^9 to 50×10^9/L. Spontaneous internal bleeding may occur with platelet counts of 10×10^9 to 20×10^9/L. Response of thrombocytopenia to therapy has been variably defined in previous studies. Complete response (CR) is most commonly defined as achieving platelet counts of 150×10^9/L for at least 30 days after splenectomy without additional therapy. Partial response (PR) results when platelet counts of at least 50×10^9/L are achieved, whereas no response (NR) is defined when counts remain less than 50×10^9/L for 30 days. Relapse occurs when thrombocytopenia recurs after achieving a normal platelet count.[1]

Idiopathic Thrombocytopenic Purpura

Idiopathic thrombocytopenic purpura (ITP), also called primary immune thrombocytopenia (PIT), is the most common hematologic disease for which splenectomy is indicated. Affected patients may be asymptomatic or may present with petechiae, ecchymosis, epistaxis, gastrointestinal bleeding, or menorrhagia. Subarachnoid or intracranial hemorrhage suggests severe thrombocytopenia. ITP is mediated by autoantibodies, typically against multiple platelet membrane glycoproteins such as IIb/IIIa, Ib/Ix, Ia/IIa, IV, and V. Splenic macrophages clear platelets coated with immunoglobulin G (IgG) autoantibodies in an accelerated fashion.[2] If compensatory platelet production is impaired or outstripped, thrombocytopenia ensues. The test for antiplatelet antibodies has a sensitivity of only 49% to 66% and a specificity of 78% to 92%.[2,3] A positive test does not definitively diagnose ITP, whereas a negative result cannot exclude it. ITP remains a clinical diagnosis of exclusion. A search for a secondary cause for thrombocytopenia should be prompted by a history of drug or toxin exposure, recent viral infections, splenomegaly on physical examination, an abnormal peripheral smear, or a hypoplastic bone marrow. Although a peripheral blood smear has been required as a diagnostic test, bone marrow aspiration is considered for patients older than age 60 years with atypical presentations and in whom other disorders are suspected and splenectomy is contemplated.[4]

The time of disease onset in childhood or adulthood determines the clinical presentation, natural history, and treatment approaches. Childhood ITP most commonly affects children between 2 and 5 years of age without a gender bias. In approximately 90% of the patients the disease manifests as acute thrombocytopenia, associated with a sudden onset of petechiae occurring 4 to 8 weeks after the prodrome of viral illness, allergies or immunizations.[5] Antibodies formed during the preceding illnesses cross-react against platelets. The natural history of childhood ITP is favorable; a vast majority (83%) spontaneously recover within 8 weeks without therapy with approximately 10% to 15% persisting as chronic ITP.[6] Therefore aggressive therapy is avoided. Typical management includes observation and avoidance of platelet-inhibiting medications and of activities predisposing to trauma. The decision to initiate any form of therapy is typically driven by a concern for the risk of intracranial hemorrhage, the development of refractory clinical symptoms, and activity restrictions that compromise a child's quality of life. First-line therapy is medical and includes intravenous immunoglobulin (IVIG), corticosteroids, anti-IgD, and platelet transfusion. Splenectomy is delayed for as long as possible.[5] However, when it is performed, response rates of 63% to 86% may be expected. The response is sustained in the long term in 45% to 60% of the patients.[7,8] Benefit from splenectomy may be predicted by preoperative response to IVIG, with positive predictive values of 74% to 91% and negative predictive values of 75% to 100%.[9,10] In the pediatric population, laparoscopic splenectomy does not compromise the response rates, can be safely performed, and allows faster recovery without increasing costs.[11]

Adult ITP has an insidious onset and affects women between 18 and 40 years of age most commonly. The natural history contrasts with that of childhood ITP, in that spontaneous remission occurs in only 2% to 9% of all patients.[12] Most patients will develop chronic ITP. Although the disease course is usually benign, those with severe or refractory thrombocytopenia face four times the risk of mortality than the general population.[13] Initiation of therapy depends on the bleeding risk, estimated from patient's age, lifestyle, platelet count, and concomitant diseases.[4] The therapeutic approach to ITP in adults has undergone dramatic change over the past decade.[14] The standard first-line therapies now include corticosteroids, IVIG, and anti-IgD. Recent studies in patients undergoing treatment with dexamethasone regimens have demonstrated up to 86% response rate, with 50% to 74% sustained response.[15,16] Multiple additional medical therapies are considered for second- and even third-line therapies, including rituximab, danazol, dapsone, azathioprine, cyclosporin A, cyclophosphamide, mycophenolate, and thrombopoietin (TPO) receptor agonists. Splenectomy is considered a second-line treatment in the most current international consensus guidelines but is also the most likely curative therapy for ITP.[14] Outcomes of splenectomy for ITP have been summarized in a systematic review by Kojouri et al. reporting on 130 articles.[1] The overall rate of platelet response to splenectomy is 67% (range, 37% to 100%), with a sustained response rate of 64% after 7 years (range, 5 to 12.75 years) of follow-up. The average relapse rate after splenectomy is 15% (range, 0% to 51%), most occurring within the first postoperative year. One single-center experience of 140 adults revealed an overall complete platelet response rate of 78% initially and 74% after 1 year.[4] Corticosteroids, danazol, and/or IVIG salvaged 81% of those who relapsed.[17] Factors predictive of successful outcome after splenectomy have also been investigated.[1,12] Younger age (<30 years) at splenectomy and previous response to glucocorticoids most consistently correlated with good response. In addition, when platelets are mainly sequestered in the spleen rather than the liver and other lymphoid organs, as identified by indium-labeled platelet scans,[4] a superior response rate has been observed; however, this modality is not currently widely available

in the United States and requires a sufficient level of circulating platelets to be harvested, radiolabeled ex vivo, and subsequently reinfused back into the patient.

Laparoscopic splenectomy has become the criterion standard of care for ITP patients. Operative mortality has decreased from 1% for open splenectomy to 0.2% for laparoscopic splenectomy. Similarly, operative morbidity has decreased from 12.9% to 9.6%.[1] Postoperative recovery is superior, with less pain and earlier hospital discharge. These benefits are realized without increased cost and without compromising hematologic response rates.[18] In debilitated patients who are unsuitable for an operation, splenic irradiation or partial splenic embolization may be considered, but the experience with this treatment is limited.

Accessory splenic tissue may be present in 16% to 29% of patients with ITP.[1] The most common locations for accessory splenic tissue include the splenic hilum, the gastrosplenic ligament, gastrocolic ligament, greater omentum, mesentery, and presacral space (Fig. 141.1).[19] A thorough search should be conducted intraoperatively whether the operative approach is open or laparoscopic because a missed accessory spleen may be the cause for relapse of ITP. The presence of residual functioning splenic

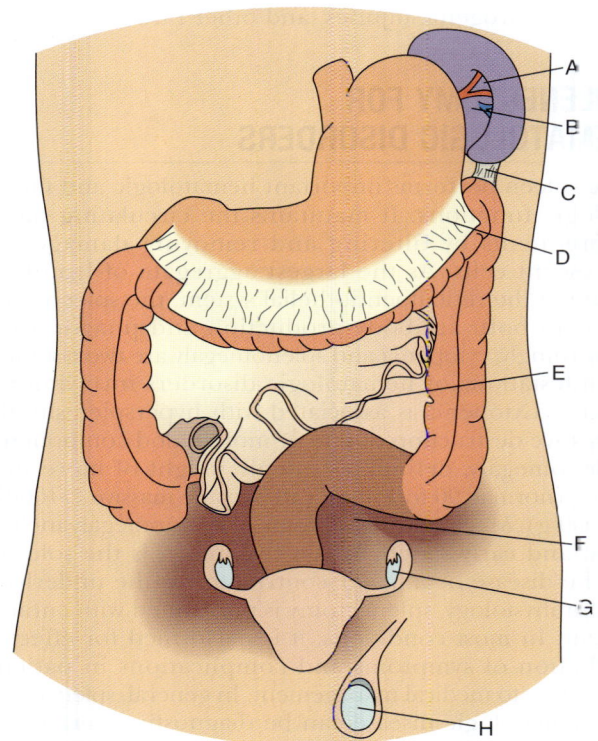

FIGURE 141.1 Common locations for accessory spleens: hilus of the spleen *(A)*; along the splenic vessels *(B)*; splenocolic ligament *(C)*; omentum *(D)*; mesentery *(E)*; presacral region *(F)*; adrenal region *(G)*; and gonads *(H)*. The weight of the dot corresponds to the frequency an accessory spleen may be found at that location. (From Martin JK. Staging laparotomy. In: Donohue J, van Heerden J, Monson J, eds. *Atlas of Surgical Oncology.* Cambridge, MA: Blackwell Science; 1995:150.)

tissue after splenectomy is indicated by the absence of Howell-Jolly bodies on a peripheral smear.

ITP occurs in every 1 to 2 per 1000 pregnancies, with or without a preexisting diagnosis. Differential diagnosis should exclude hereditary thrombocytopenia, gestational thrombocytopenia, and syndrome of hemolysis with elevated liver enzymes and low platelets. In pregnant ITP patients, bleeding risks for both the mother and the fetus must be considered because maternal IgG antibodies cross the placenta and can cause fetal thrombocytopenia. Treatment consists of careful monitoring of maternal platelet counts that typically reach a nadir in the third trimester. Intervention is generally not needed in patients with platelet counts greater than $20 \times 10^9/L$ until before delivery. A maternal count greater than $50 \times 10^9/L$ is considered safe for any mode of delivery and is the goal of therapy. Treatment options of low teratogenic risk include corticosteroids or IVIG, but their side effects may be exacerbated in pregnancy and should be carefully monitored. Splenectomy is usually avoided, but, if necessary, splenectomy should be performed during the second trimester. With maternal platelet count greater than $50 \times 10^9/L$, the incidence of fetal thrombocytopenia is 10% to 15% and that of fetal hemorrhage is less than 1%.[4,20]

Emergent intervention for ITP is indicated for patients with neurologic symptoms suggestive of intracranial bleeding, with evidence of internal or widespread mucocutaneous bleeding, and for those requiring an emergency operation for other reasons. First-line therapy consists of IVIG (1 g/kg per day for 2 days), intravenous methylprednisolone (1 g/day for 3 days), and platelet transfusions. Emergency splenectomy for refractory patients is rarely needed.[4]

Thrombotic Thrombocytopenic Purpura

Unlike ITP, thrombotic thrombocytopenic purpura (TTP) can be a highly lethal disorder. TTP is characterized by the pentad of thrombocytopenia, hemolytic anemia, fever, renal dysfunction, and less commonly, neurologic impairment. Characteristic findings include peripheral schistocytes (fragmented erythrocytes) and evidence of microvascular thrombosis. The pathophysiology of TTP involves an undefined trigger of vascular endothelial injury, leading to the release of unusually large forms of the von Willebrand factor. Abnormal platelet agglutination and marked intrasplenic phagocytosis follow. Currently, the first-line therapy consists of total plasma exchange in conjunction with corticosteroids and antiplatelet drugs such as aspirin or dipyridamole. Total plasma exchange has revolutionized the care of TTP by increasing the previously dismal survival rate to approximately 70% to 85%.[21,22] Relapse rates remain as high as 36% over 10 years.[23] TTP refractory to standard or increasing volume/frequency of plasma exchange and/or corticosteroids is most often treated with rituximab and a comprehensive evaluation of secondary causes (sepsis, drugs, etc.). Single-agent rituximab has demonstrated clinical remission in 87% to 100% of patients.[24-26] Splenectomy has been suggested for patients who remain refractory after escalating medical therapies. In several small series of patients, splenectomy induced remission of TTP in 50% of refractory patients[27] and reduced the risk of relapse by 70% to 95%.[2-28] However, the operative morbidity in

this patient population may be substantial at 17% to 39%. Only recent reports have suggested that laparoscopic splenectomy has lowered these operative risks.[28,29]

Systemic Lupus Erythematosus

Systemic lupus erythematosus (SLE) is a chronic autoimmune disease of unknown cause. Antiplatelet antibodies are demonstrable in 78% of SLE patients. These pathogenic autoantibodies and immune complexes affect virtually every body system. Destruction of antibody-coated platelets leads to severe thrombocytopenia in 8% to 20% of these patients.[30] First-line therapy involves agents aimed at reducing the pathogenic immune response: corticosteroids, rituximab, danazol, IVIG, and immunosuppressive (e.g., mycophenolate mofetil [CellCept]) and antineoplastic (e.g., cyclophosphamide, vincristine) drugs. Response rates to medical therapy have been variable and transient. Splenectomy is considered for patients who are refractory to, dependent, or intolerant of medical therapy. Despite previous concerns the operative risks of splenectomy are acceptable. The largest recent single-center experience of 25 patients undergoing splenectomy reported a 30-day mortality of 0% and morbidity of 24%, with hemorrhage and infection the most common complications.[30] The hematologic response was comparable to splenectomy for ITP, with an initial response rate of 88% and a relapse-free long-term response rate of 64%. Previously reported initial response rates ranged from 21% to 93% and prior sustained response rates were only 10% to 32%.[30] Although 36% of the patients relapsed after initial response (consistent with previously reported rates of 6% to 79%), additional medical therapy successfully salvaged 55% of these patients.[30] Because splenomegaly is typically not present, laparoscopic splenectomy is the procedure of choice in this patient population.

Human Immunodeficiency Virus

Chronic thrombocytopenia affects approximately 10% of patients infected with the human immunodeficiency virus (HIV) and 33% of those with acquired immunodeficiency syndrome (AIDS). Bleeding complications are infrequent and rarely severe even in the 1% to 5% of the patients with severe thrombocytopenia. Most patients have platelet counts higher than $50 \times 10^9/L$; some may even spontaneously correct their thrombocytopenia. The pathogenesis of HIV-thrombocytopenia involves (1) immune-mediated platelet destruction, similar to that in ITP, and (2) impaired platelet production due to infected megakaryocytes in the bone marrow.[32] Accordingly, first-line therapy consists of (1) corticosteroids, IVIG, and anti-D similar to ITP, and (2) antiviral agents such as azidothymidine (AZT) or combination highly active antiretroviral therapy to treat the primary disease.[31,33] The immunosuppressive effects of corticosteroids make them unsuitable for long-term administration. Splenectomy is indicated in patients unresponsive, refractory, or intolerant of medical therapy. Operative mortality is minimal,[4] although the complication rate approaches 24%.[35] Favorable response is achieved in 83% of HIV patients[34,36] and slightly fewer AIDS patients.[35] Splenectomy has not been shown to adversely impact the progression to AIDS, overall survival, and AIDS-free survival.[35] Despite encouraging results, the timing and

TABLE 141.1 Classification of Hereditary Spherocytosis

Variable	Trait/Carrier	Mild	Moderate	Severe
Hemoglobin, g/dL	Normal	11–15	8–12	6–8
Reticulocyte, %	<3	3–6	>6	>10
Bilirubin, μmol/L	<17	17–34	>34	>51
Spectrin per RBC, % normal	100	80–100	50–80	40–60
Splenectomy	Not indicated	Usually not indicated	Consider before puberty	Usually necessary, delay until age 6 years if possible

RBC, Red blood cell.

patient selection for splenectomy during the course of HIV infection remain controversial.

Wiskott-Aldrich Syndrome

Wiskott-Aldrich syndrome (WAS) is an X-linked immunodeficiency disorder characterized by thrombocytopenia, eczema, vasculitis, progressive immunodeficiency, and increased risk for malignancy. Its pathogenesis involves defective cytoplasmic scaffolding proteins.[37] Although phenotypic expression varies, thrombocytopenia is the most common manifestation of WAS. For patients with severe symptoms and available human leukocyte antigen (HLA)-matched donors, bone marrow transplant is performed with curative intent. For symptomatic patients without appropriate donors, splenectomy is indicated in combination with prophylactic antibiotics and immunization. Median survival of up to 25 years has been reported,[38,39] representing substantial improvement over the previously dismal median survival of less than 5 years. An IVIG may be used alone or in combination with splenectomy.

DISORDERS CAUSING ANEMIA

Hereditary Anemia

Hereditary anemias can be categorized by (1) defects of the erythrocyte membrane (e.g., hereditary spherocytosis [HS], hereditary elliptocytosis); (2) defects of an erythrocyte enzyme (e.g., pyruvate kinase deficiency, glucose-6-phosphate dehydrogenase deficiency); and (3) defects of hemoglobin synthesis (e.g., thalassemias, sickle cell anemia [SS]). All of these mutations result in abnormal erythrocyte morphology and stability and lead to increased hemolysis and phagocytosis by the spleen. The benefit and use of splenectomy vary depending on the diagnosis.

Red Blood Cell Membrane Defects. HS is the most common inherited hemolytic disorder in North America and Europe. It is transmitted mainly as an autosomal dominant trait. The pathogenesis of HS involves deficiencies in membrane structural proteins. The affected family of spectrin proteins, including β spectrin, ankyrin, band 3, and protein 4 to 2, normally forms the supportive cytoskeleton of the red blood cell (RBC). Dysfunction of these proteins results in abnormal RBC morphology, increased cell membrane fragility, and shortened life span. Clinical findings are variable and include anemia, jaundice, and splenomegaly. Pigmented gallstones form in up to 41% of patients screened with ultrasonography, and their prevalence is higher in patients who co-inherit Gilbert disease.[40] HS is distinguished from other anemias by the findings of elevated reticulocyte counts, hyperbilirubinemia, negative direct antiglobulin test (DAT), spherocytes on peripheral smear, and increased erythrocyte osmotic fragility.[41,42]

The indication for splenectomy is not based on the diagnosis of HS, per se, but on its symptoms and complications (Table 141.1).[43] For patients with mild HS and no gallstones, splenectomy has no benefit.[44] For patients with moderate or severe disease, splenectomy is indicated but usually delayed until after the sixth year of life but before puberty to minimize the risk of postsplenectomy sepsis.[45] Children with accelerating anemia, frequent hemolytic crises, transfusion dependency, or intractable leg ulcers may require earlier intervention.[41] For patients with symptomatic cholelithiasis, laparoscopic splenectomy and cholecystectomy are indicated and can be performed safely together.[45] When gallstones are asymptomatic or found incidentally, the best approach has not been established. Options include observation, cholecystotomy with stone removal, or cholecystectomy.[46]

The optimal approach for splenectomy remains controversial. Laparoscopic splenectomy offers a faster postoperative recovery in the pediatric population. It should be the approach of choice when splenomegaly is not present to increase the operative risks.[12,47] Partial (80% to 90%) open[48] or laparoscopic[49] splenectomy has been advocated for very young patients with severe disease, but preservation of splenic function must be balanced against the risks of disease recurrence. Recently, near-total splenectomy (98%) has been proposed as a means to optimize this balance.[50] Partial splenectomy has been demonstrated to be effective in resolution of hematologic parameters in the short term; however, total splenectomy has demonstrated more vigorous responses in hematologic parameters.[51,52] There have been reports of increased vascular events (arterial and venous) in patients with HS undergoing splenectomy, thought to be due to protective effects of lower hemoglobin and/or cholesterol metabolism[53] in nonsplenectomized HS patients; thus close monitoring or postoperative prophylaxis should be considered.

Hereditary elliptocytosis is a variant of HS also involving defective spectrin proteins. These patients typically have mild anemia requiring no intervention. Splenectomy does not correct the abnormal RBC morphology but is effective for the rare patient with severe transfusion-dependent anemia. HS must also be differentiated from other rare disorders of RBC membrane permeability such as hereditary stomatocytosis or cryohydrocytosis.

Splenectomy is ineffective and unwarranted and carries a high risk of postsplenectomy venous thrombosis in these patients.[41]

Red Blood Cell Enzymatic Defects. Glucose-6-phosphate dehydrogenase deficiency is the most common RBC enzymatic defect. It manifests as a mild anemia and rarely splenomegaly. Experience with splenectomy in this disease is limited. Pyruvate kinase deficiency results in reduced energy generation in RBCs. The homozygous form of this disease results in a severe anemia with splenomegaly. Splenectomy is effective in reducing transfusion requirements.[54]

Hemoglobinopathies. Sickle cell disease includes SS, hemoglobin C disease (SC), and the sickle β-thalassemia. The inherited point mutation on the sickle gene leads to an abnormal β-chain forming a hemoglobin with decreased solubility in its deoxygenated form. Pathogenesis of sickle disease results from abnormal polymerization of hemoglobin S with low cellular oxygen content. Exponential propagation of this process stiffens and distorts erythrocytes. Further compounding factors include abnormal endothelial adhesion, formation of heterocellular aggregates, dysregulation of nitric oxide–mediated vasodilation, and local inflammation. All of these factors lead to slowed RBC transit and their entrapment in the vasculature and in the spleen.[55] Microvascular occlusion results, and sickle patients suffer from end-organ damage of the eyes, kidneys, subcutaneous tissue, and bone. Splenic sequestration occurs when the RBC is trapped in the enlarged spleen, which then undergoes autoinfarction; it is observed in 7% to 30% of SS patients between 2 and 5 years of life. Acute manifestation, known as *acute splenic sequestration crisis* (ASSC), is potentially fatal. Patients present with profound acute anemia (decrease in hemoglobin by >2 g/dL), reticulocytosis, and thrombocytopenia. Acute therapy requires resuscitation by RBC transfusions. However, recurrence carries a 20% mortality rate and can occur in 50% of those who survive ASSC.[55] As a means to prevent future ASSC, elective splenectomy has been indicated in children older than 2 or 3 years of age after the first episode of ASSC. The operative mortality is 7%, and 5-year mortality is 3.4%.[56,57] The risk of postsplenectomy sepsis is approximately 2% in this patient population but increases substantially if splenectomy is performed before 4 years of age.[58-60] More recently partial splenectomy has been compared with total splenectomy in pediatric patients and has demonstrated no change in postsplenectomy hemoglobin levels in either group, underscoring the decision-making process for splenectomy which focuses on minimizing complications and improvement of quality of life. Importantly in this multiinstitutional observational study, no difference was found in the rate of postsplenectomy sepsis comparing partial to total splenectomy.[1] Splenectomy (partial or total) has not been proven to increase survival, but the benefits include reducing transfusion dependency, relief from pain from splenomegaly, and treatment of splenic abscesses resulting from splenic infarctions.[55,61]

Patients with thalassemia major (or homozygous β-thalassemia) synthesize structurally abnormal hemoglobin that deforms erythrocytes. They typically depend on multiple transfusions to maintain a hemoglobin level greater than 10 g/dL. When complications of hypersplenism develop, as measured by transfusion requirement of greater than 250 mL/kg per year and iron overload, splenectomy is indicated.[62] Splenectomy reduces the requirements for both transfusions and deferoxamine (an iron chelator) in 32% of patients.[63] More than 80% of children with thalassemia regain normal weight and growth rates after splenectomy.[64] The risk for overwhelming postsplenectomy sepsis (OPSS) is high in this patient population, approximately 10% in the long term.[65] Therefore splenectomy is usually delayed until after 6 to 8 years of age. Partial splenectomy has been advocated in younger children,[66] and laparoscopic splenectomy is definitely feasible in these patients.[67]

Acquired Hemolytic Anemia

Hemolytic anemia may result from numerous etiologies. Autoimmune hemolytic anemia (AIHA) is an IgG-mediated (so-called warm agglutinin) hemolytic anemia with a positive Coombs antiglobulin test. Erythrocyte destruction is mediated by splenic macrophages. AIHA may be idiopathic or a manifestation of a systemic disease, such as viral infection, SLE, rheumatoid arthritis, ulcerative colitis, or chronic lymphocytic leukemia (CLL). Although corticosteroids remain the first-line therapy, rituximab is favored as the initial choice of second-line therapies despite the absences of randomized data supporting this approach.[68] Splenectomy is indicated for disease refractory to corticosteroids (or other second-line therapies). It succeeds in nearly 64% of patients and reduces the steroid requirement in an additional 21% of patients.[54] The success rate is greater when AIHA is associated with systemic disease.[69] It is important for slow steroid taper postsplenectomy because rapid withdrawal can lead to acute hemolytic crises, which may mimic postoperative bleeding. In contrast, so-called cold agglutinin hemolytic anemia is mediated by IgM. Erythrocytes are sequestered and destroyed in the liver, and splenectomy therefore plays no role in this condition.

MISCELLANEOUS HEMATOLOGIC DISORDERS

Evans Syndrome

Patients with Evans syndrome present with a combination of autoimmune thrombocytopenia (ITP) and AIHA. Medical therapy typically involves multiple agents, with corticosteroids and IVIG being used most commonly.[70,71] Experience with splenectomy for this rare disease is limited.[72] Although long-term remission has been reported,[73] one study observed the median duration of response following splenectomy to be only 1 month.[70]

Felty Syndrome

Felty syndrome, defined as a combination of rheumatoid arthritis, splenomegaly, and neutropenia, affects a small subset of patients, particularly those with destructive rheumatoid arthritis, severe extraarticular symptoms, and an HLA-DR4 haplotype.[74] Neutropenic sepsis is the main cause of patient demise. First-line therapy consists of hematopoietic growth factor and often leads to rapid, favorable responses.[75] Splenectomy is indicated when the neutropenia fails to improve adequately or rapidly enough. Neutropenia is corrected by splenectomy in 80%

of patients, and active preoperative infections resolve in nearly half of patients.[75]

Autoimmune Neutropenia

Patients affected by autoimmune neutropenia, a rare disorder, usually have neutrophil counts of 500 to 1000/μL but manifest granulocyte-specific antibodies. It commonly presents in infancy as recurrent infections. When present in adults, it may be associated with underlying diseases such as viral infection, collagen vascular diseases, ITP, or AIHA. Autoimmune neutropenia is typically characterized by spontaneous disappearance of autoantibodies and does not require specific intervention. However, for acute infections or operative procedures, granulocyte colony-stimulating factors effectively improve the neutrophil counts. A total of 50% to 60% of the patients also respond to corticosteroids and IVIG.[72] Therefore the role for splenectomy is limited only to the rare patient who is refractory to medical interventions.

LYMPHOPROLIFERATIVE DISORDERS

Lymphoma

Lymphomas are categorized into two distinct types: Hodgkin disease (HD) and non-Hodgkin lymphoma (NHL). The surgeon's role in HD was intraabdominal disease staging to determine whether irradiation or chemotherapy should be the initial treatment approach. Staging laparotomy for HD has been abandoned because of the quality of dimensional imaging and positron emission tomography (PET) and because chemotherapy has become the treatment of choice for nearly all forms of HD. Splenectomy provides palliative and therapeutic benefits in several subtypes of NHL.

Non-Hodgkin Lymphoma. NHL is a diverse group of more than 20 malignancies originating from B lymphocytes (~80%), T lymphocytes (~15% to 20%), or natural killer cells (<5%). A specific NHL diagnosis requires histologic examination of lymphoid tissue plus flow cytometry and molecular marker studies. Patients with NHL frequently present with nonspecific symptoms of fever, night sweats, malaise, and weight loss. Peripheral lymphadenopathy is variably present, and lymphatic spread is often non-contiguous. The spleen is involved in 30% to 40% of NHL patients.[76] Although NHL shares the same Ann Arbor staging system as HD, clinical staging is less crucial in NHL treatment because most patients present with advanced disease. There is no role for staging laparotomy

in NHL because therapy is seldom redirected by staging information.[77]

There are three indications for splenectomy in NHL patients: (1) to correct hypersplenism and the resultant cytopenia(s), thereby allowing aggressive chemotherapy and/or independence from transfusions; (2) to relieve symptoms of splenomegaly from lymphocytic infiltration; and (3) tumor debulking when the spleen is the main site of disease involvement, either as primary treatment or for residual disease. Operative mortality ranges between 0% and 3.5%, and reported operative morbidity is higher at 11% to 37% in studies published since 1990 (Table 141.2).[78-82] The most common severe complications are venous thrombosis and subphrenic abscess. A laparoscopic splenectomy is associated with reduced morbidity but requires technical expertise, particularly when splenomegaly is present.[81] Blood counts normalize in 72% to 89% of patients with NHL within the first postoperative month. A durable response is observed in a substantial proportion of patients (see Table 141.2). Finally, these potential benefits and risks of splenectomy must be balanced against the prognosis of the primary disease. The proposed World Health Organization classification system (Box 141.1)[83] categorizes subtypes of NHL by clinical behavior: indolent subtypes have mean expected survivals measured in years, but aggressive subtypes generally have survivals measured only in months.

The spleen is the primary site of disease in several subtypes of NHL. Mantle cell lymphoma (MCL), an uncommon type, constitutes only 5% to 8% of NHL. Patients with MCL may have minimal adenopathy but prominent extranodal disease.[84] Up to 60% develop massive splenomegaly.[85] For patients with splenic-predominant MCL, splenectomy should be considered to palliate either hypersplenism or splenomegaly or both. Splenectomy may further benefit patients by stabilizing their disease, delaying the start of chemotherapy, and prolonging survival. A retrospective study of 26 patients[84] found that splenectomy is safe (no operative mortality and morbidity of 24%). Hypersplenism was corrected in 69% of patients with anemia, 90% with thrombocytopenia, and 50% of patients with both. In addition, 90% did not require chemotherapy until at least a year after splenectomy. The median survival is 5.5 years (typically 3 to 4 years), and splenectomy was the sole therapy in 15% of the patients.

The therapeutic role of splenectomy is more prominent in splenic marginal zone B-cell lymphoma (MZL). This primary lymphoma of the spleen comprises only 1%

TABLE 141.2 Experience With Splenectomy in Non-Hodgkin Lymphoma, Published Since 1990

Authors, Year	Number of Patients	Operative Technique	Operative Mortality (%)	Morbidity (%)	Initial Response (1 Month) (%)	Durable Response Follow-up (%)
Delpero et al., 1990[79]	62	Open	1.6	29	89	63 (26 months)
Lehne et al., 1994[80]	35	Open	2.9	37	72	14
Brodsky et al., 1996[78]	12	Open	0	17	80 (3 months)	N/A
Walsh and Heniford, 1999[81]	9	Laparoscopic	0	11	N/A	N/A
Xiros et al., 2000[82]	29	Open	3.5	14	88	N/A

NHL, Non-Hodgkin lymphoma; *N/A*, not available.

BOX 141.1 Proposed World Health Organization Classification of Lymphoid Neoplasms

INDOLENT LYMPHOMAS

B-Cell Neoplasms

Small lymphocytic lymphoma/B-cell chronic lymphocytic leukemia

Lymphoplasmacytic lymphoma (Waldenström macroglobulinemia)

Plasma cell myeloma/plasmacytoma

Hairy cell leukemia

Follicular lymphoma (grades I and II)

Marginal zone B-cell lymphoma

Mantle cell lymphoma

T-Cell Neoplasms

T-cell large granular lymphocyte leukemia

Mycosis fungoides

T-cell prolymphocytic leukemia

Natural Killer Cell Neoplasms

Natural killer cell large granular lymphocyte leukemia

AGGRESSIVE LYMPHOMAS

B-Cell Neoplasms

Follicular lymphoma (grade III)

Diffuse large B-cell lymphoma

T-Cell Neoplasms

Peripheral T-cell lymphoma

Anaplastic large cell lymphoma, T/null cell

HIGHLY AGGRESSIVE LYMPHOMAS

B-Cell Neoplasms

Burkitt lymphoma

Precursor B lymphoblastic leukemia/lymphoma

T-Cell Neoplasms

Adult T-cell lymphoma/leukemia

Precursor T-lymphoblastic leukemia/lymphoma

TABLE 141.3 Rai Classification of Chronic Lymphocytic Leukemia

Stage	Description
0	Lymphocytosis (WBC >150 000/mL >40% lymphocytes in bone marrow)
I	Lymphocytosis and lymphadenopathy
II	Lymphocytosis and splenomegaly/hepatomegaly
III	Lymphocytosis and anemia (hemoglobin <11 g/dL)
IV	Lymphocytosis, lymphadenopathy, anemia, and thrombocytopenia (platelet <100 000/mL)

WBC White blood cell.

CLL is the most common chronic leukemia. CLL is characterized by the accumulation of morphologically normal but functionally incompetent B lymphocytes. Patients follow either an indolent course requiring no therapy or an accelerated course with severe symptoms that require intervention.[91] Patients with CLL present with painless lymphadenopathy alone or with additional features including splenomegaly, cytopenia, and constitutional symptoms, as defined by the Rai classification (Table 141.3). Patients with stage 0 disease require no therapy, but selected patients with stage I or II disease and all patients with stage III or IV disease should receive chemotherapy, typically fludarabine.[79] Although cytopenia in CLL may result from bone marrow failure, hypersplenism, autoimmune destruction, chemotherapy, or any combination,[92] splenectomy is an efficacious method of reversing cytopenia (Table 141.4). A durable response of cytopenia in CLL is observed in at least 80% of patients, with higher response rates when splenectomy is performed for thrombocytopenia rather than for anemia.[35,92–96] However, no predicative factor of a hematologic response to splenectomy has been consistently identified.[97] The overall survival is longer in patients with a hematologic response than those who fail to respond,[95,94,97] but the survival benefit of splenectomy in patients with advanced CLL remains controversial. No significant difference in survival was observed in a case-matched study,[93] although in subgroup analysis of patients with severe anemia (hemoglobin <10 g/dL) or thrombocytopenia (platelet count <50 × 10^9/L), splenectomy did significantly prolong median survival (19 vs. 10 months and 17 vs. 4 months, respectively). These results suggest that splenectomy should be considered for all CLL patients with cytopenia, particularly those with severe anemia or thrombocytopenia.

Chronic myelogenous leukemia (CML) consists of a chronic benign phase followed by an acute blast transformation phase. Patients usually present during the chronic phase with systemic symptoms, splenomegaly, leukocytosis, and cytopenias. Chromosomal translocation t(9;22) (i.e., Philadelphia chromosome) is present in 90% of the CML patients, and treatment efficacy is monitored by decreased expression of the abnormal chromosome.[77] Therapeutic options in CML include chemotherapy (e.g., hydroxyurea or busulfan), interferon-α, and bone marrow transplant.[20] Splenectomy is used only for palliation of refractory cytopenia or painful splenomegaly. Splenectomy does not seem to increase survival or delay the onset of the acute blastic

of NHL and is characterized by massive splenomegaly, lymphocytes with villous projections, anemia, thrombocytopenia, and mild monoclonal gammopathy.[86] Reversal of cytopenia occurs in 82% to 95% of patients following splenectomy,[86–90] with a median survival of 8.5 years[87,89] and 3-year survival of 82%[88] in patients with spleen-only MZL. These results suggest that clinically localized MZL patients behave like those with localized stage I NHL. Longer overall survival correlated with prompt correction of cytopenia during the immediate postoperative period.[89] Splenectomy is a treatment of choice in patients with localized MZL.

Leukemias

Leukemia is characterized by a malignant clonal proliferation of hematopoietic stem cells. For patients with acute lymphocytic or acute myelogenous leukemia, there is consensus that splenectomy plays no role except for splenic rupture with hemorrhage.[20] For patients with chronic forms of leukemia, splenectomy may be indicated to palliate symptoms of splenomegaly or cytopenias. The survival benefit of splenectomy in patients with leukemia remains controversial.

TABLE 141.4 Experiences With Splenectomy for Chronic Lymphocytic Leukemia, Published Since 1990

Authors, Year	Number of Patients	Operative Mortality (%)	Operative Morbidity (%)	Response for Cytopenia (Response %)	Long-Term Cytopenia (Response %)	Median Survival (Months)
Thiruvengadam et al., 1990[91]	30	N/A	N/A	N/A	71–87	36 (18–62)
Neal et al., 1992[92]	50	4	26	64–77 (3 months)	84–86	36 (41, responders; 14, nonresponders)
Majumdar et al., 1992[94]	14	0	28.5	84.6 (2–3 months)	N/A	44
Pegourie-Bandelier et al., 1995[95]	29	0	34	N/A	85–100	N/A
Seymour et al., 1997[96]	55*	9	25	38–81	N/A	27 (vs. 23, P = .96)
Cusack et al., 1997[93]	77*	7.8	54	61–69	N/A	34 (vs. 24, P = .27)
Ruchlemer et al., 2002[85]	47	6.4	35	47 (3 months)	N/A	56.4

*Case matched with patients treated with fludarabine.
N/A, Not available.

transformation. Acute blastic crisis, marked by prolonged fever of unknown origin, leukocytosis, thrombocytopenia, and greater than 30% blasts in peripheral circulation, carries a grim prognosis, with median survival measured in months. Splenectomy is contraindicated during the acute phase. However, when necessary for emergency indications, a low 30-day mortality rate of 3.5% can be achieved.[91] In addition, splenectomy does not have an adverse impact on the incidence of infections, graft versus host disease, or overall survival if a bone marrow transplant is performed after splenectomy.[98]

Hairy cell leukemia (HCL) comprises 2% to 5% of leukemias and is a chronic B-lymphocyte disorder characterized by peripheral cytopenia and massive splenomegaly. The malignant cells have hairlike projections and accumulate mainly in the red pulp of the spleen but can be identified elsewhere by their positive tartrate-resistant acid phosphatase staining.[97] Cytopenia in HCL may result from hypersplenism, bone marrow failure, or other reasons. Before 1990, splenectomy was the only known effective therapy for HCL. Cytopenia improved after splenectomy in 60% to 100%,[97] with a potential survival benefit. In the early 1990s interferon-α was shown to be superior to splenectomy for cytopenia in a randomized trial.[99] Currently, medical therapies of interferon-α and purine analogues are efficacious. The indications for splenectomy in HCL are therefore limited to those patients with an uncertain diagnosis, splenic rupture, severe splenomegaly with symptomatic cytopenia, or disease refractory to chemotherapy. Resection of residual splenic disease after interferon therapy may prolong progression-free survival.[100] The contemporary experience with splenectomy for HCL is limited.

MYELOPROLIFERATIVE DISORDERS

Chronic myeloproliferative disorders are marked by abnormal clonal proliferation of hematopoietic stem cells. Myelofibrosis with myeloid metaplasia (MMM) occurs when bone marrow develops a fibrotic reaction to the stem cell disease and can be divided into agnogenic (AMM), postthrombocythemic (PTMM), and postpolycythemic (PPMM) types. PTMM and PPMM are preceded by essential thrombocythemia and polycythemic rubra vera, respectively, and splenectomy generally does not benefit these patients.[20,101,102] The AMM is characterized by peripheral cytopenia and progressive extramedullary hematopoiesis in the spleen and the liver. Associated features include painful splenomegaly, increased portal blood flow, portal hypertension from venous thrombosis (approximately 7%),[103] and cytopenia from splenic sequestration. The prognosis of AMM is poor, with median survival ranging from 3 to 5 years. Nonoperative therapy options are limited. Bone marrow transplant is frequently not an option for elderly AMM patients. Transfusions, androgens, corticosteroids, and interferon-α are largely palliative, and splenic irradiation is only transiently effective. Therefore splenectomy should be considered in symptomatic patients. Symptomatic splenomegaly, constitutional symptoms, and portal hypertension improve in 100%, 67%, and 50% of the respective patients at 1 year postsplenectomy. Among those patients with transfusion-dependent anemia, 30% remain independent of transfusions for 6 months. No benefit for splenectomy is seen with thrombocytopenic patients.[104] Despite potential benefits, splenectomy in this patient population is a high-risk procedure.[105] Before 1940, operative mortality was prohibitively high at 40%. Currently, it ranges from 8% to 11%, with postoperative morbidity ranging from 31% to 40%.[100,104,106] Hemorrhage, infection, and thrombosis are the most common nonfatal complications. Several complications characteristic of this patient population have also been described.[104] Progressive hepatomegaly develops in 12% to 29% of the patients after splenectomy; as extramedullary hematopoiesis increases in the liver, 7% develop fatal hepatic failure. Severe thrombocytosis affects 18% to 50% of AMM patients after splenectomy, particularly if the preoperative platelet count is greater than 50×10^9/L. Postsplenectomy leukemic transformation occurs in 11% to 20% of patients and manifests as an accumulation of blasts in the bone marrow and peripheral blood.[101] Whether postsplenectomy blast transformation affects overall patient survival remains controversial[1-1,102,104-107,108] and should not deter the surgeon from performing an otherwise appropriate splenectomy. The median overall postsplenectomy survival is 2.3 years.[104] The main causes of death include infection, thrombosis, bleeding, and acute leukemia. Current indications for splenectomy in patients with AMM remain palliative and include severe constitutional symptoms, mechanical symptoms of splenomegaly, portal hypertension complicated by ascites and variceal hemorrhage, and transfusion-dependent anemia.[101]

SPLENECTOMY FOR TUMORS, CYSTS, AND ABSCESSES

Tumors

Splenic masses are usually discovered incidentally. They present for surgical intervention with an unknown diagnosis, when the spleen ruptures, or when symptoms develop from their large size or associated hypersplenism.

The most common cause of a malignant splenic mass is metastasis from a primary carcinoma. Splenic metastases are present in 7% of patients dying from cancers of the breast, lung, ovary, stomach and prostate.[20] Melanoma and other skin cancers also spread to the spleen. When the spleen is the only site of metastasis, splenectomy may prolong patient survival.

Primary, nonlymphatic, malignant tumors of the spleen include angiosarcoma, hemangioendothelioma, and malignant fibrous histiocytoma. Angiosarcoma is the most common of these rare tumors. Patients present at a median age of 60 years, with abdominal pain, splenomegaly, and microangiopathic hemolytic anemia. The tumors appear as well-circumscribed nodules with central necrosis or hemorrhage. The prognosis for splenic angiosarcoma patients is dismal. Eighty-nine percent of patients die of metastatic disease, with a mean survival of 5 months.[109] Splenectomy is indicated for palliation and for splenic rupture, which may occur in 2% of patients. The rarity of the disease has hindered identification of risk factors, but exposure to thorium dioxide (Thorotrast) vinyl chloride, and anabolic steroids has been implicated in isolated reports.[109]

Benign tumors of the spleen are uncommon and include hamartoma, inflammatory pseudotumor, and vascular lesions (hemangioma, lymphangioma, peliosis). Hemangiomas are the most common benign splenic lesions and arise from the red pulp of the spleen. They can become very large, with prominent cystic components. Nonexpanding and asymptomatic hemangiomas less than 4 cm are safely observed.[110] Splenectomy may be considered to prevent or treat complications such as hypersplenism and splenomegaly. Peliosis of the spleen occurs alone or in association with peliosis of the liver. It occurs more frequently in men, is the result of the exogenous androgens and oral

contraceptives, and accompanies chronic debilitation from tuberculosis, diabetes, or a neoplasm.[20] Complications of peliosis include thrombosis and fatal hemorrhage from splenic rupture. Splenectomy is indicated when peliosis is incidentally discovered. Splenic hamartomas as large as 2 kg have been reported and require surgical intervention for diagnosis. Inflammatory pseudotumors are a poorly understood entity. Patients present with fever, night sweats, and weight loss. These tumors must be distinguished from malignant lymphoma by immunohistologic studies, making splenectomy necessary for diagnosis in many patients. Additional rare benign splenic lesions include littoral cell angioma, hemangioendothelioma, and angiomyolipoma.

Cysts

Parasitic Cysts. *Echinococcus* cysts are common in endemic disease areas but rare in the United States. Humans serve as intermediate hosts after ingestion of food contaminated with feces laden with tapeworm eggs. Hydatid cysts most commonly develop in the liver and the lungs; their daughter cysts contain multiplying larvae called *scolices*. Cysts of *Echinococcus granulosus* are unilocular, but those of *Echinococcus multilocularis* and *Echinococcus volegi* are multilocular.[12] Intervention is indicated when the disease is refractory to the antiparasitic drug albendazole or when cysts become large enough to risk rupture. Cystectomy or splenectomy should be performed with care to avoid cyst rupture or leakage. Anaphylaxis and disseminated scolices infection are serious operative complications. Administration of albendazole and instillation of hypertonic saline or ethanol before cyst manipulation have been advocated to decrease these risks.[12]

Nonparasitic Cysts. Nonparasitic splenic cysts were previously classified as true cysts (~20%) or pseudocysts (~80%) based on the presence or absence of an epithelial lining. True cysts may be epidermoid or, less commonly, dermoid in origin, resulting from splenic inclusion of embryonic tissue. They may also be associated with benign splenic hemangiomas or lymphangiomas. Pseudocysts are typically associated with antecedent splenic trauma or splenic infarction.[20] Splenic infarction occurs with hematologic disorders (most commonly sickle cell disease) in younger patients or with arterial emboli (the most common cause being atrial fibrillation) in patients older than age 40 years.[111] However, the reliability of identifying the cyst lining has been questioned. A newly proposed system classifies splenic cysts based on cause into congenital, neoplastic, true traumatic, and degenerative cysts.[112]

Intervention is not necessary for a symptomatic, small (<5 cm) splenic cysts that have imaging characteristics of a benign cyst, namely, a smooth regular cyst wall, with no solid component within the cyst interior or wall, either with or without calcification.[112] Total splenectomy is typically considered for patients with low operative risk who develop pain or early satiety because of their splenic cysts. Recently developed minimally invasive treatment options include cyst aspiration with sclerosis using alcohol or tetracycline, cyst marsupialization, and local cyst resection with or without a portion of the cyst wall contiguous with splenic parenchyma. There is significant risk of cyst recurrence with these techniques. Laparoscopic or partial splenectomy is now the preferred treatment because of their low complication and cyst recurrence rates.[113]

Abscesses

Although splenic abscess remains a rare entity, it is uniformly fatal if unrecognized or untreated. With an increasing incidence of immunosuppressive diseases and medications, splenic abscesses have become more common.[114] A high index of suspicion is required for timely diagnosis and favorable outcome. Patients able to mount an immune response present with the triad of fever, leukocytosis, and left upper quadrant pain. Chest or abdominal radiographs often show a left-sided pleural effusion, elevated hemidiaphragm, left upper quadrant mass, and extraluminal air. A computed tomography (CT) scan has a very high sensitivity and is the imaging modality of choice. A splenic abscess typically has a thick, irregular rim with a hypodense center, but multiple or miliary abscesses may be difficult to identify.

Splenic abscesses are classified by their cause.[12,114] The most common cause is primary hematogenous seeding from a distant septic source (common sources include bacterial endocarditis associated with valvular disease, intravenous drug use, bacteremia, and postoperative or primary intraabdominal infection). The most common organisms causing a splenic abscess are *Streptococcus* and *Staphylococcus* species, but *Salmonella* species, gram-negative *Escherichia coli*, and *Enterococcus* species, plus fungal infections also lead to splenic abscesses.[115] Although most splenic abscesses are solitary, multiple abscesses more frequently develop from hematogenous spread. Secondary infection of a splenic infarction is another cause of splenic abscess. Patients with an architecturally or functionally abnormal spleen are most susceptible to this type of infection. Common associated conditions include SS, lymphoproliferative and myeloproliferative diseases, trauma, and systemic arterial embolization. Patients with SS characteristically develop splenic abscesses with *Salmonella* species. The direct extension of a local septic focus may also result in a splenic abscess. These infections originate from a gastric, colonic, pancreatic, or perinephric source. Posttraumatic splenic abscesses occur after conservative management of splenic trauma or an iatrogenic intraoperative injury. Immunocompromised host accounts for up to 35% of patients with splenic abscesses. Associated conditions include malignancy, organ transplantation, chronic steroid use, and HIV/AIDS.

The treatment of choice for splenic abscess consists of broad-spectrum antibiotics, splenectomy, and drainage of the left upper quadrant. In critically ill patients unable to tolerate a surgical procedure, image-guided drainage should be attempted. When the abscess is discrete, unilocular, and filled with thin fluid, the success rate of nonoperative therapy is as high as 51%.[114] Occasionally, dense inflammatory adhesions preclude splenectomy, leaving splenotomy or surgical drainage as the only surgical options. In this setting a delayed splenectomy is necessary because intravenous antibiotics are almost never sufficient treatment for a splenic abscess. Mortality from splenic abscess still ranges from 0% to 24%. Poor outcomes occur with immunocompromised patients, delayed diagnosis, and postponed operative intervention.[114]

SPLENECTOMY FOR VASCULAR DISORDERS

SPLENIC ARTERY ANEURYSM

Splenic artery aneurysm (SAA) constitutes 60% of all visceral arterial aneurysms and is the third most common abdominal aneurysm after aortic and iliac artery aneurysms. The typical patient with SAA is a multiparous woman (in a series of 87 women, the average number of pregnancies per patient was 4.5).[116] Other associated conditions include portal hypertension, congenital vascular or connective tissue diseases, and trauma. SAA presents (1) after rupture with hemodynamic instability; (2) as a symptomatic mass; or (3) as an incidental finding. Rupture occurs most commonly in the third trimester of pregnancy and may be forewarned by a sentinel hemorrhage in 20% to 30% of patients.[117] In pregnant patients the mortality rate after rupture is 70% for the mother and approaches 100% for the fetus.[118] In nonpregnant patients the mortality rate for SAA rupture is 25%.[20] As soon as rupture is suspected, prompt resuscitation, emergent splenectomy, and resection of the aneurysm are indicated. All symptomatic aneurysms require surgical intervention. For incidental and asymptomatic aneurysms, surgical treatment is indicated if the SAA is larger than 2.5 cm in diameter and if the patient is pregnant or of childbearing potential.[20,119] Operative treatment differs by location of the SAA. Proximal SAAs are excised after proximal and distal ligation. Mid-SAAs are excluded by proximal and distal ligation of the splenic artery and all collateral vessels. The spleen blood flow is preserved by the short gastric arteries. Distal or hilar SAAs are the most common and are treated with aneurysmectomy and splenectomy.[116,118,120] For patients unable to tolerate an operation, transcatheter embolization is used. This results in splenic infarction and has the risks of distant embolization, arterial disruption, and arterial recanalization with potential future rupture.[117,119] Successful laparoscopic ligation and splenectomy have been reported.[121,122] The optimal approach to elective treatment of SAA depends on patient variables and physician expertise.

SPLENIC VENOUS THROMBOSIS

Splenic venous thrombosis (SVT) complicates acute pancreatitis and pancreatic neoplasms in 7% to 20% of patients. Nonpancreatic diseases, including primary retroperitoneal fibrosis, peptic ulcer disease, and a hypercoagulable state, may also be associated with SVT.[123] SVT results in a localized form of portal hypertension termed *sinistral portal hypertension*.[124] Collateral flow through the short gastric vessels leads to engorgement of submucosal veins of the gastric fundus (gastric varices). Esophageal varices may arise if the left gastric vein is also occluded by the thrombus. The diagnosis of SVT should be suspected in patients with upper gastrointestinal hemorrhage following pancreatitis, in patients with splenomegaly but no hepatic or hematologic disease, and when isolated gastric varices are noted on upper endoscopy. Ultrasonography, CT scan, and visceral angiography all can confirm the diagnosis. In patients presenting with hemorrhage, urgent splenectomy is indicated. The operative bleeding risk is substantial because of the perigastric varices and inflammation. To reduce this risk, some surgeons advocate preoperative splenic artery embolization.[124] In unstable patients or those not fit for an operation, endoscopic variceal sclerotherapy or banding may be performed but this is usually ineffective.[125]

In asymptomatic patients with SVT, the indication for splenectomy is controversial. Prophylactic splenectomy used to be uniformly recommended because up to 51% of asymptomatic patients with SVT were thought to develop acute variceal bleeding.[126] Studies have found a more benign natural history of SVT, with a 4% to 13% prevalence of clinical hemorrhage.[124,126] Expectant management, initially advocated by Loftus et al.,[127] has generally been adopted. Prophylactic splenectomy should be considered for noncompliant patients, those undergoing an abdominal operation for another cause, and patients who have endoscopic features, such as "red wale markings," indicating a higher risk of hemorrhage.[124,125]

PORTAL HYPERTENSION

Patients with portal hypertension often develop thrombocytopenia from platelet sequestration in the splenic sinusoids.[20] Splenectomy should be considered with a devascularization or shunting procedure when the bleeding risk from thrombocytopenia is excessive, when medical therapy cannot be administered, or when the varices are resistant to nonoperative management.[128] Portal hypertension is not an absolute contraindication to laparoscopic splenectomy, but higher conversion (9.6%) and morbidity (11%) rates have been reported.[123]

"WANDERING SPLEEN" AND SPLENIC TORSION

A "wandering spleen" occurs when the spleen is attached only by a long, loose vascular pedicle. The spleen may be ectopic on imaging studies. Wandering spleens in children arise from congenital atresia of the dorsal mesogastrium. In women between 20 and 40 years of age, wandering spleens result from an acquired tissue laxity associated with pregnancy.[129] This condition may result in acute torsion around the vascular pedicle, which manifests as acute abdominal pain, fever, vomiting, acute pancreatitis, and gastric compression. Without detorsion, splenic infarction and gangrene ensue. Chronic torsion typically causes venous congestion and splenomegaly. In children without splenic infarction the therapeutic procedure of choice is splenopexy, suturing the spleen to the diaphragm, abdominal wall, or omentum.[130] Laparoscopic splenopexy has been reported.[131] Although splenopexy allows for splenic preservation, the long-term results are unknown. For adults, splenectomy is preferred.

SPLENECTOMY FOR IATROGENIC INJURY

An iatrogenic splenic injury is an unintentional injury caused by the operator during either an interventional radiologic or surgical procedure. The surgical operations most commonly associated with iatrogenic splenic injury include distal esophageal and stomach procedures, colon surgery, left nephrectomy, and upper abdominal vascular procedures.[20] Risk factors for iatrogenic injury include a prior left upper quadrant operation, malignant or inflammatory diseases, and obese body habitus.[132] The spleen tethered by its peritoneal ligaments plus dense adhesions

is prone to injury by inappropriate traction, retractor placement, or instrumentation.

When an iatrogenic splenic injury occurs, exposure to the left upper quadrant should be optimized, blood and clots are gently removed, and severe bleeding is temporized by pressure on the splenic artery at the superior edge of the pancreas. Limited splenic capsular tears may be treated successfully by packing, by electrocautery, argon beam coagulation, or hemostatic agents such as fibrin adhesive, thrombin-soaked Gelfoam, and microfibrillar collagen. Deeper lacerations may be salvaged with argon beam coagulation, mattress sutures in the spleen with or without pledgets, wrapping the spleen in an absorbent mesh, or segmental splenectomy. If the initial attempt at repair is unsuccessful, splenectomy should be performed.[133] In patients with severe (greater than grade 4) splenic injury, hemodynamic instability, or in those requiring postoperative anticoagulation, splenectomy is indicated. Splenectomy for iatrogenic injury prolongs hospital stay and increases morbidity from 0% to 32% and from 16% to 84% in various series.[132] Whether incidental splenectomy compromises immune function and decreases survival in cancer patients is uncertain. The incidence of sepsis is low after unplanned splenectomy in adults: 1 per 545 adult-years.[15] Measures to prevent iatrogenic injury include placement of the incisions and ports to maximize exposure, gentle retraction, careful medial or downward traction on the peritoneal attachments and manipulation of stomach and colon only after dividing splenic ligaments and perisplenic adhesions.[132]

SPLENECTOMY FOR MISCELLANEOUS DISORDERS

Gaucher disease is an inherited metabolic disorder manifesting with anemia, thrombocytopenia, hepatosplenomegaly, and bone dysplasia. The genetic deficiency in lysosomal glucocerebrosidase leads to accumulation of glucosyl ceramide–laden macrophages in the reticuloendothelial cells of the liver, bone, and spleen. Enzyme replacement therapy (alglucerase or imiglucerase) effectively ameliorates symptoms of Gaucher disease.[34] Splenectomy is reserved for patients with compressive symptoms from massive splenomegaly or refractory cytopenia. The largest series to date reports operative mortality of 2.1% and morbidity of 27%.[35] In children with Gaucher disease, partial splenectomy or another spleen-preserving technique is advocated.

Splenomegaly complicates 6% of patients with sarcoidosis and is associated with anemia, neutropenia, or pancytopenia. Most patients have mild and asymptomatic splenomegaly and do not require treatment. Splenectomy is considered for massive or painful splenomegaly, refractory hypersplenism, to exclude lymphoma or other malignancy, and prophylaxis against splenic rupture. Outcome of splenectomy for sarcoidosis is favorable in isolated case reports.[136]

Amyloidosis is a systemic infiltrative disease. Splenic rupture may occur as amyloid deposits distend the capsule and increase vascular fragility.[15] Emergent splenectomy may be necessary for splenic rupture.

OPERATIVE CONSIDERATIONS FOR SPLENECTOMY

PREOPERATIVE PREPARATION

The indication for splenectomy, the underlying disease, and the patient's comorbidities, hematologic status, and previous therapy must be clearly reviewed.

Vaccinations are indicated whenever splenectomy or impaired splenic function is anticipated. The normal host defense against encapsulated organisms involves antipolysaccharide antibodies and opsonization. Splenectomy renders both processes deficient and the patient more susceptible to infection without vaccination. Vaccines should be administered at least 2 weeks before splenectomy because the vaccine immunogenicity may be reduced if given after the splenectomy.[138] If the splenectomy is emergent and preoperative vaccination is precluded, postoperative immunization is necessary. The most up-to-date recommendations regarding postsplenectomy (asplenia) vaccinations, timing of administration, and exclusion criteria can be found on the website of the Centers for Disease Control and Prevention. The current recommended regimen includes influenza, pneumococcal 13-valent conjugate (PCV13), pneumococcal polysaccharide (PPSV23), meningococcal 4-valent conjugate or polysaccharide, meningococcal B, and *Haemophilus influenzae* type b (Hib).

Patients' hematologic reserve and the operative risks must be considered. The need for blood component transfusion is anticipated. Laboratory tests (e.g., crossmatch) are performed and appropriate blood components reserved. One unit of platelets usually elevates the platelet count by $5 \times 10^9/L$, whereas one unit of erythrocytes elevates hemoglobin by 1 g/dL. In selected high-risk patients with severe thrombocytopenia (platelet count $<20 \times 10^9/L$), transfusion of six units of platelets may be considered before anesthetic induction to reduce the risk of laryngeal hematoma during endotracheal intubation. Preoperative platelet transfusion should be avoided in patients with ITP because transfused platelets will not survive splenic circulation until the splenic vessels are ligated.[20] In patients with portal hypertension and massive splenomegaly, preoperative splenic artery embolization can be performed to reduce the bleeding risk. However, its potential benefit must be balanced against the risk for pancreatitis, splenic abscess from infarction, hematoma formation, and pain.

Immediately before splenectomy, several medications are administered in the operating room. Patients on chronic steroid therapy should receive a bolus of exogenous steroid for operative stress. Prophylactic antibiotics are indicated in immunocompromised patients or when the gastrointestinal tract may be opened. In patients prone to thrombosis (e.g., myeloproliferative disorders), administration of unfractionated heparin (5000 IU subcutaneously three times daily), low-molecular-weight heparin, or antiplatelet agent (e.g., aspirin) may be beneficial.[139]

OPERATIVE CONSIDERATIONS

Splenectomy can be performed via the open, hand-assisted, or totally laparoscopic approach. The surgeon's experience and size of spleen generally determine the surgical method used. The larger the spleen, the more likely an open operation will be needed to safely remove it. Splenomegaly has been previously well defined by splenic weight and length and can be categorized as moderate splenomegaly (500 to 1500 g) or massive splenomegaly (>1500 g)[140-142] (Fig. 141.2).[140-142] This classification system corresponds to diagnosis, operative approach likelihood, and overall complications risk, which is dependent on underlying disease process as opposed to operative approach.

OPEN SPLENECTOMY

The most commonly used surgical incisions for open splenectomy are the left subcostal and the midline incisions.

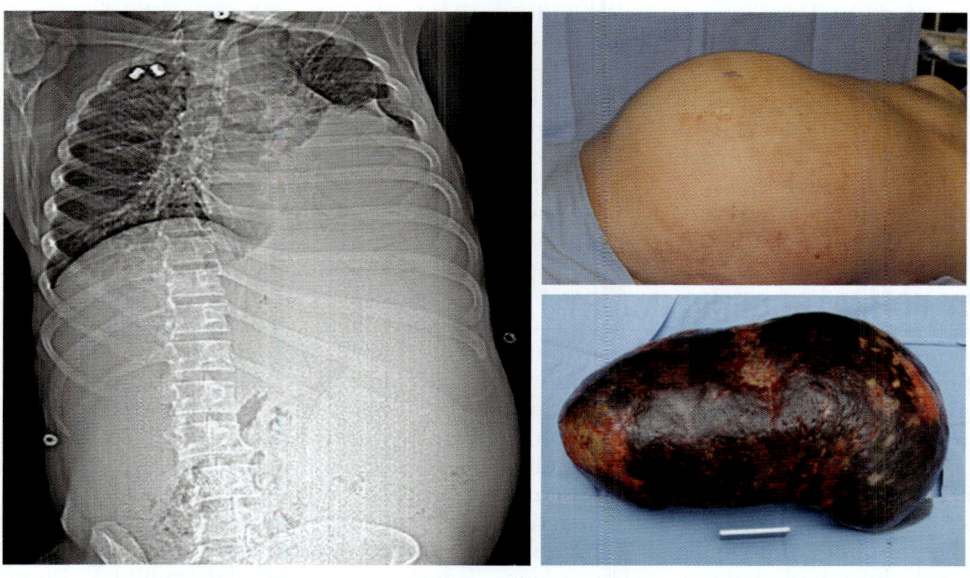

FIGURE 141.2 Massive splenomegaly. Myelofibrosis with myeloid metaplasia (48 cm, 13,085 g).

The latter is preferred for patients with narrow costal arches or with marked splenomegaly. A left thoracoabdominal incision with a midline vertical extension has been described but is rarely needed.[139] Most surgeons prefer gastric decompression via an orogastric or nasogastric tube.

The initial steps of splenectomy generally involve mobilizing the spleen. The stomach and the spleen are retracted medially to expose the splenophrenic and splenorenal ligaments. Unless mucus varices are present, the ligaments are avascular and can be divided by blunt or sharp dissection. After the spleen is freed from its posterior attachments to the diaphragm and Gerota fascia, the splenocolic ligament is divided, releasing the splenic flexure and the omentum from the inferior splenic pole. The spleen can then be lifted into the abdominal incision (Fig. 141.3). This maneuver should not be performed with excessive force, to avoid a capsular tear or avulsion of the splenic vessels. The splenogastric ligament is divided with identification, clamping, division, and ligation of the short gastric vessels. Suture ligation of these vessels on the gastric wall has been advocated by some surgeons to prevent postoperative loosening of the ligatures if the stomach becomes distended. The spleen is now attached only by the hilar vessels.

An alternative approach to splenectomy involves control of the splenic vessels at the hilum as the initial step. The gastrocolic omentum is opened lateral to the gastroepiploic arcade (Fig. 141.4A). The splenic artery is palpated along the superior border of the pancreas. Dissection of the vessels should be performed close to the splenic hilum to avoid injury to the tail of the pancreas (see Fig. 141.4B–D). The splenic artery and vein may be divided together; however, separate division is preferable to prevent the formation of an arteriovenous fistula. The splenic artery should be controlled by double ligation, with one suture ligature. The splenic vein is divided after double ligation; a continuous vascular suture or a vascular stapler is used when the vein is markedly enlarged. This approach of initial vascular control may be particularly suitable in the presence of massive splenomegaly, marked hilar lymphadenopathy, or dense perisplenic adhesions. It has also been advocated for ITP, where early ligation of the vessels allows earlier administration of platelet transfusion. Similarly, it may be preferred for splenic malignancies because it can prevent inadvertent tearing of the vessels during splenic mobilization and spillage of malignant cells.

When a partial splenectomy is considered, branches of the vasculature are identified before they enter the spleen and ligated separately. After the plane of vascular demarcation is recognized and marked, transection of the splenic parenchyma should be performed with total hilar occlusion to reduce hemorrhage on the transection surface. Placement of pledgets on through-and-through

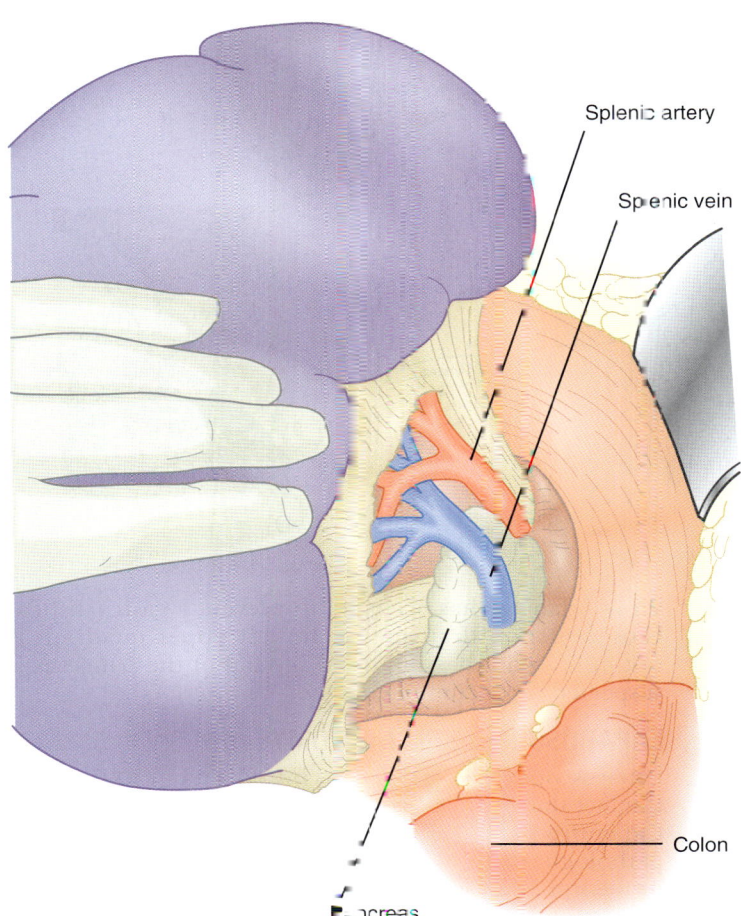

Splenic artery

Splenic vein

Colon

Pancreas

FIGURE 141.3 Mobilization of the spleen from its peritoneal ligamentous attachments. (From Scott-Conner CEH. *Chassin's Operative Strategy in General Surgery: An Exposive Atlas.* Stamford CT: Springer; 2002:736.)

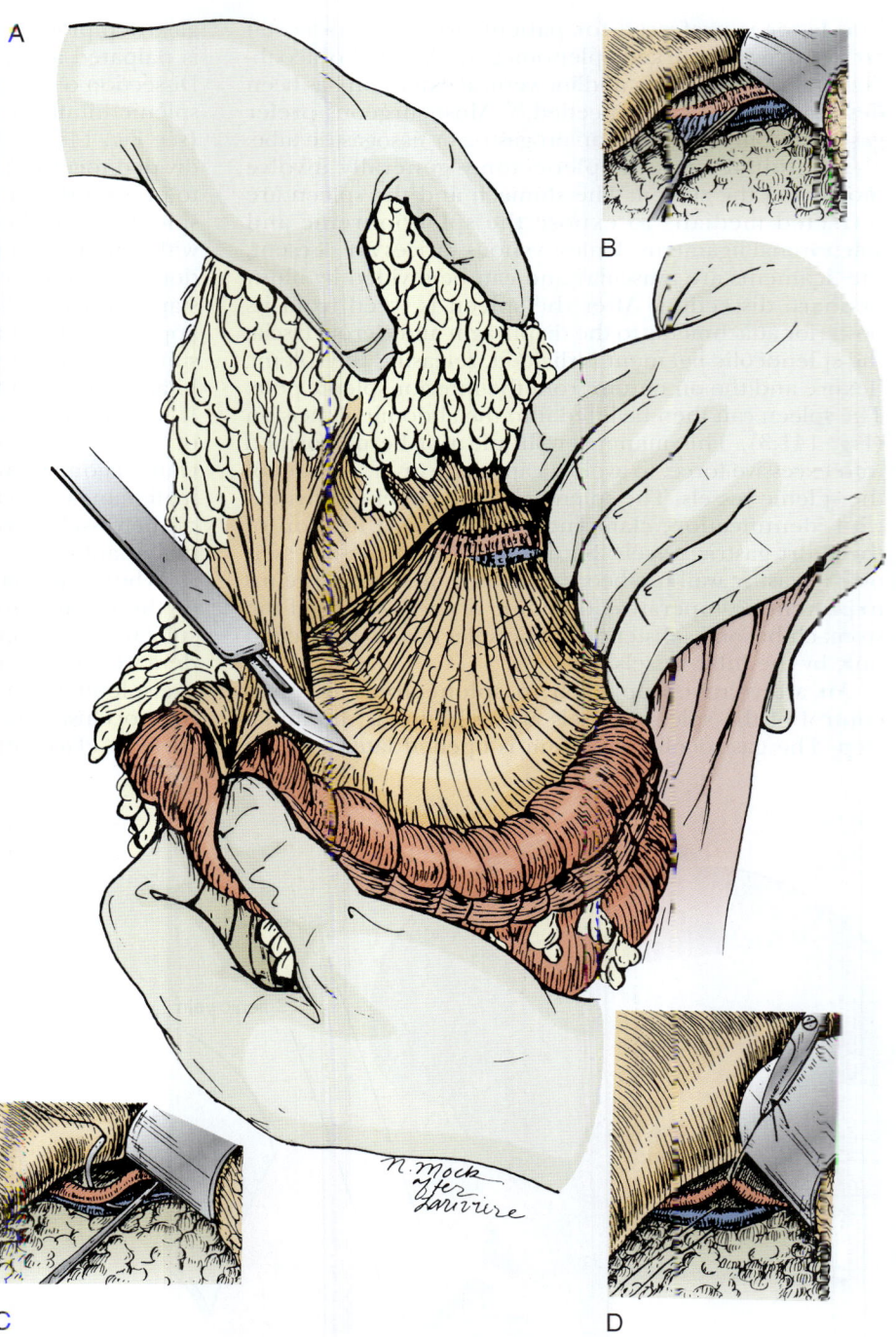

FIGURE 141.4 Approach to the splenic hilum through the lesser sac (A). Splenic vessels are identified (B) and controlled (C and D) along the superior border of the pancreas. (From Schwartz S. The spleen. In: Zinner MJ, Schwartz SI, Ellis H, eds. *Maingot's Abdominal Operations*. Stamford, CT: Appleton & Lange; 1997:2058.)

sutures with inflow occlusion reduces hemorrhage during partial splenectomy.

After removal of the spleen for hematologic diseases, the abdomen should be explored for accessory splenic tissue at the common locations (see Fig. 141.1).

Prior to closure, hemostasis in the left upper quadrant should be ascertained by inspection of the inferior surface of the diaphragm, the left cephalad retroperitoneum, the greater curvature of the stomach, and the splenic hilum. The left upper quadrant may be packed to promote hemostasis. The greater curvature of the stomach should be imbricated with interrupted Lembert sutures if any

serosal damage has occurred to prevent a gastric fistula. Closed-suction drainage of the left upper quadrant is not indicated unless injury to the tail of the pancreas is suspected or documented.

LAPAROSCOPIC SPLENECTOMY

Laparoscopic splenectomy was introduced in 1991 due to the fact that for the majority of splenectomy indications the entire intact splenic specimen was not required for pathologic examination and thus could be morcellated intracorporeally within a bag prior to removal.[143] Laparoscopic splenectomy should be considered for any spleen that is normal sized or mildly to moderately enlarged. No distinct cutoff for an upper limit of size is used, because (1) by adding a hand port, larger spleens can still be removed without a formal laparotomy and (2) in small patients, the lack of space to maneuver laparoscopically may limit the options, whereas the same-size spleen in a large patient may be amenable to laparoscopic excision. Most spleens occupying the entire left half of the abdomen or crossing the midline with the patient supine are best treated by open splenectomy. Occasionally postoperative adhesions from open operations or infection will preclude laparoscopic splenectomy. Furthermore, some patients with malignant hematologic splenic disorders may have resultant hepatomegaly and associated portal hypertension secondary to extramedullary hematopoiesis and thus may increase the operative risk with laparoscopy.

Laparoscopic splenectomy can be performed with the patient supine, in semi-right lateral decubitus or full right lateral decubitus position. The lateral or hanging spleen approach is performed with larger spleens because it is easier to manipulate the spleen anteriorly than with the patient supine.

Three ports are used, one 12-mm working port in the upper midline, which can be extended for hand port placement as indicated, a 10-mm port in the left upper quadrant for the laparoscope (this position will vary based on spleen size, ranging from near the costal margin to even in the right lower quadrant near the umbilicus with a very large spleen), and a second 12-mm port at the left anterior axillary line (the site will again vary depending on spleen size).

After port placement and inspection of the left upper quadrant, the caudal pole (splenocolic ligament) is incised with electrocautery or ultrasonic dissector while lifting the spleen. Continuing posterior to the spleen, the splenorenal and splenophrenic ligaments are divided by the dissector in the surgeon's right hand, retracting the spleen anterior with a blunt instrument in the left hand. The tissues are generally flimsy and rapidly separated once the peritoneum is divided. Care must be taken to avoid injury to the hilar vessels at this time. After switching instruments, the spleen is retracted posteriorly with the right hand and the splenogastric ligament divided from caudad to cephalad with an ultrasonic dissector. (Vessels make monopolar cautery a less suitable option with this tissue dissection.) The short gastric vessels are likewise serially divided up to the cephalad pole of the spleen. The splenic hilum is then inspected, evaluating for the location of the tail of the pancreas. After the hilar vessels are adequately skeletonized, they can be readily transected with vascular loads of a linear endoscopic stapler.

The detached spleen is placed in a specimen bag and morcellated. If a hand port has been placed, larger spleens can more readily be removed through the upper midline incision. Accessory spleens should be looked for, especially if a preoperative CT or magnetic resonance imaging (MRI) scan has not been obtained. After removal of the spleen, the left upper quadrant, in particular the hilar staple line, is inspected for hemostasis. After release of the pneumoperitoneum and removal of the cannulas, all the incisions are closed with absorbable fascial and subcutaneous sutures.

POSTOPERATIVE COURSE AND COMPLICATIONS

The highest rate of postoperative complications is anticipated in patients with massive splenomegaly (splenic weight >1500 g) or myeloproliferative diseases, where a morbidity of up to 52% has been reported.[144,145]

All patients are closely monitored during the early postoperative period for hemorrhage. Immediate postoperative bleeding most commonly arises from an unligated short gastric vessel high on the greater curvature or from small veins around the tail of the pancreas. When indicated by a fall in hemoglobin and signs of hypovolemia, exploration should be promptly performed. Another common complication, pulmonary atelectasis, can be prevented with adequate pain control and incentive spirometry. A subphrenic abscess occurs rarely but may develop with poor hemostasis and clot formation in the splenic bed or when the gastrointestinal tract is opened. Percutaneous drainage plus parenteral antibiotics is usually adequate therapy. A gastric or pancreatic fistula occurs in less than 1% of splenectomy patients and is associated with iatrogenic injury to these organs.

Leukocytosis occurs as a physiologic response to splenectomy. It may be difficult to distinguish from an infection. Traumatic splenectomy patients with white blood cell counts greater than 20×10^9/L after postoperative day 10 are more likely to harbor an infection,[146] but leukocytosis after splenectomy for nontraumatic indications has not been thoroughly investigated. Similarly, reactive thrombocytosis may occur immediately postsplenectomy, with the platelets peaking at 2 to 3 weeks postoperatively. In the absence of hemostatic or vascular complications, antiplatelet therapy is not routinely indicated for secondary thrombocytosis unless platelet counts increase to greater than 1000×10^9/L and for those who are predisposed to a higher incidence of thrombotic risk (massive splenomegaly and/or hemolytic anemia or malignant hematologic disease indications).

Venous thrombosis involving the mesenteric and portal veins is a serious complication after splenectomy. The incidence of clot formation may be as high as 50% if all patients are screened, but only 8% become symptomatic. Predisposing factors include a myeloproliferative disease or hemolytic anemia, massive splenomegaly, postoperative thrombocytosis, a previously undiagnosed systemic hypercoagulable state, and a long splenic vein stump.[147] Laparoscopic splenectomy may be associated with a higher incidence of portal and splenic vein thrombosis than the open technique (55% vs. 12% in one retrospective series).[148] Patients usually present within 10 days of splenectomy with vague symptoms, including generalized abdominal pain and distention, fever, nausea, and anorexia. The diagnosis is best obtained by contrast-enhanced abdominal CT, MRI, or ultrasonography. Systemic anticoagulation is initiated promptly and maintained for 6 months. Recannulation occurs in 90% of those on appropriate anticoagulation.[149]

All asplenic patients are at risk for OPSS. The incidence of OPSS ranges between 1% and 2.4% and is fatal in 45% to 75% of patients. The elevated risk of mortality is lifelong.[50] The majority of cases occur within 3 years of splenectomy but may occur decades later. It usually presents with either upper or lower respiratory symptoms; however, it can occur precipitously without previous symptomatology. The risk of hospitalization or death from sepsis depends on the indication for splenectomy. A Swedish registry study evaluating more than 20,000 postsplenectomy patients compared with nonsplenectomized patients found that the risk of OPSS rose significantly with lowest risk for traumatic splenectomy, moderate risk for benign hematologic disease, and the largest risk of sepsis and associated mortality in those with malignant hematologic disease.[150] Any febrile asplenic patient must be promptly evaluated and initiated on a broad-spectrum antibiotic regimen such as a third-generation cephalosporin.[138] Measures to prevent OPSS include vaccination and prophylactic antibiotics.[151] Preoperative vaccination is preferred at least 2 weeks prior to planned splenectomy. When the vaccines are administered postoperatively, although they are conventionally given on the day of dismissal to avoid confusing febrile reactions to the vaccine with a postoperative complication as well as to assure patient receipt, there are data suggesting inadequate opsonophagocytic function if administered within 2 weeks of splenectomy.[152] Current vaccine recommendations include 23-valent PPSV23 with a 5-year booster; conjugated polysaccharide *H. influenzae* (most adults already have immunity); *meningococcal* conjugate for ages 2 to 55 and polysaccharide for those greater than age 55; and annual influenza vaccine because influenza is a risk factor for severe secondary bacterial infection in asplenic patients. Prophylactic antibiotics have been advocated for highly immunocompromised patients, for previous survivors of OPSS, and for children and include two commonly used strategies. First, a daily prophylactic antibiotic is given to asplenic children (<5 years old) for the first 3 years after splenectomy. The traditional regimen has been a single daily dose of penicillin, amoxicillin, or erythromycin. Recently, antibiotics with broader spectrum, including amoxicillin/clavulanic acid, cefuroxime, and trimethoprim/sulfamethoxazole, have been used. Prophylactic antibiotics can reduce the infection rate by 47% and mortality rate by 88%.[153] Concerns of increasing pneumococcal resistance and poor patient compliance have recently brought this practice into question. Alternatively, asplenic adults are given a supply of "standby" antibiotics to be started if symptoms of infection develop. It should be emphasized that these patients seek immediate medical attention. All patients and caretakers should be educated regarding OPSS, as well as documenting the patients' asplenic state and vaccination status, plus issuing a medical alert bracelet to help recognition of OPSS.

REFERENCES

1. Kojouri K, Vesely SK, Terrell DR, George JN. Splenectomy for adult patients with idiopathic thrombocytopenic purpura: a systematic review to assess long-term platelet count responses, prediction of response, and surgical complications. *Blood.* 2004;104(9):2623-2634.
2. Cines DB, Blanchette VS. Immune thrombocytopenic purpura. *N Engl J Med.* 2002;346(13):995-1008.
3. Bell WR Jr. Role of splenectomy in immune (idiopathic) thrombocytopenic purpura. *Blood Rev.* 2002;16(1):39-41.
4. Stasi R, Provan D. Management of immune thrombocytopenic purpura in adults. *Mayo Clin Proc.* 2004;79(4):504-522.
5. Nugent DJ. Childhood immune thrombocytopenic purpura. *Blood Rev.* 2002;16(1):27-29.
6. McFarland J. Pathophysiology of platelet destruction in immune (idiopathic) thrombocytopenic purpura. *Blood Rev.* 2002;16(1):1-2.
7. El-Alfy MS, El-Tawil MM, Shahein N. 5- to 16-year follow-up following splenectomy in chronic immune thrombocytopenic purpura in children. *Acta Haematol.* 2003;110(1):20-24.
8. Kuhne T, Blanchette V, Buchanan GR, et al. Splenectomy in children with idiopathic thrombocytopenic purpura: a prospective study of 134 children from the Intercontinental Childhood ITP Study Group. *Pediatr Blood Cancer.* 2007;49(6):829-834.
9. Hemmila MR, Foley DS, Castle VP, Hirschl RB. The response to splenectomy in pediatric patients with idiopathic thrombocytopenic purpura who fail high-dose intravenous immune globulin. *J Pediatr Surg.* 2000;35(6):967-971, discussion 971–972.
10. Holt D, Brown J, Terrill K, et al. Response to intravenous immunoglobulin predicts splenectomy response in children with immune thrombocytopenic purpura. [Erratum appears in Pediatrics. 2004 Jan;113(1):184]. *Pediatrics.* 2003;111(1):87-90.
11. Hicks BA, Thompson WR, Rogers ZR, Guzzetta PC. Laparoscopic splenectomy in childhood hematologic disorders. *J Laparoendosc Surg.* 1996;6(suppl 1):S31-S34.
12. Gargiulo N III, Zenilman M. Spleen. In: Cameron J, ed. *Current Surgical Therapy.* St. Louis: CV Mosby; 2001:587.
13. Provan D, Newland A. Fifty years of idiopathic thrombocytopenic purpura (ITP): management of refractory ITP in adults. *Br J Haematol.* 2002;118(4):933-944.
14. Provan D, Stasi R, Newland AC, et al. International consensus report on the investigation and management of primary immune thrombocytopenia. *Blood.* 2010;115(2):168-186.
15. Cheng Y, Wong RS, Soo YO, et al. Initial treatment of immune thrombocytopenic purpura with high-dose dexamethasone. *N Engl J Med.* 2003;349(9):831-836.
16. Mazzucconi MG, Fazi P, Bernasconi S, et al. Therapy with high-dose dexamethasone (HD-DXM) in previously untreated patients affected by idiopathic thrombocytopenic purpura: a GIMEMA experience. *Blood.* 2007;109(4):1401-1407.
17. Kumar S, Diehn FE, Gertz MA, Tefferi A. Splenectomy for immune thrombocytopenic purpura: long-term results and treatment of postsplenectomy relapses. *Ann Hematol.* 2002;81(6):312-319.
18. Cordera F, Long KH, Nagorney DM, et al. Open versus laparoscopic splenectomy for idiopathic thrombocytopenic purpura: clinical and economic analysis. *Surgery.* 2003;134(1):45-52.
19. Donohue J, van Heerden J, Monson J. *Atlas of Surgical Oncology.* Cambridge, MA: Blackwell Science; 1995.
20. Coon WW. Surgical aspects of splenic disease and lymphoma. *Curr Probl Surg.* 1998;35(7):543-646.
21. Rock GA. Management of thrombotic thrombocytopenic purpura. *Br J Haematol.* 2000;109(3):496-507.
22. Rock GA, Shumak KH, Buskard NA, et al. Comparison of plasma exchange with plasma infusion in the treatment of thrombotic thrombocytopenic purpura. Canadian Apheresis Study Group. *N Engl J Med.* 1991;325(6):393-397.
23. Shumak KH, Rock GA, Nair RC. Late relapses in patients successfully treated for thrombotic thrombocytopenic purpura. Canadian Apheresis Group. *Ann Intern Med.* 1995;122(8):569-572.
24. de la Rubia J, Moscardó F, Gómez MJ, et al. Efficacy and safety of rituximab in adult patients with idiopathic relapsing or refractory thrombotic thrombocytopenic purpura: results of a Spanish multicenter study. *Transfus Apher Sci.* 2010;43(3):299-303.
25. Fakhouri F, Vernant JP, Veyradier A, et al. Efficiency of curative and prophylactic treatment with rituximab in ADAMTS13-deficient thrombotic thrombocytopenic purpura: a study of 11 cases. *Blood.* 2005;106(6):1932-1937.
26. Scully M, Cohen H, Cavenagh J, et al. Remission in acute refractory and relapsing thrombotic thrombocytopenic purpura following rituximab is associated with a reduction in IgG antibodies to ADAMTS-13. *Br J Haematol.* 2007;136(3):451-461.
27. Aqui NA, Stein SH, Konkle BA, Abrams CS, Strobl FJ. Role of splenectomy in patients with refractory or relapsed thrombotic thrombocytopenic purpura. *J Clin Apher.* 2003;18(2):51-54.
28. Schwartz J, Eldor A, Szold A. Laparoscopic splenectomy in patients with refractory or relapsing thrombotic thrombocytopenic purpura. *Arch Surg.* 2001;136(11):1236-1238, discussion 1239.

29. Essien FA, Ojeda HF, Salameh R, Baker KR, Rice L, Sweeney JF. Laparoscopic splenectomy for chronic recurrent thrombotic thrombocytopenic purpura. *Surg Laparosc Endosc Percutan Tech.* 2003;13(3):218-221.

30. You YN, Tefferi A, Nagorney DM. Outcome of splenectomy for thrombocytopenia associated with systemic lupus erythematosus. *Ann Surg.* 2004;240(2):286-292.

31. The Swiss Group for Clinical Studies on the Acquired Immunodeficiency Syndrome (AIDS). Zidovudine for the treatment of thrombocytopenia associated with human immunodeficiency virus (HIV). A prospective study. The Swiss Group for Clinical Studies on the Acquired Immunodeficiency Syndrome (AIDS). *Ann Intern Med.* 1988;109(9):718-721.

32. Scaradavou A. HIV-related thrombocytopenia. *Blood Rev.* 2002;16(1):73-76.

33. Hymes KB, Greene JB, Karpatkin S. The effect of azidothymidine on HIV-related thrombocytopenia. *N Engl J Med.* 1988;318(8):516-517.

34. Tyler DS, Shaunak S, Bartlett JA, Iglehart JD. HIV-1-associated thrombocytopenia. The role of splenectomy. *Ann Surg.* 1990;211(2):211-217.

35. Aboolian A, Ricci M, Shapiro K, Connors A, LaRaja RD. Surgical treatment of HIV-related immune thrombocytopenia. *Int Surg.* 1999;84(1):81-85.

36. Brown SA, Majumdar G, Harrington C, et al. Effect of splenectomy on HIV-related thrombocytopenia and progression of HIV infection in patients with severe haemophilia. *Blood Coagul Fibrinolysis.* 1994;5(3):393-397.

37. Ochs HD. The Wiskott-Aldrich syndrome. *Semin Hematol.* 1998;35(4):332-345.

38. Dupuis-Girod S, Medioni J, Haddad E, et al. Autoimmunity in Wiskott-Aldrich syndrome: risk factors, clinical features, and outcome in a single-center cohort of 55 patients. *Pediatrics.* 2003;111(5 Pt 1):e622-e627.

39. Mullen CA, Anderson KD, Blaese RM. Splenectomy and/or bone marrow transplantation in the management of the Wiskott-Aldrich syndrome: long-term follow-up of 62 cases. *Blood.* 1993;82(10):2961-2966.

40. Tamary H, Aviner S, Freud E, et al. High incidence of early cholelithiasis detected by ultrasonography in children and young adults with hereditary spherocytosis. *J Pediatr Hematol Oncol.* 2003;25(12):952-954.

41. Bolton-Maggs PH, Langer JC, Iolascon A, et al. Guidelines for the diagnosis and management of hereditary spherocytosis. *Br J Haematol.* 2004;126(4):455-474.

42. Shah S, Vega R. Hereditary spherocytosis. *Pediatr Rev.* 2004;25(5):168-172.

43. Eber SW, Armbrust R, Schroter W. Variable clinical severity of hereditary spherocytosis: relation to erythrocytic spectrin concentration, osmotic fragility, and autohemolysis. *J Pediatr.* 1990;117(3):409-416.

44. Marchetti M, Quaglini S, Barosi G. Prophylactic splenectomy and cholecystectomy in mild hereditary spherocytosis: analyzing the decision in different clinical scenarios. *J Intern Med.* 1998;244(3):217-226.

45. Caprotti R, Franciosi C, Romano F, et al. Combined laparoscopic splenectomy and cholecystectomy for the treatment of hereditary spherocytosis: is it safe and effective? *Surg Laparosc Endosc Percutan Tech.* 1999;9(3):203-206.

46. Sandler A, Winkel G, Kimura K, Soper R. The role of prophylactic cholecystectomy during splenectomy in children with hereditary spherocytosis. *J Pediatr Surg.* 1999;34(7):1077-1078.

47. Rescorla FJ, West KW, Engum SA, Grosfeld JL. Laparoscopic splenic procedures in children: experience in 231 children. *Ann Surg.* 2007;246(4):683-687, discussion 687-688.

48. de Lagausie P, Bonnard A, Berrebi M, Rorlich P, de Ribier A, Aigrain Y. Pediatric laparoscopic splenectomy: benefits of the anterior approach. *Surg Endosc.* 2004;18(1):80-82.

49. Vasilescu C, Stanciulea O, Tudor S, et al. Laparoscopic subtotal splenectomy in hereditary spherocytosis: to preserve the upper or the lower pole of the spleen. *Surg Endosc.* 2006;20(5):748-752.

50. Stoehr GA, Stauffer UG, Eber SW. Near-total splenectomy: a new technique for the management of hereditary spherocytosis. *Ann Surg.* 2005;241(1):40-47.

51. Englum BR, Rothman J, Leonard S, et al. Hematologic outcomes after total splenectomy and partial splenectomy for congenital hemolytic anemia. *J Pediatr Surg.* 2016;51(1):122-127.

52. Guizzetti L. Total versus partial splenectomy in pediatric hereditary spherocytosis: a systematic review and meta-analysis. *Pediatr Blood Cancer.* 2016;63(10):1713-1722.

53. Crary SE, Buchanan GR. Vascular complications after splenectomy for hematologic disorders. *Blood* 2009;114(14):2861-2868.

54. Coon WW. Splenectomy in the treatment of hemolytic anemia. *Arch Surg.* 1985;120(5):625-628.

55. Stuart MJ, Nagel RL. Sickle-cell disease. *Lancet.* 2004;364(9442):1343-1360.

56. al-Salem AH, Qaisaruddin S, Nasserullah Z, al Dabbous I, al Jam'a A. Splenectomy in patients with sickle-cell disease. *Am J Surg.* 1996;172(3):254-258.

57. Sorrells DL, Morrissey TB, Brown MF. Septic complications after splenectomy for sickle cell sequestration crisis. *Pediatr Surg Int.* 1998;13(2-3):100-103.

58. Emond AM, Morais P, Venugopal S, Carpenter RG, Serjeant GR. Role of splenectomy in homozygous sickle cell disease in childhood. *Lancet.* 1984;1(8368):88-91.

59. Lesher AP, Kalpatthi R, Glenn JB, Jackson SM, Hebra A. Outcome of splenectomy in children younger than 4 years with sickle cell disease. *J Pediatr Surg.* 2009;44(6):1134-1138, discussion 1138.

60. Wright JG, Hambleton IR, Thomas PW, Duncan ND, Venugopal S, Serjeant GR. Postsplenectomy course in homozygous sickle cell disease. *J Pediatr.* 1999;134(3):304-509.

61. Bar BC. Splenectomy in sickle cell disease. *J Assoc Physicians India.* 1999;47(9):890-893.

62. Graziano JH, Piomelli S, Hilgartner M, et al. Chelation therapy in beta-thalassemia major. III. The role of splenectomy in achieving iron balance. *J Pediatr.* 1981;99(5):695-699.

63. Yang XY, Qu Q, Yang TY, et al. Treatment of the thalassemia syndrome with splenectomy. *Hemoglobin.* 1988;12(5-6):601-608.

64. Hathirat P, Isarangkura P, Numbenjapon S, Opasathien P, Chuansumrit A. Results of the splenectomy in children with thalassemia. *J Med Assoc Thai* 1989;72(suppl 1):133-138.

65. Pinna AD, Argiolu F, Marongiu L, Pinna DC. Indications and results for splenectomy for beta thalassemia in two hundred and twenty-one pediatric patients. *Surg Gynecol Obstet.* 1988;167(2):109-113.

66. al-Salem AH, al-Dabbous I, Bhamidibati P. The role of partial splenectomy in children with thalassemia. *Eur J Pediatr Surg.* 1998;8(6):334-338.

67. Laopodis V, Kritikos E, Rizzotti L, Stefanidis P, Klonaris P, Tzardis P. Laparoscopic splenectomy in beta-thalassemia major patients. Advantages and disadvantages. *Surg Endosc.* 1998;12(7):944-947.

68. Salama A. Treatment options for primary autoimmune hemolytic anemia: a short comprehensive review. *Transfus Med Hemother.* 2015;42(5):294-301.

69. Akpek G, McAneny D, Weintraub L. Comparative response to splenectomy in Coombs-positive autoimmune hemolytic anemia with or without associated disease. *Am J Hematol.* 1999;61(2):98-102.

70. Mathew P, Chen G, Wang W. Evans syndrome: results of a national survey. *J Pediatr Hematol Oncol.* 1997;19(5):433-437.

71. Wang WC. Evans syndrome in childhood: pathophysiology, clinical course, and treatment. *Am J Pediatr Hematol Oncol.* 1988;10(4):330-338.

72. Bux J, Behrens G, Jaeger G, Welte K. Diagnosis and clinical course of autoimmune neutropenia in infancy: analysis of 240 cases. *Blood.* 1998;91(1):181-186.

73. Duperier T, Felsher J, Brody F. Laparoscopic splenectomy for Evans syndrome. *Surg Laparosc Endosc Percutan Tech.* 2003;13(1):45-47.

74. Campion G, Maddison PJ, Goulding N, et al. The Felty syndrome: a case-matched study of clinical manifestations and outcome, serologic features and immunogenetic associations. *Medicine (Baltimore).* 1990;69(2):69-80.

75. Rashba EJ, Rowe JM, Packman CH. Treatment of the neutropenia of Felty syndrome. *Blood Rev.* 1996;10(3):177-184.

76. Walsh RM, Brody F, Brown N. Laparoscopic splenectomy for lymphoproliferative disease. *Surg Endosc.* 2004;18(2):272-275.

77. Frederick W. Hematologic malignancies and splenic tumors. In: Feig B, Fuhrman G, eds. *The M.D. Anderson Surgical Oncology Handbook.* Philadelphia: Lippincott Williams & Wilkins; 2003:393.

78. Brodsky J, Abcar A, Styler M. Splenectomy for non-Hodgkin's lymphoma. *Am J Clin Oncol.* 1996;19(6):558-561

79. Delpero JR, Houvenaeghel G, Gastaut JA, et al. Splenectomy for hypersplenism in chronic lymphocytic leukaemia and malignant non-Hodgkin's lymphoma. [Erratum appears in Br J Surg 1990 Aug;77(8):957]. *Br J Surg.* 1990;77(4):443-449.

80. Lehne G, Hannisdal E, Langholm R, Nome O. A 10-year experience with splenectomy in patients with malignant non-Hodgkin's

lymphoma at the Norwegian Radium Hospital. *Cancer.* 1994;74(3): 933-939.

81. Walsh RM, Heniford BT. Laparoscopic splenectomy for non-Hodgkin lymphoma. *J Surg Oncol.* 1999;70(2):116-121.

82. Xiros N, Economopoulos T, Christodoulidis C, et al. Splenectomy in patients with malignant non-Hodgkin's lymphoma. *Eur J Haematol.* 2000;64(3):145-150.

83. Zelenetz A. Non-Hodgkin's Lymphoma, National Comprehensive Cancer Network. 2005;www.nccn.org.

84. Yoong Y, Kurtin PJ, Allmer C, et al. Efficacy of splenectomy for patients with mantle cell non-Hodgkin's lymphoma. *Leuk Lymphoma.* 2001;42(6):1235-1241.

85. Ruchlemer R, Wotherspoon AC, Thompson JN, Swansbury JG, Matutes E, Catovsky D. Splenectomy in mantle cell lymphoma with leukaemia: a comparison with chronic lymphocytic leukaemia. *Br J Haematol.* 2002;118(4):952-958.

86. Mulligan SP, Matutes E, Dearden C, Catovsky D. Splenic lymphoma with villous lymphocytes: natural history and response to therapy in 50 cases. *Br J Haematol.* 1991;78(2):206-209.

87. Chacon JI, Mollejo M, Muñoz E, et al. Splenic marginal zone lymphoma: clinical characteristics and prognostic factors in a series of 60 patients. *Blood.* 2002;100(5):1648-1654.

88. Hamblin T. Is chronic lymphocytic leukemia one disease? *Haematologica.* 2002;87(12):1235-1238.

89. Morel P, Dupriez B, Gosselin B, et al. Role of early splenectomy in malignant lymphomas with prominent splenic involvement (primary lymphomas of the spleen). A study of 59 cases. *Cancer.* 1993;71(1):207-215.

90. Thieblemont C, Felman P, Berger F, et al. Treatment of splenic marginal zone B-cell lymphoma: an analysis of 81 patients. *Clin Lymphoma.* 2002;3(1):41-47.

91. Thiruvengadam R, Piedmonte M, Barcos M, Han T, Henderson ES. Splenectomy in advanced chronic lymphocytic leukemia. *Leukemia.* 1990;4(11):758-760.

92. Neal TF Jr, Tefferi A, Witzig TE, Su J, Phyliky RL, Nagorney DM. Splenectomy in advanced chronic lymphocytic leukemia: a single institution experience with 50 patients. *Am J Med.* 1992;93(4):435-440.

93. Cusack JC Jr, Seymour JF, Lerner S, Keating MJ, Pollock RE. Role of splenectomy in chronic lymphocytic leukemia. *J Am Coll Surg.* 1997;185(3):237-243.

94. Majumdar G, Singh AK. Role of splenectomy in chronic lymphocytic leukaemia with massive splenomegaly and cytopenia. *Leuk Lymphoma.* 1992;7(1-2):131-134.

95. Pegourie-Bandelier B, Sotto JJ, Hollard D, Bolla M, Sarrazin R. Therapy program for patients with advanced stages of chronic lymphocytic leukemia. Chlorambucil, splenectomy, and total lymph node irradiation. *Cancer.* 1995;75(12):2853-2861.

96. Seymour JF, Cusack JD, Lerner SA, Pollock RE, Keating MJ. Case/control study of the role of splenectomy in chronic lymphocytic leukemia. *J Clin Oncol.* 1997;15(1):52-60.

97. Van Norman AS, Nagorney DM, Martin JK, Phyliky RL, Ilstrup DM. Splenectomy for hairy cell leukemia. A clinical review of 63 patients. *Cancer.* 1986;57(3):644-648.

98. Kalhs P, Schwarzinger I, Anderson G, et al. A retrospective analysis of the long-term effect of splenectomy on late infections, graft-versus-host disease, relapse, and survival after allogeneic marrow transplantation for chronic myelogenous leukemia. *Blood.* 1995;86(5):2028-2032.

99. Zakarija A, Peterson LC, Tallman MS. Splenectomy and treatments of historical interest. *Best Pract Res Clin Haematol.* 2003;16(1):57-68.

100. Barosi G, Ambrosetti A, Buratti A, et al. Splenectomy for patients with myelofibrosis with myeloid metaplasia: pretreatment variables and outcome prediction. *Leukemia.* 1993;7(2):200-206.

101. Mesa RA, Elliott MA, Tefferi A. Splenectomy in chronic myeloid leukemia and myelofibrosis with myeloid metaplasia. *Blood Rev.* 2000;14(3):121-129.

102. Mesa RA, Tefferi A. Palliative splenectomy in myelofibrosis with myeloid metaplasia. *Leuk Lymphoma.* 2001;42(5):901-911.

103. Tefferi A, Barrett SM, Silverstein MN, Nagorney DM. Outcome of portal-systemic shunt surgery for portal hypertension associated with intrahepatic obstruction in patients with agnogenic myeloid metaplasia. *Am J Hematol.* 1994;46(4):325-328.

104. Tefferi A, Mesa RA, Nagorney DM, Schroeder G, Silverstein MN. Splenectomy in myelofibrosis with myeloid metaplasia: a single-institution experience with 223 patients. *Blood.* 2000;95(7):2226-2233.

105. Lafaye F, Rain JD, Clot P, Najean Y. Risks and benefits of splenectomy in myelofibrosis: an analysis of 39 cases. *Nouv Rev Fr Hematol.* 1994;36(5):359-362.

106. Akpek G, McAneny D, Weintraub L. Risks and benefits of splenectomy in myelofibrosis with myeloid metaplasia: a retrospective analysis of 26 cases. *J Surg Oncol.* 2001;77(1):42-48.

107. Barosi G, Ambrosetti A, Centra A, et al. Splenectomy and risk of blast transformation in myelofibrosis with myeloid metaplasia. Italian Cooperative Study Group on Myeloid with Myeloid Metaplasia. *Blood.* 1998;91(10):3630-3636.

108. Mesa RA, Nagorney DS, Schwager S, Allred J, Tefferi A. Palliative goals, patient selection, and perioperative platelet management: outcomes and lessons from 3 decades of splenectomy for myelofibrosis with myeloid metaplasia at the Mayo Clinic. *Cancer.* 2006;107(2):361-370.

109. Neuhauser TS, Derringer GA, Thompson LD, et al. Splenic angiosarcoma: a clinicopathologic and immunophenotypic study of 28 cases. *Mod Pathol.* 2000;13(9):978-987.

110. Willcox TM, Speer RW, Schlinkert RT, Sarr MG. Hemangioma of the spleen: presentation, diagnosis, and management. *J Gastrointest Surg.* 2000;4(6):611-613.

111. Jaroch MT, Broughan TA, Hermann RE. The natural history of splenic infarction. *Surgery.* 1986;100(4):743-750.

112. Morgenstern L. Nonparasitic splenic cysts: pathogenesis, classification, and treatment. *J Am Coll Surg.* 2002;194(3):306-314.

113. Pachter HL, Hofstetter SR, Elkowitz A, Harris L, Liang HG. Traumatic cysts of the spleen—the role of cystectomy and splenic preservation: experience with seven consecutive patients. *J Trauma.* 1993;35(3):430-436.

114. Ooi LL, Leong SS. Splenic abscesses from 1987 to 1995. *Am J Surg.* 1997;174(1):87-93.

115. Phillips GS, Radosevich MD, Lipsett PA. Splenic abscess: another look at an old disease. *Arch Surg.* 1997;132(12):1331-1335, discussion 1335-1336.

116. Trastek VF, Pairolero PC, Bernatz PE. Splenic artery aneurysms. *World J Surg.* 1985;9(3):378-383.

117. Dave SP, Reis ED, Hossain A, Taub PJ, Kerstein MD, Hollier LH. Splenic artery aneurysm in the 1990s. *Ann Vasc Surg.* 2000;14(3):223-229.

118. Selo-Ojeme DO, Welch CC. Review: spontaneous rupture of splenic artery aneurysm in pregnancy. *Eur J Obstet Gynecol Reprod Biol.* 2003;109(2):124-127.

119. Hallett JW Jr. Splenic artery aneurysms. *Semin Vasc Surg.* 1995;8(4):321-326.

120. Abbas MA, Stone WM, Fowl RJ, et al. Splenic artery aneurysms: two decades experience at Mayo Clinic. *Ann Vasc Surg.* 2002;16(4):442-449.

121. Obuchi T, Sasaki A, Nakajima J, Nitta H, Otsuka K, Wakabayashi G. Laparoscopic surgery for splenic artery aneurysm. *Surg Laparosc Endosc Percutan Tech.* 2009;19(4):338-340.

122. Pietrabissa A, Ferrari M, Berchiolli R, et al. Laparoscopic treatment of splenic artery aneurysms. *J Vasc Surg.* 2009;50(2):275-279.

123. Han DC, Feliciano DV. The clinical complexity of splenic vein thrombosis. *Am Surg.* 1998;64(6):558-561, discussion 561-562.

124. Sakorafas GH, Sarr MG, Farley DR, Farnell MB. The significance of sinistral portal hypertension complicating chronic pancreatitis. *Am J Surg.* 2000;179(2):129-133.

125. Weber SM, Rikkers LF. Splenic vein thrombosis and gastrointestinal bleeding in chronic pancreatitis. *World J Surg.* 2003;27(11):1271-1274.

126. Heider TR, Azeem S, Galanko JA, Behrns KE. The natural history of pancreatitis-induced splenic vein thrombosis. *Ann Surg.* 2004;239(6):876-880, discussion 880-882.

127. Loftus JP, Nagorney DM, Ilstrup D, Kunselman AR. Sinistral portal hypertension. Splenectomy or expectant management. *Ann Surg.* 1993;217(1):35-40.

128. Hashizume M, Tomikawa M, Akahoshi T, et al. Laparoscopic splenectomy for portal hypertension. *Hepatogastroenterology.* 2002;49(45):847-852.

129. Desai DC, Hebra A, Davidoff AM, Schnaufer L. Wandering spleen: a challenging diagnosis. *South Med J.* 1997;90(4):439-443.

130. Cohen MS, Soper NJ, Underwood RA, Quasebarth M, Brunt LM. Laparoscopic splenopexy for wandering (pelvic) spleen. *Surg Laparosc Endosc.* 1998;8(4):286-290.

131. Peitgen K, Majetschak M, Walz MK. Laparoscopic splenopexy by peritoneal and omental pouch construction for intermittent splenic torsion ("wandering spleen"). *Surg Endosc.* 2001;15(4):413.

132. Cassar K, Munro A. Iatrogenic splenic injury. *J R Coll Surg Edinb.* 2002;47(6):731-741.

133. Holubar SD, Wang JK, Wolff BG, et al. Splenic salvage after intraoperative splenic injury during colectomy. *Arch Surg.* 2009;144(11):1040-1045.

134. Weinreb NJ, Charrow J, Andersson HC, et al. Effectiveness of enzyme replacement therapy in 1028 patients with type 1 Gaucher disease after 2 to 5 years of treatment: a report from the Gaucher Registry. *Am J Med.* 2002;113(2):112-119.

135. Fleshner PR, Aufses AH Jr, Grabowski GA, Elias R. A 27-year experience with splenectomy for Gaucher's disease. *Am J Surg.* 1991;161(1):69-75.

136. Sharma OP, Vucinic V, James LG. Splenectomy in sarcoidosis: indications, complications, and long-term follow-up. *Sarcoidosis Vasc Diffuse Lung Dis.* 2002;19(1):66-70.

137. Khan AZ, Escofet X, Roberts KM, Salman AR. Spontaneous splenic rupture—a rare complication of amyloidosis. *Swiss Surg.* 2003;9(2):92-94.

138. Brigden ML. Detection, education and management of the asplenic or hyposplenic patient. *Am Fam Physician.* 2001;63(3):499-506, 508.

139. Schwartz S. Splenectomy and splenorrhaphy. In: Baker R, Fischer J, eds. *Mastery of Surgery.* Philadelphia: Lippincott Williams & Wilkins; 2001:1691.

140. Goldstone J. Splenectomy for massive splenomegaly. *Am J Surg.* 1978;135(3):385-388.

141. Mahon D, Rhodes M. Laparoscopic splenectomy: size matters. *Ann R Coll Surg Engl.* 2003;85(4):248-251.

142. Poulin EC, Mamazza J, Schlachta CM. Splenic artery embolization before laparoscopic splenectomy. An update. *Surg Endosc.* 1998;12(6):870-875.

143. Delaitre B, Maignien B. Splenectomy by the laparoscopic approach. Report of a case. *Presse Med.* 1991;20(44):2263.

144. Arnoletti JP, Karam J, Brodsky J. Early postoperative complications of splenectomy for hematologic disease. *Am J Clin Oncol.* 1999;22(2):114-118.

145. Horowitz J, Smith JL, Weber TK, Rodriguez-Bigas MA, Petrelli NJ. Postoperative complications after splenectomy for hematologic malignancies. *Ann Surg.* 1996;223(3):290-296.

146. Rutherford EJ, Morris JA Jr, van Aalst J, Hall KS, Reed GW, Koestner A. The white blood cell response to splenectomy and bacteraemia. *Injury.* 1994;25(5):289-292.

147. Franciosi C, Romano F, Caprotti R, et al. Splenoportal thrombosis as a complication after laparoscopic splenectomy. *J Laparoendosc Adv Surg Tech A.* 2002;12(4):273-276.

148. Ikeda M, Sekimoto M, Takiguchi S, et al. High incidence of thrombosis of the portal venous system after laparoscopic splenectomy: a prospective study with contrast-enhanced CT scan. *Ann Surg.* 2005;241(2):208-216.

149. Winslow ER, Brunt LM, Drebin JA, Soper NJ, Klingensmith ME. Portal vein thrombosis after splenectomy. *Am J Surg.* 2002;184(6):631-635, discussion 635-636.

150. Edgren G, Almqvist R, Hartman M, Utter GH. Splenectomy and the risk of sepsis: a population-based cohort study. *Ann Surg.* 2014;260(6):1081-1087.

151. Working Party of the British Committee for Standards in Haematology Clinical Haematology Task Force. Guidelines for the prevention and treatment of infection in patients with an absent or dysfunctional spleen. *BMJ.* 1996;312(7028):430-434.

152. Shatz DV, Schinsky MF, Pais LB, Romero-Steiner S, Kirton OC, Carlone GM. Immune responses of splenectomized trauma patients to the 23-valent pneumococcal polysaccharide vaccine at 1 versus 7 versus 14 days after splenectomy. *J Trauma.* 1998;44(5):760-765, discussion 765-766.

153. Gaston MH, Verter JI, Woods G, et al. Prophylaxis with oral penicillin in children with sickle cell anemia. A randomized trial. *N Engl J Med.* 1986;314(25):1593-1599.

CHAPTER 142

Cysts and Tumors of the Spleen

David T. Pointer Jr. | Douglas P. Slakey

Cysts and tumors of the spleen are uncommonly encountered in clinical practice and continue to present challenges in both surgical work-up and treatment. Perhaps the continuing evolution of surgical traditions associated with splenic maladies can be partly explained by the relative rarity of these conditions. Literature references provide benchmarks to the myriad of supposed functions and attributes of the spleen as our experience and understanding of the organ continue to advance. For an excellent time line of medical and scientific inquiry into the function of the spleen, the reader is directed to the two-part review by McClusky et al. titled *Tribute to a Triad: History of Splenic Anatomy, Physiology, and Surgery.*[1] Historically it has been questioned whether the spleen is required at all for survival. It was only within the latter half of the 20th century that the spleen came to be regarded as vital. For the majority of recorded history, the spleen, although often described as having diverse functions, was regarded as wholly unnecessary. This is reflected in early surgical approaches to splenic maladies. Although the veracity of these reports has been questioned,[2] Adrian Zacarelli is thought to have performed the first splenectomy in 1549 on a 24-year-old woman who had developed splenomegaly. Later, Buliemi Ballonii (Ballonius) asked in a report of another splenectomy performed by an unknown barber-surgeon in 1578, "*Este igitur spelnatar necessarisu* [Is the spleen so necessary for life]?" Ultimately, Edwin Beer would argue in 1928 that any splenic operation must be extirpative to be considered satisfactory.[3]

Traumatic injury to the spleen provided the majority of the earliest opportunities to evaluate splenectomy as a successful treatment of splenic conditions. A testament to the rarity of splenic interventions is the observation that only 10 surgeons had followed in Zacarelli's footsteps during the next two and a half centuries. Almost invariably these reports concluded with success stories of patients returning to healthy lives. However, in 1826 Karl Quittenbaum performed an elective splenectomy on a 22-year-old female with splenomegaly, presumably from portal hypertension, that serves as the first recorded failure resulting in postoperative death. He was admonished for both his patient selection, given that the patient had ascites and anasarca, and his technique, in that a portion of the pancreas was found in the resected spleen.[2] It was the author of those admonitions, Sir Thomas Spencer Wells, who would go on to note through his own failures that the spleen may have some necessary but as yet unknown hematologic role, and that an elective total splenectomy may only be appropriate for the treatment of life-threatening leukemia. He based these speculations on the observation that enlarged spleens were often found in conjunction with an abundance of leukocytes and that by removing the spleen the surgeon

may cut off the production of these cells. His caution to those who would perform these procedures was in contrast to the long-held view of the nonnecessity of the organ. His hypothesis, although incorrect, was important to the beginning of applying methodology in evaluation of surgical treatments for conditions involving the spleen. A subsequent review of 49 splenectomies performed for the treatment of leukemia suggested an almost 90% mortality rate, and splenectomy as a treatment of choice for this condition would be later replaced by irradiation.[4]

During the 20th century clinicians continued to question the prevailing view that the spleen was unimportant. By 1952 King had observed increased rates of infection in children who had undergone splenectomy.[5] Recognition of the spleen's immunologic role and the description of overwhelming postsplenectomy infection (OPSI) encouraged surgeons to consider alternatives to extirpative surgery. Morgenstern and Shapiro are credited with the first successful open partial splenectomy for an epidermoid cyst in 1980.[6] Continuing advances in minimally invasive surgery allowed Seshadri et al. to complete the first successful laparoscopic partial splenectomy in 2000.[7] Advances in surgical technology have increased the number of management options for pathologic lesions of the spleen.[8,9] Paralleled technologic improvements in radiologic imaging, along with an increase in abdominal imaging, have led to more frequent diagnosis of splenic abnormalities, especially cystic and solid lesions.

APPROACH TO THE SPLENIC MASS

As with any medical condition, a history and physical provide the basic foundation for the evaluation of the patient with a splenic lesion. Before one determines the most appropriate treatment, the nature or type of mass must be ascertained. Splenic masses are very rare when compared with masses involving other solid organs such as the ovary, liver, or kidney, so the physician may benefit from a simplified approach that assists in the correct diagnosis and timely treatment. Patients may present to the surgeon's office with classic complaints of left upper quadrant pain or otherwise vague abdominal discomfort; however, they are frequently asymptomatic with a mass incidentally discovered in imaging obtained for other purposes. Noninvasive radiographic imaging is necessary in assisting the initial classification of the lesion as cystic or solid as well as providing size measurements. Ultrasound (US) can demonstrate the internal echoes indicative of an abscess or hematoma versus the round homogeneous, anechoic enhancing signal that is the hallmark of a cystic structure. Computed tomography (CT) scanning with intravenous contrast or magnetic resonance imaging (MRI) can better delineate the trabeculated or septated nature

TABLE 142.1 Classification of Splenic Masses

Solid Masses	Cystic Masses
LYMPHOID	PRIMARY OR "TRUE"
Hodgkin	*Parasitic*
Non-Hodgkin	*Nonparasitic*
NONLYMPHOID	Congenital
Benign	Neoplastic
Malignant (Primary or metastatic)	PSEUDOCYSTS
	Posttraumatic
	Other

of the cyst wall and wall calcification and has a superior specificity in defining whether a mass is cystic or solid. Cysts observed on CT typically demonstrate attenuation near water without rim enhancement. CT scanning may be especially useful when US views are limited by obesity or signal distortion from overlying bowel gas or the lower ribs.[10]

Both cysts and solid tumors are further divided, each into two broad categories. A cyst is classified as either a primary (true) cyst containing an epithelial lining or, more commonly, a secondary cyst (pseudocyst), which lacks an epithelial lining. True cysts are either parasitic or nonparasitic, whereas pseudocysts most commonly arise as the result of blunt abdominal trauma. Tumors of the spleen are divided into either lymphoid or nonlymphoid types. Lymphoid tumors are mainly of the Hodgkin or non-Hodgkin variety. Nonlymphoid tumors, if primary, are most commonly of vascular origin and may be either benign or malignant. Secondary nonlymphoid tumors are metastatic. This broad schema may serve as a starting point to understand the etiology of the mass and thereby provide the most appropriate course of treatment without undue risk of immunologic complication to the patient (Table 142.1).

Options for treatment include medical management with continued observation and/or surgical intervention. The varied types of intervention available include splenectomy, either complete or partial, percutaneous drainage, fenestration, or marsupialization. Management decisions will be based in part on the presentation of the patient but also by the etiology of the lesion.

CYSTIC LESIONS

Splenic cysts are most common in the second and third decades of life, although they have been noted in all age groups including infants. An asymptomatic abdominal mass is the presenting feature in 30% to 45% of cases. Abdominal symptoms such as pain or physical examination findings may present in children and adults, but symptoms are more common when cysts are larger than 6 to 8 cm. Signs may arise from the compression on adjacent structures by an enlarging mass. For example, poorly controlled hypertension may arise because of compression of the left renal artery or vague urinary complaints caused by compression and/or pressure on the left kidney or ureteropelvic junction. The pain may either be localized or referred, classically to the left shoulder. A

review of systems may yield complaints of gastrointestinal distress that are neither associated with meals nor helped by antacids. Respiratory complaints may include shortness of breath, pleuritic chest pain, or even a history of left lower lobe pneumonia. Sudden onset of abdominal pain and peritoneal signs caused by rupture may occur in previously asymptomatic patients, as the risk of rupture is 25% in cysts larger than 5 cm.[11]

Fowler is credited with the first classification system for splenic cysts after reviewing more than 400 cases. There have been attempts to simplify his system, most recently by Hansen and Moller, who collectively reviewed 800 reported cases.[9] It is important to note that the prevalence of primary versus secondary cysts differs in the United States versus other parts of the world, especially in areas endemic for *Echinococcus* such as south central Europe, South America, and Australia. Worldwide (but not in the United States) the vast majority of primary or "true" splenic cysts are parasitic, two-thirds or more being caused by echinococci, with *Echinococcus granulosus* being the most common species. The echinococcal splenic cyst is composed of an inner germinal layer and an outer laminated layer surrounded by a fibrous capsule, characteristically multilocular in appearance and filled with fluid under pressure. It may contain daughter cysts and infective scolices. Echinococcal cysts may be asymptomatic or may cause pressure symptoms when they reach a large enough size, become secondarily infected, or rupture. Diagnosis is suggested by a history of travel to an endemic area and may be confirmed by indirect hemagglutination or enzyme-linked immunosorbent assay tests, which are positive in approximately 90% of patients with echinococcal cysts. Although hepatic hydatid cysts of echinococcal disease may be treated with percutaneous drainage and systemic treatment with albendazole,[12] the treatment of choice for splenic hydatid cysts is splenectomy. However, there have been reports of limited success in small (<5 cm) single cysts with chemical sterilization with cetrimide, 3% sodium chloride, or ethanol and cyst evacuation to achieve splenic salvage.[13] Whichever method is chosen, care must be taken to avoid intraperitoneal spillage and the resultant potential for anaphylaxis and hypotension. Low morbidity rates have been reported in patients needing to undergo simultaneous surgical treatment of splenic and hepatic hydatid cysts.[14]

The remaining causes of nonparasitic primary cysts include congenital and neoplastic cysts. Congenital causes account for approximately 10% of all splenic cysts and 25% of nonparasitic cysts. Primary nonparasitic congenital cysts are seen predominantly in children and young adults. The developmental model proposed for these cysts suggests they arise as a result of invaginations of the mesothelium-lined splenic capsule and are primary in nature.[15] Neoplastic nonparasitic cysts are much less common and historically have included epidermoid, dermoid, and endodermoid cysts, the latter being the most common. Endodermoid lesions are not true cysts and include lymphangiomas and hemangiomas; they are discussed later as solid masses. Dermoid cysts are exceedingly rare and are characterized by structures derived from all three germ layers, similar to a cystic teratoma. These lesions may be observed if they are small (≤5 cm) and followed with US. Larger lesions should be surgically removed

Three-quarters of nonparasitic splenic cysts are termed *secondary cysts* (pseudocysts) and are thought to be attributed to trauma,[16] although 30% of these patients may not recall the specific event,[17] suggesting that causes other than trauma (such as splenic infarcts or infection) may play a larger role than originally thought. Secondary cysts typically occur in young and middle-aged adults. Women are more affected than men, and the reasons for this are unknown, although hormonal effects and changes during pregnancy are presumed to play a role. Secondary cysts are thought to be formed by encapsulation of a splenic hematoma, subsequent absorption of the blood, and persistence of a false cyst wall.[18] Clinically it is difficult to differentiate primary from secondary cysts, given the similarity of complaints, the overlap of the age groups, and the frequent omission of trauma from the patient's history. However, the treatment guidelines are also similar for primary and secondary cysts in that masses smaller than 5 cm may be observed and followed with serial US, whereas a surgical approach should be chosen for larger masses.

The tumor markers carcinoembryonic antigen (CEA) and carbohydrate antigen 19-9 (CA 19-9) may be elevated in primary cysts, and studies have shown immunoreactivity of the cyst's inner lining to anti-CA 19-9.[19,20] Because increased CEA or CA 19-9 levels may be from either benign or malignant processes, preoperative and postoperative levels documenting change are sometimes useful.

SOLID TUMORS

Tumors of the spleen are uncommon lesions and are categorized as either lymphoid or nonlymphoid. Lymphoid tumors of the spleen are mainly Hodgkin disease or non-Hodgkin lymphoma. As primary lesions of the spleen, these tumors are rare; however, the spleen is often the site of secondary involvement. Regardless of whether primary or secondary, lymphoid lesions are first observed in the white pulp. The process may be diffuse, as seen with nodular lymphoma, or localized with large irregular tumors, as seen with large-cell lymphomas. Surgical treatment invariably involves complete splenectomy, either as part of a staging operation in the case of Hodgkin disease or as an attempt at palliation for symptomatic splenomegaly or hypersplenism. It is notable that the usefulness of a staging laparotomy and/or a splenectomy for Hodgkin disease remains controversial and is outside the scope of this chapter.

Nonlymphoid tumors may be either primary or secondary (metastatic). It is important to distinguish benign from malignant lesions. The most common nonlymphoid primary tumors are vascular tumors consisting of benign and malignant hemangiomas, lymphangiomas, and hemangioendotheliomas. Other tumors include hamartomas, fibrosarcomas, inflammatory pseudotumors, and lipomas, although these are all rarely reported lesions. Secondary or metastatic tumors are most commonly from melanoma, breast, and lung tumors. Although the spleen is one of the most vascular organs in the body, metastatic disease is uncommon.

Hemangiomas are the most common benign tumors of the spleen. Typically, these tumors are asymptomatic, found incidentally at autopsy or in spleens removed for other reasons. They may be single, multiple, or involving

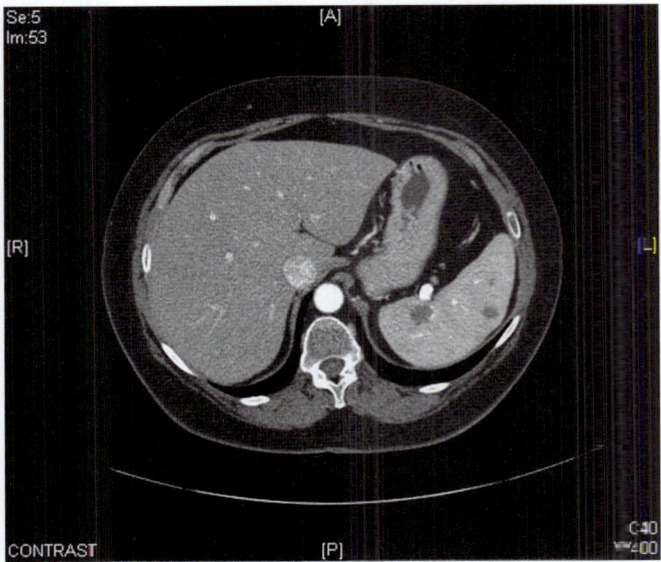

FIGURE 142.1 Multiple splenic hemangiomas demonstrated as hypoattenuating structures on computed tomography.

the entire organ. As noted, symptoms may be present when the lesion increases in size sufficient to compress adjacent structures or grows large enough to rupture spontaneously. A hematologic clue to the existence of splenic hemangioma may present as unexplained consumptive coagulopathy caused by platelet trapping. Radiographic findings can be seen as "pooling of contrast" on angiography or contrast CT, similar to hepatic hemangiomas (Fig. 142.1). Lymphangiomas are less common and are thought to be congenital malformations of the lymphatic system. These malformations may fill with eosinophilic proteinaceous material, contributing to increased weight of the spleen. These lesions usually become symptomatic because of a mass effect. They may be differentiated from the hemangiomas by the absence of the "lakes" associated with the latter. Littoral cell angioma is a rare benign tumor that arises from the cells that line the red pulp and may manifest as splenomegaly (Fig. 142.2). Treatment considerations for both benign conditions are based on symptomatology, with observation for small asymptomatic lesions and complete splenectomy for larger symptomatic hemangiomas and lymphangiomas.

Primary hemangiosarcoma, although rare, is the most common primary malignancy of the spleen. Historically, these lesions have been referred to as angiosarcomas; however, *hemangiosarcoma* is now the preferred nomenclature to distinguish them from lymphangiosarcoma. Hemangiosarcomas grow rapidly and metastasize to regional lymph nodes, liver, bone marrow, and lungs. In addition to the clinical presentation associated with splenomegaly, these patients may develop cachexia because of the aggressive nature of the malignancy. Ascites and pleural effusion are less common findings. Spontaneous rupture may be the initial presenting feature. Imaging may be similar to hemangiomas on angiography, but care must be taken to attempt differentiation, as the prognosis of hemangiosarcoma remains poor in almost all cases. Treatment, if appropriate, remains splenectomy.

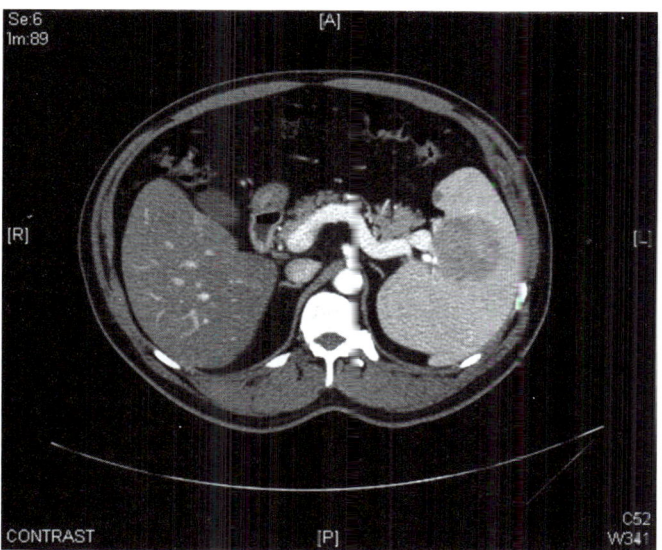

FIGURE 142.2 Littoral cell angioma, a vascular neoplasm of the spleen, demonstrated as a large heterogeneous mass on computed tomography.

The reported incidence of metastatic disease varies from 0.3% to 7.3% depending on the location of the primary tumor. Speculation as to reasons for such a relatively low rate of metastatic lesions is based on both anatomic features such as the acute angle the splenic artery presents to tumor emboli as well as a lack of afferent lymphatics, and functional peculiarities such as the rhythmic contractions of the spleen and high antitumoral activity of the splenic lymphoid tissue. The finding of metastatic disease in the spleen mandates a thorough evaluation of the rest of the body, as it is extremely rare to find the spleen as the initial site of metastasis. As in the case of other splenic lesions, symptoms are often attributable to mass effects, and the progression of disease before clinical presentation may be variable. Spontaneous rupture is a feared although exceedingly rare and devastating complication.[21] Splenectomy is the treatment of choice to assist in relieving symptoms of compression.

SURGICAL PLANNING

An algorithm for the evaluation and management of splenic lesions is shown in Fig. 142.3. Since 1952, with the demonstration of the increased mortality of splenectomized patients (mainly children) because of OFSI, there has been an interest in splenic salvage.[5] The incidence of OPSI is reported to be 0.2% to 4.3%, with a lifetime risk

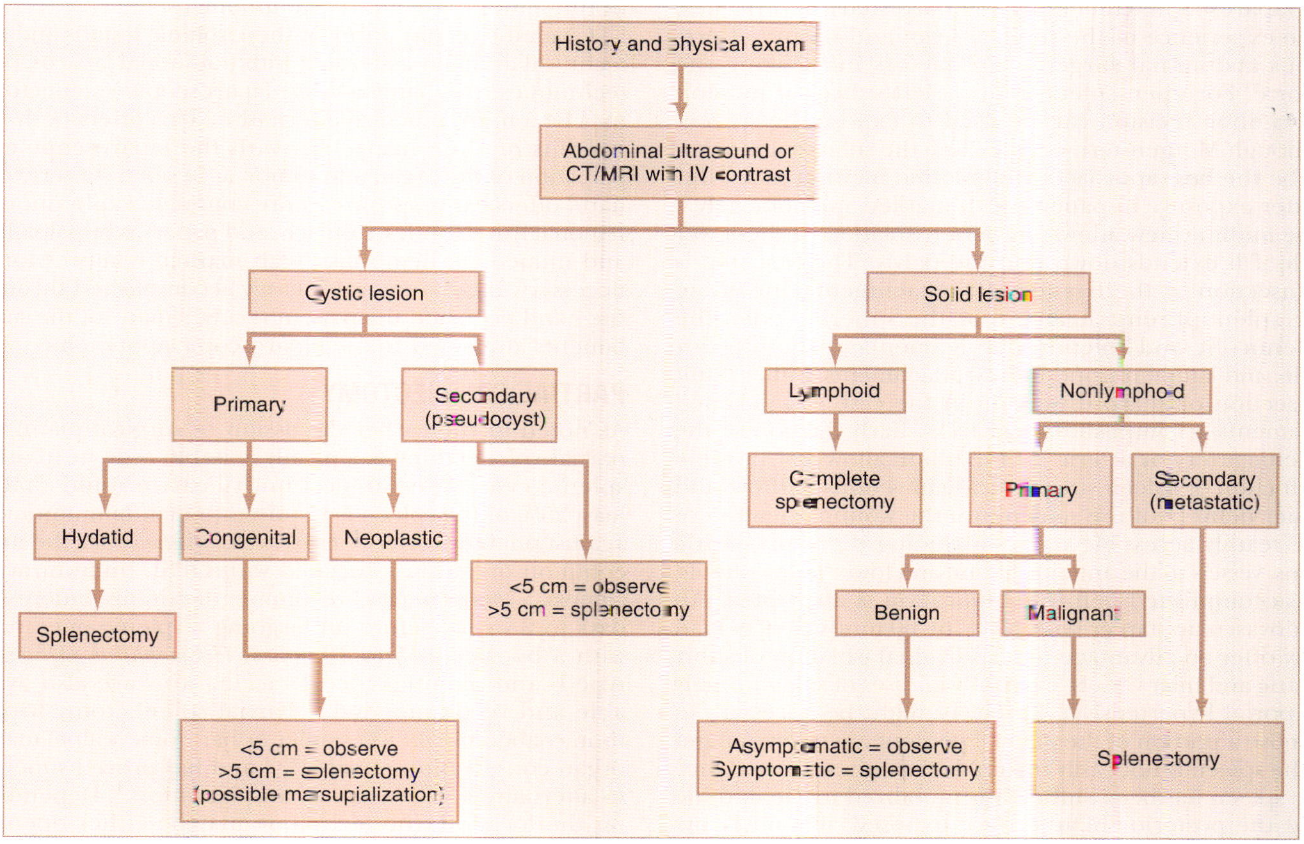

FIGURE 142.3 Algorithm for the work-up, diagnosis, and management of solid and cystic splenic lesions. *CT,* Computed tomography; *IV,* intravenous; *MRI,* magnetic resonance imaging.

of 5%.[22] Although the overall incidence may be low, the risk of developing an overwhelming infection is 200 times greater as compared with the background population.[23] The most significant organisms responsible are *Streptococcus pneumoniae, Neisseria meningitidis,* and *Haemophilus influenzae.*[24] Vaccines directed toward these three bacteria species are available in case a complete splenectomy is unavoidable.[25] Partial splenectomy has been reported only for solitary cysts of the spleen. Complete splenectomy for splenic cysts would be indicated in cases of polycystic disease.

In the case of solid tumors, sound surgical principles should be followed, meaning good exposure, removal of the entire tumor without rupture, adequate margins, and perfect hemostasis. In staging operations such as for Hodgkin disease, the risk of a negative staging error with partial splenectomy has been reported, and it is therefore advised against. Similarly, percutaneous biopsy of tumors of the spleen is not recommended because of the risks of bleeding, tumor seeding, and uncertainty of diagnosis on fine- or core-needle specimens. For primary splenic tumors, safe and effective surgical principles are best achieved with a total splenectomy. If the spleen has tumors that are clearly part of disseminated metastatic disease, splenic biopsy is sufficient, as there is no survival benefit to splenectomy to justify the risk.

COMPLETE SPLENECTOMY

Splenectomy may be performed by the traditional open or laparoscopic (including hand-assisted) approaches. The experience of the surgical team and history of previous abdominal surgeries are factors influencing the choice. For open splenectomy, a left subcostal incision or midline incision can be used to expose the spleen, although Morgenstern et al. believe the subcostal incision to be the best approach; the midline incision may offer better exposure in patients with marked splenomegaly.[26] The midline view allows for better isolation of the lower pole if it extends down into the pelvis. The first step is transection of the ligamentous attachments, including the splenophrenic ligament at the superior pole, the splenocolic and splenorenal ligaments at the inferior pole, and lateral retroperitoneal attachments. Either blunt dissection or sharp dissection in the case of thickened ligaments accomplishes these tasks. Early ligation of the splenic artery or arteries in the hilum allows for possible reduction of spleen size, decrease in venous outflow, and easier delivery of the spleen into the wound. Ligation of the readily accessible veins—including the short gastric veins, vessels to the anterior hilum, and lower pole—should be accomplished before mobilization is attempted. An endovascular stapler with a 30- or 60-mm vascular load may offer an advantage over individual isolation of short gastric and hilar vessels, especially in cases of splenomegaly or portal hypertension. Rarely, it might be necessary to remove a portion of the parietal peritoneum or diaphragm if the spleen is not easily separable from these areas. Once the spleen has been sufficiently mobilized to the midline and the posterior hilar surface exposed, it is advisable to control the large posterior splenic veins. Attempts at control of the fragile veins from the anterior approach may result in venous disruption and massive bleeding,

and an increased risk of injuring the tail of the pancreas. On removal of the spleen, attempts at sampling the hilar lymph nodes should be made. These are usually located near the major hilar vessels and may be useful in the grading of splenic tumors.[26,27]

Complete splenectomy using the laparoscopic approach for tumors has also been reported.[28,29] The principles of open tumor surgery apply for laparoscopy. In the past, opponents of laparoscopic splenectomy criticized the necessity of splenic morcellation for the removal of the spleen from the peritoneal cavity. However, with a small 3-cm extension of one of the trocar sites, most spleens can be removed intact. Carroll et al. proved that the staging surgery for Hodgkin disease could be performed entirely laparoscopically.[28] It is essential that the spleen be removed intact to avoid peritoneal dissemination of potentially malignant cells; therefore morcellation should not be done. Proponents of the laparoscopic approach believe that the spleen can be more cleanly dissected and, because of better visualization, vessels more safely ligated earlier in the course of the operation to prevent hematologic spread with manipulation of the spleen. Flowers et al. warned, however, that a learning curve of 20 laparoscopic splenectomies was usual before surgeons felt comfortable with the technique.[29] We have successfully used the hand-assisted laparoscopic technique to remove spleens as large as 25 cm. The patient is placed in a semidecubitus position with the left side elevated approximately 45 degrees. The hand port incision is made in the midline just above the umbilicus.

Given the relative rarity of these splenic lesions and the technical difficulty associated with traditional laparoscopic techniques, the hand-assisted laparoscopic splenectomy may be a more practical alternative. This offers both the benefits of close inspection with the laparoscope and palpation of the organ and tumor, as in open surgery. The hand offers easy exposure; more complete exploration of regional lymph nodes, stomach, and pancreas by palpation; and immediate hemostasis with manual compression if necessary. Intact removal is easily accomplished through the hand port, and the patient receives many of the same benefits attributed to the laparoscopic approach.

PARTIAL SPLENECTOMY

As noted in the earlier discussion of surgical planning, partial splenectomy is typically suitable only in treating splenic cysts. The surgeon must bear in mind that at least 25% of the spleen is required to maintain immunity against pneumococcus (*Streptococcus pneumoniae*), the most common organism associated with OPSI. Immunization against *S. pneumoniae* is recommended in all patients 10 days to 2 weeks before undergoing a splenic operation, with a booster in 5 to 10 years. *Haemophilus influenzae* type b and meningococcal vaccinations are also available and recommended.[22] Partial splenectomy with a thoracoabdominal (TA) stapler or harmonic scalpel makes organ conservation possible[30,31] and has proved superior to alternatives such as autotransplantation.[32] Depending on the location, the technique may be either open or laparoscopic; however, care to control the vessels supporting the cyst must be taken regardless of the chosen technique. Additionally, it is often difficult to control bleeding in a partial splenectomy. It is recommended to have an argon beam coagulator available in conjunction with commercially available hemostatic agents to effectively stop all bleeding. Excessive bleeding caused by a partial splenectomy that requires blood transfusions may negate any theoretic advantages. Surgical judgment is critical in determining when to abandon partial splenectomy in favor of total.

OTHER TECHNIQUES

When the location of the cyst is superficial, definitive treatment may be accomplished with less invasive techniques. However, care must be taken in both patient selection and the selection of the appropriate technique so as not to increase the risk of recurrence. Percutaneous laparoscopic aspiration or drainage with indwelling catheters has been suggested especially as a bridging technique in the management of pseudocysts that will eventually undergo operative resection.[33,34] Fenestration involves resection of the extrasplenic cyst wall to create a permanent opening into the peritoneum accomplished either by open or laparoscopic surgical techniques. Care must be taken to remove a large enough piece of the cyst wall to prevent recurrence, and the omentum may be attached to cover the parenchyma defect. A better alternative involves partial splenic decapsulation, also known as marsupialization. This approach involves the trocar decompression of the cyst with removal of the outer splenic capsule. A running locking suture in the splenic wall is used to ensure hemostasis, and external drainage may also be performed. One potential risk of puncture techniques is anaphylaxis if the underlying etiology is a parasite infection and cyst contents are spilled into the peritoneal cavity. This risk and the observation that a subsequent dense inflammatory reaction could make future operations for recurrence more difficult contraindicate the use of simple puncture techniques.

CONCLUSION

When faced with a splenic lesion, care must be taken to ensure that the mass is correctly identified as either cystic or solid. Fortunately, this task is easily accomplished by current imaging modalities. With the knowledge of the nature of the lesion as cystic or solid, the surgical management is greatly simplified as total splenectomy is indicated for symptomatic or potentially malignant solid tumors. For cystic structures, exposure to regions endemic for culpable parasites or a history of blunt trauma may assist in determining the appropriate treatment, which may not involve complete removal of this historically underappreciated organ. Additionally, observation alone may suffice in the case of smaller splenic cysts, sparing the patient unneeded procedures. If an operation should be indicated, laparoscopic and open techniques are equally effective and safe as long as the surgeon has the requisite experience.

REFERENCES

1. McClusky DA 3rd, Skandalakis LJ, Colborn CL, Skandalakis JE. Tribute to a triad: history of splenic anatomy, physiology, and surgery. World J Surg. 1999;23:311.
2. Wells TS. On excision of enlarged spleen, with a case in which the operation was performed. Med Times Gaz. 1866;1:2.
3. Beer E. Development and progress of surgery of the spleen. Ann Surg. 1928;88:335.
4. Johnston AB. Splenectomy. Ann Surg. 1908;88:409.
5. King H, Shumacker HB Jr. Splenic studies I. Susceptibility to infection after splenectomy performed in infancy. Ann J Surg. 1952;136:239.
6. Morgenstern L, Shapiro SJ. Partial splenectomy for non-parasitic splenic cysts. Am J Surg. 1980;139:278.
7. Seshadri PA, Poulin EC, Mamazza J, Schlachta CM. Technique for laparoscopic partial splenectomy. Surg Laparosc Endosc Percutan Tech. 2000;10:1 5.
8. Uchida H, Ohta M, Shibata K, et al. Laparoscopic splenectomy in patients with inflammatory pseudotumor of the spleen: report of 2 cases and review of the literature. Surg Laparosc Endosc Percutan Tech. 2000;6:3.
9. Hansen MB, Moller AC. Splenic cysts. Surg Laparosc Endosc Percutan Tech. 2004;4:316.
10. Robertson F, Leander P, Ekberg O. Radiology of the spleen. Eur Radiol. 2001;11:80.
11. Qureshi MA, Hafner CD, Dorchak JR. Nonparasitic cysts of the spleen: report of 14 cases. Arch Surg. 1964;39:570.
12. Khuroo MS, Wani NA, Javid G, et al. Percutaneous drainage compared with surgery for hepatic hydatid cysts. N Engl J Med. 1997;337:881.
13. Khoury G, Abiad F, Geagea T, Nabout G, Jabbour S. Laparoscopic treatment of hydatid cysts of the liver and spleen. Surg Endosc. 2000;14:243.
14. Heimarck G, Grigolia G, Loehe F, Jauch KW, Schauer RJ. Surgical management of splenic echinococcal disease. Eur J Med Res. 2009;14:165.
15. Ough YD. Mesothelial cysts of the spleen with squamous metaplasia. Am J Clin Pathol. 1981;76:666.
16. Andrews MW. Ultrasound of the spleen. World J Surg. 2000;24:183.
17. Boesby S. Spontaneous rupture of benign non-parasitic cyst of the spleen. Ugeskr Laeger. 1977;134:2546.
18. Dawes LG, Malangoni MA. Cystic masses of the spleen. Am Surg. 1986;52:333.
19. Madia C, Lumachi F, Veroux M, et al. Giant splenic epithelial cyst with elevated tumor markers CEA and CA 19-9: an incidental association? Anticancer Res. 2003;23:773.
20. Trompetas V, Panagopoulos E, Priovolou-Papaevangelou M, Ramananis G. Giant benign true cyst of the spleen with high serum levels of CA 19-9. Eur J Gastroenterol Hepatol. 2002;14:85.
21. Lam KY, Tang V. Metastatic tumors of the spleen: a twenty-five year clinicopathologic study. Arch Pathol Lab Med. 2000;124:526.
22. Davidson RN, Wall RA. Prevention and management of infections in patients without a spleen. Clin Microbiol Infect. 2001;7:657.
23. Grinblat J, Gilboa Y. Overwhelming pneumococcal sepsis 25 years after splenectomy. Am J Med Sci. 1974;270:523.
24. Sinwar PD. Overwhelming post-splenectomy infection syndrome—review study. Int J Surg. 2014;12(12) 1314-1316.
25. Smith ST, Scott DJ, Burdick JS, Rege RV, Jones DB. Laparoscopic marsupialization and hemisplenectomy for splenic cysts. J Laparoendosc Adv Surg Tech A. 2001;11:243.
26. Morgenstern L, Rosenberg J, Geller SA. Tumors of the spleen. World J Surg. 1985;9:468.
27. Schwartz SI, Cooper RA Jr. Surgery in the diagnosis and treatment of Hodgkin disease. Adv Surg. 1972;5:175.
28. Carroll BJ, Phillips EH, Semel CJ, Fallas M, Morgenstern L. Laparoscopic splenectomy. Surg Endosc. 1992;6:183.
29. Flowers JL, Lefor AT, Steers J, Heniman M, Graham SM, Imbembo AL. Laparoscopic splenectomy in patients with hematologic diseases. Ann Surg. 1996;224:19.
30. Uranüs S, Kronberger L, Kraft-Kine J. Partial splenic resection with a TA-stapler. Am J Surg. 1994;168:49.
31. Sardi A, Ojeda HF, King D Jr. Laparoscopic resection of a benign true cyst of the spleen with the harmonic scalpel producing high levels of CA 19-9 and carcinoembryonic antigen. Am Surg. 1994;64:1159.
32. Balzan SM, Riedner CE, Santos LM, Pazzinatto MC, Fontes PR. Posttraumatic splenic cysts and partial splenectomy: report of a case. Surg Today. 2001;31:262.
33. Pachter HL, Hofstetter SR, Elkowitz A, et al. Traumatic cysts of the spleen-the role of cystectomy and splenic preservation: experience with seven consecutive patients. J Trauma. 1993;35:430.
34. Moir C, Guttman F, Jequier S, Sorrino R, Youssef S. Splenic cysts: aspiration, sclerosis, or resection. J Pediatr Surg. 1989;24:646.

Colon, Rectum, and Anus

PART ONE

Anatomy, Physiology, and Diagnosis of Colorectal and Anal Diseases

Operative Anatomy of the Colon, Rectum, and Anus

Matthew P. Kelley | Jonathan Efron | Sandy H. Fang |

Bashar Safar | Susan Gearhart

Knowledge of the developmental anatomy of the digestive tract is the first step in understanding operative anatomy of the colon, rectum, and anus. The surgical approach to removing portions of the digestive tract requires an understanding of the anatomical planes of the abdomen. The digestive tract begins its development around the fourth week of pregnancy as an outpouching of the pharynx and stomach forming the primitive midgut.[1] Further progression is broken down into three stages (Fig. 143.1). In the first stage, a midgut loop enters the extraembryonic coelom or yolk sac and gradually elongates into a V-shaped loop that projects ventral toward the umbilicus. This physiologic herniation of the umbilicus eventually houses a large portion of the digestive tract, including the superior mesenteric artery (SMA) along with the mesentery of the bowel. The bowel resides in the umbilicus until the third trimester of pregnancy, when it gradually draws back. During this time, the intestines rotate counterclockwise around the SMA axis. During the second stage, the primitive intestine returns to the abdominal cavity. While doing so, the intestine and its mesentery rotate an additional 180 degrees counterclockwise around the SMA for a total of 270 degrees of rotation. With this rotation, the duodenum comes to lie and fuse in a location posterior to the SMA. If this rotation is incomplete, anomalies of rotation and fixation such as nonrotation, malrotation, reversed rotation, and omphalocele can occur (Figs. 143.2 and 143.3). The danger with abnormal rotation and fixation is the development of an internal hernia with entrapment of the intestine, leading to acute intestinal ischemia. The third stage marks the return and fixation of the colon and its mesentery in the abdominal cavity. The colon comes to reside with the ascending and descending mesentery fused to the right and left posterolateral abdominal cavity (retroperitoneum), forming a line known as the *line of Toldt*. This line indicates to the surgeon where a bloodless plane exists between the mesentery of the colon and the retroperitoneum. However, when a patient has portal venous thrombosis, venous collaterals can form between the colon mesentery and the retroperitoneum making this plane hazardous. The mesentery of the transverse colon fuses with the greater omentum creating the omental bursa (Fig. 143.4), an important landmark when mobilizing the colon. The cecum is the last portion of the colon to return to the abdomen. Initially it resides in the right upper quadrant; however, over time it lengthens toward the right lower quadrant, and the small bowel grows to occupy the upper and mid abdomen.

The hindgut digestive tract consists of the distal third of the transverse colon, descending and sigmoid colon, rectum, and proximal anal canal.[1] These structures share the same arterial inflow, venous and lymphatic drainage, and autonomic innervation. In the developing fetus, the hindgut structures and the allantois merge distally and empty into a dilated collection chamber, the *cloaca* (Latin for "sewer"). During the 6th to 12th weeks of pregnancy, the cloaca is divided sagittally by the urorectal septum into ventral and dorsal segments. Further enfolding from the lateral walls results in caudal advancement of the dorsal segment and simultaneous involution of adjacent ectodermal-derived body wall, known as the proctodeum (or anal pit). The proctoderm and distal cloaca fuse to become the cloacal membrane. This membrane is obliterated via apoptosis, forming the dentate (pectinate) line that represents the anatomic division of hindgut/ endoderm (proximal two-thirds) and the proctoderm/ ectoderm (distal one-third) of the anal canal.

The common disorders that affect the hindgut include disorders of atresia and duplication. In particular, the defects associated with the anus (anorectal malformations)

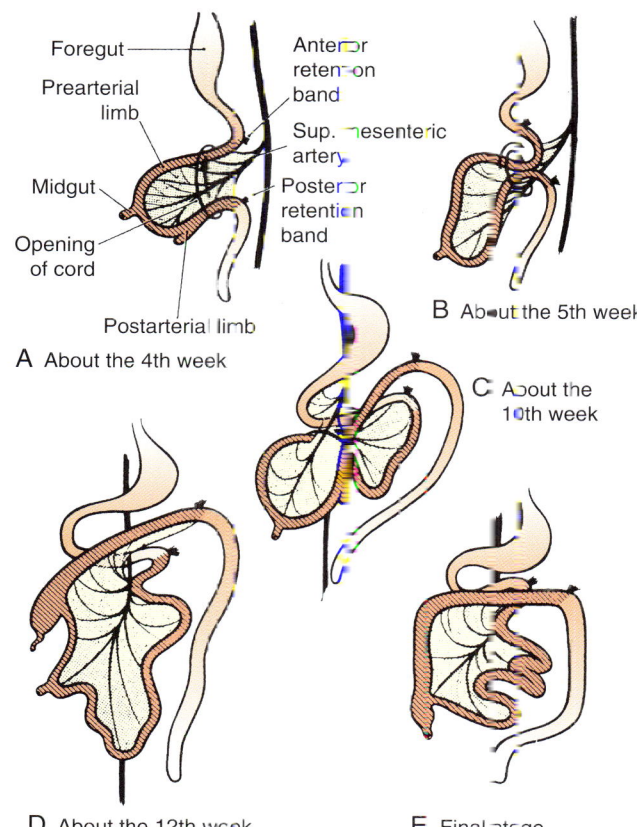

Foregut

Prearterial limb

Midgut

Opening of cord

Postarterial limb

A About the 4th week

Anterior retention band

Sup. mesenteric artery

Posterior retention band

B About the 5th week

C About the 10th week

D About the 12th week   **E** Final stage

FIGURE 143.1 Stages of the development of the primitive midgut. *Sup.,* Superior. (From Haller JD, Morgenstern L. Anomalous rotation and fixation of the left colon: embryogenesis and surgical management. *Am J Surg.* 1964;103:331.)

are classified low and high defects with regard to the relationship to the anus. In low defects, anal stenosis or atresia can present with a draining perineal fistula whereas high defects may present with obstruction. The most common duplication disorder is the finding of mesenteric cysts that are generally located in the mesocolon or mesorectum. These cysts may or may not communicate with the intestine. Although most of these cysts are benign, they may harbor foci of malignancy.[2] Fig. 143.5 is a pelvic duplication cyst found on incidental imaging. Hirschsprung disease or congenital megacolon is the result of the absence of ganglion cells in the myenteric plexus of the colon. It is thought to be secondary to an interruption of migration of the neuroenteric cells from the neural crest (described later in this chapter).[3]

When development is complete, the digestive tract allows food to travel from the mouth to the anus in a musculomembranous tube approximately 9 m long. The large intestine is approximately 165 cm long and includes the cecum and appendix, ascending, transverse, descending, sigmoid colon, and rectum. The caliber of the large intestine is largest in the cecum, with a diameter of 7.5 cm, and this gradually tapers to a 2.5-cm diameter in the sigmoid colon. The colon terminates into the rectum, which is approximately 15 cm in length, and this structure continues to the anus.

SURFACE ANATOMY

The majority of the digestive tract is contained within the abdomen. The abdomen proper differs from other great cavities of the body that are bounded by muscles and fascia, allowing it to vary in capacity and shape. The understanding of these changes and their effect on human physiology are important when performing laparoscopy. The peritoneum is a serous membrane that is applied to the abdominal wall (parietal peritoneum) and viscera (visceral peritoneum). The surface of this membrane is smooth and lubricated with serous fluid that allows the viscera to freely move within the abdominal cavity. While the transverse colon and sigmoid colon are covered with visceral peritoneum, only the ventral surfaces of the ascending and descending colon and upper rectum are covered with visceral peritoneum. Given this, these portions of the digestive tract remain relatively fixed.

The wall of the colon has characteristics that are prominent on both the internal and external surface of the bowel wall. These characteristics are important in endoscopic and minimally invasive procedures to identify portions of the digestive tract. The external wall of the colon has longitudinal bands known as *taenia*, which cause puckering of the bowel wall to form sacculations called *haustra*. There are three types of taenia, named in reference to their position on the transverse colon (most prominent segment). The taenia mesocolica connect to the mesocolon; taenia omentalis attached to the greater omentum; and the taenia libera have no attachment and are clearly visible on surface of the colon. It is between these taenia that the vasa recta brevia (small blood vessels) penetrate the colon to supply blood to the mucosa and submucosa (Fig. 143.6). A weakness or outpouching of the mucosa that develops in the wall of the colon at this intersection is known as a *diverticulum*. The location in the colon that most frequently develops diverticular disease is the sigmoid colon. The classic triangular configuration of the transverse colon as seen during colonoscopy is secondary to these prominent taenia. Small irregular stalks of fat called *appendices epiploicae* are also found on the colon. They are enveloped by peritoneum and most prevalent along the taenia libera and in the sigmoid colon. The internal lining of the colon is made up of simple columnar epithelium that lacks villi. Other landmarks that distinguish the colon from other parts of the digestive tract include the ileocecal valve, a muscular valve that separates the small bowel and colon, and the appendix.

ANATOMY OF THE COLON

Cecum

The first segment of the colon typically overlies the right iliac fossa and is covered with peritoneum. It is a saccular-shaped segment that receives the terminal ileum and serves as the origin of the appendix. In about 20% of the population the cecum is attached to an abnormally long mesentery, resulting in a cecum that is highly mobile. Excessive mobility is one underlying factor that predisposes an individual to the development of cecal volvulus. The ileum enters the cecum along its mesenteric border and is supported by two ligaments, the superior and inferior ileocecal

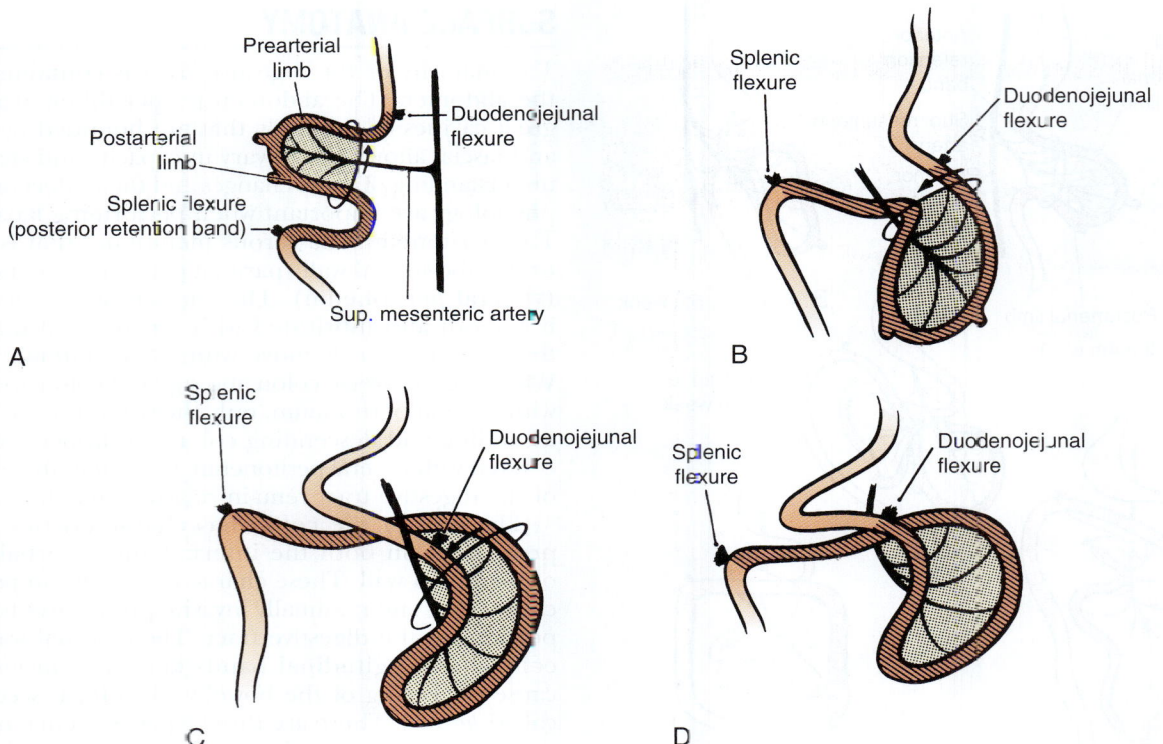

FIGURE 143.2 Mechanisms for anomalies of rotation and fixation of the colon. (A) The splenic flexure fixes to the right abdominal cavity instead of the left. (B) Correct rotation occurs, however, because the flexure is already fixed; the transverse colon comes to lie behind the superior *(Sup.)* mesentery artery (SMA). (C) The intestine reduces normally; however, the proximal colon comes to lie in front of all other structures. (D) The duodenum reduces after rotation late and then comes to rest above the SMA. (From Haller JD, Morgenstern L. Anomalous rotation and fixation of the left colon: embryogenesis and surgical management. *Am J Surg.* 1964;108;331.)

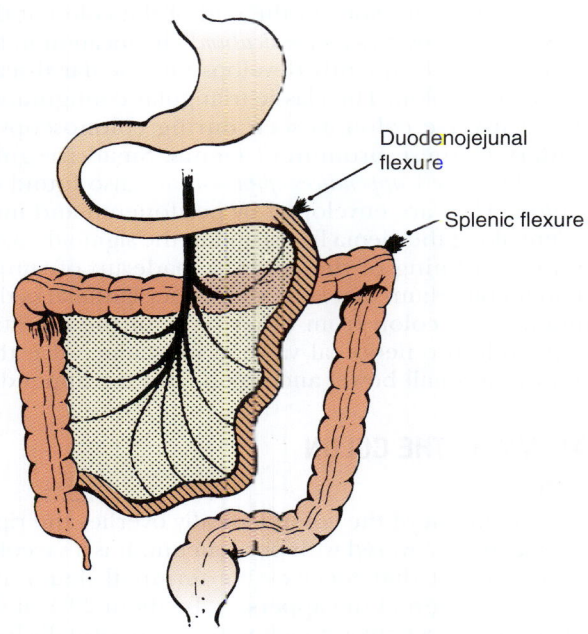

FIGURE 143.3 Reversed rotation. The transverse colon comes to lie beneath the SMA, while the duodenum lies above. (From Haller JD, Morgenstern L. Anomalous rotation and fixation of the left colon: embryogenesis and surgical management. *Am J Surg.* 1964;108:331.)

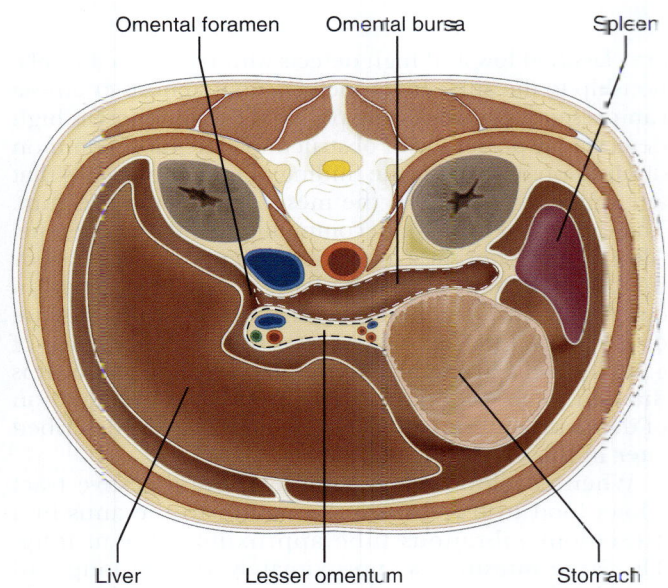

FIGURE 143.4 Development of the omental bursa by fusion of the transverse colon mesentery to the greater omentum.

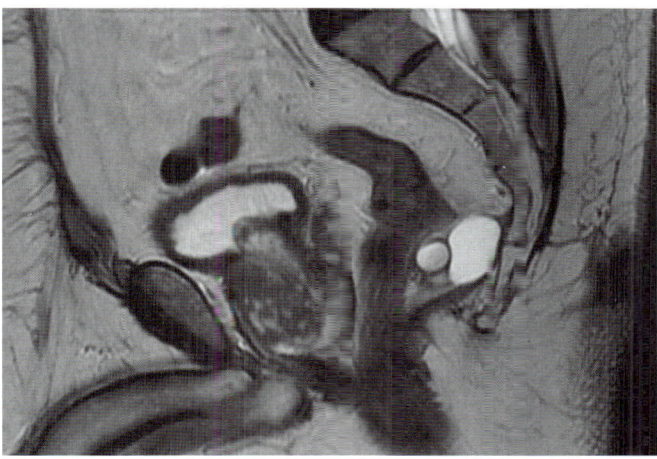

FIGURE 143.5 T2-weighted magnetic resonance image of presacral rectal duplication cyst.

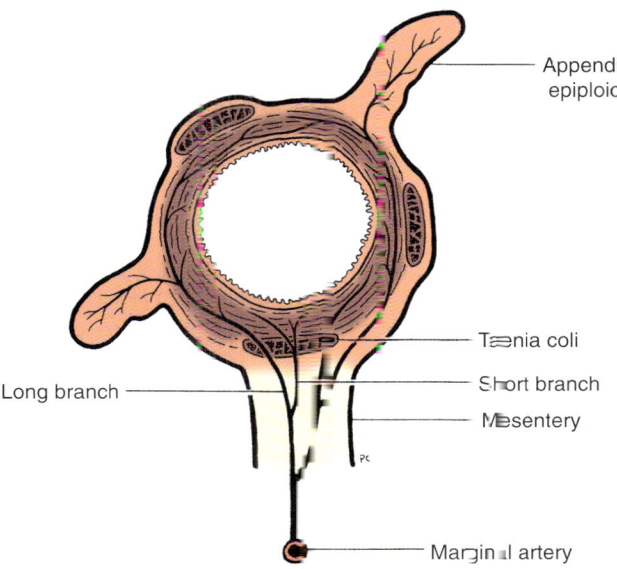

FIGURE 143.6 Surface anatomy of the wall of the colon. (From Keighley MRB, Williams NS. *Surgery of the Anus, Rectum, and Colon.* Philadelphia: Saunders; 1995.)

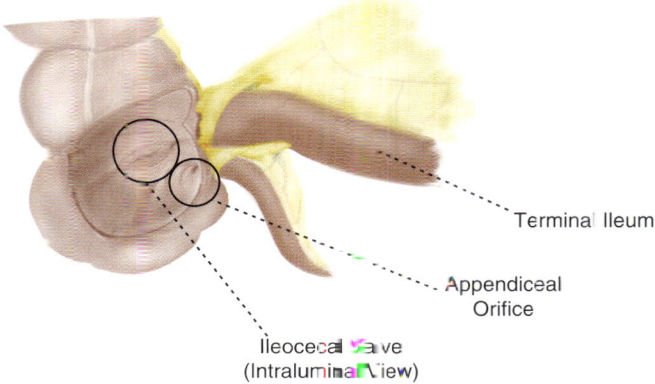

FIGURE 143.7 Anatomy of the ileocecal valve. (Courtesy Matthew P. Kelley, MD.)

ligaments (Fig. 143.7). Endoscopic view of the ileocecal valve reveals a transverse, narrow opening enclosed by two parallel curvilinear lips, forming a frenulum on both medial and lateral aspects. The function of the ileocecal valve is to delay transit from ileum to cecum, not necessarily to prevent reflux of contents from the cecum to ileum, and thus contrast enemas have indeterminate clinical significance. The method of achieving competency by the ileocecal valve is debatable. Kumar and Phillips believe the ileocolic ligaments and angulation of the ileum to the cecal wall achieve competency. Using cadaveric dissection on individuals with a proven competent valve, division of the ileocecal ligaments rendered the valve incompetent; ligaments were later repaired with subsequent restoration of competency.[4] Alternatively, Pellegrini et al. demonstrated using endoscopic and surgical biopsies of the ileocecal

region that this area contained both sphincter morphology and function.[5]

Appendix

The appendix arises most commonly (65%) from a retrocecal position and is between 8 and 10 cm in length and 5 and 10 mm in width. The posterior leaf of the ileal mesentery continues and joins the appendix, forming the mesoappendix. Appendiceal vessels are located within the mesoappendix. The appendix can be found in several common variant locations (pelvic, subcecal, preileal, and retroileal). Symptoms of acute appendicitis can vary due to the location of the appendix. Due to studies indicating that laparoscopic appendectomy reduces the length of stay and risk of postoperative wound infection, most patients undergo this approach.[6-8] As such, the difficulties of finding a subcecal appendix through a small right lower quadrant open incision no longer exist.

Ascending Colon

The ascending colon continues cephalad from the cecum and terminates at the sharp right-to-left turn of the hepatic flexure. Throughout the course it overlies the iliacus muscle, inferior pole of the right kidney, and the retroperitoneal portion of the duodenum. The relationship between the hepatic flexure and the second portion of the duodenum is critical because it can be encountered almost unexpectedly during a hasty lateral-to-medial dissection. At its origin, the ascending colon is closely related to the anterior abdominal wall; this relationship becomes increasingly disparate as it tracks superiorly. Posteriorly, it is relatively fixed to the abdominal wall and attached laterally by the peritoneal reflection or the white line of Toldt. This line serves as a guide for the surgeon during mobilization of the ascending colon. During embryologic development, the nascent mesentery, and its lymphovascular contents, migrates posteromedially. This lateral-to-medial directionality allows safe mobilization within an avascular plane of the ascending colon mesentery, both with an open and laparoscopic approach (Fig. 143.8).

Transverse Colon

The transverse colon is the longest segment of colon, averaging up to 50 cm in length. It begins at the hepatic

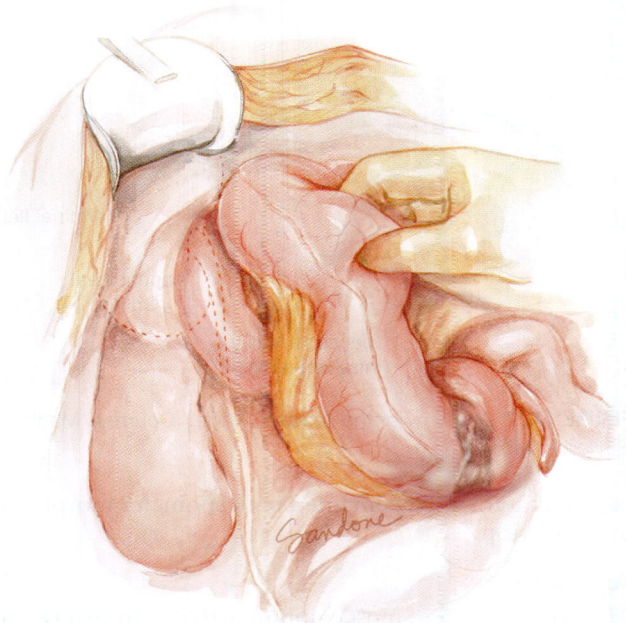

FIGURE 143.8 Following mobilization of the right colon mesentery the retroperitoneal structures are easily visualized. (Illustration from John L. Cameron, Corinne Sandone. *Atlas of Gastrointestinal Surgery*, 2nd ed. Vol. II; used with permission from People's Medical Publishing House—USA, Shelton, Connecticut.)

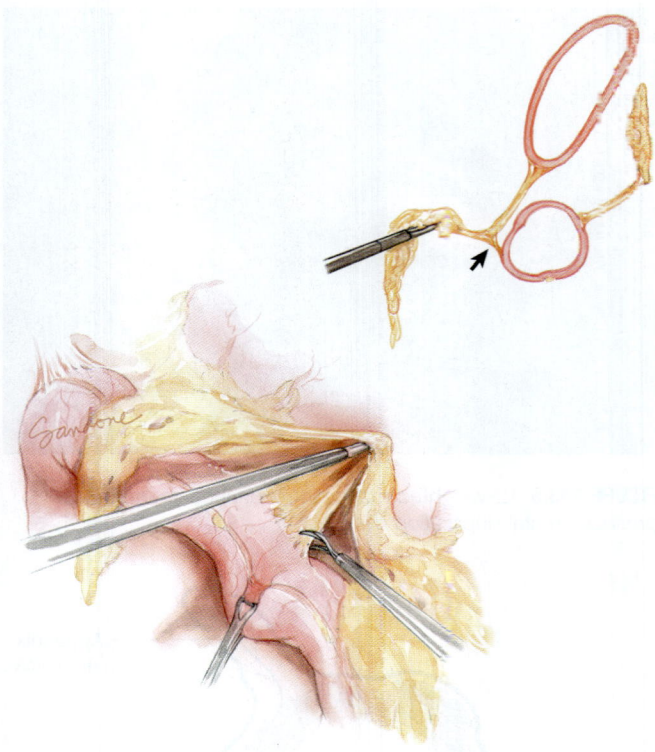

FIGURE 143.9 Mobilization of the omentum from the transverse colon and mesocolon. (Illustration from John L. Cameron, Corinne Sandone. *Atlas of Gastrointestinal Surgery*. 2nd ed. Vol. II; used with permission from People's Medical Publishing House—USA, Shelton, Connecticut.)

flexure and arcs in a slight anteroinferior direction toward the splenic flexure. It is nearly completely covered by visceral peritoneum and has a deceptively more complex mesocolon, which is often closely tethered to the omentum. Because of this, laparoscopic approaches to transverse colon malignancies can be difficult when one wants to achieve an adequate lymph node harvest.[9] The root of the mesocolon spans most of the posterior abdominal wall with attachments from the inferior pole of the right kidney to the hilum of the left kidney. The greater omentum originates from the greater curvature of the stomach, attaches to the anterosuperior transverse colon as the gastrocolic ligament, and then continues as greater omentum proper. Mobilization of the transverse colon can be accomplished by dissection of the greater omentum at the level of the gastrocolic ligament; this also provides access to the lesser sac (Fig. 143.9). The transverse colon ends with a quick upward swing, juxtaposing the spleen before its descent. At the level of the splenic flexure, two ligaments relatively fix the colon: the splenocolic and the phrenocolic ligament. The splenocolic ligament arises from the inferior pole of the spleen and should be handled with care during colon mobilization. Excess traction can result in tear of the splenic capsule. If dissection is desired, the ligament should be transected as far from the spleen as feasible. The phrenocolic ligament (sustentaculum lienis) attaches to the diaphragm at about the tenth and eleventh ribs. In addition to tethering the colon, it serves as a support for the spleen.

Descending Colon

Starting at the downward turn at the splenic flexure, the descending colon terminates at the pelvic brim, typically 25 cm in length. It descends in a gradual left-to-right direction and sits slightly more posterior than the ascending colon. It begins overlying the inferior pole of the left kidney and follows the channel between psoas and quadratus lumborum muscles. Similar to the ascending colon, peritoneum covers its anterior and lateral surfaces, and posteriorly, it is in contact with loose areolar tissue of the retroperitoneum.

Sigmoid Colon

The descending colon crosses the pelvic brim to become the sigmoid colon and terminates at the sacral promontory; this also coincides with the loss of taenia. It averages 40 to 45 cm in length and has a sigmoidal course as it descends the left pelvis, then across to the right pelvis, and finally retrograde toward the midline. It has a mobile mesocolon that is often described as V shaped and extends to the left iliac vessels (the apex of the V). Frequently it attaches to the left pelvis and forms a fold within mesocolon referred to as the *intersigmoid fossa* (Fig. 143.10). This is a critical landmark for the surgeon as this overlies the left ureter lying along the psoas muscle, which can be inadvertently collected along with the specimen if not carefully identified. Considerable variation in length and position of the

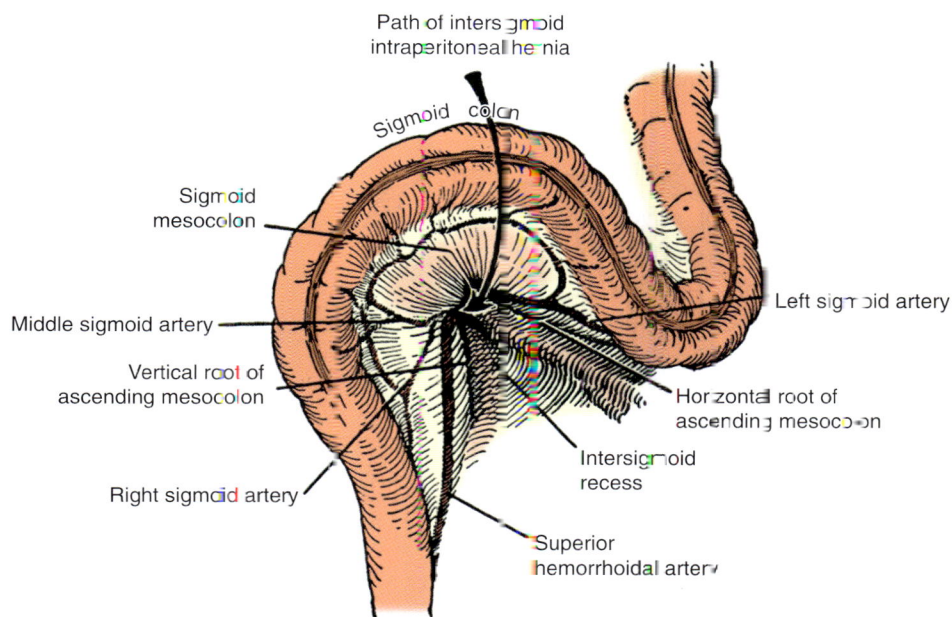

Path of intersigmoid
intraperitoneal hernia

Sigmoid colon

Sigmoid
mesocolon

Left sigmoid artery

Middle sigmoid artery

Vertical root of
ascending mesocolon

Horizontal root of
ascending mesocolon

Intersigmoid
recess

Right sigmoid artery

Superior
hemorrhoidal artery

FIGURE 143.10 Sigmoid mesocolon
and intersigmoid fossa.

sigmoid colon can occur. For instance, a redundant sigmoid colon can be seen in patients with constipation, and a long but narrow-based mesocolon is a predisposition for sigmoid volvulus. Interestingly, the incidence of sigmoid volvulus as a cause of acute obstruction is significantly higher among individuals of South American, African, Eastern European, and Asian descent (20% to 54%) than for those living in the United States, United Kingdom, and Japan (3% to 5%). The sigmoid colon is also considered the most muscular portion of the colon and has the ability to generate the highest intraluminal pressure. Given this, it is the site where diverticulosis most commonly occurs.

Arterial Supply to the Colon

The two dominant arterial systems that supply the colon and rectum are the SMA and the inferior mesenteric artery (IMA; Fig. 143.11). The SMA is responsible for the blood supply to the embryonic midgut, while the IMA delivers the blood supply to the embryonic hindgut. The SMA arises from the aorta at approximately the level of L1 vertebra and travels posterior to the pancreas and anterior to the third portion of the duodenum. The first branch, the inferior pancreaticoduodenal artery, supplies the pancreas and duodenum and is not involved in colonic perfusion. Ileal and jejunal branches come off the left side. There are three colic branches that may arise from the SMA: the right, middle, and ileocolic arteries.

- The SMA terminates into the right colic artery and the ileocolic artery. The ileocolic artery has the least anatomic variation and bifurcates into superior and inferior branches. The superior branch communicates with the descending branch of the right colic artery; the inferior branch further divides into the anterior and posterior cecal, appendicular, and ileal arteries. The right colic artery may also arise from either the ileocolic artery or the middle colic, and is absent in up to 18% of the population.

- The middle colic artery is the second branch. It originates near the inferior border of the pancreas and supplies the proximal two-thirds of the transverse colon. It divides into right and left branches that supply the right transverse colon/hepatic flexure (communicates with the superior branch of the right colic artery) and distal transverse colon, respectively. In up to 20% of cases the middle colic is absent, and less frequently there is an accessory middle colic artery.

The IMA is a branch of the aorta arising at approximately the level of L3 vertebra and typically 4 cm cephalad to the aortic bifurcation. It descends leftward toward the pelvis and divides into the left colic artery and several sigmoidal arteries; beyond the level of the left iliac vessels, the IMA terminates as the superior rectal artery (SRA).

- The left colic artery divides into ascending and descending branches. The ascending branch contributes to supply the distal third of the transverse colon and into the splenic flexure via the arcade of Riolan. The descending branch is the predominant supply of descending colon.

- The sigmoidal arteries form an arcade that supplies the sigmoid colon and collateralize with the marginal artery (of Drummond).

The location of the division of the IMA while performing a total mesorectal excision (TME) for rectal cancer remains somewhat of a debate. If the artery is ligated at the takeoff from the aorta, it is termed a "high ligation," and this site is believed to be associated with an increased number of lymph nodes harvested at a potential cost to increased hypogastric nerve damage, leading to genitourinary complication (Fig. 143.12).[10] However, this finding has yet to be seen. A low ligation of the IMA refers to the ligation of the vessel below the origin of the left colic artery. The ligation of the IMA distal to the left colic artery is often much easier to accomplish, however, and can be associated with a poorer lymph node yield

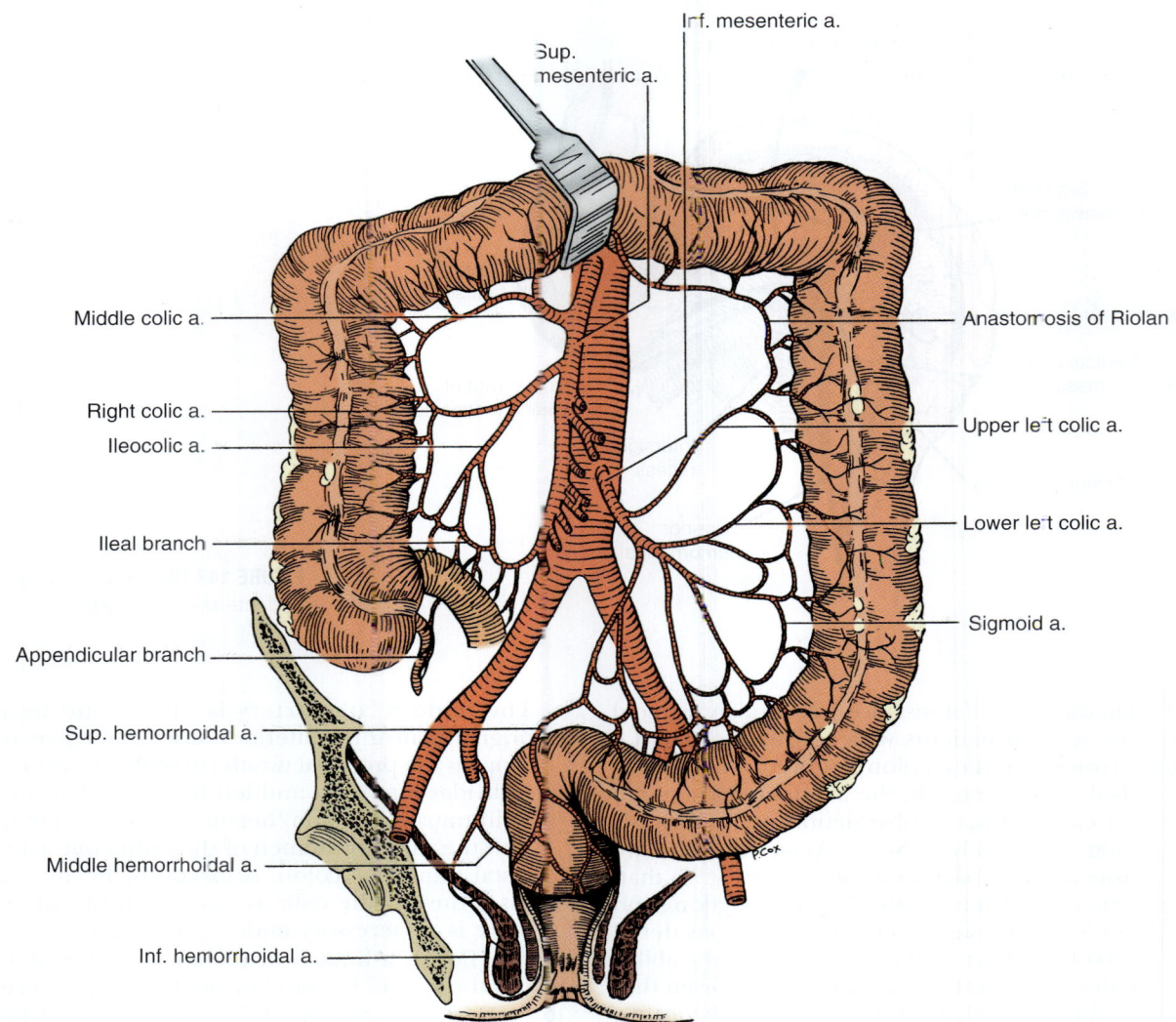

Sup.
mesenteric a.

Inf. mesenteric a.

Middle colic a.

Right colic a.

Ileocolic a.

Ileal branch

Appendicular branch

Sup. hemorrhoidal a.

Middle hemorrhoidal a.

Inf. hemorrhoidal a.

Anastomosis of Riolan

Upper left colic a.

Lower left colic a.

Sigmoid a.

FIGURE 143.11 Vascular supply to the large intestine. *a.,* Artery; *Inf.,* inferior; *Sup.,* superior. (From Keighley MRB, Williams NS. *Surgery of the Anus, Rectum, and Colon.* Philadelphia: Saunders; 1995.)

and possible mesenteric tethering, which does not allow adequate mobility for reaching the proximal colon into the pelvis following a low pelvic dissection.

Aside from the main branches of the SMA and IMA, collateral circulation extends throughout the colon and is integral in the event of an occlusion of a major mesenteric vessel or following surgical ligation. David Drummond (1852–1932) was a physician and anatomist who first demonstrated that despite ligation of the right, middle, and left colic arteries, contrast given via the ileocolic artery was seen in the sigmoidal arteries. Later termed the *marginal artery of Drummond* (MAoD), this typically small-caliber artery spans the entire colon and resides within the outer limits of the mesentery. In the event of critical stenosis or occlusion of either SMA or IMA, it dramatically enlarges to provide flow.[11,12] This collateralization is most variable, however, at the splenic flexure, as this represents the transition from midgut to hindgut. The so-called watershed area, or Griffith point, can have significant clinical implications; some sources

state that nearly 50% of patients do not have collateral circulation in this region. Because of these variations in blood flow, several novel methods have been developed to assess anastomotic viability. Most notable is the use of indocyanine green fluorescence imaging to provide real-time feedback at the time of laparoscopic resection (Fig. 143.13).[13]

The meandering mesenteric artery (MMA), also referred to as the *arc of Riolan*, is a second major collateral pathway providing flow between the middle colic artery and the proximal left colic artery. The MMA resides near the base of the mesentery in the left upper quadrant, is of moderate caliber, and can be tortuous. Similar to the MAoD, the MMA is generally appreciated when critical stenosis or occlusion of the SMA or IMA exists. Recognition of this artery is clinically significant, as ligation of a prominent MMA during left colon surgery may result in catastrophic ischemia, the location dependent upon the direction of flow. If flow is antegrade (SMA to IMA), ischemia of sigmoid colon and upper rectum may ensue. If flow is

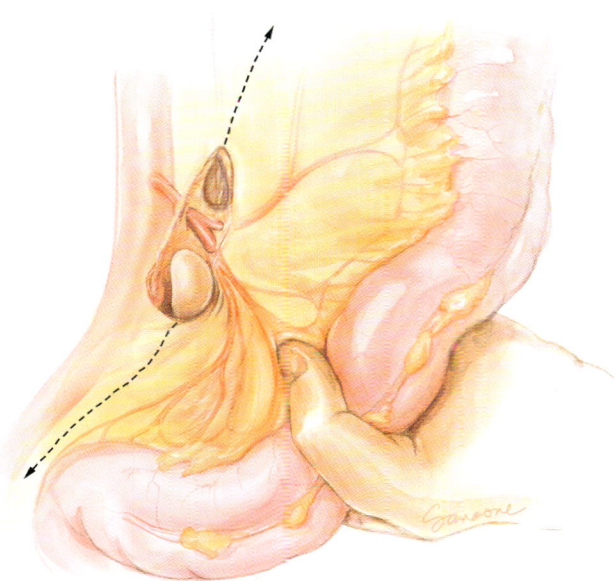

FIGURE 143.12 High ligation of the inferior mesenteric artery during resection of the colon for cancer. (Illustration from John L. Cameron, Corinne Sandone. *Atlas of Gastrointestinal Surgery*. 2nd ed. Vol. II; used with permission from People's Medical Publishing House—USA, Shelton, Connecticut.)

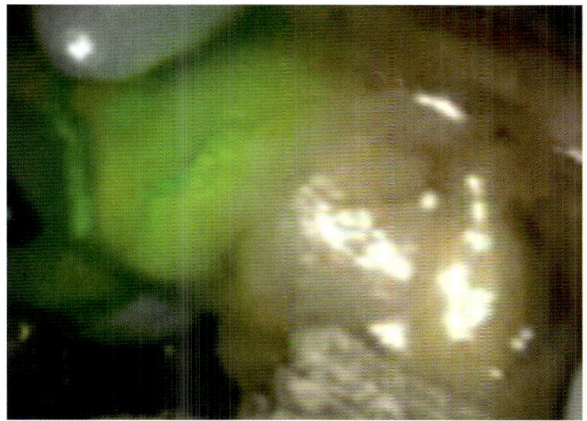

FIGURE 143.13 Demarcation of the colon demonstrating viability using indocyanine green fluorescence. The area that has fluorescence is viable.

retrograde (IMA to SMA), expect ischemia of the right colon and a majority of small bowel.

Lymphatic and Venous Drainage of the Colon

The venous drainage of the colon and rectum corresponds to its arterial supply (Fig. 143.14). The ascending colon drains via the superior mesenteric vein (SMV); blood from the descending colon, sigmoid colon, and rectum drains via the inferior mesenteric vein (IMV). Division of the IMV at a location that is more proximal along the course of the vein may greatly aid in finding more mobility in the proximal colon mesentery, to aid in reaching the pelvis following a low pelvic resection of the rectum.

There are four groups classically described for lymphatic drainage of the colon (Fig. 145.15): epiploic, paracolic, intermediate, and principal. The epiploic group is most abundant in the sigmoid colon. They are located below the peritoneum and on the bowel wall; they also can be found within appendices epiploicae. Paracolic nodes are located throughout the colon along the marginal artery and also tracking among the arcades. The principal "main" nodes parallel the course of the SMA and IMA, whereas the intermediate nodes parallel the colic arterial branches. All four nodal basins will drain into the paraaortic nodes, then cisterna chyli, and ultimately the thoracic duct.

Innervations of the Colon

Sympathetic fibers from T6 to T12 reach and synapse at the celiac, preaortic and superior mesenteric ganglia. Postganglionic fibers travel along the SMA to innervate the cecum, appendix, ascending colon, and proximal two-thirds of the transverse colon. Sympathetic preganglionic fibers of L1, L2, and L3 synapse at the preaortic nerve plexus and send postganglionic fibers as the mesenteric plexus that course along the IMA and innervate the distal one-third of the transverse colon, descending, and sigmoid colon.

Parasympathetic innervation to the cecum, appendix, ascending colon, and proximal two-thirds of the transverse colon is via preganglionic fibers from vagus nerve (right branch) and celiac plexus. These fibers follow the SMA and eventually synapse within the bowel wall to form the intrinsic neural plexuses. Parasympathetic innervation to the distal one-third of the transverse colon, descending, and sigmoid colon arise from S2, S3, and S4.

Colonic pain, as in other areas of the digestive tract, is referred pain. Nash et al. described pain following the insufflation of a balloon in various locations of the colon.[14] Pain from inflating a balloon in the cecum was referred to McBurney point and spread to the epigastrium. Pain from the insufflation in the hepatic flexure is referred to the right upper quadrant. Insufflation in the ascending, transverse, and descending colon was referred to the lower mid line abdomen. Rectosigmoid distention is referred to the suprapubic and coccygeal area.

RECTUM, ANAL CANAL, AND PERIANAL SPACES

Anatomy of the Rectum

The transition to rectum begins after the sigmoid taenia disperses and the colon reaches the sacral promontory. It is 15 cm in length and subdivided into three segments based on distance from the anal verge: lower (0 to 7 cm), middle (7 to 12 cm), and upper (12 to 15 cm). The rectum descends posteriorly in the pelvis and follows the concavity of the sacral hollow. The upper third of the rectum is covered with peritoneum anteriorly and laterally; the middle third of the rectum is covered with peritoneum anteriorly only; and the lower third is completely extraperitoneal. A thick investing layer known as Denonvillier fascia envelops the anterior rectum. This fascia separates the rectum from seminal vesicles and prostate (men) and vagina (women). Posteriorly, the rectum is closely invested with the mesorectum—thick, perirectal tissue that

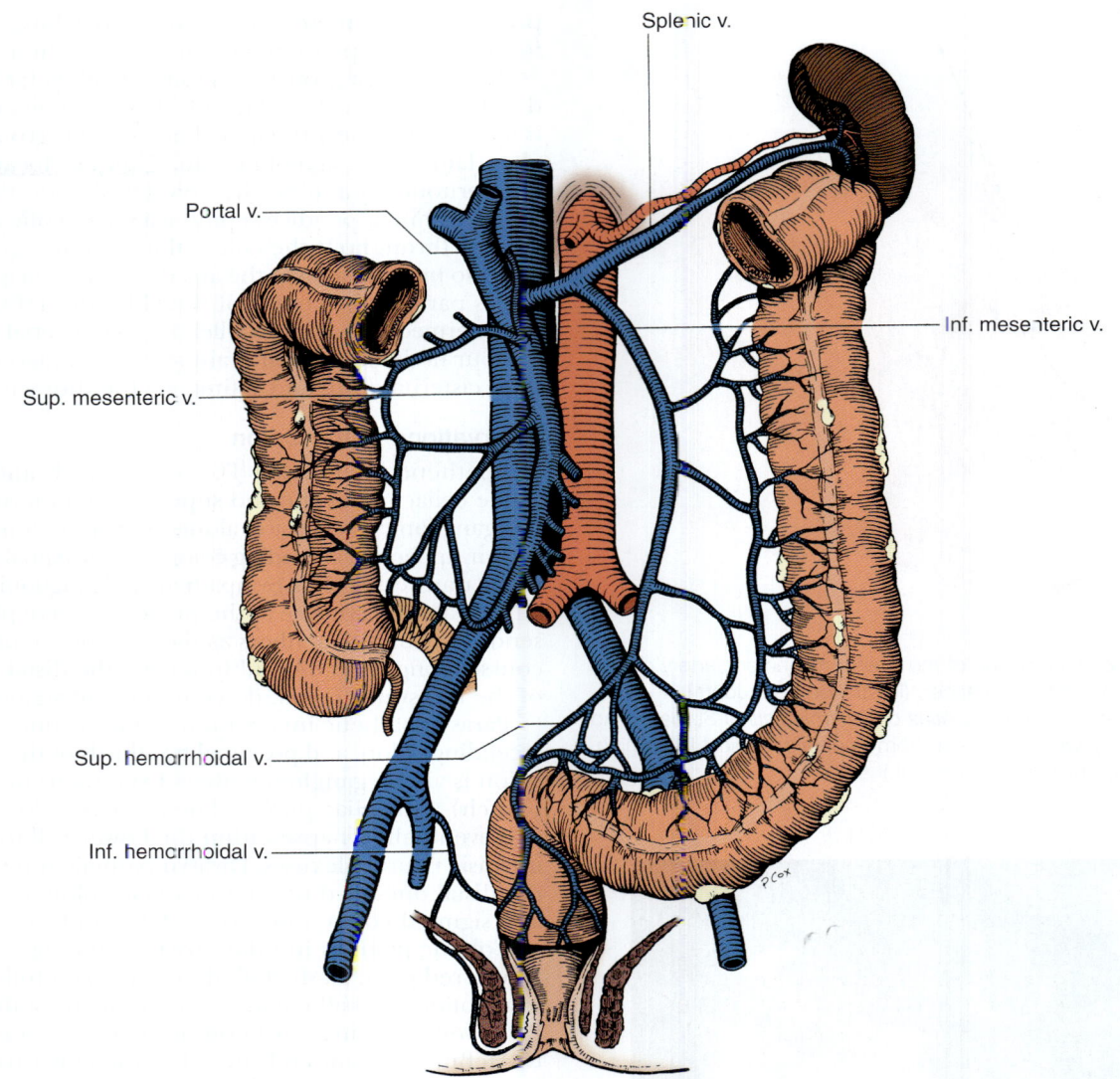

FIGURE 143.14 Venous drainage of the colon and rectum. *Inf.,* Inferior; *Sup.,* superior; *v.,* vein. (From Keighley MRB, Williams NS. *Surgery of the Anus, Rectum, and Colon.* Philadelphia: Saunders; 1995.)

contains associated vessels and lymphatics (Fig. 143.16). The mesorectum is enveloped by the fascia propria (a cephalad continuation of endopelvic fascia) that serves to separate the rectum from the presacral fascia. The term *mesorectum* is a misnomer since the "meso" refers to two layers of peritoneum that suspend an organ and the rectum is not suspended in its extraperitoneal location. In a landmark paper published in 1986, Heald popularized the concept of removal of the entire mesorectum when performing a resection of the rectum for cancer and termed it the TME.[15] Now the standard of care for surgical management of rectal cancer, TME involves circumferential dissection of the rectum along the avascular plane that separates visceral from parietal layers of endopelvic fascia with en bloc inclusion of regional lymphatics and vasculature. Sharp dissection is a critical component of TME to mitigate injury to autonomic nerves and the presacral veins that are invested into the endopelvic fascia.

Midrectum (or just caudal to it), the fascia propria condenses into lateral ligaments (lateral stalks) that anchor the rectum to the nearby endopelvic fascia. A historical topic of controversy, it was previously suggested that the middle rectal arteries were located within the lateral ligaments. Extensive literature review and cadaveric studies have demonstrated that the lateral ligaments do not contain either the middle rectal arteries or significant nerve fibers from the hypogastric plexus. Both are closely related but run underneath this ligament.[16]

The rectum contains three semilunar folds, referred to as the valves of Houston (named after the Irish-born anatomist and surgeon, John Houston [1802–1845]). Most individuals have three valves arranged in a left, right, left configuration from distal to proximal. Measuring from the anal verge, as one might with a colonoscope, the valves are located at 7 to 8 cm (left), 9 to 11 cm (right), and 12 to 13 cm (left). The middle valve (Kohlrausch

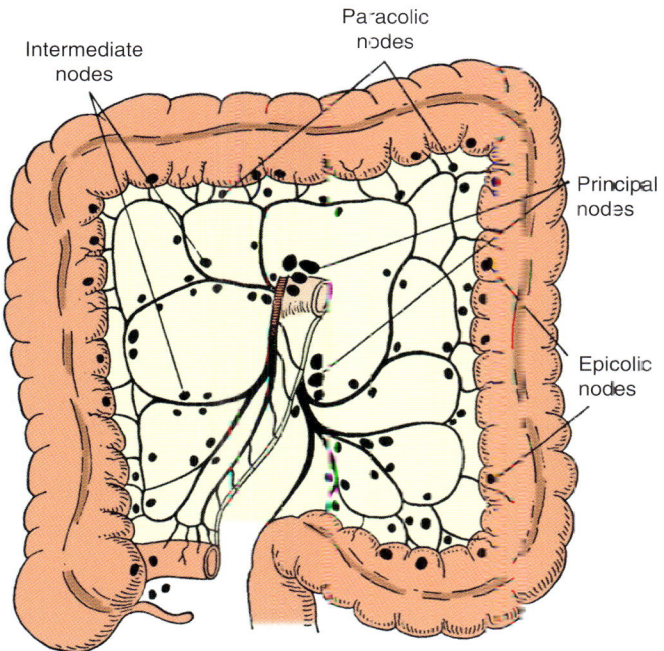

FIGURE 143.15 Lymphatic drainage of the colon and rectum. (From Grinnell RS. Lymphatic metastases of carcinoma of the colon and rectum. *Ann Surg.* 1950;131:494.)

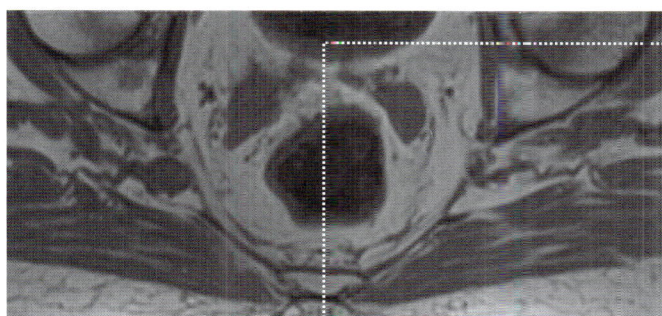

FIGURE 143.16 Axial T2-weighted magnetic resonance image of the pelvis demonstrating the rectum and surrounding mesorectum.

plica) corresponds to the anterior peritoneal reflection. Only about 45% of individuals have standard three-valve anatomy.

Anatomy of the Anal Canal

The distal rectum traverses the anorectal hiatus into the pelvis and intersects with the puborectalis, signifying the start of the anal canal. Anteriorly, the perineal body separates the anal canal from the lower vagina in women and the penile bulb in men. Posteriorly it is fixed to the coccyx via the anococcygeal ligament (Fig. 143.17). Laterally it lies within the soft tissue of the ischiorectal fossa. The "surgical" anal canal spans from the anorectal ring (proximal internal anal sphincter [IAS] and puborectalis muscle) to the anal verge. It is typically a bit longer in males than females, averaging about 4.4 cm and 4.0 cm, respectively. Within the anal mucosa, the anal transition

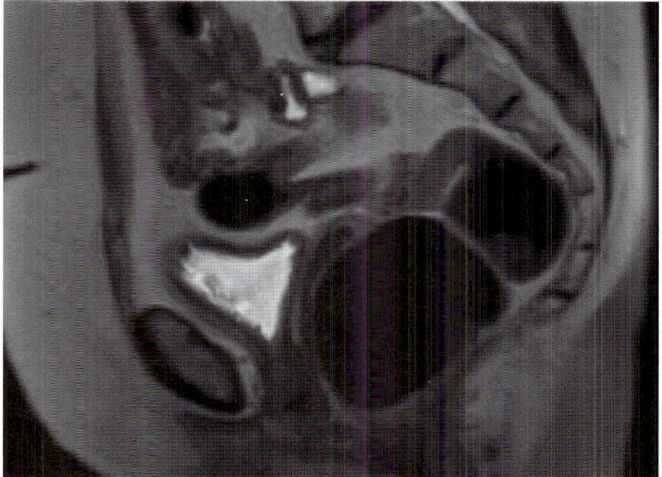

FIGURE 143.17 First valve of Houston demonstrated on sagittal T2-weighted magnetic resonance image. The anococcygeal ligament can be seen just below the valve

zone (ATZ) *begins* about 5 mm above the dentate line; it can be recognized by a visible change from the pink, columnar epithelium of the rectum to the perse squamous epithelium of the anal canal (Fig. 143.18). The histologic transition continues to the dentate line. Located at this level are redundant folds of tissue, known as the columns of Morgagni. Anal crypts form in between columns and are often associated with at least one anal gland. Anal glands are found circumferentially in this region, with preference for the posterior wall, and range between 3 and 12 in number. The majority of these glands originate from the intersphincteric plane within the conjoined longitudinal muscle (CLM); however, accessory branches from within the IAS are not uncommon.

Internal and External Anal Sphincters, Conjoined Longitudinal Muscle

The IAS is an abridgement of the circular smooth muscular layer of the rectum, typically about 2 to 3 mm thick and about 35 mm in length. It is responsible for between 50% to 85% of involuntary resting tone. The balance is from contribution of both the external anal sphincter (EAS, 25%) and anal cushions (hemorrhoids, 15%). The EAS is classically described as a tube of skeletal muscle that extends upward to meet the puborectalis and levator ani muscles. In contrast to the typical behavior of skeletal muscles, the EAS maintains an unconscious resting tone via the reflex arc. During distention of the rectum or increased abdominal pressure, the EAS contracts voluntarily up to 60 seconds to avoid incontinence. Beyond 60 seconds, the muscle becomes fatigued and continence is maintained by the IAS. Distally, the EAS extends beyond the IAS by about 1 cm where it is crossed by fibers from the *corrugator cutis ani muscle*. These fibers arise from the CLM and extend to the perianal skin. Although there are no distinct anatomic boundaries, the EAS can be divided into three components: deep (most proximal, EAS condenses with puborectalis), superficial (intermediate portion, cephalad to the distal aspect of the IAS where EAS posteriorly

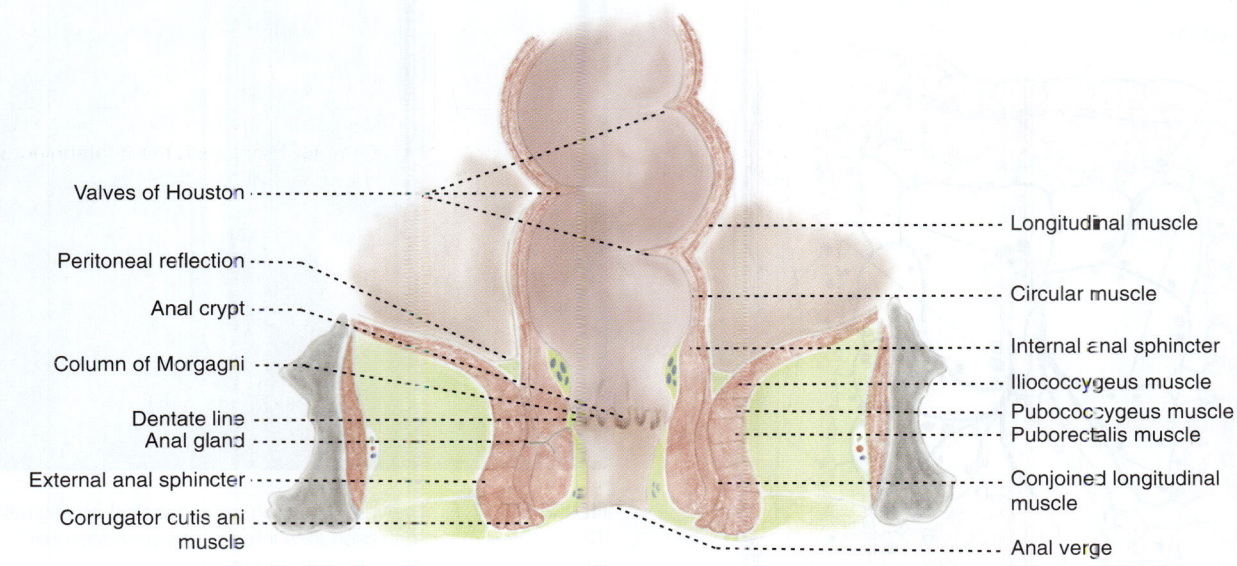

Valves of Houston

Peritoneal reflection

Anal crypt

Column of Morgagni

Dentate line
Anal gland

External anal sphincter

Corrugator cutis ani
muscle

Longitudinal muscle

Circular muscle

Internal anal sphincter

Iliococcygeus muscle

Pubococcygeus muscle

Puborectalis muscle

Conjoined longitudinal
muscle

Anal verge

FIGURE 143.18 Muscular and epithelial anatomy of the anal canal. (Courtesy Matthew P. Kelley, MD.)

attaches to coccyx), and subcutaneous (most distal). Just below the level of the puborectalis, the EAS inserts anteriorly at the perineal body, along with superficial and deep transverse perinei (TP) and bulbocavernosus (BC) muscles. Advanced magnetic resonance imaging and three-dimensional ultrasound have more accurately described these muscles as the "EAS complex muscles." The function of EAS exerts is effect in a purse-string manner with decussation anterior beyond the perineal body and possibly in continuation with the BC muscles. The clinical implication of this finding remains to be seen but should be considered when performing sphincteroplasty.

The CLM originates at the anorectal ring as a continuation of the outer longitudinal rectal muscle, located between the IAS and the EAS, up to 2 mm in thickness. At its origin, it receives minor contribution from the puborectalis muscle and, as mentioned previously, crosses the EAS distally as the *corrugator cutis ani muscle*. Oblique fibers from the midportion of the CLM merge with the IAS to form the smooth muscle component of the submucosa, historically referred to as the muscle of Treitz. The primary function of the CLM is not completely understood but is believed to play three roles. First, it functions as an anchor between the EAS and IAS; second, Haas and Fox proposed that the CLM contributes to the submucosal muscular layer and assists in maintenance of continence following surgical interruption of the anal sphincters; third, it functions as a barrier to infectious communication between adjacent perianal spaces.[17]

Perirectal and Perianal Spaces

A thorough understanding of the potential perianal and perirectal spaces is important for the diagnosis and management of both abscesses and fistula (Table 143.1, Fig. 143.19). Despite relatively distinct anatomic borders, extensive communication between them exists, as seen by the development of a horseshoe abscess in the ischiorectal (Fig. 143.20) or intersphincteric space (Fig. 143.21).

Arterial Supply to the Rectum and Anus

The rectum receives a robust blood supply from three branches: superior, middle, and inferior rectal (hemorrhoidal) arteries (Fig. 143.22). Ischemia is rarely encountered. The primary supply is via the IMA, which becomes the SRA as it crosses the left iliac vessels. Typically the SRA gives off one to two sigmoid branches, one upper rectal branch and then a terminal bifurcation into right and left branches. The internal iliac artery provides blood supply to the remainder of the rectum and anal canal via a direct branch to the middle rectal artery (MRA) and indirectly via the internal pudendal artery to the inferior rectal artery (IRA). The MRA is found bilaterally in the majority of individuals; however, it can be unilateral or absent. The IRA originates from the internal pudendal artery in the pudendal (Alcock) canal, crosses the ischiorectal fossa, and penetrates into the wall of the anal canal.

Anorectal Lymphatic and Venous Drainage

Venous drainage of the rectum occurs via the superior, middle, and inferior rectal veins. The superior rectal vein (SRV) drains the upper two-thirds of the rectum to the IMV and then portal system. The inferior one-third of the rectum and anal canal is drained by the middle and inferior rectal veins into the internal iliac veins and then inferior vena cava.

Lymphatic drainage for the proximal two-thirds follows the IMA nodal chain and ultimately the paraaortic nodes. The distal one-third of the rectum and the anal canal above the dentate line drain cephalad to the superior rectal nodes and inferior mesenteric nodes, and also laterally via the middle rectal nodal chain into internal iliac nodes. Despite being closely related, there is no communication between inferior mesenteric and internal iliac lymphatics—an important concept concerning the locoregional spread of rectal cancer. Lymphatic drainage of the anal canal below the dentate line is to ipsilateral inguinal lymph nodes.

TABLE 143.1 Potential Perianal and Perirectal Spaces

Space	Location	Notes
Perianal	Most superficial space Superior: Dentate line Lateral: EAS (superficial segment) Inferior: Perianal skin Medial: Anoderm	• Most superficial space • Communicates with the intersphincteric space
Intersphincteric (see Fig. 143.21)	Medial: IAS Lateral: EAS/Puborectalis m.	• Communicates with perianal space
Submucous	Medial: Submucosa of anal canal/rectum above dentate line Lateral: IAS	• Contains internal hemorrhoidal cushions
Ischioanal (see Fig. 143.20)	Medial: Levator ani, IAS Lateral: Obturator internus m., obturator fascia Posterior: Gluteus maximus m. Inferior: Perianal skin	• Contains perforating branches of the internal pudendal vessels, pudendal nerve • Communicates with contralateral side via deep postanal space
Supralevator	Medial: Rectum Lateral: Pelvic wall Superior: Peritoneum Inferior: Levator ani m.	—
Retrorectal	Posterior: Presacral fascia Anterior: Retrorectal fascia Lateral: Piriformis m. Inferior: Retrosacral fascia	• Common site for embryologic remnants
Postanal Superficial	Anterior: Anococcygeal ligament Posterior: Perianal skin	—
Postanal Deep	Anterior: Anococcygeal raphe Posterior: Anococcygeal ligament Lateral: Obturator internus m., obturator fascia	• Also known as retrosphincteric space of Courtney • Origin of horseshoe abscesses

EAS, External anal sphincter; *IAS*, internal anal sphincter.

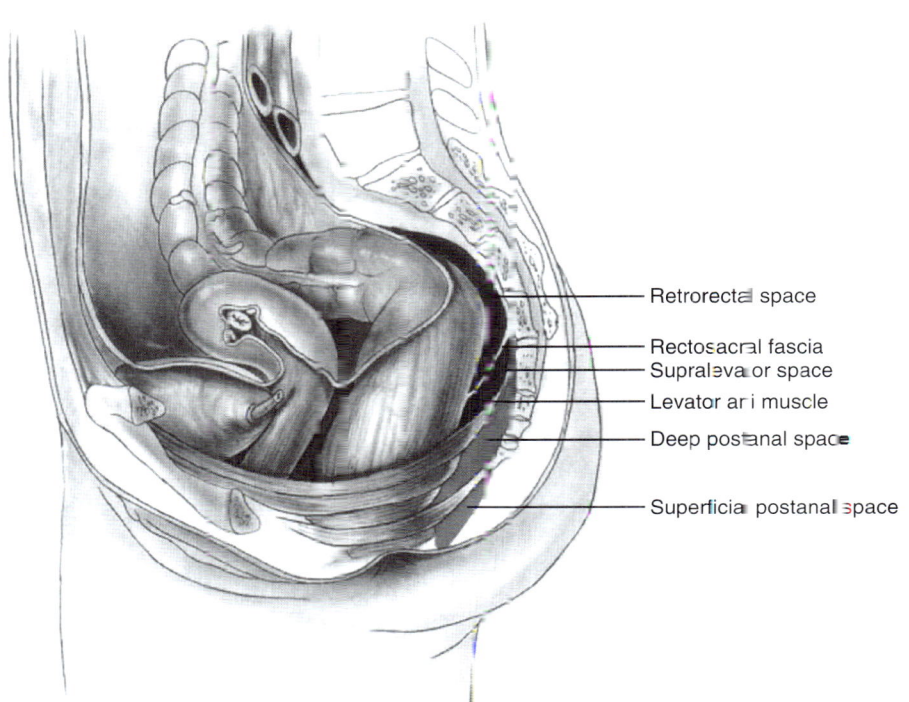

— Retrorectal space

— Rectosacral fascia
— Supralevator space
— Levator ani muscle

— Deep postanal space

— Superficial postanal space

FIGURE 143.19 Schematic of potential perianal and perirectal spaces. (From Moreira H, Wexner SD. Colectomy partial—open. In: *Essential Surgical Procedures.* Philadelphia: Elsevier; 2016:e461–e513.)

Innervation of the Rectum and Anus

The sympathetic innervation originates via preganglionic fibers of L1, L2, and L3. These fibers reach and synapse at the preaortic nerve plexus and send postganglionic fibers as the mesenteric plexus that courses along the IMA and innervates the upper rectum. Sympathetic fibers from the superior hypogastric (presacral) plexus coalesce into left and right hypogastric nerves (see Fig. 143.15). Left and right hypogastric nerves reach and synapse at the inferior hypogastric (pelvic) plexus, located on both sides of the

pelvis and adjacent to the lateral stalks. Either the left or the right hypogastric nerves must be preserved to maintain appropriate delivery of semen from the seminal vesicles to the prostatic urethra. Parasympathetic preganglionic fibers from S2, S3, and S4 are termed nervi erigentes. Nervi erigentes exit through the sacral foramina and course anterolaterally to synapse and contribute (along

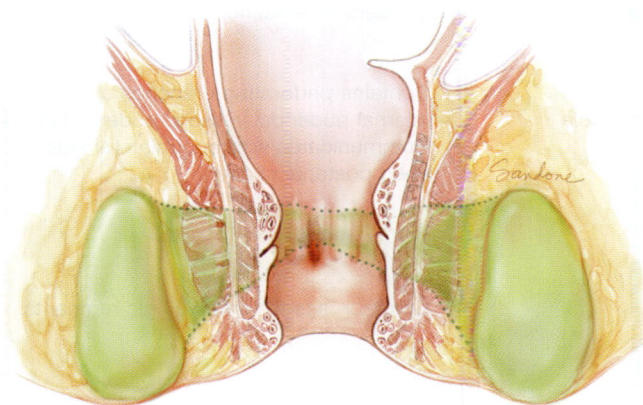

FIGURE 143.20 Ischiorectal horseshoe abscess. Illustration from John L. Cameron, Corinne Sandone. *Atlas of Gastrointestinal Surgery.* 2nd ed. Vol. II; used with permission from People's Medical Publishing House—USA, Shelton, Connecticut.)

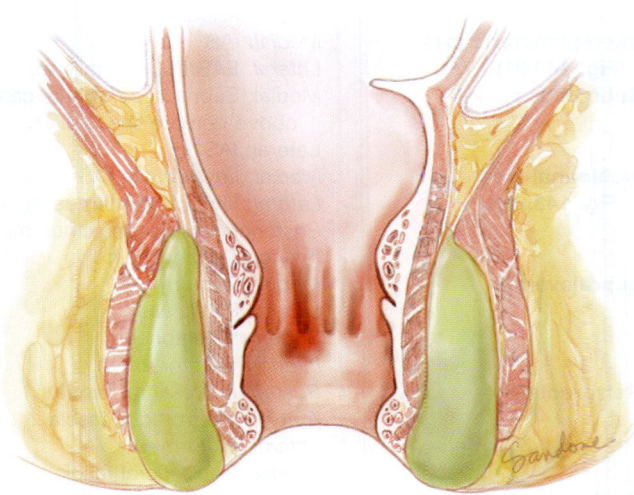

FIGURE 143.21 Intersphincteric horseshoe abscess. (Illustration from John L. Cameron, Corinne Sandone. *Atlas of Gastrointestinal Surgery.* 2nd ed. Vol. II; used with permission from People's Medical Publishing House—USA, Shelton, Connecticut.)

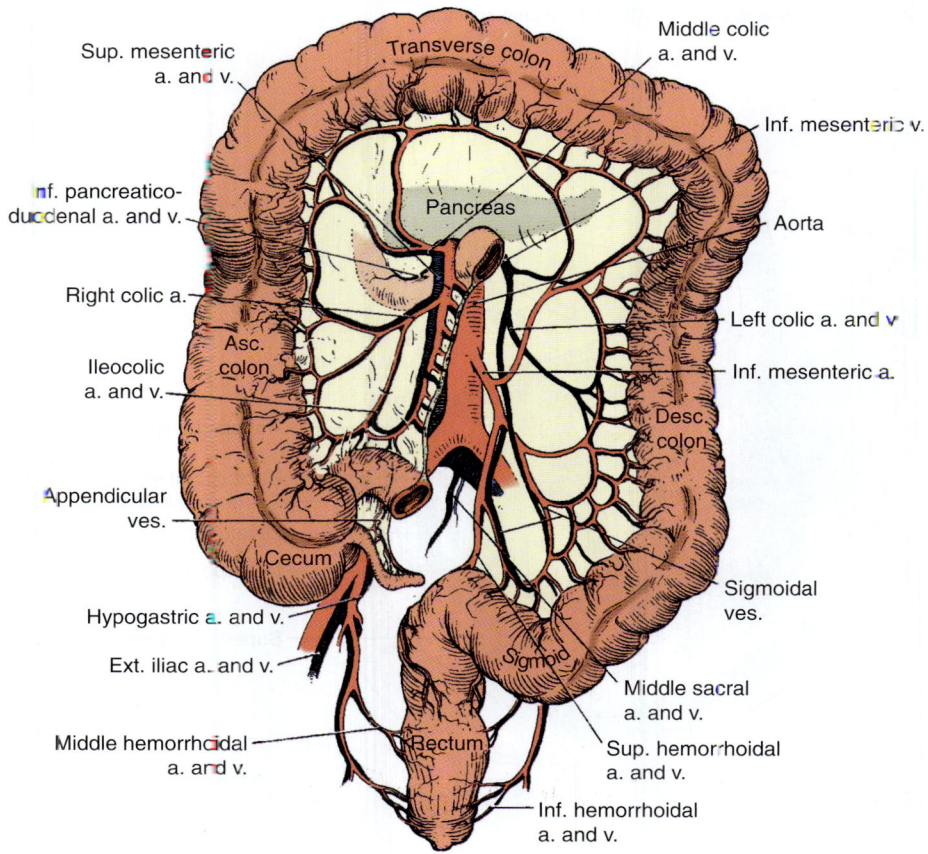

FIGURE 143.22 Vascular supply to the rectum. *a.,* Artery; *Asc.,* ascending; *Desc.,* descending; *Ext.,* external; *Inf.,* inferior; *Sup.,* superior; *v.,* vein; *ves.,* vessel. (Modified from Jones T, Shepard WC. *A Manual of Surgical Anatomy.* Philadelphia: Saunders; 1945.)

EAS receives bilateral innervation via S2 and S3 (inferior rectal branch of the pudendal nerve) and via S4 (perineal branch). The crossover of signal transmission at the spinal cord level prevents loss of EAS control during unilateral injury.

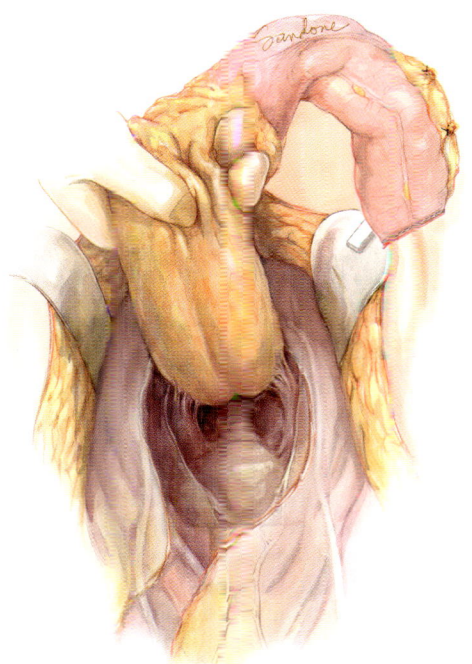

FIGURE 143.23 Intraoperative schematic of the posterior pelvis demonstrating the relationship of the hypogastric nerves to the dissection plane. (Illustration from John L. Cameron Corinne Sandone. *Atlas of Gastrointestinal Surgery*. 2nd ed. Vol. II; used with permission from People's Medical Publishing House—USA, Shelton, Connecticut)

with either hypogastric nerve to the inferior hypogastric (pelvic) plexus. Mixed autonomic postganglionic fibers innervate the rectum, anal canal, bladder, and genitals. Injury to these mixed fibers at the periprostatic plexus may result in both atonic bladder and impotence. Aggressive dissection or lateral traction of the inferior hypogastric plexus can result in sexual dysfunction, with rates of 23% to 69% in men and 19% to 62% in women undergoing surgery for rectal malignancy (Fig. 143.23).[5] Risk factors associated with increased risk of sexual dysfunction are surgery for malignancy, advanced age, use of radiotherapy, and surgical approach (i.e., abdominoperineal resection).

Sympathetic innervation of the IAS is from L5; parasympathetic innervation is from nervi er gentes. The

REFERENCES

1. Development of the Digestive System. *Grays Anatomy*. 29th ed. Tokyo, Japan: 1998:1407-1410.
2. Tan JJ, Tan K, Chew SP. Mesenteric cysts: an institutional experience over 14 years and review of the literature. *World J Surg*. 2009;33:1961.
3. Hirschsprungs H. Falle von angeborener Pylorusstenose beobactet bei Staulingen. *Jahrb Kinderh*. 1888;27:61-69.
4. Lumar D, Phillips SF. The contributions of the external ligamentous attachments to function of the ileocecal junction. *Dis Colon Rectum*. 1987;30:410-416.
5. Pelligrini E Manneschi LK, Manneschi L. The ceacocolonic junction in humans has a sphincteric anatomy and function. *Gut*. 1995;37:493.
6. Southgate E, Vousden N, Karthikeslingam A, et al. Laparoscopic vs. open appendectomy in older patients. *Arch Surg*. 2012;147:557-562.
7. Masoomi H, Mills S, Dlich MO, et al. Comparison of outcomes of laparoscopic vs open appendectomy in children: data from the Nationwide Inpatient Sample (NIS), 2006-2008. *World J Surg*. 2012;36:573-578.
8. Louhia ST Heiskanen JT, Huttunen R, et al. Long-term follow up of a randomized clinical trial of open vs. laparoscopic appendectomy. *Br J Surg*. 2010;97:1395-1400.
9. Gouvas N Pechlinvanides G, Zervakis N, Kafousi M, Xynos E. Complete mesocolic excision in colon cancer surgery a comparison between open and laparoscopic approach. *Colorectal Dis*. 2012;14:1357-1364.
10. Guraya SY Optimum level of inferior mesenteric artery ligation for the left-sided colorectal cancer. Systematic review for high and low ligation continuum. *Saudi Med J*. 2016;37:731-736.
11. Moynihan B. Remarks on the surgery of the large intestine. *Lancet*. 1913;2:1.
12. Dworkin MJ, Allen-Mersch TG. Effect of inferior mesenteric artery ligation on blood flow in the marginal artery-dependent sigmoid colon. *J Am Coll Surg*. 1996;183:357.
13. Rus F, Gines R, Cunningham C, et al. Near-infrared (NIR) perfusion angiography in minimally invasive colorectal surgery. *Surg Endosc*. 2014;28:2221-2226.
14. Nash J. *Surgical Physiology*. Springfield, IL: Charles C Thomas; 1942.
15. Heald RJ, Ryall RD. Recurrence and survival after total mesorectal excision for rectal cancer. *Lancet*. 1986;28:1479-1482.
16. Nano M, Dal Corso HM, Lanfranco G, Ferronato M, Hornung JP. Contribution to the surgical anatomy of the ligaments of the rectum. *Dis Colon Rectum*. 2000;43:1592-1598.
17. Haas PA, Fox TA Jr. The importance of the perianal connective tissue in the surgical anatomy and function of the anus. *Dis Colon Rectum*. 1977;20:303-313.
18. Chew M, Yeh Y, Lim E, Seow-Choose F. Pelvic autonomic nerve preservation in radical rectal cancer surgery: changes in the past 3 decades. *Gastroenterol Rep (Oxf)*. 2016;4:173-185.

Physiology of the Colon and Its Measurement

Adil E. Bharucha | Michael Camilleri

The human colon serves to absorb water and electrolytes, store intraluminal contents until elimination is socially convenient, and salvage nutrients after bacterial metabolism of carbohydrates that have not been absorbed in the small intestine. These functions are dependent on the colon's ability to control the distal progression of contents; in healthy adults, colonic transit normally requires several hours to almost 3 days for completion. There are differences in colonic structure and function even among mammals[1]; unless otherwise stated, this chapter will focus on the physiology of colonic function in humans. Although the colon is regarded as a single organ, there are regional differences between the right and left colon, indicated in Table 144.1. The right and left colon are derived from the embryologic midgut and hindgut, and the junction is located just proximal to the splenic flexure.

ANATOMY

GROSS ANATOMY

In adult cadavers the colon is approximately 1.5 m long. The musculature in the colonic wall is composed of outer longitudinal and inner circular layers. From the cecum to the rectosigmoid junction, the longitudinal layer is organized in three thick bands, the taeniae, with a thin layer of longitudinal muscle in between these bands.[2] At the rectosigmoid junction, the three taeniae broaden to form a uniformly thick layer throughout the rectum. In the anal canal, the longitudinal muscle layer extends into a plane between the external anal sphincter and the circular muscle layer that thickens to become the internal anal sphincter to insert on the perianal skin as the corrugator cutis ani muscle. Other than humans, only primates, horses, guinea pigs, and rabbits have taeniae coli[3]; the taeniae coli are thought to function as suspension cables upon which the circular muscle arcs are suspended, facilitating efficient contraction of the circular muscle. Thus a 17% contraction of circular muscle reduces the luminal diameter of the colon by two-thirds.[4] If the longitudinal muscles were arranged concentrically, an identical contraction of circular muscle would reduce luminal diameter by only one-third. Whether or not longitudinal and circular muscles contract synchronously during peristalsis is controversial.

The colon is suspended from the posterior abdominal wall by a mesentery. The mesentery is relatively narrow, restricting mobility of the cecum and ascending and descending colon. Around the transverse and sigmoid colon, the mesentery is broader, permitting considerable movement and contributing to the tendency in some individuals to have a pendulous transverse colon or a floppy sigmoid colon. This contributes to the looping of the colonoscope during examination.

ENTERIC NERVOUS SYSTEM

Colonic neurons, interstitial cells of Cajal (ICC), and smooth muscle work in concert to effectuate colonic contraction. The enteric nervous system possesses afferent neurons, interneurons, and motor neurons that can initiate physiologic motor activity in the absence of extrinsic input. The ICC form extensive networks in the myenteric plexus (ICC_{MY}), which is situated between longitudinal and circular muscle layers, and the submucosal plexus (ICC_{SM}) deep to the circular muscle layer (see Fig. 144.5), from where it regulates mucosal absorption. A separate layer—the intramuscular ICC (ICC_{IM})—is found in the septa that separate bundles of circular muscle cells. ICC_{MY} and ICC_{SM} form extensive networks along the colon and are electrically coupled to one another, the smooth muscle cells, and enteric motor neurons. ICC regulate colonic motility via several mechanisms. They generate electrical slow waves, which then propagate through smooth muscle cells via gap junctions[5] and influence the smooth muscle membrane potential and membrane potential gradient,[6] and they partly mediate mechanosensitivity in smooth muscle.[7] They may also mediate neurotransmission from axons of enteric motor neurons to the smooth muscle,[5] although this has recently been questioned.[8,9]

CELLULAR BASIS FOR MOTILITY

Contraction of smooth muscle results from interactions between smooth muscle, the ICC, the intrinsic or enteric nervous system, and the extrinsic nervous system. ICC are the pacemaker cells, responsible for generating slow wave activity that drives smooth muscle contraction. ICC also amplify neuronal input, act as mechanotransducers, and regulate smooth muscle membrane potential. The three basic electrical events recorded from human colonic circular smooth muscle in vitro are[10]: (1) slow wave activity with a frequency of two to four contractions/minute originating along the submucosal plexus border of the circular muscle layer; (2) membrane potential oscillations (MPOs), with a frequency of approximately 18 contractions/minute, originating in the myenteric plexus border of circular muscle; and (3) action potentials superimposed upon slow waves and MPOs.

Slow waves and MPOs summate in the central region of circular muscle producing a complex pattern of activity that regulates contractile amplitude and frequency. The predominant contractile rhythm recorded from the human colon in vitro and in vivo corresponds to the slow wave frequency of two to four/minute. Repolarization of membrane potential during slow waves results in opening of L-type calcium channels and, when a firing threshold

TABLE 144.1 Comparison of Right and Left Colon

Feature	Right Colon	Left Colon
Embryologic origin	Midgut	Hindgut
Blood supply	Superior mesenteric vessels	Inferior mesenteric vessels
EXTRINSIC NERVE SUPPLY		
Parasympathetic	Vagus	Pelvic nerves from sacral S2-S4 segments
Sympathetic	Superior mesenteric ganglion	Inferior mesenteric ganglion
Function	Mixing and storage	Conduit

is reached, action potentials. The result is Ca^{2+} influx through voltage-dependent dihydropyridine-sensitive L-type Ca^{2+} channels. Calcium phosphorylates the myosin light chains in the contractile apparatus to trigger cross-bridge cycling and smooth muscle contraction. Action potentials superimposed upon low waves greatly augment Ca^{2+} entry. Between slow waves, the open probability for Ca^{2+} channels is low, so action potentials and powerful muscle contractions do not occur. Colonic slow waves may also trigger sufficient Ca^{2+} influx to activate the contractile apparatus. Strain gauge transducers used in older studies were too insensitive to detect small contractile events.[11] L-type Ca^{2+} channels are blocked by nifedipine. In the presence of nifedipine, smooth muscle contraction is inhibited and action potentials are absent. Tonic contractions are generated by continuous action potentials. In contrast to regular cyclical contractile activity in the stomach and small intestine, colonic motility is markedly irregular. This irregularity is partly attributable to the variable frequency and duration of action potentials but is not well understood.

EXTRINSIC NERVE SUPPLY TO THE COLON

The extrinsic innervation includes sympathetic and parasympathetic components. The vagus (parasympathetic) innervates the proximal colon. The parasympathetic input to the distal colon is derived from the sacral (S2-S4) segments of the spinal cord via the pelvic plexus. After entering the colon, these fibers form the ascending colonic nerves, traveling orad in the plane of the myenteric plexus to supply a variable portion of the left colon. The sympathetic fibers originate in the paravertebral "chain" ganglion, segments from the T12 to L3 levels of the spinal cord, and are conveyed to the colon via arterial arcades of the superior and inferior mesenteric vessels. The sympathetic nervous system provides excitatory input to the sphincters and a tonic inhibitory input to nonsphincteric muscle. Norepinephrine is the major neurotransmitter released by sympathetic nerves throughout the small and large intestine. The extrinsic nerves modulate the intrinsic neural activity. For example, sympathetic nervous system exerts a tonic inhibitory input on colonic motor function, primarily via stimulation of α-adrenergic receptors, which hyperpolarize cholinergic neurons in the myenteric plexus.

Thus the α_2 agonist clonidine decreases colonic tone, whereas the α_2 antagonist yohimbine increases colonic tone in humans[12]; clonidine also enhances mucosal absorption of fluid and salt.

FUNCTIONS

REGIONAL HETEROGENEITY IN COLONIC FUNCTION

The right colon functions primarily as a reservoir for mixing and storage processes, the left colon as a conduit, and the rectum and anal canal enable defecation and continence. The ileocolonic sphincter regulates the intermittent aborad transfer of ileal contents into the colon, mainly after meals, and prevents reflux of bacteria into the ileum. The rate of delivery of liquids into the proximal colon can influence colonic transit. Thus a liquid marker injected directly into the proximal colon is emptied more rapidly than after oral ingestion of the same marker[13]. There is evidence for adaptation in these regional functions. Within 6 months after a right hemicolectomy, isotope movement from the small to large bowel normalizes in response to the augmented storage capacity in the residual transverse and descending colon.[14] In humans the ileocolonic sphincter plays only a minor role in regulating ileocolonic transit.

COLONIC FLUID AND ELECTROLYTE TRANSPORT

Under basal conditions, the healthy colon receives approximately 1500 mL of chyme over 24 hours, absorbing all but 100 mL of fluid and 1 mEq of sodium and chloride, which are lost in the feces.[15] Colonic absorptive capacity can increase to 5 to 6 L and 800 to 1000 mEq of sodium and chloride daily when challenged by larger fluid loads entering the cecum, as long as there is a slow infusion rate (i.e., 1 to 2 mL/minute). In addition to the ascending and transverse colon, the rectosigmoid may also participate in this compensatory absorptive response.[16] Absorptive mechanisms are constitutively expressed in crypt epithelial cells; secretion is regulated by one or more neurohumoral agonists released from lamina propria cells, including myofibroblasts.[17]

When the colon is perfused with a plasma-like solution, water, sodium, and chloride are absorbed, and potassium and bicarbonate are secreted into the colon.[18] Absorption of sodium and secretion of bicarbonate in the colon are active processes occurring against an electrochemical gradient. There are several different active (transcellular) processes for absorbing sodium and these show considerable segmental heterogeneity in the human colon. The regional differentiation of colonic mucosal absorption is also demonstrated by regional effects of glucocorticoids and mineralocorticoids on sodium and water fluxes. For example, in the *distal* colon, epithelial Na^+, K^+, and ATPase are activated by mineralocorticoids.[19] On the other hand, the Na^+/H^+ exchange is activated in *proximal* colonic epithelium by the mineralocorticoid aldosterone.[20] Specific channels are involved in water transport across surfaces and epithelia. These water channels, or aquaporins (AQPs), are a diverse family of proteins, of which AQP8 is expressed preferentially in colonic epithelium and small intestinal villus tip cells.

Potassium is absorbed and secreted by active processes; it is unclear if chloride is absorbed by an active process. In contrast to the small intestine, glucose and amino acids are not absorbed in the colon.

Colonic conservation of sodium is vital to fluid and electrolyte balance, particularly during dehydration, when it is enhanced by aldosterone.[21] Patients with ileostomies are susceptible to dehydration, particularly when placed on a low sodium diet or during an intercurrent illness. In addition to glucocorticoids and mineralocorticoids (aldosterone), other factors enhancing active sodium transport include somatostatin, α_2-adrenergic agents, and short-chain fatty acids (SCFAs). Clonidine mimics the effects of adrenergic innervation by stimulating α_2 receptors on colonocytes. In contrast, stimulation of mucosal muscarinic cholinergic receptors inhibits active NaCl absorption and stimulates active chloride secretion. Somatostatin, a peptide released by submucosal and myenteric nerves, also has potent antisecretory effects.

COLONIC METABOLISM

In the proximal colon, bacteria ferment organic carbohydrates to SCFAs, predominantly acetate, propionate, and butyrate.[22] There is a low, normal rate of SCFA production from malabsorbed (up to 10% of ingested) carbohydrates; diets high in fiber, beans, resistant starches, and complex carbohydrates increase the production of SCFA. SCFA are rapidly absorbed from the colon, augment sodium, chloride, and water absorption and constitute the preferred metabolic fuel for colonocytes. SCFA may also serve to regulate proliferation, differentiation, gene expression, immune function, and wound healing in the colon.

COLONIC MICROFLORA

The human intestinal tract contains a large variety of microorganisms, of which bacteria are the most dominant and diverse. Contrary to earlier estimates that suggested that the number of bacteria exceeded human cells by a factor of 100,[23] a revised estimate suggests that the number of bacteria and cells in humans is similar (i.e., approximately 39 trillion).[24] Three bacterial divisions, the Firmicutes (gram positive), Bacteroidetes (gram negative), and Actinobacteria (gram positive), dominate the adult human gut microbiota. Among other multifaceted effects, microflora can affect gastrointestinal (GI) motility by releasing bacterial substances or end products of bacterial fermentation (e.g., SCFA), affecting intestinal neuroendocrine factors, and by modulating immunity.[25] The composition of microbiota is associated with stool consistency.[26] Moreover, the profile of the colonic *mucosal* microbiota differed between constipated patients and healthy people, independent of colonic transit, and discriminated between patients with constipation and controls with 94% accuracy.[27] Genera from Bacteroidetes were more abundant in the colonic mucosal microbiota of patients with constipation. In contrast, the *fecal* microbiota were associated with colonic transit and were not different between constipation and health. Genera from Firmicutes (*Faecalibacterium, Lactococcus,* and *Roseburia*) were correlated with faster colonic transit. Perhaps this association is mediated by cholic acid, which increases the relative

abundance of Firmicutes over Bacteroidetes[28] and accelerates colonic transit, particularly in irritable bowel syndrome (IBS).[11] Alternatively, it is conceivable that faster transit is associated with lesser production of secondary bile acids, which may alter the microbiota.

Small intestinal bacterial overgrowth is a recognized complication of intestinal motility disorders (e.g., intestinal pseudoobstruction, scleroderma, radiation enteropathy). During a lactulose-hydrogen breath test, some patients with IBS have increased breath hydrogen excretion. This has erroneously been attributed to small intestinal bacterial overgrowth.[29,30] Rather, in many patients the increased breath hydrogen excretion is explained by rapid small intestinal transit, hence colon delivery, and bacterial metabolism of lactulose.[31] Thus lactulose and glucose hydrogen breath tests are not recommended for identifying small intestinal bacterial overgrowth.[32]

COLONIC MOTILITY

Assessment of Colonic Motor Function

Colonic Transit

Radiopaque Marker Methods. Since the original description by Hinton et al., there have been several refinements to the radiopaque marker technique for measuring colonic transit.[5] A widely used approach is to give a capsule containing 24 radiopaque markers on days 1, 2, and 3 and count remaining markers on a plain abdominal x-ray on days 4 and 7.[6] With this technique a total of 68 or fewer markers remaining in the colon is normal, whereas more than 68 markers is slow transit (Fig. 144.1).[6]

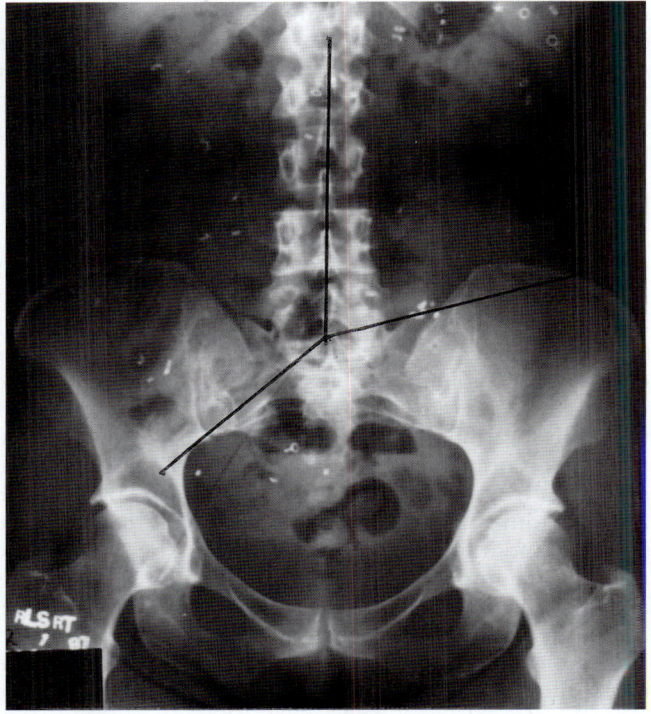

FIGURE 144.1 Abdominal radiograph demonstrating radiopaque markers and lines used to demarcate markers in the left, right, and sigmoid colon/rectum.

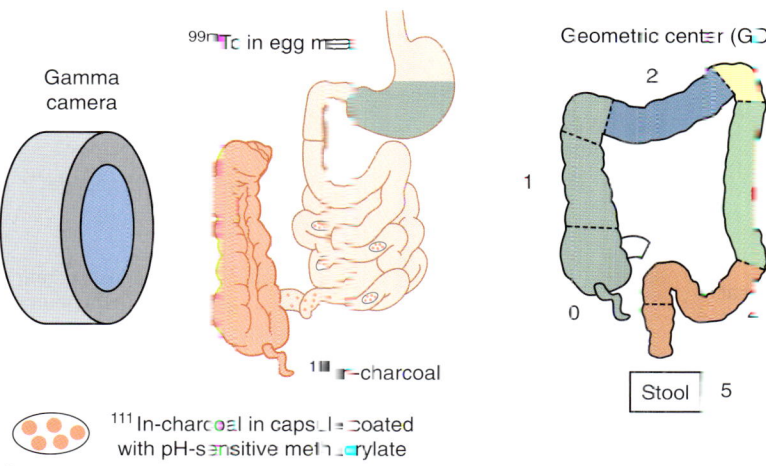

Gamma camera

^{99m}Tc in egg meal

^{111}In-charcoal

^{111}In-charcoal in capsule coated with pH-sensitive methacrylate

A

Geometric center (GC)

Stool   5

B

FIGURE 144.2 Scintigraphic assessment of gastrointestinal transit. (A) Gastric emptying and small intestinal transit are assessed with technetium 99m–labeled polystyrene pellets, whereas indium 111 (^{111}In)–labeled charcoal in delayed-release capsules measures colonic transit. (B) Proportion of ^{111}In counts in each of four colonic regions of interest and stool is multiplied by the appropriate weighting factor, ranging from 1 to 5.

Scintigraphic Techniques. Colonic transit can also be assessed by scintigraphy (Fig. 144.2).[5] To avoid dispersion of the radiolabel during passage through the GI tract, the isotope is delivered into the colon by orocecal intubation or a delayed-release capsule. The delayed-release capsule contains activated charcoal or polystrene pellets radiolabeled with technetium 99m (^{99m}Tc) or indium 111 (^{111}In) and covered with a single coating of a pH-sensitive polymer, methacrylate. The capsule dissolves at a pH between 7.2 and 7.4, generally within the distal ileum, releasing the radioisotope within the ascending colon. The colonic distribution of radioisotope on scans taken 4, 24, and 48 hours after administration of the capsule is highly sensitive and specific for identifying rapid or slow colonic transit. The proportion of counts in each of four colonic regions of interest (i.e., ascending, transverse, descending, and rectosigmoid colon) and stool is multiplied by a specific weighting factor, which ranges from 1 (for the ascending colon) to 5 (for stool). The aggregate of these products (proportion of counts × weighting factor) provides the geometric center of overall colonic transit. A low geometric center implies that most radiolabel is close to the cecum, whereas a high geometric center implies that most radiolabel is close to stool.

pH-Pressure Capsule. Colonic transit can also be recorded by an ingested capsule that measures pH, pressure, and temperature as it traverses the GI tract. The pH rises abruptly (by >2 units) when the capsule exits the stomach and drops rapidly (by >1 unit) when it crosses the ileocecal valve. In the largest studies to date, overall agreement between capsule and radiopaque markers for characterizing colonic transit was 87%.[7,8] Although the capsule can also assess gastric emptying and small intestinal transit, its sensitivity for detecting delayed gastric emptying (i.e., gastroparesis), as defined by gastric emptying measured by scintigraphy at 4 hours, is limited (i.e., 44%).[9]

In summary, allowing for differences in particle size, all three techniques probably provide comparable assessments of colonic transit. Scintigraphy and radiopaque marker techniques entail similar total body radiation exposure (i.e., 0.08 rad) for the radioactive capsule and for each abdominal radiograph. Scintigraphy is a useful research tool that allows more thorough assessment of regional colonic functions.

Colonic Motility

Recording Techniques. Colonic motor activity can be assessed by recording electrical signals or variations in luminal pressure by pressure transducers, either water perfused or solid state, or a balloon controlled by a barostat.[33,34] There are several limitations to recording colonic motor activity in humans. Intraluminal colonic recording devices can only be positioned using flexible colonoscopy, per-oral or per-nasal intubation techniques. Cleansing of the rectosigmoid and occasionally the entire colon is necessary to facilitate placement and accurate recording. Cleansing can accelerate colonic transit, but does not, with the exception of more frequent high-amplitude propagated contractions (HAPCs), fundamentally alter motor activity.[35]

Recording myoelectrical activity with serosal, mucosal, or intraluminal electrodes is fraught with technical difficulties and has fallen out of favor. Manometry can identify the colonic motor response to a meal (see later) or to a stimulatory agent, such as neostigmine or bisacodyl. However, intraluminal pressure changes may not necessarily reflect colonic contractions. Moreover, it can be challenging to assess propagation with traditional manometry catheters because of the distance, typically 10 cm, between manometric sensors. In high-resolution manometry catheters, sensors are spaced at 1-cm intervals; assessing propagation is simpler.[36]

In contrast to manometry, barostat assessments by an infinitely compliant polyethylene balloon continuously apposed to the colonic mucosa can identify colonic contraction and relaxation (Fig. 144.3). The barostat is a rigid piston within a cylinder that can adjust either the pressure or volume within the bag using a servomechanism. When the balloon is inflated to a low constant pressure, colonic contraction is accompanied by expulsion of air from the balloon into the barostat. Conversely, when the colon relaxes, the balloon volume increases to maintain a constant pressure. The advantages of the barostatic balloon over manometry are greater sensitivity for

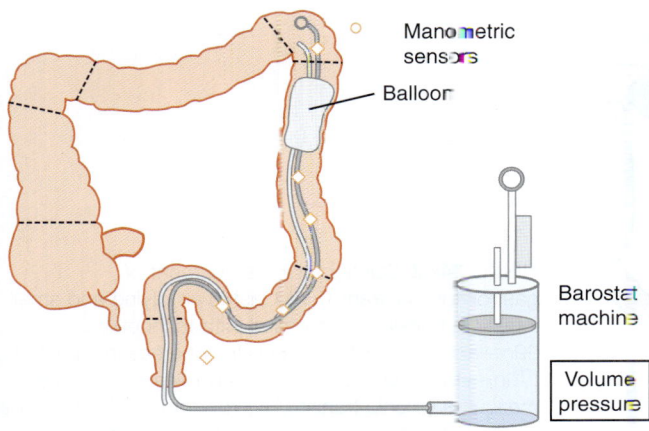

FIGURE 144.3 Barostat-manometric assembly positioned in the descending colon with polyethylene balloon in apposition with colonic mucosa.

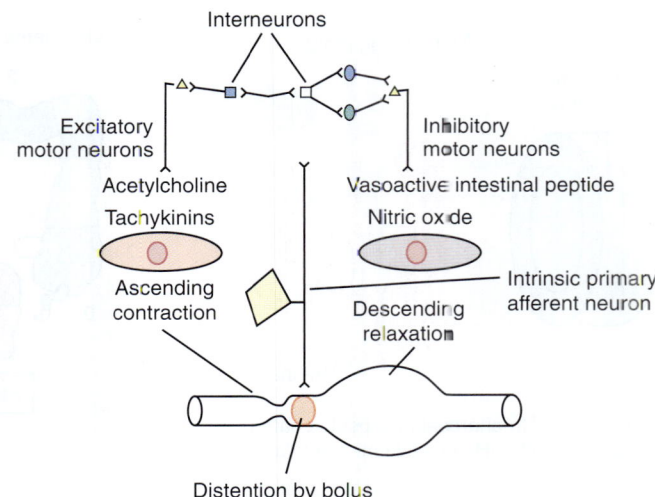

FIGURE 144.4 Schematic representation of major neurotransmitters mediating peristaltic reflex. Mechanical distention activates sensory neurons while interneurons transmit messages between sensory and motor neurons. (Modified from work by Grider and Makhlouf; Furness and Costa.)

recording contractions that do not occlude the lumen, particularly when the colonic diameter is greater than 5.6 cm.[37] Moreover, a barostat can record changes in baseline balloon volume and phasic fluctuations, coloric relaxation, and colonic pressure-volume relationships. Thus the barostat is primarily a research tool that has been introduced into clinical practice in selected centers. The barostat measurement is the only currently available technique to measure colonic tone, and it has been shown to characterize the primary motor problem in chronic megacolon.[38]

Peristalsis

Distention of a viscus evokes the peristaltic reflex, characterized by coordinated contraction of the orad segment and relaxation of the distal gut, facilitating propulsion. The neural pathways and neurotransmitters mediating this reflex are depicted in Fig. 144.4. In the human colon the principal excitatory neurotransmitter is acetylcholine, whereas in vitro studies suggest that nitric oxide and adenosine triphosphate are inhibitory neurotransmitters in the human colon.

Colonic Motor Function in Health. Contractile activity in the human colon is not cyclical. Colonic motor activity may vary from no activity or quiescence, isolated contractions, bursts of contractions, or propagated contractions. Irregular phasic activity constitutes a major proportion of colonic motor activity and probably serves to segment and mix intraluminal contents. Combined assessments of motor activity and transit in the cleansed colon of healthy subjects reveal that transit is associated with nonpropagated and propagated contractions; propagated contractions propel contents over longer distances than nonpropagated contractions.[39] However only one-third of propagated contractions are accompanied by propulsion of colonic contents. Propagated contractions are subclassified as low (5 to 40 mm Hg) or high amplitude (>75 mm Hg). In ambulatory, prolonged colonic manometry studies, HAPCs occur on an average of 6 times/day, originate predominantly in the cecum/ascending colon, and migrate over a variable distance. These HAPCs are probably responsible

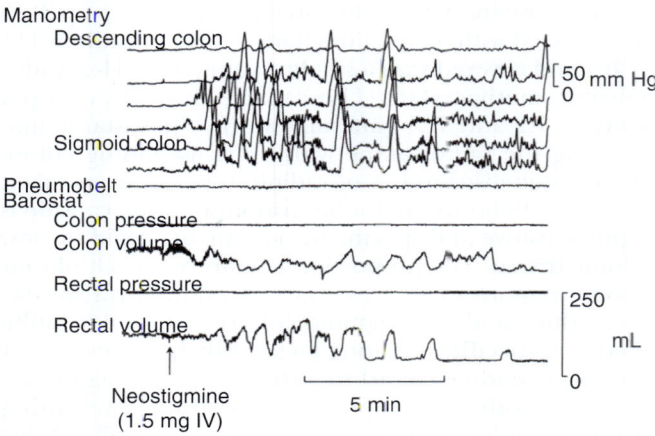

FIGURE 144.5 High-amplitude propagated contractions induced by neostigmine. (From Law NM, Bharucha AE, Undale AS, Zinsmeister AR. *Am J Physiol.* 1997;281:G1228–G1237.)

for mass movement of colonic contents. HAPCs occur more frequently after awakening and after meals and may account for the urge to defecate in healthy subjects and in patients with IBS (Fig. 144.5). The mechanisms that underlie HAPCs are poorly understood. In addition to occurring spontaneously, HAPCs can be induced by luminal distention, by the parenteral administration of cholinesterase inhibitor neostigmine, or by intraluminal stimuli (i.e., glycerol, bisacodyl, and oleic acid).

Eating is accompanied by a brisk increase in tone and phasic activity throughout the colon (Fig. 144.6).[40] Because this response is preserved even after a gastrectomy, the term "colonic motor response to eating" is preferred to "gastrocolonic reflex." The response may begin within a few seconds after eating and last, to a varying degree, for up to 2.5 hours. A biphasic response with early (first 60

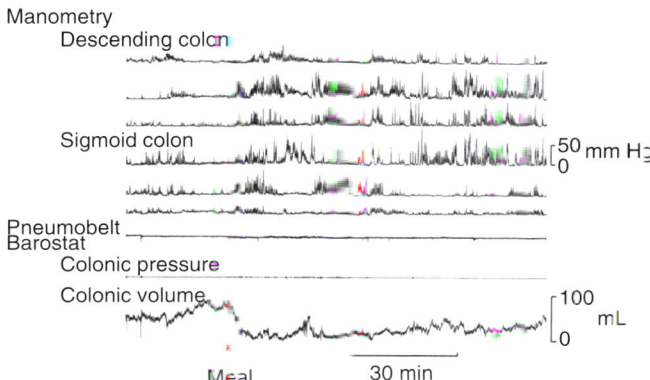

Manometry
Descending colon

Sigmoid colon
50 mm Hg
0

Pneumobelt
Barostat
Colonic pressure

Colonic volume
100 mL
0

Meal   30 min

FIGURE 144.6 Colonic motor response to a 1000-kcal meal. Note the increased phasic pressure activity recorded by manometric sensors and reduction in barostat balloon volume maintained at constant pressure, indicating increased tone.

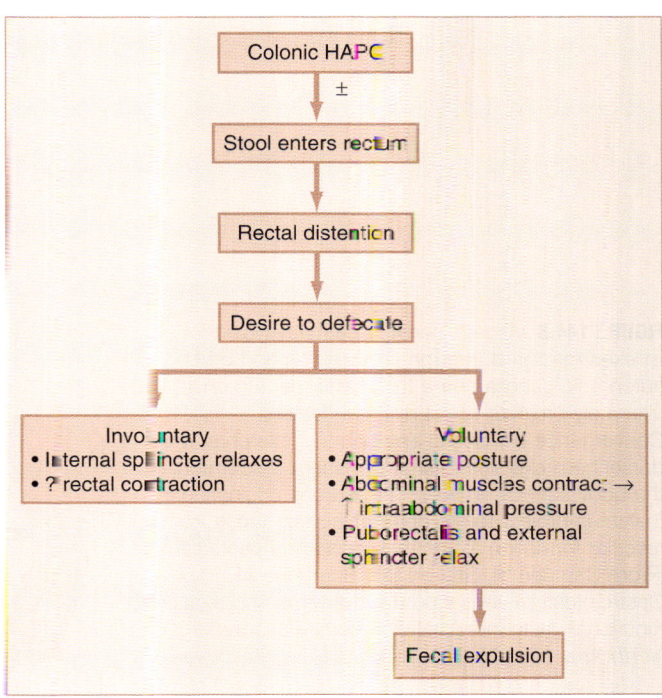

Colonic HAPC
±
Stool enters rectum

Rectal distention

Desire to defecate

Involuntary
• Internal sphincter relaxes
• ? rectal contraction

Voluntary
• Appropriate posture
• Abdominal muscles contract →
  ↑ intraabdominal pressure
• Puborectalis and external
  sphincter relax

Fecal expulsion

FIGURE 144.7 Schematic representation of events preceding defecation. *HAPCs,* High-amplitude propagated contractions.

minutes) and late (120 and 150 minutes) components has also been described.[41] Meal composition and caloric content both influence the response. A mixed meal containing greater than 500 kcal predictably elicits a response. Gastric distention and chemical stimulation by nutrients elicit comparable responses; lipids are the most potent stimuli, whereas amino acids appear to inhibit the response.[42]

The precise mechanisms mediating the response are uncertain, but neural and hormonal mechanisms have been implicated. It is conceivable that different mechanisms regulate the early and late components.[43] The early, particularly the immediate component is likely to be neurally mediated. The later component temporally coincides with arrival of chyme into the ileum and may be mediated by humoral factors, such as peptide YY, neuropeptide Y, and neurotensin released from the ileal mucosa. Although serum levels of gastrin and cholecystokinin rise after a meal, intravenous cholecystokinin actually induces colonic relaxation.[44] Atropine, naloxone, and the 5-hydroxytryptamine type 3 (5-HT₃) antagonist ondansetron inhibit the response indicating that cholinergic, opiate, and serotoninergic 5-HT₃ receptors may be involved in mediating the response.[45] There is also evidence to suggest that efferent vagal fibers contribute to the colonic motor response in primates.[46]

The colon relaxes during sleep, after intraluminal administration of SCFAs or glycerol, during balloon distention of the rectum, and in response to parenterally administered pharmacologic agents. In addition to clonidine (an α₂-adrenergic agonist), morphine, atropine, buspirone (a 5-HT₁ₐ agonist), and sumatriptan (a 5-HT₁ᴅ agonist), all reduce colonic tone in humans.[47–49] Rectal distention by a balloon to subnoxious levels induces colonic relaxation in humans.[50] Colocolonic reflexes mediated via local nervous pathways through the prevertebral ganglia and independent of central nervous system activity have been well characterized in animal preparations.[51] This propensity for colonic relaxation, particularly that induced by sympathetic stimulation and opiates, may be relevant to the pathophysiology of acute colonic dilatation or pseudoobstruction.[52] Colonic relaxation induced

by rectal distention may explain left-sided colonic transit delays in patients with obstructed defecation because restoration of normal defecation tends to restore colonic motility to normal.[53]

There are regional and age-related differences in biomechanical properties of the colon.[5] These biomechanical properties can be assessed by stress-strain relationships in vitro and by the pressure-volume relationships during balloon distention by a barostat in vivo. In ex vivo and in vivo studies, stiffness declines from the rectum to the transverse colon. These observations are probably relevant to the segmental heterogeneity in function depicted in Table 144.1 and to the pathophysiology of diverticulosis, as discussed later. Thus the compliant ascending and transverse colon are ideally suited to function as a reservoir. Conversely, the descending and sigmoid colonic segments are suited to function as conduits, tend to have lower compliances, and are the primary sites of diverticula because intraluminal pressures are transmitted to weak points in the colonic wall.

DEFECATION

In health, rectal distention evokes the desire to defecate and reflex relaxation of the internal anal sphincter (Fig. 144.7). If social circumstances are conducive, defecation is accomplished by adoption of a suitable posture and contraction of the diaphragm and abdominal muscles to raise intraabdominal pressure. Concomitant relaxation of the puborectalis and external anal sphincter, both striated muscles, enables widening of the anorectal angle by 15 degrees or more and reduction of pressure within the anal canal and perineal descent. Appropriate coordination between abdominal contraction and pelvic floor

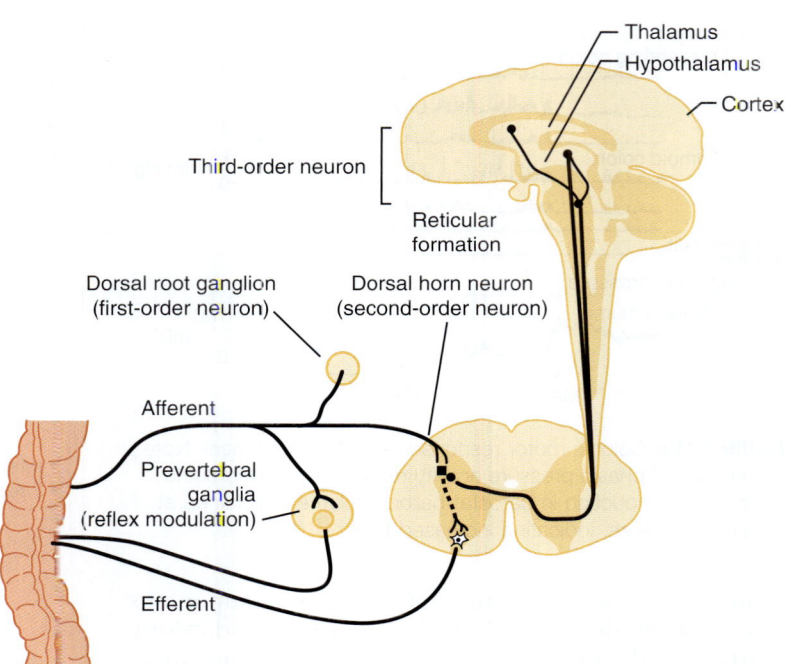

FIGURE 144.8 Visceral sensory pathways include reflexes mediated through prevertebral and other autonomic ganglia and a third-order neuron chain that ultimately projects to supraspinal centers. Convergence of visceral and somatic afferents at the dorsal horn explains referral of visceral discomfort to the body surface. Third-order neurons originating in thalamus project to the cerebral cortex; those from the reticular formation to the thalamus and hypothalamus. (From Camilleri M, Saslow SB, Bharucha AE. Gastrointestinal sensation. Mechanisms and relation to functional gastrointestinal disorders. *Gastroenterol Clin North Am.* 1996;25:247–258.)

TABLE 144.2 **Visceral Afferent Pathways**

Functions	Discriminative	Affective-Motivational
Afferent fibers	Rapidly conducting Aδ fibers	Unmyelinated C fibers
Thalamic nuclei	Lateral	Medial
Cortical area	Somatosensory cortex	Frontal, parietal, and limbic regions

relaxation is crucial to normal fecal expulsion. In addition, there is evidence to suggest that these somatic processes are integrated with visceral components such as colonic HAPCs during defecation.[54]

COLONIC SENSATION

Healthy individuals, for the most part, do not perceive physiologic processes within the gut except for the sensation of fullness and the desire to defecate. Over the past few years, it has been proposed that symptoms associated with functional GI disorders are partly related to enhanced sensory perception.[55] Visceral sensation is perceived in peripheral receptors and conveyed centrally by a three-neuron chain (Fig. 144.8).[56] Although visceral afferents can respond to one or more stimulus modality (e.g., tension, temperature, osmolarity), mechanoreceptors are particularly important in the context of functional GI diseases. Mucosal mechanoreceptors respond to mucosal pinching or stroking, whereas serosal mechanoreceptors respond to movement or strong distention of a viscus. Visceral perception is characterized by discriminative (localizing, precise) and affective motivational (diffuse, emotional) aspects, which are conveyed by discrete mechanisms, demonstrated in Table 144.2.

The predominant afferent fibers are rapidly conducting myelinated Aδ fibers and slowly conducting unmyelinated C fibers. The Aδ fibers convey the sensation of first pain, which is well localized and lasts as long as the stimulus. The C fibers convey the "second" pain, which is diffuse, lasts longer than the duration of the stimulus, and is associated with the affective-motivational aspects of pain. In the spinal cord, visceral afferents project centrally via spinothalamic, spinoreticular tracts, and a nociceptive dorsal column. The spinothalamic tracts project to the medial and lateral thalamic nuclei, which are associated with affective-motivational and discriminative aspects of pain, respectively. These thalamic nuclei project to the cortical areas indicated in Table 144.2. Descending (chiefly serotoninergic and adrenergic) pathways originating in the frontal cortex, hypothalamus, and brainstem reticular formation inhibit spinal cord dorsal horn neurons, thereby reducing pain perception.

In humans, colonic (and rectal) perception is assessed during balloon distention. The rate and pattern of balloon distention are important parameters. Perception is assessed by asking subjects to indicate when they perceive a given sensation (i.e., first threshold, desire to defecate, or discomfort). The contractile response is more pronounced during fast than during slow distention. It is conceivable that this partly explains why rapid rectal distention is more likely than slow distention to be perceived in healthy subjects and to evoke visceral hypersensitivity in IBS.[57,58]

An alternative method involves asking patients to rate the intensity of perception during balloon distentions of standardized intensity delivered in random order.[59] Perceptual intensity is recorded on separate visual analog scales for gas, desire to defecate, and discomfort. Subjective perceptual ratings are proportional to the intensity of the stimulus. Psychologic stress[60] and meals[61,62] increase perception of colonic distention and may explain why

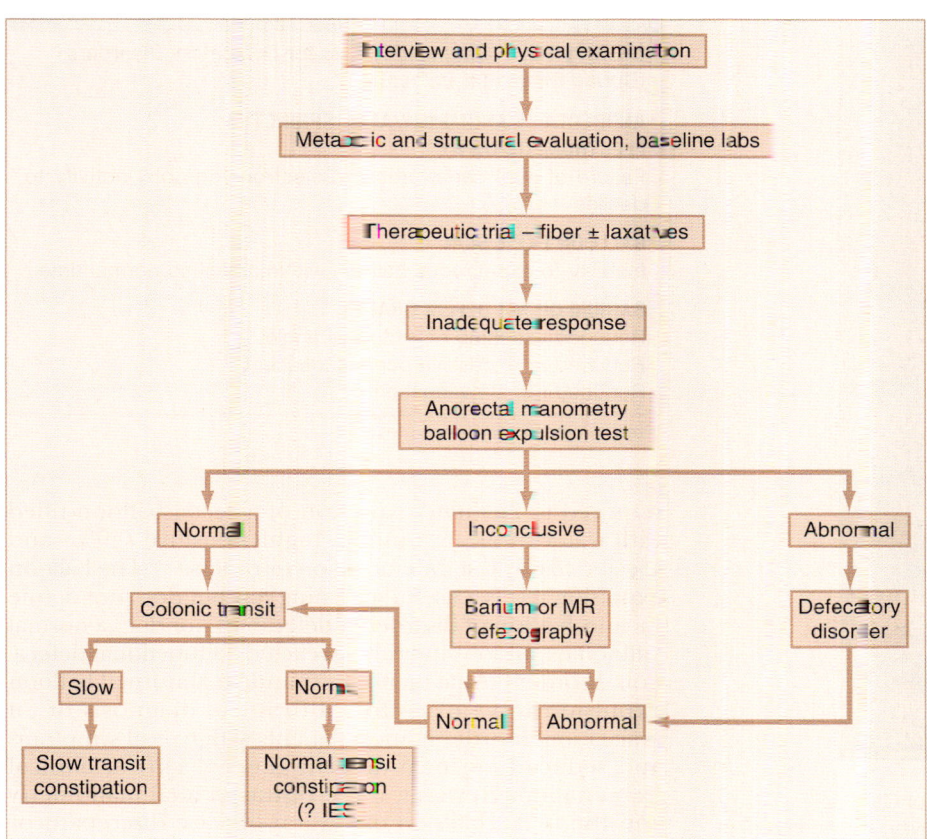

FIGURE 144.9 Diagnostic tests in management of constipated patients in clinical practice. Note these simple tests permit categorization of patients and choice of therapy. *IBS*, Irritable bowel syndrome; *MR*, magnetic resonance. (From Bharucha AE, Dorn SD, Lembo A, Pressman A. American Gastroenterological Association Medical position statement on constipation. *Gastroenterology.* 2013;144:211–217.)

these factors induce symptoms in IBS. Conversely, mental relaxation reduced perception of colonic distention in healthy people.[59] In humans balloon distention of the left colon evokes abdominal discomfort in the midline or left iliac fossa. The rectum is more sensitive than the colon and can distinguish between flatus and feces. Rectal distention induces rectal or sacral discomfort, akin to the desire to defecate or urgency. The anal canal is exquisitely sensitive, with sensitivity to touch, pain, and temperature comparable to the dorsum of the hand.

PERTURBATIONS OF COLONIC PHYSIOLOGY IN DISEASE STATES

The following are examples of illnesses that derange colonic physiology.

Constipation

Constipation may result from slow colonic transit and/or pelvic floor function, also known as defecatory disorders (DDs) (Fig. 144.9).[63,64] Among constipated patients who have not responded to simple laxatives, anorectal functions should be evaluated, generally with an anorectal manometry and a rectal balloon expulsion test (see Fig. 144.9). Colonic transit may be delayed not only due to colonic motor dysfunction but also in patients with DDs. Hence colonic transit is assessed only after excluding or managing DDs.

Patients with normal transit constipation usually respond to dietary fiber supplementation[65]; those with slow transit constipation frequently require judiciously administered

laxatives, and pelvic floor retraining is necessary to reverse pelvic floor dysfunction in patients with DDs. Colonic motor assessments should be considered in patients with medically refractory chronic constipation, particularly when surgery (i.e., total colectomy with ileorectostomy) is considered. Intraluminal measurements are useful for confirming or excluding severe colonic motor dysfunction, manifest as a reduction in the number of colonic HAPCs, and/or a reduced colonic motor response to eating.[66] In patients who have the most severe dysfunction, responses to such a stimulant as bisacodyl or neostigmine are also blunted (i.e., colonic inertia).[5] The primary reason to consider colonic motility testing instead of colonic transit times is that barostat assessments of colonic tone reveal reduced fasting colonic tone and/or postprandial colonic tonic responses in many patients with normal transit and normal motor responses in many patients with isolated slow transit constipation.[67] Moreover, some patients with chronic constipation, particularly those with constipation-predominant IBS, have increased colonic motor activity, especially in the sigmoid colon.[57,68] Increased sigmoid colonic phasic pressure activity ("spastic colon") has been implicated to retard colonic transit in chronic constipation.[69,70] Detailed histopathologic studies with special stains reveal a marked loss of nerves and ICC throughout the colon in slow transit constipation and megacolon (Fig. 144.10).[71] Rarely, constipation may be the presenting manifestation of a generalized GI motility disorder resulting from a paraneoplastic syndrome (e.g., due to small cell carcinoma of the lung).[72]

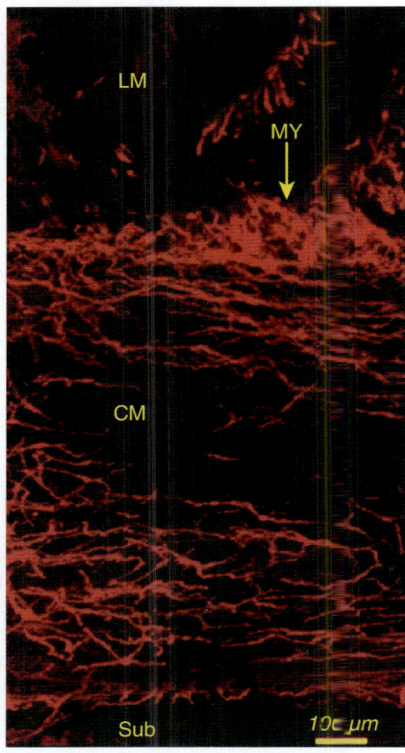

FIGURE 144.10 Distribution of interstitial cells of Cajal as demonstrated by c-Kit–positive immunoreactivity, shown in *red*, in the normal human sigmoid colon. Sections were cut parallel to the longitudinal muscle layer for both panels. *CM,* Circular muscle; *LM,* longitudinal muscle; *MY,* myenteric plexus region; *Sub,* submucosal border.

Defecatory Disorders

Patients with DDs strain excessively to overcome the functional obstruction caused by inadequate relaxation of the external anal sphincter and/or puborectalis muscle sling.[73] Dyssynergic defecation, anismus, and puborectalis dysfunction are some other terms used to describe this condition. Such symptoms as excessive straining, a sensation of incomplete evacuation, dyschezia, and digital evacuation of feces suggest but cannot be used to conclusively diagnose DDs.[74] The physical examination may reveal high resting anal sphincter tone, failure of puborectalis relaxation, and/or perineal descent during simulated defecation, or anatomic abnormalities, such as anal fissure or rectocele. The latter may occur alone or may be accompanied by pelvic floor laxity and organ prolapse (descending perineum syndrome). The clinical impression can be corroborated by objective assessments of pelvic floor function, beginning with anal manometry and a rectal balloon expulsion test (Box 144.1). With anal manometry or sphincter electromyography, paradoxical sphincter contraction or anismus can be observed in a substantial proportion of healthy subjects with no symptoms of DDs. This underscores the importance of considering clinical features and not basing the diagnosis of DDs on manometry alone.[75,76]

The rectal balloon expulsion test, performed by measuring the time required to expel, or external traction

---

BOX 144.1 Diagnostic Tests for Defecatory Disorders (During Simulated Defecation)*

ANORECTAL MANOMETRY/ANAL SPHINCTER ELECTROMYOGRAPHY
Failure of anal canal pressure/electromyography activity to decline

BALLOON EXPULSION
Inability to expel rectal balloon within specified normal time

BARIUM OR MR DEFECOGRAPHY
Reduced widening of rectoanal angle
Reduced or excessive perineal descent
Reduced rectal evacuation

*Precise criteria vary among tests.

---

required to facilitate expulsion of a rectal balloon filled with water or air, is a useful, highly sensitive (89%) and specific (84%) test for evacuation disorders.[77,78] The balloon expulsion test is a useful screening test but does not define the mechanism of disordered defecation nor does a normal balloon expulsion study always exclude a functional defecation disorder.[79] Anal manometry and an abnormal balloon expulsion test suffice to confirm the diagnosis of an evacuation disorder in most patients with typical symptoms and reduced perineal descent (i.e., <1 cm) at clinical examination. However, if the results of anal manometry and the rectal balloon expulsion test are discrepant or conflict with the clinical impression, then evaluation of rectal and pelvic floor motion during attempted defecation by barium or magnetic resonance (MR) defecography may be necessary to clarify the diagnosis. Defecography can detect structural abnormalities (rectocele, enterocele, rectal prolapse) and assess functional parameters (anorectal angle at rest and during straining, perineal descent, anal diameter, indentation of the puborectalis in the posterior aspect of the rectoanal junction, degree of rectal emptying).[80,81] The diagnostic value of defecography has been questioned primarily because normal ranges for quantified measures are inadequately defined and because some parameters, such as the anorectal angle, cannot be measured reliably because of anatomic variations in rectal contour and location (e.g., in the presence of perianal discomfort). Magnetic resonance imaging (MRI) is the only imaging modality that can visualize both anal sphincter anatomy and global pelvic floor motion (anterior, middle, and posterior compartments) in real time without radiation exposure. Dynamic MRI depicts the heterogeneity in functional defecation disorders and may be useful for clarifying the diagnosis in selected patients.[82,83] Patients with obstructed defecation may also have delayed left colonic transit, attributable to obstruction of luminal contents by retained stool, colonic motor dysfunction unrelated to obstructed defecation, rectocolonic inhibition, or decreased colonic motor response to a meal. The latter is reversible after biofeedback therapy.[53]

Acute Colonic Pseudoobstruction (Ogilvie Syndrome)

In *acute megacolon* (Ogilvie syndrome), colonic dilatation is attributed to a sympathetically mediated reflex response to a number of serious medical or surgical conditions in older patients.[52] Cholinesterase inhibitors such as neostigmine, enhance colonic contractility, reducing colonic distention in patients with acute colonic pseudoobstruction by increasing the availability of acetylcholine in myenteric plexus and neuromuscular junction.[84]

Chronic Megacolon

Chronic megacolon may be congenital (due to Hirschsprung disease; lack of distal or total colonic myenteric nerve plexus and presents as toxic megacolon in infancy or adult severe constipation due to a short segment of denervated internal sphincter) or may present later in life after a long history of refractory constipation. Confirming the diagnosis, plain or contrast radiographs or a colonic barostat study may reveal colonic distention.[38] The initial treatment for Hirschsprung disease is surgery. In chronic idiopathic megacolon, such medical measures as colonic evacuation with enemas, fiber supplementation, and laxatives do not usually suffice; if severe motor dysfunction is confined to the colon a subtotal colectomy with an ileorectal anastomosis or an ileostomy may be necessary. Chronic megacolon may also result from multiple endocrine neoplasia type 2B (MEN2B), which is associated with ganglioneuroma formation in the colon.[85]

Functional Diarrhea or Diarrhea-Predominant Irritable Bowel Syndrome

The etiopathogenesis of IBS is still incompletely understood. There is considerable evidence for peripheral disturbances, such as low-grade, microscopic inflammation that persists after acute gastroenteritis.[86] A role for intraluminal intestinal irritants, such as maldigested carbohydrates (producing SCFAs) or fats, an excess of bile acids, and gluten intolerance; alterations in the microbiome; enteroendocrine cell products and genetic susceptibility to inflammation or altered bile acid synthesis has also been implicated. These luminal and mucosal irritants can alter mucosal permeability and cause immune activation or inflammation, which in turn activates local reflexes that alter intestinal motility or secretion. The irritants also stimulate sensory mechanisms, leading to visceral hypersensitivity and pain. Psychosocial issues (e.g., anxiety, depression, stress, and abuse) are also important. In a prospective study, hypochondriasis or a recent stressful life event predicted which patients would have abnormal colonic physiology and IBS symptoms after an attack of acute gastroenteritis.[87]

A subset of patients with IBS have accelerated proximal colonic transit,[88] more frequent HAPCs,[89] and an exaggerated colonic motor response to eating. These result in postprandial abdominal discomfort and urgency to defecate in some patients with diarrhea-predominant IBS. Other studies have shown that approximately 50% of patients with diarrhea-predominant IBS have rectal hypersensitivity or project sensation to a wider cutaneous area during balloon distention. Although the significance of visceral hypersensitivity during balloon distention to symptoms in patients with IBS is unclear,[90] visceral hypersensitivity has been associated with abdominal pain and bloating.[91] However, rectal hypersensitivity does not accurately predict the response to therapy. Because bile

acids can induce colonic secretion and propulsive contractions and increase epithelial permeability, bile acid malabsorption may contribute to diarrhea after cholecystectomy and in patients with idiopathic bile acid malabsorption.[92,93] Small intestinal bacterial overgrowth, as detected by breath hydrogen testing, has also been implicated as a cause for IBS. However, using a standard definition of bacterial overgrowth i.e., $\geq 10^5$ colonic organisms/mL in jejunal cultures), only 4% of IBS patients and asymptomatic controls had small intestinal bacterial overgrowth.[31] Of unclear significance, a higher proportion of IBS patients than controls (43% vs. 12%) had mildly increased bacterial counts ($\geq 5 \times 10^3$/mL). Controlled studies suggest that a short course of antibiotics (e.g., rifaximin) may be beneficial in patients with IBS.[94] The therapeutic benefit was modest (e.g., 40.2% of the rifaximin group vs. 30.3% of placebo reported adequate relief of bloating at 3 months after a 2-week course of treatment). However, the data have been replicated in two phase III randomized controlled studies.[95] Further studies evaluating the long-term risk-benefit ratio of repeating antibiotic therapy need to be evaluated.

OTHER DIARRHEAL ILLNESSES

In carcinoid syndrome, there is accelerated small intestinal transit and increased jejunal secretion. However, there is also evidence for altered colonic physiology. Increased delivery of contents to the colon is compounded by reduced capacitance in the ascending colon and an exaggerated colonic motor response to eating, causing rapid proximal colonic emptying.[56] 5-HT$_3$ antagonists, such as ondansetron and aldosterone, reduce the colonic tonic response to eating and the rate of emptying, respectively, suggesting that 5-HT$_3$ receptors may partly mediate the motor dysfunction in these patients.[45]

Disturbances in motility and NaCl absorption have been described in patients with *ulcerative colitis*. Patients with active proctitis have a stiff, noncompliant rectum, which may explain the enhanced sensation of urgency prior to defecation.[97]

Diarrhea after *ileal resection* of less than 100 cm is induced by the secretory effects of bile acids, associated with mild steatorrhoea (<20 g/day) and responsive to cholestyramine (4 to 6 g/day).[98] After more extensive ileal resection (>100 cm) steatorrhea is severe (>20 g fat/day) and attributable to fat maldigestion and malabsorption secondary to low jejunal concentrations of bile acids. Cholestyramine will not ameliorate and may aggravate diarrhea in these patients.

Clonidine ameliorates the diarrhea related to *diabetic neuropathy* by restoring the α_2-mediated sympathetic "brake" (i.e., promoting intestinal and colonic absorption of NaCl, and inhibiting motility).[99]

DIVERTICULOSIS

Considerations relevant to the pathophysiology of diverticulosis include the orientation of taenia coli, the course taken by perforating arteries supplying the colonic wall, and changes in the biomechanical properties of the colon that accompany diverticulosis. Colonic diverticula are mucosal pouches that are pushed out between arcs of circular muscle at weak points (i.e., where arteries pierce the muscularis propria in the spaces between the mesenteric taenia and the two antimesenteric taeniae). Thus diverticula do not occur where the taeniae fuse to form a longitudinal muscle layer surrounding the rectum.[100]

Thickening of the colonic circular and longitudinal muscle layers, partly due to elastin deposition with shortening of taenia coli, may narrow the colonic lumen in diverticulosis. Studies also reveal colonic motor disturbances (i.e., more propulsive activity, more 2 to 3 cycles/minute regular, phasic, nonpropagated activity) and heightened perception of colonic distention in patients with uncomplicated, symptomatic diverticulosis.[101] Thus it is conceivable that increased motor activity, particularly rhythmic contractions, may lead to mucosal outpouching and formation of diverticula, particularly when the colon is less compliant and/or narrower (e.g., in the sigmoid colon or in the presence of long-standing disorders of defecation). These motor disturbances may be partly attributable to cholinergic hypersensitivity.[102] It has been speculated that a low residue diet with diminished fecal bulk predisposes to colonic luminal narrowing and ultimately diverticulosis. However, there is no direct evidence to corroborate a cause and effect relationship between lack of dietary fiber and luminal narrowing or elastin deposition in the taenia coli.

IMPLICATIONS OF COLONIC PHYSIOLOGY FOR SURGICAL PRACTICE

It is crucial to treat pelvic floor dysfunction in patients with severe constipation prior to considering colectomy in those with delayed colonic transit. A colectomy with ileorectostomy is the preferred procedure for patients with intractable constipation and adequate anal sphincter function.[103] Assessment of gastric and small intestinal transit or motor activity may permit recognition of patients with generalized gut dysmotility disorders in whom long-term success rates after a colectomy for constipation are lower than in patients with selective colonic dysmotility. Left-sided colectomy may result in postoperative colonic transit delays in the unresected segment; this likely represents parasympathetic denervation because ascending intramural fibers travel in retrograde manner from the pelvis to the ascending colon. The sigmoid colon and rectum are also supplied by descending fibers that run along the inferior mesenteric artery.[104] A long denervated segment is more likely to be associated with nonpropagated colonic pressure waves and delayed colonic transit than a short denervated segment. In addition to colonic denervation, a low anterior resection may also damage the anal sphincter and reduce rectal compliance[105]; in contrast to anal sphincter injury, rectal compliance may recover with time.[106] Physiologic assessments confirm clinical observations suggesting that colonic motor function recovers more rapidly after laparoscopic-assisted compared with open sigmoid colectomy.[107]

Surgeons should also be aware of the fluid absorptive capacity of the colon and its importance in fluid and electrolyte homeostasis. The retention of a segment of colon can make an enormous difference to the postoperative management of short bowel syndrome after massive resection for mesenteric vascular thrombosis or Crohn disease.

Motor disorders of the colon may be manifest with colonic dilatation; not all dilatation is secondary to obstruction and, in the presence of comorbidity or electrolyte imbalance, megacolon should be considered early, particularly because it can be treated medically or endoscopically without resorting to resection.

Finally, the colorectal surgeon, like the gastroenterologist, will encounter many patients in his or her practice in whom the diagnosis is functional diarrhea, constipation, or fecal retention. These patients deserve a compassionate, careful appraisal and advice on how to restore normal colonic physiology. Avoidance of unnecessary colonic or other surgery is the best course of management—primum non nocere.

ACKNOWLEDGMENTS

This study was supported in part by USPHS NIH Grants R01 DK78924 (AEB) and RO1 DK92179 (MC) from National Institutes of Health.

REFERENCES

1. Christensen J. *Colonic Motility.* Bethesda: American Physiological Society; 1989.
2. Fraser ID, Condon RE, Schulte WJ, DeCosse JJ, Cowles VE. Longitudinal muscle of muscularis externa in human and nonhuman primate colon. *Arch Surg.* 1981;116:61-63.
3. Pace J. The anatomy of the haustra of the human colon. *Proc R Soc Med.* 1968;61:934-935.
4. Whiteway J, Morson BC. Pathology of the ageing—diverticular disease. *Clin Gastroenterol.* 1985;14:829-846.
5. von der Ohe M, Camilleri M. Measurement of small bowel and colonic transit: indications and methods. *Mayo Clin Proc.* 1992;67:1169-1179.
6. Metcalf AM, Phillips SF, Zinsmeister AR, MacCarty RL, Beart RW, Wolff BG. Simplified assessment of segmental colonic transit. *Gastroenterology.* 1987;92:40-47.
7. Rao SS, Kuo B, McCallum RW, et al. Investigation of colonic and whole gut transit with wireless motility capsule and radioopaque markers in constipation. *Clin Gastroenterol Hepatol.* 2009;7:537-544.
8. Camilleri M, Thorne NK, Ringel R, et al. Wireless pH-motility capsule for colonic transit: prospective comparison with radiopaque markers in chronic constipation. *Neurogastroenterol Motil.* 2010;22:874-882, e233.
9. Kuo B, McCallum RW, Koch KL, et al. Comparison of gastric emptying of a nondigestible capsule to a radio-labelled meal in healthy and gastroparetic subjects. *Aliment Pharmacol Ther.* 2008;27:186-196.
10. Rae MG, Fleming N, McGregor DB, Sanders KM, Keef KD. Control of motility patterns in the human colonic circular muscle layer by pacemaker activity. *J Physiol.* 1998;510:309-320.
11. Sadik R, Abrahamsson H, Ung KA, Stotzer PO. Accelerated regional bowel transit and overweight shown in idiopathic bile acid malabsorption. *Am J Gastroenterol.* 2004;99:711-718.
12. Bharucha AE, Camilleri M, Zinsmeister AR, Hanson RB. Adrenergic modulation of human colonic motor and sensory function. *Am J Physiol.* 1997;273:G997-G1006.
13. Proano M, Camilleri M, Phillips SF, Thomforde GM, Brown ML, Tucker RL. Unprepared human colon does not discriminate between solids and liquids. *Am J Physiol.* 1991;260:G13-G16.
14. Fich A, Steadman CJ, Phillips SF, et al. Ileocolonic transit does not change after right hemicolectomy. *Gastroenterology.* 1992;103:794-799.
15. Phillips SF, Giller J. The contribution of the colon to electrolyte and water conservation in man. *J Lab Clin Med.* 1973;81:733-746.

16. Hammer J, Phillips SF. Fluid loading of the human colon: effects on segmental transit and stool composition. *Gastroenterology*. 1993; 105:988-998.

17. Singh SK, Binder HJ, Boron WF, Geibel J. Fluid absorption in isolated perfused colonic crypts. *J Clin Invest*. 1995;96:2373-2379.

18. Sandle GI. Salt and water absorption in the human colon: a modern appraisal. *Gut*. 1998;43:294-299.

19. Binder HJ, McGlone F, Sandle GI. Effects of corticosteroid hormones on the electrophysiology of rat distal colon: implications for Na+ and K+ transport. *J Physiol*. 1989;410:425-441.

20. Cho JH, Musch MW, Bookstein CM, McSwine RL, Rabenau K, Chang EB. Aldosterone stimulates intestinal Na+ absorption in rats by increasing NHE3 expression of the proximal colon. *Am J Physiol*. 1998;274:C586-C594.

21. Binder H, Sandle G. *Electrolyte Transport in the Mammalian Colon*. 3rd ed. New York: Raven Press; 1994.

22. Cook SI, Sellin JH. Review article: short chain fatty acids in health and disease. *Aliment Pharmacol Ther*. 1998;12:499-507.

23. Dethlefsen L, McFall-Ngai M, Relman DA. An ecological and evolutionary perspective on human-microbe mutualism and disease. *Nature*. 2007;449:811-818.

24. Sender R, Fuchs S, Milo R. Revised estimates for the number of human and bacteria cells in the body. *PLoS Biol*. 2016;14:e1002533. http://dx.doi.org/10.1101/036103. Accessed 14 October 2016.

25. Barbara G, Stanghellini V, Brandi G, et al. Interactions between commensal bacteria and gut sensorimotor function in health and disease. *Am J Gastroenterol*. 2005;100:2560-2568.

26. Vandeputte D, Falony G, Vieira-Silva S, Tito RY, Joossens M, Raes J. Stool consistency is strongly associated with gut microbiota richness and composition, enterotypes and bacterial growth rates. *Gut*. 2016;65:57-62.

27. Parthasarathy G, Chen J, Chen X, et al. Relationship between microbiota of the colonic mucosa vs feces and symptoms, colonic transit, and methane production in female patients with chronic constipation. *Gastroenterology*. 2016;150:367-379, e1-e61.

28. Islam KB, Fukiya S, Hagio M, et al. Bile acid is a host factor that regulates the composition of the cecal microbiota in rats. *Gastroenterology*. 2011;141:1773-1781.

29. Pimentel M. An evidence-based treatment algorithm for IBS based on a bacterial/SIBO hypothesis: part 2. *Am J Gastroenterol*. 2010;105: 1227-1230.

30. Pimentel M. Evaluating a bacterial hypothesis in IBS using a modification of Koch's postulates: part 1. *Am J Gastroenterol*. 2010; 105:718-721.

31. Posserud I, Stotzer PO, Björnsson ES, Abrahamsson H, Simrén M. Small intestinal bacterial overgrowth in patients with irritable bowel syndrome. *Gut*. 2007;56:802-808.

32. Sellin JH. A breath of fresh air. *Clin Gastroenterol Hepatol*. 2016;14: 209-211.

33. Bassotti G, Iantorno G, Fiorella S, Bustos-Fernandez L, Bilder CR. Colonic motility in man: features in normal subjects and in patients with chronic idiopathic constipation. *Am J Gastroenterol*. 1999;94: 1760-1770.

34. Camilleri M, Ford M. Review article: colonic sensorimotor physiology in health, and its alteration in constipation and diarrhoeal disorders. *Aliment Pharmacol Ther*. 1998;12:287-302.

35. Lemann M, Flourié B, Picon L, Coffin B, Jian R, Rambaud JC. Motor activity recorded in the unprepared colon of healthy humans. *Gut*. 1995;37:649-653.

36. Dinning PG, Wiklendt L, Maslen L, et al. Colonic motor abnormalities in slow transit constipation defined by high resolution, fibre-optic manometry. *Neurogastroenterol Motil*. 2015;27:379-388.

37. von der Ohe M, Hanson R, Camilleri M. Comparison of simultaneous recordings of human colonic contractions by manometry and a barostat. *Neurogastroenterol Motil*. 1994;6:213-222.

38. O'Dwyer RH, Acosta A, Camilleri M, Burton D, Busciglio I, Bharucha AE. Clinical features and colonic motor disturbances in chronic megacolon in adults. *Dig Dis Sci*. 2015;60:2398-2407.

39. Cook I, Furukawa Y, Panagopoulos V, Collins PJ, Dent J. Relationships between spatial patterns of colonic pressure and individual movements of content. *Am J Physiol*. 2000;278:G329-G341.

40. Ford MJ, Camilleri M, Wiste JA, Hanson RB. Differences in colonic tone and phasic response to a meal in the transverse and sigmoid human colon. *Gut*. 1995;37:264-269.

41. Narducci F, Bassotti G, Granata MT, et al. Colonic motility and gastric emptying in patients with irritable bowel syndrome. Effect

of pretreatment with octylonium bromide. *Dig Dis Sci*. 1986;31: 241-246.

42. Wiley J, Tatum D, Keinath R, Chung OY. Participation of gastric mechanoreceptors and intestinal chemoreceptors in the gastrocolonic response. *Gastroenterology*. 1988;94:1144-1149.

43. Snape WJ Jr, Wright SH, Battle WM, Cohen S. The gastrocolic response: evidence for a neural mechanism. *Gastroenterology*. 1979;77: 1235-1240.

44. Coffin B, Fossati S, Flourié B, et al. Regional effects of cholecystokinin octapeptide on colonic phasic and tonic motility in healthy humans. *Am J Physiol*. 1999;276:G767-G772.

45. von der Ohe MR, Camilleri M, Kvols LK. A 5HT3 antagonist corrects the postprandial colonic hypertonic response in carcinoid diarrhea. *Gastroenterology*. 1994;106:1184-1189.

46. Lapoigny M, Cowles VE, Zhu YR, Condon RE. Vagal influence on colonic motor activity in conscious nonhuman primates. *Am J Physiol*. 1992;262:G231-G236.

47. Steadman CJ, Phillips SF, Camilleri M, Talley NJ, Haddad A, Hanson R. Control of muscle tone in the human colon. *Gut*. 1992;33:541-546.

48. Coulie B, Tack J, Gevers A, et al. Influence of the sumatriptan-induced colonic relaxation on the perception of colonic distention in man. *Gastroenterology*. 1997;112:A715.

49. Coulie B, Tack J, Vos R, et al. Influence of the 5-HT1A agonist buspirone on rectal tone and the perception of rectal distention in man. *Gastroenterology*. 1998;114:G3046.

50. Law N-M, Bharucha A. Phasic rectal distention induces colonic relaxation in humans. *Gastroenterology*. 1998;114:G3233.

51. Freulen DL, Szurszewski JH. Reflex pathways in the abdominal prevertebral ganglia: evidence for a colo-colonic inhibitory reflex. *J Physiol*. 1979;295:21-32.

52. Phillips S. *Megacolon*. 1st ed. New York: Raven Press; 1991.

53. Mollen RM, Salvioli B, Camilleri M, et al. The effects of biofeedback on rectal sensation and distal colonic motility in patients with disorders of rectal evacuation: evidence of an inhibitory rectocolonic reflex in humans? *Am J Gastroenterol*. 1999;94:751-756.

54. Bharucha AE. High amplitude propagated contractions. *Neurogastroenterol Motil*. 2012;24:977-982.

55. Mertz H, Naliboff B, Munakata J, Niazi N, Mayer EA. Altered rectal perception is a biological marker of patients with irritable bowel syndrome. *Gastroenterology*. 1995;109:40-52 [Erratum appears in *Gastroenterology*. 1997;113(3):1054.]

56. Camilleri M, Saslow SB, Bharucha AE. Gastrointestinal sensation. Mechanisms and relation to functional gastrointestinal disorders. *Gastroenterol Clin North Am*. 1996;25:247-258.

57. Bharucha AE, Hubmayr RD, Ferber I, Zinsmeister AR. Viscoelastic properties of the human colon. *Am J Physiol Gastrointest Liver Physiol*. 2001;281:G459-G466.

58. Corsetti M, Cesana B, Bhoori S, et al. Rectal hypersensitivity to distention in patients with irritable bowel syndrome: role of distention rate. *Clin Gastroenterol Hepatol*. 2004;2:49-56.

59. Ford MJ, Camilleri M, Zinsmeister AR, Hanson RB. Psychosensory modulation of colonic sensation in the human transverse and sigmoid colon. *Gastroenterology*. 1995;109:1772-1780.

60. Posserud I, Agerforz P, Ekman R, Björnsson ES, Abrahamsson H, Simrén M. Altered visceral perceptual and neuroendocrine response in patients with irritable bowel syndrome during mental stress. *Gut*. 2004;53:1102-1108.

61. Simrén M, Abrahamsson H, Björnsson ES. Lipid-induced colonic hypersensitivity in the irritable bowel syndrome: the role of bowel habit, sex and psychologic factors. *Clin Gastroenterol Hepatol*. 2007;5:201-208.

62. Törnblom H, Van Oudenhove L, Tack J, Simrén M. Interaction between preprandial and postprandial rectal sensory and motor abnormalities in IBS. *Gut*. 2014;63:1441-1449.

63. Bharucha AE, Pemberton JH, Locke GR 3rd. American Gastroenterological Association technical review on constipation. *Gastroenterology*. 2013;144:218-238.

64. Bharucha AE, Locke GR, Pemberton JH. AGA practice guideline on constipation: technical review. *Gastroenterology*. 2013;144:218-238.

65. Voderholzer WA, Schatke W, Mühldorfer BE, Klauser AG, Birkner B, Müller-Lissner SA. Clinical response to dietary fiber treatment of chronic constipation. *Am J Gastroenterol*. 1997;92:95-98.

66. O'Brien MD, Camilleri M, von der Ohe MR, et al. Motility and tone of the left colon in constipation: a role in clinical practice? *Am J Gastroenterol*. 1996;91:2532-2538.

67. Ravi K, Bharucha AE, Camilleri M, Rhoten D, Bakken T, Zinsmeister AR. Phenotypic variation of colonic motor functions in chronic constipation. *Gastroenterology.* 2010;138:89-97.

68. Hasler WL, Saad RJ, Rao SS, et al. Heightened colon motor activity measured by a wireless capsule in patients with constipation: relation to colon transit and IBS. *Am J Physiol Gastrointest Liver Physiol.* 2009;297:G1107-G1114.

69. Chaudhary NA, Truelove SC. Human colonic motility: a comparative study of normal subjects, patients with ulcerative colitis, and patients with the irritable colon syndrome: I. Resting patterns of motility. *Gastroenterology.* 1961;40:1-17.

70. Connell AM. The motility of the pelvic colon. Part II. Paradoxical motility in diarrhea and constipation. *Gut.* 1962;3:342-348.

71. Lyford GL, He CL, Soffer E, et al. Pan-colonic decrease in interstitial cells of Cajal in patients with slow transit constipation. *Gut.* 2002;51:496-501.

72. Jun S, Dimyan M, Jones KD, Ladabaum U. Obstipation as a paraneoplastic presentation of small cell lung cancer: case report and literature review. *Neurogastroenterol Motil.* 2005;17:16-22.

73. Bharucha AE. Obstructed defecation: don't strain in vain. *Am J Gastroenterol.* 1998;93:1019-1020.

74. Ratuapli S, Bharucha AE, Noelting J, et al. Phenotypic identification and classification of functional defecatory disorders using high resolution anorectal manometry. *Gastroenterology.* 2013;144:314-322.

75. Grossi U, Carrington EV, Bharucha AE, Horrocks EJ, Scott SM, Knowles CH. Diagnostic accuracy study of anorectal manometry for diagnosis of dyssynergic defecation. *Gut* 2016;65:447-455

76. Lee TH, Bharucha AE. How to perform and interpret a high-resolution anorectal manometry test. *J Neurogastroenterol Motil.* 2016; 22:46-59.

77. Minguez M, Herreros B, Sanchiz V, et al. Predictive value of the balloon expulsion test for excluding the diagnosis of pelvic floor dyssynergia in constipation. *Gastroenterology.* 2004;126:57-62.

78. Ratuapli S, Bharucha AE, Harvey D, Zinsmeister AR. Comparison of rectal balloon expulsion test in seated and left lateral positions. *Neurogastroenterol Motil.* 2013;25:e813-e820.

79. Rao SS, Mudipalli RS, Stessman M, Zimmerman B. Investigation of the utility of colorectal function tests and Rome II criteria in dyssynergic defecation (Anismus). *Neurogastroenterol Motil.* 2004;16:589-596.

80. Ekberg O, Mahiew PHG, Bartram CI, Piloni V. Defecography: dynamic radiological imaging in proctology. *Gastroenterol Int.* 1990;3:93-99.

81. Shorvon PJ, McHugh S, Diamant NE, Somers S, Stevenson GW. Defecography in normal volunteers: results and implications. *Gut.* 1989;30:1737-1749.

82. Bharucha AE, Fletcher JG, Seide B, Riederer SJ, Zinsmeister AR. Phenotypic variation in functional disorders of defecation. *Gastroenterology.* 2005;128:1199-1210.

83. Karlbom U, Påhlman L, Nilsson S, Graf W. Relationships between defecographic findings, rectal emptying, and colonic transit time in constipated patients. *Gut.* 1995;36:907-912.

84. Ponec RJ, Saunders MD, Kimmey MB. Neostigmine for the treatment of acute colonic pseudo-obstruction. *N Engl J Med.* 1999;341:137-141.

85. Gibbons D, Camilleri M, Nelson AD, Eckert D. Characteristics of chronic megacolon among patients diagnosed with multiple endocrine neoplasia type 2B. *United European Gastroenterol J.* 2016; 4:449-454.

86. Camilleri M. Peripheral mechanisms in irritable bowel syndrome. *N Engl J Med.* 2013;368:578-579.

87. Spiller RC. Postinfectious irritable bowel syndrome. *Gastroenterology.* 2003;124:1662-1671.

88. Vassallo M, Camilleri M, Phillips SF, Brown ML, Chapman NJ, Thomforde GM. Transit through the proximal colon influences stool weight in the irritable bowel syndrome. *Gastroenterology.* 1992;102:102-108.

89. McKee DP, Quigley EM. Intestinal motility in irritable bowel syndrome: is IBS a motility disorder? Part 1. Definition of IBS and colonic motility. *Dig Dis Sci.* 1993;38:1761-1772.

90. Whitehead WE, Palsson OS. Is rectal pain sensitivity a biological marker for irritable bowel syndrome: psychological influences on pain perception. *Gastroenterology.* 1998;115:1263-1271.

91. Posserud I, Syrous A, Lindström L, Tack J, Abrahamsson H, Simrén M. Altered rectal perception in irritable bowel syndrome is associated with symptom severity. *Gastroenterology.* 2007;133:1113-1123.

92. Odunsi-Shiyanbade ST, Camilleri M, McKinzie S, et al. Effects of chenodeoxycholate and a bile acid sequestrant, colesevelam, on intestinal transit and bowel function. *Clin Gastroenterol Hepatol.* 2010;8:159-165.

93. Wedlake L, A'Hern R, Russell D, Thomas K, Walters JRF, Andreyev HJN. Systematic review: the prevalence of idiopathic bile acid malabsorption as diagnosed by SeHCAT scanning in patients with diarrhoea-predominant irritable bowel syndrome. *Aliment Pharmacol Ther.* 2009;30:707-717.

94. Pimentel M, Park S, Mirocha J, Kane SV, Kong Y. The effect of a nonabsorbed oral antibiotic (rifaximin) on the symptoms of the irritable bowel syndrome: a randomized trial. *Ann Intern Med.* 2006;145:557-563. [Summary for patients in *Ann Intern Med.* 2006;145(8):I24; PMID: 17043334].

95. Pimentel M, Lembo A, Chey WD, et al. Rifaximin treatment for 2 weeks provides acute and sustained relief over 12 weeks of IBS symptoms in non-constipated irritable bowel syndrome: results from 2 North American phase 3 trials (target 1 and target 2). *Gastroenterology.* 2010;138:S64-S65.

96. von der Ohe MR, Camilleri M, Kvols LK, Thomforde GM. Motor dysfunction of the small bowel and colon in patients with the carcinoid syndrome and diarrhea. *N Engl J Med.* 1993;329:1073-1078. [Erratum appears in *N Engl J Med.* 1993;329(21):1592.]

97. Farthing MJ, Lennard-Jones JE. Sensibility of the rectum to distension and the anorectal distension reflex in ulcerative colitis. *Gut.* 1978;19:64-69.

98. Hofmann AF, Poley JR. Role of bile acid malabsorption in pathogenesis of diarrhea and steatorrhea in patients with ileal resection. I. Response to cholestyramine or replacement of dietary long chain triglyceride by medium chain triglyceride. *Gastroenterology.* 1972;62:918-934.

99. Fedorak RN, Field M, Chang EB. Treatment of diabetic diarrhea with clonidine. *Ann Intern Med.* 1985;102:197-199.

100. Painter N, Truelove S, Ardran E, Tuckey M. Segmentation and the localisation of intraluminal pressures in the human colon with special reference to the pathogenesis of colonic diverticula. *Gastroenterology.* 1965;49:169-177.

101. Bassotti G, Battaglia E, De Roberto G, Morelli A, Tonini M, Villanacci V. Alteration in colonic motility and relationship to pain in colonic diverticulosis. *Clin Gastroenterol Hepatol.* 2005;3:248-253.

102. Golder M, Burleigh DE, Belai A, et al. Smooth muscle cholinergic denervation hypersensitivity in diverticular disease. *Lancet.* 2003;361:1945-1951.

103. Nyam DC, Pemberton JH, Ilstrup DM, Rath DM. Long-term results of surgery for chronic constipation. *Dis Colon Rectum.* 1997;40:273-279. [Erratum appears in *Dis Colon Rectum.* 1997;40(5):529.]

104. Koda K, Saito N, Seike K, Shimzu K, Kosugi C, Miyazaki M. Denervation of the neorectum as a potential cause of defecatory disorder following low anterior resection for rectal cancer. *Dis Colon Rectum.* 2005;48:210-217.

105. Batignani G, Monaci I, Ficari F, Tonelli F. What affects continence after anterior resection of the rectum? *Dis Colon Rectum.* 1991;34:329-335.

106. Williamson ME, Lewis WG, Finan PJ, et al. Recovery of physiologic and clinical function after low anterior resection of the rectum for carcinoma: myth or reality? *Dis Colon Rectum.* 1995;38:411-418.

107. Kasparek MS, Muller MH, Glatzle J, et al. Postoperative colonic motility in patients following laparoscopic-assisted and open sigmoid colectomy. *J Gastrointest Surg.* 2003;7:1073-1081.

Diagnostic and Therapeutic Colonoscopy

Shaun R. Brown | Terry C. Hicks | Charles B. Whitlow

Since its acceptance for clinical use in 1970, colonoscopy has become the mainstay in the prevention, diagnosis, and treatment of colonic pathology. Even with the development of new diagnostic technologies, such as computed tomography (CT) colonography, only colonoscopy allows for direct visualization of the colonic mucosa combined with the potential for tissue biopsy, removal, or destruction. Colonoscopy also is used to diagnose and treat lower gastrointestinal (GI) bleeding and obstruction. At present colonoscopic polypectomy is the most effective visceral cancer prevention tool available in clinical practice.[1]

Improved bowel preparation and anesthesia techniques have led to a wider acceptance of colonoscopy by patients. Performed properly, the complication rate is low and the cecum is reached in greater than 90% of procedures.[2]

INDICATIONS

Advances in endoscopic techniques have expanded the role of colonoscopy for the diagnosis and treatment of various disease processes. There are several indications for colonoscopy to include screening for colorectal carcinoma, treatment and surveillance of colorectal polyps, and surveillance of inflammatory bowel disease. Colonoscopy is also a therapeutic option for lower GI bleeding, colonic volvulus detorsion, and colonic decompression for colonic pseudoobstruction.

CONTRAINDICATIONS

Patients who are either unwilling to give consent or are unable to be safely sedated should not undergo colonoscopy. Relative contraindications include patient with a known or suspected bowel perforation, megacolon or toxic colitis who are considered to be at higher risk of perforation.[3]

BOWEL PREPARATION

Bowel preparation is a key component of a successful colonoscopy and significantly affects the quality of the examination. Inadequate preparation can result in both missed pathologic lesions and canceled procedures.

Inadequate bowel preparation may occur in as many as 20% of scheduled procedures,[4] and only 3% of patients with an inadequate colonic preparation reported a failure to follow preparation instructions. Several factors may contribute to inadequate prep, such as later start time, reported failure to follow instructions, inpatient status, procedural indication of constipation, tricyclic antidepressants, male gender, and history of stroke or dementia.[4] Although it is intuitive that the quality of colonic cleansing

would directly relate to the quality of colonoscopy, a multicenter observation trial demonstrated a direct link between quality of bowel prep and polyp detection rate with an odds ratio (OR) of 1.46 in the high-quality group compared with low-quality group.[5] From an economic standpoint, poor bowel preparation can increase the cost of colonoscopy by up to 22% due to prolonged procedures and the need for shorter surveillance intervals.[5]

The ideal preparation for colonoscopy should empty the colon of all fecal material with little to no alterations to colonic mucosa. In addition, the preparations should be well tolerated by the patient and not cause any significant electrolyte alterations or fluid shifts. Unfortunately, there is no perfect bowel preparation. There are several options regarding preparation, with the majority falling within three main categories: osmotic agents, stimulants, and polyethylene glycol (PEG) solutions. Osmotic agents, such as sodium phosphate, increase the passage of extracellular fluid across the cell wall. However due to severe electrolyte derangement associated with sodium phosphate preps, the US Food and Drug Administration (FDA) issued an alert regarding renal injury, which has resulted in a significant decrease in use.[7,8] Sodium sulfate acts similarly to sodium phosphate, is commonly used outside of the United States, and is approved for use in the United States. It may be used alone or in combination with magnesium citrate.[9] Magnesium citrate is another hyperosmotic agent that has the added effect of stimulating the release of cholecystokinin. This results in fluid secretion and stimulation of peristalsis. Magnesium citrate has been used in combination with other agents but, as a sole agent, has typically been less effective.[10] Stimulants such as senna or Dulcolax increase bowel wall contraction through smooth muscle stimulation, which can result in significant cramping for the patient and are often used as adjuncts to other preparations.[11] PEG-based preparations, an osmotically balanced laxative that results in minimal water loss, are frequently prescribed and often well tolerated. However, 5% to 15% of patients may not complete the preparation due to either poor taste or the large volume (up to 4 L).[12]

An alternative preparation strategy is to split the dose of preparation into half the volume the day prior to the examination and the other half the morning of the procedure. This results in improved tolerance and quality of the bowel preparation.[13] In addition, split preparation results in improved polyp detection rates, specifically adenoma detection rates (ADRs).[14]

SEDATION

Although colonoscopy remains the procedure of choice for screening the colon and rectum, the procedure is not without fear and anxiety for many patients. These barriers may result in an unwillingness for patients to undergo initial screening, and a poor experience may prevent future examinations. Subramanian et al. surveyed 210 consecutive outpatients presenting for colonoscopy and demonstrated that of the eight statements about sedation the highest valuation to patients was "I don't want to feel any pain" and "I want to go to sleep and not wake up until the procedure is over."[15] Because of this, it is in the best interest of the patient to provide them with a safe and comfortable experience.

Therefore it is not surprising that the vast majority (98%) of colonoscopies performed in the United States are done in conjunction with some form of sedation.[16] The endoscopist should be familiar with the various options and associated risks and benefits of each. Two things to consider is whether the sedation is endoscopist administered or anesthesia administered and the intended level of sedation associated with each medication. The American Society of Anesthesiologists has described different levels of sedation based on patient responsiveness, ability to protect the airway, spontaneous ventilation, and cardiovascular function.[17]

Most patients currently receive a combination of a benzodiazepine (midazolam) and a narcotic (fentanyl).[18,19] The goal of this combination, which is usually endoscopist administered, is to provide a moderate level of sedation for the patient.

Propofol has been used in increasing numbers of patients, accounting for 20% to 25% of colonoscopies performed in 2012.[20] For endoscopic procedures, propofol is frequently equated with deep sedation and is usually anesthesia administered.

When compared with midazolam/fentanyl, propofol results in a decreased recovery time, time to discharge, and improved patient satisfaction.[20] One of the disadvantages of propofol is that it is often administered by an anesthesiology provider, resulting in a 20% increase in cost for the procedure.[21] In addition, there is evidence it may result in increased complications related to the level of sedation (deep vs. moderate). Cooper et al. compared complications in more than 165,000 colonoscopies performed with anesthesia assistance versus those without. The authors found overall complications were higher in the anesthesia-assisted group (0.22% vs. 0.16%), as was the rate of aspiration (0.14% vs. 0.10%). Perforations and splenic injuries were similar between the two populations. Multivariate analysis confirmed that anesthesia services was associated with an increased risk of complication, and the authors concluded that this was likely related to depth of sedation.[22]

As previously stated, propofol is often administered by an anesthesiology provider, and there is an FDA package insert stating that propofol should be "administered only by persons trained in the administration of general anesthesia and not involved in the conduct of the surgical/diagnostic procedure." Despite these issues, there is ample evidence that nonanesthesiologist-administered propofol can be safely accomplished.[23–25] A cost-effectiveness analysis concluded that the economic benefit of implementing the practice of endoscopist-administered propofol in the United States would result in a 10-year savings of $3.2 billion.[26]

Finally, some patients may elect to undergo an unsedated colonoscopy. The advantages of unsedated colonoscopy are multiple: decreased cost, it eliminates the risks of sedation, immediate resumption of normal activity, and decreased inconvenience to patients. Requirements for unsedated colonoscopy include a motivated patient and a skilled endoscopist. However, anatomic factors may prevent successful completion without addition of sedation. The data available, although limited, demonstrate that a cecal intubation rate was 82%, which increased to 97% when on-demand sedation was administered.[27] Although this may be a viable option for some, it is likely this will remain an uncommon practice for the majority of patients.

ANTIBIOTICS

There are approximately 14 million colonoscopies performed annually in the United States, and only approximately 25 cases of infectious endocarditis (IE) have been reported with any association with endoscopic procedures.[28–30] In 2007 the American Heart Association (AHA) released guidelines for prophylaxis of IE, which stated that the administration of prophylactic antibiotics solely to prevent IE was no longer recommended for patients undergoing GI endoscopy.[31]

Similarly patients with synthetic vascular grafts or other nonvalvular cardiovascular devices are often considered at increased risk of infection. However, according to the 2003 AHA recommendations there is no evidence that microorganisms associated with GI endoscopy cause infections of nonvalvular cardiac devices. Therefore routine antibiotic prophylaxis is not recommended for those patients undergoing colonoscopy.[31]

Another group of patients sometimes felt to require prophylaxis antibiotics are those patients with orthopedic prosthesis. However, infection of prosthetic joints related to GI endoscopy is extremely rare, and the few case reports are related to invasive upper endoscopy and not colonoscopy.[32–34] The American Society of Gastrointestinal Endoscopy (ASGE) recommends against antibiotic prophylaxis for patients with orthopedic prosthesis undergoing GI endoscopy.[35]

Peritoneal dialysis patients are at increased risk of peritonitis following endoscopy,[36] and the risk of peritonitis after colonoscopy may be as high as 6.3%.[37] These patients may benefit from prophylactic antibiotics administered either intravenously the day of the procedure or intraperitoneally the night before colonoscopy.[35]

There is no evidence to support the use of prophylactic antibiotics in immunocompromised patients with normal neutrophil counts (human immunodeficiency virus [HIV]-positive patients, organ transplant), whereas the use in severe immunosuppressed patients (absolute neutrophil count <500 cells/μL) should be individualized.[38]

ANTICOAGULATION

Anticoagulation therapy is commonly prescribed to patients with such conditions as atrial fibrillation (AF), deep vein thrombosis (DVT), and acute coronary syndrome (ACS) in an attempt to decrease the risk of thromboembolic events. However, this therapy is not without inherent risks,

TABLE 145.1 American Society of Gastrointestinal Endoscopy Procedure Risk for Bleeding

Higher-Risk Procedures	Low-Risk Procedures
Polypectomy	Diagnostic (EGD, colonoscopy,
Biliary or pancreatic	flexible sigmoidoscopy)
sphincterotomy	including mucosal biopsy
Treatment of varices	ERCP with stent (biliary or
PEG placement*	pancreatic) placement or
Therapeutic balloon-	papillary balloon dilation
assisted enteroscopy	without sphincterotomy
EUS with FNA[†]	Push enteroscopy and
Endoscopic hemostasis	diagnostic balloon-assisted
Tumor ablation	enteroscopy
Cystgastrostomy	Capsule endoscopy
Ampullary resection	EUS without FNA
EMR	Argon plasma coagulation
ESD	Barrett ablation
Pneumatic or bougie dilation	Argon plasma coagulation
PEJ	Barrett ablation
	Enteral stent deployment

*PEG on aspirin or clopidogrel therapy is low risk. Does not apply to dual antiplatelet therapy.
[†]EUS-FNA of solid masses on aspirin/nonsteroidal antiinflammatory drugs is low risk.
EGD, Esophagogastroduodenoscopy; *EMR,* endoscopic mucosal resection; *ERCP,* endoscopic retrograde cholangiopancreatography; *ESD,* endoscopic submucosal dissection; *EUS,* endoscopic ultrasound; *FNA,* fine-needle aspiration; *PEG,* percutaneous endoscopic gastrostomy; *PEJ,* percutaneous endoscopic jejunostomy.

which include GI bleeding, and the use of these medications increases the risk of hemorrhage after endoscopic interventions.[39,40] The number of patients taking these medications is increasing, and the development of new therapies poses a unique challenge for the endoscopist.

When a patient on antithrombotic therapy requires colonoscopy, the endoscopist must consider several factors, such as the urgency of the procedure, bleeding risk associated with the procedure, effects of the antithrombotic medication on the bleeding risks, and risk of stopping the antithrombotic therapy (Abraham bleeding risk and strategies).[41]

According to the ASGE 2016 guidelines, a diagnostic colonoscopy and flexible sigmoidoscopy including mucosal biopsy is considered a low-risk procedure, whereas a polypectomy, endoscopic mucosal resection (EMR), and endoscopic submucosal dissection (ESD) are considered high-risk procedures (Table 145.1).[42] Overall, the risk of bleeding after polypectomy ranges from 0.3% to 10%, depending on the polyp size, location, morphology (nonpolypoid, sessile, pedunculated), and resection technique. There are data to support the use of cold snare rather than hot snare in those patients anticoagulated with warfarin. Cold snare resulted in less delayed bleeding requiring intervention.[43]

The risk of hemorrhage peaks at 4 to 6 days following the procedure and may last up to 14 days. In general, the morbidity of a thromboembolic event is greater than the risk of hemorrhage. Therefore resuming anticoagulation as soon as possible following colonoscopy is our current practice.

INSERTION AND WITHDRAWAL

Typically, patients are placed in the left lateral position, and sedation if desired, is administered. Some authors advocate starting the exam with the patient supine or in the right lateral position.[44] Air is most commonly used for insufflation, but some recommend the routine use of CO_2 because pain in the immediate periprocedural time is decreased with CO_2 insufflation.[45] No increase in complication has been demonstrated with CO_2, but there is some additional cost due to the need for a gas regulator and the cost of CO_2. For patients with suspected obstruction or intestinal distention preprocedurally, CO_2 is an excellent option.[46] It may also have benefit in prolonged cases, such as those with advanced polyp resection techniques (EMR, ESD). It is crucial to the performance of intraoperative colonoscopy. There is also a small group of enthusiasts for water-aided colonoscopy in which water instillation replaced air or CO_2 insufflation. This may be particularly beneficial in redundant colons

For the majority of patients a standard colonoscope is acceptable. Patients with difficult colons due to acute angulation may benefit from the use of a pediatric colonoscope or even a gastroscope—both of these have a smaller diameter and tighter turning radius than an adult colonoscope.[45,47] The scope should initially be placed in a neutral position with a gentle loop. The portion of the scope that connects from the handle to the processor should also be positioned without any looping. Inspection of the perianal skin is performed, followed by a thorough digital rectal exam. The left colon is the most difficult part of the colon to traverse in the majority of patients. Ideally, direct visualization of the lumen is maintained throughout the procedure, using a combination of torque on the insertion tube and angulation of the tip. Although clockwise torque is the predominant direction applied, there are some cases in which counterclockwise torque will be needed. Looping of the scope is common in the left side of the colon, but efforts to reduce looping should be made any time a relatively straight portion of the colon is encountered. A combination of slow withdrawal, aspiration of air, and torque all performed simultaneously while keeping the lumen in view with the angulation knobs is an effective loop-reducing technique. Abdominal pressure, use of an adjustable stiffness colonoscope, and positional changes are other adjuncts to allow for successful cecal intubation. Although there are instances in which a "slide by" technique may be necessary, insertion against fixed resistance should not be performed (the concept of primum non nocere is apropos in screening colonoscopy). After the cecum is intubated, photodocumentation should be obtained. It should be stressed that cecal intubation means entering into the cecum, proximal to the ileocecal valve and not simply visualizing the appendiceal orifice when the scope is distal to the valve. Thorough inspection of the cecum requires distending it and pulling back on the scope while torqueing or angulating the tip downward to expose the area immediately proximal to the valve—in this area aspiration of gas may be necessary. Intubation of the ileocecal valve, while not technically possible in all cases, is important in evaluating patients with bleeding and inflammatory bowel disease; routinely attempting

TABLE 145.2 Digital Chromoendoscopy Technologies

Technology	Manufacturer	Mechanism
Narrow band imaging	Olympus (Tokyo, Japan)	Optical filter. Mucosal vessels highlighted because of absorption of green and blue wavelengths in hemoglobin
Fujinon intelligent color enhancement	Fujinon (Tokyo, Japan)	Computerized digital manipulation of images using wavelength combinations
iScan	Pentax (Tokyo, Japan)	Computerized enhanced images of the mucosal surface and the blood vessels through postimage processing

this will develop the skill so that the endoscopist is able to perform it when needed. Retroflexion in the cecum can be performed and is sometimes necessary to remove ascending colon polyps.

Withdrawal of the scope is performed in a methodical manner. Thorough exam of all mucosal surfaces requires cleansing the colon wall with water and aspirating pools of liquid. Skillful maneuvering of the scope tip combined with strategic insufflation or aspiration allows adequate inspection of difficult folds and turns. Polypectomy and mucosal biopsies are typically done at this time, but small polyps seen on insertion are addressed if they are not going to be easily identified later in the exam. Some endoscopists routinely move patients to the supine position for withdrawal because this allows fluid to accumulate in the dependent portions of the colon (cecum, flexures, rectum), which aids in localization. Slow withdrawal of the scope gives the endoscopist adequate time for visual processing of the mucosa to minimize missed lesions. Flat polyps are more common in the right colon and require a heightened awareness. Areas of severe angulation or suboptimal visualization should be examined with multiple back and forth passes of the scope. Repositioning of the patient may be required to obtain an adequate examination. Some endoscopists routinely retroflex in the rectum, whereas others perform this maneuver selectively but obtain a thorough exam of the distal rectum and anal canal by 360-degree maneuvering of the scope.

IMPROVING NEOPLASIA DETECTION

The intent of screening colonoscopy is to detect early cancer and to detect and destroy or remove adenomas, thus preventing colorectal cancer development. Aggressive colonoscopic screening has produced a reduction in colorectal cancer (CRC) mortality, but interval cancers account for up to 6% of CRCs.[48] Adenoma miss rates of up to 24% have been reported, with a 2% miss rate for adenomas greater than 10 mm.[49,50] These limitations have led to the development of image-enhancing technologies, including high-definition colonoscopies, dye-based chromoendoscopy (referred to as chromoendoscopy here), and several electronic image-enhancing technologies referred to sometimes as digital chromoendoscopy. High-definition colonoscopy increases magnification up to 35 times but has only slightly improved adenoma detection.[51] The other technologies described later have not been adopted into widespread use for screening colonoscopy.

In dye-based chromoendoscopy the dye (indigo carmine, methylene blue, or crystal violet) is sprayed onto the colonic mucosa to enhance examination with standard or high-definition (HD) white-light colonoscopy. Screening population studies to date demonstrate a slight increase in ADR with chromoendoscopy, with most of the increase coming from diminutive, flat, and serrated lesions.[52] No data on improvement in interval cancers exist. Prolonged examination time is a drawback of chromoendoscopy. Several studies have demonstrated improved detection of dysplasia using chromoendoscopy (compared with standard white light colonoscopy) in patients with long-standing ulcerative colitis.[53,54]

Digital chromoendoscopy technologies are commercially available from different colonoscopy manufacturers and involve the use of optical filters or digital image manipulation (Table 145.2; Fig. 145.1). These technologies do not appear to increase ADR in screening populations nor have they shown superiority to standard or HD colonoscopy in detecting dysplasia in at-risk chronic ulcerative colitis patients.

Other devices for improving adenoma detection include cap-fitting, Third Eye Retroscope (Avantis Medical Systems, Sunnyvale, California), and Full Spectrum Endoscopy (Fuse) (Endochoice, Atlanta, Georgia). Cap-fitted colonoscopy involves placing a plastic cap on the end of the colonoscope. Several studies, including a randomized tandem examination study, have shown an increase in adenoma detection with cap fitting.[55] Time to cecum has also been shorter with cap-fitting in some studies. The Third Eye Retroscope has also been shown to increase adenoma detection. It is placed through the biopsy channel and therefore has to be removed to remove any polyps identified. The Fuse colonoscope has a 330-degree field of view compared with 170 degrees for a standard colonoscope. There are no data on the ADR benefits of Fuse.

NEOPLASIA REMOVAL

Because the majority of colon cancers are thought to arise via the adenoma to carcinoma sequence, polyps should generally be removed if possible. Diminutive hyperplastic rectal polyps can be left in situ. Polyps with features consistent with malignancy, such as ulceration, induration, or failure to lift with submucosal saline injection, should not be removed endoscopically. Polyp morphology and pit pattern have also been used as predictors of neoplasia and, in some instances, differentiating benignity from

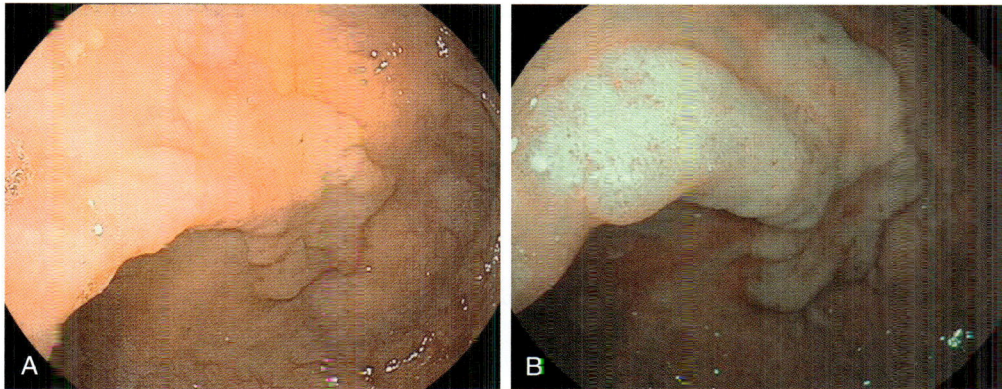

FIGURE 145.1 (A) Lesion seen with high-definition white light colonoscopy. (B) Same lesion with narrow band imaging.

TABLE 145.3 Paris Classification of Superficial Neoplastic Lesions

Class	Features
Ip	Pedunculated
Is	Sessile
IIa	Slightly raised
IIb	Nonpolypoid, flat
IIc	Nonpolypoid, slightly depressed
III	Nonpolypoid, excavated

malignancy. The Paris classification categorizes polyps by gross morphology (Table 145.3).[56] Although some evidence indicates that this morphology schema correlates with risk of malignancy, one study demonstrated only moderate interobserver agreement and therefore questions the reliability and value of this method of classification. Kudo described pit patterns in polyps viewed under colonoscopic magnification (Table 145.4).[57] A meta-analysis demonstrated that assessment of pit patterns is a highly accurate method for assessing a polyp as neoplastic or nonneoplastic.[58] The goal is to remove all neoplastic tissue safely, keeping in mind that the risk of malignancy and the risk of complications increase with polyp size.

For all polyps, maneuvering the scope so that the polyp resides in the 5 o'clock to 7 o'clock position facilitates removal because of the location of the colonoscopy biopsy channel. Pedunculated polyps are typically removed using a cautery snare. The use of coagulation mode decreases the likelihood of immediate bleeding from the stalk. Care should be taken to keep the tip of the snare off of the adjacent colon wall when applying the coagulation current to avoid unintended thermal injury.

Polypectomy for sessile polyps depends on several features, including size and location. Polyps less than 5 mm are removed by cold biopsy forceps, which are available in standard and jumbo sizes. The polyp is grasped, and the catheter quickly pulled back. The mucosa should be examined for complete removal of neoplasia, and additional passes may be required. Minor bleeding is common but rarely requires any treatment. The forceps

is removed from the biopsy channel and tissue retrieved. Hot biopsy forceps are also available. After grasping the polyp, coagulation is applied to the tissue until blanching occurs and a firm pull applied to the catheter. The amount of coagulation is imprecise, and this technique is being used less commonly because of the risk of perforation and delayed postpolypectomy bleeding. It may still be useful for removing residual neoplasia from an incomplete polypectomy or the case of a difficult to remove small polyp in which the endoscopist feels complete polypectomy will not otherwise be possible.

Sessile polyps larger than 5 mm most commonly are removed with a snare. A variety of snare shapes and sizes are available. Cold snares can be used for lesions up to 8 mm, with the expectation that acute bleeding requiring treatment will not be any higher than using a hot snare (Fig. 145.2). Coagulation, cut, and blended modes are available for hot snares. No data exist demonstrating a single electrosurgical mode or generator as superior over others in performing hot snare polypectomy, but the tradeoff is a higher rate of acute bleeding with cutting current and a higher rate of delayed bleeding and perforation with coagulation. Larger polyps and flatter polyps pose a challenge for snare polypectomy. Piecemeal excision may be performed or saline-lift polypectomy (EMR, Fig. 145.3). Saline is injected into the submucosal plane prior to placing the snare around the polyp. Failure to lift is a contraindication to EMR (Fig. 145.4). The injection should start on the proximal aspect of the lesion to push the polyp toward the scope. At this point, snare polypectomy and EMR are similar. As the snare is tightened, the tip of the catheter is moved toward the distal extent of the polyp. Gentle aspiration of gas may also be helpful. Coordinated closure of the snare by the assistant simultaneous with application of current completes the transection. Polyps that are not amenable to these techniques should be considered for laparoscopic-assisted polypectomy, segmental colectomy, or referral to an endoscopist trained in performing ESD. This technique involves the use of a needle knife to aid dissection under the entire polyp (Fig. 145.5). It had higher acceptance in the esophagus and stomach and is not widely available in the United States. However, if it is a consideration, it is best to not

TABLE 145.4 Pit Pattern Classification of Polyps

Type	Schematic	Endoscopic	Description	Suggested Pathology	Ideal Treatment
I			Round pits	Nonneoplastic	Endoscopic or none
II			Stellar or papillary pits	Nonneoplastic	Endoscopic or none
III$_S$			Small tubular or round pits that are smaller than the normal pit	Neoplastic	Endoscopic
III$_L$			Tubular or roundish pits that are larger than the normal pits	Neoplastic	Endoscopic
IV			Branch-like or gyrus-like pits	Neoplastic	Endoscopic
V$_I$			Irregularly arranged pits with type IIIs, IIIt, type IV pit patterns	Neoplastic (invasive)	Endoscopic or surgical
V$_N$			Nonstructural pits	Neoplastic (massive submucosal invasive)	Surgical

attempt any resection of the polyp initially because the fibrosis caused by attempted polypectomy decreases the chances of successful ESD.

COMPLICATIONS

Complications arising from colonoscopy are uncommon. In a systematic review of 12 studies totaling 57,742 patients who underwent average-risk screening, the overall adverse rate was 2.8 per 1000 procedures. However, 85% of the serious complications were reported in patients undergoing colonoscopy with polypectomy, producing a reported complication rate ranging from 0.7% to 3%.[59,60]

In reviewing the literature on colonic complications, the reader must be cognizant that the studies generally represent the best of experiences at high-volume expert centers and may not reflect the true incidences of complications.[61]

Perforation is the most serious common complication of colonoscopy and often results in medical-legal action against the endoscopist. Prompt identification and appropriate management minimize the morbidity and mortality of these complications.

Diagnostic perforations most commonly occur during intubation. It is usually the result of forceful passage through a loop that splits the bowel at the intestinal narrowing (most commonly in the sigmoid colon). These constricted areas are often a result of diverticular disease or adhesions from previous pelvic surgeries. It is rare for the tip of the scope to perforate the bowel except when unhealthy tissue is present, such as ischemia, ulcer, or inflammation. Traumatic perforations are usually identified

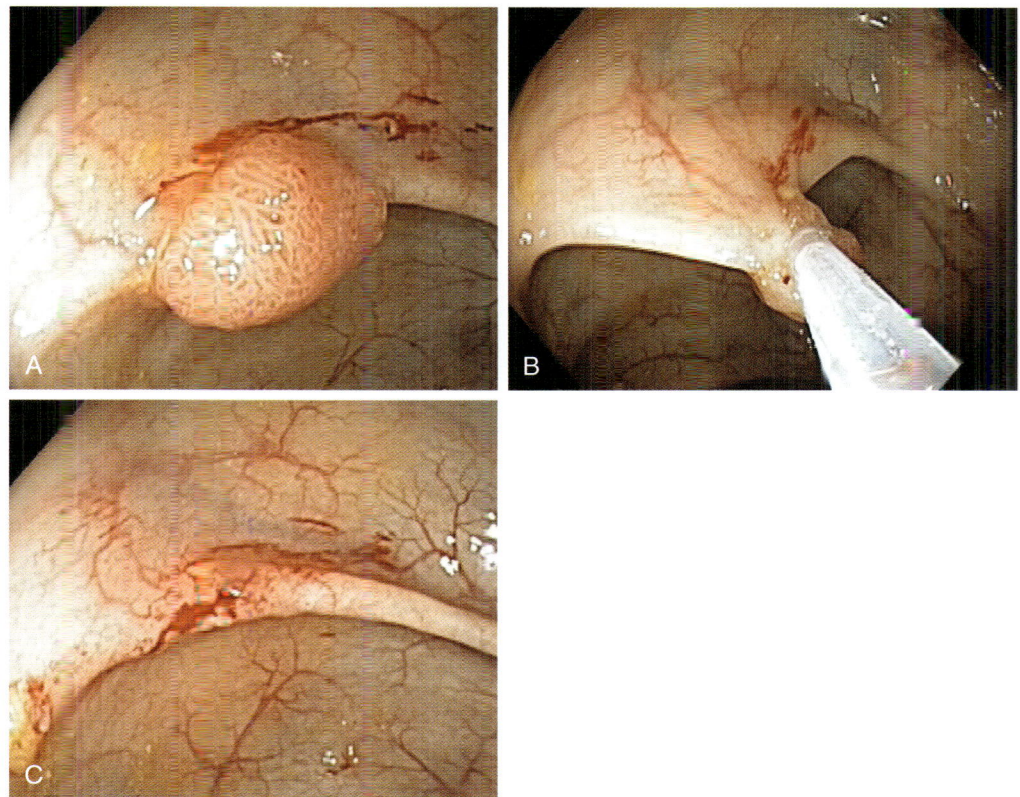

FIGURE 145.2 Cold snare polypectomy.

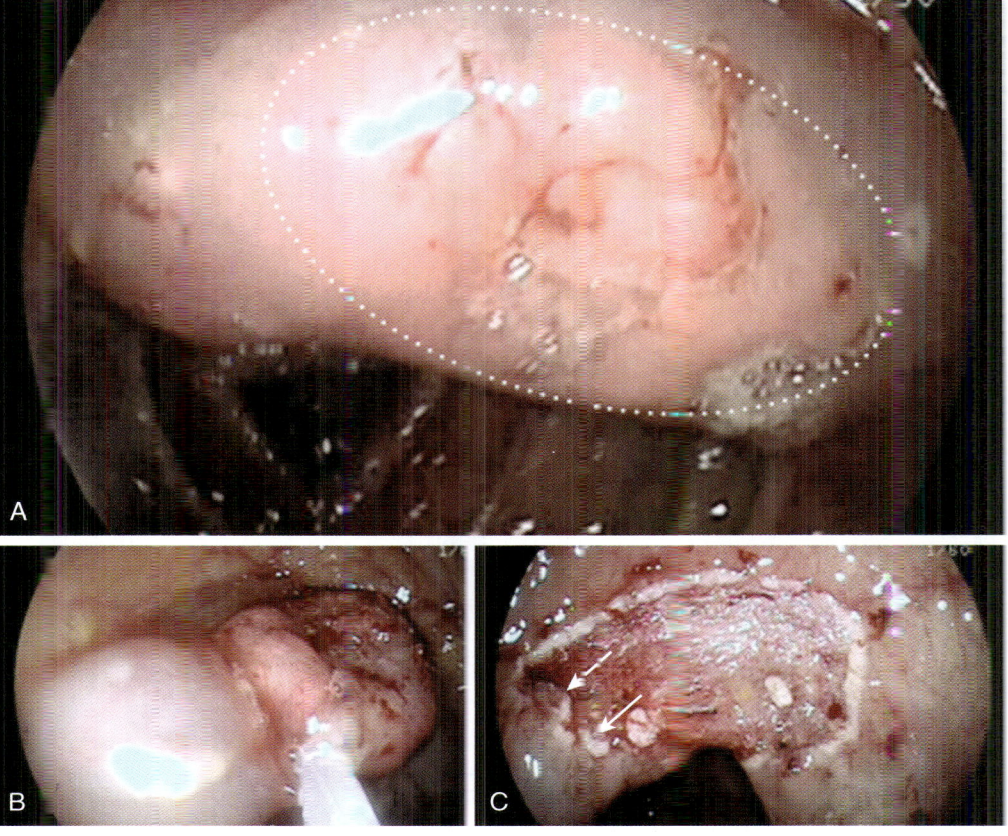

FIGURE 145.3 Endoscopic mucosal resection.

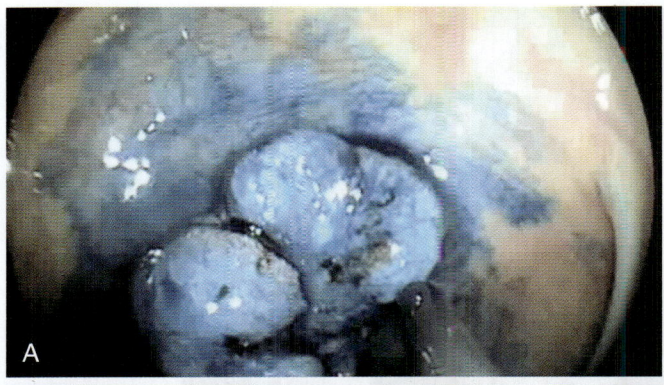

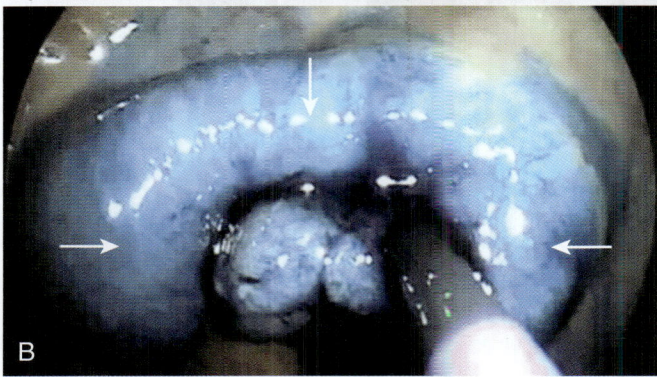

FIGURE 145.4 Nonlifting sign. *Arrows* demonstrate area of lifted mucosa with central lesion failing to lift.

intraprocedurally by the visualization of extracolonic fat, gaseous distention of the abdominal cavity, or pain. Urgent radiography may confirm the diagnosis by the presence of free intraperitoneal air.[62] If surgical intervention is timely, a primary repair of the bowel can be considered. If the surgeon encounters generalized peritonitis, resection with diversion is the safest approach.

Colonoscopic polypectomy complications include postpolypectomy syndrome, perforation, and postpolypectomy hemorrhage. Polypectomy perforation may be appreciated intraprocedurally or may occur up to 10 days postprocedure when the necrotic patch of colon at the biopsy site sloughs. Transmural injury from electrocautery is routinely the nidus for this complication. Surgical intervention has historically been the gold standard. However, an increasing number of case reports describe the feasibility of using endoscopic clipping devices to repair the perforation.[63]

Postpolypectomy syndrome is the result of electrocautery-induced perforation of the colonic wall that has sealed. The patients often present 1 to 5 days after the procedure with localized tenderness, fever, and leukocytosis but without gross peritonitis or radiographic evidence of a perforation. The incidence is reported to range from 0.003% to 0.1%.[59] Hospitalization with intravenous hydration, bowel rest, and broad-spectrum parenteral antibiotics usually resolve the symptomatology. If the injury progresses

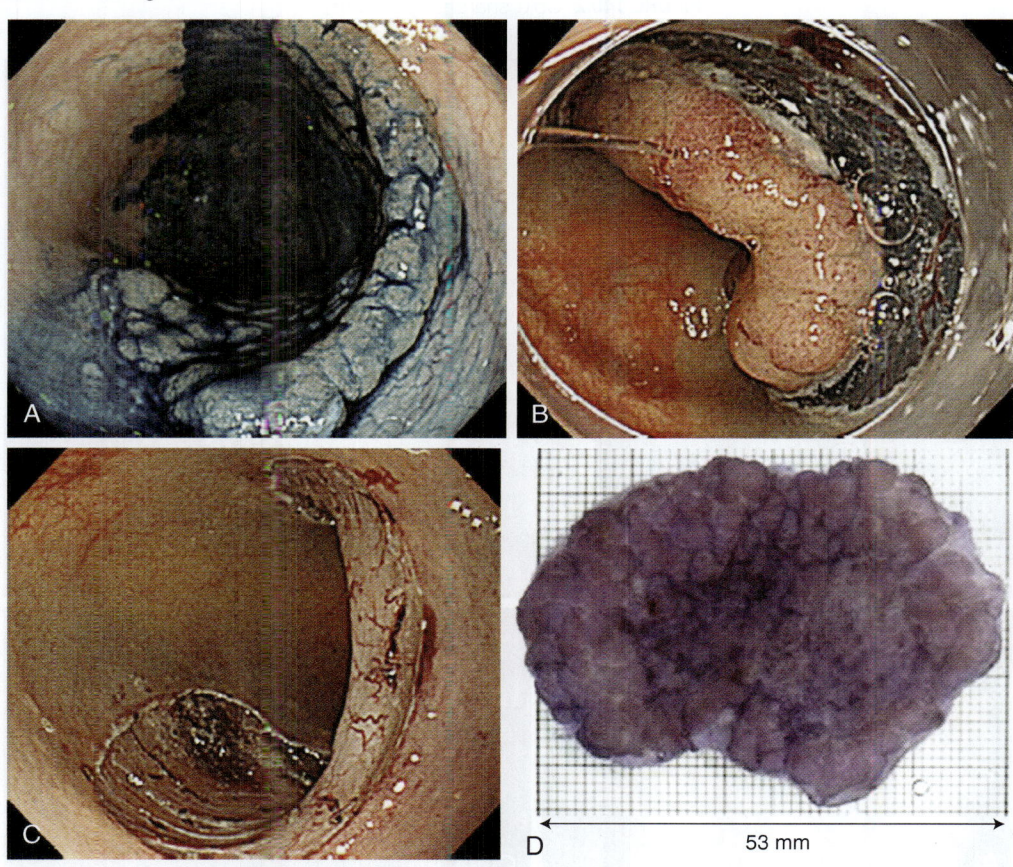

FIGURE 145.5 Example of colorectal endoscopic submucosal dissection.

53 mm

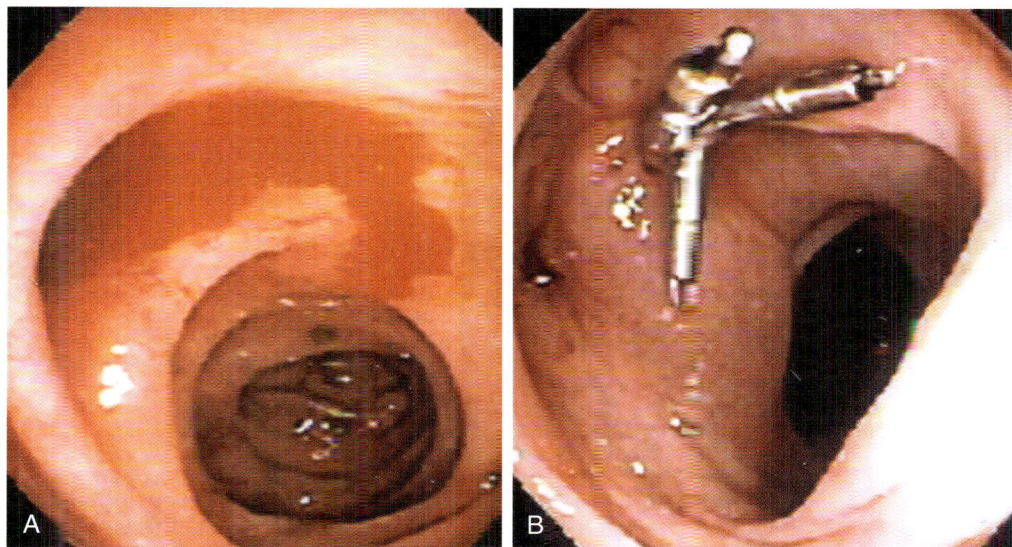

FIGURE 145.6 Endoscopic placement of clips for colonic bleeding.

to an intraabdominal abscess, it can be potentially managed with CT-guided percutaneous drainage.[64]

Colonoscopic-induced bleeding is usually associated with polypectomy and may occur immediately or can be delayed for several weeks.[65] Postprocedure risk factors for hemorrhage include large polyp size and proximal colonic location.[66] Anticoagulation use may be an independent risk factor. Immediate bleeding from a polypectomy can often be controlled with the same techniques used for acute diverticular bleeding, including injection of a diluted epinephrine solution to the site, hemoclips, or electrocoagulation (Fig. 145.6).[67] If the polyp is pedunculated, another option is to resnare the site, occluding the remaining stalk, for 15 minutes without the use of electrocoagulation.

Delayed bleeding usually presents as passage of large-volume bloody bowel movements. The initial management includes fluid resuscitation, confirming if the bleeding is still active, review of possible anticoagulation use, and review of the endoscopy note. Although up to two-thirds of patients have ceased passing bloody movements at their initial presentation, they should be placed in observation. This is especially true if they are frail, have significant comorbidities, or do not have easy access to hospital care.

In the setting of massive bleeding, visualization of colonic lumen is limited and endoscopic control may be challenging. After resuscitating the patient, computerized tomographic angiography (CTA) can be performed to identify the site of bleeding and to confirm that there is active ongoing bleeding. A positive CTA can be followed by selective arteriography and possible embolization of the bleeding vessel. If interventional therapeutic angiography and endoscopic control fail to control the bleeding, exploratory celiotomy becomes necessary.[68]

MISCELLANEOUS COMPLICATIONS

Miscellaneous complications of colonoscopy are rare but can be associated with significant morbidity. There are

case reports including splenic rupture,[69] small bowel obstructions,[70,71] acute appendicitis,[72] acute pancreatitis,[73] diverticulitis,[74] subcutaneous emphysema,[75] and tearing of mesenteric vessels with intraabdominal hemorrhage.

REFERENCES

1. Toliver KA, Rex DK. Colonoscopic polypectomy. *Gastroenterol Clin North Am*. 2008;37:229-251.
2. Niratvongs S. How to teach colonoscopy. *Clin Colon Rectal Surg*. 2001;14:387-392.
3. Minoli G, Meucci G, Bortoli A, et al. The ASGE guidelines for the appropriate use of colonoscopy in an open access system. *Gastrointest Endosc*. 2000;52:39-44.
4. Ness RM, Manam R, Hoen H, Chalasani N. Predictors of inadequate bowel preparation for colonoscopy. *Am J Gastroenterol*. 2001;96:1797-1802.
5. Froehlich F, Wietlisbach V, Gonvers JJ, Burnand B, Vader JP. Impact of colonic cleansing on quality and diagnostic yield of colonoscopy: the European Panel of Appropriateness of Gastrointestinal Endoscopy European multicenter study. *Gastrointest Endosc*. 2005;61:378-384.
6. Rex DK, Imperiale TF, Latinovich DR, Bratcher LL. Impact of bowel preparation on efficiency and cost of colonoscopy. *Am J Gastroenterol*. 2002;97:1696-1700.
7. Markowitz GS, Stokes MB, Radhakrishnan J, D'Agati VD. Acute phosphate nephropathy following oral sodium phosphate bowel purgative: an underrecognized cause of chronic renal failure. *J Am Soc Nephrol*. 2005;16:3389-3396.
8. Markowitz GS, Perazella MA. Acute phosphate nephropathy. *Kidney Int*. 2009;76:1027-1034.
9. Regev A, Fraser G, Delpre G, et al. Comparison of two bowel preparations for colonoscopy: sodium picosulphate with magnesium citrate versus sulphate-free polyethylene glycol lavage solution. *Am J Gastroenterol*. 1998;93:1478-1482.
10. Voiosu T, Ratiu I, Voiosu A, et al. Time for individualized colonoscopy bowel-prep regimens? A randomized controlled trial comparing sodium picosulphate and magnesium citrate versus 4-liter split-dose polyethylene glycol. *J Gastrointestin Liver Dis*. 2013;22:129-134.
11. Hookey LC, Depew WT, Vanner SJ. A prospective randomized trial comparing low-dose oral sodium phosphate plus stimulant laxatives with large volume polyethylene glycol solution for colon cleansing. *Am J Gastroenterol*. 2004;99:2217-2222.
12. Marshall JB, Pineda JJ, Barthel JS, King PD. Prospective, randomized trial comparing sodium phosphate solution with polyethylene glycol-electrolyte lavage for colonoscopy preparation. *Gastrointest Endosc*. 1993;39:631-634.

13. Kilgore TW, Abdinoor AA, Szary NM, et al. Bowel preparation with split-dose polyethylene glycol before colonoscopy: a meta-analysis of randomized controlled trials. *Gastrointest Endosc.* 2011;73:1240-1245.

14. Enestvedt BK, Tofani C, Laine LA, Tierney A, Fennerty MB. 4-Liter split-dose polyethylene glycol is superior to other bowel preparations, based on systematic review and meta-analysis. *Clin Gastroenterol Hepatol.* 2012;10:1225-1231.

15. Subramanian S, Liangpunsakul S, Rex DK. Preprocedure patient values regarding sedation for colonoscopy. *J Clin Gastroenterol.* 2005;39:516-519.

16. Rex DK, Khalfan HK. Sedation and the technical performance of colonoscopy. *Gastrointest Endosc Clin N Am.* 2005;15:661-672.

17. American Society of Anesthesiologists. Continuum of depth of sedation definition of general anesthesia and levels of sedation/analgesia. http://wwwasahqorg/publicationsAndServices/standards/20pdf/. Accessed 31 May 2016.

18. Childers RE, Williams JL, Sonnenberg A. Practice patterns of sedation for colonoscopy. *Gastrointest Endosc.* 2015;82:503-511.

19. Cohen LB, Wecsler JS, Gaetano JN, et al. Endoscopic sedation in the United States: results from a nationwide survey. *Am J Gastroenterol.* 2006;101:967-974.

20. Singh H, Poluha W, Cheung M, Choptain N, Baron KI, Taback SP. Propofol for sedation during colonoscopy. *Cochrane Database Syst Rev.* 2008;(4):CD006268.

21. Khiani VS, Soulos P, Gancayco J, Gross CP. Anesthesiologist involvement in screening colonoscopy: temporal trends and cost implications in the Medicare population. *Clin Gastroenterol Hepatol.* 2012;10:58-64.e1.

22. Cooper GS, Kou TD, Rex DK. Complications following colonoscopy with anesthesia assistance: a population-based analysis. *JAMA Intern Med.* 2013;173:551-556.

23. Vargo JJ, Cohen LB, Rex DK, Kwo PY. Position statement: nonanesthesiologist administration of propofol for GI endoscopy. *Hepatology.* 2009;50:1683-1689.

24. Ulmer BJ, Hansen JJ, Overley CA, et al. Propofol versus midazolam/fentanyl for outpatient colonoscopy: administration by nurses supervised by endoscopists. *Clin Gastroenterol Hepatol.* 2003;1:425-432.

25. Hansen JJ, Ulmer BJ, Rex DK. Technical performance of colonoscopy in patients sedated with nurse-administered propofol. *Am J Gastroenterol.* 2004;99:52-56.

26. Hassan C, Rex DK, Cooper GS, Benamouzig R. Endoscopist-directed propofol administration versus anesthesiologist assistance for colorectal cancer screening: a cost-effectiveness analysis. *Endoscopy.* 2012;44:456-464.

27. Petrini JL, Egan JV, Hahn WV. Unsedated colonoscopy: patient characteristics and satisfaction in a community-based endoscopy unit. *Gastrointest Endosc.* 2009;69:567-572.

28. Sekino Y, Fujisawa N, Suzuki K, et al. A case of recurrent infective endocarditis following colonoscopy. *Endoscopy.* 2010;42:E217.

29. Yu-Hsien L, Te-Li C, Chien-Pei C, Chen-Chi T. Nosocomial *Acinetobacter* genomic species 13 TU endocarditis following an endoscopic procedure. *Intern Med.* 2008;47:799-802.

30. Malani AN, Aronoff DM, Bradley SF, Kauffman CA. *Cardiobacterium hominis* endocarditis: two cases and a review of the literature. *Eur J Clin Microbiol Infect Dis.* 2006;25:587-595.

31. Wilson W, Taubert KA, Gewitz M, et al. Prevention of infective endocarditis: guidelines from the American Heart Association: a guideline from the American Heart Association Rheumatic Fever, Endocarditis, and Kawasaki Disease Committee, Council on Cardiovascular Disease in the Young, and the Council on Clinical Cardiology, Council on Cardiovascular Surgery and Anesthesia, and the Quality of Care and Outcomes Research Interdisciplinary Working Group. *Circulation.* 2007;116:1736-1754.

32. Scott NA, Tweedle DE. Pyogenic arthritis of the knee following Nd:YAG laser destruction of an esophageal cancer. *Gastrointest Endosc.* 1990;36:545-546.

33. Vanderhooft JE, Robinson RP. Late infection of a bipolar prosthesis following endoscopy. A case report. *J Bone Joint Surg Am.* 1994;76:744-746.

34. Zimmerli W, Trampuz A, Ochsner PE. Prosthetic-joint infections. *N Engl J Med.* 2004;351:1645-1654.

35. ASGE Standards of Practice Committee, Khashab MA, Chithadi KV, et al. Antibiotic prophylaxis for GI endoscopy. *Gastrointest Endosc.* 2015;81:81-89.

36. Poortvliet W, Selten HP, Raasveld MH, Klemt-Kropp M. CAPD peritonitis after colonoscopy: follow the guidelines. *Neth J Med.* 2010;68:377-378.

37. Yip T, Tse KC, Lam MF, et al. Risks and outcomes of peritonitis after flexible colonoscopy in CAPD patients. *Perit Dial Int.* 2007;27:560-564.

38. Bianco JA, Pepe MS, Higano C, Applebaum FR, McDonald GB, Singer JW. Prevalence of clinically relevant bacteremia after upper gastrointestinal endoscopy in bone marrow transplant recipients. *Am J Med.* 1990;89:134-136.

39. Jneid H, Anderson JL, Wright RS, et al. 2012 ACCF/AHA focused update of the guideline for the management of patients with unstable angina/non-ST-elevation myocardial infarction (updating the 2007 guideline and replacing the 2011 focused update). A report of the American College of Cardiology Foundation/American Heart Association Task Force on Practice Guidelines. *J Am Coll Cardiol.* 2012;60:645-681.

40. Wallentin L, Becker RC, Budaj A, et al. Ticagrelor versus clopidogrel in patients with acute coronary syndromes. *N Engl J Med.* 2009;361:1045-1057.

41. Abraham NS, Hartman C, Richardson P, Castillo D, Street RL Jr, Naik AD. Risk of lower and upper gastrointestinal bleeding, transfusions, and hospitalizations with complex antithrombotic therapy in elderly patients. *Circulation.* 2013;128:1869-1877.

42. ASGE Standards of Practice Committee, Acosta RD, Abraham NS, et al. The management of antithrombotic agents for patients undergoing GI endoscopy. *Gastrointest Endosc.* 2016;83:3.

43. Horiuchi A, Nakayama Y, Kajiyama M, Tanaka N, Sano K, Graham DY. Removal of small colorectal polyps in anticoagulated patients: a prospective randomized comparison of cold snare and conventional polypectomy. *Gastrointest Endosc.* 2014;79:417-423.

44. Vergis N, McGrath AK, Stoddart CH, Hoare JM. Right or left in COLonoscopy (ROLCOL)? A randomized controlled trial of right-versus left-sided starting position in colonoscopy. *Am J Gastroenterol.* 2015;110:1576-1581.

45. Bourke MJ, Rex DK. Tips for better colonoscopy from two experts. *Am J Gastroenterol.* 2012;107:1467-1472.

46. Wu J, Hu B. The role of carbon dioxide insufflation in colonoscopy: a systematic review and meta-analysis. *Endoscopy.* 2012;44:128-136.

47. Chen PJ, Shih YL, Chu HC, Chang WK, Hsieh TY, Chao YC. A prospective trial of variable stiffness colonoscopes with different tip diameters in unsedated patients. *Am J Gastroenterol.* 2008;103:1365-1371.

48. Bressler B, Paszat LF, Chen Z, Rothwell DM, Vinden C, Rabeneck L. Rates of new or missed colorectal cancers after colonoscopy and their risk factors: a population-based analysis. *Gastroenterology.* 2007;132:96-102.

49. Rex DK, Cutler CS, Lemmel GT, et al. Colonoscopic miss rates of adenomas determined by back-to-back colonoscopies. *Gastroenterology.* 1997;112:24-28.

50. van Rijn JC, Reitsma JB, Stoker J, Bossuyt PM, van Deventer SJ, Dekker E. Polyp miss rate determined by tandem colonoscopy: a systematic review. *Am J Gastroenterol.* 2006;101:343-350.

51. East JE, Stavrindis M, Thomas-Gibson S, Guenther T, Tekkis PP, Saunders BP. A comparative study of standard vs. high definition colonoscopy for adenoma and hyperplastic polyp detection with optimized withdrawal technique. *Aliment Pharmacol Ther.* 2008;28:768-776.

52. Bartel MJ, Picco MF, Wallace MB. Chromocolonoscopy. *Gastrointest Endosc Clin N Am.* 2015;25:243-260.

53. Subramanian V, Mannath J, Ragunath K, Hawkey CJ. Meta-analysis: the diagnostic yield of chromoendoscopy for detecting dysplasia in patients with colonic inflammatory bowel disease. *Aliment Pharmacol Ther.* 2011;33:304-312.

54. Wu L, Li P, Wu J, Cao Y, Gao F. The diagnostic accuracy of chromoendoscopy for dysplasia in ulcerative colitis: meta-analysis of six randomized controlled trials. *Colorectal Dis.* 2012;14:416-420.

55. Horiuchi A, Nakayama Y, Kajiyama M, Kato N, Ichise Y, Tanaka N. Benefits and limitations of cap-fitted colonoscopy in screening colonoscopy. *Dig Dis Sci.* 2013;58:534-539.

56. Lambert R. Endoscopic Classification Review Group. Update on the Paris classification of superficial neoplastic lesions in the digestive tract. *Endoscopy.* 2005;37:570-578.

57. Kudo S, Tamura S, Nakajima T, Yamano H, Kusaka H, Watanabe H. Diagnosis of colorectal tumorous lesions by magnifying endoscopy. *Gastrointest Endosc.* 1996;44:8-14.

58. Li M, Ali SM, Umm-a-OmarahGilani S, Liu J, Li YQ, Zuo XL. Kudo's pit pattern classification for colorectal neoplasms: a meta-analysis. *World J Gastroenterol.* 2014;20:12649-12656.

59. Ko CW, Dominitz JA. Complications of colonoscopy: magnitude and management. *Gastrointest Endosc Clin N Am.* 2010;20:659-671.

60. ASGE Standards of Practice Committee, Fisher DA, Maple JT, et al. Complications of colonoscopy. *Gastrointest Endosc.* 2011;74: 745-752.

61. Church J. Complications of colonoscopy. *Gastroenterol Clin North Am.* 2013;42:639-657.

62. Orsoni P, Berdah S, Verrier C, et al. Colonic perforation due to colonoscopy: a retrospective study of 48 cases. *Endoscopy.* 1997;29: 160-164.

63. Trecca A, Gaj F, Gagliardi G. Our experience with endoscopic repair of large colonoscopic perforations and review of the literature. *Tech Coloproctol.* 2008;12:315-321; discussion 322.

64. Nivatvongs S. Complications in colonoscopic polypectomy. An experience with 1,555 polypectomies. *Dis Colon Rectum.* 1986;29: 825-830.

65. Singaram C, Torbey CF, Jacoby RF. Delayed postpolypectomy bleeding. *Am J Gastroenterol.* 1995;90:146-147.

66. Sorbi D, Norton I, Conio M, Balm R, Zinsmeister A, Gostout CJ. Postpolypectomy lower GI bleeding: descriptive analysis. *Gastrointest Endosc.* 2000;51:690-696.

67. Parra-Blanco A, Kaminaga N, Kojima T. Hemoclipping for post-polypectomy and postbiopsy colonic bleeding. *Gastrointest Endosc.* 2000;51:37-41.

68. Barnert JA, Messmann H. Diagnosis and management of lower gastrointestinal bleeding. *Nat Rev Gastroenterol Hepatol.* 2009;6: 637-646.

69. Kamath AS, Iqbal CW, Sarr MG, et al. Colonoscopic splenic injuries: incidence and management. *J Gastrointest Surg.* 2009;13: 2136-2140.

70. Walner M, Allinger S, Wiesinger H, Pischl FC, Kramar R, Knoflauch P. Small-bowel ileus after diagnostic colonoscopy. *Endoscopy.* 1994; 26:329.

71. Hunter IA, Sarkar R, Smith AM. Small bowel obstruction complicating colonoscopy: a case report. *J Med Case Rep.* 2008;2:179.

72. Hirata K, Noguchi J, Yoshikawa I, et al. Acute appendicitis immediately after colonoscopy. *Am J Gastroenterol.* 1996;91:2239-2240.

73. Thomas AW, Mitre RJ. Acute pancreatitis as a complication of colonoscopy. *J Clin Gastroenterol.* 1994;19:177.

74. Ko CW, Dominitz JA. Complications of colonoscopy: magnitude and management. *Gastrointest Endosc Clin N Am.* 2010;20:659-671.

75. Bahler J, van Kersen F, Bellaar SJ. Pneumopericardium and pneumomediastinum after polypectomy. *Endoscopy.* 1991;23:46.

Magnetic Resonance Imaging Staging of Rectal Cancer

Warren E. Lichliter | Gregory dePrisco | James W. Fleshman |

Andrew H. Lichliter

The management of rectal cancer has changed dramatically in the last 5 years. Review of national databases has clearly outlined the wide variations in overall survival rates, rates of local recurrence, and rates of permanent colostomies. Championed by many in Western Europe, most notably by Drs. Quirk, Heald, and Brown, the multidisciplinary treatment of rectal cancer has been shown to result in significant improvement in all aspects of care. Because of these continued advances this process is rapidly gaining acceptance in the United States. The multidisciplinary team (MDT) approach is recognized by the OSTRiCh consortium, the American Cancer Society, and the American College of Surgeons Commission on Cancer, the latter of which has devised pilot programs that have adopted practices considered essential for certification for centers of excellence.[1-6] Beyond the development of the MDT, the area of care that has provided the most dramatic change in rectal cancer care has been magnetic resonance imaging (MRI) refinement for rectal cancer evaluation. Accurate local staging and restaging is increasingly possible, with the ability to better avoid the over- or undertreatment of cancer thereby achieving optimal oncologic outcomes while preserving quality of life. MRI has now largely replaced endorectal ultrasound in the evaluation of local staging. MRI is able to accurately define the T category, (to quantify depth of invasion), the extramural venous invasion (EMVI), the circumferential radial margin (CRM) status, the peritoneal reflection position relative to tumor positions in the rectum, and the lymph node involvement.[7] In addition, MRI is becoming an integral part of evaluating postneoadjuvant staging and guiding potential "watch and wait" strategies. This chapter will address the use of MRI in initial staging, postneoadjuvant restaging, and for recurrent disease.

MAGNETIC RESONANCE IMAGING INDICATIONS

MRI is now an essential component of the management of rectal cancer. Indications for MRI are focused on the initial evaluation and staging of rectal cancer, the former arising as the standard of care. Restaging rectal cancer following neoadjuvant therapy is a key component in identifying surgical strategies, especially when there are threatened margins noted on pretreatment staging examinations. MRI is now considered essential in determining decisions related to "watch and wait" strategies and is the preferred follow-up imaging for these patients.[8] However, MRI is not routinely used in surveillance follow-up after definitive management, unless surgical complications arise, such as fistula, or in cases of recurrent tumor to guide further possible surgical management. Although the incidence of local recurrence is now less than 5%, MRI has been invaluable in defining the extent of recurrence and determining resectability. When resection is considered, MRI has demonstrated value in predicting negative margins

MAGNETIC RESONANCE IMAGING— RECTAL CANCER TECHNIQUE

A standardized protocol has been validated and can be referenced in the MERCURY experience,[9] the foundation being high-resolution small field-of-view (FOV) T2 images perpendicular to the long axis of the rectum. The angles of the axial oblique slices are determined from sagittal images of the tumor with annotation by the radiologist for the technologist (Fig. 146.1A). This angulation allows for precise determination of the tumor with origin from the rectal wall (see Fig. 146.1B). MRI is not used as a screening exam for rectal cancer. The precise angulation of the slices is predicated on the knowledge of the exact tumor location, including the distance from the anal verge, tumor morphology, and radial location discovered on endoscopy or physical exam; thus, this location must be available at the time the exam is performed. Acquisition and interpretation of MRI exams without foreknowledge of tumor location may result in both understaging and overstaging lesions. For example, in the case of low rectal tumors, in addition to the standard imaging evaluation, an additional image series coronally oriented with respect to the anal canal is obtained to accurately assess the tumor's relationship to the sphincteric complex and intersphincteric plane (Fig. 146.2). MRI exams may be performed on a 1.5 or 3 T MRI scanner; neither one is proven to demonstrate superiority.[10] Recommended protocols for scanners from various manufacturers are available on the website of the Society of Abdominal Radiology.[11]

Of note, the technique does not include the use of intravenous (IV) contrast. Based on the initial experience at our institution, IV contrast creates a tendency to overstage rectal tumors. Importantly, fat saturation techniques on T2 imaging, which are commonly used when evaluating most pelvic pathology, are to be avoided when performing exams for routine staging and restaging rectal cancer. These fat saturation techniques preclude accurate assessment of the tumor in relation to the mesorectal fascia and peritoneal reflection. To decrease motion artifact related to bowel peristalsis, antispasmodics are routinely given, typically

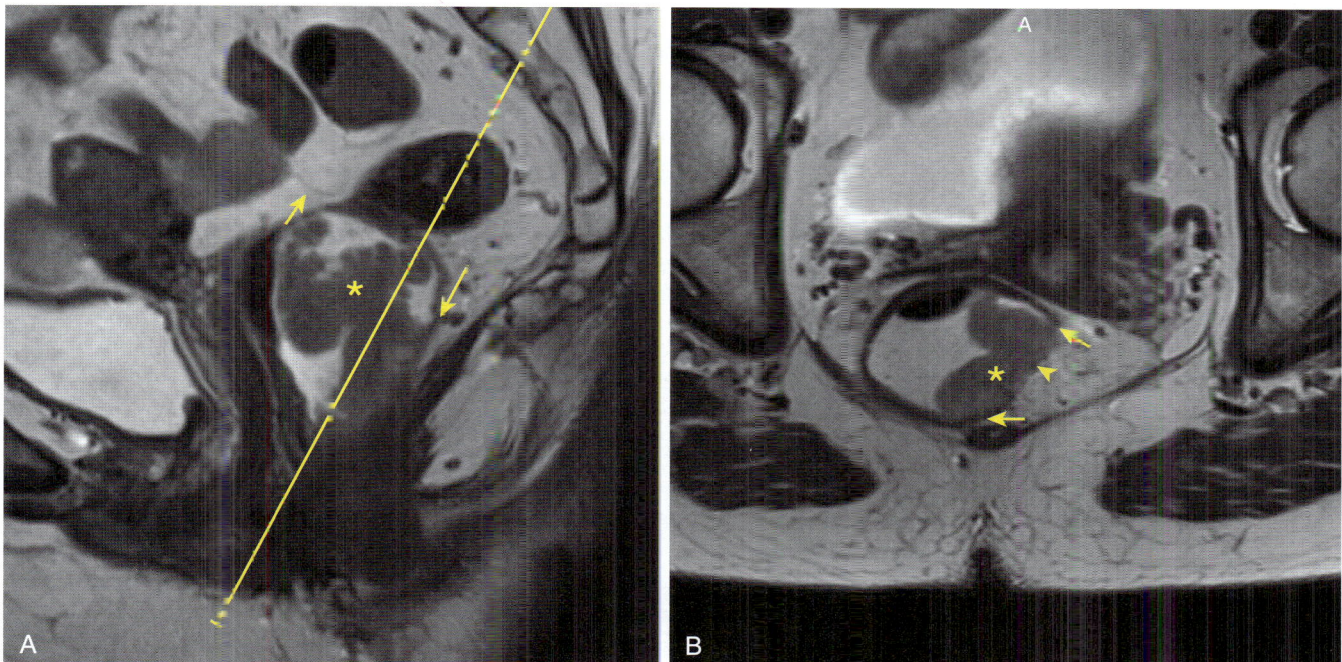

FIGURE 146.1 (A) Sagittal T2 image demonstrating a polypoid low rectal tumor arising from a broad-based in the posterior low rectum (*asterisk*). The *yellow line* present is parallel to the posterior rectal wall at the level of the stalk (*large arrow*) and proscribes the angle for the axial oblique images to assess the stalk. The tumor base is below the peritoneal reflection (*small arrow*) indicating that a transanal excision could be considered. (B) Axial oblique T2 image demonstrating the base along the left lateral aspect of the rectal wall (*asterisk*), extending the full thickness of the muscularis but not extending deeply into the mesorectal fat (*arrowhead*), compatible with a T2/T3a (<1 mm invasion into the mesorectal fat). Observe the replacement of the low signal intensity muscularis propria by intermediate tumor signal compared to the normal muscularis (*small arrows*) anterior and posterior to the tumor.

glucagon (1 mg) in the United States, although buscopan is given in much of Europe. This medication may be given intramuscularly or IV just prior to the start of the examination. Glucagon is not given if there is a patient history of pheochromocytoma or glucagon allergy. The drug has been given in patients with diabetes mellitus.

The initial use of endorectal coil MRI has been supplanted by the quality of present imaging techniques. The use of an endorectal coil is not recommended. Enema prep is not required. An indwelling rectal stent typically results in some degree of imaging artifact, but diagnostic information can often still be obtained (Fig. 146.3). Ideally, the patient receives pre- and posttreatment examinations with the exact same parameters and protocol. In today's common practice, patients may not have a pretreatment MRI, or it may have been performed using a different technique prior to care being transferred to a high-volume center. Reproducibility of the technique will continue to improve with the move to centers of excellence and the standardization of care.

Although accurate disease characterization hinges on appropriate image acquisition, synoptic reporting of findings is necessary to ensure that all elements of pathology are captured in the report. Multiple synoptic reporting templates are publically available for both the staging and restaging of rectal cancer; the Cancer Care Ontario, Society of Abdominal Radiology, and Royal Marsden Hospital[12-16] have all published similar templates, the common features of which are discussed later. Importantly,

the incorporation of MRI findings into the MDT conference has enabled the surgeon, oncologist, pathologist, radiologist, and all members of the MDT to develop treatment strategies based on accurate local staging. Discussions surrounding the threatened or positive CRM, local tumor management, "watch and wait," and recurrent disease and its management have been the main focus of these conferences and most of these discussions are based on MRI findings. Comparison of the preoperative MRI with the final pathology specimen provides an opportunity for quality assurance of surgery, pathology, and radiology (Fig. 146.4). This precise radiologic-pathologic correlation requires the pathology specimen to be processed in a "breadloaf" technique as put forth by Quirk. If the rectum is "flayed open" along the organ's long axis, point-to-point MRI to pathology correlation is not feasible. Notably, rather than longitudinally opening a rectal specimen to assure an adequate distal margin, a pathologist should be summoned to gently partially evert the rectum and measure the margin.

MAGNETIC RESONANCE IMAGING—INITIAL STAGING

Staging the patient with rectal cancer using tumor, node, metastasis (TNM) methodology put forth by the American Joint Committee on Cancer (AJCC) involves an assessment of the local tumor extent with regard to the bowel wall (T category), clinical lymph node status (N category),

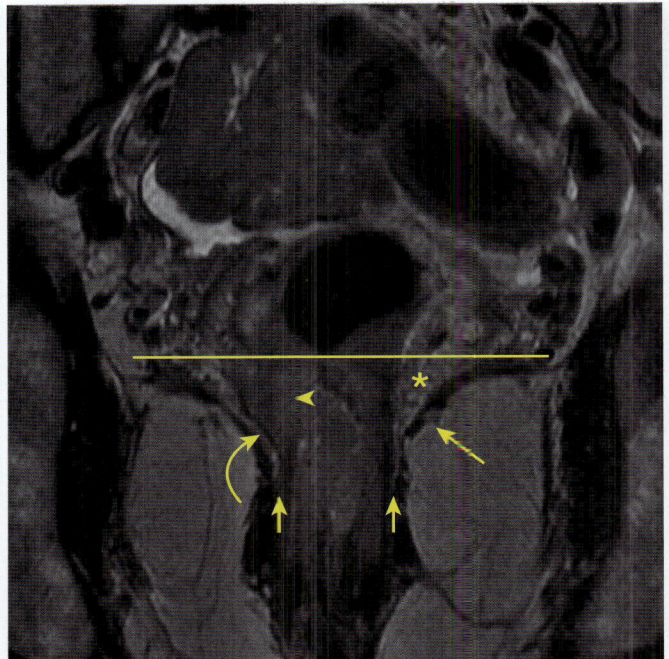

FIGURE 146.2 Coronal T2-weighted image demonstrating the surgical low rectum, which starts where the mesorectal fat decreases sharply in volume around the levator ani muscle. Below the horizontal line, observe the normal tapering of bright mesorectal fat on the left *(asterisk)* separating the low rectum from the adjacent normal dark fibers of the levator ani muscle *(large arrow)*. In this case, the tumor *(arrowhead)* is at the level of tapering and is therefore low. Note also the back intact muscularis propria *(curved arrow)*, indicating a T2 tumor. The intersphincteric plane *(small arrows)* is clear. Although the tumor encroaches on the sphincter complex, a sphincter-saving procedure could be considered.

TABLE 146.1	Low Rectal Cancer Staging
Stage	**Low Rectal Cancer as Seen on Magnetic Resonance Imaging**
1	Confined to bowel wall but does not extend through full thickness; intact outer muscle coat
2	Replaces muscle coat but does not extend into intersphincteric plane
3	Invades intersphincteric plane or lies within 1 mm of levator muscle
4	Invades external anal sphincter and is within 1 mm and beyond levators with or without invading adjacent organs

and the presence of metastatic disease (M category). The mucosa, submucosa and muscularis propria can be distinguished on high-resolution MRI (Fig. 146.5). MRI has been validated by multiple studies to accurately assess mural and direct extramural tumor spread and lymph node status. The MERCURY Trial confirmed MRI as the preferred modality of local evaluation.[17] The following parameters are part of the standard reporting system for rectal cancer imaging.

1. The primary tumor is evaluated based on its morphology (semiannular [Fig. 146.6], annular, polypoid [see Fig. 146.1]) and for the presence of mucinous features. The recognition of the tumor morphology is important because a common diagnostic pitfall leading to overstaging is confusing the raised, rolled tumor edge of a semiannular endoluminal tumor or the large endoluminal component of a polypoid tumor to be the invasive component of the tumor. Mucinous tumors are known to be a poor prognostic feature in rectal cancer. The presence of mucinous features can be reliably detected at MRI.

2. The height of the tumor from the anal verge and sphincteric complex and the radial location of the tumor are reported. Based on imaging, the tumor is in the upper third when its lowest margin is greater than 10 cm from the anal verge, and in the middle third when its lowest margin is 5 to 10 cm. The lower third is defined as less than 5 cm from the anal verge. Perhaps a more surgically relevant distinction of the low rectum is where the levator muscles converge medially, resulting in the sharp tapering of mesorectal fat, which can be observed on Fig. 146.2. This distinction is critical as it is known that low rectal tumors are more challenging to stage and treat. Indeed, a separate staging schema has been proposed for low rectal cancer (Table 146.1).[18]

3. The T stage and depth of invasion (DOI) are assessed (see Fig. 146.4). MRI estimation of DOI is accurate to less than 0.5 mm of the final pathologic specimen, as demonstrated by the MERCURY experience.[9] T2–T4 tumors need MRI for more accurate evaluation.[19,20] Small tumors, less than 2 cm, may still benefit from more precise characterization with transrectal ultrasound (TRUS). The presence of a DOI greater than 5 mm beyond the bowel wall can be detected and can help identify the need for radiation treatment planning. The ability to accurately identify T4 lesions and their invasion into the vagina, uterus, prostate, seminal vesicles, and bladder has also been helpful in pretreatment care planning (Figs. 146.7 and 146.8; see also Fig. 146.3). When measuring DOI, it is important to take into account the tumor morphology. For semiannular tumors, the DOI is measured at the midpoint of the tumor between the raised tumor edges, if present. For polypoid tumors, the DOI is measured at the tumor stalk (see Fig. 146.1 and Table 146.1).

4. The extent of the tumor and its relationship to the mesorectal fascia as determined by MRI has been shown to correlate to the pathologic margin, allowing assessment of the CRM prior to surgery.[21,22] The primary tumor, extramural vascular invasion, metastatic nodes, and tumor deposits may all involve the CRM. By MRI criteria, the CRM is taken to be positive if one of these entities is less than 1 mm from the mesorectal fascia, and the CRM is considered threatened when less than 2 mm (Fig. 146.9). For low rectal tumors, violation of the intersphincteric plane is considered a positive CRM.

5. The peritoneal reflection is an important landmark for defining tumor location (Fig. 146.10). It can be accurately identified in greater than 90% of cases.[23,24] A tumor that is present below the peritoneal reflection is considered a low rectal tumor. Knowledge of the tumor location relative to the peritoneal reflection is necessary

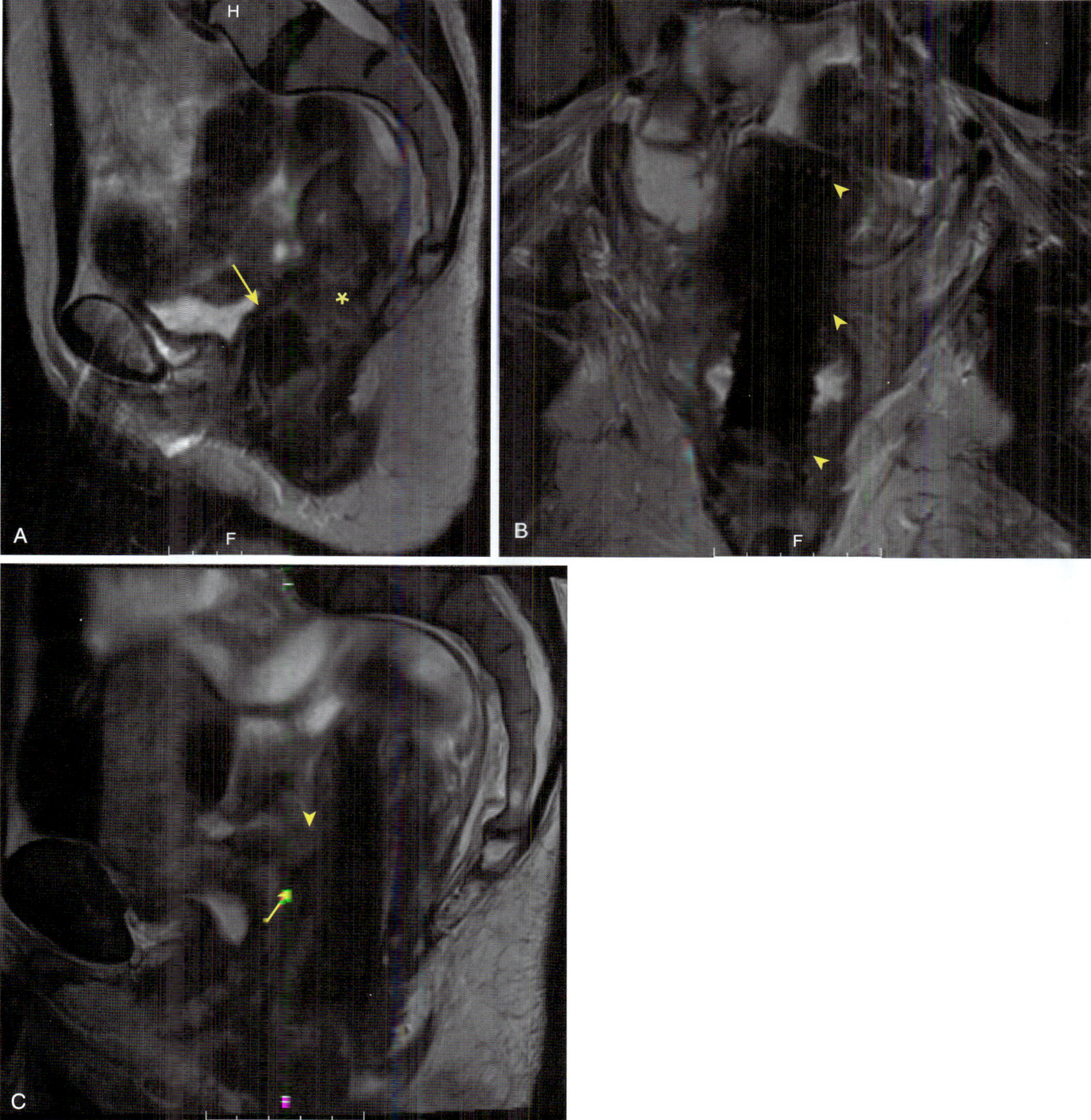

FIGURE 146.3 (A) Long-segment tumor in the mid- to low rectum *(asterisk)* invading the posterior wall of the vaginal cuff *(arrow)*. The patient developed obstructive symptoms and a rectal stent was deployed. (B) Coronal image taken from follow-up exam 3 months later demonstrating low signal intensity rectal stent with geometric borders *(arrowheads)*. The stent results in little artifact. (C) Sagittal image from the repeat exam demonstrating enlargement of the tumor involving the vaginal cuff *(arrowhead)* with a hypointense gas-filled track between the mass and the rectum *(arrow)*. A neoplastic rectovaginal fistula was confirmed at pathology.

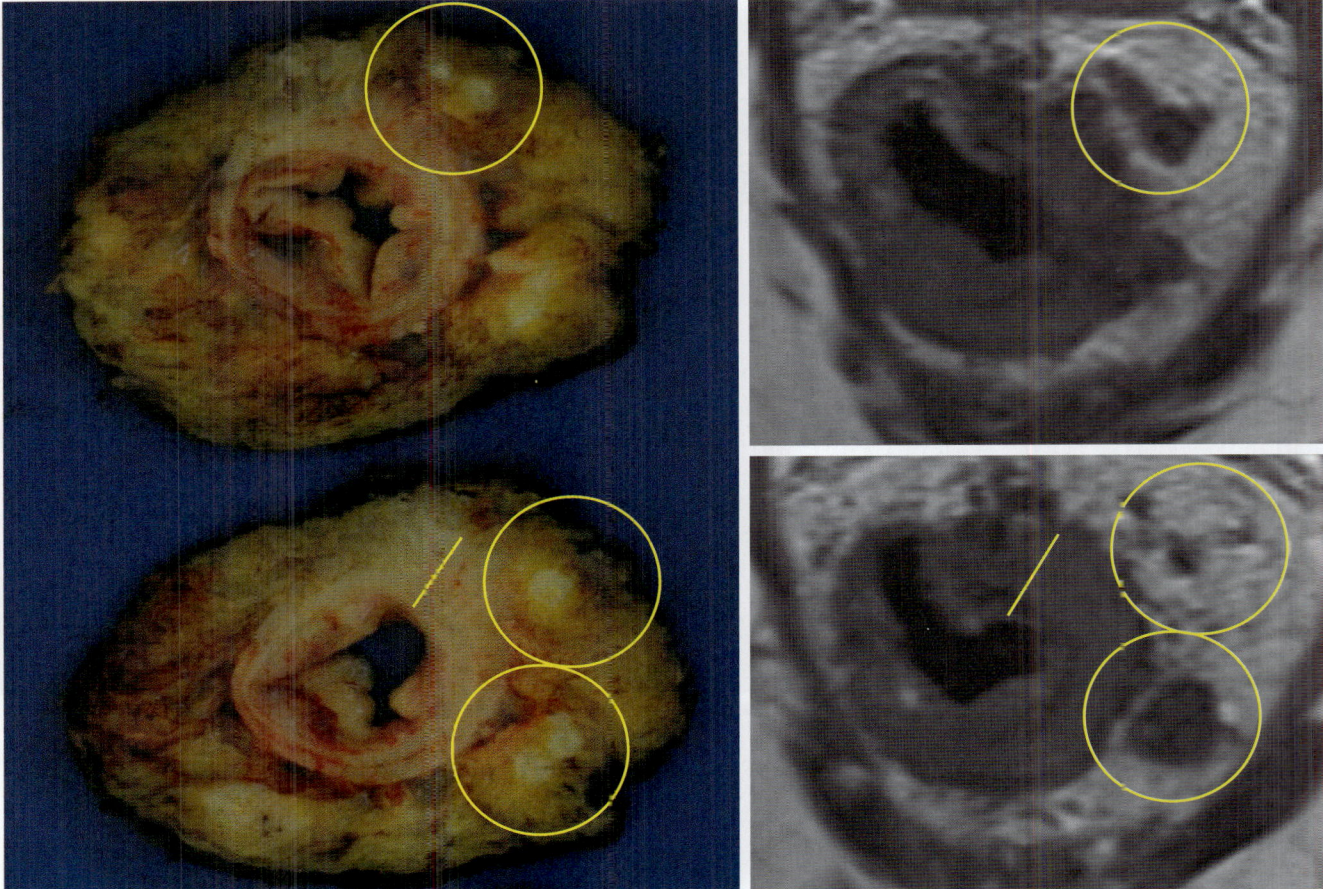

FIGURE 146.4 Axial oblique sections from a mid-rectal tumor specimen with corresponding magnetic resonance imaging slices. The *lower panel* images demonstrate the tumor arising from the left anterior rectal wall with lines drawn along the most invasive component of the tumor, nicely demonstrating concordance of the depth of invasion in this T3b tumor. Metastatic lymph nodes in the left mesorectum greater than 2 mm from the mesorectum are indicative of a negative circumferential radial margin, which is confirmed on pathology.

if considering TAMIS (transanal minimally invasive surgery) or TEMS (transanal endoscopic microsurgery) procedures (see Fig. 146.1).

6. The presence of EMVI is readily detectable on noncontrast MRI and is now a part of the standardized report for rectal cancer (see Fig. 146.9). EMVI is prevalent in 30% to 40% of patients with rectal cancer.[25] Imaging findings of EMVI include irregularity or expansion of vessels, loss of normal vascular flow void, and intraluminal intermediate tumor signal intensity contiguous or separate from the main tumor.[26] MRI is more sensitive at detecting EMVI than evaluating the pathologic specimen, as multiplanar assessment of the mesorectal fat and pelvic sidewall in their entirety is possible. Pathologic evaluation of EMVI is limited based on the slices taken and the single plane of analysis. Accurate assessment of EMVI requires pathologists to reference the MRI findings to direct their search. If EMVI is not initially confirmed on hematoxylin and eosin staining, elastin staining can be of benefit to confirm diagnosis.[27] Some new data suggest that IV contrast administration may increase reader confidence with EMVI detection, but noncontrast imaging remains the standard.[27] These findings underscore the importance of MRI in the evaluation of EMVI, given its prognostic indication of local recurrence and distant metastatic disease rather than nodal disease—the latter with a five-fold increased risk compared to patients without EMVI.[25]

7. The accurate assessment of lymph node status is becoming more predictable. Although metastatic nodes are generally larger than benign counterparts, metastasis can be present in very small nodes. Nodes larger than 8 mm short axis are virtually all neoplastic, but using this size threshold alone is insensitive for detecting metastatic nodes. Short-axis size cutoffs for suspected malignancy are not as useful as nodal morphologic features in predicting malignancy. Irregular node border and mixed signal intensity are the most reliable predictors of nodal metastases.[28] The precise relationship of perirectal nodes to the mesorectal fascia can be determined (see Figs. 146.9 and 146.10). MRI also identifies nodes outside of the mesorectum (see Fig. 146.7). Posttreatment MRI evaluation of lymph node status and pathologic correlation with the breadloafing of specimens allows node for node evaluation (see Figs. 146.4 and 146.11).[29,30]

8. MRI reporting should identify the distal tumor edge and the encroachment of the tumor on the pelvic

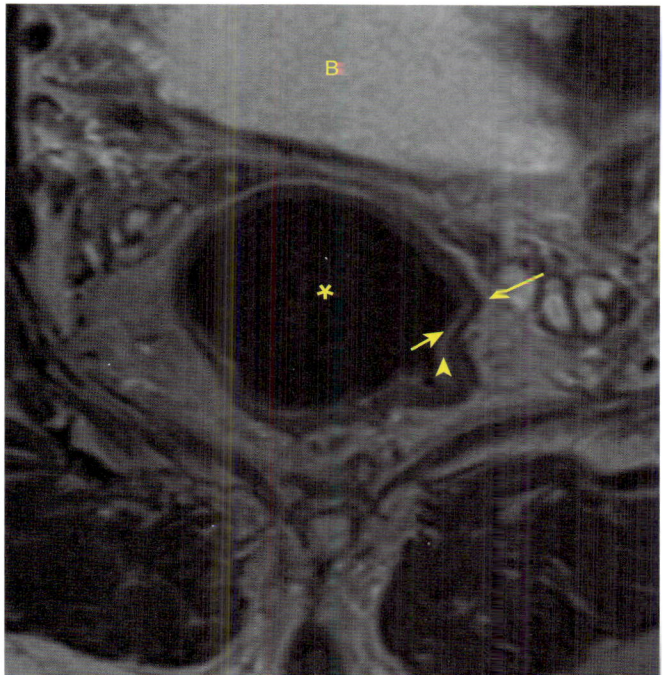

FIGURE 146.5 T2 axial oblique image of a normal rectum. The rectal lumen *(asterisk)* containing air appears black, and is located posterior to the normal bright urinary bladder (B). The mucosa is visible as a thin, dark band contacting the lumen *(small arrow,)*. The submucosa is the bright layer between the mucosa and submucosa *(arrowhead,)*. The muscularis is the dark ring *(large arrow)* deep to the submucosa.

muscle floor (see Figs. 146.2 and 146.6). This also helps to distinguish candidates for sphincter-saving procedures from those requiring abdominal perineal resection (APR) for complete clearance of the tumor.[31]

SUMMARY OF INITIAL STAGING

MRI is now an essential clinical component of the initial treatment planning during presentations for discussion at the MDT conference. The local status of the tumor in the mesorectum, the DOI, the possible T4b lesions, and the threatened margins can now be correlated with the need for neoadjuvant therapy. Avoiding neoadjuvant radiation with primary surgery for rectal cancer without threatening features has been demonstrated in Western Europe. Initial evaluation of the pelvic floor involvement with the tumor using MRI is also helpful in surgical planning. The need for an extralevator dissection during APR may be best defined by MRI imaging. The need for beyond TME approaches such as exenteration to remove multiple organs in the pelvis can be defined by MRI. The MRI can assess the encroachment of the levator floor; however, currently, it is still difficult to assess the need for low anterior resection (LAR), coloanal, or TaTME based solely on imaging.

MAGNETIC RESONANCE IMAGING RESTAGING

Control of the primary tumor site in patients with locally advanced tumors can be achieved after neoadjuvant therapy

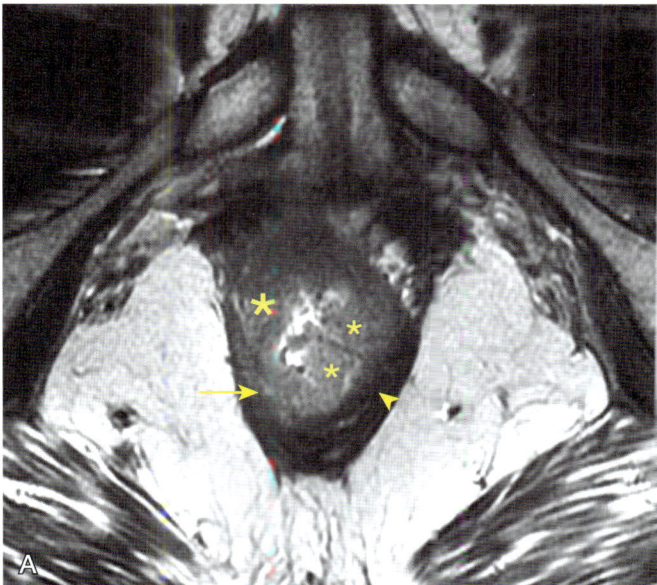
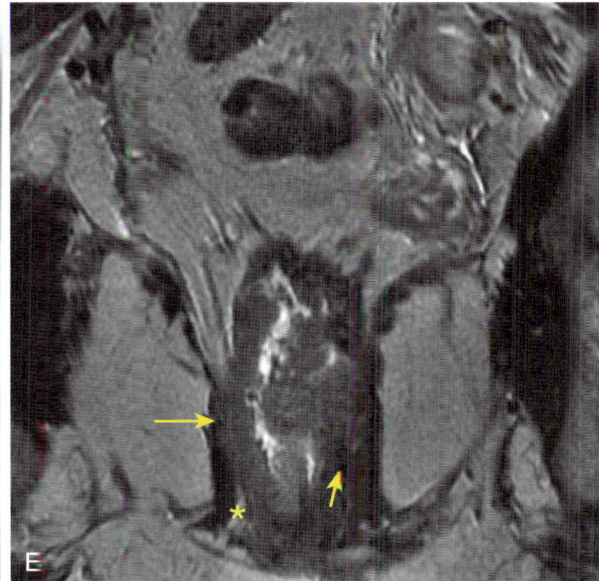

FIGURE 146.6 (A) Axial oblique T2-weighted magnetic resonance image showing a semiannular low rectal tumor arising from the right lateral rectal wall *(large asterisk)* with large raised rolled edges filling the rectal lumen and converging on the left side of the rectum *(small asterisks)*. The invasive component on the right invades the internal anal sphincter *(arrow)* with sparing of the left internal sphincter *(arrowhead)*. (B) Coronal T2 image showing the intact right intersphincteric plane inferiorly *(asterisk)* with intermediate signal tumor invading through the right mid- and upper intersphincteric plane into the external anal sphincter *(large arrow)*. Observe effacement of the normal bright signal of the thin left intersphincteric fat superior to the *small arrow*. On the basis of intersphincteric plane invasion, this lesion meets criteria for a positive circumferential margin.

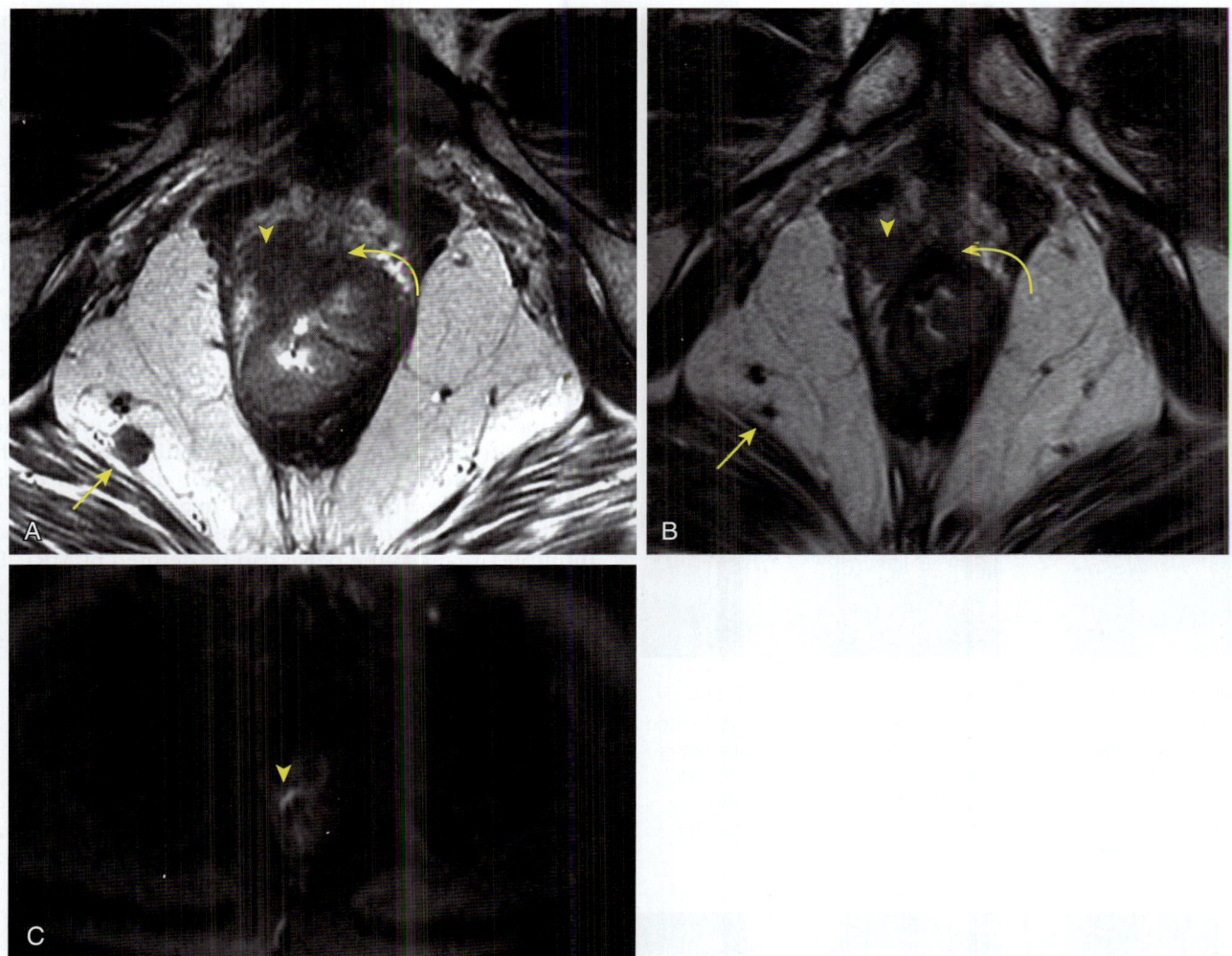

FIGURE 146.7 (A) Baseline axial oblique T2-weighted magnetic resonance (MR) image showing a semiannular low rectal tumor *(curved arrow)* with intermediate signal in the right anterior rectum with invasion of the prostate apex *(arrowhead)*. A metastatic lymph node in the right ischiorectal fossa *(straight arrow)* has a heterogeneous signal and irregular borders. (B) Axial oblique T2-weighted MR image showing the same tumor postneoadjuvant chemoradiation therapy. Observe the predominantly dark fibrosis in the mural component of the tumor with little intermediate signal *(curved arrow)*, suggesting tumor regression grade 2, but a residual intermediate-signal viable tumor invades the prostate apex *(arrowhead)* indicating tumor regression grade 4. The treated metastatic lymph node is now less than 5 mm, and has a dark signal typical of fibrosis without evidence of residual tumor *(straight arrow)*. (C) Axial large field-of-view diffusion-weighted magnetic resonance image showing residual viable tumor at the site of prostate invasion with persistent diffusion abnormality *(arrowhead)*. Final pathology confirmed a T4b lesion invading the right prostate apex.

and surgical management. Defining the response to therapy with local staging MRI, correlation with clinical exam, and discussion at MDT conference helps to develop the optimal surgical approach for each individual patient.[32]

Adequate restaging parameters include changes in T category, DOI, EMVI, lymph node status, and CRM. The response of the primary tumor can be assessed based upon the degree of tumor volume reduction, the magnetic resonance tumor regression grade (mrTRG), and evaluation of the tumor on diffusion-weighted imaging. A greater than 80% volume of tumor reduction is indicative of a favorable response following neoadjuvant therapy. The mrTRG is a Likert scale that compares the proportion of treatment-related fibrosis with dark signal intensity with the amount of gray intermediate residual tumor signal (see Figs. 146.7 and 146.11). Treated tumors with solely dark fibrotic signal have an mrTRG of 1, and treated lesions with only persistent intermediate tumor signal (even if it has decreased >80% in volume) have an mrTRG of 5, with mixtures of fibrotic and intermediate signal falling in between (Table 146.2). These findings have been shown to correlate with pathologic findings more often than the clinical exam in assessing the patient with a possible complete response (CR).[33] Diffusion-weighted imaging (DWI) is a technique that, in part, characterizes tissue on the basis of cellularity. Diffusion imaging may be of benefit in assessing residual tumor following therapy (see Fig. 146.7).[34] It should be noted that the presence of mucin, hemorrhage, and artifacts (e.g., related to biopsy or surgical staples) can render diffusion imaging nondiagnostic.[35]

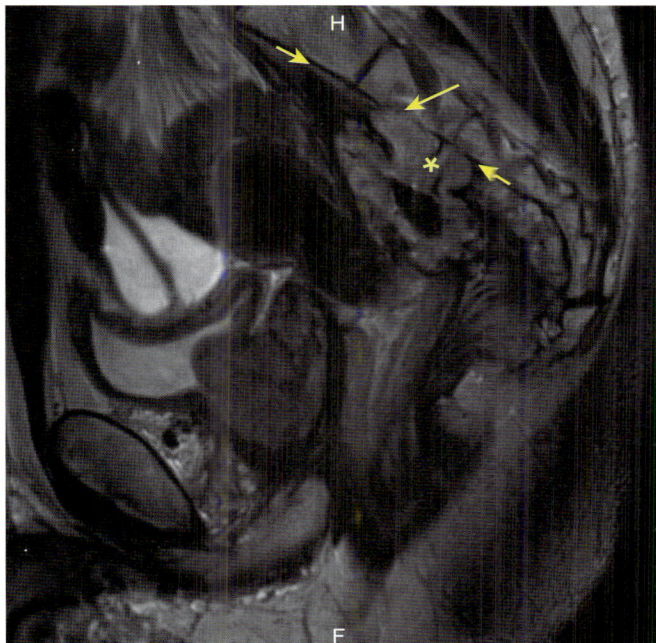

FIGURE 146.8 Large recurrent rectal tumor *(asterisk)* arising from a colorectal anastomosis invading the sacrum. Observe the destruction of the anterior sacral cortex in the mid-S2 segment that is normally a thin dark line cranial and caudal to the tumor *(short arrows)*, which has been replaced with intermediate tumor signal *(long arrow)*.

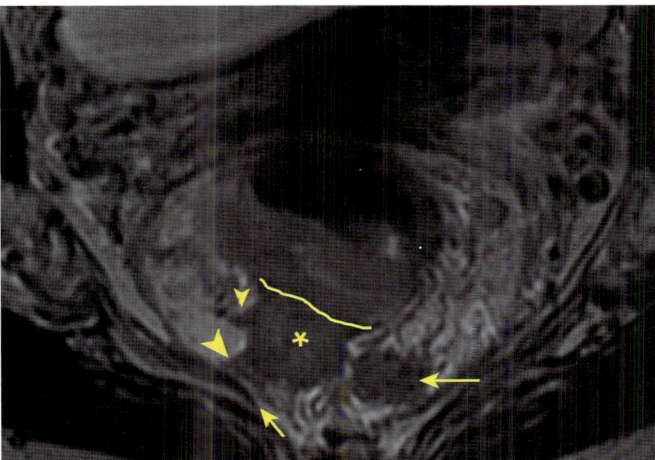

FIGURE 146.9 Axial oblique T2-weighted image showing a T3 semiannular low rectal tumor with invasive edge along the right posterior wall *(asterisk)* with greater than 15-mm extramural spread beyond the expected location of the outer border of the muscularis propria *(curved line)* indicating T3d disease. Extramural vascular invasion *(large arrowhead)* expands a vein along the posterior right aspect of the tumor coming within 1 mm of the thin, linear, dark band of mesorectal fascia *(small arrow)*, indicating a positive circumferential radial margin. An additional expansile tumor is in a vein along the right lateral wall *(small arrowhead)*. A heterogeneous signal metastatic node with irregular borders in the left posterior mesorectum *(long arrow)* is 2 mm from the mesorectal fascia, resulting in a threatened radial margin.

TABLE 146.2 Magnetic Resonance Tumor Regression Grade

Grade	Proportion of Tumor With Fibrotic Low Signal Intensity Compared to Remaining Residual Intermediate Signal Intensity
1	Predominance of fibrosis with no residual intermediate signal
2	Predominance of fibrosis with minimal residual intermediate signal
3	Substantial tumor signal present, but does not predominate the fibrosis
4	Predominance of tumor with minimal low-signal fibrosis
5	Tumor appears unchanged from baseline

Patients with an initially involved or threatened circumferential resection margin in particular may benefit from restaging MRI. A recent analysis of posttreatment staging modalities demonstrated a 50% incidence of stage change in posttreatment MRI staging with a 4% change in surgical management.[36] In this study, many of the MRI changes posttreatment had no change in CRM status. These patients had either no threatened margin or findings that determined surgical management at the outset of treatment. Although this study would argue routine MRI restaging is unnecessary for patients with an uninvolved CRM, up to 20% to 30% of patients will have a pathologic CR to neoadjuvant therapy. In these patients, further surgery will not be beneficial and the multiple risks of surgery may outweigh any potential benefit. Predicting the pathologic CR based upon MRI and physical exam findings is improving and has resulted in increasing interest in "watch and wait" approaches (see later). This option is attractive for patients wishing to defer surgery. MRI postneoadjuvant therapy is currently not a part of the American College of Surgeons (ACS) National Accreditation Program for Rectal Cancer MDT protocol.

The evaluation of extramural vascular invasion at restaging has been shown to be useful for risk stratification. Those patients who initially have documented EMVI on staging MRI who have persistent EMVI on restaging remain at a heightened risk for distant metastatic disease.[37] Certainly, the unfortunate patient who develops de novo EMVI in the course of neoadjuvant therapy has an aggressive tumor with a poor prognosis. On the other hand, patients initially having EMVI at the time of staging, which resolves on the restaging MRI, have been shown to have a similar risk of distant metastatic disease and local recurrence as the cohort of patients who were initially EMVI negative. These data can be incorporated in the MDT discussion of potential further chemotherapy treatment options.

Both benign and malignant nodes can decrease in size following neoadjuvant therapy (see Figs. 146.7 and 146.11). Nodes initially seen to be metastatic on the basis of signal heterogeneity and irregular borders, which decrease to less than 5 mm in size, are considered to be treated nodes. Lymph nodes with intermediate T2 signal intensity on the staging exam may become T2 hyperintense after treatment, which has been shown to reflect mucinous change. The acellular mucin found in such nodes has been shown to correlate with a favorable treatment response. On the other hand, T2 hyperintense mucinous metastatic lymph

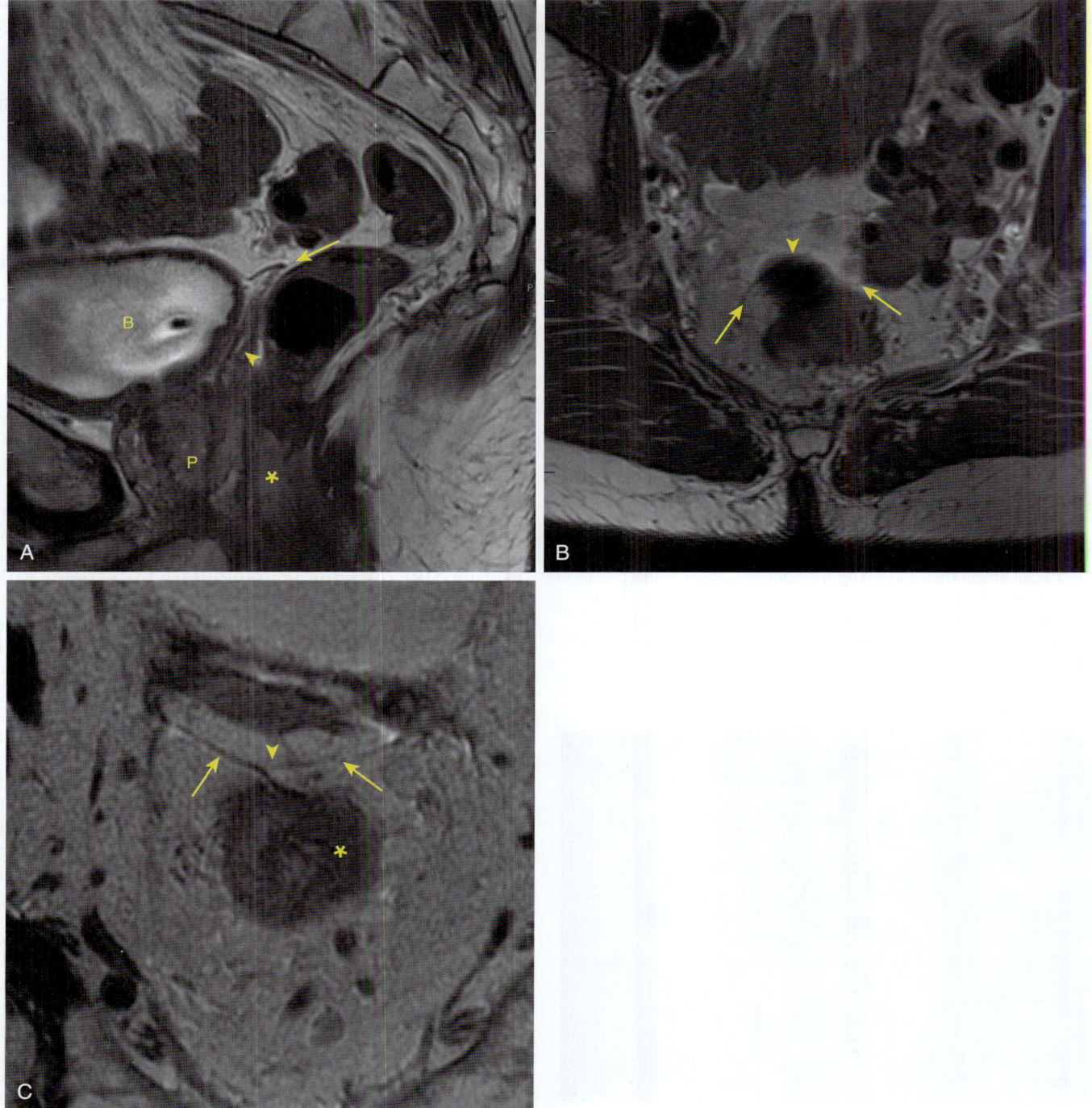

FIGURE 146.10 (A) A sagittal image demonstrating the normal appearance of the peritoneal reflection, a thin dark line *(arrow)* at the posterior aspect of the bladder dome immediately above the seminal vesicles *(arrowhead)*. The bladder (B) and prostate (P) are noted. A tumor in the anterior low rectum extends into the internal sphincter *(asterisk)*. (B) An axial oblique image in the same patient showing the right and left aspects of the peritoneal reflection *(arrows)* converging on the anterior rectal wall *(arrowhead)*. (C) A more typical gull-wing appearance *(arrowhead)* of the peritoneal reflection in another patient. The right and left aspects of the peritoneal reflection are thin, uninvolved by tumor *(arrows)*. The patient has a circumferential T3 tumor straddling the peritoneal reflection *(asterisk)*. On the basis of these images, the peritoneum does not appear to be penetrated, indicating that T4a disease is not present.

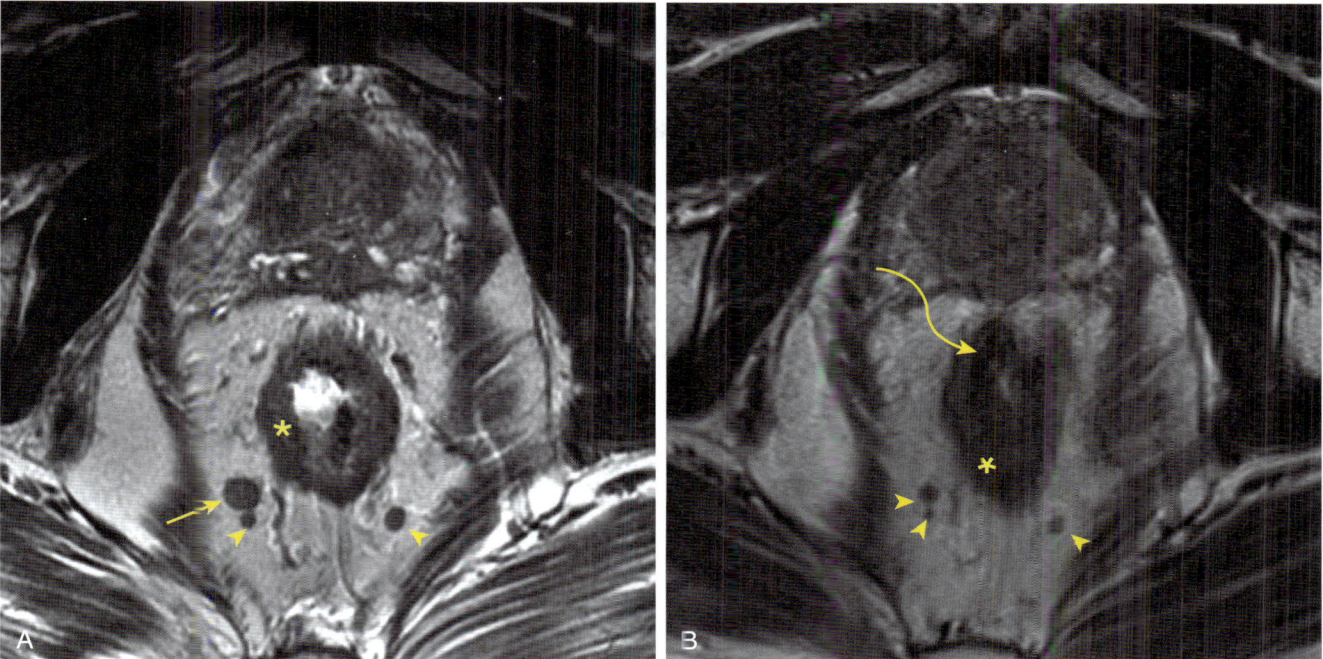

FIGURE 146.11 (A) An axial oblique T2-weighted magnetic resonance image showing a near circumferential T3 annular low rectal tumor *(asterisk)* with a metastatic heterogeneous signal perirectal lymph nodes *(arrow)* with two additional smaller suspicious nodes *(arrowheads)*. (B) An axial oblique T2-weighted magnetic resonance image showing the primary tumor persists, with equal amounts of gray intermediate signal tumor *(asterisk)* and dark hypointense fibrosis *(curved arrow)* compatible with tumor regression grade 3. The same nodes postneoadjuvant therapy *(arrowheads)* have decreased in size, but have a persistent intermediate signal supporting viable tumor, which was confirmed at pathology.

nodes on initial staging, which persist on restaging, are considered to harbor a viable tumor.[30] A recent study revealed lymph nodes identifiable on diffusion weighted imaging at initial staging that disappear on restaging exams have 100% negative predictive value for tumor, although this finding is seen in approximately 10% of cases.[30a]

A change in the level of the distal edge of the tumor on MRI, along with a clinical exam, can help to determine the feasibility of achieving a sphincter-saving procedure or the continued need for APR.[31] All posttreatment MRI parameters are considered in the context of a clinical exam and findings on endoscopy, and are discussed at the MDT conference.

MAGNETIC RESONANCE IMAGING— WATCH AND WAIT

Up to 30% of patients treated with neoadjuvant therapy will ultimately have a CR and will not benefit from major surgery and the creation of a possible ostomy. The approach was originally pioneered by Dr. Habr-Gama during the late 1980s in Brazil. Local excision to confirm complete clinical response after neoadjuvant therapy is rarely necessary because MRI has improved local staging. The potential nonsalvageability in patients with recurrent disease after local resection has also been demonstrated secondary to the disruption of the total mesorectal excision (TME). Thus a "watch and wait" strategy has been incorporated in several institutions using MRI and endoscopic criteria.[8]

The selection of patients appropriate for this treatment is difficult and controversial outside of a trial setting. Posttreatment excisional biopsies have been used to provide data to help make this decision. An assessment with restaging MRI (with mrTRG tumor grading and diffusion evaluation), a posttreatment clinical exam, and a presentation for review at the MDT expanded the role of the "watch and wait" approach, with nonsurgery and close clinical and MRI assessment over time, instead of local excision of the primary tumor site or radical excision.[38-41] As this concept has evolved and the term has been increasingly used, discussions of recurrence after "watch and wait" has been referred to as tumor progression instead of tumor recurrence, as it is assumed that there was not a pathologic CR. Surveillance protocols vary, but endoscopy at 3-month intervals along with MRI exams at 3- to 6-month intervals during the first follow-up year have been performed, with intervals extended if no tumor progression is observed. Certainly, ongoing prospective studies of the "watch and wait" paradigm include the TRIGGER and OPRA trials.

MAGNETIC RESONANCE IMAGING AFTER SURGERY

MRI after surgery is not a part of routine posttreatment imaging. That being said, correlation of the presurgical MRI and final pathologic specimen in an MDT format is a critical driver of MDT improvement. Scrutiny of the MRI and the breadloafed pathologic specimen can sharpen radiologists' interpretation of presurgical exams and can increase pathologists' sensitivity in reporting EMVI. The pathology analysis of the postsurgical specimen by breadloafing of the specimen is a quality metric in rectal cancer care, and helps to grade the quality of the surgeon and TME dissection. Correlation of the MRI findings at the sight of an incomplete resection margin can allow the radiologist to better direct the surgeon in the future.

Complications after surgery are usually assessed with computed tomography (CT), hypaque enema or fistulograms. MRI can be useful in evaluating pelvic fluid collections and fistulas, noting such exams are best performed without an with contrast. MRI is also useful in evaluating a patient for possible recurrence suspected on other imaging or based on patient symptoms. As the "watch and wait" approach is increasingly used, MRI may be a part of this follow-up.

MAGNETIC RESONANCE IMAGING RECURRENCE

Unfortunately, some patients, despite all of the advances in rectal cancer care, develop recurrent disease. Achieving a diagnosis of recurrence is sometimes difficult. The use of MRI is helpful in making a diagnosis of recurrent disease in patients whose recurrence is difficult to biopsy. Diffusion-based MRI has shown some value in increasing specific recurrent tumor diagnosis.[42]

Once a diagnosis of recurrence is made, pelvic MRI is helpful in determining the extent of recurrence, which includes adjacent spread into the anterior, posterior, and lateral compartments, as well as the degree of superior and inferior tumor extension. Detection of involvement in adjacent organs (vagina, uterus, bladder, ureters, prostate, or seminal vesicles) can help plan an exenteration procedure.

Documentation of the involvement of the sacrum and the determination of the sacral level involved can facilitate the planning for resection and the prediction of expected dysfunction based on nerve root involvement and sacral instability (see Fig. 146.8).[43-45]

The pelvic sidewall is difficult to evaluate with other imaging modalities. MRI can accurately assess extramesorectal involvement.[46] Evaluation of potentially involved vascular or neural structures guides surgical approach. Lateral pelvic sidewall and extensive extramesorectal fascia involvement indicates those patients that would be unable to undergo a planned R0 resection. Surgery with palliative intent and residual margins in rectal cancer has not been shown to be effective in symptom relief or in improvement in quality of life scores.[47] MRI, therefore, plays an important role in identifying the lack of benefit for these patients. In rare circumstances, a wider resection plane, directed by MRI findings, may suffice to achieve R0 resection.

MAGNETIC RESONANCE IMAGING LIMITATIONS

MRI imaging for rectal cancer has the same limitations as any study using magnetic resonance. Contraindications for MRI imaging include patients with pacemakers, cochlear implants, some older cardiac valves, and multiple other medical implants. Gastrointestinal stents are not typically a contraindication (see Fig. 146.3). Any implanted device's MR compatibility, as stated by the manufacturer, should be assessed prior to performing a study. Standard rectal cancer protocol uses no intravenous contrast and no fat suppression—both of which can decrease sensitivity for fistula. If fistula is clinically suspected, the addition of fistula protocol images without and with contrast along with routine rectal tumor protocol should be considered.

The most common barrier to obtaining high-quality MR images in daily practice is claustrophobia. Given the confines of the MRI scanner, premedication, (commonly with benzodiazepines) is often used in patients with claustrophobia. Severely claustrophobic patients, and those in severe tumor-related pain, may require general endotracheal anesthesia to complete the exam, which requires scanning in a hospital setting, although these contingencies are rare. Apart from claustrophobic patients who decline MRI scanning entirely, the anxiety associated with scanning often results in unwanted patient motion. The latter also commonly arises due to pain, especially in the setting of higher stage locally advanced disease.

A barrier for MR imaging for rectal cancer is the radiology department's failure to adhere to the technical aspects of the procedure. Specifically, ordering a rectal cancer protocol MRI with small FOV axial oblique imaging will help assure the exam is performed correctly. If the ordering surgeon does not have a preexisting working relationship with someone in the MRI department, embarking on one can reduce confusion and the need for patient call-backs for repeat imaging. Knowledge of the clinical location of the tumor relative to the anal verge is invaluable in obtaining diagnostic images. When the precise location of the tumor is not provided at the time of MRI, improper staging is more likely. Accurate interpretation of rectal cancer MRI exams requires radiologists dedicated to learning how to interpret these complex exams. The radiologist's systematic review of MRI findings at the MDT both pretreatment and posttreatment is critical for accurate staging and treatment planning.

Currently, limited numbers of centers have a fully functional MDT. A major focus of working groups and the ACS Commission on Cancer is to develop recommendations for the National Accreditation Program for Rectal Cancer, which will incorporate standards, processes, outcome metrics, and the accreditation of centers to improve rectal cancer care in North America. The American College of Radiology (ACR) has a project underway to credential radiologists in the interpretation of MRI exams for rectal cancer. This will help to standardize the entire MDT process, which will drive improvement in the staging, surgery, and pathologic analysis of rectal cancer.

MAGNETIC RESONANCE IMAGING— THE FUTURE

Rapid advances in the management of rectal cancer have been made in the last 5 to 10 years. Much of this has been related to the accurate staging of MRI relative to other imaging. It has largely replaced TRUS. Further improvements are anticipated. Dynamic contrast enhancement and quantitative apparent diffusion coefficient (ADC) values have some potential use, but are not widely applicable at this time due to poor reproducibility and interobserver variability with respect to placing the "regions of interest" (ROI) and the postprocessing time requirements of these techniques. PET-MRI is currently used in some centers, and studies of this modality will investigate possible staging and restaging benefits of this procedure.

Improving the ability to characterize polyps and to define the level of invasion with early T1–T2 tumors—the former of which is the aim of the MINSTRIL trial—may further decrease the need for TRUS, which is operator dependent.

Improving the accuracy of pre- and posttreatment nodal status will help determine the adequacy of TAMIS or TEMS local procedures that do not result in pathologic nodal evaluation.

Defining the peritoneal reflection has been shown to be accurate for surgical planning. Unfortunately, to date, imaging has been unable to define the dentate line. The continued pursuit of a means to identify the dentate line, instead of relying on the anal verge, may result in a better determination of the appropriateness for a sphincter-saving procedure.

Lastly, the ability to define the complete responder with negative nodal status will reduce the number of patients undergoing major surgery that results in detrimental long-term change in quality-of-life measures for no benefit in the ultimate cure of the cancer.

REFERENCES

1. Monson JRT, Probst CP, Wexner SD, et al. Failure of evidence-based cancer care in the United States. *Ann Surg.* 2014;260(4):625-630.
2. Abbas MA, Chang GJ, Rothenberger DA, et al. Optimizing rectal cancer care management: analysis of current evidence. *Dis Colon Rectum.* 2014;57:252-259.
3. Dietz DW. Consortium for Optimizing Surgical Treatment of Rectal Cancer. Multidisciplinary management of rectal cancer: the OSTRiCE. *J Gastrointest Surg.* 2013;17:1863-1868.
4. Augestad KM, Lindsetmo RO, Stulberg J, et al. International preoperative rectal cancer management: staging, neoadjuvant treatment, and impact of multidisciplinary teams. *World J Surg.* 2010;34(11):2689-2700.
5. Glasgow SC, Morris AM, Baxter NN, et al. Development of the American Society of Colon and Rectal Surgeon's Rectal Cancer Surgery Checklist. *Dis Colon Rectum.* 2016;59:601-606.
6. Rickles AS, Dietz DW, Chang GJ, et al. High rate of positive circumferential margins following rectal cancer surgery: a call to action. *Ann Surg.* 2015;262:891-898.
7. dePrisco G. MRI Staging and restaging in rectal cancer. *Clin Colon Rectal Surg.* 2015;28(3):194-200.
8. Habr-Gama A, Sabbaga J, Gama-Rodrigues J, et al. Watch and wait approach following extended neoadjuvant chemoradiation for distal rectal cancer: are we getting closer to anal cancer management? *Dis Colon Rectum.* 2013;56:1109-1117.
9. Patel UB, Blomqvist LK, Taylor F, et al. MRI after treatment of locally advanced rectal cancer: how to report tumor response—the MERCURY trial experience. *AJR Am J Roentgenol.* 2012;199(1):W55-W42.
10. Maas M, Lambregts DM, Lahaye MJ, et al. T-staging of rectal cancer: accuracy of 3.0 Tesla MRI compared with 1.5 Tesla. *Abdom Imaging.* 2012;37(3):475-481.
11. http://c.ymcdn.com/sites/www.abdominalradiology.org/resource/resmgr/education_cfp/rectal_cancer/MR_Protocols.pdf.
12. Taylor FG, Swift RI, Blomqvist L, Brown G. A systematic approach to the interpretation of preoperative staging MRI for rectal cancer. *Am J Roentgenol.* 2008;191:1827-1835.
13. MRI Rectal Staging Template 2015. Cancer Care Ontario. https://www.cancercare.on.ca/common/pages/UserFile.aspx?fileId=353643. Updated 2015. Accessed 29 October 2017.
14. MRI Primary Rectal Cancer Staging Template SAR Rectal Cancer DFP 2016. Society of Abdominal Radiology. http://http://c.ymcdn.com/sites/www.abdominalradiology.org/resource/resmgr/docs/UPDATEDmri_primary_rectal_ca.pdf. Updated 2016. Accessed 29 October 2017.
15. Taylor F, Mangat N, Swift IR, Brown G. Proforma-based reporting in rectal cancer. *Cancer Imaging.* 2010;10(1A):S142-S150.
16. Nougaret S, Reinhold C, Mikhael HW, Fouanet P, Bibeau F, Brown G. The use of MRI imaging in treatment planning for patients with rectal cancer: have you checked the "DISTANCE"? *Radiology.* 2013;268(2):330-344.
17. MERCURY Study Group. Extramural depth of tumor invasion at thin-section MR in patients with rectal cancer: results of the MERCURY study. *Radiology.* 2007;243:132-139.
18. Battersby NJ, How P, Moran B, et al. Prospective validation of a low rectal cancer magnetic resonance imaging staging system and development of a local recurrence risk stratification model: the MERCURY II study. *Ann Surg.* 2016;263(4):751-760.
19. Brown G, Davies S, Williams GT, et al. Effectiveness of preoperative staging in rectal cancer: digital rectal examination, endoluminal ultrasound or magnetic resonance imaging? *Br J Cancer.* 2004;91(1):23-29.
20. Fernandez-Esparrach G, Ayuso-Colella JR, Sendino O, et al. EUS and magnetic resonance imaging in the staging of rectal cancer: a prospective and comparative study. *Gastrointest Endosc.* 2011;74(2):347-354.
21. Taylor FG, Quirke P, Heald RJ, et al. Preoperative magnetic resonance imaging assessment of circumferential margins predicts disease-free survival and local recurrence: 5-year follow up results of the MERCURY study. *J Clin Oncol.* 2014;2:34-43.
22. Simpson GS, Eardley N, McNicol F, Healey P, Hughes M, Rooney PS. Circumferential resection margin (CRM) positivity after MRI assessment and adjuvant treatment in 189 patients undergoing rectal cancer resection. *Int J Colorectal Dis.* 2014;29(5):585-590.
23. Gollub MJ, Maas M, Beets GL, et al. Recognition of the anterior peritoneal reflection at rectal MRI. *AJR Am J Roentgenol.* 2013;201:97-101.
24. Jung EJ, Ryu CG, Kim G, et al. Is rectal MRI beneficial for determining the location of rectal cancer with respect to the peritoneal reflection? *Radiol Oncol.* 2012;46(4):296-301.
25. Siddiqui MRS, Simillis C, Hunter C, et al. A meta-analysis comparing the risk of metastases in patients with recta. cancer and MRI-detected extramural vascular invasion (mrEMVI) vs mrEMVI-negative cases. *Br J Cancer.* 2017;116(12):1513-1519.
26. Smith NJ, Shihab O, Arnaout A, Swift RI, Brown G. MRI for detection of extramural vascular invasion in rectal cancer. *AJR Am J Roentgenol.* 2008;191(5):1517-1522.
27. Jhaveri KS, Hosseini-Nik H, Thipphavong S, et al. MRI detection of extramural venous invasion in rectal cancer: correlation with histopathology using elastin stain. *AJR Am.* 2016;206:747-755.
28. Brown G, Richards CJ, Bourne MW, et al. Morphologic predictors of lymph node status in rectal cancer with use of high-spatial-resolution MR imaging with histopathologic comparison. *Radiology.* 2003;227(2):371-377.
29. Kim DJ, Kim JH, Ryu YH, Jeon TJ, Yu JS, Chung JJ. Nodal staging of rectal cancer: high-resolution pelvic versus F-FDGPET/CT. *J Comput Assist Tomogr.* 2011;35(5):531-534.
30. Park JS, Jang YJ, Choi GS, et al. Accuracy of preoperative MRI in predicting pathology stage in rectal cancers: node-for-node matched histopathology validation of MRI features. *Dis Colon Rectum.* 2014;57(1):32-38.
30a. van Heeswijk MM, et al. DWI for assessment of rectal cancer nodes after chemoradiotherapy: Is the absence of nodes at DWI proof of a negative nodal status? *AJR Am J Roentgenol.* 2017;208(3):W79-W84.
31. Shihab OC, How P, West N, et al. Can a novel MRI staging system for low rectal cancer aid surgical planning? *Dis Colon Rectum.* 2011;54(10):1260-1264.
32. McGlone ES, Shah V, Lowdell C, Blunt D, Cohen P, Dawson PM. Circumferential resection margins of rectal tumors post-radiotherapy: how can MRI aid surgical planning? *Tech Coloproctol.* 2014;18(10):937-943.
33. Bhoday J, Smith F, Siddqui MR, et al. Magnetic resonance tumor regression grade and residual mucosal abnormality as predictors for pathologic complete response in rectal cancer postneoadjuvant chemoradiotherapy. *Dis Colon Rectum.* 2016;59:925-933.

34. Lambregts DM, Vandecaveye V, Barbaro B, et al. Diffusion-weighted MRI for selection of complete responders after chemoradiation for locally advanced rectal cancer: a multicenter study. *Ann Surg Oncol.* 2011;18(8):2224-2231. doi:10.1245/s10434-011-1607-5.

35. Lambregts DM, van Heeswijk MM, Delli Pizzi A, et al. Diffusion-weighted MRI to assess response to chemoradiotherapy in rectal cancer: main interpretation pitfalls and their use for teaching. *Eur Radiol.* 2017; Apr 13 [Epub ahead of print].

36. Schneider Daniel A, Akhurst TJ, Ngan SY, et al. Relative value of restaging MRI, CT, and FDG-PET scan after preoperative chemoradiation for rectal cancer. *Dis Colon Rectum.* 2016;59:179-186.

37. Yu SK, Tait D, Chau I, Brown G. MRI predictive factors for tumor response in rectal cancer following neoadjuvant chemoradiation therapy—implications for induction chemotherapy? *Int J Radiat Oncol Biol Phys.* 2013;87(3):505-511.

38. Dalton RS, Velinemi R, Osborne ME, et al. A single-centre experience of chemoradiotherapy for rectal cancer: is there potential for nonoperative management? *Colorectal Dis.* 2012;14:567-571.

39. Maas M, Beets-Tan RG, Lambregts DM, et al. Wait-and-see policy for clinical complete responders after chemoradiation for rectal cancer. *J Clin Oncol.* 2011;29:4633-4640.

40. Smith JD, Ruby JA, Goodman KA, et al. Nonoperative management of rectal cancer with complete clinical response after neoadjuvant therapy. *Ann Surg.* 2012;256(6):965-972.

41. Lai CL, Lai MJ, Wu CC, Jao SW, Hsiao CW. Rectal cancer with complete clinical response after neoadjuvant chemotherapy, surgery or "watch and wait. *Int J Colorectal Dis.* 2016;31(2):413-419.

42. Lambregts DM, Cappendijk VC, Maas M, Beets GL, Beets-Tan RG. Value of MRI and diffusion-weighted MRI for diagnosis of locally recurrent rectal cancer. *Eur Radiol.* 2011;21:1250-1258.

43. Brown WE, Koh CE, Badgery-Parker T, Solomon MJ. Validation of MRI and surgical decision making to predict a complete resection in pelvic exenteration for recurrent rectal cancer. *Dis Colon Rectum.* 2017;60(2):144-151.

44. Dresen RC, Kusters M, Daniels-Gooszen AW, et al. Absence of tumor invasion into pelvic structures in locally recurrent rectal cancer: prediction with preoperative MR imaging. *Radiology.* 2010;256:143-150.

45. Geogiou PA, Tekkis PP, Constantinides VA, et al. Diagnostic accuracy and value of magnetic resonance imaging (MRI) in planning exenterative pelvic surgery for advanced colorectal cancer. *Eur J Cancer.* 2013;49:72-81.

46. MERCURY Study Group, Shihab OC, Taylor F, et al. Relevance of magnetic resonance imaging-detected pelvic sidewall lymph node involvement in rectal cancer. *Br J Surg.* 2011;98(12):1798-1804.

47. Quyn Aaron J, Solomon MJ, Lee PM, Badgery-Parker T, Masya LM, Young JM. Palliative pelvic exenteration: clinical outcomes and quality of life. *Dis Colon Rectum.* 2016;59:1005-1010.

Ultrasonographic Diagnosis of Anorectal Disease

Elisa Birnbaum

Endorectal and endoanal ultrasound (ERUS and EAUS, respectively) examinations are used to diagnose benign and malignant abnormalities of the rectum and anus. ERUS has been used extensively for local staging of rectal cancer and continues to have a significant role in preoperative staging of rectal tumors. Ultrasound plays less of a role in the evaluation of tumors after chemoradiation. One of the main uses of EAUS has been in the evaluation of anal sphincter injuries in patients with fecal incontinence. It has also been used for the evaluation of complex anorectal abscess/fistulas. The procedures can be done in the office setting with portable equipment and no sedation. Minimal preparation is required, tolerance by patients is high, and the results are readily available. The cost of ERUS is significantly less than other radiologic tests, often with equivalent results. This chapter discusses the use of ERUS and EAUS for the evaluation of malignant and benign abnormalities of the rectum and anus.

ENDORECTAL ULTRASOUND TECHNIQUE FOR THE EVALUATION OF RECTAL CANCER

ERUS can be performed in the office setting with minimal patient preparation. Patients are instructed to use one or two enemas prior to the office visit because fecal material within the rectum causes image artifacts. Examinations are performed in the kneeling prone or left lateral position, depending on practitioner preference. Initial proctoscopic examination is done prior to the ERUS for evaluation of rectal tumors. Any residual fecal material and enema effluent can be suctioned out to decrease image artifacts. The distance from the tumor to the anal verge is measured, the location of the tumor on the rectal wall and the size of the rectal lumen through the tumor are noted. Ideally the ultrasound probe needs to be passed proximal to the lesion for complete evaluation because adenopathy is typically found proximal to the rectal cancers. A narrow lumen and a fixed, stenotic lesion will not allow passage of the rigid ultrasound probe easily causing patient discomfort and decreasing the accuracy of imaging.

There are several ultrasound probes that rotate 360 degrees to give a radial image of the rectum, perirectal tissues, and the anal canal. Older probes have fixed crystals at the end of the probe. A balloon is used to cover the crystal at the end of a fixed probe. These probes are rigid and are advanced through a proctoscope, allowing accurate placement above tumors. The length of the proctoscope and probe limit tumor evaluation to the rectum. The proctoscope is passed proximal to the tumor, and the lubricated probe (with balloon covering the transducer crystal) is passed through the proctoscope to a point above the lesion (ideally 15 to 20 cm from the verge to completely evaluate the mesorectum). After the probe is in place, the proctoscope is pulled back slightly and the balloon is filled with degassed fluid to distend the lumen of the bowel. Probes with stationary crystals require approximately 60 mL of liquid to distend the balloon at the end of the probe. It is important to ensure that there are no air bubbles in the balloon because the air causes accustic impedance (with bright white scattering).Both probe and proctoscope are withdrawn through the rectum to obtain images. Blind insertion of the ultrasound probe is possible, but it may be difficult to advance the probe proximal to the lesion and may cause the patient significant discomfort

Newer probes have a crystal that moves within a portion of the distal shaft of the probe. A long balloon is fitted over the probe, which is passed through a specialized proctoscope. The proctoscope is partially withdrawn, exposing the area on the probe where the crystal moves and locked into place. The balloon is filled with degassed liquid, distending it along the entire length of the probe. The balloon covering the probe is large and requires more than 200 mL to distend it and rectal wall adequately. The operator moves the crystal up and down the shaft by pressing controls on the probe. Images can be obtained and stored in real time. The crystal travels approximately 7 cm, so it may be necessary to pull the proctoscope and probe lower and perform a second pass to completely evaluate the length of the rectum.

Flexible endoscopes with mounted ultrasound tips are available and allow evaluation of lesions proximal to 15 cm. These are typically used by gastroenterologists and will not be discussed in this chapter.

The fixed ultrasound probes have interchangeable crystals with several transducer capabilities. A 7-MHz transducer provides a focal length of 2 to 5 cm and is used to evaluate deeper structures (perirectal lymph nodes). A 10-MHz transducer has a focal length of 1 to 4 cm and is the probe that is more commonly used (to evaluate the rectal wall and anal sphincter). The movable probes have multifrequency transducers, which allow the investigator to change frequency to improve visualization without needing to replace the crystal at the end of the probe.

Older machines are two dimensional, which allows for video recording and photodocumentation of static images. Three-dimensional (3D) ERUS produces high-resolution, multiplanar images. These images can be rotated and viewed from different angles in an attempt to improve the diagnostic accuracy of the ERUS. Tumor volume can be measured and the relationship between the tumor and contiguous structures better understood.

Images are generated depending on the transducer model used. The stationary probe and proctoscope are withdrawn slowly through the rectum in an effort to

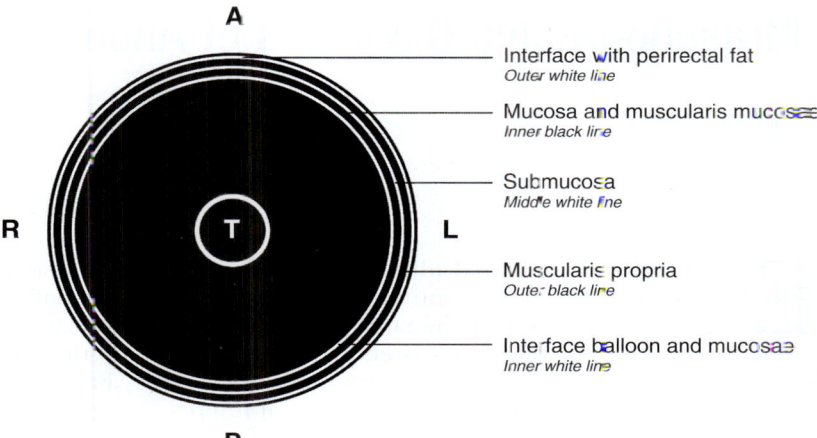

FIGURE 147.1 Five-layer anatomic model for interpretation of endorectal ultrasonographic scans. Three hyperechoic *(white)* layers and two hypoechoic *(black)* layers. *A,* Anterior; *L,* left; *P,* posterior; *R,* right; *T,* transducer.

identify perirectal lymph nodes and the tumor depth in the rectal wall. The image can be frozen to get still images of representative levels for chart documentation. Real time video documentation may also be obtained, saved, and reviewed. The movable crystal allows the probe to stay stationary above the tumor while the crystal advances through the tumor-generating images. The continuous 3D images can be stored, reviewed, and still images generated.

NORMAL ENDORECTAL ULTRASOUND RECTAL ANATOMY

Ultrasound imaging is based on echogenicity of the tissues imaged. Tissues that have a higher fluid content appear black while interfaces and tissues with less fluid density appear white. Smooth muscle with a high fluid content appears black and skeletal muscle appears white. Beynon et al. described a five-layer model for interpreting imaging of the rectal wall in 1986, and it continues to be used today as seen in Fig. 147.1.[1] The transducer appears in the center of the image. The fluid-filled balloon is the central large black image surrounding the transducer. The first hyperechoic white line is the interface between the balloon and the mucosa. The inner hypoechoic black line represents the muscularis mucosae. The middle hyperechoic white line represents the submucosa. The next hypoechoic black line is the muscularis propria, and the outer hyperechoic white line is the interface between the muscularis propria and the perirectal fat. Fig. 147.2 shows the ultrasound appearance of a normal rectal wall. Blood vessels can be seen in the surrounding tissues and appear as hypoechoic circular structures, which can elongate as the probe is withdrawn. Lymph nodes tend to be more irregular shaped and can have mixed echogenicity. Seminal vesicles are seen anterior and appear as bilateral structures.

ENDORENAL ULTRASOUND STAGING OF RECTAL CANCER

Digital rectal examination (DRE), ERUS, computed tomography (CT) scanning, and magnetic resonance

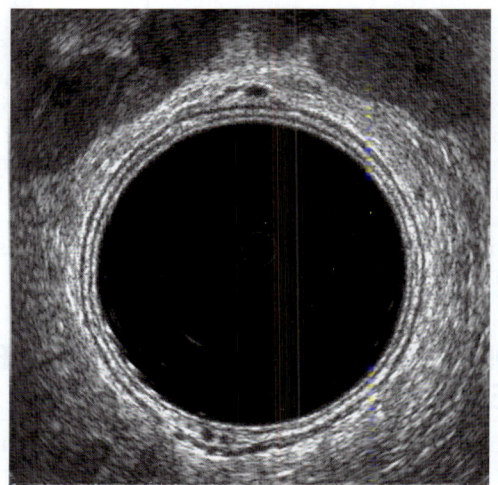

FIGURE 147.2 Normal rectal wall. Hypoechoic lines *(black)* represent the inner muscularis mucosae and the outer muscularis propria. Hyperechoic lines *(white)* represent the interfaces between the balloon (inner), submucosa (middle), and perirectal fat (outer). The seminal vesicles are seen anteriorly as bilateral hypoechoic *(black)* structures.

imaging (MRI) are commonly used for staging of rectal cancers. Each of these modalities has its proponents and detractors. DRE is useful for evaluation of the fixation of low rectal cancers but cannot assess middle level and upper level tumors. ERUS is more accurate in assessment of the depth of wall invasion and lymph node involvement when compared with DRE.[2,3] Zhou et al. performed a meta-analysis looking at studies of ERUS in the evaluation of rectal cancer. The pooled diagnostic sensitivity and specificity were 95% and 80%. Lymph node sensitivity and specificity were 58% and 80%.[4]

CT scanning is useful for evaluating distant metastatic disease and involvement of contiguous organs but is less accurate for assessment of T stage of rectal cancers. MRI is becoming more popular in the assessment of circumferential resection margins (CRMs). MRI T stage accuracy and lymph node (LN) accuracy improve with the use of endorectal coil (T, 81%; LN, 63%) and is

TABLE 147.1 Ultrasound Staging Classification (Ultrasonographic Staging of Tumor, Node, and Metastasis) for Rectal Cancer

Classification	Criteria
uT0	Noninvasive lesion confined to the mucosa
uT1	Tumor confined to the submucosa
uT2	Tumor invades into but not through the muscularis propria, remains confined to the rectal wall
uT3	Tumor penetrates through the entire thickness of the rectum and invades the perirectal fat
uT4	Tumor invades an adjacent organ/structure
uN0	No evidence of lymph node metastasis (no definable lymph nodes by ultrasound)
uN1	Evidence of lymph node metastasis (ultrasonographically apparent lymph nodes)

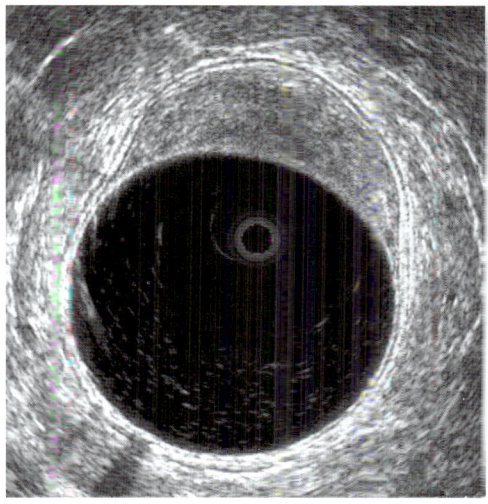

FIGURE 147.3 Benign villous tumor of the rectum (uT0). The *middle white line* is intact, indicating that the submucosa is not involved. (From Wong WD, Orrom WJ, Jensen LL. Preoperative staging of rectal cancer with endorectal ultrasonography. *Perspect Colon Rectal Surg.* 1990;3:315.)

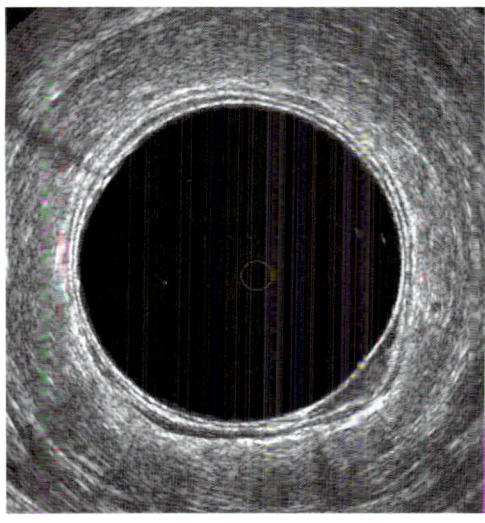

FIGURE 147.4 uT1 lesion. The *middle white line* is thickened and irregular but not disrupted, indicating invasion into but not through the submucosa.

comparable with ERUS.[5,6] Li et al. reported on a recent meta-analysis evaluating ERUS, CT, and MRI in patients not receiving preoperative chemoradiotherapy.[7] They showed similar accuracy, but none of the tests provided reliable evaluation of lymph node metastases. Accuracy for early stage tumors (T0 to T1) and later stage tumors (T3 to T4) is high when staged by ERUS (97% and 88%, respectively). Identification of T2 lesions is poor (37%), with 21% overstaged, indicating that ERUS may not be useful for evaluating patients for a tailored surgical approach.[8–10]

The phased array coil MRI has been shown to be highly accurate in the prediction of CRM in the MERCURY trial.[11] These MRIs are an arrangement of multiple external coils and fast T2-weighted sequences, which are very accurate in prediction of CRM but have a low accuracy in predicting lymph node involvement.[12,13] Several small studies compared ERUS and MRI for accuracy in determining CRM and found that the two modalities are similarly accurate.[14,15] Accuracy of pretreatment staging may improve with multimodal imaging (MRI and ERUS).[16]

ERUS can be done in the outpatient setting, it is portable and less expensive than CT and MRI. The accuracy of ERUS is operator dependent but has been reported to be as high as 95% for T staging and 80% for staging of lymph node metastases.[4,7] Tumors appear as hypoechoic or mixed echogenic masses, which disrupt the layers of the rectal wall.

Ultrasound staging (prefix *u*) of rectal cancers is a modification of the tumor, node, metastasis (TNM) staging system (pathology staging prefix *p*) and was introduced in 1985 by Hildebrandt and Feifel.[17] Table 147.1 lists the uTNM stage and correlating criteria for staging.

uT0 lesions are confined to the rectal mucosa and are noninvasive (Fig. 147.3). The middle white line (submucosa) remains intact. Tubulovillous adenomas are benign uT0 lesions that can be seen expanding the mucosal layer (the first black line).

uT1 lesions invade the mucosa and submucosa but do not invade the muscularis propria (second black line). The middle white line (submucosa) is seen as thickened and irregular but not broken (Fig. 147.4). If there is a break in the submucosa the muscularis propria is considered invaded and the lesion is staged as a uT2. Lymph node involvement can occur in 10% to 20% of T1 rectal cancers and ERUS may help to identify this subgroup of patients for whom local resection would be contraindicated. Staging accuracy varies from 47% to 96% for uT1 lesions.[18,19]

uT2 lesions cause disruption of the middle white line (submucosa) and expansion of the outer black line (muscularis propria). The outer black line (perirectal fat) is intact. There may be scalloping of the outer white layer, which may lead to overstaging of these lesions (Fig. 147.5). The accuracy of uT2 staging is approximately 68%.[19] Lymph node metastases can occur in up to 30% of T2 lesions[20,21] and probably account for why there is a

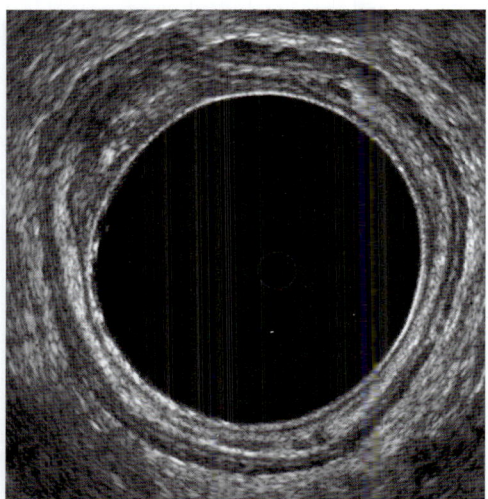

FIGURE 147.5 uT2 lesion. The *middle white line* is disrupted and there is expansion of the *outer black line*, indicating invasion of the tumor through the submucosa and into the muscularis propria. The *outer white line* is intact, indicating that the tumor is confined to the rectal wall.

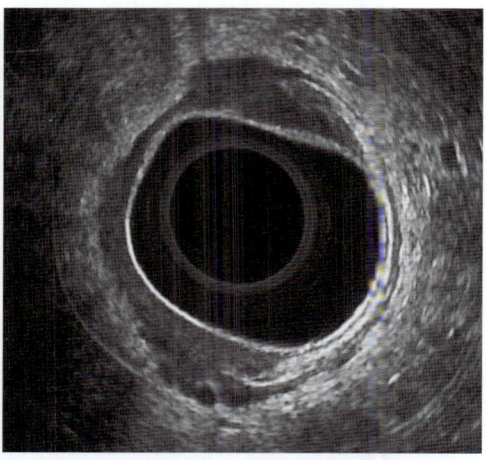

FIGURE 147.6 uT3 lesion. The *outer white line* is irregular and interrupted, indicating tumor invasion into the perirectal fat.

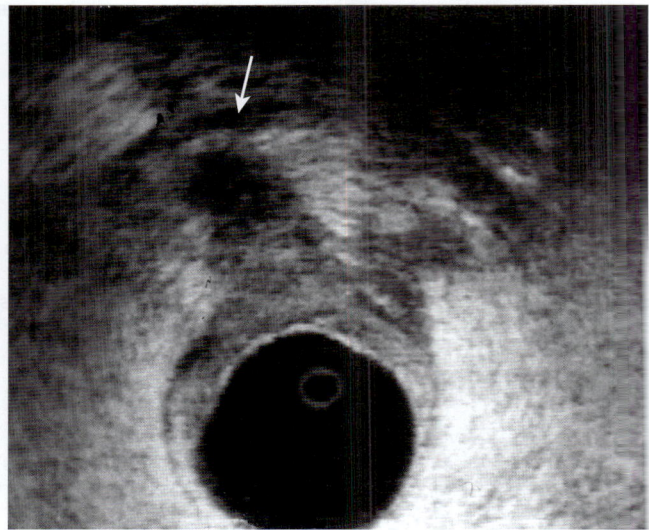

FIGURE 147.7 uT4 lesion. Tumor invades the posterior vaginal wall *(arrow)*.

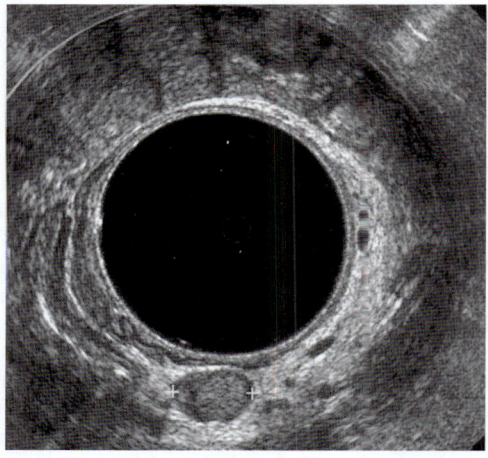

FIGURE 147.8 Posterior hypoechoic lesion outside of the rectal wall (1.2 cm), indicating metastatic lymph node.

high local recurrence rate in T2 lesions treated by local therapy alone.

uT3 lesions involve the full thickness of the rectal wall and invade the perirectal fat, disrupting the outer white layer on ultrasound imaging (Fig. 147.6). ERUS accuracy can be as high as 80% in diagnosing T3 rectal cancers.[19] Lymph node metastases can occur in up to 66% of T3 rectal cancers.[22]

uT4 lesions invade contiguous structures such as the vagina, prostate, or seminal vesicles. The hyperechoic interface between these structures and the rectal wall is disrupted if there is invasion by tumor (Fig. 147.7).

NODAL INVOLVEMENT

Normal lymph nodes are generally not seen on ultrasound. Micrometastases are not detected by ultrasound because

microscopic tumor deposits do not change the echogenic character of the nodes. Metastatic lymph nodes that have been replaced by tumor appear round and hypoechoic and have distinct borders. They are typically seen near the primary tumor or proximal to the primary in the upper mesorectum (Fig. 147.8). Hypoechoic lesions larger than 5 mm may be metastatic in up to 70%,[23] whereas those measuring 3 to 5 mm may be metastatic in up to 50%.[24,25] Small, hypoechoic spots may be seen in mesorectal lesions less than 3 mm and may represent small metastases.[26] The accuracy of ERUS staging of lymph nodes is variable and is less than the accuracy of T staging and ranges from 64% to 83%[19,27] Overstaging of nodal status is common and may be caused by enlarged, inflammatory nodes, hypoechoic blood vessels, and extensions from the primary tumor. Understaging occurs when the lymph nodes are involved with micrometastases or they are beyond the range of the transducer (either deep in the mesorectum or more proximal than can be safely evaluated). In a study by Landmann et al. the overall accuracy of ERUS for nodal staging was 70%, with a 16% false-positive rate and a 14% false-negative rate.[28] This study noted a relationship between nodal staging accuracy and T stage. The ultrasound nodal stage was 80% accurate for pT3 lesions and less than 50% accurate for pT1 lesions.

LIMITATIONS IN THE EVALUATION OF RECTAL CANCER

ERUS is operator dependent for the performance and interpretation of images. There is a learning curve, and T stage accuracy improves over time.[29] In addition to inexperience, there are other factors that affect accuracy. Stool and liquid within the rectal vault may produce artifacts obscuring accurate visualization. Biopsies of the lesion prior to ERUS may cause the lesion to be overstaged. It is recommended that the ERUS be done prior to biopsy for improved accuracy. Overstaging has been reported in the range of 11% to 18%. Understaging ranges from 5% to 13% but is more serious because it may result in inadequate management.[18,19]

ERUS after treatment with radiation and chemoradiation is inaccurate and results in a high rate of overstaging.[30] These treatments cause inflammation, edema, and fibrosis of the tumor and surrounding tissue, making it difficult to determine the difference between residual tumor and the fibrosis of treated disease. A recent meta-analysis done by Zhao et al. found overstaging to be common and a low accuracy for T restaging after chemoradiation.[30] Accuracy for restaging higher T stages (T3 to T4) was better than for T0 to T2 lesions. The specificity of N staging was high, but the sensitivity was low. Similarly, a meta-analysis done by Memon et al. reviewed restaging MRI and restaging ERUS studies.[31] They found that restaging MRI was more accurate in evaluating the circumferential resection margin but was essentially equivalent to ERUS for T stage accuracy (52% vs. 65%).

ENDOANAL ULTRASOUND TECHNIQUE FOR THE EVALUATION OF ANAL CANAL

EAUS is the procedure of choice for evaluation of the anatomy of the internal and external anal sphincters. It is used in the identification of anal sphincter defects in patients with fecal incontinence and can be useful for evaluation of complex anal fistulas, as well as tumors within the anal canal. The procedure is well tolerated and similar to a DRE.

DREs, EAUS, and MRI have been used to identify anal sphincter defects. Although the identification of a complete disruption of the anal sphincter and loss of perineal body is obvious on all three examinations, DRE has poor specificity for detecting anal sphincter defects identified on EAUS.[32]

EAUS done for fecal incontinence may be done in conjunction with anal manometry. A kneeling prone position or lateral decubitus position can be used. A simple DRE to ensure that there is no formed fecal material in the rectal vault may be all that is necessary. A hard cap is used over the end of the probe with the stationary crystal. A gel-filled balloon is placed over the probe with the movable crystal when evaluating the anal canal. The lubricated ultrasound probe is placed directly through the anal canal without the use of a proctoscope and advanced above the anal canal. The top of the anal canal is identified by the large U-shaped puborectalis muscle. The entire length of the anal canal is evaluated by withdrawal of the stationary probe or withdrawal of the movable crystal through the probe. When evaluating anal sphincter defects in women, it is often useful to place an index finger within the vagina to get a better determination of the width of the perineal body. Documentation is done with static images along the anal canal and/or video documentation.

NORMAL ENDOANAL ULTRASOUND ANATOMY

Although the ultrasound images of the anal canal may be taken continuously, the anal anatomy is examined in the upper, middle, and distal anal canal. Skeletal muscle (puborectalis and external anal sphincter) appears hyperechoic and smooth muscle (internal anal sphincter), which has a higher fluid content, appears hypoechoic. After placement of the probe above the pelvic floor, it is pulled out slowly until the puborectalis is visualized at the top of the anorectal junction. The puborectalis is the primary structure evaluated in the upper anal canal. It appears as a striated hyperechoic posteriorly based U-shaped structure and is not present in the anterior quadrant (Fig. 147.9). The external anal sphincter is seen in the middle anal canal as a continuation of the puborectalis and forms a complete hyperechoic ring around the anal canal (Fig. 147.10). The internal anal sphincter is also seen quite well in the middle anal canal as a dark, hyperechoic ring. The internal anal sphincter ends before the distal anal canal, where only the hyperechoic external anal sphincter and surrounding soft tissue are seen. It is useful to measure the perineal body in the middle and distal anal canal. The examiner's index finger is placed into the patient's vagina as the probe or crystal is withdrawn. The perineal body is the distance between the interface of the index finger and vagina and the interface between the probe and the anal sphincter (Fig. 147.11). Normal perineal

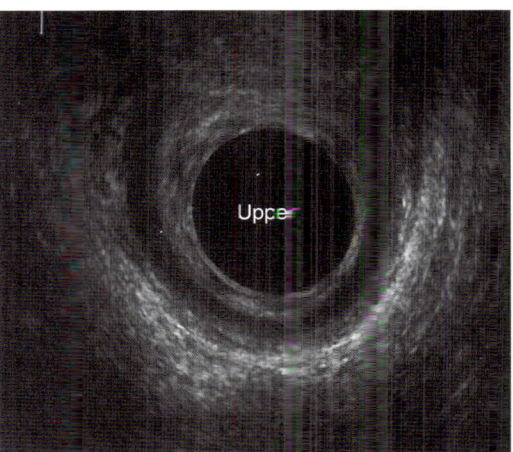

FIGURE 147.9 Upper anal canal. The puborectalis is seen as a posteriorly based, U-shaped hyperechoic structure.

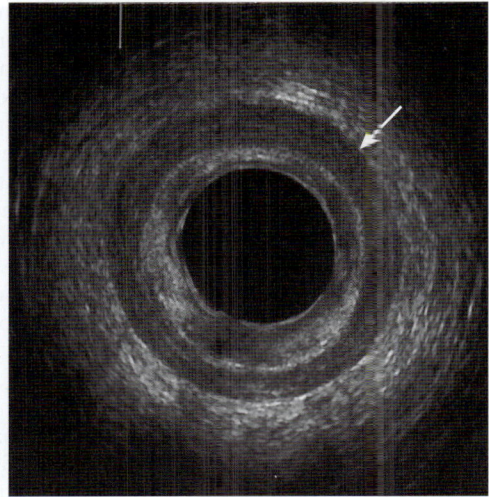

FIGURE 147.10 Midanal canal. The internal anal sphincter is a black, hypoechoic *(arrow)* ring. The external anal sphincter is a white, hyperechoic ring surrounding the internal anal sphincter. The external anal sphincter is a continuation of the puborectalis and is a complete ring in the mid anal canal.

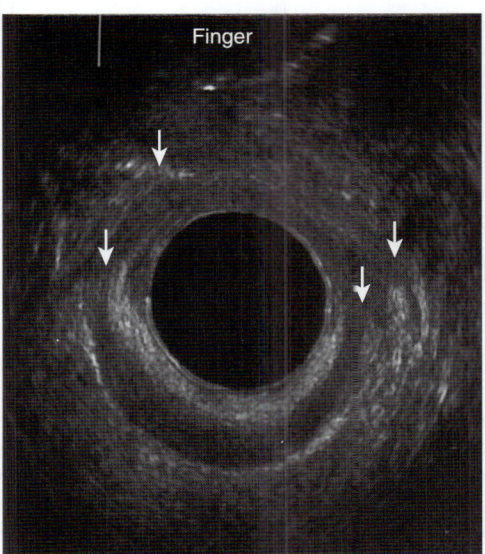

FIGURE 147.12 Anterior anal sphincter defect. There is a wide anterior separation of both the internal and external anal sphincters *(arrows)*. When cut, the internal anal sphincter contracts posteriorly.

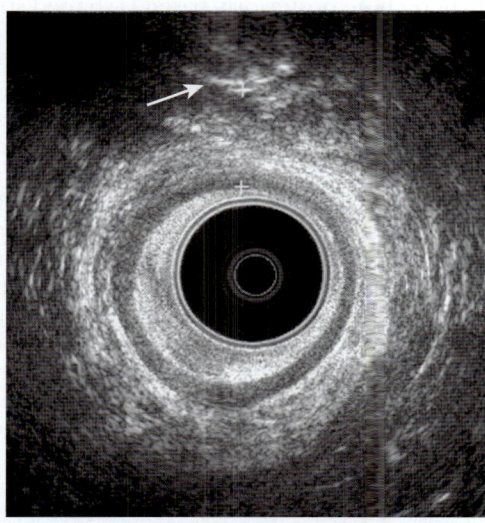

FIGURE 147.11 Perineal body measurement. The perineal body is the distance from the hyperechoic reflection of the examiner's finger *(arrow)* and the inner aspect of the internal anal sphincter.

body thickness is approximately 15 mm and is measured from the hyperechoic edge of the examiner's finger to the inner edge of the internal anal sphincter.[33]

ENDOANAL ULTRASOUND EVALUATION OF ANAL SPHINCTER DEFECTS

EAUS helps to detect anatomic mechanical defects of the internal and external anal sphincter in patients being evaluated for fecal incontinence.[34-36] Although obstetric trauma is the primary cause of fecal incontinence, anorectal surgery (lateral sphincterotomy, fistulotomy, hemorrhoidectomy, etc.), perineal trauma, and congenital defects may also

be contributing factors. Fourth-degree episiotomies occur when the episiotomy extends from the vaginal wall full thickness through the internal and external anal sphincter. Third-degree episiotomies do not extend through the rectal wall and may damage the external anal sphincter while leaving the internal anal sphincter intact. Occult sphincter injuries are common (as high as 30%) in primiparous women even if a sphincterotomy is not done.[37-39] Not all of these women develop fecal incontinence, despite the presence of occult anal sphincter injuries.

Defects of the internal anal sphincter are the easiest to identify and are the result of surgical trauma (lateral internal sphincterotomy, hemorrhoidectomy) or fourth-degree episiotomies. Because the internal anal sphincter is a muscle that is contracted at rest, when it is divided the edges retract and the remaining muscle contracts. There is an obvious separation of the hypoechoic ring at the point of division.

Defects of the external anal sphincter appear as a hypoechoic disruption of the hyperechoic ring. When both the internal and external anal sphincters are disrupted there is an obvious separation of the internal (hypoechoic) and external (hyperechoic) rings. Fig. 147.12 shows the wide separation of both the external anal sphincter and internal anal sphincter. The remaining internal sphincter is easily seen contracted posteriorly as a thickened hypoechoic structure. In Fig. 147.12 there is a thickened scar between the probe and the index finger image, indicating a normal perineal body but injured anal sphincter. Some patients have very thin perineal bodies or near cloacal defects. Ultrasound images of cloacal defects show images of the index finger within the vagina in close proximity to the probe with minimal tissue between the image of the finger and the probe. Oftentimes, there is only a partial injury to the external anal sphincter. Normal perineal body thickness is 10 to 15 mm in the middle anal canal

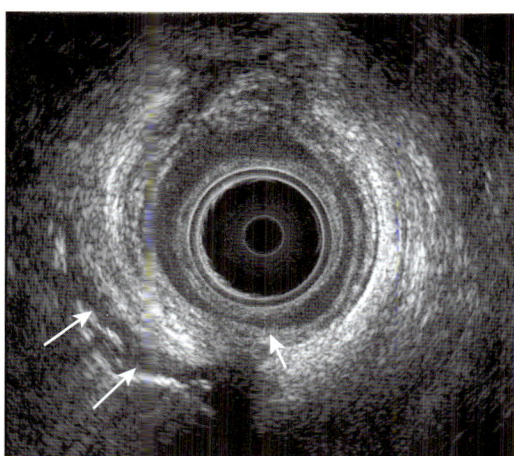

FIGURE 147.13 Fistula-in-ano. The fistula tract appears hypoechoic *(long arrows)*. The internal opening is identified in the posterior midline *(short arrow)*.

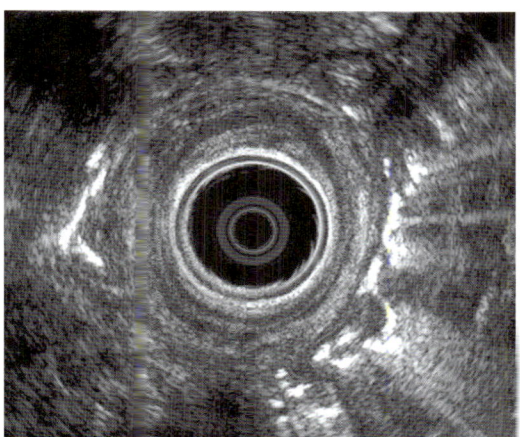

FIGURE 147.14 Fistula-in-ano. Hydrogen peroxide injected into the external opening of the fistula appears brightly hyperechoic and outlines the fistula tract.

Measurements less than 10 mm indicate a probable anal sphincter defect.[5]

False-positive rates can be as high as 25%.[40] In the upper anal canal the puborectalis is absent in the anterior quadrants, and there may be some confusion as to where the external anal sphincter starts. Limiting the evaluation to the middle and lower anal canal (distal 1.5 cm) may improve accuracy.

EVALUATION OF FISTULA AND ABSCESS DISEASE

Although perianal abscesses are typically easy to identify on DRE or under anesthesia, there are times when they may not be readily identified. 3D EAUS can accurately identify the abscess, identify the internal opening, and detect secondary extensions.[41,42] An intrasphincteric abscess may appear as a hypoechoic area between the internal and external anal sphincter. EAUS has been used more commonly for the identification of complex anorectal

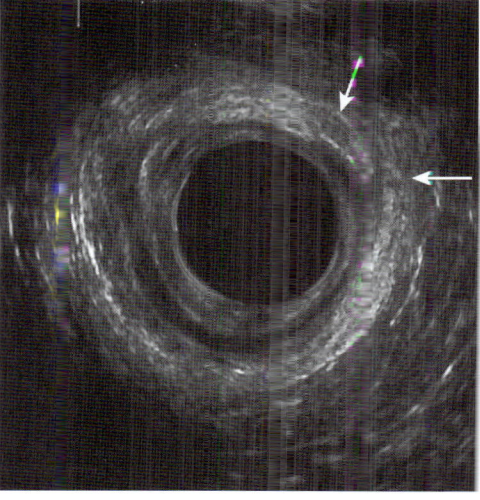

FIGURE 147.15 Intact overlapping anal sphincter repair. The spiral overlapping external sphincter is visualized anteriorly *(arrows)*.

fistulas. These fistula tracts are typically hypoechoic and can be followed through the anal canal to determine location (Fig. 147.13). Hydrogen peroxide injection into the tracts may assist in identification of complex fistulas. Hyperechoic images are seen where the peroxide bubbles release oxygen (Fig. 147.14).

3D EAUS may assist in identification of secondary fistula tracts which, if missed, might be a risk factor for recurrence.[43] In addition, 3D EAUS may help in preoperative assessment and surgical management of anterior transsphincteric fistulas by quantifying the length of muscle to be transected.[44]

EAUS is valuable in the preoperative assessment and surgical planning for patients with rectovaginal fistulas. It helps to identify patients with anterior sphincter injuries that may need to be repaired at the same time as sliding flap.[45] Patients with persistent fecal incontinence after anal sphincter reconstruction may be reevaluated with EAUS to ensure that the repair is intact. Fig. 147.15 shows an intact overlapping anal sphincter repair.

REFERENCES

1. Beynon J, Foy DM, Temple LN, Channer JL, Virjee J, Mortensen NJ. The endosonic appearances of normal colon and rectum. *Dis Colon Rectum*. 1986;28:810.
2. Rafaelsen SR, Kronberg O, Fenger C. Digital rectal examination and transrectal ultrasonography in staging of rectal cancer. *Acta Radiol*. 1994;35:300.
3. Starck M, Bohe M, Fork FT, Lindström C, Sjöberg S. Endoluminal ultrasound and low-field magnetic resonance imaging are superior to clinical examination in the preoperative staging of rectal cancer. *Eur J Surg*. 1995;161:841.
4. Zhou Y, Shao W, Lu W. Diagnostic value of endorectal ultrasonography for rectal carcinoma: a meta-analysis. *J Cancer Res Ther*. 2014;10(suppl):319.
5. Kim NK, Kim MJ, Yun SH, Sohn SK, Min JS. Comparative study of transrectal ultrasonography, pelvic computerized tomography, and magnetic resonance imaging in preoperative staging of rectal cancer. *Dis Colon Rectum*. 1999;42:770.
6. Kim NK, Kim MJ, Park JK, Park SI, Min JS. Preoperative staging of rectal cancer with MRI: accuracy and clinical usefulness. *Ann Surg Oncol*. 2000;7:732.

7. Li XT, Sun YS, Tang L, Cao K, Zhang XY. Evaluating local lymph node metastasis with magnetic resonance imaging, endoluminal ultrasound and computed tomography in rectal cancer: a meta-analysis. *Colorectal Dis.* 2015;17:129.

8. Restivo A, Zorcolo L, Marongiu L, Scintu F, Casula G. Limits of endorectal ultrasound in tailoring treatment of patients with rectal cancer. *Dig Surg.* 2015;32:129.

9. Mondal D, Betts M, Cunningham C, Mortensen NJ, Lindsey I, Slater A. How useful is endorectal ultrasound in the management of early rectal carcinoma? *Int J Colorectal Dis.* 2014;29:1101.

10. Kolev NY, Tonev AY, Ignatov VL, et al. The role of 3-D endorectal ultrasound in rectal cancer: our experience. *Int Surg.* 2014;99:106.

11. Mercury Study Group. Diagnostic accuracy of preoperative magnetic resonance imaging in predicting curative resection of rectal cancer: prospective observational study. *BMJ.* 2006;333:779.

12. Taylor FG, Swift RI, Blomqvist L, Brown G. A systematic approach to the interpretation of preoperative staging MRI for rectal cancer. *AJR Am J Roentgenol.* 2008;191:1827.

13. Lahaye MJ, Engelen SM, Kessels AG, et al. USPIO-enhanced MR imaging for nodal staging in patients with primary rectal cancer: predictive criteria. *Radiology.* 2008;246:804.

14. Granero-Castro P, Munoz E, Frasson M, et al. Evaluation of mesorectal fascia in mid and low anterior rectal cancer using endorectal ultrasound is feasible and reliable: a comparison with MRI findings. *Dis Colon Rectum.* 2014;57:709.

15. Phang PT, Goluub MJ, Loh BD, et al. Accuracy of endorectal ultrasound for measurement of the closest predicted radial mesorectal margin for rectal cancer. *Dis Colon Rectum.* 2012;55:59.

16. Heo SH, Kim JW, Shin SS, Jeong YY, Kang HK. Multimodal imaging evaluation in staging of rectal cancer. *World J Gastroenterol.* 2014;20:4244.

17. Hildebrandt U, Feifel G. Preoperative staging of rectal cancer by intrarectal ultrasound. *Dis Colon Rectum.* 1985;28:42.

18. Kwok H, Bissett IP, Hill GL. Preoperative staging of rectal cancer. *Int J Colorectal Dis.* 2000;15:9.

19. Garcia-Aguilar J, Pollack J, Lee S-K, et al. Accuracy of endorectal ultrasonography in preoperative staging of rectal tumors. *Dis Colon Rectum.* 2002;45:10.

20. Rasheed S, Bowley DM, Aziz O, et al. Can depth of tumour invasion predict lymph node positivity in patients undergoing resection for early rectal cancer? A comparative study between T1 and T2 cancers. *Colorectal Dis.* 2008;10:231.

21. Kajiwara Y, Ueno H, Hashiguchi Y, Mochizuki H, Hase K. Risk factors of nodal involvement in T2 colorectal cancer. *Dis Colon Rectum.* 2010;53:1393.

22. Sitzler PJ, Seow-Choen F, Ho YH, Leong AP. Lymph node involvement and tumor depth in rectal cancers: an analysis of 805 patients. *Dis Colon Rectum.* 1997;40:1472.

23. Sunouchi K, Sakaguchi M, Higuchi Y, Namiki K, Muto T. Limitation of endorectal ultrasonography: what does a low lesion more than 5 mm in size correspond to histologically? *Dis Colon Rectum.* 1998;41:761.

24. Akasu T, Sugihara K, Moriya Y, Fujita S. Limitations and pitfalls of transrectal ultrasonography for staging of rectal cancer. *Dis Colon Rectum.* 1997;40:S10-S15.

25. Katsura Y, Yamada K, Ishizawa T, Yoshinaka H, Shimazu H. Endorectal ultrasonography for the assessment of wall invasion and lymph node metastasis in rectal cancer. *Dis Colon Rectum.* 1992;35:362.

26. Sunouchi K, Sakaguchi M, Higuchi Y, Namiki K, Muto T. Small spot sign of rectal carcinoma by endorectal ultrasonography: histologic relation and clinical impact on postoperative recurrence. *Dis Colon Rectum.* 1998;41:649.

27. Beynon J. An evaluation of the role of rectal endosonography in rectal cancer. *Ann R Coll Surg Engl.* 1989;71:131.

28. Landmann RG, Wong WD, Hoepfl J, et al. Limitations of early rectal cancer nodal staging may explain failure after local excision. *Dis Colon Rectum.* 2007;50:1520.

29. Patel RK, Sayers AE, Kumar P, Khulusi S, Razack A, Hunter IA. The role of endorectal ultrasound and magnetic resonance imaging in the management of early rectal lesions in a tertiary center. *Clin Colorectal Cancer.* 2014;13:245.

30. Zhao YL, Cao DM, Yang N, Yao HL. Accuracy of endorectal endoscopic ultrasound (EUS) for locally advanced rectal cancer (LARC) restaging after neoadjuvant chemoradiotherapy (NAT): a meta-analysis. *Hepatogastroenterology.* 2014;61:978.

31. Memon S, Lynch AC, Bressel M, Wise AG, Heriot AG. Systematic review and meta-analysis of the accuracy of MRI and endorectal ultrasound in the restaging and response assessment of rectal cancer following neoadjuvant therapy. *Colorectal Dis.* 2015;17:748.

32. Jeppson PC, Paraiso MF, Jelovsek JE, Barber MD. Accuracy of the digital anal examination in women with fecal incontinence. *Int Urogynecol J.* 2012;23:765.

33. Oberwalder M, Thaler K, Baig MK, et al. Anal ultrasound and endosonographic measurement of perineal body thickness: a new evaluation for fecal incontinence in females. *Surg Endosc.* 2004;18:650.

34. Rostaminia G, White D, Quiroz LH, Shobeiri SA. 3D pelvic floor ultrasound findings and severity of anal incontinence. *Int Urogynecol J.* 2014;25:623.

35. Norderval S, Markskog A, Rossaak K, Vonen B. Correlation between anal sphincter defects and anal incontinence following obstetric sphincter tears: assessment using scoring systems for sonographic classification of defects. *Ultrasound Obstet Gynecol.* 2008;31:78.

36. Titi MA, Jenkins JT, Urie A, Molloy RG. Correlation between anal manometry and endosonography in females with faecal incontinence. *Colorectal Dis.* 2008;10:131.

37. Johnson JK, Lindow SW, Duthie GS. The prevalence of occult obstetric anal sphincter injury following childbirth—literature review. *J Matern Fetal Neonatal Med.* 2007;20:547.

38. Oberwalder M, Connor J, Wexner SD. Meta-analysis to determine the incidence of obstetric anal sphincter damage. *Br J Surg.* 2003;90:1333.

39. Albuquerque A. Endoanal ultrasonography in fecal incontinence: current and future perspectives. *World J Gastrointest Endosc.* 2015;10:575.

40. Sentovich SM, Wong WD, Blatchford GJ. Accuracy and reliability of transanal ultrasound for anterior anal sphincter injury. *Dis Colon Rectum.* 1998;41:1000.

41. Brillantino A, Iacobellis F, Di Sarno G, et al. Role of tridimensional endoanal ultrasound (3D-EAUS) in the preoperative assessment of perianal sepsis. *Int J Colorectal Dis.* 2015;30:535.

42. Kim Y, Park YJ. Three-dimensional endoanal ultrasonographic assessment of an anal fistula with and without H_2O_2 enhancement. *World J Gastroenterol.* 2009;15:4810.

43. Visscher AP, Schuur D, Slooff RA, Meijerink WJ, Deen-Molenaar CB, Felt-Bersma RJ. Predictive factors for recurrence of cryptoglandular fistulae characterized by preoperative three-dimensional endoanal ultrasound. *Colorectal Dis.* 2016;18:503.

44. Murad-Regadas SM, Regadas FS, Rodrigues LV, Holanda Ede C, Barreto RG, Oliveira L. The role of 3-dimensional anorectal ultrasonography in the assessment of anterior transsphincteric fistula. *Dis Colon Rectum.* 2010;53:1035.

45. Tsang CB, Madoff RD, Wong WD, et al. Anal sphincter integrity and function influences outcome in rectovaginal fistula repair. *Dis Colon Rectum.* 1998;41:1141.

PART TWO

Benign Colon, Rectal, and Anal Conditions

Diagnosis and Management of Fecal Incontinence

Janet T. Lee | Sarah A. Vogler | Robert D. Madoff

Fecal incontinence (FI) is the inability to maintain voluntary control of the passage of gas, liquid, or solid stool through the anus. Although FI is not a life-threatening condition, it is certainly a life-altering condition. The associated embarrassment, subsequent coping mechanisms, and behavioral changes can lead to a dramatic decrease in quality of life (QoL) and social isolation. The prevalence of FI is difficult to determine because of potential misdiagnosis, underdiagnosis, or variations in definition and the population under study. Community prevalence has been estimated to range from 0.5% to 11%.[1] A Wisconsin telephone survey reported that 2.2% of the general population experienced FI of varying degrees.[2] The prevalence increases to 13.4% in outpatients seeing their primary care physicians and 26% in outpatients seeing their gastroenterologist.[3] The highest rates of incontinence are seen in institutionalized individuals; a survey of 18,000 Wisconsin nursing home residents found that 47% had FI.[4] Overall, the prevalence is much higher in women, the elderly, and nursing home residents.

EVALUATION

The underlying cause of FI can be from a variety of mechanisms and can be divided into three main categories: anatomic, neurologic, or mechanical. Examples of anatomic causes of FI include obstetric injury to the sphincter or iatrogenic injury from sphincterotomy. Neurologic causes include nerve injury, diabetes, and spinal cord injury. Mechanical etiologies of FI may be related to a normal mechanism being overwhelmed by high-output liquid stool (e.g., secretory tumors or diarrhea) or prolapsing tissue through the anal canal leading to constant seepage. Oftentimes, the underlying cause of FI may be related to a combination of factors (Box 148.1).

Initial evaluation should consist of a detailed history and physical examination. This is usually sufficient to diagnose FI, and occasionally special testing is needed to identify the underlying cause. This can include imaging, laboratory tests, stool testing, colonoscopy, or anal physiology testing.

HISTORY

History taking is a vital step in the diagnosis of FI. Embarrassment and shame from these symptoms can make the history difficult to obtain. Oftentimes, it may be beneficial to conduct the history face-to-face and sitting down with the patient. Patients may downplay frequency or severity of symptoms or even be reluctant to admit that they have problems with bowel control. For example, patients may present with complaints of "diarrhea" when they actually are experiencing involuntary passage of liquid stool. Questions should be focused on understanding when and if the patient gets an urge or warning before passing gas or stool and how frequently this occurs. It is important to ask about stool consistency and if there is a change in bowel habits. The Bristol Stool Scale can be helpful in objectively understanding stool consistency.[5] Asking the patient to keep a diary to record stool frequency, urgency, and consistency allows for a better understanding of FI severity (Fig. 148.1). During the history taking, the past medical history should be focused on specific risk factors for FI, such as previous anorectal procedures[6]; vaginal deliveries,[7] particularly with episiotomies, tears or difficult extractions; pelvic radiation[8,9] diabetes mellitus; chronic diarrhea; congenital conditions[10] such as imperforate anus and spina bifida; urinary incontinence; or complaints of rectal prolapse or anal protrusion.[11,12]

Validated scoring systems and questionnaires are helpful to objectively measure frequency and severity of FI. Various scoring systems or severity indices exist and are widely used, although no one scoring system is universally accepted.[13,14] An ideal instrument will measure the frequency of accidents and nature of the leakage (gas, liquid, solid) at minimum. Use of devices (i.e., pad or tissue paper), coping methods, or urgency are also included in some measurement tools. Commonly used scoring systems include Fecal Incontinence Severity Index (FISI)[15] and Wexner.[16] The FISI is increasingly being used because its scores were derived from both patient- and colorectal surgeon-based weighting of severity.[15]

Measurement of QoL is an important tool for understanding how a disease process impacts an individual's

BOX 148.1 Causes of Fecal Incontinence

NORMAL PELVIC FLOOR
Diarrheal states
    Infectious diarrhea
    Inflammatory bowel disease
    Short gut syndrome
    Laxative abuse
    Radiation enteritis
Overflow
    Impaction
    Encopresis
    Rectal neoplasms
Neurologic conditions
    Congenital anomalies (e.g., myelomeningocele)
    Multiple sclerosis
    Dementia, strokes, tabes dorsalis
    Neuropathy (e.g., diabetes)
    Neoplasms of brain, spinal cord, cauda equina

ABNORMAL PELVIC FLOOR
Congenital anorectal malformation
Trauma
Accidental injury (e.g., impalement, pelvic fracture)
Anorectal surgery
Obstetric injury
Aging

PELVIC FLOOR DENERVATION (IDIOPATHIC NEUROGENIC INCONTINENCE)
Vaginal delivery
Chronic straining at stool
Rectal prolapse
Descending perineum syndrome

From Madoff RD, Williams JG, Caushaj PF. Fecal incontinence. *N Engl J Med.* 1992;326:1002–1007.

health. In patients with FI, the impact of the disease on QoL is used to guide clinical decision-making and determine efficacy of treatment. Use of QoL instruments in managing patients with FI is especially important because FI is fundamentally a QoL issue. General QoL scales may be used, as well as more specific QoL scales, in the FI population. Specific FI scales often include questions on overall health and well-being, behavioral modifications related to FI episodes or fear of loss of control, use of devices, ability to perform usual daily activities, social activities, and urgency. However, studies have shown that the scales may not always be applicable for certain patient populations or have undergone standardized rigorous psychometric testing to be deemed "reliable."[14] In addition, these QoL instruments may be cumbersome for the patient to fill out and for the physician to interpret. Various scales have attempted to create a single summary score, but these may not accurately capture the disease severity and impact on a patient's QoL. There is no one preferred scale for measuring FI and various testing and reformulation of existing scales is ongoing. One validated scale that is frequently used in the literature is the FI-specific QoL (FIQL) score, although studies have shown it is not the most sensitive to change and it does not include a specific urgency component.[12,17]

PHYSICAL EXAMINATION

After a thorough history, physical examination is the next step in diagnosis of FI. Exam begins with external inspection of the perianal area. Signs of moisture or bowel leakage can be evident upon examination of the area. Use of a pad or diaper can also be noticed. Excess moisture from leakage or soilage can lead to irritation and excoriation of perianal skin. Presence of external skin tags or hemorrhoids may also be a clue to factors that may be contributing to FI or leakage. The examiner should also look for any scars from trauma or previous surgery. If the patient has had previous anorectal surgery for an anal fissure or fistula, special attention should be paid to evaluate for presence of a "keyhole deformity" in the anal canal, particularly in the posterior midline. This defect can lead to seepage of stool or mucus from a previous sphincterotomy, fissurectomy, or fistulotomy. Female patients with previous obstetric injury may have a thin perineal body, rectovaginal fistula, or cloaca visible on exam. Visualization of the anus may reveal an asymmetric appearance from potential sphincter defects or previous trauma. This appearance may be exaggerated when eliciting the anocutaneous reflex. This spinal reflex results in contraction of the anal sphincter, commonly referred to as "anal wink," when the perianal skin is stroked and is mediated by afferent and efferent pathways in the pudendal nerve. It will be absent in patients where S4 has been transected.

A patulous anus can be seen in patients with rectal prolapse and may be more evident with traction of the buttocks. Additional physical exam findings may be evident if the patient is asked to bear down. A full-thickness rectal prolapse, mucosal prolapse, or hemorrhoidal prolapse may be visible. This can be done with the patient in the left lateral or prone position. However, the best position to assess presence and severity of prolapse is with the patient bearing down while seated on a commode.

Digital exam is useful for assessing resting sphincter tone, strength of squeeze, abnormal masses, and appropriateness of relaxation of the pelvic floor musculature with Valsalva. Presence of hard stool in the rectal vault can be suggestive of fecal impaction, leading to overflow incontinence. The examiner should palpate for defects or holes in the anterior rectum consistent with rectovaginal fistula, particularly in patients with history of obstetric trauma. Female patients who have had an obstetric injury may have a small perineal body due to retraction of the sphincter muscle posterolaterally. Redundancy or a bulge anteriorly may be detected in patients with rectocele or weakening of the rectovaginal septum. A large rectocele may cause the posterior wall of the vagina to be pushed out of the introitus.

The patient should be asked to squeeze on the examiner's finger during digital rectal exam, as if trying to hold in a bowel movement, then relax, and then push, as if having a bowel movement. Patients with diminished tone or weak pelvic floor muscles may try to compensate with strong contraction of the gluteal muscles. The external sphincter should fatigue to basal level after maximal contraction within 3 minutes. Patients with a weakened sphincter may have a more rapid fatigue.[18] On digital exam,

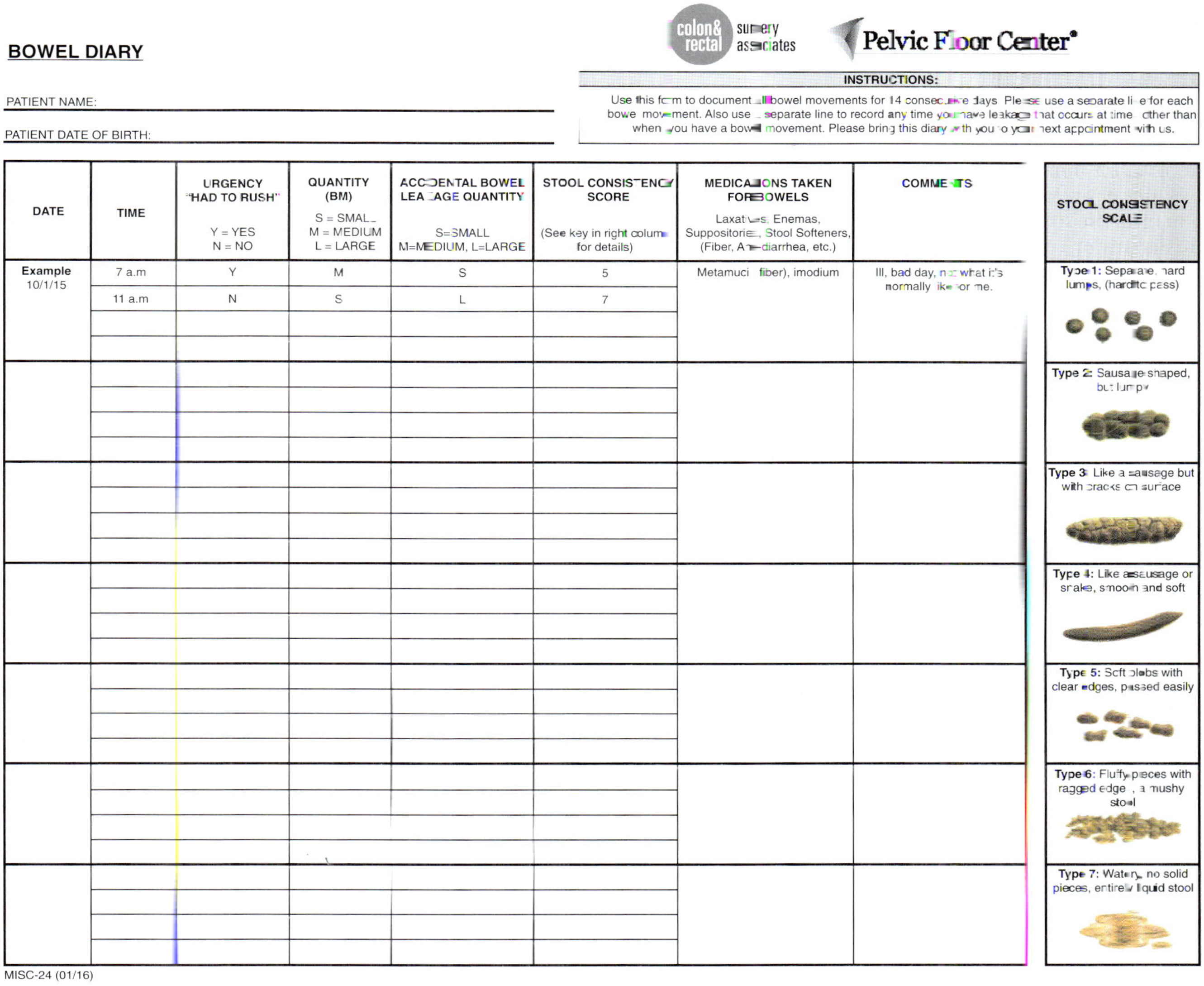

BOWEL DIARY

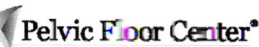

PATIENT NAME:

PATIENT DATE OF BIRTH:

INSTRUCTIONS:
Use this form to document all bowel movements for 14 consecutive days. Please use a separate line for each bowel movement. Also use a separate line to record any time you have leakage that occurs at times other than when you have a bowel movement. Please bring this diary with you to your next appointment with us.

DATE	TIME	URGENCY "HAD TO RUSH" Y = YES N = NO	QUANTITY (BM) S = SMALL M = MEDIUM L = LARGE	ACCIDENTAL BOWEL LEAKAGE QUANTITY S=SMALL M=MEDIUM, L=LARGE	STOOL CONSISTENCY SCORE (See key in right column for details)	MEDICATIONS TAKEN FOR BOWELS Laxatives, Enemas, Suppositories, Stool Softeners, (Fiber, Anti-diarrhea, etc.)	COMMENTS	STOOL CONSISTENCY SCALE
Example 10/1/15	7 a.m	Y	M	S	5	Metamucil (fiber), imodium	Ill, bad day, not what it's normally like for me.	**Type 1:** Separate, hard lumps, (hard to pass)
	11 a.m	N	S	L	7			
								Type 2: Sausage-shaped, but lumpy
								Type 3: Like a sausage but with cracks on surface
								Type 4: Like a sausage or snake, smooth and soft
								Type 5: Soft blobs with clear edges, passed easily
								Type 6: Fluffy pieces with ragged edges, a mushy stool
								Type 7: Watery, no solid pieces, entirely liquid stool

MISC-24 (01/16)

FIGURE 148.1 Bowel diary. (Courtesy Colon & Rectal Surgery Associates, Ltd., St. Paul, Minnesota.)

the puborectalis muscle can be examined by hooking one's finger posteriorly. With contraction of the puborectalis, the examiner's finger should be lifted or should feel tightening at the top of the anal canal. Conversely, when asked to push, the puborectalis should relax allowing the anorectal angle to widen.

Anoscopy should be included in the physical examination of a patient with FI. Prolapsing polyps or hemorrhoids, scarring in the anal canal from previous surgery or trauma, internal fistula openings, keyhole deformities, or mucosal inflammation may be seen during anoscopy. Further examination with a flexible sigmoidoscopy can also reveal evidence of proctitis, malignancy, or other neoplasm. Full colonoscopy may be indicated if the patient has symptoms of diarrhea.

ANORECTAL PHYSIOLOGY TESTING

The appropriate medical and/or surgical treatment can be determined for the majority of patients with FI with just a thorough history and physical exam. Additional anorectal physiology testing may be helpful in patients with unusual symptoms or an unclear diagnosis or those who have failed initial medical or surgical treatment. This testing can document the degree of anorectal dysfunction, clarify anatomy, and identify certain pathology.[13-21] The most frequently used tests include anal manometry, rectal distention testing, electromyography (EMG), ultrasound, and defecography.

Anal Manometry

Anal manometry measures pressure zones in the anal canal and distal rectum, providing an assessment of internal and external anal sphincter strength and function. There are multiple techniques of manometry, some using microtransducers, water-perfused catheters, or solid-state catheters. The pressure or resistance of flow of fluid from the catheters is measured either in a continuous pull-through method or at various predetermined spots within the anal canal ("stationary" technique). Measurements obtained from anorectal manometry include resting pressure, squeeze pressure, length of the high-pressure zone, rectal sensation, and the rectoanal inhibitory reflex. Resting pressure is a good reflection of internal anal sphincter tone because it is responsible for 55% to 85% of the resting pressure. The external anal sphincter contributes less to resting pressure.[22] Typical resting pressure in a healthy volunteer is 40 to 60 mmHg. A patient with low resting pressure may have an underlying problem with the internal anal sphincter.

Squeeze pressure can be measured by asking the patient to maximally squeeze, as if holding in a bowel movement. This is under voluntary control and reflects the external anal sphincter function. If a patient is unable to comply with directions, this pressure reading may be inaccurate. The resting and squeeze pressures are typically higher in males compared with females, and pressures decrease with age.[23,24] The length of the high-pressure zone is measured during anorectal manometry and is defined as the area where pressures are greater than half of the maximal resting pressure. This zone is typically shorter in women (2 to 3 cm) compared with men (2.5 to 3.5 cm).[23,24]

To measure rectal sensation, a balloon is inserted in the rectum and slowly inflated with air to distend the rectum. The volume at which the patient first feels the balloon, feels the urge to defecate, and feels a maximum tolerable volume are measured. Patients with lower than expected values during rectal distention testing have hyperacute sensation. This can be seen in patients with urge FI or those with poor rectal compliance. Poor compliance can be secondary to chronic inflammation, radiation changes, or postoperative changes. In such conditions the rectum cannot distend appropriately, thus leading to problems with FI, as the reservoir function of the rectum has been lost. Conversely, patients with higher than expected volumes during rectal distention measurements are felt to have blunted sensation in the rectum. This can result in overfilling and stretching of the rectum and subsequent overflow incontinence. This can be seen in patients with chronic constipation or neurogenic problems.

The rectoanal inhibitory reflex, also known as the "sampling" reflex, is a contraction of the external sphincter with subsequent internal anal sphincter relaxation in response to rectal distention. This relaxation of the internal anal sphincter allows exposure of the anal canal sensory mucosa to the distal rectal contents. Through this "sampling" of the rectal contents, the patient is then able to distinguish if the cause of the distention is gas, liquid, or solid stool and react accordingly.[22] It is a normal reflex and is notably absent in patients with Hirschsprung disease, Chagas disease, dermatomyositis, and scleroderma. It may also be absent in patients immediately after rectal resection with coloanal anastomosis or reduced in patients with megarectum or very low resting pressures.

Electromyography

EMG measures the electrical activity of sphincter muscles and pelvic floor muscles under voluntary control. Patients may be asked to squeeze, relax, and push during the EMG testing. The EMG should show an increase in electrical activity with squeeze and return to baseline with relaxing.[25] When asked to push, as if having a bowel movement, the EMG should actually show a decrease in electrical activity if the patient is relaxing their pelvic floor musculature appropriately. Patients with obstructed defecation or

problems with pelvic floor relaxation may have a paradoxic increase in electrical activity when asked to push.

Endoanal Ultrasound

Endoanal ultrasound is the best method for assessing the anatomy of the internal and external anal sphincters. Length of the sphincters and presence of defects, fistulas, or other anatomic abnormalities can be assessed (Fig. 148.2). The endoanal ultrasound uses a 360-degree rotating transducer probe and is generally well tolerated by patients. Two-dimensional (2D) and three-dimensional (3D) ultrasound models exist and are fairly easy to use. Patients with an obstetric injury to the anal sphincters will have an anterior disruption present on ultrasound. Endoanal ultrasound is very useful in evaluating patients with iatrogenic or traumatic sphincter injuries to determine the degree of injury. Magnetic resonance imaging (MRI) has also been described as a means of imaging the anal sphincters but may be less accurate at detection of internal anal sphincter defects.[26]

Fluoroscopic Defecography

Defecography involves dynamic imaging of the pelvic floor during the process of defecation. Contrast is inserted into the rectum using a thick barium paste and can also be inserted into the vagina. The anatomy of the pelvic floor during defecation is well visualized. The patient sits on a commode and is asked to empty their rectum under fluoroscopy, thus producing a dynamic image of defecation. Patients with severe FI may be unable to retain the barium paste in the rectum from the very beginning of the exam, and involuntary leakage can easily be visualized. Patients may also be asked to squeeze, which helps in showing the amount of upward pelvic motion that they can generate. Completeness of evacuation and sensation of complete evacuation can be assessed at the conclusion of the study. The presence of perineal descent, enterocele, rectocele, rectal intussusception, pelvic floor hernia, and rectal prolapse can be identified. In addition, coordination of pelvic floor movement during defecation and the change in the anorectal angle can be seen during defecography.[27]

Magnetic Resonance Imaging Defecography

Dynamic MRI has been increasingly used for the evaluation of pelvic floor disorders. Similar to fluoroscopic defecography, MRI allows for evaluation of pelvic floor muscle coordination and identification of internal pelvic organ prolapse. A major drawback of this technique is that image acquisition typically occurs with the patient supine rather than sitting, thus not in the normal position assumed during defecation.[28] There is limited reported experience with open MRI scanners that permit evacuation with the patient seated upon a commode.

Pudendal Nerve Terminal Motor Latency

The pudendal nerve provides motor innervation to the external anal sphincter and sensory innervation to the perineum. Pudendal nerve injury is caused by traction on the nerve during straining (as seen during childbirth or prolonged efforts at defecation), and it results in denervation and subsequent reinnervation of the external anal sphincter and pelvic floor musculature.

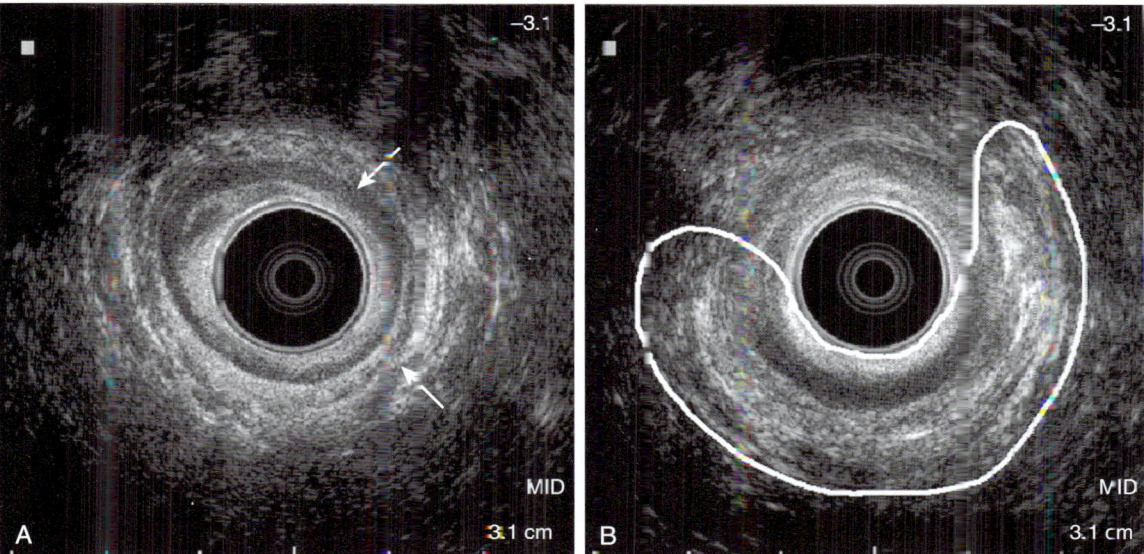

FIGURE 148.2 Endorectal ultrasound. (A) Normal sphincter, mid-anal canal: the *arrow at the 1 o'clock position* indicates the internal anal sphincter, and the *arrow at the 4 o'clock position* points to the external anal sphincter. (B) Disruption of anterior internal and external anal sphincter muscles with posterior retraction of muscles. The *line* indicates retracted muscle.

Pudendal nerve integrity can be assessed by determination of pudendal nerve terminal motor latency (PNTML) using a finger-mounted St. Mark's pudendal electrode (Medtronic; Minneapolis, Minnesota). The electrode stimulates the pudendal nerve at the level of the ischial spine and records the conduction time to the sphincter.[29] Patients with pudendal neuropathy will have prolonged PNTML times.[29] The test is affected by the skill of the examiner and body habitus of the patient; therefore the significance of an undetectable PNTML is uncertain. Some investigators have found an abnormal PNTML to be highly predictive of failure after sphincteroplasty,[30,31] but many others have observed no such correlation.[32,33] Because of the variability in test accuracy and lack of useful information from PNTML, this test has fallen out of favor in anorectal physiology testing.

Benefits and Limitations of Physiology Testing for Incontinence

Several new and less invasive treatment options for patients with FI have improved patient outcomes and changed the evaluation and treatment algorithm for this disorder. These newer treatment options include sacral nerve stimulation (SNS), injectable biomaterials, magnetic anal sphincter, and ventral rectopexy. The clinical details that are most crucial in determining the appropriate treatment are obtained from a thorough history and physical exam. Identifying the appropriate treatment option for a patient cannot be solely determined with anorectal physiology testing. Furthermore, anal manometry, EMG, PNTML, and ultrasound testing do not predict effectiveness or success of certain treatment options.[34–36] For example, a sphincter defect may be suspected based on clinical history but can be difficult to confirm through history and physical exam alone, especially if the defect is subtle. Endoanal ultrasound can reliably detect the presence of a sphincter defect and manometry may show diminished resting and squeeze

pressures. However, these test results do not influence clinical decision-making as greatly as patient age, medical comorbidities, and severity of incontinence symptoms.

There is some evidence that defecography in evaluation of FI can identify internal pelvic organ prolapse and can help to guide surgical decision-making.[37–39] Patients who are found to have a rectocele or mucosal prolapse from rectal intussusception on exam commonly have concomitant weakness or prolapse of other pelvic compartments or structures.[38] Thus identifying simultaneous vaginal prolapse or enterocele in combination with rectal intussusception may result in recommending a combined repair of this pelvic prolapse with either ventral rectopexy or sacrocolpopexy with rectopexy.[40–42] This combined approach may minimize the patient's risk of recurrent symptoms or prolapse. Identifying prolapse on defecography may also impact the effectiveness of other treatment options for FI in this scenario, such as SNS.[43]

Overall, the clinical impact of anorectal physiology testing on patients with FI is changing as new treatment options are developed. Defecography may be the most helpful in guiding decision-making and predicting success of certain treatments. Anorectal physiology testing may be most helpful in patients who fail initial attempts at treatment for their FI or those who present with unusual symptoms associated with FI.

TREATMENT

MEDICAL THERAPY

For initial therapy of mild to moderate incontinence, medical therapy aimed at treating the potential underlying etiology or affecting stool consistency can be effective. Stool consistency can greatly impact incontinence and urgency. Many patients have more problems with leakage of liquid stool and gas but decreased difficulty with solid stool. Patients with chronic diarrhea should be evaluated for an underlying cause of diarrhea, such as malabsorption, inflammatory bowel disease, microscopic colitis, food intolerance, infection, or irritable bowel syndrome. Dietary changes in patients with a food intolerance (e.g., lactose intolerance, gluten intolerance) can greatly improve the consistency of stools, decrease excessive flatulence, and decrease symptoms of urgency or incontinence. Patients with FI to liquid stool should be advised to increase dietary fiber intake, with a target of 20 to 25 g/day. The addition of fiber, whether through supplements or diet changes, should occur gradually so as to diminish potential side effects of constipation, bloating, or gas pains. Addition of bulking agents such as psyllium or antimotility agents such as loperamide can be effective at reducing FI episodes in patients with FI to liquid stool.[44]

Loperamide decreases intestinal motility and secretion, thus allowing more time for water absorption and decreased watery stools. It also can cause an increase in sphincter pressure and improved control, unlike other antimotility agents such as diphenoxylate with atropine.[45] Diphenoxylate with atropine has a mode of action similar to that of other related narcotics, such as morphine, and can also slow down intestinal transit, allowing for more water absorption. Antimotility drugs are often best used prophylactically and can be fit into a patient's routine to prevent accidents. For example, patients may take a dose every morning prior to leaving the house for work, in the evening before going to a social activity, or at night if they have difficulty with nocturnal incontinence.

Other strategies or coping mechanisms that can improve symptoms in patients with mild seepage of liquid stool include the use of tap water enemas after bowel movements to evacuate retained stool. Use of a barrier cream can help to protect the skin and decrease symptoms of irritation or excoriation of perianal skin. Placement of a 100% cotton wick in the perianal area can also help to absorb small amounts of seepage of mucous or liquid stools, keeping the perianal area dry as well. Patients who have a strong association between eating and FI episodes may benefit from adjusting their meal schedule to coincide with when they will be at home or have convenient access to a bathroom.

Improvement in FI symptoms with optimizing medical management can be recorded in a bowel diary. If a patient's symptoms fail to improve or their coping mechanisms become lifestyle limiting (e.g., not leaving the house in the morning or not eating until after work), then other treatment options should be pursued.

BIOFEEDBACK

Biofeedback describes a class of techniques that uses monitoring devices to provide information regarding a physiologic function so an individual may voluntarily alter or control that function. In the case of the anorectum, patients attempting to activate their sphincter mechanisms receive feedback confirming the extent to which muscle contraction is actually occurring. Interestingly, although much biofeedback training is directed at improving voluntary sphincter contraction, successful results appear to correlate more with improved sensation[46,47] than improved motor function.[48,49]

Incontinent patients are candidates for biofeedback if they are adequately motivated and intellectually capable of following instructions. It is commonly held that they should have some ability to contract their anal sphincter and at least some rectal sensation, but these latter qualifications are vague and poorly substantiated in the literature. The cause of incontinence does not appear to affect the outcome of therapy, although patients with keyhole deformities or deep rectal intussusception do poorly because of continued stool leakage secondary to anatomic defect.[46,50]

The literature shows mixed results as to the effectiveness of biofeedback in treating FI. A systematic review of biofeedback and pelvic floor exercises for treating FI in adults identified 46 studies involving 1364 patients.[51] In this review, 49% of patients were reported cured and 72% improved or cured. However, only 8 of the 46 studies reviewed included a control group, and the majority of individual reports are subject to criticism due to small patient numbers, short follow-up periods, heterogeneous patient groups, poor quantification of incontinence severity, and the addition of concurrent therapy (e.g., dietary counseling) and physician encouragement, each of which alone may lead to clinical improvement. A randomized controlled trial questioned the efficacy of biofeedback because it showed no benefit when biofeedback was added to standard medical care (advice from a nurse specialist or standard care plus sphincter exercises.[52] However, a more recent randomized controlled trial showed that biofeedback was more effective than pelvic floor exercises alone for treating FI.[53]

Despite some caveats, most experts continue to believe that biofeedback is an effective treatment option for certain patients with FI. Indeed, there are few contraindications to a trial of biofeedback, and the technique is painless and risk free. It plays a particularly important role in the treatment of patients with suspected overflow incontinence who have poor relaxation of the pelvic floor during defecation. Biofeedback has also been shown to be useful to improve the function of patients with suboptimal results after sphincteroplasty.[54]

SURGERY

Surgical treatment options for FI vary based on the clinical situation and typically are reserved for patients who have failed conservative treatments. Newer and more effective treatment options have been developed. Thus the surgical treatment algorithm for FI has been changing as more is understood about the degree of efficacy and the invasiveness of newer procedures.

Sacral Nerve Stimulation

SNS is a minimally invasive surgical approach to the management of FI (Fig. 148.3). The technology and technique was initially devised for urinary incontinence. This treatment involves two outpatient procedures that can be done under local anesthesia and light sedation. During the first procedure, percutaneous placement of a lead with electrodes through the third sacral foramina (S3) is performed. Because the sacral nerves also contribute fibers to the nerves of the lower extremity, it is not surprising that their stimulation leads to the contraction of both

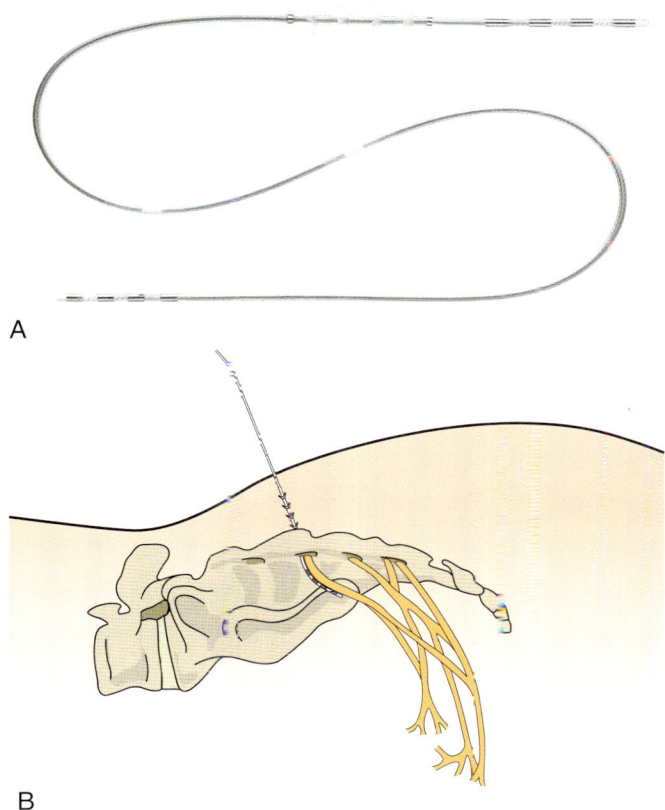

FIGURE 148.3 Sacral nerve stimulation. (A) A lead containing four electrodes is used for sacral nerve stimulation. (Copyright Medtronics, Inc.) (B) The sacral foramina are identified; in most cases, insertion through the third sacral foramen is the optimal choice for stimulation. The quadripolar lead is shown in position. (From Baxter NN, Madoff RD. Motility disorders. In: Souba WW, Fink MJ, Jurkovich GJ, et al., eds. *ACS Surgery: Principles and Practice.* New York: WebMD; 2005.)

the pelvic floor and various leg and foot muscles. The S3 sacral foramen provides electrode exposure to nerves that have maximal pelvic floor and minimal lower extremity stimulation. To confirm appropriate placement of the lead, stimulation is tested and should result in flexion of the great toe and a bellows-like contraction of the anal area. After the lead has been placed, patients undergo a test period of stimulation with an external pulse generator. If their episodes of FI have improved by 50% or greater at the end of the test period, then implantation of the permanent pulse generator is performed.

The clinical use of SNS was pioneered by Matzel et al.[55] in Erlangen. In a more recent multicenter prospective trial of 120 patients who underwent SNS, 83% of patients achieved a 50% reduction in incontinent events at 12 months, including 41% who became fully continent. These results appeared durable up for a least 3 years.[56]

The mechanism of improvement after SNS remains unknown. Manometry testing shows no consistent effect demonstrated on anal tone or squeeze strength. Other possible alternatives include a decrease in gastrointestinal transit, decrease in rectal contractility, a tered rectal sensation, and improved coordination of sensorimotor

function. Lundby et al.[57] previously demonstrated focal brain activation in response to SNS in patients immediately and 2 weeks following institution of stimulation. However, in a systematic review of the literature it appears most evidence shows that SNS affects anorectal function through effects at a pelvic afferent or central level.[58]

Injectable Biomaterials

Several studies have investigated the role of injectable biomaterials in the management of FI.[59,60] Injected materials have included autologous fat, crosslinked collagen, silicone Bioplastique (Bioplasty; St. Paul, Minnesota), and carbon-coated beads. Graf et al.[61] performed a randomized, double-blind, sham-controlled trial of intraanal injection of dextranomer in stabilized hyaluronic acid (DSHA) for FI. Fifty-two percent of treated patients met the study's primary endpoint (a 50% decrease in the number of incontinent episodes) versus 31% of controls ($P = .0089$).

Potential advantages of injection therapy include simplicity and the ability to offer treatment in an outpatient setting. A successful result can require repeated injections and migration of the injected material is reported. Manometric pressures are not significantly altered. Additional controlled trials with long-term follow-up are needed.

Sphincter Reconstruction

After an acute sphincter disruption from obstetric injury or isolated trauma, direct sphincter repair can be performed with simple sphincter apposition. Even after immediate repair in obstetric injury patients, up to 70% of women will have persistent sphincter defects and 50% will have incontinence.[62] In the blunt or penetrating trauma setting, if the patient is unstable, there are multiple associated pelvic injuries, or there is excessive contamination, immediate repair should be deferred and a proximal stoma and débridement performed instead. Sphincter repair should be delayed at least 3 to 6 months until inflammation and edema have resolved. A delayed surgical approach (>3 to 6 months) is preferable in patients with unrecognized sphincter injuries, failed primary repairs, or iatrogenic injury after anorectal surgery.

Overlapping sphincteroplasty is the standard approach for sphincter repair in the delayed setting (Fig. 148.4). Patients should have the sphincter mechanisms imaged with endoanal ultrasound to confirm size of defect and location. A mechanical bowel preparation is recommended preoperatively. In the operating room the patient is positioned in the prone jackknife position with the buttocks taped apart. General or regional anesthesia may be used. For anterior defects, a curved circumanal incision is made across the perineal body, along the border of the external anal sphincter and extended laterally over the ischiorectal fossae. A flap of anoderm is raised from the underlying tissues. Next, the external anal sphincter is identified and isolated, dissecting the two end free from the surrounding subcutaneous fat. Great care should be taken to preserve all muscle fibers. Use of a needle point cautery can help to facilitate this meticulous dissection. The sphincter muscle and rectum should be dissected free from the vagina anteriorly and laterally until the retracted, scarred ends of the external anal sphincter can be overlapped to form the repair. Posterior dissection of the sphincter

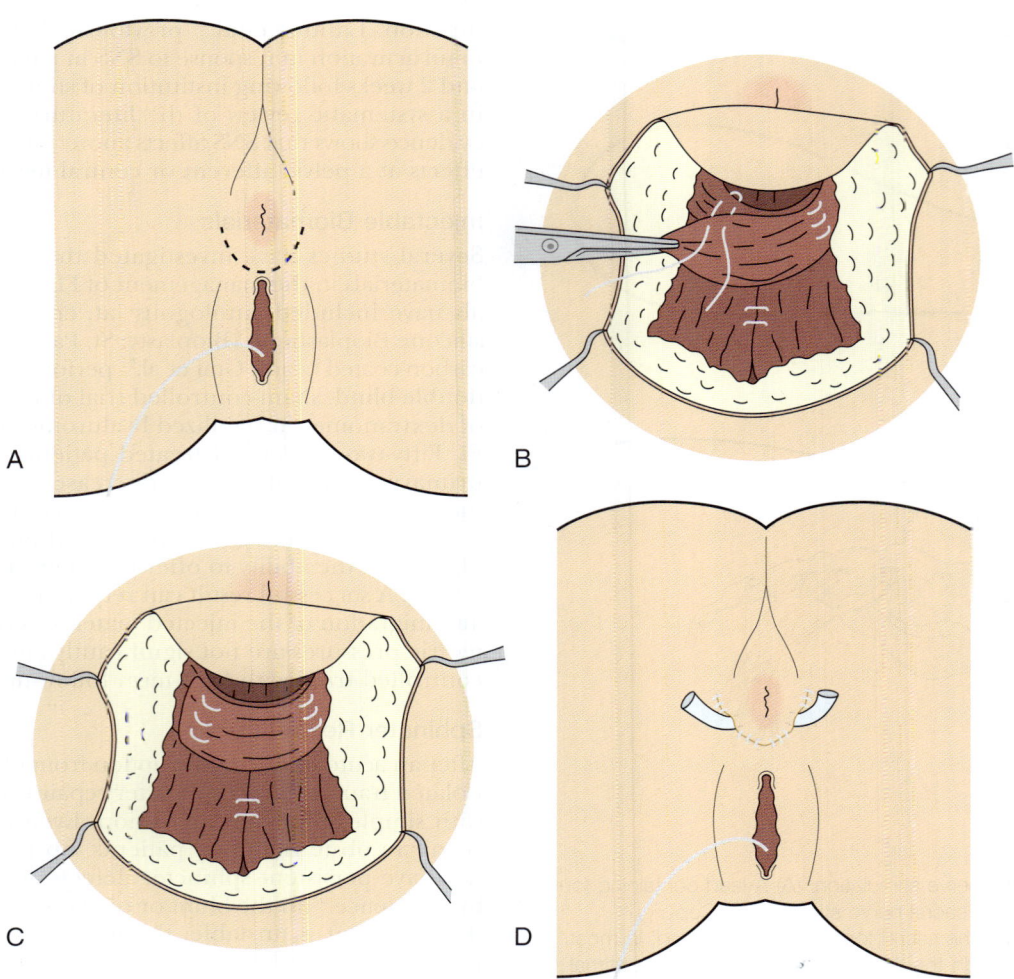

FIGURE 148.4 Overlapping sphincteroplasty. (A) With the patient in the prone jackknife position, a curvilinear incision is made. Inferior rectal nerves cross the ischiorectal fossa posterolaterally. (B) Anterior levatorplasty is performed, and overlapping sphincter repair is then initiated. (C) Sphincter repair is completed. (D) The incision is closed, with drains in place (optional), and V-Y pasty is done to restore the perineal body. (From Baxter NN, Madoff RD. Motility disorders. In: Souba WW, Fink MJ, Jurkovich GJ, et al, eds. *ACS Surgery: Principles and Practice.* New York: WebMD Professional Publishing; 2005.)

muscle should not extend beyond the mid-lateral line to avoid potential injury to the pudendal nerves, which enter the sphincter posterolaterally. Proximal dissection continues until a proximal nonscarred plane is reached or the inferior fibers of the puborectalis are encountered as they run anteriorly to the pubis. The scar connecting the two ends of sphincter muscle is divided but not excised to minimize the risk of suture pull-through. The two ends of the mobilized sphincter muscle are overlapped to create a wrap and then sutured in place with interrupted 2–0 polydiaxanone horizontal mattress sutures. Most surgeons perform a "mass" overlap of the combined internal and external sphincter muscles. Others advocate individual dissection and repair of the internal and external sphincter muscles, but the hypothetical superiority of this approach remains to be clinically demonstrated.[30] The tissue defect in the perineal body is closed in layers and the skin closed in a T-shaped configuration, allowing a small opening for drainage. A Penrose drain can be left in place. Vaginal packing can be inserted to help with hemostasis and

should be removed in the first 1 to 2 days after surgery. Patients are typically hospitalized postoperatively for 3 to 5 days or until they have return of bowel function. A daily bowel regimen that ensures soft stool consistency, and regularity is important during postoperative recovery.

Results of sphincter reconstruction surgery are widely variable. For many years the reported results after overlapping sphincteroplasty were remarkably consistent: approximately 60% to 75% of patients achieved a "good to excellent" surgical outcome, which in practice entailed perfect or near-perfect control of solid stool, occasional difficulties with control of liquid stool, and episodic "minor" accidents such as seepage or uncontrolled passage of flatus. An additional 15% to 20% of patients achieved less degrees of improvement, whereas the remaining 15% to 20% were unchanged or, rarely, worse.[30,32,54,52] However, more recent studies have raised questions about the quality and durability of results following sphincteroplasty.[63–66] Karoui et al.[63] found that 49% of patients were completely continent 3 months after sphincteroplasty, but only 28% were completely continent 40 months after surgery. Halverson and Hull[64] reported that 54% of patients were incontinent to liquid or solid stool 69 months after sphincteroplasty, and only 14% were completely continent. Maouf et al.[65] found that no patients were fully continent 77 months after sphincteroplasty; 84% had fecal urgency, and 79% had passive soiling. Bravo Gutierrez et al.[66] reviewed 191 consecutive patients after sphincteroplasty and at 10-year follow-up, found that 6% were completely continent, 57% were incontinent of solid stool, and 16% were incontinent of gas only; results worsened significantly between 3 and 10 years after the procedure. In a systematic review of long-term outcomes, there was a decline in continence with time, but this did not correlate with QoL, with most patients reporting high satisfaction in the long term.[67]

Because of the unreliable durability of an overlapping sphincter repair and the fact that less invasive surgical treatment options, especially SNS, have proven successful in patients with sphincter defects, there has been a trend away from sphincteroplasty as the initial treatment of choice for FI. Indeed, choosing the most appropriate treatment option for a patient needs to be individualized. Patients who will benefit greatly from a sphincteroplasty include those with a cloaca or rectovaginal fistula because this repair will reconstruct the perineal anatomy. Conversely, patients without noticeable anatomic defects or those who develop FI several years after childbirth may benefit most from SNS, which has good long-term results and is less invasive.

Rectal Prolapse

FI can be caused by full-thickness rectal prolapse, deep rectal intussusception, or mucosal prolapse. These abnormalities prevent closure of the anal canal, and this results in a wide range of symptoms, from seepage of mucous to incontinence of formed stool. Full-thickness rectal prolapse and mucosal prolapse can typically be seen on physical exam when asking the patient to bear down while seated on a commode. However, deep rectal intussusception may only be visible on defecography. Multiple different surgical treatment options exist for treating rectal prolapse and are discussed in more detail in the complete rectal prolapse chapter.

Repair of pelvic organ prolapse has been shown to improve or cure symptoms of FI. Watadani et al.[40] found a significant improvement in FISI scores after treating rectal prolapse or rectal intussusception and middle compartment prolapse with combined sacrocolpopexy and rectopexy, and 82% of incontinence patients reported either cure or improvement. Other treatment options for FI, such as SNS, have been shown to have lower efficacy in patients with rectal intussusception. Prapasrivorakul et al.[43] found that SNS test stimulation was successful in 86% of patients without evidence of high-grade rectal intussusception but only in 69% of patients with rectal intussusception (P = .03). Thus treatment of rectal prolapse may improve or cure FI or allow other treatment options for FI to be maximally effective.

Implantable Sphincter

The artificial anal sphincter was the original alternative option for patients with severe refractory FI. However, this device is no longer available for surgical implantation. It was an implantable device composed of a silicone elastomer that maintained continence via a fluid-filled cuff that surrounds and compresses the anal canal. The patient controls the device via a pump placed in the scrotum or labia. Squeezing the pump 9 to 12 times forces the fluid from the cuff into a reservoir balloon, which is implanted in the space of Retzius. This deflates the cuff and opens the anal canal, allowing the passage of stool. The cuff then automatically slowly reinflates and occludes the anal canal, providing continence until defecation is again desired. This device had a high rate of complications, especially wound infection and erosion, that led to a high explantation rate.

The newest US Food and Drug Administration (FDA)-approved implantable device is the FENIX Continence Restoration System (Torax Medical Inc., Shoreview, Minnesota; Fig. 148.5). It has been approved for use in patients who have failed previous medical and surgical options. It consists of an implant containing a series of titanium beads with magnetic cores that form a ring. The magnetic attraction of the beads helps to augment sphincter function to reduce episodes of FI, as the device has been shown to increase resting pressure and squeeze pressure.[68] The device comes in a variety of lengths and must be sized appropriately at time of implantation. It is contraindicated in patients with titanium allergy. The device is not MRI compatible. In an early study of 18 patients, 76% of patients had a reduction in FI episodes by 50% or greater at more than 12 months postoperatively.[68] The study also showed an improvement in QoL measures of depression, self-perception, and embarrassment. Complications included postoperative pain in 29% and erythema and swelling of the gluteal regions after implantation in another 29%, but no overt infections were reported. No devices required explantation.

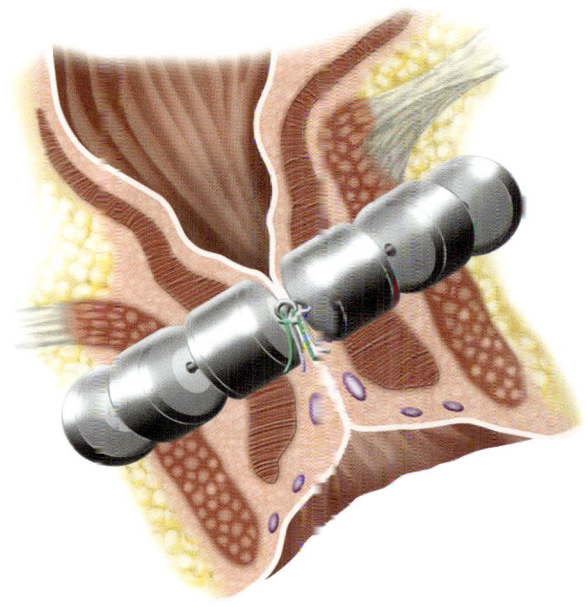

FIGURE 148.5 FENIX magnetic sphincter. (Copyright Torax Medical Inc.)

Fecal Diversion

Despite the broad range of medical and surgical therapies available to patients with FI, some patients remain with debilitating symptoms or who are not candidates for major surgery. Fecal diversion may be the best option in terms of symptom management for such patients. Although many patients initially reject the notion of having a stoma, many come to recognize with counseling that a pouchable stoma is generally preferable to what is in effect an unpouchable stoma between the buttocks—an incontinent anus. Available data are quite limited, but one questionnaire study of patients who underwent colostomy for FI documented marked improvement in subjective QoL assessment after surgery.[51] The most common choice of stoma is sigmoid end colostomy. Preoperative counseling with an enterostomal therapist and preoperative stoma site marking is essential in obtaining the best possible functional outcome for the patient. Patients may also benefit from preoperative education and discussions with patients who have undergone the procedure.

CONCLUSION

FI is a common disorder with a variety of underlying causes. Its prevalence increases with age and although it is not life threatening, it can greatly impact an individual's QoL and emotional well-being. Careful history and physical exam is needed to obtain a diagnosis, potentially identify underlying etiology, and select the appropriate initial therapy. A suggested treatment algorithm is shown in Fig. 148.6. Initial nonoperative treatment options include medical management with dietary modification,

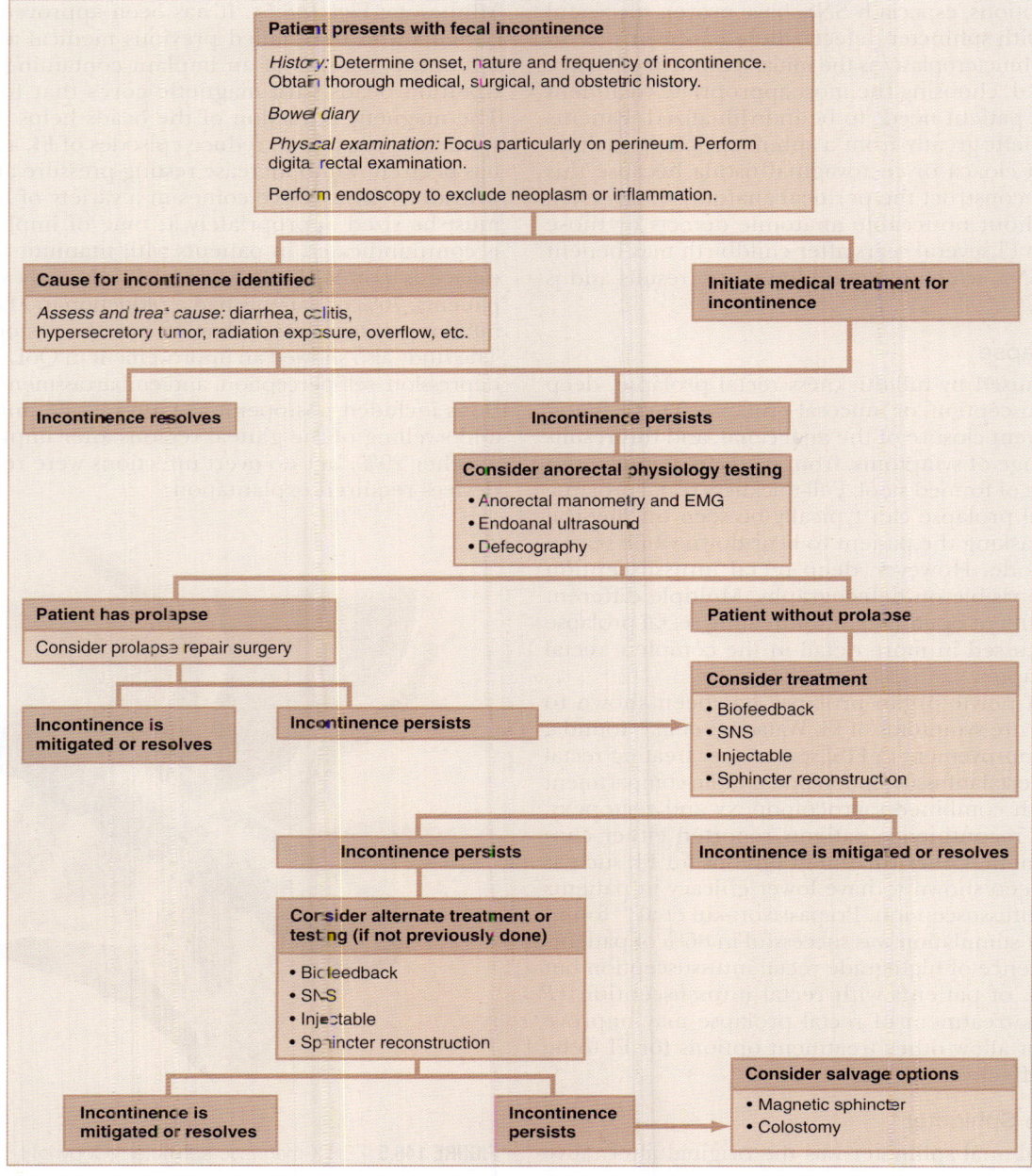

FIGURE 148.6 Suggested fecal incontinence treatment algorithm. *EMG,* Electromyography; *SNS,* sacral nerve stimulation.

fiber supplementation, and motility agents, to improve stool consistency and regularity. Biofeedback can also be considered as a nonoperative treatment option. If nonoperative treatment has been ineffective then surgical treatment options include SNS, injectable biomaterials, prolapse repair, and sphincteroplasty. Second line surgical treatment options include the magnetic anal sphincter or creation of a stoma. In select patients, anorectal physiology testing may be helpful, especially in identifying causes for incontinence that are not evident on exam, such as rectal intussusception or multicompartment pelvic prolapse. The current availability of minimally invasive surgical treatment options for FI has improved treatment success and allowed for a more individualized approach to treatment selection for patients.

ACKNOWLEDGMENT

We thank Dr. Susan C. Parker for her work on previous versions of this chapter.

REFERENCES

1. Nelson R. Epidemiology and incidence of anal incontinence: magnitude of the problem. *Semin Colon Rectal Surg.* 1997;8(2):80-83.
2. Nelson R, Norton N, Cautley E, Furner S. Community-based prevalence of anal incontinence. *JAMA.* 1995;274(7):559-561.
3. Johanson JF, Lafferty J. Epidemiology of fecal incontinence: the silent affliction. *Am J Gastroenterol.* 1996;91(1):33-36.
4. Nelson R, Furner S, Jesudason V. Fecal incontinence in Wisconsin nursing homes: prevalence and associations. *Dis Colon Rectum.* 1998;41(10):1226-1229.
5. Lewis SJ, Heaton KW. Stool form scale as a useful guide to intestinal transit time. *Scand J Gastroenterol.* 1997;32(9):920-924. doi:10.3109/00365529709011203; [PMID 9299672]
6. Garcia-Aguilar J, Belmonte Montes C, Perez JJ, Jensen L, Madoff RD, Wong WD. Incontinence after lateral internal sphincterotomy: anatomic and functional evaluation. *Dis Colon Rectum.* 1998;41(4):423-427.
7. Sultan AH, Kamm MA, Hudson CN, Thomas JM, Bartram CI. Anal-sphincter disruption during vaginal delivery. *N Engl J Med.* 1993;329(26):1905-1911.
8. Montana GS, Fowler WC. Carcinoma of the cervix: analysis of bladder and rectal radiation dose and complications. *Int J Radiat Oncol Biol Phys.* 1989;16(1):95-100.
9. Kimose HH, Fischer L, Spjeldnaes N, Wara P. Late radiation injury of the colon and rectum. Surgical management and outcome. *Dis Colon Rectum.* 1989;32(8):684-689.
10. Pena A. Anorectal malformations. *Semin Pediatr Surg.* 1995;4(1):35-47.
11. Williams JG, Wong WD, Jensen L, Rothenberger DA, Goldberg SM. Incontinence and rectal prolapse: a prospective manometric study. *Dis Colon Rectum.* 1991;34(3):209-216.
12. Madoff RD, Williams JG, Wong WD, Rothenberger DA, Goldberg SM. Long-term functional results of colon resection and rectopexy for overt rectal prolapse. *Am J Gastroenterol.* 1992;87(1):101-104.
13. Baxter NN, Rothenberger DA, Lowry AC. Measuring fecal incontinence. *Dis Colon Rectum.* 2003;46(12):1591-1605.
14. Lee JT, Madoff RD, Rockwood TH. Quality of life measures in fecal incontinence: is validation valid? *Dis Colon Rectum.* 2015;58(3):352-357.
15. Rockwood TH, Church JM, Fleshman JW, et al. Patient and surgeon ranking of the severity of symptoms associated with fecal incontinence: the fecal incontinence severity index. *Dis Colon Rectum.* 1999;42(12):1525-532.
16. Jorge JM, Wexner SD. Etiology and management of fecal incontinence. *Dis Colon Rectum.* 1993;36:77-97.
17. Rockwood TH, Church JM, Fleshman JW, et al. Fecal Incontinence Quality of Life Scale: quality of life instrument for patients with fecal incontinence. *Dis Colon Rectum.* 2000;43(1):9-17.
18. Marcello PW, Barrett RC, Coller JA, et al. Fatigue rate index as a new measurement of external sphincter function. *Dis Colon Rectum.* 1998;41(3):336-343.
19. Rao SS, Patel RS. How useful are manometric tests of anorectal function in the management of defecation disorders? *Am J Gastroenterol.* 1997;92(3):469-475.
20. Falk PM, Blatchford GJ, Cali RL, Christensen MA, Thorson AG. Transanal ultrasound and manometry in the evaluation of fecal incontinence. *Dis Colon Rectum.* 1994;37(5):468-472.
21. Farouk R, Bartolo DC. The clinical contribution of integrated laboratory and ambulatory anorectal physiology assessment in faecal incontinence. *Int J Colorectal Dis.* 1993;8(2):60-65.
22. Henry M, Swash M, eds. *Coloproctology and the Pelvic Floor.* 2nd ed. Oxford: Butterworth Heinemann; 1992.
23. Read NW, Harford WV, Schmulen AC, Read MG, Santa Ana C, Fordtran JS. A clinical study of patients with fecal incontinence and diarrhea. *Gastroenterology.* 1979;76(4):747-756.
24. Matheson DM, Keighley MR. Manometric evaluation of rectal prolapse and faecal incontinence. *Gut.* 1981;22(2):126-129.
25. Neill ME, Swash M. Increased motor unit fibre density in the external anal sphincter muscle in ano-rectal incontinence: a single fibre EMG study. *J Neurol Neurosurg Psychiatry.* 1980;43(4):343-347.
26. Malouf AJ, Williams AB, Halligan S, Bartram CI, Dhillon S, Kamm MA. Prospective assessment of accuracy of endoanal MR imaging and endosonography in patients with fecal incontinence. *AJR Am J Roentgenol.* 2000;175(3):741-745.
27. Bremmer S, Mellgren A, Holmstrom B, Uden R. Peritoneocele and enterocele formation and transformation during rectal evacuation as studied by means of defaeco-peritoneography. *Acta Radiol.* 1998;39(2):167-175.
28. Dann EW. Magnetic resonance defecography: an evaluation of obstructed defecation and pelvic floor weakness. *Semin Ultrasound CT MR.* 2008;29(6):414-419.
29. Laurberg S, Swash M, Snooks SJ, Henry MM. Neurologic cause of idiopathic incontinence. *Arch Neurol.* 1988;45(11):1250-1253.
30. Gilliland R, Altomare DF, Moreira H Jr, Oliveira L, Gilliland JE, Wexner SD. Pudendal neuropathy is predictive of failure following anterior overlapping sphincteroplasty. *Dis Colon Rectum.* 1998;41(12):1516-1522.
31. Sangwan YP, Coller JA, Barrett RC, et al. Unilateral pudendal neuropathy. Impact on outcome of anal sphincter repair. *Dis Colon Rectum.* 1996;39(6):686-689.
32. Engel AF, Kamm MA, Sultan AH, Bartram CI, Nicholls RJ. Anterior anal sphincter repair in patients with obstetric trauma. *Br J Surg.* 1994;81(8):1231-1234.
33. Karakousis CP, Cheng C, Udobi K, Lascola RJ. Abdominoinguinal incision in melanocarcinoma of the sigmoid or cecum: report of two cases. *Dis Colon Rectum.* 1998;41(10):1322-1327.
34. Leroi AM, Parc Y, Lehur PA, Mion F, Barth X, Rullier E, et al. Efficacy of sacral nerve stimulation for fecal incontinence: results of a multicenter double-blind crossover study. *Ann Surg.* 2005;242:662-669.
35. Tjandra JJ, Chan MKY, Yeh CH, Murray-Green C. Sacral nerve stimulation is more effective than optimal medical therapy for severe fecal incontinence: a randomized, controlled study. *Dis Colon Rectum.* 2008;51:494-502.
36. Sorensen J, Thomsen F. Sacral nerve stimulation increases rectal sensitivity in patients with faecal incontinence: results of a randomised double-blinded crossover study (Abstract number 437). *Proceedings of the Joint Meeting of the International Continence Society (ICS) and the International Urogynecological Association,* 2010. Aug 23-27 Toronto, Canada, August 23–27, 20102010.
37. Agachan F, Pfeifer J, Wexner SD. Defecography and proctography. Results of 744 patients. *Dis Colon Rectum.* 1996;39:899-905.
38. Mellgren A, Bremmer S, Johansson C, et al. Defecography. Results of investigations in 2816 patients. *Dis Colon Rectum.* 1994;37:1133-1141.
39. van Dam JH, Ginai AZ, Gosselink MJ, et al. Role of defecography in predicting clinical outcome of rectocele repair. *Dis Colon Rectum.* 1997;40:201-217.
40. Watadani Y, Vogler SA, Warshaw JS, et al. Sacrocolpopexy with rectopexy for pelvic floor prolapse improves bowel function and quality of life. *Dis Colon Rectum.* 2013;56:1415-1422.
41. van der Hagen SJ, van Gemert WG, Soeters PB, de Wet H, Baeten CG. Transvaginal posterior colporrhaphy combined with laparoscopic ventral mesh rectopexy for isolated Grade III rectocele: a prospective study of 27 patients. *Colorectal Dis.* 2012;14:1398-1402.
42. Sagar PM, Thekkinkattil DK, Heath RM, Woodfield J, Gonsalves S, Landon CR. Feasibility and functional outcome of laparoscopic sacrocolporectopexy for combined vaginal and rectal prolapse. *Dis Colon Rectum.* 2008;51:1414-1420.

43. Prapasrivorakul S, Gosselink MP, Gorissen KJ, et al. Sacral neuro-modulation for faecal incontinence: is the outcome compromised in patients with high-grade internal rectal prolapse? *Int J Colorectal Dis.* 2015;30:229-234.

44. Markland AD, Burgio KL, Whitehead WE, et al. Loperatmide versus psyllium fiber for treatment of fecal incontinence: the fecal incontinence prescription (Rx) management (FIRM) randomized clinical trial. *Dis Col Rectum.* 2015;58:983-993

45. Buie W. Nonoperative medical management of fecal incontinence. *Semin Colon Rectal Surg.* 1997;8(2):73-79.

46. Reboa G, Frascio M, Zanolla R, Pitto G, Rizoli EB. Biofeedback training to obtain continence in permanent colostomy. Experience of two centers. *Dis Colon Rectum.* 1985;28(6):419-421.

47. Miner PB, Donnelly TC, Read NW. Investigation of mode of action of biofeedback in treatment of fecal incontinence. *Dig Dis Sci.* 1990;35(10):1291-1298.

48. MacLeod JH. Management of anal incontinence by biofeedback. *Gastroenterology.* 1987;93(2):291-294.

49. Wald A. Biofeedback therapy for fecal incontinence. *Ann Intern Med.* 1981;95:146.

50. Hwang YH, Person B, Choi JS, et al. Biofeedback therapy for rectal intussusception. *Tech Coloproctol.* 2006;10(1):11-15.

51. Norton C, Kamm MA. Anal sphincter biofeedback and pelvic floor exercises for faecal incontinence in adults—a systematic review. *Aliment Pharmacol Ther.* 2001;15(8):1147-1154.

52. Norton C, Chelvanayagam S, Wilson-Barnett J, Redfern S, Kamm MA. Randomized controlled trial of biofeedback for fecal incontinence. *Gastroenterology.* 2003;125(5):1320-1329.

53. Heymen S, Scarlett Y, Jones K, Ringel Y, Drossman D, Whitehead WE. Randomized controlled trial shows biofeedback to be superior to pelvic floor exercises for fecal incontinence. *Dis Colon Rectum.* 2009;52(10):1730-1737.

54. Jensen LL, Lowry AC. Biofeedback improves functional outcome after sphincteroplasty. *Dis Colon Rectum.* 1997;40(2):197-200.

55. Matzel KE, Stadelmaier U, Hohenfellner M, Gall FP. Electrical stimulation of sacral spinal nerves for treatment of faecal incontinence. *Lancet.* 1995;346(8983):1124-1127.

56. Matzel KE, Kamm MA, Stosser M, et al. Sacral spinal nerve stimulation for faecal incontinence: multicentre study. *Lancet.* 2004;363(9417):1270-1276.

57. Lundby L, Moller A, Buntzen S, et al. Relief of fecal incontinence by sacral nerve stimulation linked to focal brain activation. *Dis Colon Rectum.* 2011;54:318-323.

58. Carrington EV, Evers J, Grossi U, et al. A systematic review of sacral nerve stimulation mechanisms in the treatment of fecal incontinence and constipation. *Neurogastroenterol Motil.* 2014;26:1222-1237.

59. Kumar D, Benson MJ, Bland JE. Glutaraldehyde cross-linked collagen in the treatment of faecal incontinence. *Br J Surg.* 1998;85:978-979.

60. Kenefick NJ, Vaizey CJ, Malouf AJ, Norton CS, Marshall M, Kamm MA. Injectable silicone biomaterial for faecal incontinence due to internal anal sphincter dysfunction. *Gut.* 2002;51:225-228.

61. Graf W, Mellgren A, Matzel KE, Hull T, Johansson C, Bernstein M. Efficacy of dextranomer in stabilised hyaluronic acid for treatment of faecal incontinence: a randomised, sham-controlled trial. *Lancet.* 2011;377(9770):997-1003.

62. Zetterstrom J, Lopez A, Holmstrom B, et al. Obstetric sphincter tears and anal incontinence: an observational follow-up study. *Acta Obstet Gynecol Scand.* 2003;82(10):921-928.

63. Karoui S, Leroi AM, Koning E, Menard JF, Michot F, Denis P. Results of sphincteroplasty in 86 patients with anal incontinence. *Dis Colon Rectum.* 2000;43(6):813-820.

64. Halverson AL, Hull TL. Long-term outcome of overlapping anal sphincter repair. *Dis Colon Rectum.* 2002;45(3):345-348.

65. Malouf AJ, Norton CS, Engel AF, Nicholls RJ, Kamm MA. Long-term results of overlapping anterior anal-sphincter repair for obstetric trauma. *Lancet.* 2000;355(9200):260-265.

66. Bravo Gutierrez A, Madoff RD, Lowry AC, Parker SC, Buie WD, Baxter NN. Long-term results of anterior sphincteroplasty. *Dis Colon Rectum.* 2004;47(5):727-731, discussion 731-722.

67. Glasgow SC, Lowry AC. Long-term outcomes of anal sphincter repair for fecal incontinence: a systematic review. *Dis Colon Rectum.* 2012;55:482-490.

68. Pakravan F, Helmes C. Magnetic anal sphincter augmentation in patients with severe fecal incontinence. *Dis Colon Rectum.* 2015;58:109-114.

69. Norton C. Patients' views of a colostomy for faecal incontinence. *Neurourol Urodyn.* 2003;22:403-404

Surgical Treatment of Dysmotility Disorders of the Colon

David J. Maron | Steven D. Wexner

Constipation is one of the most frequently experienced gastrointestinal complaints and one of the most common indications for medical consultation.[1] It is estimated that more than 4 million patients in North America suffer from constipation, and laxatives are annually prescribed for 2 million individuals, at a cost of more than $800 million.[2,3] In the United States, more than 90,000 patients are hospitalized each year for constipation-related problems.[4] Constipation has been shown to be more prevalent in persons of a lower socioeconomic background,[4,5] females,[6] and the elderly.[4]

The definition of constipation includes both subjective and objective aspects. In addition to decreased frequency of defecation, patients may present complaining of incomplete or difficult evacuation, abdominal or rectal pain, hard stools, decreased stool bulk or caliber, straining for evacuation, nausea, bloating, and tenesmus. Whitehead et al.[7] proposed that at least two of the following criteria need to be met in a patient who has not used laxatives for at least 12 months: (1) straining during more than 25% of bowel movements; (2) feeling of incomplete evacuation after more than 25% of bowel movements; (3) hard stool on more than 25% of bowel movements; and (4) bowel movement frequency of less than two per week with or without symptoms of constipation. Agachan et al from Cleveland Clinic Florida[8] proposed a scoring system (Cleveland Clinic Florida Constipation Score) that includes frequency of bowel movements, painful evacuation, incomplete evacuation, abdominal pain, length of time per attempts, assistance for defecation, unsuccessful attempts for evacuation per 24 hours, and duration of constipation. After evaluating more than 230 patients, the authors concluded that a score of 15 or greater represents constipation.[8] The widely used Rome III criteria defines constipation as two or more of the following abnormalities occurring for 3 months (with onset of symptoms more than 6 months prior to diagnosis): (1) less than three bowel movements per week, (2) sensation of incomplete evacuation, (3) feeling of anorectal obstruction, (4) hard or lumpy stool, (5) need for straining, or (6) need of manual disimpaction or pelvic floor support.[9]

ETIOLOGY

Numerous diseases can cause constipation. Therefore, before attributing constipation to functional or idiopathic reasons, causative etiologies (Box 149.1) must be excluded.

EVALUATION

HISTORY AND PHYSICAL EXAMINATION

The significant and critical information obtained from a highly detailed clinical history is mandatory. Surveys to measure constipation have been created. The Cleveland Clinic Florida Constipation Score was developed as a scoring system of constipation to evaluate patients' improvement following medical or surgical treatment (Table 149.1).[8] Thorough abdominal and perineal examinations must be undertaken, with an inspection of the anal region, including a digital examination, anoscopy, and a rigid or flexible sigmoidoscopy. The abdominal examination should identify any masses, distention, scars, or tenderness. A digital examination can exclude distal obstructive causes of constipation and detect the presence of any hard stool in the rectum. This latter finding may be common in patients who present with irritable bowel syndrome, inadequate fiber intake, or adequate fiber intake with suboptimal fluid ingestion.

DIAGNOSTIC STUDIES

Barium Enema/Colonoscopy

No patient who complains of constipation should be considered to have a functional cause until all mechanical and extracolonic causes are excluded. Colonoscopy has the advantage of direct visualization of the colon and the ability to biopsy or remove any pathologic lesion; however, it may be technically challenging due to the redundancy of the colon in patients with chronic constipation. Instead, sigmoidoscopy or proctoscopy can be supplemented by a double-contrast barium enema. A barium enema gives the physician a view of the anatomic configuration of the colon, including its size and length.[10] Constipated patients may present with a large, dilated colon (megacolon) and dolichocolon (Fig. 149.1).

CLINICAL APPROACH

Before beginning invasive and potentially expensive physiologic testing, all anatomic and extracolonic causes of constipation must be excluded. Therefore, after the initial office evaluation and colonoscopy or air-contrast barium enema, the aim of the general evaluation should be to exclude all of the extracolonic entities listed in Box 149.1. After such exclusion, a 6-month course of fiber supplementation, dietary measures, and exercise should eliminate patients who have inadequate fiber or water

---

BOX 149.1 **Classification of Constipation**

CONGENITAL
Hirschsprung disease

ACQUIRED
Chagas disease

MECHANICAL (OBSTRUCTIVE)
Neoplasia
Adhesions
Hernia
Volvulus
Endometriosis
Severe sigmoid diverticulitis
Anal stenosis

FUNCTIONAL
Inadequate fiber intake
Irritable bowel syndrome

IDIOPATHIC
Colonic
    Inertia
    Dolichocolon
Pelvic
    Intussusception/rectal prolapse
    Rectocele
    Sigmoidocele
    Descending perineum
    Paradoxical puborectalis contraction
    Perineal hernia

EXTRAINTESTINAL
Pharmacologic
    Analgesics
    Anesthetics
    Anticholinergics
    Anticonvulsants
    Antidepressants
    Antiparkinsonian agents
    Antacids
    Barium sulfate
    Diuretics
    Ganglionic blockers
    Iron

    Hypotensives
    Laxative abuse
    Metallic intoxication (arsenic, lead, phosphorus)
    Monoamine oxidase inhibitors
    Opiates
    Paralytic agents
    Parasympatholytics
    Phenothiazines
    Psychotherapeutic
Metabolic and endocrine
    Amyloidosis
    Diabetes
    Hypercalcemia
    Hyperparathyroidism
    Hypokalemia
    Hypopituitarism
    Hypothyroidism
    Pheochromocytoma
    Porphyria
    Pregnancy
    Scleroderma
    Uremia

NEUROGENIC
Peripheral
Autonomic neuropathy
Von Recklinghausen disease
Multiple endocrine neoplasia 2b
Spinal
    Cauda equina tumor
    Iatrogenic
    Meningocele
    Multiple sclerosis
    Paraplegia
    Resection of nervi erigentes
    Shy-Drager syndrome
    Tabes dorsalis
    Trauma
Central
    Parkinson disease
    Stroke
    Tumors

---

intake as the source for their constipation.[11] The patient should strive to develop regular bowel habits and try to have a bowel movement in the morning or after meals to take advantage of the gastrocolic reflex. The prompt discontinuation of any stimulant laxative is generally advised because the earlier mentioned measures should suffice. If laxatives must be prescribed, stool softeners and lubricants are the preferred choices (Box 149.2).

The failure of such measures should prompt physiologic investigation. Constipated patients should undergo a colonic transit time study, anorectal manometry, defecography, and anal electromyography (EMG). The distinction between colonic inertia and a pelvic outlet obstruction syndrome is crucial because it will have a direct influence on therapy.

PHYSIOLOGY LABORATORY

Colonic Transit

Colonic motility studies have demonstrated that electrical activity occurs in the colon as rhythmic or sporadic nonpropagating bursts and sporadic propagating bursts (mass movements) that occur approximately 6 times per day.[12] Colonic motility is modulated by parasympathetic and sympathetic innervation, as well as gastrointestinal hormones such as gastrin, serotonin, vasoactive intestinal peptide, and substance P, as well as by a number of local colon reflexes.

The measurement of colonic transit through the ingestion of radiopaque markers has been used and often modified since 1981.[13-16] In its most "user-friendly" form, the test

TABLE 149.1 Constipation Scoring System (Minimum Score 0, Maximum Score 30)

Symptom	Score
FREQUENCY OF BOWEL MOVEMENTS	
1–2 times per 1–2 days	0
2 times per week	1
Once per week	2
Less than once per week	3
Less than once per month	4
DIFFICULTY: PAIN EVACUATION EFFORT	
Never	0
Rarely	1
Sometimes	2
Usually	3
Always	4
COMPLETENESS: FEELING INCOMPLETE EVACUATION	
Never	0
Rarely	1
Sometimes	2
Usually	3
Always	4
ABDOMINAL PAIN	
Never	0
Rarely	1
Sometimes	2
Usually	3
Always	4
TIME: MINUTES IN LAVATORY PER ATTEMPT	
<5	0
5–10	1
>10–20	2
>20–30	3
>30	4
ASSISTANCE: TYPE OF ASSISTANCE	
Without assistance	0
Stimulant laxatives	1
Digital assistance or enemas	2
FAILURE: UNSUCCESSFUL ATTEMPTS FOR EVACUATION PER 24 HOURS	
Never	0
1–3	1
>3–6	2
>6–9	3
>9	4
HISTORY: DURATION OF CONSTIPATION (YEARS)	
<1	0
1–5	1
>5–10	2
>10–20	3
>20	4

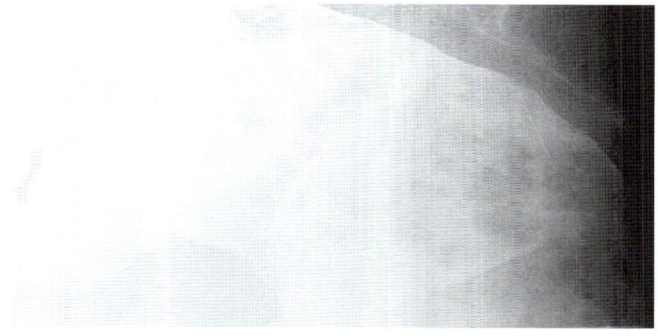

FIGURE 149.1 Barium enema of a patient with chronic constipation. Typical findings of megacolon include a very elongated and redundant colon.

BOX 149.2 General Classification of Laxatives

Bulk-Forming Agents
  Dietary
  Synthetic or processed
  Methylcellulose
  Polycarbophil
  Psyllium
Lubricants
  Mineral oil
Emollients
  Docusate calcium, sodium, or potassium
Saline Laxatives (osmotic agents)
  Magnesium-containing compounds (citrate, hydroxide, sulfate)
  Sodium phosphate
  Lactulose
  Lactitol
  Sorbitol
Stimulant (irritant)
  Bisacodyl
  Senna
  Phenolphthalein
  Danthron
  Casanthranol
  Castor oil
  Cascara

From Wexner SD, Bartolo DCC. *Constipation: Etiology, Evaluation, and Management.* Oxford: Butterworth-Heinemann; 1995.

---

includes the ingestion of a single capsule containing 24 radiopaque markers (Sitzmarks [Konsyl Pharmaceuticals, New York, New York]) followed by radiographs taken on the third and fifth days after the capsule ingestion. All laxatives, enemas, and suppositories must be discontinued prior to the examination. The diagnosis of colonic inertia is made if 20% or more of the markers are found to be diffusely scattered throughout the colon by the fifth day

(Fig. 149.2).[1] Pelvic retention of the markers is more consistent with the diagnosis of pelvic outlet obstruction.

Advantages of this method determining colonic transit are simplicity, reproducibility, and low cost. Nam and associates[18] studied a group of 51 patients with chronic idiopathic constipation, each of whom underwent a colonic transit study on two separate occasions. Patients were divided into three groups: colonic inertia, anismus, and chronic idiopathic constipation. In 35 patients (69%) the results were equal between the two studies, and in 16 patients (31%) the results were disparate (gamma correlation coefficient [CC] = 0.53; $P < .01$). When the tests were repeated within 1 year, the CC was 0.33 ($P < .05$), whereas for periods of more than 1 year, the CC was

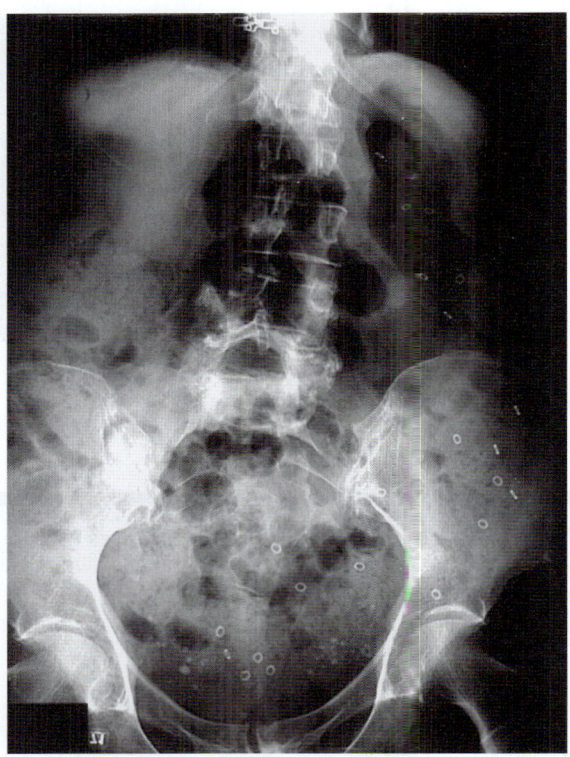

FIGURE 149.2 The radiograph shows the markers distributed diffusely throughout the colon on the fifth postingestion day. The diagnostic finding is consistent with colonic inertia.

0.79 ($P < .01$). The authors concluded that colonic transit studies are reproducible, despite the duration between tests. In an attempt to study segmental colonic transit, some authors have used different types of markers administered on successive days, with plain abdominal films taken either serially[13,15] or on a single day.[15] However, because there is no evidence that segmental colonic resection is an appropriate option in the treatment of colonic inertia, the determination of segmental transit does not justify the increased complexity of this approach.

Scintigraphy can also be applied to the measurement of colonic transit. A method of delivery by orocecal intubation was devised to avoid dispersion of the radiolabeled material (indium-111–labeled diethylenetriaminepentaacetic acid [^{111}In-DTPA]) during its passage through the stomach and small intestine.[19] However, the need for orocecal intubation is eliminated when labeled pellets are incorporated into a gelatin capsule coated with a methacrylate polymer[20] or activated charcoal.[21] Images can be obtained at three time points: 28, 52, and 60 hours after ingestion.[22] Disadvantages of this method include less-than-ideal image resolution and the difficult interpretation of the anatomy of the colon.

Small Bowel Transit

Studies have indicated that there may be a subset of constipated patients in whom orocecal transit time is delayed.[23] When surgical treatment for constipation is being contemplated, measurement of small bowel transit is important to distinguish between isolated colonic inertia and panenteric inertia. The first group of patients is known

to benefit from colectomy; the second group may remain symptomatic even after colectomy.[24]

The hydrogen breath test was first described in 1975 by Bond et al.[25] to measure orocecal transit time. This test is based on the principle that the bacterial metabolism in the colon produces hydrogen. Hydrogen is insoluble in water and highly diffusible; therefore it is promptly absorbed by the intestinal mucosa, transported to the lungs, and then exhaled. An expiratory breath specimen is measured by means of a gas chromatograph analyzer after the patient ingests a dose of 10 g of lactulose diluted in 100 mL of water; breath samples are taken every 10 minutes for a minimum of 2 hours. The time between the ingestion of the lactulose and the first breath hydrogen peak should represent the time of arrival of the substrate to the colon. This test can be altered by smoking or exercise,[26] as well as by small bowel bacterial overgrowth.

A standard meal labeled with mTc-DTPA can also be used to measure gastric emptying and small bowel transit. The patient must ingest the meal after an overnight fast, and a gamma camera is used to obtain the images until the meal arrives in the cecum. The actual small bowel transit is determined as the time between 10% gastric emptying and the appearance of scintigraphic activity in the cecum. Apart from the exposure to radiation generated by this examination, the major disadvantage of this method is the difficulty in identifying cecal filling due to the overlap of small bowel loops. Bonapace et al.[27] evaluated 73 patients with chronic constipation using whole-gut transit scintigraphy. Nineteen percent of patients were found to have delayed gastric emptying, and 7% had delayed small bowel transit time.

The detection of plasma sulfapyridine after the ingestion of sulfasalazine has also been described and corresponds to orocecal transit.[28] This technique has not been widely accepted due to its complexity and cost and the requirement for a nuclear camera. The use of a barium-labeled test meal to assess small bowel transit is not recommended, because alterations in small bowel physiology can be caused by barium; moreover, radiation exposure can be significant.

Anorectal Manometry

Anorectal manometry measures intraanal and intrarectal pressures by means of a transanally inserted catheter. Measurements can be taken in either a stationary pull-through or a motorized continuous withdrawal technique. We use a water-perfused catheter and measure pressures at 1-cm increments, in a proximal-to-distal orientation. With this method, one can establish the anal canal length (high-pressure zone), resting and squeeze pressures, and rectal capacity volume to first sensation. Most important in constipated patients, one can evaluate the rectoanal inhibitory reflex (RAIR). Because of the diversity of methods used in performing anorectal manometry, normal values do not always coincide among institutions; however, these parameters should remain identical within the same laboratory.[29]

Despite pressure variations, the absence of the RAIR is abnormal. The lack of this reflex in patients with chronic constipation may suggest Hirschsprung disease. In addition, absence can also be noted in patients with Chagas disease and should be suspected in patients from endemic countries. An abnormal reflex may also be encountered in patients with dermatomyositis or scleroderma and after any coloanal or ileoanal anastomosis[30]; elicitation of the RAIR is qualitative and not quantitative.

Defecography

Defecography is a method to assess simulated evacuation under direct real-time fluoroscopic visualization.[31–34] The rectum is filled with a radiopaque material similar in consistency to stool and the patient is seated on a water-filled commode. The evacuation process is then observed under fluoroscopic guidance. Radiographs and videos are taken during four distinct activities: at rest, during squeeze, while pushing, and after evacuation. The radiographs allow the measurement of the anorectal angle, perineal descent, and puborectalis length. Because the study is dynamic, one of the criticisms has been the reproducibility of the test. However, Pfeifer et al.[35] confirmed an 83% accuracy rate for the examination when four independent observers used the same definition for each of the pathologic findings.

Under normal circumstances, the rectum is emptied during straining within 8 to 12 seconds, depending on the viscosity of the contrast medium.[35] Even though the examination may disclose multiple abnormalities, such as rectocele and sigmoidocele, intussusception, or perineal descent, one should be cautious to not attribute clinical significance to normal anatomic variants.[36] Jorge et al.[37] found that because defecography has the ability to detect associated abnormalities, it was superior to anal EMG in the diagnosis of nonrelaxing puborectalis syndrome.

The failure to eliminate rectal contents during defecography may not be due to obstructed defecation but rather to the patient's inhibition to evacuate in the presence of an audience. To overcome potentially false-positive results, other methods have been devised, such as attempting the evacuation of a balloon from the rectum.[38–40] Radioactive isotopes can also be used to quantitatively assess evacuation.[41] The introduction of a radiolabeled artificial stool into the rectum is followed by the capture of images with a standard gamma camera, and the percentage of emptying is calculated using an equation. Even though this test provides good qualitative information about the percentage of rectal content evacuated, the low resolution of scintigraphic defecography does not permit the detection of abnormalities such as intussusception, mucosal prolapse, or many rectoceles.[42]

Dynamic pelvic magnetic resonance (MR) imaging has been used to diagnose pelvic floor disorders.[43–45] Matsuoka et al.[43] compared MR defecography with conventional videoproctography. Although all 22 patients preferred MR defecography to videoproctography due to greater comfort, MR defecography was inferior in detecting rectoceles, rectoanal intussusception, and perineal descent. The authors concluded that the routine use of MR defecography in the evaluation of constipated patients could not be justified by the high cost of the test. Elshazly et al[45] evaluated 40 patients with obstructed defecation with MR defecography and found that the results altered the management in more than 50% of the patients.

Electromyography and Pudendal Nerve Terminal Motor Latency

EMG assessment of the pudendal nerve can be helpful to analyze the neurologic status of the striated component of the anal sphincter muscles and its neural supply, respectively. The Single-Fiber Density test is based on the concept of the motor unit, which consists of an anterior horn cell, its axon and axonal branches, motor end plates, and muscle fibers innervated by that cell. The examination is undertaken with the patient in the left lateral decubitus position. The Single-Fiber Density is calculated for a single motor unit in the external sphincter using a single-fiber needle EMG to study the four quadrants. A density of motor units (upstrokes of the motor unit potential), recorded in the area of muscle normally innervated by a single nerve, if greater than 2, indicates ingrowth of other nerves to compensate for injury to the pudendal nerve.

A disposable anal plug electrode may also be used for anal EMG to detect muscle activity during cough, squeeze, straining, rest and simulated defecation. This technique has the advantage of being less invasive however, it is not as accurate as the needle examination. The electrical activity of the muscular action potentials is recorded and analyzed by means of a computer-assisted system.

The number of muscle fibers in the anal sphincter innervated by each axon is small due to its continuously contracted activity. Continuous electrical activity may be seen even at rest,[46] with an increase in its activity during squeezing and coughing; it should return to its resting pattern during evacuation. Its role in the evaluation of constipation is that it can help to diagnose paradoxical puborectalis contraction (PPC), and it can be used as a tool in its treatment.[47,48]

The pudendal nerve terminal motor latency (PNTML) technique, first described by Kiff and Swash in 1984,[49] can be measured with an electrode mounted on the examiner's finger and introduced into the rectum. The examiner's index finger is positioned so that the stimulating electrode is brought into contact with one of the ischial spines. The time between the application of the electric stimulus to the pudendal nerve in the Alcock canal and the external sphincter contraction is called the *terminal motor latency of the pudendal nerve*. A PNTML greater than 2.2 msec indicates injury to the large, fast conducting fibers in the nerve due to nerve stretch. Initially, in small series, some authors argued for a correlation between the chronic straining encountered in constipated patients and abnormally prolonged PNTML.[50–52] However, significantly larger series have not substantiated this theoretical correlation between increased perineal descent and pudendal neuropathy.[53]

Two techniques have been described to assess the sensory components of the anal canal: temperature sensation[54] and mucosal electrosensitivity.[55] The first modality consists of a water-perfused thermode to assess the thermal sensitivity of the anorectum. Even though the ability to discriminate temperature has been implicated in fecal continence, no studies have shown any aberration in constipation. For the assessment of mucosal electrosensitivity, a specially constructed probe that generates constant current is applied to the upper anal canal. The stimulus is increased until the patient feels a tingling sensation,

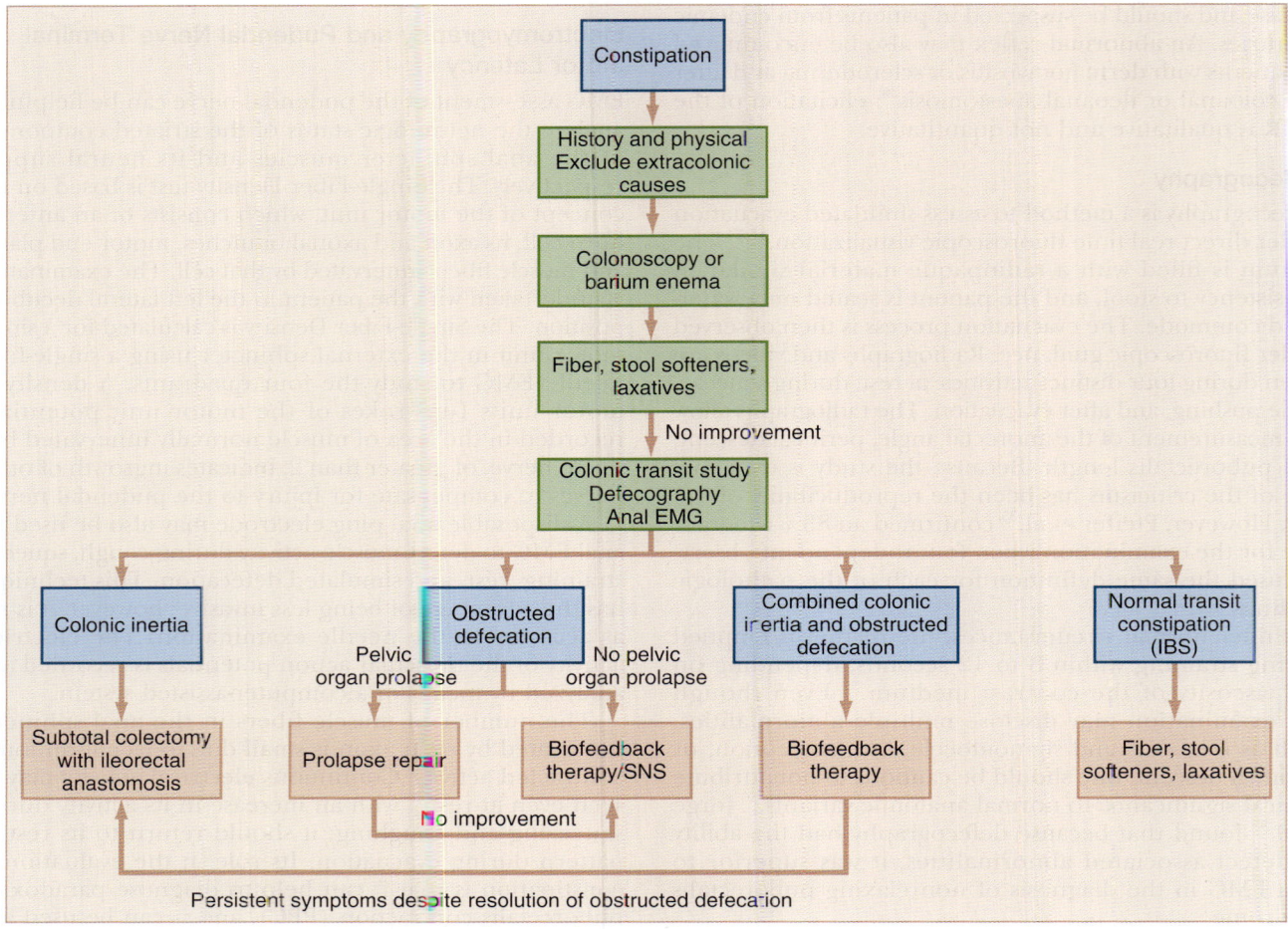

FIGURE 149.3 Evaluation and treatment algorithm of patients with chronic constipation. *EMG,* Electromyography; *IBS,* irritable bowel syndrome; *SNS,* sacral nerve stimulation.

which is recorded as the threshold of sensation. The use of rectal electrosensitivity in constipation[56] is based on the fact that rectal sensation may be decreased in these patients, although this observation may be due to damage to sensory innervation of the surrounding muscles or to feces that prevent optimal mucosal contact.[57]

INTERPRETATION OF RESULTS

The aim of the diagnostic evaluation is to determine whether the patient who presents with constipation has any objective abnormalities. As previously mentioned, the initial strategy should therefore be to exclude extracolonic and structural disorders with a barium enema or colonoscopy. If no cause for constipation is identified, a colonic transit study should be performed. If transit is normal, an assessment of the pelvic floor should be undertaken with defecography and EMG. Recurrent volvulus, Hirschsprung or Chagas disease, and systemic sclerosis must be excluded in patients who present with megabowel.

After completing the diagnostic evaluation, functional constipation can be categorized as follows:

1. Colonic causes—colonic inertia, idiopathic megabowel, adult Hirschsprung disease
2. Pelvic outlet obstruction—pelvic floor dysfunction, PPC, combined pelvic floor dysfunction and PPC

3. Combined colonic inertia with pelvic outlet obstruction
4. Normal transit constipation (usually as a result of irritable bowel syndrome)

TREATMENT

Management of patients with constipation is based on the findings of the colonic transit test and pelvic floor studies. An evaluation and treatment algorithm is detailed in Fig. 149.3.

SURGICAL APPROACH

Colonic Inertia

Patients with abnormal colonic transit and normal pelvic floor physiology who do not respond to conservative therapy are candidates for surgery. Surgical management for clinically intractable constipation was first attempted more than a century ago.[58,59] Three surgical techniques have been described to treat colonic inertia: subtotal colectomy with ileorectal anastomosis (IRA), ileosigmoid anastomosis, and cecorectal anastomosis (CRA). Many series have been reported, with variable results (Table 149.2). Despite early suboptimal results, the development and availability of anorectal physiologic testing have made

TABLE 149.2 Results of Subtotal Colectomy for Constipation

Authors, Year	Number of Patients (% Female)	Mean Age (Years)	Follow-up (Years)	Barium Enema	Biopsy	NO MEGACOLON n	NO MEGACOLON Success Rate (%)	MEGACOLON n	MEGACOLON Success Rate (%)
Watkins, 1966[59]	3[a] (100)	43	0.7	Yes	Yes	—	—	3	100
Lane and Todd, 1977[60]	3[a] (33)	45	2.2	Yes	Yes[b]	—	—	3	33
Smith et al., 1977[61]	1[a] (100)	18	3	Yes	Yes	—	—	1	100
McCready and Beart, 1979[62]	6[a] (65)	52	2.4	Yes[b]	Yes[b]	—	—	6	100
Hughes et al., 1981[63]	17[a] (94)	35	—	Yes	Yes	10	80	7	100
Belliveau et al., 1982[64]	9[a]	—	5.4	Yes[b]	—	—	—	7	78
Klatt, 1983[65]	9[c] (100)	39	2.1	Yes	—	3	100	6	100
Gilbert et al., 1984[66]	6[a] (86)	36	0.7	Yes	—	—	—	6	100
Keighley and Shouler, 1984[67]	10[a] (100)	27	—	Yes	—	10	90	—	—
Preston et al., 1984[68]	8[a] (100)	26	5.7	Yes	Yes	8	63	—	—
Krishnamurthy et al., 1985[69]	12[a] (100)	33	—	—	—	12	100	—	—
Todd, 1985[70]	16[a]	—	—	—	—	16	88	—	—
Barnes et al., 1986[71]	6[a] (43)	38	5	Yes	Yes	—	—	6	67
Roe et al., 1986[55]	7[a]	—	0.7	Yes	Yes	7	71	—	—
Beck et al., 1989[72]	14[a] (100)	41	1.2	Yes	Yes[b]	14	100	—	—
Gasslander et al., 1987[73]	6[a] (86)	37	2	Yes	Yes[b]	6	100	—	—
Leon et al., 1987[74]	13[a] (100)	31	2.6	Yes[b]	Yes	13	77	—	—
Walsh et al., 1987[75]	19[a] (86)	—	3.2	Yes[b]	Yes[b]	17	65	2	50
Akervall et al., 1988[76]	12[a] (100)	39	3.4	Yes	—	12	66	—	—
Kamm et al., 1988[77]	33[a] (100)	34	2	Yes	Yes	33	50	—	—
Vasilevsky et al., 1988[78]	51[a] (94)	45	4	Yes	—	24	71	14	93
Yoshioka et al., 1989[79]	40[d] (98)	35	3	Yes	Yes	32	58[e]	8	58[e]
Zenilman et al., 1989[80]	12[a] (100)	35	2	Yes[b]	Yes[b]	12	100	—	—
Coremans, 1990[81]	11[a] (100)	46	3.8	Yes	Yes	10	60	1	100
Kuijpers, 1990[82]	12[a]	42	—	—	—	12	50	—	—
Stabile et al., 1991[83]	11[a] (64)	43	7	Yes	—	—	—	11	100
Tajana et al., 1990[84]	7[a]	—	—	Yes	—	5	100	2	100
Pemberton et al., 1991[85]	38[a] (84)	40	—	Yes	—	38	100	—	—
Wexner et al., 1991[86]	16[a] (92)	45	1.2	Yes	Yes	16	94	—	—
Mahendrarajah et al., 1994[87]	9[a] (100)	38	1.3	—	—	9	88	—	—
Stewart et al., 1994[88]	1[a]	11	2	—	—	—	—	1	100
Takahashi et al., 1994[89]	38[a]	—	3	Yes	Yes	37	97	—	—
Piccirillo et al., 1995[90]	54[a] (78)	49	2.2	Yes	Yes	54	94	—	—
Redmond et al., 1995[91]	34[a] (92)	43	7.5	Yes	—	34	90[g]	13	—
Lubowski et al., 1996[92]	59[a] (55)	42.3	3.6	—	Yes[b]	—	35	—	96
Nyam et al., 1997[93]	74[a] (68)	43	5	Yes[b]	—	—	72	—	96
Bernini et al., 1998[94]	106[a] (98)	41	6.5	Yes	—	106	74	—	—
Pikarsky et al., 2001[95]	30[a] (21)	—	9.8	—	—	30	100	—	—
Fan and Wang, 2000[96]	24 (79)	37	1.9	Yes	—	24	87.5	—	—
Sarli et al., 2001[97]	26[h]	40	1	—	—	10	100	—	—
Verne et al., 2002[98]	13[a]	42.9	—	Yes	Yes	13	92	—	—
FitzHarris et al., 2003[99]	75	—	3.9	—	—	75	92	—	—
Glia et al., 2004[24]	14	46	5	Yes	Yes[b]	14	100	—	—
Thaler et al., 2005[100]	17 (100)	47	4.8	—	—	17	100[f]	—	—
Hassan et al., 2006[101]	110 (95)	40	11	Yes[b]	Yes[b]	104	98	—	—
Zutshi et al., 2007[102]	69 (97)	48	11	—	—	69	77	—	—
Hsiao et al., 2008[103]	44 (100)	49	1	—	—	39	88	—	—
Reshef et al., 2013[104]	144 (99)	40	3.5	—	—	128	89	—	—
Li et al., 2014[105]	72 (81)	49	5.25	—	—	63	87.5	—	—

[a]Ileorectal or ileosigmoid anastomosis.
[b]Not all patients.
[c]Ileosigmoid anastomosis.
[d]Thirty-four ileosigmoid anastomoses, five cecorectal anastomoses, and one ileorectal anastomosis.
[e]Cecorectal anastomosis.
[f]For colonic inertia.
[g]For gastrointestinal disease.
[h]Overall success.
Modified from Pfeifer J, Agachan F, Wexner SD: Surgery for constipation: A review. *Dis Colon Rectum* 1996;39:444.

better results possible during the past several decades. Subtotal colectomy with IRA has been established as the current procedure of choice for the treatment of colonic inertia. Pikarsky and associates[95] assessed by telephone interview a group of 30 patients who underwent IRA at a minimum of a 5-year follow-up. All 30 patients rated their outcome as excellent, although during this period, 6 patients (20%) required hospitalization for small bowel obstruction, of whom 3 (10%) required laparotomy. In this series, two patients (6%) still required assisted bowel movements, one patient used laxatives, and two patients needed antidiarrheals to control frequency. FitzHarris et al.[99] reported on 75 patients who underwent IRA. Eighty-one percent were at least somewhat pleased with their bowel movement frequency; however, 41% had persistent abdominal pain and 21% reported incontinence. The results appear to persist in long-term follow-up.[101,102] At a median follow-up of 11 years, Hassan et al.[101] found that 85% of patients were satisfied with their bowel function.

Subtotal colectomy with CRA has the theoretical advantage of retaining the ileocecal valve to improve the absorption of water. However, patients who undergo this procedure may suffer from persistent cecal dilation.[70] Most series reporting results of CRA have been small. Yoshioka and Keighley[79] compared results of 5 patients who underwent CRA with 34 patients who underwent IRA and found no difference in the success rate. Sarli et al.[106] reported the results of 26 patients. At 1-year follow-up, the mean number of bowel movements per day was 1.7 and all 26 patients were satisfied with the results of their surgery. Marchesi et al.[107] reported results of 29 patients who underwent CRA and found similar results to published results of patient who underwent IRA.

Because some patients may experience diarrhea or frequent bowel movements after subtotal colectomy with IRA, some authors have proposed segmental colectomy to avoid these unwanted side effects. However, the results of these procedures have been less impressive, with an overall success rate of less than 70%. In addition, up to half of patients will develop megabowel of the remaining colon.

The use of laparoscopic surgery has become commonplace for many diseases of the colon and rectum. Several authors have reported on the use of laparoscopy in the treatment of colonic inertia.[105,108–112] Ho et al.[109] compared 7 patients who underwent laparoscopic-assisted colectomy with 17 patients who underwent open colectomy. Operative time was significantly longer in the laparoscopic group, but functional outcome was equal in both groups. Complications and length of stay were also equal in both groups; however, patients who underwent open surgery were less satisfied with the cosmetic outcome. Other authors have reported functional outcomes, which are similar to reported outcomes for open colectomy.

Regardless of the type of surgery selected to treat constipation, patients must understand the risks. In addition to the standard risks, such as anastomotic leak and postoperative bowel obstruction, problems specific to colectomy for constipation also exist. Specifically, although frequency of bowel movements will likely improve, bloating, pain, nausea, and other constitutional symptoms may persist or even worsen. Furthermore, patients without these symptoms preoperatively may develop them following

surgery. No patient should undergo colectomy for constipation without understanding that the operation will not help to ameliorate these associated symptoms. In addition, patients must also be aware of the possible need for a stoma at any time following surgery.[113,114] Patients with unrealistic psychologic expectations, no matter how well suited by physiologic testing for surgery, are not surgical candidates.

In patients who wish to avoid resectional surgery, another option is the use of antegrade colonic enemas (ACEs). This procedure involves the creation of an appendicostomy or a tubularized cecal conduit through which the patient delivers water enemas (up to 2 L/day). This procedure was first described in pediatric patients and for the use of fecal incontinence but has since also been used in constipation.[115] Worsoe et al.[116] evaluated 41 patients who underwent the ACE procedure and found that after a follow-up of 3 years, 61% were satisfied or very satisfied with the results. Other authors have found similar results; however, a fair number of patients may develop leakage at the stoma site or stomal stenosis leading to failure.[117,118]

Pelvic Outlet Obstruction

Sigmoidocele may account for symptoms of obstructed defecation, particularly in patients who have previously undergone hysterectomy. The mechanism of pelvic outlet obstruction is believed to be caused by collapse of the rectal wall as a result of extrinsic compression of the hernia contents and stasis of the sigmoid loop. Jorge et al.[113] defined the classification system for sigmoidoceles based on the degree of descent of the lowest portion of the sigmoid: first degree, above the pubococcygeal line; second degree, below the pubococcygeal line and above the ischiococcygeal line; and third degree, below the ischiococcygeal line (Fig. 149.4). First- and second-degree sigmoidoceles may represent normal anatomic variants, although a nonemptying sigmoidocele can be the cause of sensation of incomplete evacuation. Patients with first- and second-degree sigmoidocele can be treated conservatively with biofeedback therapy, whereas third-degree sigmoidoceles may benefit from operative therapy.

Jorge et al.[119] reported their experiences with nine patients who had first-degree sigmoidocele, seven patients with second-degree, and eight patients who had third-degree sigmoidocele. Impaired rectal emptying was present in 16 patients (67%). Five of eight patients with third-degree sigmoidocele underwent colonic resection with or without rectopexy, whereas the other three patients were managed conservatively. One of seven patients with second-degree sigmoidocele underwent colectomy, and the other six were managed conservatively, as were all nine patients with first-degree sigmoidocele. Posttreatment improvement was noted in all patients who underwent resection, but in only 6 (33%) of 18 patients treated conservatively. Furthermore, the clinical significance of third-degree sigmoidocele is supported by the fact that all five of the patients with third-degree sigmoidocele who underwent colonic resection reported symptomatic improvement at a mean follow-up period of 23 months.

Rectocele is a protrusion of the rectal wall into the vagina during defecation. It may be commonly seen in

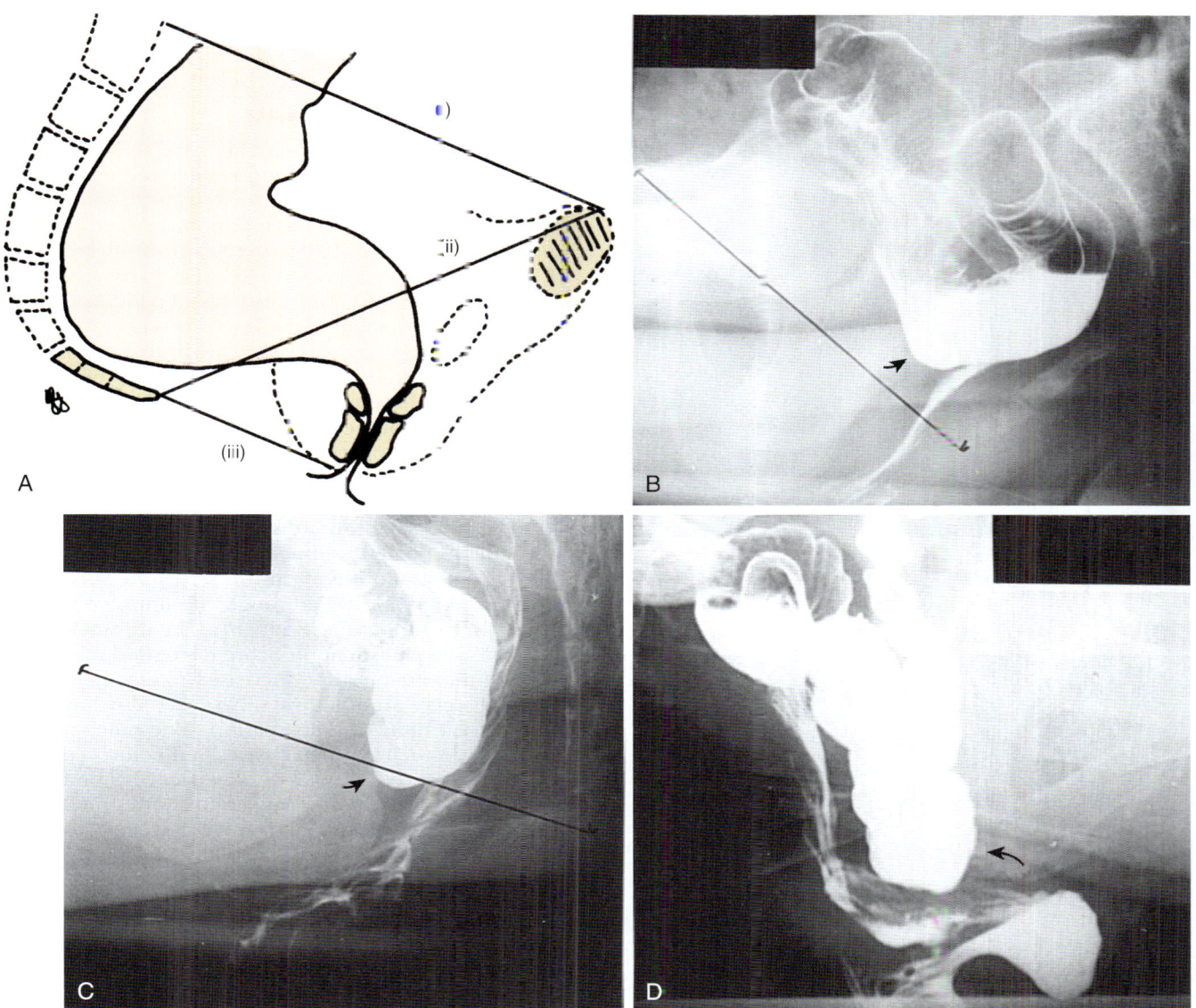

FIGURE 149.4 (A) Schematic of the three degrees of sigmoidocele: (i) pubosacral line, (ii) pubococcygeal line, and (iii) ischiococcygeal line. (B) First-degree sigmoidocele is the descent of the lowest portion of the sigmoid to above the pubococcygeal line. (C) The second degree is to below the pubococcygeal line but above the ischiococcygeal line. (D) The third degree is below the ischiococcygeal line.

healthy women[120] but is also associated with multiparity,[21] obstetric damage, and the presence of PPC.[12] Rectoceles can be classified as high level (usually due to stretching or disruption of the upper third of the vaginal wall and the cardinal and uterosacral ligaments), mid level (usually caused by loss of pelvic floor support secondary to parturition), or low level (usually the consequence of perineal body defects).

The clinical significance of rectoceles is uncertain. Rectoceles may cause mild to severe anorectal symptoms, such as perineal pressure, the sensation of a pouch in the vagina, or incomplete evacuation requiring rectal or vaginal digitation.[5] In our institution, patients are chosen for surgery according to the size of the rectocele (>2 cm), the inability to empty the rectocele at defecography, and the use of digitation or perineal support to empty the

rectum (Fig 149.5). Rectoceles can be repaired via a transvaginal[23,124] or transrectal[125–127] approach. Overall success rates range from 65% to 100%.

Rectal intussusception is an infolding of the rectum into but not beyond the anal verge. Although rectal intussusception is a common finding in defecography (Fig. 149.6), it does not usually cause constipation. Treatment should consist of adequate fiber intake and the use of enemas or laxatives to assist in evacuation as well as biofeedback therapy. Surgical repair including rectopexy has had poor long-term results.[128,129] Choi et al.[130] compared patients with large rectal intussusception treated with conservative dietary therapy, biofeedback, or surgery. Although 60% reported subjective improvement following surgery, half of these patients developed new symptoms, such as rectal bleeding or pain, incomplete evacuation, or liquid stools.

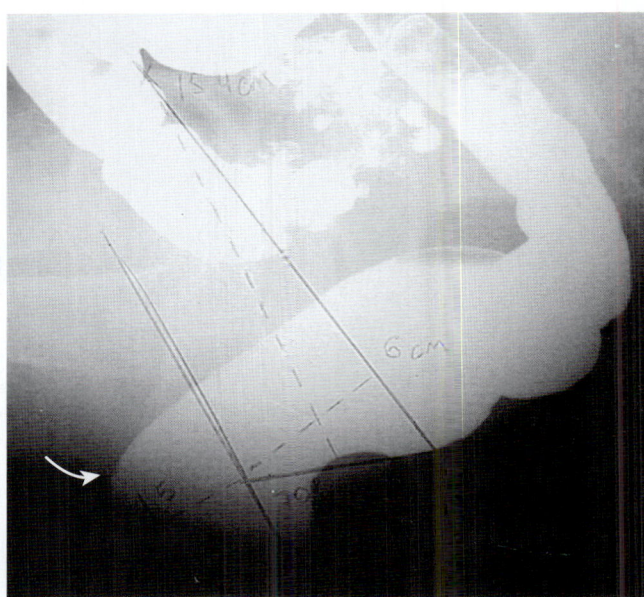

FIGURE 149.5 A nonemptying anterior rectocele is shown *(arrow)*.

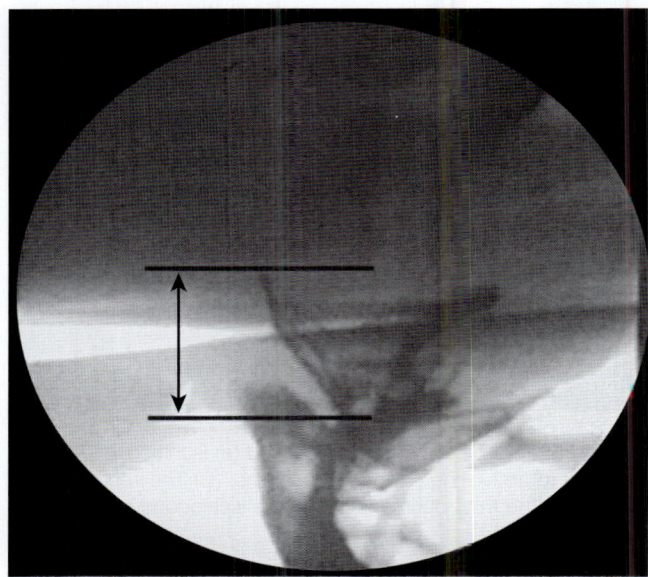

FIGURE 149.6 Rectoanal intussusception is shown.

In addition, biofeedback showed a significant improvement in number of bowel movements per week when compared with a high-fiber dietary regimen alone.

In 1998 Longo introduced a technique to surgically treat obstructed defecation, the stapled transanal rectal resection (STARR). The STARR procedure is designed to resect any internally prolapsed rectum, anatomically to correct a rectocele (if present), and to reestablish continuity of the rectal wall. This is intended to restore normal anatomy, reduce rectal volume, and restore normal compliance. It involves the use of a circular stapler fired twice, plicating both the anterior and posterior rectal walls.

Boccasanta et al.[131] evaluated 90 patients who underwent the STARR procedure. After 1 year of follow-up, 81 patients were satisfied and only 4 had poor results. The most common complications observed were urgency (17.8%), incontinence to flatus (8.9%), urinary retention space (5.5%), bleeding space (4.4%), and anal stenosis (3.3%). Ommer et al.[132] reported good results and a significant reduction in constipation scores at a mean follow-up of 19 months in 14 consecutive patients. A retrospective study that evaluated 123 patients who underwent the STARR procedure was performed by Gagliardi et al.[133] At a median follow-up of 17 months, 65% of patients reported subjective improvement. However, recurrence of rectocele was 29% and recurrence of internal intussusception was 28%, and reoperation was required in 19% of patients. Other authors have reported similar results.[134–136]

Stuto et al. published data on 2171 patients who underwent the STARR procedure for obstructed defecation. The authors demonstrated a significant improvement ($P < .0001$) in several constipation and quality-of-life scoring systems at 12 months of follow-up.[137] Kohler and colleagues evaluated its use in 80 patients, with a median follow-up of 39 months.[138] In this series the success rate was reported as 77.5%, although the improvement did not persist in 18% of these patients. The mean Cleveland Clinic Florida Constipation Score decreased from 9.3 to 4.6 at 24 months but then increased to 6.5 after 4 years.

Sacral nerve stimulation (SNS) has also been used for the treatment of constipation. The mechanism of action on the pelvic floor muscles and colorectal transit time is not entirely clear. The effects of SNS on chronic constipation were observed in patients with simultaneous urinary incontinence.[139] Ganio and colleagues[140] reported benefits in patients with difficulty in rectal emptying and incomplete evacuation, independent of bowel frequency. Ten patients underwent placement of sacral nerve stimulators. The authors found significant reduction in difficulty of evacuation, number of unsuccessful visits to the toilet, and in the time necessary to evacuate. All these improvements disappeared after removal of the electrodes. Kenefick and colleagues[141] included patients with slow bowel frequency and straining and found a significant improvement in frequency of bowel movements and quality of life. The results of these studies suggest application of SNS and improvement of symptoms for these two different types of constipation.

Thomas and colleagues conducted a retrospective review of 68 patients who had undergone SNS for constipation. There was an initial significant improvement in the Cleveland Clinic Florida Constipation Score of patients from a mean of 17 to 10.2 at first follow-up.[142] Success rates among other series range from 42% to 95%.[143–147] Constipation is currently not a US Food and Drug Administration (FDA)-approved indication for SNS in the United States.

Paradoxical Puborectalis Contraction

The normal evacuatory mechanism includes the voluntary relaxation of the external anal sphincter and the pelvic floor muscles, thus increasing the anorectal angle. However, failure of relaxation or paradoxical contraction of the puborectalis muscle during evacuation is responsible for

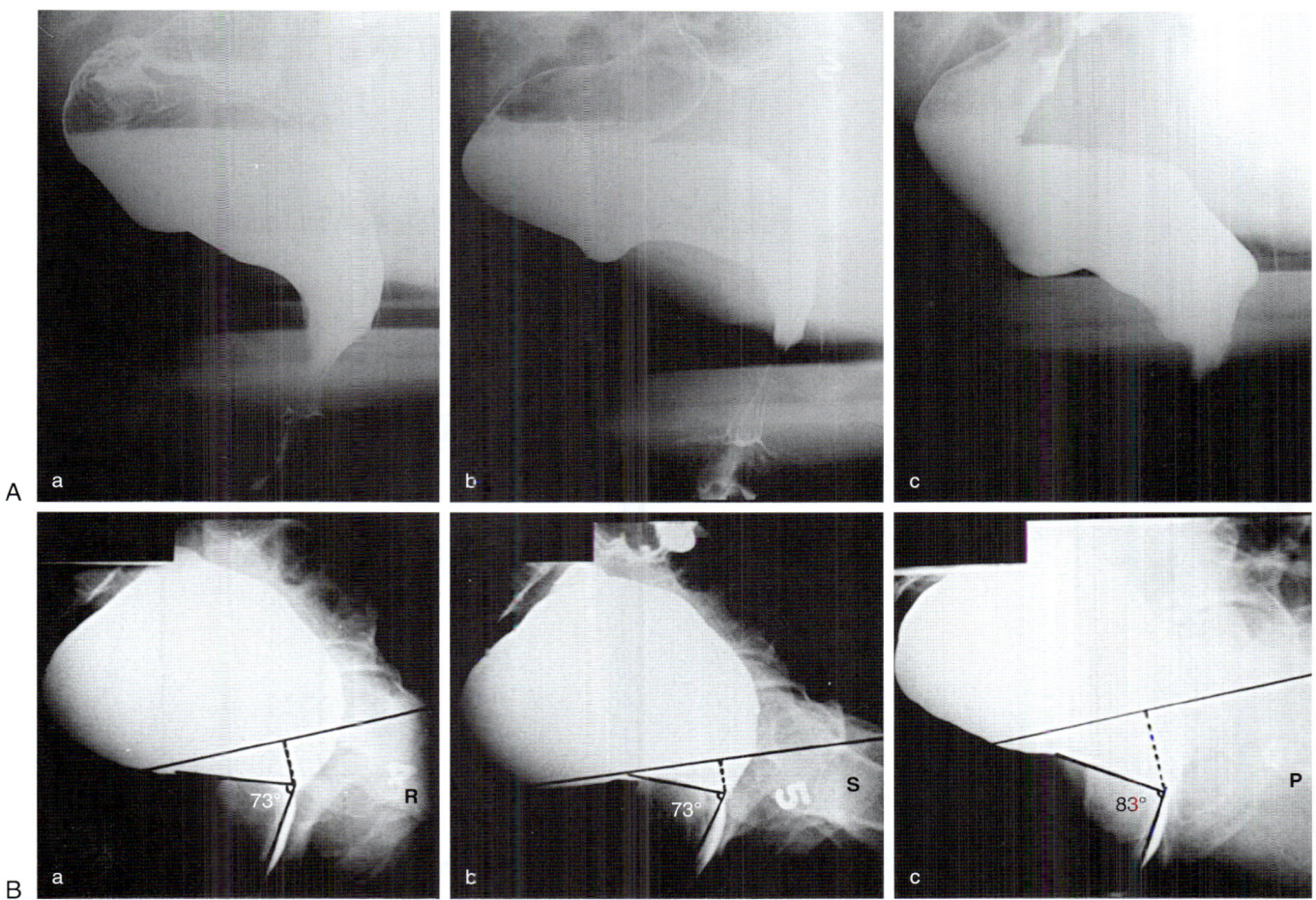

FIGURE 149.7 *Top Row* (A); normal cinedefecogram sequence at rest (a), squeeze (b), and attempted evacuation (c). *Bottom Row* (B); cinedefecogram shows paradoxical puborectalis contraction at rest (a), squeeze (b), and attempted evacuation (c). By contrasting these cinedefecograms, it can be seen that a normal sequence includes shortening of the anal canal and flattening of the anorectal angle with evacuation of barium contents. In comparison, paradoxical puborectalis contraction includes maintenance of the length of the closed anal canal and the anorectal angle or, in some instances, accentuation of these features by an even longer, more closed anal canal and an even more acute anorectal angle.

obstructed defecation,[148] a condition that is termed PPC. This syndrome has also been termed *anismus, nonrelaxing puborectalis syndrome, spastic pelvic floor syndrome,* and *rectal dyschezia.* The cause of this entity is unclear and may involve a generalized pelvic floor disorder with a strong psychologic component.[149] Patients typically complain of straining, tenesmus, and the sensation of incomplete evacuation, as well as the frequent need for suppositories, enemas, or digitation.

Diagnosis is achieved with a combination of defecography (Fig. 149.7) and EMG (Fig. 149.8) to assess the function of the puborectalis muscle. The use of one test does not always ensure a diagnosis (the patients' inhibition may lead to nonrelaxation of the pelvic floor during defecography),[148] and pain may have the same effect during EMG,[67] both of which will lead to false-positive results. Jorge and associates[37] prospectively assessed the role of defecography and EMG in the diagnosis of PPC in 112 constipated patients. In this series, EMG had a sensitivity of 67%, a positive predictive value of 70%, and a specificity

of 83%, whereas the values for defecography were 70%, 66%, and 80%, respectively. The authors concluded that although these parameters are suboptimal for both examinations, defecography may be a superior test due to its ability to detect associated abnormalities. Moreover, the inability to relax the puborectalis muscle has been demonstrated in normal control subjects[150]; therefore the diagnosis of PPC must be consistent with the clinical findings and the results of more than one physiologic test.

Because of the intense psychologic component in PPC, the treatment of choice for these patients is pelvic floor retraining with biofeedback. The success rate for this modality of treatment applied to PPC ranges from 29% to 100%, depending on the series and the techniques that are used (Table 149.3). Attempts have been made to treat PPC through surgical division of the puborectalis muscle. Independent of the site of division on the muscle, either posteriorly or laterally, symptoms of obstructed defecation did not improve and adverse results including fecal incontinence occurred in a high number of patients.[77,177]

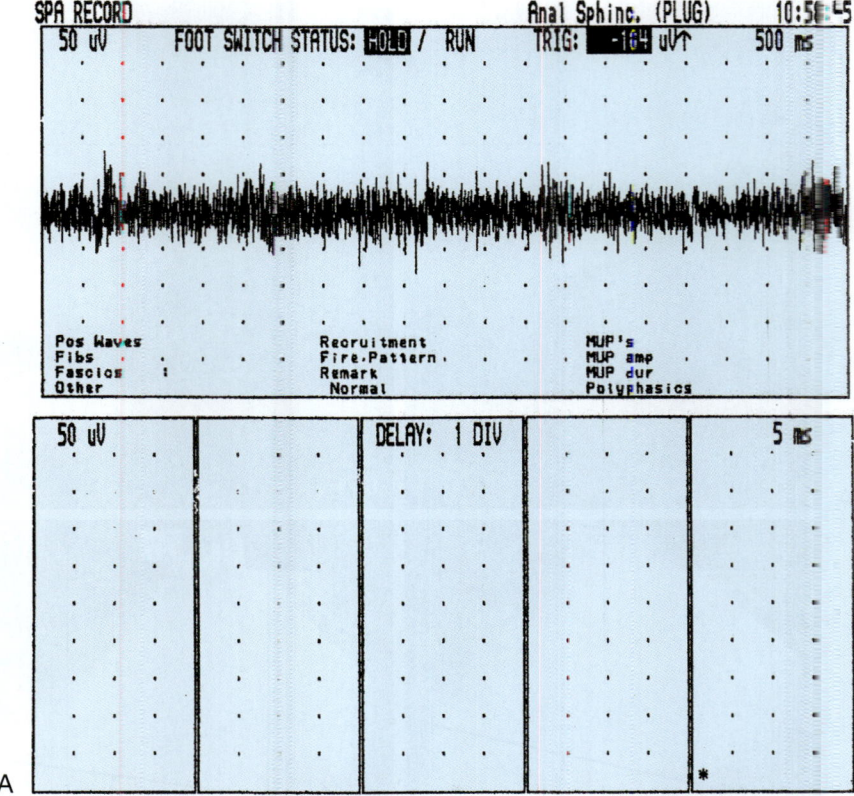

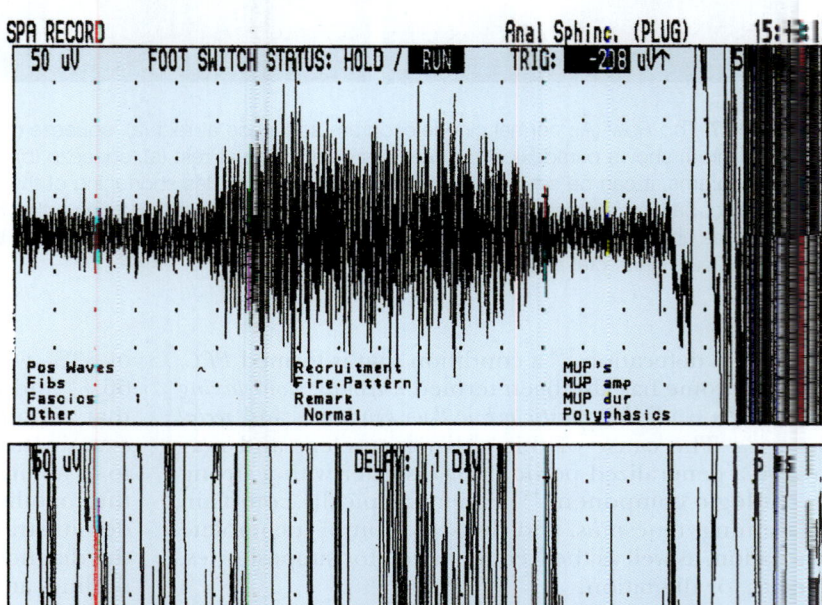

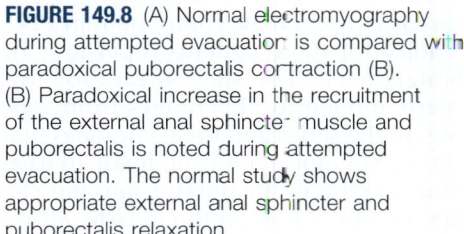

FIGURE 149.8 (A) Normal electromyography during attempted evacuation is compared with paradoxical puborectalis contraction (B). (B) Paradoxical increase in the recruitment of the external anal sphincter muscle and puborectalis is noted during attempted evacuation. The normal study shows appropriate external anal sphincter and puborectalis relaxation.

TABLE 149.3 Success of Biofeedback for Pelvic Floor Dysfunction

Authors, Year	Number of Patients	Mean Age or Range (Years)	Diagnosis	Method of Treatment	Success Rate (%)
Wald et al., 1987[151]	9	6–15	PPC	Manometry	67
Bleijenberg and Kuijpers, 1987[152]	10	19–48	PPC	EMG	70
Keren et al., 1988[153]	12	8.3	PPC	Manometry	100
Loening-Baucke, 1990[154]	22	5–16	Encopresis	EMG	77
Loening-Baucke, 1991[155]	38	6–15	Encopresis	EMG	37
Lestar et al., 1991[156]	16	42	PPC	Manometry/balloon	44
Kawimbe et al., 1991[157]	15	45	PPC	EMG	87
Dahl et al., 1991[158]	14	6–60	PPC	EMG/balloon	93
Turnbull and Ritvo, 1992[159]	7	29–42	PPC	Manometry	71
Wexner et al., 1992[160]	18	67	PPC	EMG	89
Benninga et al.,1993[161]	29	5–16	Encopresis	Manometry	55
Bleijenberg and Kuijpers, 1994[162]	11	35	PPC	EMG	73
Papachrysostomou et al., 1994[163]	22	42	PPC	EMG/balloon	86
Cox et al., 1994[164]	13	7	Encopresis	EMG	90
Siproudhis et al., 1995[165]	27	46	PPC	Manometry/balloon	52
Gilliland et al., 1997[166]	194	71	PPC	EMG	29
Karlbom et al., 1997[167]	29	46	PPC	EMG/balloon	43
Glia et al., 1997[168]	26	55	PPC	EMG/balloon	58
Weisel et al., 2000[169]	13	38	PPC	EMG/balloon	38
Lau et al., 2000[170]	108	66	PPC	EMG	55
Battaglia et al., 2004[171]	24	27–54	PPC	EMG	50
Chiarioni et al., 2006[172]	54	33	PPC	EMG	90
Heymen et al., 2007[173]	30	50	PPC	EMG	70
Rao et al., 2010[174]	26	48	PPC	EMG	50
Faried et al., 2010[175]	20	40	PPC	Manometry/balloon	50
Hart et al., 2012[176]	21	50	PPC	Manometry/balloon	*

*Improvement in constipation severity scores by 35%.
EMG, Electromyography; PPC, paradoxical puborectalis contraction.

PELVIC FLOOR RETRAINING AND BIOFEEDBACK

Biofeedback is based on the concept that patients can be taught to recognize bodily functions of which they were not previously aware. Achieving control of such functions can be translated into visual or auditory stimuli by means of different electronic devices. Electrical and hydrostatic information is displayed in such a way that patients can better understand the contraction and relaxation process. Both pressure-based (manometry) and electrical signal-based (EMG) systems have been used[151,153,159,178] Heymen et al.[179] performed a meta-analysis and found that the mean success rate of pressure-based biofeedback was 78%, whereas the success rate for EMG feedback was only 70%. In addition, there was no significant difference between the success rates, using either intraanal sensors or perianal EMG sensors. These modalities have also been combined with rectal sensation training,[1-1,173] in which patients with a poor recognition of the rectal urge were taught to perceive progressively decreasing volumes of distention. In addition to these methods, portable units are available for use at home, which allows training in a friendly, familiar environment.[56,157,159,160]

Biofeedback training consists of 3 to 10 1-hour-long sessions under the supervision of a biofeedback therapist. The patients are also instructed to keep a daily record of bowel movements, medications, and the use of enemas, laxatives, or digitation. The training is done on an outpatient basis, with the patient dressed and seated on a chair after insertion of the anal plug. Patients are taught to recognize three events: rest, push, and squeeze. The push exercises are done only under supervision during the biofeedback session, whereas the squeeze and rest exercises (Kegel maneuvers) should be practiced at home as well. Discharge conditions include the demonstration of control of pelvic floor musculature as shown with EMG, a reduction in the use of cathartics, and objective resolution of constipation as indicated in a bowel habit diary. Gilliland et al.[66] reviewed the outcome of 194 patients who underwent biofeedback therapy; patients who self-discharged from therapy had a success rate of only 29% compared with patients who were discharged by the therapist, who had a 63% success rate (P < .0001). In this multivariate analysis, which included duration of symptoms, age, gender, and multiple other variables, the self-discharge rate was the only predictor of successful outcome. The results of biofeedback are dependent both on the expectations of the patient and the expertise of the therapist.

Although several small studies have demonstrated improvement in patients following biofeedback therapy, a recent meta-analysis of 17 studies in which 931 patients were treated with biofeedback for chronic constipation and obstructed defecation failed to show sufficient evidence to confirm efficacy.[180] Many of the trials were of poor methodologic quality, highlighting the need for well-designed randomized controlled trials with validated outcome measures and long-term follow-up. Nevertheless, biofeedback therapy should be considered first-line therapy for patients with constipation secondary to pelvic floor disorders.

For the subset of patients who do not benefit from biofeedback, the use of *Clostridium botulinum* type A (BTX-A) in the treatment of PPC has been reported.[181-184] This potent neurotoxin causes paralysis of muscles through presynaptic inhibition of acetylcholine release. Joo and associates[182] treated a group of four patients diagnosed with intractable constipation due to PPC with BTX-A injections for a maximum of three sessions during a 3-month period. Under EMG guidance the BTX-A was injected into the left and right sides of the puborectalis muscle. All patients were relieved of constipation between 2 and 4 days after BTX-A injection, without any local or systemic side effects. However, 3 months after BTX-A injection, two of the four patients experienced symptomatic recurrence. Maria et al.[185] reported improvement in 15 of 15 patients treated with injection of 30 units of BTX-A. However, improvement was maintained for a mean of only 5 months, requiring reinjection of the toxin.

CONCLUSION

Although only a very few patients may benefit from surgical intervention, the evaluation of potential patients must be extensive to ensure both the inclusion of appropriate candidates, as well as the exclusion of inappropriate candidates.[185] In addition, the psychological status of these patients requires thorough assessment and often requires treatment. Through careful testing and selection, satisfactory results can be obtained in more than 90% of patients. However, patients must understand that although bowel frequency will improve and dependence on laxatives will be eliminated or significantly reduced, other symptoms, such as abdominal bloating and pain, may persist, develop anew, or become exacerbated. Patients must also understand that they may eventually require a stoma.

REFERENCES

1. Sonnenberg A, Koch TR. Physician visits in the United States for constipation: 1958 to 1986. *Dig Dis Sci.* 1989;34:606-611.
2. Faigel DO. A clinical approach to constipation. *Clin Cornerstone.* 2002;4:11-21.
3. Lembo A, Camilleri M. Chronic constipation. *N Engl J Med.* 2003;349:1360-1368.
4. Sonnenberg A, Koch TR. Epidemiology of constipation in the United States. *Dis Colon Rectum.* 1989;32:1-8.
5. Sandler RS, Jordan MC, Shelton BJ. Demographic and dietary determinants of constipation in the US population. *Am J Public Health.* 1990;80:185-189.
6. Everhart JE, Go VLW, Johannes RS, Fitzsimmons SC, Roth HP, White LR. A longitudinal survey of self-reported bowel habits in the United States. *Dig Dis Sci.* 1989;34:1153-1162.
7. Whitehead WE, Chaussade S, Corazziari E, Kumar D. Report of an international workshop on management of constipation. *Int Gastroenterol.* 1991;4:99-113.
8. Agachan F, Chen T, Pfeifer J, Reissman P, Wexner SD. A constipation scoring system to simplify evaluation and management of constipated patients. *Dis Colon Rectum.* 1996;39:681-685.
9. Longstreth GF, Thompson WG, Chey WD, Houghton LA, Mearin F, Spiller RC. Functional bowel disorders. *Gastroenterology.* 2006;130:1480-1491.
10. Patriquin H, Martelli H, Devroede G. Barium enema in chronic constipation: is it meaningful? *Gastroenterology.* 1978;75:619-622.
11. Burkitt DP, Walker AR, Painter NS. Effect of dietary fibre on stools and the transit-times, and its role in the causation of disease. *Lancet.* 1972;2:1408-1412.
12. Bassotti G, Gaburri M, Imbimbo BP, et al. Colonic mass movements in idiopathic chronic constipation. *Gut.* 1988;29:1173-1179.
13. Arhan P, Devroede G, Jehannin B. Segmental colonic transit time. *Dis Colon Rectum.* 1981;24:625-629.
14. Bouchoucha M, Devroede G, Arhan P, et al. What is the meaning of colorectal transit time measurement? *Dis Colon Rectum.* 1992;35:773-782.
15. Chaussade S, Roche H, Khyari A, Couturier D, Guerre J. Measurement of colonic transit time: description and validation of a new method. *Gastroenterol Clin Biol.* 1986;10:385-389.
16. Metcalf AM, Phillips SF, Zinsmeister AR, MacCarty RL, Beart RW, Wolff BG. Simplified assessment of segmental colonic transit. *Gastroenterology.* 1987;92:40-47.
17. Hinton JM, Lennard-Jones JE, Young AC. A new method for studying gut transit times using radioopaque markers. *Gut.* 1969;10:842-847.
18. Nam YS, Pikarsky AJ, Wexner SD, et al. Reproducibility of colonic transit study in patients with chronic constipation. *Dis Colon Rectum.* 2001;44:86-92.
19. Krevsky B, Malmud LS, D'Ercole F, Maurer AH, Fisher RS. Colonic transit scintigraphy. A physiologic approach to the quantitative measurement of colonic transit in humans. *Gastroenterology.* 1986;91:1102-1112.
20. Proano M, Camilleri M, Phillips SF, Thomforde GM, Brown ML, Tucker RL. Unprepared human colon does not discriminate between solids and liquids. *Am J Physiol.* 1991;260:G13-G16.
21. Cheng KY, Tsai SC, Lin WY. Gallium-67 activated charcoal: a new method for preparation of radioactive capsules for colonic transit study. *Eur J Nucl Med Mol Imaging.* 2003;30:907-911.
22. Notghi A, Hutchinson R, Kumar D, Smith NB, Harding LK. Simplified method for the measurement of segmental colonic transit time. *Gut.* 1994;35:976-981.
23. Cann PA, Read NW, Brown C, Hobson N, Holdsworth CD. Irritable bowel syndrome: relationship of disorders in the transit of a single solid meal to symptom patterns. *Gut.* 1983;24:405-411.
24. Glia A, Akerlund JE, Lindberg G. Outcome of colectomy for slow-transit constipation in relation to presence of small-bowel dysmotility. *Dis Colon Rectum.* 2004;47:96-102.
25. Bond JH Jr, Levitt MD, Prentiss R. Investigation of small bowel transit time in man utilizing pulmonary hydrogen (H2) measurements. *J Lab Clin Med.* 1975;85:546-555.
26. Thompson DG, Binfield P, De Belder A, O'Brien J, Warren S, Wilson M. Extra intestinal influences on exhaled breath hydrogen measurements during the investigation of gastrointestinal disease. *Gut.* 1985;26:1349-1352.
27. Bonapace ES, Maurer AH, Davidoff S, Krevsky B, Fisher RS, Parkman HP. Whole gut transit scintigraphy in the clinical evaluation of patients with upper and lower gastrointestinal symptoms. *Am J Gastroenterol.* 2000;95:2838-2847.
28. Kellow JE, Borody TJ, Phillips SF, Haddad AC, Brown ML. Sulfapyridine appearance in plasma after salicylazosulfapyridine. Another simple measure of intestinal transit. *Gastroenterology.* 1986;91:396-400.
29. Mavrantonis C, Wexner SD. A clinical approach to fecal incontinence. *J Clin Gastroenterol.* 1998;27:108-121.
30. Le Blanc I, Michot F, Duparc F, et al. Anorectal manometry and ileo-anal anastomosis: pre- and postoperative manometric comparison. *Ann Chir.* 1994;48:183-187.
31. Bartolo DC, Bartram CI, Ekberg O, et al. Symposium. Proctography. *Int J Colorectal Dis.* 1988;3:67-89.
32. Jorge JM, Habr-Gama A, Wexner SD. Clinical applications and techniques of cinedefecography. *Am J Surg.* 2001;182:93-101.
33. Kuijpers HC, Strijk SP. Diagnosis of disturbances of continence and defecation. *Dis Colon Rectum.* 1984;27:658-662.
34. Mahieu P, Pringot J, Bodart P. Defecography: I. Description of a new procedure and results in normal patients. *Gastrointest Radiol.* 1984;9:247-251.
35. Pfeifer J, Oliveira L, Park UC, Gonzalez A, Agachan F, Wexner SD. Are interpretations of video defecographies reliable and reproducible? *Int J Colorectal Dis.* 1997;12:67-72.
36. Bartram CI, Turnbull GK, Lennard-Jones JE. Evacuation proctography: an investigation of rectal expulsion in 20 subjects without defecatory disturbance. *Gastrointest Radiol.* 1988;13:72-80.

37. Jorge JM, Wexner SD, Ger GC, Salanga VD, Nogueras JJ, Jagelman DG. Cinedefecography and electromyography in the diagnosis of nonrelaxing puborectalis syndrome. *Dis Colon Rectum.* 1993;36:668-676.

38. Fleshman JW, Dreznik Z, Cohen E, Fry RD, Kodner IJ. Balloon expulsion test facilitates diagnosis of pelvic floor outlet obstruction due to nonrelaxing puborectalis muscle. *Dis Colon Rectum.* 1992;35:1019-1025.

39. Minguez M, Herreros B, Sanchiz V, et al. Predictive value of the balloon expulsion test for excluding the diagnosis of pelvic floor dyssynergia in constipation. *Gastroenterology.* 2004;126:57-62.

40. Wexner SD, Jorge JM. Colorectal physiological tests: use or abuse of technology? *Eur J Surg.* 1994;160:167-174.

41. Pezim M, Pemberton J, Phillips S. The immobile perineum: pathophysiologic implications in severe constipation. *Dig Dis Sci.* 1987;32:924.

42. Hutchinson R, Mostafa AB, Grant EA, et al. Scintigraphic defecography: quantitative and dynamic assessment of anorectal function. *Dis Colon Rectum.* 1993;36:1132-1138.

43. Matsuoka H, Wexner SD, Desai ME, et al. A comparison between dynamic pelvic magnetic resonance imaging and videoproctography in patients with constipation. *Dis Colon Rectum.* 2001;44:571-576.

44. Roos JE, Weishaupt D, Wildermuth S, Willmann JK, Marincek B, Hilfiker PR. Experience of 4 years with open MR defecography: pictorial review of anorectal anatomy and disease. *Radiographics.* 2002;22:817-832.

45. Elshazly WG, El Nekady Ael A, Hassan H. Role of dynamic magnetic resonance imaging in management of obstructed defecation case series. *Int J Surg.* 2010;8:274-282.

46. Sherrington CS. Notes on the arrangement of some motor fibres in the lumbo-sacral plexus. *J Physiol.* 1892;13:621-772, 617.

47. Preston DM, Lennard-Jones JE. Anismus in chronic constipation. *Dig Dis Sci.* 1985;30:413-418.

48. Yeh CY, Pikarsky A, Wexner SD, et al. Electromyographic findings of paradoxical puborectalis contraction correlate poorly with cinedefecography. *Tech Coloproctol.* 2003;7:77-81.

49. Kiff ES, Swash M. Slowed conduction in the pudendal nerves in idiopathic (neurogenic) faecal incontinence. *Br J Surg.* 1984;71:614-616.

50. Ger GC, Wexner SD, Jorge JM, Salanga VD. Anorectal manometry in the diagnosis of paradoxical puborectalis syndrome. *Dis Colon Rectum.* 1993;36:816-825.

51. Jones PN, Lubowski DZ, Swash M, Henry MM. Is paradoxical contraction of puborectalis muscle of functional importance? *Dis Colon Rectum.* 1987;30:667-670.

52. Snooks SJ, Barnes PR, Swash M, Henry MM. Damage to the innervation of the pelvic floor musculature in chronic constipation. *Gastroenterology.* 1985;89:977-981.

53. Kiff ES, Barnes PR, Swash M. Evidence of pudendal neuropathy in patients with perineal descent and chronic straining at stool. *Gut.* 1984;25:1279-1282.

54. Miller R, Bartolo DC, Cervero F, Mortensen NJ. Anorectal temperature sensation: a comparison of normal and incontinent patients. *Br J Surg.* 1987;74:511-515.

55. Roe AM, Bartolo DC, Mortensen N. New method for assessment of anal sensation in various anorectal disorders. *Br J Surg.* 1986;73:310-312.

56. Kamm MA, Lennard-Jones JE. Rectal mucosal electrosensory testing—evidence for a rectal sensory neuropathy in idiopathic constipation. *Dis Colon Rectum.* 1990;33:419-423.

57. Meagher AP, Kennedy ML, Lubowski DZ. Rectal mucosal electrosensitivity—what is being tested? *Int J Colorectal Dis.* 1996;11:29-33.

58. Lane WA. Remarks on the results of the operative treatment of chronic constipation. *Br Med J.* 1908;1:126-130.

59. Watkins GL. Operative treatment of acquired megacolon in adults. *Arch Surg.* 1966;93:620-624.

60. Lane RH, Todd IP. Idiopathic megacolon: a review of 42 cases. *Br J Surg.* 1977;64:307-310.

61. Smith B, Grace RH, Todd IP. Organic constipation in adults. *Br J Surg.* 1977;64:313-314.

62. McCready RA, Beart RW Jr. The surgical treatment of incapacitating constipation associated with idiopathic megacolon. *Mayo Clin Proc.* 1979;54:779-783.

63. Hughes ES, McDermott FT, Johnson WR, Polglase AL. Surgery for constipation. *Aust N Z J Surg.* 1981;51:144-148.

64. Beliveau P, Goldberg SM, Rothenberger DA, Nivatvongs S. Idiopathic acquired megacolon: the value of subtotal colectomy. *Dis Colon Rectum.* 1982;25:118-121.

65. Klatt GR. Role of subtotal colectomy in the treatment of incapacitating constipation. *Am J Surg.* 1983;145:623-625.

66. Gilbert KP, Lewis FG, Billingham RP, Sanderson E. Surgical treatment of constipation. *West J Med.* 1984;140:569-572.

67. Keighley MR, Shouler P. Outlet syndrome: is there a surgical option? *J R Soc Med.* 1984;77:559-563.

68. Preston DM, Hawley PR, Lennard-Jones JE, Todd IP. Results of colectomy for severe idiopathic constipation in women (Arbuthnot Lane's disease). *Br J Surg.* 1984;71:547-552.

69. Krishnamurthy S, Schuffler MD, Rohrmann CA, Pope CE 2nd. Severe idiopathic constipation is associated with a distinctive abnormality of the colonic myenteric plexus. *Gastroenterology.* 1985;88:26-34.

70. Todd IP. Constipation: results of surgical treatment. *Br J Surg.* 1985;72(suppl):S12-S13.

71. Barnes PR, Lennard-Jones JE, Hawley PR, Todd IP. Hirschsprung's disease and idiopathic megacolon in adults and adolescents. *Gut.* 1986;27:534-541.

72. Beck DE, Fazio VW, Jagelman DG, Lavery IC. Surgical management of colonic inertia. *South Med J.* 1989;82:305-309.

73. Gasslander T, Larsson J, Wetterfors J. Experience of surgical treatment for chronic idiopathic constipation. *Acta Chir Scand.* 1987;153:553-555.

74. Leon SH, Krishnamurthy S, Schuffler MD. Subtotal colectomy for severe idiopathic constipation. A follow-up study of 13 patients. *Dig Dis Sci.* 1987;32:1249-1254.

75. Walsh PV, Peebles-Brown DA, Watkinson G. Colectomy for slow transit constipation. *Ann R Coll Surg Engl.* 1987;69:71-75.

76. Akervall S, Fasth S, Nordgren S, Oresland T, Hulten L. The functional results after colectomy and ileorectal anastomosis for severe constipation (Arbuthnot Lane's disease) as related to rectal sensory function. *Int J Colorectal Dis.* 1988;3:96-101.

77. Karim MA, Hawley PR, Lennard-Jones JE. Lateral division of the puborectalis muscle in the management of severe constipation. *Br J Surg.* 1988;75:661-663.

78. Vasilevsky CA, Nemer FD, Balcos EG, Christensen CE, Goldberg SM. Is subtotal colectomy a viable option in the management of chronic constipation? *Dis Colon Rectum.* 1988;31:679-681.

79. Yoshioka K, Keighley MR. Clinical results of colectomy for severe constipation. *Br J Surg.* 1989;76:600-604.

80. Zenilman ME, Dunnegan DL, Soper NJ, Becker JM. Successful surgical treatment of idiopathic colonic dysmotility. The role of preoperative evaluation of coloanal motor function. *Arch Surg.* 1989;124:947-951.

81. Coremans GE. Surgical aspects of severe chronic non-Hirschsprung constipation. *Hepatogastroenterology.* 1990;37:588-595.

82. Kuijpers HC. Application of the colorectal laboratory in diagnosis and treatment of functional constipation. *Dis Colon Rectum.* 1990;33:35-39.

83. Stabile G, Kamm MA, Hawley PR, Lennard-Jones JE. Colectomy for idiopathic megarectum and megacolon. *Gut.* 1991;32:1538-1540.

84. Tajana A, Mori G, Micheletto G. Current status of surgery for severe idiopathic constipation. *Coloproctology.* 1990;6:340.

85. Pemberton JH, Rath DM, Ilstrup DM. Evaluation and surgical treatment of severe chronic constipation. *Ann Surg.* 1991;214:403-411 [discussion 411-403].

86. Wexner SD, Daniel N, Jagelman DG. Colectomy for constipation: physiologic investigation is the key to success. *Dis Colon Rectum.* 1991;34:851-856.

87. Mahendrarajah K, Van der Schaaf AA, Lovegrove FT, Mendelson R, Levitt MD. Surgery for severe constipation: the use of radioisotope transit scan and barium evacuation proctography in patient selection. *Aust N Z J Surg.* 1994;64:183-186.

88. Stewart J, Kumar D, Keighley MR. Results of anal or low rectal anastomosis and pouch construction for megarectum and megacolon. *Br J Surg.* 1994;81:1051-1053.

89. Takahashi T, Fitzgerald SD, Pemberton JH. Evaluation and treatment of constipation. *Rev Gastroenterol Mex.* 1994;59:133-138.

90. Piccirillo MF, Reissman P, Wexner SD. Colectomy as treatment for constipation in selected patients. *Br J Surg.* 1995;82:898-901.

91. Redmond JM, Smith GW, Barofsky I, Ratych RE, Goldsborough DC, Schuster MM. Physiological tests to predict long-term outcome of total abdominal colectomy for intractable constipation. *Am J Gastroenterol.* 1995;90:748-753.

92. Lubowski DZ, Chen FC, Kennedy ML, King DW. Results of colectomy for severe slow transit constipation. *Dis Colon Rectum.* 1996;39:23-29.

93. Nyam DC, Pemberton JH, Ilstrup DM, Rath DM. Long-term results of surgery for chronic constipation. *Dis Colon Rectum.* 1997;40:273-279.

94. Bernini A, Madoff RD, Lowry AD, et al. Should patients with combined colonic inertia and nonrelaxing pelvic floor undergo subtotal colectomy? *Dis Colon Rectum.* 1998;41:1363-1366.

95. Pikarsky AJ, Singh JJ, Weiss EG, Nogueras JJ, Wexner SD. Long-term follow-up of patients undergoing colectomy for colonic inertia. *Dis Colon Rectum.* 2001;44:179-183.

96. Fan CW, Wang JY. Subtotal colectomy for colonic inertia. *Int Surg.* 2000;85:309-312.

97. Sarli L, Costi R, Sarli D, Roncoroni L. Pilot study of subtotal colectomy with antiperistaltic cecoproctostomy for the treatment of chronic slow-transit constipation. *Dis Colon Rectum.* 2001;44:1514-1520.

98. Verne GN, Hocking MP, Davis RH, et al. Long-term response to subtotal colectomy in colonic inertia. *J Gastrointest Surg.* 2002;6:738-744.

99. FitzHarris GP, Garcia-Aguilar J, Parker SC, et al. Quality of life after subtotal colectomy for slow-transit constipation: both quality and quantity count. *Dis Colon Rectum.* 2003;46:433-440.

100. Thaler K, Dinnewitzer A, Oberwalder M, et al. Quality of life after colectomy for colonic inertia. *Tech Coloproctol.* 2005;9:133-137.

101. Hassan I, Pemberton JH, Young-Fadok TM, et al. Ileorectal anastomosis for slow transit constipation: long-term functional and quality of life results. *J Gastrointest Surg.* 2006;10:1330-1336, discussion 1336-1337.

102. Zutshi M, Hull TL, Trzcinski R, Arvelakis A, Xu M. Surgery for slow transit constipation: are we helping patients? *Int J Colorectal Dis.* 2007;22:265-269.

103. Hsiao KC, Jao SW, Wu CC, Lee TY, Lai HJ, Kang JC. Hand-assisted laparoscopic total colectomy for slow transit constipation. *Int J Colorectal Dis.* 2008;23:419-424.

104. Reshef A, Alves-Ferreira P, Zutshi M, Hull T, Gurland B. Colectomy for slow transit constipation: effective for patients with coexistent obstructed defecation. *Int J Colorectal Dis.* 2013;28:841-847.

105. Li F, Fu T, Tong W, et al. Effect of different surgical options on curative effect, nutrition, and health status of patients with slow transit constipation. *Int J Colorectal Dis.* 2014;29:1551-1556.

106. Sarli L, Costi R, Iusco D, Roncoroni L. Long-term results of subtotal colectomy with antiperistaltic cecoproctostomy. *Surg Today.* 2003;33:823-827.

107. Marchesi F, Sarli L, Percalli L, et al. Subtotal colectomy with antiperistaltic cecorectal anastomosis in the treatment of slow-transit constipation: long-term impact on quality of life. *World J Surg.* 2007;31:1658-1664.

108. Athanasakis H, Tsiaoussis J, Vassilakis JS, Xynos E. Laparoscopically assisted subtotal colectomy for slow-transit constipation. *Surg Endosc.* 2001;15:1090-1092.

109. Ho YH, Tan M, Eu KW, Leong A, Choen FS. Laparoscopic-assisted compared with open total colectomy in treating slow transit constipation. *Aust N Z J Surg.* 1997;67:562-565.

110. Schiedeck TH, Schwandner O, Bruch HP. Laparoscopic therapy of chronic constipation. *Zentralbl Chir.* 1999;124:818-824.

111. Iannelli A, Fabiani P, Mouiel J, Gugenheim J. Laparoscopic subtotal colectomy with cecorectal anastomosis for slow-transit constipation. *Surg Endosc.* 2006;20:171-173.

112. Sample C, Gupta R, Bamehriz F, Anvari M. Laparoscopic subtotal colectomy for colonic inertia. *J Gastrointest Surg.* 2005;9:803-808.

113. Scarpa M, Barollo M, Keighley MR. Ileostomy for constipation: long-term postoperative outcome. *Colorectal Dis.* 2005;7:224-227.

114. El-Tawil AM. Reasons for creation of permanent ileostomy for the management of idiopathic chronic constipation. *J Gastroenterol Hepatol.* 2004;19:844-846.

115. Hill J, Stott S, MacLennan I. Antegrade enemas for the treatment of severe idiopathic constipation. *Br J Surg.* 1994;81:1490-1491.

116. Worsoe J, Christensen P, Krogh K, Buntzen S, Laurberg S. Long-term results of antegrade colonic enema in adult patients: assessment of functional results. *Dis Colon Rectum.* 2008;51:1523-1528.

117. Gerharz EW, Vik V, Webb G, Leaver R, Shah PJ, Woodhouse CR. The value of the MACE (Malone antegrade colonic enema) procedure in adult patients. *J Am Coll Surg.* 1997;185:544-547.

118. Rongen MJ, van der Hoop AG, Baeten CG. Cecal access for antegrade colon enemas in medically refractory slow-transit constipation: a prospective study. *Dis Colon Rectum.* 2001;44:1644-1649.

119. Jorge JM, Yang YK, Wexner SD. Incidence and clinical significance of sigmoidoceles as determined by a new classification system. *Dis Colon Rectum.* 1994;37:1112-1117.

120. Shorvon PJ, McHugh S, Diamant NE, Somers S, Stevenson GW. Defecography in normal volunteers: results and implications. *Gut.* 1989;30:1737-1749.

121. Sehapayak S. Transrectal repair of rectocele: an extended armamentarium of colorectal surgeons. A report of 355 cases. *Dis Colon Rectum.* 1985;28:422-433.

122. Johansson C, Nilsson BY, Holmstrom B, Dolk A, Mellgren A. Association between rectocele and paradoxical sphincter response. *Dis Colon Rectum.* 1992;35:503-509.

123. Mellgren A, Anzén B, Nilsson BY, et al. Results of rectocele repair. A prospective study. *Dis Colon Rectum.* 1995;38:7-13.

124. Rao GN, Carr ND, Beynon J, Francis HC. Endorectal repair of rectocoele revisited. *Br J Surg.* 1997;84:1034.

125. Janssen LW, van Dijke CF. Selection criteria for anterior rectal wall repair in symptomatic rectocele and anterior rectal wall prolapse. *Dis Colon Rectum.* 1994;37:1100-1107.

126. Sullivan ES, Leaverton GH, Hardwick CE. Transrectal perineal repair: an adjunct to improved function after anorectal surgery. *Dis Colon Rectum.* 1968;11:106-114.

127. Tjandra JJ, Ooi BS, Tang CL, Dwyer P, Carey M. Transanal repair of rectocele corrects obstructed defecation if it is not associated with anismus. *Dis Colon Rectum.* 1999;42:1544-1550.

128. Bartolo DC, Roe AM, Virjee J, Mortensen NJ. Evacuation proctography in obstructed defaecation and rectal intussusception. *Br J Surg.* 1985;72(suppl):S111-S116.

129. Christiansen J, Zhu BW, Rasmussen OO, Sorensen M. Internal rectal intussusception: results of surgical repair. *Dis Colon Rectum.* 1992;35:1026-1028, discussion 1028-1029.

130. Choi JS, Hwang YH, Salum MR, et al. Outcome and management of patients with large rectoanal intussusception. *Am J Gastroenterol.* 2001;96:740-744.

131. Boccasanta P, Venturi M, Stuto A, et al. Stapled transanal rectal resection for outlet obstruction: a prospective, multicenter trial. *Dis Colon Rectum.* 2004;47:1285-1296, discussion 1296-1287.

132. Ommer A, Albrecht K, Wenger F, Walz MK. Stapled transanal rectal resection (STARR): a new option in the treatment of obstructive defecation syndrome. *Langenbecks Arch Surg.* 2006;391:32-37.

133. Gagliardi G, Pescatori M, Altomare DF, et al. Results, outcome predictors, and complications after stapled transanal rectal resection for obstructed defecation. *Dis Colon Rectum.* 2008;51:186-195, discussion 195.

134. Dodi G, Pietroletti R, Milito G, Binda G, Pescatori M. Bleeding, incontinence, pain and constipation after STARR transanal double stapling rectotomy for obstructed defecation. *Tech Coloproctol.* 2003;7:148-153.

135. Pescatori M, Boffi F, Russo A, Zbar AP. Complications and recurrence after excision of rectal internal mucosal prolapse for obstructed defaecation. *Int J Colorectal Dis.* 2006;21:160-165.

136. Wolff K, Marti L, Beutner U, Steffen T, Lange J, Hetzer FH. Functional outcome and quality of life after stapled transanal rectal resection for obstructed defecation syndrome. *Dis Colon Rectum.* 2010;53:881-888.

137. Stuto A, Renzi A, Carriero A, et al. Stapled trans-anal rectal resection (STARR) in the surgical treatment of the obstructed defecation syndrome: results of STARR Italian Registry. *Surg Innov.* 2011;18:248-253.

138. Kohler K, Stelzner S, Hellmich G, et al. Results in the long-term course after stapled transanal rectal resection (STARR). *Langenbecks Arch Surg.* 2012;397:771-778.

139. Kollner TG, Schnee C, Gershenzon J, Degenhardt J. The sesquiterpene hydrocarbons of maize (*Zea mays*) form five groups with distinct developmental and organ-specific distributions. *Phytochemistry.* 2004;65:1895-1902.

140. Ganio E, Masin A, Ratto C, et al. Short-term sacral nerve stimulation for functional anorectal and urinary disturbances: results in 40 patients: evaluation of a new option for anorectal functional disorders. *Dis Colon Rectum.* 2001;44:1261-1267.

141. Kenefick NJ, Nicholls RJ, Cohen RG, Kamm MA. Permanent sacral nerve stimulation for treatment of idiopathic constipation. *Br J Surg.* 2002;89:882-888.

142. Thomas GP, Dudding TC, Rahbour G, Nicholls RJ, Vaizey CJ. Sacral nerve stimulation for constipation. *Br J Surg.* 2013;100:174-181.

143. Holzer B, Rosen HR, Novi G, et al. Sacral nerve stimulation in patients with severe constipation. *Dis Colon Rectum.* 2008;51:524-529 [discussion 529-530].

144. Kamm MA, Dudding TC, Melenhorst J, et al. Sacral nerve stimulation for intractable constipation. *Gut.* 2012;59:333-340.

145. Kenefick NJ. Sacral nerve neuromodulation for the treatment of lower bowel motility disorders. *Ann R Coll Surg Engl.* 2006;88:617-623.

146. Malouf AJ, Wiesel PH, Nicholls T, Nicholls RJ, Kamm MA. Short-term effects of sacral nerve stimulation for idiopathic slow transit constipation. *World J Surg.* 2002;26:166-170.

147. Knowles CH, Thin N, Gill K, et al. Prospective randomized double-blind study of temporary sacral nerve stimulation in patients with rectal evacuatory dysfunction and rectal hyposensitivity. *Ann Surg.* 2012;255:643-649.

148. Kuijpers HC, Bleijenberg G, de Morree H. The spastic pelvic floor syndrome. Large bowel outlet obstruction caused by pelvic floor dysfunction: a radiological study. *Int J Colorectal Dis.* 1986;1:44-48.

149. Miller R, Duthie GS, Bartolo DC, Roe AM, Locke-Edmunds J, Mortensen NJ. Anismus in patients with normal and slow transit constipation. *Br J Surg.* 1991;78:690-692.

150. Womack NR, Williams NS, Holmfield JH, Morrison JF, Simpkins KC. New method for the dynamic assessment of anorectal function in constipation. *Br J Surg.* 1985;72:994-998.

151. Wald A, Chandra R, Gabel S, Chiponis D. Evaluation of biofeedback in childhood encopresis. *J Pediatr Gastroenterol Nutr.* 1987;6:554-558.

152. Bleijenberg G, Kuijpers HC. Treatment of the spastic pelvic floor syndrome with biofeedback. *Dis Colon Rectum.* 1987;30:108-111.

153. Keren S, Wagner Y, Heldenberg D, Golan M. Studies of manometric abnormalities of the rectoanal region during defecation in constipated and soiling children modification through biofeedback therapy. *Am J Gastroenterol.* 1988;83:827-831.

154. Loening-Baucke V. Modulation of abnormal defecation dynamics by biofeedback treatment in chronically constipated children with encopresis. *J Pediatr.* 1990;116:214-222.

155. Loening-Baucke V. Persistence of chronic constipation in children after biofeedback treatment. *Dig Dis Sci.* 1991;36:153-160.

156. Lestar B, Penninckx F, Kerremans R. Biofeedback defaecation training for anismus. *Int J Colorectal Dis.* 1991;6:202-207.

157. Kawimbe BM, Papachrysostomou M, Binnie NR, Clare N, Smith AN. Outlet obstruction constipation (anismus) managed by biofeedback. *Gut.* 1991;32:1175-1179.

158. Dahl J, Lindquist BL, Tysk C, Leissner P, Philipson L, Järnerot G. Behavioral medicine treatment in chronic constipation with paradoxical anal sphincter contraction. *Dis Colon Rectum.* 1991;34:769-776.

159. Turnbull GK, Ritvo PG. Anal sphincter biofeedback relaxation treatment for women with intractable constipation symptoms. *Dis Colon Rectum.* 1992;35:530-536.

160. Wexner SD, Cheape JD, Jorge JM, Heymen S, Jagelman DG. Prospective assessment of biofeedback for the treatment of paradoxical puborectalis contraction. *Dis Colon Rectum.* 1992;35:145-150.

161. Benninga MA, Buller HA, Tamminiau JA. Biofeedback training in chronic constipation. *Arch Dis Child.* 1993;68:126-129.

162. Bleijenberg G, Kuijpers HC. Biofeedback treatment of constipation: a comparison of two methods. *Am J Gastroenterol.* 1994;89:1021-1026.

163. Papachrysostomou M, Smith AN. Effects of biofeedback on obstructive defecation—reconditioning of the defecation reflex? *Gut.* 1994;35:252-256.

164. Cox DJ, Sutphen J, Borowitz S, Dickens MN, Singles J, Whitehead WE. Simple electromyographic biofeedback treatment for chronic pediatric constipation/encopresis: preliminary report. *Biofeedback Self Regul.* 1994;19:41-50.

165. Siproudhis L, Dautrème S, Ropert A, et al. Anismus and biofeedback: who benefits? *Eur J Gastroenterol Hepatol.* 1995;7:547-552.

136. Gilliland R, Heymen S, Altomare DF, et al. Outcome and predictors of success of biofeedback for constipation. *Br J Surg.* 1997;84:1123-1126.

167. Karlbom U, Hallden M, Eeg-Olofsson KE, Pahlman L, Graf W. Results of biofeedback in constipated patients: a prospective study. *Dis Colon Rectum.* 1997;40:1149-1155.

168. Glia A, Gylin M, Gullberg K, Lindberg G. Biofeedback retraining in patients with functional constipation and paradoxical puborectalis contraction: comparison of anal manometry and sphincter electromyography for feedback. *Dis Colon Rectum.* 1997;40:889-895.

169. Wiesel PH, Norton C, Roy AJ, Storrie JB, Bowers J, Kamm MA. Gut focused behavioural treatment (biofeedback) for constipation and faecal incontinence in multiple sclerosis. *J Neurol Neurosurg Psychiatry.* 2000;69:240-243.

170. Lau CW, Heymen S, Alabaz O, Iroatulam AJ, Wexner SD. Prognostic significance of rectocele, intussusception, and abnormal perineal descent in biofeedback treatment for constipated patients with paradoxical puborectalis contraction. *Dis Colon Rectum.* 2000;43:478-482.

171. Battaglia E, Serra AM, Buonafede G, et al. Long-term study on the effects of visual biofeedback and muscle training as a therapeutic modality in pelvic floor dyssynergia and slow-transit constipation. *Dis Colon Rectum.* 2004;47:90-95.

172. Chiarioni G, Whitehead WE, Pezza V, Morelli A, Bassotti G. Biofeedback is superior to laxatives for normal transit constipation due to pelvic floor dyssynergia. *Gastroenterology.* 2006;130:657-664.

173. Heymen S, Scarlett Y, Jones K, Ringel Y, Drossman D, Whitehead WE. Randomized, controlled trial shows biofeedback to be superior to alternative treatments for patients with pelvic floor dyssynergia-type constipation. *Dis Colon Rectum.* 2007;50:428-441.

174. Rao SS, Valestin J, Brown CK, Zimmerman B, Schulze K. Long-term efficacy of biofeedback therapy for dyssynergic defecation: randomized controlled trial. *Am J Gastroenterol.* 2010;105:890-896.

175. Faried M, El Nakeeb A, Youssef M, Omar W, El Monem HA. Comparative study between surgical and non-surgical treatment of anismus in patients with symptoms of obstructed defecation: a prospective randomized study. *J Gastrointest Surg.* 2010;14:1235-1243.

176. Hart SL, Lee JW, Berian J, Patterson TR, Del Rosario A, Varma MG. A randomized controlled trial of anorectal biofeedback for constipation. *Int J Colorectal Dis.* 2012;27:459-466.

177. Barnes PR, Hawley PR, Preston DM, Lennard-Jones JE. Experience of posterior division of the puborectalis muscle in the management of chronic constipation. *Br J Surg.* 1985;72:475-477.

178. Weber J, Ducrotte P, Touchais JY, Roussignol C, Denis P. Biofeedback training for constipation in adults and children. *Dis Colon Rectum.* 1987;30:844-846.

179. Heymen S, Jones KR, Scarlett Y, Whitehead WE. Biofeedback treatment of constipation: a critical review. *Dis Colon Rectum.* 2003;46:1208-1217.

180. Woodward S, Norton C, Chiarelli P. Biofeedback for treatment of chronic idiopathic constipation in adults. *Cochrane Database Syst Rev.* 2014 (3):CD008486.

181. Hallan RI, Williams NS, Melling J, Waldron DJ, Womack NR, Morrison JF. Treatment of anismus in intractable constipation with botulinum A toxin. *Lancet.* 1988;2:714-717.

182. Joo JS, Agachan F, Wolff B, Nogueras JJ, Wexner SD. Initial North American experience with botulinum toxin type A for treatment of anismus. *Dis Colon Rectum.* 1996;39:1107-1111.

183. Maria G, Brisinda G, Bentivoglio AR, Cassetta E, Albanese A. Botulinum toxin in the treatment of outlet obstruction constipation caused by puborectalis syndrome. *Dis Colon Rectum.* 2000;43:376-380.

184. Shafik A, El-Sibai O. Botulin toxin in the treatment of nonrelaxing puborectalis syndrome. *Dig Surg.* 1998;15:347-351.

185. Pfeifer J, Agachan F, Wexner SD. Surgery for constipation: a review. *Dis Colon Rectum.* 1996;39:444-460.

Pelvic Floor Dysfunction

Matthew Silviera | Deborah S. Keller

The pelvic floor is the anatomic region bounded anteriorly by the pubis, posteriorly by the sacrum, laterally by the ischial and iliac bones, superiorly by the peritoneum, and inferiorly by the levator ani and coccygeus muscles, which form the pelvic diaphragm.[1] Functionally, the pelvic floor supports the pelvic viscera, helps maintain optimal intraabdominal pressure, and provides storage and maintenance of continence as part of the urinary and bowel systems.[2]

Pelvic floor dysfunction is a broad term that covers all conditions impacting normal defecation, bowel storage, continence, or causes perineal pain. This constellation includes pelvic organ prolapse, dysfunctional bowel and/or bladder storage and evacuation, and chronic regional pain. The pelvic floor has three compartments: anterior (bladder, urethra), middle (vagina, cervix, uterus), and posterior (rectum). The complex network of muscles and fascia that form the pelvic floor supports all three compartments; damage to one or more of these myofascial elements can lead to generalized pelvic floor dysfunction. There are identifiable causes of injury and risk factors for pelvic floor dysfunction, including pregnancy and childbirth, aging, obesity, menopause, hypoestrogenism, genetic factors, smoking, prior pelvic surgery, and medical conditions that cause nerve injury to the musculature of the pelvic floor.[3–5]

The exact prevalence of pelvic floor disorders is unknown, because of underreporting, misdiagnosis, and the lack of consistent definitions. It has been reported that up to 67% of women have at least one pelvic floor disorder, with many having disorders in more than one compartment.[6] Furthermore, pelvic floor dysfunction is not limited to women, with the incidence reported in approximately 5% of men.[5] The prevalence of each subtype has been estimated as up to 24% for fecal incontinence, 50% for urinary incontinence, 33% for slow transit constipation, and 27% for obstructed defecation.[5–10] With the difficulties in reporting and diagnosis, the need for multispecialty evaluation and care is highlighted, as isolated evaluation can lead to the diagnosis and management of one component of what is a multisystem process.

EVALUATION

Evaluation of pelvic floor dysfunction requires a multidisciplinary approach from colorectal, gynecologic, radiologic, and urologic teams. As with any evaluation, this begins with a detailed history and physical examination.

HISTORY (BOX 150.1)

The history should include details of presenting symptoms, onset, duration, frequency, severity, and any exacerbating or relieving factors. A complete past medical, obstetric (for women), and surgical history should be obtained. The obstetric history should include current pregnancy status, future pregnancy plans, birth history with child size, traumatic deliveries, and need for episiotomy or repair. The patient's body mass index (BMI) should be documented, as well as any recent weight gain or loss. Current medication regimens should be documented. A social history, including psychiatric illness, sexual and physical abuse must be obtained, because they are associated with defecation difficulties and impact patient perception of symptoms.[10] The pattern of bowel function needs to be documented in detail, including frequency of evacuation, length of time spent for each evacuation, straining at stool, rectal pain, posturing and digitations, and the trend of any problems over time. Stool consistency influences the severity of incontinence and constipation and can be graded using the Bristol Stool Scale (Fig. 150.1).[11] Validated scoring systems add subjective and objective measures to the clinical history and include the Cleveland Clinic Incontinence (Wexner) score, Cleveland Clinic Constipation score, American Society of Colon and Rectal Surgeons (ASCRS) Fecal Incontinence score, ASCRS Fecal Incontinence Quality of Life score, St. Mark's Incontinence score, the PAC-SYM Patient Assessment of Constipation, the Fecal Incontinence Quality of Life Scale, and many others.[12–18]

One of the most important issues to define while taking a history from this group of patients is to learn exactly why the patient is seeking help and how much their problem is affecting their quality of life. Specific items one must ask about when eliciting a pelvic floor history are seen in Box 150.2.

Continence is maintained from a complex interaction of stool volume, stool consistency, rectal sensation, rectal capacity, and the resting tone of the anal canal. Any disturbance to these elements can result in fecal incontinence. It is important to understand that fecal incontinence is a sign or a symptom of another disease, not a definitive diagnosis. Fecal incontinence can result from a myriad of different causes, including obstetric injury, postmenopausal changes, anorectal surgery, neurological disorders, constipation, diarrhea, and inflammatory bowel diseases.[19–21] Urge incontinence results from an inability of the rectum to store stool. This can be from a sudden overwhelming bolus of stool or a rectum that is not compliant and will not hold the stool. Patients can have a combination of both problems, and a careful history is needed to differentiate what is occurring during defecation. The history should elicit a disturbance in any of the elements that maintain continence. Dietary changes, recent changes in weight, medications, and gastrointestinal surgery can impact stool volume and consistency. Low spinal cord injury, trauma, and anorectal

---

BOX 150.1 Elements of the Pelvic Floor History

- Present illness
- Duration of symptoms and inciting events
- Medical
- Surgical
- Obstetric history and trauma
- Social/psychiatric/sexual
- Detailed bowel patterns and function
- Appropriate validated scoring systems for quality of life and symptoms

---

BOX 150.2 Pelvic Floor Specific Questions for the History

- Pelvic pressure?
- Pelvic discomfort?
- Feeling as if something's falling out?
- Difficulty emptying bladder?
- Urine leakage?
- Need to wear a pad?
- Hesitance to leave the house?
- Need to strain?
- Need to manually push perineum/vaginal wall?
- Difficulty emptying rectum?
- Incontinence to gas, liquid, and/or solid stool?
- Looseness or discomfort during sex?
- Coexistent morbidities?
- Unable to perform normal daily activities?

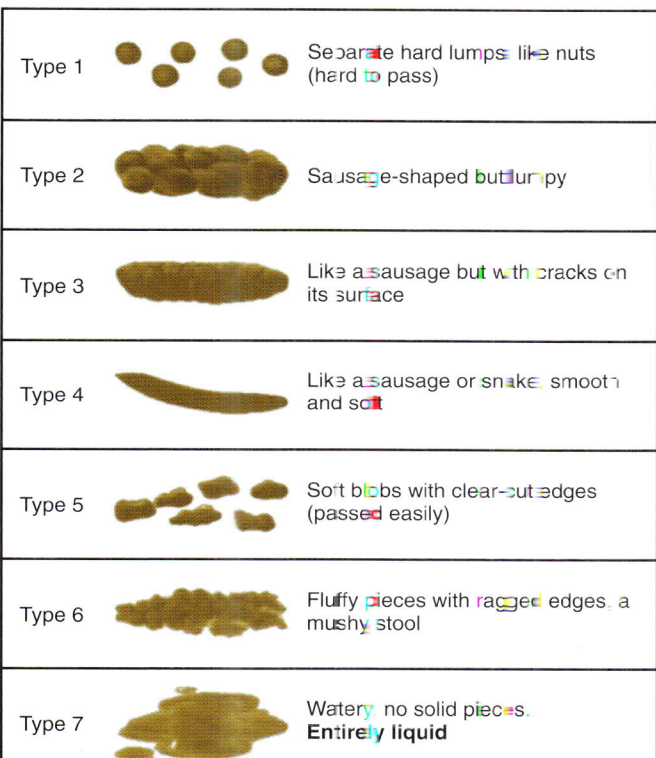

Type 1	Separate hard lumps like nuts (hard to pass)
Type 2	Sausage-shaped but lumpy
Type 3	Like a sausage but with cracks on its surface
Type 4	Like a sausage or snake, smooth and soft
Type 5	Soft blobs with clear-cut edges (passed easily)
Type 6	Fluffy pieces with ragged edges, a mushy stool
Type 7	Watery, no solid pieces. **Entirely liquid**

FIGURE 150.1 Bristol stool chart. (From Lewis SJ, Heaton KW Stool form scale as a useful guide to intestinal transit time. *Scand J Gastroenterol*. 1997;32:920.)

BOX 150.3 Rome III Diagnostic Criteria for Functional Constipation

SYMPTOMS ≥3 MONTHS; ONSET ≥6 MONTHS PRIOR TO DIAGNOSIS

Straining*
Lumpy or hard stools*
Sensation of incomplete evacuation*
Sensation of anorectal obstruction/blockage*
Manual maneuvers to facilitate defecation*
<3 defecations/week
Loose stools rarely present without the use of laxatives
Insufficient criteria for irritable bowel syndrome (constipation subtype)

*Symptoms present greater than 25%.
Based on Longstreth GF, Thompson WG, Chey WD, Houghton LA, Mearin F, Spiller RC. Functional bowel disorders. *Gastroenterology*. 2006;130:1480.

---

surgical procedures can impact rectal sensation. Rectal capacity can be impaired from normal aging, pelvic radiation, low anterior resection, inflammation, and anorectal surgery. Baseline resting pressure can be reduced with vaginal delivery, muscular trauma, and hemorrhoid issues. When investigating incontinence, the physician needs to assure there is no mass or infection is being masked by incontinence symptoms. Most patients with severe fecal incontinence will require an endoanal ultrasound (EUS) to define the sphincter muscle anatomy and physiological testing to define sensation, tone, and function.

Constipation is a common complaint, affecting an estimated 20% of Americans.[22] Physicians define constipation by frequency, with less than three spontaneous bowel movements per week as diagnostic, while patients may define constipation based on stool consistency, feelings of incomplete emptying, straining, or urge for defecation.[23–25] As constipation is a symptom-based disorder and its definition is mainly subjective, the history is especially important.[25,26] It can stem from functional, structural, or metabolic issues with the colon or anorectum. Colonic obstruction from processes such as malignancy or Hirschsprung disease must be ruled out before diagnosing constipation. In patients with constipation, the type should be stratified into slow transit, from irregularities in colonic motility, or outlet obstruction, from dysfunction of the anorectal mechanism for defecation. The Rome criteria were established to standardize the definition of constipation with consensus-derived criteria, with diagnostic questions sensitive and specific for the diagnosis of many functional gastrointestinal disorders.[26–28] The Rome III criteria for constipation requires having at least two of the following: (1) straining during ≥25% defecation; (2) lumpy or hard stools in ≥25% of defecation; (3) sensation of incomplete evacuation in ≥25% of defecation; (4) sensation of anorectal obstruction/blockage in ≥25% of defecation; (5) need for manual maneuvers to facilitate in ≥25% of defecation; and (6) fewer than three defecations per week (Box 150.3). The Rome IV diagnostic questionnaire was recently validated, and further excludes patients with opioid-induced constipation and irritable bowel syndrome from the diagnosis of functional constipation.[28] Patients presenting with constipation can have a multitude of symptoms; the investigations should be guided by the symptoms described and recent medical/surgical events in formulating a treatment plan. A bowel diary focused on dietary intake, defecation frequency, stool consistency, and any associated symptoms can be helpful to both the patient and the medical provider to formulate a treatment plan. Those with recent change in bowel habits or bleeding per rectum, especially if over age 50, should be considered for a colonoscopy.

PHYSICAL EXAMINATION (BOX 150.4)

Following a meticulous history, a physical exam should be performed in a stepwise manner. The general exam should be undertaken to detect any systemic disease that may be contributing to the patient's symptoms, including palpation of the patient's lymph node basins and assessment of the thyroid gland. Blood work, including a complete metabolic panel, calcium, blood glucose, and thyroid hormone levels is recommended.

An abdominal examination including documenting previous surgical scars should be performed. Abdominal distention or the presence of a mass may be noted.

Simple inspection of the perineal area can be informative. Inspect for scarring, excoriation, erythema, soiling, anal sphincter shape, the bulk of the perineal body, any skin tags or signs of inflammatory bowel disease, flattering of the perineum, hemorrhoids, or overt rectal prolapse. Ask the patient to strain and assess for pelvic floor descent and for prolapse. To fully evaluate prolapse, the patient should simulate evacuation on the toilet or commode.

Vaginal examination, both at rest and with strain, should be completed. Prolapse of pelvic organs should be elicited with strain and graded using a validated instrument such as the Pelvic Organ Prolapse Quantification System (POPQ) or the Baden-Walker system.[29]

Examination of the anus includes observation of scars and assessment of tone. Digital assessment should note any obvious anal pathology such as a mass, sphincter tone (at rest and squeeze), and muscle mass and any palpable sphincter defects.

Rectal examination should involve a clinical evaluation of resting tone and the ability to voluntarily contract and relax the anal sphincter. Evaluation for pelvic floor dysfunction such as perineal descent with straining, the presence of a rectocele or cystocele, and the volume and consistency of stool in the rectal vault should be noted. Stool load and consistency should also be documented.

BOX 150.4 Elements of the Physical Exam

- General
- Abdominal
- Perineum
- Vagina
- Anus
- Rectum

Levator ani and puborectalis muscles can also be assessed. It is important to differentiate sphincter contraction from puborectalis movement. Proctoscopy should be performed to help exclude neoplasia or undiagnosed inflammatory conditions and may also identify solitary rectal ulcers, hemorrhoids, and fissures. Anoscopy and sigmoidoscopy are options that can be performed to help confirm a diagnosis based on physical exam findings.

EVALUATIONS

Pregnancy testing is considered for all women of childbearing age before any invasive testing is carried out. Thyroid and calcium levels are evaluated for metabolic etiology of bowel disorders. Colonoscopy and gastrointestinal contrast studies should be considered to rule out functional etiologies, inflammatory bowel disease, and malignancy. Stool microscopy and cultures, colonoscopy, and gastroenterologist referral can be considered for patients with diarrhea.

Anorectal Manometry

Anorectal manometry (ARM) is a technique for measuring existing pressures and reflexes in the rectum and anus at rest and when elicited by stimulation. The indications for ARM are evaluation of incontinence to determine whether a sphincter defect exists and can be quantified, assessment of constipation and chronic pelvic pain syndromes to determine whether abnormal pressures exist, diagnosis of Hirschsprung disease, where loss of the rectoanal inhibitory reflex (RAIR) is pathognomonic, and to establish a baseline before an anorectal procedure or low pelvic anastomosis. Usefulness of ARM in clinical practice is currently debated due to operator dependency and inconsistent interpretation of results. Balloon expulsion provides the best current modality for the diagnosis of dyssynergic defecation.[30] The technique to perform the evaluation is either a "station" or continuous pull-through.

Equipment. The ARM equipment consists of several essential components: the catheter probe, the transducers, the recorder, and the hydraulic pump for water infusion methods. The system, catheters, and techniques used to perform ARM vary, but all elicit common parameters to evaluate the pelvic floor. ARM is performed using either water perfusion or solid-state catheter probes. The catheters are also either open-tipped or side opening. The most popular type is the water-perfusion side opening catheter probe, which is relatively inexpensive, durable, and easy to use. With this probe catheter, water is slowly perfused through the side holes, and pressure resistance of the sphincter is exerted against the holes. The simplest catheters have four holes at the same level on the probe; this circumferential array will show asymmetry within the anal canal. A balloon is attached to the catheter tip, and the balloon is inflated from a central channel in the tube to elicit rectal reflexes or sensation. Each of the side holes has an individual channel that can be connected to a transducer, and the mechanical water pressure is transmitted to the transducer. For the solid-state catheter probe, the sensors are located at the same level on the catheter, and a balloon is attached to the tip. When inflated, the sensor located at the tip within the balloon measures the pressures within the rectum. The sensors are wired to a computer for digital and graphical readout of the pressure measurements. The steady state is expensive and fragile, but it gives the most accurate, reproducible results. Transducers are an essential part of the water-perfusion system, where the mechanical water pressure is changed to electrical signals in the transducer. Each perfusion channel has a side channel that connects to a transducer, and when water is perfused through the side channels, it also transmits pressures back to individual transducers. In the water perfusion method, the water-perfusion machine is an integral component. The water is driven through each of the individual side channels in the tube at a chosen rate; as the water flows through the holes near the tip pressure changes are measured. The recorder is typically a computerized system with a small amplifier. A monitor is attached to observe the tracings as the procedure is performed, and specialized software displays the results through charts, tables, and graphical printouts.

Readings. ARM is focused on the distal 5 cm of the anorectum, which contains the sphincter muscles. The variables most frequently measured are the resting, squeeze, and strain anal pressure; RAIR; rectal sensation and compliance; and the balloon expulsion tests to look for baseline strength and strength with effort, sensation, discrimination, compliance, fatigue, and paradox. It is not possible to separate the puborectalis muscle from the external anal sphincter (EAS). However, the internal sphincter and the external sphincter may be individually analyzed based on the pressures represented by the resting tone and the squeeze pressure. The resting pressure reflects the internal sphincter function, as this muscle contributes between 55% and 85% of resting pressure, and the squeeze pressure reflects external sphincter function.[31] Because of the lack of methodological standardization, normal ranges vary between laboratories; however, a normal baseline resting pressure can be accepted as 40 mm Hg, and a normal squeeze pressure as double the resting pressure, or 80 mm Hg (Fig. 150.2). Rectal sensation can be recorded by using a balloon inserted into the rectum and recording the volume of first sensation as the balloon is filled (rectal sensory threshold), sensation of fullness (first urge to defecate), and maximum tolerated volume (how much volume can be placed into the balloon where the patient feels they can stand no more). Rectal sensation can be altered by pathologies such as inflammation or radiation therapy, which decrease rectal compliance and tolerated volumes. Increased tolerable volumes can be found in disorders such as megarectum or neurogenic abnormalities. Rectal sensory threshold has been shown to be valuable for determining whether biofeedback will be successful.[32]

The RAIR is normally elicited by inflating a balloon in the rectum while measuring anal manometry. Normally rapid rectal distention will lead to a brief increase in anal tone followed by a reflex internal anal sphincter (IAS) relaxation. This reflex is absent in Hirschsprung disease and immediately postoperatively following a low anterior resection or coloanal anastomosis. In the presence of a megarectum, a greater volume of rectal distention is required to elicit the reflex, which can lead to false-negative results.

The balloon expulsion test is usually performed using a 50-mL water-filled balloon and provides a simple baseline

Resting average (mm Hg)

	Post	Right	Anter.	Left	Max	Mean	HPZ
60cm	53	70	41	62	70	57	X
50cm	61	69	34	65	69	57	X
40cm	59	62	32	58	62	53	X
30cm	65	70	47	60	70	60	X
20cm	69	98	83	99	99	87	X
10cm	55	87	70	82	87	73	X

Squeeze increase (mm Hg)

	Post	Right	Anter.	Left	Max	Mean
60cm	67	60	43	56	67	57
50cm	48	30	30	35	48	36
40cm	57	52	51	52	57	53
30cm	57	29	25	43	57	38
20cm	29	42	34	32	42	34
10cm	39	50	38	45	50	43

Squeeze overall (mm Hg)

	Post	Right	Anter.	Left	Max	Mean
60cm	121	133	86	119	133	115
50cm	109	100	66	101	109	94
40cm	120	117	84	113	120	109
30cm	122	97	72	103	122	98
20cm	90	130	107	84	130	113
10cm	103	144	108	85	144	120

FIGURE 150.2 Normal anorectal manometry readings.

test for defecation. If the patient can expel the balloon in less than 1 minute, then it is less likely that defecatory dysfunction exists, although the test has been reported to have a sensitivity of about 97%.[33] Balloon expulsion testing can also validate the diagnosis of pelvic floor outlet obstruction caused by nonrelaxation of the puborectalis muscle.[34]

Neurophysiologic Assessment

Neurophysiologic assessment is made with electromyography (EMG) to evaluate neuromuscular activity of striated muscles (Fig. 150.3). EMG is performed using a recording needle electrode inserted into the muscle or surface electrodes placed on the surface of the muscle to evaluate accessory activity. EMG can highlight neuropathic or myopathic injury of the EAS and levator ani muscles. In sphincter injury, when muscle is replaced by scar tissue, no insertional activity is encountered. Furthermore, in denervation injury, the maximum voluntary activity is diminished.[35] EMG has also been found to help predict outcomes of surgery for fecal incontinence.[36] Gee et al. found in patients undergoing surgery for fecal incontinence, those with an increased jitter on EMG—a measure of progressive denervation and reinnervation—were associated with a poor surgical outcome compared with patients with normal jitter.[36] EMG of the pelvic floor can provide complementary information for the pelvic floor dysfunction evaluation, and is a specific test for identifying muscle injury.

Pudendal Nerve Motor Terminal Latency

Pudendal nerve motor terminal latency (PNMTL) measures the nerve conduction time along the terminal portion of the pudendal nerve, quantifying the time it takes for the external sphincter to contract after stimulation of

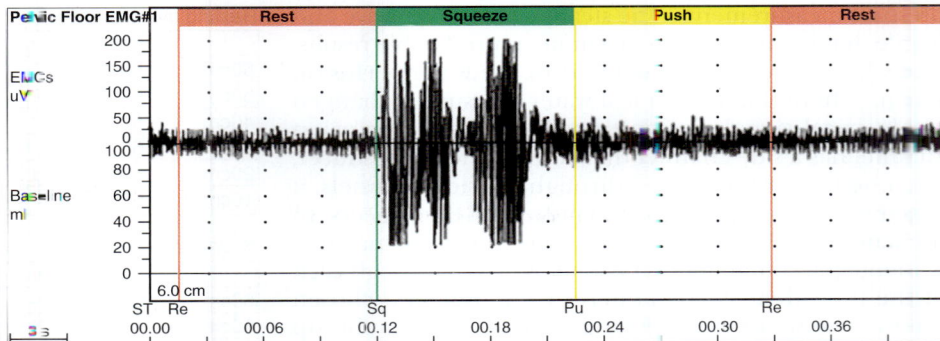

FIGURE 150.3 Normal electromyography study.

the pudendal nerve. The PNMTL test is performed by stimulating the pudendal nerve at the ischial spine with a finger-mounted St. Mark's electrode and recording the conduction time to the sphincter.[37] The technique described by Kiff and Swash entails a square wave stimulus of 50 V and 8 mA with a duration of 0.1 ms delivered to both the right and left pudendal nerves to elicit external sphincter contraction; five latencies were recorded for each nerve.[38] Normal PNTML established at less than 2.4 ms and prolongation is reflective of nerve damage. Abnormal PNTML has been associated with an underlying neuropathy in fecal incontinence patients and predictive of failure after sphincteroplasty.[38–40] However, the overall value of PNTML has been questioned. As the test evaluates the function of the fastest remaining nerve fiber, incomplete nerve injuries can be missed with this study, and the significance of an undetectable PNTML is uncertain. The authors recommend the test in conjunction with other studies for the best diagnostic picture.

Endoanal Ultrasound

While combinations of studies are used for the most accurate diagnosis of pelvic floor dysfunction, EUS may be the most valuable single tool. With EUS, the anatomy, integrity, and function of the pelvic floor can be evaluated. The technique of EUS was first described in 1989, where the sonographic anatomy of five layers of the anal canal were described: mucosa submucosa, IAS, intersphincteric plane, and EAS.[41] On ultrasound, highly reflective tissues give a white hyperechoic image, and poorly reflective tissues give a black, hypoechoic appearance. The internal sphincter contains a large amount of water and allows the ultrasound waves to easily pass through, appearing black (hypoechoic), while the EAS appears white (hyperechoic). Several studies have defined the normal sonographic anatomy, and divisions of the anal canal on EUS, which can be used as a benchmark for abnormal studies.[42–45] The anal canal is divided into three levels: the upper level is defined by the presence of the puborectalis muscle, a horseshoe-shaped mixed-echogenic structure in the posterolateral portion (Fig. 150.4). The middle anal canal has both the hypoechoic external sphincter and hyperechoic internal sphincter muscles. Perineal body measurements can be made at the level by placing the right index finger into the vagina against the rectovaginal septum and ultrasound probe (Fig. 150.5). The distance between the hyperechoic ultrasound reflection of the

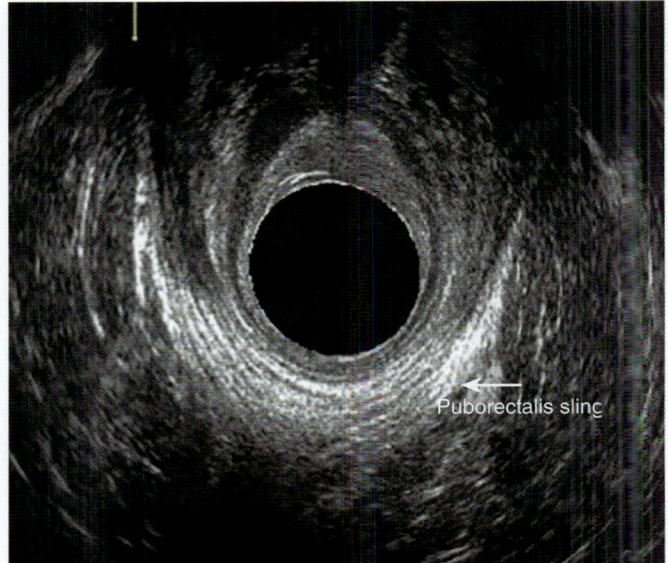

FIGURE 150.4 Endoanal ultrasound of the upper anal canal demonstrating the puborectalis muscle.

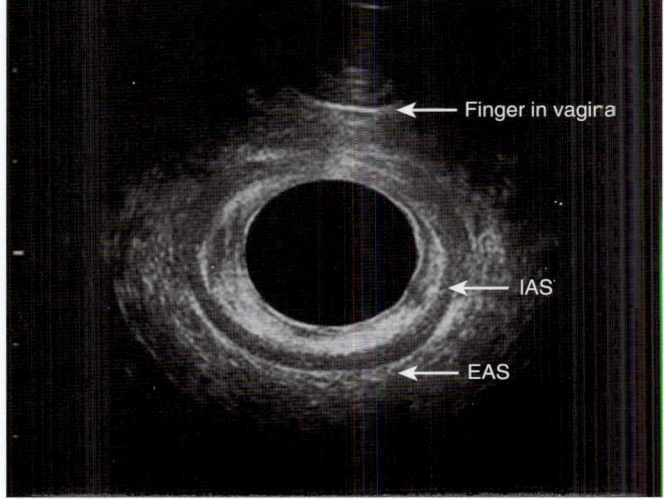

FIGURE 150.5 Endoanal ultrasound of midanal canal measuring perineal body thickness. *EAS,* External anal sphincter; *IAS,* internal anal sphincter.

finger and the inner aspect of the IAS represents the perineal body thickness (PBT); the normal range is from 10 to 12 mm.[46] The length of the anal canal varies from an average of 25 mm for women to 33 mm for men.[47] In the lower canal, the IAS is no longer seen; only the most distal portion of the hyperechoic EAS is visualized. Age changes the anatomy of the anal sphincters. The normal IAS is 2 to 3 mm thick but tends to become thicker with age,[45] while the normal EAS is 7 to 9 mm thick and becomes thinner with age.[48] Additionally, there are gender-specific differences in EUS; the sonographer should be aware of these to avoid inaccurate interpretation of images. For instance, in women, the anterior part of the EAS is shorter and slopes downward, which could lead to the incorrect diagnosis of an anterior sphincter defect.[48] The anococcygeal ligament appears as a hypoechoic triangular structure posteriorly and can be confused as a posterior sphincter defect in both men and women.

EUS results have been found to correlate well with clinical, manometric, operative and histologic findings.[49] Using histologic anatomy as the "gold standard," Sultan et al. validated the sonographic images of EAS defects as 100% accurate when compared with clinical assessment by colorectal surgeons (50%), manometry (75%), and EMG (75%).[48] Specific sphincter injuries found on ultrasound have been found to be highly associated with manometric findings, with EAS defects manifesting as lower anal squeeze pressures and IAS defects with lower resting pressures.[49] The validity of EUS images were also proven by evaluating IAS defects before and after lateral internal sphincterotomy.[50]

Several variations of EUS are available. With standard two-dimensional EUS (2DUS), assessment can be made of the EAS and IAS complex integrity, the puborectalis muscle, length, thickness, and any asymmetry and sphincter defects. 2DUS is usually performed with the patient in the left lateral decubitus or prone position using a 7- or 10-MHz rotating endoprobe scanner, providing a 360-degree view of the anal canal.[51-52] The probe is inserted to approximately 6 cm and then withdrawn down the anal canal while cross-sectional images are obtained. 2DUS only generates cross-sectional images in the axial plane but remains the mainstay of sphincter evaluation.[41] With three-dimensional ultrasonography (3DUS), a functional and anatomic assessment is seen, showing the downward displacement of pelvic organs on strain, the development of prolapse, the opening of fascial or muscular defects and the effect of a contraction and Valsalva on the levator hiatus (Fig. 150.6). Studies are limited but have demonstrated that the sensitivity of detecting both internal and external sphincter defects is comparable between the 2D and 3D studies, but interobserver variation is decreased and diagnostic accuracy is increased with the 3D imaging.[53] Additionally, Gold et al. created 3D reconstructions in 20 controls and 24 patients suffering fecal incontinence with sphincter injuries seen on regular EUS, finding that 3DUS could demonstrate the radial angle of the IAS and EAS defects better than with standard 2DUS.[45] 3DUS has become more widely available in recent years and may further the value of ultrasound for pelvic floor assessment. Dynamic transperineal ultrasound (TPUS) also provides a functional and anatomic assessment, combining sagittal

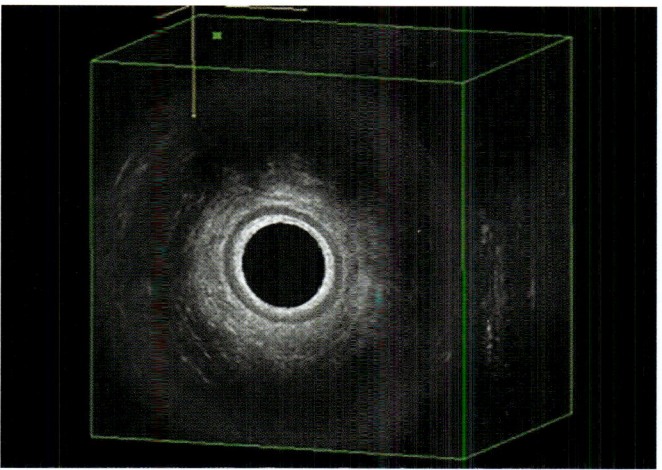

FIGURE 150.6 Three-dimensional endoanal ultrasound of the midanal canal.

and transverse transperineal images to assess evacuatory disorders and pelvic floor dysfunction. TPUS is usually performed with the patient placed in the dorsal lithotomy position, with the hips flexed and abducted, and the convex transducer positioned on the perineum between the mons pubis and the anal sphincter.[4] This modality visualizes the pelvic floor and perineum both at rest and with straining, allowing easy identification of the anal sphincters, puborectalis contraction, the anorectal angle, and any rectoceles, enteroceles, or rectoanal intussusceptions that previously required both EUS and defecography.[54] Studies have demonstrated the sensitivity of detecting both internal and external sphincter defects is comparable between the 2DUS and TPUS,[52,55] and TPUS may add value in cases of active perianal pathology or an equivocal 2DUS study.[56,57]

Defecography

Defecography is a dynamic test performed by instilling contrast into the rectum (and occasionally orally and per vagina and/or bladder) and taking video and still films at rest, during strain, and during the act of defecation. The patient is seated on a special commode behind a screen. The radiographs can be taken through the screen for this study while the patient performs the aforementioned acts of defecation. Measurements can include the anorectal angle (the angle between the longitudinal axis of the anal canal and the posterior wall of the lower part of the rectum), the ability to fully empty the rectum, the degree of perineal descent, rectoceles, enteroceles, sigmoidoceles anismus, and intussusception. There is a large amount of overlap in the findings between what is considered normal and abnormal, and all findings need to be considered in the setting of clinical symptoms (Figs. 150.7 to 150.10). As defecography facilitates visualization of the mechanism of defecation it aids identifying outlet obstruction disorders of defecation, such as nonrelaxing puborectalis, intussusception, or a large rectocele, enterocele, or sigmoidocele.[58] Four-contrast defecography (vagina, bladder, small intestine, rectum, and cul de sac as needed) defines each compartment of the pelvis.

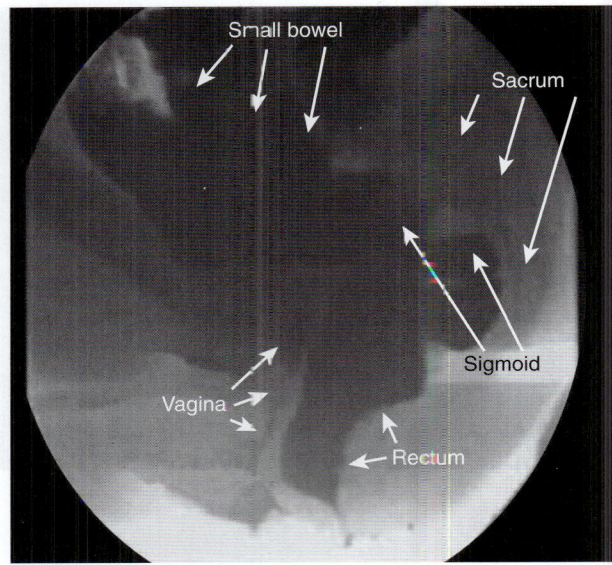

FIGURE 150.7 Defecogram showing normal anatomy. (With permission from Cleveland Clinic.)

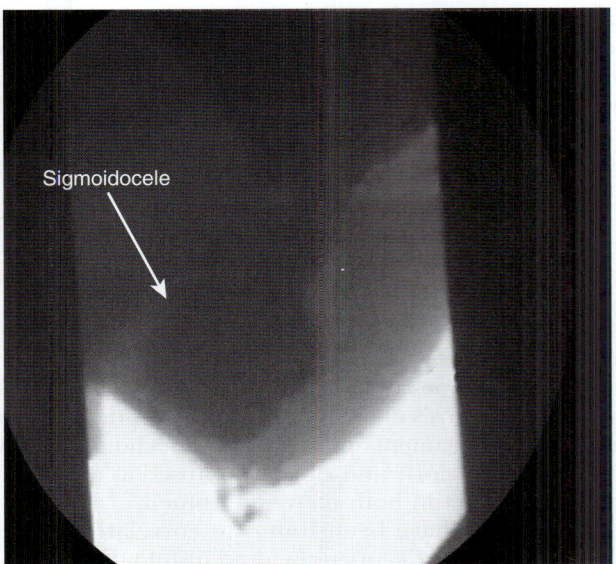

FIGURE 150.9 Defecogram demonstrating a sigmoidocele. (With permission from Cleveland Clinic.)

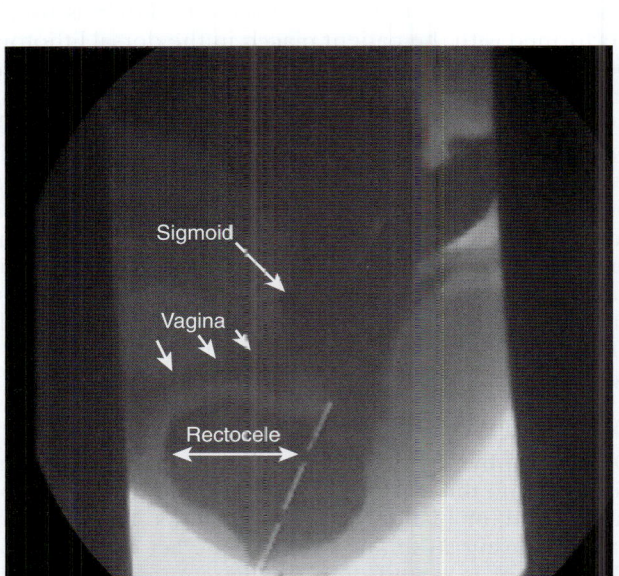

FIGURE 150.8 Defecogram demonstrating a rectocele. (With permission from Cleveland Clinic.)

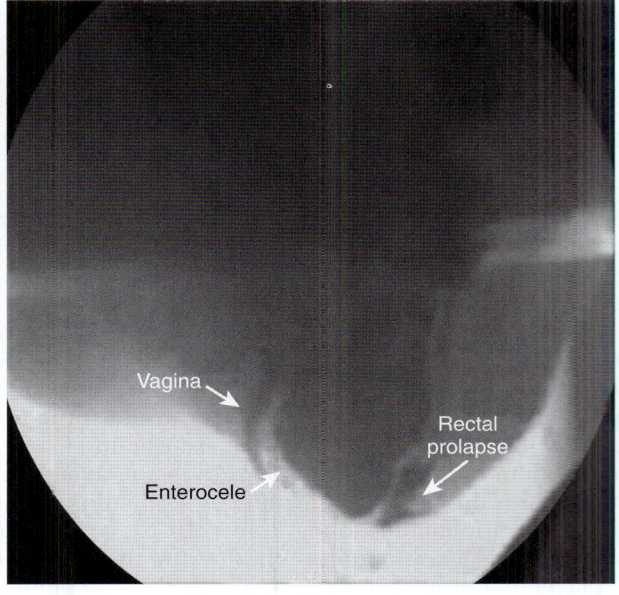

FIGURE 150.10 Defecogram demonstrating an enterocele and rectal prolapse. (With permission from Cleveland Clinic.)

Magnetic Resonance Imaging

Magnetic resonance imaging (MRI) is a promising, comprehensive tool to assess the structure and function of pelvic floor disorders. MRI may provide insights into the mechanisms of normal and dysfunctional pelvic floor anatomy and function.[39] Superior soft tissue contrast resolution allows direct visualization of the pelvic organs and their supportive structures in a single noninvasive examination. Studies have shown MRI is as accurate as EUS for identifying defects and thinning of the internal sphincter and may be better at identifying thinning of the external sphincter and puborectalis, which may correlate

with poor results after sphincteroplasty (Fig. 150.11).[60–62] MRI offers the added value of allowing visualization of all three pelvic floor compartments before undergoing pelvic floor surgery, benefiting patients who have symptoms in multiple compartments.

Dynamic Magnetic Resonance Imaging

An extension of the MRI study is dynamic MRI—also known as MR defecography (MRD) or MRI proctography. While MRI can be used for static studies to assess anatomy, dynamic studies can be used to also assess pelvic floor function. Dynamic MRI can be a valuable alternative to

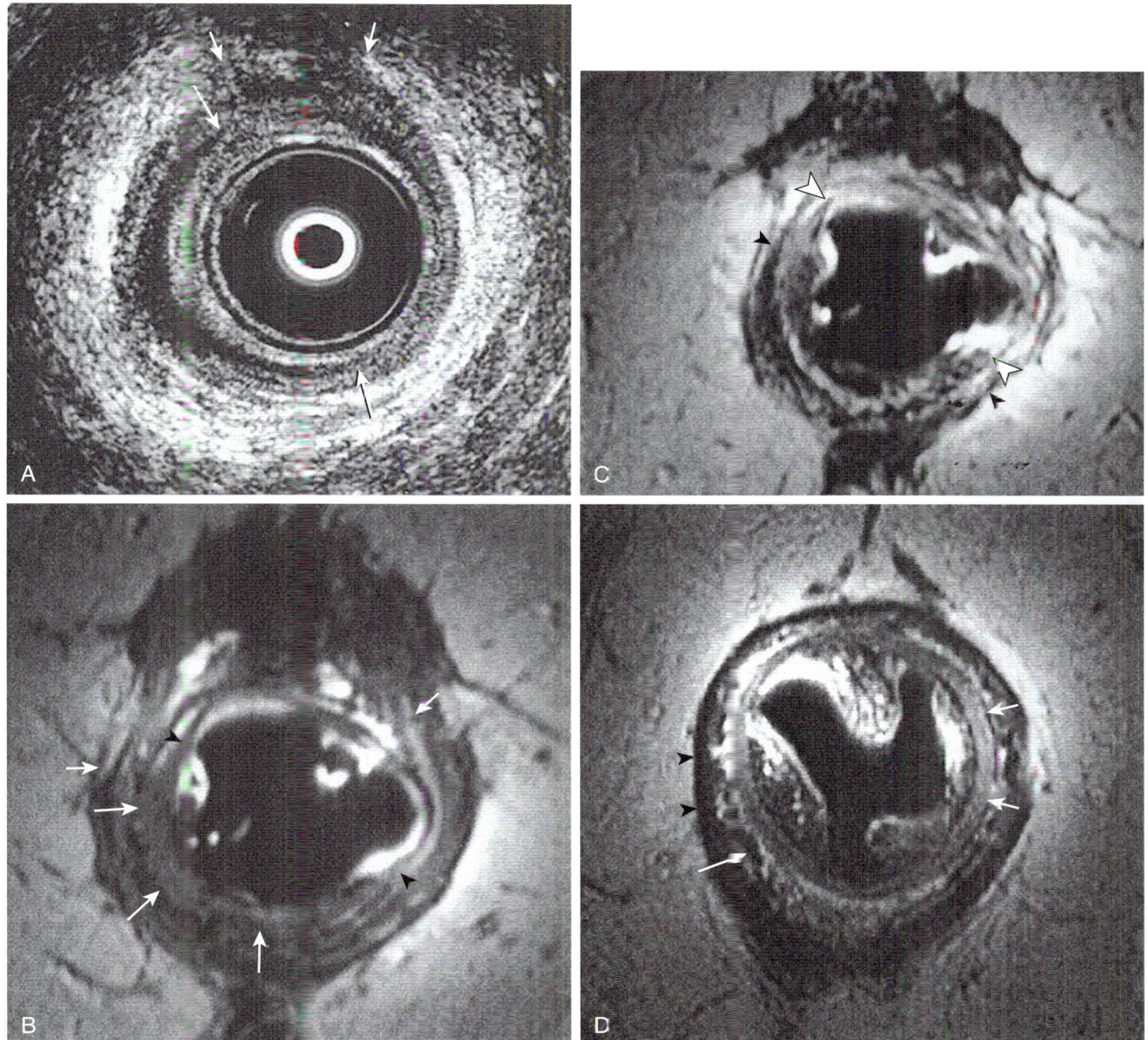

FIGURE 150.11 Endoanal ultrasound (A) and magnetic resonance images (MRIs) of anal sphincters (B to D). (A) The internal anal sphincter is thin and partially torn between 10 o'clock and 5 o'clock *(long arrows)*. The external anal sphincter tear is between the *short arrows*. (B) The same defect is seen on MRI. The intact internal anal sphincter is visible *(long white arrows)*; the internal anal sphincter defect is seen between the black arrowheads; and the external anal sphincter tear is seen between 1 o'clock and 2 o'clock *(small white arrows)*. (C) Axial endoanal MRI at a more caudal level demonstrates abnormalities in the internal anal sphincter *(between large white arrowheads)* and the external anal sphincter *(between small black arrowheads)*. (D) Axial endoanal MRI demonstrating a normal study of the internal anal sphincter *(short white arrows)*, longitudinal muscle *(long white arrow)*, and external anal sphincter *(black arrowheads)*. (From Fletcher MD. Magnetic resonance imaging of anatomic and dynamic defects of the pelvic floor in defecatory disorders. *Am J Gastroenterol.* 2003;98[2]:399–411, Fig. 1BCD, p. 404; Copyright 2003 American College of Gastroenterology.)

standard defecography for the evaluation of pelvic floor anatomy and dysfunction, including prolapse, incontinence, pelvic pain, and constipation.[63,64] Dynamic MRI evaluates all compartments of the pelvic floor and pelvic motion in real time in contrast to standard single-contrast defecography, which can only visualize the posterior compartment. There is also no ionizing radiation and no bowel preparation is needed. The fast-phase sequences allow for quick evaluation with increased patient comfort, decreased complexity, and decreased invasiveness.[65] Images are taken at rest, at maximal voluntary contraction of the sphincter and pelvic floor muscles (squeezing), at straining, and at evacuation for the presence and degree of posterior compartment descent, rectal and uterovaginal prolapse, cystocele, urethral hypermobility, rectocele, rectal intussusception, and enterocele. The exam is somewhat

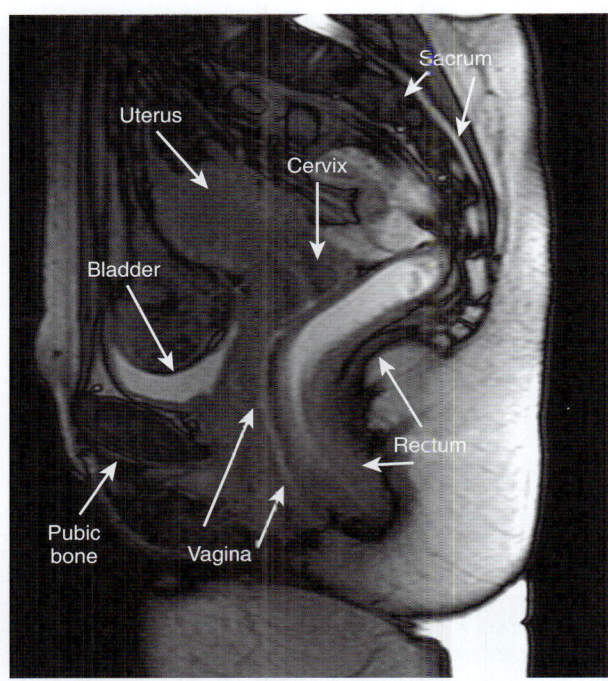

FIGURE 150.12 Normal dynamic magnetic resonance imaging. (With permission from Cleveland Clinic.)

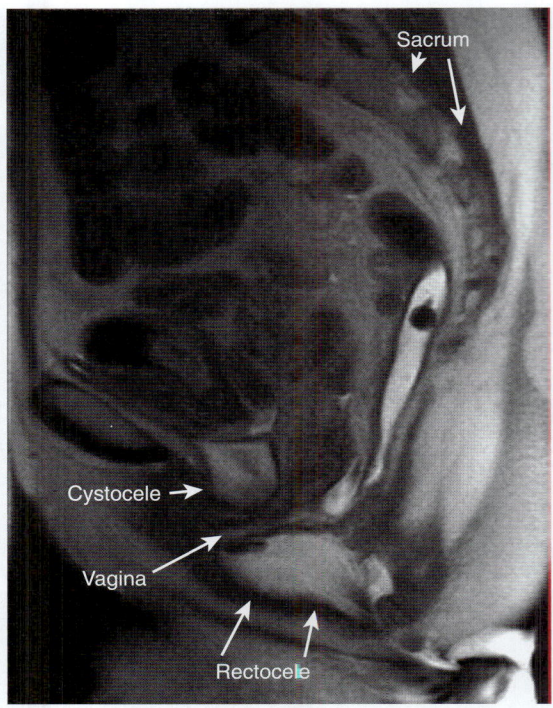

FIGURE 150.13 Dynamic magnetic resonance imaging showing a rectocele and cystocele. (With permission from Cleveland Clinic.)

limited by supine positioning of the patient. The images further allow measurement of the anorectal angle on straining, which can be used to diagnose paradoxical contraction of the puborectalis muscle (anismus). Despite the benefits, dynamic MRI is not widely used mainly due to limited availability, high cost of the test, and issues with reimbursement (Figs. 150.12 and 150.13).

Transit Studies

The mean transit time through the entire colon has been shown to be 31 hours in males and 39 hours in women.[65] Colonic transit time can be measured by using ingested radiopaque markers (SITZMARKS; Konsyl Pharmaceutials, Easton, MD). There are many protocols used to perform the study, but all essentially evaluate the number of markers that remain on simple abdominal radiographs 5 days after marker ingestion. The type of constipation can be ascertained by the pattern of marker distribution where patients with slow transit constipation will have more than 20% of ingested markers retained but scattered throughout the colon on day 5, while those with outlet obstruction constipation will have the majority of markers moved successfully to rectum and rectosigmoid area by day 5 but are unable to evacuate them. Patients with pelvic floor dysfunction can have coexisting slow transit constipation, and some authors have noted normalization in the transit time with correction of outflow problems.

Scintigraphy

Scintigraphy is an option to assess the mobility of the entire gastrointestinal system. Although not as widely available, it is useful in the assessment of transit in the colon and proximal gut. Transit times obtained through scintigraphy

are generated following consumption of a radiolabeled egg sandwich, and individual times are generated for the stomach, small bowel, and colon. These tests add value in surgical planning for slow transit constipation to ensure that the dysfunction is limited to the colon and does not affect the proximal gastrointestinal tract. Normal small bowel transit is between 90 and 120 minutes.

MANAGEMENT OF PELVIC FLOOR DISORDERS

The specific management of fecal incontinence, rectal prolapse, and constipation are discussed elsewhere in the textbook (see Chapters 148, 149, and 152).

CONCLUSION

Pelvic floor disorders are complex, common, and are overall poorly understood. A careful history and examination is essential. This initial step allows clarification of symptoms and physical findings and allows tailored investigational planning. The results of testing then can assist in planning therapy. Not all patients will be surgical candidates; however, a thoughtful work-up may increase the likelihood of symptomatic improvement after surgery.

REFERENCES

1. Segen's Medical Dictionary; 2011. http://medical-dictionary.thefreedictionary.com/pelvic+floor. Accessed 14 April 2016.
2. Daftary S, Chakravarti S. *Manual of Obstetrics*. 3rd ed. Philadelphia: Elsevier; 2011:1-16.

3. Schaffer JI, Clifford WY, Boreham M. Etiology of pelvic organ prolapse. *Clin Obstet Gynecol.* 2005;4 (3):639-647.

4. Nygaard I, Barber MD, Burgio KL, et al. Prevalence of symptomatic pelvic floor disorders in US women. *JAMA.* 2008;300 1311-1316.

5. MacLennan AH, Taylor AW, Wilson DH, Wilson D. The prevalence of pelvic floor disorders and their relationship to gender, age, parity and mode of delivery. *BJOG.* 2000;107:1460-1470.

6. Kepenekci I, Keskinkilic B, Akinsu F, et al. Prevalence of pelvic floor disorders in the female population and the impact of age, mode of delivery, and parity. *Dis Colon Rectum.* 2011;54:85-94.

7. Shamliyan T, Wyman J, Bliss DZ, Kane RL, Wilt TJ. Prevention of urinary and fecal incontinence in adults. *Evid Rep Technol Assess (Full Rep).* 2007;161:1-379.

8. Hunskaar S, Lose G, Sykes D, Voss S. The prevalence of urinary incontinence in women in four European countries. *BJU Int.* 2004;93:324-330.

9. Nelson R, Norton N, Cautley E, Furner S. Community-based prevalence of anal incontinence. *JAMA.* 1995;274:559-561.

10. Varma A, Gunn J, Gardiner A, Lindow SW, Duthie GS. Obstetric anal sphincter injury: prospective evaluation of incidence. *Dis Colon Rectum.* 1999;42:1537-1543.

11. Lewis SJ, Heaton KW. Stool form scale as a useful guide to intestinal transit time. *Scand J Gastroenterol.* 1997;32:920-924.

12. Rockwood TH, Church JM, Fleshman JW, et al. Fecal Incontinence Quality of Life Scale: quality of life instrument for patients with fecal incontinence. *Dis Colon Rectum.* 2000;43:9-16, discussion 16–17.

13. Baxter NN, Rothenberger DA, Lowry AC. Measuring fecal incontinence. *Dis Colon Rectum.* 2003;46:1591-1605.

14. Jorge JM, Wexner SD. Etiology and management of fecal incontinence. *Dis Colon Rectum.* 1993;36:77-97.

15. Frank L, Kleinman L, Farup C, Taylor L. Miner PJ. Psychometric validation of a constipation symptom assessment questionnaire. *Scand J Gastroenterol.* 1999;34:870-877.

16. Maeda Y, Vaizey CJ, Norton C. St. Mark's incontinence score. *Dis Colon Rectum.* 2007;50:2252.

17. Agachan F, Chen T, Pfeifer J, Reissman P, Wexner SD. A constipation scoring system to simplify evaluation and management of constipated patients. *Dis Colon Rectum.* 1996;39:681-685.

18. Wang JY, Varma MG. Measures for fecal incontinence, constipation, and associated quality of life. *Semin Colon Rectal Surg.* 2010;21 22.

19. Nusrat S, Gulick E, Levinthal D, Bielefeldt K. Anorectal dysfunction in multiple sclerosis: a systematic review. *ISRN Neurol.* 2012;2012:376023.

20. National Collaborating Centre for Acute Care. *Faecal Incontinence: the Management of Faecal Incontinence in Adults.* London: National Collaborating Centre for Acute Care (UK); 2007.

21. Baeten CG, Kuijpers HC. Fecal incontinence. In: Wolff BG, et al., eds. *The ASCRS Textbook of Colon and Rectal Surgery.* New York: Springer; 2007:653-664.

22. Higgins PD, Johanson JF. Epidemiology of constipation in North America: a systematic review. *Am J Gastroenterol.* 2004;99:750-759.

23. Drossman DA, Sandler RS, McKee DC, Lovitz AJ. Bowel patterns among subjects not seeking health care. Use of a questionnaire to identify a population with bowel dysfunction. *Gastroenterology.* 1982;83:529-534.

24. Heaton KW, Radvan J, Cripps H, Mountford RA, Braddon FE, Hughes AO. Defecation frequency and timing, and stool form in the general population: a prospective study. *Gut.* 1992;33:818-824.

25. Leung L, Riutta T, Kotecha J, Rosser W. Chronic constipation: an evidence-based review. *J Am Board Fam Med.* 2011;24:436-451.

26. Longstreth GF, Thompson WG, Chey WD, Houghton LA, Mearin F, Spiller RC. Functional bowel disorders. *Gastroenterology.* 2006;130:1480-1491.

27. Drossman DA. Rome III: the new criteria. *Chin J Dig Dis.* 2006;7:181-185.

28. Palsson OS, Whitehead WE, van Tilburg MA, et al. Rome IV diagnostic questionnaire and tables for investigators and clinicians. *Gastroenterology.* 2016 Feb 13 [Epub ahead of print].

29. Muir TW, Stepp KJ, Barber MD. Adoption of the pelvic organ prolapse quantification system in peer-reviewed literature. *Am J Obstet Gynecol.* 2003;189:1632-1635, discussion 1635–1636.

30. Staller K. Role of anorectal manometry in clinical practice. *Curr Treat Options Gastroenterol.* 2015;13:418-431.

31. Henry M, Swash M. *Coloproctology and the Pelvic Floor.* 2nd ed. Oxford, England: Butterworth-Heinemann; 1992.

32. Barnett JL, Hasler WL, Camilleri M. American Gastroenterological Association: medical position statement on anorectal testing techniques. *Gastroenterology.* 1999;116 732.

33. Minguez M, Herreros B, Sanchiz V, et al. Predictive value of the balloon expulsion test for excluding the diagnosis of pelvic floor dyssynergia in constipation. *Gastroenterology.* 2004;126:57-62.

34. Fleshman JW, Dreznik Z, Cohen E, Fry RD, Kodner IJ. Balloon expulsion test facilitates diagnosis of pelvic floor outlet obstruction due to nonrelaxing puborectalis muscle. *Dis Colon Rectum.* 1992;35:1019-1025.

35. Kumar A, Rao SS. Diagnostic testing in fecal incontinence. *Curr Gastroenterol Rep.* 2003;5:406-413.

36. Gee AS, Durdey P. Preoperative increase in neuromuscular jitter and outcome following surgery for faecal incontinence. *Br J Surg.* 1997;84:1265-1268.

37. Laurberg S, Swash M, Snooks SJ. Henry MM. Neurologic cause of idiopathic incontinence. *Arch Neurol* 1988;45:1250-1253.

38. Kiff ES, Swash M. Slowed conduction in the pudendal nerves in idiopathic (neurogenic) faecal incontinence. *Br J Surg.* 1984;71:614-616.

39. Barisic G, Krivokapic Z, Markovic V, Popovic M, Saranovic D, Marsavelska A. The role of overlapping sphincteroplasty in traumatic fecal incontinence. *Acta Chir Iugosl.* 2000;47:37-41.

40. Yip B, Barret RC, Coller JA, et al. Pudendal nerve terminal motor latency testing: assessing the educational learning curve: can we teach our own? *Dis Colon Rectum.* 2002;45:184-187.

41. Abdool Z, Sultan AH, Thakar R. Ultrasound imaging of the anal sphincter complex: a review. *Br J Radiol.* 2012;85:865-875.

42. Nivatvongs S, Stern HS, Fryd DS. The length of the anal canal. *Dis Colon Rectum.* 1981;24:600-601.

43. Nielsen MB, Hauge C, Rasmussen OO, Sorensen M, Pedersen JF, Christiansen J. Anal sphincter size measured by endosonography in healthy volunteers. Effect of age, sex, and parity. *Acta Radiol.* 1992;33:453-456.

44. Sultan AH, Nicholls RJ, Kamm MA, Hudson CN, Beynon J, Bartram CI. Anal endosonography and correlation with in vitro and in vivo anatomy. *Br J Surg.* 1993;80:508-511.

45. Burnett SJ, Bartram CI. Endosonographic variations in the normal internal anal sphincter. *Int J Colorectal Dis.* 1991;6:2-4.

46. Oberwalder M, Thaler K, Baig MK, et al. Anal ultrasound and endosonographic measurement of perineal body thickness: a new evaluation for fecal incontinence in females. *Surg Endosc.* 2004;18:650-654.

47. Gold DM, Bartram CI, Halligan S, Humphries KN, Kamm MA, Kmiot WA. Three-dimensional endoanal sonography in assessing anal canal injury. *Br J Surg.* 1999;86:365-370.

48. Sultan AH, Kamm MA, Hudson CN, Nicholls JR, Bartram CI. Endosonography of the anal sphincters: normal anatomy and comparison with manometry. *Clin Radiol.* 1994;49:368-374.

49. Sultan AH, Kamm MA, Bartram CI, Hudson CN. Anal sphincter trauma during instrumental delivery. *Int J Gynaecol Obstet.* 1993;43:263-270.

50. Sultan AH, Kamm MA, Nicholls RJ, Bartram CI. Prospective study of the extent of internal anal sphincter division during lateral sphincterotomy. *Dis Colon Rectum.* 1994;37:1031-1033.

51. Thakar R, Sultan AH. Anal endosonography and its role in assessing the incontinent patient. *Best Pract Res Clin Obstet Gynecol.* 2004;18:157-173.

52. Frudinger A, Bartram CI, Halligan S, Kamm M. Examination techniques for endosonography of the anal canal. *Abdom Imaging.* 1998;23:301-303.

53. Christensen AF, Nyhuus B, Nielsen MB, Christensen H. Three-dimensional anal endosonography may improve diagnostic confidence of detecting damage to the anal sphincter complex. *Br J Radiol.* 2005;78:308-311.

54. Beer-Gabel M, Teshler M, Barzilai N, et al. Dynamic transperineal ultrasound in the diagnosis of pelvic floor disorders: pilot study. *Dis Colon Rectum.* 2002;45:239-245, discussion 245–248.

55. Stewart LK, Wilson SR. Transvaginal sonography of the anal sphincter: reliable, or not? *AJR Am J Roentgenol* 1999 173:179-185.

56. Ramirez JM, Aguilella V, Martinez M, Gracia JA. The utility of endovaginal sonography in the evaluation of fecal incontinence. *Rev Esp Enferm Dig.* 2005;97:317-322.

57. Poen AC, Felt-Bersma RJ, Cuesta MA, Meuwissen GM. Vaginal endosonography of the anal sphincter complex is important in the assessment of faecal incontinence and perianal sepsis. *Br J Surg.* 1998;85:359-363.

58. Jorge JM, Wexner SD, Ger GC, Salanga VD, Nogueras JJ, Jagelman DG. Cinedefecography and electromyography in the diagnosis of nonrelaxing puborectalis syndrome. *Dis Colon Rectum*. 1993;36:668-676.

59. Fletcher JG, Busse RF, Riederer SJ, et al. Magnetic resonance imaging of anatomic and dynamic defects of the pelvic floor in defecatory disorders. *Am J Gastroenterol*. 2003;98:399-411.

60. Malouf AJ, Williams AB, Halligan S, Bartram CI, Dhillon S, Kamm MA. Prospective assessment of accuracy of endoanal MR imaging and endosonography in patients with fecal incontinence. *AJR Am J Roentgenol*. 2000;175:741-745.

61. Rociu E, Stoker J, Eijkemans MJ, Schouten WR, Lameris JS. Fecal incontinence: endoanal US versus endoanal MR imaging. *Radiology*. 1999;212:453-458.

62. Briel JW, Stoker J, Rociu E, Lameris JS, Hop WC, Schouten WR. External anal sphincter atrophy on endoanal magnetic resonance imaging adversely affects continence after sphincteroplasty. *Br J Surg*. 1999;86:1322-1327.

63. Healy JC, Halligan S, Reznek RH, et al. Dynamic MR imaging compared with evacuation proctography when evaluating anorectal configuration and pelvic floor movement. *AJR Am J Roentgenol*. 1997;169:775-779.

64. Goh V, Halligan S, Kaplan G, Healy JC, Bartram CI. Dynamic MR imaging of the pelvic floor in asymptomatic subjects. *AJR Am J Roentgenol*. 2000;174:661-666.

65. Kaufman HS, Buller JL, Thompson JR, et al. Dynamic pelvic magnetic resonance imaging and cystocolpoproctography alter surgical management of pelvic floor disorders. *Dis Colon Rectum*. 2001;44:1575-1583, discussion 1583-1584.

66. Metcalf A, Ross HM. Constipation. In: Beck DE, Wolfe BG, Fleshman JW, Pemberon JH, Wexner S, eds. *ASCRS Textbook*. 2nd ed. New York: Springer-Verlag; 2011:680.

Rectovaginal and Rectourethral Fistulas

Joshua I.S. Bleier | Robert Caleb Kovell

Fistulas between the genitourinary tract and the digestive tract present a particular conundrum for the surgeon. Not only are they uncommon, but the technical aspects of repair in conjunction with managing etiology appropriately present a multidisciplinary challenge to even the most experienced surgeon. Not only do they present particular issues with respect to quality of life but also complicated management of septic complications, management of radiated tissue, and the complicated dance of staged repair. In this chapter, we will discuss the aspects of diagnosis, classification, and management of rectovaginal and rectourethral fistulas (RUFs).

RECTOVAGINAL FISTULA

Rectovaginal fistulas (RVFs) are defined as epithelialized communications between the rectum and vagina. They are uncommon, comprising approximately 5% of all anorectal fistulas, but present a significant challenge for both the patient and the surgeon. Although they are rarely associated with mortality, they are associated with a significant degree of morbidity not only involving anatomic issues, but with a profound negative impact in quality of life from a social, psychological, and sexual point of view. Because of the rarity of RVFs, there is little well-described literature documenting systematic management, and the multiplicity of approaches highlights the fact that no single approach is uniformly successful.

ETIOLOGY

The causes of RVF are many, the most common being obstetric trauma. Approximately 2% of all vaginal deliveries are associated with advanced perineal injury, and 3% of these patients subsequently developed RVFs. These are typically associated with a prolonged second stage of labor resulting in ischemic necrosis of the rectovaginal septum. This is particularly common in developing countries where there is a lack of good obstetric care. RVFs are present in up to to 3.5 million women in Africa, with over 100,000 new cases each year.[1] Other risk factors include shoulder dystocia in the fetus, high forceps deliveries, third- and fourth-degree tears, and midline episiotomy. Worldwide, an RVF develops from every 1000 vaginal births.

Crohn disease is the next most common cause. Up to 10% of female patients with Crohn disease develop RVFs. These are associated with a very high recurrence rate, and it is not uncommon for multiple procedures to be required to help these patients. A multidisciplinary approach, including medical management to ensure quiescent anorectal disease, is critical. Other autoimmune diseases such as Behçet disease may also be associated with RVF.

Anorectal sepsis, arising from cryptoglandular infection, may also be associated with RVF. These are often a result of advanced anterior cryptoglandular infection. Other gastrointestinal (GI) infections, such as diverticulitis, may be associated with fistula to the vagina; however, these are colovaginal fistulas, arising almost exclusively in patients who have undergone hysterectomy when pelvic abscesses fistulize through the apex of the vaginal cuff. Other more rare infectious etiologies include tuberculosis, lymphogranuloma venereum, human immunodeficiency virus (HIV), and cytomegalovirus (CMV).

Iatrogenic causes of RVF are not uncommon after a variety of pelvic operations. These include sequelae of leak after low colorectal anastomosis in women, neoadjuvant radiation is a significant risk factor, and the treatment of rectal cancer is responsible for 13% of RVFs.[2] Urogynecologic procedures are also a risk factor; mesh erosion after pelvic organ prolapse repair may result in RVF. Leak after ileal J-pouch creation in the setting of ulcerative colitis or familial adenomatous polyposis (FAP) may lead to the development of a fistula. Spontaneous delayed presentation of pouch vaginal fistula is often a manifestation of previously unsuspected Crohn disease. RVF may also present as a complication of the procedure for prolapse and hemorrhoid (PPH) and the Starr procedure.

Pelvic malignancy with local invasion may also be an etiology of RVF. Often, the new development of a RVF may herald recurrent disease of cervical, rectal vaginal, or uterine cancer, especially after local radiation for palliation. This rate was as high as 18% in patients who received external beam radiotherapy using older radiation sources in addition to interstitial brachytherapy for advanced gynecologic malignancy.[3]

Other, less common causes include congenital fistula, mechanical necrosis of the rectovaginal septum due to fecal impaction and stercoral ulceration, long-standing pessary use, and trauma.

CLINICAL MANIFESTATIONS

The primary presenting symptom of RVF is the new passage of fecal material or gas through the vagina. This is often misdiagnosed as fecal incontinence or attributed to vaginal infection. Chronic urinary tract infection may also be an associated symptom. In patients who develop RVF as a result of obstetric injury, antecedent fecal incontinence is as high as 50%.[4] As a result, the presentation is often unclear, and likely a large number of these fistulas remain undiagnosed. If there are associated symptoms from the GI tract—including diarrhea, abdominal pain, or significant mucous discharge—inflammatory bowel disease may be suspected and an appropriate work-up should be undertaken. Regardless of the etiology, symptoms attributable to RVF may be ignored by the patient, and the level of suspicion in the clinical picture needs to be high.

DIAGNOSIS

Diagnosis of RVF can often be accomplished in the office, when symptoms are overt. A careful physical exam will often yield direct or circumstantial evidence of a fistula. Digital rectal exam may reveal an indurated tender fistula tract. Exam, including anoscopy, may reveal presence of stool within the vaginal vault. Anoscopic exam, accompanied by a vaginal speculum exam, may yield visible granulation tissue at the level of the tract opening. In many cases, the fistula tract is difficult to identify in the office. It is not uncommon that, due to local inflammation or prior surgery, examination under anesthesia may be required to provide patient comfort and enhance visualization. With optimal lighting and exposure, internal openings in the anal canal or low rectum may become visible. Other operative maneuvers include filling of either the rectum or vagina with liquid while simultaneously insufflating air. The site of bubbling may demonstrate a fistula site that was previously difficult to visualize.

Adjunctive testing is sometimes required. The tampon test is often successful in demonstrating subtle, hard to-identify fistulas. A tampon is placed in the vagina and a rectal enema of diluted methylene blue dye is carefully administered, to avoid overflow and leakage. The patient is then asked to ambulate for a period of 20 to 30 minutes. The tampon is then inspected, and evidence of blue staining along the length of the vagina indicates the presence of a fistula. If these tests do not yield a definitive diagnosis, a barium enema may be helpful. Clear lateral views and the use of balloon occlusion of the anal canal with positioning of the balloon as distal as possible are important.

If operative examination under anesthesia is undertaken and a fistula is identified, a seton should be placed. In addition, it is very important to assess for any evidence of local inflammation that might be associated with active Crohn disease as well as to manage any associated sepsis. It is important to inspect the entire rectovaginal septum and examine for any obvious sphincter defects, scarring, or stenosis. All of these are factors that significantly affect the plan of management.

As with complex cryptoglandular fistula disease, the goals of evaluation prior to definitive repair are to (1) identify the fistula, (2) manage any acute sepsis, (3) establish adequate drainage, (4) ascertain anatomy, including location and size of fistula as well as any surrounding injuries, and (5) determine etiology.

Once the fistula has been identified and any acute issues related to sepsis have been managed, further diagnostic studies will help in planning the surgical approach. Endoanal ultrasound is the diagnostic test of choice to identify associated sphincter injuries. The adjunctive use of hydrogen peroxide may also help to identify the anatomy of the fistula relative to the surrounding sphincter. Pelvic magnetic resonance imaging (MRI) and endorectal coil MRI are also helpful. Preferential use of ultrasound versus MRI is often institution- and practitioner-specific. Sphincter defects in association with RVF are very common. In a reported series of patients who sustained RVF after vaginal delivery, all demonstrated sphincter injury on endoanal ultrasound.[5]

Pelvic floor physiology testing including anal manometry and pudendal nerve terminal motor latency testing may also be employed. Although the results of such testing rarely affect the surgical management of RVF, pudendal nerve damage may be predictive of postoperative continence issues. The association of fecal incontinence in the setting of RVF should prompt a work-up for sphincter injury and would point to sphincter repair as an appropriate treatment even if other alternatives are available.

If malignancy is identified in the setting of RVF, appropriate staging and work-up related to the malignancy itself takes priority. Consideration for treatment of the fistula is secondary to the treatment of malignancy. Management of the fistula should be considered at the time of definitive malignancy management. It is not uncommon for a RVF to develop after treatment of locally advanced anal or cervical cancer involving the rectovaginal septum. Definitive repair should be delayed until the malignancy has been managed.

CLASSIFICATION

Accurate classification of RVFs is not merely a descriptive exercise; it also helps to inform appropriate management. RVFs are classified in several ways: When they are classified relative to the sphincter complex, they are described as either high or low. High fistulas are defined as those above the sphincter complex, and low fistulas are those at or below the level of the pelvic floor, typically at the dentate line. Low fistulas may also be referred to as anovaginal. Fistulas following traumatic obstetric injuries are almost always the low type and associated with sphincter injury. Similarly, cryptoglandular sources of RVFs are almost always low. High fistulas generally have a more complicated etiology, either iatrogenic secondary to anastomotic leak or related to inflammatory bowel disease or malignancy.

Fistulas may also be classified as either simple or complex. Simple fistulas are located in the middle or lower portion of the rectovaginal septum, are small (<2.5 cm in diameter), and are caused by local trauma or infection. Complex fistulas are either larger than 2.5 cm, located in the upper portion of the rectovaginal septum, or secondary to neoplasia, diverticulitis, or inflammatory bowel disease (Table 151.1).

TREATMENT

Conservative and Medical Management

Although the mainstay of treatment for the majority of RVFs is surgery, there are a few exceptions. On occasion, patients with small fistulas and minimal symptoms choose to pursue bowel management. A small number of fistulas due to obstetric trauma may close spontaneously in the immediate (within 3 months) postpartum period. Hyperbaric oxygen has been reported to be associated with successful healing in a small series of patients with RVFs from obstetric trauma.[6]

Medical therapy, particularly immunomodulation, has played an increasing role in the management of RVFs in patients with Crohn disease. Although the initial trial using infliximab in 1999 showed short-term healing in

TABLE 151.1 Classification of Rectovaginal Fistulas

Classification	Anatomy	Etiology
High	Above sphincter complex	Iatrogenic, irritable bowel disease (IBD), malignancy
Low (anovaginal)	Below majority of sphincter	Cryptoglandular, trauma, obstetric injury
Simple	Middle or lower part of right ventricular septum, <2.5 cm	Cryptoglandular, trauma, obstetric injury
Complex	Upper sphincter, >2.5 cm	Neoplasia, IBD, diverticular

TABLE 151.2 Etiology of Rectovaginal Fistulas

Obstetric injury	Episiotomy, third- and fourth-degree perineal lacerations
Inflammatory bowel disease	Crohn disease
Iatrogenic	Anorectal surgery (fistulotomy)
	Vaginal surgery (hysterectomy, rectocele repair)
	Abdominal surgery (hysterectomy, low anterior resection, J pouch, procedure for prolapse and hemorrhoids)
Infectious	Cryptoglandular abscess, diverticulitis, tuberculosis
Neoplastic	Anal cancer, rectal cancer, vaginal cancer, cervical cancer
Radiation-induced	External beam radiation, brachytherapy

56% to 68% of abdominal and perianal fistulas, no RVFs were included.[7] Subsequently the ACCENT II trial looked at 25 women with Crohn RVF. With infliximab, 60.7% healed initially, but long-term closure (at 14 weeks) was significantly lower, with a closure rate of 44.8%. Compared with other fistulas, the rate of RVF healing with infliximab is substantially less, and it has been suggested that this may be because of the relatively thin, nonmuscular, poorly vascularized rectovaginal septum.[9] Use of MRI has shown that although fistulas have apparent healing, they may actually simply become less symptomatic with less drainage even though tracts persist on radiographic studies. Furthermore, closure of the fistula was associated with the development of an abscess in 10% of patients, presumably because the external opening heals over before the tract has healed.[7] Poritz et al. have suggested that use of infliximab does not avoid the need for surgery in more than 70% of patients; however, such patients may be rendered relatively asymptomatic and have a reasonable quality of life before requiring surgical intervention.[10] Infliximab and other immunomodulators are increasingly used as an adjunct to surgery. In a review of 55 women with Crohn disease and RVF, use of immunomodulators such as infliximab or adalimumab in addition to 6-mercaptopurine or azathioprine within 3 months prior to surgery was associated with successful healing ($P = .009$).[11] Biologics such as infliximab are commonly used in combination with surgery for Crohn RVF and appear to improve outcome.

Preoperative Management

Preoperative preparation is according to practitioner preference as well as the type of procedure planned. Simple anal- and vaginal-based repairs require only rectal preparation with saline or phosphate enemas the morning of surgery. If a more extensive procedure is planned or if diversion will be necessary, formal bowel preparation is recommended. Perioperative antibiotics and deep venous thrombosis (DVT) prophylaxis are administered per guidelines. Smoking, recognized as a significant predictor for adverse outcome in the repair of RVF, must stop.[11,12]

Surgical Management

As with any complex anorectal procedure, conditions optimal for healing should be present prior to surgery. The goals of surgery are to preserve continence while achieving repair of the fistula.

The presence of active anorectal or anovaginal sepsis is a contraindication to definitive repair. Drainage of any abscess and establishment of definitive drainage or placement of a seton is required. We recommend delaying definitive surgery in such cases for at least 4 to 6 weeks until all sepsis and inflammation have resolved. Similarly, for treatment of RVF in the immediate postpartum period, we recommend a delay of at least 3 months to allow acute inflammation and sepsis to subside. Frequently spontaneous healing will be seen. Optimization of stool bulking is helpful, and in the setting of incontinence, sacral nerve stimulation may be an effective bridge to definitive repair. In this interval, clarification of anatomy via endoanal ultrasound or MRI can be undertaken.

The four general categories for surgical approach are transanal, transvaginal, transperineal, and transabdominal. Table 151.2 summarizes the various indications and outcomes for these approaches.

Transanal Approaches

Fistulotomy. A simple fistulotomy is the laying open of the fistula tract. This is usually approached in two stages. A seton is placed, followed by assessment of the degree of sphincter involvement. The second stage of treatment involves cutting of the remaining overlying tissue to lay open the tract. The success rate of this fistulotomy approaches 100%. However, this involves division of a varying amount of soft tissue and possibly sphincter muscle and therefore increases the risk of incontinence. In most cases, such an outcome is unacceptable; therefore simple fistulotomy alone is rarely appropriate.

Advancement Flap. The sliding-flap repair for the treatment of patients with RVF was first reported by Noble in 1902. He advocated splitting the rectovaginal septum, dissecting the lower end of the rectum from the vagina, and drawing the anterior wall down through and external to the anus. Since that time, many modifications of the sliding-flap technique have been proposed. In 1948, Laird described the use of a flap of mucosa, submucosa and some fibers of the internal sphincter.[13] Kodner et al. advocated the use of a flap similar to the Laird technique.[14] Other authors have advocated the use of a flap of mucosa, submucosa, and the full thickness of the internal sphincter. Incorporating part of the internal sphincter is generally necessary to ensure that the flap is of adequate thickness.[15] Regardless of the thickness of the flap used, the procedure is generally best for patients with simple low fistulas who have not had previous repairs. Patients with RVFs from obstetric injuries (without an associated sphincter defect) and those with Crohn RVFs without associated proctitis are good candidates for sliding-flap repair. We primarily advocate performance of the endoanal advancement flap, since this addresses the repair from the side of high pressure.

After appropriate mechanical and antibiotic bowel preparation, we typically perform this procedure with the patient in the prone jackknife position, which offers optimal exposure of the anterior rectal wall. A probe is inserted through the fistula to help identify it. A U-shaped or trapezoidal flap is outlined, with the base cephalad and twice the width of the apex. This helps to minimize the chance that the distal flap or flap edges will become ischemic. Dissection is started 1 cm distal to the fistula and consists of rectal mucosa, submucosa, and partial thickness of the underlying internal sphincter, including the fistula opening at the apex. We advocate using needle-tip cautery for precise dissection and elevation of the flap in a caudad-to-cephalad manner. The flap should

be mobilized 3 to 4 cm proximal to the fistula to ensure tension-free closure. Instillation of a dilute epinephrine solution is an option to facilitate dissection and minimize blood loss (Fig. 151.1). The fistula tract is curetted clear of all granulation tissue and the defect in the remaining internal sphincter is closed primarily with interrupted absorbable sutures. If the patient has a significant sphincter defect, a sphincteroplasty can be performed at this time.

The apex of the flap, including the fistula tract, is excised. The flap is then sutured in place at the cardinal points with full-thickness interrupted 2-0 absorbable sutures, followed by interrupted sutures in a bisecting manner until closure is achieved. The vaginal opening is left open to facilitate drainage.

Success varies considerably (29% to 100%) due to the heterogeneity of the patient groups, variations in surgical technique, and whether initial or ultimate success rates are reported.[4,14,21-27] Common causes of flap failure include ischemia of the flap and hematoma and/or the development of infection under the flap. The number of previous repairs, the presence of a concomitant sphincter defect, and the cause of the RVF all influence successful healing. If a patient has had one[19] or two[15] previous RVF repairs, the success rate with a sliding-flap repair decreases significantly. Therefore a sliding-flap repair should generally not be considered in a patient whose previous repairs

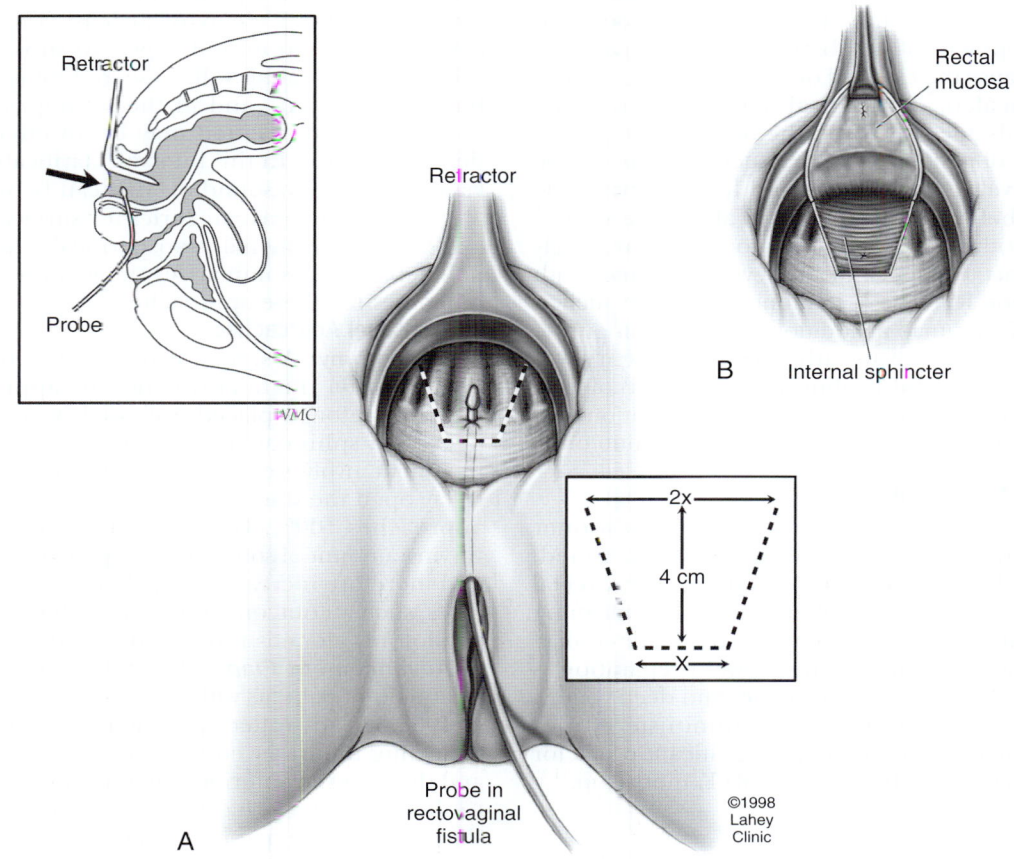

FIGURE 151.1 Endorectal sliding flap. The patient is placed in the prone jackknife position and the fistula is demonstrated (inset, arrow). (A) The flap should extend for at least 4 cm, and the base should be at least two times the width of the apex. (B) The flap should include mucosa and submucosa in addition to a portion of the internal sphincter muscle.

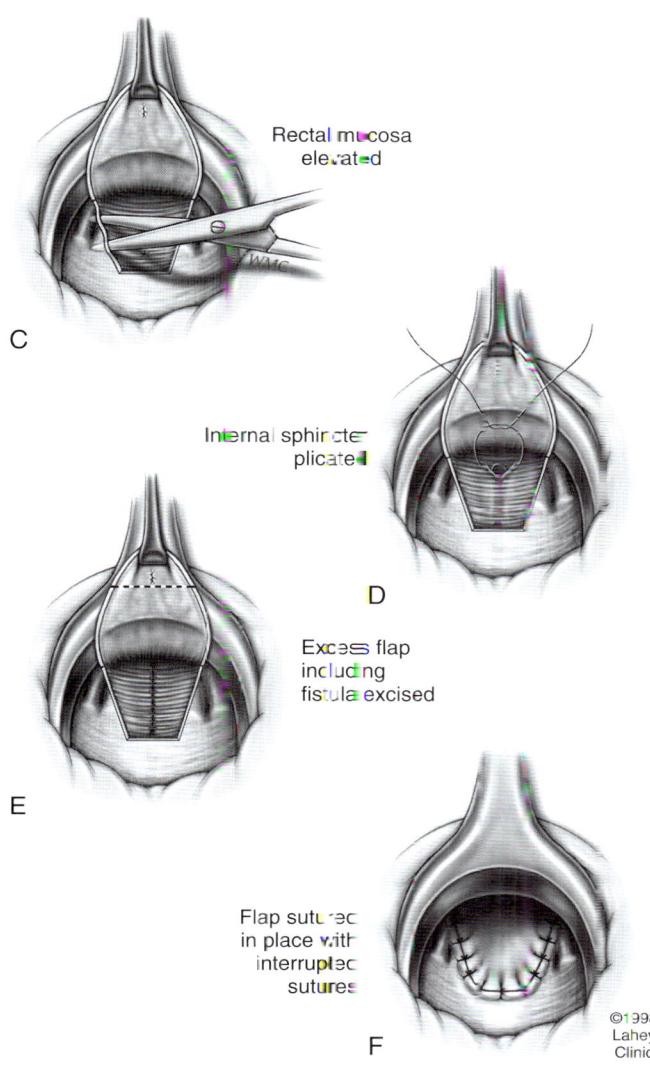

Rectal mucosa
elevated

C

Internal sphincter
plicated

D

Excess flap
including
fistula excised

E

Flap sutured
in place with
interrupted
sutures

F

©1998
Lahey
Clinic

FIGURE 151.1, cont'd C) The flap is raised and dissection is performed laterally to permit a tension-free closure. (D) The internal sphincter muscle is plicated over the area of the fistula. (E) Excess flap, including the site of the internal opening of the fistula, is trimmed. (F) The flap is secured with absorbable sutures. (Copyright 1998, Lahey Clinic, Burlington, Massachusetts.)

have failed. Sphincter function should be assessed and concomitant significant sphincter defects repaired at the time of sliding-flap procedure. The success rate for patients undergoing flap repair and sphincteroplasty with or without levatoroplasty was significantly higher than the success rate for those who underwent flap repair only (80% vs. 41%; $P < .02$).[4] As a result, some surgeons have advocated that anal ultrasonography and manometry be performed to detect occult sphincter defects in patients undergoing repair of RVFs; sphincter defects, however, in the majority of cases, can be determined by a thorough history and physical examination and then confirmed on manometry and ultrasound.[5] The underlying cause of the fistula may also determine the success of a flap repair. Patients with obstetric injuries as the cause of the RVF have a better outcome than patients with inflammatory bowel disease.

Fibrin Glue The use of fibrin glue for the repair of RVFs is limited but represents a safe approach without risk of incontinence. In this approach, the fistula tract is identified and curetted to remove granulation tissue. Fibrin glue is injected into the fistula tract from either side until it exits the secondary opening and allowed to polymerize and form a seal. The goal of fibrin glue injection is to provide a temporary mechanical obstruction of the fistula, which then will serve as a scaffold to allow autologous tissue ingrowth. Although the theory is elegant, as with complex anorectal fistulas, experience is disappointing and is almost uniformly a failure, most commonly due to extrusion of the plug due to the short length of the fistula. Modifications in the technique including closure of the internal opening and use of adhesive antibiotics have not improved the outcome.[25]

Fibrin glue has also been used as an adjunct with other procedures such as the endorectal advancement flap. In one series, fibrin glue was combined with an endorectal advancement flap in 12 patients; the failure rate was 50%, which was not significantly different from that with use of an endorectal advancement flap alone.[25] Despite initial enthusiasm, the technique is generally not used for RVFs.

Bioprosthetics. As with fibrin glue, the use of a bioprosthetic plug offers a safe approach to the treatment of RVFs. Like the fibrin glue approach, the plug is used to occlude the fistula mechanically with a bioabsorbable material designed to serve as a scaffold for autologous tissue ingrowth.

From a technical standpoint, the fistula tract is identified and curetted clean of granulation tissue. The fistula's plug or button is pulled through from the rectal side with the tapered portion coming through first until the plug is firmly lodged in place. The apex is sutured and buried in the rectal wall with an absorbable suture. The excess material is cut under tension on the vaginal side such that it countersinks slightly below the vaginal mucosa.

The reported literature is small, with success rates varying from 58% to 86% and limited follow-up. Complications are generally benign—primarily local infection and plug extrusion.[29,30]

Biologic Mesh. Bioprosthetic mesh has been used as an interposition graft to repair RVFs. In a group of 27 women with RVFs who underwent advancement flap repair and placement of an interposition graft of bioprosthetic material, there were five recurrences (19%).[31] The recurrence rate was lower than in women who underwent advancement flap repair without mesh (34%); the study was not randomized. Another small prospective nonrandomized study of mesh for closure of RVFs where the fistula was excised and the mesh was placed transvaginally in 21 patients resulted in a success rate of 75%.[32]

Transvaginal Approach—Vaginal Advancement Flap. This technique approaches the fistula from the lower-pressure vaginal side. There is a higher failure rate but it does allow for good exposure and does not put any sphincter muscle at risk. In addition, with adequate exposure, a concomitant sphincteroplasty may be performed.

The patient undergoes bowel preparation, either via oral prep or enema, and is typically approached in the lithotomy position. An incision is made in the posterior vaginal wall by the introitus, distal to the fistula. Dissection is carried down through the vaginal wall into the rectovaginal septum, exposing the fistula tract through the sphincter muscle. Adequate proximal width of the base of the flap is necessary to ensure good blood supply. The apex of the flap is trimmed to excise the fistula's opening. The defect in the sphincter is oversewn with absorbable suture, and the flap is sutured down in sections with interrupted suture. This flap has the primary advantage of the use of healthy, well-vascularized vaginal tissue, avoiding any scar or disease in the anal canal. This may be an especially attractive option in the setting of anal stenosis or in patients with Crohn disease. Using this technique, Bauer et al. reported cure of RVFs in 12 of 13 women with Crohn disease, with a mean follow-up time of 50 months.[33] A comparative analysis of 11 studies showed no statistically significant difference in the closure rates between rectal and vaginal advancement flap closures in RVFs due to Crohn disease.[34] Therefore especially when fibrostenotic disease is present in the anus or a transanal approach has failed, a transvaginal advancement flap is a viable option. Similarly, this may be the preferred procedure in the setting of pouch vaginal fistula after ileal pouch-anal anastomosis (IPAA) if approach through the anal canal is anatomically difficult.

Transperineal Approaches

Perineoproctotomy With Layered Closure. In this procedure, the fistula is converted to a fourth-degree perineal laceration by dividing all the tissue between the rectum and vagina through the perineal body. The tract is then excised, and the vagina, sphincter muscles, and rectal mucosa are identified, mobilized, and repaired in layers (Fig. 151.2). Excellent results have been reported in several series.[20,35,36] Mazier et al. reported a success rate of 100% in 38 patients who underwent perineoproctotomy.[20] Experienced clinicians have shown that, as compared with endorectal advancement flap closure, this approach yielded superior rates of healing (57.5% vs. 42.5%) as well as improved sexual function and decreased rates of fecal incontinence.[37]

Episioproctotomy and Cloacal Defects. Cloacal defects represent a severe form of obstetric trauma with essentially no perineal body, a shortened rectovaginal septum, and a retracted anal sphincter. Repair is carried out by developing the plane between the anorectal and vaginal epithelium and identifying the sphincter muscle on both sides, which is mobilized and subsequently approximated.[38,39] The procedure may also be combined with an anoplasty. Kaiser reported 12 patients with a cloacal defect who were treated using an X-flap anoplasty. Of these 12 patients, 9 healed and 3 had a persistent RVF; in 2 of these 3, it closed spontaneously. One patient subsequently required a bulbocavernosus flap.[39]

LIFT Procedure. The ligation of the intersphincteric fistulous tract (LIFT) approach involves obliteration of the fistula by ligation. First, a perineal incision is made over the intersphincteric groove. With a fistula probe traversing the tract, dissection proceeds down in the intersphincteric space. The fistula tract is identified as it traverses the rectovaginal septum and it is dissected free. A portion of the intersphincteric fistula tract is excised and the defect in the internal and external sphincter is suture-ligated with absorbable suture. The intersphincteric space is then reapproximated with interrupted absorbable suture

and the skin incision is closed with interrupted chromic. This technique was popularized in 2007 by Rojanasakul[40] and it has been employed with relative success for RVF as well. There has been little literature devoted specifically to a success rate in RVF; however, reported success rates for its use in complex fistulas range from 60% to 94%.

Sphincteroplasty. If the RVF exists in the setting of a known sphincter defect, sphincteroplasty will be an effective repair. The restoration of anatomy and sphincter function has the advantage of an autologous tissue flap repair. A perineal incision close to the anus is performed and the divided ends of the sphincter are identified and skeletonized laterally. Care must be taken not to extend the perineal incision more than 180 degrees owing to the risk of injury to the pudendal nerve. The sphincter is also dissected away from the anal mucosa and mobilized to the midline. The repair can be performed as an end-to-end approach or more commonly as an overlapping technique. The overlapped muscle is sutured in place with 20 absorbable interrupted mattress sutures. This also has the effect of lengthening the perineal body. The incision is closed loosely with interrupted sutures in a Y-configuration (Fig. 151.3). Often the center is left open for drainage. When used in the context of an advancement flap, this has been shown to increase the rate of fistula closure, as high as 100% in one series, and to restore continence in as many as 70% of patients.

Tissue Interposition Flaps. This technique employs the advantage of transposing healthy, well-vascularized tissue to buttress repair. It is commonly used in settings of failed previous repairs or in the setting of prior radiation. The most commonly used muscle grafts are the bulbocavernosus and gracilis muscles, although other grafts have been used, including the sartorius and gluteus maximus. This approach may be combined with sphincteroplasty in the setting of known sphincter injury. One of the main morbidities associated with these approaches is dyspareunia.

The bulbocavernosus flap, eponymously described by Martius in 1928,[42] was originally used for the repair of vesicovaginal fistula; however, it is also useful for radiation-induced RVF, large obstetric fistula, cases in which previous repairs have failed, and selected pouch-vaginal fistulas after restorative proctocolectomy. The Martius flap, which involves harvesting of the bulbocavernosus muscle with the overlying fat in the labia majora, is based on the perineal branch of the pudendal artery. Details of the procedure are outlined in Fig. 151.4. Since the description by Martius, Elkins et al. have shown that the bulbocavernosus muscle itself does not need to be included in the graft because the labial adipose tissue has an excellent blood supply, thus decreasing the morbidity of using the bulbocavernosus muscle and reducing the operative time.[43] Using this technique for complex fistulas, Pinedo and Phillips reported healing in 6 of 8 patients.[44] Modifications in surgical technique have been outlined by Hoskins et al.,[45] who used a full-thickness island graft from the labia majora, and Symmonds and Hill,[46] who used a full-thickness graft from the labia minora and majora. Boronow[47] reported a success rate of 84% in 5 women with RVFs. McNevin et al. reported 16 patients who underwent Martius flap for complex RVFs. The etiologies of the fistulas were obstetric (n = 9), cryptoglandular (n =

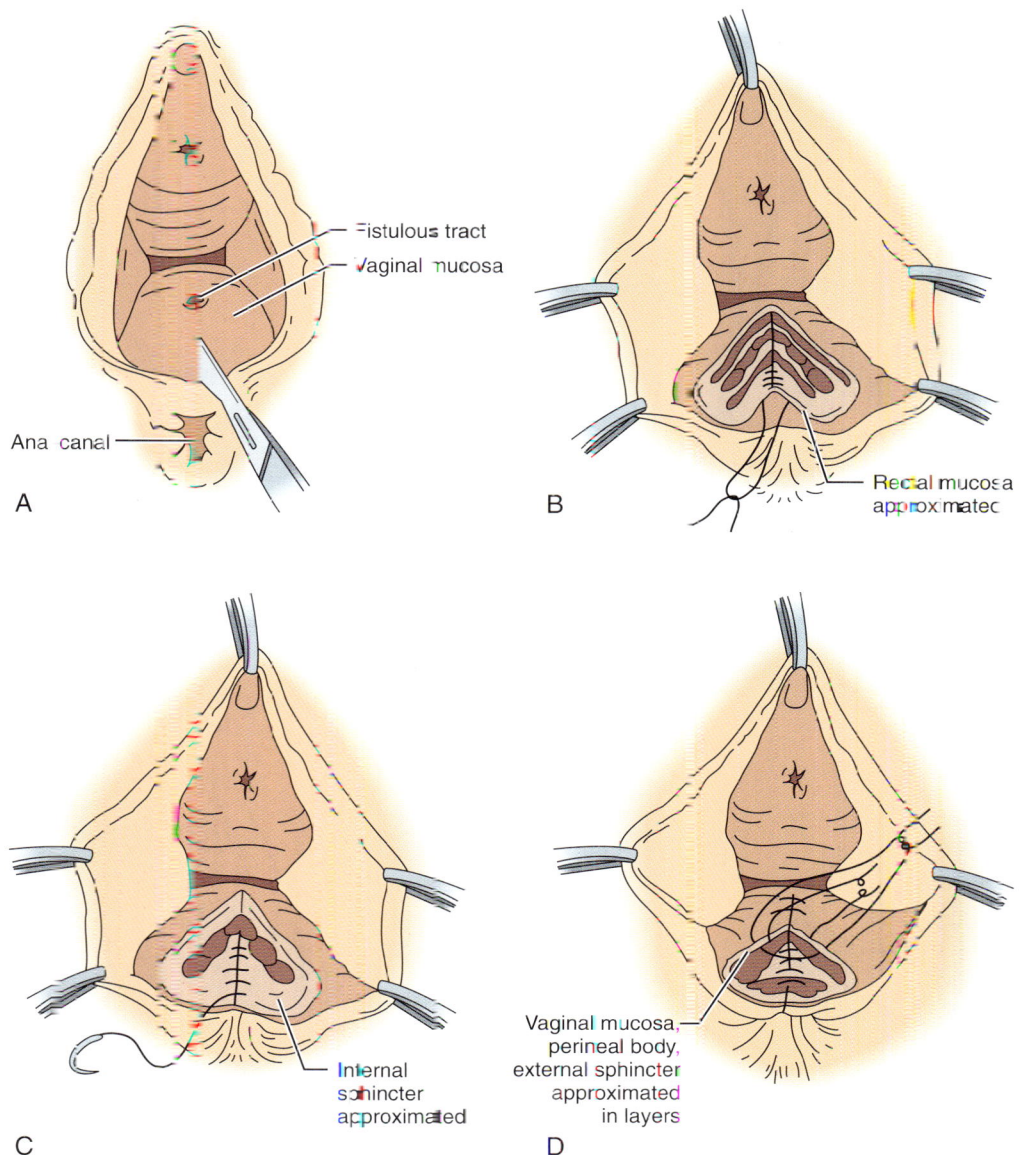

FIGURE 151.2 Perineoproctotomy. A) The patient is placed in the lithotomy position. The fistula is identified and converted into a full-thickness laceration. (B) The layers are dissected out and repaired, first repairing the rectal mucosa. (C) The repair continues, approximating the internal sphincter. D) The external sphincter is identified and repaired. Many patients will not have a discernible plane between the internal and external sphincters, in which case the internal and external sphincters may be repaired together. The vaginal mucosa is approximated.

5), and Crohn disease ($n = 2$).[48] There was one recurrent fistula and one patient had a labial wound complication. Five patients had dyspareunia (31%), whereas only one had complained of dyspareunia preoperatively. Dyspareunia, infrequently reported as an outcome variable, is a potential concern with the procedure.[47] An additional concern is the patient's self-perception of the appearance of the graft site in addition to decreased sensation or numbness of the graft site. Lee et al. found that 81% of their patients reported normal vaginal sensation; only 5% reported pain and 14% numbness. Almost 90% of patients reported no change in sexual function in responding to quality-of-life (QOL) questionnaires.[49]

The gracilis muscle may also be used to affect repair with minimal functional morbidity. The neurovascular pedicle enters the muscle in a constant location in its proximal third. The muscle can be harvested through an open or minimally invasive approach and tunneled through the subcutaneous tissue at the groin. The distal tip of the muscle is secured into the perineum and sutured over the fistula or sphincter repair. Gracilis repair of rectovaginal and pouch-vaginal fistulas has an overall healing rate per patient of 50% to 92% and a success rate per procedure of 47% to 85%.[50–54] Despite healing of the fistula in the majority of patients, quality of life and sexual function remained altered.[50] A systematic review of gracilis

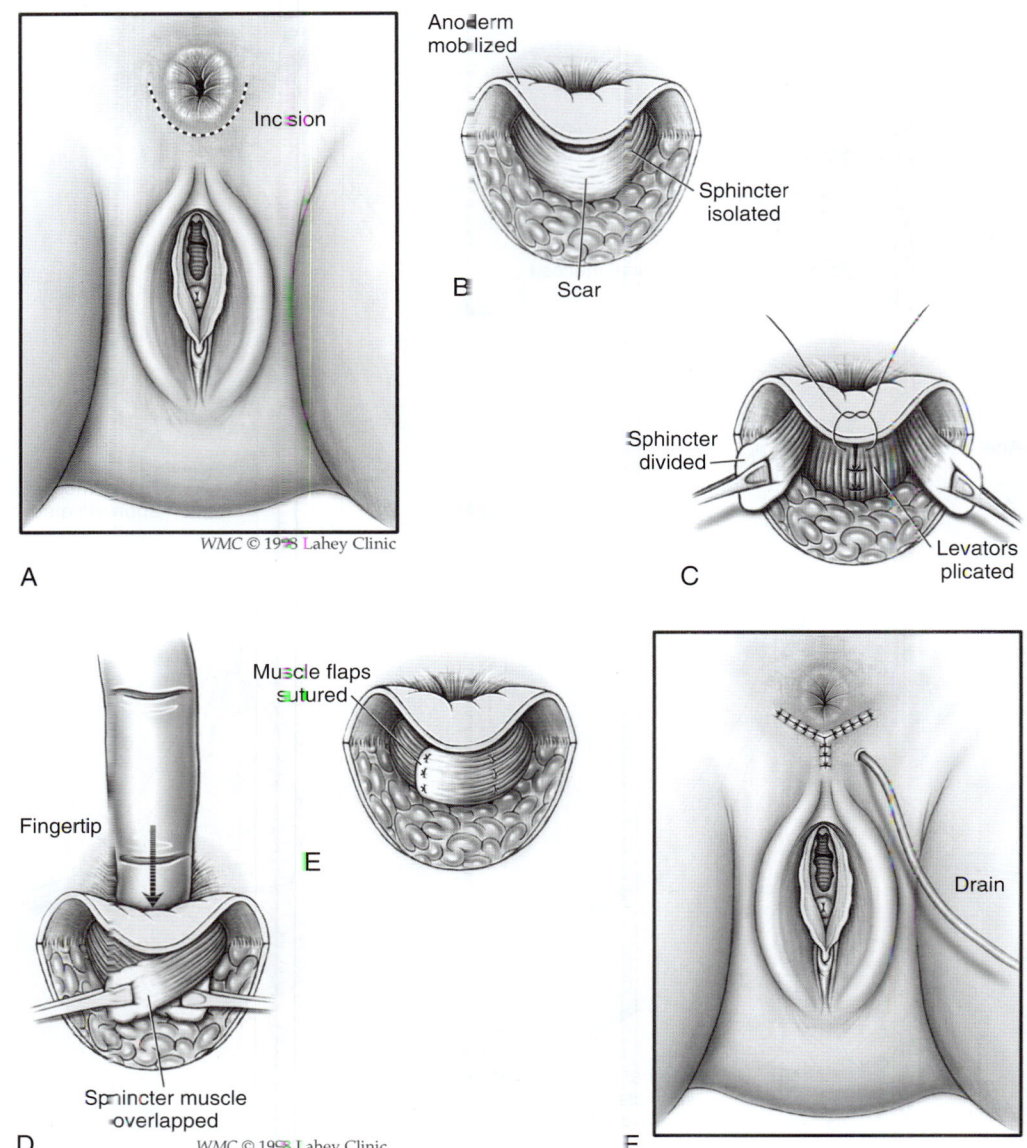

FIGURE 151.3 Overlapping sphincteroplasty. (A) The patient is placed in the prone jackknife position and a curvilinear incision is made approximately 180 degrees around the anus (B) Dissection is carried out medial to the ischiorectal fat, and the external sphincter is identified. (C) Dissection is carried up to the level of the levators, which are plicated. (D) If sufficient muscle is present, an overlapping sphincter repair is performed. If not, simple apposition of the sphincter muscle is performed. (E) The completed repair. (F) The perineal body is reconstructed, and the wound is secured in a Y configuration. A drain may be placed. (Copyright 1998, Lahey Clinic, Burlington, Massachusetts.)

interposition for RVFs performed by Hotouras concluded that this technique does have a reasonable success rate and may be considered as a first-line approach.[55]

Transabdominal Approaches. A transabdominal approach may be required for complex fistulas or those associated with a more proximal location of the fistula. Common causes of such fistulas include colovaginal fistula in the setting of complicated diverticulitis in a woman who has had a prior hysterectomy, iatrogenic bowel injury during hysterectomy, rectocele repair, anastomotic leaks after low anterior resection or prolapse procedures. In one series, RVFs occurred in 1.2% of women undergoing repair of a vaginal vault prolapse.[56] These fistulas tend to

be higher than obstetric fistulas and have surrounding tissues that are abnormal and poorly vascularized. The procedure involves mobilization of the proximal rectum, resection of the diseased distal rectum, and restoration of continuity with an anorectal anastomosis. Transabdominal approaches frequently require temporary diverting ileostomy, especially when the anastomosis is near the anal canal.

Sleeve Advancement. This approach may be required when the fistula is associated with circumferential or stricturing disease, as in radiation-associated scarring or Crohn proctitis, or anastomotic leak related to ischemia. The affected rectum must be mobilized away from the

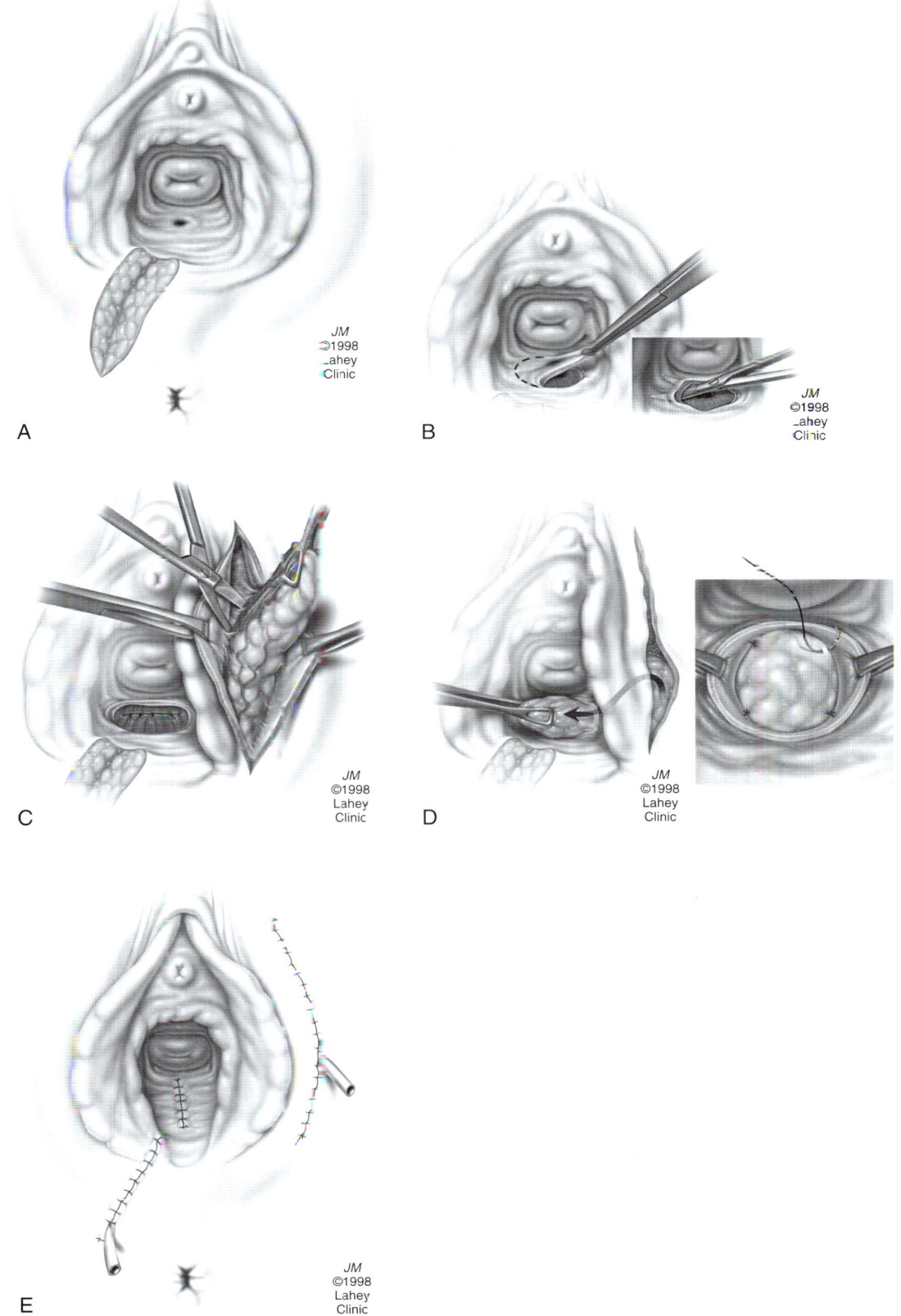

FIGURE 151.4 Bulbocavernosus (Martius) flap. (A) The patient is placed in the lithotomy position, and a mediolateral episiotomy incision is made. (B) The vaginal side of the fistula is mobilized and excised. The rectal side of the fistula is closed. (C) Along the opposite labia majora, an incision is made and the bulbocavernosus muscle and labial fat pad are mobilized. (D) The bulbocavernosus muscle and labial fat pad are brought through a subcutaneous tunnel and secured to the previously closed rectal side of the fistula (inset). (E) The vaginal defect is closed, and the incisions are closed. Drainage is effected with a Penrose or closed-suction drain. Copyright 1998, Lahey Clinic, Burlington, Massachusetts.

vagina, the fistula divided and repaired, and a healthy bowel conduit advanced distal to the fistula with subsequent anastomosis. This technique was first described by Parks et al.[57] Although Parks et al. described a distal mucosectomy followed by a coloanal anastomosis, a double-staple technique (as is used for the ileoanal pouch procedure) may also be used, and a colonic J-pouch may be added to improve neorectal function. If available, omentum is interposed between the anastomosis and the vagina. In one series, Cooke and Wellsted reported a 93% success rate in 55 patients (Fig. 151.5).[58]

Primary Repair. If the fistula is very proximal and associated with generally healthy tissue, as in the setting of colovaginal fistula from diverticulitis, a primary repair is another option. This is most commonly applied in the setting of inadvertent iatrogenic injury to the sigmoid or upper rectum. Pelvic dissection is performed to identify the site of the fistula and the fistula is divided. If the associated bowel is otherwise healthy, direct repair of the bowel and vagina can be performed. Omental interposition should be performed to buttress this repair. If the associated bowel is significantly diseased, as in the setting of chronic diverticular disease, conversion to segmental resection with primary anastomosis and omental interposition can be performed.

Bowel Diversion. In the setting of a highly symptomatic RVF in a patient with significant comorbidities or who is not a candidate for definitive repair, fecal diversion with either a loop ileostomy or colostomy can provide profound symptomatic relief and a significant improvement in the quality of life. Similarly, patients who have active Crohn disease or who have failed multiple prior repairs may be appropriate candidate for fecal diversion. As previously indicated, careful consideration should be given to temporary diversion in the setting of complicated repairs at high risk for failure. The diversion itself may not improve the success rate of repair but will mitigate the morbidity associated with anastomotic leak.

SUMMARY

The decision for the type of repair in the setting of RVF is based on a wide variety of factors including type of fistula, etiology, presence or absence of sphincter defect, the number and type of prior repair attempts, as well as comorbidities. The student clinician needs to be aware of all of the repair options as well as the factors that may influence such decisions. A proposed flow diagram is outlined in Fig. 151.6.

A successful repair can be achieved in most patients, although they should be counseled that several attempts at repair may be required. Nevertheless, even in the setting of a technically successful repair, QOL issues may remain, including fecal incontinence and dyspareunia.

RECTOURETHRAL FISTULAS

RUFs represent a significant reconstructive challenge for both patients and surgeons. Very few centers have high-volume experience with management of this condition. Utilization of a multidisciplinary approach (colorectal surgeon, urologist, and possibly a plastic surgeon) from the initial stages of management may optimize outcomes for these complex repairs.

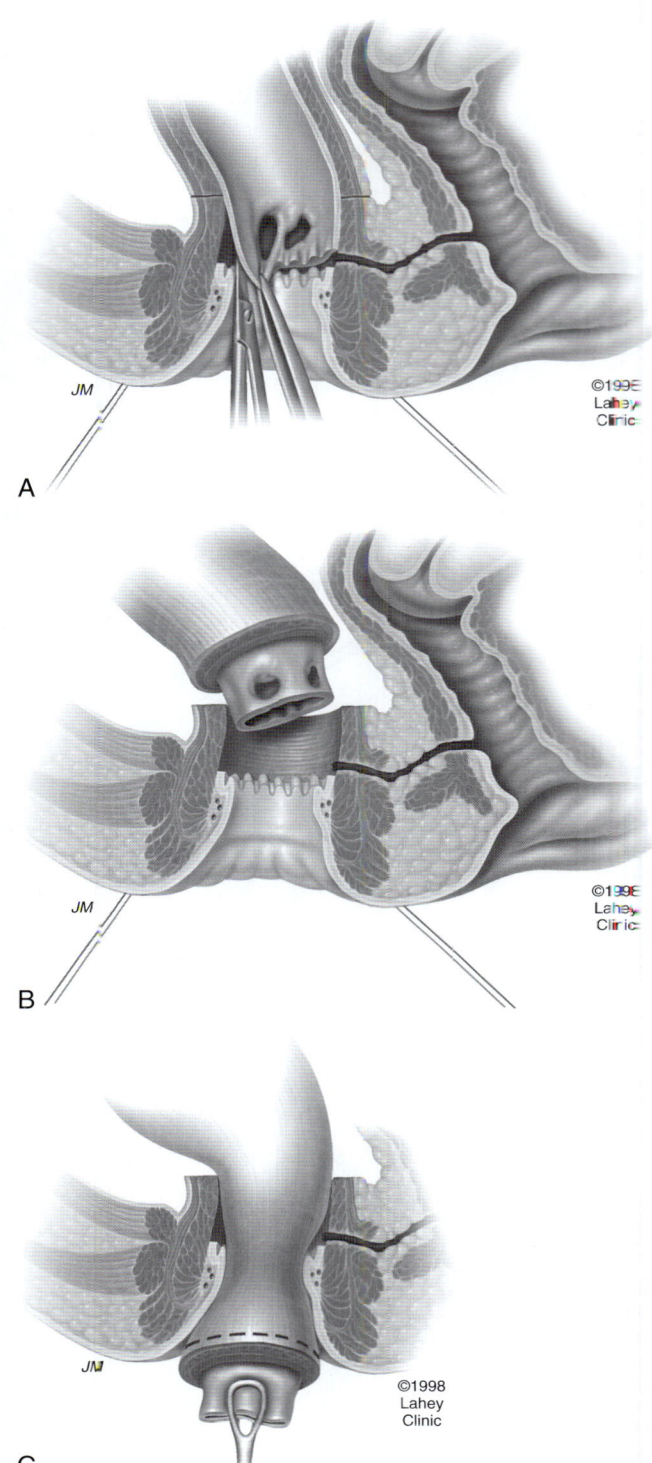

A

B

C

FIGURE 151.5 Advancement sleeve flap. (A) Commencing at the level of the dentate line, a circumferential dissection of mucosa and submucosa is performed, thus excising the ulcerated areas of the anal canal. (B) The dissection is continued cephalad and into the supralevator space, completing rectal mobilization. (C) The fistula can then be cored out and closed, and the distal cuff (*dotted line*) of the rectum is trimmed and secured to the anoderm. (Copyright 1998, Lahey Clinic, Burlington, Massachusetts.)

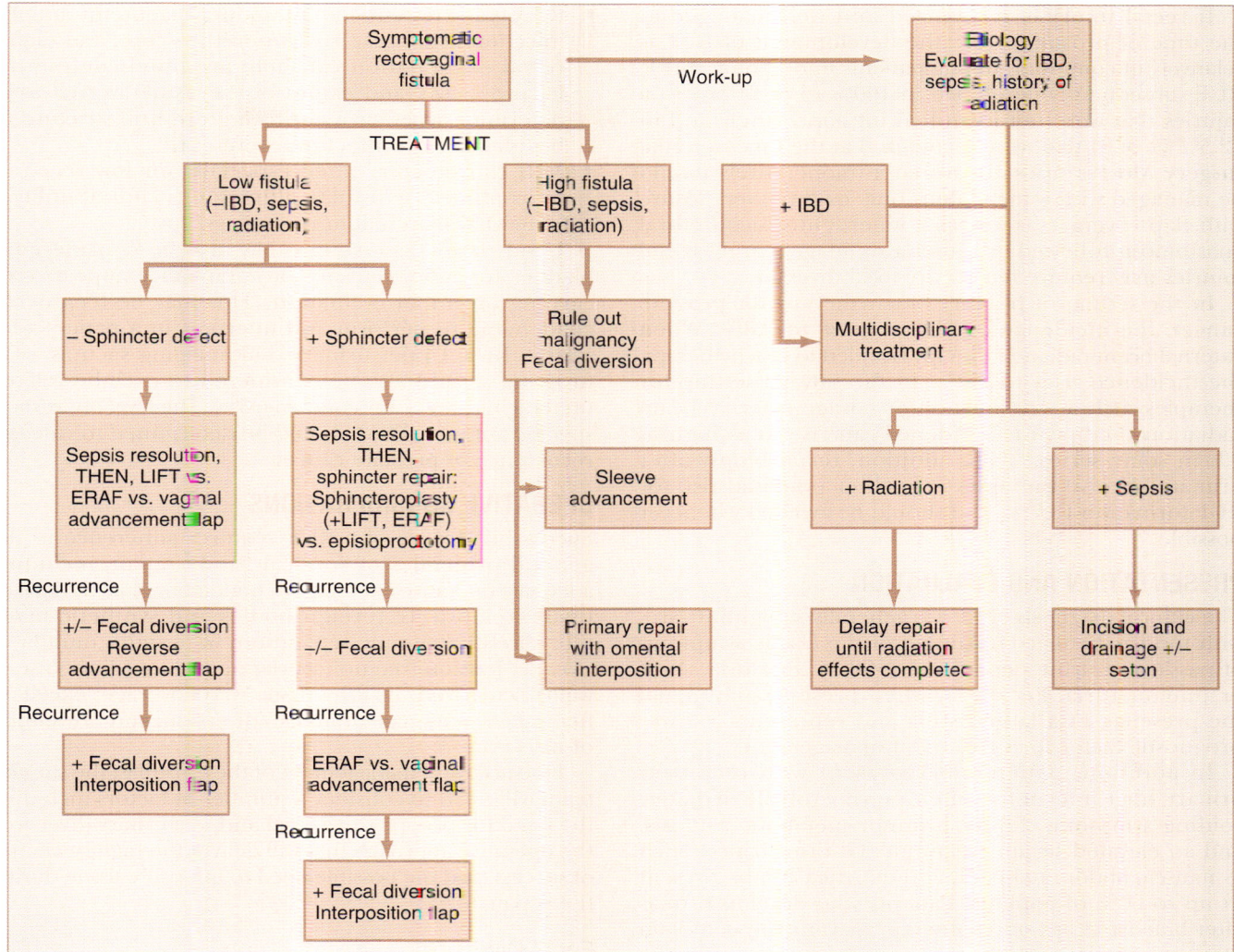

FIGURE 151.6 Proposed flow diagram for the management of rectovaginal fistulas. *ERAF,* Endorectal advancement flap; *IED,* inflammatory bowel disease; *LIFT,* ligation of the intersphincteric fistula tract.

BACKGROUND

A rectourethral fistula is an epithelialized, extraanatomic connection between the urethra (including the prostatic urethra or bladder neck) and the rectum. Acquired RUFs are uncommon and can result from any process that creates trauma, inflammation, infection, or ischaemia between the urogenital tract and rectum. Most commonly today, acquired RUFs occur as a result of surgical (open, laparoscopic, or robot-assisted radical prostatectomy [RARP]) or energy-ablative treatments (external beam radiation therapy, cryotherapy, high-intensity focused ultrasound, etc.) for prostate cancer or other pelvic malignancies. Over the last two decades, the incidence of radiation or energy-based RUF has increased, and there is a trend toward larger, increasingly complex RUFs.[59-63] Rather than simple fistula closure, the approach to RUF today often mandates utilization of urethral reconstruction with patch grafts, interposition of vascularized beds such as muscle flaps, or even completion prostatectomy.[60,63]

Conditions such as inflammatory bowel disease, blunt or penetrating pelvic trauma, pelvic abscesses, locally advanced malignancies, or surgery for benign pelvic disease can all result in RUF formation. Congenital RUFs can also be seen in the setting of other significant coloanal abnormalities, such as imperforate anus.

INCIDENCE

Rectal injury during radical prostatectomy appears to be the major risk factor for the development of surgical RUF. In a multiinstitutional review, the incidence of rectal injury during RARP was 0.17% (11 of 6650) with 72.3% (8 of 11) identified intraoperatively. Of patients with identified rectal injury from RARP, 36.4% (4 of 11) eventually developed RUFs.[64] In older case series, the incidence of rectal injury with subsequent development of RUF was reported as upward of 1% to 3.6% for open or laparoscopic radical prostatectomy and up to 11% for perineal prostatectomy.[61,65-68,69]

If rectal injury is recognized and well managed at the time of prostatectomy, the development of RUF is relatively uncommon. Among patients undergoing RARP, RUF subsequently developed in 100% (3 of 3) of rectal injuries that were not identified intraoperatively and in 12.5% (1 of 8) that were recognized at the time of initial surgery. Most injuries discovered intraoperatively should be managed with a meticulous one- or two-layer closure with flap coverage as well as a watertight vesicourethral anastomosis followed by catheter drainage. Larger rectal injuries may require temporary fecal diversion.

In the setting of primary brachytherapy for prostate cancer, the incidence of RUF is 0.4% to 0.8%. When external beam radiation therapy is added to brachytherapy, the incidence rises to 2.9%. In the salvage setting for therapies such as cryoablation or salvage external beam radiation therapy, the incidence can rise to as high as 9% in some series.[70–76] In addition, rectal biopsy after primary ablative therapies is another potential risk for RUF formation (3.7%) and should be avoided whenever possible.[77]

PRESENTATION AND EVALUATION

The clinical diagnosis of RUF is generally straightforward, with most patients complaining of the classic symptoms of passage of urine per rectum (>90%), fecaluria, and/or pneumaturia. Fecaluria, when present, may signal the presence of a large fistula and represents a worse prognostic factor for subsequent management.[68]

In addition, patients may present with recurrent urinary tract infections (often polymicrobial), irritative voiding symptoms, fevers, a minor metabolic acidosis, and an elevated serum creatinine. GI disturbances such as nausea, abdominal pain, and diarrhea can be present in up to 60% of patients. Patients who develop fistulas after brachytherapy or cryotherapy may initially complain of severe rectal pain, which generally resolves after the ischemic tissue breaks down and fistula formation occurs. These patients are also more likely to present with more significant bleeding, osteomyelitis, necrotizing infections, or even sepsis.

Preoperative evaluation will focus on obtaining a full anatomic and functional picture of the patient's lower urinary and gastrointestinal tracts to help determine the optimal options for successful fistula management. In addition to determining the size and location of the fistula, evaluation will be needed to determine the function of the anal and urethral sphincters, the size and location of any concomitant urethral stricture or bladder neck contracture, the status of the prostatic remnant (if still remaining), and the quality of tissue surrounding the fistula and tissue available for interposition as needed.

In general, endoscopy and radiology studies are the mainstay of preoperative evaluation.

- An examination under anesthesia, anoscopy, flexible sigmoidoscopy or colonoscopy, and/or barium enema can be used to identify the rectal opening of the fistulous tract, inspect the quality of the surrounding tissue, and assess the anal sphincter and rectum for evidence of intrinsic rectal disease such as inflammatory bowel disease or radiation proctitis.

- Retrograde urethrography, voiding cystourethrography, injection fistulography, cystourethroscopy, and digital rectal examination can help accurately define the location, size, and extent of the fistula as well as to determine whether a coexisting urethral stricture or bladder neck contracture is present.
- MRI can be considered especially for low rectal or transsphincteric fistulas, although its clinical utility is somewhat marginal in most cases.

Urodynamic assessment may also be considered if bladder function, capacity, or compliance appears concerning on initial evaluation. This may be technically challenging to perform and interpret in a patient with a large RUF. Upper urinary tract imaging such as a CT urogram should also be considered to exclude related ureteral injuries, if any concern exists. The level of prostate-specific antigen (PSA) should be determined to rule out recurrence of prostate cancer.

OPERATIVE CONSIDERATIONS

Successful closure of a RUF requires adherence to the general principles of surgical fistula repair, including adequate operative exposure; débridement of all devitalized tissue; removal of foreign bodies and synthetic material; careful anatomic separation; watertight, multilayer closure; tension-free nonoverlapping suture lines; use of well-vascularized, healthy tissue flap coverage; excellent hemostasis; adequate drainage/diversion; and prevention of infection.

For successful management of these fistulas, the surgical team will need to consider a number of factors including the need for preoperative fecal and/or urinary diversion, the operative approach that will deliver the highest chance of success, and the possible need to interpose tissue during the repair.

Fecal Diversion

To this point, no studies have demonstrated increased success rates of RUF closure with fecal diversion, but this should be taken with a grain of salt, given the heterogeneity of fistulas and repairs.

With small, surgically induced fistulas in the setting of urinary and fecal diversion, a small percentage of these patients may resolve spontaneously without any need for surgical therapy. In this group of patients, definitive repair without fecal diversion can also be considered if the tissue quality appears acceptable. Fecal diversion can also be undertaken, if necessary, at the time of repair.

In patients with complex fistulas (size >2 cm, radiated/ablated, prior failed repair, concomitant pelvic abscess) that will require a patch graft and muscle interposition, fecal diversion is generally considered prudent. For these more complex fistulas, delaying surgery for at least 3 months with both urinary and fecal diversion may allow for an attempt at spontaneous fistula resolution, treatment of acute infections, decreased inflammation, and optimization of tissue for future reconstruction.

In the presence of an intact anal sphincter and a compliant functional rectum, a temporary loop ileostomy, ideally performed laparoscopically, is preferable for its ease of creation and reversal. A temporary loop ileostomy prevents rectal wall distention and pressure during healing and minimizes infection, which is critical for successful complex fistula closure. In addition, it permits mobilization of the colon for colonic advancement if a proctectomy and coloanal anastomosis is required.[60] In patients with irreversible sphincter damage, an end colostomy should be considered early on in the management process.

Hanna et al. reported their outcomes in a retrospective review of 37 patients treated at one high-volume center. They found that 91% of no irradiated patients eventually had their ostomies reversed, whereas only 55% of patients in the radiated group did so.[78] These results are relatively consistent with many other studies suggesting that patients with radiation- or energy ablation–induced fistulas are much more likely to have to live with their fecal diversion permanently.

Tissue Interposition

Large fistula defects require the interposition of additional tissue to maximize healing potential, and the gracilis muscle is ideally suited for this technique. The gracilis has been used extensively in colorectal surgery for the construction of a neo-sphincter around the anus, for treatment of unhealed wounds after proctectomy for cancer or Crohn disease, for complex RVFs, and for RUFs. It is readily available and harvested with minimal morbidity in the same setting as RUF repair. It provides a well-vascularized bed to allow for wide separation of the urinary and GI tracts, closure of dead space, and improved healing of buccal mucosal grafts in the setting of complex urethral defects.

Additionally, gluteus maximus muscle flaps can be considered when a large amount of dead space coverage is required, as with fistulas that occur after abdominal perineal resection (APR), pressure-induced sacral decubitus ulcers, or large radiation defects.

OPERATIVE APPROACHES

There are a number of surgical procedures for the repair of RUFs. Historically, over 40 different types of repairs have been described in the literature, including endoscopic, transanal/transrectal, perineal, and abdominal approaches. Determining the optimal repair must take into account the complexity of the fistulas, the status of the surrounding tissues, the size of the defect, prior radiation therapy, and surgeon experience. Radiated RUF represents one of the most challenging operative cases because of the inaccessible fibrotic space, with adherent planes creating a challenging dissection and closure of the fistula. As with any complex reconstructive procedure, the first attempt at repair is generally the best chance for long-term repair.

Perineal Approach

Complex RUFs are now generally repaired via a perineal approach with gracilis muscle interposition. This approach is familiar to both the colorectal surgeon and urologist, making it appealing for combined repairs; however, limited working space can also make exposure challenging. The dissection can be performed either in the dorsal lithotomy position or prone jackknife position. This approach provides access to both the urinary tract and rectum, allowing for the concomitant repair of both as well as access to the thigh to allow for harvest of the gracilis

muscle for flap coverage. In addition, it allows exposure for concomitant management of urethral strictures or to consider prostatectomy as needed in the case of large urinary tract defects.

Under cystoscopic guidance, a catheter is initially placed across the fistula tract. An inverse "U" incision is made in the perineum following a course circumferentially anterior to the anal verge and medial to the ischial tuberosities. The ischiorectal fossa is identified and bluntly dissected bilaterally. The central perineal tendon is divided. Dissection is carried out along the anterior rectal wall until the rectourethralis muscle is encountered and divided. The prostate and urethra are separated widely from the rectum. The margins of the fistula tract are débrided until supple, healthy edges are encountered on both sides. The rectum is generally closed transversely in two layers to prevent stenosis, with an advancement flap created as needed for large defects. The small urinary tract defect is then closed primarily. The large defect requires a buccal mucosal graft patch tailored to the gracilis flap (Fig. 151.7). Concomitant urethral strictures are addressed in the same setting. In patients with extensive damage to the rectum, a proctectomy and coloanal pull-through via a separate abdominal approach may be considered.

The use of buccal mucosa as a graft material has become common practice for repairs involving radiation/energy ablative fistulas, generally being used to cover large prostatic urethral defects or to repair concomitant urethral strictures. Vanni et al. reported on their series of 39 patients with radiation/energy ablation-induced RUFs. Of these patients, 34 (87%) underwent buccal mucosa graft closure with concomitant muscle flap interposition. The prostatic urethral defect could be repaired primarily in only 3 (7.7%) patients. In addition, buccal grafts were used in 11 (28%) patients to repair urethral strictures at the time of RUF repair. Two of the patients who underwent buccal graft placement required at least one additional procedure for final closure. Although not specifically broken down into graft versus primary closure groups, an overall closure rate was achieved in 84% of these patients after a single procedure.[60]

In the largest available series to date, Harris et al. completed a retrospective review of 201 patients treated for RUF secondary to prostate cancer treatment at four large-volume centers over a 15-year period. All procedures were performed through a perineal approach, with 20% of patients requiring a combined abdominoperineal approach. They compared a cohort of 97 (48.2%) patients with surgical RUFs to 104 (51.8%) patients with radiated/ablated RUFs. Use of interposition flaps or grafts was common in both groups (>90%). Buccal mucosa grafts were used in 44.2% of patients in the radiation/energy ablation group but were required in none of the surgically induced fistulas. Successful outcomes were ultimately achieved in 99% of the surgical group and 87% of the radiated/ablated patients. In addition, postoperative urinary incontinence (35% vs. 16%) and complications (25% vs. 11%) were higher in the radiated/ablated RUF group.[69]

Transrectal Approaches

Multiple additional techniques have been used to repair small, surgically induced RUFs. The most frequently

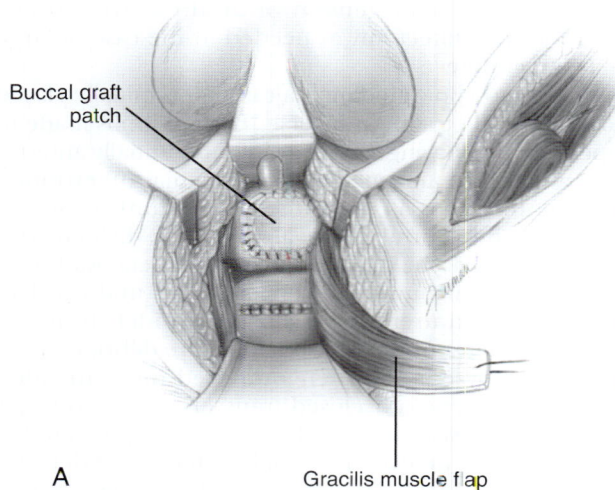

Buccal graft patch

A

Gracilis muscle flap

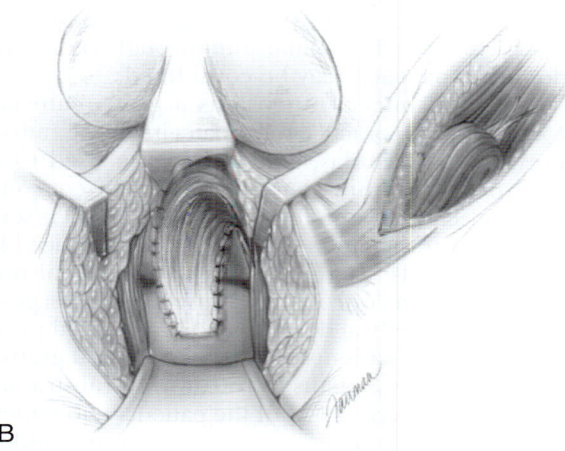

B

FIGURE 151.7 (A) Gracilis muscle interposition flap with buccal mucosal patch closure of urethra. (B) Gracilis muscle flap coverage and support of buccal graft and periurethral tissue. (Used with permission from Vanni A, Buckley JC, Zinman LN. Management of surgical and radiation induced rectourethral fistulas with an interposition muscle flap and selective buccal mucosal onlay graft. *J Urol.* 2010;184:2400.)

used transanal/transrectal techniques today include the York-Mason posterior transanosphincteric approach and minimally invasive transanal approaches.

The York-Mason procedure uses a prone jackknife position followed by posterior midline division of the sphincter muscles. The sphincter muscles are tagged for later closure. The posterior wall of the rectum is opened, providing excellent exposure of the anterior rectal wall and fistulous tract. After sharp excision of the fistula tract, the urinary tract and rectum are separated widely. The urinary tract fistula is closed primarily. In general, creation of a full-thickness rectal advancement flap allows for closure of the rectal defect with nonoverlapping suture lines. The

anal sphincter musculature is carefully reapproximated, allowing for the preservation of fecal continence (Fig. 151.8). High fistula closure rates have been reported with this approach (85% to 100%), especially in the setting of nonradiated RUF.[79,80] The advantage of relatively unscarred tissue planes must be balanced against the risk of causing anal dysfunction and the inability to repair large, complex RUFs that cannot be closed primarily.

Low, minimally complex fistulas may also be repaired by minimally invasive transanal techniques. The main advantage of such a repair is minimal morbidity and quick recovery, whereas the main disadvantage is that the high-pressure urethral side cannot be completely addressed and a period of prolonged catheter drainage may be required. Using such an approach, initial closure was achieved in 8 (67%) of 12 patients in an earlier series[81] and 12 (100%) of 12 patients using more updated techniques.[82]

ALTERNATIVE MANAGEMENT APPROACHES AND SALVAGE PROSTATECTOMY

In patients who have undergone combination energy-ablative therapies, such as external beam radiation followed by salvage cryotherapy, the prostatic remnant may have extensive necrosis and calcification. In these patients, salvage prostatectomy or even cystoprostatectomy and urinary diversion may be considered at the time of fistula management. In patients with poor performance status or limited life expectancy and large fistulas, end colostomy with concomitant suprapubic tube drainage or bilateral percutaneous nephrostomy tube drainage may be considered. In patients with severe damage or restricted capacity of the bladder from previous radiation therapy, cystoprostatetectomy and urinary diversion should also be considered at the time of fistula repair.

For patients with significant preoperative urinary incontinence or a limited likelihood of maintaining adequate continence postoperatively, there are limited data that delayed placement of an artificial urinary sphincter may be safe and effective.[83] However, early, urinary diversion may also be considered in this patient population pending discussion of their goals and the probability of a successful outcome.

CONCLUSION

Successful RUF management must be tailored to address the intricacies of both rectal and urinary function. We have included a proposed flow diagram for management (Fig. 151.9). With a shift to increasing utilization of radiation and ablative therapies, there has been a marked increase in large, complex fistulas necessitating improved and creative surgical techniques to successfully address them. A multidisciplinary approach to evaluation and management may help to optimize outcomes in these challenging cases.

ACKNOWLEDGMENTS

The authors wish to acknowledge the authors of the previous edition's chapter: Patricia Roberts, MD, and Jill C. Buckley, MD. Portions of the previous edition have been used in this chapter.

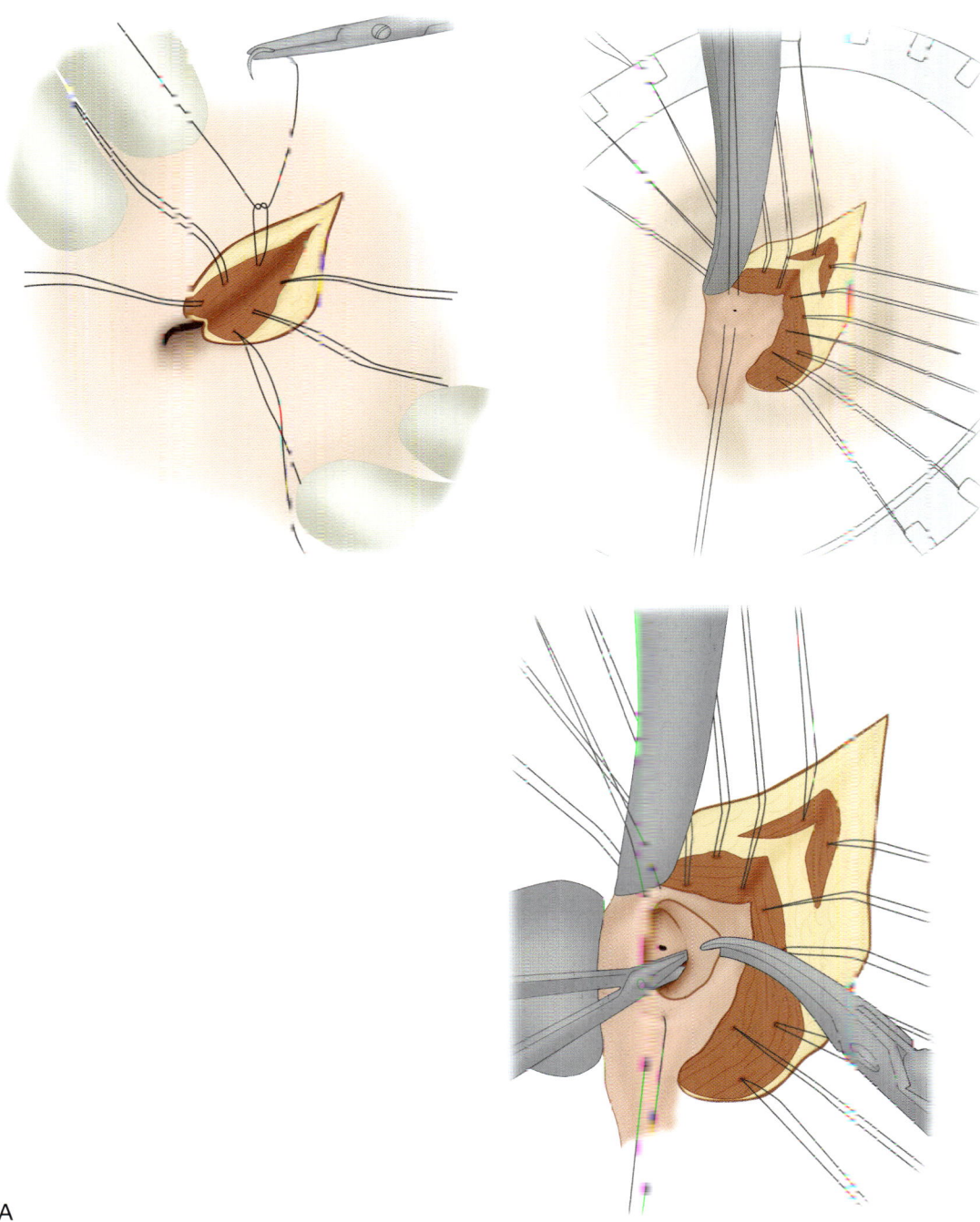

A

FIGURE 151.8 A) Positioning of patient and division through posterior rectum, exposing fistula. Layers tagged with suture.

Continued

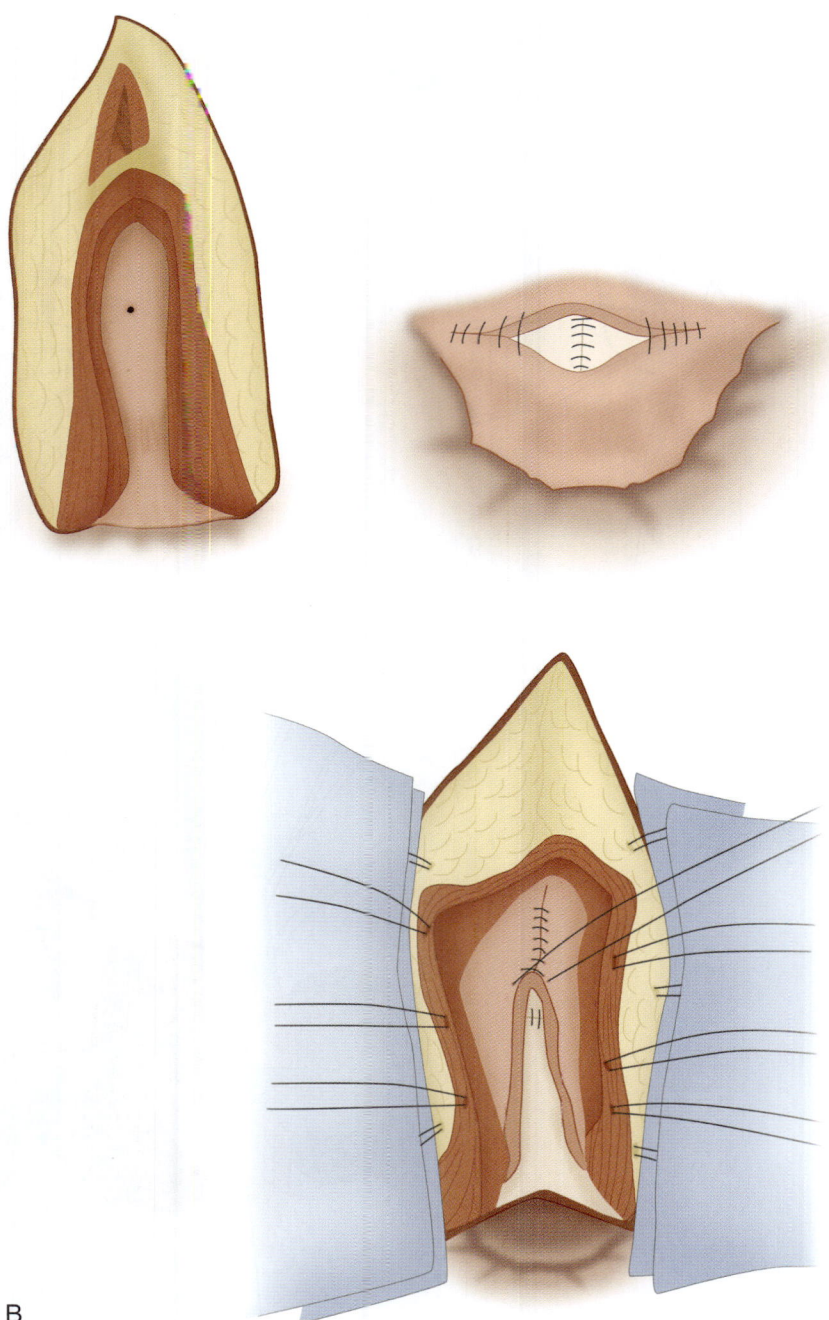

B

FIGURE 151.8, cont'd   (B) Exposure of fistula, and repair of fistula and proctotomy.

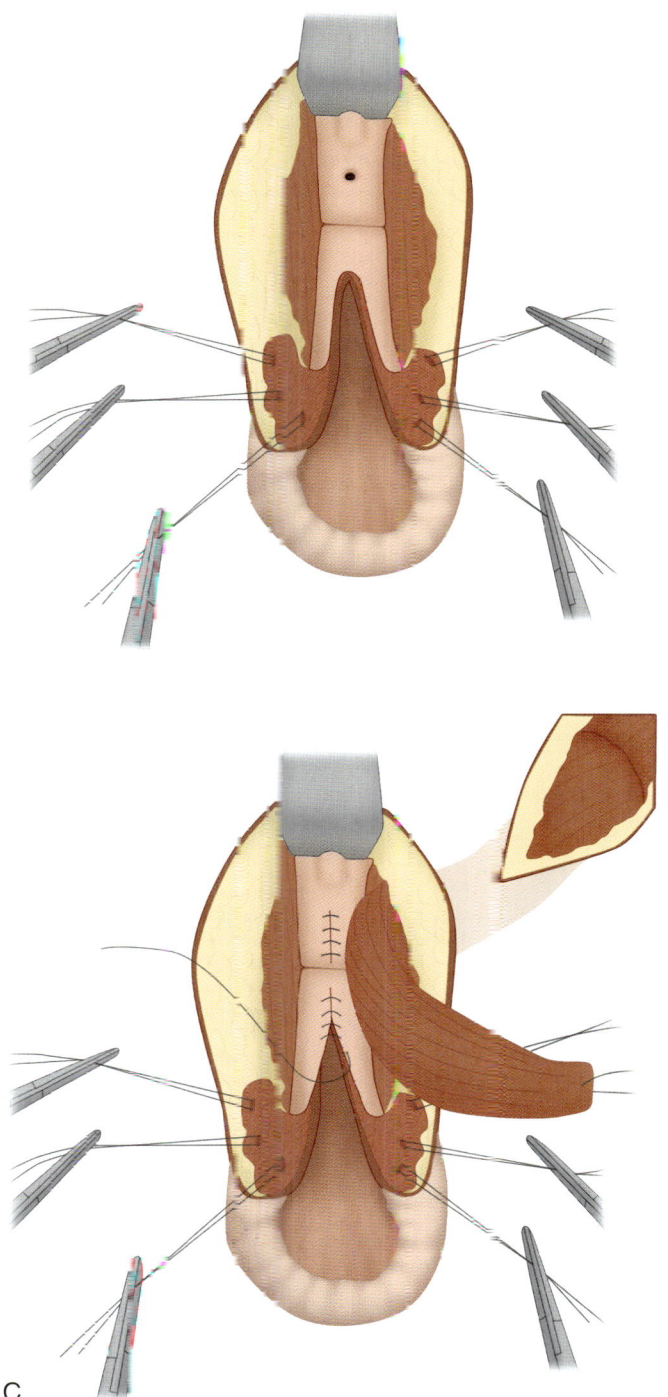

C

FIGURE 151.8 cont'd (C) Sequential layered closure of muscular layers, gracilis flap interposition.

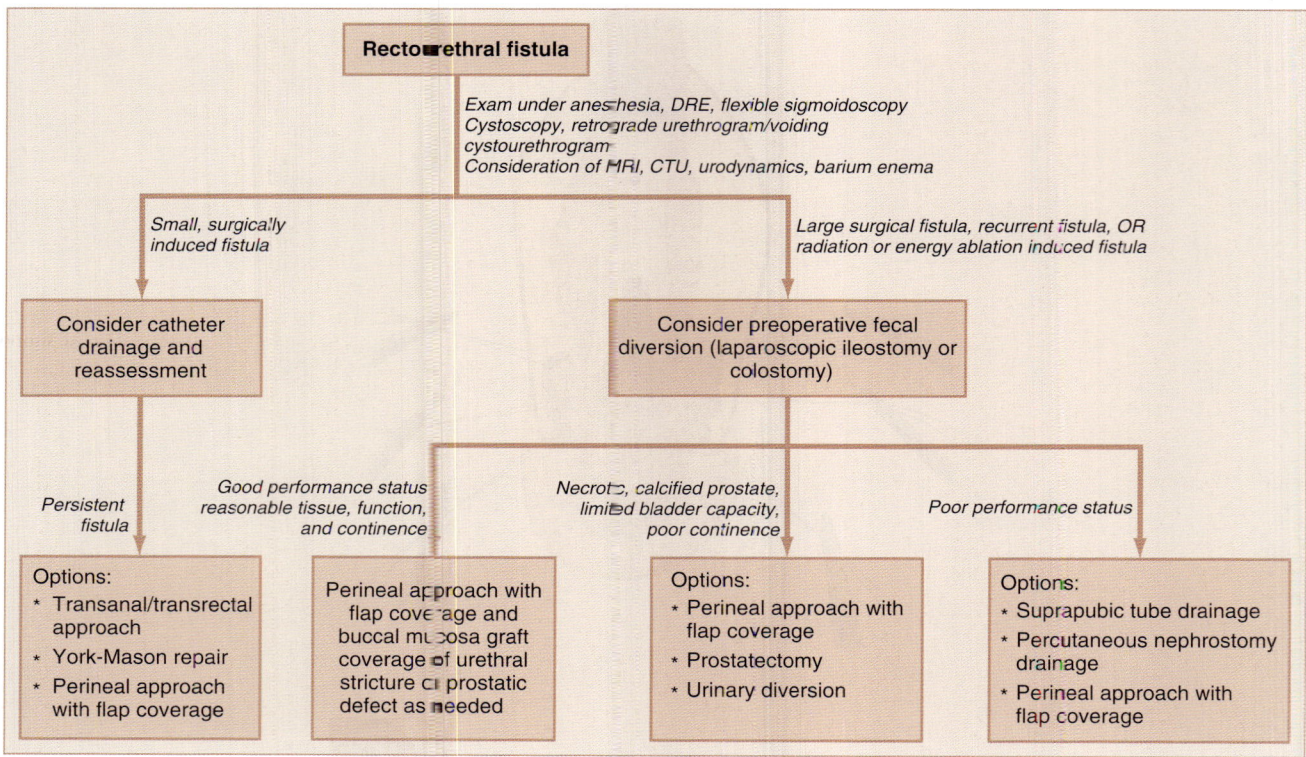

FIGURE 151.9 Proposed flow diagram for management of rectourethral fistulas. *CTU,* Core through urethrotomy; *DRE,* digital rectal examination; *MRI,* magnetic resonance imaging.

REFERENCES

1. Browning A, Allsworth JE, Wall LL. The relationship between female genital cutting and obstetric fistulae. *Obstet Gynecol.* 2010; 115(3):578-583.
2. Matthiessen P, Hansson L, Sjodahl R, Rutegård J. Anastomotic-vaginal fistula (AVF) after anterior resection of the rectum for cancer—occurrence and risk factors. *Colorectal Dis.* 2010;12(4):351-357.
3. Kasibhatla M, Clough RW, Montana GS, et al. Predictors of severe gastrointestinal toxicity after external beam radiotherapy and interstitial brachytherapy for advanced or recurrent gynecologic malignancies. *Int J Radiat Oncol Biol Phys.* 2006;65(2):398-403.
4. Tsang CB, Madoff RD, Wong WD, et al. Anal sphincter integrity and function influences outcome in rectovaginal fistula repair. *Dis Colon Rectum.* 1998;41(9):1141-1146.
5. Yee LF, Birnbaum EH, Read TE, Kodner IJ, Fleshman JW. Use of endoanal ultrasound in patients with rectovaginal fistulae. *Dis Colon Rectum.* 1999;42(8):1057-1064.
6. Dohgomori H, Arikawa K, Nobori M, Tonari M. Hyperbaric oxygenation for rectovaginal fistula: a report of two cases. *J Obstet Gynaecol Res.* 1999;25(5):343-344.
7. Present DH, Rutgeerts P, Targan S, et al. Infliximab for the treatment of fistulae in patients with Crohn's disease. *N Engl J Med.* 1999;340(18):1398-1405.
8. Sands BE, Blank MA, Patel K, van Deventer SJ. ACCENT II Study. Long-term treatment of rectovaginal fistulae in Crohn's disease: response to infliximab in the ACCENT II Study. *Clin Gastroenterol Hepatol.* 2004;2(10):912-920.
9. Andreani SM, Dang HH, Grondona P, Khan AZ, Edwards DP. Rectovaginal fistula in Crohn's disease. *Dis Colon Rectum.* 2007;50(12): 2215-2222.
10. Poritz LS, Rowe WA, Koltun WA. Remicade does not abolish the need for surgery in fistulizing Crohn's disease. *Dis Colon Rectum.* 2002;45(6):771-775.
11. El-Gazzaz G, Hull T, Mignanelli E, Hammel J, Gurland B, Zutshi M. Analysis of function and predictors of failure in women undergoing repair of Crohn's related rectovaginal fistula. *J Gastrointest Surg.* 2010;14(5):824-829.
12. Pinto RA, Peterson TV, Shawki S, Davila GW, Wexner SD. Are there predictors of outcome following rectovaginal fistula repair? *Dis Colon Rectum.* 2010;53(9):1240-1247.
13. Laird DR. Procedures used in treatment of complicated fistulae. *Am J Surg.* 1948;76(6):701-708.
14. Kodner IJ, Mazor A, Shemesh EI, Fry RD, Fleshman JW, Birnbaum EH. Endorectal advancement flap repair of rectovaginal and other complicated anorectal fistulae. *Surgery.* 1993;114(4):682-689, discussion 689–690.
15. Lowry AC, Thorson AG, Rothenberger DA, Goldberg SM. Repair of simple rectovaginal fistulae. Influence of previous repairs. *Dis Colon Rectum.* 1988;31(9):676-678.
16. Wise WE Jr, Aguilar PS, Padmanabhan A, Meesig DM, Arnold MW, Stewart WR. Surgical treatment of low rectovaginal fistulae. *Dis Colon Rectum.* 1991;34(3):271-274.
17. Khanduja KS, Yamashita HJ, Wise WE Jr, Aguilar PS, Hartmann RF. Delayed repair of obstetric injuries of the anorectum and vagina. A stratified surgical approach. *Dis Colon Rectum.* 1994;37(4):344-349.
18. Athanasiadis S, Oladeinde I, Kuprian A, Keller B. Endorectal advancement flap-plasty vs. transperineal closure in surgical treatment of rectovaginal fistulae. A prospective long-term study of 88 patients. *Chirurg.* 1995;66(5):493-502.
19. MacRae HM, McLeod RS, Cohen Z, Stern H, Reznick R. Treatment of rectovaginal fistulae that has failed previous repair attempts. *Dis Colon Rectum.* 1995;38(9):921-925.
20. Mazier WP, Senagore AJ, Schiesel EC. Operative repair of anovaginal and rectovaginal fistulae. *Dis Colon Rectum.* 1995;38(1):4-6.
21. Watson SJ, Phillips RK. Non-inflammatory rectovaginal fistula. *Br J Surg.* 1995;82(12):1641-1643.
22. Joo JS, Weiss EG, Nogueras JJ, Wexner SD. Endorectal advancement flap in perianal Crohn's disease. *Am Surg.* 1998;64(2):147-150.
23. Hyman N. Endoanal advancement flap repair for complex anorectal fistulae. *Am J Surg.* 1999;178(4):337-340.
24. Baig MK, Zhao RH, Yuen CH, et al. Simple rectovaginal fistulae. *Int J Colorectal Dis.* 2000;15(5-6):323-327.
25. Mizrahi N, Wexner SD, Zmora O, et al. Endorectal advancement flap: are there predictors of failure? *Dis Colon Rectum.* 2002;45(12):1616-1621.

26. Sonoda T, Hull T, Piedmonte MR, Fazio VW. Outcomes of primary repair of anorectal and rectovaginal fistulae using the endorectal advancement flap. *Dis Colon Rectum*. 2002;45(12):1762–1628.

27. Zimmerman DD, Gosselink MP, Hie JW, Schouten WR. The outcome of transanal advancement flap repair of rectovaginal fistulae is not improved by an additional labial fat flap transposition. *Tech Coloproctol*. 2002;6(1):37-42.

28. Singer M, Cintron J, Nelson R, et al. Treatment of fistulae-in-ano with fibrin sealant in combination with intra-adhesive antibiotics and/or surgical closure of the internal fistula opening. *Dis Colon Rectum*. 2005;48(4):799-808.

29. Gonsalves S, Sagar P, Lengyel J, Morrison C, Dunham L. Assessment of the efficacy of the rectovaginal button fistula plug for the treatment of ileal pouch-vaginal and rectovaginal fistulae. *Dis Colon Rectum*. 2009;52(11):1877-1881.

30. Gajsek U, McArthur DR, Sagar PM. Long-term efficacy of the button fistula plug in the treatment of ileal pouch-vaginal and Crohn's-related rectovaginal fistulae. *Dis Colon Rectum*. 2011;54(8):999-1002.

31. Ellis CN. Outcomes after repair of rectovaginal fistulae using bioprosthetics. *Dis Colon Rectum*. 2008;51(7):1084-1088.

32. Schwandner O, Fuerst A, Kunstreich K, Scherer E. Innovative technique for the closure of rectovaginal fistula using Surgisis mesh. *Tech Coloproctol*. 2009;13(2):135-440.

33. Bauer JJ, Sher ME, Jaffin H, Present D, Gelernt I. Transvaginal approach for repair of rectovaginal fistulae complicating Crohn's disease. *Ann Surg*. 1991;213(2):151-158.

34. Ruffolo C, Scarpa M, Bassi N, Angriman I. A systematic review on advancement flaps for rectovaginal fistula in Crohn's disease: transrectal vs transvaginal approach. *Colorectal Dis*. 2010;12(12):1183-1191.

35. Pepe F, Panella M, Arikian S, Panella P, Pepe G. Low rectovaginal fistulae. *Aust N Z J Obstet Gynaecol*. 1987;27(1):61-63.

36. Tancer ML, Lasser D, Rosenblum N. Rectovaginal fistula or perineal and anal sphincter disruption, or both, after vaginal delivery. *Surg Gynecol Obstet*. 1990;171(1):43-46.

37. Hull TL, El-Gazzaz G, Gurland B, Church J, Zutshi M. Surgeons should not hesitate to perform episioproctotomy for rectovaginal fistula secondary to cryptoglandular or obstetrical origin. *Dis Colon Rectum*. 2011;54(1):54-59.

38. Hull TL, Bartus C, Bast J, Floruta C, Lopez R. Multimedia article. Success of episioproctotomy for cloaca and rectovaginal fistula. *Dis Colon Rectum*. 2007;50(1):97-101.

39. Kaiser AM. Cloaca-like deformity with faecal incontinence after severe obstetric injury—technique and functional outcome of ano-vaginal and perineal reconstruction with X-flaps and sphincteroplasty. *Colorectal Dis*. 2008;10(8):827-832.

40. Rojanasakul A. LIFT procedure: a simplified technique for fistula-in-ano. *Tech Coloproctol*. 2009;13(3):237-240.

41. Rojanasakul A, Pattanaarun J, Sahakitrungruang C, Tantiphlachiva K. Total anal sphincter saving technique for fistula-in-ano the ligation of intersphincteric fistula tract. *J Med Assoc Thai*. 2007;90(3):581-586.

42. Martius H. Die operative Wiederherstellung der vollkommen fehlenden harnrohre und des Schliessmuskel desselben. *Zentralbl Gynak*. 1928;52:480.

43. Elkins TE, DeLancey JO, McGuire EJ. The use of modified Martius graft as an adjunctive technique in vesicovaginal and rectovaginal fistula repair. *Obstet Gynecol*. 1990;75(4):727-733.

44. Pinedo G, Phillips R. Labial fat pad grafts (modified Martius graft) in complex perianal fistulae. *Ann R Coll Surg Engl*. 1998;80(6):410-412.

45. Hoskins WJ, Park RC, Long R, Artman LE, McMahon EB. Repair of urinary tract fistulae with bulbocavernosus myocutaneous flaps. *Obstet Gynecol*. 1984;63(4):588-593.

46. Symmonds RE, Hill LM. Loss of the urethra: a report on 50 patients. *Am J Obstet Gynecol*. 1978;130(2):130-138.

47. Boronow RC. Repair of the radiation-induced vaginal fistula utilizing the Martius technique. *World J Surg*. 1986;10(2):237-248.

48. McNevin MS, Lee PY, Bax TW. Martius flap: an adjunct for repair of complex, low rectovaginal fistula. *Am J Surg*. 2007;193(5):597-599, discussion 599.

49. Lee D, Dillon BE, Zimmern PE. Martius labial fat pad procedure: technique and long-term outcomes. *Int Urogynecol J*. 2015;26(9):1395-1396.

50. Lefevre JH, Bretagnol F, Maggiori L, Alves A, Ferron M, Panis Y. Operative results and quality of life after gracilis muscle transposition for recurrent rectovaginal fistula. *Dis Colon Rectum*. 2009;52(7):1290-1295.

51. Rius J, Nessim A, Nogueras JJ, Wexner SD. Gracilis transposition in complicated perianal fistula and unhealed perineal wounds in Crohn's disease. *Eur J Surg*. 2000;166(3):218-222.

52. Zmora O, Tulchinsky H, Gur E, Goldman G, Klausner JM, Rabau M. Gracilis muscle transposition for fistulae between the rectum and urethra or vagina. *Dis Colon Rectum*. 2006;49(9):1316-1321.

53. Furst A, Schmidbauer C, Swol-Ben J, Iesalnieks I, Schwandner O, Agha A. Gracilis transposition for repair of recurrent anovaginal and rectovaginal fistulae in Crohn's disease. *Int J Colorectal Dis*. 2008;23(4):349-35.

54. Wexner SD, Ruiz DE, Genua J, et al. Gracilis muscle interposition for the treatment of rectourethral, rectovaginal, and pouch-vaginal fistulae: results in 53 patients. *Ann Surg*. 2008;248(1):39-43.

55. Hotouras A, Ribas Y, Zakeri S, Murphy J, Bhan C, Chan CL. Gracilis muscle interposition for rectovaginal and anovaginal fistula repair: a systematic literature review. *Colorectal Dis*. 2015;17(2):104-110.

56. Penalver M, Mekki Y, Lafferty H, Escobar M, Angioli R. Should sacrospinous ligament fixation for the management of pelvic support defects be part of a residency program procedure? The University of Miami experience. *Am J Obstet Gynecol*. 1998;178(2):326-329.

57. Parks AG, Allen CL, Frank JD, McPartlin JF. A method of treating post-irradiation rectovaginal fistulae. *Br J Surg*. 1978;65(6):417-421.

58. Cooke SA, Wellsted MD. The radiation-damaged rectum: resection with coloanal anastomosis using the endoanal technique. *World J Surg*. 1986;10(2):220-227.

59. Lane BR, Stein DE, Remzi FH, Strong SA, Fazio VW, Angermeier KW. Management of radiotherapy induced rectourethral fistula. *J Urol*. 2006;175(4):1382-1387, discussion 1387-1388.

60. Vanni AJ, Buckley JC, Zinman LN. Management of surgical and radiation induced rectourethral fistulae with an interposition muscle flap and selective buccal mucosal onlay graft. *J Urol*. 2010;184(6):2400-2404.

61. McLaren RH, Barrett DM, Zincke H. Rectal injury occurring at radical retropubic prostatectomy for prostate cancer: etiology and treatment. *Urology*. 1993;42(4):401-405.

62. Chrouser KL, Leibovich BC, Sweat SD, et al. Urinary fistulae following external radiation or permanent brachytherapy for the treatment of prostate cancer. *J Urol*. 2005;173(6):1953-1957.

63. Zinman L. The management of the complex recto-urethral fistula. *BJU Int*. 2004;94(9):1212-1213.

64. Wedmid A, Mendoza P, Sharma S, et al. Rectal injury during robot-assisted radical prostatectomy: incidence and management. *J Urol*. 2011;186(5):1928-1933.

65. Harpster LE, Rommel FM, Sieber PR, et al. The incidence and management of rectal injury associated with radical prostatectomy in a community-based urology practice. *J Urol*. 1995;154(4):1435-1438.

66. Yee DS, Ornstein DK. Repair of rectal injury during robotic-assisted laparoscopic prostatectomy. *Urology*. 2008;72(2):428-431.

67. Martin-Marquina Aspiunza A, Zudaire Bergera J, Sanchez Zalabardo D. Radical proctectomy. The surgical complications. *Actas Urol Esp*. 1999;23(5) e-34-e645.

68. Thomas C, Jones J, Jager W, Hampel C, Thüroff JW, Gillitzer R. Incidence, clinical symptoms and management of rectourethral fistulae after radical prostatectomy. *J Urol*. 2010;183(2):608-612.

69. Harris CR, McAninch JW, Mundy AR, et al. Rectourethral fistulae secondary to prostate cancer treatment: management and outcomes from a multi-institutional combined experience. *J Urol*. 2016;197(1):91-194.

70. Grado GL, Larson TR, Balch CS, et al. Actuarial disease-free survival after prostate cancer brachytherapy using interactive techniques with biplane ultrasound and fluoroscopic guidance. *Int J Radiat Oncol Biol Phys*. 1998;42(2):289-298.

71. Theodorescu D, Gillenwater JY, Koutrouvelis PG. Prostatourethral-rectal fistula after prostate brachytherapy. *Cancer*. 2000;89(10):2085-2091.

72. Zacharakis E, Ahmed HU, Ishaq A, et al. The feasibility and safety of high-intensity focused ultrasound as salvage therapy for recurrent prostate cancer following external beam radiotherapy. *BJU Int*. 2008;102(7):786-792.

73. Stone NN, Stock RG. Complications following permanent prostate brachytherapy. *Eur Urol*. 2002;41(4):427-433.

74. Nguyen PL, D'Amico AV, Lee AK, Suh WW. Patient selection, cancer control, and complications after salvage local therapy for postradiation prostate-specific antigen failure: a systematic review of the literature. *Cancer*. 2007;110(7):1417-1428.

75. Pisters LL, Rewcastle JC, Donnelly BJ, Lugnani FM, Katz AE, Jones JS. Salvage prostate cryoablation: initial results from the cryo on-line data registry. *J Urol*. 2008;180(2):559-563, discussion 563–564.

76. Ahmed HU, Ishaq A, Zacharakis E, et al. Rectal fistulae after salvage high-intensity focused ultrasound for recurrent prostate cancer after

combined brachytherapy and external beam radiotherapy. *BJU Int.* 2009;103(3):321-323.

77. Dinges S, Deger S, Koswig S, et al. High-dose rate interstitial with external beam irradiation for localized prostate cancer—results of a prospective trial. *Radiother Oncol.* 1998;48(2):197-202.

78. Hanna JM, Turley R, Castleberry A, et al. Surgical management of complex rectourethral fistulae in irradiated and nonirradiated patients. *Dis Colon Rectum.* 2014;57(9):1105-1112.

79. Dal Moro F, Mancini M, Pinto F, et al. Successful repair of iatrogenic rectourinary fistulae using the posterior sagittal transrectal approach (York-Mason): 15-year experience. *World J Surg.* 2006;30(1):107-113.

80. Renschler TD, Middleton RG. 30 years of experience with York-Mason repair of recto-urinary fistulae. *J Urol.* 2003;170(4 Pt 1):1222-1225, discussion 1225.

81. Garofalo TE, Delaney CP, Jones SM, Remzi FH, Fazio VW. Rectal advancement flap repair of rectourethral fistula: a 20-year experience. *Dis Colon Rectum.* 2003;46(6):762-769.

82. Nicita G, Villari D, Caroassai Grisanti S, Marzocco M, Marzi LM, Martini A. Minimally invasive transanal repair of rectourethral fistulae. *Eur Urol.* 2016;71(1):133-138.

83. Selph JP, Madden-Fuentes R, Peterson AC, et al. Long-term artificial urinary sphincter outcomes following a prior rectourethral fistula repair. *Urology.* 2015;86(3):608-612.

Current Approaches to Complete Rectal Prolapse and Internal Intussusception

Isaac Payne | Gregory Quatrino | Paul Rider | Leander Grimm Jr.

HISTORICAL PERSPECTIVE

Evidence of rectal prolapse (rectal procidentia) exists from ancient times.[1] The first described mortality from rectal prolapse was in the 4th century.[2] The initiating cause of prolapse is elusive. The path to rectal prolapse generally occurs slowly over a period of years. Suggested contributing factors include standing, constipation, colic, coughing, sneezing, weak anal sphincters and pelvic floor musculature, an abnormal cul-de-sac, and distal rectal intussusception. The proposed treatments have changed significantly over time as well. Treatments such as cauterizing the rectal mucosa, binding patient's legs together, and applying trusses have been replaced with variations of resection and rectopexy today.

PRESENTATION AND WORK-UP

Patients with rectal prolapse will often report a history of constipation and even incontinence. Women are 6 times more likely than men to suffer from prolapse. The primary presenting complaint is often of a protuberance or bulge from the anus, which is often mistaken for hemorrhoidal disease. It may spontaneously reduce or remain prolapsed, causing considerable distress. Other complaints may be a feeling of incomplete evacuation of stool, bleeding, mucus discharge, urinary incontinence, and pain.

The prolapse may be apparent on initial exam; other times it will need to be elicited by asking the patient to perform a Valsalva. At times, it is even necessary to examine the patient after having them strain while squatting on the commode. Once the prolapse is produced, it is important to differentiate true full-thickness rectal prolapse with concentric mucosal rings (Fig. 152.1) from simple hemorrhoidal disease (Fig. 152.2), which is identified by radial folds of hemorrhoidal tissue.

Colonoscopy is required in all patients considered candidates for operative repair of rectal prolapse to rule out a neoplastic lead point. On endoscopic examination, the rectal mucosa in a patient with chronic recurrent prolapse will show signs of circumferential erythema (Fig. 152.3). Other diagnostic tests of debatable significance include anal manometry, endorectal ultrasound, and defecography.[3-5] Defecography is valuable in occult, intermittent prolapse to document marked mobility of the rectosigmoid junction away from the normal point of fixation at the sacral promontory.

ACUTE TREATMENT

The immediate management of obvious prolapse is reduction. Before any attempts at reducing the prolapse, it is of utmost importance to fully assess the viability of the rectum. Ischemia or frank necrosis may be present in the neglected or demented patient. If significant full-thickness ischemia is present, reduction should be avoided and operative resection will likely be required. The majority of patients with viable prolapse will respond to continuous, steady pressure in the office setting or emergency room. At times, intravenous sedation or even general anesthesia in the operating room may be necessary for full reduction. Applying table salt or sugar to the mucosa can reduce the swelling of the incarcerated rectum and aid in reduction.[6] Another technique described for the stubborn prolapse involves encompassing the rectum with an elastic compression wrap.[7] Hyaluronidase injection into the prolapsed rectum has also been described to aid in reduction.[8]

TRANSABDOMINAL OPTIONS

Abdominal approaches to definitive repair of prolapse consistently show lower recurrence rates compared with perineal approaches. The transabdominal approach is the preferred repair in patients who can tolerate a transabdominal operation.[1,9] Ideally, the operation should be limited in morbidity and mortality, have a low recurrence rate, and address the patient's associated constipation or incontinence, if present. Care must also be given to evaluating the patient for the presence of concurrent anterior compartment prolapse to assess the feasibility of repair of these prolapsing organs as well in a combined operation.

There are two primary technical components in the abdominal approach to rectal prolapse: rectopexy and resection. The goal of rectopexy is to mobilize the rectum out of the pelvis to straighten the low rectum in the curve of the sacrum and secure it proximally at the sacral promontory so that prolapse cannot recur. In 1963, Ripstein described the posterior rectopexy: a posterior rectal dissection to the level of the coccyx and a sling of fascia lata around the rectum anchored to the proximal sacrum.[10] Modifications using biologic and synthetic meshes have come and gone over time.[11,12] Rectopexy can even be performed without the use of mesh by securing peritoneal wings of the rectum to the sacral promontory with suture or tacks. This technique, however, results in slightly higher recurrence rates than rectopexy with mesh (Table 152.1).

The extent of rectal mobilization required during rectopexy has also been an issue of debate. Circumferential mobilization may decrease the rate of prolapse recurrence[13]; however, a known drawback of rectopexy is constipation, and division of the anterolateral ligaments (parasympathetic innervations) during dissection

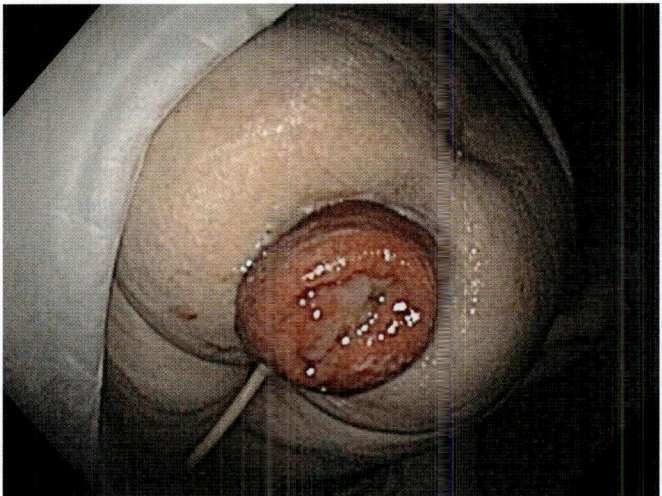

FIGURE 152.1 Full-thickness rectal prolapse with concentric rings.

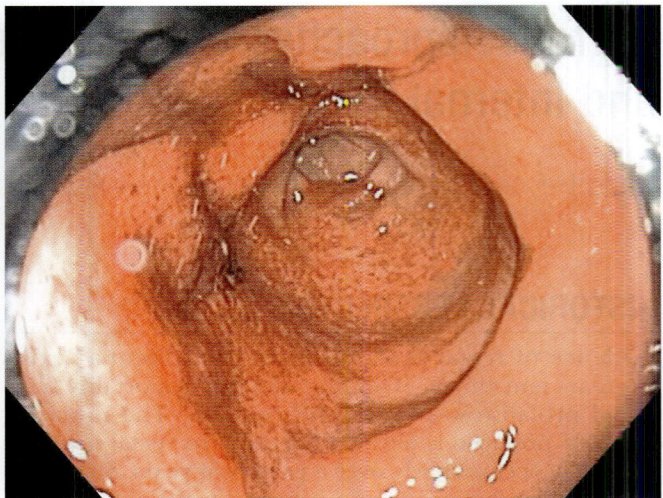

FIGURE 152.3 Inflamed circumference of rectum in chronic prolapse.

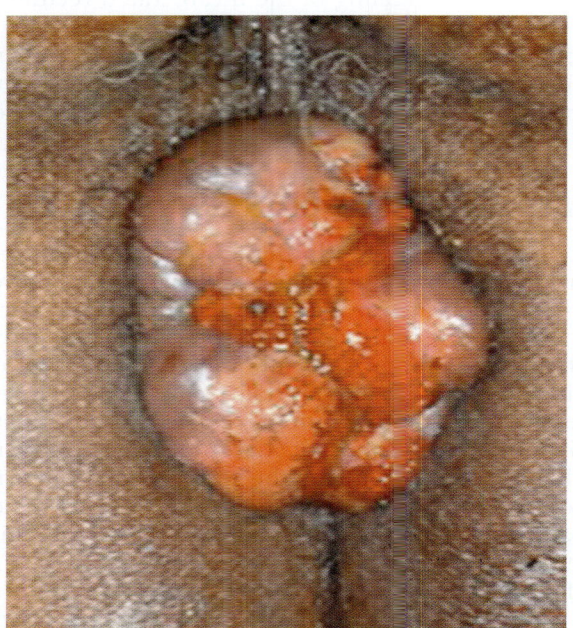

FIGURE 152.2 Radial folds of severe hemorrhoidal prolapse.

TABLE 152.1 Recurrence Rates With Abdominal Approaches[14-21]

Surgery	Recurrence (%)
Mesh rectopexy	2–5
Suture rectopexy	3–9
Resection/rectopexy	2–5
Ventral rectopexy	2–9

has been shown to increase the rate and severity of constipation.[13,14] Especially in patients with preexisting constipation, a possible solution to the increased rate of constipation is performing a concurrent resection of the redundant portion of the sigmoid colon with

primary colorectal anastomosis at the level of the sacral promontory.[15,16] Avoiding full mobilization of the splenic flexure is also recommended to avoid re-creating colonic redundancy.

The most recent addition to the abdominal operations for rectal prolapse is the ventral rectopexy that involves mobilization of the anterior portion of the rectum without a posterior or lateral dissection. Mesh shaped in the form of a "hockey stick" is then sutured from the anterior rectal wall to the sacral promontory and covered with peritoneum. This technique reduces the need for extensive posterior dissection. Some authors report lower constipation rates, while maintaining recurrence rates similar to posterior rectopexy (see Table 152.1).[17-20]

The use of laparoscopy in the repair of rectal prolapse has been studied extensively. The integrity of the repair has not been compromised with the laparoscopic approach, as recurrence rates are similar. The short-term postoperative benefits of laparoscopic surgery are realized in patients with rectal prolapse, including decreased postoperative pain, shorter hospital length of stay, and quicker return of bowel function.[21-23] These recovery benefits of laparoscopy may also allow more high-risk patients to be approached transabdominally, who may otherwise have only been considered for the less durable perineal approaches.

PERINEAL APPROACHES

While abdominal approaches for rectal prolapse have the lowest recurrence rates with better overall functional outcomes, the majority of patients with prolapse are elderly. Many of these patients have significant comorbidities that limit their ability to tolerate an abdominal approach.[24] Additionally, though a much smaller cohort, young patients, especially males, may consider a perineal approach to limit the added risk of sexual dysfunction.[25] Up to 60% of patients suffering from rectal prolapse will undergo a perineal approach.[26] When rectal prolapse recurs after an abdominal approach, a second abdominal approach can be technically difficult. In these circumstances, a perineal

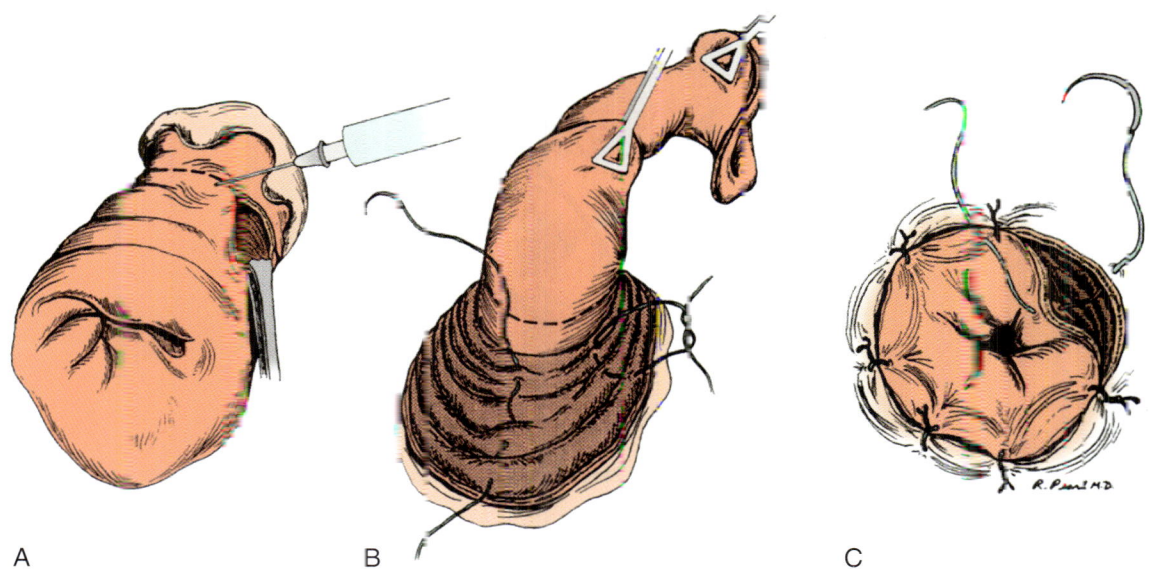

FIGURE 152.4 Perineal proctosigmoidectomy (Altemeier procedure). (From Romano G, Bianco F, Caggiano L. Modified perineal stapled rectal resection with Contour Transtar for full-thickness rectal prolapse. *Colorectal Dis* 2009;11[8]:878–881.)

approach may be a viable option. However, a perineal resection-rectopexy can spell doom if the blood supply of the rectosigmoid was previously divided, and the perineal resection leaves an ischemic segment of rectum in place.

PERINEAL PROCTOSIGMOIDECTOMY (ALTEMEIER PROCEDURE)

Perineal proctosigmoidectomy for rectal prolapse was originally introduced by Mikulicz in 1899 and popularized by Altemeier et al.[27] The procedure can be performed in lithotomy or prone jackknife position. Anesthetic options include regional or general anesthesia. The operation is begun by applying gentle retraction to the rectum so that the redundant rectum is externalized, recreating the prolapse (Fig. 152.4). The anal canal is held open with a Lone Star retractor (Lone Star Company, Frisco, Texas). The dentate line is identified. An injection of dilute epinephrine solution is administered circumferentially 1 to 2 cm proximal to the dentate line followed by a full-thickness, circumferential rectal incision with electrocautery (Fig. 152.4A). The avascular intersphincteric plane is developed up to the pelvis, and the distal rectum is pulled from the pelvis. Using either suture ligation or an energy device, the vascular supply (first laterally, then posteriorly) of the exposed bowel is then ligated as the dissection is continued proximally. The redundant rectum and sigmoid colon are extracted to the level of the left colon, and the bowel is divided under mild stretch at the point of planned coloanal anastomosis. The more bowel removed, the better. A posterior rectopexy with a postanal levatorplasty has been shown to improve anal continence.[28] The rectopexy is performed by using a nonabsorbable suture to pexy the posterior surface of the nonprolapsed bowel to the presacrococcygeal fascia. The normal anorectal angle is reconstructed with a posterior levatorplasty to restore the anorectal angle (Fig. 152.4B). A hand-sewn coloanal anastomosis is performed between left colon and dentate line (Fig. 152.4C). A stapled anastomosis can be performed using two purse strings. However, some authors report a higher probability of recurrence with a stapled anastomosis.[29] Ultimately, patients selected for a perineal proctosigmoidectomy should expect an improved continence compared with times of prolapse and decreased constipation with overall improved quality of life.[30] However, a disadvantage of the perineal proctosigmoidectomy is the increased recurrence rates of 12% to 24% compared with the abdominal approach.[29,31] This can be reduced by removing all of the redundant distal colon up to the left colon.

ANORECTAL MUCOSECTOMY WITH MUSCULAR PLICATION (DELORME PROCEDURE)

In 1900, Delorme described the anorectal mucosectomy with muscular plication for the treatment of rectal prolapse.[32] A significant advantage of the Delorme procedure is that no full-thickness bowel resection with anastomosis is performed. Similar to the Altemeier procedure, the bowel is completely prolapsed and dilute epinephrine solution is injected in a submucosal plane (Fig. 152.5). Using electrocautery, a circumferential submucosal incision is then made 1 cm proximal to the dentate line. Being careful not to violate the muscular layer of the rectal wall, a submucosal dissection is performed and extended proximally. A mucosectomy twice the length of the prolapse is performed (Fig. 152.5A). After the mucosal sleeve is excised, longitudinal plicating sutures are placed in rows along the length of the rectal wall musculature 1 cm apart. The sutures are not tied until all the sutures have been placed. As the longitudinal sutures are tied

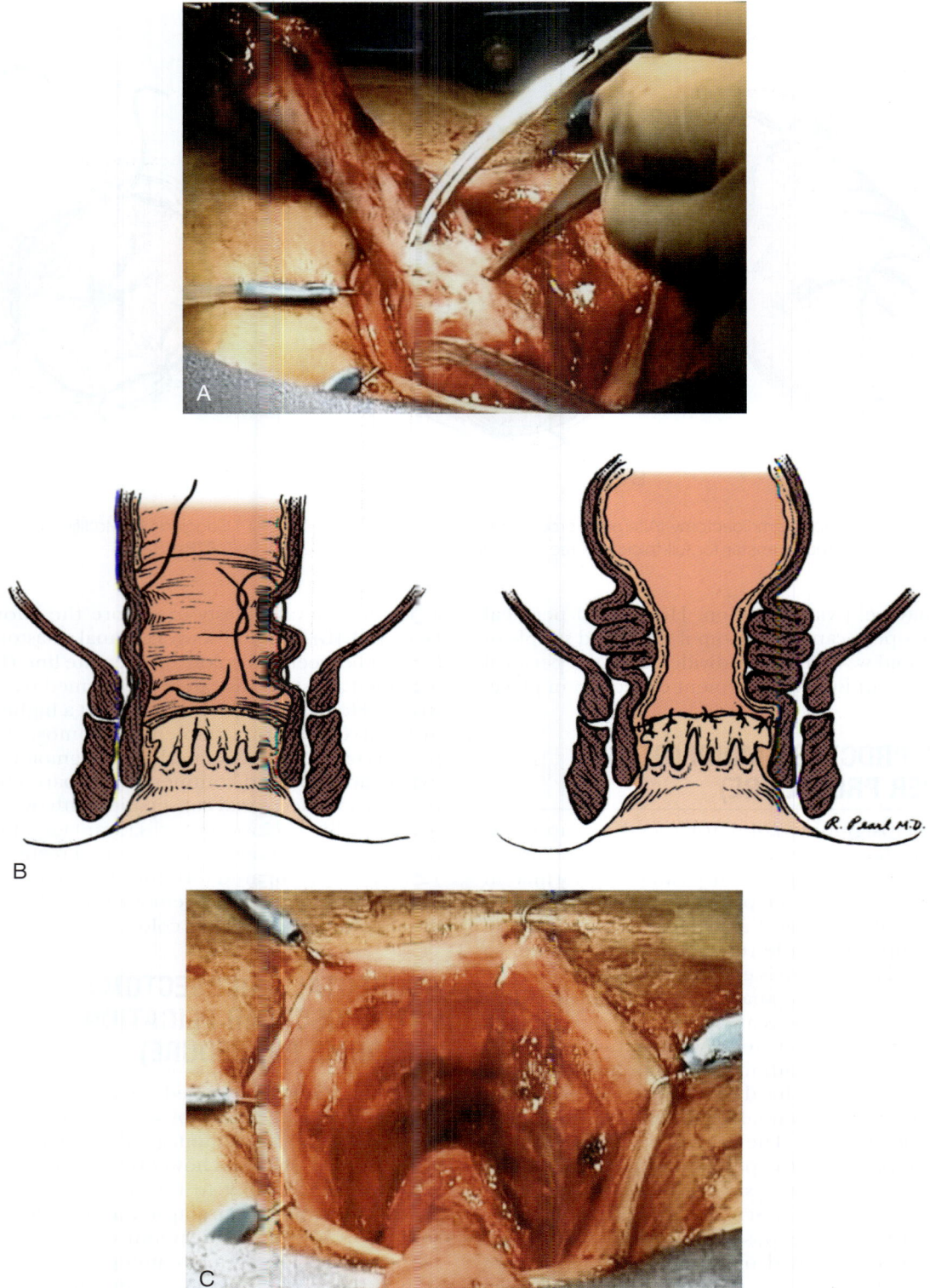

FIGURE 152.5 Anorectal mucosectomy with muscular plication (Delorme procedure). ([B] From Romano G, Bianco F, Caggiano L. Modified perineal stapled rectal resection with Contour Transtar for full-thickness rectal prolapse. *Colorectal Dis*. 2009;11[8]:878–881.)

around the circumference of the rectum the cut edge of the mucosa is brought to the level of the anal canal (Fig. 152.5B,C). Finally, the proximal and distal mucosal edges are reapproximated using absorbable sutures at the dentate line. The muscular plication and mucosal anastomosis can be alternatively performed using a circular stapler.[33] In patients with a patulous anus on physical examination and in efforts to improve continence, a posterior levatorplasty can also be performed.[34] The Delorme procedure for rectal prolapse offers patients a safe procedure, with reported low morbidity of 9.5% but reported recurrence rates of 12% to 31%.[5,35] Significant preexisting long-term constipation has been associated with higher recurrence rates, while pelvic floor repair with levatorplasty has been associated with reduced recurrence rates.[35] Patients may complain of the urge to defecate because of the reefed muscle in the anal canal.

THIERSCH PROCEDURE

Anal encirclement for the treatment of rectal prolapse was introduced in 1891 by Thiersch.[36–38] In the original description, Thiersch used a silver wire to encircle the anus in an effort to provide a mechanical replacement of the relaxed sphincter. The presence of a foreign body would incite an inflammatory reaction and create an adhesive circumferential band to create support of the perineum.[36–38] The procedure does not correct the prolapse but simply mechanically supports the anal sphincter function by narrowing the anal canal and preventing external rectal prolapse. The procedure can be performed quite quickly. With the patient in prone jackknife or lithotomy position, in reference to the center of the anus, two lateral perianal skin incisions are made 180 degrees apart (Fig. 152.6). The incisions are connected subcutaneously by tunneling through the ischiorectal fossa and perineal body. Next, a piece of polypropylene mesh or silicone roll 1.5 cm in height is tunneled circumferentially around the entire anus. The mesh is tightened to a point that allows only the passage of one finger into the anal canal, and the mesh is sutured to itself at this level of tension. Reported

complications include recurrence rates of up to 75%, anal stenosis, fecal impaction, and even erosion of the mesh or Silastic product into the anorectum.[37–39] Because of the high recurrence rates and reported complications, indications for the procedure are very narrow but include patients with mild to moderate rectal prolapse and significant life-threatening comorbidities, with anticipated short life expectancy, that prevent them from either abdominal or resective perineal approaches.

COMPARISON BETWEEN THE DIFFERENT MODALITIES

When comparing between the different treatment modalities for rectal prolapse, postoperative morbidity, recurrent rectal prolapse, fecal incontinence, and constipation are all important outcome variables to examine. Historically, elderly patients with significant comorbidities were only candidates for perineal approaches. The perineal approaches traditionally rendered less durable long-term control of prolapse compared to abdominal approaches. Comparing the Altemeier procedure to Delorme procedure, a randomized controlled study showed there were fewer recurrences after the Altemeier procedure (24% vs. 31%), but functional outcomes were similar.[31]

With abdominal rectopexy, there is no significant difference in terms of recurrence between the methods used for fixation. In investigating the degree of rectal mobilization necessary, circumferential mobilization rather than preservation of the lateral ligaments has been associated with decreased recurrent prolapse.[13] However, circumferential mobilization is also associated with increased postoperative constipation.[13,40] In comparison of resection rectopexy to rectopexy alone, lower rates of both constipation and recurrence were encountered with resection rectopexy.[21,31] Unfortunately, resection is associated with a finite anastomotic leak rate.[15,16]

Although it has been a long-held belief that perineal approaches are associated with a significantly higher recurrence rate than abdominal approaches, a 2015 Cochrane review of 15 randomized controlled trials and over 1000 patients failed to display superiority of any approach in terms of recurrence rates or quality of life.[21] Therefore the surgeon's experience and judgment are paramount to the choice of operative approach based on patient characteristics, the clinical situation, and expertise.

MANAGEMENT OF RECURRENCE

It is important to understand patient and technical factors that are associated with recurrence patterns. During perineal proctosigmoidectomy, stapled anastomosis, shorter specimen length, and severe preexisting constipation were all associated with an increased risk of recurrence. A postanal repair and levatorplasty were associated with lower recurrence rates.[29] During abdominal rectopexy, variables identified as related to recurrence included incontinence, constipation, the extent of rectal mobilization, and whether sigmoid resection was performed in the setting of constipation.[41] As mentioned in the previous section, circumferential rectal mobilization was associated

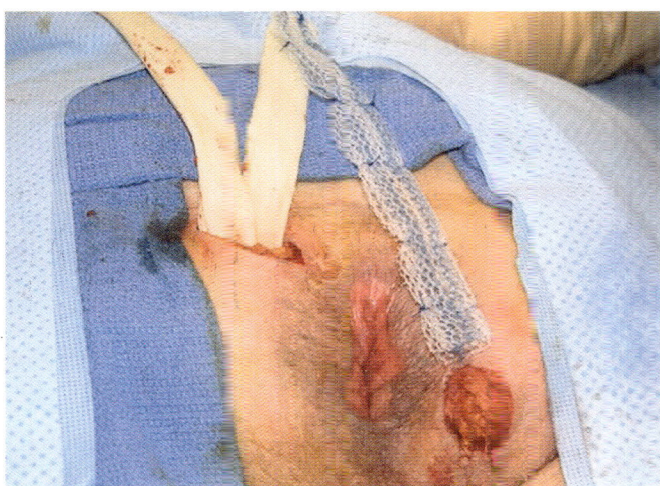

FIGURE 152.6 Thiersch anal encirclement procedure.

with decreased recurrence.[13] Overall, a high recurrence rate after either approach is likely due to technical failures such as inadequate fixation or incomplete mobilization.[42] Poor decision making and failure to recognize preexisting conditions such as colonic dysmotility in a patient undergoing rectopexy without resection will ultimately render suboptimal results.

Repair of recurrent rectal prolapse should be undertaken only after consideration of several complexities that guide choice of approach. Traditionally, if a perineal resection was initially performed, repeat perineal resection is often the safest route to avoid compromising the remaining proximal blood supply. Similarly, a recurrence after abdominal resection rectopexy should not be approached with a perineal resection, as there is great risk for rectal ischemia after ligating both the proximal and then distal rectal blood supply. However, a perineal proctosigmoidectomy is a very reasonable option if abdominal rectopexy without resection was performed as the index procedure. A second abdominal approach is often a technically difficult procedure in the pelvis that can increase the potential for added patient morbidity. Similarly, it is reasonable to consider abdominal rectopexy without resection after a recurrence from a perineal resection. Therefore, in the case of recurrent prolapse, the index procedure often dictates the reoperative surgical approach.[43] Mesh suspension may be considered if tissues were inadequate for pexy at the initial operation.

INTERNAL INTUSSUSCEPTION (INTERNAL RECTAL PROLAPSE)

Internal rectal intussusception is described as internal telescoping of the rectum that does not result in protrusion from the anal canal. When the rectum protrudes from the anal canal, rectal prolapse occurs. The Oxford grading system has been established to grade the severity of rectal prolapse based on evacuation proctography.[44] While internal intussusception has been identified in asymptomatic individuals and has historically been treated as a normal variant, evidence now suggests that patients with internal intussusception can suffer from a spectrum of disorders ranging from obstructed defecation syndrome to fecal incontinence.[45,46] As such, detailed physical examination and often extensive diagnostic imaging work-up are required.

HISTORY

Women with internal rectal intussusception commonly suffer from a range of symptoms. Historically, symptoms of internal intussusception included only symptoms of obstructive defecation; however, evidence now suggests that fecal incontinence also frequently plays a significant role in symptomatology. In fact, fecal incontinence can be the predominant complaint in patients with high-grade internal intussusception.[47] In females with internal intussusception, fecal incontinence was reported in 56%, while complaints of incomplete evacuation (45%), straining at defecation (34%), and digital assistance during defecation (34%) were also commonly reported. The majority of patients had complaints of urge incontinence, while passive incontinence and incontinence to flatus were reported less often.[47,48] During the initial clinical encounter of a patient with pelvic defecatory dysfunction, it is necessary to quantify the severity of symptoms. The subsequent success of therapy can be gauged by comparison of function before and after treatment using grading scales, which include Wexner constipation and incontinence score,[49] fecal incontinence severity index score,[50] and quality-of-life.

PATHOPHYSIOLOGY

With the association between internal intussusception, defecatory dysfunction, rectal prolapse, and fecal incontinence now better recognized, much debate remains about whether intussusception is a cause or simply a symptom of these disorders. Initial evidence pointed toward changes in the rectoanal inhibitory reflex (RAIR) caused by the intussusceptum as the source of incontinence. Reducing the intussusceptum with rectopexy, the RAIR would return to normal, and continence would be restored.[51,52] Upon evaluation with anal manometry, initial results suggested a significant reduction in the average maximum resting pressure (MRP) as the grade of rectal intussusception increased. This predicted the role of incontinence was mainly through a reduction in internal anal sphincter tone induced by the inhibitory reflex as the rectum stretched the anal canal.[53] Subsequent follow-up data, however, showed that the MRP between patients with and without intussusception did not differ, suggesting that the reduction of MRP is not permanent. Furthermore, urge incontinence associated with high-grade internal intussusception was significantly associated with a decrease in rectal sensory volume thresholds. One explanation for this observation involves the intussusceptum inciting a chronic irritation on the rectal wall, rendering a reduction in wall compliance with subsequent urge incontinence.[47,48] Unlike incontinence, constipation severity does not increase with increasing Oxford grades of internal intussusception.[54] Further research is necessary to understand the relationship between internal rectal intussusception, the development of defecatory disorders, and the need for surgical repair. The majority of mild to moderate intussusception seen on defecography is asymptomatic, and symptoms can be alleviated with the administration of dietary fiber supplements.

PHYSICAL EXAM

Performing a digital rectal examination (DRE) is a necessary initial screening tool in the work-up of patients presenting with defecatory dysfunction. Not only does the surgeon gain insight on anal sphincter pressures, but DRE also shows high positive predictive values in detecting patients with other forms of outlet obstruction such as paradoxical puborectalis contraction (PPC)[55] or increased perineal descent (IPD). Forward motion of the puborectalis shelf during attempts by the patient to push the examining finger out indicates paradoxical contraction or nonrelaxation (PPC). By having a high index of suspicion for PPC and IPD, physicians can appropriately guide therapy. A sign of intussusception during proctoscopy and anoscopy includes invagination of the circumference of the rectal wall. Low-grade intussusception remains in the rectal vault while high-grade intussusception prolapses into the anal canal without external prolapse. Valsalva maneuver can be helpful during examination to assist in diagnosis.

PHYSIOLOGIC TESTING AND DIAGNOSTIC IMAGING

Advanced physiologic and imaging procedures in the evaluation of patients suffering from defecatory dysfunction are often required. When patients have primary complaints of incontinence, anorectal manometry is often helpful. When comparing patients with internal intussusception to normal controls the MRP is no different. However, there is a statistical difference in rectal volumetric sensory measurements. There is a significant decrease in mean urge volume and mean maximum tolerable volume compared with normal controls.[48] Anal ultrasound can evaluate for sphincter injury or sphincter defects responsible for fecal incontinence. When fecal incontinence is not explained by history of anal obstetric trauma, fistulotomy abnormal anal manometry, or ultrasound further work-up is necessary. Most centers do not routinely perform evacuation defecography in patients with fecal incontinence, however, defecography is now often used in the work-up for intussusception and quite valuable in this role. Physicians must remember the most common symptom in patients suffering from internal intussusception is fecal incontinence. Using defecography, physicians have established a grading system for internal intussusception. The Oxford grading scale[44] was created to assist physicians in quantifying the severity of intussusception. The system grades intussusception according to the lowest extent reached by the apex of the prolapse, in relation to the anal canal or a rectocele. A rectocele is present in up to 83% of patients with internal intussusception.[46] Evidence supports the higher the Oxford grade of prolapse, the more significant the symptoms of urge incontinence.[7,48] The presence of intussuscepted rectum in the upper anal canal results in mucus drainage per anum.

TREATMENT

Intervention and treatment of internal rectal intussusception is afforded in two realms biofeedback therapy and surgery. Conservative measures of fiber supplementation, laxatives, and stool softeners should be trialed prior to any operative approach to management.[56] As with other forms of obstructed defecation and pelvic floor dysfunction, the cornerstone of therapy in internal intussusception is biofeedback and pelvic floor physiotherapy, from which up to 78% of patients benefit.[57,58] Biofeedback is administered by a physical therapist trained specifically in the technique, with a goal of reliable, reproducible relaxation of the puborectalis muscle.[58,59] This modality of care allows for a noninvasive approach to a complex, multifactorial problem with little risk to the patient. A high degree of efficacy can be achieved with as few as five 1-hour sessions performed in an outpatient setting. Durable effects tend to wane over

time, but retraining allows for recovery of symptomatic improvement.[58-60]

Surgery as a primary modality of treatment of internal intussusception has been met with incoming and outgoing tides of enthusiasm. This was especially the case with the introduction of the stapled transanal rectal resection (STARR) procedure. At its initial introduction, the procedure was reported to result in excellent outcomes with respect to improvement in constipation while yielding no untoward effects on rectal anatomy or physiology.[61] Subsequent reports revealed reason for concern in light of severe complications such as rectovaginal fistula, fecal incontinence, and rectal stricture.[18,62,63] While still a viable choice for internal intussusception STARR is best suited for highly selected patients who have failed medical management in conjunction with biofeedback.[58,64]

A similar wave of enthusiasm surrounds the performance of laparoscopic ventral mesh rectopexy for internal intussusception. Originally described by D'Hoore et al., the procedure is now used in both full-thickness rectal prolapse and internal intussusception.[63] The rectum is mobilized in the ventral distribution without dividing the lateral rectal attachments or performing a presacral dissection. A ventral mesh is insinuated into the rectovaginal septum after dissection of the rectovaginal plane. The mesh is affixed to the rectum, vaginal apex, and then to the sacral promontory. Care is taken to implant the mesh below a reapproximated peritoneum so as to avoid contact with bowel other than the rectum. The reported benefits over a standard rectopexy or resection rectopexy are a reduced rate of induced constipation, avoidance of anastomotic complication, and avoidance of presacral bleeding. The laparoscopic ventral rectocolpopexy affords a favorable continence profile in correcting the prolapse while subjecting the patient to less risk than a rectopexy inclusive of posterior rectal mobilization.[18,63,65,66]

CONCLUSION

Abdominal approaches for the surgical management of rectal prolapse have increasingly been used. However, recent evidence supports that perineal approaches may offer patients acceptable outcomes not clearly inferior to abdominal approaches. A major consideration for the approach taken during the index operation, or in the setting of recurrence, should then focus on the surgeon's comfort level and expertise combined with the patient's surgical history and comorbid conditions. Additionally, while biofeedback and fiber therapy remain the cornerstone of treatment in patients with internal rectal intussusception, isolated internal rectal intussusception can now be considered for surgical therapy.

REFERENCES

1. Karulf RE, Madoff RD, Goldberg SM. Rectal prolapse. *Curr Probl Surg.* 2001;38(10):771-832.
2. Ashrafian H. Erius of Alexandria (236-336 AD): the first reported mortality from rectal prolapse. *Int J Colorectal Dis.* 2014;29(4):539.
3. Felt-Bersma RJ, Tiersma ES, Cuesta MA. Rectal prolapse, rectal intussusception, rectocele, solitary rectal ulcer syndrome, and enterocele. *Gastroenterol Clin North Am.* 2008;37(3):645-668, ix.
4. Varma M, Rafferty J, Buie WD. Practice parameters for the management of rectal prolapse. *Dis Colon Rectum.* 2011;54(11):1339-1346.

5. Bordeianou L, Hicks CW, Kaiser AM, Alavi K, Sudan R, Wise PE. Rectal prolapse: an overview of clinical features, diagnosis, and patient-specific management strategies. *J Gastrointest Surg.* 2014;18(5): 1059-1069.

6. Coburn WM, Russell MA, Hofstetter WL. Sucrose as an aid to manual reduction of incarcerated rectal prolapse. *Ann Emerg Med.* 1997;30(3):347-349.

7. Sarpel U, Jacob BP, Steinhagen RM. Reduction of a large incarcerated rectal prolapse by use of an elastic compression wrap. *Dis Colon Rectum.* 2005;48(6):1320-1322.

8. Chaudhuri A. Hyaluronicase in the reduction of incarcerated rectal prolapse: a novel use. *Int J Colorectal Dis.* 1999;14(4-5):264.

9. Kim DS, Tsang CB, Wong WD, Lowry AC, Goldberg SM, Madoff RD. Complete rectal prolapse: evolution of management and results. *Dis Colon Rectum.* 1999;42(4):460-466.

10. Ripstein CB, Lanter B. Etiology and surgical therapy of massive prolapse of the rectum. *Ann Surg.* 1963;157:259-264.

11. Mcmahan JD, Ripstein CB. Rectal prolapse. An update on the rectal sling procedure. *Am Surg.* 1987;53(1):37-40.

12. Dulucq JL, Wintringer P, Mahajna A. Clinical and functional outcome of laparoscopic posterior rectopexy (Wells) for full-thickness rectal prolapse. A prospective study. *Surg Endosc.* 2007;21(12):2226-2230.

13. Speakman CT, Madden MV, Nicholls RJ, Kamm MA. Lateral ligament division during rectopexy causes constipation but prevents recurrence: results of a prospective randomized study. *Br J Surg.* 1991;78(12):1431-1433.

14. Portier G, Iovino F, Lazorthes F. Surgery for rectal prolapse: Orr-Loygue ventral rectopexy with limited dissection prevents postoperative-induced constipation without increasing recurrence. *Dis Colon Rectum.* 2006;49(8):1136-1140.

15. Luukkonen P, Mikkonen U, Järvinen H. Abdominal rectopexy with sigmoidectomy vs. rectopexy alone for rectal prolapse: a prospective, randomized study. *Int J Colorectal Dis.* 1992;7(4):219-222.

16. Mckee RF, Lauder JC, Poon FW, Aitchison MA, Finlay IG. A prospective randomized study of abdominal rectopexy with and without sigmoidectomy in rectal prolapse. *Surg Gynecol Obstet.* 1992; 174(2):145-148.

17. D'hoore A, Penninckx F. Laparoscopic ventral recto(colpo)pexy for rectal prolapse: surgical technique and outcome for 109 patients. *Surg Endosc.* 2006;20(12):1919-1923.

18. Samaranayake CB, Luo C, Plank AW, Merrie AE, Plank LD, Bissett IP. Systematic review on ventral rectopexy for rectal prolapse and intussusception. *Colorectal Dis.* 2010;12(6):504-512.

19. Boons P, Collinson R, Cunningham C, Lindsey I. Laparoscopic ventral rectopexy for external rectal prolapse improves constipation and avoids de novo constipation. *Colorectal Dis.* 2010;12(6):526-532.

20. Maggiori L, Bretagnol F, Ferron M, Panis Y. Laparoscopic ventral rectopexy: a prospective long-term evaluation of functional results and quality of life. *Tech Coloproctol.* 2013;17(4):431-436.

21. Tou S, Brown SR, Nelson RL. Surgery for complete (full-thickness) rectal prolapse in adults. *Cochrane Database Syst Rev.* 2015;(11): CD001758.

22. Purkayastha S, Tekkis P, Athanasiou T, et al. A comparison of open vs. laparoscopic abdominal rectopexy for full-thickness rectal prolapse: a meta-analysis. *Dis Color Rectum.* 2005;48(10):1930-1940.

23. Stevenson AR, Stitz RW, Lumley JW. Laparoscopic-assisted resection-rectopexy for rectal prolapse: early and medium follow-up. *Dis Colon Rectum.* 1998;41(1):46-54.

24. Sajid MS, Siddiqui MR, Baig MK. Open vs laparoscopic repair of full-thickness rectal prolapse: a re-meta-analysis. *Colorectal Dis.* 2010;12(6):515-525.

25. Yakut M, Kaymakçioğlu N, Şimşek A, Tan A, Sen D. Surgical treatment of rectal prolapse. A retrospective analysis of 94 cases. *Int Surg.* 1998;83(1):53-55.

26. Schoetz DJ. Evolving practice patterns in colon and rectal surgery. *J Am Coll Surg.* 2006;203(3):322-327.

27. Altemeier AW, Culberston WR, Schowengerdt C, Hunt J. Nineteen years' experience with the one-stage perineal repair of rectal prolapse. *Ann Surg.* 1971;173(6):993-1006.

28. Prasad ML, Pearl RK, Abcarian H, Orsay CP, Nelson RL. Perineal proctectomy, posterior rectopexy, and postanal levator repair for the treatment of rectal prolapse. *Dis Colon Rectum.* 1986;29(9):547-552.

29. Kim M, Reibetanz J, Schlegel N, et al. Recurrence after perineal rectosigmoidectomy: when and why? *Colorectal Dis.* 2014;16(11):920-924.

30. Kim M, Reibetanz J, Schlegel N, Germer CT, Jayne D, Isbert C. Perineal rectosigmoidectomy: quality of life. *Colorectal Dis.* 2013;15(8):1000-1006.

31. Senapati A, Gray RG, Middleton LJ, et al. PROSPER: a randomised comparison of surgical treatments for rectal prolapse. *Colorectal Dis.* 2013;15(7):858-868.

32. Delorme E. Sur le traitement des prolapses du rectum totaux, par L'excisoin de la muqueuse rectale or rectocolique. *Bull Mem Soc Chir Paris.* 1900;26:499-518.

33. Schütz G. Extracorporal resection of the rectum in the treatment of complete rectal prolapse using a circular stapling device. *Dig Surg.* 2001;18(4):274-277.

34. Lechaux JP, Lechaux D, Perez M. Results of Delorme's procedure for rectal prolapse. Advantages of a modified technique. *Dis Colon Rectum.* 1995;38(3):301-307.

35. Placer C, Enriquez-navascués JM, Timoteo A, et al. Delorme's procedure for complete rectal prolapse: a study of recurrence patterns in the long term. *Surg Res Pract.* 2015;2015:920154.

36. Lenormant: Prolapsus du rectum traité par la méthode de Gerard-Marchant et récidivé après trois ans: application de la méthode de Thiersch: guérison. *Bull Mem Soc Chir Paris.* 1906;32:10-17.

37. Berkowitz J. Correction of rectal procidentia; the Thiersch operation as a simple palliative procedure. *N Engl J Med.* 1953;248(17):720-722.

38. Gabriel WB. Thiersch's operation for anal incontinence and minor degrees of rectal prolapse. *Am J Surg.* 1953;86(5):583-590.

39. Hoel AT, Skarstein A, Ovrebo KK. Prolapse of the rectum, long-term results of surgical treatment. *Int J Colorectal Dis.* 2009;24(2):201-207.

40. Mollen RM, Kuijpers JH, Van Hoek F. Effects of rectal mobilization and lateral ligaments division on colonic and anorectal function. *Dis Colon Rectum.* 2000;43(9):1283-1287.

41. Bishawi M, Foppa C, Tou S, Bergamaschi R, Rectal Prolapse Recurrence Study Group. Recurrence of rectal prolapse following rectopexy: a pooled analysis of 532 patients. *Colorectal Dis.* 2016;18(8):779-784.

42. Hotouras A, Ribas Y, Zakeri S, et al. A systematic review of the literature on the surgical management of recurrent rectal prolapse. *Colorectal Dis.* 2015;17(8):657-664.

43. Ding JH, Canedo J, Lee SH, Kalaskar SN, Rosen L, Wexner SD. Perineal rectosigmoidectomy for primary and recurrent rectal prolapse: are the results comparable the second time? *Dis Colon Rectum.* 2012;55(6):666-670.

44. Lindsey I, Nugent K, Dixon T. *Pelvic Floor Disorders for the Colorectal Surgeon.* 1st ed. Oxford: Oxford University Press; 2010.

45. Shorvon PJ, Mchugh S, Diamant NE, Somers S, Stevenson GW. Defecography in normal volunteers: results and implications. *Gut.* 1989;30(12):1737-1749.

46. Collinson R, Cunningham C, D'Costa H, Lindsey I. Rectal intussusception and unexplained faecal incontinence: findings of a proctographic study. *Colorectal Dis.* 2009;11(1):77-83.

47. Wijffels NA, Jones OM, Cunningham C, Bemelman WA, Lindsey I. What are the symptoms of internal rectal prolapse? *Colorectal Dis.* 2013;15(3):368-373.

48. Bloemendaal AL, Buchs NC, Prapasrivorakul S, et al. High-grade internal rectal prolapse: does it explain so-called "idiopathic" faecal incontinence? *Int J Surg.* 2016;25:118-122.

49. Agachan F, Chen T, Pfeifer J, Reissman P, Wexner SD. A constipation scoring system to simplify evaluation and management of constipated patients. *Dis Colon Rectum.* 1996;39(6):681-685.

50. Rockwood TH, Church JM, Fleshman JW, et al. Patient and surgeon ranking of the severity of symptoms associated with fecal incontinence: the fecal incontinence severity index. *Dis Colon Rectum.* 1999;42(12):1525-1532.

51. Farouk R, Duthie GS, Macgregor AB, Bartolo DC. Rectoanal inhibition and incontinence in patients with rectal prolapse. *Br J Surg.* 1994;81(5):743-746.

52. Farouk R, Duthie GS, Bartolo DC, MacGregor AB. Restoration of continence following rectopexy for rectal prolapse and recovery of the internal anal sphincter electromyogram. *Br J Surg.* 1992;79(5):439-440.

53. Harmston C, Jones OM, Cunningham C, Lindsey I. The relationship between internal rectal prolapse and internal anal sphincter function. *Colorectal Dis.* 2011;13(7):791-795.

54. Hawkins AT, Olariu AG, Savitt LR, et al. Impact of rising grades of internal rectal intussusception on fecal continence and symptoms of constipation. *Dis Colon Rectum.* 2016;59(1):54-61.

55. Soh JS, Lee HJ, Jung KW, et al. The diagnostic value of a digital rectal examination compared with high-resolution anorectal manometry

in patients with chronic constipation and fecal incontinence. *Am J Gastroenterol.* 2015;110(8):1197-1204.

56. Ihre T. Internal procidentia of the rectum—treatment and results. *Scand J Gastroenterol.* 1972;7(7):643-646.

57. Rao SS, Valestin J, Brown CK, Zimmerman B, Schulze K. Long-term efficacy of biofeedback therapy for dyssynergic defecation: randomized controlled trial. *Am J Gastroenterol.* 2010;105(4):890-896.

58. Hwang YH, Person B, Choi JS, et al. Biofeedback therapy for rectal intussusceptions. *Tech Coloproctol.* 2006;10:11-15; discussion 15-16.

59. Hicks CW, Weinstein M, Wakamatsu M, Savitt L, Pulliam S, Bordeanou L. In patients with rectoceles and obstructed defecation syndrome, surgery should be the option of last resort. *Surgery.* 2014;155:659-667.

60. Fleshman JW, Dreznik Z, Meyer K, Fry RD, Carney R, Kodner IJ. Outpatient protocol for biofeedback therapy of pelvic floor outlet obstruction. *Dis Colon Rectum.* 1992;35:1-7.

61. Boccasanta P, Venturi M, Stuto A, et al. Stapled transanal rectal resection for outlet obstruction: a prospective, multicenter trial. *Dis Colon Rectum.* 2004;47(8):1285-1296.

62. Dodi G, Pietroletti R, Milito G, Binda G, Pescatori M. Bleeding, incontinence, pain and constipation after STARR transanal double stapling rectotomy for obstructed defecation. *Tech Coloproctol.* 2003;7:148-153.

63. D'Hoore A, Cadoni R, Penninckx F. Long-term outcome of laparoscopic ventral rectopexy for total rectal prolapse. *Br J Surg.* 2004;91:1500-505.

64. Jayne DG, Finan PJ. Stapled transanal rectal resection for obstructed defecation and evidence-based practice. *Br J Surg.* 2005;92:793-794.

65. Von Papen M, Ashari LH, Lumley JW, Stevenson AR, Stitz RW. Functional results of laparoscopic resection rectopexy for symptomatic rectal intussusception. *Dis Colon Rectum.* 2007;50:50-55.

66. Laubert T, Kleemann M, Roblick UJ, et al. Obstructive defecation syndrome: 19 years of experience with laparoscopic resection rectopexy. *Tech Coloproctol.* 2013;17:307-314.

Pilonidal Disease and Perianal Hidradenitis

Katerina Wells | Michael Pendola

PILONIDAL DISEASE

Sacrococcygeal pilonidal disease (PD) has a calculated incidence of 26 per 100,000 people and is a source of morbidity in young adults due to the chronicity of disease and extent of surgical intervention. The current understanding is that this is an acquired disease resulting in subcutaneous trauma of hair shafts. Treatment of PD ranges from simple incision and drainage to excision with flap reconstruction. Wound complications and recurrence remain high despite available therapies, making this a challenging disease process for both the patient and surgeon.

ETIOLOGY

The pathogenesis of PD has evolved since its first description by M. Hodges in 1830 as a sinus containing a nest (nidus) of hair (pilas).[1] Many theories have existed attributing PD as either a congenital or acquired condition. In 1935, Gage proposed that sinus disease was secondary to anomalous embryonic development of the medullary canal.[2] Other theories supposed that PD was caused by idiopathic invagination of integumentary structures, as evidenced by the classic sacrococcygeal dimple.

The acquired theory was supposed in World War II by Hardaway, who noted that PD was "apparently much commoner in the military service than in civilian life," attributing the difference to the predilection to young men in conditions of poor hygiene.[3] It was postulated that compression and irritation of the coccyx during field activities such as driving in jeeps was the underlying cause of PD, hence the term "jeep disease." PD was a significant source of disability and working days lost for enlisted men, stimulating the need for less morbid treatment options.[4] In 1946, Patey and Scarff further supported the acquired theory with histologic comparison of the epithelialized tracts seen in congenital dermoids with the granulation tissue–lined tracts of pilonidal sinuses, postulating that this is an "infective track" formed from surface hairs that have deeply penetrated the dermis causing a foreign-body granulomatous reaction.[5] Their observations of pilonidal sinuses in other areas such as the umbilicus and in the intertriginous folds of a barbers hands supported this theory.[6]

Further contributions by Bascom described the role of the intergluteal cleft in creating a vacuum force that directs hair foreign bodies into the subcutaneous tissue.[7] This provided the rationale behind the Bascom flap procedure, which produces effacement of the intergluteal cleft in addition to excision of sinus tissue.[8] In 1992, Karydakis theorized that three main factors underlie pathogenesis: the invasion of loose hair, the force which causes hair embedding, and the vulnerability of the affected skin.[9]

This concept motivated the Karydakis flap, wherein the sinus is excised and the intergluteal skin is replaced by more "resistant" gluteal skin through a sliding flap.[10] In more recent electron microscopy analysis of pilonidal sinus nest hair samples, the majority of embedded hair is rootless, with razor sharp ends.[11] As such, the current prevailing mechanism of action appears to be acquired and that of local irritation from embedding of loose cut hairs.

PRESENTATION

Sacrococcygeal PD is 2.2 times more common in men.[12] Presentation occurs in the second and third decades of life and rarely before the age of 15 or after the age of 40, with a median of 2 years of symptoms prior to treatment.[12,13] Risk factors include obesity, degree of hair growth, family history of PD, local trauma, and sedentary occupation.[14,15] PD is most common among white, non-Hispanic populations and rare in Asian/Pacific Islander heritage.[15] The rate is unusually high in Turkey, with a reported incidence of 6% in young adults.[16]

PD presents in an acute form as an abscess or in chronic form with single or multiple branching draining sinuses. Abscesses present with sacrococcygeal pain with progression into a fluctuant mass slightly off the midline with overlying cellulitis situated just above the gluteal cleft and cephalad to the visible midline pits (Fig. 153.1). Acute abscess is the presenting finding in approximately 50% of patients and constitutes 20% of dermatologic complaints seen in the emergency department.[17]

Following spontaneous drainage, a chronic cavity may develop which drains via a simple or complex sinus associated with one or multiple pits located in the midline. Sinus tracts characteristically contain hair debris that is easily removed with forceps.[18]

DIAGNOSIS

The characteristic appearance of PD makes this a clinical diagnosis; however, other pathologies can appear similar. Furuncle disease, hidradenitis suppurativa (HS),[19] perianal abscess or fistula, sacral osteomyelitis, syphilis, tuberculosis, and actinomycosis[20] should be excluded. Malignant degeneration is reported in 0.1% of cases, emphasizing the need for histologic examination of excised specimens.[22-24] Patients found to have PD-related malignancy have long-standing disease and are typically middle-aged and male. Histology is predominantly squamous cell carcinoma.

Histologically, the midline pits are lined with squamous epithelium. The underlying cavities are not epithelialized but lined with granulation tissue.[13] Pilonidal cavities rarely contain sweat glands or hair follicles, although hair shafts are found 75% of the time. Foreign-body giant cells associated with hair shafts are seen within a background of chronic granulation tissue[25] (Fig. 153.2).

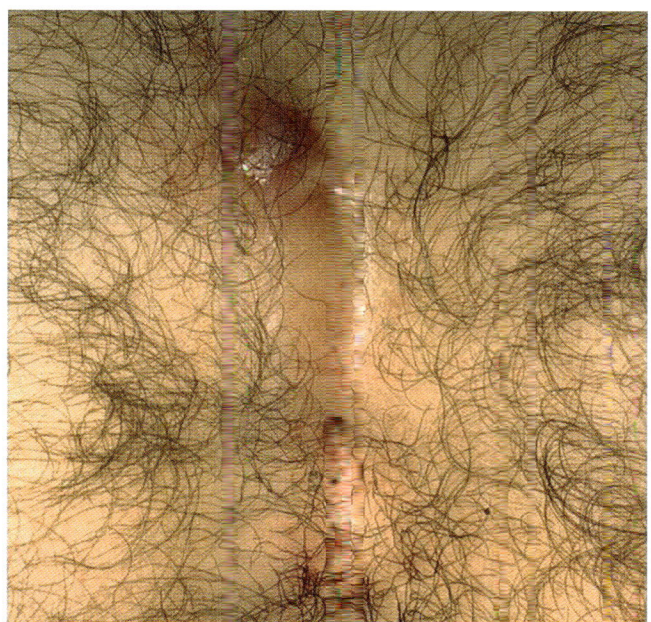

FIGURE 153.1 Sacrococcygeal pilonidal abscess and midline pit.

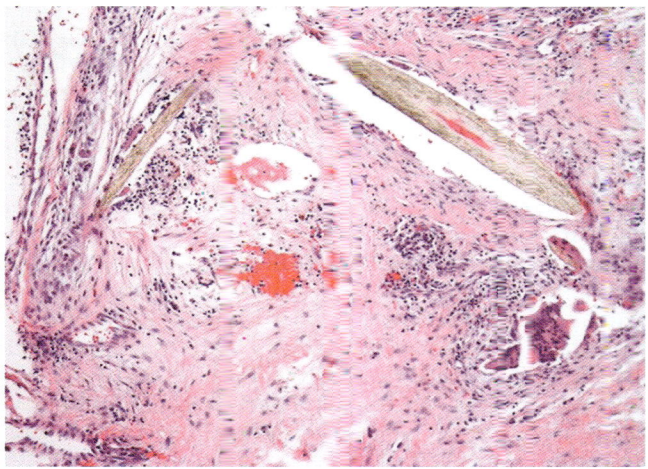

FIGURE 153.2 Histopathology: hair follicle with foreign-body giant cell reaction in a pilonidal cyst.

The microbiology of the pilonidal sinus is typically gram-negative and anaerobic organisms, with a shift toward gram-positive and aerobic bacteria in recurrent disease.[26]

TREATMENT

The evolution of pathogenesis has paralleled the treatment options. When the congenital theory prevailed, procedures were guided by the premise of complete extirpation of subcutaneous tissue to the level of the sacral fascia.[27] The need to preserve active working days for military recruits in World War II to the modern era stimulated a need for conservative excisional techniques.[4,14] With the acquired theory, complex resections with primary closure aim to address both the offending tissue and the

underlying mechanical etiology.[8,9] In recent Cochrane review comparing open approach versus primary closure, there is no clear benefit in the type of technique with regard to healing time and surgical site infection; however, primary closure techniques fare best when the incision is placed off-midline.[28] Ultimately the goal is complete wound healing with minimal patient disability and a low rate of recurrence; therefore the surgeon must individualize the approach to suit the needs and expectations of the patient.

Acute Pilonidal Abscess

Acutely, simple incision and drainage is the standard treatment to provide prompt symptom relief. In patients with acute abscess formation, a staged approach should be employed as definitive resection with abscess excision results in higher rates of recurrence.[29] This is attributed in part to contamination of tissue and tissue edema obscuring the midline sinus, leading to incomplete excision.

Technique of Drainage. Drainage procedures can be performed in the office, emergency room, or an outpatient ambulatory surgical setting. The sacrococcygeal region is best exposed in the prone jackknife position with the buttocks taped apart. A paramedian longitudinal incision is made over the abscess cavity that is large enough to allow for adequate drainage.[30] All debris and hair should be removed from the cavity. Unroofing and fulguration of all sinus tracts is supported even in the acute phase with a healing time of 5.4 ± 1.1 weeks and a low rate of recurrence of 2% at 54-month follow-up.[31] Alternative treatment with aspiration of the abscess cavity has been described as a temporizing bridge to definitive resection.[32]

Retained hair in the abscess cavity is the major factor for nonhealing and recurrence. The patient should perform sitz baths for hygiene. Weekly wound checks are recommended to ensure that the wound and surrounding skin remain free of hair and other debris during healing. Laser hair removal can be offered as an adjunctive therapy during wound healing, as well as a long-term approach to decreasing hair growth in the involved area.[33]

Chronic Pilonidal Disease

Approximately 15% to 40% of patients treated for acute abscess will progress to chronic PD.[34] Eight percent to 30% of patients with chronic PD will recur following definitive treatment, emphasizing the tenacity of this disease, despite available therapies.[34,35] Treatment options vary from nonresectional approaches, midline follicle excision and lateral drainage, incision and curettage with minimal excision followed by marsupialization or saucerization of the wound, and excision with or without primary closure. There is no clear consensus as to the preferred treatment; however, it is desirable to select an approach that can be carried out in an ambulatory setting with minimal patient inconvenience and disability. The role of antibiotics is not clear; there have been reports that have suggested antibiotics directed at anaerobic bacteria may improve healing rates.[36]

Nonresectional Approach. Armstrong and Barcia[27] advocated nonexcisional therapy consisting of meticulous hair control by shaving, good perineal hygiene, and limited lateral incision and drainage of abscesses. Hair,

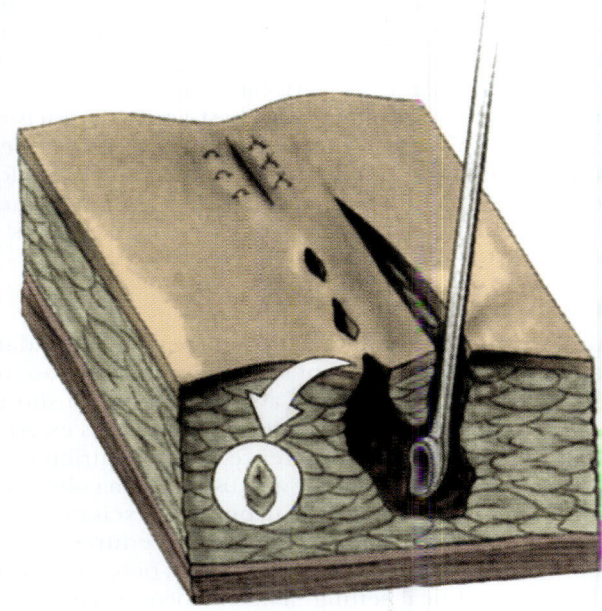

FIGURE 153.3 Treatment of pilonidal abscess by lateral incision into the abscess with curetting of granulation tissues and excision of midline pits. (From Bascom J. Pilonidal disease: origin from follicles of hairs and results of follicle removal as treatment. *Surgery*. 1980;87:567; redrawn from Nivatvongs S. Pilonidal disease. In: Gordon PH, Nivatvongs S, eds. *Principles and Practice of Surgery for the Colon, Rectum, and Anus.* 2nd ed. St. Louis: Quality Medical; 1999:293.)

when visible, should be removed. Complete healing was demonstrated in 101 consecutive cases over a 1-year period. Instillation of liquid or crystalline phenol causes an intense inflammatory reaction to promote closure of the cavity and tracts. This method has limited use due to pain and may require hospitalization for analgesia.[37,38]

Midline Follicle Excision and Lateral Drainage. Midline follicle excision and lateral drainage was described by Bascom[7] and a similar technique described by Lord and Millar[39-41] in the mid-1960s. This procedure involves a longitudinal incision off of midline for access to the chronic sinus tract. The sinus tract is débrided of necrotic material, hypergranulation tissue, and hairs. The midline epithelialized pits are also excised (Fig. 153.3). Frequently follow-up is performed for hair removal. Bascom followed 149 patients treated in this way and reported an 84% cure rate.[30] The advantage of this technique is that it can be performed in an outpatient setting with minimal morbidity and disability and short healing time, estimated at 3 weeks.

Incision and Curettage With Marsupialization or Saucerization. Laying open or deroofing and curettage of the sinus tract can be an effective way to treat chronic PD. The area is opened in the midline, followed by curettage of any debris or granulation tissue. All secondary tracts are identified with a fistula probe and similarly deroofed. Dyes and peroxide can also aid in identification of complex fistula tracts. Skin edges can be beveled (saucerization) to allow dependent drainage and easy access to the wound

(Fig. 153.4). Alternatively the skin edges can be sutured (marsupialization) to the base of the wound.[33,42-44] Meta-analysis of 13 studies involving deroofing and curettage found high success rates, low complication rates, shorter operative time, and early return to normal work by this approach.[45] This technique in general has low recurrence rates, 1% to 19%, but patients seemed to have more pain and discomfort after this procedure.[46,47] The introduction of negative pressure wound therapy with chronic wounds has helped offset this problem.[48,49] Negative pressure dressings result in increased local blood flow, upregulation of cell proliferation, decreased bacteria count, and increased wound granulation.[50] Protection from exposure and the need for less frequent dressing changes decreases the disability associated with chronic open wounds.

Excision With or Without Closure. Excision of the pilonidal cavity and associated inflammatory tissue is an extirpative approach. The wound can be closed primarily or left open to close by secondary intention. Typically the resection margin is taken down to the sacral fascia (Fig. 153.5). Meta-analysis of 18 randomized controlled trials compared the effects of open versus closed surgical treatment for pilonidal sinus.[51] Outcomes included time to heal, infection, and recurrence rates. The data suggest more rapid healing after primary closure when compared with excision without closure. In addition, there was no difference in infection rates when comparing the two techniques. There was a trend toward decreased recurrence after open healing as compared with primary closure; however patients did return to work faster after primary closure. When comparing midline closure versus off-midline closure, there was good evidence of slower healing, higher rates of infection, higher rates of recurrence, and other complications after midline primary closure compared with off-midline closure techniques.

Recurrent or Unhealed Pilonidal Disease. Recurrence rates vary and are reported as up to 40%.[46] These patients usually have extensive, complex disease and require a more radical approach. Surgeons who treat recurrent PD should have knowledge of flap techniques, as large tissue defects created by wide excision benefit from mobilization of healthy tissue to help facilitate healing.[30,52-54] Multiple procedures have been described, including Z plasty,[55] V-Y fasciocutaneous flap, rhomboid excision and Limberg flaps,[47,56] gluteal myocutaneous flaps,[55] the Karydakis operation,[57] and cleft lift procedure.[58-60] These procedures tend to carry a higher morbidity and require hospitalization. In addition, recurrence rates have been reported to be anywhere between 2% and 11%.

Technique of Cleft Lift. Bascom described this technique for a chronic nonhealing midline wound whereby the midline nonhealing wound is excised and a full-thickness skin flap is raised to overlap the skin edges of the wound on the opposite side. The end result is that the superior gluteal cleft is now eliminated and the incision line has been displaced off of midline. From a technical standpoint, this is one of the simpler flap procedures and can be performed in an outpatient ambulatory surgical setting. The patient is usually placed in jackknife position. The natural contour of the gluteal cleft and buttocks are outlined. The chronic nonhealing wound is excised in a triangular shape. The skin flap, full thickness, is then

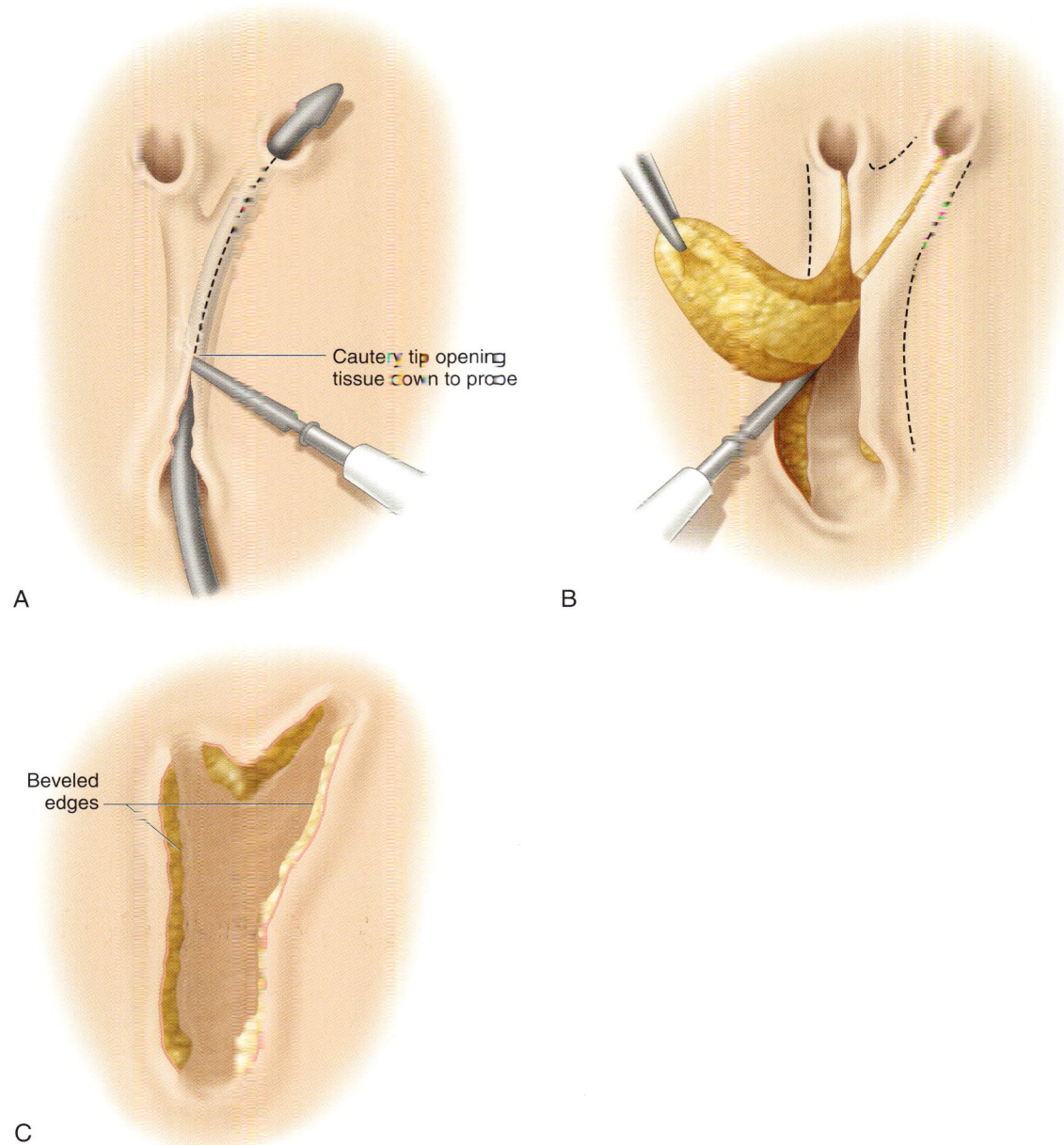

Cautery tip opening
tissue down to probe

A

B

Beveled
edges

C

FIGURE 153.4 Technique of unroofing and saucerization of pilonidal wound. (From Bailey HR. *Colorectal Surgery*. Philadelphia: Elsevier; 2012.)

developed and pulled laterally. Typically a closed-suction drain is placed in the subcutaneous tissue to help obliterate any dead space. The skin is then closed with an absorbable suture (Fig. 153.6). Recurrence rates for this technique have been reported at less than 5%.[58-60]

SUMMARY

PD is a complex chronic condition that can be a major cause of disability. The surgical approach for treatment should match the presentation of the disease. Options for treatment include simple incision, deroofing, local excision, and excision with or without complex closure. Vigilant

hair removal is a necessity to help facilitate healing and prevent recurrent disease. All effort should be made to help prevent a chronic nonhealing wound, which could be worse than the initial presenting disease itself.

PERIANAL HIDRADENITIS

Perianal HS is a debilitating condition in which recurrent inflammation arising in the apocrine glands of the perianal skin results in abscesses and chronically draining sinuses. Current understanding is that this is an acquired process secondary to occlusion of the apocrine ducts with secondary

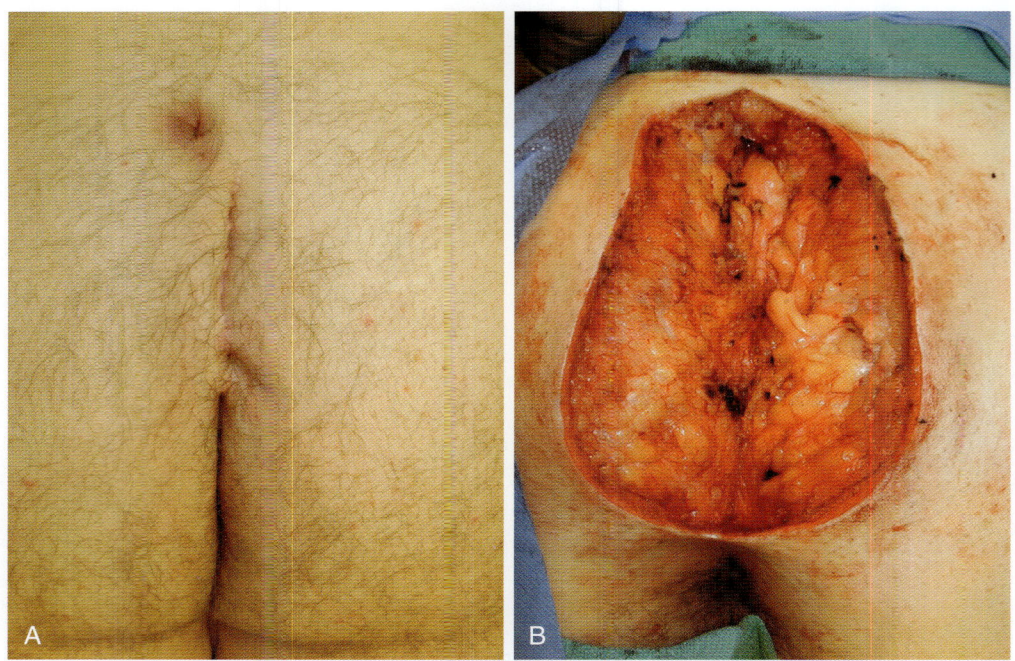

FIGURE 153.5 Recurrent pilonidal sinus shown in (A) and large wound created by excision of the "pilonidal cyst" down to the sacral fascia (B).

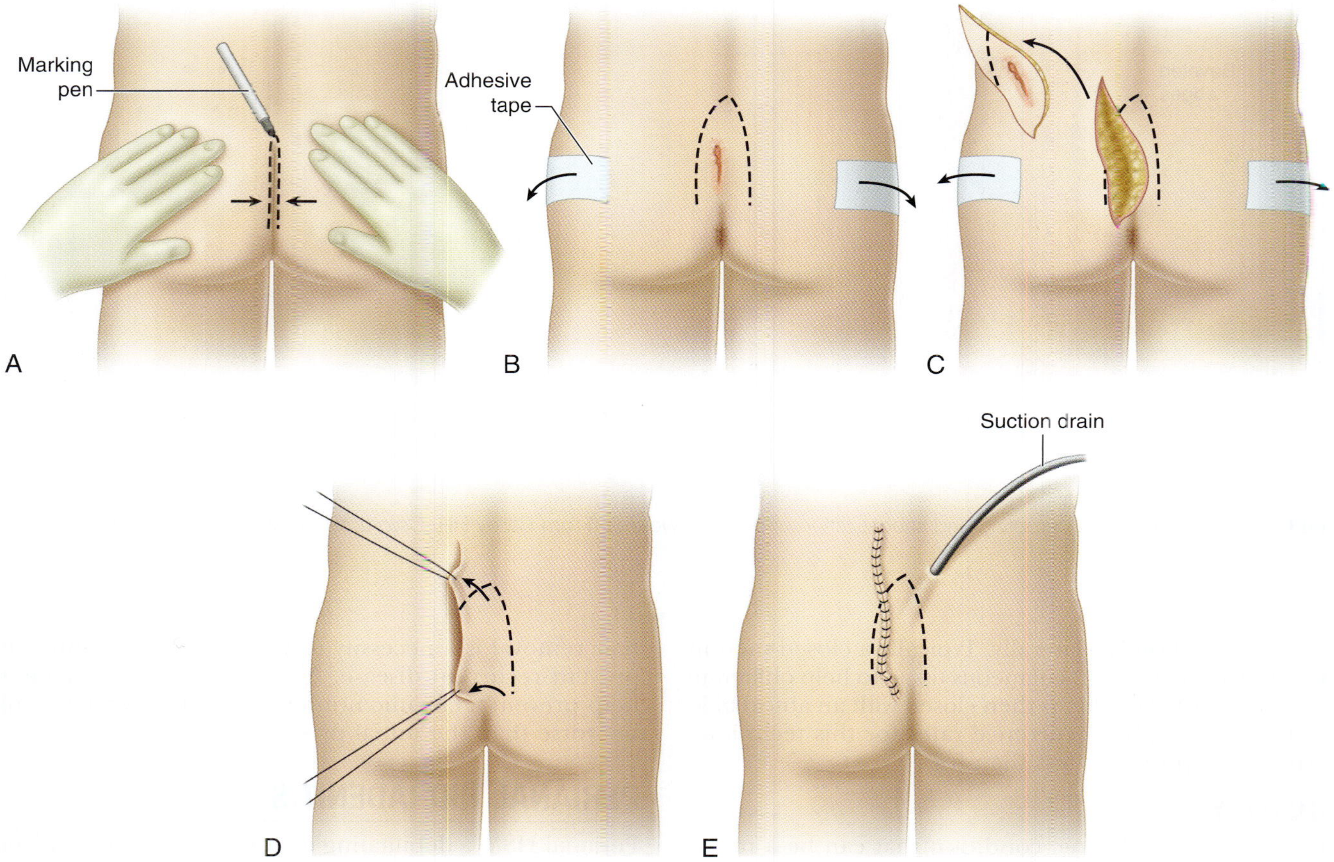

FIGURE 153.6 Cleft closure technique. (From Bascom J. Repeat pilonidal operations. *Am J Surg.* 1987;154:118; redrawn from Nivatvongs S. Pilonidal disease. In: Gordon PH, Nivatvongs S, eds. *Principles and Practice of Surgery for the Colon, Rectum, and Anus.* 2nd ed. St. Louis: Quality Medical; 1999:299.)

infection. Medical therapy is recommended for mild disease and is a useful adjunct for symptom control. Acute abscess is treated with incision and drainage. A variety of surgical approaches exist for management of chronic disease, including unroofing of sinus tracts, limited local excision, and wide excision with or without grafting or advancement flap coverage.

PATHOGENESIS

Apocrine glands are found in the axillary, inguinal, perineal, and perianal regions and are associated with hair follicles. Apocrine glands are stimulated by pain or sexual arousal to secrete an odorless fluid which subsequently becomes malodorous after interaction with skin flora.[61] First reported by Velpeau in 1859,[62] the evolution of pathogenesis supports that the inciting event is occlusion of the duct or hair follicle by keratin resulting in stasis and overgrowth of commensal microbes. Suppuration of the glands with rupture into adjacent subcutaneous tissue triggers an acute inflammatory response.[6-34] There are no specific organisms associated with HS. Wounds are polymicrobial, with coagulase-negative staphylococci and anaerobic bacteria predominating.[65]

Histologic studies have not clearly defined an anatomic glandular structure to explain susceptibility to follicular occlusion.[61] Immune dysregulation with predominance of interleukin-17 (IL-17) and tumor necrosis factor (TNF) expression may be an etiologic factor in HS inflammation.[66] There are no clear predisposing modifiable risk factors for development of HS, although obesity and smoking are strongly associated.[67,68] Contrary to popular belief, hygiene, shaving practices, and use of skin care products are not causal.[61] Hormonal imbalance, specifically androgen excess during puberty, may contribute to increase keratinization and follicular occlusion.[69] This association is further supported, as acute HS is exacerbated during menses and with the use of oral contraceptives.[70,71] Certain endocrinopathies, including Cushing disease, diabetes mellitus, and acromegaly, are highly associated with HS.[72,73] Positive family history is also seen in approximately 26% of affected patients, with familial inheritance demonstrating an autosomal dominant pattern.[74-76]

PRESENTATION

The true incidence of HS is not known; however, estimates suggest that the prevalence in the US population is 98 per 100,000 persons. The adjusted prevalence in women is more than twice that of men (137 per 100,000 vs 58 per 100,000) and highest within the third decade of life.[77] African American and biracial individuals are 2 to 7 times more susceptible than Caucasians.[77,78] Presentation occurs initially with painful subcutaneous nodules that coalesce into abscesses. Spontaneous drainage followed by spontaneous healing results in relapsing disease. In its chronic form, recurring inflammation and fibrosis causes complex cicatricial networks of subcutaneous sinus tracts. Severity of disease can range from mild localized disease to multifocal severe disease.[79] Developed in 1989, the Hurley classification is a measure of disease severity stratified into three stages.[80] Other measures, including the Acne Inversa Severity Index (AISI), consider disease severity alongside other phenotypic and quality-of-life factors.[81]

DIAGNOSIS

There are no pathognomonic features of HS, and exclusion of other pathologies should be undertaken before management. Other suppurative dermatologic conditions, including acne conglobate and perifolliculitis capitis, can appear similar.[82] Infectious diseases such as lymphogranuloma venereum, erysipelas, and tuberculosis can present with draining subcutaneous sinuses.[83] Perianal Crohn disease can also mimic severe perianal HS, and the two entities have been concomitantly described.[84,85] HS can be differentiated from perianal Crohn disease by the absence of involvement with the cryptoglandular units of the dentate line or sphincter complex.[85] Colonoscopy should be performed if there is clinical suspicion of Crohn disease, as wide excision of perianal Crohn disease would be detrimental. As mentioned in the previous section, PD and sacral osteomyelitis with fistula may present similarly. Squamous cell carcinoma has been reported in chronic wounds associated with hidradenitis, underscoring the importance of wound surveillance and histologic examination of suspicious or chronic lesions.[87-89]

TREATMENT

Medical Therapy

Topical clindamycin has been shown to be effective in a randomized, controlled trial.[90] Systemic tetracycline has similar efficacy[91]; however, no maintenance suppressive antibiotic therapy exists for long-term use.

Considering the hormonal effect on HS, suppression using synthetic gonadotropin-releasing hormone, leuprolide, has been supported.[92] Isotretinoin (Accutane), a derivative of vitamin A,[93,94] and oral cyclosporine[95] have also been used; however, these benefits must be weighed against the potential severe side effects of these medications. Newer biologic therapies including adalimumab (Humira)[96] and secukinumab (Cosentyx)[97] show promise against TNF- and IL-17–mediated HS inflammation.

Surgical Therapy

Incision and Deroofing. For acute presentations, simple incision and drainage provides prompt relief of symptoms, albeit with near-certain recurrence. More extensive drainage in which all associated tracts are deroofed with curettage of the tract epithelium is associated with lower recurrence.[86] Multiple studies report good tolerance of this approach, with recurrence between 17% and 29% in long-term follow-up.[98,99]

Limited Local Excision. In the case of limited disease, local excision of the offending tracts with primary closure of the site has been described. In report by Jemec[100] of 72 patients treated with local excision, a complete cure rate of 14.7% was achieved; however, 7.4% of patients went on to recurrence in another region.

Wide Excision. In the case of chronic or extensive disease, wide excision of apocrine gland–bearing skin to normal fascia or 0.5-cm grossly negative margins is recommended.[79] Such radically extirpative procedures require advance planning for patient expectations, postoperative pain and wound management, and attendant disability. In cases where extensive areas require excision a staged approach is recommended.

Intraoperative color-marking of sinus tracts with methylviolet solution to confirm adequate wide excision is helpful, with a 2.5% recurrence rate reported with this approach.[101] Iodine-starch testing is another useful technique for identification of apocrine glands.[61] Routine colostomy is not required, as aggressive wound care is adequate.[102] Fecal diversion can be considered in rare circumstances where proper wound care is not possible and in patients with concomitant Crohn disease.[79]

Reconstruction. The choice of closure is not predictive of recurrence[101]; therefore the approach for reconstruction should be based on the resources of the institution and fitness of the patient. There are several options for closure following wide excision: primary closure, split-thickness skin grafting (STSG), advancement flap coverage, or healing by secondary intention with or without the use of a vacuum wound management device. Closure can be performed at the time of resection or in a delayed fashion.

STSG offers the benefit of rapid coverage of the wound and greater comfort[102] at the expense of donor and graft site wound care, activity restrictions, and the risk of graft loss.[103] Skin grafting is typically performed in a delayed manner to decrease the bacterial burden and improve chances of graft incorporation. In review of 98 patients treated by this approach, 94.7% of wounds were fully grafted and closed by 30-day follow-up.[104]

Rotational fasciocutaneous flap coverage offers the benefit of early wound closure, with faster return to activity following flap healing. V-Y advancement flaps have also been described with good success.[105] Flap reconstruction restores tissue contour and cushioning compared with other techniques. Careful patient selection is required, with the complication rates approaching 25%.[106] In review by Alharbi et al., flap closure of perianal and gluteal wounds (16% of study sample) demonstrated recurrence rates of 0% in a 24-month follow-up.[107]

Healing by secondary intention avoids the complications of split-thickness skin graft and flap reconstruction.[108] This approach allows for an early return to activity at the expense of prolonged wound healing and frequent dressing changes. The use of negative pressure therapy as a bridge to primary closure or as definitive therapy accelerates healing time to an average of 2.2 months.[109] Moreover, negative pressure devices increase oxygen tension and granulation formation, and prevents shear force and painful exposure of the wound, thus improving patient comfort and decreasing wound care needs.[110] Placement can be challenging in the perianal region, due to the proximity to the anus and the high degree of motion in this area with activity.

SUMMARY

Perianal HS is a chronic condition resulting from occlusion of the apocrine glands. Management of mild disease can be performed with medical therapy and simple incision and drainage. In the case of chronic or extensive disease, wide excision of the offending area carries the lowest risk of recurrence. Options for reconstruction range from STSG, flap coverage, or healing by secondary intention.

The choice of reconstruction depends on the resources of the institution and should be individualized to the patient.

REFERENCES

1. Glenn F. Pilonidal sinus. *N Engl J Med.* 1932;207:544-546.
2. Gage M. Pilonidal sinus: an explanation of its embryologic development. *Arch Surg.* 1935;31:175-189.
3. Hardaway RM. Pilonidal cyst; neither pilonidal nor cyst. *AMA Arch Surg.* 1958;76(1):143-147.
4. Classic articles in colonic and rectal surgery. Louis A. Buie, M.D. 1890–1975: jeep disease (pilonidal disease of mechanized warfare). *Dis Colon Rectum.* 1982;25:384-390.
5. Patey DH, Scarff RW. Pathology of postanal pilonidal sinus; its bearing on treatment. *Lancet.* 1946;2(6423):484-486.
6. Patey DH, Scarff RW. Pilonidal sinus in a barber's hand with observations on postanal pilonidal sinus. *Lancet.* 1948;2(6514):13.
7. Bascom J. Pilonidal disease: origin from follicles of hairs and results of follicle removal as treatment. *Surgery.* 1980;87(5):567-572.
8. Bascom J, Bascom T. Utility of the cleft lift procedure in refractory pilonidal disease. *Am J Surg.* 2007;193(5):606-609.
9. Karydakis GE. Easy and successful treatment of pilonidal sinus after explanation of its causative process. *Aust N Z J Surg.* 1992;62(5):385-389.
10. Karydakis GE. New approach to the problem of pilonidal sinus. *Lancet.* 1973;2(7843):1414-1415.
11. Bosche F, Luedi MM, Zypen D, Moersdorf P, Krapohl B, Doll D. The hair in the sinus: sharp-ended rootless head hair fragments can be found in large amounts in pilonidal sinus nests. *World J Surg.* 2017; Jun 21 [Epub ahead of print].
12. Søndenaa K, Andersen E, Nesvik I, Søreide JA. Patient characteristics and symptoms in chronic pilonidal sinus disease. *Int J Colorectal Dis.* 1995;10(1):39-42.
13. Allen-Mersh TG. Pilonidal sinus: finding the right track for treatment. *Br J Surg.* 1990;77(2):123-132.
14. Levinson T, Sela T, Chencinski S, et al. Pilonidal sinus disease: a 10-year review reveals occupational risk factors and the superiority of the minimal surgery trephine technique. *Mil Med.* 2016;181(4):389-394.
15. Armed Forces Health Surveillance Center (AFHSC). Pilonidal cysts, active component, US Armed Forces, 2000–2012. *MSMR.* 2013;20(12):8-11.
16. Duman K, Girgin M, Harlak A. Prevalence of sacrococcygeal pilonidal disease in Turkey. *Asian J Surg.* 2016;1-4.
17. Lai-Kwon JE, Weiland TJ, Jelinek GA, Chong AH. Which patients with dermatological conditions are admitted via the emergency department? *Australas J Dermatol.* 2014;55(4):255-259.
18. de Parades V, Bouchard D, Janier M, Berger A. Pilonidal sinus disease. *J Visc Surg.* 2013;150(4):237-247.
19. Scheinfeld N. An atlas of the morphological manifestations of hidradenitis suppurativa. *Dermatol Online J.* 2014;20(4):22373.
20. Tena D, Fernández C, Lago MR, Arias M, Medina MJ, Sáez-Nieto JA. Skin and soft-tissue infections caused by *Actinobaculum schaalii*: report of two cases and literature review. *Anaerobe.* 2014;28(C):95-97.
21. Tsalis KC. Is histological examination necessary when excising a pilonidal cyst? *Am J Case Rep.* 2015;16:164-168.
22. Davis KA, Mock CN, Versaci A, et al. Malignant degeneration of pilonidal cysts. *Am Surg.* 1994;60(3):200-204.
23. De Bree E, Zoetmulder FA, Christodoulakis M, Lentrichia P. Treatment of malignancy arising in pilonidal disease. *Ann Surg Oncol.* 2001;8(1):60-64.
24. Kulaylat MN, Gong M, Doerr RJ. Multimodality treatment of squamous cell carcinoma complicating pilonidal disease. *Am Surg.* 1996;62(11):922-929.
25. Søndenaa K, Pollard ML. Histology of chronic pilonidal sinus. *APMIS.* 1995;103(4):267-272.
26. Ardelt M, Dittmar Y, Kocijan R, et al. Microbiology of the infected recurrent sacrococcygeal pilonidal sinus. *Int Wound J.* 2016;13(2):231-237.
27. Armstrong JH, Barcia PJ. Pilonidal sinus disease. The conservative approach. *Arch Surg.* 1994;129(9):914-917, discussion 917–919.
28. AL-Khamis A, McCallum I, King PM, Bruce J. Healing by primary versus secondary intention after surgical treatment for pilonidal sinus (review). *Cochrane Database Syst Rev.* 2009;(1):CD006213.

29. Almajid F, Alabdrabalnabi A, Almulhim K. The risk of recurrence of pilonidal disease after surgical management. *Saudi Med J.* 2017;38(1):70-74.

30. Bascom J. Pilonidal disease: long-term results of follicle removal. *Dis Colon Rectum.* 1983;26(12):800-807.

31. Kepenekci I, Demirkan A, Ceasin H, Gecim IE. Unroofing and curettage for the treatment of acute and chronic pilonidal disease. *World J Surg.* 2010;34(1):153-157.

32. Hussain ZI, Aghahoseini A, Alexander D. Converting emergency pilonidal abscess into an elective procedure. *Dis Colon Rectum.* 2012;55(6):640-645.

33. Oram Y, Kahraman F, Karincaoglu Y, et al. Evaluation of 60 patients with pilonidal sinus treated with laser epilation after surgery. *Dermatol Surg.* 2010;36(1):88-91.

34. Fahrni GT, Vuille-Dit-Bille RN, Leu S, et al. Five-year follow-up and recurrence rates following surgery for acute and chronic pilonidal disease: a survey of 421 cases. *Wounds.* 2016;28(1):20-26.

35. Jensen SL, Harling H. Prognosis after simple incision and drainage for a first-episode acute pilonidal abscess. *Br J Surg.* 1988;75(1):60-61.

36. Marks J, Harding KG, Hughes LE, Ribeiro CD. Pilonidal sinus excision—healing by open granulation. *Br J Surg.* 1985;72(8):637-640.

37. Dogru O, Camci C, Aygen E, Girgin M, Topuz O. P lonidal sinus treated with crystallized phenol: an eight-year experience. *Dis Colon Rectum.* 2004;47(11):1934-1938.

38. Hegge HG, Vos GA, Patka P, Hoitsma HF. Treatment of complicated or infected pilonidal sinus disease by local application of phenol. *Surgery.* 1987;102(1):52-54.

39. Edwards MH. Pilonidal sinus: a 5-year appraisal of the Millar-Lord treatment. *Br J Surg.* 1977;64(12):867-868.

40. Lord PH, Millar DM. Pilonidal sinus: a simple treatment. *Br J Surg.* 1965;52:298-300.

41. Humphries AE, Duncan JE. Evaluation and management of pilonidal disease. *Surg Clin North Am.* 2010;90(1):113-124. [table of contents].

42. Karakayali F, Karagulle E, Karabulut Z, et al. Unroofing and marsupialization vs. rhomboid excision and Limberg flap in pilonidal disease: a prospective, randomized, clinical trial. *Dis Colon Rectum.* 2009;52(3):496-502.

43. Lee SL, Tejirian T, Abbas MA. Current management of adolescent pilonidal disease. *J Pediatr Surg.* 2008;43(6):1124-1127.

44. Tejirian T, Lee JJ, Abbas MA. Is wide local excision for pilonidal disease still justified? *Am Surg.* 2007;73(10):1075-1078.

45. Garg P, Menon GR, Gupta V. Laying open (deroofing) and curettage of sinus as treatment of pilonidal disease: a systematic review and meta-analysis. *Aust N Z J Surg.* 2016;86(1-2):27-33.

46. Velasco AL, Dunlap WW. Piloridal disease and hidradenitis. *Surg Clin North Am.* 2009;89(3):689-701.

47. Eryilmaz R, Sahin M, Alimoglu O, Dasiran F. Surgical treatment of sacrococcygeal pilonidal sinus with the Limberg transposition flap. *Surgery.* 2003;134(5):745-749.

48. McGuinness JG, Winter DC, O'Connell PR. Vacuum-assisted closure of a complex pilonidal sinus. *Dis Colon Rectum.* 2003;45(2):274-276.

49. Lynch JB, Laing AJ, Regan PJ. Vacuum-assisted closure therapy: a new treatment option for recurrent pilonidal sinus disease. Report of three cases. *Dis Colon Rectum.* 2004;47(6):929-932.

50. Saxena V, Hwang CW, Huang S, Eichbaum Q, Ingber D, Orgil DP. Vacuum-assisted closure: microdeformations of wounds and cell proliferation. *Plast Reconstr Surg.* 2004;114(5):1086-1096, discussion 1097–1098.

51. McCallum IJD, King PM, Bruce J. Healing by primary closure versus open healing after surgery for pilonidal sinus: systematic review and meta-analysis. *BMJ.* 2008;336(7649):868-87 .

52. Unalp HR, Derici H, Kamer E, et al. Lower recurrence rate for Limberg vs. V-Y flap for pilonidal sinus. *Dis Colon Rectum.* 2007;50(9):1436-1444.

53. Can MF, Sevinc MM, Hancerliogullari O, Yilmaz M, Yagci G. Multicenter prospective randomized trial comparing modified Limberg flap transposition and Karydakis flap reconstruction in patients with sacrococcygeal pilonidal disease. *Am J Surg.* 2010;200(3):318-327.

54. Mahdy T. Surgical treatment of the pilonidal disease: primary closure or flap reconstruction after excision. *Dis Colon Rectum.* 2008;51(12):1816-1822.

55. Topgul K, Ozdemir E, Kilic K, Gokbayir H, Ferahkose Z. Long-term results of Limberg flap procedure for treatment of pilonidal sinus: a report of 200 cases. *Dis Color Rectum.* 2003;46(11):1545-1548.

56. Daphan C, Tekelioglu MH, Sayilgan C. Limberg flap repair for pilonidal sinus disease. *Dis Colon Rectum.* 2004;47(2):233-237.

57. Can MF, Sevinc MM, Yilmaz M. Comparison of Karydakis flap reconstruction versus primary midline closure in sacrococcygeal pilonidal disease: results of 200 military service members. *Surg Today.* 2009;39(7):580-586.

58. Senapati A, Cripps NPJ, Flashman K, Thompson MR. Cleft closure for the treatment of pilonidal sinus disease. *Colorectal Dis.* 2011;13(3):333-336.

59. Tezel E, Bostanci H, Anadol AZ, Kurukahvecioglu O. Cleft lift procedure for sacrococcygeal pilonidal disease. *Dis Colon Rectum.* 2009;52(1):135-139.

60. Abdelrazeq AS, Rahman M, Botterill ID, Alexander DJ. Short-term and long-term outcomes of the cleft lift procedure in the management of nonacute pilonidal disorders. *Dis Colon Rectum.* 2008;51(7):1100-1106.

61. Morgan WP, Hughes LE. The distribution, size and density of the apocrine glands in hidradenitis suppuritiva. *Br J Surg.* 1979;66(12):853-856.

62. Velpeau A. Dictionnaire de Medicine, un Repertoire General des Sciences Medicales sous la Rapport Theorique et Pratique. Bechet Jeune, Paris Aisselle.

63. Hoffman LK, Ghias MH, Lowes MA. Pathophysiology of hidradenitis suppurativa. *Semin Cutan Med Surg.* 2017;36(2):47-54.

64. Chen W, Plewig G. Should hidradenitis suppurativa/acne inversa best be renamed as "dissecting terminal hair folliculitis"? *Exp Dermatol.* 2017;26(6):544-547.

65. Highet AS, Warren RE, Weekes AJ. Bacteriology and antibiotic treatment of perineal suppurative hidradenitis. *Arch Dermatol.* 1988;124(7):1047-1051.

66. Lev-Tov H. Defining targets to defeat hidradenitis suppurativa. *Sci Transl Med.* 2017;9(397).

67. Wiltz O, Schoetz DJ, Murray JJ, Roberts FL, Coller JA, Veidenheimer MC. Perianal hidradenitis suppurativa. The Lahey Clinic experience. *Dis Colon Rectum.* 1990;33(9):731-734.

68. Porter ML, Kimball AB. Comorbidities of hidradenitis suppurativa. *Semin Cutan Med Surg.* 2017;36(2):55-57.

69. Harrison BJ, Kumar S, Read GF, Edwards CA, Scanlon MF, Hughes LE. Hidradenitis suppurativa: evidence for an endocrine abnormality. *Br J Surg.* 1985;72(12):1002-1004.

70. Vossen ARJV, van Straalen KR, Prens EP, et al. Menses and pregnancy affect symptoms in hidradenitis suppurativa: a cross-sectional study. *J Am Acad Dermatol.* 2017;76(1):155-156.

71. Stellon AJ, Wakeling M. Hidradenitis suppurativa associated with use of oral contraceptives. *BMJ.* 1989;298(6665):28-29.

72. Chalmers RJ, Ead RD, Beck MH, Dewis P, Anderson DC. Acne vulgaris and hidradenitis suppurativa as presenting features of acromegaly. *Br Med J (Clin Res Ed).* 1983;287(6402):1346-1347.

73. Curtis A. Cushing's syndrome and hidradenitis suppurativa. *Arch Derm Syphilol.* 1950;62(2):329-330.

74. Jemec GB. The symptomatology of hidradenitis suppurativa in women. *Br J Dermatol.* 1988;119(3):345-350.

75. Fitzsimmons S, Guilbert PR, Fitzsimmons EM. Evidence of genetic factors in hidradenitis suppurativa. *Br J Dermatol.* 1985;113(1):1-8.

76. Fitzsimmons JS, Fitzsimmons EM, Gilbert G. Familial hidradenitis suppurativa: evidence in favour of single gene transmission. *J Med Genet.* 1984;21(4):281-285.

77. Garg A, Lavian J, Lin G, et al. Incidence of hidradenitis suppurativa in the United States: a sex- and age-adjusted population analysis. *J Am Acad Dermatol.* 2017;77(1):118-122.

78. Vaidya T, Vangipuram R, Alikhan A. Examining the race-specific prevalence of hidradenitis suppurativa at a large academic center; results from a retrospective chart review. *Dermatol Online J.* 2017;23(6).

79. Parks RW, Parks TG. Pathogenesis, clinical features and management of hidradenitis suppurativa. *Ann R Coll Surg Engl.* 1997;79(2):83-89.

80. Hurley HJ. *Axillary Hyperhidrosis, Apocrine Bromhidrosis, Hidradenitis Suppurativa, and Familial Benign Pemphigus: Surgical Approach.* New York: Marcel Dekker; 1989:729-739.

81. Chiricozzi A, Faleri S, Franceschini C, Caro RD, Chimenti S, Bianchi L. AISI: a new disease severity assessment tool for hidradenitis suppurativa. *Wounds.* 2015;27(10):258-264.

82. Self SJ, Montes LF. Follicular occlusion triad. *South Med J.* 1970;63(2):156-160.

83. Church JM, Fazio VW, Lavery IC, et al. The differential diagnosis and comorbidity of hidradenitis suppurativa and perianal Crohn's disease. *Int J Colorectal Dis.* 1993;8(3):117-119.

84. Deckers IE, Benhadou F, Koldijk MJ, et al. Inflammatory bowel disease is associated with hidradenitis suppurativa: results from a multicenter cross-sectional study. *J Am Acad Dermatol*. 2017;76(1):49-53.

85. Gower-Rousseau C, Maunoury V, Colombel JF, et al. Hidradenitis suppurativa and Crohn's disease in two families: a significant association? *Am J Gastroenterol*. 1992;87(7):928.

86. Culp CE. Chronic hidradenitis suppurativa of the anal canal. A surgical skin disease. *Dis Colon Rectum*. 1983;26(10):669-676.

87. Perez-Diaz D, Calvo-Serrano M, Martinez-Hijosa E, et al. Squamous cell carcinoma complicating perianal hidradenitis suppurativa. *Int J Colorectal Dis*. 1995;10(4):225-228.

88. Shukla VK, Hughes LE. A case of squamous cell carcinoma complicating hidradenitis suppurativa. *Eur J Surg Oncol*. 1995;21(1):106-109.

89. Yon JR, Son JD, Fredericks C, et al. Marjolin's ulcer in chronic hidradenitis suppurativa: a rare complication of an often neglected disease. *J Burn Care Res*. 2017;38(2):121-124.

90. Clemmensen OJ. Topical treatment of hidradenitis suppurativa with clindamycin. *Int J Dermatol*. 1983;22(5):325-328.

91. Jemec GB, Wendelboe P. Topical clindamycin versus systemic tetracycline in the treatment of hidradenitis suppurativa. *J Am Acad Dermatol*. 1998;39(6):971-974.

92. Camisa C, Sexton C, Friedman C. Treatment of hidradenitis suppurativa with combination hypothalamic-pituitary-ovarian and adrenal suppression. A case report. *J Reprod Med*. 1989;34(8):543-546.

93. Brown CF, Gallup DG, Brown VM. Hidradenitis suppurativa of the anogenital region: response to isotretinoin. *Am J Obstet Gynecol*. 1988;158(1):12-15.

94. Hogan DJ, Light MJ. Successful treatment of hidradenitis suppurativa with acitretin. *J Am Acad Dermatol*. 1988;19(2 Pt 1):355-356.

95. Gupta AK, Ellis CN, Nickoloff BJ, et al. Oral cyclosporine in the treatment of inflammatory and noninflammatory dermatoses. A clinical and immunopathologic analysis. *Arch Dermatol*. 1990;126(3):339-350.

96. Martin-Ezquerra G, Masferrer E, Pujol RM. Use of biological treatments in patients with hidradenitis suppurativa. *G Ital Dermatol Venereol*. 2017;152(4):373-378.

97. Thorlacius L, Theut Riis P, Jemec GBE. Severe hidradenitis suppurativa responding to treatment with secukinumab: a case report. *Br J Dermatol*. 2017;doi:10.1111/bjd.15769.

98. Blok JL, Boersma M, Terra JB, et al. Surgery under general anaesthesia in severe hidradenitis suppurativa: a study of 363 primary operations in 113 patients. *J Eur Acad Dermatol Venereol*. 2015;29(8):1590-1597.

99. van der Zee HH, Prens EP, Boer J. Deroofing: a tissue-saving surgical technique for the treatment of mild to moderate hidradenitis suppurativa lesions. *J Am Acad Dermatol*. 2010;63(3):475-480.

100. Jemec GB. Effect of localized surgical excisions in hidradenitis suppurativa. *J Am Acad Dermatol*. 1988;18(5 Pt 1):1103-1107.

101. Rompel R, Petres J. Long-term results of wide surgical excision in 106 patients with hidradenitis suppurativa. *Dermatol Surg*. 2000;26(7):638-643.

102. Ramasastry SS, Conklin WT, Granick MS, et al. Surgical management of massive perianal hidradenitis suppurativa. *Ann Plast Surg*. 1985;15(3):218-223.

103. Chen E, Friedman HI. Management of regional hidradenitis suppurativa with vacuum-assisted closure and split thickness skin grafts. *Ann Plast Surg*. 2011;67(4):397-401.

104. Romanowski KS, Fagin A, Werling B, et al. Surgical management of hidradenitis suppurativa: a 14-year retrospective review of 98 consecutive patients. *J Burn Care Res*. 2017;doi:10.1097/BCR.0000000000000531.

105. Benito P, GarcIa J, De Juan A, Alcazar JA, Elena E, Cano M. Reconstruction of a perianal defect by means of a bilateral V-Y advancement flap based on the perforating arteries of the gluteus maximus shaped over a cicatricial area. *J Plast Reconstr Aesthet Surg*. 2009;62(3):412-414.

106. Buyukasik O, Hasdemir AO, Kahramansoy N, Çöl C, Erkol H. Surgical approach to extensive hidradenitis suppurativa. *Dermatol Surg*. 2011;37(6):835-842.

107. Alharbi Z, Kauczok J, Pallua N. A review of wide surgical excision of hidradenitis suppurativa. *BMC Dermatol*. 2012;12(1):1-1.

108. Burney RE. 35-Year experience with surgical treatment of hidradenitis suppurativa. *World J Surg*. 2017;doi:10.1007/s00268-017-4091-7.

109. Chen YE, Gerstle T, Verma K, Treiser MD, Kimball AB, Orgil DP. Management of hidradenitis suppurativa wounds with an internal vacuum-assisted closure device. *Plast Reconstr Surg*. 2014;133(3):370e-377e.

110. Elwood ET, Bolitho DG. Negative-pressure dressings in the treatment of hidradenitis suppurativa. *Ann Plast Surg*. 2001;46(1):49-51.

Emergent Care of the Victim of Colorectal Trauma

Michael L. Foreman | Edward R. Franko | Geoffrey A. Funk

Elective surgical philosophies and techniques are often suboptimal in the injured patient. Unlike planned colorectal operations, where hemorrhage and fecal spillage are immediately addressed, the adverse cascades of infection and shock commence at injury. This inherent delay in presentation, obscuration of tissue planes, instability without the luxury of preoperative optimization, and the requirement for impromptu but decisive operation based on minimal information differentiates trauma from elective surgery. In short, the surgeon must adapt surgical principles to treating "the patient [who has], in most cases, lost more blood than the system could conveniently space."[1]

Traumatic injury to the large intestine can occur from a number of mechanisms: blunt from acute compression or deceleration; external penetrating, most commonly from projectiles or bladed weapons; or internal penetrating from foreign bodies introduced recreationally or iatrogenically. The importance of rapid diagnosis and intervention cannot be overstated. Changes in management of colonic injuries away from mandatory diversion and the popularization of damage control laparotomy (DCL) have expanded surgical management choices in the often multiply injured and unstable patient.[2-8]

INCIDENCE

Blunt colorectal trauma is relatively rare but, compared with penetrating injury, the morbidity and mortality are quite high as a result of concomitant injuries.[9-12] Brady et al.[13] noted a less than 1% incidence of colorectal trauma, with 44% of those having blunt mechanisms, but a greater than 25% mortality rate for that subgroup. Williams et al.[14] reported that, after controlling for traumatic brain injury, colon injury predicted greater lengths of stay in both the intensive care unit (ICU) and hospital, though not mortality (Table 154.1).

Except for those caused by therapeutic or erotic misadventures via natural orifice, isolated blunt colon injuries rarely occur. In a survey of more than 200,000 blunt trauma patients, less than a third of the 1% of patients with a hollow viscus injury had colorectal involvement.[14] Of those 2152 patients with hollow viscus injury who underwent laparotomy, only 5.5% had injuries isolated to the colon. Reviewing almost 12,000 pediatric trauma admissions, Canty et al.[15] found only 17 colon injuries in the 79 patients with blunt gastrointestinal injuries. The cecum, sigmoid, and transverse colon are the most common sites of injury in blunt trauma, but mesenteric avulsion, full-thickness laceration, transection, and devascularization are seen most commonly in the ascending and descending colon.[10,16] The colon is often involved in penetrating trauma: it is the second most commonly injured organ from gunshots and the third most commonly injured from stab wounds.[17]

Due to the relatively large area of the posterior abdomen occupied by the colon, one-third of posterior stab wounds with organ injuries involve the colon.[13,19] Rectal and distal sigmoid injuries also occur more commonly in penetrating trauma.[20] The rectum is protected by the pelvis but, when injured, associated genitourinary (GU) and osseous injuries are common. Almost half of penetrating rectal injuries may have associated GU injuries.[21,22] Blunt rectal injuries are often associated with pelvic fractures, occurring in up to 25% of open pelvic fractures.[23-25]

Bowel injury from therapeutic or diagnostic enemata are well known.[26,27] Perforation from the bewildering variety of foreign bodies inserted into the rectum diagnostically and recreationally generally occurs secondary to forcible application, retention leading to necrosis, or a preexisting abnormality (e.g., stricture).[28,29]

The mandated adoption of fecal diversion during World War II was credited with marked improvement in the historically dismal outcomes of colorectal injury. Notably, this occurred in conjunction with advances in evacuation, fluid resuscitation, the availability of banked blood, and antibiotics.[2,5,30-32] Similarly, new diagnostic and operative innovations, such as damage control, have improved recent outcomes.

DIAGNOSIS

Colorectal injury is often diagnosed during operation for other emergent indications. Patients with an appropriate history of injury found to have peritonitis or unstable vital signs rarely profit from additional diagnostic procedures not performed in the operating room. Promptly addressing colon injuries is paramount to minimize morbidity and mortality. Delay in diagnosis for blunt injury greater than 5 hours is an independent risk factor for mortality,[9] as is delay to operation with penetrating injury.[33] Unfortunately, especially following blunt injury, early recognition of nonspecific, subtle, absent, or masked clinical findings from an isolated colon injury may be challenging, but certain common injury patterns (e.g., the seat belt sign) should raise suspicion.[34]

Further complicating the issue is that no imaging modalities or clinical findings are able to determine colon injury specifically, nor does any combination of findings reliably predict injury.[14] Anorectal injury is more likely to be diagnosed on examination than proximal injuries. Visualization of the perineal region for external signs of injury and digital rectal examination (DRE) for wounds, foreign bodies, or blood should be performed. Reported to miss 100% of colon injuries and 66.7% of rectal injuries, the utility of routine DRE has been questioned.[35,36] Since DRE is only 50% sensitive, a negative examination can never be regarded as conclusive, but a positive examination

TABLE 154.1 Gradation of Injuries to Colon and Rectum

Injured Structure	Grade*	Characteristics of Injury	AIS-05 Score
Colon	1	Contusion or hematoma; partial-thickness laceration	2
	2	Small (<50% of circumference) laceration	3
	3	Large (>50% of circumference) laceration	3
	4	Transection	4
	5	Transection with tissue loss; devascularized segment	4
Rectosigmoid and rectum	1	Contusion or hematoma; partial-thickness laceration	2
	2	Small (<50% of circumference) laceration	3
	3	Large (>50% of circumference) laceration	4
	4	Full-thickness laceration with perineal extension	5
	5	Devascularized segment	5

*Grade 3 and above is considered destructive.
AIS-05, Abbreviated Injury Scale Score, 2005 version.
Modified from the Abbreviated Injury Scale (AIS) 2005—update 2008. Association for the Advancement of Automotive Medicine, Barrington, IL.

may be enough to justify operation.[37] Rigid or flexible sigmoidoscopy is a useful adjunct to identify rectal injuries with 78% sensitivity,[37,38] and should be pursued if injury is suspected. Care must be exercised, as insufflation can exacerbate injury. Concomitant rectal injuries occur with GU injuries, so one should also be suspicious with hematuria or blood at the meatus.

IMAGING

While nonspecific, plain radiographs may reveal pneumoperitoneum, pelvic fractures, foreign bodies, or wound trajectories that may prompt additional studies or operation. Peritoneal fluid found by Focused Assessment with Sonography for Trauma (FAST) in an injured, unstable patient also may trigger immediate operation. Diagnostic peritoneal lavage has largely been supplanted by sonography and computed tomography (CT), but remains useful in patients with a suspicion of abdominal pathology who are too unstable for CT and who cannot be conclusively imaged sonographically or to analyze suspicious abdominal fluid on CT in the face of equivocal findings.

Multidetector CT is the predominant, if not indispensable, device for the evaluation of abdominal injuries in stable or stabilizing patients, without indication for immediate operative intervention.[1,39] Radiographic identification of isolated injury to the large intestine is difficult because of nonspecific and often subtle findings. Frequently, it is not direct radiographic findings of bowel perforation (e.g., pneumoperitoneum, extravasation of enteric contrast, intramural gas, or colon wall defects), but the presence of indirect findings (e.g., bowel wall thickening or enhancement, stranding of adjacent mesentery or mesocolon, or free intraperitoneal fluid) that prompts operation.[10,11,39] Active extravasation in the mesentery generally signals a need for operation, and may also be associated with direct injury to the colon or ischemia. Peritoneal free fluid may be from normal female physiology, preexisting ascites, transudate secondary to resuscitation, or blood from solid visceral or mesenteric injury, as well as from enteric spillage. The lack of free peritoneal fluid, however, has a high negative predictive value for bowel injury.[39] Although not uniformly present in hollow viscus rupture, pneumoperitoneum has 95%

specificity, despite 25% sensitivity.[11] Retroperitoneal air may be present as a result of perforation from the extraperitoneal colon or duodenum and may track down from or up into the chest.[11] As determining wound trajectory and depth on physical exam is difficult, one should consider CT, which can identify significant intraabdominal injuries with sensitivity and specificity greater than 90%,[40] and may identify patients suitable for observation or selective nonoperative management, and decrease nontherapeutic laparotomies. Triple-contrast imaging has been advocated to better visualize the colon, given its false-negative rate for GI injury of 1.8% and false-positive rate of 7%.[11,41,42] Rectal-contrast-enhanced CT can be quite useful, but the absence of extravasation does not exclude injury, and the enema apparatus may interfere with subtleties in the distal rectum.

TREATMENT

DAMAGE CONTROL LAPAROTOMY (DCL)

The patient with a colon injury may arrive hemodynamically unstable and with physiologic stores that are taxed or nonexistent. Recognition of the need to break the "trauma triad of death"—the downward spiral of coagulopathy, hypothermia, and acidosis contributing to deteriorating physiology[43]—changed the conventional operative approach of attempting definitive repair in favor of abbreviated laparotomy. Christened *damage control* by Rotondo et al.,[8] it references the naval term for keeping a damaged ship afloat and functional in hostile waters by any means necessary to allow survival and definitive repair under later, more favorable conditions. This paradigm shift to prioritize physiology over anatomy is the standard of care for trauma and myriad emergency surgical situations. The willingness to perform staged anastomosis and repair following stabilization has changed outcomes but also presents challenges that were unusual in the pre-DCL era.

The goals of DCL are to rapidly control bleeding and then limit contamination in severely injured patients. This necessitates expeditious entry into the abdomen with wide exposure. Hemorrhage is quickly cleared and controlled to allow brisk intraperitoneal exploration. Obvious vascular injuries that cannot be ligated or swiftly repaired may be temporarily shunted. Once bleeding is controlled and while intravascular volume is being restored, attention is turned to contamination. Coloenteric spillage should be attended to rapidly with initial clamping, temporary suture, ligation with umbilical tapes, or stapling devices. Depending on the physiologic status of the patient, definitive suture control or resection is undertaken as deemed prudent. In the unstable patient, there should be no attempt at definitive anastomosis. Instead, with the colon in discontinuity and after removing as much contamination as possible, a temporary abdominal closure is accomplished with attention to protection of the underlying bowel and resuscitation is continued in the ICU with the abdomen open. The return for definitive operation generally occurs between 24 and 48 hours and hopefully finds the patient in a clinical and metabolic state permitting reconstruction. Restoring enteric continuity with delayed anastomosis, diversion, or additional resection can then be performed in less-hurried circumstances. In the event that physiology still precludes complete resolution, the abdominal closure is again temporized with the same plan: return once stable.

Given the complexity of decision making in these patients, transfer to a higher level of care after initial lifesaving DCL should be considered.

Open Abdomen

The prolonged, repeated exposure of the viscera to a nonbiologic envelope by DCL is not benign, and the effects of the open abdomen on anastomosis and wound healing are not very well known, but there are several associated risk factors. It remains uncertain, however, if these relate to the open abdomen or are epiphenomenal to the severity of injury necessitating the technique.[44] While there is little disagreement in the advisability of initial resection and closure of colonic wounds, decisions regarding the timing for delayed anastomosis and the security of primary repair in open abdomens are controversial.[45] The open abdomen risks infection and can contribute to a sixfold increase in leak rate.[46] Resection and anastomosis from destructive injury (see Table 154.1) and delayed anastomosis result in infection and fistula more often than smaller, primary repairs.[7,47] The number of operations and time to abdominal closure are strong indicators of anastomotic complication, with 4 to 16.8 times increased risk of fistula if fascial closure is not obtained by day 5.[7,4,47-49] Similarly, complication rates from non-DCL colon repair and resection matched that of patients with delayed anastomosis who obtained fascial closure at first return, while complications rise 8- to 12-fold if more than two laparotomies were required.[47,50] Anastomotic complications were more common in more distal injuries, closure with anything other than native fascia, and vasopressor requirement.[47-49,51] Concurrent injuries leading to a higher risk of anastomotic breakdown have been noted, including injuries to the pancreas, spleen, kidney, and diaphragm.[2] Aggressive surgical attempts to close the fascial envelope at the earliest possible time while avoiding abdominal hypertension is reasonable, as duration of bowel exposure appears to be a strong indicator for the success or failure of anastomosis. Notably, there are few other modifiable risk factors. Predicting patients

who might avoid complication by fecal diversion remains difficult, as the complication rate even with colostomy remains high and is likely a proxy for injury severity and comorbidity.

DAMAGE CONTROL RESUSCITATION

While DCL changed the paradigm during and following operative intervention, damage control resuscitation (DCR) has evolved from a better understanding of the pathophysiology of exsanguination and enhances opportunities to survive to and beyond operation.[52-54] DCR attempts to mitigate the morbidity of the therapeutic vacuum between injury and meaningful intervention by minimizing blood loss with permissive hypotension prior to surgical hemostasis, using judicious volume restoration, administering antifibrinolytic agents and coagulation factor concentrates, achieving hemostatic resuscitation with early use of plasma and platelets in fixed ratio to packed red cells in goal-directed transfusion protocols, and avoiding crystalloids that can lead to a grossly edematous bowel and reduce the feasibility and outcome of delayed anastomosis following DCL.[51,53,55-58]

TREATMENT OF COLONIC INJURIES

The decision to repair or resect is influenced by a number of variables: injury mechanism, hemodynamic stability, overall injury burden, transfusion and crystalloid volume, and degree of destruction of involved tissue. Myriad algorithms have been suggested to simplify this process, resulting in three primary paths of treatment. Regardless of treatment method, all patients with suspected colonic perforation should receive immediate antibiotic coverage continued for 24 hours or less, as there is no utility in longer coverage without cause.[59]

A significant percentage of colorectal injuries result from penetrating trauma, with reports as high as 19% in general war-related series; most of those were destructive, whereas 80% to 90% are nondestructive in the civilian setting.[60] For nondestructive injuries, primary repair is a safe and preferable treatment.[61] Destructive injuries are managed with resection with anastomosis or diversion, depending on transfusion requirements and comorbidities. There remains an unsubstantiated fear of anastomotic leaks and other complications with primary repair; a review of 6817 patients with primary colon injury found that only 9% underwent diversion and indicative of the severity of injury, the patients managed with stoma formation had a mortality rate almost twice that of patients managed without diversion.[63] Diverted patients tended to be more severely injured, older, and have more ventilator, ICU, and hospital days. While uncommonly needed, colostomy and diverting ileostomy remain important and often lifesaving techniques in selected patients with complex injuries. Succinctly, diversion is preferred when the patient's overall health status cannot tolerate complication (i.e., leak, abscess, etc.).

Although operative exposure has historically revolved around laparotomy, depending on circumstance, laparoscopy may be considered.[64] Importantly, the patient must be hemodynamically able to tolerate the necessarily present pneumoperitoneum, and both surgeon and institution must have the capacity to perform the required

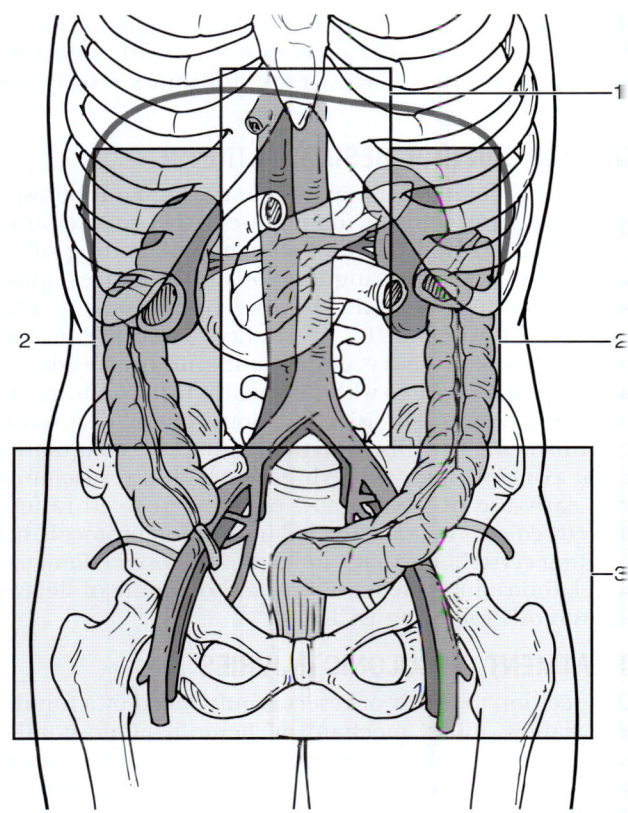

FIGURE 154.1 Abdominal zones of injury. (From Selivanov V, Chi HS, Alverdy JC, et al. Mortality in retroperitoneal hematoma. *J Trauma*. 1984;24:1022–1027, with permission.)

laparoscopic interventions. If any factor falls short, a standard laparotomy should be performed. Sources have reported missed injury rates in laparoscopy up to 4%,[65,66] but this is balanced by the ability to reduce nontherapeutic laparotomies dramatically, with rates as low as 0% when laparoscopy was used in penetrating abdominal trauma.[67] Alemayehu[68] demonstrated similar findings in a pediatric population with therapeutic intervention and no missed injuries. If there is any question as to the adequacy of exposure or completeness of laparoscopic evaluation, conversion to an open approach is mandatory.

Once the peritoneum is entered, evaluation centers upon control of life-threatening hemorrhage and only secondarily is contamination considered. While many practitioners routinely pack all quadrants irrespective of initial operative findings, an alternate and perhaps more efficient approach is selective packing of significant bleeding within the operative field after evisceration and subsequent evaluation of zones 1 and 2 (Fig. 154.1 on abdominal zones of injury). This allows for identification and treatment of great vessel injury, which a four-quadrant approach generally neglects in favor of the potential for pelvic or solid organ hemorrhage.

Given the rarity of isolated colonic injury as the impetus for exploration, the recognition of associated injuries is important. In the setting of penetrating trauma, there is an obvious advantage for the close evaluation of organs near the wound path, but much broader suspicion is required in blunt trauma due to the risk for remote multiorgan injury.[9,10,13,14]

Due to the omental coverage of the transverse colon (often broad mesenteric and retroperitoneal attachments of the descending and ascending components) and the extraperitoneal portion of the rectum, small transmural defects can be difficult to discover. Air or feculent staining under an omental or peritoneal layer may be the only finding in some cases, but should trigger a thorough evaluation. The surgeon should not hesitate to mobilize the colon along standard anatomic planes to visualize potential injury. Concerning hematomas must be explored to rule out potentially lethal occult perforation. The splenic flexure, because of its redundancy and multiple tethering attachments, is prone to missed injury and should be fully mobilized for inspection if there is concern. Similarly, the extraperitoneal rectal surfaces should be mobilized along the lateral peritoneum if there is suspicion of injury. In penetrating injuries, the *rule of two*—as entrance wounds generally have exit wounds—should lead to a search for missed injury if an odd number of wounds is encountered. While there are situations that violate this rule (e.g., projectile in the lumen of the bowel, stab wound not extending through the lumen, tangential wound tract), they should be proven as the exception. The surgeon should be able to trace the injury from its entrance into the peritoneal cavity to its conclusion. The inability to do so must be regarded as a missed injury until proven otherwise. Multiple projectiles demand even more minute attention to avoid missing inconspicuous injuries.

Whereas penetrating injuries have defined trajectories, blunt traumas typically have no such apparent injury pathways. The more diffuse distribution of energy with blunt mechanism mandates a careful, systematic evaluation of the entire colon. Small areas of partial-thickness disruptions may be imbricated, but larger areas are best resected to avoid the complications of delayed full-thickness necrosis.

If repairing primarily, nonviable edges of the wound should be débrided and single-layer closure with seromuscular Lembert sutures suffice. Adjacent through-and-through perforations are generally best managed by excising the contused segment between the wounds and converting it to a single perforation. Given the relatively large luminal size of the colon, stricture is uncommon. Formal resection and reanastomosis is generally wise for destructive injuries, especially if there is any question about vascular supply. While ardent supporters in both camps cite appropriate literature, the choice of hand-sewn versus stapled anastomoses should be left to the experience and comfort level of the surgeon.[69,70]

Although buttressing repairs or anastomoses with omentum is not effective in elective colorectal surgery, it has not been shown to be harmful, and many surgeons will likely continue using the technique.[71] It is advisable to bury repairs and anastomoses away from the midline incision, especially in situations where relaparotomy is planned, and leave them undisturbed if possible.[49]

Delayed primary anastomoses are successfully performed in civilian and military settings, but should be done before significant edema develops.[3,4,30,46,49,52] A decision for anastomosis or diversion must be made before the bowel edema, and mesenteric retraction should make the decision for the surgeon. The colon can be left in discontinuity for up to 3 days to allow for reassessment of viability and a delayed definitive operation.[30,72] Septic complications following colonic injury likely are a reflection not of the method of management, but of the severity of injury. Fecal diversion is therefore likely affected by selection bias. Avoiding an initial stoma—and the accompanying potential complications of difficult abdominal wound closure and the risk of worsening bowel and abdominal wall edema that create possible ischemic limb compromise—must be tempered by the approaching and inevitable mesenteric shortening and visceral bloat.[30,52]

Vascular Topics

Significant hemorrhage must be addressed early by clamping or packing. Once hemorrhage is mitigated and contamination is controlled, more definitive vascular investigation may proceed. If an unnamed mesenteric vessel is injured and compromises the viability of a segment of colon, ligate the vessel and resect the affected bowel. Mesenteric injury in the ileocolic and splenic flexure watershed regions should be viewed suspiciously and resection carried back to well-vascularized tissue, unless a second look to reassess viability is planned. Injuries to the superior mesenteric artery within the first, second, or third portions should never be ligated, due to the near-certain bowel ischemia and necrosis.[73] If time and patient permit, one should consider repair or, if absolutely necessary, resection of the injured segment and shunting. Similar options exist for injuries to the superior mesenteric vein, dependent on injury burden.[74] Vascular reconstruction may be necessary, even in the face of the contamination from concurrent enteric injury. Relatively few reports discuss inferior mesenteric artery or vein injury—while less common, therapeutic embolization has also been suggested.[75]

TREATMENT OF ANORECTAL INJURIES

Pelvic Anatomy for the Surgeon

Trauma to the deep pelvis and anorectum poses unique challenges to the surgeon, as access can be difficult, and problematic functional outcomes are specific concerns distinct to this region. Thus it is imperative to have a thorough grasp of the anatomic basis for such issues.

The rectum can be divided in thirds based upon peritonealization: the upper third is covered only anteriorly and laterally more distally and can be approached through the abdomen; the distal third, which is completely extraperitoneal, would be approached per the anus; and the middle third of the rectum, which is covered with peritoneum anteriorly, making the posterolateral walls extraperitoneal, is difficult to access from either approach and makes the region particularly challenging.

The rectum has a generous blood supply, which makes it more resistant to ischemia but can also make hemorrhage control difficult. The unpaired superior rectal artery is the main arterial supply of the rectum coming off the inferior mesenteric artery. The paired middle rectal artery passes into the lateral ligaments, originating off the internal iliac

artery, while the two inferior rectal arteries stem from the internal pudendal artery.

In addition, important anatomic structures are in close vicinity in this area. One must be cognizant of the course of the ureters, iliac vessels, urinary bladder, and both male and female anatomies. Most of these structures lie anteriorly, so it is safest to approach this region posteriorly.[76] Rectal dissection should be posterior to and below the superior rectal artery in the avascular presacral space. Avoiding the presacral fascia prevents disruption of presacral veins and pelvic autonomic nerves entering the pelvic side walls, but eventually wrapping anterior to be in proximity with anterior rectum at the level of the prostate or upper vagina.[77] Staying close to the rectal wall avoids injury to these structures.

Surgical Treatment of Anorectal Injuries

Anorectal traumas markedly differ from colonic traumas. For civilian injuries, evidence does not support distal rectal washout,[78,79] and it is thought that loose stool may contaminate other spaces. Likewise, diverting colostomy in intraperitoneal rectal injuries and some extraperitoneal injuries can be successfully avoided.[22,80,81] Colostomy is still advised if the injury is either not easily repaired or inaccessible.[9,82] Primary repair of extraperitoneal injury can be successful if significant dissection is not required, and associated GU injuries are approached extraabdominally.[83] Ultimately, the literature refutes routine use of presacral drainage,[82,84,85] but it should be considered for larger, inaccessible injuries or in destructive injuries with tissue loss, which are at risk for abscess formation in the retrorectal space. If normal tissue planes would be disrupted significantly, then drain placement should be avoided. Proper placement in the vicinity of injury to prevent abscess or fistula formation is key.

The patient should be in lithotomy position, and a rigid or flexible sigmoidoscope should be available. A midline laparotomy is mandatory in the unstable patient. DCL principles apply, and care should be taken, as a bladder displaced by hematoma can be injured during incision. Intraperitoneal rectal injuries can be approached similar to colon injuries. Smaller defects can be débrided and closed primarily. If relaparotomy is planned, the bowel can be left in discontinuity and the abdomen can be left open. Caution needs to be applied if the rectum requires ligation or transection, as the course of the ureters must be identified bilaterally. Insufflation via proctoscopy while the abdomen is filled with saline and the proximal bowel is occluded can help identify occult injuries. If bladder and rectal injuries are found, it is important to keep these repairs separate, using tissue to prevent rectovesical fistulas.[86]

The approach to the distal rectum will depend on location and severity of injury. In the stable patient, laparoscopy has been suggested to confirm injuries that are solely extraperitoneal.[85] Primary repair of the rectum can be performed transanally and is advocated if no extensive dissection is required.[85] Injury above the sphincter becomes increasingly difficult to access, as more proximal injuries are limited by visibility. Localizing the injury is the first goal, realizing that the initial key to treatment is to gain hemostasis and not to repair the injury, unless easily accessed. A rigid proctoscopy is usually the first choice, but with active bleeding and stool contamination, visibility may be obscured. A flexible scope has the advantages of rapid irrigation to aid in identification, as well as therapeutic use with cauterization or clip placement.

Various retractors may aid in visualization, localization, and repair. A Hill-Ferguson retractor is good for the anal canal and possibly the distal rectum, but not more proximal. A St. Mark anal retractor allows approach to the distal rectum, but not midrectum. Some angled, vaginal specula have longer reach. A Lone Star retractor can allow some visualization of both proximal and distal injuries.

Care must be taken not to overstretch the sphincter, as this may cause permanent damage. The biggest challenge is assessment and repair of any midrectal injury. In the case of massive hemorrhage, packing the rectum or using a catheter with a large inflatable balloon (30 to 60 mL) may be required and repair attempted later. In some cases, hypogastric artery ligation or embolization may be lifesaving.

Considerations for the Distal Rectum and Anus

Injury to the sphincter should be approached with caution. If injury occurs to the distal rectum without sphincter injury, the previous discussion on anorectal trauma applies. Sphincter injury, however, requires a different approach. These can result from blunt trauma such as difficult child delivery or intentional foreign body placement, or from penetrating trauma, such as impalement or assault. Third- and fourth-degree tears during delivery will involve the anus and sphincter complex but can usually be repaired primarily at the time of injury,[87] and fecal diversion is rarely necessary.[88] If a rectovaginal fistula does develop, an observation period is warranted before reattempting repair.

Blunt injuries to the anal area are commonly associated with pelvic fractures. These patients often require stabilization of the pelvis or treatment of associated injuries with subsequent treatment of sphincter and perineal injuries. Whether blunt or penetrating, judicious removal of nonviable tissue is necessary and may require multiple débridements.[89] Unlike the surrounding tissue, the sphincter itself is relatively resistant to infection. The sphincter muscle is quite vascular and only requires minimal simple débridement, whereas other nonviable tissue should be removed more liberally. With wide débridement, care is advised so as to avoid injury to the pudendal nerve, which innervates the sphincter. Likewise, either rapid simple suturing for hemostasis or repair similar to that of an obstetric injury is preferred to any extended repair, the latter of which may lead to stricture, poor functional outcome, or both.[90] Delayed repair by overlapping sphincteroplasty has been successful.[91] Fecal diversion may be avoided in simple repairs, and negative-pressure devices can aid in healing soft tissue wounds.[92] Recent wartime data on penetrating trauma show long-term results depend on degree of injury, other intraabdominal injuries, pelvic fractures, and hypogastric artery ligation. Unfortunately, even acute repair of the sphincter did not influence colostomy reversal.[93]

Foreign body removal can sometimes be performed in the emergency department (ED) if the patient can be sedated sufficiently. If the foreign body cannot be retrieved in the ED, then general anesthesia in the operating room is necessary. Further evaluation is mandatory if the patient has abdominal symptoms, and laparotomy is necessary for peritonitis. Plain X-rays may be informative, but a CT can be far more specific. Imaging should be obtained before and after attempting *any* retrieval to verify that no perforation has occurred; proctoscopic evaluation after removal is also recommended. Various reports on removal exist, but the general principle is to obtain good relaxation of the sphincter while trying to grasp the object,[94,95] though this can require novel approaches. Placing a Foley catheter alongside the object can break the vacuum seal that forms during extraction. If unsuccessful, endoscopic or laparoscopic assistance may be required.[96] Once removed, an observation period is recommended to rule out occult injury.

CONCLUSION

In addition to the significant health risks inherent in colorectal injury, the potential for therapeutic failure can lead to catastrophic outcomes. Significant variations in individual surgeon's preference and philosophy likely make an a priori decision of the right operation for the right patient unobtainable; the best answer is likely a confluence of the surgeon's experience, the demands of a multiply injured patient, and the setting in which the two meet. Ultimately, surgical judgment and experience are critical in deciding the best course of action for each patient.

ACKNOWLEDGMENT

The authors thank Jacob W. Roden-Foreman for his assistance researching, writing, and editing this chapter.

REFERENCES

1. Chisolm JJ. General treatment of gunshot wounds. In: *A Manual of Military Surgery*. 3rd ed. Dayton, OH: Morningside Press; 1864:215-221.
2. Vertrees A, Wakefield M, Pickett C, et al. Outcomes of primary repair and primary anastomosis in war-related colon injuries. *J Trauma*. 2009;66(5):1286-1291, discussion 1291–1233.
3. Weinberg JA, Griffin RL, Vandromme MJ, et al. Management of colon wounds in the setting of damage control laparotomy: a cautionary tale. *J Trauma*. 2009;67(5):929-935.
4. Kashuk JL, Cothren CC, Moore EE, Johnson JL, Biffl WL, Barnett CC. Primary repair of civilian colon injuries is safe in the damage control scenario. *Surgery*. 2009;146(4):663-668, discussion 668–670.
5. Steele SR, Maykel JA, Johnson EK. Traumatic injury of the colon and rectum: the evidence vs dogma. *Dis Colon Rectum*. 2011;54(9):1184-1201.
6. Ordoñez CA, Pino LF, Badiel M, et al. Safety of performing a delayed anastomosis during damage control laparotomy in patients with destructive colon injuries. *J Trauma*. 2011;71(6):1512-1517, discussion 1517–1518.
7. Bradley MJ, Dubose JJ, Scalea TM, et al. Independent predictors of enteric fistula and abdominal sepsis after damage control laparotomy: results from the prospective AAST open abdomen registry. *JAMA Surg*. 2013;148(10):947-954.
8. Rotondo MF, Schwab CW, McGonigal MD, et al. 'Damage control': an approach for improved survival in exsanguinating penetrating abdominal injury. *J Trauma*. 1993;35(3):375-382, discussion 382–383.
9. Malinoski DJ, Patel MS, Yakar DO, et al. A diagnostic delay of 5 hours increases the risk of death after blunt hollow viscus injury. *J Trauma*. 2010;69(1):84-87.

10. Kokabi N, Harmouche E, Xing M, et al. Specific radiological findings of traumatic gastrointestinal tract injuries in patients with blunt chest and abdominal trauma. *Can Assoc Radiol J.* 2015;56(2):158-163.

11. Bondia JM, Anderson SW, Rhea JT, Soto JA. Imaging colorectal trauma using 64-MDCT technology. *Emerg Radiol.* 2009;16(6):433-440.

12. Fakhry SM, Brownstein M, Watts DD, Baker CC, Oller D. Relatively short diagnostic delays (8 hours) produce morbidity and mortality in blunt small bowel injury: an analysis of time to operative intervention in 198 patients from a multicenter experience. *J Trauma.* 2000;48(3):408-414, discussion 414-415.

13. Brady RR, O'Neill S, Berry O, Kerssens JJ, Yalamarthi S, Parks RW. Traumatic injury to the colon and rectum in Scotland: demographics and outcome. *Colorectal Dis.* 2012;14(1):e16-e22.

14. Williams MD, Watts D, Fakhry S. Colon injury after blunt abdominal trauma: results of the EAST multi-institutional hollow viscus injury study. *J Trauma.* 2003;55(5):906-912.

15. Canty TG Sr, Canty TG Jr, Brown C. Injuries of the gastrointestinal tract from blunt trauma in children: a 12-year experience at a designated pediatric trauma center. *J Trauma.* 1999;46(2):234-240.

16. Nghiem HV, Jeffrey RB Jr, Mindelzun RE. CT of blunt trauma to the bowel and mesentery. *AJR Am J Roentgenol.* 1993;160(1):53-58.

17. Pinedo-Onofre JA, Guevara-Torres L, Sanchez-Aguilar JM. Penetrating abdominal trauma. *Cir Cir.* 2006;74(6):431-442.

18. Kong VY, Oosthuizen GV, Clarke DL. The spectrum of injuries resulting from posterior abdominal stab wounds: a South African experience. *Ann R Coll Surg Engl.* 2015;97(4):269-273.

19. Demetriades D, Rabinowitz B, Sofianos C, et al. The management of penetrating injuries of the back. A prospective study of 230 patients. *Ann Surg.* 1988;207(1):72-74.

20. Brunner RG, Shatney CH. Diagnostic and therapeutic aspects of rectal trauma. Blunt versus penetrating. *Am Surg.* 1987;53(4):215-219.

21. Pereira BM, Reis LO, Calderan TR, de Campos CC, Fraga GP. Penetrating bladder trauma: a high risk factor for associated rectal injury. *Adv Urol.* 2014;2014:385328.

22. Weinberg JA, Fabian TC, Magnotti LJ, et al. Penetrating rectal trauma: management by anatomic distinction improves outcome. *J Trauma.* 2006;60(3):508-513, discussion 513-514.

23. Hefny AF, Al-Ashaal YI, Bani-Hashem AM, Abu-Zidan FM. Seatbelt syndrome associated with an isolated rectal injury: case report. *World J Emerg Surg.* 2010;5(1):4-7922-5-4.

24. Cannada LK, Taylor RM, Reddix R, et al. The Jones-Powell classification of open pelvic fractures: a multicenter study evaluating mortality rates. *J Trauma Acute Care Surg.* 2013;74(3):901-906.

25. Ross GL, Dodd O, Lipham JC, Campbell JK. Rectal perforation in unstable pelvic fractures: the use of flexible sigmoidoscopy. *Injury.* 2001;32(1):67-68.

26. Rayner HH. Injury of the rectum caused by the faulty administration of an enema. *Br Med J.* 1932;1(3713):419-436.4.

27. de Feiter PW, Soeters PB, Dejong CH. Rectal perforations after barium enema: a review. *Dis Colon Rectum.* 2006;49(2):261-271.

28. Barkley S, Khan M, Garner J. Rectal trauma in adults. *Trauma.* 2012;15(1):3-15.

29. Goldberg JE, Steele SR. Rectal foreign bodies. *Surg Clin North Am.* 2010;90(1):173-184, Table of Contents.

30. Causey MW, Rivadeneira DE, Steele SR. Historical and current trends in colon trauma. *Clin Colon Rectal Surg.* 2012;25(4):189-199.

31. Pruitt BA Jr. Combat casualty care and surgical progress. *Ann Surg.* 2006;243(6):715-729.

32. Conrad JK, Ferry KM, Foreman ML, Gogel BM, Fisher TL, Livingston SA. Changing management trends in penetrating colon trauma. *Dis Colon Rectum.* 2000;43(4):466-471.

33. Demetriades D, Murray JA, Chan L, et al. Penetrating colon injuries requiring resection: diversion or primary anastomosis? An AAST prospective multicenter study. *J Trauma.* 2001;50(5):765-775.

34. Biswas S, Adileh M, Almogy G, Bala M. Abdominal injury patterns in patients with seatbelt signs requiring laparotomy. *J Emerg Trauma Shock.* 2014;7(4):295-300.

35. Esposito TJ, Ingraham A, Luchette FA, et al. Reasons to omit digital rectal exam in trauma patients: no fingers, no rectum, no useful additional information. *J Trauma.* 2005;59(6):1314-1319.

36. Docimo S Jr, Diggs L, Crankshaw L, Lee Y, Vinces F. No evidence supporting the routine use of digital rectal examinations in trauma patients. *Indian J Surg.* 2015;77(4):265-269.

37. Hargraves MB, Magnotti LJ, Fischer PE, et al. Injury location dictates utility of digital rectal examination and rigid sigmoidoscopy in the evaluation of penetrating rectal trauma. *Am Surg.* 2009;75(11):1069-1072.

38. Wu K, Poslazny JAJ, Branch J, et al. Trauma to the pelvis: injuries to the rectum and genitourinary organs. *Curr Trauma Rep.* 2015;1:8-15.

39. Atri M, Hanson JM, Grinblat L, Brofman N, Chughtai T, Tomlinson G. Surgically important bowel and/or mesentery injury in blunt trauma: accuracy of multidetector CT for evaluation. *Radiology.* 2008;249(2):524-533.

40. Lozano JD, Munera F, Anderson SW, Soto JA, Menias CO, Caban EM. Penetrating wounds to the torso: evaluation with triple-contrast multidetector CT. *Radiographics.* 2013;33(2):341-359.

41. Shanmuganathan K, Mirvis SE, Chiu WC, Killeen KL, Hogan GJ, Scalea TM. Penetrating torso trauma: triple-contrast helical CT in peritoneal violation and organ injury—a prospective study in 200 patients. *Radiology.* 2004;231(3):775-784.

42. Saksobhavivat N, Shanmuganathan K, Boscak AR, et al. Diagnostic accuracy of triple-contrast multi-detector computed tomography for detection of penetrating gastrointestinal injury: a prospective study. *Eur Radiol.* 2016;26(11):4107-4120.

43. Mikhail J. The trauma triad of death: hypothermia, acidosis, and coagulopathy. *AACN Clin Issues.* 1999;10(1):85-94.

44. Georgoff P, Perales P, Laguna B, Holena D, Reilly P, Sims C. Colonic injuries and the damage control abdomen: does management strategy matter? *J Surg Res.* 2013;181(2):293-299.

45. Trust MD, Brown CVR. Penetrating injuries to the colon and rectum. *Curr Trauma Rep.* 2015;1:113-118

46. Ott MM, Norris PR, Diaz JJ, et al. Colon anastomosis after damage control laparotomy: recommendations from 174 trauma colectomies. *J Trauma.* 2011;70(3):595-602.

47. Burlew CC, Moore EE, Cuschieri J, et al. Sew it up! A Western Trauma Association multi-institutional study of enteric injury management in the postinjury open abdomen. *J Trauma.* 2011;70(2):273-277.

48. Open Abdomen Advisory Panel, Campbell A, Chang M, et al. Management of the open abdomen: from initial operation to definitive closure. *Am Surg.* 2009;75(11 suppl):S1-S22.

49. Burlew CC. The open abdomen: practical implications for the practicing surgeon. *Am J Surg.* 2012;204(6):826-835.

50. Anjaria DJ, Ullmann TM, Lavery R, Livingston DH. Management of colonic injuries in the setting of damage-control laparotomy: one shot to get it right. *J Trauma Acute Care Surg.* 2014;76(3):594-598, discussion 598-600.

51. Fischer PE, Nunn AM, Wormer BA, et al. Vasopressor use after initial damage control laparotomy increases risk for anastomotic disruption in the management of destructive colon injuries. *Am J Surg.* 2013;206(6):900-903.

52. Greer LT, Gillern SM, Vertrees AE. Evolving colon injury management: a review. *Am Surg.* 2013;79(2):119-127.

53. Cotton BA, Reddy N, Hatch QM, et al. Damage control resuscitation is associated with a reduction in resuscitation volumes and improvement in survival in 390 damage control laparotomy patients. *Ann Surg.* 2011;254(4):598-605.

54. Holcomb JB, Wade CE, Michalek JE, et al. Increased plasma and platelet to red blood cell ratios improves outcome in 466 massively transfused civilian trauma patients. *Ann Surg.* 2008;248(3):447-458.

55. Pohlman TH, Walsh M, Aversa J, Hutchison EM, Olsen KP, Lawrence Reed R. Damage control resuscitation. *Blood Rev.* 2015;29(4):251-262.

56. Holcomb JB, Jenkins D, Rhee P, et al. Damage control resuscitation: directly addressing the early coagulopathy of trauma. *J Trauma.* 2007;62(2):307-310.

57. U.S. Army Institute of Surgical Research. Damage control resuscitation at level IIb/III treatment facilities. 2013. http://www.usaisr.amedd.army.mil/cpgs/Damage%20Control%20Resuscitation%20-%201%20Feb%202013.pdf. Accessed 1 May 2016.

58. Hess JR, Holcomb JB, Hoyt DB. Damage control resuscitation: the need for specific blood products to treat the coagulopathy of trauma. *Transfusion.* 2006;46(5):685-686.

59. Goldberg SR, Anand RJ, Como J, et al. Prophylactic antibiotic use in penetrating abdominal trauma: an Eastern Association for the Surgery of Trauma practice management guideline. *J Trauma Acute Care Surg.* 2012;73(5).

60. Ay N, Alp V, Aliosmanoglu I, Sevuk U, Kaya S, Dinc B. Factors affecting morbidity and mortality in traumatic colorectal injuries and reliability and validity of trauma scoring systems. *World J Emerg Surg.* 2015;10:21.

61. Sharpe JP, Magnotti LJ, Weinberg JA, et al. Applicability of an established management algorithm for colon injuries following blunt trauma. *J Trauma Acute Care Surg.* 2013;74(2):419-424, discussion 424–425.

62. Deleted in review.

63. Hatch Q, Causey M, Martin M, et al. Outcomes after colon trauma in the 21st century: an analysis of the U.S. National Trauma Data Bank. *Surgery.* 2013;154(2):397-403.

64. Zafar SN, Onwugbufor MT, Hughes K, et al. Laparoscopic surgery for trauma: the realm of therapeutic management. *Am J Surg.* 2015;209(4):627-632.

65. O'Malley E, Boyle E, O'Callaghan A, Coffey C, Walsh SR. Role of laparoscopy in penetrating abdominal trauma: a systematic review. *World J Surg.* 2013;37(1):113-122.

66. Zantut LF, Ivatury RR, Smith RS, et al. Diagnostic and therapeutic laparoscopy for penetrating abdominal trauma: a multicenter experience. *J Trauma.* 1997;42(5):825-829, discussion 829–831.

67. Lin HF, Wu JM, Tu CC, Chen HA, Shih HC. Value of diagnostic and therapeutic laparoscopy for abdominal stab wounds. *World J Surg.* 2010;34(7):1653-1662.

68. Alemayehu H, Clifton M, Santore M, et al. Minimally invasive surgery for pediatric trauma: a multicenter review. *J Laparoendosc Adv Surg Tech A.* 2015;25(3):243-247.

69. Naumann DN, Bhangu A, Kelly M, Bowley DM. Stapled versus handsewn intestinal anastomosis in emergency laparotomy: a systemic review and meta-analysis. *Surgery.* 2015;157(4):609-618.

70. Bruns B, DuBose J, Galvagno SJ, Diaz J, Scalea TM. Stapled vs handsewn: a prospective emergency surgery study (SHAPES). http://www.aast.org/Assets/377916f0-6915-4243-9d63-1f5a78174b91/635158817785370000/aastshapes-pdf; Accessed 20 January 2016.

71. Wiggins T, Markar SR, Arya S, Hanna GB. Anastomotic reinforcement with omentoplasty following gastrointestinal anastomosis: a systematic review and meta-analysis. *Surg Oncol.* 2015;24(3):181-186.

72. Govender M, Madiba TE. Current management of large bowel injuries and factors influencing outcome. *Injury.* 2010;41(1):58-63.

73. Feliciano DV, Moore EE, Biffl WL. Western Trauma Association critical decisions in trauma: management of abdominal vascular trauma. *J Trauma Acute Care Surg.* 2015;79(6):1079-1088.

74. Ball CG, Kirkpatrick AW, Smith M, Mulloy RH, Tse L, Anderson IB. Traumatic injury of the superior mesenteric vein: ligate, repair or shunt? *Eur J Trauma Emerg Surg.* 2007;33(5):540-552.

75. Uotani K, Hamanaka A, Arase M, et al. Endovascular treatment of inferior mesenteric artery avulsion caused by blunt abdominal trauma. *J Vasc Interv Radiol.* 2016;27(1):150-152.

76. Perry WB. Trauma of the colon, rectum, and anus. In: Steele SR, Hull TL, Read TE, Saclarides TJ, Senagore AJ, Whitlow CB, eds. *The ASCRS Textbook of Colon and Rectal Surgery.* 3rd ed. Cham, Switzerland: Springer International Publishing; 2016:735-747.

77. McNevin MS. Overcoming technical challenges: the pelvis. In: Ross H, Lee S, Mutch MG, Rivadeneira DE, Steele S, eds. *Minimally Invasive Approaches to Colon and Rectal Disease: Technique and Best Practices.* New York: Springer Science + Business Media; 2015:213-220.

78. Ivatury RR, Licata J, Gunduz Y, Rao P, Stahl WM. Management options in penetrating rectal injuries. *Am Surg.* 1991;57(1):50-55.

79. Velmahos GC, Gomez H, Falabella A, Demetriades D. Operative management of civilian rectal gunshot wounds: simpler is better. *World J Surg.* 2000;24(1):114-118.

80. McGrath V, Fabian TC, Croce MA, Minard G, Pritchard FE. Rectal trauma: management based on anatomic distinctions. *Am Surg.* 1998;64(12):1136-1141.

81. Gonzalez RP, Phelan H 3rd, Hassan M, Ellis CN, Rodning CB. Is fecal diversion necessary for nondestructive penetrating extraperitoneal rectal injuries? *J Trauma.* 2006;61(4):815-819.

82. Bosarge PL, Como JJ, Fox N, et al. Management of penetrating extraperitoneal rectal injuries: an Eastern Association for the Surgery of Trauma practice management guideline. *J Trauma Acute Care Surg.* 2016;80(3):546-551.

83. Levine JH, Longo WE, Pruitt C, Mazuski JE, Shapiro MJ, Durham RM. Management of selected rectal injuries by primary repair. *Am J Surg.* 1996;172(5):575-578, discussion 578–579.

84. Gonzalez RP, Falimirski ME, Holevar MR. The role of presacral drainage in the management of penetrating rectal injuries. *J Trauma.* 1998;45(4):656-661.

85. Navsaria PH, Edu S, Nicol AJ. Civilian extraperitoneal rectal gunshot wounds: surgical management made simpler. *World J Surg.* 2007;31(6):1345-1351.

86. Franko ER, Ivatury RR, Schwalb DM. Combined penetrating rectal and genitourinary injuries: a challenge in management. *J Trauma.* 1993;34(3):347-353.

87. Fowler G. Risk factors for and management of obstetric anal sphincter injury. *Obstet Gynaecol Reprod Med.* 2010;20(8):229-234.

88. Cawich S, Bambury I, Mitchell D, Plummer J, Newnham M, Christie L. Is a diverting colostomy required after repair of obstetric ano-rectal injuries? *Internet J Third World Med.* 2007;6(2).

89. Kudsk KA, Hanna MK. Management of complex perineal injuries. *World J Surg.* 2003;27(8):895-900.

90. Brill SA, Margolin DA. Anal sphincter trauma. *Semin Colon Rectal Surg.* 2004;15(2):90-94.

91. Engel AF, Kamm MA, Hawley PR. Civilian and war injuries of the perineum and anal sphincters. *Br J Surg.* 1994;81(7):1069-1073.

92. Critchlow JF, Houlihan MJ, Landolt CC, Weinstein ME. Primary sphincter repair in anorectal trauma. *Dis Colon Rectum.* 1985;28(12):945-947.

93. Glasgow SC, Heafner TA, Watson JD, Aden JK, Perry WB. Initial management and outcome of modern battlefield anal trauma. *Dis Colon Rectum.* 2014;57(8):1012-1018.

94. Lake JP, Essani R, Petrone P, Kaiser AM, Asensio J, Beart RW Jr. Management of retained colorectal foreign bodies: predictors of operative intervention. *Dis Colon Rectum.* 2004;47(10):1694-1698.

95. Barone JE, Yee J, Nealon TF Jr. Management of foreign bodies and trauma of the rectum. *Surg Gynecol Obstet.* 1983;156(4):453-457.

96. Coskun A, Erkan N, Yakan S, Yildirim M, Cengiz F. Management of rectal foreign bodies. *World J Emerg Surg.* 2013;8(1):11.

Colonic Intussusception and Volvulus

Katerina Wells

COLONIC INTUSSUSCEPTION

PATHOPHYSIOLOGY

Colonic intussusception is a rare diagnosis in adults. This process occurs when a proximal segment of intestine (intussusceptum) invaginates into a distal segment of intestine (intussuscipiens) with 86% to 90% associated with a pathologic lesion as the lead point.[1] The exact mechanism of intussusception in adults is not completely understood. It is proposed that the presence of a stimulus in the lumen of the bowel induces constriction of the bowel proximal to the stimulus and relaxation of the bowel wall distally allowing for invagination of the proximal segment. Intussusception is categorized into two discrete categories: enteric in which solely the jejunum or ileum are involved, and colonic, which includes ileocolic, colocolonic, and colorectal configurations. Often, the stimulus responsible for intussusception in adults is a gastrointestinal (GI) neoplasm with 66% of colonic intussusceptions attributed to malignancy and approximately 19% of enteric intussusceptions related to malignancy. Benign causes include benign GI neoplasms, adhesive disease, Meckel diverticulum, sprue, human immunodeficiency virus (HIV), or idiopathic intussusception.[2]

PRESENTATION

Intussusception accounts for 1% of bowel obstructions and symptoms of complete obstruction occur in fewer than 20% of cases. Unlike the presenting classic triad of abdominal pain, palpable abdominal mass, and heme-positive stools described in the pediatric population, adult patients rarely present with signs of acute obstruction. The most common presenting symptoms are crampy abdominal pain (71%), nausea and emesis (68%), abdominal distention (45%), and tenderness (60%).[3] Most patients have a history of subacute partial obstruction or intermittent obstruction occurring over days to years.[4] For this reason, misdiagnosis is common, with a majority of cases diagnosed at the time of laparotomy.[1]

DIAGNOSIS

Plain Radiography

Plain radiographs can be helpful to identify cases of enteric intussusception without colonic involvement. Contrast studies subsequently delineate the site of intussusception. In cases of enteric intussusception, upper GI series will show a "stacked coin" or "coiled spring" appearance.

Barium Enema

Barium enema can subsequently be used to identify colonic obstruction, which will demonstrate a cup shaped filling defect representing the distal extent of the intussusceptum within the lumen of the colon.[1] It is important to note that hydrostatic pressure should not be used in adults as an attempt to reduce the intussusception due to the risk of underlying malignancy and risk of perforation. Barium studies are contraindicated if there is concern for bowel perforation or ischemia.[5]

Computed Tomography

Computed tomography (CT) scan is the most accurate imaging modality for the diagnosis of intussusception and is often the imaging of choice for patients who present with the nonspecific symptoms of intussusception including obstruction or palpable abdominal mass. Characteristic findings on CT include a "target sign" in which the intussusceptum and associated mesentery is seen within the lumen of the intussuscipiens in axial view.[5] This "bowel-within-bowel" configuration where mesenteric vessels can be seen compressed between the walls of the small bowel is pathognomonic for intussusception (Fig. 155.1).[3]

Ultrasound is a readily available noninvasive method of evaluation that is typically used in diagnosis of pediatric intussusception. Ultrasound has less accuracy for the diagnosis of intussusception in adults but can identify characteristic findings including the "target" and "donut" sign when evaluating the intussusception in transverse view. The "pseudo-kidney" sign is seen when evaluating the intussusception longitudinally. The quality of ultrasound imaging may be variable depending on the experience of the operator, the body habitus of the patient, and the presence of bowel gas that may obscure underlying structures.[5]

Endoscopy

Flexible sigmoidoscopy or colonoscopy can be used in the case of subacute or chronic colonic obstruction as a means of diagnosis of a suspected colonic malignancy. In cases of chronic tissue ischemia or necrosis, biopsy or polypectomy is not recommended.

TREATMENT

Surgery is the primary treatment for adult intussusception. There is no role for nonoperative or endoscopic management given the high likelihood of malignancy as the underlying cause, especially so in patients over the age of 60.[5] Resection allows for removal of a potentially malignant lesion and prevents recurrence of intussusception. Resection should proceed as a formal oncologic resection including lymphadenectomy of the affected small bowel or colon segment.[5]

For this reason, reduction of colonic intussusception is discouraged. Care should be taken to avoid trauma to the already compromised bowel wall and prevent

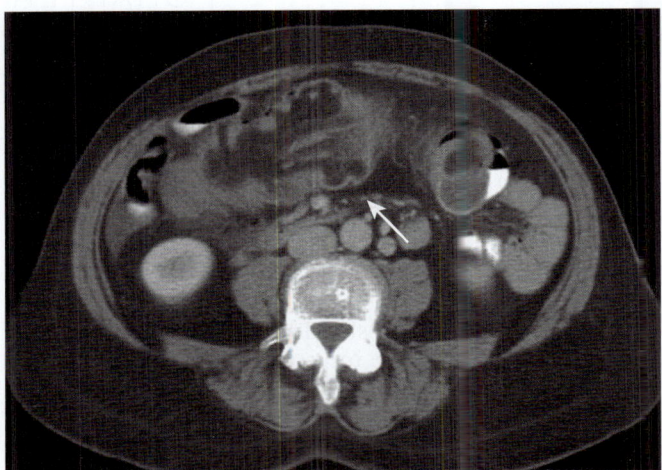

FIGURE 155.1 Intussusception on CT imaging. Axial view of intussusception, demonstrating a "bowel-within-bowel" configuration where mesenteric vessels can be seen compressed between the walls of the bowel.

perforation with seeding of the peritoneal cavity. Often the intussuscepted bowel is inflamed, edematous, or ischemic, which increases the risk of perforation. Enteric intussusception has a lower associated malignancy rate of 19% but has been reported to be up to 47% in some case series. Although some reports advocate for reduction in the setting of enteric intussusception, others recommend that reduction should be avoided unless benign etiology is confirmed or radical resection would render the patient at risk for short gut syndrome.[1,4] In cases of postoperative or adhesion related intussuception, the intussusception can be reduced as benign etiology is assumed.[2]

VOLVULUS

Colonic volvulus represents 1.9% of cases of large bowel obstruction in the United States and up to 10% to 50% of cases in Africa, the Middle East, and South America.[6,7] Volvulus occurs when a segment of colon undergoes torsion along its own mesentery (mesenterioaxial) resulting in obstruction. Torsion of 180 degrees results in clinical obstruction, and further torsion to 360 degrees causes strangulation with venous gangrene, ischemia, and eventual perforation. As the volvulized segment enlarges, it becomes trapped in the confines of the abdominal wall and is unable to spontaneously detorse. Perforation occurs in areas of necrosis at the point of torsion, within the closed loop, or in the proximal thin-walled cecum.[8]

Segments of colon that are redundant with an elongated mesentery and narrow base are more likely to undergo torsion; for this reason, the sigmoid, cecum, and the transverse colon are most commonly susceptible to volvulus

SIGMOID VOLVULUS

Pathophysiology

In both subtypes, acquired changes to the sigmoid colon and mesocolon result in lengthening of colon between two relatively close points of mesenteric fixation: the distal descending mesocolon and the mesorectum at the rectosigmoid junction.[13] In anatomic studies, Bhatnagar et al. describes the "dolichomesocolic colon," one that is vertically longer than it is wide. This anatomic configuration is more commonly found in male subjects and people over the age of 30.[14] The incidence of sigmoid volvulus peaks in the mid-70s for both men and women suggesting that this process is secondary to chronic changes. Other theories support congenital configurations that predispose to volvulus owing to its relative frequency within certain tribes and its propensity for the male gender.[15] Ultimately the exact reason for why this anatomic configuration occurs is not completely understood and may be multifactorial.

Sigmoid volvulus is also the most common cause of intestinal obstruction in pregnancy, accounting for 45% of obstructions in this group.[16] The vague presenting symptoms of sigmoid volvulus contribute to a higher rate of misdiagnosis with maternal mortality reported at 5% but up to 50% in the setting of perforation. Fetal demise approaches 30% and is secondary to reduction in placental blood flow due to mass effect from a massively dilated sigmoid.[17] Other conditions that predispose to sigmoid volvulus include postoperative adhesions and megacolon, in particular Hirschsprung disease, due to massive dilation of the colon.[18,19]

Presentation

Sigmoid volvulus is the most common form of colonic volvulus accounting for 50% to 90% of all cases of colonic volvulus.[9] Presentation of sigmoid volvulus varies by geographic region, and two distinct subtypes are described. In the United States and other westernized nations, sigmoid volvulus is uncommon, accounting for less than 5% of acute obstructions. Patients tend to be elderly, diabetic, institutionalized, and/or on psychoactive medications. In this subtype, chronic fecal loading from constipation lengthens the sigmoid colon predisposing to torsion.[10] In regions of Africa, India, the Middle East, and Latin America, the endemic subtype of sigmoid volvulus more commonly causes acute colonic obstruction with the majority of patients being young and 80% of them male.[11] It is theorized that chronic fecal loading by the high fiber diet common to these areas contributes to stretching of the sigmoid colon and lengthening along its mesentery. This theory is supported by the fact that the incidence of volvulus in these areas is decreasing as westernization in diet or migration shifts occur.[12]

Diagnosis

In the Western world, sigmoid volvulus typically presents in a delayed fashion with a mean interval between onset and presentation of 3 to 4 days. This is in part due to the comorbidities of senility or mental illness that accompany the diagnosis. Chronic constipation subtly progresses to obstipation and abdominal distention. Obstruction may be incomplete with paradoxical diarrhea. Abdominal pain is usually less severe owing to the subacuity with which the sigmoid becomes distended.[20] In younger patients and the endemic subtype, sigmoid volvulus presents as acute obstruction with abdominal pain, distention, and

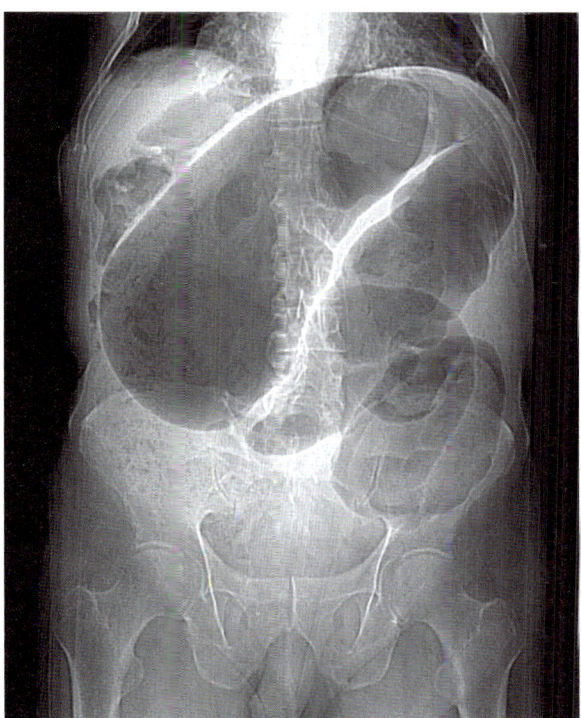

FIGURE 155.2 Plain radiograph of sigmoid volvulus demonstrating the "coffee bean" sign or omega loop.

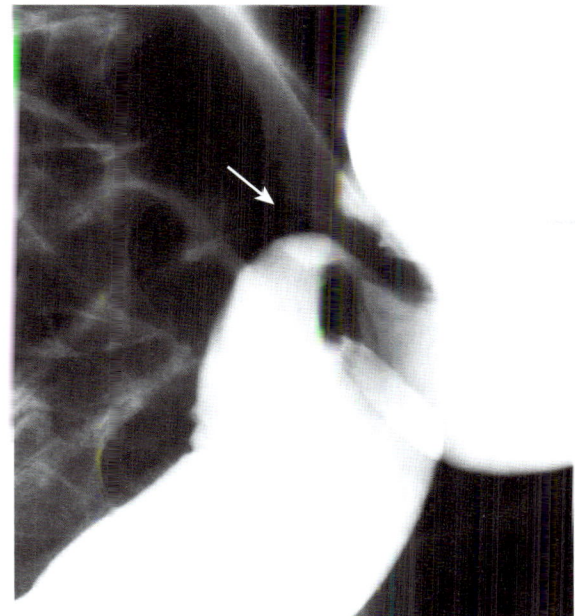

FIGURE 155.3 Contrast enema of sigmoid volvulus demonstrating the "bird's beak" sign and the point of obstruction.

obstipation with acute abdomen on examination. This is often in the setting of previous less severe episodes.

Plain Radiography. Plain radiography can be sufficient for diagnosis. The most common finding is the absence of bowel gas in the left iliac fossa due to the rotation on the sigmoid away from the left iliac fossa. The "coffee bean" sign or "omega loop" with the apex pointing to the right upper abdomen is present in 60% of cases (Fig. 155.2).[21]

Barium Enema. Lower GI contrast radiography reveals a "bird's beak" appearance representing the point of torsion and obstruction. The presence of a "bird's beak" sign in combination with characteristic findings on plain radiography carries a diagnostic accuracy of 100% (Fig. 155.3). Contrast radiography may also be therapeutic with temporary reduction of volvulus.

Computed Tomography. CT has diagnostic accuracy approaching 100% with the presence of a mesenteric twist being highly accurate for the diagnosis of volvulus. The finding of a sigmoid transition point is the most sensitive finding. The "X-marks-the-spot" sign and the "split wall" sign are also suggestive of sigmoid volvulus and represent a complete twist of adjacent sigmoid loops in a "twist-tie" configuration. These findings, though diagnostic, are seen in less than 50% of cases. Radiographic evidence of ischemia correlates poorly with clinical ischemia and clinical suspicion should supersede CT findings in the evaluation of ischemia.[21]

Treatment

Nonoperative Therapy: Endoscopic Decompression. Nonsurgical methods should not be considered definitive treatment and are contraindicated when ischemia or perforation is suspected. In the stable patient without clinical evidence of ischemia, endoscopic reduction should be attempted. Endoscopy is successful in achieving decompression of sigmoid volvulus in 60% to 90% of cases.[22] Rigid sigmoidoscopy can be performed at bedside with minimal insufflation. Insertion of the sigmoidoscope allows for visual inspection of the colonic mucosa for ischemia or the presence of an intraluminal lesion. Gentle passage through the point of torsion can allow for decompression of the proximal sigmoid and placement of a rectal tube, typically a 35-French catheter. Plain radiography should be obtained following placement of the rectal tube to confirm detorsion by decompression of the proximal colon. This catheter can maintain decompression for several days in anticipation of definitive intervention. Flexible endoscopy can similarly be used to visualize the colonic mucosa. A flexible guidewire can be inserted across the point of torsion and a rectal tube can be passed over the guidewire for colonic decompression. The time before the operation can be used to obtain screening colonoscopy and reduction of the fecal load in the proximal colon.

Recurrence following colonoscopic decompression is high, approaching 71%, and the mortality rate for recurrent sigmoid volvulus is reported to be up to 36%.[23] The interval of time between recurrent episodes of sigmoid volvulus ranges from 2 to 35 months supporting the need for expeditious operative planning.[24] Endoscopic decompression offers time during which the patient can be optimized for surgery and a colonic preparation given. Surgery should then proceed in a semielective manner during the index hospitalization. When colonoscopic decompression is unsuccessful or repeated attempts are required to maintain detorsion, urgent surgical resection is indicated.

Operative Therapy. Over the years, both resective and nonresective operative procedures have been employed in the management of sigmoid volvulus. Often, the surgeon encounters a chronically diseased sigmoid colon with loss of taenia coli, absent epiploic appendages, and a thickened and fibrotic mesentery not worth salvage. Currently, resection is the treatment of choice with 89% of patients treated with this approach. In 16% of cases, subtotal or total colectomy is required if cecal necrosis, megacolon, or colonic atony are encountered.[25,26] Stomas are still performed in approximately 50% of cases; however, resection with primary anastomosis can also be performed safely with good clinical judgment.[27] A diverting loop ileostomy should be considered over a loop colostomy because of ease of care and eventual closure.

Nonresective methods of surgical management are less commonly employed and include detorsion with or without fixation, which carries a recurrence rate of 9% to 44% with an associated mortality of 7.8%. Sigmoidopexy is associated with lower mortality rates. Sigmoidostomy is described for historical purposes and is discouraged given the high rates of recurrence and morbidity. This procedure was typically considered in only the sickest nonfunctional patients and carries a 13% mortality rate.[28] Overall mortality among patients with sigmoid volvulus is 9.4%. The presence of diffuse, feculent peritonitis, and gangrene are the highest predictors of mortality. In these cases, an end sigmoid colostomy and Hartmann stump of the rectum may be the best and safest choice. Postoperative complications such as respiratory, renal, infectious, and thromboembolic disease remain high in this population, given the attendant comorbidities.[12]

Laparoscopy has increasing application for the management of volvulus in the modern era and can be considered in younger patients with lower comorbidity scores and low expected associated mortality rates. Ideally, the abdomen is approached laparoscopically following an adequate period of endoscopic decompression whereby the dilated sigmoid colon has decreased in size, allowing for adequate working space within the insufflated abdomen. The use of laparoscopy over open surgery is not a predictor of mortality.[12]

CECAL VOLVULUS
Pathophysiology

Cecal volvulus accounts for 25% to 40% of all cases of volvulus in the United States and 1% to 1.5% of all intestinal obstructions.[29] Incomplete congenital fixation results in cecal mobility and can predispose to volvulus. Hypermobility of the cecum is congenital and occurs at the time of intestinal rotation when the cecum enters the abdominal cavity in a counterclockwise fashion to its final location in the right lower quadrant. In normal embryologic development, the right mesocolon becomes fixed to the retroperitoneum along the right paracolic gutter.[30] Congenital mobility of the cecum is not independently responsible for cecal volvulus, as this degree of mobility is common and is seen at autopsy in 11% of people.[31]

Cecal bascule is a similar condition in which the cecum folds cephalad resulting in a "flap-valve" obstruction. Outflow from the cecum is obstructed by the "flap valve"

and the cecum serves as a closed loop in the setting of a competent ileocecal valve and causes a "secondary" small bowel obstruction. Unlike cecal volvulus, the associated mesentery does not undergo torsion and ischemia is less likely, although it has been described in the dilated wall of the cecum.[32]

Presentation

Cecal volvulus affects a younger cohort compared to sigmoid volvulus, has a female predilection, and has been found to have a growing incidence of cases by 5.53% per year for the National Inpatient Sample (NIS). The incidence of cecal volvulus is biphasic: mid-40s and again in the late 70s.[12] Predisposing factors for cecal volvulus are similar to those of sigmoid volvulus including a history of chronic constipation with chronic use of cathartics, distal colonic obstruction, and psychiatric illness. A history of previous abdominal surgery is common in 30% to 70% of patients who present with cecal volvulus. It is postulated that postoperative adhesions serve as a lead point around which the cecum can then volvulize.[29] There is an association with pregnancy by which the gravid uterus displaces the cecum and stretches the ileocolic mesentery, making it more prone to torsion during or soon after delivery.[33]

The most proximal point of obstruction in cecal volvulus is the terminal ileum. Therefore presenting symptoms of cecal volvulus are consistent with those of small bowel obstruction. Onset is acute and common symptoms include abdominal pain, emesis, abdominal distention, and may progress to peritonitis in the setting of ischemia.[29] A prior history of chronic intermittent abdominal pain that is relieved with the passage of flatus can be elicited in 50% of patients who present with acute cecal volvulus. This clinical presentation is termed "mobile cecum syndrome."[30]

Diagnosis

Plain Radiography. Abdominal radiography is often the first imaging modality used for diagnosis. Characteristic findings include that of a massively dilated cecum, resembling a "kidney-bean" under the left diaphragm (Fig. 155.4). Paucity of bowel gas in the right lower quadrant correlates with deviation of the dilated cecum away from its lateral attachments. Proximal small bowel is dilated with air-fluid levels consistent with obstruction. In the case of a cecal bascule, the dilated cecum usually overlies the midabdomen or the pelvis.[32]

Barium Enema. Barium enema can identify characteristic beaking of the ascending colon. Contrast enemas are often useful in establishing this diagnosis as well as excluding any distal obstructing colon lesions as an underlying cause of cecal dilation and volvulus. Reduction using hydrostatic pressure enema is contraindicated, as these are rarely successful and carry the risk of perforation.

Computed Tomography. Characteristic findings of cecal volvulus on CT include the "whirl sign," which corresponds to torsion of engorged mesenteric vessels (Fig. 155.5). Beaking of the cecal margins with obstruction of the upstream ileum is commonly seen. In the case of cecal bascule, the folded and dilated cecum is central in the midabdomen, and a "whirl sign" is not present.[34] CT is also helpful in characterizing vascular insufficiency of the

arteriovenous communications. Greater than 90% of patients have spontaneous resolution of bleeding. Approximately 15% of patients present with massive hemorrhage.[14] Although the risks of bleeding are not well defined the number of lesions and presence of coagulopathy or bleeding disorders may predispose to bleeding episodes.

Other

Other causes of colonic bleeding include inflammatory bowel disease, infectious colitis, postpolypectomy bleeding, and ischemic colitis. A careful history will help guide the diagnostic work-up for these etiologies. Severe abdominal pain and bloody diarrhea raises suspicion for inflammatory bowel disease or infectious colitis in a young patient. A similar presentation in an older patient, especially with comorbid cardiovascular disease, would be more consistent with ischemic colitis. Ischemic colitis is the underlying etiology in approximately 7% of patients hospitalized for lower GI bleeding, and will be discussed at the end of the chapter. A history of recent colonoscopy and lower GI

BOX 156.1 Vascular Lesions of the Colon

Vascular ectasia
Hemangioma
Congenital arteriovenous malformation
Colonic varices
Telangiectasia
Syndrome-related lesions (e.g., Klippel-Trénaunay-Weber syndrome, Maffucci syndrome)
Others
   Vascular spiders and venous stars of liver disease
   Degenerative phlebectasia of older adults
   Vasculitic lesions
   Focal hypervascularity of ulcerative, Crohn, and ischemic colitis
   Neovascularity of radiation colitis
   Angiosarcoma (e.g., Kaposi sarcoma)

---

bleeding suggests postpolypectomy bleeding. Postpolypectomy bleeding occurs in 8.7 per 1000 procedures and accounts for between 2% and 8% of acute lower GI bleeding.[15]

DIAGNOSIS OF LOWER GASTROINTESTINAL BLEEDING

The diagnostic approach used in patients with evidence of lower GI bleeding varies with age, presence or absence of active bleeding, and the severity of hemodynamic compromise. All patients with lower GI bleeding require a physical examination, including a digital rectal exam. Laboratory testing is performed to evaluate the level of anemia and rule out coagulopathy. In addition, medications should be reviewed looking for nonsteroidal antiinflammatory drug (NSAID), antiplatelet, or anticoagulant use. Further evaluation is dependent on the rate of blood loss. To provide a framework for the diagnosis and treatment of lower GI bleeding based on bleeding severity, the American Society for Gastrointestinal Endoscopy (ASGE) classifies bleeding as occult bleeding, melena, scant intermittent hematochezia, and severe (Fig. 156.1).[3]

Occult Gastrointestinal Bleeding

GI bleeding is defined as occult when there is no evidence of gross bleeding. Rather, the patient presents with heme-positive stool or as iron deficiency anemia suspected to be caused by GI blood loss. Patients with occult GI bleeding should undergo colonoscopy to evaluate for colorectal neoplasia. Patients with negative colonoscopy and upper GI symptoms, iron deficiency anemia, or NSAID use should be further evaluated by upper endoscopy. Evaluation of the small bowel may be necessary in patients with continued occult bleeding after negative upper and lower endoscopy.

Melena

Melena is defined as passage of dark, black, or tarry stools. Patients with melena should first be evaluated by upper endoscopy because the majority will have an upper GI source of bleeding. A negative upper endoscopy should

---

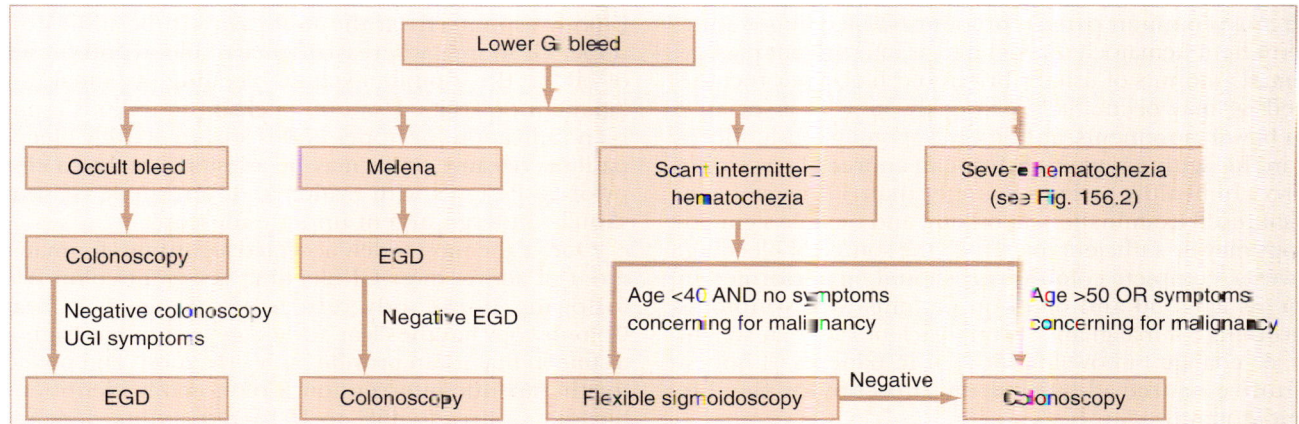

FIGURE 156.1 Diagnostic algorithm for lower gastrointestinal bleeding. *EGD,* Esophagogastroduodenoscopy; *UGI,* upper gastrointestinal. (Modified from Standards of Practice Committee of the American Society for Gastrointestinal Endoscopy. The role of endoscopy in the patient with lower GI bleeding. *Gastrointest Endosc.* 2014;79:875–885.)

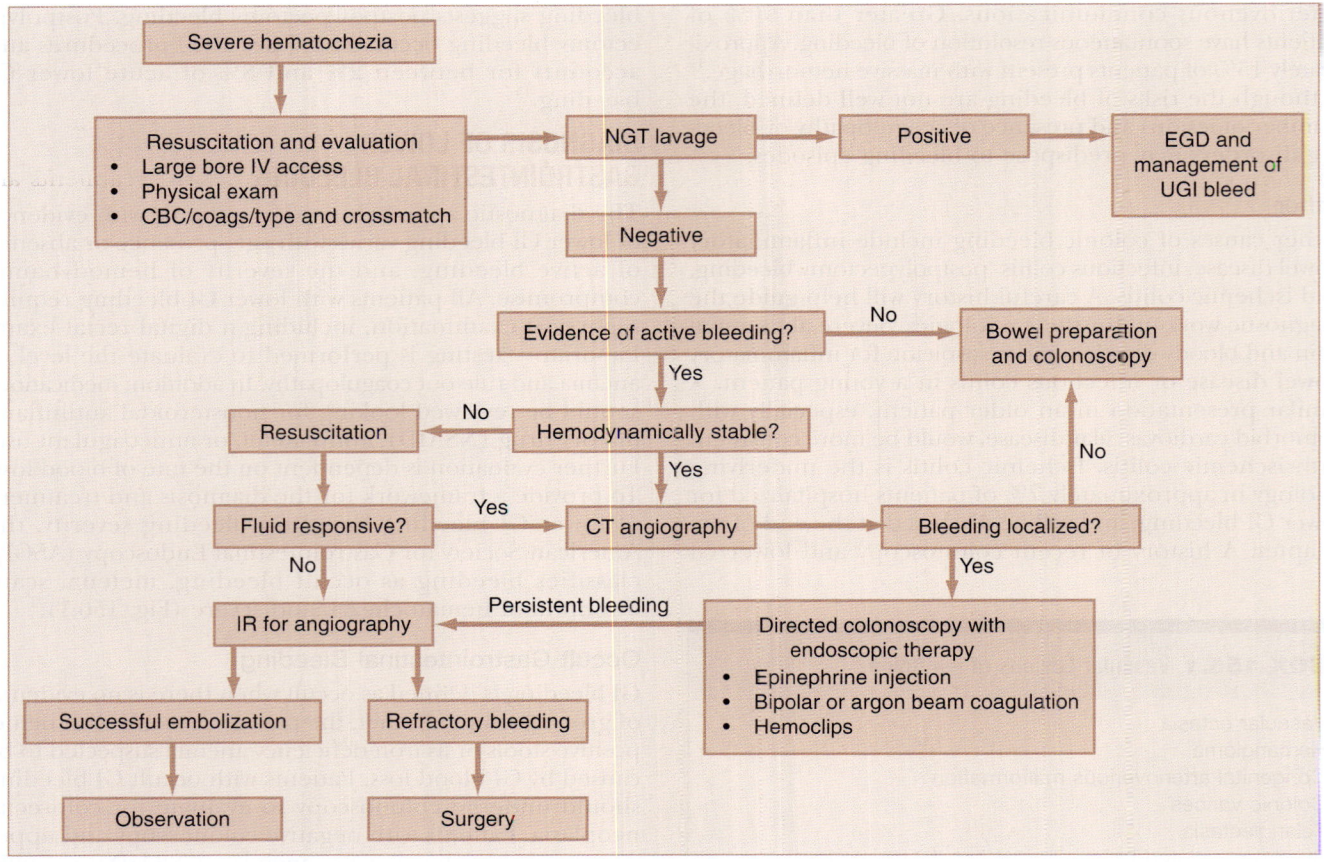

FIGURE 156.2 Treatment algorithm for severe hematochezia. *CT,* Computed tomography; *EGD,* esophagogastroduodenoscopy; *IR,* interventional radiology; *IV,* intravenous; *NGT,* nasogastric tube; *UGI,* upper gastrointestinal. (Modified from Standards of Practice Committee of the American Society for Gastrointestinal Endoscopy. The role of endoscopy in the patient with lower GI bleeding. *Gastrointest Endosc.* 2014;79:875–885.)

be followed by colonoscopy to evaluate for a colonic source. Evaluation of the small bowel may be necessary in patients with continued melena after negative upper and lower endoscopy.

Scant Intermittent Hematochezia

The most common pattern of lower GI bleeding is scant intermittent hematochezia, defined as intermittent passage of small amounts of usually bright red blood per rectum. Bleeding may occur daily or weekly, may be associated with bowel movements, and resolves spontaneously. Bleeding in this setting is typically from an anorectal or colonic source. In healthy patients younger than 40 years of age, digital rectal examination, anoscopy, and flexible sigmoidoscopy may be sufficient to identify the source of bleeding. However, complete colonoscopy should be performed in patients aged 50 and older, in patients with symptoms concerning for malignancy (iron deficiency anemia, weight loss, or change in bowel habits), or in patients without a definitive source identified on anoscopy or flexible sigmoidoscopy.

Severe Hematochezia

Severe hematochezia is defined as large-volume bright red blood per rectum. Patients with evidence of active bleeding require prompt resuscitation and hemodynamic stabilization with crystalloid intravenous (IV) fluids, blood products, and correction of coagulopathy. This should be followed by maneuvers aimed at the diagnosis and treatment of the causative lesion (Fig. 156.2). A nasogastric tube should be inserted to exclude an upper GI etiology. Bloody aspirate from the nasogastric tube indicates an upper GI source, whereas absence of blood and presence of bile in the aspirate exclude bleeding proximal to the ligament of Treitz. However, a clear, nonbilious aspirate is an indication for upper endoscopy in actively bleeding patients because there may be a lesion distal to a closed pylorus. Patients with evidence of an upper GI source should undergo urgent upper endoscopy.

One of the most widely accepted algorithms for management of active lower GI bleeding is urgent colonoscopy following nonbloody return on nasogastric lavage. Colonoscopy has the clear advantage over other diagnostic testing in that it can provide both a diagnosis and potential for therapeutic intervention. Colonoscopy identifies the bleeding source in 45% to 100% of patients, depending on the series.[16] However, the optimal timing of colonoscopy remains controversial in the literature. Most authors agree that early colonoscopy (within 8 to 24 hours of presentation) is likely to provide the most benefit in terms of enhanced diagnostic yield and therapeutic success. In addition, early colonoscopy is associated with shorter length of hospital stay and decreased hospital costs as compared with delayed (>24 hours after presentation) colonoscopy.[17] Prior to colonoscopy, colon preparation is imperative to allow for adequate visualization of the bleeding source.

It should be noted that the patient must be hemodynamically stable to undergo endoscopy. Hemodynamically unstable patients or patients with persistent bleeding despite endoscopic intervention may be better served by mesenteric angiography, with or without a preceding diagnostic radiologic study.

Scintigraphy is a noninvasive nuclear medicine study capable of identifying bleeding over a 24-hour period.[18] However, it cannot anatomically localize a bleed (i.e., distinguish between retroperitoneum, duodenum, or colon) and is unable to treat identified lesions. The radionuclide commonly used to detect intestinal bleeding is technetium 99m (^{99m}Tc)-labeled red blood cells (RBCs). ^{99m}Tc-RBCs can reliably detect active bleeding even at rates below 0.1 mL/min,[19] and serial studies can be obtained for up to 36 hours after a single injection of the radionuclide, thus detecting lesions that bleed intermittently. However, with the increasing availability, speed, and sensitivity of computed tomography angiography (CTA), the utility of scintigraphy in the acutely bleeding patient is declining.

Multidetector contrast-enhanced CTA is increasingly being used as a diagnostic tool for the active lower GI bleeding. CTA is available in most hospitals and may be rapidly performed in the emergency department. In addition, CTA can determine whether a patient is actively bleeding and identify the anatomic source, thus guiding therapeutic interventions, such as directed colonoscopy, angiographic embolization, or surgery. CTA is capable of reliably detecting GI bleeding rates of 0.5 mL/min.[20] Chua and Ridley pooled data from eight studies conducted between 1997 and 2007 comparing CT scan with other diagnostic imaging for identification of lower GI bleeding source. The authors estimated a pooled sensitivity of 86% and specificity of 95%.[21] CTA also provides information regarding etiology of the bleed, such as diverticula, tumors, or vascular ectasias. Limitations of CTA include ability to identify only active bleeding, lack of therapeutic capability, and risks of contrast allergy or contrast-induced nephropathy. The utility of CTA in the diagnosis of lower GI bleeding may be maximized by incorporation of CTA into an early branch point of a diagnostic algorithm.[22] In such an algorithm, hemodynamically stable patients with active bleeding in whom an upper GI source has been excluded would undergo CTA. A "positive" CTA reveals the location and possible etiology of lower GI bleeding, leading to a better selection of the most appropriate therapeutic step (angiography, expedited colonoscopy, or surgery). However, a "negative" CTA suggests that the bleeding may be self-limited, allowing for thorough bowel preparation prior to colonoscopy.

ENDOSCOPIC TREATMENT OF ACUTE HEMORRHAGE

In patients in whom colonoscopy has been successful and an actively bleeding lesion or fresh mucosal thrombus

(i.e., a sentinel clot) has been identified, endoscopic ablation is an effective mode of therapy. The approach of endoscopic treatment depends on the endoscopist, the location of the lesion, and the size of the lesion. It is important to recognize that the right colon is thin walled and more prone to perforation than other areas of the colon. Although a variety of endoscopic treatments are available, injection of the lesion with epinephrine solution combined with either heater probe coagulation or endoscopic clip placement is the treatment of choice for actively bleeding vascular lesions.

Other methods of endoscopic treatment include bands, injectable agents, and other forms of electrocoagulation. Although banding is more useful in gastric or small bowel lesions and not as common for colonic lesions, reports have described use selectively for the management of colonic vascular lesions.[23] Injection of sclerosing agents and argon plasma coagulation are reportedly safe and successful modalities used to treat vascular lesions of the colon.[24,25] Submucosal saline injections may prevent perforation by lifting the lesion. However, perforations can happen, with an occurrence of approximately 2% of patients treated with endoscopic coagulation.[26] A tattoo should be placed adjacent to the bleeding source when identified during colonoscopy. In the event of recurrent bleeding, tattooing facilitates identification of the bleeding site during repeat endoscopic or surgical intervention.

ANGIOGRAPHIC TREATMENT OF ACUTE HEMORRHAGE

Mesenteric angiography should be considered following unsuccessful endoscopy or in the setting of rapid ongoing bleeding. In the majority of cases, active bleeding can be at least temporarily stopped by the transcatheter infusion of vasopressin.

A selective superior mesenteric angiogram is the initial study performed because 50% to 80% of all lower GI bleeding occurs in the vascular arcade perfused by the superior mesenteric artery (SMA). Selective inferior mesenteric artery (IMA) and celiac axis (CA) studies are performed in that order if the initial superior mesenteric arteriogram does not identify the lesion. Injection of intraarterial vasopressin or selective embolization with coils, gels, or cellulose materials may be performed to obtain hemostasis in the setting of active extravasation. The likelihood of achieving successful angiographic control of hemorrhage ranges in the literature from 40% to 78%. Given the necessity for the administration of contrast, arterial access puncture, and use of the vasoconstrictor vasopressin and embolizing material, complications including renal toxicity, arterial injury, and ischemia result in a higher complication rate for angiography compared with endoscopy. This supports the algorithm for endoscopic attempts prior to angiography.[27,28]

SURGICAL TREATMENT OF ACUTE HEMORRHAGE

In patients with significant bleeding that cannot be controlled with endoscopy or angiography, operative intervention is warranted. Indications for operative intervention include hemodynamic instability, ongoing transfusion requirements, and persistent hemorrhage not responsive to other methods of treatment. Ideally, the bleeding site is preoperatively localized prior to operative intervention, thus enabling a directed segmental resection of involved bowel. As previously mentioned, localization involves either endoscopic tattooing or angiographic identification of the bleeding source. For sources of bleeding not able to be preoperatively localized, intraoperative endoscopy may be used in an attempt to identify the source. If a source is still not identified with intraoperative endoscopy, subtotal colectomy is recommended. However, in this situation there remains a small chance that the patient may continue to bleed from an unrecognized small bowel source.

COLONIC ISCHEMIA

Before 1950 colonic ischemia was considered synonymous with colonic infarction or gangrene. Since that time, colonic ischemia has become recognized as one of the more common disorders of the colon in older persons and the most common form of ischemic injury of the GI tract. Colonic ischemia is defined as hypoperfusion of the colon, whereas mesenteric ischemia refers to hypoperfusion of the small intestine. Intestinal hypoperfusion may be due to occlusive or nonocclusive obstruction of the arterial blood supply or obstruction of venous outflow. Colonic ischemia is categorized as either reversible or irreversible injury (Fig. 156.3). Reversible forms of colonic ischemia include colopathy, defined as submucosal or intramucosal hemorrhage, and colitis, where the mucosal surface develops ulcerations. Ulcerations may require several months to completely resolve, although the patient is usually asymptomatic during this time. Irreversible forms of colonic ischemia include chronic ischemic colitis, colonic gangrene, fulminant pancolitis, and stricture formation.

COLONIC CIRCULATION

The colon is normally protected from ischemia by its abundant collateral circulation. Communications between the celiac artery, SMA, IMA, and iliac artery beds are numerous. Collateral flow around small arterial branches is made possible by the multiple arcades within the bowel mesentery, and SMA or IMA occlusions are bypassed via the arch of Riolan, the central anastomotic artery, and the marginal artery of Drummond. In addition, a network of communicating submucosal vessels exists within the bowel wall, and this network maintains the viability of short segments of the colon if the extramural arterial supply is compromised.

PATHOPHYSIOLOGY OF COLONIC ISCHEMIA

What ultimately triggers the episode of colonic ischemia remains conjectural in most instances. Whether it is increased demand by colonic tissue superimposed on already marginal blood flow or whether the flow itself is acutely diminished has not been determined. Colonic ischemia tends to be a disease of older adults and may therefore result from degenerative changes in the mesenteric vasculature. Autopsy studies demonstrate abnormal musculature in the wall of the superior rectal artery in the older adult population, suggesting an age-related alteration in the mesenteric vasculature.[29] In addition, postmortem angiographic studies reveal age-related tortuosity of the longer colonic arteries, which may cause increased resistance to colonic blood flow, thus predisposing the patient to ischemia.[30]

Despite this suggestive evidence for a vascular or autonomic cause of colonic ischemia, most cases have no identifiable cause. These spontaneous episodes are thought to be the result of local nonocclusive ischemia (i.e., a low flow state) in association with small vessel disease. Occlusive ischemia secondary to thromboembolic disease is less often the cause of colonic ischemia.

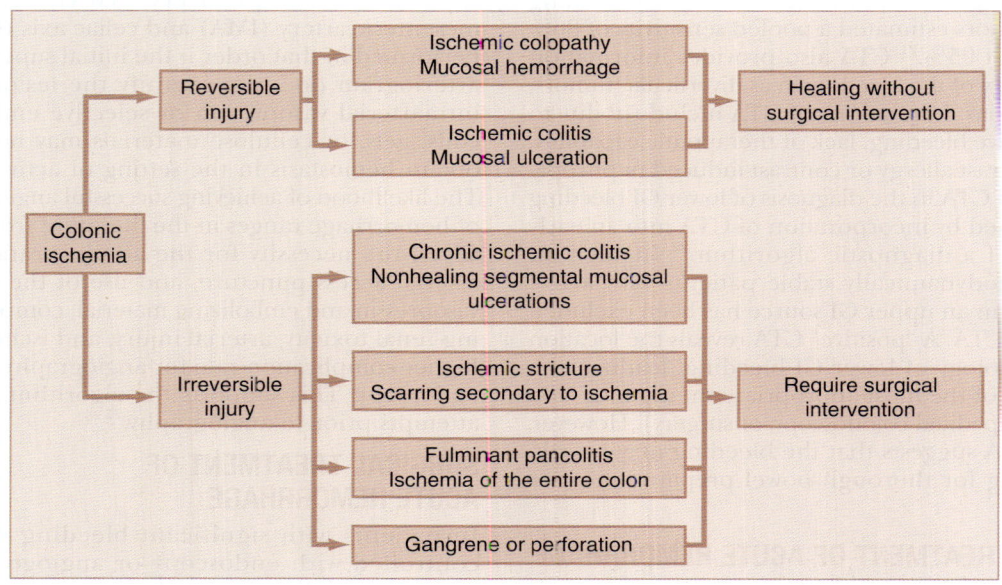

FIGURE 156.3 End results of colonic ischemia.

DEMOGRAPHICS

The diagnosis of colonic ischemia is usually made after the period of ischemia has passed and blood flow to the affected segment of colon has returned to normal. Many cases of transient or reversible ischemia are probably missed because the condition resolves before medical attention is sought or because diagnostic testing is not performed early in the course of the disease.

The published incidence of colonic ischemia ranges between 7.2 and 17.7 cases per 100,000 person-years. Colonic ischemia is more common in women, and published series report 57% to 76% of patients as female. Mortality ranges from 4% to 12%.[31,32] Many conditions, spontaneous or iatrogenic, have been associated with colonic ischemia. (Box 156.2). The most common medical comorbidities associated with colonic ischemia include cardiovascular disease, diabetes mellitus, chronic kidney disease, and chronic obstructive pulmonary disease. Irritable bowel syndrome and constipation may also increase the risk of developing colonic ischemia. Colonic ischemia is a known postoperative complication of procedures requiring ligation or exclusion of the IMA, such as aortic surgery for the treatment of aneurysmal disease and colonic resection for carcinoma.

Although most common in older adults, colonic ischemia can occur across all age groups.[33] Causes in the younger population include vasculitis (especially systemic lupus erythematosus),[34] medications (estrogens, danazol,[35]

BOX 156.2 Causes of Colonic Ischemia

Inferior mesenteric artery thrombosis
Arterial embolus
Cholesterol emboli
Cardiac failure or arrhythmias
Shock
Digitalis toxicity
Volvulus
Periarteritis nodosa
Systemic lupus erythematosus
Rheumatoid arthritis
Necrotizing arteritis
Thromboangiitis obliterans
Strangulated hernia
Drug induced (e.g., oral contraceptives, cocaine)
Polycythemia vera
Parasitic infestation
Allergy
Trauma—blunt and penetrating
Ruptured ectopic pregnancy
Iatrogenic causes
  Aneurysmectomy
  Aortoiliac reconstruction
  Gynecologic operations
  Exchange transfusions
  Colon bypass
  Lumbar aortography
  Colectomy with inferior mesenteric artery ligation

vasopressin,[36] gold,[37] psychotropic drugs[38]), sickle cell anemia,[39] coagulopathies (thrombotic thrombocytopenic purpura,[40] protein C and protein S deficiency,[41] antithrombin III deficiency[42]), competitive long-distance running,[43] and cocaine abuse.[44] Obstructing lesions of the colon, including carcinoma, stricture, and fecal impaction, may also cause colonic ischemia due to increased intracolonic pressure.[45] It is imperative that such obstructions be excluded from the differential.

CLINICAL MANIFESTATIONS

Symptoms

Colonic ischemia is usually manifested as a sudden onset of mild, crampy abdominal pain, usually localized to the lower left quadrant. Less commonly the pain is severe, or conversely, in other patients the description of pain can be elicited only retrospectively, if at all. An urgent desire to defecate frequently accompanies the pain and is followed, within 24 hours, by the passage of either bright red or maroon blood in the stool. The bleeding is not vigorous, and blood loss requiring transfusion is rare. Physical examination may reveal mild to severe abdominal tenderness elicited in the location of the involved segment of bowel.

Distribution of Colonic Ischemia

Colonic ischemia may affect any part of the colon, but the splenic flexure, descending, and sigmoid colon are the most common sites (Fig. 156.4). Segmental involvement is the most common distribution, whereas involvement of the entire colon is rare.[46] The segmental nature of colonic ischemia is due to the multiple vessels supplying the colon and rectum, specifically the SMA, the IMA, and the superior hemorrhoidal artery. Although specific causes, when identified, tend to affect defined areas of the colon, no prognostic implications can be derived from the distribution of the disease. Nonocclusive ischemic injuries generally involve watershed areas of the colon, which are regions susceptible to ischemic injury because of their location between two different main vascular pedicles. These watershed regions include the splenic flexure and the junction of the sigmoid and rectum. The rectum is very rarely involved because of its abundant dual blood supply from both the splanchnic and systemic arcades. Patients noted to have right-sided–only ischemia more commonly have atrial fibrillation, coronary artery disease, and chronic kidney disease.[47,48]

The length of bowel affected typically varies with the cause. For example, atheromatous emboli result in short segment changes, and nonocclusive injuries usually involve much longer portions of the colon. Depending on the severity and duration of the ischemic insult, fever or leukocytosis may develop. Patients with severe ischemia leading to transmural necrosis, gangrene, or perforation may develop peritonitis.

Natural History of Colonic Ischemia

Despite similarities in the initial manifestation of most episodes of colonic ischemia, the outcome cannot be predicted at its onset unless the initial physical findings indicate an unequivocal intraabdominal catastrophe. The

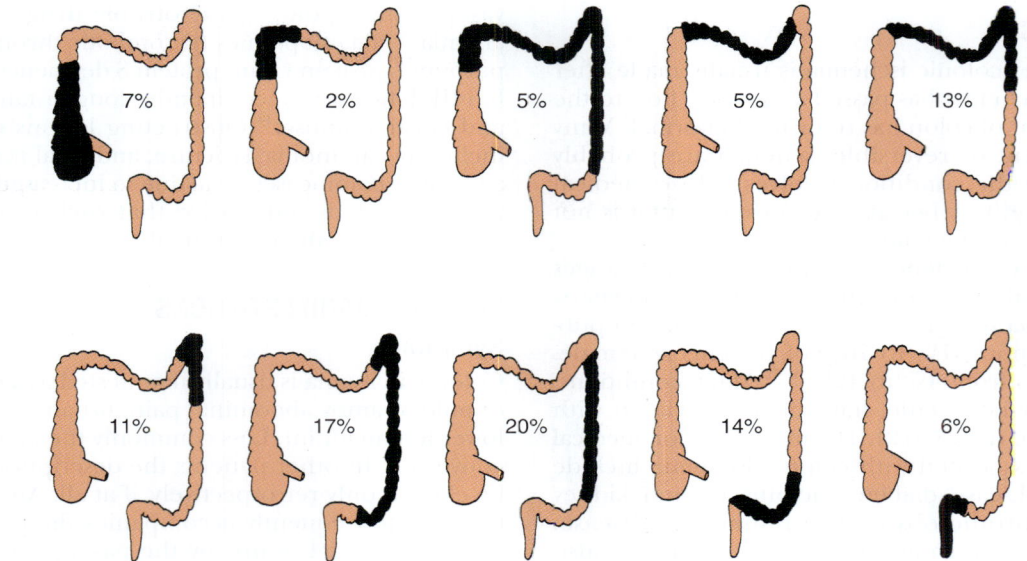

FIGURE 156.4 Distribution and length of involvement in 250 cases of colonic ischemia. More frequent involvement of the left half of the colon is apparent.

ultimate course of an ischemic insult depends on many factors: the cause (i.e., occlusive or nonocclusive), the caliber of an occluded vessel, the duration and degree of ischemia, the rapidity of onset of the ischemia, the condition of the collateral circulation, the metabolic requirements of the affected bowel, the presence and virulence of the bowel flora, and the presence of associated conditions, such as colonic distention.

Most commonly, symptoms subside within 24 to 48 hours, and clinical, radiographic, and endoscopic evidence of healing is seen within 2 weeks. More severe, but still reversible, ischemic damage may take 1 to 6 months to resolve. The majority of patients with reversible disease develop colopathy, whereas transient colitis develops in approximately one-third. Severe reversible ischemia may result in diffuse mucosal sloughing.

Severe, irreversible colonic ischemia occurs less frequently than reversible colonic ischemia. Approximately two-thirds of patients with irreversible colonic ischemia develop either chronic segmental colitis with ulceration or ischemic stricture. In the remaining third, gangrene, with or without perforation, rapidly develops within hours of the initial presentation. Patients in whom colonic ischemia develops as a complication of shock, congestive heart failure, myocardial infarction, or severe dehydration have a particularly poor prognosis.

Because the clinical course of colonic ischemia is difficult to predict, patients require serial examinations to evaluate for signs of clinical deterioration suggesting development of gangrene or perforation: rising temperature, elevated white blood cell count, worsening metabolic acidosis, hemodynamic instability, or peritonitis. Patients with diarrhea or bleeding that persists beyond the first 10 to 14 days are at risk for development of perforation or, less frequently, a protein-wasting enteropathy. Strictures may develop over a period of weeks to months and may be asymptomatic or produce progressive bowel obstruction.

Some of the asymptomatic strictures resolve spontaneously over a span of many months.

Diagnosis

Current ACG clinical guidelines recommend CT scan combined with early colonoscopy for the diagnosis of colonic ischemia.[31] Severe cases of colonic ischemia may be difficult to distinguish from acute mesenteric ischemia, whereas patients with less severe symptoms may have findings similar to those with ulcerative colitis, Crohn colitis, infectious colitis, or diverticulitis.

Historically, serial barium enema was used beginning in the 1960s to diagnose colonic ischemia. The most characteristic finding on barium enema is "thumbprinting" or "pseudotumors" corresponding to subepithelial hemorrhagic nodules or bullae. These findings either resolved on radiographs over the course of 1 to 2 weeks or evolved into segmental colitis with subsequent resolution over several months. Barium enema is now primarily used to follow the clinical course of ischemic strictures.

CT with intravenous and oral contrast is the imaging modality of choice for patients with suspected colonic ischemia. CT can demonstrate the distribution and phase of colonic ischemia as well as exclude other possible etiologies for the patient's clinical symptoms. CT findings consistent with colonic ischemia include segmental bowel wall thickening, edema, thumbprinting, pericolonic fat stranding, and occasionally ascites (Fig. 156.5). However, these signs may be seen with other etiologies of colitis, such as inflammatory bowel disease or infection, and are not specific to colonic ischemia. Findings of colonic pneumatosis or portal venous gas suggest transmural colonic infarction. CT angiography should be performed in patients with clinical suspicion for acute mesenteric ischemia.

Early colonoscopy is recommended to confirm the diagnosis of colonic ischemia and to establish the severity

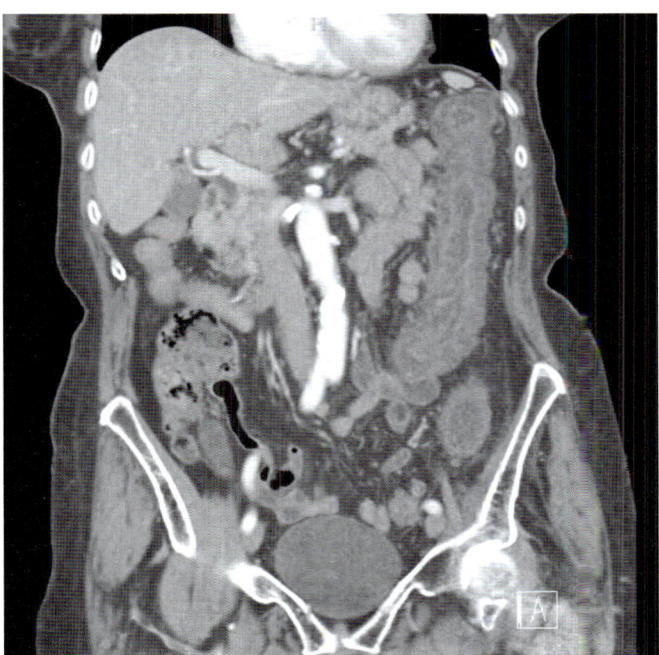

FIGURE 156.5 Computed tomography scan demonstrating left and transverse colonic ischemia. Note the thickened colonic wall with edema and fat stranding.

of the disease to guide treatment.[31] Early colonoscopy is performed within 48 hours of presentation and is typically done when CT findings are consistent with colonic ischemia. Benefits of diagnostic colonoscopy include the ability to make the diagnosis of colonic ischemia visually based on direct observation of affected tissue, as well as obtain tissue samples via biopsy. Colonoscopic findings not specific to colonic ischemia include segmental erythema, edema, friability, superficial or deep ulcerations, luminal narrowing, and intraluminal blood. Dusky, gangoic mucosa is highly suggestive of gangrene and warrants operative intervention.

Colonoscopy should be performed cautiously in the setting of colonic ischemia to decrease the risk of perforation. In patients with severe colonic ischemia, limited colonoscopy is appropriate to confirm CT findings, and the exam should be terminated at the distal extent of disease. Insufflation should be minimized. Carbon dioxide may be superior to room air because it is rapidly absorbed from the colon, thus theoretically decreasing the duration of distention and elevation of intraluminal pressure.[48] Colonoscopy should not be performed in the setting of peritonitis or irreversible ischemia (CT evidence of gangrene), as these patients warrant immediate surgical exploration.

Biopsies should be obtained, except in the case of gangrene, to rule out alternative diagnoses. Histology of biopsies from hemorrhagic nodules or bullae typically demonstrates submucosal hemorrhage, whereas biopsies of the surrounding mucosa usually show nonspecific inflammatory changes.[49] Histologic evidence of mucosal infarction is pathognomonic for ischemia.

MANAGEMENT OF COLONIC ISCHEMIA

General Principles

After the diagnosis of colonic ischemia has been established, the patient is treated expectantly with fluid resuscitation and bowel rest, unless signs and symptoms of gangrene or perforation develop. Optimization of cardiac function ensures adequate systemic perfusion. Medications that cause mesenteric vasoconstriction (e.g., digitalis and vasopressors) should be withdrawn if possible. Urine output is monitored and maintained with parenteral isotonic fluids. There is limited evidence to support the utility of administration of antibiotics; however, ACG guidelines recommend antimicrobial therapy for patients with "moderate" or "severe" disease.[31] If the colon appears distended, either clinically or radiographically, it can be decompressed with a rectal tube, with or without gentle saline irrigation. Corticosteroids are not recommended for colonic ischemia, except in cases of vasculitis.[1c]

Determination of the white blood cell count, hemoglobin, and hematocrit should be repeated frequently during the acute episode. Although rarely needed, blood products should be administered according to the patient's requirements. Serum potassium and magnesium levels must be monitored because the levels of these electrolytes are affected by the associated diarrhea and tissue necrosis. Elevated systemic levels of lactate dehydrogenase may indicate bowel ischemia but is neither sensitive nor specific for necrosis or gangrene. Patients with significant diarrhea are started on parenteral nutrition early. Narcotics should be administered judiciously. Mechanical bowel preparation is contraindicated because it may cause perforation.

Management of Reversible Ischemia

In the mildest cases of colonic ischemia, signs and symptoms of illness disappear within 24 to 48 hours and complete clinical resolution occurs within 1 to 2 weeks. No further therapy is required in these patients. More severe ischemic insults result in necrosis of the overlying mucosa with ulceration, inflammation, and the subsequent development of segmental colitis. Various amounts of mucosa may slough, which may ultimately heal over a period of several months. These patients may be clinically asymptomatic, even in the presence of persistent radiographic or endoscopic evidence of disease. Treatment includes a high-residue diet, and follow-up endoscopy is performed to confirm complete healing and exclude alternative diagnosis.

Management of Irreversible Acute and Subacute Ischemia

Acute signs of clinical deterioration during the period of observation (rising temperature, elevated white blood cell count, worsening metabolic acidosis, hemodynamic instability, or peritonitis) suggest colonic infarction and are an indication for operative intervention. Patients with persistent symptoms, such as diarrhea, rectal bleeding, or recurrent sepsis, for more than 10 to 14 days may require operative intervention. Despite a normal serosal appearance, there may be extensive mucosal injury, and the extent of resection should be guided by the distribution of disease as seen on preoperative studies rather than by the appearance of the serosal surface of the colon at the time of surgery. As in all resections for colonic ischemia, the specimen must be opened at the time of surgery to ensure normal mucosa at the margins. If at the time of surgery the segmental colitis is found to involve the rectum, a mucous fistula or Hartmann procedure with an end colostomy should be performed. Simultaneous procto-colectomy is rarely indicated but should be performed for gangrene of the rectum.

MANAGEMENT OF CHRONIC ISCHEMIA

Colonic ischemia may not be accompanied by clinical symptoms during the acute insult but may still produce chronic segmental colitis. This form of colonic ischemia may frequently be misdiagnosed if not seen during the acute episode. Barium enema studies may show a segmental colitis pattern, a stricture simulating a carcinoma, or even an area of pseudopolyposis. The clinical course of chronic colonic ischemia may be difficult to distinguish from other causes of colitis or stenosis, unless the diagnosis was made during the acute episode. Crypt abscesses and pseudo-polyposis, generally considered histologically diagnostic of ulcerative colitis, can also be seen in ischemic colitis. Regardless, de novo occurrence of a segmental area of colitis with stricture in an older patient is most likely ischemic. Elective bowel resection is indicated for patients with chronic segmental colonic ischemia and recurrent episodes of sepsis. The underlying etiology of these septic episodes is likely bacterial translocation from areas of unhealed segmental colitis.

Management of Ischemic Strictures

Stenosis or stricture of the colon may develop in patients with colonic ischemia. Strictures that produce no symptoms should be observed, and some of them will return to normal over a 12- to 24-month period with no further therapy. If, however, symptoms of obstruction develop, segmental resection is required. Endoscopic dilation of chronic colonic strictures as a result of ischemia is generally not recommended.

Management of Specific Clinical Problems

Colonic Ischemia Complicating Abdominal Aortic Surgery.
Mesenteric arterial reconstruction is not indicated in most cases of abdominal aortic surgery, but it should always be considered to prevent colonic ischemia during an open reconstruction for abdominal aortic aneurysm (aneurys-mectomy). After elective open aneurysmectomy, colono-scopic evidence of colonic ischemia is present in 3% to 7% of patients.[51,52] The incidence of colonic ischemia after repair of ruptured aortic aneurysm has been reported to be as high as 60%.[53] Clinical evidence of full-thickness colonic necrosis occurs in only 1% to 2% of patients, and when it does occur, it is responsible for approximately 10% of the deaths that take place after aortic replacement.[54] Factors that contribute to the occurrence of postoperative colonic ischemia include aneurysm rupture, perioperative hypotension, operative trauma to the colon, hypoxemia, arrhythmias, prolonged cross-clamp time, and improper management of the IMA during aneurysmectomy.

The most important aspect of management of colonic ischemia after aortic surgery is its prevention. Collateral blood flow to the left colon after occlusion of the IMA comes from the SMA via the arch of Riolan ("the meander-ing artery") or the marginal artery of Drummond and from the internal iliac arteries via the middle and inferior hemorrhoidal arteries. If these collateral pathways are intact, postoperative colonic ischemia can be minimized. Therefore obtaining an abdominal and pelvic CT angio-gram is essential before any aortic reconstruction. Digital subtraction aortography is sometimes advised to determine the patency of the CA, SMA, IMA, and internal iliac artery if the CT angiogram is inadequate. The presence of a meandering artery does not, in and of itself, allow safe ligation of the IMA because blood flow in the meandering artery frequently originates from the IMA and reconstitutes an obstructed SMA. Ligation of the IMA in the latter circumstance could be catastrophic and result in infarction of the small and large bowel (Fig. 156.6). In most cases, ligation of the IMA is safe when it has been confirmed angiographically that there is blood flow in the meandering artery from the SMA to the IMA. Reimplantation of the IMA and revascularization of the SMA are therefore required in instances in which the SMA is occluded or

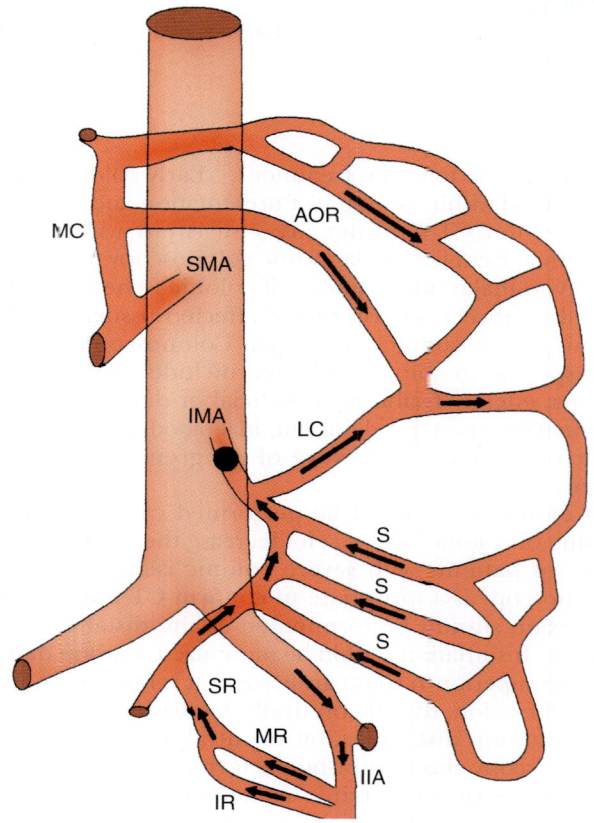

FIGURE 156.6 Collateral blood flow to the colon from the marginal artery, arch of Riolan, and internal iliac artery via the inferior and middle rectal arteries to an occluded inferior mesenteric artery. *AOR,* Arch of Riolan; *IIA,* internal iliac artery; *IMA,* inferior mesenteric artery; *IR,* inferior rectal artery; *LC,* left colic artery; *MC,* middle colic artery; *MR,* middle rectal artery; *S,* sigmoid arteries; *SMA,* superior mesenteric artery; *SR,* superior rectal artery.

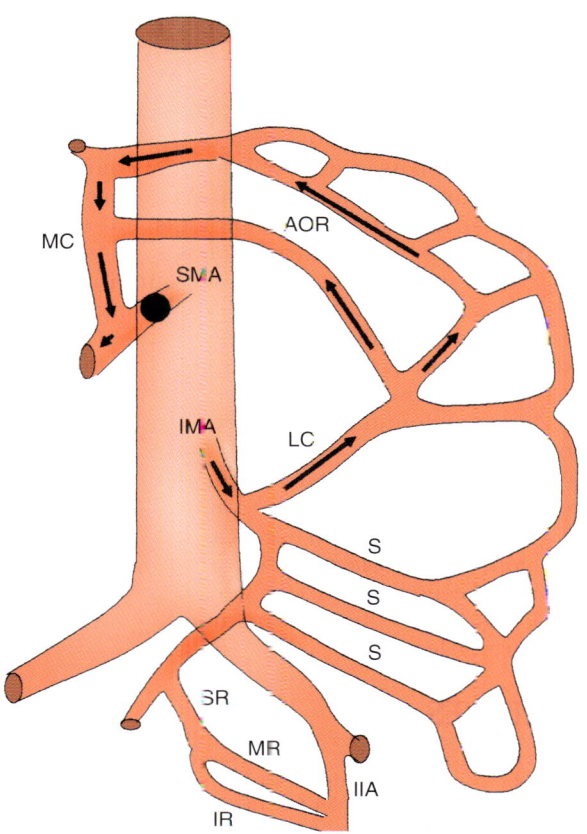

FIGURE 156.7 Collateral blood flow from the inferior mesenteric artery via the marginal artery and arch of Riolan to an occluded superior mesenteric artery. *AOR,* Arch of Riolan; *IIA,* internal iliac artery; *IMA,* inferior mesenteric artery; *IR,* inferior rectal artery; *LC,* left colic artery; *MC,* middle colic artery; *MR,* middle rectal artery; *S,* sigmoid arteries; *SMA,* superior mesenteric artery; *SR,* superior rectal artery.

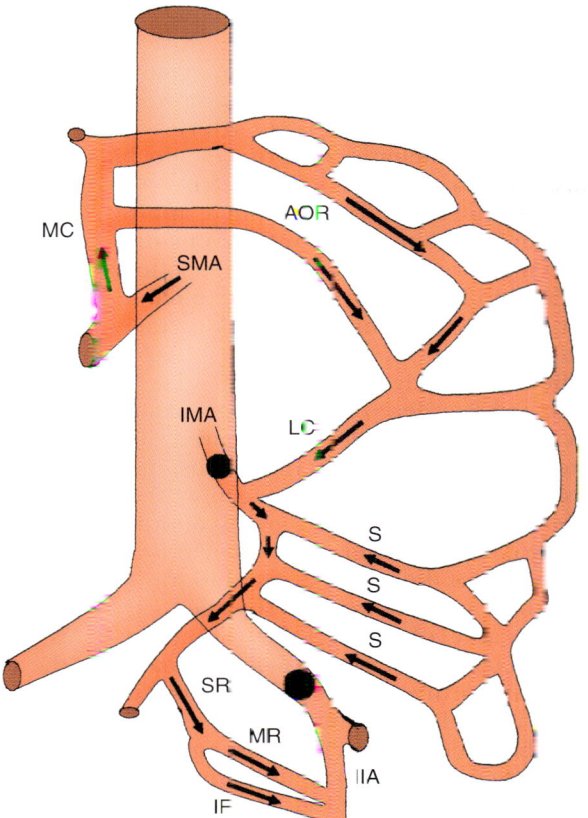

FIGURE 156.8 The entire rectal blood flow is dependent on collateral flow after occlusion of both internal iliac arteries. In this figure, the inferior mesenteric artery is also occluded, so rectal blood flow is dependent on collateral flow from the superior mesenteric artery via the arch of Riolan and the marginal artery and then via the superior rectal vessel to the middle and inferior rectal arteries. *AOR,* Arch of Riolan; *IA,* internal iliac artery; *IMA,* inferior mesenteric artery; *IR,* inferior rectal artery; *LC,* left colic artery; *MC,* middle colic artery; *MR,* middle rectal artery; *S,* sigmoid arteries; *SMA,* superior mesenteric artery; *SR,* superior rectal artery.

tightly stenosed and the IMA provides inflow to the meandering artery (Fig. 156.7). Occlusion of both hypogastric arteries on the preoperative arteriogram indicates that rectal blood flow is dependent on collateral flow from the IMA or from the SMA via the meandering artery. In this circumstance, reconstitution of flow to one or both hypogastric arteries is desirable at the time of aneurysmectomy (Fig. 156.8).

At surgery, aortic cross-clamp time should be minimized, and hypotension must be avoided. If a meandering artery is identified, it should be preserved. Because the serosal appearance of the colon is not a reliable indicator of collateral blood flow, several methods have been suggested to determine the need for IMA reimplantation. Stump pressure greater than 40 mm Hg in the transected IMA or a mean IMA stump pressure–to–mean systemic blood pressure ratio greater than 0.40 indicates adequate collateral circulation and can be reliably used to avoid IMA reimplantation.[55] The presence of Doppler ultrasound flow signals at the base of the mesentery and at the serosal surface of the colon with temporary occlusion of IMA inflow also suggests that the IMA could be ligated safely without reimplantation. However, in the presence of

superior mesenteric and internal iliac artery disease, the risk of colonic ischemia is increased, and the surgeon should have a low threshold to reimplant the IMA. Alternatively, interpositional grafts to the internal iliac arteries or reconstruction of the SMA could be performed. If the SMA is occluded, it could be revascularized with reimplantation to the aortic graft, particularly in the setting of perivisceral or pararenal aortic aneurysm repair. The simplest method of reconstructing the SMA is via a short bypass taken from the body of the aortic graft to the SMA with an end-to-side anastomosis. The second alternative is to place a bypass graft from one of the limbs in a C-shaped fashion, so that even though blood flow originates retrograde toward the SMA, the C shape allows it to be antegrade vis-à-vis the SMA.

The difficulty in accurately assessing colonic ischemia after surgery and the significant mortality rates associated with its occurrence mandate that postoperative colonoscopy be performed in high-risk patients. Patients at high risk for the development of postoperative colonic ischemia after aortic reconstruction are those with ruptured abdominal aortic aneurysms, prolonged cross-clamping time, a patent IMA on preoperative aortography, nonpulsatile flow in the hypogastric arteries at surgery, and postoperative melenic stool or hematochezia. In these cases, colonoscopy needs to be performed postoperatively, and if colonic ischemia is identified, appropriate therapy is begun before major complications develop. Clinical symptoms or signs that would suggest postoperative colonic ischemia following aortic surgery include unexplained fever, a slowly worsening metabolic acidosis, increase in fluid requirements, a widening of the Alveolar–arterial gradient, or rarely thrombocytopenia. Moreover, most patients who undergo open abdominal aortic reconstruction mobilize retained fluid acquired during operation 36 to 72 hours after operation. Thus, in the absence of worsening renal function or infection, the need for fluid or retention of fluid at this point is another harbinger of possible colonic ischemia. Clinical deterioration indicating progression of the ischemic insult to transmural necrosis necessitates reoperation. These patients should undergo resection and colostomy. Primary anastomosis is contraindicated because of potential contamination of the aortic prosthesis in the event of an anastomotic leak. If the rectum is involved, it must also be resected. Every effort should be made to protect the aortic graft from contamination; as such, the retroperitoneum overlying the graft should be reperitonealized with retroperitoneal tissues or omentum.

With the advent of endovascular techniques to repair abdominal aortic aneurysms (endovascular aortic aneurysm repair [EVAR]) the incidence of colonic ischemia appears to be decreasing as compared to the open aortic approach.[56,57] However, as in the open approach, colonic ischemia is most frequently associated with EVAR in the setting of aortic rupture and is still associated with greater than 30% mortality rate after being diagnosed. Other significant predictors of postoperative colonic ischemia are need for transfusion, renal failure, diabetes, proximal extension of the aneurysm, and female gender, not unlike the risk factors seen in open surgery. Similar to the reimplantation of the IMA during an open repair, maintaining patency of the hypogastric artery during EVAR is associated with decreasing incidence of colonic ischemia. Specifically, there are reports of postoperative colonic ischemia associated with embolization of atheromatous debris to the hypogastric artery during EVAR.[58,59] Therefore, even with endovascular approaches, all the salient open surgical principles need to be followed during an abdominal aneurysm repair, including the preoperative planning as previously discussed.

Fulminant Ischemic Pancolitis. A rare form of colonic ischemia involving all or most of the colon and rectum has been identified in a few patients. These patients experience the sudden onset of a toxic pancolitis manifested by bleeding, fever, severe diarrhea, and abdominal pain with or without peritonitis. The clinical course is rapidly progressive. Management of this condition is similar to that for other forms of fulminant colitis. Total abdominal colectomy with an ileostomy is generally required. A second-stage proctectomy may be necessary

for some patients. The histologic appearance of the resected colon is a combination of ischemic changes, severe ulcerations, and necrosis.

Colitis Associated With Colon Carcinoma. Acute ischemic colitis in patients with carcinoma of the colon has been recognized for many years.[60] This form of colitis is usually located proximal to the tumor and can occur with or without clinical obstruction. Radiologic and endoscopic appearance is typical of ischemic colitis. Clinically, patients may have symptoms of colonic ischemia or symptoms related to the primary cancer (i.e., crampy pain of a chronic nature, bleeding, or acute colonic obstruction). However, in most cases the predominant complaints are related to the ischemic episode—sudden onset of mild to moderate abdominal pain, fever, bloody diarrhea, and abdominal tenderness.

It is imperative to be aware of the frequent association of colonic ischemia and colon cancer. The diagnosis of cancer must be excluded in every case of colonic ischemia. In addition, during colectomy for carcinoma, examination of colonic resection margins for signs of ischemia is critical because poor blood flow at the anastomosis may result in stricture or leak.

REFERENCES

1. Zuckerman GR, Prakash C. Acute lower intestinal bleeding: part I: clinical presentation and diagnosis. *Gastroint Endosc.* 1998;48:606.
2. Strate LL, Ayanian JZ, Kotler G, Syngal S. Risk factors for mortality in lower intestinal bleeding. *Clin Gastroenterol Hepatol.* 2008;6:1004-1010.
3. Standards of Practice Committee of the American Society for Gastrointestinal Endoscopy. The role of endoscopy in the patient with lower GI bleeding. *Gastroint Endosc.* 2014;79:875-885.
4. Strate LL, Saltzman JR, Ookubo R, Mutinga ML, Syngal S. Validation of a clinical prediction rule for severe acute lower intestinal bleeding. *Am J Gastroenterol.* 2005;100:1821.
5. Longstreth GF. Epidemiology and outcome of patients hospitalized with acute lower gastrointestinal hemorrhage: a population-based study. *Am J Gastroenterol.* 1997;92:419.
6. Gostout CJ, Wang KK, Ahlquist DA, et al. Acute gastrointestinal bleeding. Experience of a specialized management team. *J Clin Gastroenterol.* 1992;14:260.
7. Gayer C, Chino A, Lucas C, et al. Acute lower gastrointestinal bleeding in 1,112 patients admitted to an urban emergency medical center. *Surgery.* 2009;146:600; discussion 606.
8. Peura DA, Gudmundson J, Siepman N, Pilmer BL, Freston J. Proton pump inhibitors: effective first-line treatment for management of dyspepsia. *Dig Dis Sci.* 2007;52:983.
9. McGuire HH Jr. Bleeding colonic diverticula; a reappraisal of natural history and management. *Ann Surg.* 1994;220:653-656.
10. Jensen DM, Machicado GA, Jutubha R, Kovacs TO. Urgent colonoscopy for the diagnosis and treatment of severe diverticular hemorrhage. *N Engl J Med.* 2000;342:78-82.
11. Boley SJ, Sammartano R, Adams A, DiBiase A, Kleinhaus S, Sprayregen S. On the nature and etiology of vascular ectasias of the colon. Degenerative lesions of aging. *Gastroenterology.* 1977;72:650.
12. Danesh BJ, Spiliadis C, Williams CB, Zambartas CM. Angiodysplasia—an uncommon cause of colonic bleeding: colonoscopic evaluation of 1050 patients with rectal bleeding and anaemia. *Int J Colorectal Dis.* 1987;2:218.
13. Heer M, Sulser H, Hany A. Angiodysplasia of the colon: an expression of occlusive vascular disease. *Hepatogastroenterology.* 1987;34:127.
14. Cappell MS, Gupta A. Changing epidemiology of gastrointestinal angiodysplasia with increasing recognition of clinically milder cases: angiodysplasia tends to produce mild chronic gastrointestinal bleeding in a study of 47 consecutive patients admitted from 1980–1989. *Am J Gastroenterol.* 1992;87:201.
15. Warren JL, Klabunde CN, Mariotto AB, et al. Adverse events after outpatient colonoscopy in the Medicare population. *Ann Intern Med.* 2009;150:849-857.

16. Strate LL, Naumann CR. The role of colonoscopy and radiological procedures in the management of acute lower intestinal bleeding. *Clin Gastroenterol Hepatol.* 2010;8:333-343.

17. Navaneethan U, Njei B, Venkatesh PGK, Sanaka MR. Timing of colonoscopy and outcomes in patients with lower GI bleeding: a nationwide population-based study. *Gastrointest Endosc.* 2014;79:297-306.

18. Winzelberg GG, Froelich JW, McKusick KA, Strauss HW. Scintigraphic detection of gastrointestinal bleeding: a review of current methods. *Am J Gastroenterol.* 1983;78:324.

19. Smith R, Copely DJ, Bolen FH. 99mTc RBC scintigraphy: correlation of gastrointestinal bleeding rates with scintigraphic findings. *AJR Am J Roentgenol.* 1987;148:869.

20. Kuhle WG, Sheiman RG. Detection of active colonic hemorrhage with use of helical CT: findings in a swine model. *Radiology.* 2003;228:743-752.

21. Chua AE, Ridley LJ. Diagnostic accuracy of CT angiography in acute gastrointestinal bleeding. *J Med Imaging Radiat Oncol.* 2008;52:333-338.

22. Copland A, Munroe CA, Friedland S, Triadafilopoulos G. Integrating urgent multidetector CT scanning in the diagnostic algorithm of active lower GI bleeding. *Gastrointest Endosc.* 2010 72:402-405.

23. Pishvaian AC, Lewis JH. Use of endoclips to obliterate a colonic arteriovenous malformation before cauterization. *Gastrointest Endosc.* 2006;63:865.

24. Benvenuti GA, Julich MM. Ethanolamine injection for sclerotherapy of angiodysplasia of the colon. *Endoscopy.* 1998;30:564.

25. Vargo JJ. Clinical applications of the argon plasma coagulator. *Gastrointest Endosc.* 2004;59:81.

26. Naveau S, Aubert A, Poynard T, Chaput JC. Long-term results of treatment of vascular malformations of the gastrointestinal tract by neodymium YAG laser photocoagulation. *Dig Dis Sci.* 1990;35:821.

27. Leitman IM, Paull DE, Shires GT 3rd. Evaluation and management of massive lower gastrointestinal hemorrhage. *Ann Surg.* 1989;209:175.

28. Browder W, Cerise EJ, Litwin MS. Impact of emergency angiography in massive lower gastrointestinal bleeding. *Ann Surg.* 1986;204:530.

29. Quirke P, Campbell I, Talbot IC. Ischaemic proctitis and adventitial fibromuscular dysplasia of the superior rectal artery. *Br J Surg.* 1984;71:33.

30. Binns JC, Issacson P. Age-related changes in the colonic blood supply: their relevance to ischemic colitis. *Gut.* 1978;19:384.

31. Brandt LJ, Feuerstadt P, Longstreth GF, Boley SJ. ACG clinical guideline: epidemiology, risk factors, patterns of presentation, diagnosis, and management of colon ischemia (CI). *Am J Gastroenterol.* 2015;110:18-44.

32. Suh DC, Kahler KH, Choi IS, Shin H, Kralstein J, Shetzline M. Patients with irritable bowel syndrome or constipation have an increased risk for ischemic colitis. *Aliment Pharmacol Ther.* 2007;25:681-692.

33. Cole JA, Cook SF, Sands BE, Ajene AN, Miller DP, Walker AM. Occurrence of colon ischemia in relation to irritable bowel syndrome. *Am J Gastroenterol.* 2004;99:486.

34. Tedesco FJ, Volpicelli NA, Moore FS. Estrogen- and progesterone-associated colitis: a disorder with clinical and endoscopic features mimicking Crohn's colitis. *Gastrointest Endosc.* 1982;28:247.

35. Miyata T, Tamechika Y, Toriu M. Ischemic colitis in a 33-year-old woman on danazol treatment for endometriosis. *Am J Gastroenterol.* 1988;83:1420.

36. Schmitt W, Wagner-Thiessen E, Lux G. Ischaemic colitis in a patient treated with Glypressin for bleeding oesophageal varices. *Hepatogastroenterology.* 1987;34:134.

37. Wright A, Benfield GF, Felix-Davies D. Ischaemic colitis and immune complexes during gold therapy for rheumatoid arthritis. *Ann Rheum Dis.* 1984;43:495.

38. Gollock JM, Thompson JP. Ischaemic colitis associated with psychotropic drugs. *Postgrad Med J.* 1984;26:449.

39. Gage TP, Gagnier JM. Ischemic colitis complicating sickle cell crisis. *Gastroenterology.* 1983;84:171.

40. Dubois A, Lyonnet P, Cohendy R, et al. Ischemic colitis as a manifestation of Moschkowitz's syndrome. *Ann Gastroenterol Hepatol (Paris).* 1989;25:19.

41. Blanc P, Bories P, Donadio D, et al. Colite ischemique et thromboses veineuses recidivante par deficit familial en proteine S [letter]. *Gastroenterol Clin Biol.* 1989;13:945.

42. Knot E, Tencate J, Bruin T, Iburg AH, Tytgat GN. Antithrombin III metabolism in two colitis patients with acquired antithrombin III deficiency. *Gastroenterology.* 1985;89:421.

43. Heer M, Repond F, Hany A, Sulser H, Kehl O, Jäger K. Acute ischemic colitis in a female long distance runner. *Gut.* 1987;28:896.

44. Fishel R, Hamamoto G, Barbul A, Jiji V, Efron G. Cocaine colitis: is this a new syndrome? *Dis Colon Rectum.* 1985;28:264.

45. Walker AM, Bohn RL, Cali C, Cook SF, Ajene AN, Sands BE. Risk factors for colon ischemia. *Am J Gastroenterol.* 2004;99:1333.

46. Brandt LJ, Feuerstadt P, Blaszka MC. Anatomic patterns, patient characteristics, and clinical outcomes in ischemic colitis: a study of 313 cases supported by histology. *Am J Gastroenterol.* 2010;105:2245; quiz 2253.

47. Sotiriadis J, Brandt LJ, Behin DS, Southern WN. Ischemic colitis has a worse prognosis when isolated to the right side of the colon. *Am J Gastroenterol.* 2007;102:2247.

48. Guttorson NL, Bubrick MP. Mortality from colonic ischemia. *Dis Colon Rectum.* 1989;32:469.

49. Brandt LJ, Boley SJ, Sammartano RJ. Carbon dioxide and room air insufflation of the colon. *Gastrointest Endosc.* 1986;32:324.

50. Boley SJ, Brandt LJ, Veith FJ. Ischemic disorders of the intestine. *Curr Probl Surg.* 1978;15:1.

51. Ernst CB, Hagihara PF, Daugherty ME, Sachatello CR, Griffen WO Jr. Ischemic colitis incidence following abdominal aortic reconstruction: a prospective study. *Surgery* 1976;80:417.

52. Zelenock GB, Strodel WE, Knol A, et al. A prospective study of clinically and endoscopically documented colonic ischemia in 100 patients undergoing aortic reconstructive surgery with aggressive and direct pelvic revascularization: comparison with historic controls. *Surgery.* 1989;106:771.

53. Hagihara PF, Ernst CB, Griffen WE. Incidence of ischemic colitis following abdominal aortic reconstruction. *Surg Gynecol Obstet.* 1979;149:571.

54. Kim MW, Hundahl SA, Dang CR, McNamara JJ, Straehley C, Whelan TJ Jr. Ischemic colitis following aortic aneurysmectomy. *Am J Surg.* 1983;145:392.

55. Ernst CB, Hagihara PF, Daugherty ME, Griffen WO Jr. Inferior mesenteric artery stump pressure: a reliable index for safe IMA ligation during abdominal aortic aneurysmectomy. *Ann Surg.* 1978;187:641.

56. Perry RJ, Martin MJ, Eckert MJ, Sohn VY, Steele SR. Colonic ischemia complicating open vs endovascular abdominal aortic aneurysm repair. *J Vasc Surg.* 2008;8(2):272-277.

57. Moghadamyeghaneh Z, Sgroi MD, Chen SL, Kabutey NK, Stamos MJ, Fujitani RM. Risk factors and outcomes of postoperative ischemic colitis in contemporary open and endovascular abdominal aortic aneurysm repair. *J Vasc Surg.* 2016 63(4):866-872.

58. Maldonado TS, Rockman CB, Riles E, et al. Ischemic complications after endovascular abdominal aortic aneurysm repair. *J Vasc Surg.* 2004;40(4):703-709.

59. Geraghty PJ, Sanchez LA, Rubin BG, et al. Overt ischemic colitis after endovascular repair of aortoiliac aneurysms. *J Vasc Surg.* 2004;40(3):413-418.

60. Teitjen GW, Markowitz AM. Colitis proximal to obstructing colonic carcinoma. *Arch Surg.* 1975;110:323.

Diverticular Disease Management

Rocco Ricciardi | Susannah Clark | Patricia L. Roberts

Diverticulitis is one of the most commonly diagnosed inflammatory conditions of the gastrointestinal (GI) tract. The condition was relatively uncommon a century ago, yet it now results in approximately 300,000 hospital admissions per year, placing it among the top five most costly GI tract diseases in the United States.[1-3] Yet despite how relatively common it is and the considerable cost to the nation, there remain numerous knowledge gaps and controversies in the area of pathophysiology, triggering factors for the development of diverticulitis, the most effective treatment, indications for surgery, and even the role of antibiotics for uncomplicated disease. Today, many of the commonly understood tenets of diverticulitis are being reconsidered. For example, the understanding that diverticulitis represents discrete episodes of acute colon inflammation followed by a return to an asymptomatic state is being re-evaluated.[3] Many patients have more chronic symptoms that wax and wane. It is unclear how the chronic manifestation of this disease is any different than those with more episodic disease. Lastly, patient education is a critical area of need as the materials available to patients, whether in print or online, continue to misrepresent the truth about diet and treatment indications for diverticulitis.

TERMINOLOGY

DIVERTICULOSIS

Diverticula are saccular outpocketings of the colonic wall. They may be false diverticula involving the mucosa and muscularis mucosae or true diverticula, involving all layers of the bowel wall. In Western nations, diverticula are most common in the sigmoid and left colon (95%), and represent false diverticula. In Asia, diverticula are more common on the right side of the colon and generally represent true diverticula. Diverticulosis is generally rare in populations under age 30, but increases in prevalence with age to include the majority of individuals by age 80. In industrialized nations, diverticulosis seems to be equally prevalent in men and women.[3-5] Most individuals with diverticulosis have no symptoms and are frequently unaware of the abnormality until the diagnosis is made following routine screening colonoscopy. Diverticulosis is one of the most common findings on screening colonoscopy.[3] In addition, patients are often confused by the diagnosis of diverticulosis, mistaking it for diverticulitis and erroneously concluding that they should alter their dietary habits or seek a surgeon's counsel.[6] For these reasons, patients should be reassured that in the absence of symptoms, they need not change their lifestyle.

DIVERTICULAR DISEASE

Diverticular disease characterizes any symptoms referable to the presence of diverticulosis, including diverticular bleeding, diverticulitis, segmental colitis associated with diverticula, or symptomatic uncomplicated diverticular disease (SUDD), are all manifestations of diverticular disease.

Diverticular bleeding: Diverticula can cause profuse episodic bleeding and constitute the cause of 10% to 30% of GI bleeds that require attention. Diverticular bleeds frequently manifest as life-threatening lower GI bleeding, rarely causing subtle or occult bloody bowel movements. The development of bleeding occurs with injury to a diverticulum resulting in intimal thickening, scarring, and irritation of the vasa recta. This sequence leads to bowel lining rupture, with bleeding into the colon lumen rather than into the abdominal cavity.[7] Diverticular bleeding often ceases without any intervention in most cases, but sometimes an endoluminal, radiologic, or surgical intervention is needed.

Acute diverticulitis: This occurs when there is inflammation of one or more diverticula. The condition manifests as left lower quadrant abdominal pain, malaise, low-grade fevers, and evidence of leukocytosis.[8] The condition was thought to be caused by obstruction of diverticula by particulate matter or fecaliths, leading to inflammation and microperforation.[6] This area of microperforation may cause a local process or develop into a more severe phlegmon or abscess, which can increase in size to erupt into an intraabdominal abscess. At that point, infection can spread systemically through the bloodstream to cause bacteremia or sepsis. At times, a large abscess can erode into the surrounding organs causing a fistula.[8] In addition, local inflammation and irritation may lead to an ileus, producing nausea and crampy abdominal pain.

SUDD: It is becoming increasingly recognized that diverticulitis is not simply an episodic condition with periods of inflammation and a return to periods of normal health. Some patients experience lingering symptoms that are attributable to diverticulosis despite resolution of inflammation on imaging.[3] Beyond acute diverticulitis, SUDD may represent a chronic variant of diverticular disease and may have been referred to as chronic smoldering diverticulitis or atypical diverticulitis in the past. This condition is characterized by low-grade abdominal pain that is often colicky but can also be constant.[6,9] The diagnosis is made after excluding acute diverticulitis, irritable bowel syndrome (IBS), and segmental colitis associated with diverticulosis (SCAD).[9]

SCAD: This is a subtype of chronic diverticulitis that appears to overlap with inflammatory bowel disease (IBD) and may be a precursor or variant of that entity.[3,9] The condition leads to localized inflammation of actual diverticula. It is a rare condition that is often called *diverticular colitis* and resembles chronic IBD but can also present with milder inflammatory changes.

PATHOPHYSIOLOGY AND EPIDEMIOLOGY

INCIDENCE

Diverticulitis was rarely mentioned in the medical literature before 1880 but is now the sixth most common GI outpatient diagnosis in the United States, and the most common GI diagnosis on hospital discharge.[10,11] Diverticulosis is the most commonly noted finding on routine colonoscopy, despite the fact that it isn't routinely reported by endoscopists.[3] Given the prevalence of this condition, diverticulitis creates significant morbidity, mortality and fiscal burden in the United States. As total United States hospital admissions for diverticulitis top 300,000, treatment costs are estimated at $2.5 billion annually.[1–3,12] In addition, the condition results in about 3400 deaths annually,[1,13] despite fairly well-tolerated treatment options.

Diverticulitis is more common in older patients, and the incidence of diverticular disease has also increased as the population has aged.[2,3] In a retrospective study of male Veterans Affairs patients, the authors found that for every additional 10 years of age at the time of diverticulosis diagnosis, the risk of developing diverticulitis decreased by 24%.[14] In a review of national population-based data, it was noted that hospital discharges with a diagnosis of diverticulitis had increased nearly 50% over 15 years.[4] This increased incidence is particularly evident among younger persons in whom hospitalization increased by 82% in those under 44 years of age and by 36% in patients aged 45 to 74 years.[9,15]

PATHOPHYSIOLOGY

The pathophysiology of diverticular disease remains difficult to define. We do not know whether the pathophysiology of diverticulosis and/or diverticulitis is due to varying exposure to the same causative agent, completely unrelated and distinct, or multiple defined triggers along a pathway to disease. Ultimately the development of diverticulitis may be completely separate and unrelated to the development of diverticulosis. Alternatively, the development of diverticulosis and diverticulitis are simply a continuum on a pathway to disease. Theories on the origin of diverticulosis relate to issues of colonic structure, colonic motility, and diet.[6] Other factors likely combine to bring about the inflammation found in diverticulitis, which may include diverticular obstruction, colonic dysmotility, and the alteration of bacterial flora.[6]

The classic 1969 postmortem study by Hughes demonstrated that 90% of Western patients have diverticular disease isolated to the sigmoid and descending colon, and that with increasing age, diverticula are much more likely to increase in number, incidence, and distribution, and to be found in other segments of the colon proximal to the sigmoid.[6,9,16] Interestingly, in Asia, diverticular disease is much less commonly diagnosed, and when it is, up to 70% of diverticula are identified in the right colon.[6,17,18] A number of factors have been proposed to explain these differences, yet the fact that Asians who migrate and adopt a typical Western diet develop similarly high rates of diverticulitis in the distal colon does lend strength to the theory of environment and diet.[3]

Diverticula are most commonly seen in the longitudinal plane between the mesenteric taeniae and the antimesenteric taeniae at the point where the vasa recta are closest to the mesentery. As diverticulosis becomes more prevalent, those diverticula will begin to develop in other areas such as between the two antimesenteric taeniae.[6,19] It is unclear why diverticulosis prefers to develop between the mesenteric and antimesenteric taeniae yet not between the two antimesenteric taeniae, although the presumption is that it is related to the vasculature of the colonic wall. There is a weak area at the point where large vessels perforate the colon wall, the area of the colon that is closer to the mesentery.[19]

Diet: Dietary fiber has been implicated as a major factor in the development of diverticulosis, as was initially described by Painter and Burkitt in 1971.[20] The investigators noted that diverticulosis was relatively rare in rural African populations but increasingly prevalent in First World countries and subsequently hypothesized that dietary fiber may have been the factor. The diet theory specifies that low-fiber foods are converted into smaller stools and raise intracolonic pressures as the bowel generates higher pressures to expel feces. Ultimately herniations at weak points in the colon wall develop because of the raised pressures.

The link between fiber and diverticulosis became more convincing with the advent of screening colonoscopy.[21] At this time, several large studies have shown a positive association between low fiber intake and the development of symptomatic diverticular disease.[20] In a cohort of 47,888 men between the ages 40 to 75 in the Health Professionals Follow-up Study, Aldoori et al. found a decreased risk of developing symptomatic diverticular disease in men who consumed a higher level of fiber compared with those who consumed the least.[19,20,22] Crowe et al., in their 2011 prospective study examining 47,033 men and women from the Oxford cohort of European Prospective Investigation into Cancer and Nutrition (EPIC) found an inverse association with fiber intake thus patients consuming the highest fiber diets had a 41% lower risk of hospital admission for diverticular disease than those consuming low-fiber diets.[20,21,23]

Vegetarians are thought to be at substantially lower risk of diverticulosis compared with non-vegetarians, but conclusive evidence demonstrating protection against diverticulitis is lacking.[21,24] In the previously discussed Oxford cohort of 47,033 patients, Crowe et al. found that after adjusting for a number of confounding factors, vegetarians had a 30% lower risk of developing diverticular disease than meat and fish eaters.[20,23] Similarly, Aldoori's study with a similarly large cohort found that the intake of red meat was positively associated with the risk of symptomatic diverticular disease, although no association was seen with chicken or fish.[20,22] These data seem to point to an association between diet and diverticular disease.

Although diverticulosis is a known precursor to diverticulitis, the development of diverticulitis must pass through other stages before symptomatic disease develops. Initial data from Parks' widely quoted 1975 study estimated that 10% to 25% of those with diverticulosis will progress to diverticulitis in their lifetime.[11–16] A 1947 analysis of 47,000 imaging studies of the colon for varied reasons identified diverticulosis in 8.5% of all patients and diverticulitis in 15% of the affected population. Thus only a small proportion of patients with diverticulosis develop diverticulitis. Interestingly, the trigger or triggers that lead to diverticulitis is unknown but was historically presumed to be related to a dietary item causing obstruction of diverticula. The theory that diverticulitis is caused by food is based on the idea that dense, small, particulate foods impact and obstruct the lumen of a diverticula and cause increased intraluminal pressure, weakening of the mucosal wall, diverticular inflammation, colon wall ischemia, and eventually microperforation.[3] However, a well-powered analysis examining diet by Strate et al. from the Health Professionals Follow-up Study demonstrated no association between nuts, popcorn, and corn with the development of diverticular complications. The study found that consumption of these foods was not associated with an increased risk of diverticulitis; rather, an inverse relationship between diverticulitis and nut and popcorn intake, but not corn consumption, was noted. In addition, no association was noted between corn consumption and diverticulitis or any of these foods with diverticular bleeding. The authors hypothesized that the antiinflammatory properties and high mineral content of nuts may actually be protective against diverticular complications rather than causative.[9,27] The mechanism by which nut consumption may be protective is unclear.

Properties of the colon wall: A number of physiological changes occur in patients with diverticular disease. The wall diameter of the colon thickens in patients with diverticulosis, and the circular muscle develops a corrugated appearance. Although muscular hypertrophy was initially proposed, electron and light microscopy studies by Whiteway and Morson noted neither hypertrophy nor hyperplasia in the colon muscle cells, but rather an increase in elastin deposition in the taeniae by more than 200% compared with the healthy colon.[19,28] In addition, increased collagen cross-linking leads to stiffening of the colon wall, making it less resistant to stretch forces while increasing intraluminal pressure. There are other intrinsic properties of the colon wall that predispose the colon to diverticulum. For example, the sigmoid colon is the segment of the bowel wall with the smallest radius, leading to the generation of higher intraluminal pressures.[19] Studies of intraluminal colonic pressures in the setting of diverticulosis do reveal even higher colonic pressures.[29-31] The submucosa then becomes more prone to small tears as increased intraluminal pressure provides the point of weakness for which herniation begins.[19]

Altered colon motility: Colonic motility also affects intraluminal pressure. Motility as characterized by the process of segmentation is defined by simultaneous contraction of two neighboring haustra, which can create temporarily a closed loop segment, leading to high intraluminal pressures.[6] One popular theory is that the high pressures of segmentation cause focal muscle atrophy or attenuation, which in turn permits herniation through the mucosa.[19] Others have proposed that low-volume stools noted in low-fiber diets prevalent in Western societies incur higher intraluminal pressures during colonic muscle contraction.[9]

In addition to the previously noted changes in intraluminal colonic pressures, colons with diverticular disease are considered spastic with evidence of hypermotility. The motility hypothesis is based on a lack of interstitial cells of Cajal, which are crucial for the generation and propagation of the pacemaker activity in the colon. Interstitial cells of Cajal provide the regulatory signals from the enteric nervous system to coordinate motor activity along the GI tract.[3,23] Compared with controls, patients with diverticulosis have significantly reduced numbers of interstitial cells of Cajal, as well as other enteric glial cells. The authors hypothesized that the relative paucity of these enteric cells might lead to disorganized colonic rhythmic contraction observed in patients with diverticulosis and a relative elevation of intracolonic pressures.[32]

Triggers of inflammation: There are a number of factors that are proposed to act together to lead to diverticular inflammation, including obstruction of a diverticulum, fecal stasis, alteration of bacterial flora within the colon, and local ischemia.[6] It is believed that the local inflammation brings about microperforation and serosal irritation. This microperforation may cause local irritation and develop into a phlegmon and/or abscess. Free perforation associated with a spreading inflammatory response can propagate infection spreading systemically, leading to sepsis. A fistula may also form when an abscess erodes into surrounding organs such as the bladder, another loop of bowel, skin, uterus, or vagina.[8] Complications of colovaginal fistulas are most commonly identified in those patients who have had hysterectomy.

Fecal stasis: The role of fecal stasis in the development of diverticular disease is proposed to lead to two separate phenomena: slow transit of feces through the colon and entrapment of feces within diverticula. Evidence of fecal stasis is corroborated by the specific anatomy of pathologic specimens in patients with diverticular disease. Slack's 1962 paper evaluating the specimens of patients undergoing colectomy for diverticulitis as well as autopsy specimens suggested that "there must have been some degree of obstruction to the fecal content of the bowel."[33] The fecal content of the bowel in patients with diverticular disease is likely to be related to delayed intestinal transit time in patients with diverticulosis. However, at this time, it is unclear if any associations made between transit times and diverticular disease result from the underlying condition or cause actual inflammation and disease.

Fecal stasis within diverticula is often suggested as a possible inciting factor in acute diverticulitis. Early studies have characterized the difficulty of expelling stool from colonic diverticulum, due to the fact that the diverticula are devoid of musculature.[29] The entrapped stool then produces an alteration of the intestinal flora, a local ischemia, or a mechanical breakdown of the colon wall. One theory proposes that normal fecal bacteria can penetrate the colon wall and trigger an inflammatory and immunological response of diverticulitis or diverticular bleeding.[29,34]

However, a well-performed study by Strate et al. examined the question of whether particulate matter can trigger diverticulitis by evaluating dietary intake of nuts, popcorn, and corn on the incidence of diverticular complications. The study found that consumption of these foods was not associated with an increased risk of diverticulitis; rather, an inverse relationship between diverticulitis attacks and nut and popcorn consumption was noted.[27] The Strate study rebuked the guidelines of avoiding nuts, seed, and popcorn in diverticular disease, but did not answer the question of whether fecal stasis leads to diverticulitis.

Bacterial flora: Some investigators have questioned whether a change in colonic bacterial flora, possibly due to a low-fiber diet, is the trigger for inflammation in acute or chronic diverticular disease.[35] Alteration of the native colonic bacterial populations might diminish the barrier function of the colonic mucosa, resulting in an upregulation of inflammatory cytokines, leading to chronic inflammation in the colon that in turn affects the enteric nervous system.[9,35,36] We know that the bacteria of the GI tract changes over time and can result in altered ratios of aerobic and anaerobic bacteria.[3,8] Diets that are low in insoluble fiber and high in fat have greater numbers of *Bacteroides* colonies. Alteration of the colonic bacterial population then alters the immune response of the colon itself generating inflammatory cytokines.[35,37] Although studies confirming a link between the presence of diverticula, bacterial overgrowth, and inflammation are presently lacking, this combination of factors seems to be emerging as the leading theory to the pathogenesis of diverticular disease.[34]

Age: Diverticular disease is more common in older patients; yet, traditionally, diverticulitis in the young has been viewed as a more virulent process than in older patients. However, in a systematic review of 4982 patients, the course of diverticulitis in the young was noted to not be more severe than that in older patients, but the disease tended to recur more often in younger patients.[38] In another systematic review, the relative risk for requiring urgent surgery for recurrent disease was higher in younger patients, yet the absolute risk difference was relatively small.[39] These data seem to indicate that factors other than age should be considered when identifying treatment options. Other studies suggest that the underlying problem in younger patients is not more aggressive disease but rather an issue of initial misdiagnosis or inattention to symptoms, leading to a delay in diagnosis and treatment.[40] In particular, diverticulitis should be considered in young obese males presenting with abdominal pain, low-grade fever, and leukocytosis.[41]

Obesity: Obesity is a risk factor for many human illnesses, including diverticular disease.[42] Two large cohort studies from the Swedish Mammography Cohort and the Health Professionals Follow-up Study identified an association between overweight body habitus and increased risk of diverticular disease.[11] The Swedish study demonstrated that women with body mass index (BMI) of 25 to 29.9 had a 29% increased risk of diverticular disease, and women with a BMI of 30 or greater had a 33% increased risk.[11,43] This same study also found that obesity seems to be associated with worse disease: women with a BMI of 30 or more had twice the risk of experiencing complicated diverticulitis.[11,43] Increasing waist circumference and waist-to-hip ratio were also associated with the development of diverticulitis and diverticular bleeding.[42] While the mechanism for increased risk of symptomatic diverticular disease and obesity is unknown, it has been speculated that increased levels of inflammatory cytokines secreted by adipose tissue

may play a role in inciting or exacerbating inflammatory processes in the colon.[42]

Exercise: Because physical activity is thought to reduce colonic transit time, inflammation, and colon pressure, it has been suggested that regular strenuous physical activity may have a protective effect against diverticulosis and diverticulitis.[44] The Swedish Mammography Cohort revealed that exercise for 30 minutes or less per day increased the risk of diverticular disease by 42%, compared with exercise more than 30 minutes per day.[11,43] Similarly, in the Health Professionals Follow-up Study, men with the highest level of activity had a 25% and 46% reduction in the risk of diverticulitis and diverticular bleeding, as compared with men with the lowest level of physical activity.[44] In addition, men who spent the most time sitting had a 30% increased risk of uncomplicated diverticulosis compared with men who spent less than 16 hours a week sitting.[44] It is unclear how much of the effect of exercise on diverticular disease is related to other concomitant healthy lifestyle choices.

Nonsteroidal antiinflammatory drugs (NSAIDs): A number of case-controlled studies have examined the relationship between aspirin or NSAID intake and diverticular disease, demonstrating a consistent association.[11,45] In the Health Professionals Follow-up Study, Strate et al. noted that intake of two to six 325 mg aspirin tablets weekly or 4 to 6 days a week was associated with the highest risk of diverticular bleeding. Similarly, NSAIDs increased the risk of diverticulitis and diverticular bleeding compared with nonusers of these medications.[11,45] Alterations in permeability of the colon from chronic NSAID or aspirin use may decrease the integrity of the colon wall,[11,46] leading to diverticular complications

Medications: Corticosteroids may increase the risk of perforation in diverticulitis, perhaps due to the reduction in collagen turnover that reduces colon wall integrity brought on by chronic use.[11,46] Humes et al. looked at 899 cases of perforated diverticular disease from the UK General Practice Research Database and found an almost threefold increased risk of perforation in patients currently taking corticosteroids, adjusted for comorbidity and smoking.[11,46] It is unclear as to whether the effect of steroids on diverticular complications is related to an effect on healing or reduced capacity to appreciate symptoms of diverticular disease.

Seasonal variation: There are data demonstrating increased incidence of hospital admissions for acute diverticulitis during the summer months.[2] These seasonal variations may be due to ultraviolet light exposure, the most important contributor to serum vitamin D levels.[47] In fact, geographic and seasonal variations of diverticulitis admissions were significantly higher in geographic areas with low UV light levels.[43] The apparent paradox between higher admissions in the summer, when UV light exposure is greatest may be due to a lag time between the onset of low UV light and vitamin D levels.[48]

Immune status: Diverticulitis in the immunocompromised patient is more likely to present in an atypical manner, presenting with a more smoldering course than the general population and making diagnosis more difficult.[5,9] It is also more likely to be complicated; a 1991 retrospective study of 40 immunocompromised patients diagnosed with acute diverticulitis found a greater risk of free perforation and need for surgery than in an immunocompetent population.[9,49] In addition to diagnosis, management is also more complex in the immunocompromised patient. The temptation is to rush these patients to surgery, as they have a presumably increased risk of perioperative mortality.[9] A 2010 review by Hwang et al. examined 25 papers focused on the impact of diverticulitis in transplant patients or on chronic corticosteroid therapy, and found that the mortality rate from acute diverticulitis was 23% when the disease was treated surgically and 56% when treated medically.[50,51] Although the study has the potential for selection bias, the data do point to the importance of prompt diagnosis and management of these complex patients.

Smoking: Nicotine decreases the formation of collagen, increases colonic motility and intraluminal pressure, and impairs blood flow to the colonic mucosa, which may then lead to diverticular disease.[3,52] Although the data demonstrating an increased risk of diverticulitis from smoking are equivocal, we do know that smokers have increased risk of perforation or abscess compared with nonsmokers.[3,52] Hjern et al. also found that current and past smokers had an increased risk of symptomatic diverticular disease compared with nonsmokers.[3,52]

Alcohol: Aldoori et al. noted that drinkers who had more than an ounce (30 grams) of alcohol daily were at increased risk of symptomatic diverticular disease after adjustment for age.[22] It is unclear, however, what the pathway for alcohol is in the development of diverticulitis.

Family history: Whatever factors come into play in the formation of diverticula and the development of diverticulitis, family history is proposed to increase baseline susceptibility to diverticular disease.[13] One retrospective analysis of 954 consecutive patients diagnosed with diverticulitis over a 7-year period found that a family history of diverticulitis was associated with a hazard ratio of 2.2 for recurrent disease.[51,52] A study of the Swedish Twin Registry revealed that the odds ratio of a twin developing diverticulitis after the first sibling received that diagnosis was 7.2 for monozygotic twins and 3.2 for dizygotic twins.[11,53]

DIAGNOSIS

There are a varied number of presentations attributed to diverticular disease. It is generally acknowledged that patients with diverticulosis have no symptoms attributable to the actual presence of uninflamed diverticula. However, a range of symptoms, from crampy discomfort with irritable bowels to peritonitis from perforating disease, is seen in more severe disease.

HISTORY AND PHYSICAL EXAM

As with all medical conditions, a complete history and physical exam is the first step in the diagnosis of diverticular disease. It is important to remind patients that the mere presence of diverticulosis is almost always asymptomatic, although this finding on screening colonoscopy can often lead to confusion and unnecessary concern by patients.[6] The spectrum of conditions attributed to diverticulosis is vast; thus the provider must be attuned to the potential range of symptoms. For example, diverticular bleeds will present as occult bleeding or massive hemorrhage per rectum.[54] These bleeds tend to be of a large amount, not occult, and without warning. In general, patients with diverticular bleeding rarely have abdominal pain or other associated symptoms in addition to hemorrhage; however, a rare patient may present with diverticular bleeding and pain.

The pathophysiology of SUDD is unclear. Patients who develop symptoms such as colicky or constant abdominal pain without signs of acute diverticulitis may have SUDD. This condition is characterized by attacks of usually colicky but sometimes constant abdominal pain that is often relieved by passing flatus or having a bowel movement.[6,9] Changes in bowel habits, constipation more than diarrhea, left lower quadrant tenderness sometimes with a palpable mass, and fullness or bloating are also reported.[6,9] The condition is diagnosed by excluding acute diverticulitis, as well as signs of overt colitis. The greatest challenge in diagnosis is distinguishing the condition from IBS, which similarly manifests with abdominal pain and loose stools.

Patients with diverticulitis classically present with changes in bowel habits, low-grade fevers, and left lower quadrant abdominal pain.[5,6] Fullness in the lower abdomen or rectum is also seen, a consequence of the inflammation in the sigmoid colon.[5] Stool can be guaiac positive, and the patient will describe constipation, loose stools, or mucous stools.[5,6] Anorexia, nausea, and vomiting are also often described.[13] A large number of patients have had prior bouts of diverticulitis and may thus quickly attribute their symptoms to diverticular disease.[13]

During the ascertainment of the chief complaint and medical history, it is important to elicit associated symptoms that may be related to complicated disease.[6] For example, with free perforation, the patient may describe generalized abdominal pain because of peritoneal irritation from stool leakage.[5] In addition, a reactive ileus or a phlegmon may affect the small bowel, leading to a constellation of obstructive symptoms such as abdominal distention, nausea, vomiting, and generalized abdominal pain.[6] Inflammation of the colon might also impinge on the bladder, leading to urgency and frequency.[6] Infection can also travel via mesenteric circulation back to the liver and cause hepatic abscess.[6] The condition can also progress into the hip joint and cause recurring septic arthritis of the hip as well.[6]

A small number of patients develop colonic fistulas during complicated diverticulitis, with end-organ involvement that leads to organ-specific signs and symptoms.[9,6,55] One of the most common diverticular fistulas is the colovesical fistula, which makes up about two-thirds of all fistulas attributed to diverticular disease.[9,56] Patients with colovesical fistula often report pneumaturia or fecaluria, or may describe recurrent urinary tract infection symptoms or changes in urine color.[6] Pneumaturia, which is often identified on computed tomography (CT) scan, should be considered a colovesical fistula unless instrumentation or catheterization of the bladder has recently occurred.[9,56] Colovaginal fistulas are also a consideration and are more common in women who have had hysterectomies, as the free vaginal cuff is more readily accessible, and these fistulas lead to feces or air passing from the vagina.[6] Enterocolonic fistulas are less common and usually asymptomatic but can cause diarrhea or abdominal cramps.[6] There is concern that a decrease in the rate of surgical intervention" may ultimately lead to an increased rate of fistulization or other complications, but data to support this hypothesis are lacking.

LABORATORY STUDIES

Laboratory investigation for diverticulitis should begin with a complete blood count to evaluate for leukocytosis, which is noted in 55% of patients with acute diverticulitis.[13] In addition, a basic metabolic panel is helpful to assess electrolytes and kidney function, particularly in the situation of altered fluid or nutrition intake.[13] A urinalysis can assist in the evaluation of urinary tract infection and to diagnose colovesical fistula.[6,13] There are data demonstrating that a C-reactive protein of more than 50 mg/L in conjunction with left lower quadrant tenderness and no vomiting is most consistent with acute diverticulitis.

IMAGING

The value of imaging studies is to confirm the condition and elucidate the location of the disease, the extent of inflammation, and any complications (e.g., abscess, phlegmon, fistula).[6] Although an important adjunct to the history and physical, imaging may be deferred in patients with mild symptoms if they have had confirmatory evidence in the past.[13] Imaging modalities for evaluation of diverticular disease include plain radiographs, contrast enema, ultrasound, and CT.[6] Plain films can demonstrate free air if perforation is suspected in acute diverticulitis, but these studies add little else to the diagnosis.[13]

CT scan: Abdominal and pelvic CT is the test of choice for diagnosing diverticulitis, due to its high diagnostic capacity and the ability to rule out other conditions.[6,13] A meta-analysis of eight single-center studies involving 684 patients found excellent diagnostic accuracy of CT scan in the setting of divert cular disease, with a summary sensitivity of 94% and a specificity of 99%. CT is best suited for evaluating bowel wall thickening and fat stranding, and most specific for evaluating abscesses, fascial thickening, free or intramural air, inflammation of the diverticula, intramural sinus tract, and phlegmon. CT colonography can also be considered in the nonacute setting for screening patients, following an attack of diverticulitis. Although there are many primary benefits of CT, disadvantages of CT include ionizing radiation[6,13] and expense.

Ultrasound: Ultrasonography is an acceptable alternative to CT for diagnosing diverticulitis but has disadvantages in identifying the scope of large abscesses and in identifying free air. A meta-analysis of eight single-center studies involving 684 patients found that in diagnosing acute colonic diverticulitis, the summary sensitivity of ultrasound was 92% and the summary specificity was 90%. Current available best evidence demonstrates no statistically significant difference in the accuracy of ultrasound versus CT for diagnosing acute diverticulitis.[13,57] Although our group prefers CT scans, ultrasound is a consideration for evaluating diverticulitis in pregnant patients and to avoid ionizing radiation in patients who have had many studies.

Gastrografin/barium enema: Although of limited value in diverticulitis, barium enema is a good option in the evaluation of diverticulosis. In more chronic disease states, contrast studies can help identify luminal narrowing,

bowel tethering, colonic strictures, and colonic fistulas. Unfortunately, contrast studies are less helpful at evaluating disease beyond the lumen of the colon, and the clinician should be aware of the potential for barium leak into the abdomen from a natural or iatrogenically perforated diverticulum. For these reasons, when perforation is suspected, a CT scan is the best consideration.[6] But in cases where adenocarcinoma is high on the differential list, a water-soluble contrast study may be one of the most helpful studies.[5]

Magnetic resonance imaging (MRI): MRI is another accurate and sensitive imaging modality in the diagnosis of acute diverticulitis. MRI permits more subtle delineation of soft tissue without ionizing radiation. This imaging modality is, however, associated with increased cost and imaging time, while requiring longer processing times than CT.

Cystography: In the differential diagnosis of colovesical fistula, cystography can be useful in establishing the diagnosis and ruling out other causes of fistula. No matter what, these fistulas are often difficult to visualize on any imaging study and are often best seen on CT scan, as confirmed by the presence of air in the bladder. The presence of air is generally sufficient to establish the diagnosis of colovesical fistula as long as no urinary instrumentation of the bladder has occurred.[6] Endoluminal and bladder evaluation can then be confirmatory and rule out primary bladder disease.

Endoscopy: Colonoscopy or sigmoidoscopy during an acute episode of diverticulitis is generally discouraged. The concern that flexible sigmoidoscopy or colonoscopy could cause perforation in an inflamed colon or exacerbate the disease process leads most endoscopists to defer endoscopy.[6] Once an acute attack of diverticulitis has resolved, however, colonoscopy is helpful to rule out other conditions that can present in a manner similar to diverticulitis (e.g., IBD and/or malignancy). Historical data reveal that about 3% to 5% of patients diagnosed with acute diverticulitis have other conditions such as adenocarcinoma as the actual cause of inflammation, not diverticulitis.[6]

CLASSIFICATION

Though frequently encountered, diverticular disease does not have a widely accepted and practical general classification system.[9] One of the most widely recognized classifications systems was initially proposed by Hinchey in 1978, based on the earlier clinical classification of acute diverticulitis by Hughes et al. This classification system created four stages based on clinical and surgical findings but failed to include the presence or location of intraabdominal abscesses in its categories.[3,58–66] The classification is Hinchey I—pericolic abscess or phlegmon; Hinchey II—pelvic, intraabdominal, or retroperitoneal abscess; Hinchey III—generalized purulent peritonitis; and Hinchey IV—generalized fecal peritonitis. The Hinchey system has been faulted for failing to classify individuals with less severe forms of diverticular disease who have no obvious abscess. In addition, the Hinchey classification, modified or otherwise, has never been validated prospectively against clinical outcomes, but several studies have found a significant correlation between Hinchey classification and intraoperative findings when patients with perforated diverticulitis underwent surgery.[9,60,61] In 1998, Hansen et al. proposed a classification system that has been used with great success in Germany. It includes a category for clinical diagnosis of asymptomatic diverticulosis and also grades complicated diverticulitis by severity of complications. Although it is regarded as one of the most useful classification systems in clinical practice, it has not been widely accepted in North America or in the rest of the world.[59]

Prior to the widespread adoption of CT scans, several studies found that the clinical diagnosis of acute diagnosis was quite poor. The introduction of CT scans, however, led to substantial gains in classification systems. Given that CT imaging is now the most frequently ordered diagnostic test in the diagnosis of acute diverticulitis,[59] it is not surprising that a number of new classification systems have been created. To further classify acute diverticulitis by making use of the greater detail of CT scans, several modifications based on CT imaging were suggested in the late 1990s, each with increasing levels of sophistication. The most popular of these is the Wasvary modification, which includes differentiation of the level of perforation.[58] To further improve this system, a Stage 0, representing mild clinical disease, has also been added.[59]

Although the list of classification systems proposed is numerous, none have had the capacity to do everything that might be needed by the patient, the gastroenterologist, or the surgeon. The patient may be most interested in learning what the predictors are of chronic illness or long-term quality of life. Alternatively, a classification system that accurately predicts medical treatment failure or future "complicated disease" would likely be of significant value to the internist or surgeon in educating patients about surgical indications. At this time, no such classification system exists, as long-term data for these patients are lacking.

CLINICAL FEATURES/ DIFFERENTIAL DIAGNOSIS

Diverticular disease has varied presentations that are related to the degree of disease, patient factors, and other comorbidities. Not every case of diverticulitis presents with classic symptoms, and thus it is important to keep all the potential variants of disease in mind during work-up. First and foremost is the developing perspective of diverticulitis transitioning from an episodic condition to a more chronic smoldering condition with unrelenting low-grade symptoms. The full span of symptoms and diverticular disease diagnoses is challenging to keep straight, but labeling the various conditions is not as important as understanding the potential manifestations of disease.

Almost all patients with diverticular disease (not including those with diverticular bleeding) describe some element of lower abdominal pain or pressure in the left lower quadrant. However, the sigmoid colon can be redundant and often crosses the midline, leading to right lower quadrant or pelvic pain rather than left lower quadrant discomfort.[5] Numerous other diseases that cause lower abdominal pain—IBD, pelvic inflammatory disease, IBS, nephrolithiasis, ectopic pregnancy, cystitis or urinary tract infection, colon cancer, and infectious or ischemic

---

> **BOX 157.1** Differential Diagnosis of Diverticulitis
>
> Appendicitis
> Bowel obstruction
> Colorectal cancer
> Gynecologic disease
> Kidney stones
> Ischemic colitis
> Inflammatory bowel disease
> Irritable bowel syndrome
> Urinary tract infection/Pyelonephritis
> Pneumonia
> Cystitis

colitis—must also be considered (Box 157.1).[5,6] A thorough history and physical and CT scan are thus critical in the work-up of the patient with presumed diverticulitis, at least for the initial presentation.

Acute diverticulitis: This form of diverticular disease manifests as left lower quadrant abdominal pain, malaise, low-grade fevers, and evidence of leukocytosis.[8] This area of microperforation may cause a local process or develop into a more severe phlegmon or abscess, which can increase in size to erupt into an intraabdominal abscess. At that point, infection can spread systemically through the blood-stream to cause bacteremia or sepsis.

Chronic diverticulitis: Chronic diverticulitis is distinct from acute diverticulitis, as the condition is characterized by the development of chronic symptoms that include abdominal pressure or cramping, bloating, decreased stool caliber, and at times obstruction. The symptoms are generally present for at least 2 months, and these patients rarely have classic signs and symptoms of acute diverticulitis, such as substantial abdominal tenderness, guarding, fever, or leukocytosis. The obstructive symptoms are generally from luminal narrowing, presumably caused by chronic inflammation, leading to structuring of the colon and nonmobility pericolonic tissues from inflammatory and scar tissue.[62,63] The differential diagnosis of patients with presumed chronic diverticulitis is malignancy. It is for this reason that all patients should have an endoluminal evaluation at some point following presentation.

Complicated diverticulitis: Unlike acute diverticulitis, complicated diverticulitis is characterized by abscess, fistula, obstruction, or perforation. Complicated disease can occur on first presentation, the presumed case with perforation, or with subsequent episodes. In a recent review of our institutional data, complicated recurrence (fistula, abscess, free perforation) occurred in only 3.9% of patients with a prior episode of acute uncomplicated diverticulitis at 5 years.[4] The differential for complicated disease is dependent on the type of disease. However, all perforated viscus can mimic perforated diverticulitis. In addition, there should be consideration to urinary tract infection as well as other genitourinary concerns.

Right-sided diverticulitis: A less than common condition in North America, right-sided disease can be asymptomatic or present as GI bleeding or a more classic inflammatory process. When inflammation of right-sided diverticulum occurs, appendicitis should be high on the differential.

Significant clinical findings suggestive of right-sided diverticulitis versus appendicitis include no real nausea, emesis, or anorexia accompanying right lower quadrant abdominal pain, as well as more variability in the maximum point of tenderness on exam.[64] The differential for right-sided diverticulitis should also include cholecystitis, gastritis, and peptic ulcer disease.[65]

SCAD: A 2009 review of 18 studies identified a prevalence rate of 1.3% to 3.8% for all diverticulitis cases.[66] Affected patients are more commonly male and middle-aged at the time of onset. Similar to acute diverticulitis, typical presenting symptoms include crampy abdominal pain, but the patient with SCAD also frequently describes diarrhea, tenesmus, and intermittent hematochezia,[3,36] with variable symptom duration. Evaluation by colonoscopy often reveals congested, friable, or granular luminal mucosa, with superficial ulcerations confined most often to the crests of colonic folds, sparing diverticular openings, the rectum, and areas of the colon unaffected by diverticula.[9,57] On pathology review, focal chronic colitis is seen with lymphomononuclear infiltration of the lamina propria, with crypt abscesses and distorted architecture, and prominent basal lymphoid aggregates.[3,9,57] In addition, biopsies of the rectum are normal in this disease, which is often mistakenly diagnosed as IBD.[9]

SUDD: Because diverticulitis has been traditionally considered to be a disease of discrete attacks with resolution of symptoms, management of chronic low-grade symptoms without evidence of clear pathologic changes is a fairly new problem. Clinically, SUDD is a condition that often presents with symptoms similar to IBS but in the presence of diverticulosis and occurring most commonly after an attack of acute diverticulitis.[6,9,21] It is difficult to differentiate if patients with SUDD are experiencing symptoms from their diverticular burden or if they simply have diverticulosis and IBS. It is thought that following an attack of acute diverticulitis, low-grade symptoms can impact patients' health-related quality of life, lasting well beyond the resolution of their acute symptoms.[57,68,69] Given the diagnostic challenges, not everyone is convinced of the presence of SUDD, questioning the premise that diverticulosis can be associated with chronic GI symptoms.

Crohn disease: Segmental Crohn inflammation in the same location as diverticulosis can be difficult to distinguish from acute diverticulitis. There is substantial commonality of symptoms for these two entities, including constipation, diarrhea, mucous discharge, abdominal pain, weight loss, and fever. CT scans will similarly identify segmental colon wall thickening, pericolonic stranding, and abscess/fistula.[70] Longer duration of disease is more consistent with Crohn disease. Crohn disease is also differentiated from SCAD by ongoing disease beyond diverticula, with aphthous erosions, ulcerations, and cobblestone appearance of colonic mucosa.[70] An evaluation of the small bowel is of some value in ruling out Crohn disease as well.

TREATMENT OF DIVERTICULAR DISEASE

DIVERTICULOSIS TREATMENT

There are almost no evidence-based recommendations for diverticulosis. Asymptomatic patients should be counseled about the differences between diverticulosis and active disease. Ultimately, however, no dietary changes are necessary. There should be some effort to improve daily fiber intake to reduce high colonic pressures and reduce the risk of diverticulitis.

DIVERTICULAR BLEEDING TREATMENT

As stated earlier, diverticular bleeding is the most common cause of acute lower GI bleeding in the United States. It is challenging to know exactly how often diverticulosis causes bleeding, as bleeding ceases without intervention in the vast majority of cases. When treatment is necessary, however, treatment options include endoscopic, radiologic, and surgical techniques. Endoscopic measures include clips, injections, and cautery, and have low rates of recurrence and complication.

Radiologic approaches use vasopressin and/or embolization, which has excellent success rates and low recurrence rates. However, postembolization ischemia is a concern and is reported in 5% to 10% of cases. When these techniques are unsuccessful or not available, surgical resection may be necessary. Patients with recurrent severe diverticular bleeds should be considered for surgery; however, it is unclear how many episodes of diverticular bleeding should prompt surgery. Surgical resection is most successful when the bleed can be localized, as total colectomy is a drastic option with high morbidity and mortality. Furthermore, blind segmental resection is associated with high bleeding recurrence; thus total or subtotal colectomy should be considered when bleeding cannot be localized.

MEDICAL TREATMENT

The mainstay of treatment for acute diverticulitis has consisted of antibiotics directed at the bacterial flora of the GI tract. A number of antibiotic combinations have been used and are generally administered for 7 to 10 days.

Outpatient versus inpatient treatment: Depending on the severity of disease, patients may be treated as an inpatient or outpatient. Patients with localized abdominal pain and tenderness without system signs of toxicity may be treated as outpatients. Ideal candidates for outpatient treatment are patients who are able to tolerate liquids; are reliable with no cognitive, social, or psychiatric impairment; are not immunosuppressed; and have no signs of toxicity. Dietary restriction to either clear liquids or a low residue diet is common, but not supported by evidence. The DIVER trial randomized patients older than 18 years with acute uncomplicated diverticulitis diagnosed by abdominal computed tomography to hospitalization or to outpatient treatment.[71] Patients were given the first dose of antibiotics intravenously in the emergency room and then randomized to inpatient or outpatient treatment. Overall, there were no differences in treatment failure rate among the two groups and no differences in quality of life. The overall health care costs with outpatient treatment were much less (1124 euros per patient) than patients treated as inpatients. Of the 132 patients entered into the trial, 4 patients in the inpatient group and three patients in the outpatient group failed treatment.[71] Etzioni and coworkers also looked at the role of outpatient treatment for diverticulitis. Factors associated with failure of outpatient treatment included female sex and the presence of free fluid on initial CT scans.[15]

Role of antibiotics: Antibiotics aimed at the coverage of GI flora have been the mainstay of treatment, with the prevailing wisdom that diverticulitis represents a primary bacterial infection with associated infection and/or microperforation. This presumption has been challenged by an alternate hypothesis suggesting that diverticulitis represents an inflammatory process. Several studies have looked at treatment with no antibiotics, with equivalent results to patients treated with antibiotics. The AVOD (antibiotics in uncomplicated diverticulitis) study was a multicenter study of 623 patients with uncomplicated left-sided diverticulitis diagnosed by CT scan.[72] Patients were randomized to either intravenous fluid without antibiotics or intravenous fluid and antibiotics. All patients were treated in the inpatient setting. There was no difference in outcome in patients treated with antibiotics versus those patients who were not treated with antibiotics. A subsequent Cochrane review of three randomized trials of patients with uncomplicated diverticulitis who were randomized to antibiotics or no antibiotics had the same findings.[73] An additional trial looked at 528 patients at 22 sites in the Netherlands and compared observation versus antibiotics for patients with CT-proven uncomplicated acute diverticulitis.[74] The primary end point was time to recovery in a 6 month follow-up period, and secondary end points were readmission, development of complicated, ongoing or recurrent diverticulitis, the need for sigmoid resection, mortality, and length of stay. There was no difference in the two groups in any of the end points except length of stay, and patients who were given antibiotics had a day longer length of stay (3 vs. 2 days) than patients who did not receive antibiotics. These studies challenge our conventional principles with respect to treatment of diverticulitis, and although it is not common practice at present to omit antibiotics in patients with acute uncomplicated diverticulitis, there is accumulating evidence to support this practice. The studies on omitting antibiotics have been done on inpatients, and there are no studies thus far of outpatient treatment omitting antibiotics.

Role of colonic evaluation: Colonoscopy is generally not recommended during an acute attack of diverticulitis because of the concern for insufflation of air with the scope causing perforation (or unsealing of a walled-off perforation or segment of diverticulitis). Following treatment of uncomplicated diverticulitis, the majority of patients improves and has no further diverticulitis issues. Current clinical practice guidelines recommend colonic evaluation approximately 6 to 8 weeks following recovery from an attack of diverticulitis to visualize the mucosa and exclude another diagnosis such as IBD or cancer (in patients who have not had recent colonic evaluation).[51] However, the majority of patients who have been diagnosed with diverticulitis, particularly those who have been hospitalized, have undergone a CT scan of the abdomen and pelvis and the role of additional colonic imaging has been questioned, particularly with the use of 64 and 128 slice CT scanners. More recent evidence suggests that routine colonic evaluation may not be necessary in patients with uncomplicated diverticulitis but should be performed in patients who have recovered

from complicated diverticulitis because of a high risk of underlying colorectal cancer. A recent study looked at the role of colonoscopy after treatment of Hinchey I and II left-sided diverticulitis in a cohort of 110 patients who had been diagnosed with diverticulitis and undergone CT scan as part of the evaluation. They suggested that patients only undergo follow-up colonoscopy if the CT scan suggested malignancy, if the patient has nonspecific inflammatory findings, or if the patient is otherwise due for routine screening or surveillance and not be used as routine follow-up.[75] Obviously these are small numbers, and the operating surgeon must consider the potential consequences of a missed neoplasm or error in diagnosis. It is our practice to continue to use endoscopic evaluation for proper diagnosis in these patients.

Recurrence after an attack of diverticulitis is common and in a population-based study, the risk of recurrence was 8% at 1 year, 17% at 5 years, and 22% at 10 years.[76] The risk of recurrence is increased in women and in younger individuals. In contrast, older individuals and men have an increased risk of recurrence complicated by stricture, fistula, or obstruction. Patients frequently seek advice on how to decrease the risk of subsequent attacks of diverticulitis. No studies have looked at the identification of risk factors to prevent recurrent diverticulitis; however, in keeping with the knowledge of risk factors for the first episode of diverticulitis, it is reasonable to advise patients to avoid the use of nonsteroidal antiinflammatory agents, consume a high-fiber diet, and pursue vigorous physical activity.[77] There is no evidence that nuts, corn, and popcorn cause diverticulitis, and there is no reason to advise patients against them.[3] Prophylactic medical therapy with mesalamine has not been shown to reduce the risk of recurrent diverticulitis. Rifaximin and other antibiotics are not recommended to reduce the risk of recurrent diverticulitis. In addition, there is no high-quality evidence that probiotics reduce the risk of recurrent diverticulitis.

There is increasing evidence that patients may have persistent chronic GI symptoms after resolution of an acute episode of diverticulitis. These symptoms have included abdominal pain, cramping, bloating, diarrhea, constipation, and abdominal distention. One study of patients with CT-documented acute uncomplicated diverticulitis found that 45% of patients reported persistent abdominal pain and 30% had a change in bowel habits 1 year after an episode of diverticulitis.[72] An additional retrospective cohort study noted that following an episode of diverticulitis, patients had a five times increased risk of a diagnosis of IBS and a two times risk of a diagnosis of a functional bowel or mood disorder.[79]

SURGICAL TREATMENT

Indications for surgery: Indications for surgery should be stratified by recommendations for uncomplicated versus complicated diverticulitis and by elective and emergency surgery.

Uncomplicated diverticulitis—The "traditional" recommendation for surgery was elective resection after two attacks of uncomplicated diverticulitis and after one attack of complicated diverticulitis (Fig. 157.1). The number of attacks is no longer a determinant, and currently

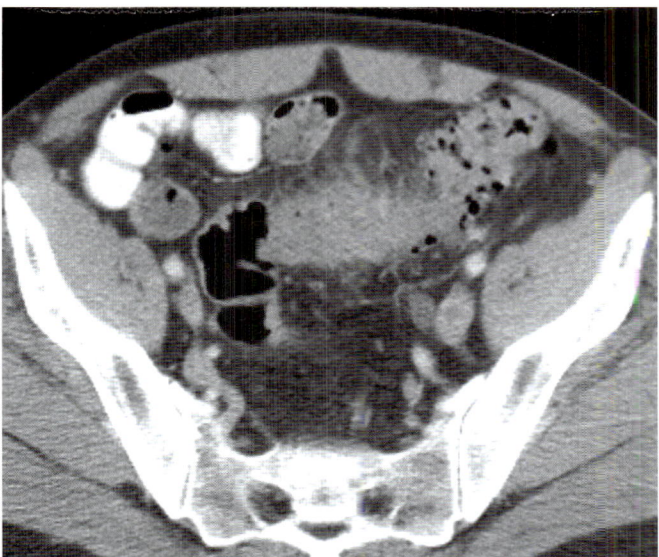

FIGURE 157.1 Computed tomography shows a long segment of uncomplicated diverticulitis with inflammation and streaky fat consistent with a phlegmon.

recommendations for surgery are individualized based on a number of patient- and disease-related factors:

- Risk of subsequent attacks of diverticulitis—long (>5 cm segment), family history
- Risk of developing complicated diverticulitis after recovery from diverticulitis—less than 5% after final episode of uncomplicated diverticulitis
- Risk of free perforation and the need for emergency surgery—immune suppression, renal failure, collagen vascular disease; severity of disease on CT
- Number of attacks and interval between attacks—greater than three episodes in 2 years

Risk of subsequent attacks of diverticulitis: Following recovery from an attack of uncomplicated diverticulitis the risk of developing a subsequent attack of diverticulitis has varied from 10% to 36%.[40] We have noted a risk of recurrence in 36% of patients who were hospitalized for diverticulitis and diagnosed by clinical criteria, with objective findings on CT scan.[4] However, the majority of patients have no further attacks of diverticulitis. Attention should be focused on identifying patients at high risk for the development of recurrent attacks of diverticulitis. Patients with a long segment of diverticulitis (>5 cm) on CT scan and those with a family history of diverticulitis are at increased risk for subsequent attacks. A cohort of patients may also have multiple attacks over a short span of time. These patients most likely have an ongoing attack of diverticulitis that has not totally resolved, or what some groups have called "smoldering diverticulitis." These patients fail to resolve symptoms despite multiple courses of antibiotics and require sigmoid resection.

Risk of developing complicated diverticulitis: The clinical course of diverticulitis appears to be determined by the first attack. Patients who present with uncomplicated diverticulitis do not necessarily progress to complicated diverticulitis. A number of large studies have noted that the risk of having a subsequent attack of complicated

diverticulitis after recovery from an attack of uncomplicated diverticulitis to be less than 5%.[81]

Risk of developing free perforation: The risk of requiring emergency surgery and stoma after recovery from an episode of uncomplicated diverticulitis is fairly low. In the past, an elective sigmoid resection was recommended after recovery from diverticulitis, to avoid an emergency resection and possible stoma. Recent data indicate that the most severe attack of diverticulitis tends to be the first attack and an emergency stoma, and/or urgent Hartmann resection is rarely required.[82] A population based study of 25,058 patients with diverticulitis from 1987 to 2001 showed that emergency operation was required in 19.6% of patients on the initial attack.[83] Of those patients who recovered, 5.5% required a subsequent emergency operation (7% of young patients). A systematic review of 85 papers showed that after recovery from one attack of diverticulitis, the risk of urgent Hartmann operation and ostomy was 1 in 2000 patient-years' follow-up.[34] Patients who are immunosuppressed, have chronic renal failure, and/or collagen vascular disease have a five times higher risk of perforation, with subsequent attacks of diverticulitis, and should be considered for early resection.[59]

Severity of disease and indications for surgery: The widespread use of CT scanning as the initial modality in patients with suspected diverticulitis in addition to history and physical examination has allowed for a more thorough assessment and grading of the severity of disease. CT findings in diverticulitis include the presence of diverticulosis, pericolic inflammation, colonic wall thickening, and abscess or fistula. The findings that correlate with severe disease include the presence of abscess, extraluminal air, and extraluminal contrast, while the findings associated with mild disease include localized sigmoid wall thickening and inflammation of the pericolic fat. The presence of any severe findings on CT scan predicts a poorer outcome with a greater chance of recurrent disease and the need for surgical intervention (Fig. 157.2).[85] In a study of 312 patients with acute left colonic diverticulitis who underwent CT scanning, the findings of abscess and extraintestinal gas 5 mm in diameter or larger correlated with unfavorable outcome of nonoperative treatment.[40]

Number and frequency of attacks: While the number of attacks of diverticulitis is no longer an indication for elective surgery, a randomized controlled trial looked at patients with three or more episodes of diverticulitis within 3 years and randomized them to laparoscopic sigmoid resection or conservative management.[86] The primary end-point was the health-related quality of life as measured by the gastrointestinal quality of life index (GIQLI). Elective sigmoid resection resulted in better quality of life in these patients compared with conservative treatment. It is therefore reasonable to recommend sigmoid resection to patients with three or more episodes of diverticulitis within a 2-year period.

ELECTIVE SURGERY

The goal of treatment for acute diverticulitis is to convert an urgent or emergent procedure into an elective procedure. After the decision has been made to proceed with elective sigmoid resection, a 4- to 6-week waiting period is generally recommended to allow the inflammatory phlegmon to

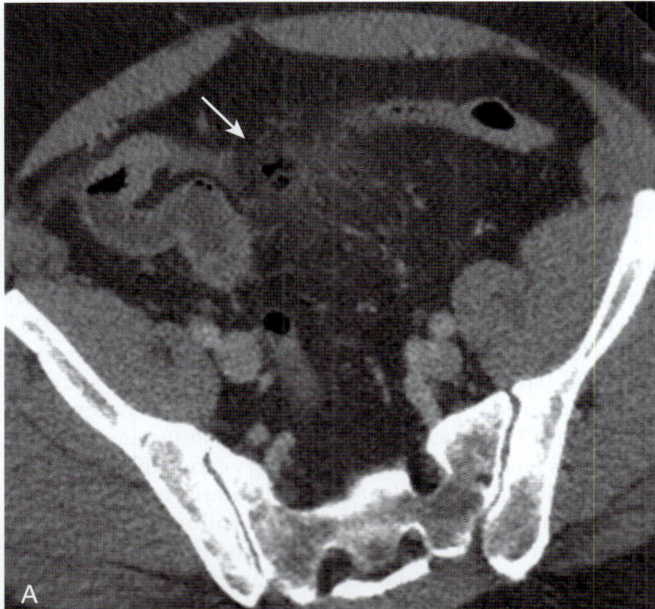

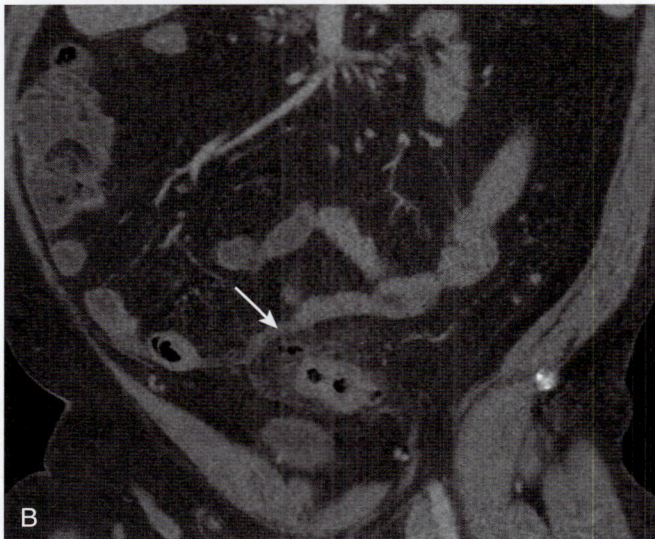

FIGURE 157.2 Computed tomography axial (A) and coronal (B) images demonstrate wall thickening and eccentric fat stranding in the mid sigmoid colon with adjacent localized perforation.

selectively and are more commonly used for reoperative surgery or in patients with an associated hydronephrosis from the inflammatory phlegmon.

While single-stage sigmoid resection may be performed by an open or laparoscopic technique, a laparoscopic technique results in shorter length of stay, quicker recovery, and less pain.[88] Increasingly, colectomy for diverticular disease is performed by a laparoscopic approach, resulting in a lower incidence of surgical site infections and sepsis, less postoperative ileus, and less adhesions. The SIGMA trial, a prospective randomized trial at five centers comparing laparoscopic and open sigmoid resection, showed a longer operating time, less blood loss, less pain, and improved quality of life (as measured by the Short Form-36 [SF-36] health questionnaire), with a laparoscopic approach and more major complications (9.6% vs. 25.0%) with an open approach.[89]

Open resection: The patient is positioned on the operating room table in lithotomy position or, if available, supine with the legs abducted on the split-leg table (to avoid prolonged lithotomy position but to allow for easy passage of the EEA stapler). A Foley catheter is inserted. The abdomen is entered through a vertical midline incision, and abdominal exploration is carried out. In the course of the dissection, the ureter and gonadal vessels are identified and preserved. Prior phlegmon or inflammation may make identification of these structures difficult; in these cases, dissecting closer to the bowel and not performing a wide resection of the mesentery mitigates the risk of injury to the ureter. If it is difficult to identify the ureter in the left lower quadrant, it may be identified more proximally away from the prior inflammatory phlegmon. Alternatively, staying close to the colon and taking the mesentery just adjacent to the colon also may decrease the risk of ureteral injury. Some studies have suggested that preservation of the superior mesenteric artery may improve blood flow and decrease the risk of anastomotic leak. Dissection is carried down to the pelvic brim/sacral promontory and distally, as needed to mobilize the rectum, to facilitate passage of a sizer and ultimately the circular stapler. The proximal rectum, which is the intended distal resection margin, is identified by the splaying of the taenia. Splenic flexure mobilization is often needed to allow for a tension free anastomosis. The proximal resection margin is soft pliable bowel that is free of diverticulitis. While the extent of resection is generally the sigmoid colon, at times inflammation of the distal descending colon requires a wider resection.

It is helpful to pass the sizer through the rectum to ensure adequate mobilization and subsequent easy passage of the circular stapler. The rectum is transected with a linear stapler and a purse-string is placed in the more proximal bowel. While a handsewn or stapled anastomosis may be performed, a stapled anastomosis is technically easier using the circular stapler. An air leak test is performed to test the integrity of the anastomosis by occluding the bowel proximal to the anastomosis and insufflating through either a proctoscope or a flexible sigmoidoscope after filling the pelvis with saline. Standard abdominal closure is performed.

Laparoscopic resection: The preoperative considerations are similar to open surgery with exceptions of consideration of prior abdominal surgery and BMI. Adhesions from

resolve and maximize the chance of an uncomplicated single-stage sigmoid resection. For patients who have not had a recent evaluation of the colon, colonoscopy is performed to evaluate the more proximal colon and exclude pathology such as an underlying colon cancer or IBD. While mechanical bowel preparation has been debated prior to elective colon surgery, recent data suggest that preparation combined with oral antibiotics decreases the risk of surgical site infection.[87] Bowel preparation also makes handling the colon easier during laparoscopic surgery and facilitates passage of the stapler through the rectum. Standard intravenous antibiotic prophylaxis is administered, as well as venous thrombosis prophylaxis. The elective diverticulitis case is ideal for use of an enhanced recovery pathway. Ureteral stents may be employed prior abdominal surgery may preclude the ability to safely perform a laparoscopic resection. Morbidly obese patients should be counseled as to a higher risk of conversion to open surgery because of the technical challenges with laparoscopic procedures (although, on occasion, a laparoscopic approach is easier than an open approach in such patients), or even the inability of such patients to physiologically tolerate the Trendelenburg position, which is needed in the course of the resection. The patient is placed on the split-leg table with the legs abducted or if such a table is not available, in modified lithotomy position. The arms are tucked and the patient is secured to the table with a beanbag and with taping around the chest.

Entry into the abdomen is either by a Hasson technique (preferred) or with a Veress needle and pneumoperitoneum is established. Port placement may vary based on patient anatomy and surgeon preference but generally includes a supraumbilical port, right and left lower quadrant ports, and a right upper quadrant port. A lateral to medial or a medial to lateral approach for mobilization of the colon may be employed, depending on surgeon preference. Many surgeons prefer to perform these procedures with a hand-assist approach. Insertion of the hand may facilitate dissection in cases with significant fibrosis or phlegmon, where the ability to use a hand to "pinch off" adhesions is helpful. Some studies have also shown a lower conversion rate with a hand-assisted technique compared with a straight laparoscopic technique.[90,91]

For a lateral to medial approach, the sigmoid and rectosigmoid are retracted medially, and incision is made along the line of Toldt and continued up toward the splenic flexure and down to the sacral promontory and the rectosigmoid junction. The ureter and gonadal vessels are identified. The peritoneum is incised and a window created to ligate the inferior mesenteric artery. The ureter can at times be confused with the superior rectal artery, and both should be identified prior to transection.

Medial to lateral mobilization allows for immediate identification of the plane between the retroperitoneum and the mesocolon. The inferior mesenteric artery is identified and transected, and the colon is then mobilized in the above place in a lateral direction toward the line of Toldt. Both the medial to lateral and the lateral to medial techniques are safe, and the surgeon should be facile with both techniques. A significant inflammatory phlegmon and foreshortened mesentery, as is seen in cases of recurrent diverticulitis, can render the medial to lateral technique difficult and at times impossible to perform. Proximal and distal resection margins are identified as outlined previously and anastomosis is performed. Air leak testing is routinely performed.

Robotic resection: Robotic-assisted sigmoid resection may be performed for sigmoid diverticulitis. The potential benefit of this technique and cost compared to laparoscopic or open resection continue to be evaluated.

COMPLICATED DIVERTICULITIS

The treatment of complicated diverticulitis is based on the type of complication—that is, abscess, fistula, obstruction, and/or perforation. Complicated diverticulitis is further subcategorized into acute complicated diverticulitis (including diverticular abscess, perforation, and obstruction) and

chronic complicated diverticulitis (including diverticular stricture and fistula). A large number of patients with complicated diverticulitis ultimately require sigmoid resection, and the goal of treating such patients is to improve quality of life and reduce further complications. It is our practice to try to convert an urgent or emergent operation into an elective procedure performed as a single stage with primary anastomosis and without the need for fecal diversion, when possible. Although prior guidelines recommended surgery after one episode of complicated diverticulitis, a more conservative approach has been recently advocated.[40,51,92]

Diverticular fistulas: Fistulas associated with diverticulitis may occur in any adjacent organ and include colovesical, colovaginal, coloenteric, and colocutaneous fistulas. Many patients with diverticular fistulas present with relatively few abdominal symptoms as the septic process has necessitated to an adjacent organ. As such, many patients may present to another specialist first, such as a woman with a colovaginal fistula presenting to a gynecologist with complaints of vaginal discharge.

There is good consensus internationally about recommendations for resection for patients with diverticular fistulas. More conservative options are available for high-risk patients including a diverting colostomy without resection or the use of antibiotics for suppression in selected patients.[93]

Colovesical fistulas are the most common type of diverticular fistula (Fig. 157.3). Presenting signs and symptoms include pneumaturia, fecaluria, and polymicrobial urinary tract infections. In taking a history from the patient there may be no obvious prior attack of diverticulitis. The best test to diagnose a colovesical fistula is a CT scan; the presence of air in the bladder in the absence of prior instrumentation is diagnostic of a fistula. While the majority of colovesical fistulas occur from diverticular disease, it is important to exclude a diagnosis of colorectal cancer (which would change the operative approach). Cystoscopy or cystogram may also be used for evaluation. Colonoscopy is helpful to visualize the mucosa and exclude the diagnosis of a perforating colon cancer. The majority of patients with a colovesical fistula may undergo a single-stage open or laparoscopic sigmoid resection where the fistula is pinched off, omentum (if available) is used to interpose between the anastomosis and the bladder, leaving a Foley catheter in place. The fistula orifice to the bladder is sutured or, if not readily apparent, left in situ without suture repair. Ureter stents are not routinely used but may be considered on a case-by-case basis, particularly in the presence of a significant inflammatory phlegmon. A cystogram is generally performed prior to removing the Foley catheter.

Colovaginal fistulas occur almost exclusively in women who have undergone prior hysterectomy (Fig. 157.4). Presenting signs and symptoms include vaginal discharge and passage of air or stool per vagina. A limited Gastrografin enema is helpful to delineate the trajectory of the fistula tract if it is not apparent on CT scan. On occasion a vaginogram is needed to delineate the fistula. A perforated colon cancer can present with similar signs and symptoms, and colonoscopy is helpful to visualize the mucosa. A similar operative approach to that of a

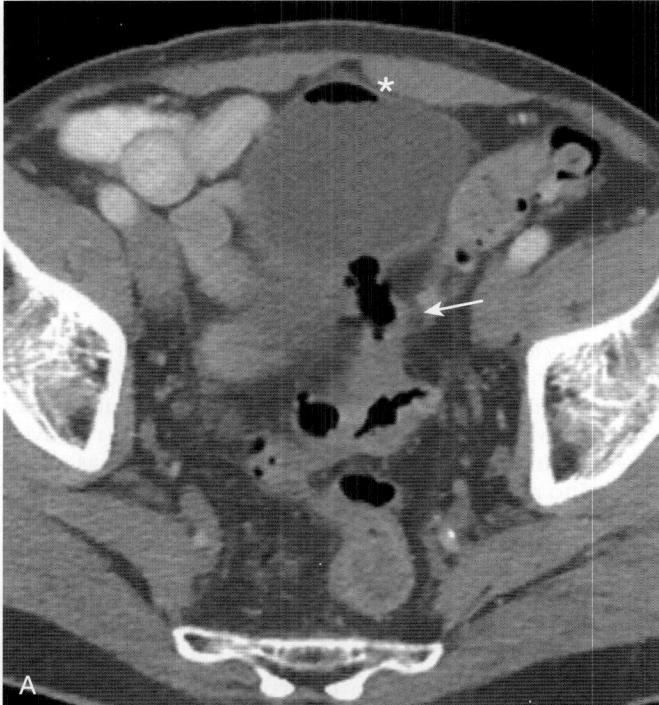

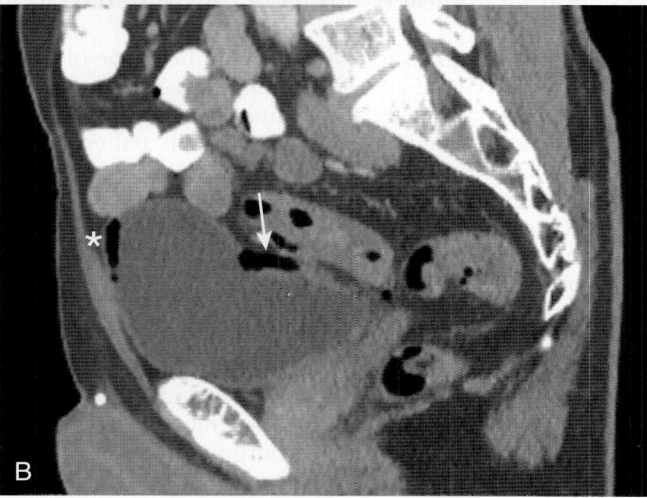

FIGURE 157.3 Contrast-enhanced axial (A) and sagittal (B) computed tomography images show colovesical fistula *(arrows)* with air in the urinary bladder *(asterisk)*.

TABLE 157.1 Hinchey Classification

Stage 1	Pericolic abscess or phlegmon
Stage II	Pelvic, intraabdominal, or retroperitoneal abscess
Stage III	Generalized purulent peritonitis
Stave IV	Generalized fecal peritonitis

MODIFIED HINCHEY CLASSIFICATION

Stage 0	Mild clinical diverticulitis
Stage Ia	Confined pericolic inflammation-phlegmon
Stage Ib	Confined pericolic abscess
Stage II	Pelvic, distant intraabdominal or retroperitoneal abscess
Stage III	Generalized purulent peritonitis
Stave IV	Generalized fecal peritonitis

Classification of perforated diverticulitis based on the original Hinchey classification.
Modified after Hinchey EJ, Schaal PG, Richards GK. Treatment of perforated diverticular disease of the colon. *Adv Surg.* 1978;12;85–109.

Diverticular stricture: Strictures and resultant partial large bowel obstruction may also occur as a result of multiple attacks of diverticulitis or potentially smoldering/chronic disease (Fig. 157.6). Many patients do not present with complete large bowel obstruction but rather with progressive constipation and obstructive symptoms. Once again, endoscopic visualization of the mucosa is helpful to exclude other diagnoses such as colon cancer, ischemic colitis, or IBD. Colonic stenting to treat large bowel obstruction from diverticular disease can be considered but is generally less successful than stenting for colon cancer.

If the obstruction is partial and resolves, an elective resection may be performed. If the obstruction is complete and unresolving, a number of options are available, including sigmoid resection with primary anastomosis (with or without diverting ileostomy), Hartmann resection, on table lavage with primary anastomosis, or colonic stenting followed by resection (which is generally challenging).

Diverticular abscess: Diverticulitis may be associated with an abscess in approximately 10% of hospitalized patients (Figs. 157.7 and 157.8). The incidence of diverticular abscess has almost doubled from 5.9% in 1995 to 9.6% in 2005 in review of the discharge data from the Nationwide Inpatient Sample.[2] This increase may be due to the increased use of imaging with CT scan for evaluation of abdominal pain with increased detection of abscess rather than a true increase in the number of patients with abscesses. A number of staging systems have been used, but the Hinchey system (with modifications thereof) remains the most commonly used (Table 157.1). Smaller abscesses (generally defined as <4 cm) may be treated with antibiotics, without the need for percutaneous drainage or repetitive CT scans (particularly if the patient is clinically improving with decreasing pain, fever, and leukocytosis). Larger abscesses or patients who do not improve on antibiotic treatment and continue to have signs and symptoms of sepsis should undergo percutaneous drainage or washout with or without resection.

The ASCRS guidelines recommend elective resection after successful treatment by percutaneous drainage but also mention the possibility of nonoperative management,

colovesical fistula is used, pinching off the fistula (the vaginal side is generally left open for drainage and not sutured) and using omentum to interpose between the vagina and the anastomosis.

Colocutaneous fistulas may occur after percutaneous drainage of a diverticular abscess or as a consequence of an anastomotic leak after a prior anastomosis (Fig. 157.5). In a large series of 93 patients with colocutaneous fistulas, residual sigmoid colon distal to an anastomosis (i.e., not performing the anastomosis between colon and soft proximal rectum) was a major risk factor for the development of such a fistula. Unsuspected Crohn disease may also manifest as a colocutaneous fistula after sigmoid resection for diverticular disease.[94]

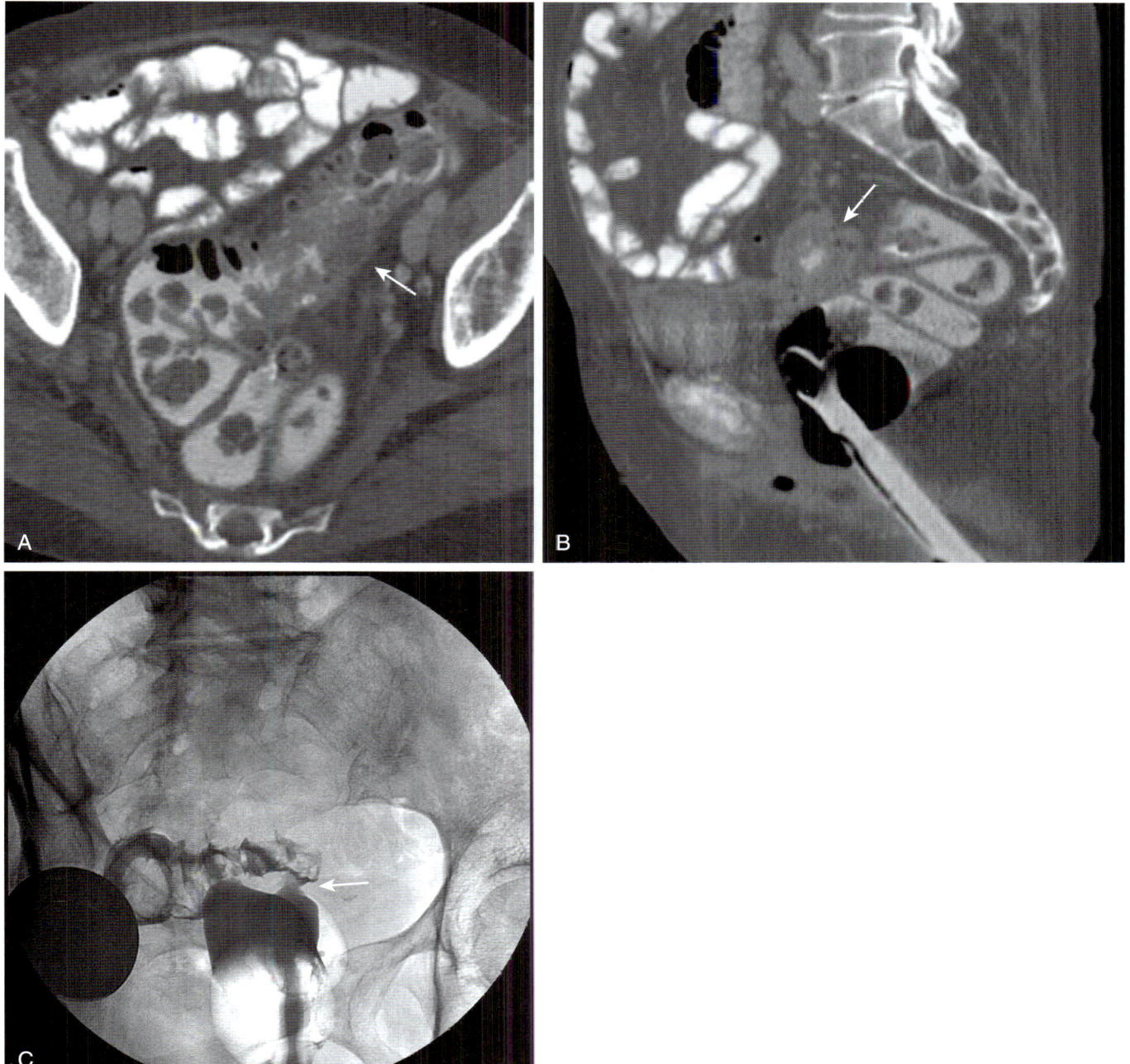

FIGURE 157.4 (A) Axial and (B) sagittal computed tomography images with intravenous, oral, and rectal contrast demonstrate marked wall thickening in the mid sigmoid colon. Colovaginal fistulas were suspected clinically but difficult to demonstrate on computed tomography *(arrows).* Follow-up vaginogram (C) clearly shows a fistulous tract from the mid sigmoid colon to the left vaginal fornix *(arrow).*

and guidelines from other organizations such as the Association of Coloproctology of Great Britain and Ireland (ACPGBI) and World Society of Emergency Surgery (WSES) recommend elective resection only for pelvic abscess.[93] In addition, others have noted that patients with pelvic abscess complicating diverticulitis have a higher rate of resection than those patients with pericolic abscess (51% vs. 71%).[95] A number of reviews assessing this heterogeneous group of patients have led to varying conclusions. A review of 218 patients who underwent

percutaneous drainage for diverticular abscess noted that 42% of patients had a single recurrence, and no patient had a second recurrence.[96] There were no late operations, and they concluded that observation was safe in these patients. Another study of 210 patients with diverticular abscess concluded that colectomy should be performed, and in this cohort 60% had a recurrent abscess, and of the 65 patients who underwent percutaneous drainage, 6% had an urgent operation and 69% had a recurrent abscess.[97] The largest review was of 22 studies with 1051 patients

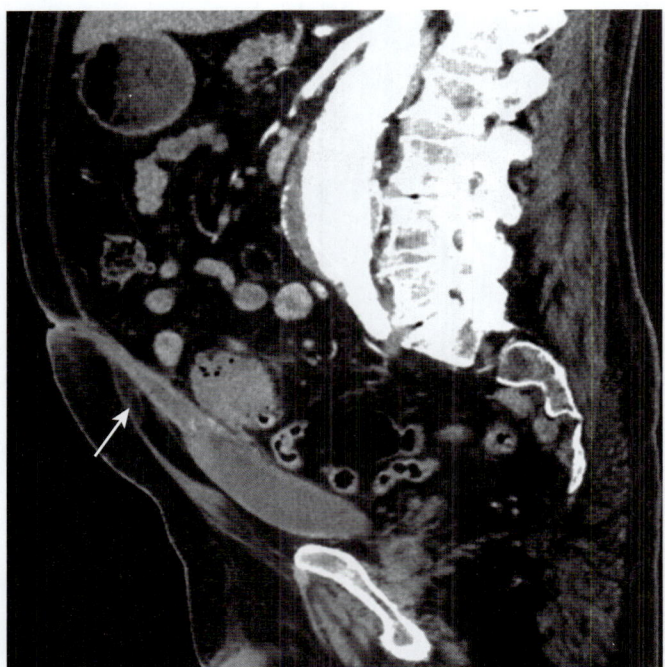

FIGURE 157.5 Colocutaneous fistula in association with diverticulitis with fistula to the abdominal wall and umbilicus. Most colocutaneous fistulas occur after surgery.

with acute diverticulitis with abscess (modified Hinchey grade Ib and II), and in this group percutaneous drainage was successful in 49% and antibiotics were successful in 14%. Only 28% of patients had no surgery and no recurrence in the follow-up period. Recurrence was most common in the first 3 to 6 months, and less than 1% who were observed developed free perforation.[98] Thus, while the presence of an abscess is not an absolute indication for ultimate elective surgery, patients with complicated diverticulitis with an associated abscess appear to have a higher rate of recurrent abscess and ongoing symptoms than patients with uncomplicated diverticulitis and should be appropriately counseled.

Free perforation of diverticulitis: The optimal treatment for free perforation of diverticulitis has undergone substantial reconsideration. Despite the increase in diagnosis of diverticular abscess, the rate of free perforation appears to be stable.[2] Options include Hartmann resection, sigmoid resection with primary anastomosis (in selected patients), sigmoid resection and primary anastomosis with proximal diversion, on-table lavage with primary anastomosis, and laparoscopic lavage without resection. Hartmann resection, a procedure initially used for rectal cancer, remains one of the most common operations performed for perforated diverticulitis but has a number of drawbacks. Approximately one-third of patients never undergo reversal of the stoma. The operation has considerable morbidity and a reported mortality of up to 18.8%. Over the years, a number of other surgical options have been proposed. Fibrin glue with suture repair and omental patching of the perforation has been reported. On-table lavage in patients with colonic emergencies has largely been abandoned, since

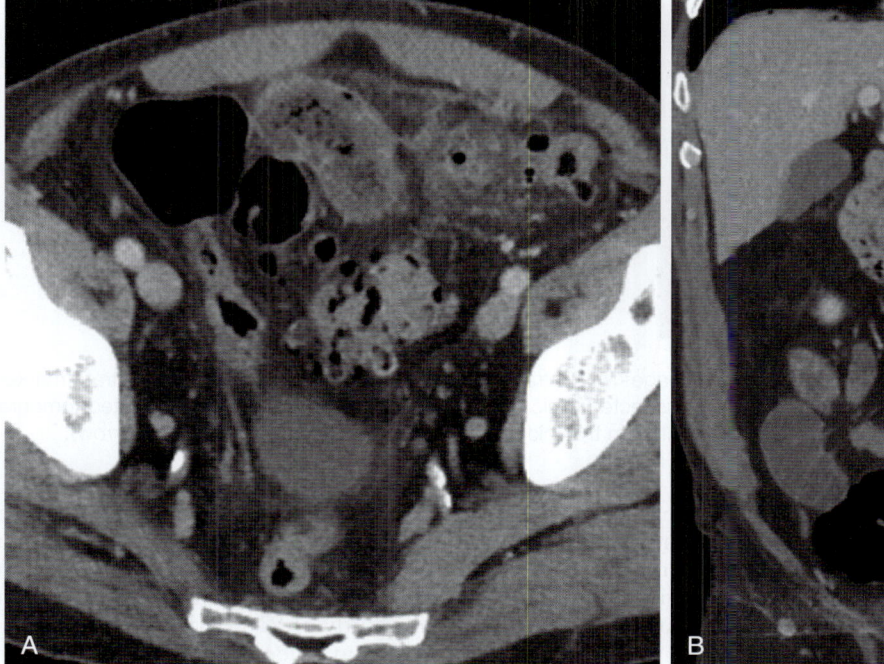

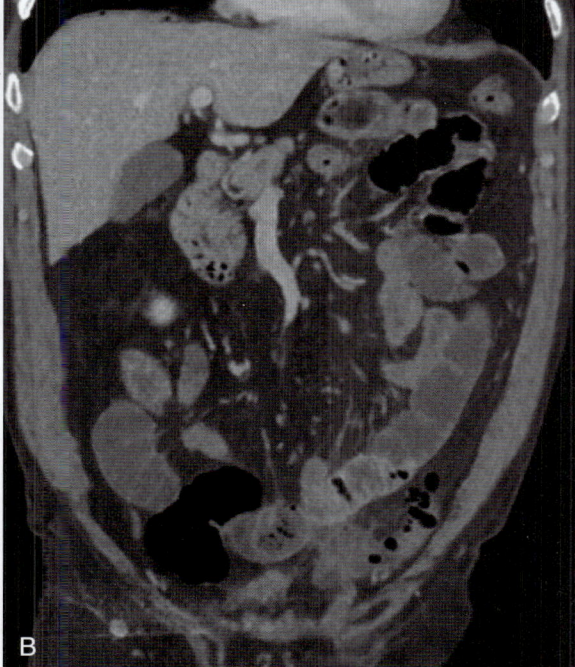

FIGURE 157.6 Computed tomography shows sigmoid diverticulitis with localized perforation and associated pericolic fat stranding and associated small bowel obstruction. Patients with diverticulitis may develop large bowel obstruction from diverticular stricture and small bowel obstruction from adherent loops of small bowel to the diverticular phlegmon.

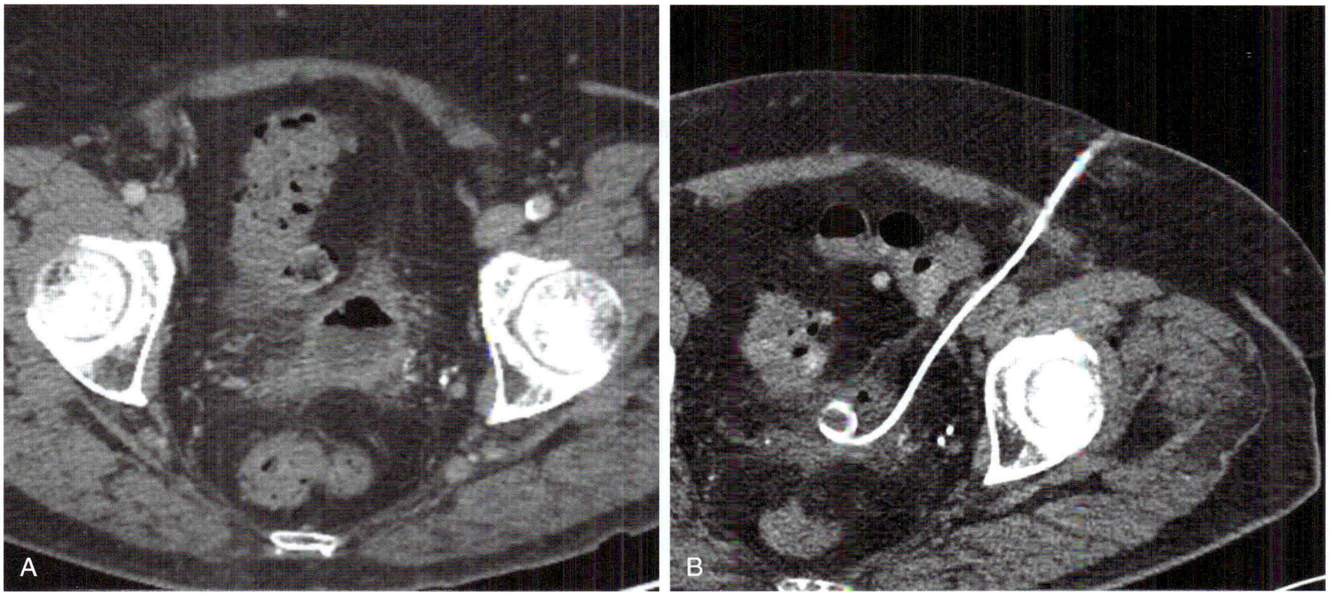

FIGURE 157.7 Pelvic abscess adjacent to the sigmoid colon and left vaginal fornix, which required percutaneous drainage.

the need for bowel preparation has been challenged by a number of reviews. A systematic review of 569 cases from 50 studies suggested that primary anastomosis with or without diversion was safe in certain patients with peritonitis, but noted a mortality of 9.9% and an anastomotic leak rate of 13.9%.[99]

An additional trial randomized a total of 62 patients with left-sided colonic perforation (Hinchey stage III or IV) to either Hartmann resection or primary anastomosis with fecal diversion (ileostomy).[100] There was no difference in outcome after initial resection, and mortality and morbidity were no different. However, the rate of stoma reversal was higher in the primary anastomosis and ileostomy group (90%) compared with the Hartmann resection group (57%). In addition, there was an increase in serious complications in the Hartmann takedown group, which led to a halt of trial accrual.

It is important to consider the necessity of surgery in all patients with evidence of perforation. The clinician must distinguish between peritonitis on physical examination and those patients who have CT findings consistent with perforation but no objective findings of toxicity or persistent leak. In the past, the finding of free air on a chest x-ray or x-ray for kidneys, ureters, and urinary bladder (KUB) was an absolute indication for laparotomy. However, the findings of free air on CT imaging do not necessarily translate into a similar recommendation. In an attempt to quantify the amount of extraluminal air, Dharmarajan and coworkers devised a predictive grading system based on size and extent of air.[101] Ultimately, the clinical status of the patient is far more important than any quantity or location of free air (Fig. 157.9).

TREATMENT OF COMPLICATED DIVERTICULITIS

Management: The majority of patients require surgery in the setting of complicated diverticulitis. However, the protocol tends to be to turn an emergent case into an elective case. Patients are placed on antibiotics, bowel rest, and supportive care.

In the setting of diverticular abscess, percutaneous techniques have helped to substantially reduce the number of emergency operations. With the widespread use of percutaneous CT drainage, patients with an abscess can now postpone surgery to a time when inflammation has largely subsided and potentially avoid stoma altogether.[51] Of patients undergoing percutaneous drainage, 2.5% experienced procedure-related complications, and 15.5% needed adjustment or replacement of the drain.[102] Today, percutaneous drainage has become the treatment of choice for the vast majority of abscesses that can be instrumented.

More recently there has been some interest in treating patients with diverticular abscess without instrumentation but rather, with antibiotics and no drainage. Considerations include abscess size, abscess location, multiplicity, patient characteristics, and other factors. A study by Siewert et al.[103] evaluated abscess size in patients with diverticulitis and demonstrated that antibiotics alone successfully managed diverticular abscesses in three-fourths of patients with abscesses less than 3 cm and half of patients with abscesses between 3 and 4 cm in size. The authors did indicate that larger abscesses were frequently treated with multiple drainage procedures. The location of the abscess in the abdomen or pelvis may also affect outcomes. Pelvic abscesses are more difficult to manage. In the study by Ambrosetti et al. of 465 patients with left-sided colonic diverticulitis, 15% of patients with mesocolic abscesses required surgery compared with 2 to 3 times more patients with pelvic abscesses.[95] Multiplicity of abscesses and/or loculated abscesses can also be a challenge to manage percutaneously. Multiple drains and needle sticks are often needed in these circumstances.

It is difficult to compare percutaneous drainage with no intervention for diverticular abscess. In a systematic review of 42 studies comparing patients treated acutely for

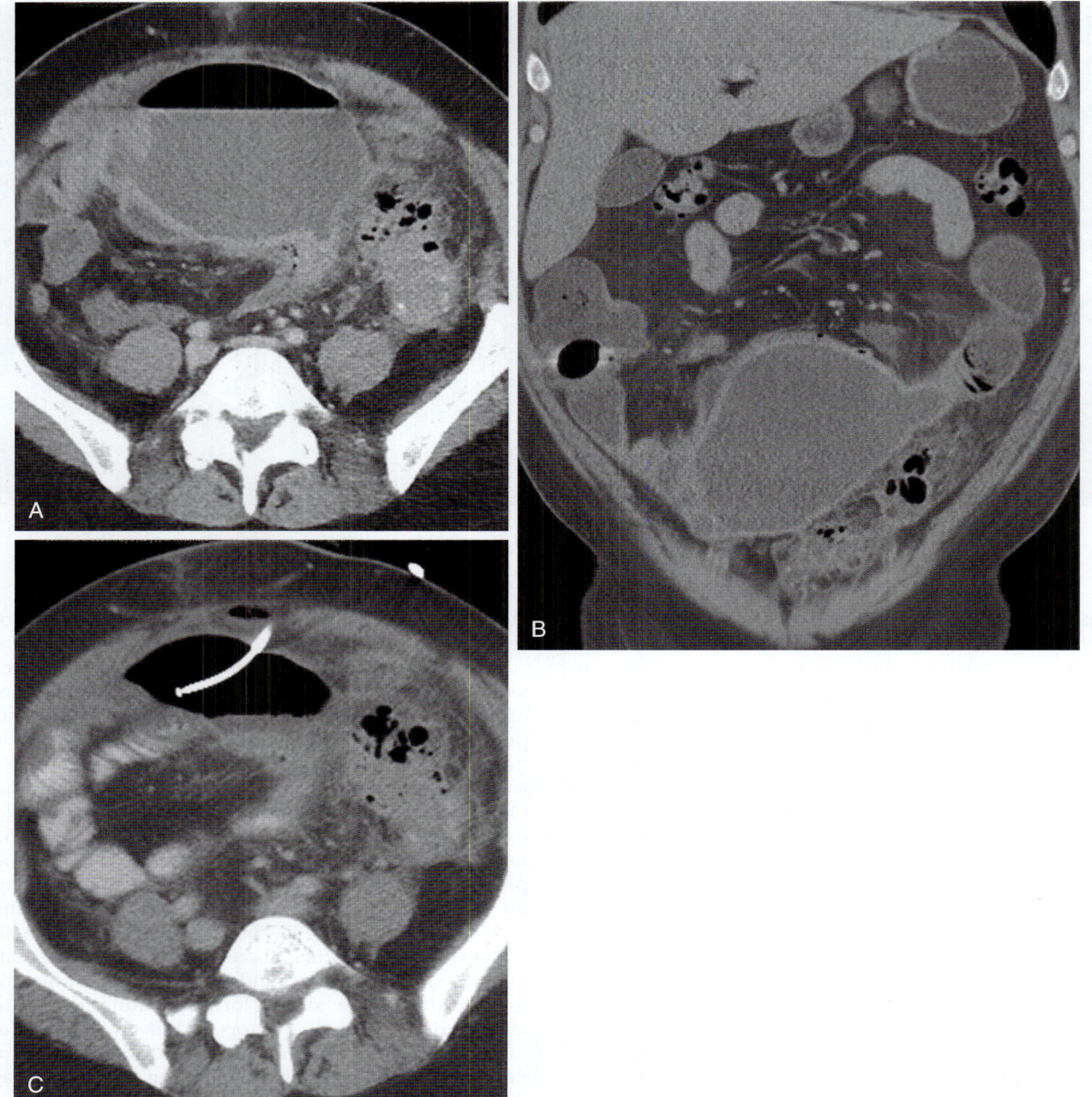

FIGURE 157.8 Axial (A) and coronal (B) computed tomography images show large abscess requiring percutaneous drainage. While small (<4 cm) abscesses may successfully be treated with antibiotics, larger abscesses require drainage (C).

Hinchey Ib and II diverticulitis, 25% of patients treated nonoperatively experienced a recurrent episode during long-term follow-up. When comparing percutaneous drainage to antibiotic treatment alone, percutaneous treatment led to substantially fewer recurrences. In addition, patients who underwent emergent surgery had increased risk of death compared with patients treated with percutaneous drainage alone.[102] At this time, the American Society of Colon and Rectal Surgeons recommends that small abscesses of 3 to 4 cm should be managed medically without percutaneous drainage unless there is a lack of response. The ASCRS also recommends percutaneous drainage for stable patients with larger diverticular abscesses.[51]

Hartmann resection: The Hartmann resection was originally described in 1923 as an alternative to abdominoperineal resection in patients with rectal cancer. The procedure quickly became the most commonly performed procedure for patients with perforated diverticulitis. In the second half of the 20th century, it gradually replaced the three-stage procedure of initial colostomy, subsequent resection, and ultimately colostomy takedown that was

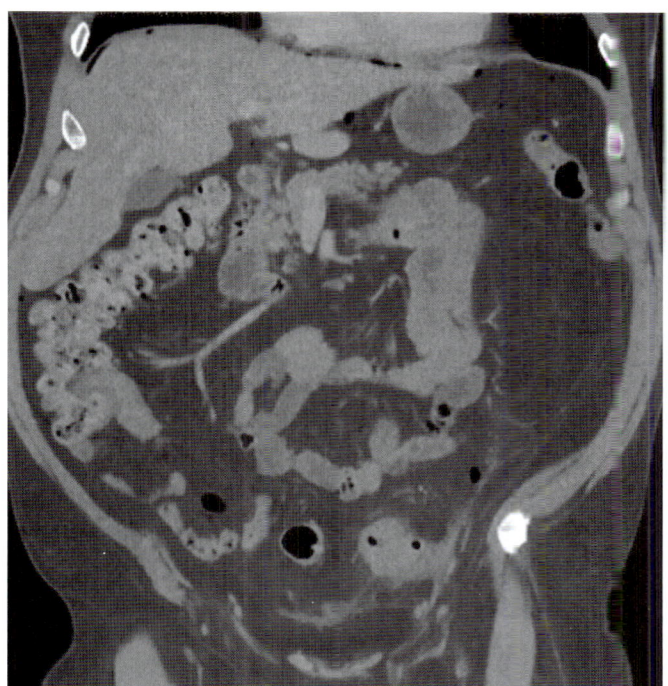

FIGURE 157.9 Perforated diverticulitis with free intraabdominal air. Depending on the clinical presentation, some patients who are stable and not septic may be treated with intravenous antibiotics.

advocated by Lockhart Mummery and by Smithwick. While a laparoscopic approach is also feasible it is more commonly done by an open approach in the emergency setting.

Primary sigmoid resection with fecal diversion: In selected urgent or emergent cases, a sigmoid resection and primary anastomosis may be performed with a diverting loop ileostomy. This procedure obviates the need for a potentially difficult Hartmann takedown in the future while mitigating the potential consequences of an anastomotic leak. If such a procedure is performed in a patient who has not had a bowel preparation, on-table lavage and cleansing of the colon should be considered.

Comparative data are lacking to guide surgical decision making in patients with free perforation of diverticulitis. However, one analysis compared primary resection and anastomosis with defunctioning stoma to Hartmann procedure in Hinchey stage III-IV perforated diverticulitis. The authors found that the probability of morbidity and mortality was lowest for Hartmann procedure and highest for primary anastomosis without diversion. However, stomas remained permanent in 27% of patients with end colostomy but in only 8% of patients with anastomosis and fecal diversion. A decision model revealed that the optimal strategy was primary anastomosis with proximal fecal diversion because of the high complication rate without diversion. However, Hartmann procedure became the optimal strategy in very high-risk patients with substantial morbidity and mortality.[104]

Laparoscopic lavage for perforated diverticulitis: There has been renewed interest in the role of laparoscopic lavage without resection for treatment of patients with perforated

diverticulitis to manage purulent peritonitis. The initial series in 1996 included eight patients with perforated diverticulitis and purulent peritonitis who underwent laparoscopic lavage as the sole treatment with no interval resection. Following lavage, patients were maintained on intravenous antibiotics.[105] At a follow-up of 12 to 48 months, no patients required subsequent resection and no patient required an emergent colostomy. The technique received little attention until the publication of a prospective multi-institutional trial in 2008 of 100 patients with perforated diverticulitis who underwent laparoscopic lavage.[106] The procedure was carried out through umbilical, suprapubic, and right lower quadrant ports, with 4 L of fluid or until the returns were clear. No attempt was made to identify and/or suture the perforation. The median patient age was 62.5 years, and follow-up was 36 months. From this total, eight patients were found to have feculent peritonitis, converted to an open Hartmann resection. Ninety-two patients were managed with laparoscopic lavage, and no patient required subsequent resection for diverticulitis. Two patients developed a pelvic abscess in the postoperative period and required drainage, and two patients presented with a subsequent attack of diverticulitis. The morbidity was 4%, and the mortality was 3%, much lower than what has historically been reported for the Hartmann procedure. Three randomized trials have recently examined the role of laparoscopic lavage in the treatment of patients with perforated diverticulitis.[107-109]

The largest trial, the SCANDIV trial, randomized patients to laparoscopic lavage versus primary resection at 21 centers in Sweden and Norway. Patients with feculent peritonitis underwent resection. The primary outcome was severe postoperative complications within 90 days, which occurred in 30.7% of patients in the laparoscopic group and 26.0% of patients in the resection group (no statistical difference). However, reoperation was much higher in the lavage group—20.3% versus 5.7% in the resection group (P = .01). The authors concluded that lavage did not reduce severe postoperative complications and led to worse outcomes. The Ladies trial looked at two groups—the LOLA group comparing laparoscopic lavage with sigmoidectomy and the DIVA group comparing Hartmann resection with sigmoidectomy and primary anastomosis. In the LOLA section of the Ladies trial, 90 patients were randomized, and the study was ultimately terminated because of an increased event rate in the lavage group. The investigators concluded that lavage was not superior to sigmoidectomy for treatment of patients with Hinchey III perforated diverticulitis (purulent peritonitis).[103] The DILALA trial compared laparoscopic lavage with resection and stoma and randomized 83 patients. Lavage resulted in no difference in mortality and morbidity, but was associated with shorter operating time and shorter hospital stay.[109]

Although the lavage data were mixed, the results do reveal some degree of comparability between lavage and resection, with significantly more postoperative abscess in the lavage group. There may be a group of patients who may best be served with lavage and do not want a stoma but need surgery to control sepsis. At this time, many questions remain. For example, which patients should be selected for lavage, should patients have subsequent resection after lavage, and what are the long-term results?

The ideal candidate for lavage has not been identified, and further classification such as use of the Mannheim peritonitis index or the peritonitis severity score may help define such patients. In addition, many series include patients initially thought to have perforated diverticulitis but ultimately noted to have perforated colon cancer, which highlights the importance of colonoscopic evaluation at some point in the postoperative period for patients in whom subsequent resection is not recommended.

A number of clinical practice guidelines have been refined to include a statement on the role of lavage. The Association of Coloproctology of Great Britain and Ireland states that "laparoscopic lavage may play a role in some patients with acute diverticulitis. Whilst this is an alternative to resection in the acute setting for some patients, it is not certain whether it is an acute alternative to delayed resection."[112] The clinical practice guidelines of the American Society of Colon and Rectal Surgeons state that "in patients with purulent or feculent peritonitis, operative therapy without resection is generally not an appropriate alternative to colectomy."[51]

Reoperative surgery: These cases can be challenging and occur for two main reasons: as a planned procedure to restore intestinal continuity after resection, stoma, and Hartmann closure of the rectum, or as an unplanned procedure to treat complications or unanticipated events after initial resection and primary anastomosis. Hartmann takedown is associated with considerable morbidity and mortality, and up to a third of patients, for a variety of reasons, never undergo stoma reversal.

Hartmann takedown (reversal): After Hartmann resection for perforated diverticulitis, most patients are eager to proceed as soon as possible with stoma reversal. These patients have often presented with free perforation as the initial manifestation of diverticulitis and never anticipated requiring a stoma for treatment. Reversal surgery may be undertaken early (<3 months from the initial surgery) or later (>3 months from the initial procedure). There are advocates of each approach and no randomized trials to guide recommendations. Proceeding with a Hartmann takedown close to the time of initial surgery has several disadvantages, predominantly due to adhesions and the acute inflammatory response after initial surgery, which may lead to a difficult dissection, potential enterotomies, and difficulty with identification of the Hartmann stump. While waiting for at least 3 months will presumably allow the patient sufficient time to heal and facilitate identification of the Hartmann stump, waiting longer may make identification of the stump more difficult secondary to fibrosis.

Prior to reversal, a Gastrografin enema through the rectum is helpful to provide an assessment of the length and configuration of the rectal segment, in addition to assessing residual sigmoid colon and/or diverticula. This protocol may be especially helpful if the surgeon reversing the Hartmann is not the same surgeon who performed the initial resection. Another advantage to this imaging study is that fecal residue may be evacuated, which ultimately helps with passing the circular stapler and the sizer. Colonoscopy or barium enema is performed through the stoma, and a mechanical bowel preparation is administered prior to surgery. The patient is placed in low lithotomy position or (preferably) on the split-leg table with the legs abducted. The procedure may be done in open or laparoscopic fashion. Initial dissection is focused on lysing adhesions of the small bowel to identify the Hartmann pouch; in the majority of cases this involves lysing the majority of the adhesions from the ligament of Treitz to the ileocecal valve. With few exceptions, there are generally small bowel adhesions or omental adhesions to the top of the Hartmann pouch. While some have advocated tacking the top of the Hartmann with a long suture, we have not found this helpful and find passing a scope or sizer per rectum more useful in identifying the Hartmann. Adhesions of the ovary and fallopian tube to the Hartmann are also quite common. Mobilization of the Hartmann pouch is carried out as needed to be able to pass the sizer. It is best to begin the rectal mobilization at the mid rectum, as the top of the Hartmann tends to be most scarred. After dissection, our preference is to re-resect the top of the Hartmann pouch. The stoma is taken down and resected and a purse-string suture placed, and the anvil of the circular stapler is secured. A circular end-to-end stapler is most commonly used, although a handsewn anastomosis may also be performed. In cases where it is difficult to pass the stapler, we prefer to staple the side of the colon to the top of the rectum. Standard air leak testing is performed.

POSTOPERATIVE CONCERNS

Risk of recurrent diverticulitis after resection: A number of patients may have persistence of abdominal symptoms following resolution of an attack of diverticulitis, and an appreciable number of patients may also have chronic or persistent abdominal pain after resection. In a study of 183 patients who had surgery for diverticulitis, 22% reported ongoing diffuse abdominal pain after resection, and 5% to 10% of patients reported no long-term relief of symptoms postoperatively.[113] The reasons for these findings are not well-defined but certainly may be related to the overlap of IBS and diverticular disease. Therefore, in approaching patients with recurrent abdominal symptoms following resection for diverticulitis, it is important to consider IBS, small bowel obstruction, anastomotic complication, and recurrent diverticulitis. Two studies have specifically addressed the risk of recurrent diverticulitis following sigmoid resection and have reported similar results. Benn and colleagues reviewed 501 patients who underwent sigmoid resection for diverticular disease at the Mayo Clinic.[114] In 321 patients, the anastomosis was performed to the distal sigmoid colon, and 12.5% of patients had recurrent diverticulitis. Anastomosis to the proximal rectum was performed in 180 patients, who had a 6.7% incidence of recurrent diverticulitis. The authors concluded that the distal resection margin should be the proximal rectum (as evidenced by the area where the taenia fan out) to decrease the risk of recurrent diverticulitis. A subsequent study at the Cleveland Clinic of 236 patients who underwent sigmoid resection for diverticular disease had similar conclusions, and the risk of recurrent diverticulitis was four times higher in patients who had a colosigmoid versus a colorectal anastomosis.[115] Of interest, there has been little focus on the proximal resection margin, and clinical practice guidelines suggest that the margin should use "soft, pliable bowel." It has also been suggested that "limited resections" have a greater tendency to develop recurrent symptoms and the ACPGBI has suggested that the splenic flexure should be routinely mobilized in patients undergoing resection for diverticulitis. As the bowel tends to be somewhat foreshortened in diverticular disease, mobilization of the splenic flexure is often necessary to perform a tension-free anastomosis.

CONCLUSION

There has been tremendous growth in knowledge and experience with diverticulitis pathophysiology, management, and surgical indications over the past few years. Yet despite these gains in knowledge, significant gaps remain in critical areas. The traditional understanding of diverticulitis as an episodic condition is now changing, and a growing body of data is noting some chronicity to the condition. In addition, information for patients regarding the role of diet, family history, and treatment need to be evidence based. With the growing focus on patient-centered outcomes, the value of colectomy in patients with diverticulitis needs to be better developed.

SUGGESTED READINGS

Connelly TM, Berg AS, Hegarty JP, et al. The TNFSF15 gene single nucleotide polymorphism rs 784647 is associated with surgical diverticulitis. Ann Surg. 2014;259:1132-1137.

Daniels L, Unlu C, de Korte N, et al. Randomized clinical trial of observational versus antibiotic treatment for a first episode of CT-proven uncomplicated acute diverticulitis. Br J Surg. 2017;104(1):52-61.

Feingold D, Steele SR, Lee S, et al. Practice parameters for the treatment of sigmoid diverticulitis. Dis Colon Rectum. 2014;57:284-294.

Penna M, Markar SR, Mackenzie H, Hompes R, Cunningham C. Laparoscopic lavage versus primary resection for acute perforated diverticulitis: review and meta-analysis. Ann Surg. 2017;doi:10.1097/SLA.0000000000002256; [Epub ahead of print].

Regenbogen SE, Hardiman KM, Hendren S, Morris AM. Surgery for diverticulitis in the 21st century. A systematic review. JAMA Surg. 2014;149(3):292-302.

REFERENCES

1. Sandler RS, Everhart JE, Donowitz M, et al. The burden of selected digestive diseases in the United States. Gastroenterology. 2002;122:1500-1511.
2. Ricciardi R, Baxter NN, Read TE, Marcello PW, Hall J, Roberts PL. Is the decline in the surgical treatment for diverticulitis associated with an increase in complicated diverticulitis? Dis Colon Rectum. 2009;52:1558-1563.
3. Strate LL, Liu YL, Syngal S, Aldoori WH, Giovannucci EL. Nut, corn, and popcorn consumption and the incidence of diverticular disease. JAMA. 2008;300:907-914.
4. Hall JF, Roberts PL, Ricciardi R, et al. Long-term follow-up after an initial episode of diverticulitis: what are the predictors of recurrence? Dis Colon Rectum. 2011;54:283-288.
5. Jacobs DO. Diverticulitis. N Engl J Med. 2007;357:2057-2066.
6. Touzios JG, Dozois EJ. Diverticulosis and acute diverticulitis. Gastroenterol Clin N Am. 2009;38:513-525.
7. Myron L. Bleeding colonic diverticula. J Clin Gastroenterol. 2008;42:1156-1158.
8. Floch MH, Bina I. The natural history of diverticulitis: fact and theory. J Clin Gastroenterol. 2004;38:S2-S7.
9. Hemming J, Floch M. Features and management of colonic diverticular disease. Curr Gastroenterol Rep. 2010;12:399-407.
10. Peery AF, Sandler R. Diverticular disease: reconsidering conventional wisdom. Clin Gastroent Hepatol. 2013;11:1532-1537.
11. Templeton AW, Strate LL. Updates in diverticular disease. Curr Gastroentero Rep. 2013;15 339.
12. Everhart JE, Khare M, Hill M, Maurer KR. Prevalence and ethnic differences in gallbladder disease in the United States. Gastroenterology. 1999;117:632-639.
13. Wilkins T, Embry K, George R. Diagnosis and management of acute diverticulitis. Am Fam Physician. 2008;87:612-620.
14. Shahedi K, Fuller G, Bolus R, et al. Long-term risk of acute diverticulitis among patients with incidental diverticulosis found during colonoscopy. Clin Gastroenterol Hepatol. 2013;11:1609-1613.
15. Etzioni DA, Chiu VY, Cannom RR, Burchette FJ, Haigh PI, Abbas MA. Outpatient treatment of acute diverticulitis: rates and predictors of failure. Dis Colon Rectum. 2010;53:861-865.
16. Hughes LE. Postmortem survey of diverticular disease of the colon. II. The muscular abnormality of the sigmoid colon. Gut. 1969;10:344-351.
17. Nakada I, Ubukata H, Goto Y, et al. Diverticular disease of the colon at a regional general hospital in Japan. Dis Colon Rectum. 1995;38:755-759.
18. Korzenik JL. Case closed? Diverticulitis: epidemiology and fiber. J Clin Gastroenterol. 2006;40:S112-S116.
19. Hobson KG, Roberts PL. Etiology and pathophysiology of diverticular disease. Clin Col Rect Surg. 2004;17:147-152.
20. Spiller RC. Changing views on diverticular disease: impact of aging, obesity, diet, and microbiota. Neurogastroenterol Motil. 2015;27:305-312.
21. Peery AF, Sandler RS, Ahnen DJ, et al. Constipation and a low-fiber diet are not associated with diverticulosis. Clin Gastroenterol and Hepatol. 2013;11:1622-1627.
22. Aldoori WH, Giovannucci EL, Rimm EB, et al. A prospective study of alcohol, smoking, caffeine and the risk of symptomatic diverticular disease in men. Ann Epidemiol. 1995;5:221-228.
23. Crowe FL, Appleby PN, Allen NE, Key TJ. Diet and risk of diverticular disease in Oxford cohort of European Prospective Investigation into Cancer and Nutrition (EPIC): prospective study of British vegetarians and non-vegetarians. BMJ. 2011;343:d4131.
24. Gear JSS, Ware A, Fursdon P, et al. Symptomless diverticular disease and intake of dietary fibre. Lancet. 1979;1:511-514.
25. Deleted in review.
26. Parks TG. Natural history of diverticulitis disease of the colon. A review of 521 cases. Br Med J. 1969;4:639.
27. Strate L, Liu Y, Syngal S, et al. Nut, corn, and popcorn consumption and the incidence of diverticular disease. JAMA. 2008;300:907-914.
28. Whiteway J, Morson BC. Elastosis in diverticular disease of the sigmoid colon. Gut. 1985 26:258-266.
29. Arfwidsson S, Knock NG, Lehmann L, Winberg T. Pathogenesis of multiple diverticula of the sigmoid colon in diverticular disease. Acta Chir Scand. 1964;342:1-68.
30. Painter NA. The aetiology of diverticulosis of the colon with special reference to the action of certain drugs on the behaviour of the colon. Ann R Coll Surg Engl. 1964;34:98-119.
31. Bassotti G, Battaglia E, Bellone G, et al. Interstitial cells of Cajal, enteric nerves, and glial cells in colonic diverticular disease. J Clin Pathol. 2005;58:973-977.
32. Bassotti G, Battaglia E, De Roberto G. Alterations in colonic motility and relationship to pain in colonic diverticulosis. Clin Gastroent Hepatol. 2005;3:248-253.
33. Slack WW. The anatomy, pathology, and some clinical features of diverticulitis of the colon. Br J Surg. 1962;50:185-190.
34. Colecchia A, Sandri L, Capodicasa S, et al. Diverticular disease of the colon: new perspectives in symptom development and treatment. World J Gastroenterol. 2003 9:1385-1389.
35. Tursi A, Brandimarte G, Giorgetti GM, Elisei W. Assessment of small intestinal bacterial overgrowth in uncomplicated acute diverticulitis of the colon. World J Gastroenterol. 2005;11:2773-2776.
36. Floch MH. The microbiome and intestinal microflora in diverticular disease. J Clin Gastroenterol. 2011;45:S12-S14.
37. Isolauri E, Sütas Y, Kankaanpää P, et al. Probiotics: effects on immunity. Am J Clin Nutr. 2001;73:444S-450S.
38. Katz LH, Guy DD, Lahat A, Gafter-Gvili A, Bar-Meir S. Diverticulitis in the young is not more aggressive than in the elderly, but it tends to recur more often: systematic review and meta-analysis. J Gastroenterol Hepatol. 2013;28:1274-1281.
39. Van de Wal BJ, Poerink JA, Draaisma WA. Diverticulitis in young versus elderly patients: a meta-analysis. Scand J Gastroenterol. 2013;48:643-651.

40. Anaya DA, Flum DR. Risk of emergency colectomy and colostomy on patients with diverticulitis disease. *Arch Surg.* 2005;140:681-685.

41. Schweitzer J, Casillas RA, Collins JC. Acute diverticulitis in the young adult is not "virulent. *Am Surg.* 2002;68:1044-1047.

42. Strate LL, Modi R, Cohen E, Spiegel BMR. Diverticular disease as a chronic illness: evolving epidemiological and clinical insights. *Am J Gastroenterol.* 2012;107:1486-1493.

43. Hjern F, Josephson T, Altman D, et al. Conservative treatment of acute colonic diverticulitis: are antibiotics always mandatory? *Scand J Gastroenterol.* 2007;42:41-47.

44. Strate LL, Liu YL, Aldoori WH, Giovannucci EL. Physical activity decreases diverticular complications. *Am J Gastroenterol.* 2009;104:1221-1230.

45. Strate LL, Liu YL, Aldoori WH, et al. Obesity increases the risks of diverticulitis and diverticular bleeding. *Gastroenterology.* 2009;136:115-122.

46. Humes DJ, Fleming KM, Spiller RC, West J. Concurrent drug use and the risk of perforated colonic diverticular diseases: a population-based case-control study. *Gut.* 2011;60:219e224.

47. Maguire LH, Song M, Strate LE, et al. Association of geographic and seasonal variation with diverticulitis admissions. *JAMA Surg.* 2015;150:74-77.

48. Maguire LH, Song M, Strate LE, et al. Higher serum levels of vitamin D are associated with a reduced risk of diverticulitis. *Clin Gastroenterol Hepatol.* 2013;11:1631-1635.

49. Tyau ES, Prystowsky JB, Joehl RJ, et al. Acute diverticulitis: a complicated problem in the immunocompromised patient. *Arch Surg.* 1991;126:855-859.

50. Hwang SS, Cannom RR, Abbas MA, Etzioni D. Deverticulitis in transplant patients and patients on chronic corticosteroid therapy: a systematic review. *Dis Colon Rectum.* 2010;53:1699-1707.

51. Feingold D, Steele SR, Lee S, et al. Practice parameters for the treatment of sigmoid diverticultis. *Dis Colon Rectum.* 2014;57:284-294.

52. Hjern F, Wolk A, Håkansson N. Obesity, physical inactivity, and colonic diverticular disease requiring hospitalisation in women: a prospective cohort study. *Am J Gastroenterol.* 2012;107:296-302.

53. Granlund J, Svensson T, Granath F, et al. Diverticular disease and the risk of colon cancer—a population-based case-control study. *Aliment Pharmacol Ther.* 2011;34:675-681.

54. Lewis M. Bleeding colonic diverticula. *J Clin Gastroenterol.* 2008;42:1156-1158.

55. Cirocchi R, Arezzo A, Renzi C, et al. Is laparoscopic surgery the best treatment in fistulas complicating diverticular disease of the sigmoid colon? A systematic review. *Int J Surg.* 2015;24(Pt A):95-100.

56. Najjar SF, Jamal MK, Savas JF, et al. The spectrum of colovesical fistula and diagnostic paradigm. *Am J Surg.* 2004;188:617.

57. Lamps LW, Knapple WL. Diverticular disease-associated segmental colitis. *Clin Gastroenterol Hepatol.* 2007;5:27-31.

58. Hinchey EJ, Schaal PG, Richards GK. Treatment of perforated diverticular disease of the colon. *Adv Surg.* 1978;12:85-109.

59. Klarenbeek BR, Samuels M, van der Wal MA, van der Peet DL, Maijerink WJ, Cuesta MA. Indications for elective sigmoid resection in diverticular disease. *Ann Surg.* 2010;251:670-674.

60. Kaiser A, Jiang J, Lake J, et al. The management of acute complicated diverticulitis and the role of computed tomography. *Am J Gastroenterol.* 2005;100:910-917.

61. Sheer AJ, Heckman JE, Schneider EB, et al. Congestive heart failure and chronic obstructive pulmonary disease predict poor surgical outcomes in older adults undergoing elective diverticulitis surgery. *Dis Colon Rectum.* 2011;54:1430-1437.

62. Morson BC, Dawson IMP. Muscular disorders. In: Morson BC, Dawson IMP, eds. *Gastrointestinal Pathology.* 2nd ed. Oxford, UK: Blackwell Scientific Publications; 1979:581-593.

63. Whitehead R, du Boulay CEH. Diverticular disease of the colon and solitary rectal ulcer syndrome. In: Whitehead R, ed. *Gastrointestinal and Oesophageal Pathology.* 2nd ed. Edinburgh, UK: Churchill Livingstone; 1991:431-437.

64. Nirula R, Greaney G. Right-sided diverticulitis: a difficult diagnosis. *Am Surg.* 1997;3:871-873.

65. Sugihara K, Muto T, Morioka Y, Asano A, Yamamoto T. Diverticular disease of the colon in Japan. A review of 615 cases. *Dis Colon Rectum.* 1984;27:531-537.

66. Mulhall AM, Mahid SS, Petras RE, Galandiuk S. Diverticular disease associated with inflammatory bowel disease-like colitis: a systematic review. *Dis Colon Rectum.* 2009;52:1072-1079.

67. Deleted in review.

68. Boles JRRS, Jordan SM. The clinical significance of diverticulos s. *Gastroenterology.* 1958;35:579-582.

69. Comparato G, Fanigliulo L, Cavallaro LG, et al. Prevention of complications and symptomatic recurrences in diverticular disease with mesalazine: a 12-month follow-up. *Dig Dis Sci.* 2007;52:2934-2941.

70. Peppercorn MA. The overlap of inflammatory bowel disease and diverticular disease. *J Clin Gastroenterol.* 2004;38:S8-S10.

71. Biondo S, Golda T, Kreisler E, et al. Outpatient versus hospitalization management for uncomplicated diverticulitis: a prospective, multicenter randomized clinical trial (DIVER trial). *Ann Surg.* 2014;259:38-44.

72. Chabok L, Påhlman F, Hjern F, Haapaniemi S, Smedh K, AVCD Study Group. Randomized clinical trial of antibiotics in acute uncomplicated diverticulitis. *Br J Surg.* 2012;99:532-539.

73. Shabanzadeh DM, Wille-Jørgensen P. Antibiotics for uncomplicated diverticulitis. *Cochrane Database Syst Rev.* 2012;14:11.

74. Daniels LUC, de Korte N. A randomized clinical trial of observational versus antibiotic treatment for a first episode of uncomplicated acute diverticulitis. *United European Gastroenterol J.* 2014;2(1S):A2.

75. Walker AS, Bingham JR, Janssen KM, et al. Colonoscopy after Hinchey I and II left-sided diverticulitis: utility or futility? *Am J Surg.* 2016;212(5):837-843.

76. Bharucha AE, Parthasarathy G, Ditah I, et al. Temporal trends in the incidence and natural history of diverticulitis: a population based study. *Am J Gastroenterol.* 2015;110:1589-1596.

77. Stollman N, Smalley W, Hirano I. American Gastroenterological Association Institute guideline on management of acute diverticulitis. *Gastroenterology.* 2015;149:1944-1949.

78. Deleted in review.

79. Cohen E, Fulller G, Bolus R, et al. Increased risk for irritable bowel syndrome after acute diverticulitis. *Clin Gastroenterol Hepatol.* 2013;11:1614-1619.

80. Deleted in review.

81. Eglinton T, Nguyen T, Raniga S, Dixon L, Dobbs B, Frizelle FA. Patterns of recurrence in patients with acute diverticulitis. *Br J Surg.* 2010;97:952-957.

82. Humes DJ, West J. Role of acute diverticulitis in the development of complicated colonic diverticular disease and 1-year mortality after diagnosis in the UK: population-based cohort study. *Gut.* 2012;61:95-100.

83. Anaya DA, Flum DR. Risk of emergency colectomy and colostomy in patients with diverticular disease. *Arch Surg.* 2005;140:681-685.

84. Janes S, Meagher A, Frizelle FA. Elective surgery after acute diverticulitis. *Br J Surg.* 2005;92:133-142.

85. Morris AM, Regenbogen S, Hardiman KM, et al. Sigmoid diverticulitis: a systematic review. *JAMA.* 2014;311:287-297.

86. Van de Wall BJM, Stam MAW, Draalsma WA, et al. Surgery versus conservative management for recurrent ad ongoing left-sided diverticulitis (DIRECT trial): an open-label, multicenter, randomized controlled trial. *Lancet Gastroenterol Hepatol.* 2017;2(1):13-22.

87. Scarborough JE, Mantyh CR, Sun Z, Migaly J. Combined mechanical and oral antibiotic bowel preparation reduces incisional surgical site infection and anastomotic leak rates after elective colorectal resection: an analysis of colectomy-targeted ACS NSQIP. *Ann Surg.* 2015;262:331-337.

88. Cirocchi R, Farinella E, Trastulli S, Sciannameo F, Audisio RA. Elective sigmoid colectomy for diverticular disease. Laparoscopic vs open surgery: a systematic review. *Colorectal Dis.* 2012;14:671-683.

89. Klarenbeek BR, Veenhof AA, Bergamaschi R, et al. Laparoscopic sigmoid resection for diverticulitis decreases major morbidity rates: a randomized control trial: short-term results of the Sigma Trial. *Ann Surg.* 2009;249:39-44.

90. Chang YJ, Marcello PW, Rusin LC, Roberts PL, Schoetz DJ. Hand-assisted laparoscopic sigmoid colectomy; helping hand or hindrance? *Surg Endosc.* 2005;19:656-661.

91. Benlice C, Costedio M, Stocchi L, Abbas MA, Gorgun E. Hand-assisted laparoscopic vs open colectomy: an assessment from the American College of Surgeons National Surgical Quality Improvement Program procedure-targeted cohort. *Am J Surg.* 2016;212:808-813.

92. Rafferty J, Shellito P, Hyman NH, Buie WD. Practice parameters for sigmoid diverticulitis. *Dis Colon Rectum.* 2006;49:939-944.

93. Vennix S, Morton DG, Hahnloser D, Lange JF, Bemelman WA. Systematic review of evidence and consensus on diverticulitis; an analysis of national and international guidelines. *Colorectal Dis.* 2014;16:866-878.

94. Fazio VW, Church JM, Jagelman DG, et al. Colocutaneous fistulas complicating diverticulitis. *Dis Colon Rectum*. 1987;30:89-94

95. Ambrosetti P, Chautems R, Soravia C, Peiris-Waser N, Terrier F. Long term outcome of mesocolic and pelvic diverticular abscesses of the left colon—a prospective study of 73 cases. *Dis Colon Rectum*. 2005;48:787-791.

96. Gaertner WB, Willis DJ, Madoff RD, et al. Percutaneous drainage of colonic diverticular abscess; is colon resection necessary? *Dis Colon Rectum*. 2013;5:622-626.

97. Devaraj B, Liu W, Tatum J, Cologne K, Kaiser AM. Medically treated diverticular abscess associated with high risk of recurrence and disease complications. *Dis Colon Rectum*. 2016;59 208-215.

98. Lamb MN, Kaiser AM. Elective resection versus observation after nonoperative management of complicated diverticulitis with abscess: a systematic review and meta-analysis. *Dis Colon Rectum*. 2014;57:1430-1440.

99. Salem L, Flum DR. Primary anastomosis or Hartmann's procedure for patients with diverticular peritonitis? A systematic review. *Dis Colon Rectum*. 2004;47:1953-1964.

100. Oberkofler CE, Rickenbacher A, Raptis DA, et al. A multicenter randomized clinical trial of primary anastomosis of Hartmann's procedure for perforated left colonic diverticulitis with purulent or fecal peritonitis. *Ann Surg*. 2012;256:819-826.

101. Dharmarajan S, Hunt SR, Birnbaum EH, Fleshman JW, Mutch MG. The efficacy of nonoperative management of acute complicated diverticulitis. *Dis Colon Rectum*. 2011;54:663-671.

102. Gregersen R, Mortensen LQ, Burcharth J, Pommergaard HC, Rosenberg J. Treatment of patients with acute colonic diverticulitis complicated by abscess formation: a systematic review. *Int J Surg*. 2016;35:201-208.

103. Siewert B, Tye G, Kruskal J, et al. Impact of CT-guided drainage in the treatment of diverticular abscesses: size matters. *AJR Am J Roentgenol*. 2006;186:680-686.

104. Constantinides VA, Heriot A, Remzi F, et al. Operative strategies for diverticular peritonitis: a decision analysis between primary resection and anastomosis versus Hartmann's procedures. *Ann Surg*. 2007;245:94-103.

105. O'Sullivan GC, Murphy D, O'Brien MG, Ireland A. Laparoscopic management of generalized peritonitis due to perforated colonic diverticula. *Am J Surg*. 1996 171:432-434.

106. Myers E, Hurley M, O'Sullivan GC, Kavanagh D, Wilson I, Winter DC. Laparoscopic peritoneal lavage for generalized peritonitis due to perforated diverticulitis. *Br J Surg*. 2008;95:97-101

107. Schultz JK, Yaqub S, Wallon S, et al. Laparoscopic lavage vs primary resection for acute perforated diverticulitis. *JAMA*. 2015;314(15):1364-1375.

108. Vennix S, Musters GD, Mulder IM, et al. Laparoscopic peritoneal lavage or sigmoidectomy for perforated diverticulitis with purulent peritonitis a multicentre, parallel-group, randomised, open-label trial. *Lancet* 2015;386(10000):1269-1277.

109. Angenete E, Thornell A, Burcharth J, et al. Laparoscopic lavage is feasible and safe for the treatment of perforated diverticulitis with purulent peritonitis: the first results from the randomized controlled trial DILALA. *Ann Surg*. 2016;263:117-122.

110. Deleted in review.

111. Deleted in review.

112. Fozard JB, Armitage NC, Schofield JB. Jones OM. Position statement on elective resection for diverticulitis colorectal surgery. *Colorectal Dis*. 2011;13:1-11.

113. Andeweg C, Peters J, Bleichrodt R, van Goor H. Incidence and risk factors of recurrence after surgery for pathology proven diverticular disease. *World J Surg*. 2008;32:1501-1506.

114. Benn PL, Wolff BG, Ilstrup DM. Level of anastomosis and recurrent colonic diverticulitis. *Am J Surg*. 1986;151:269-271.

115. Thaler K, Baig MK, Berho M, et al. Determinants of recurrence after sigmoid resection for uncomplicated diverticulitis. *Dis Colon Rectum*. 2003;46:385-388.

Hemorrhoids and Rectoceles

Skandan Shanmugan | Bradley J. Champagne | Anthony Senagore

Hemorrhoids have been referenced in ancient texts dating back 4000 years.[1,2] Included in many of these Egyptian and Greek writings are multiple recommended treatment regimens including anal dilation, topical ointments, and the intimidating red hot poker.[3,4] Although few people have died of hemorrhoidal disease, many patients wish they had, particularly after therapy, and this fact led to the sanctification of St. Fiachre, the patron saint of gardeners and hemorrhoidal sufferers.[5] This discussion will guide the practitioner in a more humane approach to hemorrhoidal disease, with the emphasis on cost-effectiveness with minimal morbidity and mortality.

ANATOMY AND ETIOLOGY

Hemorrhoids are normal vascular cushions suspended in the submucosal layer of the anal canal by longitudinal connective tissue and muscle fibers.[6] Internal hemorrhoids originate above the dentate line, while external hemorrhoids occur below this level. Mixed component hemorrhoids can occur above and below the dentate line. These vascular cushions appear predictably in the right anterior, right posterior, and left lateral positions, although there may be intervening secondary hemorrhoidal complexes that blur this classic anatomy. Their blood supply is derived from the superior rectal artery via the inferior mesenteric, the middle rectal arteries via the internal iliac arteries, and the inferior rectal arteries via the pudendal arteries that derive flow from the external iliac arteries. The venous drainage transitions from the portal venous system above the level of the dentate line to the systemic venous system below this level. The columnar epithelium of *internal hemorrhoids* is viscerally innervated and therefore not sensitive to pain, touch, or temperature. On the other hand, *external hemorrhoids* are covered by squamous epithelium anoderm, which contains an abundance of somatic pain fibers, making thrombosed external hemorrhoids extremely painful and sensitive.

The pathogenesis of symptomatic hemorrhoids is most likely due to the weakening of the connective tissue within these vascular cushions which produces bleeding, with or without prolapsing of the hemorrhoidal tissue.[7-8] These symptoms occur as a result of low-fiber dietary intake, excessive straining, chronic constipation, prolonged sitting, pregnancy, advanced age, and in patients on anticoagulation or antiplatelet therapy.[8] Many factors contribute to symptomatic hemorrhoids such as deterioration of the anchoring connective tissue that occurs with advanced age. Internal anal sphincter dysfunction may also play a role in the development of hemorrhoidal disease, and a number of investigators have demonstrated increased internal anal sphincter tone in patients with hemorrhoidal disease.[9-14] Abnormal distention or dilation of the arteriovenous formations within the hemorrhoid plexus may also play a role, although it is unclear whether this association is causal or a result of constipation and straining.[9,12]

The standard classification for hemorrhoidal diseases[13] is as follows:

- Grade I, visualized on anoscopy and may bulge into the lumen but do not prolapse below the dentate line, bleed during defecation
- Grade II, prolapse out of the anal canal with defecation or with straining but reduce spontaneously, bleed and secrete mucus
- Grade III, prolapse requiring manual reduction
- Grade IV, prolapse that cannot be manually reduced, generally mixed hemorrhoids that include internal and external components

Although this staging system tends to correlate with patients' symptoms, it is unclear that it can be completely relied on when making therapeutic decisions. Alternative anorectal pathology must be considered, such as mucosal prolapse or skin tags, to produce the symptoms.

CLINICAL EVALUATION

Only 30% of patients seen for "hemorrhoids" will actually have true hemorrhoidal disease.[15] Bleeding, protrusion, and pain are among the most common symptoms associated with hemorrhoidal disease. Hemorrhoidal bleeding from internal hemorrhoids typically results in bright red blood either on the toilet paper or may drip into the toilet at the end of defecation and is generally painless in nature. More vigorous bleeding can occur as the hemorrhoids enlarge and the hemorrhoidal complex becomes displaced and is fixed externally, allowing the blood to drip or spurt into the toilet. Patients with grade III or IV internal hemorrhoids may also complain of a sensation of fullness, fecal incontinence, and constant mucous discharge. Usually, prompt reduction of the protruding mass causes this symptom to abate. Acute thrombosed internal or external hemorrhoids are usually associated with severe pain and a palpable perianal mass or lump. These patients are generally quite uncomfortable, and the diagnosis is immediately obvious on clinical examination.

Examination of the patient with hematochezia, although tailored by the age of the patient, should include sufficient investigations to rule out a proximal source of bleeding such as inflammatory bowel disease and neoplasia. Other anorectal pathologies should also be considered as sources of pain, such as fissures, fistulas, abscesses, or neoplasm. We prefer to examine the patient in the prone jackknife position using the proctology table. This approach allows relative patient comfort and the ability to clearly inspect the perianal skin and perform anoscopy and proctosigmoidoscopy. Digital rectal examination should be performed at rest and with straining and should include palpation for masses, fluctuance, tenderness, and characterization of anal sphincter tone. Internal hemorrhoids are generally not palpable on digital examination in the absence of thrombosis. In addition, a thrombosed hemorrhoid is extremely tender to palpation, and a thrombus may be palpable within the hemorrhoid. The presence of thickening or scar in the posterior midline or roughening of the otherwise smooth anoderm is suggestive of a partially healed anal fissure. Hypertrophic, edematous eccentrically placed, and tender skin tags should raise suspicion for the underlying Crohn disease. An assessment of the sphincter tone and history of fecal incontinence should also be obtained, as this information may alter your surgical planning. In contrast, in the absence of a thrombosed external hemorrhoid, an anoscopy should be performed to evaluate the anal canal and the distal rectum. Internal hemorrhoidal bundles appear as bulging purplish-blue veins, and prolapsed internal hemorrhoids appear as dark pink, glistening, and sometimes tender masses at the anal margin. Thrombosed external hemorrhoids are acutely tender and have a purplish hue. Anoscopy has the advantage of being a quick, relatively painless, inexpensive procedure that can be performed in an unprepped patient to diagnose hemorrhoids and exclude other distal anorectal disorders.

If hemorrhoids or other pathology is not found, a colonoscopy should be done regardless of age, to rule other pathologic sources for the rectal bleeding. While performing a colonoscopy or flexible sigmoidoscopy, the distal rectum and anal verge should be inspected in retroflexion with the rectum partially insufflated. Complete insufflation should be avoided, as this causes the rectal vault to distend and stretch, thereby flattening internal hemorrhoids.

NONOPERATIVE TREATMENT

The initial and most efficacious nonoperative treatment for hemorrhoidal disease is implementation of fiber and increased liquid intake. A systematic review and meta-analysis showed significant resolution of hemorrhoidal symptoms by more than 50% at 6 weeks and incrementally more at 3 months.[16] Further randomized controlled trials of 20 g of psyllium/day versus placebo showed symptomatic relief in 84% versus 54% of the patients.[17] Patients should also be advised to implement other lifestyle modifications such as avoiding prolonged sitting or straining on the toilet, perianal hygiene, and avoiding foods or other triggers for constipation. The main goal of nonoperative treatment is to reverse the pathology of hemorrhoidal disease and to provide symptomatic relief. The downside of nonoperative therapy is that it may take several weeks to manifest and requires a great deal of patience and compliance.

Various topical agents propose to reduce hemorrhoidal symptoms, but in reality, these agents are aimed at providing symptomatic relief rather than altering the pathophysiology of hemorrhoidal disease.[15] These preparations include local anesthetics, vasoactive agents, and corticosteroids. Although these treatments are plentiful, randomized controlled trials regarding their efficacy in comparison to other modalities are sparse.

OFFICE-BASED PROCEDURES

Several office procedures are now commonly used in the management of symptomatic hemorrhoidal disease. Modalities include infrared coagulation, sclerotherapy, and rubber band ligation. Other novel techniques are constantly being introduced and evolving, but they are at their infancy and studies are lacking to reinforce their efficacy. The underlying mechanisms in all these techniques rely on tissue destruction and/or fixation.

Sclerotherapy

The use of sclerotherapy to treat symptomatic internal hemorrhoidal disease was first advocated by Mitchell in 1871[18] and typically involves injecting a sclerosing agent into the submucosa, resulting in atrophy of the tissue and scarification with fixation of the hemorrhoidal complex within its normal location in the anal canal. A variety of injecting solutions have been advocated, although it appears that sodium morrhuate and sodium tetradecyl sulfate currently predominate. This modality is most effective in situations with minimal enlargement of hemorrhoidal complexes where the primary complaint is bright red rectal bleeding.[18–20]

The procedure is performed with the patient in the left lateral decubitus or prone jackknife position. An anoscope is inserted to clearly identify the hemorrhoid complex and a 25-gauge spinal needle is used to instill the sclerosant into the submucosal space (Fig. 158.1). The syringe should be aspirated before injection to avoid a direct intravascular injection. Typically, 3 to 5 mL of sclerosant is adequate. The surgeon can inject as many locations as desired, because the procedure is essentially painless. It is important, however, not to circumferentially inject the anal canal, because this may induce stricture formation. Other described complications, although rare, include bacteremia, pelvic sepsis, prostatic abscesses, creation of rectourethral fistulas, rectal perforations, and necrotizing fasciitis.[21–26] Success rates of 75% to 89% have been reported in patients with grades I to III disease.[18–20,27–30] However, longer follow-up intervals often demonstrate a relatively higher rate of symptomatic recurrence.[?] The ideal candidates may be patients with bleeding tendencies or those on antiplatelet or anticoagulation therapy, since this provides a less invasive and perhaps less bloody alternative to excisional hemorrhoidectomy.

Bipolar Diathermy, Infrared Coagulation, Direct Current Therapy

Bipolar diathermy employs electrical current to coagulate the hemorrhoidal tissue, including the mucosa and submucosa.[31,32] The machine generates a 2-second pulse of energy to accomplish the treatment. Once again, this approach is applicable for small bleeding hemorrhoids and probably has no greater efficacy than sclerotherapy. Other variations on the use of energy to destroy internal hemorrhoids include infrared coagulation and Ultroid (direct-current) therapy.[33] Infrared coagulation uses a tungsten halogen lamp that generates heat through a covered probe in 1.5-second pulses, resulting in destruction of the mucosa and submucosa at the application site (Fig. 158.2). The depth of penetration of this injury

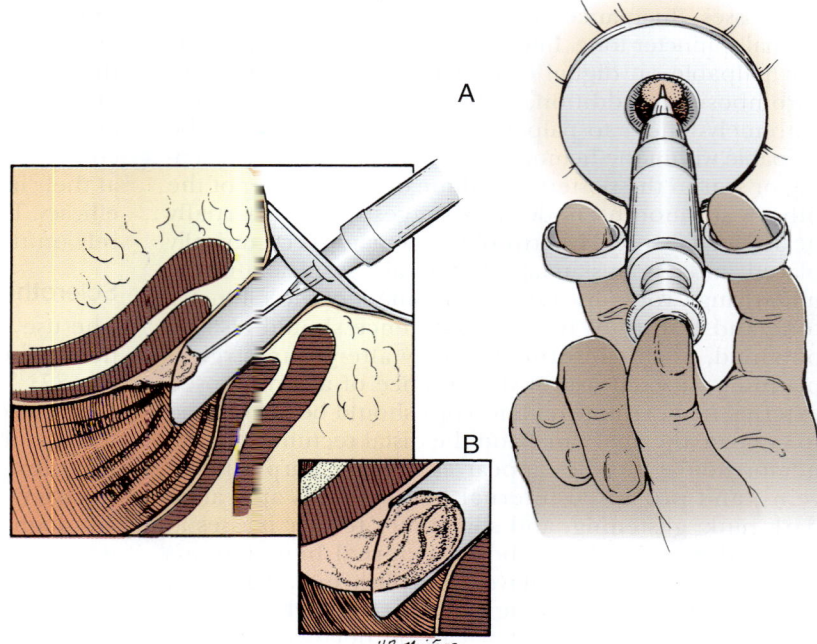

FIGURE 158.1 (A) Injection of internal hemorrhoid. (B) Postinjection striations.

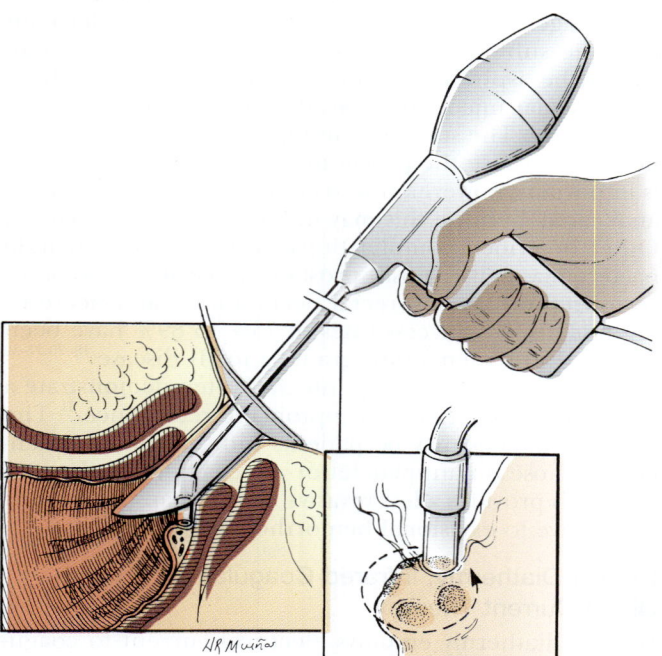

FIGURE 158.2 Infrared coagulation. *Left,* Coagulator inserted through a Hirschman anoscope. *Right,* Coagulation points.

is usually 3 mm and should clearly be applied above the dentate line. Conversely, the Ultroid uses electrical current that is applied for up to 10 minutes for each complex. Ultimately, all these modalities are a variation on the theme of local tissue destruction and fixation of the hemorrhoidal tissue at the appropriate level. There is probably no advantage of one technique over the other;

however, sclerotherapy offers an advantage to the physician since minimal instrumentation is required and is more cost effective. While earlier reports demonstrated high rates of recurrence, especially with grades III and IV hemorrhoids, recent randomized studies have demonstrated outcomes similar to rubber band ligation.[34–36]

Rubber Band Ligation

Rubber band ligation was first described by Blaisdell in 1958 and has since become the office-based procedure of choice for patients with grades I, II, and III internal hemorrhoids.[37] The procedure is generally well tolerated without the need for prescription analgesia if the band is placed above the level of the dentate line. The technique is demonstrated in Fig. 158.3 and begins with the introduction of an anoscope, identifying the hemorrhoidal pedicle, maneuvering it into the cylindrical opening of the ligator with either a forceps or suction, pushing up against the base of the hemorrhoid, and engaging the trigger to deploy the rubber band. The band causes localized ischemia and the hemorrhoid and band are passed in several days during defecation. The resultant fibrosis causes fixation of the remaining hemorrhoidal tissues, preventing further prolapse and bleeding. It is important to ask patients if they experience any pain during placement of the bander before deployment of the band. If they have pain before placement of the band, it will worsen after deployment; therefore that particular application should be altered or aborted. Discomfort immediately after band placement may be reduced by the injection of a local anesthetic agent; however, this does not appear to be a long-lasting benefit.[8]

Several instruments are commercially available for application of the rubber bands. Suction ligators allow the surgeon to draw in the hemorrhoidal tissue using

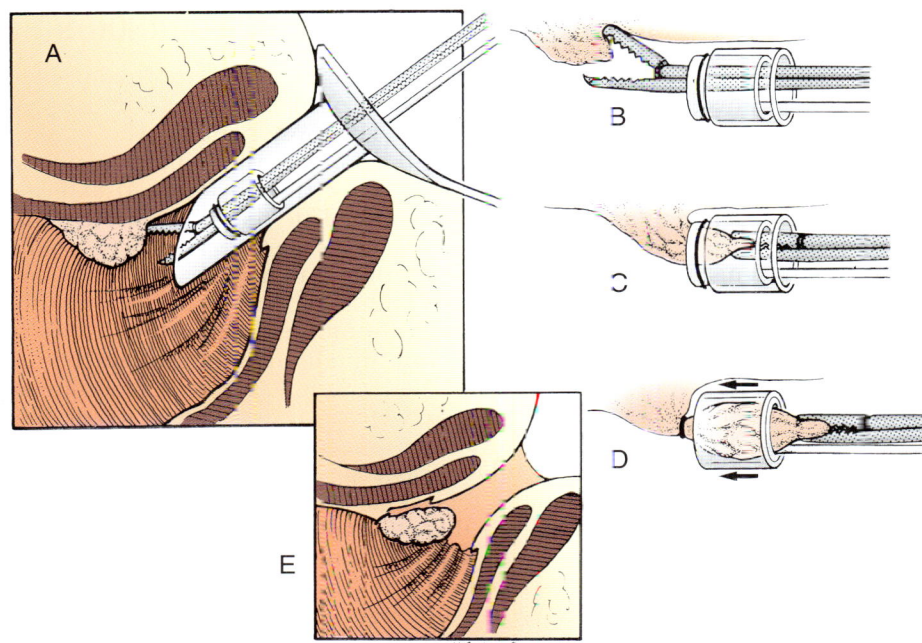

H.R. Muñoz

FIGURE 158.3 (A) Ligator in a Hirschman anoscope. (B) Internal hemorrhoid being grasped. (C) Internal hemorrhoid pulled up into drum. (D) O-ring applied to internal hemorrhoid. (E) Appearance of hemorrhoid after ligation.

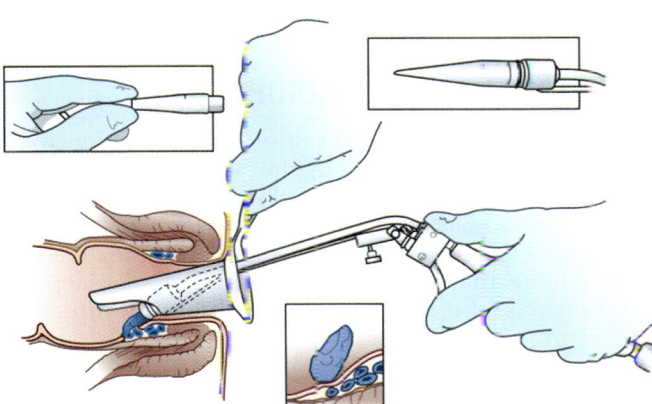

FIGURE 158.4 Rubber band ligation for an internal hemorrhoid. The band is advanced onto the end of the ligator instrument using a conical attachment (*insets*). The hemorrhoid is identified at a level proximal to the dentate; this area is tested for sensation before banding. Occluding the suction port of the ligator instrument draws the hemorrhoid into the open end of the ligator, and the instrument is fired. The banded hemorrhoid typically sloughs in 1 week. (From Beard JM, Osborn J. Common office procedures. In: Rakel RE, ed. *Textbook of Family Medicine.* Philadelphia, Elsevier, 2016:594–621.)

wall suction (Fig. 158.4). This approach is advantageous, because it allows the surgeon to position an anoscope with the nondominant hand and apply the rubber band with the other hand. Other devices require the operator to grasp the hemorrhoid with forceps and apply the rubber band with the other hand. These devices require an assistant to hold the anoscope while the surgeon is applying the rubber band. This technical disadvantage is balanced by the fact that one can usually band more tissue with the

later device. In direct comparison, suction ligation of second- and third-degree hemorrhoids was noted to be beneficial in comparison with forceps ligation in terms of pain tolerance, use of analgesics, and intraprocedural bleeding.[39]

Banding has been associated with several rare complications, including bleeding, vasovagal response, pain, and urinary retention.[40–50] Increased or excessive bleeding 5 to 10 days after placement of a rubber band correlates with the clotting cascade and is a frequent complaint that is usually self-limited. While this is usually a one-time event, ongoing bleeding may require an examination under anesthesia and suture ligation of the offending hemorrhoidal pile. A careful and detailed history should be specifically obtained from the patient regarding the presence of coagulation disorders, either intrinsic, such as those with thrombocytopenia, or acquired, as seen with antiplatelet therapy (Plavix) or anticoagulation with warfarin (Coumadin) or heparin products. In general, the performance of a banding procedure is contraindicated in this group because of the exceedingly high incidence of postprocedure bleeding. Patients should hold anticoagulants for the week after banding, if possible.

Severe pain as a complication of banding can be avoided by ensuring that the rubber band is placed well above the dentate line. When the rubber band is correctly placed, need for early removal because of pain is rare. If removal of the band is necessary, this can be accomplished with a No. 11 blade or hook, and the resultant bleeding can be tamponaded with dilute epinephrine, packing, or may require a visit to the operating room. Pelvic sepsis is an uncommon but frequently fatal complication, which is heralded by the symptoms of increasing rectal pain, fever, and inability to void.[44–47] It is essential to treat these symptoms early and aggressively with early antibiotic treatment coupled with aggressive surgical drainage and/or débridement.

Bayer et al. reported a series of 2934 patients with 79% of patients achieving complete relief of symptoms following a single session of banding at only one or two locations.[38] Placement of bands in multiple quadrants simultaneously increased the risk of pain and urinary retention.[51] Using this approach, patients required multiple sessions for control of symptoms (two sessions, 32%; three sessions, 17%; four sessions, 25%; and five or more sessions, 20%). Although the multiple sessions required are a negative aspect of this technique, only 2.1% of patients required excisional hemorrhoidectomy. It may be possible to achieve a similar outcome with a shorter duration of therapy, albeit at the expense of greater posttreatment pain, by banding all symptomatic hemorrhoidal sites at the initial visit. Banding techniques appear to be durable after initial control of symptoms, with 69% of patients maintaining long-term relief and only 7.5% ultimately requiring excisional hemorrhoidectomy.

In a meta-analysis of 18 randomized prospective studies, rubber band ligation was superior to injection sclerotherapy and infrared coagulation in the treatment of grades I, II, and III hemorrhoids in terms of the need for repeated treatments. However, the risk of complications, albeit small, and pain tended to be greater for rubber band ligation in comparison with the other modalities.[52,53] Another systematic review of randomized controlled trials found that rubber band ligation was less effective and more likely to require multiple procedures than surgical excision.[54,55] However, rubber band ligation was associated with less pain and fewer complications than the operative approach. A recent Cochrane review by the same group reported that band ligation may be the preferred choice for grade II hemorrhoids and even considered for first-line therapy in grade III hemorrhoids, whereas surgical excision may be more appropriately reserved for grade III or rubber band treatment failures.[56]

THROMBOSED EXTERNAL HEMORRHOIDS

Patients with a thrombosed external hemorrhoid present with an acutely painful purplish or blue mass in the perianal area (Fig. 158.5). For those patients who present within 72 hours from the onset of pain, with an organized superficial clot, excision of the thrombosed external hemorrhoid provides immediate relief. The preferential technique is to make a superficial elliptical incision around the clot and excise it rather than making an incision and simple evacuation of the clot.[57] The recurrence rate for a completely excised thrombosed hemorrhoid is 5% to 19%.[58] By comparison, simple incision and evacuation of the clot is associated with a 30% risk of reaccumulation and thrombosis, which may disseminate to adjacent hemorrhoidal columns. When a patient presents later in the course of the disease, conservative management alone with sitz baths, topical analgesic, and fiber is warranted. Occasionally, a thrombosed hemorrhoid will evacuate spontaneously, leaving a small ulcer with residual clot at the anal opening that will typically resolve on its own over a few weeks, although the patient may be left with a skin tag that rarely causes enough symptoms to warrant its removal.[57,59] Expression of the clot through the ulcer may give instant relief of the pain and pressure and stop the bleeding.

EXCISIONAL HEMORRHOIDECTOMY

The decision to proceed to excisional hemorrhoidectomy requires a mutual decision by the physician and patient that medical and office-based options have either failed or are not appropriate. The usual clinical symptoms that lead to surgical excision are frequent prolapsing of the internal hemorrhoids that result in discomfort and anal seepage. Alternatively, the thickened and prolapsing internal/

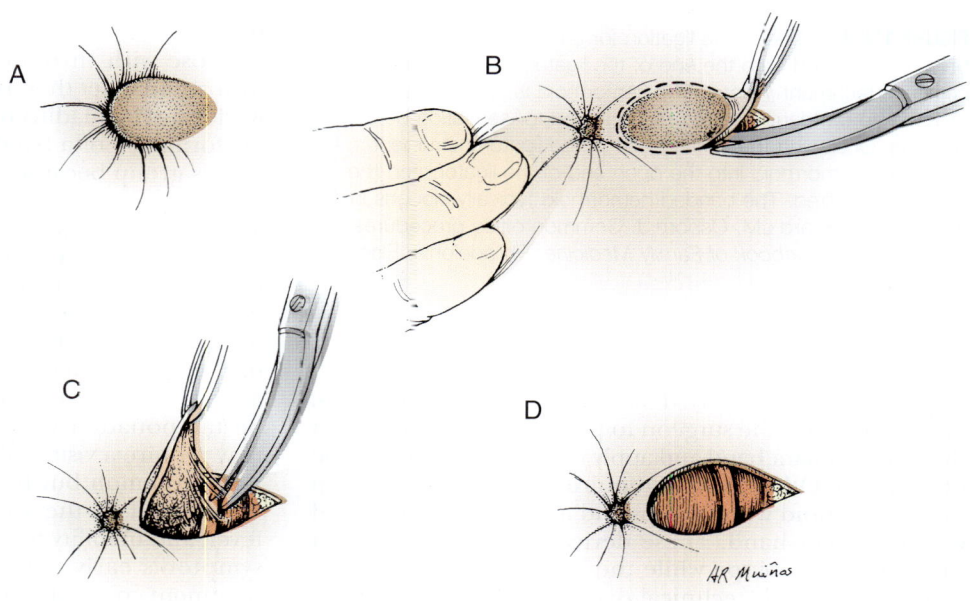

FIGURE 158.5 (A) Thrombosed external hemorrhoid in the right lateral quadrant. (B) Allis clamp applied to apex of thrombosis and elliptical incision made. (C) Thrombosis dissected free of sphincter. (D) Appearance of wound after thrombectomy.

external hemorrhoidal complexes may make anal hygiene difficult for the patient and may make excision preferable. Coagulopathic patients requiring definitive control of rectal bleeding are also candidates for surgical excision. The final indication for excisional hemorrhoidectomy, although debatable, is the development of acutely thrombosed and gangrenous internal hemorrhoids.

Preoperative preparation begins with the patient instructed to undergo a cleansing enema as a full mechanical bowel preparation is not indicated and may be counterproductive. Anesthetic selection is usually left to the anesthesiologist and patient; however, local anesthesia supplemented by the administration of intravenous narcotics and propofol is highly effective and short-acting. The use of spinal anesthesia, although effective, may increase the risk of postoperative urinary retention partially because of a higher intraoperative administration of intravenous fluids.[61] Our preference for positioning is prone jackknife, but surgery can also be accomplished in the high lithotomy position. There is a paucity of data regarding the need for antibiotic prophylaxis. A retrospective review of 852 patients demonstrated a 1.4% incidence of post-hemorrhoidectomy surgical site infection without reduction with the use of preoperative antibiotics.[62] However, patients with underlying immunosuppression or extensive cellulitis may benefit from perioperative antibiotics, such as metronidazole or a second-generation cephalosporin.

Options for excisional hemorrhoidectomy include the following techniques: Milligan-Morgan hemorrhoidectomy, Ferguson closed hemorrhoidectomy, Whitehead hemorrhoidectomy, and the more recently described stapled hemorrhoidopexy (SH) and Doppler-guided transanal devascularization. Division of tissues during excisional hemorrhoidectomy can be accomplished by a variety of means, including a scalpel, scissors, monopolar cauterization, and newer bipolar energy and ultrasonic devices.[63] The available literature does not bear out any advantage of any particular approach, but surgeons should be familiar with several different techniques and approaches.

The Milligan-Morgan or open hemorrhoidectomy, which is widely practiced in Europe, was originally described in 1937, and its efficacy has been documented in many series subsequently.[64,65] This technique includes resection of the entire enlarged internal hemorrhoid complex, ligation of the arterial pedicle, and preservation of the intervening anoderm. The distal anoderm and external skin are left open to minimize the risk of infection in the wounds (Fig. 158.6). Results from this technique have shown this to be a safe and effective means for managing advanced hemorrhoidal disease. However, the fact that the external wounds are left open for delayed healing can be a cause of considerable discomfort and prolonged morbidity after this procedure. The closed Ferguson hemorrhoidectomy was proposed as an alternative to the Milligan-Morgan technique and enjoys a similar large body of evidence regarding its safety and efficacy.[66–69] It is performed by using a hemostat or Kelly clamp to tent up the external hemorrhoid at the anal verge (Fig. 158.7). An elliptical incision is made at the base, close to the anoderm. The hemorrhoidal tissue is then dissected free from the underlying sphincter muscles, staying in the submucosal plane to avoid injury to the sphincter. After the base of the

hemorrhoid is reached, the pedicle of the hemorrhoid is suture ligated and the hemorrhoidal tissue is amputated. One of the stitches used to ligate the pedicle should be left long, because this suture can be used to close the wound in a running fashion. As the stitch is run toward the anoderm, small bites of the underlying muscle are taken to obliterate the dead space.

The Whitehead hemorrhoidectomy, described in 1882, was devised to eradicate the enlarged internal hemorrhoidal tissue in a circumferential fashion and to relocate the prolapsed dentate line that is often a component of prolapsing hemorrhoids (PPHs).[70] Although this technique enjoyed a long period of widespread application, it was subsequently largely abandoned because of the high rates of mucosal ectropion and anal stricture.[71–73] The technique has enjoyed renewed support, with several authors documenting minimal stricture rates and no occurrences of mucosal ectropion.[74–76] Despite these promising reports, the Whitehead procedure is technically demanding because of the need to accurately identify the dentate line and relocate it to its proper location.

A meta-analysis found that the long-term outcomes of excisional hemorrhoidectomy were unequivocally superior to those of office-based procedures, such as rubber band ligation. Furthermore, patients undergoing excisional hemorrhoidectomy are less likely to require multiple treatments.[52] On the other hand, excisional hemorrhoidectomy had higher associations with certain complications, such as anal stenosis and postoperative hemorrhage. Excisional hemorrhoidectomy was also associated with an increased incidence of incontinence to flatus, although this result did not reach statistical significance.

INSTRUMENTATION FOR EXCISIONAL HEMORRHOIDECTOMY

Over the past 10 to 15 years, a variety of new devices have been advocated for hemorrhoidectomy. These energy-based cutting devices have been devised to allow simultaneous tissue division and coagulation. The main advantage proposed for these devices is provision of hemostasis without need for suture ligation and therefore reduction in postoperative pain. However, these benefits must be interpreted in the context of the significant cost of acquisition of the devices as compared with the low cost of a disposable scalpel blade and suture.

The first energy cutting tool applied to hemorrhoidectomy is standard monopolar electrocautery, which surgeons generally use to replace the scalpel or Metzenbaum scissors during an open or closed hemorrhoidectomy. Surgeons using this tool have also employed various degrees of wound closure by suture, ranging from pedicle ligation only to complete wound closure.[78–80] Despite the value of hemostasis, the thermal spread leaves patients with significant postoperative pain compared with other bipolar devices and SH. The STOPP trial study group compared diathermy hemorrhoidectomy with SH in a randomized clinical trial for grade III and IV hemorrhoids. Hemorrhoidal prolapse was corrected equally by either operation at 1 year, but total pain scores were significantly higher in the first 14 days using diathermy

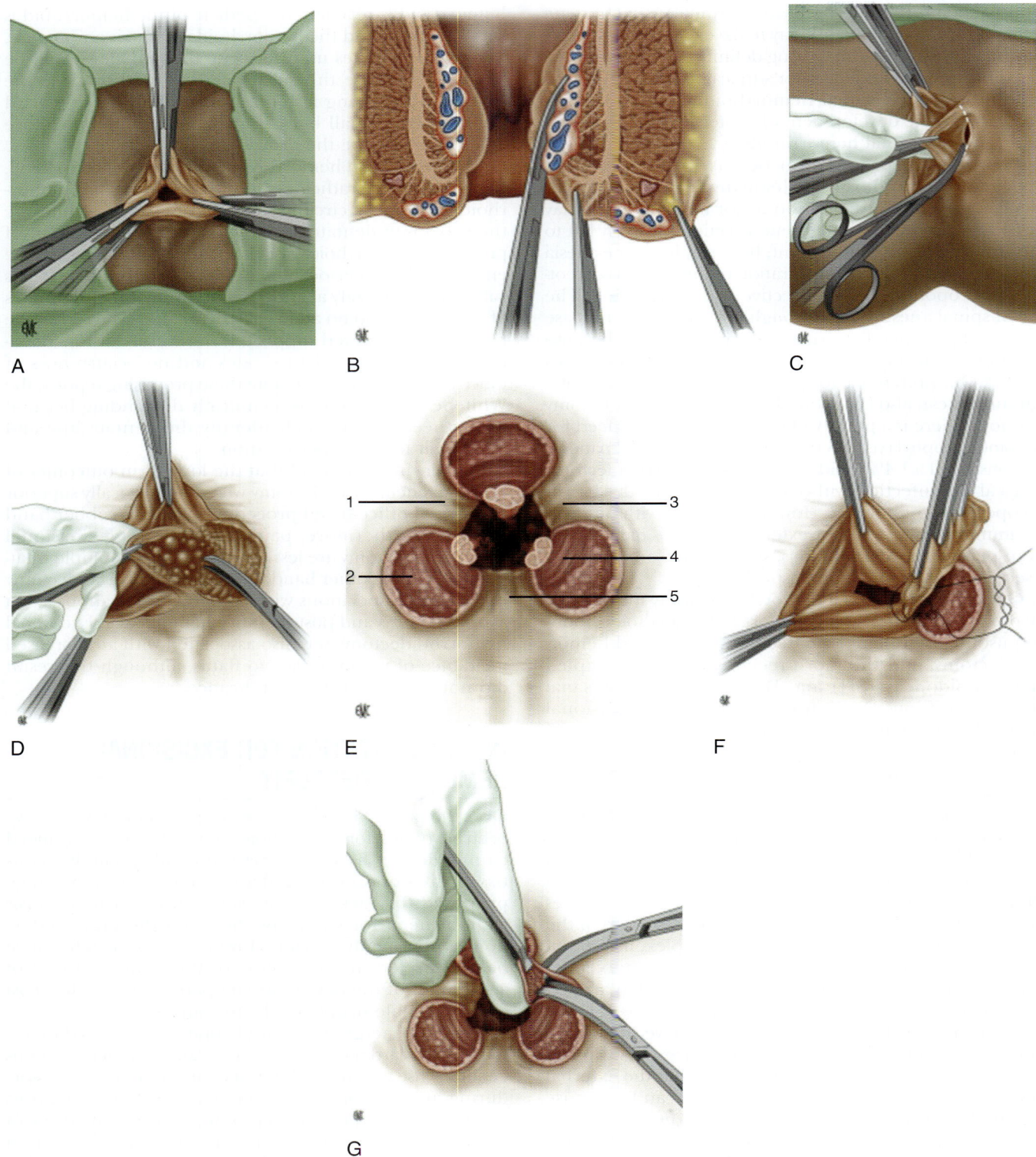

FIGURE 158.6 The open Milligan-Morgan hemorrhoidectomy. (A) Milligan-Morgan hemorrhoidectomy, position of the three sets of clamps; (B) Placement of three clamps on the hemorrhoidal group, frontal view; (C) dissection of the left hemorrhoidal group; (D) exposure of the internal sphincter after division of Parks' ligament; (E) final postoperative appearance. *1,* Left anterior mucocutaneous bridge. *2,* internal anal sphincter. *3,* posterior mucocutaneous bridge. *4,* subcutaneous fibers of the external anal sphincter. *5,* right anterior mucocutaneous bridge; (F) suture ligature of the hemorrhoidal pedicle; (G) cleaning up the mucocutaneous bridges. (From Pillant-LeMoult H, et al. Classical treatment of hemorrhoids. *J Visc Surg.* 2015;152:S3–S9).

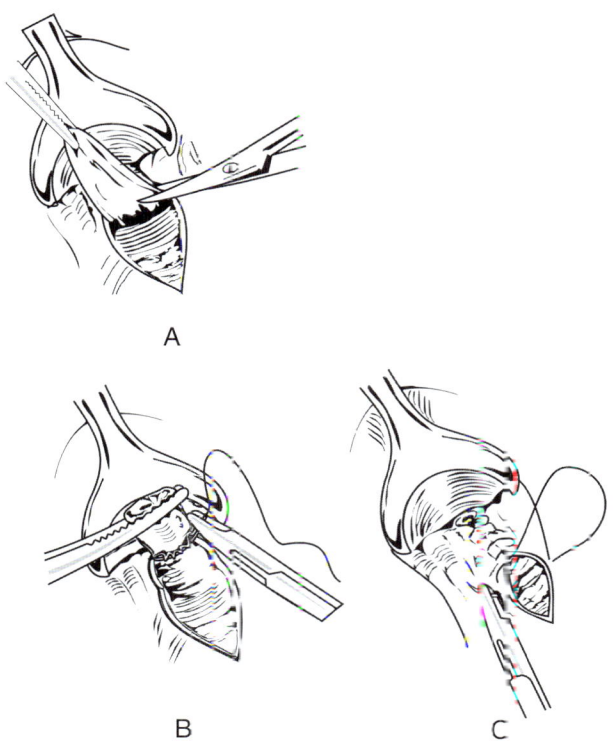

A

B

C

FIGURE 158.7 Ferguson closed hemorrhoidectomy. (A) Hemorrhoid bundle is grasped; dissection proceeds cephalad. (B) Apex is transfixed with suture; bundle is amputated. (C) Suture is used to close wound, leaving a few millimeters open for drainage. (From Rakinic J, Poola VP. Hemorrhoids and fistulas: new solutions for old problems. *Curr Probl Surg.* 2014:51[3];98-137.)

(daily: 25.2 vs. 36.8, *P* = .002; peak: 41.7 vs. 61.1, *P* < .001).[81] Similar findings were reported by Thaha et al. looking at grade II, III, and IV hemorrhoids, but the superiority of diathermal excision was related to prolapse control at 1 year (*P* = .087).[82]

A bipolar cautery device capable of simultaneous tissue division and blood vessel coagulation is the LigaSure. This device has been compared with monopolar diathermy hemorrhoidectomy, with most of the data suggesting reductions in operative time and early postoperative pain. Chung et al. compared a sutureless LigaSure technique with the standard closed Ferguson hemorrhoidectomy and confirmed a reduction in operative time and pain reduction during the first 48 hours.[83] However, there were no significant differences in wound complications or time to full recovery. In a recent meta-analysis of 12 studies with 1142 patients, the use of a bipolar energy device was found to be faster and to provide less postoperative pain in comparison with conventional hemorrhoidectomy.[84] Additionally, postoperative manometric testing and squeeze pressures were significantly decreased in the Ferguson group at the 6-week follow-up, perhaps suggesting less sphincter injury with the Ligasure device.

A competing technology is the Harmonic Scalpel, which relies on a rapidly reciprocating blade to generate heat for coagulation and tissue transection. The largest reported experience was provided by Armstrong et al. with 500 consecutive excisional hemorrhoidectomies,[85,86] and they reported a low postoperative hemorrhage rate (0.6%). The overall postoperative complication rates were low, with urinary retention in 2%, fissure in 1%, and abscess/fistula in 0.8%. Several subsequent prospective, randomized comparison of diathermy to Harmonic scalpel failed to confirm any advantages between the two tools.[87,88] A randomized controlled trial by Abo-hashem et al. compared bipolar electrocautery hemorrhoidectomy with Harmonic scalpel and found favorable results in regard to pain scores and return to work, but complications were similar, except for urine retention, which was significantly less frequent in the Harmonic scalpel group (9.4% vs. 34.4%; *P* < .05).[89]

Probably, the best guidance on this topic is the study by Chung et al., who evaluated scissor/Milligan-Morgan, Harmonic scalpel, and bipolar scissors for hemorrhoidectomy: Harmonic scalpel demonstrated superior early pain scores to scissors; however, the long-term recovery was similar between the groups.[90] Of note, the majority of these studies still not emphasize the product cost alone for any of these devices, which can range from $300 to $750 as compared with the zero product cost of conventional excisional hemorrhoidectomy. Therefore, the cumulative data suggest that patient benefits are modest for any of the energy-delivering techniques, and the cost differential is significant.

PROCEDURE FOR PROLAPSING HEMORRHOIDS

Another option for advanced hemorrhoidal disease is a nonexcisional hemorrhoidectomy or pexy procedure referred to as the procedure for PPHs or SH.[91] These procedures were first described and are arguably more suitable for mucosal prolapse. The technique (Fig. 158.8) uses a circular transanally placed purse-string suture placed 2 to 4 cm proximal to the dentate line, at the apex of the enlarged internal hemorrhoids. Suture placement too close to the dentate line will lead to chronic pain, while sutures placed deep to the submucosal layer can cause injury to the internal anal sphincter and fecal incontinence. A circular stapler head is then inserted through the purse-string and secured. The stapler is closed while maintaining moderate tension on the purse-string. The stapler is then fired and opened revealing a staple line above the hemorrhoidal tissue. Although some hemorrhoid tissue may be included in the segment of mucosa that is excised, stapled hemorrhoidectomy functions to prevent prolapse of the hemorrhoids by pexying them in the anal canal.[92]

Since the introduction of the PPH technique, there have been a large number of prospective randomized trials comparing this approach with excisional hemorrhoidectomy.[93-103] Most of the data support the concept that PPH is associated with a lesser degree of early postoperative pain and a general reduction in the duration of pain after surgery. A multicenter trial comparing PPH with Ferguson closed hemorrhoidectomy confirmed similar benefits and reported a reduction in the need for early reoperation for complications in the PPH group.[96] In addition, several meta-analyses have been published comparing PPH with the Ferguson closed hemorrhoidectomy and

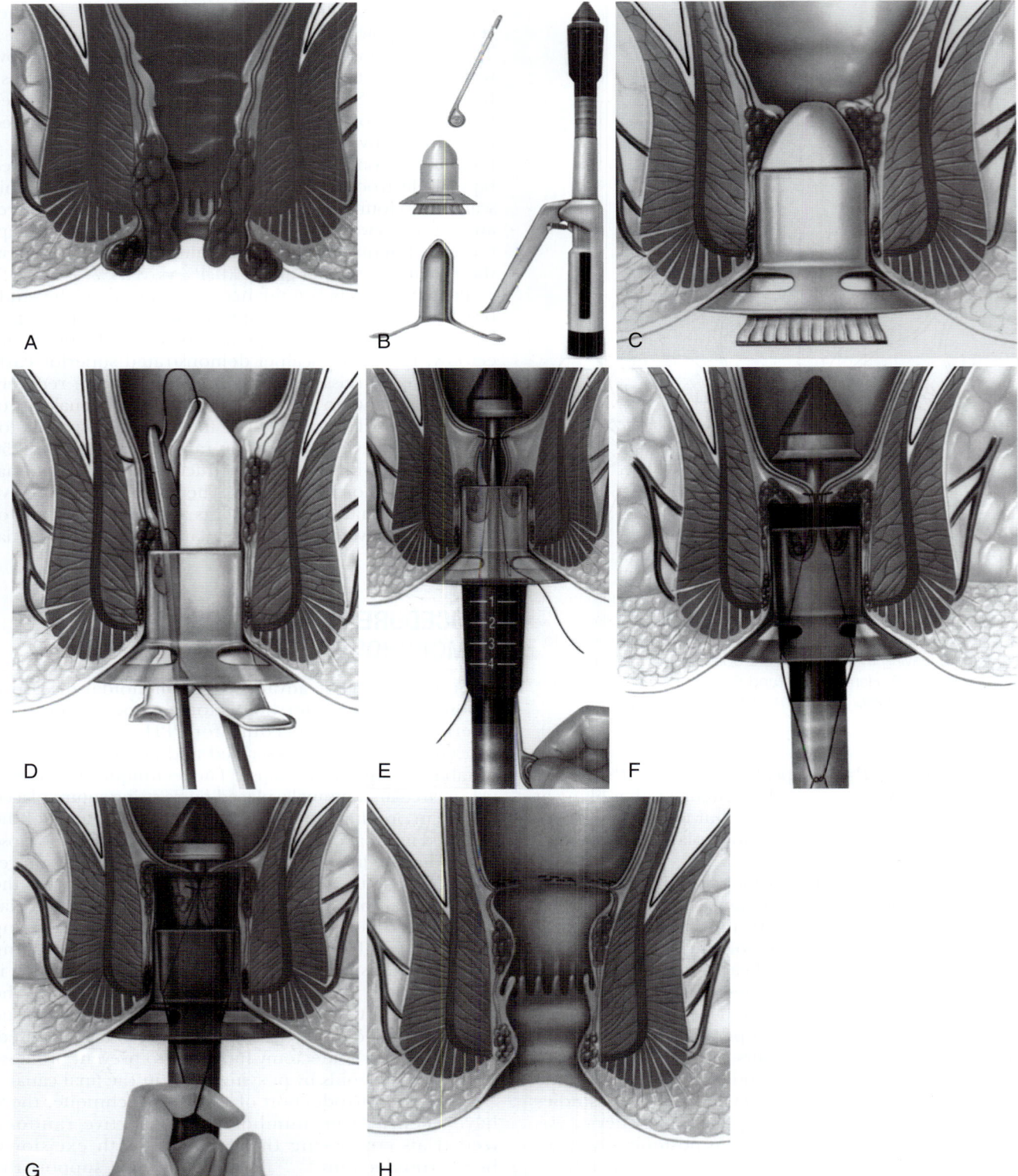

FIGURE 158.8 (A and B) Identification of the internal hemorrhoidal complexes and the instrumentation used for a stapled hemorrhoidectomy are shown. (C and D) A purse-string suture is accurately placed 4 cm above the dentate line by using an anoscope. (E–G) The purse string is tied securely around the rod of the stapling anvil, which allows the hemorrhoidal tissue to be pulled into the barrel of the stapler head. (H) The stapler is closed, fired, and held in place for 20 to 30 seconds. The staple line should be inspected and any bleeding sites suture-ligated.

the Milligan-Morgan open hemorrhoidectomy. There was significant heterogenicity of trials and follow-up was short, but early publications concluded that PPH is associated with less pain and reduced operative time and hospital stay in addition to earlier return to normal activity.

However, a more recent Cochrane review of six randomized trials with 628 patients all having follow-up greater than 1 year demonstrated no significant differences between SH and conventional hemorrhoidectomy in terms of pain, pruritus, and urgency, with higher long-term recurrences following the stapled technique.[104] These results were also confirmed in a 2004 meta-analysis, comparing SH with conventional excisional hemorrhoidectomy, which demonstrated a higher long-term recurrence rate in patients undergoing SH.[105]

Therefore, long-term data suggest that recurrence appears to be higher in PFH.[104] In the aforementioned Cochrane systematic review, randomized controlled trials from 1998 to 2006 comparing SH with conventional excisional hemorrhoidectomy were evaluated.[104] SH patients were significantly more likely to have recurrent hemorrhoids in long-term follow-up than those receiving conventional hemorrhoidectomy (seven trials, 537 patients; OR, 3.85; 95% confidence interval (CI), 1.47 to 10.07; P = .006). In trials where there was follow-up of 1 year or more, SH was associated with higher recurrence rates (five trials, 417 patients; OR, 3.60; 95% CI, 1.24 to 10.49; P = .02). A significantly higher proportion of patients with SH complained of the symptom of prolapse (eight studies, 798 patients; OR, 2.96; 95% CI, 1.33 to 6.58; P = .008). Giordano et al. looked at long-term outcome for PPH in a separate analysis looking at all randomized controlled trials that had follow-up of 1 year or longer comparing PPH with conventional hemorrhoidectomy. Fifteen articles met their inclusion criteria, for a total of 1201 patients.[101] Outcomes at 1 year showed a significantly higher rate of prolapse recurrence in the PPH group (14 studies, 1063 patients; OR, 5.5; P < 0.001), and patients were likely to undergo further treatment to correct recurrent prolapses compared with conventional hemorrhoidectomy (10 studies, 824 patients; OR, 1.9; P < .002). The authors concluded rightly that it is a matter of preference whether to accept a higher recurrence rate to take advantage of the short-term benefits of PPH. As pointed out in the Cochrane review, patients need to be educated about the pros and cons of the techniques available.

Although the bulk of the data supports the safety of this new technique, there have been several reports of complications. Early complications (6.6%) after 150 consecutive SHs by Bove et al. were five bleeding, four acute urinary retention, one external hemorrhoid thrombosis, and one hematoma of the rectal wall.[106] Late complications (10%) were five fecal urgency (improved after 6 months), six moderate asymptomatic strictures, and four persistent skin tags. Recurrences of 5.1% were in grade III and IV patients and occurred within the first 24 months. In a retrospective review, Jongen et al. looked at reoperations for 1233 patients undergoing SH over a 10-year time frame. Reoperation (10%) was also stapler-related due to recurrent/persistent hemorrhoidal symptoms or to address other anorectal issues not corrected by the circular SH procedure.[107] No life-threatening complications occurred,

and the need for both early and late reoperations decreased significantly over time (P < .05). Case reports have been published on severe pelvic sepsis after SH. Van Wensen et al. reported a case requiring exploratory laparotomy with presacral drainage and diverting ileostomy.[108] On reoperation, a digital examination revealed a dorsolateral rectal perforation, but it is unclear in their publication whether this was at the staple line or not. Martellucci et al. reported a double rectal perforation after SH. The more distal perforation was related to a staple line dehiscence, and they theorized that the more proximal perforation at the rectosigmoid junction may have been related to a sigmoidocele trapped in the stapler during the initial operation.[109] Molloy and Kingsmore reported a case of severe pelvic sepsis, likely resulting from an inadvertent rectal injury.[110] Cheetham et al. also raised concern over persistent severe anorectal pain as a possible sequela of PPH.[111] Other unique complications such as rectovaginal fistulas and staple line bleeding have been described, but overall, complication rates are similar to conventional excisional hemorrhoidectomy. A meta-analysis of almost 2000 patients found the complication rates to be 20.2% for SH versus 25.2% for conventional hemorrhoidectomy (P = .06).[112] In general, the stapled procedure is not effective for large external or thrombosed hemorrhoids, although limited data have demonstrated some success.[113]

HEMORRHOIDAL ARTERIAL LIGATION

A new technique that is gaining popularity is Doppler-guided hemorrhoidal artery ligation (HAL) or transanal hemorrhoidal dearterialization (THD). The guided reduction in arterial blood flow can be coupled with a mucosopexy when there is significant prolapse so that this aspect can be corrected and venous outflow can be improved. This technique was first described by Morinaga et al. in 1995 and is based on closure of the hemorrhoidal blood flow that feeds the hemorrhoidal plexus via the terminal branches of the superior rectal artery,[114] and a specifically designed proctoscope is used coupled with a Doppler transducer. At the distal end, there is a small window that allows suturing of the rectal mucosa 2 to 3 cm above the dentate line (Fig. 158-9). The reduction of blood flow is thought to lead to shrinkage of the hemorrhoidal complex. In addition, a mucosopexy can be performed that lifts the prolapsing tissue into its normal anatomic position. Giordano et al. published an extensive review of the current evidence on THD, looking specifically at safety and effectiveness of the technique.[115] In their review, 16 of the 17 articles that met inclusion criteria were observational studies, and the study quality ranged from low to very low. The majority of patients treated had grade II or III disease, and of the 1996 patients who were involved in these studies, the most common early postoperative event was postoperative pain (18.5%). Residual prolapse, bleeding, and fever were complications documented with an incidence higher than 3%. When the studies with a follow-up of 1 year or more were analyzed (6/17 publications), the incidence of prolapse was 10.8%, bleeding 9.7%, and pain on defecation 3.7%. Other prospective studies using Doppler-guided/assisted hemorrhoidal ligation demonstrated favorable results

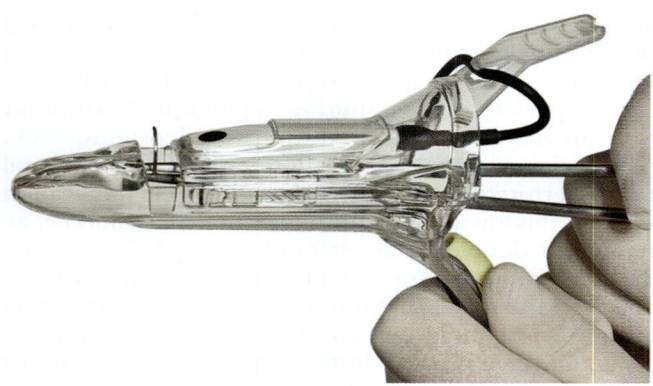

FIGURE 158.9 Image of device for transanal hemorrhoidal dearterialization. A Doppler incorporated in device is used to locate terminal branches of the hemorrhoidal arteries. Once localized, the arteries are suture ligated. A hemorrhoidopexy can be performed for prolapse repair with a running absorbable suture above the dentate line. This repair atrophies the hemorrhoidal cushions and restores prolapsed tissue to its anatomic position.

with reported control of bleeding in more than 90% of patients, with recurrence occurring in 10% to 15%.[116–118] Currently, larger studies including variations of the Doppler technique and comparisons with other methods with longer follow-up intervals are required before recommending this method over conventional surgery.[119,120]

POSTOPERATIVE MANAGEMENT AFTER HEMORRHOID SURGERY

Regardless of the excisional technique used for treatment of advanced hemorrhoidal disease, the key to effective patient management is avoidance of postoperative complications. Pain is the most frequent complication and is the most feared sequela of the procedure from the patient's perspective. A variety of analgesic regimens have been recommended, usually consisting of a combination of oral and parenteral narcotics.[121–125] The use of local infiltration of bupivacaine into the wounds and perianal skin has been variably successful in long-term pain reduction. Conversely, ketorolac has demonstrated considerable efficacy in managing posthemorrhoidectomy pain.[125] The use of alternative administration routes for narcotics either by patch or subcutaneous pump have been successful in controlling pain; however, the management of these routes of administration can be risky in the outpatient setting because of the risk of narcotic-induced respiratory depression and development of narcotic dependency. The most appropriate regimen following outpatient hemorrhoidectomy appears to be intraoperative use of ketorolac, sufficient doses of oral narcotic analgesics for home administration, and supplementation of the narcotics by an oral nonsteroidal antiinflammatory drug (NSAID). Two recent publications have supported the use of nifedipine with lidocaine ointment and glyceryl trinitrate (GTN) ointment for posthemorrhoidectomy pain. Reducing the internal sphincter spasm may contribute to the effectiveness of this therapy. Of 69 patients randomized

to receive 0.2% GTN or placebo, the patients in the GTN group experienced significantly less postoperative pain on days 1, 3, and 7 ($P < .05$), used less analgesics, and had improved wound healing compared with placebo at 3 weeks from a diathermy Ferguson hemorrhoidectomy.[126,127] Joshi et al. looked at evidence-based management of pain after hemorrhoidectomy surgery in a systemic review in 2010.[128] The findings revealed that local anesthetic infiltration as a sole technique or with general or regional anesthetic should be recommended in addition to a combination of NSAID, paracetamol, and opiates. Other medications that are recommended as analgesic adjuncts may include laxatives and oral metronidazole started before surgery.

Urinary retention is a frequent postoperative problem following hemorrhoidectomy, ranging in incidence from 1% to 52%.[129–132] A variety of strategies have been used to treat the problem, including parasympathomimetics, α-adrenergic blocking agents, and sitz baths.[133] The best approach, however, seems to be a strategy of prevention that includes limiting perioperative fluid administration to 250 mL, an anesthetic approach that avoids use of spinal anesthesia, avoidance of anal packing, and an aggressive oral analgesic regimen.[134]

Early postoperative bleeding (<24 hours) occurs in approximately 1% of cases and represents a technical error requiring return to the operating theater for resuturing of the offending wound.[135] Delayed hemorrhage occurs in 0.5% to 4% of cases of excisional hemorrhoidectomy at 5 to 10 days postoperatively.[135–138] The etiology has been held to be early separation of the ligated pedicle before adequate thrombosis in the feeding artery can occur.[139] The bleeding in this scenario is usually significant and requires some method for control of ongoing hemorrhage. Options include return to the operating theater for suture ligation or tamponade at the bedside by Foley catheter or anal packing.[139–141] The subsequent outcome after control of secondary hemorrhage is generally good, with virtually no risk of recurrent bleeding.

SUMMARY

The management of symptomatic hemorrhoidal disease should be directed at the symptom complex of the individual patient. The majority of these patients can be successfully treated by improving diet with fiber and lifestyle modifications along with time, reassurance, and patience. For persistent symptoms, either injection or banding of the internal hemorrhoids is predictably successful. In addition, only a few patients should require excisional hemorrhoidectomy by any of the described techniques. Circular SH and THD with or without mucosopexy may prove to be effective, less painful techniques to manage grade III hemorrhoids, but they will require buy-in for the product cost and time to achieve a new learning curve.

RECTOCELE

A rectocele is one of a spectrum of pelvic floor disorders resulting from the loss of pelvic floor support. Rectoceles are often associated with other pelvic organ prolapse disorders such as rectal prolapse, which will be described elsewhere. Rectoceles are more common in women due to

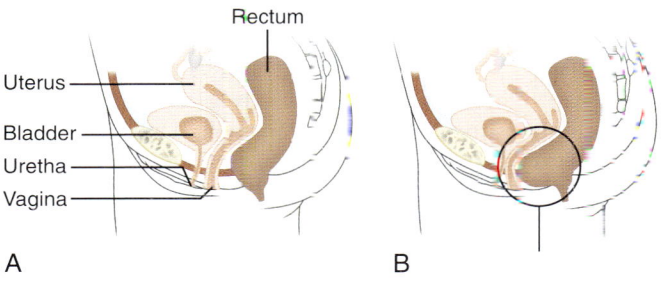

FIGURE 158.10 (A) Normal pelvic floor anatomy. (B) Rectocele.

the enlarged genital hiatus between the pubic symphysis and the levator muscles. Furthermore, the vagina and the rectum run in parallel to each other and share a common muscular wall. The back wall of the vagina and the front wall of the rectum together make up the rectovaginal septum. A rectocele then occurs when the rectovaginal septum becomes so weak that the rectum bulges forward onto the posterior wall of the vagina (Fig. 158.10). This is often described as a herniation or defect of the rectovaginal septum.[142] As a result, rectoceles are more common in elderly women and in those who have delivered children vaginally. Other risk factors for developing a rectocele include constipation, obesity, and those with collagen abnormalities. Patients with rectoceles often complain of rectal pressure, difficulty with defecation, incomplete emptying, pelvic pain, and are often confused with "hemorrhoids."[143-151]

The finding of a small rectocele on examination is very common and is of no concern if the patient does not have significant symptoms. However, when a rectocele becomes large, stool can become trapped within it, making it difficult to have a bowel movement or creating a sensation of incomplete evacuation. Symptoms are usually due to stool trapping, difficulty passing stool, and protrusion of the back of the vagina through the vaginal opening. During bowel movements, women with large, symptomatic rectoceles may describe the need to put their fingers into their vagina and push back toward the rectum to allow the stool to pass ("splinting").[152]

DIAGNOSIS

Often, a rectocele is easily recognized on physical examination in the dorsal lithotomy or upright position, at rest or with performance of various maneuvers such as a Valsalva. In instances of very large rectoceles, the back wall of the vagina may bulge out beyond the opening of the vagina. Palpation of the rectocele must be undertaken to rule out sigmoidocele or an enterocele. Imaging modalities such as video defecography and dynamic magnetic resonance imaging (MRI) can be useful in the diagnosis of a rectocele. In the presence of a rectocele, the contrast material can be seen bulging from the front of the rectum into the back of the vagina. Sometimes the contrast material stays in the rectocele while the liquid in the rectum is expelled—this is called "stasis," or stool trapping (Fig. 158.11).[153] The size of the rectocele is determined by measuring the distance between the line of the anterior border of the anal canal and the maximal point of the

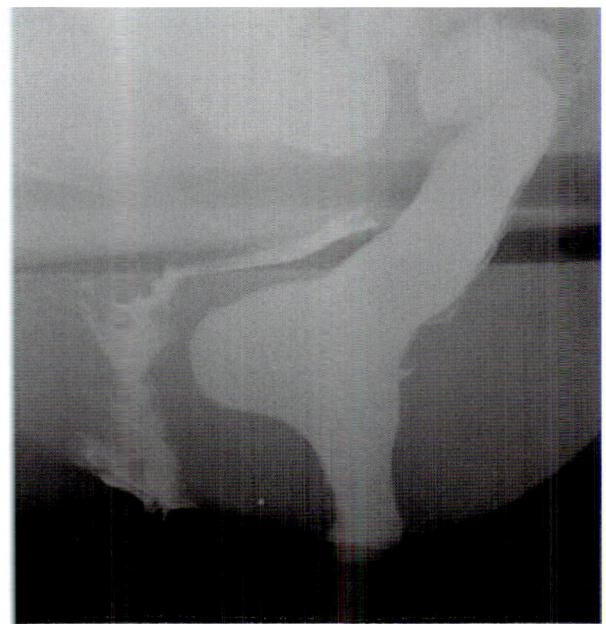

FIGURE 158.11 Rectocele on magnetic resonance imaging defecography.

bulge of the anterior rectal wall into the posterior vaginal wall. Anything less than 2 cm is considered normal, while a rectocele is considered large if the anterior rectal wall protrudes more than 3.5 cm. MRI defecography, although useful, is lacking standardization in the grading of prolapse, has high cost and relatively limited availability.[154]

TREATMENT

In the absence of severe symptoms, the recommended treatment for a rectocele is nonsurgical and focused on optimizing stool consistency to aid in the passage of stool. This often involves increasing daily fiber and liquid intake. Biofeedback, or pelvic floor physical therapy aimed at improving a patient's rectal sensation and pelvic floor muscle contraction, may also be helpful. In one trial women assigned to biofeedback prior to surgical intervention had higher scores on quality of life questionnaires and higher maximum pelvic floor muscle squeeze on manometry.[155] It may be that increasing the strength of the levator ani muscles improved support of the pelvic organ during the crucial window of postoperative healing. However, further long-term studies have not been performed to demonstrate persistent benefits of biofeedback therapy alone. Given that there are minimal adverse effects from pelvic floor muscle training, the main drawbacks are the cost of providing instruction and the investment of time patients need to make to maximize efficacy. Patients will obtain the most benefit from physical therapy by an experienced physical therapist or nurse practitioner in a supervised program, usually consisting of one to two visits per week for 8 to 12 weeks, with ongoing maintenance exercises.

When symptoms persist despite appropriate nonsurgical measures, surgical treatment may be considered. Surgical repairs of rectoceles are generally divided into transanal and transvaginal approaches. The most common transanal approach to rectocele repair is the modified Delorme procedure popularized by Sullivan et al. in which the anterior rectal wall was plicated after the mucosa was lifted up from the muscularis propria.[156] This usually involves reinforcement of the rectovaginal septum using either an approach through the rectum (as favored by most colon and rectal surgeons) or through the vagina (as favored by most gynecologists). The technique begins with the patient in a prone jackknife position with the buttocks spread and taped. The rectal mucosa proximally 1 to 2 cm proximal to the dentate line is infiltrated with local anesthetic circumferentially. A U-shaped or T incision is made in the rectal mucosa at or proximal to the dentate line. A flap is developed to a level proximal to the rectocele (usually ~7 cm in length). The rectal mucosal flap is trimmed and the rectal mucosa is closed with a running 5-0 polyglycolic acid suture. If the mucosa is not removed, plication of the rectal mucosa can lead to necrosis and postoperative infection, and some patients also complain of persistent tenesmus. The rectovaginal septum is reapproximated using vertical plication sutures with a 3-0 polyglycolic acid suture. Levator ani plication also can be done with the endorectal approach. This in essence corrects the rectal intussusception and the rectocele and lifts the rectum back into alignment in the pelvis. Transanal rectocele repair is effective in alleviating defecation dysfunction and outlet obstruction in approximately 80% of patients.[157,158] However, long-term outcomes of transanal rectocele repair are associated with a 50% recurrence rate at 5 years.[159]

Some surgeons have recently begun using a technique called the stapled transanal rectal resection (STARR) procedure, in which a surgical stapling device is used to remove a portion of the rectocele. This procedure consists of introducing the circular stapler with a disposable circular anal dilator and a purse-string suture anoscope, stapling off a portion of the rectocele and internal rectal prolapse (including mucosa, submucosa, and muscularis) first anteriorly, then posteriorly. A prospective multicenter trial reported the results of 90 patients with outlet obstruction who underwent this procedure, with significant improvement in constipation symptoms, no worsening of anal incontinence or dyspareunia, and restoration of rectal compliance.[160] However, complications included an 18% fecal urgency rate and a 3% anastomotic stenosis rate. This is a newer procedure that is not performed by all colon and rectal surgeons, and its success and complication rates are still being studied in prospective randomized controlled trials; therefore, definitive recommendations are lacking.

Transvaginal techniques of rectocele repair are primarily performed by gynecologists and can be divided into four primary techniques including rectovaginal muscularis reapproximation, site-specific repair of the rectovaginal septum, reapproximation of the rectovaginal septum to the levator ani, and posterior repair of rectovaginal defect with graft or mesh. All techniques involve an incision in the posterior wall of the vagina and separation between the rectum and the vaginal wall. Specific details of each technique are beyond the scope of this chapter, but nonetheless, the results of these procedures are more favorable than the transanal repair. This was illustrated in a meta-analysis of three randomized trials that found a significantly lower rate of objective failure for posterior colporrhaphy (10% vs. 42%; risk ratio, 0.24; 95% CI, 0.09 to 0.64).[161] Further prospective trials have reinforced this sentiment of superiority of the transvaginal approach.[162–165]

However, we must also be mindful of the potential complications such as pain, temporary urinary retention, and constipation, which are the most common. Serious but uncommon complications include development of a hematoma, infection, inclusion cyst formation, fecal impaction, and injury to the rectum with the development of a rectovaginal or a rectoperineal fistula.[166–170] Bowel and defecatory dysfunction may continue long-term, and prolapse, de novo dyspareunia, or fecal incontinence may also occur.[171–174] Utilization of mesh is associated with additional complications, such as mesh erosion, infection of the graft, and persistence of granulation tissue.[175]

In summary, rectoceles are commonly associated with other pelvic organ prolapse and may require a multidisciplinary approach with radiology, physical therapy, urology, and/or gynecology. Constipation should be corrected with dietary and lifestyle modifications along with biofeedback physiotherapy. The isolated surgical management for rectoceles can be approached via a transanal incision, but results are superior with a transvaginal repair.

REFERENCES

1. Holley CJ. History of hemorrhoidal surgery. *South Med J.* 1946;39:536.
2. Madoff RD. Biblical Management of Anorectal Disease. Presented at the Midwest Society of Colon and Rectal Surgeons. Brechenridge, Colorado; 1991.
3. Dirckx JH. The biblical plague of "hemorrhoids". An outbreak of bilharziasis. *Am J Dermatopathol.* 1985;7:341.
4. Maimonides M, Rosner F, Munter S [trans]. *Treatise on Hemorrhoids.* Philadelphia: JB Lippincott; 1969.
5. Rachochot JE, Petourand CH, Riovoire JO. Saint Fiacre: the healer of hemorrhoids and patron saint of proctology. *Am J Proctol.* 1971;22:175.
6. Thomson WH. The nature of haemorrhoids. *Br J Surg.* 1975;62:542.
7. Morgado PJ, Suarez JA, Gomez LG. Histoclinical basis for a new classification of hemorrhoidal disease. *Dis Colon Rectum.* 1988;31:474-480.
8. Burkitt DP, Graham-Steward CW. Hemorrhoid-postulated pathogenesis and proposed prevention. *Postgrad Med J.* 1975;51:631.
9. Haas PA, Fox TA Jr, Haas GP. The pathogenesis of hemorrhoids. *Dis Colon Rectum.* 1984;27:442.
10. Arab Y, Alexzander Williams J, Keighley MR. Anal pressures in hemorrhoids and anal fissure. *Am J Surg.* 1977;134:608.
11. Hancock BD. Internal sphincter and the nature of haemorrhoids. *Gut.* 1977;18:651.
12. Arscia SD. *Morphological and Physiological Aspects of Anal Continence and Defecation.* Brussels: Presses Academiquues Europeenes; 1969:150.
13. Goligher J. Haemorrhoids or piles. In: *Surgery of the Anus, Rectum and Colon.* London: Balliere Tindall; 1984:98.
14. Benyon J. *Endorectal and Anal Sonography in Surgery of the Colon, Rectum and Anus.* Philadelphia: Saunders; 1995.
15. Rivadeneira DE, Steele SR, Ternent C, et al. On behalf of the Standards Practice Task Force of the American Society of Colon and Rectal Surgeons. Practice parameters for the management of hemorrhoids (revised 2010). *Dis Colon Rectum.* 2011;54(9):1059-1064.
16. Alonso-Coello P, Mills E, Heels-Ansdell D, et al. Fiber for the treatment of hemorrhoids complications: a systematic review and metaanalysis. *Am J Gastroenterol.* 2006;101:181-188.
17. Moesgaard F, Nielsen ML, Hansen JB, et al. High fiber diet reduces bleeding and pain in patients with hemorrhoids: a double-blind trial of Vi-Siblin. *Dis Colon Rectum.* 1982;25:454-456.
18. Khoury GA, Lake SP, Lewis MC, Lewis AA. A randomized trial to compare single with multiple phenol injection treatments for haemorrhoids. *Br J Surg.* 1985;72:741-742.

19. Mann CV, Motson R, Clifton M. The immediate response to injection therapy for first-degree haemorrhoids. *J R Soc Med.* 1988;81:146-148.

20. Senapati A, Nicholls RJ. A randomized trial to compare the results of injection sclerotherapy with a bulk laxative alone in the treatment of bleeding internal haemorrhoids. *Int J Colorectal Dis.* 1988;3:124-125.

21. Murray-Lyon IM, Kirkham JS. Hepatic abscesses complicating injection sclerotherapy of haemorrhoids. *Eur J Gastroenterol Hepatol.* 2001;13:971-972.

22. Adami B, Eckhardt V, Suermann R, et al. Bacteremia after proctoscopy and hemorrhoical injection sclerotherapy. *Dis Colon Rectum.* 1981;24:373-374.

23. Gupta N, Katoch A, Lai P, Hadke NS. Rectourethral fistula after injection sclerotherapy for hemorrhoids, a rare complication. *Colorectal Dis.* 2011;13:105.

24. Kaman L, Aggarwal S, Kumar R, Behera A, Katariya RN. Necrotizing fasciitis after injection sclerotherapy for hemorroids: report of a case. *Dis Colon Rectum.* 1999;42:419-420.

25. Schulte T, Fandrich F, Kahlke V. Life-threatening rectal necrosis after injection sclerotherapy for haemorrhoids. *Int J Colorectal Dis.* 2008;23:725-726.

26. Vindal A, Lai P, Chander J, Ramleke VK. Rectal perforation after injection sclerotherapy for hemorrhoids: case report. *Indian J Gastroenterol.* 2008;27:84-85.

27. Kanellos I, Goulimaris I, Vkalis I, et al. Long-term evaluation of sclerotherapy for haemorrhoids: a prospective study. *Int J Surg Investig.* 2000;2:295-298.

28. Johanson JF, Rimm A. Optimal nonsurgical treatment of hemorrhoids: a comparative analysis of infrared coagulation, rubber band ligation, and injection sclerotherapy. *Am J Gastroenterol.* 1992;87:1600-1606.

29. Gartell PC, Sheridan RJ, McGinn FP. Out-patient treatment of haemorrhoids: a randomized clinical trial to compare rubber band ligation with phenol injection. *Br J Surg.* 1985;72:478-479.

30. Chew SS, Marshall L, Kalish L, et al. Short-term and long-term results of combined sclerotherapy and rubber band ligation of hemorrhoids and mucosa prolapse. *Dis Colon Rectum.* 2003;46:1232-1237.

31. Dennison A, Whiston RJ, Rooney S, Chadderton RD, Wherry DC, Morris DL. A randomized comparison of infrared photocoagulation with bipolar diathermy for the outpatient treatment of hemorrhoics. *Dis Colon Rectum.* 1990;33:32.

32. Hinton CP, Morris DL. A randomized trial comparing direct current therapy and bipolar diathermy in the outpatient treatment of third-degree hemorrhoids. *Dis Colon Rectum.* 1990;33:931.

33. Zinberg SS, Stern DH, Furman DS, Wittles JM. A personal experience in comparing three nonoperative techniques for treating internal hemorrhoids. *Am J Gastroenterol.* 1989;84:488.

34. Linares Santiago E, Gomez Parra M, Mendoza Olivares FJ, Pellicer Bautista FJ, Herrerias Gutierrez JM. Effectiveness of hemorrhoidal treatment by rubber band ligation and infrared photocoagulation. *Rev Esp Enferm Dig.* 2001;93:238-247.

35. Marques CF, Nahas SC, Nahas CS, Sobrado CW Jr, Habr-Gama A, Kiss DR. Early results of the treatment of internal hemorrhoid disease by infrared coagulation and elastic banding: a prospective randomized cross-over trial. *Tech Coloproctol.* 2006;10:312-317.

36. Poen AC, Felt-Bersma RJ, Cuesta MA, Deville W, Meuwissen SG. A randomized controlled trial of rubber band ligation versus infra-red coagulation in the treatment of internal haemorrhoids. *Eur J Gastroenterol Hepatol.* 2000;12:535-539.

37. Barron J. Office ligation of internal hemorrhoids. *Am J Surg.* 1963;105:563.

38. Bayer I, Myslovaty B, Picovsky BM. Rubber band ligation of hemorrhoids. Convenient and economic treatment. *J Clin Gastroenterol.* 1996;23:50.

39. Ramzisham AR, Sagap I, Nadeson S, Ali IM, Hasni MJ. Prospective randomized clinical trial on suction elastic band ligator versus forceps ligator in the treatment of haemorrhoids. *Asian J Surg.* 2005;28:241-245.

40. El Nakeeb AM, Fikry AA, Omar WH, et al. Rubber band ligation for 750 cases of symptomatic hemorrhoids out of 2200 cases. *World J Gastroenterol.* 2008;14:6525-6530.

41. Marshman D, Huber PJ Jr, Timmerman W, Simonton CT, Odom FC, Kaplan ER. Hemorrhoidal ligation. A review of efficacy. *Dis Colon Rectum.* 1989;32:369.

42. Oueidat DM, Jurjus AR. Management of hemorrhoids by rubber band ligation. *J Med Liban.* 1994;42:11.

43. Wrobleski DE. Rubber band ligation of hemorrhoids. *R I Med.* 1995;78:12.

44. Wrobleski DE, Corman ML, Veidenheimer MC, Coller JA. Long-term evaluation of rubber ring ligation in hemorrhoical disease. *Dis Colon Rectum.* 1980;23:478.

45. Alemdaroglu K, Ulualp KM. Single session ligation treatment of bleeding hemorrhoids. *Surg Gynecol Obstet.* 1993;177:62.

46. Clay LD 3rd, White JJ Jr, Davidson JT, Chandler JJ. Early recognition and successful management of pelvic cellulitis following hemorrhoidal banding. *Dis Colon Rectum.* 1986;29:579.

47. Quevedo-Bonilla G, Farkas AM, Abcarian H, Hambrick E, Orsay CP. Septic complications of hemorrhoidal banding. *Arch Surg.* 1988;123:650.

48. Russell TR, Donohue JH. Hemorrhoidal banding. A warning. *Dis Colon Rectum.* 1985;28:291.

49. Scarpa FJ, Hillis W, Sabetta JR. Pelvis cellulitis: a life-threatening complication of hemorrhoidal banding. *Surgery.* 1988;103:383.

50. Lau WY, Chow HP, Poon GP, Wong SH. Rubber band ligation of three primary hemorrhoids in a single session. A safe and effective procedure. *Dis Colon Rectum.* 1982;25:336.

51. Lee HH, Spencer RJ, Beart RW Jr. Multiple hemorrhoidal bandings in a single session. *Dis Colon Rectum.* 1994;37:37.

52. MacRae HA, McLeod RS. Comparison of hemorrhoidal treatment modalities: a meta-analysis. *Dis Colon Rectum.* 1995;38:687-694.

53. MacRae HM, McLeod RS. Comparison of hemorrhoidal treatments: a meta-analysis. *Can J Surg.* 1997;40:14-17.

54. Hardy A, Chan CL, Cohen CR. The surgical management of hemorrhoids: a review. *Dig Surg.* 2005;22:26-33.

55. Shanmugam V, Thaha MA, Rabindranath KS, Campbell KL, Steele RJ, Loudon MA. Systematic review of randomized trials comparing rubber band ligation with excisional hemorrhoidectomy. *Br J Surg.* 2005;92:1481-1487.

56. Shanmugam V, Thaha MA, Rabindranath KS, Campbell KL, Steele RJ, Loudon MA. Rubber band ligation versus excisional haemorrhoidectomy for haemorrhoids. *Cochrane Database Syst Rev.* 2005;(3):CD005034.

57. Grosz CR. A surgical treatment of thrombosed external hemorrhoids. *Dis Colon Rectum.* 1990;33:249.

58. Greenspon J, Williams SB, Young HA, Orkin BA. Thrombosed external hemorrhoids: outcome after conservative or surgical management. *Dis Colon Rectum.* 2004;47:1493.

59. Jongen J, Each S, Stübinger SH, Bock JU. Excision of thrombosed external hemorrhoid under local anesthesia: a retrospective evaluation of 340 patients. *Dis Colon Rectum.* 2003;46:1226.

60. Deleted in review.

61. Read TE, Henry SE, Hovis RM, et al. Prospective evaluation of anesthetic technique for anorectal surgery. *Dis Colon Rectum.* 2002;45(11):1553-1558.

62. Nelson DW, Champagne BJ, Rivadeneira DE, et al. Prophylactic antibiotics for hemorrhoidectomy are they really needed? *Dis Colon Rectum.* 2014;57(3):365-369.

63. Senagore A, Mazier WP, Luchtefeld MA, et al. Treatment of advanced hemorrhoidal disease: a prospective, randomized comparison of cold scalpel vs. contact Nd:YAG laser. *Dis Colon Rectum.* 1993; 36:1042.

64. Milligan ET, Morgan CN, Lord LE. Surgical anatomy of anal canal, and the operative treatment of hemorrhoids. *Lancet.* 1937;2: 1119.

65. Tajana A. Hemorrhoidectomy according to Milligan-Morgan: ligature and excision technique. *Int Surg.* 1989;74:158

66. Ferguson JA, Heaton JR. Closed hemorrhoidectomy. *Dis Colon Rectum.* 1959;2:176.

67. Ganchrow MI, Mazier WP, Friend WG, Ferguson JA. Hemorrhoidectomy revisited—computer analysis of 2,038 cases. *Dis Colon Rectum.* 1971;14:128.

68. McConnell JC, Khubchandani I. Long-term follow-up of closed hemorrhoidectomy. *Dis Colon Rectum.* 1983;26:797.

69. Muldoon JP. The completely closed hemorrhoidectomy: a reliable and trusted friend for 25 years. *Dis Colon Rectum.* 1981;24:211.

70. Whitehead W. The surgical treatment of haemorrhoids. *Br Med J.* 1882;1:148

71. Andrews E. Disastrous results following Whitehead's operation and the so-called American operation. *Columbus Med J.* 1895;15:97.

72. Andrews E. Some of the evils caused by Whitehead's operation and by its modification, the American operation. *Trans Illinois Med Soc.* 1895;433.

73. Khubchandani M. Results of Whitehead operation. *Dis Colon Rectum*. 1984;27:730.

74. Rand AA. The sliding skin-flap graft operation for hemorrhoids: a modification of the Whitehead procedure. *Dis Colon Rectum*. 1969;12:265.

75. Bonello JC. Who's afraid of the dentate line? The Whitehead hemorrhoidectomy. *Am J Surg*. 1988;156:182.

76. Wolff BG, Culp CE. The Whitehead hemorrhoidectomy. An unjustly maligned procedure. *Dis Colon Rectum*. 1988;31:587.

77. Deleted in review.

78. Andrews BT, Layer GT, Jackson BT, Nicholls RJ. Randomized trial comparing diathermy hemorrhoidectomy with the scissor dissection Milligan-Morgan operation. *Dis Colon Rectum*. 1993;36:580.

79. Ibrahim S, Tsang C, Lee YL, Eu KW, Seow-Choen F. Prospective, randomized trial comparing pain and complications between diathermy and scissors for closed hemorrhoidectomy. *Dis Colon Rectum*. 1998;41:141.

80. Quah HM, Seow-Choen F. Prospective, randomized trial comparing diathermy excision and diathermy coagulation for symptomatic, prolapsed hemorrhoids. *Dis Colon Rectum*. 2004;47:367.

81. Nystrom PO, Qvist N, Raahave D, et al. Randomized clinical trial of symptom control after stapled anopexy or diathermy excision for haemorrhoid prolapse. *Br J Surg*. 2010;97:167.

82. Thaha MA, Campbell KL, Kazmi SA, et al. Prospective randomized multi-centre trial comparing the clinical efficacy, safety and patient acceptability of circular stapled anopexy with closed diathermy haemorrhoidectomy. *Gut*. 2009;58:668.

83. Chung YC, Wu HJ. Clinical experience of sutureless closed hemorrhoidectomy. *Dis Colon Rectum*. 2003;46:87.

84. Nienhuijs S, de Hingh I. Conventional versus LigaSure hemorrhoidectomy for patients with symptomatic hemorrhoids. *Cochrane Database Syst Rev*. 2009;(1):CD006761.

85. Armstrong DN, Frankum C, Schertzer ME, et al. Harmonic Scalpel hemorrhoidectomy: five hundred consecutive cases. *Dis Colon Rectum*. 2002;45:354.

86. Armstrong DN, Ambroze WL, Schertzer ME, Ambroze WL, Orangio GR. Harmonic Scalpel vs. electrocautery hemorrhoidectomy: a prospective evaluation. *Dis Colon Rectum*. 2001;44:558.

87. Khan S, Pawlak SE, Eggenberger JC, et al. Surgical treatment of hemorrhoids: prospective, randomized trial comparing closed excisional hemorrhoidectomy and the Harmonic Scalpel technique of excisional hemorrhoidectomy. *Dis Colon Rectum*. 2001;44:845.

88. Tan JJ, Seow-Choen F. Prospective, randomized trial comparing diathermy and Harmonic Scalpel hemorrhoidectomy. *Dis Colon Rectum*. 2001;44:677.

89. Abo-hashem AA, Sarhan A, Aly AM. Harmonic Scalpel compared with bipolar electro-cautery hemorrhoidectomy: a randomized controlled trial. *Int J Surg*. 2010;8:243.

90. Chung CC, Ha JP, Tai YP, et al. Double-blind, randomized trial comparing Harmonic Scalpel hemorrhoidectomy, bipolar scissors hemorrhoidectomy, and scissors excision: ligation technique. *Dis Colon Rectum*. 2002;45:789.

91. Kohlstadt CM, Weber J, Prohm P. [Stapler hemorrhoidectomy. A new alternative to conventional methods]. *Zentralbl Chir*. 1999;124:238.

92. Boccasanta P, Venturi M, Orio A, et al. Circular hemorrhoidectomy in advanced hemorrhoidal disease. *Hepatogastroenterology*. 1998;45:969.

93. Khalil KH, O'Bichere A, Sellu D. Randomized clinical trial of sutured versus stapled closed hemorrhoidectomy. *Br J Surg*. 2000;87:1352.

94. Mehigan BJ, Monson JR, Hartley JE. Stapling procedure for haemorrhoids versus Milligan-Morgan haemorrhoidectomy: randomized controlled trial. *Lancet*. 2000;355:782.

95. Rowsell M, Bello M, Hemingway DM. Circumferential mucosectomy (stapled haemorrhoidectomy) versus conventional haemorrhoidectomy: randomized controlled trial. *Lancet*. 2000;355:779.

96. Ganio E, Altomare DF, Gabrielli F, Milito G, Canuti S. Prospective randomized multicentre trial comparing stapled with open haemorrhoidectomy. *Br J Surg*. 2001;88:669.

97. Sengore AJ, Singer M, Abcarian H, et al. Procedure for Prolapse and Hemmorrhoids (PPH) Multicenter Study Group. A prospective, randomized, controlled multicenter trial comparing stapled hemorrhoidopexy and Ferguson hemorrhoidectomy: perioperative and one-year results. *Dis Colon Rectum*. 2004;47:1824.

98. Madiba TE, Esterhuizen TM, Thomson SR. Procedure for prolapsed haemorrhoids versus excisional haemorrhoidectomy—a systematic review and meta-analysis. *S Afr Med J*. 2009;99:43.

99. Laughlan K, Jayne DG, Jackson D, Rupprecht F, Ribaric G. Stapled haemorrhoidopexy compared to Milligan-Morgan and Ferguson haemorrhoidectomy: a systematic review. *Int J Colorectal Dis*. 2009;24:335.

100. Jayaraman S, Colquhoun PH, Malthaner RA. Stapled versus conventional surgery for hemorrhoids. *Cochrane Database Syst Rev*. 2006;(4):CD005393.

101. Giordano P, Gravante G, Sorge R, Ovens L, Nastro P. Long-term outcomes of stapled hemorrhoidopexy vs conventional hemorrhoidectomy: a meta-analysis of randomized controlled trials. *Arch Surg*. 2009;144:266.

102. Burch J, Epstein D, Sari AB, et al. Stapled haemorrhoidopexy for the treatment of haemorrhoids: a systematic review. *Colorectal Dis*. 2009;11:233, discussion 243.

103. Sakr MF, Moussa MM. LigaSure hemorrhoidectomy versus stapled hemorrhoidopexy: a prospective, randomized clinical trial. *Dis Colon Rectum*. 2010;53:1161.

104. Jayaraman S, Colquhoun PH, Malthaner RA. Stapled hemorrhoidopexy is associated with a higher long-term recurrence rate of internal hemorrhoids compared with conventional excisional hemorrhoid surgery. *Dis Colon Rectum*. 2007;50:1297-1305.

105. Nisar PJ, Acheson AG, Neal KR, Scholenfield JH. Stapled hemorrhoidopexy compared with conventional hemorrhoidectomy: systematic review of randomized controlled trials. *Dis Colon Rectum*. 2004;47:1837-1845.

106. Bove A, Bongarzoni G, Palone G, et al. Effective treatment of haemorrhoids: early complication and late results after 150 consecutive stapled haemorrhoidectomies. *Ann Ital Chir*. 2009;80:299.

107. Jorgen J, Eberstein A, Bock JU, et al. Complications, recurrences, early and late reoperations after stapled haemorrhoidopexy: lessons learned from 1,233 cases. *Langenbecks Arch Surg*. 2010;395:1049.

108. Van Wensen RJ, van Leuken MH, Bosscha K. Pelvis sepsis after stapled hemorrhoidopexy. *World J Gastroenterol*. 2008;14:5924.

109. Martellucci J, Papi F, Tanzini G. Double rectal perforation after stapled haemorrhoidectomy. *Int J Colorectal Dis*. 2009;24:1113.

110. Molloy RG, Kingsmore D. Life threatening pelvic sepsis after stapled haemorrhoidectomy. *Lancet*. 2000;355:810.

111. Cheetham MJ, Mortensen NJ, Nystrom PO, Kamm MA, Phillips RK. Persistent pain and faecal urgency after stapled haemorrhoidectomy. *Lancet*. 2000;356:730.

112. Tjandra JJ, Chan MK. Systematic review on the procedure for prolapse and hemorrhoids (stapled hemorrhoidopexy). *Dis Colon Rectum*. 2007;50:878-892.

113. Wong JC, Chung CC, Yau KK, et al. Stapled technique for acute thrombosed hemorrhoids: a randomized, controlled trial with long-term results. *Dis Colon Rectum*. 2008;51:397-403.

114. Morinaga K, Hasuda K, Ikeda T. A novel therapy for internal hemorrhoids: ligation of the hemorrhoidal artery with newly devised instrument (Moricorn) in conjunction with a Doppler flowmeter. *Am J Gastroenterol*. 1995;90:610.

115. Giordano P, Overton J, Madeddu F, et al. Transanal hemorrhoidal dearterialization: a systematic review. *Dis Colon Rectum*. 2009;52:1665.

116. Ratto C, Donisi L, Parello A, Litta F, Doglietto GB. Evaluation of transanal hemorrhoidal dearterialization as a minimally invasive therapeutic approach to hemorrhoids. *Dis Colon Rectum*. 2010;53:803-811.

117. Felice C, Privitera A, Ellul E, Klaumann M. Doppler-guided hemorrhoidal artery ligation: an alternative to hemorrhoidectomy. *Dis Colon Rectum*. 2005;48:2090-2093.

118. Faucheron JL, Gangner Y. Doppler-guided hemorrhoidal artery ligation for the treatment of symptomatic hemorrhoids: early and three-year follow-up results in 100 consecutive patients. *Dis Colon Rectum*. 2008;51:945-949.

119. Infantino A, Bellomo R, Dal Monte PP, et al. Transanal haemorrhoidal artery echo Doppler ligation and anopexy (THD) is effective for II and III degree haemorrhoids: a prospective multicentric study [published online ahead of print April 15, 2009]. *Colorectal Dis*. 2010;12:804-809.

120. Dal Monte PP, Tagariello C, Sarago M, et al. Transanal haemorrhoidal dearterialisation nonexcisional surgery for the treatment of haemorrhoidal disease. *Tech Coloproctol*. 2007;11:333-338.

121. Goldstein ET, Williamson PR, Larach SW. Subcutaneous morphine pump for postoperative hemorrhoidectomy pain management. *Dis Colon Rectum*. 1993;36:439.

122. Kilbride M, Morse M, Senagore A. Transdermal fentanyl improves management of postoperative hemorrhoidectomy pain. *Dis Colon Rectum*. 1994;37:1070.

123. Kilbride MJ, Senagore AJ, Morse M. Improving patient safety with transdermal-fentanyl for post-hemorrhoidectomy pain. *Dis Colon Rectum.* 1995;38:104.

124. Kuo RJ. Epidural morphine for post-hemorrhoidectomy analgesia. *Dis Colon Rectum.* 1984;27:529.

125. O'Donovan S, Ferrara A, Larach S, Williamson P. Intraoperative use of Toradol facilitates outpatient hemorrhoidectomy. *Dis Colon Rectum.* 1994;37:793.

126. Perrotti P, Dominici P, Grossi E, Cerutti R, Antropoli C. Topical nifedipine with lidocaine ointment versus active control for pain after hemorrhoidectomy: results of a multicentre, prospective, randomized, double-blind study. *Can J Surg.* 2010;53:17.

127. Karanlik H, Akturk R, Camlica H, Asoglu O. The effect of glyceryl trinitrate ointment on posthemorrhoidectomy pain and wound healing: results of a randomized double-blind, placebo-controlled study. *Dis Colon Rectum.* 2009 52:280.

128. Joshi GP, Neugebauer EA. Evidence-based management of pain after haemorrhoidectomy surgery. *Br J Surg.* 2010;97:1155.

129. Hoff SD, Bailey HR, Butts DR, et al. Ambulatory surgical hemorrhoidectomy—a solution to postoperative urinary retention? *Dis Colon Rectum.* 1994;37:1242.

130. Leventhal A, Pfau A. Pharmacologic management of postoperative overdistention of the bladder. *Surg Gynecol Obstet.* 1978;146:347.

131. Petros JG, Bradley TM. Factors influencing postoperative urinary retention in patients undergoing surgery for benign anorectal disease. *Am J Surg.* 1990;159:374.

132. Tammela T, Kontturi M, Lukkarinen O. Postoperative urinary retention. I. Incidence and predisposing factors. *Scand J Urol Nephrol.* 1986;20:197.

133. Shafik A. Role of warm water bath in inducing micturition in postoperative urinary retention after anorectal operations. *Urol Int.* 1993;50:213.

134. Corman ML. Complications in hemorrhoid and fissure surgery. In: Ferrari BT, Ray JE, Gathright JB, eds. *Complications of Colon and Rectal Surgery: Prevention and Management.* Philadelphia: Saunders; 1985:91.

135. Kilbourne NJ. Internal haemorrhoids: comparative value of treatment by operative and by injection methods: a survey of 62,910 cases. *Ann Surg.* 1934;99:600.

136. Gabriel WB. Hemorrhoids. In: *The Principles and Practice of Rectal Surgery.* 5th ed. Springfield, IL: Charles C Thomas; 1964:110.

137. Milsom JW. Hemorrhoidal disease. In: Wexner SD, Beck DE, eds. *Fundamentals of Anorectal Surgery.* New York: McGraw-Hill; 1992 192.

138. Salvati EP, Eisenstat TE. Hemorrhoidal disease. In: Zuidema GD, Condon RE, eds. *Shackelford's Surgery of the Alimentary Tract.* Philadelphia: Saunders; 1991:294.

139. Rosen L, Sipe P, Stasik JJ, Riether RD, Trimpi HD. Outcome of delayed hemorrhage following surgical hemorrhoidectomy. *Dis Colon Rectum.* 1993;36:743.

140. Basso L, Pescatori M. Outcome of delayed hemorrhage following surgical hemorrhoidectomy. *Dis Colon Rectum.* 1994:37:288.

141. Cirocco WC, Golub RW. Local epinephrine injection as treatment for delayed hemorrhage after hemorrhoidectomy. *Surgery.* 1995; 117:235.

142. Mollen R, Van Laarhoven C, Kuijpers J. Pathogenesis and management of rectoceles. *Semin Colon Rectal Surg.* 1996;7:192-196.

143. Moalli PA, Jones Ivy S, Meyn LA, Zyczynski HM. Risk factors associated with pelvic floor disorders in women undergoing surgical repair. *Obstet Gynecol.* 2003;101:869.

144. Lukacz ES, Lawrence JM, Contreras R, Nager CW, Luber KM. Parity, mode of delivery, and pelvic floor disorders. *Obstet Gynecol.* 2006;107:1253.

145. DeLancey JO, Kearney R, Chou Q, Speights S, Binno S. The appearance of levator ani muscle abnormalities in magnetic resonance images after vaginal delivery. *Obstet Gynecol.* 2003;101:46.

146. Chen L, Ashton-Miller JA, Hsu Y DeLancey JO. Interaction among apical support, levator ani impairment, and anterior vaginal wall prolapse. *Obstet Gynecol.* 2006;108:324.

147. Swift SE, Tate SB, Nicholas J. Correlation of symptoms with degree of pelvic organ support in a general population of women: what is pelvic organ prolapse? *Am J Obstet Gynecol.* 2003;189:372.

148. Dietz HP, Clarke B. Prevalence of rectocele in young nulliparous women. *Aust N Z J Obstet Gynaecol.* 2005;45:391.

149. Moalli PA, Shand SH, Zyczynski HM, Gordy SC, Meyn LA. Remodeling of vaginal connective tissue in patients with prolapse. *Obstet Gynecol.* 2005;106:953.

150. Norton PA, Baker JE, Sharp HC, Warenski JC. Genitourinary prolapse and joint hypermobility in women. *Obstet Gynecol.* 1995;85:225.

151. Hendrix SL, Clark A, Nygaard I, Aragaki A, Barnabei V, McTiernan A. Pelvic organ prolapse in the Women's Health Initiative: gravity and gravidity. *Am J Obstet Gynecol.* 2002;186:1160.

152. Bradley CS, Zimmerman MB, Wang Q, Nygaard IE. Women's Health Initiative. Vaginal descent and pelvic floor symptoms in postmenopausal women: a longitudinal study. *Obstet Gynecol.* 2008;111:148.

153. Greenberg T, Kelvin FM, Maglinto DD. Barium trapping in rectoceles: are we trapped by the wrong definition? *Abdom Imaging.* 2001;26:587.

154. Savoye-Collet C, Savoye G, Koning E, Leroi AM, Dacher JN. Defecography in symptomatic older women living at home. *Age Ageing.* 2003;32:347.

155. Jarvis SK, Hallam TK, Lujic S, Abbott JA, Vancaillie TG. Perioperative physiotherapy improves outcomes for women undergoing incontinence and/or prolapse surgery: results of a randomised controlled trial. *Aust N Z J Obstet Gynaecol.* 2005;45:300.

156. Sullivan ES, Leaverton GH, Hardwick CE. Transrectal repair: an adjunct to improved function after anorectal surgery. *Dis Colon Rectum.* 1968;11:106-114.

157. Murthy VK, Orkin BA, Smith LA, Glassman LM. Excellent outcome using selective criteria for retocele repair. *Dis Colon Rectum.* 1996;39:374-378.

158. Khubchandani IT, Sheets JA, Stasik JJ, Hakki AR. Endorectal reapair of rectocele. *Dis Colon Rectum.* 1983 26:792-796.

159. Sehapayak S. Transrectal repair of rectocele: an extended armamentarium of colorectal surgeons. A report of 355 cases. *Dis Colon Rectum.* 1985;28:422-433.

160. Boccasanta P, Venturi M, Stuto A, et al. Stapled transanal rectal resection for outlet obstruction: a prospective, multicenter trial. *Dis Colon Rectum.* 2004;47:1285.

161. Maher C, Feiner B, Baessler K, Schmid C. Surgical management of pelvic organ prolapse in women. *Cochrane Database Syst Rev.* 2013;(4): D004014.

162. Kahn MA, Stanton SL, Kumar D Fox SD. Posterior colporrhaphy is superior to the transanal repair to treatment of posterior vaginal wall prolapse. *Neurourol Urodyn.* 1999;18:70.

163. Nieminen K, Hiltunen KM, Laitinen J, Oksala J, Heinonen PK. Transanal or vaginal approach to rectocele repair: a prospective, randomized pilot study. *Dis Colon Rectum.* 2004;47:1636.

164. Farid M, Madbouly KM, Hussein A, Mahdy T, Moneim HA, Omar W. Randomized controlled trial between perineal and anal repairs of rectocele in obstructed defecation. *World J Surg.* 2010;34:822.

165. Gustilo-Ashby AM, Paraiso MF, Jelovsek JE, Walters MD, Barber MD. Bowel symptoms 1 year after surgery for prolapse: further analysis of a randomized trial of rectocele repair. *Am J Obstet Gynecol.* 2007;197:76.e1.

166. Mellgren A, Anzén B, Nilsson BY, et al. Results of rectocele repair. A prospective study. *Dis Colon Rectum.* 1995;38:7.

167. Weber AM, Walters MD, Piedmonte MR. Sexual function and vaginal anatomy in women before and after surgery for pelvic organ prolapse and urinary incontinence. *Am J Obstet Gynecol.* 2000;182:1610.

168. Maher CF, Qatawneh AM, Baessler K, Schluter PJ. Midline rectovaginal fascial plication for repair of rectocele and obstructed defecation. *Obstet Gynecol.* 2004 104:685.

169. Cundiff GW, Weidner AC, Visco AG, Addison WA, Bump RC. An anatomic and functional assessment of the discrete defect rectocele repair. *Am J Obstet Gynecol.* 1998;179:1451.

170. Kenton K, Shott S, Brubaker L. Outcome after rectovaginal fascia reattachment for rectocele repair. *Am J Obstet Gynecol.* 1999;181:1360.

171. Porter WE, Steele A, Walsh P, Kohli N, Karram MM. The anatomic and functional outcomes of defect-specific rectocele repairs. *Am J Obstet Gynecol.* 1999;181:1353.

172. Glavind K, Madsen H. A prospective study of the discrete fascial defect rectocele repair. *Acta Obstet Gynecol Scand.* 2000;79:145.

173. Abramov Y, Gandhi S, Goldberg RP, Botros SM, Kwon C, Sand PK. Site-specific rectocele repair compared with standard posterior colporrhaphy. *Obstet Gynecol.* 2005;105:314.

174. Sung VW, Rogers RG, Schaffer JI, et al. Graft use in transvaginal pelvic organ prolapse repair: a systematic review. *Obstet Gynecol.* 2008;112:1131.

175. Murphy M. Society of Gynecologic Surgeons Systematic Review Group. Clinical practice guidelines on vaginal graft use from the Society of Gynecologic Surgeons. *Obstet Gynecol.* 2008 112:1123.

Fissure-in-Ano

Rahila Essani | Harry T. Papaconstantinou

Anal fissure (fissure-in-ano) is a common condition that usually presents as anal pain or bleeding with defecation. It is easily confused with symptomatic hemorrhoids. It can be very troubling because the severity of patient discomfort and extent of disability far exceed that which would be expected from such trivial lesion.

Bleeding is a common symptom and is usually scant, bright red, and found on the tissue when cleansing after a bowel movement. Anal fissure is described as a linear defect, or laceration, in the anoderm, located between the dentate line and the anal verge. It can be acute or chronic. An acute fissure is a simple laceration, whereas a chronic anal fissure is an ulceration with built-up scarred edges and exposed internal anal sphincter muscle fibers at its base. Additional findings may include a perianal skin tag at the external margin of the fissure and a hypertrophied papilla at the dentate line. Chronic fissure is defined by these three findings—visible muscle, a skin tag (sentinel tag), and hypertrophied papilla (Fig. 159.1). Importantly, acute and chronic anal fissures are almost always located in the midline, with the posterior location predominating. However, in 10% of women and in 1% of men, anal fissure can be seen in the anterior midline.[1] Fissures located off the midline are usually associated with more serious systemic diseases such as Crohn disease and immunodeficiency syndromes (Fig. 159.2).

ETIOLOGY

Trauma to the anal canal, because of passing hard stools, is probably the most frequent cause of fissure-in-ano. Patients will often remember the exact time the fissure developed based on the symptoms. Classically, this will almost always be associated with an episode of constipation. Anal fissure can also be a consequence of frequent defecation and diarrhea. Preexisting anal canal irritation has been postulated to lead to fissure. Scarring, stricture, and stenosis, from prior anal injury or surgery, are recognized conditions that predispose to fissure formation.[2] Because fissures occur most often in the posterior midline, various structural theories have been proposed as causes,[3–5] the most compelling of which is the vascular anatomy of the internal sphincter.

In 1989 Klosterhalfen et al.[5] reported on anatomic dissections that detailed the blood supply of the inferior hemorrhoidal artery. In the majority of cadaver specimens (85%), the posterior commissure of the anal canal was not directly perfused except by end arterioles. Branching from the sphincteric arterioles occurred at right angles to the parent vessels and coursed perpendicularly through the circular fibers of the internal sphincter. These anatomic findings established the possibility of decreased mucosal perfusion, particularly in the posterior midline.

Others have confirmed in cadaveric studies that there is a significant trend to an increasing number of arterioles posterior to anterior in the subanodermal space at all levels.[6] Furthermore, sphincter spasm and hypertonicity, which is common in this disease, may further decrease blood flow posteriorly. Schouten et al.[7,8] have shown increased anal canal pressures correlated with decreased mucosal blood flow, as measured by laser Doppler flowmetry. Reports of normal anal maximal resting pressure are highly variable, ranging from 60 to 100 cm H_2O in females and slightly higher in males; however, the measurement is defined as the maximal pressure recorded at rest.[9] The higher pressures seen in patients with anal fissures will produce a sawtooth pattern on manometry tracings. This vascular-anal hypertonic resting pressure hypothesis has prompted trials aimed at improving blood flow and lowering anal canal resting pressures. Whether sphincter hypertonia is a cause or effect is unknown.

The most common systemic conditions that are associated with atypical anal fissure/anal ulcer are Crohn disease and acquired immunodeficiency syndrome. Both of these conditions lead to an immunocompromised patient. Atypical features include fissures off the true midline, shaggy large defects with undermined edges, and granulation tissue in the base. Actual cavitation of the internal sphincter is another ominous clue to the presence of systemic disease. In the immunocompromised patient, a fissure or an ulcer and a concomitant mass should raise the question of malignancy. Lymphoma, leukemic ulcer, and anal canal epithelial tumors are often associated with surface defects. There are subtle changes, which distinguish these conditions from uncomplicated acute or chronic anal fissure.

Infections also cause fissure-in-ano. Syphilis and tuberculosis were seen frequently in the United States over the last century but are currently uncommon causes of anal fissure. Today, sexually transmitted diseases and infections associated with immunocompromised conditions may be the cause of anal fissure and include chancroid, herpes simplex virus, and cytomegalovirus. Herpes simplex infection manifests as multiple superficial ulcers and vesicles, while syphilitic ulcers are purulent and have a granular base. The treatments for these disease processes are different, and therefore it is important to recognize the differences between anal canal fissures and atypical anal canal ulcers (see Fig. 159.2).

DIAGNOSIS

A tearing or burning discomfort during defecation is by far the most common symptom of anal fissure. Bleeding is usually only detected on the toilet paper. The pain associated with anal fissure lasts for minutes to hours,

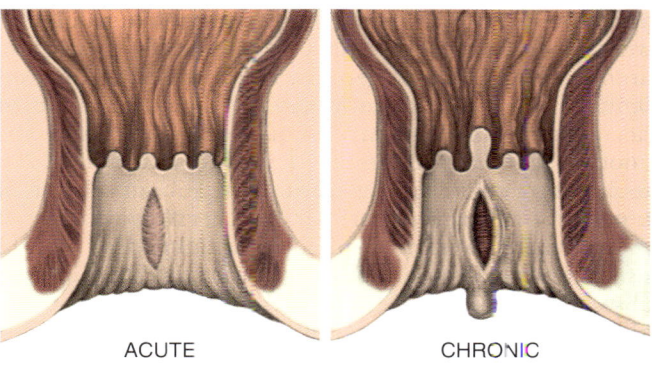

ACUTE   CHRONIC

FIGURE 159.1 Acute and chronic fissure. (Modified from Hicks TC, Ray JE. Rectal and perianal complaints. In: Polk HC Jr, Stone HH, Gardner B, eds. *Basic Surgery*. 3rd ed. Norwalk, CT: Appleton-Century-Crofts; 1987:455.)

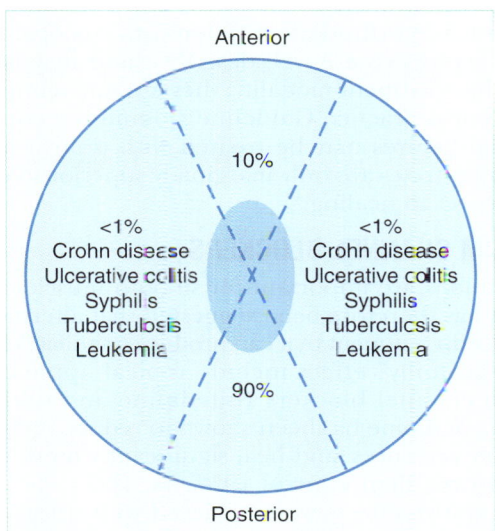

FIGURE 159.2 Diagram of the location of typical fissures and atypical fissures where a systemic illness should be suspected.

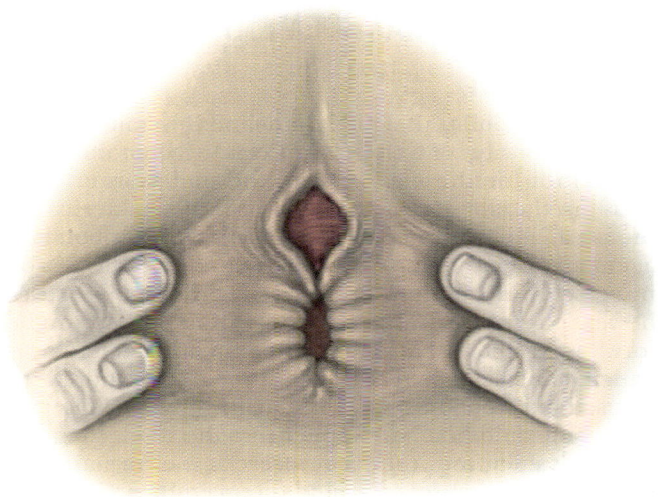

FIGURE 159.3 Inspection of fissure.

and in patients with acute anal fissure, it is most often described as a cutting or tearing sensation during the act of defecation. The patient often relates that constipation is the antecedent event, but once pain develops, the fear of the act of defecation and refusal of the call to stool can exacerbate this problem. This anxiety leads to fecal impaction, particularly in children and the elderly. Those individuals with a chronic anal fissure will present with a different symptom complex. They may complain of a lump representing the sentinel tag, drainage or discharge from the open wound, pruritus, or a combination of several symptoms. Bleeding may be absent, and pain is usually mild or absent as well. The pain of anal fissure can be differentiated from that of proctalgia fugax in that the latter produces discomfort, which usually not related to bowel action. In addition, the patient with a fissure feels the discomfort in the anal area, the pain of proctalgia fugaxis

higher in the rectum or deep pelvis and more deep-seated. Another anal condition that commonly produces pain is a thrombosed hemorrhoid. With this complaint, the patient also reports feeling a lump, which will not be present if an acute anal fissure is the cause of the pain.

Examination must be carefully performed; the pain caused by an aggressive examination of an anal fissure is not easily forgotten by the patient or examiner. Simple spreading of the buttocks to gently roll open the anal verge will usually demonstrate the fissure (Fig 159.3). Endoscopy, which must be performed as part of the complete evaluation of patients with fissure, should be postponed; a more complete anorectal examination can be better accomplished when the fissure is healed. Importantly, topical anesthetics do not facilitate pain-free examinations.

Atypical-appearing fissures require more intensive inquiry. Symptoms of inflammatory bowel disease should be sought. Sexual activity and drug history should likewise be documented. If there is cause for concern as to the true nature of the ulcer or fissure, biopsy, stool culture, serology, and gastrointestinal evaluation may be indicated. High-risk behavior for human immunodeficiency virus infection necessitates screening and may explain the presence of the atypical fissure. Syphilitic ulcers can be diagnosed with dark-field, wet prep microscopy. Tuberculous ulcer, although commonly superinfected, will show acid-fast bacilli on staining. The critical issue in patients with atypical-appearing fissures is a high index of suspicion. If an atypical fissure is treated the same way as a typical fissure, a large nonhealing wound could result.

Most diagnostic tests will not be tolerated as office procedures. Examination under anesthesia permits a thorough evaluation of the anus and rectum. Cultures, biopsies, and possible therapeutic interventions can be safely and carefully performed with anesthesia. Indeed, patients embrace the opportunity to have a pain-free evaluation under anesthesia.

NONSURGICAL MANAGEMENT

CONSERVATIVE

In 2010 the Clinical Practice Guideline Committee of the American Society of Colon and Rectal Surgeons published guidelines for the management of anal fissure.[10] The first-line therapy for patients with simple, acute fissure-in-ano includes warm-water sitz baths and stool-bulking agents. Warm-water soaks likely relieve anal discomfort by muscle relaxation, which lowers anal canal pressures; however, results from prospective studies are contradictory.[11] Nevertheless, heat provides dramatic relief to most patients with acute and chronic fissure-in-ano, and should be used in all patients. Stool-bulking agents, such as psyllium, bran, and fiber, draw water into the stool, changing its consistency, and therefore prevent the formation of hard stool that causes sustained trauma to the anal canal. Furthermore, bran has been shown to be effective in preventing recurrence of acute anal fissure.[12] Preparations containing mineral oil are not advised because of difficulty in cleansing the area following defecations and detrimental effect to the colonic mucosa. Topical creams and steroids may provide some transient relief but are not routinely recommended as management options, because these modalities do not address the underlying problem. These conservative, nonsurgical measures successfully heal 90% of acute anal fissures, but only 40% of chronic fissures. The task force concludes that nonoperative treatment continues to be safe, has few side effects, and should usually be the first step in therapy. Chronic anal fissures are managed with medications that provide a "chemical sphincterotomy," and are described later.

NITROGLYCERIN

It has been suggested that poor posterior anal canal blood flow and generalized hypertonia of the internal anal sphincter are causes of anal fissures. Therefore improvement in the blood supply and sphincter relaxation should facilitate healing. Nitric oxide is a potent smooth muscle relaxant and promotes vasodilation. Topical nitroglycerin is a nitric oxide donor that is absorbed transcutaneously, and when applied to the anus, diffuses across the mucosa causing reduction in internal anal sphincter presure.[12] This leads to improvement of anal blood flow with the consequence of increased likelihood for healing of the fissure. Indeed, nitroglycerin has become an important adjuvant treatment option in patients with fissures that do not heal with stool-bulking agents and local heat therapy.[13–15] In 2004 a meta-analysis of randomized controlled trials comparing nitroglycerin ointment to placebo for the treatment of anal fissures showed that nitroglycerin is significantly more effective than placebo in primary healing of anal fissure (46% vs. 33%; $P < .0001$).[16] In fact, several independent studies have demonstrated the therapeutic efficacy of nitroglycerin paste in 60% to 75% of patients with anal fissures.[15–21]

The dosage and strength of the nitroglycerin have varied from study to study, but there is some correlation between dose and degree of sphincter relaxation.[22] A multiinstitutional investigation was conducted in 17 centers, with the aim of determining the optimal dosage and dosing interval for the use of nitroglycerin.[22] There were no significant differences observed in fissure healing among any treatment groups, but those who received 0.4% (1.5 mg) nitroglycerin had a statistically significant decrease in pain intensity. Most of the other studies report good results with 0.2% nitroglycerin. Application of 200 to 500 mg of 0.2% nitroglycerin paste (about the size of a pea) to the anus is performed at least twice daily. It is important to inform patients that either they should use a Q-tip or a glove should be worn, to protect against absorption of the nitroglycerin through the skin on the finger. The ointment should be protected from exposure to air and light because nitroglycerin paste is volatile and will deactivate. Pain relief is nearly immediate (5 minutes) and lasts for up to 12 hours.[13,16,17] Headache is a significant side effect and limits the amount of paste that can be applied. With this therapy, healing of the fissure takes 4 to 6 weeks. Patients with fissures that fail to heal often have persistently elevated anal canal pressures despite the use of nitroglycerin. Recurrent disease after initial healing can be successfully retreated.[16,17] Other adverse effects such as orthostatic hypotension, syncopal attacks, and tachyphylaxis are well described and may limit the use of this treatment modality; they are uncommon.[16,22,23] The Clinical Practice Guideline Committee concluded that anal fissures may be treated with topical nitrates, although nitrates are only marginally superior to placebo with respect to healing.[10]

CALCIUM CHANNEL BLOCKERS

Calcium ions are important for smooth muscle contractions. It has therefore been suggested that alternatives to nitroglycerin ointment that can produce a similar "chemical sphincterotomy" effect include topical application of calcium channel blockers (nifedipine and diltiazem). Topical nifedipine has been shown to reduce resting anal sphincter pressures, and heal significantly more chronic anal fissures than control (95% vs. 16%; $P < .001$).[24] These positive effects were achieved with no significant side effects of this medication. Other calcium channel blockers, such as topical 2% diltiazem, have been shown to be as effective as nitroglycerin in the treatment of chronic anal fissures.[25,26] In fact, topical diltiazem heals between 48% and 75% of fissures that have failed to heal with nitroglycerin alone.[27,28,28a] This class of drug may ultimately supersede nitroglycerin in the treatment of chronic anal fissure, because it is equally effective in treating chronic anal fissures and has a superior side-effect profile. Oral calcium channel blockers have been used but have a lower rate of healing than topical application with a higher rate of side effects, primarily headaches.[29,30] Due to the similar healing rates between nitroglycerin and calcium channel blockers, the standards practice task force felt that anal fissures may be treated with topical calcium channel blockers, with the expectation of lower incidence of adverse effects than nitrates. However, there are insufficient data to conclude whether they are superior to placebo in healing anal fissures.[10]

BOTOX

Another alternative is botulinum toxin A, an exotoxin produced by the bacterium *Clostridium botulinum* that causes

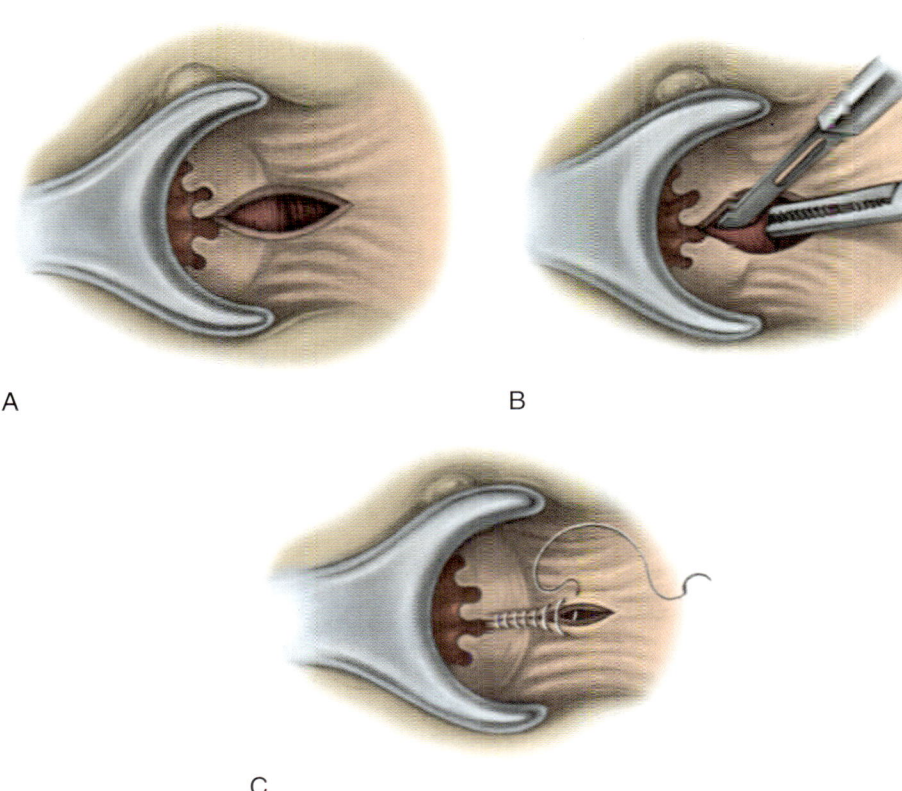

FIGURE 159.4 Lateral internal anal sphincterotomy. (A) Internal anal sphincter visible through incision. (B) Lateral division of internal anal sphincter. (C) Wound closure. (Modified from Storer EH, Goldberg SM, Nivatvongs S. Colon, rectum and anus. In: Schwartz SI, ed. *Principles of Surgery*. 4th ed. New York: McGraw-Hill; 1984:1139.)

paralysis of skeletal muscle by preventing the presynaptic release of acetylcholine. Botulinum toxin A has been shown to be efficacious in the treatment of chronic anal fissure. In one study, 73% of anal fissures were healed at 8 weeks, with no recurrences at a mean of 16 months' follow-up.[10] Results of a randomized double-blind placebo-controlled trial comparing botulinum toxin A injection to topical nitroglycerin ointment showed that at 8 weeks anal fissures were healed in 96% of patients injected with neurotoxin and 60% of those treated with nitroglycerin.[31] There was no recurrence in either group at a mean follow-up of 15 months.[32] The optimal dose and injection site of botulinum toxin A for the treatment of chronic anal fissures are unclear. There are no data to determine the optimal dose, and anywhere from 10 to 100 units have been reported. Injection of 50 units of botulinum toxin A into the internal sphincter on either side of the fissure has shown to be well tolerated.[32] Healing of posterior anal fissures are accelerated in patients injected with neurotoxin in the anterior anus when compared with posterior injection.[53] Although initial studies reported injections into the external anal sphincter recent studies have performed intersphincteric injections or injection into the internal sphincter with excellent results, with healing rates of 60% to 80%.[30,31,33–35] Complications of this form of treatment are infrequent and include transient incontinence to flatus in 18%[29] and stool in 5%[29] and perianal hematoma. Although botulinum toxin A injection has been supported as a first-line therapy for the treatment of chronic anal fissures, cost and convenience issues argue for its second-line use after failure of topical agents. The topical calcium channel blockers nifedipine and diltiazem

have become the initial first-line treatment. Although compounding is required, they are cheap, convenient, and widely available, with an excellent, low side-effect profile.

SURGICAL THERAPY

Studies have reported on the combination of Botox injection along with fissurectomy. Barnes et al. in 2015 reported the use of Botox with fissurectomy in 102 patients.[36] Fissurectomy was defined as curettage of base of the anal fissure ulcer and excision of the rolled up edges along with excision of sentinel skin tag/papilloma. They reported 95% fissure healing rate with this combination without resorting to surgical sphincterotomy.[36] The Clinical Practice Guidelines Committee comments that Botox injection has been associated with healing rates superior to that of a placebo. However, they note that there is inadequate consensus on dosage, precise site of administration, number of injections, or efficacy.[10]

The Clinical Practice Guidelines Committee of the American Society of Colon and Rectal Surgeons in 2010[10] concluded that lateral internal sphincterotomy (LIS) is the surgical treatment of choice for refractory anal fissure (Fig. 159.4) This technique requires the surgeon to be familiar with anal canal anatomy. The strategy of operative sphincterotomy is to divide the hypertonic portion of the internal anal sphincter muscle to reduce anal canal pressure and facilitate healing of the anal fissure. This procedure was originally described by Eisenhammer in 1951 as a midline posterior incision through the fissure.[4] However, subsequent studies noted problems with wound healing and the formation of a "keyhole" deformity to the anus.[3] "Keyhole" deformities are a persistent groove in the midline following sphincter division that may result in a significant degree of anal seepage or incontinence. Subsequent modifications to this procedure included repositioning the incision to the right or left lateral position, which has effectively eliminated the complication of this deformity.[5] Notaras is credited with introducing the "closed" sphincterotomy that is performed through a stab incision at the intersphincteric groove (Fig. 159.5), rather than an "open" exposure of the internal sphincter.[37,38] This closed technique can be done in the office setting with local anesthetic using either a small anoscope or a finger in the anal canal to guide division of a portion of the sphincter.[39]

LIS has produced excellent results for the treatment of chronic anal fissure, with an 85% to 100% healing rate and very low incidence of persistent or early relapse (Table 159.1).[37-45] There has been a low, but persistent, complication rate for soiling (1% to 22%) and incontinence to flatus (0% to 28%) and stool (0% to 11%). Comparing open versus closed techniques has not shown any differences of significance in postoperative pain, treatment success, complication of incontinence, or overall outcome. The length of internal sphincterotomy has been evaluated in a combined analysis. In terms of healing and incontinence, division of the sphincter limited to the length of the fissure was compared with a longer division beyond the fissure to the level of the dentate line.[45] The longer sphincterotomy was associated with a significantly lower risk of treatment failure, with no difference in postoperative incontinence rates as measured by the Wexner score.[46] Some degree of transient incontinence may be experienced by the patient in the early postoperative period, but this usually improves with time.[44] To further lower incontinence rates, a calibrated sphincterotomy has been performed. A fissure apex sphincterotomy was performed and extended using a calibrated sound to 30-mm base aperture. In three small series, this technique showed similar healing, with lower rates of incontinence compared with standard apex sphincterotomy.[46-48] Therefore, given the low but persistent rate of incontinence with LIS, this operation should be performed in select patients who have failed nonsurgical therapy. Absence of preoperative continence problems and meticulous surgical techniques are necessary to achieve good results.

Other surgical procedures for the management of chronic anal fissures exist but are performed less frequently. Fissurectomy is the excision of the anal fissure and is still performed today. This procedure results in a defect in the anoderm that can be covered with a rotation or

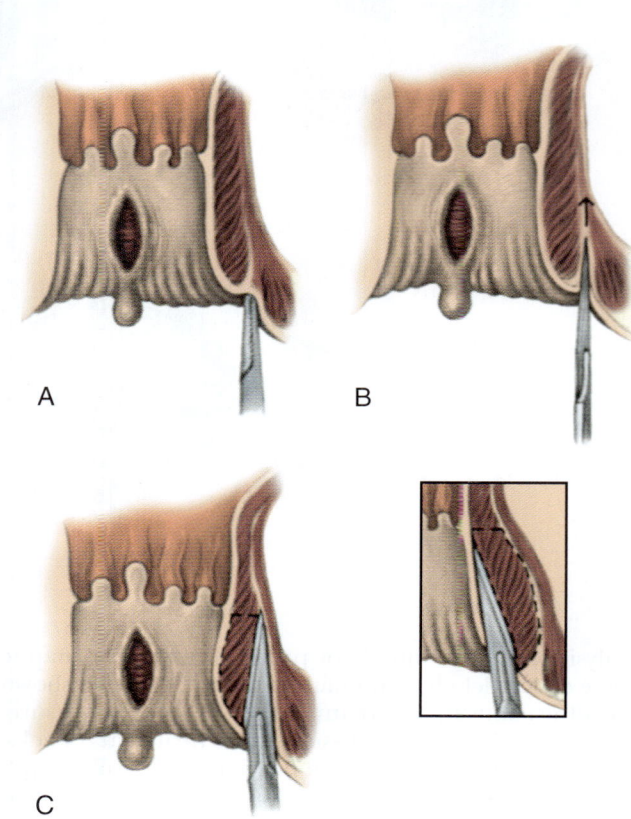

FIGURE 159.5 Blind lateral subcutaneous internal anal sphincterotomy. (A) Hemostat demonstrating intersphincteric groove. (B) Insertion of scalpel between internal and external sphincters. (C) Sphincter division by inward motion of the scalpel. *Inset,* Original Notaras technique showing outward motion of scalpel. (Modified from Notaras MJ. The treatment of anal fissure by lateral subcutaneous internal sphincterotomy: a technique and results. *Br J Surg.* 1971;58:96.)

TABLE 159.1 Impaired Anal Incontinence After Lateral Internal Sphincterotomy

Authors, Year	No. of Patients	Healed (%)	Recurrence/ Persistence (%)	IMPAIRED ANAL CONTINENCE (%)		
				Soiling	Flatus	Stool
Hoffman and Goligher, 1970[40]	99	97	3	1.0	6.1	7.1
Notaras, 1971[38]	82	100	0	1.4	2.7	5.5
Rudd, 1975[39]	200	99.5	0.5	0	0	0
Boulos and Araujo, 1984[41]	23	100	0	0	17.9	NA
Pernikoff et al., 1994[42]	500	97	3	4	3	1
Garcia-Aguilar et al., 1996[43]	549	89	11	22	28	8
Hananel and Gordon, 1997[44]	312	99	1	1	1	1
Nyam and Pemberton, 1999[45]	487	96	4	8	6	1

NA, Not available.

advancement flap to avoid a keyhole deformity and address a coincidental stricture or anal stenosis.[49] Advancement flap without fissurectomy is attractive, as theoretically there should be less risk of incontinence. One series showed a trend to better healing in the flap group; however, the recurrence rate was higher.[50] Surgical adjuncts to surgery to improve outcome have included anal papilla excision. Satisfaction was higher in those who had their papilla excised.[51] In another study, 39 patients were randomized to have the anal wound dressed open to avoid infection or sutured shut to hasten healing.[52] Wound problems occurred more often in the open group (4/17) compared with the sutured group (1/22). Healing occurred twice as fast in the sutured group.[52]

Dilation of the anal canal by four-finger insertion technique has fallen out of favor and should be discouraged, because this procedure stretches the anal canal in an uncontrolled fashion, resulting in unacceptable levels of postoperative incontinence. Furthermore, a recent meta-analysis showed that anal dilation resulted in significantly greater persistence of disease than sphincterotomy.[53] Retractors and balloon-tipped dilating catheters have been used for dilation in the treatment of chronic anal fissures.[54–57] These more controlled dilation procedures have been reported to be as efficacious as LIS.

In a recent study, patients with symptomatic chronic anal fissure were randomly assigned to pneumatic balloon dilation or LIS with anal ultrasonography and anal manometry performed before and 6 months after surgery. Anal continence, scored by using a validated continence grading scale, was evaluated preoperatively (at 1 and 6 weeks) and at 12 and 24 months postoperatively.[58] Twenty-four patients (11 males; mean age, 42 ± 8.2 years) underwent pneumatic balloon dilation, and 25 patients (10 males; mean age, 44 ± 7.3 years) underwent LIS. Fissure healing rates were 83.3% in the pneumatic balloon dilation and 92% in the LIS group. Recurrent anal fissure was observed in one patient (4%) after LIS. At anal manometry, mean resting pressure decrements obtained after pneumatic balloon dilation and LIS were 30.5% and 34.3%, respectively. After pneumatic balloon dilation, anal ultrasonography did not show any significant sphincter damage. At 24-month follow-up, the incidence of incontinence, irrespective of severity, was zero in the pneumatic balloon dilation group and 16% in the LIS group ($P < .0001$).[56] Calibrated balloon dilation may provide a method that is safe and as efficacious as sphincterotomy. As with LIS, pneumatic balloon dilation generates a high anal fissure healing rate but with a statistically significant reduction in postoperative anal incontinence.

CONCLUSION

Most acute anal fissures will heal with conservative measures, while chronic anal fissures may respond to medical therapies, or injection of botulinum toxin. Patients with persistent fissures should be considered for lateral partial internal sphincterotomy. Our approach is outlined in the algorithm (Fig. 159.6). The gratitude from a patient successfully treated after suffering with a painful anal fissure may be more immense than that from the cure of a cancer patient.

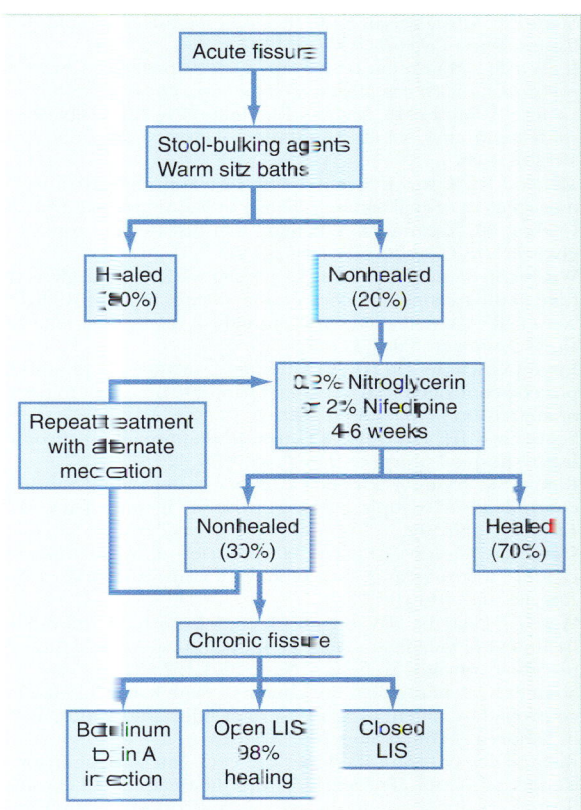

FIGURE 159.6 Algorithm for therapeutic options in decision making for managing anal fissures. *LIS,* Lateral internal sphincterotomy.

REFERENCES

1. Goligher JC. *Surgery of the Anus, Rectum and Colon.* 4th ed. New York, NY: Macmillan; 1980:136 Oh C. The role of internal sphincterotomy. *Mt Sinai J Med.* 1982;49:484.
2. Abcarian H. Surgical correction of chronic anal fissure: results of lateral internal sphincterotomy vs fissurectomy–midline sphincterotomy. *Dis Colon Rectum.* 1980;23:31.
3. Eisenhammer S. The surgical correction of chronic internal anal (sphincteric) contracture. *S Afr Med J.* 1951;25:486.
4. Eisenhammer S. The evaluation of the internal anal sphincterotomy operation with special reference to anal fissure. *Surg Gynecol Obstet.* 1959;109:583.
5. Klosterhalfen B, Vogel P, Rixen H, Mittermayer C. Topography of the inferior rectal artery: a possible cause of chronic, primary fissure. *Dis Colon Rectum.* 1989;32:43.
6. Lund JN, Binch C, McGarth J, Sparrow RA, Scholefield JH. Topographical distribution of blood supply to the anal canal. *Br J Surg.* 1999;86(4):496-498.
7. Schouten WR, Briel JW, Auwerda JJ. Relationship between anal pressure and anodermal blood flow—the vascular pathogenesis of anal fissure. *Dis Colon Rectum.* 1994;57:664.
8. Schouten WR, Briel JW, Auwerda JJ, De Graaf EJ. Ischaemic nature of anal fissure. *Br J Surg.* 1996;83:63.
9. Lowry AC, Simmang CL, Boulos P, et al. Consensus statement of definition of anorectal physiology and rectal cancer: report of the Tripartite Consensus Conference on definitions for anorectal physiology and rectal cancer, Washington D.C., May 1999. *Dis Colon Rectum.* 2001;44:915.
10. Perry WB, Dykes SL, Buie WD, Rafferty JF. Standards Practice Task Force of the American Society of Colon and Rectal Surgeons. Practice parameters for the management of anal fissures (3rd revision). *Dis Colon Rectum.* 2010;53(8):1110-1115.

11. Stein BL. Nitroglycerin and other nonoperative therapies for anal fissure. *Semin Colon Rectal Surg.* 1997;8:24.

12. Jensen SL. Maintenance therapy with unprocessed bran in the prevention of acute anal fissure recurrence. *J R Soc Med.* 1987;80:296.

13. Loder PB, Kamm MA, Nicholls RJ, Phillips RK. "Reversible chemical sphincterotomy" by local application of glyceryl trinitrate. *Br J Surg.* 1994;81:1386.

14. McLeod RS, Evans J. Symptomatic care and nitroglycerine in the management of anal fissure. *J Gastrointestinal Surg.* 2002;6(3):278-280.

15. Gorfine SR. Treatment of benign anal disease with topical nitroglycerin. *Dis Colon Rectum.* 1995;38:453.

16. Watson SJ, Kamm MA, Nicholls R, Phillips RK. Topical glyceryl trinitrate in the treatment of chronic anal fissure. *Br J Surg.* 1996;83:771.

17. Nelson R. A systematic review of medical therapy for anal fissure. *Dis Colon Rectum.* 2004;47:422.

18. Lund JN, Scholefield JH. A randomized, prospective, double-blind, placebo-controlled trial of glyceryl trinitrate ointment in treatment of anal fissure. *Lancet.* 1997;349:11.

19. Scholefield JH, Lund JN. A nonsurgical approach to chronic anal fissure hospital practice. *Hosp Pract.* 1997;32:181.

20. Kenny SE, Irvine T, Driver CP, et al. Double blind randomized controlled trial of topical glyceryl trinitrate in anal fissure. *Arch Dis Child.* 2001;85:404.

21. Oettle GJ. Glyceryl trinitrate vs. sphincterotomy for treatment of chronic fissure-in-ano: a randomized, controlled trial. *Dis Colon Rectum.* 1997;40:1318.

22. Were AJ, Palamba HW, Bilgen E, et al. Isosorbide dinitrate in the treatment of anal fissure: a randomised, prospective, double blind, placebo-controlled trial. *Eur J Surg.* 2001;167:382.

23. Sonmez K, Demirogullari B, Ekingen G, et al. Randomized, placebo-controlled treatment of anal fissure by lidocaine, EMLA, and GTN in children. *J Pediatr Surg.* 2002;37:1313.

24. Richard CS, Gregoire R, Plewes EA, et al. Internal sphincterotomy is superior to topical nitroglycerine in the treatment of chronic anal fissure: results of a randomized, controlled trial by the Canadian Colorectal Surgical Trials Group. *Dis Colon Rectum.* 2000;43:1048.

25. Altomere DF, Rinaldi M, Milito G, et al. Glyceryl trinitrate for chronic anal fissure—healing or headache? Results of a multicenter, randomized, placebo-controlled, double-blind trial. *Dis Colon Rectum.* 2000;43:174.

26. Perrotti P, Bove A, Antropoli C, et al. Topical nifedipine with lidocaine ointment versus active control for treatment of chronic anal fissure: results of a prospective, randomized, double-blind study. *Dis Colon Rectum.* 2002;45:1468.

27. Kocher HM, Steward M, Leather AJM, Cullen PT. Randomized clinical trial assessing the side-effects of glyceryl trinitrate and diltiazem hydrochloride in the treatment of chronic anal fissure. *Br J Surg.* 2002;89:413.

28. Bielecki K, Kolodziejczak M. A prospective randomized trial of diltiazem and glyceryl trinitrate ointment in the treatment of chronic anal fissure. *Colorectal Dis.* 2003;5:256.

28a. DasGupta R, Franklin I, Pitt J, Dawson PM. Successful treatment of chronic anal fissure with diltiazem gel. *Colorectal Dis.* 2002;4:20.

29. Griffin N, Acheson AG, Jonas M, Scholefield JH. The role of topical diltiazem in the treatment of chronic anal fissures that have failed glyceryl trinitrate therapy. *Colorectal Dis.* 2002;4:430.

30. Nelson RL, Thomas K, Morgan J, Jones A. Non surgical therapy for anal fissure. *Cochrane Database Syst Rev.* 2012;(2):CD003431.

31. Maria G, Cassetta E, Gui D, Brisinda G, Bentivoglio AR, Albanese A. A comparison of injections of botulinum toxin and saline for the treatment of chronic anal fissure. *N Engl J Med.* 1998;338:217.

32. Brisinda G, Maria G, Bentivoglio AR, Cassetta E, Gui D, Albanese A. A comparison of injections of botulinum toxin and topical nitroglycerine ointment for the treatment of chronic anal fissure. *N Engl J Med.* 1999;341:65.

33. Brisinda G, Albanese A, Cadeddu F, et al. Botulinum neurotoxin to treat chronic anal fissure: Results of a randomized "Botox vs. Dysport" controlled trial. *Aliment Pharmacol Ther.* 2004;19:695.

34. Maria G, Brisinda G, Bentivoglio AR, Cassetta E, Gui D, Albanese A. Influence of botulinum toxin site of injections on healing rate in patients with chronic anal fissure. *Am J Surg.* 2000;179:46.

35. Lindsey I, Jones OM, Cunningham C, George BD, Mortensen NJ. Botulinum toxin as second-line therapy for chronic anal fissure failing 0.2 percent glyceryl trinitrate. *Dis Colon Rectum.* 2003;46:361.

36. Barnes TG, Zafrani Z, Abdelrazeq AS. Fissurectomy combined with high-dose botulinum toxin is a safe and effective treatment for chronic anal fissure and a promising alternative to surgical sphincterotomy. *Dis Colon Rectum.* 2015;58(10):967-973.

37. Notaras MJ. Lateral subcutaneous sphincterotomy for anal fissure—a new technique. *Proc R Soc Med.* 1969;62:713

38. Notaras MJ. The treatment of anal fissure by lateral subcutaneous internal sphincterotomy—a technique and results. *Br J Surg.* 1971;58:96.

39. Rudd WW. Lateral subcutaneous internal sphincterotomy for chronic anal fissure, an outpatient procedure. *Dis Colon Rectum.* 1975;18:319.

40. Hoffman DC, Goligher JC. Lateral subcutaneous internal sphincterotomy in the treatment of anal fissure. *BMJ.* 1970;3:673.

41. Boulos PB, Araujo JG. Adequate internal sphincterotomy for chronic anal fissure: subcutaneous or open technique? *Br J Surg.* 1984;71:360.

42. Pernikoff BJ, Eisenstat TE, Rubin RJ, Oliver GC, Salvati EP. Reappraisal of partial lateral internal sphincterotomy. *Dis Colon Rectum.* 1994;37:1291.

43. Garcia-Aguilar J, Belmonte C, Wong WD, Lowry AC, Madoff RD. Open vs. closed sphincterotomy for chronic anal fissure: long-term results. *Dis Colon Rectum.* 1996;39:440.

44. Hananel N, Gordon PH. Lateral internal sphincterotomy for fissure-in-ano—revisited. *Dis Colon Rectum.* 1997;40 597.

45. Nyam DC, Pemberton JH. Long-term results of lateral internal sphincterotomy for chronic anal fissure with particular reference to incidence of fecal incontinence. *Dis Colon Rectum.* 1999;42:1306.

46. Nelson RL. Operative procedures for fissure in ano (Review). *Cochrane Libr.* 2010;1:1.

46a. Cho DY. Controlled lateral sphincterotomy for chronic anal fissure. *Dis Colon Rectum.* 2005;48:1037.

47. Rosa G, Lolli P, Piccinelli D, et al. Calibrated lateral internal sphincterotomy for chronic anal fissure. *Tech Coloproctol.* 2005;9:127.

48. Mentes BB, Guner MK, Leventoglu S, Akyurek N. Fine-tuning of the extent of lateral internal sphincterotomy: spasm-controlled vs. up to the fissure apex. *Dis Colon Rectum.* 2008;51:128.

49. Arnell T, Stamos MJ. Sphincterotomy for anal fissure. *Semin Colon Rectal Surg.* 1997;8:24.

50. Leong AF, Seow-Choen F. Lateral sphincterotomy compared with anal advancement flap for chronic anal fissure. *Dis Colon Rectum.* 1995;38:69.

51. Gupta PJ, Kalaskar S. Removal of hypertrophied anal papillae and fibrous anal polyps increases patient's satisfaction after anal fissure surgery. *Tech Coloproctol.* 2003;7:155.

52. Aysan E, Aren A, Ayar E. Lateral internal sphincterotomy incision: suture or not? A prospective randomized controlled trial. *Am Surg.* 2004;187:291.

53. Nelson RL. Meta-analysis of operative techniques for fissure-in-ano. *Dis Colon Rectum.* 1999;42:1424.

54. Sohn N, Eisenberg MM, Weinstein MA, Lugo RN, Ader J. Precise anorectal sphincter dilation—its role in therapy of anal fissures. *Dis Colon Rectum.* 1992;35:322.

55. Marby M, Alesander-Williams J, Buchmann P, et al. A randomized controlled trial to compare anal dilatation with lateral subcutaneous sphincterotomy for anal fissure. *Dis Colon Rectum.* 1979;22:308.

56. Oliver DW, Booth MW, Kernick VF, Irvin TT, Campbell WB. Patient satisfaction and symptom relief after anal dilatation. *Int J Colorectal Dis.* 1998;13:228.

57. Saad AM, Omer A. Surgical treatment of chronic fissure-in-ano: a prospective randomized study. *East Afr Med J.* 1992;69:107.

58. Renzi A, Izzo D, Di Sarno G, et al. Clinical, manometric and ultrasonographic results of pneumatic balloon dilatation vs. lateral internal sphincterotomy for chronic anal fissure: a prospective, randomized, controlled trial. *Dis Colon Rectum.* 2008;51:121.

Anal Fistula Management

Piyush Aggarwal | Charles A. Ternent | Alan G. Thorson

Anorectal suppurative disease may manifest itself in an acute or a chronic setting. Anal sepsis (abscess) represents the acute manifestation, and anal fistula represents the chronic form of the suppurative process. In its simplest form, an anal fistula represents a communication between an internal opening in the anal canal and an external opening through which an abscess has drained. A fistula and abscess may coexist or be associated with atypical internal openings and multiple tracts that result in a complex suppurative process.

ETIOLOGY

Foreign bodies, malignancy, trauma, tuberculosis, actinomycosis, leukemia, postoperative infection, inflammatory bowel disease, and simple skin infections have long been associated with anal sepsis. Recently an association between anal abscess-fistula and history of concurrent or recent cigarette smoking has been demonstrated.[1] This association diminishes as the history of cigarette smoking grows more remote. However, most anal sepsis is related to an infection of the anal glands and ducts. Fecal bacterial plugging of the ducts leads to obstruction and subsequent abscess formation. This process represents the cryptoglandular theory of anal sepsis. Robinson,[2] Seow-Choen,[3] and their associates have suggested that the description of the anal glands by Chiari in 1878 and the subsequent histologic studies of Parks in 1961 contributed to the acceptance of the cryptoglandular theory as the most common cause for anal sepsis.

CLASSIFICATION

ANORECTAL ABSCESSES

Anorectal abscesses are classified according to the perirectal space involved in the suppurative process; these include the perianal, ischiorectal, intersphincteric, submucosal, deep postanal, and supralevator spaces (Fig. 160.1). A given suppurative process may involve multiple perirectal spaces. For example, the classic "horseshoe" abscess originates in an infected gland in the posterior midline extending through the intersphincteric and deep postanal spaces to one or both of the ischiorectal spaces. A condition known as "floating anus" may occur with circumanal spread of intersphincteric, supralevator, or ischiorectal collections.

It is difficult to accurately assess the incidence of various abscesses because of the numerous classifications and referral patterns reflected in large series.[4–8] However, perianal abscesses account for the largest number in most series (Table 160.1).

ANAL FISTULA

Historically, anal fistulas have been classified in many different ways. However, the Parks classification introduced

in 1976 is the most comprehensive and widely used. It is derived from the cryptoglandular hypothesis and has therapeutic implications. Parks and Gordon classified fistulas into four main subgroups according to the course taken by the main tract: intersphincteric, transsphincteric, suprasphincteric, or extrasphincteric.[9] Each category can be further subclassified based on associated secondary tracts and other anatomic details (Fig. 160.2). As with abscesses, the incidence of various fistulas is difficult to quantify. However, overall, intersphincteric fistulas seem to predominate (Table 160.2).

DIAGNOSIS

ANORECTAL ABSCESS

History

Symptoms common to all abscesses include the slow, gradual onset of pain, increasing in intensity to the sensation of pressure and fullness. This is a constant nonrelieving sensation. These symptoms should always lead to the consideration of an abscess even in the absence of obvious physical findings (hidden abscesses). Approximately 20% to 33% of all patients will report a history of a previous episode of anorectal sepsis.[7,10]

Physical Examination

The physical findings associated with anorectal abscesses vary depending on the anatomic location of the abscess. The presence of pus in any of the perianal and perirectal spaces may be confirmed with needle aspiration. An examination under general anesthesia may be necessary to confirm the diagnosis.

PERIANAL ABSCESS

Localized swelling, hyperemia, induration or fluctuance, and tenderness are present adjacent to the anus. A purulent discharge may be present if spontaneous drainage has occurred. Although there usually are no systemic symptoms, the patient may have fever or malaise or be acutely ill.

ISCHIORECTAL ABSCESS

Although small collections may present with discrete localized swelling, more commonly there is a large, erythematous, and indurated mass in the buttock. Large volumes of purulent material may accumulate in the ischiorectal space. Fever and leukocytosis are common but not always present. A large ischiorectal abscess frequently represents a horseshoe extension (see later). A source in the posterior midline should be sought.

INTERSPHINCTERIC AND SUBMUCOSAL ABSCESS

The intersphincteric and submucosal abscesses usually present with no visible evidence of sepsis because these

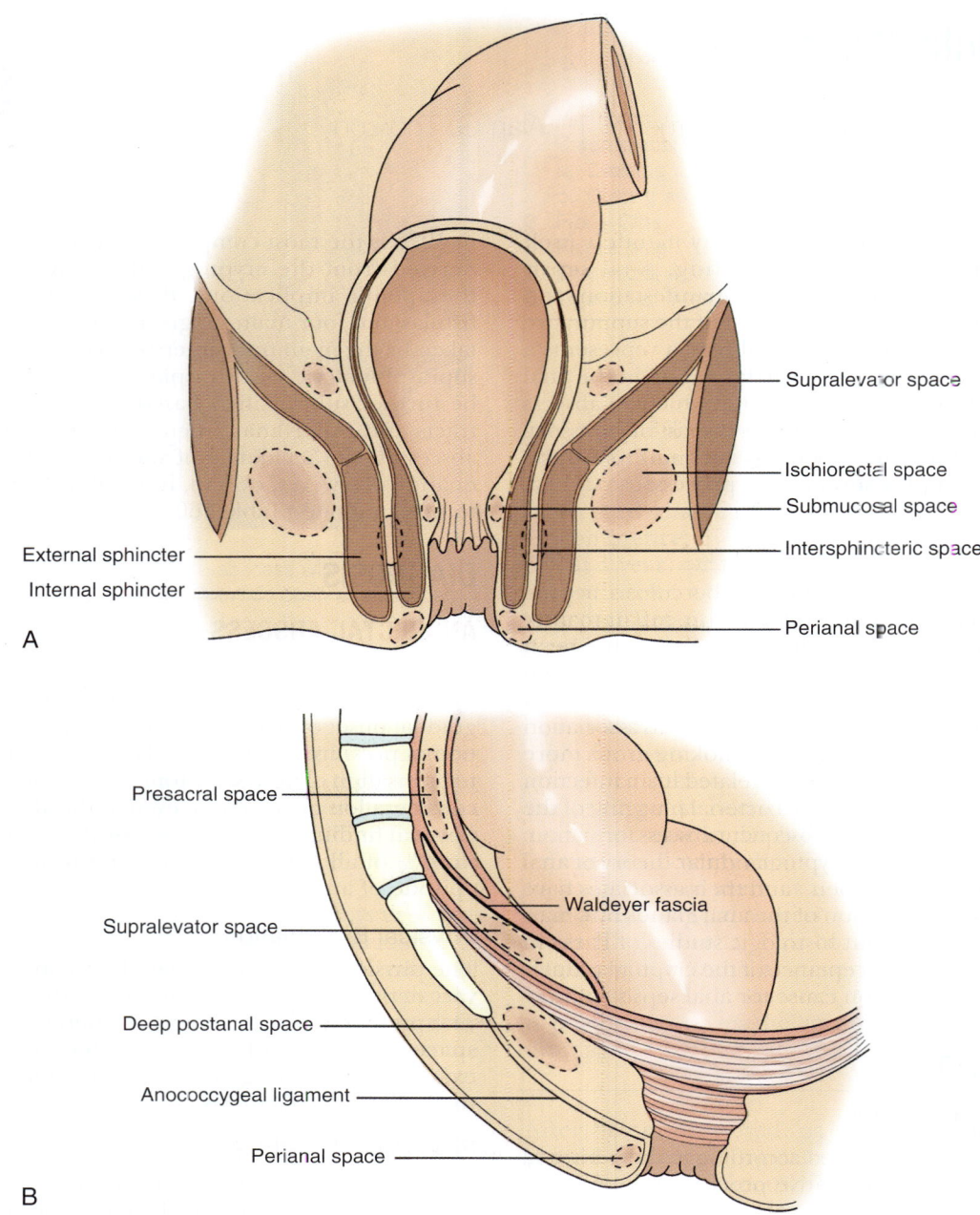

A

B

FIGURE 160.1 Classification of anorectal abscesses by location. (A) Coronal view. (B) Sagittal view.

"hidden abscesses" are confined to the anal canal. Owing to the patient's discomfort, a digital rectal examination is not always possible. In this situation, an examination under general anesthesia is warranted to identify the abscess.

SUPRALEVATOR ABSCESS

Supralevator abscess may occur as an upward extension of a collection in the distal anal canal, usually an intersphincteric abscess, or as a true pelvic abscess secondary to intraabdominal or pelvic pathology. Possibilities include appendicitis, diverticulitis, pelvic inflammatory disease, or ruptured viscus. The patient may be systemically ill. A

pelvic mass may be identified by rectal or vaginal examination.

POSTANAL ABSCESS AND HORSESHOE EXTENSION

Transsphincteric extension of an intersphincteric abscess in the posterior midline leads to the accumulation of purulent material in the deep postanal space. This space is difficult to evaluate clinically, making these the second type of hidden abscess. Inspection does not reveal any inflammatory skin changes because the abscess is deep. There may be tenderness posterior to the anus but anterior to the coccyx. The collection may be apparent only by needle aspiration or with an examination under general

TABLE 160.1 Incidence of Anorectal Abscess by Location

| Abscess Locations | NO. OF PATIENTS | | | | | TOTAL | |
	McElwain et al.[4]	Scoma et al.[7]	Vasilevsky and Gordon[3]	Schouten and van Vroonhoven[6]	Ramanujam et al.[5]	No. of Patients	%
Perianal	456	174	20	—	437	1087	44.8
Submucosal	3	—	—	—	—	3	0.1
Intermuscular	541	30	—	—	59	630	26
Intersphincteric	—	—	18	28	219	265	11
Transsphincteric	—	—	—	30	—	30	1.2
Ischiorectal	—	14	63	—	233	310	12.8
Supralevator	—	9	2	—	75	86	3.6
Retrorectal	—	5	—	—	—	5	0.2
Unclassified	—	—	—	8	—	8	0.3
Total	1000	232	103	66	1023	2424	100

TABLE 160.2 Incidence of Anal Fistulas

| Fistula Type | NO. OF PATIENTS | | | | TOTAL | |
	Parks et al.[9]	Marks and Ritchie[95]	Vasilevsky and Gordon[94]	Garcia-Aguilar et al.[95]	No. of Patients	%
Intersphincteric	180	428	67	180	855	49.5
Transsphincteric	120	167	83	108	478	27.7
Suprasphincteric	80	24	3	6	113	6.5
Extrasphincteric	20	24	0	6	50	2.9
Miscellaneous or unclassified	—	150	7	75	232	13.4
Total	400	793	160	375	1728	100

anesthesia. A horseshoe abscess is the result of a direct extension of a postanal abscess into the ischiorectal space (see section Ischiorectal Abscess). It may be unilateral or bilateral.

ANORECTAL FISTULAS

History

Most patients with a fistula-in-ano have a previous history of anorectal suppuration. The patient usually presents with complaints of intermittent or persistent purulent or serosanguineous drainage from an external opening in the perianal area. Symptoms classically consist of a buildup of pain, slight fever, and pain on defecation followed by mucopurulent drainage and abatement of the pain. Pruritic symptoms may be present because of skin irritation associated with the chronic discharge.

Physical Examination

Fistula tracts are fibrous inflammatory tubes with a diameter of 3 to 7 mm. They are lined with infected granulation tissue. Many fistulas may be palpated during a careful digital rectal examination. Essential points that should be obtained from a clinical examination were described nearly 100 years ago by Goodsall and Miles[11]; they include the identification of the external and internal openings, the course of the primary and any secondary tracts, the

tone of anal sphincters and an assessment for the presence of an underlying complicating disease.

Using an anoscope, systematic inspection and palpation can define most of these characteristics. The gentle use of a number of malleable anorectal probes and crypt hooks can help to delineate the fistula by attempting to pass these instruments via the internal or external opening. It is important not to force the passage of the probe because the development of false tracts can complicate evaluation and management. Secondary tracts may be present when induration is palpated or asymmetry is noted between the right and left sides of the anorectum. In some cases, such as recurrent, extensive, or complex fistulas, the use of sophisticated imaging techniques may yield additional information to guide successful therapy.

The external opening is identified as a small pit surrounded by scar or granulation tissue. Active seropurulent drainage may be present. Intersphincteric tracts usually open externally close to the anal verge; transsphincteric and other complicated tracts open farther away. Occasionally the external opening may be localized inside the anal canal or at the distal end of a fissure. Several external openings may be present because of multiple complex fistula tracts; this condition is known as watering can perineum (Fig. 160.3).

The internal opening may be felt as an indurated nodule, most often at the dentate line. This is consistent

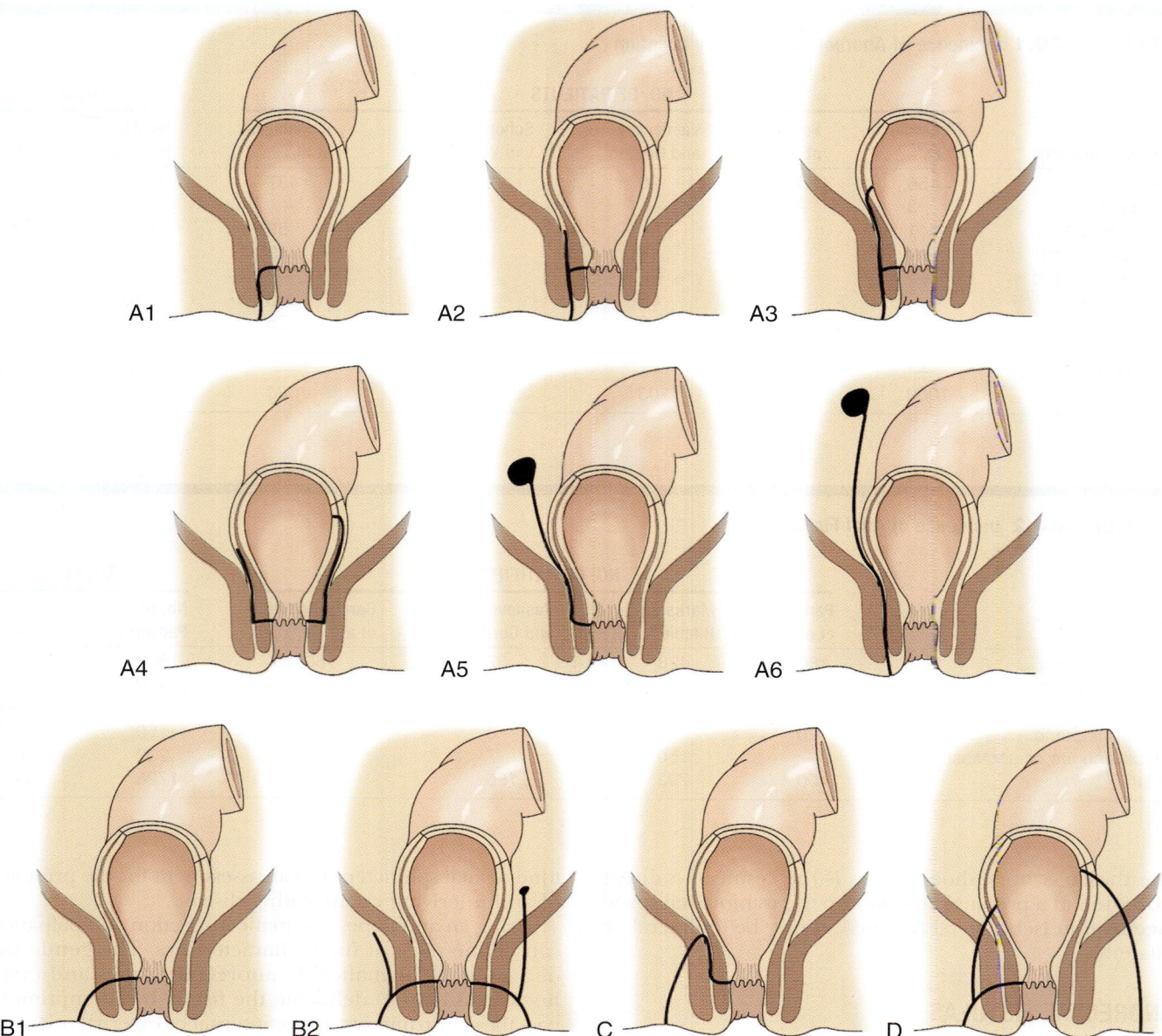

FIGURE 160.2 Classification of anal fistulas. (A) Intersphincteric: the tract remains in the intersphincteric plane. *1,* Simple. *2,* High blind tract. There is a high extension of the fistula between the internal sphincter and the longitudinal muscle of the upper anal canal. *3,* High tract with rectal opening. *4,* High intersphincteric fistula without a perineal opening. There may or may not be a rectal opening. *5,* High intersphincteric fistula with a pelvic extension. The infection spreads up to reach the true pelvic cavity lying above the levator musculature. *6,* Intersphincteric fistula secondary to pelvic disease. This fistula results from the spread of pelvic collections via the intersphincteric plane. This does not represent a true anal fistula because its origin is outside the anal area. There is no opening at the dentate line. (B) Transsphincteric: the fistula tract passes from the intersphincteric plane through the external sphincter muscle. *1,* Uncomplicated. *2,* High blind tract. The upper tract extension may go to the apex of the ischiorectal fossa or extend higher through the levator musculature into the pelvic cavity. (C) Suprasphincteric: there is an upward extension of the fistula tract in the intersphincteric plane. The tract then passes above the level of the puborectalis muscle and continues downward through the ischiorectal fossa to the perianal area. (D) Extrasphincteric: there is a tract that passes from the skin of the perineum through the ischiorectal fossa and the levator muscles before entering the rectal wall. This fistula may be a consequence of an extension of a transsphincteric fistula or secondary to trauma, anorectal disease, or pelvic inflammation.

with the cryptoglandular theory of anorectal sepsis. The use of saline, milk, dye, or dilute hydrogen peroxide as an injection into the external fistula opening has been made in an attempt to localize the internal opening. An enlarged papilla may be noted at this site. Because most of the anal glands are located in the posterior midline, it is not surprising that 61% to 69% of internal openings can be traced to this location.[3]

The Goodsall rule may be helpful in locating the internal opening. This rule states that an external opening

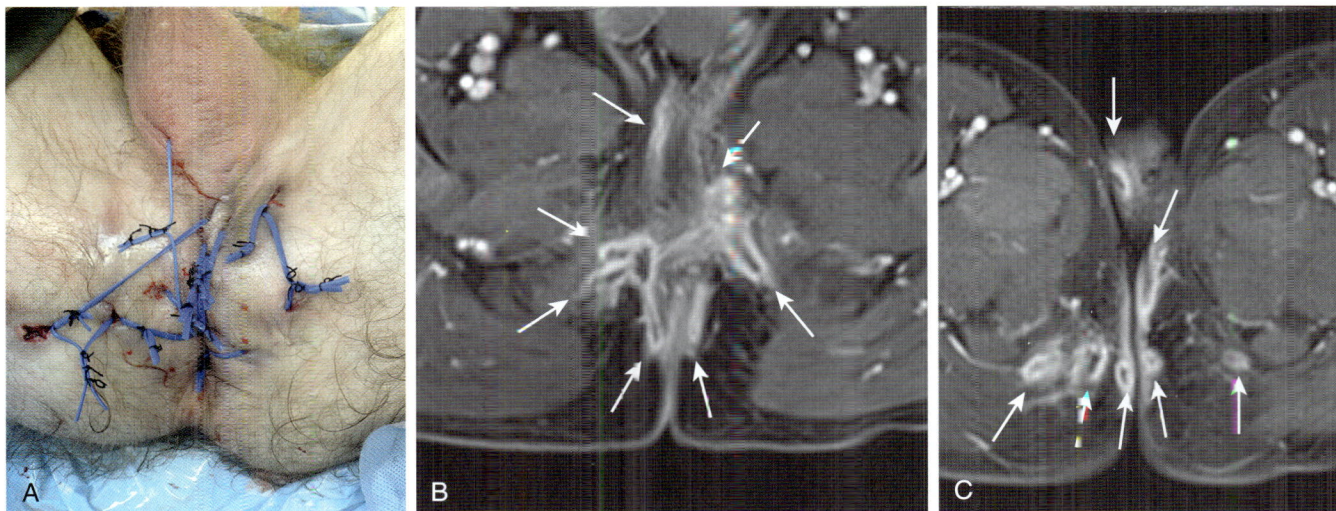

FIGURE 160.3 (A) Watering can perineum with draining setons. (B and C) Fistula tracts shown in axial T1-weighted fat-saturated gadolinium enhanced sequence. Note numerous fistula tracts (arrows) extending anteriorly to scrotum, bilaterally to ischiorectal fossas, and posterior perianal regions.

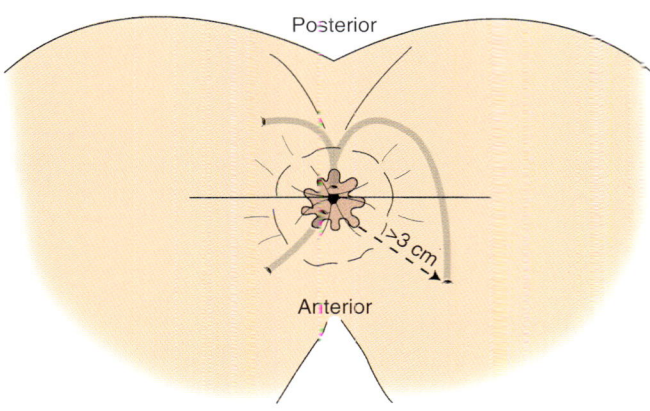

FIGURE 160.4 Goodsall rule.

anterior to an imaginary transverse anal line in the coronal plane most likely communicates with an internal opening lying at the end of a radial line drawn to the nearest crypt at the dentate line. If the external opening is posterior to this line, the internal opening will most likely be located in the posterior midline with the tract following a curved route to reach its source. Exceptions to this rule include anterior openings more than 3 cm from the anal verge and the presence of multiple external openings. In these cases, the internal opening will most likely be in the posterior midline (Fig. 160.4). However, the predictive accuracy of Goodsall rule has been challenged, especially with anterior external openings[12] or when Crohn disease or carcinoma is present.[13]

SPECIAL STUDIES

Sigmoidoscopy and Colonoscopy

Sigmoidoscopy should be performed in all patients with anorectal fistulas. The presence of associated pathology,

such as neoplasms, inflammatory bowel disease, or associated secondary tracts in the rectum, must be sought. Such findings may dictate the need for full colonoscopic evaluation.

Fistulography

Fistulography may be warranted in patients with recurrent fistulas or when a prior procedure has failed to identify the internal opening. With this technique, the external opening is cannulated with a small-caliber tube and contrast material is injected under minimal pressure while films are taken in several projections. Fistulography may be useful in identifying unsuspected pathology, planning surgical management, and demonstrating anatomic relationships. However, a study by Kuijpers and Schulpen[14] found fistulography to be unreliable compared with operative findings. They observed a prohibitively high incidence of false-positive results that could lead to unnecessary and harmful surgical exploration.

Anorectal Ultrasonography

Transanal ultrasound can delineate the muscular anatomy of the anal sphincters in relation to an abscess or a fistula. Most commonly, ultrasonographic examination of the anal canal is performed with the use of a 360-degree rotating probe using a 7-, 10-, or 13-MHz transducer with a water-filled sonolucent plastic cone over the transducer (Fig. 160.5). Fistula tracts and abscesses appear as hypoechoic defects within the muscular elements of the anal canal (Fig. 160.6). The internal opening is not distinctly identified. Although generally accurate in the localization of abscesses and fistula tracts, primary superficial, extrasphincteric, and suprasphincteric tracts or secondary supralevator or infralevator tracts may be missed.[15] The use of hydrogen peroxide injected into fistulas as an image enhancer has been shown to be safe, effective, and sometimes helpful in the detection of these complex fistulas (Fig. 160.7).[16] In addition,

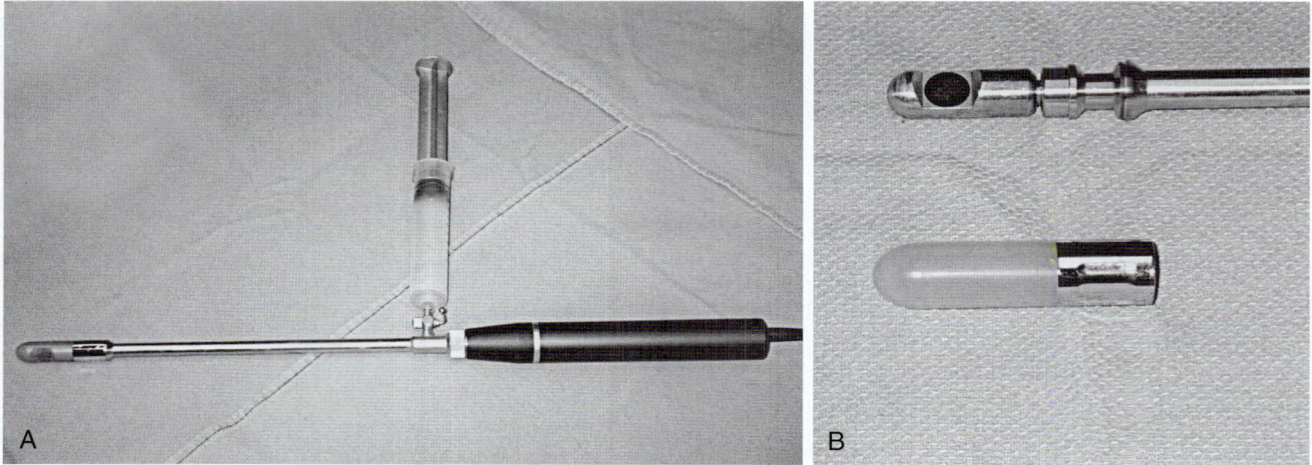

FIGURE 160.5 (A) Transanal ultrasound probe (type 1850; Brüel and Kjaer, Naerum, Denmark). (B) The rotating transducer is covered by a hard plastic sonolucent cone, which is then filled with water to provide an acoustic interphase.

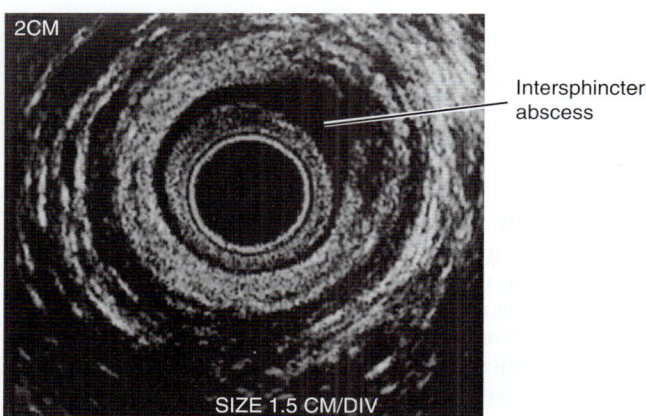

Intersphincteric abscess

FIGURE 160.6 Intersphincteric abscess as seen with the use of transanal ultrasound.

three-dimensional endoanal ultrasonography is now reliable and accurate in the diagnosis of fistula-in-ano with or without hydrogen peroxide enhancement.[17]

The use of a linear 7-MHz ultrasound device instead of a radial probe has been described and may carry the advantages of greater focal depth, improved ischiorectal and supralevator visualization, multiplanar views of complex fistulas, and less need for echo-enhancing injection.[18] Finally, it has been shown that vaginal endosonography may increase the diagnostic yield of perianal sepsis in 25% of patients and may obviate the need for uncomfortable digital or endoanal ultrasound examinations in those patients with hidden abscesses or anal stenosis.[19]

Magnetic Resonance Imaging

Another accurate method of imaging anal fistula disease is magnetic resonance imaging (MRI). A majority of anal fistulas have a single simple fistula tract that is easily identified during surgery. However, 5% to 15% of complex fistulas are often associated with recurrent fistulas and fistulas associated with underlying Crohn disease. MRI

has shown to be helpful, especially in these complex fistulas in identification of fistulous tracts, secondary extensions, and internal openings (Fig. 160.8).[20] In a study by Beets-Tan et al., preoperative MRI had a sensitivity and specificity of 100% and 86%, respectively, in identification of fistula tracts. In addition, the study found a 96% sensitivity and 90% specificity for preoperative MR detection of internal fistula openings.[20] MRI is particularly useful in the evaluation of complex fistulous disease. Combining MRI with endoanal ultrasonography and an examination under anesthesia may enhance the accuracy of these tests in determining fistula anatomy.[21]

Computed Tomography

The use of computed tomography (CT) in the evaluation of anal fistulas is limited because of poor visualization of the levators and sphincter complex. The role of CT in anal sepsis and fistula is thus limited to the assessment of associated pelvic pathology in patients with supralevator abscesses and in patients with some complex anal fistulas.

Anorectal Manometry

Anorectal manometry is an objective method for studying the contribution of the anorectal sphincter to the physiologic process of defecation. Manometry can assist in identifying patients at the greatest risk for postoperative incontinence. Surgical management can be tailored accordingly, improving clinical and functional outcome. The selective use of anorectal manometry is especially warranted in patients with suspected sphincter impairment; patients suspected of needing substantial portions of the external sphincter divided for fistula cure; and women with a history of multiparity, forceps delivery, third-degree perineal tear, high birthweight, or prolonged second stage of labor.[13] Patients with lower preoperative resting pressures have significantly poorer continence control following surgery for intersphincteric fistula when compared prospectively with patients with normal preoperative resting pressures.[22]

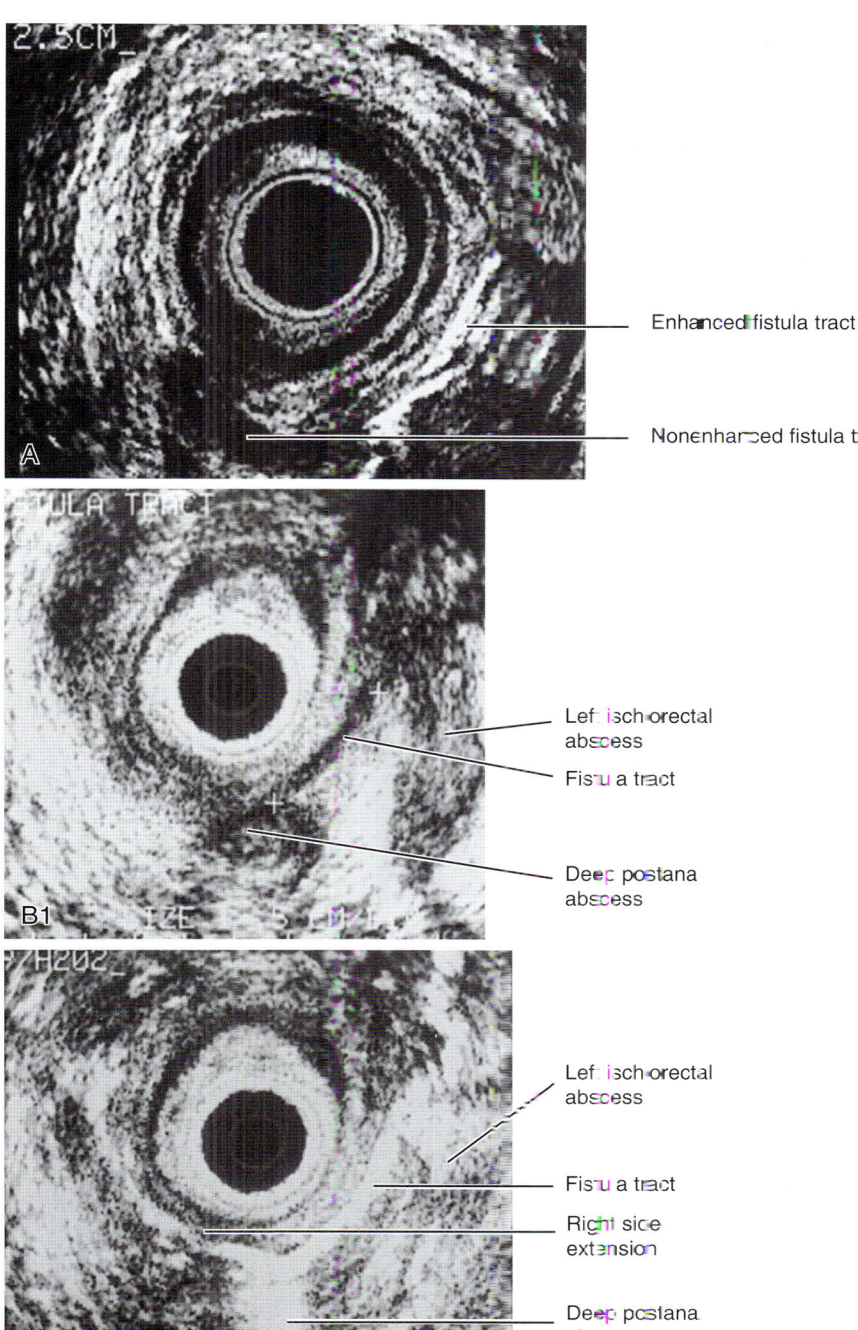

Enhanced fistula tract

Nonenhanced fistula tract

Left ischiorectal abscess

Fistula tract

Deep postanal abscess

Left ischiorectal abscess

Fistula tract

Right side extension

Deep postanal abscess

FIGURE 160.7 (A) Transsphincteric hypoechogenic tract extending toward the posterior midline. The tract is enhanced as hydrogen peroxide is injected into the external opening. (B) Complex fistula tract and collections as seen without (1) and with (2) hydrogen peroxide enhancement. Hydrogen peroxide enhancement allowed for a more precise delineation of the tracts in addition to a right-sided extension of the tract.

Fistuloscopy

Anorectal fistuloscopy using flexible ureteroscopes has been described. This is a potentially useful intraoperative technique used to identify primary fistula openings, multiple or complex tracts, and iatrogenic tracts. Modified flexible ureteroscopes are in the early developmental stages. We look forward to their evolution because they represent a novel diagnostic and therapeutic tool that may significantly improve the outcomes of complex fistula diagnosis and treatment.

TREATMENT

ANORECTAL ABSCESS

The treatment of anorectal abscesses should be considered a surgical emergency, with early drainage the mainstay of treatment. There is no place for conservative management. Treatment delay may result in chronic infection and tissue destruction with fibrosis and long-term impairment of function. The condition of the patient and the type of abscess usually determine whether drainage can be

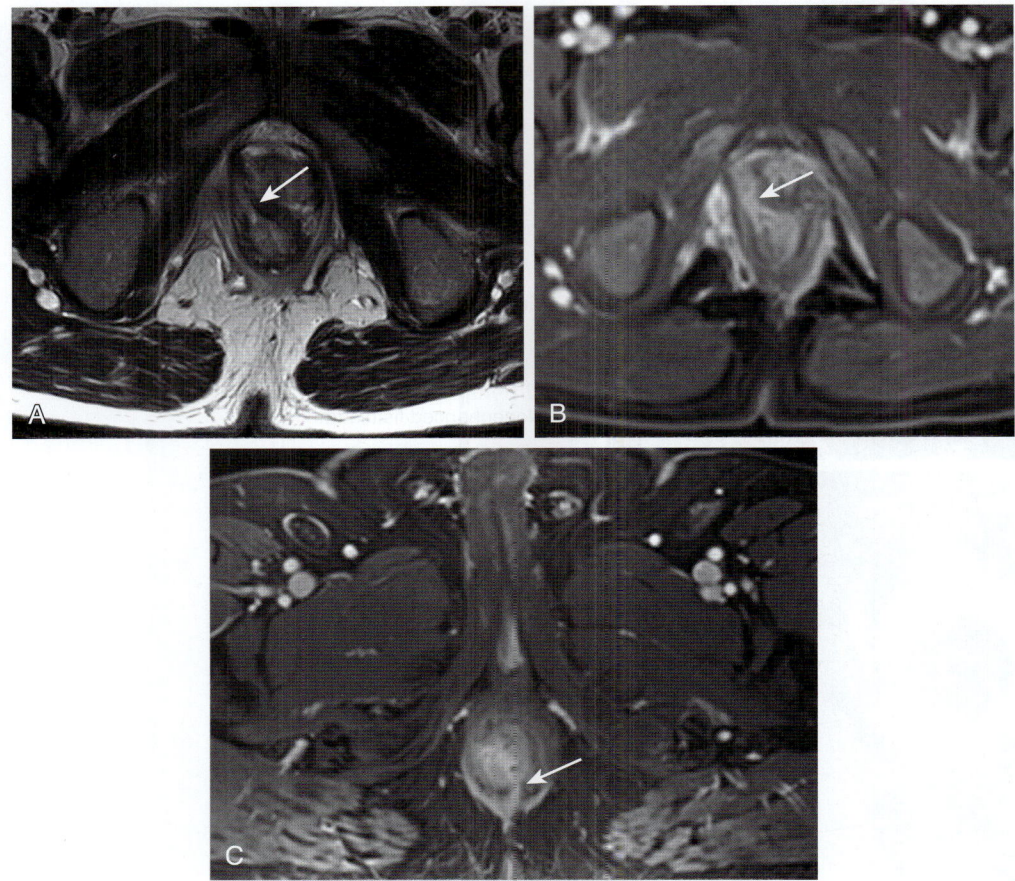

FIGURE 160.8 Transsphincteric horse-shoe anal fistula tract with internal opening anteromidline *(arrows)* axial views. (A) T1 weighted fat-saturated gadolinium enhanced sequence volumetric interpolated breath-hold examination (VIBE). (B) T2 weighted fast spin echo sequence. (C) Transsphincteric anal fistula tract with posteromidline internal fistula opening *(arrow)* axial view shown in T1 weighted fat-saturated gadolinium-enhanced sequence (VIBE).

performed in the office or emergency department or in the operating room. Antibiotics should be used as adjunctive therapy in special circumstances only; these include patients with valvular heart disease excluding mitral valve prolapse,[23] immunosuppression, extensive associated cellulitis, and diabetes.[24]

Anorectal abscesses associated with gut-derived organisms are more likely to be associated with an underlying fistula than are abscesses associated with skin-derived organisms.[25] However, the positive predictive value for this association has been found to be quite low; therefore cultures are rarely indicated.[26]

Perianal Abscess

Simple perianal abscesses can almost always be drained as an office or outpatient procedure, usually under local anesthesia. A cruciate incision is made over the most tender or fluctuant point as close to the anal verge as possible. If a fistula develops, the external opening will be close to the verge, so a fistulotomy would require division of the least amount of muscle. The skin edges are usually excised to avoid early coaptation, which could seal the cavity prematurely and lead to recurrence (Fig. 160.9).

After all loculations are broken, packing is not required; packing contributes to significant discomfort and does not allow for free drainage of the abscess cavity. Continued drainage of large cavities may be achieved with the use of a 3- to 5-mm de Pezzer or similar catheter left in situ until drainage subsides. This technique may be used in a number of different abscesses but is not suitable for use in cases of submucous or intersphincteric abscess.

Ischiorectal Abscess

After horseshoe extension is excluded by ensuring that the deep postanal space is not involved, unilateral ischiorectal abscesses may be drained through a single incision or several counterincisions over the area of maximal swelling, pain, and fluctuance but as close to the anal verge as possible. Here a de Pezzer catheter may also be used to enhance the drainage of large cavities.

Intersphincteric Abscess

An intersphincteric abscess is drained by laying open the internal sphincter (sphincterotomy) overlying the cavity. By definition, a fistulotomy is performed by destruction of the inciting anal gland. For hemostasis, adequate

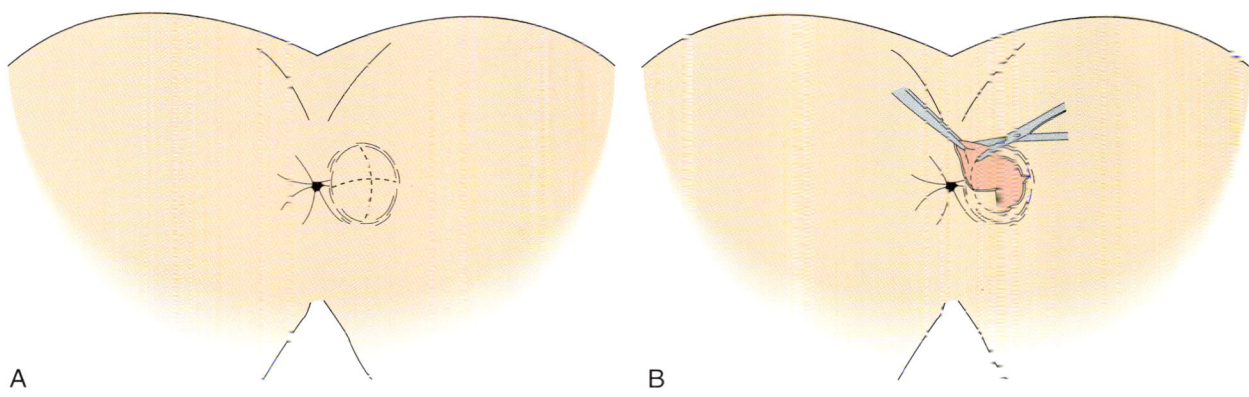

FIGURE 160.9 (A) Cruciate incision made over the most tender or fluctuant area. (B) The skin edges are excised.

drainage, and faster healing, the edges of the wound may be marsupialized.

Submucosal Abscess

Submucosal abscesses are drained internally by incising the mucosa over the abscess. The edges of the wound may be marsupialized. No packing or drainage catheter is indicated.

Supralevator Abscess

Anatomic localization of the septic origin is of paramount importance in the management of supralevator collections. Collections that result from abdominopelvic disease may be drained transrectally or transabdominally. Overall management depends on the underlying pathology. Supralevator collections that result from an upward extension of an intersphincteric abscess should be drained transrectally. Transperineal drainage through the ischiorectal fossae could result in a suprasphincteric fistula. Supralevator collections that result from the cephalad extension of a transsphincteric fistula or an ischiorectal collection should be drained transperineally through the ischioanal fossae. If erroneously drained transrectally, the result will be an extrasphincteric fistula. Transperineal drainage of this type of collection will likely result in a transsphincteric fistula that is relatively easy to manage (Fig. 160.10).

Postanal Abscess and Horseshoe Extension

Hanley first described the conservative surgical approach to a horseshoe abscess that preserved function and anatomy.[27] The abscess in the postanal space is drained by a deep posterior midline incision. All of the muscles attached to the coccyx, the superficial external sphincter, and the lower edge of the internal sphincter are divided. When the suppurative process extends to the ischiorectal spaces as a horseshoe, one or multiple secondary incisions are placed in the skin overlying the ischiorectal space. These may be connected to each other with soft drains to allow for continuous drainage. We favor a modification of Hanley's technique in which the posterior midline incision consists of only a partial distal internal sphincterotomy to include a fistulotomy with destruction of the anal gland at the dentate line. The external sphincter

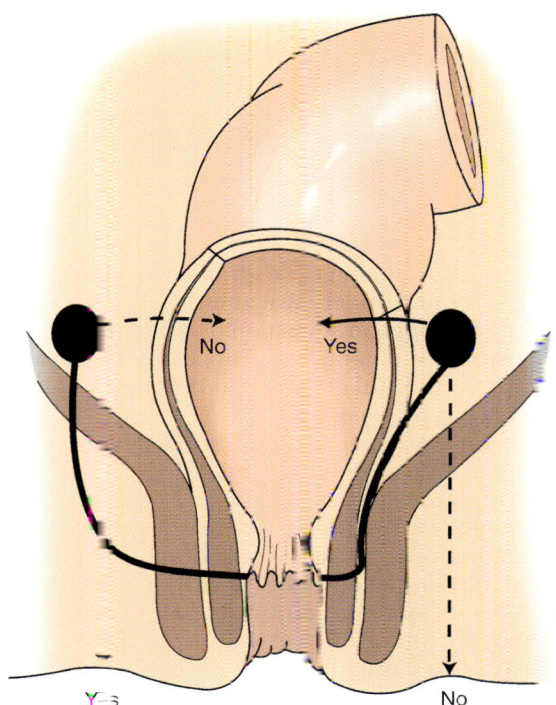

FIGURE 160.10 Appropriate type of drainage of supralevator abscesses depending on the course taken by the fistula tract.

fibers are usually splayed out thin as a result of tension from the abscess. This condition allows efficient drainage of the postanal space via a posterior sphincterotomy while maintaining the muscular attachments of the coccyx in place (Fig. 160.11). Counterincisions and drains are used for horseshoe extensions as previously described.

Primary Versus Delayed Fistulotomy

The use of primary fistulotomy when draining an abscess remains controversial. Issues surrounding this controversy include the ability to localize an internal opening at the time of an acute septic event and the effect of primary fistulotomy on recurrence and continence. Does the type of abscess affect the risk of recurrent fistula? Is a cost

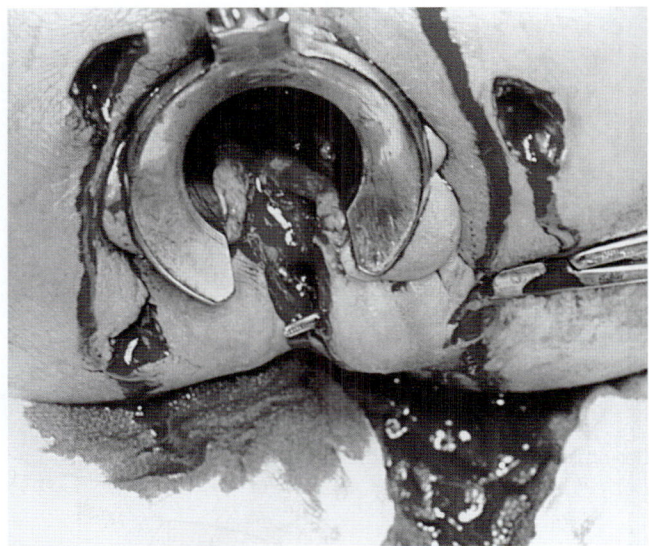

FIGURE 160.11 Drainage of a postanal abscess with horseshoe extension. The postanal space has been laid open as described by Hanley. Secondary incisions are placed in the skin overlying the ischiorectal space.

TABLE 160.3 Techniques for Management of Fistula-in-Ano

1. Fistulotomy
2. Seton placement
   a. Draining seton
   b. Cutting seton
3. Fibrin Glue
4. Fistula plug
5. Endorectal advancement flap
6. Ligation of intersphincteric fistula tract

effective to take a patient for whom an outpatient procedure is performed under local anesthesia to the operating room for a thorough examination under general anesthesia and a primary fistulotomy in the hope of avoiding a second procedure for a fistula that might develop if only simple drainage were performed?

A one-stage procedure theoretically destroys the cryptoglandular source of sepsis, decreasing the incidence of fistula formation. However, internal openings may not always be found. Attempts to define a primary opening in the setting of an acute infection may be a hazardous undertaking. Not all abscesses lead to fistulas; thus some patients would undergo an unnecessary procedure that puts them at risk for incontinence.

The reported incidence of recurrent abscess and subsequent development of anorectal fistula varies considerably. Scoma et al. found that 66% of 232 patients developed a fistula or recurrent abscess after incision and drainage alone.[4] Vasilevsky and Gordon found that 11% of 83 patients developed recurrent abscess and 37% developed a fistula after incision and drainage.[7] They noted that the greatest risk of recurrence was in patients who had ischiorectal abscesses, an observation we have also made. The subset of patients with no previous episode of anorectal suppuration had a lower incidence of recurrence. Both authors advocated incision and drainage alone for acute abscesses, reserving fistulotomy as a secondary procedure in patients with recurrence.

In contrast, several authors favor a policy of immediate fistulotomy in the treatment of anorectal abscesses. In a series of almost 800 cases, Eisenhammer described a nearly 100% cure rate obtained with a single operation.[28] McElwain et al. reported on the outcome of 1000 cases of primary fistulotomy for anorectal abscesses, including intersphincteric and postanal abscesses.[5] The recurrence

rate was 3.6%, and the disturbance of continence rate was 3.2%. This approach is further supported by a randomized prospective trial of 200 patients. Oliver et al. demonstrated that drainage with fistulotomy was safe (incontinence, 6% at 1 year) and effective (recurrence, 5% at 1 year) when compared with drainage alone (0% incontinence and 29% recurrence).[29] Ultimately this approach requires the consistent finding of an internal opening to perform fistulotomy. In general, internal openings can be identified in 34% to 88% of acute abscesses.[6,30]

In summary, a percentage of patients who have drainage alone for the treatment of anal abscess develop a recurrent abscess or subsequent fistula. A primary fistulotomy in this setting may decrease this risk but at the expense of a small increase in the risk for disturbance of continence. Primary fistulotomy should be considered in patients who have a history of previous anorectal sepsis or who present with an ischiorectal abscess with an internal opening that is readily apparent. This controversy has no impact in dealing with postanal abscesses with horseshoe extensions or intersphincteric abscesses. In these cases a fistulotomy is performed when the sphincterotomy is the primary drainage technique.

ANORECTAL FISTULAS

After being diagnosed, patients with anorectal fistulas should undergo surgical treatment. Anorectal fistulas rarely heal spontaneously. Untreated patients frequently develop chronic abscess formation and complex fistula tracts. Surgical treatment for most anorectal fistulas is best accomplished in the operating room, with good lighting and appropriate instrumentation. The patient is positioned in the most efficient way that allows adequate visualization of the external and internal fistula openings. Patients may be placed in the prone jackknife position with the buttocks taped apart; lithotomy position, which allows en face visualization of the posterior anal canal as well as genital and perineal body regions; or left lateral decubitus position in case of pregnancy in the third trimester. General, regional, or local anesthesia with intravenous sedation should be selected on the basis of individual patient characteristics.

The goals of treatment for anal fistula are to cure the disease, prevent its recurrence, and preserve continence. The common surgical techniques used for the treatment of anorectal fistulas are mentioned in Table 160.3.

Fistulotomy

Most anorectal fistulas may be adequately treated by the classic laying-open technique or fistulotomy. Recurrence rates are low, and risks for continence disturbance are minimal.[3] A fistulotomy is accomplished by passing a fistula probe via the external opening, along the tract, and through the internal opening. With the probe in place, the relationship of the fistulous tract to the external sphincter muscle can be determined. If the tract lies distal to the majority of the external muscle, then cautery is used to lay it open. Secondary tracts should be drained through the fistulotomy incision after all tracts have been curetted. Marsupialization with a running continuous absorbable suture is associated with faster healing.

Fistulotomy has been the mainstay treatment for intersphincteric and low transsphincteric fistulas. There is a direct correlation between the amount of transection of external sphincter and incontinence when the lay-open technique is used.[31,32] In patients with otherwise normal continence, the perianal skin, anal epithelium, a portion of the internal anal sphincter, and a few fibers of subcutaneous external sphincter may be divided with minimal risk of incontinence. However, in women with anterior fistulas, such a fistulotomy is associated with an unacceptably high risk of incontinence because of the intrinsic thin nature of the sphincter mechanism in this area. Therefore sphincter-preserving techniques should be used in the treatment of most anterior fistulas in women.

Seton Management

The word *seton* is derived from the Latin word *seta*, meaning "bristle." It refers to any foreign material that can be inserted into the fistula tract to encircle the sphincter muscles. These materials may include silk, Penrose drains, Silastic vessel loops, rubber bands, nylon or polypropylene, and braided steel wire. Setons are placed by securing the selected material to the end of a fistula probe after the probe has been passed through the internal opening (Fig. 160.12).

Setons are useful in the management of complex anorectal fistulas where there is an appreciable risk of incontinence or poor healing; such cases include patients with Crohn disease, immunocompromised and incontinent patients, patients with chronic diarrheal states, and anterior fistulas in women. Complete healing of selected anorectal fistulas has been reported solely with the use of long-term setons.[33]

Setons may be used for marking, draining, cutting, or staging. A marking seton is useful when it is difficult to determine the amount of muscle the fistula tract crosses. Encircling the tract with a seton allows the surgeon to assess the amount of muscle, particularly the puborectalis, after the patient is awake. If adequate muscle is present above the fistula tract, a fistulotomy may be performed without significant risk for incontinence.

A draining seton traverses a fistula tract to provide long-term drainage of a septic process. It may be used as a bridge to definitive surgical therapy or be left in place for long periods. Epithelialization of the tract prevents recurring abscesses. Long-term draining setons are tied loosely. They are particularly useful in the management of complex fistulas associated with Crohn disease. The

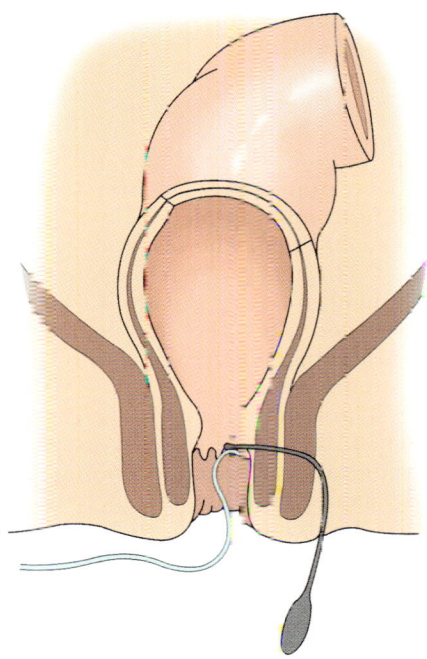

FIGURE 160.12   Insertion of a seton with the aid of a fistula probe.

combination of a draining seton and immunomodulation therapy with infliximab appears to improve outcomes while maintaining sphincter function in Crohn patients with complex anal fistulas.[34] Removal of a seton can be considered once biologic therapy dries up the fistula tract with the understanding that recurrence of an abscess or active fistula can recur depending on activity levels of the biologic therapy.[35]

A cutting seton is used to gradually transect the striated sphincter muscle. This technique promotes fibrosis in the tissue surrounding the muscle encircled by the seton. By definition the skin over the muscle must be incised in the track of the seton to allow the skin to heal over the seton. At regular, 2-week intervals the seton is progressively tightened, dividing the muscle by a process of ischemic necrosis. The cut edge of the divided muscle separates minimally because of the fibrosis that forms during the time it takes to divide the muscle. The seton can be progressively tightened with silk ligatures. Alternatively, a hemorrhoid ligator may be used to progressively tighten the seton with rubber bands. This process can be quite uncomfortable for the patient.

When a staging seton is used, the fistula tract is identified and only the most superficial portion is divided. The seton is placed through that portion of the fistula tract that traverses the sphincter, thus encircling the muscle. This portion of the tract is divided as a second procedure after adequate fibrosis occurs (usually 8 weeks). A "high" fistula may be converted to a "low" fistula by dividing only the proximal portion of the tract, leaving the distal tract encircled with a seton for division at a later date.

Whether to use a cutting seton or a staging seton with second-stage fistulotomy appears to be up to surgeon preference. In a study of 59 patients with high anal fistula, Garcia-Aguilar et al.[36] showed no difference in fistula eradication, incontinence, and patient satisfaction between 12 patients treated with cutting setons and 47 treated with two-stage seton fistulotomy.

Fibrin Glue

The use of fibrin glue in the management of anorectal fistulas has been popularized. A prepared mixture of fibrinogen and thrombin is injected into the fistula tract after it has been curetted. The resulting coagulum plugs the fistula tract. This technique represents an alternative mode of treatment in complex cases for which standard treatment has failed. The complete healing rate in one series was 60% and included patients with Crohn disease and human immunodeficiency virus (HIV)-associated anal disease.[37] Sentovich performed a two-stage fistulotomy with injection of fibrin glue into the external opening after seton removal at the second operation, with 69% success in 48 patients.[38] Buchanan et al. found only a 14% complex fistula closure rate in 22 patients.[39] Despite mixed results, fibrin glue remains a viable treatment option because of its safety, ease of application, and low risk of sphincter injury.

Fistula Plug

An anal fistula plug (AFP) is a bioprosthetic material that is placed in the fistula tract that acts as a scaffolding for native tissue ingrowth. It is inherently resistant to infection, produces no foreign body or giant cell reaction, and becomes repopulated with host cell tissue during a period of 3 months. The fistula plug is inserted into the primary opening of the fistula and secured into place with one or two interrupted stitches. Currently commercially available AFPs are either made of lyophilized porcine intestinal submucosa or of synthetic absorbable biomaterial. This intervention appears to be a safe option because it preserves anal function, is associated with a low morbidity, and has high patient tolerance. The success rate of AFP has been quite varied in different studies.[40] A review article reports overall success to be approximately 50% to 60%.[41] More recent studies have shown decreased success rates, correlating with the decreased adoption of the technique.[40]

Endorectal Advancement Flaps

Endorectal advancement flaps (ERAFs) consist of mucosa, submucosa, and part of the internal sphincter. The underlying fistula tract is débrided, and the internal opening is sutured at the level of the muscle. The edge of the elevated flap containing the internal opening is excised, and the flap is advanced and sutured over the internal defect (Fig. 160.13).

ERAFs offer the advantage of a one-stage procedure, quicker healing, limited damage to the underlying sphincter, and minimal risk of anal canal deformity.[3] Several studies have reported good success, with few complications using anorectal advancement flaps in the treatment of both simple and complex fistulas.[42] Factors such as Crohn disease,[43] smoking,[44] and multiple prior surgeries,[45,46] along with concurrent use of fibrin glue,[47] have been associated with higher risk of flap failure.

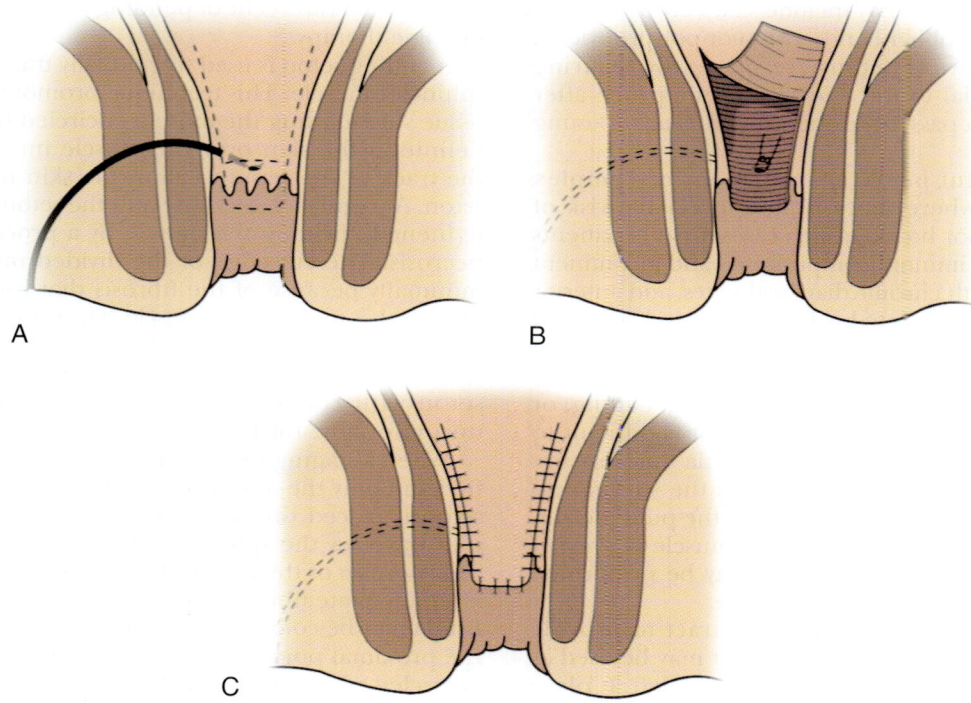

FIGURE 160.13 (A) Anorectal advancement flap for closure of the internal opening in the treatment of perianal fistulas. The base of the flap should be wider than the apex. (B) With the flap elevated, the internal opening is débrided and closed with a suture. (C) The apex of the flap is advanced and sutured over the defect.

ERAFs can result in mucosal ectropion if the flap is advanced too far. It also requires proximal anal and rectal wall suitable for mobilization. Patients with high fistulas or with prior surgical procedures can have dense scarring, which may limit the mobilization of adequate tissue. For such circumstances, anocutaneous advancement flaps have been described.[48–51] Such flaps involve mobilization of pedicled flap from the anal margin with advancement into the anal canal. However, advancing too much anoderm too far into the anal canal may result in severe pruritic symptoms.

Ligation of Intersphincteric Fistula Tract

Recently, a method termed the LIFT procedure or "ligation of the intersphincteric fistula tract" has become popular. LIFT was first described in 1993 by Phillips et al[52]; however, it was popularized by Dr. Rojanasakul from Thailand in 2007.[53] This sphincter-preserving method for fistula closure involves making an incision in the intersphincteric groove, dissection between the sphincter muscles, and identification of the fistula tract. The fistula probe is left in situ during this time to facilitate identification of the tract. The fistula tract is then dissected free and the probe removed. Next, the fistula tract is divided and ligated. The internal opening is closed with absorbable suture and the external opening curetted and left open to drain (Fig. 160.14). Recent systematic reviews of this procedure have demonstrated a success rate similar to other sphincter-preserving procedures, between 40% and 94% with pooled success of approximately 70%.[54–57]

Failure after LIFT procedure has been classified into type I—residual sinus tract from intersphincteric groove without any internal opening, type II—downstaged tract from intersphincteric groove to internal opening, and type III with complete failure that extends from previous internal opening to one or more external openings.[58] Type I failure is treated with local curettage and antibiotics, type II failure is treated with fistulotomy, and type III failure is treated with a secondary repair using other modalities or a repeat LIFT.[59] Several authors have described modifications of the LIFT procedure by adding a bioprosthetic mesh in the intersphincteric groove (Bio-LIFT) or by placing a fistula plug through the external sphincter (LIFT-plug), with better success rates.[60,61] However, long-term results are lacking. Among the sphincter-sparing procedures for fistula management, ERAF and LIFT have the highest rates of fistula cure. Two prospective trials have not shown any difference in outcomes between these two techniques.[62,63]

POSTOPERATIVE CARE

In general, most anorectal surgery is performed as an outpatient procedure.[64] Patients are instructed to consume a high-fiber diet postoperatively. No bowel confinement regimen is required for the treatment of simple conditions. For complex procedures, bowel confinement may be considered, although the evidence for this is controversial and of low grade.[65–67] Sitz baths are recommended for perianal hygiene and comfort. More complex procedures may require inpatient status for pain management and wound care. Wound healing after fistulotomy usually takes 4 to 8 weeks. Patients with an anorectal abscess should be followed closely after drainage for possible fistula development.

COMPLICATIONS

Complications after surgical intervention for anorectal suppurative disease are numerous and related to surgical technique. Urinary retention is the most common complication, occurring in up to 25% of patients.[68] Other complications include hemorrhage, acute external thrombosed hemorrhoids, cellulitis, fecal impaction, stricture, rectovaginal fistula, incontinence, and recurrence. Local wound problems and complications associated with anesthesia, such as hypotension, hypertension, and seizures, have also been reported. The issue of fistula recurrence after drainage of anorectal abscess has been discussed previously.

The rate of recurrent fistula after fistulotomy ranges from 0% to 18%,[69] although the true incidence is probably approximately 3% to 7%.[6,70] The primary causes of fistula recurrence relate to unrecognized internal openings and inadequate drainage of abscess cavities.[2] In a study of 375 patients, Garcia-Aguilar[70] found that recurrence was also associated with lateral location of internal openings and fistulas with horseshoe extension.

The rate of disorders of continence after fistulotomy ranges from 18% to 52%.[69] Factors associated with incontinence risk include increased complexity of the fistulas, female sex, division of a significant portion of the external sphincter, the use of two-stage seton or cutting seton fistulotomy (probably because of complexity of the fistula), and a history of prior fistula surgery.[70]

EMERGING TECHNOLOGIES FOR FISTULA REPAIR

Surgical treatment of high and complex anal fistulas still remains challenging, with 15% to 60% failure rates. Multiple novel techniques have been described with variable short-term success rates. Laser emitted by a radial fiber (FiLaC) has been used to destroy the fistula epithelium and simultaneously closes the tract.[71–73] Recently published case series have shown a 71% healing rate at median follow-up of 30 months.[71] A similar tract ablation under videoscopic guidance and stapled closure of the internal opening was described by Meinero in the technique named video-assisted anal fistula treatment (VAAFT).[74] This technique has an advantage of visually identifying the anatomy of fistula tract and any residual abscess cavity. Review of the results by the same author demonstrated a 70% healing rate at 6 months. Stapling of the internal opening was associated with better results when compared with suture closing.

The use of stem cells derived from autologous subcutaneous fat has been proposed for the repair of complex anal fistulas. These mesenchymal stem cells exert immunomodulatory and antiinflammatory properties by regulating functions of lymphocytes, neutrophils, natural killer (NK) cells, and monocyte-derived dendritic cells. However, in a phase I randomized control trial, healing rates at

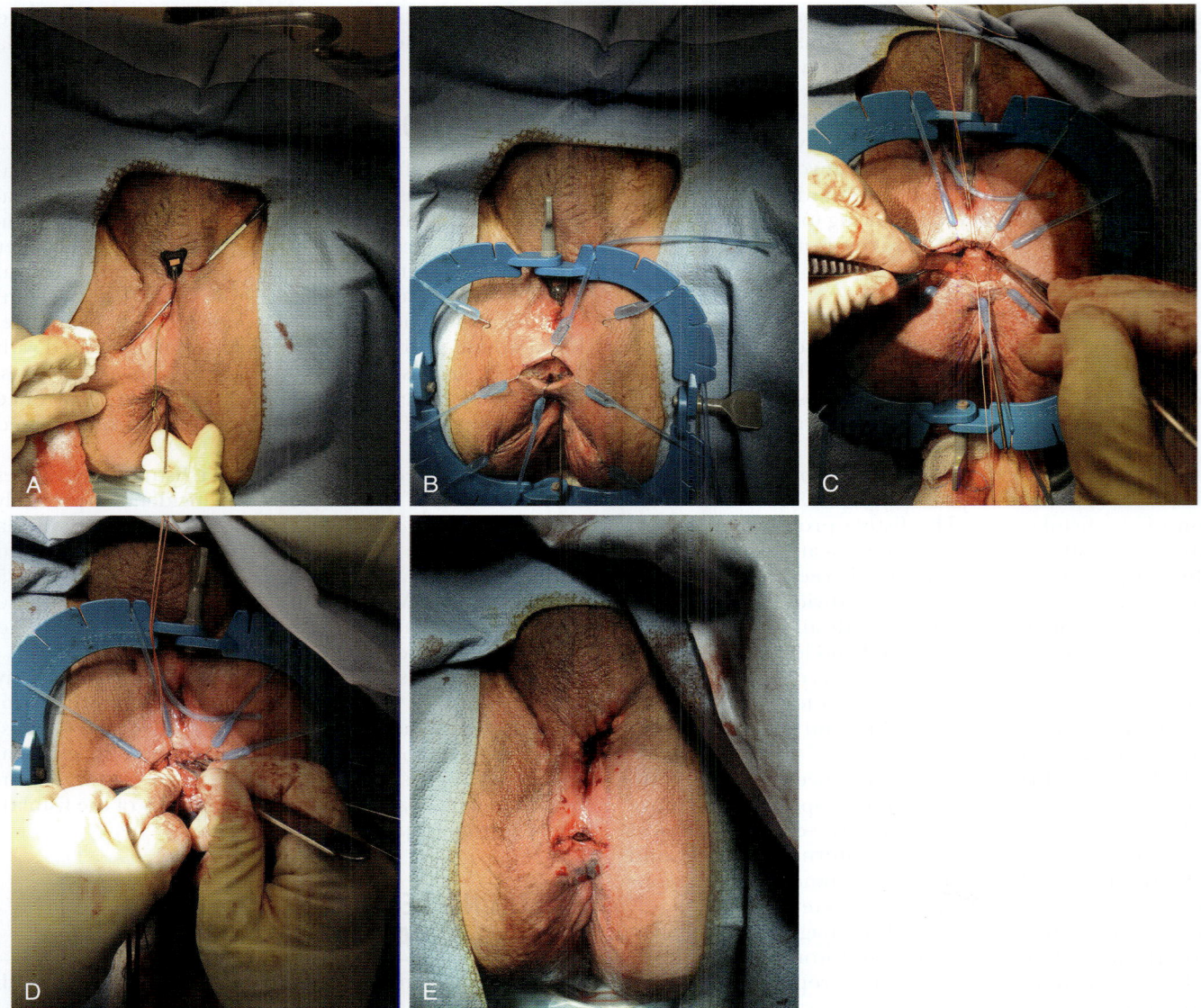

FIGURE 160.14 (A) Complex anterior transsphincteric anal fistula with extension to perineum and base of scrotum after first-stage fistulotomy and seton placement. (B) Perianal incision in intersphincteric groove for ligation of intersphincteric fistula tract with Lone Star retractor for exposure. (C) Isolation and ligation of intersphincteric fistula tract. (D) Division of the tract. (E) Ligation of intersphincteric fistula tract incision closure to allow drainage. This patient also had drainage of scrotal fistula component and marsupialization.

6 months were approximately 40% and no difference was seen when compared to fibrin glue treatment.[75]

SPECIAL CONSIDERATIONS

CROHN DISEASE

Crohn disease manifests with perianal or rectal symptoms in approximately one-third of patients. It is associated with a more disabling natural history,[76] increased extraintestinal manifestations,[77] and more steroid resistance.[78] Anorectal abscess in patients with Crohn disease should be treated with prompt drainage. Long-term catheter drainage has been found to be safe and effective and may be of benefit in preventing or delaying recurrence and the subsequent need for proctectomy.

The treatment of anorectal fistulas in patients with Crohn disease should be tailored to the specific situation encountered. Consideration should be given to the complexity of the fistula and the presence of active Crohn disease in the rectum. In general, treatment modalities should be conservative. Extensive procedures may increase the risk of incontinence and nonhealing wounds. A simple fistula in a patient with a normal rectum can be treated by primary fistulotomy with good outcome and satisfactory healing rates.[79] Complex fistulas in patients with active rectal Crohn disease remain a therapeutic challenge. These cases are better served with prolonged drainage to achieve long-term palliation. In selected cases, rectal advancement flaps, LIFT, AFP, or fibrin glue may be used with good functional results and their respective variable success rates.[80] Some patients with complex anorectal fistulas in the presence of anal Crohn may require diversion of the fecal stream for symptomatic relief. Ultimately, between 12% and 39% of patients will require proctectomy for progressive intestinal disease or intractable perianal disease.[81] Shinozaki et al., in a series of 39 patients, found that simultaneously performing a bowel resection for active Crohn disease at the time of drainage of perianal sepsis or draining seton placement led to better healing of the anal fistula.[82] It is theorized that control of the intraabdominal Crohn disease improves healing of perianal Crohn fistulas.

A monoclonal antibody to tumor necrosis factor-α (TNF-α) was approved in August 1998 by the US Food and Drug Administration for the treatment of patients with fistulizing Crohn disease. Infliximab (Remicade) is a genetically constructed murine-human chimeric immunoglobulin. It neutralizes the biologic activity of TNF-α and inhibits binding to its receptors. A randomized trial in which infliximab was used in the management of patients with Crohn fistulas (perianal and abdominal) demonstrated a 68% clinical response (defined as >50% reduction from baseline in the number of draining fistulas) and a 46% complete closure of all fistulas compared with 26% and 13%, respectively, of patients in the placebo group.[83] However, the duration of response is short-lived, and therefore chronic use of the biologic agent is usually required for a long-term beneficial effect.

FISTULA IN INFANCY

Anal fistula in infancy occurs almost exclusively in otherwise healthy boys younger than 2 years. The cause of this condition appears to be a congenital abnormality of the anal glands with abnormally deep and thick crypts of Morgagni. These factors predispose the patients to cryptitis with abscess and fistula formation. Simple fistulotomy is recommended in this patient population with expected good results. A concomitant cryptotomy has been recommended by some to decrease the likelihood of recurrence. Nonoperative management is favored by those who believe that abscess and fistula are self-limited in this population. Opponents argue that such fistula disease is seldom limited. They argue that the process is truly characterized by frequent intermittent relapse or a prolonged silent state with late recurrence requiring subsequent intervention.

MALIGNANT TRANSFORMATION IN CHRONIC ANAL FISTULA

Carcinoma arising in an anorectal fistula is a rare condition. Rosser[84] established the first association between adenocarcinoma and anal fistula. There is controversy regarding the possibility of malignancy arising from a benign anorectal fistula. A slow-growing cancer may not become evident for years, and in some cases the fistula could result from the local extension of a neoplasm. To rule out the preexistence of even the slowest growing cancer, it has been arbitrarily determined that a fistula should have been present for at least 10 years before the diagnosis of carcinoma if malignant transformation is to be considered.

Carcinoma arising in anorectal fistulas in patients with Crohn disease has been reported. The estimated incidence is 0.7%.[85] Deep biopsy samples, careful histologic examination of atypical cells obtained from ductal structures, and a high index of suspicion in cases of longstanding anorectal fistulas may provide a clue to the diagnosis of underlying carcinoma. Resection with either wide local excision or abdominoperineal resection has the potential to result in cure.

ANORECTAL SEPSIS AND FISTULA IN HUMAN IMMUNODEFICIENCY VIRUS DISEASE

Anorectal disease is a prevalent problem in the HIV-positive population, with an estimated frequency of 6% to 34%.[86] Although there is concern in performing elective anorectal surgery in this population because of the fear of poor healing, symptomatic anorectal sepsis and fistula often require surgical management. Treatment should be tailored to the patient's severity of illness. The risk for disturbed wound healing increases as the preoperative CD4+ count decreases. The presence of acquired immunodeficiency syndrome and a white blood cell count of less than 3000/mm^3 are also associated with poor wound healing.[87] In the absence of these risk factors, fistulotomy for simple fistulas may be performed with expected good results. For complex fistulas and patients with risk factors for poor healing, the liberal use of draining setons is recommended for symptomatic relief.

ANORECTAL COMPLICATIONS IN PATIENTS WITH LEUKEMIA

Anorectal complications in patients with leukemia represent a rare but potentially life-threatening problem. The incidence of concomitant symptomatic anorectal disease and leukemia has been reported to be as high as 5.8%, with acute anorectal sepsis accounting for a majority of cases.[88] Many of these patients present with fever and per anal pain without any sign of fluctuant abscess secondary to low leukocyte count. The majority of these infections are polymicrobial. The most frequently found organisms are *Escherichia coli, Enterococcus, Bacteroides*, and *Klebsiella*.[89] The mortality rate for patients with acute perianal sepsis in this population has been reported to be from 5% to 20%.[89,90] Surgical treatment of anorectal sepsis in uncontrolled acute leukemia has been avoided because of the fear that the septic process would spread and wound healing would be impaired. This led to a generally accepted policy of symptomatic care as primary treatment, with surgical management reserved for the drainage of an obviously fluctuant abscess.[91] Symptomatic care consisted of sitz baths or warm compresses, stool softeners, analgesic agents, and broad-spectrum antibiotics. Additional precautionary measures included no rectal examinations, no instrumentation and no enemas. However, other reports indicate that surgical intervention in the form of incision and drainage appears to be safe in this patient population.[88,90,92]

REFERENCES

1. Devaraj B, Khabassi S, Cosman BC. Recent smoking is a risk factor for anal abscess and fistula. *Dis Colon Rectum*. 2011;54(6):681-685.
2. Robinson AM Jr, DeNobile JW. Anorectal abscess and fistula-in-ano. *J Natl Med Assoc*. 1988;80(11):1209-1213.
3. Seow-Choen F, Nicholls RJ. Anal fistula. *Br J Surg*. 1992;79(3):197-205.
4. Ssoma JA, Susati EP, Rubin RJ. Incidence of fistulas subsequent to anal abscess. *Dis Colon Rectum*. 1974;17(3):357-359.

5. McElwain JW, MacLean MD, Alexander RM, Hoexter B, Guthrie JF. Anorectal problems: experience with primary fistulectomy for anorectal abscess, a report of 1,000 cases. *Dis Colon Rectum*. 1975; 18(8):646-649.

6. Ramanujam PS, Prasad ML, Abcarian H, Tan AB. Perianal abscesses and fistulas. A study of 1023 patients. *Dis Colon Rectum*. 1984;27(9): 593-597.

7. Vasilevsky CA, Gordon PH. The incidence of recurrent abscesses or fistula-in-ano following anorectal suppuration. *Dis Colon Rectum*. 1984;27(2):126-130.

8. Schouten WR, van Vroonhoven TJ. Treatment of anorectal abscess with or without primary fistulectomy. Results of a prospective randomized trial. *Dis Colon Rectum*. 1991;34(1):60-63.

9. Parks AG, Gordon PH, Hardcastle JD. A classification of fistula-in-ano. *Br J Surg*. 1976;63(1):1-12.

10. Buchan R, Grace RH. Anorectal suppuration: the results of treatment and the factors influencing the recurrence rate. *Br J Surg*. 1973;60(7): 537-540.

11. Goodsall DH, Miles WE. *Diseases of the Anus and Rectum*. London: Longman, Green; 1900.

12. Cirocco WC, Reilly JC. Challenging the predictive accuracy of Goodsall's rule for anal fistulas. *Dis Colon Rectum*. 1992;35(6):537-542.

13. Fazio VW. Complex anal fistulae. *Gastroenterol Clin North Am*. 1987;16(1):93-114.

14. Kuijpers HC, Schulpen T. Fistulography for fistula-in-ano. Is it useful? *Dis Colon Rectum*. 1985;28(2):103-104.

15. Choen S, Burnett S, Bartram CI, Nicholls RJ. Comparison between anal endosonography and digital examination in the evaluation of anal fistulae. *Br J Surg*. 1991;78(4):445-447.

16. Buchanan GN, Bartram CI, Williams AB, Halligan S, Cohen CR. Value of hydrogen peroxide enhancement of three-dimensional endoanal ultrasound in fistula-in-ano. *Dis Colon Rectum*. 2005;36(1):141-147.

17. Kim Y, Park YJ. Three-dimensional endoanal ultrasonographic assessment of an anal fistula with and without H_2O_2 enhancement. *World J Gastroenterol*. 2009;15(38):4810-4815.

18. Orsoni P, Barthet M, Portier F, Panuel M, Desjeux A, Grimaud JC. Prospective comparison of endosonography, magnetic resonance imaging and surgical findings in anorectal fistula and abscess complicating Crohn's disease. *Br J Surg*. 1999;86(3):360-364.

19. Poen AC, Felt-Bersma RJ, Cuesta MA, Meuwissen GM. Vaginal endosonography of the anal sphincter complex is important in the assessment of faecal incontinence and perianal sepsis. *Br J Surg*. 1998;85(3):359-363.

20. Beets-Tan RG, Beets GL, van der Hoop AG, et al. Preoperative MR imaging of anal fistulas: does it really help the surgeon? *Radiology*. 2001;218(1):75-84.

21. Schwartz DA, Wiersema MJ, Dudiak KM, et al. A comparison of endoscopic ultrasound, magnetic resonance imaging, and exam under anesthesia for evaluation of Crohn's perianal fistulas. *Gastroenterology*. 2001;121(5):1064-1072.

22. Chang SC, Lin JK. Change in anal continence after surgery for intersphincteral anal fistula: a functional and manometric study. *Int J Colorectal Dis*. 2003;18(2):111-115.

23. Wilson W, Taubert KA, Gewitz M, et al. Prevention of infective endocarditis: guidelines from the American Heart Association: a guideline from the American Heart Association Rheumatic Fever, Endocarditis, and Kawasaki Disease Committee, Council on Cardiovascular Disease in the Young, and the Council on Clinical Cardiology, Council on Cardiovascular Surgery and Anesthesia, and the Quality of Care and Outcomes Research Interdisciplinary Working Group. *Circulation*. 2007;116(15):1736-1754.

24. Steele SR, Kumar R, Feingold DL, Rafferty JL, Buie WD. Practice parameters for the management of perianal abscess and fistula-in-ano. *Dis Colon Rectum*. 2011;54(12):1465-1474.

25. Toyonaga T, Matsushima M, Tanaka Y, et al. Microbiological analysis and endoanal ultrasonography for diagnosis of anal fistula in acute anorectal sepsis. *Int J Colorectal Dis*. 2007;22(2):209-213.

26. Seow-Choen F, Leong AF, Goh HS. Results of a policy of selective immediate fistulotomy for primary anal abscess. *Aust N Z J Surg*. 1993;63(6):485-489.

27. Hanley PH. Conservative surgical correction of horseshoe abscess and fistula. *Dis Colon Rectum*. 1965;8(5):364-368.

28. Eisenhammer S. The final evaluation and classification of the surgical treatment of the primary anorectal cryptoglandular intermuscular

29. Oliver I, Lacueva FJ, Perez Vicente F, et al. Randomized clinical trial comparing simple drainage of anorectal abscess with and without fistula track treatment. *Int J Colorectal Dis*. 2003;18(2):107-110.

30. Fucini C. One stage treatment of anal abscesses and fistulas. A clinical appraisal on the basis of two different classifications. *Int J Colorectal Dis*. 1991;6(1):12-16.

31. Garcés-Albir M, García-Botello SA, Esclapez-Valero P, et al. Quantifying the extent of fistulotomy. How much sphincter can we safely divide? A three-dimensional endosonographic study. *Int J Colorectal Dis*. 2012;27(8):1109-1116.

32. Cavanaugh M, Hyman N, Osler T. Fecal incontinence severity index after fistulotomy: a predictor of quality of life. *Dis Colon Rectum*. 2002;45(3):349-353.

33. Lentner A, Wienert V. Long-term, indwelling setons for low transsphincteric and intersphincteric anal fistulas. Experience with 108 cases. *Dis Colon Rectum*. 1996;39(10):1097-1101.

34. Topstad DR, Panaccione R, Heine JA, Johnson DR, MacLean AR, Buie WD. Combined seton placement, infliximab infusion, and maintenance immunosuppressives improve healing rate in fistulizing anorectal Crohn's disease: a single center experience. *Dis Colon Rectum*. 2003;46(5):577-583.

35. Strong SA, Koltun WA, Hyman NH, Donald Buie W, the Standards Practice Task Force of the American Society of Colon and Rectal Surgeons. Practice parameters for the surgical management of Crohn's disease. *Dis Colon Rectum*. 2007;50(11):1735-1746.

36. García-Aguilar J, Belmonte C, Wong DW, Goldberg SM, Madoff RD. Cutting seton versus two-stage seton fistulotomy in the surgical management of high anal fistula. *Br J Surg*. 1998;85(2):243-245.

37. Abel ME, Chiu YS, Russell TR, Volpe PA. Autologous fibrin glue in the treatment of rectovaginal and complex fistulas. *Dis Colon Rectum*. 1993;36(5):447-449.

38. Sentovich SM. Fibrin glue for anal fistulas: long-term results. *Dis Colon Rectum*. 2003;46(4):498-502.

39. Buchanan GN, Bartram CI, Phillips RK, et al. Efficacy of fibrin sealant in the management of complex anal fistula: a prospective trial. *Dis Colon Rectum*. 2003;46(9):1167-1174.

40. Kontovounisios C, Tekkis P, Tan E, Rasheed S, Darzi A, Wexner SD. Adoption and success rates of perineal procedures for fistula-in-ano: a systematic review. *Colorectal Dis*. 2016;18(5):441-458.

41. Köckerling F, Alam NN, Narang SK, Daniels IR, Smart NJ. Treatment of fistula-in-ano with fistula plug – a review under special consideration of the technique. *Front Surg*. 2015;2:55.

42. Soltani A, Kaiser AM. Endorectal advancement flap for cryptoglandular or Crohn's fistula-in-ano. *Dis Colon Rectum*. 2010;53(4):486-495.

43. Sonoda T, Hull T, Piedmonte MR, Fazio VW. Outcomes of primary repair of anorectal and rectovaginal fistulas using the endorectal advancement flap. *Dis Colon Rectum*. 2002;45(12):1622-1628.

44. Ellis CN, Clark S. Effect of tobacco smoking on advancement flap repair of complex anal fistulas. *Dis Colon Rectum*. 2007;50(4):459-463.

45. Ozuner G, Hull TL, Cartmill J, Fazio VW. Long-term analysis of the use of transanal rectal advancement flaps for complicated anorectal/vaginal fistulas. *Dis Colon Rectum*. 1996;39(1):10-14.

46. Schouten WR, Zimmerman DD, Briel JW. Transanal advancement flap repair of transsphincteric fistulas. *Dis Colon Rectum*. 1999;42(11):1419-1422; discussion 1422–1423.

47. Ellis CN, Clark S. Fibrin glue as an adjunct to flap repair of anal fistulas: a randomized, controlled study. *Dis Colon Rectum*. 2006;49(11):1736-1740.

48. Sungurtekin U, Sungurtekin H, Kabay B, et al. Anocutaneous V-Y advancement flap for the treatment of complex perianal fistula. *Dis Colon Rectum*. 2004;47(12):2178-2183.

49. Nelson RL, Cintron J, Abcarian H. Dermal island-flap anoplasty for transsphincteric fistula-in-ano: assessment of treatment failures. *Dis Colon Rectum*. 2000;43(5):681-684.

50. Zimmerman DD, Briel JW, Gosselink MP, Schouten WR. Anocutaneous advancement flap repair of transsphincteric fistulas. *Dis Colon Rectum*. 2001;44(10):1474-1480.

51. Hossack T, Solomon MJ, Young JM. Ano-cutaneous flap repair for complex and recurrent supra-sphincteric anal fistula. *Colorectal Dis*. 2005;7(2):187-192.

52. Matos D, Lunniss PJ, Phillips RK. Total sphincter conservation in high fistula in ano: results of a new approach. *Br J Surg*. 1993;80(6):802-804.

(intersphincteric) fistulous abscess and fistula. *Dis Colon Rectum*. 1978;21(4):237-254.

53. Rojanasakul A, Pattanaarun J, Sahakitrungruang C, Tantiphlachiva K. Total anal sphincter saving technique for fistula-in-ano; the ligation of intersphincteric fistula tract. *J Med Assoc Thai* 2007; 90(3):581-586.

54. Hong KD, Kang S, Kalaskar S, Wexner SD. Ligation of intersphincteric fistula tract (LIFT) to treat anal fistula: systematic review and meta-analysis. *Tech Coloproctol*. 2014; 18(8):685-691.

55. Murugesan J, Mor I, Fulham S, Hitos K. Systematic review of efficacy of LIFT procedure in crpytoglandular fistula-in-ano. *J Coloproctol*. 2014;34(2):109-119.

56. Yassin NA, Hammond TM, Lunniss PJ, Phillips RK. Ligation of the intersphincteric fistula tract in the management of anal fistula. A systematic review. *Colorectal Dis*. 2013;15(5):527-535.

57. Zirak-Schmidt S, Perdawood SK. Management of anal fistula by ligation of the intersphincteric fistula tract—a systematic review. *Dan Med J*. 2014;61(12):A4977.

58. Liu WY, Aboulian A, Kaji AH, Kumar RR. Long-term results of ligation of intersphincteric fistula tract (LIFT) for fistula-in-ano. *Dis Colon Rectum*. 2013;56(3):343-347.

59. Tan KK, Tan IJ, Lim FS, Koh DC, Tsang CB. The anatomy of failures following the ligation of intersphincteric tract technique for anal fistula: a review of 93 patients over 4 years. *Dis Colon Rectum*. 2011;54(11):1368-1372.

60. Ellis CN. Outcomes with the use of bioprosthetic grafts to reinforce the ligation of the intersphincteric fistula tract (BioLIFT procedure) for the management of complex anal fistulas. *Dis Colon Rectum*. 2010;53(10):1361-1364.

61. Han JG, Yi BQ, Wang ZJ. Ligation of the intersphincteric fistula tract plus a bioprosthetic anal fistula plug (LIFT-Plug): a new technique for fistula-in-ano. *Colorectal Dis*. 2013;15(5):582-586.

62. Madbouly KM, El Shazly W, Abbas KS, Hussein AM. Ligation of intersphincteric fistula tract versus mucosal advancement flap in patients with high transsphincteric fistula-in-ano: a prospective randomized trial. *Dis Colon Rectum*. 2014;57(10):1202-1208.

63. Mushaya C, Bartlett L, Schulze B, Ho YH. Ligation of intersphincteric fistula tract compared with advancement flap for complex anorectal fistulas requiring initial seton drainage. *Am J Surg*. 2012;204(3):283-289.

64. Ternent CA, Fleming F, Welton ML, et al. Clinical practice guideline for ambulatory anorectal surgery. *Dis Colon Rectum*. 2015;58(10):915-922.

65. Nessim A, Wexner SD, Agachan F, et al. Is bowel confinement necessary after anorectal reconstructive surgery? A prospective, randomized, surgeon-blinded trial. *Dis Colon Rectum*. 1999;42(1):16-23.

66. Mahony R, Behan M, O'Herlihy C, O'Connell PR. Randomized, clinical trial of bowel confinement vs. laxative use after primary repair of a third-degree obstetric anal sphincter tear. *Dis Colon Rectum*. 2004;47(1):12-17.

67. Joos AK, Palma P, Jonescheit JO, Hasenberg T, Herold A. Enteral vs parenteral nutrition in reconstructive anal surgery—a prospective-randomized trial. *Colorectal Dis*. 2008;10(6):605-609.

68. Mazier WP. The treatment and care of anal fistulas: a study of 1,000 patients. *Dis Colon Rectum*. 1971;14(2):134-144.

69. Vasilevsky CA. Fistula-in-ano and abscess. In: Beck DE, Wexner SD, eds. *Fundamentals of Anorectal Surgery*. 2nd ed. WB Saunders; 1998:557.

70. Garcia-Aguilar J, Belmonte C, Wong WD, Goldberg SM, Madoff RD. Anal fistula surgery. Factors associated with recurrence and incontinence. *Dis Colon Rectum*. 1996;39(7):723-729.

71. Giamundo P, Esercizio L, Geraci M, Tibaldi L, Valente M. Fistula-tract Laser Closure (FiLaC): long-term results and new operative strategies. *Tech Coloproctol*. 2015;19(8):449-453.

72. Giamundo P, Geraci M, Tibaldi L, Valente M. Closure of fistula-in-ano with laser—FiLaC: an effective novel sphincter-saving procedure for complex disease. *Colorectal Dis*. 2014;16(2):110-115.

73. Wilhelm A. A new technique for sphincter-preserving anal fistula repair using a novel radial emitting laser probe. *Tech Coloproctol*. 2011;15(4):445-449.

74. Meinero P, Mori L. Video-assisted anal fistula treatment (VAAFT): a novel sphincter-saving procedure for treating complex anal fistulas. *Tech Coloproctol*. 2011;15(4):417-422.

75. Herreros MD, Garcia-Arranz M, Guadalajara H, De-La-Quintana P, Garcia-Olmo D. Autologous expanded adipose-derived stem cells for the treatment of complex cryptoglandular perianal fistulas: a phase III randomized clinical trial (FATT 1: Fistula Advanced Therapy Trial 1) and long-term evaluation. *Dis Colon Rectum*. 2012;55(7):762-772.

76. Beaugerie L, Seksik P, Nion-Larmurier I, Gendre JP, Cosnes J. Predictors of Crohn's disease. *Gastroenterology*. 2006;130(3):650-656.

77. Rankin GB, Watts HD, Melnyk CS, Kelley ML Jr. National Cooperative Crohn's Disease Study: extraintestinal manifestations and perianal complications. *Gastroenterology*. 1979;77(4 Pt 2):914-920.

78. Gelbmann CM, Rogler G, Gross V et al. Prior bowel resections, perianal disease, and a high initial Crohn's disease activity index are associated with corticosteroid resistance in active Crohn's disease. *Am J Gastroenterol*. 2002;97(6):1438-1445.

79. Morrison JG, Gathright JB Jr, Ray JE, Ferrari BT, Hicks TC, Timmcke AE. Surgical management of anorectal fistulas in Crohn's disease. *Dis Colon Rectum*. 1989;32(6):492-496.

80. Makowiec F, Jehle EC, Becker HD, Starlinger M. Clinical course after transanal advancement flap repair of perianal fistula in patients with Crohn's disease. *Br J Surg*. 1995;82(5):603-606.

81. Whiteford MH, Kilkenny J 3rd, Hyman N, et al. Practice parameters for the treatment of perianal abscess and fistula-in-ano (revised). *Dis Colon Rectum*. 2005;48(7):1337-1342.

82. Shinozaki M, Koganei K, Fukushima T. Simultaneous anus and bowel operation is preferable for anal fistula in Crohn's disease. *J Gastroenterol*. 2002;37(8):611-616.

83. Present DH, Rutgeerts P, Targan S. Infliximab for the treatment of fistulas in patients with Crohn's disease. *N Engl J Med*. 1999; 340(18):1398-1405.

84. Rosser C. The relation of fistula-in-ano to cancer of the anal canal. *Trans Am Proctol Soc*. 1934;35:65-71.

85. Ky A, Sohn N, Weinstein MA, Korelitz B. Carcinoma arising in anorectal fistulas of Crohn's disease. *Dis Colon Rectum*. 1998;41(8): 992-996.

86. Consten EC, Slors FJ, Noten HJ, Oosting H, Danner SA, van Lanschot J. Anorectal surgery in human immunodeficiency virus-infected patients. Clinical outcome in relation to immune status. *Dis Colon Rectum*. 1995;38(11):1169-1175.

87. Nadal SR, Manzione CR, Galvao VM, Salim VR, Speranzini MB. Healing after anal fistulotomy: comparative study between HIV+ and HIV- patients. *Dis Colon Rectum*. 1998;41(2):177-179.

88. Grewal H, Guillem JG, Quan SH, Enker WE, Cohen AM. Anorectal disease in neutropenic leukemic patients. Operative vs nonoperative management. *Dis Colon Rectum*. 1994;37(11):1095-1099.

89. Chen CY, Cheng A, Huang SY. Clinical and microbiological characteristics of perianal infections in adult patients with acute leukemia. *PLoS One*. 2013;8(4):e60624.

90. Büyükaşik Y, Ozcebe OI, Sayinalp N et al. Perianal infections in patients with leukemia: importance of the course of neutrophil count. *Dis Colon Rectum*. 1998;41(1):81-85.

91. Badgwell BD, Chang GJ, Rodriguez-Bigas MA, et al. Management and outcomes of anorectal infection in the cancer patient. *Ann Surg Oncol*. 2009;16(10):2752-2758.

92. Barnes SG, Sattler FR, Ballard JO. Perirectal infections in acute leukemia. Improved survival after incision and debridement. *Ann Intern Med*. 1984;100(4):515-518.

93. Marks CG, Ritchie JK. Anal fistulas at St Mark's Hospital. *Br J Surg*. 1977;64:84.

94. Vasilevsky CA, Gordon PH. Results of treatment of fistula-in-ano. *Dis Colon Rectum*. 1985;28:225.

95. Garcia-Aguilar J, Belmonte C, Wong WD, et al. Anal fistula surgery: factors associated with recurrence and incontinence. *Dis Colon Rectum*. 1996;39:723.

CHAPTER 161

Concepts in Inflammatory Bowel Disease Management

Evangelos Messaris | Themistocles Dassopoulos

The prototypical inflammatory bowel diseases (IBDs), ulcerative colitis (UC), and Crohn disease (CD), are idiopathic inflammatory disorders of the intestinal tract characterized by a chronic, relapsing course. UC and CD have profound effects on the life of patients and create significant challenges for the entire health care system. Research in the genetics, epidemiology, and basic mechanisms of IBD has produced a giant leap in our understanding of IBD over the past 20 years. Currently, there is no curative medical therapy for these disorders. Nonetheless, advances in our understanding of IBD pathogenesis, utilization of an expanding array of antiinflammatory agents, and application of sound surgical principles have contributed to improved health outcomes. In this chapter, we present an overview of the medical and surgical therapies of IBD, with a particular emphasis on the most current understanding of the disease and recent developments in management.

GENETICS

The familial aggregation of IBD was an important early clue to the genetic basis of IBD.[1] Indeed, the greatest risk factor for IBD is a positive family history, with first-degree relatives of IBD patients having an approximately 15-fold higher risk for IBD than the general population.[1] Additional evidence suggesting a genetic susceptibility came from observed ethnic differences in IBD incidence and prevalence, the association of IBD with other disorders with recognized genetic susceptibility (such as ankylosing spondylitis and psoriasis), and the existence of genetic syndromes (such as glycogen storage disease type 1b and Hermansky-Pudlak syndrome) with phenotypes resembling IBD.[1] Although familial and ethnic aggregation may reflect shared genetic factors, environmental factors may be shared as well. Powerful support for the contribution of both genes and the environment in IBD came from twin concordance studies. Concordance for CD among monozygotic twins ranged from 35% to 58%, whereas dizygotic twin concordance ranged from 0% to 4%.[2-4] In UC, monozygotic and dizygotic concordances were 16% to 19% and 0% to 5%, respectively.[2-4] The twin concordance studies confirmed (1) the contribution of both genes and the environment in IBD and (2) the stronger genetic influence in CD compared with UC.

A number of approaches were taken to identify IBD susceptibility genes. Linkage studies identify regions of the human genome associated with disease susceptibility by testing a series of marker alleles for cosegregation (linkage) with disease status across a number of families. In 1996 the first CD linkage study mapped a susceptibility gene to chromosome 16.[5] In 2001 two studies identified three low-frequency risk variants within the NOD2 (nucleotide-binding oligomerization domain containing 2) gene on chromosome 16.[6,7] NOD2 is an intracellular receptor that binds muramyl dipeptide (MDP), a bacterial wall peptide. The three NOD2 variants individually conferred odds ratios (ORs) of 2 to 4 in heterozygotes and 20 to 40 for homozygotes. At least one mutation was present in 30% to 40% of CD cases compared with 6% to 7% in European controls.[8] Notably, these NOD2 variants were not observed in CD patients of Japanese or Chinese ancestry. Owing to the fact that linkage studies can easily detect only highly penetrant risk loci, subsequent studies replicated only a few additional loci (6p21 [human leukocyte antigen (HLA)], 5q31, and 19p).[1,8,9]

Genome-wide association studies (GWASs) constituted the next milestone in IBD gene discovery. These studies became feasible after technologic advances allowed the mapping of the human genome using a relatively limited number of selected single nucleotide polymorphisms (SNPs) (<1 million SNPs for individuals of European ancestry), which comprehensively assayed common genetic variations across the genome.[9] Compared with linkage studies, GWASs have greater statistical power to detect loci of small to moderate effect sizes. The first GWAS, conducted in a Japanese population and published in 2005, found that polymorphisms in TNFSF15 (tumor necrosis factor superfamily, member 15) conferred susceptibility to CD.[10] TNFSF15 is involved in Th1-mediated inflammatory responses in the gut. Next, a GWAS published in 2006 identified IL23R as a susceptibility gene for both UC and CD (17068223), thereby implicating the interleukin-23 (IL-23)/IL-17–producing T-helper cell (Th17) axis in intestinal inflammation. Subsequent GWASs identified genes involved in autophagy (*ATG16L1* and *IRGM*), innate immune responses (*TLR4, CARD9, IL23R, STAT3*), and the adaptive immune system (*HLA, IRF5, PTPN22*)[1].

Further insights were provided by meta-analyses of GWAS. The largest meta-analysis, performed in cohorts of European descent (75,000 cases and controls), identified a total of 163 IBD loci, including 30 new loci.[12] There were 110 loci conferring risk to both IBD subtypes, 30 loci unique to CD, and 23 loci unique to UC.[12] This degree of sharing of genetic risk suggests that nearly all of the biologic mechanisms involved in one disease have some role in the other. With the exception of *NOD2* (OR 1.5 for CD) and *IL23R* (OR 1.5 for IBD), all other IBD loci conferred low risks (1 < OR < 1.5). Among the UC-specific loci, *HLA* conferred the highest risk (OR, 1.15). The loci identified by the meta-analysis explained only 13.6% of CD and 7.5% of UC total disease variances, suggesting that other factors, such as rarer genetic variations not captured by GWAS or environmental exposures, make substantial contributions to pathogenesis. Many of the identified IBD loci were implicated in other immune-mediated disorders, most notably ankylosing spondylitis and psoriasis. The IBD loci identified were also markedly enriched in genes involved in the primary immunodeficiencies, such as genes that correlate with reduced levels of T-cell subsets, such as Th17 cells (*STAT3*), memory T cells (*SP110*), and regulatory T cells (*STAT5B*). Finally, the IBD loci were enriched in genes leading to mendelian susceptibility to mycobacterial disease (*IL12B, IFNGR2, STAT1, IRF8, TYK2,* and *STAT3*). Additional analyses were conducted to classify the loci according to immune pathways. These analyses identified genes involved in cytokine production (*interferon-gamma [IFN-γ], IL12, tumor necrosis factor-alpha [TNF-α], IL10*); activation of T, B, and NK cells; response to molecules of bacterial origin; and the IL-17/IL-23 signaling pathway (*IL23R, IL12B, JAK2, TYK2,* and *STAT3*). There was no evidence of CD or UC specificity in any of these pathways.

The first multiethnic association study of IBD (87,000 Europeans and 10,000 individuals of East-Asian, Indian, or Iranian descent) added 38 new IBD loci (4 for UC, 7 for CD, and 27 common loci) to the 163 loci already identified by the GWAS meta-analysis, thus bringing the total of confirmed IBD loci to more than 200.[13] For most loci, the direction and magnitude of effect were consistent in European and non-European cohorts. However, there was genetic heterogeneity at several established risk loci, driven by a combination of differences in allele frequencies (*NOD2*), effect sizes (*TNFSF15, ATG16L1*), or a combination of both (*IL23R, IRGM*). It is clear that the genetic architecture of IBD varies across diverse populations.

Altogether, the identified IBD gene and genetic loci can be grouped into several pathways crucial for intestinal homeostasis, including barrier function, epithelial restitution, autophagy and other types of antimicrobial defense, regulation of innate and adaptive immunity, cytokine signaling, generation of reactive oxygen species, endoplasmic reticulum stress, and metabolic pathways associated with cellular homeostasis.[14] For all populations, *HLA* is the major risk factor for UC. Among white people, *NOD2* mutations confer by far the highest risk for CD.[12]

TABLE 161.1 Inflammatory Bowel Disease Genetics—Key Points

- UC and CD are polygenic diseases
- There is a stronger genetic influence in CD compared with UC
- There are more than 200 confirmed IBD loci
  - 37 unique to CD
  - 27 unique to UC
  - 137 common to both CD and UC
- The genetic architecture of IBD varies across diverse ethnic populations
- IBD shares susceptibility genes with other immune-mediated disorders
- For Caucasians, *NOD2* confers the higher risk for CD
- For all populations, *HLA* is the major risk factor for UC
- The identified IBD gene loci can be grouped into several important homeostatic pathways including:
  - Innate immunity
    - Autophagy (in CD)
    - Other types of antimicrobial defense
    - IL-17/-23 pathway
  - Adaptive immunity
  - Barrier function and epithelial restitution

CD, Crohn disease; *IBD,* inflammatory bowel disease; *UC,* ulcerative colitis.

It appears that, in European populations, linkage studies and GWAS have uncovered all variants with large effects (OR > 3) and frequencies greater than 1%.[11] In addition, it is probable that nearly all variants with frequencies greater than 5% and ORs greater than 1.2 have also been identified. The remaining genetic contribution is expected to arise from a combination of common variants with ever-smaller effect sizes and rare variants.[1] Whole exome sequencing (WES) has recently become a practical and cost-effective tool to identify rare variants not detected by GWAS. WES was first used in a boy who presented at 15 months with intractable CD, detecting a rare mutation affecting the regulatory function of the X-linked inhibitor of apoptosis (*XIAP*) gene.[15] *XIAP* had not previously been associated with CD but has a central role in the proinflammatory response and bacterial sensing through the NOD signaling pathway. WES has since been used to identify other rare variants implicated in the pathogenesis of very early onset IBD (VEOIBD), a nonclassic form of IBD that occurs in children less than 6 years of age.[9] VEOIBD tends to be resistant to standard medical and surgical therapies and is commonly caused by single-gene mutations (*IL-10, IL-10R, NCF2, LRBA,* and *TTC7,* among many other genes).[16]

The identification of IBD loci using linkage, genome-wide association, and sequencing studies has constituted only a first step in our understanding of IBD. A summary of the key points on the genetics of IBD is provided in Table 161.1. Fine-mapping studies and experimental work will be required to identify the causal gene variants and elucidate the disease mechanisms.

EPIDEMIOLOGY

IBD is a disease of the modern world. Isolated reports in the late 19th century and the first half of the 20th century gave way to more frequent diagnosis in the second half of the 20th century. A recent, systematic review of more than 200 population-based studies has crystallized the global IBD geography.[17] Both the prevalence (up to 0.5%) and incidence of IBD (10 to 30/100,000 per year) are highest in the Western world, namely Europe, North America, and Oceania. Within Europe, the incidence of IBD is highest in Western Europe, low in countries adjacent to the Mediterranean, and varies from low to high in Eastern Europe. Population data outside the Western world are limited to studies from Japan, China, South Korea, South America, and South Africa. In all of these countries, the incidence of IBD is significantly lower than in Western countries.[17] Interestingly, studies of people emigrating from countries of low IBD prevalence to developed countries found that the incidence of IBD increased in successive generations,[18-20] highlighting the importance of environmental factors in the development of disease.

The increase in IBD incidence in Western countries in the second half of the 20th century has long been evident and was confirmed by time-trend analysis in a systematic review.[17] Several additional temporal trends are becoming apparent. The previously observed North-South gradient in Europe appears to be fading.[17] IBD incidence is increasing in urbanized societies in East Asia (South Korea, Japan, China, and Hong Kong) and in developing countries.[17,21,22] Finally, evidence points to a disproportionate increase in childhood IBD (as compared with adult IBD) over the past few decades.[23-25]

The sequential rise of IBD in the West and then in the westernizing countries of the developing world may reflect the adoption of the high–animal fat/low-fiber Western diet. Observational studies have linked IBD with consumption of greater amounts of meat and fats, particularly polyunsaturated fatty acids (PUFAs) and omega-6 (n-6) fatty acids.[26] Conversely, diets high in fiber, fruits, and vegetables seem to be protective.[26] The results of the European Prospective Investigation into Cancer and Nutrition (EPIC) study and the Nurses' Health Study are particularly noteworthy because of their prospective design. EPIC found an association between a higher consumption of linoleic acid (an n-6 PUFA present in high concentrations in red meat, cooking oils, and margarine) with a higher incidence of UC.[27] In contrast, people who consumed higher levels of omega-3 (n-3) PUFA docosahexaenoic acid were less likely to be diagnosed with UC. In the Nurses' Health Study, a greater consumption of long-chain n-3 PUFAs and a higher ratio of n-3:n-6 PUFAs was again protective against the development of UC.[28] A higher consumption of fiber, particularly fruits, was associated with a lower risk of CD, but not UC.[29]

In addition to the Western diet, a number of other environmental factors have been implicated in IBD pathogenesis. Cigarette smoking has been the most extensively studied environmental factor. Multiple studies have demonstrated that smoking is associated with an increased risk of CD and more aggressive CD, namely stricturing and fistulizing complications, requirement for immunosuppressive therapy and surgery, earlier postoperative recurrence, and need for reoperation.[30,31] Smoking cessation is associated with decreased CD activity and a

---

TABLE 161.2 Inflammatory Bowel Disease Epidemiology—Key Points

- The prevalence and the incidence of IBD are highest in the Western world
- IBD is becoming more frequent in developing countries
- IBD is increasing disproportionately in the pediatric population
- Upwards of 1 million Americans suffer from IBD
- IBD represents a significant burden to the health care system of the United States

IBD, Inflammatory bowel disease.

---

lower risk of postoperative recurrence.[30,32] Remarkably, smoking has opposite effects in UC. Smokers have a lower risk of a UC reactivation, as well as a lower risk of colectomy.[33] The mechanisms behind the divergent effects of smoking on CD and UC are not well understood. Appendectomy before age 20 for appendicitis (but not for nonspecific abdominal pain) is associated with a lower incidence of UC.[34] Vitamin D deficiency[35] and use of nonsteroidal antiinflammatory drugs[36] have been associated with an increased risk of both UC and CD.

In the United States, IBD represents a significant burden for the health care system. A study published in 2007 used insurance claim data to estimate that 993,300 Americans were affected with IBD in 2005.[37] The prevalence of both UC and CD was lower in the South compared with the Northeast, Midwest, and West. Interestingly, IBD appeared to be more common in commercially insured individuals, compared with those insured by Medicaid.[37] Using insurance data from 2003 and 2004, one study estimated mean annual costs per patient at $8265 for CD and at $5066 for UC.[38] In both diseases, hospitalizations, outpatient care, and medications each accounted for approximately one-third of direct costs.[38] Annual direct costs in the United States were estimated at $6.3 billion ($3.6 billion for CD, $2.7 billion for UC). A follow-up study using the same claims database estimated that 1,171,000 Americans suffered from IBD in 2008 to 2009.[39] Time-trend analysis showed an increase in IBD prevalence over three successive periods (2004 to 2005, 2006 to 2007, and 2008 to 2009), likely attributable to the absence of a cure and the low disease mortality.[39] A population study from Olmsted County, Minnesota, found that the incidence of CD and UC remained stable between 1970 and 2000.[40] In contrast, a population study from Kaiser Permanente Northern California found that, between 1996 and 2006, the incidence of UC increased from 1.8 to 4.9 per 100,000 per year ($P < .001$).[41] The annual incidence of CD increased from 2.2 to 4.3 per 100,000 per year, albeit without reaching statistical significance ($P = .09$).[41] A summary of key points on IBD epidemiology is provided in Table 161.2.

ETIOPATHOGENESIS

A large number of animal IBD models were developed in the 1990s and early 2000s. Models of aberrant immunoregulation included genetically engineered mice that underexpressed ($IL2^{-/-}$, $IL10^{-/-}$, $TCR^{-/-}$) or overexpressed

($TNF1^{\Delta ARE}$, *STAT4*) immune regulatory molecules, as well as models of regulatory T-cell transfer ($CD45RB^{high} \rightarrow SCID$). In other models, IBD was induced by epithelial barrier defects (dominant-negative N-cadherin, $mdr1a^{-/-}$, $Muc2^{-/-}$) and toxins (TNBS-induced colitis). Most animal models were characterized by heightened effector cell responses or inadequate regulatory cell responses, ultimately producing either a Th1 inflammatory profile (excessive IL-12/IFN-γ/TNF-α secretion), or a Th2 profile (increased IL-4/IL-5/IL-13 secretion). CD was viewed as a Th1 disorder, whereas UC was considered an atypical Th2 disorder (characterized by enhanced production of IL-5 and IL-13 but low levels of IL-4). In the early 2000s, the Th1/Th2 paradigm was revised with the discovery of the proinflammatory Th17 cells, which are stimulated by IL-23.[42,43] IL-17 production was found to be increased in some animal models, as well as in IBD, especially CD.[43] Intriguingly, a GWAS published in 2006 identified IL23R as an IBD gene.[44]

Genetically engineered animal models had inherent limitations. In contrast to the genetic heterogeneity seen in human IBD, the animal models were characterized by single genetic defects. In addition, most models failed to recapitulate small bowel disease and its complications, such as strictures and fistulas. The greatest contribution of the early disease models came from the observation that susceptible animals did not develop IBD when raised under germ-free conditions, thus demonstrating the critical role of commensal intestinal flora in IBD pathogenesis.

Gene discovery refocused basic research in IBD. *NOD2*, the first gene definitively linked to CD, is an intracellular receptor that is expressed in several cell types, particularly intestinal monocytes and Paneth cells. NOD2 binds MDP, a bacterial wall peptide, producing a proinflammatory immune response. The discovery of *NOD2* thus reframed IBD as a disorder partly caused by an aberrant innate immune response to common bacterial motifs. More than 15 years after the identification of *NOD2* as a risk gene, there is still uncertainty as to how loss-of-function mutations of this "proinflammatory" protein could lead to inflammation. Decreases in the antibacterial activities of Paneth cells may play a role.[45] In addition, NOD2 plays a key role in autophagy, a critical innate immune response against intracellular microbes.[46] For example, *NOD2*-deficient ($NOD2^{-/-}$) mice, but not wild-type mice, were colonized by *Bacteroides vulgatus*, suggesting that *NOD2* may prevent colonization by specific commensal bacteria.[47] Finally, tantalizing clues came from a study showing that NOD2 may be tolerogenic (i.e., antiinflammatory) under certain conditions, such as chronic stimulation by MDP.[48] Hence loss-of-function mutations may abrogate the tolerogenic function of NOD2.

Besides *NOD2*, other autophagy genes confirmed to increase CD risk include *ATG16L1* and *IRGM*.[12,49-51] In vitro, animal and human studies are examining the role of impaired autophagy in IBD pathogenesis. *NOD2* and *ATG16L1* risk alleles were associated with impaired autophagy of *Salmonella* in vitro.[51,55,56] Monocytes from CD patients homozygous for the *ATG16L1* risk allele were less effective at killing adherent-invasive *Escherichia coli* when compared with monocytes from patients who were homozygous for the *ATG16L1* protective allele.[57]

ATG16L1-deficient mice displayed impaired autophagy in the ileum; decreased, aberrant, and disorganized granules within Paneth cells; defective granule exocytosis by Paneth cells; and altered expression of genes involved in regulating response to cell injury.[58] Strikingly, CD patients homozygous for the *ATG16L1* risk allele displayed Paneth cell abnormalities similar to those seen in ATG16L1-deficient mice.[58]

The intestinal microbiome represents the newest frontier in IBD research. The human intestine houses several trillions of microbial cells that express almost 10 million genes.[59] More than a billion years of mammalian-microbial coevolution has led to interdependency.[60] Not surprisingly, the intestinal microbiota contribute to a wide array of homeostatic functions, including the maturation and continued education of the host immune response, protection against pathogens, and elimination of toxins.[60] Imbalances in the composition of the intestinal microbiome (dysbiosis) have long been noted in IBD.[61-65] Dysbiosis encompasses alterations in the relative abundances of certain bacterial taxa, as well as a decrease in the diversity of the community.[66] Emerging research is uncovering the interactions between impaired autophagy and intestinal dysbiosis. For example, inflamed ileal tissue from patients homozygous for the *ATG16L1* risk allele contained increased numbers of Fusobacteriaceae, whereas inflamed ileal tissue of patients homozygous for the *ATG16L1* protective allele showed decreased numbers of Bacteroidaceae and Enterobacteriaceae and increased Lachnospiraceae.[57] The *ATG16L1* allele did not affect the bacterial composition in noninflamed ileal tissue. In addition to alterations in microbial composition, dysbiosis also encompasses alteration in the normal functions of the microbiome.[66] Intriguingly, changes in the intestinal virome were described in patients with IBD.[67] It must be emphasized that dysbiosis is not a proven cause of intestinal inflammation and that altered bacterial composition and function may be sequelae of inflammation. Moreover, there may be bidirectional interactions between intestinal bacteria and inflammation.

The recognition of intestinal dysbiosis in IBD refocused attention to diet as a cause of IBD. Dietary preferences are an established determinant of the intestinal microbiome. A seminal study found striking differences between the microbiota of European children and those of children from a rural village in Burkina Faso.[68] Similarly, a later study found pronounced differences in gut bacterial composition and bacterial functional gene repertoires of individuals living in the United States compared with individuals living in Malawi and the Amazonas State of Venezuela.[69] The dietary intake of animal protein, animal fat, and fiber modulates the gut microbiome.[70,71] Separately, consumption of fat and fiber may influence the development of IBD.[27-29] Although it is tempting to speculate that the Western diet may predispose to IBD via effects on the gut microbiome, other mechanisms are probably operable, including effects of the diet on the epithelial barrier and production of inflammatory mediators. In turn, the gut microbiome is influenced not only by diet but also other factors, including mode of birth, age, infections, antibiotic use, gut inflammation, genetics and, possibly, cigarette smoking.[72-74]

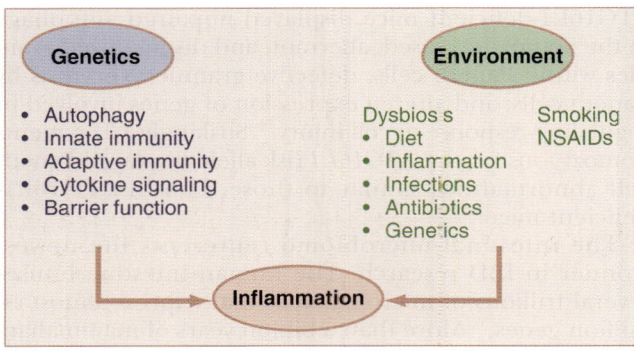

FIGURE 161.1 Pathogenesis of inflammatory bowel disease. *NSAIDs,* Nonsteroidal antiinflammatory drugs.

In summary, over the past decade, we have seen tremendous progress in our understanding of IBD pathogenesis, particularly in the areas of abnormal immune regulation (IL-17/IL-23 signaling pathway), autophagy, and intestinal dysbiosis. In parallel, more complex animal models of IBD are being developed, namely models that incorporate abnormalities in autophagy, interactions between host and specific commensal bacteria and viruses, and/or dietary interventions.[47,75–77]

Fig. 161.1 summarizes our current understanding of IBD pathogenesis. Genetic susceptibility and proinflammatory environmental factors are necessary, but not sufficient, for the development of IBD. Intestinal dysbiosis (i.e., alterations in the composition and function of intestinal bacteria) is suspected to be a major proinflammatory factor. In turn, the Western diet may select for commensal bacteria that promote the development of intestinal inflammation.

PHENOTYPIC VARIABILITY OF INFLAMMATORY BOWEL DISEASE

In the first detailed characterization of CD, Crohn, Ginsburg and Oppenheimer described 14 young adults (mean age, 32 years) with disease limited to the terminal ileum.[78] It was soon recognized that, although the disease process typically affected the terminal ileum, the more proximal small bowel and/or the colon could be involved as well. Over time, investigators recognized phenotypic variability in the age of onset and the risk of stricturing, perforating, and perianal complications. In parallel, researchers described the variable phenotype of UC. Some patients presented with nonprogressive proctitis or proctosigmoiditis, whereas others presented with extensive colitis or pancolitis, or experienced proximal extension of initially distal disease.[79–81] Younger age at diagnosis of UC was associated with a greater risk of colectomy.[82] In 2005 a consensus group codified the phenotypic variability of IBD in the Montreal classification (Table 161.3).[83] This scheme categorized IBD into three types: CD, UC, and IBD, type unclassified (IBDU). IBDU was defined as isolated colitis (i.e., no small bowel involvement) but without definitive histologic or other evidence to favor either CD or UC. CD was characterized according to age of onset,

TABLE 161.3 Montreal Classification of Inflammatory Bowel Disease

CROHN DISEASE

Age at diagnosis (A)
A1 16 years or younger
A2 17–40 years
A3 Over 40 years

Location (L)	*Upper Gastrointestinal (GI) modifier (L4)*
L1 Terminal ileum	L1 + L4 (terminal ileum and upper GI)
L2 Colon	L2 + L4 (colon and upper GI)
L3 Ileum and colon	L3 + L4 (ileocolic and upper GI)
L4 Upper GI	—
Behavior (B)	*Perianal disease modifier (p)*
B1 Nonstricturing, nonpenetrating	B1p (nonstricturing, nonpenetrating and perianal)
B2 Stricturing	B2p (stricturing and perianal)
B3 Penetrating	B3p (penetrating and perianal)

ULCERATIVE COLITIS

Disease extent (E) (defined as maximal endoscopic extent during follow-up)
E1 Ulcerative proctitis (limited to the rectum)
E2 Left-sided (limited to colon distal the splenic flexure)
E3 Extensive ulcerative colitis (disease proximal to the splenic flexure)

Disease severity (S)
S0 Clinical remission (no symptoms)
S1 Mild (passage of four or fewer stools/day (with or without blood), absence of any systemic illness, and normal inflammatory markers (erythrocyte sedimentation rate [ESR])
S2 Moderate (passage of more than four stools per day but with minimal signs of systemic toxicity)
S3 Severe (passage of at least six bloody stools daily, pulse rate of at least 90 beats/min, temperature of at least 37.5°C, hemoglobin of <10.5 g/100 mL, and ESR of at least 30 mm/h)

Modified from Silverberg MS, Satsangi J, Ahmad T, et al. Toward an integrated clinical, molecular and serological classification of inflammatory bowel disease: report of a Working Party of the 2005 Montreal World Congress of Gastroenterology. *Can J Gastroenterol.* 2005;19(suppl A):5A.

location, and luminal (stricturing or penetrating) and perianal complications. UC was characterized by disease extent and severity of individual relapses. The consensus group felt there was insufficient information to classify UC by age of diagnosis.[83] The most important criticism of the Montreal classification concerns the absence of classification according to long-term risk. Nonetheless, the development of standardized definitions was a significant step toward bringing consistency across clinical studies.

The phenotypic heterogeneity of IBD is not surprising given the multiple genetic, immunologic, microbiomic, and environmental factors involved in IBD pathogenesis. A number of consistent correlations have been observed between certain genetic and environmental factors and disease phenotype. In early studies, *NOD2* mutations correlated with small bowel CD and stricturing complications,[84] whereas the *HLA-DRB1*0103* allele was associated with severe and extensive UC.[85] A recent study of almost 30,000 IBD patients assessed the association between genotype and phenotype, including age at diagnosis and time to surgery (all IBD), disease location and behavior in CD, and disease extent in UC.[86] Three loci (*NOD2 MHC,* and *MST1 3p21*) were associated with IBD phenotype. *NOD2* was associated with CD location, behavior, and age at diagnosis. After adjusting for the other phenotypes, the association of *NOD2* with behavior was shown to derive almost entirely from its correlation with location and age at diagnosis. *HLA* was associated with age of onset, CD disease location and behavior, UC extent, and surgery. *MST1* was associated with age of IBD onset. The investigators found that little to no genetic association with disease behavior remained after conditioning on disease location and age at onset. It may be hypothesized that for a disorder like IBD with numerous low-risk alleles, the total burden of alleles may influence disease susceptibility and phenotype. Genetic risk scores that combined information from the 163 known IBD gene associations were generated and were strongly associated with disease subphenotype, even after exclusion of *NOD2, HLA,* and *MST1.* The genetic scores separated IBD into three distinctive subgroups, namely ileal CD, colonic CD, and UC (rather than the currently defined IBD types of CD and UC). The investigators concluded that disease location is in part genetically determined and that disease location (rather than genotype) is the major determinant of disease behavior.[86] A major caveat is that current studies have examined only phenotype associations with known IBD genes. It is quite plausible that genes that do not predispose to IBD per se may actually influence IBD behavior.

The only consistent environment-phenotype correlation involves cigarette smoking. As reviewed previously, cigarette smoking is associated with an increased risk of complicated CD[3] and a decreased risk of severe UC requiring colectomy.[33] Research correlating the intestinal microbiome with IBD type and behavior is at its infancy. In a study of children with CD, *Ruminococcus* was implicated in stricturing complications and *Veillonella* in penetrating complications.[87] These results will need to be replicated in other cohorts. Moreover, the microbiome may interact with genotype to produce distinct disease phenotypes.

The Montreal classification, having been developed in 2005, could have been only clinical. Since then, we have achieved a more sophisticated understanding of IBD pathogenesis. Computational methods have been developed that combine genetic, microbiomic, and inflammatory pathway markers and their interactions.[88] These methods will hopefully generate classification schemes that will integrate the system biology of IBD, provide risk stratification, and predict response to different therapeutic approaches.

VARIATION IN CARE AND QUALITY IMPROVEMENT IN INFLAMMATORY BOWEL DISEASE

Variation in care may result in differences in health care quality, outcomes, and costs and could therefore be the target of quality improvement programs. Examples of variation in care include management of anemia,[89] vaccination practices,[90] prophylaxis against venous thromboembolism

(VTE),[91,92] and testing for *Clostridium difficile.*[93] Colectomy rates for UC vary according to geographic location in the United States, with rates in the West and Midwest regions threefold higher than in the Northeast.[94] There is even variation in the care provided by IBD experts. A study from 2007 analyzed the use of five medication classes among 311 children with newly diagnosed CD followed at 10 pediatric gastroenterology centers in North America.[95] Median use was 56% for immunomodulators (range 29% to 97%), 78% for prednisone (32% to 88%), 29% for antibiotics (11% to 68%), 64% for aminosalicylates (18% to 92%), and 8% for infliximab (3% to 21%). There was statistically significant intercenter variation in use of all therapies, which remained significant even after adjustment for demographic and clinical factors.

Studies demonstrating disparities in care according to race and socioeconomic status (SES) provide additional examples of variation in care. A systematic review reported race- and SES-based disparities in the content of medical and surgical health care, use of inpatient and ambulatory medical care, adherence to medical therapy, and disease perceptions and knowledge.[96] For example, most studies found lower rates of immunomodulators and infliximab use among minority patients. Among African Americans, there was lower utilization of specialist care and lower adherence to medical therapy. In addition, several studies identified race- and SES-based disparities in outcomes for IBD, including in-hospital mortality rates and health-related quality of life.[96] Minority status and non-private health insurance were associated with lower rates of resection for CD, whereas higher median income was associated with lower mortality from surgery for CD.[97] In UC, African-American race and Hispanic ethnicity were associated with lower odds for colectomy,[94] and Medicaid (as opposed to private) insurance was associated with higher mortality from colectomy.[94,98]

Finally, differences at the health care system level may also be associated with divergent patterns and outcomes of care. Low hospital volume has been associated with increased mortality following colectomy for UC (adjusted OR of 2.42; 95% confidence interval [CI], 1.26 to 4.63).[98] In a Canadian study, UC patients hospitalized under a nongastroenterologist had higher in-hospital mortality compared with those admitted to a GI service (1.1% vs. 0.2%, *P* < .0001).[99]

The need for improvement in the quality of IBD care cannot be overemphasized. UC and CD are common diseases that result in significant morbidity and costs. Disease algorithms have become even more complex with the approval of new agents, yet studies of comparative effectiveness are lacking. Practitioners vary in their familiarity with best practices. Finally, access to care varies according to race and SES. Recognizing the opportunities for quality improvement, the American Gastroenterological Association (AGA),[100] the Crohn's and Colitis Foundation of America (CCFA),[101] and a Canadian collaborative group[102] developed indicators to measure processes and outcomes of IBD care. Common themes in these measures are summarized in Table 161.4.

Variation in IBD care may be decreasing. In a prospective study of 590 adult IBD patients followed at seven high-volume centers between 2012 and 2015, investigators

TABLE 161.4 Quality Measures in Inflammatory Bowel Disease

Process Measures	Outcome Measures
Assessment of IBD type, location, and activity	Proportion of patients with steroid-free clinical remission for 1 year
Use of steroid-sparing therapies in patients with steroid-dependent disease	Proportion of patients currently taking steroids
Assessment of bone loss among steroid-treated patients	Proportion of time lost from school/work due to IBD
Influenza and pneumococcal vaccinations	Days per year in the hospital due to IBD
Testing for latent TB and HBV before anti-TNF therapy	Days per year in the ER due to IBD
Screening and intervention for tobacco use	Proportion of patients with anemia
Testing for *Clostridium difficile* in hospitalized patients	Proportion of patients taking narcotics
Prophylaxis for venous thromboembolism in hospitalized patients	Proportion of patients with malnutrition
Assessment for postoperative recurrence of CD	

CD, Crohn disease; *HBV*, hepatitis B virus; *ER*, emergency room; *IBD*, inflammatory bowel disease; *TNF*, tumor necrosis factor; *TB*, tuberculosis.

found no variation among centers in the treatment of UC patients with immunomodulators alone, anti-TNF-α agents alone, or combination therapy. There was significant variation in the treatment of CD with immunomodulators and combination immunomodulator and anti-TNF-α therapy but not with anti-TNF-α agents alone.[103] In a study from the Allegheny General Hospital in Pittsburgh, Pennsylvania, IBD specialists performed better than general gastroenterologists on a set of IBD quality measure (73.9 vs. 66.3, $P = .001$), but both groups scored above the recommended score of 60.[104] The best example of IBD quality improvement in action has come from the Improve Care Now Network, a network of pediatric IBD centers. The collaborating centers measure and share data on quality of care and then develop and assess protocols to achieve selected goals. Using this model, the network achieved significant increases in the proportions of CD and UC patients with quiescent disease, as well as a significant increase in the proportion of CD patients not taking prednisone.[105]

CHRONIC DISEASE MANAGEMENT IN INFLAMMATORY BOWEL DISEASE

IBD is a lifelong, dynamic, multifaceted disease that requires comprehensive care. There is a plethora of treatment options and a multitude of disease- and treatment-related complications. Moreover, the disease has profound effects on the physical and emotional health of patients and on their personal aspirations. For these reasons, IBD management can be approached only through the framework of chronic disease management.

Patient empowerment and education are central to the chronic disease model. Caregivers must provide education, support, and open lines of communication. Patient trust in the physician is associated with improved adherence to IBD therapy, which is a surrogate for more prolonged remission.[106] Understanding the patient's concerns, preferences, and expectations allows for a tailored approach and deepens the therapeutic relationship. Educational resources, in the electronic web (such as the CCFA website; www.ccfa.org) or in other formats, may supplement office discussions and improve outcomes and cost of care. Two randomized controlled trials (RCTs) in UC have shown that, in comparison with standard management, patient education and self-management were associated with more prompt control of flares, fewer doctor and hospital visits, and cost savings.[107,108]

A multidisciplinary approach is critical in addressing all aspects of the patient's illness. Recognizing the importance of the multidisciplinary approach, various experts have advocated the development of IBD comprehensive care units and have proposed criteria for such units.[109,110] Involving the primary care physician is integral to overall coordination of care and may increase the implementation of preventive measures, such as vaccinations, assessment of bone health, and screening and intervention for cigarette smoking. Transitioning from pediatric to adult care is associated with nonadherence, increased emergency department use, and increased hospitalizations and should be approached in a gradual, well-planned manner.[111] Close collaboration between the gastroenterologist and the colorectal surgeon is critical in optimizing patient status before surgery and planning for medical therapy to reduce the risk of postoperative recurrence of CD. Developing a network of consultants with an interest in IBD is important in managing the extraintestinal manifestations of the disease. Nutrition experts assist in the management of malnutrition and deficiencies of vitamins and micronutrients and educate patients on proper diets according to disease state (such as active or quiescent disease, or after extensive resection). Stoma nurses provide education and support to patients and their families. As with other chronic diseases, stress, depression, and anxiety are common in IBD patients. Psychiatric comorbidity appears to be associated with poorer clinical outcomes and greater health care costs in patients with IBD.[112–114] Treatment of these disorders may improve general and emotional well-being[115,116] and may even improve IBD outcomes.[117]

An emerging trend in the care of IBD patients involves the increased use of mid-level providers. Given the need to improve care while controlling costs, specialist nurses, nurse practitioners, and physician assistants will inevitably assume greater roles in the management of patients and may even direct care in some domains. These providers can triage patients (reducing unnecessary emergency room or office visits), facilitate access to medical therapies, and make appropriate referrals to primary providers, collaborating specialists, and mental health professionals. Studies are beginning to examine the role of IBD-specialist nurses. A study from Norway reported that, in comparison with conventional follow-up, nurse-led follow-up produced similar outcomes in terms of hospitalizations, surgery, sick leave, performance of endoscopic procedures, and number of additional telephone consultations.[118] Moreover, nurse-led follow-up was associated with a significantly faster treatment upon relapse.

PRINCIPLES OF MEDICAL THERAPY

UC and CD are life-long diseases with a relapsing and remitting course. Consequently, induction of clinical remission followed by maintenance of remission emerged as the main goals of therapy. Additional goals include improved quality of life, prevention of disease- and treatment-related complications (including opioid dependence[119-121] and excessive exposure to diagnostic radiation),[122-124] restoration and maintenance of optimal nutritional status, optimization of preoperative status, and, in the case of CD, prevention of postoperative recurrence

Traditionally, the selection of inductive therapy has been based on symptoms and laboratory indicators. This approach is endorsed by all existing guidelines.[125-130] In clinical practice, disease activity is classified qualitatively. In UC for example, activity is classified as mild, moderate or severe, according to the Truelove-Witts criteria (see Table 161.3).[33,131] Similarly the American College of Gastroenterology developed operational definitions for CD activity.[125] Activity is categorized into four states: (1) remission: asymptomatic disease off steroids; (2) mild-moderate disease: mild symptoms without manifestations of dehydration, systemic toxicity, abdominal tenderness, painful mass, intestinal obstruction, or greater than 10% weight loss; (3) moderate-severe disease: prominent symptoms of fever, significant weight loss, abdominal pain or tenderness, intermittent nausea or vomiting but without obstruction, or significant anemia; and (4) severe-fulminant disease: persistent symptoms despite the introduction of conventional corticosteroids or biologic agents as outpatients, or high fevers, persistent emesis, cachexia, significant peritoneal signs, or evidence of obstruction or abscess.

These classification schemes were inadequate for regulatory purposes. Therefore disease activity indices had to be developed and validated for therapeutic trials.[132,133] These indices incorporated symptoms, signs, laboratory results, and, sometimes, endoscopic activity. The Crohn's Disease Activity Index (CDAI) was for many years the preferred instrument to assess CD activity in the context of clinical trials. However, it has long been known that the CDAI correlates poorly with endoscopic activity.[134-137] Endoscopy offers the most objective assessment of UC severity as well. As a result, there is now broad consensus that assessment of drug efficacy in clinical trials must incorporate endoscopic response.

The lack of correlation between CDAI and endoscopic severity is not surprising to clinicians who frequently see coexistent irritable bowel syndrome masquerading as active CD. Consequently, endoscopy is necessary not only in clinical trials but also in daily practice to objectively assess the inflammatory burden. The situation is somewhat different for UC, where symptoms generally correlate well with endoscopic activity.[138-141] Hence treating most patients based on symptoms (i.e., without endoscopic assessment) seems appropriate in clinical practice.

TABLE 161.5 Current and Evolving Principles of Medical Therapy

- Inflammatory bowel disease therapy consists of two phases:
  - Induction of clinical remission
  - Maintenance of clinical remission
- The selection of inductive therapy is based on the severity of the active disease (mild, moderate, severe)
- Endoscopic healing is emerging as an important treatment goal
- Risk stratification will likely be incorporated in future therapy algorithms

Numerous studies have shown that, regardless of the agent used, endoscopic healing is associated with improved long-term outcomes in both UC and CD, including sustained clinical remission, steroid-free remission, and reduced hospitalizations and surgeries.[142-146] However, even with potent therapies, such as the combination of an immunomodulator and an anti-TNF-α agent, endoscopic healing occurs only in a minority of patients. The achievability of healing may also be limited by the nature of the disease process. For example, CD of longer duration responds less well to anti-TNF-α therapy than newly diagnosed disease.[129] Finally, even if achievable, endoscopic healing would be desirable only insofar as it was cost effective. Notwithstanding these issues, there is growing consensus that endoscopic healing, besides being a trial endpoint, should also be a treatment goal in standard clinical practice.

Traditionally, the selection of therapy has been based solely on the severity of symptoms in real time. This approach does not take into account long-term risks, such as stricturing and fistulizing complications in CD and colectomy in UC. To this effect, the AGA has added long-term risk in its clinical decision tools for both CD and UC.[147,148] For example, immunomodulators and/or biologics are recommended in patients with severe endoscopic disease activity (regardless of symptoms). Similarly, the European Crohn's and Colitis Organization (ECCO) has incorporated risk in some recommendations.[129] For example, ECCO advocates early immunomodulator or anti-TNF therapy in patients with markers of poor prognosis, such as young age at diagnosis, extensive disease, requirement for steroids at diagnosis, or perianal disease at diagnosis. Future guidelines will likely incorporate endoscopic severity (a predictor of both short- and long-term risk) and other predictors of long-term risk in decision making. Current and evolving principles of medical therapy are summarized in Table 161.5.

CLASSES OF MEDICAL THERAPIES

An ever-expanding number of agents are available for the therapy of UC and CD. Some agents are used for both UC and CD, whereas others are effective for only one of the two diseases. For each medication, it is important to understand its relative positioning in the induction and maintenance phases of therapy, as well as to recognize potential adverse effects (Tables 161.6 to 161.8).

TABLE 161.6 Therapies for Ulcerative Colitis

	Induction of Remission	Maintenance of Remission
Mesalamine	Mild to moderate UC	After successful induction with mesalamine or budesonide
Steroids	Budesonide for mild to moderate UC Prednisone for moderate UC IV steroids for severe UC	No efficacy
Cyclosporine	Severe UC after failure of IV steroids	No efficacy
Thiopurines* (azathioprine, mercaptopurine)	No efficacy	Maintenance of remission induced by prednisone, IV steroids or IV cyclosporine
Anti-TNF-α* (infliximab, adalimumab, golimumab)	• Moderate UC (first-line therapy) • Moderate UC that is steroid-dependent or steroid-refractory UC, or has failed thiopurine • Infliximab for severe UC (first-line therapy or after failure of IV steroids)	After successful anti-TNF-α induction
Vedolizumab	• Moderate UC (first-line therapy) • Moderate UC that is steroid-dependent, or steroid-refractory UC, or has failed thiopurine or anti-TNF-α	After successful vedolizumab induction

*Anti-TNF-α therapy combined with a thiopurine is more efficacious than anti-TNF-α monotherapy in inducing remission in UC. The addition of methotrexate probably also increases the efficacy of anti-TNF-α induction by decreasing immunogenicity. No maintenance data are available, but the combination of an immunomodulator (thiopurine or methotrexate) and anti-TNF-α is probably more effective than anti-TNF-α monotherapy in maintaining remission.
IV, Intravenous; *TNF-α,* tumor necrosis factor alpha; *UC,* ulcerative colitis.

TABLE 161.7 Therapies for Crohn Disease

	Induction of Remission in Luminal Disease	Maintenance of Remission in Luminal Disease	Perianal Disease	Prevention of Postoperative Recurrence
Steroids	+	No efficacy	No efficacy	No efficacy
Antibiotics	No efficacy	No efficacy	+*	+
Thiopurines†	No efficacy	−	+	+
Methotrexate†	No efficacy	−	No data	No data
Anti-TNF-α† (infliximab, adalimumab, certolizumab pegol)	+	−	+	+
Vedolizumab	+	−	No data	No data
Ustekinumab	+	−	No data	No data

*Ciprofloxacin and metronidazole do not heal fistulas but reduce fistula drainage and are used as adjuncts to anti-TNF-α agents.
†Anti-TNF-α therapy combined with a thiopurine or methotrexate is more efficacious than anti-TNF-α monotherapy in inducing and maintaining remission in CD.
CD, Crohn disease; *TNF-α,* tumor necrosis factor-α.

MEDICAL THERAPIES

ULCERATIVE COLITIS

Aminosalicylates

The aminosalicylates, sulfasalazine (SASP), and mesalamine (or 5-aminosalicylic acid or 5-ASA) constitute first-line treatment for both the induction of remission and the maintenance of remission in patients with mild to moderate UC.

The mechanism of action involves several pathways, including inhibition of nuclear factor κB (NF-κB) activation,[149] inhibition of prostaglandin synthesis,[150] and scavenging of free radicals.[151] SASP (4 to 6 g/day), the prototype aminosalicylate formulation, contains a sulfapyridine moiety linked by an azo bond to the 5-ASA moiety. SASP is absorbed minimally by the small intestine, remaining intact until reaching the colon, where bacteria cleave the azo bond to release free sulfapyridine and 5-ASA. In effect, sulfapyridine functions as a carrier, delivering the 5-ASA moiety to the colon, where luminal 5-ASA exerts its activity directly onto inflamed mucosa. Although 5-ASA can produce diarrhea and nephrotoxicity, the sulfapyridine moiety is responsible for most SASP adverse effects, including nausea, dyspepsia, headaches, and sperm abnormalities. To circumvent these issues, oral, sulfa-free formulations were developed that deliver and release the 5-ASA to the colon using pH-dependent or time-dependent mechanisms.

A recent systematic review encompassed 11 RCTs ($n = 2086$) comparing 5-ASA versus placebo for the induction of remission in mild to moderately active UC.[152] Remission rates were 39.7% for 5-ASA versus 19.8% for placebo. No differences in efficacy were observed among different

TABLE 161.8 Toxicities of Main Inflammatory Bowel Disease Therapies

Mesalamine	Diarrhea, headache, pancreatitis, interstitial nephritis
Ciprofloxacin	*Clostridium difficile* infection, tendinopathy and tendon rupture, photosensitivity, seizures
Metronidazole	Metallic taste, nausea, yeast vaginitis, peripheral neuropathy, seizures
Steroids	Infections, suppression of hypothalamic-pituitary-adrenal axis, growth suppression in children, osteoporosis, osteonecrosis, hypertension, hyperglycemia, dyslipidemia, myopathy, psychiatric/cognitive disturbances, cataracts, glaucoma
Cyclosporine	Nephrotoxicity, hypertension, hyperkalemia, hypomagnesemia, infection, hepatotoxicity, hyperlipidemia, hirsutism, gingival hyperplasia, tremor, seizures
Thiopurines	Leukopenia, abnormal liver chemistries, nausea, fatigue, fever, pancreatitis, infections, lymphoma, non-melanoma skin cancer
Methotrexate	Nausea, fatigue, abnormal liver chemistries, hepatic fibrosis, pneumonitis, infections
Anti-tumor necrosis factor-alpha	Infusion or injection reactions, infections, hepatotoxicity, worsening of congestive heart failure, melanoma, drug-induced lupus, demyelinating syndromes (multiple sclerosis and optic neuritis)
Vedolizumab	Infusion reactions, infections
Ustekinumab	Infusion/injection reactions, infections

5-ASA formulations. Remission rates were similar for low (2.0 to 2.5 g/day) versus 5-ASA high doses (>2.5 g/day). Nonetheless, RCTs and clinical experience are consistent with a dose-response curve, particularly in patients with moderately severe UC, with a maximal effect seen at 4.0 to 4.8 g/day.[153] The same systematic review also assessed 11 RCTs (n = 1502) that compared 5-ASA versus placebo in maintaining remission. Relapse rates at 6 to 12 months were 40.3% on 5-ASA versus 52.6% on placebo. As with active UC, there were no differences in efficacy depending on the type of 5-ASA formulation. A maintenance dose of 2 g/day or greater was more efficacious than a dose less than 2 g/day. These findings are congruent with anecdotal experience that higher doses (3.6 to 4.8 g/day) are more effective than lower doses (2.4 g/day) in maintaining remission. In clinical practice, the maintenance dose is usually the same as the inductive dose.

Rectal 5-ASA formulations, either as monotherapy or in conjunction with oral therapies, are indicated in patients with distal UC, as well as in patients with more extensive disease but prominent distal symptoms (tenesmus and urgency). 5-ASA suppositories deliver drug to the distal 10 cm of the rectum, whereas enemas deliver drug up to the splenic flexure. Remission rates in distal UC using rectal formulations are in the order of 50% to 75%, superior to the rates observed with oral 5-ASA monotherapy or with topical steroids.[154] The combination of rectal and oral 5-ASA was more efficacious than either agent alone in the treatment of distal colitis.[155] Combination of rectal/oral 5-ASA was more efficacious than oral 5-ASA alone in patients with mild-moderate extensive UC as well.[156] Moreover, the combination of oral 5-ASA and twice-weekly 5-ASA enemas was superior to oral 5-ASA alone in maintaining remission in patients who had disease beyond the rectum and a history of multiple relapses.[157]

Owing to their limited systemic absorption, the 5-ASA agents are extremely well tolerated. Side effects include watery diarrhea in 2%, headaches and, rarely, pancreatitis and interstitial nephritis. Common errors in the use of 5-ASA include (1) not maximizing the oral dose, particularly in patients with moderately severe UC; (2) not using rectal therapies in patients with active distal disease, or in patients with more extensive disease with prominent distal symptoms; (3) not assessing whether the patient is adequately retaining the rectal agent (rectal therapy may not be retained by patients with severe distal disease); (4) using formulations that require a higher burden of pills, thus potentially compromising compliance; and (5) mistaking 5-ASA–induced diarrhea for a symptom of colitis.

Corticosteroids

Corticosteroids are used for the induction of remission in patients with mild-moderate distal UC (topical steroids), moderate disease (oral steroids), or severe disease (intravenous [IV] steroids).

The 1955 landmark study by Truelove and Witts provided initial evidence of the efficacy of corticosteroids in UC.[131] A recent systematic review and meta-analysis identified only five suitable RCTs (n = 445). Failure to achieve remission was seen in 54% of subjects randomized to oral steroids versus 79% of those randomized to placebo. The likelihood of failure to achieve remission was significantly reduced with steroids (relative risk [RR] = 0.65; 95% CI, 0.45 to 0.93), with a number-needed-to-treat (NNT) of 3. Extended-release budesonide is effective for the induction of remission in patients with active, mild to moderate UC.[158,159] The formulation (budesonide embedded in a multimatrix of hydrophilic and lipophilic excipients) was designed to deliver the agent to the colon and thus minimize systemic absorption.

IV steroids are first-line therapy for hospitalized patients with severe UC. A systematic review of 32 cohort studies and controlled trials published between 1974 and 2006 assessed short-term colectomy rates in patients with severe UC treated with IV steroids.[160] In the pooled analysis, 581 of 1991 patients required colectomy (weighted mean, 27%; 95% CI, 26% to 28%). Meta-regression analysis showed that the colectomy rates had not changed between 1974 and 2006. Meta-regression analysis also showed no dose-colectomy response for methylprednisolone doses greater than 60 mg daily. Common predictors of IV steroid failure include the disease extent, stool frequency, temperature, heart rate, C-reactive protein, albumin, and radiologic evidence of colonic dilation.[160] Severe endoscopic disease is probably a predictor of poor prognosis as well.[161] Currently, there are no validated predictive indices for IV steroid failure.

Prednisone is used in patients with moderately severe UC at doses of 40 to 60 mg/day until clinical remission is achieved, typically after 7 to 14 days. Doses higher than 60 mg do not translate to better response and are accompanied by greater toxicity. In general, prednisone is tapered by 5 to 10 mg each week to a dose of 15 to 20 mg/day, then by 2.5 to 5 mg each week. *However, one cannot overemphasize the importance of individualizing the prednisone taper according to the rapidity and degree of patient response.* Oral budesonide is approved at doses of 9 mg/day for up to 8 weeks.

Rectal corticosteroids are used in patients with distal or left-sided UC or in those with prominent distal symptoms. Available formulations include hydrocortisone foam (900 mg of 10% hydrocortisone acetate containing 80 mg of hydrocortisone), budesonide foam (supplied in canisters containing 14 metered doses, 2 mg budesonide per dose), and hydrocortisone enemas (100 mg hydrocortisone in one 60-mL enema).

For hospitalized patients with severe UC, accepted IV steroid therapies include methylprednisolone 20 mg every 8 hours, hydrocortisone 100 mg every 8 hours, or prednisolone 30 mg every 12 hours. There is no difference between IV bolus delivery and 24-hour continuous infusions.[162] The response to IV steroids should be assessed by the third day.[130,163] Responders are continued on IV steroids and are switched to prednisone once rectal bleeding has resolved and stool frequency has decreased to 1 to 2 bowel movements above baseline. Treatment should be given for a defined period because extending therapy beyond 7 to 10 days carries no additional benefit. Options for nonresponders include cyclosporine, infliximab, or surgery.

Corticosteroids have numerous, well-known toxicities, including suppression of the hypothalamic-pituitary-adrenal (HPA) axis, cushingoid appearance, growth suppression in children, osteoporosis, osteonecrosis, fluid retention, hypertension, hyperglycemia, dyslipidemia, myopathy, psychiatric and cognitive disturbances, cutaneous effects, cataracts, and glaucoma. The risk of severe infection is sometimes not appreciated. Serious, opportunistic, and postoperative infections may occur.[164–167] Severe joint pain should raise concern for osteonecrosis. Rectal steroids may be absorbed systemically and suppress the HPA axis.

Common errors when prescribing steroids include (1) using excessive doses; (2) tapering steroids too rapidly or too slowly; (3) using steroids inappropriately, for example mistaking irritable bowel syndrome for active UC; and (4) not educating patients about steroid toxicities and about proper tapering (as opposed to abrupt termination) of therapy.

It must be emphasized that *the requirement for systemic (oral or IV) steroids in UC constitutes a sentinel event predicting an aggressive course.* In a population-based, inception cohort study of 63 patients with UC diagnosed between 1970 and 1993 and treated with steroids, outcomes 1 year after initiation of steroids were prolonged response in 49%, steroid dependence in 22%, and colectomy in 29%.[168] Therefore most steroid-treated patients should be treated with steroid-sparing therapies, such as thiopurines, anti-TNF-α agents, or vedolizumab. Only select patients

with milder disease (such as patients with moderate UC and a swift response to prednisone) are transitioned to 5-ASA maintenance.

Cyclosporine

Cyclosporine is a calcineurin inhibitor used as rescue therapy in patients with severe UC failing 5 to 7 days of IV corticosteroids. In the seminal study by Lichtiger et al., 82% of patients with severe, steroid-refractory UC treated with IV cyclosporine avoided colectomy in the short term.[169] Based on pooled data from controlled and uncontrolled trials, approximately 80% of patients respond to IV cyclosporine and avoid colectomy in the short term.[170] Unless started on thiopurine therapy, most responders eventually require colectomy. Even when thiopurine therapy is started, 20% to 50% of patients require colectomy within 12 to 18 months.[171,172] Cyclosporine is also effective as first-line therapy in severe UC (in lieu of IV steroids). In a double-blind RCT, IV cyclosporine was as effective as IV methylprednisolone (response rates of 64% and 53%, respectively).[173]

Cyclosporine is also effective as first-line therapy in severe UC (in lieu of IV steroids). In a double-blind RCT, IV cyclosporine was as effective as IV methylprednisolone (response rates of 64% and 53%, respectively).[173] Colectomy is recommended if there is no improvement following 4 to 7 days of salvage therapy.[130]

The place of cyclosporine in the treatment of severe, steroid-refractory UC has been reassessed with the advent of infliximab. A systematic review and meta-analysis identified studies that compared these agents as rescue therapies in patients with acute, severe, steroid-refractory UC. Among three RCTs, no significant differences were seen with regard to treatment response and 3- or 12-month colectomy. Among 13 nonrandomized studies, infliximab was associated with a significantly higher rate of treatment response (OR, 2.96; 95% CI, 2.12 to 4.14) and a lower 12-month colectomy rate (OR, 0.42; 95% CI, 0.22 to 0.83), with no significant differences in the 3-month colectomy rate (OR, 0.53; 95% CI, 0.22 to 1.28) compared with cyclosporine. The meta-analysis found no significant differences between the two agents with regard to adverse drug-related events, postoperative complications, or mortality. A recent study reported that, among 115 patients with acute steroid-refractory UC randomized to cyclosporine or infliximab and also started on azathioprine (AZA), rates of colectomy-free survival at 5 years were 62% (95% CI, 49% to 74%) and 65% (95% CI, 52% to 78%), respectively.[174]

Cyclosporine is administered by continuous IV infusion at a dose of 2 mg/kg per day, adjusted to target serum concentrations of 150 to 250 ng/mL.[175] After successful induction with IV cyclosporine, the patient is converted to the oral formulation and started on a thiopurine. Patients must receive prophylaxis against *Pneumocystis jiroveci* with trimethoprim-sulfamethoxazole or dapsone. Adverse effects include nephrotoxicity, hypertension, hyperkalemia, hypomagnesemia, infection, hepatotoxicity, hyperlipidemia, hirsutism, gingival hyperplasia, tremor, and seizures. The risk of seizures is increased in the setting of hypomagnesemia and hypocholesterolemia. Given the significant toxicities of cyclosporine and the need for intensive clinical and laboratory monitoring, cyclosporine is typically reserved for compliant patients managed by experts with extensive experience in its use.

Small, open-label studies of tacrolimus, another calcineurin inhibitor, showed effectiveness in preventing colectomy in the short term in two-thirds of patients with refractory UC.[176,177] In a randomized, placebo-controlled trial of oral tacrolimus in hospitalized patients with steroid-refractory UC, tacrolimus therapy improved clinical response at week 2 (50% vs. 13%; $P = .003$) and mucosal healing (44% vs. 13%; $P = .012$).[178]

Thiopurines

The thiopurines, 6-mercaptopurine (6-MP), and its prodrug AZA, modulate immune responses through several mechanisms, including inhibition of DNA and RNA synthesis and apoptosis of activated T cells.[179] These drugs are metabolized via two competing pathways one pathway generates the active, 6-thioguanine nucleotide (6-TGN) metabolites. High 6-TGN concentrations correlate with leukopenia. The other pathway generates the inactive 6-MMPN metabolites via the enzyme thiopurine methyltransferase (TPMT) (20932143). TPMT activity is under genetic control by high ($TPMT^H$) and low activity ($TPMT^L$) alleles (7191632). Normal TPMT metabolizers (89% of the population) carry two high-activity alleles ($TPMT^H/TPMT^H$), produce relatively greater amounts of the 6-MMPN metabolites, and are treated at standard doses (6-MP 1 to 1.5 mg/kg per day or AZA 2.0 to 3.0 mg/kg per day). Eleven percent of individuals are intermediate metabolizers ($TPMT^H/TPMT^L$), produce 6-TGN in excess of 6-MMPN, and will develop leukopenia at standard thiopurine doses. Intermediate metabolizers are therefore treated at half the standard doses (6-MP 0.5 mg/kg per day or AZA 1.0 mg/kg per day). One in 300 individuals has absent TPMT ($TPMT^H/TPMT^L$). When exposed to drug, these patients shunt metabolism entirely to 6-TGN and develop life-threatening leukopenia. Measurement of TPMT activity is therefore mandatory before initiating thiopurine therapy.[180]

RCTs have found thiopurines effective in maintaining steroid-free remission in patients with steroid-dependent UC.[181-183] Thiopurines are also appropriate for patients with mild to moderate disease activity who have experienced early or frequent relapses while taking mesalamine at optimal doses or who are intolerant to mesalamine.[150] Thiopurines are appropriate maintenance therapy for hospitalized patients who responded to IV steroids or IV cyclosporine.[126,130,148,163] Thiopurines enhance the efficacy of anti-TNF-α agents as induction therapy in UC, likely via suppression of anti-drug antibodies (ADAs). In a randomized, double-blind trial that compared AZA monotherapy, infliximab monotherapy, and combination therapy in adults with moderate to severe UC, rates of steroid-free remission at week 16 were 24%, 22%, and 40%, respectively ($P = .03$).[184] Mucosal healing at week 16 occurred in 63% of patients receiving AZA plus infliximab, compared with 55% of those receiving infliximab ($P = .295$) and 37% of those receiving AZA ($P = .001$).[184] No RCTs have assessed combination therapy for the maintenance of remission. However, the addition of a thiopurine decreases ADA and, analogous to CD,[185] likely enhances the efficacy of anti-TNF in maintaining remission. Due to their slow

on et of action, the thiopurines are ineffective as inductive therapies.

Therapeutic drug monitoring guides decision making in patients failing thiopurine therapy.[186] Low 6-TGN and 6-MMPN concentrations indicate noncompliance or inadequate dosing. Low 6-TGN concentrations and high 6-MMPN concentrations are consistent with preferential synthesis of the 6-MMPN metabolites, which can be abrogated by the addition of allopurinol. Finally, therapeutic 6-TGN concentrations are consistent with thiopurine-refractory disease and mandate switching to a drug with a different mechanism of action.[186]

Leukopenia and transaminitis each occur in 10% to 15% of patients and resolve with dose adjustments. Nausea, emesis, and malaise are not uncommon. High fever and pancreatitis (which occurs in 2% of patients, typically in the first 6 to 8 weeks of treatment) are the only absolute contraindications to using the alternate thiopurine. Other risks include bacterial infections in the setting of leukopenia, shingles, lymphoma,[187,188] and non-melanoma skin cancer.[189] The highest estimate of lymphoma risk on thiopurine therapy is 1.37 per 1000 per year (vs. 0.26 per 1000 per year in untreated controls).[188,190] Decision models have shown that the benefits far outweigh the risks of therapy.[191]

Anti-Tumor Necrosis Factor-α Therapies

The anti-TNF-α monoclonal antibodies (mAbs) exert their effects through several mechanisms, which include neutralization of soluble and membrane-bound TNF-α, apoptosis of T cells and monocytes, antibody-dependent cell-mediated cytotoxicity, complement-dependent cytotoxicity, and reverse (outside-to-inside) signaling via membrane-bound TNF.[192] Three anti-TNF-α agents are approved for the induction and maintenance of remission of moderate to severe UC in the United States: infliximab (Remicade; Janssen Biotech, Horsham, Pennsylvania), adalimumab (Humira; Abbvie, North Chicago, Illinois), and golimumab (Simponi; Janssen Biotech, Horsham, Pennsylvania). Infliximab is a chimeric mAb consisting of a human constant region immunoglobulin G1 linked to a mouse variable region and is administered IV. Both adalimumab and golimumab are humanized mAbs consisting of a human constant region immunoglobulin G1 and a human-derived variable region and are administered subcutaneously (SC). In clinical practice, these agents are used in patients with (1) moderate to severe UC as first-line therapy in lieu of steroids; (2) steroid-dependent disease (including steroid-dependent disease failing thiopurines); and (3) steroid-refractory disease. However, long-term efficacy is compromised by the development of ADAs and accompanying loss of response. ADAs reduce the effectiveness of anti-TNF-α agents by neutralizing drug and by increasing drug clearance.[193]

In two large, phase III RCTs, infliximab 5 mg/kg led to 64% to 69% response rates at 8 weeks, versus 29% to 37% for placebo.[194] This benefit was maintained through 54 weeks, with a 45% response rate in infliximab-treated patients vers us 20% in the placebo arm. RCTs showed that adalimumab[195,196] and golimumab[197,198] were also efficacious in inducing and maintaining remission in patients with moderate-severe UC. Adalimumab was more efficacious in infliximab-naïve compared with infliximab-experienced patients.[195] There are no head-to-head comparisons of anti-TNF-α mAbs in UC. Comparative effectiveness studies have not found any significant differences between infliximab and adalimumab.[199–202]

Anti-TNF-α mAbs may be combined with immunomodulators. Combination infliximab-AZA therapy was more efficacious than infliximab monotherapy in inducing clinical remission at week 16 (40% vs. 22%).[184] Similar results were seen with combination therapy for CD induction (20393175) and reflect the reduced formation of ADA in patients who receive concomitant AZA. However, the combination of a thiopurine and an anti-TNF-α mAb incurs an even higher risk of lymphoma than AZA alone.[187,188] Methotrexate (like the thiopurines) reduces the formation of ADA[203] but does not increase the risk of lymphoma. Although the combination of methotrexate and an anti-TNF-α mAb is not supported by data in UC, it is expected to be similarly effective to thiopurine–anti-TNF-α combination therapy without increasing the background risk of lymphoma.

Owing to its rapid onset, infliximab (but not adalimumab or golimumab) is also used in hospitalized patients with severe UC failing IV steroids. In a double-blind RCT, 45 patients were randomized to a single infusion of infliximab 5 mg/kg versus placebo. Rates of colectomy at 3 months were 7 of 24 and 14 of 21 in the infliximab and placebo arms, respectively (OR, 4.9; 95% CI, 1.4 to 17).[204] By 3 years of follow-up, 12 of 24 (50%) patients given infliximab and 16 of 21 (76%) given placebo had required colectomy (P = .012).[205] Infliximab may also be used in hospitalized patients with severe disease as first-line therapy (i.e., in lieu of IV corticosteroids).[206] As reviewed in the cyclosporine section, infliximab and cyclosporine are similarly effective in preventing colectomy short-term and long-term in patients with severe disease failing IV steroids.

Therapeutic drug monitoring guides decision making in patients who lose response to anti-TNF-α therapy.[207] Low trough drug concentrations in the absence of ADA indicate increased clearance and dictate dose escalation. Low trough concentrations in the presence of high titers of ADA indicate increased, ADA-mediated clearance and necessitate switching to an alternate anti-TNF-α agent. Finally, therapeutic trough concentrations are consistent with anti-TNF-α–refractory disease and mandate switching to an agent with a different mechanism of action.[207]

The anti-TNF-α agents share the same toxicity profile. Adverse effects include acute and delayed infusion/injection reactions, infections, hepatotoxicity, worsening of heart failure, drug-induced lupus, and demyelinating disorders, such as multiple sclerosis and optic neuritis. Bacterial, mycobacterial, and fungal infections may occur. Patients require screening for latent tuberculosis and hepatitis B because these infections may be reactivated on anti-TNF-α therapy.

Vedolizumab

The migration of leukocytes to inflamed intestine is highly regulated. Gut-specific lymphocytes express the $\alpha_4\beta_7$ integrin, which binds to mucosal addressin-cell adhesion molecule 1 (MAdCAM-1), expressed on the intestinal endothelium. Inhibition of lymphocyte trafficking to the gut therefore held the promise of ameliorating intestinal inflammation. Indeed, natalizumab, an anti-α4 mAb, demonstrated efficacy in CD.[208–210] By means of blocking the binding of leukocyte-expressed $\alpha_4\beta_1$ integrin with vascular cell adhesion molecule-1 (VCAM-1) on brain endothelium, natalizumab also proved efficacious for multiple sclerosis. Unfortunately, this mechanistic property of natalizumab is linked to a high risk of progressive multifocal leukoencephalopathy (PML), a usually fatal brain infection. Vedolizumab (Entyvio; Takeda Pharmaceuticals America, Deerfield, Illinois), a humanized mAb that targets the $\alpha_4\beta_7$ integrin, blocks lymphocyte trafficking to the gut only, and would not be expected to cause PML. Two RCTs showed that vedolizumab was more effective than placebo in inducing and maintaining remission in UC.[211]

Vedolizumab is used in patients with (1) moderate to severe UC as first-line therapy in lieu of steroids, (2) steroid-dependent disease, (3) steroid-refractory disease, and (4) inadequate response, loss of response, or intolerance to anti-TNF-α agent or thiopurine. Therapy is more effective in anti-TNF-α–naïve compared with anti-TNF-α–experienced patients.[212,213] Some patients require dose escalation from every 8 to every 4 weeks.[214] Adverse effects include infusion reactions (≤5%)[215] and infections. However, long-term studies have not identified any clinically important safety signals and no cases of PML have been reported.[215]

Other Therapies

An Israeli study found that methotrexate at a weekly oral dose of 12.5 mg was not better than placebo in inducing or maintaining remission in UC.[216] A double-blind trial compared parenteral methotrexate (25 mg weekly for 24 weeks) with placebo in patients with steroid-dependent UC. There were no differences in the primary end-point of combined clinical and endoscopic remission off steroids at 16 weeks (methotrexate 31.7%, vs. placebo 19.6%; P = .15).[217] Controlled trials of antibiotics have demonstrated no therapeutic benefit when added to IV steroids.[218,219] However, broad-spectrum antibiotics have been advocated for patients with severe UC and signs of toxicity.[126] There is no evidence to support the use of oral antibiotics in outpatients with mild or moderate disease. Fecal microbiota transplantation (FMT) has been studied with mixed results.[220,221] Guidelines recommend against using FMT in UC.[128] Studies with probiotics have produced mixed results, so that guidelines recommend against their use.[128] Although transdermal nicotine reduces symptoms in active UC, it is ineffective as maintenance therapy, produces frequent side effects, and is not recommended in any guidelines.[126,222–224] Antidiarrheal agents are useful in decreasing diarrhea but are contraindicated in severe disease given the risk of toxic megacolon. There are no guidelines regarding diet in UC patients. Physicians may advise patients to avoid foods that aggravate symptoms and to limit their consumption of red meat and margarine.[225] Because controlled studies of total parenteral nutrition (TPN) in patients with severe colitis have shown no benefit, TPN is limited to patients who are unable to eat or have significant malnutrition.[226,227]

Approach to Therapy in Ulcerative Colitis

The selection of therapy is based on disease severity (Table 161.9).[126,129,130,148] Patients with mild proctitis/proctosigmoiditis are typically treated with oral and/or rectal mesalamine. Combination rectal and oral 5-ASA is more efficacious than either oral or rectal 5-ASA monotherapy in distal UC.[155] Patients with mild extensive disease are typically treated with oral 5-ASA, with or without rectal 5-ASA. Combination rectal and oral 5ASA is more efficacious than oral 5-ASA monotherapy in extensive UC.[156,128] Successfully induced patients with distal disease are maintained on oral and/or rectal 5-ASA. Successfully induced patients with disease extending above the sigmoid colon are maintained on oral 5-ASA, with or without rectal 5-ASA. Again, combination therapy is more efficacious than oral 5-ASA alone in maintaining remission.[157]

Oral budesonide may be used instead of oral 5-ASA. Rectal steroids may be used but are probably less effective than rectal 5-ASA[154] and may be accompanied by side effects from systemic absorption. The choice of rectal formulation depends on the extent of the distal disease: suppositories are used for distal proctitis (up to 10 cm from the anus), foams for proctitis (up to 20 cm from the anus), and enemas for left-sided disease extending to 40 to 60 cm from the anus. Patients who enter remission are maintained on oral mesalamine, with or without rectal mesalamine. Patients with mild disease who do not respond to the aforementioned therapies are treated as patients with moderate disease.

Patients with moderate disease have several options for inductive therapy. Budesonide may be used for patients with less severe disease. After successful budesonide induction, these patients are transitioned to mesalamine. Patients with more severe disease may be treated with prednisone, an

anti-TNF-α agent, or vedolizumab. After successful induction with prednisone, patients typically receive thiopurine maintenance therapy, although an anti-TNF-α agent (with or without a thiopurine) or vedolizumab are viable options as well. After successful anti-TNF-α induction, the patient continues on the anti-TNF-α agent to maintain remission. A thiopurine (or methotrexate) may be added to decrease immunogenicity and improve long-term effectiveness. Although vedolizumab may be used for induction, its onset of action is somewhat delayed, and concomitant steroids are often required. After successful induction, the patient continues on vedolizumab to maintain remission. Some patients with moderate UC experience persistent symptoms of distal disease and require rectal therapies.

Hospitalized patients with severe UC are typically treated with IV steroids. After successful induction, maintenance options include a thiopurine, an anti-TNF-α agent (with or without a thiopurine), or vedolizumab. Alternatively, in lieu of IV steroids, these patients may be treated with infliximab. Following successful induction, infliximab is continued, either alone or in combination with a thiopurine. If the patient fails 5 days of IV steroids, then options for rescue therapy include infliximab or IV cyclosporine. If rescue therapy fails, then colectomy is preferred. Trying the alternate rescue agent (i.e., cyclosporine if infliximab fails, or the converse) is associated with significant risks of severe infection and death.[48,163]

CROHN DISEASE

Steroids

Two RCTs found standard corticosteroids more effective than placebo for the induction of CD remission.[229,230] A meta-analysis found budesonide superior to placebo for inducing remission (RR of no remission = 0.73; 95% CI, 0.63 to 0.84) but not in preventing relapse.[231] Standard

---

TABLE 161.9 Medical Therapy of Ulcerative Colitis

	Disease Activity	Induction	Maintenance
Mild	Ulcerative proctitis or sigmoiditis	Oral 5-ASA* and/or rectal 5-ASA[†,‡,§]	Oral 5-ASA and/or rectal 5-ASA
	Left-sided and extensive UC	Oral 5-ASA* with or without rectal 5-ASA[§,I]	Oral 5-ASA with or without rectal 5-ASA[¶]
Moderate		Budesonide	Oral 5-ASA
		Prednisone	Thiopurine, anti-TNF-α (with or without thiopurine), or vedolizumab
		Anti-TNF-α	Anti-TNF-α (with or without thiopurine)
		Vedolizumab	Vedolizumab
Severe		IV steroids	Thiopurine, anti-TNF-α, or vedolizumab
		Infliximab (first line or after failure of IV steroids)	Infliximab (with or without thiopurine)
		Cyclosporine (after failure of first-line IV steroids)	Thiopurine, anti-TNF-α (with or without thiopurine), or vedolizumab

*Budesonide may be used instead of oral 5-ASA.
[†]Rectal 5-ASA is first-line therapy for distal UC.
[‡]Combination rectal and oral 5-ASA is more efficacious than either oral or rectal 5-ASA monotherapy in mild distal UC.
[§]Rectal steroids may be used instead of rectal 5-ASA.
[I]Combination oral-rectal 5-ASA is more efficacious than oral 5-ASA alone in mild extensive UC.
[¶]Combination oral-rectal 5-ASA is more efficacious than oral 5-ASA alone in maintaining remission in extensive UC.
5-ASA, 5-Aminosalicylic acid; IV, intravenous; TNF-α, tumor necrosis factor-alpha; UC, ulcerative colitis.

steroids were superior to budesonide for inducing remission (RR of no remission = 0.82; 95% CI, 0.68 to 0.98) but had more adverse effects (RR = 1.54; 95% CI, 1.34 to 2.00).[231]

Parenteral corticosteroids have been the mainstay of therapy for severe inflammatory CD. In a retrospective study of 49 patients with severe inflammatory CD who were treated with IV prednisolone, 76% achieved remission.[232] No dose-ranging studies have been performed to define the optimal dose. Most clinicians administer parenteral corticosteroids equivalent to 40 to 60 mg of prednisone in divided doses or as a continuous infusion (hydrocortisone 300 mg/day, methylprednisolone 40 mg/day). IV adrenocorticotropic hormone (ACTH) can be used instead of IV corticosteroids but is potentially complicated by adrenal hemorrhage.[233] In a randomized, double-blind trial of continuous IV infusion of ACTH 120 U/day of versus hydrocortisone 300 mg/day in hospitalized patients, the rates of response after 10 days of therapy were 82% and 93%, respectively (not significant [NS]).[234] IV steroids may be used in patients with bowel obstruction that is attributed to inflammatory (as opposed to stricturing) disease on the basis of appropriate clinical characteristics (fever, night sweats, elevated C-reactive protein). Parenteral corticosteroids were safe and effective in an uncontrolled study of 24 patients with CD and inflammatory masses.[235] Corticosteroids should not be used when an abscess is suspected on the basis of high fever or suspicious imaging findings. There is no role for steroids in the management of internal or perianal fistulizing CD. With the advent of infliximab, IV steroids are nowadays restricted to patients presenting acutely with suspected but unconfirmed inflammatory CD, or as bridge therapy until infliximab is initiated.

It must be emphasized that *the requirement for systemic steroids in CD constitutes a sentinel event predicting an aggressive course.* In a population-based inception cohort study of 74 patients diagnosed with CD between 1970 and 1993 and treated with steroids, outcomes 1 year after initiation of steroids were prolonged response in 33%, steroid dependence in 28%, and bowel resection in 38% (1% was lost to follow-up).[168] Therefore steroid-treated CD patients should be treated with steroid-sparing therapies.

Antibiotics

There is no established role for antibiotics in luminal CD.[129,147] However, ciprofloxacin and metronidazole are used in the treatment of perianal fistulas.[236,237] A meta-analysis of three trials reported a statistically significant benefit in reducing fistula drainage (RR = 0.8; 95% CI, 0.66 to 0.98).[238] Two double-blind RCTs found that ciprofloxacin combined with infliximab[239] or adalimumab[240] was superior to the respective anti-TNF agent alone in reducing fistula drainage. Although useful as adjunctive therapies, antibiotics do not heal perianal fistulas. Antibiotics reduce the risk of clinical and endoscopic recurrence postoperatively by approximately 50%.[241,242] However, the nitroimidazoles (metronidazole and ornidazole) are significantly inferior to anti-TNF agents and probably modestly inferior to thiopurines as well.[243] In addition, nitroimidazoles are accompanied by frequent side effects. Therefore the AGA guidelines suggest metronidazole prophylaxis only

in patients with intolerance of, or preference against, thiopurines and anti-TNF-α agents.[243] Antibiotics are also used to treat small intestinal bacterial overgrowth and septic complications.

Thiopurines

Due to their slow onset of action, thiopurines are not effective for the induction of remission in CD.[127,244] However, early initiation of therapy may produce long-term benefits. In a seminal, placebo-controlled, pediatric trial, mercaptopurine therapy (1.5 mg/kg per day) commenced within 8 weeks of CD diagnosis, was steroid sparing and resulted in fewer relapses at 18 months (9% vs. 47%; *P* = .007).[245] In contrast, AZA conferred no long-term benefits in two RCTs in adults with newly diagnosed CD.[246,247] The thiopurines are effective in maintaining steroid-induced remission.[244] They are first-line therapy in steroid-dependent disease and should also be considered in CD patients who have required their first course of steroids.[127,129]

When added to an anti-TNF-α agent, thiopurines decrease anti-TNF-α immunogenicity and enhance its effectiveness.[185] However, the combination of a thiopurine and an anti-TNF-α mAb incurs an even higher risk of lymphoma than AZA alone.[190] Methotrexate (like the thiopurines) reduces the formation of ADA[203] but does not increase the risk of lymphoma. Although long-term data are lacking, methotrexate may be used in lieu of a thiopurine in patients with CD who want to maximize the effectiveness of anti-TNF-α therapy without incurring the risk of lymphoma.

The thiopurines are modestly effective for perianal disease,[236,237] but their use has been superseded by the introduction of anti-TNF-α agents. Although the thiopurines are more effective than placebo in preventing postoperative CD recurrence,[243] a network meta-analysis found that anti-TNF-α agents were superior to thiopurines in this setting.[241] As with UC, the initial thiopurine dose is based on the baseline TPMT enzyme activity and management of nonresponders is guided by measurement of the thiopurine metabolite concentrations.

Methotrexate

Methotrexate was designed to treat cancer by inhibiting dihydrofolate reductase and other folate-dependent enzymes. This agent is also used in CD and other inflammatory disorders but at doses that are up to two log orders lower than those used in cancer chemotherapy. Surprisingly, there has been little research on the mechanism of action of methotrexate in CD. A working hypothesis is that methotrexate stimulates release of adenosine, which suppresses the inflammatory functions of neutrophils, macrophage/monocytes, dendritic cells, and lymphocytes.[248,249]

Two RCTs compared methotrexate with placebo for the induction of remission.[250,251] Doses and routes of administration of (intramuscular [IM] vs. oral) differed between the two studies, and methotrexate may have been underdosed in one study.[251] In addition, there were differences in disease severity among the populations. In a meta-analysis using a random effects model, there was no statistically significant benefit of methotrexate over placebo (RR, 0.82; 95% CI, 0.65 to 1.03).[244] The AGA guidelines suggest *against* methotrexate for the induction of remission in CD.[127]

A Cochrane systematic review found that methotrexate at a weekly dose of 15 mg intramuscularly is significantly more effective than placebo in maintaining remission in CD (RR, 1.67; 95% CI, 1.05 to 2.67).[252] Methotrexate is endorsed as steroid-sparing maintenance therapy by the AGA[127] and ECCO.[149] There are no data on methotrexate for perianal CD[236,247] or the prevention of postoperative recurrence.[242] Methotrexate reduces ADA in patients receiving anti-TNF-α therapy.[253] Since ADAs predict loss of response to anti-TNF-α, cotherapy with methotrexate is expected to enhance the long-term effectiveness of the anti-TNF-α agent.

Anti-Tumor Necrosis Factor-α Agents

Three anti-TNF-α agents are approved for the induction and maintenance of remission of moderate to severe CD in the United States: infliximab (Remicade; Janssen Biotech, Horsham, Pennsylvania), adalimumab (Humira; Abbvie, North Chicago, Illinois), and certolizumab pegol (Cimzia; UCB, Smyrna, Georgia). Certolizumab pegol is an SC-administered polyethylene glycosylated (PEGylated) antigen-binding fragment of a humanized anti-TNF-α mAb. Lacking an Fc region, certolizumab pegol cannot mediate antibody-dependent cell-mediated cytotoxicity and complement-dependent cytotoxicity, which are mechanistic properties of both infliximab and adalimumab. Infliximab is also approved for perianal fistulizing disease, whereas adalimumab is also approved for uveitis and hidradenitis suppurativa. Regardless of approved indication, all three agents are used for perianal fistulas and extraintestinal manifestations of IBD. Anti-TNF mAbs induce mucosal healing and decrease the risks of hospitalizations and surgeries in CD.[254] Efficacy and toxicity profiles are similar, so that agent selection often depends on availability, route of delivery, patient preference, and cost.

No randomized trials have compared anti-TNF-α mAbs in CD. In one comparative effectiveness study the likelihood of nonresponse was higher with adalimumab than infliximab (OR, 1.62; 95% CI, 1.21 to 2.17).[201] However, there was no difference in CD-related surgery, hospitalizations, or prednisone use within 1 year of starting therapy.[201] A study of US Medicare data from 2006 through 2010 found that, after 26 weeks of treatment, 49% of patients receiving infliximab remained on drug, compared with 47% of those receiving adalimumab (OR, 0.98; 95% CI, 0.81 to 1.19). Fewer patients treated with infliximab underwent surgery, but this difference did not reach statistical significance (5.5 vs. 6.9 surgeries per 100 person-years; hazard ratio, 0.79; 95% CI, 0.60 to 1.05). Rates of hospitalization did not differ between groups (hazard ratio, 0.88; 95% CI, 0.72 to 1.07). A network meta-analysis of RCTs found that infliximab (OR, 2.1; 95% CI, 0.98 to 5.5) and adalimumab (OR, 2.1; 95% CI, 1.0 to 4.6) were more effective than certolizumab in inducing remission in CD.[25448924] Similarly, infliximab (OR, 1.4; 95% CI, 0.77 to 2.6) and adalimumab (OR, 2.5; 95% CI, 1.4 to 4.6) were more effective than certolizumab in maintaining remission.[255]

Best results are obtained by combining an anti-TNF-α mAb with a thiopurine. SONIC was a pivotal RCT that compared infliximab monotherapy, AZA monotherapy,

and combination therapy in 508 adults with moderate to severe CD who were naïve to immunosuppressants and biologics.[185] Rates of steroid-free remission at 26 weeks were 56.8% on combination therapy, versus 44.4% on infliximab (P = .02) and 30.0% on AZA (P < .001 for the comparison with combination therapy and P = .006 for the comparison with infliximab). Mucosal healing was observed in 43.9% of subjects on combination therapy, versus 30.1% on infliximab (P = .06) and 16.5% on AZA (P < .001 for the comparison with combination therapy and P = .02 for the comparison with infliximab). The superiority of combination therapy over infliximab monotherapy likely owed to AZA's efficacy as an antiinflammatory agent, as well its suppression of ADAs to infliximab were detected in only 0.9% of patients who received combination therapy versus 14.6% of those who received infliximab alone. Rates of serious infections were similar across all arms (3.9% to 5.6%).[185] Combination therapy was explored in another RCT, which compared methotrexate plus infliximab to infliximab alone in CD patients who had started prednisone inductive therapy within the preceding 6 weeks.[253] There was no difference in the primary outcome of treatment failure at week 50 (30.6% in the combination arm vs. 29.8% in the infliximab arm; P = .63). However, the frequency of ADA (a harbinger of loss of response) was lower on combination therapy (4% vs. 20%; P = .01).[253]

Using the GRADE scheme, the AGA guidelines made a conditional recommendation for thiopurine–anti-TNF-α combination therapy over anti-TNF-α monotherapy for the induction of remission (24267474). Patient preferences are critical in selecting the appropriate approach. Individuals who place a higher value on avoiding the risk of lymphoma and a relatively lower value on attaining and maintaining remission may choose to be treated with an anti-TNF-α agent only. Combination therapy is favored in patients with poor prognosis, or patients who have failed a prior anti-TNF-α mAb due to the development of ADA. Citing the lack of data, the AGA guidelines made no recommendation regarding combination therapy vs. anti-TNF-α monotherapy in the maintenance of remission. Combination therapy probably reduces the risk of loss of response to the anti-TNF-α agent but is accompanied by an increased risk of lymphoma.

Infliximab and adalimumab are effective in reducing clinical and endoscopic recurrence postoperatively,[241,256-261] and appear superior to the thiopurines in this regard.[241,258,260] Although not approved for the prevention of CD recurrence after surgery, anti-TNF-α agents received a conditional recommendation from the AGA for preventing postoperative recurrence.[243]

As in UC, therapeutic drug monitoring guides decision making in patients who lose response to therapy.[207]

Vedolizumab

Vedolizumab, a humanized mAb that targets the $\alpha_4\beta_7$ integrin, is effective in inducing and maintaining remission in moderately severe CD.[262] This agent was also studied in a CD population that consisted of patients who had previously failed one or more anti-TNF-α therapies.[253] No differences were seen between the vedolizumab and placebo arms in the primary outcome of proportion of patients in clinical remission at week 6 (15.2% vs. 12.1%).

However, a benefit emerged at week 10, when remission rates were 26.6% and 12.1% in the vedolizumab and placebo groups, respectively ($P = .001$). These results are congruent with real world experience, where vedolizumab appears to have a delayed onset of action. This observation is likely explained by the fact that vedolizumab inhibits the recruitment of additional inflammatory cells to the gut but probably has minimal effects on resident immune cells. Vedolizumab induces mucosal healing[213,264] and has a favorable safety profile.[213,215] The positioning of vedolizumab vis-à-vis the anti-TNF-α agents in the treatment of CD remains to be determined, but it appears that the drug will be more useful in patients with less severe disease.

Ustekinumab

Ustekinumab (Stelara; Janssen Biotech, Inc., Horsham, Pennsylvania) is a fully human mAb that targets the p40 subunit of the IL-12 (p35/p40) and IL-23 (p19/p40) heterodimeric cytokines. IL-12 and IL-23 play a key role in T-helper cell and innate lymphocyte cell differentiation and expansion.[265] Before receiving US Food and Drug Administration (FDA) approval for CD in September 2016, ustekinumab had been approved for psoriasis in 2009 and psoriatic arthritis in 2013. Ustekinumab is effective in the induction and maintenance of remission in patients with moderate to severe CD, including patients who have failed anti-TNF-α therapy.[266,267] In CD the drug is administered as a single, initial, weight-based, IV dose (≤55 kg, 260 mg; >55 to 85 kg, 390 mg; >85 kg, 520 mg), followed by a maintenance dose of 90 mg administered subcutaneously every 8 weeks. Adverse reactions include infections and rare hypersensitivity reactions. In the CD trials, adverse events, serious adverse events, and infections occurred at similar frequencies in the ustekinumab and placebo arms. Moreover, ustekinumab has an excellent safety record in psoriasis.[268] Postmarketing studies will be needed to assess long-term safety, immunogenicity, and (possible) loss of response to therapy. Presently, ustekinumab is primarily used in CD patients who have failed anti-TNF-α therapy. Patients with concomitant psoriasis or anti-TNF-α–induced psoriasis are ideal candidates. The high cost of the drug in the United States limits its use as primary therapy.

Other Therapies

The role of 5-ASA in the management of CD has declined over the past 2 decades. A systematic review and network meta-analysis found that 5-ASA was not superior to placebo for inducing or maintaining remission.[269] A Cochrane systematic review concluded that sulfasalazine is only modestly effective with a trend toward benefit over placebo and is inferior to steroids for the treatment of mild to moderate CD.[270] Reflecting these data, recent CD guidelines do not endorse 5-ASA for the induction or maintenance of remission.[129] Mesalamine produces a very modest reduction in clinical recurrence after surgery (RR, 0.86; 95% CI, 0.74 to 0.99; NNT = 13).[271] Moreover, 5-ASA therapy does not reduce postoperative endoscopic recurrence.[241]

IV cyclosporine has been effective anecdotally in patients with severe inflammatory and perianal fistulizing disease.[272-274] However, there are no controlled data, and IV cyclosporine for CD has been superseded by infliximab. A meta-analysis concluded that low-dose oral cyclosporine (5 mg/kg per day) is ineffective for the induction of remission of CD.[275]

Approach to Therapy in Crohn Disease

Three observations have contributed to a drastic shift in the approach to luminal CD over the past decade: (1) symptoms in CD correlate poorly with endoscopic activity; (2) more severe endoscopic activity predicts worse outcomes; and (3) endoscopic healing is associated with improved short- and long-term outcomes. There is emerging consensus that the goals of therapy should include endoscopic, as well as clinical, remission. Mesalamine and antibiotics are not effective in inducing clinical and endoscopic remission and are not recommended in the most updated guidelines.[130,147] Similarly, although steroids induce clinical remission, they do not effect endoscopic healing. Although the thiopurines and methotrexate are ineffective as inductive therapies, these agents are good options for the maintenance of steroid-induced remission, prevention of anti-TNF-α immunogenicity, and augmentation of anti-TNF-α effectiveness. The thiopurines are less effective than anti-TNF-α mAbs in achieving endoscopic healing,[185] whereas methotrexate is least effective in that regard.[276]

The anti-TNF-α agents have emerged as the most effective therapies in inducing and maintaining clinical remission, achieving endoscopic healing, and decreasing hospitalizations and surgeries in CD.[255,277] With the recognition that therapy for CD is more effective in disease of shorter duration,[129] there has been trend toward using the anti-TNF-α mAbs earlier in the course of CD. This approach is supported by RCTs demonstrating that early anti-TNF-α therapy in unselected patients was associated with better outcomes compared with the "conventional" approach of sequential therapy (steroids, followed by immunomodulators, followed by anti-TNF agents).[278,279] However, under this paradigm, patients with less aggressive CD will be treated unnecessarily with potentially toxic and expensive therapies. Risk stratification is therefore poised to inform future guidelines. It should be emphasized that risk depends not only on current inflammatory burden (e.g., the presence of deep ulcers on endoscopy) but also on longitudinal disease characteristics.[147] For example, a patient with a history of fistulizing complications should be considered for anti-TNF therapy, even if clinically well at the time of evaluation.

The AGA has developed a clinical decision support tool for the assessment and medical therapy of CD (Fig. 161.2).[147] Central to this approach is the joint assessment of current inflammatory burden and markers of longitudinal risk. Current inflammatory burden is based on symptoms and the results of laboratory, endoscopic, and imaging tests. Longitudinal risk is based on several factors, including age at diagnosis, extent of anatomic involvement and history of surgical resection, strictures, and/or penetrating behavior. Based on inflammatory burden and long-term risk factors, the patient is stratified as low-risk or moderate/high-risk. Low-risk patients are treated with budesonide or prednisone, with or without AZA. High-risk patients are treated with either anti-TNF-α monotherapy or

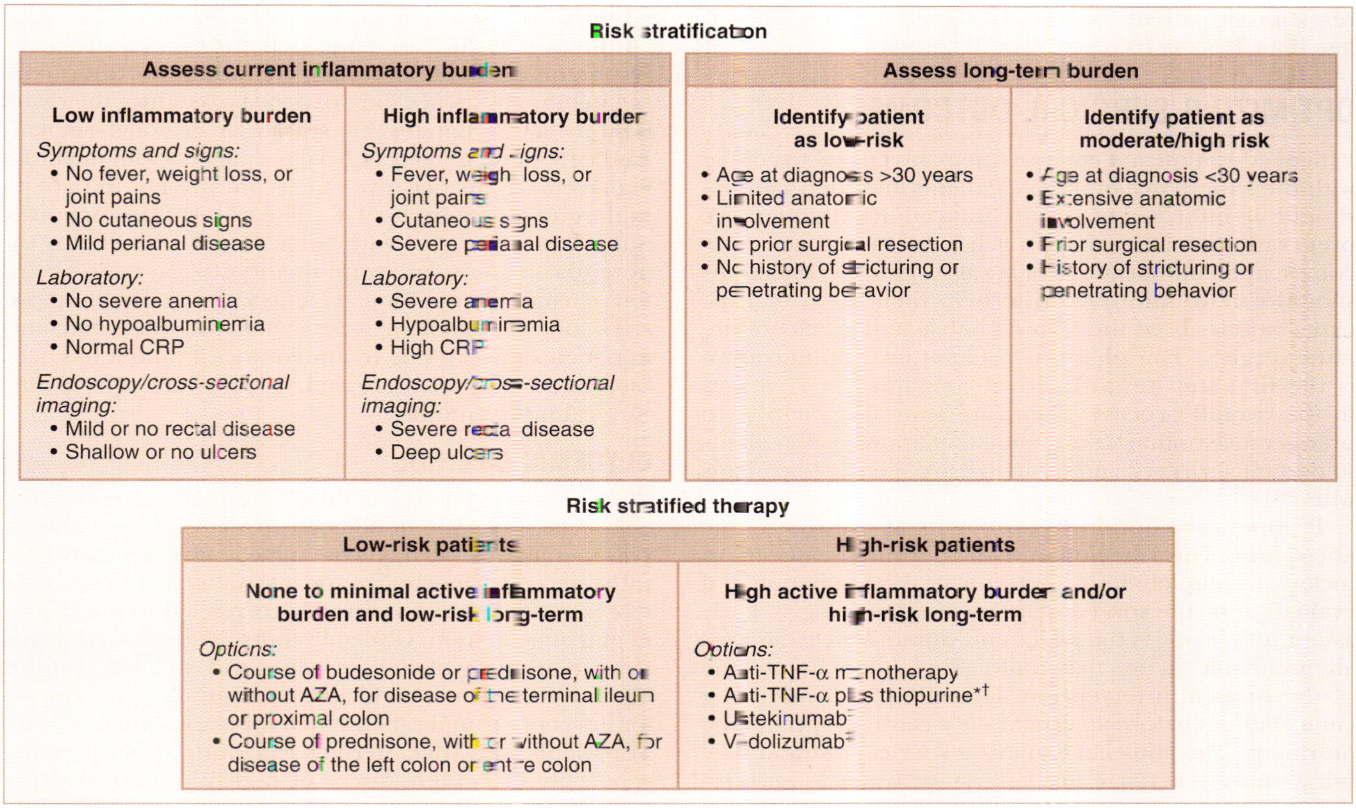

Risk stratification

Assess current inflammatory burden		Assess long-term burden	
Low inflammatory burden	**High inflammatory burden**	**Identify patient as low-risk**	**Identify patient as moderate/high risk**
Symptoms and signs: • No fever, weight loss, or joint pains • No cutaneous signs • Mild perianal disease *Laboratory:* • No severe anemia • No hypoalbuminemia • Normal CRP *Endoscopy/cross-sectional imaging:* • Mild or no rectal disease • Shallow or no ulcers	*Symptoms and signs:* • Fever, weight loss, or joint pains • Cutaneous signs • Severe perianal disease *Laboratory:* • Severe anemia • Hypoalbuminemia • High CRP *Endoscopy/cross-sectional imaging:* • Severe rectal disease • Deep ulcers	• Age at diagnosis >30 years • Limited anatomic involvement • No prior surgical resection • No history of stricturing or penetrating behavior	• Age at diagnosis <30 years • Extensive anatomic involvement • Prior surgical resection • History of stricturing or penetrating behavior

Risk stratified therapy

Low-risk patients	High-risk patients
None to minimal active inflammatory burden and low-risk long-term	**High active inflammatory burden and/or high-risk long-term**
Options: • Course of budesonide or prednisone, with or without AZA, for disease of the terminal ileum or proximal colon • Course of prednisone, with or without AZA, for disease of the left colon or entire colon	*Options:* • Anti-TNF-α monotherapy • Anti-TNF-α plus thiopurine*† • Ustekinumab‡ • Vedolizumab‡

FIGURE 161.2 Medical therapy of inflammatory luminal Crohn disease.[147] *The combination of a thiopurine and infliximab is the most effective inductive therapy. The American Gastroenterological Association (AGA) gave combination therapy a conditional recommendation over anti-tumor necrosis factor (TNF)-α monotherapy for the induction of remission. The AGA made no recommendation regarding combination therapy versus anti-TNF monotherapy for the maintenance of remission. Combination therapy likely offers improved durability due to the suppression of anti-drug antibodies against the anti-TNF-α agent but also incurs a higher risk of lymphoma. Combination therapy should be considered in patients requiring their second or third anti-TNF-α. †Use methotrexate for patients who do not tolerate thiopurine. ‡Comparative effectiveness studies will be needed to determine the relative positioning of vedolizumab and ustekinumab vis-à-vis the anti-TNF-α agents. *AZA,* Azathioprine *CRP,* C-reactive protein

thiopurine–anti-TNF-α combination therapy. Methotrexate is recommended for patients who are intolerant to thiopurines. Comparative effectiveness studies will be needed to determine the relative positioning of vedolizumab and ustekinumab vis-à-vis the anti-TNF-α agents in the treatment of CD.

PRINCIPLES OF SURGICAL MANAGEMENT

Although UC is primarily treated medically, approximately 20% to 30% of patients with severe or complicated disease will require colectomy.[280] In CD, 50% of patients will require some kind of surgical procedure during their lifetime.[281] The key difference between the two disorders lies in surgical intent. In patients with CD, surgery treats the potentially life-threating complications of obstruction and contained sepsis. In contrast, colectomy in UC is curative.

INDICATIONS FOR SURGERY

Surgery in CD is indicated for complications, including obstruction, free perforation, abscesses, symptomatic

fistulas, and cancer. With advances in pharmacotherapy, surgery is nowadays less frequently performed for medically refractory disease. The main surgical indications in UC include medical refractory disease and dysplasia/carcinoma. Less frequently, patients require colectomy for toxic megacolon, uncontrolled hemorrhage, perforation, obstruction, or stricture that raises concern for malignancy and, in children, failure to thrive. A recent Danish population-based study compared the risk for surgery of CD patients over 3 decades. Over the decades the study group treatment changed significantly with decrease in 5-ASA compounds and steroids and increase in the use of biologics. The investigators demonstrated that the risk of first major surgery in CD decreased over calendar time. This was observed within the first year and also 5 years and 9 years after diagnosis. Likewise, the cumulative probability of undergoing first major surgery was lowest in the treated-with-biologic cohorts within the first year, 5 years, and 9 years after diagnosis (overall *P* = .004).[282] Similar results were found for patients with UC. Risk of first major surgery decreased significantly over calendar time and the decrease was found at 1, 5, and 9 years after diagnosis. In this study the risk for surgical resection in patients with UC in the era of biologics was less than 10% at 10 years from diagnosis.[282]

OPTIMIZING SURGICAL OUTCOMES

Patient education and empowerment are critical to coping with the experience of illness. Patients and their families should be informed about the indications, preoperative preparations, technical approach, recovery process, outcomes, and complications of surgery. Moreover, patients should receive information to help them form realistic expectations about their bowel habits and quality of life after surgery. The phase of preoperative optimization is the first step toward actively engaging the patient in the overall process. There are several principles to preoperative optimization, some that apply to all patients undergoing surgery, and some that are specific to patients with IBD.[283,284]

Preoperative optimization begins at the first clinic encounter. The key elements of the initial assessment include a complete history and physical examination and evaluation by the surgeon and an anesthesiologist. Early assessment provides the patient maximum time to address all modifiable factors that could affect the final outcome of the surgical intervention. Detecting and modifying comorbidities before an operation is central for reducing morbidity. The clinician can assess surgical risk and take initial steps to manage this risk via measures to improve the patient's general condition and organ function. The preoperative assessment should be focused on the following key areas: smoking cessation, glycemic control, correction of anemia, optimization of nutrition, review of medications, and management of any intraabdominal infection.

SMOKING CESSATION

Tobacco use is associated with worse outcomes after colorectal surgery. The amount of daily tobacco use correlates linearly with the severity of complications after gastrointestinal surgery. Tobacco use is an independent risk factor for respiratory failure, admission to the intensive care unit, pneumonia, laryngospasm, and increased use of respiratory therapy services after the administration of general anesthesia.[285] In a large study of adult patients undergoing major surgery, current smoking was associated with an increased risk of myocardial infarction, stroke, respiratory events, and death.[286] In all surgical patients, smoking cessation has been proven to provide better postoperative outcomes. The US Preventive Services Task Force recommends that all adult smokers be provided tobacco cessation interventions before surgery.[287] The American Society of Anesthesiologists recommends that all patients should abstain from smoking for as long as possible both before and after surgery, and they should be supported by their physicians to achieve complete smoking cessation. There are two effective approaches to smoking cessation: behavioral techniques and medical therapy (such as nicotine replacement therapy and varenicline). A Cochrane review[288] showed that when such preoperative interventions were delivered intensively with multisession face-to-face counseling, smokers were 10 times more likely to quit smoking (RR = 10.8; 95% CI, 4.6 to 25.5). The optimal timing of smoking cessation before surgery was

investigated in a systematic review of 25 studies.[289] Smoking abstinence for at least 4 weeks before surgery reduced respiratory and wound healing complications. Short-term (<4 weeks) abstinence did not appear to reduce the risk of postoperative respiratory complications. Although smoking has been found to be beneficial for patients with medically managed UC, its negative effects are present in patients undergoing surgery for UC. The adverse postoperative outcomes associated with tobacco use overwhelm the potential benefit for symptomatic disease control that tobacco may offer in some patients with UC. Furthermore, it is known that smoking is associated with worse outcomes in patients undergoing treatment for CD and it has been associated with an increased risk for having repeated surgical interventions.[290]

GLYCEMIC CONTROL

Postoperative hyperglycemia is frequent after elective colorectal surgery in nondiabetic patients.[291] Even a single postoperative elevated glucose value is adversely associated with increased morbidity and mortality after colorectal resection.[292] The risk is directly correlated to the degree of glucose elevation. Glycemic control before surgery and strict monitoring of glucose values and early intervention after surgery even in nondiabetic patients decrease the risk for infectious complications.[293] Steroids are commonly used in patients with IBD. Steroids can cause hyperglycemia, especially in circumstances of high physiologic stress, such as a surgical resection. Minimizing steroid exposure in IBD patients can limit episodes of hyperglycemia and consequently the risk of infectious wound complications.

ANEMIA

Anemia is the most common hematologic complication of IBD.[294] The main causes of anemia in IBD include deficiencies of iron and vitamin B_{12} and chronic inflammation.[295] Anemia is more common in CD than in UC and is usually undertreated.[296] One-third of IBD patients have a hemoglobin less than 12 g/dL.[294] Not surprisingly, the frequency and severity of the anemia are related to disease activity in patients with IBD. Establishing the cause of anemia is key to proper management, such as administration of iron or vitamin B_{12}, or blood transfusion. For perioperative patients, transfusion is usually needed for hemoglobin levels less than 7 g/dL. Blood should be transfused 1 to 2 days before surgery to maximize oxygen transport to the tissues. Moreover, transfusing the patient on the day of operation entails the risk of a transfusion reaction that will lead to postponement of surgery.

NUTRITIONAL STATUS

The definition of malnutrition varies among studies in the literature. Data suggest that malnutrition affects a large portion of patients with IBD, estimated in 65% to 75% of patients with CD and in 18% to 62% of patients with UC. Based on body mass index (BMI) analysis, malnutrition prevalence seems to be higher in CD compared to UC, although several authors reported similar prevalence of malnutrition in both conditions. Therefore it is difficult to estimate the prevalence of malnutrition in surgical patients with IBD.[297] Several processes contribute to malnutrition, including malabsorption as a result of small bowel disease or short bowel syndrome, increased energy expenditures, and diminished oral intake due to anorexia or postprandial symptoms.[298] Harries et al. used anthropometric measurements to determine the prevalence of malnutrition in patients with IBD compared to healthy controls.[299] All anthropometric measures were significantly reduced in those with CD as compared with those with UC or the healthy controls. More recently Mijac et al. assessed the nutrition status of patients with IBD over time and found that 67% of patients with active IBD experienced significant weight loss over 6 months.[300] Using the Nationwide Inpatient Sample, Nguyen et al. found that protein-calorie malnutrition was significantly more common in hospitalized patients with IBD compared with other hospitalized patients.[301] In addition to malnutrition, patients with IBD may develop micronutrient deficiencies, even in the presence of adequate intake. Patients may have a normal BMI and appear well nourished, yet have deficiencies of vitamins A, C, K, B_{12}, D, and magnesium, iron, zinc, and calcium.[297] All these deficiencies have been associated with several postoperative complications after IBD surgery.[297] Conversely, preoperative nutritional optimization improves outcomes.[302] The mechanisms by which nutrition support improves outcomes have not been fully elucidated. There is some evidence that nutritional optimization with either enteral or parenteral nutrition when needed alters the gut microbiome and changes the genes associated with membrane transport, sulfur reduction, and nutrient biosynthesis.[303] Furthermore, preoperative nutritional support can increase skeletal muscle mass, protein mass, and decrease resting energy expenditure, whereas in patients treated with exclusive preoperative elemental diet, mesenteric adipocytes were larger and expressed fewer inflammatory cytokines.[304]

Preoperative nutritional optimization may reduce the inflammatory response.[302,305,306] Preoperative management of malnutrition including nutritional therapy can decrease postoperative morbidity, but it remains controversial whether it can decrease the risk for an unnecessary fecal diversion.[307]

Nutritional replacement may occur through the enteral or the parenteral route. It has been shown that enteral nutrition enhances mucosal healing, controls local inflammation, and confers benefits for growth and overall nutritional status. RCTs estimate an overall remission rate of 60% in patients with CD and specific enteral nutrition as the sole treatment.[305] Although enteral nutrition is the evidence-based, preferred route of alimentation in IBD patients with malnutrition, patients with strictures may not tolerate oral diet. Moreover, patients with high-output enterocutaneous fistulas, perforation, or toxic megacolon should be made nil per os. Although enteral nutrition is preferred when the gastrointestinal tract is accessible and functional, parenteral nutrition is a suitable alternative when enteral nutrition is not feasible. For these patients, TPN may optimize the patient in the preoperative period. TPN risks include line thrombosis and infection, hyperglycemia, electrolyte disturbances, and hepatotoxicity.[301] Perioperative TPN offers a potential adjunctive treatment to surgery; however whether it improves surgical outcomes, disease severity, or nutrition status remains under debate. The evidence for benefits

from preoperative TPN remains inconclusive. On the other hand, there is no evidence of inferiority of TPN, either in the preoperative or postoperative periods.[306] Although several retrospective studies showed that perioperative TPN significantly reduced the risk of postoperative complications, a large RCT has not been done to show whether there is significant difference in postoperative complications between subjects who receive perioperative TPN and those who do not. Older studies indicated that perioperative TPN may be associated with a significant decrease in the length of resected small bowel.[308] Other studies found that preoperative TPN was associated with increased total postoperative complications, when IV line infections were accounted for.[309] In the preoperative period TPN is a good adjunct in the treatment of patients with severe disease and protein-caloric malnutrition who cannot tolerate enteral nutrition.[310]

PREOPERATIVE MEDICATIONS

A thorough review of all prescribed medications, over-the-counter drugs, supplements, and herbal remedies is required in all surgical candidates. The surgeon should provide clear advice on which medicines should be continued and which should be stopped. The use of steroids for more than 3 months has been associated with wound dehiscence and postoperative infectious complications, especially in patients with CD. Numerous studies, mostly retrospective, have assessed whether preoperative steroid use leads to poor perioperative outcomes.[311,312] A meta-analysis demonstrated a 1.7-fold increased risk of postoperative infectious complications and 1.4-fold increased risk of overall complications in patient using steroids.[311] A study that used data from the National Surgical Quality Improvement Program found that the use of preoperative steroids was associated with VTE in both CD and UC.[313] It is possible that corticosteroids are a marker of disease severity, which is a risk factor for VTE, but it has also been shown that steroids may also have an independent thrombogenic effect.[314] It is therefore key to reduce the dose or even discontinue steroids before surgery. For patients who received a short course of steroids, the risk for a complication is minimal. The risk is much higher for long-term users. For these patients, a two-stage procedure with creation of a temporary ostomy mitigates risk. The ostomy can be taken down after steroids are discontinued.

Anti-TNF-α agents are now initiated early in the course of IBD, so that a large proportion of surgical patients are receiving these therapies. Most studies have shown no differences in outcomes,[312,315-317] but some authors have suggested either increased infectious or total postoperative complications in patients treated with anti-TNF-α agents preoperatively.[318-320] Meta-analyses have also yielded contradictory results. Rosenfeld et al. included six studies and found no significant differences in the rates of postoperative complication of infliximab-treated versus nontreated patients.[321] A meta-analysis of 21 studies found that anti-TNF-α–treated patients had an increased risk of postoperative complications (OR, 1.25; 95% CI, 1.02 to 1.53) and infectious postoperative complications (OR, 1.45; 95% CI, 1.03 to 2.05).[320] A drug window, with the purpose of drug washout, may minimize the potential influence of immunosuppressive therapy on the risk of infections after surgery. There are limited data on biologics other than the anti-TNF-α agents. Vedolizumab, an anti-$\alpha_4\beta_7$ integrin mAb, may theoretically influence the risk of infectious anastomotic complications. A retrospective study of 94 patients reported more frequent infectious adverse events in patients treated with vedolizumab versus those treated with anti-TNF-α therapy.[322] In the study 37% of patients who received vedolizumab within 30 days of a major abdominal operation experienced a 30-day postoperative surgical site infections, significantly higher than patients receiving TNF-α inhibitors or no biologic therapy.

INTRAABDOMINAL INFECTION

The presence of intraabdominal sepsis is associated with higher postoperative morbidity. The presence of intraabdominal sepsis is an independent predictor of postoperative intraabdominal infectious complications.[323–325] Preoperative use of antibiotics and drainage of any intraabdominal collections are the initial steps for control of sepsis, until surgical resection can achieve complete control of the disease and the source of the sepsis.[324] If no other risk factors such as malnutrition or chronic steroid use are present, then primary anastomosis is a safe option. In high-risk patients the surgeon should consider a two-stage procedure. Patients with CD and an intraabdominal abscess have been successfully treated in our center with percutaneous drainage of the abscess, IV steroids, TPN for 1 to 2 weeks, and surgical removal of the septic source with primary anastomosis of the gastrointestinal tract, without diversion.[326] The alternative approach would include drainage of the abscess, fecal diversion if needed, and then surgical resection weeks later.[327]

For patients undergoing elective surgical resection, education in ostomy care by a certified wound ostomy care nurse should be provided during the preoperative period. Patient education decreases stoma-related complications and unplanned readmissions after surgery.[328–330]

SURGICAL CONSIDERATIONS

ONE-, TWO-, MODIFIED TWO-, OR THREE-STAGE ILEAL POUCH–ANAL ANASTOMOSIS

Improvements in the medical management of severe UC over the past decade have led to a decrease in the number of emergent colectomies for toxic colitis and an increase in the number of colectomies performed for medically refractory disease.[282] The colorectal surgeon has four options for patients with UC requiring surgery: one-stage total proctocolectomy with ileal pouch–anal anastomosis (IPAA); two-stage approach with total proctocolectomy with formation of IPAA and a diverting loop ileostomy, followed by takedown of ileostomy; a modified two-stage procedure involving a total abdominal colectomy with end ileostomy as the first stage and then completion proctectomy with IPAA (without ostomy) as the second stage; and, finally, a three-stage approach, starting with a total abdominal colectomy and end ileostomy, proceeding to completion

proctectomy with IPAA at the second-stage operation, and reversal of ileostomy at a third operation. Any of these approaches to IPAA can be pursued by minimally invasive techniques.

One-stage procedures are relatively rare because of their potential for high morbidity, hence only a very highly selected patient population undergoes this procedure.[331,332] The two-stage procedure also carries significant morbidity, causing many centers to use the three-stage approach preferentially.[333] Two centers have presented their experience with two-stage versus modified two-stage procedures.[334,335] In one study from Canada, 223 patients underwent traditional two-stage IPAA and 237 patients received the modified two-stage procedure. The modified two-stage group had a lower rate of anastomotic leak following IPAA (4.6% vs. 15.7%; $p < .01$). Multivariate analysis confirmed that the modified approach was associated with a lower risk of anastomotic leak (OR, 0.27; 95% CI, 0.12–0.57). In another study from Hershey Medical Center, interval IPAA reconstruction without a stoma (two-stage modified procedure) after colectomy was functionally equivalent to the traditional three-stage protocol in terms of clinical outcome. However, it had the advantage of overall lower hospital costs and a shorter length of hospital stay.[334] Overall, the modified two-stage approach is a safe alternative to the traditional two- and three-stage approaches because it decreases the risk for an anastomotic complication without increasing the cost or the number of surgeries the patient has to undergo.

LIVER TRANSPLANTATION AND ILEAL POUCH–ANAL ANASTOMOSIS

Patients with UC can have concomitant primary sclerosing cholangitis (PSC) (10%), but the majority of the patients with PSC suffer from UC. No effective medical treatment exists for advanced PSC, and orthotopic liver transplantation is the only surgical option for cure. Occasionally, patients will require a total proctocolectomy with an IPAA before, at the same time, or even after transplantation. The group from Mayo Clinic reported on 32 patients who underwent IPAA either before or after the liver transplantation. There were no deaths or increased morbidity from the procedures. More than 75% of the patients developed pouchitis after the IPAA, and 40% were alive at 4 years.[336] Another multicenter study demonstrated that proctocolectomy-IPAA can be performed safely after liver transplantation.[337] IPAA or liver transplantation are not mutually exclusive in patients with UC and PSC.

SPECIAL CONSIDERATIONS IN CROHN DISEASE

MANAGEMENT OF PERIANAL DISEASE

Perianal CD is an aggressive and disabling form of the disease that is present in nearly a third of the patients with CD. Since the introduction of anti-TNF-α agents, the need for aggressive surgical intervention, such as proctectomy, has significantly decreased.[338] Level I evidence from two randomized trials using anti-TNF-α agents demonstrated up to 50% 1-year fistula closure rate for CD with perianal fistulas.[339,340]

The key to successful treatment of patients with perianal disease is the close collaboration between the gastroenterologist and the surgeon.[341] Initial assessment of the patient should include a thorough history and physical exam with documentation of the location of all the external openings of the fistulas in the perineum. A colonoscopy and computed tomography or magnetic resonance enterography are warranted to detect luminal disease. The mucosa of the mid and distal rectum needs to be thoroughly examined to determine the extent and severity of disease activity. A magnetic resonance study of the pelvis[342] or a high-resolution endorectal ultrasound can map out the perineal disease.[343] The use of ultrasound is usually limited by the patient's ability to tolerate probe insertion into a highly inflamed perineum. Finally, an exam under anesthesia will complement the previous studies and allow the surgeon to delineate the extent of the sphincter muscle involvement by the fistulas. Drainage of any undrained infection and placement of noncutting seton drains will provide some symptomatic relief to the patient. The seton drain will preserve the integrity of the anal sphincter, drain the fistula tracts and limit the chances of abscess formation or perineal sepsis during medical therapy.[341]

Currently the use of biologics is highly recommended for patients with perineal disease. The healing rate at 12 months ranges from 30% to 70%.[338] The anti-TNF-α agents have been proven to be superior to immunomodulators for the treatment of perianal CD.[338] Data on managing perianal disease with newer biologics, such as vedolizumab, are limited. It has been shown that the presence of active perianal disease when vedoluzimab is initiated is a predictor of decreased response to the medication and lower chances for clinical remission.[213]

Within 12 months from treatment initiation the rectum should be reexamined and if no luminal disease is present, then complex fistulas should be considered for repair. Most common procedure used is the endorectal advancement flap with healing rates ranging between 55% and 72%.[344] More recently the technique of ligation of intersphincteric fistula tract (LIFT) has been used for complex fistula-in-ano with CD. The small studies have demonstrated up to 60% healing rate.[345] For complex fistulas injection of allogenic or native stem cells into the tract is an emerging alternative to surgical repair of perianal Crohn-related fistulas. Success rate is less than 50% in 1 year.[346] Simple superficial fistulas can be treated with simple fistulotomy.

STRICTUREPLASTY FOR BOWEL PRESERVATION

Strictureplasty is a bowel-sparing procedure that avoids resection and preserves intestinal absorptive capacity in patients with obstructing CD.[347] Most of the surgical techniques currently used for strictureplasty were initially applied for gastric and duodenal strictures from either peptic ulcer disease or upper gastrointestinal tract CD, essentially in cases where resection would be difficult. The principle of all strictureplasty techniques involves incising the stricture and reapproximating surrounding bowel to preserve intestinal length while enlarging luminal diameter. Traditional strictureplasty techniques include

the Heineke-Mikulicz (most commonly used), Finney, and Jaboulay.[348] These techniques can be used for short, up to 5-cm (Heineke-Mikulicz) strictures or longer, up to 20-cm strictures (Finney or Jaboulay). Other techniques for long strictures include the isoperistaltic, side-to-side strictureplasty.[349]

Strictureplasty is applied in cases where extensive resection needs to be avoided to avert the risk for short bowel syndrome and severe malabsorption. Several studies have demonstrated that strictureplasty is as safe and effective as resection. Meta-analysis of 3529 small bowel strictureplasties in more than 1000 patients demonstrated a 15% morbidity.[350] Infectious complications such as anastomotic leak, fistula, and abscess occurred in 4%, which is similar to that of patients undergoing ileocolonic resection for CD. Patient undergoing resection and patients undergoing strictureplasty have similar symptomatic CD recurrence rates that range from 30% to 50% at 5 years post surgery. The decision as to whether the surgeon should proceed with a resection versus a strictureplasty is individualized for each patient and is based on several factors such as patient's age (younger patients favor strictureplasty for bowel preservation), disease severity (combination of stricturing and penetrating disease favors resection), disease location (isolated small bowel disease favors strictureplasty), disease duration (long-standing, >20 years' disease favors resection to rule out malignancy at the area of stricture), history of previous resections (previous resections favor strictureplasty for bowel length preservation), length of diseased bowel (shorter segments favor strictureplasty), and distance between strictured bowel segments (short distance between several strictures favors resection). There are cases where both techniques may be incorporated into the same operation.

PREVENTION OF POSTOPERATIVE RECURRENCE

Postoperative CD recurrence can be defined as histologic, endoscopic, radiographic, clinical, or surgical. Clinical and endoscopic recurrence rates are most commonly reported. Clinical recurrence is defined by symptoms, such as diarrhea, weight loss and abdominal pain, and measured with the CDAI.[351] Endoscopic recurrence is defined by the Rutgeerts score, which predicts clinical and surgical recurrence.[352] Endoscopic recurrence has been reported in 54% of patients at 5 years,[352] and clinical recurrence follows endoscopic recurrence with a prevalence of 28% to 45%.

Recurrence of the disease after surgery is influenced by several factors, some modifiable. Young age at diagnosis, young age at first surgical intervention, short disease duration until the first surgical resection, penetrating disease, perianal disease, prior operations, multiple sites of the disease, and NOD2/CARD15 gene mutation are risk factors for early recurrence of the disease.[353] None of these factors can be modified. In contrast, cigarette smoking, surgical technique (need for negative gross surgical margin), the presence of significant postoperative complications, and the initiation of appropriate medical treatment are modifiable parameters.[354-35] Smoking cessation is critical in preventing disease recurrence.[357,358] Patients who quit before surgery have similar recurrence rates to nonsmokers and significantly reduced rates when compared with smokers.[357] The presence of positive microscopic resection margins does not increase risk for early recurrence but does increase the risk of an infectious complication after surgery that can lead to extremely delayed initiation of medical treatment to prevent recurrence.[359]

In a placebo-controlled, randomized trial of only 20 patients, Regueiro et al. found that endoscopic recurrence at 1 year occurred significantly less frequently in the infliximab arm (9.1% vs. 84.6%; $P = .0006$).[256] In a large, multicenter trial, patients were randomized to infliximab versus placebo in the first 45 days after surgery. Infliximab was not superior to placebo in preventing clinical recurrence up to 76 weeks after resection. However, infliximab did reduce endoscopic recurrence (30% vs. 60%; $P < .001$).[261] The American Gastroenterological Association recently published a systematic review and guidelines on the medical prophylaxis of postoperative recurrence.[243] The patients were divided into low and high risk for disease recurrence based on their disease history and operative findings. Currently, postoperative risk stratification for early recurrence based on known risk factors is the safest guide to determine postoperative "preventive" treatment. Low-risk patients who have long-standing CD, with first surgery for a short stricture should be closely observed. Moderate-risk patients with less than 10 years of CD, long stricture, or inflammatory phenotype of CD should be placed on nonbiologic maintenance treatment. Finally, high-risk patients with penetrating CD, with two or greater surgeries should receive biologics to prevent endoscopic recurrence. For the majority of CD patients with surgically induced remission, early pharmacologic prophylaxis is recommended over endoscopy-guided pharmacologic treatment. For a small portion of lower risk of recurrence patients, who place a higher value on avoiding the small risks of adverse events from pharmacologic prophylaxis and a lower value on the potential risk of early disease recurrence, selecting endoscopy-guided pharmacologic treatment is reasonable. For patients who are in surgically induced remission of CD, the use of anti-TNF-α therapy and/or thiopurines over other agents is recommended.[243] The use of mesalamine (or other 5-aminosalicylates), budesonide, or probiotics is not recommended.[243] All patients should have endoscopic surveillance of the disease 6 to 12 months after surgery. If asymptomatic disease is present on surveillance endoscopy then initiating or optimizing anti-TNF-α and/or thiopurine therapy over continued monitoring alone is recommended.[243]

CONCLUSION

The management of CD and UC requires a collaborative effort between specialized gastroenterologists and colon and rectal surgeons. Medical therapy is evolving based on increasing discovery of new mechanism based therapies. The patient benefits from the presence of an IBD center, where immediate experts are available for the medical and surgical aspects of the disease management.[360] Expert surgical care allows the patient to retain quality of life, avoid life-threatening complications, and enjoy a prolonged disease-free period, always with the joint effort of the IBD GI specialist.

REFERENCES

1. Bonen DK, Cho JH. The genetics of inflammatory bowel disease. *Gastroenterology*. 2003;124:521.
2. Orholm M, Binder V, Sorensen TI, Rasmussen LP, Kyvik KO. Concordance of inflammatory bowel disease among Danish twins. Results of a nationwide study. *Scand J Gastroenterol*. 2000;35:1075.
3. Halfvarson J, Bodin L, Tysk C, Lindberg E, Järnerot G. Inflammatory bowel disease in a Swedish twin cohort: a long-term follow-up of concordance and clinical characteristics. *Gastroenterology*. 2003;124:1767.
4. Spehlmann ME, Begun AZ, Burghardt J, Lepage P, Raedler A, Schreiber S. Epidemiology of inflammatory bowel disease in a German twin cohort: results of a nationwide study. *Inflamm Bowel Dis*. 2008;14:968.
5. Hugot JP, Laurent-Puig P, Gower-Rousseau C, et al. Mapping of a susceptibility locus for Crohn's disease on chromosome 16. *Nature*. 1996;379:821.
6. Hugot JP, Chamaillard M, Zouali H, et al. Association of NOD2 leucine-rich repeat variants with susceptibility to Crohn's disease. *Nature*. 2001;411:599.
7. Ogura Y, Bonen DK, Inohara N, et al. A frameshift mutation in NOD2 associated with susceptibility to Crohn's disease. *Nature*. 2001;411:603.
8. Mathew CG, Lewis CM. Genetics of inflammatory bowel disease: progress and prospects. *Hum Mol Genet*. 2004;13(Spec1):R161.
9. McGovern DP, Kugathasan S, Cho JH. Genetics of inflammatory bowel diseases. *Gastroenterology*. 2015;149:1163.
10. Yamazaki K, McGovern D, Ragoussis J, et al. Single nucleotide polymorphisms in TNFSF15 confer susceptibility to Crohn's disease. *Hum Mol Genet*. 2005;14:3499.
11. Liu JZ, Anderson CA. Genetic studies of Crohn's disease: past, present and future. *Best Pract Res Clin Gastroenterol*. 2014;28:373.
12. Jostins L, Ripke S, Weersma RK, et al. Host-microbe interactions have shaped the genetic architecture of inflammatory bowel disease. *Nature*. 2012;491:119.
13. Liu JZ, van Sommeren S, Huang H, et al. Association analyses identify 38 susceptibility loci for inflammatory bowel disease and highlight shared genetic risk across populations. *Nat Genet*. 2015;47:979.
14. Khor B, Gardet A, Xavier RJ. Genetics and pathogenesis of inflammatory bowel disease. *Nature*. 2011;474:307.
15. Worthey EA, Mayer AN, Syverson GD, et al. Making a definitive diagnosis: successful clinical application of whole exome sequencing in a child with intractable inflammatory bowel disease. *Genet Med*. 2011;13:255.
16. Uhlig HH. Monogenic diseases associated with intestinal inflammation: implications for the understanding of inflammatory bowel disease. *Gut*. 2013;62:1795.
17. Molodecky NA, Soon IS, Rabi DM, et al. Increasing incidence and prevalence of the inflammatory bowel diseases with time, based on systematic review. *Gastroenterology*. 2012;142:46.
18. Carr I, Mayberry JF. The effects of migration on ulcerative colitis: a three-year prospective study among Europeans and first- and second-generation South Asians in Leicester (1991–1994). *Am J Gastroenterol*. 1999;94:2918.
19. Li X, Sundquist J, Hemminki K, Sundquist K. Risk of inflammatory bowel disease in first- and second-generation immigrants in Sweden: a nationwide follow-up study. *Inflamm Bowel Dis*. 2011;17:1784.
20. Benchimol EI, Mack DR, Guttmann A, et al. Inflammatory bowel disease in immigrants to Canada and their children: a population-based cohort study. *Am J Gastroenterol*. 2015;110:553.
21. Ng WK, Wong SH, Ng SC. Changing epidemiological trends of inflammatory bowel disease in Asia. *Intest Res*. 2016;14:111.
22. Victoria CR, Sassak LY, Nunes HR. Incidence and prevalence rates of inflammatory bowel diseases, in midwestern of Sao Paulo State, Brazil. *Arq Gastroenterol*. 2009;46:20.
23. Benchimol EI, Guttmann A, Griffiths AM, et al. Increasing incidence of paediatric inflammatory bowel disease in Ontario, Canada: evidence from health administrative data. *Gut*. 2009;58:1490.

24. Benchimol EI, Fortinsky KJ, Gozdyra P, et al. Epidemiology of pediatric inflammatory bowel disease: a systematic review of international trends. *Inflamm Bowel Dis.* 2011;17:423.

25. Malmborg P, Grahnquist L, Lindholm J, Montgomery S, Hildebrand H. Increasing incidence of paediatric inflammatory bowel disease in northern Stockholm County, 2002-2007. *J Pediatr Gastroenterol Nutr.* 2013;57:29.

26. Hou JK, Abraham B, El-Serag H. Dietary intake and risk of developing inflammatory bowel disease: a systematic review of the literature. *Am J Gastroenterol.* 2011;106:563.

27. IBD in EPIC Study Investigators, Tjonneland A, Overvad K, et al. Linoleic acid, a dietary n-6 polyunsaturated fatty acid, and the aetiology of ulcerative colitis: a nested case-control study within a European prospective cohort study. *Gut.* 2009;58: 606.

28. Ananthakrishnan AN, Khalili H, Konijeti GG, et al. Long-term intake of dietary fat and risk of ulcerative colitis and Crohn's disease. *Gut.* 2014;63:776.

29. Ananthakrishnan AN, Khalili H, Konijeti GG, et al. A prospective study of long-term intake of dietary fiber and risk of Crohn's disease and ulcerative colitis. *Gastroenterology.* 2013;145:97.

30. Cosnes J, Carbonnel F, Beaugerie L, Le Quintrec Y, Gendre JP. Effects of cigarette smoking on the long-term course of Crohn's disease. *Gastroenterology.* 1996;110:424.

31. Ananthakrishnan AN. Environmental risk factors for inflammatory bowel diseases: a review. *Dig Dis Sci.* 2015;60:290.

32. Cosnes J, Beaugerie L, Carbonnel F, Gendre JP. Smoking cessation and the course of Crohn's disease: an intervention study. *Gastroenterology.* 2001;120:1093.

33. Cosnes J. Smoking and diet: impact on disease course? *Dig Dis.* 2016;34:72.

34. Andersson RE, Olaison G, Tysk C, Ekbom A. Appendectomy and protection against ulcerative colitis. *N Engl J Med.* 2001;344:808.

35. Ananthakrishnan AN, Khalili H, Higuchi LM, et al. Higher predicted vitamin D status is associated with reduced risk of Crohn's disease. *Gastroenterology.* 2012;142:482.

36. Ananthakrishnan AN, Higuchi LM, Huang ES, et al. Aspirin, nonsteroidal anti-inflammatory drug use, and risk for Crohn disease and ulcerative colitis: a cohort study. *Ann Intern Med.* 2012; 156:350.

37. Kappelman MD, Rifas-Shiman SL, Kleinman K, et al. The prevalence and geographic distribution of Crohn's disease and ulcerative colitis in the United States. *Clin Gastroenterol Hepatol.* 2007;5:1424.

38. Kappelman MD, Rifas-Shiman SL, Porter CQ, et al. Direct health care costs of Crohn's disease and ulcerative colitis in US children and adults. *Gastroenterology.* 2008;135:1907.

39. Kappelman MD, Moore KR, Allen JK, Cook SF. Recent trends in the prevalence of Crohn's disease and ulcerative colitis in a commercially insured US population. *Dig Dis Sci.* 2013;58:519.

40. Loftus CG, Loftus EV Jr, Harmsen WS, et al. Update on the incidence and prevalence of Crohn's disease and ulcerative colitis in Olmsted County, Minnesota, 1940-2000. *Inflamm Bowel Dis.* 2007;13:254.

41. Abramson O, Durant M, Mow W, et al. Incidence, prevalence, and time trends of pediatric inflammatory bowel disease in Northern California, 1996 to 2006. *J Pediatr.* 2010;157:233.

42. McGovern D, Powrie F. The IL23 axis plays a key role in the pathogenesis of IBD. *Gut.* 2007;56:1333.

43. de Souza HS, Fiocchi C. Immunopathogenesis of IBD. Current state of the art. *Nat Rev Gastroenterol Hepatol.* 2016; 3:13.

44. Duerr RH, Taylor KD, Brant SR, et al. A genome-wide association study identifies IL23R as an inflammatory bowel disease gene. *Science.* 2006;314:1461.

45. Wehkamp J, Harder J, Weichenthal M, et al. NOD2 (CARD15) mutations in Crohn's disease are associated with diminished mucosal alpha-defensin expression. *Gut.* 2004;53:1658.

46. Boyle JP, Parkhouse R, Monie TP. Insights into the molecular basis of the NOD2 signalling pathway. *Open Biol.* 2014;4: 12).

47. Ramanan D, Tang MS, Bowcutt R, Loke P, Cadwell K. Bacterial sensor Nod2 prevents inflammation of the small intestine by restricting the expansion of the commensal *Bacteroides vulgatus.* *Immunity.* 2014;41:311.

48. Hedl M, Li J, Cho JH, Abraham C. Chronic stimulation of Nod2 mediates tolerance to bacterial products. *Proc Natl Acad Sci USA.* 2007;104:19440.

49. Wellcome Trust Case Control Consortium. Genome-wide association study of 14,000 cases of seven common diseases and 3,000 shared controls. *Nature.* 2007;447:661.

50. Hampe J, Franke A, Rosenstiel P, et al. A genome-wide association scan of nonsynonymous SNPs identifies a susceptibility variant for Crohn disease in ATG16L1. *Nat Genet.* 2007;39:207.

51. Rioux JD, Xavier RJ, Taylor KD, et al. Genome-wide association study identifies new susceptibility loci for Crohn disease and implicates autophagy in disease pathogenesis. *Nat Genet.* 2007;39:596.

52. Parkes M, Barrett JC, Prescott NJ, et al. Sequence variants in the autophagy gene IRGM and multiple other replicating loci contribute to Crohn's disease susceptibility. *Nat Genet.* 2007;39:830.

53. McCarroll SA, Huett A, Kuballa P, et al. Deletion polymorphism upstream of IRGM associated with altered IRGM expression and Crohn's disease. *Nat Genet.* 2008;40:1107.

54. Prescott NJ, Dominy KM, Kubo M, et al. Independent and population-specific association of risk variants at the IRGM locus with Crohn's disease. *Hum Mol Genet.* 2010;19:1828.

55. Kuballa P, Huett A, Rioux JD, Daly MJ, Xavier RJ. Impaired autophagy of an intracellular pathogen induced by a Crohn's disease associated ATG16L1 variant. *PLoS One.* 2008;3:e3391.

56. Homer CR, Richmond AL, Rebert NA, Achkar JP, McDonald C. ATG16L1 and NOD2 interact in an autophagy-dependent antibacterial pathway implicated in Crohn's disease pathogenesis. *Gastroenterology.* 2010;139:1630.

57. Sadaghian Sadabad M, Regeling A, de Goffau MC, et al. The ATG16L1-T300A allele impairs clearance of pathosymbiont in the inflamed ileal mucosa of Crohn's disease patients. *Gut.* 2015;64:1546.

58. Cadwell K, Liu JY, Brown SL, et al. A key role for autophagy and the autophagy gene Atg16l1 in mouse and human intestinal Paneth cells. *Nature.* 2008;456:259.

59. Li J, Jia H, Cai X, et al. An integrated catalog of reference genes in the human gut microbiome. *Nat Biotechnol.* 2014;32:834.

60. Lynch SV, Pedersen O. The human intestinal microbiome in health and disease. *N Engl J Med.* 2016;375:2369.

61. Seksik P, Rigottier-Gois L, Gramet G, et al. Alterations of the dominant faecal bacterial groups in patients with Crohn's disease of the colon. *Gut.* 2003;52:237.

62. Ott SJ, Musfeldt M, Wenderoth DF, et al. Reduction in diversity of the colonic mucosa associated bacterial microflora in patients with active inflammatory bowel disease. *Gut.* 2004;53:685.

63. Manichanh C, Rigottier-Gois L, Bonnaud E, et al. Reduced diversity of faecal microbiota in Crohn's disease revealed by a metagenomic approach. *Gut.* 2006;55:205.

64. Gophna U, Sommerfeld K, Gophna S, Ford Doolittle W, Veldhuyzen van Zanten SJO. Differences between tissue-associated intestinal microfloras of patients with Crohn's disease and ulcerative colitis. *J Clin Microbiol.* 2006;44:4136.

65. Frank DN, St Amand AL, Feldman RA, et al. Molecular-phylogenetic characterization of microbial community imbalances in human inflammatory bowel diseases. *Proc Natl Acad Sci USA.* 2007;104:13780.

66. Kostic AD, Xavier RJ, Gevers D. The microbiome in inflammatory bowel disease: current status and the future ahead. *Gastroenterology.* 2014;146: 1489.

67. Norman JM, Handley SA, Baldridge MT, et al. Disease-specific alterations in the enteric virome in inflammatory bowel disease. *Cell.* 2015;160:447.

68. De Filippo C, Cavalieri D, Di Paola M, et al. Impact of diet in shaping gut microbiota revealed by a comparative study in children from Europe and rural Africa. *Proc Natl Acad Sci USA.* 2010;107: 14691.

69. Yatsunenko T, Rey FE, Manary MJ, et al. Human gut microbiome viewed across age and geography. *Nature.* 2012;486:222.

70. Wu GD, Chen J, Hoffmann C, et al. Linking long-term dietary patterns with gut microbial enterotypes. *Science.* 2011;334:105.

71. Zimmer J, Lange B, Frick JS, et al. A vegan or vegetarian diet substantially alters the human colonic faecal microbiota. *Eur J Clin Nutr.* 2012;66:53.

72. Lee D, Albenberg L, Compher C, et al. Diet in the pathogenesis and treatment of inflammatory bowel diseases. *Gastroenterology.* 2015;148: 1087.

73. Lewis JD, Chen EZ, Baldassano RN, et al. Inflammation, antibiotics, and diet as environmental stressors of the gut microbiome in pediatric Crohn's disease. *Cell Host Microbe.* 2015;18:489.

74. Biedermann L, Zeitz J, Mwinyi J, et al. Smoking cessation induces profound changes in the composition of the intestinal microbiota in humans. *PLoS One.* 2013;8:e59260.

75. Cadwell K, Patel KK, Maloney NS, et al. Virus-plus-susceptibility gene interaction determines Crohn's disease gene Atg16L1 phenotypes in intestine. *Cell.* 2010;141:1135.

76. Bloom SM, Bijanki VN, Nava GM, et al. Commensal *Bacteroides* species induce colitis in host-genotype-specific fashion in a mouse model of inflammatory bowel disease. *Cell Host Microbe.* 2011;9:390.

77. Desai MS, Seekatz AM, Koropatkin NM, et al. A dietary fiber-deprived gut microbiota degrades the colonic mucus barrier and enhances pathogen susceptibility. *Cell.* 2016;167:1339.

78. Crohn BB, Ginzburg L, Oppenheimer GD. Landmark article Oct 15, 1932. Regional ileitis. A pathological and clinical entity. By Burril B. Crohn, Leon Ginzburg, and Gordon D. Oppenheimer. *JAMA.* 1984;251:73.

79. Farmer RG. Long-term prognosis for patients with ulcerative proctosigmoiditis (ulcerative colitis confirmed to the rectum and sigmoid colon). *J Clin Gastroenterol.* 1979;1:47.

80. Powell-Tuck J, Ritchie JK, Lennard-Jones JE. The prognosis of idiopathic proctitis. *Scand J Gastroenterol.* 1977;12:727.

81. Farmer RG, Easley KA, Rankin GB. Clinical patterns, natural history, and progression of ulcerative colitis. A long-term follow-up of 1116 patients. *Dig Dis Sci.* 1993;38:1137.

82. Solberg IC, Hoivik ML, Cvancarova M, Moum B. IBSEN Study Group: Risk matrix model for prediction of colectomy in a population-based study of ulcerative colitis patients (the IBSEN study). *Scand J Gastroenterol.* 2015;50:1456.

83. Silverberg MS, Satsangi J, Ahmad T, et al. Toward an integrated clinical, molecular and serological classification of inflammatory bowel disease: report of a Working Party of the 2005 Montreal World Congress of Gastroenterology. *Can J Gastroenterol.* 2005;(19 supplA):5A.

84. Economou M, Trikalinos TA, Loizou KT, Tsianos EV, Ioannidis JP. Differential effects of NOD2 variants on Crohn's disease risk and phenotype in diverse populations: a metaanalysis. *Am J Gastroenterol.* 2004;99:2393.

85. Ahmad T, Marshall SE, Jewell D. Genetics of inflammatory bowel disease: the role of the HLA complex. *World J Gastroenterol.* 2006;12:3628.

86. Cleynen I, Boucher G, Jostins L, et al. Inherited determinants of Crohn's disease and ulcerative colitis phenotypes: a genetic association study. *Lancet.* 2016;387:156.

87. Kugathasan S, Denson LA, Walters TD, et al. Prediction of complicated disease course for children newly diagnosed with Crohn's disease: a multicentre inception cohort study. *Lancet.* 2017;389:1710.

88. Li J, Wei Z, Hakonarson H. Application of computational methods in genetic study of inflammatory bowel disease. *World J Gastroenterol.* 2016;22:949.

89. Hou JK, Gasche C, Drazin NZ, et al. Assessment of gaps in care and the development of a care pathway for anemia in patients with inflammatory bowel diseases. *Inflamm Bowel Dis.* 2017;23:35.

90. Wasan SK, Coukos JA, Farraye FA. Vaccinating the inflammatory bowel disease patient: deficiencies in gastroenterologists' knowledge. *Inflamm Bowel Dis.* 2011;17:2536.

91. Tinsley A, Naymagon S, Trindade AJ, Sachar DB, Sands BE, Ullman TA. A survey of current practice of venous thromboembolism prophylaxis in hospitalized inflammatory bowel disease patients in the United States. *J Clin Gastroenterol.* 2013;47:e1.

92. Sam JJ, Bernstein CN, Razik R, Thanabalan R, Nguyen GC. Physicians' perceptions of risks and practices in venous thromboembolism prophylaxis in inflammatory bowel disease. *Dig Dis Sci.* 2013;58:46.

93. Krishnarao A, de Leon L, Bright R, et al. Testing for *Clostridium difficile* in patients newly diagnosed with inflammatory bowel disease in a community setting. *Inflamm Bowel Dis.* 2015;21:564.

94. Nguyen GC, Laveist TA, Gearhart S, Bayless TM, Brant SR. Racial and geographic variations in colectomy rates among hospitalized ulcerative colitis patients. *Clin Gastroenterol Hepatol.* 2006;4:1507.

95. Kappelman MD, Bousvaros A, Hyams J, et al. Intercenter variation in initial management of children with Crohn's disease. *Inflamm Bowel Dis.* 2007;13:890.

96. Sewell JL, Velayos FS. Systematic review: the role of race and socioeconomic factors on IBD healthcare delivery and effectiveness. *Inflamm Bowel Dis.* 2013;19:627.

97. Nguyen GC, Bayless TM, Powe NR, Laveist TA, Brant SR. Race and health insurance are predictors of hospitalized Crohn's disease patients undergoing bowel resection. *Inflamm Bowel Dis.* 2007;13:1408.

98. Kaplan GG, McCarthy EP, Ayanian JZ, Korzenik J, Hodin R, Sands BE. Impact of hospital volume on postoperative morbidity and mortality following a colectomy for ulcerative colitis. *Gastroenterology.* 2008;134:680.

99. Murthy SK, Steinhart AH, Tinmouth J, Austin PC, Nguyen GC. Impact of gastroenterologist care on health outcomes of hospitalised ulcerative colitis patients. *Gut.* 2012;61:1410.

100. Allen JI, Dassopoulos T. American Gastroenterological Association. Adult Inflammatory Bowel Disease Physician Performance Measures Set, 2011. http://www.gastro.org/practice/quality-initiatives/IBD_Measures.pdf. Accessed 10.03.17.

101. Melmed GY, Siegel CA, Spiegel BM, et al. Quality indicators for inflammatory bowel disease: development of process and outcome measures. *Inflamm Bowel Dis.* 2013;19:662.

102. Nguyen GC, Devlin SM, Afif W, et al. Defining quality indicators for best-practice management of inflammatory bowel disease in Canada. *Can J Gastroenterol Hepatol.* 2014;28:275.

103. Ananthakrishnan AN, Kwon J, Raffals L, et al. Variation in treatment of patients with inflammatory bowel diseases at major referral centers in the United States. *Clin Gastroenterol Hepatol.* 2015;13:1197.

104. Bilal M, Singh S, Lee H, Khosa K, Ehehra R, Clarke K. Bridges to excellence quality indicators in inflammatory bowel disease (IBD): differences between IBD and non-IBD gastroenterologists. *Ann Gastroenterol.* 2017;30:192.

105. Crandall WV, Margolis PA, Kappelman MD, et al. Improved outcomes in a quality improvement collaborative for pediatric inflammatory bowel disease. *Pediatrics.* 2012;129:e1030.

106. Nguyen GC, LaVeist TA, Harris ML, Datta LW, Bayless TM, Brant SR. Patient trust-in-physician and race are predictors of adherence to medical management in inflammatory bowel disease. *Inflamm Bowel Dis.* 2009;15:1233.

107. Robinson A, Thompson DG, Wilkin D, Roberts C. Northwest Gastrointestinal Research Group: Guided self-management and patient-directed follow-up of ulcerative colitis: a randomised trial. *Lancet.* 2001;358:976.

108. Elkjaer M, Shuhaibar M, Burisch J, et al. E-health empowers patients with ulcerative colitis: a randomised controlled trial of the web-guided 'Constant-care' approach. *Gut.* 2010;59:1652.

109. Calvet X, Panes J, Alfaro N, et al. Delphi consensus statement: quality indicators for inflammatory bowel disease comprehensive care units. *J Crohns Colitis.* 2014;8:240.

110. Louis E, Dotan I, Ghosh S, Mlynarsky L, Reenaers C, Schreiber S. Optimising the inflammatory bowel disease unit to improve quality of care: expert recommendations. *J Crohns Colitis.* 2015;9:685.

111. Trivedi I, Holl JL, Hanauer S, Keefer L. Integrating adolescents and young adults into adult-centered care for IBD. *Curr Gastroenterol Rep.* 2016;18:21.

112. Bitton A, Sewitch MJ, Peppercorn MA, et al. Psychosocial determinants of relapse in ulcerative colitis: a longitudinal study. *Am J Gastroenterol.* 2003;98:2203.

113. Mittermaier C, Dejaco C, Waldhoer T, et al. Impact of depressive mood on relapse in patients with inflammatory bowel disease: a prospective 18-month follow-up study. *Psychosom Med.* 2004;66:79.

114. Persoons P, Vermeire S, Demyttenaere K, et al. The impact of major depressive disorder on the short- and long-term outcome of Crohn's disease treatment with infliximab. *Aliment Pharmacol Ther.* 2005;22:101.

115. Boye B, Lundin KE, Jantschek G, et al. INSPIRE study: does stress management improve the course of inflammatory bowel disease and disease-specific quality of life in distressed patients with ulcerative colitis or Crohn's disease? A randomized controlled trial. *Inflamm Bowel Dis.* 2011;17:1863.

116. Diaz Sibaja MA, Comeche Moreno MI, Mas Hesse B. [Protocolized cognitive-behavioural group therapy for inflammatory bowel disease]. *Rev Esp Enferm Dig.* 2007;99:593.

117. Goodhand JR, Greig FI, Koodun Y, et al. Do antidepressants influence the disease course in inflammatory bowel disease? A retrospective case-matched observational study. *Inflamm Bowel Dis.* 2012 18:1232.

118. Jelsness-Jorgensen LP, Bernklev T, Henriksen M, Torp R, Moum B. Is patient reported outcome (PRO) affected by different follow-up regimens in inflammatory bowel disease (IBD)? A one year prospective, longitudinal comparison of nurse-led versus conventional follow-up. *J Crohns Colitis.* 2012;6:837.

119. Hanson KA, Loftus EV Jr, Harmsen WS, Diehl NN, Zinsmeister AR, Sandborn WJ. Clinical features and outcome of patients with inflammatory bowel disease who use narcotics: a case-control study. *Inflamm Bowel Dis.* 2009;15:772.

120. Long MD, Barnes EL, Herfarth HH, Drossman DA. Narcotic use for inflammatory bowel disease and risk factors during hospitalization. *Inflamm Bowel Dis*. 2012;18:869.

121. Targownik LE, Nugent Z, Singh H, Bugden S, Bernstein CN. The prevalence and predictors of opioid use in inflammatory bowel disease: a population-based analysis. *Am J Gastroenterol*. 2014;109:1613.

122. Kroeker KI, Lam S, Birchall I, Fedorak RN. Patients with IBD are exposed to high levels of ionizing radiation through CT scan diagnostic imaging: a five-year study. *J Clin Gastroenterol*. 2011;45:34.

123. Fuchs Y, Markowitz J, Weinstein T, Kohn N, Choi-Rosen J, Levine J. Pediatric inflammatory bowel disease and imaging-related radiation: are we increasing the likelihood of malignancy? *J Pediatr Gastroenterol Nutr*. 2011;52:280.

124. Chatu S, Subramanian V, Pollok RC. Meta-analysis: diagnostic medical radiation exposure in inflammatory bowel disease. *Aliment Pharmacol Ther*. 2012;35:529.

125. Lichtenstein GR, Hanauer SB, Sandborn WJ, et al. Management of Crohn's disease in adults. *Am J Gastroenterol*. 2009;104:465.

126. Kornbluth A, Sachar DB. Practice Parameters Committee of the American College of Gastroenterology: Ulcerative colitis practice guidelines in adults: American College of Gastroenterology, Practice Parameters Committee. *Am J Gastroenterol*. 2010;105:501.

127. Terdiman JP, Gruss CB, Heidelbaugh JJ, et al. American Gastroenterological Association Institute guideline on the use of thiopurines, methotrexate, and anti-TNF-alpha biologic drugs for the induction and maintenance of remission in inflammatory Crohn's disease. *Gastroenterology*. 2013;145:1459.

128. Bressler B, Marshall JK, Bernstein CN, et al. Clinical practice guidelines for the medical management of nonhospitalized ulcerative colitis: the Toronto consensus. *Gastroenterology*. 2015;148:1035.

129. Gomollon F, Dignass A, Annese V, et al. 3rd European evidence-based consensus on the diagnosis and management of Crohn's disease 2016. Part 1: diagnosis and medical management. *J Crohns Colitis*. 2017;11:3.

130. Harbord M, Eliakim R, Bettenworth D, et al. Third European evidence-based consensus on diagnosis and management of ulcerative colitis. Part 2: current management. *J Crohns Colitis*. 2017;Jan 28 [Epub ahead of print].

131. Truelove SC, Witts LJ. Cortisone in ulcerative colitis; final report on a therapeutic trial. *Br Med J*. 1955;2:1041.

132. Sandborn WJ, Feagan BG, Hanauer SB, et al. A review of activity indices and efficacy endpoints for clinical trials of medical therapy in adults with Crohn's disease. *Gastroenterology*. 2002;122:512.

133. D'Haens G, Sandborn WJ, Feagan BG, et al. A review of activity indices and efficacy end points for clinical trials of medical therapy in adults with ulcerative colitis. *Gastroenterology*. 2007;132:763.

134. Modigliani R, Mary JY, Simon JF, et al. Clinical, biological, and endoscopic picture of attacks of Crohn's disease. Evolution on prednisolone. Groupe d'Etude Therapeutique des Affections Inflammatoires Digestives. *Gastroenterology*. 1990;98:811.

135. Cellier C, Sahmoud T, Froguel E, et al. Correlations between clinical activity, endoscopic severity, and biological parameters in colonic or ileocolonic Crohn's disease. A prospective multicentre study of 121 cases. The Groupe d'Etudes Therapeutique des Affections Inflammatoires Digestives. *Gut*. 1994;35:231.

136. Daperno M, D'Haens G, Van Assche G, et al. Development and validation of a new, simplified endoscopic activity score for Crohn's disease: the SES-CD. *Gastrointest Endosc*. 2004;60:505.

137. Rutgeerts P, Diamond RH, Bala M, et al. Scheduled maintenance treatment with infliximab is superior to episodic treatment for the healing of mucosal ulceration associated with Crohn's disease. *Gastrointest Endosc*. 2006;63:433.

138. Higgins PD, Schwartz M, Mapili J, Zimmermann EM. Is endoscopy necessary for the measurement of disease activity in ulcerative colitis? *Am J Gastroenterol*. 2005;100:355.

139. Dhanda AD, Creed TJ, Greenwood R, Sands BE, Probert CS. Can endoscopy be avoided in the assessment of ulcerative colitis in clinical trials? *Inflamm Bowel Dis*. 2012;18:2056.

140. Lewis JD, Chuai S, Nessel L, Lichtenstein GR, Aberra FN, Ellenberg JH. Use of the noninvasive components of the Mayo score to assess clinical response in ulcerative colitis. *Inflamm Bowel Dis*. 2008;14:1660.

141. Bewtra M, Brensinger CM, Tomov VT, et al. An optimized patient-reported ulcerative colitis disease activity measure derived from the Mayo score and the simple clinical colitis activity index. *Inflamm Bowel Dis*. 2014;20:1070.

142. Froslie KF, Jahnsen J, Moum BA, Vatn MH, Group IBSEN. Mucosal healing in inflammatory bowel disease: results from a Norwegian population-based cohort. *Gastroenterology*. 2007;133:412.

143. Ardizzone S, Cassinotti A, Duca P, et al. Mucosal healing predicts late outcomes after the first course of corticosteroids for newly diagnosed ulcerative colitis. *Clin Gastroenterol Hepatol*. 2011;9:483.

144. Colombel JF, Rutgeerts P, Reinisch W, et al. Early mucosal healing with infliximab is associated with improved long-term clinical outcomes in ulcerative colitis. *Gastroenterology*. 2011;141:1194.

145. Shah SC, Colombel JF, Sands BE, Narula N. Systematic review with meta-analysis: mucosal healing is associated with improved long-term outcomes in Crohn's disease. *Aliment Pharmacol Ther*. 2016;43:317.

146. Shah SC, Colombel JF, Sands BE, Narula N. Mucosal healing is associated with improved long-term outcomes of patients with ulcerative colitis: a systematic review and meta-analysis. *Clin Gastroenterol Hepatol*. 2016;14:1245.

147. Sandborn WJ. Crohn's disease evaluation and treatment: clinical decision tool. *Gastroenterology*. 2014;147:702.

148. Dassopoulos T, Cohen RD, Scherl EJ, Schwartz RM, Kosinski L, Regueiro MD. Ulcerative colitis care pathway. *Gastroenterology*. 2015;149:S8.

149. Rousseaux C, Lefebvre B, Dubuquoy L, et al. Intestinal antiinflammatory effect of 5-aminosalicylic acid is dependent on peroxisome proliferator-activated receptor-gamma. *J Exp Med*. 2005;201:1205.

150. Sharon P, Ligumsky M, Rachmilewitz D, Zor U. Role of prostaglandins in ulcerative colitis. Enhanced production during active disease and inhibition by sulfasalazine. *Gastroenterology*. 1978;75:638.

151. Ahnfelt-Ronne I, Nielsen OH, Christensen A, Langholz E, Binder V, Riis P. Clinical evidence supporting the radical scavenger mechanism of 5-aminosalicylic acid. *Gastroenterology*. 1990;98:1162.

152. Ford AC, Achkar JP, Khan KJ, et al. Efficacy of 5-aminosalicylates in ulcerative colitis: systematic review and meta-analysis. *Am J Gastroenterol*. 2011;106:601.

153. Hanauer SB, Sandborn WJ, Kornbluth A, et al. Delayed release oral mesalamine at 4.8 g/day (800 mg tablet) for the treatment of moderately active ulcerative colitis: the ASCEND II trial. *Am J Gastroenterol*. 2005;100:2478.

154. Cohen RD, Woseth DM, Thisted RA, Hanauer SB. A meta-analysis and overview of the literature on treatment options for left-sided ulcerative colitis and ulcerative proctitis. *Am J Gastroenterol*. 2000;95:1263.

155. Safdi M, DeMicco M, Sninsky C, et al. A double-blind comparison of oral versus rectal mesalamine versus combination therapy in the treatment of distal ulcerative colitis. *Am J Gastroenterol*. 1997;92:1867.

156. Marteau P, Probert CS, Lindgren S, et al. Combined oral and enema treatment with Pentasa (mesalazine) is superior to oral therapy alone in patients with extensive mild/moderate active ulcerative colitis: a randomised, double blind, placebo controlled study. *Gut*. 2005;54:960.

157. d'Albasio G, Pacini F, Camarri E, et al. Combined therapy with 5-aminosalicylic acid tablets and enemas for maintaining remission in ulcerative colitis: a randomized double-blind study. *Am J Gastroenterol*. 1997;92:1143.

158. Sandborn WJ, Travis S, Moro L, et al. Once-daily budesonide MMX(R) extended-release tablets induce remission in patients with mild to moderate ulcerative colitis: results from the CORE I study. *Gastroenterology*. 2012;143:1218.

159. Travis SP, Danese S, Kupcinskas L, et al. Once-daily budesonide MMX in active, mild-to-moderate ulcerative colitis: results from the randomised CORE II study. *Gut*. 2014;63:433.

160. Turner D, Walsh CM, Steinhart AH, Griffiths AM. Response to corticosteroids in severe ulcerative colitis: a systematic review of the literature and a meta-regression. *Clin Gastroenterol Hepatol*. 2007;5:103.

161. Carbonnel F, Gargouri D, Lemann M, et al. Predictive factors of outcome of intensive intravenous treatment for attacks of ulcerative colitis. *Aliment Pharmacol Ther*. 2000;14:273.

162. Bossa F, Fiorella S, Caruso N, et al. Continuous infusion versus bolus administration of steroids in severe attacks of ulcerative colitis: a randomized, double-blind trial. *Am J Gastroenterol*. 2007;102:601.

163. Bitton A, Buie D, Enns R, et al. Treatment of hospitalized adult patients with severe ulcerative colitis: Toronto consensus statements. *Am J Gastroenterol*. 2012;107:179.

164. Afif W, Loftus EV Jr. Safety profile of IBD therapeutics: infectious risks. *Gastroenterol Clin North Am.* 2009;38:691.

165. Lichtenstein GR, Feagan BG, Cohen RD, et al. Serious infection and mortality in patients with Crohn's disease: more than 5 years of follow-up in the TREAT registry. *Am Gastroenterol.* 2012;107:1409.

166. Brassard P, Bitton A, Suissa A, Sinyavskaya L, Patenaude V, Suissa S. Oral corticosteroids and the risk of serious infections in patients with elderly-onset inflammatory bowel diseases. *Am J Gastroenterol.* 2014;109:1795.

167. Nguyen GC, Elnahas A, Jackson TD. The impact of preoperative steroid use on short-term outcomes following surgery for inflammatory bowel disease. *J Crohns Colitis.* 2014;8:1661.

168. Faubion WA Jr, Loftus EV Jr, Harmsen WS, Zinsmeister AR, Sandborn WJ. The natural history of corticosteroid therapy for inflammatory bowel disease: a population-based study. *Gastroenterology.* 2001;121:255.

169. Lichtiger S, Present DH, Kornbluth A, et al. Cyclosporine in severe ulcerative colitis refractory to steroid therapy. *N Engl J Med.* 1994;330:1841.

170. Van Assche G, Vermeire S, Rutgeerts P. Management of acute severe ulcerative colitis. *Gut.* 2011;60:130.

171. Moskovitz DN, Van Assche G, Maenhout B, et al. Incidence of colectomy during long-term follow-up after cyclosporine-induced remission of severe ulcerative colitis. *Clin Gastroenterol Hepatol.* 2006;4:760.

172. Cohen RD, Stein R, Hanauer SB. Intravenous cyclosporin in ulcerative colitis: a five-year experience. *Am J Gastroenterol.* 1999;94:1587.

173. D'Haens G, Lemmens L, Geboes K, et al. Intravenous cyclosporine versus intravenous corticosteroids as single therapy for severe attacks of ulcerative colitis. *Gastroenterology.* 2001;120:1323.

174. Laharie D, Bourreille A, Branche J, et al. Long-term outcome of patients with steroid-refractory acute severe UC treated with ciclosporin or infliximab. *Gut.* 2017;Jan 4 [Epub ahead of print].

175. Van Assche G, D'Haens G, Noman M, et al. Randomized, double-blind comparison of 4 mg/kg versus 2 mg/kg intravenous cyclosporine in severe ulcerative colitis. *Gastroenterology.* 2003;125:1025.

176. Fellermann K, Tanko Z, Herrlinger KR, et al. Response of refractory colitis to intravenous or oral tacrolimus (FK506). *Inflamm Bowel Dis.* 2002;8:317.

177. Hogenauer C, Wenzl HH, Hinterleitner TA, Petritsch W. Effect of oral tacrolimus (FK 506) on steroid-refractory moderate/severe ulcerative colitis. *Aliment Pharmacol Ther.* 2003;18:415.

178. Ogata H, Kato J, Hirai F, et al. Double-blind, placebo-controlled trial of oral tacrolimus (FK506) in the management of hospitalized patients with steroid-refractory ulcerative colitis. *Inflamm Bowel Dis.* 2012;18:803.

179. Atreya I, Neurath MF. Azathioprine in inflammatory bowel disease: improved molecular insights and resulting clinical implications. *Expert Rev Gastroenterol Hepatol.* 2008;2:23.

180. Ha C, Dassopoulos T. Thiopurine therapy in inflammatory bowel disease. *Expert Rev Gastroenterol Hepatol.* 2010;4:575.

181. Ardizzone S, Maconi G, Russo A, Imbesi V, Colombo E, Bianchi Porro G. Randomised controlled trial of azathioprine and 5-aminosalicylic acid for treatment of steroid dependent ulcerative colitis. *Gut.* 2006;55:47.

182. Mantzaris GJ, Sfakianakis M, Archavlis E, et al. A prospective randomized observer-blind 2-year trial of azathioprine monotherapy versus azathioprine and olsalazine for the maintenance of remission of steroid-dependent ulcerative colitis. *Am J Gastroenterol.* 2004;99:1122.

183. Sood A, Midha V, Sood N, Kaushal V. Role of azathioprine in severe ulcerative colitis: one-year, placebo-controlled, randomized trial. *Indian J Gastroenterol.* 2000;19:14.

184. Panaccione R, Ghosh S, Middleton S, et al. Combination therapy with infliximab and azathioprine is superior to monotherapy with either agent in ulcerative colitis. *Gastroenterology.* 2014;146:392.

185. Colombel JF, Sandborn WJ, Reinisch W, et al. Infliximab, azathioprine, or combination therapy for Crohn's disease. *N Engl J Med.* 2010;362:1383.

186. Dassopoulos T, Sninsky CA. Optimizing immunomodulators and anti-TNF agents in the therapy of Crohn disease. *Gastroenterol Clin North Am.* 2012;41:393.

187. Herrinton LJ, Liu L, Weng X, Lewis JD, Hutfless S, Allison JE. Role of thiopurine and anti-TNF therapy in lymphoma in inflammatory bowel disease. *Am J Gastroenterol.* 2011;106:2146.

188. Beaugerie L, Brousse N, Bouvier AM, et al. Lymphoproliferative disorders in patients receiving thiopurines for inflammatory bowel disease: a prospective observational cohort study. *Lancet.* 2009;374:1617.

189. Long MD, Herfarth HH, Pipkin CA, Porter CQ, Sandler RS, Kappelman MD. Increased risk for non-melanoma skin cancer in patients with inflammatory bowel disease. *Clin Gastroenterol Hepatol.* 2010;8:268.

190. Dassopoulos T, Sultan S, Falck-Ytter YT, Inadomi JM, Hanauer SB. American Gastroenterological Association Institute technical review on the use of thiopurines, methotrexate, and anti-TNF-alpha biologic drugs for the induction and maintenance of remission in inflammatory Crohn's disease. *Gastroenterology.* 2013;145:1464.

191. Lewis JD, Schwartz JS, Lichtenstein GR. Azathioprine for maintenance of remission in Crohn's disease: benefits outweigh the risk of lymphoma. *Gastroenterology.* 2000;118:1018.

192. Dassopoulos T, Sorrentino D. Infliximab vs adalimumab for Crohn's disease: perhaps too early to call it a tie. *Clin Gastroenterol Hepatol.* 2014;12:818.

193. Ordas I, Feagan BG, Sandborn WJ. Therapeutic drug monitoring of tumor necrosis factor antagonists in inflammatory bowel disease. *Clin Gastroenterol Hepatol.* 2012;10:1079.

194. Rutgeerts P, Sandborn WJ, Feagan BG, et al. Infliximab for induction and maintenance therapy for ulcerative colitis. *N Engl J Med.* 2005;353:2462.

195. Sandborn WJ, van Assche G, Reinisch W, et al. Adalimumab induces and maintains clinical remission in patients with moderate-to-severe ulcerative colitis. *Gastroenterology.* 2012;142:257.

196. Reinisch W, Sandborn WJ, Hommes DW, et al. Adalimumab for induction of clinical remission in moderately to severely active ulcerative colitis: results of a randomised controlled trial. *Gut.* 2011;60:780.

197. Sandborn WJ, Feagan BG, Marano C, et al. Subcutaneous golimumab maintains clinical response in patients with moderate-to-severe ulcerative colitis. *Gastroenterology.* 2014;146:96.

198. Sandborn WJ, Feagan BG, Marano C, et al. Subcutaneous golimumab induces clinical response and remission in patients with moderate-to-severe ulcerative colitis. *Gastroenterology.* 2014;146:85.

199. Singh S, Andersen NN, Andersson M, et al. Comparison of infliximab and adalimumab in biologic-naive patients with ulcerative colitis: a nationwide Danish cohort study. *Clin Gastroenterol Hepatol.* 2017;15(8):1218-1225.

200. Singh S, Heien HC, Sangaralingham LR, et al. Comparative effectiveness and safety of infliximab and adalimumab in patients with ulcerative colitis. *Aliment Pharmacol Ther.* 2016;43:994.

201. Ananthakrishnan AN, Cagan A, Cai T, et al. Comparative effectiveness of infliximab and adalimumab in Crohn's disease and ulcerative colitis. *Inflamm Bowel Dis.* 2016;22:880.

202. Sandborn WJ, Sakuraba A, Wang A, et al. Comparison of real-world outcomes of adalimumab and infliximab for patients with ulcerative colitis in the United States. *Curr Med Res Opin.* 2016;32:1233.

203. Qiu Y, Mao R, Chen BL, et al. Effects of combination therapy with immunomodulators on trough levels and antibodies against tumor necrosis factor antagonists in patients with inflammatory bowel disease: a meta-analysis. *Clin Gastroenterol Hepatol.* 2017;15(9):1359-1372.

204. Jarnerot G, Hertervig E, Friis-Liby I, et al. Infliximab as rescue therapy in severe to moderately severe ulcerative colitis: a randomized, placebo-controlled study. *Gastroenterology.* 2005;128:1805.

205. Gustavsson A, Jarnerot G, Hertervig E, et al. Clinical trial: colectomy after rescue therapy in ulcerative colitis—3-year follow-up of the Swedish-Danish controlled infliximab study. *Aliment Pharmacol Ther.* 2010;32:984.

206. Ochsenkuhn T, Sackmann M, Goke B. Infliximab for acute, not steroid-refractory ulcerative colitis: a randomized pilot study. *Eur J Gastroenterol Hepatol.* 2004;16:1167.

207. Steenholdt C, Bendtzen K, Brynskov J, Ainsworth MA. Optimizing treatment with TNF inhibitors in inflammatory bowel disease by monitoring drug levels and antidrug antibodies. *Inflamm Bowel Dis.* 2016;22:1999.

208. Ghosh S, Goldin E, Gordon FH, et al. Natalizumab for active Crohn's disease. *N Engl J Med.* 2003;348:24.

209. Sandborn WJ, Colombel JF, Enns R, et al. Natalizumab induction and maintenance therapy for Crohn's disease. *N Engl J Med.* 2005;353:1912.

210. Targan SR, Feagan BG, Fedorak RN, et al. Natalizumab for the treatment of active Crohn's disease: results of the ENCORE Trial. *Gastroenterology.* 2007;132:1672.

211. Feagan BG, Rutgeerts P, Sands BE, et al. Vedolizumab as induction and maintenance therapy for ulcerative colitis. *N Engl J Med*. 2013;369:699.

212. Feagan BG, Rubin DT, Danese S, et al. Efficacy of vedolizumab induction and maintenance therapy in patients with ulcerative colitis, regardless of prior exposure to tumor necrosis factor antagonists. *Clin Gastroenterol Hepatol*. 2017;15:229.

213. Dulai PS, Singh S, Jiang X, et al. The real-world effectiveness and safety of vedolizumab for moderate-severe Crohn's disease: results from the US VICTORY Consortium. *Am J Gastroenterol*. 2016;111:1147.

214. Loftus EV Jr, Colombel JF, Feagan BG, et al. Long-term efficacy of vedolizumab for ulcerative colitis. *J Crohns Colitis*. 2017;11:400.

215. Colombel JF, Sands BE, Rutgeerts P, et al. The safety of vedolizumab for ulcerative colitis and Crohn's disease. *Gut*. 2017;66:839.

216. Oren R, Arber N, Odes S, et al. Methotrexate in chronic active ulcerative colitis: a double-blind, randomized, Israeli multicenter trial. *Gastroenterology*. 1996;110:1416.

217. Carbonnel F, Colombel JF, Filippi J, et al. Methotrexate is not superior to placebo for inducing steroid-free remission, but induces steroid-free clinical remission in a larger proportion of patients with ulcerative colitis. *Gastroenterology*. 2016;150:380.

218. Chapman RW, Selby WS, Jewell DP. Controlled trial of intravenous metronidazole as an adjunct to corticosteroids in severe ulcerative colitis. *Gut*. 1986;27:1210.

219. Mantzaris GJ, Hatzis A, Kontogiannis P. Triadaphillou G: Intravenous tobramycin and metronidazole as an adjunct to corticosteroids in acute, severe ulcerative colitis. *Am J Gastroenterol*. 1994;89:43.

220. Moayyedi P, Surette MG, Kim PT, et al. Fecal microbiota transplantation induces remission in patients with active ulcerative colitis in a randomized controlled trial. *Gastroenterology*. 2015;149:102.

221. Rossen NG, Fuentes S, van der Spek MJ, et al. Findings from a randomized controlled trial of fecal transplantation for patients with ulcerative colitis. *Gastroenterology*. 2015;149:110.

222. Pullan RD, Rhodes J, Ganesh S, et al. Transdermal nicotine for active ulcerative colitis. *N Engl J Med*. 1994;330:811.

223. Thomas GA, Rhodes J, Mani V, et al. Transdermal nicotine as maintenance therapy for ulcerative colitis. *N Engl J Med*. 1995;332:988.

224. Sandborn WJ, Tremaine WJ, Offord KP, et al. Transdermal nicotine for mildly to moderately active ulcerative colitis. A randomized, double-blind, placebo-controlled trial. *Ann Intern Med*. 1997;126:364.

225. Richman E, Rhodes JM. Review article: evidence-based dietary advice for patients with inflammatory bowel disease. *Aliment Pharmacol Ther*. 2013;38:1156.

226. Dickinson RJ, Ashton MG, Axon AT, Smith RC, Yeung CK, Hill GL. Controlled trial of intravenous hyperalimentation and total bowel rest as an adjunct to the routine therapy of acute colitis. *Gastroenterology*. 1980;79:1199.

227. McIntyre PB, Powell-Tuck J, Wood SR, et al. Controlled trial of bowel rest in the treatment of severe acute colitis. *Gut*. 1986;27:481.

228. Probert CS, Dignass AU, Lindgren S, Oudkerk Pool M, Marteau P. Combined oral and rectal mesalazine for the treatment of mild-to-moderately active ulcerative colitis: rapid symptom resolution and improvements in quality of life. *J Crohns Colitis*. 2014;8:200.

229. Summers RW, Switz DM, Sessions JT Jr, et al. National Cooperative Crohn's Disease Study: results of drug treatment. *Gastroenterology*. 1979;77:847.

230. Malchow H, Ewe K, Brandes JW, et al. European Cooperative Crohn's Disease Study (ECCDS): results of drug treatment. *Gastroenterology*. 1984;86:249.

231. Ford AC, Bernstein CN, Khan KJ, et al. Glucocorticosteroid therapy in inflammatory bowel disease: systematic review and meta-analysis. *Am J Gastroenterol*. 2011;106:590.

232. Shepherd HA, Barr GD, Jewell DP. Use of an intravenous steroid regimen in the treatment of acute Crohn's disease. *J Clin Gastroenterol*. 1986;8:154.

233. Kornbluth AA, Salomon P, Sachar DB, et al. ACTH-induced adrenal hemorrhage: a complication of therapy masquerading as an acute abdomen. *J Clin Gastroenterol*. 1990;12:371.

234. Chun A, Chadi RM, Korelitz BI, et al. Intravenous corticotrophin vs. hydrocortisone in the treatment of hospitalized patients with Crohn's disease: a randomized double-blind study and follow-up. *Inflamm Bowel Dis*. 1998;4:177.

235. Felder JB, Adler DJ, Korelitz BI. The safety of corticosteroid therapy in Crohn's disease with an abdominal mass. *Am J Gastroenterol*. 1991;86:1450.

236. Gecse KB, Bemelman W, Kamm MA, et al. A global consensus on the classification, diagnosis and multidisciplinary treatment of perianal fistulising Crohn's disease. *Gut*. 2014;63:1381.

237. Gionchetti P, Dignass A, Danese S, et al. 3rd European evidence-based consensus on the diagnosis and management of Crohn's disease 2016. Part 2: surgical management and special situations. *J Crohns Colitis*. 2017;11:135.

238. Khan KJ, Ullman TA, Ford AC, et al. Antibiotic therapy in inflammatory bowel disease: a systematic review and meta-analysis. *Am J Gastroenterol*. 2011;106:661.

239. West RL, van der Woude CJ, Hansen BE, et al. Clinical and endosonographic effect of ciprofloxacin on the treatment of perianal fistulas in Crohn's disease with infliximab: a double-blind placebo-controlled study. *Aliment Pharmacol Ther*. 2004;20:1329.

240. Dewint P, Hansen BE, Verhey E, et al. Adalimumab combined with ciprofloxacin is superior to adalimumab monotherapy in perianal fistula closure in Crohn's disease: a randomised, double-blind, placebo controlled trial (ADAFI). *Gut*. 2014;63:292.

241. Singh S, Garg SK, Pardi DS, Wang Z, Murad MH, Loftus EV Jr. Comparative efficacy of pharmacologic interventions in preventing relapse of Crohn's disease after surgery: a systematic review and network meta-analysis. *Gastroenterology*. 2015;148:64.

242. Regueiro M, Velayos F, Greer JB, et al. American Gastroenterological Association Institute Technical review on the management of Crohn's disease after surgical resection. *Gastroenterology*. 2017;152:277.

243. Nguyen GC, Loftus EV Jr, Hirano I, et al. American Gastroenterological Association Institute guideline on the management of Crohn's disease after surgical resection. *Gastroenterology*. 2017;152:271.

244. Khan KJ, Dubinsky MC, Ford AC, Ullman TA, Talley NJ, Moayyedi P. Efficacy of immunosuppressive therapy for inflammatory bowel disease: a systematic review and meta-analysis. *Am J Gastroenterol*. 2011;106:630.

245. Markowitz J, Grancher K, Kohn N, Lesser M, Daum F. A multicenter trial of 6-mercaptopurine and prednisone in children with newly diagnosed Crohn's disease. *Gastroenterology*. 2000;119:895.

246. Cosnes J, Bourrier A, Laharie D, et al. Early administration of azathioprine vs conventional management of Crohn's disease: a randomized controlled trial. *Gastroenterology*. 2013;145:758.

247. Panes J, Lopez-Sanroman A, Bermejo F, et al. Early azathioprine therapy is no more effective than placebo for newly diagnosed Crohn's disease. *Gastroenterology*. 2013;145:766.

248. Egan LJ, Sandborn WJ. Methotrexate for inflammatory bowel disease: pharmacology and preliminary results. *Mayo Clin Proc*. 1996;71:69.

249. Cronstein B. How does methotrexate suppress inflammation? *Clin Exp Rheumatol*. 2010;28:S21.

250. Feagan BG, Rochon J, Fedorak RN, et al. Methotrexate for the treatment of Crohn's disease. The North American Crohn's Study Group Investigators. *N Engl J Med*. 1995;332:292.

251. Oren R, Moshkowitz M, Odes S, et al. Methotrexate in chronic active Crohn's disease: a double-blind, randomized, Israeli multicenter trial. *Am J Gastroenterol*. 1997;92:2203.

252. Patel V, Wang Y, MacDonald JK, Chande N. Methotrexate for maintenance of remission in Crohn's disease. *Cochrane Database Syst Rev*. 2014;(8):CD006884.

253. Feagan BG, McDonald JW, Panaccione R, et al. Methotrexate in combination with infliximab is no more effective than infliximab alone in patients with Crohn's disease. *Gastroenterology*. 2014;146:681.

254. Singh S, Pardi DS. Update on anti-tumor necrosis factor agents in Crohn disease. *Gastroenterol Clin North Am*. 2014;43:457.

255. Hazlewood GS, Rezaie A, Borman M, et al. Comparative effectiveness of immunosuppressants and biologics for inducing and maintaining remission in Crohn's disease: a network meta-analysis. *Gastroenterology*. 2015;148:344.

256. Regueiro M, Schraut W, Baidoo L, et al. Infliximab prevents Crohn's disease recurrence after ileal resection. *Gastroenterology*. 2009;136:441.

257. Yoshida K, Fukunaga K, Ikeuchi H, et al. Scheduled infliximab monotherapy to prevent recurrence of Crohn's disease following ileocolic or ileal resection: a 3-year prospective randomized open trial. *Inflamm Bowel Dis*. 2012;18:1617.

258. Savarino E, Bodini G, Dulbecco P, et al. Adalimumab is more effective than azathioprine and mesalamine at preventing postoperative recurrence of Crohn's disease: a randomized controlled trial. *Am J Gastroenterol*. 2013;108:1731.

259. Regueiro M, Kip KE, Baidoo L, Swoger JM, Schraut W. Postoperative therapy with infliximab prevents long-term Crohn's disease recurrence. *Clin Gastroenterol Hepatol.* 2014;12:1494.

260. De Cruz P, Kamm MA, Hamilton AL, et al. Efficacy of thiopurines and adalimumab in preventing Crohn's disease recurrence in high-risk patients—a POCER study analysis. *Aliment Pharmacol Ther.* 2015;42:867.

261. Regueiro M, Feagan BG, Zou B, et al. Infliximab reduces endoscopic, but not clinical, recurrence of Crohn's disease after ileocolonic resection. *Gastroenterology.* 2016;150:1568.

262. Sandborn WJ, Feagan BG, Rutgeerts P, et al. Vedolizumab as induction and maintenance therapy for Crohn's disease. *N Engl J Med.* 2013;369:711.

263. Sands BE, Feagan BG, Rutgeerts P, et al. Effects of vedolizumab induction therapy for patients with Crohn's disease in whom tumor necrosis factor antagonist treatment failed. *Gastroenterology.* 2014;147:618.

264. Noman M, Ferrante M, Bisschops R, et al. Vedolizumab induces long term mucosal healing in patients with Crohn's disease and ulcerative colitis. *J Crohns Colitis.* 2017;Mar 24 [Epub ahead of print].

265. Niederreiter L, Adolph TE, Kaser A. Anti-IL-12/23 in Crohn's disease: bench and bedside. *Curr Drug Targets.* 2013;14:1379.

266. Sandborn WJ, Gasink C, Gao LL, et al. Ustekinumab induction and maintenance therapy in refractory Crohn's disease. *N Engl J Med.* 2012;367:1519.

267. Feagan BG, Sandborn WJ, Gasink C, et al. Ustekinumab as induction and maintenance therapy for Crohn's disease. *N Engl J Med.* 2016;375:1946.

268. Papp K, Gottlieb AB, Naldi L, et al. Safety surveillance for ustekinumab and other psoriasis treatments from the Psoriasis Longitudinal Assessment and Registry (PSOLAR). *J Drugs Dermatol.* 2015;14:706.

269. Moja L, Danese S, Fiorino G, Del Giovane C, Bonovas S. Systematic review with network meta-analysis: comparative efficacy and safety of budesonide and mesalazine (mesalamine) for Crohn's disease. *Aliment Pharmacol Ther.* 2015;41:1055.

270. Lim WC, Wang Y, MacDonald JK, Hanauer S. Aminosalicylates for induction of remission or response in Crohn's disease. *Cochrane Database Syst Rev.* 2016;(7):CD008870.

271. Ford AC, Khan KJ, Talley NJ, Moayyedi P. 5-Aminosalicylates prevent relapse of Crohn's disease after surgically induced remission: systematic review and meta-analysis. *Am J Gastroenterol.* 2011;106:413.

272. Present DH, Lichtiger S. Efficacy of cyclosporine in treatment of fistula of Crohn's disease. *Dig Dis Sci.* 1994;39:374.

273. Hanauer SB, Smith MB. Rapid closure of Crohn's disease fistulas with continuous intravenous cyclosporin A. *Am J Gastroenterol.* 1993;88:646.

274. Egan LJ, Sandborn WJ, Tremaine WJ. Clinical outcome following treatment of refractory inflammatory and fistulizing Crohn's disease with intravenous cyclosporine. *Am J Gastroenterol.* 1998;93:442.

275. McDonald JW, Feagan BG, Jewell D, Brynskov J, Stange EF, Macdonald JK. Cyclosporine for induction of remission in Crohn's disease. *Cochrane Database Syst Rev.* 2005;(2):CD000297.

276. Laharie D, Reffet A, Belleannee G, et al. Mucosal healing with methotrexate in Crohn's disease: a prospective comparative study with azathioprine and infliximab. *Aliment Pharmacol Ther.* 2011; 33:714.

277. Cholapranee A, Hazlewood GS, Kaplan GG, Peyrin-Biroulet L, Ananthakrishnan AN. Systematic review with meta-analysis: comparative efficacy of biologics for induction and maintenance of mucosal healing in Crohn's disease and ulcerative colitis controlled trials. *Aliment Pharmacol Ther.* 2017;45:1291.

278. D'Haens G, Baert F, van Assche G, et al. Early combined immunosuppression or conventional management in patients with newly diagnosed Crohn's disease: an open randomised trial. *Lancet.* 2008;371:660.

279. Khanna R, Bressler B, Levesque BG, et al. Early combined immunosuppression for the management of Crohn's disease (REACT): a cluster randomised controlled trial. *Lancet.* 2015;386:1825.

280. Leijonmarck CE, Persson PG, Hellers G. Factors affecting colectomy rate in ulcerative colitis: an epidemiologic study. *Gut.* 1990;31:329.

281. Thia KT, Sandborn WJ, Harmsen WS, Zinsmeister AR, Loftus EV Jr. Risk factors associated with progression to intestinal complications of Crohn's disease in a population-based cohort. *Gastroenterology.* 2010;139:1147.

282. Rungoe C, Langholz E, Andersson M, et al. Changes in medical treatment and surgery rates in inflammatory bowel disease: a nationwide cohort study 1979–2011. *Gut.* 2014;63:1607.

283. Patel KV, Darakhshan AA, Griffin N, Williams AB, Sanderson JD, Irving PM. Patient optimization for surgery relating to Crohn's disease. *Nat Rev Gastroenterol Hepatol.* 2016;13:707.

284. Nickerson TP, Merchea A. Perioperative considerations in Crohn disease and ulcerative colitis. *Clin Colon Rectal Surg.* 2016;29:80.

285. Warner DO. Perioperative abstinence from cigarettes: physiologic and clinical consequences. *Anesthesiology.* 2006;104:356.

286. Musallam KM, Rosendaal FR, Zaatari G, et al. Smoking and the risk of mortality and vascular and respiratory events in patients undergoing major surgery. *JAMA Surg.* 2013;148:755.

287. U. S. Preventive Services Task Force. Counseling and interventions to prevent tobacco use and tobacco-caused disease in adults and pregnant women: U.S. Preventive Services Task Force reaffirmation recommendation statement. *Ann Intern Med.* 2009;150:551.

288. Thomsen T, Villebro N, Moller AM. Interventions for preoperative smoking cessation. *Cochrane Database Syst Rev.* 2014;(3):CD002294.

289. Wong J, Lam DP, Abrishami A, Chan MT, Chung F. Short-term preoperative smoking cessation and postoperative complications: a systematic review and meta-analysis. *Can J Anaesth.* 2012;59:268.

290. Breuer-Katschinski BD, Hollander N, Goebell H. Effect of cigarette smoking on the course of Crohn's disease. *Eur J Gastroenterol Hepatol.* 1996;8:225.

291. Kwon S, Thompson R, Dellinger P, Yanez D, Farrohki E, Flum D. Importance of perioperative glycemic control in general surgery: a report from the Surgical Care and Outcomes Assessment Program. *Ann Surg.* 2013;257:8.

292. Jackson RS, Amdur RL, White JC, Macsata RA. Hyperglycemia is associated with increased risk of morbidity and mortality after colectomy for cancer. *J Am Coll Surg.* 2012;214:68.

293. Kiran RP, Turina M, Hammel J, Fazio V. The clinical significance of an elevated postoperative glucose value in nondiabetic patients after colorectal surgery: evidence for the need for tight glucose control? *Ann Surg.* 2013;258:599.

294. Burisch J, Vegh Z, Katsanos KH, et al. Occurrence of anaemia in the first year of inflammatory bowel disease in a European population-based inception cohort—an ECCO-EpiCom study. *J Crohns Colitis.* 2017;May 31 [Epub ahead of print].

295. Murawska N, Fabisiak A, Fichna J. Anemia of chronic disease and iron deficiency anemia in inflammatory bowel diseases: pathophysiology, diagnosis, and treatment. *Inflamm Bowel Dis.* 2016;22:1198.

296. Koutroubakis IE, Ramos-Rivers C, Regueiro M, et al. Five-year period prevalence and characteristics of anemia in a large US inflammatory bowel disease cohort. *J Clin Gastroenterol.* 2016;50:638.

297. Scaldaferri F, Pizzoferrato M, Lopetuso LR, et al. Nutrition and IBD. Malnutrition and/or sarcopenia? A practical guide. *Gastroenterol Res Pract.* 2017;2017:8646495.

298. Forbes A, Escher J, Hebuterne X, et al. ESPEN guideline: clinical nutrition in inflammatory bowel disease. *Clin Nutr.* 2017; 36:321.

299. Harries AD, Jones LA, Heatley RV, Rhodes J. Malnutrition in inflammatory bowel disease: an anthropometric study. *Hum Nutr Clin Nutr.* 1982;36:307.

300. Mijac DD, Jankovic GL, Jorga J, Krstić MN. Nutritional status in patients with active inflammatory bowel disease: prevalence of malnutrition and methods for routine nutritional assessment. *Eur J Intern Med.* 2010;21:315.

301. Nguyen DL, Parekh N, Bechtold ML, Jamal MM. National trends and in-hospital outcomes of adult patients with inflammatory bowel disease receiving parenteral nutrition support. *JPEN J Parenter Enteral Nutr.* 2016;40:412.

302. Grass F, Pache B, Martin D, Hahnloser D, Demartines N, Hübner M. Preoperative nutritional conditioning of Crohn's patients—systematic review of current evidence and practice. *Nutrients.* 2017;9(6):562.

303. Quince C, Ijaz UZ, Loman N, et al. Extensive modulation of the fecal metagenome in children with Crohn's disease during exclusive enteral nutrition. *Am J Gastroenterol.* 2015;110:1718.

304. Feng Y, Li Y, Mei S, et al. Exclusive enteral nutrition ameliorates mesenteric adipose tissue alterations in patients with active Crohn's disease. *Clin Nutr.* 2014;33:850.

305. Nguyen DL, Limketkai B, Medici V, Saire Mendoza M, Palmer L, Bechtold M. Nutritional strategies in the management of adult patients with inflammatory bowel disease: dietary considerations

from active disease to disease remission. *Curr Gastroenterol Rep.* 2016;18:55.

306. Schwartz E. Perioperative parenteral nutrition in adults with inflammatory bowel disease: a review of the literature. *Nutr Clin Pract.* 2016;31:159.

307. Zhu W, Guo Z, Zuo L, et al. CONSORT. Different end-points of preoperative nutrition and outcome of bowel resection of Crohn disease: a randomized clinical trial. *Medicine (Baltimore).* 2015;94:e1175.

308. Lashner BA, Evans AA, Hanauer SB. Preoperative total parenteral nutrition for bowel resection in Crohn's disease. *Dig Dis Sci.* 1989;34:741.

309. Salinas H, Dursun A, Konstantinidis I, et al. Does preoperative total parenteral nutrition in patients with ulcerative colitis produce better outcomes? *Int J Colorectal Dis.* 2012;27:1479.

310. Jacobson S. Early postoperative complications in patients with Crohn's disease given and not given preoperative total parenteral nutrition. *Scand J Gastroenterol.* 2012;47:170.

311. Huang W, Tang Y, Nong L, Sun Y. Risk factors for postoperative intra-abdominal septic complications after surgery in Crohn's disease: a meta-analysis of observational studies. *J Crohns Colitis.* 2015;9:293.

312. Fumery M, Seksik P, Auzolle C, et al. Postoperative complications after ileocecal resection in Crohn's disease: a prospective study from the REMIND group. *Am J Gastroenterol.* 2017;112:337.

313. Wallaert JB, De Martino RR, Marsicovetere PS, et al. Venous thromboembolism after surgery for inflammatory bowel disease: are there modifiable risk factors? Data from ACS NSQIP. *Dis Colon Rectum.* 2012;55:1138.

314. Magro F, Soares JB, Fernandes D. Venous thrombosis and prothrombotic factors in inflammatory bowel disease. *World J Gastroenterol.* 2014;20:4857.

315. Colombel JF, Loftus EV Jr, Tremaine WJ, et al. Early postoperative complications are not increased in patients with Crohn's disease treated perioperatively with infliximab or immunosuppressive therapy. *Am J Gastroenterol.* 2004;99:878.

316. Kunitake H, Hodin R, Shellito PC, Sands BE, Korzenik J, Bordeianou L. Perioperative treatment with infliximab in patients with Crohn's disease and ulcerative colitis is not associated with an increased rate of postoperative complications. *J Gastrointest Surg.* 2008;12:1730.

317. Canedo J, Lee SH, Pinto R, Murad-Regadas S, Rosen L, Wexner SD. Surgical resection in Crohn's disease: is immunosuppressive medication associated with higher postoperative infection rates? *Colorectal Dis.* 2011;13:1294.

318. Kopylov U, Ben-Horin S, Zmora O, Eliakim R, Katz LH. Anti-tumor necrosis factor and postoperative complications in Crohn's disease: systematic review and meta-analysis. *Inflamm Bowel Dis.* 2012;18:2404.

319. Yang ZP, Hong L, Wu Q, Fan DM. Preoperative infliximab use and postoperative complications in Crohn's disease: a systematic review and meta-analysis. *Int J Surg.* 2014;12:224.

320. Billioud V, Ford AC, Tedesco ED, Colombel JF, Roblin X, Peyrin-Biroulet L. Preoperative use of anti-TNF therapy and postoperative complications in inflammatory bowel diseases: a meta-analysis. *J Crohns Colitis.* 2013;7:853.

321. Rosenfeld G, Qian H, Bressler B. The risks of post-operative complications following pre-operative infliximab therapy for Crohn's disease in patients undergoing abdominal surgery: a systematic review and meta-analysis. *J Crohns Colitis.* 2013 7:868.

322. Lightner AL, Raffals LE, Mathis KL, et al. Postoperative outcomes in vedolizumab-treated patients undergoing abdominal operations for inflammatory bowel disease. *J Crohns Colitis.* 2017;11:185.

323. Wilson MZ, Connelly TM, Hollenbeak CS, Messaris E. Organ space infection following ileocolectomy for Crohn's disease: a National Surgical Quality Improvement Project study. *Am J Surg.* 2014;208:749.

324. Kanazawa A, Yamana T, Okamoto K, Sahara R. Risk factors for postoperative intra-abdominal septic complications after bowel resection in patients with Crohn's disease. *Dis Colon Rectum.* 2012;55:957.

325. Crowell KT, Messaris E. Risk factors and implications of anastomotic complications after surgery for Crohn's disease. *World J Gastrointest Surg.* 2015;7:237.

326. Sangster W, Berg AS, Choi CS, et al. Outcomes of early ileocolectomy after percutaneous drainage for perforated ileocolic Crohn's disease. *Am J Surg.* 2016;212:728.

327. Bellolio F, Cohen Z, Macrae HM, et al. Outcomes following surgery for perforating Crohn's disease. *Br J Surg.* 2013;100:1344.

328. Stokes AL, Tice S, Follett S, et al. Institution of a preoperative stoma education group class decreases rate of peristomal complications in new stoma patients. *J Wound Ostomy Continence Nurs.* 2017;44(4):363-367.

329. Forsmo HM, Pfeffer F, Rasdal A, Sintonen H, Körner H, Erichsen C. Pre- and postoperative stoma education and guidance within an enhanced recovery after surgery (ERAS) program reduces length of hospital stay in colorectal surgery. *Int J Surg.* 2016;36:121.

330. Younis J, Salerno G, Fanto D, Hadjipavlou M, Chellar D, Trickett JP. Focused preoperative patient stoma education, prior to ileostomy formation after anterior resection, contributes to a reduction in delayed discharge within the enhanced recovery programme. *Int J Colorectal Dis.* 2012;27:43.

331. Sugerman HJ, Sugerman EL, Meador JG, Newsome HH Jr, Kellum JM Jr, DeMaria EJ. Ileal pouch-anal anastomosis without ileal diversion. *Ann Surg.* 2000;232:530.

332. McGuire BB, Brannigan AE, O'Connell PR. Ileal pouch-anal anastomosis. *Br J Surg.* 2007;94:812.

333. Mege D, Figueiredo MN, Manceau G, Maggiori L, Bouhnik Y, Panis Y. Three-stage laparoscopic ileal pouch-anal anastomosis is the best approach for high-risk patients with inflammatory bowel disease: an analysis of 185 consecutive patients. *J Crohns Colitis.* 2016;10:898.

334. Swenson BR, Hollenbeak CS, Poritz LS, Koltun WA. Modified two-stage ileal pouch-anal anastomosis: equivalent outcomes with less resource utilization. *Dis Colon Rectum.* 2005;48:256.

335. Zittan E, Wong-Chong N, Ma GW, McLeod RS, Silverberg MS, Cohen Z. Modified two-stage ileal pouch-anal anastomosis results in lower rate of anastomotic leak compared with traditional two-stage surgery for ulcerative colitis. *J Crohns Colitis.* 2016;10:766.

336. Mathis KL, Dozois EJ, Larson DW, et al. Ileal pouch-anal anastomosis and liver transplantation for ulcerative colitis complicated by primary sclerosing cholangitis. *Br J Surg.* 2008;95:882.

337. Cho CS, Dayton MT, Thompson JS, Koltun WA, Heise CP, Harms BA. Proctocolectomy-ileal pouch-anal anastomosis for ulcerative colitis after liver transplantation for primary sclerosing cholangitis: a multi-institutional analysis. *J Gastrointest Surg.* 2008;12:1221.

338. de Groof EJ, Sahami S, Lucas C, Ponsioen CY, Bemelman WA, Buskens CJ. Treatment of perianal fistula in Crohn's disease: a systematic review and meta-analysis comparing seton drainage and anti-tumour necrosis factor treatment. *Colorectal Dis.* 2016;18:667.

339. Present DH, Rutgeerts P, Targan S, et al. Infliximab for the treatment of fistulas in patients with Crohn's disease. *N Engl J Med.* 1999;340 1398.

340. Colombel JF, Sandborn WJ, Rutgeerts P, et al. Adalimumab for maintenance of clinical response and remission in patients with Crohn's disease: the CHARM trial. *Gastroenterology.* 2007;132:52.

341. Choi CS, Berg AS, Sangster W, et al. Combined medical and surgical approach improves healing of septic perianal Crohn's disease. *J Am Coll Surg.* 2016;223:506.

342. Sheedy SP, Bruining DH, Dozois EJ, Faubion WA, Fletcher JG. MR imaging of perianal Crohn disease. *Radiology.* 2017;282:628.

343. Bezzio C, Bryant RV, Manes G, Maconi G, Saibeni S. New horizons in the imaging of perianal Crohn's disease: transperineal ultrasonography. *Expert Rev Gastroenterol Hepatol.* 2017;11:523.

344. Jarrar A, Church J. Advancement flap repair: a good option for complex anorectal fistulas. *Dis Colon Rectum.* 2011;54:1537.

345. Gingold DS, Murrell ZA, Fleshner PR. A prospective evaluation of the ligation of the intersphincteric tract procedure for complex anal fistula in patients with Crohn's disease. *Ann Surg.* 2014; 260:1057

346. Panes J, Garcia-Olmo D, Van Assche G, et al. Expanded allogeneic adipose-derived mesenchymal stem cells (Cx601) for complex perianal fistulas in Crohn's disease: a phase 3 randomised, double-blind controlled trial. *Lancet.* 2016;388:1281.

347. Fichera A, Hurst RD, Michelassi F. Current methods of bowel-sparing surgery in Crohn's disease. *Adv Surg.* 2003;37:231.

348. Hurst RD, Michelassi F. Strictureplasty for Crohn's disease: techniques and long-term results. *World J Surg.* 1998;22:359.

349. Michelassi F. Side-to-side isoperistaltic strictureplasty for multiple Crohn's strictures. *Dis Colon Rectum.* 1996;39:345.

350. Yamamoto T, Fazio VW, Tekkis PP. Safety and efficacy of strictureplasty for Crohn's disease: a systematic review and meta-analysis. *Dis Colon Rectum.* 2007;50:1968.

351. Best WR, Becktel JM, Singleton JW, Kern F Jr. Development of a Crohn's disease activity index. National Cooperative Crohn's Disease Study. *Gastroenterology.* 1976;70:439.

352. Rutgeerts P, Geboes K, Vantrappen G, Beyls J, Kerremans R, Hiele M. Predictability of the postoperative course of Crohn's disease. *Gastroenterology.* 1990;99:956.

353. Alvarez-Lobos M, Arostegui JI, Sans M, et al. Crohn's disease patients carrying Nod2/CARD15 gene variants have an increased and early need for first surgery due to stricturing disease and higher rate of surgical recurrence. *Ann Surg.* 2005;242:693.

354. De Cruz P, Kamm MA, Prideaux L, Allen PB, Desmond PV. Postoperative recurrent luminal Crohn's disease: a systematic review. *Inflamm Bowel Dis.* 2012;18:758.

355. de Barcelos IF, Kotze PG, Spinelli A, et al. Factors affecting the incidence of early endoscopic recurrence after ileocolonic resection for Crohn's disease: a multicentre observational study. *Colorectal Dis.* 2017;19:O39.

356. Yamamoto T. Factors affecting recurrence after surgery for Crohn's disease. *World J Gastroenterol.* 2005;11:3971.

357. Nunes T, Etchevers MJ, Garcia-Sanchez V, et al. Impact of smoking cessation on the clinical course of Crohn's disease under current therapeutic algorithms: a multicenter prospective study. *Am J Gastroenterol.* 2016;111:411.

358. Reese GE, Nanidis T, Borysiewicz C, Yamamoto T, Orchard T, Tekkis PP. The effect of smoking after surgery for Crohn's disease: a meta-analysis of observational studies. *Int J Colorectal Dis.* 2008; 23:1213.

359. Guo Z, Cao L, Guo F, et al. The presence of postoperative infectious complications is associated with the risk of early postoperative clinical recurrence of Crohn's disease. *World J Surg.* 2017;41(9): 2372-2377.

360. Koltun WA. Better together: improved care of the IBD patient using the multi-disciplinary IBD center. *Expert Rev Gastroenterol Hepatol.* 2017;11:491.

Operative Therapy for Ulcerative Colitis: A Minimally Invasive Approach

Katerina Wells | Scott A. Strong | Matthew Mutch

Proctocolectomy with ileal pouch–anal anastomosis (IPAA) has become the standard restorative procedure for patients requiring surgery for ulcerative colitis. Since the operation's introduction in 1978 by Sir Alan Parks, several refinements have occurred as new medications and technologies have come into practice. New biologic therapies have become a standard in medical management, and they have forced the surgeon to better understand the physiologic state of the patient and reconsider the optimal timing of surgery. Advances in stapling technology and emergence of the double-stapled anastomosis have allowed for more efficient pouch construction and improved functional outcomes, respectively. Minimally invasive procedures have gained support because of more rapid recovery, better cosmesis, and potential long-term benefits. The procedure continues to carry the risk of complications, such as pelvic sepsis and delayed onset of Crohn disease, which influence long-term pouch function and durability. Careful preoperative evaluation and timely postoperative intervention are critical to improving surgical outcomes. This chapter will focus on two- and three-stage restorative proctocolectomy via straight and hand-assisted laparoscopic approaches. Alternative procedures to the IPAA will also be discussed.

INDICATIONS FOR ELECTIVE SURGERY

FAILURE OF MEDICAL THERAPY

Patients with ulcerative colitis may require surgery either because they have failed to respond to medical therapy or because the risks of medical therapy outweigh its benefits. Furthermore, the disease can cause debilitating symptoms and lead to a poor quality of life despite appropriate medical treatment. Acute colitis that cannot be controlled is the most common presentation of failed medical management, but chronic issues such as persistent anemia, malnutrition, and protein-losing enteropathy may also prompt consideration of surgical intervention. Close consultation between the patient, gastroenterologist, and surgeon is important to ensure the most appropriate timing for surgery. Delayed operative intervention for patients with acute severe ulcerative colitis is associated with an increased risk for postoperative complications.[1,2] Patients must be counseled about the short- and long-term risks and benefits of the medical and surgical options so that an informed decision can be derived. It is also important to consider the value of each treatment modality. Patients who undergo definitive surgery for ulcerative colitis have reduced direct medical costs in the 2 years after surgical

recovery, and surgical intervention is associated with long-term economic benefit.[3,4]

PRESENCE OF CANCER AND DYSPLASIA

Patients with ulcerative pancolitis for more than 8 years are at increased risk of colorectal cancer, approximating 0.5% to 1% per year.[5–7] Those persons with primary sclerosing cholangitis as a complication of their ulcerative colitis have been shown to have an even higher incidence of dysplasia and cancer. Colonoscopic surveillance with random and chromoscopic-directed biopsies has been recommended in patients with long-standing ulcerative colitis. An obstructing lesion and unresectable dysplasia generally warrant surgery. Historically, high-grade dysplasia and multifocal low-grade dysplasia were widely accepted as clear indications for colectomy because of the high rate of an occult malignancy within the colon.[8,9] However, there are circumstances in which dysplastic lesions within a field of normal colonic mucosa can be adequately managed endoscopically.[10] This is an evolving area of management that requires a clear understanding of the lesion itself, the patient's disease course, and the comfort of the treating physicians.

INDICATIONS FOR EMERGENCY SURGERY

SEVERE COLITIS

Patients with a severe attack of ulcerative colitis should be resuscitated and medically treated if signs of life-threatening hemorrhage or perforation are absent. Deterioration of the patient's condition and failure to improve within a predetermined time period are indications for surgical intervention. Patients initially managed with corticosteroids should improve after 3 days. Rescue therapy includes treatment with cyclosporin or infliximab, and improvement with these agents should occur within 5 to 7 days. Intervention for failed therapy should take the form of colectomy with preservation of the rectum and creation of an end ileostomy. The rectosigmoid stump can be closed and left intraperitoneally, brought up as a closed stump in the subcutaneous tissue, or matured as a mucous fistula above skin level.

TOXIC MEGACOLON

Toxic megacolon, which is dilation (5 to 6 cm) of the colon, due to inflammation-induced paralysis of the colon or obstruction proximal to severe disease, is a potentially life-threatening condition. Patients are very ill and often manifest high fever, abdominal pain and tenderness, tachycardia, and leukocytosis. Prompt resuscitation and medical therapy are essential. Early decision to operate is life saving.

HEMORRHAGE, PERFORATION, AND OBSTRUCTION

Massive hemorrhage is uncommon and accounts for less than 10% of emergency colectomies in patients with ulcerative colitis. Perforation of the colon is a clear indication for surgery. If it occurs in the absence of megacolon, the possibility of Crohn disease should be considered. High doses of corticosteroids often mask these symptoms and signs. Strictures causing an obstruction in patients with chronic ulcerative colitis are uncommon and represent malignant lesions until proven otherwise.

IMPACT OF BIOLOGIC AGENTS

A significant number (30%) of patients who undergo surgery have had some exposure to biologic agents.[4,11–13] Anti–tumor necrosis factor (TNF)-α therapies may increase infectious complications, compromised pouch function, and even pouch loss.[14–19] Controversy persists regarding their use, timing of surgery, and risk for complications of surgery.[20–22] In a meta-analysis by Selvaggi et al. patients receiving biologic agent therapy prior to restorative proctocolectomy were at higher risk of developing short-term, local pelvic complications (odds ratio [OR] 4.12; 95% confidence interval [CI] 2.3 to 7.1).[23,24] However, studies included in this analysis demonstrated heterogeneity in reporting of procedures and complications that may contribute to variable outcomes between biologic agent and nonbiologic agent comparison groups.[19,25–29]

The Crohn's and Colitis Foundation of America published a position statement regarding anti-TNF-α therapy management for inflammatory bowel disease (IBD).[4] This position statement supports the safety of total colectomy with end ileostomy in the setting of anti-TNF-α therapy as part of a three-stage approach to restorative proctocolectomy. Use of a two-stage technique is associated with increased risk of postoperative complications, and it is recommended that a two-stage approach may be used only in selected patients. Anti-TNF-α therapy is considered an absolute contraindication to single-stage restorative proctocolectomy, based on limited data.

Fortunately, as operative experience in the setting of current and novel biologic agent therapies matures, greater understanding of the impact of these therapies on operative outcomes will guide the surgeon's ability to make decisions.

RESTORATIVE PROCTOCOLECTOMY WITH ILEAL POUCH–ANAL ANASTOMOSIS

OVERVIEW OF THE OPERATION

Restorative procotocolectomy with IPAA is usually performed in two or three stages based on the patient's physiology and the surgeon's judgment. In a two-stage operation, the abdominal colon is mobilized, a nerve-sparing rectal dissection is used, and the proctocolectomy specimen is removed in its entirety. The ileum is preserved and dissected free of its retroperitoneal and duodenal

attachments to allow for a tension-free IPAA. Typically, an ileal J pouch is created using 30 to 45 cm of distal ileum, with each limb of the pouch measuring 15 to 20 cm in length. The IPAA is performed by either mucosectomy with a handsewn technique or preservation of the anal transitional zone (ATZ) with a stapled technique, depending upon indication for surgery or surgeon's preference. A temporary ileostomy is created to protect the ileal pouch and the anastomosis. The ileostomy is closed approximately 12 weeks later, following confirmation of proper pouch healing with contrast enema and digital examination.

In a three-stage operation, the abdominal colon is removed to the distal sigmoid colon or upper rectum, and an end ileostomy is matured. The superior hemorrhoidal artery may be left intact to maintain positioning of the rectal stump and preserve anatomic planes of dissection at the time of future proctectomy. Following medical and nutritional optimization of the patient, the second stage of restoration consists of a nerve-sparing completion proctectomy followed by takedown of the end ileostomy and mobilization of the small bowel mesentery from its retroperitoneal and duodenal attachments. An ileal pouch is created as previously described, and a diverting loop ileostomy is brought up through the existing ileostomy aperture.

MINIMALLY INVASIVE APPROACH TO THE ILEAL POUCH–ANAL ANASTOMOSIS

Laparoscopic surgery appeals to patients due to the potential benefit of reduced disability, enhanced recovery, and better cosmesis. The majority of reports tout the benefits of laparoscopy over open surgery, including reduced major and minor complications, decreased narcotic use, and lower rate of intraoperative transfusion, at the expense of longer operative times.[30–32] Length of stay is similar between the laparoscopic and open groups owing to the need for ileostomy education before discharge, but the laparoscopic approach has fewer postoperative complications and better cosmesis.[33,34] Studies have failed to show a significant difference in the quality of life associated with the two operative approaches.[35–37] Several single institutional reports demonstrate the safety of laparoscopic colectomy in the setting of acute ulcerative colitis.[38,39] The minimally invasive approach preserved fertility and decreased the incidence of incisional hernia.[40,41] Laparoscopic, hand-assisted, single-port, or robotic-assisted approaches are not different.[42–44] A randomized trial comparing hand-assisted laparoscopic with open restorative proctocolectomy found no difference in postoperative narcotic use, morbidity, length of stay, or quality of life at 3 months after surgery.[45,46] Hand-assisted laparoscopy approach is associated with a 55-minute reduction in operative time compared with straight laparoscopy, with no difference in short-term outcomes.[47,48] Robotic IPAA is possible with minimal complications.[49,50]

Further consideration should be given to surgical approach based on the indication for the procedure in light of a randomized controlled trial comparing laparoscopic versus open proctectomy for rectal cancer that failed to demonstrate noninferiority of pathologic outcomes following laparoscopic proctectomy.[51,52] Oncologic principles of resection are required, and careful consideration of operative approach should be given to the colitis patient with rectal cancer.

OPERATIVE TECHNIQUE: TWO-STAGE LAPAROSCOPIC ILEAL POUCH–ANAL ANASTOMOSIS

The patient is placed in dorsal lithotomy positioning with adequate space left between the legs to allow for access to the anus and operator standing room. A bean bag with chest wrap can be used to secure the patient during steep Trendelenburg positioning. The patient's arms are padded and tucked at the sides. The hips are positioned with 0 degrees of flexion to help keep the thighs out of the way during dissection in the upper quadrants.

The peritoneum is entered via a periumbilical incision using either an open or closed insertion technique. A 12-mm port should be ideally placed in the midline, halfway between the pubis symphysis and the xiphoid process, which allows for the camera to be at the apex of the 12-mm Hg pneumoperitoneum. A 10-mm, 0- or 30-degree laparoscope can be used. In one of the more commonly used approaches, at least three 5-mm working ports are placed (see figures).

Extraction of the specimen is possible through a planned ileostomy site, periumbilical site, Pfannenstiel incision, or left lower quadrant muscle-splitting incision.

Our sequence of procedures follows right colon mobilization, opening the lesser sac and transverse colon mobilization, ligation of the right and transverse colon mesentery, mobilization of the left colon, and ligation of its mesentery and the rectal dissection. Right colon mobilization starts with accessing the retroperitoneum, followed by mobilization of the right colon off the retroperitoneum, division of the lateral attachments, entering the lesser sac, and ligation of the mesentery. Regardless of a posterior, medial to lateral, or lateral approach, the steps are the same, but the order in which they are performed are different. The posterior approach will be presented in this chapter.

The abdomen is explored (including small bowel evaluation to look for Crohn disease), the patient is placed in a steep Trendelenburg position so the small bowel can be placed in the right upper quadrant. The posterior aspect of the small bowel mesentery is exposed from the fourth portion of the duodenum to the cecum. The right hand grasper elevates the small bowel mesentery to expose the fourth portion of duodenum. The energy source is in the left hand (for a left-handed surgeon), and the peritoneum is incised. The duodenum is swept away from the right colon mesentery, which is elevated off the retroperitoneum in a medial to lateral direction. The patient is then placed right side up to allow the small bowel to fall into the left side of abdomen. The lateral attachments are finally divided from the cecum toward the hepatic flexure.

The patient is placed in reverse Trendelenburg position, and the lesser sac is entered through the gastrocolic ligament, separating the lesser omentum from its attachments to the transverse colon mesentery. The major challenge with this maneuver is to avoid dissecting into the transverse colon mesentery. Therefore the cut edge of the lesser omentum is elevated to expose its avascular attachments to the transverse colon and its mesentery.

Near the pylorus, the lesser omentum and transverse colon mesentery appear fused, but with careful dissection under tension, the omentum and mesocolon can be separated. The lesser omentum is then divided toward the splenic flexure, which fully exposes the lesser sac and facilitates exposure of the transverse colon mesentery.

The mesenteric vessels can now be ligated. The ileocecal junction is grasped and pulled to the right lower quadrant to facilitate exposure of the ileocolic pedicle. The ileocolic pedicle is ligated at the superior mesenteric artery (SMA) away from the second portion of the duodenum. The transverse colon mesentery is elevated to expose the bare area to the left of the middle colic vessels. The peritoneum is incised toward the right branch of the middle colic vessels and the previously cut edge of the right colic mesentery. The middle colic vessels are free to be isolated and ligated.

Attention is now turned to the mobilization of the left colon. The patient is placed in a steep Trendelenburg and right side down position to facilitate placement of the small bowel to the right upper quadrant. The left colon is mobilized in a medial to lateral approach. The retroperitoneum can be accessed either at the level of the sacral promontory or medial to the inferior mesenteric vein. At the sacral promontory the superior rectal vessels are elevated and the peritoneum is incised while avoiding damage to the sympathetic nerves. The wider the incision and bigger the window created, the greater the mobility of the vessel and exposure of the retroperitoneum. After the left ureter is identified and swept free into the retroperitoneum, the inferior mesenteric artery is isolated and ligated at its origin. The inferior mesenteric artery can also be divided distal to the vessel's branching. The inferior mesenteric vein is elevated off the retroperitoneum, isolated, and transected near the inferior border of the pancreas. The first assistant elevates the cut edge of the transverse colon mesentery, and the surgeon elevates the ligated inferior mesenteric vein pedicle, exposing the remaining colonic mesentery. Depending upon the extent of transverse colon mesentery divided during the right-sided mobilization, only a few vascular pedicles on the left transverse mesocolon remain for division. The left colon mesentery is released from the retroperitoneum beyond the lateral aspect of the colon, from the level of the sigmoid colon to the splenic flexure. The lateral attachments are incised starting at the pelvic brim during medial traction on the sigmoid colon. The prior plane of dissection is entered and the lateral attachments are divided to the splenic flexure. Any intact omental adhesions are divided, and the mesenteric attachments along the inferior border of the pancreas can be cut to finish mobilization of the abdominal colon.

The rectal dissection can be the most technically challenging aspect of the procedure because of the confined space of the pelvis, limited angling of the instruments, stapling difficulties at the pelvic floor, and mesenteric inflammation from the proctitis. It is easiest to perform the dissection immediately outside the fascia propria of the mesorectum, but care must be taken to avoid injury to the sympathetic and parasympathetic nerves. Given the limited space of the pelvis and the angles of visualization, achieving adequate exposure and tension can be difficult.

Conceptually, the rectum and mesorectum form a cylinder within the cylinder of the pelvis. The dissection is achieved with curvilinear sweeping incisions in the areolar tissue plane following the curves of the pelvis. Ideal tension is achieved when traction is perpendicular to the point of dissection (i.e., anterior to posterior, medial to lateral) rather than pulling the rectum out of the pelvis. Small changes in the force vectors of retraction can profoundly impact tension and exposure. The dissection begins with entering the presacral plane by retracting the rectum directly anterior. As the dissection moves laterally, the angle of retraction is rotated to the contralateral side to maintain tension and exposure.

The posterior dissection is carried down to the pelvic floor, and at the tip of the coccyx, the plane of dissection sweeps anterior to the pelvic outlet. The peritoneum on the lateral aspects of the mesorectum is divided all the way to the anterior peritoneal reflection, which exposes the anterior and deep lateral planes. The lateral dissection on both sides of the pelvis progresses by retracting the rectum medially and superiorly so the plane can be dissected in a posterior to anterior fashion. The anterior dissection begins, after completion of the lateral dissection, by pulling the peritoneum overlying the cervix or posterior bladder/prostate in an anterior direction and the rectum in a posterior fashion. The rectum is rotated to the contralateral side to maintain the tension in a plane that is perpendicular to the point of dissection. A laparoscopic stapler is directed into the pelvis to divide the rectum in a single firing, if possible. It is best to divide the rectum with three or fewer staplings oriented in the same direction. A right lower quadrant port or suprapubic port or a Pfannenstiel incision can be accessed to divide the rectum.

Prior to extraction of the specimen through an abdominal wall incision, it is important to ensure that the colon is anterior to the small bowel to avoid avulsion of the small bowel mesentery, or a volvulus of the small bowel mesentery. Proper orientation of the ileum during extraction of the specimen facilitates construction of the ileal pouch. After construction of the pouch (see later), a circular stapling anvil is secured in the apex of the ileal pouch and the pouch is returned to the abdomen. The extraction site is closed, and the IPAA is completed under direct laparoscopic visualization. A proximal loop of ileum is matured into a diverting loop ileostomy in the right lower quadrant. The stoma should be brought through the stoma aperture under direct laparoscopic vision to ensure proper orientation. A closed suction drain may be placed into the pelvis through the left lower quadrant port site to facilitate evacuation of blood and fluid that can lead to pelvic fibrosis and impact pouch compliance.

OPERATIVE TECHNIQUE: HAND-ASSISTED TWO-STAGE ILEAL POUCH–ANAL ANASTOMOSIS

Alternatively, a hand-assisted technique via a 6- to 8-cm Pfannenstiel or lower midline incision can be considered. Use of the hand-assisted approach is a matter of surgeon's preference, and based on the previous data, it offers the surgeon another tool for their toolbox.

The sequence of the proctocolectomy is the same as described previously, but this section will describe how the

hand is used for the procedure. The camera port should be placed in the supraumbilical position so that the skirt of the hand port does not interfere with the camera. A 5-mm working port is placed on the right and left side, lateral to the rectus muscle and midway between the camera and hand port. Additional 5-mm working ports can be placed in the right and left upper quadrants as needed. The posterior approach is used for mobilization of the right colon. The surgeon stands on the patient's left side with her/his left hand in the abdomen, and the right hand holds the energy device. With the patient in steep Trendelenburg and the small bowel reflected to the right upper quadrant, the posterior aspect of the small bowel mesentery is exposed. The mesentery is grasped and elevated with the middle finger and thumb. The index finger is used to further expose the fourth portion of the duodenum (Fig. 162.1).

The base of the terminal ileal mesentery is incised from the third portion of the duodenum to the cecum. After the retroperitoneum is entered, the hand is placed palm down into the retroperitoneum to elevate the right colon mesentery so the duodenum and retroperitoneal structures can be pushed posteriorly with the instrument in the right hand (Fig. 162.2). The dissection is extended beneath the hepatic flexure and ascending colon. To divide the lateral attachments, the patient is tilted right side up so the small bowel is displaced to the left side of the abdomen, exposing the lateral attachments and hepatic flexure. The hand is placed into the retroperitoneum, under the right colon mesentery, and the colon is retracted medially to expose the lateral attachments at the level of the cecum. The first assistant then divides the lateral attachments toward the hepatic flexure. The lesser sac is entered, and the lesser omentum is divided toward the splenic flexure as far as possible (Fig. 162.3).

The ileocecal angle is grasped and retracted to the right lower quadrant to expose the ileocolic pedicle for isolation and ligation at the level of the SMA (Fig. 162.4).

The middle colic vessels are exposed by passing the hand through the mesenteric defect, created by ligation

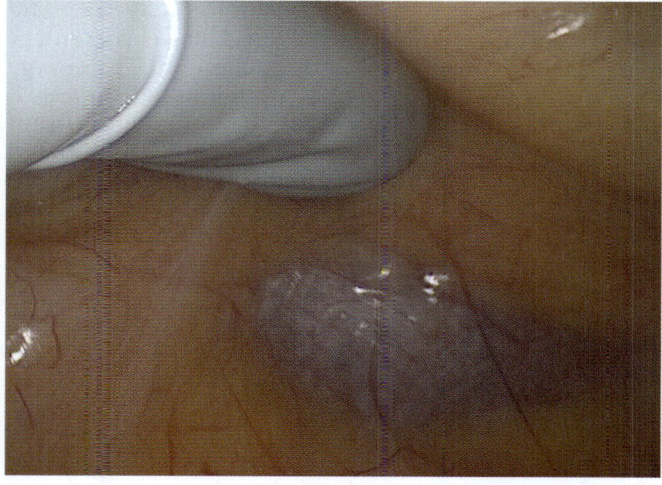

FIGURE 162.1 Exposure of the fourth portion of the duodenum.

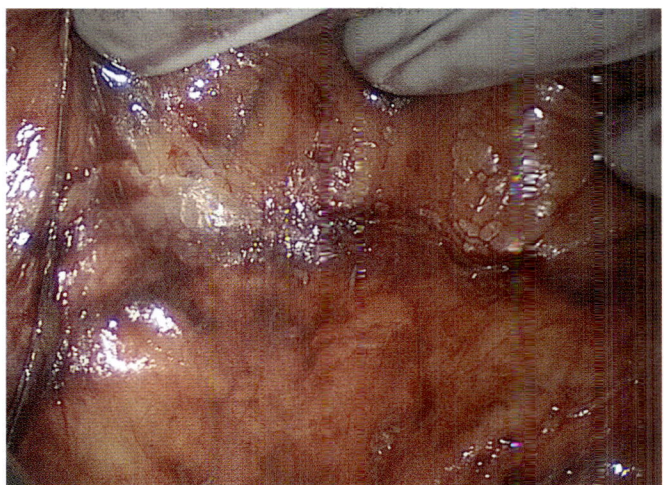

FIGURE 162.2 Dissection of the right colon mesentery off of the retroperitoneum.

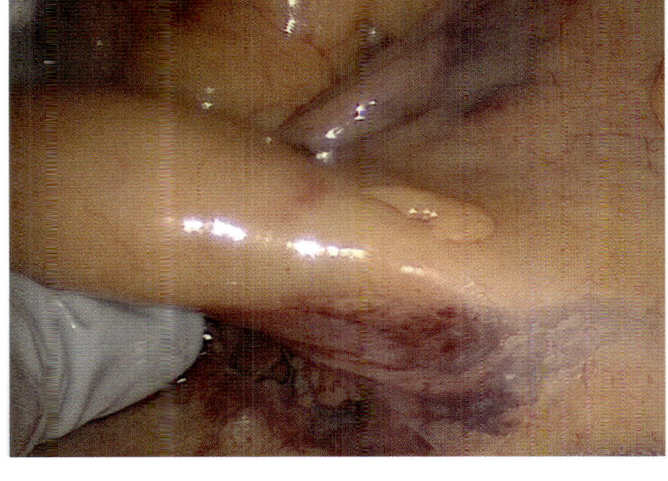

FIGURE 162.4 Identification of the ileocolic pedicle.

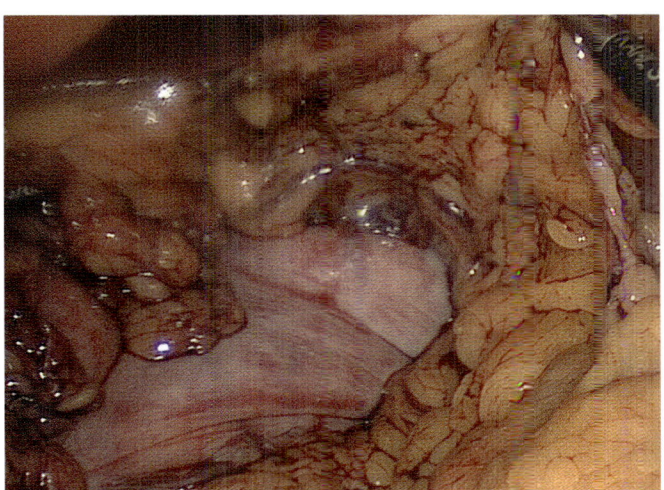

FIGURE 162.3 Exposure of the lesser sac.

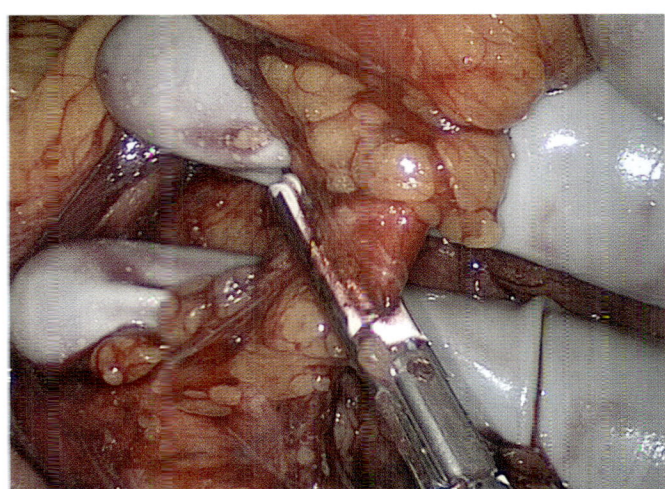

FIGURE 162.5 Ligation of the inferior mesenteric artery.

of the ileocolic pedicle, and into the lesser sac. The fingers encircle the base of the middle colic vessels. The peritoneum is scored over the bare area adjacent to the ligament of Treitz and the vessels are isolated, sealed, and divided. As long as the vessels are ligated anterior to the pancreas, there is no risk of injuring the superior mesenteric vessels.

For resection of the left colon and rectum, the left-handed surgeon stands on the patient's right side with her/his right hand in the abdomen and left hand on the energy source. The right-handed surgeon also stands on the right side, with the left hand in the abdomen and right hand on the energy source in the right lower quadrant port. The patient is in steep Trendelenburg and left side up to keep the small bowel in the right upper quadrant. The retroperitoneum can be accessed either at the level of the sacral promontory or medial to the inferior mesenteric vein. Starting at the sacral promontory, the superior rectal vessels are grasped and elevated, and the retroperitoneum

is entered. With the left ureter identified and safely swept into the retroperitoneum, the index finger with the pad toward the anterior abdominal wall elevates and applies tension on the superior rectal vessels. The middle finger then sweeps free all the tissue adjacent and lateral to the vessels. This maneuver allows exposure of the bare area cephalad to the inferior mesenteric artery and medial to the inferior mesenteric vein. The peritoneum medial to and along the inferior mesenteric vein is incised allowing entry into the retroperitoneal plane of dissection. Once it has been confirmed that the left ureter is away from the course of the inferior mesenteric artery, the artery can be safely divided (Fig. 162.5). The inferior mesenteric vein is then isolated near the inferior border of the pancreas in the same manner described for the artery (Fig. 162.6). When ligating the inferior mesenteric vein, the index and middle fingers are placed into the retroperitoneal space to isolate the vessel, while the fourth and fifth fingers remain in the peritoneal space covering the small bowel to prevent the energy source injury. The remaining

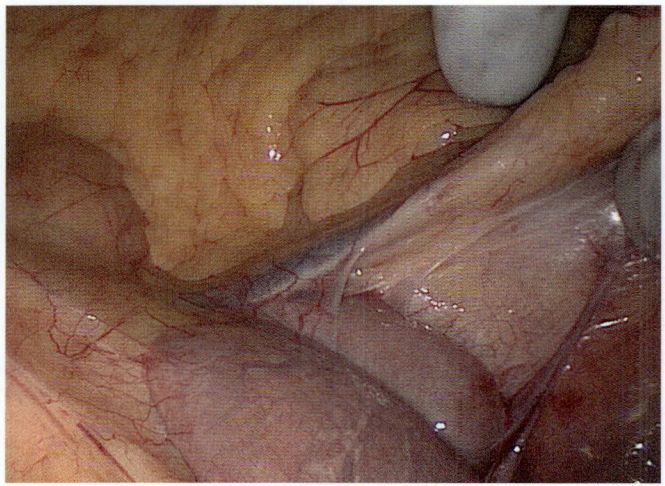

FIGURE 162.6 Identification of the inferior mesenteric vein.

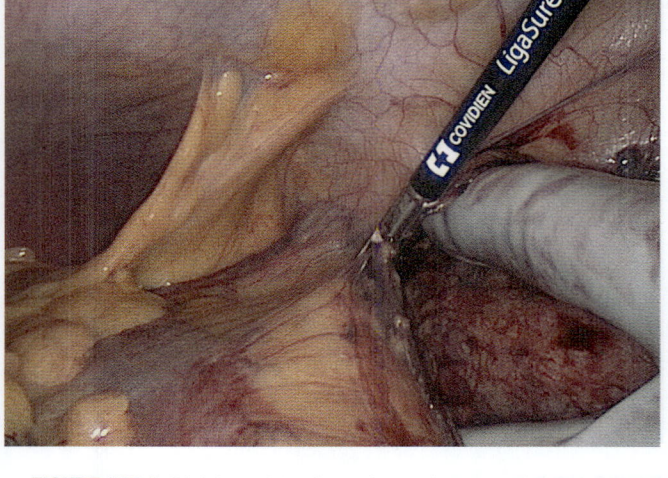

FIGURE 162.8 Division of the lateral attachments of the colon.

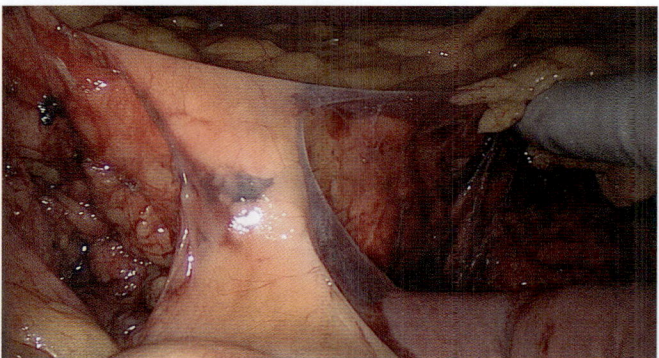

FIGURE 162.7 Maneuver to expose remaining colonic mesentery.

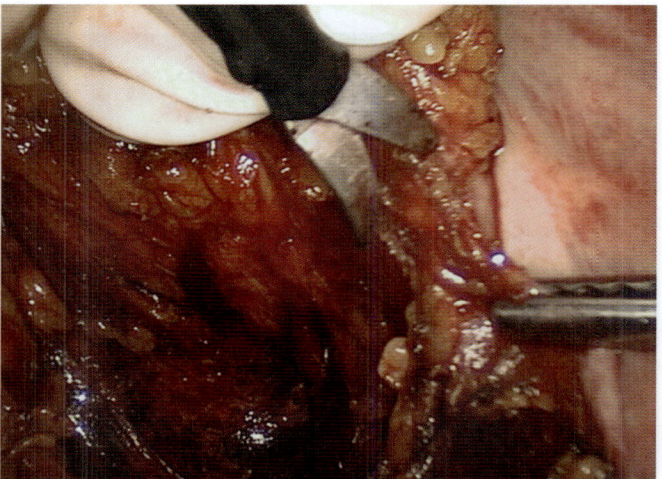

FIGURE 162.9 Hand-assisted posterior dissection.

transverse colon mesentery is divided in the same fashion as described previously (Fig. 162.7).

Mobilization of the descending and sigmoid colon mesenteries is facilitated by using the hand placed palm down to elevate the mesentery and an instrument to downward sweep the retroperitoneum. By creating the greatest tension safely possible, this dissection is carried beyond the lateral colon. The lateral attachments of the sigmoid colon are incised and the prior plane of dissection is entered. The hand is placed through this defect, and the remaining attachments are divided toward the splenic flexure (Fig. 162.8).

At the splenic flexure, the lesser sac is entered and the medial cut edge of the lesser sac from the transverse colon dissection is identified. Division of the remaining omentum completely opens the lesser sac, leaving only the peritoneal attachments along the inferior border of pancreas. The right-handed surgeon stands between the legs to mobilize the splenic flexure. The left hand lifts the colon toward the midline, and the colon is released from the kidney and spleen using the energy source through the left lower quadrant port. The final attachments to the pancreas are exposed by bringing the hand into the retroperitoneal space from a lateral direction and

pulling the transverse colon caudally, which allows the first assistant to divide this remaining tissue.

For the pelvic dissection, the left-handed surgeon stays in the same position with her/his right hand through the port. The dissection begins by entering the avascular plane between the presacral fascia and fascia propria of the mesorectum. The hand is pronated so the palm is up and the right thumb is pointing to the patient's right side. In this position, the hand anteriorly retracts the upper rectum to expose the plane of dissection. The fingers are creating tension as close to the plane of dissection as possible (Fig. 162.9). The right-handed surgeon places the left hand through the suprapubic port, which lifts the rectum. The right hand uses the energy source through the right lower quadrant port to dissect the rectum from the pelvis, as described earlier for straight laparoscopy.

This maneuver allows for tactile feedback as to the appropriate plane. The dissection is carried from sidewall to sidewall, and the hand is rotated right and left to maintain tension as the dissection is carried out toward the opposite sidewall. As the dissection continues deeper into the pelvis, better exposure is gained and tension is created by flexing the fingers rather than pulling the hand and mesorectum out of the pelvis. The lateral dissection is completed by incising the lateral peritoneal attachments down to the anterior peritoneal reflection. The anterior dissection begins with incising the anterior peritoneal reflection as the hand is pronated as described previously to anteriorly retract the bladder/prostate or the uterus/cervix while the first assistant posteriorly displaces the rectum. As the dissection moves deeper into the pelvis, the first assistant rotates the rectum in the direction contralateral to the dissection. For example, as the dissection is carried to the left, the rectum is retracted in a posterior and right direction to keep the tension perpendicular to the plane of dissection. If there is difficulty completing the pelvic dissection in this manner, the procedure can be completed using open instruments introduced through the hand port.

With the pelvic dissection completed to the level of the pelvic floor, the colon needs to be extracted. This is accomplished by passing the small bowel underneath the colon so the cecum can be delivered, which allows the small bowel to be oriented so it is on the patient's left side and the cut edge of the mesentery is facing the patient's right side. Starting in the left upper quadrant, the colon is elevated, and the small bowel is fed underneath the colon. As this maneuver progresses, the patient is tilted left side down to allow gravity to facilitate passing the small bowel to the left upper quadrant. At the conclusion, the hand should have worked its way to the cecum, which is extracted through the hand port, allowing the terminal ileum and its mesentery to be divided. The remaining colon is then easily extracted. The rectum can be divided through the hand access port sleeve with a single transverse staple line at the pelvic floor. Before firing the stapler to divide the rectum, it is best to ensure the anterior tissue in a male and the posterior wall of the vagina in a female are free from the stapler. The construction of the ileal pouch is described later.

OPERATIVE TECHNIQUE: THREE-STAGE ILEAL POUCH–ANAL ANASTOMOSIS: STRAIGHT LAPAROSCOPIC AND HAND-ASSISTED

The three-stage restorative proctocolectomy begins with removal of the abdominal colon and creation of an end ileostomy. After the patient has mentally and physiologically recovered from the first operation, they undergo completion proctectomy with creation of ileal pouch with anastomosis and diverting loop ileostomy. The third stage is completed with closure of the loop ileostomy.

The technical steps of the total abdominal colectomy are exactly the same as described previously. The only significant variation is the management of the rectal stump. Given the presence of acute colitis, possible immunosuppression, and state of the patient, a real concern exists related to breakdown of the rectal stump staple line. Therefore various alternatives to managing the rectal stump and its vasculature should be considered. The first option is to ligate the inferior mesenteric artery at its origin as described previously, and divide the rectum and mesorectum just below the rectosigmoid junction.

Dissection below the sacral promontory should be minimized to preserve this plane as much as possible. A large (34 French) rectal drain is left in the rectum for a few days to decompress the rectum and reduce the risk of "stump blowout." The second option involves preserving the superior rectal artery and leaving a long enough rectosigmoid stump to reach the anterior abdominal wall. The rectal stump is then secured in a subcutaneous position through the hand port or extraction site. This option preserves all of the pelvic planes and minimizes injury to the sympathetic nerves, and disruption of the stump becomes an easily controlled mucous fistula. In a retrospective review of 204 patients undergoing laparoscopic colectomy comparing these two approaches, no difference was found in the number of stump leaks in each group (5 intraperitoneal vs. 10 subcutaneous; $P = .23$). All stump leaks in the subcutaneous group were locally managed without the need for reoperation. However, this group had higher rates of wound infection. Five patients with intraperitoneal stump leak required antibiotic therapy or computed tomography (CT)-guided drainage and one patient required reexploration. No predisposing risk factors for stump leak among these patients were noted.[1,3-55]

The second stage or completion proctectomy can be approached via the same approach as described previously (Figs. 162.10–162.14).

MANEUVERS FOR INCREASING REACH OF THE ILEAL POUCH

There are occasions when the ileal J pouch will not reach the pelvic floor even after lysis of all adhesions and complete mobilization of the small bowel mesentery over the duodenum. Five maneuvers can be used to create extra length to improve reach of the pouch into the pelvis. First, if the ileocolic pedicle was not divided during colectomy, it can be ligated and a window of peritoneum

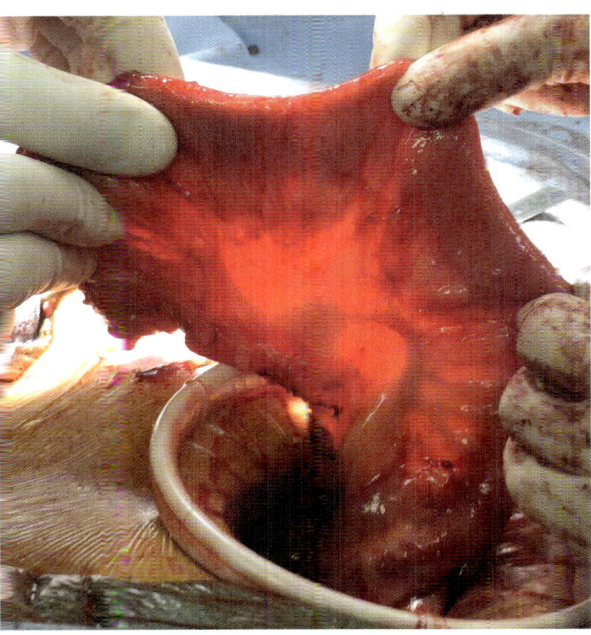

FIGURE 162.10 The vascular arcade of the ileal pouch

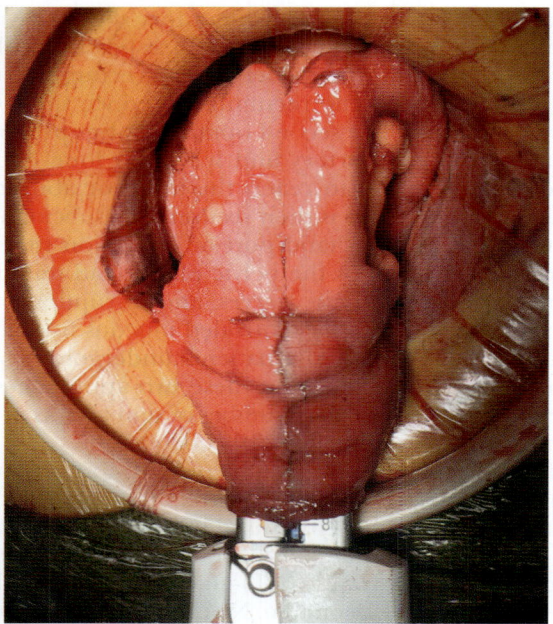

FIGURE 162.11 Construction of the ileal pouch.

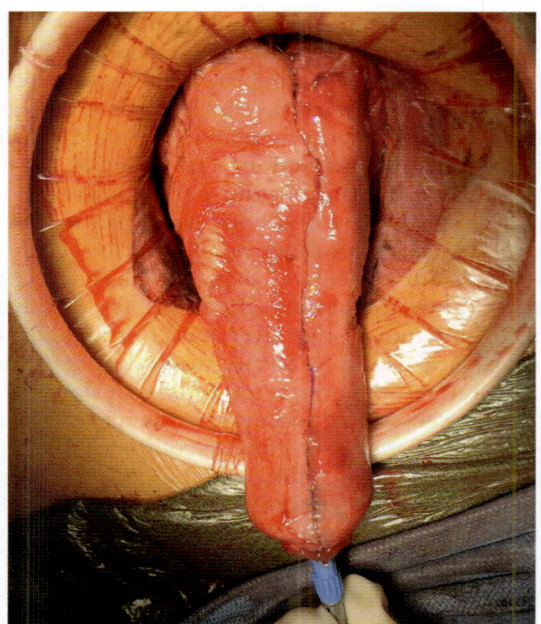

FIGURE 162.13 Completed pouch.

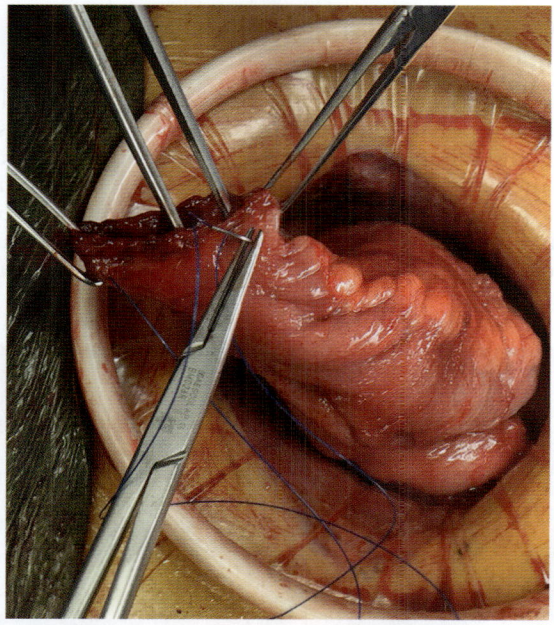

FIGURE 162.12 Purse-string suture around the common enterotomy.

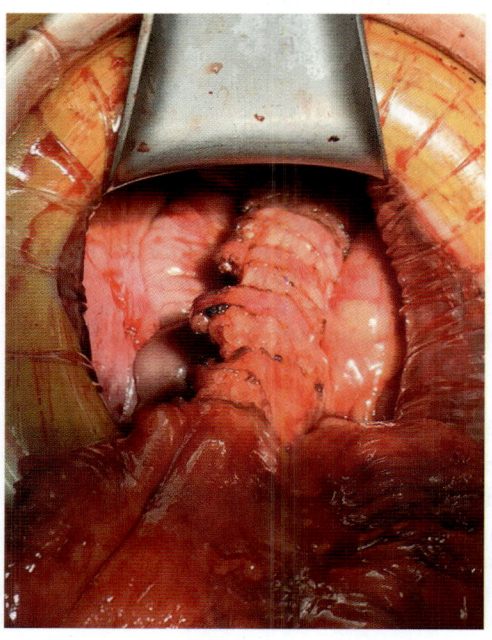

FIGURE 162.14 Scoring of the peritoneum over the superior mesenteric artery pedicle.

excised to increase length. Second, the anterior and posterior peritoneum overlying the superior mesenteric vessels can be incised transversely at multiple levels. This maneuver risks injury to the blood supply of the pouch and can result in hematoma. The denuded mesentery can be easily avulsed, which can result in a devastating mesenteric hematoma and ileal pouch loss. Third, the mesentery can be transilluminated and selective division of secondary arcade mesenteric vessels to the apex of

pouch can be performed. The arcade to the distal ileum must be preserved. The peritoneum over the arcade is incised, and the individual branches are divided. Division of the secondary arcade vessels typically results in one-for-one increase in length (i.e., every centimeter of transverse incision results in a centimeter of longitudinal lengthening). Fourth, an S pouch can be created. The near-normal orientation of the mesentery and a 2-cm efferent limb allow for extra reach. The details for creating

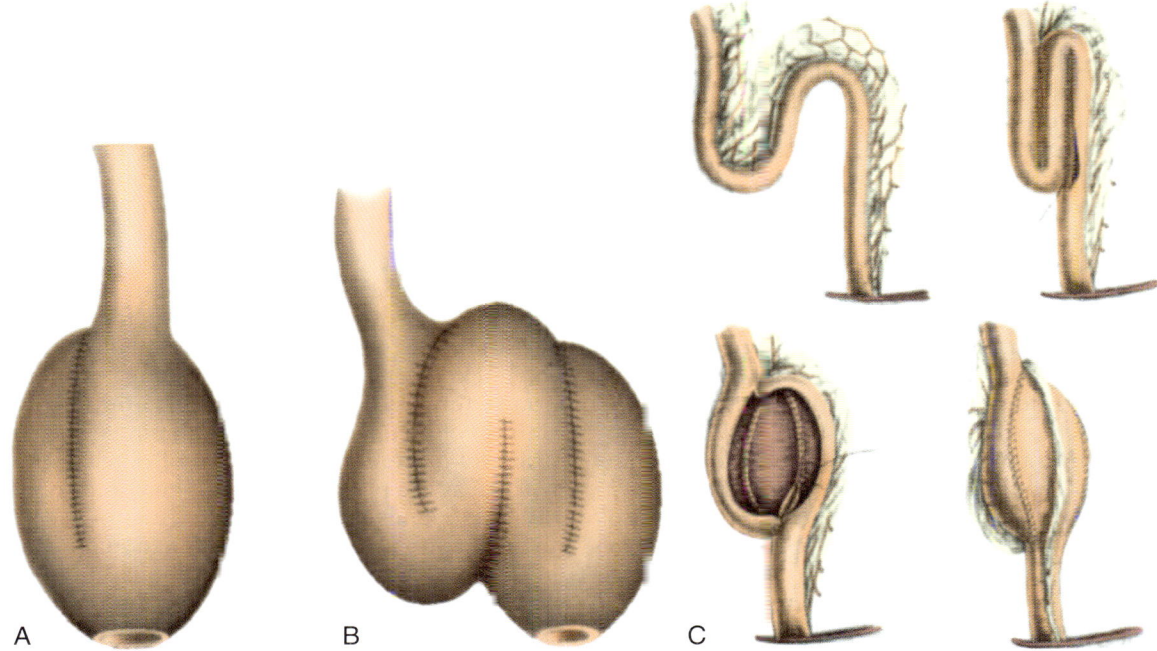

FIGURE 162.15 Ileal pouch designs. (A) J-pouch configuration; (B) W-pouch configuration; (C) S-pouch configuration.

an S pouch are described later. Finally, when despite all of these maneuvers, a tension-free ileoanal anastomosis is not possible, the created pouch can be left suspended in the pelvis as the distal end of a loop ileostomy. The pouch outlet must be closed prior to placing the pouch in the pelvis, and the pouch can be anchored to the pelvic floor with a suture. This maneuver will require another operation to create the anastomosis and can be complicated by reperitonealization of the pelvic floor and rectal stump.

CONSTRUCTION OF THE ILEAL POUCH

Various configurations are described for construction of the ileal pouch. The J, S, and W pouch configurations are well described (Fig. 162.15). Functional outcomes are similar across all of these designs. The choice of pouch configuration is dictated by the experience of the surgeon and the body habitus of the patient.[3]

Two-Limbed Pelvic Ileal Reservoir—J Pouch

Originally described by Utsunomiya et al. in 1980,[5] the ileal J pouch is the most commonly used configuration. The J pouch is a two-limbed folded ileal pouch. The apex of the pouch must reach the anal canal without tension and is determined as the most dependent part of the reservoir. The length of the pouch is typically 15 to 20 cm, and no functional difference exists between J pouches constructed from two 15-cm limbs or two 20-cm limbs.[59] The reservoir is created by making an enterotomy at the portion of the terminal ileum that most easily reaches below the pubis. A linear stapler is passed up either limb, the antimesenteric borders of the afferent and efferent limbs are aligned, and the stapler fired to create the reservoir. Multiple firings may be required to complete the length

of the pouch. Each subsequent stapler is placed into the pouch and the pouch is telescoped onto the stapler so the end of the previous staple line is at the crotch of the stapling device. Seromuscular sutures can be placed between the antimesenteric aspects of each limb to prevent torque on the staple line. The anvil of the circular stapler is fitted into the apex of the ileal pouch and secured with a handsewn purse-string suture in preparation for the IPAA.

ALTERNATIVE POUCH CONFIGURATIONS: THE S POUCH AND W POUCH

Alternatives to the J pouch design include the three-limbed S pouch and four-limbed W pouch. The S pouch configuration described in the original restorative procedures is an adaptation of the Kock continent ileostomy reservoir (see Fig. 162.15).[61,62] The distal 30 to 45 cm of ileum are folded in an S shape and anastomosed to create a reservoir with a remaining efferent limb. Each of the three limbs is approximately 10 cm in length with a 2-cm efferent limb that is handsewn to the dentate line in the anal canal. Because of its configuration, the three "seams" of the pouch must be handsewn. Interrupted or running seromuscular sutures are placed to create the outer back wall of the ileal pouch, and the "pouch" is opened by making an enterotomy along the entire length of the S shape directly antimesenteric. Starting at the apex of each bend of the S shape, a running full-thickness suture line is created with an absorbable, monofilament material. The two sutures are carried onto the front wall of the ileal pouch until they meet in the middle of the pouch. This suture line is inbricated with interrupted or running seromuscular sutures. The S pouch is placed in a supralevator location, and the efferent limb serves as a neoanal canal. The S pouch is typically considered only when it is anticipated that a J pouch is unable to reach into the pelvis. The S pouch configuration usually provides sufficient length for a tension-free anastomosis. However, if the efferent limb is too long (>2 cm) or a long rectal cuff is retained, outflow obstruction can occur and self-catheterization may be required. Spontaneous lengthening of the efferent limb can also occur over time as a result of chronic distention of the pouch. Efferent limbs of 4 to 5 cm have been found at the time of revision in pouches originally constructed with a 1-cm efferent limb.[16,63] The efficiency of evacuation of S pouches is inferior to the J and W pouch. The need for self-catheterization is higher with an S pouch.[11,12,64,65] Outflow obstruction commonly leads to stasis, bacterial overgrowth, distention, and atony of the pouch.[12,66]

Local approaches to shorten the pouch outlet include transanal stapling of the septum between the efferent limb and the pouch without the need for proximal diversion.[14] Transanal sleeve advancement of the efferent limb is also reported, but success with local approaches is somewhat limited.[67] A transabdominal mobilization of the ileal pouch is usually required, wherein the efferent limb is transected at the desired level and the pouch-anal anastomosis recreated. Alternatively, the triplicated pouch can be converted to a J pouch or the efferent limb can be entirely excised and anastomosis performed via a stapled technique to the base of the ileal reservoir. Unfortunately, only 50% of these patients eventually report good function.[16,68]

The four-limbed W pouch was introduced in 1985 by Nicholls and Pezim in an effort to address the outflow complications seen in the S pouch and improve the functional result of the J pouch.[18,69] The W pouch is created from four 12-cm lengths of ileum in a W configuration. The apex of the pouch is the site of the IPAA so there is no efferent limb with this pouch configuration. Once again, this configuration requires a handsewn construction and follows similar technical steps as described for the S pouch. The four-limbed construction makes this a capacious and bulky pouch that offers increased reservoir akin to the native rectal ampulla. However, the size and bulk can be problematic within the confines of a narrow pelvis. In a narrow pelvis, design of the reservoir may be modified such that the distal two limbs are each 11 to 12 cm in length and the more proximal two limbs are 9 to 10 cm long, effectively making the reservoir out of two J pouches that are offset from one another (see Fig. 162.15).

COMPARATIVE STUDIES OF POUCH DESIGN AND FUNCTIONAL OUTCOME

The W pouch is associated with lower daytime and nighttime frequency of defecation and less use of antidiarrheal medication compared with the J pouch.[20,70] However, this benefit is only demonstrated in short-term follow-up, with similar function seen in both pouch configurations at 9-year follow-up.[23,71] This short-term benefit does not completely justify the complexity in construction required of the W pouch, and routine use of the J pouch configuration is generally favored.[25,72–74]

Frequency of defecation correlates inversely with the capacity of the reservoir.[30,64,73,74] A balance exists between adequate capacity of the ileal pouch to allow for acceptable

frequency and prevention of pouch overdistention with associated outflow obstruction and atony. Patients with a mature ileal pouch pass approximately 600 to 700 mL of semiformed stool each day. Loperamide reduces intestinal motility and thus may improve intestinal absorption, reduce the volume of stool, and decrease the frequency of bowel action. Although dietary discretion and stool-bulking agents play a major role in addressing urgency of defecation and perianal irritation by increasing stool consistency, these measures seem to have minimal effect on stool volume. Studies have shown little difference in the efficiency of evacuation of pouches according to the consistency of stool, which implies that measures to alter the thickness of stool will have minimal influence on ileal pouch function.[33,75] Function is maintained long term with very little, if any, deterioration in terms of frequency of bowel movements, efficiency of evacuation, and fecal leakage as the pouch matures. The choice of ileal pouch design depends on the characteristics of the patient and the surgeon's preference. The functional outcome varies little between different configurations, and most patients will find that they will have bowel movements between 4 and 7 times per 24 hours with perhaps one nocturnal evacuation. The majority of patients will experience a normal urge to defecate and will be able to defer defecation and discriminate between flatus and feces.

ILEOANAL ANASTOMOSIS: COMPARISON OF HANDSEWN VERSUS STAPLED

Two techniques of IPAA have been described: transanal mucosectomy with handsewn anastomosis technique and a stapled anastomosis technique. Mucosectomy in theory removes all diseased mucosa. However, this is a time-consuming and technically challenging procedure that risks anal trauma and incontinence. Stapling is quicker and easier to perform, with minimal anal trauma, but the retained mucosa is at risk for dysplasia or symptomatic cuffitis.

The risk of dysplasia in the retained anorectal mucosa after double-stapled anastomosis is low and rarely progresses to carcinoma with regular endoscopic surveillance.[38,76] In the case of mucosectomy, residual mucosa can be present 14% of the time within the rectal cuff that is excluded from endoscopic surveillance.[64,77,78]

The anorectal cuff created after mucosectomy can be a source of perianastomotic abscess. Comparison of handsewn versus stapled IPAA demonstrated that handsewn IPAA is associated with higher rates of anastomotic disruptions, peripouch abscess, pouch removal, postoperative anastomotic stricture, and small bowel obstruction.[19,42,47,63]

Double-stapled anastomosis is associated with better fine control of continence due to preservation of the richly innervated ATZ. Simple passage of the stapling device decreases trauma to the anus.[35,79] After a mean follow-up of 7.1 years, Kirat et al. reported that a handsewn IPAA anastomosis was associated with worse incontinence, seepage, pad usage, and dietary/work restrictions. Quality of life metrics were significantly greater in those who underwent a stapled anastomosis.[47,63]

In a recent comparison of 91 patients with ulcerative colitis undergoing handsewn versus stapled IPAA, older patients with handsewn anastomoses had higher rates of fecal soiling and frequency of bowel movements. However, no significant differences in functional and quality-of-life measures were noted at 3 years.[49,80] In a meta-analysis of 4183 patients, the functional disadvantage of handsewn anastomosis is clear, with anal rest and squeeze pressures and increased nocturnal incontinence.[45,65]

TRANSANAL MUCOSECTOMY: OPERATIVE TECHNIQUE

The table is positioned in the Trendelenburg position, and the hips are placed in flexion to adequately expose the anus. A self-retaining anal retractor is used to evert the anus and expose the dentate line. A circumferential incision is made through the mucosa at the dentate line, and the more proximal submucosal plane is infiltrated with a solution of 1 : 100,000 epinephrine The mucosa is dissected off the underlying rectal wall with scissors or cautery, with the dissection continued to a level above the anorectal ring, at which point the rectal wall is incised and the proctectomy is completed. The specimen is either transabdominally or transanally removed, and the apex of the pouch is delivered to the level of the sphincter. Prior to delivering the pouch into the anal canal, four or more full-thickness sutures incorporating the anal mucosa and internal sphincter are placed at regular intervals around the circumference of the canal to begin the anastomosis. A ring or atraumatic clamp is passed through the anal canal into the pelvis to grasp the pouch in proper orientation (small bowel mesenteric edge to the patient's right, body of pouch in curve of sacrum) and deliver it to the distal canal. The previously placed sutures are passed through the full thickness of the pouch wall to secure the pouch into place. Finally, the anastomosis is completed with interrupted, full-thickness sutures such that no defects are identified. The spacing between each suture and the total number of sutures is at the surgeon's discretion (Fig. 162.16).

STAPLED ILEOANAL ANASTOMOSIS: OPERATIVE TECHNIQUE

After the rectum is circumferentially mobilized, the surgeon must determine the level of rectal transaction with a linear stapler. Rectal transection within 1.5 cm above the dentate line offers good functional results while minimizing the length of retained mucosa.[5,53–55,81] The level of transection can be confirmed with a digital examination through the anus to a distance at some point between the distal and middle phalangeal joint. Alternatively, the stapler is placed within 3 cm of the anal verge. Getting the stapler to the pelvic floor can be difficult in a patient with a long or narrow pelvis so perineal pressure can be applied to help bring the distal rectum into the pelvis for stapling.

One of the major shortcomings encountered with laparoscopic proctectomy is the technical challenge of rectal division at the appropriate level above the dentate line. For this reason, some surgeons advocate for rectal division with a linear stapler through an extended port site or Pfannenstiel incision. After the rectum is divided, the circular stapling device is inserted into the anorectal stump and the central spike is advanced through the transecting staple line. The shaft of the anvil previously secured in the apex of the pouch is mated to stapler spike,

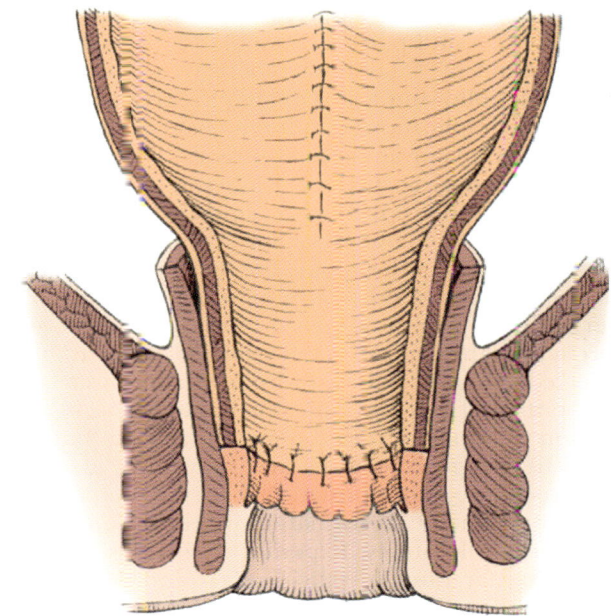

FIGURE 162.16 Handsewn ileoanal anastomosis.

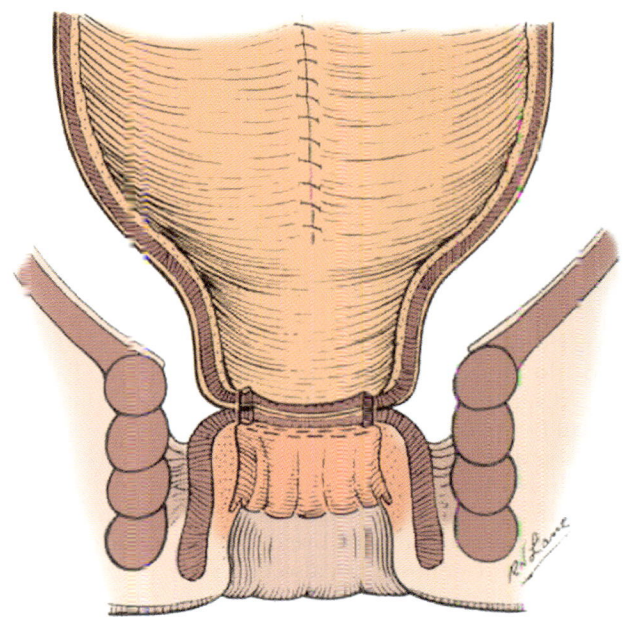

FIGURE 162.17 Stapled ileoanal anastomosis.

and the distal staple line is gently effaced against the head of the stapler. Any surrounding tissue is retracted, and the stapler is closed under direct visualization to ensure no torsion of the ileal pouch has occurred. The pouch orientation is ensured. A leak test of the anastomosis is recommended (Fig. 162.17).

Rectal eversion is associated with a decrement in manometric parameters.[56,82] However, the effect on long-term functional outcomes is mixed.[57,58,60,83,84]

Pelvic sepsis following an IPAA results in a pouch failure rate of 20%[61,85] and poor functional outcomes when the pouch is retained.[63,85] Lower rates of pelvic septic complications occur following a three-stage procedure, without additional complications despite the patient undergoing an additional major abdominal surgery. The association between high-dose corticosteroids (equivalent to ≥40 mg of daily prednisone) and pelvic sepsis is supported and should be a consideration in staging.[64,65,84,86] These data can be interpreted to both support the safety of a three-stage approach in the case of the immunocompromised or emergently ill patient and argue the use of a two-stage approach in the appropriately selected patients.[66,86] In a selected group of patients who have optimized nutrition, control of any extraintestinal manifestations, and cessation of corticosteroid therapy for at least 3 months after a first-stage colectomy and ileostomy, a second-stage procedure is performed that includes completion proctectomy and IPAA formation without the inclusion of a diverting ileostomy. Experience with this approach reports similar rates of pelvic sepsis and comparable functional outcomes during short-term follow-up. A shorter preoperative duration of illness was associated with a higher rate of complications, likely attributable to the severity of disease in patients who required surgery soon after diagnosis. In a cost analysis, this modified two-stage approach was significantly less costly by $14,206 per patient.[68,87]

Experience with a single-stage pouch is reported by several centers, with rates of postoperative complications equivalent to those seen with two- and three-stage ileal pouch procedures.[69,87] Careful patient selection and a low threshold for intervention is required as a significantly higher proportion of these patients require emergency laparotomy for management of septic complications compared with diverted patients.[70,88] This is an appealing option considering that the creation and closure of a diverting loop ileostomy contributes to postoperative morbidity, with 21% of small bowel obstructions occurring at the site of the ileostomy takedown following IPAA. Patients with a diverting ileostomy have significantly higher rates of small bowel obstruction at 11.4% versus 5.2% in those without a diversion.[71,89]

High stoma output is also a common cause of dehydration, requiring readmission. Local problems, including peristomal skin breakdown, stoma prolapse, retraction, and stenosis, can also be a source of morbidity. Ultimately discretion of the surgeon and the patient's willingness to accept risk dictate the appropriate approach to staging.

MANAGEMENT OF POUCH-SPECIFIC POSTOPERATIVE COMPLICATIONS

INVESTIGATION

Early postoperative complications following restorative proctocolectomy approach 19% to 33%, with a reported mortality rate of 0.1%.[72–74,90–93] Awareness of the common postoperative complications and a systematic approach to identifying underlying causes are necessary for prompt diagnosis and intervention (Table 162.1).

TABLE 162.1 Assessment of Dysfunction of the Ileal Pouch

Clinical examination	Inspection	Fecal seepage
		External fistulas
		Anal fissures/abrasions
		Excoriation
		Mucosal prolapse
	Digital examination	Anastomotic stenosis
		Perianal induration
		Height of anastomosis above dentate line
Endoscopy	Anoscopy	Cuffitis
		Mucosal prolapse
	Pouchoscopy	Mucosal inflammation
		Distensibility of pouch
		4-quadrant biopsies
	Flexible pouchoscopy	Prepouch inflammation
		Small bowel Crohn disease
	Examination under anesthesia	Identification of anastomosis defect
		Need for procedure (Drainage/dilation/biopsy)
Imaging	CT	Suspicion of pelvic sepsis
	MR	Assessment of fistulas
	Water-contrast enema	Structural abnormality of the pouch
		Small bowel Crohn disease
Anal assessment	Anal manometry	Fecal seepage/soilage

CT, Computed tomography; *MR,* magnetic resonance.

PELVIC SEPSIS

The most common sources of pelvic sepsis are related to an anastomotic leak. Pouch ischemia, inflammation, or infection can also present with a similar constellation of clinical and physical findings.

The incidence of pelvic sepsis following IPAA ranges from 5% to 19%.[38,64,73,74,82,94,95] In a series from Heuschen et al. fistulas accounted for 76% of septic events (56% ileal pouch–anal anastomotic, 13% ileal pouch–vaginal, 7% proximal pouch), with anastomotic separation (16%) and parapouch abscesses (8%) constituting the remainder of cases of pelvic sepsis.[75,96]

Presentation of pelvic sepsis can be acute, manifested by abdominal pain, fever, and general or local peritonitis. Subacute scenarios can present, with indolent pelvic pain and pouch dysfunction, and are sometimes asymptomatic, only to be diagnosed at the time of water-contrast enema prior to ileostomy reversal.

DIAGNOSIS

CT imaging is the best diagnostic tool to identify pelvic sepsis because it typically will reveal a pelvic collection or inflammation and thickening of the ileal pouch. The most common site of disruption is the circular staple line, but disruption can also occur at the "blind end of the J" or within the longitudinal staple lines of the pouch.[79,97] A contrast pouchogram, examination under anesthesia, and percutaneous drainage with fistulagram are potential options used to identify the site of disruption. A pelvic collection may also spontaneously discharge through the anastomosis, with subsequent formation of a fistula that will help identify the location of the internal opening.

INTERVENTION

Treatment options for pelvic sepsis depend on the extent of and patient response to the sepsis. Experience from the Mayo Clinic of 1508 patients undergoing IPAA reports the outcome of 73 (4.8%) patients with pelvic sepsis. The rate of transabdominal operative intervention in these patients was 55% and the rate of local intervention was 8%. Of the remaining patients nonoperatively managed, 15% of abscesses resolved with antibiotics alone and 22% required CT-guided drainage, with all but three patients healing without the need for subsequent operation. Pouch failure occurred in 20% of patients developing pelvic sepsis.[76-98] In the case of an organized pelvic abscess, drainage can be performed via a transanal or percutaneous approach. Transanal drainage is generally preferred if an anastomotic leak is suspected. Careful evaluation of the anastomotic suture line may reveal a dehiscence. In this case, a small mushroom-tipped catheter, usually 10 or 12 French, can be placed into the collection through the area of dehiscence and sutured to the wall of the ileal pouch at the site of the defect. The perineum and vagina should be closely inspected for evidence of fistula, but primary perineal or transvaginal drainage is discouraged, given the high incidence of resultant complicated fistulas. Percutaneous drainage can take a transabdominal or transgluteal approach but may result in an extrasphincteric fistula in ano if an anastomotic leak is present.

In cases of uncontrolled sepsis or failure of nonoperative management, abdominal exploration with pelvic washout is required. The ileal pouch must be endoscopically evaluated. If the patient is not diverted, a loop ileostomy should be created to salvage the pouch. In some cases, the site of perforation can be repaired and widely drained. Pouch ischemia is an absolute indication for ileal pouch excision. If there is complete pouch separation but no communication to the peritoneal cavity, the pouch should be left in situ to facilitate pouch revision in the future. Prompt diagnosis and treatment are essential to minimize inflammation and the fibrosis that ultimately leads to pouch dysfunction or loss.

RISK FACTORS FOR DEVELOPMENT OF PELVIC SEPSIS

A clear association exists between high-dose corticosteroids (equivalent to ≥40 mg of daily prednisone) and pelvic septic complications.[64,78,82] The effect of infliximab and other biologic agents may be an independent risk factor for postoperative infectious complications, as already discussed.[15,17,19,99,100] Obesity (body mass index [BMI] >30 kg/m^2) and intraoperative blood transfusion are markers for technically challenging pelvic surgery and are also independent risk factors for pelvic sepsis.[65-101] Technical factors are related to construction of the IPAA. If lengthening maneuvers that involve manipulating the mesentery lead to ischemia, anastomotic healing will be compromised.

Tension is the most common and underappreciated risk factor for anastomotic disruption. When the pouch is connected to the anal canal, the tension is in cephalad to caudad direction, but with a short mesentery or thick abdominal wall, delivery of the stoma above the skin level will create an anterior direction in the force vector and result in further tension on the anastomosis. This tension can be alleviated by choosing a more proximal segment of bowel as the site of diverting stoma.

Pouch sepsis resulted in increased stool frequency, the need for antidiarrheal medication, day and nighttime incontinence, decreased stool/gas discrimination, and sexual dysfunction.[63,102] Risk of pouch excision approaches 40% in patients who have experienced pelvic sepsis at the time of pouch creation. Among those patients able to be treated with a nonoperative approach, function is acceptable in more than 90%.[86,103]

POSTOPERATIVE HEMORRHAGE

Postoperative hemorrhage is rare, occurring in 1.5% to 3.5% of patients. The site of hemorrhage is most often intraluminal along staple lines or at the ileostomy. Hemorrhage can also occur at an extraluminal site in the pelvis or peritoneal cavity.[81,104]

Visual inspection of the IPAA and linear staple lines with intraoperative pouchoscopy may help to identify sites of anastomotic bleeding and any anastomotic defects.

The vast majority of staple line bleeding is self-limited, and site of bleeding is often difficult to identify. When minor bleeding or multiple points of bleeding are encountered, endoscopy and clipping or cautery of the bleeding site or irrigation of the pouch with a dilute epinephrine solution is effective in 80% of cases.[81,105] Delayed pouch bleeding is uncommon and should raise the suspicion for anastomotic complications. An examination under anesthesia may reveal foci of anastomotic dehiscence that can be managed with transanal drain placement or oversewing as tissue integrity permits.[82,106]

Intraabdominal bleeding most commonly occurs in the pelvis or from the ileal-pouch mesentery. In severe cases, packing of the pelvis or detachment of the pouch and careful inspection may be required to control the bleeding.[83,10-]

STRICTURE AT THE ILEAL POUCH–ANAL ANASTOMOSIS

The rate of stricture formation is higher following a handsewn anastomosis compared with the stapled technique. However, use of a small-diameter circular stapler can create a narrow circular opening that is also prone to stenosis as it heals. Larger diameter staplers are less frequently associated with the long-term development of an anastomotic stricture. Symptoms of an anastomotic stricture include incomplete evacuation with straining, defecatory urgency, and frequent watery stools. The time interval from IPAA construction to the development of an anastomotic stricture ranges from 6 to 9 months.[84,107] All patients should undergo a digital examination to assess the patency of the anastomosis prior to closure of the ileostomy. This allows for dilation of stenosis and may also detect subclinical anastomotic disruption. Following mucosectomy, the narrowing is often longer.[85] Digital dilation should be gently performed and pressure distributed in a radial fashion rather than focused to a single area to avoid disruption of the anastomosis. Short soft strictures due to a web formation at circular staple lines are adequately dilated in a single session because daily bowel function will help prevent recurrence. Longer, more fibrotic strictures will require more frequent dilatation. Hegar dilators can be used to sequentially dilate the anastomosis in the clinic or operative setting. An average of 1.5 dilations (range, 1 to 7) is required for treatment. Self-dilation can be prescribed for maintenance of patency. Dilation alone is successful in 95% of nonfibrotic strictures and only 45% of fibrotic strictures. Among patients who respond well to dilation, pouch function is normal.

Strictures refractory to dilation more commonly occur as a consequence of pelvic sepsis with resultant fibrosis. In a study of 1884 restorative proctocolectomy patients treated at Mayo Clinic, 11.2% of patients with anastomotic stricture required operative intervention. Excision of a short segmental stricture with mucosal advancement was performed in five patients, the pouch was redone in three patients, and excision of the pouch with permanent ileostomy was performed in nine patients. All nine excised pouches were associated with perianastomotic complications, including abscess, fistula, or pouch retraction.

POUCH-VAGINAL FISTULAS

The average interval from restorative proctocolectomy to formation of a pouch-vaginal fistula is 21 months (range, 1 to 132 months).[86] Fistulas related to septic complications occur earlier than fistulas without an obvious septic etiology. In a retrospective review by Shah et al., patients with early presentation of a pouch-vaginal fistula typically had faster rates of healing (within 6 months) following repair compared with late fistulas.[86] Delayed or refractory fistulizing disease may represent a delayed presentation of Crohn disease, have significantly lower rates of primary healing, and often require a combination of prolonged fecal diversion in combination with medical therapy.[86] Presenting symptoms of an ileal pouch–vaginal fistula include feculent vaginal drainage or transvaginal passage of flatus. A water-soluble contrast enema or instillation of methylene blue into the pouch with an indicator tampon in the vagina can confirm the diagnosis of a fistula. Pouchoscopy and speculum examination with instillation of methylene blue or hydrogen peroxide solution into the suspected fistula can help localize the defect and define the extent and relationship of the fistula to anastomotic suture lines. A biopsy is indicated if Crohn disease is suspected.

A number of operative approaches have been used in the management of pouch-vaginal fistula. The use of a noncutting seton for control of sepsis is a good initial measure. A significant anterior sphincter defect must often be addressed to achieve healing. Fistulas located at or distal to the ileoanal anastomosis are typically managed with a local procedure and fistulas located above the anastomosis usually require a transabdominal approach.[87]

In a recently published experience with pouch-vaginal fistulas by the Cleveland Clinic, the incidence of pouch-vaginal fistula was 2.9%, with an overall pouch failure rate of 33% at a median follow-up of 83 months (range, 5 to 480 months). A redo-ileal pouch procedure was performed in 19 patients, with a pouch retention rate of 40%. An ileal pouch advancement was associated with a healing rate of 42% when performed as an initial procedure, and 66% when performed after a failed prior repair. Transvaginal repair was associated with a healing rate of 55% when performed as a primary procedure, and 40% when performed as a secondary procedure.[87] Transvaginal repair is a way to limit anal sphincter trauma in a group of patients at already high risk for anal incontinence.[88]

Use of a diverting ileostomy was not demonstrated to reduce the risk of pouch-vaginal fistula nor improve the success of repair. However, the benefit of diversion in reducing the extent of pelvic sepsis would suggest a theoretical risk reduction of sepsis–related fistulas. Regardless, diversion is often performed for complex fistula repair and in part offers respite from symptoms.[89]

SMALL BOWEL OBSTRUCTION

Small bowel obstruction is a common complication following restorative proctocolectomy and occurs in 20% to 40% of patients. Adhesive disease accounts for the majority of cases of small bowel obstructions. In review of 460 patients treated at the Lahey Clinic, 94 patients (20%) had 109 episodes of obstruction, with 40 episodes occurring after the creation of the pouch, 29 episodes after closure of the ileostomy, and 40 episodes in the subsequent follow-up period.[91] Operative intervention was required only 7% of the time, with the source of obstruction identified at the site of ileostomy takedown in 52% of cases. In 12% of cases, adhesions from the afferent limb of the pouch to the sacral hollow result in sharp angulation with obstruction. The typical presentation in this scenario is recurrent episodes of small bowel obstruction with plain radiography or CT imaging demonstrating small bowel dilation to the level of the pouch. A preoperative water-soluble contrast enema may confirm the inlet obstruction. Operative intervention should be used as with any patient who has a bowel obstruction, but caution is needed to understand the anatomy and avoid injury to the proximal pouch or intervening mesentery. If there is extensive scarring in the pelvis and the afferent limb cannot be reduced into the abdomen, an enteroenteral bypass with pouchopexy can be performed to alleviate the obstruction.[92]

Laparoscopy has not borne out as an effective method of reducing postoperative obstructive adhesions. In a comparison of operative outcomes between laparoscopic and open restorative proctocolectomy by Fichera et al., no difference was seen in the incidence of small bowel obstruction (12.7% open vs. 15.1% laparoscopic; $P = .66$) or the need for surgical correction of an obstruction (4.7% open vs. 9.6% laparoscopic; $P = .226$) between the groups.[93]

LONG-TERM COMPLICATIONS

CUFFITIS

Retention of a few centimeters of rectal mucosa following construction of a double-stapled IPAA can result in symptomatic inflammation in up to 15% of cases.[90] Presenting symptoms include fecal frequency, outlet bleeding, and pelvic pain, which are some of the same symptoms seen with pouchitis. The treatments for cuffitis and pouchitis are different, so it is important to distinguish between these processes using endoscopy. Cuffitis is typified by a normal-appearing ileal pouch, rectal cuff erythema and friability, and histologic features of ulceration with inflammatory cell infiltration. The exact opposite endoscopic findings are seen with pouchitis.

Treatment of cuffitis with topical corticosteroids or 5-aminosalicylic suppositories or enemas offers a significant reduction in symptoms, with approximately 92% of patients experiencing resolution of outlet bleeding.[94] If cuffitis persists despite topical therapy, systemic agents can be considered. This is rare, and a high index of suspicion for other etiologies such as chronic pelvic sepsis or Crohn disease should be entertained. In the absence of other etiologies, cuffitis that is resistant to medical therapy can be treated with mucosectomy and pouch advancement to prevent sequelae of stricture, pouch dysfunction, and pouch failure.[82] The mucosectomy is performed via a perineal approach with submucosal infiltration of a solution of 1:100,000 epinephrine. A mucosal resection is performed from the level of the dentate line to the stapled IPAA. The anastomosis is excised and the dissection is continued cephalad into the peripouch space to allow tension-free delivery of the ileal pouch to the level of the anal verge. A new IPAA is created with interrupted sutures. Induration and friability of the mucosa and pouch makes this a technically challenging procedure. Lack of adequate pouch mobility may require transabdominal mobilization of the ileal pouch to allow for a tension-free anastomosis. In cases of severe inflammation, a permanent end ileostomy may be required and the patient must be counseled regarding this possibility.[95]

RISK FOR NEOPLASIA

The retained rectal mucosa following a double-stapled IPAA is also subject to dysplasia and malignant transformation. In a prospective review by Remzi et al. 289 patients with IPAA were surveyed with serial biopsies of the ATZ. After a minimum 10-year follow-up, dysplasia developed in only eight patients, at a median of 9 months (range, 4 to 123 months) after surgery with no cancers identified during the study period. Based on these findings, surveillance recommendations for patients without preexisting dysplasia of their rectum or other neoplasia risk factors include pouchoscopy and biopsy of the IPAA 1 year after surgery and every 2 to 3 years thereafter. Patients with preexisting dysplasia in the upper two-thirds of the rectum or other risk factors for neoplasia should be surveyed annually with pouchoscopy and biopsy. The only widely accepted indication for mucosectomy is the presence of cancer or dysplasia in the rectum. However, little data are available to support this practice because there appears to be minimal risk of development of adenocarcinoma in the anal canal with or without a mucosectomy.[15,17,38] Stapled IPAA is an acceptable technique in this setting, but regular surveillance of the retained rectal cuff is paramount.[38] A stapled IPAA should be strongly considered in obese or elderly patients or those with preoperative low sphincter pressures, due to the higher risk of incontinence following mucosectomy and handsewn anastomosis. In the setting of preoperative diagnosis of dysplasia, surveillance pouchoscopy and biopsy should begin 6 months following surgery and continue on an annual basis based on findings. Findings of low-grade

dysplasia on postoperative surveillance should be closely followed with repeat biopsies every 6 months for up to 3 years. Mucosectomy with ileal pouch advancement is indicated in patients with persistent low-grade dysplasia or progression to high-grade dysplasia.

POUCHITIS

Pouchitis is one of the most common complications following restorative proctocolectomy, with an incidence of 16% to 48%. This incidence increases over time, with 40% of patients reporting at least one episode of pouchitis at 10 years and 70% at 20 years.[5]

Pathogenesis

Pouchitis is an idiopathic disorder with multiple risk factors predisposing to its development. In a meta-analysis comparing familial adenomatous polyposis versus ulcerative colitis managed by restorative proctocolectomy, ulcerative colitis was associated with a substantially higher risk of pouchitis (5.5% vs. 30.1%: OR 6.44; 95% CI, 3.21 to 12.9; $P < .001$).[97] Pouchitis is also more common in ulcerative colitis patients with primary sclerosing cholangitis compared with those without the disease. Other extraintestinal manifestations are associated with a 10-fold increase in risk for the development of pouchitis after 5-year follow-up (48% vs. 4.6%; $P = .01$) suggesting that pouchitis is mediated by the same proinflammatory process underlying the primary diagnosis.[98] Other risk factors for the development of pouchitis include postoperative septic complications, older age, nonsmoking status, and postoperative use of nonsteroidal antiinflammatory drugs (NSAIDs).[82]

Some evidence suggests that pouchitis is infectious in nature, with stasis and bacterial overgrowth resulting in morphologic changes in the pouch mucosa. Villous atrophy and crypt hyperplasia are classified as colonic metaplasia and may represent a response to inflammation. In a histologic study of pouch biopsy specimens from patients with and without pouchitis, colonic metaplasia and inflammation scores were higher among patients with pouchitis, suggesting that these architectural changes are a reparative response to inflammation.[99]

The pouch microbiome also differs between patients with pouchitis compared with unaffected patients, with higher concentrations of anaerobes and aerobes and a reduced ratio of anaerobes to aerobes. The effectiveness of antibiotic therapy directed to anaerobic flora supports this association.[100] Other causative factors include mucosal ischemia, immune deficiency, nonspecific IBD, and occult Crohn disease. In addition, a wide spectrum in the severity and frequency of pouchitis is appreciated and the clinical scenario appears to be dictated by its underlying mechanism. For example, isolated, acute bouts of pouchitis are more likely related to the microbiome of the ileal pouch. Conversely, chronic, medication-dependent pouchitis appears to be more inflammatory mediated.

Diagnosis of Pouchitis

Patients with pouchitis experience an increase in fecal frequency. Bowel consistency is looser secondary to exudative inflammation with blood staining or mucus. Pelvic discomfort and low-grade fever with malaise often accompany the change in bowel habits. Extraintestinal manifestations, including erythema nodosum, uveitis, and arthritis, may also reactivate in the setting of pouchitis. Endoscopic evaluation is significant for inflamed and friable pouch mucosa with ulceration and exudate. Histopathologic assessment reveals an acute inflammatory infiltrate and the presence of neutrophils and villous atrophy with crypt abscesses. However, the association between endoscopic and histologic appearance of the pouch inconsistently correlates with the patient's clinical symptoms.

In the clinical setting, a diagnosis of pouchitis is not dictated by strict diagnostic criteria, but a spectrum of disease exists. The Pouchitis Disease Activity Index (PDAI) is a useful tool for quantifying disease severity using clinical, endoscopic, and histologic features in a scoring system, and pouchitis is defined as a total score greater than 7 (Table 162.2).

TABLE 162.2 Pouchitis Disease Activity Index

Criteria	Score
CLINICAL	
Stool Frequency	
Usual postoperative BM	0
1–2 BM more than usual	1
3+ more than usual	2
Rectal Bleeding	
None	0
Present daily	1
Fecal Urgency or Cramps	
None	0
Occasional	1
Usual	2
Fever	
Absent	0
Present	1
ENDOSCOPIC INFLAMMATION	
Edema	1
Granularity	1
Friability	1
Loss of vascular pattern	1
Mucous exudate	1
Ulceration	1
ACUTE HISTOLOGIC INFLAMMATION	
Leukocyte Infiltration	
Mild	1
Moderate with crypt abscess	2
Severe with crypt abscess	3
Ulceration Per Low-Power Field (Mean)	
<25%	1
25%–50%	2
>50%	3

Note: Pouchitis is defined as a total score greater than 7 points.
BM, Bowel movement.
From Sandborn WJ, Tremaine WJ, Batts KP, Pemberton JH, Phillips SF. Pouchitis after ileal pouch–anal anastomosis: a Pouchitis Disease Activity Index. *Mayo Clin Proc.* 1994;69:409.

The PDAI is an easy-to-use and accurate measure of pouchitis symptoms, with significantly greater scores seen in patients with clinical features of pouchitis compared with asymptomatic patients.[101]

TREATMENT OF ACUTE POUCHITIS

Oral metronidazole at a dose of 750 to 1500 mg/day for 7 to 14 days is effective with resolution of symptoms generally seen within 3 days of starting therapy. A randomized, double-blind, placebo-controlled crossover trial in 13 patients confirmed the long-held view of the efficacy of this form of treatment. The side effects of oral therapy can be avoided by topical therapy, in which serum concentrations of metronidazole are very low. Patients who are unresponsive to metronidazole may respond to cyclic courses of three or four antibiotics, such as ciprofloxacin, amoxicillin/clavulanic acid, erythromycin, and tetracycline, given at weekly intervals. Budesonide suppositories (1.5 mg/day) have also been shown to be efficacious. Frequent relapses of pouchitis require treatment with long-term, low-dose suppressive metronidazole therapy.

Stool studies suggest that the fecal concentration of lactobacilli and bifidobacteria is significantly decreased in patients with pouchitis. A randomized, double-blind, placebo-controlled trial evaluated use of the probiotic VSL#3, which consists of eight bacterial strains, in the prevention of recurrence of pouchitis. In the treatment group, 17 of 20 patients were still in remission at 9 months, as compared with 0 of 20 patients treated with placebo. However, all patients who received VSL#3 relapsed within 4 months of discontinuing their treatment. The fecal concentrations of lactobacilli and bifidobacteria were significantly increased in the treatment group during the study period but returned to baseline 1 month after completion of the study.[102] It remains unclear whether multiple bacterial strains are required to induce remission. A Cochrane analysis of the treatment and prevention of pouchitis reviewed 11 randomized controlled trials that fulfilled the inclusion criteria with evaluation of 10 different pharmacologic agents. Ciprofloxacin was more effective at inducing remission in acute pouchitis than metronidazole, but neither rifaximin nor lactobacillus GG was more effective than placebo. VSL#3 was more effective than placebo in maintaining remission in chronic pouchitis and in preventing pouchitis.[103]

Chronic antibiotic-refractory pouchitis (CARP) is uncommon and may represent underlying viral infection, structural/functional pathologies, or autoimmune-mediated disease. Fecal bacterial culture and sensitivity testing is a good first measure for pouchitis that is refractory to commonly used empiric antibiotics. Cytomegalovirus infection should be evaluated and requires treatment with the antiviral ganciclovir therapy.[104] *Clostridium difficile*–associated infection requires treatment with oral metronidazole or vancomycin.[105] NSAID use and structural/functional issues, including fistula, ischemia, and stricture, should be excluded. Immune-mediated pouchitis is a newly described disorder that may underlie CARP. The association between patients with CARP and other autoinflammatory disorders, such as primary sclerosing cholangitis and autoimmune thyroid disease, has been described.[106] Empiric treatment includes topical or systemic corticosteroids, immunomodulators, or even anti-TNF-α agents.[104] The efficacy of infliximab has been studied in the treatment of chronic refractory pouchitis complicated after restorative proctocolectomy. The long-term efficacy of infliximab in patients with refractory pouch complications such as luminal inflammation or pouch fistulas was evaluated in 28 patients, and 88% of patients with refractory luminal inflammation showed clinical response, whereas 86% of patients showed fistula response.[107]

Prepouch ileitis can also occur concurrent with pouchitis. In a study by McLaughlin et al. prepouch ileitis was diagnosed concurrent with pouchitis in 34 (5.7%) of 742 patients undergoing pouchoscopy. The clinical implications of prepouch ileitis are unknown, but this finding does not appear to imply missed Crohn disease or increase the risk of pouch failure.[108] Combination antibiotic therapy (Cipro 500 mg twice daily and flagyl 500 mg three times daily) appears to be effective in reducing the length of prepouch inflammation and inducing symptomatic remission in most patients.

Irritable pouch syndrome is a functional disorder in patients with an IPAA that causes symptoms in the absence of structural or inflammatory abnormalities of the pouch. It resembles other functional disorders, such as irritable bowel syndrome, that are characterized by visceral hypersensitivity. Similarly, irritable pouch syndrome is characterized by sensation of gas, urge to defecate, and pain.[94]

CROHN DISEASE

The clinical presentation of ulcerative colitis can have significant overlap with indeterminate colitis, as well as Crohn disease. Crohn disease is an independent predictor of pouch failure, with up to 50% of pouch failures attributed to this diagnosis.[109]

In a retrospective review of 790 patients treated by IPAA at the Lahey Clinic, 4.1% of patients were identified as having a postoperative diagnosis of Crohn disease. The median time to diagnosis was 19 months (range, 0 to 188 months). Complications occurred in 93% of patients, including anorectal abscess/fistula, refractory pouchitis, and anal stricture, and 29% of patients underwent diversion or pouch excision at a median of 66 months (range, 6 to 187 months). Among patients with a functional IPAA, 60% of patients admitted to leakage, 45% required pad use, and 50% required medical therapy for disease control. These findings demonstrate the significant morbidity associated with Crohn disease affecting an ileal reservoir.[109]

Despite this compelling evidence, Regimbeau et al. have suggested that restorative proctocolectomy can be offered to a selected group of patients with isolated colonic disease in whom proctocolectomy with permanent end ileostomy would be the only alternative.[110] Based on experience with 41 patients fitting these criteria, disease-related complication rates were considered acceptably low at 27% after 2-year follow-up. Seven patients developed pouch-perineal fistulas surgically managed. In a subset of 20 patients with follow-up greater than 10 years, 35% had experienced disease-related complications, but pouch excision was required in only two patients. It is unclear whether the outcomes reported here are more favorable due to the presence of indeterminate colitis in this select group.

Others have reported acceptable outcomes in patients with indeterminate colitis or Crohn disease of the colon and no evidence of small bowel disease or anoperineal disease.[111,112] Certainly, use of IPAA in patients with limited Crohn disease is controversial and deserves further scrutiny.

OTHER COMPLICATIONS

Polyps may develop within a pouch as in the rest of the small bowel. Inflammatory polyps may occur in up to 20% of patients with ulcerative colitis. Inflammatory fibroid polyps, although rare, may cause bleeding or obstruction. Such polyps may occasionally sufficiently grow to fill the lumen of the pouch and require pouch resection with conversion to a permanent ileostomy.

Alopecia has been rarely reported after IPAA, and one study reported a somewhat surprising incidence of 38% in a series of 24 patients.[113] Fortunately, it is a temporary phenomenon, but female patients in particular should be forewarned and reassured if this occurs.

Ileal pouch prolapse is another rare complication with no obvious predisposing factors. A series of 3176 patients identified 11 patients in whom either full-thickness ($n = 7$) or mucosal ($n = 4$) prolapse developed. Although mucosal prolapse was found to respond to either stool bulking or a local procedure, full-thickness prolapse required definitive surgery and was associated with pouch loss.[114]

MALE SEXUAL FUNCTION

Many patients who undergo a restorative proctocolectomy are young, sexually active, and concerned about their sexual function after pelvic surgery. Pelvic surgery may cause male sexual problems, such as erectile dysfunction, absence of ejaculation, or retrograde ejaculation. Only a small percentage (2% to 4%) of male patients suffer severe sexual problems after surgery. Sexual function of males has been examined in a systematic manner by means of a validated scoring system, the International Index of Erectile Function. The scoring system was used to study 127 males who underwent restorative proctocolectomy between 1995 and 2000, with comparison of results before and after IPAA. A statistically significant improvement was reported in erectile function, sexual desire, intercourse satisfaction, and overall satisfaction, with patients having improved scores after surgery compared with before surgery. Overall psychometric sexual satisfaction and sexual quality of life were increased, most likely because of enhanced general health. This study would suggest that male patients undergoing IPAA can be counseled that their sexual function is likely to be retained after surgery.[115] Although the application of the laparoscopic approach to the restorative proctocolectomy may be predicted to further improve sexual function and body image, a comparison of 100 laparoscopic and 189 open operations reported excellent body image and high cosmetic and quality-of-life scores regardless of operative approach. However, orgasmic function scores were lower in men who underwent laparoscopic restorative proctocolectomy compared with the open group.[116] Any male of an age who wishes to have children should be counseled regarding sperm banking in case there is any level of resultant sexual dysfunction.

FEMALE SEXUAL FUNCTION

In an interview-based study by Damgaard et al., sexual function and frequency of intercourse in women following IPAA improved in 35% and 16% experienced an increase in the quality of orgasm. Dyspareunia does increase following restorative proctocolectomy and may be due to alterations in pelvic anatomy or the formation of adhesions. Because the most systematic physical reaction to sexual stimulation is an increase in vaginal vasocongestion, sexual dysfunction may also be associated with autonomic pelvic nerve damage or partial devascularization of the vagina. Studies are mixed regarding persistence of dyspareunia in long-term follow-up.[117,118]

FEMALE REPRODUCTIVE HEALTH

Menses following restorative proctocolectomy is not significantly affected, with the majority of women reporting no change in menstrual cycle. In a small percentage of patients, transient irregularity is reported but is noted to resolve after 2 years of follow-up.[119] However, a clear association exists between restorative proctocolectomy and infertility. In recent meta-analysis, the risk of infertility following IPAA was estimated to be approximately 50% compared with 15% among medically treated patients.[120] Given these data, many surgeons advocate for a three-stage procedure in which subtotal colectomy with end ileostomy is performed and IPAA is deferred until childbearing is completed.[121]

The etiology of infertility following restorative proctocolectomy is thought to be postoperative adhesions to the pelvis with occlusion of fallopian tubes. In a study by Oresland et al., hysterosalpingograms obtained in 21 patients following restorative proctocolectomy discovered fallopian tube occlusion in 52% and adherence of the fallopian tubes to the pelvic floor in 48% of patients.[122] These were largely among patients treated with open procedures that increase the likelihood of adhesion formation. Recent data that consider the formation of pelvic adhesions following laparoscopic surgery suggest that a laparoscopic approach results in fewer pelvic and adnexal adhesions. In an observational study of pelvic and adnexal adhesions at the time of ileostomy takedown, patients who underwent laparoscopic restorative proctocolectomy had significantly lower adhesion scores.[123] In a cross-sectional survey–based study of 179 restorative proctocolectomy patients, laparoscopic IPAA was associated with better preservation of fertility and a higher rate of postoperative pregnancy. A trend toward shorter time to pregnancy was also seen, with 56% of laparoscopic patients achieving conception within 12 months compared with 30% in the open group, suggesting that laparoscopy may be the preferable approach in female patients of childbearing age.[41]

Pregnancy in the patient who has undergone a restorative proctocolectomy remains a topic of controversy, and variability exists regarding the recommended mode of delivery for these patients. In a cross-sectional survey study, most obstetricians recommend vaginal delivery as the mode of delivery, whereas the majority of colorectal surgeons recommend cesarean section, voicing concerns for anal sphincter and pudendal nerve injury resulting in fecal incontinence.[124] Nevertheless, vaginal delivery remains a safe option and does not appear to directly influence pouch function.[117] Until consensus is reached, both methods of delivery are supported.

AGE-RELATED SURGICAL RESULTS AND FUNCTIONAL OUTCOME

Prior to the advent of effective stapling devices that limit the need for prolonged anal dilation and trauma, restorative proctocolectomy was not recommended for older patients. However, the basis for this recommendation is limited, and several studies support restorative proctocolectomy in older patients with minor limitations in postoperative function and quality of life. Farouk et al. found that incontinence and nocturnal frequency was higher in patients who underwent restorative proctocolectomy over the age of 45 years and dysfunction of the pouch deteriorated over time compared with young controls. However, the older patients had better postoperative satisfaction despite dysfunction.[125]

In a prospective study of functional outcome and quality of life in 1895 patients stratified by age with 1-, 3-, 5-, and 10-year follow-up after IPAA, incontinence and nighttime seepage was more common in older patients. However, there was no difference in daytime stool frequency at 5-year follow-up. Nighttime frequency was worse at 1-year follow-up but decreased over 5- and 10-year follow-up. Quality of life, health, energy, and happiness were similar across strata with a slight benefit in the younger group. At all times in the study, at least 95% of patients in each group stated that they would undergo their surgery again and would recommend IPAA to someone else with the same diagnosis.[126]

The effect of the aging process itself on functional outcome and the quality of life of patients with IPAA were studied by the Mayo Clinic group, with the functional and quality-of-life outcomes of 409 patients being assessed at 5, 10, and 15 years. Over this time frame, little change in daytime stool frequency was noted, whereas nighttime frequency increased from one stool to two stools per night. Incontinence to gas and stool increased from 1% to 10% during the day and from 2% to 24% at night over the 15-year period. After 15 years, more than 90% of patients were in the same job, and social activities, recreational sports, long-distance travel, and sexual activity all improved after surgery and did not show deterioration over time.[127]

ALTERNATIVES TO ILEAL POUCH–ANAL ANASTOMOSIS

TOTAL ABDOMINAL COLECTOMY WITH ILEORECTAL ANASTOMOSIS

Before the introduction of IPAA as a procedure, total colectomy with ileorectal anastomosis was considered in patients with minimal rectal disease interested in maintaining intestinal continuity. Ileorectal anastomosis avoids the need for a stoma and reduces the risk of damage to the pelvic nerves. Fecal frequency is less compared with IPAA, with patients typically having 2 to 4 liquid daytime bowel movements daily and occasional nocturnal bowel movements.[128] Ileorectal anastomosis is still a reasonable alternative for high-risk patients, with reasonable rectal compliance in whom IPAA is unsuitable. This procedure can also be offered as a temporizing procedure for selected young patients interested in returning to school or work requirements without a stoma or in suitable young women of childbearing age who are interested in preserving fertility, as outlined previously. Interval proctectomy may be required in up to 40% of patients, and the risk for rectal cancer is approximately 15% after 30 years, emphasizing the importance of regular endoscopic surveillance.

Ileorectal anastomosis should not be offered to patients with severe proctitis, poor rectal compliance, fecal incontinence, or anoperineal disease. Preservation of the rectum is also contraindicated if dysplasia or carcinoma is present.

TOTAL PROCTOCOLECTOMY WITH END ILEOSTOMY

Total proctocolectomy with end ileostomy is an extirpative procedure that "cures" the patient of ulcerative colitis. The proctectomy is completed with an intersphincteric dissection and layered closure of the levator muscles, puborectalis, and external anal sphincter relegating the patient to a permanent ileostomy and precluding possibility of a future restorative procedure. The risk associated with this procedure is lower than restorative procedures, owing to the absence of surgical anastomosis. However, patients remain at risk for pelvic neuropathy following pelvic dissection, stoma complications, and perineal wound complications. In patients who are considered high risk for perineal complications, the rectal stump can be divided at the level of the levators, with perineal proctectomy completed at a later date.[1-9]

KOCK CONTINENT ILEOSTOMY

The Kock pouch consists of an ileal pouch, a valve created by intussuscepting the terminal ileum into the reservoir, and an exit spout. The pouch is emptied intermittently by intubation.[130] This option has the advantage of allowing the patient to control drainage of effluent, and an external appliance is not needed. The Kock pouch carries a high complication rate, with reoperation common due to prolapse and slipping of the valve. The application of the Kock pouch is limited and is probably restricted to patients who have undergone proctocolectomy and wish to have control over their ileostomy effluent and those people undergoing restorative proctocolectomy in whom a structural problem leads to initial or subsequent anastomotic failure.

CONCLUSION

The development of proctocolectomy with IPAA has led to significant advances in the surgical treatment of ulcerative colitis. IPAA is safe and successful in most patients. Minimally invasive approaches to IPAA are gaining widespread application, and patient demand has made this approach a standard of care. The J pouch with double-stapled IPAA is the most widely preferred operative technique. Appropriate staging of this restorative procedure is motivated by disease-, patient-, and surgeon-dependent factors. Patients benefit from low postoperative mortality, acceptable postoperative morbidity, and good long-term function. Postoperative short- and long-term

complications must be aggressively managed to prevent pouch dysfunction and ultimate pouch loss. Nevertheless, laparoscopic restorative proctocolectomy is an established procedure associated with safe disease eradication and good quality of life.

ACKNOWLEDGMENT

The authors give credit to Dr. Peter M. Sagar and Dr. John H. Pemberton for their authorship of the 7th edition Chapter 160: Surgery for Inflammatory Bowel Disease: Chronic Ulcerative Colitis, from which some content is adapted.

REFERENCES

1. Gu J, Stocchi L, Remzi F, Kiran RP. Intraperitoneal or subcutaneous: does location of the (colo) rectal stump influence outcomes after laparoscopic total abdominal colectomy for ulcerative colitis? *Dis Colon Rectum.* 2013;56:615-621.
2. Randall J, Singh B, Warren BF, Travis SP, Mortensen NJ, George BD. Delayed surgery for acute severe colitis is associated with increased risk of postoperative complications. *Br J Surg.* 2010;97: 404-409.
3. Sagar PM, Taylor BA. Pelvic ileal reservoirs: the options. *Br J Surg.* 1994;81:325-332.
4. Holubar SD, Holder-Murray J, Flasar M, Lazarev M. Anti-tumor necrosis factor-α antibody therapy management before and after intestinal surgery for inflammatory bowel disease. *Inflamm Bowel Dis.* 2015;21:2658-2672.
5. Utsunomiya J, Iwama T, Imajo M, et al. Total colectomy, mucosal proctectomy and ileoanal anastomosis. *Dis Colon Rectum.* 1980;23:459-466.
6. Ekbom A, Helmick C, Zack M, Adami HO. Ulcerative colitis and colorectal cancer. A population-based study. *N Engl J Med.* 1990;323: 1228-1233.
7. Prior P, Gyde SN, Macartney JC, Thompson H, Waterhouse JA, Allan RN. Cancer morbidity in ulcerative colitis. *Gut.* 1982;23:490-497.
8. Thomas T, Abrams KA, Robinson RJ, Mayberry JF. Meta-analysis: cancer risk of low-grade dysplasia in chronic ulcerative colitis. *Aliment Pharmacol Ther.* 2007;25:657-668.
9. Farraye FA, Odze RD, Eaden J, et al. AGA medical position statement on the diagnosis and management of colorectal neoplasia in inflammatory bowel disease. *Gastroenterology.* 2010;138:738-745. doi:10.1053/j.gastro.2009.12.037
10. Laine L, Kaltenbach T, Barkun A, et al. SCENIC international consensus statement on surveillance and management of dysplasia in inflammatory bowel disease. *Gastrointes Endosc.* 2015;81(3): 489-501.
11. Wu X-R, Kiran RP, Mukewar S, Remzi FH, Shen B. Diagnosis and management of pouch outlet obstruction caused by common anatomical problems after restorative proctocolectomy. *J Crohns Colitis.* 2014;8:270-275. doi:10.1016/j.crohns.2013.08.012.
12. Sagar PM, Holdsworth PJ, Godwin PG, Quirke P, Smith AN, Johnston D. Comparison of triplicated (S) and quadruplicated (W) pelvic ileal reservoirs. Studies on manovolumetry, fecal bacteriology, fecal volatile fatty acids, mucosal morphology, and functional results. *Gastroenterology.* 1992;102:520-528.
13. Bressler B, Marshall JK, Bernstein CN, et al. Clinical practice guidelines for the medical management of nonhospitalized ulcerative colitis: the Toronto Consensus. *Gastroenterology.* 2015;148:1035-1058.
14. Schoetz DJ, Coller JA, Veidenheimer MC. Can the pouch be saved? *Dis Colon Rectum.* 1988;31:671-675.
15. Selvasekar CR, Cima RR, Larson DW, et al. Effect of infliximab on short-term complications in patients undergoing operation for chronic ulcerative colitis. *J Am Coll Surg.* 2007;204:956-962.
16. Galandiuk S, Scott NA, Dozois RR, et al. Ileal pouch-anal anastomosis. Reoperation for pouch-related complications. *Ann Surg.* 1990;212: 446-452; discussion 452-454.
17. Schluender SJ, Ippoliti A, Dubinsky M, et al. Does infliximab influence surgical morbidity of ileal pouch-anal anastomosis in patients with ulcerative colitis? *Dis Colon Rectum.* 2007;50:1747-1753.
18. Nicholls RJ, Lubowski DZ. Restorative proctocolectomy: the four loop (W) reservoir. *Br J Surg.* 1987;74:564-566.

19. Mor IJ, Vogel JD, da Luz Moreira A, Shen B, Hammel J, Remzi FH. Infliximab in ulcerative colitis is associated with an increased risk of postoperative complications after restorative proctocolectomy. *Dis Colon Rectum.* 2008;51:1202-1210.

20. Nicholls RJ, Pezim ME. Restorative proctocolectomy with ileal reservoir for ulcerative colitis and familial adenomatous polyposis: a comparison of three reservoir designs. *Br J Surg.* 1985;72:470-474.

21. Ehteshami-Afshar S, Nikfar S, Rezaie A, Abdollahi M. A systematic review and meta-analysis of the effects of infliximab on the rate of colectomy and post-operative complications in patients with inflammatory bowel disease. *Arch Med Sci.* 2011;6:1000-1012.

22. Narula N, Charleton D, Marshall JK. Meta-analysis: peri-operative anti-TNFα treatment and post-operative complications in patients with inflammatory bowel disease. *Aliment Pharmacol Ther.* 2013;37:1057-1064.

23. McCormick PH, Guest GD, Clark AJ, et al. The ideal ileal-pouch design. *Dis Colon Rectum.* 2012;55:1251-1257.

24. Selvaggi F, Pellino G, Canonico S, Sciaudone G. Effect of preoperative biologic drugs on complications and function after restorative proctocolectomy with primary ileal pouch formation. *Inflamm Bowel Dis.* 2015;21:79-92.

25. Johnston D, Williamson ME, Lewis WG, Miller AS, Sagar PM, Holdsworth PJ. Prospective controlled trial of duplicated (J) versus quadruplicated (W) pelvic ileal reservoirs in restorative proctocolectomy for ulcerative colitis. *Gut.* 1996;39:242-247.

26. Coquet-Reinier B, Berdah SV, Grimaud J-C, et al. Preoperative infliximab treatment and postoperative complications after laparoscopic restorative proctocolectomy with ileal pouch–anal anastomosis: a case-matched study. *Surg Endosc.* 2010;24:1866-1871.

27. Ferrante M, D'Hoore A, Vermeire S, et al. Corticosteroids but not infliximab increase short-term postoperative infectious complications in patients with ulcerative colitis. *Inflamm Bowel Dis.* 2009;15:1062-1070.

28. Nørgård BM, Nielsen J, Qvist N, Gradel KO, de Muckadell OB, Kjeldsen J. Pre-operative use of anti-TNF-α agents and the risk of post-operative complications in patients with ulcerative colitis—a nationwide cohort study. *Aliment Pharmacol Ther.* 2012;35(11): 1301-1309.

29. Gu J, Remzi FH, Shen B, Vogel JD, Kiran RP. Operative strategy modifies risk of pouch-related outcomes in patients with ulcerative colitis on preoperative anti-tumor necrosis factor-α therapy. *Dis Colon Rectum.* 2013;56:1243-1252.

30. O'Connell PR, Pemberton JH, Brown ML, Kelly KA. Determinants of stool frequency after ileal pouch-anal anastomosis. *Am J Surg.* 1987;153:157-164.

31. Wu X-J, He X-S, Zhou X-Y, Ke J, Lan P. The role of laparoscopic surgery for ulcerative colitis: systematic review with meta-analysis. *Int J Colorectal Dis.* 2010;25:949-957.

32. Telem DA, Vine AJ, Swain G, et al. Laparoscopic subtotal colectomy for medically refractory ulcerative colitis: the time has come. *Surg Endosc.* 2010;24:1616-1620.

33. Ambroze WL, Pemberton JH, Bell AM, Brown ML, Zinsmeister AR. The effect of stool consistency on rectal and neorectal emptying. *Dis Colon Rectum.* 1991;34:1-7.

34. Fleming FJ, Francone TD, Kim MJ, Gunzler D, Messing S, Monson JR. A laparoscopic approach does reduce short-term complications in patients undergoing ileal pouch-anal anastomosis. *Dis Colon Rectum.* 2011;54:176-182.

35. Tuckson W, Lavery I, Fazio V, Oakley J, Church J, Milsom J. Manometric and functional comparison of ileal pouch anal anastomosis with and without anal manipulation. *Am J Surg.* 1991;161(1):90-95; discussion 95–96.

36. Dunker MS, Bemelman WA, Slors J. Functional outcome, quality of life, body image, and cosmesis in patients after laparoscopic-assisted and conventional restorative proctocolectomy. *Dis Colon Rectum.* 2001;44:1801-1807.

37. Singh P, Bhangu A, Nicholls RJ, Tekkis P. A systematic review and meta-analysis of laparoscopic vs open restorative proctocolectomy. *Colorectal Dis.* 2013;15(7):e340-e351.

38. Remzi FH, Fazio VW, Delaney CP, et al. Dysplasia of the anal transitional zone after ileal pouch-anal anastomosis: results of prospective evaluation after a minimum of ten years. *Dis Colon Rectum.* 2003;46:6-13.

39. Chung TP, Fleshman JW, Birnbaum EH, et al. Laparoscopic vs. open total abdominal colectomy for severe colitis: impact on recovery and subsequent completion restorative proctectomy. *Dis Colon Rectum.* 2009;52:4-10.

40. Pecorelli N, Greco M, Amodeo S, Braga M. Small bowel obstruction and incisional hernia after laparoscopic and open colorectal surgery: a meta-analysis of comparative trials. *Surg Endosc.* 2017;31(1):85-99.

41. Bartels SAL, D'Hoore A, Cuesta MA, Bensdorp AJ, Lucas C, Bemelman WA. Significantly increased pregnancy rates after laparoscopic restorative proctocolectomy. *Ann Surg.* 2012;256:1045-1048.

42. Ziv Y, Fazio VW, Church JM, Lavery IC, King TM, Ambrosetti P. Stapled ileal pouch anal anastomoses are safer than handsewn anastomoses in patients with ulcerative colitis. *Am J Surg.* 1996;171: 320-323.

43. Larson DW, Dozois EJ, Piotrowicz K, Cima RR, Wolff BG, Young-Fadok TM. Laparoscopic-assisted vs open ileal pouch-anal anastomosis: functional outcome in a case-matched series. *Dis Colon Rectum.* 2005;48(10):1845-1850.

44. Geisler DP, Condon ET, Remzi FH. Single incision laparoscopic total proctocolectomy with ileopouch anal anastomosis. *Colorectal Dis.* 2009;12:941-943.

45. Lovegrove RE, Constantinides VA, Heriot AG, et al. A comparison of hand-sewn versus stapled ileal pouch anal anastomosis (IPAA) following proctocolectomy. *Ann Surg.* 2006;244:18-26.

46. Maartense S, Dunker MS, Slors JF, et al. Hand-assisted laparoscopic versus open restorative proctocolectomy with ileal pouch anal anastomosis. *Ann Surg.* 2004;240:984-992.

47. Kirat HT, Remzi FH, Kiran RP, Fazio VW. Comparison of outcomes after hand-sewn versus stapled ileal pouch-anal anastomosis in 3,109 patients. *Surgery.* 2009;146:723-730.

48. Marcello PW, Fleshman JW, Milsom JW, et al. Hand-assisted laparoscopic vs. laparoscopic colorectal surgery: a multicenter, prospective, randomized trial. *Dis Colon Rectum.* 2008;51:818-826; discussion 826–828.

49. Ishii H, Kawai K, Hata K, et al. Comparison of functional outcomes of patients who underwent hand-sewn or stapled ileal pouch-anal anastomosis for ulcerative colitis. *Int Surg.* 2015;100:1169-1176.

50. McLemore EC, Cullen J, Horgan S, Talamini MA, Ramamoorthy S. Robotic-assisted laparoscopic stage II restorative proctectomy for toxic ulcerative colitis. *Int J Med Robot.* 2011;8:178-183.

51. Annibali R, Hultén L, Öresland T. Does the level of stapled ileoanal anastomosis influence physiologic and functional outcome? *Dis Colon Rectum.* 1994;37(4):321-329.

52. Fleshman J, Branda M, Sargent DJ, et al. Effect of laparoscopic-assisted resection vs open resection of stage II or III rectal cancer on pathologic outcomes. *JAMA.* 2015;314:1346.

53. Wexner SD, James K, Jagelman DG. The double-stapled ileal reservoir and ileoanal anastomosis. A prospective review of sphincter function and clinical outcome. *Dis Colon Rectum.* 1991;34:487-494.

54. Church JM, Saad R, Schroeder T, et al. Predicting the functional result of anastomoses to the anus: the paradox of preoperative anal resting pressure. *Dis Colon Rectum.* 1993;36(10):895-900.

55. Choi H-J, Saigusa N, Choi J-S, et al. How consistent is the anal transitional zone in the double-stapled ileoanal reservoir? *Int J Colorectal Dis.* 2003;18:116-120.

56. Williamson ME, Lewis WG, Miller AS, Sagar PM, Holdsworth PJ, Johnston D. Clinical and physiological evaluation of anorectal eversion during restorative proctocolectomy. *Br J Surg.* 1995;82: 1391-1394.

57. DeFriend DJ, Mughal M, Grace RH, Schofield PF. Effect of anorectal eversion on long-term clinical outcome of restorative proctocolectomy. *J R Soc Med.* 1997;90:375-378.

58. Huntington JT, Boomer LA, Pepper VK, Diefenbach KA, Dotson JL, Nwomeh BC. Minimally invasive ileal pouch-anal anastomosis with rectal eversion allows for equivalent outcomes in continence in pediatric patients. *J Laparoendosc Adv Surg Tech A.* 2016;26:222-225.

59. Liljeqvist L, Lindquist K, Ljungdahl I. Alterations in ileoanal pouch technique, 1980 to 1987. Complications and functional outcome. *Dis Colon Rectum.* 1988;31:929-938.

60. Hicks CW, Hodin RA, Savitt L, Bordeianou L. Does intramesorectal excision for ulcerative colitis impact bowel and sexual function when compared with total mesorectal excision? *Am J Surg.* 2014;208: 499e4-504e4.

61. Kiely JM, Fazio VW, Remzi FH, Shen B, Kiran RP. Pelvic sepsis after IPAA adversely affects function of the pouch and quality of life. *Dis Colon Rectum.* 2012;55:387-392.

62. Parks AG, Nicholls RJ. Proctocolectomy without ileostomy for ulcerative colitis. *Br Med J.* 1978;2(6130):85-88.

63. Selvaggi F, Sciaudone G, Limongelli P, et al. The effect of pelvic septic complications on function and quality of life after ileal

pouch-anal anastomosis: a single center experience. *Am Surg.* 2010;76:428-435.

64. Heuschen UA, Hinz U, Allemeyer EH, et al. Risk factors for ileoanal J pouch-related septic complications in ulcerative colitis and familial adenomatous polyposis. *Ann Surg.* 2002;235:207-216.

65. Kiran RP, da Luz Moreira A, Remzi FH, et al. Factors associated with septic complications after restorative proctocolectomy. *Ann Surg.* 2010;251:436-440.

66. Pandey S, Luther G, Umanskiy K, et al. Minimally invasive pouch surgery for ulcerative colitis: is there a benefit in staging? *Dis Colon Rectum.* 2011;54(3):306-310.

67. Nicholls RJ, Gilbert JM. Surgical correction of the efferent ileal limb for disordered defaecation following restorative proctocolectomy with the S ileal reservoir. *Br J Surg.* 1990;77:152-154.

68. Swenson BR, Hollenbeak CS, Poritz LS, Koltun WA. Modified two-stage ileal pouch-anal anastomosis: equivalent outcomes with less resource utilization. *Dis Colon Rectum.* 2005;48:256-261.

69. Sagar PM, Lewis W, Holdsworth PJ, Johnston D. One-stage restorative proctocolectomy without temporary defunctioning ileostomy. *Dis Colon Rectum.* 1992;35:582-588.

70. Williamson ME, Lewis WG, Sagar PM, Holdsworth PJ, Johnston D. One-stage restorative proctocolectomy without temporary ileostomy for ulcerative colitis: a note of caution. *Dis Colon Rectum.* 1997;40:1019-1022.

71. MacLean AR, Cohen Z, MacRae HM, et al. Risk of small bowel obstruction after the ileal pouch-anal anastomosis. *Ann Surg.* 2002;235:200-206.

72. Fazio VW, Kiran RP, Remzi FH, et al. Ileal pouch anal anastomosis: analysis of outcome and quality of life in 3707 patients. *Ann Surg.* 2013;257:679-685.

73. Meagher AP, Farouk R, Dozois RR, Kelly KA, Pemberton JH. J ileal pouch-anal anastomosis for chronic ulcerative colitis: complications and long-term outcome in 1310 patients. *Br J Surg.* 1998;85:800-803.

74. Pemberton JH, Kelly KA, Beart RW, Dozois RR, Wolff BG, Ilstrup DM. Ileal pouch-anal anastomosis for chronic ulcerative colitis. Long-term results. *Ann Surg.* 1987;206:504-513.

75. Heuschen UA, Allemeyer EH, Hinz U, Lucas M, Herfarth C, Heuschen G. Outcome after septic complications in J pouch procedures. *Br J Surg.* 2002;89:194-200.

76. Farouk R, Dozois RR, Pemberton JH, Larson D. Incidence and subsequent impact of pelvic abscess after ileal pouch-anal anastomosis for chronic ulcerative colitis. *Dis Colon Rectum.* 1998;41:1239-1243.

77. O'Connell PR, Pemberton JH, Weiland LH, et al. Does rectal mucosa regenerate after ileoanal anastomosis? *Dis Colon Rectum.* 1987;30:1-5.

78. Cohen Z, McLeod RS, Stephen W, Stern HS, O'Connor B, Reznick R. Continuing evolution of the pelvic pouch procedure. *Ann Surg.* 1992;216:506-511; discussion 511-512.

79. Kirat HT, Kiran RP, Oncel M, et al. Management of leak from the tip of the "J" in ileal pouch-anal anastomosis. *Dis Colon Rectum.* 2011;54:454-459.

80. Scott NA, Dozois RR, Beart RW Jr, Pemberton JH, Wolff BG, Ilstrup DM. Postoperative intra-abdominal and pelvic sepsis complicating ileal pouch-anal anastomosis. *Int J Colorectal Dis.* 1988;3(3):149-152.

81. Lian L, Serclova Z, Fazio VW, Kiran RP, Remzi F, Shen B. Clinical features and management of postoperative pouch bleeding after ileal pouch-anal anastomosis (IPAA). *J Gastrointest Surg.* 2008;12:1991-1994.

82. Francone TD, Champagne B. Considerations and complications in patients undergoing ileal pouch anal anastomosis. *Surg Clin North Am.* 1998;92:107-143.

83. Bach SP, Mortensen NJ. Revolution and evolution: 30 years of ileoanal pouch surgery. *Inflamm Bowel Dis.* 2006;12:131-145.

84. Prudhomme M, Dozois RR, Godlewski G, Mathison S, Fabbro-Peray P. Anal canal strictures after ileal pouch-anal anastomosis. *Dis Colon Rectum.* 2003;46:20-23.

85. Lewis WG, Kuzu A, Sagar PM, Holdsworth PJ, Johnston D. Stricture at the pouch-anal anastomosis after restorative proctocolectomy. *Dis Colon Rectum.* 1994;37:120-125.

86. Shah NS, Remzi F, Massmann A, Baixauli J, Fazio VW. Management and treatment outcome of pouch-vaginal fistulas following restorative proctocolectomy. *Dis Colon Rectum.* 2003;46:911-917.

87. Mallick IH, Hull TL, Remzi FH, Kiran RP. Management and outcome of pouch-vaginal fistulas after IPAA surgery. *Dis Colon Rectum.* 2014;57:490-496.

88. Burke D, van Laarhoven CJ, Herbst F, Nicholls RJ. Transvaginal repair of pouch-vaginal fistula. *Br J Surg.* 2001;88:241-245.

89. Lolohea S, Lynch AC, Robertson GB, Frizelle FA. Ileal pouch-anal anastomosis-vaginal fistula: a review. *Dis Colon Rectum.* 2005;48:802-1810.

90. Chambers WM, McC Mortensen NJ. Should ileal pouch-anal anastomosis include mucosectomy? *Colorectal Dis.* 2007;9:384-392.

91. Marcello PW, Roberts PL, Schoetz DJ Jr. Obstruction after ileal pouch-anal anastomosis: a preventable complication? *Dis Colon Rectum.* 1993;36:1105-1111.

92. Read TE, Schoetz DJ Jr, Marcello PW. Afferent limb obstruction complicating ileal pouch-anal anastomosis. *Dis Colon Rectum.* 1997;40:566-569.

93. Fichera A, Silvestri MT, Hurst RD, Rubin MA, Michelassi F. Laparoscopic restorative proctocolectomy with ileal pouch anal anastomosis: a comparative observational study on long-term functional results. *J Gastrointest Surg.* 2008;12:526-532.

94. Shen B, Achkar J-P, Lashner BA, et al. Irritable pouch syndrome: a new category of diagnosis for symptomatic patients with ileal pouch-anal anastomosis. *Am J Gastroenterol.* 2002;97:972-977.

95. Fazio VW, Tjandra JJ. Transanal mucosectomy. Ileal pouch advancement for anorectal dysplasia or inflammation after restorative proctocolectomy. *Dis Colon Rectum.* 1994;37:1008-1011.

96. Hahnloser D, Pemberton JH, Wolff BG, Larson DR, Crownhart BS, Dozois RR. Results at up to 20 years after ileal pouch-anal anastomosis for chronic ulcerative colitis. *Br J Surg.* 2007;94:333-340.

97. Lovegrove RE, Tilney HS, Heriot AG, et al. A comparison of adverse events and functional outcomes after restorative proctocolectomy for familial adenomatous polyposis and ulcerative colitis. *Dis Colon Rectum.* 2006;49:1293-1306.

98. Hata K, Watanabe T, Shinozaki M, Nagawa H. Patients with extraintestinal manifestations have a higher risk of developing pouchitis in ulcerative colitis: multivariate analysis. *Scand J Gastroenterol.* 2003;38:1055-1058.

99. Fruin AB, El-Zammer O, Stucchi AF, O'Brien M, Becker JM. Colonic metaplasia in the ileal pouch is associated with inflammation and is not the result of long-term adaptation. *J Gastrointest Surg.* 2003;7:246-253; discussion 253-254.

100. Ruisma J, Mentula S, Luukkonen P, et al. Factors associated with ileal mucosa morphology and inflammation in patients with ileal pouch-anal anastomosis for ulcerative colitis. *Dis Colon Rectum.* 2003;46:1473-1483.

101. Sandborn WJ, Tremaine WJ, Batts KP, Pemberton JH, Phillips SF. Pouchitis after ileal pouch-anal anastomosis: a pouchitis disease activity index. *Mayo Clin Proc.* 1994;69:409-415.

102. Gionchetti P, Rizzello F, Venturi A, et al. Oral bacteriotherapy as maintenance treatment in patients with chronic pouchitis: a double-blind, placebo-controlled trial. *Gastroenterology.* 2000;119:305-309.

103. Holubar SD, Cima RR, Sandborn WJ, Pardi DS. Treatment and prevention of pouchitis after ileal pouch-anal anastomosis for chronic ulcerative colitis. *Cochrane Database Syst Rev.* 2010;(6): CD001176.

104. Shen B. Pouchitis: what every gastroenterologist needs to know. *Clin Gastroenterol Hepatol.* 2013;11:1538-1549.

105. Mann SD, Pitt J, Springall RG, Thillainayagam AV. *Clostridium difficile* infection—an unusual cause of refractory pouchitis: report of a case. *Dis Colon Rectum.* 2003;46(2):267-270.

106. Seril DN, Yao Q, Lashner BA, Shen B. Autoimmune features are associated with chronic antibiotic-refractory pouchitis. *Inflamm Bowel Dis.* 2015;21:110-120.

107. Ferrante M, D'Haens G, Dewit O, et al. Efficacy of infliximab in refractory pouchitis and Crohn's disease-related complications of the pouch: a Belgian case series. *Inflamm Bowel Dis.* 2010;16:243-249.

108. McLaughlin SD, Clark SK, Bell AJ, Tekkis PP, Ciclitira PJ, Nicholls RJ. Incidence and short-term implications of prepouch ileitis following restorative proctocolectomy with ileal pouch-anal anastomosis for ulcerative colitis. *Dis Colon Rectum.* 2009;52:879-883.

109. Braveman JM, Schoetz DJ Jr, Marcello PW, et al. The fate of the ileal pouch in patients developing Crohn's disease. *Dis Colon Rectum.* 2004;47:1613-1619.

110. Regimbeau JM, Panis Y, Pocard M, et al. Long-term results of ileal pouch-anal anastomosis for colorectal Crohn's disease. *Dis Colon Rectum.* 2001;44:769-778.

111. Melton GB, Fazio VW, Kiran RP, et al. Long-term outcomes with ileal pouch-anal anastomosis and Crohn's disease. *Transact Meet Am Surg Assoc.* 2008;126:251-259.

112. Murrell ZA, Melmed GY, Ippoliti A, et al. A prospective evaluation of the long-term outcome of ileal pouch-anal anastomosis in patients with inflammatory bowel disease-unclassified and indeterminate colitis. *Dis Colon Rectum.* 2009;52:872-878.

113. Thompson JS. Alopecia after ileal pouch-anal anastomosis. *Dis Colon Rectum.* 1989;32:457-465.

114. Joyce MR, Fazio VW, Hull TT, et al. Ileal pouch prolapse: prevalence, management, and outcomes. *J Gastrointest Surg.* 2010;14:993-997.

115. Gorgun E, Remzi FH, Montague DK, et al. Male sexual function improves after ileal pouch anal anastomosis. *Colorectal Dis.* 2005; 7:545-550.

116. Larson DW, Davies MM, Dozois EJ, et al. Sexual function, body image, and quality of life after laparoscopic and open ileal pouch-anal anastomosis. *Dis Colon Rectum.* 2008;51:392-396.

117. Wax JR, Pinette MG, Cartin A, Blackstone J. Female reproductive health after ileal pouch anal anastomosis for ulcerative colitis. *Obstet Gynecol Surv.* 2003;58:270-274.

118. Damgaard B, Wettergren A, Kirkegaard P. Social and sexual function following ileal pouch-anal anastomosis. *Dis Colon Rectum.* 1995;38:286-289.

119. Bharadwaj S, Philpott JR, Barber MD, Graff LA, Shen B. Women's health issues after ileal pouch surgery. *Inflamm Bowel Dis.* 2014; 20:2470-2482.

120. Waljee A, Waljee J, Morris AM, Higgins PD. Threefold increased risk of infertility: a meta-analysis of infertility after ileal pouch anal anastomosis in ulcerative colitis. *Gut.* 2006;55:1575-1580. doi:10.1136/gut.2005.090316.

121. Cima RR. Impact of ileal-pouch anal anastomosis on fertility. *Inflamm Bowel Dis.* 2007;13:1310-1311.

122. Oresland T, Palmblad S, Ellstrom M, Berndtsson I, Crona N, Hultén L. Gynaecological and sexual function related to anatomical changes in the female pelvis after restorative proctocolectomy. *Int J Colorectal Dis.* 1994;9:77-81.

123. Hull TL, Joyce MR, Geisler DP, Coffey JC. Adhesions after laparoscopic and open ileal pouch-anal anastomosis surgery for ulcerative colitis. *Br J Surg.* 2011;99:270-275.

124. Bradford K, Melmed GY, Fleshner P, Silverman N, Dubinsky MC. Significant variation in recommendation of care for women of reproductive age with ulcerative colitis postileal pouch–anal anastomosis. *Dig Dis Sci.* 2014;59:1115-1120.

125. Farouk R, Pemberton JH, Wolff BG, Dozois RR, Browning S, Larson D. Functional outcomes after ileal pouch-anal anastomosis for chronic ulcerative colitis. *Ann Surg.* 2000;231:919-926.

126. Delaney CP, Fazio VW, Remzi FH, et al. Prospective, age-related analysis of surgical results, functional outcome, and quality of life after ileal pouch-anal anastomosis. *Ann Surg.* 2003;238:221-228.

127. Hahnloser D, Pemberton JH, Wolff BG, Larson DR, Crownhart BS, Dozois RR. The effect of ageing on function and quality of life in ileal pouch patients: a single cohort experience of 409 patients with chronic ulcerative colitis. *Ann Surg.* 2004;240:615-621; discussion 621–623.

128. Newton CR, Baker WN. Comparison of bowel function after ileorectal anastomosis for ulcerative colitis and colonic polyposis. *Gut.* 1975;16:785-791.

129. Bohl JL, Sobba K. Indications and options for surgery in ulcerative colitis. *Surg Clin North Am.* 2015;95:1211-1232, vi.

130. Kock NG. Intra-abdominal "reservoir" in patients with permanent ileostomy. Preliminary observations on a procedure resulting in fecal "continence" in five ileostomy patients. *Arch Surg.* 1969;99:223-231.

Surgery for Crohn Disease: Personalizing the Operation

Amy L. Lightner | Heidi Chua | John H. Pemberton

Crohn disease (CD) is a chronic inflammatory disease of the intestinal tract with an unknown etiology and an unknown cure. The characteristic transmural inflammation can progress to refractory inflammatory disease, stricturing disease, and fistulizing disease—all potential indications for surgery when medical management has been exhausted. An important tenet to remember is that surgery is not curative but is rather an adjunct to maximal medical therapy. Thus bowel preservation is imperative because up to two-thirds of patients will require subsequent operations in their lifetime.

MEDICAL TREATMENT OF CROHN DISEASE

Because there is no cure for CD, medical management is used with the intent of symptom control and, ideally, maintaining disease remission. With such vast number of medications now approved for the treatment of CD, management can be compartmentalized by phenotype and severity of disease. The three classic phenotypes include inflammatory, fibrotic, or fistulizing disease. And within each of these subtypes, disease may be mild to moderate, moderate to severe, severe, or refractory.

In the setting of mild to moderate disease, patients are often treated with 5-aminosalicylate products, such as sulfasalazine, oral mesalamine (Pentasa, Asacol), and rectal mesalamine (Rowasa). For ileal, ileocolonic, and colonic disease, sulfasalazine as a 3- to 6-g daily divided dose is effective treatment.[1] Multiple trials across the United States and Europe have demonstrated its benefits over placebo.[1] However, its ability to induce or maintain remission is significantly less than corticosteroids, and sulfasalazine and mesalamine are significantly less effective than corticosteroids in managing active CD. In contrast, budesonide is equally as effective as conventional oral corticosteroids in the treatment of mild to moderate ileal and right colonic disease.[1] However, controlled-release formulations of budesonide (9 mg/day) are limited to treatment of disease in the ileum and right colon and are not effective for treating disease in the proximal small bowel or rectum.

For patients with moderate to severe disease, corticosteroids are the cornerstone of medical management until symptoms resolve. Patients may require up to 40 to 60 mg daily until clinical improvement is seen. Alternatives to steroid therapy effective for inducing remission and closing fistulas include azathioprine at 2 to 3 mg/kg per day and 6-mercaptopurine at 1.5 mg/kg per day. In steroid-dependent or refractory CD, methotrexate at 25 mg/week may be effective.

Since the US Food and Drug Administration (FDA) approval of infliximab in 1998 for the treatment of CD,

we have entered a new era of biologic medical therapy, which has largely supplanted the aforementioned classes of medications or certainly added to the armamentarium. Anti–tumor necrosis factor (TNF) monoclonal antibodies (infliximab, adalimumab, certolizumab) were the first class to be introduced and are the most commonly prescribed. Additional biologic therapies have since been introduced for patients with contraindications, complications, or loss of response to the anti-TNF-α class. These include antibodies that target integrins (natalizumab, vedolizumab) and interleukin (IL)-12/23 (ustekinumab). Initially, biologic agents were only given to patients with severe disease, half of whom had already required surgery for complications, and a third of whom had failed to respond to thiopurines.[2] However, post hoc analysis of the large randomized controlled trials found that overall remission rates with biologics were greater when administered to patients within 2 years of diagnosis.[3] Thus the preferred patient for introducing biologics is one with active disease, prior to the development of strictures, who is at higher risk of complications. Unfortunately, up to 60% of patients experience recurrence of symptoms after induced remission with anti-TNF-α agents.[4] With more and more biologic classes being FDA approved, these patients, rather than going to surgery, are now often given an alternative class of biologic therapy. Thus, patients are generally arriving to the operating room with more advanced disease activity and a longer duration of immunosuppression. However, it is worth noting that in the prebiologic era, up to 30% of CD patients who underwent surgery would require another operation within 5 to 10 years, and now in the era of biologic therapy, only 10% of CD patients will require another operation within 8 years of the index case.[5] Furthermore, meta-analyses have shown that biologic therapy, although not without complication, has a significant impact on preventing disease recurrence.[6]

Although biologics have significantly enhanced medical management, they are not without potential morbidity and significant cost. Patients are at increased risk of opportunistic infection or reactivation of latent infections, malignancy (especially lymphoma), worsening of congestive heart failure, and eczematous skin lesions.[7] Thus treatment must be individualized, and careful consideration given to patients with significant comorbidities or of advanced age.

INDICATIONS FOR SURGERY

Despite making significant advances in medical therapy, up to 70%[8,9] of patients eventually require an operation. The leading indication for surgery is disease that is refractory to medical management. The end result presents as obstruction, fistulas, abscesses, gastrointestinal bleeding, or perforation.[10] In addition, less common indications for surgery include growth retardation in children, toxic megacolon, and fulminant colitis.

It is important to remember that a multidisciplinary approach is central to the management of this patient population. The patient, gastroenterologist, and surgeon should be in close communication as the patient's disease severity increases and surgery becomes increasingly likely. Before exhausting all medical options, a patient should at least have had a surgical consultation to understand the risks and benefits of an operation versus ongoing medical management. Ideally, a consensus will be reached by all parties involved before the patient is taken to the operating room. At that time, careful preoperative planning in a joint fashion should ensue.

PREOPERATIVE CONSIDERATIONS

The decision to operate is made in the context of the patient's preoperative nutritional status, immunosuppressive regimen, and any undrained sources of infection. The patient's nutritional status is often compromised by severe disease and long-standing poor nutrition. Total parenteral nutrition (TPN) may be indicated if the patient is severely malnourished (defined as loss of more than 5% of body weight in 1 month or 10% in 6 months, a body mass index less than 19 kg/m^2, or an albumin level <3 g/dL) to achieve improvement in wound healing and prevention of anastomotic leaks.[11] This finding was demonstrated in a study of 395 malnourished patients who received 1 week of TPN before surgery and had significantly fewer noninfectious complications as compared with the controls (5% vs. 43%).[12]

The impact of immunosuppressive medications on postoperative complications remains controversial. Recently, there has been a significant focus on whether biologic therapy increases postoperative complications. A previous series from our institution concluded that anti-TNF-α therapy did not increase the rate of postoperative complications after surgery for CD.[13] However, recent meta-analyses including up to 18 studies concluded infliximab does increase the rate of postoperative complications, especially postoperative infectious complications, which are reported to occur at a rate of 15% to 17%.[14,15] Thus the timing of surgery as it relates to the most recent dose of biologic therapy becomes important to consider.

Patients with abscesses should be drained nonoperatively prior to going to the operating room, unless contraindicated due to need for emergent surgery. Interventional radiology can be used to drain intraabdominal abscesses, and examination under anesthesia can be used to drain perirectal abscesses. For intraabdominal abscesses, adequate drainage may obviate the need for surgery altogether; if not, it at least minimizes the degree of intraabdominal inflammation, allowing for a more limited bowel resection.[16,17] If infection or abscesses are present at the time of the operation, the surgeon should consider postoperative antibiotic therapy and delayed closure of operative incisions.

After it is decided that the patient will proceed with surgery, the surgical plan should incorporate detailed information from imaging, endoscopy, and prior operative reports. Cross-sectional imaging with computed tomography (CT) or magnetic resonance (MR) enterography provides important information about the distribution and extent of disease, any undrained fluid collections, anatomic location of fistulizing disease, alteration in anatomy due to prior operations, and an estimate of remaining small bowel length.[15,19] MR enterography has the added advantage of no radiation, with improved anatomic detail, especially important in this young population who will likely require several repeat abdominal images over the course of their lifetime. Thus it is has largely supplanted fluoroscopic imaging, which is now primarily used for complex fistulizing disease requiring careful preoperative planning, and assessment of distal patency prior to stoma reversal.

A final important step prior to taking a patient to the operating room is a discussion regarding the potential need of a permanent or temporary stoma. Because anxiety around stoma formation is common among CD patients, early comprehensive education and support from an enterostomal therapist is important. In addition, it is important to consider preoperative stoma marking if the patient has any suspicion of requiring a stoma, especially in complex reoperative CD in which unexpected intraoperative findings or technical difficulties may mandate stoma construction.

INITIAL OPERATION

After patient optimization and preoperative planning are completed, the initial operation for CD should focus on bowel preservation, careful measurement and description of remaining bowel, and how to maximize a minimally invasive approach. Because surgery is not curative and the dreaded fear of short bowel is real, more conservative operative approaches have been adopted over time. Resections are performed to macroscopically uninvolved rather than microscopically uninvolved bowel, and more aggressive use of long stricturoplasty to preserve bowel may be used. When confronted with challenging cases in the operating room, it is important to keep in mind that when more than 70% of the small bowel is resected supplemental parenteral nutrition is nearly always required. If less than 50% of the small bowel is resected, patients can still experience malabsorption of fat-soluble vitamins and lactose.

There are at least three aspects of the index operation that can aid any subsequent operations. The first is the measurement and dictation of the length of remaining small bowel. To do this, the bowel is kept in a relaxed state and a suture of known length, usually a 60-cm silk suture, is manually used to measure the small bowel from the ligament of Treitz to the ileocolonic anastomosis or ileostomy. Second, a laparoscopic approach should be used whenever safe and feasible to prevent adhesive disease formation. Studies have found laparoscopy to be safe in both index and reoperative CD cases, with added benefits including reduction of adhesive disease, earlier return of bowel function, decreased length of hospital stay, improved cosmetic satisfaction, and decreased rates of small bowel obstruction.[20,21] One of the main indications to convert a laparoscopic approach to an open one in CD patients is the thickened, vascularized mesentery. If this is encountered, a laparoscopic approach will likely need to be abandoned. Third, the use of antiadhesion barriers, such as Seprafilm, reduces pelvic and abdominal adhesive disease[22,23] and may make the next operation easier and safer when entering the abdomen or reversing a stoma.

OPERATIVE CONSIDERATIONS BASED ON PHENOTYPE

STRICTURING CROHN DISEASE

Indications for an operation in the setting of stricturing CD include persistent obstructive symptoms that do not resolve with maximal escalation of medical therapy, chronic requirement for steroids, weight loss, or the need for chronic narcotic pain medication. Repeated episodes of inflammation, remodeling, and scarring of the bowel wall occur more often in small bowel than the colon. Regardless of the location, the normal pliable tissue is replaced with thickened nondistensible segments that narrow the lumen.

The length of the stricture, number of strictures, number of prior operations, and remaining small bowel length all contribute to the intraoperative decision making of bowel resection versus stricturoplasty. At an initial operation, a long-segment stricture may be resected if the remaining small bowel looks healthy. However, if there are multiple segments or the remaining small bowel has areas of narrowing, stricturoplasty should be considered due to the concern for bowel shortening.

On initial exploration in the setting of known obstructive disease, the entire bowel should be examined for any evidence of disease. Obvious strictures should be marked with sutures. If there are any questionable areas of narrowing during visual and tactile examination of the bowel, a sizing device can be run through the small bowel to assess diameter and distensibility. A balloon-tipped catheter may be passed through an enterotomy made at an obvious stricture site and advanced through the bowel looking for additional strictures (Fig. 163.1). Our preference is the use of surgical steel balls of varying diameter that pass through the bowel much easier and with less manipulation. As the balls are passed through the bowel each additional area of narrowing is marked with a suture, and assessment of bowel length and the number and spacing of required stricturoplasty is assessed to determine which surgical approach will be used. Fortunately stricturoplasty is appropriate to perform at any place along the length of bowel, including the duodenum, jejunum, ileum, and even colon. However, it should not be performed if there is an associated phlegmon or perforation.

The first reported stricturoplasty for the treatment of CD was by Lee and Papaioannou in 1982.[24] Since then, many techniques for stricturoplasty have been described, and more surgeons are advocating the use of stricturoplasty in place of resection for first-time ileocolic disease.[25] For strictures less than 4 to 5 cm in length, a Heineke-Mikulicz technique can be used, opening the stricture longitudinally and closing the bowel wall transversely (Fig. 163.2). Two sutures are placed at the midpoint of the stricture, to be

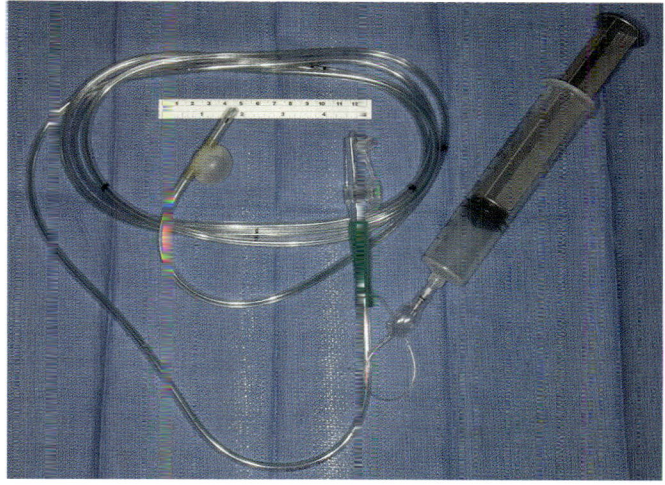

FIGURE 163.1 The Baker tube used to help to identify areas of small bowel strictures not easily identified on inspection and palpation of the bowel. The bowel is inflated with 15 mL of normal saline to achieve a diameter of 1 cm.

used as stay sutures to open the stricturoplasty. An antimesenteric longitudinal incision is made over the stricture using cautery and extended onto normal bowel of equal distance in both directions. If the patient has had long-standing inflammation or the stricture has been present more than 5 years, biopsy of the mucosa may be prudent to rule out dysplasia or malignancy intraoperatively because this would change the operation performed. The enterotomy is then closed in a transverse, two-layered hand sewn fashion. For strictures longer than 4 to 5 cm in length, a Finney stricturoplasty can be used to prevent narrowing at the inlet or tension on the transverse closure. A Finney stricturoplasty is similar to a side-to-side anastomosis and is useful in the setting of a single long stricture or multiple short-segment strictures in close proximity. Two options exist. First, if the strictured area is mildly stenotic and the bowel has remaining pliability, the strictured area can be opened and sutured to normal bowel in a hand sewn side-to-side fashion. The second option is to exclude the strictured segment. If the segment is severely narrowed and nonpliable, normal bowel proximal and distal to the strictured segment can be overlapped and sewn together in a side-to-side fashion, effectively bypassing the area of strictured bowel. The concerns with this technique are the possible complications, including bacterial overgrowth and malignant degeneration of the excluded segment of bowel.

Significant dilation proximal to a strictured segment that results in significant size discrepancy between the normal proximal and distal bowel discourages a Heineke-Mikulicz stricturoplasty. In this much less common scenario, a Hoskel-Walske-Neumayer stricturoplasty can be performed. The stricture is opened along the antimesenteric border as a Y-shaped enterotomy with the Y portion in the dilated bowel just proximal to the stricture. The strictured segment is then pulled apart and the antimesenteric segment of the proximal bowel is advanced into the strictured area and closed in a transverse fashion with

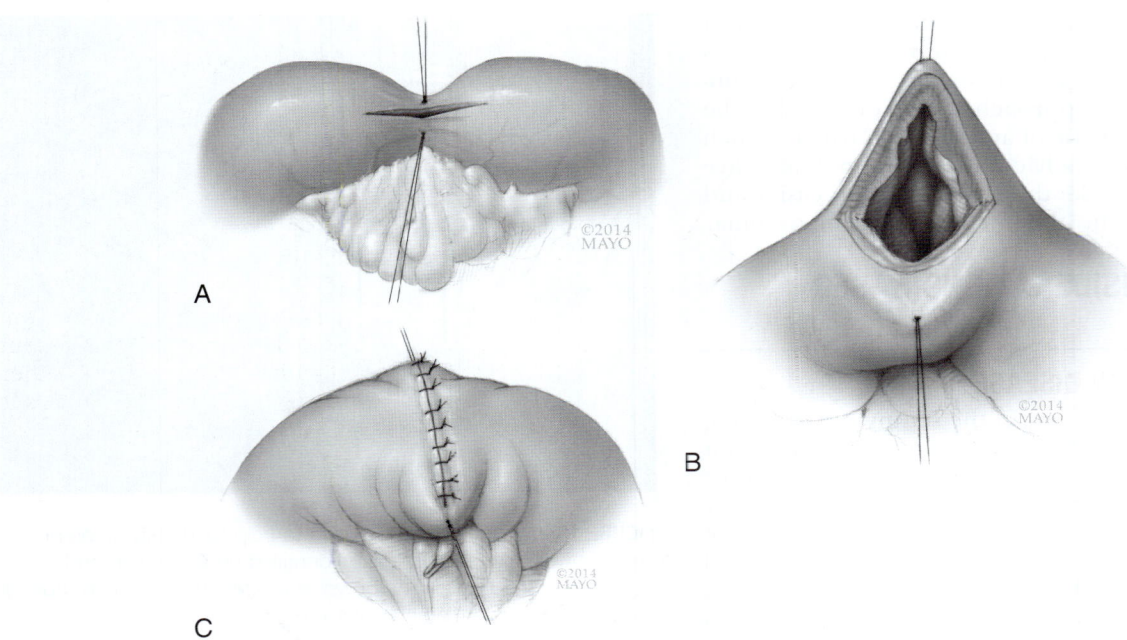

A

B

C

FIGURE 163.2 A Heineke-Mikulicz strictureplasty is performed by opening the small bowel along the antimesenteric border of the stricture and then closed transversely. (Copyright Mayo Clinic 2014.)

one side of the closure being normal bowel along the entire length and the other being the two strictured bowel edges.

The most difficult type of stricture to address is the very long, greater than 20 cm, stricture or series of strictures in close proximity. Due to the length of compromised bowel, resection is not recommended. Fortunately, Michelassi developed and published a unique technique to address this anatomic challenge.[26] A side-to-side isoperistaltic strictureplasty is made by completely dividing the bowel transversely in the middle of the strictured segment. The mesentery is then divided perpendicular to the long axis of the bowel to permit the now two segments of strictured bowel to lay side by side along the entire length of strictured bowel (Fig. 163.3). Both strictured segments are then opened along the antimesenteric border and sewn to one another in an isoperistaltic fashion. This technique does not exclude any bowel but rather incorporates all strictured areas. Shatari et al. published an initial series of 21 patients describing this technique as safe for long-segment strictures.[27] A meta-analysis of 148 patients followed; this technique did not increase postoperative morbidity. The largest series of 184 patients across six international centers found the technique safe, with 11% morbidity and 0% mortality, and effective, with only 23% of patients requiring reoperation at 5 years.[28]

As strictureplasty has become more widely adopted, several analyses regarding safety and efficacy have been published. Dietz et al. reported an overall morbidity of 18% and a septic complication rate of 5% among 314 patients with 1124 strictureplasties.[29] Tichansky et al. found that 90% of strictures in their series of 506 patients across 15 articles were less than 10 cm in length, of which 85% were successfully treated with a Heineke-Mikulicz technique. Interestingly, the authors found a trend toward

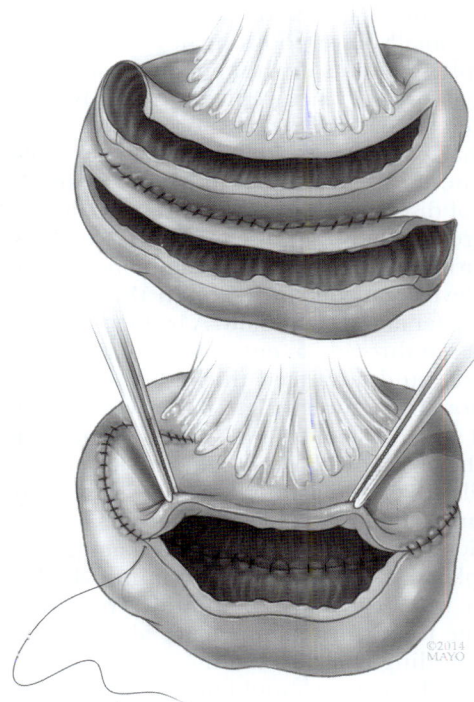

FIGURE 163.3 The isoperistaltic side-to-side strictureplasty is used to treat long strictures or multiple strictures that are very close to one another. The diseased segment is divided in the center of the area and overlapped. The antimesenteric border is opened in both segments and then the divided bowel segments are sutured together to construct a common lumen. (Copyright Mayo Clinic 2014.)

lower recurrence with the Finney technique.[30] Yamamoto et al. found a 4% rate of septic complications among 1112 patients who underwent 3259 strictureplasties and a site-specific recurrence rate of only 3%.[31] Campbell et al. compared the type of strictureplasty performed and found no difference in immediate- and long-term complication rates between the conventional Heineke-Mikulicz and nonconventional Finney and Michelassi technique among 1516 patients with 4538 strictureplasties.[32] Putting these results together, regardless of the operative technique used, bowel can be safely preserved with a low recurrence rate at the site of strictureplasty.

FISTULIZING CROHN DISEASE

Ongoing transmural inflammation can result in fistula formation between loops of bowel, bowel to bladder, bowel to abdominal wall, or bowel to any other structure or organ in the abdomen and pelvis. Historically, intra-abdominal CD fistulas were treated with bowel rest, intravenous nutrition, proximal diversion, and occasional resection. The introduction of infliximab in 1998 changed the paradigm of operative indication given its efficacy in closing abdominal wall and perianal fistulas.[33] In the initial multicenter, double blind, randomized trial assessing the efficacy of infliximab for fistulizing CD, 55% of all patients had closure of their fistulas and 70% had a reduction in the number of actively draining fistulas.[33] In the follow-up trial of long-term outcomes, 36% of patients had complete absence of fistulas at 1 year compared with 19% in the placebo.[34] Another more recent study found a third of patients with enterocutaneous fistulas achieved closure within 3 months of infliximab initiation.[35] Following these studies, patients now undergo a 3-month trial of infliximab prior to operating for fistulizing disease, in hopes of healing the fistula without an operation.

After it has been decided an operation is needed to address the fistulizing disease, the type of operation performed depends on the anatomic location of the fistula and degree of associated sepsis. For enterocutaneous fistula, the goal is to resect the bowel and skin communicating via the fistula. This should be attempted only after the patient has exhausted maximal medical therapy, the skin surrounding the fistula is soft and pliable, sepsis related to the fistula has been adequately drained, and the patient demonstrates adequate nutritional parameters. At this stage, interventional radiology may be required to drain any intraabdominal sources of infection, TPN may be necessary to improve a patient's nutrition prior to a major operation, and preoperative planning for potential mesh placement with loss of abdominal domain is imperative. The operation is performed in an open manner, taking care to lyse adhesions without inadvertent enterotomies. When resecting the small bowel, the consistent principles of bowel conservation should be kept in mind. The bowel is resection often with a primary anastomosis, and the skin and abdominal wall are excised back to healthy tissue. If the abdominal wall cannot be closed, mesh can be inserted. Prosthetic material, such as Prolene or Gore-Tex, is contraindicated due to infection risk, but biologic meshes, now abundantly available, can be used. Biologic mesh has the advantage of slow tissue ingrowth, decreased adhesion formation, and the ability

to not becoming chronically infected in the setting of local contamination. The mesh should be placed as an underlay with normal surrounding tissue and drains placed under any flaps to prevent seroma formation. If the mesh is left exposed, a wound vacuum closure device can be used with continuous drainage to facilitate tissue ingrowth, or transition to placement of a skin graft.

Entero-enteral fistulas may not be clinically significant unless a large segment of bowel is bypassed. If found preoperatively, preoperative planning should include imaging to best delineate the anatomy before an operation. When an operation is undertaken, often only one segment of bowel is actively involved with CD, whereas the other is a bystander and is not actively inflamed. When this is seen, the actively inflamed segment with fistula should be resected while the other can be repaired primarily following fistula takedown. This allows for increased bowel preservation with minimal morbidity and mortality.[36]

PERIANAL DISEASE

Perianal disease is a particularly morbid manifestation of CD affecting up to 20% of patients, with a lifetime risk of 20% to 40%.[37,38] Fistulas can tract from the rectum to the perianal skin, vagina, or sphincter complex. Initially, drainage of any active infection or abscess is undertaken, and placement of a seton (vessel loop or suture) through the fistula tract can promote ongoing source control while more aggressive medical and surgical managements ensue. Unfortunately, there is no available data concerning the ideal time to remove the seton, and this is performed on empirical basis, reported to range between 3 and 58 months by some authors.[39] If an early removal may intuitively lead to abscess formation, a prolonged stay in situ can result in fibrosis of the fistulous tract, leading to persistent incapability to heal after seton removal. Furthermore, disappointing results can be expected in the long term, with symptomatic recurrences occurring in more than 30% of patients after removal.[39] However, placing a seton loosely is a safe and useful strategy before attempting a definitive approach, without continence disturbances.

Unfortunately, definitive treatment of perianal disease is notoriously difficult, and despite several pharmacologic and surgical options, one-fifth of these patients will end up requiring proctectomy and a permanent end ileostomy due to the persistent morbidity associated with the disease. Infliximab heals only half of perianal fistulas at 1 year; adalimumab and certolizumab have even worse results and are not recommended in place of infliximab. Seton placement can be permanent, and additional surgical options carry a risk of incontinence due to sphincter impairment. A more invasive option of diversion with a temporary loop ileostomy does work to quiet perianal disease when combined with medical therapy. However, after being reversed and intestinal continuity is restored, 70% to 80% of patients with this have recurrence of symptoms despite biologic therapy, making this treatment option temporary and limited.[40,41] Newer treatment modalities, including adipose-derived mesenchymal stem cells (MSCs) and Gore plugs (Gore Medical, Flagstaff, Arizona), have improved clinical and radiographic healing rates, but widespread adoption of these treatment modalities has yet to be adopted.[42,43]

INFLAMMATORY CROHN DISEASE

SEGMENTAL COLITIS

In the setting of segmental medically refractory colitis, we believe patients should also be approached with the same bowel-preserving perspective unless there is multifocal dysplasia or malignancy, in which case subtotal colectomy (STC) or total proctocolectomy should be considered. This is largely for two reasons; first, the rate of colonic malignancy in CD is quite low,[44] and, second, no studies have shown the need to resect to histologically negative margins.[45,46] Thus, in the setting of segmental colonic colitis, we recommend excision and primary anastomosis of the grossly affected segment. At the time of surgery, a sigmoidoscope or colonoscope should be available in case the extent of mucosal disease should be evaluated prior to making a primary anastomosis. After surgery, resumption of CD medications remains nonstandardized. In general, most patients are surveilled 3 to 6 months after surgery with colonoscopy, and at that time, depending on the severity of disease, medication may be restarted or a new class initiated. If, at the time of resection, a significant burden of disease was noted, biologics may be resumed 2 to 4 weeks after surgery.

PANCOLITIS WITH RECTAL SPARING

In the case of rectal-sparing Crohn colitis, two options are available: (1) STC with ileorectal anastomosis (IRA) or (2) total proctocolectomy with end ileostomy. Given the pouch morbidity and significant increased rates of pouch failure in the setting of CD, an ileal pouch-anal anastomosis (IPAA) is rarely performed in this patient population. In the case of rectal-sparing Crohn colitis, STC with IRA can be safely performed, with nearly 70% still functioning at 5 years. Since the introduction of biologic therapy, our own data support even better outcomes with this operation, with a 0% failure rate at 1, 3, and 5 years (unpublished data).

When the rectum is not spared and medical management has been exhausted, total proctocolectomy and end ileostomy are performed. Some select centers will offer an IPAA to a patient with CD with no small bowel involvement and no perianal disease, but these centers are limited and the number of patients who meet those criteria is exceedingly small. At our institution we generally do not offer an IPAA to patients with CD.

ISOLATED PROCTITIS

In patients with isolated proctitis, without colonic involvement, two options remain. Either the patient may be diverted with a loop ileostomy and medical therapy maximized, or the patient may be offered a proctectomy. In the patient with significant perianal disease, in which an abdominal perineal resection would leave a significant perianal defect, a combination of these surgical approaches may be used. A diversion may first be performed to quiet and minimize the perianal fistulizing disease, followed by a proctectomy with closure of the anus and ability to retain the sphincter complex in the anal canal.

Unfortunately, in patients diverted for severe perianal disease with associated proctitis, the stomal reversal rate is only 22%, even in the era of biologic therapy; for proctitis alone the stomal reversal rate is slightly improved at 50%. The most important factors associated with stoma reversal are the presence of proctitis and number of prior setons placed, reflecting the severity of perianal disease.[47] Thus, although diversion may be attempted, in the majority of patients with severe proctitis, proctectomy will eventually be required. Again, bowel preservation is at the forefront of managing these patients. Therefore, without colonic involvement or neoplasia, the colon may be preserved in this patient population.

OPERATIVE CONSIDERATIONS AND DISEASE-SPECIFIC SCENARIOS

TYPE OF ANASTOMOSIS

As with all gastrointestinal anastomoses performed, an anastomosis in CD should not be performed under tension, should have good blood flow, and should ideally not be performed in a contaminated field. Outside of these basic principles, the type of anastomosis, hand sewn versus stapled, and configuration of a side-to-side versus end-to-end have been widely studied without definitive preference in terms of leak or recurrence rate. Although no anastomotic type has been found to be superior to another in patients with CD,[48–51] a few basic principles should still be kept in mind and applied when appropriate. The first is staple height. There are two staple sizes—3.6 and 4.8 mm. When the bowel wall is thickened, a 4.8-mm staple height may be best for the bowel wall, but at the expense of decreased hemostasis achieved compared with the 3.6-mm stapler. Thus both bowel wall thickness and hemostasis must be weighed intraoperatively. The second is bowel lumen size discrepancy. In the setting of significant size discrepancy, an end-to-end anastomosis may be more challenging to perform than a side-to-side one. Fortunately, early postoperative outcomes are comparable with regard to anastomotic leak rate and surgical site infection.[51] Third, when considering that 20% of patients who undergo ileocolic resection will develop symptomatic stenosis after their initial surgery and 45% of those patients will require surgery, the evaluation of disease recurrence associated with the type of anastomosis performed becomes important.[52] To date, none of the commonly performed anastomotic techniques can be favored with regard to recurrence of CD at the anastomotic site.[48] With no reported differences in leak or recurrence rates, the type of anastomosis constructed can be individualized at the time of the operation based on intraoperative findings.

Techniques to potentially minimize risk of recurrence are currently under development. The Kono-S is one such novel technique. This technique uses a linear stapler-cutter to transversely divide the tissue for resection. The corners of the two stapled lines are sutured together and antimesenteric longitudinal enterotomies are created on both sides. The enterotomies are then closed transversely in two layers, resulting in an antimesenteric functional end-to-end anastomosis. This technique has shown promise in a small cohort of 18 patients, 43% of whom have undergone follow-up endoscopic surveillance with an average Rutgeert score of 0.7 (0-3) at a mean of 6.8 months.[53]

LAPAROSCOPIC OPERATIONS

Laparoscopic surgery is ideally suited for patients with CD, a young cohort with high lifetime potential need for reoperation. Both randomized and nonrandomized studies have demonstrated safety and decreased morbidity and mortality with laparoscopic versus open resection in patients with CD.[20,54-60] Additional studies have shown decreased length of stay, shorter time to return of bowel function, decreased cost, improved postoperative complication rate, and decreased small bowel obstructions with laparoscopic surgery (35% vs. 11%) for small bowel and ileocolonic CD.[20,54-61,62] Unfortunately, despite 75% of patients being potential candidates for a laparoscopic approach,[61] only 6% of resections are being done laparoscopically as of 2009.[56] Hopefully, as more surgeons become familiar and facile with laparoscopic technique, this percentage will continue to increase.

However, patient selection is again important. A thickened mesentery, fistulizing disease, and fixed masses surrounding abscess cavities present challenges to safely performing a case laparoscopically. Thus, again, patient selection and intraoperative decision making becomes key.

RESECTION MARGIN

Margin status used to be a more controversial topic in CD surgery. Retrospective reviews had shown that disease-free margins of 4 cm[63] or "radical" disease-free margins of 10 cm compared with placebo had lower recurrence rates[63,64] and even improved quality of life.[63] However, later larger studies[65] and prospective studies[66] showed no difference in recurrence rate. More recent data, looking at the importance of microscopic disease-free margins, have not found a difference in recurrence based on microscopic margins.[45,46] In the only randomized study to date, Fazio et al.[66] evaluated recurrence in 131 ileocolectomy patients randomized to undergo resections with proximal margins either 2 or 12 cm from the macroscopically diseased tissue followed up for median of 56 months. Clinical recurrence was demonstrated in 33% versus 29% of those with limited and extended resections, respectively, and no relationship was found between microscopic CD found at the resection margin and disease recurrence. Thus current standard practice is to resect all gross macroscopically involved bowel and leave "positive margins" with microscopically involved bowel in place; again, this underscores the concept of bowel preservation among patients with CD.

DUODENAL CROHN DISEASE

Gastroduodenal CD is rare, occurring in only 0.5% to 4% of all CD patients.[67] Similar to any other location in the gastrointestinal tract, treatment is a combination of medical, endoscopic, and surgical intervention. Given the challenging anatomic location and increased major surgical morbidity in nearly one-third of patients,[68] medical therapy should be exhausted before surgery is undertaken. The most common indication for surgery is obstruction. Patients may also present with pancreatitis due to local invasion into the pancreas or pancreatic duct or duodenoenteric fistulas resulting for distal obstruction.

In the setting of obstructive-like symptoms, TPN should be considered before an operation in the case of long-standing obstruction and weight loss of greater than 10%. In addition, iron supplementation should be given and vitamin D and calcium considered. In cases in which there is a short stricture length of less than 2 cm, endoscopic balloon dilation is a viable alternative to surgery. However, as the length of the stricture increases, so does the risk of perforation, limiting the use of endoscopic intervention.

Up to 40% of patients with duodenal CD will eventually become medically refractory and ultimately require surgery.[69] When patients have duodenal narrowing or obstruction, bypass procedures, such as gastrojejunostomy and Roux-en-Y duodenojejunostomy, can be undertaken when absolutely necessary. However, morbidity need for reoperation due to marginal ulceration, obstruction of the afferent limb, and duodenal fistula approaches one-third of patients.[68,70,71] When feasible, strictureplasty can be used as a safe option to preserve bowel.[72] Lesions most amenable to this intervention are those that are short, fibrous strictures, but these remain limited in number.[73]

When patients present with fistulizing disease from adjacent organs, the involved bowel (e.g., ileum or colon) should be resected and the duodenum repaired primarily. Before primary repair, the duodenal edges should be cleaned.

RECTOVAGINAL FISTULAS

Rectovaginal fistulas (RVFs) are a particularly distressing complication of CD that affects 2% of women with CD. Fortunately, most fistulas are very distal and have no associated symptoms. Surgical intervention is reserved for patients who have failed medical management and continue to experience symptoms with an unacceptable quality of life. For patients who undergo surgical repair, the disease should be quiescent and the rectum distensible. Proximal diversion prior to surgical repair may be required to achieve these goals. In general, for a very distal RVF in which less than 15% of the internal sphincter is involved, a simple fistulotomy may be performed. Alternatives include an endorectal advancement flap or noncutting setons in patients who do not have active rectal inflammation.[74,75] Joo et al.[74] reported sustained closure in 74% of 26 patients with fistulizing CD treated with an endorectal advancement flap, and Hull and Fazio[76] reported 68% ultimate healing. Few others have reported such good outcomes, and, in our hands, endorectal advancement flap yields unpredictable results at best.

COLORECTAL DYSPLASIA OR CANCER

As stated earlier, colorectal cancer related to CD remains rare, and the 5-year survival and local recurrence rate, stage for stage, remain similar to that of sporadic cancer.[77] However, all patients with CD longer than 10 years should undergo annual surveillance colonoscopy due to an increased risk of colorectal cancer over the general population.[78] At the time of colonoscopy, chromoendoscopy or white light may be used to increase visualization of small, irregular lesions. Regardless of the technology used, four random biopsies are taken every 10 cm throughout the colon and rectum in addition to any abdominal mucosal lesions. When dysplasia is found on endoscopy, the histology should always be confirmed by a second pathologist before discussion of surgical intervention. Patients with unifocal low-grade dysplasia (LGD) can continue surveillance. Patients with multifocal LGD or high-grade dysplasia (HGD) should undergo surgical intervention. If patients have rectal-sparing disease and are reliable for ongoing endoscopic surveillance, an STC with IRA is reasonable to perform. If there is rectal dysplasia, long-standing chronic inflammation in the setting of colonic dysplasia, or an unreliable patient who will likely be lost from ongoing surveillance, total proctocolectomy and end ileostomy is the operation of choice. In the setting of a colon or rectal cancer, a total proctocolectomy and end ileostomy is also the operation of choice, and the surgeon should be mindful of high vessel ligation and adequate lymph node sampling, not a common concern in inflammatory bowel disease surgery.

DISEASE RECURRENCE AND REOPERATIVE CROHN DISEASE

Within 1 year of surgery, subclinical endoscopic recurrence occurs at the anastomosis in 90% of patients with CD, symptomatic clinical recurrence occurs in 30%, and 5% of patients will require another operation.[79–81] Over time, approximately 70% of patients who have had operations need further surgery.[8,82] Smoking, perforating disease, and previous resection have been identified individually from retrospective studies as risk factors for earlier postoperative recurrence, but these factors have not been used to tailor postoperative initiation of medical therapy.[48,83–85] Recurrent mucosal disease after an operation typically precedes any clinical symptoms, and its severity predicts the subsequent clinical disease.[80] Therefore early endoscopy might be useful in earlier initial and more aggressive use of postoperative medical therapy.[86,87]

From a medical point of view, there are conflicting data regarding the use of postoperative prophylaxis.[88] In general, patients considered high risk (e.g., smokers, perforating disease) should resume anti-TNF-α therapy. Patients who have few risk factors may benefit from 3 months of antibiotics and followed with endoscopy at 1 year. Those with no risk factors are generally rescoped at 1 year to assess mucosal disease. Methods to stratify patients into high- and low-risk populations combined with prophylaxis tailored to endoscopic recurrence would be ideal but remains undefined. Thus, for most patients, a decision to give medical prophylaxis after resection needs to be individualized.

The most common indication for reoperative CD is recurrent inflammatory or stricturing disease and less often, fistulizing disease. A few preoperative actions can be used to assist with the expected difficulty of the case. First, liberal placement of bilateral ureteral stents to help to identify the ureters during the operation can be quite helpful in the setting of retroperitoneal inflammation and a reoperative field. Second, the patient should be placed in the combined position if the case has any potential to involve the rectum or left colon; this allows improved access to the pelvis and perineum. Third, a flexible endoscope should be available in the room to allow for intraoperative mucosal or anastomotic evaluation.

CROHN DISEASE OF THE POUCH

CD of the ileoanal pouch is an exceedingly common diagnosis given rather liberally to patients complaining of pouch dysfunction and remains a challenging diagnosis with a large differential. Patient symptoms, physical exam, pouchoscopy, and radiographic imaging are all used in making the diagnosis and distinguishing it from technical complications of the IPAA, such as a leak or sepsis, chronic pouchitis, and pouch dysfunction. CD of the pouch may be overdiagnosed if timing of the diagnosis in relation to IPAA is not considered. For example, an early fistula or chronic sinus tract may be the result of an operative misadventure or leak rather than CD, and an anastomotic stricture may be related to relative ischemia at the time of IPAA rather than CD. Thus timing of the onset of the complication must be used to distinguish CD from operation-related complications. If symptoms begin immediately after surgery, or a patient has a leak following IPAA, or a patient experiences a stricture within 6 months following an IPAA, these are likely related to technical details of the pouch operation. If fistulizing and stricturing disease occur late, after 6 months to a year following IPAA, then CD becomes a more likely cause. After a patient is given the diagnosis of CD of the pouch, adalimumab has some utility, with up to 70% of patients showing an improvement in symptoms at 8 weeks.[89] If the disease causes significant pouch dysfunction, eventual diversion or pouch excision may be required; this occurs in up to 18% of patients with CD of the pouch.[89]

SUMMARY

A wide range of indications for surgery exist in patients with CD. Many sophisticated techniques are available, and all should be in the surgeon's armamentarium. Considering that CD cannot be cured, indications for surgery have to be strict and surgery should be performed in as limited and minimally invasive form as possible. Maintaining close collaboration between surgeons and gastroenterologists will ultimately serve these patients best due to the highly complex nature of the disease and difficulty in determining when to escalate medical therapy versus taking the patient to the operating room.

ACKNOWLEDGMENTS

The authors acknowledge David W. Larson, MD, and Bruce G. Wolff, MD, for their contribution to this chapter in the previous edition, which was the basis for this rewrite.

REFERENCES

1. Lichtenstein GR, Hanauer SB, Sandborn WJ. Practice Parameters Committee of American College of Gastroenterology. Management of Crohn's disease in adults. *Am J Gastroenterol.* 2009;104(2):465-483; quiz 464, 484.
2. Hanauer SB, Feagan BG, Lichtenstein GR, et al. Maintenance infliximab for Crohn's disease: the ACCENT I randomised trial. *Lancet.* 2002;359(9317):1541-1549.

3. Cornillie F, Hanauer SB, Diamond RH, et al. Postinduction serum infliximab trough level and decrease of C-reactive protein level are associated with durable sustained response to infliximab: a retrospective analysis of the ACCENT I trial. *Gut.* 2014;63(11):1721-1727.

4. Karmiris K, Paintaud G, Noman M, et al. Influence of trough serum levels and immunogenicity on long-term outcome of adalimumab therapy in Crohn's disease. *Gastroenterology.* 2009;137(5):1628-1640.

5. Riss S, Schuster I, Papay P, et al. Surgical recurrence after primary ileocolic resection for Crohn's disease. *Tech Coloproctol.* 2014;18(4):365-371.

6. De Cruz P, Kamm MA, Hamilton AL, et al. Crohn's disease management after intestinal resection: a randomised trial. *Lancet.* 2015;385(9976):1406-1417.

7. Arora Z, Shen B. Biological therapy for ulcerative colitis. *Gastroenterol Rep (Oxf).* 2015;3(2):103-109.

8. Bernell O, Lapidus A, Hellers G. Risk factors for surgery and postoperative recurrence in Crohn's disease. *Ann Surg.* 2000;231(1):38-45.

9. Peyrin-Biroulet L, Harmsen WS, Tremaine WJ, Zinsmeister AR, Sandborn WJ, Loftus EV Jr. Surgery in a population-based cohort of Crohn's disease from Olmsted County, Minnesota (1970–2004). *Am J Gastroenterol.* 2012;107(11):1693-1701.

10. Andrews HA, Keighley MR, Alexander-Williams J, Allan RN. Strategy for management of distal ileal Crohn's disease. *Br J Surg.* 1991;78(6):679-682.

11. Semrad CE. Use of parenteral nutrition in patients with inflammatory bowel disease. *Gastroenterol Hepatol (N Y).* 2012;8(6):393-395.

12. Perioperative total parenteral nutrition in surgical patients. The Veterans Affairs Total Parenteral Nutrition Cooperative Study Group. *N Engl J Med.* 1991;325(8):525-532.

13. Nasir BS, Dozois EJ, Cima RR, et al. Perioperative anti–tumor necrosis factor therapy does not increase the rate of early postoperative complications in Crohn's disease. *J Gastrointest Surg.* 2010;14(12):1859-1865; discussion 1865-1866.

14. Kopylov U, Ben-Horin S, Zmora O, Eliakim R, Katz LH. Anti-tumor necrosis factor and postoperative complications in Crohn's disease: systematic review and meta-analysis. *Inflamm Bowel Dis.* 2012;18(12):2404-2413.

15. Yang ZP, Hong L, Wu Q, Wu KC, Fan DM. Preoperative infliximab use and postoperative complications in Crohn's disease: a systematic review and meta-analysis. *Int J Surg.* 2014;12(3):224-230.

16. Gutierrez A, Lee H, Sands BE. Outcome of surgical versus percutaneous drainage of abdominal and pelvic abscesses in Crohn's disease. *Am J Gastroenterol.* 2006;101(10):2283-2289.

17. Sahai A, Belair M, Gianfelice D, Cote S, Gratton J, Lahaie R. Percutaneous drainage of intra-abdominal abscesses in Crohn's disease: short and long-term outcome. *Am J Gastroenterol.* 1997;92(2):275-278.

18. Allen BC, Leyendecker JR. MR enterography for assessment and management of small bowel Crohn disease. *Radiol Clin North Am.* 2014;52(4):799-810.

19. Sinha R, Trivedi D, Murphy PD, Fallis S. Small-intestinal length measurement on MR enterography: comparison with in vivo surgical measurement. *AJR Am J Roentgenol.* 2014;203(3):W274-W279.

20. Bergamaschi R, Pessaux P, Arnaud JP. Comparison of conventional and laparoscopic ileocolic resection for Crohn's disease. *Dis Colon Rectum.* 2003;46(8):1129-1133.

21. Tan JJ, Tjandra JJ. Laparoscopic surgery for Crohn's disease: a meta-analysis. *Dis Colon Rectum.* 2007;50(5):576-585.

22. Becker JM, Dayton MT, Fazio VW, et al. Prevention of postoperative abdominal adhesions by a sodium hyaluronate-based bioresorbable membrane: a prospective, randomized, double-blind multicenter study. *J Am Coll Surg.* 1996;183(4):297-306.

23. Diamond MP. Reduction of adhesions after uterine myomectomy by Seprafilm membrane (HAL-F): a blinded, prospective, randomized, multicenter clinical study. Seprafilm Adhesion Study Group. *Fertil Steril.* 1996;66(6):904-910.

24. Lee EC, Papaioannou N. Minimal surgery for chronic obstruction in patients with extensive or universal Crohn's disease. *Ann R Coll Surg Engl.* 1982;64(4):229-233.

25. de Buck van Overstraeten A, Vermeire S, Vanbeckevoort D, et al. Modified side-to-side isoperistaltic strictureplasty over the ileocaecal valve: an alternative to ileocaecal resection in extensive terminal ileal Crohn's disease. *J Crohns Colitis.* 2016;10(4):437-442.

26. Michelassi F. Side-to-side isoperistaltic strictureplasty for multiple Crohn's strictures. *Dis Colon Rectum.* 1996;39(3):345-349.

27. Fhatari T, Clark MA, Yamamoto T, et al. Long strictureplasty is as safe and effective as short strictureplasty in small-bowel Crohn's disease. *Colorectal Dis.* 2004;6(6):438-441.

28. Michelassi F, Taschieri A, Tonelli F, et al. An international, multicenter, prospective, observational study of the side-to-side isoperistaltic strictureplasty in Crohn's disease. *Dis Colon Rectum.* 2007;50(3):277-284.

29. Dietz DW, Remzi FH, Fazio VW. Strictureplasty for obstructing small-bowel lesions in diffuse radiation enteritis—successful outcome in five patients. *Dis Colon Rectum.* 2001;44(12):1772-1777.

30. Tichansky D, Cagir B, Yoo E, Marcus SM, Fry RD. Strictureplasty for Crohn's disease: meta-analysis. *Dis Colon Rectum.* 2000;43(7):911-919.

31. Yamamoto T, Fazio VW, Tekkis PP. Safety and efficacy of strictureplasty for Crohn's disease: a systematic review and meta-analysis. *Dis Colon Rectum.* 2007;50(11):1968-1986.

32. Campbell L, Ambe R, Weaver J, Marcus SM, Cagir B. Comparison of conventional and nonconventional strictureplasties in Crohn's disease: a systematic review and meta-analysis. *Dis Colon Rectum.* 2012;55(6):714-726.

33. Present DH, Rutgeerts P, Targan S, et al. Infliximab for the treatment of fistulas in patients with Crohn's disease. *N Engl J Med.* 1999;340(18):1398-1405.

34. Sands BE, Anderson FH, Bernstein CN, et al. Infliximab maintenance therapy for fistulizing Crohn's disease. *N Engl J Med.* 2004;350(9):876-885.

35. Amiot A, Setakhr V, Seksik P, et al. Long-term outcome of enterocutaneous fistula in patients with Crohn's disease treated with anti-TNF therapy: a cohort study from the GETAID. *Am J Gastroenterol.* 2014;109(9):1443-1449.

36. Michelassi F, Stella M, Balestracci T, Giuliante F, Marogna P, Block GE. Incidence, diagnosis, and treatment of enteric and colorectal fistulae in patients with Crohn's disease. *Ann Surg.* 1993;218(5):660-666.

37. Rankin GB, Watts HD, Melnyk CS, Kelley ML Jr. National Cooperative Crohn's Disease Study: extraintestinal manifestations and perianal complications. *Gastroenterology.* 1979;77(4 Pt 2):914-920.

38. Schwartz DA, Loftus EV Jr, Tremaine WJ, et al. The natural history of fistulizing Crohn's disease in Olmsted County, Minnesota. *Gastroenterology.* 2002;122(4):875-880.

39. Buchanan GN, Owen HA, Torkington J, Lunniss PJ, Nicholls RJ, Cohen CR. Long-term outcome following loose-seton technique for external sphincter preservation in complex anal fistula. *Br J Surg.* 2004;91(4):476-480.

40. Hong MK, Craig Lynch A, Bell S, et al. Faecal diversion in the management of perianal Crohn's disease. *Colorectal Dis.* 2011;13(2):171-176.

41. Mennigen R, Heptner B, Senninger N, Rijcken E. Temporary fecal diversion in the management of colorectal and perianal Crohn's disease. *Gastroenterol Res Pract.* 2015;2015:286315.

42. Garcia-Olmo D, Garcia-Arranz M, Herreros D, Pascual I, Peiro C, Rodriguez-Montes JA. A phase I clinical trial of the treatment of Crohn's fistula by adipose mesenchymal stem cell transplantation. *Dis Colon Rectum.* 2005;48(7):1416-1423.

43. Garcia-Olmo D, Herreros D, Pascual I, et al. Expanded adipose-derived stem cells for the treatment of complex perianal fistula: a phase II clinical trial. *Dis Colon Rectum.* 2009;52(1):79-86.

44. Freeman HJ. Colorectal cancer risk in Crohn's disease. *World J Gastroenterol.* 2008;14(12):1810-1811.

45. Bordeianou L, Stein SL, Ho VP, et al. Immediate versus tailored prophylaxis to prevent symptomatic recurrences after surgery for ileocecal Crohn's disease? *Surgery.* 2011;149(1):72-78.

46. Malireddy K, Larson DW, Sandborn WJ, et al. Recurrence and impact of postoperative prophylaxis in laparoscopically treated primary ileocolic Crohn disease. *Arch Surg.* 2010;145(1):42-47.

47. Gu J, Valente MA, Remzi FH, Stocchi L. Factors affecting the fate of faecal diversion in patients with perianal Crohn's disease. *Colorectal Dis.* 2015;17(1):66-72.

48. McLeod RS, Wolff BG, Ross S, Parkes R, McKenzie M, Investigators of the CAST Trial. Recurrence of Crohn's disease after ileocolic resection is not affected by anastomotic type: results of a multicenter, randomized, controlled trial. *Dis Colon Rectum.* 2009;52(5):919-927.

49. Neutzling CB, Lustosa SA, Proenca IM, da Silva EM, Matos D. Stapled versus handsewn methods for colorectal anastomosis surgery. *Cochrane Database Syst Rev.* 2012;(2):CD003144.

50. Scarpa M, Angriman I, Barollo M, et al. Role of stapled and hand-sewn anastomoses in recurrence of Crohn's disease. *Hepatogastroenterology.* 2004;51(58):1053-1057.

51. Zurbuchen U, Kroesen AJ, Knebel P, et al. Complications after end-to-end vs. side-to-side anastomosis in ileocecal Crohn's disease—early postoperative results from a randomized controlled multi-center trial (ISRCTN-45665492). *Langenbecks Arch Surg.* 2013;398(3):467-474.

52. Yamamoto T. Factors affecting recurrence after surgery for Crohn's disease. *World J Gastroenterol.* 2005;11(26):3971-3979.

53. Fichera A, Zoccali M, Kono T. Antimesenteric functional end-to-end handsewn (Kono-S) anastomosis. *J Gastrointest Surg.* 2012;16(7):1412-1416.

54. Duepree HJ, Senagore AJ, Delaney CP, Brady KM, Fazio VW. Advantages of laparoscopic resection for ileocecal Crohn's disease. *Dis Colon Rectum.* 2002;45(5):605-610.

55. Larson DW, Pemberton JH. Current concepts and controversies in surgery for IBD. *Gastroenterology.* 2004;126(6):1611-1619.

56. Lesperance K, Martin MJ, Lehmann R, Brounts L, Steele SR. National trends and outcomes for the surgical therapy of ileocolonic Crohn's disease: a population-based analysis of laparoscopic vs. open approaches. *J Gastrointest Surg.* 2009;13(7):1251-1259.

57. Milsom JW, Hammerhofer KA, Bohm B, Marcello P, Elson P, Fazio VW. Prospective, randomized trial comparing laparoscopic vs. conventional surgery for refractory ileocolic Crohn's disease. *Dis Colon Rectum.* 2001;44(1):1-8; discussion 8–9.

58. Nguyen SQ, Teitelbaum E, Sabnis AA, Bonaccorso A, Tabrizian F, Salky B. Laparoscopic resection for Crohn's disease: an experience with 335 cases. *Surg Endosc.* 2009;23(10):2380-2384.

59. Reissman P, Salky BA, Pfeifer J, Edye M, Jagelman DG, Wexner SD. Laparoscopic surgery in the management of inflammatory bowel disease. *Am J Surg.* 1996;171(1):47-50; discussion 50–51.

60. Soop M, Larson DW, Malireddy K, Cima RR, Young-Fadok TM, Dozois EJ. Safety, feasibility, and short-term outcomes of laparoscopically assisted primary ileocolic resection for Crohn's disease. *Surg Endosc.* 2009;23(8):1876-1881.

61. Holubar SD, Dozois EJ, Privitera A, et al. Laparoscopic surgery for recurrent ileocolic Crohn's disease. *Inflamm Bowel Dis.* 2010;16(8):1382-1386.

62. Holubar SD, Wolff BG. Advances in surgical approaches to Crohn's disease: minimally invasive surgery and biologic therapy. *Expert Rev Clin Immunol.* 2009;5(4):463-470.

63. Softley A, Myren J, Clamp SE, Bouchier IA, Watkinson G, de Dombal FT. Factors affecting recurrence after surgery for Crohn's disease. *Scand J Gastroenterol Suppl.* 1988;144:31-34.

64. Krause U, Ejerblad S, Bergman L. Crohn's disease. A long-term study of the clinical course in 186 patients. *Scand J Gastroenterol.* 1985;20(4):516-524.

65. Raab Y, Bergstrom R, Ejerblad S, Graf W, Pahlman L. Factors influencing recurrence in Crohn's disease. An analysis of a consecutive series of 353 patients treated with primary surgery. *Dis Colon Rectum.* 1996;39(8):918-925.

66. Fazio VW, Marchetti F, Church M, et al. Effect of resection margins on the recurrence of Crohn's disease in the small bowel. A randomized controlled trial. *Ann Surg.* 1996;224(4):563-571; discussion 571–573.

67. Reynolds HL Jr, Stellato TA. Crohn's disease of the foregut. *Surg Clin North Am.* 2001;81(1):117-135, viii.

68. Shapiro M, Greenstein AJ, Byrn J, et al. Surgical management and outcomes of patients with duodenal Crohn's disease. *J Am Coll Surg.* 2008;207(1):36-42.

69. Nugent FW, Roy MA. Duodenal Crohn's disease: an analysis of 89 cases. *Am J Gastroenterol.* 1989;84(3):249-254.

70. Murray JJ, Schoetz DJ Jr, Nugent FW, Coller JA, Veidenheimer MC. Surgical management of Crohn's disease involving the duodenum. *Am J Surg.* 1984;147(1):58-65.

71. Ross TM, Fazio VW, Farmer RG. Long-term results of surgical treatment for Crohn's disease of the duodenum. *Ann Surg.* 1983;197(4):399-406.

72. Worsey MJ, Hull T, Ryland L, Fazio V. Strictureplasty is an effective option in the operative management of duodenal Crohn's disease. *Dis Colon Rectum.* 1999;42(5):596-600.

73. Dehn TC, Kettlewell MG, Mortensen NJ, Lee EC, Jewell DP. Ten-year experience of strictureplasty for obstructive Crohn's disease. *Br J Surg.* 1989;76(4):339-341.

74. Joo JS, Weiss EG, Nogueras JJ, Wexner SD. Endorectal advancement flap in perianal Crohn's disease. *Am Surg.* 1998;64(2):147-150.

75. Makowiec F, Jehle EC, Starlinger M. Clinical course of perianal fistulas in Crohn's disease. *Gut.* 1995;37(5):696-701.

76. Hull TL, Fazio VW. Surgical approaches to low anovaginal fistula in Crohn's disease. *Am J Surg.* 1997;173(2):95-98.

77. Kiran RP, Khoury W, Church JM, Lavery IC, Fazio VW, Remzi FH. Colorectal cancer complicating inflammatory bowel disease: similarities and differences between Crohn's and ulcerative colitis based on three decades of experience. *Ann Surg.* 2010;252(2):330-335.

78. Mattar MC, Lough D, Pishvaian MJ, Charabaty A. Current management of inflammatory bowel disease and colorectal cancer. *Gastrointest Cancer Res.* 2011;4(2):53-61.

79. Olaison G, Smedh K, Sjodahl R. Natural course of Crohn's disease after ileocolic resection: endoscopically visualised ileal ulcers preceding symptoms. *Gut.* 1992;33(3):331-335.

80. Rutgeerts P, Geboes K, Vantrappen G, Beyls J, Kerremans R, Hiele M. Predictability of the postoperative course of Crohn's disease. *Gastroenterology.* 1990;99(4):956-963.

81. Rutgeerts P, Geboes K, Vantrappen G, Kerremans R, Coenegrachts JL, Coremans G. Natural history of recurrent Crohn's disease at the ileocolonic anastomosis after curative surgery. *Gut.* 1984;25(6):665-672.

82. Landsend E, Johnson E, Johannessen HO, Carlsen E. Long-term outcome after intestinal resection for Crohn's disease. *Scand J Gastroenterol.* 2006;41(10):1204-1208.

83. Binder V, Hendriksen C, Kreiner S. Prognosis in Crohn's disease—based on results from a regional patient group from the county of Copenhagen. *Gut.* 1985;26(2):146-150.

84. Reese GE, Nanidis T, Borysiewicz C, Yamamoto T, Orchard T, Tekkis PP. The effect of smoking after surgery for Crohn's disease: a meta-analysis of observational studies. *Int J Colorectal Dis.* 2008;23(12):1213-1221.

85. Simillis C, Yamamoto T, Reese GE, et al. A meta-analysis comparing incidence of recurrence and indication for reoperation after surgery for perforating versus nonperforating Crohn's disease. *Am J Gastroenterol.* 2008;103(1):196-205.

86. Van Assche G, Vermeire S, Noman M, et al. Infliximab administered with shortened infusion times in a specialized IBD infusion unit: a prospective cohort study. *J Crohns Colitis.* 2010;4(3):329-333.

87. Rutgeerts P, Van Assche G. What is the role of endoscopy in the postoperative management of Crohn's disease? *Inflamm Bowel Dis.* 2008;14(suppl 2):S179-S180.

88. Vaughn BP, Moss AC. Prevention of post-operative recurrence of Crohn's disease. *World J Gastroenterol.* 2014;20(5):1147-1154.

89. Shen B, Remzi FH, Lavery IC, et al. Administration of adalimumab in the treatment of Crohn's disease of the ileal pouch. *Aliment Pharmacol Ther.* 2009;29(5):519-526.

Appendix

Geoffrey Fasen | Bruce Schirmer | Traci L. Hedrick

ACUTE APPENDICITIS

Acute appendicitis is one of the most common problems encountered by a general surgeon, accounting for approximately 1% of all surgical operations.[1] Historically the appendix has been identified as a potential source of right lower quadrant pain and disease for centuries, with a scattering of case reports through the early 19th century describing abscesses and evidence of inflammation of the appendix in autopsies. The first description of an appendectomy stems from 1735 when Dr. Claudius Amyand removed one during treatment of a scrotal hernia, yielding the description of the eponymous inguinal hernia containing the appendix. The first suggestion of appendectomy to treat typhlitis stems from 1827. The coalescence of the appendix as the source of disease, as well as appendectomy as therapy for it, did not fully mature until 1886, when it was presented in a paper from Reginald Fitz.[2] The incidence in the United States is estimated to be 9.38/10,000 per year, a slight increase over the past 20 years. Approximately 300,000 appendectomies are performed annually. The most common age group to be afflicted is 10 to 19 years, with that age decile accounting for 23% of all diagnosed cases; more than 50% of cases occur before the age of 30.[3] Among teenagers and young adults the male-to-female ratio is approximately 3:2. After age 25 years, the ratio gradually declines until the sex ratio is equal by the mid-30s.

PATHOPHYSIOLOGY

The common end point for the different etiologies of appendicitis is the translocation of bacteria across the mucosa of the appendix, leading to suppurative appendicitis. The classic teaching is that luminal obstruction, secondary to fecalith, lymphoid hyperplasia, or malignancy is the main initiator of this process. The proposed pathway is that obstruction of the lumen leads to accumulation of mucus in the appendix, creating increased intraluminal pressure. The lack of luminal drainage leads to bacterial overgrowth while the increased pressure leads to mucosal ischemia with impaired venous and lymphatic drainage. This combination of factors then leads to bacterial invasion of the appendiceal wall and development of acute appendicitis, which, left unchecked, can lead to gangrenous and perforated appendicitis.

However, this teaching has been challenged by a number of studies, demonstrating low frequency of obstructing lesions, such as fecolith, tumor, or lymphoid hyperplasia in pathologic specimens and their relative frequency in normal appendices.[4,5] In addition, normal intraluminal pressures were found when measured in vivo on patients undergoing appendectomy.[5] The differing incidences of appendicitis in developing and developed countries also suggest that there may be environmental factors, including diet, infection, and gut flora, that contribute to the development of appendicitis.[7] Genetic factors also appear to play a role, with an increased risk of appendicitis in families.[8] This different understanding of the progression of appendicitis has made itself relevant through new methods of treating appendicitis, namely nonoperative management

CLINICAL PRESENTATION

SYMPTOMS

Irrespective of the etiology, the symptomatic progression of appendicitis often follows a typical course. The initial stages of appendiceal inflammation correspond with the development of periumbilical, visceral type pain. This is accompanied by anorexia (92%), nausea (78%), and vomiting (67%).[1] When vomiting does occur, it is rarely persistent and most commonly occurs after the onset of pain. As the appendiceal inflammation progresses, it leads to irritation of the nearby parietal peritoneum, leading to localized pain that manifests as migration of the visceral pain from the periumbilical region to the right lower quadrant somatic pain where the appendix typically lies. This pattern of pain progression is found in approximately 75% of patients with acute appendicitis.[1] Differences in presentation of abdominal pain can be secondary to abnormal appendiceal location with retrocecal appendices leading to diffuse right flank pain, or pelvic location of the appendix causing poorly localized hypogastric discomfort, or tenesmus. The presentation of atypical pain is more common in the very young and older patients. The early course of appendicitis is often not accompanied by a fever because it remains a localized process. The presence of constipation or diarrhea is generally not helpful in the diagnosis of appendicitis.

SIGNS

Combined with the patient's history, the physical examination can be sufficient to make a diagnosis of appendicitis, especially in men where the differential diagnosis is not as extensive as in women. The typical signs of acute appendicitis include localized right lower quadrant tenderness, abdominal wall guarding and rebound tenderness. A flushed facial appearance can be present, with fever more often than not being absent if the patient has an acute uncomplicated appendicitis.

ABDOMINAL EXAM

Pain with pressure over McBurney point, or two-thirds the distance between the umbilicus and anterior superior iliac spine, is the physical exam finding in the vast majority of patients (91%) and corresponds with an inflamed appendix lying within the typical location in the right lower quadrant.[1] For patients with an atypical position of the appendix, such as retrocecal or deep pelvic, pressure in this location may not elicit the typical exam findings. In the case of a retrocecal appendix the pain may be localized over the right flank, elicited by an extension of the hip (*psoas sign*), or may not be well localized on physical exam at all. An *obturator sign* may be present with appendicitis located in the deep pelvis. A *Rosving sign* consists of pain in the right lower quadrant with palpation in the left lower quadrant. Jostling the bed or striking the heel of the extended right leg can lead to right lower quadrant pain. Similarly the patient may be asked to bounce or attempt to jump, producing pain in the area. Although these findings are typical for an uncomplicated appendicitis, perforation can lead to a more generalized peritonitis, with involuntary diffuse guarding, high fever, and hemodynamic changes.

An abdominal mass on physical exam is rarely present and, when present, may be difficult to appreciate due to discomfort with deep palpation and increased abdominal wall thickness. The presence of a mass is suggestive of an abscess or phlegmon, reflecting a rupture of the appendix with adherence of omentum and surrounding bowel to the inflamed appendix. After patients are adequately treated with pain medication or when asleep after initiation of anesthesia, a mass can sometimes be palpated in children or thin patients.

DIAGNOSIS

PELVIC EXAMINATION

Pelvic examination is essential in all women of childbearing age presenting with appendicitis. A speculum examination of the cervix is undertaken to evaluate for purulent drainage caused by gynecologic infection. In addition, a bimanual examination can be performed to palpate for the adnexal structures.

LABORATORY EVALUATION

Blood tests are of limited use in the diagnosis of an uncomplicated acute appendicitis because of their lack of specificity but can help to confirm a suspicion based on history and physical exam. As many as 50% of patients with acute appendicitis can present with a normal leukocyte count, with the variance attributable to both age and ethnic factors.[9-11] In uncomplicated appendicitis the leukocytosis is typically mild, with an average value of 14.2×10^9/L.[11] Attempts have been made to make a more sensitive test for appendicitis by including the leukocyte differential or C-reactive protein (CRP) values. A left shift (increased percentage of neutrophils to greater than 74%) is present irrespective of the presence of leukocytosis in up to 87% of patients. When all three variables are used together, they are quite effective in ruling out appendicitis. A physical exam suggestive of appendicitis in the setting of normal white blood cell (WBC) count, differential, and CRP is quite rare.

Urinalysis, pregnancy tests, and sexually transmitted disease (STD) evaluation are all useful in identifying other potential causes for lower abdominal pain but do not contribute directly to a diagnosis of appendicitis.

RADIOGRAPHIC EVALUATION

Plain abdominal radiograph is of little utility in the diagnosis of appendicitis, except when it identifies another source for abdominal pain or is able to identify a radiopaque fecolith, which is uncommon. Computed tomography (CT) and ultrasound (US) imaging are the preferred imaging modalities for diagnosis of abdominal pain and appendicitis. Studies comparing the two modalities for appendicitis reveal increased accuracy with CT over US,[12] and in equivocal cases have demonstrated CT to be more accurate.[13] For most adult patients with abdominal pain and suspected appendicitis, the abdominal CT has become the main diagnostic imaging study with an accuracy of greater than 94%.[14,15] Typical findings of acute appendicitis on CT imaging include the presence of a dilated appendix greater than 6 mm, periappendiceal fat stranding, phlegmon, or abscess in the area (Fig. 164.1). Inflammatory changes of the cecum or terminal ileum with a normal-appearing appendix is insufficient for diagnosis and should prompt evaluation for additional pathology, such as inflammatory or infectious bowel disease.

US has a reported diagnostic accuracy of greater than 90%.[16] The size criteria for diagnosing appendicitis with US is a size cutoff of greater than or equal to 6 mm appendiceal diameter; 7 mm is used in some centers to increase specificity because 23% of normal appendices can have a diameter of 6 mm or greater.[17] A noncompressible lumen, increased vascularity, and increased wall thickness to greater than 2 mm are also used as diagnostic criteria for appendicitis.[16,18,19] Inability to visualize the appendix has been noted to have as high as 90% negative predictive value.[20] US has found increased utility in the pediatric population and in most children's hospitals is now the most commonly used imaging modality.[21] Accuracy is operator and patient-variability dependent.

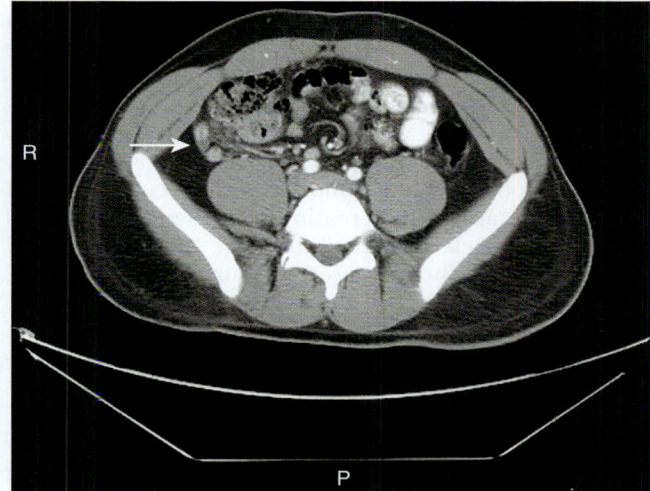

FIGURE 164.1 Computed tomography demonstrating findings consistent with acute appendicitis (*white arrow*), including fat stranding of the appendiceal mesentery located between the cecum and the appendix, as well as an enhancing appendiceal wall consistent with hyperemia and enlarged appendiceal diameter of 8 mm.

Magnetic resonance imaging (MRI) as a diagnostic study is used primarily in pregnant women. The size criteria remain the same as with CT and US, with appendiceal diameter usually greater than 6 mm. There is typically high signal intensity fluid in the appendiceal lumen on T2-weighted imaging. Its accuracy is similar to that of CT, with sensitivity reported in between 90% and 100%, with specificity of 94% to 98%. Its ability to visualize a normal appendix is markedly improved compared with US at 87% versus 2%, which is useful in evaluating abdominal pain in the pregnant patient.[22]

SPECIAL POPULATIONS

INFANTS AND TODDLERS

As noted previously, the clinical history and examination can be the most important diagnostic tool for diagnosing appendicitis. In pediatric patients, particularly those of a preschool age range, the ability to provide an accurate history may be impaired, leading to delayed or incorrect diagnosis. Typical signs, such as anorexia, guarding, and focal right lower quadrant pain, are more often absent in this population than adults.[23] The most common presenting symptoms are diffuse abdominal pain, nausea, and vomiting, which are unfortunately quite nonspecific and can indicate a host of abdominal pathologies. Most patients will have had symptoms for 3 days by the time of evaluation, with children less than 4 years of age averaging 4 days of symptoms.[24] As a result, an increased number of pediatric patients present with perforated appendicitis, with 50% of patients under the age of 5 presenting with a perforated appendicitis. This rate goes up as patients become younger, with 66% perforated below age 3, and almost 100% of patients presenting with perforation in children younger than 1 year of age.[24,25]

OLDER ADULTS

Approximately 5% of appendicitis cases occur in patients age 70 and older.[3] Morbidity and mortality are increased in older patients with appendicitis compared with a younger population. This has been attributed both to the increased number of comorbidities in older patients, as well as delay in diagnosis. The delay in diagnosis can be due in part to milder signs at time of presentation but also due to a delay in presentation.[26] As a result, 25% to 44% of older patients will present with a perforated appendicitis.[27,28] Diagnostic delay has decreased with more liberal use of CT imaging and operative morbidity has decreased with wider use of laparoscopy.

PREGNANCY

The risk of appendicitis in pregnancy mirrors the risk of developing appendicitis of the patient's normal age range. However, the consequences of a delay or missed diagnosis are markedly higher due to the increased mortality to the fetus. Rates of fetal loss are as high as 8% in ruptured appendicitis, compared with 2% in uncomplicated appendicitis.[29] The risk of rupture is slightly higher in the pregnant population, owing to atypical presentation caused by displacement of the appendix by the enlarging uterus. In addition, diagnosis is often delayed when nonspecific symptoms, such as nausea, vomiting, and abdominal discomfort, are mistakenly attributed to the pregnancy. However, during the third trimester the enlarging uterus tends to displace the appendix laterally or cephalad, leading to atypical pain location and lack of focal peritonitis in some cases. As noted, the typical diagnostic imaging of CT is often avoided to reduce the risk of ionizing radiation. MRI and US are the preferred modalities for diagnosis; although, given the high rate of prematurity or fetal loss, the use of CT when MRI is not available may be justified, especially after the first trimester.

DIAGNOSTIC ALGORITHMS

In 1986 the first algorithm was developed as a scoring system (Alvarado score), which used eight factors: focal right lower quadrant (RLQ) tenderness, leukocytosis, migratory pain, left shift, fever, anorexia, nausea/vomiting, and rebound tenderness.[30] More recently the appendicitis inflammatory response (AIR) score incorporates more factors, such as CRP and gradation of RLQ pain.[31] When compared head to head, the AIR score had a greater specificity, as well as positive predictive value, than the Alvarado score and performed better at discriminating patients with both high- and low-risk of appendicitis.[32,33] The utility of these scoring systems in reducing unnecessary imaging studies has been suggested, with avoidance of up to 33% of CT scans and 58% of USs.[34]

DIFFERENTIAL DIAGNOSIS

The diseases in children that are most frequently encountered on the differential for acute appendicitis include Meckel diverticulum, mesenteric lymphadenitis, intussusception, and acute gastroenteritis. In the adolescent age group, gynecologic issues begin to arise in young women, including endometriosis, ectopic pregnancy, pelvic inflammatory disease, mittelschmerz, and salpingitis. For older patients the risk of malignancy, diverticulitis, and inflammatory bowel disease can all masquerade as appendicitis as well.

TREATMENT

After a diagnosis of acute appendicitis has been made, the most commonly accepted course of treatment is appendectomy, although there is increasing research into nonoperative management. Preoperative preparation typically consists of intravenous (IV) fluid administration, pain medication, and antibiotic therapy with a broad-spectrum antibiotic, such as cefoxitin, ampicillin/sulbactam, or the combination of cefazolin and metronidazole. A single prophylactic dose is all that is necessary for uncomplicated appendicitis. In most cases, surgery can be safely delayed for up to 12 hours without any evidence of negative impact on patient outcomes.[35,36]

Laparoscopic appendectomy—One of the earliest general surgery operations to be undertaken laparoscopically, laparoscopic appendectomy is currently the most common method for performing appendectomy in the United States. It is associated with an overall decrease in complications compared with an open approach, particularly in obese patients.[37,38]

Our preferred technique begins with the placement of the camera port in a supraumbilical location. Port placement may be modified based on prior abdominal surgery or other complicating factors, such as pregnancy. A Hasson technique works well in thin patients, and a Veress needle technique is beneficial in morbidly obese patients. The suprapubic and left lower quadrant are typical locations for working ports. A right upper quadrant 5-mm port is also helpful for retraction. Care must be taken to avoid the bladder with placement of the suprapubic port. The patient is then placed in the Trendelenburg position, with the table tilted to the left, to help to clear omentum and small bowel from the right lower quadrant. The patient must be adequately secured to the table with a deflatable bean bag, a foam pad, or straps to prevent shifting during the case. The typical finding is an inflamed, engorged appendix. After being identified, the appendix is traced back to its base at the cecum. If the appendix is not acutely inflamed at this site, a window can be dissected in the base of the mesoappendix. The mesoappendix can then be divided using either a laparoscopic stapler, harmonic scalpel or other sealing device, or clips. The appendix is transected at its base with an Endo GIA stapler and then placed into a retrievable bag and removed from the abdominal cavity. We then inspect the staple lines for hemostasis and aspirate any spilled blood or fluid free from the pelvis and operative site. Thorough cleansing of the pelvis and abdominal gutters of any fluid will decrease the incidence of postoperative abscess. Irrigation does not necessarily decrease the rate of postoperative abscess.[39–41] Laparoscopic appendectomy was associated with a higher rate of postoperative intraabdominal abscess compared with an open approach in the early randomized controlled trials. The *overall* rate of surgical site infection remained lower with the laparoscopic approach.[42] This may have resulted from inexperience and inadequate cleansing of the pelvis and abdomen. More recent retrospective studies demonstrate equivalent rates of intraabdominal abscess formation after laparoscopic and open appendectomies.[43,44]

Open appendectomy—There are several approaches to incision orientation and location for an appendectomy. The Rockey-Davis incision (transverse) and McBurney incision (oblique following skin lines) are the two most common incision types. The length of the incision is dependent in part on the patient's body habitus. In thin patients and children a smaller incision is often sufficient, whereas in obese patients the incision may have to be up to 10 cm in length. The incision should typically be centered over the location of the most intense pain identified during physical exam. When dividing the external and internal oblique aponeuroses, it can be beneficial to place clamps on the fascial edges to aid in identification and closure of these layers at the end of the case (Fig. 164.2).

After the peritoneum is opened, the appendix can be identified by first locating the ascending colon or cecum. After the anterior taenia is located on these structures, it can be followed to the base of the appendix. Loose adhesions between the inflamed appendix and the surrounding ileum or abdominal wall can be broken up with gentle blunt dissection. In the case of a retrocecal appendix, the lateral peritoneal reflection may need to be incised to mobilize the appendix sufficiently into the operative field. When doing this, it is important to protect the right ureter because it often runs in close proximity to the retrocecal appendix.

After the appendix has been sufficiently mobilized into the operative field, the next step is to divide the mesoappendix and appendiceal artery. This can be accomplished by dividing the mesoappendix immediately adjacent to the appendiceal base between clamps or by sequentially clamping, dividing, and ligating the mesoappendix in parallel to the appendix until the base is reached. After being free of its mesentery, a hemostat or Kocher clamp is placed across the base of the appendix, crushing the tissue and ensuring there is no fecalith at that location. The clamp is then moved just distal, and an absorbable suture is tied around the crushed base (2-0 Vicryl or 2-0 polydiaxanone suture). The appendix is transected just proximal to the clamp. This is typically sufficient for closure of the appendiceal base; however, some surgeons continue to invert the base of the appendix using a Z-stitch or purse-string suture.

Nonoperative management—There is a growing body of evidence regarding the safety and efficacy of nonoperative management, stemming from early reports of nonoperative management in patients aboard submarines.[45,46] The first randomized studies were reported in the 1990s and demonstrated successful early therapy but a high rate of recurrence and need for surgery within the next year.[47] Subsequent randomized studies confirmed the safety of initial antibiotic therapy with successful nonoperative management in 89% to 91% of patients within the first 30 days. However, in the following year, there was a relatively high recurrence rate requiring appendectomy at 1 year, between 14% and 36%.[48–52] Table 164.1 outlines the specific details of the randomized trials. Currently, surgery remains the gold standard for treating patients presenting with appendicitis. Attempts at nonoperative management should be undertaken only for patient contraindications to surgery or as part of a clinical trial.

Gangrenous or perforated appendicitis—Cross-sectional imaging will demonstrate evidence of an abscess, phlegmon, or free perforation in the setting of complicated appendicitis. The presence of complicated appendicitis is often suspected based on an evidence of sepsis at presentation. Given the heterogeneity of presentation for these patients, clear-cut recommendations cannot be made regarding conservative versus operative management. In general, patients presenting with diffuse peritonitis, overt sepsis, or specific populations, such as pregnant patients or immunosuppressed patients, should undergo urgent operative exploration and appendectomy. Antibiotic treatment should cover gram-negative rods and anaerobic organisms. The Study To Optimize Peritoneal Infection Therapy (STOP-IT) trial in patients with complicated intraabdominal infection after adequate source control, randomized patients to a fixed course of antibiotics (4 days) versus antibiotics until 2 days after resolution of clinical signs of infection (up to a maximum of 10 days).[53] There was no difference in the two groups in terms of intraabdominal infection, indicating earlier stoppage of antibiotics is appropriate.

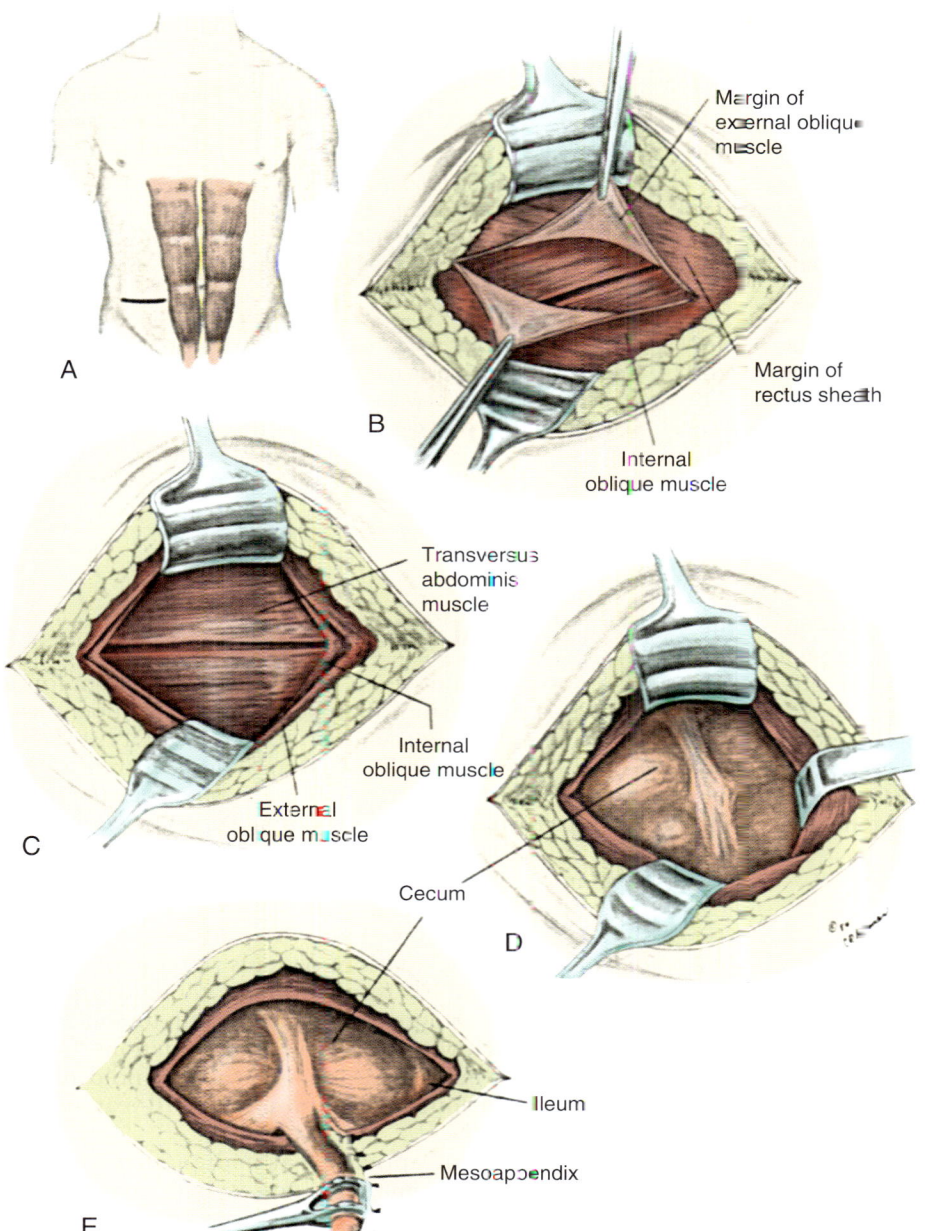

FIGURE 164.2 Steps in exposing the appendix for an appendectomy through a transverse incision. (A) Placement of the skin incision. (B and C) External and internal oblique and transversus abdominis muscles are divided in the direction of their fibers. (D) After incision of the peritoneum, the cecum is exposed and the appendix is located by following the anterior cecal taeria inferiorly. (E) The cecum is mobilized into the wound through incision of its lateral peritoneal reflections. (From Moody FG, Carey L, Jones RS, et al. *Surgical Treatment of Digestive Diseases.* Chicago: Year Book; 1986.)

Patients presenting with a phlegmon, well-contained abscess, or localized peritonitis can safely undergo operative intervention, although it should be cautioned that they are at higher risk for complication or iatrogenic injury to surrounding structures, such as bowel or ureter, and are at higher risk for postoperative complications, such as abscess or wound infection.[54] These patients are also more likely to require conversion to an open approach, an ileocolic resection, and in the most extreme cases, a stoma. Nonoperative management is generally most successful in patients with a drainable fluid collection in the absence of a fecalith. Nonoperative management in these patients consists of IV antibiotics and percutaneous drainage of any abscess present. The success rate of nonoperative therapy in these patients approaches 75%.[31,55,56] Such factors as smoking, generalized abdominal tenderness, tachycardia, small undrainable (<5 cm) abscess size, appendicolith, and small bowel obstruction have been noted to be predictive of failure of nonoperative management.[5,57,58]

Operative approach should be tailored to the patient's presentation and the surgeon's preference. A lower midline incision may be preferred in patients presenting with a diffuse peritonitis to gain access to the rest of the abdomen if necessary. Laparoscopy can also be used, and is our method of choice, with conversion to an open operation

TABLE 164.1 Randomized Controlled Trials Comparing Antibiotics to Appendectomy for the Management of Acute Appendicitis

Study	Inclusion Criteria	No. of Patients	Antibiotic Used	Failed Antibiotic Therapy (%; Includes Immediate Failures and Within 1 Yr)
Eriksson et al.[47] (Sweden)	• >18 y • Clinical diagnosis	Surgery: 20 Antibiotic: 20	IV: cefotaxime and tinidazole Oral: ciproflaxacin plus metronidazole	8/20 (40)
Styrud et al.[52] (Sweden)	• 18–50 y • Clinical diagnosis and CRP > 10 mg/L • Women excluded	Surgery: 124 Antibiotic: 128	IV: cefotaxime plus metronidazole Oral: ciprofloxacin plus metronidazole	31/128 (24)
Hansson et al.[49] (Sweden)	• >18 • Clinical diagnosis	Surgery: 167 Antibiotic: 202	IV: cefotaxime plus metronidazole Oral: ciprofloxacin plus metronidazole	111/202 (55)
Vons et al.[51] (France)	• >18 y • CT imaging • Included pts with fecalith	Surgery: 119 Antibiotic: 120	IV: amoxicillin plus clavulanic acid Oral: amoxicillin plus clavulanic acid	44/120 (37)
Salminen et al.[50] (Finland)	• 18–60 y • CT imaging uncomplicated	Surgery: 273 Antibiotic: 257	IV: ertapenem Oral: levofloxacin	70/257 (27)

CRP, C-reactive protein; *CT*, computed tomography; *IV*, intravenous.

if needed. The surrounding inflammation will make the dissection more difficult in the setting of perforated appendicitis. Gentle blunt dissection is often effective at releasing the appendix from the surrounding structures and the retroperitoneum. If this is not easily accomplished, it can be helpful to mobilize the right colon in an area, where there may be less inflammation. Occasionally the drainage of abscesses, irrigation, and placement of drains is all that can be safely achieved.

INTERVAL APPENDECTOMY

Historically, interval appendectomy was recommended after nonoperative management, due to concern for recurrent appendicitis. More recent data demonstrate that it is safe to defer appendectomy altogether. Only 5% of patients with recurrence required surgical intervention in a longitudinal population-based study.[59] Children have a low risk of recurrent appendicitis.[60]

The risk to foregoing appendectomy includes the failure to identify an underlying neoplasm. Malignancy has been reported in 4% to 29% of adult patients presenting with complicated appendicitis in which appendectomy is delayed in the acute setting.[61–63] Patients' age 40 and older managed nonoperatively with complicated appendicitis should undergo colonoscopic evaluation, followed by an interval appendectomy to evaluate for a possible underlying malignancy.

Negative appendectomy rates of 20% were accepted as necessary in the past to avoid perforated appendicitis.[64] Cross-sectional imaging has reduced the negative appendectomy rates to 1.7% to 7%.[65–68] If a normal appendix is found during exploration, the abdomen and pelvis should be carefully evaluated for the source of pain, including ovarian cysts, colonic diverticulitis, tuboovarian abscess, mesenteric adenitis, Meckel diverticulum, and malignancy.[68,69] It is reasonable to remove a normal appendix in a patient with chronic abdominal pain to reduce the risk of diagnostic confusion in the future.

APPENDICEAL NEOPLASMS

The most common type of appendiceal neoplasm found incidentally at the time of appendectomy for appendicitis is a carcinoid or neuroendocrine tumor (NET) (0.3%).[70] NETs account for 88% of all appendiceal tumors and are the most frequent site of gastrointestinal (GI) tract carcinoid tumors (38%), compared with small bowel (29%) and colon (13%).[71] Appendiceal carcinoid tumors smaller than 2 cm, not involving the mesoappendix, and remote from the base have been historically treated with simple appendectomy alone.[70] Reports of a higher rate of lymph node metastasis in patients with tumors greater than 1 cm in size has resulted in recommendation for a right hemicolectomy in young patients with tumors greater than 1 cm.[72] However, these recommendations are soft because even malignant appendiceal carcinoid tumors have excellent long-term survival, with 10-year survival approaching 90%.[73]

Other types of appendiceal malignancies include mucinous cystadenoma, mucinous cystadenocarcinoma, goblet cell carcinoid, and colonic-type adenocarcinoma. Mucinous cystadenoma and cystadenocarcinoma are typically indistinguishable prior to resection when confined to the appendix and should be resected without rupturing the appendix to reduce the risk of peritoneal seeding and development of pseudomyxoma peritonei. When suspected preoperatively or encountered intraoperatively, many surgeons will convert from a laparoscopic to open approach to avoid potential rupture; a right hemicolectomy is advised if it is suspected preoperatively or identified intraoperatively. Goblet cell carcinoid and colonic-type adenocarcinoma are more aggressive tumor types and should be treated in a similar fashion as a colon cancer, including the right colon resection and adjuvant chemotherapy.[74]

ACKNOWLEDGMENTS

We thank Matthew I. Goldblatt, Gordon L. Telford, and James R. Wallace for their previous work on this chapter.

REFERENCES

1. Lewis FR, Holcroft JW, Boey J, Dunphy E. Appendicitis. A critical review of diagnosis and treatment in 1,000 cases. *Arch Surg.* 1975;110(5):677-684.

2. Williams GR. Presidential address: a history of appendicitis. With anecdotes illustrating its importance. *Ann Surg.* 1983;197(5):495-506.

3. Buckius MT, McGrath B, Monk J, Grim R, Bell T, Ahuja V. Changing epidemiology of acute appendicitis in the United States: study period 1993–2008. *J Surg Res.* 2012;175(2):185-190.

4. Andreou P, Blain S, Du Boulay CE. A histopathological study of the appendix at autopsy and after surgical resection. *Histopathology.* 1990;17(5):427-431.

5. Chang FC, Hogle HH, Welling DR. The fate of the negative appendix. *Am J Surg.* 1973;126(6):752-754.

6. Arnbjornsson E, Bengmark S. Role of obstruction in the pathogenesis of acute appendicitis. *Am J Surg.* 1984;147(3):390-392.

7. Bhangu A, Soreide K, Di Saverio S, Assarsson JH, Drake FT. Acute appendicitis: modern understanding of pathogenesis, diagnosis, and management. *Lancet.* 2015;386(10000):1278-1287.

8. Ergul E. Heredity and familial tendency of acute appendicitis. *Scand J Surg.* 2007;96(4):290-292.

9. Hubbell DS, Barton WK. Leukocytosis in appendicitis in older persons. *J Am Med Assoc.* 1961;175:139-141.

10. Hyman P, Westring DW. Leukocytosis in acute appendicitis. Observed racial difference. *J Am Med Assoc.* 1974;229(12):1630-1631.

11. Yang HR, Wang YC, Chung PK, Chen WK, Jeng LB, Chen RJ. Laboratory tests in patients with acute appendicitis. *ANZ J Surg.* 2006;76(1-2):71-74.

12. Terasawa T, Blackmore CC, Bent S, Kohlwes RJ. Systematic review: computed tomography and ultrasonography to detect acute appendicitis in adults and adolescents. *Ann Intern Med.* 2004;141(7):537-546.

13. Pieper R, Kager L, Nasman P. Acute appendicitis: a clinical study of 1018 cases of emergency appendectomy. *Acta Chir Scand.* 1982;148(1):51-62.

14. Fuchs JR, Schlamberg JS, Shortsleeve MJ, Schuler JG. Impact of abdominal CT imaging on the management of appendicitis: an update. *J Surg Res.* 2002;106(1):131-136.

15. Holloway JA, Westerbuhr LM, Chain J, et al. Is appendiceal computed tomography in a community hospital useful? *Am J Surg.* 2003;186(6):682-684; discussion 684.

16. Yacoe ME, Jeffrey RB Jr. Sonography of appendicitis and diverticulitis. *Radiol Clin North Am.* 1994;32(5):899-912.

17. Rettenbacher T, Hollerweger A, Macheiner P, et al. Outer diameter of the vermiform appendix as a sign of acute appendicitis: evaluation at US. *Radiology.* 2001;218(3):757-762.

18. Brown MA. Imaging acute appendicitis. *Semin Ultrasound CT MR.* 2008;29(5):293-307.

19. Rybkin AV, Thoeni RF. Current concepts in imaging of appendicitis. *Radiol Clin North Am.* 2007;45(3):411-422, vii.

20. Kessler N, Cyteval C, Gallix B, et al. Appendicitis: evaluation of sensitivity, specificity, and predictive values of US, Doppler US, and laboratory findings. *Radiology.* 2004;230(2):472-478.

21. Saito JM, Yan Y, Evashwick TW, Warner BW, Tarr PI. Use and accuracy of diagnostic imaging by hospital type in pediatric appendicitis. *Pediatrics.* 2013;131(1):e37-e44.

22. Pedrosa I, Lafornara M, Pandharipande PV, Goldsmith JD, Rofsky NM. Pregnant patients suspected of having acute appendicitis: effect of MR imaging on negative laparotomy rate and appendiceal perforation rate. *Radiology.* 2009;250(3):749-757.

23. Becker T, Kharbanda A, Bachur R. Atypical clinical features of pediatric appendicitis. *Acad Emerg Med.* 2007;14(2):124-129.

24. Sakellaris G, Tilemis S, Charissis G. Acute appendicitis in preschool-age children. *Eur J Pediatr.* 2005;164(2):80-83.

25. Stone HH, Sanders SL, Martin JD Jr. Perforated appendicitis in children. *Surgery.* 1971;69(5):673-679.

26. Owens BJ, Hamit HF. Appendicitis in the elderly. *Ann Surg.* 1978;187(4):392-396.

27. Korner H, Sondenaa K, Soreide JA, et al. Incidence of acute nonperforated and perforated appendicitis: age-specific and sex-specific analysis. *World J Surg.* 1997;21(3):313-317.

28. Paranjape C, Dalia S, Pan J, Horattas M. Appendicitis in the elderly: a change in the laparoscopic era. *Surg Endosc.* 2007;21(5):777-781.

29. Gilo NB, Amini D, Landy HJ. Appendicitis and cholecystitis in pregnancy. *Clin Obstet Gynecol.* 2009;52(4):586-596.

30. Alvarado A. A practical score for the early diagnosis of acute appendicitis. *Ann Emerg Med.* 1986;15(5):557-564.

31. Andersson M, Andersson RE. The appendicitis inflammatory response score: a tool for the diagnosis of acute appendicitis that outperforms the Alvarado score. *World J Surg.* 2008;32(8):1843-1849.

32. de Castro SM, Unlu C, Steller EP, van Wagensveld BA, Vrouenraets BC. Evaluation of the appendicitis inflammatory response score for patients with acute appendicitis. *World J Surg.* 2012;36(7):1540-1545.

33. Kollar D, McCartan DP, Bourke M, Cross KS, Dowdall J. Predicting acute appendicitis? A comparison of the Alvarado score, the Appendicitis Inflammatory Response Score and clinical assessment. *World J Surg.* 2015;39(1):104-109.

34. Scott AJ, Mason SE, Arunakirinatham M, Reissis Y, Kinross JM, Smith J. Risk stratification by the appendicitis inflammatory response score to guide decision-making in patients with suspected appendicitis. *Br J Surg.* 2015;102(5):563-572.

35. Sauvain MO, Slankamenac K, Muller MK, et al. Delaying surgery to perform CT scans for suspected appendicitis decreases the rate of negative appendectomies without increasing the rate of perforation nor postoperative complications. *Langenbecks Arch Surg.* 2016;401:643-649.

36. Sivit CJ, Newman KD, Boenning DA, et al. Appendicitis: usefulness of US in diagnosis in a pediatric population. *Radiology.* 1992;185(2):549-552.

37. Masoomi H, Nguyen NT, Dolich MO, Mills S, Carmichael JC, Stamos MJ. Laparoscopic appendectomy trends and outcomes in the United States: data from the Nationwide Inpatient Sample (NIS), 2004–2011. *Am Surg.* 2014;80(10):1074-1077.

38. Dasari BV, Baker J, Markar S, Gardiner K. Laparoscopic appendectomy in obese is associated with improvements in clinical outcome: systematic review. *Int J Surg.* 2015;13:250-256.

39. Cho J, Park I, Lee D, Sung K, Baek J, Lee J. Risk factors for postoperative intra-abdominal abscess after laparoscopic appendectomy: analysis for consecutive 1,817 experiences. *Dig Surg.* 2015;32(5):375-381.

40. St Peter SD, Adibe OO, Iqbal CW, et al. Irrigation versus suction alone during laparoscopic appendectomy for perforated appendicitis: a prospective randomized trial. *Ann Surg.* 2012;256(4):581-585.

41. Snow HA, Choi JM, Cheng MW, Chan ST. Irrigation versus suction alone during laparoscopic appendectomy; a randomized controlled equivalence trial. *Int J Surg.* 2016;28:91-96.

42. Laschinski T, Mosch C, Eikermann M, Neugebauer EA. Laparoscopic versus open appendectomy in patients with suspected appendicitis: a systematic review of meta-analyses of randomised controlled trials. *BMC Gastroenterol.* 2015;15:48.

43. Asarias JR, Schlussel AT, Cafasso DE, et al. Incidence of postoperative intraabdominal abscesses in open versus laparoscopic appendectomies. *Surg Endosc.* 2011;25(8):2678-2683.

44. Nataraja RM, Teague WJ, Galea J, et al. Comparison of intraabdominal abscess formation after laparoscopic and open appendicectomies in children. *J Pediatr Surg.* 2012;47(2):317-321.

45. Adams ML. The medical management of acute appendicitis in a nonsurgical environment: a retrospective case review. *Mil Med.* 1990;155(8):345-3–7.

46. Gurin NN, Slobodchuk Iu S, Gavrilov Iu F. The efficacy of the conservative treatment of patients with acute appendicitis on board ships at sea. *Vestn Khir Im I I Grek.* 1992;148(5):144-150.

47. Eriksson S, Granstrom L. Randomized controlled trial of appendicectomy versus antibiotic therapy for acute appendicitis. *Br J Surg.* 1995;82(2):166-169.

48. Di Saverio S, Sibilio A, Giorgini E, et al. The NOTA Study (Non Operative Treatment for Acute Appendicitis): prospective study on the efficacy and safety of antibiotics (amoxicillin and clavulanic acid) for treating patients with right lower quadrant abdominal pain and long-term follow-up of conservatively treated suspected appendicitis. *Ann Surg.* 2014;260(1):109-117.

49. Hansson J, Korner U, Khorram-Manesh A, Solberg A, Lundholm K. Randomized clinical trial of antibiotic therapy versus appendicectomy as primary treatment of acute appendicitis in unselected patients. *Br J Surg.* 2009;96(5):473-481.

50. Salminen P, Paajanen H, Rautio T, et al. Antibiotic therapy vs appendectomy for treatment of uncomplicated acute appendicitis: the APPAC randomized clinical trial. *J Am Med Assoc.* 2015;313(23):2340-2348.

51. Vons C, Barry C, Maitre S, et al. Amoxicillin plus clavulanic acid versus appendicectomy for treatment of acute uncomplicated

appendicitis: an open-label, non-inferiority, randomised controlled trial. *Lancet.* 2011;377(9777):1573-1579.

52. Styrud J, Eriksson S, Nilsson I, et al. Appendectomy versus antibiotic treatment in acute appendicitis. A prospective multicenter randomized controlled trial. *World J Surg.* 2006;30(6):1033-1037.

53. Sawyer RG, Claridge JA, Nathens AB, et al. Trial of short-course antimicrobial therapy for intraabdominal infection. *N Engl J Med.* 2015;372(21):1996-2005.

54. Blakely ML, Williams R, Dassinger MS, et al. Early vs interval appendectomy for children with perforated appendicitis. *Arch Surg.* 2011;146(6):660-665.

55. Maxfield MW, Schuster KM, Bokhari J, McGillicuddy EA, Davis KA. Predictive factors for failure of nonoperative management in perforated appendicitis. *J Trauma Acute Care Surg.* 2014;76(4):976-981.

56. Vargas HI, Averbook A, Stamos MJ. Appendiceal mass: conservative therapy followed by interval laparoscopic appendectomy. *Am Surg.* 1994;60(10):753-758.

57. Shindoh J, Niwa H, Kawai K, et al. Predictive factors for negative outcomes in initial non-operative management of suspected appendicitis. *J Gastrointest Surg.* 2010;14(2):309-314.

58. Talishinskiy T, Limberg J, Ginsburg H, Kuenzler K, Fisher J, Tomita S. Factors associated with failure of nonoperative treatment of complicated appendicitis in children. *J Pediatr Surg.* 2016;51(7):1174-1176.

59. Kaminski A, Liu IL, Applebaum H, Lee SL, Haigh PI. Routine interval appendectomy is not justified after initial nonoperative treatment of acute appendicitis. *Arch Surg.* 2005;140(9):897-901.

60. Puapong D, Lee SL, Haigh PI, Kaminski A, Liu IL, Applebaum H. Routine interval appendectomy in children is not indicated. *J Pediatr Surg.* 2007;42(9):1500-1503.

61. Carpenter SG, Chapital AB, Merritt MV, Johnson DJ. Increased risk of neoplasm in appendicitis treated with interval appendectomy: single-institution experience and literature review. *Am Surg.* 2012;78(3):339-343.

62. Furman MJ, Cahan M, Cohen P, Lambert LA. Increased risk of mucinous neoplasm of the appendix in adults undergoing interval appendectomy. *JAMA Surg.* 2013;148(8):703-706.

63. Lugo JZ, Avgerinos DV, Lefkowitz AJ, et al. Can interval appendectomy be justified following conservative treatment of perforated acute appendicitis? *J Surg Res.* 2010;164(1):91-94.

64. Cantrell JR, Stafford ES. The diminishing mortality from appendicitis. *Ann Surg.* 1955;141(6):749-758.

65. Drake FT, Florence MG, Johnson MG, et al. Progress in the diagnosis of appendicitis: a report from Washington State's Surgical Care and Outcomes Assessment Program. *Ann Surg.* 2012;256(4):586-594.

66. Raja AS, Wright C, Sodickson AD, et al. Negative appendectomy rate in the era of CT: an 18-year perspective. *Radiology.* 2010;256(2):460-465.

67. Rao PM, Rhea JT, Rattner DW, Venus LG, Novelline RA. Introduction of appendiceal CT: impact on negative appendectomy and appendiceal perforation rates. *Ann Surg.* 1999;229(3):344-349.

68. Soyer P, Dohan A, Eveno C, et al. Pitfalls and mimickers at 64-section helical CT that cause negative appendectomy: an analysis from 1057 appendectomies. *Clin Imaging.* 2013;37(5):895-901.

69. Seetahal SA, Bolorunduro OB, Sookdeo TC, et al. Negative appendectomy: a 10-year review of a nationally representative sample. *Am J Surg.* 2011;201(4):433-437.

70. Moertel CG, Weiland LH, Nagorney DM, Dockerty MB. Carcinoid tumor of the appendix: treatment and prognosis. *N Engl J Med.* 1987;317(27):1699-1701.

71. Ellis L, Shale MJ, Coleman MP. Carcinoid tumors of the gastrointestinal tract: trends in incidence in England since 1971. *Am J Gastroenterol.* 2010;105(12):2563-2569.

72. Mullen JT, Savarese DM. Carcinoid tumors of the appendix: a population-based study. *J Surg Oncol.* 2011;104(1):41-44.

73. McCusker ME, Cote TR, Clegg LX, Sobin LH. Primary malignant neoplasms of the appendix: a population-based study from the Surveillance, Epidemiology and End Results program, 1973–1998. *Cancer.* 2002;94(12):3307-3312.

74. Rossi RE, Luong TV, Caplin ME, et al. Goblet cell appendiceal tumors—management dilemmas and long-term outcomes. *Surg Oncol.* 2015;24(1):47-53.

PART FOUR

Neoplastic Disease

Inherited Colorectal Cancer and the Genetics of Colorectal Cancer

Matthew F. Kalady | C. Richard Boland | James M. Church

Colorectal cancer (CRC) is a complex heterogeneous disease with a variety of factors influencing genetic and epigenetic changes that drive tumor initiation and progression. Alterations in the intricate system of biological checks and balances can lead to a malignant change of the normal colorectal mucosa. The underlying changes, whether inherited or sporadic, influence the genotype and phenotype of that particular cancer and patient. Understanding CRC in this context, and grouping patients based on the underlying cancer pathway, helps to study the disease and provide more precise clinical management. This chapter provides an overview of the underlying changes in colorectal carcinogenesis and the hereditary CRC syndromes.

GENETIC BASIS OF COLORECTAL CANCER

MULTISTEP CARCINOGENESIS IN COLORECTAL CANCER

Cancer is fundamentally a genetic disease as tumors develop through genetic or epigenetic *somatic* alterations in cells. A relatively small proportion of gastrointestinal (GI) cancer, probably less than 5%, develops as a consequence of a highly penetrant *germline mutation* in one gene, resulting in a familial GI polyposis or cancer syndrome. The tumors that develop in these syndromes then follow the same evolutionary paths as sporadic tumors, but the risk for cancer is greatly elevated in the mutation carrier, the tumors have a substantially earlier median age of onset, and the patients are at risk for multiple metachronous tumors. An understanding of the biological basis of sporadic CRCs has provided insight into the special instances of the familial syndromes, all of which are quite distinct genetically and clinically.

There are multiple signaling pathways that regulate cell growth. Consequently, there are multiple possible pathways for tumorigenesis, which explains why CRCs—and the cancer syndromes—are heterogeneous genetically and clinically.[1] However, there is a discrete number of parallel regulatory pathways, which crosstalk with one another, and the function of any pathway can be altered by a defect in any one of the serial links.

There are three classes of genes involved in the evolution of cancer: *proto-oncogenes*, which become activated through mutation, amplification, or chromosomal rearrangement; *tumor suppressor genes*, which become inactivated through mutation, chromosomal deletion, or promoter methylation; and genes involved in maintaining *genomic stability*, which become dysregulated—usually by inactivation—leading to genomic instability and the rapid accumulation of more mutations. Moreover, without some form of genomic instability, it would take a very long time to accumulate mutations in these specific genes that drive cancer development.

CLASSIC CHROMOSOMAL INSTABILITY

We can classify CRCs into three broad classes of genetic or epigenetic instability, but there is some overlap among them, which can be initially confusing. The first is manifested by chromosomal instability (CIN), and was first proposed in 1990 by Vogelstein in the context of multistep carcinogenesis.[2] The first step in the CIN pathway is inactivation of the WNT signaling pathway, followed, in sequence, by activating mutations in key growth-stimulating genes, such as *KRAS, CDC4, PIK3CA,* and others, followed by disruption of the negative growth regulatory network of transforming growth factor (TGF)-3 signaling (typically through inactivation of one or more of the SMAD genes), and the cataclysmic conversion of benign to malignant behavior by mutations and allelic losses of the *p53* (TP53) gene, which abrogates the G1/S cell cycle checkpoint and permits the accumulation of chromosomal rearrangement and aneuploidy.[3] This pathway is illustrated in Fig. 165.1. More than half of all CRCs develop through this pathway. There is considerable heterogeneity in the evolution of this pathway, and only three of these, *APC, KRAS* and *p53,* are mutated in greater than 11% of all CRCs.

The initial genetic alteration in the classic pathway is inactivation of the WNT signaling pathway, which is a key concept for understanding familial adenomatous polyposis (FAP). This usually occurs by biallelic inactivation of the *APC* gene, removing the protein that regulates the intracellular concentration of β-catenin, which is a transcription factor that helps turn on the growth program, and it is also involved in the intercellular adhesion complex that holds colonic epithelial cells together. However, the same

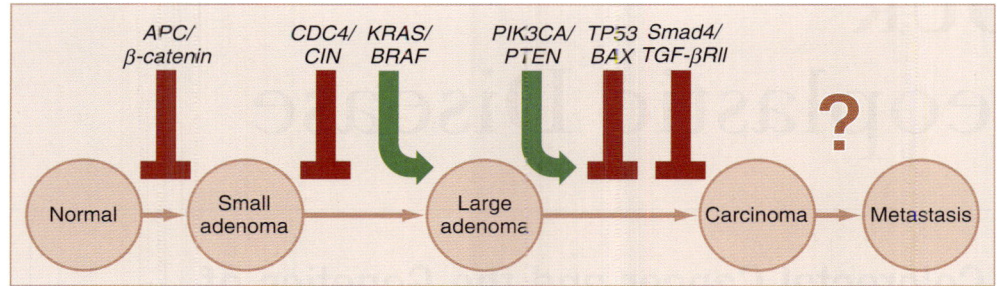

FIGURE 165.1 Classic chromosomal instability *(CIN)* and multistep carcinogenesis. The classic multistep carcinogenesis model proposed in 1990 has been repeatedly confirmed over the decades. The initial step is the disruption of WNT signaling, either by loss of adenomatous polyposis coli *(APC)* or a "downstream" event that achieves the same result. The adenoma can remain small indefinitely, but if it acquires additional mutations that activate proto-oncogenes, they become larger and more dysplastic. The loss of p53 is the most common event at the adenoma-to-carcinoma transition. Initially, colorectal cancers *(CRCs)* may have minimal ability to metastasize, but the accumulation of additional mutations or other alterations eventually permits tumor cells to escape the primary tumor mass and grow at a distant site. *TGF-β*, Transforming growth factor beta. (From Jones S, Chen WD, Parmigiani G, et al. Comparative lesion sequencing provides insights into tumor evolution. *Proc Natl Acad Sci U S A.* 2008;105:4283–4288.)

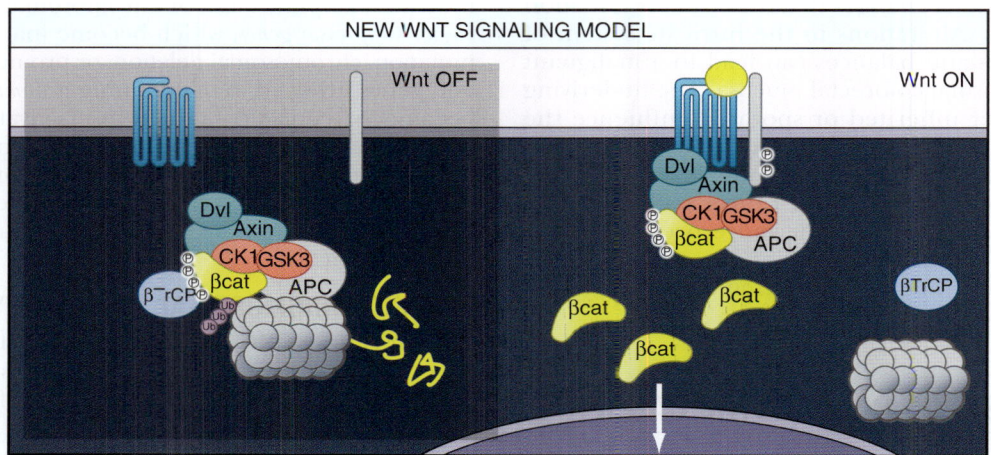

FIGURE 165.2 Wnt signaling. *On the left*, when there is no Wnt ligand interacting with the 7-transmembrane spanning receptor (unnamed here but termed "frizzled" in lower organisms), Wnt signaling is off, APC interacts with β-catenin leading to its phosphorylation and degradation, and the proliferative program is inactive. (*Wnt* derived its name from a conflation of the wingless gene in flies–wt—and the Int-1 proto-oncogene; there are 19 human Wnt genes.) *On the right*, the yellow Wnt ligand is secreted by an adjacent cell, binds to the receptor complex, which prevents APC from interacting with β-catenin, permitting its intracellular concentration to rise, triggering a growth program and inhibiting the differentiation program.[4] Dysregulation of Wnt signaling is seen in almost all colorectal neoplasms, and germline mutations in APC cause FAP. *β-cat*, β-catenin; *βTrCP*, β-transducin repeats-containing proteins (a ubiquitin ligase subunit involved in the degradation of β-catenin in the proteasome); *APC*, adenomatous polyposis coli gene; *Axin*, part of the APC-containing complex; *CK1*, casein kinase-1 (together with GSK3, phosphorylates β-cat at multiple sites, which leads to its destruction); *Dvl*, disheveled; *GSK3*, glycogen synthase kinase-3. (From Clevers H, Nusse R. Wnt/beta-catenin signaling and disease. *Cell.* 2012;149:1192–1205.)

effect can be achieved through a stabilizing mutation in the β-catenin gene that renders the protein incapable of being degraded by the adenomatous polyposis coli (APC) protein. Indeed, additional downstream events involving T-cell factor/lymphoid enhancer-binding factor (TCF or LEF) proteins can do this as well.[4] The WNT signaling pathway is depicted in Fig. 165.2.

Once WNT signaling is dysregulated, the colonic epithelial cell can undergo uncontrolled divisions and fails to differentiate. The colorectal adenoma is a collection of epithelial cells that continue to grow outside of the colonic crypt, do not fully differentiate, and form a mass

lesion. The actual "drivers" of the process are the β-catenin gene (now upregulated), and eventually, other activated oncogenes. CIN begins in benign adenomas, which can remain stable for decades, or grow slowly. But once the *p53* gene is lost (typically by one inactivating mutation and loss of the other allele), there is an increase in the accumulation of abnormal chromosomal rearrangements, which results in large numbers of deleted, duplicated, and rearranged genes. These changes synergize to drive the neoplastic process forward. Because of the very large number of specific genetic alterations that can contribute to the process, CRCs that evolve through the classic pathway can be quite heterogeneous in appearance and clinical behavior.

Most families with FAP have a germline mutation in the *APC* gene. Occasional families with FAP have no detectable mutation in *APC*, however, there are no convincing examples of germline mutations in any other gene that cause typical FAP. Even a mutation that results in the deletion of a long-range promoter sequence in *APC* (literally over 46,000 bases upstream of the start codon) can cause full-blown FAP.

Since biallelic mutations in APC are required for neoplastic colonic epithelial cell growth to occur, the phenotype in a person with a germline mutation in *APC* is normal at birth, but over time, losses of the other "wild type" allele occurs in individual epithelial cells, which results in adenomas. Over time, unregulated growth predisposes the adenoma to the accumulation of more mutations in the multistep pathway. Illustrating the long time frame in which this occurs, the median age for the first adenoma in FAP is 16, but the median age for cancer is 39. There are no instances of inheriting biallelic APC germline mutations as that phenotype is embryonically lethal.

CPG ISLAND METHYLATOR PHENOTYPE

The second CRC pathway involves the inactivation of tumor suppressor genes through hypermethylation of gene promoters, a normal physiologic process for silencing genes that becomes accelerated through a process that is not completely understood.[5] The sequences in the promoters that are hypermethylated are C-G dinucleotide pairs (called CpG sequences, in which the *p* stands for the phosphodiester bond between the C and G). These sequences are infrequent in the genome except in gene promoters (the on–off switch or rheostat for gene expression), and they occur in clusters called CpG islands. When there is an excess of promoter methylation in the cancer genome, this is the CpG island methylator phenotype, or *CIMP*. This occurs as a predominant epigenetic "lesion" in about 32% of CRCs, but increased CpG methylation is also seen in many other CRCs, so the methylation must be quantitated at selected promoters for the CRC to be categorized as CIMP. CIMP often (but not always) occurs in association with a mutation in the *BRAF* gene (V600E), and this is associated with more aggressive, lethal CRCs compared with tumors arising from the other pathways.

Tumors in the CIMP pathway are thought to begin as sessile serrated adenomas (SSAs) rather than as typical adenomatous polyps; consequently, this has been called the serrated carcinoma pathway. Both SSAs and CIMP CRCs occur predominantly in the proximal colon. The genetic or epigenetic events that drive the SSA from a benign, nonneoplastic-appearing lesion to CRC are not specifically known, although the genes that commonly undergo promoter methylation in CIMP include *p16*, *CDKN2A*, *THBS1*, *HPP1*, and *MLH1*. The underlying "instability" involves excessive promoter methylation, whereas it is the silencing of tumor suppressor genes that acts as the "driver" of carcinogenesis in CIMP-related tumors. Additionally, a number of microRNAs, which are key regulators of gene expression, are silenced by methylation in cancer, and are an increasingly important part of the driving force in

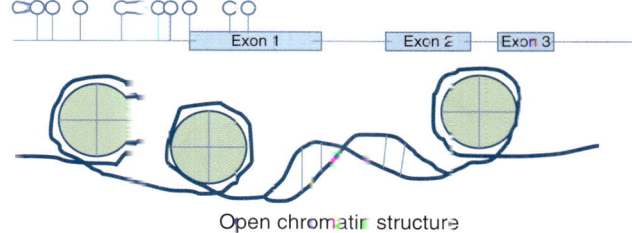

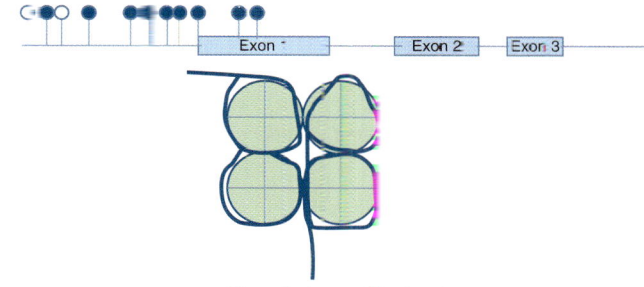

FIGURE 165.3 CIMP and methylation-induced silencing of genes. A gene is depicted as a line with three (*blue*) exons and multiple CpG sites indicated by circles on sticks; white circles are unmethylated cytosines and blue circles are methylated. The CpG sites are clustered just to the left of the start site of the gene and in the first exon. At the top, the unmethylated CpG sites leave the chromatin "open" and available to transcription factors for gene expression. After the methylation of the cytosines in a CIMP-CRC (*lower panel*), the closed chromatin structure silences gene expression. Only the CpG clusters in the promoter and first exon are important for gene silencing as shown here.[6] *β-cat*, β-catenin; *βTrCP*, β-transducin repeats-containing proteins; *APC*, adenomatous polyposis coli gene; *Axin*, part of the APC-containing complex; *CK1*, casein kinase-1; *Dvl*, disheveled; *GSK3*, glycogen synthase kinase-3. (Image source: Lao W, Grady WM. Epigenetics and colorectal cancer. *Nat Rev Gastroenterol Hepatol.* 2011;8:686–700.)

CIMP-mediated carcinogenesis. Fig. 165.3 illustrates the CIMP and methylation-mediated gene silencing.

MICROSATELLITE INSTABILITY

The third pathway for colorectal carcinogenesis is a *secondary consequence* of either CIN (in the setting of Lynch syndrome) or CIMP, and is called "*microsatellite instability*" or MSI. The nucleus has multiple enzyme systems that monitor DNA for damage, and either repair the mutation or prevent the cell from replicating. One of these is mainly an S-phase monitor for errors introduced by DNA polymerase (also playing a role outside of DNA synthesis), called the DNA mismatch repair (MMR) system. During DNA replication, DNA polymerases are prone to errors while copying the correct number of nucleotides at simple

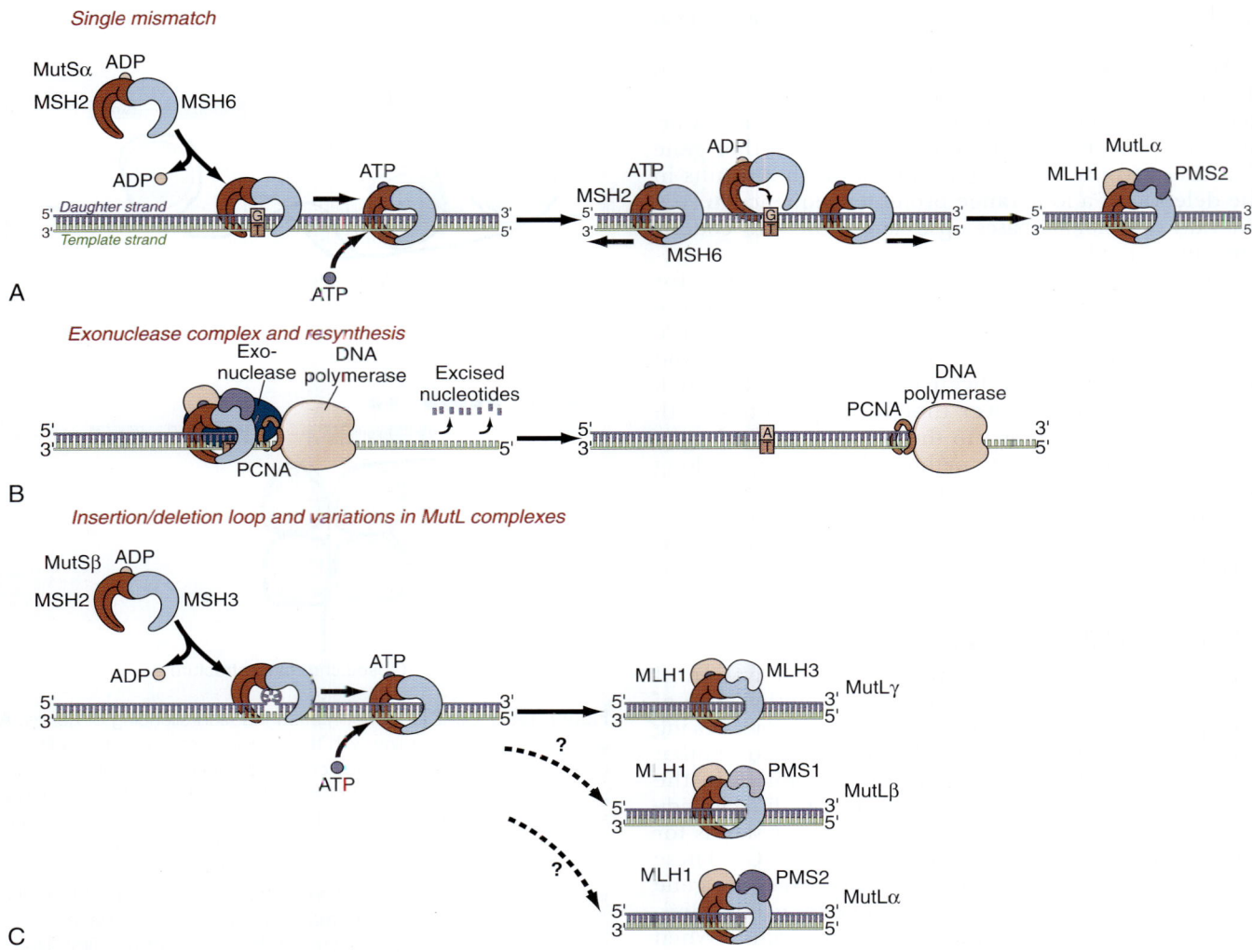

FIGURE 165.4 DNA mismatch repair (MMR). The DNA MMR system involves a series of cooperating enzymes. (A) The heterodimer of MSH2 and MSH6 proteins make up the MutSα mismatch recognition complex as shown. MutSα binds to DNA at random locations (with an exchange of ADP for ATP) and slides along the nascent DNA strand until it encounters a DNA mismatch, at which time the MutLα complex (made up of MLH1 and PMS2 proteins) is recruited. MutSα preferentially recognizes single base-pair mismatches and single base insertion-deletion lesions. (B) Exonuclease is recruited to the mismatch by MutSα and nucleotides are serially excised specifically from the daughter strand and the mismatch is excised. Then DNA polymerase resynthesizes the daughter strand. (C) The human MMR system broadens its specificity for mismatch recognition when MSH2 heterodimerizes with the MSH3 protein, forming MutSβ, which has additional specificity to recognize larger insertion-deletion loops containing 2 to 6 nucleotides. Also, MLH1 can heterodimerize with PMS1 (forming MutLβ) or MLH3 (forming MutLγ), but the precise roles of these complexes is incompletely understood. *ADP*, Adenosine diphosphate; *ATP*, adenosine triphosphate. (From Boland CR, Goel A. Microsatellite instability in colorectal cancer. *Gastroenterology*. 2010;138:2073–2087, e2073.)

repetitive sequences (mono-, di-, tri-, and tetra-nucleotide repeats) called microsatellites. The DNA MMR system identifies these small DNA copying errors and removes the faulty sequences, which permits the cell to resynthesize the sequence correctly. In the absence of DNA MMR activity, there is greater than 100-fold increase in synthetic errors in microsatellite sequences, which is where the term MSI was derived.[7] The DNA MMR system is shown in Fig. 165.4.

CRCs with MSI can occur in three circumstances. First, approximately 12% of all CRCs begin as CIMP tumors, but when methylation occurs at both alleles of one of the

DNA MMR genes (*MLH1*), MSI ensues and overwhelms the CIMP background, as the accumulation of mutations occurs rapidly. These tumors have a background of CIMP, but are recognized as MSI tumors because of this overwhelming phenotype, and often have an activating mutation in *BRAF*. If they do not have a mutation in *BRAF*, the prognosis is better than for CIN or pure CIMP CRCs.

Second, about 3% of CRCs occur in the setting of Lynch syndrome (previously referred to as hereditary nonpolyposis CRC [HNPCC]), of which most have MSI. There is evidence that neoplasms in Lynch syndrome arise initially as otherwise ordinary adenomatous polyps, and then develop MSI when there is loss of the wild-type allele of the DNA MMR gene responsible for the Lynch syndrome.[8] However, it is possible that some neoplasms may arise directly from a nonneoplastic colonic crypt with defective DNA MMR activity, which is present in large numbers in the nonneoplastic epithelium of the colon.[9] Once there is a DNA MMR-deficient cell, the progeny accumulate mutations at DNA sequences that encode mononucleotide repeat nucleotides (i.e., C_n, T_n, G_n, or A_n where $n = 6$ to 10). There are about 30 genes in the human genome that have microsatellites in coding sequences, and these include a number of critical tumor suppressor genes (such as TGF-β receptor 2, BAX, Caspase-5, and others) that are frequently mutated at the microsatellite by deletion or insertion of one base pair in the sequence, which inactivates the gene. As such, these microsatellite-encoding genes are the actual "drivers" of carcinogenesis once mutated.

Third, a very small proportion of CRCs begin in the CIN pathway, and develop biallelic mutations at one of the DNA MMR genes, after which MSI ensues, which rapidly overtakes the prior phenotype. This is called "Lynch-like syndrome."[6] Curiously, it can be familial, which is not understood.

MSI can occur in the context of CIMP, in which approximately 90% of the tumors are in the proximal colon, and the patients are on average about 5 years older than those with sporadic CRCs. It can also occur in the context of Lynch syndrome, in which case about two-thirds of the tumors are in the proximal colon and the patients are 15 to 20 years younger than others with CRC. It can also occur due to biallelic somatic mutations in DNA MMR genes, and will masquerade as Lynch syndrome.

WHY COLORECTAL CANCERS ARE SO HETEROGENEOUS

Because the "driver" mutations are different for each of these pathways, the clinical behavior of the tumors is different for each group. Importantly, however, the CIN or classic pathway is the sequence seen in the disease FAP, which is always associated with a germline mutation in the APC gene. The MSI pathway is present in essentially all CRCs that occur in Lynch syndrome, which is caused by germline mutations in one of the four DNA MMR genes (MLH1, MSH2, MSH6, and PMS2). However, most CRCs with MSI are not Lynch syndrome, but are a consequence of methylation-induced silencing of MLH1, or less commonly, Lynch-like syndrome. There has been no identifiable form of a familial CIMP syndrome.

The hamartomatous polyposis syndromes are quite distinct from either FAP or Lynch syndrome. In these instances, the germline mutations cause benign lesions to develop in the small and/or large intestine, usually in the context of a unique, identifiable phenotype. However, all of the hamartoma syndromes are associated with a variety of cancers in the gut and elsewhere because of the dysregulation of growth they cause. These are discussed later in this chapter.

INHERITED COLORECTAL CANCER SYNDROMES

POLYPOSIS SYNDROMES

There are several hereditary syndromes of CRC predisposition that are associated with a strong tendency toward multiple colorectal polyps. Polyposis simply means "lots of polyps," but in practical terms it is defined as more than 100 polyps at one examination. Fewer numbers of polyps, from 10 to 100, are often referred to as attenuated polyposis or "oligopolyposis." Polyposis syndromes also can be classified according to polyp histology (the phenotype) and according to the gene that is mutated in the patient's germline (genotype). The various syndromes, along with their clinical and genetic criteria, are listed in Table 165.1. Management of the polyposis syndromes involves diagnosis, evaluation, and management with the goals to (1) prevent death from cancer and (2) maintain adequate quality of life.

Familial Adenomatous Polyposis

Epidemiology and Genetics. FAP is rare, with an incidence of approximately 1 in 10,000 live births. Prevalence is estimated at 1 in 24,000 to 1 in 60,000[10] and depends on the average size of families in a country or region, and the completeness of registration of the disease. FAP affects all races and both genders equally. The expression of the disease may vary according to genotype and vary even within patients who share the same mutation, due to modifying factors, such as gender.[11] FAP is caused by a germline APC mutation, which results in a generalized growth disorder expressed as benign and malignant tumors in a variety of tissues.[12] Manifestations associated with the mutation are summarized in Table 165.2. The severity of the growth disorder and the risks and age at onset of cancer vary between and within families.

Diagnosis. Most patients with FAP are diagnosed based on family history. For a dominantly inherited syndrome with close to 100% penetrance, the family history of CRC and other manifestations of the APC mutation is compelling. Children of an affected parent usually undergo genetic testing at puberty and, if affected, start colonoscopy at that time.[13] Testing in infancy is generally discouraged because of the possible effect of a positive result on the parent's attitude to their affected children, but this fear may not be borne out in practice. However, the possibility of hepatoblastoma, a rare manifestation of the germline APC mutation, is a reason to perform genetic testing of newborns and then hepatoblastoma screening (6-monthly liver ultrasound and alpha fetoprotein) until the age of 7.

Approximately 25% of patients with FAP have no knowledge of a family history of the disease. Reasons for this include adoption, deliberate withholding of information by affected family members, nonpaternity, germline mosaicism, and a de novo mutation at conception. These patients are unaware of the risk posed by the unsuspected germline mutation and usually present with symptoms of their polyposis or cancer, such as rectal bleeding, abdominal pain, and diarrhea. They have a high chance of having CRC at diagnosis.[14]

TABLE 165.1 The Hereditary Colorectal Polyposes

Syndrome	Polyp Histology	Gene(s)	Number of Polyps for Diagnosis	Inheritance Pattern
Familial adenomatous polyposis	Adenoma	APC	Severe/profuse: >1000 Mild: 100–1000 Attenuated: <100	Dominant
MutYH-associated polyposis	Adenoma	MutYH	Any	Recessive
NTHL1-associated polyposis	Adenoma	NTHL1	Any	Recessive
Polymerase proofreading-associated polyposis	Adenoma	POLD, POLE	Any	Dominant
Lynch syndrome	Adenoma	MLH1, MSH2, MSH6, PMS2 EPCAM	>10	Dominant
Serrated polyposis	Serrated polyp	?	>20 of any size and location >5 proximal to the sigmoid, 2 >10-mm diameter	?
Hereditary mixed polyposis syndrome	Adenoma, serrated polyp, hamartoma	GREM1	>5, at least 1 juvenile polyp	Dominant (Ashkenazi Jews)
PTEN hamartoma tumor syndrome	Juvenile polyp, hamartoma, lipoma, fibroma, neurofibroma, serrated polyp	PTEN	—	Dominant
Juvenile polyposis	Juvenile polyp	SMAD4 BMPR1A	>5 >1 plus a family history of juvenile polyposis	Dominant
Peutz-Jeghers polyposis	Peutz-Jeghers polyp	STK11	>1 plus a family history of Peutz-Jegher polyposis	Dominant

TABLE 165.2 Manifestations of the Germline _APC_ Mutation in Patients With Familial Adenomatous Polyposis

Organ	Benign	Malignant
Colon and rectum	Adenoma	Carcinoma
Stomach	Adenoma Fundic gland polyp	Carcinoma
Small intestine	Adenoma	Carcinoma
Thyroid	—	Papillary carcinoma
Adrenal gland	Adenoma	Carcinoma
Bone	Osteoma	—
Skin	Epidermoid cyst	—
Teeth	Extra teeth	—
Fibroblasts	Desmoid disease	—
Brain	—	Medulloblastoma
Liver	—	Hepatoblastoma

Clinical diagnosis of FAP is usually made on colonoscopy followed by efforts to establish a genetic diagnosis so that the family can be triaged. The odds of identifying an _APC_ mutation are greater than 80% in patients with greater than 100 adenomas. If a germline _APC_ mutation is found, then all at-risk relatives can be offered screening. Other genetic mechanisms may cause FAP and include deletion of the _APC_ promoter 1B,[15] chromosomal loss (often associated with reduced mental capacity),[16] and _APC_ haploinsufficiency.[17] If genetic testing is negative, sometimes extracolonic manifestations can be used to predict an affected relative.

Initial Evaluation and Management. Care of patients with FAP and their families is best given by centers of experience and excellence.[18] Such centers are scattered around the world, and are often linked by organizations such as the Collaborative Group of the Americas for Inherited CRC (cgaicc.com) and the International Society for Gastrointestinal Hereditary Tumors (InSiGHT). Patients and their families who enroll in a registry benefit at least from enhanced survival due to organized surveillance.

CRC is the main risk in patients with FAP and is the most common cause of death.[19] In classic FAP (>100 synchronous adenomas), the average age at cancer diagnosis is 39 years, with much younger onset in patients with profuse polyposis. The most effective way of preventing cancer is to remove the colon, and thus thought should be given regarding the timing of prophylactic surgery once a diagnosis is established. Symptomatic patients should undergo colectomy using an oncologic technique as occult cancer risk is elevated in these patients. For patients who do not require a colectomy around the time of diagnosis, annual colonoscopy should be performed with removal of larger polyps and continued thoughtfulness of the timing of surgery.

Almost all patients with FAP develop fundic gland polyps in the stomach, and adenomas in the duodenum.[20] Duodenal cancers are the third most common cause of death in FAP (after CRC and desmoid disease) and upper GI surveillance begins at 20 to 25 years old. An esophagoduodenoscopy should be done with a side-viewing duodenoscope so that the duodenal ampulla can be examined.

Timing of Prophylactic Colectomy. CRC is rare in FAP patients younger than 20 years old.[21] For patients diagnosed in their teenage years, the timing of surgery depends primarily on the severity of the polyposis. Factors governing the timing of colectomy are shown in Table 165.3. While the top priority is to avoid cancer or to remove it as early as possible, lifestyle concerns are real and need to be considered. Many FAP patients are in their teen or twenties when faced with the prospect of surgery, and are often asymptomatic. They have academic, financial, social, and developmental concerns, and the idea of a stoma or the chance of a complication is scary. This is especially the case where other members of the family have had unfortunate outcomes. Therefore, appropriate surgery selection is key to decrease the cancer risk, maintain the quality of life, and minimize the complications. Note that increased risk of desmoid disease is listed as an indication to defer surgery as long as possible in Table 165.3. This is because approximately 10% of desmoid disease in FAP develops after abdominal surgery, presumably secondary to the intervention.[22]

Choice of Surgery. There are three main options for prophylactic surgery in patients with FAP: colectomy with ileorectal anastomosis (IRA), total proctocolectomy with ileal pouch–anal anastomosis (IPAA), and total procto-colectomy with end ileostomy (TPC-EI). These surgeries can be done by open or minimally invasive techniques, and the IPAA can be done with a stapled anastomosis or with a mucosectomy and handsewn anastomosis. Tables 165.4 and 165.5 show the factors that favor or disfavor the different surgeries. An oncologic technique with high ligation of the feeding vessels and removal of the mesentery and the omentum should always be used because unsuspected cancer may be found in the specimen.[23]

TABLE 165.3 Timing of Prophylactic Colectomy

Urgency	Timing	Indication
Immediate	Next available list	Cancer
		Symptoms
		Complications of colonoscopy
Soon	Within 3 months	Profuse polyposis (>1000 adenomas)
		Multiple large (>1 cm) adenomas
		High-grade dysplasia in an adenoma
Sometime	On a year-by-year basis	Mild polyposis (100–1000 adenomas)
		Asymptomatic
		Social, intellectual, academic, financial, family factors
Defer	Put off as long as possible	High risk of desmoid disease
		High comorbidity

TABLE 165.4 Analysis of the Advantages and Disadvantages Indications and Contraindications of the Three Main Colorectal Surgical Options of Patients With Familial Adenomatous Polyposis

	Advantages	Disadvantages	Indications	Contraindications
Ileorectal anastomosis	Quick, safe, uncomplicated Good quality of life Bowel function acceptable Controls colonic polyposis Avoids any ileostomy Surveillance easy	Risk of rectal cancer Surveillance required	<20 rectal adenomas <1000 colonic adenomas	Rectal cancer
Ileal pouch–anal anastomosis	Controls most colorectal polyposis Avoids permanent ileostomy Reasonable quality of life	High complications Bowel function unpredictable Ileostomy needed Risk of pouch polyposis Risk of ATZ cancer Quality of life unpredictable Surveillance can be difficult	>20 rectal adenomas Rectal cancer	High desmoid risk Lack of surgical expertise <20 rectal adenomas
Proctocolectomy and ileostomy	Least risk of complications Complete removal of cancer risk in lower GI tract	Permanent ileostomy	Low rectal cancer IPAA impossible Poor anal sphincter function	Good sphincters No rectal cancer
Minimally invasive	Less trauma, less pain, reduced length of stay, quicker recovery, minimal scars	Expertise required, slower, may cause issues with IPAA	Slim, young patients Expertise available	Severe desmoid risk IPAA
Open	Less operative time	More pain, longer recovery, scar	Best for IPAA patients with high desmoid risk	Patients where cosmesis is an issue, high morbidity

ATZ, Anal transition zone; *GI*, gastrointestinal tract; *IPAA*, ileal pouch–anal anastomosis.

TABLE 165.5 A Staging System for Intraabdominal Desmoid Disease

Stage	Size	Symptoms	Growth
I	<10 cm	None	None
II	<10 cm	Mild	<25% in 6 months
III	11–20 cm	Moderate	25% to 50% in 6 months
IV	>20 cm	Severe	>50% in 6 months

Note: Many patients have multiple desmoids. The worst stage is taken for treatment planning.

In practical terms, the decision for IRA or IPAA is driven by the severity of the polyposis: the more severe the polyposis the higher the risk of metachronous rectal polyposis and/or rectal cancer. Church et al. showed that when there were 5 or fewer rectal adenomas and 1000 or fewer colonic polyps, no patient needed a subsequent proctectomy. When there were 6 to 20 rectal adenomas, 15% of patients needed later proctectomy; however, with 20 or more rectal adenomas, the incidence of later proctectomy was more than 50%.[24] Recently this "rule" has been stretched in favor of a conservative approach.[25] Teenagers who might otherwise need proctectomy and a pouch have been treated with a laparoscopic IRA, for the benefits of a quicker, safe surgery, better bowel function, lower risk of desmoid disease, no stoma, and quicker recovery.[26] These are considerable benefits for young, active patients; however, annually, careful proctoscopy is needed to keep the rectal polyposis in check.

Colectomy and Ileorectal Anastomosis. The need for postoperative surveillance should be considered when planning the surgery. The ideal length of the rectum is 15 cm, which provides reasonable bowel function while still allowing easy endoscopic evaluation. With an IRA at 15 cm from the anal verge, patients on average have between 4 and 5 semiformed bowel movements without urgency or incontinence. A diverting stoma is not routine and recovery is quick, particularly after a laparoscopic approach. Preoperatively, all large rectal polyps must be removed to assure there is not cancer. Small (<5 mm) polyps may be left for future surveillance and removal as needed. Postoperatively, the rectal polyp burden may spontaneously reduce, likely because of the different types of stool the mucosa encounters.[27] The IRA itself can be tricky to construct because of the disparity in luminal diameter between the ileum and the rectum. A technical point to limit this disparity is to resect the terminal ileum flush with the ileocecal valve to preserve the "trumpet-like" flare of the bowel just before it reaches the cecum. The ileal mesentery can also be a source of trouble as the mesenteric defect can allow an internal hernia, which could cause small bowel obstruction. Small mesenteric defects should be closed.

Proctocolectomy With Ileal Pouch–Anal Anastomosis. The main differences between IRA and IPAA are (1) the loss of the rectum; (2) the extent of surgery that requires deep pelvic dissection; and (3) the different physiology of an ileal pouch. If the low rectum is relatively free of adenomas, a stapled IPAA can be performed with an ileal J pouch. This gives decent function with the expectation of an average of 5 to 6 daily bowel movements and good control with the ability to defer the movement for 1 to 2 hours.[28] If the anal transition zone (ATZ) and the low rectum are carpeted by adenoma, then mucosectomy and handsewn IPAA should be performed. An S pouch is the preferred configuration under these circumstances.[29] A handsewn IPAA is prone to stricture and leak, and has a higher rate of seepage and a need for the patients to wear pads.[30] Surgeons performing IPAA should be familiar with either anastomotic technique, and be able to perform the operation open as well as laparoscopically. Taking the pouch down to the anus without twists is critical to good function, as even a twist of 90 degrees can cause shelves in the pouch that hinder defecation. A diverting loop ileostomy is routine. However, if the IPAA procedure is stapled, the operation goes well, the stapler donuts are intact, and the leak test on the anastomosis is negative, then omitting the temporary loop ileostomy may be considered.

Total Proctocolectomy With End Ileostomy. For patients who prefer an operation that completely removes the chance of large bowel cancer, and who do not mind an EI, this is the best choice. It is critical that the ileostomy be well positioned and well constructed, with a 2-cm spout, so that pouching is easy and the skin-protective appliance lasts 3 to 4 days.

Postoperative Surveillance. Patients with an IRA and an IPAA need surveillance of their rectum or pouch, as adenomas and cancers can occur. Adenomas and cancers can also occur on an EI, although cancer takes at least 15 years to develop. Surveillance of the rectum and ileal pouch is performed yearly, usually as an office procedure without sedation, after two fleet enemas. The terminal ileum above the IRA or pouch is examined for at least 15 cm. The anastomosis itself is checked and the body of the pouch or rectum is examined for adenomas.[31] Polyps may be hyperplastic or lymphoid follicles, and pouch adenomas can be quite subtle. Because the ileal mucosa has villi, the adenomas tend to blend into the surrounding epithelium. Ulcers may be seen at the IRA and at the entry of the ileum into the pouch. They should be biopsied, but they are common and do not have any clinical significance in asymptomatic patients. The ATZ is a "hot spot" for adenomas. Whereas pouch adenomas usually take several years to form (42% of pouches have adenomas by 7 years follow-up),[32] ATZ adenomas may be there at the time of surgery and can sprout quite quickly. They are twice as common after a stapled IPAA as after a handsewn IPAA and, if not dealt with, can turn to cancer.[33] They can often be simply snared, but carpeting with villous adenoma requires stripping of the ATZ and a handsewn reanastomosis if possible. Sometimes this needs a formal redo of the IPAA with transabdominal pouch mobilization; the preferred technique is to do this transanally, with half the circumference done initially and the other half after the ATZ has healed from the first procedure. Pouch cancer is rare.[33] EIs should be checked once a year and the patient educated in the appearance of adenomas on the stoma.

Chemoprevention. Chemoprevention in FAP means treating colorectal, ileal, and duodenal adenoma risk with medications to suppress the neoplasia, as an alternative to surgery and polypectomy, or at least to postpone it. Many studies have tested a variety of agents in patients with FAP, mostly because the accelerated adenoma to carcinoma sequence in FAP allows the effects of putative chemotherapeutic agents to become obvious relatively quickly. The most tested drug is sulindac (Clinoril), a nonsteroidal antiinflammatory agent with cyclooxygenase (COX)-1 and COX-2 inhibiting activity.[34] However, sulindac can cause GI distress, bleeding, intestinal ulceration, and renal effects, and is not tolerated in 20% of patients.[35] That being said, a dose of 150 to 200 mg twice daily suppresses colorectal adenomas and desmoid disease,[36,37] but its effectiveness depends on strict compliance with taking the drug. There is a concern that cancers can still develop in patients whose adenomas have been suppressed for years.[38] For this reason, and because no chemotherapeutic agent has been shown to be completely effective in FAP, we do not favor chemoprevention as a routine option for colorectal adenomas in FAP. However, chemoprevention with sulindac is reasonable in FAP patients with pouch polyposis as the surgical alternative is pouch removal and likely an EI. Other agents that have shown some effect include difluoromethylornithine (DFMO) and celecoxib (Celebrex), although neither is used in standard practice. For duodenal adenomas in FAP, the epidermal growth factor receptor inhibitor erlotinib (Tarceva), in combination with sulindac, has recently shown great promise in the treatment of duodenal adenomas in FAP.[39] Combination chemotherapy, whereby multiple pathways to cancer are targeted at once, holds great promise for the future.

Desmoid Disease in Familial Adenomatous Polyposis.

Desmoid disease is a manifestation of the *APC* mutation that is found in 30% of FAP patients, mostly in the abdominal wall, in the small bowel mesentery, and in the retroperitoneum. It is an abnormal proliferation of fibroblasts that can produce tumors, or hard white sheets. Desmoid tumors can grow rapidly and be fatal, while even desmoid sheets can pucker adjacent organs, causing bowel or ureteric obstruction, and enterocutaneous fistulas.[40–43] The clinical behavior of desmoid disease varies from patient to patient and even within a patient, becoming less aggressive over time. Overall, about 12% regress, 7% are lethal, and the remainder never disappear, but rather grow and shrink to a small extent while remaining relatively asymptomatic.[44] There is no predictably effective treatment for desmoid disease and thus, for patients at high risk (see later), deferring its onset by avoiding abdominal surgery needs consideration. Desmoid disease can interfere with plans for an IPAA by restricting the length of the small intestinal mesentery so that the pouch will not reach the anus. A recent Cleveland Clinic study of patients undergoing proctectomy after an initial IRA showed that desmoid disease was present in 26 of 67 patients. Although proctectomy can still be completed in nearly all patients, desmoid disease prevented a planned IPAA in 8 of 62 patients.[45] This possibility should be discussed with patients preoperatively.

Desmoid Disease Risk Factors.

The risk factors predicting the possibility of desmoid disease include sex (females twice as likely as males), family history of desmoids, extracolonic manifestations of Gardner syndrome (epidermoid cysts, osteomas, extra teeth), and genotype. Traditionally, the location of the *APC* mutation was believed to determine

TABLE 165.6 Treatment of Intraabdominal Desmoid Disease in Familial Adenomatous Polyposis, According to Stage

Stage	Treatment	Surveillance
I	Nothing, or sulindac 150–200 mg by mouth twice a day	Repeat scan in 1 year
II	Sulindac 150–200 mg twice a day with raloxifene 60 mg by mouth twice a day	Repeat scan in 6 months
III	Methotrexate/vinorelbine or sorafenib	Repeat scan in 3 months
IV	Doxil/Adriamycin	Repeat scan in 3 months

the likelihood of an FAP patient to develop desmoid disease, but a recent Cleveland Clinic study showed that the location of the mutation does not predict the occurrence of desmoids, but rather predicts their severity; tumors in patients with mutations at the 3 prime end of codon 1400 tend to have more severe disease.[46] Church et al. have proposed a staging system for desmoid tumors based on size, symptoms, and pattern of growth, as summarized in Table 165.6.[47,48]

Treatment of Desmoids. While there is no predictably successful treatment for desmoid disease, a staging system can be used to triage patients for the various options (Table 165.6). Since complete eradication of desmoid disease is unlikely, the achievable therapy goal is to stabilize the disease and render the patient asymptomatic. For early-stage desmoid disease, sulindac is effective, but the response may take up to 2 years to be clinically evident.[37] Sulindac is usually given in combination with systemic estrogen-modifying agents such as tamoxifen or raloxifene.[49] For higher stage, more symptomatic patients, a quicker response is sought and chemotherapy may be used. Methotrexate and vinorelbine is effective in about 30% of cases,[50] while doxorubicin (Doxil) is perhaps even more effective.[51] Doxorubicin and dacarbazine are the most toxic options, but they do have the highest rate of regression or disappearance.[52]

Surgery is usually reserved to treat symptoms or to treat or preempt complications. Studies reporting the results of surgery for desmoid tumors rarely separate FAP-related tumors from sporadic tumors. Results for mixed populations of patients need to be reviewed carefully as the presence of a germline mutation may well influence recurrence rates, and FAP-related desmoids are often multiple. Abdominal wall desmoids can be resected with success, often requiring abdominal wall repair with mesh. Local recurrence occurs in about one-third of cases. Intraabdominal desmoids are less often resectable because of their predilection to occur in the retroperitoneum and the small bowel mesentery. However, desmoids in the distal mesentery away from the root vessels are often resectable, but have a local recurrence rate ranging from 57% to 80%.[53,54] These are challenging cases and can be technically difficult, resulting in large volume blood loss.[55] In some cases, when there are no other options, a complete enterectomy can be considered with small bowel transplant. Although desmoid tumors may be sensitive to radiation, this is not an option for intraabdominal desmoids due to the proximity of the small bowel.

Upper Gastrointestinal Tract in Familial Adenomatous Polyposis. Almost all patients with FAP have fundic gland polyps in the stomach, and adenomas in the duodenum.[20] Duodenal cancers are the third most common (10%) cause of death in FAP after CRC and desmoid disease.[56] Surveillance with esophagogastroduodenoscopy (EGD) using a side-viewing duodenoscope begins for patients at 20 to 25 years old. The duodenal ampulla must be examined. The density of duodenal adenomas tends to be centered on the duodenal ampulla, establishing a relationship between bile exposure and duodenal neoplasia risk where every epithelial cell carries a mutation in *APC*. Fifty percent of normal-appearing ampullas have epithelial dysplasia, although the significance of this is questionable.[20]

Fundic gland polyps are nonneoplastic, hyperplastic polyps of gastric mucosa. However, they can be numerous, and when proliferative can hide an underlying carcinoma. Low-grade dysplasia has been found in up to 40% of random biopsies and a low threshold for concern is appropriate.[57] Gastric adenomas occur in approximately 10% of FAP patients. They are frequently located in the antrum and may develop as a result of bile reflux into the stomach. As they may be precursors to gastric cancer, removal is recommended.[58] Duodenal adenomas are more common with a near 100% incidence, and they have a tendency to progress to cancer. The severity of duodenal adenomatosis predicts the chances of duodenal cancer, and can be described using the Spigelman staging system that is based on adenoma number, size, and histology (Table 165.7).[59] Patients with stage 0 disease (no adenomas) can be surveyed again in 5 years. Stage I patients can be surveyed in 3 years; stage II in 1 year; stage III in 6 months; and stage IV is an indication to consider surgery. Groves et al. from St. Mark's Hospital showed that 36% of patients with stage IV duodenal adenomas developed cancer.[60] In such patients, a pancreas-preserving duodenectomy is effective in preventing cancer without the full range of morbidity and lifestyle change incurred after a pancreaticoduodenectomy (Whipple procedure). A Whipple is indicated for a duodenal cancer that is definitively operable. Duodenal adenomas can be treated by snare polypectomy or by transduodenal polypectomy. Ampullary adenomas can be treated by endoscopic mucosal resection or surgical ampullectomy. All of these lesser procedures have lower morbidity than duodenectomy but have much higher recurrence rates.[61–63]

Other Extracolonic Manifestations of Familial Adenomatous Polyposis. Several other organs are affected by FAP and can develop a range of benign and malignant tumors. The cluster of manifestations referred to as Gardner syndrome includes osteomas (usually in the head and face), epidermoid cysts, extra teeth, and desmoids. The osteomas and cysts should be removed if they become symptomatic. Papillary thyroid cancer is approximately 7 times more common in FAP than in the general population, and is twice as common in women as in men with FAP.[64] Annual thyroid ultrasound is recommended for surveillance. It is quick, noninvasive, and effective as a screening test. Cleveland Clinic has shown that thyroid cancers detected on screening are smaller than incident cancer and have a better outcome.[64] Adrenal adenomas are often seen incidentally on computed tomography (CT) scans obtained to investigate desmoid disease. They are rarely symptomatic and even more rarely functional, and can be observed as long as they are less than 5 cm in diameter.[65] Turcot syndrome refers to the association of brain tumors with hereditary CRC and medulloblastoma is most common. The risk is relatively low but is higher than that in the general population. Hepatoblastoma is a potentially lethal liver tumor that is rare but is associated with FAP in infants. If found early, it is curable with surgery, making the case for screening infants to age 7 with ultrasound and α-fetoprotein.[66]

Attenuated Familial Adenomatous Polyposis. Attenuated FAP (aFAP) describes a subset of patients with a germline *APC* mutation in whom the colorectal phenotype is weak, or "attenuated." These patients are clinically defined as having less than 100 synchronous colorectal adenomas. They present at a later age than patients with classical FAP and develop CRC 10 to 20 years older.[67] *APC* mutations associated with attenuated polyposis tend to be at either extremity of the gene. With extreme 3 prime mutations there is a predilection for severe desmoid disease, and sometimes there are no colorectal adenomas at all (hereditary desmoid disease). Patients with aFAP are at the same, if not greater, risk of upper GI polyposis as those with classical FAP. Desmoid disease is common in those with 3 prime mutations but can also happen with 5 prime mutations. Colorectal surgery tends to occur later and is almost always colectomy and IRA. Patients with very mild colorectal polyposis may be treated with colonoscopy every year rather than colectomy. There is an overlap in phenotype between aFAP and *MutYH*-associated polyposis (MAP), and with otherwise undefined oligopolyposis.

MutYH-Associated Polyposis and *NTHL1*-Associated Polyposis

MutYH and *NTHL1* are genes involved in DNA base excision repair, a pathway that repairs oxidative damage to DNA. Oxidation causes guanine to mispair with thymine during replication, creating CG:TA transversions that produce mutations in a range of genes.[68] *MutYH* and *NTHL1* are two of a series of genes that corrects this problem and prevents the mutations from occurring. Recessive inheritance of mutations in both copies of these genes causes CRC predisposition and usually an

---

TABLE 165.7 Spigelman Staging System for Duodenal Adenomas

	1 Point	2 Points	3 Points
Polyp number	1–4	5–20	>20
Polyp size	1–4	5–10	>10
Polyp histology	Tubular	Tubulovillous	Villous
Degree of dysplasia	Low	Moderate*	High

*Now combined with low-grade dysplasia.
Stage 0 = 0 points; stage I = 1–4 points; stage II = 5–6 points; stage III = 7–8 points; stage IV = 9–12 points.

attenuated form of adenomatous polyposis resembling aFAP.[68,69] This is likely because *APC* is frequently affected by unrepaired oxidation. The incidence of MAP is very rare (<1% of all CRCs), while only an *NTHL1*-associated polyposis (NAP) is even more rare with only a few families described to date.

Since these diseases are recessively inherited, a mutated copy from each parent must be passed on for the offspring to develop the syndrome. In that situation, both parents must be at least carriers (i.e., one mutated allele and one normal allele) and the odds of a child inheriting both copies is 1 in 4. If one parent has the disease and the other parent is a carrier, the odds of the children developing the disease are 1 in 2. The population frequency of the carrier state (monoallelic mutation) is about 2%. There has been some debate about the risk to carriers for developing CRC. There is an approximately twofold CRC risk compared with the general population in *MutYH* mutation carriers, and thus some recommend colorectal surveillance commensurate with guidelines for people with similar risk, such as people with one affected first-degree relative. Lefevre et al. describe a similar risk of cancer for both monoallelic and biallelic mutation carriers who both have polyposis, suggesting that even in these monoallelic carriers gene expression is significantly reduced, leading to the phenotype.[70]

Clinical Features. MAP can present in many different ways, mimicking almost all other syndromes of hereditary CRC.[71] Classic MAP phenotypically resembles aFAP with less than 100 synchronous adenomas and a young age of onset of microsatellite stable (MSS) CRC. However, various reports in the literature show that cancers in patients with biallelic *MutYH* mutations can be solitary (no polyposis), and can occur in either very young or older patients and in patients with no family history. The polyps may develop early or late, and can include adenomas and serrated polyps. Cancers can be microsatellite unstable. Church and Kravochuck recently reported rectal "studding" as a possible pathognomonic sign of MAP.[72] Although the family history is classically recessive, with unaffected parents and affected second-degree relatives, sometimes a dominant inheritance pattern or even no family history of CRC is seen. Patients with suspicion for MAP, or patients thought to have FAP but who do not have an *APC* mutation, should be tested for *MutYH* mutations. The advent of panel testing allows more screening for *MutYH* mutations and the identification of atypical cases. Testing of patients for *NTHL1* mutations is not yet commercially available.

Extracolonic Manifestations. MAP seems to have a spectrum of extracolonic manifestations similar to that found with classical FAP. There are reports of gastric and duodenal adenomas, small bowel carcinomas, desmoid tumors, and thyroid cancer. The phenotypic spectrum of patients with *NTHL1* mutations has yet to be defined.

Clinical Management. Management depends on the severity of colorectal polyposis and the age of the patient at presentation. If the colorectal neoplasia is controllable by colonoscopy, this is a reasonable option, especially when expert colonoscopy is available and the patient is compliant. Rules for endoscopic management of patients with MAP include a high quality, uncompromising colonoscopy with excellent bowel preparation. If no polyps are seen,

the exam can be repeated in 3 to 5 years. If neoplasia is found, all adenomas greater than 5 mm diameter should be removed. The exam is repeated at an interval appropriate for the polyp number, size, and degree of dysplasia, but no longer than 1 to 2 years. Colectomy is reserved for patients with an uncontrolled polyp burden or for CRC. The risk of developing CRC in biallelic carriers is approximately 75%. If a colon cancer is present, and there is a known MAP diagnosis, an extended colectomy and IRA is recommended. If an MAP patient presents more like classical FAP, with greater than 1000 adenomas, they are treated as if they had FAP.

Extracolonic surveillance includes thyroid screening with ultrasound, and EGD, starting at presentation and continuing at intervals appropriate for the findings. Without findings, the exam is repeated every 3 to 5 years. There are no recommendations for the treatment of NAP, and, indeed, the syndrome is so new and the number of families so small that the phenotype of the syndrome has not yet been established.

Polymerase Proofreading-Associated Polyposis

DNA replication is a key event occurring during cell division, and multiple biologic systems are designed to maximize the fidelity of replication. One key system is the DNA proofreading domains of DNA polymerase. Failure of these proofreading domains can lead to a dominantly inherited syndrome of colorectal and endometrial cancer predisposition.[73] Such a failure of proofreading creates a mutator phenotype where mistakes in DNA replication persist in daughter cells and lead to secondary mutations in other genes. When these genes are drivers of colorectal carcinogenesis, tumors occur. The polymerases shown to be involved are *POLD1* and *POLE*. The syndrome is characterized by oligoadenomatous polyposis and early age of onset CRC, and endometrial cancer in patients with a *POLE* mutation. Recent studies show that POLE mutations can be associated with both MSS and unstable CRCs, and so polymerase proofreading-associated polyposis is among the differential diagnoses of Lynch syndrome. There are few families reported with this syndrome, so the full picture of the phenotype is lacking. However, a young age of onset CRC, and multiple, advanced adenomas are suggestive. Patients must be treated according to their presentation, although in those already diagnosed who present with a cancer, extended surgery seems reasonable. In patients with an early age of onset CRC and oligoadenomatous polyposis, germline mutations in *POLD1/POLE* can be sought via panels offered by various commercial laboratories.

HAMARTOMATOUS POLYPOSIS SYNDROMES

Hamartomatous polyps are benign, localized overgrowths of mature epithelial cells. The hamartomatous polyp syndromes are rare entities that include juvenile polyposis syndrome (JS), Peutz-Jeghers syndrome (PJS), and *PTEN* hamartoma tumor syndrome (PHTS), which includes Cowden syndrome (CS) and Bannayan-Riley-Ruvalcaba syndrome (BRRS). Less than 1% of all CRC is associated with hamartomatous polyposis syndromes. Knowledge of these syndromes allows the appropriate genetic counseling and testing, the assessment of cancer risk, and the screening recommendations.

Juvenile Polyposis Syndrome

Solitary juvenile polyps are the most frequent colorectal polyps in children. They are bright red, usually pedunculated, and histologically are hamartomas that feature an inflammatory infiltrate with large mucus-filled spaces distributed in an expanded lamina propria and a prominent inflammatory infiltrate. Isolated juvenile polyps are not inherited and are not premalignant. However, multiple juvenile polyps raise the possibility of JPS.

Diagnosis and Genetics. Diagnostic criteria for diagnosis of JPS include any juvenile polyp in a patient with a family history of juvenile polyposis, or greater than 4 synchronous juvenile polyps in the large intestine. The polyps are usually found in the colon and rectum, but they may also be found in the stomach, duodenum or small bowel, and occasionally diffusely throughout the GI tract. The estimated incidence of JPS ranges from 1 in 50,000 to 1 in 100,000. JPS is genetically heterogeneous, and is associated with germline mutations in *SMAD4* and *BMPR1A* genes, two members of the TGF-β superfamily. Germline mutations in the *SMAD4* suppressor gene, located on chromosome 18q21.1, account for 18% to 50% of JPS cases. This gene encodes a cytoplasmic mediator involved in the TGF-β signal transduction pathway. The finding of JPS kindred with *BMPR1A* mutations further supports the importance of TGF-β superfamily mutations in this syndrome. It is inherited in an autosomal dominant manner with variable penetrance. Approximately 20% to 50% of cases have a family history of JPS. In sporadic cases, the condition may represent a new mutation or incomplete penetrance of the gene, but it also may result from environmental factors.

Clinical Features. Polyp growth begins in the first decade of life and there are variable numbers, usually between 50 and 200.[74] Macroscopically, the polyps are 5 to 50 mm in size, red to brown in color, spherical or lobulated, and pedunculated, often with superficial ulceration. The cut surface shows cystic spaces, and microscopically, the characteristic feature is dilated cystic glands lined by tall columnar epithelium. The lamina propria is expanded and consists of an inflammatory infiltrate consisting of neutrophils, eosinophils, and a few lymphocytes.[74] Polyps are distributed throughout the GI tract, but most commonly are in the colon. Hofting et al. described the following distribution of polyps in 262 cases of juvenile polyposis: colorectum 98%, stomach 13.6%, duodenum 2.3%, and jejunum and ileum 6.5%.[75] As the upper GI tract has not often been screened adequately, the rate of upper GI tract involvement may be higher. The colorectal polyps appear to be evenly distributed throughout the large bowel. Isolated polyposis involving only the stomach has been described.

Sachatello et al. subdivided JPS into three categories based upon clinical presentation and disease course[76]: (1) juvenile polyposis of infancy; (2) juvenile polyposis coli; and (3) generalized juvenile polyposis. Juvenile polyposis of infancy is an extremely rare syndrome in which the entire GI tract is usually affected. Patients present with bloody diarrhea, protein-losing enteropathy, intussusception, and rectal prolapse. The prognosis is unfavorable and is related to the severity and extent of GI involvement. The common manifestations lead to anemia, hypoproteinemia, anasarca, failure to thrive, and finally death within 2 years of life in 90% of infants.

In juvenile polyposis coli, as the name implies, the juvenile polyps are limited to the colon and rectum, while in generalized JPS, the polyps occur anywhere from the stomach to the rectum. Presentation of both these subtypes usually occurs in the first and second decades of life, and almost always by 30 years of age. In a review examining 218 patients with JPS, Coburn et al. found that juvenile polyposis coli patients usually presented between the ages of 5 to 15 years, while patients with generalized JPS presented at age 12. The most common manifestations are rectal bleeding and anemia, which may occur in as many as 75% of patients. Other frequent symptoms are prolapse of either a polyp or the rectum itself, abdominal cramps or pain, and diarrhea. Some patients may present with clubbing of the fingers. Besides anemia, laboratory findings may include hypoproteinemia, hypokalemia, and a skin test anergy. Different clinical subtypes of JPS can exist in the same kindred, suggesting variable penetrance, and making the distinction between subtypes somewhat arbitrary.

Patients with juvenile polyposis may have extraintestinal morphologic abnormalities. Congenital anomalies were described in up to 20% of cases and have included macrocephaly, mental retardation, atrial and ventricular septal defects, pulmonary arteriovenous malformations, pulmonary stenosis, Meckel diverticulum, malrotation, cryptorchidism, hypertelorism, and telangiectasia.

Genotype/phenotype correlations in JPS patients have emerged. The results are consistent with the suggestions that some carriers of *SMAD4* mutations may have higher cancer risk than patients without *SMAD4* mutations.[77] *SMAD4* families were found to have more upper GI juvenile polyps when compared with *BMPR1A*-mutation positive or no-mutation families, and so it seems that *SMAD4* mutations predispose to generalized JPS, while *SMAD4*-mutation negative cases are more likely to have a juvenile polyposis coli phenotype. In addition, *SMAD4* mutation carriers seem to be the patients prone to hereditary hemorrhagic telangiectasia (HHT).[78] The association is strong enough to suggest that patients with JPS and an *SMAD4* mutation should undergo HHT screening before surgery.

Malignant Potential in Juvenile Polyposis Syndrome. While CRC was the first to be described, and is the most frequent malignancy seen in JPS patients, carcinoma of the stomach, pancreas, duodenum, and small intestine occurs. CRC cases have been reported in patients with both colorectal and generalized juvenile polyposis, as well as in sporadic forms and in familial ones. Howe et al. reported that 55% of affected members of a large Iowa JPS kindred developed GI cancer; 38% had CRC and 21% had gastric cancer.[79] A similar risk for CRC was reported by Brosens et al.[80] The mean age for diagnosing GI cancer in JPS is around 35 years in different series, but the range is wide (4 to 60 years). Carcinomas can develop 1 to 25 years (average 15 years) after the onset of symptoms or the diagnosis.

Jass et al. suggested a more aggressive behavior of CRCs in JPS patients. In 18 of 80 (22%) patients who developed CRC, 5 patients were not resectable for cure, and tumors from 9 of these patients showed mucinous features and/or poor differentiation.[81] A hamartoma-adenoma-dysplasia-carcinoma sequence in JPS patients is proposed by several authors. There are not enough data to support a transition of juvenile polyps into adenocarcinoma, although juvenile polyps with adenomatous areas, mixed juvenile adenomatous polyps, and purely adenomatous polyps can be found in affected colons. Kinzler and Vogelstein have postulated that the overgrowth of the stromal/mesenchymal elements leads to the production of a microenvironment, which influences or "landscapes" the epithelial element of the hamartomatous polyps.[82] Jass and colleagues retrospectively studied the pathologic findings of 1032 polyps from 80 JPS patients.[81] A total of 840 polyps were typical juvenile polyps, whereas 169 differed in being multilobulated or showed villous configuration. Of the latter, 47% contained foci of epithelial dysplasia (with a tendency toward a higher degree of moderate to marked epithelial dysplasia), whereas only 9% of typical polyps were dysplastic (typically mild dysplasia).

Clinical Management: Screening and Surveillance. For kindred in which a gene mutation is known, other potentially affected individuals can be diagnosed by genetic testing. Screening by colonoscopy should begin at age 12 to 15, or earlier if symptoms are present. If no neoplasia is seen, colonoscopy should be repeated in 2 to 3 years. If polyps are present, they should be removed at colonoscopy and examined histologically, with repeat colonoscopy annually until the exam is clear. If that is achieved, the interval can be pushed back to every 2 to 3 years. Upper GI screening should be done by EGD and begin between the ages of 15 and 25 or earlier if symptoms develop. If a mutation is not identified in the proband, first-degree relatives should be screened as mentioned earlier. Diffuse or symptomatic polyposis may need colectomy or gastrectomy.

Clinical Management: Surgery. In a symptomatic JPS patient, initial management includes correction of anemia, electrolyte imbalance, and nutritional deficits. After complete evaluation of the extent of the disease, surgery is considered. Indications for surgery in JPS patients are controversial. For children with generalized juvenile polyposis and hypoproteinemia, failure to thrive, or instances of intussusception, surgery is recommended. Other troublesome symptoms, such as bleeding and diarrhea may also be an indication for surgery. Surgery is indicated for patients with any suspicion of dysplasia or cancer. Because of the high risk of CRC, most authors believe that all polyps, symptomatic or not, should be removed endoscopically or surgically. Currently, there are insufficient data from JPS patients to justify performing a routine prophylactic colectomy in asymptomatic patients, solely for the risk of colorectal carcinoma. Colonoscopic polypectomy followed by colonoscopic surveillance is a reasonable alternative, as long as polyp clearance is possible and patient compliance is good. Factors in favor of prophylactic colectomy due to presumably increased potential for CRC include multiple polyps that cannot be controlled by snaring, adenomatous elements in polyps that have been snared, and those cases where CRC is a feature of the family history. Unlike FAP, a patient's age at prophylactic colectomy is variable, reflecting both the heterogeneous phenotype of the disease and the varying recommendations for prophylactic colectomy. The

percentage of JPS patients who will eventually have surgery is difficult to estimate as most reported series are small. Coburn et al. reviewed 218 cases published in the English literature and found that 99 (45%) patients underwent 138 surgical procedures.[83] Of these, 121 were colorectal operations, including 41 partial colectomies, 56 subtotal or total colectomies, 7 restorative proctocolectomies, 3 total proctocolectomies with ileostomy, 2 abdominoperineal resections (APRs), and 12 operative polypectomies. The remaining 17 operations involved the stomach in 12 cases, and the small bowel in 5 cases. Almost all patients who did not have surgery were treated with endoscopic polypectomy.

The surgical choices for managing large bowel disease in JPS are similar to those for FAP: colectomy and IRA or proctocolectomy with ileal pouch–anal anastomosis. When choosing the surgical procedure, the balance between the morbidity of the procedure and the need for lifetime surveillance of any remaining colon and rectum should be considered. Partial colectomy does not seem to be an appropriate procedure due to the high probability for recurrent polyps and cancer in the remaining colon. In general, colectomy and IRA might be recommended in those cases in which surgery is necessary, and the rectum can be cleared endoscopically. A TPC is required for significant involvement of both the colon and rectum. However, as opposed to FAP, the number of preoperative rectal polyps may not be a good indicator of the need for proctectomy. Oncel and associates reported that 5 of 10 patients whose rectums were spared at the initial procedure subsequently underwent proctectomy for rectal polyposis. Four of the remaining five patients required multiple endoscopic polypectomies. No correlation between the initial number of rectal polyps and the need for subsequent proctectomy was noted.[84] Two of eight patients who underwent ileal pouch procedures required endoscopic or surgical excision of polyps in the pouch. Hence, follow-up after both procedures is necessary due to the high recurrence rates of juvenile polyps in either the remnant rectum or the pouch. The role of mucosectomy while performing a pouch procedure for JPS patients is not well discussed in the literature.

Prior to colon surgery for JPS, an EGD and small bowel evaluation should be performed. Alternatively, upper endoscopy including small bowel visualization can be performed at the time of surgical exploration. In the future, capsule endoscopy may have a place in preoperative evaluation and surveillance of the small bowel in JPS patients. Managing polyps of the stomach is more challenging than those of the colon, for these are usually diffuse and cannot be removed endoscopically. These patients often have severe anemia and will eventually require subtotal or total gastrectomy. Gastric resection is also the treatment of choice for dysplasia or carcinoma. In patients with duodenal or small bowel polyps, enterotomy should be performed at the time of surgery and the polyps excised because these polyps may harbor a carcinoma. More extensive resection may be necessary in case of diffuse polyposis or malignancy.

Surveillance after surgery for involvement of either part of the GI tract should be resumed and include periodic upper and lower GI tract examinations. Anecdotally, in two patients who had removal of recurrent polyps from ileal pouches after a pouch procedure, sulindac therapy was associated with further long-term polyp-free pouches,[84] but future studies are needed to determine the role of sulindac in the management of JPS patients.

Peutz-Jeghers Syndrome

Diagnosis and Genetics. PJS is diagnosed using clinical criteria, which includes the presence of ≥2 Peutz-Jeghers polyps anywhere in the GI tract, or at least one intestinal Peutz-Jeghers polyp in a patient that has a family history of PJS or the classic finding of mucocutaneous pigmentation. In the absence of Peutz-Jeghers polyps, a diagnosis can still be made when there is a family history of the disease and typical pigmentations. As many as 50% of affected individuals are new cases and have no family history of the disease. When inherited, it is with a dominant inheritance pattern, with a reported incidence of 1 in 120,000 live births.[85] It is caused by genetic alterations in a serine threonine kinase gene (*STK11*, also known as *LKB1*), located on chromosome 19. Mutations in *STK11* are found in up to 69% of carefully selected individuals.

Clinical Features. PJS is characterized by diffuse hamartomatous polyposis. The polyps can arise anywhere in the GI tract, but the small intestine is the most common site, being involved in greater than 75% of individuals.[85] Polyps affect the colon in 42% of cases, the stomach in 38%, and the rectum in 28%. Less common locations for tumors include the upper respiratory, biliary, and urinary tracts. Peutz-Jeghers polyps are typically different from juvenile polyps in that they have smooth muscle bundles within the lamina propria of the stalk and head of the polyp, and do not have dilated cystic-filled spaces pathognomonic for juvenile polyps. The other characteristic finding in PJS is the characteristic pigmented melanin macules on the skin or mucous membranes, which can be identified in over 95% of patients. The lips and perioral region (94%), hands (74%), and feet (62%) are most commonly affected. The macules increase in intensity from infancy and early childhood but often fade in adult life with complete disappearance in some cases. Pigmented spots on the buccal mucosa are present in over two-thirds of individuals, but unlike the skin macules, the buccal lesions usually persist throughout life.

Abdominal discomfort and distention are the most common presenting symptoms, and small bowel obstruction due to intussusception is the presenting feature in nearly half of individuals. One-third of PJS patients become symptomatic during the first decade of life and nearly half experience symptoms that require an operation for bowel obstruction by the age of 20 years. Recurrent obstruction requiring relaparotomy is common and is performed between 1 and 4 times per patient.[86] Polyps may also cause GI bleeding which, depending on its severity and chronicity, may be occult, overt, or associated with an iron deficiency anemia.

Risk of Cancer. PJS is a cancer predisposition syndrome. This risk of cancer was first appreciated in the original family described by Peutz. The age of death in affected family members was substantially younger (38 years) when compared with that in unaffected members (69 years) and was usually due to intestinal obstruction and cancer. Spigelman et al. reported that 48% of PJS patients

died of malignancy by the age of 57 years.[87] There is a substantial risk of both GI and non-GI cancers with a combined occurrence of any sort of cancer up to 93% by age 65 years.[88,89] The intestinal cancer risks included colon (39%), pancreas (36%), stomach (29%), small bowel (13%), and esophagus (0.5%). Nondigestive organs at risk for cancer include breast (54%), ovary (21%), lung (15%), and uterus (9%). Cancers of the biliary tree and gallbladder have also been reported. Unusual genital tract tumors including adenoma malignum of the cervix, ovarian sex cord tumors with annular tubules (SCTAT), or testicular tumors resembling SCTAT (also referred to as *large cell calcifying Sertoli cell tumors*) also occur.

Clinical Management. As multiple organ systems are affected in PJS, screening and surveillance protocols are complex and aim to reduce cancer risk and symptomatic disease. For the GI tract, this equates to minimizing the risk of bowel obstruction, GI bleeding, or cancer, but the efficacy of surveillance in reducing cancer incidence or mortality is unknown.[90] Although recommendations on the age to begin surveillance and frequency of exams vary, most guidelines advocate upper endoscopy and complete small bowel evaluation every second year starting at age 10 years, and colonoscopy every 2 to 3 years from the age of 25.

Upper endoscopy, small bowel enteroscopy, and polypectomy are the cornerstone of management of proximal small bowel polyposis in PJS. An aggressive approach to the diagnosis and resection of small bowel polyps is mandatory to minimize the need for emergency surgery. Small bowel radiography has been the traditional method for the detection of small bowel polyps, but capsule endoscopy is more accurate and should supplant small bowel radiograph.[91] Polyps detected on capsule endoscopy lead to surgery in at least 50% of patients.[92] The imaging capsule is safe to use in individuals who have had previous bowel resection and in those with mild symptoms due to small bowel polyposis. Patients with symptoms suggesting complications of small bowel polyposis or asymptomatic patients who have polyps greater than 1 to 1.5 cm in size detected on capsule endoscopy should undergo laparotomy or laparoscopy with intraoperative endoscopy. The goal of the combined endoscopic and surgical approach is to clear *all* small bowel polyps, not just those causing symptoms. There are several reports suggesting that that the combined approach with clearance of all polyps may delay the time between operations.[86] Intraoperative enteroscopy is required because external palpation of the small bowel and small bowel transillumination may not detect all polyps that require polypectomy. Asymptomatic gastric or colonic polyps greater than 1 cm should be removed endoscopically.

For extraintestinal screening in PJS, the National Comprehensive Cancer Network (NCCN) recommends males should undergo annual testicular physical examination starting at the age of 10 years, and females should undergo annual pelvic examination and Papanicolaou stain starting at the age of 18 to 20 years. Women should have breast physical examinations every 6 months and yearly mammogram and breast magnetic resonance imaging starting at the age of 25 years. Pancreatic cancer screening involves endoscopic ultrasound or magnetic resonance cholangiopancreatography along with serum CA19-9 every 1 to 2 years starting at the age of 25 to 30 years.[64] Other screening regimens have been proposed by other authors.[93–95]

PTEN Hamartoma Tumor Syndromes

PHTS represents a spectrum of rare hereditary syndromes characterized by hamartomatous polyps in the GI tract and abnormalities of the skull, skeleton, and skin. This extremely rare group of syndromes includes CS, BRRS, Gorlin syndrome, and Proteus syndrome. CS and BRRS are the more common syndromes and are associated with an increased risk of CRC. The phenotypes are often overlapping.

Genetics. *PTEN* is a tumor suppressor gene that encodes a phosphatase in the PI3K/AKT signaling pathway. It plays a key role in apoptosis and acts as a tumor suppressor gene. *PTEN* mutations are found in association with a variety of sporadic and hereditary tumors affecting multiple organs, including the colon and rectum, uterus, brain, thyroid, breast, skin, and prostate. CS and BRRS are both autosomally dominant inherited disorders associated with a *PTEN* mutation. Approximately 80% of patients who meet the diagnostic criteria for CS, and 60% of patients with BRRS, have *PTEN* mutations.[96,97] Now that *PTEN* is included in most gene panels offered by commercial laboratories, the diagnosis of PHTS may be made more often.

Cowden Syndrome. Patients with CS develop multiple hamartomas and are at risk of multiple benign and malignant tumors. The International Cowden Consortium developed clinical CS diagnostic criteria and include major and minor criteria.[94,98] Major criteria include breast cancer, thyroid cancer (especially follicular), macrocephaly, endometrial cancer, and Lhermitte-Duclos disease. Minor features include benign thyroid changes (e.g., goiter), mental retardation, hamartomatous intestinal polyps, fibrocystic changes in the breast, lipomas, fibromas, genito-urinary tumors (such as kidney cancer or uterine fibroids), or malformations. If a patient has either macrocephaly or Lhermitte-Duclos disease and one other major feature, a CS diagnosis is made. CS diagnosis is also present if one major feature and three minor features, or at least four minor features are met. Common skin manifestations associated with CS include trichilemmomas and papillomatous papules, and macrocephaly is common. Colorectal features include hamartomas, but also serrated or hyperplastic polyps, inflammatory polyps, adenomas, and ganglioneuromas. A germline *PTEN* mutation supports the clinical diagnosis.

Malignancy risk in CS is significant outside the GI tract. Women have a 50% lifetime risk of developing breast cancer and a 5% to 10% lifetime risk of developing endometrial cancer. Men and women with CS have a 10% lifetime risk of developing epithelial thyroid cancer. Other malignancies described in association with CS include transitional carcinoma of the bladder, melanoma, and renal cell carcinoma.

The main colorectal feature of CS is colorectal polyps with a variety of histology. Most of these are of subepithelial origin and include fibromas, lipomas, neuromas, ganglioneuromas, and neurofibromas. There are also adenomas, serrated polyps, and juvenile-like hamartomas.[99] The polyps can be numerous but rarely carpet the colon. Until recently there was not thought to be an increased risk of CRC in

CS. However, Heald et al. reported on 69 *PTEN* mutation carriers who met relaxed criteria for CS; 64 had colorectal polyps,[99] 24 had both upper GI and colorectal polyps, and 9 (13%) had CRC. The standardized incidence ratio for CRC was 224.1 (95% confidence interval, 109.3 to 411.3; P < .0001). Other groups have supported a 9% to 16% lifetime risk for CRC.[100–102] It is uncertain if the cancers develop from the hamartomatous or adenomatous polyps. In the upper GI tract, gastric and duodenal polyps are common and can include hyperplastic polyps, hamartomas, and adenomas.

As the cancer risk spans many organs, the CS screening regimen is complex and includes the following: (1) physical exam starting at 18 years of age, or 5 years before the earliest cancer was diagnosed in the family; (2) breast screening with monthly self-examinations and an annual clinical examination starting at age 18 years; mammography starting at 30 years of age, or 5 years younger than the earliest family breast cancer; (3) thyroid ultrasound starting at age 18, every 1 to 2 years; (4) colonoscopy starting at age 20 and repeated every 1 to 3 years depending on the findings at the examination; (5) EGD starting at age 30, repeated every 3 to 5 years depending on the findings; (6) endometrial cancer screening by pelvic ultrasound at the age of 35 to 40 years, or five years prior to the earliest family case of endometrial cancer; and (7) dermatologic exam to screen for melanoma.[103]

Bannayan-Riley-Ruvalcaba Syndrome. BRRS, like CS, is an autosomal dominant disorder characterized by multiple phenotypic abnormalities and hamartomas in the intestine and other tissues. Specific diagnostic criteria for BRRS are not established, but patients with macrocephaly, hamartomatous colonic polyposis, lipomas, and pigmented macules of the glans penis should be considered for genetic testing.[104] Less common manifestations include Hashimoto thyroiditis, vascular malformations, and mental retardation. The series of case reports in the literature suggest that patients with BRRS have a similar colorectal phenotype to those with CS. The intestinal polyps are most commonly juvenile polyps, which develop early in life and may contain adenomatous dysplasia. BRRS is not often associated with an increased cancer risk, although the multiple colorectal polyps may be symptomatic (intussusception and obstruction). While surgery for CRC is rare in patients with BRRS, patients may need a colectomy or at least a polypectomy for the symptoms caused by the polyps. The possibility of adenomatous dysplasia in the juvenile polyps suggests that regular surveillance is indicated.

Other Clinical Syndromes Associated With *PTEN* Mutations. Proteus syndrome ("Elephant Man" syndrome) and Gorlin syndrome (nevoid basal cell carcinoma syndrome) are rare syndromes without any obvious colorectal involvement. However, it seems reasonable to follow such patients with colonoscopy after a baseline exam of upper and lower GI tracts, as the germline *PTEN* mutation may produce epithelial and subepithelial polyps. There are a paucity of data on these syndromes, and much of the available information is from small series or case reports.

Hereditary Mixed Polyposis Syndrome

Hereditary mixed polyposis syndrome (HMPS) is an autosomal dominantly inherited syndrome, which was originally reported in an Ashkenazi Jewish family and is characterized by the finding of colorectal polyps of multiple histologies.[105] In particular, adenomas, serrated polyps, and juvenile hamartomas are found in the same colon, and there is an increased risk for CRC. In the original family, 42 family members developed either colorectal polyps or CRC.[105] No patient in this family had more than 15 polyps, and 13 patients developed CRC. There did not seem to be a risk for extracolonic cancers. The mutation in this family was identified as a deletion in *GREM1*.[106] A similar syndrome has been found in other Jewish families, and in one non-Jewish family; however, not all of these families have had *GREM1* sequencing analysis. The management goal of HMPS is to control the CRC risk in the least invasive way possible. Colonoscopy with polypectomy may suffice, but if cancer is diagnosed then an extended resection should be considered.

NONPOLYPOSIS COLORECTAL CANCER

Overview

The term nonpolyposis CRC syndromes was introduced to distinguish from the previously better characterized polyposis syndromes. As more is learned about the underlying genetics that cause these syndromes, a more precise definition is being formed. As such, it is important to distinguish these syndromes to assign more precise risk stratification. Historically, nonpolyposis syndromes were generically called HNPCC. Current understanding defines HNPCC as a clinical diagnosis based on cancer patterns within a family defined by the Amsterdam II criteria, which include the following[107]: (1) within a family, there should be at least three relatives with an HNPCC-associated cancer (cancer of the colorectum, endometrium, ovaries, small bowel, stomach, ureter or renal pelvis, pancreas, brain, skin); (2) one should be a first-degree relative to the other two; (3) at least two successive generations should be affected; (4) at least one cancer should be diagnosed before age 50; and (5) FAP is excluded. Patients with a heritable deleterious or pathogenic genetic variant in one of the MMR genes are defined as having Lynch syndrome, regardless of the clinical context or family history. As described earlier, approximately 93% of patients with Lynch syndrome have microsatellite unstable tumors. Patients who meet Amsterdam criteria, but have MSS tumors are given a diagnosis of familial CRC type X (FCC X).[108,109] As expected, in addition to having MSS tumors, patients with FCC X do not have a causative MMR gene mutation. Approximately 50% of patients with Lynch syndrome do not meet Amsterdam criteria.[110] This is an important distinction as the colorectal and extracolonic risks are different for Lynch syndrome and FCC X. Lastly, there is a subset of patients who have microsatellite unstable tumors and with loss of MMR protein expression, but do not have an identifiable MMR gene germline defect. These patients have more recently been defined as Lynch-like, or Tumor-Lynch. Each of these classifications has unique risk profiles and thus has different management recommendations.

Lynch Syndrome

Lynch syndrome is defined as the inherited cancer-predisposing disease caused by a germline mutation in one of the DNA MMR genes: *MLH1*, *MSH2*, *MSH6*, and *PMS2*. Additionally, there are cases of Lynch syndrome caused by germline deletions of *EPCAM*. Lynch syndrome patients develop colorectal and extracolonic cancers at a young age. It accounts for approximately 3% of all CRCs, and 10% to 19% of CRCs diagnosed before age 50.[110-112] Lynch syndrome is an autosomal dominant condition, and thus all first-degree relatives of an affected patient have a 50% chance of also carrying the mutation. Therefore, identification of individuals who potentially have Lynch syndrome has implications for both the patient and their families.

Screening and Diagnosis. Clinical characteristics such as Amsterdam criteria and Bethesda criteria[113] are used to identify patients who should undergo further testing for Lynch syndrome. Several histologic features such as poor differentiation, signet cell histology, abundance of extracellular mucin, tumor-infiltrating lymphocytes, and a lymphoid host response to tumor are associated with microsatellite instability, which is a molecular hallmark of Lynch syndrome. These factors should trigger testing for microsatellite instability or evaluation of MMR protein expression by immunohistochemistry. In Lynch syndrome-associated CRC, up to 91% exhibit MSI-H,[114] and approximately 83% have loss of expression for one of the four MMR proteins.[114] These test results guide genetic counseling and testing for germline mutations in a specific gene.

To combat the lack of adequate sensitivity in targeted screening programs, several groups have recently endorsed universal screening for Lynch syndrome on all CRCs.[115] The Evaluation of Genomic Applications in Practice and Prevention (EGAPP) Working Group recommended that all newly diagnosed CRCs undergo MSI and/or immunohistochemistry (IHC) as screening for Lynch syndrome.[114,116] The NCCN recommends universal screening of all CRCs under age 70 and those older than 70 that meet Bethesda guidelines.[117] Ideally, preoperative testing is done on the cancer biopsy before surgery in which Lynch syndrome is suspected, which would provide an opportunity for definitive diagnosis and would guide surgical management. However, this is not always practical as some patients do not want to delay surgery to wait for genetic testing results. MSI-H or loss of MMR protein expression do not confirm a Lynch syndrome diagnosis. The majority of MSI-H CRCs arise via acquired methylation of the *MLH1* promoter.[118,119] Therefore, if MMR screening reveals loss of MLH1 protein expression, further analysis is required to determine the cause. As the majority of non-Lynch MLH1-deficient tumors harbor *BRAF* mutations and are methylated at the MLH1 promoter, *BRAF* mutation and/or *MLH1* methylation testing should be done.[108] A wild-type *BRAF* or methylated *MLH1* promoter suggest a sporadic MSI-H cancer. If IHC reveals *MSH2*, *MSH6*, or *PMS2* are lost, Lynch syndrome is suspected and germline confirmation is pursued for those specific genes. Several predictive models have been developed to help identify patients to be screened for Lynch syndrome. For patients without a personal history of CRC, but with a family history suggestive of Lynch syndrome, the use of readily available prediction models such as $PREMM_{1,2,6}$ (http://premm.dfci.harvard.edu/) or MMRpro (http://

www4.utsouthwestern.edu/breasthealth/cagene/) may be useful.

Colorectal Cancer and Extracolonic Cancer Risks.

CRC risk for Lynch syndrome patients varies according to the underlying genetic etiology. For *MLH1*, *MSH2*, and *PMS2* mutation carriers, the lifetime risk is 50% to 74%, while *MSH6* carriers have 10% to 22% risk.[10,120-123] Lynch syndrome CRCs occur earlier in life than sporadic cancer with a mean age at diagnosis between 44 and 61 years.[125,126]

Endometrial cancer represents the highest extracolonic cancer risk with rates as high as 44% in women with *MSH6* and *MSH2* mutations.[123,127] *PMS2* mutation carriers have the lowest endometrial lifetime risk at 15% to 20%.[122,124] Like CRC, endometrial cancers develop at a younger age than sporadic cancer with the mean age between 48 and 62 years. Synchronous endometrial and ovarian cancers have been reported in 7% to 21% of the women with Lynch syndrome.[129]

Multiple other organs are at increased risk of malignancy compared with the general population. The more common sites include the urinary tract, stomach, small bowel, brain, skin, pancreas, prostate, and breast.[130] Prostate and breast cancer risk continue to be debated and studied. Compared with the general population, patients with Lynch syndrome have nearly twice as much risk to develop prostate cancer,[131] and possibly elevated risks for breast cancer.[130,132]

Clinical Management: Surveillance.

The best evidence for surveillance and intervention as a risk-reducing strategy is for colonoscopy. The purpose of surveillance in patients with Lynch syndrome is to detect and remove premalignant polyps before they develop into cancer. Surveillance colonoscopy can reduce CRC incidence by 62% reduction and reduce the CRC-related mortality by 72% in Lynch syndrome patients.[133] Due to early-age onset and a shortened adenoma to carcinoma interval,[121,134] patients with Lynch syndrome should undergo colonoscopy every 1 to 2 years starting at age 20 to 25 years.[108,121]

The benefit of screening for extracolonic cancers in Lynch syndrome is less established in the literature, but is established based on clinical expert opinion weighing risks and benefits. As endometrial cancer represents the second highest lifetime risk for women with Lynch syndrome, most experts recommend annual screening, including pelvic examination and transvaginal ultrasound with endometrial biopsy.[135] Clinicians and patients must be aware of warning symptoms of endometrial cancer, such as abnormal uterine bleeding or pelvic pain so that early evaluation is performed. Due to the high risk of endometrial and ovarian cancers, prophylactic hysterectomy and bilateral salpingo-oophorectomy should be considered in Lynch syndrome women who have completed childbearing. Urinalysis and cytology have been considered for screening for urothelial cancers.[136] While this is noninvasive and relatively inexpensive, these tests are not particularly sensitive nor specific. Upper endoscopy may be used to screen for gastric and small bowel cancers, but there is no evidence regarding their cost effectiveness. Annual or biannual dermatologic exams for patients with Lynch syndrome can be considered for the detection of sebaceous skin neoplasms.[6,121]

Clinical Management: Chemoprevention.

The Colorectal Adenoma/Carcinoma Prevention Programme 2 (CAPP2) trial was a 2 × 2 design, large multicenter, double-blind, randomized study comparing the effect of 600 mg aspirin daily versus placebo, or resistant starch versus placebo, on the development of CRC in Lynch syndrome patients.[137] Lynch syndrome patients who took aspirin for at least 2 years had an almost 60% decrease in CRC incidence compared with those patients who took a placebo. It is important to note that a statistical benefit was not realized until 10 years after entry into the study, even after stopping the aspirin. At least 2 years of aspirin use was also associated with a 55% reduction in other cancers associated with Lynch syndrome. The tested dose of aspirin (600 mg) used in CAPP2 is not a standard formulation in the United States. Currently, the evidence is not sufficiently mature to recommend the routine use of high-dose aspirin in Lynch syndrome patients.[108,121] There is an ongoing CAPP3 trial that aims to establish the best effective dose and duration of aspirin treatment in Lynch patients.[138]

Clinical Management: Surgery for Colorectal Cancer.

CRC management in Lynch syndrome patients requires thoughtful decision making that balances the risk of metachronous CRC against expected postoperative quality of life. Surgery is based on the oncologic principles of obtaining adequate margins, high vascular ligation and appropriate regional lymphadenectomy. However, unlike patients with sporadic CRC, Lynch syndrome patients have a significant risk of developing metachronous CRC in any residual colorectal tissue. Thus, expert opinion recommends the extended resection of colon cancer to include a total colectomy with IRA.[108,121,139] Multiple retrospective studies have demonstrated a higher rate of metachronous CRC following segmental colectomy compared with extended colectomy with risks after segmental colectomy between 11% and 45%, at a follow-up of 8 to 13 years.[140-142] In a large international study from the Colon Cancer Family Registries, the cumulative risk of metachronous CRC after segmental colectomy was 16%, 41%, and 62% at 10, 20, and 30 years, respectively.[143] Although colectomy and IRA removes most mucosa at risk for cancer, the risk of metachronous rectal cancer is between 3% and 12% at 10 to 12 years, which underscores the importance of continued surveillance of the remaining rectum. Annual surveillance by flexible proctoscopy, which can be performed in the office setting without sedation is recommended.

Reduction in metachronous cancer risk must be balanced against the bowel functional expectations after an extended colectomy. A study from the Netherlands compared outcomes of Lynch syndrome patients who underwent a total abdominal colectomy and IRA compared with a segmental colectomy.[144] Patients who underwent subtotal or total colectomy had a higher stool frequency, and a worse score on stool-related aspects and social impact. However, this did not equate to any difference in perceived quality of life based on the Short Form-36 survey. The authors concluded that although functional outcomes are worse after subtotal colectomy than after partial colectomy, generic quality of life does not differ after the two different surgeries in Lynch syndrome. Surgical decision making should be done after an educational conversation with the patient considering the family history, the patient's individual situation, the patient's feelings on risk aversion, other medical comorbidities, and life expectancy.

Despite the relative incidence of proximal colonic lesions in Lynch syndrome, rectal cancer is common. Approximately 20% to 30% of patients with Lynch syndrome will develop rectal cancer, including 15% to 24% with rectal cancer as their initial presentation.[145–147] As with colon cancer, there are many factors to consider when planning surgical management of rectal cancer in a Lynch syndrome patient. Surgical options include a proctectomy in the form of a low anterior resection (LAR) or APR, depending on sphincter involvement; or an extended resection that removes all at-risk colorectum in the form of a TPC and EI or more commonly a restorative IPAA. When determining the extent of resection, the surgeon must consider the risk of metachronous colon cancer, bowel function, quality of life, and patient comorbidities.

The risk of colon cancer after proctectomy alone in Lynch syndrome is between 15% and 54% at about 10 to 15 years' follow-up.[145,146,148,149] In a study from the Colon Cancer Family Registries, the cumulative risk of metachronous colon cancer after proctectomy was 19% at 10 years, 47% at 20 years, and 69% at 30 years.[149] However, there are functional implications after a TPC compared with a proctectomy alone. As there are no prospective trials data evaluating bowel function after IPAA for rectal cancer in Lynch syndrome, data can be extrapolated from pouch function and quality of life studied in other diseases, and that information can be applied to Lynch syndrome patients. Proctectomy alone with colorectal anastomosis yields less frequent bowel movements and more normal function (less incontinence and seepage) than after an IPAA.[150] The consistency of stool is looser, and function may be worse in patients with baseline weak anal sphincter tone.[151] However, this does not discount that IPAA can result in good functional outcomes. In FAP patients, TPC and IPAA is often done to reduce CRC risk, while maintaining acceptable bowel function with comparable results in terms of bowel movements per day, urgency, seepage, and incontinence.[152]

TPC for rectal cancer in Lynch syndrome remains debated, and several factors, including the patient's age, medical comorbidities, rectal cancer stage, sphincter function, and compliance with surveillance regimens, should be evaluated with the patient in the larger clinical picture. Given the high risk of metachronous neoplasia after a segmental proctectomy, many experts recommend TPC with an IPAA.

Variations of Lynch Syndrome

Muir-Torre Syndrome. Muir-Torre syndrome is a clinical variant of Lynch syndrome characterized by skin sebaceous gland neoplasms (sebaceous adenomas and carcinomas) and/or hair follicle neoplasms (keratoacanthomas) in addition to other Lynch-associated tumors. Sebaceous adenomas on the trunk or extremities are the most common presentation.[153,154] It is most commonly associated with an *MSH2* mutation.[155] The clinical presentation of sebaceous adenomas should raise suspicion for Muir-Torre syndrome and prompt the obtaining of a detailed family history and referral to genetic counseling.

Turcot Syndrome. Turcot syndrome is characterized by the presence of CRC and a brain tumor. It is associated with an MMR gene mutation in Lynch syndrome, or it also can be associated with an *APC* mutation. Turcot syndrome with an MMR gene mutation is commonly associated with glioblastoma,[156] while cases associated with an *APC* mutation more commonly are associated with anaplastic astrocytoma, ependymoma or medulloblastoma.

Constitutional Mismatch Repair Deficiency. Constitutional mismatch repair deficiency (CMMRD) is a rare variant of Lynch syndrome caused by biallelic inheritance of MMR genetic variations. Patients exhibit a distinct phenotype with the development of CRC at very young ages (before age 20), multiple adenomatous polyps numbering between 10 and 100, café-au-lait skin lesions, hematologic malignancies, and brain tumors.[157] The mean age of first cancer diagnosis is 16 years.[157] The reader is referred to a recently published Multisociety Taskforce comprehensive review on CRC in CMMRD.[157]

FAMILIAL COLORECTAL CANCER TYPE X

FCC X is a clinical diagnosis given to patients from families who satisfy Amsterdam criteria, but whose CRC is an MSS tumor.[109,158,159] Approximately 40% of patients meeting Amsterdam I criteria have MSS tumors. The genetic causes of FCC X are not delineated, and it is likely that this group represents a heterogeneous population genetically. Although these patients do not have the same cancer risk as Lynch syndrome patients, they do have an approximately twofold increased CRC risk compared with the general population.[109,159] The mean age of CRC diagnosis is 61 years, which is between that of Lynch syndrome patients and sporadic cancer patients. Screening by colonoscopy is recommended at age 45, or 10 years younger than the youngest CRC in that family. If no pathology is found on that exam, the colonoscopy should be repeated every 5 years. For FCC X patients who develop CRC, a segmental rather than total colectomy is recommended as the metachronous CRC risk is not completely defined, and there is no evidence that extended colectomy significantly decreases subsequent CRCs. Another important distinction between FCC X and Lynch syndrome is the lack of increased extracolonic cancer risk in FCC X patients. Thus, extracolonic screening is not recommended.[109,159,160]

LYNCH-LIKE OR TUMOR LYNCH

There is a more recently defined subset of patients distinct from Lynch syndrome and FCC X. The practice of universal screening of CRCs for MSI-H and MMR protein deficiency has increasingly identified patients with tumor characteristics suggestive of Lynch syndrome. However, when germline testing for the causative mutation is explored, some patients have no identified genetic variant. This group of patients with a tumor profile suggesting Lynch syndrome, but without an explained germline variant in any of the major MMR genes, has been called Tumor Lynch, Lynch-like syndrome,[6,161,162] suspected Lynch syndrome,[163] or mutation-negative Lynch syndrome.[164] There are multiple reasons why a germline mutation is not found in these situations.[6,165,166] Recently, studies have reported that up to 69% of these patients can be explained by biallelic somatic mutations within the tumor.[161,165,166]

These patients do not have Lynch syndrome, and thus, neither the individual nor their family have an increased risk of colorectal or extracolonic cancers based on genetics. These patients and families should be managed according to their family history and other risk factors. Importantly, 50% of these cases of Tumor Lynch are still not defined. In this situation, a family history is even more critical to help assess likely risk. If Lynch syndrome cannot be eliminated from the diagnosis, these patients should be managed as if they have Lynch syndrome, especially if they have a suspicious family history. This clinical situation is being actively researched, and nomenclature and risk assessments are evolving.

REFERENCES

1. Cancer Genome Atlas Network. Comprehensive molecular characterization of human colon and rectal cancer. *Nature*. 2012;487(7407):330-337.
2. Fearon ER, Vogelstein B. A genetic model for colorectal tumorigenesis. *Cell*. 1990;61(5):759-767.
3. Drost J, van Jaarsveld RH, Ponsioen B, et al. Sequential cancer mutations in cultured human intestinal stem cells. *Nature*. 2015;521(7550):43-47.
4. Clevers H, Nusse R. Wnt/beta-catenin signaling and disease. *Cell*. 2012;149(6):1192-1205.
5. Lao VV, Grady WM. Epigenetics and colorectal cancer. *Nat Rev Gastroenterol Hepatol*. 2011;8(12):686-700.
6. Rodriguez-Soler M, Perez-Carbonell L, Guarinos C, et al. Risk of cancer in cases of suspected Lynch syndrome without germline mutation. *Gastroenterology*. 2013;144(5):926-932 e921 quiz e913-924.
7. Boland CR, Goel A. Microsatellite instability in colorectal cancer. *Gastroenterology*. 2010;138(6):2073-2087, e2073.
8. Yurgelun MB, Goel A, Hornick JL, et al. Microsatellite instability and DNA mismatch repair protein deficiency in Lynch syndrome colorectal polyps. *Cancer Prev Res (Phila)*. 2012;5(4):574-582.
9. Kloor M, Huth C, Voigt AY, et al. Prevalence of mismatch repair-deficient crypt foci in Lynch syndrome: a pathological study. *Lancet Oncol*. 2012;13(6):598-606.
10. Jarvinen HJ. Epidemiology of familial adenomatous polyposis in Finland: impact of family screening on the colorectal cancer rate and survival. *Gut*. 1992;33(3):357-360.
11. Lucci-Cordisco E, Risio M, Venesio T, Genuardi M. The growing complexity of the intestinal polyposis syndromes. *Am J Med Genet A*. 2013;161A(11):2777-2787.
12. Galiatsatos P, Foulkes WD. Familial adenomatous polyposis. *Am J Gastroenterol*. 2006;101(2):385-398.
13. Septer S, Lawson CE, Anant S, Attard T. Familial adenomatous polyposis in pediatrics: natural history, emerging surveillance and management protocols, chemopreventive strategies, and areas of ongoing debate. *Fam Cancer*. 2016;15(3):477-485.
14. Ripa R, Bisgaard ML, Bulow S, Nielsen FC. De novo mutations in familial adenomatous polyposis (FAP). *Eur J Hum Genet*. 2002;10(10):631-637.
15. Snow AK, Tuohy TM, Sargent NR, Smith LJ, Burt RW, Neklason DW. APC promoter 1B deletion in seven American families with familial adenomatous polyposis. *Clin Genet*. 2015;88(4):360-365.
16. Herrera L, Kakati S, Gibas L, Pietrzak E, Sandberg AA. Gardner syndrome in a man with an interstitial deletion of 5q. *Am J Med Genet*. 1986;25(3):473-476.
17. Venesio T, Balsamo A, Rondo-Spaudo M, et al. APC haploinsufficiency, but not CTNNB1 or CDH1 gene mutations, accounts for a fraction of familial adenomatous polyposis patients without APC truncating mutations. *Lab Invest*. 2003;83(12):1859-1866.
18. Vasen HF, Velthuizen ME, Kleibeuker JH, Varesco L, Risio M, Ranzani GN. Hereditary cancer registries improve the care of patients with a genetic predisposition to cancer: contributions from the Dutch Lynch syndrome registry. *Fam Cancer*. 2016;15(3):429-435.
19. de Campos FG, Perez RO, Imperiale AR, Seid VE, Nahas SC, Cecconello I. Evaluating causes of death in familial adenomatous polyposis. *J Gastrointest Surg*. 2010;14(12):1943-1949.
20. Church JM, McGannon E, Hull-Boiner S, et al. Gastroduodenal polyps in patients with familial adenomatous polyposis. *Dis Colon Rectum*. 1992;35(12):1170-1173.
21. Church JM, McGannon E, Burke C, Clark B. Teenagers with familial adenomatous polyposis: what is their risk for colorectal cancer? *Dis Colon Rectum*. 2002;45(7):887-889.
22. Hartley JE, Church JM, Gupta S, McGannon E, Fazio VW. Significance of incidental desmoids identified during surgery for familial adenomatous polyposis. *Dis Colon Rectum*. 2004;47(3):334-338, discussion 339-340.
23. Liang J, Church JM. Rectal cancers in patients with familial adenomatous polyposis. *Fam Cancer*. 2013;12(4):749-754.
24. Church J, Burke C, McGannon E, Pastean O, Clark B. Predicting polyposis severity by proctoscopy: how reliable is it? *Dis Colon Rectum*. 2001;44(9):1249-1254.
25. Church JM. Controversies in the surgery of patients with familial adenomatous polyposis and Lynch syndrome. *Fam Cancer*. 2016;15(3):447-451.
26. Ziv Y, Church JM, Oakley JR, McGannon E, Fazio VW. Surgery for the teenager with familial adenomatous polyposis: ileo-rectal anastomosis or restorative proctocolectomy? *Int J Colorectal Dis*. 1995;10(1):6-9.
27. Feinberg SM, Jagelman DG, Sarre RG, et al. Spontaneous resolution of rectal polyps in patients with familial polyposis following abdominal colectomy and ileorectal anastomosis. *Dis Colon Rectum*. 1988;31(3):169-175.
28. Hassan I, Chua HK, Wolff BG, et al. Quality of life after ileal pouch-anal anastomosis and ileorectal anastomosis in patients with familial adenomatous polyposis. *Dis Colon Rectum*. 2005;48(11):2032-2037.
29. Wu XR, Kirat HT, Kalady MF, Church JM. Restorative proctocolectomy with a handsewn IPAA: S-pouch or J-pouch? *Dis Colon Rectum*. 2015;58(2):205-213.
30. Lovegrove RE, Constantinides VA, Heriot AG, et al. A comparison of hand-sewn versus stapled ileal pouch anal anastomosis (IPAA) following proctocolectomy: a meta-analysis of 4183 patients. *Ann Surg*. 2006;244(1):18-26.
31. Hurlstone DP, Saunders BP, Church JM. Endoscopic surveillance of the ileoanal pouch following restorative proctocolectomy for familial adenomatous polyposis. *Endoscopy*. 2008;40(5):437-442.
32. Parc YR, Olschwang S, Desaint B, Schmitt G, Parc RG, Tiret E. Familial adenomatous polyposis: prevalence of adenomas in the ileal pouch after restorative proctocolectomy. *Ann Surg*. 2001;233(3):360-364.
33. Church J. Ileoanal pouch neoplasia in familial adenomatous polyposis: an underestimated threat. *Dis Colon Rectum*. 2005;48(9):1708-1713.
34. Cruz-Correa M, Hylind LM, Romans KE, Booker SV, Giardiello FM. Long-term treatment with sulindac in familial adenomatous polyposis: a prospective cohort study. *Gastroenterology*. 2002;122(3):641-645.
35. Park GD, Spector R, Headstream T, Goldberg M. Serious adverse reactions associated with sulindac. *Arch Intern Med*. 1982;142(7):1292-1294.
36. Winde G, Schmid KW, Brandt B, Müller O, Osswald H. Clinical and genomic influence of sulindac on rectal mucosa in familial adenomatous polyposis. *Dis Colon Rectum*. 1997;40(10):1156-1168, discussion 1168-1159.
37. Tsukada K, Church JM, Jagelman DG, et al. Noncytotoxic drug therapy for intra-abdominal desmoid tumor in patients with familial adenomatous polyposis. *Dis Colon Rectum*. 1992;35(1):29-33.
38. Lynch HT, Thorson AG, Smyrk T. Rectal cancer after prolonged sulindac chemoprevention. A case report. *Cancer*. 1995;75(4):936-938.
39. Samadder NJ, Neklason DW, Boucher KM, et al. Effect of sulindac and erlotinib vs placebo on duodenal neoplasia in familial adenomatous polyposis: a randomized clinical trial. *JAMA*. 2016;315(12):1266-1275.
40. Quintini C, Ward G, Shatnawei A, et al. Mortality of intra-abdominal desmoid tumors in patients with familial adenomatous polyposis: a single center review of 154 patients. *Ann Surg*. 2012;255(3):511-516.
41. Xhaja X, Church J. Small bowel obstruction in patients with familial adenomatous polyposis related desmoid disease. *Colorectal Dis*. 2013;15(12):1489-1492.
42. Joyce M, Mignanelli E, Church J. Ureteric obstruction in familial adenomatous polyposis-associated desmoid disease. *Dis Colon Rectum*. 2010;53(3):327-332.
43. Xhaja X, Church J. Enterocutaneous fistulae in familial adenomatous polyposis patients with abdominal desmoid disease. *Colorectal Dis*. 2013;15(10):1238-1242.

44. Church J, McGannon E, Ozuner G. The clinical course of intra-abdominal desmoid tumours in patients with familial adenomatous polyposis. *Colorectal Dis.* 1999;1(3):168-173.

45. Church JM, Xhaja X, Warrier SK, et al. Desmoid tumors do not prevent proctectomy following abdominal colectomy and ileorectal anastomosis in patients with familial adenomatous polyposis. *Dis Colon Rectum.* 2014;57(3):343-347.

46. Church J, Xhaja X, LaGuardia L, O'Malley M, Burke C, Kalady M. Desmoids and genotype in familial adenomatous polyposis. *Dis Colon Rectum.* 2015;58(4):444-448.

47. Church J, Berk T, Boman BM, et al. Staging intra-abdominal desmoid tumors in familial adenomatous polyposis: a search for a uniform approach to a troubling disease. *Dis Colon Rectum.* 2005;48(8):1528-1534.

48. Church J, Lynch C, Neary P, LaGuardia L, Elayi E. A desmoid tumor-staging system separates patients with intra-abdominal, familial adenomatous polyposis-associated desmoid disease by behavior and prognosis. *Dis Colon Rectum.* 2008;51(6):897-901.

49. Quast DR, Schneider R, Burdzik E, Hoppe S, Möslein G. Long-term outcome of sporadic and FAP-associated desmoid tumors treated with high-dose selective estrogen receptor modulators and sulindac: a single-center long-term observational study in 134 patients. *Fam Cancer.* 2016;15(1):31-40.

50. Toiyama Y, Konishi N, Inoue Y, et al. Successful treatment of ileal pouch desmoids using multimodal chemotherapy with low-dose vinblastine and methotrexate in a patient with familial adenomatous polyposis. *Clin J Gastroenterol.* 2009;2(3):170-174.

51. Bertagnolli MM, Morgan JA, Fletcher CDM, et al. Multimodality treatment of mesenteric desmoid tumours. *Eur J Cancer.* 2008;44(16):2404-2410.

52. Gega M, Yanagi H, Yoshikawa R, et al. Successful chemotherapeutic modality of doxorubicin plus dacarbazine for the treatment of desmoid tumors in association with familial adenomatous polyposis. *J Clin Oncol.* 2006;24(1):102-105.

53. Rodriguez-Bigas MA, Mahoney MC, Karakousis CP, et al. Desmoid tumors in patients with familial adenomatous polyposis. *Cancer.* 1994;74(4):1270-1274.

54. Latchford AR, Sturt NJH, Neale K, Rogers PA, Phillips RK. A 10-year review of surgery for desmoid disease associated with familial adenomatous polyposis. *Br J Surg.* 2006;93(10):1258-1264.

55. Clark SK, Neale KF, Landgrebe JC, Phillips RK. Desmoid tumours complicating familial adenomatous polyposis. *Br J Surg.* 1999;86(9):1185-1189.

56. Galle TS, Juel K, Bulow S. Causes of death in familial adenomatous polyposis. *Scand J Gastroenterol.* 1999;34(8):808-812.

57. Bianchi LK, Burke CA, Bennett AE, Lopez R, Hasson H, Church JM. Fundic gland polyp dysplasia is common in familial adenomatous polyposis. *Clin Gastroenterol Hepatol.* 2008;6(2):180-185.

58. Ngamruengphong S, Boardman LA, Heigh RI, Krishna M, Roberts ME, Riegert-Johnson DL. Gastric adenomas in familial adenomatous polyposis are common, but subtle, and have a benign course. *Hered Cancer Clin Pract.* 2014;12:4.

59. Spigelman AD, Williams CB, Talbot IC, Domizio P, Phillips RK. Upper gastrointestinal cancer in patients with familial adenomatous polyposis. *Lancet.* 1989;2(8666):783-785.

60. Groves CJ, Saunders BP, Spigelman AD, Phillips RK. Duodenal cancer in patients with familial adenomatous polyposis (FAP): results of a 10 year prospective study. *Gut.* 2002;50(5):636-641.

61. Johnson MD, Mackey R, Brown N, Church J, Burke C, Walsh RM. Outcome based on management for duodenal adenomas: sporadic versus familial disease. *J Gastrointest Surg.* 2010;14(2):229-235.

62. Latchford AR, Neale KF, Spigelman AD, Phillips RK, Clark SK. Features of duodenal cancer in patients with familial adenomatous polyposis. *Clin Gastroenterol Hepatol.* 2009;7(6):659-663.

63. Skipworth JR, Morkane C, Raptis DA, et al. Pancreaticoduodenectomy for advanced duodenal and ampullary adenomatosis in familial adenomatous polyposis. *HPB (Oxford).* 2011;13(5):342-349.

64. Feng X, Milas M, O'Malley M, et al. Characteristics of benign and malignant thyroid disease in familial adenomatous polyposis patients and recommendations for disease surveillance. *Thyroid.* 2015;25(3):325-332.

65. Smith TG, Clark SK, Katz DE, Reznek RH, Phillips RK. Adrenal masses are associated with familial adenomatous polyposis. *Dis Colon Rectum.* 2000;43(12):1739-1742.

66. Aretz S, Koch A, Uhlhaas S, et al. Should children at risk for familial adenomatous polyposis be screened for hepatoblastoma and children with apparently sporadic hepatoblastoma be screened for APC germline mutations? *Pediatr Blood Cancer.* 2006;47(6):811-818.

67. Knudsen AL, Bulow S, Tomlinson I, et al. Attenuated familial adenomatous polyposis: results from an international collaborative study. *Colorectal Dis.* 2010;12(10 Online):e243-e249.

68. Sampson JR, Dolwani S, Jones S, et al. Autosomal recessive colorectal adenomatous polyposis due to inherited mutations of MYH. *Lancet.* 2003;362(9377):39-41.

69. Weren RD, Ligtenberg MJ, Kets CM, et al. A germline homozygous mutation in the base-excision repair gene NTHL1 causes adenomatous polyposis and colorectal cancer. *Nat Genet.* 2015;47(6):668-671.

70. Lefevre JH, Parc Y, Svrcek M, et al. APC, MYH, and the correlation genotype-phenotype in colorectal polyposis. *Ann Surg Oncol.* 2009;16(4):871-877.

71. Church J, Heald B, Burke C, Kalady M. Understanding MYH-associated neoplasia. *Dis Colon Rectum.* 2012;55(3):359-362.

72. Church J, Kravochuck S. The "studded" rectum: phenotypic evidence of MYH-associated polyposis. *Dis Colon Rectum.* 2016;59(6):565-569.

73. Palles C, Cazier JB, Howarth KM, et al. Germline mutations affecting the proofreading domains of POLE and POLD1 predispose to colorectal adenomas and carcinomas. *Nat Genet.* 2013;45(2):136-144.

74. Latchford AR, Neale K, Phillips RK, et al. Juvenile polyposis syndrome: a study of genotype, phenotype, and long-term outcome. *Dis Colon Rectum.* 2012;55(10):1038-1043.

75. Hofting I, Pott G, Stolte M. [The syndrome of juvenile polyposis]. *Leber Magen Darm.* 1993;23(3):107-108, 111–102.

76. Sachatello CR, Hahn IS, Carrington CB. Juvenile gastrointestinal polyposis in a female infant: report of a case and review of the literature of a recently recognized syndrome. *Surgery.* 1974;75(1):107-114.

77. Aytac E, Sulu B, Heald B, et al. Genotype-defined cancer risk in juvenile polyposis syndrome. *Br J Surg.* 2015;102(1):114-118.

78. O'Malley M, LaGuardia L, Kalady MF, et al. The prevalence of hereditary hemorrhagic telangiectasia in juvenile polyposis syndrome. *Dis Colon Rectum.* 2012;55(8):886-892.

79. Howe JR, Mitros FA, Summers RW. The risk of gastrointestinal carcinoma in familial juvenile polyposis. *Ann Surg Oncol.* 1998;5:751-756.

80. Brosens LA, van Hattem A, Hylind LM, et al. Risk of colorectal cancer in juvenile polyposis. *Gut.* 2007;56(7):965-967.

81. Jass JR, Williams CB, Bussey HJ, Morson BC. Juvenile polyposis—a precancerous condition. *Histopathology.* 1988;13(6):619-630.

82. Kinzler KW, Vogelstein B. Landscaping the cancer terrain. *Science.* 1998;280(5366):1036-1037.

83. Coburn MC, Pricolo VE, DeLuca FG, Bland KI. Malignant potential in intestinal juvenile polyposis syndromes. *Ann Surg Oncol.* 1995;2(5):386-391.

84. Oncel M, Church JM, Remzi FH, Fazio VW. Colonic surgery in patients with juvenile polyposis syndrome: a case series. *Dis Colon Rectum.* 2005;48(1):49-55, discussion 55-46.

85. McGarrity TJ, Kulin HE, Zaino RJ. Peutz-Jeghers syndrome. *Am J Gastroenterol.* 2000;95(3):596-604.

86. Oncel M, Remzi FH, Church JM, Connor JT, Fazio VW. Benefits of 'clean sweep' in Peutz-Jeghers patients. *Colorectal Dis.* 2004;6(5):332-335.

87. Spigelman AD, Murday V, Phillips RK. Cancer and the Peutz-Jeghers syndrome. *Gut.* 1989;30(11):1588-1590.

88. Giardiello FM, Brensinger JD, Tersmette AC, et al. Very high risk of cancer in familial Peutz-Jeghers syndrome. *Gastroenterology.* 2000;119(6):1447-1453.

89. Giardiello FM, Welsh SB, Hamilton SR, et al. Increased risk of cancer in the Peutz-Jeghers syndrome. *N Engl J Med.* 1987;316(24):1511-1514.

90. McGrath DR, Spigelman AD. Preventive measures in Peutz-Jeghers syndrome. *Fam Cancer.* 2001;1(2):121-125.

91. Parsi MA, Burke CA. Utility of capsule endoscopy in Peutz-Jeghers syndrome. *Gastrointest Endosc Clin N Am.* 2004;14(1):159-167.

92. Schulmann K, Schmiegel W. Capsule endoscopy for small bowel surveillance in hereditary intestinal polyposis and non-polyposis syndromes. *Gastrointest Endosc Clin N Am.* 2004;14(1):149-158.

93. Calva D, Howe JR. Hamartomatous polyposis syndromes. *Surg Clin North Am.* 2008;88(4):779-817.

94. Zbuk KM, Eng C. Hamartomatous polyposis syndromes. *Nat Clin Pract Gastroenterol Hepatol.* 2007;4(9):492-502.

95. Giardiello FM, Trimbath JD, Giardiello FM, et al. Peutz-Jeghers syndrome and management recommendations. *Clin Gastroenterol Hepatol.* 2006;4(4):408-415.

96. Marsh DJ, Dahia PL, Caron S, et al. Germline PTEN mutations in Cowden syndrome-like families. *J Med Genet.* 1998;35(11):881-885.

97. Marsh DJ, Dahia PL, Coulon V, et al. Allelic imbalance, including deletion of PTEN/MMAC1, at the Cowden disease locus on 10q22-23, in hamartomas from patients with Cowden syndrome and germline PTEN mutation. *Genes Chromosomes Cancer.* 1998;21(1):61-69.

98. Gustafson S, Zbuk KM, Scacheri C, Eng C. Cowden syndrome. *Semin Oncol.* 2007;34(5):428-434.

99. Heald B, Mester J, Rybicki L, Orloff MS, Burke CA, Eng C. Frequent gastrointestinal polyps and colorectal adenocarcinomas in a prospective series of PTEN mutation carriers. *Gastroenterology.* 2010;139(6):1927-1933.

100. Stanich PP, Owens VL, Sweetser S, et al. Colonic polyposis and neoplasia in Cowden syndrome. *Mayo Clin Proc.* 2011;86(6):489-492.

101. Tan MH, Mester JL, Ngeow J, Rybicki LA, Orloff MS, Eng C. Lifetime cancer risks in individuals with germline PTEN mutations. *Clin Cancer Res.* 2012;18(2):400-407.

102. Riegert-Johnson DL, Gleeson FC, Roberts M, et al. Cancer and Lhermitte-Duclos disease are common in Cowden syndrome patients. *Hered Cancer Clin Pract.* 2010;8(1):6.

103. Syngal S, Brand RE, Church JM, et al. ACG clinical guideline: genetic testing and management of hereditary gastrointestinal cancer syndromes. *Am J Gastroenterol.* 2015;110(2):223-262, quiz 263.

104. Gorlin RJ, Cohen MM Jr, Condon LM, et al. Bannayan-Riley-Ruvalcaba syndrome. *Am J Med Genet.* 1992;44(3):307-314.

105. Whitelaw SC, Murday VA, Tomlinson IP, et al. Clinical and molecular features of the hereditary mixed polyposis syndrome. *Gastroenterology.* 1997;112(2):327-334.

106. Jaeger E, Leedham S, Lewis A, et al. Hereditary mixed polyposis syndrome is caused by a 40-kb upstream duplication that leads to increased and ectopic expression of the BMP antagonist GREM1. *Nat Genet.* 2012;44(6):699-703.

107. Vasen HF, Watson P, Mecklin JP, Lynch HT. New clinical criteria for hereditary nonpolyposis colorectal cancer (HNPCC, Lynch syndrome) proposed by the International Collaborative group on HNPCC. *Gastroenterology.* 1999;116(6):1453-1456.

108. Giardiello FM, Allen JI, Axilbund JE, et al. Guidelines on genetic evaluation and management of Lynch syndrome: a consensus statement by the US Multi-Society Task Force on Colorectal Cancer. *Am J Gastroenterol.* 2014;109(8):1159-1179.

109. Lindor NM, Rabe K, Petersen GM, et al. Lower cancer incidence in Amsterdam-I criteria families without mismatch repair deficiency: familial colorectal cancer type X. *JAMA.* 2005;293(16):1979-1985.

110. Hampel H, Frankel WL, Martin E, et al. Screening for the Lynch syndrome (hereditary nonpolyposis colorectal cancer). *N Engl J Med.* 2005;352(18):1851-1860.

111. Aaltonen LA, Sankila R, Mecklin JP, et al. A novel approach to estimate the proportion of hereditary nonpolyposis colorectal cancer of total colorectal cancer burden. *Cancer Detect Prev.* 1994;18(1):57-63.

112. de la Chapelle A. The incidence of Lynch syndrome. *Fam Cancer.* 2005;4(3):233-237.

113. Umar A, Boland CR, Terdiman JP, et al. Revised Bethesda Guidelines for hereditary nonpolyposis colorectal cancer (Lynch syndrome) and microsatellite instability. *J Natl Cancer Inst.* 2004;96(4):261-268.

114. Teutsch SM, Bradley LA, Palomaki GE, et al. The Evaluation of Genomic Applications in Practice and Prevention (EGAPP) Initiative: methods of the EGAPP Working Group. *Genet Med.* 2009;11(1):3-14.

115. Beamer LC, Grant ML, Espenschied CR, et al. Reflex immunohistochemistry and microsatellite instability testing of colorectal tumors for Lynch syndrome among US cancer programs and follow-up of abnormal results. *J Clin Oncol.* 2012;30(10):1058-1063.

116. Weissman SM, Burt R, Church J, et al. Identification of individuals at risk for Lynch syndrome using targeted evaluations and genetic testing: National Society of Genetic Counselors and the Collaborative Group of the Americas on Inherited Colorectal Cancer joint practice guideline. *J Genet Couns.* 2012;21(4):484-493.

117. Genetic/Familial High-Risk Assessment: Colorectal. NCCN Clinical Practice Guidelines in Oncology. 2014.

118. Aaltonen LA, Peltomaki P, Leach FS, et al. Clues to the pathogenesis of familial colorectal cancer. *Science.* 1993;260(5109):812-816.

119. Kim H, Jen J, Vogelstein B, Hamilton SR. Clinical and pathological characteristics of sporadic colorectal carcinomas with DNA replication errors in microsatellite sequences. *Am J Pathol.* 1994;145(1):148-156.

120. Barrow E, Hill J, Evans DG. Cancer risk in Lynch syndrome. *Fam Cancer.* 2013;12(2):229-240.

121. Vasen HF, Blanco I, Aktan-Collan K, et al. Revised guidelines for the clinical management of Lynch syndrome (HNPCC): recommendations by a group of European experts. *Gut.* 2013;62(6):812-823.

122. Goodenberger ML, Thomas BC, Riegert-Johnson D, et al. PMS2 monoallelic mutation carriers: the known unknown. *Genet Med.* 2016;18(1):13-19.

123. Baglietto L, Lindor NM, Dowty JG, et al. Risks of Lynch syndrome cancers for MSH6 mutation carriers. *J Natl Cancer Inst.* 2010;102(3):193-201.

124. Senter L, Clendenning M, Sotamaa K, et al. The clinical phenotype of Lynch syndrome due to germ-line PMS2 mutations. *Gastroenterology.* 2008;135(2):419-428.

125. Aarnio M, Sankila R, Pukkala E, et al. Cancer risk in mutation carriers of DNA-mismatch-repair genes. *Int J Cancer.* 1999;81(2):214-218.

126. Hampel H, Stephens JA, Pukkala E, et al. Cancer risk in hereditary nonpolyposis colorectal cancer syndrome: later age of onset. *Gastroenterology.* 2005;129(2):415-421.

127. Stoffel E, Mukherjee B, Raymond VM, et al. Calculation of risk of colorectal and endometrial cancer among patients with Lynch syndrome. *Gastroenterology.* 2009;137(5):1621-1627.

128. Deleted in review.

129. Pal T, Permuth-Wey J, Sellers TA. A review of the clinical relevance of mismatch-repair deficiency in ovarian cancer. *Cancer.* 2008;113(4):733-742.

130. Win AK, Young JP, Lindor NM, et al. Colorectal and other cancer risks for carriers and noncarriers from families with a DNA mismatch repair gene mutation: a prospective cohort study. *J Clin Oncol.* 2012;30(9):958-964.

131. Raymond VM, Mukherjee B, Wang F, et al. Elevated risk of prostate cancer among men with Lynch syndrome. *J Clin Oncol.* 2013;31(14):1713-1718.

132. Buerki N, Gautier L, Kovac M, et al. Evidence for breast cancer as an integral part of Lynch syndrome. *Genes Chromosomes Cancer.* 2012;51(1):83-91.

133. Jarvinen HJ, Aarnio M, Mustonen H, et al. Controlled 15-year trial on screening for colorectal cancer in families with hereditary nonpolyposis colorectal cancer. *Gastroenterology.* 2000;118(5):829-834.

134. Vasen HF, Tomlinson I, Castells A. Clinical management of hereditary colorectal cancer syndromes. *Nat Rev Gastroenterol Hepatol.* 2015;12(2):88-97.

135. Reitamo J. The desmoid tumor. IV. Choice of treatment, results, and complications. *Arch Surg.* 1983;118(11):1318-1322.

136. Mork M, Hubosky SG, Roupret M, et al. Lynch syndrome: a primer for urologists and panel recommendations. *J Urol.* 2015;194(1):21-29.

137. Burn J, Gerdes AM, Macrae F, et al. Long-term effect of aspirin on cancer risk in carriers of hereditary colorectal cancer: an analysis from the CAPP2 randomised controlled trial. *Lancet.* 2011;378(9809):2081-2087.

138. Burn J, Mathers JC, Bishop DT. Chemoprevention in Lynch syndrome. *Fam Cancer.* 2013;12(4):707-718.

139. Kalady MF. Surgical management of hereditary nonpolyposis colorectal cancer. *Adv Surg.* 2011;45:265-274.

140. Fitzgibbons RJ Jr, Lynch HT, Stanislav GV, et al. Recognition and treatment of patients with hereditary nonpolyposis colon cancer (Lynch syndromes I and II). *Ann Surg.* 1987;206(3):289-295.

141. Kalady MF, McGannon E, Vogel JD, Manilich E, Fazio VW, Church JM. Risk of colorectal adenoma and carcinoma after colectomy for colorectal cancer in patients meeting Amsterdam criteria. *Ann Surg.* 2010;252(3):507-511, discuss on 511-503.

142. Natarajan N, Watson P, Silva-Lopez E, Lynch HT. Comparison of extended colectomy and limited resection in patients with Lynch syndrome. *Dis Colon Rectum.* 2010;53(1):77-82.

143. Parry S, Win AK, Parry B, et al. Metachronous colorectal cancer risk for mismatch repair gene mutation carriers: the advantage of more extensive colon surgery. *Gut.* 2011;60(7):950-957.

144. Haanstra JF, de Vos Tot Nederveen Cappel WH, Gopie JP, et al. Quality of life after surgery for colon cancer in patients with Lynch syndrome: partial versus subtotal colectomy. *Dis Colon Rectum.* 2012;55(6):653-659.

145. Kalady MF, Lipman J, McGannon E, Church JM. Risk of colonic neoplasia after proctectomy for rectal cancer in hereditary nonpolyposis colorectal cancer. *Ann Surg.* 2012;255(6):1121-1125.

146. Lee JS, Petrelli NJ, Rodriguez-Bigas MA. Rectal cancer in hereditary nonpolyposis colorectal cancer. *Am J Surg*. 2001;181(3):207-210.

147. Moslein G, Nelson H, Thibodeau S, Dozois RR. Rectal carcinomas in HNPCC. *Langenbecks Arch Chir Suppl Kongressbd*. 1998;115:1467-1469.

148. Cirillo L, Urso ED, Parrinello G, et al. High risk of rectal cancer and of metachronous colorectal cancer in probands of families fulfilling the Amsterdam criteria. *Ann Surg*. 2013;257(5):900-904.

149. Win AK, Parry S, Parry B, et al. Risk of metachronous colon cancer following surgery for rectal cancer in mismatch repair gene mutation carriers. *Ann Surg Oncol*. 2013;20(6):1829-1836.

150. Fazio VW, Kiran RP, Remzi FH, et al. Ileal pouch anal anastomosis: analysis of outcome and quality of life in 3707 patients. *Ann Surg*. 2013;257(4):679-685.

151. Fazio VW, O'Riordain MG, Lavery IC, et al. Long-term functional outcome and quality of life after stapled restorative proctocolectomy. *Ann Surg*. 1999;230(4):575-584, discussion 584–576.

152. Erkek AB, Church JM, Remzi FH. Age-related analysis of functional outcome and quality of life after restorative proctocolectomy and ileal pouch-anal anastomosis for familial adenomatous polyposis. *J Gastroenterol Hepatol*. 2007;22(5):710-714.

153. Roberts ME, Riegert-Johnson DL, Thomas BC, et al. Screening for Muir-Torre syndrome using mismatch repair protein immunohistochemistry of sebaceous neoplasms. *J Genet Couns*. 2013;22(3):393-405.

154. Cesinaro AM, Ubiali A, Sighinolfi P, et al. Mismatch repair proteins expression and microsatellite instability in skin lesions with sebaceous differentiation: a study in different clinical subgroups with and without extracutaneous cancer. *Am J Dermatopathol*. 2007;29(4):351-358.

155. Lazar AJ, Lyle S, Calonje E. Sebaceous neoplasia and Torre-Muir syndrome. *Curr Diagn Pathol*. 2007;13(4):301-319.

156. Hamilton SR, Liu B, Parsons RE, et al. The molecular basis of Turcot's syndrome. *N Engl J Med*. 1995;332(13):839-847.

157. Durno CA, Holter S, Sherman PM, Gallinger S. The gastrointestinal phenotype of germline biallelic mismatch repair gene mutations. *Am J Gastroenterol*. 2010;105(11):2449-2456.

158. Giardiello FM, Allen JI, Axilbund JE, et al. Guidelines on genetic evaluation and management of Lynch syndrome: a consensus statement by the US Multi-Society Task Force on Colorectal Cancer. *Gastroenterology*. 2014;147(2):502-526.

159. Lindor NM, Petersen GM, Hadley DW, et al. Recommendations for the care of individuals with an inherited predisposition to Lynch syndrome: a systematic review. *JAMA*. 2006;296(12):1507-1517.

160. Shiovitz S, Copeland WK, Passarelli MN, et al. Characterisation of familial colorectal cancer Type X, Lynch syndrome, and non-familial colorectal cancer. *Br J Cancer*. 2014;111(3):598-602.

161. Carethers JM. Differentiating Lynch-like from Lynch syndrome. *Gastroenterology*. 2014;146(3):602-604.

162. Boland CR. The mystery of mismatch repair deficiency: Lynch or Lynch-like? *Gastroenterology*. 2013;144(5):868-870.

163. Buchanan DD, Rosty C, Clendenning M, Spurdle AB, Win AK. Clinical problems of colorectal cancer and endometrial cancer cases with unknown cause of tumor mismatch repair deficiency (suspected Lynch syndrome). *Appl Clin Genet*. 2014;7:183-193.

164. You YN, Vilar E. Classifying MMR variants: time for revised nomenclature in Lynch syndrome. *Clin Cancer Res*. 2013;19(9):2280-2282.

165. Haraldsdottir S, Hampel H, Tomsic J, et al. Colon and endometrial cancers with mismatch repair deficiency can arise from somatic, rather than germline, mutations. *Gastroenterology*. 2014;147(6):1308-1316, e1301.

166. Mensenkamp AR, Vogelaar IP, van Zelst-Stams WA, et al. Somatic mutations in MLH1 and MSH2 are a frequent cause of mismatch-repair deficiency in Lynch syndrome-like tumors. *Gastroenterology*. 2014;146(3):643-646, e648.

Basic Principles of the Operative Treatment of Colorectal Cancer

Martin R. Weiser | Julio Garcia-Aguilar

Despite recent advances in understanding the biology of cancer that have resulted in new targeted and biological therapies, surgery is still the primary treatment for most patients with colorectal cancer. While the overall treatment plan may be different for colon and rectal cancers, the principles that guide the surgical procedures to treat them are similar. These principles, based on the Halstedian concept of tumor progression from the primary site to the regional nodes, were first introduced over a century ago. While the ideas about tumor progression have evolved and the concept of orderly tumor progression from the primary site along the lymphatic vessels to progressively more central nodal stations has been challenged, the basic principles of the operative treatment have remained unaltered due to the need to remove a minimum number of nodes for accurate staging. In addition, there is evidence that the excision of the bowel and its mesentery along anatomical planes established during embryologic development is associated with lower risk of local recurrence and improved survival. In this chapter, we will review the basic principles of colorectal resections and the specific technical details for interventions performed to treat tumors located in different segments of the large bowel.

GENERAL PRINCIPLES

Curative-intent surgery for colon and rectal cancers is aimed at removing the tumor-bearing segment of the bowel with adequate margins and excising en bloc the mesentery containing the feeding vessels and regional lymph nodes. The extent of the resection depends on the location of the primary tumor, which determines lymphatic drainage. Lymphatic capillaries are primarily located in the submucosal and subserosal layers of the bowel wall. Lymphatic flow is primarily circumferential in the colon, with longitudinal spread along the bowel wall being generally less than 1 cm in each direction. Therefore, a 5-cm margin of normal bowel on either side of the primary tumor is considered sufficient to avoid anastomotic recurrence. The length of the terminal ileum resected in patients with cecal cancer does not influence the risk of anastomotic recurrence. Since longitudinal lymphatic flow is primarily upward in the rectum, cancer cells do not generally spread distally along the bowel wall more than 1 cm from the macroscopic distal end of the tumor. Therefore, a 2-cm margin of normal bowel distal to the tumor, or an even smaller margin in patients treated with neoadjuvant therapy, is considered appropriate for an oncologically safe resection.[1] This margin may be insufficient in rectal cancer patients with extensive nodal metastasis that could block the lymphatic channels in the bowel wall and the mesorectum and redirect the lymphatic flow distally.

The regional lymph nodes of the colon are classified into four main groups on the basis of their proximity to the bowel and its blood supply: epicolic, paracolic, intermediate, and apical (Fig. 166-1). Epicolic lymph nodes are located in the bowel wall under the peritoneum, often close to the epiploic appendices; paracolic nodes are found along the marginal vessels; intermediate nodes are in the middle of the mesentery; and apical (or central) nodes are located close to the root of the mesentery, in the vicinity of the origin of the named vessels. Although colorectal cancer generally spreads sequentially from paracolic to apical lymph nodes, nodal metastases sometimes skip one of the nodal groups.[2] Therefore an oncologic resection should include all nodal groups.

The application of the principles of the sentinel node used extensively in breast cancer and melanoma surgery remains controversial in colon and rectal cancer surgery.[3] The injection of isosulfan blue or radioactive dye in the periphery of the tumor to identify the apical node was found to improve staging and to modify the extent of the resection in several retrospective case series.[4] These results have not been replicated in prospective trials.[5,6] Therefore, the principle of sentinel node sampling is rarely used in colon and rectal cancer surgery today.

The extent of mesenteric resection for colon cancer is determined by the need to remove all the lymph nodes draining the corresponding segment of the bowel, including the central lymph nodes. Since in most cases a tumor is located between two named vascular pedicles, both pedicles should be resected at their origin. When central nodes are suspected of being involved by the tumor, they should be marked on the specimen, as they have negative prognostic information. Because lymphatic drainage does not always follow an orderly pattern, lymph nodes located away from the feeding vessels and suspected of tumor involvement should be removed during surgery and analyzed.[4,7] If metastatic lymph nodes are not removed during surgery, the resection is considered incomplete.

In addition to achieving safe oncologic margins and adequate lymphadenectomy, ensuring sufficient blood supply to the bowel ends and maintaining tension-free anastomosis in order to avoid anastomotic complications are also important goals of surgical resection for colorectal cancer.

A locally advanced tumor attached to adjacent organs should be removed en bloc with the contiguously involved structures. Since inflammatory adhesions cannot be distinguished clinically or radiographically from tumor infiltration, en bloc resection of the affected organ avoids the risk of disseminating cancer cells associated with the separation of structures infiltrated by the tumor. Intraoperative tumor perforation has negative prognostic implications. The relative completeness of the resection

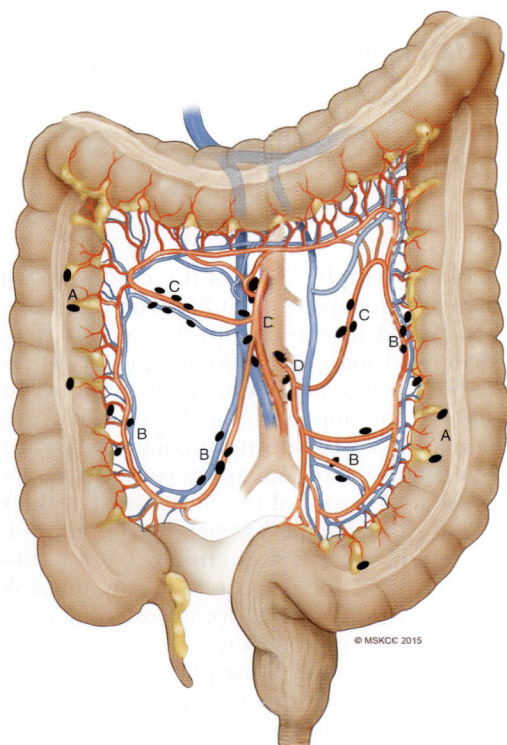

FIGURE 166.1 Anatomy of the colon. Epicolic (A), paracolic (B), intermediate (C), and apical (central) (D) lymph nodes are indicated. (Copyright 2017, Memorial Sloan Kettering Cancer Center.)

(R0, R1, or R2), combining clinical and pathologic information, is important for determining the risk of locoregional recurrence and long-term prognosis.

The no-touch technique, in which the vascular supply is controlled before the tumor is manipulated in order to avoid releasing cancer cells into the bloodstream, has not been shown to improve oncologic outcomes.[8] However, for minimally invasive colorectal surgery, early vascular control with medial-to-lateral dissection of the mesentery, before mobilization of the colon, is the preferred approach because it helps identify all vascular and retroperitoneal structures.

Proper surgical technique is crucial for achieving optimal results. For rectal cancer, a total mesorectal excision (TME) using sharp dissection along normal anatomical planes to remove the rectum along with its mesorectal envelope is associated with a low risk of local tumor recurrence.[9,10] Likewise, a complete mesocolic excision (CME), with removal of all the lymph node-bearing mesentery along embryologic planes and central ligation of the named blood vessels, has been associated with a low risk of local tumor recurrence in colon cancer patients.[11] A recent study from Denmark showed that, in patients with stage I–III colon adenocarcinoma, CME resulted in longer disease-free survival than conventional resection.[12] Differences in the completeness of TME and CME probably contribute to the variation in oncologic outcomes between surgeons and between institutions.

LOCALIZED COLON CANCER

COLECTOMY

Resection is indicated for biopsy-proven adenocarcinoma of the colon without evidence of distant metastasis and without contraindications to major surgery. The extent of a resection depends on the location of the primary tumor. For tumors in the cecum and ascending colon, a right hemicolectomy is used, with division of the ileocolic, right colic, and sometimes the right branch of the middle colic vessels (Fig. 166.2A). The portion of the omentum attached to the removed segment of the colon should be resected en bloc with the colon and mesentery. For tumors located at the hepatic flexure or in the right portion of the transverse colon, an extended right colectomy is used, which in addition to division of the ileocolic and right colic vessels, involves division of the middle colic vessels at their origin (Fig. 166.2B). For tumors in the middle portion of the transverse colon, either an extended right colectomy or a transverse colectomy is employed. A transverse colectomy divides only the middle colic vessels, but to ensure a tension-free anastomosis, both the hepatic flexure and the splenic flexure are often mobilized (Fig. 166.2C). For tumors in the distal transverse colon, splenic flexure, or proximal descending colon, either an extended right colectomy (Fig. 166.2D) or a left hemicolectomy (Fig. 166.2E) is used. The latter procedure involves division of the left branches of the middle colic vessels and the left colic artery and vein at the point where the left colic vein joins the inferior mesenteric vein.

Because locally advanced tumors in the transverse colon can metastasize to the regional lymph nodes located along the greater omentum and the gastroepiploic arcades, an omentectomy with division of the gastroepiploic vessels at their origin may be necessary for complete nodal control.[13] However, the benefit of such an extended lymphadenectomy is subject to debate.

For tumors in the sigmoid colon, a sigmoid colectomy, including the superior rectal artery and its takeoff from the inferior mesenteric artery, is performed (Fig. 166.2F).

Patients with synchronous tumors, which occur in up to 5% of patients with colorectal cancer, should be investigated for hereditary colorectal cancer syndromes or other predisposing conditions. In patients without hereditary predisposition, and depending on the location of the primary tumors, either separate resections or an extended resection incorporating both lesions can be used.[14] When more than one segmental resection is performed, care must be taken to preserve the blood supply to the intermediate segment of colon in order to avoid ischemia and the associated perioperative complications. In patients with hereditary nonpolyposis colorectal cancer, synchronous tumors are indications for a subtotal or total colectomy.

MINIMALLY INVASIVE APPROACHES

Several prospective clinical trials have shown that laparoscopic colectomy for cancer is associated with short-term advantages and leads to equivalent long-term oncologic outcomes compared with the traditional open surgical approach. The advantages of laparoscopic surgery include

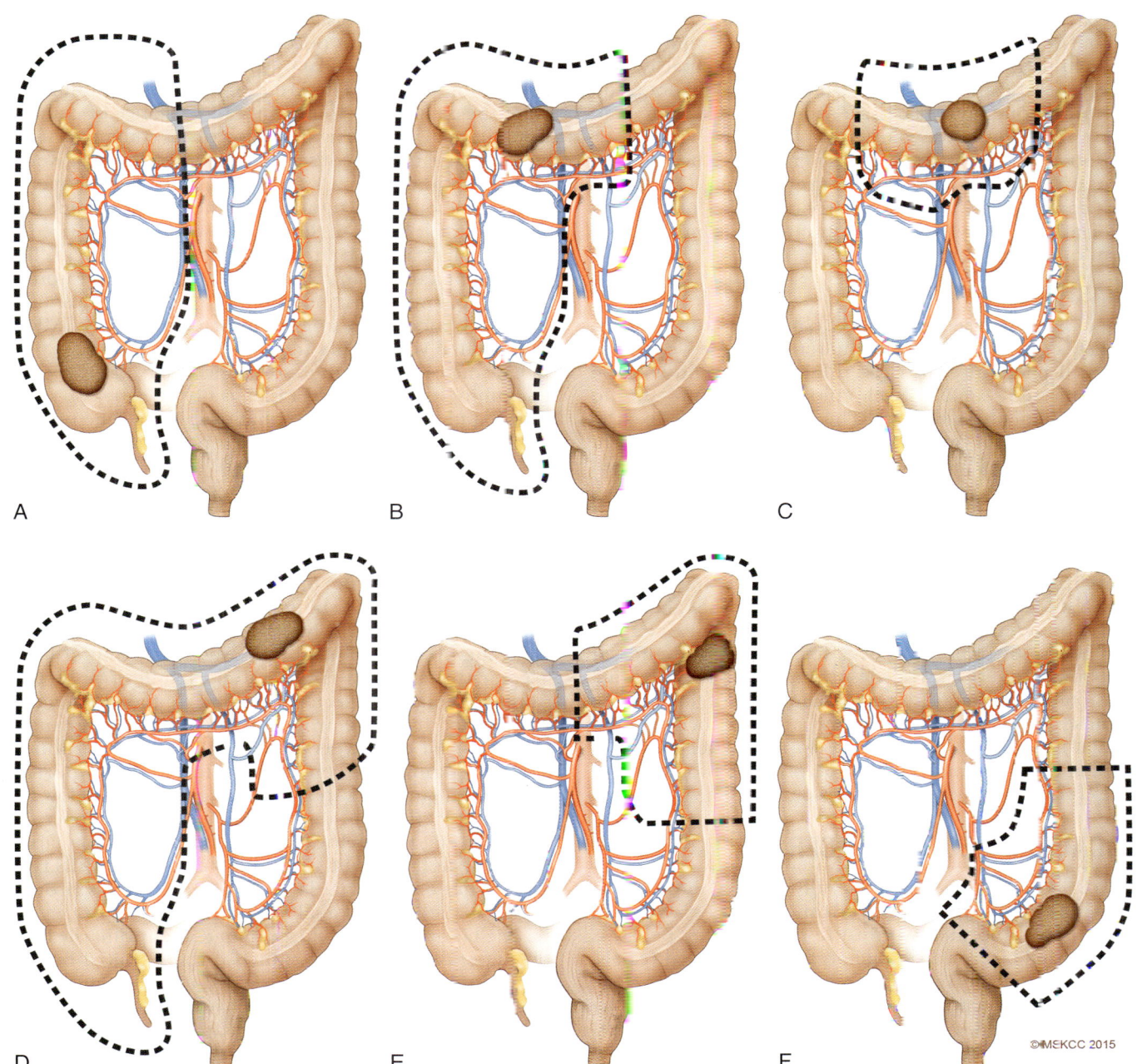

FIGURE 166.2 Segmental colonic resection. (A) Right colectomy; (B) right colectomy extended to transverse colon; (C) transversectomy; (D) right colectomy extended to the splenic flexure; (E) left colectomy; (F, sigmoidectomy. (Copyright 2017, Memorial Sloan Kettering Cancer Center.)

less postoperative pain, earlier return of bowel function, shorter hospital stay, and decreased rate of complications. However, laparoscopic surgery is technically challenging and takes time to master. In addition, the presence of multiple adhesions from previous surgery, locally advanced disease, or obesity may make laparoscopy particularly difficult. Early or preemptive conversion from laparoscopic to open surgery is associated with complication rates similar to those for open surgery, but complications are more frequent for late (reactive) conversion.[15]

Laparoscopic colectomy is typically performed using three to five ports and a specimen extraction site. With growing expertise, fewer ports, smaller instruments, and shorter incisions are now being used. Thus, in single-port laparoscopic surgery (SPLS), performed through a small port at the specimen extraction site, the camera and the operating ports are all positioned through the SPLS device.

A recent systematic review of 38 case series, including 565 patients who underwent SPLS, found that the procedure is feasible but technically challenging. Evidence regarding the safety of SPLS was limited.[16] After comparing the results of that review with the results from a Cochrane Review of 3526 patients treated with conventional laparoscopic colectomy, the authors concluded that SPLS did not result in less postoperative pain or a shorter hospital stay than conventional laparoscopic surgery.[16]

Robotic platforms have further enhanced the visualization and dexterity available to the surgeon. Compared with conventional laparoscopy, robotic colon resection is associated with lower conversion rates and similar short-term outcomes but higher costs.[17]

ANASTOMOTIC TECHNIQUES

After a colon resection, bowel continuity can be reestablished using different techniques, but a few common surgical principles must be followed. The ends to be anastomosed—small bowel, colon, or rectum—should have an intact blood supply. The terminal ileum, like the rest of the small bowel, has a plexiform rich blood supply. The colon has a more segmental blood supply provided by the vasa recta branching individually from the marginal arcade. Ideally, the last segmental artery of the segment of the colon to anastomose should have an intact arterial pulse. The end of the bowel to anastomose should be mobilized enough to allow a tension-free anastomosis. Finally, the stitches or staples should include the submucosa of the bowel, the layer with the highest collagen content and the most important layer for holding the ends of the bowel together. The description of the individual anastomotic techniques is beyond the scope of this chapter. Handsewn and stapled anastomoses are associated with similar complication rates in the normal bowel. However, the handsewn techniques may be preferred for suturing thick, edematous, or fibrotic bowel.

LOCALIZED RECTAL CANCER

Rectal cancer surgery is generally more complex and more challenging than colon cancer surgery, because the rectum is located within the narrow bony pelvis; is surrounded by the urogenital organs, large blood vessels, and autonomic nerves; and is close to the anal sphincters. As a result, rectal cancer surgery is more likely to be associated with perioperative complications and is often followed by a permanent reduction in the quality of life, stemming from the loss of urinary, sexual, and/or bowel function. Rectal cancer is also associated with a higher rate of local recurrence after curative-intent surgery. On the other hand, because most of the rectum is located below the peritoneal reflection and is close to the anal orifice, the rectum is accessible to exploratory methods (such as digital rectal examination and endorectal ultrasound) and interventions (such as external beam radiation therapy, brachytherapy, and local excision) not currently available for colon cancer.

ANATOMY

The rectum represents the distal portion of the large bowel, extending from the rectosigmoid junction to the anorectal ring, which corresponds to the imprint of the puborectalis muscle on the bowel wall. The anal canal extends from the anorectal ring to the anal verge, the palpable groove between the distal edge of the internal sphincter and the subcutaneous portion of the external sphincter (Fig. 166.3). For practical purposes and standardization, the rectum is defined in terms of distance in centimeters from the anal verge. To measure the distance of a tumor from the anal verge, a rigid proctoscope is commonly used, as it allows simultaneous visualization of the anal verge and the centimeter marks on the outside of the scope. In European countries, tumors with the distal edge located within the last 15 cm of the large bowel are categorized as rectal cancer; in the United States, the limit is 12 cm. The location of a tumor in relation to the anterior peritoneal reflection, and its distance from the anal verge, can also be determined by magnetic resonance imaging (MRI), with sagittal views being the most useful.

The mesorectum is the visceral mesentery of the rectum containing the terminal branches of the superior rectal vessels and the rectum's lymphatic drainage. The portion of the rectum above the anterior peritoneal reflection is covered with peritoneum in the front and on both sides and has a posterior mesorectum attached to the concavity of the sacrum, which is a continuation of the mesentery of the sigmoid colon. Below the peritoneal reflection, the rectum is completely extraperitoneal and fully surrounded by the mesorectum. The mesorectum is covered by a thin, glistening membrane called mesorectal fascia (MRF). Posteriorly, the mesorectum is separated from the presacral fascia by an avascular plane of loose areolar tissue, which is the natural plane of dissection during a radical proctectomy. Anteriorly, the mesorectum is separated from the urogenital organs by a remnant of the fusion of two layers of the embryologic peritoneal cul-de-sac known as Denonvilliers fascia—an important anatomical landmark in rectal cancer surgery. Below the peritoneal reflection, the lateral ligaments connect the mesorectum to the pelvic sidewall. The mesorectum tapers off distally as the rectum funnels toward the anorectal ring, where the longitudinal layer of the muscularis propria becomes the internal anal sphincter.

The blood supply of the rectum comes primarily from the superior rectal artery, which is the terminal branch of the inferior mesenteric artery after it gives off the left colic artery. The superior rectal vein follows a parallel course to its homonymous artery and joins the left colic vein to form the inferior mesenteric vein draining into the splenic vein. The lower portion of the rectum and the anal canal also receive blood supply from the internal iliac vessels through the middle rectal artery, an inconsistent branch of the inferior vesical artery; the inferior rectal artery is a branch of the pudendal artery. The middle and inferior rectal vessels anastomose with the upper rectal vessels, supplying enough blood to the entire rectum. As in other locations, the middle and inferior rectal veins follow the course of the homonymous arteries, draining into systemic circulation through the internal iliac veins.

Because the autonomic pelvic nerve system is very close to the planes of dissection during different parts of the operation, the surgeon must take great care to avoid damaging the nerves involved in urinary and/or sexual function. The hypogastric plexus, located in front of the aorta, contains predominantly preganglionic sympathetic fibers originating from the lumbar sympathetic trunk.

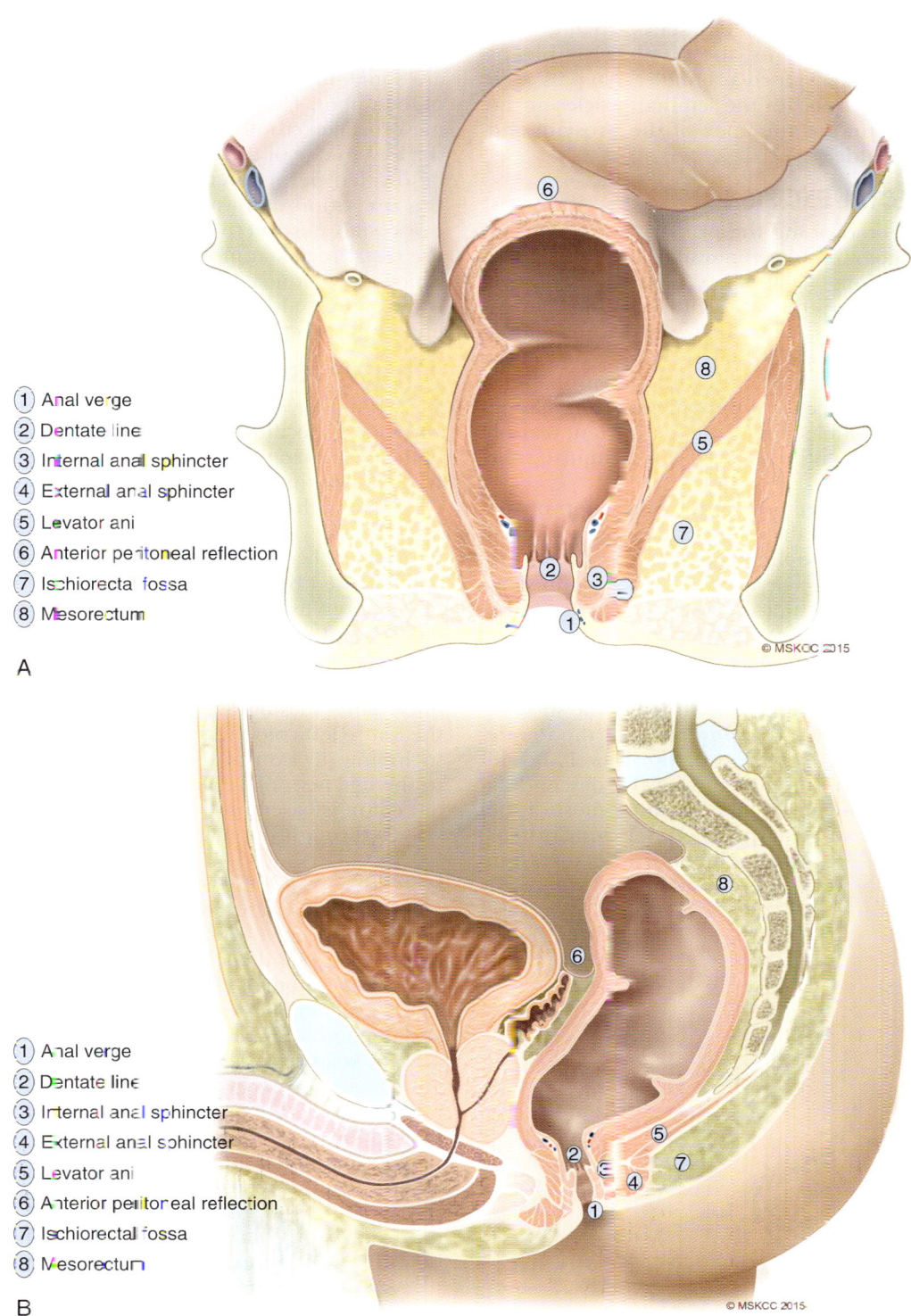

① Anal verge
② Dentate line
③ Internal anal sphincter
④ External anal sphincter
⑤ Levator ani
⑥ Anterior peritoneal reflection
⑦ Ischiorectal fossa
⑧ Mesorectum

© MSKCC 2015

A

① Anal verge
② Dentate line
③ Internal anal sphincter
④ External anal sphincter
⑤ Levator ani
⑥ Anterior peritoneal reflection
⑦ Ischiorectal fossa
⑧ Mesorectum

© MSKCC 2015

B

FIGURE 166.3 Anatomy of the rectum. (Copyright 2015, Memorial Sloan Kettering Cancer Center.)

The fibers of the hypogastric plexus converge at the level of the aortic bifurcation into well-defined hypogastric nerves, which course laterally and anteriorly over the internal iliac vessels toward the lateral pelvic sidewall. There they join the splanchnic pelvic nerves, containing primarily postganglionic parasympathetic fibers from the anterior rami of S2, S3, and S4, to form the pelvic plexus. Branches of the pelvic plexus provide innervation to the distal ureter, vas deferens, seminal vesicles, urinary bladder, and prostate. Branches of the pelvic plexus also provide innervation to the distal rectum, passing through the lateral rectal ligaments, or lateral stalks. Finally, distal to the lateral rectal ligaments, the distal pelvic plexus forms the urogenital neurovascular bundles that pass close to the posterolateral aspect of the seminal vesicles or the vagina, extending toward the apex of the prostate and the neck of the bladder.

TOTAL MESORECTAL EXCISION

TME is aimed at eradicating the primary tumor and its lymphatic drainage by en bloc removal of the rectum and the mesorectum, along well-defined anatomical planes. A TME dissection proceeds under direct vision along the areolar tissue plane situated between the mesorectal fascia and presacral fascia (Fig. 166.4). A sharp dissection along this plane is associated with a higher probability of achieving a negative circumferential resection margin (CRM), a lower risk of bleeding from inadvertent tearing of the presacral veins, and a reduced risk of injuring the hypogastric nerves.[9]

Adequate lymphadenectomy requires division of the lymphovascular pedicle at the origin of the superior rectal vessels, distal to the branching of the left colic artery from the inferior mesenteric artery (usually defined as low tie). In patients with clinically suspicious nodes at the origin of the inferior mesenteric artery, lymphovascular control should be extended proximally by dividing the inferior mesenteric artery close to the origin (high tie). Since the sigmoidal branches are included in the surgical specimen in both the high-tie approach and the low-tie approach, the proximal division of the bowel should ideally be performed at the junction of the descending colon and the sigmoid colon, incorporating most of the sigmoid colon in the surgical specimen.[18] As distal tumor extension along the rectal wall is limited, a distal margin of 2 cm of normal bowel wall is considered adequate for most tumors. However, in patients with extensive nodal metastasis, distal spread in the mesorectum may extend farther than intramural spread, and mesorectal deposits are sometimes found 3 to 4 cm distal to the lower edge of the tumor. Therefore, for tumors of the upper rectum, mesorectal excision should be extended to 5 cm distal to the lower edge of the tumor, and the mesorectum should be divided perpendicular to the axis of the rectum. In this operation, known as tumor-specific TME, some of the distal mesorectum is left in the pelvis along with the distal rectal stump, in contrast to standard TME, in which dissection is carried to the pelvic floor, the rectum is divided distal to the end of the mesorectum, and the entire mesorectum is included in the surgical specimen.[1]

SPHINCTER-SAVING PROCEDURES

The sphincter can be preserved in both standard TME and tumor-specific TME by anastomosing the divided end of the descending or the sigmoid colon to the rectal stump. In this operation, known as low anterior resection (LAR), (Fig. 166.5), the rectum is divided distal to the tumor using a stapling device that simultaneously staples and divides the rectum, leaving a short rectal stump. The anastomosis is completed by connecting the end of the colon to the rectal stump using a circular stapler. The continuity of the large bowel can be reestablished by suturing the colon to the anal canal, in a procedure referred to as coloanal anastomosis. A tension-free, well-vascularized low colorectal or coloanal anastomosis requires complete mobilization of the entire left colon with takedown of the splenic flexure, including division of the inferior mesenteric vein close to the ligament of Treitz. The blood supply to the entire left colon is based on the left branch of the middle colic vessels through the marginal artery.

Creating a Colonic Reservoir

Many patients undergoing a sphincter-saving procedure report high bowel frequency, urgency, soiling, and an inability to defer defecation for 15 minutes.[19] This constellation of symptoms is commonly known as LAR syndrome.[20] The frequency and severity of these symptoms are variable and depend to some degree on the location of the tumor and the anastomosis, the patient's prior bowel function, and the use of neoadjuvant or adjuvant therapy.[21] Pelvic irradiation, before or after surgery, significantly increases the risk of bowel dysfunction.[22,23]

The anatomical and physiologic factors that contribute to LAR syndrome are not completely understood. Anal sphincter pressure in patients with LAR syndrome is no different from that in other patients. What appears to be different is an exaggerated anal sphincter relaxation to even small volumes of stool within the neorectum.[24] Surgeons have tried to overcome the low capacitance of the neorectum—which is associated with end-to-end anastomosis—by creating a colonic reservoir in the form of either a colonic J-pouch or a side-to-end anastomosis (Fig. 166.6).

Several studies have compared straight end-to-end anastomosis and the J-pouch in terms of functional outcomes. A systematic review of nine trials that randomized 473 rectal cancer patients to either the J-pouch procedure or end-to-end anastomosis found that short-term bowel

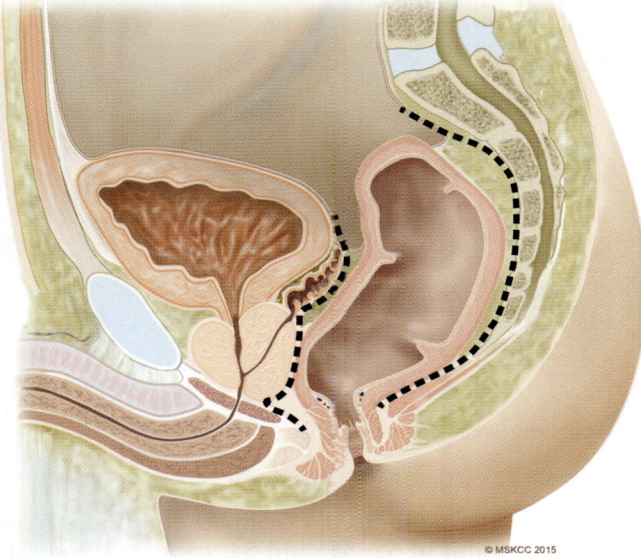

FIGURE 166.4 Planes of dissection for total mesorectal excision. (Copyright 2017, Memorial Sloan Kettering Cancer Center.)

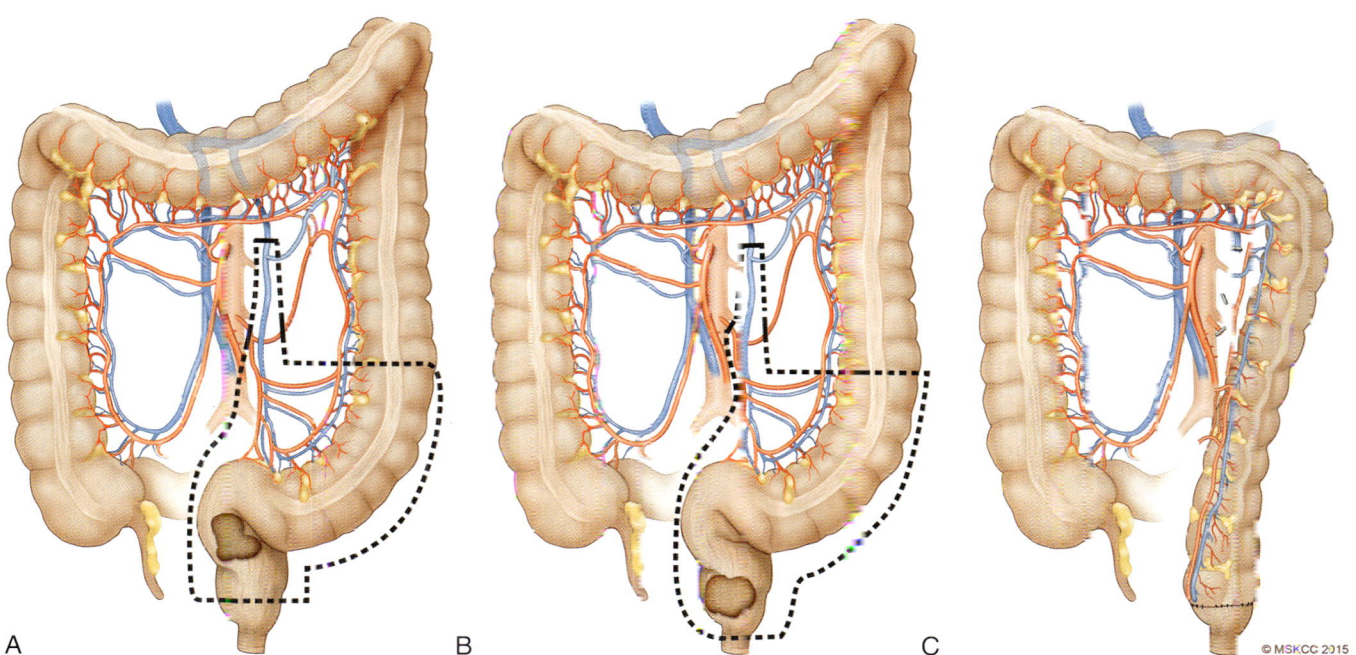

FIGURE 166.5 (A) Low anterior resection in the distal third of the rectum (candidate for colorectal anastomosis). (B) Low anterior resection above the sphincteric complex (candidate for coloanal anastomosis). (C) Colorectal anastomosis. (Copyright 2017, Memorial Sloan Kettering Cancer Center.)

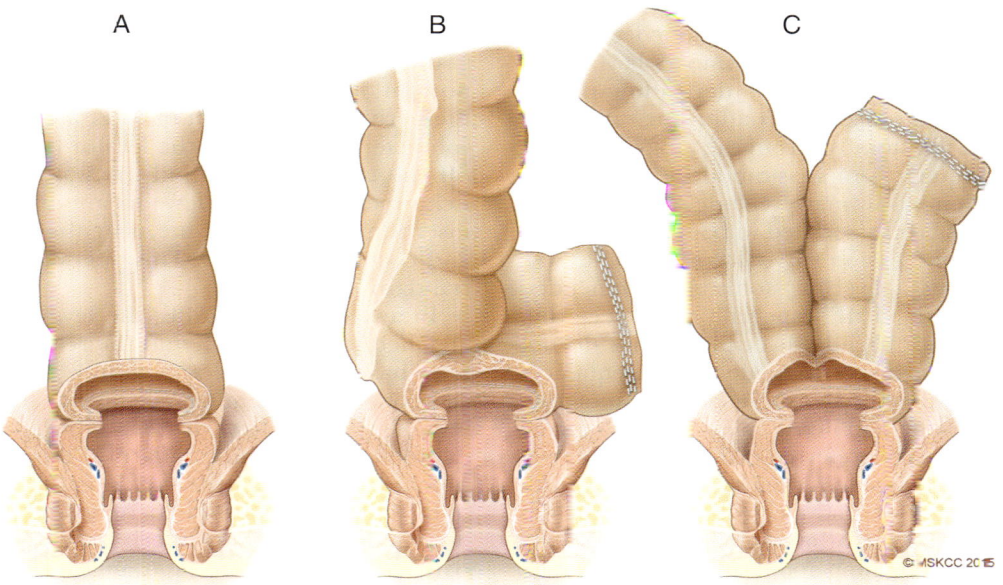

FIGURE 166.6 Reconstructive options after low anterior resection. (A) End-to-end anastomosis; (B) end-to-side anastomosis; (C) J-pouch anastomosis. (Copyright 2017, Memorial Sloan Kettering Cancer Center.)

function was better in the J-pouch patients.[25] Frequency and urgency were less prevalent in patients with a J-pouch, but the rates of fecal incontinence in the two groups were similar.

The only two trials that followed patients long-term found that the J-pouch was associated with a short-term improvement in frequency and urgency but provided no apparent long-term benefit compared with end-to-end anastomosis. The rates of anastomotic leak or other complications did not differ between the J-pouch and end-to-end anastomosis groups. Of note, almost one-third of patients with colonic J-pouches often complained of long-term difficulty emptying the rectum, requiring the use of laxatives or suppositories.[26,27] In view of the fact that these symptoms are more prevalent with larger pouches, pouch size should be limited to 5 to 6 cm.[28,29]

Side-to-end anastomosis can also potentially increase the reservoir capacity of the anastomosis. This procedure entails the insertion of the anvil of a circular stapler 3 to 4 cm from the end of the mobilized descending colon. Side-to-end anastomosis produces similar functional results but is easier to construct than the J-pouch. However, like the J-pouch, side-to-end anastomosis is also associated with defecatory problems.[30] A transverse coloplasty proximal to an end-to-end anastomosis can help increase the capacity of the neorectum, but this procedure is associated with a higher anastomotic leak rate.[25]

In summary, colonic reservoirs are associated with a temporary improvement in bowel frequency and urgency but also carry the risk of long-term defecatory problems. In general, we prefer end-to-end anastomosis using the larger descending colon, rather than the sigmoid colon, for the creation of the neorectum.

Reducing the Risk of Anastomotic Leak

The integrity of the anastomosis should be tested intraoperatively with a pneumatic test consisting of distending the bowel while submerging the anastomosis in saline. If an air leak is detected, the defect may be treated with suture repair, redo of the anastomosis, and/or the creation of a proximal diverting stoma. The endoscopic visualization of a colorectal anastomosis helps to identify bleeding or other abnormalities that could be repaired while the patient is under anesthesia. The testing of the integrity of the anastomosis during surgery has been shown to reduce the risk of clinical postoperative anastomotic leak.[31]

Low colorectal and coloanal anastomoses have a risk of leakage ranging from 3% to 34%, depending on the patient population, the use of neoadjuvant radiation, the distance of the anastomosis from the anal verge, and the surgical technique.[32,33] An anastomotic leak can cause pelvic sepsis, which not only may preclude sphincter preservation but also has been associated with an increased risk of local recurrence and poorer survival.[34] To prevent these possible complications, a diverting stoma is recommended for patients undergoing TME, especially those receiving neoadjuvant radiation.[35] While diverting stomas do not prevent complications, they do mitigate the consequences of a leak and reduce the need for urgent reoperation due to a leak.[36,37] Because a loop ileostomy is easier to create and remove, it is generally preferred over a transverse loop colostomy.[38] However, loop ileostomies are associated with postoperative dehydration and electrolyte abnormalities often requiring hospital readmission.[39] With adequate patient education and training about stoma management, these complications can be prevented.

ABDOMINOPERINEAL EXCISION

In many cases, when a tumor is located in the distal rectum, particularly when the levator muscles or the anal sphincter is infiltrated, the sphincter cannot be preserved if an oncologically safe circumferential and/or distal resection margin is to be achieved. In such cases, an R0 resection requires TME with en bloc excision of the levator muscles and the anal canal, and the creation of a permanent end colostomy. This operation is known as abdominoperineal excision (APE) (Fig. 166.7). The abdominal component of the procedure—proximal lymphovascular control, division

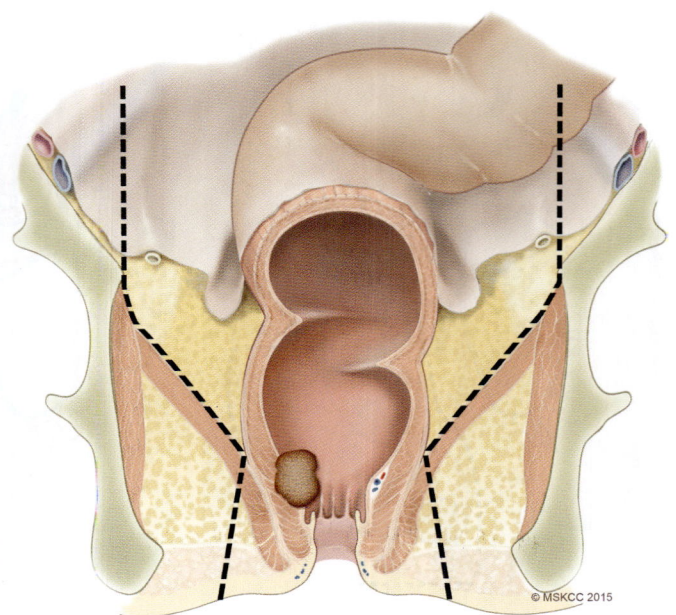

FIGURE 166.7 Standard abdominoperineal excision. (Copyright 2017, Memorial Sloan Kettering Cancer Center.)

of the colon, and dissection along the mesorectal plane—is similar to LAR, except that the mesorectal dissection stops at the upper level of the levators, to avoid disturbing the portion of the rectum resting on the levator muscles. In the perineal component of APE, the anal canal with the sphincter complex and the levator muscles are dissected off the ischiorectal fat, all the way to the apex of the ischiorectal fossa. The levators are divided close to their insertion in the white line near the obturator internus and coccygeus muscles. This operation is referred to as standard APE.[40]

In an extralevator APE, the levator muscles are left attached to the rectum, and the resulting surgical specimen has a cylindrical appearance (Fig. 166.8).[41] Some surgeons recommend removing only the portion of the levators required to clear the tumor. The choice between extralevator APE and standard APE is controversial. The potential oncologic benefit of larger tissue removal needs to be weighed against the increased morbidity potentially associated with a larger perineal defect, particularly in patients treated with neoadjuvant therapy.[42] A recent meta-analysis of 949 patients from one randomized trial, one prospective case-control study, and six retrospective case series found that patients who underwent extralevator APE had lower rates of intraoperative rectal perforation, positive CRM, and local recurrence but similar complication rates compared with patients who underwent standard APE.[43] However, the benefit of extralevator APE over standard APE has not been proven conclusively, and it is possible that the two techniques are equivalent as long as an R0 resection, with an intact rectal specimen, is achieved.

APE is often performed with the patient in a modified lithotomy position (also known as the Lloyd-Davies position), which provides relatively good access to the

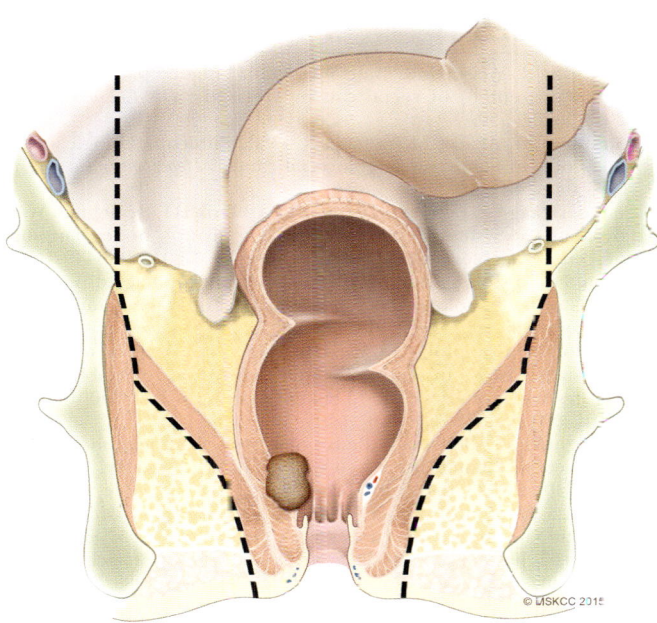

FIGURE 166.8 Extralevator abdominoperineal excision. (Copyright 2017, Memorial Sloan Kettering Cancer Center.)

perineum and allows two teams to work simultaneously on the abdominal and the perineal portions of the procedure. Some surgeons perform the abdominal part with the patient in the supine position and the perineal part with the patient prone over a hip roll and padding of the bony prominences. The prone position provides better exposure of the perineum and facilitates assistance and teaching. The disadvantages of the prone position are that it requires additional time for turning the patient and it does not allow a two-team approach. Results seem to be similar for the two approaches, and the choice between them depends on the surgeon's preference.[44]

MINIMALLY INVASIVE APPROACHES

Open surgery for rectal cancer requires long abdominal incisions. An APE can be performed through a midline infraumbilical or low transverse incision. Most sphincter-preserving procedures require a long midline incision, extending from the epigastrium to the symphysis of the pubis, in order to permit access to the entire left side of the large bowel from the splenic flexure to the lower rectum. Such abdominal incisions cause patient discomfort and are associated with short- and long-term morbidity.

Laparoscopic Total Mesorectal Excision

The goal of minimally invasive surgery for rectal cancer is to reduce the size of the abdominal incision, thus expediting recovery, without compromising the completeness of the mesorectal excision or the oncologic outcomes. Several retrospective case series and small randomized controlled trials found that, compared with open TME, laparoscopic TME produces less postoperative pain and is associated with less surgical morbidity and shorter length of hospital stay but offers no apparent benefit in

the amount of time required, CRM positivity, or the rate of local recurrence.[45-47] Even though laparoscopic TME has been shown to be feasible, less than 20% of all rectal cancer operations in the United States are performed laparoscopically,[48] likely due in part to the difficulty of working in the relatively deep and narrow pelvic space using long, rigid, nonarticulated instruments.

Three large multi-institutional prospective randomized trials have compared open TME and laparoscopic TME for rectal cancer.[49-51] The combined experience of these trials indicates that laparoscopic TME results in less blood loss, faster bowel recovery, and shorter hospital stay than open TME. Operative mortality, intraoperative and postoperative complications, and CRM positivity in patients who underwent laparoscopic TME did not differ from those in patients who underwent open TME. However, the rates of conversion and CRM positivity in patients who underwent laparoscopic surgery varied widely between the studies. These differences may stem from differences in trial design, inclusion criteria, randomization, and the use of neoadjuvant therapy. In the two trials that reported 3-year oncologic outcomes, the rates of local recurrence, distant metastasis, and survival after laparoscopic surgery did not differ from those after open surgery. While these findings appear to justify the use of laparoscopy in rectal cancer, it is prudent to wait for the results of larger trials before endorsing laparoscopy as the preferred surgical approach for locally advanced rectal cancer.

Many surgeons currently use a hybrid approach, consisting of laparoscopic lymphovascular control and colon mobilization and open mesorectal dissection and anastomosis through a lower abdominal transverse incision. The hybrid approach facilitates the most technically challenging portion of the operation: dissection of the distal rectum and creation of an anastomosis. With this approach, the size of the abdominal wall incision is smaller than in a fully open procedure but larger than in a fully laparoscopic procedure. Although there is some evidence of short-term advantages of the hybrid approach,[52] no long-term benefits have been reported.

Robotic Total Mesorectal Excision

The da Vinci robotic platform was added to the surgical armamentarium to facilitate minimally invasive prostatectomy, hysterectomy, and TME, which require optimal visualization and dexterity in the narrow pelvic space. The latest evidence from retrospective institutional case series indicates that robotic TME is equivalent to laparoscopic TME in terms of completeness of the mesorectal excision, CRM positivity, and short-term oncologic outcomes. Conversion rates appear to be lower than for laparoscopic TME, but hospital charges are higher.[53]

Transanal-Transabdominal Total Mesorectal Excision

For patients with a narrow pelvis, a transanal-transabdominal proctectomy (or down-to-up TME) offers a minimally invasive approach, using conventional transabdominal laparoscopy for lymphovascular control, the entire colonic mobilization, and dissection.[53-55] The dissection of the distal rectum is performed through the anus, using conventional transanal equipment for very distal tumors or endoscopic equipment for higher tumors. The rectal wall is incised circumferentially, distal to the tumor, and the mesorectal fascia is identified. The lumen of the colon is closed with a purse-string suture to avoid contamination. The dissection proceeds cephalad in the proper plane until the abdominal field is reached. The specimen is then removed, and anastomosis is performed through the anus.

Transanal-transabdominal proctectomy is particularly useful for very distal rectal tumors treated with chemoradiation, when the surgeon working in the pelvis has no anatomical cues about where to transect the rectum in order to achieve a negative distal margin. The transanal approach allows the surgeon to choose precisely the point for transecting the rectum while visualizing the distal edge of the tumor. The advantages of the down-to-up approach for higher rectal cancers that could be treated with a conventional transabdominal dissection and double-stapled anastomosis are unclear.

LOCAL EXCISION

Stage I rectal tumors localized to the bowel wall (T1 or T2) without involvement of mesorectal nodes (N0) can potentially be cured with a local excision (LE) of the portion of the rectal wall containing the tumor. This operation avoids most of the negative consequences of TME, such as mortality; morbidity; and bowel, urinary, and sexual dysfunction. However, meticulous patient selection is essential in order for LE to succeed. Since LE does not include the removal or inspection of the mesorectum for pathologic nodal staging (unlike most colorectal cancer surgeries), it should be performed only if nodal metastasis is unlikely. The selection criteria for LE are tumor size less than 3 cm, involvement of less than 30% of the circumference of the rectum, mobility on digital rectal examination, localization to the submucosa on endorectal ultrasound, no evidence of metastatic lymph nodes as determined by endorectal ultrasound and computed tomography or MRI, and no high-risk histologic features (i.e., grade 3 or 4, lymphovascular or perineural invasion).[56]

In the past, only tumors located in the distal rectum could be treated with conventional transanal excision, and LE was recommended only for tumors located within 8 cm from the anal verge. With the use of endoscopic instrumentation and large operating proctoscopes or single-port devices, LE now can be easily performed for tumors located in the mid- and upper rectum. While LE offers a significant benefit for patients with very distal tumors that otherwise would require a low anastomosis or a permanent stoma, the benefit of LE for tumors in the upper rectum is a matter of debate.

To avoid local recurrence, a full-thickness excision of the portion of the bowel wall involved by the tumor, with a 1-cm negative margin, is required. The final decision regarding the suitability of LE is made after the pathologic evaluation of the surgical specimen. If the resection margins are positive, the depth of invasion is beyond the submucosa (T stage ≥2), or the histology reveals high-risk features (grade 3 or 4, lymphovascular or perineural invasion), the evidence suggests that a proactive elective TME shortly after LE results in better oncologic outcomes compared with a salvage procedure after a local recurrence.

REFERENCES

1. Monson JR, Weiser MR, Buie WD, et al. Practice parameters for the management of rectal cancer (revised). *Dis Colon Rectum.* 2013;56:535-550.
2. Shiozawa M, Akaike M, Yamada R, et al. Clinicopathological features of skip metastasis in colorectal cancer. *Hepatogastroenterology.* 2007;54:81-84.
3. van der Zaag ES, Bouma WH, Tanis PJ, Ubbink DT, Bemelman WA, Buskens CJ. Systematic review of sentinel lymph node mapping procedure in colorectal cancer. *Ann Surg Oncol.* 2012;19:3449-3459.
4. Saha S, Johnston G, Korant A, et al. Aberrant drainage of sentinel lymph nodes in colon cancer and its impact on staging and extent of operation. *Am J Surg.* 2013;205:302-305, discussion 305-306.
5. Redston M, Compton CC, Miedema BW, et al. Analysis of micrometastatic disease in sentinel lymph nodes from resectable colon cancer: results of Cancer and Leukemia Group B Trial 80001. *J Clin Oncol.* 2006;24:878-883.
6. Bertagnolli M, Miedema B, Redston M, et al. Sentinel node staging of resectable colon cancer: results of a multicenter study. *Ann Surg.* 2004;240:624-628, discussion 628-630.
7. Toyota S, Ohta H, Anazawa S. Rationale for extent of lymph node dissection for right colon cancer. *Dis Colon Rectum.* 1995;38:705-711.
8. Wiggers T, Jeekel J, Arends JW, et al. No-touch isolation technique in colon cancer: a controlled prospective trial. *Br J Surg.* 1988;75:409-415.
9. Heald RJ. The 'Holy Plane' of rectal surgery. *J R Soc Med.* 1988;81:503-508.
10. MacFarlane JK, Ryall RD, Heald RJ. Mesorectal excision for rectal cancer. *Lancet.* 1993;341:457-460.
11. Hohenberger W, Weber K, Matzel K, Papadopoulos T, Merkel S. Standardized surgery for colonic cancer: complete mesocolic excision and central ligation—technical notes and outcome. *Colorectal Dis.* 2009;11:354-364, discussion 364-365.
12. Bertelsen CA, Neuenschwander AU, Jansen JE, et al. Disease-free survival after complete mesocolic excision compared with conventional colon cancer surgery: a retrospective, population-based study. *Lancet Oncol.* 2015;16:161-168.
13. Kessler H, Hohenberger W. Extended lymphadenectomy in colon cancer is crucial. *World J Surg.* 2013;37:1789-1798.
14. Noshc K, Kure S, Irahara N, et al. A prospective cohort study shows unique epigenic, genetic, and prognostic features of synchronous colorectal cancers. *Gastroenterology.* 2009;137:1609–1620.e1–e3.
15. Yang C, Wexner SD, Safar B, et al. Conversion in laparoscopic surgery: does intraoperative complication influence outcome? *Surg Endosc.* 2009;23:2454-2458.
16. Fung AK, Aly EH. Systematic review of single-incision laparoscopic colonic surgery. *Br J Surg.* 2012;99:1353-1364.
17. Kim CW, Kim CH, Baik SH. Outcomes of robotic-assisted colorectal surgery compared with laparoscopic and open surgery: a systematic review. *J Gastrointest Surg.* 2014;18:816-830.
18. Lange MM, Buunen M, van de Velde CJ, Lange JF. Level of arterial ligation in rectal cancer surgery: low tie preferred over high tie. A review. *Dis Colon Rectum.* 2008;51:1139-1145.
19. Zotti P, Del Bianco P, Serpentini S, et al. Validity and reliability of the MSKCC Bowel Function instrument in a sample of Italian rectal cancer patients. *Eur J Surg Oncol.* 2011;37:589-596.
20. Emmertsen KJ, Laurberg S. Low anterior resection syndrome score: development and validation of a symptom-based scoring system for bowel dysfunction after low anterior resection for rectal cancer. *Ann Surg.* 2012;255:922-928.
21. Emmertsen KJ, Laurberg S. Bowel dysfunction after treatment for rectal cancer. *Acta Oncol.* 2008;47:994-1003.
22. Lundby L, Krogh K, Jensen VJ, et al. Long-term anorectal dysfunction after postoperative radiotherapy for rectal cancer. *Dis Colon Rectum.* 2005;48:1343-1349, discussion 1349-1352; author reply 1352.
23. Chen TY, Wiltink LM, Nout RA, et al. Bowel function 14 years after preoperative short-course radiotherapy and total mesorectal excision for rectal cancer: report of a multicenter randomized trial. *Clin Colorectal Cancer.* 2015;14:106-114.
24. Lewis WG, Martin IG, Williamson ME, et al. Why do some patients experience poor functional results after anterior resection of the rectum for carcinoma? *Dis Colon Rectum.* 1995;38:259-263.
25. Brown CJ, Fenech DS, McLeod RS. Reconstructive techniques after rectal resection for rectal cancer. *Cochrane Database Syst Rev.* 2008;(2):CD006040.

26. Parc R, Tiret E, Frileux P, Moszkowski E, Loygue J. Resection and colo-anal anastomosis with colonic reservoir for rectal carcinoma. *Br J Surg.* 1986;73:139-141.

27. Seow-Choen F, Goh HS. Prospective randomized trial comparing J colonic pouch-anal anastomosis and straight coloanal reconstruction. *Br J Surg.* 1995;82:608-610.

28. Hida J, Yasutomi M, Fujimoto K, et al. Functional outcome after low anterior resection with low anastomosis for rectal cancer using the colonic J-pouch. Prospective randomized study for determination of optimum pouch size. *Dis Colon Rectum.* 1996;39:986-991.

29. Lazorthes F, Gamagami R, Chiotasso P, Istvan G, Muhammad S. Prospective, randomized study comparing clinical results between small and large colonic J-pouch following coloanal anastomosis. *Dis Colon Rectum.* 1997;40:1409-1413.

30. Machado M, Nygren J, Goldman S, Ljungqvist O. Functional and physiologic assessment of the colonic reservoir or side-to-end anastomosis after low anterior resection for rectal cancer: a two-year follow-up. *Dis Colon Rectum.* 2005;48:29-36.

31. Daams F, Wu Z, Lahaye MJ, Jeekel J, Lange JF. Prediction and diagnosis of colorectal anastomotic leakage: a systematic review of literature. *World J Gastrointest Surg.* 2014;6:14-26.

32. Jones OM, John SK, Horseman N, Lawrance RJ, Fozard JB. Low anastomotic leak rate after colorectal surgery: a single-centre study. *Colorectal Dis.* 2007;9:740-744.

33. Eberl T, Jagoditsch M, Klingler A, Tschmelitsch J. Risk factors for anastomotic leakage after resection for rectal cancer. *Am J Surg.* 2008;196:592-598.

34. McArdle CS, McMillan DC, Hole DJ. Impact of anastomotic leakage on long-term survival of patients undergoing curative resection for colorectal cancer. *Br J Surg.* 2005;92:1150-1154.

35. Matthiessen P, Hallbook O, Andersson M, Rutegård J, Sjödah R. Risk factors for anastomotic leakage after anterior resection of the rectum. *Colorectal Dis.* 2004;6:462-469.

36. Tan WS, Tang CL, Shi L, Eu KW. Meta-analysis of defunctioning stomas in low anterior resection for rectal cancer. *Br J Surg.* 2009;96:462-472.

37. Machado M, Hallbook O, Goldman S, Nyström PO, Järhult J, Sjödahl R. Defunctioning stoma in low anterior resection with colonic pouch for rectal cancer: a comparison between two hospitals with a different policy. *Dis Colon Rectum.* 2002;45:940-945.

38. Rondelli F, Reboldi P, Rulli A, et al. Loop ileostomy versus loop colostomy for fecal diversion after colorectal or coloanal anastomosis: a meta-analysis. *Int J Colorectal Dis.* 2009;24:479-488.

39. Chun LJ, Haigh PI, Tam MS, Abbas MA. Defunctioning loop ileostomy for pelvic anastomoses: predictors of morbidity and nonclosure. *Dis Colon Rectum.* 2012;55:167-174.

40. Perdawood SK, Lund T. Extralevator versus standard abdominoperineal excision for rectal cancer. *Tech Coloproctol.* 2015 19-3: 145-152.

41. Marr R, Birbeck K, Garvican J, et al. The modern abdominoperineal excision: the next challenge after total mesorectal excision. *Ann Surg.* 2005;242:74-82.

42. Musters GD, Buskens C, Bemelman WA, Tanis PJ. Perineal wound healing after abdominoperineal resection for rectal cancer: a systematic review and meta-analysis. *Dis Colon Rectum.* 2014;57:1129-1139.

43. Yu HC, Peng H, He XS, Zhao RS. Comparison of short- and long-term outcomes after extralevator abdominoperineal excision and standard abdominoperineal excision for rectal cancer: a systematic review and meta-analysis. *Int J Colorectal Dis.* 2014;29:183-191.

44. de Campos-Lobato LF, Stocchi L, Dietz DW, Lavery IC, Fazio VW, Kalady MF. Prone or lithotomy positioning during an abdominoperineal resection for rectal cancer results in comparable oncologic outcomes. *Dis Colon Rectum.* 2011;54:939-946.

45. Lujan J, Valero G, Hernandez Q, Sanchez A, Frutos MD, Parrilla P. Randomized clinical trial comparing laparoscopic and open surgery in patients with rectal cancer. *Br J Surg.* 2009;96:982-989.

46. Ng KH, Ng DC, Cheung HY, et al. Laparoscopic resection for rectal cancers: lessons learned from 579 cases. *Ann Surg.* 2009;249:82-86.

47. Greenblatt DY, Rajamanickam V, Pugely AJ, Heise CP, Foley EF, Kennedy GD. Short-term outcomes after laparoscopic-assisted proctectomy for rectal cancer: results from the ACS NSQIP. *J Am Coll Surg.* 2011;212:844-854.

48. Yeo H, Niland J, Milne D. et al. Incidence of minimally invasive colorectal cancer surgery at National Comprehensive Cancer Network centers. *J Natl Cancer Inst.* 2015;107:362.

49. Jayne DG, Thorpe HC, Copeland J, Quirke P, Brown JM, Guillou PJ. Five-year follow-up of the Medical Research Council CLASICC trial of laparoscopically assisted versus open surgery for colorectal cancer. *Br J Surg.* 2010;97:1638-1645.

50. Jeong SY, Park JW, Nam BH, et al. Open versus laparoscopic surgery for mid-rectal or low-rectal cancer after neoadjuvant chemoradiotherapy (COREAN trial): survival outcomes of an open-label, non-inferiority, randomised controlled trial. *Lancet Oncol.* 2014;15:767-774.

51. van der Pas MH, Haglind E, Cuesta MA, et al. Laparoscopic versus open surgery for rectal cancer (COLOR II): short-term outcomes of a randomised, phase 3 trial. *Lancet Oncol.* 2013;14:210-218.

52. Vithiananthan S, Cooper Z, Betten K, et al. Hybrid laparoscopic flexure takedown and open procedure for rectal resection is associated with significantly shorter length of stay than equivalent open resection. *Dis Colon Rectum.* 2001;44:927-935.

53. Xiong B, Ma L, Zhang C, Cheng Y. Robotic versus laparoscopic total mesorectal excision for rectal cancer: a meta-analysis. *J Surg Res.* 2014;188:404-414.

54. de Lacy AM, Rattner DW, Adelsdorfer C, et al. Transanal natural orifice transluminal endoscopic surgery (NOTES) rectal resection: "down-to-up" total mesorectal excision (TME)—short-term outcomes in the first 20 cases. *Surg Endosc.* 2013;27:3165-3172.

55. Rouanet P, Mourregot A, Azar CC, et al. Transanal endoscopic proctectomy: an innovative procedure for difficult resection of rectal tumors in men with narrow pelvis. *Dis Colon Rectum.* 2013;56:408-415.

56. National Comprehensive Cancer Network. NCCN Clinical Practice Guidelines in Oncology—Rectal Cancer; 2015. www.nccn.org. Accessed February 2017.

Transanal Approaches to Early Rectal Cancers: Transanal Minimally Invasive Surgery

Matthew R. Albert | Joseph M. Plummer | Lawrence L. Lee

The realization that local excision may result in equivalent oncologic outcomes for histologically favorable rectal cancer is not a recent development.[1] Conventional transanal excision (TAE) using traditional anorectal retractors has been associated with substantial margin positivity and tumor fragmentation.[2] This has resulted in significantly higher local recurrence rates and worse long-term survival as compared with transabdominal resection for these lesions.[3]

The development of advanced endoscopic platforms has significantly improved the resection quality for local excision. These platforms allow access to lesions located in the upper two-thirds of the rectum. Better visibility and improved operating ergonomics yields higher quality local excision compared with traditional TAE. In 1984, Dr. Gerhard Buess[4] introduced transanal endoscopic microsurgery (TEM) local excision, which resulted in significantly higher rates of R0 and en bloc resections compared with traditional TAE.[2] A single randomized trial comparing TEM with radical resection for early rectal cancer demonstrated no difference in oncologic outcomes.[3,5]

Transanal minimally invasive surgery (TAMIS) was first reported in 2010 by Atallah et al.[6] using standard skills and equipment already available to laparoscopic surgeons through a flexible transanal port. TAMIS has a shorter learning curve, greater luminal access, and visibility of lesions, and patients can be placed in the dorsal lithotomy position regardless of lesion location.[7]

PATIENT SELECTION AND PREOPERATIVE INVESTIGATIONS

Cure rates for early rectal cancer, defined as histologically favorable (i.e., well-differentiated, absence of lympho-vascular, or perineural invasion), with invasion into the superficial submucosa (sm1) only (T1N0M0) are high after treatment with radical surgery. Local excision of early rectal cancer should offer cure rates comparable to radical surgery with a goal of improved functional outcomes and reduced morbidity. Appropriate patient selection is critical, and every effort must be made to select patients with minimal risk of lymph node involvement for curative local excision.[8] The National Comprehensive Cancer Network (NCCN) rectal cancer guidelines state that patients with mobile cT1N0 well to moderately differentiated lesions that are less than 3 cm in diameter with no lymphovascular or perineal invasion are appropriate candidates for local excision. Lesions larger than 3 cm may also be eligible for local excision but have poorer outcomes. Complete pathologic

evaluation with substaging of T1 lesions using the Kikuchi classification is critical for accurate risk stratification. Lesions that demonstrate invasion deeper than the first third of the submucosa (i.e., sm2/3) are also at higher risk of lymph node metastases and should be strongly considered for transabdominal resection. Strict adherence to these criteria should result in equivalent oncologic outcomes for local excision compared with radical surgery. An analysis of the Surveillance, Epidemiology, and End Results database reported comparable cancer-specific survival between local excision and transabdominal resection,[9] and a meta-analysis comparing TEM local excision and radical surgery for T1 rectal cancer also demonstrated equivalent 5-year overall survival.[3]

Patients should be counseled that final pathologic analysis may unexpectedly demonstrate high-risk features, which requires a radical surgery for cure. An individualized discussion should be performed considering the patient's desires and risk tolerance. Comorbidities, ability to tolerate surgery, and reliability to undergo intensive surveillance should be considered. Similarly, lesions with diagnostic uncertainty (i.e., T1 vs. T2) on preoperative evaluation can be offered TAMIS local excision as an "excisional biopsy," with further management dictated by the final pathology of the lesion. Lesions that invade the muscularis propria (i.e., pT2) should be offered radical surgery due to the high risk of lymph node metastases.

There are emerging indications for TAMIS local excision for more advanced lesions for patients who are unwilling or unable to tolerate radical surgery. These patients must be presented at a multidisciplinary tumor board for consideration of chemotherapy and/or radiation in addition to TAMIS local excision. Patients who are medically able to tolerate surgery but are unwilling to accept the functional impairments or risk of permanent ostomy from radical surgery must be advised that local excision in these cases results in oncologically inferior outcomes, and every effort must be made to offer the patient curative radical surgery. Rarely, TAMIS local excision can be performed for palliation of symptoms in patients with extreme comorbidities or in the setting of metastatic diseases. TAMIS can also be performed following definitive neoadjuvant chemoradiotherapy. Wound dehiscence is common in this setting and is associated with significant pain, hospital readmission, and need for fecal diversion.[7]

Lesions that are located within 3 cm of the anal verge may be hidden from access by TAMIS due to the length of operating port (37 to 44 mm in length). The TEM rectoscope also presents difficulties in obtaining a proper seal for very distal lesions. A hybrid approach is possible using Parks retractors to dissect the distal lesion and then introducing the TAMIS port to finish the proximal dissection. This approach allows for the advantages of the advanced endoscopic platforms to be applied for lesions that would otherwise be at high risk of R1 resection and fragmentation by traditional TAE.

Preoperative evaluation begins with a detailed history, including disease-specific and associated symptoms, family history, performance status, functional capacity, fecal continence, and physical examination with particular attention paid to digital rectal examination. Lesions that can be palpated by digital rectal exam should be assessed as to whether they are firm, mobile, or fixed. Full endoscopic evaluation of the colon must be performed to rule out synchronous lesions that may change the management strategy. Rigid proctosigmoidoscopy by the operating surgeon clarifies tumor size, location within the lumen, distance of the lower and upper extent of the tumor from the anal verge, and circumferential extent.

Transrectal ultrasound and pelvic magnetic resonance imaging (MRI) with rectal cancer protocol may be used individually or in combination to stage the tumor locally. Computed tomography of the chest, abdomen, and pelvis and carcinoembryonic antigen level completes the staging evaluation. Routine laboratory investigations and positron emission tomography scans are not necessary. Once the preoperative evaluation is complete, patients should be presented at a multidisciplinary tumor board to arrive at a consensus management plan.

TECHNICAL ASPECTS/OPERATIVE TECHNIQUE FOR TRANSANAL MINIMALLY INVASIVE SURGERY

A full mechanical bowel preparation, or more commonly a limited left-sided bowel preparation with the use of enemas, ensures a clear operative field and limits contamination in case of rectal perforation. Antibiotic and venous thromboembolism (VTE) prophylaxis are given in accordance with guidelines for colonic surgery. Foley catheterization may be of benefit in males due to the high incidence of urinary retention.[10]

The patients can be placed in lithotomy position regardless of lesion position within the rectal lumen. The main operative monitor is placed at the head of the bed, and both surgeon and assistant (camera holder) are seated between the legs of the patient. Basic laparoscopic instruments (including graspers, monopolar cautery, and needle drivers) can be used. A 5-mm angled (30- to 45-degree) scope is preferable, as it offsets the operating surgeon's hands to minimize instrument collision, facilitates assessment of the lateral and proximal margins, and can improve visualization around the rectal valves. Simple monopolar cautery, combined suction-cautery instruments, as well as energy devices can all be used for dissection and hemostasis.

TAMIS is performed using the SILS Port (Medtronic, Minneapolis, Minnesota), the GelPOINT Path (Applied Medical, Rancho Santa Margarita, California), Triport (Olympus), and SSL (Ethicon, Somerville, New Jersey). Exposure of the anal canal can be improved with the Lone Star retractor system (CooperSurgical, Trumbull

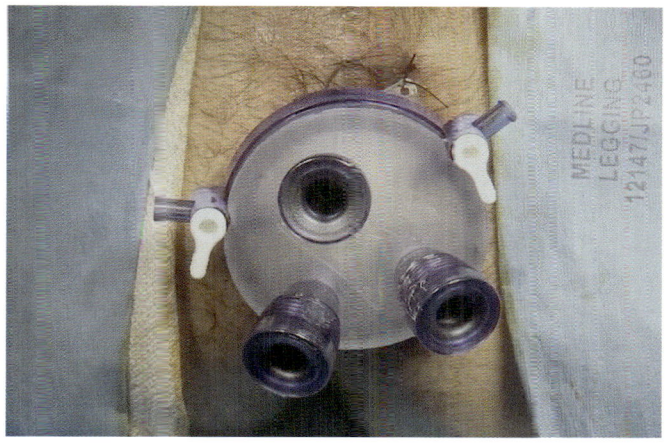

FIGURE 167A.1 GelPOINT path with cap and trocars—one of two FDA-approved platforms for transanal minimally invasive surgery.

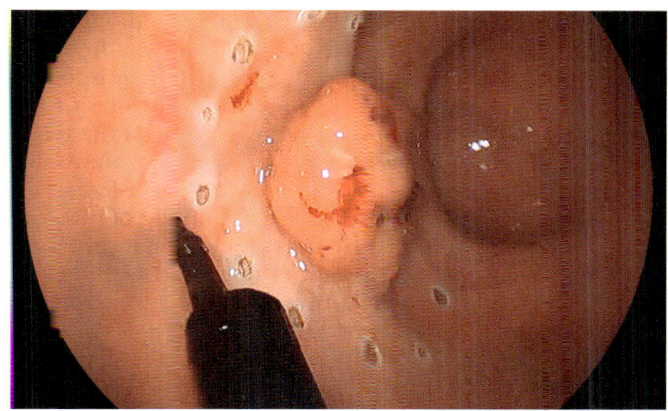

FIGURE 167A.2 Lesion being marked out during transanal minimally invasive surgery local excision. Monopolar cautery device is used to score the rectal mucosa with a 1 cm circumferential margin.

Connecticut) is required (Fig. 167A.1). The 5-mm camera, hook electrocautery, suction irrigator, and grasper are introduced through the Gel cap and the operation commenced. Setup time averaged 1.9 minutes in the initial publications of the TAMIS procedure.[10] Pneumorectum is created with carbon dioxide insufflation kept at 15 to 18 mm Hg and can be increased up to 20 mm Hg if required in patients with morbid obesity. A suction device is important to facilitate smoke evacuation. Recently, new insufflators have been developed (AirSeal Insufflation System; ConMed, Inc. Utica, New York), providing improved stability of pneumorectum at lower pressures and dramatically reduce intraluminal smoke, the two most vexing problems found by early TAMIS users.

A nonfragmented, full-thickness, margin-negative tumor resection is mandatory. Submucosal dissection, which may be used for benign polyps to minimize risk of wound complications has no role in early rectal cancer. The procedure begins by marking out a 1-cm circumferential margin using electrocautery (Fig. 167A.2). Full-thickness perpendicular incision of the rectal wall, distal to the

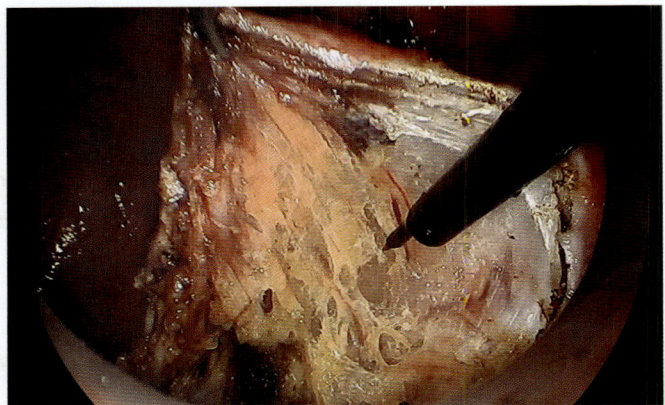

FIGURE 167A.3 Full-thickness excision. Note the mesorectal fat underneath the lesion, signifying that entire rectal wall has been transected.

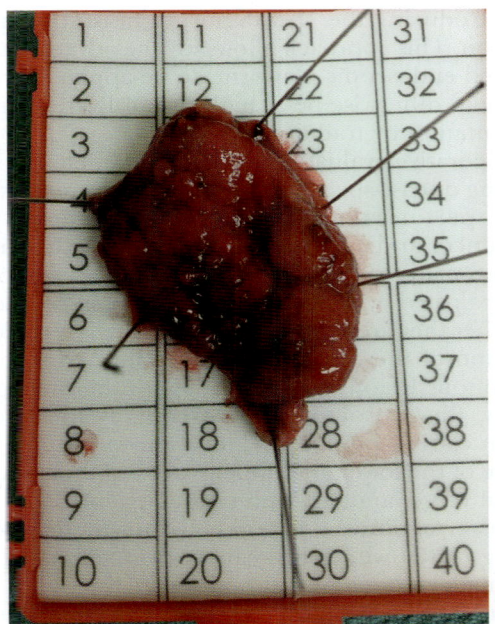

FIGURE 167A.4 Specimen removed by transanal minimally invasive surgery is pinned and oriented.

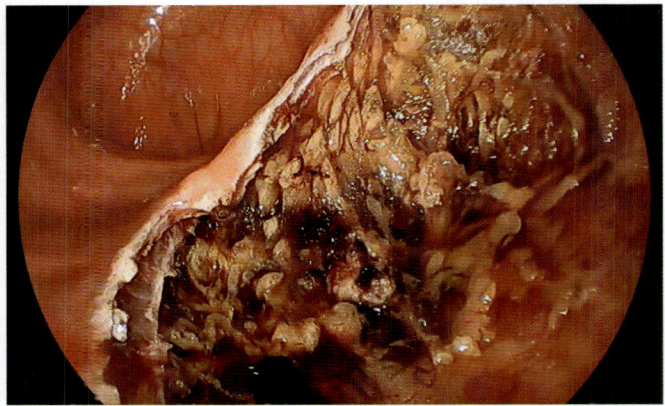

FIGURE 167A.5 Rectal wall defect after being irrigated with dilute povidone-iodine (Betadine), prior to closure.

lesion, allows manipulation of the specimen without direct contact of the tumor. Mesorectal fat serves as the deep margin (Fig. 167A.3). The specimen should be grasped on the edge of normal mucosa or underneath the lesion on the mesorectal fat to minimize fragmentation of the tissue and tumor. Some surgeons advocate en bloc removal of mesorectal fat beneath a posteriorly placed lesion in an attempt to retrieve lymph nodes. The sampling of involved lymph nodes may alter treatment recommendations. Care must be taken to avoid breaching the mesorectal fascial envelope to minimize disruption of the anatomic planes should proctectomy become necessary.[7]

Anterior lesions are still best accessed in the lithotomy position, in contrast to conventional TAE or TEM where the prone jackknife position is necessary. Injury to the prostate or vagina is possible anteriorly where the mesorectum is much thinner, but this has not been reported in any series of TAMIS. Familiarity with the anatomic planes and surrounding critical structures is important. Peritoneal entry is a known risk (4%) in patients with anterior tumors located in the mid and upper rectum.[11] Closure of the rectal wall must be performed by first closing the peritoneum and then the rectal wall. However, transient loss of pneumorectum may occur. Rarely, laparoscopic access is required to cleanse the pelvis, facilitate wall closure, or perform a leak test. In our experience of more than 250 TAMIS procedures, conversion to transabdominal laparoscopic closure occurred more frequently within our first 100 procedures and may have been associated with failure to maintain stable pneumorectum to permit safe endoluminal closure. Peritoneal entry has not been associated with increased pelvic infection or worse oncologic outcomes. Informed consent in patients at risk of peritoneal entry should be strongly considered.

The specimen should be oriented (Fig. 167A.4), pinned out and sent to the pathologist as a fresh, nonpreserved specimen to facilitate margin evaluation. Strong consideration should be given to reexcision of a positive margin or formal radical oncologic surgery.

It is easy to irrigate the rectum with povidone-iodine (Betadine) and can potentially minimize bacteria and tumor contamination. The best method of handling the defect in the rectal wall is debatable (Fig. 167A.5). All full-thickness defects are closed with interrupted or continuous suturing. Hahnloser et al. reported outcomes from 75 TAMIS excisions performed at three centers and found no difference in complications between defects that were closed and those that were left open.[12] The rectal defect is closed transversely so as not to narrow the lumen. During the suturing process, it is best to reduce the intraluminal pressure to 8 to 10 mm Hg to reduce tension on the suture lines. A running closure beginning in the lateral portion of the incision can be achieved but is technically more challenging. The use of a V-Loc suture (Covidien, Mansfield, Massachusetts) can expedite continuous closure by maintaining tension and negating the need for knot tying (Fig. 167A.6). Conversely, closure can be performed in an interrupted fashion with knot tying facilitated by laparoscopic knot pushers. The use

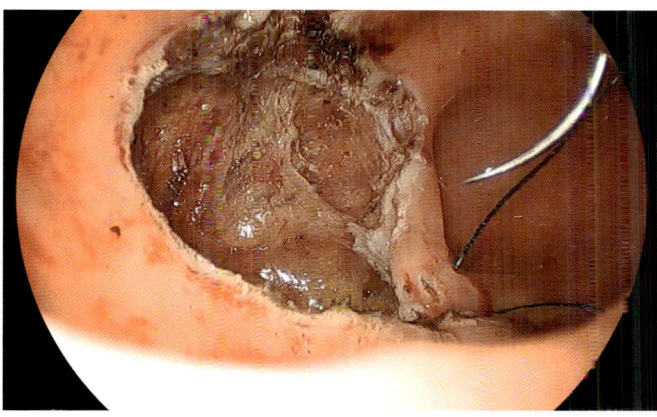

FIGURE 167A.6 Rectal wall defect being closed using continuous V-Loc suture.

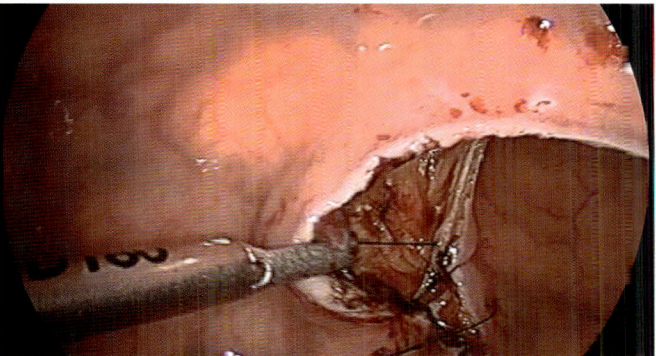

FIGURE 167A.7 Commercially available automated laparoscopic suturing device that can be used in transanal minimally invasive surgery (LSI Solution, TK).

of modern suturing devices can significantly shorten the learning curve at the expense of increased procedural costs. Laparoscopic knot tying devices and methods are available (Fig. 167A.7). A rigid or flexible sigmoidoscopy can also be performed at the end of the procedure to access the luminal diameter.

TAMIS has been performed robotically with good success.[13,14] However, robot docking time, which can be up to 36 minutes,[14] and the additional costs incurred by the use of the robot equipment (up to 1000 Euro per patient, excluding capital expenditure on the robot system and its maintenance), limit the applicability of robotic TAMIS.

POSTOPERATIVE CARE

TAMIS has been shown to be feasible on an outpatient basis. In patients with advanced age, significant comorbidities, or at increased risk of bleeding, selective overnight admission can be considered. In our experience of over 260 patients, nearly 80% underwent same-day discharge. All patients must be counseled on the signs of early and late postoperative hemorrhage and pelvic sepsis. Transient rectal discharge and short-term change in bowel habits is expected. A regular diet is initiated once recovered from

anesthesia. Narcotics are frequently unnecessary, except in tumors where the incision or closure abuts the dentate line. Postoperative antibiotics are not recommended.

COMPLICATIONS

TAMIS has a fairly low complication rate with low severity. Bleeding is the most common complication associated with TAMIS and is usually self-limited. Bleeding can occur early or be delayed, related to suture line dehiscence, and can be successfully managed without further intervention. Endoscopic evaluation with injection or coagulation, or examination under anesthesia with oversewing of the offending vessel is usually successful.

Examination after 30 days nearly always demonstrates complete healing regardless of whether the defect was closed or not. Suture line dehiscence after peritoneal entry has the obvious potential to lead to more significant complications such as pelvic sepsis. TAMIS following neoadjuvant therapy is associated with a high incidence of wound breakdown, severe pain readmission, and may even require fecal diversion. In a series by Marks et al., morbidity following patients who underwent neoadjuvant chemoradiation followed by TEM, a 25.6% wound complication rate was reported with one patient requiring diversion.[15] Perez et al. reported suture line dehiscence rates of 50.9% with 43.3% of patients requiring readmission, and have since abandoned this approach.[16]

Fever has been reported following TAMIS, which may be caused by transient bacteremia. Observation is generally safe and antibiotics are usually not necessary. However, persistence of or high fever and other signs of a systemic inflammatory response mandates further evaluation. As with most any anorectal operation, urinary retention requiring catheterization has been reported with TAMIS but is uncommon, and it is hypothesized to be exacerbated by compression of the resectoscope against the anterior rectal wall and urethra. Minimal pressure is applied to these structures in TAMIS, as the TAMIS ports are softer than the TEM resectoscope and deploy below the level of the prostate. Resolution following catheterization should be expected. More serious urologic complications, such as rectourethral fistula, have not been reported with TAMIS but could result from any ureteral injury following deep dissection of an anterior lesion. In our series, one patient developed scrotal emphysema-pneumoscrotum without peritoneal entry, which resolved spontaneously.

Transient fecal incontinence may occur following TAMIS. Anal dilatation from the 4-cm access channel, loss of rectal volume, subsequent poor rectal compliance, and increased mucous production in the healing rectum are likely causative factors. Incontinence is temporary, with restoration of normal function and manometric parameters at 6 months. Karakayali et al.[17] evaluated anorectal function after TAMIS for rectal tumors in 10 patients and found no difference between preoperative and 3-week postoperative anorectal manometry. Only mean minimal sensory volumes were lower after surgery. Cleveland Clinic Incontinence Scores were also normal in all patients at 6 weeks. Versveld et al.[18] reported no detrimental impact of TAMIS on quality of life or anorectal function in 24 patients.

FOLLOW-UP

Close clinical and endoscopic follow-up is vital to detection of local and systemic recurrence. In accordance with the NCCN guidelines, patients should undergo a history, physical examination, rigid proctoscopy, and serum carcinoembryonic antigen (CEA) level every 3 months for 2 years and then every 6 months for a total of 5 years after excision of a malignant lesion. A full colonoscopy at 1 and 3 years following resection should be performed and every 5 years thereafter to identify metachronous lesions. It is the authors' practice to supplement the radiologic evaluation with a pelvic MRI to identify suspicious lymph nodes every 6 months for the first 2 years following resection.

OUTCOME/CURRENT RESULTS

Since its introduction in 2009, there have been over 500 published TAMIS cases for local excision of rectal neoplasia.[12,19,20] Perioperative outcomes are excellent, as morbidity and mortality after TAMIS are low. The overall complication rate was 7.4% with no mortality in a systematic review of 390 TAMIS cases. There also does not appear to be any impairments in anorectal function or quality of life after TAMIS.[18,21] In our own experience of over 250 TAMIS procedures for local excision of rectal neoplasia, of which 55% were performed for malignancy, 93% of patients have an R0 resection and 95% of patients had an en bloc resection. Overall, 6% of patients experienced a local recurrence after a mean follow-up of 14.4 months, but only 1% of patients experienced curatively resected invasive disease. Keller et al.[20] reported TAMIS in 75 patients, 6.6% positive margins, less than 1% fragmented tumors, and local recurrence of 5.8% after mean follow-up of 36.5 months. These data compare favorably with traditional TAE and TEM.[2,22] There are no data specifically comparing TAMIS and radical surgery, and thus much of the data are extrapolated from TEM.[3]

CONCLUSION

The management of patients with early rectal cancer involves a delicate balance between cure and the complication and functional morbidities that occur with radical surgery. Selected patients who would have traditionally undergone radical surgery for early rectal cancer may now be managed via local excision for curative intent. TAMIS is an advanced endoscopic platform that may be used for curative excision for select patients with early rectal cancer. We have described the indications, surgical technique, perioperative care, and potential complications of this technique. Current data suggest that resection quality and local recurrence rates are comparable to TEM. For carefully selected patients, TAMIS for local excision of rectal neoplasia is a valid option with low morbidity that maintains the advantages of organ preservation.

REFERENCES

1. Morson BC, Bussey HJ, Samoorian S. Policy of local excision for early cancer of the colorectum. *Gut.* 1977;18(12):1045-1050.
2. Clancy C, Burke JP, Albert MR, O'Connell PR, Winter DC. Transanal endoscopic microsurgery versus standard transanal excision for the removal of rectal neoplasms: a systematic review and meta-analysis. *Dis Colon Rectum.* 2015;58(2):254-261.
3. Kidane B, Chadi SA, Kanters S, Colquhoun PH, Ott MC. Local resection compared with radical resection in the treatment of T1N0M0 rectal adenocarcinoma: a systematic review and meta-analysis. *Dis Colon Rectum.* 2015;58(1):122-140.
4. Buess G, Hutterer F, Theiss J, Bobel M, Isselhard W, Pichlmaier H. A system for a transanal endoscopic rectum operation. *Chirurg.* 1984;55(10):677-680.
5. Winde G, Nottberg H, Keller R, Schmid KW, Bunte H. Surgical cure for early rectal carcinomas (T1). Transanal endoscopic microsurgery vs. anterior resection. *Dis Colon Rectum.* 1996;39(9):969-976.
6. Atallah S, Albert M, Larach S. Transanal minimally invasive surgery: a giant leap forward. *Surg Endosc.* 2010;24(9):2200-2205.
7. de Beche-Adams T, Nassif G. Transanal minimally invasive surgery. *Clin Colon Rectal Surg.* 2015;28(3):176-180.
8. Glasgow SC, Bleier JI, Burgart LJ, Finne CO, Lowry AC. Meta-analysis of histopathological features of primary colorectal cancers that predict lymph node metastases. *J Gastrointest Surg.* 2012;16(5):1019-1028.
9. Bhangu A, Brown G, Nicholls RJ, Wong J, Darzi A, Tekkis P. Survival outcome of local excision versus radical resection of colon or rectal carcinoma: a Surveillance, Epidemiology, and End Results (SEER) population-based study. *Ann Surg.* 2013;258(4):563-569, discussion 569-571.
10. Sumrien H, Dadnam C, Hewitt J, McCarthy K. Feasibility of transanal minimally invasive surgery (TAMIS) for rectal tumours and its impact on quality of life—the Bristol series. *Anticancer Res.* 2016;36(4):2005-2009.
11. Burke JP, Atallah S, Albert MR. Transanal endoscopic resection with peritoneal entry: a word of reason. *Tech Coloproctol.* 2015;19(10):663-664.
12. Hahnloser D, Cantero R, Salgado G, Dindo D, Rega D, Delrio P. Transanal minimal invasive surgery for rectal lesions: should the defect be closed? *Colorectal Dis.* 2015;17(5):397-402.
13. Atallah S, Drake J, Martin-Perez B, Kang C, Larach S. Robotic transanal total mesorectal excision with intersphincteric dissection for extreme distal rectal cancer: a video demonstration. *Tech Coloproctol.* 2015;19(7):435.
14. Hompes R, Rauh SM, Ris F, Tuynman JB, Mortensen NJ. Robotic transanal minimally invasive surgery for local excision of rectal neoplasms. *Br J Surg.* 2014;101(5):578-581.
15. Marks JH, Valsdottir EB, DeNittis A, et al. Transanal endoscopic microsurgery for the treatment of rectal cancer: comparison of wound complication rates with and without neoadjuvant radiation therapy. *Surg Endosc.* 2009;23(5):1081-1087.
16. Perez RO, Habr-Gama A, Sao Juliao GP, Proscurshim I, Scanavini Neto A, Gama-Rodrigues J. Transanal endoscopic microsurgery for residual rectal cancer after neoadjuvant chemoradiation therapy is associated with significant immediate pain and hospital readmission rates. *Dis Colon Rectum.* 2011;54(5):545-551.
17. Karakayali FY, Tezcaner T, Moray G. Anorectal function and outcomes after transanal minimally invasive surgery for rectal tumors. *J Minim Access Surg* 2015;11(4):257-262.
18. Verseveld M, Barendse RM, Gosselink MP, Verhoef C, de Graaf EJ, Doornebosch PG. Transanal minimally invasive surgery: impact on quality of life and functional outcome. *Surg Endosc.* 2016;30(3):1184-1187.
19. Martin-Perez B, Andrade-Ribeiro GD, Hunter L, Atallah S. A systematic review of transanal minimally invasive surgery (TAMIS) from 2010 to 2013. *Tech Coloproctol.* 2014;18(9):775-788.
20. Keller DS, Tahilramani RN, Flores-Gonzalez JR, Mahmood A, Haas EM. Transanal minimally invasive surgery: review of indications and outcomes from 75 consecutive patients. *J Am Coll Surg.* 2015;222(5):814-822.
21. Schiphorst AH, Langenhoff BS, Maring J, Pronk A, Zimmerman DD. Transanal minimally invasive surgery: initial experience and short-term functional results. *Dis Colon Rectum.* 2014;57(8):927-932.
22. Arezzo A, Passera R, Saito Y, et al. Systematic review and meta-analysis of endoscopic submucosal dissection versus transanal endoscopic microsurgery for large noninvasive rectal lesions. *Surg Endosc.* 2014;28(2):427-438.

Transanal Approaches to Early Rectal Cancer: Transanal Endoscopic Microsurgery and Conventional Transanal Excision

Marco E. Allaix | Alessandro Fichera

Widespread introduction of screening programs has resulted in a significant increase in the early detection of rectal cancers. In addition, staging tools and treatment modalities for rectal cancer have greatly improved. As a consequence, there is an increasing interest in multimodal organ-preserving strategies in patients with early rectal cancer (ERC), including the use of local excision (LE)[1] and chemoradiation therapy (CRT).[2]

Until the 1990s, conventional transanal excision (TAE) with retractors was considered an oncologically adequate alternative to radical rectal resection for the treatment of ERC.[3] However, the advent of the total mesorectal excision (TME) and the implementation of new endoscopic techniques, including transanal endoscopic microsurgery (TEM), have challenged the role of conventional TAE even in T1 rectal cancer patients. To date, abdominal rectal resection combined with TME is the current standard for the surgical treatment of rectal cancer. TEM is an attractive option in selected T1N0 cancer patients because it avoids the morbidity and the functional sequelae associated with radical surgery. Recently, its use in association with neoadjuvant CRT has been proposed in selected T2-N0 rectal cancer patients.

The aim of this chapter is to review surgical techniques and short- and long-term oncologic outcomes of TAE and TEM for ERC.

EARLY RECTAL CANCER: DEFINITION

There is no consensus regarding how to define an ERC (Table 167B.1). Some classifications define ERC based on the degree of submucosal infiltration; the Haggitt levels estimate the submucosal invasion in pedunculated tumors,[4] whereas the Kikuchi classification[5] describes the depth of submucosal invasion in nonpedunculated lesions by dividing the submucosa in three parts: sm1, sm2, and sm3 T1 cancers.

The Paris classification of superficial neoplastic lesions[6] and its revised edition[7] represent the most recent attempt to classify ERC from a pathologic point of view. A tumor is defined as superficial when the depth of tumor infiltration is limited to the submucosa. A polypoid lesion may be pedunculated (0-Ip), sessile (0-Is), or with a mixed pattern (0-Isp). Nonpolypoid lesions are either slightly elevated (0-IIa, with elevation <2.5 mm above the level of the mucosa), completely flat (0-IIb), or slightly depressed (0-IIc). The mixed types include elevated and depressed lesions (0-IIa + IIc), depressed and elevated (0-IIc + IIa), and sessile and depressed (0-Is + IIc). The nondepressed types (i.e., 0-IIa, 0-IIb) might progress to polypoid or laterall-spreading tumors.

Even though ERC is considered as a rectal cancer with low risk of lymph node metastases (T1-2N0),[8] this definition does not thoroughly reflect the clinical impact of ERC on both treatment and survival. Therefore a clinical definition has recently been proposed: ERC is a rectal cancer with good prognostic features that might be safely removed preserving the rectum, and that will have a very limited risk of relapse after LE.[9]

CONVENTIONAL TRANSANAL EXCISION/ TRANSANAL ENDOSCOPIC MICROSURGERY

PREOPERATIVE WORK-UP

The preoperative work-up includes

- Clinical evaluation including digital rectal examination
- Complete colonoscopy to rule out the presence of synchronous colonic lesions
- Rigid proctoscopy to locate the lesion along the circumference and to measure the distance of the upper and lower limits from the anal verge
- Endoscopic ultrasound (EUS) to assess the depth of invasion of the tumor in the rectal wall
- Pelvic magnetic resonance imaging (MRI) to detect potential lymph node metastases
- Chest and abdominal computed tomography to rule out distant metastases
- Serum carcinoembryonic antigen (CEA) assay

PATIENT PREPARATION

Candidates for TEM/TAE of an ERC should be on a low-fiber diet the week before surgery and undergo a rectal enema 12 and 2 hours preoperatively. If violation of the peritoneal cavity is expected, a full bowel preparation with oral antibiotics is administered. Intravenous antibiotics, such as a second-generation cephalosporin and metronidazole, are administered before starting the operation and continued on the first postoperative day. Deep venous thrombosis prophylaxis is not routinely administered.

CONVENTIONAL TRANSANAL EXCISION

INDICATIONS

- T1N0 tumors located in the lower rectum (<10 cm from the anal verge)

TABLE 167B.1 Definitions of Early Rectal Cancer

Classification	Description
Haggitt classification (pedunculated T1 cancers)[4]	*Level 1*: invasion of submucosa limited to polyp head *Level 2*: invasion of submucosa of the polyp neck *Level 3*: invasion of submucosa of the polyp stalk *Level 4*: invasion of submucosa beyond the stalk
Kikuchi classification (nonpedunculated T1 cancers)[5]	*sm1*: invasion less than 1 mm *sm2*: intermediate between sm1 and sm3 *sm3*: invasion near to the muscularis propria
The Paris classification of superficial neoplastic lesions and its revised edition[6,7]	A *polypoid* lesion may be • Pedunculated (0-Ip) • Sessile (0-Is) • With a mixed pattern (0-Isp) *Nonpolypoid* lesions are • Slightly elevated (0-IIa, with elevation less than 2.5 mm above the level of the mucosa) • Completely flat (0-IIb) • Slightly depressed (0-IIc) *Mixed* types are • Elevated and depressed lesions (0-IIa + IIc) • Depressed and elevated (0-IIc + IIa) • Sessile and depressed (0-Is + IIc)
EAES Consensus Conference[9]	Early rectal cancer is a rectal cancer with good prognostic features that might be safely removed preserving the rectum, and that will have a very limited risk of relapse after local excision.

EAES, European Association for Endoscopic Surgery.

- Mobile and polypoid lesions
- Tumors involving less than 1/3 of rectal circumference
- Tumors less than 3 cm in diameter
- G1-2 tumors
- No evidence of lymphovascular invasion (even though the preoperative evaluation of this parameter is challenging)

SURGICAL TECHNIQUE

- With posterior lesions, the patient is usually placed in high lithotomy, whereas with anterior lesions the patient is placed in the prone jackknife position to allow the surgeon to look down on the tumor while operating.
- A Lone Star retractor may be placed to evert the anus and improve the exposure of the surgical field.
- A self-retaining retractor is then positioned in the anus to identify the tumor.
- The mucosa is scored circumferentially by using conventional monopolar electrocautery to adequately define the resection margin (at least 0.5 cm).
- A retraction suture placed at the apex of the tumor might be useful in the presence of a proximal tumor to bring the lesion out of the anus as the dissection progresses.

- A full-thickness excision of the tumor is performed down to the perirectal fatty tissue; during dissection, the rectal mass should be lifted away from the underlying fatty tissue to resect the tumor en bloc including surrounding perirectal tissue and adequate free resection margins.
- The procedure ends with closure of the rectal wall defect using interrupted resorbable sutures. If the defect is too wide to obtain closure without tension, the opening is left to heal by secondary intention.

POSTOPERATIVE COMPLICATIONS

- Rectal bleeding
- Perirectal infection
- Pain in case of resection reaching the dentate line
- Anorectal stenosis
- Prostate or vagina injury in case of anterior rectal tumors

TRANSANAL ENDOSCOPIC MICROSURGERY

CURRENT INDICATIONS (IN ADDITION TO THOSE LISTED FOR CONVENTIONAL TRANSANAL EXCISION)

- Tumor located in higher and mid-rectum (limited to experienced surgeons)
- T2 N0 rectal cancers responding to CRT in the setting of study protocols or in patients unfit for abdominal surgery

SURGICAL TECHNIQUE

Equipment

To date, there are two different platforms used to perform transanal endoscopic surgery for ERC: the TEM and the transanal endoscopic operation (TEO) platforms. Both platforms allow removal of lesions in the mid and upper rectum that cannot be accessed with conventional TAE, with better visualization of the rectal lumen than TAE.

TEM (Richard Wolf, Knittlingen, Germany) equipment (Fig. 167B.1) was originally conceived by Gerhard Buess in the early 1980s and includes the following:

- An operating proctoscope that is 4 cm in diameter and is available in three different lengths with correspondent obturators that allow insertion of the proctoscope
- A working adapter and a working insert to connect the proctoscope to working instruments, the camera, and the insufflator
- A Martin arm to fix the proctoscope to the operating table
- A light source and a stereoscopic angled telescope, which allows dissection under microsurgical conditions with three-dimensional (3D) visualization through ocular lenses
- Instruments including suction and irrigation tubes, curved and straight monopolar grasping forceps, suture clips forceps, electrocautery, and a needle holder

TEO Instrumentation by Karl Storz GmbH (Tuttlingen, Germany) (Fig. 167B.2) is an alternative to the TEM platform that is gaining acceptance worldwide.

TEO instrumentation includes a 7- or 15-cm proctoscope (4 cm in diameter) with three working channels (12, 5,

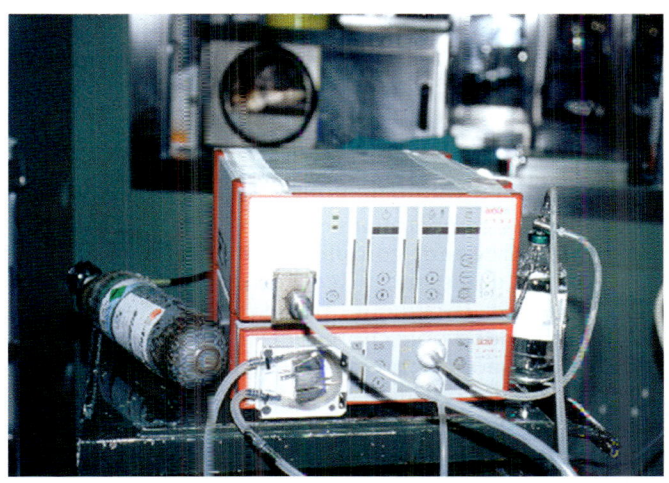
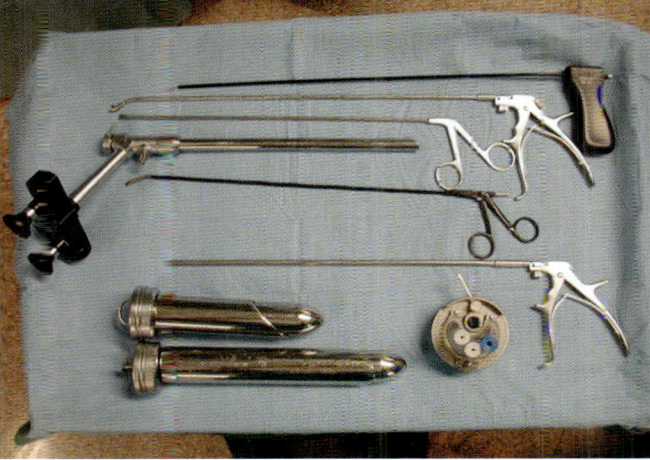

FIGURE 167B.1 Transanal endoscopic microsurgery equipment.

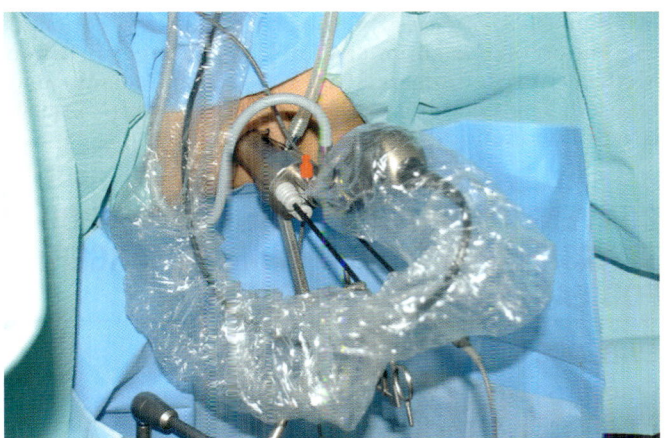

FIGURE 167B.2 Transanal endoscopic operation equipment.

and 5 mm) for dedicated or conventional laparoscopic instruments, and a 5-mm channel for a 30-degree, two-dimensional (2D) camera. The shape of the TEO proctoscope tip allows manipulation and suturing of the rectal wall on a 360-degree surface. A standard laparoscopic camera unit is used with this system, with the imaging displayed on a screen.

An underpowered, randomized controlled trial comparing 34 patients undergoing TEM or TEO for early rectal tumors failed to show any significant difference in intraoperative and postoperative outcomes. TEO platform costs were significant lower than TEM platform.[10]

Positioning of the Patient on the Operating Table

The TEM procedure can be performed under general or spinal anesthesia. A recent report of a prospective series of 50 patients treated via the TEO platform for rectal tumors, showed that TEO under spinal anesthesia is safe and feasible. No intraoperative complications occurred, and no procedure required conversion to general anesthesia. The median duration of operation was 60 (range, 20 to 165) minutes. No opioids were administered during the perioperative or postoperative period. The median

postoperative pain score was 0 at 4, 8, 24, and 48 hours after surgery. No significant postoperative changes were observed in hemodynamic parameters.[11]

The patient is placed either prone or supine to keep the lesion as close to the 6 o'clock position as possible. Patients with posterior lateral rectal tumors are placed in the supine position. If the lesion is located on the anterolateral wall (12 to 3 o'clock position or 9 to 12 o'clock position) or close to the peritoneal reflection, the prone position is used. The prone jackknife position removes small bowel loops from the surgical field and reduces air leakage through the bowel wall opening above its peritoneal reflection into the peritoneal cavity, thus facilitating suture of the peritoneal opening.

A Foley catheter is inserted before starting the procedure and is usually kept in place for the first 24 hours.

Step 1: Dissection

- The surgeon is seated between the patient's legs, while the assistant is to the left of the surgeon. The monitor is placed in front of the surgeon.
- The proctoscope is inserted into the rectum and fixed after identification of the rectal lesion. The proctoscope position might be adjusted during the procedure, thus ensuring optimal visualization and clear access to the tumor margins.
- Carbon dioxide (CO_2) inflation is maintained at an 8-mm Hg endorectal pressure, which in some cases might be increased up to 16 mm Hg.
- The operation starts by marking the lesion circumferentially with the electrocautery, thus ensuring at least 5-mm clear circumferential margins (Fig. 167B.3).
- The dissection begins at the right lower border of the tumor (Fig. 167B.4A), and continues proximally around and under the tumor until a circumferential dissection is achieved and the tumor is excised en bloc (see Fig. 167B.4B and C). Tumor excision can be safely performed using monopolar electrocautery. Ultrasonic shears or an electrothermal bipolar vessel sealing system might be useful in difficult cases to complete the dissection. Due to the limited accuracy of the preoperative staging tools, a full-thickness excision down to the

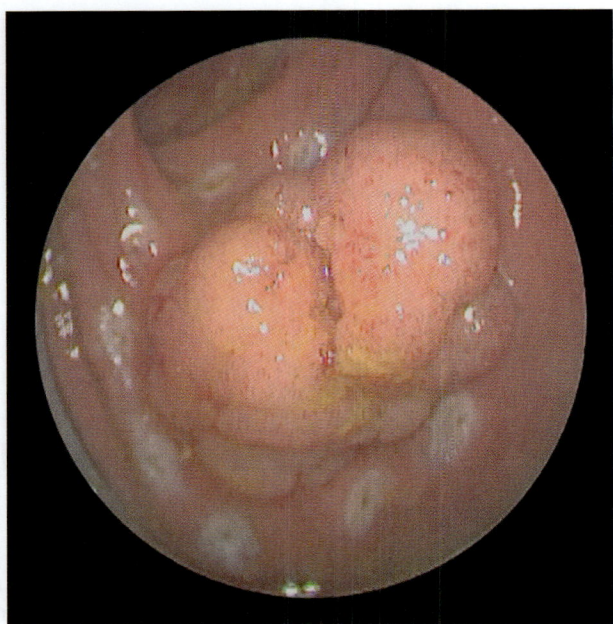

FIGURE 167B.3 Marking the margins of resection.

perirectal fatty tissue should be routinely performed. Females with a thin rectovaginal septum and males with prior prostatectomy, who undergo a TEM/TEO procedure for an anteriorly located rectal tumor, are at higher risk of developing a rectovaginal or rectovesical fistula, respectively.

- The specimen is then retrieved transanally and is oriented and pinned to a corkboard to preserve the margins of normal rectal mucosa surrounding the tumor.
- In cases where the peritoneum is entered, the surgeon's experience greatly influences the ability to complete the procedure transanally. In our experience, the prone position of the patient on the operating table and the shape of the tip of the TEO proctoscope help the surgeon close the rectal wall defect. The risk of conversion to open surgery or the need for a stoma is minimized.

Step 2: Wall Defect Suturing

The technical advantages of TEM/TEO to close the rectal wall defect compared to classic transanal excision can reduce the risks of postoperative local infection and sepsis. This also translates to fewer complications in the case of subsequent rectal resection with TME in patients with recurrence or unfavorable pathology on the LE specimen.

- The wall defect is first irrigated with iodopovidone solution to reduce septic complications and the risk of tumor cell implantation.
- The rectal wall defect is then closed with one or more monofilament absorbable running sutures, usually from right to left (Fig. 167B.5A). For large wall defects, a midline stitch is placed to approximate proximal and distal margins, thus reducing the tension of the suture. Dedicated silver clips are used to secure the suture because knot tying during the procedure is challenging.

Suturing devices such as Endo Stitch can be used to suture the rectal wall as an alternative to the clips.
- At the end of the procedure, patency of the rectal lumen is carefully checked through the TEM/TEO proctoscope (see Fig. 167B.5B).

Postoperative Complications

Postoperative complications occur in up to 15% of patients. The most frequent complications are rectal bleeding and suture dehiscence. Rectal bleeding is self-limiting in most cases. Treatment options include blood transfusions and endoscopic clipping. Dehiscence of the suture line occurs more frequently after neoadjuvant radiation therapy usually in patients preoperatively staged as cT2N0. Patients with suture dehiscence experience severe rectal pain, tenesmus, and fever. Endoscopy or cross-sectional imaging is performed to evaluate the suture line and the size of the perirectal collection for possible drainage. Conservative treatment includes intravenous antibiotics and 10% iodine solution enemas and leads to healing in about 90% of cases.[12] Other treatment tools such as the endoscopic vacuum system (Endosponge, B Braun Medical BV, Melsungen AG, Tuttlingen, Germany) may be used. The need for a stoma creation to control sepsis is very uncommon.

CONVENTIONAL TRANSANAL EXCISION OR TRANSANAL ENDOSCOPIC MICROSURGERY FOR EARLY RECTAL CANCER?

EVIDENCE

Comparison of TEM and TAE for T1N0 rectal cancers has revealed significantly higher rates of tumor fragmentation and positive resection margins after TAE than TEM. The result is higher (and unacceptable) local recurrence rates after TAE.[13] Langer et al.[14] reviewed 38 T1 rectal cancer patients treated by TAE (18 patients) or TEM (20 patients). The rates of positive or indeterminate resection margins were higher after TAE than TEM (37% vs. 19%, positive; 16% vs. 5%, indeterminate). Christoforidis et al.[15] compared 42 stage 1 (T1-2) rectal cancer patients treated by TEM and 129 treated by TAE. TAE was found to have significantly higher rates of positive resection margins than TEM (16% vs. 2%; P = .017). A recent systematic review and meta-analysis of studies comparing TAE and radical resection for T1N0M0 rectal cancer showed that TAE had higher local recurrence rates and poorer 5-year survival.[16] The evidence that TAE compromises survival in patients with ERC has led to a decrease in the use of this approach during the last 15 years, favoring the adoption of TEM.[17,18]

TEM does not jeopardize the long-term survival in low-risk T1 carcinoma according to Hermanek criteria.[19] Comparison of patients who had a TEM or TME for a T1 low-risk cancer had no difference in local recurrence (4% vs. 3%, respectively), whereas higher local recurrence rates were observed after TEM than TME in high-risk rectal cancer patients (33% vs. 18%).[20] Local recurrence rates in 52 patients treated by TEM and in 17 patients who underwent rectal resection with TME for G1 or G2

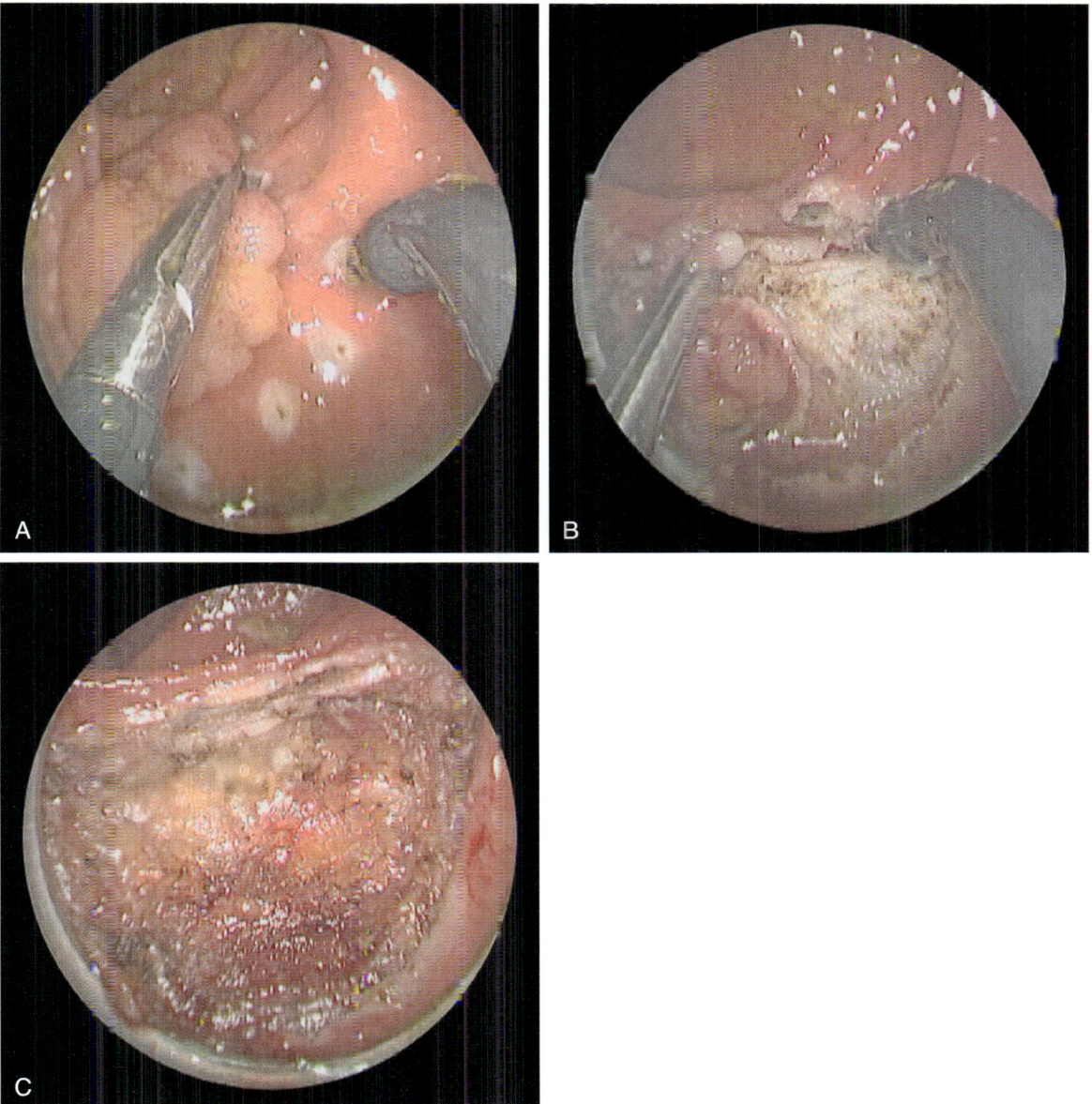

FIGURE 167B.4 (A) Dissection starting at the right lower border of the tumor. (B) Dissection continued proximally around and under the lesion. (C) Perirectal fatty tissue after removal of the tumor.

rectal cancers were similar (4% vs. 0%; $P = .05$). Recurrence rates and 10-year cancer-free survival in pT1 cancer patients treated by TEM differ based on low- and high-risk designations. Local recurrence rates have been reported as 6% after R0 TEM in low-risk and 39% in high-risk patients.[21] The recurrence rate was significantly reduced to 6% in those high-risk patients who underwent an immediate reoperation ($P = .015$).[22]

Submucosal tumor invasion is a strong prognostic factor for long-term survival in rectal cancer patients undergoing TEM for T1N0 rectal cancer.[23,24] T1 rectal cancers with a submucosal tumor invasion less than 1000 μm (T1sm1) have the lowest risk of recurrence and sm2-3 T1 and T2 rectal cancers have similar recurrence rates.[23] Local

recurrence rate should be less than 5% for pT1 Sm1 rectal cancers with no evidence of lymphovascular invasion and a diameter of 3 cm or less.

TEM was initially developed for the treatment of tumors located in the mid and lower rectum. In the treatment of high rectal ERCs, TEM has shown no increased short-term morbidity or mortality and no adverse oncologic outcomes, even in the case of inadvertent peritoneal opening.[25–30] The experience of the surgeon is key in the decision-making process for the treatment strategy to be adopted when the peritoneum is entered.[31]

TEM does not impair anorectal function and quality of life in ERC patients. Although a transient reduction in anal resting and squeeze pressures is observed at 3

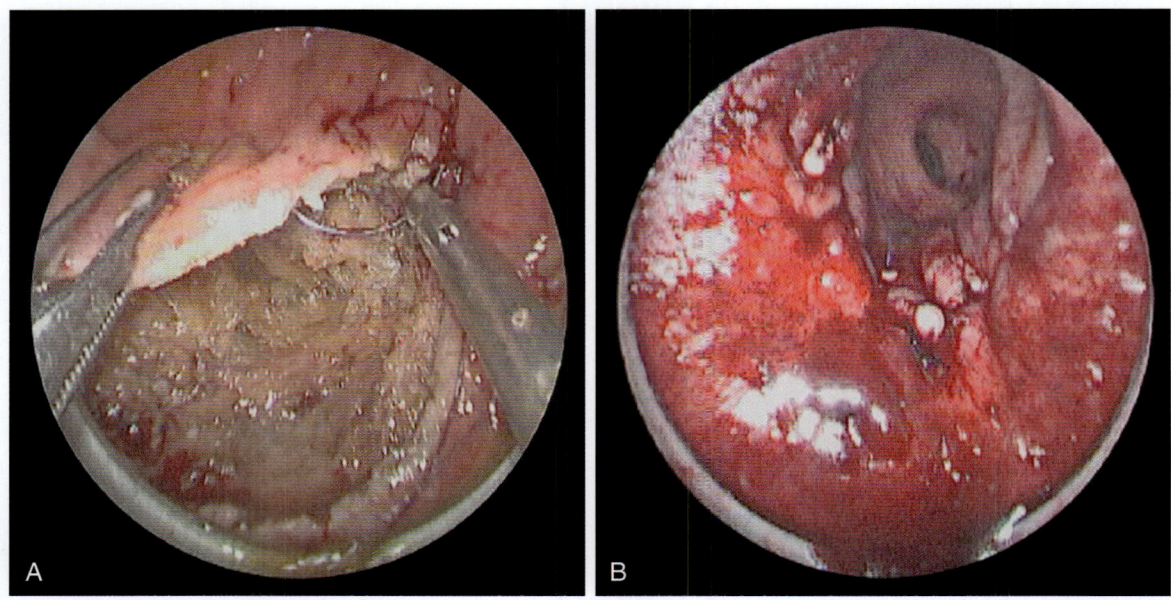

FIGURE 167B.5 (A) Closure of the rectal wall defect with a running suture. (B) Control of the patency of the rectal lumen.

months after surgery, normal values are recorded within 1 year after TEM. A similar trend is reported in rectal sensitivity thresholds that leads to increased rates of urgency and to a slight increase in the Wexner score for fecal continence. A return to preoperative values can be anticipated within 1 year after surgery.[32]

In conclusion, TAE should be abandoned for the treatment of ERC. TEM should be considered in selected T1 (sm1) rectal cancer patients, thus avoiding unnecessary rectal resection without compromising survival.

TRANSANAL ENDOSCOPIC MICROSURGERY FOR T2N0 RECTAL CANCER

The assessment of perirectal lymph node status is the main challenge of LE for rectal cancer. The risk of lymph node metastases increases with tumor T and Sm stage: from 0% to 3% for T1 sm1, to 15% for T1 sm2-3 and to 25% for T2 rectal cancers.[33,34] As a consequence, high-risk T1 and T2 rectal cancer patients have a significantly higher risk of recurrence after LE alone than after radical surgery.

During the last decade, a multimodal organ-preserving approach, including neoadjuvant CRT followed by LE, has been proposed in selected T1-2N0 rectal cancer patients to avoid the postoperative morbidity and mortality associated with rectal resection and TME without affecting survival.[35–38] A review of 7378 patients undergoing LE and 36,116 patients treated with major rectal resection for T0-2N0M0 rectal cancer revealed that LE had similar oncologic outcomes compared to abdominal surgery in T0-1 rectal cancer patients. Poor results were obtained with LE alone in T2 rectal cancer patients.[36] Poor results were obtained with LE alone in T2 rectal cancer patients. Neoadjuvant therapy followed by LE for T2 rectal cancer yielded outcomes similar to those patients treated with abdominal surgery.

The impact of a multidisciplinary strategy including neoadjuvant CRT followed by TEM for the treatment of T2N0M0 is gaining increasing interest in the surgical community, because preliminary oncologic results are promising.[2,21,39,40] A randomized controlled trial has shown cancer-related and overall survival rates to be similar in 50 patients treated by TEM compared with 50 patients undergoing rectal resection, both after long-course CRT: G1-G2 tumors, T2N0M0, smaller than 3 cm, within 6 cm of the anal verge (89% vs. 94% (P= .687), and 72% versus 80% (P= .609).[2] In both groups, local or distant recurrences were reported only in partial or nonresponders to neoadjuvant CRT. The prospective phase 2 ACOSOG Z6041 trial showed that 3-year disease-free survival in 72 patients with T2N0 rectal cancer treated by neoadjuvant CRT followed by TAE or TEM was 86.9% (95% confidence interval [CI], 79.3% to 95.3%). LE after neoadjuvant CRT may be considered as an organ-preserving alternative in carefully selected patients with clinically staged T2N0 tumors who refuse, or are not fit for, radical rectal resection.[41]

However, this strategy has some potential drawbacks. Significant rectal wound-related morbidity (up to 70%) has been reported in patients undergoing neoadjuvant treatment followed by TEM.[12,42,43] Wound complication has been reported in 25.6% of patients receiving radiotherapy before TEM compared to none in patients treated by TEM alone (P= .015).[12] Rectal suture dehiscence occurred more frequently in radiated patients and readmission increased (70% vs. 23%; P= .03) (43% vs. 7%; P= .02).[42]

Suturing irradiated tissue could be the reason for the high incidence of rectal wall dehiscence observed in patients undergoing TEM after neoadjuvant radiation therapy. Optimal management of the rectal wall defect following TEM after neoadjuvant radiation therapy remains controversial.

This combined surgery and CRT approach is also associated with poor functional outcomes that are similar to those observed after radical rectal resection.[44,45] Functional outcomes at 1 year after LE and CRT compared to radical resection for TME have been similar.[44] Thirty-eight percent of patients after LE and CRT claimed anorectal dysfunction affecting their quality of life. Sexual life was impaired in 19% of men and 20% of women.

A multimodality strategy should be proposed only in the setting of clinical trials while awaiting the long-term results of large randomized controlled trials.[9] The TEM after Chemoradiotherapy for Rectal Cancer (CARTS) trial is investigating the outcomes of TEM performed 8 to 10 weeks after preoperative long-course CRT.[45] The TEM and Radiotherapy in Early Rectal Cancer (TREC)[47] trial is an ongoing phase II open, multicenter randomized controlled trial that compares radical rectal resection by TME with short-course radiotherapy followed by delayed (8 to 10 weeks) TEM for ERC. The TREC and CARTS groups have combined their phase II protocols (STAR-TREC) to produce a single phase III trial that will randomize patients to (1) radical surgery, (2) short-course radiotherapy followed by TEM, or (3) CRT followed by TEM.

CONCLUSION

TEM is the procedure of choice for LE of selected low-risk T1N0 rectal cancers, because morbidity and mortality rates are significantly lower than rates after rectal resection with TME and long-term survival is similar. TAE should be limited to a few cases of highly selected distal ERCs if TEM is not feasible for technical reasons. The role of neoadjuvant CRT followed by TEM in highly selected T2 N0 rectal cancer is still under evaluation.

REFERENCES

1. You YN, Baxter NN, Stewart A, Nelson H. Is the increasing rate of local excision for stage I rectal cancer in the United States justified? a nationwide cohort study from the National Cancer Database. *Ann Surg.* 2007;245:726-733.
2. Lezoche E, Baldarelli M, Lezoche G, Paganini AM, Gesuita R, Guerrieri M. Randomized clinical trial of endoluminal locoregional resection versus laparoscopic total mesorectal excision for T2 rectal cancer after neoadjuvant therapy. *Br J Surg.* 2012;99:1211-1218.
3. Steele GD Jr, Herndon JE, Bleday R, et al. Sphincter-sparing treatment for distal rectal adenocarcinoma. *Ann Surg Oncol.* 1999;6:433-441.
4. Haggitt RC, Glotzbach RE, Soffer EE, Wruble LD. Prognostic factors in colorectal carcinomas arising in adenomas: implications for lesions removed by endoscopic polypectomy. *Gastroenterology.* 1985;89:328-336.
5. Kikuchi R, Takano M, Takagi K, et al. Management of early invasive colorectal cancer. Risk of recurrence and clinical guidelines. *Dis Colon Rectum.* 1995;38:1286-1295.
6. Participants in the Paris Workshop. The Paris endoscopic classification of superficial neoplastic lesions: esophagus, stomach, and colon: November 30 to December 1, 2002. *Gastrointest Endosc.* 2003;58:S3-S43.
7. Endoscopic Classification Review Group. Update on the Paris classification of superficial neoplastic lesions in the digestive tract. *Endoscopy.* 2005;37:570-578.
8. Kitajima K, Fujimori T, Fujii S, et al. Correlations between lymph node metastasis and depth of submucosal invasion in submucosal invasive colorectal carcinoma: a Japanese collaborative study. *J Gastroenterol.* 2004;39:534-543.
9. Morino M, Risio M, Bach S, et al. Early rectal cancer: the European Association for Endoscopic Surgery (EAES) clinical consensus conference. *Surg Endosc.* 2015;29:755-773.
10. Serra-Aracil X, Mora-Lopez L, Alcantara-Moral M, Caro-Tarrago A, Navarro-Soto S. Transanal endoscopic microsurgery with 3-D (TEM) or high-definition 2-D transanal endoscopic operation (TEO) for rectal tumors. A prospective, randomized clinical trial. *Int J Colorectal Dis.* 2014;29:605-610.
11. Arezzo A, Cortese G, Arolfo S, et al. Transanal endoscopic operation under spinal anaesthesia. *Br J Surg.* 2016;103(7):916-920. doi 10.1002/bjs.10082.
12. Marks JH, Valsdottir EB, DeNittis A, et al. Transanal endoscopic microsurgery for the treatment of rectal cancer: comparison of wound complication rates with and without neoadjuvant radiation therapy. *Surg Endosc.* 2009;23:1081-1087.
13. Clancy C, Burke JP, Albert M, O'Connell PR, Winter DC. Transanal endoscopic microsurgery versus standard transanal excision for the removal of rectal neoplasms: a systematic review and meta-analysis. *Dis Colon Rectum.* 2015;58:254-261.
14. Langer C, Liersch T, Süss M, et al. Surgical cure for early rectal carcinoma and large adenoma: transanal endoscopic microsurgery (using ultrasound or electrosurgery) compared to conventional local and radical resection. *Int J Colorectal Dis.* 2003;18:222-229.
15. Christoforidis D, Cho HM, Dixon MR, Mellgren AF, Madoff RD, Finne CO. Transanal endoscopic microsurgery versus conventional transanal excision for patients with early rectal cancer. *Ann Surg.* 2009;249:776-782.
16. Kidane B, Chadi SA, Kanters S, Colquhoun PH, Ott MC. Local resection compared with radical resection in the treatment of T1N0M0 rectal adenocarcinoma: a systematic review and meta-analysis. *Dis Colon Rectum.* 2015;58:122-140.
17. Atallah S, Keller D. Why the conventional Parks transanal excision for early stage rectal cancer should be abandoned. *Dis Colon Rectum.* 2015;58:1211-1214.
18. Gillern SM, Mahmoud NN, Paulson EC. Local excision for early stage rectal cancer in patients over age 65 years: 2000-2009. *Dis Colon Rectum.* 2015;58:172-178.
19. Hermanek P, Gall FP. Early (microinvasive) colorectal carcinoma. Pathology, diagnosis, surgical treatment. *Int J Colorectal Dis.* 1986;1:79-84.
20. Heintz A, Morschel M, Junginger T. Comparison of results after transanal endoscopic microsurgery and radical resection for T1 carcinoma of the rectum. *Surg Endosc.* 1998;12:1145-1148.
21. Lee W, Lee D, Choi S, Chun H. Transanal endoscopic microsurgery and radical surgery for T1 and T2 rectal cancer. *Surg Endosc.* 2003;17:1283-1287.
22. Borschitz T, Heintz A, Junginger T. The influence of histopathologic criteria on the long-term prognosis of locally excised pT1 rectal carcinomas: results of local excision (transanal endoscopic microsurgery) and immediate reoperation. *Dis Colon Rectum.* 2006;49:1492-1506.
23. Bach SP, Hill J, Monson JR, Association of Coloproctology of Great Britain and Ireland Transanal Endoscopic Microsurgery (TEM) Collaboration, et al. A predictive model for local recurrence after transanal endoscopic microsurgery for rectal cancer. *Br J Surg.* 2009;96:280-290.
24. Morino M, Allaix ME, Caldart M, Scozzari G, Arezzo A. Risk factors for recurrence after transanal endoscopic microsurgery for rectal malignant neoplasm. *Surg Endosc.* 2011;25:3683-3690.
25. Gavagan JA, Whiteford MH, Swanstrom LL. Full-thickness intraperitoneal excision by transanal endoscopic microsurgery does not increase short-term complications. *Am J Surg.* 2004;187:630-634.
26. Ramwell A, Evans J, Bignell M, Mathias J, Simson J. The creation of a peritoneal defect in transanal endoscopic microsurgery does not increase complications. *Colorectal Dis.* 2009;11:964-966.
27. Baatrup G, Borschitz T, Cunningham C, Qvist N. Perforation into the peritoneal cavity during transanal endoscopic microsurgery for rectal cancer is not associated with major complications or oncological compromise. *Surg Endosc.* 2009;23:2680-2683.
28. Morino M, Allaix ME, Famiglietti F, Caldart M, Arezzo A. Does peritoneal perforation affect short- and long-term outcomes after transanal endoscopic microsurgery? *Surg Endosc.* 2013;27:181-188.
29. Eyvazzadeh DJ, Lee JT, Madoff RD, Mellgren AF, Finne CO. Outcomes after transanal endoscopic microsurgery with intraperitoneal anastomosis. *Dis Colon Rectum.* 2014;57:438-441.

30. Marks JH, Frenkel JL, Greenleaf CE, D'Andrea AP. Transanal endoscopic microsurgery with entrance into the peritoneal cavity: is it safe? *Dis Colon Rectum*. 2014;57:1176-1182.

31. Salm R, Lampe H, Bustos A, Matern U. Experience with TEM in Germany. *Endosc Surg Allied Technol*. 1994;2:251-254.

32. Allaix ME, Rebecchi F, Giaccone C, Mistrangelo M, Morino M. Long-term functional results and quality of life after transanal endoscopic microsurgery. *Br J Surg*. 2011;98:1635-1643.

33. Yamamoto S, Watanabe M, Hasegawa H, et al. The risk of lymph node metastasis in T1 colorectal carcinoma. *Hepatogastroenterology*. 2004;51:998-1000.

34. Saraste D, Gunnarsson U, Janson M. Predicting lymph node metastases in early rectal cancer. *Eur J Cancer*. 2013;49:1104-1108.

35. Garcia-Aguilar J, Shi Q, Thomas CR Jr, et al. A phase II trial of neoadjuvant chemoradiation and local excision for T2N0 rectal cancer: preliminary results of the ACOSOG Z6041 trial. *Ann Surg Oncol*. 2012;19:384-391.

36. Bhangu A, Brown G, Nicholls RJ, Wong J, Darzi A, Tekkis P. Survival outcome of local excision versus radical resection of colon or rectal carcinoma: a Surveillance, Epidemiology, and End Results (SEER) population-based study. *Ann Surg*. 2013;258:563-569.

37. Pucciarelli S, De Paoli A, Guerrieri M, et al. Local excision after preoperative chemoradiotherapy for rectal cancer: results of a multicenter phase II clinical trial. *Dis Colon Rectum*. 2013;56:1349-1356.

38. Shaikh I, Askari A, Ourû S, Warusavitarne J, Athanasiou T, Faiz O. Oncological outcomes of local excision compared with radical surgery after neoadjuvant chemoradiotherapy for rectal cancer: a systematic review and meta-analysis. *Int J Colorectal Dis*. 2015;30:19-29.

39. Allaix ME, Arezzo A, Giraudo G, Morino M. Transanal endoscopic microsurgery vs. laparoscopic total mesorectal excision for T2N0 rectal cancer. *J Gastrointest Surg*. 2012;16:2280-2287.

40. Sajid MS, Farag S, Leung P, Sains P, Miles WF, Baig MK. Systematic review and meta-analysis of published trials comparing the effectiveness of transanal endoscopic microsurgery and radical resection in the management of early rectal cancer. *Colorectal Dis*. 2013;16:2-16.

41. Garcia-Aguilar J, Renfro LA, Chow OS, et al. Organ preservation for clinical T2N0 distal rectal cancer using neoadjuvant chemoradiotherapy and local excision (ACOSOG Z6041): results of an open-label, single-arm, multi-institutional, phase 2 trial. *Lancet Oncol*. 2015;16:1537-1546.

42. Perez RO, Habr-Gama A, São Julião GP, Proscurshim I, Scanavini Neto A, Gama-Rodrigues J. Transanal endoscopic microsurgery for residual rectal cancer after neoadjuvant chemoradiation therapy is associated with significant immediate pain and hospital readmission rates. *Dis Colon Rectum*. 2011;54:545-551.

43. Arezzo A, Arolfo S, Allaix ME, et al. Results of neoadjuvant short-course radiation therapy followed by transanal endoscopic microsurgery for T1-T2 N0 extraperitoneal rectal cancer. *Int J Radiat Oncol Biol Phys*. 2015;92:299-306.

44. Gornicki A, Richter P, Polkowski W, et al. Anorectal and sexual functions after preoperative radiotherapy and full-thickness local excision of rectal cancer. *Eur J Surg Oncol*. 2014;40:723-730.

45. Restivo A, Zorcolo L, D'Alia G, et al. Risk of complications and long-term functional alterations after local excision of rectal tumors with transanal endoscopic microsurgery (TEM). *Int J Colorectal Dis*. 2016;31:257-266.

46. Verseveld M, de Graaf EJ, Verhoef C, et al. Chemoradiation therapy for rectal cancer in the distal rectum followed by organ-sparing transanal endoscopic microsurgery (CARTS study). *Br J Surg*. 2015; 102:853-860.

47. TREC study http://www.controlled-trials.com/isrctn 14422743.

Operations for Rectal Cancer: Low Anterior Resection—Open, Laparoscopic or Robotic, taTME, Coloanal Anastomosis

Anthony P. D'Andrea | Marta Jiménez-Toscano | Ana Otero-Piñeiro

Raquel Bravo-Infante | Antonio M. Lacy | Patricia Sylla

The management of rectal cancer has evolved over the past century. Since the first description of radical abdominoperineal resection (APR) by Miles in 1908, surgery for rectal cancer has moved toward less aggressive approaches to reduce morbidity and mortality while making sphincter preservation a priority.[1,2] APR involves both abdominal and perineal dissection to remove the anorectal complex en bloc with the rectum followed by creation of a permanent end-colostomy. Although this became the oncologic approach of choice for patients with rectal cancer, APR has been well known to have a profound negative impact on patients' quality of life and body image. Fast-forwarding to 1979, the concept of total mesorectal excision (TME) in conjunction with rectal resection, was introduced by Heald et al. and ultimately became the standard of care with or without neoadjuvant treatment.[3,4] TME involves precise and sharp, rather than blunt, dissection in the avascular areolar plane surrounding the mesorectum with removal of the specimen as a whole while preserving the inferior hypogastric nerve plexuses. Adoption of the surgical principles of TME led to a decrease in local recurrence rates from 20% to 45% prior to the 1990s, to 5% to 10% in more contemporary series.[5,6] These results also reflect the impact of neoadjuvant treatment, which has been demonstrated to markedly lower local recurrence in rectal cancer in multiple randomized controlled trials (RCTs).[7-9] Because of the substantial downstaging effect that can be achieved with current neoadjuvant therapies, sphincter preservation can be achieved in a large proportion of patients with low rectal cancers with acceptable oncologic and functional outcomes. The introduction of laparoscopy in the 1990s with advances in surgical technique and instrumentation further improved outcomes of rectal surgery by minimizing surgical trauma as reflected by reduced hospital length of stay (LOS) and recovery time while providing equivalent short- and long-term oncologic results.[6,10]

In an effort to further improve maneuverability and visualization during minimally invasive pelvic surgery, robotic-assisted surgery was introduced, which has lagged in adoption by colorectal surgeons relative to other urologic and gynecologic applications. Compared to laparoscopy, the robot provides a stable camera platform, enhanced 3D visualization of the pelvic anatomy, and additional degrees of freedom to facilitate fine, tremor-free dissection. Despite these benefits and the well-demonstrated ergonomic advantages of the robotic platform, global adoption of robotics in colorectal surgery has been limited by prohibitively high costs of the platform, especially in light of the lack of evidence supporting clinical benefits relative to laparoscopic surgery.

Most recently, the growing interest in natural orifice transluminal surgery (NOTES) has facilitated the development of transanal natural orifice and minimally invasive surgery. Local transanal excision has played an important role in the management of early rectal cancer, and innovations have included development of the rigid multiport transanal endoscopic microsurgery (TEM) platform by Buess et al. in 1983 (Richard Wolf, Vernon Hills, IL), followed by the transanal endoscopic operation (TEO) system (Karl Storz, Tuttlingen, Germany). Most recently, adoption of transanal endoscopic surgery (TES) has been accelerated by the development of disposable transanal endoscopic platforms, namely transanal minimally invasive surgery (TAMIS) platforms in 2010.[11,12] Through the use of adapted multiport transanal platforms and standard laparoscopic instrumentation, submucosal excision of benign rectal lesions and full-thickness excision of low-risk early-stage rectal tumors can be performed with low morbidity and acceptable local recurrence rates in carefully selected cases with no high-risk histopathologic features. In parallel to the evolution of local excision techniques for early rectal cancer, further developments in traditional proctectomy have set the stage for the most recent evolution in TME, namely transanal TME. The transabdominal and transanal (TATA) approach described by Marks et al. in 1984 combined a limited transanal intersphincteric resection (ISR) to complete the abdominal TME and facilitate sphincter-preserving proctectomy for low-lying rectal cancer.[13] Further advances took advantage of the superior transanal endoscopic access provided by TEM to perform the entire TME using a transanal approach, a technique subsequently called taTME.[14-16] The feasibility and reproducibility of this approach was demonstrated first in swine survival experiments and then in human cadaver series.[17-22] This hybrid transabdominal and transanal approach to complete a radical proctectomy offers technical advantages beyond the ability to remove the specimen transanally.[23-27] Transanal rectal and mesorectal dissection is greatly facilitated by CO_2 insufflation and direct endoscopic visualization provided by transanal endoscopic platforms, which permits accurate identification of the distal resection margin and exposure of perirectal dissection planes, greatly facilitating completion of TME, particularly for low tumors in patients with a narrow pelvis, significant visceral obesity, and when sphincter preservation is intended.[4,23]

This chapter reviews the various surgical approaches for the curative resection of rectal cancer, including the different techniques for completing a proctectomy with sphincter preservation. Open low anterior resection (LAR), laparoscopic LAR, robotic LAR, and laparoscopic-assisted taTME are reviewed. The benefits and limitations of each surgical approach are reviewed, as well as post-operative complications and oncologic and functional outcomes.

ANATOMIC HIGHLIGHTS

A thorough understanding of the anatomy of the colon, rectum, and pelvis is essential when performing surgery for rectal cancer regardless of the technique. The goal is to achieve adequate oncologic resection to reduce the risk of recurrence and minimize intraoperative complications, including pelvic autonomic nerve injury, to expedite recovery and provide the best quality of life with respect to urinary, sexual, and defecatory function. Mastery of pelvic anatomy allows the surgeon to recognize key anatomic landmarks and understand the pitfalls inherent in each step performed during rectal cancer surgery. Of particular importance in these procedures is the understanding of fascial planes, pelvic nerve plexuses, and their relationship to the surgical planes of dissection. To preserve sexual and bladder function after TME, it is important to identify the pelvic autonomic plexus and neurovascular bundles and avoid inadvertent injury during deep pelvic dissection.[28,29]

The rectum is located along the curved sacrum and is approximately 12 to 15 cm in length. The ischial tuberosities and iliac wings form the boundaries of the pelvic cavity forming a very narrow and deep space, especially at the level of the anorectal junction. The mesorectum of the distal rectum starts to thin out and is almost absent starting approximately 2 cm above the levator ani muscles, where only the rectal wall remains. The rectum and the mesorectum are encased in the embryologically derived endopelvic fascia. The mesorectum is enveloped by the proper rectal fascia, which is separate from the parietal presacral fascia or Waldeyer fascia. This fascia is dorsal to the hypogastric nerves and ventral to the presacral venous plexus and pelvic splanchnic nerves. The prehypogastric nerve fascia can be identified between them. The Denonvilliers fascia is present between the anterior surface of the mesorectum and the prostate or vagina.[29,30]

The superior hypogastric plexus located around the inferior mesenteric artery (IMA) descends along the sacral promontory and bifurcates into the hypogastric nerves. The paired hypogastric nerves run 1 to 2 cm medial to the ureters and enter the pelvis by crossing the common iliac arteries at the level of the sacrum. They then run along the posterolateral wall of the pelvis.[29-31] The superior

hypogastric plexus may be damaged during lymph node dissection or high ligation of the IMA at its origin. The hypogastric nerves are also at risk of being injured during mobilization of the rectosigmoid colon from the gonadal vessels and ureters or during posterior dissection of the mesorectum. Injury may lead to urinary incontinence, retrograde ejaculation in men, and decreased orgasmic intensity in women. The pelvic (inferior hypogastric) plexus extends inferiorly as a mesh composed of the hypogastric and pelvic splanchnic nerves at the lateral pelvic wall. The neurovascular bundles descend to the urogenital organ at the lateral corner of the seminal vesicle in the 10 and 2 o'clock directions. Its damage may lead to voiding, erection, ejaculation, or lubrication dysfunction.

The cavernous nerve is included within the neurovascular bundles and runs through the prostate surface of the Denonvilliers fascia and continues to the periprostatic plexus. This nerve provides parasympathetic innervation to the prostate, seminal vesicles, cavernous bodies, and the last portion of the vas deferens. Injury of these bundles results in sexual dysfunction with disturbances in erection, ejaculation, and/or vaginal lubrication.

PREOPERATIVE STAGING

Accurate preoperative staging is essential when planning the most appropriate treatment for rectal cancer. A complete medical and surgical history is obtained with assessment of performance status as well as baseline urinary, sexual, and defecatory function. A comprehensive physical examination is performed including digital rectal exam (DRE). For low rectal tumors, DRE helps determine tumor location and extent along the rectal wall, relationship to the anal sphincters and anorectal ring, fixity, and sphincter tone and squeeze. A complete colonoscopy with biopsies is required for tissue diagnosis, as well as rigid proctoscopy to determine the exact location and distance of the tumor from the anal verge. Laboratory studies include a complete blood count, serum chemistries, liver function tests, and baseline serum carcinoembryonic antigen level.

Radiologic tumor staging includes computed tomography (CT) scans of the chest, abdomen, and pelvis to rule out distant metastases and magnetic resonance imaging (MRI) of the pelvis with or without endorectal ultrasound (ERUS) to evaluate the local extent of the neoplasm. Preoperative MRI has a sensitivity of 0.97 (95% confidence interval [CI], 0.96 to 0.98) and specificity of 0.97 (95% CI, 0.96 to 0.98) for determining invasion into the muscularis propria and adjacent organs, and therefore has a relatively high diagnostic accuracy for preoperative T staging and assessment of the circumferential radial margin (CRM).[32,33] All radiologic imaging modalities are fraught with relatively low sensitivity with respect to lymph node assessment. Relative to ERUS, pelvic MRI is more accurate in its ability to detect lymph node involvement as it is able to view the entire mesorectum and pelvic sidewall.[32,33]

For early rectal tumors and/or malignant polyps that may be eligible for local excision, ERUS is the most accurate imaging modality to confirm T1 staging given its superior resolution and definition of infiltration depth.[34] That being said, modern MRI can assess depth of spread accurately to within 1 mm of histopathology assessments.[34]

NEOADJUVANT TREATMENT

Exact tumor location and accurate preoperative lymph node staging play a crucial role in preoperative and surgical planning. Rectal cancers located in the upper third of the rectum are typically treated like rectosigmoid tumors and are exempt from neoadjuvant treatment. Standard treatment of clinical stage II and III mid and lower rectal cancer includes neoadjuvant treatment with either long-course chemoradiation therapy (CRT) or preoperative short-course radiotherapy (SCRT), which not only reduces local recurrence rates relative to radical surgery alone, but also downstages a substantial proportion of tumors, potentially enabling sphincter preservation for very low rectal tumors. Long-course CRT, with 5-fluorouracil-based chemotherapy and concomitant 50.4 Gy of radiation delivered over 5 weeks can achieve up to 20% rates of complete pathologic response.[9,34-36] Radical resection with TME is typically performed 6 to 12 weeks after completion of CRT, which allows for additional downstaging of chemosensitive tumors.[5,7,34-39] SCRT can be used as an alternative to long-course CRT when chemotherapy cannot be administered or in special situations such as resectable synchronous metastases or synchronous tumors in the colon.[37] TME is typically performed 1 week after completion of SCRT.[37]

It is important to note that pelvic radiation is associated with significant deleterious long-term effects on anorectal, urinary, and sexual function. In addition, radiation is associated with increased rates of cardiovascular disease, pelvic fractures, and increased risk of secondary malignancies 10 years after radiation. Therefore, the potential benefits of preoperative radiotherapy in reducing local recurrence rates need to be weighed against the risks of increased long-term morbidity when determining the appropriate treatment for patients with rectal cancer.[8,34,38-40]

In an effort to avoid overtreatment of low-risk rectal tumors with neoadjuvant treatment, more recent recommendations are based on improved prognostication of rectal tumors using high-resolution MRI. Currently, it is increasingly recommended that the use of CRT and SCRT be limited to rectal tumors deemed at high risk for local recurrence based on staging by pelvic MRI, including cT3b-d tumors located less than 1 mm from the mesorectal fascia, cT4 and cN1 tumors, and tumors with evidence of extramural vascular invasion (EMVI) or infiltration of the internal or external sphincter or intersphincteric space. On the other hand, tumors deemed at low risk for local recurrence based on staging MRI including cT2/T3a, cN0, and with no evidence of infiltration of the internal sphincter, should proceed directly to radical resection without administration of neoadjuvant treatment.[8,34] These most recent recommendations rely on high-quality surgical resection being achieved, namely a complete TME with negative margins and CRM. TME specimen quality is critical with the majority of local recurrences reflecting inadequate mesorectal resection.[34]

PREOPERATIVE PREPARATION

Preoperative preparation of rectal cancer patients who commonly present with chronic cardiovascular or respiratory conditions includes a comprehensive medical assessment and "prehabilitation" when possible to improve baseline performance status and optimize postoperative outcomes. Prehabilitation is a multimodal strategy that includes a nutritional assessment, control of anemia, and an adapted program of exercises to improve the patient's cardiologic and respiratory function. Fertility options should be discussed with patients of childbearing age. Patients in whom a permanent or temporary stoma is planned should be evaluated by an enterostomal therapist for preoperative teaching and stoma site marking.

On the day prior to surgery, patients undergo oral mechanical bowel preparation and many practitioners also routinely administer several doses of oral antibiotics (metronidazole and neomycin or erythromycin). This is based on a recent analysis of the 2012 Colectomy-Targeted American College of Surgeons National Surgical Quality Improvement Program (ACS NSQIP) database, where a decrease in the rate of surgical site infections, anastomotic leakage, and procedure-related hospital readmissions were demonstrated in patients who received combined mechanical and oral antibiotic preparation relative to patients who received no preoperative preparation or patients who received either mechanical or oral antibiotic preparation alone.[41] Many practitioners also supplement mechanical bowel preparation with enemas to maximize clearance of the rectosigmoid and facilitate transanal access for tumor identification, rectal transection, and colorectal anastomosis.

If open surgery is planned or if conversion to open surgery is likely, epidural anesthesia is planned for improved pain control. Parenteral prophylactic antibiotics are administered prior to surgical incision as per routine, usually a second-generation cephalosporin, metronidazole, or clindamycin with a cephalosporin, ciprofloxacin or gentamicin, based on preference or allergy to penicillin or depending on patients' allergies and/or sensitivities.[42] Other perioperative preventive measures against surgical site infection include tight glucose control in diabetics, hair removal using clippers, and maintenance of normothermia and adequate oxygenation during anesthesia.[42] Deep venous thromboembolic prophylaxis with unfractionated heparin or low-molecular-weight heparin should be administered starting prior to surgical incision. In addition to standard prepping of the abdomen and perineum, the rectum is typically irrigated with a 1% dilute iodine solution.

Postoperatively, enhanced recovery protocols are usually followed that include early mobilization, transition to oral pain control, and resumption of oral food intake. The Foley catheter is typically removed 48 hours postoperatively, taking into account a higher risk of urinary retention in male patients with benign prostatic hyperplasia. Patients are discharged when tolerating an oral diet with resumption of bowel function, when adequate pain control with an oral regimen is achieved, and when short-term complications have been ruled out or resolved.

SURGICAL MANAGEMENT OF RECTAL CANCER

The oncologic principles guiding completion of radical proctectomy for rectal cancer, whether performed open or using a minimally invasive approach, are highlighted in the original description of TME.[3] Dissection of the areolar plane surrounding the visceral fascia that envelops the rectum and mesorectum should be carried out sharply, which maximizes the likelihood of obtaining a negative CRM and mitigates the chance for local recurrence. Identification and preservation of the autonomic nerve plexuses that control urinary and sexual function should be ensured to preserve function and quality of life. Preservation of the anal sphincter and pelvic floor with restoration of gastrointestinal continuity should be applied when oncologically feasible, in highly motivated patients with realistic expectations regarding short- and long-term postoperative defecatory function and fecal continence. The various approaches to TME will be reviewed including the detailed surgical techniques, benefits and limitations, complications, and functional and oncologic outcomes.

OPEN LOW ANTERIOR RESECTION

SURGICAL TECHNIQUE

Operative Setup

Regardless of the approach, LAR and APR require patients to be positioned in a Lloyd Davis position with the legs carefully padded in stirrups, both arms tucked at the side, and with the patient secured carefully to the operating table to minimize sliding while in steep Trendelenburg position or extreme lateral tilt. In case of APR for low rectal tumors abutting the dentate line, or when ISR with partial or complete resection of the internal anal sphincter is planned, a transanal setup is needed including a transanal scrub technician, transanal instrumentation with anorectal tray, anoscopes, a Lone Star retractor (Cooper Surgical, Trumbull, Connecticut), a headlight, and either absorbable sutures or a circular end-to-end anastomosis (EEA) stapler depending on how the coloanal anastomosis is completed. Of note, an indocyanine green (ICG) fluorescence imaging system may be used to assess vascular perfusion prior to proximal colon transection, prior to completion of colorectal anastomoses, and/or following anastomoses. Open LAR requires an adequate set of abdominal and pelvic retractors, a headlight, and a long instrument tray.

Procedural Steps

Open LAR is performed through a vertical midline laparotomy incision followed by abdominal exploration to rule out peritoneal disease and liver metastasis, vascular mobilization, mesenteric dissection, TME, rectal transection, colon resection, and colorectal or coloanal reconstruction.

After completing abdominal exploration, the patient is positioned in Trendelenburg with the right side down. The small bowel is carefully retracted out of the pelvis and to the right. A lateral-to-medial approach is used to mobilize the rectosigmoid colon. Mobilization proceeds along the white line of Toldt to mobilize the left colon and sigmoid colon. The left gonadal vessels and ureter are identified as they cross the pelvic brim and travel downward into the pelvis. The peritoneum overlying the left common iliac artery is incised and this peritoneal incision is extended further into the pelvis until reaching the avascular plane between the rectosigmoid mesentery and retroperitoneum. At this point, dissection should not proceed further and attention is returned to the proximal left colon. The lateral attachments of the proximal left colon are divided heading up toward the splenic flexure, which is then mobilized. This is followed by high ligation of the IMA, below the origin of the left colic artery. This part of the operation can also be performed using a medial-to-lateral approach, first by scoring the peritoneum at the base of the sigmoid mesentery, just above the sacral promontory, and extending this incision to the right and toward the right posterolateral region of the pelvis, with high ligation of the IMA near its origin. Dissection then moves toward the lateral attachments of the left colon, which are divided as they head up toward the splenic flexure. Pelvic dissection of the rectum is then carried out anteriorly toward the peritoneum overlying the pouch of Douglas in women and the Denonvilliers fascia in men. Anterior dissection is carried out with visualization of the seminal vesicles and prostate in men or the posterior wall of the vagina in women. Posteriorly, dissection is carried out along the plane between the Waldeyer fascia and the mesorectal fascia, with care to preserve the integrity of the mesorectum according to the principles of a TME.

In the case of a low or ultra LAR, posterior dissection between the mesorectal fascia and Waldeyer fascia is extended down toward the levators. Care should be taken to avoid injury to the pelvic autonomic nerves, specifically the superior hypogastric nerves, as they enter into the pelvis above the sacral promontory and the nervi erigentes as they travel along the pelvic sidewalls to join the inferior hypogastric plexus forming the pelvic plexus. With innervation to the prostate, genitalia, and bladder, injury to these structures may lead to erectile and urinary dysfunction.

Following complete TME with mobilization of the rectum and mesorectum well below the level of the tumor, the rectum is clamped below the tumor with a distal margin 2 cm or greater when possible, although a distal margin 0.5 cm or greater following chemoradiation is deemed oncologically acceptable.[43-45] The rectum is then transected, and either a stapled colorectal or handsewn anastomosis is performed based on the level of rectal transection. A diverting loop ileostomy is often performed depending on the height of the anastomosis and whether the patient was treated with radiation preoperatively. The various types of coloanal reconstruction are reviewed in the laparoscopic LAR section of this chapter.

BENEFITS AND LIMITATIONS

The oncologic goals of radical resection for rectal cancer are to achieve cure and to minimize locoregional recurrence. Wide adoption of the TME principles and technique has resulted in significant reduction in local recurrence rates.[46] However, achievement of good-quality TME is not only dependent on adequate training and technical expertise of the surgeons, but also depends on tumor- and body habitus-related factors. The adequacy of the TME can be complicated by unfavorable anatomy and tumor-related factors such as low rectal tumors in a deep and narrow male pelvis with significant visceral obesity. This scenario often presents as an insurmountable obstacle to achieving adequate exposure to perform a complete rectal and mesorectal dissection under direct vision, preserve the anal sphincters, and secure adequate distal and radial margins. Deep pelvic dissection is particularly challenging when carried out down to the levators, where visualization of the distal-most portion of the rectum is severely hindered. This difficulty is reflected in the traditionally high reported rates of APR for rectal cancers located 5 cm or less from the anal verge, ranging from 7% to 27%.[47-51] In addition, open LAR procedures are associated with significant morbidity including relatively high incidence of wound-related complications such as wound infection, incisional pain, prolonged LOS and recovery, and incisional hernia. It is not surprising that the adoption of laparoscopy in colorectal surgery was driven by efforts to reduce morbidity and mortality. Although adoption of laparoscopy for rectal cancer resection was delayed due to the steep learning curve and concerns over oncologic safety relative to the open approach, laparoscopy has helped overcome some of the limitations of open surgery, specifically by improving exposure of the narrow male pelvis, in patients with visceral obesity and high body mass index (BMI).[52,53]

LAPAROSCOPIC, HAND-ASSISTED, AND SINGLE PORT LOW ANTERIOR RESECTION

SURGICAL TECHNIQUE

Operative Setup

Patient preparation and positioning is similar to that described for open LAR. An ergonomically sound laparoscopic setup requires two monitors to be placed on either side of the patient. Ideally, monitors are moveable on a swivel to allow for ample maneuverability rather than fixed to the laparoscopic towers. When possible, procedures are performed with two assistants, one camera assistant, and a second assistant for effective retraction, particularly during the pelvic portion of the dissection. Laparoscopic towers, energy platforms, high-flow insufflator, and smoke evacuation systems are routinely used. An ICG fluorescence imaging system may be used to assess vascular perfusion prior to completion of colorectal anastomoses.

Procedural Steps

Pneumoperitoneum is achieved using a Veress needle inserted periumbilically or in the left upper quadrant, an OptiView trocar in the left upper quadrant, or using a Hasson technique with cut-down at the umbilicus to introduce a 12-mm trocar. After insertion of a 5- or 12-mm trocar at the umbilicus, a 5- or 10-mm, 30-degree-angled high definition (HD) laparoscope is inserted with placement of four or more additional trocars under direct laparoscopic visualization. Care should be taken to avoid

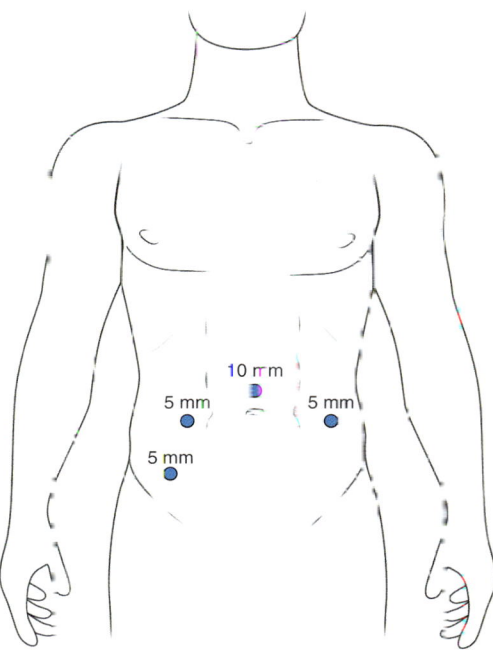

FIGURE 168.1 Standard laparoscopic low anterior resection trocar positioning.

injury to the inferior epigastric vessels when placing the trocars. Common trocar locations include the marked ileostomy site, the suprapubic region, the right and left upper quadrants, and the right lower quadrant (Fig. 168.1). If a single port technique is used, a 4-cm vertical midline periumbilical incision is needed to introduce the single port device. Following trocar placement, the abdominal cavity is explored to rule out occult peritoneal carcinomatosis, hepatic metastases, or other unsuspected abdominal pathology. The table is tilted in steep Trendelenburg with the right side down, and the small bowel is retracted out of the pelvis superiorly and to the right. The sigmoid colon is retracted superiorly to place the mesentery under tension and highlight the inferior mesenteric pedicle. Adequate exposure for a medial-to-lateral approach includes visualizing the sacral promontory, right iliac vessel and right ureter, and the takeoff the IMA pedicle off the aorta. There may be instances when a lateral-to-medial approach is preferred, such as during reoperative surgery, in the setting of inflammation, adhesions, or significant visceral obesity, when difficulties identifying the correct retromesenteric plane or the left ureter are anticipated or encountered. The peritoneum overlying the base of the sigmoid mesentery, starting on the right of the inferior mesenteric pedicle, is incised with monopolar cautery and the plane between the sigmoid mesentery and the retroperitoneum is dissected using a combination of sharp and blunt dissection. The left ureter is typically identified coursing over the left common iliac artery and alongside the left gonadal vessels, heading down and laterally toward the pelvis (Fig. 168.2). After identification of the left ureter, the IMA and inferior mesenteric vein (IMV) are dissected separately, and the IMA is divided 1 cm from its origin with a vessel-sealing device, a vascular load of the EndoGIA stapler, or scissors

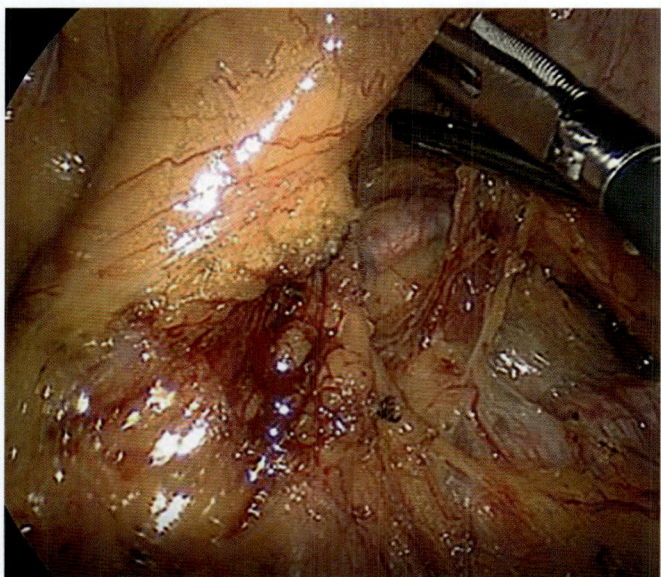

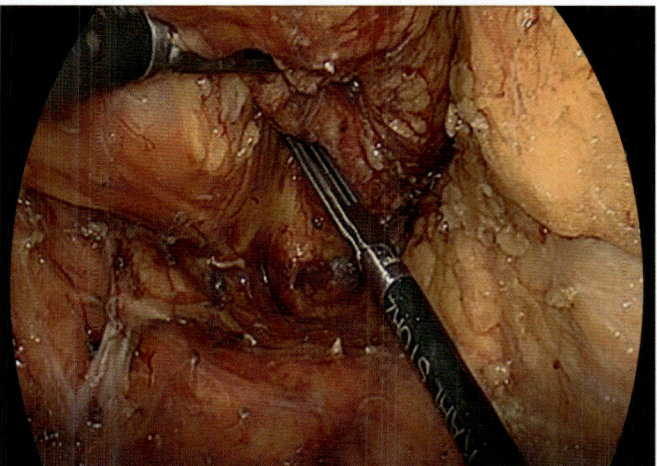

FIGURE 168.3 Laparoscopic total mesorectal excision dissection proceeding posteriorly along the sacrum with care taken to avoid injury to the ureters, hypogastric nerves, and pelvic plexus.

FIGURE 168.2 Identification of the left ureter prior to division of the inferior mesenteric artery pedicle during laparoscopic low anterior resection with total mesorectal excision.

following clipping. The left colic artery may be preserved to improve perfusion of the proximal colon in patients with a low rectal tumor. The IMV is divided just inferior to the pancreas to maximize the subsequent reach of the proximal colon down toward the pelvis. After mobilizing the left colon and sigmoid mesentery off the retroperitoneum, the lateral attachments of the left colon, sigmoid, and rectosigmoid are divided. In most cases of low or very low rectal cancer, complete mobilization of the splenic flexure is necessary, which may require placement of an additional trocar and is facilitated by the operator standing between the patient's legs. The splenic flexure is mobilized from its attachments to the spleen and to the left kidney over the Gerota fascia. The splenic flexure may be approached by elevating the omentum and dissecting off from the transverse colon. This approach allows access to the lesser sac, exposure to the stomach, pancreas, and retroperitoneum, and provides a direct approach. After complete mobilization of the sigmoid and descending colon with takedown of the splenic flexure, attention is turned to the pelvic dissection. With the assistant providing upward retraction on the rectum, the plane between the mesorectum and the sacral promontory is identified and dissected sharply, preserving the parietal layer, and keeping within the avascular TME plane between the fascia propria of the rectum and Waldeyer fascia. The middle sacral artery is divided, and the TME dissection continues inferiorly along the retrorectal space (Fig. 168.3). During the posterior and posterolateral TME dissection, care is taken to avoid injury to bilateral hypogastric nerves, and more laterally and distally to the bilateral ureters and the pelvic nerve plexus. Laterally, care is taken to identify and avoid dissection of the pelvic plexuses. Anteriorly, the peritoneal reflection is incised and the rectovesical pouch in men or the rectovaginal pouch in women is incised, exposing the Denonvilliers fascia. Posterior

mesorectal dissection continues through the rectosacral ligament at the S4 level, toward the levator ani muscle of the pelvic floor. Following complete circumferential dissection of the rectum and mesorectum down to the pelvic floor, the rectum is prepared for transection. The exact level of planned distal rectal transection is based on the exact tumor location, which can be confirmed by laparoscopic palpation, transanal manipulation, or endoscopy. The rectum is then transected with a laparoscopic reticulating linear stapler. In the case of very low rectal tumors, a perineal ISR is required to achieve a negative distal resection margin. The intersphincteric plane is subsequently connected to the abdominal TME plane followed by transanal or transabdominal extraction of the specimen.[54,55]

With a hand-assisted laparoscopic approach, a hand-port is inserted through a 4.5- to 7-cm-long Pfannenstiel, vertical midline periumbilical, or vertical midline suprapubic incision, depending on the surgeon's hand size. A hand-assisted laparoscopic approach can be used from the start of the operation to facilitate or expedite colon retraction during mesenteric dissection or splenic flexure takedown, or later to facilitate the pelvic phase of the operation. This approach has been demonstrated to be safe and associated with the same benefits of conventional laparoscopy.[56,57]

A number of operators commonly use a hybrid approach and will complete the distal TME and transect the rectum under direct open visualization through a lower vertical midline or Pfannenstiel incision using a curved stapler. The same incision will then be used for exteriorizing the specimen and creating the anastomosis. This hybrid approach was commonly used by surgeons in the laparoscopic arm of the ACOSOG Z6051 laparoscopic versus open rectal cancer trial.[50] Stapled colorectal or handsewn coloanal anastomosis is subsequently performed, depending on the height of the anorectal stump from the anal verge. Laparoscopic LAR for tumors 5 cm or more from the anal verge is usually followed by intracorporeal stapled anastomosis under laparoscopic visualization.

Colorectal/Coloanal Anastomosis

Following TME and distal rectal transection, the specimen is most commonly extracted through an abdominal incision—peri umbilical, lower vertical midline, or Pfannenstiel—using a wound protector. The proximal colon is prepared for intracorporeal colorectal anastomosis by checking adequate reach toward the pelvis without undue tension. Stapled or handsewn anastomosis can be performed either end-to-end or side-to-end, although side-to-end anastomosis is favored due to improved defecatory function.[58] Coloanal J pouch and transverse coleplasty are strongly recommended for coloanal reconstruction based on improved short-term outcomes with respect to functional outcomes.[58,59]

After securing the anvil onto the proximal colon, which is returned to the abdominal cavity, the circular stapler is introduced transanally under laparoscopic guidance followed by firing of the stapler and completion of the anastomosis. If a hand-port or open lower abdominal incision is used, the surgeon can manually connect both sides of the stapler by hand, with good control of the tissues and surrounding organs. For tumors that are less than 5 cm from the anal verge, ISR is often performed followed by transanal extraction of the specimen and handsewn end-to-end, side-to-end coloanal anastomosis, or using coloanal J pouch reconstruction or transverse coloplasty. A Lone Star retractor greatly facilitates coloanal anastomosis, which is performed using interrupted absorbable sutures. As for open LAR, creation of a temporary diverting loop ileostomy, placement of a pelvic drain, and placement of a rectal drain across the anastomosis are based on the surgeon's preference.

BENEFITS AND LIMITATIONS

The establishment of laparoscopic surgery, along with the description of TME, may have been the greatest advance in rectal cancer treatment of recent decades. Initial adoption was challenged by early concerns over the oncologic safety of this approach, but results from the CLASICC, COLOR II, and COREAN laparoscopic versus open TME RCTs demonstrated superiority of the laparoscopic approach with respect to short-term postoperative outcomes and noninferiority of short- and long-term oncologic outcomes relative to open TME (Tables 168.1 and 168.2).[3,60-66] Although the laparoscopic approach required longer operative times, there was less intraoperative blood loss and patients enjoyed a faster postoperative recovery. Additionally, the TME quality was comparable to that of open surgery as demonstrated by the similar locoregional recurrence rates. Long-term oncologic results at 3, 5, and 10 years demonstrate equivalent recurrence rates and disease-free and overall survival.[48,62-66] Based on these results, the surgical community concluded that when performed by a skilled surgeon in appropriately selected patients with rectal cancer, laparoscopic TME is associated with improved postoperative outcomes including faster return of bowel function, shorter LOS, and shorter recovery compared to open TME with similar morbidity and oncologic safety with respect to resection margins and completeness of the TME.

Nevertheless, there remains skepticism regarding wide adoption of laparoscopy for rectal cancer. Two recent noninferiority comparative laparoscopic versus open TME RCTs were published, the Australian ALaCaRt and American ACOSOG Z6051 that confirmed the short-term postoperative benefits provided by the laparoscopic approach, but failed to show noninferior oncologic outcomes as demonstrated by the slightly higher rates of positive circumferential margins in patients undergoing laparoscopic TME (12.1% vs. 10.0% in the ACOSOG and 7% vs. 3% in ALaCaRt).[50,51] In addition, relative to the rising rates of adoption of laparoscopy for right and left colectomy for benign and malignant diseases, the adoption of laparoscopic TME has remained limited due to the difficulty of the pelvic dissection as reflected by relatively high reported conversion rates (17%, 11.3% and 9% in the COLOR II, ACOSOG, and ALaCaRt trials, respectively), the steep learning curve to achieve expertise, and the lack of demonstrated benefits over open TME with respect to morbidity or functional outcomes.[67] Morbidity rates for laparoscopic and open TME are similar (30% to 50%) and include a 5% to 12% incidence of urinary dysfunction, 10% to 35% incidence of sexual dysfunction, and 20% to 30% incidence of fecal incontinence. In addition, despite the benefits conferred by the laparoscopic approach with regard to short-term postoperative outcomes and improved visualization of pelvic structures, the laparoscopic approach still requires an abdominal extraction site with wound-related complications such as incisional pain, superficial and deep wound infection, incisional hernia, and prolonged recovery.[68]

The single-port technique for laparoscopic surgery was developed in an effort to further minimize surgical trauma from required skin incisions and reduce overall morbidity. Unfortunately, single incision laparoscopic colectomy is technically challenging with significant restrictions in hand movement and triangulation. The technical challenge is amplified when single-incision laparoscopy is applied to the narrow confines of the pelvis. Although single-incision surgery has been demonstrated to be oncologically safe with acceptable rates of morbidity and mortality, this is only the case in patients with normal weight and rectal tumors limited to the rectal wall.[69,70] At this time and based on the very limited experience to date, single-incision laparoscopic surgery for rectal cancer should only be used by highly experienced operators in specialized centers and for carefully selected patients.

ROBOTIC-ASSISTED LOW ANTERIOR RESECTION

SURGICAL TECHNIQUE

Two approaches are routinely used to perform robotic-assisted laparoscopic TME. The hybrid robotic approach involves laparoscopic mobilization of the sigmoid and left colon, ligation of the IMA and IMV, and splenic flexure takedown. This is followed by docking of the robot to complete the pelvic dissection robotically. In the totally robotic approach, the entire procedure is performed robotically with transanal extraction of the specimen, intracorporeal placement of the anvil into the lumen of proximal colon, followed by stapled or handsewn coloanal anastomosis. There are benefits and challenges with either

TABLE 168.1 Patient Characteristics of Published Randomized Controlled Trials Comparing Open Versus Laparoscopic Total Mesorectal Excision for Rectal Cancer

Study	N Open	N Lap	TUMOR LOCATION (cm) Open	TUMOR LOCATION (cm) Lap	PREOPERATIVE STAGE Open	PREOPERATIVE STAGE Lap	NEOADJUVANT CRT Open	NEOADJUVANT CRT Lap
MRC CLASICC[49,60,63]	268	526	Colon (140), Rectum (128)	Colon (273), Rectum (253)	NR	NR	NR	NR
COLOR II[47,62]	345	699	<5 cm (93), 5–10 cm (136), 10–15 cm (116)	<5 cm (203), 5–10 cm (273), 10–15 cm (223)	I (96), II (107), III (126), missing data (16)	I (201), II (209), III (257), missing data (32)	348	608
Hong Kong Study[64,65]	200	203	>5 cm	>5 cm	I (28), II (73), III (69), IV (30)	I (31), II (72), III (64), IV (36)	0	0
COREAN Trial[48,66]	170	170	<9 cm	<9 cm	cT3, N0-2, M0	cT3, N0-2, M0	170	170
ACOSOG Z6051[50]	222	240	High (28), Middle (95), Low (116)	High (33), Middle (85), Low (124)	I (3), IIA (92), IIIA (11), IIIB (114), IIC (19)	I (2), IIA (99), IIIA (11), IIIB (114), IIIC (16)	238	239
ALaCaRT[51]	237	238	High (50), Middle (102), Low (83)	High (53), Middle (103), Low (82)	T1 (11), T2 (68), T3 (155), N0 (125), N1 (30), N2 (30), M1 (10)	T1 (18), T2 (68), T3 (151), N0 (107), N1 (92), N2 (37), M1 (10)	116	119

APR, Abdominoperineal resection; *CRT*, chemoradiation therapy; *CRM*, circumferential resection margin; *DRM*, distal resection margin; *Lap*, laparoscopic; *LAR*, low anterior resection; *LHC*, left hemicolectomy; *NR*, not reported; *PME*, partial mesorectal excision; *RHC*, right hemicolectomy; *TME*, total mesorectal excision.

TABLE 168.2 Postoperative Outcomes of Published Randomized Controlled Trials Comparing Open Versus Laparoscopic Total Mesorectal Excision for Rectal Cancer

Study	N Open	N Lap	MEAN LOS (d) Open	MEAN LOS (d) Lap	INTRAOPERATIVE COMPLICATIONS (n) Open	INTRAOPERATIVE COMPLICATIONS (n) Lap	FOLLOW-UP PERIOD (months) Open	FOLLOW-UP PERIOD (months) Lap
MRC CLASICC[49,60,63]	268	526	11	9	29 (11%)	67 (13%)	36.8	36.8
COLOR II[47,62]	345	699	9.0	8.0	49 (14%)	81 (12%)	36	36
Hong Kong Study[64,65]	200	203	8.7	8.2	NR	NR	49.2 (35.4 median)	52.7 (38.9 median)
COREAN Trial[48,66]	170	170	9 (8.0–12.0)	8 (7.0–12.0)	NR	NR	46 (median)	48 (median)
ACOSOG Z6051[50]	222	240	7.0	7.3	17 (8%)	26 (11%)	NR	NR
ALaCaRT[51]	237	238	8 (median)	8 (median)	NR	NR	NR	NR

EORTC QLQ-C30, European Organisation for Research and Treatment of Cancer Quality of Life questionnaire, version 3; *GI,* gastrointestinal; *GU,* genitourinary; *LOS,* length of hospital stay; *Lap,* laparoscopic; *NR,* not reported.

TABLE 168.1 Patient Characteristics of Published Randomized Controlled Trials Comparing Open Versus Laparoscopic Total Mesorectal Excision for Rectal Cancer—cont'd

RESECTION TYPE			NO. OF LYMPH NODES COLLECTED		TME QUALITY	POSITIVE DRM		POSITIVE CRM	
Open	Lap	Conversions	Open	Lap	Open	Open	Lap	Open	Lap
LAR (96), RHC (63), LHC (23) sigmoidectomy (33), APR (34), other (8)	LAR (196), RHC (125), LHC (36), sigmoidectomy (56), APR (63), other (21)	143 (29%)	NR	NR	NR	NR	NR	6 (5%) colon, 14 (14%) rectum	16 (7%) colon, 30 (16%) rectum
PME (35), TME (230), APR (80)	PME (72), TME (418), APR (200), Missing data (9)	121 (17%)	14 (median)	13 (median)	Incomplete 9 (3%)	NR	NR	30 (10%)	56 (10%)
LAR	LAR	47 (23%)	12.1	11.1	NR	NR	NR	NR	NR
LAR (146), APR (24)	LAR (151), APR (19)	2	18 (13–24)	17 (12–22)	Complete (127), nearly complete (23)	NR	NR	7 (4%)	5 (3%)
LAR (182), APR (57)	LAR (187), APR (55)	27 (11%)	16.5 (SD 34)	17.9 (SD 10.1)	Complete (187), nearly complete (30) incomplete (11)	0	0	17 (10%)	29 (12%)
LAR (218), APR (17)	LAR (220), APR (18)	21 (9%)	NR	NR	Complete (216)	2 (1%)	3 (1%)	9 (3%)	16 (7%)

TABLE 168.2 Postoperative Outcomes of Published Randomized Controlled Trials Comparing Open Versus Laparoscopic Total Mesorectal Excision for Rectal Cancer—cont'd

OVERALL MORBIDITY RATE			DISEASE-FREE SURVIVAL		LOCAL RECURRENCE		DISTANT METASTASIS	
Open	Lap	Functional Outcomes	Open	Lap	Open	Lap	Open	Lap
113 (42%)	246 (47%)	EORTC QLQ-C30 scores return to baseline at 3 months in both groups	58.6%	55.3%	8.7%	10.8%	20.6%	21.0%
128 (37%)	278 (40%)	NR	70.8%	74.8%	15 (5.0%)	31 (5.0%)	22.1%	19.1%
45	40	NR	78.3% (3.7%)	75.3% (3.7%)	7 (4.1%)	11 (6.6%)	30 (18.0%)	26 (15.3%)
40 (24%)	36 (21%)	At 3 months, lap group with better physical functioning, less fatigue, and fewer GI and GU problems.	72.5%	79.2%	4	2	35	27
129 (58%)	137 (57%)	NR	NR	NR	NR	NR	NR	NR
NR	NR	NR	NR	NR	NR	NR	NR	NR

method and more data are needed to compare the efficacies of each approach.[71]

Operative Setup

Patient preparation and positioning is identical to that described for open and laparoscopic LAR. A large foam mat is placed on the operating room table directly beneath and in contact with the patient to prevent sliding during steep Trendelenburg, and the thorax is taped to prevent patient movement during extreme lateral positional changes. As for open and laparoscopic LAR, the perineum is prepped if transanal extraction or anastomosis is anticipated. Rectal irrigation with a dilute povidone-iodine (Betadine) solution is performed. Ureteral stents are placed only if deemed necessary by the operating surgeon. Anoscopy and/or flexible sigmoidoscopy is performed to confirm the tumor location as needed. Unless ISR is performed first, the abdominal portion of the procedure is initiated.

Pneumoperitoneum is established with a Veress needle below the left costal margin at the midclavicular line. Alternatively, laparoscopic access is obtained using an OptiView trocar or a Hasson technique. A 12-mm camera port is placed in the periumbilical area, typically located 20 cm above the pubic symphysis and slightly to the left of the umbilicus, through which a 0- or 30-degree 10-mm robotic camera is inserted. The minimum distance between robotic trocars typically is 8 to 10 cm to avoid robotic arm collision. Three additional robotic trocars are inserted under direct laparoscopic visualization including arm 1 trocar (R1), which consists of an 8-mm robotic trocar inserted through a 12-mm laparoscopic trocar inserted in the right midclavicular line halfway between the umbilicus and right anterior superior iliac spine. If an ileostomy is expected, all attempts should be made to place R1 through the lateral aspect of the marked area. Arm 2 trocar (R2) consists of an 8-mm robotic trocar inserted in the left midclavicular line halfway between the umbilicus and left anterior superior iliac spine, and arm 3 trocar (R3) is an 8-mm robotic trocar located approximately 5 cm above the umbilical camera port and 8 to 10 cm lateral to R2 in the anterior axillary line over the left flank. This port is critical for providing cranial retraction and exposure during the deep portion of the pelvic dissection. Following insertion of the robotic trocars in the configuration described, the robot is docked in a lateral position over the patient's left hip rather than between the legs to provide enough space between the legs for intraoperative digital or endoscopic examinations, transanal specimen extraction, or transanal surgery, particularly ISR or APR. One of two laparoscopic trocars may be inserted in the right upper quadrant along the right midclavicular line (L1) and halfway between the right midclavicular line and the midline (L2) to provide assistance with retraction and suction during robotic-assisted LAR. When the robotic cart is docked over the left hip, the camera port should be aligned with the left hip and the contralateral right shoulder (Fig. 168.4).

Procedural Steps

In a hybrid robotic-assisted LAR, the initial steps are identical to that of a laparoscopic LAR using laparoscopic

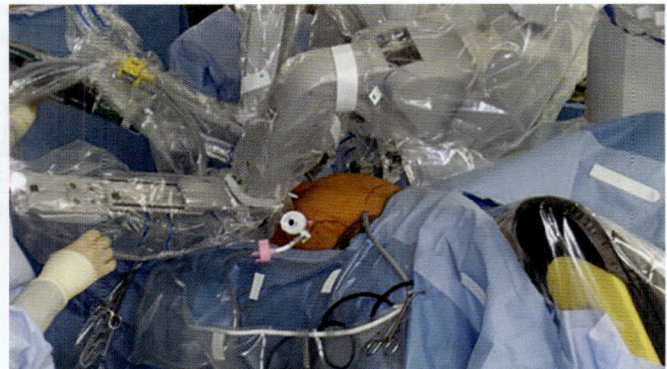

FIGURE 168.4 Standard operative setup for robotic low anterior resection

or robotic trocars, including diagnostic laparoscopy, identification of the left ureter, ligation of the IMA and IMV, mobilization of the sigmoid colon, descending colon, and splenic flexure. After upsizing laparoscopic trocars to robotic trocars, the robot is then docked to start the pelvic dissection. In a total robotic-assisted LAR, following diagnostic laparoscopy and placement of all robotic trocars, the robot is docked over the left hip making sure that the camera port is aligned with the left hip and the contralateral right shoulder. All robotic ports and the laparoscopic assistant port(s) are typically used during the case for fine dissection and tissue retraction. R1 is equipped with a monopolar hook or scissors. R2 is used for fine tissue retraction with a bipolar fenestrated grasper. R3 is usually equipped with an atraumatic bowel grasper and used for more effective tissue retraction for structures such as the sigmoid colon, anterior peritoneal reflection, or uterus. The same surgical steps described for laparoscopic LAR are followed. Medial-to-lateral dissection of the IMA pedicle is then performed. Following identification of the left ureter, the pedicle is divided with the robotic vessel sealer or a standard laparoscopic vessel sealer. The three-dimensional (3D) visualization of the robotic camera system allows identification of the hypogastric plexuses, which are preserved prior to the transection of the vessels. Mobilization of the sigmoid colon is achieved by dissecting the lateral peritoneal reflection at the white line of Toldt with monopolar hook cautery through the R1 port. Meanwhile, graspers through R2 and R3 are used to retract the sigmoid medially. Blunt retromesenteric dissection is carried out cephalad to the Gerota fascia until the splenic flexure is reached and care should be taken to avoid injury to the tail of the pancreas. The inferior mesenteric vein is divided followed by takedown of the splenic flexure. R3 is then undocked from the left flank port and repositioned through the right upper quadrant robotic trocar in preparation for the pelvic dissection.

For both hybrid and total robotic-assisted pelvic phase of the TME, dissection starts at the sacral promontory, and as previously described for open and laparoscopic TME, a plane of dissection within the avascular presacral space is developed with R1 and R2 while retraction is maintained by R3. The grasper in port R3 should be passed underneath the rectosigmoid junction and used to "hook" the colon laterally and cranially for retraction. Monopolar hook or scissors with minimal use of cautery are preferred until the hypogastric nerves and both ureters are identified. Dissection should progress along the posterior mesorectal space and not the presacral space to avoid presacral venous bleeding and injury to the hypogastric nerves. Once the plane between the presacral Waldeyer fascia and mesorectal fascia is identified, the dissection may proceed posteriorly while retracting the sigmoid colon anteriorly. The rectosacral fascia is then entered distally at approximately the level of S3, and dissection advances caudally to the level of the levator muscles. Anterior dissection is initiated by incising the peritoneum between the rectum and vagina or the seminal vesicles and prostate. In the case of large anterior tumors, the rectovesical fascia is resected en-bloc with the rectum. R3 is the ideal anterior retractor during this part of the operation. Dissection of the mesorectal plane should be performed circumferentially from proximal to distal and the hypogastric nerves are found laterally along the pelvic sidewall. The lateral stalks are divided close to the rectum to avoid nerve injury.

After adequate circumferential dissection of the rectum, a DRE, flexible sigmoidoscopy, or anoscopy can be performed to confirm the appropriate level of rectal transection. The mesorectum is divided off the rectal wall and the rectum is transected with an articulating laparoscopic or robotic linear stapler inserted through the R1 trocar. Given that studies have shown that the risk of anastomotic leak increases with the number of stapler firings, rectal transection is completed with a single stapler firing if possible.[72] Otherwise, the stapler is fired sequentially with care taken to avoid crossing previous staple lines. Alternatively, for tumors located deep in the bony pelvis, rectal transection may need to be performed vertically using a suprapubic trocar.

The benefit of a totally robotic approach is that it allows the proximal transection and placement of a purse-string intracorporeally. For distal malignancies, a transanal extraction may be used particularly if a handsewn coloanal anastomosis is planned. Care should be taken to ensure that the planned specimen is not too bulky to fit through the anal canal.

The specimen is exteriorized through the ileostomy site, through a small suprapubic Pfannenstiel incision, a vertical midline suprapubic incision, or transanally. A wound protector should be placed prior to specimen extraction. The mesocolon is ligated at the proximal edge of the specimen, and the colon is divided and the specimen is passed off the field. In a totally robotic approach where transanal extraction of the specimen is planned, care must be taken to ensure that the rectosigmoid is not too bulky for extraction through the anal orifice. Depending on the level of rectal transection, the purse-string and positioning of the anvil in the proximal colon is performed intracorporeally if the rectal stump is relatively high, or transanally if the rectal stump is relatively low, with planned handsewn anastomosis. Of note, near-infrared imaging with ICG fluorescence may be used to assess vascular perfusion of the proximal and distal ends of the colon prior to transection of the proximal colon. This can be performed whether the LAR is performed open, laparoscopically, or robotically, by injecting intravenous ICG. The proximal colon is subsequently prepared for colorectal or coloanal stapled or handsewn anastomosis as previously described. The anastomosis is evaluated endoscopically by flexible sigmoidoscopy and with an air-leak test to confirm the mechanical integrity of the anastomosis. If the integrity of the anastomosis is compromised, the decision must be made to reinforce with sutures, reconstruct the anastomosis proximally, or divert with a loop ileostomy when not previously planned. ICG can also be reinjected intravenously to assess the perfusion of the proximal and distal aspects of the anastomosis, which may impact further intervention including reconstruction of the anastomosis.

BENEFITS AND LIMITATIONS

Given the overall limited adoption of laparoscopic TME, further stalled recently in light of recent oncologic data from two RCTs that failed to demonstrate noninferiority of the laparoscopic approach relative to open TME, robotic surgery has been held as a potential enabling technology that can facilitate completion and adoption of minimally invasive TME. Despite initial skepticism over the true benefits of robotic surgery over laparoscopy, especially in the setting of increased costs, robotic-assisted laparoscopic TME for rectal cancer has become increasingly adopted by colorectal surgeons. The quoted advantages of the robotic platform are especially compelling when applied to low pelvic dissection, particularly in the narrow male pelvis with visceral obesity. The improved optics with stable 3D visualization of pelvic structures, combined with fully wristed instrumentation that provides tremor-free 360-degree range of motion, improved ergonomics, and three actionable robotic arms for traction, countertraction, and dissection, make robotic surgery particularly attractive for TME.

The first robotic-assisted LAR for rectal cancer was performed by Pigazzi et al. in 2006,[73] who compared six robotic-assisted LARs to six case-matched laparoscopic-assisted LARs with no conversion in the robotic group, autonomic nerve preservation in all cases, and no significant differences in operative and pathologic data, complications, and hospital stay relative to the laparoscopic group.[73] Since then, several large series of robotic-assisted TMEs have demonstrated procedural and oncologic safety with adequate lymph node harvest, TME quality, and rate of negative distal and radial margins achieved, as well as lower conversion rates than historical conversion rates with laparoscopic TME.[74-78]

The most recent comparative studies on robotic versus laparoscopic TME with sample size in the robotic arm ranging from 33 to 133 are included in Tables 168.3 and 168.4.[71,75,76,79-84] Cumulatively, across 9 published comparative series, 536 patients underwent robotic-assisted TME for low and mid-rectal cancers and 3 patients underwent robotic-assisted partial mesorectal excision (PME) for tumors located in the upper rectum. Hybrid robotic-assisted TME was performed in four of nine series, and total robotic-assisted TME was performed in five series. Overall, 2.8% (15/536) of robotic TME cases were performed

TABLE 168.3 Patient Characteristics of Comparative Studies on Robotic Versus Laparoscopic Total Mesorectal Excision for Rectal Cancer

Study	N Rob	N Lap	TUMOR LOCATION (cm) Rob	TUMOR LOCATION (cm) Lap	PREOPERATIVE STAGE Rob	PREOPERATIVE STAGE Lap	NEOADJUVANT CRT Rob	NEOADJUVANT CRT Lap
Park et al. (2015)[79]	133	84	Low (33), Mid (60), Upper (40)	Low (16), Mid (37), Upper (31)	Stage I-III	Stage I-III	15 (11.3%)	10 (11.9%)
Baek et al. (2011)[76]	41	41	Lower (15), Mid (21), Upper (5)	Lower (10), Mid (18), Upper (13)	Stage I-III	Stage I-III	33 (75%)	18 (43.9%)
Patriti et al. (2009)[80]	29	37	5.9 ± 4.2	11 ± 4.5	Stage I (11), II (9), III (7), IV (2)	Stage I (17), II (8), III (10), IV (2)	7 (24.1%)	2 (5.4%)
Feroci et al. (2016)[81]	53	58	8 (4–12)	8 (3–12)	Stage I-III	Stage I-III	26 (49.1%)	25 (43.1%)
Kim and Kang (2010)[71]	100	100	Low (32), Mid (49), Upper (19)	Low (19), Mid (64), Upper (17)	NR	NR	14 (14.0%)	7 (7.0%)
Park et al. (2010)[82]	41	82	5.7 ± 2.0	5.9 ± 2.2	T1 (3), T2 (14), T3 (24)	T1 (3), T2 (30), T3 (49)	14 (34.1%)	17 (20.7%)
Kwak et al. (2011)[84]	59	59	Upper (6), Mid (29), Low (24)	Upper (6), Mid (29), Low (24)	Stage 0 (3), I (16), II (23), III (13), IV (4)	Stage 0 (3), I (16), II (23), III (12), IV (5)	8 (13.6%)	5 (8.5%)
Kim, YS 2016[83]	33	66	5.41 ± 1.9	5.57 ± 2.1	Stage 0 (3), I (8), II (10), III (12)	Stage 0 (8), I (12), II (20), III (26)	33 (100%)	66 (100%)
D'Annibale et al. (2013)[75]	50	50	Upper (8), Middle (9), Lower (33)	Upper (21), Middle (12), Lower (17)	pT0 (11), T1 (2), T2 (14), T3 (20), T4 (3), pN0 (35), N1 (10), N2 (7)	pT0 (5), T1 (10), T2 (14), T3 (17), T4 (4), pN0 (35), N1 (10), N2 (5)	34 (68.0%)	28 (56.0%)

APR, Abdominoperineal resection; *CAA*, coloanal anastomosis; *CRT*, chemoradiation therapy, *CRM*, circumferential resection margin; *DRM*, distal resection margin; *ISR*, intersphincteric resection; *Lap*, laparoscopic; *LAR*, low anterior resection; *PME*, partial mesorectal excision; *Rob*, robotic; *TME*, total mesorectal excision.

TABLE 168.3 Patient Characteristics of Comparative Studies on Robotic Versus Laparoscopic Total Mesorectal Excision for Rectal Cancer—cont'd

TYPE OF RESECTION		OPERATING TIME (min)		CONVERSIONS		NO. OF LYMPH NODES COLLECTED		POSITIVE DRM		POSITIVE CRM	
Rob	Lap	Rob	Lap	Rob	Lap	Rob	Lap	Rob	Lap	Rob	Lap
LAR	LAR	205.7 (109–505)	208.8 (94–407)	0 (0.0%)	6 (7.1%)	16.34 (2–43)	16.63 (2–49)	0	0	9 (6.8%)	6 (7.1%)
LAR (33) CAA (2) APR (6)	LAR (33) CAA (2) APR (6)	296 (150–520)	315 (174–584)	3 (7.3%)	9 (22.0%)	13.1 (3–33)	16.2 (5–39)	0	0	1 (2.4%)	2 (4.9%)
PME (3) TME (18) APR (5) ISR (5)	PME (24) TME (8) APR (3) CAA (2)	202 ± 12	208 ± 7	0 (0.0%)	7 (18.9%)	10.3 ± 4	11.2 ± 5	0	0	NR	NR
LAR	LAR	342 (249–536)	192 (90–335)	2 (3.8%)	1 (1.7%)	18 (4–49)	11 (3–27)	1	1	0	1
LAR (98) APR (2)	LAR (99) APR (1)	385.3 ± 102.6	297.3 ± 83.7	2 (2.0%)	3 (3.0%)	14.7 ± 9.7	16.6 ± 9.1	0	0	3	2
LAR (29) CAA (12) APR (0)	LAR (63) CAA (18) APR (1)	231.9 ± 61.4	168.6 ± 49.3	0 (0.0%)	0 (0.0%)	17.3 ± 7.7	14.2 ± 8.9	0	0	2 (4.9%)	3 (3.7%)
LAR (54) ISR (5) APR (0)	LAR (52) ISR (6) APR (1)	270 (241–325)	228 (177–254)	0 (0.0%)	2 (3.4%)	20 (12–27)	21 (14–28)	0	0	1 (1.7%)	0
LAR (31) APR (2)	LAR (61) Hartmann's (1) APR (4)	377 ± 88	277	2 (6.1%)	0 (0.0%)	22.3 ± 11.7	21.6 ± 11.0	0	0	5 (16.1%)	4 (6.7%)
LAR	LAR	270 (240–315)	275 (240–335)	0 (0.0%)	6 (12.0%)	16.5 ± 7.1	13.8 ± 6.7	0	0	0	6 (12.0%)

TABLE 168.4 Postoperative Outcomes of Published of Comparative Studies on Robotic Versus Laparoscopic Total Mesorectal Excision for Rectal Cancer

Study	N		LENGTH OF STAY (d)		INTRAOPERATIVE COMPLICATIONS (n)		FOLLOW-UP PERIOD (months)	
	Rob	Lap	Rob	Lap	Rob	Lap	Rob	Lap
Park et al. (2015)[79]	133	84	5.9 (4–14)	6.5 (3–25)	Bladder injury (1), anastomosis disruption (1)	Bladder injury (1)	58 (4–80)	58 (4–80)
Baek et al. (2011)[76]	41	41	6.5 (2–33)	6.6 (3–20)	NR	NR	NR	NR
Patriti et al. (2009)[80]	29	37	11.9 (6–29)	9.6 (5–37)	NR	NR	18.7	29.2
Feroci et al. (2016)[81]	53	58	6	8	NR	NR	37.4 (2–85)	37.4 (2–85)
Kim and Kang (2010)[71]	100	100	11.7 ± 6.7	14.4 ± 10.0	NR	NR	NR	NR
Park et al. (2010)[82]	41	82	9.9 ± 4.2	9.4 ± 2.9	NR	NR	NR	NR
Kwak et al. (2011)[84]	59	59	NR	NR	NR	NR	17 (11–25)	13 (9–22)
Kim et al. (2016)[83]	33	66	10.9 ± 6.2	13.1 ± 12.8	NR	NR	NR	NR
D'Annibale et al. (2013)[75]	50	50	8 (7–11)	10 (8–14)	NR	NR	NR	NR

DR, Distal recurrence; *IPSS*, International Prostate Symptom Score; *Lap*, laparoscopic; *LR*, local recurrence; *NR*, not reported; *Rob*, robotic.

TABLE 168.4 Postoperative Outcomes of Published of Comparative Studies on Robotic Versus Laparoscopic Total Mesorectal Excision for Rectal Cancer—cont'd

OVERALL MORBIDITY RATE		FUNCTIONAL OUTCOMES		RECURRENCE		COST	
Rob	Lap	Rob	Lap	Rob	Lap	Rob	Lap
33 (25%)	24 (29%)	NR	NR	LR (3) DR (16)	LR (1), DR (14)	12,742.5 + 3509.9	10,101.30 ± 2804.80
9 (22%)	11 (27%)	NR	NR	NR	NR	$33,915	$62,601
16 (55%)	16 (43%)	Erectile dysfunction (1), fecal incontinence (2), constipation (4)	Erectile dysfunction (3), fecal incontinence (1), constipation (3)	Local (0%)	Local (5.4%),	—	—
17 (32.1%)	26 (44.3%)	NR	NR	LR 1 (1.9%) DR 9 (17.4%)	LR 3 (5.2%) DR 5 (8.6%)	—	—
20 (20%)	27 (27%)	NR	NR	NR	NR	—	—
12 (29.3%)	19 (23.2%)	NR	NR	NR	NR	—	—
NR	NR	NR	NR	LR (1) DR (2)	LR (1) DR (2)	—	—
15 (45.6%)	26 (39.4%)	NR	NR	NR	NR	—	—
5 (10.0%)	11 (22.0%)	IPSS and erectile function worse 1 month after surgery but restored completely 1 year after surgery	IPSS and erectile function worse 1 month after surgery but restored completely and partially 1 year after surgery	NR	NR	—	—

with APR and 97.2% as part of sphincter-preserving LAR. Most robotic TMEs were performed for nonobstructing, resectable tumors including preoperatively staged T1, T2, and T3, N0 or N1 cancers. Negative distal resection margins were achieved in 99.8% (535/536) and negative CRM in 96.1% (515/536) with an average 10 to 22 lymph nodes harvested. These results were not significantly different than those from the laparoscopic cohorts. Operative times were similar between robotic and laparoscopic groups in five of the nine studies. Although four studies reported longer operative times for robotic TME compared to laparoscopic TME, the required time for robotic TME decreased after a learning curve was achieved by the surgeons. Although the overall rate of conversion to open surgery was higher in the laparoscopic versus robotic TME group (5.4% vs. 1.7%), this difference was not statistically significantly different in any of the comparative studies. Overall morbidity rates were also equivalent between the groups (26.5% vs. 30.1% in the robotic and laparoscopic group respectively). Average LOS in the robotic group was 8.9 days (range 2 to 33) compared to 9.7 days (range 1 to 37) in the laparoscopic group.

Regarding long-term oncologic and functional outcomes, only four series reported results with follow-up ranging 2 to 85 months. Two of the series reported no significant differences in functional outcomes between robotic and laparoscopic TME with respect to fecal incontinence and erectile dysfunction.[75,80] Regarding long-term oncologic outcomes, no statistically significant differences were found in local recurrence rates (0.9% vs. 1.0%), or distal recurrence rates (5.0% vs. 3.5%) between the groups.[79-81,84] The average time to recurrence after surgery was not reported. Regarding procedural costs, three series reported substantially higher average hospital costs for robotic TME relative to laparoscopic TME.[76,79]

Although there has been a recent increase in adoption of robotic surgery in the management of rectal cancer, retrospective and case-matched comparative studies thus far have only demonstrated outcomes comparable to those of laparoscopy. Short-term clinical and oncologic outcomes are not significantly different, and while long-term results are now being published, similar rates for overall survival, disease-free survival, and recurrence are being shown. Operative times are potentially longer for robotic TME and the average monetary cost for robotic TME is consistently and significantly higher than laparoscopic TME. Additionally, the overall experience for robotic TME, including the recently completed ROLARR robotic versus laparoscopic RCT, has not demonstrated a significant reduction in the rate of conversion to open surgery as originally anticipated. There is insufficient data to justify or invalidate the adoption of the robotic system over laparoscopy. For the additional costs of robotic-assisted surgery to be justified, there must be significant improvements in one or more outcomes in addition to equivalence to standard laparoscopic surgery. With regard to rectal cancer surgery, the most important factor is the long-term oncologic outcomes, and the surgical community awaits the results from two ongoing multicenter randomized trials comparing robotic versus laparoscopic surgery for rectal cancer, the ROLARR and COLRAR trials.[85,86]

TRANSANAL TOTAL MESORECTAL EXCISION

SURGICAL TECHNIQUE

taTME may be performed in a hybrid fashion with laparoscopic or robotic transabdominal assistance or in a pure transanal endoscopic fashion. Although pure transanal TME has been reported in several small case series, this approach is only feasible in a minority of patients in whom a complete splenic flexure takedown is not required. Given the current limitations in the laparoscopic and endoscopic equipment, a pure NOTES transanal TME is not currently recommended outside of expert centers with extensive taTME experience, and in carefully selected patients. In the hybrid approach, two surgical teams, a transanal and transabdominal team, may work simultaneously or a single team may perform the abdominal and transanal portions sequentially. Transabdominal assistance is used to perform high ligation of the inferior mesenteric vessels, mobilize the splenic flexure takedown, and complete the superior portion of the TME not completed from the transanal approach.

Operative Setup

Preoperative preparation for taTME is similar to that previously described for open and laparoscopic LAR. Complete mechanical bowel preparation is essential given that transanal endoscopic access is needed to perform the TME. Mechanical preparation is often supplemented with enemas the day prior to surgery to maximize rectal clearance. In the operating room, following positioning in lithotomy position, rectal irrigation is performed with dilute Betadine until all gross fecal material has been evacuated. As for APR, the abdomen and perineum are prepped and draped to allow simultaneous or sequential access during hybrid transanal procedures.

The operating room setup needs to be adapted to accommodate two scrub technicians, abdominal and transanal instrument tables, two laparoscopic towers, energy platforms, and suction machines. There should be enough space for one to two surgeons to operate transanally, depending on the transanal platform used. Video monitors should have a moveable screen on swivel, with one located between the legs facing the transanal team at eye level without obstructing the operative field of the abdominal team. The abdominal team requires one video monitor on the right and another on the left side of the patient.

Standard laparoscopic or robotic instrumentation is used for the abdominal portion, and the transanal procedure requires standard anorectal tray anoscopes, Lone Star retractor, headlight, transanal endoscopic surgery platform of choice (TAMIS, TEO, or TEM), monopolar cautery with hook or spatula, bipolar or ultrasonic device, and a high flow insufflator with smoke evacuation system of choice, suction, and irrigation. A bariatric-length 10-mm camera is used if a TAMIS platform is used, and a circular stapler is used if stapled anastomosis is performed. An ICG fluorescence imaging system may also be used if the perfusion is to be assessed intraoperatively.

Procedural Steps

Whether performing the taTME with a one-team or two-team approach, the abdominal dissection is performed using the same steps as described for laparoscopic and robotic LAR with ligation of the IMA at its origin, division of the IMV just under the pancreas, complete splenic flexure takedown, and mobilization of the left colon, sigmoid, and proximal rectum. Pelvic dissection extends down to just above the peritoneal reflection anteriorly and to below the sacral promontory posteriorly. If performing the surgery with a single team, that team would transition to the transanal approach when dissection of the deep mesorectum becomes technically difficult. Occasionally, the transanal dissection may be initiated first and then followed by abdominal access and dissection.

The transanal portion of the surgery begins with confirmation of the exact location of the tumor with digital and visual inspection via anoscopy. The transanal platform may also be placed if it offers better visualization

of the tumor. At this point, the surgeon is able to judge the appropriate distal margin. If the tumor is located above the anorectal ring, a purse-string suture with 2-0 Prolene or Vicryl is placed 0.5 to 1.0 cm distal to the rectal tumor. This is performed either directly through a standard anoscope or endoscopically through a transanal platform. The purse-string suture must be airtight to prevent distention of the proximal colon and spillage of fecal material or tumor cells into the operative field during rectal insufflation (Fig. 168.5).

After successful purse-string occlusion of the rectum followed by insertion of the transanal platform, the rectum is insufflated with CO_2 to a pressure of 10 to 12 mm Hg. With monopolar cautery, the rectum is scored circumferentially and followed by full-thickness rectal and mesorectal mobilization (Fig. 168.6). Transanal TME is then carried out circumferentially in a sequential and even pattern. Care should be taken to avoid dissection too far along any given plane to prevent distortion of the other

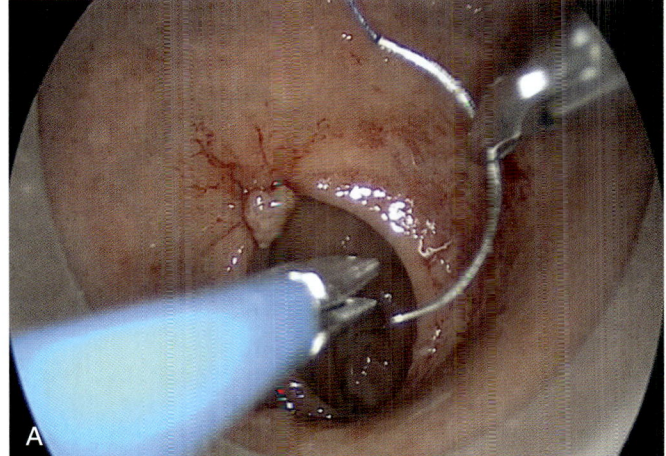 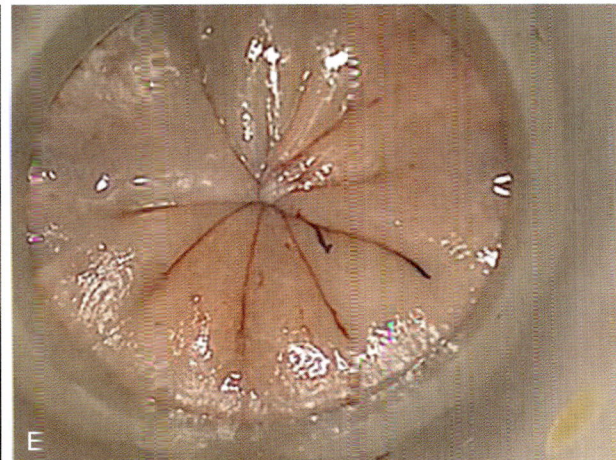

FIGURE 168.5 (A) Purse-string suture placement during transanal total mesorectal excision to achieve airtight occlusion of the rectum below the rectal tumor (B).

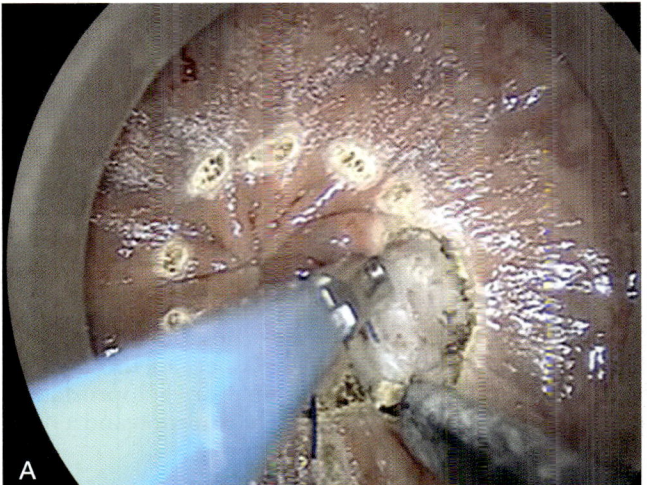 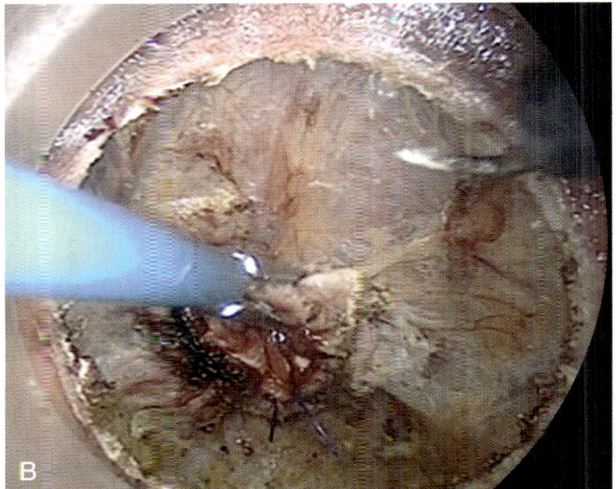

FIGURE 168.6 (A) Transanal total mesorectal excision circumferential rectal mucosal scoring followed by full-thickness rectal and mesorectal dissection (B).

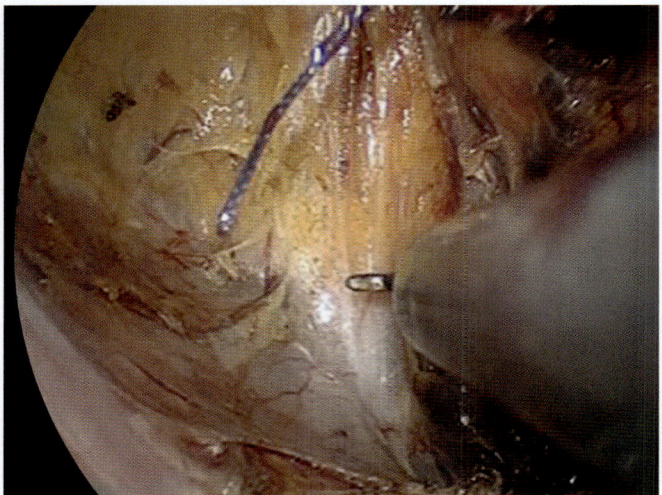

FIGURE 168.7 Transanal total mesorectal excision posterior mesorectal dissection performed in the avascular plane between the mesorectal fascia and the sacrum.

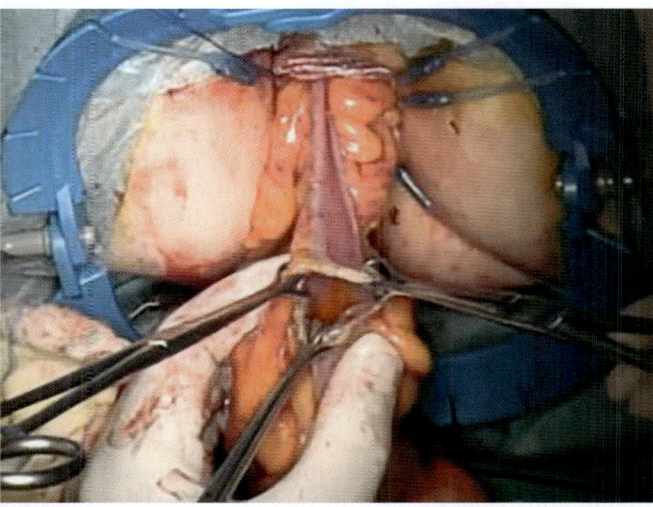

FIGURE 168.8 Transanal total mesorectal excision specimen extraction followed by preparations for stapled colorectal anastomosis.

planes. Posterior mesorectal dissection is performed in the avascular plane between the mesorectal fascia and the sacrum (Fig. 168.7). Technically this is the easiest portion of the mesorectal excision because the main landmarks, namely the presacral fascia and mesorectal fascia, are readily identifiable. During lateral mesorectal dissection, care must be taken to avoid dissection of the pelvic sidewall with subsequent damage to the pelvic plexus. As the dissection progresses anterolaterally, care must be taken to avoid injury to the neurovascular bundles that are located in the 10 and 2 o'clock positions. Anterior dissection is then carried out between the rectovaginal or retroprostatic fascia. Oftentimes, it is difficult to identify the posterior aspect of the vagina or prostate. The neurovascular bundles may serve as landmarks during these situations. Anterior dissection is carried out cephalad until the peritoneal reflection is reached. Posteriorly, the dissection extends up to the sacral promontory. At this point, the procedure is best performed with two teams working simultaneously to complete the rectal mobilization and merge the abdominal and transanal dissection planes. Peritoneal entry is typically performed transanally with laparoscopic visualization from above. One should avoid premature peritoneal entry until complete circumferential TME has been extended as far cephalad as possible to prevent loss of pneumorectum. After the rectum and sigmoid colon have been completely mobilized, the TME specimen is exteriorized transanally or through an abdominal incision if the specimen is too bulky or if there is concern of too much tension on the proximal mesentery during transanal extraction. The specimen is transected and the decision is made to proceed with stapled or handsewn colorectal/coloanal anastomosis as described previously (Figs. 168.8 to 168.10). In the case when a stapled colorectal anastomosis is planned, a double purse-string circular stapled anastomosis is used with end-to-end, side-to-end, coloanal J pouch, or transverse coloplasty.[87] A protective loop ileostomy may be constructed with placement of pelvic drains based on the surgeon's preference.

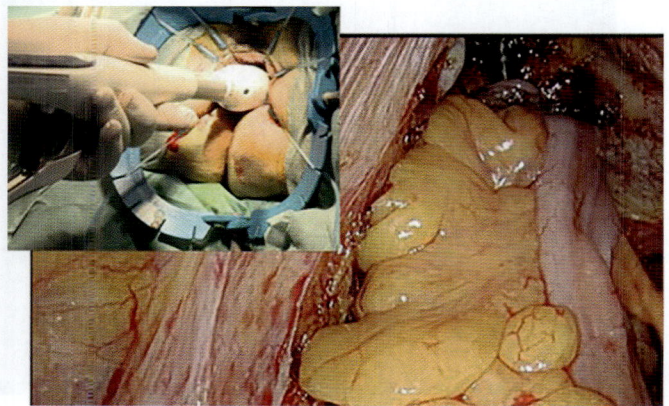

FIGURE 168.9 Transanal and transabdominal views of completion of stapled colorectal anastomosis following transanal total mesorectal excision dissection.

For very distal tumors abutting the dentate line where ISR is performed with either partial or complete resection of the internal anal sphincter, intersphincteric dissection is performed in an open fashion using a Lone Star retractor until the puborectalis and bottom of the mesorectum are reached posteriorly and the rectovaginal or retroprostatic plane is exposed anteriorly. A purse-string suture is then placed to close the anorectal stump and the transanal platform is inserted. Further dissection is required posteriorly through the anococcygeal raphe to access the presacral space. taTME then proceeds as described previously after identification of the inferior aspect of the mesorectum posteriorly and the rectovaginal or rectoprostatic plane anteriorly, followed by specimen extraction and a handsewn coloanal anastomosis.

BENEFITS AND LIMITATIONS

Since the first reported case of a laparoscopic-assisted taTME in 2010 for a mid-rectal T2N1 cancer treated with

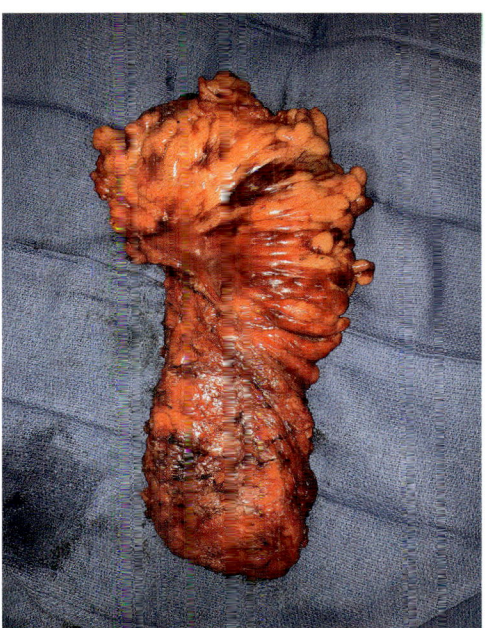

FIGURE 168.10 Complete total mesorectal excision specimen following transanal total mesorectal excision.

neoadjuvant therapy, a growing number of case series have been published worldwide demonstrating technical feasibility and preliminary oncologic safety in carefully selected patients with upper, mid, and low rectal cancers. All case series with a sample size of 15 patients or more undergoing taTME in pure fashion or with laparoscopic, single port, or robotic abdominal assistance are presented in Tables 168.5 and 168.6.[8-102] Cumulatively, among the 14 relevant series, 594 patients underwent taTME. Sample sizes ranged from 16 to 140 cases with 7% (42/594) being performed as part of an APR and 93% as part of sphincter-preserving LAR. Selected patients typically had resectable, nonobstructing tumors clinically staged T1, T2, T3, N0, and N1

Circumferential resection margins were negative in 96% of patients and the mesorectum was complete or near complete in 98%. The average number of harvested lymph nodes was 15.1. The intraoperative complication rate was 2% and included eight cases of significant intraoperative bleeding, three perforations, four urethral injuries, one ureteral injury, one vaginal wall injury, and one prostatic injury. Intraoperative complications were more likely to occur early in the surgeon's experience with taTME, but it was noted that laparoscopic assistance with a two-team approach helped to identify and avoid critical anatomic structures. Conversion to laparotomy occurred in 3% of cases. The average LOS was 7.8 days (range, 5 to 14). The rate of postoperative morbidity was 30% and included transient urinary retention, ileus, small bowel obstruction, anastomotic leak, and pelvic abscess. Follow-up ranged from 5 to 32 months. Functional outcomes were reported in 5 of the 14 series with an average Wexner score of 6.9 (range, 3 to 18). Oncologic outcomes were reported in 9 of the 14 series with 46 local and distal recurrences. The time to recurrence ranged from 5 to 24 months.

In all case series, it was unanimously reported that the transanal approach was particularly beneficial in patients who were anticipated to have a high risk of conversion to open surgery and an incomplete mesorectal specimen because of difficulties negotiating staplers in the low pelvis from an abdominal approach. These patients were typically male, with substantial visceral obesity, a narrow pelvis, and a distally located rectal tumor.

The overall experience with taTME is preliminary and based on single-institutional case series with no randomized trial comparing taTME with open or laparoscopic TME. However, there have been six retrospective studies that compare the outcomes of matched cohorts of patients undergoing taTME versus laparoscopic TME.[97-99,102-104] Cumulatively they did not demonstrate a significant difference with respect to quality of the mesorectal specimen, lymph node harvest, resection margins, or intraoperative complications.

Most recently, an international taTME registry was launched by the Pelican Cancer Foundation to further assess the safety and efficacy of taTME in the wider surgical population. This registry is an international database with collaboration among 66 surgical units in 23 different countries.[105] Their initial report of 720 taTME cases is the largest cohort published to date with a caseload distribution described as follows: 0 to 5, 6 to 10, 11 to 20, and greater than 30 cases in 33 (50%), 12 (18%), 8 (12%), and 13 (20%) surgical units. Results from this report are encouraging and quite similar to those demonstrated from the smaller cohorts mentioned previously. The rate of conversion from laparoscopic to open abdominal surgery was 6.3%. A completely intact TME specimen was achieved in 85% and TME specimens with minor defects in 11%. Intraoperative complications included 39.3% related to technical problems, 7.8% dissection into the wrong plane, 6.9% pelvic bleeding, and 1.5% visceral injury. Visceral injuries during perineal dissection included five urethral injuries, two bladder injuries, one vaginal perforation, one unilateral resection of hypogastric nerves, and two rectal perforations. The rate of positive CRM was 2.4%. Postoperative morbidity was 32.6% with complications including anastomotic leak, ileus, urinary tract infection, and abdominal or pelvic abscess. Risk factors for R1 resection or poor TME specimen included positive CRM on staging MRI, low rectal tumor less than 2 cm from the anorectal junction, and laparoscopic transabdominal posterior dissection to less than 4 cm from the anal verge. Interestingly, patient characteristics such as increased BMI or male sex were not significant risk factors for poor histologic results, suggesting that the transanal approach may overcome patient characteristics that traditionally would create a difficult pelvic dissection from the laparoscopic or open abdominal approach.

The initial results from the international taTME registry demonstrate short-term safety and feasibility with acceptable clinical outcomes. Long-term results will be reported after 3 years' follow-up with oncologic results as well as functional outcomes and quality of life after taTME. It is important to note that although small cohorts from single centers are of limited value, registry data also have limitations including the lack of validation of self-reported data. A well-stratified randomized controlled trial is needed

TABLE 168.5 Patient Characteristics of Published Clinical Series of Transanal Total Mesorectal Excision for Rectal Cancer

Series	N	BMI (kg/m²)	Tumor Location	Neoadjuvant CRT	Operative Technique	Transanal Platform
Veltcamp Helbach et al. (2015)[88]	80	27.5 (19.5–40)	5.3 (1–10) cm from DL	Yes (65) No (15)	LA, SILS	SILS Port (Covidien USA); Gelpoint (Applied Medical)
Lacy et al. (2015)[89]	140	25.2 ± 3.9	7.6 ± 3.6 cm from AV	Yes (94) No (46)	LA	Gelpoint (Applied Medical)
Tuech et al. (2015)[90]	56	27 (20–42)	4.0 (0–5) cm from AV	Yes (47) No (9)	LA (41), SILS (8), laparotomy (4), RA (1)	Endorec (Aspide) (42), SILS Port (Covidien) (11), Gelpoint (Applied Medical) (3)
Muratore et al. (2015)[91]	26	26.2 (16.9–38.2)	4.4 (3–6) cm from AV	Yes (19) No (7)	LA, SILS	SILS Port (Covidien)
Serra-Aracil et al. (2015)[92]	32	25 (20–35)	8.0 (5–10) cm from AV	Yes (16) No (16)	LA	TEO (Storz)
Rouanet et al. (2013)[93]	30	26.0 (21.0–32.4)	<5 cm from AV (20), 5–10 cm from AV (10)	Yes (29) No (1)	LA	TEO (Storz)
Burke et al. (2016)[94]	50	26.0 (22.7–31.2)	4.4 (3.0–5.5) cm from AV	Yes (43) No (7)	Open (4), LA (14), HA (19), RA (10)	Gelpoint (Applied Medical)
Chouillard et al. (2014)[95]	16	27.9 (21–38)	Mid- or low-rectal tumors	NR	SILS, Pure	SILS Port (Covidien)
Chen et al. (2015)[96]	50	24.2 (16–37)	5.8 (2–10) cm from AV	Yes (50)	LA, SILS	Gelpoint (Applied Medical)
De'Angelis et al. (2015)[98]	32	25.13	4.0 (2.5–5) cm from AV	Yes (27) No (5)	LA	Gelpoint (Applied Medical)
Perdawood et al. (2015)[99]	25	28 (18–46)	8.0 (4–10) cm from AV	Yes (7) No (18)	LA	Gelpoint (Applied Medical)
Buchs et al. (2016)[100]	20	27.1 (17.4–38.4)	2.0 (0–7) cm from anorectal junction	Yes (6) No (14)	LA, RA	Gloveport (4), Gelpoint (Applied Medical) (16)
Kang et al. (2015)[101]	20	22.2 (16.7–27.5)	6.1 (3–12) cm from AV	Yes (6) No (14)	LA, SILS, Pure	SILS Port (Covidien)
Marks et al. (2016)[102]	17	26.4 (20.1–32.3)	0.9 (−2.0 to 3.0)	Yes (17)	LA	Gelpoint (Applied Medical), SILS Port (Coviden)

APR, Abdominoperineal resection; *AV*, anal verge; *BMI*, body mass index; *CRM*, circumferential resection margin; *CRT*, chemoradiation therapy, *DRM*, distal resection margin, *DL*, dentate line, *ELAPE*, extralevator abdominoperineal excision; *IPAA*, ilial pouch-anal anastomosis; *LA*, laparoscopic-assisted; *LAR*, low anterior resection; *NR*, not reported; *PA*, robot-assisted; *SILS*, single incision laparoscopic surgery; *TATA*, transanal abdominal transanal resection; *TEO*, transanal endoscopic operation; *TME*, total mesorectal excision; tumor staging: *CR*, complete response; *M*, metastasis; *N*, node; *p*, pathologic; *T*, tumor; *y*, neoadjuvant therapy administered.

TABLE 168.5 Patient Characteristics of Published Clinical Series of Transanal Total Mesorectal Excision for Rectal Cancer—cont'd

Type of Resection	Operating Time (min)	Final Stage (n)	No. of Lymph Nodes Collected	TME Quality	Positive DRM	Positive CRM
LAR 65, APR 15	204 (91–447)	ypT0 (6), ypT1 (3), ypT2 (29), ypT3 (42), N0 (44), N1 (21), N2 (15)	14 (6–30)	71 Complete, 7 near complete, 2 incomplete	0	2
LAR 138, 2 proctocolectomy with IPAA	166 (60–360)	Complete response (15), stage I (34), II (43), III (39), IV (9)	14.7 ± 6.8	136 Complete, 3 near complete, 1 incomplete	NR	9 (6.4%)
APR 4, LAR 52	270 (150–495)	NR	12 (7–29)	47 Complete, 9 nearly complete	NR	3
LAR 25, APR 1	241 (150–360)	pT0 (5), pT1 (7), pT2 (6), pT3 (8), pN+ (7)	10 (median 8)	23 Complete, 3 near complete	0	0
LAR 32	240 (165–360)	Stage 0 (2), I (7), II (10), III (12), IV (1)	NR	30 Complete, 2 near complete	0	0
LAR 30	304 (120–432)	pCR 0, pT1 (1), pT2 (8), pT3 (18), pT4 (3), pN0 (14), pN1 (13), pN2 (3)	13 (8–32)	30 Complete	0	4
APR 7, LAR 43	267 (227–331)	pCR (12), pT1 (2), pT2 (11), pT3 (21), pT4 (4), N0 (34), N1 (8), N2 (8)	18 (12–24)	36 Complete, 13 near complete 1 incomplete	1 (2%)	2 (4%)
LAR 14, APR 2	265 (155–440)	pTy (1), pT1 (3), pT2 (4), pT3 (7), pT4 (1), N0 (11), N1 (4), N2 (1)	17 (12–81)	16 Complete	0	0
LAR 50	182.1 ± 55.4	ypT1/T2N0 (13), ypT3/T4N0 (12), ypTanyN1-2 (17), pCR (8)	16 (6–42)	NR	0	2 (4%)
LAR 32	195	pT1 (3), ypT2 (12), ypT3 (11), ypT4 (2), N0 (27), N1 (5), N2 (0)	17 (7.14)	27 Complete, 3 near complete, 2 incomplete	2 (6.2%)	1 (3.1%)
LAR 18, APR 7	NR	T0 (0), T1 (0), T2 (8), T3 (16), T4 (1), N0 (14), N1 (8), N2 (3)	21 (9–42)	20 Complete, 5 near complete	0	1 (4%)
LAR 16, ELAPE 2, completion proctectomy 1, APR 1	315.3 ± 77.1	T0 (4), T1 (0), T2 (8), T3 (5), T4 (0), N0 (10), N1 (5), N2 (2)	23 (11–45)	16 Complete, 1 near complete	0	1 (5.9%)
LAR 20	200 (70–420)	Complete response (2), Tis (2), stage I (10), II (4), III (2)	12 (1–20)	18 Complete, 2 near complete	0	0
TATA 12, APR 5	421.7	NR	7.5	15 Complete, 2 near complete	0	0

TABLE 168.6 Postoperative Outcomes of Published Clinical Series of Transanal Total Mesorectal Excision for Rectal Cancer

Series	Length of Stay (d)	Intraoperative Complications (n)	Follow-up Period (months)	Morbidity Rate (%)	Early Postoperative Complications (n)	Late Postoperative Complications (n)	Functional Outcomes	Recurrence
Veltcamp Helbach et al. (2015)[88]	8 (3–41)	Laparotomy (4), bleeding (2), perforation (3), abdominal incision for extraction (7)	24	39	Anastomotic leakage, ischemia of proximal limb of colon, small bowel laceration, revision of colostomy, small bowel obstruction, hematoma, full-thickness ischemia of mucosa distal to anastomosis	NR	NR	LR(2)
Lacy et al. (2015)[89]	7.8 (3–39)	None	15.0 ± 9.1	34	Adhesive obstruction (1), anastomotic leak (12), ileostomy obstruction/ileus (11), intraabdominal collection (4), bleeding (5), anastomotic bleed (3), high ileostomy output (2), acute pancreatitis (1), urinary retention (3), fever (5), blood transfusion (3), ascites (1)	Anastomotic stricture (6); colitis (4); high ileostomy output (3); ileostomy obstruction (2); intestinal obstruction (1), rectovaginal fistula (1)	NR	LR(1), DR(8), both(2)
Tuech et al. (2015)[90]	10 (6–21)	3 conversion, 6 delayed coloanal anastomosis	29 (18–52)	26	Anastomotic leak not requiring reoperation (3), pelvic sepsis without evidence of anastomotic leak (3), transient urinary disorders (5), blood transfusion (2), cerebral infarction (1)	NR	Wexner 5 (3–18)	LR(1), DR(2)
Muratore et al. (2015)[91]	7 (3–25)	0	23 (16–30)	27	Myocardial infarction (1), asymptomatic anastomotic leak (2), transient urinary retention (1), lymphorrhea (1), intestinal obstruction (2)	NR	NR	DR(2)
Serra-Aracil et al. (2015)[92]	8 (4–20)	0	NR	31	Nosocomial infection (3), SSI (3), anastomotic leakage (3), SBO requiring reintervention (1), necrosis of descending colon due to injury of marginal artery (1)	NR	NR	NR

Study							Median Wexner score	LR or DR
Rouanet et al. (2013)[93]	14 (8–25)	2 urethral injury (due to anterior bulky tumor and concurrent prostatic tumor), 1 air embolism	21 (10–41)	30	Sepsis (2), bowel obstruction (1), anastomotic leak (1)	NR	11	DR (14)
Burke et al. (2016)[94]	4.5 (4–8)	3 (6%), 1 urethral injury, 1 ureteral injury, 1 injury to iliac vessels,	15.1 (7.0–23.2)	36	Ileus (9), pelvic abscess (4), anastomotic leak (3), urinary retention (2), pneumonia (1), SSI (1), reoperations (6)	NR	NR	LR(2), DR(0)
Chouillard et al. (2014)[95]	10.4 (4–29)	0	9 (3–29)	19	Intestinal obstruction (2), pelvic abscess (1)	NR	—	0
Chen et al. (2015)[96]	7.4 (5–18)	2 presacral bleeding, 1 vaginal wall injury	—	20	UTI (1), pelvic abscess (3), rectovaginal fistula (1), anastomosis defect (3), pseudomembranous colitis (1), bleeding (1)	NR	NR	NR
De'Angelis et al. (2015)[98]	7.8	0	32.6	25	Urinary disorder (1), urinary infection (1), wound infection (1), anastomosis leak causing pelvic abscess (2), transfusion (1), anastomotic leak medically managed (1), anastomotic leak requiring surgical drainage (1)	NR	Wexner score 9	LR(1), DR(1)
Perdawood et al. (2015)[99]	5 (2–43)	2 bleeding	NR	52	Anastomotic leakage requiring readmission (2), high ileostomy output (2), stoma necrosis (1), mechanical obstruction from adhesions (2)	NR	Wexner 4.5 (0–7)	NR
Buchs et al. (2016)[100]	7 (3–36)	1 (5%)	10 (6–21)	30	High ileostomy output, anastomotic leak	Delayed pelvic sepsis secondary to a contained anastomotic leak (1)	NR	DR(1)
Kang et al. (2015)[101]	NR	1 (5%) massive bleeding, 1 (5%) prostate and urethra injury	5 (1–8)	20	Urethral injury (1), urinary retentions (2), anastomotic hemorrhage (1), mild anastomotic leak (1)	NR	Wexner 5.0 (3–11)	0
Marks et al. (2016)[102]	5	0	10.5	26	Neorectal prolapse (1), postoperative ileus (3)	NR	NR	LR(1), DR(0)

DR, Distal recurrence; *LR,* local recurrence; *NR,* not reported; *SBO,* small bowel obstruction; *SSI,* surgical site infection; *UTI,* urinary tract infection.

to truly confirm the purported benefits of taTME. At present, two international RCTs are underway including COLOR III and GRECCAR, where eligible patients with low and mid-rectal cancers are randomized to taTME or laparoscopic TME.[106,107] In addition, there is firm consensus among taTME experts that safe implementation of taTME requires prior expertise in laparoscopic or robotic TME, expertise in transanal endoscopic surgery (TAMIS, TEO, or TEM), and experience with TATA/ISR techniques. Structured training on cadavers is an essential component of taTME training, and proctorship of initial cases is strongly recommended to ensure safe adoption and minimize procedural complications.[108,109]

COMPLICATIONS OF LOW ANTERIOR RESECTION

The most effective way to prevent intraoperative and postoperative complications is by anticipating them during each step of the procedure. Regardless of the surgical approach used, the surgical steps of LAR are similar, as are the relative incidence of intraoperative and postoperative complications.

INTRAOPERATIVE COMPLICATIONS

Hemorrhage is uncommon and usually related to poor hemostasis during vascular ligation of the IMA, IMV, or the rectosigmoid mesentery. Presacral hemorrhage during transabdominal or transanal TME can occur during posterior mobilization of the mesorectum along the incorrect plane overly close to the sacrum. It can usually be controlled by applying pressure or packing, and/or by using monopolar cautery or topical hemostatic agents. Rarely, thumbtacks need to be applied to the sacrum to control persistent severe hemorrhage. Periprostatic bleeding can also occur during anterior mesorectal dissection performed transabdominally or transanally, when the plane of dissection is incorrect and overly close to the prostate or seminal vesicles. It can usually be controlled using monopolar and/or bipolar or ultrasonic energy. Anastomotic bleeding rarely requires a revision of the anastomosis. When reachable through an anoscope, it can usually be controlled with suture ligation. Otherwise, it may require endoscopic intervention with clipping.

Rectal perforation can result from traumatic laparoscopic or robotic instrument retraction of the rectum during TME or from cautery-related injury when dissection is carried out close to the rectal wall. It may be identified and repaired at the time of surgery but may present in a delayed fashion as an abscess, leak, or fistula. By limiting the need for proximal colon and rectal retraction with rigid instruments, the incidence of rectal perforation may be reduced, although there are no data to date to support this assumption. Besides rectal perforation, other organ injuries that are infrequently reported during LAR include small bowel, colon perforation, vaginal and bladder perforation, vascular injury such as injury to the iliac vessels, and ureteral injury. Although routine use of ureteral stents is not strictly advocated during open, laparoscopic, robotic, or transanal TME, selective use may help in identifying ureters early in cases where difficulties

with the pelvic dissection are anticipated, and will alert the surgeon to an injury if it occurs. Depending on the exact location of the injury along the ureter, primary end-to-end suture repair (ureteroureterostomy) may be possible rather than reimplantation to the contralateral ureter (transureteroureterostomy) or bladder (psoas hitch or Boari flap).

Organ injury is the most common reason for conversion to open surgery during laparoscopic, robotic, or transanal TME, when repair cannot be safely performed using a minimally invasive approach. Other reasons include hemorrhage and failure to progress when difficulties with exposure and identification of the correct dissection planes and of key anatomic landmarks cannot be overcome.

Urethral injury has emerged as an unusual morbidity specific to taTME. Although it is reported as a rare complication of the perineal phase of an APR with an estimated incidence of 1% to 2%, it has not been reported in open or laparoscopic TME. There have been 4 cases of urethral injury out of the more than 500 described cases of taTME, and 5 urethral injuries (0.7%) out of the 720 cases from the LOREC registry.[93,94,97,100,105,110,111] The risk of urethral injury seems to be highest early during the surgeon's learning curve, during difficult anterior dissection for very low rectal tumors, and in patients with bulky anterior rectal tumors or an enlarged prostate, which can distort the anatomy and make recognition of the correct rectoprostatic plane more difficult. It is imperative that the urethral injury be recognized intraoperatively and repaired primarily at the time of the injury, ideally by a urology specialist, with or without temporary urinary diversion. This is especially true in patients who have received preoperative radiation. Urethral repair is performed using a perineal approach, or a transabdominal open, laparoscopic, or robotic approach.[112]

POSTOPERATIVE COMPLICATIONS

Anastomotic complications include anastomotic leaks with pelvic sepsis and anastomotic strictures. Small leaks that are relatively well contained in a patient without overt signs of sepsis may be managed conservatively with parenteral antibiotics, delay in oral intake, and percutaneous drainage of the pelvic abscess when present. In a patient with sepsis, reexploration with washout, wide drainage, and ileostomy or colostomy creation is required. Transanal endoscopic evaluation at the time of reoperation may allow visualization of a focal anastomotic defect with suture repair in selected cases. Anastomotic strictures are typically the result of ischemia with management ranging from serial endoscopic balloon dilations to stricturoplasty, permanent fecal diversion, or redo-colorectal anastomosis.

With respect to functional outcomes following LAR, transient urinary dysfunction, including urinary retention and urinary incontinence, is common with incidence ranging from 0% to 27%.[113,114] This is usually treated with temporary urinary drainage using a catheter for up to several weeks. Sexual dysfunction includes erectile dysfunction, absence of ejaculation, or retrograde ejaculation in males, and diminished vaginal lubrication, dyspareunia, and inability or difficulty achieving orgasm in females.[28] Globally, sexual dysfunction has been described to range in incidence from 11% to 55% following TME for rectal cancer.[113-117]

Defecatory dysfunction following proctectomy ranges from mild disturbances to severe LAR syndrome and debilitating fecal incontinence, tenesmus, and fecal urgency.

Up to 90% of patients will suffer symptomatology related to LAR syndrome, which negatively influences their quality of life and can be worse in patients previously treated with radiation or where partial or complete ISR was performed for low rectal tumors.[118,119] Most symptoms improve after 6 to 12 months, but a group of patients will have symptoms that persist for a longer period of time. The etiology of these symptoms is multifactorial and can include colonic dysmotility, decreased rectal sensibility, disappearance of the anorectal reflex, reduction of rectal tone, and damage to the pelvic nerves or internal sphincter.

Diagnosis requires meticulous assessment and the implementation of different scores such as the Low Anterior Resection Syndrome (LARS) score or Wexner score, and other validated questionnaires assessing fecal incontinence and defecatory dysfunction. Treatment should be multimodal. Fecal incontinence following LAR is usually managed conservatively starting with dietary recommendations, antimotility agents, and fiber supplements. Low resting anal sphincter tone and squeeze can be improved with pelvic floor strengthening exercises and biofeedback, which have been demonstrated to result in fewer episodes of incontinence, decreased severity of incontinence, and better quality of life.[120]

Regarding sacral nerve stimulation for the cure of postoperative fecal incontinence, there is a heterogeneity of single-center studies that show improvement in symptomatology and quality of life by decreasing the number of incontinence episodes and providing the ability to delay defecation. At this time, larger studies with better patient selection are needed to further investigate the effect of sacral nerve stimulation in rectal cancer patients undergoing LAR.[121,122]

ONCOLOGIC OUTCOMES

The oncologic objective of radical oncologic resection for rectal cancer includes the complete removal of the primary tumor and tumor deposits in the mesorectum. A complete TME consists of an R0 resection with negative circumferential, distal, and proximal margins. A negative CRM is of particular importance because it was shown to serve as an independent prognostic factor for the risk of local recurrence following rectal cancer resection.[123]

As previously described and as demonstrated in the majority of RCTs comparing open and laparoscopic TME for rectal cancer, laparoscopic TME was shown to result in equivalent short- and long-term oncologic outcomes with respect to rates of negative margins achieved, number of lymph nodes retrieved, and quality and grade of TME specimens.[47-49,62-64,57,68] This is with the exception of the recent ACOSOG Z6051 and the ALaCaRt trials that failed to demonstrate noninferiority of the laparoscopic approach when using a composite endpoint based on TME quality and margin status.[50,51] The preliminary results of the ROLARR trial demonstrated equivalent short-term oncologic results of robotic-assisted versus laparoscopic TME.[85] Although RCT data of taTME versus laparoscopic TME are lacking, preliminary results from registry and

moderate-sized series also suggest equivalence relative to laparoscopic TME.[94-101,105]

Long-term oncologic outcomes from several RCTs comparing laparoscopic and open TME have demonstrated no difference of 3-, 5-, and 10-year overall survival and disease-free survival.[48,62-54] Long-term oncologic results of the ROLARR trial are needed, as well as short- and long-term outcomes from COLRAR, GRECCAR 11, and COLOR III trials comparing robotic or transanal TME versus laparoscopic TME. Thus far, the evidence suggests that in the hands of expert laparoscopic surgeons, similar oncologic results can be obtained whether TME is performed open or laparoscopically.

Interestingly, there are a few series in which the overall survival at 5 years was better in the laparoscopic than in the open group, especially in stage III tumors.[124-126] The potential impact of laparoscopic surgery on survival is not clear, but the role of the immunologic response has been suggested. Levels of inflammatory mediators such as TNF-α, IL 1-6, and C reactive protein are lower after laparoscopic compared to open colorectal surgery. An inflammatory response facilitates septic complications and neoplastic cell proliferation, and the degree of inflammation may correspond to the level of surgical stress. Laparoscopic surgery may improve either overall or cancer-free survival by limiting the degree of surgical stress and its corresponding immunologic response. This positive impact of laparoscopy is probably marginal but could explain why it is observed that the risk of cancer-related mortality is significantly lower in stage III cancers.[124-126] The long-term results of larger comparative trials are needed to better clarify if the laparoscopic approach is associated with improved survival in this subgroup of patients.

FUNCTIONAL OUTCOMES

Meaningful assessment of the impact of LAR on defecatory, urinary, and sexual function requires the administration of questionnaires at several time points during the patient's care. These opportunities include (1) at baseline and prior to any rectal cancer treatment, (2) 2 to 3 months postoperatively or following ileostomy closure, and (3) 1 year postoperatively or following ileostomy closure, for long-term functional assessment. Questionnaires should be validated and include quality-of-life metrics.[162,127] Defecatory function is typically assessed using the Wexner score and LAR Syndrome Score.[118,127] Sexual function should be evaluated with the International Index Erectile Function (IIE-5) questionnaire in males and the Female Sexual Function Index (FSFI).[128,129] Urinary dysfunction is measured by the International Prostate Symptom Score (IPSS) questionnaire or the International Consultation on Incontinence Modular Questionnaire (ICIQ).[129,130] With respect to quality-of-life surveys, there are two types of questionnaires that should be given, the first to assess overall quality of life, and the second to assess quality of life as it relates to colorectal cancer. An example is the 36-Item Short Form Survey (SF-36) or the European Organization for Research and Treatment of Cancer (EORTC) QLQ-C 30 to evaluate quality of life related to oncologic patients and the EORTC QLQ-CR29, which is specific for colorectal cancer.[131,132]

It was presumed that improved pelvic visualization provided by the laparoscopic and robotic approach may result in more accurate dissection and improved sparing of autonomic nerves, which would in turn result in a lower incidence of urinary and sexual dysfunction. However, no significant differences in functional outcomes between open and laparoscopic TME have been demonstrated.[30,49] Regarding laparoscopic and robotic TME, the long-term functional outcomes have been comparable overall, although faster recovery of sexual and urinary function has been demonstrated in few case-matched series.[30,75,80,133,134] At this time, further clinical studies are needed to obtain high-level evidence demonstrating this possible benefit of robotic surgery. As described earlier, only a few taTME series have reported on functional outcomes following TME, and those series have short follow-up and variability in the type of questionnaires and time points.[97,98,100,135] Overall, long-term functional outcomes following LAR need to be assessed more consistently across studies, using the same validated questionnaires and similar time points, in order to understand the impact of various surgical approaches on functional outcomes and quality of life.

HIGH VERSUS LOW LIGATION OF THE INFERIOR MESENTERIC ARTERY

The level at which the IMA should be ligated has been controversial. The high-tie technique involves dividing the IMA 1 cm distal to its origin, while the low-tie technique recommends dividing the IMA distal to the takeoff of the left colic artery. With high ligation, a more complete D3 lymphadenectomy may be performed, which has been advocated by many as associated with lower local recurrence rates and improved overall survival. However, the oncologic superiority of high ligation of the IMA and D3 lymphadenectomy has not been proven, hence the controversy. On the other hand, low ligation of the IMA improves the perfusion of the proximal colon and of the colorectal anastomosis, therefore possibly lowering the risk for anastomotic failure. Low ligation may also be protective against the risk of superior hypogastric nerve injury and may lower the risk of genitourinary dysfunction. Future studies comparing low versus high IMA ligation and the impact on short- and long-term results are needed before definitive recommendations can be made.[136]

ASSESSMENT OF BOWEL PERFUSION

The specific etiology of anastomotic leaks is multifactorial with several well-known risk factors (level of anastomosis, tobacco use, preoperative radiation, etc.). In addition to the mechanical integrity of colorectal anastomosis, adequate bowel perfusion plays a critical role with ischemia being an important risk factor for anastomotic leak in colorectal and other gastrointestinal anastomoses. Adequate perfusion of the resection margins and the anastomosis is usually determined using clinical judgment alone. The surgeon observes the color of the tissue, checks for bleeding from the cut edges, palpates for arterial pulses, and evaluates for peristalsis. This method of assessment is subjective, difficult to quantify, and can be inaccurate, making it

a poor predictor of the risk of anastomotic leakage. A current trend in the literature on open and minimally invasive gastrointestinal surgery is the use of ICG fluorescence imaging to assess the adequacy of tissue perfusion prior to making a decision regarding the level of bowel transection and the segment of bowel to be used for the anastomosis.[137,138]

Several ICG fluorescence imaging systems are currently commercially available to assess bowel perfusion with real-time endoscopic HD and near-infrared fluorescence imaging. Laparoscopic or robotic systems include a laparoscope optimized for vision/infrared illumination and imaging with a camera head that mounts to the laparoscopic eyepiece and an endoscopic video processor illuminator that provides infrared illumination to the surgical laparoscope. ICG, which is approved for human use by the United States Food and Drug Administration, is a sterile, water-soluble, tricarbocyanine compound that can be administered intravenously or intraarterially. It absorbs infrared light and emits fluorescence. This compound rapidly and extensively binds to plasma proteins and is therefore confined to the intravascular compartment with minimal leakage into the interstitium. It is cleared by the liver in 3 to 5 minutes into bile with no known metabolites.[137,139] Either before or after transection of the proximal colon, 5 to 10 mg of ICG are injected intravenously and the proximal colon and rectum are evaluated for perfusion in the fluorescence mode. A second dose of ICG is typically given following completion of the anastomosis to assess perfusion.

To date, a few studies have evaluated the impact of ICG fluorescence perfusion assessment on surgeons' change in decision making in the operating room and subsequent incidence of anastomotic leak. Preliminary studies suggest that fluorescence imaging during colorectal procedures provides important additional information regarding the adequacy of bowel perfusion at the planned colonic transection site that can lead to a change in the level of colon transection.[137,140] This technology may ultimately improve our subjective and inaccurate methods of assessing perfusion at the anastomosis and thus decrease anastomotic leak rates.

CONCLUSION

The treatment of rectal cancer has undergone remarkable transformation over the last 50 years. Although APR was the standard of care for the first half of the 20th century, it was associated with significant morbidity, mortality, and largely suboptimal oncologic outcomes. The introduction of the TME technique by Heald revolutionized the standards and practice of rectal cancer surgery with substantial improvement in local recurrence rates and improved survival. Subsequent breakthroughs included the introduction of transanal endoscopic surgery by Buess, advances in neoadjuvant therapies in conjunction with the technique of TATA and intersphincteric techniques that allowed increasing rates of sphincter preservation for very low rectal tumors. Over the last two decades, additional seminal events have included the worldwide adoption of laparoscopy, soon followed by robotics, and most recently taTME, the latest innovation born from combining TES and TATA to perform TME from a transanal approach with hybrid abdominal assistance. Overall, recent minimally invasive TME techniques have thus far matched the oncologic standards of open TME, although randomized trials with long-term oncologic and functional data are needed to clearly establish the role that each of these approaches should play in the arsenal of surgical treatments for rectal cancer.

REFERENCES

1. Miles W. A method of performing abdomino-perineal excision for carcinoma of the rectum and of the terminal portion of the pelvic colon. *Lancet.* 1908;2:1312-1813.
2. Abel A. The modern treatment of cancer of the rectum. *Milwaukee Proc.* 1931;296-300.
3. Heald R, Moran B, Ryall R, Sexton R, MacFarlane J. Rectal cancer: the Basingstoke experience of total mesorectal excision, 1978-1997. *Arch Surg.* 1998;133:894-899.
4. Weiser M, Quah H, Shia J, et al. Sphincter preservation in low rectal cancer is facilitated by preoperative chemoradiation and intersphincteric dissection. *Ann Surg.* 2009;249(2):236-242.
5. Tytherleigh M, McC Mortensen N. Options for sphincter preservation in surgery for low rectal cancer. *Br J Surg.* 2003;90(8):922-933.
6. Boutros M, Hippalgaonkar N, Silva E, Allende D, Wexner S, Berho M. Laparoscopic resection of rectal cancer results in higher lymph node yield and better short-term outcomes than open surgery: a large single-center comparative study. *Dis Colon Rectum.* 2013;56(6):679-688.
7. Swedish Rectal Cancer Trial, Cedermark B, Dahlberg M, et al. Improved survival with preoperative radiotherapy in resectable rectal cancer. *N Engl J Med.* 1997;336(14):980-987.
8. van Gijn W, Marijnen C, Nagtegaal I, et al. Preoperative radiotherapy combined with total mesorectal excision for resectable rectal cancer: 12-year follow-up of the multicentre, randomised controlled TME trial. *Lancet Oncol.* 2011;12(6):575-582.
9. Sauer R, Becker H, Hohenberger W, et al. Preoperative versus postoperative chemoradiotherapy for rectal cancer. *N Engl J Med.* 2004;351(17):1731-1740.
10. Agha A, Benseler V, Hornung M, et al. Long-term oncologic outcome after laparoscopic surgery for rectal cancer. *Surg Endosc.* 2014;28(4):1119-1125.
11. Buess G, Theiss R, Günther M, Hutterer F, Pichlmaier H. Endoscopic surgery in the rectum. *Endoscopy.* 1985;17(1):31-35.
12. Atallah S, Albert M, Larach S. Transanal minimally invasive surgery: a giant leap forward. *Surg Endosc.* 2010;24(9):2200-2205.
13. Marks J, Frenkel J, D'Andrea A, Greenleaf C. Maximizing rectal cancer results: TEM and TATA techniques to expand sphincter preservation. *Surg Oncol Clin N Am.* 2011;20(3):501-520.
14. D'Hoore A, Wolthuis M. Laparoscopic low anterior resection and transanal pull-through for low rectal cancer: a Natural Orifice Specimen Extraction (NOSE) technique. *Colorectal Dis.* 2011;20(13):7.
15. Atallah S, Albert M, DeBeche-Adams T, Nassif G, Polavarapu H, Larach S. Transanal minimally invasive surgery for total mesorectal excision (TAMIS-TME): a stepwise description of the surgical technique with video demonstration. *Tech Coloproctol.* 2013;17(3):321-325.
16. Zorron R, Phillipps H, Coelho D, Flach L, Lemos F, Vassallo R. Perirectal NOTES access: "down-to-up" total mesorectal excision for rectal cancer. *Surg Innov.* 2012;19(1):11-19
17. Sylla P, Bordeianou L, Berger D, Han K, Lauwers G, Sahani D, et al. A pilot study of natural orifice transanal endoscopic total mesorectal excision with laparoscopic assistance for rectal cancer. *Surg Endosc.* 2013;27(9):3396-3405.
18. Trunzo J, Delaney C. Natural orifice proctectomy using a transanal endoscopic microsurgical technique in a porcine model. *Surg Innov.* 2010;17(1):48-52.
19. Sohn D, Jeong S, Park J, et al. Comparative study of NOTES rectosigmoidectomy in a swine model: E-NOTES vs. P-NOTES. *Endoscopy.* 2011;43(6):526-532.
20. Telem D, Berger D, Bordeianou L, Rattner D, Sylla P. Update on transanal NOTES for rectal cancer: transitioning to human trials. *Minim Invasive Surg.* 2012;2012:287613.
21. Telem D, Han K, Kim M, et al. Transanal rectosigmoid resection via natural orifice transluminal endoscopic surgery (NOTES) with total

22. mesorectal excision in a large human cadaver series. *Surg Endosc.* 2013;27(1):74-80.
22. Bhattacharjee H, Kirschniak A, Storz P, Wilhelm P, Kunert W. Transanal endoscopic microsurgery-based transanal access for colorectal surgery: experience on human cadavers. *J Laparoendosc Adv Surg Tech A.* 2011;29(9):835-840.
23. Tuech J, Bridoux V, Kianifard B, et al. Natural orifice total mesorectal excision using transanal port and laparoscopic assistance. *Eur J Surg Oncol.* 2011;37(4):334-335.
24. Lacy A, Rattner D, Adelsdorfer C, et al. Transanal natural orifice transluminal endoscopic surgery (NOTES) rectal resection: 'down-to-up' total mesorectal excision (TME)—short-term outcomes in the first 20 cases. *Surg Endosc.* 2013;27(9):3165-3172.
25. Lacy A, Adelsdorfer C, Delgado S, Sylla P, Rattner D. Minilaparoscopy-assisted transrectal low anterior resection (LAR): a preliminary study. *Surg Endosc.* 2013;27(1):339-346.
26. Dumont F, Goéré D, Honoré C, Elias D. Transanal endoscopic total mesorectal excision combined with single-port laparoscopy. *Dis Colon Rectum.* 2012;55(9):996-1001.
27. Funahashi K, Shiokawa H, Teramoto T, Koike J, Kaneko H. Clinical outcome of laparoscopic intersphincteric resection combined with transanal rectal dissection for T3 low rectal cancer in patients with a narrow pelvis. *Int J Surg Oncol.* 2011;2011:901574.
28. Kim N. Anatomic basis of sharp pelvic dissection for curative resection of rectal cancer. *Yonsei Med J.* 2005;46(6):737-749.
29. Kinugasa Y, Murakami G, Suzuki D, Sugihara K. Histological identification of fascial structures posterolateral to the rectum. *Br J Surg.* 2007;94(5):620-626.
30. Kim N, Kim Y, Cho M. Total mesorectal excision for rectal cancer with emphasis on pelvic autonomic nerve preservation: expert technical tips for robotic surgery. *Surg Oncol.* 2015;24(3):172-180.
31. Hollabaugh RJ, Steiner M, Sellers K, Samm B, Dmochowski R. Neuroanatomy of the pelvis: implications for colonic and rectal resection. *Dis Colon Rectum.* 2000;43(10):1390-1397.
32. Zhang G, Cai Y, Xu G. Diagnostic accuracy of MRI for assessment of T category and circumferential resection margin involvement in patients with rectal cancer: a meta-analysis. *Dis Colon Rectum.* 2016;59(8):789-799.
33. Al-Sukhni E, Milot L, Fruitman M, et al. Diagnostic accuracy of MRI for assessment of T category, lymph node metastases, and circumferential resection margin involvement in patients with rectal cancer: a systematic review and meta-analysis. *Ann Surg Oncol.* 2012;19(7):2212-2223.
34. Lutz M, Zalcberg J, Glynne-Jones R, et al. Second St. Gallen European Organisation for Research and Treatment of Cancer Gastrointestinal Cancer Conference: consensus recommendations on controversial issues in the primary treatment of rectal cancer. *Eur J Cancer.* 2016;63:11-24.
35. Bosset J, Collette L, Calais G, et al. Chemotherapy with preoperative radiotherapy in rectal cancer. *N Engl J Med.* 2006;355(11):1114-1123.
36. Roh M, Colangelo L, O'Connell M, et al. Preoperative multimodality therapy improves disease-free survival in patients with carcinoma of the rectum: NSABP R-03. *J Clin Oncol.* 2009;27(31):5124-5130.
37. Bujko K, Nowacki M, Nasierowska-Guttmejer A, Michalski W, Bebenek M, Kryj M. Long-term results of a randomized trial comparing preoperative short-course radiotherapy with preoperative conventionally fractionated chemoradiation for rectal cancer. *Br J Surg.* 2006;93(10):1215-1223.
38. Sebag-Montefiore D, Stephens R, Steele R, et al. Preoperative radiotherapy versus selective postoperative chemoradiotherapy in patients with rectal cancer (MRC CR07 and NCIC-CTG C016): a multicentre, randomised trial. *Lancet.* 2009;373(9666):811-820.
39. Gérard J, Conroy T, Bonnetain F, et al. Preoperative radiotherapy with or without concurrent fluorouracil and leucovorin in T3-4 rectal cancers: results of FFCD 9203. *J Clin Oncol.* 2006;24(28):4620-4625.
40. Pollack J, Holm T, Cedermark B, et al. Late adverse effects of short-course preoperative radiotherapy in rectal cancer. *Br J Surg.* 2006;93(12):1519-1525.
41. Scarborough J, Mantyh C, Sun Z, Migaly J. Combined mechanical and oral antibiotic bowel preparation reduces incisional surgical site infection and anastomotic leak rates after elective colorectal resection: an analysis of colectomy-targeted ACS NSQIP. *Ann Surg.* 2015;262(2):331-337.
42. Poggio J. Perioperative strategies to prevent surgical-site infection. *Clin Colon Rectal Surg.* 2013;26(3):168-173.

43. Kang D, Kwak H, Sung N, et al. Oncologic outcomes in rectal cancer patients with a ≤1-cm distal resection margin. *Int J Colorectal Dis.* 2017;32(3):325-332.
44. Moore H, Riedel E, Minsky B, et al. Adequacy of 1-cm distal margin after restorative rectal cancer resection with sharp mesorectal excision and preoperative combined-modality therapy. *Ann Surg Oncol.* 2003;10(1):80-85.
45. Bujko K, Rutkowski A, Chang G, Michalski W, Chmielik E, Kusnierz J. Is the 1-cm rule of distal bowel resection margin in rectal cancer based on clinical evidence? A systematic review. *Ann Surg Oncol.* 2012;19(3):801-808.
46. Law W, Chu K. Anterior resection for rectal cancer with mesorectal excision: a prospective evaluation of 622 patients. *Ann Surg.* 2004;240(2):260-268.
47. van der Pas M, Haglind E, Cuesta M, et al. Laparoscopic versus open surgery for rectal cancer (COLOR II): short-term outcomes of a randomised, phase 3 trial. *Lancet Oncol.* 2013;14(3):210-218.
48. Jeong S, Park J, Nam B, et al. Open versus laparoscopic surgery for mid-rectal or low-rectal cancer after neoadjuvant chemoradiotherapy (COREAN trial): survival outcomes of an open-label, non-inferiority, randomised controlled trial. *Lancet Oncol.* 2014;15(7):767-774.
49. Guillou P, Quirke P, Thorpe H. Short-term endpoints of conventional versus laparoscopic-assisted surgery in patients with colorectal cancer (MRC CLASICC trial): multicentre, randomised controlled trial. *Lancet.* 2005;365(9472):1718-1726.
50. Fleshman J, Branda M, Sargent D, et al. Effect of laparoscopic-assisted resection vs open resection of stage II or III rectal cancer on pathologic outcomes: the ACOSOG Z6051 randomized clinical trial. *JAMA.* 2015;314(13):1356-1364.
51. Stevenson A, Solomon M, Lumley J, et al. Effect of laparoscopic-assisted resection vs open resection on pathological outcomes in rectal cancer: the ALaCaRT randomized clinical trial. *JAMA.* 2015;314(13):1356-1363.
52. Ogiso S, Yamaguchi T, Hata H, et al. Evaluation of factors affecting the difficulty of laparoscopic anterior resection for rectal cancer: "narrow pelvis" is not a contraindication. *Surg Endosc.* 2011;25(6):1907-1912.
53. Akiyoshi T, Kuroyanagi H, Oya M, et al. Factors affecting the difficulty of laparoscopic total mesorectal excision with double stapling technique anastomosis for low rectal cancer. *Surgery.* 2009;146(3):483-489.
54. Nagtegaal I, van de Velde C, Marijnen C, et al. Low rectal cancer: a call for a change of approach in abdominoperineal resection. *J Clin Oncol.* 2005;23(36):9257-9264.
55. Saito N, Sugito M, Ito M, et al. Oncologic outcome of intersphincteric resection for very low rectal cancer. *World J Surg.* 2009;33(8):1750-1756.
56. Cima R, Pendlimari R, Holubar S, et al. Utility and short-term outcomes of hand-assisted laparoscopic colorectal surgery: a single-institution experience in 1103 patients. *Dis Colon Rectum.* 2011;54(9):1076-1081.
57. Pyo D, Huh J, Park Y, et al. A comparison of hand-assisted laparoscopic surgery and conventional laparoscopic surgery in rectal cancer: a propensity score analysis. *Surg Endosc.* 2016;30(6):2449-2456.
58. Hallböök O, Påhlman L, Krog M, Wexner S, Sjödahl R. Randomized comparison of straight and colonic J pouch anastomosis after low anterior resection. *Ann Surg.* 1996;224(1):58-65.
59. Heriot A, Tekkis P, Constantinides V, et al. Meta-analysis of colonic reservoirs versus straight coloanal anastomosis after anterior resection. *Br J Surg.* 2006;93(1):19-32.
60. Jayne D, Guillou P, Thorpe H, et al. Randomized trial of laparoscopic assisted resection of colorectal carcinoma 3 year results of the UK MRC CLASICC Trial Group. *J Clin Oncol.* 2007;25(21):3061-3068.
61. Green B, Marshall H, Collinson F, et al. Long-term follow-up of the Medical Research Council CLASICC trial of conventional versus laparoscopically assisted resection in colorectal cancer. *Br J Surg.* 2013;100(1):75-82.
62. Bonjer H, Deijen C, Abis G, et al. A randomized trial of laparoscopic versus open surgery for rectal cancer. *N Engl J Med.* 2015;372(4):1324-1332.
63. Jayne D, Thorpe H, Copeland J, Quirke P, Brown J, Guillou P. Five-year follow-up of the Medical Research Council CLASICC trial of laparoscopically assisted versus open surgery for colorectal cancer. *Br J Surg.* 2010;97(11):1638-1645.
64. Ng S, Leung K, Lee J, Yiu R, Li J, Hon S. Long-term morbidity and oncologic outcomes of laparoscopic-assisted anterior resection for upper rectal cancer: ten-year results of a prospective, randomized trial. *Dis Colon Rectum.* 2009;52(4):558-566.
65. Leung K, Kwok S, Lam S, et al. Laparoscopic resection of rectosigmoid carcinoma: prospective randomised trial. *Lancet.* 2004;363(9416):1187-1192.
66. Kang S, Park J, Jeong S, et al. Open versus laparoscopic surgery for mid or low rectal cancer after neoadjuvant chemoradiotherapy (COREAN trial): short-term outcomes of an open-label randomised controlled trial. *Lancet Oncol.* 2010;11(7):637-645.
67. Lee G, Sylla P. Shifting paradigms in minimally invasive surgery: applications of transanal natural orifice transluminal endoscopic surgery in colorectal surgery. *Clin Colon Rectal Surg.* 2015;28(3):181-193.
68. Pamela D, Roberto C, Francesco L, et al. Trocar site hernia after laparoscopic colectomy: a case report and literature review. *ISRN Surg.* 2011;2011:725601.
69. Bulut O, Aslak K, Rosenstock S. Technique and short-term outcomes of single-port surgery for rectal cancer: a feasibility study of 25 patients. *Scand J Surg.* 2013;103(1):26-33.
70. Makino T, Milsom J, Lee S. Feasibility and safety of single-incision laparoscopic colectomy: a systematic review. *Ann Surg.* 2012;255(4):667-676.
71. Kim N, Kang J. Optimal total mesorectal excision for rectal cancer: the role of robotic surgery from an expert's view. *J Korean Soc Coloproctol.* 2010;26(6):377-387.
72. Ito M, Sugito M, Kobayashi A, Nishizawa Y, Tsunoda Y, Saito N. Relationship between multiple numbers of stapler firings during rectal division and anastomotic leakage after laparoscopic rectal resection. *Int J Colorectal Dis.* 2008;23(7):703-707.
73. Pigazzi A, Ellenhorn J, Ballantyne G, Paz I. Robotic-assisted laparoscopic low anterior resection with total mesorectal excision for rectal cancer. *Surg Endosc.* 2006;20(10):1521-1525.
74. Young M, Pigazzi A. Total mesorectal excision: open, laparoscopic or robotic. *Recent Results Cancer Res.* 2014;203:47-55.
75. D'Annibale A, Pernazza G, Monsellato I, et al. Total mesorectal excision: a comparison of oncological and functional outcomes between robotic and laparoscopic surgery for rectal cancer. *Surg Endosc.* 2013;27(6):1887-1895.
76. Baek J, Pastor C, Pigazzi A. Robotic and laparoscopic total mesorectal excision for rectal cancer: a case-matched study. *Surg Endosc.* 2011;25(2):521-525.
77. Baik S, Kwon H, Kim J, et al. Robotic versus laparoscopic low anterior resection of rectal cancer: short-term outcome of a prospective comparative study. *Ann Surg Oncol.* 2009;16(6):1480-1487.
78. Du X, Shen D, Li R, et al. Robotic anterior resection of rectal cancer: technique and early outcome. *Chin Med J.* 2013;126(1):51-54.
79. Park E, Cho M, Baek S, et al. Long-term oncologic outcomes of robotic low anterior resection for rectal cancer: a comparative study with laparoscopic surgery. *Ann Surg.* 2015;261(1):129-137.
80. Patriti A, Ceccarelli G, Bartoli A, Spaziani A, Biancafarina A, Casciola L. Short- and medium-term outcome of robot-assisted and traditional laparoscopic rectal resection. *JSLS.* 2009;13(2):176-183.
81. Feroci F, Vannucchi A, Bianchi P, et al. Total mesorectal excision for mid and low rectal cancer: laparoscopic vs robotic surgery. *World J Gastroenterol.* 2016;22(13):3602-3610.
82. Park J, Choi G, Lim K, Jang Y, Jun S. Robotic-assisted versus laparoscopic surgery for low rectal cancer: case-matched analysis of short-term outcomes. *Ann Surg Oncol.* 2010;17(12):3195-3202.
83. Kim Y, Kim M, Park S, et al. Robotic versus laparoscopic surgery for rectal cancer after preoperative chemoradiotherapy: case-matched study of short-term outcomes. *Cancer Res Treat.* 2016;48(1):225-231.
84. Kwak J, Kim S, Kim J, Son D, Baek S, Cho J. Robotic vs laparoscopic resection of rectal cancer: short-term outcomes of a case-control study. *Dis Colon Rectum.* 2011;54(2):151-156.
85. Collinson F, Jayne D, Pigazzi A, et al. An international, multicentre, prospective, randomised, controlled, unblinded, parallel-group trial of robotic-assisted versus standard laparoscopic surgery for the curative treatment of rectal cancer. *Int J Colorectal Dis.* 2012;27(2):233-241.
86. Choi G, Kim N, Kim S. A trial to assess robot-assisted surgery and laparoscopy-assisted surgery in patients with mid or low rectal cancer (COLRAR); 2013. http://www.clinicaltrials.gov/show/NCT01423214. Accessed 25 May 2017.

87. Penna M, Knol J, Tuynman J, Tekkis P, Mortensen N, Hompes R. Four anastomotic techniques following transanal total mesorectal excision (TaTME). *Tech Coloproctol.* 2016;20(3):185-191.

88. Veltcamp Helbach M, Deijen C, Velthuis S, Bonjer H, Tuynman J, Sietses C. Transanal total mesorectal excision for rectal carcinoma: short-term outcomes and experience after 80 cases. *Surg Endosc.* 2016;30(2):464-470.

89. Lacy A, Tasende M, Delgado S, et al. Transanal total mesorectal excision for rectal cancer: outcomes after 140 patients. *J Am Coll Surg.* 2015;221(2):415-423.

90. Tuech J, Karoui M, Lelong B, et al. A step toward NOTES total mesorectal excision for rectal cancer: endoscopic transanal proctectomy. *Ann Surg.* 2015;261(2):228-233.

91. Muratore A, Mellano A, Marsanic P, De Simone M. Transanal total mesorectal excision (taTME) for cancer located in the lower rectum: short- and mid-term results. *Eur J Surg Oncol.* 2015;41(4):478-483.

92. Serra-Aracil X, Mora-López L, Casalots A, Pericay C, Guerrero R, Navarro-Soto S. Hybrid NOTES: TEO for transanal total mesorectal excision: intracorporeal resection and anastomosis. *Surg Endosc.* 2016;30(1):346-354.

93. Rouanet P, Mourregot A, Azar C, et al. Transanal endoscopic proctectomy: an innovative procedure for difficult resection of rectal tumors in men with narrow pelvis. *Dis Colon Rectum.* 2013;56(4):408-415.

94. Burke J, Martin-Perez B, Khan A, et al. Transanal total mesorectal excision for rectal cancer: early outcomes in 50 consecutive patients. *Colorectal Dis.* 2016;18(6):570-577.

95. Chouillard E, Chahine E, Khoury G, et al. NOTES total mesorectal excision (TME) for patients with rectal neoplasia: a preliminary experience. *Surg Endosc.* 2014;28(11):3150-3157.

96. Chen T, Emmertsen K, Laurberg S. What are the best questionnaires to capture anorectal function after surgery in rectal cancer? *Curr Colorectal Cancer Rep.* 2015;11:37-43.

97. Chen C, Lai Y, Jiang J, et al. Transanal total mesorectal excision versus laparoscopic surgery for rectal cancer receiving neoadjuvant chemoradiation: a matched case-control study. *Ann Surg Oncol.* 2015;23(4):1169-1176.

98. de'Angelis N, Portigliotti L, Azoulay D, Brunetti F. Transanal total mesorectal excision for rectal cancer: a single center experience and systematic review of the literature. *Langenbecks Arch Surg.* 2015;400(8):945-959.

99. Perdawood S, Al Khefagie G. Transanal vs laparoscopic total mesorectal excision for rectal cancer: initial experience from Denmark. *Colorectal Dis.* 2016;18(1):51-58.

100. Buchs N, Nicholson G, Yeung T, et al. Transanal rectal resection: an initial experience of 20 cases. *Colorectal Dis.* 2016;18(1):45-50.

101. Kang L, Chen W, Luo S, et al. Transanal total mesorectal excision for rectal cancer: a preliminary report. *Surg Endosc.* 2016;30(6):2552-2562.

102. Marks J, Montenegro G, Salem J, Shields M, Marks G. Transanal TATA/TME: a case-matched study of taTME versus laparoscopic TME surgery for rectal cancer. *Tech Coloproctol.* 2016;20(7):467-473.

103. Fernández-Hevia M, Delgado S, Castells A, et al. Transanal total mesorectal excision in rectal cancer: short-term outcomes in comparison with laparoscopic surgery. *Ann Surg.* 2015;261(2):221-227.

104. Velthuis S, Nieuwenhuis D, Ruijter T, Cuesta M, Bonjer H, Sietses C. Transanal versus traditional laparoscopic total mesorectal excision for rectal carcinoma. *Surg Endosc.* 2014;28(12):3494-3499.

105. Penna M, Hompes R, Arnold S, et al. Transanal total mesorectal excision: international registry results of the first 720 cases. *Ann Surg.* 2017;266(1):111-117.

106. Deijen C, Velthuis S, Tsai A, et al. COLOR III: a multicentre randomised clinical trial comparing transanal TME versus laparoscopic TME for mid and low rectal cancer. *Surg Endosc.* 2016;30(8):3210-3215.

107. Dominique G, Sandra C, Lelong B. A multicentric randomised trial to evaluate efficacy, morbidity and functional outcome of endoscopic tranAnal proctectomy versus standard transabdominal laparoscopic proctectomy for low lying rectal cancer (ETAP-GRECCAR 11); 2015. https://clinicaltrials.gov/ct2/show/NCT02584985. accessed 28 July 2017.

108. Penna M, Hompes R, Mackenzie H, Carter F, Francis N. First international training and assessment consensus workshop on transanal total mesorectal excision (taTME). *Tech Coloproctol.* 2016;20(6):343-352.

109. McLemore E, Harnsberger C, Broderick R, et al. Transanal total mesorectal excision (taTME) for rectal cancer: a training pathway. *Surg Endosc.* 2016;30(9):4130-4135.

110. Ng K, Ng D, Cheung H, et al. Laparoscopic resection for rectal cancers: lessons learned from 579 cases. *Ann Surg.* 2009;249(1):82-86.

111. Andersson A, Bergdahl L. Urologic complications following abdominoperineal resection of the rectum. *Arch Surg.* 1976;111(9):969-971.

112. Zinman L, Vanni A. Surgical management of urologic trauma and iatrogenic injuries. *Surg Clin North Am.* 2016;96(3):425-439.

113. Pocard M, Zinzindohoue F, Haab F, Caplin S, Parc R, Tiret E. A prospective study of sexual and urinary function before and after total mesorectal excision with autonomic nerve preservation for rectal cancer. *Surgery.* 2002;131(4):368-372.

114. Maurer C, Z'Graggen K, Renzulli P, Schilling M, Netzer P, Büchler M. Total mesorectal excision preserves male genital function compared with conventional rectal cancer surgery. *Br J Surg.* 2001;88(11):1501-1505.

115. Kim N, Aahn T, Park J, et al. Assessment of sexual and voiding function after total mesorectal excision with pelvic autonomic nerve preservation in males with rectal cancer. *Dis Colon Rectum.* 2002;45(9):1178-1185.

116. Nagawa H, Muto T, Sunouchi K, Higuchi Y, Tsurita G, Watanabe T, et al. Randomized, controlled trial of lateral node dissection vs. nerve-preserving resection in patients with rectal cancer after preoperative radiotherapy. *Dis Colon Rectum.* 2001;44(9):1274-1280.

117. Quah H, Jayne D, Eu K, Seow-Choen F. Bladder and sexual dysfunction following laparoscopically assisted and conventional open mesorectal resection for cancer. *Br J Surg.* 2002;89(12):1551-1556.

118. Ridolfi T, Berger N, Ludwig K. Low anterior resection syndrome: current management and future directions. *Clin Colon Rectal Surg.* 2016;29(5):239-245.

119. Juul T, Ahlberg M, Biondo S, Espin E, Jimenez L, Matzel K, et al. Low anterior resection syndrome and quality of life: an international multicenter study. *Dis Colon Rectum.* 2014;57(5):585-591.

120. Kim K, Yu C, Yoon Y, Yoon S, Lim S, Kim J. Effectiveness of biofeedback therapy in the treatment of anterior resection syndrome after rectal cancer surgery. *Dis Colon Rectum.* 2011;54(9):1107-1113.

121. Thomas C, Bradshaw E, Vaizey C. A review of sacral nerve stimulation for faecal incontinence following rectal surgery and radiotherapy. *Colorectal Dis.* 2015;17(11):939-942.

122. Ramage L, Qiu S, Kontovounisios C, Tekkis P, Rasheed S, Tan E. A systematic review of sacral nerve stimulation for low anterior resection syndrome. *Colorectal Dis.* 2015;17(9):762-771.

123. Quirke P, Durdey P, Dixon M. Williams N. Local recurrence of rectal adenocarcinoma due to inadequate surgical resection. Histopathological study of lateral tumour spread and surgical excision. *Lancet.* 1986;1(2):996-999.

124. Laurent C, Leblanc F, Wütrich P, Scheffler M, Rullier E. Laparoscopic versus open surgery for rectal cancer: long-term oncologic results. *Ann Surg.* 2009;250(1):54-61.

125. Morino M, Allaix M, Giraudo G, Corno F, Garrone C. Laparoscopic versus open surgery for extraperitoneal rectal cancer: a prospective comparative study. *Surg Endosc.* 2005;19(11):1460-1467.

126. Lacy A, García-Valdecasas J, Delgado S, et al. Laparoscopy-assisted colectomy versus open colectomy for treatment of non-metastatic colon cancer: a randomised trial. *Lancet.* 2002;359(9325):2224-2229.

127. Rockwood T, Church J, et al. Fecal incontinence quality of life scale: quality of life instrument for patients with fecal incontinence. *Dis Colon Rectum.* 2000;43(1):9-16.

128. Rosen R, Brown C, Heiman J, et al. The Female Sexual Function Index (FSFI): a multidimensional self-report instrument for the assessment of female sexual function. *J Sex Marital Ther.* 2000;26(2):191-208.

129. Rosen R, Riley A, Wagner G, Osterloh I, Kirkpatrick J, Mishra A. The international index of erectile function (IIEF): a multidimensional scale for assessment of erectile dysfunction. *Urology.* 1997;49(6):822-830.

130. Breukink S, van der Zaag-Loonen H, Bouma E, et al. Prospective evaluation of quality of life and sexual functioning after laparoscopic total mesorectal excision. *Dis Colon Rectum.* 2007;50(2):147-155.

131. Sprangers M, te Velde A, Aaronson N. The construction and testing of the EORTC colorectal cancer-specific quality of life questionnaire module (QLQ-CR38). European Organization for Research and Treatment of Cancer Study Group on Quality of Life. *Eur J Cancer.* 1999;35(2):238-247.

132. Stiggelbout A, Kunneman M, Baas-Thijssen M, et al. The EORTC QLQ-CR29 quality of life questionnaire for colorectal cancer: validation of the Dutch version. *Qual Life Res.* 2016;25(7):1853-1858.

133. Park S, Choi G, Park J, Kim H, Ryuk J, Yun S. Urinary and erectile function in men after total mesorectal excision by laparoscopic or robot-assisted methods for the treatment of rectal cancer: a case-matched comparison. *World J Surg.* 2014;38(7):1834-1842.

134. Kim J, Kim N, Lee K, Hur H, Min B, Kim J. A comparative study of voiding and sexual function after total mesorectal excision with autonomic nerve preservation for rectal cancer: laparoscopic versus robotic surgery. *Ann Surg Oncol.* 2012;19(8):2485-2493.

135. Elmore U, Fumagalli Romario U, Vignali A, Sosa M, Angiolini M, Rosati R. Laparoscopic anterior resection with transanal total mesorectal excision for rectal cancer: preliminary experience and impact on postoperative bowel function. *J Laparoendosc Adv Surg Tech A.* 2015;25(5):364-369.

136. Mari G, Maggioni D, Costanzi A, et al. High or low inferior mesenteric artery ligation in laparoscopic low anterior resection: study protocol for a randomized controlled trial (HIGHLOW trial). *Trials.* 2015;16:21.

137. Jafari M, Wexner S, Martz J, et al. Perfusion assessment in laparoscopic left-sided/anterior resection (PILLAR II): a multi-institutional study. *J Am Coll Surg.* 2015;220(1):82-92.

138. Cahill R, Mortensen N. Intraoperative augmented reality for laparoscopic colorectal surgery by intraoperative near-infrared fluorescence imaging and optical coherence tomography. *Minerva Chir.* 2010;65(4):451-462.

139. Alander J, Kaartinen I, Laakso A, et al. A review of indocyanine green fluorescent imaging in surgery. *Int J Biomed Imaging.* 2012;2012:940585.

140. Hellan M, Spinoglio G, Pigazzi A, Lagares-Garcia J. The influence of fluorescence imaging on the location of bowel transection during robotic left-sided colorectal surgery. *Surg Endosc.* 2014;28(5):1695-1702.

Abdominoperineal Resection for Rectal Cancer

Jason Bingham | Matthew Dyer | Scott R. Steele

A bdominoperineal resection (APR) is the operation of choice for low-lying rectal cancers, as well as for many recurrent rectal cancers, and as salvage therapy for anal cancers. In very select circumstances, APR may also be appropriate for benign disease, such as in patients with severe refractory anorectal Crohn disease. Finally, APR may be used in both benign and malignant disease in patients whose underlying disease would otherwise allow restoration of continuity but are plagued by problems with continence. The procedure involves the complete removal of the anus (including the sphincter complex), rectum, and distal colon using both anterior abdominal and perineal incisions, resulting in a permanent colostomy. Both open and laparoscopic approaches are commonly used, although there has been some controversy regarding the oncologic equivalence of minimally invasive approaches for locally advanced rectal cancer, and this is an area of active investigation.[1–4]

Since originally popularized by Miles more than 100 years ago, APR has undergone significant evolution in both application and technique to develop into the modern operation we describe here. Overall, the fundamental principle of the APR is to attain locoregional control of disease through complete tumor resection with negative circumferential margins (CFMs). As the vast majority of regional disease spread is contained within the mesorectum, complete resection of the rectum and mesorectum as a single unit is the goal of curative resection.[5–10] Thus total mesorectal excision (TME) with autonomic nerve preservation has become an important cornerstone of rectal cancer surgery.

Perhaps too often APR is thought of as an operation of last resort to be applied only when there are no sphincter-preserving options available. This has led to trends favoring more aggressive and arguably overzealous attempts for sphincter preservation. Although the conservation of intestinal continuity is clearly preferable, it is only justifiable if based on sound oncologic principles. It has been suggested that tumors less than 5 cm from the anal verge may represent a more biologically aggressive disease than those of the more proximal rectum.[7] Low rectal tumors have been shown to carry a lower 5-year survival rate compared with midrectal tumors, as well as have a higher incidence of mesorectal and lateral lymph node involvement and higher rate of local recurrence. In addition, more aggressive pathologic findings, such as poor differentiation and neurovascular invasion have been demonstrated in low rectal cancers.[6,8,11] Therefore APR should not be thought of as simply a procedure of last resort but rather the appropriate and necessary surgery for select distal rectal cancers and conditions that merit its use.

TUMOR-SPECIFIC APPROACHES

Clearly not all low rectal cancers are equal, and a tailored surgical approach is necessary to achieve the appropriate oncologic resection while simultaneously limiting patient morbidity. APR is first and foremost a procedure that is focused on curative resection. This is especially important at the level of the levator ani, where separation of the mesorectum from the pelvic floor can be particularly challenging. Imperfect technique at this level can occasionally lead to tumor perforation, positive resection margins, and higher rates of local recurrence. This can be demonstrated on magnetic resonance imaging (MRI) as a threatened margin. As a result, many have questioned the extent of perineal (i.e., muscle) resection required at the level of the levators for optimal oncologic outcomes.

In general, the surgeon's options for perineal dissection during APR include (1) the "traditional," or so-called standard APR, in which the resection margin is "coned in" at the level of the levators, thus preserving pelvic floor structure without compromising the margins (Fig. 169.1); or (2) the extended or extralevator APR (ELAPE) or cylindrical APR, wherein the abdominal mobilization of the mesorectum is stopped at the lateral margins of the pelvic floor and wide transection of the levators is performed, resulting in a cylinder of tissue around the tumor (Fig. 169.2). This debate is often referred to as the *waist* versus *cylinder* resection due to the appearance of the resected specimen (Fig. 169.3). Some have advocated for more liberal application of ELAPE, arguing the technique results in lower rates of positive resection margins and decreased incidence of tumor perforation.[12] However, there are several problems with this approach preventing its more widespread application. The more extensive levator resection translates to higher rates of perineal wound complications, and as the entire levator plate is removed with this technique, tissue transfer or mesh reconstruction is almost mandatory (Fig 169.4). Moreover, there should theoretically be no advantage to wide excision of the levators where there is no risk of direct tumor involvement using a standard approach. Indeed, when the literature is looked at on the whole, there does not appear to be significantly improved oncologic outcomes when routine ELAPE is compared with tumor-specific excision of the levators (Table 169.1).[12–17] Thus we recommend limiting the use of such a technique to distal tumors with circumferential invasion through the external sphincter or involving the levators, especially when the margin is threatened on MRI. For noncircumferential invasion, it seems reasonable to avoid coning in on the levators in the region where the tumor is located and

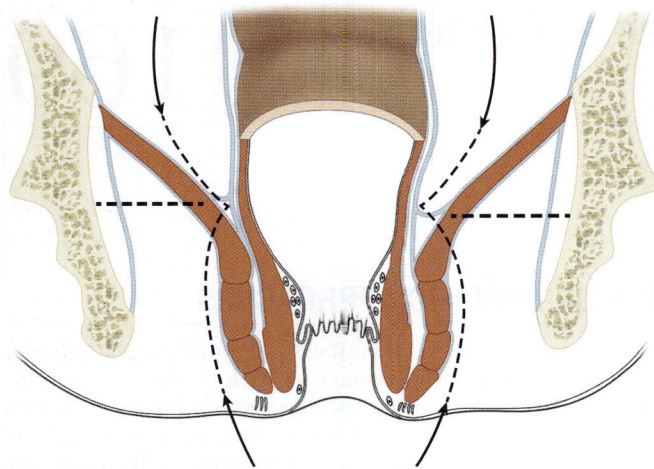

FIGURE 169.1 Traditional abdominoperineal resection. Note the potential for coning in on the resection margin at level of levators.

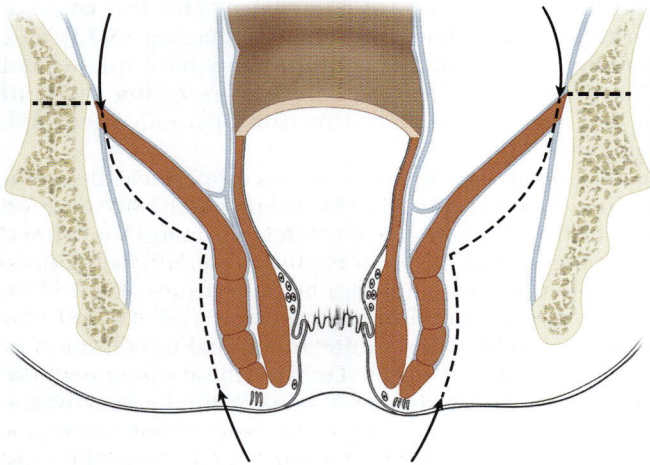

FIGURE 169.2 Extended abdominoperineal resection. Wider transection of the levators, resulting in a cylinder of tissue around the tumor but leaving a larger pelvic floor defect.

sparing extensive resection of the levators where appropriate. This results in an asymmetric specimen with the entire tumor covered in an R0 resection. However, compromising oncologic principles and resulting in a positive CFM for any lesion, especially for the primary purpose of leaving levator muscle for closure, is unacceptable.

In select circumstances, a more radical ischioanal resection may be required, such as when there is ischioanal involvement of the tumor or when there are significant associated fistulas or abscesses (Fig. 169.5). Alternatively, when APR is done for benign disease, or when performed due to preexisting fecal incontinence in patients with upper rectal tumors, an intersphincteric perineal dissection may be more appropriate (Fig. 169.6). Overall, the surgeon must balance the oncologic need for a particular approach with resultant morbidity, mortality, and functional outcome in each individual patient. There simply is no "one size fits all" approach to treating these challenging distal lesions.

SURGICAL ANATOMY

BONES AND FASCIA

The bony pelvis is made up of the sacrum, ileum, ischium, and pubis. The pelvic brim marks the transition from the greater (false) and lesser (true) pelvis. A plane through the sacral promontory, arcuate and pectineal lines, and the upper margin of the pubic symphysis delineates the level of the pelvic brim. The rectum and anal canal lie within the bony pelvis and form the most distal portion of the large intestine. The beginning of the rectum can be marked by the point at which the taeniae coli bands splay to form the outer longitudinal muscle layer. Peritoneum covers the upper two-thirds of the rectum anteriorly but only one-third posteriolaterally, thus leaving the lower one-third of the rectum with no peritoneal covering. Rather, it is enveloped in the endopelvic fascia. Anteriorly in males, Denonvilliers fascia separates the rectum from the prostate and seminal vesicles. This structure is analogous to the rectovaginal fascia in females. Posteriorly, there is a strong layer of fascia known as Waldeyer fascia, which connects the rectum to the anterior sacrum at about the level of S4 (Fig. 169.7).

PELVIC FLOOR MUSCULATURE

Composed of a funnel-shaped sling of fascia and muscle (levator ani), the pelvic diaphragm forms the inferior border of the abdominopelvic cavity. It extends from the pubic symphysis to the coccyx and to the bilateral pelvic sidewalls. The muscles of the pelvic floor are organized into superficial and deep layers. The superficial muscle layers include the external anal sphincter, perineal body, and transverse perinei muscles. The deep pelvic floor muscles consist of individual muscles that comprise the levator ani: the ileococcygeus, pubococcygeus, and puborectalis (Fig. 169.8). The puborectalis forms the superior external anal sphincter and marks the top of the anorectal ring. The anorectal ring encompasses the internal anal sphincter and is formed by the levator ani muscles proximally and the superficial external anal sphincters more distally.

ANATOMIC SPACES

There are a number of anatomic spaces around the anorectum that are surgically important. Laterally, the external sphincter is contiguous with the ischioanal (ischiorectal) space. Posterior to the anal canal is the superficial postanal space, which ends at the coccyx. Above the superficial postanal space and deep to the anococcygeal ligament is the deep postanal space. This space is continuous with the ischioanal (ischiorectal) spaces laterally. The supralevator space is located above the levator ani between the rectum and the sacrum. Waldeyer fascia separates this space from the retrorectal space, which can continue into the retroperitoneum (Fig. 169.9).

PELVIC ARTERIAL BLOOD SUPPLY

The arterial blood supply to the rectum and anus is derived from both the inferior mesenteric artery and the internal iliac arteries. The terminal branch of the inferior mesenteric artery, the superior rectal artery,

TABLE 169.1 Comparison of Oncologic Results of Extralevator Abdominoperineal Resection Versus Traditional Abdominoperineal Resection

Author	Year	Study Type	Number of Patients	Local Recurrence	Overall Survival	Tumor Perforation
Han	2012	Randomized control trial	67	Decreased with ELAPE [2.8% vs. 13.8%; P = .048]	NS	NS
Krishna	2013	Systemic review	8 studies	NS	NS	NS
Prytz	2015	Prospective observational	1397	Increased with ELAPE [OR = 4.91]	NS	Increased with ELAPE [OR = 3.90]
Zhou	2015	Meta-analysis	7 studies	NS	—	NS
Shen	2015	Prospective observational	69	Decreased with ELAPE [0% vs. 15.2%; P = .034]	NS	—

APR, Abdominoperineal resection; *ELAPE,* extralevator abdominoperineal resection; *NS,* not significant; *OR,* odds ratio.

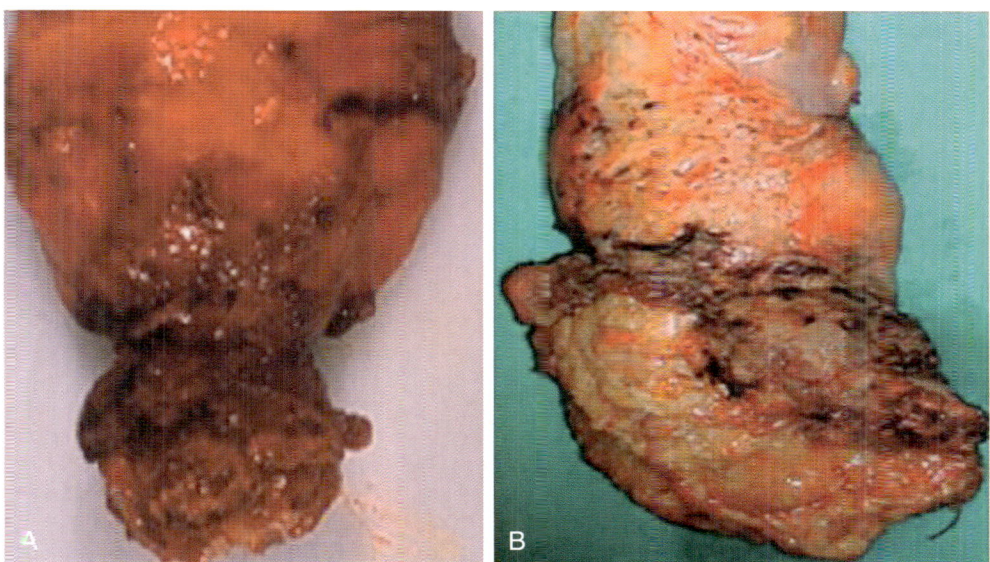

FIGURE 169.3 (A) Waist versus (B) cylinder resection.

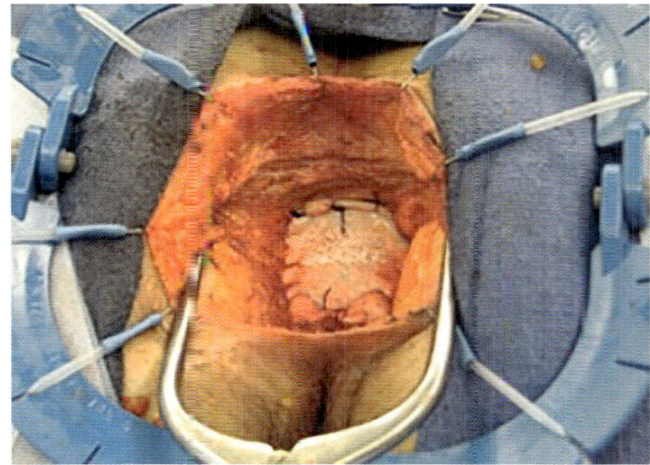

FIGURE 169.4 Pelvic floor reconstruction with porcine dermal collagen following extralevator abdominoperineal resection.

supplies the rectum and upper one-third of the anal canal. The middle rectal arteries branch from the internal iliac arteries and the inferior rectal arteries arise from the internal pudendal arteries (themselves a branch of internal iliac arteries).

PELVIC NERVES

The anatomic course of the autonomic nerve plexuses of the pelvis are of particular concern to surgeons because they can be easily damaged during pelvic surgery, resulting in urinary incontinence and sexual dysfunction. Sympathetic nerves arising from the L1 to L5 spinal cord levels extend from the preaortic plexus (superior hypogastric plexus) at the aortic bifurcation to the mesenteric plexus before reaching the upper rectum. The sympathetic fibers then bifurcate and travel laterally along the pelvis to join with parasympathetic fibers from the S2 to S4 nerve roots to create the pelvic plexus (inferior hypogastric plexus). The pelvic plexus is located superior to the levator ani muscles in the midportion of the lateral stalks and provides autonomic innervation to the rectum and urogenital organs (Fig. 169.10).

PROCEDURE AND OPERATIVE TIPS

APR can be performed either with simultaneous abdominal and perineal dissections through a two-team approach or with a sequential approach, in which the abdominal dissection is performed first, followed by perineal resection. Regardless of which method is used, many surgeons prefer placing the patient in modified lithotomy position with moderate Trendelenburg and the surgeon positioned on the patient's left for the abdominal portion. Although

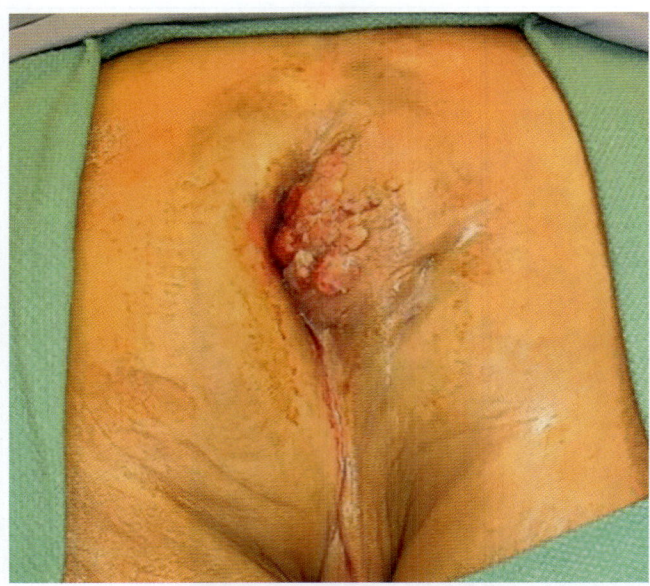

FIGURE 169.5 Low rectal tumor with extensive ischioanal involvement.

generally not routinely required, placement of ureteral stents may be done to facilitate intraoperative identification and protection of the ureters during pelvic dissection. A Foley catheter and an orogastric tube is placed (the latter to be removed at the end of the operation). Appropriate prophylactic parenteral antibiotics and subcutaneous heparin are administered, and sequential compression devices are used for deep vein thrombosis prevention. The anus is sutured closed, if desired, following enema with a povidone-iodine solution to prevent contamination, and the lower abdomen and perineum are prepped and draped.

ABDOMINAL COMPONENT

The procedure begins with either a midline incision extending from the umbilicus to the pubic symphysis or

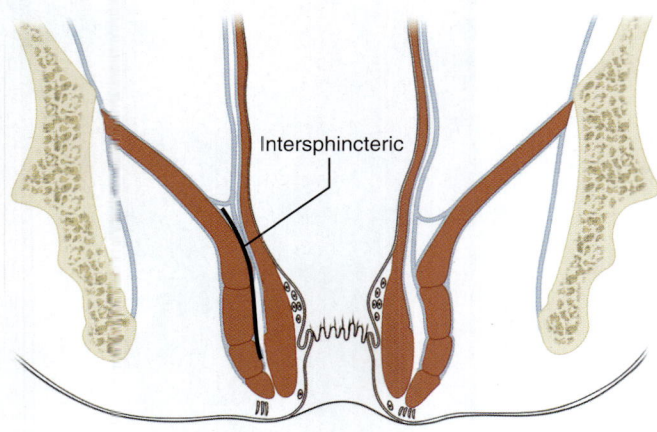

FIGURE 169.6 Intersphincteric approach.

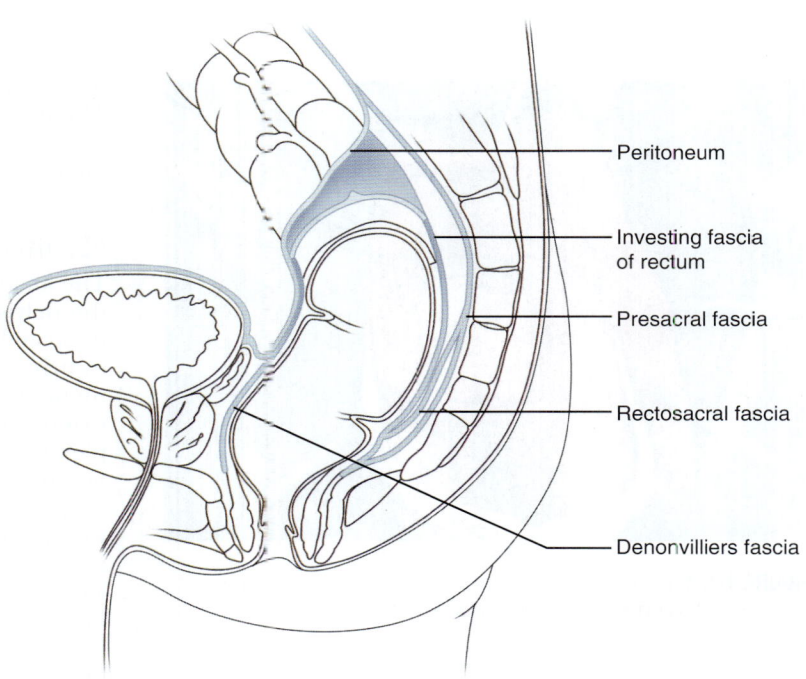

FIGURE 169.7 Pelvic floor fascia. (Redrawn with permission from Barleben A, Mills S. Anorectal anatomy and physiology. *Surg Clin North Am.* 2010;90:1–15.)

through a periumbilical 10- to 12-mm Hasson trocar. With a laparoscopic approach, port placements are as pictured (Fig. 169.11), and we prefer a 10-mm 30-degree camera. Alternatively, a hand port may be placed in a low-midline or via Pfannensteil position. It is important to note that laparoscopic resection of rectal cancer remains controversial. Although several series have demonstrated the safety and feasibility of laparoscopic resection, as well as many short-term benefits, the long-term oncologic equivalence to open surgery demands further validation through well-designed randomized studies.[18–22] Regardless of the approach, the fundamental principles and exposures remain exactly the same as the open resection (Table 169.2).

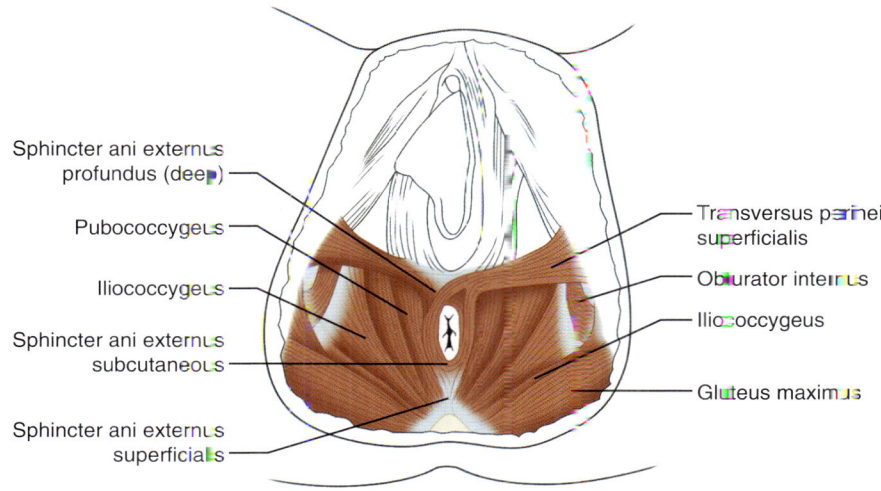

FIGURE 169.8 Pelvic floor musculature. (Redrawn with permission from Barleben A, Mills S. Anorectal anatomy and physiology. *Surg Clin North Am.* 2010;90:1–15.)

Sphincter ani externus profundus (deep)
Pubococcygeus
Iliococcygeus
Sphincter ani externus subcutaneous
Sphincter ani externus superficialis

Transversus perinei superficialis
Obturator internus
Iliococcygeus
Gluteus maximus

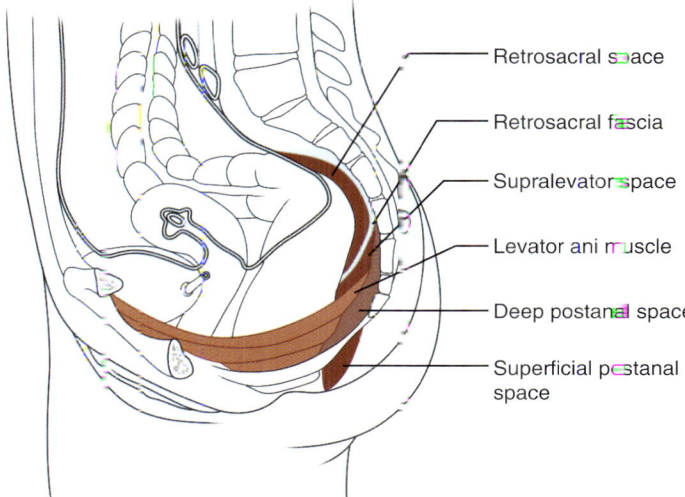

Retrosacral space
Retrosacral fascia
Supralevator space
Levator ani muscle
Deep postanal space
Superficial postanal space

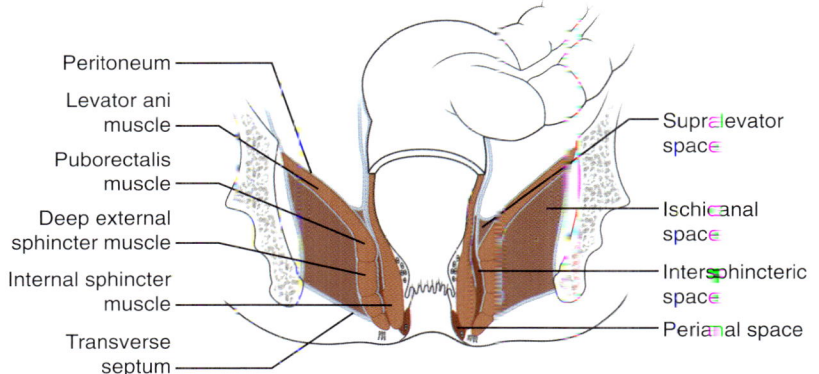

FIGURE 169.9 Anatomic spaces of the pelvis. (Redrawn with permission from Barleben A, Mills S. Anorectal anatomy and physiology. *Surg Clin North Am.* 2010;90:1–15.)

Peritoneum
Levator ani muscle
Puborectalis muscle
Deep external sphincter muscle
Internal sphincter muscle
Transverse septum

Supralevator space
Ischioanal space
Intersphincteric space
Perianal space

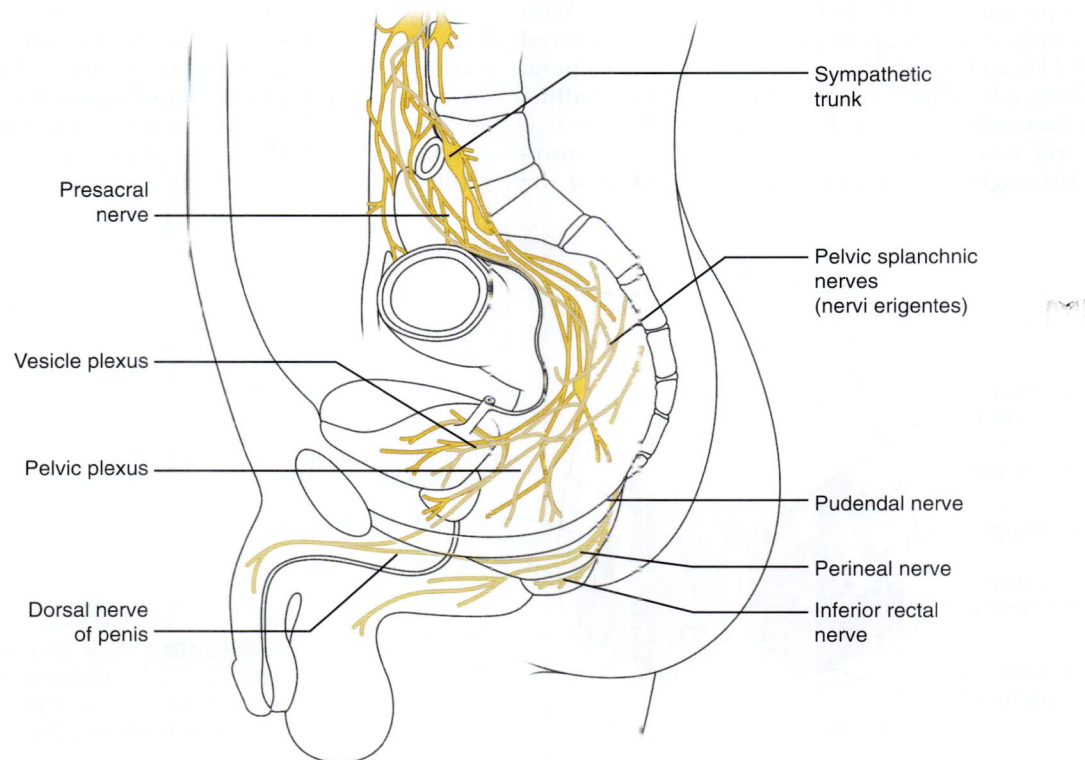

FIGURE 169.10 Pelvic nerves. (Redrawn with permission from Barleben A, Mills S. Anorectal anatomy and physiology. *Surg Clin North Am.* 2010;90:1–15.)

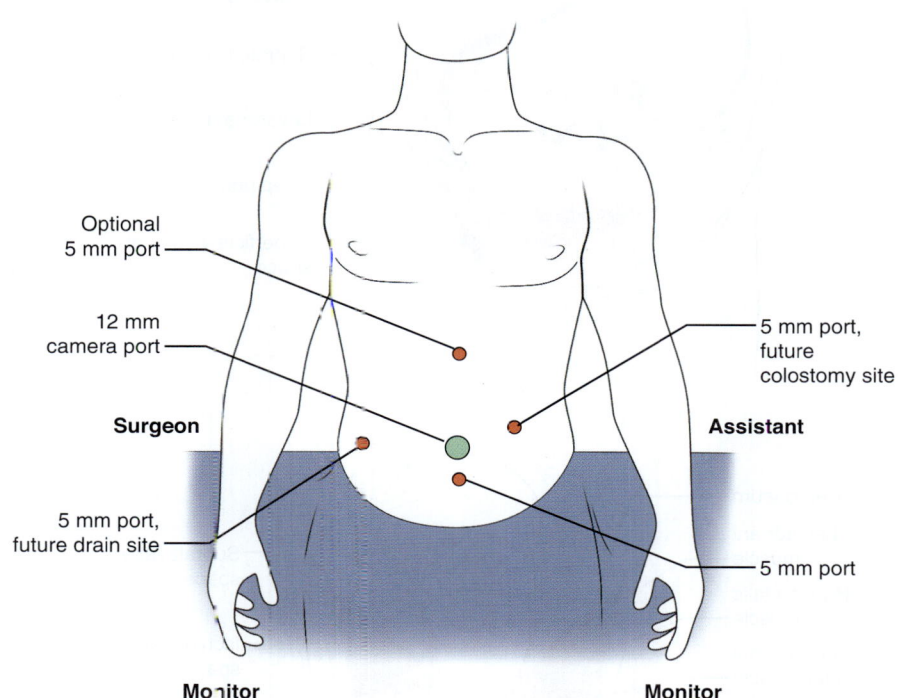

FIGURE 169.11 Port placement for a laparoscopic abdominoperineal resection.

TABLE 169.2 Laparoscopic Rectal Cancer Resection Series

Author	Year	n	LAR/APR	Conversion (%)	LOS (days)	Recurrence/Survival (%)
Franklin	1996	200	74/26	4	5.7	12/87
Fleshman	1999	42	0/42	21	7	19/69
Hartley	2001	28	21/7	33	—	7/—
Anthuber	2003	101	77/24	3	14	3/—
Morino	2003	100	98/—	12	11.4	3.2/80
Leung	2004	203	203/—	23	8.2	7/76
Barlehner	2005	143	127/16	1	7	6.7/66.3
CLASSICC	2005	259	196/63	34	10	—
Kim	2006	312	214/44	2.6	11	2.9/—
Law	2006	98	98/0	12	7	3.3/55.5
Brachet	2014	132	116/16	5.3	—	4.1/83
Zhou	2014	122	98/34	8.8	7	14.1/87.1
Fleshman	2015	486	373/113	11.3	7.3	—

APR, Abdominal perineal resection; *CLASSICC,* conventional versus laparoscopic-assisted surgery in patients with colorectal cancer trial; *LAR,* low anterior resection; *LOS,* length of stay.

First, the abdomen is initially explored for evidence of metastasis, and any suspicious lesions may then be biopsied. The small bowel is then retracted superiorly and to the right and held in place with moist laparotomy pads. Alternatively, the patient is placed in a steep Trendelenburg position and rotated to the right to allow the small bowel to fall into the right upper quadrant with the aid of gravity. Initial placement of the omentum over the top of the transverse colon and into the upper abdomen may help with small bowel contain issues, especially in the morbidly obese. Next, the redundant sigmoid colon is removed from the pelvis to ensure proper orientation. Using a lateral approach the sigmoid colon is grasped and mobilized medially by dividing the lateral attachments anchoring it to the left pelvic wall. The avascular plane along the line of Toldt is divided, mobilizing the left colon. Blunt-nosed scissors may be placed beneath the posterior parietal peritoneum and used to carefully separate the underlying gonadal vessels and ureter and protect them from injury. The peritoneum is incised down to the cul-de-sac on the left side (Fig. 169.12). It is crucial to identify and protect the left ureter at this time because it may course in close proximity to the root of the mesentery of the rectosigmoid, and can be easily damaged or transected during dissection. If preoperative ureteral stents have been placed, the ureter can often be easily and frequently palpated to ensure it remains retracted to the left side of the pelvis and out of the dissection plane. Alternatively, the ureter can be identified as it crosses the pelvic brim over the left common iliac artery bifurcation (Fig. 169.13). Peristaltic waves can be seen if the ureter is pinched with forceps or laparoscopic atraumatic grasper.

Approaching from the left, the surgeon's hand can be passed behind the sigmoid colon, mobilizing it from the underlying pelvic brim. The sigmoid is then retracted toward the left, and the right-sided peritoneal reflection is tented from underneath with the surgeon's hand, thus separating it from the underlying right ureter and allowing for safe division of the reflection down to the cul-de-sac (Fig. 169.14). The incision is made lateral to the inferior

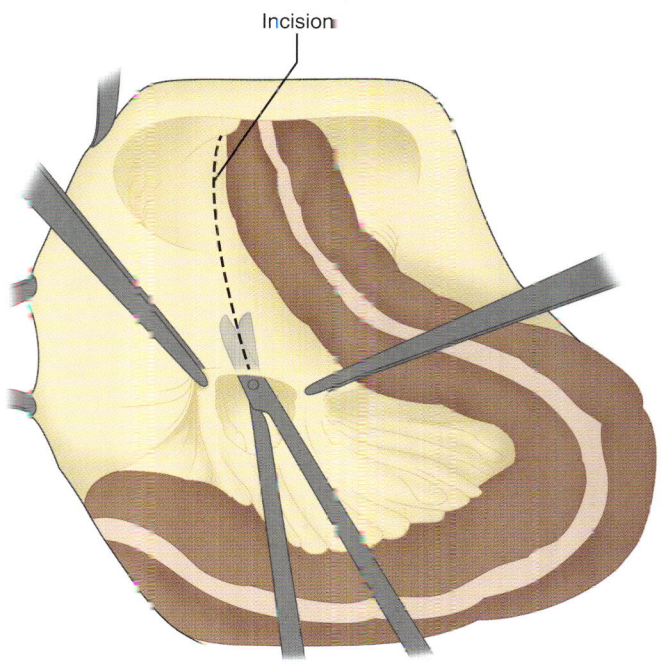

FIGURE 169.12 Lateral mobilization and opening the left pelvis via an open approach. (Redrawn with permission from Zollinger RM Jr, Ellison EC, eds. *Zollinger's Atlas of Surgical Operations.* 9th ed. New York: McGraw-Hill Medical; 2011.)

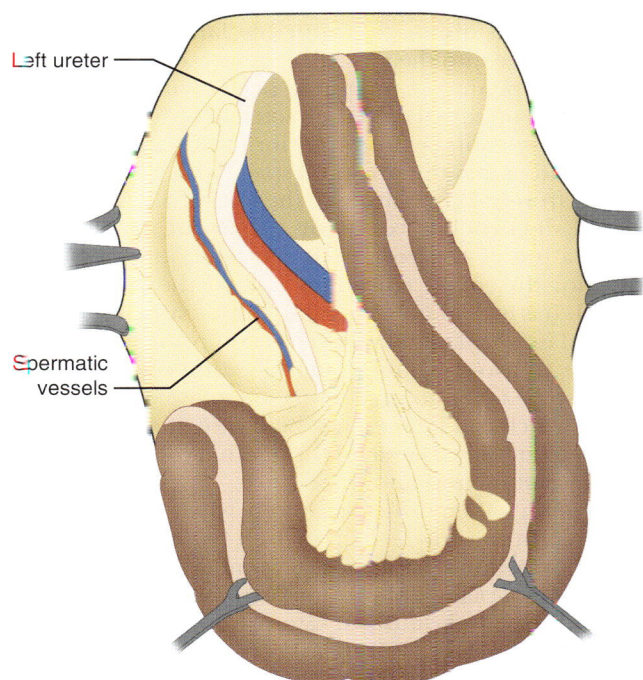

FIGURE 169.13 Location of the left ureter as it crosses the pelvic brim. (Redrawn with permission from Zollinger RM Jr, Ellison EC, eds. *Zollinger's Atlas of Surgical Operations.* 9th ed. New York: McGraw-Hill Medical; 2011.)

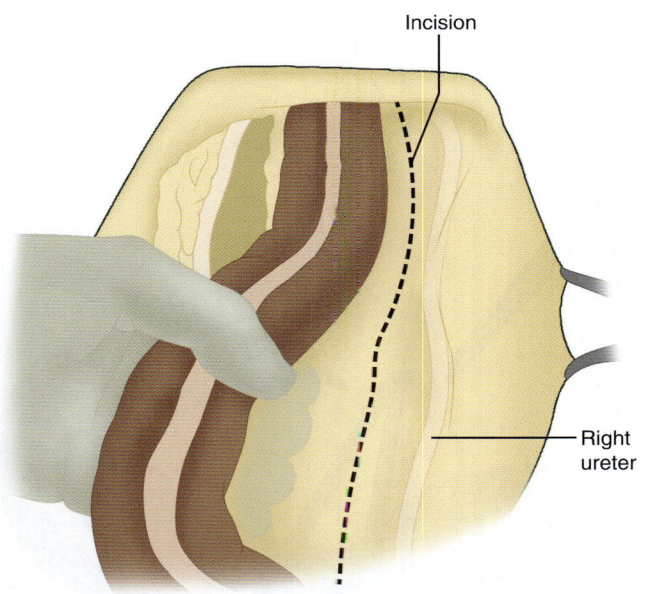

FIGURE 169.14 Opening the right pelvis from the left side. (Redrawn with permission from Zollinger RM Jr, Ellison EC, eds. *Zollinger's Atlas of Surgical Operations.* 9th ed. New York: McGraw-Hill Medical; 2011.)

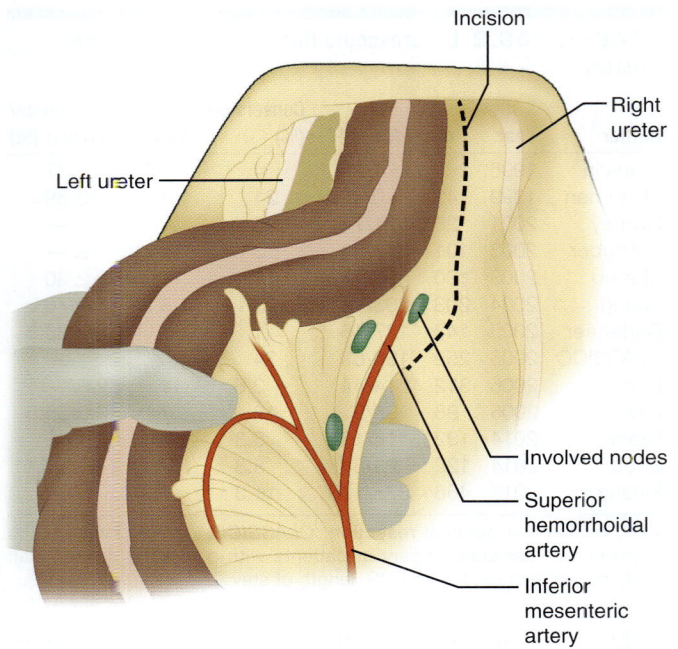

FIGURE 169.15 Division of the peritoneal reflections with entry under the inferior mesenteric artery and medial to the right ureter. (Redrawn with permission from Zollinger RM Jr, Ellison EC, eds. *Zollinger's Atlas of Surgical Operations.* 9th ed. New York: McGraw-Hill Medical; 2011.)

mesenteric and superior rectal vessels. It is important to identify the right ureter, expose it carefully, and protect it from accidental injury when dividing the peritoneal reflections (Fig. 169.15). Identification of the sacral promontory is also a reproducible landmark that will allow entrance into the avascular presacral plane and help the initial opening of the pelvic peritoneum.

With the proximal colon retracted anteriorly and laterally, the dissection begins posterior to the superior rectal vessels and enters the presacral space with sharp division of the retrorectal fascia at about the level of S2. A fiberoptic lighted deep pelvic retractor is helpful in providing visualization as the rectum is retracted anteriorly and posterior dissection continues toward the coccyx (Fig. 169.16). It is important to visualize the sacral veins beneath parietal fascia and maintain a dissection plane just anterior to these to avoid troublesome bleeding. Extreme care must also be taken to prevent damage to the hypogastric nerves, which can be seen just below the iliac vessels and ureters bilaterally. Damage to these nerves can result in bladder dysfunction and impotence.

Attention is then turned anteriorly, where the peritoneal reflection in the cul-de-sac is incised behind the bladder in men or behind the uterus in women. Dissection then proceeds in a plane anterior to Denonvilliers fascia until the seminal vessels and prostate or rectovaginal septum is encountered (Fig. 169.17).

Lateral dissection must be performed cautiously as the autonomic nerve plexus, middle rectal vessels, and ureters can easily be damaged as dissection is carried down to the level of the levator musculature (Fig. 169.18). The rectum must be carefully separated from the parietal fascia overlying the lateral pelvic wall structures. The

autonomic nerve plexus can be seen coursing close to the rectum at the level of the prostate or upper vagina. Damage in this area will result in a mixed parasympathetic and sympathetic injury. The middle rectal vessels may be encountered bilaterally within an area of fused mesorectal tissue. These vessels may be ligated with the use of electrocautery, an energy device, or require suture ligation. Once again, one must continuously be mindful of the course of the ureter throughout the abdominal portion of the procedure to prevent iatrogenic injury.

Next, the blood supply to the rectosigmoid is divided (Fig. 169.19). We prefer to use an energy device, although a stapler with a vascular load or clamps and suture ligation may also be used. Ideally, the inferior mesenteric artery is ligated just distal to the origin of the left colic artery (Fig. 169.20). Conversely, some prefer to divide the inferior mesenteric artery near its point of origin at the aorta. This will also help with gaining additional length for cases in which the bowel needs to reach the anterior abdominal wall. Although this may be safely accomplished, one must be aware that this leaves the portion of the sigmoid that will be used as a colostomy dependent on collateral flow from the marginal artery of Drummond.

High ligation of the inferior mesenteric artery also puts the preaortic sympathetic nerve plexus at risk for damage, which results in retrograde ejaculation in the male. These nerve fibers can be swept back onto the aorta to protect them. The point of proximal transection must be planned to allow adequate oncologic margins while ensuring the rectal stump is short enough to be tucked into the pelvic cavity and allow closure of the overlying

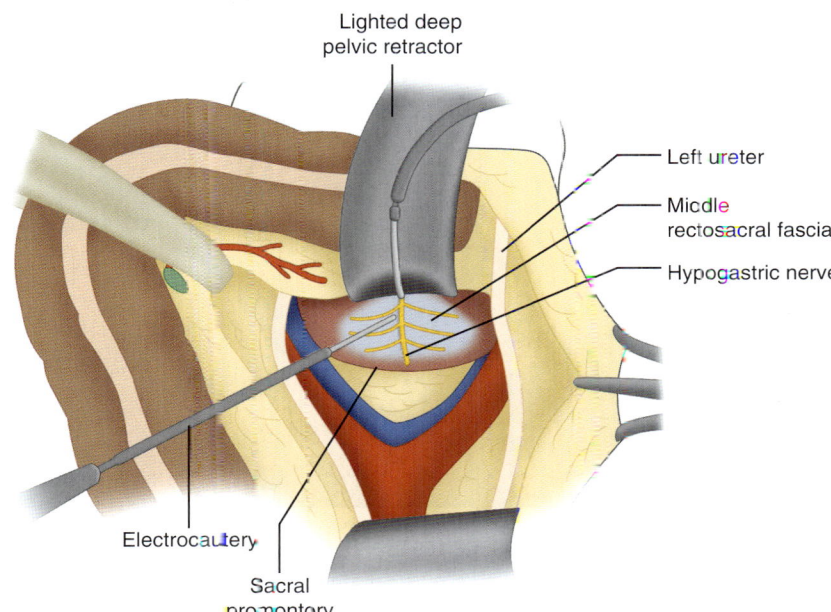

FIGURE 169.16 Posterior dissection in the avascular plane. (Redrawn with permission from Zollinger RM Jr, Ellison EC eds. *Zollinger's Atlas of Surgical Operations.* 9th ed. New York: McGraw-Hill Medical; 2011.)

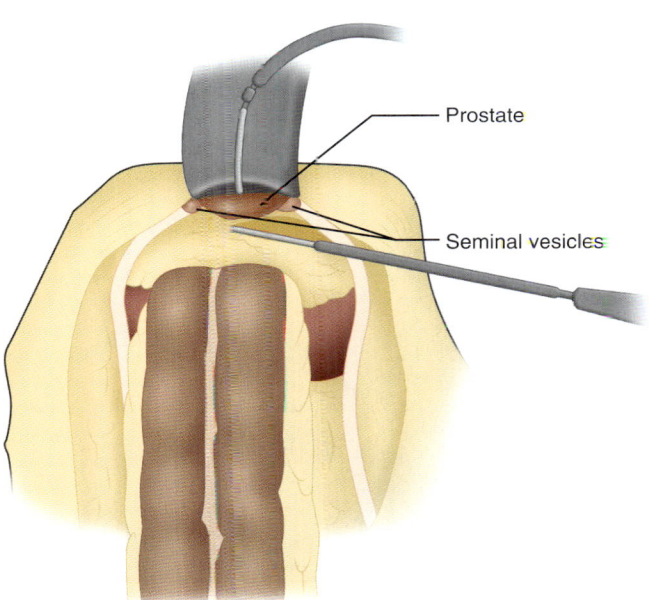

FIGURE 169.17 Dissection of the anterior plane. (Redrawn with permission from Zollinger RM Jr, Ellison EC, eds. *Zollinger's Atlas of Surgical Operations.* 9th ed. New York: McGraw-Hill Medical; 2011.)

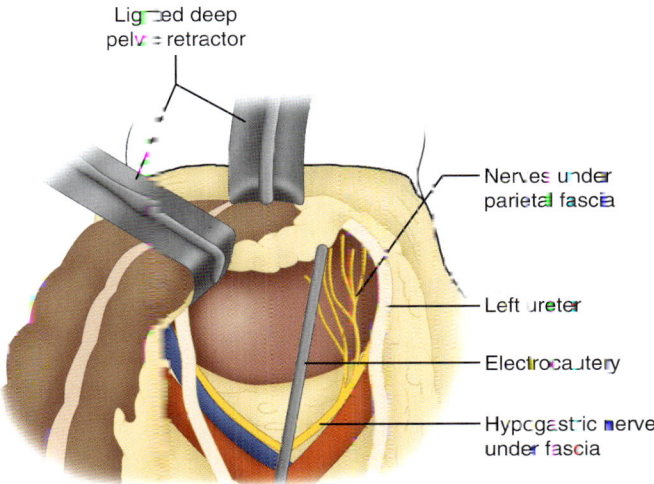

FIGURE 169.18 Lateral dissection of the pelvic during a total mesorectal excision. (Redrawn with permission from Zollinger RM Jr, Ellison EC, eds. *Zollinger's Atlas of Surgical Operations.* 9th ed. New York: McGraw-Hill Medical; 2011.)

pelvic peritoneum. The redundant sigmoid is retracted upward, and the proximal transection point is determined, which will provide adequate blood flow and allow tension-free reach of the proximal bowel to the skin surface for use as a permanent colostomy. The sigmoid is then transected at this point with a GIA linear cutting stapler.

Following this, the peritoneal floor can be mobilized and closed, under the discretion of the surgeon. If desired, toothed forceps are used to grasp the peritoneum and the margins are bluntly freed with the surgeon's hand.

Although it is sometimes possible to close the pelvic peritoneum in a straight line, a radial closure is more often needed to avoid tension on the suture line. Any gap in the suture line risks capturing a loop of small intestine as an internal hernia and small bowel obstruction. During closure, the location of the ureters should be frequently assessed to avoid inadvertent ligation. After pelvic closure, the table is leveled and the omentum is positioned over the suture line.

Attention is then turned to the creation of the end colostomy. Ideally, the location should be marked preoperatively, within the left lower quadrant rectus muscle, in consultation with an enterostomal therapist. A 3-cm circular

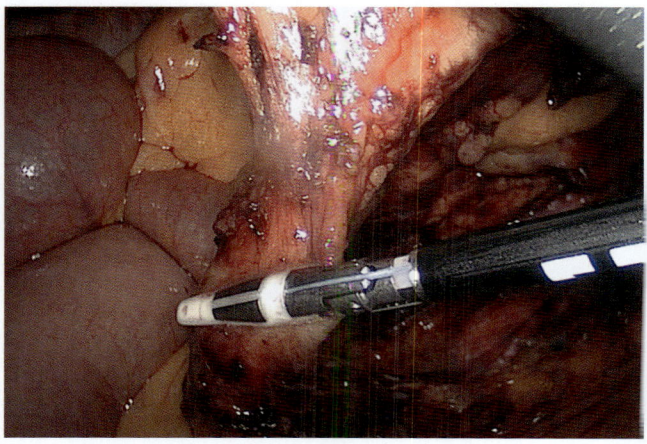

FIGURE 169.19 Laparoscopic ligation of the inferior mesenteric artery using energy device.

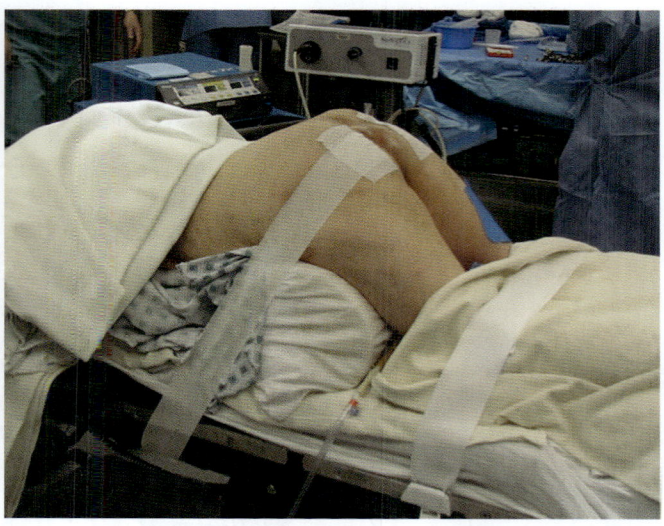

FIGURE 169.21 Prone-jackknife position.

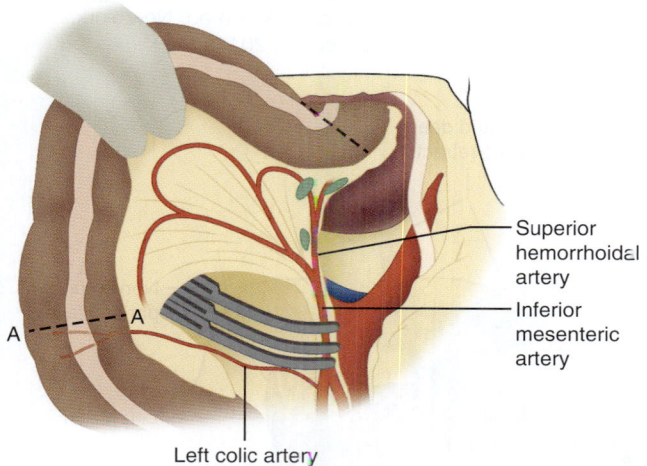

Superior hemorrhoidal artery

Inferior mesenteric artery

Left colic artery

FIGURE 169.20 Left colic artery and point of division of the bowel. (Redrawn with permission from Zollinger RM Jr, Ellison EC, eds. *Zollinger's Atlas of Surgical Operations*. 9th ed. New York: McGraw-Hill Medical; 2011.)

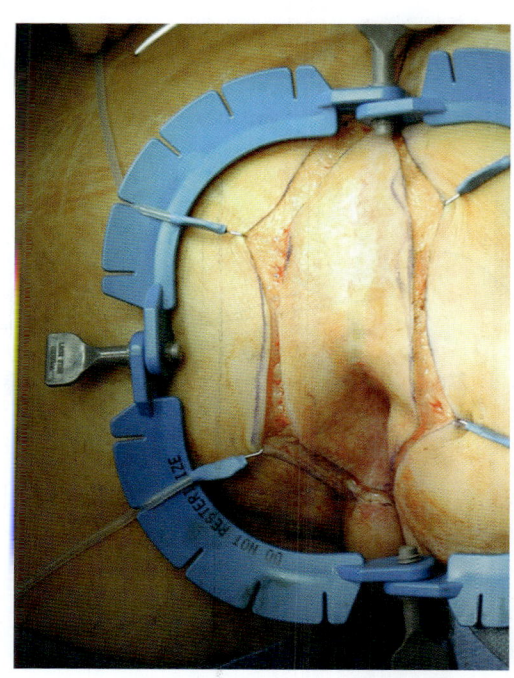

FIGURE 169.22 Perineal incision.

skin opening is created, and a two-fingerwide fascial incision is made. The colon is grasped with a Babcock forcep and brought through the opening, ensuring there is no undue tension or rotation of mesenteric blood flow. The midline abdominal fascia and skin (or port sites) are closed in the usual fashion and the incision is protected with sterile dressing prior to opening the staple line and maturing the colostomy.

PERINEAL PORTION

The perineal resection may be performed either simultaneously with the abdominal portion of the procedure as part of a two-team approach, or it may be done sequentially following abdominal closure and colostomy creation. Typically, the patient remains in the modified lithotomy position for this portion of the operation. However, if done sequentially following abdominal closure, some prefer to reposition the patient in the prone-jackknife

position (Fig. 169.21). The latter often provides better exposure for a cross-table assistant and visualization of the anterior attachments, which are often the more difficult portion of the procedure.

The perineal dissection is begun by first identifying key superficial landmarks: the perineal body, the coccyx, and the ischial tuberosities. An elliptical incision is planned that extends from the perineal body to the coccyx and laterally to the tuberosities (Fig. 169.22). It is important to remember the location and size of the tumor when planning the initial incision to ensure the greatest odds of achieving negative pathologic margins. Occasionally, en bloc resection of adjacent organs is required for locally advanced tumors (Fig. 169.23). If extensive excision is

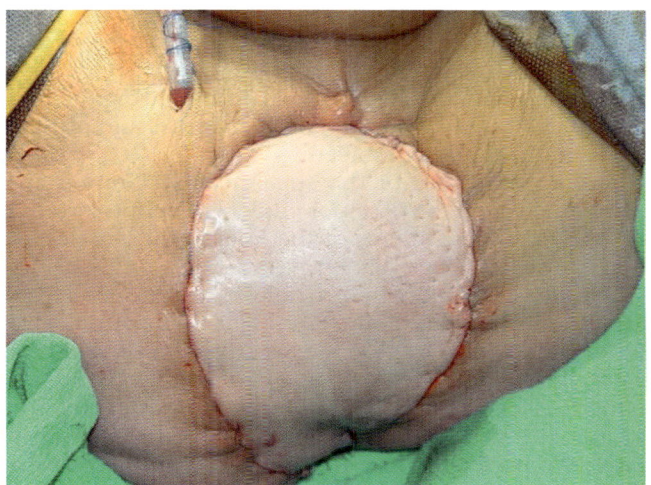

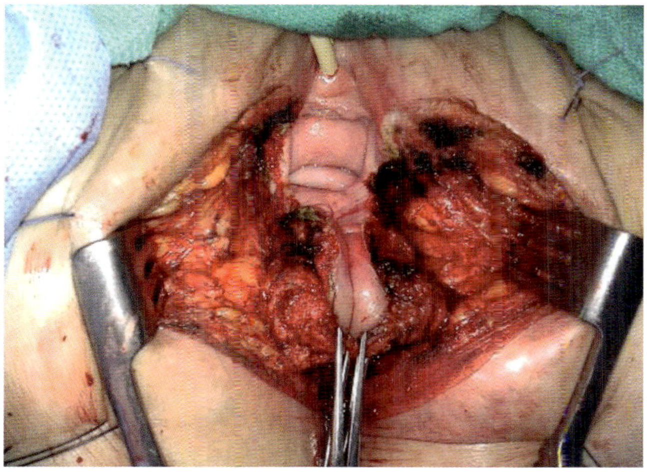

FIGURE 169.23 Posterior vaginectomy as part of resection for invasive rectal tumor.

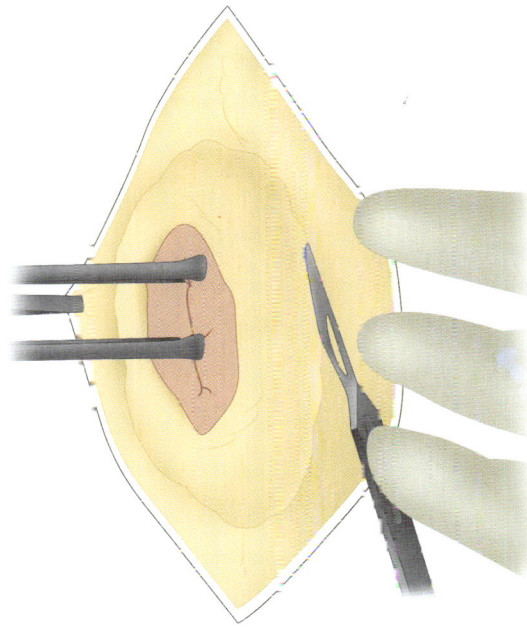

FIGURE 169.25 Continued subcutaneous dissection from the perineum. (Redrawn with permission from Zollinger RM Jr, Ellison EC, eds. *Zollinger's Atlas of Surgical Operations.* 9th ed. New York: McGraw-Hill Medical; 2011.)

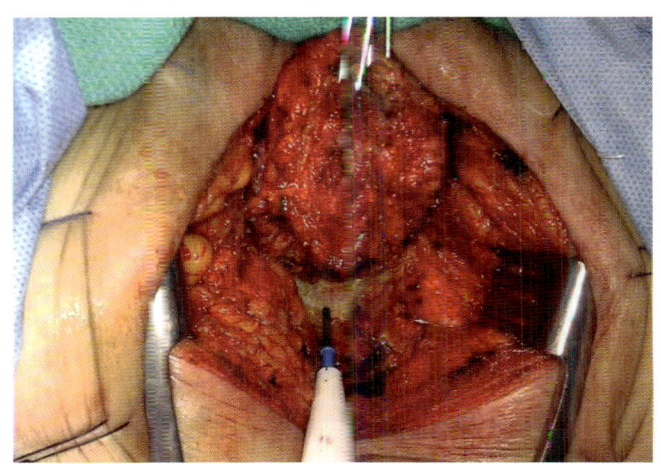

FIGURE 169.26 Division of anococcygeal raphe.

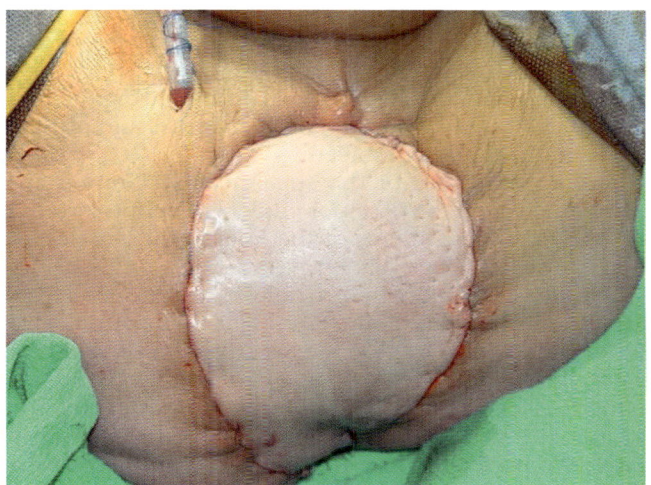

FIGURE 169.24 Myocutaneous flap reconstruction of perineal wound.

anticipated, preoperative consultation with a plastic surgeon is advised because myocutaneous flap reconstruction may be needed (Fig. 169.24).

The skin is incised at least 2 cm from the closed anal orifice and dissection is carried through the subcutaneous tissue. The perianal skin and skin surrounding the anal orifice may be grasped with several Allis clamps to aid with retraction as the subcutaneous tissue is further divided with electrocautery (Fig. 169.25).

Dissection continues posteriorly directly over the coccyx, and the anococcygeal raphe is identified and sharply divided (Fig. 169.26). Waldeyer fascia is then divided and the presacral space is entered. The superficial fascia laterally is divided, and the ischiorectal fossa is entered bilaterally. Throughout lateral dissection, it is important to visualize the boundaries of the ischiorectal fossa: those being the ischial tuberosity and obturator fascia laterally, the fascia of the levator ani and sphincter muscles medially, the transverse perinei superficialis and profunda muscles

anteriorly, and the fascia of the gluteus maximus muscle posteriorly. Care must be taken in the upper part of the ischiorectal fossa in identifying and suture ligating the inferior rectal vessels including the pudendal artery and nerve as they enter the external sphincter posterolaterally. If inadvertently transected during dissection, these vessels may retract only to cause bleeding at a later time.

The posterior dissection is continued by elevating the anal canal away from the sacrum and dividing the areolar tissue between the rectal fascia and presacral fascia, thus progressively elevating the rectum off the presacral fascia. The curve of the rectum should be conceptualized as the dissection proceeds and care should be taken not to dissect too closely to the sacrum, to avoid the bleeding

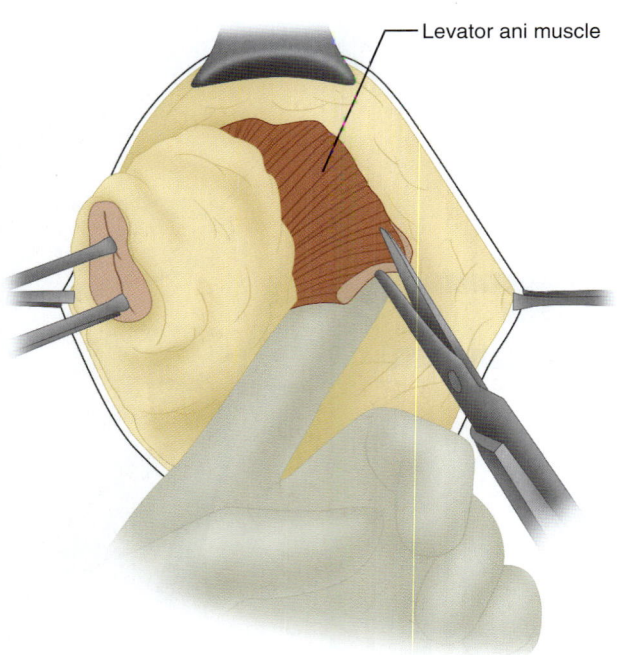

FIGURE 169.27 Division of the levators. (Redrawn with permission from Zollinger RM Jr, Ellison EC, eds. *Zollinger's Atlas of Surgical Operations.* 9th ed. New York: McGraw-Hill Medical; 2011.)

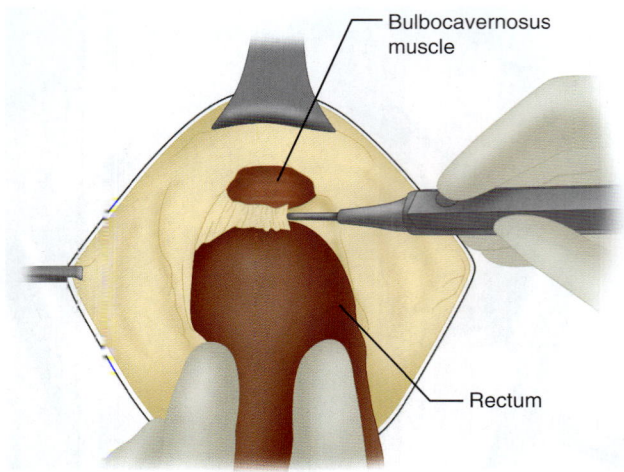

FIGURE 169.28 Division of the anterior plane from the perineum. (Redrawn with permission from Zollinger RM Jr, Ellison EC, eds. *Zollinger's Atlas of Surgical Operations.* 9th ed. New York: McGraw-Hill Medical; 2011.)

from presacral veins. The iliococcygeus muscle is then palpated by placing an index finger into the presacral space and sweeping laterally. The muscle is exposed bilaterally and divided sequentially with either electrocautery or curved Metzenbaum scissors (Fig. 169.27). The surgeon may choose to apply curved clamps prior to transection of the muscle to provide opportunity to control any bleeding vessels prior to them retracting out of reach. Dissection is continued anteriorly onto the pubococcygeal and puborectalis muscles. This dissection may be facilitated by tension placed between the ischiorectal fat laterally and rectum medially using malleable retractors.

After the levator ani muscles have been successfully transected, the anterior dissection proceeds. This is generally considered the most difficult portion of the perineal dissection, particularly in male patients. The membranous urethra, prostate, and seminal vesicles are all closely adhered to the anterior wall of rectum and anal sphincters. The perineal skin is retracted anteriorly while the anus and rectum are pulled inferiorly and posteriorly to facilitate exposure. The space between the rectum, and prostate is developed by dividing the rectourethralis and the remaining anterior attachments are progressively thinned (Fig. 169.28). It is important to avoid dissecting too far anteriorly because this may result in urethral injury. Frequent palpation of the Foley catheter and prostate can assist the surgeon in maintaining the proper plane of dissection. Alternatively, the patient may be placed prone for this portion of the procedure to help in identification of the proper dissection plane. In the female, the dissection between the vagina and rectum is easier. However, care should be taken to avoid inadvertent injury to the posterior vaginal wall. It is also important to use

gentle retraction and support the rectum during the final stages of dissection as avulsion off the urethra and prostate can result in injury and bleeding.

The sigmoid end of the specimen is clamped and delivered through the posterior end of the perineal wound, and the final attachments of the levator ani muscles are then transected (Fig. 169.29).

The pelvic cavity is then irrigated and inspected for hemostasis. Bleeding points are controlled with electrocautery and suture ligation. Persistent venous oozing can generally be controlled by packing of the cavity with dry sponges. After hemostasis is confirmed, one to two closed-suction drains are generally placed in the presacral space. We prefer to close the wound in multiple layers. The levator ani muscles are approximated with 2-0 and 3-0 Vicryl sutures (Fig. 169.30), and the subcutaneous tissue and skin are loosely approximated with vertical mattress sutures (Fig. 169.31).

COMPLICATIONS

Perineal wound complications are common and occur in as many as 36% to 80% of patients following APR.[23] Prior pelvic radiation is a key contributing factor, along with malnutrition, smoking history, and obesity. There are many reconstructive options developed to facilitate perineal wound healing and decrease the incidence of wound complications. As discussed previously, myocutaneous flaps, such as the vertical rectus abdominis myocutaneous (VRAM) flap, rotational anterolateral thigh flaps, and the gracilis myocutaneous flap, are occasionally required for perineal reconstruction. Myocutaneous flaps have the major advantage of providing well-vascularized soft tissue volume with excellent blood supply and associated skin coverage for the perineum. Several comparative studies of flap reconstruction versus primary closure have demonstrated decreased perineal wound complications utilizing flap reconstruction.[24–26]

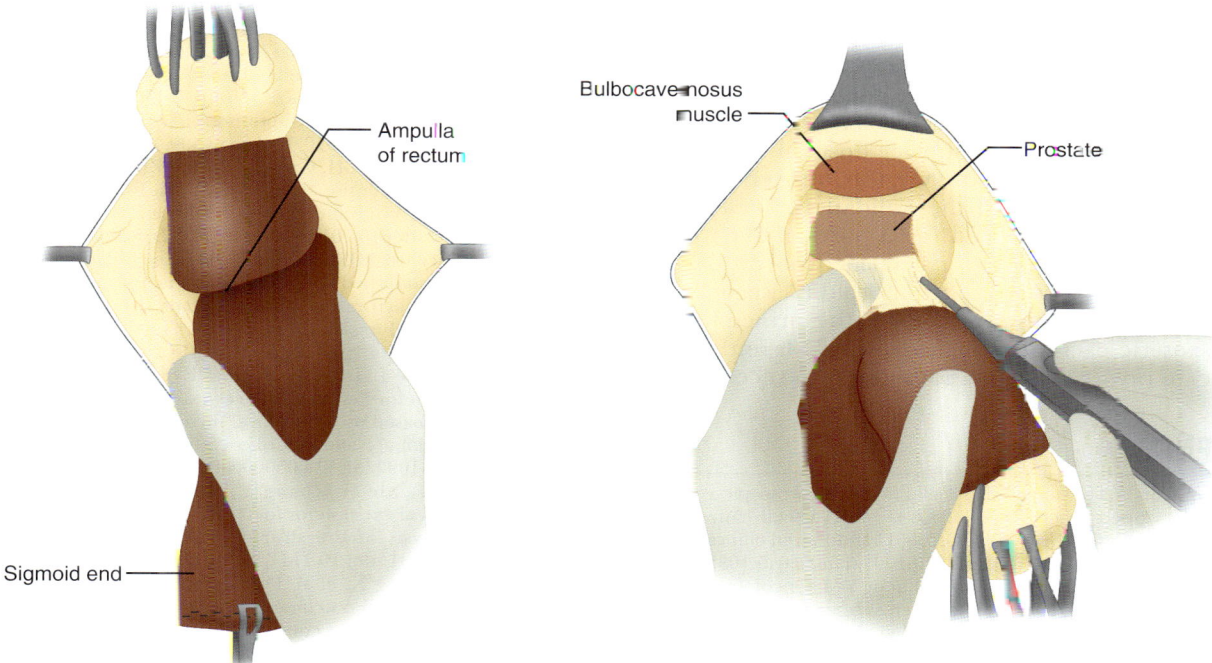

FIGURE 169.29 Division of the final anterior attachments. (Redrawn with permission from Zollinger RM Jr, Ellison EC, eds. *Zollinger's Atlas of Surgical Operations.* 9th ed. New York: McGraw-Hill Medical; 2011.)

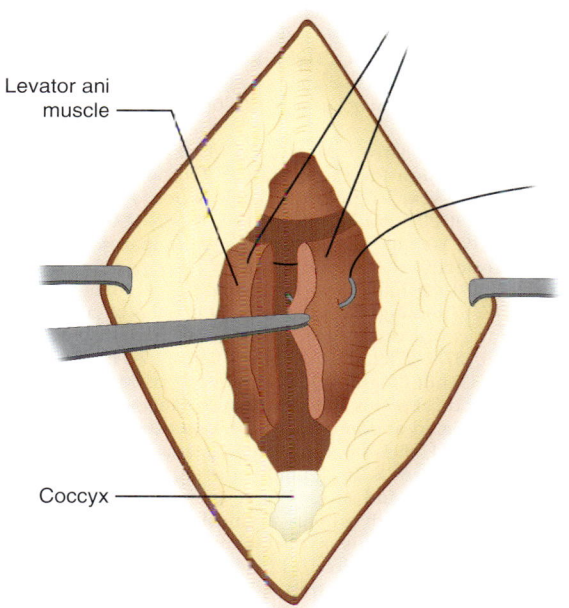

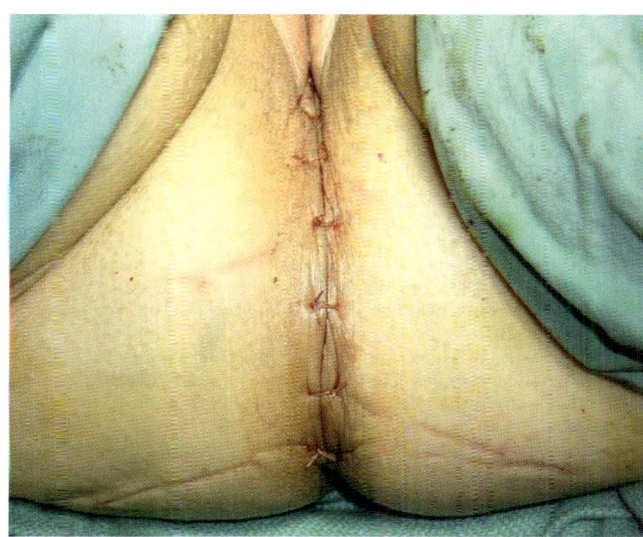

FIGURE 169.31 Closed perineal wound.

FIGURE 169.30 Closure of the levator ani. (Redrawn with permission from Zollinger RM Jr, Ellison EC, eds. *Zollinger's Atlas of Surgical Operations.* 9th ed. New York: McGraw-Hill Medical; 2011.)

Autonomic nerve preservation requires an understanding of the anatomy of the pelvic nerves. Injury to the pelvic autonomic nerves can be associated with significant genitourinary dysfunction and morbidity. Damage to the sympathetic hypogastric nerves can result in increased bladder tone and reduced bladder capacity, as well as with impaired ejaculation in men. Damage to the parasympathetic system can result in voiding difficulties from increased tone in the bladder neck, as well as with erectile dysfunction in men and impaired vaginal lubrication in women. Management of urinary complications requires prolonged bladder drainage with a Foley catheter and in some cases follow-up with urologic surgeons. All complications involving the male reproductive system should include referral or opinions of urologic colleagues.

SUMMARY

APR is a technically driven operation and is often the oncologically necessary procedure for low-lying rectal tumors. Minimally invasive approaches may offer decreased postoperative morbidity and shorter hospital stays over traditional open resection; however, the long-term oncologic equivalence requires further validation. The extent of perineal resection needed for a particular patient requires a tailored approach to achieve adequate oncologic resection and limit postoperative morbidity. Regardless of the particular technical approach, the principles of total mesenteric excision with negative CFMs and autonomic nerve preservation are paramount to success.

REFERENCES

1. Fleshman J, Branda M, Sargent D, et al. Effect of laparoscopic-assisted resection vs open resection of stage II or III rectal cancer on pathologic outcomes: the ACOSOG Z6051 randomized clinical trial. *JAMA.* 2015;314(13):1346-1355. doi:10.1001/jama.2015.10529.

2. Liang J-T, Huang K-C, Lai H-S, Lee P-H, Jeng Y-M. Oncologic results of laparoscopic versus conventional open surgery for stage II or III left-sided colon cancers: a randomized controlled trial. *Ann Surg Oncol.* 2007;14(1):109-117. doi:10.1245/s10434-006-9135-4.

3. Ng SSM, Leung KL, Lee JFY, et al. Laparoscopic-assisted versus open abdominoperineal resection for low rectal cancer: a prospective randomized trial. *Ann Surg Oncol.* 2008;15(9):2418-2425. doi:10.1245/s10434-008-9895-0.

4. Row D, Weiser MR. An update on laparoscopic resection for rectal cancer. *Cancer Control.* 2010;17(1):16-24. http://www.ncbi.nlm.nih.gov/pubmed/20010515. Accessed 14 December 2015.

5. Nagtegaal ID, van de Velde CJH, Marijnen CAM, van Krieken JHJM, Quirke P. Low rectal cancer: a call for a change of approach in abdominoperineal resection. *J Clin Oncol.* 2005;23(36):9257-9264. doi:10.1200/JCO.2005.02.9231.

6. Enker WE, Thaler HT, Cranor ML, Polyak T. Total mesorectal excision in the operative treatment of carcinoma of the rectum. *J Am Coll Surg.* 1995;181(4):335-346. http://www.ncbi.nlm.nih.gov/pubmed/7551328. Accessed 21 December 2015.

7. Enker WE, Havenga K, Polyak T, Thaler H, Cranor M. Abdominoperineal resection via total mesorectal excision and autonomic nerve preservation for low rectal cancer. *World J Surg.* 1997;21(7):715-720. http://www.ncbi.nlm.nih.gov/pubmed/9276702. Accessed 21 December 2015.

8. Hida J, Yasutomi M, Maruyama T, Fujimoto K, Uchida T, Okuno K. Lymph node metastases detected in the mesorectum distal to carcinoma of the rectum by the clearing method: justification of total mesorectal excision. *J Am Coll Surg.* 1997;184(6):584-588. http://www.ncbi.nlm.nih.gov/pubmed/9179114. Accessed 21 December 2015.

9. Reynolds JV, Joyce WP, Dolan J, Sheahan K, Hyland JM. Pathological evidence in support of total mesorectal excision in the management of rectal cancer. *Br J Surg.* 1996;83(8):1112-1115. http://www.ncbi.nlm.nih.gov/pubmed/8869320. Accessed 30 December 2015.

10. Havenga K, Enker WE, Norstein J, et al. Improved survival and local control after total mesorectal excision or D3 lymphadenectomy in the treatment of primary rectal cancer: an international analysis of 1411 patients. *Eur J Surg Oncol.* 1999;25(4):368-374. doi:10.1053/ejso.1999.0659.

11. Hida J, Yasutomi M, Tokoro T, Kubo R. Examination of nodal metastases by a clearing method supports pelvic plexus preservation in rectal cancer surgery. *Dis Colon Rectum.* 1999;42(4):510-514. http://www.ncbi.nlm.nih.gov/pubmed/10215053.

12. West NP, Anderin C, Smith KJE, Holm T, Quirke P. Multicentre experience with extralevator abdominoperineal excision for low rectal cancer. *Br J Surg.* 2010;97(4):588-599. doi:10.1002/bjs.6916.

13. Han JG, Wang ZJ, Wei GH, Gao ZG, Yang Y, Zhao BC. Randomized clinical trial of conventional versus cylindrical abdominoperineal resection for locally advanced lower rectal cancer. *Am J Surg.* 2012;204(3):274-282. doi:10.1016/j.amjsurg.2012.05.001.

14. Krishna A, Rickard MJFX, Keshava A, Dent OF, Chapuis PH. A comparison of published rates of resection margin involvement and intra-operative perforation between standard and "cylindrical" abdominoperineal excision for low rectal cancer. *Colorectal Dis.* 2013;15(1):57-65. doi:10.1111/j.1463–1318.2012.03167.x.

15. Prytz M, Angenete E, Bock D, Haglind E. Extralevator abdominoperineal excision for low rectal cancer-extensive surgery to be used with discretion based on 3-year local recurrence results: a Registry-based, Observational National Cohort Study. *Ann Surg.* 2016;263(3):516-521. doi:10.1097/SLA.0000000000001237.

16. Zhou X, Sun T, Xie H, Zhang Y, Zeng H, Fu W. Extralevator abdominoperineal excision for low rectal cancer: a systematic review and meta-analysis of the short-term outcome. *Colorectal Dis.* 2015·17(6):474-481. doi:10.1111/codi.12921.

17. Shen Z, Ye Y, Zhang X, et al. Prospective controlled study of the safety and oncological outcomes of ELAPE procure with definitive anatomic landmarks versus conventional APE for lower rectal cancer. *Eur J Surg Oncol.* 2015;41(4):472-477. doi:10.1016/j.ejso.2015.01.017.

18. Ahmad NZ, Racheva G, Elmusharaf H. A systematic review and meta-analysis of randomized and non-randomized studies comparing laparoscopic and open abdominoperineal resection for rectal cancer. *Colorectal Dis.* 2013;15(3):269-277. doi:10.1111/codi.12007.

19. Zhou T, Zhang G, Tian H, Liu Z, Xia S. Laparoscopic rectal resection versus open rectal resection with minilaparotomy for invasive rectal cancer. *J Gastrointest Oncol.* 2014;5(1):36-45. doi:10.3978/j.issn.2078–6891.2013.052.

20. Kim S-H, Park I-J, Joh Y-G, Hahn K-Y. Laparoscopic resection for rectal cancer: a prospective analysis of thirty-month follow-up outcomes in 312 patients. *Surg Endosc.* 2006;20(8):1197-1202. doi:10.1007/s00464-005-0599-2.

21. Brachet Contul R, Grivon M, Fabozzi M, et al. Laparoscopic total mesorectal excision for extraperitoneal rectal cancer: long-term results of a 18-year single-centre experience. *J Gastrointest Surg.* 2014;18(4):796-807. doi:10.1007/s11605-013-2441-9.

22. Fleshman JW, Wexner SD, Anvari M, et al. Laparoscopic vs. open abdominoperineal resection for cancer. *Dis Colon Rectum.* 1999;42(7):930-939. http://www.ncbi.nlm.nih.gov/pubmed/10411441.

23. Schiller DE, Cummings BJ, Rai S, et al. Outcomes of salvage surgery for squamous cell carcinoma of the anal canal. *Ann Surg Oncol.* 2007;14(10):2780-2789. doi:10.1245/s10434-007-9491-8.

24. Butler CE, Gündeslioglu AO, Rodriguez-Bigas MA. Outcomes of immediate vertical rectus abdominis myocutaneous flap reconstruction for irradiated abdominoperineal resection defects. *J Am Coll Surg.* 2008;206(4):694-703. doi:10.1016/j.jamcollsurg.2007.12.007.

25. Sunesen KG, Buntzen S, Tei T, Lindegaard JC, Nørgaard M, Laurberg S. Perineal healing and survival after anal cancer salvage surgery: 10-year experience with primary perineal reconstruction using the vertical rectus abdominis myocutaneous (VRAM) flap. *Ann Surg Oncol.* 2009;16(1):68-77. doi:10.1245/s10434-008-0208-4.

26. Tei TM, Stolzenburg T, Buntzen S, Laurberg S, Kjeldsen H. Use of transpelvic rectus abdominis musculocutaneous flap for anal cancer salvage surgery. *Br J Surg.* 2003;90(5):575-580. doi:10.1002/bjs.407.

Minimally Invasive Approaches to Colon Cancer

Jennifer L. Paruch | Todd D. Francone

Laparoscopic colectomy was first described more than three decades ago, following the success of laparoscopic approaches to biliary surgery and appendicitis in the 1980s. Jacobs et al.[1] described their first 20 laparoscopic colectomies for benign and malignant conditions. The paper was fairly modern, with operative times (170 minutes for sigmoid and 155 minutes for right colectomy) and lengths of stay (3 to 5 days for right, 3 to 8 days for sigmoid) comparable to more recent randomized trials. The authors concluded that the procedure "will become as accepted as laparoscopic cholecystectomy."

Although initial reports were promising, adoption of laparoscopic colectomy for cancer was met with early controversy. A report published by Johnstone et al. in 1996 documented 35 port site recurrences in patients undergoing laparoscopic colon cancer surgery.[2] Other similar reports emerged, creating growing concerns over the safety of laparoscopic colectomy.[3,4] As a result, a series of randomized trials were undertaken to compare outcomes between laparoscopic and open colectomy for cancer. These trials are described in detail later and represent one of the most comprehensive bodies of literature to evaluate the safety and efficacy of an emerging surgical technique.

Despite the evidence supporting laparoscopic colectomy, widespread adoption has been slow. Moghadamyeghaneh et al.[5] reviewed the National Inpatient Sample between 2009 and 2012 and found that 49% of elective colectomies for cancer were performed laparoscopically, with the rate of laparoscopy increasing over that time period. Other studies have reported similar numbers, with higher rates at academic centers, suggesting that there is still opportunity for increased utilization.[6,7] Reasons for low adoption rates may include lack of specialized training, low surgeon or hospital volume, underreporting related to reliance on billing codes, or limitations of administrative data in capturing contraindications to laparoscopy.

This chapter will review the trials comparing laparoscopic and open colectomy for cancer and discuss the key technical components of these procedures. It should be noted that laparoscopy is a technique and that it should be used when the surgeon has determined that an equivalent operation can be performed with regard to patient safety and oncologic outcome. Many of the trials included later excluded patients with locally advanced disease, perforation, or obstruction at the time of presentation.

SHORT-TERM OUTCOMES

Many authors comparing laparoscopic to open colectomy for cancer published early papers focusing on short-term outcomes. All of these reported longer operative times for laparoscopic procedures (Table 170.1) with differences ranging from 30 to 84 minutes. The rate of conversion to open varies widely across studies, ranging from 3% to 25% (see Table 170.1). The CLASICC study reported the highest conversion rate (25%) but did note that the rate decreased over the course of the study suggesting that this may be more reflective of the learning curve.[10]

One of the most universal advantages of laparoscopic colon resection across trials is a decreased length of stay (see Table 170.1). This difference ranges from a 1-day in the COST study[9] to a 5-day difference reported by Liang et al.[14] Interestingly, Basse et al.[12] published a study comparing laparoscopic and open colectomy in the setting of a universal fast-track surgery protocol and showed a 2-day length of stay in both groups. This raises the question of whether some advantages of laparoscopy may be blunted as more centers adopt enhanced recovery protocols.

The majority of studies did not find any significant differences in short-term morbidity or mortality between the laparoscopic and open groups (see Table 170.1). Lacy et al.[8] and Braga et al.[13] demonstrated lower overall rates of postoperative complications in the laparoscopic group. In both studies, this seemed to be driven primarily by lower rates of wound infection.

RETURN OF BOWEL FUNCTION

Although there is heterogeneity across studies in the definition of return of bowel function (flatus, bowel movement, oral tolerance), there is a consistent earlier return of bowel function in the laparoscopic group (Table 170.2). This is hypothesized to be the result of gentler tissue handling, and to account for the consistent decrease in length in the laparoscopic group. Interestingly, the Basse et al.[12] study, which compared laparoscopic and open colectomy with a fast-track protocol, found no difference in length of stay or time to return of bowel function between the groups. This further supports the hypothesis that the benefit of laparoscopy in decreasing length of stay may be related to shortened ileus.

POSTOPERATIVE PAIN

Postoperative pain is measured differently across trials, likely because of the challenges with quantifying this outcome (Table 170.3). Most studies used some measure of narcotic use as a surrogate for pain and found a benefit in the laparoscopic group in either duration of narcotic use or percent of patients requiring narcotics. This difference may be more beneficial than was understood at the time of publication of these papers, as surgical fields come under increasing political pressure to decrease the prescription of opiates.[7]

TABLE 170.1 Short-Term Outcomes After Colon Resection

Trial	Sample Size	LOS (DAYS)		MORTALITY		OPERATIVE TIME (MINUTES)		POSTOPERATIVE COMPLICATIONS		Conversion Rates	LYMPH NODE HARVEST	
		Lap	Open	Lap	Open	Lap	Open	Lap	Open		Lap	Open
Lacy et al., 2002[8]	219	5.2	7.9*					12%	31%†	11%	No difference	
COST, 2004[9]	872	5	6†	No difference		150	95†			21%		
CLASICC, 2005[10]	794	No difference		No difference		180	135	No difference		25%	No difference	
COLOR, 2005[11]	1248	8.2	9.3‡	No difference		145	115‡	No difference		17%	No difference	
Basse et al., 2005[12]	60	No difference				215	131§			10%		
Braga et al., 2005[13]	391	9.4	12.7‡					17.9%	36.3%ᴵ	4.2%		
Liang et al., 2007[14]	269	9	14†			224	184†	No difference		3%		
ALCCaS, 2008[15]	592	7	8	No difference				No difference		14.6%		
Braga et al., 2010[16]	268	7	8.7¶			213	174†	No difference		5.2%		

*P = .005
†P < .001
‡P < .0001
§P < .05
ᴵP = .0005
¶P = .002
lap, Laparoscopic; *LOS*, length of stay.

TABLE 170.2 Return of Bowel Function After Colon Resection

Trial	Sample Size	TIME TO FLATUS		DAYS TO BOWEL MOVEMENT		TIME TO PO TOLERANCE		LENGTH OF ILEUS	
		Lap	Open	Lap	Open	Lap	Open	Lap	Open
Lacy et al., 2002[8]	219	36 h	55 h*			54 h	84 h*		
COLOR, 2005[11]	1248			3.6	4.6†	2.9 days	3.8 days†		
CLASICC, 2005[10]	794			5	6	No difference			
Basse et al., 2005[12]	60			No difference					
Liang et al., 2007[14]	269							48 h	96 h*
ALCCaS, 2008[15]	592	3 days	3 days‡	4	5§				

*P = .001
†P < .0001
‡P = .27
§P < .011
PO, Per os; *Lap*, laparoscopic.

TABLE 170.3 Postoperative Pain Control After Colon Resection

Trial	Sample Size	Measurement	Outcome
COST, 2004[9]	872	Days of parenteral narcotics	3 days laparoscopic vs. 4 days open (P < .001)
		Days of oral analgesics	1 day lap vs. 2 days open (P = .02)
COLOR, 2005[11]	1248	Percent of patients using opiates POD#1-3	POD#1: No difference POD#2: 41% lap vs. 49% open (P = .008) POD#3: 26% lap vs. 37% open (P = .0003)
Liang et al., 2007[14]	269	Visual analog scale (POD#1)	3.5 laparoscopic vs. 8.6 open (P < .001)

h, Hours; *POD*, postoperative day.

LONG-TERM OUTCOMES

ONCOLOGIC OUTCOMES

As mentioned earlier, one of the key motivating factors for these studies was to demonstrate equivalent oncologic outcomes between laparoscopic and open colectomy. Since their initial publication, several trials have continued to publish updates (out to 10 years) to provide a definitive answer to this question. Table 170.4 summarizes the results from these studies. In every case, groups found no significant difference in overall survival, disease-free survival, wound recurrence, or overall recurrence between laparoscopic and open colectomy. The only study showing any type of oncologic difference, reported by Lacy et al.,[8] showed an advantage for laparoscopic colectomy group in cancer-related mortality. This collective body of data has demonstrated that laparoscopic colectomy is noninferior to open colectomy in appropriately selected cancer patients.

TABLE 170.4 Long-Term Outcomes After Colon Resection

Trial	Follow-Up	Overall Survival	Disease-Free Survival	Wound Recurrence	Recurrence	Incisional Hernia	Small Bowel Obstruction
COST, 2004[9]	3 years	No difference		No difference	No difference		
COST, 2007[18]	5 years	No difference		No difference	No difference		
CLASICC, 2007[19]	3 years	No difference	No difference	No difference	No difference		
CLASICC, 2010[20]	5 years	No difference	No difference		No difference		
CLASICC, 2010[21]	3 years					No difference	No difference
CLASICC, 2013[22]	10 years	No difference	No difference		No difference		
COLOR, 2009[23]	5 years	No difference	No difference		No difference		
COLOR, 2011[24]	5 years						No difference
Lacy et al., 2008[25]	Median 95 months	No difference			No difference		
Braga et al, 2010[16]	5 years	No difference	No difference	No difference		No difference	No difference
LAFA, 2014[26]	5 years	No difference			No difference	10% lap, 17% open (P = .022)	2.4% lap, 7.3% open (P = .039)
Liang et al., 2007[14]	Median 40 months			No difference	No difference		
ALCCaS, 2012[15]	5 years	No difference	No difference		No difference		

Lap, Laparoscopic.

INCISIONAL HERNIA AND ADHESIVE BOWEL OBSTRUCTION

In addition to survival, many long-term studies included data on rates of incisional hernia and adhesive small bowel obstruction. Although one may hypothesize that smaller incisions and decreased tissue handling associated with laparoscopic surgery would decrease the risk of these complications, that has not been clearly supported by the literature (see Table 170.4). The majority of groups found no difference, with the exception being the LAFA study, which showed decreases in both outcomes in the laparoscopic group.[26] It may be possible that longer-term follow-up is needed to detect differences between the groups.

QUALITY OF LIFE

Quality of life (QoL) is a challenging outcome to compare between procedures. There are numerous instruments available, and their use varies widely across studies. Many trials hypothesized that QoL would be improved in the laparoscopic group and invested considerable resources into collecting these data. Overall, most found at least some short-term QoL benefit in the laparoscopic group.

The COST group published two papers focusing on QoL.[27,28] They used a Symptom Distress Scale (SDS), QoL index, and single-item global scale. They found slightly better global QoL rating at 2 weeks in the laparoscopic group; however, no other comparisons out to 2 months reached significance. At 18 months, they found a modest benefit in the laparoscopic group for global QoL, but no differences for activity, daily living, health, or support.

Other groups have studied differences in QoL with mixed results.[10,26,19-29] Braga et al.[13] looked at QoL at 12, 24, and 36 months using the Short Form-36. They found significantly better general health and physical and social

functioning in the laparoscopic group at 12 months. However, this difference disappeared at 48 months.

Taken together, the literature suggests that certain QoL domains are improved in laparoscopic compared with open colectomy and that these differences are probably the most significant in the first 6 to 12 months after surgery.

COST

The cost of the operation itself is higher for laparoscopic colectomy than for open colectomy. Liang et al.[14] reported significantly higher overall costs for laparoscopic compared with open colectomy ($194,442 vs. $136,420; P < .001). These differences were largely driven by increased equipment and disposable instrument costs. The CCLOR group reported higher cost of operation (€1171; P < .001), higher cost of admission (€1556; P = .015), and higher cost to the healthcare system (€2244; P = .018) for laparoscopic colectomy. However, when they took into account total cost to society (time off of work), they found no difference between laparoscopic and open colectomy at 12 months.[30]

ADDITIONAL CONSIDERATIONS

ROBOTICS

Early studies on robotic colectomy were published in 2002.[31,32] The three-dimensional view, improved articulation, and multiinstrument platform provide an advantage for many surgical specialties performing complex minimally invasive procedures. Although robotics is gaining more attention for proctectomy,[33-35] studies have been published comparing robotic with laparoscopic colectomy. Park et al.[37] randomized 70 patients to robotic versus laparoscopic right colectomy for cancer. They demonstrated equivalent length of stay, pain scores, complications, margins, and lymphadenectomy for both groups. The robotic group had longer operative times (195 vs. 130 minutes; $P < .001$) and increased operative costs ($12,235 vs. $10,320; $P = .013$). The increased cost of robotics and who should be responsible for this (patient, hospital, surgeon) remain a limitation for robotic colectomy.

SINGLE INCISION

Single-incision laparoscopic colectomy (SILC) increases the complexity of laparoscopic colectomy, with the goal of limiting the incision size to only that needed for specimen extraction. Early case reports established its feasibility as an approach for both cancer and inflammatory bowel disease.[38-40] More recently, two randomized trials have been published comparing SILC with standard laparoscopic colectomy.[41,42] Results from these trials have demonstrated similar operating times, complication rates, and lymph node harvests, along with a decreased length of stay by 1 day in one of the studies. This remains a promising and challenging technique, with similar outcomes to standard laparoscopy for appropriately selected patients.

COMPLETE MESOCOLIC EXCISION

Complete mesocolic excision (CME) with central vascular ligation is hypothesized to provide an oncologic benefit. This is based on the premise that metastases as determined by the primary tumor with cancer progression occurs in a stepwise pattern. CME therefore improves outcomes by removing the mesocolon in one package with high ligation of the feeding vessels.[43,44] Data suggest improved short- and long-term oncologic outcomes.[45,46] Improved outcomes are thought to be related to strict adherence to oncologic principles including dissection through the proper plane, central vascular ligation, and length of proximal and distal margins. CME has been shown to achieve an en bloc removal of the disease lesion with increased amounts of colonic mesentery. It is a technically challenging operation due to high ligation of the vascular pedicles with dissection along the aorta and mobilization of the splenic flexure.

Numerous recent publications have demonstrated the feasibility of laparoscopic CME with short-term outcomes similar to those of open surgery.[47,48] Operative times are typically longer with the laparoscopy, with majority of studies demonstrating equivalent morbidity and mortality when compared with open CME groups. The conversion to an open CME ranges between 2% and 10%.

TECHNIQUE AND PEARLS OF WISDOM

Minimally invasive surgery, both laparoscopic and robotic, have become increasingly used both for benign and malignant disease processes. Based on the underlying disease and sequelae of such processes, it is essential to be familiar with various approaches (i.e., medial to lateral, lateral to medial, superior to inferior, etc.) resulting in optimal exposure, as well as safer, quicker, and a more reproducible dissection. This is without a doubt facilitated by a fundamental understanding of the surgical anatomy, allowing the surgeon the ability to proceed in a safe manner, perform an appropriate oncologic resection, and allow for additional diagnostic and therapeutic maneuvering.

LAPAROSCOPIC RIGHT COLECTOMY FOR COLON CANCER

With either laparoscopic or robotic techniques, the patient is in the supine position. If the location of the tumor is unclear based on prior review of diagnostic imaging, the patient should be placed in the modified lithotomy or split-leg position to facilitate an intraoperative endoscopic evaluation. The preferred laparoscopic and robotic port placements are demonstrated in Fig. 170.1. The patient is placed in a Trendelenburg position with the operating table inclined toward the left. Once pneumoperitoneum is established, a thorough evaluation of the abdomen is critical to understand the anatomy, evaluate for disseminated disease, and assess the feasibility of an R0 resection. The omentum is retracted superiorly over the transverse colon and liver, and the small bowel is mobilized out of the pelvis. Grasping either the cecum or mesentery close to the cecum anteriorly or ventrally will highlight the ileocolic artery branching off the superior mesenteric artery. A tenting or bowstringing effect will be noted, with the mesenteric vasculature acting as the scaffold (Fig. 170.2).

The medial-lateral approach is our preferred approach, with early ligation of the ileocolic pedicle. This is generally first performed by creating an opening in the peritoneum parallel to the vessels and then encircling the vessels superiorly. Some mobilization of the mesocolon from the retroperitoneal structures may be necessary and can be performed with gentle blunt sweeping motions dorsally. When doing so, care must be taken both to visualize the right ureter as well as the duodenum. Once these structures are well visualized and out of harm's way, a high ligation of the vessel can be performed. The medial-to-lateral dissection can then be continued with retroperitoneal attachments safely dissected away from the right colon and its mesentery, either sharply or with gentle brush movements. Care must be taken to stay in the appropriate plane and not injure the duodenum or more laterally, not mobilize the kidney (Fig. 170.3).

For hepatic flexure and proximal transverse colon tumors, further distal dissection of the mesentery is performed to the level of the middle colic vessels. The middle colic vessel is the primary blood supply to the proximal two-thirds of the transverse colon. Care must be taken to use precise technique in this retroperitoneal space because the pancreaticoduodenal and gastroepiploic veins may cause significant hemorrhage if excess tension or shearing occurs. After the middle colic vessel is identified, the right branch of the middle colic vessel is then divided after isolation.

At this point the right colon will now be held in place only by lateral avascular attachments to the abdominal sidewall, hepatic flexure, and gastrocolic attachments, including the omentum to the transverse colon. These can generally be easily divided by dissecting energy devices. Dissection is carried out proximally, dividing the hepatic flexure attachments and then distally toward the pelvis. The gastrocolic attachments to the transverse colon need to be divided oftentimes with entry into the lesser sac. For right colectomies, the distal extent of dissection is generally around the falciform ligament or in line with

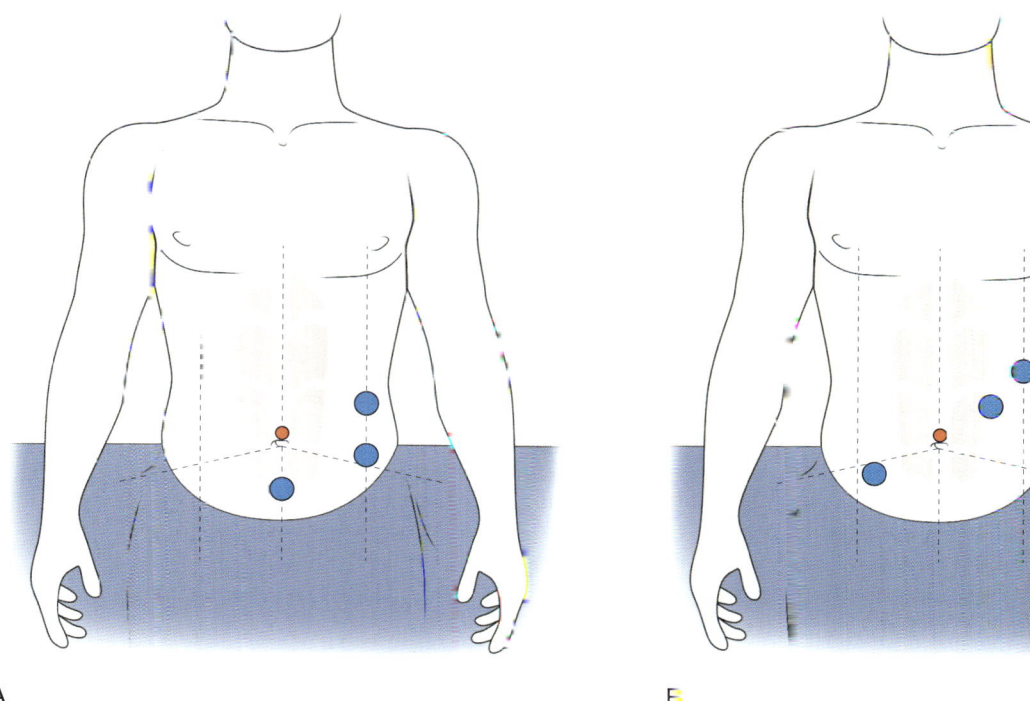

A

B

FIGURE 170.1 (A) Four-port technique for laparoscopic right colectomy. Extraction site is through the midline or surgeon preference. (B) Four-arm technique for robotic right colectomy using the DaVinci Xi. Extraction site is through the midline or surgeon preference.

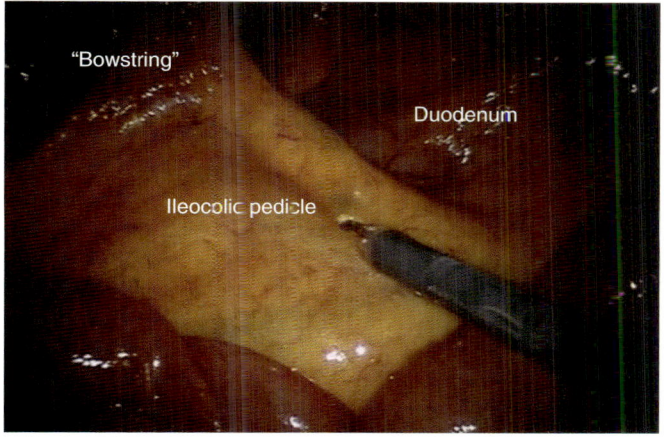

FIGURE 170.2 Grasping the cecum or its mesentery and lifting anterolateral to the abdominal wall will create a tenting or "bowstring" effect with a distinct crease coursing parallel to the vessel.

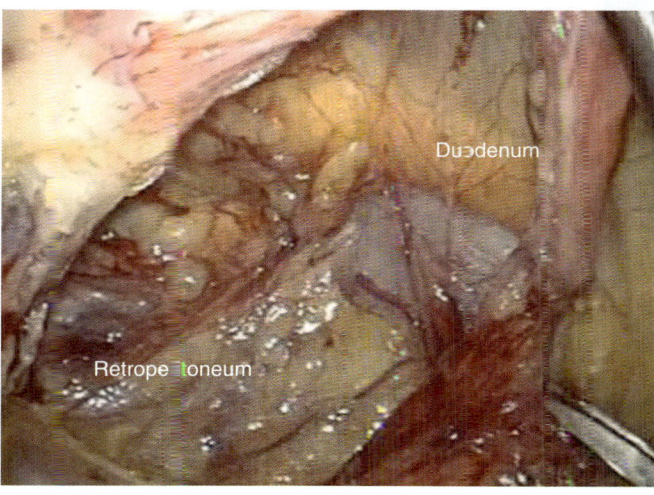

FIGURE 170.3 Medial-to-lateral mobilization highlighting duodenum and white line of Toldt.

the middle colic vessels. It is sometimes best to start at this point and work retrograde toward the hepatic flexure.

Hepatic flexure and proximal transverse colon tumors can be quite challenging due to the surrounding anatomy including the duodenum, pancreas, gallbladder, and kidney (Fig. 170.4). Potential involvement of these structures should instigate a cascade of diagnostic and endoscopic evaluations with involvement of the appropriate surgical teams, whether approaching it minimally invasive or open.

In the presence of a hepatic flexure or proximal colon tumor, the omentum may be involved and should remain attached to the colon to ensure an en bloc resection. Entry into the lesser sac can often be helpful in the event there is potential involvement of retroperitoneal structures. The lesser sac is entered, and the proximal transverse mesocolon can then be sharply dissected from the other abdominal and retroperitoneal structures (Fig. 170.5), including the duodenum and pancreas. Another point

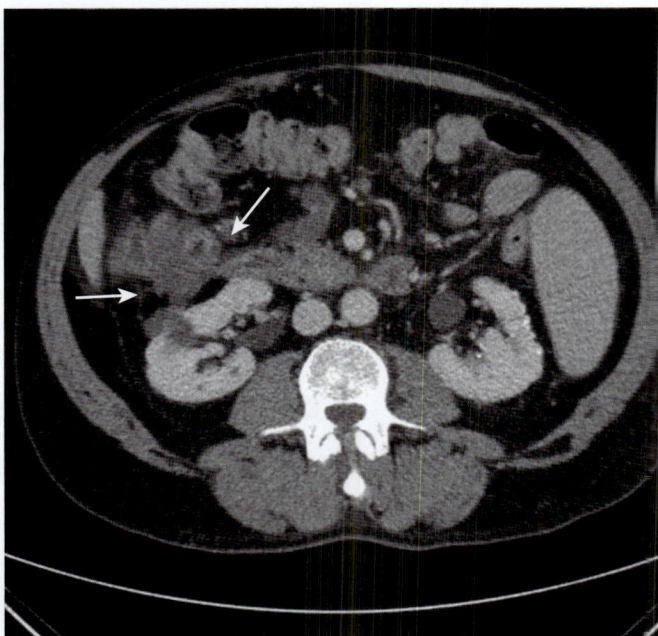

FIGURE 170.4 Hepatic flexure tumor *(arrows)* involving the right kidney and duodenum.

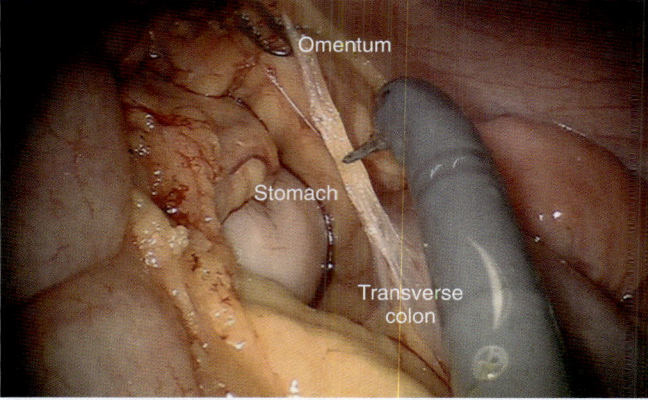

FIGURE 170.5 Accessing the lesser sac through the omentum (gastrocolic ligament); early entry into the lesser sac is key to facilitating mobilization of the transverse colon.

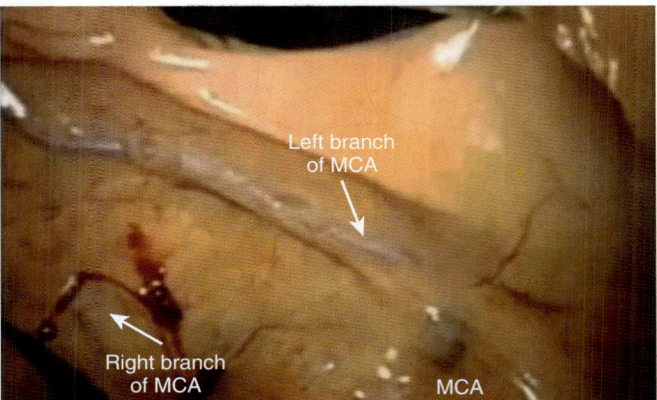

FIGURE 170.6 The classic "Y" pattern of the middle colic vessels is not always straightforward. Often both the right and left branch course to the patient's right. The right branch courses off the head of the pancreas and the duodenum; the left branch makes a sharp upward turn and then veers to the left, as shown here. *MCA,* Middle colic artery.

of entry into the lesser sac will be the fusion or attachment of the gallbladder dome to the transverse colon or mesocolon.

Once completely dissected, the right colon and mesentery should be able to be mobilized and expressed as a midline structure. Division of the intestines and subsequent anastomosis can now be performed either intracorporeally via laparoscopy or in an open fashion once extracorporealized through an extraction incision.

TRANSVERSE COLECTOMY AND THE MIDDLE COLIC VESSELS

In cases requiring resection of the transverse colon, the middle colic vessel will need to be ligated and divided, sometimes in a high fashion (Fig. 170.6). Rather than isolating the right branch of the middle colic vessel, the entire middle colic vessel may be divided. This can be challenging due to the truncated length of the middle colic vessels. It may be isolated by gently retracting the mesentery of the transverse colon superiorly. The middle colic artery and its right and left branches will be identified. A window can be created around the middle colic vessels and divided in a retrograde left-to-right fashion.

LAPAROSCOPIC LEFT COLECTOMY/SIGMOID RESECTION FOR COLON CANCER

Left colectomy refers to resection of the descending and/or splenic flexure with anastomosis of the distal transverse colon to the sigmoid colon, whereas sigmoid resection refers to removal of the sigmoid colon with restoration of intestinal continuity between the descending colon and the rectum. As mentioned previously, there are potentially no absolute contradictions to proceeding with an oncologic resection minimally invasive; however, those patients with a suspected T4 tumor should have the appropriate multidisciplinary surgical teams involved in the event a more extensive resection is required for an R0 oncologic resection. In particular, sigmoid colon cancers may involve the ureter or bladder, and as such a urologist should be involved for possible partial cystectomy or ureteral reimplantation. If the resection is considered extensive, the surgeon should have a low threshold for conversion to an alternative approach, such as an open procedure, to optimize exposure and facilitate the dissection.

All patients are placed in modified lithotomy (legs in slight hip flexion) or split-leg position with both arms tucked at the sides. Positioning in this manner affords the surgeons numerous advantages including exposure to the anus/rectum for intraoperative colonoscopy if needed. This can be particularly useful for a tumor that may not have been preoperatively tattooed and localized. The

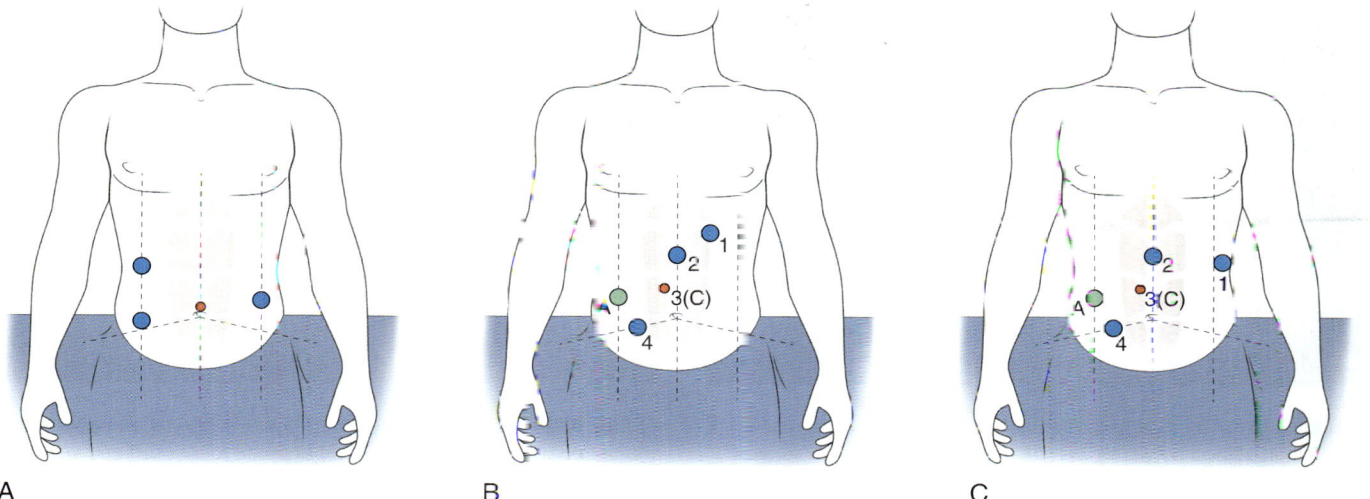

FIGURE 170.7 (A) Four-port technique for laparoscopic left colectomy. Extraction site is through the midline or Pfannenstiel incision. (B) Standard proposed port placement for a robotic sigmoidectomy using the DaVinci X. Notice the camera port is slightly off midline. This allows dissection of the splenic flexure and upper pelvis. C) Our preferred port placement for a robotic sigmoid resection or low anterior resection using the DaVinci Xi. The "hockey stick" formation allows access to the splenic flexure as well as the pelvis with no need to redock the arms.

preferred laparoscopic port placement is demonstrated in Fig. 170.7A. When performing a left colectomy or sigmoid resection, it is customary to divide the bowel (and potentially the major vascular structures) with an endomechanical linear stapling device of various staple heights. For this reason, a 12-mm port is used in the right lower quadrant (RLQ). When performing a robotic approach, ports are spaced evenly in a straight line from the anterior superior iliac spine in the RLQ to the mid-clavicle in the left upper quadrant (LUQ) (see Fig. 170.7B and C).

Prior to any mobilization or resection, inspect the abdominal and pelvic cavity to evaluate for any altered anatomy (phlegmon or occult metastatic processes) not previously appreciated or identified on preoperative imaging. In oncologic procedures, the liver is carefully inspected on both anterior and posterior surfaces, and the peritoneum, omentum, and mesentery are examined for metastatic studding. If the latter is identified, biopsy and surgical judgment will dictate how next to proceed—and whether any further resection is necessary or prudent. During diagnostic laparoscopy the surgeon often identifies the pathology. In the setting of a colonic neoplasm, the pathology's location should often be marked with an endoscopic tattoo. Ideally, the location is marked in three to four quadrants such that the tattoo is clearly visible on the antimesenteric surface. Marking the lesion in only one quadrant may pose some difficulty in identification if the tattoo lies on the mesenteric border or in a difficult location such as the splenic or hepatic flexures. In this event, an intraoperative CO_2 endoscopy may be performed. CO_2 insufflation allows for quick resolution of bowel distention and continued laparoscopy during or following the endoscopic evaluation.

Once the pathology has been localized, adjustments to the preoperative surgical plan may be required. In the setting of malignancy, the location of the tumor will determine resection margins and vessel ligation. For cancers in the left colon, oncologic margins should be 5 cm proximal and distal to the tumor. A high ligation of the inferior mesenteric artery (IMA) pedicle is often performed to ensure adequate mobilization and appropriate lymph node harvesting. Pathology located in the proximal sigmoid colon or distal descending colon may necessitate mobilization of the splenic flexure for appropriate tension-free anastomosis. For lesions in the proximal descending colon, a high ligation of the inferior mesenteric vein (IMV) may also be necessary to allow mobilization and approximation of the proximal colon to the upper rectum to create an intestinal anastomosis without tension.

Similar to a right colectomy, the initial dissection involves the development of the avascular plane between the parietal peritoneum overlying the retroperitoneum and the visceral peritoneum encompassing the mesentery of the left colon. There are multiple approaches to achieve this task including medial to lateral and lateral to medial. We prefer a medial-to-lateral approach for a left colectomy. The initial step for this approach requires initial identification of the IMA pedicle. The mesenteric fold containing the IMA can be found overlying and cephalad to the sacral promontory. Ventral retraction of the sigmoid and left colon mesentery will assist in outlining the IMA pedicle entering into the pelvis to form the superior rectal artery, in a similar bowstring effect noted with the ileocolic pedicle (Fig. 170.8). In the event that division of these adhesions does not allow for a clear "bowstring" of the IMA pedicle, then an alternative approach, such as a lateral to medial, should be considered to avoid injury to underlying structures such as the ureter, hypogastric nerves, and iliac vessels (Fig. 170.9).

After the key retroperitoneal structures have been identified, the IMA may be divided to facilitate the pelvic

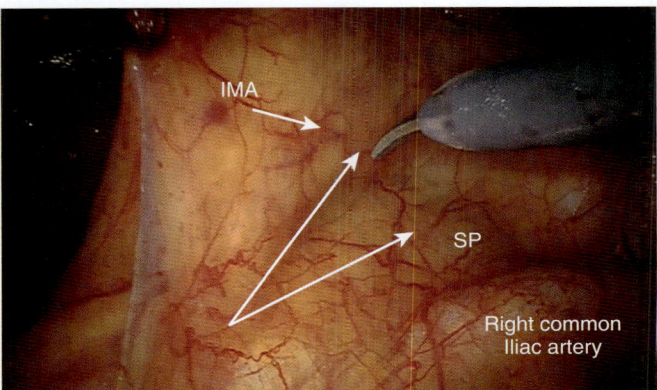

FIGURE 170.8 The outline of the inferior mesenteric artery (IMA) can be visualized by gentle ventral retraction of the pedicle as it courses over the sacral promontory (SP). The space between the IMA and the SP has been termed the *critical angle* and marks the avascular plane between the retroperitoneum and the colon mesentery.

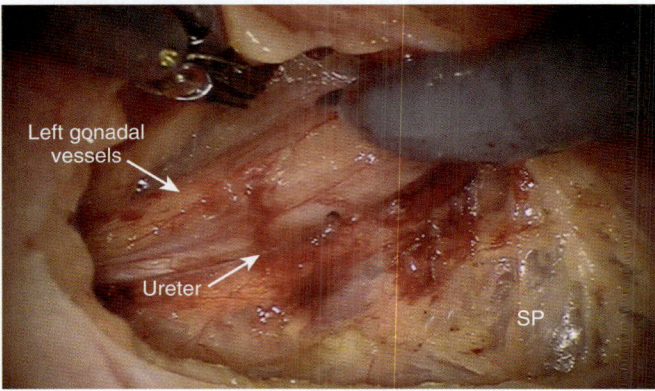

FIGURE 170.9 Care is taken to identify and avoid the left ureter, left gonadal vessels, and the hypogastric nerve plexus. *SP*, Sacral promontory.

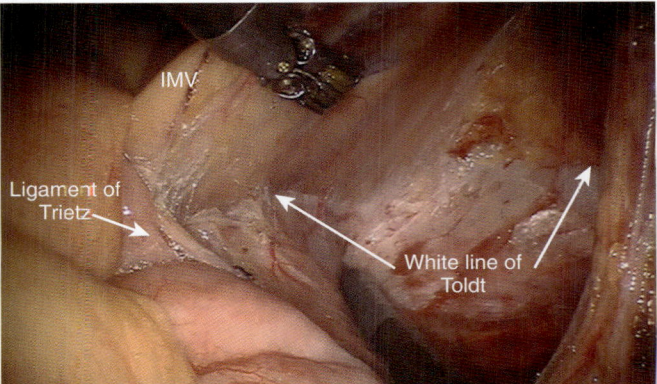

FIGURE 170.10 Continued medial-to-lateral mobilization between the inferior mesenteric artery (IMA) and inferior mesenteric vein (IMV) will facilitate mobilization of the splenic flexure.

dissection. The medial-to-lateral mobilization is performed similar to that done on the right side. The dissection proceeds cephalad to the level of the superior pole of the kidney and may continue to the inferior aspect of the spleen. After medial-to-lateral mobilization is completed, the remaining avascular lateral attachments of the colon to the omentum, spleen, and abdominal and retroperitoneal sidewalls should be divided. Remember, when performing a resection of a tumor in the transverse colon, the omentum should be left on the colon and resected with the specimen to ensure adequate margins and an R0 resection.

In the presence of a descending colon or distal transverse colon mass, splenic flexure mobilization will be required. Splenic flexure mobilization is generally performed using a combination of approaches. The patient is placed in a reverse Trendelenburg position with the table inclined toward the right. Typically, if an adequate medial-to-lateral mobilization is performed of the left colon and IMV, then mobilization of the splenic flexure is reduced to division of the lateral attachments of the phrenocolic ligaments

(Fig. 170.10). Laterally, the attachments to the abdominal sidewall and spleen are carefully divided while being mindful not to injure the splenic capsule.

A critical step in left colectomy is identification of a distal transection point. Distal transection localization is dependent upon both anatomic and physiologic entities. Appropriate mesenteric vascular supply must be accounted for, as well as distal resection margins in the setting of malignancy. For a sigmoid or distal left colectomy, division is generally performed at the level of the proximal rectum, past the splaying of the taenia coli on the antimesenteric surface. Further dissection and transection may be required to get appropriate distal margins. In general, at least a 5-cm distal margin is required for colonic malignancies. After the point of transection is selected, the mesentery is divided. Division of the upper rectum is generally performed with an endomechanical stapling device through the RLQ port.

The colon is then extracted. Options for an extraction site include extension of the periumbilical incision, creation of a Pfannenstiel incision, or extension of the RLQ incision. After the abdominal wall is opened appropriately and the peritoneal cavity entered, a wound protector is inserted to protect the skin and soft tissue from contamination during externalization and creation of anastomosis. Through the wound protector, the distal stapled end of the colon and the proximal mobilized colon and mesentery are extracorporealized. The proximal dissection point is predicated upon a number of issues. In the setting of malignancy, at least a 5-cm margin is required. In all cases, appropriate maintenance of vascular supply must be ensured to minimize risk of ischemia of the anastomosis.

Double-stapled end-end or end-side technique is often used during a left or sigmoid colectomy. It is recommended by the American Society of Colon and Rectal Surgeons that all left-sided anastomoses be tested for leakage. Once confident the anastomosis is secure and viable, the extraction sites and all port sites 10 mm or greater in size are closed.

COMPLETE MESOCOLIC EXCISION

When performing a CME for right colon tumor located in the cecum approximately, the right branches of the middle colic artery and vein are ligated in addition to the ileocolic vessels. It is imperative to ligate the vessels just as they take off the superior mesenteric artery (SMA). For lesions located in the hepatic flexure and proximal transverse colons, an extended right colectomy is performed with the middle colic artery and vein ligated.[49] Omentectomy is performed just below the gastroepiploic vessels and unless infiltrated by the tumor, the right gastroepiploic vessels are preserved. When performing a CME for a left colon tumor located in the proximal descending colon, the IMA is preserved and the left colic artery and superior rectal artery are ligated at their origin. For mid-descending and sigmoid colon cancers, the root of the IMA is ligated and the IMV is ligated just below the lower border of the pancreas.[50]

CONCLUSION

Ongoing evidence supports the feasibility and safety of a minimally invasive surgery approach for colon cancer. To date, laparoscopy remains the most widely used minimally invasive technique with robotic surgery gaining momentum despite unsubstantiated evidence for cost-effectiveness in the treatment of both colon cancer and rectal cancer. It cannot be overstated that minimally invasive surgery is a technique or a "tool" that a surgeon may use to successfully remove pathology. It should be used when the surgeon has determined that an equivalent operation can be performed with regard to patient safety and oncologic outcome when compared with an open approach.

REFERENCES

1. Jacobs M, Verdeja JC, Goldstein HS. Minimally invasive colon resection (laparoscopic colectomy). *Surg Laparosc Endosc.* 1991;1(3):144-150.
2. Johnstone PA, Rohde DC, Swartz SE, Fetter JE, Wexner SD. Port site recurrences after laparoscopic and thoracoscopic procedures in malignancy. *J Clin Oncol.* 1996;14(6):1950-1956.
3. Berends FJ, Kazemier G, Bonjer HJ, Lange JF. Subcutaneous metastases after laparoscopic colectomy. *Lancet.* 1994;344(8914):58.
4. Reilly WT, Nelson H, Schroeder G, Wieand HS, Bolton J, O'Connell MJ. Wound recurrence following conventional treatment of colorectal cancer. A rare but perhaps underestimated problem. *Dis Colon Rectum.* 1996;39(2):200-207.
5. Moghadamyeghaneh Z, Carmichael JC, Mills S, Pigazzi A, Nguyen NT, Stamos MJ. Variations in laparoscopic colectomy utilization in the United States. *Dis Colon Rectum.* 2015;58(10):950-956.
6. Yeo HL, Isaacs AJ, Abelson JS, Milsom JW, Sedrakyan A. Comparison of open, laparoscopic, and robotic colectomies using a large national database: outcomes and trends related to surgery center volume. *Dis Colon Rectum.* 2016;59(6):535-542.
7. Bardakcioglu O, Khan A, Aldridge C, Chen J. Growth of laparoscopic colectomy in the United States: analysis of regional and socioeconomic factors over time. *Ann Surg.* 2013;258(2):270-274.
8. Lacy AM, García-Valdecasas JC, Delgado S, et al. Laparoscopy-assisted colectomy versus open colectomy for treatment of non-metastatic colon cancer: a randomised trial. *Lancet.* 2002;359(9325):2224-2229.
9. Nelson H, Sargent DJ, Wieand HS, et al. A comparison of laparoscopically assisted and open colectomy for colon cancer. *N Engl J Med.* 2004;350(20):2050-2059.
10. Guillou PJ, Quirke P, Thorpe H, et al. Short-term endpoints of conventional versus laparoscopic-assisted surgery in patients with colorectal cancer (MRC CLASICC trial): multicentre, randomised controlled trial. *Lancet.* 2005;365(9472):1718-1726.
11. Veldkamp R, Kuhry E, Hop WC, et al. Laparoscopic surgery versus open surgery for colon cancer: short-term outcomes of a randomised trial. *Lancet Oncol.* 2005;6(7):477-484.
12. Basse L, Jakobsen DH, Bardram L, et al. Functional recovery after open versus laparoscopic colonic resection: a randomized, blinded study. *Ann Surg.* 2005;241(3):416-423.
13. Braga M, Frasson M, Vignali A, Zuliani W, Civelli V, Di Carlo V. Laparoscopic vs. open colectomy in cancer patients: long-term complications, quality of life, and survival. *Dis Colon Rectum.* 2005;48(12):2217-2223.
14. Liang JT, Huang KC, Lai HS, Lee PH, Jeng YM. Oncologic results of laparoscopic versus conventional open surgery for stage II or III left-sided colon cancers: a randomized controlled trial. *Ann Surg Oncol.* 2007;14(1):109-117.
15. Hewett PJ, Allardyce RA, Bagshaw PF, et al. Short-term outcomes of the Australasian randomized clinical study comparing laparoscopic and conventional open surgical treatments for colon cancer: the ALCCaS trial. *Ann Surg.* 2008;245(5):728-738.
16. Braga M, Frasson M, Zuliani W, Vignali A, Pecorelli N, Di Carlo V. Randomized clinical trial of laparoscopic versus open left colonic resection. *Br J Surg.* 2010;97(8):1180-1186.
17. Waljee JF, Li L, Brummett CM, Englesbe MJ. Iatrogenic opioid dependence in the United States: are surgeons the gatekeepers? *Ann Surg.* 2017;265(4):728-730.
18. Fleshman J, Sargent DJ, Green E, et al. Laparoscopic colectomy for cancer is not inferior to open surgery based on 5-year data from the COST Study Group trial. *Ann Surg.* 2007;246(4):655-662 discussion 62-654.
19. Jayne DG, Guillou PJ, Thorpe H, et al. Randomized trial of laparoscopic assisted resection of colorectal carcinoma: 3-year results of the UK MRC CLASICC Trial Group. *J Clin Oncol.* 2007;25(21):3061-3068.
20. Jayne DG, Thorpe HC, Copeland J, Quirke P, Brown JM, Guillou PJ. Five-year follow-up of the Medical Research Council CLASICC trial of laparoscopically assisted versus open surgery for colorectal cancer. *Br J Surg.* 2010;97(11):1638-1645.
21. Taylor GW, Jayne DG, Brown SR, et al. Adhesions and incisional hernias following laparoscopic versus open surgery for colorectal cancer in the CLASICC trial. *Br J Surg.* 2010;97(1):70-78.
22. Green BL, Marshall HC, Collinson F, et al. Long-term follow-up of the Medical Research Council CLASICC trial of conventional versus laparoscopically assisted resection in colorectal cancer. *Br J Surg.* 2013;100(1):75-82.
23. Buunen M, Veldkamp R, Hop WC, et al. Survival after laparoscopic surgery versus open surgery for colon cancer: long-term outcome of a randomised clinical trial. *Lancet Oncol.* 2009;10(1):44-52.
24. Sholin J, Buunen M, Hop W, et al. Bowel obstruction after laparoscopic and open colon resection for cancer: results of 5 years of follow-up in a randomized trial. *Surg Endosc.* 2011;25(12):3755-3760.
25. Lacy AM, Delgado S, Castells A, et al. The long-term results of a randomized clinical trial of laparoscopy-assisted versus open surgery for colon cancer. *Ann Surg.* 2008;248(1):1-7.
26. Bartels SA, Vlug MS, Hollmann MW, et al. Small bowel obstruction, incisional hernia and survival after laparoscopic and open colonic resection (LAFA study). *Br J Surg.* 2014;101(9):1153-1159.
27. Weeks JC, Nelson H, Gelber S, Sargent D, Schroeder G, Clinical Outcomes of Surgery (COST) Study Group. Short-term quality-of-life outcomes following laparoscopic-assisted colectomy vs open colectomy for colon cancer: a randomized trial. *JAMA.* 2002;287(3):321-328.
28. Stucky CC, Pockaj BA, Novotny PJ, et al. Long-term follow-up and individual item analysis of quality of life assessments related to laparoscopic-assisted colectomy in the COST trial 93-46-53 (INT 0146). *Ann Surg Oncol.* 2011;18(9):2422-2431.
29. Basse L, Jakobsen DH, Bardram L, et al. Functional recovery after open versus laparoscopic colonic resection: a randomized blinded study. *Ann Surg.* 2005;241(3):416-423.
30. Janson M, Björholt I, Carlsson P, et al. Randomized clinical trial of the costs of open and laparoscopic surgery for colonic cancer. *Br J Surg.* 2004;91(4):409-417.
31. Marola S, Weber P, Wasielewski A, Ballantyne GH. Comparison of laparoscopic colectomy with and without the aid of a robotic camera holder. *Surg Laparosc Endosc Percutan Tech.* 2002;12(1):46-51.
32. Weber PA, Merola S, Wasielewski A, Ballantyne GH. Telerobotic-assisted laparoscopic right and sigmoid colectomies for benign disease. *Dis Colon Rectum.* 2002;45(12):1689-1694, discussion 1695-1696.
33. Bianchi PP, Ceriani C, Locatelli A, et al. Robotic versus laparoscopic total mesorectal excision for rectal cancer: a comparative analysis of oncological safety and short-term outcomes. *Surg Endosc.* 2010;24(11):2888-2894.

34. Allemann P, Duvoisin C, Di Mare L, Hübner M, Demartines N, Hahnloser D. Robotic-assisted surgery improves the quality of total mesorectal excision for rectal cancer compared to laparoscopy: results of a case-controlled analysis. *World J Surg.* 2016;40(4):1010-1016.

35. Ghezzi TL, Luca F, Valvo M, et al. Robotic versus open total mesorectal excision for rectal cancer: comparative study of short and long-term outcomes. *Eur J Surg Oncol.* 2014;40(9):1072-1079.

36. Collinson FJ, Jayne DG, Pigazzi A, et al. An international, multicentre, prospective, randomised, controlled, unblinded, parallel-group trial of robotic-assisted versus standard laparoscopic surgery for the curative treatment of rectal cancer. *Int J Colorectal Dis.* 2012;27(2):233-241.

37. Park JS, Choi GS, Park SY, Kim HJ, Ryuk JP. Randomized clinical trial of robot-assisted versus standard laparoscopic right colectomy. *Br J Surg.* 2012;99(9):1219-1226.

38. Merchant AM, Lin E. Single-incision laparoscopic right hemicolectomy for a colon mass. *Dis Colon Rectum.* 2009;52(5):1021-1024.

39. Law WL, Fan JK, Poon JT. Single incision laparoscopic left colectomy for carcinoma of distal transverse colon. *Colorectal Dis.* 2010;12(7):698-701.

40. Law WL, Fan JK, Poon JT. Single-incision laparoscopic colectomy: early experience. *Dis Colon Rectum.* 2010;53(3):284-288.

41. Huscher CG, Mingoli A, Sgarzini G, et al. Standard laparoscopic versus single-incision laparoscopic colectomy for cancer: early results of a randomized prospective study. *Am J Surg.* 2012;204(1):115-120.

42. Poon JT, Cheung CW, Fan JK, Lo OS, Law WL. Single-incision versus conventional laparoscopic colectomy for colonic neoplasm: a randomized, controlled trial. *Surg Endosc.* 2012;26(10):2729-2734.

43. Klein CA. Parallel progression of primary tumours and metastases. *Nat Rev Cancer.* 2009;9(4):302-312.

44. Søndenaa K, Quirke P, Hohenberger W, et al. The rationale behind complete mesocolic excision (CME) and a central vascular ligation for colon cancer in open and laparoscopic surgery: proceedings of a consensus conference. *Int J Colorectal Dis.* 2014;29(4):419-428.

45. Bertelsen CA, Neuenschwander AU, Jansen JE, et al. Disease-free survival after complete mesocolic excision compared with conventional colon cancer surgery: a retrospective, population-based study. *Lancet Oncol.* 2015;16(2):161-168.

46. Hohenberger W, Weber K, Matzel K, Papadopoulos T, Merkel S. Standardized surgery for colonic cancer: complete mesocolic excision and central ligation—technical notes and outcome. *Colorectal Dis.* 2009;11(4):354-364, discussion 364–355.

47. Bae SU, Saklani AP, Lim DR, et al. Laparoscopic-assisted versus open complete mesocolic excision and central vascular ligation for right-sided colon cancer. *Ann Surg Oncol.* 2014;21(7):2288-2294.

48. Kitano S, Inomata M, Mizusawa J, et al. Survival outcomes following laparoscopic versus open D3 dissection for stage II or III colon cancer (JCOG0404): a phase 3, randomised controlled trial. *Lancet Gastroenterol Hepatol.* 2017;2(4):261-268.

49. Cho MS, Baek SJ, Hur H, Soh Min B, Baik SH, Kyu Kim N. Modified complete mesocolic excision with central vascular ligation for the treatment of right-sided colon cancer: long-term outcomes and prognostic factors. *Ann Surg.* 2015;261(4):708-715.

50. Kim NK, Kim YW, Han YD, et al. Complete mesocolic excision and central vascular ligation for colon cancer: principle, anatomy, surgical technique, and outcomes. *Surg Oncol.* 2016;25(3):252-262.

Recurrent and Metastatic Colorectal Cancer

Kellie L. Mathis

There are approximately 40,000 new diagnoses of rectal cancer in the United States each year.[1] Developments such as total mesorectal excision (TME) and neoadjuvant chemoradiotherapy (NACXRT) as well as international guidelines have improved the prognosis of primary rectal cancer. But despite these advances, local recurrence after surgery remains a significant issue. Historically, local recurrence and metastatic disease signified an incurable condition, but there has increasingly been a shift from a palliative approach to a multimodal treatment approach with curative intent. Good outcomes from salvage surgery within a multidisciplinary approach have been demonstrated.

TUMOR RELAPSE

INCIDENCE OF RECURRENT DISEASE

In the modern series, the incidence of local recurrence after rectal cancer surgery ranges from 5% to 15%, and this number appears to be decreasing.[2,3] Approximately half of patients who present with locally recurrent rectal cancer (LRRC) will be considered candidates for curative resection. The likelihood of relapse was historically believed to be highest within the first 2 years after primary resection, but recent reports suggest that the median time to recurrence is increasing, especially for rectal cancers, and surveillance beyond 5 years may be necessary.[4]

Prior to the widespread adoption of TME technique, most recurrences were extraluminal in the lymph node bearing tissue. Now that TME is the standard of care, there is a higher percentage of intraluminal recurrences, up to 30% to 50% of recurrences in several published series,[5,6] as well as extraluminal recurrences, even in patients who were lymph node negative at the original operation.

FACTORS THAT INFLUENCE RECURRENCE

A large number of risk factors have been associated with relapses of colorectal cancer (Table 171.1).

Tumor Stage

The extent of disease, or tumor stage, is to date the single most important predictor of relapse and survival. The American Joint Committee on Cancer (AJCC) Colorectal Cancer Staging system is shown in Table 171.2. The risk of local recurrence is increased when the tumor has invaded beyond the confines of the bowel wall (T3 to T4 or involves nodes (N+) and is highest in patients with both.

Other Tumor Factors

Certain histologic features have been correlated with aggressive behavior, including poor tumor differentiation,

high tumor grade, mucin production, and venous, lymphatic, and perineural invasion. Involvement of the circumferential radial margin (CRM) is also prognostic for both colon and rectal carcinoma.[7] Other high-risk features include bowel obstruction, perforation, and tumor adherence to local organs.[8,9] A long disease-free interval between primary tumor resection and LRRC may also indicate more favorable tumor biology.

Molecular Features

High microsatellite instability phenotype which is present in approximately 20% of colorectal cancers, has been associated with an improved prognosis. Conversely, the presence of low microsatellite instability has been associated with a worse prognosis.[10,11]

Technical Factors

Technical factors also influence rates of local recurrence and overall survival. Local recurrence rates range from 4% to 40%, which is at least partially dependent on the individual operating surgeon. Some authors have shown increased local recurrence rates when tumors are in the distal rectum, possibly related to increased technical difficulty. At a minimum, it is vital that wide anatomic resection of the tumor in all dimensions (mesorectal, distal, circumferential, and en bloc resection of adherent organs) is achieved.

In 2000, a consensus panel was convened to discuss surgical guidelines for colon and rectal cancer to combine the best evidence to balance oncologic results with functional outcomes. In summary, all margins should be negative. For rectal cancers, a minimum distal margin of 2 cm is ideal and a margin of more than 1 mm is acceptable where the tumor is not locally advanced, after neoadjuvant therapy and abdominoperineal resection (APR) is the only alternative. Circumferential margins should be as wide as possible, ideally greater than 2 mm.[12]

Total mesorectal clearance should be routine. Sharp dissection should be performed in the areolar tissue behind the mesentery, just in front of the sacrum and particularly at the level of Waldeyer fascia. The fascia propria should be removed intact with proper rectal dissection. Therefore a TME is advised for all cancers of the distal rectum for which APR or low anterior resection and coloanal anastomosis are planned. In the management of more proximal rectal cancers, it seems reasonable to use a margin of approximately 5 cm of distal mesorectum as a benchmark, because tumor deposits in the mesorectum are rarely reported 4 cm beyond the tumor. Despite optimization of surgical techniques, adjuvant radiation treatment remains an independent factor for reducing the incidence of local relapse.[13]

TABLE 171.1 Factors Associated With a High Risk of Relapse for Colorectal Cancer

TUMOR FACTORS

Disease stage
High-grade tumor (poorly differentiated)
Tumor location (more distal)
Obstruction/perforation
Lymphovascular invasion
Perineural invasion
Mucin production
Diminished stromal immune reaction
Low microsatellite instability

TECHNICAL FACTORS

Inadequate resection margins (circumferential radial, distal, mesorectal)
Implantation of exfoliated cells
Anastomotic leak
Tumor location (tumors in pelvis and splenic flexure are anatomically and technically more difficult)

TABLE 171.2 American Joint Committee on Cancer TNM Cancer Staging for Colorectal Cancer, Seventh Edition

PRIMARY TUMOR (T)

TX primary tumor cannot be assessed
T0 no evidence of primary tumor
Tis carcinoma in situ: intraepithelial or invasion of lamina propria
T1 tumor invades submucosa
T2 tumor invades muscularis propria
T3 tumor invades through the muscularis propria into peri-colorectal tissues
T4a tumor penetrates to the surface of the visceral peritoneum
T4b tumor directly invades or is adherent to other organs or structures

REGIONAL LYMPH NODES (N)

NX regional lymph nodes cannot be assessed
N0 no regional lymph node metastasis
N1 metastasis in 1–3 regional lymph nodes
N1a metastasis in one regional lymph node
N1b metastasis in 2–3 regional lymph nodes
N1c tumor deposit(s) in the subserosa, mesentery, or nonperitonealized pericolic or perirectal tissues without regional nodal metastasis
N2 metastasis in 4 or more regional lymph nodes
N2a metastasis in 4–6 regional lymph nodes
N2b metastasis in 7 or more regional lymph nodes

DISTANT METASTASIS (M)

M0 no distant metastasis
M1 distant metastasis
M1a metastasis confined to one organ or site (e.g., liver, lung, ovary, nonregional node)
M1b metastases in more than one organ/site or the peritoneum

TNM, Tumor-node-metastasis.

Other Factors

Failure to administer neoadjuvant chemoradiation therapy (NACXRT) or postoperative adjuvant therapy, when it is indicated, is a risk factor for recurrence.

Routine clearance of the lateral pelvic sidewall lymph nodes during primary rectal cancer surgery is not standard in the United States due to the difficulty of the procedure and the associated sexual and urinary morbidity. When lateral lymph nodes are presumed positive before neoadjuvant therapy and then not removed, the risk of lateral compartment recurrence is increased.[14] The Japanese JCOG0212 trial randomized patients to TME with routine lateral compartment lymph node dissection versus TME alone for primary stage II–III rectal cancer, but survival results have not yet been reported.[15]

Anastomotic leak following primary surgery has been shown in some studies to be associated with LRRC but not distant recurrence.[16] Inadequate lymph node harvest may also be a risk factor, but this remains controversial as lymph node (LN) counts are often low following neoadjuvant therapy.[17]

DETECTION OF RELAPSE

Key to the detection of relapse is the implementation of surveillance guidelines. Detection of the recurrence is the first step and then confirmatory tests are used to delineate the extent of disease and the suitability for resection and adjuvant therapies. Historically, 90% of recurrences occur within the first 5 years, but Coco et al. found that when primary rectal cancer was treated with NACXRT, 30% of the LRRCs were found greater than 5 years later (while 90% of the distant metastases presented within 5 years).[13] Similar results have been reported by others.[19]

Surveillance Guidelines

A 2007 Cochrane review of eight randomized trials that investigated the impact of intensive surveillance strategies confirmed a significant survival advantage at 5 years in patients participating in more intensive surveillance after curative resection of colorectal cancer. Moreover, the group with more intensive follow-up had more frequent operations with curative intent as well. Additional meta-analyses of these trials have confirmed reduction in death rates and cost-effectiveness of intensive surveillance strategies in some cases.[20] Unfortunately, each of the surveillance strategies within the eight trials was unique, and it is not clear which specific component(s) of the proposed surveillance programs is most responsible for improving survival. Several cancer and specialty societies, including the American Society of Colon and Rectal Surgeons (ASCRS), the American Society of Clinical Oncology (ASCO), and the National Cancer Comprehensive Network (NCCN) have published guidelines for surveillance strategies. Each strategy is unique, but there are several generalities, including frequent physical examinations with serum carcinoembryonic antigen (CEA) measurement, at least annual chest and abdominal imaging for 3 to 5 years, and colonoscopy. Current ASCRS guidelines for surveillance after rectal cancer surgery include an office visit and CEA every 3 to 6 months for 2 years and then every 6 months until 5 years; computed tomography (CT) of the chest, abdomen, and pelvis annually for 5 years; colonoscopy 1 year after surgery and every 3 to 5 years thereafter; and proctoscopy every 6 to 12 months for patients with a rectal anastomosis.[21]

History and Physical Examination

Patients should be asked about pain (abdominal, pelvic, perineal), change in bowel habits, symptoms of obstruction, anorexia or weight loss, malaise, and bleeding or discharge. Physical examination should include abdomen, rectal and vaginal/perineal, and lymph node basins. The history and physical exam also provides valuable information on the general health status of the patient, which is vital in determining suitability for aggressive resection.

Laboratory and Imaging Studies

CEA is the only known tumor marker for colorectal cancer, and it is simple to obtain. It has been shown to be effective in detecting the presence of local and liver recurrences before the disease is clinically apparent. In a meta-analysis of 20 studies, the overall sensitivity and specificity of CEA for detecting colorectal cancer recurrence was 64% and 90%, respectively.[22]

The Cochrane review suggested a survival benefit in patients who underwent liver imaging with those who did not,[20] so routine CT scans of the abdomen and pelvis have been adopted by all societies.

Endoscopy

The aim of endoscopy is the detection of anastomotic recurrences and metachronous lesions, the latter being more common. Full colonoscopy is required to detect metachronous lesions, but the frequency of surveillance colonoscopies remains the subject of debate. For average-risk patients, a colonoscopy at 1 and 5 years seems the most common practice. ASCRS guidelines suggest colonoscopy at 3- to 5-year intervals.[21] For patients with genetic susceptibilities, the interval should be 1 to 2 years depending on the certainty and magnitude of the risk. Also, patients who did not receive a preoperative colonoscopy (because of emergency presentation and obstruction) should undergo colonoscopy as early as 3 to 6 months after resection.

For patients with rectal anastomoses, it is reasonable to perform more frequent examinations of the anastomosis using flexible sigmoidoscopy.

Positron Emission Tomography

Positron emission tomography (PET), an imaging modality based on the detection of 2-(^{18}F)-fluoro-2-deoxyglucose, is not recommended for routine use in colorectal cancer surveillance. PET may play a greater role as a confirmatory study in verifying the presence of a recurrence in the setting of a rising CEA or equivocal imaging studies. However, as discussed later a positive finding on PET scan is not equivalent to histology and is not sufficient evidence to proceed to surgical exploration. PET may also be used to confirm that metastases are limited to a single site prior to operative therapy, for example, prior to major liver resection.

Conclusion

The aim of any postoperative surveillance strategy should be early detection of resectable disease. These efforts should be focused on identifying tumors of favorable prognosis; sites of disease amenable to resection for cure (i.e., locoregional, hepatic, and pulmonary); and patients who are a good risk, vigorous and motivated who would be suitable for extensive resection.

LOCOREGIONAL RECURRENCE

This section focuses on LRRC, because the strategies for diagnosis and management of recurrent colon cancer can be similarly applied.

Patients with untreated LRRC live a median of 5 months. Symptoms are often debilitating and difficult to palliate, including pain, bleeding, and fistula drainage. Nonoperative therapy is not curative,[23] and radiation with or without chemotherapy but absent surgery can palliate symptoms and extend survival by only 12 to 14 months.[24] In contrast, complete resection of LRRC can be accomplished in some patients with mean survival times of 38 to 59 months and a 5-year overall survival rate of 30%.[25]

Patients with LRRC without demonstrable extrapelvic disease present a challenge because of the technical difficulty achieving adequate exposure and surgical access in the pelvis. These recurrences typically involve multiple organs and structures, which require extensive resection to achieve histologically negative margins. A number of factors must be carefully considered, including the overall health status of the patient, the status of extrapelvic disease, and the extent of the local recurrence.

Preoperative Evaluation and Patient Selection

A multidisciplinary team including at a minimum a colorectal surgeon, a radiation oncologist, and a medical oncologist is essential for planning and implementing care. Additional surgeons (e.g., urologist, gynecologic surgeon, orthopedic surgeon, and plastic surgeon) and other providers (e.g., enterostomal therapist and social worker) may also be required. Consideration should be given to discussion of the patient with LRRC at the local Tumor Board to obtain additional opinions and insight.

General Health

The patient must be informed of the extent and magnitude of the treatment plan. The ideal patient is motivated and understands the associated morbidities and potential impacts on quality of life (QOL) by radical surgery and adjuvant therapies. Medical, cardiac, and pulmonary clearance is essential.

Exclusion of Extrapelvic Disease

Once it is determined that the patient is suitable for surgery, the next step is to confirm that the LRRC is isolated. This requires a CT scan of the chest, abdomen, and pelvis. Any indeterminate or nondiagnostic liver disease seen on CT can be further characterized with ultrasound, magnetic resonance imaging (MRI), and/or PET scan. The identification of small indeterminate pulmonary nodules is common; PET can also be useful in these patients.

Evaluation of the Presence and Extent of Local Disease

Evaluation begins with a physical examination, particularly of the rectum and vagina, followed by endoscopy to determine the intraluminal extent and location. Histologic evidence may be obtained from a luminal or mucosal aspect of the recurrence, although this presentation is least common. Extraluminal lesions that are palpable through the perineum/rectum/vagina may be biopsied transrectally or transvaginally. All other tumors are generally amenable to biopsy with CT guidance. Occasionally, pelvic disease is suspected because of a rising CEA level with no obvious recurrence by imaging. In such situations, histologic proof should be sought prior to considering surgery. Exploratory pelvic surgery should be discouraged in the absence of imaging findings, because the CEA elevation could be due to extrapelvic disease or unrelated to LRRC. Furthermore, the only way to exclude a pelvic recurrence is to explore the entire pelvis down to the level of the pelvic floor, which is often an extraordinary task and even when possible, it is difficult to distinguish scar from tumor even using frozen-section histology. Some tumors produce nodular or discrete recurrences, whereas others can have ill-defined limits and be infiltrative or sheet-like in nature; the determination of borders and resectability can, accordingly, be difficult. Histologic evidence of recurrence and radiographic imaging suitable for defining the extent and boundaries of a pelvic recurrence are essential.

Imaging to determine resectability in the setting of LRRC is best done with MRI. MRI of the pelvis (high-resolution, phase-arrayed with reconstructions) read by an experienced radiologist has been shown in at least one study to have positive predictive value of 53% to 100% and negative predictive value of 93% to 100% when used to predict tumor invasion into local pelvic structures in LRRC. Agreement among interpreters was reasonable at 64% to 99%. As expected, interpretation of diffuse fibrosis was the most difficult.[26,27]

Resectability

Locoregional recurrences can extend anteriorly, posteriorly, laterally, or in a combination of directions. In addition, any of the organs in and around the pelvis may be involved, including intestinal, urologic, gynecologic, bony, and vascular structures. When assessing locoregional recurrences, two factors are important: fixation and anatomic location. The combination of these two factors determines resectability. Anteriorly fixed lesions may require a hysterectomy and/or a partial or complete cystectomy, and in lesions with posterior fixation, a sacrectomy may be necessary.

Some indicators predict that curative surgery with negative resection margins is not likely (Table 171.3). For example, unless there is infiltration of the trigone of the bladder at the insertion of the ureters to the bladder, bilateral ureteric obstruction usually indicates a bulky tumor that has invaded the lateral pelvic sidewalls. This indicates that disease is present at the level of the pelvic inlet, suggesting circumferential disease, and generally, the large circumferential tumor that extends to the pelvic sidewall, or a tumor with extensive lateral sidewall involvement alone, should be considered unresectable. For relapses that involve the sacrum, lesions that are central and distal to S2 can be removed with a distal sacrectomy. Nerve root involvement of S1 or S2 or evidence of invasion of the sacrum at the level of S1 and S2 typically indicates unresectable disease. Sacrectomy proximal to

TABLE 171.3 Relative Contraindications to Resection of Locally Recurrent Rectal Cancer

Extrapelvic disease (exception may be patient with resectable oligometastasis)
Predicted R2 resection margin
Sciatic pain
Bilateral ureteral obstruction (exception may be involvement of the trigone)
Circumferential or extensive pelvic sidewall involvement
Tumor extension through the greater sciatic notch
Tumor encasement of the common or external iliac vessels
S1 or S2 involvement (bony and/or neural)
Poor patient fitness and surgical risk (ASA classifications IV or V, rare ASA III)

ASA, American Society of Anesthesiologists.

S2 results in sacroiliac joint instability, and although it is technically feasible to internally fix this, it is not widely performed for cases of LRRC. Lesions above S2 and unilateral are occasionally treated with resection of the anterior sacral table. Some of these contraindications have been challenged.

Trimodality Therapy

The cornerstone of treatment for LRRC with a curative intent is surgery. However, surgery alone results in a high local and systemic failure rate. This has been the rationale for a multimodality approach to the treatment using neoadjuvant radiation therapy with concomitant chemotherapy, maximal resection for local control, and adjuvant chemotherapy to address the possibility of systemic failure.

Preoperative Radiation Therapy and Chemotherapy

Although it provides symptomatic relief, radiation therapy alone does not result in any significant chance of cure. When combined, radiation therapy and surgery reduce local recurrence rates and increase resectability.[13] Similarly, when used in the scenario of LRRC, radiation therapy has been shown to improve results. Chemoradiation is associated with better local control than radiation alone for primary rectal cancer[28] and chemotherapy added to radiation for re-irradiated patients with LRRC has been shown to be associated with improved survival.[29] As an added modality to avoid or reduce dose-related toxicity while improving local control, we combine external beam radiation therapy (EBRT) plus chemotherapy with intraoperative radiation therapy (IORT). IORT offers the advantages of tumor-directed therapy with limited normal tissue exposure and single-fraction, high biologic equivalence with improved local control in high-risk sites.

A full course of external beam radiation (5040 cGy) with protracted venous infusion 5-fluorouracil (5-FU) chemotherapy (225 mg/m^2 per 24 hours) or oral capecitabine is administered preoperatively to patients who have not had previous pelvic radiation. Patients who have received previous radiotherapy in the treatment of their primary tumor are treated again with 1000 to 3000 cGy of preoperative radiation plus 5-FU-based chemotherapy when possible. For patients receiving a full course of treatment with doses of approximately 5040 cGy, a 6- to 8-week rest period before surgery and IORT is standard. Restaging is performed before the procedure is undertaken with CT scans of the chest, abdomen, and pelvis.

The safety and feasibility of re-radiation to the pelvis has been established.[30,31] Susko et al. studied the toxicity associated with re-irradiation of the pelvis in the setting of LRRC in 33 patients; they found improvement in symptoms and low rates of toxicity and a high rate of R0 resection in the group that went on to surgery.[32] The use of multifield intensity modulated radiation therapy with three-dimensional (3D) conformal imaging to plan the treatment has improved the accuracy and reduced the toxicity of the use of re-irradiation.

Operative Procedures

It is imperative that the first step in planning for surgery of this magnitude includes an extensive discussion and explanation of the planned procedure with the patient and relatives. Sphincter-saving surgery is often not indicated in cases of LRRC but may be considered when adequate margins are achievable, there is no involvement of pelvic floor by tumor or fibrosis, and the patient has an anticipated reasonable functional outcome. The high risk of local recurrence after radical pelvic surgery makes sphincter-sparing reconstruction a difficult choice when the ultimate outcome is obstruction at the level of the pelvis.

Patients undergo a mechanical and antibiotic bowel preparation the night before surgery. At our institution, all patients with LRRCs are scheduled for surgery in a dedicated IORT suite. This suite houses the standard operating room equipment, a linear accelerator, and special anesthetic equipment that allows movement of the anesthetized patient from operating to radiating stations (Fig. 171.1). In addition, remote controls allow monitoring of the patient outside the suite in a lead-shielded room while radiation is delivered.

The patient is placed in the combined position. Special care is taken to ensure that the calves are not resting on the stirrups, because prolonged operating times can result in compartment syndrome or venous thrombosis.

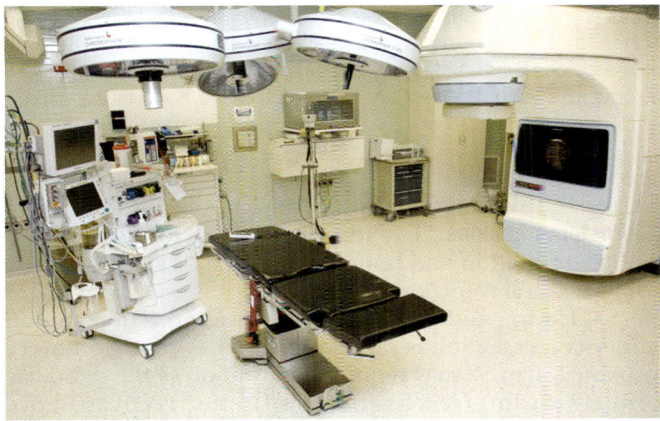

FIGURE 171.1 The intraoperative electron radiation therapy suite, showing the equipment, operating room table, and linear accelerator.

Nearly all patients receive ureteral stents. On occasion, direct bladder invasion is detected cystoscopically; this information can help guide the extent of surgery. No. 5 French ureteral stents are inserted using the 30-degree cystoscope, and these are secured to a Foley catheter.

A lower midline incision is used to provide optimal pelvic exposure and to facilitate the possible use of rectus abdominis myocutaneous flap. Care is exercised to preserve the inferior epigastric vessels when it is anticipated that a transpelvic rectus abdominis flap may be used. Exploration includes an examination of the liver, peritoneum, omentum, ovaries, retroperitoneum, and wound to confirm the absence of extrapelvic disease, because this would contraindicate radical resection. Very rarely, exceptions may be made in very young patients who have limited pelvic and liver disease where the pelvic recurrence and liver metastases are each synchronously resected for curative potential (R0). We use a self-retaining ring retractor. After adhesiolysis, the small bowel is packed superiorly for pelvic exposure. Because these operations are lengthy, care must be taken to avoid pressure from a retractor on the retroperitoneal/pelvic tissues; femoral nerve injuries have been described, implicating prolonged retractor pressure as a causative factor. Because pelvic fibrosis is the rule, the dissection starts at the bifurcation of the aorta so a safe fascial plane is found to guide the posterior dissection down to the pelvic floor (Fig 171.2A). The iliac arteries and veins are coursed from the aorta and cava to the branching of the internal and external branches. Below the common and external branches of the iliac arteries, the vessels can be ligated without concern for ischemia. Knowledge of the location of these vessels prevents most of the risk for exsanguination and the need for vascular bypass, and it facilitates identification of the safest posterior and lateral planes. Similarly, the ureters are identified from the pelvic brim and followed by anterior dissection to the level of their insertion into the bladder. It is usually necessary to trace the ureters right to their insertion into the bladder so the lateral dissection can be performed safely. Ureter dissection is more extensive when a cystectomy or sacrectomy is contemplated; it is essential for the construction of an ileal conduit and for the prevention of injury during the posterior dissection, respectively.

Fig. 171.3A–F shows examples of LRRC by areas of fixation.

Central Nonfixed Lesions. A central recurrence after a local excision or low anterior resection may require nothing more than a completion APR. The main difference between this and the standard APR is the added difficulty in dissection due to fibrosis and postoperative changes in anatomy. Distinction between fibrosis and tumor infiltration is difficult at best. In such circumstances, particularly when it occurs outside the realm of planned resection (sacral promontory and lateral pelvic sidewalls), frozen-section histology should be performed. If tumor cells are seen within the samples of diffuse or extensive "fibrosis," complete resection with negative margins is not feasible.

Anterior Lesions. Anterior lesions demonstrate the greatest diversity between men and women. In women, anterior fixation may require little more than en bloc resection

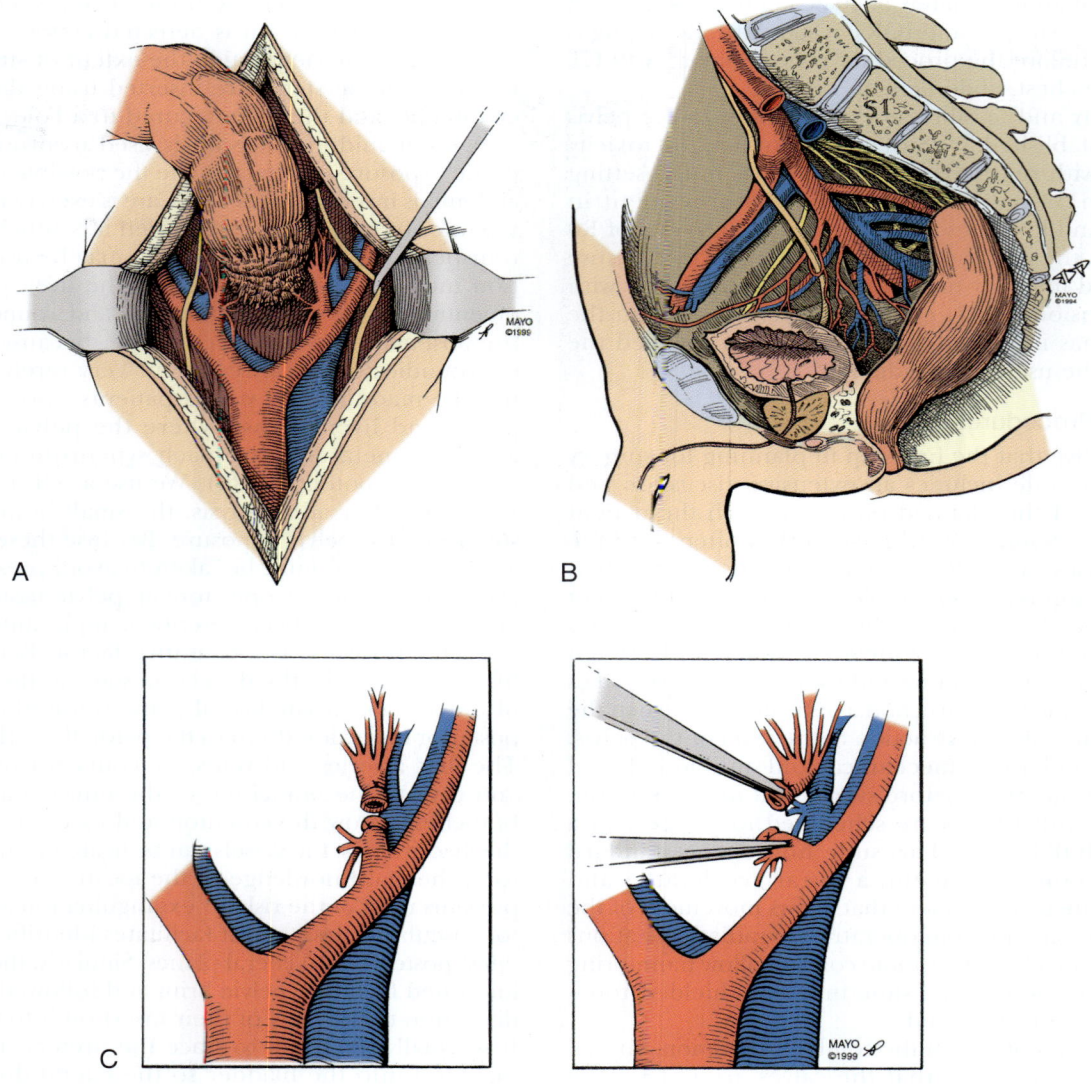

FIGURE 171.2 (A) Broad view of pelvic dissection. The iliac vessels are dissected from the level of the aortic bifurcation to at least the origin of the internal iliac branches. The ureters are located and followed from the pelvic brim to their insertion into the bladder. Once the vessels and ureters are located, it is safe to proceed with the posterior dissection, commencing at the sacral promontory. (B) Anterior approach (operative anatomy of pelvic structures). The anterior procedure provides assurance that no extrapelvic disease is present and provides several preparatory steps for the sacral resection, including anterior and lateral dissection, proximal sacral margin delineation, parasacral vascular ligation, gastrointestinal and/or urinary stoma formation, and omental or rectus abdominis flap creation. (C) Bilateral internal iliac artery and vein ligation is performed if sacral transection proximal to S3–S4 is expected. The artery typically must be ligated and divided to provide exposure to the internal iliac vein. The vein can be ligated without transection. (Copyright Mayo Foundation, 1999.)

of the rectum, uterus, and posterior wall of the vagina. In contrast, anterior fixation in a narrow male pelvis is more likely to require cystectomy or cystoprostatectomy. Caution should be exercised for lesions that are directly invading the trigone or prostate, because these are often circumferential and "after the fact" found not to be resectable for cure. Pelvic MRI or PET-CT fusion studies show promise for better delineation of tumor extent in these cases.

For anterior lesions, partial cystectomy may be sufficient in some cases to accomplish negative margins. However, it may be preferable to perform total cystectomy and ileal conduit for heavily irradiated bladders where tissues are unlikely to allow for proper healing and acceptable postoperative functional results.

Posterior Lesions. The ideal procedure for tumors with posterior fixation and bone involvement is a distal sacrectomy. If sacral resection is considered it should be distal to S2–S3. Having said that, true sacral invasion is uncommon and sacral resection is rarely indicated. A resection more proximal than S2 may require stabilization of the sacroiliac joints with internal fixation and other reconstructive methods and is rarely indicated. Furthermore, by limiting the resection to the S2–S3 level, the preservation of one S3 root is generally possible. This is usually sufficient to preserve bladder function.

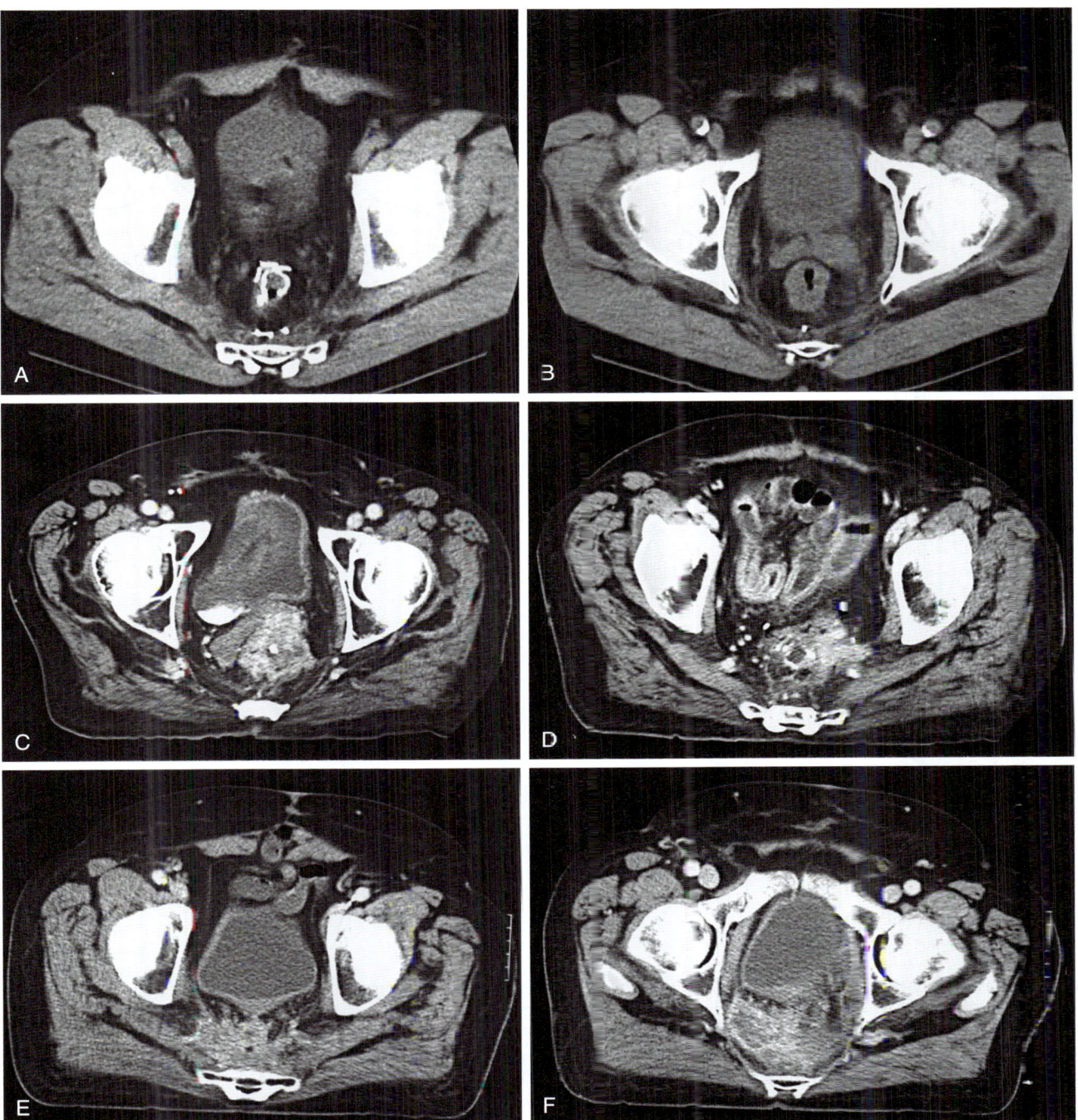

FIGURE 171.3 Classification of local recurrence according to fixation. (A and B) Examples of no fixation (FO). (A) The stapled low anterior anastomosis is easily visualized on CT scan. (B) Distal to the anastomosis is a perianastomotic recurrence; there is no evidence of fixation to local organs or structures. Complete resection with negative margins would be anticipated. (C and D) Examples of fixed resectable (FR). (C) Single-site fixation to anterior structures such as the bladder, as illustrated, or gynecologic structures can typically be resected with negative margins. (D) Lateral pelvic sidewall fixation can be resected, but margins will often be close or microscopically positive. (E and F) Examples of fixed and not resectable (FNR). These two images from the same patient illustrate posterior fixation (E) and anterior fixation (F) in addition to lateral sidewall involvement, rendering this recurrence unresectable.

Distal sacrectomy consists of four stages: (1) the anterior resection procedures, (2) the posterior resection procedures, (3) IORT, and (4) pelvic reconstruction. Anterior procedures are performed with the patient in the lithotomy position. As described earlier, to minimize the

risk of inadvertent injury due to anatomic displacement, dissection of the ureters and iliac vessels begins at the level of the aortic bifurcation (see Fig. 171.2A and B) and progresses deep into the pelvis. The posterior plane is generally the safest place to begin but is limited to the

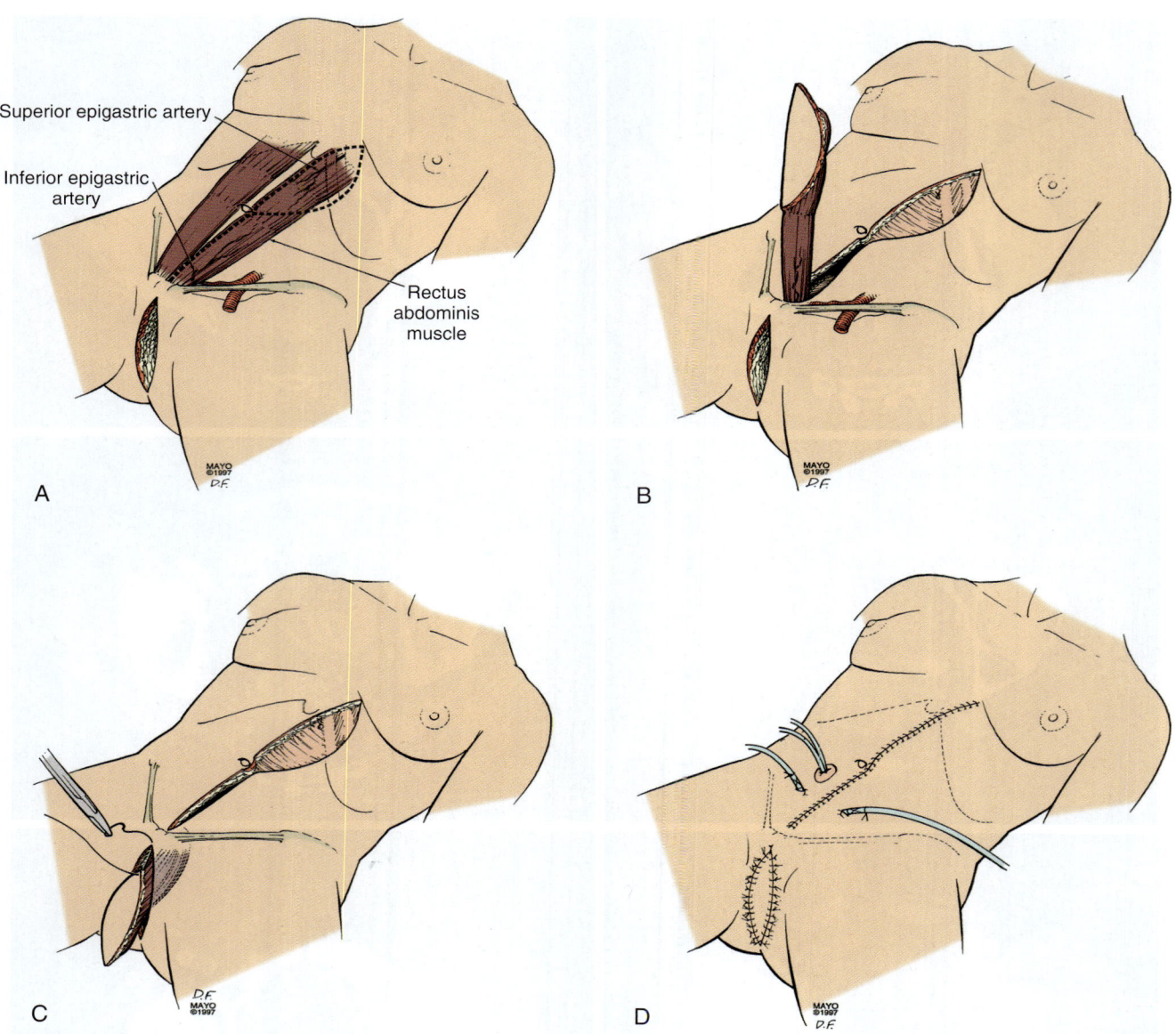

FIGURE 171.4 Rectus abdominis myocutaneous flap pelvic closure. This series of drawings illustrates the perineal positioning of a rectus flap. The same technique is used for sacrectomy wounds—only that the flap is left in the pelvis at the end of the anterior (abdominal) procedures and pulled through the posterior defect and sutured after the sacrectomy and intraoperative electron radiation therapy are completed. (A) Once perineal resection is complete, the skin paddle is designed to match the size of the defect. The harvest site for the skin paddle is determined based on the direct perforators from the underlying rectus abdominis muscle. (B) The myocutaneous flap and associated skin paddle are raised and include the anterior fascia of the rectus sheath. The blood supply is provided by the inferior epigastric artery. (C) The flap is delivered through the pelvis to the perineal defect. Care is taken to avoid stretching or torsion on the inferior epigastric blood supply. (D) The skin paddle is secured with interrupted sutures, and the abdominal fascia and skin are reapproximated. (Copyright Mayo Foundation, 1997.)

level of the tumor. Anterior and lateral resection planes are dissected with adherent organs, and structures are removed en bloc leaving the tumor attached only to the sacrum posteriorly. A frozen-section biopsy at the level of posterior fixation ensures that a negative sacral margin is achievable. The top of the sacral resection margin is scored, a maneuver that facilitates identification of the level of posterior sacral transection. The internal iliac artery and veins are ligated bilaterally if sacral transection proximal to S3–S4 is anticipated (see Fig. 171.2C); this reduces blood

loss during sacrectomy. Either an omental or a rectus abdominis flap (Fig. 171.4) is mobilized and transposed into the pelvis for subsequent retrieval and reconstruction during the posterior procedure. The gastrointestinal or urinary stomas are fashioned before closure of the abdomen. This completes the anterior procedures.

On the same day or as a planned procedure for the next operative day, the patient is repositioned prone, and a posterior midline incision is made over the lower lumbars and sacrum to the coccyx. If sacrectomy is performed

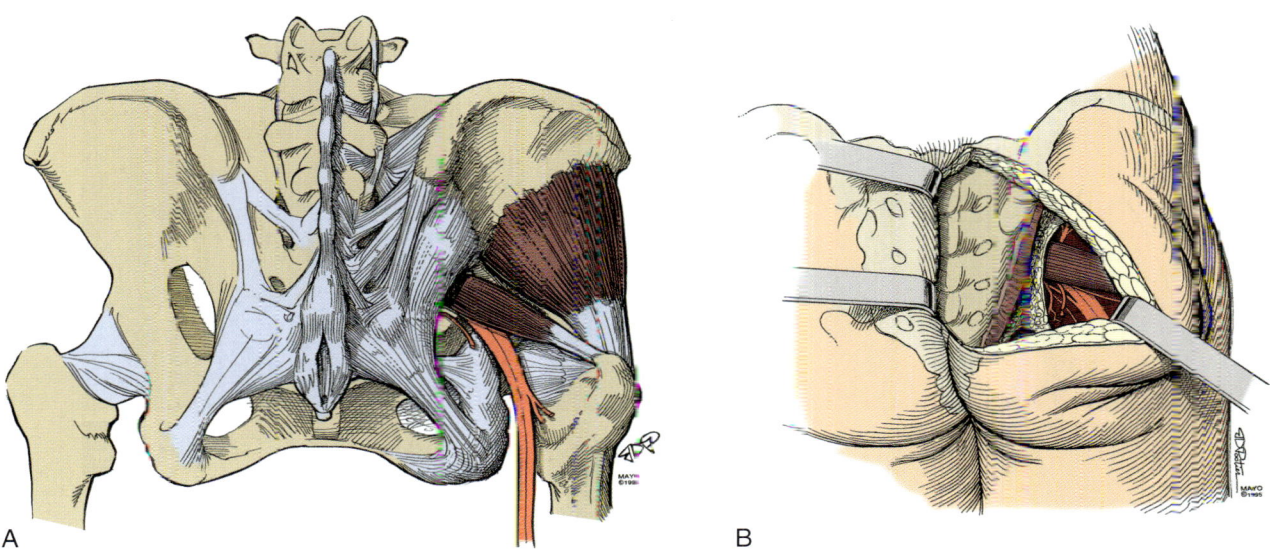

FIGURE 171.5 Operative techniques, posterior approach showing (A) anatomic relationships and (B) operative anatomy. To remove the sacral tumor posteriorly, the gluteus must be dissected from the sacrum, and the sciatic nerve identified. The sacrotuberous and sacrospinous ligaments, piriformis muscle, and endopelvic fascia are divided, and then the dural sac is ligated and sacrum transected. (Copyright Mayo Foundation, 1994.)

simultaneous with APR en bloc, then the elliptical anal excision is incorporated with the proximal sacrum incision. The gluteus is dissected to expose the entire sacrum. This exposure facilitates the division of the sacrotuberous and sacrospinous ligaments (Fig. 171.5A). With care taken to protect the sciatic and pudendal nerves, the piriformis muscle is divided (see Fig. 171.5B). Division of this muscle allows the endopelvic fascia to be entered. Once the pelvic floor is opened, palpation from behind allows identification of the level of sacral transection as previously determined by frozen sections that confirmed the absence of tumor. The orthopedic surgeon next performs the laminectomy, dural sac ligation, and bony transection. The pelvic surgeon assists in completing the lateral pelvic sidewall dissection, taking care to protect the ureters, bladder, and urethra. Intraoperative irradiation, as described later, is performed next, followed by wound closure with or without flap reconstruction.

High sacrectomy has been described at our institution[33] in addition to other institutions.[25,34–36] A subcortical sacrectomy has also been described when the sacral invasion is superficial.[37]

Lateral Lesions. Lesions that are fixed laterally are approached the same way with proximal control of the ureters and iliac vessels. A ureteric resection is often necessary and expected preoperatively. The internal iliac vessels may be ligated on the side of the tumor to decrease vascularity. The obturator nerve should be preserved when possible.

Intraoperative Delivery of Electron Beam Radiation Therapy

Once the specimen is resected, it is reviewed by the pathologist, surgeon, and radiation oncologist to determine margins and the need for IORT. As indicated, additional biopsies may be required to define sites of marginal resection. When IORT is required, a Lucite applicator is positioned in the pelvis to target the tissues at risk (Fig. 171.6). The applicator is selected for size (typically 5 to 8 cm in diameter) and shape (typically circular and 30 degrees beveled). The patient is then positioned under the linear accelerator. Between 1000 and 2000 cGy is delivered depending on the extent of margin involvement and the dose of preoperative EBRT. If full-dose preoperative EBRT of 5040 cGy was achieved, a dose of 1000 to 1250 cGy is recommended for R0 (clear margins) or R1 (microscopic residual disease) margins and 1500 to 2000 cGy for R2 (gross residual disease) margins. These single-dose radiation treatments are biologically equivalent to 1.5 to 2.5 times the same quantity of EBRT fractions.[38] If the preoperative EBRT dose was limited because of prior EBRT, the IORT dose ranges from 1500 to 2000 cGy to account for some of the dose that could not be delivered with EBRT. IORT doses of less than 1250 cGy are less likely to cause long-term side effects such as motor and sensory neuropathies but usually are not feasible in retreatment situations.

Perineal Wound Closure

Because the residual defects are generally sizable and the tissue quality poor because of prior irradiation, flaps are usually required to partition the pelvis, obliterate the dead space, and deliver nonirradiated, vascularized, well-oxygenated tissues to the area. Perineal wound complication rates as high as 41% have been reported after EBRT and APR.[39] If the omentum is not of suitable size or consistency, the vertical rectus abdominis myocutaneous (VRAM) flap is preferred, especially for sacrectomy wounds (see Fig. 171.4).[40] The rectus is versatile and can be used to reconstruct a narrowed or shortened vagina after extensive resection; a vaginal tube can be constructed from a spiral configuration of the rectus attached to a short

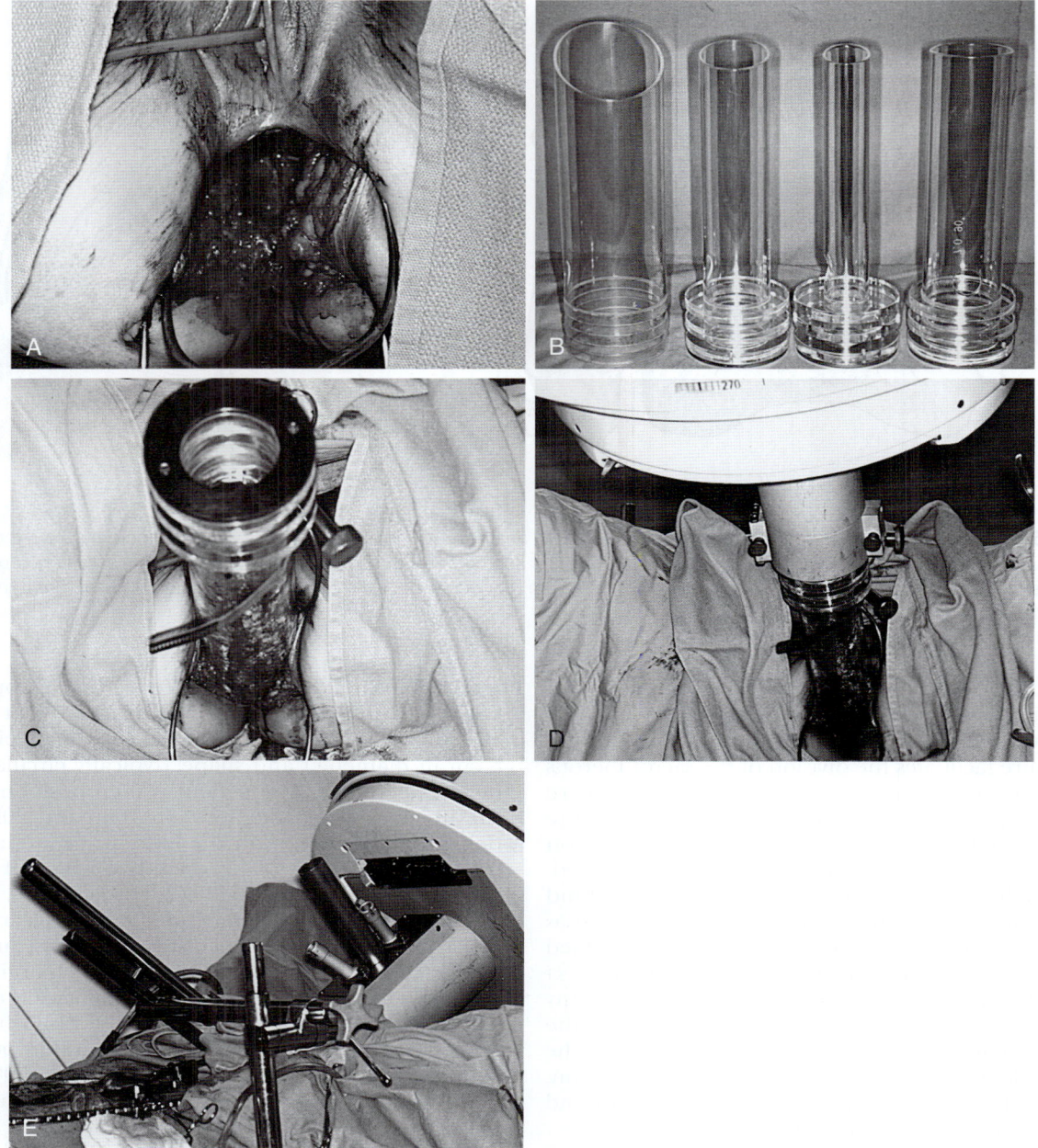

FIGURE 171.6 Intraoperative delivery of radiation therapy. (A) Once the tumor is resected, the pathologist, surgeon, and radiation oncologist examine the closest margins and determine the site and extent of tumor bed risk. Sites of recurrence deep in the pelvis are often best approached with a perineal port for radiation therapy. (B) A Lucite applicator is selected to fit the surgical field at risk for failure of local control. Several sizes and shapes are available with varying degrees of bevel to accommodate the field of radiation. (C to E) The applicator is placed into the field, stabilized to the operating table, and connected to the linear accelerator.

cuff at the introitus or from a folded flap reconstructing the anterior or posterior defects. Sexual function can be acceptable after flap-vaginal reconstruction.[41] Patients undergoing VRAM reconstruction have fewer wound complications (abscess, wound dehiscence) than those undergoing primary closure or thigh flaps. Abdominal wall complications are rare after VRAM harvest.[42] Vastus lateralis muscle flaps have also been described when a VRAM is not available.[43]

RESULTS OF TRIMODALITY TREATMENT FOR LOCALLY RECURRENT DISEASE

In the largest experience with long-term follow-up reported to date, 607 patients with LRRCs were treated at our institution between 1981 and 2008 with the multimodality approach we have described. All patients underwent maximal resection with the administration of IORT. The margins were histologically negative (R0) in 227 cases

(37%), microscopically positive (R1) in 224 patients (37%), and grossly involved (R2) in 156 (26%). Follow-up was complete until death or for a median of 44 months for the 194 surviving patients. At multivariable analysis, only treatment era (better survival for more recently treated patients), no prior chemotherapy, and margin status (R0 better than R1 better than R2) were statistically significant.[25]

Morbidity

In the Haddock et al. series, 30-day mortality occurred in one patient (0.2%), and five additional patients (0.8%) died from treatment-related complications within 3 to 22 months of surgery. Overall morbidity (combining short- and long-term throughout follow-up period) was 50%. The most frequent causes of morbidity were wound-related complications in 20% of patients, gastrointestinal obstruction or fistula in 14%, ureteral obstruction in 10%, and peripheral neuropathy in 7%.[25]

Additional reports of patients undergoing similar multimodality therapy for recurrent rectal cancers describe rates of short-term morbidity (17% to 100%) and mortality (0% to 3%).[44,45]

Cancer Outcomes

In the study by Haddock et al., the median survival was 36 months, and the 5- and 10-year survival estimates were 30% and 16%, respectively. Patients undergoing potentially curative resection (R0) had longer 5-year overall survival compared with patients with residual disease (R1 and R2). Central relapse (within the IORT field) occurred in only 14% of patients at 5 years. Local relapse within the external beam radiation field was observed in 28% of patients at 5 years, and distant relapse had occurred in 53% by 5 years. All forms of relapse were more common in patients with subtotal resection (R1 and R2) than in patients with R0 resection.[25] Although the highly selected use of IORT precludes definitive conclusions regarding its specific contribution to cancer outcomes, the encouraging cancer outcomes in this series of patients support its continued use.

You et al. described results from 229 patients undergoing salvage surgery for LRRC. IORT was given to 36% for margins less than 2 mm or R1 margins. An R0 resection was accomplished in 80%. Overall survival at 3 and 5 years was 62% and 42%, respectively; disease-free survival at 3 and 5 years was 67% and 47%, respectively. Independent predictors of decreased overall survival were R1 resection margin and secondary failure, which occurred in 55% of patients at a median of 19 months.[46]

In almost all studies reported, margin status is the greatest predictor of outcome. This highlights the importance of obtaining a negative margin when possible and adding IORT when margins are close or positive.[47] The degree of R0 is also relevant. Alberda et al. found that when the tumor-free margin was greater than 2 mm as compared with 0 to 2 mm, the 5-year local recurrence rate was 80% versus 62% and overall survival was 60% versus 37%. A close R0 was still better than a positive margin with R1 resections having a 16% overall survival and R2 resections only 5%.[48]

Tanis et al. performed a systematic review of 3767 patients within 55 cohort studies undergoing curative attempts for LRRC. They found a lot of variability in neoadjuvant treatment with the use of radiation ranging from 12% to 100% between series. Overall, R0 resection rate was 56% and 5-year overall survival (OS) was 25% to 41%. Survival improved over time within the entire cohort.[49]

Table 171-1 highlights the series in the literature with at least 70 patients undergoing multimodality therapy for LRRC.

Quality of Life

You et al. performed a QOL assessment in 105 patients treated for LRRC (59% curative surgery, 12% noncurative surgery, and 28% nonsurgical management). Baseline pain at presentation was predictive of overall survival and the pain persisted among most long-term survivors.[61] Another report studied QOL among 75 patients undergoing pelvic exenteration (for both primary and recurrent rectal cancer). They found that long-term survivors had comparable mental component summary scores to the general population; physical component scores were decreased.[62] Dozois et al. reported that 89% of patients after high sacrectomy could ambulate independently or with the assistance of a walking aid.[33]

Surveillance After Trimodality Treatment

Guidelines are scarce for surveillance after curative treatment of LRRC. The TME Collaborative is a consensus document with 51 summary statements about the management of primary and recurrent rectal cancer. This document suggests that, at a minimum, patients should undergo an annual pelvic MRI and annual CT scans of the chest, abdomen, and pelvis and serial serum CEA.[63]

RE-RECURRENT RECTAL CANCER

Additional salvage procedures for locally re-recurrent rectal cancer in highly selected patients have been described.[46,64,65]

LOCALLY RECURRENT COLON CARCINOMA

It is estimated that approximately 10% to 20% of patients with resected colon cancer present with an isolated locoregional recurrence amenable to surgical resection. The role of multimodality treatment for this specific indication is not considered as standard of care. However, in one study of 73 patients with locally recurrent colon carcinoma treated with a combination of chemotherapy, EBRT, and surgical excision followed by IORT, there was a 5-year survival of 24.7% (R0 resection, 37.4%).[66] Although this specific treatment strategy and, in particular, the use of IORT cannot be easily applied on a widespread basis, these data demonstrate again the validity of an aggressive approach to treat locally recurrent colon carcinoma in select patients.

SUMMARY

Patients who otherwise enjoy good health and who present with isolated LRRCs may be candidates for trimodality therapy with EBRT, chemotherapy (concomitant with EBRT and maintenance following resection), repeat resection, and IORT. The possibility of cure and the extent of resection, including anterior and posterior exenteration, are determined by the anatomic location and degree of

TABLE 171.4 Published Series (With >70 Patients) Reporting Multidisciplinary Surgical Management of Locally Recurrent Rectal Cancer

References	No. Patients	% Receiving Intraoperative Radiation Therapy	% With R0 Resection	Follow-up Time (Months)	5-Year Local Recurrence Rate	5-Year Disease-Free Survival	5-Year Overall Survival	RFs for Decreased Overall Survival	MVA FOR DISEASE-FREE SURVIVAL RFs for Decreased Disease-Free Survival
Haddock et al.[25]	607	100	37	44	62		30	Prior chemotherapy Earlier timeframe of the study Margin positive	NR
Harris et al.[50]	533	100	59				28	Lack of preoperative chemotherapy and radiation	NR
You et al.[46]	229	36	80			47	42	Margin positive Recurrence	NR
Kusters et al.[51]	170	98	54	35	46		41*	Posterior tumor location	NR
Dresen et al.[8]	147	100	57		54	34	32	Margin positive Lack of EBRT	Lack of EBRT
Wiig et al.[52]	107	55	41	43	48		30	Margin positive	NR
Salo et al.[53]	103	52	69	23			24	Elevated CEA Recurrence beyond the bowel	NR
Kanemitsu et al.[54]	101	18	60		35		32*	NR	Upper sacral/lateral invasive type Extrapelvic disease Hydronephrosis High-grade lymphatic or venous invasion of the primary tumor
Shoup et al.[55]	100	100	64	23			39	Margin positive Vascular invasion	Margin positive Vascular invasion
Roeder et al.[56]	97	54	37	51	59		30	Margin positive	Margin positive
Rahbari et al.[57]	92	68	59	23	25		47*	APR or exenteration	NR
Bedrosian et al.[58]	85	44	76	43	49		36	Elevated CEA Margin positive	NR
Martinez-Monge et al.[59]	80	100	0	48	74		6	Lack of postoperative EBRT Margin positive	NR
Sole et al.[60]	143 (rectal CA = 72)	100	100	48	53	44	46	Margin positive Disease-free interval <24 months High-grade tumor	Lack of EBRT Margin positive Disease-free interval <24 months Fragmentation of the surgical specimen

*Indicates cancer-specific survival.

APR, Abdominoperineal resection; *CA,* cancer; *CEA,* carcinoembryonic antigen; *DFS,* disease-free survival; *EBRT,* external beam radiation therapy; *IORT,* intraoperative radiation therapy; *LRRC,* locally recurrent rectal cancer; *MVA,* multivariable analysis; *NR,* not reported; *OS,* overall survival; *R0,* negative resection margin.

tumor fixation. When achievable with negative margins or microscopic residual disease, the use of resection and trimodality therapy that includes IORT is associated with reasonable 5-year survival rates and acceptable morbidity.

PULMONARY METASTASIS

The liver is the most common site of colorectal metastasis, and the management of hepatic lesions is discussed separately. The lung is the second most common site of colorectal cancer metastasis. Less than 10% of patients with pulmonary metastases have disease isolated to the lungs and only 2% of patients with colorectal lung metastases are candidates for metastasectomy. The basic management is described here. In general, favorable outcomes can be anticipated when lesions are isolated or in only one lung lobe and can be completely resected in an otherwise healthy individual. Patients with low-volume disease may have favorable tumor biology.

PATIENT SELECTION

No formal guidelines exist regarding pulmonary surveillance after resection of colorectal carcinoma. A CT scan of the thorax is necessary to evaluate the resectability of the lesion and to detect other smaller lesions, and a metastatic work-up with PET scan should be done to exclude extrathoracic lesions. General guidelines for pulmonary resection for metastatic disease include the following: disease should be limited, preferably three or fewer lesions, all less than 3 cm; all disease must be amenable to complete resection; and patients must be in good health with good pulmonary function and pulmonary reserve. Additionally, there should be no extrathoracic disease with the exception of maybe limited hepatic metastases and the primary site should be controlled.

RESULTS OF PULMONARY RESECTION

Pulmonary resection for metastasis can be performed with low mortality[67,68] and high success rates, with contemporary 5-year survival rates in the range of 50%.[69,70] Analogous to hepatic metastases, there is an inverse relationship between the number of metastases and survival outcomes.[69] Other prognostic factors include maximal size of the largest lesion,[71] mediastinal or thoracic lymph node involvement,[69] disease-free interval,[72] and prethoracotomy CEA level.[71] In the Mayo Clinic series of 139 patients, 71% had solitary lesions. The authors reported an operative mortality rate of 1.4%, a 5-year survival rate of 31%, and a 20-year survival rate of 16%.[67] In the report by Onaitis et al., there was no difference in oncologic outcomes between those treated with thoracoscopic procedures versus standard thoracotomy.[73] The role of adjuvant therapy after resection of pulmonary metastasis is not established, because there is no evidence that systemic therapies reduce the high risk of subsequent relapse in these patients. Guerrera et al. found that patients with multiple metastases (>3) had improved survival with the addition of adjuvant therapy.[39] Repeat resection of recurrent pulmonary metastasis has been described, with survival being very similar to that for the first resection.[69,74] Nonsurgical options include radiofrequency ablation and stereotactic ablative radiotherapy (SABR).

ISOLATED METASTASES—OTHER SITES

The bone and brain are much less often involved with focal metastatic lesions. These lesions typically manifest in the setting of diffuse disease and are rarely curable. Bone metastases are usually treated with internal fixation as required for stabilization and irradiation for palliation of pain and to control disease. In cases of solitary brain metastases in a nonvital region, resection and postoperative irradiation are reasonable. When surgical resection is not indicated, steroids plus irradiation serve to palliate the process.

Peritoneal carcinomatosis is present in approximately 10% of patients presenting with colorectal cancer, and median survival is 7 months.[75] It was previously considered to be an incurable disease and treated with palliative therapies only. In the last decade, cytoreductive surgery followed by hyperthermic intraperitoneal chemotherapy (HIPEC) has been used with some success. A phase III randomized trial comparing maximal cytoreductive surgery and HIPEC to systemic chemotherapy with palliative surgery for colorectal cancer with peritoneal carcinomatosis showed improved survival in the HIPEC group (median survival, 22.3 vs. 12.6 months).[76] The United States Military Cancer Institute in conjunction with the American College of Surgeons Oncology Group is conducting a phase III protocol comparing overall survival in patients with peritoneal carcinomatosis from colorectal cancer undergoing either cytoreductive surgery with HIPEC versus systemic chemotherapy. The Dutch Colorectal Cancer Group is also performing a randomized trial of patients with T4 or perforated colorectal cancers (without obvious carcinomatosis). Patients will be randomized to standard care (surgery with systemic adjuvant chemotherapy) versus surgery with adjuvant HIPEC followed by adjuvant systemic chemotherapy. They anticipate a reduction in the absolute risk of carcinomatosis from 25% with standard treatment to 0% with the addition of HIPEC.[77]

DIFFUSE METASTASES

In the presence of diffuse disease, no curative options are available. However, the importance and complexity of palliative therapies should not be overlooked or underestimated. Management should be refocused toward the short-term goals of improving QOL and prolonging life where appropriate. Toward the end of life, the physician should facilitate the family and individual in coping with chronic illness and the concept of death while alleviating disabling symptoms.

CONCLUSION

Colorectal cancer relapse, although often complex in presentation, can best be considered and categorized as resectable for a possible cure. Where the former is possible, long-term survival can be achieved, specifically for isolated lesions in the liver, lungs, and locoregional sites. For relapses in local and regional sites, results appear to be improved with the use of a multispecialty approach, including EBRT plus concomitant 5-FU-based chemotherapy (even in previously irradiated patients), in addition to maximal resection and IORT. This approach can be done safely and can lead to long-term disease-free and overall survival. These results may be further enhanced by the introduction of new systemic adjuvant therapies with different mechanisms of actions that are aimed at reducing the risk of systemic failure. When re-recurrence occurs, salvage may be possible. R0 resection remains the primary determinant of outcome. When presented with cases of diffuse disease, clinical efforts should not be abandoned but rather refocused on improving QOL.

REFERENCES

1. Siegel RL, Miller KD, Jemal A. Cancer statistics, 2015. *CA Cancer J Clin.* 2015;65:5-29.
2. Bakx R, Visser O, Josso J, Meijer S, Slors JF, van Lanschot JJ. Management of recurrent rectal cancer: a population based study in greater Amsterdam. *World J Gastroenterol.* 2008;14:6018-6023.
3. Palmer G, Martling A, Cedermark B, Holm T. A population-based study on the management and outcome in patients with locally recurrent rectal cancer. *Ann Surg Oncol.* 2007;14:447-454.
4. Platell CF. Changing patterns of recurrence after treatment for colorectal cancer. *Int J Colorectal Dis.* 2007;22:1223-1231.
5. Park JK, Kim YW, Hur H, et al. Prognostic factors affecting oncologic outcomes in patients with locally recurrent rectal cancer: impact of patterns of pelvic recurrence on curative resection. *Langenbecks Arch Surg.* 2009;394:71-77.
6. Klose J, Tarantino I, Schmidt T, et al. Impact of anatomic location on locally recurrent rectal cancer: superior outcome for intraluminal tumour recurrence. *J Gastrointest Surg.* 2015;19:1123-1131.
7. Porter GA, Soskolne CL, Yakimets WW, Newman SC. Surgeon-related factors and outcome in rectal cancer. *Ann Surg.* 1998;227:157-167.
8. Dresen RC, Gosens MJ, Martijn H, et al. Radical resection after IORT-containing multimodality treatment is the most important determinant for outcome in patients treated for locally recurrent rectal cancer. *Ann Surg Oncol.* 2008;15:1937-1947.
9. Stocchi L, Nelson H, Sargent DJ, et al. Impact of surgical and pathologic variables in rectal cancer: a United States community and cooperative group report. *J Clin Oncol.* 2001;19:3895-3902.
10. Kohonen-Corish MR, Daniel JJ, Chan C, et al. Low microsatellite instability is associated with poor prognosis in stage C colon cancer. *J Clin Oncol.* 2005;23:2318-2324.
11. Soreide K, Janssen EA, Soiland H, Körner H, Baak JP. Microsatellite instability in colorectal cancer. *Br J Surg.* 2006;93:395-406.
12. Nelson H, Petrelli N, Carlin A, et al. Guidelines 2000 for colon and rectal cancer surgery. *J Natl Cancer Inst.* 2001;93:583-596.
13. Kapiteijn E, Marijnen CA, Nagtegaal ID, et al. Preoperative radiotherapy combined with total mesorectal excision for resectable rectal cancer. *N Engl J Med.* 2001;345:638-646.
14. Shihab OC, Taylor F, Bees N, et al. Relevance of magnetic resonance imaging-detected pelvic sidewall lymph node involvement in rectal cancer. *Br J Surg.* 2011;298:1798-1804.
15. Fujita S, Akasu T, Mizusawa J, et al. Postoperative morbidity and mortality after mesorectal excision with and without lateral lymph node dissection for clinical stage II or stage III lower rectal cancer (JCOG0212): results from a multicentre, randomised controlled, non-inferiority trial. *Lancet Oncol.* 2012;13:616-621.
16. Mirnezami A, Mirnezami R, Chandrakumaran K, Sasapu K, Sagar P, Finan P. Increased local recurrence and reduced survival from colorectal cancer following anastomotic leak: systematic review and meta-analysis. *Ann Surg.* 2011;253:890-899.
17. Govindarajan A, Gonen M, Weiser MR, et al. Challenging the feasibility and clinical significance of current guidelines on lymph node examination in rectal cancer in the era of neoadjuvant therapy. *J Clin Oncol.* 2011;29:4568-4573.
18. Coco C, Valentini V, Manno A, et al. Long-term results after neoadjuvant radiochemotherapy for locally advanced resectable extraperitoneal rectal cancer. *Dis Col Rectum.* 2006;49:311-318.
19. Zitt M, DeVries A, Thaler J, et al. Long-term surveillance of locally advanced rectal cancer patients with neoadjuvant chemoradiation and aggressive surgical treatment of recurrent disease: a consecutive single-centre experience. *Int J Colorectal Dis.* 2015;30:1705-1714.
20. Jeffery M, Hickey BE, Hider PN. Follow-up strategies for patients treated for non-metastatic colorectal cancer. *Cochrane Database Syst Rev.* 2007;(1):CD002200.
21. Steele SR, Chang GJ, Hendren S, et al. Practice guideline for the surveillance of patients after curative treatment of colon and rectal cancer. *Dis Colon Rectum.* 2015;58:713-725.
22. Tan E, Gouvas N, Nicholls RJ, et al. Diagnostic precision of carcinoembryonic antigen in the detection of recurrence of colorectal cancer. *Surg Oncol.* 2009;18:15-24.
23. Schurr P, Lentz E, Block S, et al. Radical redo surgery for local rectal cancer recurrence improves overall survival: a single center experience. *J Gastrointest Surg.* 2008;12:1232-1238.
24. Ito Y, Ohtsu A, Ishikura S, et al. Efficacy of chemoradiotherapy on pain relief in patients with intrapelvic recurrence of rectal cancer. *Jpn J Clin Oncol.* 2003;33:180-185.
25. Haddock MG, Miller RC, Nelson H, et al. Combined modality therapy including intraoperative electron irradiation for locally recurrent colorectal cancer. *Int J Radiat Oncol Biol Phys.* 2011;79:143-150.
26. Dresen RC, Kusters M, Daniels-Gooszen AW, et al. Absence of tumor invasion into pelvic structures in locally recurrent rectal cancer: prediction with preoperative MR imaging. *Radiology.* 2010;256:143-150.
27. Messiou C, Chalmers AG, Boyle K, Wilson D, Sagar P. Pre-operative MR assessment of recurrent rectal cancer. *Br J Radiol.* 2008;81:468-473.
28. Bosset JF, Collette L, Calais G, et al. Chemotherapy with preoperative radiotherapy in rectal cancer. *N Engl J Med.* 2006;355:1114-1123.
29. Yu SK, Bhangu A, Tait DM, Tekkis P, Wotherspoon A, Brown G. Chemoradiotherapy response in recurrent rectal cancer. *Cancer Med.* 2014;3:111-117.
30. Das P, Delclos ME, Skibber JM, et al. Hyperfractionated accelerated radiotherapy for rectal cancer in patients with prior pelvic irradiation. *Int J Radiat Oncol Biol Phys.* 2010;77:60-65.
31. van der Meij W, Rombouts AJ, Rutten H, Bremers AJ, de Wilt JH. Treatment of locally recurrent rectal carcinoma in previously (chemo) irradiated patients: a review. *Dis Colon Rectum.* 2016;59:148-156.
32. Susko M, Lee J, Salama J, et al. The use of re-irradiation in locally recurrent, non-metastatic rectal cancer. *Ann Surg Oncol.* 2016;23:3609-3615.
33. Dozois EJ, Privitera A, Holubar SD, et al. High sacrectomy for locally recurrent rectal cancer: can long-term survival be achieved? *J Surg Oncol.* 2010;103:105-109.
34. Milne T, Solomon MJ, Lee P, et al. Sacral resection with pelvic exenteration for advanced primary and recurrent pelvic cancer: a single-institution experience of 100 sacrectomies. *Dis Colon Rectum.* 2014;57:1153-1161.
35. Milne T, Solomon MJ, Lee P, Young JM, Stalley P, Harrison JD. Assessing the impact of a sacral resection on morbidity and survival after extended radical surgery for locally recurrent rectal cancer. *Ann Surg.* 2013;258:1007-1013.
36. Bhangu A, Ali SM, Cunningham D, Brown G, Tekkis P. Comparison of long-term survival outcome of operative vs nonoperative management of recurrent rectal cancer. *Colorectal Dis.* 2013;15:156-163.
37. Shaikh I, Holloway I, Aston W, et al. High subcortical sacrectomy: a novel approach to facilitate complete resection of locally advanced and recurrent rectal cancer with high (S1–S2) sacral extension. *Colorectal Dis.* 2016;18:386-392.
38. Okunieff P, Scala S, Cheng SW. Biology of large dose per fraction irradiation. In: Gunderson LL, ed. *Intraoperative Irradiation: Techniques and Results.* New Jersey: Humana Press Inc; 2000:25-46.
39. Bullard KM, Trudel JL, Baxter NN, Rothenberger DA. Primary perineal wound closure after preoperative radiotherapy and abdominoperineal resection has a high incidence of wound failure. *Dis Colon Rectum.* 2005;48:438-443.
40. Radice E, Nelson H, Mercill S, Farouk R, Petty P, Gunderson L. Primary myocutaneous flap closure following resection of locally advanced pelvic malignancies. *B J Surg.* 1999;86:349-354.
41. D'Souza DN, Pera M, Nelson H, Finical SJ, Tran NV. Vaginal reconstruction following resection of primary locally advanced and recurrent colorectal malignancies. *Arch Surg.* 2003;138:1340-1343.
42. Butler CE, Gundeslioglu AO, Rodriguez-Bigas MA. Outcomes of immediate vertical rectus abdominis myocutaneous flap reconstruction for irradiated abdominoperineal resection defects. *J Am Coll Surg.* 2008;206:694-703.
43. Wong S, Garvey P, Skibber J, Yu P. Reconstruction of pelvic exenteration defects with anterolateral thigh-vastus lateralis muscle flaps. *Plast Reconstr Surg.* 2009;124:1177-1185.

44. Heriot AG, Byrne CM, Lee P, et al. Extended radical resection: the choice for locally recurrent rectal cancer. *Dis Colon Rectum.* 2008;51:284-291.

45. Yang TX, Morris DL, Chua TC. Pelvic exenteration for rectal cancer: a systematic review. *Dis Colon Rectum.* 2013;56:519-531.

46. You YN, Skibber JM, Hu CY, et al. Impact of multimodal therapy in locally recurrent rectal cancer. *B J Surg.* 2016;103(6):753-762.

47. Alberda WJ, Verhoef C, Nuyttens JJ, et al. Intraoperative radiation therapy reduces local recurrence rates in patients with microscopically involved circumferential resection margins after resection of locally advanced rectal cancer. *Int J Radiation Oncol Biol Phys.* 2014;88:1032-1040.

48. Alberda WJ, Verhoef C, Schipper ME, et al. The importance of a minimal tumor-free resection margin in locally recurrent rectal cancer. *Dis Colon Rectum.* 2015;58:677-685.

49. Tanis PJ, Doeksen A, van Lanschot JJ. Intentionally curative treatment of locally recurrent rectal cancer: a systematic review. *Can J Surg.* 2013;56(2):135-144

50. Harris CA, Solomon MJ, Heriot AG, et al. The outcomes and patterns of treatment failure after surgery for locally recurrent rectal cancer. *Ann Surg.* 2015;364:323-329.

51. Kusters M, Dresen RC, Martijn H, et al. Radicality of resection and survival after multimodality treatment is influenced by subsite of locally recurrent rectal cancer. *Int J Radiat Oncol Biol Phys.* 2009;75:1444-1449.

52. Wiig JN, Tveit KM, Poulsen JP, Olsen DR, Giercksky KE. Preoperative irradiation and surgery for recurrent rectal cancer. Will intraoperative radiotherapy (IORT) be of additional benefit? A prospective study. *Radiother Oncol.* 2002;62:207-213.

53. Salo JC, Paty PB, Guillem J, Minsky BD, Harrison LB, Cohen AM. Surgical salvage of recurrent rectal carcinoma after curative resection: a 10-year experience. *Ann Surg Oncol.* 1999;6:171-177.

54. Kanemitsu Y, Hirai T, Komori K, Kato T. Prediction of residual disease or distant metastasis after resection of locally recurrent rectal cancer. *Dis Colon Rectum.* 2010;53:779-789.

55. Shoup M, Guillem JG, Alektiar KM, et al. Predictors of survival in recurrent rectal cancer after resection and intraoperative radiotherapy. *Dis Colon Rectum.* 2002;45:585-592.

56. Roeder F, Goetz JM, Habl G, et al. Intraoperative Electron Radiation Therapy (IOERT) in the management of locally recurrent rectal cancer. *BMC Cancer.* 2012;12:592.

57. Rahbari NN, Ulrich AB, Bruckner T, et al. Surgery for locally recurrent rectal cancer in the era of total mesorectal excision: is there still a chance for cure? *Ann Surg.* 2011;253:522-533.

58. Bedrosian I, Giacco G, Pederson L, et al. Outcome after curative resection for locally recurrent rectal cancer. *Dis Colon Rectum.* 2006;49:175-182.

59. Martinez-Monge R, Nag S, Martin EW. Three different intraoperative radiation modalities (electron beam, high-dose-rate brachytherapy, and iodine-125 brachytherapy) in the adjuvant treatment of patients with recurrent colorectal adenocarcinoma. *Cancer.* 1999;86:236-247.

60. Sole CV, Calvo FA, Lizarraga S, et al. Single-institution multidisciplinary management of locoregional oligo-recurrent Pelvic Malignancies: Long-Term Outcome Analysis. *Ann Surg Oncol.* 2015;22(suppl 3):S1247-S1255.

61. You YN, Habiba H, Chang GJ, Rodriguez-Bigas MA, Skibber JM. Prognostic value of quality of life and pain in patients with locally recurrent rectal cancer. *Ann Surg Oncol.* 2011;18:989-996.

62. Austin KK, Young JM, Solomon MJ. Quality of life of survivors after pelvic exenteration for rectal cancer. *Dis Colon Rectum.* 2010;53:1121-1126.

63. Beyond TME Collaborative. Consensus statement on the multidisciplinary management of patients with recurrent and primary rectal cancer beyond total mesorectal excision planes. *B J Surg.* 2013;100:E1-E33.

64. Colibaseanu DT, Mathis KL, Abdelsattar ZM, Larson DW, Haddock MG, Dozois EJ. Is curative resection and long-term survival possible for locally re-recurrent colorectal cancer in the pelvis? *Dis Colon Rectum.* 2013;56:14-19.

65. Harji DP, Sagar PM, Boyle K, Maslekar S, Griffiths B, McArthur DR. Outcome of surgical resection of second-time locally recurrent rectal cancer. *B J Surg.* 2013;100:403-409.

66. Taylor WE, Donohue JH, Gunderson LL, et al. The Mayo Clinic experience with multimodality treatment of locally advanced or recurrent colon cancer. *Ann Surg Oncol.* 2002;9:177-185.

67. McAfee MK, Allen MS, Trastek VF, Ilstrup DM, Deschamps C, Pairolero PC. Colorectal lung metastases: results of surgical excision. *Ann Thorac Surg.* 1992;53:780-785.

68. Salah S, Ardissone F, Gonzalez M, et al. Pulmonary metastasectomy in colorectal cancer patients with previously resected liver metastasis: pooled analysis. *Ann Surg Oncol.* 2015;22:1844-1850.

69. Guerrera F, Mossetti C, Ceccarelli M, et al. Surgery of colorectal cancer lung metastases: analysis of survival, recurrence and re-surgery. *J Thorac Dis.* 2016;8:1764-1771.

70. McCormack PM, Burt ME, Bains MS, Martini N, Rusch VW, Ginsberg RJ. Lung resection for colorectal metastases. 10-year results. *Arch Surg.* 1992;127:1403-1406.

71. Koga R, Yamamoto J, Saiura A, Yamaguchi T, Hata E, Sakamoto M. Surgical resection of pulmonary metastases from colorectal cancer: four favourable prognostic factors. *Jpn J Clin Oncol.* 2006;36:643-648.

72. Brister SJ, de Varennes B, Gordon PH, Sheiner NM, Pym J. Contemporary operative management of pulmonary metastases of colorectal origin. *Dis Colon Rectum.* 1998;31:786-792.

73. Onaitis MW, Petersen RP, Haney JC, et al. Prognostic factors for recurrence after pulmonary resection of colorectal cancer metastases. *Ann Thoracic Surg.* 2009;87:1684-1688.

74. Salah S, Watanabe K, Park JS, et al. Repeated resection of colorectal cancer pulmonary oligometastases: pooled analysis and prognostic assessment. *Ann Surg Oncol.* 2013;20:1955-1961.

75. Jayne DG, Fook S, Loi C, Seow-Choen F. Peritoneal carcinomatosis from colorectal cancer. *B J Surg.* 2002;89:1545-1550.

76. Verwaal VJ, van Ruth S, Witkamp A, Boot H, van Slooten G, Zoetmulder FA. Long-term survival of peritoneal carcinomatosis of colorectal origin. *Ann Surg Oncol.* 2005;12:65-71.

77. Klaver CE, Musters GD, Bemelman WA, et al. Adjuvant hyperthermic intraperitoneal chemotherapy (HIPEC) in patients with colon cancer at high risk of peritoneal carcinomatosis; the COLOPEC randomized multicentre trial. *BMC Cancer.* 2015;15:428.

Management of Metastatic Colorectal Cancer to the Liver

Keith M. Cavaness | William C. Chapman

Colorectal cancer is the third most common cancer diagnosed in both males and females in the United States. As of January 2016 there are an estimated 1.4 million men and women living with a diagnosis of colorectal cancer, with an expected 134,490 new diagnoses and 49,190 deaths that same year.[1] Of the projected new cases diagnosed in 2016, approximately 50% to 60% of those patients will develop metastases to the liver.[2,3] It has been estimated that more than 50% of patients who die of colorectal cancer have liver metastases at autopsy and 35% have isolated hepatic metastases. Metastatic liver disease is the cause of death in most patients.[4] The majority of patients develop metachronous metastatic lesions. However, 20% to 34% of patients present with metastatic disease to the liver at the time of diagnosis and carry a worse prognosis.[5] Hepatic resection for colorectal metastases is the treatment of choice for patients with resected or resectable primary and regional disease if all liver disease can be treated.

In this chapter, we will focus on the management of liver metastases from colorectal cancer. Our primary aim will be to provide practical treatment strategies for various clinical situations encountered by surgeons. Within this overview we will review the approach to liver resection and the supporting data. We will also outline nonresection treatment therapies that can be used in the management of metastases.

EVOLUTION OF TREATMENT FOR COLORECTAL METASTASIS

The principal spread of metastatic colorectal cancer is through the portal circulation to the liver. Weiss et al. analyzed the metastatic patterns of colorectal cancer in 1541 necropsies and proposed a cascade hypothesis that describes the occurrence of liver metastases through seeding from the portal venous system.[6] These secondary hepatic metastases seed the lungs to form tertiary pulmonary metastases. The tertiary pulmonary metastases then spread through the arterial system to form quaternary metastases in other organs. In 2004 Wang et al. described the liver as a filter that prevents metastatic spread to distant sites.[7] In a study led by Uetsuji et al. metastases were noted in patients without cirrhosis (46 of 210), whereas those patients with cirrhosis had no evidence of metastasis (0 of 40).[8] The authors concluded that decreased portal flow in the cirrhotic liver limited the exposure to metastatic cells.

Untreated colorectal cancer with metastases to the liver has classically shown dismal outcomes. The median survival of this patient population is just 5 to 10 months, with a 3-year survival that is rarely reported.[9] The prognosis is closely linked to both the metastatic burden and the timing of metastasis. In 2015 Adam et al. reported a standardized definition of metastases. Liver metastases detected at or before diagnosis of the primary tumor are defined as synchronous liver metastases. Early metachronous metastases are those detected within 12 months after diagnosis or surgery of the primary, whereas late metachronous metastases are those detected more than 12 months after diagnosis or surgery of the primary. Their review suggests that synchronous metastases have less favorable cancer biology and synchronicity is a sign of poor prognosis.[10]

With a better understanding of hepatic physiology and recent advances in chemotherapy, targeted surgical strategies have been used to successfully treat liver metastases. To date, numerous studies have demonstrated that liver resection for colorectal liver metastases (CRLMs) is safe, with some reporting a 5-year survival of greater than 50%.[11] Based on these studies, liver resection has now become the standard treatment for metastatic colorectal cancer to the liver.

PATIENT SELECTION

Many controversies arise when discussing the treatment of liver metastases from colorectal cancer. Some of these include the use of neoadjuvant or adjuvant chemotherapy, the timing of resection for synchronous metastases, how to approach disappearing lesions, the best methods to treat bilobar disease, the treatment of recurrent metastases, and the operative indications for extrahepatic disease (EHD).[12] To select the patients who would benefit most from surgery, a multidisciplinary approach should be used. At our center, patients are presented at a multidisciplinary tumor conference including specialized surgeons, medical oncologists, pathologists, radiologists, and key ancillary staff. Through multidisciplinary discussion, therapeutic options can be discussed and an optimal treatment plan formulated.

Selection of patients for hepatic resection includes the patient's medical fitness for major laparotomy, the stage of the primary tumor, the extent of the hepatic metastases, and the intent of the resection. The morbidity associated with hepatic resection is directly related to patient selection. Although multiple factors are considered in surgical decision making, a study of 747 hepatectomies revealed that the incidence of postoperative complications was significantly influenced by the American Society of Anesthesiologists (ASA) score, the presence of hepatic steatosis, the extent of resection, and an associated extrahepatic procedure.[13] Kamiyama et al. reviewed 793 consecutive hepatectomies and reported that independent relative risk for morbidity was influenced by an operative time greater than 360 minutes, blood loss greater than 400 mL, and serum albumin less than 3.5 g/dL.[14] Thus the patient's clinical performance status and comorbidities of major organ systems should allow them to undergo a major resection with an expected mortality risk of less than 5%.

The extent of hepatic metastatic disease affects patient selection for liver resection. Historically, adequate hepatic reserve in patients without chronic liver disease requires at least two remaining anatomically adjacent segments after resection (with normal vascular inflow and outflow, and normal biliary drainage). If cirrhosis is present, the extent of resection is reduced dramatically and ablation may assume a larger therapeutic role. Extensive hepatic steatosis without cirrhosis also limits the extent of hepatic resection.

Technical advances in both liver and colonic surgery have enabled simultaneous resection of the primary colorectal cancer and liver metastases in carefully selected patients with synchronous tumors. Undertaking concurrent resection of the primary colorectal cancer and hepatic metastases requires thorough preoperative hepatic imaging, thus allowing for evaluation of the intrahepatic extent of disease and also to exclude EHD. A publication by de Haas et al. suggests that combining colorectal resection with limited hepatectomy is safe in patients with synchronous tumors and is associated with less cumulative morbidity than a delayed liver resection procedure.[15] Extensive liver metastases, including multiple bilobar metastases require careful planning for the optimal approach These cases often require a combination of resection and nonresectional therapies to address all liver disease Involvement of the afferent or efferent vasculature may require advanced vascular resections, whereas involvement of both the afferent and efferent vasculature may be a contraindication to resection.

Hepatic resection for metastases should rarely be undertaken if extensive extrahepatic metastases exist, exclusive of regional lymph node or limited (usually solitary) pulmonary metastases. Although resection of focal EHD that is concurrently resectable with the primary has been reported to show long-term control, it has not been shown to be curative. Current contraindications to resection of hepatic metastases in the setting of extrahepatic metastases include distant metastases, including peritoneal carcinomatosis, osseous or brain metastases, extraabdominal lymph node metastases, and multiple unresectable pulmonary metastases.

PROGNOSTIC DETERMINANTS

Traditionally it had been suggested that survival rates for patients with metastases from colorectal cancer could be improved through careful selection of operative candidates and the use of neoadjuvant therapy to help with downstaging. However, there continues to be a wide range of oncologic characteristics of the tumors, leading to a variable degree of aggressiveness. Although useful, markers such as tumor number, size, bilobar disease, and high serum carcinoembryonic antigen (CEA) are not as clinically predictive as was once thought.[16,17] With the evolution of more potent and targeted chemotherapy, emerging determinants include the radiologic and pathologic response of the tumor to chemotherapy, disease-free interval, and synchronicity, as well as the genetic mutational status of the tumor. Poultsides et al. evaluated the pathologic response

to preoperative chemotherapy. Even though tumor size may decrease on imaging, this does not always correlate with tumor regression. They suggested that fibrosis is the main determinant of treatment response and that the degree of tumor fibrosis noted in the liver resection specimen correlated with disease-specific survival.[3]

Tumor progression while on neoadjuvant chemotherapy is associated with a poor outcome.[19] Radiologic response has also played a role in evaluating tumor response to chemotherapy. Traditionally the RECIST criteria have been used to evaluate tumor response on imaging[20]; however, newer morphologic characteristics have been noted in response to chemotherapy that correlate more closely with pathologic response. Shindoh et al. reported on the texture of the tumor noted on computed tomography (CT) and concluded that optimal morphologic response following preoperative chemotherapy correlated with improved overall survival.[21]

With improved techniques in mutational analysis, the identification of specific mutations has also been linked to prognosis. RAS oncogene status is a strong predictor of response to antiepidermal growth factor receptor agents. Some have suggested that KRAS mutational status is associated with aggressive tumor biology.[22] In a recent study, Mise et al. reported that RAS mutational status can be used as a prognostic indicator for those undergoing liver resection for CRLMs. They concluded that major pathologic responses were more common in patients with wild-type RAS in comparison to those with RAS mutations (59.9% vs. 36.8%, respectively; P = .015).[23]

FACTORS DETERMINING RESECTABILITY

ONCOLOGIC EVALUATION

Traditionally complete resection of all viable disease is essential to achieve the best long-term outcomes. Preoperative evaluation of the surgical candidate should include the tumor response to chemotherapy, the mutational status of the tumor, and the presence of EHD. Current contraindications to resection of hepatic metastases include diffuse peritoneal carcinomatosis, osseous or brain metastases, extraabdominal lymph node metastases, and multiple, unresectable pulmonary metastases. Focal extrahepatic peritoneal disease that is concurrently resectable was previously thought to be a contraindication to resection but is now considered an option in appropriately selected patients.

Overall number of extrahepatic metastases resected has a stronger prognostic effect than the location.[24] Carpizo et al. presented their series of 127 patients who underwent hepatectomy with concurrent resection of EHD. They reported a 5-year survival of 26% compared with 49% for those resected without EHD. They concluded that the presence of limited and resectable EHD should not be a contraindication to resection and could be associated with long-term survival.[25] A noticeable feature of their analysis showed that 95% of the patients recurred after complete resection, indicating that concurrent resection of hepatic metastases and EHD is not considered curative. Leung et al. developed an EHD risk scoring system. The score was prognostic of overall and recurrence-free survival.[26] In general, appropriately selected patients with limited

EHD could be resected with the expectation of reasonable long-term control with the use of newer adjuvant chemotherapies.

Patients who successfully underwent downstaging with neoadjuvant chemotherapy and then resection have similar survival rates as those patients who were resectable at their initial presentation. This neoadjuvant approach also provides an insight into the response of the tumor, thus revealing its biologic activity or tumor biology. Some have even suggested that in the era of modern chemotherapy, tumor biology is a more important factor in survival than surgical margin clearance.[27] With the use of modern systemic chemotherapy (SC), progression during preoperative treatment is relatively rare. However, progression (with or without the development of new lesions) during preoperative chemotherapy should be regarded as a marker of poor prognosis and an indication for second line chemotherapy before surgery is considered.[28]

Although the neoadjuvant approach can be effective, it is not without risk. As Vauthey et al. have shown, there is a 20% incidence of steatohepatitis in association with irinotecan-based chemotherapy and a 19% incidence of sinusoidal injury after treatment with oxaliplatin. Steatohepatitis was associated with an increased 90-day mortality.[29] Ribero et al. also found that the addition of bevacizumab reduced the incidence and severity of oxaliplatin-related sinusoidal injury while improving clinical response to the chemotherapy.[30] Other series have reported a higher rate of sinusoidal injury and an increase in perioperative blood transfusions and surgical complications in patients who received preoperative chemotherapy than those who did not.[31]

TECHNICAL EVALUATION FOR RESECTABILITY

The extent of resection depends on the burden of metastases, the intrahepatic site, and the relationship of the tumor to major vasculature and bile ducts. Historically, evaluation for resection was based on resection of all viable disease with (1) preservation of at least two contiguous hepatic segments with (2) adequate vascular inflow and outflow, with biliary drainage and (3) the ability to preserve an adequate future liver remnant (FLR) (>20% in healthy normal liver, >25% for most cases as a minimum FLR).[32]

With advances in resection techniques the development of volumetric and functional measurements has been established to allow a more detailed evaluation of the FLR. As a greater volume of diseased liver is resected, the incidence of postoperative hepatic insufficiency (PHI) increases. The basis of volumetric measurements relies on the use of mutliplanar imaging to assess the volume of the FLR in comparison with the whole liver volume. When considering resection, minimal FLR volume has been set at greater than 20% for a normal liver, greater than 30% in a damaged liver after extensive treatment, and greater than 40% for a cirrhotic liver.[33] A strong correlation between FLR size and PHI, morbidity, and mortality has been shown.

Another method of determining an adequate remnant volume is by assessing the regenerative capacity of the liver. This can be measured with volume of hypertrophy, as well as rate of hypertrophy defined as the kinetic growth rate (KGR); a KGR of 2% per week reduces hepatic complications and liver failure–related death.[34] This typically is in conjunction with portal vein embolization (PVE) or staged hepatectomy. A third measure of overall hepatic regenerative capacity is indocyanine green clearance[35] and hepatic scintigraphy.[36] Both methods effectively estimate the metabolic function of the liver and can be used to accurately assess the FLR.

RISK SCORING SYSTEMS

To aid in determining who will benefit most from surgical intervention, several clinical risk scoring (CRS) systems have been developed. The aims of these scoring systems are to optimize patient selection for hepatic resection and to stratify patients for the need of adjuvant therapies. Independent risk factors, such as CEA level, tumor size, and tumor number, have been reported to predict outcome after resection of CRLMs. Different authors have used different variables and cutoff values to discriminate between patient groups with different prognoses.

Nordlinger et al., through a national collective registry of 1568 patients, developed a prognostic scoring system based on seven identified risk factors: (1) age more than 60 years, (2) primary cancer extending into serosa, (3) positive regional lymph nodes, (4) liver metastases confirmed within 24 months of the primary cancer, (5) CEA levels, (6) size of metastasis more than 5 cm, and (7) less than 1-cm resection margin of the metastases.[16] Three risk groups were defined: low risk (zero to two risk factors), intermediate risk (three to four risk factors), and high risk (five to seven risk factors).

In a similar method, Fong et al. through a single institution study of 1001 patients, devised a CRS system based on: (1) nodal status of primary, (2) disease-free interval from the primary to discovery of liver metastases less than 12 months, (3) number of tumors greater than 1, (4) size of the largest tumor greater than 5 cm, and (5) preoperative CEA level greater than 200 ng/mL. Each positive criterion is assigned a point, with the total score out of 5 being predictive of outcome.[37] The Fong prognostic scoring system has been validated by numerous independent databases and shows a significant survival difference between groups scoring 0 to 2 when compared with groups that scored 3 to 5. Merkel et al. compared the three score systems of Nordlinger, Fong, and the extended TNM classification. They identified the CRS system developed by Fong to be the most important tool for estimating prognosis and selecting patients for surgical resection.[38] This CRS system has also been helpful in selecting patients that could benefit from neoadjuvant therapy or be stratified into clinical trials. Fong et al. demonstrated that use of this CRS was shown to be useful in guiding preoperative evaluation of the patient with metastatic colorectal cancer, including when to use positron emission tomography (PET)/CT and diagnostic laparoscopy to prevent unneeded laparotomy.

PRETHERAPEUTIC IMAGING EVALUATION

COMPUTED TOMOGRAPHY

Contrast-enhanced CT (ce-CT) has become the primary tool used for evaluation of CRLMs. Chest, abdomen, and pelvis can all be evaluated in a matter of minutes. This modality identifies CRLMs as hypovascular lesions when compared with surrounding normal liver parenchyma. Although CRLMs can often be identified on ce-CT imaging, the timing of the contrast is vital to identify these hypovascular lesions. A ce-CT that includes arterial, portal venous, and delayed venous phases will help to define the burden of disease and relevant anatomy and aid in preoperative planning. Although ce-CT can be quick and relatively inexpensive, it does expose the patient to radiation and potential contrast allergies and has a limited ability to evaluate lesions less than 10 mm in size.

MAGNETIC RESONANCE IMAGING

Historically, magnetic resonance imaging (MRI) has been used as a problem-solving modality in lesions that are equivocal on ce-CT or ultrasound imaging. CRMs often appear hypointense on T1-weighted images and hyperintense on T2- and diffusion-weighted sequences. In 2014 Zech et al. evaluated the efficacy of gadoxetic acid–enhanced MRI (Eovist) compared with conventional MRI with extracellular contrast medium (ECCM) and ce-CT in detecting CRLMs.[39] They concluded that Eovist MRI is superior as a first line imaging modality in detecting CRLMs. They noted that the use of Eovist imaging in preoperative planning was associated with the lowest proportion of patients for whom the surgical plan had to be changed at the time of surgery. They also noted that when used to help to better define ce-CT imaging characteristics, it prevented unnecessary surgery and clarified metastatic characteristics, allowing patients to undergo successful hepatic resection. Although Eovist imaging is more sensitive and specific for detecting CRLMs, it is also associated with a higher cost and lower patient compliance and is not readily available in all institutions.

POSITRON EMISSION TOMOGRAPHY

PET relies on the activity of hypermetabolic malignant tissue to take up radiolabeled glucose molecules. This modality is often combined with CT to better define areas of concern. In evaluating liver tumors, it has been shown to be less sensitive than MRI or CT; however, it can be useful for defining radiologically occult EHD. PET/CT is not currently recommended as a staging or baseline modality except in those circumstances in which previous imaging has revealed surgically resectable metastatic disease and the patient needs to be evaluated for unrecognized metastatic disease that would preclude surgical management.

GENERAL PRINCIPLES FOR RESECTION

Resection or ablation of metastases should never put the liver at risk for irreversible dysfunction. The extent of resection will depend on the size of the metastases, intrahepatic site, and on the relationship of the tumor to major afferent and efferent vasculature and bile ducts. In patients with deeply seated metastases, formal anatomic resections are indicated. Moreover, metastatic disease manifesting indistinct margins mandates formal resection. A negative margin is vital to reduce the risk of intrahepatic recurrence at the margins of resection. However, margins of resection should never risk damage to major hepatic

vasculature. The afferent and efferent vasculature of the liver remnant must be protected. The liver parenchyma can be transected by a variety of methods: compression (finger fracture or clamp fracture), contact (Cavitron Ultrasonic Aspirator [Cavitron, Long Island, New York]), thermal (electrocautery, laser, radiofrequency ablation [RFA], LigaSure, Harmonic scalpel), or stapled techniques. Each approach has advantages and disadvantages and are often selected based on surgeon preference. Most methods disrupt parenchyma to expose vessels and bile ducts for ligation, whereas newer methods including TissueLink (TissueLink Medical, Dover, New Hampshire), Harmonic scalpel (Ethicon Endo-Surgery, Cincinnati, Ohio), and LigaSure (Covidien Ltd., Dublin, Ireland) fuse small vessels and ducts while transecting parenchyma. Although the extent of parenchymal necrosis adjacent to the transection plane varies among techniques, such devitalized parenchyma is not clinically significant. Vessels or ducts of diameter larger than 2 mm generally require ligation with suture or clips. Major hepatic or portal veins are best occluded securely with the use of vascular staples or alternatively a running monofilament permanent suture.

ANATOMY

Safe hepatic resection depends on a clear understanding of the hepatic anatomy. Although hepatic regenerative capacity and metabolic reserve permit many types of resections, resection based on preservation of residual anatomic integrity best reduces the operative risk and optimizes function. Couinaud's[40] description of hepatic anatomy highlights the anatomic features of the liver relevant to resection and in adults provides anatomic terminology that is clinically useful. Fig. 172.1 details the functional divisions of the liver, according to Couinaud's nomenclature. Although the regenerative capacities and metabolic reserve of the liver are important, hepatic resection based on anatomic considerations reduces operative risk and optimizes postoperative liver function. In general, anatomic resections are the oncologically approved method to ensure cancer-free margins and to lower the risk of potential sites for intrahepatic spread. The major anatomic features of the liver relevant to resection have been detailed elsewhere.[40]

The hilar plate is the extension of a vasobiliary sheath that is particularly relevant to hepatic resection (Fig. 172.2). The vasobiliary sheath represents a fusion of the endoabdominal fascia around the bile ducts, portal vein, and hepatic artery at the porta hepatis. These fibrous sheaths invest the components of the pedicles from the portal vein bifurcation to the sinusoids. By contrast, the hepatic veins lack endoabdominal fascial investment and, consequently, are more fragile than their portal counterparts. The density of the vasculobiliary sheaths decreases as the pedicles extend intrahepatically. At the hepatic hilus, these sheaths fuse to form plates that surround the portal pedicles, both anteriorly and posteriorly. Three primary hepatic plates are recognized: the cystic, the hilar, and the umbilical plates (Fig. 172.3). Recognition of the vasculobiliary sheaths and the hepatic plates facilitates precise access to the hilar structures. Division of these plates is needed to expose and mobilize the portal pedicle during resection.

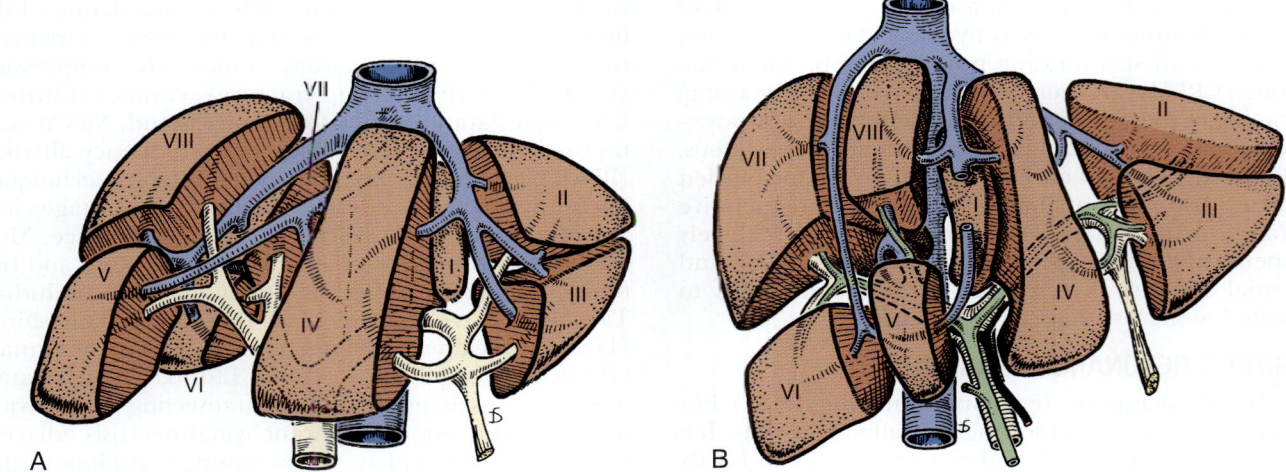

FIGURE 172.1 The functional division of the liver and of the liver segments according to Couinaud's nomenclature. (A) As seen in the patient. (B) In the ex vivo position. (From Blumgart LH, ed. *Video Atlas: Liver, Biliary & Pancreatic Surgery*. Philadelphia: Saunders; 2011; with laparoscopic video contributions from Carlos U. Corvera. Figure 1.9.)

NUMBER OF METASTASES

The number of metastases is no longer a contraindication to resection provided an adequate FLR remains and all metastases are ultimately completely resected or ablated. Kokudo et al. concluded that resection in patients with four or more CRM can achieve long-term survival and that the number of hepatic metastases alone should not be used as a sole contraindication to resection.[41] Similarly, although long-term prognosis in patients with metastases to lymph nodes is unfavorable, hepatic resection combined with lymphadenectomy may be beneficial in occasional patients whose disease has been downstaged or completely eliminated clinically by chemotherapy and can be resected completely. Timing of resection in patients presenting with synchronous disease should allow for liver resection before lung resection to permit complete pulmonary function prior to lung resection. In addition, hepatic resection before lung resection allows for surgical inspection of the abdomen, ruling out advanced disease. Extensive peritoneal metastases are considered by most advanced centers to be a contraindication to surgical resection. Although there are limited data reporting a small survival advantage of combined resection and hyperthermic intraperitoneal chemotherapy (HIPEC), this is not standard of care and is usually practiced in the setting of clinical trials.

MARGINS

Although a 1- to 2-cm margin has historically been considered appropriate to reduce the risk of intrahepatic recurrence, there have been variable data suggesting that margins less than 1 cm might be sufficient. Recent data suggest that more effective chemotherapy and microscopically free resection margins continue to allow for improved survival when compared with positive margins. Vandeweyer et al. reviewed 261 consecutive primary liver resections for CRLMs.[42] They noted no significant difference in patient survival or disease-free survival with margins greater than 1 mm. When comparing the groups with margins 1 mm or less and those with margins greater than 1 mm, there was

a significant 5-year survival difference of 25% versus 43%, respectively ($P < .04$). They concluded that a margin of greater than 1 mm is associated with an improved 5-year overall survival. Kokudo et al. examined the relationship of measured margins of hepatic resection to survival and local recurrence and suggested that a smaller margin (1 mm) may be as effective.[43] Histopathology of resected specimens showed that micrometastases in the surrounding liver were present in 2% of patients and were found within 4 mm of the margin. The incidence of definitive recurrence at the surgical margin was 13.3%, 2.8%, and 0% if the margin was less than 2 mm, 2 to 4 mm, and 5 mm or wider, respectively. It is important to remember that margins, no matter how close, should never risk damage to vital hepatic structures. In addition, resection margins can be extended with the use of adjuvant therapies such as RFA or cryoablation, provided the ablation zone does not affect major ducts or vessels. Although data with respect to the optimal surgical margin are variable, a margin of 0.5 to 10 mm is generally preferred.

DISAPPEARING LIVER METASTASES

Despite the evidence favoring hepatectomy after short-course chemotherapy, many patients continue long-term SC, resulting in small residual nodules without uptake on PET/CT or complete disappearance of the lesions.[44] There is some debate over whether to resect these lesions based on pretreatment localization or to observe closely and only resect areas of defined recurrence.

Benoist et al.[45] examined whether a complete radiographic response indicated a cure of CRLMs. In their series, they identified 38 of 586 patients with CRLMs who had disappearance of at least one metastasis following chemotherapy. These 38 patients had 183 metastases, of which 66 disappeared on CT imaging. Pathologic examination of 15 of these sites showed viable cancer cells. Other lesions that were not found at the time of surgery but were noted on CT were left in place and followed. At 1 year they showed recurrence at those sites. Overall,

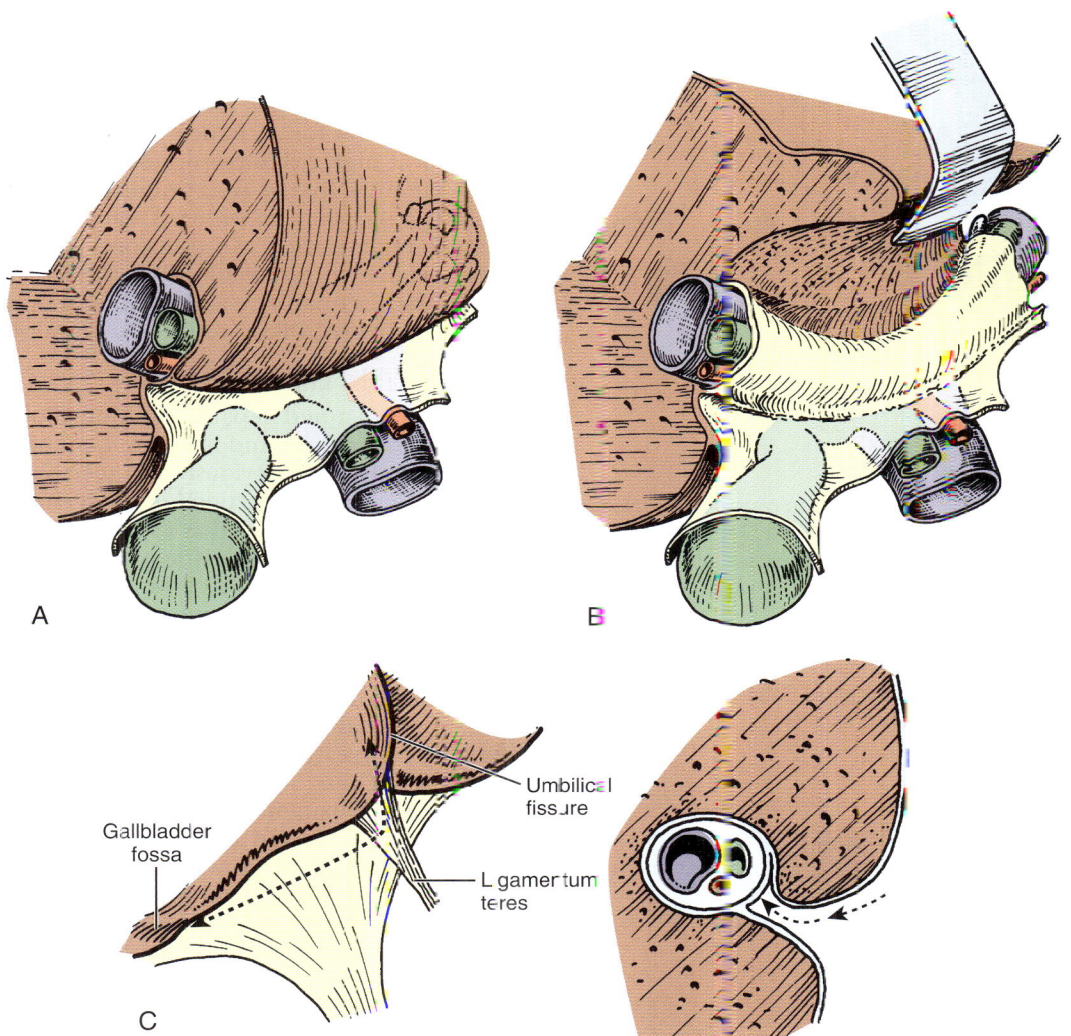

FIGURE 172.2 (A) Relationship between the posterior aspect of the quadrate lobe and the biliary confluence. The hilar plate is formed by the fusion of the connective tissue enclosing the biliary and vascular elements with Glisson capsule. (B) Biliary confluence and left hepatic duct exposed by lifting the quadrate lobe upward after incision of Glisson capsule at its base. This technique (lowering of the hilar plate) generally is used to display a dilated bile duct above an iatrogenic stricture or hilar cholangiocarcinoma. (C) Line of incision *(left)* to allow extensive mobilization of the quadrate lobe. This maneuver is of particular value for high bile duct stricture and in the presence of liver atrophy or hypertrophy. The procedure consists of lifting the quadrate lobe upward (see [A] and [B]), then not only opening the umbilical fissure, but also incising the deepest portion of the gallbladder fossa. *Right,* Incision of Glisson capsule to gain access to the biliary system *(arrow).* (From Blumgart LH, ed. *Video Atlas: Liver, Biliary & Pancreatic Surgery.* Philadelphia: Saunders; 2011; with laparoscopic video contributions from Carlos U. Corvera. Figure 1.26.)

they noted persistent disease or early recurrence in 83% of patients who had a complete response on imaging.

Chapman et al. evaluated disappearing CRLMs with Eovist, which is known to be the most sensitive imaging modality for detecting CRLMs.[46] In 23 patients they detected 200 CRLMs; 77 of the 200 CRLMs were determined to have disappeared on baseline Eovist imaging (38.5%). At surgical pathology or 1-year follow-up, 55% were noted to have viable tumor or recurrence. They observed that the odds for 1 or more disappearing CRLMs is 11.25 times greater in synchronous versus metachronous lesions (Fig. 172.4). They concluded that with the use of Eovist MRI imaging, 38.5% of CRLMs disappeared, and of those, 55% were noted to have viable tumor or recurrence.

Although a complete radiographic response was once thought to be an indicator of cure, the data have shown that a complete radiographic response does not equate to a complete pathologic response. In the group determined to have a complete radiographic response, the subgroup of complete pathologic response has been reported between 17% and 65%. When patients with a complete pathologic response undergo resection, 5-year survival rates have been reported up to 75%, by two independent groups.[31]

STRATEGIES TO IMPROVE RESECTABILITY

Strategies for improving resectability are based on the clinical response to neoadjuvant chemotherapy to downstage disease and increase postresection hepatic reserve.

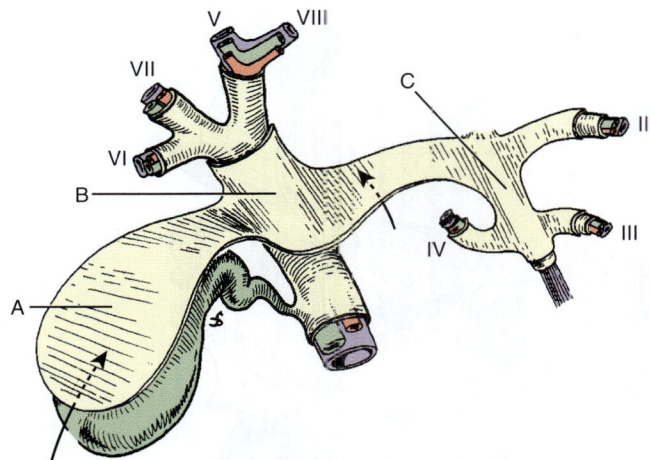

FIGURE 172.3 Sketch of the anatomy of the plate system. Note the cystic plate *(A)* above the gallbladder, the hilar plate *(B)* above the biliary confluence and at the base of the quadrate lobe, and the umbilical plate *(C)* above the umbilical portion of the portal vein. *Arrows* indicate the plane of dissection of the cystic plate during cholecystectomy and of the hilar plate during approaches to the left hepatic duct. (From Blumgart LH, ed. *Video Atlas: Liver, Biliary & Pancreatic Surgery*. Philadelphia; Saunders; 2011; with laparoscopic video contributions from Carlos U. Corvera. Figure 1.25.)

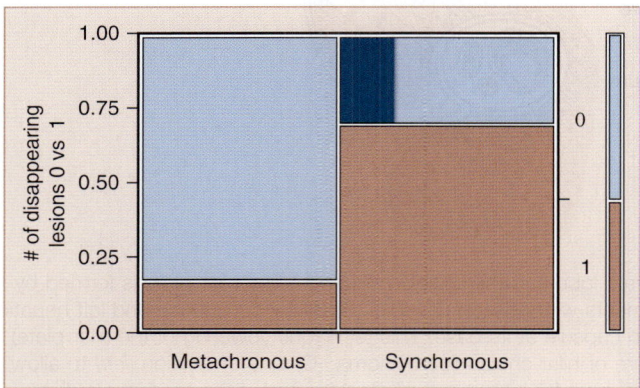

FIGURE 172.4 Mosaic plot—Contingency analysis demonstrates that the odds for 1 or more disappearing lesions within the synchronous group are 11.25 times greater than in the metachronous group (odds ratio, 11.25; *P* = .0064). (From Owen JW, Fowler KJ, Doyle MB, et al. Colorectal liver metastases: disappearing lesions in the era of Eovist hepatobiliary magnetic resonance imaging. *HPB [Oxford]*. 2016;18:296–303.)

Cytodestructive modalities such as RFA, cryoablation, and irreversible electroporation (IRE) can be used in combination with chemotherapy and surgery to completely address disease burden. Novel chemotherapeutic regimens combining 5-fluorouracil (5-FU), folinic acid, and oxaliplatin or irinotecan with or without biologic agents such as bevacizumab have been demonstrated to increase both patient survival and quality of life. Indeed, response to chemotherapy before hepatic resection has become a major selection factor for resection. Tumor stabilization or a decrease in tumor burden during chemotherapy

was associated with long-term survival. Five-year survival was 37%, 30%, and 8% for patients with objective tumor response, tumor stabilization, and tumor progression, respectively. Control of metastatic disease before surgery may be crucial for a chance of prolonged remission in patients at high risk for progression after resection.

If the anticipated functional hepatic volume after hepatic resection is considered marginal, strategies using hepatic regeneration can transform some patients from unresectable to resectable. PVE, staged resection, and associating liver partition and portal vein ligation for staged hepatectomy (ALPPS) are three treatment modalities.

PORTAL VEIN EMBOLIZATION

PVE of the planned hepatic resection allows hypertrophy of the remnant liver and has been demonstrated to allow more patients with previously unresectable liver tumors to undergo successful resection.[47] PVE is generally considered when the functional FLR is estimated at less than 25% to 30% of initial functional hepatic volume (high risk of postoperative death). PVE of the side of planned resection induces contralateral compensatory hypertrophy of the hepatic remnant, thus decreasing the risk of postoperative liver failure. After hypertrophy of the remnant liver volume has plateaued, usually 4 to 6 weeks after the procedure, hepatic resection can be performed. Preresectional selective PVE may increase the rate of resection in such patients by 20%.[48] Their 5-year survival is 40%, similar to the survival rate of patients who did not require selective PVE. Some have suggested that inducing liver hypertrophy may promote tumor growth and lead to a higher recurrence. A large review including 6 studies and 668 patients determined that PVE does not have an adverse effect on postoperative recurrence or overall survival.[49]

TWO-STAGE HEPATECTOMY

Two-stage hepatectomy consists of sequentially resecting hepatic metastases that would otherwise be unresectable because of insufficient hepatic reserve. This option is usually reserved for patients with multiple bilobar metastases responsive to chemotherapy. The initial hepatic resection for metastases is performed on the planned remnant liver, which allows it to hypertrophy in the absence of metastasis. The second hepatic resection for metastases is performed after restaging at 6 weeks from original hepatectomy to allow the early regeneration of the remnant liver. Postoperative chemotherapy, consisting of the same proven chemotherapy that the patient responded to previously, is continued for further response. The second hepatectomy should generally only be performed if there is no interim tumor progression and significant hepatotoxicity from chemotherapy has not occurred. A total of 1104 of 1439 patients (77%) with CRLMs who were initially unresectable were treated with combination chemotherapy consisting of 5-FU, leucovorin combined with oxaliplatin, irinotecan, or both.[50] Of the 1104 patients treated, 138 patients (12.5%) were considered good responders and underwent hepatic resection after an average of 10 cycles. Liver resection was combined with PVE, ablative treatment, or second-stage hepatectomy in 42 patients (30%), and resection of EHD was performed in 41 patients (30%). Operative mortality was less than

1% and after a mean follow-up of 48.7 months, 111 of the 138 patients (80%) developed tumor recurrence. Of the 111 patients, some developed isolated hepatic recurrence ($n = 40$), isolated extrahepatic recurrence ($n = 12$), or both hepatic and extrahepatic recurrence ($n = 59$). Isolated hepatic recurrences were treated by repeat hepatectomy, whereas patients with extrahepatic tumors underwent resection. Overall treatment of the 138 patients included 223 hepatectomies, 42 specific procedures to allow resectability, and 77 extrahepatic surgical procedures. Overall survival was 52%, 33%, and 23% at 3, 5, and 10 years, respectively. Disease-free survival was 30%, 22%, and 17% at 3, 5, and 10 years, respectively. Patients whose hepatic metastases were initially resectable had 3-, 5-, and 10-year overall survival of 66%, 48%, and 30%, respectively. Downstaging of metastatic disease and modalities to induce selective hypertrophy of the remnant liver can now permit hepatic resection with curative intent in selective responsive patients.

SURGICAL APPROACH

PREOPERATIVE PREPARATION AND CARE

The preoperative preparation for patients undergoing hepatic resection is similar to that undertaken for any major pancreaticobiliary procedure. Coagulation profiles (rarely needed) are corrected, and prophylactic antibiotics directed at upper gastrointestinal tract flora are administered at the time of surgery. Importantly, if jaundice or cholangitis and bile duct obstruction are present (rarely present in patients with CRLMs), biliary decompression by endoscopic or percutaneous intubation is preferred to improve hepatic function and control infection. Biliary drainage is established for the anticipated hepatic remnant. In general, major hepatic resection is not undertaken unless the total serum bilirubin is nearly normal and clinical infection is controlled.

Intraoperative management of the patient is critical to the success of the procedure. The maintenance of low central venous pressure (5 to 7 mm Hg) reduces parenchymal blood loss via hepatic venous sources.[51] Large-bore intravenous access for rapid transfusion is also essential.

The major pitfalls or danger points with hepatic resection include hemorrhage from hepatic veins, portal veins, or hepatic arteries; air embolism from hepatic venous injury; injury to the biliary ductal system with postoperative obstruction or fistula formation; portal or hepatic vein compromise with subsequent ischemia or postsinusoidal portal hypertension; prolonged vascular inflow occlusion leading to refractory hepatic ischemia or hepatic injury; and injury to the diaphragm, inferior vena cava, or intestine.

INCISION AND EXPOSURE

Whether performing the resection laparoscopically or open, obtaining adequate exposure is critical to safe resection. Laparoscopic liver resections are covered elsewhere and will not be discussed.

A bilateral subcostal incision or a right subcostal incision with a vertical extension to the xiphoid process affords

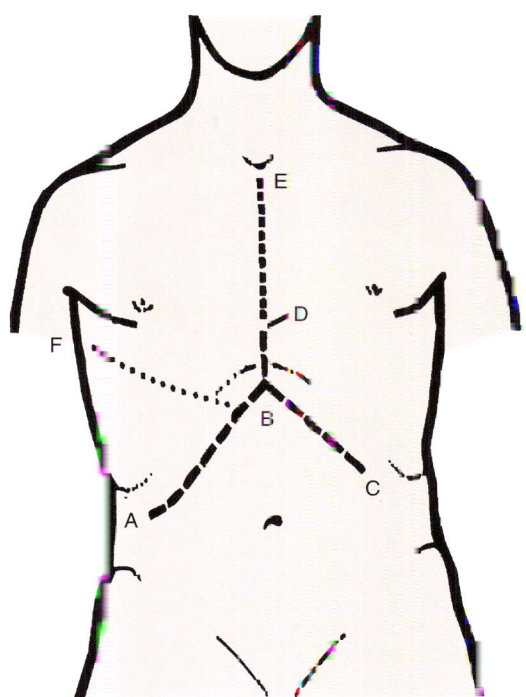

FIGURE 172.5 Incisions used for partial hepatectomy. Most often an extended right subcostal incision (*ABD*) is adequate *ABC*, Rooftop incision with vertical extension; *DE*, median sternotomy; *F*, right thoracic extension. (From Blumgart LH, ed. *Video Atlas. Liver, Biliary & Pancreatic Surgery*. Philadelphia: Saunders; 2011; with laparoscopic video contributions from Carlos U. Corvera. Figure 2.15.)

wide exposure for any open hepatic resection (Fig. 172.5). A long midline incision provides a satisfactory alternative, particularly for limited resections of segments I through VI or if the patient has a narrow or acute costal angle. Tumors that involve segments VII or VIII or extended lobar resections are approached more safely through a bilateral subcostal incision, which permits better exposure and control of the hepatic vein/inferior vena cava junction. Rarely, a right thoracic extension (thoracoabdominal incision) may be necessary for safe exposure of large bulky tumors that involve segments VII and VIII or those that require inferior caval reconstruction. All perihepatic adhesions are divided. Any adherent diaphragm is excised with the metastasis. The liver is mobilized by complete division of the appropriate ligamentous attachments (i.e., coronary, falciform, and triangular ligaments). Fig. 172.6 shows division of the left triangular ligament when planning for a left hepatectomy. The thin gastrohepatic omentum is incised adjacent to the hepatoduodenal ligament. The foramen of Winslow is opened in anticipation of subsequent inflow vascular occlusion. In our practice, a Thompson retractor is used to elevate the rib cage anteriorly and cephalad while retracting the remaining viscera caudally.

PARENCHYMAL TRANSECTION

The hepatic parenchyma is transected by the method of personal preference. Each method disrupts the parenchyma

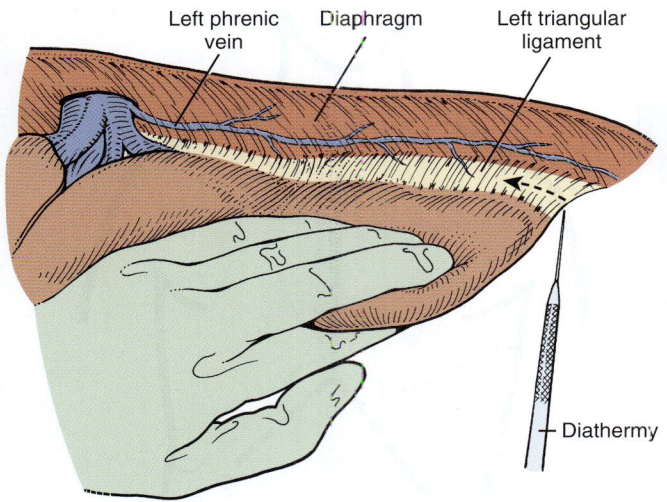

FIGURE 172.6 The left triangular ligament is exposed and divided with the cautery. Care should be taken not to injure the left phrenic vein. (From Blumgart LH, ed. *Video Atlas: Liver, Biliary & Pancreatic Surgery*. Philadelphia: Saunders; 2011; with laparoscopic video contributions from Carlos U. Corvera. Figure 2.18)

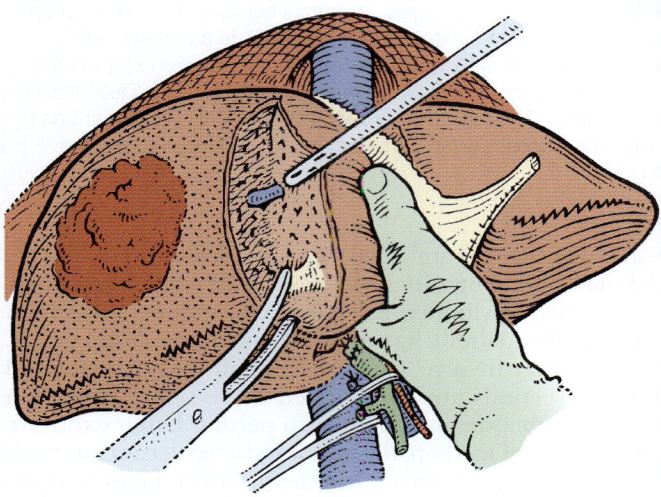

FIGURE 172.7 Parenchymatous transection of the liver tissue by a fracture or crushing technique using a clamp. The portal triad to the right liver has been divided, and a line of demarcation has developed. The liver tissue is opened in this line. The operator opens the liver tissue, crushing the parenchyma between clamps. The parenchymal transection is done with a vessel loop occluding the hilar vessels (Pringle maneuver). (From Blumgart LH, ed. *Video Atlas: Liver, Biliary & Pancreatic Surgery*. Philadelphia: Saunders; 2011; with laparoscopic video contributions from Carlos U. Corvera. Figure 3.10A.)

to expose vessels or ducts for ligation or cauterization. Hemorrhage is reduced by digital compression of the liver on each side of the transection plane. Both the surgeon and the assistant compress the parenchyma on opposing sides of the transection plane (Fig. 172.7). Typically, the assistant surgeon maintains hemostasis by electrocautery or clips. An additional assistant maintains field exposure

by suctioning bile or blood from the transection interface. Bile ducts or vessels with diameter larger than 2 mm are clamped with metal clips or ligated with suture. Suture ligation of remnant vessels or ducts reduces artifacts during postoperative imaging. After local hemostasis and bile stasis are obtained, the abdomen is closed. Closed, low-pressure suction drainage is optional and tends to be used based on surgeon preference.

TYPES OF SURGICAL TREATMENT FOR HEPATIC METASTASIS

Multiple terms have been used to describe various hepatic resections. The current recommendations for formal terminology have been proposed and are referenced for review.[52]

WEDGE RESECTIONS

Wedge resections typically are subsegmental and frequently cross intersegmental planes and are well tolerated by the liver because they are used for small peripheral, nonhilar tumors. Wedge resections are usually performed with a minimum of blood loss, typically without inflow vascular occlusion.

ANATOMIC UNISEGMENTAL AND POLYSEGMENTAL RESECTIONS

Anatomic resections of a single liver segment or multiple contiguous liver segments require identification and ligation of the segmental vascular biliary pedicles for accurate anatomic demarcation of the segment or segments. Portal and segmental pedicles are best approached by dissection from the hilus to the appropriate pedicle or by direct rapid parenchymal transection along an estimated intersegmental plane with ultrasound guidance. Dissection from the hilum is most applicable for anterior liver segments. Dissection along an intersegmental plane is more appropriate for ligation of the posterior hepatic segments II, VII, and VIII. Both approaches are facilitated by temporary inflow vascular occlusion to reduce hemorrhage and by the use of the ultrasonic aspirator to rapidly expose the pedicles through the intervening parenchyma. Alternatively, some have proposed injection of methylene blue into the segmental or portal pedicle using ultrasound guidance, which provides visual identification of the anatomic segmental or sectoral anatomy. Total vascular isolation of the liver may be required rarely for large tumors. If so, the infrahepatic suprarenal and suprahepatic inferior vena cava are encircled during the initial dissection to permit occlusion by vascular clamps or tapes.

SECTIONAL RESECTIONS

Sectional resections are polysegmental resections based on the primary right and left portal pedicles and include left lateral sectionectomy, left hemisectionectomy, right hemihepatectomy, right anterior sectionectomy, and right posterior sectionectomy. The risk of blood loss is reduced significantly by ligation of the appropriate lobar hepatic arterial and portal venous branches before parenchymal transection. In addition, ligation of the corresponding hepatic vein before parenchymal transection

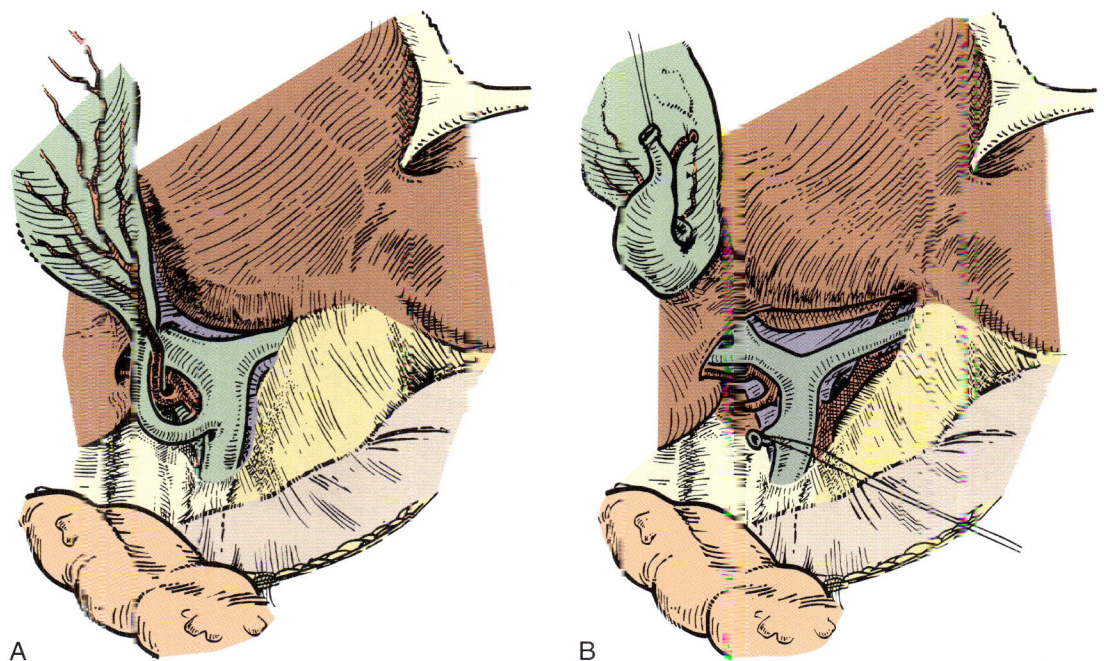

FIGURE 172.8 (A) The peritoneum overlying the common bile-duct and extending up into Calot triangle is incised. (B) The cystic duct and cystic artery are secured. A tie is left on the cystic duct for later retraction. The hilar plate is lowered to expose the left hepatic duct and the confluence of the bile ducts. (From Blumgart LH, ed. *Video Atlas: Liver, Biliary & Pancreatic Surgery*. Philadelphia: Saunders; 2011; with laparoscopic video contributions from Carlos U. Corvera. Figure 3.1.)

further reduces blood loss. Major lobar resections can be extended either anatomically or nonanatomically. Anatomic extensions are performed by resecting the involved liver segments adjacent to the principal plane and nonanatomic extensions by subsegmentectomy; for example, an extended right hepatectomy can include segment IV, along with segment V to VIII (also known as a right trisectionectomy).

The liver is mobilized fully for all hemihepatectomy resections. Cholecystectomy is performed either en bloc with the resected lobe (if adherent to the tumor) or before parenchymal transection to facilitate exposure of the hilar structures (Fig. 172.8). The corresponding hepatic artery is ligated initially. The right hepatic artery generally traverses the triangle of Calot. Hilar lymph nodes are excised to further expose the bile duct, portal vein, and hepatic artery and for staging. For a right hepatectomy, the right lateral aspect of the hepatoduodenal ligament is incised longitudinally just posterior to the bile duct, allowing exposure to the hepatic artery and portal vein (Fig. 172.9). The right hepatic artery, regardless of the origin, is always found lateral to the common hepatic duct or inferior to the right main hepatic duct, where it enters the liver parenchyma.

The left hepatic artery is approached through the lesser sac through the left lateral aspect of the hepatoduodenal ligament after division of the gastrohepatic omentum. The main left hepatic artery is generally found just inferior to the base of the round ligament as it enters the left lobe between segments III and IV anterior to segment I (Fig. 172.10). When present, an accessory left hepatic artery arising from the left gastric artery courses through

the gastrohepatic omentum and is often divided during division of the gastrohepatic omentum for resections of the left lobe. Lymphatic vessels around the hepatic arteries are ligated before division to reduce postoperative lymphatic drainage. Regardless of the type of liver resection performed, the artery that supplies that portion to be resected can be occluded temporarily, whereas the artery to the opposite lobe is palpated to ensure patency of the arterial supply to the FLR. After blood flow to the hepatic remnant is appropriately confirmed, the artery supplying the portion to be resected can be doubly ligated with heavy silk and divided.

A similar approach is used for right hepatic artery ligation, although the right hepatic artery is exposed to the right aspect of the hepatoduodenal ligament. The bile duct is retracted anteriorly with a vein retractor to expose the portal venous bifurcation. Again the right portal vein is exposed to the right of the hepatoduodenal ligament, and the left portal vein is exposed to the left of the hepatoduodenal ligament. The main left portal vein branch always bifurcates from the right main branch at an approximately 90-degree angle and courses anterolaterally.

Occasionally, two major branches of the right portal vein—anterior and posterior—may arise separately without a common trunk, resulting in a portal vein trifurcation. The appropriate major portal vein branch is freed from the surrounding lymphoareolar tissue and is ligated with a vascular stapler or a running vascular suture after division between clamps (see Fig. 172.9). A simple suture ligature is not used on the portal vein because accidental slipping of the ligature can result in immediate life-threatening hemorrhage. After division of the blood supply, a clear

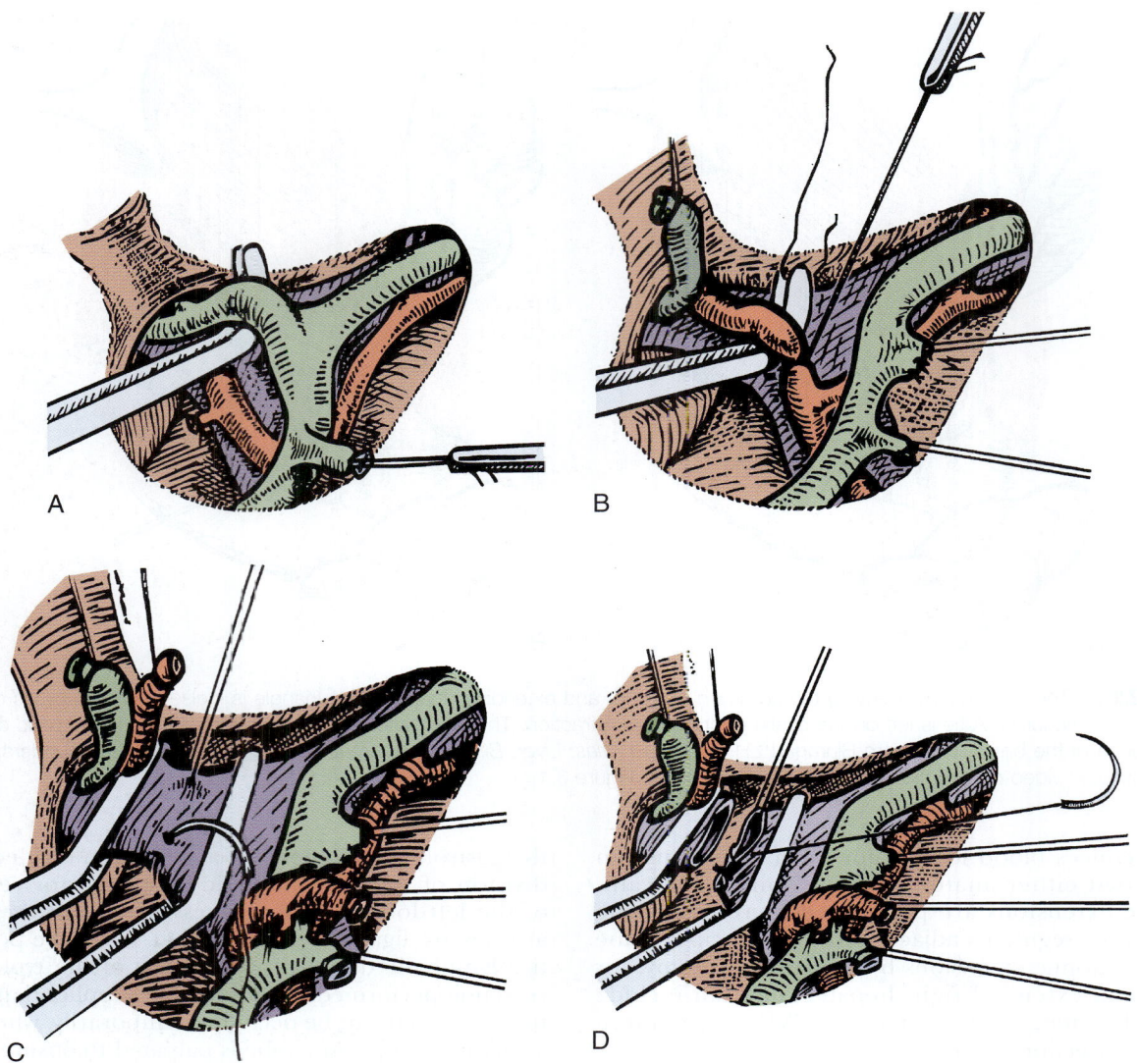

FIGURE 172.9 (A) The right hepatic duct is dissected (we now, more often than not, leave the right hepatic duct for intrahepatic control during parenchymal transection; see text). The confluence of the hepatic ducts is shown. (B) The right hepatic duct has been transfixed with absorbable suture material, divided, and ligated or oversewn. Alternatively, it may simply be divided under direct vision and then oversewn. Traction on the sutures attached to the cystic duct and the right hepatic duct stump allows retraction of the common hepatic duct and common bile duct to the left and assists in displaying the vessels beneath. The right hepatic artery is dissected, ligated, and divided, usually to the right (as shown) but sometimes to the left of the common hepatic duct. (C) The right portal vein is dissected, and forceps are gently passed beneath it. Special care is taken not to damage the first (caudate branch) of the right portal vein. This branch is sought initially and ligated and divided or avoided (see text). Straight-bladed vascular clamps are applied to the right portal vein. (D) The vein is divided, and its proximal stump is oversewn. (From Blumgart LH, ed. *Video Atlas: Liver, Biliary & Pancreatic Surgery*. Philadelphia: Saunders; 2011; with laparoscopic video contributions from Carlos U. Corvera. Figure 3.2.)

line of vascular demarcation along the principal hepatic plane for resection confirms appropriate and complete vascular ligation (Fig. 172.11). Alternatively, the portal venous branch(es) to the portion of the liver to be resected can be left intact and divided intraparenchymally during the course of the resection. Parenchymal transection can be initiated at this time or after ligation of the hepatic vein (depending on the size of the tumor and the tumor–hepatic vein relationship). After the blood supply to the liver has been controlled, the hepatic veins may be approached safely.

During a right hepatectomy, multiple short retrohepatic veins between the inferior vena cava and the paracaval segments are ligated to prevent avulsion during anterior retraction of the liver. Ligation starts caudally and proceeds cephalad. Occasionally, a large right inferior hepatic vein enters the inferior vena cava from the posterior aspect of segment VI. Either staples or a running suture closure for secure ligation of this vein is preferred to simple ligature. To expose the main right hepatic vein, the hepatocaval ligament bridging segments I and VII is divided (Fig. 172.12). A moderate-sized vein frequently traverses this ligament,

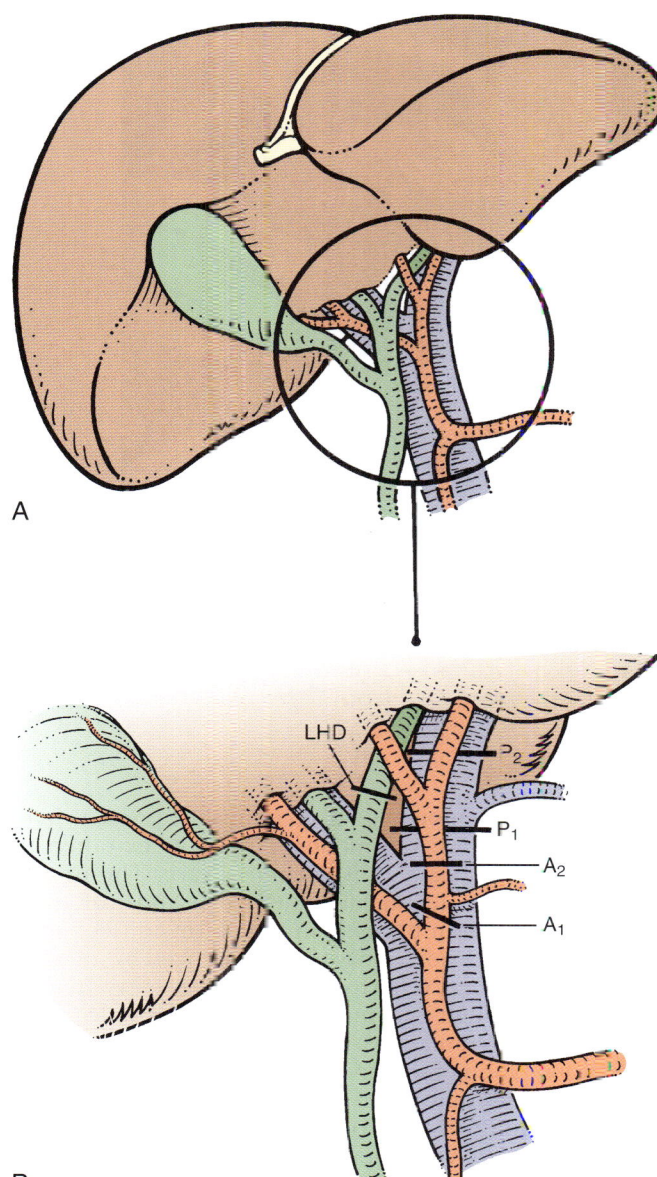

A

B

FIGURE 172.10 (A) Dissection for left hepatectomy at the base of the umbilical fissure. (B) Left hepatic duct *(LHD)* is divided at the base of the umbilical fissure. *A1,* Point of division of the left hepatic artery for concomitant removal of caudate lobe; *A2,* point of division of left hepatic artery for left hepatectomy; *P1,* point of division of the left portal vein for left hepatectomy and caudate lobectomy; *P2,* point of division of left portal vein for left hepatectomy alone. (From Blumgart LH, ed. *Video Atlas: Liver, Biliary & Pancreatic Surgery.* Philadelphia: Saunders; 2011 with laparoscopic video contributions from Carlos U. Corvera. Figure 4.1.)

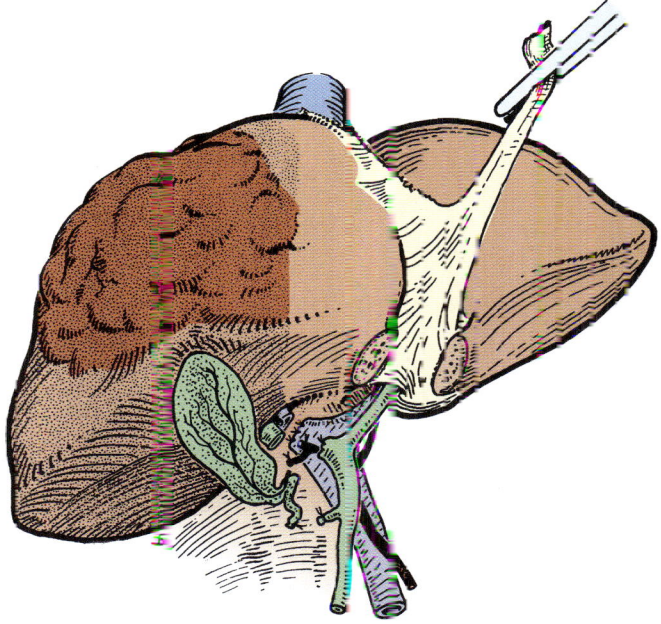

FIGURE 172.11 The bridge of liver tissue has been divided. (From Blumgart LH, ed. *Video Atlas: Liver, Biliary & Pancreatic Surgery.* Philadelphia: Saunders; 2011; with laparoscopic video contributions from Carlos U. Corvera. Figure 3.13.)

transection. Alternatively, clamps can be placed and the divided vessel oversewn directly if it is not possible to safely use a surgical stapler.

During left hepatectomy or left lateral sectionectomy, ligation of the main left hepatic vein, which usually joins the middle hepatic vein before entering the vena cava, can be deferred until parenchymal transection is complete because extrahepatic exposure is technically more difficult. Although the middle hepatic vein can be ligated during either right or left lobectomy, preservation reduces postoperative hepatic congestion and the volume of postoperative serous drainage. Alternatively, compression of the left hepatic vein at the confluence of the middle and left hepatic veins by a vascular clamp can be used to reduce hemorrhage from the hepatic venous branches along the interface of the liver during transection.

The parenchymal transection is guided by the zone of vascular demarcation and intraoperative ultrasonography. Parenchyma is transected by the surgeon's method of choice. Major bile ducts are ligated with permanent suture. Injection of the cystic duct stump or main bile duct can be performed with saline or a dilute methylene blue solution to exclude occult bile leaks along the transection interface. Bile leaks are closed with sutures or clips. After parenchymal transection, topical hemostatic agents are used as needed.

In general, persistent, diffuse interface hemorrhage or oozing results from elevated central venous pressure due to excessive intraoperative crystalloid, colloid, and blood product transfusion or, rarely, due to various causes of right heart failure. Compression of the transection interface and reduction in the central venous pressure by vasodilators or by decreasing the rate of fluid infusion

and its presence should be anticipated before division. The main right hepatic vein, which has an extrahepatic component of 1 to 2 cm, is dissected from the inferior vena cava and the overlying liver. Unless large metastases preclude access, the right hepatic vein can almost always be transected with a vascular stapler before parenchymal

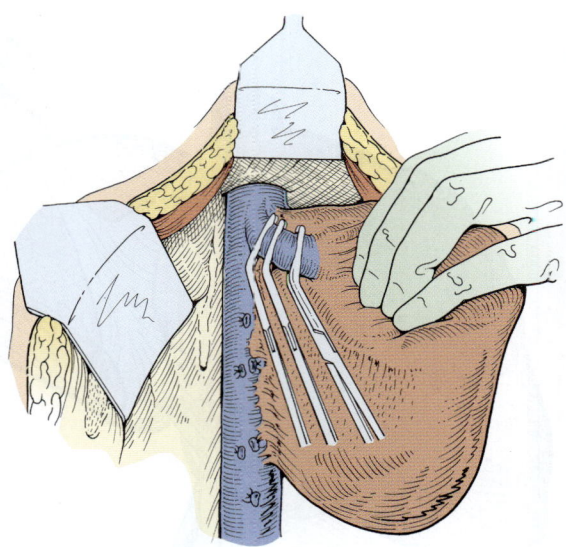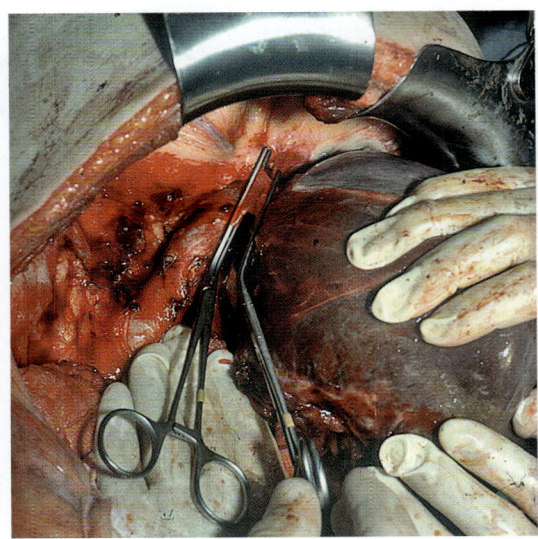

FIGURE 172.12 Approach to the right hepatic vein. The right liver has been extensively mobilized and the inferior vena cava exposed up to the right hepatic vein. The right hepatic vein is dissected (see text), and a vascular clamp is applied on the caval side. An additional clamp is placed on the hepatic side, although this is not essential because if the vein is divided after the portal triad at the hilus, bleeding from the exposed venous orifice can be readily controlled with a suture after division of the vein. A second clamp should be applied on the caval side before division of the vein. (From Blumgart LH, ed. *Video Atlas: Liver, Biliary & Pancreatic Surgery.* Philadelphia: Saunders; 2011; with laparoscopic video contributions from Carlos U. Corvera. Figure 3.8.)

and diuresis will reduce such hemorrhage. Development of a coagulopathy requires blood component therapy, liver packing, and normothermia. The divided falciform ligament may be reapproximated to prevent torsion of a small left lobe hepatic remnant and postoperative vascular compression of the left hepatic vein. The abdomen is closed in a standard fashion.

POSTOPERATIVE CARE

Postoperative care generally involves appropriate fluid administration. The addition of albumin to standard crystalloid solutions reduces postoperative weight gain and maintains adequate urine output. Most hepatic resections are associated with a mild acidosis and coagulation abnormalities in the immediate postoperative period. Neither acid-based abnormalities nor coagulation deficits are corrected postoperatively unless they are clinically significant. Urinary output is monitored until hemodynamic stability has been maintained for 24 hours. Postoperative epidural analgesia markedly improves pulmonary function and pain control.

SURGICAL OUTCOMES AND COMPLICATIONS

INTRAOPERATIVE COMPLICATIONS

Hemorrhage is the most common intraoperative complication. It results from major vessel trauma along the transection interface or from coagulopathy. Inflow occlusion or total hepatic vascular isolation has dramatically reduced abrupt life-threatening hemorrhage from trauma to the major hepatic vasculature. A simple Pringle maneuver with an appropriate-sized vascular clamp or loop snare

easily controls hemorrhage from either the portal vein or the hepatic arteries. Traumatic injury to the extrahepatic bile duct from a vasculature clamp is rare. The noncirrhotic liver tolerates warm ischemia periods for more than 1 hour without permanent long-term consequence. Ischemia/reperfusion injury may be reduced by intermittent occlusion (e.g., reperfusion of the liver every 10 to 15 minutes). Although ischemic hepatic injury is reflected by elevations of serum aspartate transaminase and bilirubin and prolongation of the prothrombin time, these changes usually reverse to normal within 7 to 10 days.

Diffuse hemorrhage from the transection interface usually results from elevation of the central venous pressure greater than 12 to 15 mm Hg. Continuous intraoperative monitoring of the central venous pressure and volume replacement to maintain central venous pressures between 5 and 8 mm Hg reduces this operative risk of hemorrhage but allows the maintenance of adequate systemic hemodynamics. Vasodilators may also be required. Persistent interface hemorrhage is treated best by coagulation with electrocautery, the argon beam coagulator, bipolar cautery, or compression with laparotomy pads and topical hemostatic agents. Should interface bleeding persist after the use of these techniques, intraoperative evaluation for coagulopathy must be undertaken. An intraoperative thromboelastogram (TEG) should be obtained, and abnormal coagulation profiles should be corrected with blood products, as indicated.

The last significant intraoperative complication is air embolus from hepatic vein damage. Although a potentially life-threatening source of cardiac arrhythmias and ventilation/perfusion defects, early recognition is possible through careful anesthetic monitoring. The techniques for anesthetic monitoring for venous air embolism include precordial Doppler sonography, right heart catheterization, capnography from mass spectroscopy, transcutaneous oxygen probes, and transesophageal echocardiography (TEE). Doppler sonography and TEE are the most sensitive, whereas abnormalities of capnographic mass spectrometry provide the most practical recognition of venous air embolism. With an increasing volume of air embolism, initial gas exchange abnormalities are supplanted by deteriorating systemic hemodynamics. Venous air embolism should be suspected initially by decreases in arterial oxygen tension, transcutaneous oxygen pressure, and fractional end-tidal concentrations of carbon dioxide and an increase in fractional end-tidal concentration of nitrogen. If undetected, the arterial carbon dioxide tension and transcutaneous carbon dioxide pressures will increase rapidly. Treatment consists of placing the patient in a Trendelenburg position, suture closure of the hepatic vein, and aspiration of the intracardiac air through a central venous pressure catheter with positive-pressure ventilation.

PERIOPERATIVE MORBIDITY AND MORTALITY

Postoperative hemorrhage usually arises from displaced vascular clips or ligatures. Recognition should be obvious by depressed hemodynamics or sanguineous abdominal drainage. Any concurrent coagulopathy should be at least partially corrected before reoperation for control of hemorrhage. If abdominal drains are placed, serosanguineous drainage is expected postoperatively. The volume of drainage may vary widely. Large-volume drainage may require isotonic fluid replacement to maintain fluid and electrolyte balance in the postoperative period. In general, abdominal drains can be removed safely regardless of the volume unless the drainage is bilious. Usually, even high-output drainage volumes are resorbed rapidly through the peritoneum without the formation of focal fluid collections or ascites. In patients with cirrhosis, drains should be avoided after hepatic resection because of protracted ascitic fluid drainage. Moreover, secondary infection of the ascites, which is associated with prolonged drainage, will be avoided.

Bilious drainage through the intraabdominal drains or after puncture of loculated perihepatic fluid collections is indicative of a biliary injury. Most injuries are best managed conservatively by continuous closed-suction drainage until they resolve. Minor fistulas (<100 mL/day) usually resolve with continuous suction drainage. Major fistulas (>200 mL/day) warrant cholangiographic evaluation and biliary stenting to speed resolution. Major fistulas may rarely require Roux-en-Y hepaticojejunostomy for definitive repair. Reoperation for repair of biliary fistula is indicated when there has been complete disruption of the major bile duct from the remnant liver and a complete absence of bilioenteric bile flow.

A perihepatic intraabdominal abscess may occur after any hepatic resection. Careful hemostasis and bile stasis after resection will reduce perihepatic fluid accumulation and the risk of infection. Percutaneous drainage of abscesses is the treatment of choice.

Finally, hepatic insufficiency or failure can occur after hepatic resection. Hepatic failure usually occurs in patients with chronic hepatic diseases and cirrhosis or after extended polysegmental resection. The most common

cause of hepatic insufficiency after hepatic resection is inadequate residual functional reserve. The treatment of this cause of hepatic failure is simply supportive. Preoperative PVE is indicated in patients in whom small hepatic remnants are anticipated (<30% of total liver volume). Orthotopic liver transplantation provides the only curative solution for refractory postoperative hepatic failure caused by inadequate reserve. However, even in selected patients, the risk associated with orthotopic liver transplantation for the salvage of hepatic failure induced by resection is exceedingly high and contraindicated in the presence of metastatic cancer, albeit resected.

Correctable causes of hepatic insufficiency should be sought postoperatively. Correctable causes of hepatic failure postoperatively include major bile duct obstruction and efferent or afferent vascular compromise as a result of vascular thrombosis or vessel narrowing. Bile duct obstruction should be suspected by steadily increasing total and direct serum bilirubin levels. Endoscopic retrograde or magnetic resonance cholangiography best defines the location and extent of the injury, but only the former technique permits therapeutic intervention. Percutaneous transhepatic cholangiography is less useful postoperatively because of delayed proximal bile duct dilation and altered hepatic position after resection.

Potentially correctable major hepatic vasculature injuries include portal and hepatic vein thromboses. Color flow Doppler ultrasonography is the best screening technique if suspected. Definitive imaging by angiography, MRI, or CT angiography further defines the extent and vascular damage caused by thrombus. After thromboses are recognized, reoperation for thrombectomy and repair of the venous damage that precipitated the thrombus are indicated. Systemic thrombolytic agents are contraindicated because of recent operative intervention. Anticoagulants (heparin and warfarin [Coumadin]) are useful to prevent recurrent thrombosis.

Additional aspects important to mention in the surgical resection of hepatic colorectal metastases are sinusoidal obstruction syndrome (SOS) and chemotherapy-associated steatohepatitis (CASH). Specifically, oxaliplatin has been shown to be associated with sinusoidal dilation, whereas irinotecan is associated with steatohepatitis, the latter of which is associated with increased operative risk and mortality. Thus the extent of resection, as well as other patient factors and chemotherapy administered, should be taken into account prior to liver resection.[29]

NONRESECTIONAL TREATMENT FOR HEPATIC METASTASIS

HEPATIC ARTERY INFUSION THERAPY

Hepatic artery infusion (HAI) therapy is a regional therapy targeting patients with liver-only or liver-predominant metastatic disease. The theoretical rationale for regional or hepatic artery infusional chemotherapy is based on the nearly exclusive arterial blood supply of the metastases from the hepatic artery and first pass drug clearance kinetics, which support high local hepatic concentrations of the drug with reduced systemic toxicity. 5-Flurodeoxyuridine

(5-FUDR) is the deoxyribonucleoside derivative of 5-FU and functions as a thymidylate synthetase inhibitor. Multiple studies have compared the use of regional HAI of 5-FUDR, showing high first pass extraction and tumoral levels of 400 times greater than that of systemic administration of 5-FU.[53] In 1980 Buchwald et al. reported the use of a totally implantable, percutaneously refillable infusion pump.[54] Since that time, pumps have become significantly more complex, allowing effective administration of regional therapy to provide maximal benefit.

Although many groups report the insertion of HAI pumps through minimally invasive techniques, the currently accepted implantation technique is with laparotomy. Patients are selected on their burden of disease and absence of extrahepatic metastases. Other factors to consider are greater than 30% tumor-free hepatic parenchyma, stable hepatic function with no evidence of portal hypertension, and a good performance status. The pump catheter is inserted into the gastroduodenal artery (GDA) and secured with permanent sutures. Great caution is taken to ligate all small branches proximal to the origin of the GDA and distally to the branch point of the left and right hepatic arteries, to prevent accidental chemoinfusion of the duodenum and stomach. The tubing is then brought through the abdominal wall and connected to a subcutaneously placed pump.

Complications of intrahepatic arterial chemotherapy can be divided into pump-related complications and chemotherapy-related complications.[6] Pump-related complications can include pump malfunctions, pump site infections, a pump that flips in the pocket, catheter thrombosis, or arterial thrombosis or dissection. Pump-related complications have been reported in 12% to 41% of patients, with the majority of complications occurring greater than 30 days after implantation.[55] Chemotherapy-related complications can include hematologic and gastrointestinal toxicities. Gastrointestinal toxicity typically manifests as nausea, vomiting, and diarrhea, which occur infrequently with HAI of 5-FUDR. The most common problems of HAI therapy are gastroduodenal ulceration and hepatotoxicity. Ulcer disease usually results from misperfusion of the stomach and duodenum via small collateral branches of the hepatic artery or the right gastric artery that were not divided during pump placement. Hepatobiliary toxicity can be a problematic toxicity. The bile ducts are particularly sensitive to regional therapy because they derive their blood supply almost exclusively from the hepatic artery. Clinically, biliary toxicities manifest as an elevation in the aspartate aminotransferase, alkaline phosphatase, and bilirubin levels, as well as cholangiographic biliary sclerosis mimicking sclerosing cholangitis. Dose reduction of 5-FUDR and concurrent corticosteroid perfusion through the pump may reduce hepatobiliary toxicity.

The most notable data for adjuvant HAI therapy following resection for colorectal metastases were reported in 1999 by Kemeny et al.[56] They observed an 86% overall 2-year survival in the patients treated with systemic plus HAI therapy (combined group) as compared with 72% in the group treated with systemic therapy alone. They reported an improved median survival, progression-free survival, and reduced risk ratio of death for the combined group. The

combination of HAI with systemic therapy improves the outcome at 2 years. Other trials have shown that objective tumor response rates are significantly greater for regional 5-FUDR than for systemic 5-FU treatment[57]; however, there is minimal improvement in overall survival. The use of regional infusional chemotherapy in unresectable patients improved median survival by only 3.2 months compared with SC. The data from individual trials may bias outcomes because many patients randomized to regional therapy did not complete therapy because of technical problems with the infusion pump or toxicity. Subset analyses of the patients who actually received regional therapy suggest improved survival compared with those treated systemically. Further trials of regional infusion of 5-FUDR are being carried out in an attempt to reduce associated toxicity and to address the role of concurrent SC as an adjunct after the resection of metastases. Trials are also evaluating the role of HAI therapy as a downstaging technique to convert patients with unresectable disease to resectable disease.[58]

CRYOABLATION

Cryoablation uses rapid freeze-thaw cycles, cooling tumor tissue to extremely low temperatures. The freeze cycles interrupt cell metabolism, causing apoptosis and vascular thromboses resulting in coagulative necrosis. To achieve a total cell kill, tissue temperatures of less than $-50°C$ are required. Repetitive freeze-thaw cycles increase the probability of complete tissue destruction. Thawing should be completed before the onset of the next freeze cycle for maximum cytotoxic potential. Cryoablation offers a technically sound and biologically rational approach for the treatment of such liver metastases.[59] The reported advantages of cryoablation versus resection of hepatic metastases are the avoidance of the inherent risks of resection over the technical ease and safety of the cryoablation with its potentially similar efficacy.

Intraoperative ultrasonography is essential for effective cryoablation. Ultrasonography provides (1) accurate positioning of cryoprobes within the metastases to avoid injury to major bile ducts and vessels, (2) accurate monitoring of the freeze-thaw process with a clear demonstration of the freeze-front, and (3) detection of occult hepatic metastases. For large tumors, multiple concurrent probes speed treatment.

Cryoablation of larger tumors can be associated with significant bleeding as the ice fractures the liver parenchyma and then thaws. There have also been reports, in cirrhotic livers, of a systemic inflammatory response known as cryoshock that leads to significant morbidity and mortality. Other potential complications include accidental freezing of adjacent tissues, bleeding due to the introduction of trotter probes, hypothermia and related cardiac arrhythmias, nitrogen embolism, bile duct or major vascular injury, and renal failure from myoglobinuria. Insulation of the diaphragm, bowel, and skin from the liver with laparotomy packs prevents accidental cryoinjury to adjacent structures. Bleeding from the probe tract is rarely a problem and can be easily controlled by packing the cryotract with hemostatic material. Large vessels tolerate cryotherapy extremely well without rupture or occlusion because of the continued dissipation of thermal energy by the flow of blood. In contrast, large bile ducts are extremely vulnerable to cryoinjury, and caution should be exercised in treating tumors located near the hilum. After cryosurgery, a transient elevation of liver enzymes and a mild leukocytosis may occur, but they should normalize within 1 week.

Survival rates after cryoablation for unresectable metastases approach 60% at 2 years with median survival times of 25 to 32 months.[59,60] To date, the outcome of cryoablation alone for hepatic metastases from colorectal carcinoma has been variable. Survival rates have ranged from 15% to 35% at 5 years. Whether survival after cryoablation will be equivalent to resection is yet undetermined.

RADIOFREQUENCY ABLATION

RFA is a therapy used to treat malignant tumors with the application of alternating electrical current that causes tissue coagulation through frictional heating. A standard treatment results in local tissue temperatures greater than 100°C, which produce coagulative necrosis of both the tumor and surrounding tissue. As necrosis develops, the tissue impedance rises, leading to reduced and eventual cessation of flow from the generator.[61]

The use of RFA, as either a primary or adjunct modality, has proven the most versatile of ablative techniques.[62] It can be used either percutaneously or laparoscopically or at laparotomy. Five-year overall survival rates in patients treated with RFA for unresectable CRMs have been reported at 21% to 36%.[63,64] Solbiati et al. reported a 5-year survival of 48% and a 10-year survival of 18%.[65] In 2016 van Amerongen et al. reported on their series of 638 patients who underwent partial hepatectomy with RFA ($n = 98$) or resection only ($n = 534$). They observed a local recurrence rate of 15.1% in the partial hepatectomy with RFA group (CG) and a 7.2% local recurrence in the resection only group (ROG). The 5-year overall survival was 42% and 62.2% for the CG and ROG, respectively.

One of the main disadvantages of RFA is the inability to treat tumors next to major vascular or biliary structures. When treating tumors close to major vascular structures, convective cooling (the heat sink effect) prohibits reaching target temperatures and inducing complete coagulative necrosis. With convective cooling and inadequate necrosis, residual viable tumor cells would be left behind increasing the rate of local recurrence. The heat from the probe can also cause thermal injury to vascular and biliary structures, resulting in unwanted thrombosis, ischemia, biliary strictures, and infection. As mentioned earlier, the rise in impedance reduces the flow of current through desiccated tissue. As the tumor size increases, so does the local recurrence rate. Currently the standard is to treat lesions less than 3 cm in size.[66] RFA is used primarily as an adjunct to resection or as primary therapy when resection is prohibitive or lesions are small, with minimal morbidity and mortality.

EMBOLIZATION

Transarterial therapy is a percutaneous technique used to access the arterial supply to malignant tumors in an affected organ. Although the liver derives the majority of its blood supply from the portal system, colorectal metastases are known to be vascular tumors that obtain their blood supply through branches of the hepatic artery.

This provides a unique opportunity to access the feeding arterial branches and subsequently administer targeted chemotherapy or radiation therapy and then effectively occlude the supplying artery to cause stasis and tumor death. This selective technique allows targeted therapy to the tumor while sparing the remainder of the liver from exposure to hepatotoxic therapy. Two therapies that are gaining popularity are transarterial chemoembolization with drug-eluting beads (TACE-DEB) and radioembolization with yttrium-90 microspheres (Y-90).

Most treatments are targeted to patients who are not surgical candidates and who have failed first line and often second line therapy. Martin et al. presented 55 patients who had received prior SC and underwent a total of 99 TACE-DEB treatments.[67] They noted response rates of 66% at 6 months and 75% at 12 months. The reported overall survival was 19 months, with a progression-free survival of 11 months. Fiorentini et al. presented their series of 74 patients who were randomized to TACE-DEB or SC.[68] At 50 months they reported a longer median survival (20 vs. 15 months) and progression-free survival (7 vs. 4 months) for the TACE-DEB and SC groups, respectively ($P = .006$). In 2015 Abbott et al. reported on 68 patients who had received radioembolization with Y-90 for CRLM.[69] They reported a median and 2-year overall survival of 11.6 months and 34%. They noted that the overall survival was directly related to the hepatic disease burden (hdb). The 2-year overall survival for patients with an hdb less than 25% versus greater than 25% was 42% and 0%, respectively. Although the initial data for transarterial therapy have been encouraging, subsequent studies have shown no advantage over resection. As transarterial therapies continue to evolve, more studies are needed to define their role in the treatment of CRLMs.

MICROWAVE ABLATION

Microwave ablation (MWA) was first described by Tabuse et al. in 1985.[70] It targets malignant lesions with multiple antennas that simultaneously emit electromagnetic waves, in the microwave frequency, to create a uniform zone of coagulation necrosis. As opposed to RFA, MWA has been shown to create a more consistent heat zone in larger tumors (>3 cm) that results in a faster ablation time with no heat sink effect.[71] Stattner et al. reported their experience in 28 patients with combined MWA and hepatectomy for unresectable CRLMs. They observed a local recurrence rate of 3.5%, with an estimated 1-, 3- and 5-year overall survival of 85%, 45%, and 18%, respectively.[72] Bhardwaj et al. reported similar outcomes in their series of 31 patients with 39 liver tumors. They observed a local tumor recurrence rate of 2%, with a 3-year median survival of 40%.[73] MWA is a safe and effective treatment. Although good long-term data are lacking, the technology continues to improve, giving it the potential to become the thermal ablative therapy of choice in the future.

IRREVERSIBLE ELECTROPORATION

IRE applies high-voltage, direct current through electrical pulses generated by parallel electrodes. The electrodes are positioned around the tumor, and the high-voltage current causes irreversible cellular membrane disruption, creating large pores that lead to cell death.[74] This treatment modality is nonthermal and so efficacy is not altered by proximity to blood vessels causing convective cooling. It is effective at targeting unresectable tumors close to connective tissue structures that could be at risk for thermal injury, such as arteries, veins, and bile ducts. Although this is a promising technique, long-term outcomes are lacking. Kingham et al. reported their series of 28 patients with a total of 65 tumors. The median size of the tumor was 1 cm or less. Tumors were 1 cm or less from a major hepatic vein in 57% of cases and 40% of tumors were 1 cm or less from a portal pedicle. At 6 months they observed three local recurrences and one tumor with persistent disease, for a combined local failure rate of 7.5%.[75] Others have reported efficacy ranging from 55% to 93%.[76] Currently, IRE is reserved for select patients with relatively small tumors abutting major vascular structures or portal pedicles, where RFA is considered less effective.

STEREOTACTIC WHOLE BODY RADIATION THERAPY

Stereotactic whole body radiation therapy (SBRT) is a system for delivering conformal high-dose radiation to the tumor in a few fractions while limiting the dose to surrounding critical tissues.[77] This allows treatment of the affected area and prevention of radiation-induced liver disease. In 2010 van der Pool et al. reported their results on 20 patients with 31 lesions. They observed a local control rate at 1 and 2 years of 100% and 74%, respectively.[78] In 2016 Scorsetti et al. treated 42 patients with 52 liver metastases, with a slightly higher dose of 75 Gy in three fractions. They reported a 1-, 2-, and 3-year local control rate of 95%, 91%, and 85%, respectively. They observed that local control did not correlate with the size of the lesion (<3 or >3 cm).[79] The best candidates for SBRT are oligometastatic patients with a good performance status, controlled or absent extrahepatic disease, number of hepatic lesions 3 or less, size of lesions 3 cm or less, lesion distance from organs at risk greater than 8 mm, and liver volume greater than 1000 mL.[77] Although SBRT is not currently recommended as a first line treatment for metastatic colorectal cancer to the liver, it can provide local control and improved survival in those patients who are not candidates for resection. Prospective randomized trials are needed to confirm clinical efficacy and long-term results.

RECURRENCE AND REPEAT HEPATIC RESECTION

Recurrence (or reappearance) of tumor after potentially curative liver resection usually involves the liver, lungs, and peritoneal cavity. In the French multicenter study, 1013 of 1569 patients (65%) with accessible follow-up data developed recurrent disease. The liver was involved in 63% of patients with recurrences, which included nearly 47% of patients with recurrent disease limited to the liver. Metastatic disease after hepatectomy occurred in 70% of the 607 patients from the US Registry of Hepatic Metastases.[62] A total of 316 patients had recurrence in a single organ: 149 (47%) in the liver, 73 (23%) in the lung, 30 (10%) local, and 61 (19%) in other sites. These patterns of recurrence after hepatic resection for metastatic colorectal cancer have been confirmed repeatedly. Given

the frequency of isolated hepatic progression, repeat hepatic resection has been often performed.[80–82] Interestingly, reports have consistently shown that survival after repeat resection is equal to that after the initial hepatic resection, and predictors of survival are similar to those for the first hepatic operation: 5-year survival rates of 25% to 30% can be expected after repeat hepatic resection. These findings warrant assessment for resection in all patients with recurrent hepatic metastases after hepatic resection.

The main cause of unresectability is achieving a balance between resection of the entire tumor burden while leaving sufficient residual functional liver parenchyma (at least 30% of initial liver parenchyma) for survival. The definition of unresectability depends on many factors, not the least of which is the surgical expertise and support care at the medical facility. Theoretical prognostic factors and technical factors of unresectability of hepatic metastases are essentially determined by factors that affect the amount of postresection functional hepatic mass; the most important of these are tumor location, number of metastases, and bilobar disease.

CONCLUSION

The management of CRLMs has made significant changes in the past decade. With thorough staging and targeted therapies, a 5-year survival of greater than 40% can be expected. Selection of the appropriate surgical candidate should include the ability to tolerate a major laparotomy and assessment of the regenerative capacity of the liver. Minimal FLR volume has been set at greater than 20% for a normal liver, greater than 30% in a damaged liver after extensive treatment, and greater than 40% for a cirrhotic liver.[33] The goals of surgical management should include a margin negative resection with the preservation of an adequate FLR. Strategies for improving resection include PVE, two-staged hepatectomy, neoadjuvant chemotherapy to assess the tumor biology, and local ablative techniques that control the disease burden while preparing for resection. Hepatic resection for CRLMs is the standard of care for patients with resectable disease.

ACKNOWLEDGMENTS

The authors thank Dr. Sara Boostrom, Dr. David Nagorney, and Dr. Florencia Que for their contributions to the chapter.

REFERENCES

1. Miller KD, Siegel RL, Lin CC, et al. Cancer treatment and survivorship statistics, 2016. *CA Cancer J Clin.* 2016;66(4):271-289. doi:10.3322/caac.21349.
2. Van Cutsem E, Nordlinger B, Adam R, et al. Towards a pan-European consensus on the treatment of patients with colorectal liver metastases. *Eur J Cancer.* 2006;42(14):2212-2221. doi:10.1016/j.ejca.2006.04.012.
3. Yoo PS, Lopez-Soler RI, Longo WE, Cha CH. Liver resection for metastatic colorectal cancer in the age of neoadjuvant chemotherapy and bevacizumab. *Clin Colorectal Cancer.* 2006;6(3):202-207. doi:10.3816/CCC.2006.n.036.
4. Foster JH. Treatment of metastatic disease of the liver: a skeptic's view. *Semin Liver Dis.* 1984;4(2):170-179. doi:10.1055/s-2008-1040656.
5. Tsai M-S, Su Y-H, Ho M-C, et al. Clinicopathological features and prognosis in resectable synchronous and metachronous colorectal liver metastasis. *Ann Surg Oncol.* 2007;14(2):786-794. doi:10.1245/s10434-006-9215-5.

6. Weiss L, Grundmann E, Torhorst J, et al. Haematogenous metastatic patterns in colonic carcinoma: an analysis of 1541 necropsies. *J Pathol.* 1986;150(3):195-203. doi:10.1002/path.1711500308.

7. Wang J, Yang M, Hoffman RM. Visualizing portal vein metastatic trafficking to the liver with green fluorescent protein-expressing tumor cells. *Anticancer Res.* 2004;24(6):3699-3702.

8. Uetsuji S, Yamamura M, Yamamichi K, Okuda Y, Takada H, Hioki K. Absence of colorectal cancer metastasis to the cirrhotic liver. *Am J Surg.* 1992;164(2):176-177.

9. Norstein J, Silen W. Natural history of liver metastases from colorectal carcinoma. *J Gastrointes Surg.* 1997;1(5):398-407.

10. Adam R, de Gramont A, Figueras J, et al. Managing synchronous liver metastases from colorectal cancer: a multidisciplinary international consensus. *Cancer Treat Rev.* 2015;41(9):729-741. doi:10.1016/j ctrv.2015.06.006.

11. Pawlik TM, Scoggins CR, Zorzi D, et al. Effect of surgical margin status on survival and site of recurrence after hepatic resection for colorectal metastases. *Ann Surg.* 2005;241(5):715-722; discussion 722-724.

12. Minagawa M, Yamamoto J, Kosuge T, Matsuyama Y, Miyagawa S-I Makuuchi M. Simplified staging system for predicting the prognosis of patients with resectable liver metastasis: development and validation. *Arch Surg.* 2007;142(3):269-276; discussion 277. doi:10.1001/ archsurg.142.3.269.

13. Belghiti J, Hiramatsu K, Benoist S, Massault P, Sauvanet A, Farges O. Seven hundred forty-seven hepatectomies in the 1990s: an update to evaluate the actual risk of liver resection. *J Am Coll Surg* 2000;191(1):38-46.

14. Kamiyama T, Nakanishi K, Yokoo H, et al. Perioperative management of hepatic resection toward zero mortality and morbidity: analysis of 793 consecutive cases in a single institution. *J Am Coll Surg* 2010;211(4):443-449. doi:10.1016/j.jamcollsurg.2010.06.005.

15. de Haas RJ, Adam R, Wicherts DA, et al. Comparison of simultaneous or delayed liver surgery for limited synchronous colorectal metastases *Br J Surg.* 2010;97(8):1279-1289. doi:10.1002/bjs.7106.

16. Nordlinger B, Guiguet M, Vaillant JC, et al. Surgical resection of colorectal carcinoma metastases to the liver. A prognostic scoring system to improve case selection, based on 1568 patients. Association Francaise de Chirurgie. *Cancer.* 1996;77(7):1254-1262.

17. Minagawa M, Makuuchi M, Torzilli G, et al. Extension of the frontiers of surgical indications in the treatment of liver metastases from colorectal cancer: long-term results. *Ann Surg.* 2000;231(4):487-499

18. Poultsides GA, Bao F, Servais EL, et al. Pathologic response to preoperative chemotherapy in colorectal liver metastases: fibrosis not necrosis, predicts outcome. *Ann Surg Oncol.* 2012;19(9):2797-2804 doi:10.1245/s10434-012-2335-1.

19. Adam R, Pascal G, Castaing D, et al. Tumor progression while on chemotherapy: a contraindication to liver resection for multiple colorectal metastases? *Ann Surg.* 2004;240(6):1052-1064.

20. Eisenhauer EA, Therasse P, Bogaerts J, et al. New response evaluation criteria in solid tumours: revised RECIST guideline (version 1.1) *Eur J Cancer.* 2009;45(2):228-247. doi:10.1016/j.ejca.2008.10.026.

21. Shindoh J, Loyer EM, Kopetz S, et al. Optimal morphologic response to preoperative chemotherapy: an alternate outcome end point before resection of hepatic colorectal metastases. *J Clin Oncol* 2012;30(36):4566-4572. doi:10.1200/JCO.2012.45.2854.

22. Andreou A, Aloia TA, Brouquet A, et al. Margin status remains an important determinant of survival after surgical resection of colorectal liver metastases in the era of modern chemotherapy. *Ann Surg.* 2013;257(6):1079-1088. doi:10.1097/SLA.0b013e318283a4d1.

23. Mise Y, Zimmitti G, Shindoh J, et al. RAS mutations predict radiologic and pathologic response in patients treated with chemotherapy before resection of colorectal liver metastases. *Ann Surg Oncol.* 2015;22(3):834-842. doi:10.1245/s10434-014-4042-6.

24. Elias D, Liberale G, Vernerey D, et al. Hepatic and extrahepatic colorectal metastases: when resectable, their localization does not matter, but their total number has a prognostic effect. *Ann Surg Oncol.* 2005;12(11):900-909. doi:10.1245/ASO.2005.01.010.

25. Carpizo DR, Are C, Jarnagin W, et al. Liver resection for metastatic colorectal cancer in patients with concurrent extrahepatic disease: results in 127 patients treated at a single center. *Ann Surg Oncol.* 2009;16(8):2138-2146. doi:10.1245/s10434-009-0521-5.

26. Leung U, Gonen M, Allen PJ, et al. Colorectal cancer liver metastases and concurrent extrahepatic disease treated with resection. *Ann Surg.* 2016;doi:10.1097/SLA.0000000000001624; [Epub ahead of print].

27. Truant S, Sequier C, Leteurtre E, et al. Tumour biology of colorectal liver metastasis is a more important factor in survival than surgical margin clearance in the era of modern chemotherapy regimens. *HPB (Oxford).* 2015;17(2):176-184. doi:10.1111/hpb.12316

28. Nordlinger B, Sorbye H, Glimelius B, et al. Perioperative chemotherapy with FOLFOX4 and surgery versus surgery alone for resectable liver metastases from colorectal cancer (EORTC Intergroup trial 40983): a randomised controlled trial. *Lancet.* 2008 371(9617):1007-1016. doi:10.1016/S0140-6736(08)60455-9.

29. Vauthey J-N, Pawlik TM, Ribero D, et al. Chemotherapy regimen predicts steatohepatitis and an increase in 90-day mortality after surgery for hepatic colorectal metastases. *J Clin Oncol.* 2006;24(13):2065-2072. doi:10.1200/JCO.2005.05.3074.

30. Ribero D, Wang H, Donadon M, et al. Bevacizumab improves pathologic response and protects against hepatic injury in patients treated with oxaliplatin-based chemotherapy for colorectal liver metastases. *Cancer.* 2007;110(12):2761-2767. doi:10.1002/ cncr.23099.

31. Thomay AA, Charpentier KP. Optimizing resection for "responding" hepatic metastases after neoadjuvant chemotherapy. *J Surg Oncol.* 2010;102(8):1002-1008. doi:10.1002/jso.21696.

32. Charnsangavej C, Clary B, Fong Y, Grothey A, Pawlik TM, Choti MA. Selection of patients for resection of hepatic colorectal metastases: expert consensus statement. *Ann Surg Oncol.* 2006;13(10):1261-1268. doi:10.1245/s10434-006-9023-y

33. Shindoh J, Tzeng C-WD, Aloia TA, et al. Optimal future liver remnant in patients treated with extensive preoperative chemotherapy for colorectal liver metastases. *Ann Surg Oncol.* 2013;20(8):2493-2500. doi:10.1245/s10434-012-2864-7.

34. Shindoh J, Truty MJ, Aloia TA, et al. Kinetic growth rate after portal vein embolization predicts posthepatectomy outcomes: toward zero liver-related mortality in patients with colorectal liver metastases and small future liver remnant. *J Am Coll Surg.* 2013;216(2):201-209. doi:10.1016/j.jamcollsurg.2012.10.018.

35. Fan ST. Liver functional reserve estimation: state of the art and relevance for local treatments: the Eastern perspective. *J Hepatobil Pancreat Sci.* 2010;17(4):380-384. doi:10.1007/s00534-009-0229-9.

36. de Graaf W, van Lienden KP, Dinant S, et al. Assessment of future remnant liver function using hepatobiliary scintigraphy in patients undergoing major liver resection. *J Gastrointest Surg.* 2010;14(2):369-378. doi:10.1007/s11605-009-1085-2.

37. Feroci F, Fong Y. Use of clinical score to stage and predict outcome of hepatic resection of metastatic colorectal cancer. *J Surg Oncol.* 2010;102(8):914-921. doi:10.1002/jso.21715

38. Merkel S, Bialecki D, Meyer T, Muller V, Papadopoulos T, Hohenberger W. Comparison of clinical risk scores predicting prognosis after resection of colorectal liver metastases. *J Surg Oncol.* 2009;100(5):349-357. doi:10.1002/jso.21346.

39. Zech CJ, Korpraphong P, Huppertz A, et al. Randomized multicentre trial of gadoxetic acid-enhanced MRI versus conventional MRI or CT in the staging of colorectal cancer liver metastases. *Br J Surg.* 2014;101(6):613-621. doi:10.1002/bjs.9465.

40. Couinaud C. *Surgical Anatomy of the Liver Revisited.* Paris (15, rue Spontini, 75116): C. Couinaud; 1989.

41. Kokudo N, Imamura H, Sugawara Y, et al. Surgery for multiple hepatic colorectal metastases. *J Hepatobiliary Pancreat Surg.* 2004;11(2):84-91. doi:10.1007/s00534-002-0754-2.

42. Vandeweyer D, Neo EL, Chen JWC, Maddern GJ, Wilson TG, Padbury RTA. Influence of resection margin on survival in hepatic resections for colorectal liver metastases. *HPB (Oxford).* 2009;11(6):499-504. doi:10.1111/j.1477-2574.2009.00092.x.

43. Kokudo N, Miki Y, Sugai S, et al. Genetic and histological assessment of surgical margins in resected liver metastases from colorectal carcinoma: minimum surgical margins for successful resection. *Arch Surg.* 2002;137(7):833-840.

44. Adams RB, Haller DG, Roh MS. Improving resectability of hepatic colorectal metastases: expert consensus statement by Abdalla et al. *Ann Surg Oncol.* 2006;13(10):1281-1283. doi:10.1245/s10434-006-9149-y.

45. Benoist S, Brouquet A, Penna C, et al. Complete response of colorectal liver metastases after chemotherapy: does it mean cure? *J Clin Oncol.* 2006;24(24):3939-3945. doi:10.1200/JCO.2005.05.8727.

46. Owen JW, Fowler KJ, Doyle MB, Saad NE, Linehan DC, Chapman WC. Colorectal liver metastases: disappearing lesions in the era of Eovist hepatobiliary magnetic resonance imaging. *HPB (Oxford).* 2016;18(3):296-303. doi:10.1016/j.hpb.2015.10.009.

47. Abulkhir A, Limongelli P, Healey AJ, et al. Preoperative portal vein embolization for major liver resection: a meta-analysis. *Ann Surg.* 2008;247(1):49-57. doi:10.1097/SLA.0b013e31815f6e5b.

48. Azoulay D, Castaing D, Smail A, et al. Resection of nonresectable liver metastases from colorectal cancer after percutaneous portal vein embolization. *Ann Surg.* 2000;231(4):480-486.

49. Giglio MC, Giakoustidis A, Draz A, et al. Oncological outcomes of major liver resection following portal vein embolization: a systematic review and meta-analysis. *Ann Surg Oncol.* 2016;23(11):3709-3717. doi:10.1245/s10434-016-5264-6.

50. Adam R, Delvart V, Pascal G, et al. Rescue surgery for unresectable colorectal liver metastases downstaged by chemotherapy: a model to predict long-term survival. *Ann Surg.* 2004;240(4):644-648.

51. Hughes MJ, Ventham NT, Harrison EM, Wigmore SJ. Central venous pressure and liver resection: a systematic review and meta-analysis. *HPB (Oxford).* 2015;17(10):863-871. doi:10.1111/hpb.12462.

52. Pang YY. The Brisbane 2000 terminology of liver anatomy and resections. HPB 2000; 2:333-339. *HPB (Oxford).* 2002;4(2):99; author reply 99-100. doi:10.1080/136518202760378489.

53. Dizon DS, Schwartz J, Kemeny N. Regional chemotherapy: a focus on hepatic artery infusion for colorectal cancer liver metastases. *Surg Oncol Clin North Am.* 2008;17(4):759-771, viii. doi:10.1016/j.soc.2008.04.009.

54. Buchwald H, Grage TB, Vassilopoulos PP, Rohde TD, Varco RL, Blackshear PJ. Intraarterial infusion chemotherapy for hepatic carcinoma using a totally implantable infusion pump. *Cancer.* 1980;45(5):866-869.

55. Allen PJ, Nissan A, Picon AI, et al. Technical complications and durability of hepatic artery infusion pumps for unresectable colorectal liver metastases: an institutional experience of 544 consecutive cases. *J Am Coll Surg.* 2005;201(1):57-65. doi:10.1016/j.jamcollsurg.2005.03.019.

56. Kemeny N, Huang Y, Cohen AM, et al. Hepatic arterial infusion of chemotherapy after resection of hepatic metastases from colorectal cancer. *N Engl J Med.* 1999;341(27):2039-2048. doi:10.1056/NEJM199912303412702.

57. Piedbois P, Buyse M, Kemeny N, et al. Reappraisal of hepatic arterial infusion in the treatment of nonresectable liver metastases from colorectal cancer. *J Natl Cancer Inst.* 1996;88(5):252-258.

58. Ammori JB, Kemeny NE, Fong Y, et al. Conversion to complete resection and/or ablation using hepatic artery infusional chemotherapy in patients with unresectable liver metastases from colorectal cancer: a decade of experience at a single institution. *Ann Surg Oncol.* 2013;20(9):2901-2907. doi:10.1245/s10434-013-3009-3.

59. Ravikumar TS. The role of cryotherapy in the management of patients with liver tumors. *Adv Surg.* 1996;30:281-291.

60. Korpan NN. Hepatic cryosurgery for liver metastases. Long-term follow-up. *Ann Surg.* 1997;225(2):193-201.

61. Curley SA. Radiofrequency ablation of malignant liver tumors. *Oncologist.* 2001;6(1):14-23.

62. Hughes KS, Simon R, Songhorabodi S, et al. Resection of the liver for colorectal carcinoma metastases: a multi-institutional study of patterns of recurrence. *Surgery.* 1986;100(2):278-284.

63. Hamada A, Yamakado K, Nakatsuka A, et al. Radiofrequency ablation for colorectal liver metastases: prognostic factors in non-surgical candidates. *Jpn J Radiol.* 2012;30(7):567-574. doi:10.1007/s11604-012-0089-0.

64. Gillams AR, Lees WR. Five-year survival in 309 patients with colorectal liver metastases treated with radiofrequency ablation. *Eur Radiol.* 2009;19(5):1206-1213. doi:10.1007/s00330-008-1258-5.

65. Solbiati L, Ahmed M, Cova L, Ierace T, Brioschi M, Goldberg SN. Small liver colorectal metastases treated with percutaneous radiofrequency ablation: local response rate and long-term survival with up to 10-year follow-up. *Radiology.* 2012;265(3):958-968. doi:10.1148/radiol.12111851.

66. Ziemlewicz TJ, Wells SA, Lubner MG, Brace CL, Lee FTJ, Hinshaw JL. Hepatic tumor ablation. *Surg Clin North Am.* 2016;96(2):315-339. doi:10.1016/j.suc.2015.12.006.

67. Martin RCG, Joshi J, Robbins K, et al. Hepatic intra-arterial injection of drug-eluting bead, irinotecan (DEBIRI) in unresectable colorectal liver metastases refractory to systemic chemotherapy: results of multi-institutional study. *Ann Surg Oncol.* 2011;18(1):192-198. doi:10.1245/s10434-010-1288-5.

68. Fiorentini G, Aliberti C, Tilli M, et al. Intra-arterial infusion of irinotecan-loaded drug-eluting beads (DEBIRI) versus intravenous therapy (FOLFIRI) for hepatic metastases from colorectal cancer: final results of a phase III study. *Anticancer Res.* 2012;32(4):1387-1395.

69. Abbott AM, Kim R, Hoffe SE, et al. Outcomes of therasphere radioembolization for colorectal metastases. *Clin Colorectal Cancer.* 2015;14(3):146-153. doi:10.1016/j.clcc.2015.02.002.

70. Tabuse K, Katsumi M, Kobayashi Y, et al. Microwave surgery: hepatectomy using a microwave tissue coagulator. *World J Surg.* 1985;9(1):136-143.

71. Harari CM, Magagna M, Bedoya M, et al. Microwave ablation: comparison of simultaneous and sequential activation of multiple antennas in liver model systems. *Radiology.* 2016;278(1):95-103. doi:10.1148/radiol.2015142151.

72. Stattner S, Primavesi F, Yip VS, et al. Evolution of surgical microwave ablation for the treatment of colorectal cancer liver metastasis: review of the literature and a single centre experience. *Surg Today.* 2015;45(4):407-415. doi:10.1007/s00595-014-0879-3.

73. Bhardwaj N, Strickland AD, Ahmad F, et al. Microwave ablation for unresectable hepatic tumours: clinical results using a novel microwave probe and generator. *Eur J Surg Oncol.* 2010;36(3):264-268. doi:10.1016/j.ejso.2009.10.006.

74. Scheffer HJ, Vroomen LGPH, Nielsen K, et al. Colorectal liver metastatic disease: efficacy of irreversible electroporation—a single-arm phase II clinical trial (COLDFIRE-2 trial). *BMC Cancer.* 2015;15:772. doi:10.1186/s12885-015-1736-5.

75. Kingham TP, Karkar AM, D'Angelica MI, et al. Ablation of perivascular hepatic malignant tumors with irreversible electroporation. *J Am Coll Surg.* 2012;215(3):379-387. doi:10.1016/j.jamcollsurg.2012.04.029.

76. Scheffer HJ, Melenhorst MCAM, Echenique AM, et al. Irreversible electroporation for colorectal liver metastases. *Tech Vasc Interv Radiol.* 2015;18(3):159-169. doi:10.1053/j.tvir.2015.06.007.

77. Scorsetti M, Clerici E, Comito T. Stereotactic body radiation therapy for liver metastases. *J Gastrointest Oncol.* 2014;5(3):190-197. doi:10.3978/j.issn.2078-6891.2014.039.

78. van der Pool AEM, Mendez Romero A, Wunderink W, et al. Stereotactic body radiation therapy for colorectal liver metastases. *Br J Surg.* 2010;97(3):377-382. doi:10.1002/bjs.6895.

79. Scorsetti M, Comito T, Tozzi A, et al. Final results of a phase II trial for stereotactic body radiation therapy for patients with inoperable liver metastases from colorectal cancer. *J Cancer Res Clin Oncol.* 2015;141(3):543-553. doi:10.1007/s00432-014-1833-x.

80. Fernandez-Trigo V, Shamsa F, Sugarbaker PH. Repeat liver resections from colorectal metastasis. Repeat Hepatic Metastases Registry. *Surgery.* 1995;117(3):296-304.

81. Nordlinger B, Vaillant JC. Repeat resections for recurrent colorectal liver metastases. *Cancer Treat Res.* 1994;69:57-61.

82. Tanaka K, Shimada H, Ohta M, et al. Procedures of choice for resection of primary and recurrent liver metastases from colorectal cancer. *World J Surg.* 2004;28(5):482-487. doi:10.1007/s00268-004-7214-x.

Neoplasms of the Anus: High-Grade Squamous Intraepithelial Lesions and Cancer

Mark Lane Welton | Imran Hassan

The perianal region includes the (1) anal canal, (2) perianus, and (3) perianal skin. This chapter will review the definition and anatomy of the anal canal and perianus and discuss the diagnosis and management of neoplasms that occur in these regions. Malignancies of the anal canal and perianus are uncommon and account for 2% of all lower gastrointestinal tract cancers. The most common malignancies include squamous cell carcinoma (SCC) of the anal canal and perianus, squamous intraepithelial lesions (SILs), as well as uncommon neoplasms such as adenocarcinoma, melanoma, Buschke-Löwenstein tumors (verrucous carcinoma), Paget disease, and basal cell carcinomas (BCCs).

ANATOMY

The anal canal starts at the pelvic floor where the rectum enters the puborectalis muscle at the superior most aspect of the sphincter complex and ends where the stratified squamous epithelium becomes continuous with the perianal skin (Fig. 173.1). On digital examination, this corresponds to the palpable anorectal ring superiorly and the intersphincteric groove, the outermost boundary of the internal sphincter inferiorly.[1] It includes columnar epithelium above the dentate line, squamous epithelium below the dentate line, and the anal transition zone (ATZ). The ATZ is a region 1 to 12 mm in length at the dentate line where there is a "transitional urothelium-like" epithelium. This is considered to be a variant of squamous epithelium and includes cloacogenic, transitional, and basaloid epithelium instead of the columnar epithelium of the rectum. The "transformation zone" refers to the squamous metaplasia that can involve the proximal anal canal above the dentate line that is usually lined with columnar epithelium.[1] The average length of the anal canal is longer in men (3 to 6 cm) than in women (2 to 4 cm).

Anal canal lesions cannot be visualized at all or are incompletely visualized with gentle traction placed on the buttocks. The perianus extends from the inferior boundary of the anal canal to approximately a radius of 5 cm around the anus and represents a region and not a distinct anatomic boundary. This region was previously referred to as the anal margin, but under the current accepted nomenclature, lesions of the perianus are referred to as perianal lesions. It is characterized by stratified squamous epithelium as well as skin appendages such as apocrine glands and hair. Perianal lesions are easily visible and are within a 5-cm radius of the anal canal when gentle traction is placed on the buttocks. Finally, skin lesions fall outside of the 5-cm radius of the perianus (see Fig. 173.1).[1] This distinction is important to determine the exact location

of lesions because the management of anal canal and lesions of the perianus and skin can be different.

The anal canal and perianal region has a diverse number of cell types and therefore a variety of different cancers can originate from this region. The most frequent malignancy is SCC that can be nonkeratinizing or keratinizing. Lesions originating from the ATZ include cloacogenic, transitional, basaloid, and mucoepidermoid carcinomas. These distinctions are not clinically important anymore as they are grouped under SCCs because their treatment and prognosis are similar to anal SCC. The second most common malignancy of the anal canal are adenocarcinomas. Other uncommon malignancies include melanoma, verrucous carcinoma, Paget disease, and BCC.

ANAL SQUAMOUS CELL CARCINOMA

EPIDEMIOLOGY

Anal SCC is relatively uncommon, representing only 0.5% of all new cancers diagnosed annually in the United States. There were just over 8200 estimated cases in 2017, accounting for approximately 1100 deaths, representing 0.2% of cancer deaths.[2]

In the United States the incidence of anal cancer has increased in men and women by 2.2% per year during the last decade, with the incidence being higher in women (2 per 100,000) than men (1.5 per 100,000).[1] The median age of diagnosis is 60 years, and the overall 5-year disease-specific survival (DSS) is 66%. Patients with early-stage disease American Joint Committee on Cancer (AJCC stage I and II) have a 5-year DSS of approximately 80%, but for patients with locally advanced disease, nodal disease (AJCC stage III), or distant disease (AJCC stage IV) the 5-year DSS is significantly worse, being 60% and 15%, respectively.[2] Risk factors for anal SCC include female gender, infection with human papillomavirus (HPV) and human immunodeficiency virus (HIV), anal receptive intercourse, multiple sexual partners, HPV-related cancers such as vulvar and cervical cancer, smoking, and immunosuppression after organ transplantation. Men who have sex with men (MSM) are approximately 20 times more likely than heterosexual men to develop anal SCC. The incidence of anal SCC in HIV-positive patients has itself increased since the introduction of highly active antiretroviral therapy (HAART) possibly because it has prolonged the survival of patients with HIV. Studies have shown that the anal cancer incidence rates are 30 times as high for HIV-positive patients compared with the general population, although the incidence rates vary widely from 18 to 149 per 100,000 person years.[3]

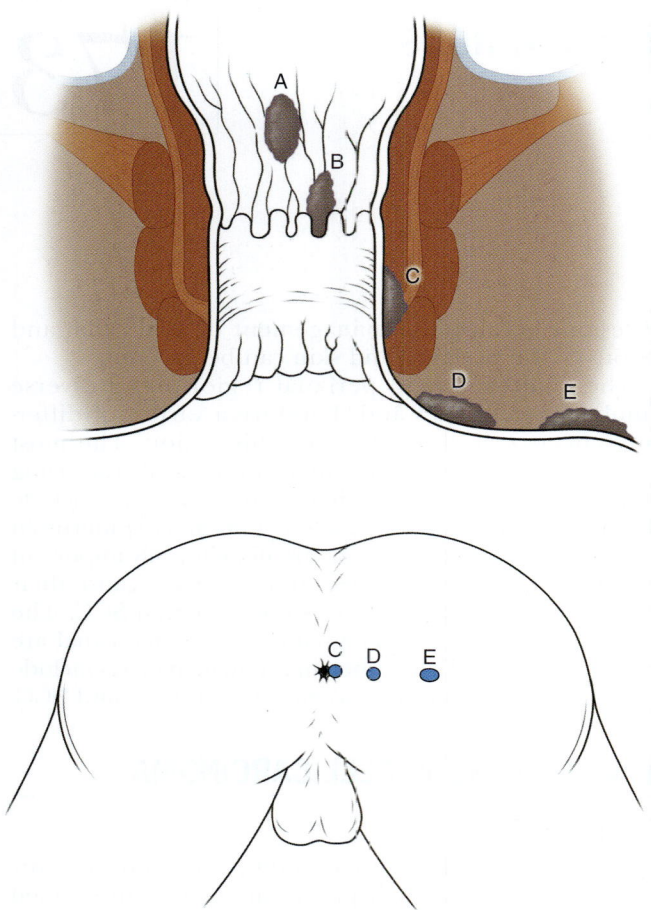

FIGURE 173.1 Anal canal and perianal anatomy. Anal cancer (A, B, and C), perianal cancer (D). Skin cancer (E) as visualized with gentle traction on the buttocks. (From Welton ML, Steele SR, Goodman KA. Anus. In: Amin MB, Edge S, Greene F, et al., eds. *AJCC Cancer Staging Manuel*. 8th ed. Berlin: Springer; 2016:275–284.)

The highest rates have been observed in HIV-positive MSM. HIV-positive heterosexual men may have a higher incidence than HIV-positive women, although this is not consistent across studies.[3]

Based on clinical, epidemiologic, and laboratory data, HPV infection is considered the underlying etiology in approximately 95% of anal SCC and as a result, the risk factors for both are similar. The most common HPV strain associated with anal SCC is HPV-16, which has been seen in 89% of cases.[1] The carcinogenic effects of HPV are mediated through oncoproteins E6 and E7, which interact with tumor suppressor proteins such as p53 and pRB, and disrupt the cell cycle, resulting in uncontrolled cell division.[4] There is no definite association of anal SCC with dietary habits, chronic inflammatory conditions, and symptomatic hemorrhoidal disease.[5]

PRESENTATION AND DIAGNOSIS

The common presenting symptoms are anal pain, bleeding, anal discharge, irritation, and discomfort. Patients may report anal leakage or soiling and can also develop fecal

incontinence and tenesmus if the sphincter complex is involved. In patients with locally advanced disease, there may be signs and symptoms of perianal sepsis and fistulous disease. Patients can also be asymptomatic or be incidentally diagnosed after excision of anal lesions or after hemorrhoid surgery. Due to the nonspecific nature of these presenting symptoms, patients are frequently misdiagnosed as having a benign anorectal pathology. In patients with a nonhealing anal fissure, chronic ulcer, or fistula that is not responsive to therapy, it is important to rule out an underlying malignancy with a tissue diagnosis.

The initial work-up of a patient with anal SCC should include a complete history including assessment of risk factors for anal cancer and a physical examination with emphasis on the inguinal lymph nodes, a digital rectal examination, and anoscopic examination with biopsy. It is important to note the location and size of the lesion, its relationship to the sphincter complex, and evidence of invasion into surrounding structures such as the vagina, urinary bladder/urethra, and pelvic sidewalls. Although this can all be performed with the patient awake in the office, it is usually uncomfortable for the patient. Therefore an exam under anesthesia provides a better opportunity to thoroughly examine the patient, as well as obtain a tissue diagnosis.

DIAGNOSTIC IMAGING

The clinical assessment of the primary disease and inguinal nodes is helpful in the clinical staging of the disease, whereas radiologic evaluation is more accurate and reliable in determining the nature and extent of local, nodal, and distant disease. Because the definitive treatment for anal cancer is chemoradiation, there are few data to validate the accuracy and reliability of radiologic staging of local and nodal disease, as there is no pathologic correlation or comparable referent stage. The most frequent staging modality used to evaluate metastatic disease is a contrast computed tomography (CT) scan because it can reliably evaluate for distant disease in the liver and lungs, as well as abnormal lymphadenopathy in the inguinal region and the pelvis. For local staging purpose, endorectal ultrasound (ERUS) allows visualization of the anal canal and can accurately assess the depth of tumor penetration and extension to surrounding structures, including sphincter complex involvement. However, ERUS is of limited value in assessing mesorectal and pelvic lymphadenopathy, and therefore its routine use is not recommended. Magnetic resonance imaging (MRI) provides accurate assessment of the primary lesion, in particular the extent and nature of involvement of surrounding organs, and is also more reliable than ERUS in evaluating lymph nodes in the mesorectum and inguinal regions and as a result should be used to complement CT scan findings.

FLUORODEOXYGLUCOSE POSITRON EMISSION TOMOGRAPHY–COMPUTED TOMOGRAPHY

PET/CT with fluorodeoxyglucose (FDG) has the ability to evaluate lymph node involvement and distant metastases because the majority of these cancers are FDG avid. It can also detect lymph nodes with metastatic disease that have increased uptake but are normal size. In early-stage disease (T size <3 cm) the risk of inguinal node involvement is less than 5%, whereas in clinical stages T3 (>5 cm) and T4 (involvement of adjacent structures such as bladder or vagina) the probability of metastatic lymph node disease is almost 20%. Clinical examination and imaging with CT scans along with fine-needle aspiration is considered the standard to determine nodal involvement.[6] This strategy likely understages a proportion of patients because almost half of involved lymph nodes are less than 5 mm in size and would not be clinically palpable or detected by CT scan,[6] which usually has a size threshold of 8 mm.

Overall, the data would suggest that FDG-PET/CT alters the stage in approximately 20% of cases, with a trend toward upstaging, and results in modification of treatment intent in 3% to 5% of patients.[7] As a result, PET/CT has been advocated to be incorporated into the staging work-up because it may be able to identify positive lymph nodes that may not necessarily be identified by CT scan or physical examination.[8,9] The current National Comprehensive Cancer Network Clinical Practice Guidelines in Oncology (NCCN Guidelines) have included PET/CT as a part of the routine diagnostic work-up.

STAGING

SCC of the anal canal can spread by (1) direct extension and invasion of adjacent structures such as the vagina in women, the bladder, and urethra; (2) lymphatic spread through the perirectal, pelvic, and inguinal lymph nodes; and (3) hematogenously to distant organs such as the liver and lung.[4] This relatively wide and variable range of spread is due to the unique lymphatic and venous drainage of the anal canal. As a result, metastases can occur to the inguinal and pelvic lymph nodes and to the liver by the portal system or to the lung via the systemic circulation, depending on the location of the SCC. The part of the anal canal above the dentate line drains through the superior rectal vessels to the inferior mesenteric lymph nodes and vein and laterally to the internal iliac lymph nodes. The anal canal below the dentate line, as well as the perianus, drains primarily into the inguinal lymph nodes and the internal iliac vein through the inferior rectal vein but could also involve the inferior and superior rectal lymph nodes.

Tumors of the anus and perianus that are discussed in this chapter are staged according to the unified AJCC/International Union against Cancer (UICC) staging system, eighth edition, which incorporates tumor size (T), lymph node status (N), and distant metastasis. The T stage is based on size of the cancer and extent of involvement of surrounding structures, and the N stage is based on presence or absence of nodal disease (Table 173.1). Mesorectal, superficial and deep inguinal, superior rectal, and external and internal iliac nodes are considered regional lymph nodes, whereas all other nodal groups represent distant metastasis (Fig. 173.2).[1]

TREATMENT

The management of anal SCC is dependent on the stage of the disease at presentation. Early-stage and locally advanced

TABLE 173.1 American Joint Committee on Cancer Eighth Edition Classification of Anal Canal Squamous Cell Carcinoma

PRIMARY TUMOR (T)

TX	Tumor cannot be assessed
T0	No evidence of primary tumor
Tis	High-grade intraepithelial squamous lesion
T1	Tumor less than 2 cm in greatest dimension
T2	Tumor 2–5 cm in greatest dimension
T3	Tumor greater than 5 cm in greatest dimension
T4	Tumor invades deep structures (muscle, bone, cartilage)

NODAL STATUS (N)

Nx	Regional lymph nodes cannot be assessed
N0	No regional lymph node metastasis
N1	Metastasis in inguinal, mesorectal or internal iliac or external lymph nodes
N1a	Metastasis in inguinal, mesorectal or internal iliac
N2b	Metastasis in external iliac lymph nodes
N3c	Metastasis in external lymph nodes with any N1a lymph nodes

DISTANT METASTASIS (M)

Mx	Distant metastasis cannot be assessed
M0	No distant metastasis
M1	Distant metastasis present

STAGES

Stage 0	Tis	N0	M0
Stage 1	T1	N0	M0
Stage 2a	T2	N0	M0
Stage 2b	T3	N0	M0
Stage 3a	T1,2	N1	M0
Stage 3b	T4	N0	M0
Stage 3c	T3,4	N1	M0
Stage 4	Any Y	Any N	M1

From Welton ML, Steele SR, Goodman KA. Anus. In: Amin MB, Edge S, Greene F, et al., eds. *AJCC Cancer Staging Manual*. 8th ed. Berlin: Springer; 2016:275–284.

SCC is treated with the combination of concurrent chemotherapy and radiation. In patients with metastatic disease, chemoradiation can be used for symptom control if the primary disease is symptomatic, whereas asymptomatic patients can receive palliative chemotherapy. The primary goal of curative treatment for anal SCC is to achieve local control of the disease while preserving patient quality of life (QoL). Prior to 1970 anal SCC was treated with radical surgery that included an abdominoperineal resection (APR). This treatment was associated with an overall 5-year survival rate of between 40% and 70% and required the patient to have a permanent colostomy, along with its associated morbidity and impact on QoL. Local or regional nodal recurrence occurred in 20% to 50% of patients within 2 years and was associated with an adverse prognosis. Norman Nigro introduced the use of radiotherapy with concurrent chemotherapy in the neoadjuvant setting prior to surgical resection. In his initial report of three patients, it was observed that two patients did not have any residual disease in the resected surgical specimens, whereas the third patient who refused to have surgery was disease free after 14 months. This treatment

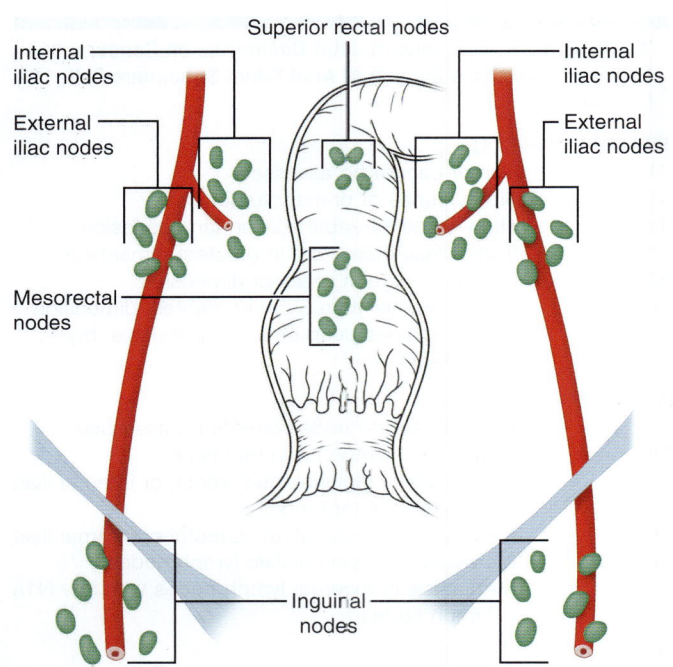

Internal iliac nodes

External iliac nodes

Superior rectal nodes

Internal iliac nodes

External iliac nodes

Mesorectal nodes

Inguinal nodes

FIGURE 173.2 Regional lymph nodes of the anal canal. (From Welton ML, Steele SR, Goodman KA. Anus. In: Amin MB, Edge S, Greene F, et al., eds. *AJCC Cancer Staging Manuel*. 8th ed. Berlin: Springer; 2016:275–284.)

regimen included 30 Gy of external beam radiation, a 5-day infusion of 5-fluorouracil, and a single injection of mitomycin C; it became known as the "Nigro protocol" and represented a major advance in the management of patients with anal SCC.[10] This regimen was further modified in terms of radiation dose and chemotherapy agents and most of the subsequent studies, including six randomized trials (EORTC 22861, ACT I, ACT II, RTOG 87-04, RTOG 98-11, and ACCORD 03), used a "modified" form of the classic Nigro protocol for comparison.[5]

Out of these six randomized trials, two trials (EORTC 22861 and ACT I) were designed to compare the effectiveness of chemoradiation and radiation alone and the other four trials evaluated chemoradiation with different regimens of concurrent/neoadjuvant or adjuvant chemotherapy (Table 173.2).

Based on the data from these trials, radiation alone can lead to adequate local control even for locally advanced SCC in approximately 45% to 56% of patients. To increase the efficacy of radiation, chemotherapy can be administered before radiation (neoadjuvant or induction), concurrently with radiation, or after radiation (consolidation or maintenance). However, only concurrent chemoradiation was shown to positively impact disease-free survival (DFS) and colostomy-free survival. The three cytotoxic agents that have been studied in these clinical trials include fluorouracil (5-FU), mitomycin C, and cisplatin, either alone or in combination, and although the regimens were similar the doses were highly variable.[11] Among these agents, cisplatin has been associated with higher serious toxicities with no significant positive impact on

TABLE 173.2 Summary of Randomized Trials of Chemoradiation in Patients With Anal Squamous Cell Carcinoma

Trial Name (Years)	Number of Patients	Design	Primary Endpoint	Complete Response Rate	Local Failure Rate	Colostomy-Free Survival	Overall Survival
ACT I (1996)	577	RT vs. RT with 5-FU	Local failure	30% vs. 39% at 6 weeks	57% vs. 32%	37% vs. 47% at 5 years	53% vs. 58% at 5 years
EORTC 22861 (1997)	110	RT vs. RT with 5-FU/MMC	Disease-free survival	54% vs. 80% at 6 weeks	50% vs. 32%	Estimated improvement in colostomy-free survival by 32%	54% vs. 58%
RTOG-87-04 (1988–1991)	291	5-FU with RT vs. 5-FU/MMC with RT	Loco-regional control	Path CR (biopsy) at 4–6 weeks 86% vs. 92%	16% at 4 years	59% vs. 71%	71% vs. 78%
RTOG 98-11 (1998–2005)	641	NACT cisplatin/5-FU vs. 5-FU/MMC	Disease-free survival	Data not provided	25% vs. 33%	Colostomy rate: 10% vs. 19%	75% vs. 70%
UKCCCR ACT II (2001–2008)	940	CRT (5-FU/MMC) vs. 5-FU/cisplatin ± maintenance CT 5-FU/cisplatin	Relapse-free survival	94% vs. 95% at 18 weeks	11% vs. 13%	Colostomy rate was same in both arms: 5% with maintenance vs. 4% without maintenance	85% with maintenance and 85% without maintenance at 3 years
ACCORD-03 (1999–2005)	307	NACT and CRT (5-FU/cisplatin) ± HDRT	Colostomy-free survival	Overall 79% at 2 months post boost	28%–12% between different arms	70%–82% between different arms	79%–89% between different arms

Modified from Ahmed S, Eng C. Optimal treatment strategies for anal cancer. *Curr Treat Options Oncol*. 2014;15(3):443–455.

oncologic outcomes. As a result the standard treatment of anal SCC consists of concurrent chemoradiation using fluoropyramidines (including oral and infusional 5-FU) and mitomycin C with conventional doses of radiation between 50 and 60 Gy in standard fractionated schedules of 1.8 to 2 Gy per fraction. The radiation fields usually include the primary tumor as well as the inguinal lymph nodes, even in the absence of definite involvement This is due to the fact that the risk of nodal involvement increases with increasing tumor stage, with up to 20% involvement with T3 tumors. In certain situations, this regimen may be modified based on patient and disease characteristics. In immunosuppressed patients or patients with limited physiologic and functional reserve, chemotherapy can be omitted. Also in patients with a limited survival due to medical comorbidities and/or age, consideration to not giving chemotherapy can be made because there was no definite advantage on long-term overall survival.

INTENSITY-MODULATED RADIATION THERAPY

Intensity-modulated radiation therapy (IMRT) has been found to be effective in other tumor sites that show a marked dose-response but are in close proximity to critical structures. In case of anal SCC, IMRT allows delivery and modulation of radiation doses to the tumor while avoiding normal surrounding structures such as the perianal skin, the external genitalia, the bladder, and small bowel, as well as osseous structures such as the pelvis, sacrum, and femoral head and neck. By avoiding these structures, acute gastrointestinal, genitourinary, hematologic, and dermatologic toxicities can be minimized, leading to fewer treatment disruptions and shorter overall treatment time, both factors that have been associated with better prognosis. The RTOG 0529 was a phase II trial that was designed to see if IMRT could reduce treatment-related

toxicities compared with the RTOG 98-11, which was a randomized trial that used conventional 3D pelvic radiation to compare concurrent 5FU and Mitomycin C to induction chemotherapy using 5 FU and cisplatin.[12] The primary endpoint was a 15% reduction in grade 2 or higher genitourinary and gastrointestinal toxicity. Although this could not be reached, there was a significant decrease in acute grade 2 or greater hematologic toxicity and grade 3 or greater dermatologic and gastrointestinal toxicity. There have been several other retrospective studies that have compared the toxicities and outcomes of patients with conventional three-dimensional (3D) conformal radiation and IMRT. Most of the studies have shown a significant reduction in grade 3 toxicities, including less gastrointestinal and dermatologic toxicity. These studies have also shown equivalent oncologic outcomes with regard to locoregional control, colostomy-free survival, and overall survival (OS) (Table 173.3).[4] As a result of these data suggesting reduced toxicity, IMRT has become the standard in administration of radiation in patients undergoing treatment for anal SCC.[4]

PROGNOSIS AND PROGNOSTIC FACTORS

The locoregional failure rate with standard chemoradiation therapy is approximately 40%, and the colostomy-free survival rate is 15% to 36%. Disease-related factors including nodal involvement and large tumors, are the most significant prognostic factors because patients with N1 disease and tumors greater than 5 cm in size have only a 30% probability of being disease free at 3 years.[13] The DFS that is sometimes referred to as relapse-free survival is between 56% and 75% at 3 years, depending on studies, with the overall 5-year OS ranging between 67% and 91%. The 5-year OS for stage I is 77%, stage II is 67%, IIIA 58%, IIIB is 51%, and stage IV is 15%. These oncologic outcomes are influenced by patient-, disease-, and treatment-related factors. Male gender, African-American ethnicity, and

TABLE 173.3 Studies Evaluating Outcomes of Intensity-Modulated Radiotherapy-Based Chemoradiation for Anal Squamous Cell Carcinoma

	Follow-Up (months)	Number of Patients	Acute Grade >3 GI Toxicity	Acute Grade >3 Dermatologic Toxicity	Acute Grade >3 Hematologic Toxicity	Overall Survival	Progression-Free Survival	Colostomy Free Survival
Milano et al (2005)	20.3	17	0	0	–	91%*	35%	82%
Salama et al (2007)	14.5	53	15%	38%	30% leukopenia and 34% neutropenia	93%	84% (local PFS) 93% (distant PFS)	84%
Pepek et al (2010)	14	29	9%	0%	7% leukopenia and 2% thrombocytopenia	100%	100% (distant PFS)	91%
Bazan et al (2011)	26			21%		87.8%	84%	
Kachnic et al (2012)	24	43	7%	10%	51%	94%	82%	90%
DeFoe et al (2012)	16	78	28%	29%	13%	86.9%	84% (local PFS) 82% (distant PFS)	81%
Mitchell et al (2013)	19	65	9%			96%	36%	
Mitchell et al (2013)	26.5	52	9.6%	11.5%		91%†	82%	91%
RTOG 0529	27	52	21%	23%		86%		
RTOG-98-11	N/A	649	36%	49%		78%		72%

*At 2 years.
†At 3 years.
GI, Gastrointestinal; PFS, progress on-free survival.
Modified from Glynne-Jones R, Lim F. Anal cancer: an examination of radiotherapy strategies. *Int J Radiat Oncol Biol Phys.* 2011 79(5):1290–1301.

age greater than 65 years have been considered to be associated with adverse prognosis, whereas HPV infection is considered to be a favorable prognostic characteristic. Chemoradiation including 5-FU in combination with mitomycin C or cisplatin are equally effective regimens, but breaks in treatment and inability to complete treatment, particularly in HIV-positive patients, negatively impact outcomes.[14]

MANAGEMENT IN HUMAN IMMUNODEFICIENCY VIRUS–POSITIVE PATIENTS

Despite the benefits of HAART in the treatment of HIV and restoring immune function, there is a 55-fold increase in prevalence of anal SCC in HIV-positive patients compared with HIV-negative patients.[14,15] Studies from the pre-HAART era had observed an increase in acute toxicities with chemoradiation requiring treatment interruption and dose reduction, as well as worse clinical outcomes in HIV-positive patients.[16-19] As a result, all of the aforementioned trials did not include patients with HIV. With the increased use of HAART in the 1990s resulting in restoration of the immune system with effective suppression of the viral load and elevation of CD4 counts, a decrease in chemoradiation-related side effects in HIV-positive patients was observed.

Wexler et al.[19] reported the oncologic outcomes of 32 HIV-positive patients treated between 1997 and 2005 with standard chemoradiation. The 5-year locoregional relapse rate, DSS, and OS were 16%, 75%, and 65%, respectively. More than two-thirds of patients required treatment interruption due to toxicities. In another retrospective analysis of 36 HIV-positive patients treated between 1997 and 2012 with standard chemoradiation (median radiation dose, 54 Gy; 5-FU and mitomycin C), the 5-year local control, colostomy-free survival, cancer-specific survival, and OS were 72%, 87%, 77%, and 74%, respectively. This is comparable to patients who are HIV negative.[20] Therefore, in the HAART era, in patients with CD4 counts of greater than 200/mm^3, the standard chemoradiation for anal SCC can be safely and effectively used with similar oncologic outcomes.[21]

FOLLOW-UP AND SURVEILLANCE

Anal SCC has a slow rate of regression that continues even after chemoradiation. It is estimated that by 12 weeks following completion of treatment, a maximal response should be seen. Current NCCN Guidelines suggest that patients should be evaluated at an 8- and 12-week interval after completion of treatment and classified as (1) complete responders, (2) stable but persistent disease, and (3) progressive disease. From a practical standpoint, most patients do not tolerate an exam before 3 months and should therefore be examined after at least that time period. The initial response to treatment has been considered to be an independent prognostic factor, with patients having a complete response having a better outcome as compared with patients who did not respond. Routine biopsy following completion of therapy is not currently recommended based on NCCN Guidelines, although a strategy of routine biopsy at a 3-month interval has been proposed versus a selective

approach to biopsying only suspicious lesions.[22] Biopsy can be associated with nonhealing ulcers and pain and can lead to significant morbidity, particularly if an APR becomes necessary for symptom control. Therefore limited targeted biopsies to establish a tissue diagnosis of lesions that appear to progress is a more conservative approach to avoid these complications. Patients with persistent disease and nonprogressive disease can be followed in 4-week intervals because tumor regression can continue for several more months. The majority of recurrences occur in the first 3 years following treatment; therefore these patients should be followed closely. Current guidelines suggest a history and physical examination including evaluation of the anal canal with a digital rectal examination (DRE) and anoscopy and inguinal nodes every 3 to 6 months for 5 years (usually every 3 months for 2 years and every 6 months for 3 years). Routine cross-sectional imaging with CT is recommended only for patients with advanced disease.

SALVAGE SURGERY

Chemoradiation results in long-term disease control in a majority of patients, yet 15% to 40% of patients will experience residual or recurrent locoregional disease.[20,23-25] Treatment options in these patients include either repeat radiation or surgery. In the Intergroup trial[26] patients with biopsy-proven persistent disease after chemoradiation, an external beam boost was attempted as salvage treatment. Twenty-five patients were treated, and of the 22 patients who underwent posttreatment biopsies, 12 (55%) were negative. Overall, 50% of patients were alive without disease at 4 years, but half of the surviving patients underwent an APR. Currently most patients who have persistent or recurrent disease undergo salvage APR. Patients undergoing salvage APR have a 5-year survival of 40% to 60% compared with a 3-year OS of 5% for patients who do not undergo surgery.[24]

In analysis of 105 patients with persistent (42 patients), recurrent (55 patients) disease or a contradiction to radiation (7 patients), the OS and DFS was 61% and 48%, respectively. Recurrence occurred in almost 43% of patients, with the type of recurrence (local, inguinal, or metastatic) not influencing survival. In the adjusted analyses, tumor stage (T3 and T4), positive margins in the surgical specimen, and the presence of metastatic disease were associated with an adverse prognosis. The indication for the APR, gender, HIV infection, and the need for a flap reconstruction did not have an impact on the OS and DFS.[27] Mullen et al.[28] identified the most significant prognostic factor after salvage APR was a negative margin (R0 resection). In their study the median survival for patients with negative and positive margin after salvage surgery was 33 months versus 14 months, respectively.[28]

Salvage APR for recurrent or persistent anal SCC involves a wider lateral margin extending to the ischial tuberosities on each side. If the lesion is close to the vaginal wall, then an en bloc resection of the posterior vaginal wall may be needed. As a result of the larger perineal defect, a reconstructive tissue flap with a vertical rectus abdominis myocutaneous (VRAM) flap or a gracilis flap is necessary, but the former is preferred given its size and bulk.[29] There is a significant amount of wound morbidity associated with these surgeries, and a multidisciplinary approach is preferred. Patients with an inguinal recurrence, who have not received radiation to the inguinal regions, can be salvaged with chemoradiation. However, if there is inguinal recurrence after groin radiation, a deep and superficial inguinal lymph node dissection should be performed in patients who are symptomatic, whereas asymptomatic patients may be given palliative chemotherapy, although this is usually associated with a poor prognosis.

SQUAMOUS INTRAEPITHELIAL LESIONS

The lesions under this term have been previously known as Bowen disease, anal intraepithelial neoplasia (AIN) I, II, and III, anal dysplasia, and SCC in situ.[30] Based on current guidelines,[30] it has been recommended that these should be classified as either (1) low-grade squamous intraepithelial lesions (LSILs) or (2) high-grade squamous intraepithelial lesions (HSILs). The difference between LSIL and HSIL is based on histologic features, including nuclear-to-cytoplasmic ratio and relationship of the atypical cells with the basement membrane. Based on its current definition, LSIL includes AIN I, as well as anal and perianal condylomas, and HSIL includes Bowen disease, AIN II and AIN III, as well as SCC in situ. The exact prevalence of HSIL is not known and is considered to be less than 1%, but its incidence appears to be increasing. Certain factors are associated with a high risk of HSIL and include HIV, systemic immunosuppression, long-term steroid use a history of cervical and vulvar intraepithelial neoplasia (CIN and VIN), and extensive condylomatous disease. The incidence of HSIL in MSM is 35 per 100,000, and this doubles in the same population that is HIV positive. The prevalence of HSIL in nonimmunocompromised patients such as women with VIN and CIN, is approximately 5% whereas it is reported to be approximately 3% to 5% in renal allograft patients.[31]

The natural history of HSIL is not clearly established with progression to invasive cancer reported to be approximately 10% in 5 years, with several factors impacting this rate, including the immune status of the patient and how HSIL is managed.[31] The incidence of progression in HIV-positive and immunocompromised patients is probably higher, based on the fact that there is a higher incidence of anal SCC in these patient groups. The theoretical progression of HSIL to anal SCC is considered to be approximately 1 in 600 per year in HIV-positive MSM and 1 in 4000 per year in HIV-negative MSM.[32]

The clinical features of HSIL are relatively non specific and most patients are asymptomatic with the diagnosis being made during surgical excision of perianal lesions including anal condylomas. The incidence of HSIL in patients who undergo excision of condylomas is between 28% and 35% but can be as high as 60% in HIV-positive patients. In symptomatic patients, HSIL of the perianus can be associated with plaques, erythema, and/or pigmentation and may present with perianal irritation or pain.

The primary objective of treating HSIL is to prevent its progression to anal SCC, preserve anorectal function and minimize treatment-related morbidity. There are several treatment modalities available for treating HSIL

including surgical excision, electrocautery ablation, topical imiquimod, and topical 5-FU. However, the efficacy and benefit of any one therapy over the other is limited by the lack of high-quality data. Although surgery involving wide local excision with negative margins was considered the standard treatment, it is associated with significant wound morbidity, adverse functional outcomes (incontinence, anal stenosis), and high rates of local recurrence. There also does not appear to be a significant impact on decreasing the progression to invasive disease. As a result, less radical approaches have been considered and available evidence suggests that high-resolution anoscopy (HRA) is the optimal treatment approach. This technique allows for targeted destruction of HSIL with minimal wound and functional morbidity with lower rates of progression to invasive disease than other reported approaches.

In HRA the anal canal and perianus is coated with 3% acetic acid and then examined using an operating microscope. Areas that are affected by HPV turn white and have characteristic vascular patterns. Lugol iodine may then be applied to areas of concern that may lack the classic vascular changes; areas of HSIL do not absorb the Lugol iodine and turn yellow, whereas areas of LSIL and normal tissue turn brown/black. The area of suspected HSIL should be biopsied to confirm the diagnosis and then ablated with either electrocautery or infrared coagulation, with the goal of achieving a superficial burn in the areas of HSIL and preserving uninvolved regions. Using this approach, HSIL can be eradicated, even in immunocompromised patients, although multiple treatments may be required initially.[5,34]

An alternative treatment for HSIL is immunomodulators such as 5% imiquimod (Aldara) cream, topical 5% 5-FU, or a combination of the two. In a randomized trial, 388 HIV-positive MSM were screened for HSIL by HRA, of which 246 patients who were diagnosed with HSIL were randomly assigned to receive imiquimod, topical 5-FU, or ablation with electrocautery. Although electrocautery was superior to the other two regimens more than half of the patients recurred regardless of the treatment agent.[35] These finding are similar to those from a large retrospective cohort analysis of 456 HIV-positive and 271 HIV-negative MSM treated for HSIL with ablation. After a follow-up of 3 years, 77% of the HIV- positive and 66% of the HIV-negative patients developed recurrent HSIL.[36] Despite the high risk of recurrence and regardless of the treatment strategy, HIV-positive patients and/or MSM should be closely monitored for recurrent HSIL and be treated as this approach minimizes the risk of progression to anal SCC.

ANAL CANAL ADENOCARCINOMAS

Adenocarcinoma of the anal canal is the second most common anal canal malignancy and accounts for 10% to 20% of anal canal cancers but is more aggressive as compared with SCC of the anal canal. Unlike adenocarcinomas of the rectum, which arise from the mucosa, anal canal adenocarcinomas usually arise from the columnar epithelium lining the anal glands, which open into the transitional zone of the anal canal but can also arise from the mucosa de novo.[37] It can be challenging to differentiate anal canal adenocarcinomas from distal rectal adenocarcinomas that extend into the anal canal. Risk factors for developing anal canal adenocarcinomas include chronic inflammation, anal fistulous disease, and Crohn disease. The incidence of fistula-related anal cancers associated with Crohn disease is 0.3% to 0.7%, which is higher than the general population. The most common histologic type is adenocarcinoma followed by SCC. Metastatic disease occurs more frequently than with other primary anal canal tumors, and the DFS is between 20% and 60%, depending on the stage at presentation and treatment regimen.[38] Due to its relative rarity, treatment regimens have not been well established and include primary surgical resection, definitive chemoradiation or neoadjuvant chemoradiation, and surgical resection.[37,38] Neoadjuvant chemoradiation followed by APR is associated with the greatest 5-year survival, with tumor stage and differentiation being significant prognostic factors.[37,38]

PERIANAL LESIONS

Perianal neoplasms are uncommon and account for approximately 3% to 4% of all anorectal neoplasms. These lesions involve the perianus, which anatomically extends from the inferior most aspect of the internal sphincter to approximately a radius of 5 cm around the anus and represents a region and not a distinct anatomic boundary (this region was previously described as the anal margin). The perianus is characterized by stratified squamous epithelium, as well as skin appendages such as apocrine gland and hair. Commonly seen lesions include SCC, Buschke-Löwenstein tumors (verrucous carcinoma), Paget disease, and BCC.

PERIANAL CANCERS

SCCs of the perianus are similar to SCCs of the skin, and therefore their management is similar to cutaneous SCC. The key issue in diagnosing perianal SCC is the location of the lesion in relation to the anal canal. In particular, it is important to rule out an anal cancer that is extending outward and therefore should be managed as an anal canal SCC.

These lesions can present without symptoms or can be symptomatic causing irritation, bleeding, and discomfort. On examination, these may be firm, erythematous lesions that may have a central ulcer and/or heaped up edges. The diagnosis of a perianal SCC is usually established from a biopsy, where they can be differentiated from anal canal SCC based on the presence of skin appendages, keratinization, and location. Perianal SCCs most commonly metastasize to the inguinal lymph nodes, the risk of which is proportional to the size of the primary lesion.[39] The evaluation of perianal SCC includes confirming its location, a physical examination with attention to the inguinal lymph nodes, and radiologic assessment with a CT scan of the chest, abdomen, and pelvis.

The management is based on the size and location. Small perianal cancers (T1, N0) are treated like cutaneous SCC with wide local excision with 1-cm margins. Lesions that involve the anal sphincter may result in compromise of fecal continence with wide local excision and can be

managed with chemoradiation as an alternative to an APR. Larger lesions or lesions involving the inguinal lymph nodes and/or the sphincter complex require chemoradiation. Lesions that are larger than 2 cm should receive radiation to the inguinal region, whereas the pelvic lymph nodes should be involved in the radiation field for lesions greater than 5 cm in size.[39]

ANORECTAL MELANOMA

Anorectal melanoma accounts for less than 1% of all malignant melanomas and fewer than 4% of anal canal and perianal malignancies. The anorectal region is the most common site of malignant melanoma in the gastrointestinal tract. It is more common in women, with a median age of presentation of 60 years. Sixty-five percent of cases are located within the anal canal or perianus, with the remaining being found in the distal rectum.[40] The presenting symptoms are relatively nonspecific and similar to other benign anorectal conditions and include bleeding, irritation, and discomfort. As a result, they are often managed as a benign condition such as hemorrhoids. It is particularly challenging to diagnose anorectal melanoma in situations when the lesion is amelanotic, which can occur in up to 25% of cases.[40,41] In a proportion of patients the diagnosis is incidentally made following excision of benign anorectal lesions such as hemorrhoids or anal skin tags. The overall survival is less than 20%, with most patients dying from metastatic disease, which can be present at initial presentation in almost half of the patients.[41] The diagnostic work-up is similar to melanoma elsewhere in the body and includes radiologic imaging with appropriate cross-sectional imaging.

Anorectal melanomas are radioresistant and chemoresistant, and therefore surgery has been the mainstay of treatment, but the optimal surgery is controversial. In majority of the published studies in the literature, a comparison of oncologic outcomes between APR and local excisions has been unable to identify a significant survival advantage between either modality. In a meta-analysis that included 31 studies with 1006 patients, there was no difference in OS and DFS after APR and local excision.[41] Patients undergoing an APR had a lower rate of local recurrence compared with patients undergoing local excision, with most local recurrences being accompanied by distant metastases. Because patients with local recurrence can be salvaged with an APR if necessary, local excision is considered the first line of treatment because it avoids the short and long morbidity of an APR and its impact on patient QoL. Recent years have seen significant advances in the treatment of cutaneous melanomas with targeted therapies and immune checkpoint inhibitors. However, mucosal melanomas, including anorectal melanomas, are uniquely different with respect to their etiology and pathogenesis, as well as their genetic configuration.[42] Although the incidence of activating mutations in the BRAF oncogene is common in cutaneous melanoma, it is rare in mucosal melanoma, with an estimated incidence of 10%, although it may be more common in anorectal melanomas. There also appears to be a higher incidence of activating mutations in the KIT oncogene, with an estimated rate to be approximately 25% to 39%.[42] Most clinical trials looking at novel therapies in melanoma have excluded patients with noncutaneous melanomas, but even with the limited data available no systemic chemotherapy has shown to improve survival.[42] Several smaller studies have investigated the efficacy of tyrosine kinase inhibitors (imatinib) and anti-CTLA-4 monoclonal antibodies (ipilimumab) in patients with metastatic disease.[42] The results have been considered encouraging, and more data are necessary to validate a proven benefit. Given the poor prognosis of patients with anorectal melanoma, these patients should be referred for enrollment in clinical trials with these therapies.

BUSCHKE-LÖWENSTEIN TUMORS

Buschke-Löwenstein tumors are also known as verrucous carcinoma or giant condylomata acuminata. These lesions are related to HPV, with HPV-6 and HPV-11 being the most frequent strains identified.[1] Like condylomatous disease, they affect the anogenital region, but they can grow to a significant size in the perianal region and present as large cauliflower-like lesions. They are characterized by an endophytic and exophytic growth pattern, which distinguishes them from ordinary condyloma acuminatum. However, the endophytic growth could be growth along preexisting cryptoglandular fistula tracts rather than actual invasion. Rarely, a large lesion can undergo malignant degeneration and develop invasive disease, particularly if associated with HIV infection. These lesions are usually managed with wide local excision, with the resultant skin defect being allowed to heal by secondary intention or covered with a split-thickness skin graft or rotational and advancement flaps. In cases of large lesions in close proximity to sphincter complex or development of invasive disease, an APR is required, often with rectus flap coverage of the resultant perineal defect. There also have been several case reports documenting regression of these lesions with chemotherapy and radiation.[43]

PAGET DISEASE

Perianal Paget disease is an intraepithelial adenocarcinoma that is thought to originate from apocrine glands or pleuripotent keratinocyte stem cells.[44] It is commonly seen in older men and women and can be associated with other malignant conditions, although this association may not be as strong as it is for mammary Paget.[45] It usually presents as chronic erythematous or scaling rashlike lesions with well-demarcated borders in the perianal region. The diagnosis is established with a biopsy, and the treatment is based on the extent of the disease and if there is an underlying malignancy. Like other uncommon lesions of the perianal region, there is no clear consensus on how to manage this disease and whether local excision versus radical surgery is necessary. Wide local excision with negative microscopic margins is the most common surgical treatment in the absence of invasive disease. The recurrence rates are high (up to 50%),[44,46] and it is also not possible to achieve negative margins without creating large perianal skin defects that can be difficult to manage. In situations in which there is extensive perianal disease or invasive disease, an APR may be necessary. Radiation

and combined chemoradiation can be considered as alternatives to surgery. Other treatment modalities include Mohs microscopic surgery, photodynamic therapy, systemic chemotherapy, and topical agents such as 5-FU and imiquimod.[45] However, the evidence supporting all these modalities is limited to case reports and small case series. The treatment strategy therefore should balance disease control against the high risk of recurrence despite surgery and its impact on patient morbidity, long-term function, and QoL.

BASAL CELL CARCINOMAS

BCCs of the perianal region account for less than 1% of all BCCs, despite being the most common malignancy in the human body. It is important to distinguish them from basaloid SCCs of the anal canal because they can have overlapping histologic features It is more common in men in their sixth decade of life. There is an association with other skin lesions and should mandate a complete clinical examination. These lesions are not aggressive and can be adequately managed with wide local excision. Recurrence rates of up to 30% have been reported, but cancer specific survival is 100%.[47] Deeper invasion into the anal canal is uncommon and requires an APR, whereas local recurrences can be treated with repeat excision or radiation.

REFERENCES

1. Welton ML, Steele SR, Goodman KA. Anus. In: Amin MB, Edge S, Greene F, Byrd DR, Brookland RK, et al., eds. *AJCC Cancer Staging Manuel.* 8th ed. Berlin: Springer; 2016:275-284.
2. https://seer.cancer.gov/statfacts/html/anus.html. Accessed 31 July 2017.
3. Silverberg MJ, Lau B, Justice AC, et al. Risk of anal cancer in HIV-infected and HIV-uninfected individuals in North America. *Clin Infect Dis.* 2012;54(7):1026-1034
4. Shridhar R, Shibata D, Chan E, Thomas CR. Anal cancer: current standards in care and recent changes in practice. *CA Cancer J Clin.* 2015;65(2):139-162.
5. Glynne-Jones R, Renehan A. Current treatment of anal squamous cell carcinoma. *Hematol Oncol Clin North Am.* 2012;26(6):1315-1350.
6. Gerard JP, Chapet O, Samiei F, et al. Management of inguinal lymph node metastases in patients with carcinoma of the anal canal: experience in a series of 270 patients treated in Lyon and review of the literature. *Cancer.* 2001;92(1):77-84.
7. Glynne-Jones R, Nilsson PJ, Aschele C, et al. Anal cancer: ESMO-ESSO-ESTRO clinical practice guidelines for diagnosis, treatment and follow-up. *Eur J Surg Oncol.* 2014;40(10):1165-1176.
8. Cotter SE, Grigsby PW, Siegel BA, et al. FDG-PET/CT in the evaluation of anal carcinoma. *Int J Radiat Oncol Biol Phys.* 2006;65(3):720-725.
9. Trautmann TG, Zuger JH. Positron emission tomography for pretreatment staging and posttreatment evaluation in cancer of the anal canal. *Mol Imaging Biol.* 2005;7(4):309-313.
10. Osborne MC, Maykel J, Johnson EK, Steele SR. Anal squamous cell carcinoma: an evolution in disease and management. *World J Gastroenterol.* 2014;20(36):13052-13059.
11. Vinayan A, Glynne-Jones R. Anal cancer—What is the optimum chemoradiotherapy? *Best Pract Res Clin Gastroenterol.* 2016;30(4):641-653.
12. Kachnic LA, Winter K, Myerson RJ, et al. RTOG 0529: a phase 2 evaluation of dose-painted intensity modulated radiation therapy in combination with 5-fluorouracil and mitomycin-C for the reduction of acute morbidity in carcinoma of the anal canal. *Int J Radiat Oncol Biol Phys.* 2013;86(1):27-33.
13. Lim F, Glynne-Jones R. Chemotherapy/chemoradiation in anal cancer: a systematic review. *Cancer Treat Rev.* 2011;37(7):520-532.
14. Egger M, May M, Chene G, et al. Prognosis of HIV-1-infected patients starting highly active antiretroviral therapy: a collaborative analysis of prospective studies. *Lancet.* 2002;360(9327):119-129

15. Silverberg MJ, Chao C, Leyden WA, et al. HIV infection, immunodeficiency, viral replication, and the risk of cancer. *Cancer Epidemiol Biomarkers Prev.* 2011;20(12):2551-2559.

16. Holland JM, Swift PS. Tolerance of patients with human immunodeficiency virus and anal carcinoma to treatment with combined chemotherapy and radiation therapy. *Radiology.* 1994;193(1):251-254.

17. Kim JH, Sarani B, Orkin BA, et al. HIV-positive patients with anal carcinoma have poorer treatment tolerance and outcome than HIV-negative patients. *Dis Colon Rectum.* 2001;44(10):1496-1502.

18. Place RJ, Gregorcyk SG, Huber PJ, Simmang CL. Outcome analysis of HIV-positive patients with anal squamous cell carcinoma. *Dis Colon Rectum.* 2001;44(4):506-512.

19. Wexler A, Berson AM, Goldstone SE, et al. Invasive anal squamous-cell carcinoma in the HIV-positive patient: outcome in the era of highly active antiretroviral therapy. *Dis Colon Rectum.* 2008;51(1):73-81.

20. Gunderson LL, Winter KA, Ajani JA, et al. Long-term update of US GI intergroup RTOG 98-11 phase III trial for anal carcinoma: survival, relapse, and colostomy failure with concurrent chemoradiation involving fluorouracil/mitomycin versus fluorouracil/cisplatin. *J Clin Oncol.* 2012;30(35):4344-4351.

21. Hoffman R, Welton ML, Klencke B, Weinberg V, Krieg R. The significance of pretreatment CD4 count on the outcome and treatment tolerance of HIV-positive patients with anal cancer. *Int J Radiat Oncol Biol Phys.* 1999;44(1):127-131.

22. Steele SR, Varma MG, Melton GB, et al. Practice parameters for anal squamous neoplasms. *Dis Colon Rectum.* 2012;55(7):735-749.

23. James RD, Glynne-Jones R, Meadows HM, et al. Mitomycin or cisplatin chemoradiation with or without maintenance chemotherapy for treatment of squamous-cell carcinoma of the anus (ACT II): a randomised, phase 3, open-label, 2 x 2 factorial trial. *Lancet Oncol.* 2013;14(6):516-524.

24. Renehan AG, Saunders MP, Schofield PF, O'Dwyer ST. Patterns of local disease failure and outcome after salvage surgery in patients with anal cancer. *Br J Surg.* 2005;92(5):605-614.

25. Alamri Y, Buchwald P, Dixon L, et al. Salvage surgery in patients with recurrent or residual squamous cell carcinoma of the anus. *Eur J Surg Oncol.* 2016;42(11):1687-1692.

26. Flam M, John M, Pajak TF, et al. Role of mitomycin in combination with fluorouracil and radiotherapy, and of salvage chemoradiation in the definitive nonsurgical treatment of epidermoid carcinoma of the anal canal: results of a phase III randomized intergroup study. *J Clin Oncol.* 1996;14(9):2527-2539.

27. Lefevre JH, Corte H, Tiret E, et al. Abdominoperineal resection for squamous cell anal carcinoma: survival and risk factors for recurrence. *Ann Surg Oncol.* 2012;19(13):4186-4192.

28. Mullen JT, Rodriguez-Bigas MA, Chang GJ, et al. Results of surgical salvage after failed chemoradiation therapy for epidermoid carcinoma of the anal canal. *Ann Surg Oncol.* 2007;14(2):478-483.

29. Sunesen KG, Buntzen S, Tei T, Lindegaard JC, Norgaard M, Laurberg S. Perineal healing and survival after anal cancer salvage surgery: 10-year experience with primary perineal reconstruction using the vertical rectus abdominis myocutaneous (VRAM) flap. *Ann Surg Oncol.* 2009;16(1):68-77.

30. Darragh TM, Colgan TJ, Thomas Cox J, et al. The lower anogenital squamous terminology standardization project for HPV-associated lesions: background and consensus recommendations from the College of American Pathologists and the American Society for Colposcopy and Cervical Pathology. *Int J Gynecol Pathol.* 2013;32(1):76-115.

31. Scholefield JH, Harris D, Radcliffe A. Guidelines for management of anal intraepithelial neoplasia. *Colorectal Dis.* 2011;13(suppl 1):3-10.

32. Machalek DA, Poynten M, Jin F, et al. Anal human papillomavirus infection and associated neoplastic lesions in men who have sex with men: a systematic review and meta-analysis. *Lancet Oncol.* 2012;13(5):487-500.

33. Pineda CE, Berry JM, Jay N, Palefsky JM, Welton ML. High resolution anoscopy in the planned staged treatment of anal squamous intraepithelial lesions in HIV-negative patients. *J Gastrointest Surg.* 2007;11(11):1410-1415, discussion 1415–1416.

34. Pineda CE, Berry JM, Jay N, Palefsky JM, Welton ML. High-resolution anoscopy targeted surgical destruction of anal high-grade squamous intraepithelial lesions: a ten-year experience. *Dis Colon Rectum.* 2008;51(6):829-835, discussion 835–827.

35. Richel O, de Vries HJ, van Noesel CJ, Dijkgraaf MG, Prins JM. Comparison of imiquimod, topical fluorouracil, and electrocautery for the treatment of anal intraepithelial neoplasia in HIV-positive men who have sex with men: an open-label, randomised controlled trial. *Lancet Oncol.* 2013;14(4):346-353.

36. Goldstone SE, Johnstone AA, Moshier EL. Long-term outcome of ablation of anal high-grade squamous intraepithelial lesions: recurrence and incidence of cancer. *Dis Colon Rectum.* 2014;57(3):316-323.

37. Anwar S, Welbourn H, Hill J, Sebag-Montefiore D. Adenocarcinoma of the anal canal—a systematic review. *Colorectal Dis.* 2013;15(12):1481-1488.

38. Chang GJ, Gonzalez RJ, Skibber JM, Eng C, Das P, Rodriguez-Bigas MA. A twenty-year experience with adenocarcinoma of the anal canal. *Dis Colon Rectum.* 2009;52(8):1375-1380.

39. Jiang Y, Ajani JA. Anal margin cancer: current situation and ongoing trials. *Curr Opin Oncol.* 2012;24(4):448-453.

40. Belic DM, Smyth E, Perez D, et al. Anal versus rectal melanoma: does site of origin predict outcome? *Dis Colon Rectum.* 2013;56(2):150-157.

41. Matsuda A, Miyashita M, Matsumoto S, et al. Abdominoperineal resection provides better local control but equivalent overall survival to local excision of anorectal malignant melanoma: a systematic review. *Ann Surg.* 2015;261(4):670-677.

42. Roy AC, Wattchow D, Astill D, et al. Uncommon Anal Neoplasms. *Surg Oncol Clin N Am.* 2017;26(1):143-161.

43. Haque W, Kelly E, Dhingra S, Carpenter LS. Successful treatment of recurrent Buschke-Lowenstein tumor by radiation therapy and chemotherapy. *Int J Colorectal Dis.* 2010;25(4):539-540.

44. Perez DR, Trakarnsanga A, Shia J, et al. Management and outcome of perianal Paget's disease: a 6-decade institutional experience. *Dis Color Rectum.* 2014;57(6):747-751.

45. Rajendran S, Koh CE, Solomon MJ. Extramammary Paget's disease of the perianal region: a 20-year experience. *ANZ J Surg.* 2017;87(3):132-137.

46. Isik O, Aytac E, Brainard J, Valente MA, Abbas MA, Gorgun E. Perianal Paget's disease: three decades experience of a single institution. *Int J Colorectal Dis.* 2016;31(1):29-34.

47. Leonard D, Beddy D, Dozois EJ. Neoplasms of anal canal and perianal skin. *Clin Colon Rectal Surg.* 2011;24(1):54-63.

Retrorectal Tumors

Amit Merchea | Eric J. Dozois

R etrorectal tumors comprise an uncommon group of lesions, originating from one or more of the three germ cell layers that occupy the retrorectal or presacral space. The reported incidence of less than 1% likely represents an underestimate, given the indolent nature of these tumors with often vague and nonspecific symptoms. Tumors are often heterogeneous and are more often congenital than acquired.[1-3] Given the complexity of pelvic anatomy and the frequent involvement of multiple pelvic structures, a multidisciplinary surgical team is often required for safe and effective management. Appropriate surgical planning with the aid of preoperative imaging and selective biopsy of these lesions has allowed for safe use of neoadjuvant chemoradiation. This, coupled with the employment of multidisciplinary teams, has led to generally favorable outcomes in these patients.

ANATOMY

Given the bony confines of the pelvis and its complex gastrointestinal, genitourinary, neurologic, and vascular anatomy, tumors arising in the retrorectal space often involve multiple structures (Fig. 174.1). Retrorectal tumors can grow to fill the pelvis and lead to displacement of pelvic organs. The mesorectum forms the anterior border of this space, and the anterior aspect of the sacrum forms the posterior border. Superiorly, the space extends to the peritoneal reflection and inferiorly to the rectosacral fascia. Laterally, the retrorectal space is bounded by the lateral ligaments, the ureters, and the iliac vessels. The retrorectal space itself contains loose connective tissue, the middle sacral artery, superior hemorrhoidal vessels, and branches of sympathetic and parasympathetic nerves. Vascular and neural structures originate or traverse in proximity to this area and may give rise to, or be involved by, retrorectal tumors (Fig. 174.2).

Vascular involvement can often be managed by either ligation or reconstruction, with little clinical sequelae. Management of neural involvement may be more complex and requires knowledge of sacral root function to counsel patients adequately regarding potential functional deficits. If all sacral roots are sacrificed unilaterally, normal anorectal function is preserved, and a sphincter-sparing operation may be considered if oncologically appropriate. Similarly, if the upper three sacral roots (S1 to S3) remain intact on either side of the sacrum, the patient will still maintain spontaneous defecation and control of anorectal function. If bilateral S3 roots are sacrificed or damaged, anal incontinence and poor defecatory function will result, and a permanent colostomy should be considered.[4]

Pelvic surgery may also result in sexual or urologic dysfunction. Injury to the hypogastric nerves may result in retrograde ejaculation and/or bladder dysfunction. The risk for injury is highest during ligation of the inferior mesenteric artery at its origin, and during mobilization of the rectum near the sacral promontory. The nervi erigentes course anteriorly within the lateral stalks of the rectum and contain parasympathetic fibers from S2 to S4. Injury to these nerves will lead to erectile dysfunction. Finally, the pudendal nerve (S2 to S4) extends inferiorly to the perineum and has two branches—a sensory branch supplying the skin of the penis and glans and a motor branch innervating the external anal sphincter. Unilateral pudendal nerve injuries generally do not result in incontinence, as there is cross innervation at the level of the spinal cord.[5,6]

Sacrectomy may be required if there is bony involvement by the tumor or in some circumstances, to gain access to the pelvis for complete resection. This requires the surgical team be familiar with the anatomy of the sacrotuberous and sacrospinous ligaments (Fig. 174.3), sciatic nerve, piriformis muscle (Fig. 174.4), and the thecal sac and sacral nerve roots (Fig. 174.5). In our practice, we incorporate the skills of both an oncologic orthopedic surgeon and a spine surgeon to assist in operations requiring sacrectomy. When the majority of the sacrum is removed, pelvic stability can be maintained if more than half of the S1 vertebral body is preserved. Because stress fractures to this remnant may occur if preoperative radiation has been used, preservation of spinopelvic stability may require fusion.

CLASSIFICATION OF RETRORECTAL TUMORS

These tumors have been comprehensively classified according to each potential cell line.[7] This has been previously modified by Dozois et al. to further classify these tumors into malignant and benign status because this has significant clinical implications (Box 174.1). In general, the majority of tumors are congenital in origin of which most are developmental cysts.[8] These may originate from any of the three germ layers and include epidermoid and dermoid cysts, enterogenous cysts, tailgut cysts (TGCs), and teratomas. Cystic lesions are seen most commonly in women, and most solid lesions are either chordomas or sarcomas.[8] Malignancy is more common in men, even though the majority of retrorectal tumors occur in women.

CLINICAL PRESENTATION AND DIAGNOSIS

HISTORY AND PHYSICAL EXAMINATION

Symptoms associated with retrorectal tumors are often vague and ill defined. Tumors may be discovered incidentally on routine pelvic or rectal examination. Symptoms may include pelvic or low back pain, constipation, a palpable mass, or obstructive type symptoms. Classically, this pain is aggravated by sitting and ameliorated by standing or walking. However, pain is an ominous sign and has been described as being present more commonly when the lesion is malignant than benign (88% vs. 39%).[2] One should be concerned about a potentially more advanced tumor when symptoms include urinary or fecal incontinence and sexual dysfunction because sacral nerve involvement may be present.

Occasionally, patients may have persistent perianal discharge and have been misdiagnosed with chronic perianal fistula or pilonidal disease. Circumstances that should alert the examiner to the possibility of a retrorectal cystic lesion as a cause of this presentation include repeated operations for "anal fistula," inability to uncover a primary source of infection at the dentate line, recurrent infection of the retrorectal space without obvious cause, presence of a postanal dimple, and fullness and fixation of the precoccygeal area.[8]

A careful and focused perineal and anorectal physical examination is necessary. Although rare, the presence of a postanal dimple should alert the clinician to the possibility of an underlying retrorectal mass. The majority of patients have a palpable mass on digital rectal examination because the rectum tends to be displaced anteriorly. The overlying rectal mucosa is usually smooth and mobile; absence of this feature overlying the mass is suggestive of prior infection of a cystic lesion that has discharged through the rectum or of advanced malignancy. The rectal examination is also important in evaluating for fixation and determining the level of the tumor in relation to the coccyx and other structures such as the prostate. A complete neurologic evaluation should be completed and focused on the sacral nerves and musculoskeletal reflexes, impairment of which may indicate the presence of sacral nerve involvement.

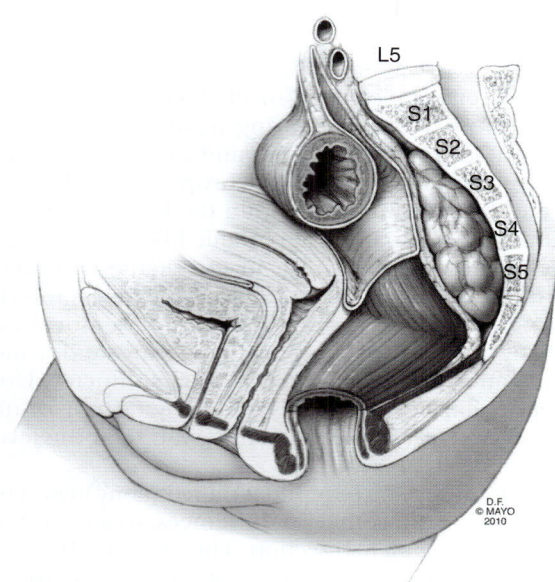

FIGURE 174.1 Retrorectal mass displacing pelvic organs. (Used with permission of Mayo Foundation for Medical Education and Research. All rights reserved.)

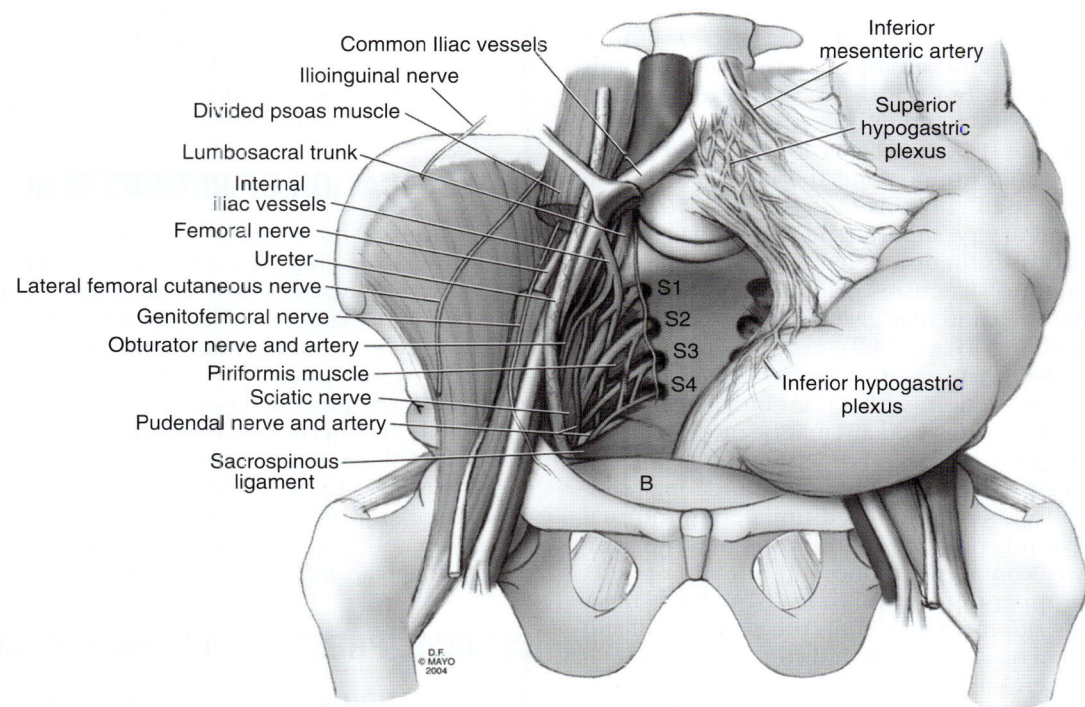

FIGURE 174.2 Vascular and neural anatomy of retrorectal space. *B,* Bladder. (Used with permission of Mayo Foundation for Medical Education and Research. All rights reserved.)

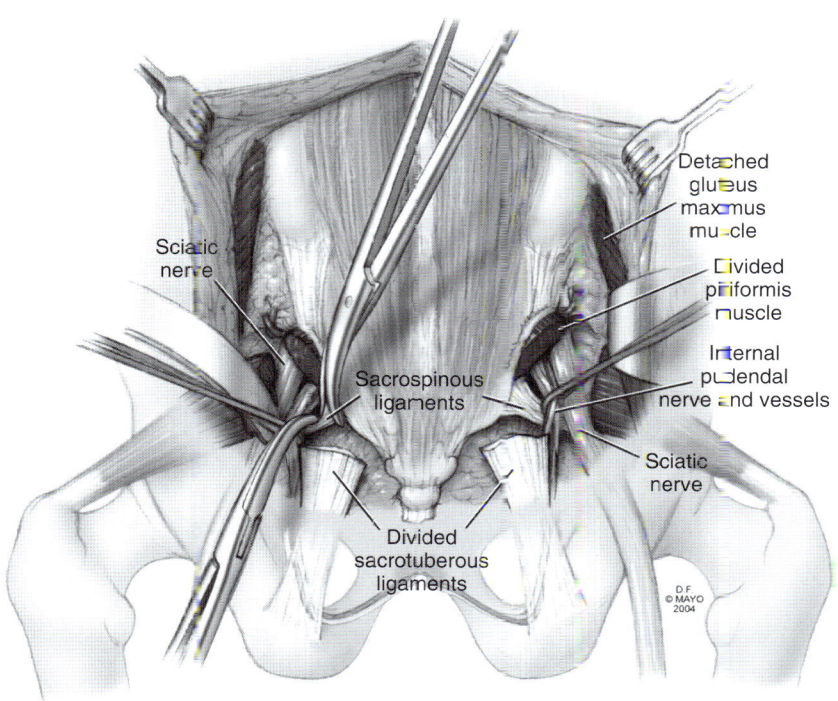

FIGURE 174.3 Anatomy of posterior sacrum: sacrotuberous and sacrospinous ligaments. (Used with permission of Mayo Foundation for Medical Education and Research. All rights reserved.)

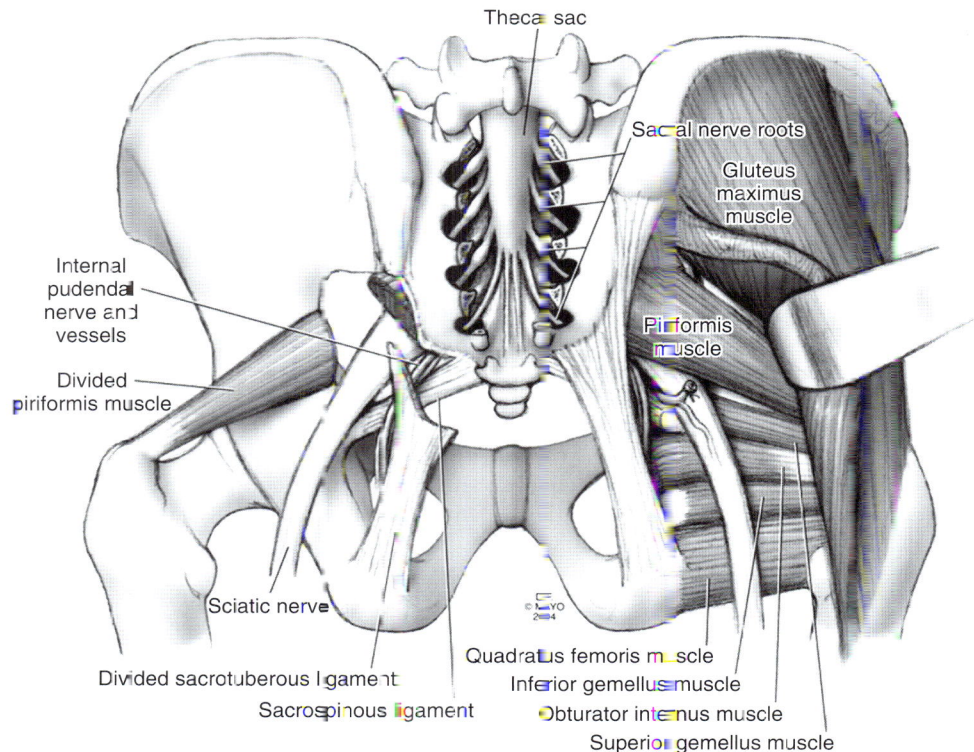

FIGURE 174.4 Anatomy of posterior sacrum: piriformis muscle and sciatic and pudendal nerves. (Used with permission of Mayo Foundation for Medical Education and Research. All rights reserved.)

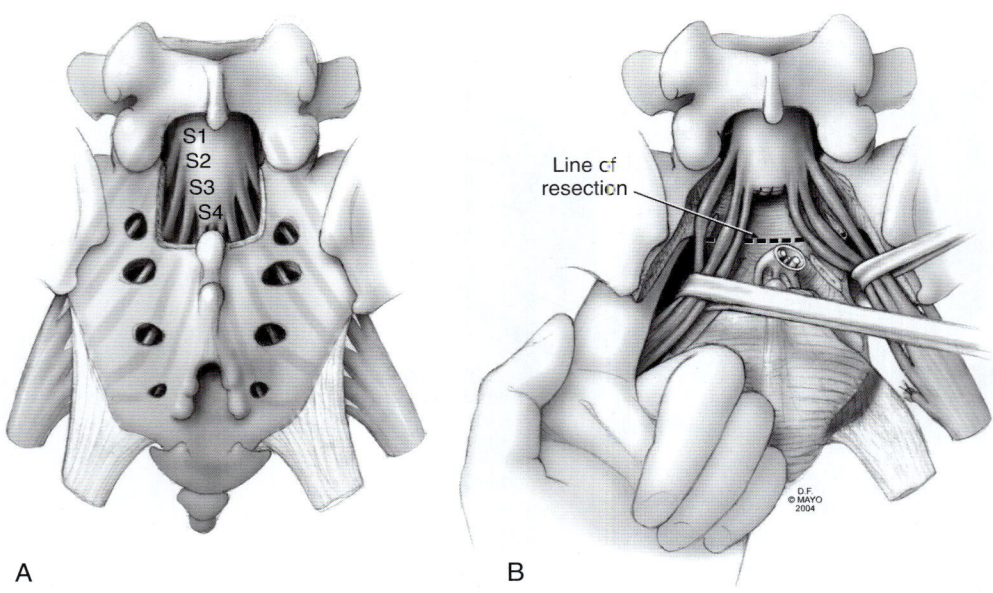

A　　　　　　　　　　　　　　　　　B

FIGURE 174.5 Anatomy of posterior sacrum: thecal sac (A) and nerve roots (B). (Used with permission of Mayo Foundation for Medical Education and Research. All rights reserved.)

WORK-UP

Retrorectal masses should undergo a focused physical examination, high-resolution cross-sectional imaging, and percutaneous biopsy of solid or heterogeneous tumors.[9] Plain radiographs of the sacrum are of limited use and computed tomography (CT) and/or magnetic resonance imaging (MRI) should be used preferentially. However, when obtained, plain films may identify bone destruction, calcification, and soft tissue–occupying masses—features commonly seen with chordoma, giant cell tumors, neurilemoma, aneurysmal bone cysts, and osteochondroma.[2] A "scimitar" sign on sacral views (or sickle-shaped sacrum) is a classic feature seen in association with anterior sacral meningocele, a diagnosis that must be confirmed with myelography or contrast-enhanced MRI.

Cross-sectional imaging, particularly with CT, allows for defining tumors as cystic, solid, or heterogeneous (solid and cystic components). It is important to evaluate if other pelvic structures, such as the bladder, uterus, ureters, or rectum, are involved. CT best demonstrates cortical bone destruction, whereas MRI is superior in evaluation of marrow involvement. Moreover, we find MRI, due to a high degree of soft tissue resolution, is helpful in defining the complete extent of the tumor and involvement of adjacent structures and assists greatly in surgical planning. Spinal imaging is best performed by MRI, which may demonstrate meningocele, nerve root, and foraminal involvement by tumor and thecal sac compression. MR angiogram or venogram may add additional information regarding vascular involvement and, if present, should prompt the involvement of a vascular surgeon. Based on several studies, MRI appears to be more accurate than CT imaging in determining malignant from benign lesions.[9,10]

ROLE OF PREOPERATIVE BIOPSY

The role of preoperative biopsy in the management of retrorectal tumors remains controversial. Opposition to biopsy has generally been fueled by the lack of information available on these rare tumors. Some experts believe that preoperative biopsy is contraindicated in any presacral tumor considered resectable,[2,11,12] whereas others have stated that all solid or heterogeneous tumors should be percutaneously biopsied prior to surgical intervention.[9] Rationale for biopsy includes (1) potential impact upon the operative approach, for example, en bloc resection for malignant tumors versus marginal resection for benign ones, (2) application of direct neoadjuvant chemotherapy or radiation therapy in sensitive tumors, and (3) obtaining more complete information to better counsel the patient prior to operative intervention. Thus biopsy serves an important role as knowledge of the tumor histology impacts the overall treatment algorithm.

Simple cystic lesions, which are uniformly benign, do not need to be biopsied because results will not alter management. Patients with tumors responsive to neoadjuvant chemoradiation (e.g., certain sarcoma variants—Ewing sarcoma, osteogenic sarcoma, and neurofibrosarcoma) may benefit from neoadjuvant therapy, and a tissue diagnosis is critical in assisting in decision making. Malignant tumors that reach a considerable size, filling the pelvis, may be more readily excised if some degree of tumor regression is obtained with radiation (Fig. 174.6). In our opinion, the most important role of biopsy, apart from determining the need for neoadjuvant therapy, is for surgical planning. Malignant lesions may require extensive oncologic resection, including multivisceral resection, sacrectomy, and/or lower extremity amputation. In these situations,

BOX 174.1 Classification of Retrorectal Tumors

CONGENITAL
Benign
    Developmental cysts (teratoma, epidermoid, dermoic, mucus secreting)
    Duplication of rectum
    Anterior sacral meningocele
    Adrenal rest tumor
Malignant
    Chordoma
    Teratocarcinoma

NEUROGENIC
Benign
    Neurofibroma
    Neurilemoma (Schwannoma)
    Ganglioneuroma
Malignant
    Neuroblastoma
    Ganglioneuroblastoma
    Ependymoma
    Malignant peripheral nerve sheath tumors

OSSEOUS
Benign
    Giant cell tumor
    Osteoblastoma
    Aneurysmal bone cyst
Malignant
    Osteogenic sarcoma
    Ewing sarcoma
    Myeloma
    Chondrosarcoma

MISCELLANEOUS
Benign
    Lipoma
    Fibroma
    Leiomyoma
    Hemangioma
    Endothelioma
    Desmoid
    Hemangiopericytoma
Malignant
    Liposarcoma
    Fibrosarcoma/malignant fibrous histiocytoma
    Leiomyosarcoma
    Metastatic carcinoma
Other
    Ectopic kidney
    Hematoma
    Abscess

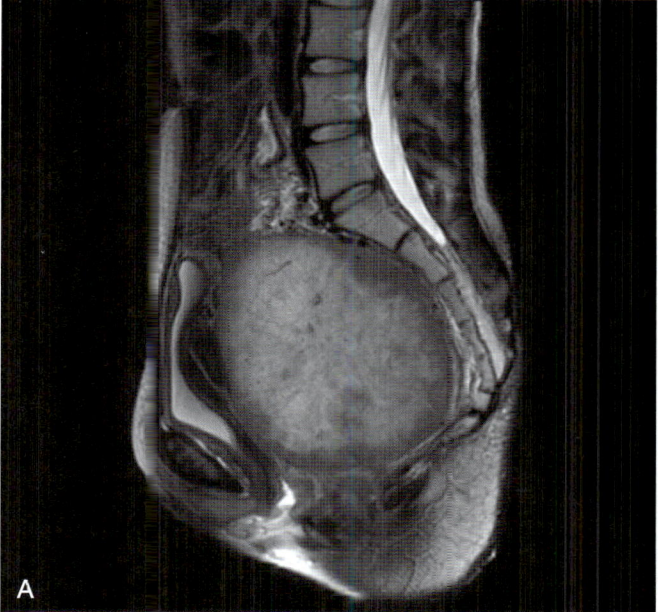
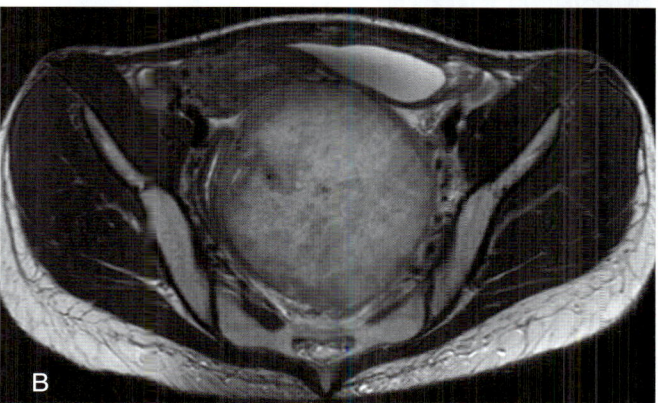

FIGURE 174.6 Sagittal T2-weighted magnetic resonance image of massive presacral pelvic tumor filling the pelvis (A) The tumor displaces the uterus and bladder anteriorly. (B) The rectum is displaced laterally.

when compared with postoperative pathology 90% of the time, compared with 40% of those patients diagnosed on imaging alone. The sensitivity and specificity of biopsy to predict malignant disease was 96% and 100%, respectively. This compared with 83% sensitivity and 81% specificity for imaging to predict malignant disease. There were no reports of tumor seeding along the biopsy tract.[9]

When a biopsy is to be performed, a transperineal or parasacral approach within the field of the resection is used so that the needle tract may be excised if necessary (Fig. 174.7). Transrectal or transvaginal biopsy should never be done for several reasons—if malignancy is present, excision of the rectum and/or vagina may not be necessary but becomes mandated if the biopsy tract traverses these organs. In cystic lesions, transrectal biopsy introduces the risk of infection, rendering subsequent attempts at excision more difficult because of distortion of embryologic tissue planes, which in turn increase the

multidisciplinary team planning and discussion with the patient regarding prognosis and quality of life depend heavily on the preoperative diagnosis obtained by biopsy.

The experience with preoperative biopsy has been reported by Mayo Clinic and demonstrated that biopsy was safe and highly concordant with postoperative pathology compared with imaging alone. For those patients undergoing percutaneous biopsy, the diagnosis was correct

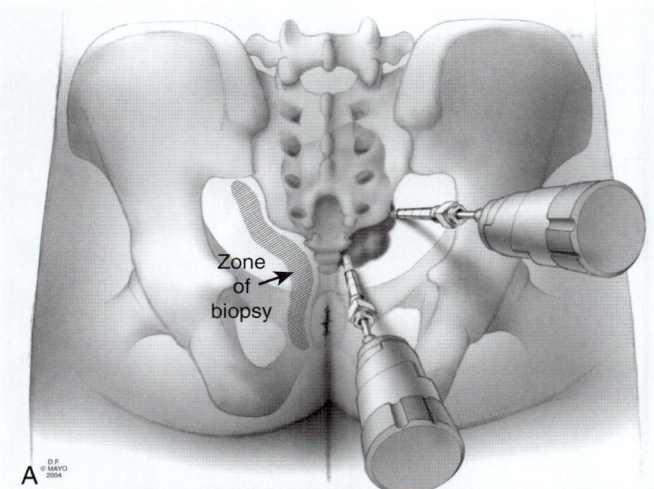

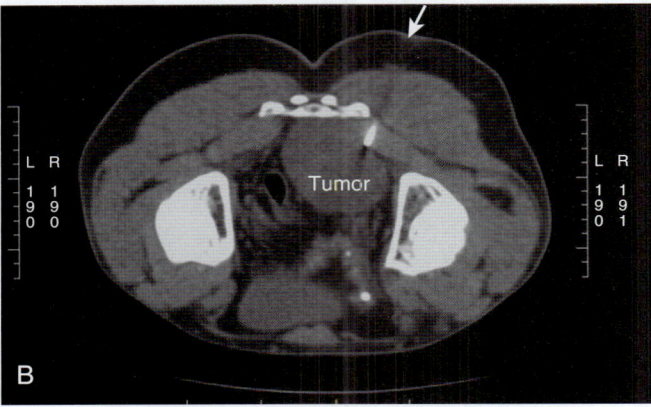

FIGURE 174.7 Preoperative biopsy technique showing ideal zone of needle path (A) and computed tomography scan demonstrating appropriate direction of biopsy tract (B). ([A] Used with permission of Mayo Foundation for Medical Education and Research. All rights reserved; [B] from Dozois EJ, Jacofsky DJ, Dozois RR. Presacral tumors. In: Wolff BG, Fleshman JW, Beck DE, et al., eds. *The ASCRS Textbook of Colon and Rectal Surgery*. New York: Springer; 2007:511.)

risk of recurrence and collateral injury. Finally, inadvertent biopsy of a meningocele may result in the catastrophic complication of meningitis and potential death.

TUMOR-SPECIFIC FEATURES

DEVELOPMENTAL CYSTS

Epidermoid and Dermoid Cysts

These cysts result from abnormal closure of the ectodermal tube of the fetus and are more commonly found in females. Often, these lesions are associated with a postanal dimple or sinus.[13] Epidermoid and dermoid cysts both exhibit keratinizing stratified squamous epithelium, whereas epidermoid cysts bear no skin appendages (Table 174.1). Dermoid cysts may exhibit characteristic sweat glands, hair follicles, or sebaceous cysts and have an intraspinal component.[14]

These lesions may become infected up to 30% of the time and present as a pelvic or perirectal abscess. Furthermore, patients may be misdiagnosed with fistula in ano if a communication between an abscess and a postanal dimple exists.

Enterogenous Cysts

Enterogenous cysts (duplication cysts of the rectum) result from sequestration of the developing hindgut. They may be lined by squamous epithelium (like dermoid and epidermoid cysts) or columnar epithelium (like TGC). They differ from these other entities by having a well-defined muscular wall with a myenteric plexus. Villi or crypts are also commonly found in intestinal duplications but not TGC, and malignancy has been reported.[15]

Tailgut Cysts

TGCs are also referred to as cystic hamartomas, and postanal gut cysts arise from remnants of the embryonic primitive gut that extends into the transient true tail, which develops between 35 and 56 days of gestation before regressing.[15] These lesions are often multicystic and multilocular (Fig. 174.8). The lining is often composed of a combination of squamous, glandular columnar, or

TABLE 174.1 Features of Retrorectal Cysts

Cyst Type	Tissue Type	Distinguishing Features	Mechanism of Formation	Female (F): Male (M) Ratio
Dermoid cyst	Keratinizing stratified squamous epithelium	± Sweat glands, hair follicles, sebaceous cysts	Failure of separation of cutaneous ectoderm from neural ectoderm	F > M
Epidermoid cyst	Keratinizing stratified squamous epithelium	No skin appendages	Failure of separation of cutaneous ectoderm from neural ectoderm	F > M
Enterogenous cyst (duplication cyst)	Squamous or columnar epithelium	Well-defined muscular wall with myenteric plexus; ± villi or crypts	Sequestration of the developing hindgut	F > M
Tailgut cyst	Squamous or glandular columnar or transitional or mixture	Smooth muscle may be present, but not well defined; no myenteric plexus	Remnants of embryonic primitive gut	3:1
Teratoma	Contains tissue from each of the germ layers	May contain hair, bone, teeth		F > M

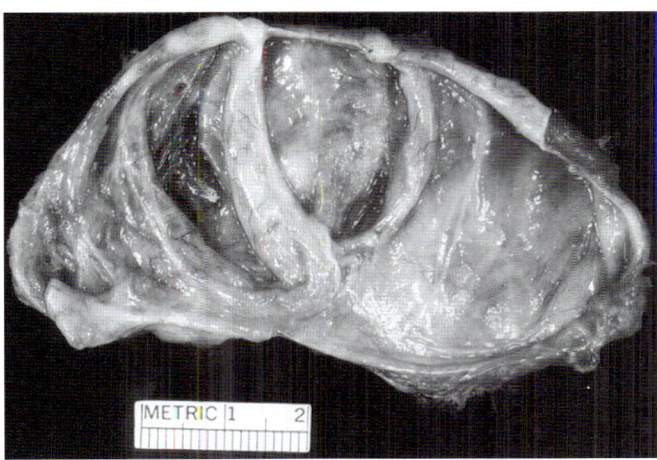

FIGURE 174.8 Gross pathologic specimen of a tailgut cyst revealing multicystic, multiloculated appearance.

transitional epithelium.[16] The presence of glandular or transitional epithelium excludes the diagnosis of dermoid and epidermoid cysts, which contain squamous epithelium only. Unlike duplication cysts, there should be no evidence of a well-defined muscular wall with myenteric plexus. The majority of TGCs have been reported in adults, with few reports of these lesions being detected in neonates.[17] Although the presence of calcification on imaging is uncommon with TGCs and is most often seen with teratomas, this may still occur in the presence of malignant degeneration.[15] CT imaging reveals a well-defined, homogeneous mass, with preservation of adjacent fat planes and often keratinous debris within the cysts.[18]

Historically, malignancy was thought to rarely develop in TGCs (approximately 2)[15]; however, a more contemporary series of 31 patients from the Mayo Clinic demonstrated that malignancy of TGCs was identified in 13%.[19] In this series, complete cyst excision was achieved in all patients, using a posterior (20/31), anterior (9/31), or combined (2/31) approach. A fistula to the rectum was found in four patients (13%). One benign recurrence was detected during follow-up. This series also demonstrated that coccygectomy was not routinely required, despite the historical beliefs, and that recurrence was lower when coccygectomy was performed (approximately 6% in patients with follow-up of at least 1 year). The author's approach has been to preserve the coccyx, unless resection is mandated secondary to malignancy or the cyst is densely adherent to the coccyx. The majority of reported malignancies have been adenocarcinomas.[15,16,20–22] Presacral carcinoid tumors have also been described in association with TGC,[23,24] leading to the speculation that these carcinoids arise from neuroendocrine cells in presacral hindgut rests.[25]

NEUROGENIC TUMORS

Neurogenic tumors have an estimated incidence of 1 in 250,000 to 800,000 hospital visits and include schwannoma, ganglioneuroma, ganglioneuroblastoma, neurofibroma, neuroblastoma, ependymoma, and malignant peripheral nerve sheath tumors (neurofibrosarcoma, malignant schwannomas, neurogenic sarcomas). As these tumors

grow, significant neurologic sequelae may result, leading to sensory, motor, anorectal, or urogenital dysfunction. A previously published Mayo Clinic series of neurogenic tumors of the pelvis demonstrated that schwannomas were the most common benign tumor and malignant peripheral nerve sheath tumors, the most common malignant lesions.[26] Benign schwannomas are typically solitary, well-circumscribed, encapsulated tumors.[27] Malignant transformation of schwannomas is rare.[28] Differentiating between benign and malignant neurogenic tumors preoperatively can be challenging without a tissue biopsy as imaging alone is not adequate for this differentiation, and in these patients, a preoperative biopsy is paramount to guide operative approach (nerve sparing vs. nerve resection).

Among the largest surgical series reported to date of pelvic neurogenic tumors included several in the presacral space.[26] In this series, 89 patients were identified, 44 were male. Median age was 38 years. Lesions were determined to be malignant in 43 patients (48%). Schwannomas were the most common benign tumor (61%) and malignant peripheral nerve sheath tumors the most common malignant lesion (51%). Malignant tumors had histopathologic evidence of infiltration of surrounding structures in 49% of cases. Intralesional resection was the most common surgical technique used, regardless of presence of malignancy. The 5-year local recurrence rates for benign and malignant lesions were 35.9% and 35.0%, respectively. Survival in those with malignant lesions at 1, 5, and 10 years was 79.5%, 47.9%, and 29.6%, respectively. Five-year disease-free survival for malignant tumors was 25.9%.

The Mayo Clinic published their experience on the treatment of benign presacral neurogenic tumors.[29] It is our practice to use a nerve- and function-sparing resection technique in the resection of these tumors. Thus confirmation of benign nature via preoperative biopsy is important. Over a 6-year period, 17 consecutive patients with benign tumors were identified and surgically treated. The most common presenting symptom was pain (most commonly sciatalgia). Twelve patients were found to have a schwannoma, and five had neurofibroma. Only one patient developed neurologic dysfunction postoperatively (foot drop), which was transient. At a median follow-up of 34 months, 15 patients were alive and 2 had died of unrelated reasons. Our approach to the treatment of these tumors is outlined in the illustrated algorithm (Fig. 174.9).

SACROCOCCYGEAL CHORDOMAS

Sacrococcygeal chordomas are the most frequently encountered malignant tumor of the retrorectal space. They are believed to originate from the primitive notochord tissue either from the nuclei pulposi or from abnormal rests. This explains their location anywhere along the spinal column with a predilection for the sphenooccipital and the retrorectal regions.

Chordomas tend to have a male predominance and are rarely identified before the age of 30 years. Patients may be asymptomatic or present with a long-standing history of vague pain mostly in the perineal area, characteristically aggravated by sitting and ameliorated by standing or walking.[30–32] Advanced, large tumors may cause anorectal

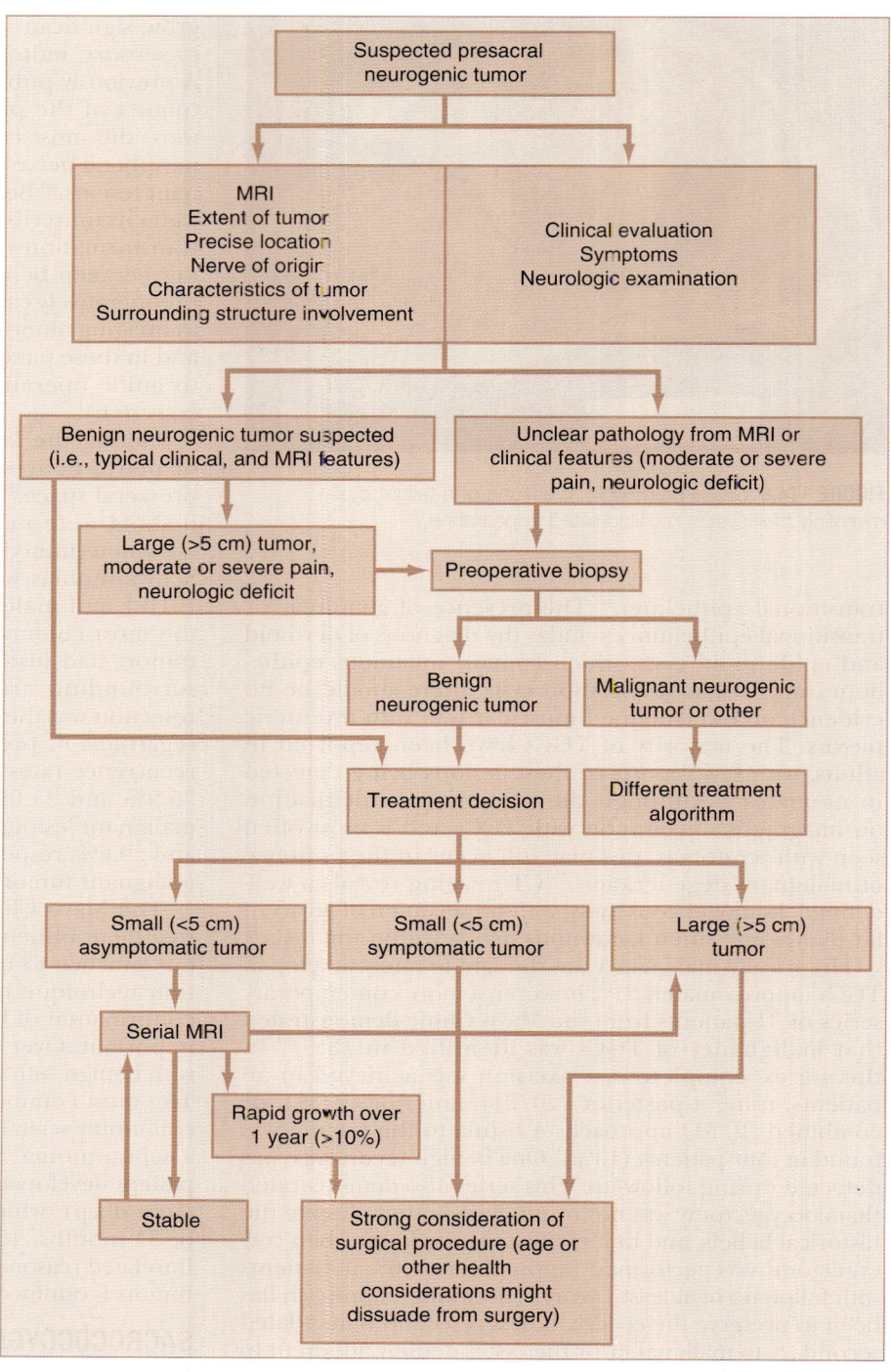

FIGURE 174.9 Algorithm for the management of neurogenic tumors. *MRI*, Magnetic resonance imaging.

or urogenital dysfunction (constipation, fecal and urinary incontinence, and sexual dysfunction). Anterior and lateral plain radiographs of the sacrum often demonstrate bone destruction and a soft tissue–occupying mass. Other tumors that may cause bony destruction but are less likely, include giant cell tumors, schwannomas, aneurysmal bone cysts, and osteochondromas.[30]

Outcomes following surgical resection are entirely dependent upon the ability to obtain a negative margin resection. Kaiser et al. found that local recurrence rate increased from 28% to 64% if the tumor was violated in patients with chordomas.[33]

Fuchs et al. have reported one of the largest series of sacral chordoma.[34] Fifty-two patients underwent surgical treatment for sacrococcygeal chordoma over a 21-year period. Most patients had symptoms present for an average duration of 27 months, most tumors were large (average diameter of 9 cm), and nearly two-thirds had extended cephalad to S3. At an average follow-up of 7.8 years, 23 patients were alive with no evidence of disease.

Twenty-three patients (44%) had local recurrence. The rate of recurrence-free survival was 59% at 5 years and 46% at 10 years. The overall survival rates were 74%, 52%, and 47% at 5, 10, and 15 years, respectively. The most important predictor of survival was a wide negative margin.

TERATOMA AND TERATOCARCINOMA

Presacral teratoma is the most common teratoma seen in infancy and has a female predominance.[35] Presacral teratomas typically contain tissue from each germ layer, although the degree of differentiation may vary. Tumors demonstrating greater differentiation, with recognizable hair, bone or teeth, are more likely to be benign. As with other retrorectal masses, benign lesions are usually cystic, whereas malignant degeneration is generally indicated by solid or heterogeneous components.

Sacrococcygeal teratomas are externally visible in 90% of infants. In contrast, teratomas in adults are most commonly intrapelvic, explaining their later discovery.[35] Altman classified these tumors into four types depending on the relative representation of external and intrapelvic components (Fig. 174.10).[35] These differences in presentation explain why more than 50% of infants were diagnosed on the day of birth in a series from 1974; 18% were not diagnosed within the first 6 months of life. This impacted significantly on the rate of malignancy at diagnosis because the development of malignancy correlates strongly with age in infants only 7% of girls and 10% of boys presented with malignancy prior to 2 months, but these rates rose to 48% and 67%, respectively, after 2 months.[35] The current trend toward widespread use of ultrasound monitoring during pregnancy would be anticipated to greatly increase the rate of prenatal diagnosis and reduce the risk of malignancy.

A series by the Mayo Clinic recently reported on the surgical outcomes of benign and malignant sacrococcygeal teratomas.[36] Twenty-six patients were identified over a 33-year period. Five patients (19%) were found to have malignant tumors. Preoperative biopsy had a 100% concordance with final surgical pathology. For the majority of patients, a posterior surgical approach was sufficient for complete resection. All patients with

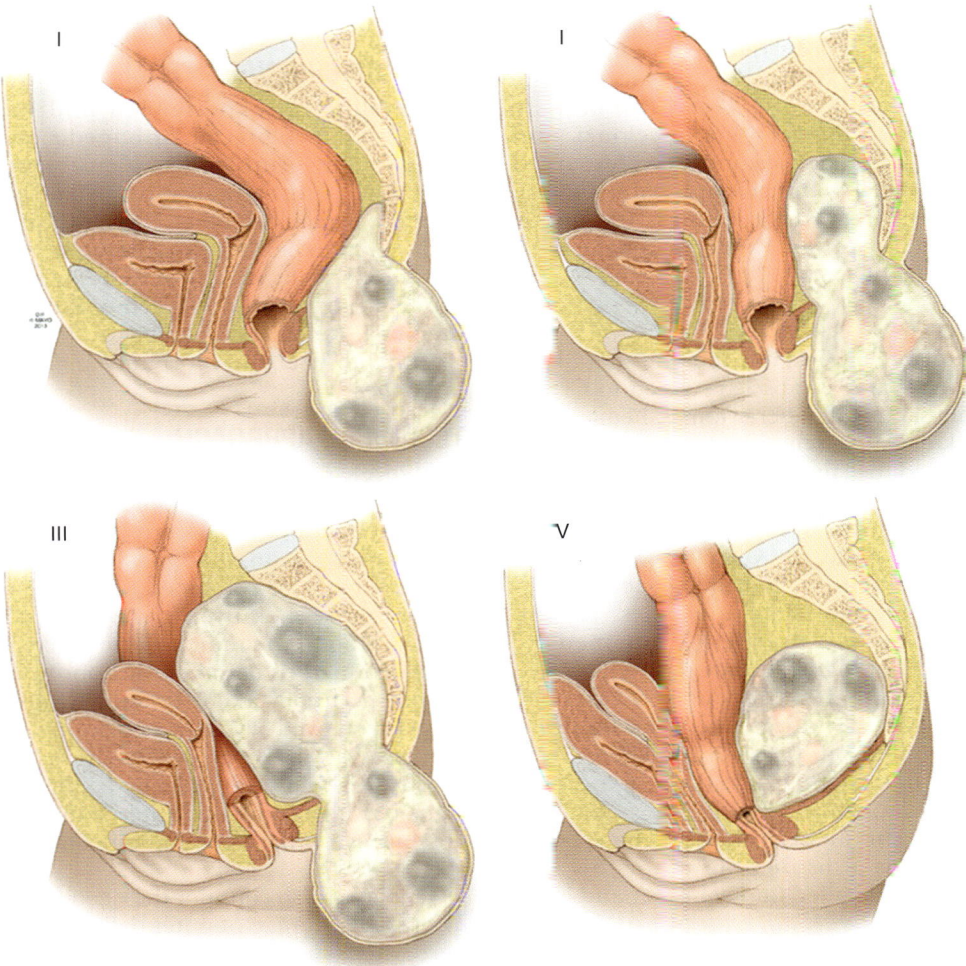

FIGURE 174.10 Classification of sacrococcygeal teratomas. Type I is predominantly external tumor, type II is external tumor with intrapelvic extension, type III is predominantly intrapelvic with external extension, and type IV is a presacral tumor. (Used with permission of Mayo Foundation for Medical Education and Research. All rights reserved.)

malignant lesions underwent distal sacrectomy and had an R0 resection; however, only 57% of patients with benign lesions required sacral or coccygeal resection. There was no short-term mortality, and 30-day morbidity was 60% (with the minority, 19%, with Clavien-Dindo grade III or greater). In those patients with benign lesions, median follow-up was 23 months, and recurrence (which was malignant) was noted in one patient at 6 years. In those five patients with malignant tumors, three ultimately died of metastatic disease at a median follow-up of 20 months. Adjuvant therapy for the treatment of malignant tumors is not universal, and there are no consensus guidelines for the treatment of the adult population. Our practice has been extrapolated from the pediatric population—surgery followed by etoposide, bleomycin, and cisplatin chemotherapy as necessary. Preoperative radiation for tumors with malignant degeneration to adenocarcinoma or squamous cell carcinoma can shrink the mass of tumor, potentially provide clear resection margins, and may reduce local recurrence rates. Sarcomatous lesions may also benefit from radiation therapy depending on cell type.

OSSEOUS LESIONS

Most osseous lesions of the presacral space are metastatic; however, primary osseous lesions remain the next most common retrorectal mass after neurogenic tumors. There is a male predominance of 2:1, and half of these masses are malignant: Ewing sarcoma, myeloma, and osteogenic sarcoma.[2] Malignant lesions are represented by such tumors as giant cell tumor, aneurysmal bone cyst, and osteochondroma.[2] Bone destruction is frequently seen accompanying such tumors. Pain remains the most common presenting feature.

MISCELLANEOUS LESIONS

Miscellaneous lesions in this region include metastatic lesions, inflammatory changes/abscess related to Crohn disease or diverticulitis, hemangiopericytomas, hematomas, and pelvic ectopic kidneys. Carcinoid tumors are unusual but have been reported, but most represent direct extension or metastatic spread from rectal carcinoids.[37]

Rarely, presacral tumors will present as part of a congenital syndrome, such as the Currarino syndrome, which is characterized by the triad of presacral mass, anorectal malformations, and sacral anomalies.[38] In the Currarino syndrome the most frequent component of the presacral mass is meningocele, but teratomas have been identified in 20% to 40% of reported cases.[39,40] The mutation causing this syndrome has been localized to the HLXB9 gene on chromosome 7q36. There likely exists some genetic heterogeneity and the expressed phenotype is variable. In sporadic cases, differing mutations have been identified. The identification of the specific sacral anomaly, which is a distinct entity for this syndrome, should prompt a detailed family history and gene testing.[41,42]

In a review of retrorectal sarcomas at our institution, 37 patients underwent resection, 84% had an R0 margin, and 16% an R1.[43] Overall, 76% of the patients required en bloc resection of adjacent pelvic organs and bony structures. The most frequent sarcomas found were malignant peripheral nerve sheath tumors and chondrosarcomas.

Intraoperative radiation therapy was administered to 22% of patients. Overall survival at 2, 5, and 10 years was 75%, 55%, and 47%, respectively. Disease-free survival at 5 years was 51%.

SURGICAL INTERVENTION AND APPROACH

RATIONALE

Once identified, retrorectal tumors should be treated surgically. This recommendation is based on the fact that a reasonable proportion of these tumors may be malignant or progress to malignancy from a benign state. Anterior sacral meningoceles may become infected and result in meningitis if left untreated. Cystic lesions are also at risk of becoming infected, which renders subsequent excision more difficult and increases the risk of recurrence. Retrorectal masses in young women may continue to grow and result in dystocia. Furthermore, locoregional symptoms often have significant impact upon patient's function and quality of life. Oncologic and functional outcomes can be optimized, whether the tumor is malignant or benign, if an experienced, multidisciplinary team approaches these tumors in a systematic, thoughtful fashion.[43]

MULTIDISCIPLINARY TEAM

Assembling an experienced multidisciplinary team composed of colorectal, orthopedic oncologic surgeons, spine surgeons, urologists, vascular surgeons, and plastic surgeons ensures that appropriate expertise exists to optimize patient outcomes. Preoperatively, members should include an experienced radiologist, medical oncologist, radiation oncologist, and anesthesiologist. Postoperatively, the team may also require the skills of a rehabilitation therapist. Referral of patients to experienced centers is essential to decrease morbidity and maximize oncologic outcomes.

TECHNICAL APPROACH

The surgical approach is dependent upon the location of the tumor within the pelvis. There are three possible approaches to the resection of a retrorectal tumor: anterior-only (transabdominal), posterior-only (perineal or parasacral), or combined anterior-posterior approach. Accurate preoperative imaging is vital in defining the relationship of the tumor to the sacrum and the margins of resection, thus defining the appropriate approach that should be undertaken. Lesions lying entirely below S3 may be removed with a posterior-only approach through a parasacral/paracoccygeal incision. Tumors extending above S3 should be approached either from the abdomen alone or with a combined anterior and posterior approach, depending on the need for concomitant sacral resection (Fig. 174.11).

One must also consider the need for reconstruction and soft tissue coverage of potentially large pelvic defects. It is here where the plastic surgeon plays a vital role. A rectus abdominis myocutaneous flap is a versatile option and is often the flap of choice. Occasionally, a gracilis flap or gluteal advancement flap may be used. Whichever flap is contemplated, appropriate planning for positioning and skin preparation must be considered.

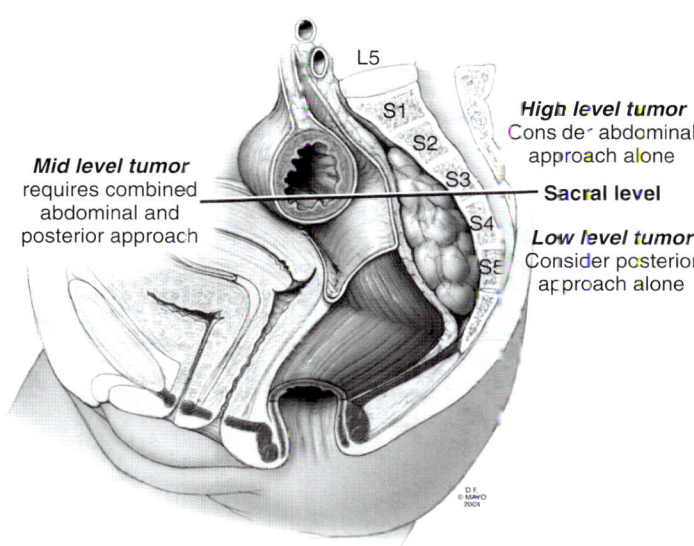

Mid level tumor
requires combined
abdominal and
posterior approach

L5

S1
S2
S3
S4
S5

High level tumor
Consider abdominal
approach alone

— **Sacral level**

Low level tumor
Consider posterior
approach alone

D.F.
© MAYO
2004

FIGURE 174.11 Determination of anterior, posterior, or combined anterior-posterior approach based on level of tumor in relation to sacral bodies. (Used with permission of Mayo Foundation for Medical Education and Research. All rights reserved.)

Tumors Located Below S3—The Posterior Approach

The patient is placed in the prone jackknife position, and the buttocks are taped apart. An incision is made over the lower sacrum and coccyx down to the anoderm, avoiding damage to the sphincter complex. Coccygectomy or distal sacrectomy can facilitate exposure to the pelvis and resection of large tumors but is not mandated unless malignancy is present with involvement of these structures. The lesion can then be dissected in a plane between the retrorectal fat and the tumor. A pseudocapsule is often encountered that facilitates safe dissection from the surrounding tissues, including the rectal wall. In the case of very small lesions, especially if cystic, the surgeon may use the nondominant hand and, with the index finger in the anal canal and lower rectum, push the lesion outward, away from the depths of the wound (Fig. 174.12). This technique facilitates dissection of the lesion away from the wall of the rectum without entry into the rectal lumen. Prior infection of a cystic lesion may obliterate the plane between the cyst wall and the rectum. A portion of the rectal wall may be excised with the specimen and the defect closed in two layers.

Combined Anterior-Posterior Approach

If the tumor extends above the level of S3, a combined anterior-posterior approach is preferred. The patient is usually positioned in the supine position and the dissection begins transabdominally. If resection of the rectum is to be combined with reestablishment of bowel continuity, a carefully padded, combined synchronous (modified dorsal lithotomy) position is used. Other positions, such as the "sloppy lateral" position have also been described to facilitate a two-team approach to the combined anterior and posterior resection.

The abdominal cavity is entered through a lower midline incision and the peritoneal cavity is carefully explored to rule out disseminated disease. After mobilization of

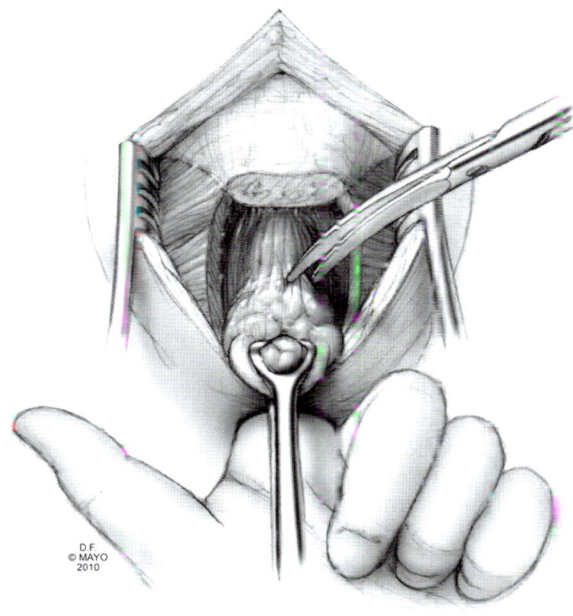

D.F.
© MAYO
2010

FIGURE 174.12 Use of finger to assist tumor extraction off rectum via perineal approach. (Used with permission of Mayo Foundation for Medical Education and Research. All rights reserved.)

the lower sigmoid, the presacral space is entered just below the sacral promontory and the posterior mesorectum dissected off the sacral fascia down to the upper extension of the tumor. If the tumor can be separated safely from the posterior rectum, the lesion is dissected free in a plane anterior to the mass between its capsule and the mesorectum. Posterior to the tumor, if a plane exists between the lesion and the sacrum, this too is carefully developed. Isolated tumors, without invasion of adjacent organs, may be dissected free circumferentially in this manner and removed. If the tumor is bulky, it may compress or displace the rectum, making attempts at separating the tumor and the rectum risky. In this scenario, we tend to perform an en bloc excision of the rectum with the tumor. Reestablishment of bowel continuity may be considered (particularly with benign tumors), with a protective diverting loop ileostomy if indicated (anastomosis below the anterior peritoneal reflection and/or preoperative irradiation). If the tumor extends high on the sacrum, with evidence of invasion so that both S3 roots and even S2 nerve roots will need to be sacrificed, the patient will be rendered incontinent. Thus excision of the rectum en bloc with the mass may facilitate resection and avoids tumor cell spillage. In this situation the upper rectum is transected above the level of the tumor, using a cutting stapler and distally its anterior and lateral attachments are completely freed to the level of the pelvic floor, with subsequent removal of the anus and entire sphincter complex if necessary. An end sigmoid colostomy is then created.

Resection of large complex tumors may result in substantial blood loss. This may occur from friable, irradiated pelvic vessels, involvement of pelvic vasculature by the tumor, or the sacrectomy itself. Thus, when a major sacrectomy is contemplated, ligation of the middle sacral artery and the internal iliac vessels and its branches may help reduce blood loss. Efforts should be undertaken to preserve the anterior division of the internal iliac artery, which gives off the inferior gluteal artery. This reduces the risk of potential perineal and gluteal necrosis. The assistance of a vascular surgeon is invaluable for this step, especially in the presence of an irradiated field. It is helpful to mobilize the ureters, together with supporting tissues, and suspend them laterally away from the planned margin of the sacrectomy.

In patients requiring extended sacral resection, especially when radiation has been an integral part of the treatment, a well-vascularized musculocutaneous flap derived from the rectus abdominis can be used to close the perineum to limit the risk of perineal wound complications. The flap can be mobilized at this point in the procedure and placed in the deep pelvis to be accessed later via the perineal wound and used for closure. To protect both the flap and other vital structures during the perineal portion of the procedure, a barrier of thick plastic sheeting or laparotomy pads is placed immediately in front of the sacrum, to be removed after resection of the sacrum.

Prior to transitioning the patient to the prone position, the abdominal incision is closed and the ostomy (if required) is created. A midline incision is made over the sacrum and coccyx down to the anus, the anococcygeal ligament is transected and the levators retracted bilaterally. If the rectum is to be preserved, its posterior aspect is separated from the tumor. The orthopedic surgeon can then proceed with dissection of the gluteus maximus muscles on both sides, transection of the sacrospinous and sacrotuberous ligaments, and division of the piriformis

muscles to expose the sciatic nerves. An osteotomy is then carried out at the S3 level or even higher after exposing and preserving if at all possible at least one S3 nerve root. The neural sac may need to be ligated. In this fashion, the tumor can be removed en bloc with the attached sacrum, coccyx, and involved sacral nerve roots, with or without the rectum.

Minimally Invasive Approaches for Presacral Tumor Resection. Recently, there have been reports using minimally invasive (laparoscopic or robotic) techniques as an approach for presacral tumor resection.[44-46] Most current reports have limited this to highly selected tumors that are benign and can be approached through an entirely transabdominal approach. Minimally invasive techniques should decrease the morbidity of the overall operation significantly. Lengyel et al. described a laparoscopic approach to treat advanced rectal cancer with a similar surgical approach to the malignant presacral tumor laparoscopic resection.[46] It was performed in two phases: a laparoscopic abdominal phase with the patient in the modified Lloyd-Davies position, followed by a transsacral phase with the patient in the prone jackknife position. The key features of the abdominal (laparoscopic) component were lateral-to-medial mobilization of the rectum, ligation of the inferior mesenteric vessels, careful identification and preservation of the pelvic nerves and sacral nerve roots, and division of the colon with construction of the colostomy and completion of the proctectomy. A more recent series by Fong et al. reported 10 patients undergoing laparoscopic resection of benign tumors. There was no reported major intraoperative or postoperative morbidity. Median tumor size was 8 cm.[47] The fundamental goal in approaching these patients in a minimally invasive manner should be to limit morbidity. However, most importantly, one must not compromise the surgical resection of malignant disease in an effort to preserve cosmesis.

PATIENT FOLLOW-UP CONSIDERATIONS

For patients with benign tumors, our practice has been to assess for recurrence with an annual visit that includes a digital rectal examination. If digital rectal examination reveals a palpable mass, cross-sectional pelvic imaging is obtained. Furthermore, we recommend a baseline CT at 1 year following surgery and then repeated at every 5 years, even if the physical examination is normal.

Patients with malignant tumors are followed more intensely, with particular attention to locoregional recurrence and pulmonary metastasis. An annual abdominopelvic MRI and chest CT scan are performed for the first 5 years. If the patient has the rectum in place, an annual digital rectal examination with possible endoscopic evaluation is performed. Patients are offered repeat resection for locally advanced tumors and for pulmonary metastasis if all disease can be removed operatively.

ALGORITHM

At our institution, we have established a decision-making algorithm to guide the management of retrorectal tumors (Fig. 174.13).

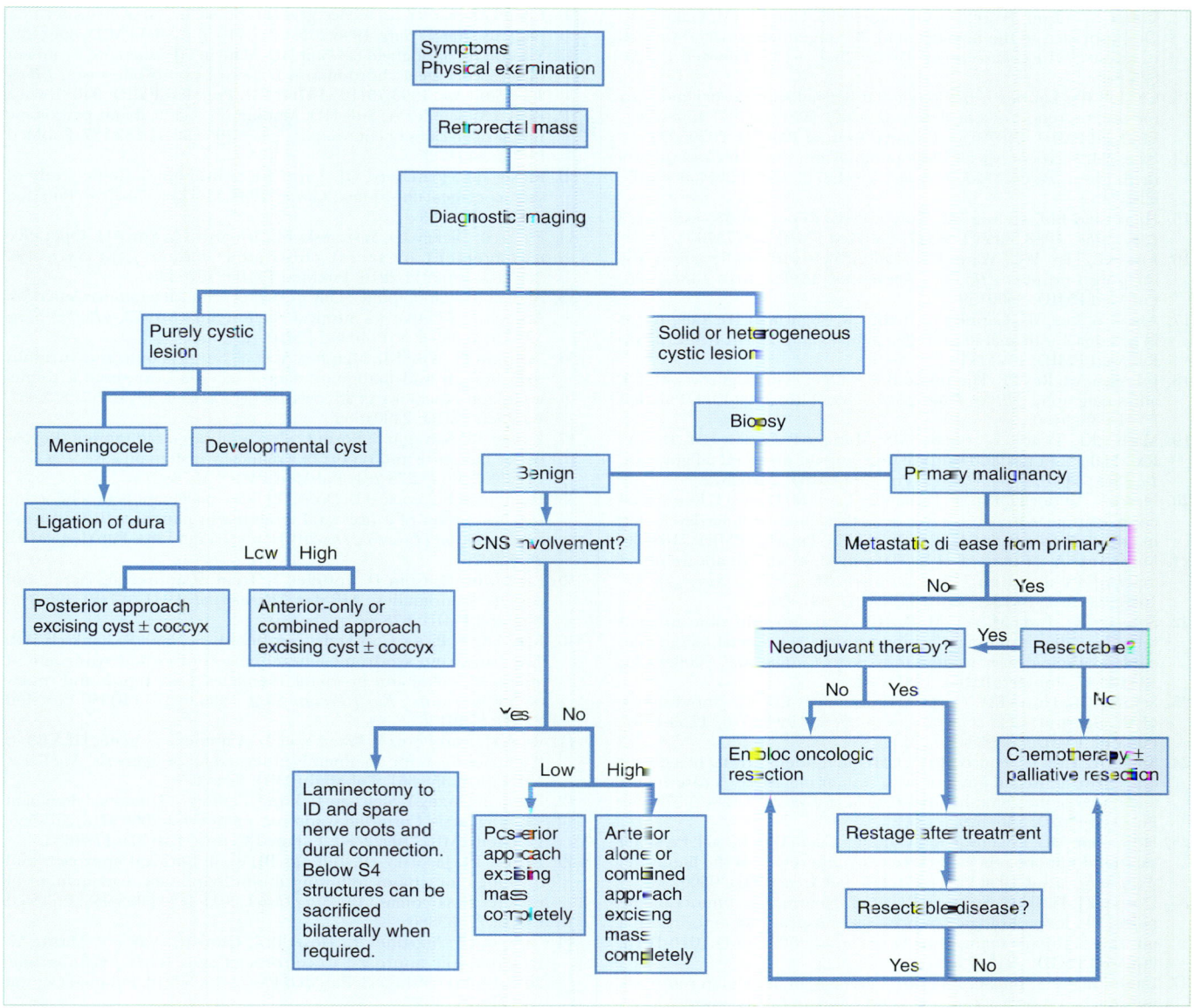

FIGURE 174.13 Algorithm to guide the management of retrorectal tumors. *CNS*, Central nervous system. (From Dozois EJ, Jacofsky DJ, Dozois RR. Presacral tumors. In: Wolff BG, Fleshman JW, Beck DE, et al., eds. *The ASCRS Textbook of Colon and Rectal Surgery.* New York: Springer; 2007:512.)

REFERENCES

1. Whittaker LD, Pemberton JD. Tumors ventral to the sacrum. *Ann Surg.* 1938;107(1):96-106. PubMed PMID: 17857121. Pubmed Central PMCID: 1386919.
2. Jao SW, Beart RW Jr, Spencer RJ. Reiman HM, Ilstrup DM. Retrorectal tumors. Mayo Clinic experience, 1960–1979. *Dis Color Rectum.* 1985;28(9):644-652. PubMed PMID: 2996861.
3. Glasgow SC, Birnbaum EH. Lowney JK, et al. Retrorectal tumors: a diagnostic and therapeutic challenge. *Dis Colon Rectum.* 2005;48(8):1581-1587. PubMed PMID: 15937630.
4. Gunterberg B, Kewenter J, Petersen I, Stener B. Anorectal function after major resections of the sacrum with bilateral or unilateral sacrifice of sacral nerves. *Br J Surg.* 1976;63(7):546-554. PubMed PMID: 953450.
5. Bauer JJ, Gelernt IM, Salky B, Kreel I. Sexual dysfunction following proctocolectomy for benign disease of the colon and rectum. *Ann Surg.* 1983;197(3):363-367. PubMed PMID: 6830342. Pubmed Central PMCID: 1352742.

6. Bernstein WC, Bernstein EF. Sexual dysfunction following radical surgery for cancer of the rectum. *Dis Colon Rectum.* 1966;9(5):328-332. PubMed PMID: 5959686.
7. Uhlig BE, Johnson RL. Presacral tumors and cysts in adults. *Dis Colon Rectum.* 1975;18(7):581-589. PubMed PMID: 1181152.
8. Singer MA, Cintron JR, Martz JE, Schoetz DJ, Abcarian H. Retrorectal cyst: a rare tumor frequently misdiagnosed. *J Am Coll Surg.* 2003;196(6):880-886. PubMed PMID: 12788424.
9. Merchea A, Larson DW, Hubner M, Wenger DE, Rose PS, Dozois EJ. The value of preoperative biopsy in the management of solid presacral tumors. *Dis Colon Rectum.* 2013;56(6):756-760. PubMed PMID: 23652750.
10. Hopper L, Eglinton TW, Wakeman C, Dobbs BR, Dixon L, Frizelle FA. Progress in the management of retrorectal tumours. *Colorectal Dis.* 2016;18(4):410-417. PubMed PMID: 26367385.
11. Lev-Chelouche D, Gutman M, Goldman G, et al. Presacral tumors: a practical classification and treatment of a unique and heterogeneous group of diseases. *Surgery.* 2003;133(5):473-478. PubMed PMID: 12773974.

12. Bohm B, Milsom JW, Fazio VW, Lavery IC, Church JM, Oakley JR. Our approach to the management of congenital presacral tumors in adults. *Int J Colorectal Dis.* 1993;8(3):134-138. PubMed PMID: 8245668.

13. Cardell BS, Laurance B. Congenital dermal sinus associated with meningitis: report of a fatal case. *Br Med J.* 1951;2(4747):1558-1561. PubMed PMID: 14879150. Pubmed Central PMCID: 2070503.

14. Bale PM. Sacrococcygeal developmental abnormalities and tumors in children. *Perspect Pediatr Pathol.* 1984;8(1):9-56. PubMed PMID: 6366733.

15. Hjermstad BM, Helwig EB. Tailgut cysts. Report of 53 cases. *Am J Clin Pathol.* 1988;89(2):139-147. PubMed PMID: 3277378.

16. Lim KE, Hsu WC, Wang CR. Tailgut cyst with malignancy: MR imaging findings. *AJR Am J Roentgenol.* 1998;170(6):1488-1490. PubMed PMID: 9609159.

17. Antao B, Lee AC, Gannon C, Arthur R, Sugarman ID. Tailgut cyst in a neonate with anal stenosis. *Eur J Pediatr Surg.* 2004;14(3):212-214. PubMed PMID: 15211416.

18. Johnson AR, Ros PR, Hjermstad BM. Tailgut cyst: diagnosis with CT and sonography. *AJR Am J Roentgenol.* 1986;147(6):1309-1311. PubMed PMID: 3535460.

19. Mathis KL, Dozois EJ, Grewal MS, Metzger P, Larson DW, Devine RM. Malignant risk and surgical outcomes of presacral tailgut cysts. *Br J Surg.* 2010;97(4):575-579. PubMed PMID: 20169572.

20. Marco V, Autonell J, Farre J, Fernandez-Layos M, Doncel F. Retrorectal cyst-hamartomas. Report of two cases with adenocarcinoma developing in one. *Am J Surg Pathol.* 1982;6(8):707-714. PubMed PMID: 7168459.

21. Maruyama A, Murabayashi K, Hayashi M, et al. Adenocarcinoma arising in a tailgut cyst: report of a case. *Surg Today.* 1998;28(12):1319-1322. PubMed PMID: 9872560.

22. Schwarz RE, Lyda M, Lew M, Paz IB. A carcinoembryonic antigen-secreting adenocarcinoma arising within a retrorectal tailgut cyst: clinicopathological considerations. *Am J Gastroenterol.* 2000;95(5):1344-1347. PubMed PMID: 10811351.

23. Schnee CL, Hurst RW, Curtis MT, Friedman ED. Carcinoid tumor of the sacrum: case report. *Neurosurgery.* 1994;35(6):1163-1167. PubMed PMID: 7885566.

24. Song DE, Park JK, Hur B, Ro JY. Carcinoid tumor arising in a tailgut cyst of the anorectal junction with distant metastasis: a case report and review of the literature. *Arch Pathol Lab Med.* 2004;128(5):578-580. PubMed PMID: 15086297.

25. Horenstein MG, Erlandson RA, Gonzalez-Cueto DM, Rosai J. Presacral carcinoid tumors: report of three cases and review of the literature. *Am J Surg Pathol.* 1998;22(2):251-255. PubMed PMID: 9500228.

26. Dozois EJ, Wall JC, Spinner RJ, et al. Neurogenic tumors of the pelvis: clinicopathologic features and surgical outcomes using a multidisciplinary team. *Ann Surg Oncol.* 2009;16(4):1010-1016. PubMed PMID: 19194756.

27. Daneshmand S, Youssefzadeh D, Chamie K, et al. Benign retroperitoneal schwannoma: a case series and review of the literature. *Urology.* 2003;62(6):993-997. PubMed PMID: 14665342.

28. Woodruff JM, Selig AM, Crowley K, Allen PW. Schwannoma (neurilemoma) with malignant transformation. A rare, distinctive peripheral nerve tumor. *Am J Surg Pathol.* 1994;18(9):882-895. PubMed PMID: 8067509.

29. Hebert-Blouin MN, Sullivan PS, Merchea A, Leonard D, Spinner RJ, Dozois EJ. Neurological outcome following resection of benign presacral neurogenic tumors using a nerve-sparing technique. *Dis Colon Rectum.* 2013;56(10):1185-1193. PubMed PMID: 24022536.

30. Chandawarkar RY. Sacrococcygeal chordoma: review of 50 consecutive patients. *World J Surg.* 1996;20(6):717-719. PubMed PMID: 8662159.

31. Samson IR, Springfield DS, Suit HD, Mankin HJ. Operative treatment of sacrococcygeal chordoma. A review of twenty-one cases. *J Bone Joint Surg Am.* 1993;75(10):1476-1484. PubMed PMID: 8408136.

32. Rich TA, Schiller A, Suit HD, Mankin HJ. Clinical and pathologic review of 48 cases of chordoma. *Cancer.* 1985;56(1):182-187. PubMed PMID: 2408725.

33. Kaiser TE, Pritchard DJ, Unni KK. Clinicopathologic study of sacrococcygeal chordoma. *Cancer.* 1984;53(11):2574-2578. PubMed PMID: 6713355.

34. Fuchs B, Dickey ID, Yaszemski MJ, Inwards CY, Sim FH. Operative management of sacral chordoma. *J Bone Joint Surg Am.* 2005;87(10):2211-2216. PubMed PMID: 16203885.

35. Altman RP, Randolph JG, Lilly JR. Sacrococcygeal teratoma: American Academy of Pediatrics Surgical Section Survey-1973. *J Pediatr Surg.* 1974;9(3):389-398. PubMed PMID: 4843993.

36. Simpson PJ, Wise KB, Merchea A, et al. Surgical outcomes in adults with benign and malignant sacrococcygeal teratoma: a single-institution experience of 26 cases. *Dis Colon Rectum.* 2014;57(7):851-857. PubMed PMID: 24901686.

37. Luong TV, Salvagni S, Bordi C. Presacral carcinoid tumour. Review of the literature and report of a clinically malignant case. *Dig Liver Dis.* 2005;37(4):278-281. PubMed PMID: 15788213.

38. Pendlimari R, Leonard D, Dozois EJ. Rare malignant neuroendocrine transformation of a presacral teratoma in patient with Currarino syndrome. *Int J Colorectal Dis.* 2010;25(11):1383-1384. PubMed PMID: 20532537.

39. Currarino G, Coln D, Votteler T. Triad of anorectal, sacral, and presacral anomalies. *AJR Am J Roentgenol.* 1981;137(2):395-398. PubMed PMID: 6789651.

40. Kochling J, Pistor G, Marzhauser Brands S, Nasir R, Lanksch WR. The Currarino syndrome—hereditary transmitted syndrome of anorectal, sacral and presacral anomalies. Case report and review of the literature. *Eur J Pediatr Surg.* 1996;6(2):114-119. PubMed PMID: 8740138.

41. Ross AJ, Ruiz-Perez V, Wang Y, et al. A homeobox gene, HLXB9, is the major locus for dominantly inherited sacral agenesis. *Nat Genet.* 1998;20(4):358-361. PubMed PMID: 9843207.

42. Lynch SA, Wang Y, Strachan T, Burn J, Lindsay S. Autosomal dominant sacral agenesis: Currarino syndrome. *J Med Genet.* 2000;37(8):561-566. PubMed PMID: 10922380. Pubmed Central PMCID: 1734652.

43. Dozois EJ, Jacofsky DJ, Billings BJ, et al. Surgical approach and oncologic outcomes following multidisciplinary management of retrorectal sarcomas. *Ann Surg Oncol.* 2011;18(4):983-988. PubMed PMID: 21153886.

44. Gunkova P, Martinek L, Dostalik J, Gunka I, Vavra P, Mazur M. Laparoscopic approach to retrorectal cyst. *World J Gastroenterol.* 2008;14(42):6581-6583. PubMed PMID: 19030218. Pubmed Central PMCID: 2773352.

45. Konstantinidis K, Theodoropoulos GE, Sambalis G, et al. Laparoscopic resection of presacral schwannomas. *Surg Laparosc Endosc Percutan Tech.* 2005;15(5):302-304. PubMed PMID: 16215494.

46. Lengyel J, Sagar PM, Morrison C, Gonsalves S, Lee P, Phillips N. Multimedia article. Laparoscopic abdominosacral composite resection. *Dis Colon Rectum.* 2009;52(9):1662-1664. PubMed PMID: 19690498.

47. Fong SS, Codd R, Sagar PM. Laparoscopic excision of retrorectal tumours. *Colorectal Dis.* 2014;16(11):O400-O403. PubMed PMID: 25204730.

Rare Colorectal Malignancies

Scott R. Steele | Yuxiang Wen | Gregory D. Kennedy

R are tumors of the colon and rectum account for 5% of all colorectal malignancy and can be broadly separated into four categories: epithelial (Fig. 175.1), lymphoid, mesenchymal, or other (Table 175.1). In this chapter we will describe the presentation, diagnosis, and treatment of these different tumor types.

EPITHELIAL TUMORS

NEUROENDOCRINE TUMORS

Carcinoid tumors are neuroendocrine cells in origin, and stain silver with an external reducing agent. They were first observed in 1907 by Oberndorfer, initially because they were observed to have a more indolent course and different behavior than adenocarcinomas.[1] The neuroendocrine cells can take up various amine precursors and produce end products such as neuropeptides, neurotransmitters, as well as hormones that exhibit local and systemic effects.[2]

Neuroendocrine tumor (NET) is the official umbrella term adopted by the World Health Organization (WHO) to represent different neuroendocrine neoplasms, including carcinoid tumors. According to the 2003 study based on the Surveillance, Epidemiology, and End Results (SEER) Program, NETs are most commonly seen within the gastrointestinal (GI) tract (67%) and bronchopulmonary system (25%).[3] In the United States there is a significant correlation between tumor location and race, with primary lung NETs most commonly seen in white patients (30%), and primary rectal NETs more commonly seen in Asian/Pacific Islanders (41%), American Indian/Alaskan Native (32%), and African Americans (26%).[4]

In addition to the racial differences noted in tumor location, the incidence of NETs also varies by location in the GI tract. There has been an increase in the incidence of NETs, with the most remarkable increase in stomach and rectum. The most common location for carcinoid tumors in the GI tract is the appendix (38%), followed by the small intestine (29%) and large intestine (21%).[4] However, NETs continued to comprise less than 2% of all the GI tumors in 2000–2006. NETs are extremely rare in the large intestine, accounting for 0.92% of all colonic tumors and 0.49% of all rectal tumors.[5] There is a slight female predominance over male (52% vs. 48%), and most tumors occur the fifth and sixth decade of age.[4] Patients diagnosed with primary appendiceal NETs tend to be younger with a median age of 47 years at diagnosis. However, patients with primary NETs of the rectum, colon, and cecum tend to be slightly older at 56, 65, and 68 years.[4]

CLASSIFICATION OF NEUROENDOCRINE TUMORS

Gastrointestinal NETs are classified into three major categories (WHO criteria) based on the degree of differentiation and histologic features: grade 1 (low grade, well differentiated), grade 2 (intermediate grade, well differentiated) and grade 3 (high grade, poorly differentiated).[6,7] The distinction between well-differentiated and poorly differentiated NETs facilitates understanding the clinical behavior of the two categories and promotes appropriate treatment strategies. *Carcinoid tumor* or *neuroendocrine tumor* refers to low- and intermediate-grade tumors that are well differentiated, whereas *neuroendocrine carcinoma* is reserved for high-grade tumors that are poorly differentiated (Table 175.2).

PATHOLOGY

The typical benign carcinoid tumor is a small, well-circumscribed submucosal, yellow lesion with high lipid content, often multicentric and composed of small round cells that contain dense, microscopic, neurosecretory granules. Neuroendocrine carcinomas are associated with increased cellular atypia, high mitotic activity, or necrosis.[8] Serotonin in the neurosecretory granules reduces silver salts into metallic silver in the cytoplasm.

Argentaffin staining is pathognomonic of NETs. Argyrophilic-stained tumors are those that lack the ability to reduce silver in the absence of a reducing agent. Midgut NETs are often argentaffin positive, whereas 85% to 90% of hindgut NETs contain only 8% to 16% argentaffin-positive cells.

Immunohistochemical markers, including serum chromogranin synaptophysin, and neuron-specific enolase, are important tools for diagnosis of NETs and surveillance following treatment. Serum chromogranin A is a useful marker to follow up patients' response to treatment with metastasis or after surgery.[9,10]

COLORECTAL NEUROENDOCRINE TUMORS

Local growth of carcinoid tumors causes obstruction, distant metastasis, and production of bioactive substances leading to local and systemic effects. The classic carcinoid syndrome occurs in 10% to 18% of patients with carcinoid tumors.[11] Carcinoid syndrome includes episodic flushing, wheezing, nonbloody watery diarrhea, abdominal pain, and right-sided heart failure, which are usually precipitated by serotonin-containing foods such as chocolate, caffeine, and alcohol.[8] Serum levels of serotonin produce the symptoms of hypermotility of the intestinal tract including abdominal cramping and diarrhea. Kallikrein is associated with wheezing and flushing.

The clinical presentation of carcinoid syndrome depends on the tumor location. Midgut tumors are more likely to present with abdominal pain (40%). Hindgut tumors tend to have a more indolent course. No primary GI tumor is responsible for carcinoid syndrome because the portal venous system delivers the hormones to the liver where they are metabolized. Therefore, patients who have carcinoid syndrome must have liver metastasis or a

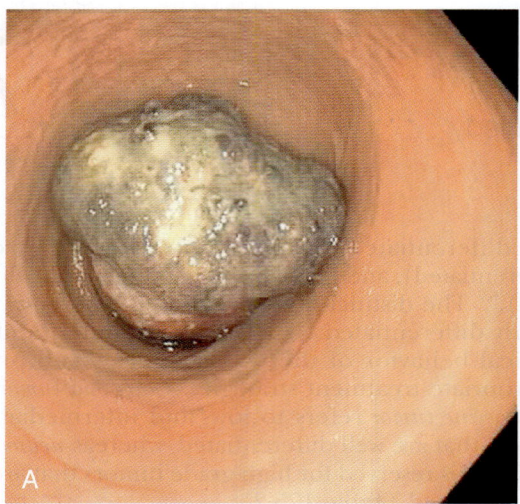
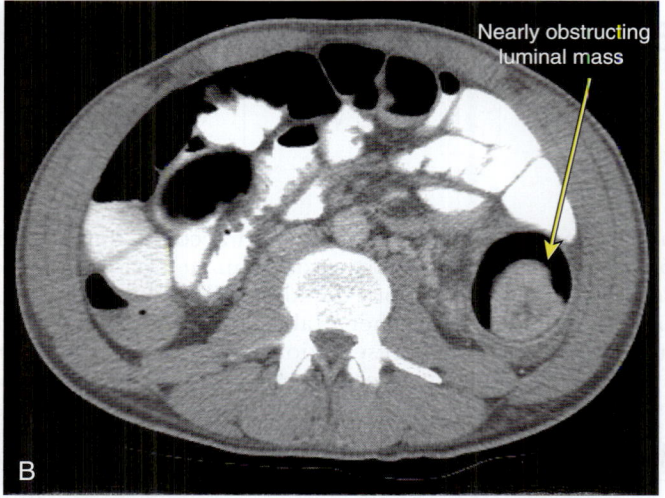

Nearly obstructing luminal mass

FIGURE 175.1 The patient is a 25-year-old man who presented with obstructive symptoms and blood in his stool. Colonoscopy demonstrated an intraluminal, necrotic-appearing mass (A). Computed tomography colonography confirmed the intraluminal mass (B) and revealed no other colonic lesions. Final pathology demonstrated an undifferentiated epithelial tumor.

TABLE 175.1 Classification of Primary Rare Colorectal Tumors

Epithelial	Lymphoid	Mesenchymal	Others
Neuroendocrine tumor	Lymphoma	Gastrointestinal stromal tumor	Kaposi sarcoma
Squamous cell carcinoma	Extramedullary plasmacytoma	Leiomyosarcoma	
		Liposarcoma	
		Malignant fibrous histiocytoma	
		Schwannoma	
		Fibrosarcoma	
		Rhabdomyosarcoma	

Modified from Corman ML. *Colon and Rectal Surgery*. 4th ed. Philadelphia: Lippincott Williams & Wilkins; 1998.

TABLE 175.2 2010 World Health Organization Classification and Grading System of Gastroenteropancreatic–Neuroendocrine Tumor

	Grade 1 (G1)	Grade 2 (G2)	Grade 3 (G3)
WHO/ENETs nomenclature	NET, Grade 1	NET, Grade 2	Neuroendocrine carcinoma (large cell or small cell type)
Traditional nomenclature	Carcinoid, islet cell tumor	(Atypical) carcinoid, islet cell tumor	Small cell carcinoma, large cell neuroendocrine carcinoma
Differentiation	Well differentiated	Well differentiated	Poorly differentiated
Mitotic feature	Mitoses <2 per 10 HPF	Mitoses 2–20 per 10 HPF	Mitoses >20 per 10 HPF
Ki-67 index	<3%	3%–20%	>20%

HPF, High-power field; *NET*, neuroendocrine tumor.
Modified from Bosman FT, Carneiro F, Hruban RH, Theise ND. *WHO Classification of Tumours of the Digestive System*. 4th ed. World Health Organization; 2010; and Klimstra DS, Modlin IR, Coppola D, Lloyd RV, Suster S. The pathologic classification of neuroendocrine tumors: a review of nomenclature, grading, and staging systems. *Pancreas*. 2010;39(6):707–712.

---

tumor with systemic venous drainage. It is recommended that patients have a thorough work-up to evaluate for synchronous (40%) and metastatic (25%) disease at the time of diagnosis.

IMAGING

Colonoscopy and biopsy are the most reliable tools for evaluating and diagnosing colorectal NETs. Endoscopic ultrasound may be useful to assess tumor size, depth of invasion, and nodal involvement. A computed tomography (CT) or magnetic resonance imaging (MRI) are often needed to evaluate for the presence of metastatic disease for lesions that are greater than 2 cm or when there is high-grade histology. Small tumors of less than 2 cm rarely metastasize.[12–14] Somatostatin receptor scintigraphy may be useful in the setting of a known metastatic tumor to determine the presence of bioactive tumor and to evaluate for tumor burden.[15]

Tumor Markers

The 24-hour urine 5-hydroxyindoleacetic acid (5-HIAA; breakdown product of serotonin) measurement is the most common tool for confirming the diagnosis (sensitivity 73%, specificity 100%).[16] Ingestion of serotonin-rich foods, such as bananas, pineapples, aged cheese, and red wine, will result in false elevation of 5-HIAA levels. Chromogranin A is a very sensitive and useful tool for follow-up of GI carcinoids.

TREATMENT OF PRIMARY TUMORS

Surgical resection of colonic carcinoid tumors following all oncologic principles is the standard of care. In highly selected patients with small intramucosal tumors (<1 cm), endoscopic resection may be appropriate.[17,18] However, endoscopic submucosal dissection is associated with higher rates of incomplete non-R0 resection and complications.[19] For localized disease, 5-year survival rates range from 44% to 76%, whereas patients with metastatic disease experience a 5-year survival rate of 30%.[3]

In contrast to patients with colonic tumors, patients with rectal carcinoids are often candidates for local excision because rectal NETs are usually small and follow an indolent course. They are commonly diagnosed as an incidental finding during other procedures. Tumor size (>1 cm), depth of invasion, and lymphovascular involvement are important risk factors that predict a worse outcome.[20,21] Patients with high-risk lesions should be carefully counseled on the risk for recurrence associated with local excision and may be candidates for total mesorectal excision. In fact, patients with tumors larger than 2 cm are at increased risk of metastasis and may experience a 5-year survival rate of 44% with lymph node involvement and 7% if distant disease is present.[3,14] Small localized rectal NETs carry a favorable prognosis with overall 5-year survival rate up to 88% and may be candidates for rectal-sparing local excision.[3] Several local excision techniques are available. For example, endoscopic management with endoscopic mucosal resection (EMR) or endoscopic submucosal dissection (ESD) may be appropriate for the treatment of small rectal lesions.[3,22,23] ESD is considered superior to EMR with better R0 resection rates and similar complication and recurrence rates.[23] In addition, transanal endoscopic microsurgery (TEM) or transanal minimally invasive surgical (TAMIS) resection may be useful tools for local excision of rectal carcinoids. These techniques may be considered for primary resection for tumors less than 2 cm, and for resection after prior incomplete colonoscopic excision.[24]

Full oncologic resection with total mesorectal excision should be performed in patients with high-risk rectal lesions (Table 175.3). Adjuvant chemotherapy or radiotherapy is generally not considered.

FOLLOW-UP

There is no standard guideline for the follow-up of NETs. For low-risk carcinoid tumors, routine radiologic imaging follow-up is not necessary. For more aggressive and advanced lesions, radiologic surveillance and routine serum marker evaluation may be useful for detecting

TABLE 175.3 High-Risk Features of Rectal Carcinoid Tumors

Size >2 cm
Lymphovascular invasion
Perineural invasion
Invasion into muscularis propria
Lymph node involvement by endoscopic ultrasound

recurrence. Serum chromogranin A levels on a regular basis (6 months) can monitor for a change in activity and guide the use of CT scanning or octreotide scanning and endoscopy to look for metachronous or metastatic disease.

TREATMENT OF METASTATIC DISEASE

The treatment of metastatic colorectal NETs is limited. Current data from clinical trials are based on metastatic NETs from primary tumors of various sites. Systemic therapy usually involves somatostatin analogues, interferon-α, biologic agents, and hepatic arterial embolization.

Somatostatin analogues are primarily used for the treatment of carcinoid syndrome related to the hormonal effect in the metastatic disease. A recent randomized controlled multicenter trial from Europe (CLARINET trial) demonstrated that the somatostatin analogue lanreotide is associated with significantly prolonged progression-free survival.[25]

NEUROENDOCRINE CARCINOMAS

High-grade NETs are considered neuroendocrine carcinomas (NECs). These are extremely rare in the colon and rectum and are associated with a very poor prognosis. The NORDIC NEC study found that patients with high-grade NECs in the GI tract had quite poor survival.[26] These observations were supported by a retrospective review of 126 cases from Memorial Sloan Kettering Cancer Center that demonstrated a median survival of 13.2 months, and 3-year overall survival was 5% and 18% of patients with and without metastatic disease, respectively.[27] Another series of 100 patients with high-grade NECs of the colon and rectum found a median survival of 14.7 months, and 2-year and 5-year overall survival (OS) rates of 22% and 8%, respectively.[28] Absence of metastatic disease and response to chemotherapy are predictive of better overall survival. With the aggressive nature of this disease, multimodal systemic treatment is suggested for advanced or metastatic disease (Fig. 175.2A–D).[27,28] Aggressive surgical clearance of abdominal disease may offer the patient disease-free intervals.

SQUAMOUS CELL CARCINOMA

Squamous cell carcinoma (SCC) is extremely rare in the colon and rectum and has a reported incidence of 0.25% to 0.85% of all colorectal malignancies.[29] It is important to rule out extension of anal SCC (can be found up to 15 cm above the anal canal), metastasis from other sites to the colon and rectum, and SCC originating from the external side of a fistula tract.[30-35] The pathogenesis is poorly understood and might be related to chronic inflammatory response or viral infection including human

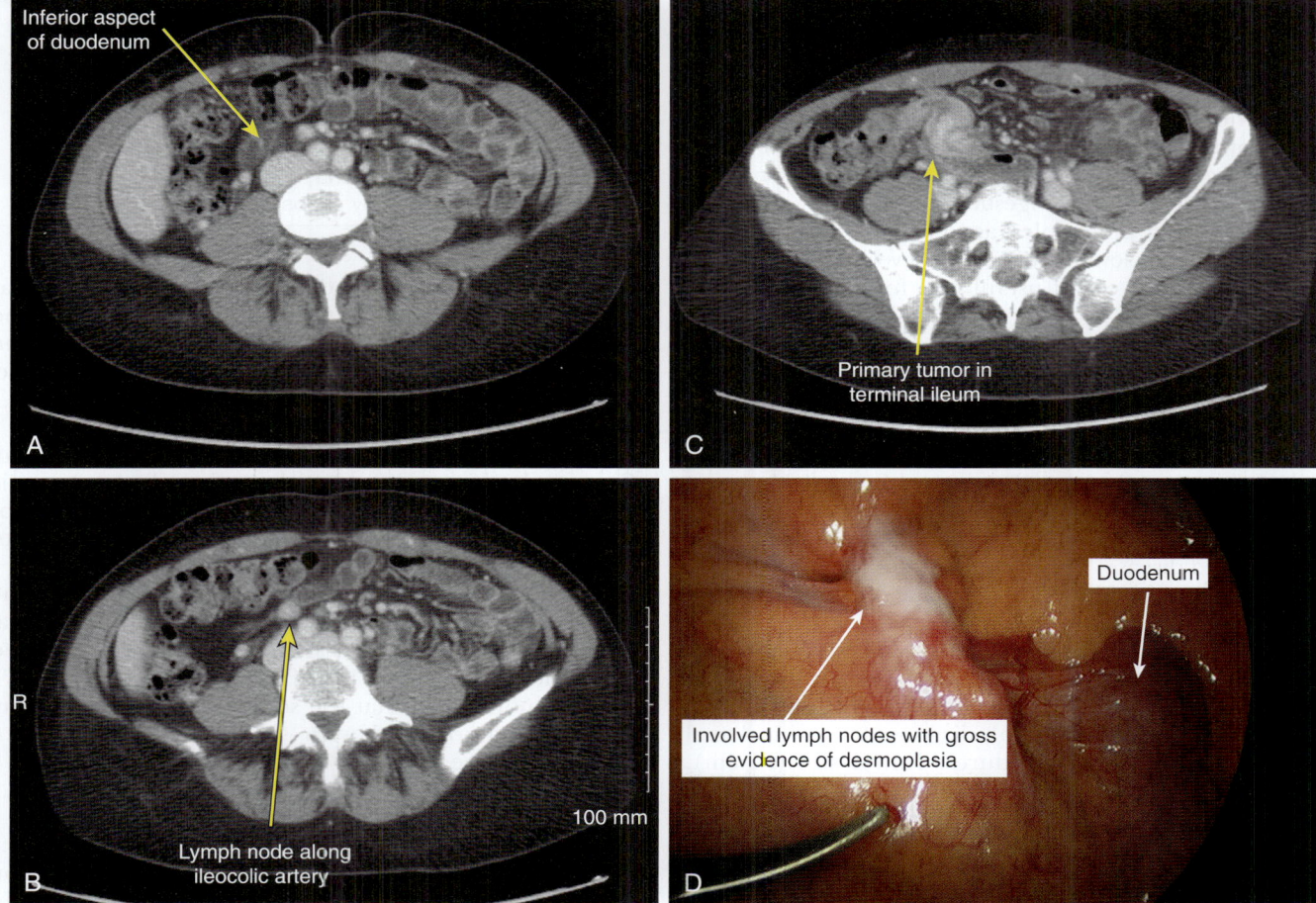

FIGURE 175.2 Patient with a neuroendocrine carcinoma of the terminal ileum. The patient had several months of obstructive-like symptoms. (A–C) Representative computed tomography images. (D) Intraoperative photograph from her laparoscopic right hemicolectomy.

immunodeficiency virus (HIV) or human papillomavirus (HPV) infection.[34] Standard treatment of this disease is still controversial; however, surgery remains the cornerstone of the treatment algorithm. Concomitant chemoradiation might be an effective adjunct for SCCs of the rectum.[35–37] In general, patients with SCC of the colon and rectum have an extremely poor prognosis.[38]

LYMPHOID TUMORS OF THE COLON AND RECTUM

PRIMARY LYMPHOMA

Primary colorectal lymphoma is rare, with a reported incidence of 0.2% to 0.6% of all large bowel cancers.[39] When the diagnosis of lymphoma of the large intestine is made, one must rule out systemic lymphoma with GI involvement because the GI tract is the most common extranodal site of involvement. Dawson criteria are used to label primary GI tract lymphoma and are summarized in Table 175.4.[40]

Several factors increase the risk for the development of colorectal lymphoma including the use of

---

TABLE 175.4 Dawson Criteria for Identifying Primary Gastrointestinal Lymphoma

1. Absence of peripheral lymphadenopathy at the time of presentation
2. Lack of enlarged mediastinal lymph nodes
3. Normal total and differential white blood cell count
4. Predominance of bowel lesion at the time of laparotomy with lymph nodes obviously affected only in the immediate vicinity
5. No lymphomatous involvement of liver and spleen

---

immunosuppressives, inflammatory bowel disease, and HIV infection.[41,42] Symptoms are generally nonspecific and may include weight loss and abdominal pain with or without change in bowel movement. CT, endoscopic ultrasonography, and colonoscopy are useful imaging modalities for the diagnosis of primary lymphoma. Endoscopic classification of primary GI tract lymphoma consists of three subtypes: ulcerative, polypoid, and massive type.[43] Biopsy can be confirmatory.

Treatment primarily involves surgical resection to achieve local tumor control. Chemotherapy could be used as adjuvant therapy for advanced disease. However, with the rarity of this disease, there is limited evidence to guide optimal therapy and compare outcomes of different treatment strategies. Prognosis is determined by location and stage of the tumor with 5-year overall survival as high as 57%.[44]

PLASMACYTOMA

The diagnosis of solitary extramedullary plasmacytoma is made after exclusion of metastasis from primary multiple myeloma. This is most commonly performed by measuring the urinary Bence-Jones protein, checking serum electrophoresis, and bone marrow biopsy. Final diagnosis relies on the histologic and immunohistochemical findings with monoclonal plasma cell proliferation. There is no consensus on the treatment guidelines. Because plasma cells are radio sensitive, radiation therapy has proven to provide local control, but regional recurrence could occur outside of the radiation fields.[45,46] Surgery is also an option for cure.[47] Conversion to multiple myeloma occurs in about one-third of patients with 5-year follow-up.[45,46]

MESENCHYMAL TUMORS

Gastrointestinal Stromal Tumors

Gastrointestinal stromal tumor (GIST) is the most common type of the mesenchymal tumors, accounting for 82% of all mesenchymal tumors.[48,49] Other mesenchymal tumors include liposarcoma, leiomyoma, leiomyosarcoma, rhabdomyosarcoma, malignant fibrous histiocytoma, angiosarcoma, fibrosarcoma, and schwannoma.

GISTs originate from interstitial cells of Cajal, and stain positive for CD117, which is a product of c-kit protooncogene.[49] The c-kit protooncogene is a tyrosine kinase receptor that participates in the regulation of cellular proliferation. One theory of the pathogenesis of GIST involves mutation of c-kit leading to unchecked cellular proliferation. About 60% to 70% of GISTs are also positive for CD34, which is a hematopoietic progenitor cell antigen. In addition, 30% to 40% of GISTs also stain positive for smooth muscle actin (SMA).[50] The diagnosis of GIST is made histologically with immunohistochemical confirmation. The positive expression of CD117 is the major diagnostic criteria with high specificity.[50] CD34 positivity is more associated with colorectal and esophageal GISTs, whereas SMA positivity is most commonly seen in small bowel lesions.[50,51]

GISTs occur throughout the entire GI tract, but are most commonly found in the stomach (51%) and small bowel (36%). Only 15% of GISTs occur in the colon and rectum.[52] In rare cases, they can also occur in the omentum, mesentery, and retroperitoneum.

Colorectal GISTs present with rectal bleeding, pain, tenesmus, and obstructive symptoms, or they may be asymptomatic. On endoscopic evaluation, they may present as an intraluminal or a submucosal mass. Multimodal imaging with CT, MRI, and endoscopic ultrasound (EUS) is helpful to evaluate tumor size, morphology, depth of invasion, and metastasis to other sites. GIST tumors commonly present with distant disease (47%).[49] Positron

emission tomography (PET) is a useful test for both the identification of metastasis and monitoring response to medical therapy. Biopsies with immunohistochemical analysis are crucial for accurate diagnosis, designing neoadjuvant therapy, and surgical planning.

Surgical resection is the cornerstone of the treatment algorithm for localized tumors. Because GISTs do not spread through lymphatics, lymph node dissection is unnecessary but should be included if lymph node involvement is suspected at the time of surgery. Local excision or segmental resections with clean margins are important to prevent recurrence. Tumor size, R0 resection, and c-kit positivity are important prognostic factors.[49,52,53] Generally, a 2-cm margin is required to achieve clear margin and R0 resection. However, the local recurrence rate in patients with localized tumors who undergo R0 resection can still be as high as 35%.[49]

For advanced and metastatic lesions, neoadjuvant and adjuvant therapy have demonstrated good therapeutic results. The small-molecule tyrosine kinase inhibitors selectively block c-kit function and halt excessive proliferation. Imatinib mesylate and sunitinib are tyrosine kinase inhibitors approved for use in advanced and metastatic GISTs. For metastatic patients, the partial response rate to imatinib is reported to be 83.5% in patients with a specific c-kit mutation at exon 11 and only 47.8% in patients with a c-kit mutation at exon 9.[54] For patients with advanced primary GIST lesions without distant metastases, the use of imatinib in the adjuvant setting has been shown to improve recurrence-free survival compared to placebo after primary surgical resection at 1-year follow-up.[55] The long-term results of adjuvant imatinib are equally satisfying, with 5-year overall survival rate of 83% and 5-year recurrence-free survival rate of 40%.[56] Recurrence after imatinib treatment is associated with high tumor mitotic rate, tumor location, large tumor size, age, and adjuvant imatinib for 12 months.[56,57] Resistance to imatinib therapy has also been shown to develop over time and to be associated with new mutations.[58] Switching therapy to another tyrosine kinase receptor inhibitor such as sunitinib could further slow tumor progression.[59] Side effects include fatigue, diarrhea, skin discoloration, and nausea, but have generally been reported to be tolerable. PET/CT is recommended for surveillance of tumor response and guidance in decisions for maintenance therapy as well as change in therapy. Radiation therapy is not suggested because it is not effective for GISTs.

By definition, benign GISTs have no evidence of local invasion and have low mitotic activity, thus prognosis is favorable with local excision alone. Patients with malignant GISTs have an overall 5-year survival rate of only 45%.[49] In fact, the recurrence rate has been shown to be 40% to 42% at 2 years from surgery even after early excision.[49,60,61] Patients with tumors less than 2 cm have a 5% recurrence rate and patients with tumors 2 to 5 cm a recurrence rate of 25%, usually locally or in the liver.[62]

LEIOMYOMA AND LEIOMYOSARCOMA

Leiomyoma and leiomyosarcoma arise from the smooth muscle of muscularis mucosa, are negative for CD117 or CD34 staining but positive for desmin and SMA staining. They are the second most common GI mesenchymal tumors and account for less than 0.1% of all rectal tumors.

Lesions in the colon and rectum are generally discovered incidentally at the time of routine colonoscopy, especially because most patients are asymptomatic. These often appear as a polypoid lesion or submucosal tumor with normal overlying mucosa. Further work-up might include CT or MRI for lesions in the colon to determine the size and exact location within the wall of the colon. EUS may be helpful in assessing rectal lesions to determine the exact location within the rectal wall. Increased size, irregularity, foci of necrosis, and heterogeneous echogenicity have been shown to be associated with increased risk of malignancy.[63]

Benign lesions can be effectively managed with local excision, especially those arising from muscularis mucosa, and rarely recur after excision with snare polypectomy.[62,64,65] In general, resection of these lesions should be planned based on tumor grade. Low-grade lesions, or those with fewer than 50 mitoses per high-power field, may be excised with a 1-cm margin, whereas high-grade leiomyosarcomas should be resected with a 4-cm margin. For tumors in the rectum, sphincter preservation might be feasible with local excision and adjuvant radiotherapy.[66,67] Sarcomas require higher doses of radiation to achieve response, which leads to increased rates of toxicity and wound complications. Complex reconstructive techniques, such as vertical rectus abdominus muscle (VRAM) flaps, should be considered after radiation and resection of the pelvic floor and external sphincter, such as with pleomorphic undifferentiated sarcoma.

MALIGNANT FIBROUS HISTIOCYTOMA

The malignant fibrous histiocytoma (MFH), now known as the pleomorphic undifferentiated sarcoma (PUS), is very rare, with only 23 case reports of colorectal involvement. The clinical presentation of MFH/PUS is nonspecific, including abdominal pain, diarrhea, tenesmus, or weight loss.[68–71] Histologically, these tumors are composed of large, pleomorphic giant cells as well as spindle cells, arranged in a fascicular and storiform pattern mixed with inflammatory cells.[69] They generally stain negative for c-kit and positive for α_1-antitrypsin and CD68. This immunohistochemical pattern clearly differentiates the MFH from a GIST, which is c-kit positive.

Treatment of PUS requires surgical resection. Adjuvant radiation may be considered in bulky lesions that have been resected with a close or positive margin as MFHs.[72] However, there is still a lack of evidence on the local control effect and optimal timing for radiation.[73] Chemotherapy is not indicated because these tumors are chemoresistant. However, apatinib, a new-generation tyrosine kinase inhibitor, has been reported to trigger partial response in advanced disease.[74]

LIPOSARCOMA

Liposarcoma is a rare mesenchymal tumor of the GI tract. There are only few case reports in the literature, and common symptoms include abdominal pain and mass. CT imaging is helpful for evaluation of the tumor location, invasion, and multifocality.[75–78] Anatomic distribution and prognosis have both been correlated with histologic

TABLE 175.5 Histologic Variant of Liposarcoma in Disease-Specific Survival

Histology	5-Year DSS Rate	Primary Anatomic Site	12-Year DSS Rate
Well-differentiated	93%	Upper extremity	87%
Differentiated	44%	Lower extremity	82%
Myxoid	92%	Truncal	77%
Round cell	74%	Retroperitoneal —no organ resection	53%
Pleomorphic	59%	Retroperitoneal —require organ resection	32%

DSS, Disease-specific survival.
From Dalal KM, Kattan MW, Antonescu CR, Brennan MF, Singer S. Subtype specific prognostic nomogram for patients with primary liposarcoma of the retroperitoneum, extremity, or trunk. *Ann Surg.* 2006;244(3):381–391.

subtypes (Table 175.5).[76,79] High myxoid content is considered a predictor of poor outcome with 5-year survival rates of 50%. By comparison, patients with atypical lipomatous tumor or well-differentiated liposarcoma (ALT/WD) have the most favorable outcomes with 5-year survival rates from 75% to 100%.[79] Surgery with wide excision is usually enough for cure, and the extent of surgery is closely related to survival.[80,81] The role of chemotherapy is not well established, but doxorubicin or ifosfamide may provide some survival benefits.[79,81] These need to be differentiated from benign lipomas that are more commonly found in the GI tract (Fig. 175.3A–E).

RHABDOMYOSARCOMA

Rhabdomyosarcomas (RMSs) are rare tumors in children and even less common in adults. The clinical presentation is nonspecific, usually due to late mass effect. Therefore, prognosis is usually poor with delayed diagnosis and worse for adults.[82]

The pathophysiology of RMS is poorly understood. There is an association with Li-Fraumeni syndrome (p53 mutation), neurofibromatosis type 1, Costello syndrome (HRAS mutation), Beckwith-Wiedemann syndrome, and Noonan syndrome. Exposure to certain prenatal drugs and X-rays has been suggested as risk factors for pediatric RMS. However, there is no study on the etiology of adult RMS.

Diagnosis is based on biopsy, immunohistochemistry, or electron microscopy. Histologically, RMS is composed of small blue round cells. The detection of markers such as α-actin, myoD, myogenin, and desmin is helpful in differentiating RMS from other tumors.[82] CT or MRI are useful in defining the size of the tumor, proximity to adjacent vital structures, bony or lymph node involvement, and aid in surgical planning. PET/CT are also used in more accurate staging and restaging of RMS.

There are no established guidelines for treating adult RMS. Multidisciplinary management of both primary and metastatic RMS includes discussion of chemotherapy, radiation, and surgical resection with wide margins. RMS of childhood often is treated with vincristine, actinomycin D, and cyclophosphamide (VAC). However, adult patients are often treated with combination therapy consisting of cyclophosphamide, doxorubicin, and vincristine.

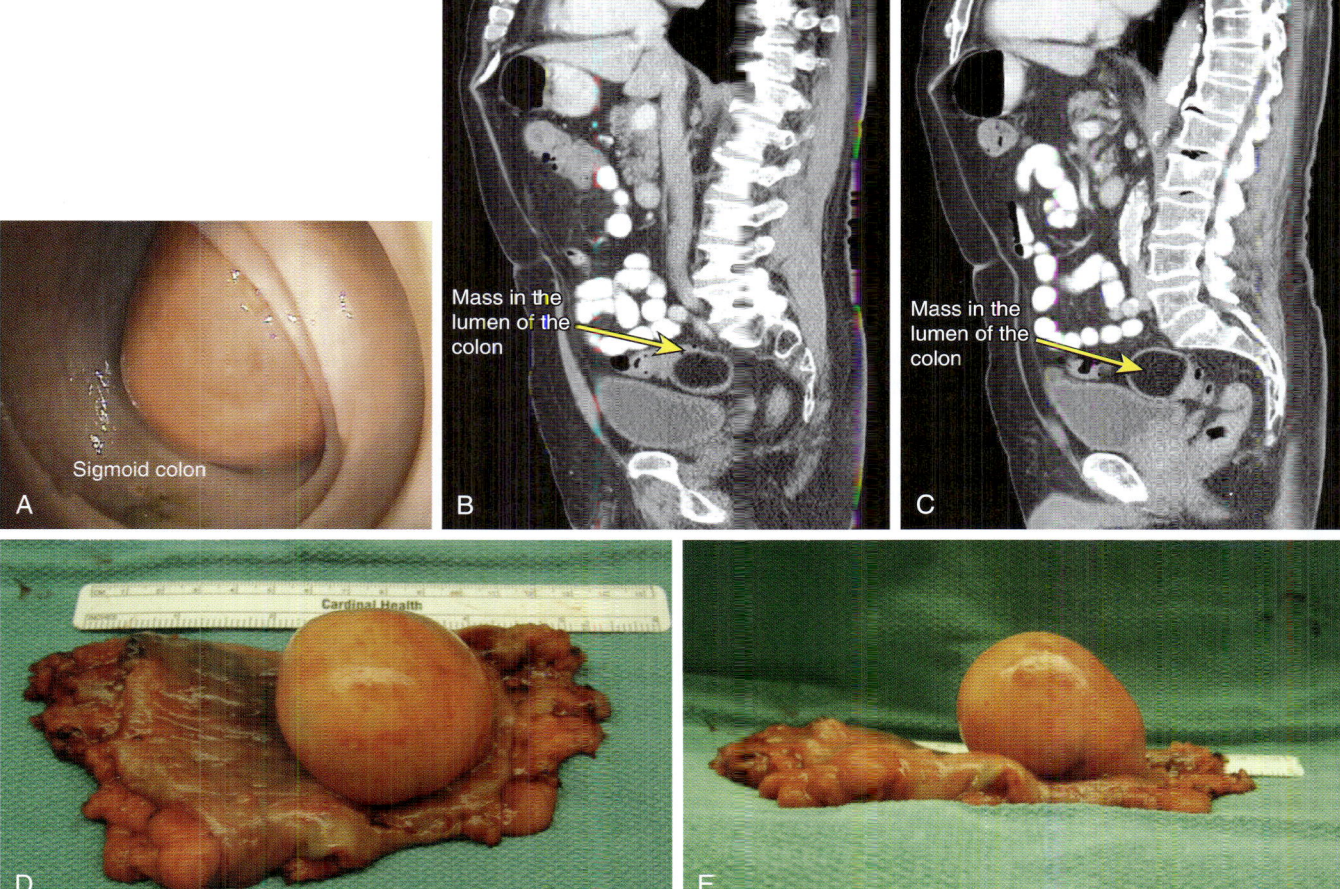

FIGURE 175.3 The patient is an 80-year-old man who presented with new onset of obstructive-type symptoms. Colonoscopy demonstrated an intraluminal mass (A). CT demonstrated a submucosal lesion consistent with a lipoma (B and C). Figures D and E are ex vivo pictures of what turned out to be a benign lipoma of the colon.

Doxorubicin, ifosfamide, and dacarbazine have also been used without major effect on survival.[83] After completion of chemotherapy, patients should be reevaluated for need of surgery or radiation. Surgical resection with a 1-cm margin is ideal. Radiation therapy (50.4 Gy) is important for patients with unresectable, residual disease or nodal involvement, but may be toxic for abdominal or pelvic lesions. Intensity-modulated radiation therapy (IMRT) or proton beam radiation may improve functional outcomes with more precise dose delivery.[82,84,85]

SCHWANNOMA OF COLON AND RECTUM

Schwannomas arise from neural sheath cells. The stomach is the most commonly involved GI organ and primary lesions of the colon and rectum are extremely rare. They usually present with an asymptomatic polyp or submucosal mass, bleeding secondary to mucosal ulceration, or colonic obstruction and abdominal pain secondary to a large mass.[86–90] These tumors are strongly positive for S-100 protein and generally have few mitoses per high-power field. Resection of the involved segment of large intestine

is generally adequate treatment and local recurrences have not been described.[91]

OTHER MISCELLANEOUS TUMORS

KAPOSI SARCOMA

In patients with untreated HIV and acquired immunodeficiency syndrome (AIDS), Kaposi sarcoma (KS) is common. However, the wide adoption of highly active antiretroviral therapy (HAART) has significantly decreased the incidence of KS.[92] KS is part of the differential diagnosis for HIV-patients with anal lesions. The small round purplish lesions are often mistaken for hemorrhoids. It is rare.[93] Surgery does not play a significant role in the treatment of KS. Chemotherapy in addition to HAART reduces disease progression in patients with severe or progressive KS. Commonly used chemotherapeutics include liposomal doxorubicin, liposomal daunorubicin, and paclitaxel, but no significant improvement in mortality has been documented.[94]

SUMMARY

Tumors that rarely occur in the GI tract are often diagnosed after the onset of symptoms. Surgery is the primary treatment of most of these tumors because they are often resistant to standard chemotherapeutic regimens. Multidisciplinary management teams are key to the successful diagnosis, treatment, and follow-up of patients with these rare tumors.

REFERENCES

1. Oberndorfer S. Carcinoid tumors of the small intestine. *Frankf Z Pathol.* 1907;1:426-432.
2. Beck DE, Roberts PL, Saclarides TJ, Senagore AJ, Stamos MJ, Nasseri Y, eds. *The ASCRS Textbook of Colon and Rectal Surgery.* Springer Science & Business Media; 2011.
3. Modlin IM, Lye KD, Kidd M. A 5-decade analysis of 13,715 carcinoid tumors. *Cancer.* 2003;97(4):934-959.
4. Ellis L, Shale MJ, Coleman MP. Carcinoid tumors of the gastrointestinal tract: trends in incidence in England since 1971. *Am J Gastroenterol.* 2010;105(12):2563-2569.
5. Hauso O, Gustafsson BI, Kidd M, et al. Neuroendocrine tumor epidemiology: contrasting Norway and North America. *Cancer.* 2008;113(10):2655-2664.
6. Yao JC, Hassan M, Phan A, et al. One hundred years after carcinoid: epidemiology of and prognostic factors for neuroendocrine tumors in 35,825 cases in the United States. *J Clin Oncol.* 2008;26(18):3063-3072.
7. Bosman FT, Carneiro F, Hruban RH, Theise ND, eds. *WHO Classification of Tumours of the Digestive System.* 4th ed. World Health Organization; 2010.
8. Klimstra DS, Modlin IR, Coppola D, Lloyd RV, Suster S. The pathologic classification of neuroendocrine tumors: a review of nomenclature, grading, and staging systems. *Pancreas.* 2010;39(6):707-712.
9. Eriksson B, Oberg K, Stridsberg M. Tumor markers in neuroendocrine tumors. *Digestion.* 2000;62(suppl 1):33-38.
10. Modlin IM, Oberg K, Chung DC, et al. Gastroenteropancreatic neuroendocrine tumours. *Lancet Oncol.* 2008;9(1):61-72.
11. Tichansky DS, Cagir B, Borrazzo E, et al. Risk of second cancers in patients with colorectal carcinoids. *Dis Colon Rectum.* 2002;45(1):91-97.
12. Landry CS, Brock G, Scoggins CR, McMasters KM, Martin RC 2nd. Proposed staging system for colon carcinoid tumors based on an analysis of 2,459 patients. *J Am Coll Surg.* 2008;207(6):874-881.
13. Landry CS, Brock G, Scoggins CR, McMasters KM, Martin RC 2nd. A proposed staging system for rectal carcinoid tumors based on an analysis of 4701 patients. *Surgery.* 2008;144(3):460-466.
14. Anthony LB, Strosberg JR, Klimstra DS, et al. The NANETS consensus guidelines for the diagnosis and management of gastrointestinal neuroendocrine tumors (NETs): well-differentiated NETs of the distal colon and rectum. *Pancreas.* 2010;39(6):767-774.
15. Bombardieri E, Maccauro M, De Deckere E, Savelli G, Chiti A. Nuclear medicine imaging of neuroendocrine tumours. *Ann Oncol.* 2001;12(suppl 2):S51-S61.
16. Nikou GC, Lygidakis NJ, Toubanakis C, et al. Current diagnosis and treatment of gastrointestinal carcinoids in a series of 101 patients: the significance of serum chromogranin-A, somatostatin receptor scintigraphy and somatostatin analogues. *Hepatogastroenterology.* 2005;52(63):731-741.
17. Al Natour RH, Saund MS, Sanchez VM, et al. Tumor size and depth predict rate of lymph node metastasis in colon carcinoids and can be used to select patients for endoscopic resection. *J Gastrointest Surg.* 2012;16(3):595-602.
18. Chung TP, Hunt SR. Carcinoid and neuroendocrine tumors of the colon and rectum. *Clin Colon Rectal Surg.* 2006;19(2):45-48.
19. Chen T, Yao LQ, Xu MD, et al. Efficacy and safety of endoscopic submucosal dissection for colorectal carcinoids. *Clin Gastroenterol Hepatol.* 2016;14(4):575-581.
20. Shields CJ, Tiret E, Winter DC. Carcinoid tumors of the rectum: a multi-institutional international collaboration. *Ann Surg.* 2010;252(5):750-755.
21. Fahy BN, Tang LH, Klimstra D, et al. Carcinoid of the rectum risk stratification (CaRRS): a strategy for preoperative outcome assessment. *Ann Surg Oncol.* 2007;14(2):396-404.
22. Park HW, Byeon JS, Park YS, et al. Endoscopic submucosal dissection for treatment of rectal carcinoid tumors. *Gastrointest Endosc.* 2010;72(1):143-149.
23. Zhong DD, Shao LM, Cai JT. Endoscopic mucosal resection vs endoscopic submucosal dissection for rectal carcinoid tumours: a systematic review and meta-analysis. *Colorectal Dis.* 2013;15(3):283-291.
24. Kumar AS, Sidani SM, Kolli K, et al. Transanal endoscopic microsurgery for rectal carcinoids: the largest reported United States experience. *Colorectal Dis.* 2012;14(5):562-566.
25. Caplin ME, Pavel M, Ćwikła JB, et al. Lanreotide in metastatic enteropancreatic neuroendocrine tumors. *N Engl J Med.* 2014;371(3):224-233.
26. Sorbye H, Welin S, Langer W, et al. Predictive and prognostic factors for treatment and survival in 305 patients with advanced gastrointestinal neuroendocrine carcinoma (WHO G3): the NORDIC NEC study. *Ann Oncol.* 2013;24(1):152-160.
27. Smith JD, Reidy DL, Goodman KA, Shia J, Nash GM. A retrospective review of 126 high-grade neuroendocrine carcinomas of the colon and rectum. *Ann Surg Oncol.* 2014;21(9):2956-2962.
28. Conte B, George B, Overman M, et al. High-grade neuroendocrine colorectal carcinomas: a retrospective study of 100 patients. *Clin Colorectal Cancer.* 2016;15(2):e1-e7.
29. Kiran RP, Tripodi G, Frederick W, Dudrick SJ. Adenosquamous carcinoma of the colon: a rare tumor. *Am Surg.* 2006;72(8):754-755.
30. Williams GT, Blackshaw AJ, Morson BC. Squamous carcinoma of the colorectum and its genesis. *J Pathol.* 1979;129(3):139-147.
31. Yeh J, Hastings J, Rao A, Abbas MA. Squamous cell carcinoma of the rectum: a single institution experience. *Tech Coloproctol.* 2012;16(5):349-354.
32. Hickey WF, Corson JM. Squamous cell carcinoma arising in a duplication of the colon: case report and literature review of squamous cell carcinoma of the colon and of malignancy complicating colonic duplication. *Cancer.* 1981;47(3):602-609.
33. Ozuner G, Aytac E, Gorgun E, Bennett A. Colorectal squamous cell carcinoma: a rare tumor with poor prognosis. *Int J Colorectal Dis.* 2015;30(1):127-130.
34. Coghill AE, Shiels MS, Rycroft RK, et al. Rectal squamous cell carcinoma in immunosuppressed populations: is this a distinct entity from anal cancer? *AIDS.* 2016;30(1):105-112.
35. Tronconi MC, Carnaghi C, Bignardi M, et al. Rectal squamous cell carcinoma treated with chemoradiotherapy: report of six cases. *Int J Colorectal Dis.* 2010;25(12):1435-1439.
36. Jeong BG, Kim DY, Kim SY. Concurrent chemoradiotherapy for squamous cell carcinoma of the rectum. *Hepatogastroenterology.* 2013;60(123):512-516.
37. Wang ML, Heriot A, Leong T, Ngan SY. Chemoradiotherapy in the management of primary squamous-cell carcinoma of the rectum. *Colorectal Dis.* 2011;13(3):296-301.
38. Ozuner G, Aytac E, Gorgun E, Bennett A. Colorectal squamous cell carcinoma: a rare tumor with poor prognosis. *Int J Colorectal Dis.* 2015;30(1):127-130.
39. Glass AG, Karnell LH, Menck HR. The national cancer data base report on non-Hodgkin's lymphoma. *Cancer.* 1997;80(12):2311-2320.
40. Dawson IM, Cornes JS, Morson BC. Primary malignant lymphoid tumours of the intestinal tract. Report of 37 cases with a study of factors influencing prognosis. *Br J Surg.* 1961;49:80-89.
41. Dionigi G, Annoni M, Rovera F, et al. Primary colorectal lymphomas: review of the literature. *Surg Oncol.* 2007;16:169-171.
42. Jones JL, Loftus EV. Lymphoma risk in inflammatory bowel disease: is it the disease or its treatment? *Inflamm Bowel Dis.* 2007;13(10):1299-1307.
43. Yu H, Wang Y, Peng L, Lia A, Zhang Y. Endoscopic manifestations of primary colorectal lymphoma. *Hepatogastroenterology.* 2014;61(129):76-78.
44. Drolet S, Maclean AR, Stewart DA, Dixon E, Paolucci EO, Buie WD. Primary colorectal lymphoma-clinical outcomes in a population-based series. *J Gastrointest Surg.* 2011;15(10):1851-1857.
45. Liebross RH, Ha CS, Cox JD, Weber D, Delasalle K, Alexanian R. Clinical course of solitary extramedullary plasmacytoma. *Radiother Oncol.* 1999;52(3):245-249.
46. Chao MW, Gibbs P, Wirth A, Quong G, Guiney MJ, Liew KH. Radiotherapy in the management of solitary extramedullary plasmacytoma. *Intern Med J.* 2005;35(4):211-215.
47. Hashiguchi K, Iwai A, Inoue T, et al. Extramedullary plasmacytoma of the rectum arising in ulcerative colitis: case report and review. *Gastrointest Endosc.* 2004;59(2):304-307.

48. Perez EA, Livingstone AS, Franceschi D, et al. Current incidence and outcomes of gastrointestinal mesenchymal tumors including gastrointestinal stromal tumors. *J Am Coll Surg.* 2006;202(4):623-629.

49. DeMatteo RP, Lewis JJ, Leung D, Mudan SS, Woodruff JM, Brennan MF. Two hundred gastrointestinal stromal tumors: recurrence patterns and prognostic factors for survival. *Ann Surg.* 2000;231(1): 51-58.

50. Fletcher CD, Berman JJ, Corless C, et al. Diagnosis of gastrointestinal stromal tumors: a consensus approach. *Hum Pathol.* 2002;33(5):459-465.

51. Miettinen M, Sobin LH, Sarlomo-Rikala M. Immunohistochemical spectrum of GISTs at different sites and their differential diagnosis with a reference to CD117 (KIT). *Mod Pathol.* 2000;13(10):1134-1142.

52. Tran T, Davila JA, El-Serag HB. The epidemiology of malignant gastrointestinal stromal tumors: an analysis of 1,458 cases from 1992 to 2000. *Am J Gastroenterol.* 2005;100(1):162-168.

53. Krajinovic K, Germer CT, Agaimy A, Wünsch PH, Isbert C. Outcome after resection of one hundred gastrointestinal stromal tumors. *Dig Surg.* 2010;27(4):313-319.

54. Heinrich MC, Corless CL, Demetri GD, et al. Kinase mutations and imatinib response in patients with metastatic gastrointestinal stromal tumor. *J Clin Oncol.* 2003;21(23):4342-4349.

55. Dematteo RP, Ballman KV, Antonescu CR, et al. Adjuvant imatinib mesylate after resection of localised, primary gastrointestinal stromal tumour: a randomised, double-blind, placebo-controlled trial. *Lancet.* 2009;373(9669):1097-1104.

56. DeMatteo RP, Ballman KV, Antonescu CR, et al. Long-term results of adjuvant imatinib mesylate in localized, high-risk, primary gastrointestinal stromal tumor (GIST): ACOSOG Z9000 (Alliance) intergroup phase 2 trial. *Ann Surg.* 2013;258(3):422-459.

57. Joensuu H, Eriksson M, Hall KS, et al. Risk factors for gastrointestinal stromal tumor recurrence in patients treated with adjuvant imatinib. *Cancer.* 2014;120(15):2325-2333.

58. Gounder MM, Maki RG. Molecular basis for primary and secondary tyrosine kinase inhibitor resistance in gastrointestinal stromal tumor. *Cancer Chemother Pharmacol.* 2011;67(1):25-43.

59. Demetri GD, van Oosterom AT, Garrett CR, et al. Efficacy and safety of sunitinib in patients with advanced gastrointestinal stromal tumour after failure of imatinib: a randomised controlled trial. *Lancet.* 2006; 368(9544):1329-1338.

60. Reddy RM, Fleshman JW. Colorectal gastrointestinal stromal tumors: a brief review. *Clin Colon Rectal Surg.* 2006;19(2):69-77.

61. McGrath PC, Neifeld JP, Lawrence W Jr, Kay S, Horsley JS 3rd, Parker GA. Gastrointestinal sarcomas. Analysis of prognostic factors. *Ann Surg.* 1987;206(6):706-710.

62. Miettinen M, Furlong M, Sarlomo-Rikala M, Burke A, Sobin LH, Lasota J. Gastrointestinal stromal tumors, intramural leiomyomas, and leiomyosarcomas in the rectum and anus: a clinicopathologic, immunohistochemical, and molecular genetic study of 144 cases. *Am J Surg Pathol.* 2001;25(9):1121-1133.

63. Lee SH, Ha HK, Byun JY, et al. Radiological features of leiomyomatous tumors of the colon and rectum. *J Comput Assist Tomogr.* 2000;24(3):407-412.

64. Yeh CY, Chen HH, Tang R, Tasi WS, Lin PY, Wang JY. Surgical outcome after curative resection of rectal leiomyosarcoma. *Dis Colon Rectum.* 2000;43(11):1517-1521.

65. Walsh TH, Mann CV. Smooth muscle neoplasms of the rectum and anal canal. *Br J Surg.* 1984;71(8):597-599.

66. Grann A, Paty PB, Guillem JG, Cohen AM, Minsky BD. Sphincter preservation of leiomyosarcoma of the rectum and anus with local excision and brachytherapy. *Dis Colon Rectum.* 1999;42(10):1296-1299.

67. Minsky BD, Cohen AM, Hajdu SI, Nori D. Sphincter preservation in rectal sarcoma. *Dis Colon Rectum.* 1990;33(4):319-322.

68. Bosmans B, de Graaf EJ, Torenbeek R, Tetteroo GW. Malignant fibrous histiocytoma of the sigmoid: a case report and review of the literature. *Int J Colorectal Dis.* 2007;22(5):549-552.

69. Azizi R, Mahjoubi B, Shayanfar N, Anaraki F, Zahedi-Shoolami L. Malignant fibrous histiocytoma of rectum: report of a case. *Int J Surg Case Rep.* 2011;2(6):111-113.

70. Verma P, Chandra U, Bhatia PS. Malignant histiocytoma of the rectum: report of a case. *Dis Colon Rectum.* 1979;22(3):179-182.

71. Singh MS. Malignant fibrous histiocytoma of the rectum. *Malaysian J Med Sci.* 2006;13.

72. Henderson MT, Hollmig ST. Malignant fibrous histiocytoma: changing perceptions and management challenges. *J Am Acad Dermatol.* 2012; 67(6):1335-1341.

73. El-Absi E, Farrokhyar F, Sharma R, et al. A systematic review and meta-analysis of oncologic outcomes of pre- versus postoperative radiation in localized resectable soft-tissue sarcoma. *Ann Surg Oncol.* 2010;17(5):1367-1374.

74. G, Hong L, Yang P. Successful treatment of advanced malignant fibrous histiocytoma of the right forearm with apatinib: a case report. *Onco Targets Ther.* 2016;9:643-647.

75. Lutsu E, Ghelrim G, Gagauz I, Mishin I, Iakovleva I. Liposarcoma of the colon: a case report and review of literature. *J Gastrointest Surg.* 2006;10(5):652-656.

76. Dalal KM, Kattan MW, Antonescu CR, Brennan MF, Singer S. Subtype specific prognostic nomogram for patients with primary liposarcoma of the retroperitoneum, extremity, or trunk. *Ann Surg.* 2006;244(3): 381-391.

77. Chen KT. Liposarcoma of the colon: a case report. *Int J Surg Pathol.* 2004;12(3):281-285.

78. Chen Z, Wang S. Fu L, et al. Therapeutic experience with primary liposarcoma from the sigmoid mesocolon accompanied with well-differentiated liposarcomas in the pelvis. *Surg Today.* 2014;44(10): 1863-1868.

79. Gebhard S, Condre JM, Michels JJ, et al. Pleomorphic liposarcoma: clinicopathologic, immunohistochemical, and follow-up analysis of 53 cases: a study from the French Federation of Cancer Centers Sarcoma Group. *Am J Surg Pathol.* 2002;26(5):601-616.

80. Singer S, Maki RG, O'sullivan B. Soft tissue sarcoma. In: DeVita VT, Lawrence TS, Rosenberg SA, eds. *Cancer: Principles and Practice of Oncology.* 9th ed. Philadelphia, PA: Lippincott Williams & Wilkins; 2011:1533-1577.

81. Singer S, Antonescu CR, Riedel E, Brennan ME. Histologic subtype and margin of resection predict pattern of recurrence and survival for retroperitoneal liposarcoma. *Ann Surg.* 2003;238(3):358-370; discussion 370-371.

82. Ruiz-Mesa C, Goldberg JM, Coronado Munoz AJ, Dumont SN, Trent JC. Rhabdomyosarcoma in adults: new perspectives on therapy. *Curr Treat Options Oncol.* 2015;16(6):1-42.

83. Antman K, Crowley J, Balcerzak SP, et al. An intergroup phase III randomized study of doxorubicin and dacarbazine with or without ifosfamide and mesna in advanced soft tissue and bone sarcomas. *J Clin Oncol.* 1993;11(7):1276-1285.

84. Lin C, Donaldson SS, Meza JL, et al. Effect of radiotherapy techniques (IMRT vs. 3D-CRT) on outcome in patients with intermediate-risk rhabdomyosarcoma enrolled in COG D9803—a report from the Children's Oncology Group. *Int J Radiat Oncol Biol Phys.* 2012;82(5): 1764-1770.

85. Ladra MM, Edgington SK, Mahajan A, et al. A dosimetric comparison of proton and intensity modulated radiation therapy in pediatric rhabdomyosarcoma patients enrolled on a prospective phase II proton study. *Radiother Oncol.* 2014;113(1):77-83.

86. Trivedi A, Ligato S. Microcystic/reticular schwannoma of the proximal sigmoid colon: case report with review of literature. *Arch Pathol Lab Med.* 2013;137(2):284-288.

87. de Mesquita Neto JW, Lima Verde Leal RM, de Brito EV, Cordeiro DF, Costa ML. Solitary schwannoma of the cecum: case report and review of the literature. *Case Rep Oncol.* 2013;6(1):62-65.

88. Fotiadis CI, Kouerinis IA, Papandreou I, Zografos GC, Agapitos G. Sigmoid schwannoma: a rare case. *World J Gastroenterol.* 2005;11(32): 5079-5081.

89. Braumann C, Guenther N, Menenakos C, Junghans T. Schwannoma of the colon mimicking carcinoma: a case report and literature review. *Int J Colorectal Dis.* 2007;22(12):1547-1548.

90. Miettinen M, Shekitka KM, Sobin LH. Schwannomas in the colon and rectum: a clinicopathologic and immunohistochemical study of 20 cases. *Am J Surg Pathol.* 2001;25(7):846-855.

91. Wang WB, Chen WB, Lin JJ, Xu JH, Wang JH, Sheng QS. Schwannoma of the colon: a case report and review of the literature. *Oncol Lett.* 2016;11(4):2580-2582.

92. Gates AE, Kaplan LD. AIDS malignancies in the era of highly active antiretroviral therapy. *Oncology (Williston Park, NY).* 2002;16(4):441-451, 456, 459.

93. Yuhan R, Orsay C, DelPino A, et al. Anorectal disease in HIV-infected patients. *Dis Colon Rectum.* 1998;41(11):1367-1370.

94. Gbabe OF, Okwundu CI, Dedicoat M, Freeman EE. Treatment of severe or progressive Kaposi's sarcoma in HIV-infected adults. *Cochrane Database Syst Rev.* 2014;(8):CD003256

Adjuvant and Neoadjuvant Therapy for Colorectal Cancer: Molecular-Based Therapy

Yvonne Coyle

Colorectal cancer (CRC) is the third most common cancer and the fourth most common cancer cause of death worldwide. The incidence of CRC is low at ages younger than 50 years but increases significantly with age.[1] Although the T (tumor size), N (presence of malignant lymph nodes), and M (presence of distant metastases) classification of disease at diagnosis provides a strong prognostic assessment to help direct treatment for CRC, research has shown that integrating existing knowledge of relevant clinicopathologic and molecular markers in CRC may provide a more accurate assessment of prognosis and response to therapy for this disease.[2,3] Molecular markers used to predict prognosis and therapy response in patients with CRC have been derived from our current understanding of the molecular pathogenesis of CRC.

The pathogenesis of CRC is a very complex and diverse process influenced by multiple factors, some of which may be related to diet and lifestyle, whereas others are related to genetic predisposition. Another risk factor for CRC is the presence of long-standing inflammatory bowel disease (IBD), either Crohn disease or ulcerative colitis.[4] Research over the past 30 years has increased our understanding of the mechanisms involved in the initiation and development of CRC. These findings demonstrate the existence of at least three pathways that define CRC pathogenesis: (1) chromosomal instability (CIN), (2) microsatellite instability (MSI), and (3) CpG island methylator phenotype (CIMP).

MOLECULAR PATHWAYS INVOLVED IN COLORECTAL CANCER

CHROMOSOMAL INSTABILITY PATHWAY OF COLORECTAL CANCER

Fearon and Vogelstein originally theorized that CRC formation was a multistep process and that most, if not all, CRCs arose from benign tumors or adenomas.[5] During this multistep process, initially mutational inactivation of tumor suppressor genes occurred followed by mutational activation of oncogenes that result in CIN and eventual creation of CRC. Fearon and Vogelstein also theorized that mutations in at least four to five genes are required for the formation of a tumor.[5] The development of CRC via the CIN pathway has been referred to as the classic adenoma-carcinoma sequence. CRC often progresses over 10 years, beginning with dysplastic adenomas or polyps as the most common premalignant precursor lesion.[6] A key step in this process is the early mutation of the adenomatous polyposis coli (APC) gene. APC is a tumor suppressor gene involved in both sporadic CIN and, when germ line mutated, in all persons with familial adenomatous polyposis (FAP). Sporadic CIN occurs in approximately 60% to 70% of adenomas that progress to carcinomas.[7] The adenoma-carcinoma process is enhanced further by mutations that activate the Kirsten rat sarcoma viral oncogene homolog (KRAS) oncogene and inactivate the tumor protein 53 (TP53) tumor suppressor gene.[8] These gene mutations are associated with CIN and promote tumor cell proliferation and invasiveness. Other gene alterations found in the CIN pathway affect CIN, such as loss of heterozygosity (LOH) of the long arm of chromosome 18 (18q), which inactivates tumor suppressor genes. Other genetic changes include extreme hypomethylation of the LINE-1 (long interspersed nucleotide element-1) gene, changes in the kinetochore, a multiprotein complex essential for normal segregation during mitosis, and overexpression of hypoxia-inducible factor 1α (HIF1α), which regulates the HIF1 and HIF2 genes mediating the cellular response to hypoxia. These genetic and epigenetic changes in the genome increase expression of genes involved in angiogenesis, cell survival, and glucose metabolism, as well as influencing different pathways to promote cellular growth of the tumor.[9]

MICROSATELLITE INSTABILITY PATHWAY

The MSI pathway represents a form of genomic instability that is found in approximately 15% of sporadic CRCs and in almost all cases of hereditary nonpolyposis colorectal cancer (HNPCC) syndrome, which represents 2% to 5% of all CRC.[10] MSI is caused by inactivity of the DNA mismatch repair (MMR) system. When the DNA MMR system is not active, there is a 100-fold increase in the mutation rate in colorectal mucosa cells.[11] In cases of sporadic CRC the MMR defect is caused primarily by hypermethylation of the MutL homolog 1 (MLH1) gene promoter due to senescence, which results in altered gene expression. In CRC occurring in Lynch syndrome patients, the MMR defect is caused primarily by germ-line mutations in one of the MMR genes (MLH, MutS protein homolog 2 [MSH2], MSH6, and PSM1 homolog 2 [PMS2]).

The MMR system is highly conserved and involves a number of genes, MLH1, MSH2, MSH6, and PMS2, whose products interact and are actively engaged in identifying and correcting DNA mismatches created during DNA replication.[11-13] Microsatellites are short tandem sequences of nucleotides (one to six base pairs [bps]) that are repeated from 5 to 50 times in regions within the DNA sequence. They are distributed throughout the genome, and they are especially prone to replication errors. If DNA replication errors occur and are not repaired due to a deficient MMR system, protein synthesis is disrupted due to frameshift mutations as a consequence of insertions and deletions of nucleotides in the DNA sequence. Therefore an accumulation of frameshift mutations in microsatellites results in genetic instability. However, most importantly, a deficient MMR system has tumorigenic potential, particularly when it alters the function of key genes that regulate cellular growth and apoptosis.

Immunohistochemical (IHC) staining of tissues is a simple, fast, and inexpensive method to detect high-level MSI (MSI-H), which is defined as the absence of expression in one or more of the MMR proteins (MLH1, MSH2, PMS2, and MSH6).[14] IHC in the case of a normal pattern of MMR protein staining, provides good sensitivity (>90%), excellent specificity (100%), and a 96.7% predictive value of a microsatellite stable (MSS) phenotype.[15] In the case of an abnormal pattern of protein expression, there is a 100% predictive value of MSI phenotype. However, normal IHC staining may not entirely exclude all MSI cases because certain mutations in the MMR genes can lead to the production of a nonfunctional protein that retains antigenicity (results in normal IHC staining but does not function). The polymerase chain reaction (PCR)–based method has become the gold standard for MSI testing. Currently, the PCR-based method uses a five quasimonomorphic mononucleotide (one base) repeats: BAT-25, BAT-26, NR21, NR24, and NR27 as a panel to identify MSI. Contrary to most microsatellites that are polymorphic (more than one base), these mononucleotides are called quasimonomorphic because they are characterized in normal DNA by a one nucleotide repeat of 20 to 30 bps that is variable or polymorphic in the population but is almost identical in size between individuals. This means that one can determine MSI in tumor tissue without having to analyze matched DNA from normal tissues. The MSI-H phenotype is defined by the presence of at least two unstable markers among the five analyzed (or >30% of unstable markers if a larger panel is used), whereas those with instability at one marker or showing no instability are defined as MSI-low (MSI-L) and MSS tumors, respectively.[14]

In sporadic settings, MSI-H CRCs are due to the epigenetic silencing of the *hMLH1* gene promoter. The resulting mutant phenotype, as in the case of HNPCC, leads to inactivation of target genes, in particular those that regulate cellular growth and apoptosis. Most MSI-H CRC cases harbor the *V600E* mutation of the B-RAF protooncogene. *BRAF*, a member of the *RAF* gene family, makes a serine/threonine kinase called B-Raf, which is involved in the RAS/MAPK pathway in the cell. B-Raf is involved in cell growth and division, apoptosis, and cell migration. In the case of the V600E mutation, the *BRAF* gene is constitutively active, meaning tumor cells undergo dysregulated growth and division. MSI-H sporadic CRCs also display CIMP features, and this will be described in the CIMP pathway of CRC section.

CRC that develops as a consequence of the MSI pathway (hereditary and sporadic) has distinct clinical features; the malignancy is often located in the proximal colon, with a poorly differentiated and mucinous or medullary histologic subtype, and frequently includes intense peritumoral and intratumoral lymphocytic infiltrations.[16] It is thought that the high density of tumor-infiltrating lymphocytes is due to a heightened host immune system

response that not only recognizes tumor antigens but also novel tumor antigens that arise due to the frameshift mutations in the DNA sequence as a consequence of MSI. In general, the prognosis and survival of patients affected by MSI-H CRC is better and longer than survival of patients with CRC derived from CIN.[17]

CPG ISLAND METHYLATOR PHENOTYPE AND SERRATED PATHWAY OF COLORECTAL CANCER

A third pathway responsible for carcinogenesis in the colon is the CIMP.[18,19] The CIMP phenotype is due to the aberrant hypermethylation of CpG islands, regions with a high incidence of CpG sites located in the promoter regions of genes involved in cell cycle regulation, apoptosis, angiogenesis, DNA repair, cell invasion, and adhesion. CpG islands are at least 200 bps in length, with a GC percentage higher than 50%. Hypermethylation of these CpG islands in the promoter region of genes causes loss of gene expression and thereby loss of function. CIMP is found in 20% to 30% of CRC cases, and the clinical features of CIMP CRC are similar to CRCs that are MSI-H.[20]

Based on the numbers of methylated markers, CRC with the CIMP phenotype can be divided into CIMP-high and CIMP-low. A mutation in the *BRAF* protooncogene often is identified in CIMP-high CRCs. CRCs containing *BRAF* mutations are associated with increased cell growth, progression of carcinogenesis, and high CRC-specific mortality. CRCs with mutations in the *BRAF* gene are a negative prognostic factor for overall survival (OS) in early-stage CRC due to its association with poor survival after relapse.[3,21–26] It is important to determine the tumor MSI status in a *BRAF*-mutated CRC and the anatomic location of the tumor.[22,24] As mentioned previously, MSI-H sporadic CRCs are a result of epigenetic silencing of the *hMLH1* gene promoter in the MSI pathway and early-stage MSI-H right-sided CRCs containing *BRAF* mutations have a more favorable prognosis than the MSS left-sided colon tumors.[3,24,25]

Mutations in the *BRAF* gene are found in 90% of CRC cases with sessile serrated adenomas (SSAs), but they are never present in conventional adenomas. *BRAF* mutations are an early event in the serrated pathway that leads to cancer. These mutations are present in early hyperplastic (serrated precursors) polyps and in advanced dysplastic serrated polyps, confirming its role in CRC neoplastic progression. SSA polyps with *BRAF* mutations frequently have CIMP-high and MSI-H features; thus researchers have surmised that in sporadic settings CIMP-high, MSI-H CRCs arise from the serrated pathway of carcinogenesis.[27]

BRAF and *KRAS* gene mutations are considered mutually exclusive in CRC.[28] Researchers have found that when a *KRAS* mutation is present in a CRC, this cancer is CIMP-negative.[29] *KRAS* mutation–positive, CIMP-low CRCs are also frequently associated with mutations in the DNA repair gene, *methylguanine methyltransferase (MGMT)* that likely contributes to the development of mutations in the phosphatidylinositol-4,5-bisphosphate 3-kinase catalytic subunit alpha *(PIK3CA)* gene.[30–32] Therefore CIMP-low CRCs appear to have a different phenotype than CIMP-high CRCs. An "alternative serrated pathway" has been described, in which CIMP-low CRCs are the result of a hybrid carcinogenesis pattern observed for both adenomatous and serrated polyps. It has been hypothesized that CRC derived from these types of polyps that carry the *KRAS* mutation represent only 2% of CRC cases, and they have the potential to be extremely aggressive due to the inactivation of the *MGMT* gene.[30]

INFLAMMATORY PATHWAY

Patients with IBD are at an increased risk for developing CRC.[33] The high risk for acquiring CRC in the setting of IBD increases with length of duration of IBD, as well as the extent and degree of tissue inflammation, family history of CRC, and the coexistence of primary sclerosing cholangitis.[33] The pathogenesis of IBD-associated CRC is poorly understood. Many of the genetic changes associated with the initiation of sporadic CRC (such as CIN, MSI, and CIMP) also play roles in the incidence of IBD-related CRC. However, unlike sporadic CRC, which develops from colon tissue dysplasia in one or two foci of the colon or rectum, cancer that arises from chronically inflamed mucosa usually develops from multifocal areas of dysplasia, indicating that a "field cancerization defect" may come into play.[34] The result of chronic inflammation, such as the induction of cyclooxygenase *(COX)-2* gene expression and increased levels of inflammatory cytokines and chemokines, may play a role in the pathogenesis of IBD-related CRC. Nonsteroidal antiinflammatory drugs (NSAIDs) have been shown to decrease the risk of CRC in IBD patients by 40% to 50%.[35,36] NSAIDs exert their effects through inhibition of the activity of COX enzymes. Among the three isoforms of the *COX* enzyme, COX-1, -2, and -3, COX-2 expression is enhanced by inflammation and its levels are elevated in 50% of colorectal adenomas and in 85% of colorectal adenocarcinomas.[37,38] COX-2 protein overexpression occurs earlier in colorectal neoplasia originating in IBD, which may explain why CRC develops in patients with IBD at a younger age.[39] In addition, oxidative stress develops in inflammatory states where inflammatory cells, activated neutrophils, and macrophages produce large amounts of reactive oxygen and nitrogen species (RONs).[40-42] Active IBD-affected mucosa shows increased expression of nitric oxide synthase and RONs.[40,43,44] RONs can promote mutations in genes that are key in carcinogenic pathways associated with CRC, such as the *TP53* and *MMR* genes.[41]

CONCLUSIONS

Identifying the different molecular pathways that cause the development of CRC has helped us to better understand how CRC initiates and progresses. However, more importantly, a better understanding of the pathogenesis of CRC gives us a guide for identifying the molecular markers that predominantly influence this disease's behavior, as well as its prognosis and response to treatments.

ADJUVANT TREATMENT IN STAGE II AND III COLON CANCER

Fluorouracil (5-FU) and oxaliplatin combination chemotherapy is the current standard of care after resection of stage III colon cancer (CC). The benefit for adding oxaliplatin to 5-FU or capecitabine was demonstrated in three landmark clinical trials showing an approximately 20% relative risk reduction for disease-free survival (DFS),[45-47] as well as a similar improvement in OS[48] for stage III CC. However, it remains uncertain whether patients with stage II CC derive any clinically meaningful benefit from adjuvant chemotherapy, when considering the associated toxicity, inconvenience, and cost.[49,50] The decision about which stage II CC patients may derive a clinically meaningful benefit from adjuvant chemotherapy has relied on using clinicopathologic factors associated with a poor prognosis. These clinicopathologic factors are (1) T4 stage (tumor penetrates to the surface of the visceral peritoneum or invades or is adherent to other organs and structures), (2) tumor perforation or obstruction, (3) indeterminate or positive surgical margins, (4) poorly differentiated histology (excluding those whose tumors harbor MSI), (5) lymphovascular or perineural invasion, or (6) less than 12 lymph nodes in retrieved specimen.[49,51-53] However, even though these factors are of prognostic significance, there is no evidence to indicate that they hold any predictive importance for recurrence in patients with stage II CC. Therefore there is a need to add prognostic and predictive value to the current TNM staging system for CC with the use of validated molecular biomarkers. Biomarkers for CC need to be developed separately for the nonmetastatic and metastatic settings because research has already shown that not all agents with proven benefit for CC in the metastatic setting have improved clinical outcomes for patients with CC in the adjuvant setting.[54-56] A simple explanation may be that nonmetastatic CC is not dependent on the same mechanisms for survival as is metastatic CC.

MOLECULAR BIOMARKERS IN COLON CANCER

The two major biologic domains of molecular biomarkers for need for chemotherapy in stage II CC are the patient and their tumor characteristics (Fig. 176.1). For the patient, there are potentially three areas from which these biomarkers can be derived: germ-line genetic mutations, genetic polymorphisms, and immunologic disorders. For the tumor, tumor-specific mutations and tumor-specific expression are two areas to investigate for the identification of biomarkers. Currently, molecular biomarkers for nonmetastatic CC that may determine adjuvant therapy benefit are the presence of tumor MSI, *BRAF* or *KRAS* gene mutations, *CDX2* expression, gene expression profiling, and *TYMPS*, *DPD*, and excision repair cross-complementing group 1 *(ERCC1)* and x-ray repair cross-complementing group 1 *(XRCC1)* gene polymorphisms in the patient.

MICROSATELLITE INSTABILITY

As mentioned earlier, defective DNA MMR is a prognostic marker validated for use in patients with CC. The presence of MSI-H in the tumor has a positive impact on survival, and it is more pronounced in earlier stage disease. MSI-H stage II CC patients have low recurrence rates and good clinical outcomes without adjuvant treatment.[57,58] In addition, distant recurrences were not reduced with 5-FU–based adjuvant treatment in MSI-H stage II CC patients.[59]

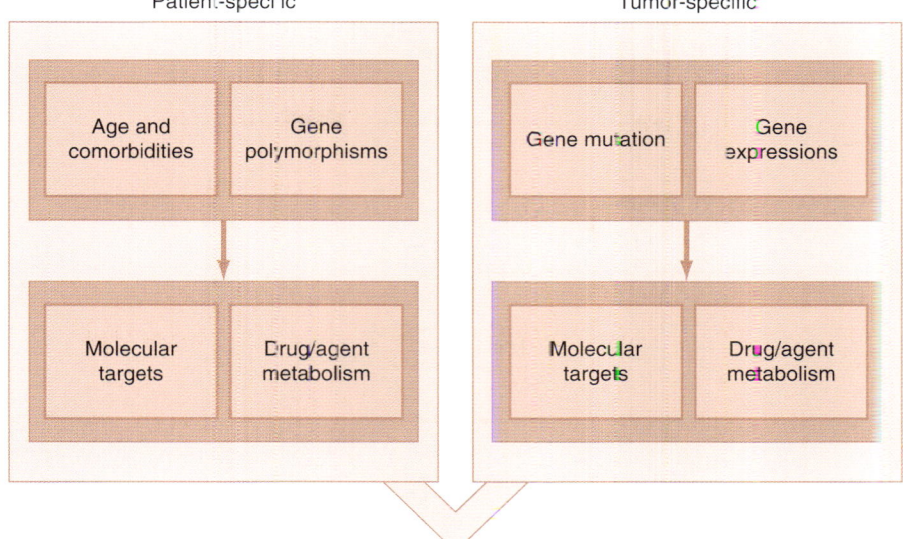

Patient-specific

Tumor-specific

- Age and comorbidities
- Gene polymorphisms
- Molecular targets
- Drug/agent metabolism

- Gene mutation
- Gene expressions
- Molecular targets
- Drug/agent metabolism

FIGURE 176.1 Molecular-based predictors of response to treatment.

Furthermore, in one report, patients with MSI-H stage II CC that were treated with 5-FU–based chemotherapy had a significant reduction in OS, but this finding has yet to be confirmed.[60] Results from some preclinical and clinical trials have suggested that MSI tumors are more responsive to irinotecan.[61,62] Results of one trial showed that patients with MSI-H stage III CC who received adjuvant treatment with irinotecan, 5-FU, and leucovorin had a significantly longer DFS compared with patients who received adjuvant treatment with 5-FU and leucovorin alone, but this effect became marginal in an updated report.[61,63] The lack of significant correlation between MSI status and irinotecan treatment was corroborated in a recent clinical trial.[64] Moreover, in a randomized clinical trial of stage II and III CC patients with MSI, those who received adjuvant therapy with 5-FU, leucovorin, and oxaliplatin (FOLFOX) and bevacizumab derived a significantly longer OS compared to the control patients who received adjuvant therapy with FOLFOX alone.[65] However, the benefit of bevacizumab was not noted in MSI stage II and III CC patients who received bevacizumab together with capecitabine or capecitabine alone.[66] Therefore there are no data to support the use of adjuvant treatment in MSI stage II patients.

MSI stage III patients did derive benefit from adjuvant therapy with 5-FU– or oxaliplatin-based regimens, similar to the response of patients with MSS stage III CC.[22,57,67] An algorithm for using microsatellite status along with the clinical pathologic features of stage II and III CC to inform adjuvant therapy decision is helpful (Fig. 176.2).

BRAF GENE MUTATIONS

BRAF mutation in CC has been validated as an independent poor prognostic factor for OS in patients with early-stage CC.[3,21–23,25,26] However, this is due primarily to this mutation's association with poor survival after relapse.[3,25] Interpretation of the presence of a *BRAF* mutation in a colorectal tumor as a risk factor for OS has to be made in the context of MSI status and tumor location. This mutation's largest impact for predicting prognosis is seen in tumors that are MSS and located in the left side of the colon; in this setting the presence of *BRAF* mutations in a tumor confers a worse DFS.[3,25] Studies have shown up to a sixfold increase in risk of death in patients with CC that contains a *BRAF* mutation, is MSS, and located in the left colon.[3] Even though the general prognostic value of having a *BRAF* mutation in a tumor seems to be affected by MSS status and location of the tumor, some studies suggest that this mutation may have an adverse effect on the prognosis for patients with MSI-H CC.[3,22] Still, the protective effect of MSI-H status in patients with early-stage CC overrides the poor prognosis conferred by *BRAF* mutated tumors, and as a result the CC patient with a MSI *BRAF*-mutated early-stage tumor has a favorable prognosis.[3,24]

KRAS GENE MUTATIONS

The presence of a *KRAS* mutation in *BRAF* wild-type CC confers a worse prognosis for patients: reduced DFS and OS, as compared with *KRAS* wild-type CC.[68–71] The poor prognostic effect of the *KRAS* mutation in tumors with *BRAF* wild-type stage II and III CC is greatest for *KRAS* mutations in codon 12 and in left-sided tumors.[26,68,69,71] Interestingly, KRAS mutations in codon 12 or 13 negate the effect of cetuximab, an anti–epidermal growth factor–receptor agent, in the adjuvant setting.[26,72] Cetuximab was actually associated with a detrimental effect in OS in stage II CC patients with *KRAS* wild-type tumors.[26]

CDX2 GENE EXPRESSION

Dalerba et al. identified 16 genes in 2115 poorly differentiated CC specimens, one of which was *CDX2*.[73] *CDX2* is a master regulator of intestinal development and oncogenesis, and its expression is highly specific for intestinal epithelium.[74–75] CCs showing no *CDX2* expression by IHC are associated with an increased likelihood for aggressive features, such as advanced stage, poor differentiation, vascular invasion, *BRAF* mutation, and CIMP. Lack of *CDX2* expression identified a subgroup of patients with

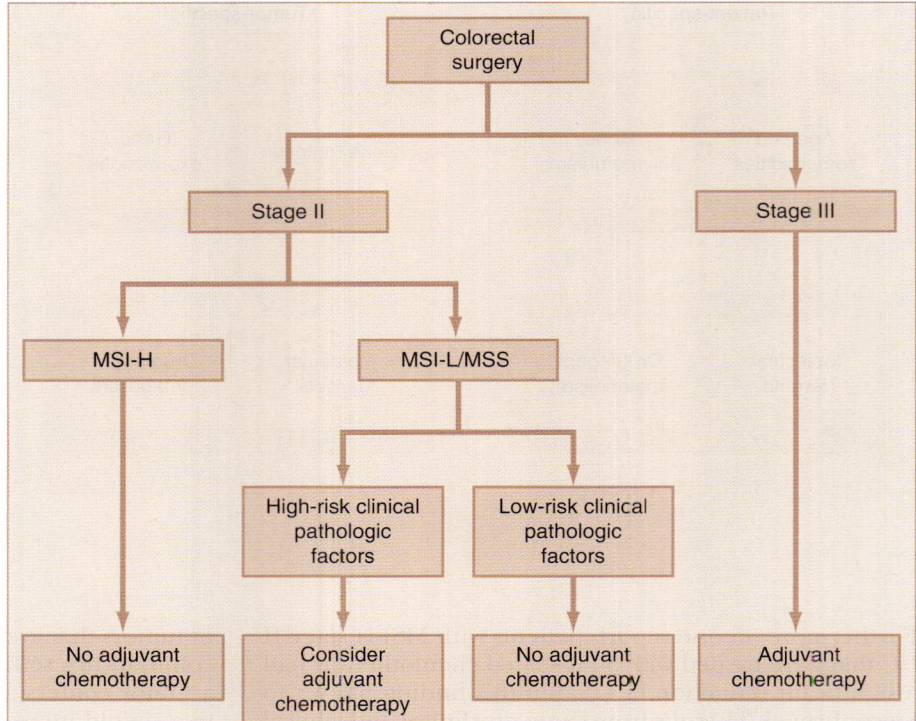

FIGURE 176.2 Algorithm for using microsatellite instability in conjunction with clinical pathologic factors in stage II and III colorectal cancer to determine potential benefit for adjuvant chemotherapy. *MSI-H*, High microsatellite instability; *MSI-L*, low microsatellite instability; *MSS*, microsatellite stable. (Modified from Van Schaeybroeck S, Kyula JN, Fenton A, et al. Oncogenic KRAS promotes chemotherapy-induced growth factor shedding via ADAM17. *Cancer Res*. 2011;71:1071–1080.)

high-risk stage II CC who appeared to benefit from adjuvant chemotherapy.[73]

GENE EXPRESSION PROFILING

With the advent of high-throughput technologies, assessment of the whole tumor genome has become possible. Not only has high-throughput genotyping enabled the efficient analysis of genes, such as *KRAS* and *BRAF* in individual colon tumors, but also gene expression profiling can be used to identify and validate genetic prognostic and predictive biomarkers for CC. As a result, using retrospective data, several gene and microRNA expression signatures have been developed for stage II and III CC to assess a patient's risk for relapse.[36,77–84] However, although there appears to be little overlap in the genes selected for the different gene signatures predictive for recurrence, they all add prognostic value to the traditional clinicopathologic risk factors when assessing a patient's prognosis. The lack of overlap for the genes selected for these different gene panels is not unexpected, because many of these genes come from highly correlated functional groups. Currently, further testing and validation of these gene panels is in progress, but to date, none of the genetic signatures that predict stage II and III CC patient prognosis are able to predict benefit from adjuvant therapy. Ideally, prognostic information provided by these gene signatures may have the greatest clinical utility when used as a complement to T stage and microsatellite status, especially for patients who have pT3 MSS stage II disease.

TYMPS GENE POLYMORPHISM

The antitumor effect of 5-FU has been ascribed to a number of mechanisms, including competitive inhibition of the thymidylate synthase (TS) enzyme.[85–87] TS is an enzyme encoded by the *TYMPS* gene that directs synthesis of thymidine by methylating deoxyuridine monophosphate to form thymidine monophosphate or thymidine, which is later converted to thymine. Thymine is one of the four bases that make up the structure of DNA, and, with low levels of thymine, DNA synthesis is inhibited. 5-FU is called an antimetabolite because it inhibits DNA synthesis by blocking TS activity through competitive binding. Because blocking the action of TS causes a scarcity in thymine, rapidly dividing cancerous cells undergo cell death via what has been called a "thymineless death."[88] 5-FU has remained the mainstay of therapeutic regimens used in the treatment of CRC with single-agent response rates of 20% to 25% in the metastatic setting. Pharmacogenetics has become a well-studied area to personalize treatment for individual patients being treated with 5-FU to maximize clinical outcomes and reduce toxicity.[89] Initially, studies showed that there was variation in intratumoral TS levels in CRC, which was presumed to be due to germ-line polymorphisms in the *TYMPS* gene. In addition, TS expression in cultures of cancer cells was shown to be a determinant of their response to fluoropyrimidines.[90,91] As a result of this finding in vitro, clinical studies that followed showed that higher intratumoral levels of TS were associated with a lower OS in patients with advanced and localized CRC.[92] A systemic review and meta-analysis of studies investigating the relationship between TS expression and survival in patients with localized and metastatic CRC showed that tumors with high levels of TS were associated with a poorer OS compared with tumors expressing low levels.[93] However, even though most studies of CRC in the metastatic setting demonstrated that higher intratumoral TS levels predict nonresponsiveness to 5-FU, as well as a worse prognosis,[93] a benefit for adjuvant therapy with 5-FU among CC patients with lower intratumoral TS levels was not always apparent.[94–99] Due to the lack of reproducibility of intratumoral TS levels to predict response to 5-FU in CRC, other genetic factors were examined to determine their prognosis for determining the response of CRC to 5-FU treatment.

Some studies find there may be a relationship between *TP53* gene mutation in CRC, microsatellite status, and TS tumor expression because TS expression is significantly higher in MSI tumors compared with MSS tumors, and CRC cells with high TS levels are more likely to overexpress *TP53*. However, no clinical studies to date have been able to predict a clinical response to 5-FU on the basis of MSI, *TP53* gene mutation, and TS status.[100,101]

DIHYDROPYRIMIDINE DEHYDROGENASE GENE POLYMORPHISM

Even though CRC response to 5-FU is very important, just as important are the toxicities associated with 5-FU treatment. DPD is an enzyme encoded by the *DPYD* gene that is responsible primarily for pyrimidine catabolism, deactivating more than 80% to 90% of the administered 5-FU and the oral 5-FU prodrug capecitabine. Treatment with fluoropyrimidines, such as 5-FU and capecitabine, is generally well tolerated, except in 5% to 10% of the treated population, who develop severe, potentially life-threatening toxicity early on in treatment.[102–104] Intolerance to fluoropyrimidines is most commonly associated with deficiency of DPD.[105] True deficiency of DPD affects approximately 5% of the overall population, with the *DPYD* gene polymorphism, *DPYD*2A* being the most clinically relevant mutation associated with this toxicity. A study showed that genotyping upfront for the *DPYD*2A* polymorphism is feasible and improves the safety of fluoropyrimidine therapy.[106]

ERCC1 AND XRCC1 GENE POLYMORPHISMS

Oxaliplatin is a platinum-based chemotherapeutic agent that when used in combination with 5-FU (FOLFOX regimen) significantly improved progression-free survival (PFS) and the response rate for patients with metastatic CRC.[107] In a recent study, the addition of oxaliplatin to 5-FU to adjuvant chemotherapy improved clinical outcome for patients with stage III CC by reducing the risk of disease recurrence and increasing OS.[45,108] However, in this study, FOLFOX failed to eradicate micrometastatic disease in approximately one-third of the stage III CC patients. Oxaliplatin exerts its action by forming DNA-platinum monoadducts that inhibit DNA replication and transcription and subsequently induces apoptosis. Investigations to identify gene polymorphisms to enhance DNA repair efficiency are ongoing.

Oxaliplatin-induced adducts are not recognized by the MMR system but are repaired predominantly by the nucleotide excision repair (NER) and base excision repair (BER) pathways.[109,110] Several studies reported that single nucleotide polymorphisms in genes that repair DNA, such as the *ERCC1*[111] and *XRCC1* genes,[112,113] or genes involved in drug metabolism, such as glutathione S-transferase *P1* (*GSTP1*) gene,[114–116] may predict clinical outcomes for patients receiving oxaliplatin-based chemotherapy. The ability of these gene polymorphisms to predict clinical

TABLE 176.1 Molecular Biomarkers for Use in Nonmetastatic Colorectal Cancer

Molecular Biomarker	Predictive	Prognostic
TUMOR		
MSI	Yes	Yes
KRAS gene	No	Yes
BRAF gene	No	Yes
CDX2 gene	Unclear	Unclear
Gene Expression Profiling	Yes	No
PATIENT GENE POLYMORPHISMS		
TYMPS gene	Unclear	Yes
ERCC1 gene	Unclear	Unclear
XRCC1 gene	Unclear	Unclear

BRAF, v-Raf murine sarcoma viral oncogene homolog B; *CDX2*, caudal-type homeobox 2; *ERCC1*, excision repair cross-complementation group 1; *KRAS*, Kirsten rat sarcoma viral oncogene homolog; MSI, microsatellite instability; *TYMPS*, thymidine phosphorylase; *XRCC*, x-ray repair cross-complementing protein.

outcome for patients treated with oxaliplatin-based adjuvant chemotherapy is limited. *ERCC1* and *XRCC1* polymorphisms, but not the *GSTP1* polymorphisms, improved DFS of stage III CC patients treated with FOLFOX adjuvant therapy.[117] However, these findings need to be confirmed in future independent prospective studies.

CONCLUSIONS

Although the use of adjuvant chemotherapy resulted in dramatic improvements in the clinical outcomes of patients with CC, matching the patient to the right therapeutic regimen, in addition to balancing the relative benefits and risks of these treatments, is key to achieving the most favorable treatment outcomes. As presented previously in the studies to date, most have focused primarily on the development of single genes or tumor phenotypes as candidate prognostic and predictive molecular biomarkers (Table 176.1). The presence of tumor MSI is the only molecular biomarker, thus far that can be used to guide treatment in patients with stage II CC. Although there are many other biomarkers still under investigation (*KRAS*, *BRAF*, *CDX2* gene expression, *TYMPS*, *DPYD*, *ERCC1*, and *XRCC1* gene polymorphisms), no single biomarker predicts benefit from adjuvant therapy in patients with CC. There have been no prospective studies to demonstrate use of molecular biomarkers for the prediction of response to adjuvant therapy in CC (see Fig. 176.2).

NEOADJUVANT TREATMENT IN RECTAL CANCER

Up to 70% of patients with nonmetastatic rectal cancer present with locally advanced disease (T3N0 or T any] N1-2) or stage III disease.[118]

Neoadjuvant therapy with chemoradiotherapy (CRT) is an integral part of successful treatment of rectal cancer. However, there needs to be more selection of patient and tumor-specific treatment. The use of total mesorectal excision (TME) has significantly decreased local recurrence (LR) rates for rectal cancer.[119-123] Magnetic resonance imaging (MRI) for determining the effects of neoadjuvant therapy and for surgical planning has contributed significantly to decreased LR and improved OS rates for patients with rectal cancer. MRI provides a 92% specificity for predicting a negative circumferential resection margin (CRM) that has been shown to result in a 5-year 67.2% DFS in patients with MRI-clear CRMs compared with a 47.3% DFS in patients with MRI-involved CRMs.[124,125] As a result, MRI has become the preferred imaging modality for evaluating patients with stage III rectal cancer.[53]

The current standard of care in the United States for the treatment of stage III rectal cancer is neoadjuvant chemoradiation followed by radical resection with TME and then adjuvant chemotherapy. Due to the complexity of decision making for CRC, particularly rectal cancer, a multidisciplinary team including representation from colorectal surgery, medical oncology, radiation oncology, radiology, and pathology should have input on the patient's course of treatment.[126,127] The assessment by a multidisciplinary team has been associated with a reduced rate of positive CRMs for rectal cancer.[128] Multidisciplinary teams have reduced perioperative mortality for patients with rectal cancer; however, there was no effect observed on OS.[129]

Neoadjuvant treatment with long-course radiotherapy combined with chemotherapy or CRT is generally recommended for patients with stage III rectal cancer. Radiotherapy can be administered using a short-course radiotherapy (SCRT) or CRT. In the United States and some European countries, CRT is preferred, whereas in other countries (e.g., Sweden, Norway, and Netherlands) SCRT is used primarily.[130] In general, SCRT is followed by surgery within 7 days; potential benefits of this approach are a shorter treatment duration, more efficient use of resources, and reduced cost compared with long-course CRT. There have been concerns that SCRT increases the risk for delayed toxicity and results in lower tumor regression.[131,132] SCRT followed by surgery and adjuvant chemotherapy compared with CRT followed by TME and adjuvant chemotherapy has not been shown to increase the risk for LR or OS.[133-136]

The substitution of the oral prodrug, capecitabine (converted to 5-FU by intracellular thymidine phosphorylase) for the continuous venous infusion (CVI) of 5-FU is attractive because it is more convenient for patients than the use of 5-FU CVI.[137] CRT with capecitabine was not found to be inferior to CRT with CVI 5-FU with respect to 5-year OS; it was even superior to CRT with CVI 5-FU in 3-year OS.[138] Finally, although trials with neoadjuvant chemotherapy (FOLFOX or capecitabine and oxaliplatin) without radiotherapy for the treatment of stage III rectal cancer appear promising, further study is required to prove efficacy for this treatment approach.[139-141]

Although the incorporation of targeted therapy with inhibitors of the epidermal growth factor receptor and vascular endothelial growth factor for treatment of stage III rectal cancer has been tested in phase II clinical trials, particularly as radiosensitizers for radiotherapy, these studies did not yield the results needed for advancement into phase III trials.[142-145] Therefore targeted therapies

currently play no role in neoadjuvant treatment of patients with stage III rectal cancer outside of the clinical trial setting. Profiles of predictive molecular biomarkers for tumor response in patients receiving neoadjuvant chemoradiation are also clinically relevant, and, although research has been conducted to identify these types of profiles, none of this work is ready for clinical practice.[146]

ADJUVANT TREATMENT IN RECTAL CANCER

In the past, in patients with stage III rectal cancer, LR was the primary problem. Currently, more patients develop distant rather than local relapse. Patients with stage III rectal cancer treated with neoadjuvant radiotherapy or radiotherapy in combination with chemotherapy followed by TME currently undergo postoperative chemotherapy independent of the response to neoadjuvant therapy.[147] A meta-analysis of 21 randomized clinical trials that included patients with T(any), N(any), or M0 rectal cancer concluded that postoperative 5-FU therapy improved DFS and OS; however, only a few of these studies focused their analyses on stage III rectal cancer patients alone.[148] Therefore the current recommendations for the use of 5-FU–based adjuvant therapy in patients with stage III rectal cancer treated with CRT and TME is based, in part, on data from this meta-analysis, as well as extrapolation from CC data.[48,149]

SUMMARY

Personalizing treatment for nonmetastatic CRC will require refining our approach to defining patients at risk for recurrence of disease combined with the best treatment options based on the use of molecular biomarkers. Just as important, development of new neoadjuvant and adjuvant therapies for CRC will involve identifying biologically driven events in the various tumor types defined by their molecular signature. In addition, we need to identify the molecular biomarkers unique to the patient's biologic makeup that predict their response to treatment.

REFERENCES

1. Ferlay J, Shin HR, Bray F, Forman D, Mathers C, Parkin DM. Estimates of worldwide burden of cancer in 2008: GLOBOCAN 2008. *Int J Cancer*. 2010;127(12):2893-2917.
2. Roth AD, Delorenzi M, Tejpar S, et al. Integrated analysis of molecular and clinical prognostic factors in stage II/III colon cancer. *J Natl Cancer Inst*. 2012;104(21):1635-1646.
3. Lochhead P, Kuchiba A, Imamura Y, et al. Microsatellite instability and BRAF mutation testing in colorectal cancer prognostication. *J Natl Cancer Inst*. 2013;105(15):1151-1156.
4. Xie J, Itzkowitz SH. Cancer in inflammatory bowel disease. *World J Gastroenterol*. 2008;14(3):378-389.
5. Fearon ER, Vogelstein B. A genetic model for colorectal tumorigenesis. *Cell*. 1990;61(5):759-767.
6. Jass JR. Classification of colorectal cancer based on correlation of clinical, morphological and molecular features. *Histopathology*. 2007;50(1):113-130.
7. Boland CR, Thibodeau SN, Hamilton SR, et al. A National Cancer Institute Workshop on Microsatellite Instability for cancer detection and familial predisposition: development of international criteria for the determination of microsatellite instability in colorectal cancer. *Cancer Res*. 1998;58(22):5248-5257.
8. Fearon ER. Molecular genetics of colorectal cancer. *Annu Rev Pathol*. 2011;6:479-507.

9. Lengauer C, Kinzler KW, Vogelstein B. Genetic instability in colorectal cancers. *Nature*. 1997;386(6625):623-627.

10. Boland CR, Goel A. Microsatellite instability in colorectal cancer. *Gastroenterology*. 2010;138:2073-2087.e3.

11. Thomas DC, Umar A, Kunkel TA. Microsatellite instability and mismatch repair defects in cancer. *Mutat Res*. 1996;350(1):201-205.

12. Fishel R. Mismatch repair, molecular switches, and signal transduction. *Genes Dev*. 1998;12(14):2096-2101.

13. Grilley M, Holmes J, Yashar B, Modrich P. Mechanisms of DNA-mismatch correction. *Mutat Res*. 1990;236(2-3):253-267.

14. Buecher B, Cacheux W, Rouleau E, Dieumegard B, Mitry E, Lièvre A. Role of microsatellite instability in the management of colorectal cancers. *Dig Liver Dis*. 2013;45(6):441-449.

15. Lindor NM, Burgart LJ, Leontovich O, et al. Immunohistochemistry versus microsatellite instability testing in phenotyping colorectal tumors. *J Clin Oncol*. 2002;20(4):1043-1048.

16. Lanza G, Gafà R, Maestri I, Santini A, Matteuzzi M, Cavazzini L. Immunohistochemical pattern of MLH1/MSH2 expression is related to clinical and pathological features in colorectal adenocarcinomas with microsatellite instability. *Mod Pathol* 2002;15(7):741-749.

17. Sinicrope FA, Sargent DJ. Molecular pathways: microsatellite instability in colorectal cancer: prognostic, predictive, and therapeutic implications. *Clin Cancer Res*. 2012;18(6):1506-1512.

18. Samowitz WS, Albertsen H, Herrick J, et al. Evaluation of a large, population-based sample supports a CpG island methylator phenotype in colon cancer. *Gastroenterology*. 2005;129(3):837-845.

19. Shen L, Toyota M, Kondo Y, et al. Integrated genetic and epigenetic analysis identifies three different subclasses of colon cancer. *Proc Natl Acad Sci USA*. 2007;104(47):18654-18659.

20. Ogino S, Odze RD, Kawasaki T, et al. Correlation of pathologic features with CpG island methylator phenotype (CIMP) by quantitative DNA methylation analysis in colorectal carcinoma. *Am J Surg Pathol*. 2006;30(9):1175-1183.

21. Roth AD, Tejpar S, Delorenzi M, et al. Prognostic role of KRAS and BRAF in stage II and III resected colon cancer: results of the translational study on the PETACC-3, EORTC 40993, SAKK 60-00 trial. *J Clin Oncol*. 2010;28(3):466-474.

22. Gavin PG, Colangelo LH, Fumagalli D, et al. Mutation profiling and microsatellite instability in stage II and III colon cancer: an assessment of their prognostic and oxaliplatin predictive value. *Clin Cancer Res*. 2012;18(23):6531-6541.

23. Ogino S, Shima K, Meyerhardt JA, et al. Predictive and prognostic roles of BRAF mutation in stage III colon cancer: results from intergroup trial CALGB 89803. *Clin Cancer Res*. 2012;18(3):890-900.

24. Popovici V, Budinska E, Bosman FT, Tejpar S, Roth AD, Delorenzi M. Context-dependent interpretation of the prognostic value of BRAF and KRAS mutations in colorectal cancer. *BMC Cancer*. 2013;13:439.

25. Sinicrope FA, Mahoney MR, Smyrk TC, et al. Prognostic impact of deficient DNA mismatch repair in patients with stage III colon cancer from a randomized trial of FOLFOX-based adjuvant chemotherapy. *J Clin Oncol*. 2013;31(29):3664-3672.

26. Sinicrope FA, Yoon HH, Mahoney MR, et al. Overall survival result and outcomes by KRAS, BRAF, and DNA mismatch repair in relation to primary tumor site in colon cancers from a randomized trial of adjuvant chemotherapy: NCCTG (Alliance) N0147. *J Clin Oncol*. 2014;32(suppl):abstr 3525.

27. Kambara T, Simms LA, Whitehall VL, et al. BRAF mutation is associated with DNA methylation in serrated polyps and cancers of the colorectum. *Gut* 2004;53(8):1137-1144.

28. Phipps AI, Limburg PJ, Baron JA, et al. Association between molecular subtypes of colorectal cancer and patient survival. *Gastroenterology*. 2015;148:77-87.e2.

29. Petko Z, Ghiassi M, Shuber A, et al. Aberrantly methylated CDKN2A, MGMT, and MLH1 in colon polyps and in fecal DNA from patients with colorectal polyps. *Clin Cancer Res*. 2005;11(3):1203-1209.

30. East JE, Saunders BP, Jass JR. Sporadic and syndromic hyperplastic polyps and serrated adenomas of the colon: classification, molecular genetics, natural history, and clinical management. *Gastroenterol Clin North Am*. 2008;37(1):25-46, v.

31. Ogino S, Kawasaki T, Kirkner GJ, Suemoto Y, Meyerhardt JA, Fuchs CS. Molecular correlates with MGMT promoter methylation and silencing support CpG island methylator phenotype-low (CIMP-low) in colorectal cancer. *Gut*. 2007;56(11):1564-1571.

32. Shima K, Morikawa T, Baba Y, et al. MGMT promoter methylation, loss of expression and prognosis in 855 colorectal cancers. *Cancer Causes Control*. 2011;22(2):301-309.

33. Kim ER, Chang DK. Colorectal cancer in inflammatory bowel disease: the risk, pathogenesis, prevention and diagnosis. *World J Gastroenterol*. 2014;20(29):9872-9881.

34. Slaughter DP, Southwick HW, Smejkal W. Field cancerization in oral stratified squamous epithelium; clinical implications of multicentric origin. *Cancer*. 1953;6(5):963-968.

35. Smalley WE, DuBois RN. Colorectal cancer and nonsteroidal anti-inflammatory drugs. *Adv Pharmacol*. 1997;39:1-20.

36. Azer SA. Overview of molecular pathways in inflammatory bowel disease associated with colorectal cancer development. *Eur J Gastroenterol Hepatol*. 2013;25(3):271-281.

37. Marnett LJ, DuBois RN. COX-2: a target for colon cancer prevention. *Annu Rev Pharmacol Toxicol*. 2002;42:55-80.

38. Elzagheid A, Emaetig F, Alkikhia L, et al. High cyclooxygenase 2 expression is associated with advanced stages in colorectal cancer. *Anticancer Res*. 2013;33(8):3137-3143.

39. Agoff SN, Brentnall TA, Crispin DA, et al. The role of cyclooxygenase 2 in ulcerative colitis-associated neoplasia. *Am J Pathol*. 2000;157(3):737-745.

40. Hussain SP, Amstad P, Raja K, et al. Increased p53 mutation load in noncancerous colon tissue from ulcerative colitis: a cancer-prone chronic inflammatory disease. *Cancer Res*. 2000;60(13):3333-3337.

41. Kraus S, Arber N. Inflammation and colorectal cancer. *Curr Opin Pharmacol*. 2009;9(4):405-410.

42. Ullman TA, Itzkowitz SH. Intestinal inflammation and cancer. *Gastroenterology*. 2011;140(6):1807-1816.

43. Rachmilewitz D, Stamler JS, Bachwich D, Karmeli F, Ackerman Z, Podolsky DK. Enhanced colonic nitric oxide generation and nitric oxide synthase activity in ulcerative colitis and Crohn's disease. *Gut*. 1995;36:718-723.

44. Kimura H, Hokari R, Miura S, et al. Increased expression of an inducible isoform of nitric oxide synthase and the formation of peroxynitrite in colonic mucosa of patients with active ulcerative colitis. *Gut*. 1998;42(2):180-187.

45. André T, Boni C, Mounedji-Boudiaf L, et al. Oxaliplatin, fluorouracil, and leucovorin as adjuvant treatment for colon cancer. *N Engl J Med*. 2004;350(23):2343-2351.

46. Haller DG, Tabernero J, Maroun J, et al. Capecitabine plus oxaliplatin compared with fluorouracil and folinic acid as adjuvant therapy for stage III colon cancer. *J Clin Oncol*. 2011;29(11):1465-1471.

47. Yothers G, Sargent DJ, Wolmark N, et al. Outcomes among black patients with stage II and III colon cancer receiving chemotherapy: an analysis of ACCENT adjuvant trials. *J Natl Cancer Inst*. 2011;103(20):1498-1506.

48. André T, Boni C, Navarro M, et al. Improved overall survival with oxaliplatin, fluorouracil, and leucovorin as adjuvant treatment in stage II or III colon cancer in the MOSAIC trial. *J Clin Oncol*. 2009;27:3109-3116.

49. Benson AB 3rd, Schrag D, Somerfield MR, et al. American Society of Clinical Oncology recommendations on adjuvant chemotherapy for stage II colon cancer. *J Clin Oncol*. 2004;22(16):3408-3419.

50. O'Connor ES, Greenblatt DY, LoConte NK, et al. Adjuvant chemotherapy for stage II colon cancer with poor prognostic features. *J Clin Oncol*. 2011;29(25):3381-3388.

51. Zaniboni A, Labianca R, Gruppo Italiano per lo Studio e la Cura dei Tumori del Digerente. Adjuvant therapy for stage II colon cancer: an elephant in the living room? *Ann Oncol*. 2004;15:1310-1318.

52. Labianca R, Nordlinger B, Beretta GD, et al. Early colon cancer: ESMO Clinical Practice Guidelines for diagnosis, treatment and follow-up. *Ann Oncol*. 2013;24(suppl 6):vi64-vi72.

53. Benson AB 3rd, Venook AP, Bekaii-Saab T, et al. Rectal cancer, version 2.2015. *J Natl Compr Canc Netw*. 2015;13(6):719-728; quiz 728.

54. Saltz LB, Niedzwiecki D, Hollis D, et al. Irinotecan fluorouracil plus leucovorin is not superior to fluorouracil plus leucovorin alone as adjuvant treatment for stage III colon cancer: results of CALGB 89803. *J Clin Oncol*. 2007;25:3456-3461.

55. Van Cutsem E, Labianca R, Bodoky G, et al. Randomized phase III trial comparing biweekly infusional fluorouracil/leucovorin alone or with irinotecan in the adjuvant treatment of stage III colon cancer: PETACC-3. *J Clin Oncol*. 2009;27(19):3117-3125.

56. Ychou M, Raoul JL, Douillard JY, et al. A phase III randomised trial of LV5FU2 + irinotecan versus LV5FU2 alone in adjuvant high-risk colon cancer (FNCLCC Accord02/FFCD9802). *Ann Oncol.* 2009;20(4):674-680.

57. Hutchins G, Southward K, Handley K, et al. Value of mismatch repair, KRAS, and BRAF mutations in predicting recurrence and benefits from chemotherapy in colorectal cancer. *J Clin Oncol.* 2011;29(10):1261-1270.

58. Sargent D, Shi Q, Yothers G, et al. Prognostic impact of deficient mismatch repair (dMMR) in 7,803 stage II/III colon cancer (CC) patients (pts): a pooled individual pt data analysis of 17 adjuvant trials in the ACCENT database. *J Clin Oncol.* 2014;32(suppl):abstr 3507.

59. Sinicrope FA, Foster NR, Thibodeau SN, et al. DNA mismatch repair status and colon cancer recurrence and survival in clinical trials of 5-fluorouracil-based adjuvant therapy. *J Natl Cancer Inst.* 2011;103(11):863-875.

60. Sargent DJ, Marsoni S, Monges G, et al. Defective mismatch repair as a predictive marker for lack of efficacy of fluorouracil-based adjuvant therapy in colon cancer. *J Clin Oncol.* 2010;28(20):3219-3226.

61. Shiovitz S, Bertagnolli MM, Renfro LA, et al. CpG island methylator phenotype is associated with response to adjuvant irinotecan-based therapy for stage III colon cancer. *Gastroenterology.* 2014;147(3):637-645.

62. Vilar E, Tabernero J. Molecular dissection of microsatellite instable colorectal cancer. *Cancer Discov.* 2013;3(5):502-511.

63. Bertagnolli MM, Niedzwiecki D, Compton CC, et al. Microsatellite instability predicts improved response to adjuvant therapy with irinotecan, fluorouracil, and leucovorin in stage III colon cancer: Cancer and Leukemia Group B Protocol 89803. *J Clin Oncol.* 2009;27(11):1814-1821.

64. Klingbiel D, Saridaki Z, Roth AD, Bosman FT, Delorenzi M, Tejpar S. Prognosis of stage II and III colon cancer treated with adjuvant 5-fluorouracil or FOLFIRI in relation to microsatellite status: results of the PETACC-3 trial. *Ann Oncol.* 2015;26(1):126-132.

65. Pogue-Geile K, Yothers G, Taniyama Y, et al. Defective mismatch repair and benefit from bevacizumab for colon cancer: findings from NSABP C-08. *J Natl Cancer Inst.* 2013;105(13):989-992.

66. Midgley RS, Love S, Tomlinson I, et al. Final results from QUASAR2, a multicentre, international randomised phase III trial of capecitabine (CAP) +/- bevacizumab (BEV) in the adjuvant setting of stage II/III colorectal cancer (CRC). *Ann Oncol.* 2014;25:v1-v41, LBA12.

67. Flejou J-F, André T, Chibaudel B, et al. Effect of adding oxaliplatin to adjuvant 5-fluorouracil/leucovorin (5FU/LV) in patients with defective mismatch repair (dMMR) colon cancer stage II and III included in the MOSIAC study. *J Clin Oncol.* 2013;31:abstr 3524.

68. Imamura Y, Morikawa T, Liao X, et al. Specific mutations in KRAS codons 12 and 13, and patient prognosis in 1075 BRAF wild-type colorectal cancers. *Clin Cancer Res.* 2012;18(17):4753-4763.

69. Blons H, Emile JF, Le Malicot K, et al. Prognostic value of KRAS mutations in stage III colon cancer: post hoc analysis of the PETACC8 phase III trial dataset. *Ann Oncol.* 2014;25(12):2378-2385.

70. Reyngold M, Niland J, ter Veer A, et al. Neoadjuvant radiotherapy use in locally advanced rectal cancer at NCCN member institutions. *J Natl Compr Canc Netw.* 2014;12:235-243.

71. Yoon HH, Tougeron D, Shi Q, et al. KRAS codon 12 and 13 mutations in relation to disease-free survival in BRAF-wild-type stage III colon cancers from an adjuvant chemotherapy trial (N0147 alliance). *Clin Cancer Res.* 2014;20(11):3033-3043.

72. Taieb J, Tabernero J, Mini E, et al. Oxaliplatin, fluorouracil, and leucovorin with or without cetuximab in patients with resected stage III colon cancer (PETACC-8): an open-label, randomised phase 3 trial. *Lancet Oncol.* 2014;15(8):862-873.

73. Dalerba P, Sahoo D, Paik S, et al. CDX2 as a prognostic biomarker in stage II and stage III colon cancer. *N Engl J Med.* 2016;374(3):211-222.

74. Chawengsaksophak K, James R, Hammond VE, Köntgen F, Beck F. Homeosis and intestinal tumours in Cdx2 mutant mice. *Nature.* 1997;386(6620):84-87.

75. Werling RW, Yaziji H, Bacchi CE, Gown AM. CDX2, a highly sensitive and specific marker of adenocarcinomas of intestinal origin: an immunohistochemical survey of 476 primary and metastatic carcinomas. *Am J Surg Pathol.* 2003;27(3):303-310.

76. Beck F, Stringer EJ. The role of Cdx genes in the gut and in axial development. *Biochem Soc Trans.* 2010;38(2):353-357.

77. Jiang Y, Casey G, Lavery IC, et al. Development of a clinically feasible molecular assay to predict recurrence of stage II colon cancer. *J Mol Diagn.* 2008;10(4):346-354.

78. Kennedy RD, Bylesjo M, Kerr P, et al. Development and independent validation of a prognostic assay for stage II colon cancer using formalin-fixed paraffin-embedded tissue. *J Clin Oncol.* 2011;29(35):4620-4626.

79. Gray RG, Quirke P, Handley K, et al. Validation study of a quantitative multigene reverse transcriptase-polymerase chain reaction assay for assessment of recurrence risk in patients with stage II colon cancer. *J Clin Oncol.* 2011;29(35):4611-4619.

80. Salazar R, Roepman P, Capella G, et al. Gene expression signature to improve prognosis prediction of stage II and III colorectal cancer. *J Clin Oncol.* 2011;29(1):17-24.

81. Venook AP, Niedzwiecki D, Lopatin M, et al. Biologic determinants of tumor recurrence in stage II colon cancer: validation study of the 12-gene recurrence score in Cancer and Leukemia Group B (CALGB) 9581. *J Clin Oncol.* 2013;31(14):1775-1781.

82. Yothers G, O'Connell MJ, Lee M, et al. Validation of the 12-gene colon cancer recurrence score in NSABP C-07 as a predictor of recurrence in patients with stage II and III colon cancer treated with fluorouracil and leucovorin (FU/LV) and FU/LV plus oxaliplatin. *J Clin Oncol.* 2013;31:4512-4519.

83. Zhang JX, Song W, Chen ZH, et al. Prognostic and predictive value of a microRNA signature in stage II colon cancer: a microRNA expression analysis. *Lancet Oncol.* 2013;14(13):1295-1306.

84. Di Narzo AF, Tejpar S, Rossi S, et al. Test of four colon cancer risk-scores in formalin fixed paraffin embedded microarray gene expression data. *J Natl Cancer Inst.* 2014;106.

85. Danenberg PV, Langenbach RJ, Heidelberger C. Structures of reversible and irreversible complexes of thymidylate synthetase and fluorinated pyrimidine nucleotides. *Biochemistry.* 1974;13(5):926-933.

86. Kufe DW, Major PP, Egan EM, Loh E. 5-Fluoro-2'-deoxyuridine incorporation in L1210 DNA. *J Biol Chem.* 1981;256(17):8885-8888.

87. Danenberg PV, Heidelberger C, Mulkins MA, Peterson AR. The incorporation of 5-fluoro-2'-deoxyuridine into DNA of mammalian tumor cells. *Biochem Biophys Res Commun.* 1981;102(2):654-658.

88. Longley DB, Harkin DP, Johnston PG. 5-Fluorouracil: mechanisms of action and clinical strategies. *Nat Rev Cancer.* 2003;3(5):330-338.

89. Meyerhardt JA, Mayer RJ. Systemic therapy for colorectal cancer. *N Engl J Med.* 2005;352(5):476-487.

90. Berger SH, Jenh CH, Johnson LF, Berger FG. Thymidylate synthase overproduction and gene amplification in fluorodeoxyuridine-resistant human cells. *Mol Pharmacol.* 1985;28(5):461-467.

91. Johnston PG, Drake JC, Trepel J, Allegra CJ. Immunological quantitation of thymidylate synthase using the monoclonal antibody TS 106 in 5-fluorouracil-sensitive and -resistant human cancer cell lines. *Cancer Res.* 1992;52(16):4306-4312.

92. Sulzyc-Bielicka V, Bielicki D, Binczak-Kuleta A, et al. Thymidylate synthase gene polymorphism and survival of colorectal cancer patients receiving adjuvant 5-fluorouracil. *Genet Test Mol Biomarkers.* 2013;17(11):799-806.

93. Popat S, Matakidou A, Houlston RS. Thymidylate synthase expression and prognosis in colorectal cancer: a systematic review and meta-analysis. *J Clin Oncol.* 2004;22(3):529-536.

94. Leichman CG, Lenz HJ, Leichman L, et al. Quantitation of intratumoral thymidylate synthase expression predicts for disseminated colorectal cancer response and resistance to protracted-infusion fluorouracil and weekly leucovorin. *J Clin Oncol.* 1997;15(10):3223-3229.

95. Iacopetta B, Grieu F, Joseph D, Elsaleh H. A polymorphism in the enhancer region of the thymidylate synthase promoter influences the survival of colorectal cancer patients treated with 5-fluorouracil. *Br J Cancer.* 2001;85(6):827-830.

96. Edler D, Glimelius B, Hallström M, et al. Thymidylate synthase expression in colorectal cancer: a prognostic and predictive marker of benefit from adjuvant fluorouracil-based chemotherapy. *J Clin Oncol.* 2002;20(7):1721-1728.

97. Kawakami K, Watanabe G. Identification and functional analysis of single nucleotide polymorphism in the tandem repeat sequence of thymidylate synthase gene. *Cancer Res.* 2003;63(18):6004-6007.

98. Tsuji T, Hidaka S, Sawai T, et al. Polymorphism in the thymidylate synthase promoter enhancer region is not an efficacious marker for tumor sensitivity to 5-fluorouracil-based oral adjuvant chemotherapy in colorectal cancer. *Clin Cancer Res.* 2003;9:3700-3704.

99. Prall F, Ostwald C, Schiffmann L, Barten M. Do thymidylate synthase gene promoter polymorphism and the C/G single nucleotide polymorphism predict effectiveness of adjuvant 5-fluorouracil-based chemotherapy in stage III colonic adenocarcinoma? *Oncol Rep* 2007;18(1):203-209.

100. Popat S, Wort R, Houlston RS. Inter-relationship between microsatellite instability, thymidylate synthase expression, and p53 status in colorectal cancer: implications for chemoresistance. *BMC Cancer* 2006;6:150.

101. Kristensen MH, Weidinger M, Bzorek M, Pedersen PL, Mejer J. Correlation between thymidylate synthase gene variants, RNA and protein levels in primary colorectal adenocarcinomas. *J Int Med Res*. 2010;38(2):484-497.

102. Hoff PM, Ansari R, Batist G, et al. Comparison of oral capecitabine versus intravenous fluorouracil plus leucovorin as first-line treatment in 605 patients with metastatic colorectal cancer: results of a randomized phase III study. *J Clin Oncol*. 2001;19(8):2282-2292.

103. Van Cutsem E, Twelves C, Cassidy J, et al. Oral capecitabine compared with intravenous fluorouracil plus leucovorin in patients with metastatic colorectal cancer: results of a large phase III study. *J Clin Oncol*. 2001;19(21):4097-4106.

104. Koopman M, Antonini NF, Douma J, et al. Sequential versus combination chemotherapy with capecitabine, irinotecan, and oxaliplatin in advanced colorectal cancer (CAIRO): a phase III randomised controlled trial. *Lancet*. 2007;370(9582):135-142.

105. Tuchman M, Stoeckeler JS, Kiang DT, O'Dea RF, Ramnaraine ML, Mirkin BL. Familial pyrimidinemia and pyrimidinuria associated with severe fluorouracil toxicity. *N Engl J Med*. 1985;313(4):245-249.

106. Deenen MJ, Meulendijks D, Cats A, et al. Upfront genotyping of DPYD*2A to individualize fluoropyrimidine therapy: a safety and cost analysis. *J Clin Oncol*. 2016;34(3):227-234.

107. de Gramont A, Figer A, Seymour M, et al. Leucovorin and fluorouracil with or without oxaliplatin as first-line treatment in advanced colorectal cancer. *J Clin Oncol*. 2000;18:2938-2947.

108. Kuebler JP, Wieand HS, O'Connell MJ, et al. Oxaliplatin combined with weekly bolus fluorouracil and leucovorin as surgical adjuvant chemotherapy for stage II and III colon cancer: results from NSABP C-07. *J Clin Oncol*. 2007;25:2198-2204.

109. Chaney SG, Campbell SL, Bassett E, Wu Y. Recognition and processing of cisplatin- and oxaliplatin-DNA adducts. *Crit Rev Oncol Hematol* 2005;53(1):3-11.

110. Zaanan A, Meunier K, Sangar F, Fléjou JF, Praz F. Microsatellite instability in colorectal cancer: from molecular oncogenic mechanisms to clinical implications. *Cell Oncol (Dordr)*. 2011;34(3):155-176.

111. Yin M, Yan J, Martinez-Balibrea E, et al. ERCC1 and ERCC2 polymorphisms predict clinical outcomes of oxaliplatin-based chemotherapies in gastric and colorectal cancer: a systemic review and meta-analysis. *Clin Cancer Res*. 2011;17(6):1632-1640.

112. Stoehlmacher J, Ghaderi V, Iobal S, et al. A polymorphism of the XRCC1 gene predicts for response to platinum based treatment in advanced colorectal cancer. *Anticancer Res*. 2001;21(4B):3075-3079.

113. Lv H, Li Q, Qiu W, et al. Genetic polymorphism of XRCC1 correlated with response to oxaliplatin-based chemotherapy in advanced colorectal cancer. *Pathol Oncol Res*. 2012;18(4):1009-1014.

114. Stoehlmacher J, Park DJ, Zhang W, et al. Association between glutathione S-transferase P1, T1, and M1 genetic polymorphism and survival of patients with metastatic colorectal cancer. *J Natl Cancer Inst*. 2002;94(12):936-942.

115. Stoehlmacher J, Park DJ, Zhang W, et al. A multivariate analysis of genomic polymorphisms: prediction of clinical outcome to 5-FU/oxaliplatin combination chemotherapy in refractory colorectal cancer. *Br J Cancer*. 2004;91(2):344-354.

116. Chen YC, Tzeng CH, Chen PM, et al. Influence of GSTP1 105V polymorphism on cumulative neuropathy and outcome of FOLFOX-4 treatment in Asian patients with colorectal carcinoma. *Cancer Sci* 2010;101(2):530-535.

117. Zaanan A, Dalban C, Emile JF, et al. ERCC1, XRCC1 and GSTP1 single nucleotide polymorphisms and survival of patients with colon cancer receiving oxaliplatin-based adjuvant chemotherapy. *J Cancer*. 2014;5(6):425-432.

118. Berardi R, Maccaroni E, Onofri A, et al. Locally advanced rectal cancer: the importance of a multidisciplinary approach. *World J Gastroenterol*. 2014;20(46):17279-17287.

119. Heald RJ, Ryall RD. Recurrence and survival after total mesorectal excision for rectal cancer. *Lancet*. 1986;1(8496):1479-1482.

120. Arbman G, Nilsson E, Hallböök O, Sjödahl R. Local recurrence following total mesorectal excision for rectal cancer. *Br J Surg*. 1996;83(3):375-379.

121. Kapiteijn E, Putter H, van de Velde CJ. Impact of the introduction and training of total mesorectal excision on recurrence and survival in rectal cancer in The Netherlands. *Br J Surg*. 2002;89(9):1142-1149.

122. Wibe A, Møller B, Norstein J, et al. A national strategic change in treatment policy for rectal cancer—implementation of total mesorectal excision as routine treatment in Norway. A national audit. *Dis Colon Rectum*. 2002;45(7):857-866.

123. Martling A, Holm T, Rutqvist LE, et al. Impact of a surgical training programme on rectal cancer outcomes in Stockholm. *Br J Surg*. 2005;92(2):225-229.

124. MERCURY Study Group. Diagnostic accuracy of preoperative magnetic resonance imaging in predicting curative resection of rectal cancer: prospective observational study. *BMJ*. 2006;333(7572):779.

125. Taylor FG, Quirke P, Heald RJ, et al. Preoperative magnetic resonance imaging assessment of circumferential resection margin predicts disease-free survival and local recurrence: 5-year follow-up results of the MERCURY study. *J Clin Oncol*. 2014;32(1):34-43.

126. Brenner H, Kloor M, Pox CP. Colorectal cancer. *Lancet*. 2014; 383(9927):1490-1502.

127. Richardson B, Preskitt J, Lichliter W, et al. The effect of multidisciplinary teams for rectal cancer on delivery of care and patient outcome: has the utilization of multidisciplinary teams for rectal cancer affected the utilization of available resources, proportion of patients meeting the standard of care, and does this translate into changes in patient outcome? *Am J Surg*. 2016;211(1):46-52.

128. Burton S, Brown G, Daniels IR, et al. MRI directed multidisciplinary team preoperative treatment strategy: the way to eliminate positive circumferential margins? *Br J Cancer*. 2006;94(3):351-357.

129. Wille-Jørgensen P, Sparre P, Glenthøj A, et al. Result of the implementation of multidisciplinary teams in rectal cancer. *Colorectal Dis*. 2013;15(4):410-413.

130. Sauer R, Liersch T, Merkel S, et al. Preoperative versus postoperative chemoradiotherapy for locally advanced rectal cancer: results of the German CAO/ARO/AIO-94 randomized phase III trial after a median follow-up of 11 years. *J Clin Oncol*. 2012;30(16):1926-1933.

131. Kapiteijn E, Marijnen CA, Nagtegaal ID, et al. Preoperative radiotherapy combined with total mesorectal excision for resectable rectal cancer. *N Engl J Med*. 2001;345(9):638-646.

132. Peeters KC, van de Velde CJ, Leer JW, et al. Late side effects of short-course preoperative radiotherapy combined with total mesorectal excision for rectal cancer: increased bowel dysfunction in irradiated patients—a Dutch colorectal cancer group study. *J Clin Oncol*. 2005;23(25):6199-6206.

133. Bujko K, Nowacki MP, Nasierowska Guttmejer A, Michalski W, Bebenek M, Kryj M. Long-term results of a randomized trial comparing preoperative short-course radiotherapy with preoperative conventionally fractionated chemoradiation for rectal cancer. *Br J Surg*. 2006;93(10):1215-1223.

134. Ngan SY, Burmeister B, Fisher RJ, et al. Randomized trial of short-course radiotherapy versus long-course chemoradiation comparing rates of local recurrence in patients with T3 rectal cancer: Trans-Tasman Radiation Oncology Group trial 01.04. *J Clin Oncol*. 2012;30:3827-3833.

135. Bujko K. Short-course preoperative radiotherapy for low rectal cancer. *J Clin Oncol*. 2013;31(14):1799.

136. Tan D, Glynne-Jones R. But some neoadjuvant schedules are more equal than others. *J Clin Oncol*. 2013;31(14):1799-1800.

137. Fernández-Martos C, Nogué M, Cejas P, Moreno-García V, Machengs AH, Feliu J. The role of capecitabine in locally advanced rectal cancer treatment: an update. *Drugs*. 2012;72(8):1057-1073.

138. Hofheinz RD, Wenz F, Post S, et al. Chemoradiotherapy with capecitabine versus fluorouracil for locally advanced rectal cancer: a randomised, multicentre, non-inferiority, phase 3 trial. *Lancet Oncol*. 2012;13(6):579-588.

139. Chau I, Brown G, Cunningham D, et al. Neoadjuvant capecitabine and oxaliplatin followed by synchronous chemoradiation and total mesorectal excision in magnetic resonance imaging-defined poor-risk rectal cancer. *J Clin Oncol*. 2006;24(4):668-674.

140. Fernández-Martos C, Pericay C, Aparicio J, et al. Phase II, randomized study of concomitant chemoradiotherapy followed by surgery and adjuvant capecitabine plus oxaliplatin (CAPOX) compared with

induction CAPOX followed by concomitant chemoradiotherapy and surgery in magnetic resonance imaging–defined, locally advanced rectal cancer: Grupo Cancer de Recto 3 study. *J Clin Oncol.* 2010;28(5):859-865.

141. Schrag D, Weiser MR, Goodman KA, et al. Neoadjuvant chemotherapy without routine use of radiation therapy for patients with locally advanced rectal cancer: a pilot trial. *J Clin Oncol.* 2014;32(6): 513-518.

142. Nogué M, Salud A, Vicente P, et al. Addition of bevacizumab to XELOX induction therapy plus concomitant capecitabine-based chemoradiotherapy in magnetic resonance imaging–defined poor-prognosis locally advanced rectal cancer: the AVACROSS study. *Oncologist.* 2011;16(5):614-620.

143. Dewdney A, Cunningham D, Tabernero J, et al. Multicenter randomized phase II clinical trial comparing neoadjuvant oxaliplatin, capecitabine, and preoperative radiotherapy with or without cetuximab followed by total mesorectal excision in patients with high-risk rectal cancer (EXPERT-C). *J Clin Oncol.* 2012;30(14): 1620-1627.

144. Dipetrillo T, Pricolo V, Lagares-Garcia J, et al. Neoadjuvant bevacizumab, oxaliplatin, 5-fluorouracil, and radiation for rectal cancer. *Int J Radiat Oncol Biol Phys.* 2012;82(1):124-129.

145. Torino F, Sarmiento R, Gasparini G. The contribution of targeted therapy to the neoadjuvant chemoradiation of rectal cancer. *Crit Rev Oncol Hematol.* 2013;87(3):283-305.

146. Maring ED, Tawadros PS, Steer CJ, Lee JT. Systematic review of candidate single-nucleotide polymorphisms as biomarkers for responsiveness to neoadjuvant chemoradiation for rectal cancer. *Anticancer Res.* 2015;35(7):3761-3766.

147. Benson AB 3rd, Bekaii-Saab T, Chan E, et al. Rectal cancer. *J Natl Compr Canc Netw.* 2012;10(12):1528-1564.

148. Peterson SH, Harling H, Kirkeby L, Wille-Jørgensen P, Mocellin S. Postoperative adjuvant chemotherapy in rectal cancer operated for cure. *Cochrane Database Syst Rev.* 2012;3:CD4078.

149. West NP, Finan PJ, Anderin C, Lindholm J, Holm T, Quirke P. Evidence of the oncologic superiority of cylindrical abdominoperineal excision for low rectal cancer. *J Clin Oncol.* 2008;26(21):3517-3522.

150. Van Schaeybroeck S, Kyula JN, Fenton A, et al. Oncogenic KRAS promotes chemotherapy-induced growth factor shedding via ADAM17. *Cancer Res.* 2011;71(3):1071-1080.

Prevention, Diagnosis, and Management of Anastomotic Leak

Walter R. Peters Jr. | Nathan Smallwood | Neil H. Hyman

INCIDENCE AND CONSEQUENCES OF ANASTOMOTIC LEAK

Anastomotic leak is perhaps the most physiologically significant and psychologically devastating complication that commonly occurs following operations for colon or rectal disease. The reported incidence of anastomotic leak following colorectal surgery has varied from 1% to 30%, largely based on the criteria for diagnosis and the length of follow-up; the highest leak rate is seen with anastomoses involving the distal rectum.[1,2] Leaks account for one-third of all deaths following low anterior resection, with even higher mortality rates observed with intraperitoneal leaks.[2] Anastomotic leaks are associated with dramatically increased perioperative morbidity and mortality, prolonged length of stay, higher readmission rates the potential need for multiple operative interventions in a hostile surgical environment and unintended permanent stomas. This results in significantly increased hospital costs and resource use, decreased quality of life, and potentially worse oncologic outcomes.[3–7]

DEFINITION OF ANASTOMOTIC LEAK

Historically, studies of the incidence and etiology of anastomotic leak have been hindered by a lack of a consensus definition of anastomotic leak. There are a broad array of clinical scenarios that could reasonably be described as representing or caused by an overt or occult disruption/imperfection in the anastomotic site e.g., postoperative abscess).[8] This has often made comparative analyses between institutions and among surgeons a largely arbitrary and unreliable exercise. In 2010 the International Study Group of Rectal Cancer proposed a uniform definition of anastomotic leak as a defect at the anastomotic site leading to a communication between the intraluminal and extraluminal compartments. This communication can be confirmed radiographically, endoscopically, or intraoperatively. A pelvic abscess in close proximity to the anastomosis is also considered an anastomotic leak. The group also defined the severity of anastomotic leaks based upon the clinical management required. Grade A leaks

are those managed without an invasive intervention, grade B leaks are those managed with invasive intervention other than a laparotomy (e.g., percutaneous drainage), and grade C leaks are those requiring laparotomy.[9]

PREVENTION

Discussion of anastomotic leak prevention has generally centered around risk factors associated with anastomotic leak and/or mechanical means to increase anastomotic strength. Both of these areas of inquiry have contributed to only a limited understanding of the actual mechanism by which leaks occur and how best to prevent them. The reported risk factors vary greatly from study to study, and it can be challenging to know which clinical features are simply associated with a greater tendency for a leak and which may serve as a surrogate for some other factor that is of pathogenic importance.

For decades, studies have focused on the technical aspects of anastomotic creation, considering such issues as sutures versus staples versus compression, single- versus two-layer construction, inverted versus everted technique, and the merits of a wide variety of mechanical devices designed to strengthen or protect the anastomosis, usually finding minimal impact on the incidence of anastomotic leaks. This structural framework of understanding has not appreciably moved the needle in preventing this devastating complication; it seems clear that new paradigms are needed. In this light, the possible role of the microbiome and collagenolytic bacteria in causing anastomotic leaks is intriguing.[10] Certainly the historical admonitions of attention to detail, avoidance of tension, and assurance of adequate blood supply seem prudent, but the fact remains that anastomotic leaks still most commonly occur in anastomoses that have no evidence of ischemia, are under no tension, and have been carefully tested for structural defects.

PREOPERATIVE AND PERIOPERATIVE ENTERAL NUTRITION

Preoperative malnutrition has been identified as a major risk factor for anastomotic leaks, whether defined generally by low preoperative serum albumin and total protein or more specifically by weight loss of 10% or more, serum albumin less than 3.5 g/dL, and serum protein less than 5.5 g/dL.[11–14] Identifying those patients with diminished nutritional status and treating them perioperatively with nutritional repletion may reduce the risk of, and the morbidity and mortality from, anastomotic leakage.[11]

INTRAOPERATIVE ASSESSMENT

Laser Fluorescence Angiography

Adequate blood supply has long been highlighted as critical for proper healing of an anastomosis. Less obvious is the amount of blood flow that represents a critical threshold for adequate healing to occur. Traditionally, perfusion has been assessed through visual inspection for color and bleeding of the cut edges, fluorescein dye angiography with a Wood lamp, or presence of pulsatile flow identified by palpation or Doppler ultrasound. More recently, the use of intraoperative laser fluorescence angiography with indocyanine green dye (ICG-FA) has been used by surgeons to assess tissue perfusion. ICG-FA is performed by administering indocyanine green intravenously, then assessing tissue perfusion with a near-infrared imaging system. Perfusion may be assessed before transecting the bowel or after completion of the anastomosis.

Currently, assessment of fluorescence intensity is subjective, and it may be unclear when a change in the surgical plan is appropriate based on the image. This may be no small matter in selected circumstances, such as a low pelvic anastomosis where further resection to an area of "improved" perfusion may require extensive additional mobilization and potentially result in the unintended consequence of increased tension on the anastomosis. A systematic review of 12 different randomized studies suggested that ICG-FA may reduce the risk of anastomotic leakage; however, given the heterogeneity of study designs and lack of high-quality evidence, the review was considered inconclusive for the existence of any actual clinical benefit.[15] Data assessing the potential benefit of ICG-FA will be forthcoming from a randomized controlled, parallel, multicenter study assessing perfusion outcomes in patients with rectal cancer undergoing a low anterior resection (PILLAR III trial).

Air Leak Test

Air leak testing involves filling the pelvis with warm saline followed by distention of the newly created anastomosis with air. A randomized controlled study supports the use of air leak testing; the leak rate was reduced from 14% to 4%, presumably by identifying and remediating technically imperfect anastomoses.[16] Based upon the results of a large cohort study of 825 patients, patients with positive air leak tests treated with suture repair had higher clinical leak rates (12.2%) than patients who received a diverting stoma (0%) or underwent reanastomosis (0%).[17] The key in this setting is a sober and objective assessment of the problem and the prospects for repair. If a well-localized and clearly defined defect is identified in an otherwise healthy anastomosis, suture repair with repeat testing of the anastomosis is appropriate. However, when exposure is suboptimal and the defect cannot be clearly visualized to enable an accurate repair, the anastomosis should be redone and/or the patient diverted.

Dye Test

A dye test can be performed by injecting a mixture of sterile water and blue dye or povidone-iodine (Betadine) through a large-bore catheter placed transanally, while clamping the proximal bowel. A volume of 180 to 240 mL is usually required to adequately distend the anastomosis. One study has shown that the dye test allowed for the easier detection and localization of leaks than air leak testing.[18]

Endoscopy

Intraoperative endoscopic visualization of the anastomosis allows surgeons to assess for mucosal viability, staple line disruptions, or bleeding and provides the ability to intervene immediately if necessary. Although intraoperative endoscopy provides a useful adjunct to air leak testing, there is currently no evidence that its use alone results in fewer anastomotic complications.[19] As with ICG-FA, objective endoscopic criteria are lacking to assess the quality of the anastomosis and guide intraoperative decision making.[20]

DRAINS

The use of prophylactic intraperitoneal drains has been extensively debated. An accurate assessment of benefit has been difficult due to variation in the types of drains used, their location, and the duration of their use. There is extensive evidence that draining an intraperitoneal anastomosis is of no benefit.[21] However, as compared with the abdominal cavity, fluid is much more likely to accumulate in the dependent area of the pelvis, and using pelvic drains after low anterior resection may be of greater utility because the nonperitonealized pelvic floor fails to absorb fluid efficiently.[22,23] However, it remains unclear how effectively pelvic drains manage to remove this fluid and whether they really provide any benefit. Current evidence suggests that routine prophylactic drainage does not reduce postoperative anastomotic complications.[24,25] Another suggested benefit of placing drains near a pelvic anastomosis is the early detection of an anastomotic leak prior to the onset of symptoms. Unfortunately, many leaks do not present themselves through a surgical drain, and surgeons often remove drains early in the postoperative period, before a leak might manifest itself.[26]

DIVERTING STOMAS

Benefits of Diversion

Fecal diversion through the creation of a proximal loop colostomy or loop ileostomy is commonly used in patients felt to be at a high risk for an anastomotic leak. The precise indications for a diverting stoma to protect a distal anastomosis continue to be actively debated. A Cochrane review has shown that fecal diversion does indeed reduce the risk of clinically symptomatic leaks and the need for urgent reoperation in patients undergoing anterior resection for rectal cancer.[27] The incidence of clinical leak was reduced from 19.6% to 6.3% in diverted patients, with an even greater reduction in the need for urgent reoperation. Proximal diversion has been shown to reduce the risk of severe septic complications in cancer patients undergoing coloanal anastomosis but also increased the risk of acute renal failure.[28]

Complications of Diversion

Despite the acknowledged potential benefits, a diverting stoma significantly impacts quality of life and subjects patients to significant potential morbidity, including skin problems, dehydration, electrolyte abnormalities, and mechanical obstruction. Indeed, a 17% readmission rate has been observed in patients with a diverting stoma following low anterior resection.[29] Ostomies can be particularly problematic in certain subsets of patients, including those with morbid obesity, chronic renal insufficiency, or an inability to care for a stoma due to diminished vision or dexterity. Stoma-related complications have been shown to delay the initiation of adjuvant chemotherapy or necessitate the need for dose reduction. In addition, there is a 15% to 20% complication rate with ostomy closure. All of these issues have been shown to increase the average cost of a routinely diverted patient by $43,000.[30–32]

Decision to Divert

Because of the morbidity, cost, and dissatisfaction associated with diverting ostomies, it would be highly desirable to be able to identify those anastomoses that have a risk of leak sufficient to justify the creation of a stoma. The decision to create a diverting stoma must weigh the potentially devastating consequences of a leak with the morbidity associated with an ostomy. The appropriate decision for an individual patient should balance the surgeon's assessment of the risk of a leak, the potential for complications related to a stoma, and the anticipated consequence of a leak should one occur.

MECHANICAL BOWEL PREPARATION AND ORAL ANTIBIOTICS

Mechanical bowel preparation (MBP) alone does not impact the incidence of anastomotic leaks in elective colon resections.[33] Less certainty exists concerning the effectiveness of MBP alone in rectal resections. Although some studies have shown that MBP can be safely omitted in rectal resections, most studies have excluded patients with a rectal anastomosis.[34–36] However, there is a growing body of evidence that MBP, when given in combination with oral antibiotics, does significantly decrease the incidence of infectious complications after colectomy, including anastomotic leak.[37–39]

There is no direct evidence to support the use of oral antibiotics alone because no trials have directly studied whether oral antibiotics given without MBP decrease the risk of infectious complications or anastomotic leak. The most familiar antibiotic regimen is that proposed by Condon, consisting of neomycin (1 g) and erythromycin (1 g) at 1:00, 2:00, and 10:00 pm.[40] Some have subsequently substituted metronidazole for erythromycin; erythromycin was initially chosen because of its activity against *Bacteroides fragilis* and its poor absorption leading to high intraluminal concentrations.[41] Although concerns have been raised that oral antibiotics might increase the occurrence of *Clostridium difficile* infections postoperatively, the majority

of studies have not shown this to be the case and actually have suggested a decreased incidence.[42–45]

OMENTOPLASTY

The use of an omental pedicle graft to protect a rectal anastomosis was described by Goldsmith in 1977.[46] Experimental studies have demonstrated the unique ability of the omentum to adhere to and effectively bridge the anastomosis, while also allowing for absorption of fluid.[47–49] A meta-analysis demonstrated a benefit to omental reinforcement of esophageal anastomoses, but no benefit has been found in colorectal anastomoses.[49] This may be due to inclusion of colocolic, as well as colorectal, anastomoses in the constituent studies; omental reinforcement may provide greater benefit for an extraperitoneal rectal anastomosis. In addition, the technique used has varied in these studies with inconsistent emphasis placed on suture fixation of the flap.[49–52] Further studies evaluating standardized techniques of omental reinforcement as originally described by Goldsmith would seem appropriate.

STAPLE-LINE REINFORCEMENT

Permanent, semiabsorbable, and absorbable materials have been used to reinforce the staple line and buttress a colonic anastomosis. However, neither Seamguard (W.L. Gore & Associates, Flagstaff, Arizona) nor meshed AlloDerm (Lifecell, Bridgewater, New Jersey) have been shown to improve the anastomotic strength experimentally.[53,54] Clinical data evaluating the use of such tissue-bolstering devices for a colorectal anastomosis are limited; two recent randomized controlled trials (RCTs) evaluating reinforcement with bioabsorbable material did not show any benefit in reducing anastomotic leaks.[55,56]

TRANSANAL DECOMPRESSION DEVICES

Transanal intraluminal devices have been proposed to prevent or reduce anastomotic leakage. Large-diameter rectal tubes made of soft rubber are placed above the anastomosis for 5 to 7 days in an attempt to decrease intraluminal pressure.[57] Although nonrandomized studies assessing transanal tube placement suggested a possible advantage, no benefit was seen when RCTs were performed.[57–59]

DIAGNOSIS

Early diagnosis of an anastomotic leak allows for timely management that may minimize the morbidity from septic complications.[60,61] Alves et al. found that the mortality rate increased from 0% to 18% if the diagnosis of a leak was made after the fifth postoperative day.[62] Studies using routine imaging or with a low threshold for endoscopic assessment of the anastomosis have suggested that most leaks could be diagnosed by the fifth postoperative day.[63]

A subset of patients with anastomotic leak present with the classic signs and symptoms of severe abdominal pain, diffuse peritonitis, and hemodynamic instability; the diagnosis of an anastomotic leak may be straightforward and readily apparent in this setting. However, anastomotic leaks more often present with a diverse array of cardiovascular, pulmonary, and gastrointestinal (GI) symptoms that are commonly seen in patients without a leak and which overlap clinically with a broad range of other postoperative complications. Signs and symptoms such as fever and leukocytosis, which may be considered indicative of a leak, are actually very common after colectomy. Indeed, the positive predictive value of abnormal vital signs after colon resection is only 4% to 11%.[64] Operatively placed drains may provide early clues to a leaking anastomosis but have never been proven to be able to reliably diagnose leaks.[26] Because signs and symptoms are nonspecific and often take time to progress, leaks may present clinically until weeks after the index operation. Up to 42% of patients are diagnosed only upon readmission after initial hospital discharge and may even be diagnosed months later in asymptomatic patients.[65,66]

After a patient has been diagnosed with a leak, it is often easy to point to a variety of suggestive factors in hindsight, but this really does not accurately capture and reflect the nuances and variability of the postoperative patient after colectomy. There is a critical need for more sensitive, specific, and predictive diagnostic markers that will enable earlier diagnosis and intervention.

IMAGING

The use of water-soluble contrast enemas has fallen out of favor due to the reported variability in sensitivity and overall accuracy in diagnosing leaks.[66] Computed tomography (CT) has assumed a major role in the diagnosis of postoperative complications, abscesses, and other fluid collections following abdominal and pelvic surgery. However, the sensitivity of CT in diagnosing anastomotic leakage may be as low as 68%.[67] When there is demonstrable extravasation of enteric contrast, the diagnosis is generally secure, but the ubiquitous finding of residual air and fluid collections in the postoperative patient reduces the accuracy of CT. Perianastomotic air/fluid levels appear to be the most reliable finding other than extravasation of contrast.[68–70]

Contrast extravasation on diagnostic CT scans in the setting of a colonic anastomotic leak can be as low as 15% to 17%.[67] Contrast extravasation on CT is more often identified in the setting of a rectal anastomotic leak, with a sensitivity and specificity of 83% and 97%, respectively.[67] The use of rectal contrast can reduce the number of false-negative or indeterminate CTs and the mean time to reoperation by almost 2 days.[68] As such, CT investigation of a rectal anastomosis for a suspected anastomotic leak should generally be performed with rectal contrast. The accurate assessment of more proximal anastomoses with or without enteric contrast remains more difficult.

BIOMARKERS

C-reactive protein (CRP) has been the most extensively studied biomarker. CRP is an inflammatory-induced marker with peak levels observed on the second postoperative day. Based upon a meta-analysis of 11 studies in more than 2500 patients, CRP values below specific cutoffs on postoperative days (PODs) 3 and 5 are rarely associated with an anastomotic leak. Unfortunately, cutoff levels have varied (range, 100 to 190 mg/L) between studies or between postoperative days within the same study. This lack of consistency detracts from the clinical utility of this marker. Furthermore, although low values may reliably

exclude a leak, the overall positive predictive value appears to be low (20.7%).[71] As such, higher levels of postoperative CRP require further investigation to confirm the presence of a leak.

Procalcitonin (PCT) is the prohormone of calcitonin with physiologic serum concentrations below 0.5 ng/mL; values in patients studied in the face of sepsis vary over an enormous range. A threshold of 2.0 ng/mL has been suggested as strongly indicative of sepsis.[72] PCT has a shorter induction period (4 to 12 hours) than CRP, and microbial infection stimulates the release of PCT from a wide variety of tissues for a sustained half-life of 22 to 35 hours.[72–75] PCT levels have been extensively studied and used in a wide variety of clinical scenarios, particularly in the critical care setting and for the monitoring of sepsis. Only recently have PCT levels been evaluated for use in colorectal surgery.

A recent meta-analysis demonstrated that low PCT levels on PODs 3 and 5 had high negative predictive values similar to CRP, and reliably excluded anastomotic leak.[71] As with CRP, the use of varying cutoff levels between studies and on different postoperative days within the same study diminishes the clinical utility of PCT monitoring. The importance of a single PCT level may be of far less significance than the changes in these levels over time, referred to as PCT kinetics. Studies have shown that the magnitude of decrease in PCT levels from admission through hospital days 3 to 5 could accurately predict survival in patients with sepsis and septic shock.[76–81] The predictive capabilities of PCT kinetics instead of isolated levels offers a potential area for future studies assessing the utility of PCT in the diagnosis of anastomotic leaks.

POSTOPERATIVE ENDOSCOPY

Endoscopy has become a commonly used diagnostic tool in evaluating an esophageal anastomosis for leak in the immediate postoperative period. Performance of endoscopy in the early postoperative period does not result in anastomotic complications or worsening of anastomotic dehiscence and appears superior to the use of contrast imaging.[82–84] In colorectal surgery, the use of postoperative endoscopy has been primarily limited to the treatment of known or suspected anastomotic leaks identified on imaging studies.

The safety and efficacy of endoscopic examination of colorectal anastomoses in the early postoperative period have been described by Ikeda.[63] In this study, endoscopic anastomotic evaluation was not routinely performed, but the authors had a low threshold for its use in any patient who was felt to have deviated from the normal postoperative course. Endoscopic examinations were performed in 41 out of 191 patients; an anastomotic leak was correctly diagnosed in 18 of 19 patients, resulting in a sensitivity, specificity, positive predictive value, and negative predictive value of 0.94, 0.95, 0.94, and 0.95, respectively. Endoscopic examination resulted in an early diagnosis of leak (POD 4) and was useful in the determination of subsequent therapeutic strategies.[63] The missed leak in this study underscores our limited knowledge and understanding of the normal appearance and changes that occur in colorectal anastomoses during the postoperative period. A better understanding of the "normal" healing process, as well as the distinguishing features that characterize an "at risk" anastomosis, would be of great value. Indeed, the anastomosis is typically the most important "wound" in a patient undergoing bowel resection; the practice of avoiding visual assessment of this wound for many weeks after the index procedure may need to be revisited.

MANAGEMENT

INITIAL RESUSCITATION OF THE SEPTIC PATIENT WITH A LEAK

A quantitative resuscitation protocol targeting specific physiologic goals, including urine output, mean arterial pressure, and serum lactate, should begin within 6 hours of the diagnosis of sepsis-induced tissue hypoperfusion. This type of resuscitation has been referred to as early goal-directed therapy (EGDT) and has been shown to significantly reduce mortality rates in patients with severe sepsis or septic shock.[35,86]

ANTIMICROBIAL THERAPY

In recognition of evidence that mortality rates continue to increase for every hour effective antimicrobial therapy is delayed, the 2012 Surviving Sepsis Guidelines recommended that antimicrobial therapy be started within the first hour following the diagnosis of severe sepsis or septic shock.[85] Appropriate empiric therapy is determined by the type, location, and severity of the involved infection, the pathogens most likely involved, and the presence of any risk factors associated with major resistance patterns. Anastomotic leaks are a type of hospital-acquired (nosocomial) infection that require broad-spectrum antimicrobials due to the increasing rates of multidrug-resistant organisms, including enterococci, *Pseudomonas*, and extended-spectrum β-lactamase–producing Enterobacteriaceae (ESBL-E).[85,87] The use of monotherapy often provides inadequate coverage; superior outcomes have been associated with combination therapy (≥2 different classes of antibiotics).[88,89] Combination therapy with imipenem or meropenem and amikacin was most recently recommended in the 2015 French Clinical Practice Guidelines.[88] Guidelines now also recommend the use of antifungal agents in patients with severe sepsis or septic shock and a postoperative intraabdominal infection.[85,83]

SOURCE CONTROL

Source control is defined as any intervention that is used to remove the focus of infection, prevent further contamination, and restore anatomic and physiologic function. Inadequate source control has a profound impact on patient survival following an anastomotic leak.[89,90] Failure to achieve source control is more likely to occur in patients with advanced age (>70 years), multiple comorbidities, higher severity of illness (APACHE II ≤15), and a greater degree of peritoneal involvement.[91] Early source control improves mortality by minimizing the duration of severe sepsis or septic shock and preventing the progression to multiple organ failure.[91] *Based upon current guidelines, it is recommended that an intervention to obtain source control be initiated within the first 12 hours after the diagnosis of severe sepsis or septic shock where possible.*[85]

Postoperative peritonitis most commonly occurs in patients with an anastomotic leak, although only a minority of leaks present in this manner. Patients with generalized peritonitis and/or signs of severe sepsis or septic shock typically require laparotomy with washout, débridement, and drainage to obtain source control. Some surgeons perform planned relaparotomies in patients with intra-abdominal sepsis because of the increased mortality seen in patients with inadequate source control. However, current evidence supports the use of relaparotomy only if it becomes clinically warranted. Unfortunately, there are very few reliable indicators of the need for repeat laparotomy very early in the postoperative period other than persistent peritonitis and continued severe sepsis or septic shock.[92,93] Patients in whom a relaparotomy was performed within 48 hours of their initial operation had lower mortality rates (28% vs. 77%) compared with patients whose relaparotomy was performed after 48 hours.[92]

Patients in whom source control cannot be achieved, and those with severe physiologic derangements or with hemodynamic instability, are best treated with an abbreviated laparotomy and temporary abdominal closure. This prevents further physiologic deterioration and allows for resuscitation in the intensive care setting. Definitive operation can then be performed at a later time under more favorable physiologic conditions.[94] Abbreviated laparotomies require that some form of temporary abdominal closure be used during the postoperative period. It is important that the method used for temporary abdominal closure protects the abdominal contents, prevents the formation of fistulas, continuously drains the peritoneal cavity, and facilitates the eventual definitive closure.[95]

Negative pressure wound therapy (NPWT) has become the most commonly used method of temporary closure and consists of a perforated plastic sheet covering the intestines with a polyurethane sponge placed between the fascial edges. The wound is covered with transparent draping to provide an airtight seal and a centrally applied suction drain is connected to a suction unit with a fluid collection system. Data from a number of prospective comparative studies have shown that compared with other methods of temporary abdominal closure, NPWT results in decreased mortality, increased fascial closure rates, and no increased risk of enteric fistula formation.[96,97]

ANASTOMOTIC SALVAGE VERSUS TAKEDOWN

Source control also includes measures to prevent further contamination from the anastomotic defect and restore anatomic structure and physiologic function. Management of the leaking anastomosis has been predominantly based on the surgeon's own personal experience because little evidence exists to help guide management. The most common approach consists of resecting the anastomosis and creating an end ostomy. This strategy results in a 2.5-fold increase in the rate of permanent fecal diversion when compared with anastomotic salvage using either a loop ostomy alone or in conjunction with repair or revision of the anastomosis.[98,99]

Based upon current evidence, patients with an intraperitoneal anastomosis that has a minor anastomotic defect (≤¼ circumference) and without purulent or feculent peritonitis may be safely managed with anastomotic salvage in combination with proximal loop diversion.[99] Some anastomotic leaks may lend themselves to resection and reanastomosis, with or without proximal diversion. The choice of technique should be made based on the location and extent of the anastomotic defect, the degree of peritonitis, and the physiologic condition of the patient.

A larger body of evidence supports the use of anastomotic salvage and loop diversion in patients with an extraperitoneal anastomosis (i.e., a low pelvic anastomosis). Reoperations for anastomotic leak typically take place in a hostile abdomen in the setting of a severe inflammatory response and are usually encumbered by the dense adhesions of the early postoperative period. In addition, the inflammatory reaction around the anastomotic leak commonly precludes safe surgical dissection. In these situations, the anastomosis should be left in place with drains placed in close proximity and a proximal diverting ostomy created. Anastomotic salvage with loop diversion resulted in statistically fewer postoperative deaths, recurrent sepsis, reoperations, and permanent stomas than anastomotic takedown.[98–101] There has been an associated increase in mortality when anastomotic repair is used without proximal diversion and therefore is not recommended for low pelvic anastomoses.[98,101]

NONOPERATIVE INTERVENTIONS

Between one-third to one-half of patients with leaks can be successfully treated without an operative intervention.[98,102] Patients who successfully undergo nonoperative management are more likely those who have lower severity leaks, have been previously diverted, and/or have an extraperitoneal anastomosis.[98,101,102] It should be noted that a protective stoma placed at the time of the initial operation may reduce the incidence of clinical leakage but is not significantly associated with decreased mortality rates in those patients who develop an anastomotic leak.[103,104]

It has been shown that in patients who receive nonoperative management, an interventional drainage procedure significantly lowers mortality rates as compared with medical treatment alone.[105] Percutaneous drainage, if technically feasible, is an effective therapy in many patients with anastomotic leaks who are hemodynamically stable and do not have signs of diffuse peritonitis, resulting in lower hospital costs and shorter hospital stays compared with surgical management. Unsuccessful outcomes are more likely in patients whose leaks are diagnosed early in the postoperative period, those associated with multiple abscesses, and those found to have a residual collection after initial percutaneous drainage.[106,107] Percutaneous transgluteal drainage of deep pelvic abscesses may be used but is often associated with significant discomfort both during the procedure and as long as the drain remains in place, a tendency for the catheter to kink in the supine patient, and the potential for development of gluteal abscesses.[108] Some collections located within the pelvis and inaccessible to a percutaneous abdominal approach are amenable to transanastomotic drainage, which may be often preferred over transgluteal drainage.

REESTABLISHING INTESTINAL CONTINUITY

Even with adequate source control and fecal diversion, many low pelvic leaks do not heal, leaving a chronic sinus tract and resulting in a permanent stoma in more than half of patients.[3] Leaks that do ultimately close are often associated with poor rectal function owing to chronic inflammation and fibrosis, resulting in loss of reservoir capacity.[109]

There is very little consensus regarding the optimal approach to restoring intestinal continuity in the setting of a chronic anastomotic sinus. Many surgeons continue to rely on a wait-and-see approach and follow the anastomosis expectantly. One potential drawback of this approach is that definitive treatment of the leak will be delayed in the patients whose leaks do not close on their own. This approach has been challenged by the emergence of therapies that may more actively promote closure of the leak.

ENDOLUMINAL VACUUM THERAPY

Endoscopic vacuum (E-Vac) therapy has been proposed as a method to overcome the limitations of conventional drainage therapy. E-Vac therapy provides for continuous and effective drainage of the perianastomotic abscess cavity, resulting in granulation tissue formation and wound contraction, which over time leads to closure of the cavity and defect. The Endo-Sponge (B Braun Melsungen AG, Melsungen, Germany) is a device that has been commercially available in Europe for more than a decade and has been used to treat GI leaks. It is not currently available in the United States. Others have modified the current Wound V.A.C. (Lifecell, Bridgewater, New Jersey) for off-label use as an internal negative pressure dressing, as first described by Weidenhagen in 2008.[110–116]

E-Vac therapy for cavities associated with anastomotic leaks involving the rectum has resulted in impressive closure rates (85.7%) and low permanent stoma rates (18.9%). The highest closure rates and lowest permanent stoma rates were seen in patients with proximal diverting stomas and/or early treatment (<6 weeks postoperatively). No deaths related to E-Vac therapy or anastomotic leak occurred following the initiation of therapy. Complications thought to be related to E-Vac therapy were infrequent and included recurrent abscesses, fistulas, and bleeding.[110–116] Unfortunately, the use of E-Vac is very time and resource intensive, requiring considerable patience and tenacity both on the part of the surgical endoscopist and the patient; patients should be counseled and informed of the expected number of endoscopic changes (7 to 11) and treatment duration (18 to 34 days) required for leak closure.[110–116] E-Vac therapy can be combined with marsupialization of the sinus tract or posterior extrarectal cavity to eventually heal the anastomotic area but only in the diverted patient. The end result is a diverticulum in the rectal wall, proximal to the anastomotic suture line, but this rarely impacts defecatory function.

STENTS

Although covered stents have been successfully used in the treatment of esophageal anastomotic leaks, the reported experience with their use in the lower GI tract has been relatively sparse. In the largest series to date, fully covered colonic stents were used in the treatment of 19 of 22 patients with colorectal anastomotic leaks.[117] In the remaining three patients, uncovered colonic stents were placed. The stents were placed with the lower end at least 1 cm above the dentate line to avoid postoperative rectal pain or tenesmus. Complete closure of the leak occurred in 19 of the 22 patients (86%), allowing for closure of the ostomy in all patients. In 15 patients, leaks were closed after an average time of 3 months; four additional patients required a second stent. All 19 patients initially experienced incontinence that eventually resolved after an average of 14 weeks.[117] Other studies have shown varying degrees of success in the use of stents to treat colorectal anastomotic leaks.[118,119] Unfortunately, migration remains an issue and in the vast majority of patients, additional procedures to provide drainage are needed.[117–119]

REOPERATIVE SURGERY

Reoperative surgery is often required in patients who have suffered an anastomotic leak to restore intestinal continuity, often by resecting and then creating a new anastomosis. In patients with an anastomotic leak or fistula that have failed other therapies, reoperation has been successful in restoring intestinal continuity in up to 78% of patients.[100,120–122] Reconstructive surgery is typically very challenging even for the experienced surgeon and is associated with substantial risk of intraoperative and postoperative morbidity, for which further surgical intervention is required in 10% of patients.[100,120–122] Therefore reoperative surgery should only be considered in patients with few comorbidities who would be at a low risk of postoperative mortality. Patients need to be highly motivated to have their ostomy closed and must have a complete understanding of the risk of complications the potential need for further surgery, and the possibility of poor bowel function. Finally, reconstructive surgery after a failed low pelvic anastomosis is technically demanding and requires familiarity with an array of advanced techniques needed to mobilize the colon to achieve adequate length and to create a new anastomosis, including Turnbull-Cutait delayed anastomosis or the Soave procedure.[120–122]

SUMMARY

Anastomotic leaks have significant consequences for patients and the surgeons who care for them. Prevention of anastomotic leaks will require improved understanding of the actual mechanisms by which they occur. Early detection, perhaps by more aggressive use of endoscopy or biomarkers of inflammation, may diminish the deleterious effects of a leak and allow for greater use of nonsurgical treatments. Reduction in the frequency and severity of complications due to anastomotic leak may eventually allow surgeons to move away from the current liberal use of "temporary" diverting stomas, which are, in and of themselves, a source of substantial physical and psychological morbidity and expense.

REFERENCES

1. Kingham TP, Pachter HL. Colonic anastomotic leak: risk factors, diagnosis, and treatment. *J Am Coll Surg.* 2009;208(2):269-278.
2. Snijders HS, Wouters M, Van Leersum NJ, et al. Meta-analysis of the risk for anastomotic leakage, the postoperative mortality caused by leakage in relation to the overall postoperative mortality. *Eur J Surg Oncol.* 2012;38(11):1013-1019.

3. Lindgren R, Hallböök O, Rutegård J, Sjödahl R, Matthiessen P. What is the risk for a permanent stoma after low anterior resection of the rectum for cancer? A six-year follow-up of a multicenter trial. *Dis Colon Rectum.* 2011;54(1):41-47.
4. Ogilvie JW Jr, Dietz DW, Stocchi L. Anastomotic leak after restorative proctosigmoidectomy for cancer: what are the chances of a permanent ostomy? *Int J Colorectal Dis.* 2012;27(10):1259-1266.
5. Nesbakken A, Nygaard K, Lunde OC. Outcome and late functional results after anastomotic leakage following mesorectal excision for rectal cancer. *Br J Surg.* 2001;88(3):400-404.
6. Paun BC, Cassie S, MacLean AR, Dixon E, Buie WD. Postoperative complications following surgery for rectal cancer. *Ann Surg.* 2010; 251(5):807-818.
7. Hammond J, Lim S, Wan Y, Gao X, Patkar A. The burden of gastrointestinal anastomotic leaks: an evaluation of clinical and economic outcomes. *J Gastrointest Surg.* 2014;18(6):1176-1185.
8. Bruce J, Krukowski ZH, Al-Khairy G, Russell EM, Park KGM. Systematic review of the definition and measurement of anastomotic leak after gastrointestinal surgery. *Br J Surg.* 2001;88(9):1157-1168.
9. Rahbari NN, Weitz J, Hohenberger W, et al. Definition and grading of anastomotic leakage following anterior resection of the rectum: a proposal by the International Study Group of Rectal Cancer. *Surgery.* 2010;147(3):339-351.
10. Shogan BD, Belogortseva N, Luong PM, et al. Collagen degradation and MMP9 activation by *Enterococcus faecalis* contribute to intestinal anastomotic leak. *Sci Transl Med.* 2015;7(286):286ra68.
11. Frasson M, Granero-Castro P, Rodriguez JLR, et al. Risk factors for anastomotic leak and postoperative morbidity and mortality after elective right colectomy for cancer: results from a prospective, multicentric study of 1102 patients. *Int J Colorectal Dis.* 2015;31(1): 105-114.
12. Telem DA, Chin EH, Nguyen SQ, Divino CM. Risk factors for anastomotic leak following colorectal surgery: a case-control study. *Arch Surg.* 2010;145(4):371-376.
13. Golub R, Golub RW, Cantu R Jr, Stein HD. A multivariate analysis of factors contributing to leakage of intestinal anastomoses. *J Am Coll Surg.* 1997;184(4):364-372.
14. Jie B, Jiang Z-M, Nolan MT, Zhu S-N, Yu K, Kondrup J. Impact of preoperative nutritional support on clinical outcome in abdominal surgical patients at nutritional risk. *Nutrition.* 2012;28(10):1022-1027.
15. Degett TH, Andersen HS, Gögenur I. Indocyanine green fluorescence angiography for intraoperative assessment of gastrointestinal anastomotic perfusion: a systematic review of clinical trials. *Langenbecks Arch Surg.* 2016;401:1-9.
16. Beard JD, Nicholson ML, Sayers RD, Lloyd D, Everson NW. Intraoperative air testing of colorectal anastomoses: a prospective, randomized trial. *Br J Surg.* 1990;77(10):1095-1097.
17. Ivanov D, Cvijanovic R, Gvozdenovic L. Intraoperative air testing of colorectal anastomoses. *Srp Arh Celok Lek.* 2011;139(5-6):333-338.
18. Chen CW, Chen MJ, Yeh YS, Tsai HL, Chang YT, Wang JY. Intraoperative anastomotic dye test significantly decreases incidence of anastomotic leaks in patients undergoing resection for rectal cancer. *Tech Coloproctol.* 2013;17(5):579-583.
19. Nachiappan S, Askari A, Currie A, Kennedy RH, Faiz O. Intraoperative assessment of colorectal anastomotic integrity: a systematic review. *Surg Endosc.* 2014;28(9):2513-2530.
20. Ghole S, Nguyen A, Jafari M, et al. Going beyond the air leak test—our initial experience with a new grading system utilizing flexible endoscopy for the intraoperative evaluation of rectal anastomoses. *Dis Colon Rectum.* 2013;56:e28 -e282.
21. Karliczek A, Jesus EC, Matos D, Castro AA, Atallah AN, Wiggers T. Drainage or nondrainage in elective colorectal anastomosis: a systematic review and meta-analysis. *Colorectal Dis.* 2006;8(4):259-265.
22. Nisar PJ, Lavery IC, Kiran RP. Influence of neoadjuvant radiotherapy on anastomotic leak after restorative resection for rectal cancer. *J Gastrointest Surg.* 2012;16(9):1750-1757.
23. Tsujinaka S, Kawamura YJ, Konishi F, Maeda T, Mizokami K. Pelvic drainage for anterior resection revisited: use of drains in anastomotic leaks. *ANZ J Surg.* 2008;78(6):461-465.
24. Urbach DR, Kennedy ED, Cohen MM. Colon and rectal anastomoses do not require routine drainage: a systematic review and meta-analysis. *Ann Surg.* 1999;229(2):174.
25. Zhang HY, Zhao CL, Xie J, et al. To drain or not to drain in colorectal anastomosis: a meta-analysis. *Int J Colorectal Dis.* 2016; 31(5):951-960.

26. Tsujinaka S, Konishi F. Drain vs no drain after colorectal surgery. *Indian J Surg Oncol.* 2011;2(1):3-8.

27. Montedori A, Cirocchi R, Farinella E, Sciannameo F, Abraha I. Covering ileo- or colostomy in anterior resection for rectal carcinoma. *Cochrane Libr.* 2010;(5):CD006878.

28. Nurkin S, Kakarla VR, Ruiz DE, Cance WG, Tiszenkel HI. The role of faecal diversion in low rectal cancer: a review of 1791 patients having rectal resection with anastomosis for cancer, with and without a proximal stoma. *Colorectal Dis.* 2013;15(6):e309-e316.

29. Messaris E, Sehgal R, Deiling S, et al. Dehydration is the most common indication for readmission after diverting ileostomy creation. *Dis Colon Rectum.* 2012;55(2):175-180.

30. Robertson JP, Wells CI, Vather R, Bissett IP. Effect of diversion ileostomy on the occurrence and consequences of chemotherapy-induced diarrhea. *Dis Colon Rectum.* 2016;59(3):194-200.

31. Bakx R, Busch ORC, Bemelman WA, Veldink GJ, Slors JFM, Van Lanschot JJB. Morbidity of temporary loop ileostomies. *Dig Surg.* 2004;21(4):277-281.

32. Stey AM, Brook RH, Keeler E, Harris MT, Heimann T, Steinhagen RM. Outcomes and cost of diverted versus undiverted restorative proctocolectomy. *J Gastrointest Surg.* 2014;18(5):995-1002.

33. Cao F, Li J, Li F. Mechanical bowel preparation for elective colorectal surgery: updated systematic review and meta-analysis. *Int J Colorectal Dis.* 2012;27(6):803-810.

34. Bretagnol F, Alves A, Ricci A, Valleur P, Panis Y. Rectal cancer surgery without mechanical bowel preparation. *Br J Surg.* 2007;94(10): 1266-1271.

35. Vlot EA, Zeebregts CJ, Gerritsen JJ, Mulder HJ, Mastboom WJ, Klaase JM. Anterior resection of rectal cancer without bowel preparation and diverting stoma. *Surg Today.* 2005;35(8):629-633.

36. Bretagnol F, Panis Y, Rullier E, et al. Rectal cancer surgery with or without bowel preparation: the French GRECCAR III multicenter single-blinded randomized trial. *Ann Surg.* 2010;252(5): 863-868.

37. Kiran RP, Murray AC, Chiuzan C, Estrada D, Forde K. Combined preoperative mechanical bowel preparation with oral antibiotics significantly reduces surgical site infection, anastomotic leak, and ileus after colorectal surgery. *Ann Surg.* 2015;262(3):416-425.

38. Scarborough JE, Mantyh CR, Sun Z, Migaly J. Combined mechanical and oral antibiotic bowel preparation reduces incisional surgical site infection and anastomotic leak rates after elective colorectal resection. *Ann Surg.* 2015;262(2):331-337.

39. Moghadamyeghaneh Z, Hanna MH, Carmichael JC, et al. Nationwide analysis of outcomes of bowel preparation in colon surgery. *J Am Coll Surg.* 2015;220(5):912-920.

40. Clarke JS, Condon RE, Bartlett JG, et al. Preoperative oral antibiotics reduce septic complications of colon operations: results of prospective, randomized, double-blind clinical study. *Ann Surg.* 1977;186(3): 251-259.

41. Matheson DM, Arabi Y, Baxter-Smith D, Alexander-Williams J, Keighley MRB. Randomized multicentre trial of oral bowel preparation and antimicrobials for elective colorectal operations. *Br J Surg.* 1978;65(9):597-600.

42. Lewis RT. Oral versus systemic antibiotic prophylaxis in elective colon surgery: a randomized study and meta-analysis send a message from the 1990s. *Can J Surg.* 2002;45(3):173.

43. Englesbe MJ, Brooks L, Kubus J, Luchtefeld M, Lynch J, Senagore A, et al. A statewide assessment of surgical site infection following colectomy: the role of oral antibiotics. *Ann Surg.* 2010;252(3): 514.

44. Hata H, Yamaguchi T, Hasegawa S, et al. Oral and parenteral versus parenteral antibiotic prophylaxis in elective laparoscopic colorectal surgery (JMTO PREV 07-01): a phase 3, multicenter, open-label, randomized trial. *Ann Surg.* 2016;263(6):1085-1091.

45. Kim EK, Sheetz KH, Bonn J, et al. A statewide colectomy experience: the role of full bowel preparation in preventing surgical site infection. *Ann Surg.* 2014;259(2):310-314.

46. Goldsmith H. Protection of low rectal anastomosis with intact omentum. *Surg Gynecol Obstet.* 1977;144(4):584-586.

47. Moreaux J, Horiot A, Barrat F, Mabille J. Obliteration of the pelvic space with pedicled omentum after excision of the rectum for cancer. *Am J Surg.* 1984;148(5):640-644.

48. Merad F, Hay JM, Fingerhut A, Flamant Y, Molkhou JM, Laborde Y. Omentoplasty in the prevention of anastomotic leakage after colonic or rectal resection: a prospective randomized study in 712 patients. French Associations for Surgical Research. *Ann Surg.* 1998;227(2):179.

49. Tocchi A, Mazzoni G, Lepre L, et al. Prospective evaluation of omentoplasty in preventing leakage of colorectal anastomosis. *Dis Colon Rectum.* 2000;43(7):951-955.

50. Wiggins T, Markar SR, Arya S, Hanna GB. Anastomotic reinforcement with omentoplasty following gastrointestinal anastomosis: a systematic review and meta-analysis. *Surg Oncol.* 2015;24(3):181-186.

51. Topor B, Acland RD, Kolodko V, Galandiuk S. Omental transposition for low pelvic anastomoses. *Am J Surg.* 2001;182(5):460-464.

52. Ozben V, Aytac E, Liu X, Ozuner G. Does omental pedicle flap reduce anastomotic leak and septic complications after rectal cancer surgery? *Int J Surg.* 2016;27:55-57.

53. Fajardo AD, Chun J, Stewart D, Safar B, Fleshman JW. 1.5:1 meshed AlloDerm bolsters for stapled rectal anastomoses does not provide any advantage in anastomotic strength in a porcine model. *Surg Innov.* 2011;18:21-28.

54. Fajardo AD, Amador-Ortiz C, Chun J, Stewart D, Fleshman JW. Evaluation of bioabsorbable seamguard for staple line reinforcement in stapled rectal anastomoses. *Surg Innov.* 2012;19(3):288-294.

55. Senagore A, Lane FR, Lee E, et al. Bioabsorbable staple line reinforcement in restorative proctectomy and anterior resection: a randomized study. *Dis Colon Rectum.* 2014;57(3):324-330.

56. Placer C, Enríquez-Navascués JM, Elorza G, et al. Preventing complications in colorectal anastomosis: results of a randomized controlled trial using bioabsorbable staple line reinforcement for circular stapler. *Dis Colon Rectum.* 2014;57(10):1195-1201.

57. Ha GW, Kim HJ, Lee MR. Transanal tube placement for prevention of anastomotic leakage following low anterior resection for rectal cancer: a systematic review and meta-analysis. *Ann Surg Treat Res.* 2015;89(6):313-318.

58. Bülow S, Bulut O, Christensen IJ, Harling H. Transanal stent in anterior resection does not prevent anastomotic leakage. *Colorectal Dis.* 2006;8(6):494-496.

59. Xiao L, Zhang W, Jiang P, et al. Can transanal tube placement after anterior resection for rectal carcinoma reduce anastomotic leakage rate? A single-institution prospective randomized study. *World J Surg.* 2011;35(6):1367-1377.

60. Hyman NH. Managing anastomotic leaks from intestinal anastomoses. *Surgeon.* 2009;7(1):31-35.

61. Murrell ZA, Stamos MJ. Reoperation for anastomotic failure. *Clin Colon Rectal Surg.* 2006;19(4):213-216.

62. Alves A, Panis Y, Trancart D, Regimbeau JM, Pocard M, Valleur P. Factors associated with clinically significant anastomotic leakage after large bowel resection: multivariate analysis of 707 patients. *World J Surg.* 2002;26(4):499-502.

63. Ikeda T, Kumashiro R, Taketani K, et al. Endoscopic evaluation of clinical colorectal anastomotic leakage. *J Surg Res.* 2015;193(1):126-134.

64. Erb L, Hyman NH, Osler T. Abnormal vital signs are common after bowel resection and do not predict anastomotic leak. *J Am Coll Surg.* 2014;218(6):1195-1199.

65. Hyman N, Manchester TL, Osler T, Burns B, Cataldo PA. Anastomotic leaks after intestinal anastomosis: it's later than you think. *Ann Surg.* 2007;245(2):254-258.

66. Daams F, Wu Z, Lahaye MJ, Jeekel J, Lange JF. Prediction and diagnosis of colorectal anastomotic leakage: a systematic review of literature. *World J Gastrointest Surg.* 2014;6(2):14-26.

67. Kornmann VN, Treskes N, Hoonhout LH, Bollen TL, van Ramshorst B, Boerma D. Systematic review on the value of CT scanning in the diagnosis of anastomotic leakage after colorectal surgery. *Int J Colorectal Dis.* 2013;28(4):437-445.

68. Huiberts AA, Dijksman LM, Boer SA, Krul EJ, Peringa J, Donkervoort SC. Contrast medium at the site of the anastomosis is crucial in detecting anastomotic leakage with CT imaging after colorectal surgery. *Int J Colorectal Dis.* 2015;30(6):843-848.

69. Kauv P, Benadjaoud S, Curis E, Boulay-Coletta I, Loriau J, Zins M. Anastomotic leakage after colorectal surgery: diagnostic accuracy of CT. *Eur Radiol.* 2015;25(12):3543-3551.

70. Nicksa GA, Dring RV, Johnson KH, Sardella WV, Vignati PV, Cohen JL. Anastomotic leaks: what is the best diagnostic imaging study? *Dis Colon Rectum.* 2007;50(2):197-203.

71. Cousin F, Ortega-Deballon P, Bourredjem A, Doussot A, Giaccaglia V, Fournel I. Diagnostic accuracy of procalcitonin and C-reactive protein for the early diagnosis of intra-abdominal infection after elective colorectal surgery: a meta-analysis. *Ann Surg.* 2016;264: 252-256.

72. Becker KL, Snider R, Nylen ES. Procalcitonin assay in systemic inflammation, infection, and sepsis: clinical utility and limitations. *Crit Care Med.* 2008;36(3):941-952.

73. Meisner M. Pathobiochemistry and clinical use of procalcitonin. *Clin Chim Acta.* 2002;323(1):17-29.

74. Reinhart K, Karzai W, Meisner M. Procalcitonin as a marker of the systemic inflammatory response to infection. *Intensive Care Med.* 2000;26(9):1193-1200.

75. Becker KL, Nylen ES, White JC, Muller B, Snider RH Jr. Procalcitonin and the calcitonin gene family of peptides in inflammation, infection, and sepsis: a journey from calcitonin back to its precursors. *J Clin Endocrinol Metab.* 2004;89(4):1512-1525.

76. Karlsson S, Heikkinen M, Pettila V, et al. Predictive value of procalcitonin decrease in patients with severe sepsis: a prospective observational study. *Crit Care.* 2010;14(6):R205.

77. Charles PE, Tinel C, Barbar S, Aho S, Prin S, Doise JM, et al. Procalcitonin kinetics within the first days of sepsis: relationship with the appropriateness of antibiotic therapy and the outcome. *Crit Care.* 2009;13(2):1.

78. Guan J, Lin Z, Lue H. Dynamic change of procalcitonin, rather than concentration itself, is predictive of survival in septic shock patients when beyond 10 ng/mL. *Shock.* 2011;36(6):570-574.

79. Seligman R, Meisner M, Lisboa TC, et al. Decreases in procalcitonin and C-reactive protein are strong predictors of survival in ventilator-associated pneumonia. *Crit Care.* 2006;10(5):1.

80. Boussekey N, Leroy O, Alfandari S, Devos P, Georges H, Guery B. Procalcitonin kinetics in the prognosis of severe community-acquired pneumonia. *Intensive Care Med.* 2006;32(3):469-472.

81. Lipińska-Gediga M, Mierzchała-Pasierb M, Durek G. Procalcitonin kinetics—prognostic and diagnostic significance in septic patients. *Arch Med Sci.* 2016 12(1):112-119.

82. Page RD, Asmat A, McShane J, Russell GN, Pennefather SH. Routine endoscopy to detect anastomotic leakage after esophagectomy. *Ann Thorac Surg.* 2013;95(1):292-298.

83. Maish MS, DeMeester SR, Choustoulakis E, et al. The safety and usefulness of endoscopy for evaluation of the graft and anastomosis early after esophagectomy and reconstruction. *Surg Endosc Interv Tech.* 2005;19(8):1093-1102.

84. Schaible A, Sauer P, Hartwig W, et al. Radiologic versus endoscopic evaluation of the conduit after esophageal resection: a prospective, blinded, intraindividually controlled diagnostic study. *Surg Endosc.* 2014;28(7):2078-2085.

85. Dellinger RP, Levy MM, Rhodes A, et al. Surviving sepsis campaign: international guidelines for management of severe sepsis and septic shock. *Crit Care Med.* 2013;41(2):580-637.

86. Rivers E, Nguyen B, Havstad S, et al. Early goal-directed therapy in the treatment of severe sepsis and septic shock. *N Engl J Med.* 2001;345(19):1368-1377.

87. Augustin P, Kermarrec N, Muller-Serieys C, et al. Risk factors for multidrug resistant bacteria and optimization of empirical antibiotic therapy in postoperative peritonitis. *Crit Care.* 2010;14(1):R20.

88. Montravers P, Dupont H, Leone M, et al. Guidelines for management of intra-abdominal infections. *Anaesth Crit Care Pain Med.* 2015;34(2):117-130.

89. Schein M, Marshall JC. *Source Control: A Guide to the Management of Surgical Infections.* Berlin. Heidelberg: Springer—Verlag; 2003.

90. Sartelli M, Viale P, Catena F, et al. 2013 WSES guidelines for management of intra-abdominal infections. *World J Emerg Surg.* 2013;8(1):3.

91. Rüttinger D, Kuppinger D, Hölzwimmer M, et al. Acute prognosis of critically ill patients with secondary peritonitis: the impact of the number of surgical revisions, and of the duration of surgical therapy. *Am J Surg.* 2012;204(1):28-36.

92. van Ruler O, Mahler CW, Boer KR, et al. Comparison of on-demand vs planned relaparotomy strategy in patients with severe peritonitis: a randomized trial. *JAMA.* 2007;298(8):865-872.

93. Lamme B, Boermeester MA, Reitsma JB, Mahler CW, Obertop H, Gouma DJ. Meta-analysis of relaparotomy for secondary peritonitis. *Br J Surg.* 2002;89(12):1516-1524.

94. Person B, Dorfman T, Bahouth H, Osman A, Assalia A, Kluger Y. Abbreviated emergency laparotomy in the non-trauma setting. *World J Emerg Surg.* 2009;4(1):41.

95. Schein M, Saadia R, Jamieson JR, Decker GA. The "sandwich technique" in the management of the open abdomen. *Br J Surg.* 1986;73(5):369-370.

96. Cheatham ML, Demetriades D, Fabian TC, et al. Prospective study examining clinical outcomes associated with a negative pressure wound therapy system and Barker's vacuum packing technique. *World J Surg.* 2013;37(9):2018-2030.

97. Roberts DJ, Zygun DA, Grendar J, et al. Negative-pressure wound therapy for critically ill adults with open abdominal wounds: a systematic review. *J Trauma Acute Care Surg.* 2012;73(3):629-639.

98. Krarup PM, Jorgensen LN, Harling H. Management of anastomotic leakage in a nationwide cohort of colonic cancer patients. *J Am Coll Surg.* 2014;218(5):940-949.

99. Fraccalvieri D, Biondo S, Saez J, et al. Management of colorectal anastomotic leakage: differences between salvage and anastomotic takedown. *Am J Surg.* 2012;204(5):671-676.

100. Maggiori L, Bretagnol F, Lefèvre JH, Ferron M, Vicaut E, Panis Y. Conservative management is associated with a decreased risk of definitive stoma after anastomotic leakage complicating sphincter-saving resection for rectal cancer: conservative management is associated with a decreased risk of definitive stoma. *Colorectal Dis.* 2011;13(6):632-637.

101. Parc Y, Frileux P, Schmitt G, Dehni N, Ollivier JM, Parc R. Management of postoperative peritonitis after anterior resection: experience from a referral intensive care unit. *Dis Colon Rectum.* 2000;43(5):579-587; discussion 587-589.

102. Cong ZJ, Hu LH, Bian ZQ, et al. Systematic review of anastomotic leakage rate according to an international grading system following anterior resection for rectal cancer. *PLoS One.* 2013;8(9):e75519.

103. Kulu Y, Ulrich A, Bruckner T, et al. Validation of the International Study Group of Rectal Cancer definition and severity grading of anastomotic leakage. *Surgery.* 2013;153(6):753-761.

104. Matthiessen P, Hallböök O, Rutegård J, Simert G, Sjödahl R. Defunctioning stoma reduces symptomatic anastomotic leakage after low anterior resection of the rectum for cancer: a randomized multicenter trial. *Ann Surg.* 2007;246(2):207-214.

105. Burke LMB, Bashir MR, Gardner CS, et al. Image-guided percutaneous drainage vs. surgical repair of gastrointestinal anastomotic leaks: is there a difference in hospital course or hospitalization cost? *Abdom Imaging.* 2015;40(5):1279-1284.

106. Kassi F, Dohan A, Soyer P, et al. Predictive factors for failure of percutaneous drainage of postoperative abscess after abdominal surgery. *Am J Surg.* 2014;207(6):915-921.

107. Okita Y, Mohri Y, Kobayashi M, et al. Factors influencing the outcome of image-guided percutaneous drainage of intra-abdominal abscess after gastrointestinal surgery. *Surg Today.* 2015;43(10):1095-1102.

108. van Doesburg IA, Boerma D, Bollen TL, van Ramshorst B, Wiezer MJ. Large gluteal abscesses as a complication of transgluteal drainage of pelvic abscesses: analysis of three cases and a search of the literature. *Dig Surg.* 2009;26(4):329-332.

109. Ashburn JH, Stocchi L, Kiran RP, Dietz DW, Remzi FH. Consequences of anastomotic leak after restorative proctectomy for cancer: effect on long-term function and quality of life. *Dis Colon Rectum.* 2013;56(3):275-280.

110. Weidenhagen R, Gruetzner EU, Wiecken T, Spelsberg F, Jauch KW. Endoscopic vacuum-assisted closure of anastomotic leakage following anterior resection of the rectum: a new method. *Surg Endosc.* 2008;22(8):1818-1825.

111. Kuehn F, Janisch F, Schwandner F, et al. Endoscopic vacuum therapy in colorectal surgery. *J Gastrointest Surg.* 2016;20(2):328-334.

112. Nerup N, Johansen JL, Alkhefagie GAA, Maina P, Jensen KH. Promising results after endoscopic vacuum treatment of anastomotic leakage following resection of rectal cancer with ileostomy. *Dan Med J.* 2013;60(4):A4604.

113. Strangio G, Zullo A, Ferrara EC, et al. Endo-sponge therapy for management of anastomotic leakages after colorectal surgery: a case series and review of literature. *Dig Liver Dis.* 2015;47(6):465-469.

114. Riss S, Stift A, Kienbacher C, et al. Recurrent abscess after primary successful endo-sponge treatment of anastomotic leakage following rectal surgery. *World J Gastroenterol.* 2010;16(36):4570-4574.

115. Arezzo A, Verra M, Passera R, Bullano A, Rapetti L, Morino M. Long-term efficacy of endoscopic vacuum therapy for the treatment of colorectal anastomotic leaks. *Dig Liver Dis.* 2015;47(4):342-345.

116. von Bernstorff W, Glitsch A, Schreiber A, Partecke LI, Heidecke CD. ETVARD (endoscopic transanal vacuum-assisted rectal drainage) leads to complete but delayed closure of extraperitoneal rectal anastomotic leakage cavities following neoadjuvant radiochemotherapy. *Int J Colorectal Dis.* 2009;24(7):819-825.

117. Lamazza A, Sterpetti AV, De Cesare A, Schillaci A, Antoniozzi A, Fiori E. Endoscopic placement of self-expanding stents in patients with symptomatic anastomotic leakage after colorectal resection for cancer: long-term results. *Endoscopy.* 2015;47(3):270-272.

118. Amrani L, Ménard C, Berdah S, et al. From iatrogenic digestive perforation to complete anastomotic disunion: endoscopic stenting as a new concept of "stent-guided regeneration and re-epithelialization." *Gastrointest Endosc.* 2009;69(7):1282-1287.

119. DiMaio CJ, Dorfman MP, Gardner GJ, et al. Covered esophageal self-expandable metal stents in the nonoperative management of postoperative colorectal anastomotic leaks. *Gastrointest Endosc.* 2012;76(2):431-435.

120. Genser L, Manceau G, Karoui M, et al. Postoperative and long-term outcomes after redo surgery for failed colorectal or coloanal anastomosis: retrospective analysis of 50 patients and review of the literature. *Dis Colon Rectum.* 2013;56(6):747-755.

121. Picel S, Lefèvre JH, Tiret E, Chafai N, Parc Y. Redo coloanal anastomosis: a retrospective study of 66 patients. *Ann Surg.* 2012;256(5):806-810; discussion 810-811.

122. Patsouras D, Yassin NA, Phillips RKS. Clinical outcomes of colo-anal pull-through procedure for complex rectal conditions. *Colorectal Dis.* 2014;16(4):253-258.

Ostomy Construction and Management: Personalizing the Stoma for the Patient

David E. Beck

More than a million patients in North America live with some type of intestinal stoma.[1] These stomas are typically constructed as one of the last components of a long and challenging surgical procedure. Stomal construction is important because their function will have significant impact on the ostomate's life. Stomal creation is a technical exercise that if done correctly will result in good function and minimal complications for the remainder of the ostomate's life. Conversely, if created poorly, stoma complications are common and can lead to years of misery. Intestinal stomas are in fact enterocutaneous anastomoses, and all the principles that apply to creation of any anastomosis (i.e., using healthy intestine, avoiding ischemia and undue tension) are important in stoma creation. This chapter reviews construction and management of ileostomies and colostomies

INDICATIONS

Stomas are created either as a temporary means of fecal diversion when an anastomosis is unsafe or unwise, or as permanent orifices for the passage of stool or urine when surgical resection prohibits the body's normal orifices from accomplishing these tasks.

Permanent colostomies are usually created from the sigmoid or descending colon, usually in association with distal bowel resection. Colostomies proximal to the splenic flexure function poorly, are often placed in locations difficult for ostomates to manage, and are at high risk for complications. If a permanent colostomy is contemplated using the transverse or ascending colon, the surgeon should strongly consider resecting the remaining large bowel and creating an end ileostomy.[1] Common indications for a colostomy are listed in Box 178.1.

With the development and general acceptance of the ileal pouch–anal anastomosis (IPAA), permanent ileostomies are currently less common. Nonetheless, permanent ileostomies are created for inflammatory bowel disease, familial adenomatous polyposis, multiple synchronous colorectal cancers, and a variety of other miscellaneous disorders. Poor anal function, comorbid diseases, or quality of life considerations may make an ileostomy preferable to more complex reconstructive options in selected patients.

Temporary diverting stomas are usually created in association with distal bowel resections when anastomosis is unsafe or to protect a distal anastomosis when operative conditions or comorbidities make proximal diversion of the fecal stream prudent. Three types of diverting stomas predominate: end sigmoid colostomy, loop colostomy, and loop ileostomy.

PREOPERATIVE CONSIDERATIONS

Patients undergoing either elective or emergency surgery in which the creation of an abdominal stoma is a possibility should have adequate preparation preoperatively. Emergent surgery dictates a more rapid preparation than elective surgery, but stoma considerations must not be neglected.

Many patients lack knowledge of intestinal stomas. A few minutes of preoperative education by the surgeon combined with printed material is very helpful. In addition, if available, all patients should meet with a wound ostomy care nurse (WOCN) or enterostomal therapist (ET). The WOCN can provide specific information regarding stoma appliances, dietary and clothing alterations, and pouch management. Most importantly, the WOCN will help to select the appropriate abdominal wall site for the future stoma. Appropriate stoma placement decreases postoperative complications and may improve the ostomate's well-being. Bass et al. showed that preoperative counseling and marking by an ET prior to surgery improves postoperative quality of life.[2]

In addition to meeting with a WOCN, patients scheduled for stomal surgery often benefit from the opportunity to meet with other ostomates. Patients who have adjusted to life with a stoma provide an excellent, nonmedical source of information and are often glad to share their experience with new ostomates. In addition, local chapters of the United Ostomy Association of America and the Crohn's and Colitis Foundation may be of benefit in this area.

Patients should have their stoma site marked prior to surgery. An abdominal surgeon should be able to locate and mark stoma sites. In most circumstances, marking is simple, straightforward, and requires only a few minutes. Three abdominal wall landmarks outline the ostomy triangle (Fig. 178.1): the anterior superior iliac spine, pubic tubercle, and umbilicus. The stoma should lie within this triangle overlying the rectus muscle, generally at the site of an infraumbilical bulge in the abdominal wall. A site should be located on a flat segment of the abdominal wall 5 cm away from bony prominences, the umbilicus, prior surgical scars, or skin folds. After the site has been selected and marked, the patient should sit up to ensure any new skin folds do not interfere with the stoma site. The patient's belt line should be identified and avoided if possible because this decreases postoperative clothing restrictions.

Special circumstances may require additional consideration. In obese individuals, a large pannus may preclude stoma placement below the umbilicus. The pannus is often thicker in this area and may also hide the stoma from the patient's vision, making management difficult. Patients

BOX 178.1 **Common Indications for Permanent Colostomy**

Rectal cancer
Radiation proctopathy
Incontinence
Refractory anorectal Infection
Ischemia
Crohn disease
Diverticular disease
Sacral decubitus

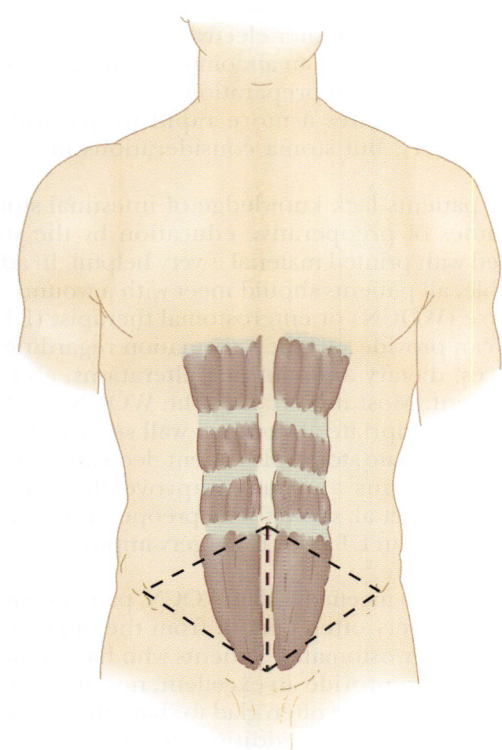

FIGURE 178.1 The ostomy triangle is defined by the anterior superior iliac spine, the umbilicus, and the pubic tubercle on the right and left sides of the abdominal wall for ileostomy and colostomy placement, respectively.

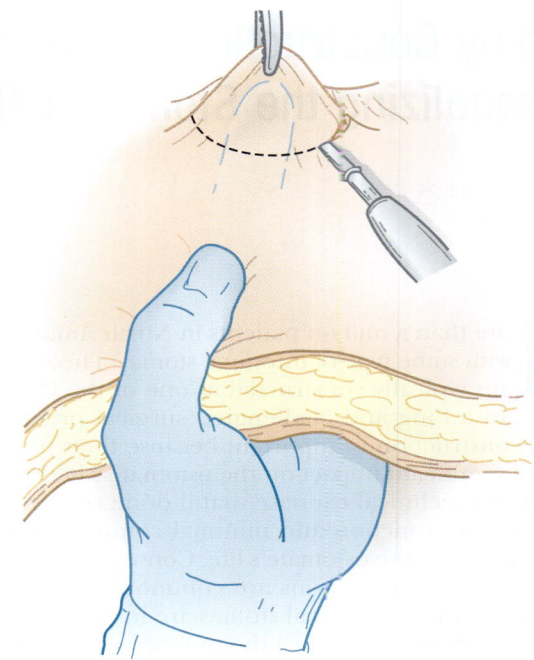

FIGURE 178.2 A disc of skin is excised at the stoma site.

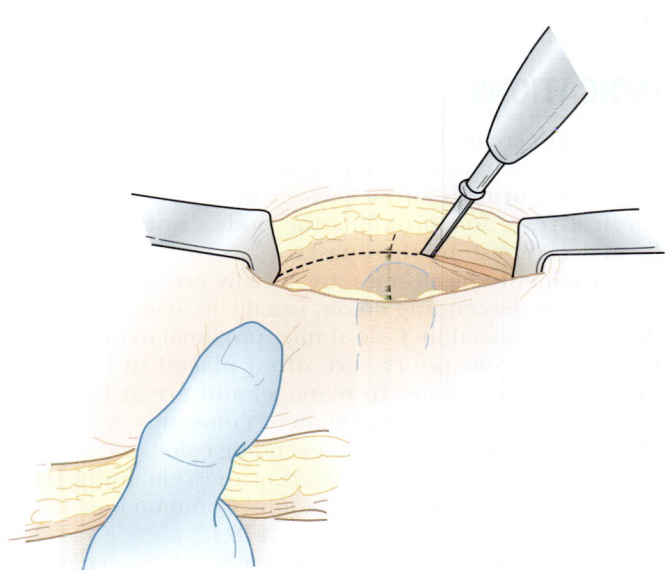

FIGURE 178.3 The anterior rectus sheath is opened vertically.

confined to a wheelchair should be marked while in their chair to avoid unanticipated postoperative difficulties. As mentioned, despite these restrictions, the stoma should pass through the rectus abdominal muscle to decrease the complications of parastomal hernia and stomal prolapse. In complex or potentially problematic cases, a stoma site can be marked and the stoma appliance left in place for 24 hours to determine the accuracy of preoperative placement. Other challenges can be addressed with such procedures as abdominal wall contouring (described later).

OPERATIVE TECHNIQUES

END STOMAS

End ileostomies are routinely performed in association with either partial or total colorectal resections. Exposure

is generally through a midline incision, and the stoma is created after performing the indicated bowel resection. The premarked stoma site (usually in the right lower quadrant) is excised (Fig. 178.2). A skin disc the size of a quarter is removed, sparing all subcutaneous fat because this fat is helpful to support the stoma in the postoperative period. The fat is then separated with cautery to expose the anterior rectus sheath. The sheath is incised vertically with cautery for 3 to 4 cm (Fig. 178.3). The rectus abdominis muscle is split in the direction of its fibers to expose the posterior sheath. With the nondominant hand protecting the underlying viscera, the posterior sheath is opened

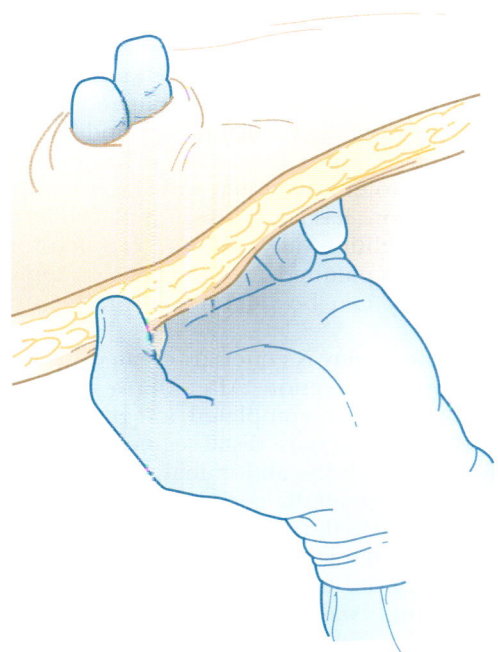

FIGURE 178.4 The stoma site admits two fingers.

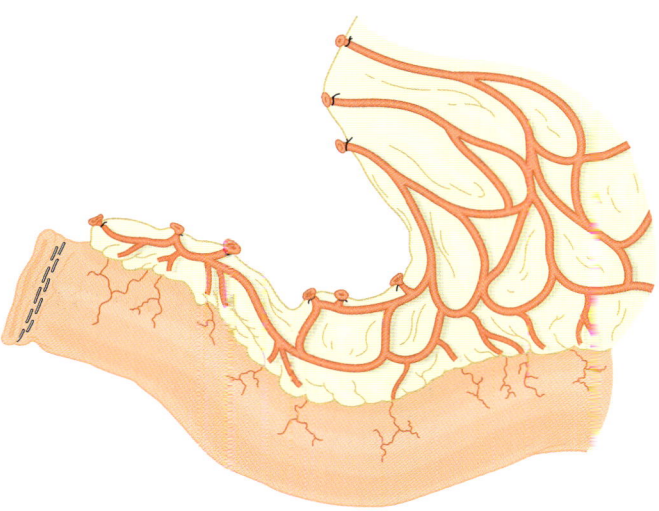

FIGURE 178.5 The ileum is prepared for ileostomy creation.

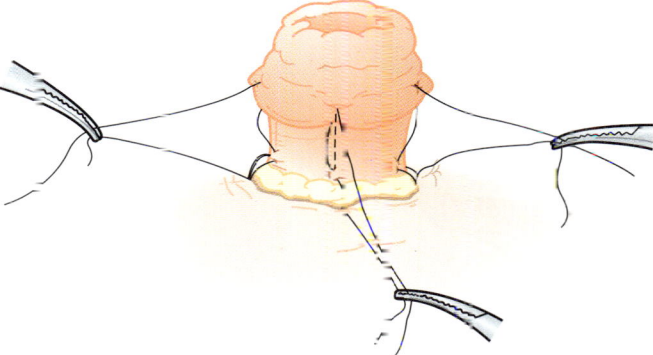

FIGURE 178.6 Tripartite bites between the dermis, the seromuscular layer of the bowel wall at the fascial level, and full thickness of the cut edge evert the stoma.

with cautery and the defect is enlarged to admit two fingers (Fig. 178.4)

After the abdominal wall defect has been created, the ileum is prepared. Any residual retroperitoneal attachments are divided to facilitate passage of the bowel through the abdominal wall without tension. The mesentery may be cleared from the terminal 5 to 6 cm of the ileum. However, care is taken to leave at least a 1-cm strip of mesentery with the ileum as this generally carries a vessel paralleling the ileal wall and will prevent stomal ischemia (Fig. 178.5). The ileum is then oriented with the cut mesenteric edge cephalad and passed through the previously created defect in the abdominal wall. The ileum should protrude 5 to 6 cm beyond skin level and appear pink and well perfused.

The lateral ileal gutter may be closed if desired to prevent small bowel obstruction secondary to small bowel rotating around the ileostomy. This is done by suturing the free edge of the ileal mesentery (taking care to avoid blood vessels feeding the stoma) to the abdominal wall lateral to the midline incision up to the falciform ligament. There is no need to suture the ileum to the posterior fascia of the abdominal wall because this has not been shown to decrease the risk of prolapse or hernia. The abdominal incision is then closed in routine fashion including the skin.

The incision is protected to prevent contamination with intestinal contents and the staple line removed from the ileum. Ileostomies must be everted and matured to prevent serositis and skin irritation because of the caustic nature of the ileal effluent. This is accomplished by tripartite sutures containing dermis the seromuscular layer of the bowel at the fascial level, and full-thickness bites of the cut edge of the ileum (Fig. 178.6). Three or four of these everting sutures are placed at the ordinals without tying. General traction on these sutures facilitates eversion of the ileum. After the stoma has been everted, the enterocutaneous anastomosis is completed with sutures between the cut edge of the ileum and dermis. These additional sutures (4 to 8) approximate the bowel mucosa to the dermis. The bowel should appear pink and protrude 2 to 3 cm beyond the abdominal skin.

As previously discussed, left-sided **end colostomies** are usually created in association with distal colorectal resection. The lateral attachments of the colon are transected along the white line of Toldt until sufficient colon is mobilized to create a colostomy that protrudes from the abdominal wall and can be matured without tension. After the colon has been sufficiently mobilized, the stoma site is prepared and the abdominal wall defect created similar to that described for end ileostomy. The only differences are that the premarked stoma site is usually in the lower left quadrant and the cutaneous and fascial openings may need to be slightly larger to facilitate unrestricted passage of the colon through the abdominal wall.

After the ostomy site has been successfully created, the colon is oriented without twisting and passed through the abdominal wall. Again, the colon should protrude beyond the abdominal skin and appear well perfused.

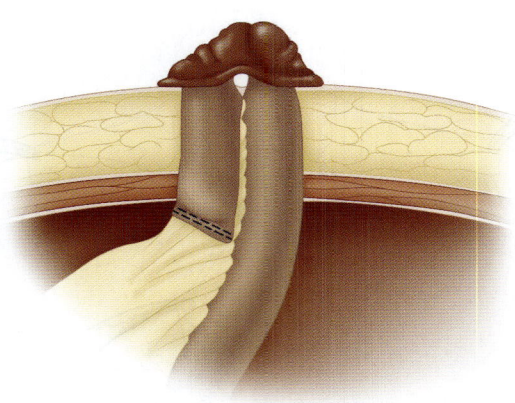

FIGURE 178.7 Creation of a loop end stoma.

There is no need to close the lateral gutter or to suture the colon to the posterior abdominal fascia as neither of these maneuvers has been shown to prevent parastomal hernia or prolapse. Alternatively, a retroperitoneal colostomy can be created by tunneling the colon under the posterolateral peritoneum and exiting through the previously created stoma site. This has been associated with decreased rates of parastomal herniation and prolapse, but the increased technical demands with its creation have limited its utility.

After the abdominal incision has been closed and protected, the colostomy can be matured. Colostomies may be sutured with minimal eversion because distal colonic contents are not irritating to the surrounding skin.

Meagher et al. have devised a technique helpful in creating an end sigmoid colostomy in patients with a thick abdominal wall.[3] The stoma site is created in standard fashion. A small wound protector (used in laparoscopic specimen extraction) is then inserted into the stoma trephine and opened maximally. The bowel is then passed through the wound protector. The inner ring of the wound protector is transected and removed. The remaining wound protector is brought out externally. The authors suggest this technique decreases spillage and minimizes bowel trauma during stoma exteriorization, particularly in the obese patient.[3]

A variation of end stomas is the loop end stoma. This type of stoma is useful in obese patients or those with a shortened or thickened mesentery. In these patients, it is difficult to get the stoma to reach the skin or the bowel's blood supply may be questionable.[4] A distal loop of bowel is selected and using an umbilical tape for traction, the loop end (close to the bowel end) is brought through the abdominal wall without dividing the mesentery (Fig. 178.7). A stomal rod is helpful in maintaining traction, and the bowel is matured as in a traditional loop stoma (see next section). This type of stoma can be made from ileum or colon.

LOOP STOMAS

As previously mentioned, diverting or loop stomas are created to divert the fecal stream away from the "downstream" intestine. Diverting stomas consist of three types: loop ileostomy, loop colostomy, and end loop stomas. In the past, the most common loop stoma created was the transverse loop colostomy, popularized for the treatment of complicated diverticular disease and for protection of distal anastomoses. The transverse loop colostomy is often a poorly tolerated stoma with high complication rates and therefore has largely been replaced by the loop ileostomy. In addition, anywhere a loop ileostomy or a loop colostomy is planned, an end loop ileostomy or end loop colostomy can be performed at the surgeon's discretion.

The **loop ileostomy** is generally created in association with distal bowel resection. After the resection and/or anastomosis have been completed, a segment of terminal ileum is selected. The most distal segment of the terminal ileum that will reach the abdominal wall without tension is selected. This generally corresponds to a segment 15 to 30 cm proximal to the ileocecal valve or from an ileoanal reservoir. The ileum is encircled with a Penrose drain or umbilical tape after its mobility has been ensured.

An abdominal wall defect is created as previously described for an end ileostomy. The defect may need to be slightly larger to accommodate both loops of bowel, which, by necessity, pass through the abdominal wall in a loop stoma. Before passing the ileum through the abdominal wall, proper orientation is ensured and the distal end is marked with a suture to prevent maturation of the incorrect segment after the abdominal incision has been closed. The ileal loop is passed through the abdominal wall without twisting and should protrude 4 to 5 cm beyond the abdominal skin. The midline incision is closed appropriately and protected with a cutaneous drape. The distal aspect of the ileum just above the abdominal wall is transected along approximately 80% of its circumference (from mesentery to mesentery). The distal end is then matured with simple sutures between the full-thickness terminal bowel and dermis. These sutures are placed close to one another to reserve the majority of the stoma site for the functional, proximal stoma.

After the distal end has been sewn to the abdominal skin, the proximal end is everted. Three tripartite bites are taken between the dermis, the seromuscular layer of the ileum 5 cm proximal to the transected end, and a full-thickness bite of the open end of the ileum. After the three sutures have been placed, they are tied with gentle traction applied within the lumen to facilitate eversion. Maturation is completed with two additional sutures between the dermis and the full thickness of the terminal ileum (Fig. 178.8). The loop stoma should protrude adequately, with its functional end occupying approximately 80% of the trephine circumference. Unless undue tension is present, a support rod is generally not necessary.

A **loop sigmoid colostomy** may be created to prevent the fecal stream from reaching the rectum and anus in cases of incontinence, severe anorectal infection, or for proximal protection after complex anal reconstruction. This stoma is essentially created in identical fashion to that of a loop ileostomy, with the exception that the stoma is commonly placed in the left lower quadrant. Eversion is not strictly necessary because of the noncaustic nature of the effluent from the left colon. However, in many

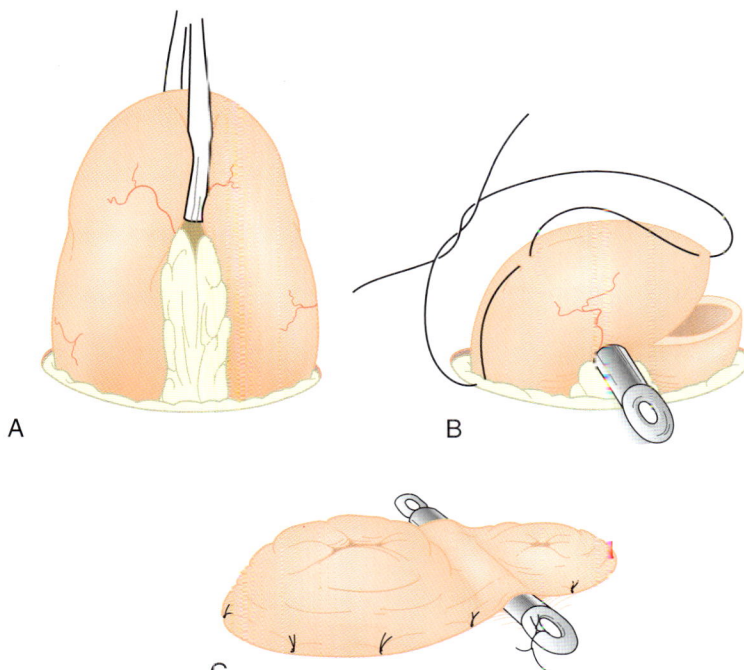

A

B

C

FIGURE 178.8 Creation of a loop ileostomy with support rod. (A) A 4- to 5-cm loop of distal ileum is brought through abdominal aperture with no twist. (B) A stoma rod is passed through the mesentery. The ileum is opened toward the nonfunctioning limb and a tripartite suture is placed. (C) The rod is sutured to the skin and the remainder of the ileostomy is matured with sutures.

circumstances, an end loop or divided loop stoma, as described in the following section, is easier to create and functions better than the standard loop colostomy.[5]

There are three types of **end loop stomas**: end loop ileostomy, end loop colostomy, and end loop ileocolostomy. These stomas have three main benefits: (1) they often make stoma management easier in the postoperative period because they appear very similar to end stomas, (2) they can be created with remote sections of the intestine, such as an end loop ileotransverse colostomy, and (3) they do not require formal laparotomy for stoma takedown. The end loop ileostomy and end loop colostomy can be created in any situation in which a standard loop ileostomy or loop colostomy might be performed. End loop ileocolostomies can be created in association with intestinal resection. For example, a right colectomy may be performed for right colon trauma or for right colon ischemia and an anastomosis is deemed unwise. In this situation, the ileostomy and the transected edge of the proximal transverse colon can be brought through one single stoma site, avoiding the need for a second stoma and laparotomy at the time of stoma takedown.

Following intestinal resection and creation of an appropriate abdominal wall defect, the **end loop** or **divided loop ileostomy** is created as follows: A small defect is created in the mesentery at the preselected ileal stomal site. The bowel is then transected with a linear stapling device. The proximal or functional end of the ileostomy is brought through the abdominal wall as for a standard end ileostomy. The nonfunctional segment can be managed in several ways. It can be brought through the fascia and sutured to the functional bowel or scarpa fascia. This method completely diverts the bowel. Another option is to bring the antimesenteric corner of the distal nonfunctional bowel through the same stoma site. The incision is closed appropriately. The antimesenteric corner of the

distal staple line is transected, and the small opening in the distal bowel is matured to the abdominal wall without eversion. The remainder of the staple line lies buried in the subcutaneous tissue. The proximal bowel is then everted and matured in a similar fashion to any end ileostomy (Fig. 178.9). A single suture between the proximal end ileostomy and the distally matured segment connects the two and completes the maturation. These stomas completely divert the fecal stream and appear almost identical to end ileostomies.

The **end loop colostomy** is created with a preselected segment of the sigmoid colon. It is mobilized appropriately and passed through the previously created abdominal wall defect similar to that of an end loop ileostomy. The abdominal incision is closed appropriately. The end colostomy is matured in a similar fashion to that of the end loop ileostomy. As previously mentioned for loop colostomies, the proximal end may be everted but a flush colostomy may also be created.

An **end loop ileocolostomy** can be performed in association with resection of the right colon when an anastomosis is unsafe. Following resection, the terminal ileum is prepared as for any routine end ileostomy. Often a stoma site will have to be created in the right upper quadrant to facilitate passage of the ileostomy and the distal transverse colon through the same abdominal aperture. After the stoma site has been created, the terminal ileum is brought through the abdominal wall, similar to an end ileostomy. The stapled-off end of the proximal transverse colon is brought through the abdominal wall defect. The mesenteric defect can be closed as with any standard colon resection.

Following this, the abdominal incision is closed in routine fashion. The antimesenteric corner of the transverse colon staple line is then transected and matured without eversion to the abdominal wall stoma site.

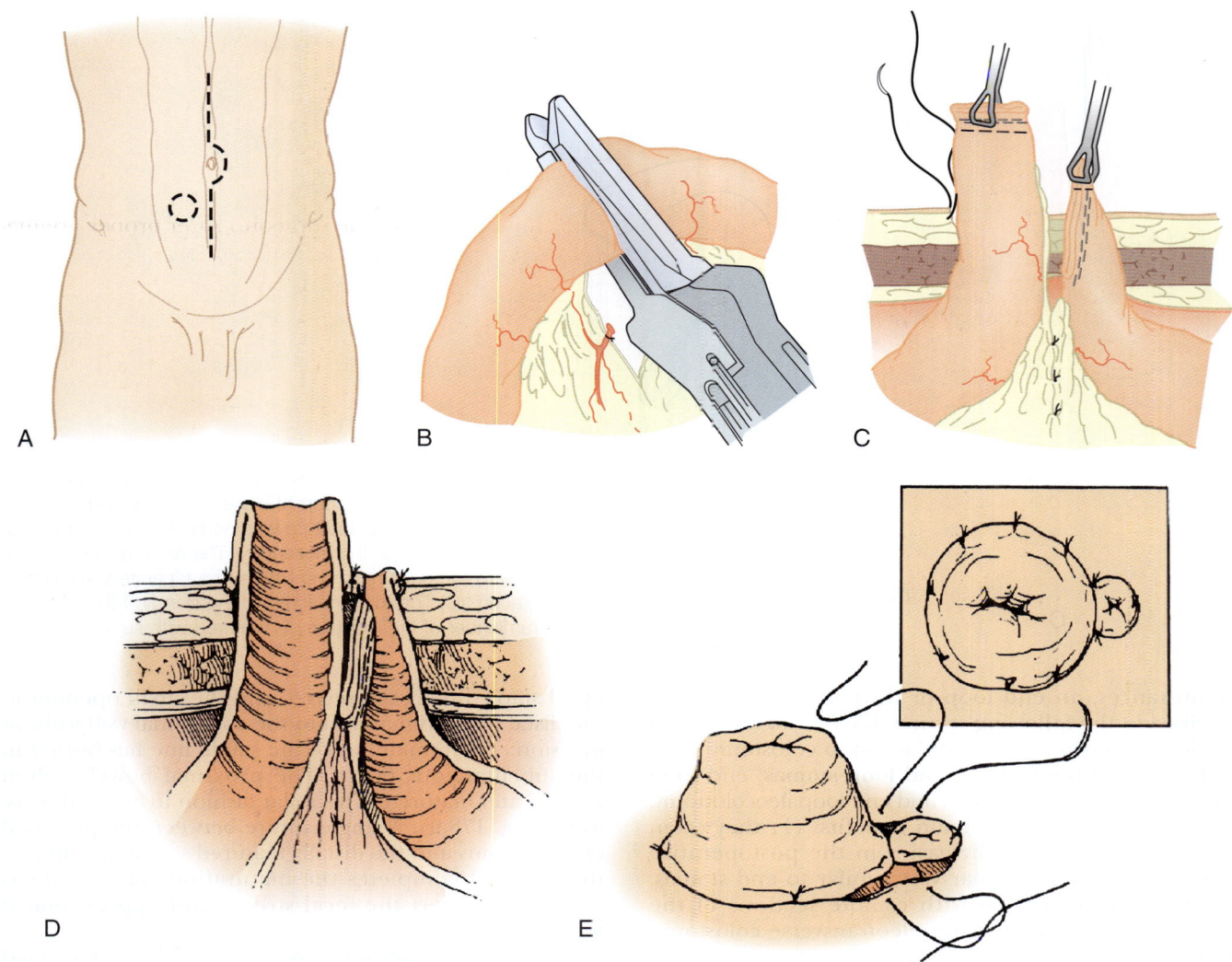

FIGURE 178.9 Creation of an end loop ileostomy. (A) The abdomen is explored through a midline incision and the ostomy opening is created as previously described (see Figs. 178.2 to 178.4). (B) A segment of ileum that will reach the abdominal wall is selected and divided with a liner cutting stapler. (C) Divided ends of the ileum are brought through the ostomy aperture (functional end is marked with a suture). (D) The staples of the functional end are excised and the bowel is matured producing a 2 cm spout. Staples at the antimesenteric end of the nonfunctioning end are excised, and the small end is sutured to the deep dermis and medial edge of functioning stoma. (Sagittal view.) (E) Completed ileostomy.

Cutaneous sutures should be placed in proximity to save the majority of the stoma site for the ileostomy. After this has been completed, the staple line is resected from the terminal ileum and the ileum matured as for a standard end ileostomy (Fig. 178.10). The final suture between transverse colon and the ileum is placed to complete the maturation.

This stoma has the previously mentioned advantages of avoiding a second stoma site for a mucous fistula. In addition, because the terminal ileum and transverse colon are in close approximation through the same stoma site, stoma takedown can be later performed directly through a parastomal incision without the need for a formal laparotomy. This may significantly decrease subsequent morbidity and recovery time after the subsequent stoma takedown.

LAPAROSCOPIC STOMAS

If an ileostomy is needed in conjunction with a laparoscopic bowel resection (protection of a low anastomosis) or an ileostomy alone is needed (diversion proximal to complex anovaginal fistula repair or anal canal reconstruction), it can be created laparoscopically. Principles that apply to open ileostomy creation also apply when the operation is performed laparoscopically. The site should be selected according to the patient's body habitus and functional needs. If a colectomy in conjunction with the ileostomy is essential, then ileostomy siting should be considered at the time of trochar placement. A trochar can certainly be placed through the future stoma trephine, but sites adjacent to the trephine within the footprint of the stoma appliance should be avoided. Trochars in place for the

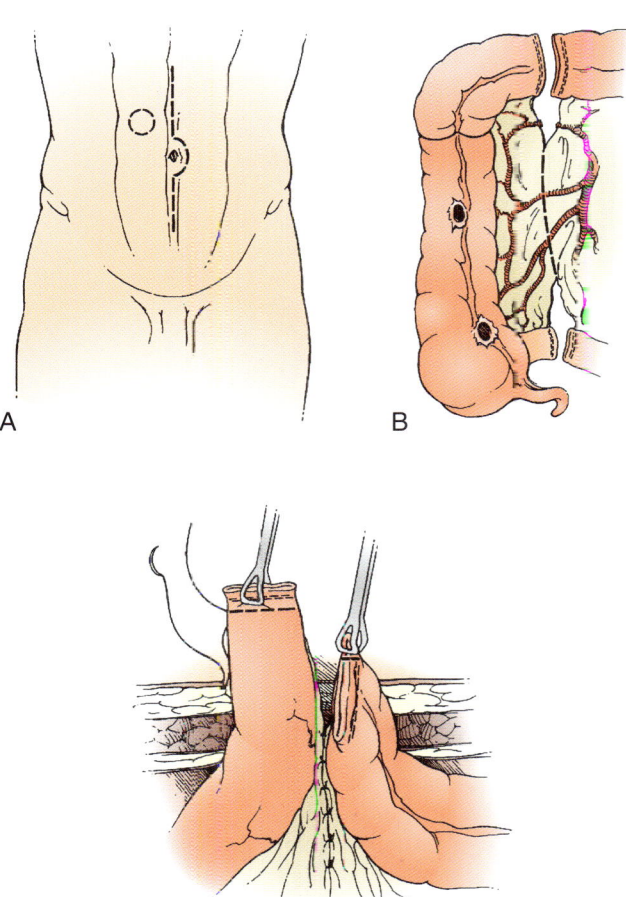

FIGURE 178.10 Creation of an end loop ileocolostomy. (A) Abdomen is explored via midline incision. (B) Terminal ileum and right colon are resected. (C) Functional end of ileum and end of nonfunctional colon are brought through the ostomy aperture. Ostomy is matured as in Fig. 178.9D and E.

colectomy or proctectomy can be used to perform the intracorporeal components of the ileostomy creation.

If the ileostomy is created without any additional abdominal surgery, then only two ports are commonly necessary: one at the umbilicus for the camera and a second through the stoma site to manipulate the terminal ileum. Under either circumstance, the operative principles are similar.

The terminal ileum is located just proximal to the ileocecal valve. The bowel is followed retrograde until a segment that easily reaches the abdominal wall at the stoma site is identified. Pneumoperitoneum should be deflated when assessing ileal length, as the abdomen will not be distended when the ileostomy is created or in use. Ileal mobilization is rarely required. Extreme care should be taken to ensure proper orientation of the bowel. The proper loop of bowel is grasped with a grasper through the stoma trephine and proximal and distal bowels carefully identified. If an additional port is available, the tip of a marking pen is grasped with a laparoscopic grasper and the distal end marked just beyond the grasper. (This is not possible if the two-port technique is used.)

Pneumoperitoneum is released and the stoma trephine is created in standard fashion around the grasper. The loop is then eviscerated carefully without twisting. After this is done, pneumoperitoneum is reestablished and proper orientation is confirmed. This is *essential* because creating an ileostomy from the distal limb is highly problematic for the patient [because it can lead to an unanticipated mechanical small bowel obstruction] and very embarrassing for the surgeon.) After proper orientation is confirmed, the stoma can be matured in standard fashion. A loop, end loop, or end ileostomy can be created as indicated based on the clinical setting. After completion of stoma maturation, pneumoperitoneum is reestablished, proper orientation confirmed, and the abdominal cavity is checked for bleeding.

Similar to ileostomy, all types of colostomies can be performed laparoscopically. Sigmoid colostomy is most common. Techniques are very similar to the creation of laparoscopic ileostomies. If trocars have been placed for rectosigmoid resection, no additional ports will be needed. If a colostomy is performed without other abdominal surgery, then three or four ports may be necessary. A camera port is placed through the umbilicus. Two ports are placed in the right midabdomen and the right lower quadrant, respectively. A fourth port may be placed through the previously marked stoma site if colonic mobilization is required. If the colostomy is created in conjunction with an abdominoperineal resection or sigmoid resection, mobilization is often already completed at this point. Occasionally, additional descending colon mobilization is necessary to create a stoma without tension.

If no colonic resection has been performed, then the sigmoid and descending colon will require mobilization. The sigmoid colon is retracted medially through the right midabdomen port, and the lateral peritoneal reflection is retracted laterally through the stoma port. The lateral attachments are then taken down with scissors or cautery through the right lower quadrant port. After mobilization is complete, pneumoperitoneum is released and the colon checked for length. Again, the distal end is marked with a marker tip attached to a grasper (if distal resection has not been performed) after orientation has been carefully confirmed.

Pneumoperitoneum is then decompressed, and the stoma trephine created in standard fashion. The colon is brought through the abdominal wall defect without twisting and the stoma matured with standard technique. As with ileostomy, end, end loop, or loop colostomy can all be created laparoscopically. After stoma completion, pneumoperitoneum is reestablished, orientation confirmed, and the abdominal wall cavity checked for bleeding.

MODIFIED ABDOMINOPLASTY (ABDOMINAL WALL CONTOURING)

Patients who may benefit from these techniques include those with stomal retraction (especially those who have bowel limitations, e.g., continent ileostomies, dense intraabdominal adhesions or short gut; prolapse; large peristomal hernias; abdominal wall laxity, usually resulting from major weight loss) and peristomal skin problems, such as pyodermia. In many of these patients, stomal relocation may not be the best option.

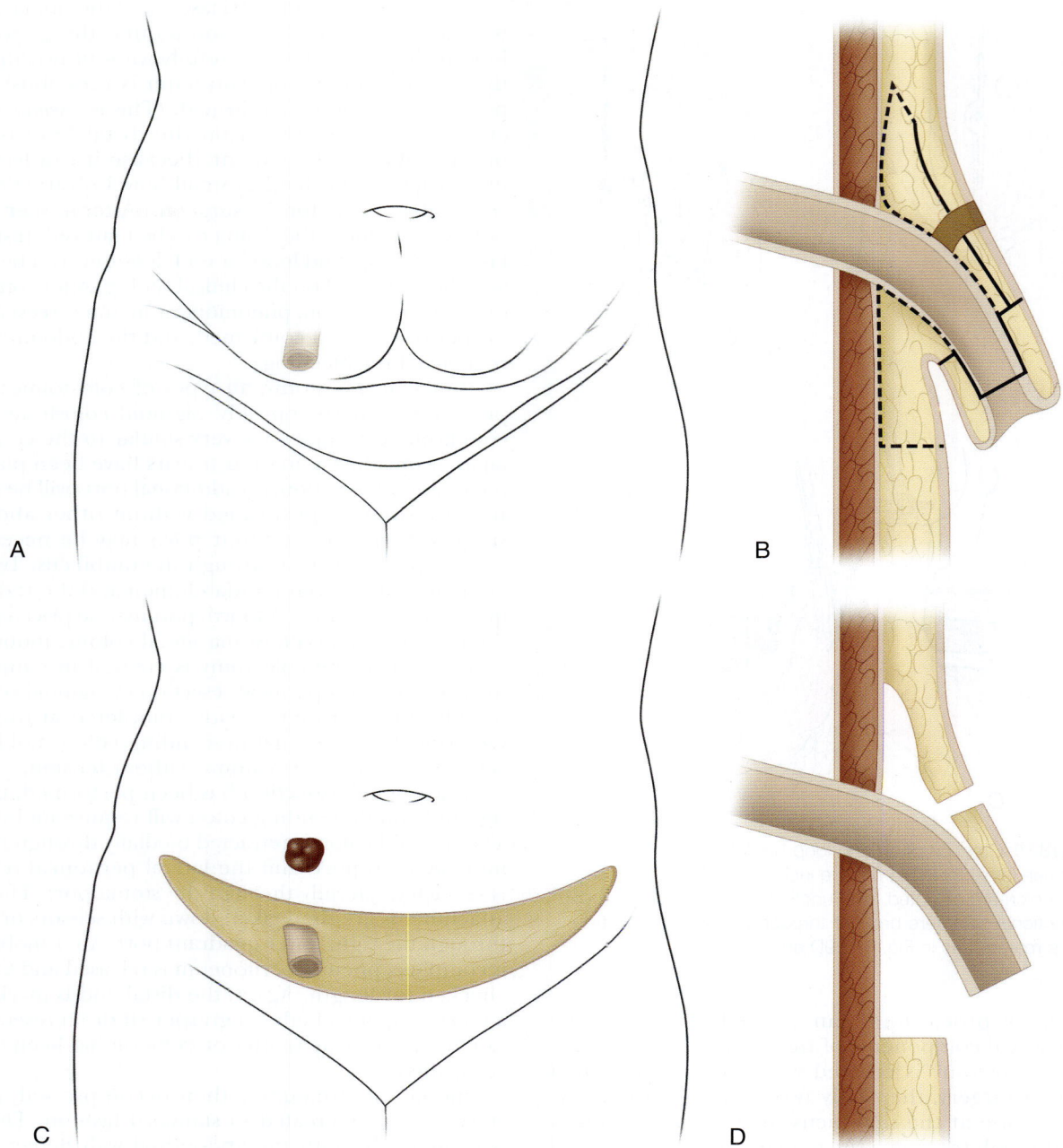

FIGURE 178.11 Modified abdominoplasty. Redundant abdominal wall folds of skin associated with ileostomy retraction. (A) Frontal view. (B) Sagittal section demonstrating skin and subcutaneous fat incisions. (C) Excess skin and subcutaneous fat have been excised (frontal view) and (D) sagittal section.

The technique is similar to that used by plastic surgeons.[6] A low curvilinear transverse incision is made at the inferior abdominal fold or 2 to 3 cm above the pubis and anterior superior iliac spines (Fig. 178.11) and carried down to the fascia. A flap of skin and subcutaneous tissue is created by electrocautery dissection in a cranial direction, just above the fascia. Perforating vessels are identified and ligated or cauterized. As the dissection continues, the stoma will be encountered. With the flap on traction, the intestine is separated from the skin and subcutaneous tissue. Care is taken to avoid injury to the bowel or its blood supply. The dissection should err on leaving additional subcutaneous fat attached to the intestine. This can be carefully resected later. A similar maneuver may be performed at the umbilicus if the surgeon and patient prefer to preserve it in its normal location. Again, care is taken to preserve the tissue's blood supply. If the umbilicus is not to be maintained, it can be amputated at the fascial level. The flap dissection is continued cranially just above the fascia until enough laxity or length is

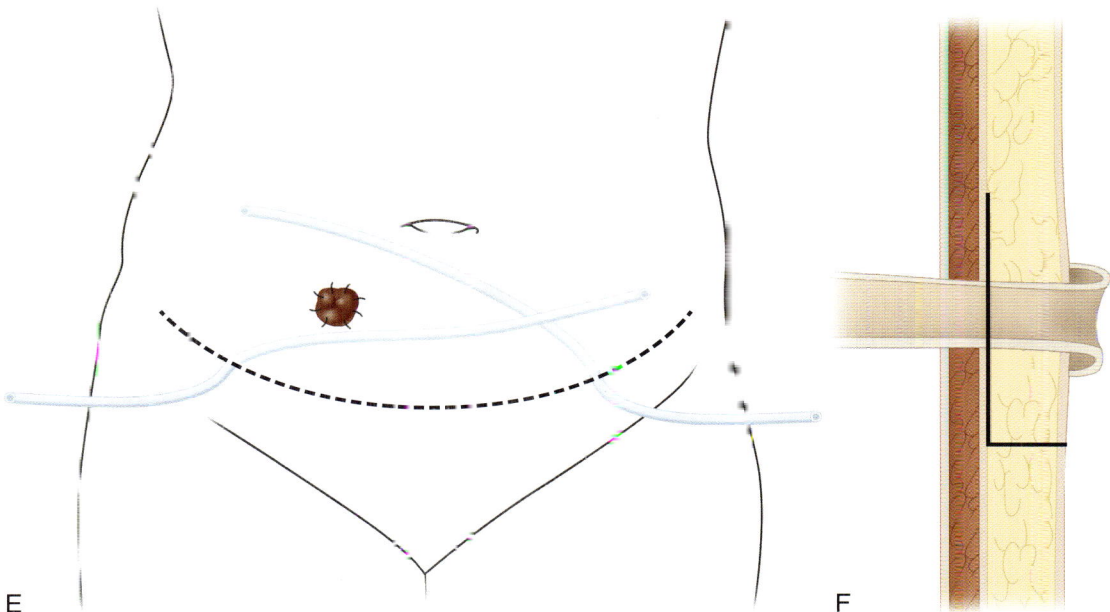

E   F

FIGURE 178.11, cont'd (E) Ileostomy relocated through upper flap and skin incisions closed. Closed-suction drains placed below flaps. (F) Sagittal section.

obtained in the upper flap for the upper edge of the previous stomal opening to reach the inferior portion of the incision without excessive tension or to the costal margins. Any associated peristomal hernia can be repaired at this time with suture repair of the fascia and/or mesh (synthetic or biologic) reinforcement.

As the flap is retracted inferiorly, new sites for the ostomy and, if desired, the umbilicus are selected and openings created in the flap. Excess subcutaneous fat can be carefully removed to thin the flap. Fortunately, there is usually less subcutaneous fat above the umbilicus compared with below it. The excess, distal portion of the flap is excised (see Fig. 178.11). The intestine and umbilicus are brought through the respective flap openings and matured with interrupted absorbable sutures. Excess bowel or umbilical tissue can be carefully excised. Closed-suction drains are placed below the flap to avoid seromas and the inferior incision is closed in layers. Because intraabdominal dissections are avoided with this technique, patients usually recover quickly. Morbidity is usually associated with infection, flap ischemia, or seromas. These are managed with wound care.

Several types of flaps can be used to modify the abdominal wall around the stomas. Most involve peristomal dissections and removal of skin and subcutaneous fat. The medial approach starts with an incision through the midline incision down to the fascia (Fig. 178.12A). Dissection is carried laterally just above the fascia until the stoma is reached. The ostomy is dissected free of the skin and subcutaneous tissue as described previously. After the stoma is freed, lateral dissection to the flanks will provide enough laxity to advance the previous stoma site to the midline (advancement flap). As above, a new ostomy opening, in fresh skin, is created. Excess fat may be excised around the stoma, and redundant midline skin is resected.

If the skin flap is not redundant enough to advance the original ostomy opening to the midline, the subcutaneous fat can be excised and the stoma returned to its original skin opening through the thinned flap. Either method is performed in such a manner to leave a smooth, flat, thinned flap that provides a flat surface to site the appliance. The stoma is matured, and the midline incision is closed. Subcutaneous closed-suction drains are placed above and below the stoma. A similar technique can be used through an inferior or inferolateral peristomal incision.

Rapid and significant weight gain in ostomy patients may produce stomal retraction. If attempts at weight loss have not been successful and stomal revision is not desirable or feasible (e.g., continent ileostomy or short gut patients), liposuction is an excellent option. This method is preferred if there is no associated stomal stenosis or hernia. Experienced plastic surgeons can carefully use liposuction techniques to remove subcutaneous fat around the stoma. Obviously, care must be taken to not injure the stoma during the procedure and to leave a flat smooth peristomal skin surface for the ostomy faceplate. After the fatty tissue is removed, it will not be redeposited despite additional weight gain.

ANTIADHESION BARRIERS AND STOMAS

Some authors have advocated the use of carboxymethyl cellulose (CMC) and sodium hyaluronate (Seprafilm; Genzyme, Cambridge, Massachusetts) when creating temporary loop stomas to facilitate ostomy reversal.[78] Very little is known about this, and it has not been subject to the rigors of a clinical trial. Authors suggest that wrapping the ileum at the time of stoma creation will minimize adhesions between the stoma and the abdominal wall, making stoma takedown easier. One study by Kawamura

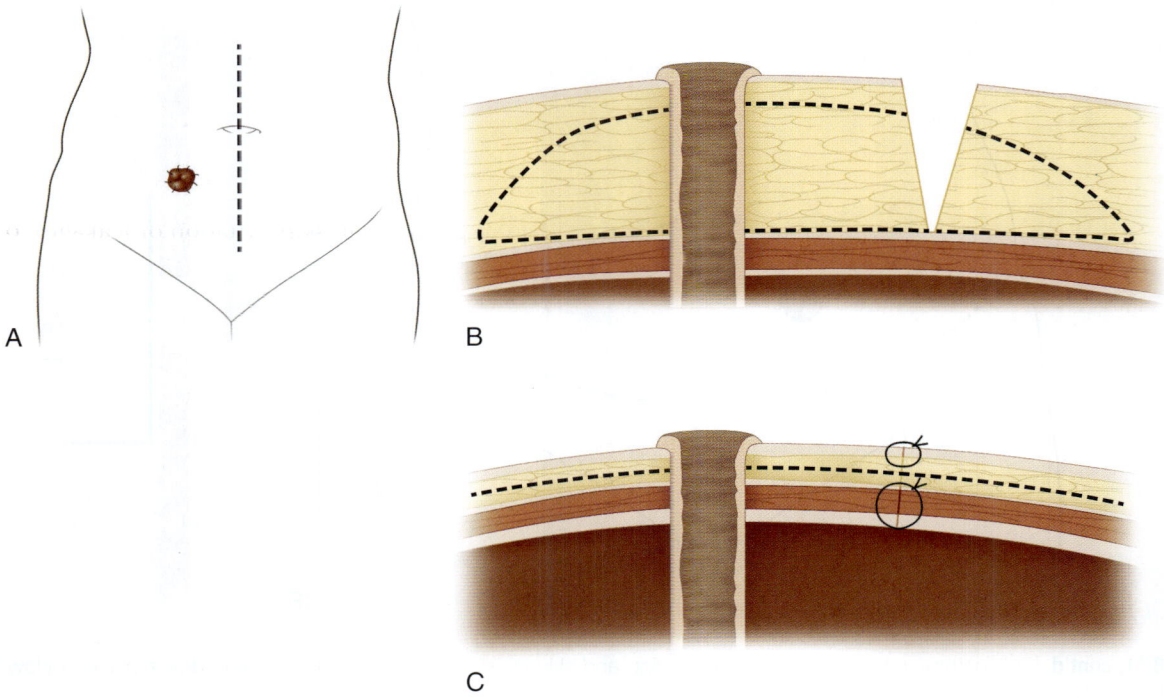

FIGURE 178.12 Medial approach. (A) Frontal view with skin incisions marked. (B) Cross section demonstrating midline incision and areas of subcutaneous fat excision. (C) After removal of excess subcutaneous tissue, incision is closed, flaps attached to fascia, and stoma matured with adequate eversion.

et al. suggests shorter operative times in the antiadhesion group.[7] Another study by Salum et al. found fewer stomal adhesions when an antiadhesion product was used.[8]

The technique is described as follows. The loop selected is eviscerated and a sheet of CMC is cut in half. The proximal and distal limbs of the bowel and their adjacent mesentery are wrapped in a sushi roll style. After the barrier has adhered, the loop is brought through the abdominal wall at the preselected site and the stoma matured in standard fashion. The utility of this technique has been difficult to prove, but minimizing adhesions between the ileum and the abdominal wall should, in concept, make dissection at the time of ileostomy takedown easier.

ENTEROSTOMAL THERAPY

A dedicated WOCN or ET's contribution to the long-term quality of life of an ostomate is simply immeasurable. Such therapists provide preoperative counseling, early postoperative education and guidance, and act as a long-term resource for individuals with stomas. They supply information on appliance choices, local support groups such as the United Ostomy Associations of America and the Crohn's and Colitis Foundation, suggest dietary or clothing modifications that may alleviate stoma-related problems, and aid in the management of skin problems, parastomal hernias, prolapse, and other complications. In most situations, an ET or surgical nurse will provide detailed postoperative education for a new ostomate. However, if this support is unavailable, it is the surgeon's

responsibility to ensure the patient is educated in appliance management.

The appliance must be emptied frequently enough to avoid overfilling and dislodgement of the pouch. This is determined by the location of the stoma and the patient's natural bowel pattern. Ileostomies are usually emptied four to six times per day, with colostomies emptied once or twice per day or even once every other day. The entire appliance only needs to be changed every 4 to 7 days. The exact details vary from individual to individual, but a common technique for changing a typical one-piece system is explained in Box 178.2.

Pouches should generally be changed when the stoma is least active, which is often after a period of fasting. The time will vary from individual to individual, but changing the appliance when the stoma is less active avoids the need to control fresh output during the procedure.

The noise and odor of gas emitted from a stoma are a major concern to most ostomates. Anything that causes gas before creation of the stoma is likely to create gas following its construction. Gas comes from two sources: swallowed air and bacterial breakdown of ingested foodstuffs, particularly carbohydrates. The amount of swallowed air can be minimized by avoiding the use of straws, excessive talking while eating, chewing gum, and smoking. Each individual can best identify which foods lead to gas production, but beans, broccoli, onions, Brussels sprouts, beer, and dairy products in lactose-deficient individuals are common culprits. Avoiding these foods is a personal choice but will decrease the quantity and odor of stomal flatus. Yogurt, parsley, and orange juice have been

---

BOX 178.2 Stoma Care

1. Gather all supplies.
2. Gently remove soiled pouch by pushing down on skin while lifting up on pouch. Discard soiled pouch in odor-proof plastic bag. *Save tail closure.*
3. Clean stoma and peristomal skin with water; pat dry. *If indicated,* shave or clip peristomal hair.
4. Use stoma-measuring guide or established pattern to determine size of stoma. *Presized pouch:* Check to be sure pouch opening is correct size. Order new supplies if indicated. *Cut-to-fit-pouch:* Trace correctly sized pattern onto back of barrier or pouch surface and cut stoma opening to match pattern. After stomal shrinkage is complete, this step may be omitted and preparation of the clean pouch may be completed before the soiled pouch is removed.
5. Apply skin barrier paste or skin sealant to skin. Allow to dry.
6. Remove paper backing from pouch or barrier to expose adhesive surface; center pouch opening over stoma and press into place. Attach closure.

From Lavery IC, Erwin-Toth P. Stoma therapy. In: Cataldo P, MacKeigan J, eds. *Intestinal Stomas.* New York: Marcel Dekker; 2004:65.

---

associated with decreased odor. Odor-proof pouches, charcoal filters, and pouch deodorants (such as commercial deodorants, mouthwash, and perineal deodorants) may also help. Orally ingested deodorants are also available and include bismuth subgalate and chlorophyllin complex. However, the most important key to preventing odor is good peristomal hygiene and creating a leak-proof seal at the time of appliance change.

A period of adjustment occurs in all ostomates, but attention to detail at the time of appliance change, combined with minor dietary and clothing modifications, should make a stoma completely unnoticeable to all except the ostomate's closest acquaintances. In addition, abdominal stomas should not preclude participation in almost any physical activity.

COMPLICATIONS

Despite modest advances in surgical technique and enterostomal therapy, complications after stoma creation remain extremely common. The rate of stoma-specific complications in the literature varies quite widely, ranging from 10% to 70%, depending on the methodology of the study, the length of follow-up, and the definition of a complication.[9-13] For example, virtually all ostomates will have at least transient episodes of minor peristomal irritation, and skin irritation is often the most commonly reported stoma complication. Studies reporting only problems that require revisional surgery will obviously indicate a much lower rate of complications. As such, the relative incidence and frequency of the specific complications vary substantially from series to series.

Stoma-related complications may be classified as those that occur early (within 1 month of surgery) or late (more than 1 month postoperatively). The most common early complications are peristomal skin irritation, leakage, high output, and ischemia. The most commonly reported late complications include parastomal hernia, prolapse, obstruction, and stenosis.

INCIDENCE

In the absence of a universally accepted definition of what constitutes a stomal complication, adverse events may be mild (e.g., transient skin irritation or leakage), or require major revisional surgery (parastomal hernia or necrosis). In a 20-year retrospective review of 1615 patients in the Cook County Hospital database, Park et al. reported a 34% incidence of complications, 28% being early and 6% classified as late.[9] The most common early complications were skin irritation (12%), pain associated with poor stoma location (7%), and partial necrosis (5%). The most common late complications were also skin irritation (6%), prolapse (2%), and stenosis (2%). Of note, complications varied greatly by service, with ostomies created by general surgeons associated with a 47% complication rate, whereas the complication rate for colorectal surgeons was 32%. Duchesne et al. retrospectively reviewed 164 ostomates cared for at Charity Hospital in New Orleans.[10] The overall complication rate was 25%; 38% of the complications were early and 62% were late. As is typically the case, ileostomies were associated with a higher complication rate than colostomies. The most common complications were necrosis (22%), prolapse (22%), skin irritation (17%), and stenosis (17%). Risk factors for complications included inflammatory bowel disease, ischemic colitis, and increased body mass index. As others have observed, obesity markedly increased the risk of skin irritation.[11] Of particular note was the sixfold decrease in stoma complications when an ET was involved in the patient's care.

SKIN IRRITATION AND LEAKAGE

Skin irritation is very common among patients with a stoma. In a review of 610 patients, it was by far the most common early local complication.[11] The problem is far more commonly seen in patients with an ileostomy owing to the liquid, caustic effluent[14]; this highlights the need for proper technique when an ileostomy is created.

Although a minor degree of skin irritation on occasion is probably inevitable, most significant cases of skin irritation are potentially preventable. Preoperative marking by an ET can help to ensure proper siting and a secure fit. Appropriate location and careful appliance fitting minimize the noxious, irritating effect that can be associated with leakage or unprotected peristomal skin (Fig. 178.13). Patients also need to be monitored for allergic reactions to the components of the appliance.

Particular attention must be paid to older patients who may have limitations in eyesight or dexterity. Patients with a high-output stoma are at particular risk for skin irritation and ulceration if they do not have an appropriately fitted appliance. Obesity has been frequently reported to be associated with an increased risk of skin irritation, likely owing to technical problems with stoma construction.[15] Consideration should be given to placing the stoma in the upper abdomen, where there is typically much less subcutaneous fat and the patient can see it much more readily.

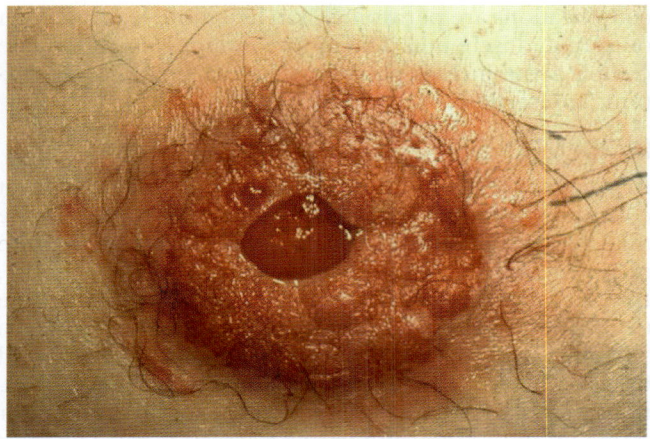

FIGURE 178.13 Skin irritation around the stoma site from a poorly fitting appliance.

The patient should be instructed to avoid creams or ointments that may interfere with the adherence of their appliance. In the postoperative period, a stoma will tend to become less edematous and the abdomen becomes less distended. As such, it is quite common to need to downsize the appliance at the first postoperative visit to minimize exposed skin. Changing a stoma too frequently may lead to excessive wear and tear on the parastomal skin; on the other hand, too long an interval between changing the appliance may be associated with erosion of the protective barrier.

Even with the help of an excellent ET, specific skin infections may occur. Fungal overgrowth is evident when there is a bright red rash around the stoma with associated satellite lesions. This is typically easily treated by dusting the parastomal skin with an appropriate antifungal powder or an oral agent in refractory cases. If the dermatitis conforms precisely to the outline of the stoma appliance, then an allergic reaction to the wafer or other component of the appliance is likely the culprit. Peristomal skin irritation may also be associated with reactivation of inflammatory bowel disease.

Fortunately, most cases of skin irritation and leakage are readily managed by conservative means. However, a redundant pannus, surgical scars, or creases with poor stoma siting may result in the need for revisional surgery. Revising the site of the stoma or combined abdominal wall recontouring and stoma revision may be necessary.[6,16]

HIGH-OUTPUT STOMAS

For obvious reasons, a high-output state is typically described in association with an ileostomy rather than a colostomy. Marked diarrhea and dehydration occur in 5% to 20% of ileostomy patients, with the greatest risk occurring in the early postoperative period. An ileostomy usually functions by the third or fourth postoperative day.[17] The output typically peaks on the fourth postoperative day, with an output of up to 3.2 L reported. Because the ostomy effluent is rich in sodium, hyponatremia can be a problem. The particular window of vulnerability for dehydration appears to be between the third and eighth postoperative day. In time, the small bowel typically adapts

with mucosal hyperplasia and there is a steady decrease in ostomy output. However, patients with an ileostomy, particularly those who have had concomitant small bowel resection, are at risk to become dehydrated. Most often, this is easily managed by oral rehydration with one of the commonly available sports drinks. However, patients who have lost considerable absorptive surface owing to previous bowel resection and/or those with recurrent/residual Crohn disease are at particular risk. In addition to the loss of absorptive surface area, ileal resection also removes the fat or complex carbohydrate stimulation of the so-called ileal brake, which slows gastric emptying and small bowel transit.[18] Fluid and electrolyte maintenance in these patients may require a period of parenteral hydration and nutrition.

Clostridium difficile enteritis is an increasingly reported cause of ileostomy diarrhea, especially in patients who have had a total colectomy for inflammatory bowel disease.[19] The typical presentation is ileostomy diarrhea followed by ileus. This condition has been associated with a high mortality, although early recognition and treatment appears to be associated with better outcomes.[20]

Ileostomy diarrhea may be treated in its milder forms with oral fiber supplements or cholestyramine, which can thicken secretions. Histamine receptor antagonists or proton pump inhibitors are often useful in reducing gastric fluid secretion, especially in the first 6 months after surgery when hypergastrinemia is most severe.[21] Often, antimotility agents (e.g., loperamide or diphenoxylate) or opiates (e.g., codeine or tincture of opium) may be required to slow intestinal transit. In refractory cases, somatostatin analogue has been used with some success. Somatostatin reduces salt and water excretion and slows gastrointestinal tract motility. However, its clinical use has met with variable results.[22] Special mention is made of patients with an anastomotic small bowel leak. Good results have been reported with exteriorizing the leak and reinfusing the ostomy effluent into the downstream limb until gastrointestinal continuity can be restored. This has led to weaning parenteral nutrition in a substantial number of patients.[23]

A related problem in patients with an ileostomy is the development of urinary stones. The obligatory loss of fecal water, sodium, and bicarbonate reduces urinary pH and volume.[24] Whereas approximately 4% of the general population develop urinary stones, the incidence in patients with an ileostomy is approximately twice that. Whereas uric acid stones comprise less than 10% of the calculi in the general population, they comprise 60% of stones in ileostomy patients. There is also an increase in the incidence of calcium oxalate stones.[25]

BOWEL OBSTRUCTION

Life table analyses suggest that bowel obstruction is a rather common complication of ostomy creation. Twenty-three percent of patients with an ileostomy ultimately develop bowel obstruction.[26] Adhesions are probably the most common cause, but small bowel volvulus or internal hernia may be the culprit. Although it is frequently mentioned that suture of the mesentery to the lateral abdominal wall may prevent volvulus or obstruction, retrospective analyses have not shown any benefit to this maneuver.[26] Treatment is not dissimilar to other patients presenting with a mechanical small bowel obstruction.

However, special note must be made of food bolus obstruction. Many patients with an ileostomy may develop signs and symptoms of bowel obstruction owing to the accumulation of poorly digested foodstuffs (e.g., popcorn, peanuts, and fresh fruits and vegetables). A careful history may reveal dietary indiscretions. Furthermore, the possibility of a food bolus obstruction should be considered in any patient with an ileostomy who has radiologic evidence of a distal obstruction. A red rubber catheter may be inserted gently into the ostomy and saline irrigation initiated. If suspicious concretions begin to pass into the stoma, the irrigations may be carefully repeated until the obstruction is relieved.

ISCHEMIA

Edema and venous congestion are very common after stoma creation, owing to mechanical trauma and compression of the small mesenteric venules as they traverse the abdominal wall. This is typically self-limiting and requires no treatment.[27] However, ischemia may be related to tension on the mesentery or excessive mesenteric division, particularly in obese patients or those undergoing emergency surgery.[28] A common error is dividing the sigmoidal vessels to obtain the length to allow a colostomy to reach the skin. In these cases, the inferior mesenteric vessels should instead be divided proximally and/or the splenic flexure mobilized, preserving the sigmoid arcades.

If ischemia becomes apparent, a glass test tube or flexible endoscope may be inserted into the stoma. If the stoma is viable at fascial level, then the patient may be carefully observed. However, if there is question about the viability of the stoma at the fascial level, immediate laparotomy and stoma revision is required. Early ischemia is seen in 1% to 10% of colostomies and 1% to 5% of ileostomies.[29]

PARASTOMAL HERNIA

Parastomal hernia is probably the most common stoma complication requiring operative intervention (Fig. 178.14). A parastomal hernia develops in 2% to 28% of patients with an end ileostomy and 4% to 48% with an

end colostomy.[30] The occurrence of these hernias increases with time[31]; as such, the reported incidence depends greatly on the length of follow-up. Most patients with a parastomal hernia can be managed expectantly or with a belted appliance; however patients with unrelenting pain, obstruction, or difficulty maintaining an appliance generally require surgical repair.

Patient-specific factors such as obesity, advanced age, and chronic obstructive pulmonary disease appear to increase the risk of parastomal herniation.[13] From the technical standpoint, making the smallest possible opening in the abdominal wall without making the stoma ischemic seems prudent. However, many of the other preventive measures, such as lateral space closure, fascial fixation, or stoma placement through the rectus muscle, appear to have no effect on the incidence of these hernias. The use of prosthetic mesh prophylactically, especially in the sublay position, may reduce the risk of parastomal herniation.[32-34]

Unfortunately, the results of surgical correction have historically been poor, highlighting the importance of careful patient selection and prudent attempts at conservative management in patients without clear indications for surgery. In one of the largest reported series, 33% of patients developed a recurrent hernia and 63% had at least one complication.[35] The most commonly described techniques are direct repair, stoma relocation, and mesh repair. The recurrence rate with mesh repairs (0% to 33%) clearly appears to be lower than that of direct repair (46% to 100%) or stoma relocation (76%).[30,36,37]

A wide variety of mesh repairs have been described, but it remains uncertain what type of mesh should be used and what the optimal position is for placement. The intraperitoneal or underlay mesh repair, championed by Sugarbaker, has probably been associated with the most encouraging results.[38] Intraabdominal pressure tends to keep the mesh in place. One benefit of the intraperitoneal technique is that a concomitant incisional hernia may be repaired at the same time. Various laparoscopic techniques have been successfully used for intraperitoneal mesh placement.[39–41] Concerns have been expressed about the long-term risk of mesh erosion, prompting interest in the use of biologic mesh materials.[37,42]

Mesh may also be placed using an extraperitoneal fascial onlay technique.[43,44]

A curvilinear lateral incision is made outside the outline of the stoma wafer. The hernia sac is entered, and omentum and bowel are reduced. An onlay mesh is secured to the fascial defect. The advantage of this technique is that it avoids a major intraperitoneal procedure, making it attractive in patients who are poor candidates for laparoscopy/laparotomy. However, the recurrence rate with this procedure is undoubtedly much higher than with underlay placement of the mesh.

STENOSIS

Stoma stenosis may result from ischemia, excessive tension, retraction, or recurrent inflammatory bowel disease. The reported incidence is typically less than 10%.[27] Mild asymptomatic stenosis does not require any treatment. Skin-level stenosis is readily treated with local procedures such as a Z- or W-plasty, whereas those associated with

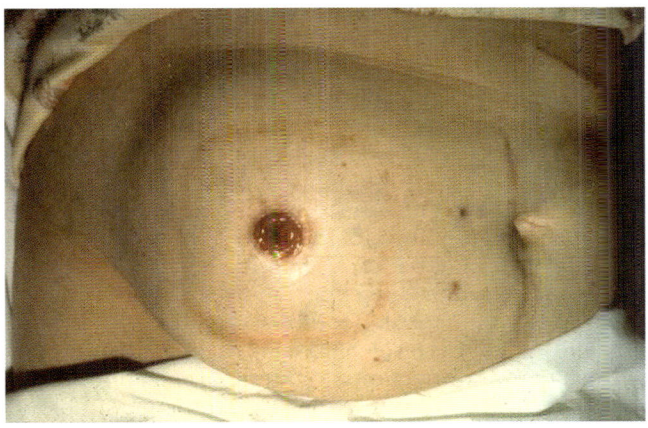

FIGURE 178.14 Large parastomal hernia.

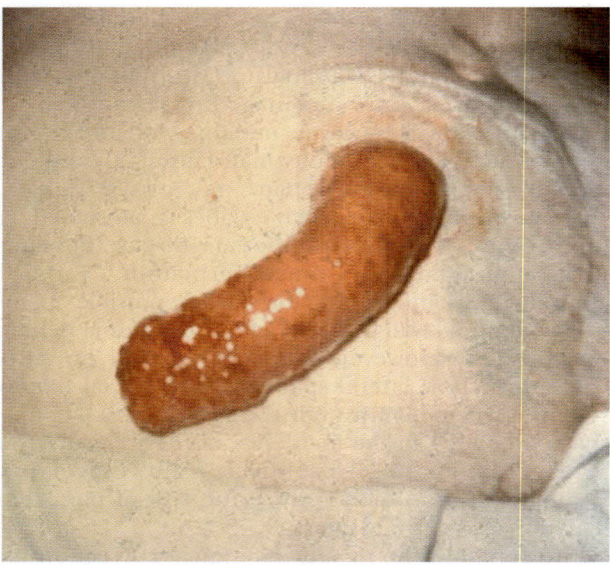

FIGURE 178.15 Prolapsed ileostomy.

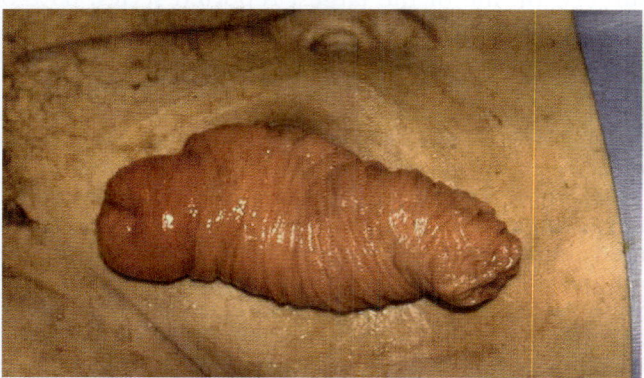

FIGURE 178.16 Large prolapse of a transverse loop colostomy.

Crohn disease usually require formal bowel resection.[45] Timing of surgery is an important consideration in patients with a retracted and/or stenotic stoma. Fourteen percent of colostomies and 12% of ileostomies develop retraction within 3 weeks of surgery; many of these will develop a stenosis, ultimately requiring revision.[46] With good enterostomal therapy (e.g., use of a convex pouch) and temporizing measures, such as gentle digital dilation, the acute inflammatory response is permitted to subside. This facilitates the ability to perform a local revision at a later date when the bowel and mesentery are less friable and rigid.

PROLAPSE

The risk of stoma prolapse has been reported to be 11.8% at 13 years (Fig. 178.15).[47] Transverse loop colostomies are especially notorious for prolapse (Fig. 178.16); the efferent limb is virtually always the offending cause. This is one of the reasons why loop ileostomy is commonly preferred to loop colostomy for temporary fecal diversion.[48] Although often advocated, mesenteric fixation or lateral

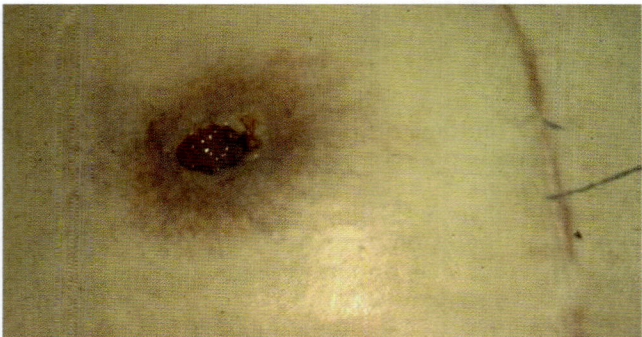

FIGURE 178.17 The characteristic blue hue of peristomal varices is visible only after removing the stoma appliance.

space closure do not appear to reduce the incidence of stoma prolapse.

Although the prolapse is often unsettling to the patient or health care providers, asymptomatic prolapse requires no treatment, especially if the stoma is temporary. When the prolapse causes ischemia, obstruction, or pouching problems, surgical intervention is warranted and usually straightforward. The stoma is freed up from the abdominal wall and the bowel delivered until taut. The redundant bowel is amputated and the mucocutaneous border reestablished. In cases of incarcerated prolapse without advanced ischemia, sugar can be applied as a desiccant to facilitate reduction and obviate the need for urgent surgery.[49]

PERISTOMAL VARICES

Stomal varices may cause life-threatening hemorrhage. The varices occur at the level of the mucocutaneous border of the ostomy secondary to the anastomoses between the high-pressure portal venous system and the low-pressure subcutaneous veins of the abdominal wall.[50] The diagnosis is suspected in ostomates with serious liver disease and confirmed by the typical purplish hue or "caput medusae" of the peristomal skin. Common scenarios include extensive liver metastases after abdominoperineal resection for rectal cancer or sclerosing cholangitis in a patient who has undergone total proctocolectomy with ileostomy for ulcerative colitis. A high index of suspicion is critical, and the stoma wafer must be removed to allow for skin inspection (Fig. 178.17).[51]

Patients with an acute bleed are managed with local pressure with epinephrine-soaked gauze or suture ligation and minimizing local trauma to the ostomy site. Additional therapy is directed at lowering the portal pressure by such procedures as transjugular intrahepatic portosystemic shunting (TIPS). Unfortunately, TIPS has a limited duration of action, usually 6 to 12 months. Percutaneous coil embolization may be another option.[52] Because many patients have a short life expectancy (e.g., extensive liver metastases), a mucocutaneous disconnection (the stoma is freed up to the level of fascia, thereby dividing the portosystemic connections) or stomal relocation may be considered. Unfortunately, these are difficult and bloody procedures, and the portosystemic anastomoses typically reform within 1 year. Long-term success may require a liver transplantation, based on the patient's life expectancy and the status of the associated liver disease.

ACKNOWLEDGMENT

Portions of this chapter were adapted from the previous edition by Cataldo and Hyman.

SUGGESTED READINGS

Carne PW, Robertson GM, Frizelle FA. Parastomal hernia. *Br J Surg.* 2003;90:784.

Cottam J, Richards K, Halsted A, Blackman A. Results of a nationwide prospective audit of stoma complications within three weeks of surgery. *Colorectal Dis.* 2007;9:834.

Israelsson LA. Parastomal hernias. *Surg Clin North Am.* 2008;88:113.

Lavery IC, Erwin-Toth P. Stoma therapy. In: Cataldo P, MacKeigan J, eds. *Intestinal Stomas.* New York: Marcel Dekker; 2004:65.

REFERENCES

1. Cataldo P, Hyman N. Ostomy management. In: Yeo CJ, Matthews JB, McFadden DW, eds. *Shackelford's Surgery of the Alimentary Tract.* 7th ed. Philadelphia: Saunders; 2012:2248-2261.
2. Bass EM, Pino AD, Tan A, Pearl RK, Orsay CP, Abcarian H. Does preoperative stoma marking and education by the enterostomal therapist affect outcome? *Dis Colon Rectum.* 1997;40:440.
3. Meagher AP, Owen G, Gett R. Multimedia article. An improved technique for end stoma creation in obese patients. *Dis Colon Rectum.* 2009;52:531.
4. Strong SA. The difficult stoma: challenges and strategies. *Clin Colon Rectal Surg.* 2016;29:152-159.
5. Unti JA, Abcarian H, Pearl RK, et al. Rodless end-loop stomas—a seven year experience. *Dis Colon Rectum.* 1991;34:999.
6. Beck DE. Abdominal wall modification for the difficult stoma. *Clin Colon Rectal Surg.* 2008;20:71-75.
7. Kawamura YJ, Kakizawa N, Tan KY, et al. Sushi-roll wrap of Seprafilm for ileostomy limbs facilitates ileostomy closure. *Tech Coloproctol.* 2009;13:211.
8. Salum M, Wexner SD, Nogueras JJ, et al. Does sodium hyaluronate-and carboxymethylcellulose-based bioresorbable membrane (Seprafilm) decrease operative time for loopileostomy closure? *Tech Coloproctol.* 2006;10:187-191.
9. Park JJ, Del Pino A, Orsay CE, et al. Stoma complications: the Cook County Hospital experience. *Dis Colon Rectum.* 1999;42:1575.
10. Duchesne JC, Wang YZ, Weintraub SL, Boyle M, Hunt JF. Stoma complications: a multivariate analysis. *Ann Surg.* 2002;68:961.
11. Pearl RK, Prasad LM, Orsay CP, Abcarian H, Tan AB, Melzl MT. Early local complications from intestinal stomas. *Arch Surg.* 1985;120:1145.
12. Saghir JH, McKenzie FD, Leckie DM. Factors that predict complications after construction of a stoma: a retrospective study. *Br J Surg.* 2001;167:531.
13. Arumugam PJ, Bevan L, MacDonald L, et al. A prospective audit of stomas—analysis of risk factors and complications and their management. *Colorectal Dis.* 2003;5:49.
14. Makela JT, Turku PH, Laitinen ST. Analysis of late stomal complications following ostomy surgery. *Ann Chir Gynaecol.* 1997;86:305.
15. Leenen LPH, Kuypers JH. Some factors influencing the outcome of stoma surgery. *Dis Colon Rectum.* 1989;32:500.
16. Evans JP, Brown MH, Wilkes GH, Cohen Z, McLeod RS. Revising the troublesome stoma: combined abdominal wall recontouring and revision of stomas. *Dis Colon Rectum.* 2003;46:122.
17. Tang CL, Yunos A, Leong AP, Seow-Choen F, Goh HS. Ileostomy output in the early postoperative period. *Br J Surg.* 1995;82:607.
18. Nehra V, Camilleri M, Burton D, Oenning L, Kelly DG. An open trial of octreotide long-acting release in the management of short bowel syndrome. *Am J Gastroenterol.* 2001;96:1494.
19. Wood M, Hyman N, Heber J, Blaszyk H. Catastrophic *Clostridium difficile* enteritis in a pelvic pouch patient. *J Gastrointest Surg.* 2008;1:350.
20. Lundeen SJ, Otterson MF, Binion DG, Carman ET, Peppard WJ. *Clostridium difficile* enteritis: an early postoperative complication in

21. Buchman AL, Scolapio J, Fryer J. AGA technical review on short bowel syndrome and intestinal transplantation. *Gastroenterology.* 2003;124:111.
22. Szilagyi A, Shrier I. Systematic review: the use of somatostatin or octreotide in refractory diarrhea. *Aliment Pharmacol Ther.* 2003;15:1889.
23. Calicis B, Parc Y, Caplin S, et al. Treatment of postoperative peritonitis of small bowel origin with continuous enteral nutrition and succus entericus refusion. *Arch Surg.* 2002;137:296.
24. Christie PM, Knight GS, Hill GL. Comparison of relative risks of urinary stone formation after surgery for ulcerative colitis: conventional ileostomy *vs.* J-pouch. A comparative study. *Dis Colon Rectum.* 1996;39:50.
25. Christie PM, Knight GS, Hill GL. Metabolism of body water and electrolytes after surgery for ulcerative colitis: conventional ileostomy versus J-pouch. *Br J Surg.* 1990;77:149.
26. Leong AP, Londono-Schimmer EE, Phillips RK. Life table analysis of stomal complications following ileostomy. *Br J Surg.* 1994;81:727.
27. Cottam J, Richards K, Hasted A, Blackman A. Results of a nationwide prospective audit of stoma complications within 3 weeks of surgery. *Colorectal Dis.* 2007;9:834.
28. Robertson I, Eung E, Hughes D, et al. Prospective analysis of stoma related complications. *Colorectal Dis.* 2005;7:279.
29. Shellito PC. Complications of abdominal stoma surgery. *Dis Colon Rectum.* 1998;41:1562.
30. Carne PW, Robertson GM, Frizelle FA. Parastomal hernia. *Br J Surg.* 2003;90:784.
31. Mylonakis E, Scarpa M, Barolla M, Yarnoz C, Keighley MR. Life table analysis of hernia following end colostomy construction. *Colorectal Dis.* 2001;3:334.
32. Janes A, Cengiz Y, Israelsson LA. Randomized clinical trial of the use of a prosthetic mesh to prevent parastomal hernia. *Br J Surg.* 2004;91:280.
33. Gögenur I, Mortensen J, Harvald T, Rosenberg J, Fischer A. Prevention of parastomal hernia by placement of a polypropylene mesh at the primary operation. *Dis Colon Rectum.* 2006;46:1131.
34. Hansson BM, Slater NJ, van der Velden AS, et al. Surgical techniques for parastomal hernia repair: a systematic review of the literature. *Ann Surg.* 2012;255(4):685-695.
35. Rubin MS, Schoetz DJ Jr, Matthews JB. Parastomal hernia. Is stoma relocation superior to fascial repair? *Arch Surg.* 1994;129:413.
36. Cheung M, Chia NH, Chiu WY. Surgical treatment of parastomal hernia complicating sigmoid colostomies. *Dis Colon Rectum.* 2001;44:266.
37. Steele SR, Lee P, Martin MJ, Mullenix PS, Sullivan ES. Is parastomal hernia repair with polypropylene mesh safe? *Am J Surg.* 2003;185:436.
38. Sugarbaker PH. Peritoneal approach to prosthetic mesh repair of paraostomy hernias. *Ann Surg.* 1985;201:344.
39. Stelzner S, Hellmich G, Ludwig K. Repair of paracolostomy hernias with a prosthetic mesh in the intraperitoneal onlay position: modified Sugarbaker technique. *Dis Colon Rectum.* 2004;47:185.
40. Hansson BME, Bleichrodt RP, de Hingh IH. Laparoscopic parastomal hernia repair using a keyhole technique results in a high recurrence rate. *Surg Endosc.* 2009;23:1456.
41. Mancini G, McClusky DA 3rd, Khaitan L, et al. Laparoscopic parastomal hernia repair using a nonslit mesh technique. *Surg Endosc.* 2007;21:1487.
42. Ellis CN. Short-term outcomes with the use of bioprosthetics for the management of parastomal hernias. *Dis Colon Rectum.* 2008;46:1118.
43. Hansson BME, van Nieuwenhoven EJ, Bleichrodt RP. Promising new technique in the repair of parastomal hernia. *Surg Endosc.* 2003;17:1789.
44. Amin SN, Armitage NC, Abercrombie JF, Scholefield JH. Lateral repair of parastomal hernia. *Ann R Coll Surg Engl.* 2001;83:206.
45. Beraldo S, Titley G, Allan A. Use of W-plasty in stenotic stoma: a new solution for an old problem. *Colorectal Dis.* 2006;8:715.
46. Londono-Schimmer EE, Leong AP, Phillips RK. Life table analysis of stomal complications following colostomy. *Dis Colon Rectum.* 1994;37:916.
47. Edwards DP, Leppington-Clarke A, Sexton R, Heald RJ, Moran BJ. Stoma-related complications are more frequent after transverse

colostomy than loop ileostomy: a prospective randomized clinical trial. *Br J Surg.* 2001;88:360.

48. Rondelli F, Reboldi P, Rulli A, et al. Loop ileostomy versus loop colostomy for fecal diversion after colorectal or coloanal anastomosis: a meta-analysis. *Int J Colorectal Dis.* 2009;24:479.

49. Shapiro R, Chin EH, Steinhagen RM. Reduction of an incarcerated, prolapsed ileostomy with the assistance of sugar as a desiccant. *Tech Coloproctol.* 2010;14:269.

50. Fucini CF, Wolff BG, Dozois RR. Bleeding from peristomal varices: perspectives on prevention and treatment. *Dis Colon Rectum.* 1991;34:1073.

51. Spier BJ, Fayyad AA, Lucey MR, et al. Bleeding stomal varices: case series and systematic review of the literature. *Clin Gastroenterol Hepatol.* 2008;6:346.

52. Naidu SG, Castle EP, Kriegshauser JS, Huettl EA. Direct percutaneous embolization of bleeding stomal varices. *Cardiovasc Intervent Radiol.* 2010;33:201.

Reducing the Risk of Infection in the Elective and Emergent Colectomy Patient

Emmanouil P. Papadou | Ravi P. Kiran

Colorectal surgery is associated with a greater risk for infections than most other surgical specialties and is considered an outlier for surgical site infections (SSIs). In addition to SSI, as with other types of surgical operations patients undergoing colectomy are at risk for respiratory, urinary tract, and line-related infections, as well as the development of *Clostridium difficile*. Perioperative measures can reduce the occurrence of these complications and improve outcomes.

SURGICAL SITE INFECTION

Colorectal surgery continues to have one of the highest rates of SSI among surgical procedures, with reported rates between 5% and 30%.[-6] SSIs are the most frequent adverse event after colorectal surgery and comprise a spectrum of infections occurring at the surgical site, ranging from a mild superficial infection to deep-seated abdominal cavity infections on the other side of the spectrum. The US Centers for Disease Control and Prevention (CDC) has developed criteria that define SSI as infection related to an operative procedure that occurs at or near the surgical incision within 30 days of the procedure or within a year if prosthetic material is implanted at surgery.[7] SSIs are divided anatomically into three categories of superficial, deep, and organ/space infections (Table 179.1). Superficial infections involve the skin and subcutaneous tissues, deep infections involve the muscle and fascia, and organ/space infections arise in the abdominal cavity. The CDC diagnostic criteria of SSIs have become the accepted national standard and are followed by medical staff, hospitals, health care organizations, and surveillance and quality control programs.[8-10]

SSIs in colorectal surgery are associated with significant morbidity, mortality, and increased health care costs, frequently requiring prolonged hospitalization, readmission, or even reoperation during the course of treatment. A study analyzing the impact of SSIs on hospital use and treatment costs using the Healthcare Cost and Utilization Project National Inpatient Sample (HCUP NIS) database found that SSIs extend the length of stay by an average of 9.7 days, while increasing costs by $20,842 per admission.[11] Because of the frequency and severity of their impact, many methods to prevent and reduce SSIs have been implemented. Preventing SSIs is a multidisciplinary endeavor; involving the entire health team, including nurses, surgical staff, and physicians, is critical. It may involve taking measures at every step of the care process, ranging from preoperative optimization, to the operating room and postoperative care, combined with audit and surveillance of SSI rates and providing feedback, as well as education to health care personnel when appropriate.[12-16]

PATHOGENESIS AND MICROBIOLOGY OF SURGICAL SITE INFECTIONS IN COLORECTAL SURGERY

SSIs in colorectal surgery originate in the majority of cases from contamination of the surgical site with the patient's endogenous flora, with the colonic lumen being the major (>90%) source of bacterial contamination. The colon is a repository of a large number of gram-negative and gram-positive aerobic as well as anaerobic bacteria, with counts as high as 10^{12} per gram of content, containing more than 600 different species of bacteria.[17] The higher the number of contaminating bacteria at the surgical site (inoculum), the higher the probability of developing an SSI because the quantity of bacterial contamination may exceed the capacity of the host for clearance.[18,19] *Escherichia coli* and *Bacteroides fragilis* are the most likely organisms to be encountered at the contaminated site, *B. fragilis* being the organism with the highest density in the left colon and rectosigmoid but inconsistently cultured because of its obligate anaerobic nature.[20] Aerobic (*E. coli*) and anaerobic (*B. fragilis*) colonic species can have a synergistic relationship that enhances their virulence when both species are concurrently present at a critical inoculum at the surgical site.[21] *Klebsiella pneumoniae* and *Enterococcus* species are common in the colon but infrequent causes of SSIs. *Pseudomonas aeruginosa*, *Serratia* species, and *Acinetobacter* species can be encountered in SSIs after colorectal surgery, especially in patients with prior antibiotic exposure or prolonged hospital stay resulting in alteration of the normal native microflora.[20]

Skin colonization can be a source for a smaller percentage (<20%) of infections. SSIs may originate from exogenous sources brought within the sterile field, such as the operating room environment, infected instruments and materials, or members of the surgical team. *Staphylococcus* species (e.g., *S. aureus* including methicillin-resistant *S. aureus* and coagulase-negative staphylococci) are responsible for the majority of SSIs caused by skin or operating room environmental contaminants.[22,23]

Another variable that may lead to SSIs after colorectal surgery is the patient's (host's) responsiveness to eradicating microbes. Innate or acquired immunodeficiency and chronic conditions, such as diabetes and liver, kidney, or lung insufficiency, as well as cancer, impair the host responsiveness and are associated with increased SSI rates in colorectal surgery.

TABLE 179.1 Classification and Definition of a Surgical Site Infection

SUPERFICIAL INCISIONAL SSI

Infection occurs within 30 days after the operation, and infection involves only skin or subcutaneous tissue of the incision and at least ONE of the following:

1. Purulent drainage, with or without laboratory confirmation, from the superficial incision.
2. Organisms isolated from an aseptically obtained culture of fluid or tissue from the superficial incision.
3. At least one of the following signs or symptoms of infection: pain or tenderness, localized swelling, redness, or heat AND superficial incision is deliberately opened by surgeon, UNLESS incision is culture negative.
4. Diagnosis of superficial incisional SSI by the surgeon or attending physician.

DEEP INCISIONAL SSI

Infection occurs within 30 days after the operation if no implant is left in place or within 1 year if implant is in place and the infection appears to be related to the operation, and infection involves deep soft tissues (e.g., fascial and muscle layers) of the incision and at least ONE of the following:

1. Purulent drainage from the deep incision but not from the organ/space component of the surgical site.
2. A deep incision spontaneously dehisces or is deliberately opened by a surgeon when the patient has at least one of the following signs or symptoms: fever (>38°C), localized pain, or tenderness, unless site is culture negative.
3. An abscess or other evidence of infection involving the deep incision is found on direct examination, during reoperation, or by histopathologic or radiologic examination.
4. Diagnosis of a deep incisional SSI by a surgeon or attending physician.

Notes

1. Report infection that involves both superficial and deep incision sites as deep incisional SSI.
2. Report an organ/space SSI that drains through the incision as a deep incisional SSI.

ORGAN/SPACE SSI

Infection occurs within 30 days after the operation if no implant is left in place or within 1 year if implant is in place and the infection appears to be related to the operation, and the infection involves any part of the anatomy (e.g., organs or spaces), other than the incision, which was opened or manipulated during an operation and at least one of the following:

1. Purulent drainage from a drain that is placed through a stab wound into the organ/space. If the area around a stab wound becomes infected, it is not an SSI. It is considered a skin or soft tissue infection, depending on its depth into the organ/space.
2. Organisms isolated from an aseptically obtained culture of fluid or tissue in the organ/space.
3. An abscess or other evidence of infection involving the organ/space that is found on direct examination, during reoperation, or by histopathologic or radiologic examination.
4. Diagnosis of an organ/space SSI by a surgeon or attending physician.

SSI, Surgical site infection.

Modified from Mangram AJ, Horan TC, Pearson ML, Silver LC, Jarvis WR. Guideline for prevention of surgical site infection. *Infect Control Hosp Epidemiol.* 1999;20:247–280.

Environmental and technical factors may contribute to SSIs in colorectal surgery, even with reduced bacterial counts; hematomas or necrotic tissue at the surgical site that provide a rich supply of nutrients, foreign bodies that cannot be cleaned by the host's phagocytes, and the presence of dead space that provides an aqueous environment for bacterial growth all enhance microbial replication and accordingly increase SSIs.[25–27] In addition, stool spillage during colorectal resection may seed the peritoneal cavity with high amounts of microbial contaminants that cannot be eradicated by the innate host response, leading to accumulation of colonic contents in areas of dependent drainage in the abdominal cavity, such as the pelvis or the paracolic gutters, leading to an abscess.[28]

Another important factor for development of SSIs, especially organ/space SSIs, following colorectal resection is the development of an anastomotic leak.[29] Anastomotic leak rates between 2% and 20% have been reported after colorectal surgery, with rates being higher for rectal surgery.[30–32] Patient factors such as age, sex, obesity, comorbidities, radiation and chemotherapy, as well as other determinants such as surgical technique and experience have all been shown to be important determining factors of anastomotic leak risk.

PREOPERATIVE MEASURES FOR PREVENTION OF SURGICAL SITE INFECTIONS IN COLORECTAL SURGERY

MALNUTRITION

Preoperative malnutrition is commonly observed in patients undergoing colorectal surgery, with reported rates as high as 30% to 50%.[33] Preoperative malnutrition is a major risk factor for increased postoperative morbidity and mortality. Hypoalbuminemia, with levels below 3.5 g/dL, especially in colorectal cancer patients significantly contributes to postoperative morbidity.[34] Although currently there is insufficient data to suggest that preoperative nutritional supplementation prevents SSIs, data from limited studies suggest that preoperative nutritional assessment and support may prove to be helpful in wound healing.[34–37]

ACTIVE INFECTION

If active infection is already present in the surgical site, it is considered to be a dirty wound. A near-linear relationship of escalating wound classification and subsequent SSIs has been demonstrated in the literature, with SSI rates as high as 40% for dirty wounds.[38,39] The presence of infection impairs the wound healing process because bacteria produce inflammatory mediators that inhibit the inflammatory phase of wound healing and prevent epithelialization.[40] Therefore it is recommended to allow healing of an active wound at the surgical site, if possible, before proceeding with elective colorectal surgery.

SMOKING CESSATION AND NICOTINE REPLACEMENT THERAPY

Cigarette smoking interferes with primary wound healing, possibly secondary to constriction of peripheral blood vessels, leading to tissue hypovolemia and hypoxia.[41] Smoking has been associated with poor perineal wound healing and deep SSIs after colorectal surgery.[42,43] In 2003 a randomized controlled trial demonstrated that abstinence from smoking for as little as 4 weeks significantly reduced SSIs.[44] No difference between transdermal nicotine patch and placebo was found. Based on these findings, smoking cessation and nicotine replacement therapy should be strongly recommended before elective colorectal resection.

PROLONGED PREOPERATIVE HOSPITALIZATION

Preoperative hospitalization of as little as 2 to 4 days has been associated with increased incidence of SSI rates and other hospital-acquired infections.[45,46] It is likely that colonization with resistant skin or colonic flora may lead to the increased resistance to preventive antibiotics and thus high SSI rates. Prolonged hospitalization is also a surrogate for patient and case complexity, resulting in higher complication rates.

PREOPERATIVE CLEANSING OF THE SURGICAL SITE

Preoperative showering and scrubbing of the surgical site with antiseptic soap or antiseptics has been proposed as a means of reducing SSIs.[47] It is unclear whether reducing skin microflora leads to a lower incidence of SSIs. In a meta-analysis including 10,157 participants, bathing with chlorhexidine compared with placebo did not result in a statistically significant reduction in SSIs.[48] Given that the major source of SSIs after colorectal surgery is from the colon, it is unlikely that aggressive skin cleansing will have a major impact on SSIs. However, almost all enhanced recovery programs include preoperative and postoperative skin-cleansing protocols.

BOWEL PREPARATION

Considerable current evidence supports the use of mechanical bowel preparation (MBP) in combination with oral antimicrobial prophylaxis as a method to facilitate the delivery of intraluminal antibiotics and reduce SSIs. The colorectal surgery literature has come full circle on this topic, first supporting the combined use of MBP and oral antibiotics for reduction of SSIs, later abandoning its use, until more recent clinical evidence overwhelmingly supported the use of combined preoperative MBP with oral antibiotics in reducing SSIs by nearly half.[49]

In the 1940s and 1950s it was known that an MBP alone did not reduce the high inoculum of bacteria within the colon lumen, therefore orally administered, poorly absorbed sulfa antibiotics were introduced to reduce the concentration of colonic bacteria.[50] Initial data in the early 1970s showed a remarkable reduction in SSI rates following MBP along with the oral administration of nonabsorbed oral antibiotics, which was shown to be associated with a reduction of the concentration of intraluminal colonic bacteria.[51,52] The original preparation described by Nichols et al. used a combination of oral erythromycin with neomycin, which led to reduction of SSI rates in randomized patients. A subsequent rush of prospective randomized trials in later years reported no benefit from MBP alone, and therefore colon resection with preoperative bowel preparation and oral antibiotics

was abandoned and even professional societies advised against its use.[53,54] However, more recent data including retrospective cohort studies, prospective randomized trials, and meta-analyses have confirmed a statistically significant reduction of SSIs by combining oral antibiotics and systemic antibiotics compared with systemic antibiotics alone.[49,55–59] Thus the weight of clinical evidence currently supports the use of MBP in combination with oral antibiotic bowel preparation and in conjunction with systemic preoperative antibiotics in preventing SSIs.

It is important to note that administering oral antibiotics independently of MBP is of unproven benefit. Timing is also of importance because administration of the oral antibiotics before the mechanical preparation is complete will likely result in the antibiotics passing through the colon with no benefit to the patient. In patients undergoing elective colon resection, we suggest the use of an MBP combined with oral antibiotics. MBP at our institution is accomplished with 238 g of polyethylene glycol solution mixed with 64 ounces of clear liquid, followed by 1 g of neomycin and 500 mg of metronidazole taken at 1 pm, 2 pm, and 10 pm.

INTRAOPERATIVE MEASURES FOR PREVENTION OF SURGICAL SITE INFECTIONS IN COLORECTAL SURGERY

PROPHYLACTIC ANTIBIOTICS

Use of intravenous prophylactic antibiotics is widely considered to be the most significant method for reducing SSIs in colorectal surgery. Timing of administration to optimize tissue concentration at the time of surgery and appropriate antibiotic selection are two key components of systemic antimicrobial prophylaxis.

Regarding the influence of timing of antibiotic prophylaxis, pioneering data from the 1970s demonstrated a statistically significant reduction in SSI rates in colorectal surgery with administration of antibiotics before incision; furthermore it was shown that initiation of antibiotics after wound closure had no impact on SSI rates.[60–62] Further data including a meta-analysis of randomized trials in colorectal surgery validated that only preoperative antibiotics are necessary for reduction of SSIs and that prolonged use of systemic antibiotics does not reduce SSIs.[63,64] Following closure of the wound, the dead space is promptly filled with fibrin, creating a dense protein matrix that is functionally ischemic, excluding the possibility of effective antibiotic delivery.

Optimal time for administration of parenteral antibiotics is believed to be 30 to 60 minutes prior to incision or within 2 hours before incision if vancomycin or floroquinolones are required for prophylaxis. Another consideration is the biologic elimination or half-life of antibiotic. Short half-life antibiotics may be cleared rapidly from the bloodstream and no surgical protection may be available if operations are extended beyond the second half-life of the antibiotics. Thus long half-life antibiotics, such as cefotetan, are preferred, and timely redosing of short half-life antibiotics is recommended to extend the duration of the effect after the procedure is initiated.

TABLE 179.2 Antimicrobial Prophylaxis Choices Currently Recommended for Colorectal Surgery by the Surgical Care Improvement Project

Recommended Agents	Alternative Agents in Patients With β-Lactam Allergy
1. Cefazolin + metronidazole, OR cefoxitin, OR cefotetan, OR ampicillin-sulbactam*	1. Clindamycin + aminoglycoside‡ OR aztreonam OR fluoroquinolone§
2. Ceftriaxone + metronidazole,† OR ertapenem	2. Metronidazole + aminoglycoside‡ OR fluoroquinolone§

For most patients, a mechanical bowel preparation combined with oral neomycin sulfate plus oral erythromycin base or with oral neomycin sulfate plus oral metronidazole should be given in addition to intravenous pro-phylaxis.

The antimicrobial agent should be started within 60 min before surgical incision (120 min for vancomycin or fluoroquinolones).

Although single-dose prophylaxis is usually sufficient, the duration of prophylaxis for all procedures should be less than 24 h.

If an agent with a short half-life is used (e.g., cefazolin, cefoxitin), it should be readministered if the procedure duration exceeds the recommended redosing interval. Readministration may also be warranted if prolonged or excessive bleeding occurs or if there are other factors that may shorten the half-life of the prophylactic agent (e.g., extensive burns). Readministra-tion may not be warranted in patients in whom the half-life of the agent may be prolonged (e.g., patients with renal insufficiency or failure).

*Due to increasing resistance of *E. coli* to fluoroquinolones and ampicillin-sulbactam, local population susceptibility profiles should be reviewed prior to use.

†Where there is increasing resistance to first- and second-generation cephalosporins among gram-negative isolates from surgical site infections, a single dose of ceftriaxone plus metronidazole may be preferred over the routine use of carbapenems.

‡Gentamicin or tobramycin.

§Due to increasing resistance of *E. coli* to fluorocuinolones and ampicillin-sulbactam, local population susceptibility profiles should be reviewed prior to use. Ciprofloxacin or levofloxacin. Fluoroquinolones are associated with an increased risk of tendonitis and tendon rupture in all ages. However, this risk would be expected to be quite small with single-dose antibiotic prophylaxis. Although the use of fluoroquinolones may be necessary for surgical antibiotic prophylaxis in some children, they are not drugs of first choice in the pediatric population, due to an increased incidence of adverse events as compared with controls in some clinical trials.

Modified from Bratzler DW, Dellinger EP, Olsen KM, et al. Clinical practice guidelines for antimicrobial prophylaxis in surgery. *Am J Health Syst Pharm*. 2013;70(3):195–283.

Appropriate selection of antibiotics that have activity against the likely pathogens of the surgical site is also important.[65] It is important to target the likely pathogens that cause SSIs. The currently recommended prophylactic antibiotic choices by the US Surgical Care Improvement Project (SCIP) are shown in Table 179.2. Combination antibiotics, such as a first-generation cephalosporin (e.g., cefazolin), along with anaerobic coverage, such as a metronidazole, is the preferred approach at our institution, and clindamycin and a fluoroquinolone or metronidazole and a fluoroquinolone may be another choice. Each hospital pharmacy and therapeutics committee will have a recommended list of "institution appropriate" prophylaxis.

Another issue for which there is paucity of data is appropriate dosage of antibiotics. Traditionally the same dosing has been used for all patients. However, for bariatric patients and patients with a body mass index greater than 30 kg/m², consideration to increase the conventional antibiotic dose is recommended to achieve adequate incisional concentrations. Lastly, no studies have examined the use of methicillin-resistant *Staphylococcus aureus* (MRSA) coverage for colorectal patients. MRSA decontamination or coverage is currently not recommended for elective colon surgery; however, in patients who have had recent prolonged hospitalization, in nursing home patients, or patients who have been recently exposed to antibiotics, consideration for broader spectrum antibiotics should be made.

HAIR REMOVAL

Preoperative hair removal, especially when razors are used for shaving, has been associated with an increased rate of SSIs in the majority of studies and should be avoided.[66,67] If necessary, hair removal can be performed with clippers or depilatory agents just prior to incision.[39,68] In a meta-analysis that included 11 randomized trials, there were nonsignificant trends toward higher rates of SSI in patients who had their hair shaved, compared with those who did not or those who used a depilatory cream. More SSIs occurred in patients who underwent hair removal through shaving compared with clipping, suggesting that if hair needs to be removed, it should be clipped rather than shaved.[39]

SKIN ANTISEPSIS

Routine application of antiseptic solutions to the skin should be performed prior to surgery to reduce the burden of skin flora.[66] The three most commonly used topical antiseptic agents are chlorhexidine, povidone iodine, and isopropyl alcohol. Isopropyl alcohol has the best antibacterial activity but is also flammable and has been associated with fires in the operating room. Chlorhexi-dine solution has been associated with lower SSI rates compared with povidone iodine.[70,71] Chlorhexidine may be superior to iodine because chlorhexidine is not inac-tivated by blood or serum.[72] Recently, chlorhexidine-alcohol combinations have been used. The alcohol evaporation ensures timely drying of the chlorhexidine, and the mixture has been shown to be superior compared with povidone iodine alone in a randomized trial of 849 patients undergo-ing clean-contaminated surgery.[73]

SURGICAL HAND HYGIENE, TECHNIQUE AND USE OF MINIMALLY INVASIVE SURGERY

Although there is general agreement that hand hygiene and proper surgical technique reduces the risk of SSIs, evidence-based studies are lacking. In a recent review that analyzed the results of 14 trials, no evidence was found for one type of hand antisepsis being better than another in reducing SSIs. It is unclear whether the use of nail picks or brushes have a differential impact on the number of colony-forming units remaining on the hand.[74]

Minimizing tissue injury during surgery, ensuring adequate hemostasis, and gentle handling of the tissues including at the incision and within the abdomen are believed to be important in preventing SSIs. Excessive traction or pressure creates local inflammation that may lead to tissue necrosis and may result in increased SSI rates. The minimally invasive approach has been independently associated with a reduced SSI when compared with open surgery and should, when feasible, be considered for colon and rectal operations.[75,76] Steroid use, length of operation, prior radiation, creation of ostomy, and intraoperative need for blood transfusion have all been identified as technical and intraoperative risk factors for SSIs.[8,28,77,78] Colon and rectal surgeries differ with regard to incidence and risk factors for developing superficial, deep, and organ/space SSIs.[23] SSI rates in rectal surgery have been reported in some studies to be nearly twice as high compared with colon surgery with creation of a colostomy, preoperative radiation and preoperative use of steroids identified as independent risk factors.[78] Prophylactic use of intraabdominal drains after colorectal surgery, especially after complex pelvic surgery, may decrease the development of pelvic collections; however, it is not clear whether drains influence the rates of SSIs.[79] A meta-analysis of 11 randomized trials, which included 1803 patients, demonstrated that routine use of prophylactic drainage after creation of a colorectal anastomosis does not reduce complications, including SSIs.[80] Suture material coated with antibacterial or antiseptic products, such as triclosan, has been theorized to prevent SSIs and has been shown to reduce bacterial growth in vivo; however, clinical studies have shown conflicting results in reducing SSIs.[81,82] The use of surgical safety checklists has also been demonstrated to decrease the rates of postoperative complications, including SSIs.[83,84] Preventive SSI bundles in colorectal surgery, which may include various measures, such as changes in gown and gloves, redraping, wound lavage, and new sets of instruments for closure, may also be associated with a decrease in surgical adverse events, but it is possible that many of the positive changes associated with the use of the bundles are due to temporal changes, confounding factors, and publication bias.[15,74,85]

WOUND PROTECTORS AND WOUND IRRIGATION

Wound protectors are devices that are placed into a surgical wound to protect it from contamination and provide atraumatic tissue retraction. They also provide a barrier to keep the wound edges from drying out. Wound protectors are available for incisions in both laparoscopic and open cases. A meta-analysis of six randomized controlled trials, representing 1008 patients, evaluating the use of wound protectors in gastrointestinal surgical procedures found that the use of a wound protector was associated with nearly a 50% decrease in SSIs (relative risk [RR] = 0.55; 95% confidence interval [CI] = 0.31 to 0.98 P = .04).[86] However, multicenter randomized trials from the United Kingdom and Germany did not demonstrate a significant reduction of SSIs with the use of wound protectors.[87,88]

Irrigation of the surgical site with saline, antiseptic, or antimicrobial agents has been proposed to reduce bacterial wound contamination and the risk of SSIs. A meta-analysis of 41 randomized controlled trials covering more than 9000 patients compared intraoperative wound irrigation (IOWI) using any solution with no irrigation, and it revealed a significant benefit in the reduction of SSI rates with irrigation ([odds ratio] OR = 0.54, 95% CI = 0.42; 0.69, P < .0001).[89] Subgroup analysis showed that this effect was strongest in colorectal surgery and that IOWI with antibiotic solutions had a stronger effect than irrigation with povidone iodine or saline. However, all of the included trials were at considerable risk of bias according to the quality assessment.

INCREASED OXYGEN DELIVERY

Several experimental and clinical studies have documented the potential benefits of increasing intraoperative oxygen delivery in the prevention of SSIs following bacterial contamination.[90,91] In a randomized trial of 500 patients undergoing elective open colorectal resection, administration of 80% of inspired oxygen during the operation and for 2 hours afterward led to a statistical reduction in SSIs.[91] A meta-analysis of randomized controlled trials, which included 8093 patients, also demonstrated that high fraction of inspired oxygen (FiO_2) had a statistically significant benefit in reducing SSIs in patients undergoing colorectal surgery, with a risk ratio of 0.735 (95% CI, 0.573 to 0.944 P = .016).[92] Additional studies are needed to clarify the optimal inspired oxygen concentration, the benefits, and perhaps the risks of this preventive method. An analysis demonstrated that supplemental oxygen had no influence on long-term mortality in the surgical population or in patients having cancer surgery.[93]

PRESERVATION OF NORMOTHERMIA

Mild perioperative hypothermia, which is common during major surgery, has been hypothesized to predispose patients to SSIs by triggering thermoregulatory vasoconstriction, which may decrease the partial pressure of oxygen in tissues, impair oxidative killing by neutrophils, and interfere with collagen deposition, resulting in impaired wound healing.[94] In a randomized trial of 200 patients undergoing colorectal surgery, patients who were randomized to be maintained at normothermia (36.7°C) intraoperatively had a lower rate of SSIs and shorter hospitalizations compared with patients who were allowed to have their core temperatures decline to as low as 34.7°C. SSIs occurred in 19% of hypothermic patients versus 6% of the normothermic patients (P = .009), and the duration of hospitalization was prolonged by 2.6 days (approximately 20%) in the hypothermia group (P = .01).[95] This led to the adoption of maintaining normothermia as a process measure by the SCIP. However, this notion was challenged in subsequent studies, which concluded that intraoperative hypothermia is not a predictive factor of SSIs on multivariate analyses.[96,97] Further randomized trials are necessary to validate the role of normothermia in reducing SSIs in colorectal surgery.

POSTOPERATIVE MEASURES FOR PREVENTION OF SURGICAL SITE INFECTIONS IN COLORECTAL SURGERY

GLYCEMIC CONTROL

Studies have consistently shown that hyperglycemia causes immunosuppression.[98] Postoperative hyperglycemia has been associated with increased risk of SSIs in all operations, including colorectal resections.[99–101] Treating hyperglycemia has become a target of many enhanced recovery after surgery programs developed for colorectal procedures.[102] A retrospective review of 5145 patients (1072 were diabetic) undergoing colorectal operations showed an increased risk of superficial SSI (OR = 1.53; P = .03), sepsis (OR = 1.61; P < .01), and death (OR = 2.26; P < .01), in the setting of postoperative serum hyperglycemia (blood glucose >180 mg/dL) only in nondiabetic patients. The study concluded that hyperglycemia and not diabetes is associated with development of SSIs.[103] Even a single postoperative elevated glucose value has been shown to be adversely associated with morbidity and mortality after colorectal surgery.[104] In the future, specific pathways and vigorous postoperative assessment of blood glucose levels for patients at risk for perioperative hyperglycemia may address this specific issue.

DRESSINGS AND WOUND CARE

Dressings used on primarily closed wounds may be removed 24 hours after closure, because a fibrin seal is already present. Daily wound probing and use of wicks with modified primary closure have been shown in small studies to be associated with reduction of SSIs in contaminated wounds.[105,106] Furthermore, trials investigating the role of incisional negative pressure wound therapy in decreasing the morbidity and costs associated with the development of SSI in colorectal patients are underway.[107]

Future research in the biology of SSIs and novel therapeutic measures will be instrumental in providing evidence-based methods to further reduce SSIs and their associated consequences.

REDUCING THE RISK OF OTHER INFECTIONS

URINARY TRACT INFECTIONS

More than 4% of patients undergoing colorectal surgery develop postoperative urinary tract infection (UTI).[108,109] In an analysis of National Surgical Quality Improvement Program data, independent predictors of UTI after colorectal surgery included female sex (OR = 1.705), open procedure (OR = 1.419), rectal procedure (OR = 1.267), older than 65 years (OR = 1.322), nonindependent functional status (OR = 1.609), steroid use (OR = 1.524), higher anesthesia class, and longer operative time.[110] Patients with UTI had longer hospital stays (7 vs. 12 days), higher reoperation rates (11.9% vs. 5.1%), and higher 30-day mortality (3.3% vs. 1.7%). Postoperative UTI correlated with other complications, including sepsis, SSIs, and pulmonary embolism (P < .001).

Early urinary catheter removal after colorectal surgery reduces UTI rates significantly while only slightly increasing the risk of urinary retention and has been promoted as a part of the national SCIP. Enhanced recovery after surgery protocols often include catheter removal on postoperative day 1, and some studies have noted a significantly reduced postoperative UTI rate compared with conventional patient groups.[111] For nonpelvic colorectal resections, the evidence supports removal of the catheter on postoperative day 1.[112] Most enhanced recovery protocols recommend removal of the catheter in the immediate recovery period after routine colectomy. For mid-to-low rectal surgery, the risk of urinary retention is increased, and catheter removal

on day 3 to day 6 is recommended. Nagle et al. found that sterile intraoperative placement of urinary catheters and a daily electronic prompt requiring justification for catheters postoperatively reduced UTI rates from 6.9% to 0.8% in their colorectal patient cohort.[113]

RESPIRATORY TRACT INFECTIONS

Pneumonia occurs in approximately 6% of patients after colorectal surgery and is a major cause of perioperative death, especially in older adults, in patients with comorbidities, and after emergency colorectal procedures.[114,115] A multidisciplinary approach is often necessary to prevent respiratory tract infections and involves patient and family education, preoperative smoking cessation, early postoperative mobilization, pulmonary care with use of incentive spirometry, coughing and deep breathing, oral care, and head-of-bed elevation.[116,117]

CLOSTRIDIUM DIFFICILE INFECTION

C. difficile is a spore-forming, anaerobic, gram-positive rod that produces a toxin that injures the colonic mucosa. Antibiotic administration prompts transmission of these spores into active bacteria, which are pathogenic. *C. difficile* toxin A (an enterotoxin) and toxin B (a cytotoxin) classically produce a colitis in humans. Usual symptoms are crampy abdominal pain and diarrhea. A diagnosis of *C. difficile* should be considered in symptomatic patients who have been on antibiotics in the previous 3 months, been hospitalized, or develop diarrhea within 48 hours of admission. Predisposing factors for *C. difficile* colitis include antibiotic therapy, proton pump inhibitors, older age, immunosuppression, organ transplantation, and hospitalization. Diagnosis is typically by genetic testing for the *C. difficile* toxin by polymerase chain reaction (PCR) or stool culture. *C. difficile* infection occurs at a high incidence (5% to 7%) in patients who have undergone surgery involving the gastrointestinal tract.[118] Preoperative oral antibiotics, metallic colonic stent insertion, and age 60 have been identified as risk factors after colorectal surgery.[119,120] Metronidazole orally is the drug of choice for mild colitis. For severe disease, oral vancomycin is used. Several randomized trials suggest that fidaxomicin is superior to vancomycin and associated with improved survival, lower rates of recurrence, and less diarrhea.[121–123] Rarely, in immunocompromised patients, acute fulminant colitis requires total abdominal colectomy.

CONCLUSION

Prevention of SSIs can be achieved by several methods, including optimized preoperative patient preparation, perioperative bowel preparation, strict adherence to antibiotic prophylaxis guidelines, proper tissue handling during operation, increased intraoperative oxygen delivery, wound irrigation, maintenance of intraoperative normothermia, and postoperative glycemic control. Prevention of UTIs can be achieved by early urinary catheter removal and sterile intraoperative catheter placement. Respiratory infections can be prevented by smoking cessation, early postoperative mobilization, pulmonary care with use of incentive spirometry, coughing and deep breathing, oral care, and head-of-bed elevation. Future research in the biology of SSIs and novel therapeutic measures should provide evidence-based methods to further reduce postoperative infections.

REFERENCES

1. Itani KM, Wilson SE, Awad SS, Jensen EH, Finn TS, Abramson MA. Ertapenem versus cefotetan prophylaxis in elective colorectal surgery. *N Engl J Med.* 2006;355(25):2640-2651.
2. Serra-Aracil X, Garcia-Domingo MI, Pares D, et al. Surgical site infection in elective operations for colorectal cancer after the application of preventive measures. *Arch Surg.* 2011;146(5):606-612.
3. Tang R, Chen HH, Wang YL, et al. Risk factors for surgical site infection after elective resection of the colon and rectum: a single-center prospective study of 2,809 consecutive patients. *Ann Surg.* 2001;234(2):181-189.
4. National Nosocomial Infections Surveillance (NNIS) System report, data summary from October 1986–April 1998, issued June 1998. *Am J Infect Control.* 1998;26(5):522-533.
5. Kobayashi M, Mohri Y, Inoue Y, Okita Y, Miki C, Kusunoki M. Continuous follow-up of surgical site infections for 30 days after colorectal surgery. *World J Surg.* 2008;32(6):1142-1146.
6. Wick EC, Vogel JD, Church JM, Remzi F, Fazio VW. Surgical site infections in a high outlier institution: are colorectal surgeons to blame? *Dis Colon Rectum.* 2009;52(3):374-379.
7. Horan TC, Gaynes RP, Martone WJ, Jarvis WR, Emori TG. CDC definitions of nosocomial surgical site infections, 1992: a modification of CDC definitions of surgical wound infections. *Infect Control Hosp Epidemiol.* 1992;13(10):606-608.
8. Consensus paper on the surveillance of surgical wound infections. The Society for Hospital Epidemiology of America; The Association for Practitioners in Infection Control; The Centers for Disease Control; The Surgical Infection Society. *Infect Control Hosp Epidemiol.* 1992;13(10):599-605.
9. Draft guideline for the prevention of surgical site infection, 1998—CDC. Notice. *Fed Regist.* 1998;63(116):33168-33192.
10. Berrios-Torres SI. Evidence-based update to the U.S. Centers for Disease Control and Prevention and Healthcare Infection Control Practices advisory committee guideline for the prevention of surgical site infection: developmental process. *Surg Infect.* 2016;17(2):256-261.
11. de Lissovoy G, Fraeman K, Hutchins V, Murphy D, Song D, Vaughn BB. Surgical site infection: incidence and impact on hospital utilization and treatment costs. *Am J Infect Control.* 2009;37(5):387-397.
12. Mangram AJ, Horan TC, Pearson ML, Silver LC, Jarvis WR. Guideline for prevention of surgical site infection, 1999. Hospital Infection Control Practices Advisory Committee. *Infect Control Hosp Epidemiol.* 1999;20(4):250-278; quiz 279-280.
13. Jamtvedt G, Young JM, Kristoffersen DT, O'Brien MA, Oxman AD. Audit and feedback: effects on professional practice and health care outcomes. *Cochrane Database Syst Rev.* 2006;(2):CD000259.
14. Nair BG, Newman SF, Peterson GN, Wu WY, Schwid HA. Feedback mechanisms including real-time electronic alerts to achieve near 100% timely prophylactic antibiotic administration in surgical cases. *Anesth Analg.* 2010;111(5):1293-1300.
15. Tanner J, Padley W, Assadian O, Leaper D, Kiernan M, Edmiston C. Do surgical care bundles reduce the risk of surgical site infections in patients undergoing colorectal surgery? A systematic review and cohort meta-analysis of 8,515 patients. *Surgery.* 2015;158(1):66-77.
16. Yamamoto T, Morimoto T, Kita R, et al. The preventive surgical site infection bundle in patients with colorectal perforation. *BMC Surg.* 2015;15:128.
17. Ahmed S, Macfarlane GT, Fite A, McBain AJ, Gilbert P, Macfarlane S. Mucosa-associated bacterial diversity in relation to human terminal ileum and colonic biopsy samples. *Appl Environ Microbiol.* 2007;73(22):7435-7442.
18. Robson MC, Krizek TJ, Heggers JP. Biology of surgical infection. *Curr Probl Surg.* 1973;1-62.
19. Krizek TJ, Robson MC. Evolution of quantitative bacteriology in wound management. *Am J Surg.* 1975;130(5):579-584.
20. Owens CD, Stoessel K. Surgical site infections: epidemiology, microbiology and prevention. *J Hosp Infect.* 2008;70(suppl 2):3-10.
21. Onderdonk AB, Bartlett JG, Louie T, Sullivan-Seigler N, Gorbach SL. Microbial synergy in experimental intra-abdominal abscess. *Infect Immun.* 1976;13(1):22-26.
22. Hidron AI, Edwards JR, Patel J, et al. NHSN annual update: antimicrobial-resistant pathogens associated with healthcare-associated infections: annual summary of data reported to the National Healthcare Safety Network at the Centers for Disease Control and Prevention, 2006–2007. *Infect Control Hosp Epidemiol.* 2008;29(11):996-1011.
23. Fry DE, Barie PS. The changing face of *Staphylococcus aureus*: a continuing surgical challenge. *Surg Infect (Larchmt).* 2011;12(3):191-203.
24. Fry DE, Fry RV. Surgical site infection: the host factor. *AORN J.* 2007;86(5):801-810; quiz 811-4.
25. Fry DE. The prevention of surgical site infection in elective colon surgery. *Scientifica (Cairo).* 2013;2013:896297.
26. Poggio JL. Perioperative strategies to prevent surgical-site infection. *Clin Colon Rectal Surg.* 2013;26(3):168-173.
27. Polk HC Jr, Miles AA. Enhancement of bacterial infection by ferric iron: kinetics, mechanisms, and surgical significance. *Surgery.* 1971;70(1):71-77.
28. Adelaide Murray AC, Pasam R, Estrada D, Kiran RP. Risk of surgical site infection varies based on location of disease and segment of colorectal resection for cancer. *Dis Colon Rectum.* 2016;59(6):493-500.
29. Rickles AS, Iannuzzi JC, Kelly KN, et al. Anastomotic leak or organ space surgical site infection: what are we missing in our quality improvement programs? *Surgery.* 2013;154(4):680-687; discussion 687–689.
30. Trencheva K, Morrissey KP, Wells M, et al. Identifying important predictors for anastomotic leak after colon and rectal resection: prospective study on 616 patients. *Ann Surg.* 2013;257(1):108-113.
31. Frasson M, Flor-Lorente B, Rodríguez JL, et al. Risk factors for anastomotic leak after colon resection for cancer: multivariate analysis and nomogram from a multicentric, prospective, national study with 3193 patients. *Ann Surg.* 2015;262(2):321-330.
32. Daams F, Wu Z, Lahaye MJ, Jeekel J, Lange JF. Prediction and diagnosis of colorectal anastomotic leakage: a systematic review of literature. *World J Gastrointest Surg.* 2014;6(2):14-26.
33. Truong A, Hanna MH, Moghadamyeghaneh Z, Stamos MJ. Implications of preoperative hypoalbuminemia in colorectal surgery. *World J Gastrointest Surg.* 2016;8(5):353-362.
34. Hu WH, Cajas-Monson LC, Eisenstein S, Parry L, Cosman B, Ramamoorthy S. Preoperative malnutrition assessments as predictors of postoperative mortality and morbidity in colorectal cancer: an analysis of ACS-NSQIP. *Nutr J.* 2015;14:91.
35. Kabata P, Jastrzębski T, Kąkol M, et al. Preoperative nutritional support in cancer patients with no clinical signs of malnutrition—prospective randomized controlled trial. *Support Care Cancer.* 2015;23(2):365-370.
36. Jie B, Jiang ZM, Nolan MT, Zhu SN, Yu K, Kondrup J. Impact of preoperative nutritional support on clinical outcome in abdominal surgical patients at nutritional risk. *Nutrition.* 2012;28(10):1022-1027.
37. Arnold M, Barbul A. Nutrition and wound healing. *Plast Reconstr Surg.* 2006;117(7 suppl):42S-58S.
38. Culver DH, Horan TC, Gaynes RP, et al. Surgical wound infection rates by wound class, operative procedure, and patient risk index. National Nosocomial Infections Surveillance System. *Am J Med.* 1991;91(3B):152S-157S.
39. Cruse PJ, Foord R. The epidemiology of wound infection. A 10-year prospective study of 62,939 wounds. *Surg Clin N Am.* 1980;60(1):27-40.
40. Bowler PG, Duerden BI, Armstrong DG. Wound microbiology and associated approaches to wound management. *Clin Microbiol Rev.* 2001;14(2):244-269.
41. Turan A, Mascha EJ, Roberman D, et al. Smoking and perioperative outcomes. *Anesthesiology.* 2011;114(4):837-846.
42. Wilson MZ, Dillon PW, Stewart DB, Hollenbeak CS. Timing of postoperative infections after colectomy: evidence from NSQIP. *Am J Surg.* 2016;212(5):844-850.
43. Althumairi AA, Canner JK, Gearhart SL, et al. Risk factors for wound complications after abdominoperineal resection: analysis of the ACS NSQIP database. *Colorectal Dis.* 2016;18(7):O260-O266.
44. Sorensen LT, Karlsmark T, Gottrup F. Abstinence from smoking reduces incisional wound infection: a randomized controlled trial. *Ann Surg.* 2003;238(1):1-5.
45. Vogel TR, Dombrovskiy VY, Lowry SF. In-hospital delay of elective surgery for high volume procedures: the impact on infectious complications. *J Am Coll Surg.* 2010;211(6):784-790.
46. Cruse PJ, Foord R. A five-year prospective study of 23,649 surgical wounds. *Arch Surgery.* 1973;107(2):206-210.

47. Murray BW, Huerta S, Dineen S, Anthony T. Surgical site infection in colorectal surgery: a review of the nonpharmacologic tools of prevention. *J Am Coll Surg.* 2010;211(6):812-822.

48. Webster J, Osborne S. Preoperative bathing or showering with skin antiseptics to prevent surgical site infection. *Cochrane Database Syst Rev.* 2015;(2):CD004985.

49. Kiran RP, Murray AC, Chiuzan C, Estrada D, Forde K. Combined preoperative mechanical bowel preparation with oral antibiotics significantly reduces surgical site infection, anastomotic leak, and ileus after colorectal surgery. *Ann Surg.* 2015;262(3):416-425; discussion 423–425.

50. Firor WM, Jonas AF. The use of sulfanilylguanidine in surgical patients. *Ann Surg.* 1941;114(1):19-31.

51. Nichols RL, Broido P, Condon RE, Gorbach SL, Nyhus LM. Effect of preoperative neomycin-erythromycin intestinal preparation on the incidence of infectious complications following colon surgery. *Ann Surg.* 1973;178(4):453-462.

52. Nichols RL, Condon RE, DiSanto AR. Preoperative bowel preparation. Erythromycin base serum and fecal levels following oral administration. *Arch Surg.* 1977;112(12):1493-1496.

53. Cao F, Li J, Li F. Mechanical bowel preparation for elective colorectal surgery: updated systematic review and meta-analysis. *Int J Colorectal Dis.* 2012;27(6):803-810.

54. Eskicioglu C, Forbes SS, Fenech DS, McLeod RS, Best Practice in General Surgery Committee. Preoperative bowel preparation for patients undergoing elective colorectal surgery: a clinical practice guideline endorsed by the Canadian Society of Colon and Rectal Surgeons. *Can J Surg.* 2010;53(6):385-395.

55. Cannon JA, Altom LK, Deierhoi RJ, et al. Preoperative oral antibiotics reduce surgicl site infection following elective colorectal resections. *Dis Colon Rectum.* 2012;55(11):1160-1166.

56. Bellows CF, Mills KT, Kelly TN, Gagliardi G. Combination of oral non-absorbable and intravenous antibiotics versus intravenous antibiotics alone in the prevention of surgical site infections after colorectal surgery: a meta-analysis of randomized controlled trials. *Tech Coloproctol.* 2011;15(4):385-395.

57. Lewis RT. Oral versus systemic antibiotic prophylaxis in elective colon surgery: a randomized study and meta-analysis send a message from the 1990s. *Can J Surg.* 2002;45(3):173-180.

58. Morris MS, Graham LA, Chu DI, Cannon JA, Hawn MT. Oral antibiotic bowel preparation significantly reduces surgical site infection rates and readmission rates in elective colorectal surgery. *Ann Surg.* 2015;261(6):1034-1040.

59. Nelson RL, Gladman E, Barbateskovic M. Antimicrobial prophylaxis for colorectal surgery. *Cochrane Database Syst Rev.* 2014;(5):CD001181.

60. Polk HC Jr, Lopez-Mayor JF. Postoperative wound infection: a prospective study of determinant factors and prevention. *Surgery.* 1969;66(1):97-103.

61. Stone HH, Haney BB, Kolb LD, Geheber CE, Hooper CA. Prophylactic and preventive antibiotic therapy: timing, duration and economics. *Ann Surg.* 1979;189(6):691-699.

62. Stone HH, Hooper CA, Kolb LD, Geheber CE, Dawkins EJ. Antibiotic prophylaxis in gastric, biliary and colonic surgery. *Ann Surg.* 1976;184(4):443-452.

63. McDonald M, Grabsch E, Marshall C, Forbes A. Single- versus multiple-dose antimicrobial prophylaxis for major surgery: a systematic review. *Aust N Z J Surg.* 1998;68(6):388-396.

64. Song F, Glenny AM. Antimicrobial prophylaxis in colorectal surgery: a systematic review of randomized controlled trials. *Br J Surg.* 1998;85(9):1232-1241.

65. Bratzler DW, Dellinger EP, Olsen KM, et al. Clinical practice guidelines for antimicrobial prophylaxis in surgery. *Am J Health Syst Pharm.* 2013;70(3):195-283.

66. Anderson DJ, Podgorny K, Berríos-Torres SI, et al. Strategies to prevent surgical site infections in acute care hospitals: 2014 update. *Infect Control Hosp Epidemiol.* 2014;35(suppl 2):S66-S88.

67. Mishriki SF, Law DJ, Jeffery PJ. Factors affecting the incidence of postoperative wound infection. *J Hosp Infect.* 1990;16(3):223-230.

68. Seropian R, Reynolds BM. Wound infections after preoperative depilatory versus razor preparation. *Am J Surg.* 1971;121(3):251-254.

69. Tanner J, Woodings D, Moncaster K. Preoperative hair removal to reduce surgical site infection. *Cochrane Database Syst Rev.* 2006;(3):Cd004122.

70. Dumville JC, McFarlane E, Edwards P, Lipp A, Holmes A, Liu Z. Preoperative skin antiseptics for preventing surgical wound infections after clean surgery. *Cochrane Database Syst Rev.* 2015;(4):CD003949.

71. Lee I, Agarwal RK, Lee BY, Fishman NO, Umscheid CA. Systematic review and cost analysis comparing use of chlorhexidine with use of iodine for preoperative skin antisepsis to prevent surgical site infection. *Infect Control Hosp Epidemiol.* 2010;31(12):1219-1229.

72. Brown TR, Ehrlich CE, Stehman FB, Golichowski AM, Madura JA, Eitzen HE. A clinical evaluation of chlorhexidine gluconate spray as compared with iodophor scrub for preoperative skin preparation. *Surg Gynecol Obstet.* 1984;158(4):363-366.

73. Darouiche RO, Wall MJ Jr, Itani KM, et al. Chlorhexidine-alcohol versus povidone-iodine for surgical-site antisepsis. *N Engl J Med.* 2010;362(1):18-26.

74. Ghuman A, Chan T, Karimuddin AA, Brown CJ, Raval MJ, Phang PT. Surgical site infection rates following implementation of a colorectal closure bundle in elective colorectal surgeries. *Dis Colon Rectum.* 2015;58(11):1078-1082.

75. Kiran RP, El-Gazzaz GH, Vogel JD, Remzi FH. Laparoscopic approach significantly reduces surgical site infections after colorectal surgery: data from National Surgical Quality Improvement Program. *J Am Coll Surg.* 2010;211(2):232-238.

76. Pasam RT, Esemuede IO, Lee-Kong SA, Kiran RP. The minimally invasive approach is associated with reduced surgical site infections in obese patients undergoing proctectomy. *Tech Coloproctol.* 2015;19(12):733-743.

77. Kirby JP, Mazuski JE. Prevention of surgical site infection. *Surg Clin North Am.* 2009;89(2):365-389, viii.

78. Konishi T, Watanabe T, Kishimoto J, Nagawa H. Elective colon and rectal surgery differ in risk factors for wound infection: results of prospective surveillance. *Ann Surg.* 2006;244(5):758-763.

79. Puleo FJ, Mishra N, Hall JF. Use of intra-abdominal drains. *Clin Colon Rectal Surg.* 2013;26(3):174-177.

80. Zhang HY, Zhao CL, Xie J, et al. To drain or not to drain in colorectal anastomosis: a meta-analysis. *Int J Colorectal Dis.* 2016; 31(5):951-960.

81. Wang ZX, Jiang CP, Cao Y, Ding YT. Systematic review and meta-analysis of triclosan-coated sutures for the prevention of surgical-site infection. *Br J Surg.* 2013;100(4):465-473.

82. Chang WK, Srinivasa S, Morton R, Hill AG. Triclosan-impregnated sutures to decrease surgical site infections: systematic review and meta-analysis of randomized trials. *Ann Surg.* 2012;255(5):854-859.

83. de Jager E, McKenna C, Bartlett L, Gunnarsson R, Ho YH. Postoperative adverse events inconsistently improved by the World Health Organization surgical safety checklist: a systematic literature review of 25 studies. *World J Surg.* 2016;40(8):1842-1858.

84. Bergs J, Hellings J, Cleemput I, et al. Systematic review and meta-analysis of the effect of the World Health Organization surgical safety checklist on postoperative complications. *Br J Surg.* 2014; 101(3):150-158.

85. Keenan JE, Speicher PJ, Thacker JK, Walter M, Kuchibhatla M, Mantyh CR. The preventive surgical site infection bundle in colorectal surgery: an effective approach to surgical site infection reduction and health care cost savings. *J Am Med Assoc Surg.* 2014; 149(10):1045-1052.

86. Edwards JP, Ho AL, Tee MC, Dixon E, Ball CG. Wound protectors reduce surgical site infection: a meta-analysis of randomized controlled trials. *Ann Surg.* 2012;256(1):53-59.

87. Pinkney TD, Calvert M, Bartlett DC, et al. Impact of wound edge protection devices on surgical site infection after laparotomy: multicentre randomised controlled trial (ROSSINI Trial). *Br Med J.* 2013;347:f4305.

88. Mihaljevic AL, Schirren R, Özer M, et al. Multicenter double-blinded randomized controlled trial of standard abdominal wound edge protection with surgical dressings versus coverage with a sterile circular polyethylene drape for prevention of surgical site infections: a CHIR-Net trial (BaFO; NCT01181206). *Ann Surg.* 2014;260(5): 730-737; discussion 737–739.

89. Mueller TC, Loos M, Haller B, et al. Intra-operative wound irrigation to reduce surgical site infections after abdominal surgery: a systematic review and meta-analysis. *Langenbecks Arch Surg.* 2015;400(2):167-181.

90. Knighton DR, Halliday B, Hunt TK. Oxygen as an antibiotic. A comparison of the effects of inspired oxygen concentration and antibiotic administration on in vivo bacterial clearance. *Arch Surg.* 1986;121(2):191-195.

91. Greif R, Akça O, Horn EP, Kurz A, Sessler DI, Outcomes Research Group. Supplemental perioperative oxygen to reduce the incidence of surgical-wound infection. *N Engl J Med.* 2000;342(3):161-167.

92. Yang W, Liu Y, Zhang Y, Zhao QH, He SF. Effect of intra-operative high inspired oxygen fraction on surgical site infection: a meta-analysis of randomized controlled trials. *J Hosp Infect*. 2016;93(4): 329-338.

93. Podolyak A, Sessler DI, Reiterer C, et al. Perioperative supplemental oxygen does not worsen long-term mortality of colorectal surgery patients. *Anesth Analg*. 2016;122(6):1907-1911.

94. Sessler DI, Rubinstein EH, Moayeri A. Physiologic responses to mild perianesthetic hypothermia in humans. *Anesthesiology*. 1991;75(4):594-610.

95. Kurz A, Sessler DI, Lenhardt R. Perioperative normothermia to reduce the incidence of surgical-wound infection and shorten hospitalization. Study of Wound Infection and Temperature Group. *N Engl J Med*. 1996;334(19):1209-1215.

96. Melton GB, Vogel JD, Swenson BR, Remzi FH, Rothenberger DA, Wick EC. Continuous intraoperative temperature measurement and surgical site infection risk: analysis of anesthesia information system data in 1008 colorectal procedures. *Ann Surg*. 2013;258(4): 606-612; discussion 612-613.

97. Lehtinen SJ, Onicescu G, Kuhn KM, Cole DJ, Esnaola NF. Normothermia to prevent surgical site infections after gastrointestinal surgery: holy grail or false idol? *Ann Surg*. 2010;252(4):696-704.

98. Turina M, Fry DE, Polk HC Jr. Acute hyperglycemia and the innate immune system: clinical, cellular, and molecular aspects. *Crit Care Med*. 2005;33(7):1624-1633.

99. Sehgal R, Berg A, Figueroa R, et al. Risk factors for surgical site infections after colorectal resection in diabetic patients. *J Am Coll Surg*. 2011;212(1):29-34.

100. Kwon S, Thompson R, Dellinger P, Yanez D, Farrokhi E, Flum D. Importance of perioperative glycemic control in general surgery: a report from the Surgical Care and Outcomes Assessment Program. *Ann Surg*. 2013;257(1):8-14.

101. Ramos M, Khalpey Z, Lipsitz S, et al. Relationship of perioperative hyperglycemia and postoperative infections in patients who undergo general and vascular surgery. *Ann Surg*. 2008;248(4):585-591.

102. Thompson RE, Broussard EK, Flum DR, Wisse BE. Perioperative glycemic control during colorectal surgery. *Curr Diab Rep*. 2016;16(3): 32.

103. Mohan S, Kaoutzanis C, Welch KB, et al. Postoperative hyperglycemia and adverse outcomes in patients undergoing colorectal surgery: results from the Michigan surgical quality collaborative database. *Int J Colorectal Dis*. 2015;30(11):1515-1523.

104. Kiran RP, Turina M, Hammel J, Fazio V. The clinical significance of an elevated postoperative glucose value in nondiabetic patients after colorectal surgery: evidence for the need for tight glucose control? *Ann Surg*. 2013;258(4):599-604; discussion 604-605.

105. Towfigh S, Clarke T, Yacoub W, et al. Significant reduction of wound infections with daily probing of contaminated wounds: a prospective randomized clinical trial. *Arch Surg*. 2011;146(4): 448-452.

106. Kim BJ, Aloia TA. An inexpensive modified primary closure technique for class IV (dirty) wounds significantly decreases superficial and deep surgical site infection. *J Gastroint Surg*. 2016; 20(11):1904-1907.

107. Chadi SA, Vogt KN, Knowles S, et al. Negative pressure wound therapy use to decrease surgical nosocomial events in colorectal resections (NEPTUNE): study protocol for a randomized controlled trial. *Trials*. 2015;16:322.

108. Attaluri V, Kiran RP, Vogel J, Remzi F, Church J. Risk factors for urinary tract infections in colorectal compared with vascular surgery: a need to review current present-on-admission policy? *J Am Coll Surg*. 2011;212(3):356-361.

109. Regenbogen SE, Read TE, Roberts PL, Marcello PW, Schoetz DJ, Ricciardi R. Urinary tract infection after colon and rectal resections: more common than predicted by risk-adjustment models. *J Am Coll Surg*. 2011;213(6):784-792.

110. Sheka AC, Tevis S, Kennedy GD. Urinary tract infection after surgery for colorectal malignancy: risk factors and complications. *Am J Surg*. 2016;211(1):31-39.

111. Miller TE, Thacker JK, White WD, et al. Reduced length of hospital stay in colorectal surgery after implementation of an enhanced recovery protocol. *Anesth Analg*. 2014;118(5):1052-1061.

112. Hendren S. Urinary catheter management. *Clin Colon Rectal Surg*. 2013;26(3):178-181.

113. Nagle D, Curran T, Anez-Bustillos L, Poylin V. Reducing urinary tract infections in colon and rectal surgery. *Dis Colon Rectum*. 2014;57(1):91-97.

114. Longo WE, Virgo KS, Johnson FE, et al. Risk factors for morbidity and mortality after colectomy for colon cancer. *Dis Colon Rectum*. 2000;43(1):83-91.

115. McGillicuddy EA, Schuster KM, Davis KA, Longo WE. Factors predicting morbidity and mortality in emergency colorectal procedures in elderly patients. *Arch Surg*. 2009;144(12):1157-1162.

116. McAlister FA, Bertsch K, Man J, Bradley J, Jacka M. Incidence of and risk factors for pulmonary complications after nonthoracic surgery. *Am J Respir Crit Care Med*. 2005;171(5):514-517.

117. Schmid M, Sood A, Campbell L, et al. Impact of smoking on perioperative outcomes after major surgery. *Am J Surg*. 2015;210(2): 221-229, e1.

118. Kent KC, Rubin MS, Wroblewski L, Hanff PA, Silen W. The impact of *Clostridium difficile* on a surgical service: a prospective study of 374 patients. *Ann Surg*. 1998;227(2):296-301.

119. Yeom CH, Cho MM, Baek SK, Bae OS. Risk factors for the development of *Clostridium difficile*-associated colitis after colorectal cancer surgery. *J Korean Soc Coloproctol*. 2010;26(5):329-335.

120. Wren SM, Ahmed N, Jamal A, Safadi BY. Preoperative oral antibiotics in colorectal surgery increase the rate of *Clostridium difficile* colitis. *Arch Surg*. 2005;140(8):752-756.

121. Crook DW, Walker AS, Kean Y, et al. Fidaxomicin versus vancomycin for *Clostridium difficile* infection: meta-analysis of pivotal randomized controlled trials. *Clin Infect Dis*. 2012;55(suppl 2):S93-S103.

122. Cornely OA, Crook DW, Esposito R, et al. Fidaxomicin versus vancomycin for infection with *Clostridium difficile* in Europe, Canada, and the USA: a double-blind, non-inferiority, randomised controlled trial. *Lancet Infect Dis*. 2012;12(4):281-289.

123. Louie TJ, Miller MA, Mullane KM, et al. Fidaxomicin versus vancomycin for *Clostridium difficile* infection. *N Engl J Med*. 2011;364(5): 422-431.

Reoperative Pelvic Surgery

David W. Dietz | Feza H. Remzi

Mastering the challenges of reoperative pelvic surgery requires preparation, a thorough understanding of pelvic anatomy, the ability to think several steps ahead, considerable experience, and no small measure of courage on the part of the surgeon. This chapter covers the anatomy of the reoperative pelvis, common pitfalls encountered during reoperative pelvic surgery, the preoperative preparation of the patient, useful technical tips, and finally a discussion of the most common clinical scenarios that lead to reoperative pelvic surgery—namely, reversal of Hartmann procedure, redo pelvic pouch surgery, salvage of colorectal and coloanal anastomotic complications, and recurrent rectal cancers.

ANATOMY AND PITFALLS OF THE REOPERATIVE PELVIS

The difficulty of pelvic surgery in general relates to the narrow and deep confines of this anatomical compartment that is rigidly bound by bone, connective tissue, and muscle and contains many vital structures in close proximity to one another that are at risk of inadvertent damage. The challenges of adequate visualization and precise dissection are compounded in the reoperative patient, as scarring from previous surgery often further limits exposure and obliterates the normal anatomical planes. In addition, structures such as the ureters, pelvic nerves, and blood vessels may be displaced into unusual positions where they are more prone to injury.

The reoperative surgeon's understanding of the fascial planes within the pelvis is critical for the success of any endeavor. The pelvis is lined by a parietal fascia, which then extends to cover the pelvic organs as the visceral fascia. Overlying the sacrum, the presacral fascia constitutes a thickening and condensation of the parietal endopelvic fascia, where it protects the underlying presacral venous plexus. The vast majority of pelvic surgeries should be conducted in a plane anterior to this presacral fascia between it and the parietal fascia investing the mesorectum. Only rarely is violation of the presacral fascia indicated in the resection of a locally advanced or recurrent rectal cancer that involves this layer. Dissection deep to the presacral fascia, often blunt and due to lack of exposure, will invariably result in injury to the presacral veins. These vascular structures are prone to bleed precipitously due to the fact that they are avalvular and communicate directly with the basivertebral veins. Controlling bleeding from the presacral veins is especially challenging, as injury often results in an end-on venotomy rather than one on the lateral wall of the vessel. The special techniques used to deal with this complication are discussed later in the chapter, but precise anatomical dissection and avoidance

of presacral venous injury is the best approach. Even in the reoperative situation, the plane between the presacral fascia and the mesentery of the ileal J pouch or colonic neorectum is usually present and can be identified.

The anterior counterpart to the presacral fascia is the fascia of Denonvilliers. This fascial layer separates the rectum and the base of the bladder and serves to protect the underlying seminal vesicles, prostate gland, and parasympathetic nerves that are involved in sexual function. Damage to these nervi erigentes will lead to erectile dysfunction in the male patient. Only in the case of an anterior rectal tumor that is closely opposed to Denonvilliers fascia should this plane be knowingly violated to ensure a clear radial margin.

The distal half of the ureters are also at risk during reoperative pelvic surgery when they may be displaced medially due to prior mobilization or concealed by scar tissue. Injury can occur at any location but is most common where the ureter crosses the pelvic brim or close to its insertion into the bladder. Injury in the former location is usually due to overaggressive and early lateral dissection, whereas damage in the latter instance typically results from inadequate exposure and visualization. Ureter injuries are inevitable in a high-volume reoperative pelvic surgery practice, but the keys to minimizing their occurrence and consequence are the liberal use of ureteric stents and maintenance of a high index of suspicion so that injuries can be immediately recognized and repaired. Ureter injuries that are dealt with at the time of surgery rarely have adverse consequences, whereas those that go unrecognized and present later in the postoperative period often lead to significant morbidity. One of the first steps in a reoperative pelvic surgery should be identification of the course of the ureters, either by palpation of previously placed plastic stents or by dissection and tagging with vessel loops. In the case of overt injury, enlisting the aid of an experienced urologist for repair or reimplantation is vital. If occult injury is suspected, the administration of methylene blue or indocyanine green intravenously may aid in identification.

One of the most dramatic intraoperative complications of reoperative pelvic surgery is injury to the internal iliac artery or vein as they course along the pelvic sidewall. These injuries can be extremely difficult to control and may lead to massive and life-threatening bleeding. Less commonly, the common or external iliac vessels may be injured. This problem is even more difficult, as control of bleeding must not jeopardize perfusion to the lower extremities. In the event of significant bleeding from any of these vessels, the first step should be pressure at the bleeding site with either the surgeon's finger or a peanut sponge. The latter is preferable, as this can then be passed to the assistant, freeing the surgeon to gain proximal control of the vessel. The anesthesia team should be notified of impending blood loss so that blood products can be ordered and administered. Only when the patient is resuscitated and stabilized should an attempt be made to either ligate or definitively repair the vascular injury. Additional suction catheters can be useful to keep the field cleared of blood for adequate visualization. Blindly placed sutures are discouraged because they risk further vascular injury, especially in the case of venous bleeding or inadvertent ligation of the adjacent ureter. Obtaining the help of a vascular surgeon in this situation can be invaluable.

Finally, the surgeon must often deal with small bowel loops that are adhesed within the pelvis after previous proctectomy, hysterectomy, or in the worst scenario, cystectomy. The small bowel loops should be mobilized en masse from the pelvis using sharp dissection in a plane between the small bowel serosa or mesentery and the endopelvic fascia. Keeping the dissection flush with the small bowel will minimize the risk of injuring adjacent structures such as the ureter or pelvic sidewall vessels. Any serosal tears or enterotomies created should be either immediately repaired or tagged with sutures to facilitate identification and repair prior to completion of surgery.

TIMING OF SURGERY

The proper timing of reoperative pelvic surgery may be one of the most critical components for its success. It is our practice to wait a minimum of 6 months from the last laparotomy before attempting procedures such as redo ileal pouch- or coloanal anastomosis and Hartmann reversal. In the interim and if necessary, pelvic sepsis can usually be controlled with percutaneous drains. If proximal fecal diversion is necessary, then a limited upper abdominal laparotomy will usually allow the creation of a loop jejunostomy or ileostomy while avoiding the hostile lower abdomen or pelvis. Such patients can then be maintained on total parenteral nutrition until reoperation is safe. In cases where the previous laparotomy was extremely difficult due to dense adhesions, delaying reoperation for 12 months may be wise. A crude but effective method to determine whether the patient is ready for reoperative surgery is the "abdominal mobility test." With the patient lying supine and relaxed, abdominal wall palpation should reveal movement of the intraabdominal contents, independent of the abdominal wall. This is a highly subjective measure and must be informed by experience, but it can be quite useful and is commonly employed by us. Other criteria that should be met prior to reoperation are restoration of the patient's nutritional status and resolution of sepsis. Abdominal wounds should also be healed.

On the other hand, if an anastomotic complication has been recognized in the early postoperative period, then surgery may be undertaken for repair at that time since intraabdominal adhesions are not usually limiting within the first 7 to 10 days. Early recognition and treatment of complications can alleviate the disability associated with the complication and the need for prolonged courses of parenteral nutrition, wound care, and skilled nursing facility stays.

PREPARATION FOR SURGERY

Measures taken to prepare for reoperative pelvic surgery involve both the patient and the surgeon. Patients should undergo a thorough preoperative medical clearance evaluation in order to identify and correct any underlying cardiopulmonary risk factors. In some extremely high-risk patients, the patient and surgeon may choose to manage the existing complication conservatively rather than embark on a high-risk reoperative procedure. In these circumstances, the patient's current quality of life must be weighed against the chances for success, the degree of potential improvement and the inherent risks of surgery. Patients must have a thorough understanding of the magnitude of the surgery, length of hospital stay, risk of complications, and the possible need for rehabilitation after hospital discharge. The preoperative consent process should also include a realistic and clear discussion of the goals of surgery. Bowel function, risk of sexual dysfunction, and anticipated quality of life should all be clearly articulated so that expectations are realistic. Patients should also understand that in some cases the goals of surgery cannot be achieved without undue risk and that the operation may need to be aborted.

Records related to previous surgery should be thoroughly reviewed so that the surgeon has an understanding of the anatomical alterations that may be encountered. If unclear, abdominopelvic computed tomography (CT) scans and/or contrast studies of the pelvic viscera may be helpful. In cases of recurrent cancer, a positron emission tomography (PET) scan to exclude extrapelvic metastatic disease and a pelvic magnetic resonance imaging (MRI) to delineate involvement of adjacent structures and determine resectability should be obtained. Endoscopy is often performed to exclude occult neoplasia and to examine the length and condition of the rectal stump in the case of Hartmann reversal or to assess the size and health of the ileal J pouch in the case of a redo ileal pouch–anal anastomosis (IPAA).

Sufficient time should be scheduled for the operation, and it may be best to avoid additional surgical cases on these days. Any subspecialists that may be needed should be informed. It is much better to have a urologist, gynecologist, or vascular surgeon listed on the operative schedule and not needed than to be left scrambling for an intraoperative operative consult late in the day.

Immediately prior to surgery, the patient should be marked for a stoma in all four quadrants of the abdomen, blood products should be reserved, and appropriate antibiotics and deep venous thrombosis prophylaxis should be administered. Reoperative pelvic surgery cases are usually prolonged and contaminated affairs, and the patients are subsequently at high risk for thromboembolic complications and wound infections.

SURGICAL TECHNIQUE

PATIENT POSITIONING AND EQUIPMENT

Proper patient positioning is critical in reoperative surgery cases. The surgeon should always have access to the perineum, and therefore the legs should be elevated and

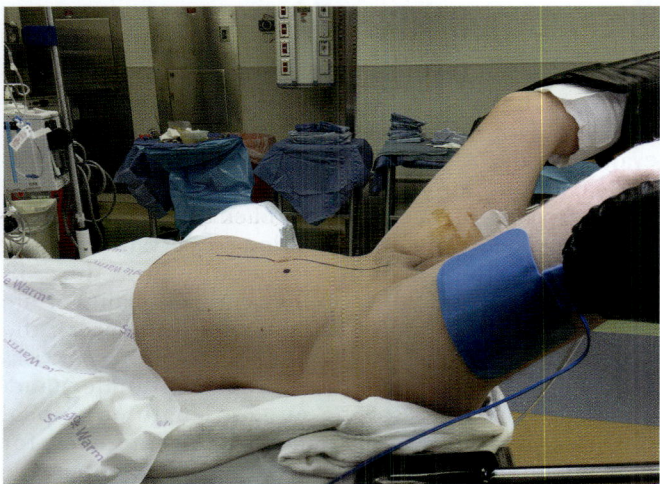

FIGURE 180.1 The modified lithotomy position provides access to the abdominal cavity, pelvis, and perineum during reoperative pelvic surgery.

spread in the modified lithotomy position (Fig. 180.1). We routinely use yellow fin stirrups for this purpose and take great care to provide sufficient padding to the posterior and lateral aspect of the calf near the fibular head. Prolonged pressure at this point can result in superficial peroneal neuropathy with resultant loss of dorsiflexion and eversion of the foot. Injuries to the sciatic and femoral nerves have also been described after lithotomy positioning. The latter may occur after improper placement of a pelvic Balfour or Bookwalter retractor. The lower edge of the buttocks should also protrude slightly from the bottom of the operating table to provide adequate access to the perineum. As steep Trendelenburg position is frequently required to facilitate pelvic exposure, we prefer to secure the patient to the table with a chest strap or beanbag to prevent them from sliding cephalad. After adequate intravenous access has been established, the arms should be tucked at the patient's side. Leaving the arms extended outward on arm boards can sometimes limit the surgeon's mobility when working in the pelvis. The skin should be prepared from the nipple line to the perineum, and in cases in which vascular reconstruction is anticipated, the groins should be prepared bilaterally. Draping should maintain access to the perineum.

Several pieces of equipment are especially useful during reoperative pelvic surgery. A foot pedal Bovie control coupled with the extender tip will provide adequate reach into the deepest pelvis. Likewise, long instruments such as forceps, needle drivers, and clamps along with suction catheter tips are essential. A set of lighted deep pelvic retractors is crucial for gaining adequate exposure, and a headlamp can also be complementary. The retractor set pictured in Fig. 180.2 contains a lighted BriteTrac (VitalCor Inc., Westmont, Illinois), along with Deaver and curved deep pelvic retractors with narrow, medium, and wide blades (Electrosurgical Instruments, Rochester, New York). The Deaver retractor is typically used to elevate the bladder and provide anterior exposure early in the pelvic dissection. The BriteTrac provides anterior retraction of the rectum and mesorectum for dissection of the mesial

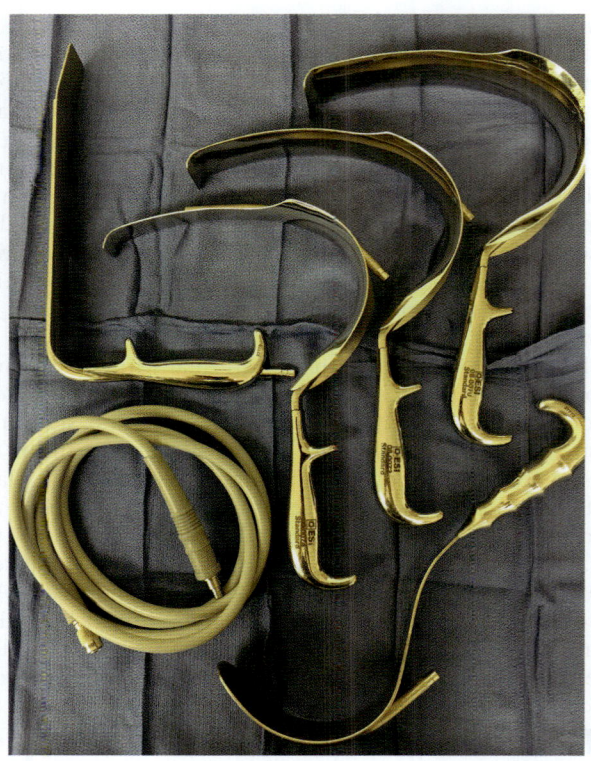

FIGURE 180.2 A set of lighted pelvic retractors greatly facilitates reoperative pelvic surgery. *Clockwise from upper left*: straight-blade retractor; narrow, medium, and wide curved deep pelvic retractors; Deaver retractor.

rectal plane and is also useful for exposing the anterolateral junction of the perirectal tissues and the pelvic sidewall and seminal vesicles. The curved deep pelvic retractors are used for both posterior and anterior exposure in the deepest phase of pelvic dissection.

ABDOMINAL ENTRY AND ADHESIOLYSIS

A generous midline incision is advised for reoperative pelvic surgery, extending from the pubis to the epigastrium. Small bowel adherent to the undersurface of the prior midline scar should be anticipated in all cases, and initial entry to the peritoneal cavity is usually safest in the upper abdomen. Once the fascia is encountered, the application of gentle pressure with the bevel of the scalpel blade, rather than a cutting stroke, is used to breach the peritoneum. Using this technique, it is usually possible to recognize an adherent bowel loop before enterotomy occurs.

In the most favorable scenario, intraabdominal adhesions will be few in number and soft in character. In the worst cases, the peritoneal cavity will be totally obliterated by scar tissue. An orderly and systematic approach to adhesiolysis is advised in these instances. First, the underside of the midline scar is cleared so that the entire length of the incision can be opened. Next, adhesions to the abdominal wall are dissected laterally until both paracolic gutters are reached. This will allow the placement of a self-retaining retractor (Balfour is our preference) to facilitate exposure. Particularly severe adhesions that defy identification of the bowel and peritoneal surfaces, the so-called frozen abdomen, may be injected with saline through a fine-gauge needle to separate the surfaces and thus facilitate adhesiolysis. Attention is then turned to the pelvis where the most difficult adhesions are often encountered. Rather than separating individual bowel loops at this stage, the small bowel residing in the pelvis should be mobilized "en masse" by lysing adhesions to the pelvic structures in an anterior to posterior manner in order to roll the whole of the intestine up and out of the pelvis. In some instances, individual loops that are adherent in the deepest recesses of the pelvis must be mobilized individually. Isolating both the afferent and efferent limbs and using gentle traction with a gauze sponge can expose the apex of the loop. Sharp dissection flush with the serosal surface will allow the loop of the bowel to be dissected off of the endopelvic fascia without injury to underlying structures. The final portion of this stage of the operation involves mobilizing the plane between the small bowel mesentery and the retroperitoneum until the duodenum is encountered. Only at this point, and if justified by the indication for surgery, are all adhesions between individual bowel loops lysed in order to free the entire length of the small intestine. The bowel is then inspected for any coexisting pathology and for enterotomies or serosal tears created in the course of mobilization. These are repaired with inverting seromuscular sutures. In some instances, adhesions are so severe or the anatomy is distorted to such a degree that the operation must be abandoned. It is important for the surgeon to recognize this point and to back away before becoming fully committed by devascularizing a portion of the bowel or creating enterotomies in a loop that is not able to be mobilized for repair. Planning for a reoperative pelvic surgery should always include a well–thought out strategy for abandoning the operation if needed. An example would be the creation of a high-loop jejunostomy in the case of a patient with a frozen abdomen and chronic pelvic sepsis due to a coloanal anastomotic leak. Surgery can then be deferred further until adhesions have softened, or referral to a more experienced reoperative pelvic surgeon can be made.

IDENTIFYING PELVIC STRUCTURES

One of the most difficult aspects of reoperative pelvic surgery can be the identification of pelvic structures. Prior surgery, pelvic sepsis, and pelvic radiation therapy can conspire to severely distort the anatomy and in some cases hide the rectal stump, bladder, vagina, and ureters under a thick layer of pelvic peritoneum. The inexperienced surgeon may, in fact, encounter what appears to be an empty pelvis, and only through bimanual examination can the presence of a rectal stump or vaginal cuff be confirmed. The following maneuvers can be helpful to identify structures in the reoperative pelvis.

URETERS

As mentioned previously, one of the cardinal sins of any pelvic surgery is an unrecognized ureter injury. In the case of the reoperative pelvis, ureter injury is much more likely, and great care must be taken to identify the ureters early in the course of surgery to avoid this complication. Ureteric stents should be placed at the time of surgery when possible. Stents can help facilitate and

hasten the identification of the ureters by palpation and can also alert the surgeon to inadvertent injury. In some cases, however, stents cannot be placed due to strictures or angulations of the ureter due to previous surgeries. In these circumstances we prefer to identify the ureter within the retroperitoneum before entering the pelvis. The ureter can be tagged with a Silastic vessel loop for identification and then referred back to intermittently as the pelvic dissection proceeds. Dissection within the pelvis should be done sharply and without cautery whenever possible, and should hug the surface of the organ being mobilized in order to minimize the risk of ureter injury.

BLADDER

As the bladder is an anterior and relatively superficial structure, it is usually readily identified during reoperative pelvic surgery. There are several points in time, however, where bladder injury can occur. The first is during completion of the caudal-most aspect of the midline incision at the level of the pubic symphysis. In some instances the bladder will have been previously mobilized and found to be densely adherent to the undersurface of the lower abdominal wall. If care is not taken when dividing the fascia, the bladder can be entered. It is our practice to immediately look for the prevesical fat after dividing the lowermost aspect of the fascia and to then push the bladder downward as the remainder of the fascia is opened. If injury occurs during this phase of the operation, it usually involves the bladder dome and can easily be repaired with absorbable seromuscular sutures. A Foley catheter is then left in place for 5 days postoperatively and a cystogram obtained to confirm healing before removal.

The base of the bladder can also be injured during reoperative pelvic surgery, especially during the later phases of pelvic dissection. It is common to encounter a dense fibrous band at the bladder base in patients who have been treated with previous radiation therapy and who have suffered low colorectal or coloanal anastomotic leaks. This band can often severely limit exposure within the deep pelvis and can restrict the blood supply to a colon pull-through. Radial incisions made with cautery into this band of scar can open the pelvic outlet and facilitate exposure. While this is often a useful maneuver, great care must be taken, as the bladder base or even the ureteral insertions can be injured. Injury to the trigone region of the bladder should be addressed by a urologist, as repair is complicated and must often be performed through a cystotomy in the bladder dome.

RECTAL STUMP

Identification of the rectal stump in the reoperative pelvis can be straightforward at times and nearly impossible at others. During Hartmann procedure for perforated diverticulitis, the upper rectum or distal sigmoid colon is typically divided with the linear stapler. This results in a relatively long rectal stump that in some cases can even be secured to the underside of the lower abdominal wall. On the other hand, when a true "perforectomy" is performed, a significant length of the distal sigmoid colon can be left adherent within the pelvis. Realization of this situation is

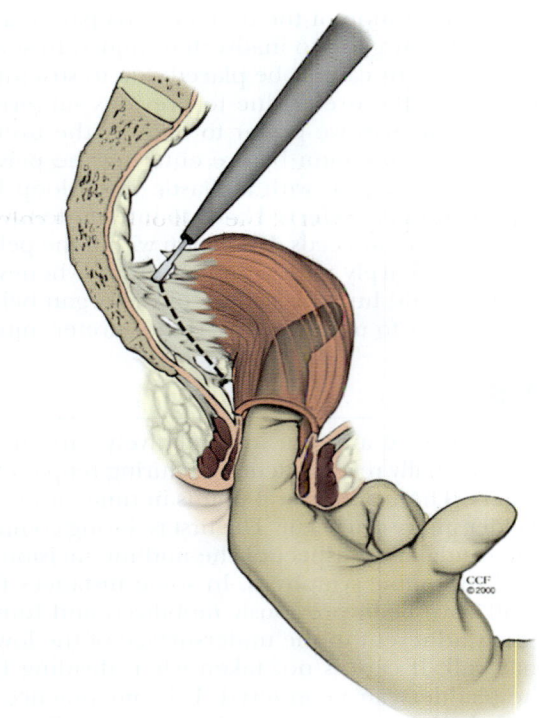

FIGURE 180.3 Bimanual examination by the surgeon can help to locate the rectal stump and facilitate dissection. Cautery dissection should be initiated in the posterior midline plane and then carried laterally for short distances to avoid injury to the ureters or pelvic sidewall structures. (Copyright 2000, Cleveland Clinic Foundation.)

important to avoid an anastomosis to retained sigmoid colon that may be involved with diverticular disease and predisposes the patient to a high risk of recurrence. This should always be expected and the upper rectum mobilized fully to confirm the location of the anterior peritoneal reflection. Full mobilization of the rectum will also aid in the passage of the circular stapler for creation of the colorectal anastomosis. Conversely, if a rectal perforation or colorectal anastomotic leak has resulted in resection of the majority of the rectum and a very short remaining Hartmann stump, it can be extremely difficult to identify the rectal remnant. Use of a bougie, EEA sizer, or bimanual examination by the surgeon can help locate the rectal stump and facilitate dissection (Fig. 180.3). As a general rule, the midline posterior plane between the mesorectal fascia and the presacral fascia should first be identified. A narrow, posterior midline dissection is then carried down to the level of the pelvic floor and only then is the dissection extended laterally. By limiting the dissection to the midline initially, the ureters, autonomic nerves, and iliac vessels can be identified and swept away as the dissection proceeds toward the pelvic sidewall. Lateral attachments are then mobilized once these vital structures have been protected. Finally, the anterior plane between the rectal wall and the vagina or prostate gland can be developed. This dissection should be carried out flush with the serosal surface of the rectum to minimize the risk of violating Denonvilliers fascia and injuring the

parasympathetic nervi erigentes. For extremely short rectal stumps, grasping the apex with a Babcock clamp or a heavy suture can provide upward retraction that can facilitate dissection. In a female patient with a prior hysterectomy, the vaginal cuff can be densely adherent to a short rectal stump, and similar maneuvers directed there can help separate these structures.

VAGINA

As stated previously, the vagina is at risk for injury during reoperative pelvic surgery, especially in women who have previously undergone hysterectomy. Inadvertent injury to the apex of the vaginal cuff is easily repaired with absorbable sutures. In the case of injuries involving the anterior wall and extending toward the pelvic floor, repair can be more difficult. These "injuries" are often purposeful en bloc resections of the anterior wall during proctectomy for primary or recurrent rectal cancers, or if a colovaginal fistula has resulted from a stapled colonic or ileal pouch–anal anastomosis that incorporated the vaginal wall. Relatively narrow defects can be closed primarily through the perineal wound. If possible, an omental pedicle graft should be placed over the vaginal repair or interposed between it and the new bowel anastomosis. Larger defects, and those occurring after pelvic radiation therapy, typically require flap closure. A vaginal closure that fails after proctectomy can be the source of prolonged and disabling perineal wound drainage.

BLEEDING

Significant pelvic bleeding during reoperative pelvic surgery is often the result of blind and blunt dissection in the wrong surgical plane. This most commonly occurs posteriorly in the pelvis when the presacral fascia is inadvertently breached and withdrawal of the surgeon's hand is followed by brisk venous bleeding. This can be a difficult situation, as the rate of bleeding and the fact that posterior dissection has just begun may make it impossible to identify and expose the source. The first step should be to apply direct pressure to the area of bleeding, either with carefully placed packs or the surgeon's finger. The anesthesia team is then notified, and blood transfusion can be initiated. A second suction device should be employed and long instruments obtained. If the presacral space can be packed and the bleeding tamponaded, then attention should be directed to further mobilization of the rectum or neorectum so that the presacral area can be adequately exposed. At a minimum, the lateral stalks should be dissected, but if the anastomosis can be reached and taken down to allow the surgeon to completely remove the bowel segment from the pelvis, then this is best. Efforts to blindly address presacral venous bleeding before good exposure is obtained will usually result in worsening hemorrhage due to tearing of the veins during attempts at suture ligation or development of coagulopathy as bleeding persists. Once the area of bleeding has been adequately exposed, more precise control of bleeding can be achieved by applying point pressure with a gauze "peanut" on a long Kelly clamp. A careful attempt to ligate the bleeding vein can then be made with a 2-0 Prolene suture fixed to a deeply curved

"UR-type" needle. If this fails to control bleeding on the first or second attempt, the surgeon should not persist with attempts at ligation but should instead move to an alternate approach. These secondary measures usually rely on tamponade of the bleeding vein with either synthetic materials (sterile thumbtacks, sacral pins, or surgical pledgets) or autologous patches of rectus muscle.

Other sites of bleeding during reoperative pelvic surgery are often unavoidable. Anterior bleeding from the periprostatic vessels and bleeding from the pelvic sidewall can occur, as the rectum or neorectum may be fused to these vessels as a consequence of chronic pelvic sepsis or radiation therapy. Anterior bleeding usually ceases with packing and application of direct pressure. Lateral bleeding, on the other hand, typically requires suture ligation and is the result of injury to branches of the internal iliac artery or vein. If pelvic sidewall dissection is anticipated (e.g., recurrent rectal cancer), it is wise to first dissect and encircle the internal iliac vessels at their origins with Silastic vessel loops. This will allow for quick occlusion should bleeding be encountered. Often one of the earliest steps in the resection of a tumor that is invading the pelvic sidewall is ligation and division of the internal iliac vessels just distal to their bifurcation from the common iliacs. This maneuver provides direct access to the plane lateral to these vessels that must be dissected in order to achieve an R0 resection. Use of a handheld energy device is helpful in this plane to minimize bleeding from small venous and arterial branches.

DRAINS

Dead space can be a major problem in the reoperated pelvis due to the effects of previous radiation therapy and the absence of organs that typically fill this space such as the rectum, bladder, and uterus. In addition, the raw surface created by extensive pelvic dissection along with the likelihood of ongoing postoperative bleeding make fluid accumulation likely and placement of pelvic drains advised. We use either a 10-mm Jackson-Pratt or Atraum drain placed through a stab incision in the left or right lower quadrant and lateral to the rectus muscle. If bleeding is anticipated or significant contamination occurred during surgery, an irrigating sump drain is placed. Drains are removed when output has decreased below 30 mL/day.

Omental pedicle grafts are also routinely used to help obliterate pelvic dead space and to buttress anastomoses. It is also advisable to interpose omentum between bowel anastomosis and other nearby suture lines such as vaginal cuff repairs and ureteroneocystostomies. The graft is usually based on the left gastroepiploic vessels and is brought to the pelvis along the left paracolic gutter. The apex of the graft is held in place with a suture.

SPECIFIC INDICATIONS/PROCEDURES

HARTMANN REVERSAL

Reversal of Hartmann procedure for diverticulitis with creation of a colorectal anastomosis is a common reoperation performed by many general and colorectal surgeons

that can at times involve considerable pelvic dissection. There are several critical steps necessary for creation of a safe anastomosis and to minimize the risk of recurrent diverticulitis. To ensure the latter, the entirety of the high-pressure zone of the sigmoid and descending colon should be resected and the anastomosis constructed with the true rectum. The proximal extent of resection is defined by careful palpation of the wall of the left colon, with the goal being removal of the entire segment that bears muscular hypertrophy and wall thickening. The distal line of transection must be in the upper rectum, as evidenced by disappearance or coalescence of the taenia coli. Failure to include the uppermost aspect of the rectum in the resection will increase the risk of recurrent diverticulitis by twofold.[1] As mentioned previously, the surgeon must also be vigilant so as not to miss "hidden" sigmoid colon adherent in a very difficult pelvis and thus construct an anastomosis between the descending colon and the midsigmoid colon. This scenario is not uncommon and can lead to anastomotic leak due to poor blood supply, continued colonic obstruction or pelvic sepsis if the area of stricture or prior perforation in the distal sigmoid colon is not resected.

It is also important to sufficiently mobilize the proximal colon to allow for a tension-free colorectal anastomosis. This usually requires complete mobilization of the splenic flexure and often high ligation of the inferior mesenteric artery and vein near their origins. Blood supply to the proximal aspect of the anastomosis is then provided by the left branch of the middle colic artery via the ascending branch of the left colic artery and the marginal artery. It is wise to "flash" the marginal artery adjacent to the cut end of the colon to confirm pulsatile bleeding prior to vessel ligation. In cases where reach to the pelvis cannot be achieved after these maneuvers, the right branches of the middle colic vessels can be divided and a retroileal colorectal anastomosis constructed. This will often result in sacrifice of a portion of the descending and distal transverse colons, but typically allows for a tension-free anastomosis to be constructed.

Creation of the anastomosis can be challenging as well, and the surgeon should be facile in several different anastomotic techniques. Ideally, a stapled colorectal anastomosis can be constructed, using either a double-stapled or double-pursestring technique. The former is sometimes made difficult by angulation or tethering of the midrectum at the level of the anterior peritoneal reflection that prevents transanal passage of the stapler. Further rectal mobilization and gentle and sequential dilation using EEA sizers will often allow the stapler to be passed. A second area of difficulty can be encountered at the apex of a long Hartmann pouch where the head of the stapler will not adequately efface the end of the rectal stump. This "concertina" effect can result in an incomplete anastomotic ring if the issue is forced. Inspissated mucus can also become trapped between the head of the stapler and the apex of the rectal stump if adequate rectal irrigation has not been performed, and this can cause the same problem. No matter the cause, further attempts to force the stapler should be abandoned rather than risk rectal perforation. Our practice in this circumstance is to resect the apex of the rectal stump and

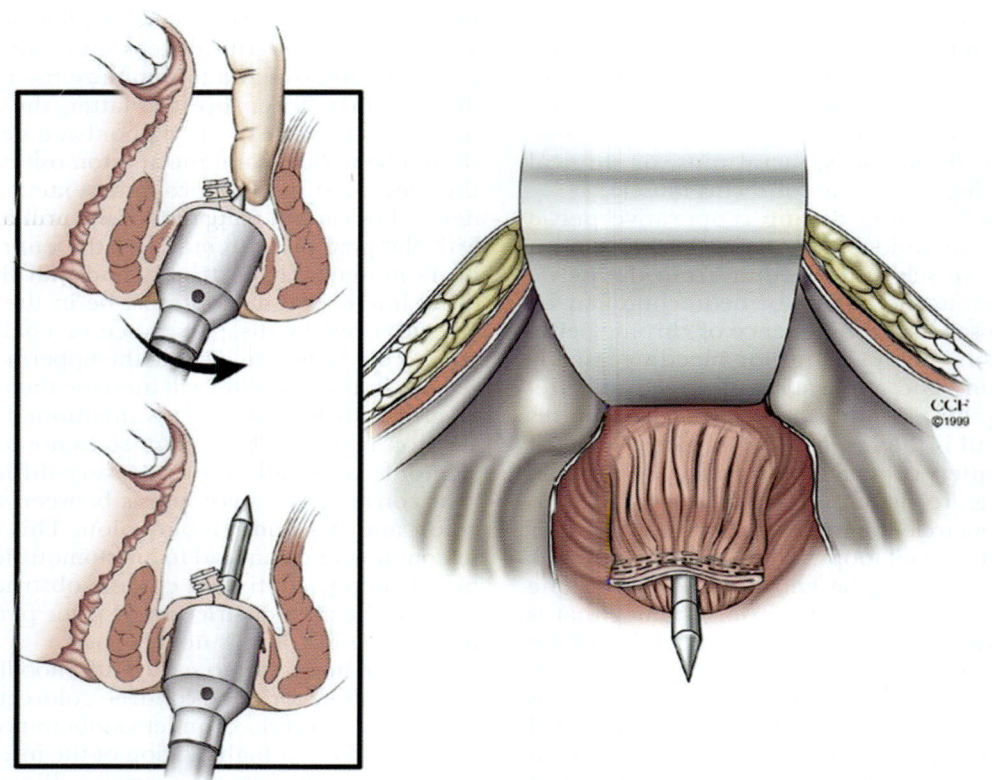

FIGURE 180.4 Construction of a double-stapled coloanal anastomosis *(counterclockwise from upper left)*. The surgeon's finger supports the apex of the rectal stump as the stapler is inserted. The spike of the stapler is brought out posterior to the transverse staple line. Both maneuvers may prevent inadvertent injury to the rectal stump that can greatly complicate Hartmann reversal. (Copyright 1999, Cleveland Clinic Foundation.)

to perform either a double-pursestring stapled anastomosis or a handsewn colorectal anastomosis. The head of the stapler can usually be guided out of the open end of the stump without difficulty, and any obstructing mucus or stool can be removed with forceps.

In some cases, the previous operation has included pelvic dissection with removal of a portion of the rectum proper, and these cases can be more challenging. The shorter the rectal stump, the more likely that the surgeon will have difficulty identifying, mobilizing, and preparing the rectal remnant for anastomosis. The maneuvers described previously (bimanual exam and use of transanal dilators) will be helpful in this circumstance. Once the stump has been prepared, the surgeon's fingers should be placed against the apex of the stump before the assistant inserts the stapler through the anal canal. This simple move can prevent the tremendous difficulties that ensue if the stapler is inadvertently pushed through the apex of the stump. Once the stapler has been successfully placed, the pin is brought out posterior to the transverse rectal staple line. The staple line then acts to support the pin if the assistant applies undue downward force to their end of the stapler and prevents splitting of the anterior rectal wall, a complication that may force a handsewn coloanal anastomosis (CAA) as the last resort (Fig. 180.4).

After completion, all colorectal and coloanal anastomoses should be leak tested using either povidone-iodine (Betadine) instilled into the rectum or air insufflation with the pelvis filled with saline solution. Liberal use of a diverting loop ileostomy for low anastomoses (<6 cm from the anal verge) or when construction of the anastomosis has been difficult is strongly advised.

REDO ILEAL POUCH–ANAL ANASTOMOSIS

While primary IPAA is successful in approximately 95% of patients with ulcerative colitis, some patients suffer postoperative complications that put maintenance of intestinal continuity at risk. While Crohn disease can develop in the pouch or anal canal after restorative proctocolectomy for presumed ulcerative colitis, it is a rare but often overblamed cause of IPAA failure. The vast majority of problems that threaten the IPAA are technical errors made at the time of primary surgery. As pelvic pouch surgery has expanded outward from high-volume centers, problems such as chronic presacral abscess due to posterior IPAA leaks, afferent limb syndrome and refractory proctitis due to excessive rectal length distal to the IPAA, and ischemic pouchitis resulting from inadequate mobilization of the small bowel mesentery or twisting of the pouch during anastomosis are becoming more common. In some cases, several of these problems coexist in the same patient.

Fortunately, many failing IPAAs can be salvaged. In our published experience of more than 500 transabdominal redo IPAAs, the overall success rate was 80%.[2] And in rare instances, even failed *redo* IPAAs can be salvaged with further surgical procedures. Critical to the success of these endeavors, however, is both a highly experienced expert surgeon as well as an extremely motivated patient.

Many of the technical aspects described previously are important in reoperative pelvic pouch surgery. Mobilization of the existing pouch should begin by establishing the posterior midline plane between the pouch mesentery and the presacral fascia at the level of the sacral promontory. The ureters and the iliac vessels should be identified and kept lateral. Ureteric stents are important in these cases because they can help facilitate identification of the ectopic ureters and aid in the recognition of injuries. Lateral and anterior dissection are typically carried out flush with the serosal surface of the pouch to avoid injury to pelvic sidewall structures and the anterior parasympathetic nerves that control aspects of sexual function. This dissection is done sharply with scissors because extensive use of cautery can damage the pouch and render it unusable for redo IPAA. Once the dissection reaches the level of the failed IPAA, the anastomosis is divided sharply, ideally on the distal side, to include the previous staple line with the pouch. The pouch can then be brought out of the pelvis for inspection. In our previously reported experience, the existing pouch was able to be used when constructing the redo IPAA in 60% of cases. In the remainder, primary pouch pathology, surgical trauma, and anatomical problems such as abnormally small volume necessitated pouch excision and creation of a neo-ileal J pouch. This can be facilitated if the previously created diverting loop ileostomy was made thoughtfully and placed approximately 20 cm proximal to the pouch, allowing the stapler to be introduced through this enterotomy for creation of the 15 to 20 cm linear pouch staple line. The failed pouch is then resected by dividing the afferent limb where it enters the pouch (Fig. 180.5). This staple line will then become the tip of the new J pouch. Reach of the new pouch to the anus is usually not an issue, as long as the small bowel mesentery is completely mobilized to its origin and all interloop small bowel adhesions are divided. If reach is difficult, creation of an S pouch will add several centimeters of length, although care must be taken to keep the efferent limb less than 2 cm in length to avoid the potential of outlet obstruction. In our experience with redo ileal pouch surgery, creation of an S pouch rather than the standard J configuration is required in only 10% of patients.[2]

In the case of chronic presacral abscess due to IPAA leak, the presacral scar and granulation tissue should be excised completely to prevent postoperative pelvic sepsis. Anal canal mucosectomy is then performed from the perineal approach beginning just above the dentate line. Care must be taken to resect all remaining proximal anal canal and low rectal mucosa, including the previous IPAA staple line if it was not included in resection of the pouch. Finally, the apex of the existing or new pouch is brought through the anal canal with a long Babcock clamp and a handsewn neo-IPAA is fashioned using interrupted 3-0 absorbable sutures. A new diverting loop ileostomy is created, typically using the existing stoma aperture, and a presacral drain is placed.

As stated previously, overall outcomes following redo ileal pouch surgery are excellent, with the vast majority of patients successfully salvaged. Postoperative morbidity is common, however, with anastomotic leaks, pelvic sepsis, and bowel obstruction occurring in 8%, 10%, and 16% of patients, respectively. Several factors have been identified that are independently associated with failure of redo pouch surgery, and these include pouch vaginal fistula as the indication for redo IPAA, pathology consistent with Crohn disease involving the failed primary pouch, and postoperative pelvic sepsis. Bowel function after redo pouch surgery is characterized by six daytime and two nighttime bowel movements per 24 hours with approximately 50% of patients admitting to seepage and pad usage. More that 90% of patients state that they would undergo redo pouch surgery again and would recommend the surgery to others if needed.[2]

REDO COLOANAL ANASTOMOSIS, INCLUDING TURNBULL-CUTAIT PROCEDURE

Reoperative surgeries for complications related to low colorectal and coloanal anastomoses are similar to those undertaken for IPAA problems. While many of the principles described previously also apply to these patients, some additional factors are common in this setting and require special consideration. In many cases, the primary operation that led to the anastomotic complication was related to rectal cancer, and the presence of recurrent disease should be excluded. This can be difficult, however, as there is often significant pelvic fibrosis as a consequence of the anastomotic leak, combined with effects of neoadjuvant radiation therapy. It is our practice to first examine these patients under anesthesia in an attempt to exclude locally recurrent cancer and to assess the patient's candidacy for redo CAA. Biopsies of the fibrotic perianastomotic tissues are obtained using a core biopsy needle introduced through the anus. Endoscopy is performed to assess the viability and distensibility of the neorectum, and digital exam defines the status of the anal canal and sphincters as well as the degree of fibrosis surrounding the neorectum and the capacity of the pelvic outlet to accommodate a pulled-through segment of the colon and its mesocolon. Dense pelvic fibrosis that is likely to render the newly created neorectum nondistensible or a tightly narrowed pelvic outlet that will lead to ischemia of the pulled-through colon are contraindications to redo CAA. In comparison to patients presenting for redo IPAA, those seeking redo CAA tend to be much older and with a higher incidence of significant comorbidities. A thorough preoperative medical evaluation is critical so that the risks of surgery can be considered against potential benefits. In some cases, the best decision is for takedown of the failed CAA, completion intersphincteric proctectomy, and creation of an end colostomy. In cases where operative risk is extremely high, colostomy creation alone may be the only option. This is not ideal, however, as the patient will still suffer with chronic pelvic pain and purulent anal drainage.

In most cases, we use the "Turnbull-Cutait pull-through procedure" when attempting redo CAA. The defining component of this procedure is the delayed CAA described by Dr. Rupert Turnbull and colleagues in the 1960s for the treatment of rectal cancer and Hirschprung disease,[3] and it was used by Dr. Daher Cutait for the

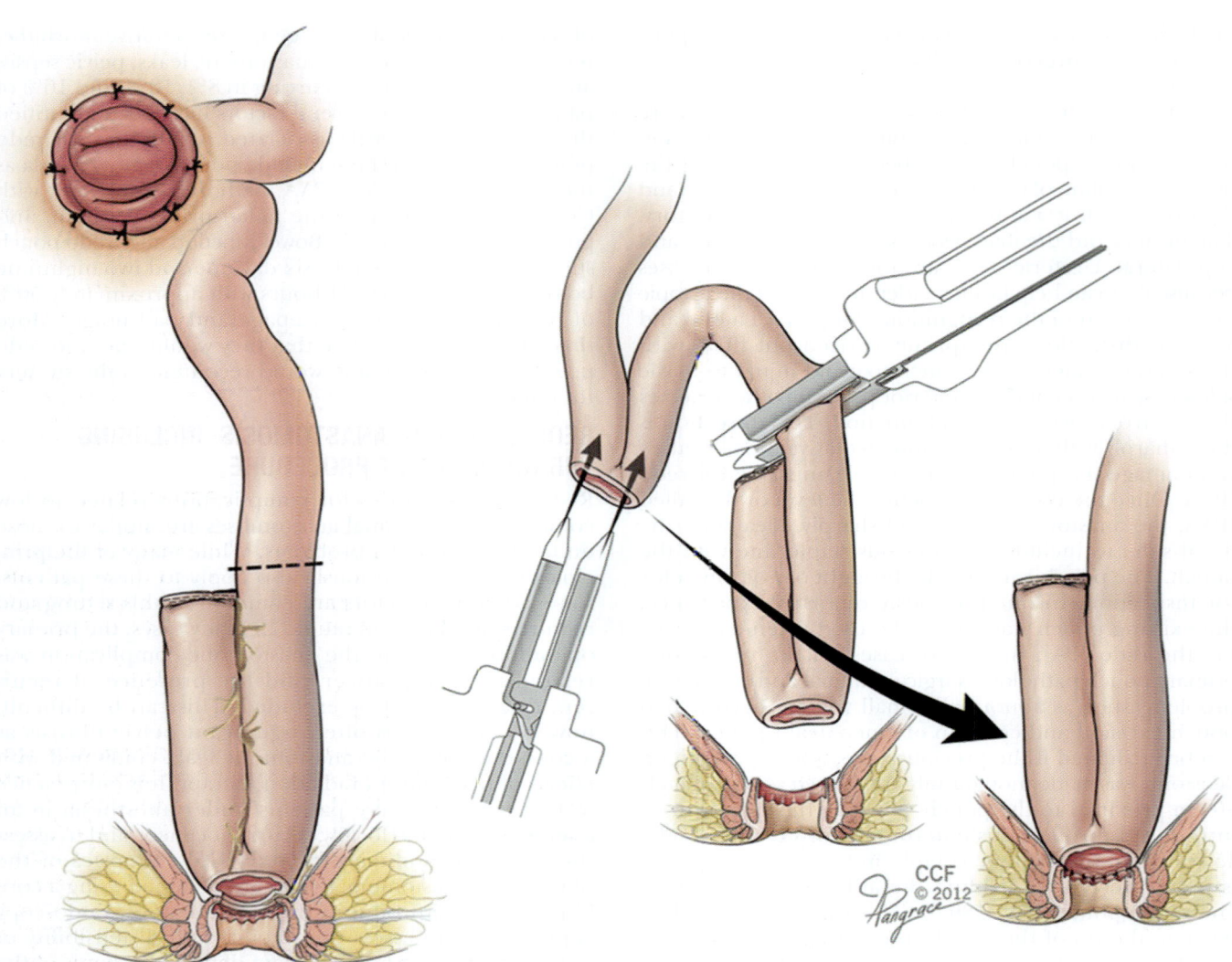

FIGURE 180.5 Resection of a failed pelvic pouch and creation of a neo-ileal J pouch anal anastomosis *(left to right)*. If a diverting loop ileostomy is created prior to redo ileal pouch anal anastomosis surgery, it should be placed approximately 20 cm proximal to the pouch. In the event that excision of the failed pouch is necessary, this will facilitate creation of the new J pouch as illustrated. (Copyright 2012, Cleveland Clinic Foundation.)

treatment of Chagas disease in the 1980s.[4] The theoretical advantage of this approach over a primary CAA is that by allowing the exteriorized colon to become adherent to the anal canal during the first postoperative week before constructing the CAA, the anastomosis is less likely to fail with retraction of the neorectum back into the pelvis.

The Turnbull-Cutait procedure is performed in two stages. In the first stage, the patient is placed in the modified lithotomy position to allow access to both the abdomen and perineum, and bilateral ureteric stents are inserted. A generous midline abdominal incision extending caudally to the symphysis pubis is opened, and pelvic dissection is performed as noted previously to disconnect the failed CAA and remove the neorectum from the pelvis. If present, the chronic pelvic abscess cavity is excised or débrided using cautery. In many cases the pelvic outlet will be stenotic due to a rim of dense scar tissue at the base of the bladder. If not addressed, this can constrict the exteriorized colon, leading to venous ischemia, necrosis, and failure of the redo CAA. Careful radial incisions into this fibrotic ring using cautery can help dilate the pelvic outlet and provide sufficient room for the pulled-through colon. Great care must be taken, however, to avoid injury to the distal ureters and bladder base during this maneuver.

Attention is then turned to the perineum where four to six perineal eversion sutures are placed to facilitate exposure of the distal anal canal and the mucosectomy is completed as described previously for redo IPAA. Eight deep sutures of 2-0 or 3-0 polyglactic acid, each incorporating the mucosa, submucosa, and superficial aspect of the internal sphincter, are then placed along the circumference of the distal anal canal margin. The needles are left attached to allow the anastomosis to be matured at a later date.

The remaining left colon is then fully mobilized, the splenic flexure is taken down, and the distal end is grasped

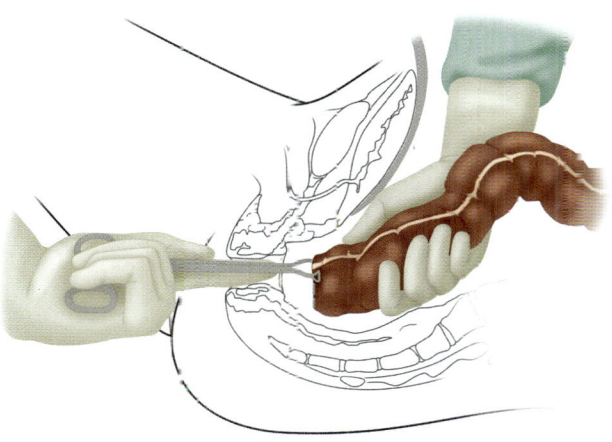

FIGURE 180.6 Turnbull-Cutait pull-through: first stage. After resection of the failed coloanal anastomosis, the distal end of the colon is grasped with a long Babcock clamp and is pulled through the anal canal. (Copyright Cleveland Clinic Foundation.)

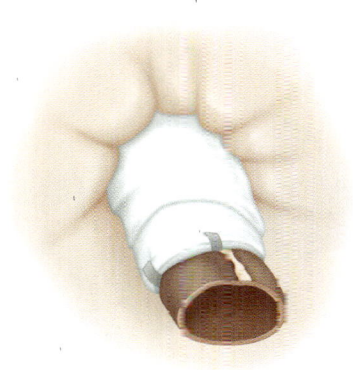

FIGURE 180.7 Turnbull-Cutait pull-through: first stage. The exteriorized colon is then wrapped in gauze and the gauze roll is secured to the distal colon with metal clips. This will prevent the colon from retracting back into the pelvis during the postoperative period. (Copyright Cleveland Clinic Foundation.)

with a long Babcock clamp passed transanally (Fig. 180.6). The colon is pulled through the anal canal and exteriorized for a distance of approximately 10 to 15 cm, after which its viability is confirmed by cutting the most distal edge to demonstrate active arterial bleeding. The colon will subsequently lie directly over the aorta, with the mesocolon oriented posteriorly at the anus. In patients with urethral or vaginal defects from anastomotic fistulas, the colon can be partially rotated so that the mesentery covers the injury. The exteriorized colon is then wrapped in gauze along with the eight sutures and attached needles, and the gauze roll is secured to the distal colon with metal clips (Fig. 180.7). Finally, a presacral drain is placed and a loop ileostomy created prior to abdominal closure.

The second stage of the Turnbull-Cutait procedure occurs 7 to 10 days later in the lithotomy position under general anesthesia. The gauze wrap is removed and the eight previously placed anal canal sutures are unraveled and arranged (Fig. 180.8). The exteriorized colon is then amputated several centimeters distal to the anal verge. It is best to err on the side of leaving behind more rather than less exteriorized colon, as the morbidity of anastomotic dehiscence or stricture far outweighs a mucosal ectropion, which can be easily excised at a later date. CAA is then completed using the previously placed sutures (Fig. 180.9).

Two groups have recently reported their results in patients undergoing the Turnbull-Cutait pull-through procedure, the majority of which were performed for failed low colorectal or coloanal anastomoses.[5,6] The success rate, defined as freedom from a stoma, was approximately 80% in each study, with the mean length of follow-up ranging from 2.5 to nearly 6 years. Functional outcomes were similar to those in patients undergoing primary CAA, with three daytime and one nighttime bowel movements per 24 hours. Twenty percent of patients admitted to a significant degree of fecal incontinence, while one-third experienced fecal urgency and used pads.[5]

RECURRENT RECTAL CANCER

Operations for recurrent rectal cancer can be the most challenging of all reoperative pelvic surgery cases. Over the past 30 years, the attitude of surgeons confronted with these patients has evolved from one of trepidation and reluctance to that of optimism and a much more aggressive approach. This has largely been aided by technological advances in preoperative imaging, neoadjuvant and intraoperative radiation therapy, improved surgical techniques, and better intensive care unit care, and the traditional long list of contraindications to resection of a recurrent cancer has been whittled down to only a few. Modern recurrent rectal cancer surgeons accept only three strict contraindications to surgical resection: unresectable extrapelvic metastatic disease, comorbidities precluding major surgery, and inability to achieve a negative margin (R0) resection based on assessment by preoperative imaging. Recent reports from expert centers suggest that nearly 50% of patients with recurrent rectal cancer qualify for an attempted curative resection. In addition, one-third of all surgically treated patients will survive 5 years, 60% of operated patients achieve an R0 resection, and the 5-year survival rate for this group is 50%, the surgical mortality rate has decreased to less than 2%, and quality of life of these patients after surgery is similar to that of primary rectal cancer patients.[7–9]

The keys to achieving good outcomes in patients with recurrent rectal cancer are proper patient selection, a multidisciplinary team approach, technical expertise, and commitment of the surgeon to the necessary operation to attain an R0 resection. Preoperative evaluation should include a PET-CT of the chest, abdomen, and pelvis to exclude unresectable extrapelvic metastatic disease and a high-quality pelvic MRI to assess resectability and to define the planes that will need to be dissected to obtain clear margins. An examination under anesthesia

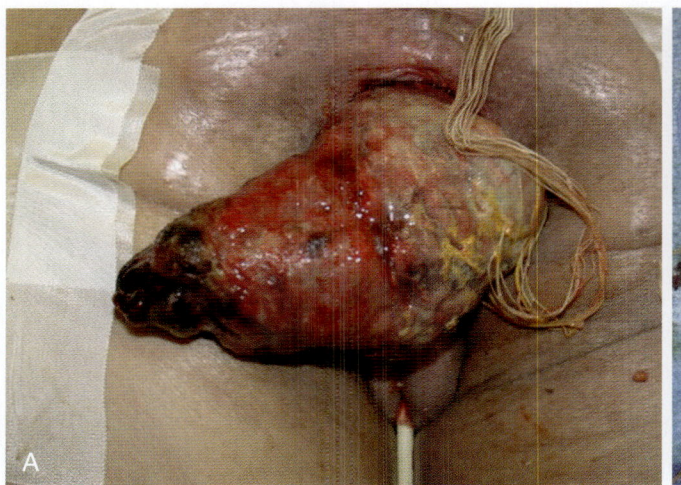 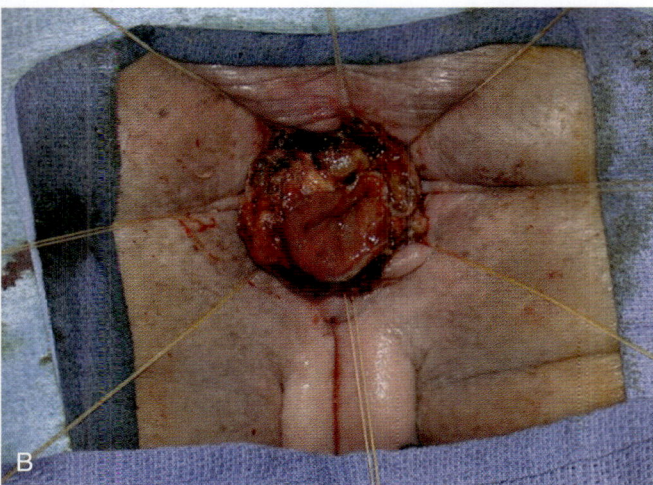

FIGURE 180.8 Turnbull-Cutait pull-through: second stage. (A) The gauze wrap has been removed from the exteriorized colon on postoperative day 7. (B) The eight previously placed sutures are unraveled and arranged in preparation for coloanal anastomosis.

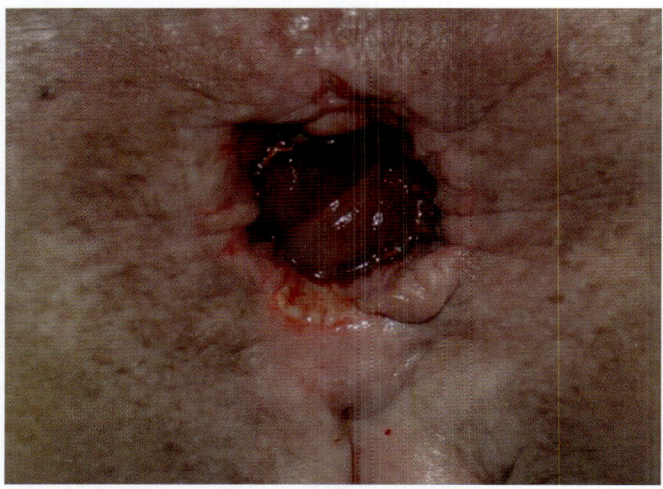 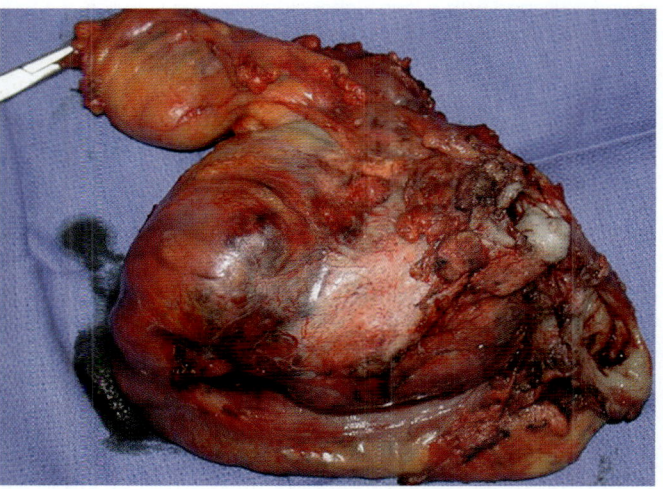

FIGURE 180.9 Turnbull-Cutait pull-through: second stage. Completed coloanal anastomosis. The resulting mucosal ectropion will usually resolve prior to loop ileostomy closure.

FIGURE 180.10 Anterior pelvic exenteration for recurrent rectal cancer in a male patient. The operative specimen consists of the colon, rectum, and bladder removed in en bloc fashion.

can be an important adjunct to these imaging studies, especially if bladder, prostate, or vaginal involvement is suspected. All imaging should be reviewed in the context of a multidisciplinary team conference so that an individualized treatment plan can be constructed for each patient. Decisions regarding neoadjuvant and intraoperative radiation therapy, sacrectomy, vascular resection and grafting, urologic and gynecologic surgery involvement, and plastic surgery reconstruction are made at this time, and appropriate arrangements are made well in advance.

A detailed discussion of the entire spectrum of surgery for recurrent rectal cancer is beyond the scope of this chapter; however, a few general points regarding surgical technique can be made. As previously stated, the ultimate goal in any such operation is the achievement of an R0 resection. To this end, the surgeon must stay committed to the idea of being "one plane deeper" than the lateral-, posterior-, and anterior-most extent of the tumor. This often requires the en bloc resection of adjacent structures

such as the urinary bladder and prostate gland in men, the vagina in women, internal iliac vessels, and the sacrum. While resection of these structures adds additional morbidity and quality-of-life issues to an already difficult procedure, ill-advised attempts to "shave" tumor off of these structures in an attempt to preserve them does the patient a disservice as the median survival time in patients undergoing a grossly positive-margin resection (R2) is no different from that of patients not taken to surgery.[10]

The location of pelvic recurrence is a strong predictor of the likelihood of R0 resection. Axial recurrences have the greatest chance of being removed with clear margins and are often located at the prior anastomosis or in residual mesorectum. Axial recurrences are usually the result of poor primary surgery, with either an inadequate distal resection margin or an incomplete mesorectal excision. Anterior recurrences also have a high chance of R0 resection, but typically require exenteration of the anterior pelvic organs in an en bloc fashion with the tumor (Fig. 180.10). While anterior pelvic exenteration in the

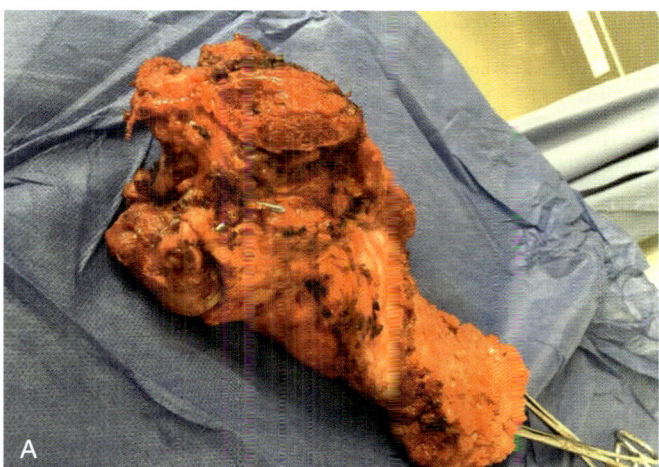

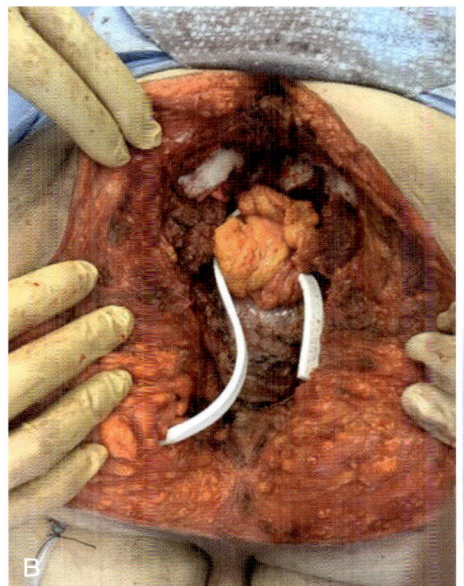

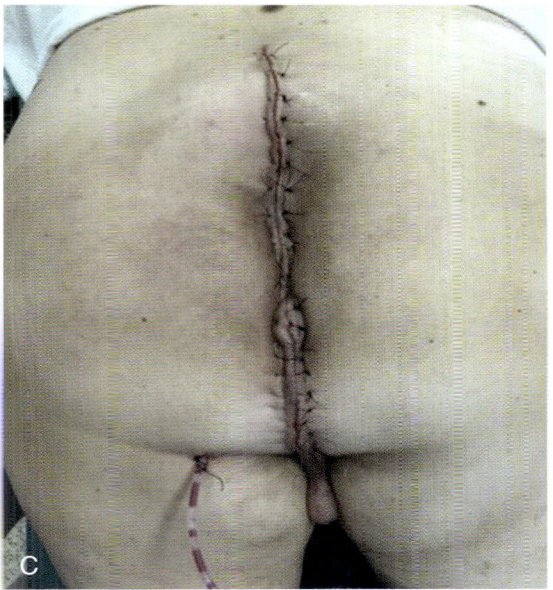

FIGURE 180.11 Resection of recurrent rectal cancer with en bloc sacrectomy. (A) Operative specimen. (B) Resultant perineal defect with lower edge of sacrum posteriorly and prostate gland anteriorly. Pelvic drain and omental pedicle flap are visible. (C) The perineal wound is closed with vertical mattress sutures.

male patient is a complex operation from the standpoint of urologic reconstruction, it is also the most common procedure performed for recurrent rectal cancer at most centers and has a high likelihood of success. Posterior recurrences often require en bloc partial sacrectomy to achieve a clear radial margin (Fig. 180.11). Sacral resection at or below the level of S3 are well accepted and carry minimal morbidity, aside from possible urinary and sexual dysfunction. "High" sacral resections, involving the S1 or S2 sacral body, are more controversial and can lead to considerable disability. Lateral recurrences, defined as those involving the pelvic sidewall structures, are the most difficult to cure, although a recent study has reported a 50% R0 resection rate in a group of these patients treated with en bloc iliac vessel resection. These authors emphasize that the key to achieving such outcomes is a methodical approach to pelvic sidewall dissection that uses the plane lateral to the internal iliac vessels to expose the obturator internus and piriformis muscles, sacrotuberous

and sacrospinous ligaments, and sacral nerve roots for potential en bloc resection.[8]

REFERENCES

1. Benn PL, Wolff BG, Ilstrup DM. Level of anastomosis and recurrent colonic diverticulitis. *Am J Surg.* 1986;151:269-271.
2. Remzi FH, Aytac E, Ashburn J, et al. Transabdominal redo ileal pouch surgery for failed restorative proctocolectomy. Lessons learned in over 500 patients. *Ann Surg.* 2015;262:675-682.
3. Turnbull RB Jr. Pull-through resection of the rectum, with delayed anastomosis, for cancer or Hirschprung's disease. *Surgery.* 1966;59:498-502.
4. Cutait DE, Cutait R, Ioshimoto M, Hypólito da Silva J, Manzione A. Abdominoperineal endoanal pull-through resection. A comparative study between immediate and delayed colorectal anastomosis. *Dis Colon Rectum.* 1985;28:294-299.
5. Remzi FH, El Gazzaz G, Kiran RP, Kirat HT, Fazio VW. Outcomes following Turnbull-Cutait abdominoperineal pull-through compared with coloanal anastomosis. *Br J Surg.* 2009;96:424-429.
6. Maggiori L, Blanche J, Harnoy Y, Ferron M, Panis Y. Redo-surgery by transanal colonic pull-through for failed anastomosis associated

with chronic pelvic sepsis or rectovaginal fistula. *Int J Colorectal Dis.* 2015;30:543-548.

7. Heriot AG, Byrne CM, Lee P, et al. Extended radical resection: the choice for locally recurrent rectal cancer. *Dis Colon Rectum.* 2008;51:284-291.

8. Austin KK, Solomon MJ. Pelvic exenteration with en bloc iliac vessel resection for lateral pelvic wall involvement. *Dis Colon Rectum.* 2009;52:1223-1233.

9. Austin KK, Young JM, Solomon MJ. Quality of life of survivors after pelvic exenteration for rectal cancer. *Dis Colon Rectum.* 2010;53:1121-1126.

10. Bhangu A, Ali SM, Darzi A, et al. Meta-analysis of survival based on resection margin status following surgery for recurrent rectal cancer. *Colorectal Dis.* 2012;15:156-163.

Evidence-Based Decision Making in Colon and Rectal Surgery

Najjia N. Mahmoud | Emily Carter Paulson

Evidence-based surgical practice is rapidly becoming synonymous with "quality" care. The topics of evidence-based care in colorectal surgery are immense and diverse, and many have been covered in other chapters of this textbook. In the following pages, we attempt to highlight areas of interest in colorectal surgery, not previously covered, that involve evidence-based care of the colorectal surgery patient.

ENHANCED RECOVERY PATHWAYS

During the past decade there has been much interest in postoperative recovery pathways designed to streamline and codify postoperative care following a variety of procedures. Although these protocols differ from hospital to hospital, there are basic elements that are included in most enhanced recovery pathways (ERPs) (Table 181.1).[1] The most common elements include preoperative counseling, avoidance of bowel preparation (see discussion later), no preoperative fasting, opioid-sparing analgesia and midthoracic epidurals, antibiotic prophylaxis, short incisions, no nasogastric tubes, normothermia, operative and postoperative fluid restrictions, no abdominal drains, oral diet at will, and early mobilization.

An early review by Wind et al., published in 2006, included six studies, three randomized controlled trials (RCTs), and three single-arm controlled clinical trials, published between 1998 and 2005.[2] These were single-institution studies, and the number of ERP elements included ranged from 4 to 12, although all studies induced early mobilization and diet. In five of six studies hospital stay was significantly shorter in the ERP patients, and in pooled analysis the ERP patients had a hospital stay almost 2 days shorter than patients in a traditional pathway (TP). There was no difference seen in the rate of readmissions. One study reported significantly lower morbidity in the ERP group, especially cardiovascular and pulmonary complications. In pooled analysis, this trend was also observed. There was no difference seen in rates of anastomotic leakage or mortality. Postoperative ileus (PCI), measured by time to first bowel movement (BM) and tolerance of a solid diet, was reduced in the ERP group. There were mixed results regarding the outcomes of pain and fatigue, with some studies reporting no difference between ERP and TP groups, whereas others reported increased pain and fatigue in the TP group compared with the ERP group. These authors concluded that ERP programs result in improved recovery after surgery, with a reduction in morbidity rates and hospital stay. These findings were confirmed by a review published in 2009, by Gouvas et al., which evaluated 11 studies—four RCTs

and seven controlled clinical trials—comparing ERP with TP.[3] These authors conclude that ERPs contribute to a quicker recovery of patients after colorectal surgery and result in lower morbidity and shorter hospital stays.

Two more recent meta-analyses have further examined the impact of ERPs in colorectal surgery. In 2013 Zhuang et al. analyzed 13 studies (1910 patients) comparing ERP with TP.[4] The mean number of enhanced recovery after surgery (ERAS) elements incorporated in each study was 11. The ERPs were associated with significantly decreased length of primary stay (−2.4 days, $P < .001$), total days in hospital (including readmission, −2.39 days; $P < .001$), and overall complications (relative risk [RR] = 0.68; $F = .0006$). There were no differences noted in readmission rates, surgery-specific complications, or mortality.

In 2014 Greco et al. performed a meta-analysis of 16 RCTs that included 2376 patients.[5] In 11 of the 16 studies, at least 10 ERP elements were included in the ERPs; the most common elements included early postoperative feeding and mobilization, no postoperative nasogastric tube, epidural analgesia, and no preoperative fasting. Their analysis demonstrated a reduction in overall morbidity (RR = 0.60, 95% confidence interval [CI], 0.46 to 0.76) and length of stay (−2.28 days; 95% CI, −3.09 to −1.47 days) associated with ERP.

Although the individual elements differ among studies, the existing evidence is robust that a codified ERP can reduce length of stay and morbidity following colorectal surgery. Interestingly, many of the early studies in ERP were performed when open surgery was more common. The benefit associated with ERPs has been questioned in the setting of laparoscopic procedures, which are becoming increasingly common. Several studies have addressed this specific question. In 2011, Vlug et al. randomized 427 patients into four treatment arms—open colectomy with TP, open colectomy with ERP, laparoscopic colectomy with TP, and laparoscopic colectomy with ERP.[6] The shortest length of primary hospital stay (median, 5 days) was noted in the laparoscopic/ERP group. In the laparoscopic/TP group, median length of stay was 6 days ($P < .001$). A similar and significant difference was noted for total hospital stay (including readmission days). These authors concluded that optimal treatment for colorectal patients is laparoscopy in conjunction with ERP.

In 2012 Haverkamp et al. compared ERP and TP in 185 patients undergoing only laparoscopic colectomies.[7] The median length of stay in the ERP cohort was 4 days compared with 6 days for the TP patients ($F = .007$). Return to bowel function was noted 1 day earlier in the ERP group (2 vs. 3 days; $P < .001$). No differences were noted in postoperative complications, readmission, or

TABLE 181.1 Components of a Standard Enhanced Recovery Pathway for Colorectal Surgery

Enhanced Recovery Pathway Components	Level of Evidence*
Preoperative counseling	Grade B
Preoperative feeding—minimization of fasting	Grade A
Synbiotics	Not discussed in consensus review
No bowel preparation	Grade A
No premedication	Grade A
Fluid restriction	Grade A
Perioperative high O_2 concentrations	Not discussed in consensus review
Active prevention of hypothermia	Grade A
Epidural analgesia	Grade A
Minimally invasive/transverse incisions	Grade B
No routine use of nasogastric tubes	Grade A
No use of drains above peritoneal reflection	Grade A
Enforced postoperative mobilization	Grade B
Enforced early postoperative feeding	Grade A
Balanced analgesia—multimodal, low/no opioids	Grade A
Standard laxatives and antiemetics	Grade B
Early removal of urinary catheter	Not discussed in consensus review

Grade A, Based on at least two good-quality randomized controlled trials (RCTs) or one meta-analysis of RCTs with homogeneity; *Grade B,* consensus recommendations based on the best available evidence.
*Level of evidence from Lassen K, Soop M, Nygren J, et al. Consensus review of optimal perioperative care in colorectal surgery: Enhanced Recovery After Surgery (ERAS) Group recommendations. *Arch Surg.* 2009;144(10):961–969.

mortality. Again, these authors conclude that ERPs are beneficial even in the setting of laparoscopic approaches to resection.

In 2014 Kennedy et al. reported the results of the EnRol (ENhanced Recovery Open versus Laparoscopic) trial, an RCT of 204 patients randomized to either open surgery or laparoscopic resection within an ERP.[8] There was no difference in the primary outcome, physical fatigue at 1-month postoperatively, between the two groups, nor was there any difference in complications or other patient-reported outcomes. The total hospital stay was significantly shorter in the laparoscopy cohort (median, 5 days vs. 7 days; $P = .033$). Based on these results, the authors conclude that, within an ERP, laparoscopy can significantly reduce length of hospital stay.

Finally, two meta-analyses published in 2015 attempted to clarify overlapping benefits of laparoscopy and ERP. Zhuang et al. analyzed five RCTs, including 598 patients, to look at the benefit of laparoscopy when all patients are enrolled in an ERP.[9] The authors noted that the overall quality of existing evidence was low to moderate, with several of the included trials using suboptimal ERPs. They concluded that total hospital stay following laparoscopic resection in the setting of an ERP was reduced compared with open resection but that more robust evidence is needed to truly prove that laparoscopy provides other benefits in the setting of optimal ERPs.

Spanjersberg et al., analyzed three RCTs and six controlled clinical trials in an attempt to answer two questions: (1) does laparoscopy offer benefit within an ERP, and (2) does ERP offer an advantage when all patients get laparoscopic resection.[10] In the laparoscopic patients, the length of stay was shorter in patients enrolled in an ERP (-2.3 days; $P = .001$). In the ERP patients, postoperative morbidity was lower in the laparoscopic group than the open ([odds ratio] OR $= 0.42$; $P = .006$). As with the previously mentioned review, the quality of the included studies was graded to be moderate to poor. Despite this, the authors conclude that both ERP and laparoscopy are associated with independent benefit but that better designed trials are needed to more definitively answer these questions.

Overall, there has been a great deal of effort put into designing ERPs based on the best evidence available. In general, there are elements supported by extremely strong evidence, such as early initiation of diet and mobilization, and antibiotic prophylaxis (see discussion later), whereas other elements are less well supported. In 2009 the ERAS Group published a consensus review of optimal perioperative care in colorectal surgery.[1] They reviewed the evidence for and made recommendations about 20 ERP elements. Again, although the evidence is not robust for all elements, this remains a good summary of the most common elements of standard ERPs for colorectal surgery. A more recent set of guidelines drew from these recommendations and was reviewed in 2013 by Gustafsson et al., as part of the ERAS Society.[11] The strength of recommendations ranged from low to high for individual elements of the pathway. Although adherence to all elements is difficult and requires multidisciplinary coordination in the perioperative period, there is evidence to suggest that increasing compliance with ERPs is associated with reduced hospital stays and possibly, fewer complications (ERAS Compliance Group). In the 2013 review the authors concluded that there was high-quality evidence that ERPs result in shorter length of hospital stay following colorectal resections. However, the existing evidence suggesting that ERPs result in fewer complications and hospital readmission was deemed to be low.

MECHANICAL BOWEL PREPARATION

Mechanical bowel preparation before elective colorectal resection remains a common practice among general and colorectal surgeons. However, its use over the past decade has been decreasing, primarily in response to many RCTs and meta-analyses that have not only failed to show a benefit to mechanical bowel preparation but also have demonstrated an increase in complications following bowel preparation.

Two of the earliest RCTs to examine this issue were performed in 1994 by Burke et al. and Santos et al.[12,13] In both of these studies the authors concluded that bowel preparation does not influence outcome after elective colorectal surgery. Since that time, continued controversy over the use of bowel preparation has spawned several more RCTs. In 2007 Pena-Soria et al. examined the relationship between bowel preparation and surgical-site infection and anastomotic leak in 97 patients.[14] They found no difference in surgical site infection between the two groups, but a higher rate of anastomotic dehiscence in the non-prepped group (8.3% vs. 4.1%; $P = .05$). The largest RCT examining this question was published in 2007 by Contant et al. and included more than 1400 patients at 13 hospitals.[15] Patients were consented to receive either no bowel preparation, which included a regular diet the day before surgery versus a bowel preparation of either polyethylene glycol or sodium phosphate and a clear liquid diet the day before surgery. In this study the rate of anastomotic leak, 4.8% in patients who received bowel prep and 5.4% in patients who did not, did not differ significantly between groups ($P = .69$). Patients who had mechanical bowel preparation did have fewer abscesses after anastomotic leak than those who did not (0.3% vs. 2.5%; $P = .001$). Other complications, such as fascial dehiscence, superficial infection, and mortality, did not differ between groups. These authors concluded that mechanical bowel preparation before elective colorectal surgery can safely be abandoned. Several studies supported these conclusions for left-sided colon and rectal resections as well.[16,1]

Further buttressing the argument against mechanical bowel prep were multiple large meta-analyses synthesizing the results from the almost 20 years of trials examining this issue. In 2004, Slim et al. analyzed the results of seven randomized trials, including 1454 patients, comparing bowel preparation with no preparation in colorectal surgery.[18] They reported significantly higher rates of anastomotic leak after bowel preparation (5.6% vs. 3.2%; $P = .032$). All other end points (wound infection, other septic complications, and nonseptic complications also favored the no-preparation regimen. In 2010 Zhu et al. specifically analyzed five RCTs that compared mechanical bowel preparation with polyethylene glycol with no preparation.[19] They found no significant differences in rates of surgical site infection, organ/space infection, mortality, or anastomotic leak between the groups. Finally, the largest and most thorough meta-analysis was published by Guenaga et al. in 2009.[17] These authors analyzed 13 RCTs, including 4777 patients, comparing bowel preparation with no bowel preparation. They found that rates of anastomotic leakage, although slightly higher in the bowel preparation groups, were not significantly different following either low anterior or rectal resections or colonic resections. Rates of secondary complications, such as wound infection and extraabdominal complications, were not different between the two groups. They concluded that there was no statistically significant evidence that patients benefit from mechanical bowel preparation.

Based on this robust body of evidence, many surgeons began to reduce their use of bowel preparation prior to colorectal surgery. However, interestingly, new evidence is emerging that mechanical bowel preparation with oral antibiotic administration is beneficial prior to elective colorectal surgery. In almost all of the trials mentioned previously, oral antibiotics were not included as part of the mechanical bowel preparation pathway. Many investigators believe that the benefit from bowel preparation stems from the delivery of the oral antibiotics to the colon lumen and mucosa, a process that is enhanced by the mechanical colon cleanse. In light of these concerns regarding the existing bowel preparation literature, a new series of studies have been published evaluating the efficacy of bowel preparations that include oral antibiotics. The results of these studies, which are discussed in more detail later, indicate that, although mechanical preparation alone may not be of benefit, mechanical preparation with oral antibiotics is beneficial in reducing surgical site infection and anastomotic leak following colorectal surgery.

In 2012 Cannon et al. evaluated almost 10,000 patients undergoing elective colorectal surgery within the Veterans Administration Health System.[20] They compared patients receiving no bowel prep to those receiving mechanical-only bowel prep, mechanical bowel prep plus oral antibiotics, or oral antibiotics alone. They reported that oral antibiotics plus mechanical bowel preparation was associated with a 57% decrease in surgical site infection occurrence compared with no bowel prep (OR = 0.43; 95% CI, 0.34 to 0.55).

Following that study, in 2013 Toneva et al. reported on the association between oral antibiotic bowel preparation and length of stay and readmissions in a similar Veterans Administration Health System cohort of 8140 patients.[21] They report that oral antibiotic bowel preparation was associated with a significantly reduced length of stay, as well as a significant reduction in the number of readmissions, due mostly to a reduction in readmission for infection.

In 2014 Kim et al. used the Michigan Surgical Quality Collaborative data to examine almost 1000 pairs of patients undergoing elective colectomy who differed only by administration of bowel preparation.[22] The bowel preparation group received mechanical bowel preparation with nonabsorbable oral antibiotics, and the control group received no bowel prep. These authors found that patients receiving full preparation were less likely to have any surgical site infection (5.0% vs. 9.7%; $P = .0001$), organ/space infection (1.6% vs. 3.1%; $P = .024$), and superficial surgical site infection (3.0% vs. 6.0%; $P = .001$). They were also less likely to develop postoperative *Clostridium difficile* colitis (0.5% vs. 1.8%; $P = .01$).

In 2015 four retrospective studies using American College of Surgeons National Surgical Quality Improvement Program–targeted colectomy data were published.[23–26] Meghadamyerhaneh et al. reported on just more than 5000 patients undergoing elective colorectal resections between 2012–2013.[23] They reported no difference in postoperative morbidity between patients receiving no preparation and either mechanical preparation alone or oral antibiotic preparation alone. Multivariable analysis revealed that the combination of oral antibiotics and mechanical bowel preparation significantly reduced the risk of overall morbidity (OR = 0.63; $P < .01$), surgical site infection (OR = 0.31; $P < .01$), and anastomotic disruption (OR = 0.14; $P < .01$), especially following left-sided resections. Morris et al. examined 8145 patients undergoing elective colon and rectal resections.[24] They found that patients receiving oral antibiotics had a significantly lower risk of surgical site infection than either those patients receiving no bowel preparation or those receiving mechanical preparation only. This was consistent for both open and minimally invasive approaches and for both colon and rectal resections. Scarborough et al. reported on the outcome of almost 5000 patients undergoing elective colorectal resections.[25] Again, they found that patients receiving oral antibiotics combined with mechanical preparation had the lowest rate of surgical site infection, anastomotic leak, and procedure-related readmission. There was no difference noted among the no preparation, oral antibiotic alone preparation, or mechanical preparation alone groups. Finally, Kiran et al. reported on 8442 patients undergoing elective colorectal procedures.[26] After their multivariable analysis, mechanical bowel preparation with oral antibiotics was independently associated with reduced surgical site infection (OR = 0.40; 95% CI, 0.31 to 0.53), anastomotic leak (OR = 0.57; 95% CI, 0.35 to 0.94), and ileus (OR = 0.71, 95% CI, 0.56 to 0.90).

All of these studies have countered the increasingly held belief that bowel preparation prior to elective colorectal surgery is not necessary and may be harmful. Each of these provides retrospective evidence that oral antibiotic administration in combination with a mechanical bowel preparation can have significant beneficial effects for colorectal surgery patients, including decreased risks of wound infection, anastomotic leak, ileus, and readmission. Based on this body of evidence, many providers are routinely using the combination of oral antibiotics and mechanical bowel preparation for their colorectal surgery patients. Randomized controlled data would add to this ample body of retrospective data as the debate around the appropriate use of preoperative bowel preparation continues to evolve.

ANTIBIOTIC PROPHYLAXIS

It has long been recognized that antibiotic prophylaxis for patients undergoing surgery on the large intestine reduces the risk of postoperative wound infection. In 1981 Baum et al. published the results of a meta-analysis evaluating a series of studies comparing the rate of wound infection in patients receiving antibiotic prophylaxis to patients receiving no prophylaxis.[27] They concluded that the risk of wound infection was so diminished in the prophylaxis group that, in the future, studies investigating prophylactic antibiotic use could not ethically include a no-treatment group. Since that time, the use of preoperative antibiotics has become routine, but the choice of antibiotic, the timing of antibiotic dosing, and the use of postoperative therapy continues to defy easy standardization.

There have been hundreds of studies looking at the type of antibiotic used, the timing of antibiotic dosing, and the need for intraoperative redosing and postoperative dosing. These are too numerous to describe in detail in this text. Based on these innumerable studies, the current Clinical Practice Guidelines for Antimicrobial Prophylaxis in Surgery were published in 2013 as a collaboration between several infectious disease, surgical infection, pharmacy, and epidemiology societies.[28] In addition, a recent, extensive meta-analysis, published in 2014, sought to distill the results of the RCTs into several coherent conclusions for the colorectal surgery population.[29] Available evidence was combined and analyzed to address the need for prophylaxis, the spectrum of bacterial coverage needed, and the optimal timing and route of antibiotic administration.

Most surgeons, based on reviews of practice patterns, recognize that prophylactic antibiotic dosing is beneficial in patients undergoing large bowel surgery. This practice is clearly supported by a large body of evidence, including 10 placebo-controlled trials in the 1980s. The combined analysis of these trials indicates that prophylactic antibiotics reduce the wound infection rate from 39% to 10%, with all 10 trials individually finding a significant or nearly significant benefit in favor of prophylaxis. There is no debate that antibiotic prophylaxis is standard of care for elective clean-contaminated colorectal surgery procedures.

Both the 2013 guidelines and the 2014 meta-analysis conclude that, for the majority of intravenous (IV) antibiotics, the optimal time for administration is within 60 minutes before surgical incision. However, the use of postoperative antibiotics and the need for intraoperative redosing is more controversial. In particular, many prescribe 24 hours of postoperative prophylactic antibiotics or favor redosing of IV antibiotics during lengthy cases. Nelson's meta-analysis evaluated 33 trials that compared a single preoperative dose of antibiotics to longer duration of dosing. There was no evidence that longer duration of antibiotic dosing reduced the risk of wound infection more than a single preoperative dose (RR = 1.10; CI, 9.93 to 1.30; P = .26). These results are supported by the Clinical Practice Guidelines, which recommend stopping antibiotics when the procedure is completed and the incision is closed. The guidelines state that, at most, antibiotics should be continued for no more than 24 hours postoperatively.

Conflicting recommendations regarding intraoperative redosing of antibiotics also exist. In a 2014 meta-analysis, Nelson et al. concluded based on a review of nine studies that evidence is lacking to support intraoperative redosing of antibiotics. This is in contradiction to several published studies and the 2013 practice guidelines. In a study by Morita et al. in 2005, wound infection was double in patients who underwent procedures greater than 4 hours and who did not get redosing of antibiotics compared to those patients who did receive a second intraoperative dose (P = .008).[30] The 2013 Clinical Practice Guidelines, based on review of multiple trials, recommends intraoperative redosing of the IV antibiotic if the length of the operation exceeds two half-lives of the antibiotic or if there is excessive blood loss.

The spectrum of antibiotics used for prophylaxis is another area in which practice patterns vary widely. However, there are many studies indicating that treatment with antibiotics covering both aerobic and anaerobic bacteria provides the greatest benefit in the reduction of postoperative wound infection. Based on the meta-analysis of existing randomized trials, the addition of anaerobic coverage to a regimen including aerobic coverage reduced wound infections by 43% (RR = 0.47; P = .0004). Similarly, adding aerobic coverage to a regimen of anaerobic coverage reduced wound infection by more than 45% (RR = 0.44; P = .0002).

Based on an evaluation of 260 randomized studies that included almost 44,000 patients, Nelson et al. made several conclusions regarding the use of prophylactic antibiotics for colorectal surgery.[29] Not surprisingly, they found that there is overwhelming evidence to support the use of antibiotic prophylaxis in patients undergoing colorectal surgery. They also concluded that the antibiotics used should cover both anaerobic and aerobic bacteria. In addition, the evidence indicates that preoperative dosing of IV antibiotics, preferably approximately 1 hour prior to incision, is imperative. They found no evidence supporting redosing of antibiotics during long cases or the routine administration of postoperative antibiotics following uncomplicated, elective colorectal surgery. Finally, based on the evidence reviewed in this analysis, it appears that the combination of oral (discussed previously) and IV antibiotics provides the optimal prophylactic regimen in patients receiving a bowel preparation. For the most part the current clinical practice guidelines mirror these findings with one key exception. The published guidelines do recommend intraoperative redosing of IV antibiotics, as discussed previously.

POSTOPERATIVE ORAL INTAKE

Resumption of oral intake following colorectal surgery is often the prime factor limiting patient's discharge from the hospital. Traditionally, oral intake has been withheld until patients demonstrate return of bowel function, either by passing flatus or having a BM. Following this conservative pathway, the average patient tolerates a regular diet on day 5 following colorectal resection. Although there is little evidence to support this approach, many still use it to guide postoperative diet management. In reality, there are numerous studies that support the idea that early oral nutrition following colorectal surgery has no deleterious effect on patient outcome and, in fact, can be beneficial in terms of patient satisfaction and length of hospital stay.

More than 20 years ago, Binderow et al. performed a small RCT in patients undergoing laparotomy and colon resection, comparing traditional diet advancement with allowance of regular diet on postoperative day 1.[31] These investigators found that a slightly higher percentage of the early diet patients required replacement of a nasogastric tube but that bowel function as evidenced by return of flatus or BM still occurred at the same time in both groups. In addition, in patients who tolerated early oral intake, there was a trend toward shorter hospitalizations. This seminal, small study concluded that early oral intake is possible after laparotomy and colorectal resection.

Several years later, Hartsell et al. performed another randomized study, again comparing early institution of oral intake to traditional diet management.[32] In this trial, early oral intake consisted of liquids on postoperative day 1, followed by regular diet as soon as the patient could tolerate a liter of fluid during the day, regardless of flatus or BM. No significant differences were seen in rates of nausea and vomiting or nasogastric tube replacement. There was also no difference noted in length of hospital stay.

In 2007 a randomized trial by Han-Geurts et al. compared early institution of oral intake as tolerated by the patient (a "free diet" group) with traditional advancement of diet based on return of bowel function.[33] They observed that more patients in the free diet group required reinsertion of a nasogastric tube (20% vs. 10%; $P = .213$) but that this was not statistically significant. There was no difference observed in the complication rate, and the return of gastrointestinal (GI) function was similar in both groups. A normal diet was tolerated after a median of 2 days in the free diet group compared with 5 days in

the conventional group ($P < .001$). These authors again showed that early resumption of oral intake does not lead to a significantly increased rate of nasogastric tube reinsertion or complications. The lack of traditional markers of GI functional recovery, namely flatus and BMs, did not affect the tolerance of oral diet. They concluded that there is no reason to withhold oral intake in the early postoperative period following open colorectal surgery.

In 2009 a meta-analysis was published evaluating RCTs published through 2006, which compared traditional diet advancement with early oral intake following colorectal surgery.[34] These authors included 13 RCTs, with a total of 1173 patients. Overall, there were few differences noted between the two treatment groups in terms of complications. There was a trend toward fewer anastomotic dehiscences and shorter hospital stays, by approximately 1 day, in the early oral intake groups, although these did not reach significance. There was a slightly higher incidence of vomiting noted across the trials in the patients treated with early initiation of oral intake, but again, return of bowel function, recorded as flatus or BM, was unaffected. The conclusion of this meta-analysis, the largest to date, was that there is no advantage to the traditional conservative management of oral intake following colorectal surgery. In 2018 a meta-analysis of seven RCTs and almost 600 patients, confirmed this conclusion. In this analysis, early feeding was associated with reduced length of stay (−1.58 days; $P = .009$) and fewer postoperative complications (RR = 0.70; $P = .04$).[35]

MU-OPIOID RECEPTOR ANTAGONISTS

Peripherally acting mu-opioid receptor antagonists are a class of agents that specifically block the action of opiates on intestinal mu receptors, thereby mitigating the effects of opioid-induced constipation. The most commonly used US Food and Drug Administration (FDA)–approved drug in this class is alvimopan. Alvimopan was approved in May 2008 as an orally administered drug for the treatment of POI. It is a novel, selective, peripherally active mu-opioid receptor antagonist that works by blocking the mu-opioid receptor, minimizing the paralytic effect opiates have on the intestines, while, because it does not cross the blood-brain barrier, having little effect on analgesia. The promise of pharmaceutical reduction of POI has spurred great interest in this and other mu-opioid antagonists

In 2004 an RCT of 451 patients undergoing bowel resection was performed by Wolff et al.[36] Patients were randomized to receive 6 mg of alvimopan, 12 mg of alvimopan, or placebo 2 hours preoperatively and twice a day postoperatively. The time to GI recovery, defined as tolerance of regular food and passage of a BM, was accelerated with 6 or 12 mg of alvimopan, with a mean difference of 15 hours ($P < .005$) and 22 hours ($P < .001$), respectively, compared with placebo. In the 12-mg group, time to hospital discharge was also improved by an average of 22 hours compared with placebo ($P = .003$). Complications and adverse reactions were not different among the groups. These authors concluded that alvimopan was well tolerated and accelerated GI recovery and time to hospital discharge compared with placebo in patients undergoing bowel resection.

Two subsequent RCTs by Delaney et al. and Viscusi et al., respectively, confirmed the findings from this initial trial.[37,38] A pooled analysis of these three trials was performed in 2007 by Delaney et al.[39] This pooled analysis included more than 1100 patients randomized to 6 mg or 12 mg of alvimopan or placebo in patients who underwent laparotomy and bowel resection. In pooled analysis, alvimopan reduced the time to GI recovery by 12 to 18 hours in both the 6- and 12-mg alvimopan groups compared to placebo. Additionally, the time to placement of a discharge order was reduced by 16 hours ($P < .001$) in the 6-mg group and 18 hours ($P < .001$) in the 12-mg group. There was no significant difference in opioid use between the groups. In addition, the rate of adverse effects was lower in the alvimopan group, with lower rates of nausea and POI.

Two RCTs in 2008 confirmed the efficacy and safety of alvimopan. Ludwig et al. compared 12-mg alvimopan to placebo administered before surgery and twice per day afterward in 629 patients undergoing laparotomy and bowel resection.[40] All patients were managed postoperatively with standard ERPs that included early ambulation and early institution of oral feeding. In this study, the mean times to recovery of GI function and hospital discharge were accelerated by 20 hours ($P < .001$) and 17 hours ($P < .001$), respectively, in the alvimopan group compared with placebo. In addition, significantly fewer patients who received alvimopan remained in the hospital for 7 postoperative days or longer (18% vs. 30.8%; $P < .001$). Alvimopan patients were almost 60% less likely to develop a POI and more than 40% less likely to require nasogastric tube insertion. Opioid consumption did not differ significantly between the two groups.

In the same year, Buchler et al. published the results of another RCT evaluating the safety and efficacy of alvimopan (6 and 12 mg every 12 hours) compared with placebo in patients undergoing laparotomy and either small or large bowel resection.[41] Overall, unlike the prior studies, they did not show a significant reduction in time to tolerate solid food and first BM or flatus, although the trend was in favor of alvimopan. However, patients in this trial received either opioid patient-controlled analgesia (PCA) or opioids without PCA delivery. In the other trials, all patients received opioid analgesia via a PCA. In this study, the opioid use differed significantly between the PCA and non-PCA patient groups. For example, in the placebo patients the PCA group received an average of 92.1 morphine sulfate equivalents (MSEs), whereas the non-PCA group received only 45.3 MSEs. Differences were similar in the alvimopan treatment groups. In the PCA group, return of bowel function and time to first BM were significantly accelerated in the alvimopan treatment groups compared with placebo, whereas in patients treated with intermittent morphine and no PCA, no reductions in mean time to GI recovery were observed. This trial offered a unique perspective on alvimopan use, suggesting that alvimopan, although safe in all patients, is most useful in patients receiving opioid analgesia in higher total quantities via a PCA.

Despite the apparent efficacy of alvimopan, its use has not been widespread. One factor likely curtailing its use is its relatively high cost. However, several studies in the past 5 years have examined the cost effectiveness of alvimopan following bowel resection. In 2011 Poston et al. performed a retrospective matched-cohort study of 480 alvimopan patients and 960 matched controls.[42] They found that there was a $1040 reduction in hospital cost in the alvimopan group ($P = .03$), most likely due to the shorter length of stay in the alvimopan group (5.6 days vs. 6.5 days; $P < .001$). A retrospective study of patients undergoing segmental colectomy in the University Health System Consortium from 2008–2009 was published by Simorov et al. in 2014.[43] These authors found that regardless of approach (laparoscopic or open), alvimopan was associated with shorter length of stay (4.4 days vs. 5.9 days; $P < .001$) and reduced hospital costs ($9974.00 vs. $11,303.00; $P < .001$). Another study by Adam et al. in 2016 compared 197 colorectal surgery patients receiving alvimopan to 463 colorectal surgery patients not receiving alvimopan.[44] Alvimopan was again associated with faster return of bowel function, lower incidence of ileus, and shorter length of stay. These benefits translated into a cost savings of $1492.00 per patients treated with alvimopan ($P = .01$). In 2016 Ehlers et al. reported on more than 14,000 patients undergoing elective colorectal surgery[45]; 11% of the patients received alvimopan. In the alvimopan cohort, length of stay was 1.8 days shorter ($P < .01$) and costs were $2017.00 lower ($P < .01$) than the cohort not receiving alvimopan.

Finally, a meta-analysis by Earnshaw et al. in 2015 combined data from several bowel resection trials and specifically examined the efficacy and cost of alvimopan in the setting of an ERP.[46] They found that the incidence of ileus was significantly reduced (7% vs. 15%; $P < .0001$) and that the time to discharge was also shorter (8.4 days vs. 11.1 days; $P < .0001$) in the alvimopan cohort. The average hospital costs were more than $700.00 less in the alvimopan patients.

POSTOPERATIVE ANALGESIA

There has been debate over the years as to the optimal postoperative analgesia regimen for patients undergoing colon resection, both following laparotomy and laparoscopy. It has long been recognized that IV opioids, although effective for pain relief, can prolong POI, delaying return of bowel function and possibly tolerance of a regular diet. As such, there has been interest in using epidural analgesia in the postoperative period. There have been numerous randomized trials comparing epidural and IV analgesia following open colon resection. A few of the largest of these trials, as well as a meta-analysis evaluating 16 of these RCTs, are discussed briefly later. In addition, there have been a few studies and reviews examining the same issue following laparoscopic colon resection. These are also discussed briefly at the end of this section.

One of the early randomized trials evaluating the efficacy and safety of epidural analgesia versus IV analgesia following colorectal resection was published in 2001 by Carli et al.[47] In this study, patients received either morphine PCA or a bupivacaine and fentanyl infusion via an epidural catheter for 4 days postoperatively. Analgesia was discontinued on postoperative day 4, and acetaminophen and codeine were then used orally as needed. Diet (in this study, liquid and protein drinks were started on all patients on postoperative day 1) and mobilization were the same between the two groups. The cumulative pain score (measured by the visual analog scale [VAS]) was significantly improved in the epidural patients with rest, coughing, and movement on the first 3 postoperative days. Pain scores were the same between groups by day 4. There was no difference in the incidence of postoperative nausea and vomiting between the two groups, but the time from surgery to first flatus and BM was significantly shorter in the epidural group. Twelve of 21 epidural patients passed flatus and 7 of 21 had a BM during the first 2 postoperative days, compared with 4 of 21 (P = .001) and 1 of 21 (P = .005), respectively, in the PCA group. Length of stay and rate of complications were the same between the two groups.

A trial published by Zutshi et al. in 2005 evaluated epidural versus IV analgesia in patients undergoing laparotomy and bowel resection, all of whom were enrolled in an enhanced recovery program including early ambulation and oral intake.[58] Postoperatively, patients in the epidural group received a continuous infusion of bupivacaine and fentanyl supplemented by a patient-controlled bolus. The epidural was removed on postoperative day 2, and oral pain medications were offered. Patients in the IV group received a PCA that delivered IV analgesia on demand and were switched to oxycodone starting 48 hours after surgery. There was no difference in length of stay between the two groups. Although patients in the epidural group passed stool earlier than the PCA group (2 days vs. 4 days), there was no difference in time to tolerance of a regular diet. The epidural patients did have a lower pain score during the first 2 days (mean score, 2.46 vs. 3.33; P = .01). In addition, there was no significant difference between groups for quality of life, satisfaction with hospital stay, or return to normal activities at discharge or at postoperative days 10 and 30. These authors concluded that for patients undergoing bowel resection who are enrolled in an ERP following surgery, epidural anesthesia offers no benefit.

In 2007 Marret et al. published a meta-analysis evaluating 16 randomized trials comparing epidural analgesia versus IV opioid analgesia after colorectal surgery.[49] More than 800 patients were included in the study, 406 in the epidural group and 400 in the IV group. Length of stay was not significantly different in the two groups across the 13 trials that measured this outcome. Interestingly, in the later studies that used an ERP for all patients, length of stay was generally significantly shorter than in studies using a more traditional recovery pathway. As in the previously discussed study, the use of epidural analgesia in patients treated with an enhanced pathway did not shorten length of stay compared with the IV analgesia group. Pain relief, as measured by the VAS in 11 studies, was improved in the epidural groups at 24 and 48 hours. In addition, in 15 studies, POI was shortened in the epidural groups by an average of 36 hours. The rate of major postoperative complications was the same between groups, but there was a higher rate of complications, such as hypotension and urinary retention in the epidural groups. Overall, this meta-analysis concluded that epidural analgesia does decrease VAS pain score and the duration of ileus, which results in improved patient comfort and

facilitates more prompt resumption of oral intake. Despite these benefits, the use of epidural analgesia does not shorten length of hospital stay. Based on this meta-analysis, the authors conclude that hospital stay is most affected by "fast-track postoperative care," regardless of analgesia method used.

Until recently, there were very few studies examining the efficacy of epidural versus IV analgesia in patients undergoing laparoscopic colectomy. An article published in 2010 by Levy et al. reviewed the eight studies that examined analgesia regimens specifically following laparoscopic colorectal resections.[50] Based on the three randomized trials included, there was no difference in length of stay between the epidural and IV analgesia groups. Although there was heterogeneity in the studies, the average time to tolerance of a regular diet was approximately 1 day shorter in the epidural group (2.8 vs. 3.9 days). The one randomized trial that included time to passage of flatus found the epidural group to have a significantly shorter time to passing flatus (2 vs. 3 days). Similarly, the two RCTs that looked at time to first BM found that this was shorter in the patients receiving epidural analgesia. Both RCTs that evaluated pain as an outcome reported that the visual analog pain scores (1-10) were significantly lower in the epidural groups (2.5 vs. 5.4). Overall, there was no difference in the rates of complications and readmissions between the two groups. These authors concluded that there is still a paucity of data assessing the most appropriate analgesia regimen following laparoscopic colon resection.

A more recent meta-analysis was published in 2013 examining the effect of epidural analgesia on bowel function in laparoscopic colorectal surgery. These authors evaluated six RCTs published between 1999–2011. Time to first BM and pain scores were significantly better in the epidural patients, but there was no difference in hospital stay. Adverse effects were also not different between the groups. Another meta-analysis by Liu et al. was published in 2014[51] and reviewed seven RCTs specifically evaluating thoracic epidural analgesia in the setting of laparoscopic colectomy. Short-term pain scores were improved in the epidural patients with no difference in complications, length of stay, or return of bowel function.

The ERAS Society commented on the use of epidural anesthesia in their 2013 Guidelines for Perioperative Care in Elective Colonic Surgery.[1] They recommend, based on a high level of evidence, that midthoracic epidurals be used for open colorectal surgery. There is less evidence supporting the benefits of epidural analgesia in laparoscopic colorectal surgery. Based on moderate-grade evidence, they recommended opioid-PCA or spinal analgesia in the setting of laparoscopic colorectal resection.

VENOUS THROMBOEMBOLIC PROPHYLAXIS

Venous thromboembolic (VTE) events, including deep vein thrombosis (DVT) and pulmonary embolus (PE) are relatively common complications after major abdominal surgery, and VTE prevention is a common focus of patient safety measures. Following colorectal surgery, the incidence of postoperative VTE, even with appropriate prophylaxis, has been reported to be as high as 9% to 10%.[52,53] There is little controversy around the use of postoperative VTE prophylaxis in the inpatient setting. Based on the most recent CHEST guidelines, there is solid evidence (grade 1B) to support postoperative prophylaxis with both intermittent pneumatic compression devices and also pharmacologic prophylaxis with low-molecular-weight heparin or low-dose unfractionated heparin.[54] In a 2015 study, it was reported that in-hospital, postoperative VTE prophylaxis was used in 91.4% of patient undergoing colorectal resections by 2011.[55]

More controversial is the use of postdischarge, extended VTE prophylaxis. Many of the studies and subsequent recommendations stem from a pivotal study published in 2002 in the *New England Journal of Medicine*.[56] This randomized trial found that enoxaparin prophylaxis for 4 weeks after surgery for abdominal/pelvic cancer was safe and reduced the incidence of venographically demonstrated venous thrombosis compared with only 1 week of enoxaparin treatment. In 2014 a similar study was performed specifically in patients undergoing laparoscopic colorectal cancer surgery.[52] In this study of 301 colorectal cancer patients, the 3-month incidence of VTE was 9.7% in the group randomized to 1 week of prophylaxis and 0.9% in the extended prophylaxis group ($P = .001$), with no difference in bleeding complications.

Based on these and other studies, multiple societies have published guidelines regarding the use of extended (postdischarge) VTE prophylaxis, although none target colorectal surgery patients directly. The CHEST guidelines published in 2012 recommend that patients at high risk for VTE undergoing abdominal or pelvic surgery for cancer receive extended-duration, postoperative pharmacologic prophylaxis (4 weeks) with low-molecular-weight heparin.[54] The American Society of Clinical Oncology guidelines published in 2014 also recommend that extended prophylaxis (4 weeks) be used in high-risk patients undergoing major cancer surgery, such as those with restricted mobility, obesity, and history of VTE. Despite the evidence and existing guidelines, the use of extended prophylaxis in postoperative colorectal cancer patients is not as common as its use in the inpatient setting. In the 2015 study by the Colorectal Writing Group, only 11.7% of colorectal surgery patients were discharged on extended prophylaxis.[55] Although the exact numbers were not reported, the majority of these patients had a diagnosis of malignancy.

Although most of the evidence and guidelines regarding use of extended prophylaxis involves cancer patients, there is evidence that other indications for colorectal surgery may carry as high, or higher, risk of VTE. The use of extended prophylaxis in these patients remains an active area of investigation. Several studies report a higher rate of postoperative VTE in patients undergoing surgery for inflammatory bowel disease compared with those undergoing cancer resection.[55,57,58] In addition, many studies report a high incidence of postdischarge VTE, even for noncancer colorectal surgery patients.[57–59] There are currently no guidelines regarding the use of extended prophylaxis in the noncancer colorectal surgery population. Future studies are clearly needed to clarify the risk of postoperative VTE in all colorectal surgery patients and to help answer the questions regarding

the use of extended VTE prophylaxis in this diverse population.

REFERENCES

1. Lassen K, Soop M, Nygren J, et al. Consensus review of optimal perioperative care in colorectal surgery: Enhanced Recovery After Surgery (ERAS) Group recommendations. *Arch Surg*. 2009;144(10): 961-969.
2. Wind J, Polle SW, Fung Kon Jin PH, et al. Systematic review of enhanced recovery programmes in colonic surgery. *Br J Surg*. 2006; 93(7):800-809.
3. Gouvas N, Tan E, Windsor A, Xynos E, Tekkis PP. Fast-track vs standard care in colorectal surgery: a meta-analysis update. *Int J Colorectal Dis*. 2009;24(10):1119-1131.
4. Zhuang CL, Ye XZ, Zhang XD, Chen BC, Yu Z. Enhanced recovery after surgery programs versus traditional care for colorectal surgery: a meta-analysis of randomized controlled trials. *Dis Colon Rectum*. 2013;56(5):667-678.
5. Greco M, Capretti G, Beretta L, Gemma M, Pecorelli N, Braga M. Enhanced recovery program in colorectal surgery: a meta-analysis of randomized controlled trials. *World J Surg*. 2014;38(6):1531-1541.
6. Vlug MS, Wind J, Hollmann MW, et al. Laparoscopy in combination with fast track multimodal management is the best perioperative strategy in patients undergoing colonic surgery: a randomized clinical trial (LAFA-study). *Ann Surg*. 2011;254(6):868-875.
7. Haverkamp MP, de Roos MA, Ong KH. The ERAS protocol reduces the length of stay after laparoscopic colectomies. *Surg Endosc*. 2012;26(2):361-367.
8. Kennedy RH, Francis EA, Wharton R, et al. Multicenter randomized controlled trial of conventional versus laparoscopic surgery for colorectal cancer within an enhanced recovery programme: EnROL. *J Clin Oncol*. 2014;32(17):1804-1811.
9. Zhuang CL, Huang DD, Chen FF, et al. Laparoscopic versus open colorectal surgery within enhanced recovery after surgery programs: a systematic review and meta-analysis of randomized controlled trials. *Surg Endosc*. 2015;29(8):2091-2100.
10. Spanjersberg WR, van Sambeeck JD, Bremers A, Rosman C, van Laarhoven CJ. Systematic review and meta-analysis for laparoscopic versus open colon surgery with or without an ERAS programme. *Surg Endosc*. 2015;29(12):3443-3453.
11. Gustafsson UO, Scott MJ, Schwenk W, et al. Guidelines for perioperative care in elective colonic surgery: Enhanced Recovery After Surgery (ERAS) Society recommendations. *World J Surg*. 2013;37(2):259-284.
12. Burke P, Mealy K, Gillen P, Joyce W, Traynor O, Hyland J. Requirement for bowel preparation in colorectal surgery. *Br J Surg*. 1994;81(6): 907-910.
13. Santos JC Jr, Batista J, Sirimarco MT, Guimaraes AS, Levy CE. Prospective randomized trial of mechanical bowel preparation in patients undergoing elective colorectal surgery. *Br J Surg*. 1994;81(11):1673-1676.
14. Pena-Soria MJ, Mayol JM, Anula-Fernandez R, Arbeo-Escolar A, Fernandez-Represa JA. Mechanical bowel preparation for elective colorectal surgery with primary intraperitoneal anastomosis by a single surgeon: interim analysis of a prospective single-blinded randomized trial. *J Gastrointest Surg*. 2007;11(5):562-567.
15. Contant CM, Hop WC, van't Sant HP, et al. Mechanical bowel preparation for elective colorectal surgery: a multicentre randomised trial. *Lancet*. 2007;370(9605):2112-2117.
16. Bucher P, Gervaz P, Soravia C, Mermillod B, Erne M, Morel P. Randomized clinical trial of mechanical bowel preparation versus no preparation before elective left-sided colorectal surgery. *Br J Surg*. 2005;92(4):409-414.
17. Guenaga KK, Matos D, Wille-Jorgensen P. Mechanical bowel preparation for elective colorectal surgery. *Cochrane Database Syst Rev*. 2009;(1):CD001544.
18. Slim K, Vicaut E, Panis Y, Chipponi J. Meta-analysis of randomized clinical trials of colorectal surgery with or without mechanical bowel preparation. *Br J Surg*. 2004;91(9):1125-1130.
19. Zhu QD, Zhang QY, Zeng QQ, Yu ZP, Tao CL, Yang WJ. Efficacy of mechanical bowel preparation with polyethylene glycol in prevention of postoperative complications in elective colorectal surgery: a meta-analysis. *Int J Colorectal Dis*. 2010;25(2):267-275.
20. Cannon JA, Altom LK, Deierhoi RJ, et al. Preoperative oral antibiotics reduce surgical site infection following elective colorectal resections. *Dis Colon Rectum*. 2012;55(11):1160-1166.

21. Toneva GD, Deierhoi RJ, Morris M, et al. Oral antibiotic bowel preparation reduces length of stay and readmissions after colorectal surgery. *J Am Coll Surg.* 2013;216(4):756-762; discussion 762-763.

22. Kim EK, Sheetz KH, Bonn J, et al. A statewide colectomy experience: the role of full bowel preparation in preventing surgical site infection. *Ann Surg.* 2014;259(2):310-314.

23. Moghadamyeghaneh Z, Hanna MH, Carmichael JC, et al. Nationwide analysis of outcomes of bowel preparation in colon surgery. *J Am Coll Surg.* 2015;220(5):912-920.

24. Morris MS, Graham LA, Chu DI, Cannon JA, Hawn MT. Oral antibiotic bowel preparation significantly reduces surgical site infection rates and readmission rates in elective colorectal surgery. *Ann Surg.* 2015;261(6):1034-1040.

25. Scarborough JE, Mantyh CR, Sun Z, Migaly J. Combined mechanical and oral antibiotic bowel preparation reduces incisional surgical site infection and anastomotic leak rates after elective colorectal resection: an analysis of colectomy-targeted ACS NSQIP. *Ann Surg.* 2015;262(2):331-337.

26. Kiran RP, Murray AC, Chiuzan C, Estrada D, Forde K. Combined preoperative mechanical bowel preparation with oral antibiotics significantly reduces surgical site infection, anastomotic leak, and ileus after colorectal surgery. *Ann Surg.* 2015;262(3):416-425; discussion 423-425.

27. Baum ML, Anish DS, Chalmers TC, Sacks HS, Smith H Jr, Fagerstrom RM. A survey of clinical trials of antibiotic prophylaxis in colon surgery: evidence against further use of no-treatment controls. *N Engl J Med.* 1981;305(14):795-799.

28. Bratzler DW, Dellinger EP, Olsen KM, et al. Clinical practice guidelines for antimicrobial prophylaxis in surgery. *Am J Health Syst Pharm.* 2013;70(3):195-283.

29. Nelson RL, Gladman E, Barbateskovic M. Antimicrobial prophylaxis for colorectal surgery. *Cochrane Database Syst Rev.* 2014;(5):CD001181.

30. Morita S, Nishisho I, Nomura T, et al. The significance of the intraoperative repeated dosing of antimicrobials for preventing surgical wound infection in colorectal surgery. *Surg Today.* 2005;35(9):732-738.

31. Binderow SR, Cohen SM, Wexner SD, Nogueras JJ. Must early postoperative oral intake be limited to laparoscopy? *Dis Colon Rectum.* 1994;37(6):584-589.

32. Hartsell PA, Frazee RC, Harrison JB, Smith RW. Early postoperative feeding after elective colorectal surgery. *Arch Surg.* 1997;132(5):518-520; discussion 520-521.

33. Han-Geurts IJ, Hop WC, Kok NF, Lim A, Brouwer KJ, Jeekel J. Randomized clinical trial of the impact of early enteral feeding on postoperative ileus and recovery. *Br J Surg.* 2007;94(5):555-561.

34. Lewis SJ, Andersen HK, Thomas S. Early enteral nutrition within 24 h of intestinal surgery versus later commencement of feeding: a systematic review and meta-analysis. *J Gastrointest Surg.* 2009;13(3):569-575.

35. Zhuang CL, Ye XZ, Zhang CJ, Dong QT, Chen BC, Yu Z. Early versus traditional postoperative oral feeding in patients undergoing elective colorectal surgery: a meta-analysis of randomized clinical trials. *Dig Surg.* 2013;30(3):225-232.

36. Wolff BG, Michelassi F, Gerkin TM, et al. Alvimopan, a novel, peripherally acting mu opioid antagonist: results of a multicenter, randomized, double blind, placebo-controlled, phase III trial of major abdominal surgery and postoperative ileus. *Ann Surg.* 2004;240(4):728-734; discussion 734-735.

37. Delaney CP, Weese JL, Hyman NH, et al. Phase III trial of alvimopan, a novel, peripherally acting, mu opioid antagonist, for postoperative ileus after major abdominal surgery. *Dis Colon Rectum.* 2005;48(6):1114-1125; discussion 1125-1126; author reply 1127-1129.

38. Viscusi ER, Goldstein S, Witkowski T, et al. Alvimopan, a peripherally acting mu-opioid receptor antagonist, compared with placebo in postoperative ileus after major abdominal surgery: results of a randomized, double-blind, controlled study. *Surg Endosc.* 2006;20(1):64-70.

39. Delaney CP, Wolff BG, Viscus ER, et al. Alvimopan, for postoperative ileus following bowel resection: a pooled analysis of phase III studies. *Ann Surg.* 2007;245(3):355-363.

40. Ludwig K, Enker WE, Delaney CP, et al. Gastrointestinal tract recovery in patients undergoing bowel resection: results of a randomized trial of alvimopan and placebo with a standardized accelerated postoperative care pathway. *Arch Surg.* 2008;143(11):1098-105.

41. Buchler MW, Seiler CM, Monson JR, et al. Clinical trial: a vimopan for the management of post-operative ileus after abdominal surgery: results of an international randomized, double-blind multicentre placebo-controlled clinical study. *Aliment Pharmacol Ther.* 2008;28(3):312-325.

42. Poston S, Broder MS, Gibbons MM, et al. Impact of alvimopan (entereg) on hospital costs after bowel resection: results from a large inpatient database. *P T.* 2011;36(4):209-220.

43. Simorov A, Thompson J, Oleynikov D. Alvimopan reduces length of stay and costs in patients undergoing segmental colonic resections: results from multicenter national administrative database. *Am J Surg.* 2014;208(6):919-925; discussion 925.

44. Adam MA, Lee LM, Kim J, et al. Alvimopan provides additional improvement in outcomes and cost savings in enhanced recovery colorectal surgery. *Ann Surg.* 2016;264(1):141-146.

45. Colorectal Writing Group for the SCOAP-CERTAIN Collaborative, Ehlers AP, Simianu VV, et al. Alvimopan use, outcomes, and costs: a report from the surgical care and outcomes assessment program comparative effectiveness research translation network collaborative. *J Am Coll Surg.* 2016;222(5):870-877.

46. Earnshaw SR, Kauf TL, McDade C, et al. Economic impact of alvimopan considering varying definitions of postoperative ileus. *J Am Coll Surg.* 2015;221(5):941-950.

47. Carli F, Trudel JL, Belliveau P. The effect of intraoperative thoracic epidural anesthesia and postoperative analgesia on bowel function after colorectal surgery: a prospective, randomized trial. *Dis Colon Rectum.* 2001;44(8):1083-1089.

48. Zutshi M, Delaney CP, Senagore AJ, et al. Randomized controlled trial comparing the controlled rehabilitation with early ambulation and diet pathway versus the controlled rehabilitation with early ambulation and diet with preemptive epidural anesthesia/analgesia after laparotomy and intestinal resection. *Am J Surg.* 2005;189(3):268-272.

49. Marret E, Remy C, Bonnet F, Postoperative Pain Forum Group. Meta-analysis of epidural analgesia versus parenteral opioid analgesia after colorectal surgery. *Br J Surg.* 2007;94(6):665-673.

50. Levy BF, Tilney HS, Dowson HM, Rockall TA. A systematic review of postoperative analgesia following laparoscopic colorectal surgery. *Colorectal Dis.* 2010;12(1):5-15.

51. Liu H, Hu X, Duan X, Wu J. Thoracic epidural analgesia (TEA) vs. patient controlled analgesia (PCA) in laparoscopic colectomy: a meta-analysis. *Hepatogastroenterology.* 2014;61(133):1213-1219.

52. Vedovati MC, Becattini C, Rondelli F, et al. A randomized study on 1-week versus 4-week prophylaxis for venous thromboembolism after laparoscopic surgery for colorectal cancer. *Ann Surg.* 2014;259(4):665-669.

53. McLeod RS, Geerts WH, Sniderman KW, et al. Subcutaneous heparin versus low-molecular-weight heparin as thromboprophylaxis in patients undergoing colorectal surgery: results of the Canadian colorectal DVT prophylaxis trial: a randomized, double-blind trial. *Ann Surg.* 2001;233(3):438-444.

54. Gould MK, Garcia DA, Wren SM, et al. Prevention of VTE in nonorthopedic surgical patients: antithrombotic therapy and prevention of thrombosis, 9th ed: American College of Chest Physicians evidence-based clinical practice guidelines. *Chest.* 2012;141(2 suppl):e227S-e277S.

55. Colorectal Writing Group for Surgical Care and Outcomes Assessment Program-Comparative Effectiveness Research Translation Network (SCOAP-CERTAIN) Collaborative, Nelson DW, Simianu VV, et al. Thromboembolic complications and prophylaxis patterns in colorectal surgery. *JAMA Surg.* 2015;150(8):712-720.

56. Bergqvist D, Agnelli G, Cohen AT, et al. Duration of prophylaxis against venous thromboembolism with enoxaparin after surgery for cancer. *N Engl J Med.* 2002;346(13):975-980.

57. Moghadamyeghaneh Z, Alizadeh RF, Hanna MH, et al. Post-hospital discharge venous thromboembolism in colorectal surgery. *World J Surg.* 2016;40(5):1255-1263.

58. Wilson MZ, Connelly TM, Tinsley A, Hollenbeak CS, Koltun WA, Messaris E. Ulcerative colitis is associated with an increased risk of venous thromboembolism in the postoperative period: the results of a matched cohort analysis. *Ann Surg.* 2015;261(6):1160-1166.

59. Davenport DL, Vargas HD, Kasten MW, Xenos ES. Timing and perioperative risk factors for in-hospital and post-discharge venous thromboembolism after colorectal cancer resection. *Clin Appl Thromb Hemost.* 2012;18(6):569-575.

Index

Page numbers followed by "*f*" indicate figures, "*t*" indicate tables, and "*b*" indicate boxes.

Caustic esophageal injury (Continued)
  initial investigations in, 517–520
  intermediate phase, 521–522
  long-term considerations to, 523
  management of, 517–520
  medical management of, 520–521
  nutritional support for, 521
  pathophysiology of, 515–516
  reconstruction for, 522–523
  resection or bypass of strictures for, 522
  stricture prophylaxis for, 521–522
  surgical management of, 521
Cavernous hemangioma, 1532, 1533t
Cavernous nerve, 2006
CBD. see Common bile duct
CCK. see Cholecystokinin
CCK-stimulated hepatoiminodiacetic acid
    (CCK-HIDA) nuclear scintigraphy, for
    biliary dyskinesia, 1294–1295
CD. see Crohn disease
CDP. see Contractile deceleration point
CDX2 gene expression, in colorectal cancer,
    2129–2130
CEA. see Carcinoembryonic antigen
Cecal bascule, 1810
Cecal volvulus, 1810–1811, 1811f
Cecocolic malrotation, 970
Cecorectal anastomosis (CRA), subtotal
    colectomy with, 1740
Cecum, 1663–1665
Celiac artery, 823, 1027–1028
Celiac artery aneurysms, 1049–1050
  branch, 1050–1051, 1050f–1051f
Celiac axis
  in mesenteric circulation, 1014,
      1016–1018
  superior mesenteric artery and, 1019
Celiac nodes, 826f
Celiac plexus neurolysis, endoscopic
    ultrasound-guided, 1317
Celiac sprue, 760
Celiac trunk, 824f
  nodes, 431
Celiomesenteric artery, 1018
Cell differentiation, in small intestine
    embryology, 817, 819f
α-cells, 1062–1063
β-cells, 1062–1063
  differentiation of, oxygen tension and,
      1071
Cellular injury, in liver chemistry tests,
    1398–1399
Centers for Disease Control and Prevention
    (CDC)
  surgical site infection and, 2163
  wound classification, 548
Central pancreatectomy, for neuroendocrine
    tumors, 1203
Central splenorenal shunt, in Budd-Chiari
    syndrome, 1522
Central venous catheters, 1132
Central visceral adiposity, in increased risk
    of Barrett esophagus, 338
Centrocyte, 1596t
Cephalic phase, of digestion, 644
Cerebral edema, ammonia and, 1508
Certolizumab pegol, for Crohn disease,
    871–872
Cervical anastomosis, 441–442, 454–455,
    475
  in removing esophagus, 408
Cervical dysphagia, upper esophageal
    sphincter and, 4

Cervical esophagus, 31–33, 35f, 35f
  anatomy of, 368
  recurrent laryngeal nerves in, 33, 35f
  spine and, 33, 35f
  trachea and, 33, 35f
  upper esophageal sphincter and, 31–33
Cervical node dissection, 432, 434t
Cervical perforations, surgical approach for,
    541, 542f
Cetuximab, for colorectal cancer metastases,
    to liver, 1566
CHA. see Common hepatic artery
Chagas disease, esophagram and, 65
Charité Onkologie 001 (CONKO-001) trial,
    1146
Charlson Comorbidity Index, 1281
Chemoprophylaxis, for Barrett esophagus,
    340–341
Chemoradiation therapy (CRT)
  for esophageal cancer, 411, 471–472
  for gastric adenocarcinoma, 715
  neoadjuvant, in esophageal cancer
    chemotherapy versus, 398–400, 399t
    as definitive therapy, 400–401, 401t
    in local/regional control, 396
    survival benefit of, 400
    in systemic control, 397
    toxicity in, 397–398
  for rectal cancer, 2007
  for T2 N0 rectal cancer, 2002
Chemotherapy
  for colorectal cancer, metastasis to liver
    and, 1566–1567, 1567t, 2087–2088
  cytotoxic, for Zollinger-Ellison syndrome,
      709
  for esophageal cancer, 411
  for gastric adenocarcinoma, 715
  for intrahepatic cholangiocarcinoma,
      1559
  palliative, for gastric adenocarcinoma, 717
  for pancreatic and periampullary cancer,
      1146–1147
  perioperative, in esophageal cancer,
      391–394
    chemoradiation versus, 398–400, 399t
    in pre- or postoperative setting, 394
    survival of patients, 391–393
    triplet versus doublets regimen, 393–394
  for primary pancreatic lymphoma, 1177
  systemic, 948
Chest pain
  in achalasia, 184
  in esophageal perforation, 526
  in GERD, 46, 197
  in splenic cysts, 1655
Chest radiography
  for congenital diaphragmatic hernia, 564,
      564f
  esophageal, after esophagectomy, 72
  for gastric volvulus, 855
CHI. see Congenital hyperinsulinism;
    Congenital hyperinsulinism (CHI)
Chicago Classification, for esophageal
    motility disorders, 11
Chief cells, 640–641
Child-Pugh score, 1459, 1459t, 1549–1550,
    1581t
Children
  biliary atresia in, 1361–1366
    classification of, 1362, 1362f
    diagnosis of, 1361
    etiology of, 1361–1362
    liver transplantation in, 1365

Children (Continued)
    operative management of, 1362–1363,
        1364t
    outcomes in, 1365
    postoperative management of,
        1363–1365
  foreign body ingestion in, 750
  gastrointestinal stromal tumor in, 957
  pancreatic problems in, 1215–1225
    acute and chronic pancreatitis in,
        1219–1220, 1220f
    annular pancreas in, 1215, 1215f–1217f
    congenital hyperinsulinism in,
        1215–1218, 1218f
    endoscopic retrograde
        cholangiopancreatography in,
        1222–1223, 1223f
    other tumors in, 1221, 1221f
    pancreas divisum in, 1218–1220, 1219f
    pancreatoblastoma in, 1220–1221, 1220f
    primitive neuroectodermal tumor in,
        1221
    proximal versus distal duct injuries in,
        1222
    pseudocyst drainage, options for, 1222,
        1222f
    solid pseudopapillary tumor in, 1221,
        1221f
    trauma in, 1221–1222, 1222f
    tumors in, 1220–1221
  small intestine of, surgical conditions of,
      970–990
    duodenal atresia in, 972–973, 974f–975f
    duplication cysts in, 977–978, 978f
    intussusception in, 985–986, 986f–988f
    jejunoileal atresia in, 973–973,
        975f–977f
    malrotation in, 970–972, 971f–973f
    Meckel diverticulum in, 981, 981f, 983f
    meconium disorders in, 978–981
    necrotizing enterocolitis in, 983–985,
        984f–985f
    omphalomesenteric remnants in,
        981–983, 981f–982f
  splenic trauma in, 1626–1634
    evaluation of, 1626–1628
    nonoperative management of,
        1628–1632, 1629t
    operative management of, 1628
    outcomes in, 1632–1633
    spleen anatomy and physiology of,
        1626, 1627f
Child-Turcotte-Pugh Scoring, 1495–1496,
    1496t
Chimeric antigen receptor T cells (CARTs),
    967
China, prevalence of GERD, 198–199
Chlorhexidine, SSIs in colorectal surgery
    and, 2166
Cholangiocarcinoma, 1136, 1328–1337
  adjuvant therapy for, 1334
  diagnosis of, 1329–1331, 1330f–331f
  distal, 1335
  epidemiology of, 1328–1329
  hilar, 1332–1333
  intrahepatic, 1331, 1556–1560, 1557f,
      1558t
  palliation for, 1334–1335
  pathology of, 1329
  presentation of, 1329
  primary sclerosing cholangitis associated
      with, 1308–1309
  pyogenic liver abscess and, 1451, 1431f

Cicatrization phase, of caustic esophageal injury, 516, 516t

CIM. *see* Cardia intestinal metaplasia

Ciprofloxacin, for Crohn disease, 871

Circular myotomy, in peroral endoscopic myotomy, 193, 193f

Circular staplers, 1009, 1009f

Circulation, fetal, congenital diaphragmatic hernia and, 561–562

Cirrhosis
  ascites and, 1587
  drug-induced, 1529
  hemodynamics in, 1491
  hepatocellular carcinoma and, 1541–1543, 1580
  in liver transplantation, 1488
  pathophysiology of, 1410–1413
  portal hypertensive bleeding in, 1492
  pulmonary issues in, 1491, 1492b

Cisplatin
  anthracycline and, 393
  for esophageal cancer, 393
  for gastric adenocarcinoma, 717

Cisterna chyli, 826f

CITR. *see* Collaborative Islets Transplant Registry (CITR)

C-KIT mutation, in gastrointestinal stromal tumor, 952

Classic achalasia, 120t

Classic chromosomal instability, in colorectal cancer, 1959–1961, 1960f

Classic malrotation, 970

Claustrophobia, magnetic resonance imaging and, 1710

CLE. *see* Confocal laser endomicroscopy

Cleft lift, technique of, in pilonidal disease, 1792–1793, 1794f

Clinical bile gastritis, 727

Clinical stage, endoscopic esophageal ultrasonography and, 102–107
  determination of computed tomography classification in, 99–100, 102–105, 103f–105f
  determination of M classification in, 107, 108f
  determination of N classifications in, 105–106, 106f–107f

CLIP. *see* Cancer of the Liver Italian Program

CLL. *see* Chronic lymphocytic leukemia

Cloacal defects, in rectovaginal fistula, 1766

Clonal expansion, in progression of Barrett esophagus, 332–333

Clonidine, sodium transport and, 1678

Closed Ferguson hemorrhoidectomy, 1853, 1855

Closed-loop obstruction, in SBO, 845–847

Clostridium difficile enteritis, after ileostomy, 2158

Clostridium difficile infection, SSIs in colorectal surgery and, 2168

CMI. *see* Chronic mesenteric ischemia

C-mixed triglyceride breath test, in chronic pancreatitis, 1089

Coagulation proteins, production of, in liver, 1511

Coagulopathy
  contraindication to
    intubation of stomach and small intestine, 665
    laparoscopic splenectomy, 1604
  liver and biliary tract disease and, 1412

Code, Charles, 206

Codivilla, Alessandro, 1181

Coffee bean sign, in sigmoid volvulus, 1809, 1809f

Coil embolization, for splenic artery aneurysms, 1046–1047, 1047f

Cold snare polypectomy, 1693–1694, 1695f

Colectomy
  bowel preparation in, 2187
  and ileorectal anastomosis, 1966
  for localized colon cancer, 1982, 1983f

Colic artery aneurysms, 1051–1052

Colitis
  associated with colon carcinoma, 1824
  indeterminate, 1935

Collaborative Islets Transplant Registry (CITR), 1234

Collagenolysis, 1005

Collateral blood flow, mesenteric, 1028

Collateral pathways, in mesenteric circulation, 1018–1019, 1020f

Collis gastroplasty
  in failed fundoplications, 272t, 273
  in laparoscopic paraesophageal hernia repair, 288
  in Nissen fundoplication, 243–244
  for short esophagus, 305–307
    outcome with, 306–307
    transthoracic, 306
    wedge fundectomy, 305–306

Collis-Nissen gastroplasty, for paraesophageal hernia, 293, 294f

Coloanal anastomosis, 2011
  redo, 2179–2181

Colocolic anastomosis, 454

Colocutaneous fistulas, 1838, 1840f

Cologastric anastomosis, 454, 455f

Colon, 451–458
  advantages and disadvantages of right and left, 453t
  anatomy of, 1663–1669, 1981, 1982f
    arterial supply to, 1667–1669, 1668f
    innervations of, 1669
    lymphatic drainage of, 1669, 1670f–1671f
    surface, 1665f
    venous drainage of, 1669, 1670f
  anomalies of, 1664f
  dysmotility disorders of. *see* Constipation
  indocyanine green fluorescence for, 1669f
  interposition, 454, 454f
    technique of, 452–455, 453f, 455f
  lateral attachments of, 1924f
  lymphoid tumors of, 2120–2123
  measurement of, 1676–1688
  modalities for, 452f
  outcomes of, 456–458, 457f
  physiology of, 1676–1688
    acute colonic pseudo-obstruction and, 1684–1685
    anatomy and, 1676–1677
    chronic megacolon and, 1685
    colon fluid and electrolyte transport in, 1677–1678
    colonic metabolism and, 1678
    colonic microflora and, 1678
    colonic motor function, assessment of, 1678–1679
    colonic sensation and, 1682–1683, 1682f, 1682t
    constipation and, 1683, 1683f–1684f
    defecatory disorders and, 1684, 1684b
    diverticulosis and, 1685–1686

Colon *(Continued)*
  function and, 1677–1686
  functional diarrhea or diarrhea-predominant irritable bowel syndrome and, 1685
  implications of, for surgical practice, 1686
  peristalsis and, 1680–1681, 1680f
  perturbations of, in disease states, 1683–1685
  pH-pressure capsule, for assessment, of colonic transit, 1679
  radiopaque marker methods, for assessment, of colonic transit, 1678, 1678f
  recording techniques for, 1679–1680, 1680f
  regional heterogeneity in colonic function and, 1677
  right and left, comparison of, 1677t
  scintigraphic techniques, for assessment, of colonic transit, 1679, 1679f
  preoperative management of, 452
  proximal part of, 454
  radiation enteritis and, 914
  reversed, 1664f
  SSIs in colorectal surgery and, 2163
  variations of, 455–453, 457f
  vascularization of, 451f
  volvulus of, 1808–1812
    cecal, 1810–1811, 1811f
    ileosigmoid knotting in, 1812
    sigmoid, 1808–1810, 1809f
    transverse, 1811–1812
  wall of, diverticulitis and, 1828

Colon cancer. *see also* Colorectal cancer
  complete mesocolic excision, 2052, 2056–2057
  laparoscopic
    left colectomy for, 2054–2057, 2055f–2056f
    right colectomy for, 2052–2054, 2053f–2054f
  minimally invasive approaches to, 2049–2058
    bowel function, return of, 2049, 2050t
    bowel obstruction, adhesive, 2051
    cost of, 2051
    incisional hernia, 2051
    life, quality of, 2051
    long-term outcomes, 2050–2051, 2051t
    oncologic outcomes, 2050
    postoperative pair, 2049, 2050t
    short-term outcomes, 2049, 2050t
    technique and pearls of wisdom, 2052–2054
  sigmoid resection for, 2054–2057
  transverse colectomy for, 2054, 2054f

Colon carcinoma, locally recurrent, 2069

Colon graft, in vagal-sparing esophagectomy, 423

Colon interposition
  in removing esophagus, 408–409
  in vagal-sparing esophagectomy, 421

Colon resection, low anterior
  complications of, 2028–2029
  functional outcomes in, 2029–2030
  hand-assisted, 2009–2011
  laparoscopic, 2009–2011, 2009f–2010f, 2012t, 2016t, 2013t
  oncologic outcomes in, 2029
  open, 2008–2009, 2012t
  robotic-assisted, 2011–2020, 2014f, 2016t, 2013t
  single port, 2009–2011

F

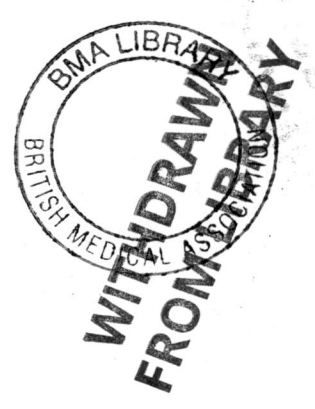

BMA LIBRARY
BRITISH MEDICAL ASSOCIATION

WITHDRAWN
FROM LIBRARY